W9-DEU-627

PART EIGHT   INFECTIOUS DISEASES

I   BASIC PRINCIPLES, 1334

II   LABORATORY AND DIAGNOSTIC TESTS, 1366

III   CLINICAL SYNDROMES, 1375

IV   ORGANISMS INFECTIVE TO HUMANS, 1483

Viral Diseases, 1483

Chlamydial Diseases, 1534

Rickettsial Diseases, 1541

Bacterial Diseases, 1546

Enterococcal Diseases, 1560

Fungal Diseases, 1651

Protozoal Diseases, 1671

Helminthic Diseases, 1696

PART NINE   ENDOCRINOLOGY, METABOLISM, AND GENETICS

I   BASIC PRINCIPLES, 1708

II   LABORATORY AND DIAGNOSTIC TESTS, 1732

III   SPECIFIC DISEASE ENTITIES, 1748

IV   SPECIFIC ENDOCRINE, METABOLIC, AND GENETIC DISORDERS, 1773

V   METABOLIC DISORDERS IN ADULTS, 1903

PART TEN   ALIMENTARY TRACT, LIVER, BILIARY TREE, AND PANCREAS

ALIMENTARY TRACT, 1976

I   BASIC PRINCIPLES, 1976

II   LABORATORY AND DIAGNOSTIC TESTS, 1993

III   SPECIFIC DISEASE ENTITIES, 2008

LIVER, BILIARY TREE, AND PANCREAS, 2118

I   BASIC PRINCIPLES, 2118

II   LABORATORY AND DIAGNOSTIC TESTS, 2134

III   SPECIFIC DISEASE ENTITIES, 2147

PART ELEVEN   SPECIAL TOPICS IN INTERNAL MEDICINE

APPENDIX   IMMUNIZATION SCHEDULE FOR ADULTS, 2315

Internal Medicine

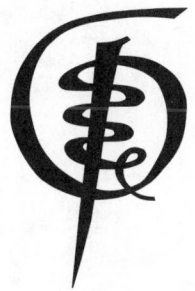

Internal Medicine

Editor-in-Chief

JAY H. STEIN, M.D.

Section Editors

John M. Eisenberg, M.D.
John J. Hutton, M.D.
John H. Klippel, M.D.
Peter O. Kohler, M.D.
Nicholas F. LaRusso, M.D.
Robert A. O'Rourke, M.D.
Herbert Y. Reynolds, M.D.
Martin A. Samuels, M.D.
Merle A. Sande, M.D.
Nathan J. Zvaifler, M.D.

*with **1177** illustrations and **172** full-color illustrations*

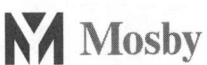 Mosby

St. Louis Baltimore Boston Carlsbad Chicago Minneapolis New York Philadelphia Portland
London Milan Sydney Tokyo Toronto

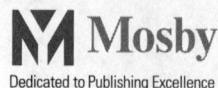

Mosby
Dedicated to Publishing Excellence

A Times Mirror
Company

Editor: Richard Furn
Senior Developmental Editor: Sandra Clark Brown
Project Manager: Patricia Tannian
Project Specialist: Ann E. Rogers
Manufacturing Manager: David Graybill
Book Design Manager: Gail Morey Hudson
Cover Design: Teresa Breckwoldt

FIFTH EDITION
Copyright © 1998 by Mosby, Inc.

All rights reserved. No part of this publication may be reproduced, stored in a retrieval system, or transmitted, in any form or by any means, electronic, mechanical, photocopying, recording, or otherwise, without prior written permission from the publisher.

Permission to photocopy or reproduce solely for internal or personal use is permitted for libraries or other users registered with the Copyright Clearance Center, provided that the base fee of $4.00 per chapter plus $.10 per page is paid directly to the Copyright Clearance Center, 222 Rosewood Drive, Danvers, MA 01923. This consent does not extend to other kinds of copying, such as copying for general distribution, for advertising or promotional purposes, for creating new collected works, or for resale.

NOTE: The indications for and dosages of medications recommended conform to practices at the present time. References to specific products are incorporated to serve only as guidelines; they are not meant to exclude a practitioner's choice of other, comparable drugs. Many oral medications may be given with more scheduling flexibility than implied by the specific time intervals noted. Individual drug sensitivity and allergies must be considered in drug selection. Adult doses are provided as a gauge of the maximum dose commonly used.

Every effort has been made to ensure accuracy and appropriateness. New investigations and broader experience may alter present dosage schedules, and it is recommended that the package insert of each drug be consulted before administration. Often there is limited experience with established drugs for neonates and young children. Furthermore, new drugs may be introduced, and indications for use may change. This rapid evolution is particularly noticeable in the use of antibiotics and cardiopulmonary resuscitation. The clinician is encouraged to maintain expertise concerning appropriate medications for specific conditions.

Printed in the United States of America
Composition by The Clarinda Company
Printing/binding by World Color Book Group
Color separation and film by Top Graphics, Inc.

Mosby, Inc.
11830 Westline Industrial Drive
St. Louis, Missouri 63146

Library of Congress Cataloging in Publication Data

Internal medicine/editor-in-chief, Jay H. Stein; section editors,
   John M. Eisenberg . . . [et al.].—5th ed.
      p.   cm.
   Includes bibliographical references and index.
   ISBN 0-8151-8698-3 (hardcover)
   1. Internal medicine. I. Stein, Jay H.
   [DNLM: 1. Internal Medicine.   WB 115 I605 1998]
RC46.I475   1998
616—dc21
DNLM/DLC
for Library of Congress   97-51786
                                  CIP

98 99 00 01 02 / 9 8 7 6 5 4 3 2 1

EDITORS

Editor-in-Chief

JAY H. STEIN, M.D.
Senior Vice President and Vice Provost for Health Affairs
The University of Rochester Medical Center
Chief Executive Officer
University of Rochester Medical Center and Strong Health
Professor of Medicine
University of Rochester School of Medicine and Dentistry
Rochester, New York
Renal and Electrolyte Disorders

Section Editors

JOHN M. EISENBERG, M.D.
Administrator, Agency for Health Care Policy and Research
United States Department of Health and Human Services
Rockville, Maryland
Formerly, Department of Medicine
Georgetown University Medical Center
Washington, DC
Introduction to Modern Medical Practice
Special Topics in Internal Medicine

JOHN JAMES HUTTON, M.D.
Christian R. Holmes Professor and
Dean, College of Medicine
University of Cincinnati
Cincinnati, Ohio
Hematology and Oncology

JOHN H. KLIPPEL, M.D.
Clinical Director
National Institute of Arthritis and Musculoskeletal and Skin
Diseases
National Institutes of Health
Bethesda, Maryland
Clinical Immunology, Rheumatology, and Dermatology

PETER O. KOHLER, M.D.
President, Oregon Health Sciences University
Portland, Oregon
Endocrinology, Metabolism, and Genetics

NICHOLAS F. LaRUSSO, M.D.
Professor of Medicine and Biochemistry and Molecular Biology
Chairman, Division of Gastroenterology
Mayo Medical School, Clinic and Foundation
Rochester, Minnesota
Alimentary Tract, Liver, Biliary Tree, and Pancreas

ROBERT A. O'ROURKE, M.D.
Charles Conrad Brown Distinguished Professor in Cardiovascular
Disease
Department of Medicine/Cardiology
The University of Texas Health Sciences Center at San Antonio
San Antonio, Texas
Diseases of the Heart and Blood Vessels

HERBERT Y. REYNOLDS, M.D.
Professor and Chair, Department of Medicine
Milton S. Hershey Medical Center
The Pennsylvania State University College of Medicine
Hershey, Pennsylvania
Pulmonary and Critical Care Medicine

MARTIN A. SAMUELS, M.D.
Professor of Neurology, Harvard Medical School
Neurologist-in-Chief
Chairman, Department of Neurology
Brigham and Women's Hospital
Boston, Massachusetts
Neurologic Disorders

MERLE A. SANDE, M.D.
Professor and Chairman, Department of Internal Medicine
University of Utah School of Medicine
Salt Lake City, Utah
Infectious Diseases

NATHAN J. ZVAIFLER, M.D.
Professor of Medicine
Division of Rheumatology
Department of Medicine
University of California, San Diego
La Jolla, California
Clinical Immunology, Rheumatology, and Dermatology

To
Dr. T. Franklin Williams
the father of modern geriatric medicine
with admiration

PREFACE

In this fifth edition of *Internal Medicine,* we have sharpened and refined the basic format that has been praised by reviewers and has proven tremendously valuable to students, house officers, and practicing physicians. The book is organized by clinical subspecialty, and each subspecialty is divided into three primary sections: an introductory section on the basic principles of a given organ system; a section on laboratory tests, including a review of the differential diagnoses; and a detailed section on various disease entities.

Although we have preserved this basic structure, the book is new and innovative in many ways. There are three new section editors and 160 new contributors to the fifth edition. Of the more than 1100 photos, illustrations, and algorithms, nearly 400 are new. The book's generous use of tables and algorithms—regarded as "fabulous additions to the writing" in *JAMA's* review of the fourth edition—help convey the most essential information quickly and clearly. While *Internal Medicine* is encyclopedic, it is also built to be readable and rapidly usable.

Also new in this edition is the "When to Refer" box in nearly every chapter on specific disease entities. This feature offers guidance and criteria for when a patient should be referred to a specialist—a valuable resource for house staff as well as practicing physicians. As an ancillary to the book, we will offer a CD-ROM version that incorporates a host of extra information, including drug prescribing information from Mosby's GenRX, diagnostic algorithms, and patient education information.

Internal Medicine remains a tool for use at the forefront of daily practice. To strengthen its utility, we begin this edition with a new section entitled Introduction to Modern Medical Practice, with chapters on Managed Care, Implementing Clinical Practice Guidelines, Clinical Bioethics, Medical Informatics, and other topics.

In Part Two, Diseases of the Heart and Blood Vessels, we have included a new chapter on interventional cardiac catheterization techniques that discusses the usefulness, advantages, and complications associated with these interventional techniques frequently used for treating patients with single or multiple coronary artery stenoses. Nine of the 25 chapters in Part Two have been rewritten by new authors, and all chapters have been updated considerably to reflect recent advances in the diagnosis and treatment of patients with cardiovascular disease.

In Part Three, Pulmonary and Critical Care Medicine, clinical decision pathways have been added for pulmonary embolism, a solid pulmonary nodule or mass, and for common respiratory symptoms such as wheezing cough and dyspnea. For the treatment of lung diseases, many innovations and new treatments are described. These include different types of ventilatory support such as pressure controlled, inverse ratio ventilation and permissive hypercapnia; immunomodulation of various cytokines to suppress inflammation, to treat asthma, or to enhance activity against infectious agents; and nitric oxide to treat pulmonary hypertension or acute lung injury or to assess responsiveness of chemoreceptors.

Part Four, Hematology and Oncology, continues to provide balanced coverage of both Hematology and Oncology. In Hematology, particular attention is paid to abnormal bleeding and clotting—an area in which our understanding has advanced dramatically over the past decade. Risk factors predisposing to venous thromboembolism are better defined, as is the effectiveness of various therapies. In Oncology, there are new chapters on the Genetics of Cancer, Principles of Cancer Treatment, and Complications of Cancer and Cancer Therapy. The Oncology section outlines recent advances in our understanding of the causes of cancer, the mechanisms of action of drugs used to treat cancer, and the ways we can improve our support of patients during therapy. All chapters on diagnosis and management of specific malignancies have been updated, with particular attention to those in which medical therapy plays a key role such as breast cancer, prostate cancer, and the hematologic malignancies.

Part Five, Renal and Electrolyte Disorders, continues to stress the pathophysiology of renal and electrolyte disorders. The chapters on the Nephrotic Syndrome, Nephrolithiasis, Disorders of Acid-Base Balance, Renal Manifestations of Dysproteinemias, and Drug- and Chemical-Induced Nephropathy have been substantially revised by new authors. The chapter on Chronic Renal Failure includes an expanded section on renal transplantation.

Part Six, Neurologic Disorders, reflects the many important advances in the field. The use of several new antiepileptic drugs is discussed, as well as the new, potent, and less toxic dopamine receptor agonists now available for the treatment of Parkinson's disease. Treatment of acute stroke with recombinant tissue plasminogen activator, as well as new, sensitive neuroimaging techniques such as diffusion-weighted imaging, is discussed as the first real treatment for acute cerebral infarction.

In Part Seven, Clinical Immunology, Rheumatology, and Dermatology, the chapters on Rheumatology have been extensively revised to cover recent advances in immunogenetics, cytokine biology, and regulation of the immune response. A new chapter on Primary Immunodeficiency Disorders provides a striking example of the potential of understanding—at a molecular and genetic level—the dysfunctions of the immune system that underlie the clinical consequences of the disease. Similar progress is reflected in chapters on common inflammatory and immune-mediated disorders of the musculoskeletal system and skin, such as rheumatoid arthritis and psoriasis.

Part Eight, Infectious Diseases, includes 53 revised chapters. The Acquired Immunodeficiency Syndrome chapter is of particular importance and contains completely updated information.

In Part Nine, Endocrinology, Metabolism, and Genetics, every chapter has been updated to reflect new knowledge in each area. One new chapter has been added on Benign Disorders of the Breast.

In Part Ten, Alimentary Tract, Liver, Biliary Tree, and Pancreas, each chapter has been substantially updated to include new information about the pathogenesis and the biology of the hollow and solid components of the digestive tract, as well as the major developments in the detection and treatment of digestive diseases. The result is the most comprehensive collection of information on the science and clinical practice regarding the digestive system ever assembled in a textbook of medicine.

We conclude the book with Part Eleven, Special Topics in Internal Medicine. This section emerged out of the realization that all of patient care cannot be described within a format that is organized according to organ systems and pathophysiology. This section includes valuable chapters on The Periodic Health Examination, Prevention and Control of Injuries, Gerontology, Chronic Fatigue Syndrome, Women's Health, and more.

Acknowledgments

Publishing a book of this size and scope is a monumental task requiring the talents of hundreds of people. We are indebted to each of them for the care and attention they have given this book through every step of the publishing process. We would especially like to express our gratitude to Christopher DiFrancesco for his editorial oversight of the book, and Sandy Clark Brown at Mosby for her outstanding work in the development of the manuscript. In addition we would like to acknowledge the superb work of Ann Rogers at Mosby in shepherding the manuscript through the production process, and Susan Crawford, Pamela Derish, and Jackie Gandre for their editorial assistance to the section editors.

Jay H. Stein

CONTRIBUTORS

SHELLEY ALBERT, M.D.
Assistant Professor of Medicine
Division of Surgical Research
Hospital for Sick Children
Toronto, Ontario, Canada
124 *Tubulointerstitial Renal Diseases*

JOSEPH S. ALPERT, M.D.
Professor and Department Head
Department of Medicine
University of Arizona Health Sciences Center
Tucson, Arizona
29 *Pulmonary Hypertensive Heart Disease*

WILLIAM D. ANDERSON, M.D.
Assistant Professor of Medicine/Cardiology
Andreas Gruentzig Cardiovascular Center of Emory University
Emory University Hospital
Atlanta, Georgia
15 *Interventional Cardiac Catheterization*

GRANT J. ANHALT, M.D.
Professor of Dermatology
Acting Chairman of Dermatology
Johns Hopkins University School of Medicine
Baltimore, Maryland
213 *Bullous Diseases*

FREDERICK R. APPELBAUM, M.D.
Director, Clinical Research Division
Fred Hutchinson Cancer Research Center
Seattle, Washington
77 *Hematopoietic Stem Cell Transplantation*
90 *Bone Marrow Failure and Myelodysplasia*

JANE APPLEBY, M.D.
Assistant Professor
Department of Medicine
Division of General Medicine
The University of Texas Health Sciences Center at San Antonio
San Antonio, Texas
369 *Preoperative Evaluation*

MICHAEL D. APSTEIN, M.D.
Assistant Professor of Medicine
Harvard Medical School
Associate Physician
Division of Gastroenterology
Brigham and Women's Hospital
Boston, Massachusetts
Chief of Clinical Gastroenterology
Brockton West Roxbury VA Medical Center
West Roxbury, Massachusetts
345 *Diverticular and Other Intestinal Diseases*
364 *Biliary Tract Stones and Associated Diseases*

SHREERAM ARADHYE, M.D.
Assistant Professor of Medicine
Renal-Electrolyte and Hypertension Division
Hospital of the University of Pennsylvania
Philadelphia, Pennsylvania
124 *Tubulointerstitial Renal Diseases*

EURICO ARRUDA, M.D.
Assistant Professor
Department of Parasitology, Microbiology and Immunology
University of São Paulo School of Medicine
Rebeirao Preto, São Paulo, Brazil
251 *Paramyxovirus (Parainfluenza, Mumps, Measles, and Respiratory Syncytial Virus), Rubella Virus, Coronavirus, and Adenovirus Infections*

JOHN P. ATKINSON, M.D.
Professor of Medicine and Molecular Microbiology
Washington University School of Medicine
St. Louis, Missouri
178 *Complement Measurements*
186 *Inherited Complement Deficiencies*

VICKI V. BAKER, M.D.
Chief, Division of Gynecologic Oncology
George W. Morley Professor of Obstetrics and Gynecology
University of Michigan Medical Center
Ann Arbor, Michigan
96 *Gynecologic Cancers*

GEORGE L. BAKRIS, M.D., F.A.C.P., F.C.P.
Vice Chairman of Preventive Medicine
Associate Professor of Preventive and Internal Medicine
Director, Rush University Hypertension Training Program
Rush Presbyterian/St. Luke's Medical Center
Chicago, Illinois
101 *Principles of Renal Physiology*
125 *Renovascular Diseases*

DAVID BANGSBERG, M.D.
Assistant Adjunct Professor of Medicine
Center for AIDS Prevention
Department of Epidemiology and Biostatistics
Division of Infectious Diseases
San Francisco General Hospital
University of California–San Francisco
San Francisco, California
269 *Infections Caused by* Salmonella *and* Shigella *Species*
274 *Infections Caused by Spirochetes*

H. VERDAIN BARNES, M.D., F.A.C.P.
Professor and Chair
Department of Medicine
Associate Dean for Information Technology
Eastern Virginia Medical School
Norfolk, Virginia
294 *Disorders of Adolescent Growth and Development*

RICHARD J. BAROHN, M.D.
Associate Professor of Neurology
University of Texas Southwestern Medical Center at Dallas
Dallas, Texas
131 *Electromyography*

FRANCOISE BASSET, M.D.
Faculté de Médecine Xavier Bichat
Paris, France
55 *Langerhans' Cell Granulomatosis (Histiocytosis X, Eosinophilic Granuloma)*

LAURENCE H. BECK, M.D.
Professor of Medicine
Chief, Division of General Internal Medicine
Georgetown University Medical Center
Washington, DC
5   *Quality of Care*

RICHARD C. BECKER, M.D.
Associate Professor of Medicine
Cardiovascular Thrombosis Research Center
Division of Cardiovascular Medicine
University of Massachusetts Medical School
Worcester, Massachusetts
20   *Hypotension and Cardiogenic Shock*

WILLIAM S. BECKETT, M.D., M.P.H.
Professor, Environmental Medicine
University of Rochester School of Medicine
Rochester, New York
57   *Occupational Lung Diseases*

NORMAN H. BELL, M.D.
Professor of Medicine and Pharmacology
Medical University of South Carolina
Staff Physician
Charleston Veterans Administration Medical Center
Charleston, South Carolina
317   *Osteomalacia and Disorders of Vitamin D Metabolism*

RODNEY D. BELL, M.D.
Professor of Neurology
Director
Cerebral Vascular Center
Thomas Jefferson University Hospital
Philadelphia, Pennsylvania
130   *Electroencephalography and Evoked Responses*

GEORGE A. BELLER, M.D.
Chief, Cardiovascular Division
Ruth C. Heede Professor of Cardiology
Professor and Vice-Chairman
Department of Medicine
The University of Virginia Health Sciences Center
Charlottesville, Virginia
13   *Cardiac Noninvasive Techniques*

WILLIAM M. BENNETT, M.D.
Professor of Medicine and Pharmacology
Department of Medicine
Division of Nephrology, Hypertension and Clinical Pharmacology
Oregon Health Sciences University
Portland, Oregon
119   *Drug- and Chemical-Induced Nephropathy*

MERRILL D. BENSON, M.D.
Chairman, Department of Medical and Molecular Genetics
Indiana University School of Medicine
Indianapolis, Indiana
210   *Amyloidoses*

MICHELLE BERLIN, M.D., M.P.H.
Assistant Professor of Obstetrics and Gynecology and
   Epidemiology
University of Pennsylvania
Philadelphia, Pennsylvania
371   *Women's Health*

GORDON R. BERNARD, M.D.
Professor, Division of Allergy, Pulmonary and Critical Care
   Medicine
Vanderbilt University School of Medicine
Nashville, Tennessee
48   *Pulmonary Edema*

ADIL E. BHARUCHA, M.D.
Assistant Professor of Medicine
Division of Gastroenterology and Hepatology
Mayo Clinic and Foundation
Rochester, Minnesota
358   *Primary Biliary Cirrhosis, Primary Sclerosing Cholangitis,*
   and Other Cholangiopathies

ROGER D. BIES, M.D.
Associate Director of Cardiology
Department of Medicine
University of Colorado Health Sciences Center
Veterans Administration Medical Center
Denver, Colorado
10   *Molecular Biology of the Cardiovascular System*

TIMOTHY D. BIGBY, M.D.
Associate Professor of Medicine
University of California, San Diego
Chief, Pulmonary and Critical Care
Department of Veterans Affairs Medical Center
San Diego, California
188   *Asthma*

JOHN P. BILEZIKIAN, M.D.
Professor of Medicine and of Pharmacology
Chief, Division of Endocrinology
Columbia University
College of Physicians and Surgeons
New York, New York
312   *Hypercalcemia*
313   *Hypocalcemia*
322   *Primary Hyperparathyroidism*

ANDREW B. BINDMAN, M.D.
Associate Professor of Medicine and Epidemiology & Biostatistics
University of California, San Francisco
San Francisco, California
8   *Managed Care*

PETER M. BLACK, M.D., Ph.D.
Franc C. Ingraham Professor of Neurosurgery
Harvard Medical School
Neurosurgeon-in-Chief
Brigham and Women's Hospital
Children's Hospital
Boston, Massachusetts
155   *Head Trauma*

JOSEPH R. BLOOMER, M.D.
Professor of Medicine
Director, Liver Center
University of Alabama
Birmingham, Alabama
311   *Disorders of Porphyrin Metabolism*

HARRY G. BLUESTEIN, M.D.
Professor of Medicine
Director, Division of Rheumatology
University of California, San Diego Medical Center
San Diego, California
190   *Periarticular Rheumatic Complaints*

DAVID H. BOLDT, M.D.
Professor of Medicine
Chief, Division of Hematology
University of Texas Health Sciences Center at San Antonio
San Antonio, Texas
80   *Abnormal Nucleated Blood Cell Counts*
81   *Lymphadenopathy and Splenomegaly*
91   *Abnormalities of Phagocytes, Eosinophils, and Basophils*

DAVID BORSOOK, M.D., Ph.D.
Massachusetts General Hospital
Department of Anesthesia
Wang Ambulatory Care Center
Boston, Massachusetts
161 *Neuroendocrinology*

PITER J. BOSMA, Ph.D.
Academic Medical Center
Universiteit van Amsterdam
Amsterdam, The Netherlands
353 *Jaundice and Disorders of Bilirubin Metabolism*

JULIE R. BRAHMER, M.D.
Medical Oncology Fellow
Department of Medical Oncology
Johns Hopkins Hospital
Baltimore, Maryland
273 *Tuberculosis and Nontuberculous Mycobacterial Infections*

KENNETH D. BRANDT, M.D.
Professor of Medicine and Head
Rheumatology Division
Indiana University School of Medicine
Director, Indiana University Multipurpose Arthritis and
    Musculoskeletal Diseases Center
Indianapolis, Indiana
206 *Osteoarthritis*

GLENN D. BRAUNSTEIN, M.D.
Chairman, Department of Medicine
Professor of Medicine
UCLA School of Medicine
Los Angeles, California
295 *Disorders of the Hypothalamus and Anterior Pituitary*

KENNETH L. BRIGHAM, M.D.
The Ralph and Lulu Owen Professor of Pulmonary Medicine
Director, Center for Lung Research
Division of Allergy, Pulmonary and Critical Care Medicine
Vanderbilt University School of Medicine
Nashville, Tennessee
48 *Pulmonary Edema*

LYNN S. BRODERICK, M.D.
Assistant Professor of Radiology
Indiana University School of Medicine
Indianapolis, Indiana
43 *Pulmonary Diagnostic Imaging*

ROY G. BROWER. M.D.
Associate Professor of Medicine
Johns Hopkins University
Baltimore, Maryland
38 *Pulmonary Blood Flow*

ROBERT H. BROWN, Jr., M.D., Ph.D.
Associate Professor of Neurology
Harvard Medical School
Associate in Neurology
Director, Day Neuromuscular Research Laboratory
Massachusetts General Hospital
Charlestown, Massachusetts
149 *Muscle Disease*

RICHARD E. BRYANT, M.D.
Head, Division of Infectious Diseases
Oregon Health Sciences University
Portland, Oregon
241 *Skin and Subcutaneous Infections*

BOOKER T. BUSH, M.D.
Assistant Professor of Medicine
Harvard Medical School
Beth Israel–Deaconess Medical Center
Boston, Massachusetts
374 *Substance Abuse*

JEAN-PAUL BUTZLER, M.D., Ph.D.
Department of Clinical Microbiology
St. Pierre University Hospital
Brussels, Belgium
267 *Infections Caused by* Campylobacter *and* Helicobacter *Species*

T. EDWARD BYNUM, M.D.
Private Practice
Marlborough, Massachusetts
335 *Abdominal Pain*
342 *Intestinal Obstruction and Peritonitis*
344 *Vascular Diseases of the Intestine*

LEONARD H. CALABRESE, D.O. F.A.C.P.
Vice Chairman
Head, Section of Clinical Immunology
Department of Rheumatic and Immunologic Diseases
Cleveland Clinic Foundation
Cleveland, Ohio
195 *Vasculitic Syndromes*

LOUIS R. CAPLAN, M.D.
Professor and Chair of Neurology
Tufts University School of Medicine
Neurologist
New England Medical Center
Boston, Massachusetts
144 *Cerebrovascular Disease (Stroke)*

MARTIN C. CAREY, M.D., D.Sc., F.R.C.P.I., A.M. (Harv.), LL.D. (N.U.I.), M.R.I.A. (Hon)
Professor of Medicine
Professor of Health Sciences and Technology
Harvard Medical School
Brigham and Women's Hospital
Boston, Massachusetts
349 *Bile Production and Secretion*

DENNIS A. CARSON, M.D.
Professor of Medicine
University of California, San Diego
San Diego, California
182 *Rheumatoid Factors*

JOHN E. CARTER, M.D.
Associate Professor
Department of Medicine
Division of Neurology
The University of Texas Health Sciences Center at San Antonio
San Antonio, Texas
158 *Ocular Manifestations of Neurologic Disorders*

ROBERT H. CARTER, M.D.
Assistant Professor of Medicine
Department of Medicine
University of Alabama at Birmingham
Birmingham, Alabama
175 *Complement System and Immune Complex Diseases*
178 *Complement Measurements*
186 *Inherited Complement Deficiencies*

JOSEPH M. CASH, M.D.
Department of Rheumatic and Immunologic Diseases
Chairman, Department of General Internal Medicine
Cleveland Clinic Foundation
Cleveland, Ohio
205 *Antirheumatic Drugs*

AGUSTIN CASTELLANOS, M.D.
Professor of Medicine
Director, Clinical Electrophysiology
Department of Medicine
Division of Cardiology
University of Miami School of Medicine
Miami, Florida
18 *Cardiac Arrhythmias and Conduction Disturbances*

SIMON C. CHAKKO, M.D.
Associate Professor of Medicine
University of Miami School of Medicine
Chief, Cardiology Section
Veterans Administration Medical Center
Miami, Florida
18 *Cardiac Arrhythmias and Conduction Disturbances*

CHARLES K. CHAN, M.D., F.R.C.P.(C), F.C.C.P., F.A.C.P.
Associate Professor of Medicine
Consultant Staff in Respiratory Medicine
The Toronto Hospital
The Princess Margaret Hospital
The Wellesley Hospital
University of Toronto
Toronto, Ontario, Canada
63 *Pulmonary Thromboembolism*

MICHAEL R. CHARLTON, M.D.
Assistant Professor of Medicine
Division of Gastroenterology & Hepatology
Mayo Clinic and Foundation
Rochester, Minnesota
340 *Diseases of Small Bowel Absorption*

KANU CHATTERJEE, M.D., F.R.C.P. (London), F.R.C.P. (Scotland)
Professor of Medicine
Lucie Stern Professor of Cardiology
University of California, San Francisco
San Francisco, California
22 *Ischemic Heart Disease*

MELVIN D. CHEITLIN, M.D.
Professor of Medicine, Emeritus
San Francisco General Hospital
San Francisco, California
33 *Cardiac Tumors: Cardiac Manifestations of Endocrine, Collagen Vascular, and HIV Disease; and Traumatic Injury of the Heart*

NEIL S. CHERNIACK, M.D.
Director of Clinical Affairs
Professor of Medicine and Physiology
New Jersey Medical School
Newark, New Jersey
36 *Abnormalities of the Control of Breathing*

MICHAEL R. CHICOINE, M.D.
Skull Base Fellow
University of Cincinnati
Department of Neurosurgery
Washington University
St. Louis, Missouri
240 *Brain Abscess and Perimeningeal Infections*

ANTHONY W. CHOW, M.D.
Professor of Medicine
Division of Infectious Diseases
University of British Columbia
Vancouver Hospital Health Sciences Center
Vancouver, British Columbia, Canada
271 *Infections Caused by* Bacteroides *and Other Nonsporulating* Anaerobes

STEVEN L. CHUCK, M.D.
Assistant Professor, Molecular Medicine Unit
Department of Medicine
Beth Israel Deaconess Medical Center
Boston, Masschusetts
252 *Rabies*

MELISSA CLARK, M.D.
Division of Pulmonary & Critical Care Medicine
Vanderbilt University
Nashville, Tennessee
47 *Multiple Organ Dysfunction in the Context of ARDS*

DANIEL J. CLAUW, M.D.
Associate Professor of Medicine
Chief, Division of Rheumatology, Immunology and Allergy
Georgetown University Medical Center
Washington, DC
375 *Chronic Fatigue Syndrome*

WILLIAM E. CLUTTER, M.D.
Associate Professor of Medicine
Department of Internal Medicine
Washington University School of Medicine
St. Louis, Missouri
304 *Hypoglycemia*

C. GLENN COBBS, M.D.
Chief, Medical Service
Veterans Affairs Medical Center
Birmingham, Alabama
245 *Gram-Negative Bacteremia and the Sepsis Syndrome*

BERNARD A. COHEN, M.D.
Director, Pediatric Dermatology
Johns Hopkins Children's Center
Baltimore, Maryland
220 *Superficial Fungal Infections*

DEWEY J. CONCES, Jr., M.D.
Professor of Radiology
Department of Radiology
Indiana University School of Medicine
Indiana University Hospital
Indianapolis, Indiana
43 *Pulmonary Diagnostic Imaging*

J. ALLEN D. COOPER, Jr., M.D.
Professor of Medicine
Pulmonary Division
The University of Alabama
Birmingham, Alabama
58 *Adverse Pulmonary Reactions to Drugs and Other Therapeutic Modalities*

CONSTANTINO COSTARANGOS, M.D.
Dermatology Resident
Johns Hopkins University School of Medicine
Baltimore, Maryland
220 *Superficial Fungal Infections*

WILLIAM G. COUSER, M.D.
Head of Division of Nephrology
Belding H. Scribner Professor of Medicine
University of Washington
Seattle, Washington
116 *Glomerular Diseases*

DAVID W. CRABB, M.D.
Professor of Medicine and of Biochemistry and Molecular Biology
Indiana University
Indianapolis, Indiana
357 *Alcoholic Liver Diseases and Nonalcoholic Steatohepatitis*

TIMOTHY J. CRAIG, D.O.
Assistant Professor
Division of Allergy–Immunology
Department of Internal Medicine
University of Iowa College of Medicine
Iowa City, Iowa
54 *Hypersensitivity Pneumonitis*

JAMES M. CRAWFORD, M.D., Ph.D.
Associate Professor of Pathology
Yale University School of Medicine
New Haven, Connecticut
349 *Bile Production and Secretion*

WILLIAM F. CROWLEY, Jr., M.D.
Professor of Medicine
Harvard Medical School
Director of the Reproductive Endocrine Sciences Center
National Center for Infertility Research
Massachusetts General Hospital
Boston, Massachusetts
291 *Amenorrhea*
300 *Disorders of the Ovary*

PHILIP E. CRYER, M.D.
Irene E. and Michael M. Carl Professor of Endocrinology and
  Metabolism
Department of Internal Medicine
Washington University School of Medicine
St. Louis, Missouri
304 *Hypoglycemia*

JOHN J. CURTIS, M.D.
Professor of Medicine
Department of Medicine
University of Alabama at Birmingham
Birmingham, Alabama
110 *Chronic Renal Failure*

ALBERT J. CZAJA, M.D.
Professor of Medicine
Mayo Medical School
Consultant in Gastroenterology
Mayo Clinic
Rochester, Minnesota
351 *Evaluation of Hepatobiliary Diseases*

RALPH G. DACEY, Jr., M.D.
Schwartz Professor and Chairman
Department of Neurosurgery
Washington University
St. Louis, Missouri
240 *Brain Abscess and Perimeningeal Infections*

JAMES E. DALEN, M.D., M.P.H.
Vice President for Health Sciences
Dean, College of Medicine
The University of Arizona
Tucson, Arizona
29 *Pulmonary Hypertensive Heart Disease*

WALTER J. DALY, M.D.
Dean Emeritus
Indiana University School of Medicine
Indianapolis, Indiana
35 *Respiratory Pathophysiology*

JAMES H. DAUBER, M.D.
Professor of Medicine
Director, Pulmonary Transplantation
University of Pittsburgh Medical Center
Pittsburgh, Pennsylvania
66 *Pulmonary Transplantation*

JOHN DAVENPORT, M.D., C.M.
Staff Neurologist
Veterans Administration Medical Center
Assistant Professor of Neurology
University of Minnesota Medical School
Minneapolis, Minnesota
141 *Epilespy*

NICHOLAS O. DAVIDSON, M.D.
Department of Medicine
The University of Chicago
Chicago, Illinois
331 *Evaluation of Intestinal Disease*

PAMELA B. DAVIS, M.D., Ph.D.
Professor of Pediatrics and Medicine
Case Western Reserve University
Pediatric Pulmonary Division
Rainbow Babies and Children's Hospital
Cleveland, Ohio
59 *Cystic Fibrosis and Bronchiectasis*

DAVID M. DAWSON, M.D.
Professor of Neurology
Brigham and Women's Hospital
Boston, Massachusetts
145 *Demyelinating Diseases*

LOUIS J. DELL'ITALIA, M.D.
Department of Medicine
University of Alabama at Birmingham
Birmingham, Alabama
16 *Chest Pain*

PETER DENSEN, M.D.
Professor of Internal Medicine
Department of Internal Medicine
Associate Dean, Office of Student Affairs and Curriculum
University of Iowa College of Medicine
Iowa City, Iowa
229 *Basic Principles of Infectious Disease*
230 *Host Defense Against Infection: The Roles of Antibody, Complement, and Phagocytic Cells*

EMMANUEL N. DESSYPRIS, M.D.
Professor of Medicine
Medical College of Virginia
Virginia Commonwealth University
Chief, Hematology/Oncology Section
H.H. McGuire DVA Medical Center
Richmond, Virginia
79 *Abnormal Hematocrit*

STEPHEN DEUTSCH, M.D.
Medical Director
Cedars-Sinai Medical Care Foundation
Associate Clinical Professor of Medicine
Department of Medicine
University of California–Los Angeles
Los Angeles, California
6 *Implementing Clinical Practice Guidelines*

GERALD F. DIBONA, A.B., M.D.
Professor and Vice Chairman
Department of Internal Medicine
University of Iowa College of Medicine
Chief of Medicine
Veterans Administration Medical Center
Iowa City, Iowa
121   *Glomerular and Interstitial Hereditary Nephropathies*

SUSAN R. DIGIOVANNI, M.D.
Assistant Professor of Medicine
Medical College of Virginia
Richmond, Virginia
115   *Disorders of Acid-Base Balance*

JEREMIAH P. DONOVAN, M.D.
Associate Professor of Medicine
Department of Internal Medicine
Medical Director of Hepatic Transplantation
University of Nebraska Medical Center
Omaha, Nebraska
363   *Liver Transplantation*

R. GORDON DOUGLAS, Jr., M.D.
Adjunct Professor of Medicine
Cornell University Medical College
Attending Physician
The New York Hospital
New York, New York
250   *Common Viral Infections: Picornavirus and Orthomyxovirus Infections (Rhinovirus, Enterovirus, and Influenza)*

IAN R.G. DOWDESWELL, M.B., B.S.
Associate Professor of Medicine
Assistant Chief of Medicine
Veterans Administration Medical Center
Indiana University Medical School
Indianapolis, Indiana
64   *Pleural Diseases*
65   *Diseases of the Mediastinum*

THOMAS A. DRAKE, M.D.
Department of Pathology and Laboratory Medicine
University of California–Los Angeles
Los Angeles, California
233   *Use of Laboratory Tests in Infectious Diseases*

FRANK W. DRISLANE, M.D.
Department of Neurology
Beth Israel Hospital
Boston, Massachusetts
166   *Neuropulmonology*

GEORGE F. DUNA, M.D.
Staff Rheumatologist
Kelsey-Seybold Clinic
Clinical Assistant Professor
Baylor College of Medicine
Houston, Texas
195   *Vasculitic Syndromes*

TERRI DUNN, M.D.
Dermatology Resident
Johns Hopkins University School of Medicine
Baltimore, Maryland
222   *Cutaneous Manifestations of Internal Malignancy*

HERBERT L. DUPONT, M.D.
H. Irving Schweppe Jr. Chair in Internal Medicine
Vice-Chairman, Department of Internal Medicine
Baylor College of Medicine
Mary W. Kelsey Professor of Medical Sciences
The University of Texas Health Sciences Center
Chief, Internal Medicine
St. Luke's Episcopal Hospital
Houston, Texas
242   *Gastrointestinal Infections*

DAVID T. DURACK, M.D., D.Phil.
Consulting Professor of Medicine
Duke University
Durham, North Carolina
Worldwide Medical Director
Becton Dickinson Microbiology Systems
Baltimore, Maryland
259   *Rickettsial Infections*
266   *Infections Caused by* Haemophilus *Species*

RONALD DWORKIN, M.D.
Assistant Director, Medical Education
Providence Portland Medical Center
Assistant Professor of Medicine
Oregon Health Sciences University
Portland, Oregon
263   *Gram-Positive Bacillary Infections and Clostridial Infections*

FRANCES M. DYRO, M.D.
Private Practice
Maine Medical Center
Portland, Maine
159   *Neurology of the Lower Urinary Tract*

J. DONALD EASTON, M.D.
Professor and Chairman of Neurology
Rhode Island Hospital
Brown University
Providence, Rhode Island
136   *Faintness and Syncope*

GREGORY L. EASTWOOD, M.D.
President, State University of New York
Health Science Center at Syracuse
Syracuse, New York
332   *Gastrointestinal Bleeding*
337   *Gastritis and Other Gastric Diseases*

JOHN EDMEADS, M.D., F.R.C.P, F.A.C.P.
Physician-in-Chief
Department of Medicine
Sunnybrook Health Science Centre
Toronto, Ontario, Canada
137   *Headache and Facial Pain*

JOHN E. EDWARDS, Jr., M.D.
Professor of Medicine
University of California at Los Angeles
School of Medicine
Chief of Infectious Diseases
Harbor/UCLA School of Medicine
Los Angeles, California
277   *Infections Caused by* Candida, Actinomyces, *and* Nocardia *Species*

JOHN M. EISENBERG, M.D.
Administrator, Agency for Heath Care Policy and Research
United States Department of Health and Human Services
Rockville, Maryland
Formerly, Department of Medicine
Georgetown University Medical Center
Washington, DC
2 *Principles of Diagnostic Testing*

M. JOYCELYN ELDERS, M.D.
Professor of Pediatric Endocrinology
University of Arkansas School of Medicine
Little Rock, Arkansas
307 *Lipodystrophies*

RONALD P.J. OUDE ELFERINK, Ph.D.
Universiteit van Amsterdam
Amsterdam, The Netherlands
353 *Jaundice and Disorders of Bilirubin Metabolism*

GEORGE M. ELIOPOULOS, M.D.
Department of Medicine
Beth Israel Deaconess Medical Center
Boston, Massachusetts
231 *Principles of Antiinfective Therapy*

JACK ENDE, M.D.
Chief, Department of Medicine
Presbyterian Medical Center
University of Pennsylvania Health System
Philadelphia, Pennsylvania
1 *Physician-Patient Encounter*

MURRAY EPSTEIN, M.D.
Professor of Medicine
University of Miami School of Medicine
Veterans Administration Medical Center
Miami, Florida
113 *Disorders of Sodium Balance*

MATS ESTONIUS, M.D., Ph.D.
Professor of Medicine and of Biochemistry and Molecular Biology
Indiana University
Division of Gastroenterology/Hepatology
Riley Hospital for Children
Indianapolis, Indiana
357 *Alcoholic Liver Diseases and Nonalcoholic Steatohepatitis*

MARK D. FABER, M.D.
Senior Staff Physician
Division of Nephrology
Co-Director, Continually Ambulatory Peritoneal Dialysis
Henry Ford Hospital
Detroit, Michigan
112 *Disorders of Water Balance*

MICHAEL FARRELL, M.D.
Resident
Head and Neck Fellow
Department of Otolaryngology—Head and Neck Surgery
University of Cincinnati Medical Center
College of Medicine
Cincinnati, Ohio
98 *Head and Neck Cancer*

GEORGE M. FELDMAN, M.D.
McGuire Veterans Administration Medical Center
Richmond, Virginia
115 *Disorders of Acid-Base Balance*

STEVEN R. FELDMAN, M.D., Ph.D.
Associate Professor of Dermatology and Pathology
Bowman Gray School of Medicine
Wake Forest University
Winston-Salem, North Carolina
225 *Cutaneous Manifestations of Sarcoidosis*

WILLIAM F. FINN, M.D.
University of North Carolina
School of Medicine
Chapel Hill, North Carolina
119 *Drug- and Chemical-Induced Nephropathy*

SUZANNE W. FLETCHER, M.D. M.Sc.
Professor of Ambulatory Care and Prevention
Harvard Medical School and Harvard Pilgrim Health Care
Professor of Epidemiology
Harvard School of Public Health
Boston, Massachusetts
368 *The Periodic Health Examination*

DAVID A. FLOCKHART, M.D., Ph.D.
Assistant Professor of Medicine and Pharmacology
Director, Analytical Core Laboratory
Georgetown University Medicine Center
Washington, DC
378 *Drug Interactions and Adverse Effects*

BARRY S. FOGEL, M.D.
Adjunct Professor of Community Health
Brown University Medical School
Lecturer in Psychiatry
Harvard Medical School
Neuropsychiatrist
Brigham Behavioral Neurology Group
Brigham and Womens Hospital
Boston, Massachusetts
151 *Anxiety*
152 *Mood Disorders*
153 *Personality Disorders, Maladaptive Illness Behavior, and Somatization*
154 *Thought Disorders*

MARVIN FORLAND, M.D.
Associate Dean for Clinical Affairs
Professor of Medicine
University of Texas Health Sciences Center at San Antonio
San Antonio, Texas
102 *Urinalysis and Renal Function Tests*
106 *Dysuria*

GEORGE R. FOURNIER, Jr., M.D.
Atlanta, Georgia
246 *Urinary Tract Infections*

ROBERT I. FOX, M.D., Ph.D.
Division of Rheumatology
Scripps Clinic and Research Foundation
La Jolla, California
193 *Sjögren's Syndrome*

GARY S. FRANCIS, M.D.
Professor of Medicine
Ohio State University
Columbus, Ohio
Director, Coronary Intensive Care
The Cleveland Clinic Foundation
Cleveland, Ohio
19 *Congestive Heart Failure*

ROY FREEMAN, M.D.
Department of Neurology
Harvard Medical School
Director, Autonomic and Peripheral Nerve Laboratory
Beth Israel Deaconess Hospital
Boston, Massachusetts
133 *Autonomic Nervous System*
150 *Behavioral Neurology*

MARK E. FRISSE, M.D., M.S., M.B.A.
Associate Professor of Medicine
Department of Internal Medicine
Associate Dean, Director
Bernard Becker Medical Library
Washington University School of Medicine
St. Louis, Missouri
7 *Medical Informatics*

MARVIN J. FRITZLER, M.D., Ph.D.
Department of Medicine
University of Calgary
Calgary, Alberta, Canada
181 *Autoantibodies*

JACK D. FULMER, M.D.†
Division of Pulmonary and Critical Care
University of Alabama at Birmingham
Birmingham, Alabama
52 *Interstitial Lung Disease*

WILLIAM H. GAASCH, M.D.
Professor of Medicine
University of Massachusetts Medical Center
Director, Cardiovascular Research
Lahey Hitchcock Medical Center
Burlington, Massachusetts
14 *Cardiac Catheterization and Angiography*

ALAN J. GARBER, M.D., Ph.D.
Professor of Medicine, Biochemistry and Cell Biology
Baylor College of Medicine
Houston, Texas
303 *Diabetes Mellitus*
305 *Heritable Disorders of Carbohydrate Metabolism*
309 *Lysosomal Storage Diseases*

J. BERNARD L. GEE, M.D.
Professor of Medicine, Emeritus
Department of Internal Medicine
Pulmonary and Critical Care Section
Yale University School of Medicine
New Haven, Connecticut
57 *Occupational Lung Diseases*

THOMAS DAVID GELEHRTER, M.D.
Professor and Chairman
Department of Human Genetics
Professor of Internal Medicine
University of Michigan Medical School
Ann Arbor, Michigan
310 *Phakomatoses*

JAMES N. GEORGE, M.D.
Professor of Medicine
Chief, Hematology-Oncology Section
The University of Oklahoma Health Sciences Center
Oklahoma City, Oklahoma
69 *Hemostasis and Fibrinolysis*
75 *Evaluation of Hemostasis and Thrombosis*
82 *Excessive Bleeding and Clotting*

JULIE LOUISE GERBERDING, M.D.
San Francisco General Hospital
San Francisco, California
248 *Acquired Immunodeficiency Syndrome*

MEGHAN GERETY, M.D.
Department of Medicine
University of Texas Medical School at San Antonio
San Antonio, Texas
373 *Gerontology and Geriatric Medicine*

BERNARD J. GERSH, M.B., Ch.B., D.Phil., F.R.C.P.
W. Proctor Harvey Teaching Professor of Cardiology
Georgetown University Medical Center
Washington, D.C.
23 *Acute Myocardial Infarction*

ABRAHAM A. GHIATAS, M.D.
Athens, Greece
103 *Imaging of Renal Disorders*

JAMES L. GILMAN, M.D.
Deputy Commander for Clinical Services
Darnall Army Community Hospital
Fort Hood, Texas
21 *Sudden Cardiac Death*

JACK L. GLUCKMAN, M.D.
Professor and Chairman
Department of Otolaryngology–Head and Neck Surgery
University of Cincinnati Medical Center
College of Medicine
Cincinnati, Ohio
98 *Head and Neck Cancer*

STANLEY GOLDFARB, M.D.
Senior Vice Chair for Clinical Affairs
Department of Medicine
Professor of Medicine
University of Pennsylvania Health System
Philadelphia, Pennsylvania
111 *Nephrolithiasis*
117 *Diabetic Nephropathy*
122 *Disorders of Renal Transport*
314 *Disorders of Phosphate Homeostasis*
315 *Disorders of Magnesium Homeostasis*

ALAN GOLDFIEN, M.D.
Professor Emeritus
Departments of Medicine, Obstetrics, Gynecology and Reproductive
    Sciences and the Cardiovascular Research Institute
University of California at San Francisco
San Francisco, California
299 *Disorders of the Adrenal Medulla*

NORA GOLDSCHLAGER, M.D.
Professor of Clinical Medicine
Department of Medicine
University of California, San Francisco
Director, Coronary Care Unit
San Francisco General Hospital
San Francisco, California
12 *Electrocardiography*

GREGORY J. GORES, M.D., F.A.C.P.
Professor of Medicine
Division of Gastroenterology
Center for Basic Research in Digestive Diseases
Mayo Medical School, Clinic, and Foundation
Rochester, Minnesota
362 *Hepatic Tumors*

---

†Deceased.

PETER D. GOREVIC, M.D.
Division of Rheumatology
State University of New York at Stony Brook
Stony Brook, New York
202 *Cryoglobulinemia*

RAJ K. GOYAL, M.D.
Mallinckrodt Professor of Medicine
Harvard Medical School
Boston, Massachusetts
ACOS for Research and Development
Veterans Administration Medicial Center
West Roxbury, Massachusetts
324 *Alimentary Tract Motor Function*

CHRISTOPHER J. GRACE, M.D.
Fletcher Allen Health Care
Burlington, Vermont
272 *Infections Caused by Legionellae*

REUBEN MICHAEL GRANICH, M.D.
Department of Medicine
California Pacific Medical Center
San Francisco, California
275 *Infections with* Mycobacterium leprae *(Leprosy)*

JARED J. GRANTHAM, M.D.
Professor of Medicine
University of Kansas Medical Center
Kansas City, Kansas
120 *Cystic Diseases of the Kidney*

JOHN R. GRAYBILL, M.D.
Professor, Department of Medicine
Chief, Infectious Diseases
University of Texas Health Sciences Center at San Antonio
South Texas Medical Hospital
Audie L. Murphy Division
San Antonio, Texas
276 *Infections Caused By Common Fungi*

C. JEFFREY GRIFFIN, M.D.
Ambulatory Care
Audie L. Murphy Memorial Veterans Hospital
San Antonio, Texas
369 *Preoperative Evaluation*

JEANE ANN GRISSO, M.D., M.Sc.
Associate Professor of Medicine
Division of General Internal Medicine
Center for Clinical Epidemiology and Biostatistics
University of Pennsylvania Medical Center
Philadelphia, Pennsylvania
371 *Women's Health*

JOANNA L. GRODEN, Ph.D.
Assistant Professor
Department of Molecular Genetics, Biochemistry & Microbiology
University of Cincinnati
College of Medicine
Cincinnati, Ohio
70 *The Genetics of Cancer*

THOMAS M. GROGAN, M.D.
Professor of Pathology
Assistant Director of Hematology Lab
Co-Director of Clinical Immunopathology Lab
University of Arizona College of Medicine
Tucson, Arizona
93 *Hodgkin's Disease and Non-Hodgkin's Lymphoma*

ALLEN B. GRUBER, M.D.
Private Practice
St. Rose Medical Office Building
San Antonio, Texas
131 *Electromyography*

SCOTT M. GRUNDY, M.D., Ph.D.
Center for Human Nutrition
University of Texas Southwestern Medical Center at Dallas
Dallas, Texas
306 *Disorders of Lipids and Lipoproteins*

RICHARD L. GUERRANT, M.D.
Thomas H. Hunter Professor of International Medicine
Chief, Division of Geographic and International Medicine
Director, Office of International Health
Division of Geographic and International Medicine
Department of Internal Medicine
University of Virginia School of Medicine
Charlottesville, Virginia
268 *Infections Caused by* Vibrio *Species*

PAUL A. GUTIERREZ, M.D.
Assistant Chief of Spinal Cord Injury Service
Long Beach Veterans Administration Medical Center
Professor of Medicine
Department of Neurology
University of California–Irvine
Irvine, California
156 *Spinal Cord Injury*

JACK M. GWALTNEY, Jr., M.D.
Professor, Internal Medicine
Head, Division of Epidemiology and Virology
University of Virginia Health Sciences Center
Charlottesville, Virginia
237 *Respiratory Tract Infections*

VAN HA, M.D.
Resident
Johns Hopkins Outpatient Clinic
Baltimore, Maryland
223 *Cutaneous Manifestations of Gastrointestinal Diseases*

STEPHEN B. HANAUER, M.D.
Professor of Medicine and Clinical Pharmacology
University of Chicago
Pritzker School of Medicine
Chicago, Illinois
341 *Idiopathic Inflammatory Bowel Disease*

ALLAN J. HANCE, M.D.
Facultè de Mèdecine Xavier Bichat
Paris, France
55 *Langerhans' Cell Granulomatosis (Histiocytosis X, Eosinophilic Granuloma)*

EARL H. HARLEY, M.D.
Associate Professor of Otolaryngology
Department of Otolaryngology–Head and Neck Surgery
Georgetown University Medical Center
Washington, DC
377 *Common Ear, Nose, and Throat Problems*

STEPHEN CRANE HAUSER, M.D.
Assistant Professor of Medicine
Harvard Medical School
Director of Gastroenterology Clinics
Brigham and Women's Hospital
Boston, Massachusetts
360 *Hepatic Veno-Occlusive Disease*
365 *Other Diseases of the Gallbladder and Biliary Tree*

FREDERICK G. HAYDEN, M.D.
Stuart S. Richardson Professor of Clinical Virology
Professor of Internal Medicine and Pathology
University of Virginia School of Medicine
Charlottesville, Virginia
251   *Paramyxovirus (Parainfluenza, Mumps, Measles, and*
      Respiratory Syncytial Virus), Rubella Virus, Coronavirus, and
      Adenovirus Infections

J. OWEN HENDLEY, M.D.
Professor of Pediatrics
Head, Division of Pediatric Infectious Diseases
Department of Pediatrics
University of Virginia Health Sciences Center
Charlottesville, Virginia
270   *Infections Caused by* Brucella, Francisella tularensis,
      Pasteurella, Yersinia *Species, and* Bordetella pertussis
      (Whooping Cough)

NANCY K. HENRY, M.D., Ph.D.
Associate Professor of Pediatrics
Consultant, Department of Pediatrics and Adolescence Medicine
Mayo Clinic and Foundation
Rochester, Minnesota
270   *Infections Caused by* Brucella, Francisella tularensis,
      Pasteurella, Yersinia *Species, and* Bordetella pertussis
      (Whooping Cough)

DANIEL B. HIER, M.D.
Head, Department of Neurology
Professor of Neurology
University of Illinois College of Medicine
Chicago, Illinois
140   *Disorders of Speech and Language*

BRIAN D. HOIT, M.D.
Professor of Medicine
Division of Cardiology
University of Cincinnati
College of Medicine
Cincinnati, Ohio
27   *Pericardial Disease and Pericardial Heart Disease*

ANTOINETTE F. HOOD, M.D.
Professor, Departments of Pathology and Dermatology
Indiana University School of Medicine
Indianapolis, Indiana
221   *Cutaneous Manifestations of Drug Reactions*

EDWARD W. HOOK, III, M.D.
Professor of Medicine
Division of Infectious Diseases
University of Alabama at Birmingham
Birmingham, Alabama
265   Neisseria gonorrhoeae *Infections*

THOMAS D. HORN, M.D.
Professor of Dermatology and Pathology
Chairman, Department of Dermatology
University of Arkansas for Medical Sciences
Little Rock, Arkansas
226   *Cutaneous Manifestations of Human Immunodeficiency*
      Virus Infection

EDWARD S. HORTON, M.D.
Vice President, Director of Clinical Research
Joslin Diabetes Center
Boston, Massachusetts
288   *Obesity*

ANASTACIO M. HOYUMPA, M.D.
Professor of Medicine
Department of Medicine
Division of Gastroenterology and Nutrition
University of Texas Health Sciences Center at San Antonio
San Antonio, Texas
354   *Principal Complications of Liver Failure*

LEONARD D. HUDSON, M.D.
Professor of Medicine
Head, Division of Pulmonary and Critical Care Medicine
University of Washington
Harborview Medical Center
Seattle, Washington
46   *Acute Respiratory Failure*

RUSSELL D. HULL, M.B.B.S
Co-Director, Thrombosis Research Unit
Professor of Medicine, General Internal Medicine
University of Calgary
Calgary, Alberta, Canada
85   *Thrombosis and Anticoagulation*

GARY W. HUNNINGHAKE, M.D.
Professor and Director
Pulmonary Disease Division
Department of Medicine
Iowa City, Iowa
53   *Sarcoidosis*

JOHN J. HUTTON, M.D.
Christian R. Holmes Professor and Dean
College of Medicine
University of Cincinnati
Cincinnati, Ohio
92   *The Leukemias and Polycythemia Vera*

STEVEN E. HYMAN, M.D.
Molecular Neurobiology Laboratory
Massachusetts General Hospital East
Boston, Massachusetts
161   *Neuroendocrinology*

MICHAEL C. IANNUZZI, M.D.
Senior Staff Physician
Division of Pulmonary and Critical Care Medicine
Associate Professor of Internal Medicine
Case Western Reserve University
Henry Ford Hospital
Detroit, Michigan
60   *Neoplasms of the Lung*

MICHAEL D. INFELD, M.D.
Pediatric Pulmonary Division
Rainbow Babies and Children's Hospital
Cleveland, Ohio
59   *Cystic Fibrosis and Bronchiectasis*

DAVID H. INGBAR, M.D.
Associate Professor of Medicine
Pulmonary and Critical Care Medicine Division
Department of Medicine
University of Minnesota School of Medicine
Director, Medical Intensive Care Unit
Co-Medical Director, Respiratory Care
University of Minnesota Hospital and Clinic
Minneapolis, Minnesota
49   *Respiratory Therapy and Monitoring*

ROBERT D. INMAN, M.D.
Director, Rheumatology
The Toronto Hospital Western Division
Toronto, Ontario, Canada
200   *Spondyloarthropathies*

RICHARD S. IRWIN, M.D.
Director of Pulmonary, Allergy, and Critical Care Medicine
Professor of Medicine
University of Massachusetts Medical School
Worcester, Massachusetts
29 *Pulmonary Hypertensive Heart Disease*

M. COLIN JORDAN, M.D.
Professor of Medicine and Microbiology
Director, Division of Infectious Diseases
University of Minnesota Medical School
Minneapolis, Minnesota
255 *Herpesvirus Infections (Herpes Simples Virus, Varicella-Zoster Virus, Cytomegalovirus, and Epstein-Barr Virus)*

RICHARD M. JORDAN, M.D.
Professor of Medicine
Chief, Division of Endocrinology
Associate Chief, Department of Medicine
James H. Quillen College of Medicine
East Tennessee State University
Chief, Medical Service
Veterans Administration Medical Center
Mountain Home, Tennessee
282 *Principles of Endocrine Physiology*
285 *Laboratory Diagnosis in Endocrinology*
287 *Weight Loss*

RAFAEL L. JURADO, M.D.
Assistant Chief, Medical Service VAMC
Decatur, Georgia
Associate Professor (Infectious Disease)
Department of Medicine
Emory University School of Medicine
Atlanta, Georgia
249 *Fever in the Hospitalized Patient*

MARTIN F. KAGNOFF, M.D.
Professor of Medicine
Director, Laboratory of Mucosal Immunology
University of California–San Diego
San Diego, California
327 *Intestinal Immunity*

ASHWANI KAPILA, M.D.
Professor of Radiology
University of Texas Health Sciences Center
San Antonio, Texas
132 *Neuroradiologic Studies*

NORMAN M. KAPLAN, M.D.
Professor of Internal Medicine
University of Texas Southwestern Medical Center
Dallas, Texas
32 *Arterial Hypertension*

ADOLF W. KARCHMER, M.D.
Chief, Division of Infectious Diseases
Beth Israel Deaconess Medical Center
Professor of Medicine
Harvard Medical School
Boston, Massachusetts
203 *Infections of the Joints*

MICHAEL KATZ, M.D.
Department of Medicine
University of Texas Medical School at San Antonio
San Antonio, Texas
373 *Gerontology and Geriatric Medicine*

BALAKUNTALAM S. KASINATH, M.D.
Associate Professor of Medicine
University of Texas Health Sciences Center at San Antonio
Chief, Renal Section
Audie L. Murphy Veterans Administration Hospital
San Antonio, Texas
104 *Hematuria*
105 *Proteinuria*
107 *Acute Nephritic Syndrome*
108 *Nephrotic Syndrome*

DAVID A. KATZENSTEIN, M.D.
Division of Infectious Diseases
Stanford University Medical Center
Stanford, California
255 *Herpesvirus Infections (Herpes Simplex Virus, Varicella-Zoster Virus, Cytomegalovirus, and Epstein-Barr Virus)*

SANJIV KAUL, M.B.B.S.
Professor of Medicine
Division of Cardiology
University of Virginia Health Sciences Center
Charlottesville, Virginia
13 *Cardiac Noninvasive Techniques*

DONALD KAYE, M.D.
Klinghoffer Professor of Medicine
Executive Vice President for Health Affairs
Allegheny University of the Health Sciences
President and CEO
Allegheny Health, Education and Research Foundation, Eastern Region
Philadelphia, Pennsylvania
246 *Urinary Tract Infections*

ARTHUR L. KELLERMAN, M.D., M.P.H.
Professor and Director
Center for Injury Control, Rollins School of Public Health
Emory University
Atlanta, Georgia
370 *Prevention and Control of Injuries*

JOHN KENDALL, M.D.
Professor of Medicine
Oregon Health Sciences University
Distinguished Physician
Portland Veterans Affairs Medical Center
Portland, Oregon
298 *Disorders of the Adrenal Cortex*

KENNETH M. KESSLER, M.D.
Professor of Medicine
Associate Director, Division of Cardiology
University of Miami School of Medicine
Chief, Section of Cardiology
Veterans Administration Medical Center
Miami, Florida
18 *Cardiac Arrhythmias and Conduction Disturbances*

L. LYNDON KEY, Jr., M.D.
Professor of Pediatrics
Medical University of South Carolina
Charleston, South Carolina
317 *Osteomalacia and Disorders of Vitamin D Metabolism*

SPENCER B. KING, III, M.D.
Professor of Medicine
Emory University School of Medicine
Atlanta, Georgia
15 *Interventional Cardiac Catheterization*

BARBARA J. KIRCHER, M.D.
Private Practice
Baltimore, Maryland
62 *Pulmonary Hypertension: Primary and Secondary Causes*

SAULO KLAHR, M.D.
Simon Professor of Medicine
Washington University School of Medicine
Barnes–Jewish Hospital
St. Louis, Missouri
123 *Obstructive Uropathy*

IRWIN L. KLEIN, M.D.
Professor of Medicine
New York University School of Medicine
Chief of Endocrinology
North Shore University Hospital
Manhasset, New York
297 *Disorders of the Thyroid*

JARED KLEIN, M.D.
Assistant Professor of Medicine
Section of Medical Oncology and Hematology
Department of Medicine
Wayne State University School of Medicine
Detroit, Michigan
100 *Cancer of Unknown Primary Site*

JOHN H. KLIPPEL, M.D.
Clinical Director
National Institute of Arthritis and Musculoskeletal and Skin
  Diseases
National Institutes of Health
Bethesda, Maryland
194 *Systemic Lupus Erythematosus*
201 *Uncommon Arthropathies*

SIDNEY KOBRIN, M.D.
Associate Professor
Renal Electrolyte and Hypertension Division
University of Pennsylvania Medical Center
University of Pennsylvania School of Medicine
Philadelphia, Pennsylvania
122 *Disorders of Renal Transport*
315 *Disorders of Magnesium Homeostasis*

SUSAN E. KOCH, M.D.
Assistant Professor of Dermatology
Director, Pigmented Lesion Clinic
Johns Hopkins University School of Medicine
Baltimore, Maryland
215 *Melanoma*
224 *Cutaneous Manifestations of Endocrine Disorders*

PETER O. KOHLER, M.D.
President
Oregon Health Sciences University
Portland, Oregon
282 *Principles of Endocrine Physiology*
285 *Laboratory Diagnosis in Endocrinology*
287 *Weight Loss*

DONALD P. KOTLER, M.D.
Associate Professor of Medicine
Department of Medicine
Columbia University College of Physicians and Surgeons
St. Luke's Roosevelt Hospital Center
New York, New York
346 *Gastrointestinal Manifestations of HIV Infection and AIDS*

KRIS V. KOWDLEY, M.D., F.A.C.P.
Associate Professor of Medicine
Division of Gastroenterology/Hepatology
University of Washington School of Medicine
Seattle, Washington
359 *Hemochromatosis, Wilson's Disease, and Other Genetic Liver*
  Diseases Affecting the Adult

STEPHEN M. KRANE, M.D.
Chief and Physician
Arthritis Unit, Massachusetts General Hospital
Persis, Cyrus and Marlow B. Harrison Professor of Medicine
Harvard Medical School
Boston, Massachusetts
211 *Heritable and Developmental Disorders of Connective Tissue*

MARGO J. KRASNOFF, M.D.
State University of New York at Buffalo
Buffalo, New York
371 *Women's Health*

G. GOPAL KRISHNA, M.D.
Private Practice
Selena, California
112 *Disorders of Water Balance*

SATISH KUMAR, M.D.
Associate Professor of Medicine
University of Oklahoma Health Sciences Center
Oklahoma City, Oklahoma
109 *Acute Renal Failure*

ROBERT C. KURTZ, M.D.
Director, Gastrointestinal Endoscopy Unit
Gastroenterology-Nutrition Service
Memorial Sloan-Kettering Cancer Center
New York, New York
338 *Tumors of the Stomach*

S. LUKE KUSMIREK, M.D.
Fellow in Hypertension
Department of Preventative Medicine
Rush University
Presbyterian/St. Luke's Medical Center
Chicago, Illinois
125 *Renovascular Diseases*

ROBERT A. KYLE, M.D.
Professor of Medicine and Laboratory Medicine
Hematology and Internal Medicine
Mayo Clinic
Rochester, Minnesota
74 *Evaluation of Monoclonal Proteins in Serum and Urine*
94 *Multiple Myeloma and the Dysproteinemias*

SUSAN D. LAMAN, M.D.
Assistant Professor
Department of Dermatology
Johns Hopkins University School of Medicine
Baltimore, Maryland
222 *Cutaneous Manifestations of Internal Malignancy*
223 *Cutaneous Manifestations of Gastrointestinal Diseases*

STANFORD I. LAMBERG, M.D.
Associate Professor of Dermatology
The Johns Hopkins Medical Institutions
Baltimore, Maryland
228 *Mycosis Fungoides and Sézary's Syndrome*

VALERIE A. LAWRENCE, M.D., M.Sc.
Division of General Medicine
University of Texas Health Sciences Center at San Antonio
San Antonio, Texas
369 *Preoperative Evaluation*

JAMES LEGGETT, M.D.
Assistant Director, Medical Education
Providence Portland Medical Center
Associate Professor of Medicine
Oregon Health Sciences University
Portland, Oregon
263 *Gram-Positive Bacillary Infections and Clostridial Infections*

GERALD S. LEVEY, M.D.
Provost, Medical Sciences
Dean, UCLA School of Medicine
Los Angeles, California
297 *Disorders of the Thyroid*

MATTHEW E. LEVISON, M.D.
Professor of Medicine
Chief, Division of Infectious Diseases
Department of Medicine
Allegheny University of the Health Sciences
Medical College of Pennsylvania
Hahnemann School of Medicine
Philadelphia, Pennsylvania
238 *Intraabdominal Infections*

JAY A. LEVY, M.D.
Professor of Medicine
Division of Hematology/Oncology
University of California–San Francisco
San Francisco, California
256 *Human Retrovirus Infections*

MARTIN M. LeWINTER, M.D.
Professor of Medicine
Director, Cardiology Unit
University of Vermont College of Medicine
Fletcher Allen Health Care/MCHV Campus
Burlington, Vermont
9 *Cardiovascular Physiology*

DAVID R. LICHTENSTEIN, M.D., F.A.C.G.
Director of Endoscopy
Department of Medicine–Gastroenterology Division
Boston Medical Center
Boston University School of Medicine
Boston, Massachusetts
361 *Liver Abscesses and Cysts*

CHARLES J. LIGHTDALE, M.D.
Professor of Clinical Medicine
Columbia University, College of Physicians and Surgeons
Director, Clinical Gastroenterology
Columbia-Presbyterian Medical Center
New York, New York
343 *Tumors of the Small and Large Intestines*

ALDO A.M. LIMA, M.D.
University of Virginia School of Medicine
Charlottesville, Virginia
268 *Infections Caused by* Vibrio *Species*

PETER K. LINDENAUER, M.D.
Division of General Internal Medicine
University of California at San Francisco
San Francisco, California
235 *Fever and Rash*

KEITH D. LINDOR, M.D.
Associate Professor of Medicine
Division of Gastroenterology and Hepatology
Mayo Clinic and Foundation
Rochester, Minnesota
358 *Primary Biliary Cirrhosis, Primary Sclerosing Cholangitis, and Other Cholangiopathies*

M. KATHRYN LISZEWSKI, M.D.
Laboratory Manager
Division of Rheumatology
Department of Internal Medicine
Washington University School of Medicine
St. Louis, Missouri
178 *Complement Measurements*
186 *Inherited Complement Deficiencies*

EDWARD V. LOFTUS, Jr., M.D.
Senior Associate Consultant
Division of Gastroenterology and Hepatology
Mayo Clinic and Foundation
Rochester, Minnesota
340 *Diseases of Small Bowel Absorption*

ERIC L. LOGIGIAN, M.D.
Associate Professor of Neurology
Harvard Medical School
Director, Clinical Neurophysiology Laboratory
Brigham and Women's Hospital
Boston, Massachusetts
147 *Diseases of Peripheral Nerve and Motor Neurons*

JACOB S.O. LOKE, M.D.
Clinical Professor of Medicine
Yale University School of Medicine
New Haven, Connecticut
35 *Respiratory Pathophysiology*
41 *Pulmonary Function Testing*

D. LYNN LORIAUX, M.D., Ph.D.
Chairman, Department of Medicine
Oregon Health Sciences University
Portland, Oregon
290 *Hirsutism*
298 *Disorders of the Adrenal Cortex*

JAMES S. LOUIE, M.D.
Chief of Rheumatology
Harbor-UCLA Medical Center
Professor, UCLA School of Medicine
Torrance, California
203 *Infection of the Joints*

ROBERT G. LUKE, M.D., F.A.C.P.
Chairman
Department of Internal Medicine
University of Cincinnati Medical Center
Cincinnati, Ohio
110 *Chronic Renal Failure*

JAMSON S. LWEBUGA-MUKASA, M.D., Ph.D.
Associate Professor of Medicine
Director, Division of Pulmonary and Critical Care
Buffalo General Hospital
State Univeristy of New York at Buffalo
School of Medicine and Biomedical Sciences
Buffalo, New York
40 *Mechanisms of Lung Injury and Repair*

WENDY LYNCH, M.B., Bch., B.A.O., M.R.C.P.I., M.R.C.P.
Dermatology Resident
Johns Hopkins Medical Institutions
Baltimore, Maryland
212 *Cutaneous Manifestations of Connective Tissue Diseases*

JOHN S. MacGREGOR, M.D., Ph.D.
Director, Cardiac Catheterization Laboratory
San Francisco General Hospital
Assistant Professor of Medicine
University of California–San Francisco
San Francisco, California
33   *Cardiac Tumors; Cardiac Manifestations of Endocrine, Collagen Vascular, and HIV Disease; and Traumatic Injury of the Heart*

JON T. MADER, M.D.
Department of Internal Medicine
The University of Texas Medical Branch
Galveston, Texas
243   *Osteomyelitis*

R. ELLEN MAGENIS, M.D.
Oregon Health Sciences University
Portland, Oregon
284   *Principles of Genetic Disorders*

BARRY J. MAKE, M.D.
Director, Emphysema Center
Pulmonary Sciences and Critical Care Medicine Division
National Jewish Medical and Research Center
Professor
University of Colorado School of Medicine
Denver, Colorado
50   *Pulmonary Rehabilitation*

JUAN-R. MALAGELADA, M.D.
Chief, Digestive Diseases
Hospital General Vall D'Hebron
Barcelona, Spain
336   *Peptic Ulcer Disease*

HARTMUT H. MALLUCHE, M.D.
Professor and Chief
Division of Nephrology, Bone and Mineral Metabolism
Department of Internal Medicine
University of Kentucky Medical Center
Lexington, Kentucky
321   *Renal Bone Disease*

GERALD L. MANDELL, M.D.
Professor of Medicine
Owen R. Cheatham Professor of the Sciences
Chief, Division of Infectious Diseases
University of Virginia Health Sciences Center
Charlottesville, Virginia
230   *Host Defense Against Infection: The Roles of Antibody, Complement, and Phagocytic Cells*

R. MAÑON-ESPAILLAT, M.D.
Clinical Associate Professor
Department of Neurology
Thomas Jefferson University
Philadelphia, Pennsylvania
130   *Electroencephalography and Evoked Responses*

DAVID MARCANTONIO, M.D.
Assistant Professor
Director, Musculoskeletal Imaging
Department of Radiology
University of Texas Southwestern Medical Center
Dallas, Texas
184   *Imaging Evaluation of Patients With Arthritis*

DIANA L. MARQUARDT, M.D.
Associate Professor of Medicine
University of California–San Diego
San Diego, California
189   *Anaphylaxis*

LIAM MARTIN, M.B., M.R.C.P.I., F.R.C.P.C.
Associate Professor
Faculty of Medicine
Division of Rheumatology
University of Calgary
Calgary, Alberta, Canada
181   *Autoantibodies*

CIRO R. MARTINS, M.D.
Assistant Professor
Department of Dermatology
Johns Hopkins Medical Institutions
Johns Hopkins University
Baltimore, Maryland
226   *Cutaneous Features of the Human Immunodeficiency Virus Infection*

JOHN MARSHALL, M.D., Ph.D.
Professor of Medicine
Director, Center for Research in Reproduction
University of Virginia Health Sciences Center
Charlottesville, Virginia
292   *Impotence and Altered Libido*
293   *Gynecomastia*

FREDERICK A. MASOUDI, M.D.
Cardiology Fellow
The University of Colorado Health Sciences Center
Denver, Colorado
12   *Electrocardiography*
24   *Infective Endocarditis*

R. MICHAEL MASSANARI, M.D.
Professor of Medicine
Wayne State University
Director for the Center of Healthcare Effectiveness Research
Wayne State University/Detroit Medical Center
Detroit, Michigan
232   *Hospital Infection Control*

JEAN K. MATHESON, M.D.
Assistant Professor of Clinical Neurology
Harvard Medical School
Co-Director, Sleep Disorders Center
Beth Israel Hospital
Boston, Massachusetts
134   *Sleep and Sleep Disorders*

RICHARD A. MATTHAY, M.D.
Boehringer Ingelheim Professor of Medicine
Associate Director, Department of Medicine
Pulmonary and Critical Care Section
Yale University School of Medicine
New Haven, Connecticut
63   *Pulmonary Thromboembolism*

SUZANNE M. MATSUI, M.D.
Assistant Professor
Department of Medicine
Stanford University School of Medicine
Stanford, California
Staff Physician
Department of Medicine
VA Palo Alto Health Care System
Palo Alto, California
254   *Rotavirus and Norwalk-Like Virus Infections*

RICHARD W. McCALLUM, M.D., F.A.C.P., F.R.A.C.P.C.(Aust), F.A.C.G.
Professor of Medicine
Chief, Division of Gastroenterology and Hepatology
Department of Medicine
University of Kansas Medical Center
Kansas City, Kansas
334 *Nausea, Vomiting, and Anorexia*

DANIEL J. McCARTY, M.D.
Will and Cava Ross Professor of Medicine, Emeritus
Director, Arthritis Institute
Medical College of Wisconsin
Milwaukee, Wisconsin
208 *Arthritis Associated with Calcium-Containing Crystals*

JAMES M. McGILL, M.D.
Assistant Professor of Medicine
Department of Medicine
Indiana University School of Medicine
Indianapolis Veterans Administration Medical Center
Indianapolis, Indiana
367 *Diseases of the Peritoneum, Mesentery, and Omentum*

JOHN E. McGOWAN, Jr., M.D.
Professor of Pathology and Laboratory Medicine
Professor of Epidemiology
Emory University
Atlanta, Georgia
249 *Fever in the Hospitalized Patient*

T. DWIGHT McKINNEY, M.D.
Executive Director, Clinical Pharmacology
Lilly Laboratory for Clinical Research
Professor of Medicine
Indiana University School of Medicine
Indianapolis, Indiana
102 *Urinalysis and Renal Function Tests*
126 *Renal Cell Carcinoma*

GEOFFREY McLENNAN, M.D.
Associate Professor
Department of Medicine
The University of Iowa Hospitals
Iowa City, Iowa
53 *Sarcoidosis*

ROBERT T. MEANS, Jr., M.D.
Associate Professor of Medicine and Director
Diagnostic Hematology Laboratory
Division of Hematology/Oncology
University of Cincinnati College of Medicine
Assistant Chief for Experimental Hematology/Oncology
Hematology/Oncology Section
Department of Veterans Affairs Medical Center
Cincinnati, Ohio
86 *Iron Deficiency Anemia, Anemia of Chronic Disease, Sideroblastic Anemia, and Iron Overload*
87 *Megaloblastic Anemia*

THOMAS A. MEDSGER, Jr., M.D.
Gerald P. Rodnan Professor of Medicine
Department of Medicine
Division of Rheumatology and Clinical Immunology
University of Pittsburgh Medical Center
Pittsburgh, Pennsylvania
197 *Systemic Sclerosis*

SHLOMO MELMED, M.D.
Director, Cedars-Sinai Research Institute
Department of Endocrinology and Metabolism
Cedars Sinai–UCLA School of Medicine
Los Angeles, California
295 *Disorders of the Hypothalamus and Anterior Pituitary*

JAY E. MENITOVE, M.D.
Executive Director and Medical Director
Community Blood Center of Greater Kansas City
Clinical Professor of Internal Medicine
Kansas University School of Medicine
University of Missouri–Kansas City
School of Medicine
Kansas City, Kansas
76 *Blood Transfusion*

JONATHAN H. MERMIN, M.D.
Division of General Internal Medicine
Department of Medicine
San Francisco General Hospital
San Francisco, California
275 *Infections With* Mycobacterium leprae *(Leprosy)*

LAURENCE J. MILLER, M.D.
Professor of Medicine and Biochemistry/Molecular Biology
Mayo Medical School
Center for Basic Research in Digestive Diseases
Rochester, Minnesota
350 *Pancreatic Secretion*

STANLEY J. MILLER, M.D.
Assistant Professor of Dermatology
Department of Dermatology
The Johns Hopkins Medical Institutions
Baltimore, Maryland
214 *Cutaneous Malignancies: Basal Cell Carcinoma and Squamous Cell Carcinoma*

THOMAS P. MILLER, M.D.
Professor of Medicine
University of Arizona
Arizona Cancer Center
Tucson, Arizona
93 *Hodgkin's Disease and Non-Hodgkin's Lymphoma*

PROFESSOR JOHN MILLS, B.S. Hons (Chicago), M.D. Hon (Harvard), F.R.A.C.P., F.A.C.P.
Director, Macfarlane Burnet Centre for Medical Research
Fairfield, Australia
258 *Mycoplasmal Infections*

BEVERLY S. MITCHELL, M.D.
Professor and Division Chief
School of Medicine
University of North Carolina–Chapel Hill
Associate Director of Lineberger Cancer Center
Chapel Hill, North Carolina
71 *Principles of Cancer Treatment*

CHARLOTTE E. MODLY, M.D.
Clinical Assistant Professor
University of Maryland Medical Center
Baltimore, Maryland
218 *Acne Vulgaris*

ROBERT C. MOELLERING, Jr., M.D.
Shields Warren-Mallinckrodt Professor of Medical Research
Harvard Medical School
Boston, Massachusetts
Associate Physician-in-Chief
Beth Israel Deaconess Medical Center
Boston, Massachusetts
231 *Principles of Antiinfective Therapy*

MARIE-CLAUDE MONIER-FAUGERE, M.D.
Associate Research Professor
Division of Nephrology, Bone and Mineral Metabolism
Department of Internal Medicine
University of Kentucky Medical Center
Lexington, Kentucky
321 *Renal Bone Disease*

WARWICK L. MORISON, M.B., B.S., M.D., M.R.C.P.
Professor of Dermatology
Johns Hopkins University
Baltimore, Maryland
216 *Psoriasis*
219 *Photodermatoses*

ROBB E. MOSES, M.D.
Chairman Professor
Molecular and Medical Genetics
Oregon Health Sciences University
Portland, Oregon
284 *Principles of Genetic Disorders*

ANNE W. MOULTON, M.D.
Associate Professor of Medicine
Brown University School of Medicine
Associate Physician
Division of General Internal Medicine
Rhode Island Hospital
Providence, Rhode Island
371 *Women's Health*

ANANTH V. MUDGIL, M.D.
Senior Resident
Department of Ophthalmology
Brown University School of Medicine
The Rhode Island Hospital
Providence, Rhode Island
376 *Common Eye Problems*

LOUIS A. MULIERI, Ph.D.
Research Associate Professor
Department of Molecular Physiology and Biophysics
University of Vermont College of Medicine
Burlington, Vermont
9 *Cardiovascular Physiology*

GREGORY R. MUNDY, M.D.
Heyser Professor of Bone and Mineral Metabolism
Program Director, Frederic C. Bartter Clinical Research Unit
Professor and Head
Department of Medicine
Division of Endocrinology
University of Texas Health Sciences Center at San Antonio
San Antonio, Texas
283 *Physiology of Bone and Mineral Homeostasis*
286 *Diagnostic Approach to Bone and Mineral Disorders*
319 *Osteopetrosis*
320 *Fibrous Dysplasia*
323 *Malignant Disease and the Skeleton*

JOSEPH P. MURGO, M.D., F.A.C.C.
CEO/Medical Director
Heart and Vascular Institute of Texas
San Antonio, Texas
14 *Cardiac Catheterization and Angiography*

JOCK MURRAY, M.D.
Professor of Medical Humanity
Director, Dalhousie University Multiple Sclerosis Research Unit
Halifax, Nova Scotia, Canada
127 *Neurologic History and Examination*

ROBERT J. MYERBURG, M.D.
Professor of Medicine and Physiology
Director, Division of Cardiology
University of Miami School of Medicine
Miami, Florida
18 *Cardiac Arrhythmias and Conduction Disturbances*

GERALD V. NACCARELLI, M.D.
Professor of Medicine
Chief, Division of Cardiology
Director, Penn State Cardiovascular Center
The Pennsylvania State University College of Medicine
Hershey, Pennsylvania
21 *Sudden Cardiac Death*

KENNETH K. NAKANO, M.D., M.P.H., F.R.C.P.(C)
Neurologist
Straub Clinic
Honolulu, Hawaii
138 *Neck and Back Pain*
165 *Neurorheumatology*

ROBERT G. NARINS, M.D.
Division Head
Division of Nephrology and Hypertension
Henry Ford Hospital
Detroit, Michigan
112 *Disorders of Water Balance*
114 *Disorders of Potassium Balance*

ERIC G. NEILSON, M.D.
C. Mahlon Kline Professor of Medicine
Chief, Renal-Electrolyte and Hypertension Division
Hospital of the University of Pennsylvania
Philadelphia, Pennsylvania
124 *Tubulointerstitial Renal Diseases*

DAVID L. NELSON, M.D.
Chief, Immunophysiology Section
Metabolism Branch, DCS, NCI
National Institutes of Health
Bethesda, Maryland
185 *The Primary Immunodeficiency Disorders*

LINDA NICI, M.D.
Assistant Professor of Medicine
Pulmonary and Critical Care Division
Brown University School of Medicine
The Rhode Island Hospital
Providence, Rhode Island
49 *Respiratory Therapy and Monitoring*

CHARLES R. NOLAN, M.D.
Associate Professor of Medicine
University of Colorado Health Sciences Center
Denver, Colorado
102 *Urinalysis and Renal Function Tests*

HOSSEIN C. NOUSARI, M.D.
Fellow in Dermatoimmunology
Department of Dermatology
Johns Hopkins University
Baltimore, Maryland
213 *Bullous Diseases*

DAVID R. NUNLEY, M.D.
Senior Fellow
Division of Critical Care Medicine
University of Pittsburgh Medical Center
Pittsburgh, Pennsylvania
66 *Pulmonary Transplantation*

THOMAS B. NUTMAN, M.D.
Head, Helminth Immunology Section
Laboratory of Parasitic Diseases
National Institutes of Health
Bethesda, Maryland
174 *Cellular Immunity, Cytokines, and Immunoregulation*

KATHRYN ANN O'CONNELL, M.D., Ph.D.
Assistant Professor of Dermatology
Johns Hopkins University School of Medicine
Baltimore, Maryland
227 *Kaposi's Sarcoma*

G. RICHARD OLDS, M.D.
Charles H. Rammelkamp Jr. Professor and
Chairman of Medicine
Department of Medicine
Metro Health Medical Center
Case Western Reserve University
Cleveland, Ohio
281 *Infections Caused by Helminths*

MARGARET O'NEILL, M.D.
Dermatology Resident
Johns Hopkins University School of Medicine
Baltimore, Maryland
214 *Cutaneous Malignancies: Basal Cell Carcinoma and Squamous Cell Carcinoma*

DIANE J. ORLINSKY, M.D.
Clinical Fellow
Johns Hopkins Medical Center
Baltimore, Maryland
224 *Cutaneous Manifestations of Endocrine Disorders*

ROBERT A. O'ROURKE, M.D.
Charles Conrad Brown Distinguished Professor in Cardiovascular Disease
Department of Medicine/Cardiology
The University of Texas Health Sciences Center at San Antonio
San Antonio, Texas
17 *Palpitations*
30 *Diseases of the Aorta*
136 *Faintness and Syncope*

C. KENT OSBORNE, M.D.
Professor of Medicine
Chief, Division of Medical Oncology
The University of Texas Health Sciences Center at San Antonio
San Antonio, Texas
95 *Breast Cancer*

JOHN J. O'SHEA, M.D.
Chief, Lymphocyte Cell Biology Section
Arthritis and Rheumatism Branch
National Institute of Arthritis, Musculoskeletal and Skin Diseases
National Institutes of Health
Bethesda, Maryland
174 *Cellular Immunity, Cytokines, and Immunoregulation*
179 *Evaluation of Cellular Immune Function*

GEORGE OSOL, Ph.D.
Professor
Department of Obstetrics and Gynecology
University of Vermont
Burlington, Vermont
9 *Cardiovascular Physiology*

J. DONALD OSTROW, M.D., M.Sc.
Gastrointestinal and Liver Department
Academic Medical Center
University of Amsterdam
Amsterdam, Netherlands
353 *Jaundice and Disorders of Bilirubin Metabolism*

STEPHEN W. PARKER, M.D.
Assistant Professor of Neurology
Harvard Medical School
Director of Otoneurology
Department of Neurology
Massachusetts General Hospital
Boston, Massachusetts
139 *Otoneurology*

THOMAS F. PATTERSON, M.D.
Associate Professor of Medicine
Department of Medicine
University of Texas Health Sciences Center at San Antonio
San Antonio, Texas
276 *Infections Caused by Common Fungi*
278 *Cryptococcus neoformans Infections*

DOUGLAS J. PEARCE, M.D.
Private Practice
Nashville, Tennessee
16 *Chest Pain*

JOHN R. PERFECT, M.D.
Professor
Department of Medicine
Duke University
Durham, North Carolina
266 *Infections Caused by* Haemophilus *Species*

ROGER M. PERLMUTTER, M.D., Ph.D.
Senior Vice President
Merck Research Laboratories
Rahway, New Jersey
173 *Antibodies: Structure and Genetics*

WILLIAM P. PETERS, M.D., Ph.D.
Director and Chief Executive Officer
Barbara Ann Karmanos Cancer Institute
Detroit, Michigan
100 *Cancer of Unknown Primary Site*

BRET T. PETERSEN, M.D.
Consultant in Gastroenterology
Director, Advanced Endoscopy Fellowship
Division of Gastroenterology and Hepatology
Mayo Clinic
Rochester, Minnesota
328 *Gastrointestinal Endoscopy*

CAROLYN PETERSEN, M.D.
Assistant Professor of Medicine
San Francisco General Hospital
San Francisco, California
279 *Infections Caused by Protozoa*

WALTER L. PETERSON, M.D.
Professor of Medicine
Veterans Affairs Medical Center
Dallas, Texas
330 *Evaluation of Gastroduodenal Diseases*

GRAHAM F. PINEO, M.D.
Professor of Medicine
University of Calgary
Calgary, Alberta, Canada
85 *Thrombosis and Anticoagulation*

JOANN PINKERTON, M.D.
Associate Professor of Medicine
Director, MidLife Health
University of Virginia Health Sciences Center
Charlottesville, Virginia
302 *Benign Breast Diseases*

C.S. PITCHUMONI, M.D., F.R.C.P.(C) M.P.H.
Professor of Medicine
Professor of Community and Preventive Medicine
New York Medical College
Director of Medicine
Chief of Gastroenterology and Clinical Nutrition
Our Lady of Mercy Medical Center
Bronx, New York
352 *Evaluation of Pancreatic Diseases*
366 *Pancreatic Diseases*

PAUL H. PLOTZ, M.D.
Chief, Arthritis and Rheumatism Branch, NIAMS
Bethesda, Maryland
199 *Inflammatory Myopathies*

FRISSO A. POTTS, M.D.
Neurology Service
Brockton-West Roxbury
Veterans Administration Medical Center
Brockton, Massachusetts
146 *Myelopathies*

SUMANTH D. PRABHU, M.D.
Assistant Professor of Medicine
Department of Medicine
The University of Texas Health Sciences Center at San Antonio
San Antonio, Texas
17 *Palpitations*
136 *Faintness and Syncope*

THOMAS T. PROVOST, M.D.
Professor
Department of Dermatology
Johns Hopkins Medical Institutions
Baltimore, Maryland
212 *Cutaneous Manifestations of Connective Tissue Diseases*

AMY A. PRUITT, M.D.
Department of Neurology
University of Pennsylvania Medical Center
Philadelphia, Pennsylvania
160 *Neurooncology*

WILLIAM E.M. PRYSE-PHILLIPS, M.D.
Department of Neurology
Memorial University of Newfoundland
Health Sciences Center
St. John's, Newfoundland, Canada
128 *Psychologic Testing*

SHAHBUDIN H. RAHIMTOOLA, M.B., F.R.C.P., M.A.C.P.
Distinguished Professor
George C. Griffith Professor of Cardiology
Chairman, Griffith Center
Professor of Medicine
University of Southern California
Los Angeles, California
25 *Valvular Heart Disease*

LAWRENCE G. RAISZ, M.D.
Program Director, General Clinical Research Center
University of Connecticut Health Center
Farmington, Connecticut
316 *Osteoporosis*

JORGE RAKELA, M.D.
Professor of Medicine
Division of Gastroenterology and Hepatology
University of Pittsburgh
Pittsburgh, Pennsylvania
355 *Acute and Chronic Viral Hepatitis*

JOHN A. RANKIN, M.D.
Associate Clinical Professor of Medicine
Yale University School of Medicine
New Haven, Connecticut
Pulmonary and Critical Care Section
West Haven Veterans Administration Medical Center
West Haven, Connecticut
42 *Invasive Diagnostic Techniques*

GARY E. RASKOB, M.Sc.
Associate Professor
Department of Biostatistics & Epidemiology & Medicine
University of Oklahoma Health Sciences Center
Oklahoma City, Oklahoma
85 *Thrombosis and Anticoagulation*

JEAN-PIERRE RAUFMAN, M.D.
Jerome Levy Professor of Medicine
Director, Division of Gastroenterology
Department of Medicine
University of Arkansas for Medical Sciences
Chief, Digestive Diseases and Nutrition
McClellan Memorial Veterans Hospital
Little Rock, Arkansas
325 *Gastric Secretion*

CHARLES A. REASNER II, M.D.
Department of Medicine
Division of Endocrinology and Metabolism
University of Texas Health Sciences Center at San Antonio
San Antonio, Texas
283 *Physiology of Bone and Mineral Homeostasis*
286 *Diagnostic Approach to Bone and Mineral Disorders*
319 *Osteopetrosis*
323 *Malignant Disease and the Skeleton*

GUY S. REEDER, M.D.
Professor of Medicine
Director, Coronary Care Unit
Mayo Clinic and Foundation
Rochester, Minnesota
23 *Acute Myocardial Infarction*

MICHAEL F. REIN, M.D.
Professor of Medicine
Associate Chair for Undergraduate Medical Education
University of Virginia School of Medicine
Charlottesville, Virginia
244 *Sexually Transmitted Diseases (Urethritis, Vaginitis, Cervicitis, Proctitis, Genital Lesions)*
274 *Infections Caused by Spirochetes*

JAMES A. REINARZ, M.D.
Director of Infectious Disease
JPS Health Network
Fort Worth, Texas
264 Neisseria meningitidis *Infections*

DONALD L. RESNICK, M.D.
Professor of Radiology
University of California–San Diego
Chief of Osteoradiology
VAMC San Diego
San Diego, California
184 *Imaging Evaluation of Patients with Arthritis*

HERBERT Y. REYNOLDS, M.D.
Professor and Chair
Department of Medicine
Milton S. Hershey Medical Center
The Pennsylvania State University College of Medicine
Hershey, Pennsylvania
39 *Host Defense Mechanisms in the Respiratory Tract*
45 *Approach to the Patient with Respiratory System Disease*
54 *Hypersensitivity Pneumonitis*

ROBERT R. RICH, M.D.
Distinguished Service Professor
Department of Microbiology and Immunology
Baylor College of Medicine
Houston, Texas
171 *Human Immune Response*

JEAN E. RINALDO, M.D.
Chief, Pulmonary Medicine
Veterans Administration Medical Center
Division of Pulmonary/Critical Care Medicine
Vanderbilt University
Nashville, Tennessee
47 *Multiple Organ Dysfunction in the Context of ARDS*

ROBERT ROBERTS, M.D.
Section of Cardiology
Baylor College of Medicine
Houston, Texas
10 *Molecular Biology of the Cardiovascular System*

GARY L. ROBERTSON, M.D.
Professor of Medicine and Neurology
Center for Endocrinology, Metabolism, and Nutrition
Northwestern University Medical School
Chicago, Illinois
296 *Disorders of the Posterior Pituitary*

DUDLEY F. ROCHESTER, M.D.
Professor Emeritus
University of Virginia Health Sciences Center
Charlottesville, Virginia
37 *Respiratory Muscles and Respiratory Muscle Failure*

ALLAN H. ROPPER, M.D.
Chief of Neurology
St. Elizabeth's Medical Center
Professor of Neurology
Tufts University School of Medicine
Boston, Massachusetts
163 *Principles of Coma and Neurologic Emergencies*

PHILIP J. ROSENTHAL, M.D.
Associate Professor of Medicine
Department of Medicine
University of California–San Francisco
San Francisco General Hospital
San Francisco, California
247 *Infections in Travelers*

ROBIN D. ROTHSTEIN, M.D.
Assistant Professor of Medicine
Department of Gastroenterology
University of Pennsylvania Hospital
Philadelphia, Pennsylvania
339 *Diarrhea, Constipation, and Irritable Bowel Syndrome*

LEWIS J. RUBIN, M.D.
Head, Division of Pulmonary and Critical Care Medicine
Professor of Medicine and Physiology
University of Maryland
School of Medicine
Baltimore, Maryland
62 *Pulmonary Hypertension: Primary and Secondary Causes*

LAWRENCE M. RYAN, M.D.
Professor of Medicine
Will and Cava Ross Professor
Chief, Division of Rheumatology
Medical College of Wisconsin
Milwaukee, Wisconsin
208 *Arthritis Associated with Calcium-Containing Crystals*

SEYMOUR M. SABESIN, M.D.
Dyrenforth Professor of Medicine
Director, Division of Digestive Diseases
Rush-Presbyterian-St. Luke's Medical Center
Rush Medical College
Chicago, Illinois
348 *Hepatic Metabolism*

SHARON SAFRIN, M.D.
Director, Clinical Research
Gilead Sciences Inc.
Associate Professor of Clinical Medicine and Epidemiology
University of California–San Francisco
San Francisco, California
280 *Pneumocystis carinii Infection*

STEPHEN M. SAGAR, M.D.
Department of Neurology
University of California–San Francisco
Mount Zion Medical Center
San Francisco, California
162 *Metabolic and Toxic Disorders*

MARTIN A. SAMUELS, M.D.
Professor of Neurology
Harvard Medical School
Neurologist-in-Chief
Chairman, Department of Neurology
Brigham and Women's Hospital
Boston, Massachusetts
129 *Spinal Fluid Examination*
135 *Coma and Related Disorders*
164 *Neurocardiology*
166 *Neuropulmonology*
167 *Neurogastroenterology*
168 *Neurohepatology*
169 *Neurohematology*
170 *Neuronephrology*

MERLE A. SANDE, M.D.
Professor and Chairman
Department of Internal Medicine
University of Utah
School of Medicine
Salt Lake City, Utah
24 *Infective Endocarditis*
229 *Basic Principles of Infectious Diseases*
235 *Fever and Rash*
248 *Acquired Immunodeficiency Syndrome*
269 *Infections Caused by Salmonella and Shigella Species*
273 *Tuberculosis and Nontuberculous Mycobacterial Infections*

CHARLES E. SANDERS, Jr., M.D.
Lifelink Transplantation Institution
Tampa, Florida
110 *Chronic Renal Failure*

LISA ISTORICO SANDERS, M.D.
Assistant Professor
Division of Infectious Diseases
University of South Florida
Tampa, Florida
245 *Gram-Negative Bacteremia and the Sepsis Syndrome*

PAUL W. SANDERS, M.D.
Associate Professor of Medicine
University of Alabama at Birmingham
Birmingham, Alabama
118 *Renal Manifestations of Dysproteinemias*

RICHARD J. SANTEN, M.D.
Professor of Medicine
Department of Medicine
University of Virginia Health Sciences Center
Charlottesville, Virginia
301 *Disorders of the Testis*
302 *Benign Breast Diseases*

DAVID J. SARTORIS, M.D.
Professor of Radiology
School of Medicine
University of California–San Diego
San Diego, California
184 *Imaging Evaluation of Patients with Arthritis*

JULIUS SCHACHTER, Ph.D.
University of California–San Francisco
San Francisco, California
257 *Chlamydial Infections*

ANDREW I. SCHAFER, M.D.
WA and Deborah Moncrief, Jr. Professor and Acting Chairman
Department of Medicine
Baylor College of Medicine
Acting Chief, Internal Medicine Service
The Methodist Hospital
Houston, Texas
83 *Thrombocytopenia and Disorders of Platelet Function*

MICHAEL SCHATZ, M.D.
Staff Allergist
Department of Allergy
Kaiser-Permanente Medical Center, San Diego
Clinical Professor
Department of Medicine
University of California–San Diego
School of Medicine
San Diego, California
187 *Rhinitis*

W. MICHAEL SCHELD, M.D.
Professor of Internal Medicine and Neurosurgery
Associate Chair for Residency Programs
Director, Residency Programs in Internal Medicine
University of Virginia Health Sciences Center
Charlottesville, Virginia
239 *Acute Meningitis*

STEVEN SCHENKER, M.D.
Professor of Medicine and Pharmacology
Chief, Division of Gastroenterology and Nutrition
University of Texas Health Sciences Center at San Antonio
San Antonio, Texas
354 *Principal Complications of Liver Failure*

ROBERT C. SCHLANT, M.D.
Professor of Medicine (Cardiology)
Emory University School of Medicine
Chief of Cardiology
Grady Memorial Hospital
Atlanta, Georgia
28 *Congenital Heart Disease*

CHARLES J. SCHLEUPNER, M.D.
Professor and Associate Chairman
Department of Internal Medicine
University of Florida Health Sciences Center
Jacksonville, Florida
253 *Unusual Viral Infections: Arenavirus, Colorado Tick Fever Virus, Parvovirus, Bunyavirus, and Togavirus (Ebola)*

KEVIN SCHULMAN, M.D.
Associate Professor of Medicine
Director of Clinical Economics Research Unit
Georgetown University Medical Center
Washington, DC
4 *Costs and Outcomes*

KONRAD S. SCHULZE-DELRIEU, M.D.
Professor
Division of Gastroenterology-Hepatology
Department of Internal Medicine
University of Iowa Hospital and Clinic
Iowa City, Iowa
329 *Evaluation of Esophageal Disease*
333 *Esophageal Diseases*

HAROLD R. SCHUMACHER, M.D.
Medical Director, Hematology Service
Alliance Laboratory Services
Director, Hematopathology Fellowship Program
University Hospital, Inc.
Cincinnati, Ohio
73 *Molecular Diagnostics*

BENJAMIN D. SCHWARTZ, M.D., Ph.D.
Searle Research and Development
Monsanto Company
St. Louis, Missouri
172 *Human Leukocyte Antigen Complex*

STEPHEN C. SCHWARTZ, M.D.
Assistant Professor of Medicine
Section of Medical Oncology and Hematology
Department of Medicine
Wayne State University School of Medicine
Detroit, Michigan
100 *Carcinoma of Unknown Primary Site*

J. EDWIN SEEGMILLER, M.D.
Professor of Medicine, Emeritus
Department of Medicine
Associate Director of Stein Institute for Research on Aging
University of California–San Diego
School of Medicine
La Jolla, California
209 *Ochronosis and Alkaptonuria*

MARJORIE E. SEYBOLD, M.D.
Director, EMG Laboratory
Veterans Administration San Diego Health Care System
Adjunct Professor of Neurosciences
University of California–San Diego
Director, Medical Services
Quintiles CNS Therapeutics
San Diego, California
148 *Diseases of the Neuromuscular Junction*

PRAVIN M. SHAH, M.D.
Professor of Medicine/Cardiology
Director of Academic Program
Loma Linda University Medical Center
Loma Linda, California
26 *Cardiomyopathies*

BHAGWAN T. SHAHANI, M.D., D.Phil (Oxon), F.A.C.P.
Professor of Neurology
Professor and Chairman
Department of Rehabilitation Medicine & Restorative Medical
Sciences
University of Chicago College of Medicine
Chicago, Illinois
157 *Principles of Neurorehabilitation*

MRINAL SHARMA, M.D.
Assistant Professor of Medicine
Associate Director, Coronary Care Unit
Director, Clinical Trials Section
Cardiovascular Thrombosis Research Center
University of Massachusetts Medical School
Worcester, Massachusetts
20 *Hypotension and Cardiogenic Shock*

JAMES A. SHAVER, M.D
Professor of Medicine
Director, Cardiovascular Fellowship Program
University of Pittsburgh Medical Center
Pittsburgh, Pennsylvania
11 *Physical Examination of the Cardiovascular System*

JOHN N. SHEAGREN, M.D.
Professor
Rush Medical College
Chair
Department of Internal Medicine
Illinois Masonic Medical Center
Chicago, Illinois
260 *Staphylococcal Infections*

RICHARD M. SILVER, M.D.
Professor of Medicine
Director, Division of Rheumatism and Immunology
Medical University of South Carolina
Charleston, South Carolina
196 *Raynaud's Phenomenon*
198 *Diffuse Fasciitis with Eosinophilia*

EVA SIMMONS-O'BRIEN, M.D.
Department of Dermatology
Johns Hopkins Medical Institutions
Baltimore, Maryland
212 *Cutaneous Manifestations of Connective Tissue Diseases*

ANDREA J. SINGER, M.D.
Department of General Internal Medicine
Georgetown University Medical Center
Washington, DC
372 *Medical Disorders During Pregnancy*

FREDERICK R. SINGER, M.D.
Director, Endocrine/Bone Disease Program
John Wayne Cancer Institute at Saint John's Health Center
Clincal Professor
UCLA School of Medicine
Los Angeles, California
318 *Paget's Disease of Bone*

NAV T. SINGH, M.D.
Assistant Professor of Medicine
Department of Pulmonary Medicine
University of Connecticut Health Center
Farmington, Connecticut
56 *Primary Granulomatous Pulmonary Vasculitis*

GORDON L. SNIDER, M.D.
Chief, Medical Service
Boston Veterans Administration Medical Center
Vice Chairman and Professor of Medicine
Boston University School of Medicine
Boston, Massachusetts
51 *Chronic Obstructive Pulmonary Disease*

AKSHAY SOOD, M.D.
Pulmonary Associates
Las Vegas, Nevada
57 *Occupational Lung Diseases*

MICHAEL F. SORRELL, M.D.
Robert L. Grissom Professor of Medicine
Medical Director
Liver Transplant Program
University of Nebraska Medical Center
Omaha, Nebraska
363 *Liver Transplantation*

IRFAN SOYKAN, M.D.
Division of Gastroenterology & Hepatology
University of Ankara School of Medicine
Sihhiye, Ankara, Turkey
334 *Nausea, Vomiting, and Anorexia*

JOHN A. SPITTELL, Jr., M.D.
Assistant Professor of Medicine
Mayo Medical School
Consultant
Department of Internal Medicine
Division of Cardiovascular Diseases
Mayo Medical Center
Rochester, Minnesota
31 *Diseases of the Peripheral Arteries and Veins*

PETER C. SPITTELL, M.D.
Consultant, Division of Cardiovascular Diseases
Mayo Clinic
Rochester, Minnesota
31 *Diseases of the Peripheral Arteries and Veins*

JOHN L. STAUFFER, M.D.
Professor of Medicine
The Milton S. Hershey Medical Center
The Pennsylvania State University
Hershey, Pennsylvania
45 *Approach to the Patient with Respiratory System Disease*

JAY H. STEIN, M.D.
Senior Vice President and Vice Provost for Health Affairs
The University of Rochester Medical Center
Chief Executive Officer
University of Rochester Medical Center and Strong Health
Professor of Medicine
University of Rochester School of Medicine and Dentistry
Rochester, New York
101 *Principles of Renal Physiology*
109 *Acute Renal Failure*

ALFRED D. STEINBERG, M.D.
Mitretek Systems
McLean, Virginia
Potomac, Maryland
177 *Tolerance and Autoimmunity*

MARTIN H. STEINBERG, M.D.
Associate Chief of Staff for Research
Professor of Medicine
Veterans Administration Medical Center
Jackson, Mississippi
88 *Hemoglobinopathies and Thalassemias*

RICHARD H. STERNS, M.D.
Professor of Medicine
University of Rochester School of Medicine
Chief of Medicine
Rochester General Hospital
Rochester, New York
114 *Disorders of Potassium Balance*

DENNIS L. STEVENS, M.D., Ph.D.
Chief, Infectious Disease Section
Veterans Administration Medical Center
Boise, Idaho
Professor of Medicine
University of Washington
Seattle, Washington
261 *Streptococcus pyogenes Infections*

LYNNE WARNER STEVENSON, M.D.
Associate Professor of Medicine
Harvard Medical School
Clinical Director
Cardiomyopathy/Heart Failure Program
Brigham and Women's Hospital
Boston, Massachusetts
34 *Cardiac Transplantation*

LARRY JAMES STRAUSBAUGH, M.D.
Hospital Epidemiologist and Staff Physician
Veterans' Affairs Medical Center
Portland, Oregon
Professor of Medicine
School of Medicine
Oregon Health Sciences University
Portland, Oregon
262 *Enterococcal and Non–Group A Streptococcal Infections*

LEWIS R. SUDARSKY, M.D.
Assistant Professor of Neurology
Harvard Medical School
Boston, Massachusetts
Assistant Chief Neurology Service
Veterans Administration Medical Center
West Roxbury, Massachusetts
143 *Parkinsonism and Movement Disorders*

STEPHEN B. SULAVIK, M.D.
Professor Emeritus of Medicine
University of Connecticut School of Medicine
Clinical Professor of Medicine
Yale University School of Medicine
New Haven, Connecticut
56 *Primary Granulomatous Pulmonary Vasculitis*

THOMAS Y. SULLIVAN, M.D.
Medical Director
Pulmonary Function and Sleep Disorders Center
Methodist Hospital
Indianapolis, Indiana
61 *Solitary Pulmonary Tumor*

DANIEL P. SULMASY, M.D., Ph.D.
Associate Professor of Medicine
Center for Clinical Bioethics
Georgetown University Medical Center
Washington, DC
3 *Clinical Bioethics*

ROBERT W. SUMMERS, M.D.
Professor of Internal Medicine
Division of Gastroenterology-Hepatology
University of Iowa College of Medicine
Iowa City, Iowa
329 *Evaluation of Esophageal Disease*
333 *Esophageal Diseases*

J. T. SYLVESTER, M.D.
David Marine Professor of Medicine
Division of Pulmonary and Critical Care Medicine
Johns Hopkins University School of Medicine
Baltimore, Maryland
38 *Pulmonary Blood Flow*

ANGELO TARANTA, M.D.
Department of Medicine
Cabrini Medical Center
New York, New York
204 *Rheumatic Fever*

ROBERT D. TARVER, M.D.
Professor of Radiology
Indiana University School of Medicine
Wishard Memorial Hospital
Indianapolis, Indiana
43 *Pulmonary Diagnostic Imaging*

MARTIN G. TÄUBER, M.D.
Chief, Infectious Diseases
Co-Director, Institute for Medical Microbiology
University of Berne
Berne, Switzerland
234 *Fever of Unknown Origin*

ANTHONY S. TAVILL, M.D. F.A.C.P., F.R.C.P.
Professor of Medicine and Nutrition
Case Western Reserve University
Mathile and Morton J. Stone Professor of Digestive and Liver
  Disorders
Mount Sinai Medical Center
Cleveland, Ohio
359 *Hemochromatosis, Wilson's disease, and Other Genetic Liver
  Diseases Affecting the Adult*

ABDELLATIF TAZI, M.D., Ph.D.
Professor of Medicine
Service de Pneumologie
Hôpital Avicenne
Bobigny, France
55 *Langerhans' Cell Granulomatosis (Histiocytosis X,
  Eosinophilic Granuloma)*

ROBERT A. TERKELTAUB, M.D.
Chief of Rheumatology
San Diego Veterans Administration Medical Center
Associate Professor of Medicine
University of California–San Diego
San Diego, California
207 *Gout and Hyperuricemia*

JESS G. THOENE, M.D.
Professor of Pediatrics
Director of the Division of Biochemical Genetics and Metabolism
Associate Professor of Biological Chemistry
University of Michigan
Ann Arbor, Michigan
308 *Disorders of Amino Acid Metabolism*

GALEN B. TOEWS, M.D.
Professor of Internal Medicine
Department of Internal Medicine
Chief of the Division of Pulmonary and Critical Care Medicine
University of Michigan Medical Center
Ann Arbor, Michigan
60 *Neoplasms of the Lung*

JERRY S. TRIER, M.D.
Professor of Medicine
Department of Medicine
Harvard Medical School
Brigham and Women's Hospital
Boston, Massachusetts
326 *Intestinal Absorption*

WILLIAM G. TSIARAS, M.D.
Chairmain
Department of Ophthalmology
Brown University School of Medicine
The Rhode Island Hospital
Providence, Rhode Island
376 *Common Eye Problems*

ALLAN R. TUNKEL, M.D., Ph.D.
Associate Chair for Education
Associate Professor of Medicine
Allegheny University of the Health Sciences
MCP Hahnemann School of Medicine
Philadelphia, Pennsylvania
239 *Acute Meningitis*
246 *Urinary Tract Infections*

MANUEL VALDIVIESO, M.D.,
Director
Cancer Center of Excellence
Oakwood Healthcare System
Dearborn, Mighican
Adjunct Professor of Internal Medicine
University of Michigan
Ann Arbor, Michigan
99 *Lung Cancer*

MANJERI A. VENKATACHALAM, M.B.B.S.
Professor
Department of Pathology
University of Texas Health Sciences Center at San Antonio
San Antonio, Texas
105 *Proteinuria*

DAVID L. VESELY, M.D., Ph.D., F.A.C.P., F.A.C.E.
Chief of Endocrinology and Metabolism
Director of Atrial Natriuretic Peptides Laboratories
James A. Haley Veterans Hospital
Professor of Internal Medicine, Physiology, and Biophysics
University of South Florida Health Sciences Center
Tampa, Florida
289 *Weakness*

RAKISH VINAYEK, M.D.
Clinical Fellow
University of Pittsburgh Medical Center
Pittsburgh, Pennsylvania
355 *Acute and Chronic Viral Hepatitis*

DAVID H. WALKER, M.D.
Chairman, Department of Pathology
Director, WHO Collaborating Center for Tropical Diseases
University of Texas Medical Branch
Galveston, Texas
259 *Rickettsial Infections*

THOMAS M. WALSHE III, M.D.
Assistant Professor
Harvard University
Associate Chief, Neurology Service
Veterans Administration Medical Center
Brockton, Massachusetts
142 *Cognitive Failure Dementia*

STEPHEN I. WASSERMAN, M.D.
The Helen M. Ranney Professor and Chair
Department of Medicine
University of California–San Diego
San Diego, California
176 *Immediate Hypersensitivity*
180 *Laboratory Methods in Immediate Hypersensitivity*
188 *Asthma*

DAVID L. WEINBAUM, M.D.
Associate Professor of Medicine
University of Pittsburgh
Chief, Infectious Diseases
West Penn Hospital
Staff Physician
Allegheny General Hospital
Pittsburgh, Pennsylvania
230 *Host Defense Against Infection: The Roles of Antibody, Complement, and Phagocytic Cells*

SCOTT R. WEINGARTEN, M.D., M.P.H.
Director, Health Services Research
Cedars-Sinai Health System
Associate Professor of Medicine
UCLA School of Medicine
Los Angeles, California
6 *Implementing Clincal Practice Guidelines*

MICHAEL H. WEISMAN, M.D.
Professor of Medicine
University of California–San Diego School of Medicine
La Jolla, California
Attending Physician
University of California–San Diego Medical Center
San Diego, California
203 *Infections of the Joints*

GEOFFREY R. WEISS, M.D.
Professor of Medicine
The University of Texas Health Sciences Center at San Antonio
San Antonio, Texas
97 *Cancer of the Prostate and Testis*

FREDERICK G. WENZEL IV, M.D.
Resident, Dermatology Department
Johns Hopkins Medical Institutions
Baltimore, Maryland
216 *Psoriasis*
219 *Photodermatoses*

RICHARD P. WENZEL, M.D.
Professor and Chairman
Department of Internal Medicine
Virginia Commonwealth University
Richmond, Virginia
232 *Hospital Infection Control*

ELLIOT WESER, M.D.
Professor and Deputy Chairman
Department of Medicine
The University of Texas Health Sciences Center at San Antonio
San Antonio, Texas
347 *Nutrition and Internal Medicine*

ARTHUR P. WHEELER, M.D.
Vanderbilt Medical Center
Nashvillle, Tennessee
48 *Pulmonary Edema*

GILBERT C. WHITE II, M.D.
Professor of Medicine and Pharmacology
University of North Carolina School of Medicine
Chapel Hill, North Carolina
84 *Disorders of Blood Coagulation*

S. ELIZABETH WHITMORE, M.D.
Assistant Professor, Department of Dermatology
Johns Hopkins University
Baltimore, Maryland
217 *Dermatitis*

HERBERT P. WIEDEMANN, M.D.
Chairman, Department of Pulmonary and Critical Care Medicine
Cleveland Clinic Foundation
Cleveland, Ohio
44 *Intensive Care Monitoring and Mechanical Ventilation*

LAUREL A. WIEGAND, M.D.
Associate Professor of Medicine
Pulmonary/Critical Care Division
College of Medicine
University Hospital-Children's Hospital
The Milton S. Hershey Medical Center
Hershey, Pennsylvania
67 *Sleep-Related Respiratory Disorders*

PENNY A. WILLIAMS, M.D.
Assistant Professor of Medicine
University of Pittsburgh Medical Center
Pittsburgh, Pennsylvania
66 *Pulmonary Transplantation*

DAVID A. WILLIAMS, M.D.
Frieda and Albrecht Kipp Professor of Pediatrics
Professor of Medical Molecular Genetics
Indiana University School of Medicine
Associate Investigator
Howard Hughes Medical Institute
Indianapolis, Indiana
68 *Molecular and Cellular Biology of Hematopoiesis*

MARY E. WILSON, M.D.
Professor of Medicine
Departments of Internal Medicine and Microbiology
University of Iowa College of Medicine
Iowa City, Iowa
268 *Infections Caused by* Vibrio *Species*

WALTER R. WILSON, M.D.
Professor of Medicine
Chief, Division of Infectious Diseases
Mayo Clinic
Rochester, Minnesota
270 *Infections Caused by* Brucella, Francisella tularensis,
   Pasteurella, Yersinia *Species and* Bordetella pertussis
   (Whooping Cough)

JOHN C. WINKELMANN, M.D.
Herbert F. Koch Professor of Internal Medicine
Director, Division of Hematology/Oncology
Department of Internal Medicine
University of Cincinnati
College of Medicine
Cincinnati, Ohio
72 *Evaluation of Peripheral Blood and Bone Marrow Cells*
89 *Hemolytic Anemia*

WASHINGTON C. WINN, Jr., M.D., M.B.A.
Professor of Pathology
University of Vermont College of Medicine
Director, Clinical Microbiology Laboratory
Fletcher Allen Health Care
Burlington, Vermont
272 *Infections Caused by Legionellae*

BIRGIT WINTHER, M.D.
Assistant Professor
Department of Otolaryngology, Head and Neck Surgery
University of Virginia Medical Center
Charlottesville, Virginia
237 *Respiratory Tract Infections*

ELEANOR ANNE YOUNG, Ph.D., R.D./L.D. (retired)
formerly
Professor of Medicine
Department of Medicine
The University of Texas Health Sciences Center at San Antonio
San Antonio, Texas
347 *Nutrition and Internal Medicine*

K. RANDALL YOUNG, Jr., M.D.
The Ben V. Branscomb Professor of Medicine
Director, Division of Pulmonary and Critical Care Medicine
The University of Alabama at Birmingham
Birmingham, Alabama
51 *Interstitial Lung Disease*

LOWELL S. YOUNG, M.D.
Clinical Professor of Medicine
University of California–San Francisco
Chief, Division of Infectious Diseases
Director, Kuzell Institute
California Pacific Medical Center
San Francisco, California
236 *Fever in the Compromised Host*

ROBERT R. YOUNG, M.D.
Professor and Vice Chairman
Department of Neurology
University of California–Irvine
Irvine, California
156 *Spinal Cord Injury*

MIGUEL ZABALGOITIA, M.D
Director of Echocardiography
Associate Professor of Medicine
The University of Texas Health Sciences Center at San Antonio
San Antonio, Texas
30 *Disease of the Aorta*

SARA L. ZAKNOEN, M.D.
Assistant Professor of Medicine
Division of Hematology/Oncology
Department of Medicine
University of Cincinnati Hospital
The Barrett Center for Cancer Prevention, Treatment and Research
Cincinnati, Ohio
78 *Complications of Cancer and Cancer Therapy*

ROBERT S. ZEIGER, M.D., Ph.D.
Chief of Allergy
Kaiser Permanente Medical Center
Clinical Professor of Pediatrics
University of California–San Diego
San Diego, California
187 *Rhinitis*

HYMAN J. ZIMMERMAN, M.D.
Professor of Medicine, Emeritus
George Washington University
Washington, DC
356 *Drug- and Toxic-Induced Liver Disease*

FUAD N. ZIYADEH, M.D.
Associate Professor of Medicine
Renal-Electrolyte and Hypertension Division
University of Pennsylvania
Philadelphia, Pennsylvania
117 *Diabetic Nephropathy*
314 *Disorders of Phosphate Homeostasis*

NATHAN J. ZVAIFLER, M.D.
Professor of Medicine
Division of Rheumatology
Department of Medicine
University of California, San Diego
La Jolla, California
183 *Synovial Fluid Analysis*
191 *Evaluation of Joint Complaints*
192 *Rheumatoid Arthritis*
201 *Uncommon Arthropathies*

CONTENTS

PART ONE
INTRODUCTION TO MODERN MEDICAL PRACTICE

1 **Physician-Patient Encounter,** 2
Jack Ende

2 **Principles of Diagnostic Testing,** 5
John M. Eisenberg

3 **Clinical Bioethics,** 9
Daniel P. Sulmasy

4 **Costs and Outcomes,** 14
Kevin Schulman

5 **Quality of Care,** 16
Laurence H. Beck

6 **Implementing Clinical Practice Guidelines,** 23
Scott Weingarten and Stephen Deutsch

7 **Medical Informatics,** 26
Mark. E. Frisse

8 **Managed Care,** 29
Andrew B. Bindman

PART TWO
DISEASES OF THE HEART AND BLOOD VESSELS

I   BASIC PHYSIOLOGY AND MOLECULAR BIOLOGY

9 **Cardiovascular Physiology,** 36
Martin M. LeWinter, Louis A. Mulieri, and George Osol

10 **Molecular Biology of the Cardiovascular System,** 49
Roger D. Bies and Robert Roberts

II   LABORATORY TESTS AND DIAGNOSTIC METHODS

11 **Physical Examination of the Cardiovascular System,** 63
James A. Shaver

12 **Electrocardiography,** 81
Frederick A. Masoudi and Nora Goldschlager

13 **Cardiac Noninvasive Techniques,** 91
George A. Beller and Sanjiv Kaul

14 **Cardiac Catheterization and Angiography,** 107
William H. Gaasch and Joseph P. Murgo

15 **Interventional Cardiac Catheterization,** 116
Spencer B. King, III, and William D. Anderson

III   CLINICAL SYNDROMES

16 **Chest Pain,** 125
Louis J. Dell'Italia and Douglas J. Pearce

17 **Palpitations,** 130
Sumanth D. Prabhu and Robert A. O'Rourke

18 **Cardiac Arrhythmias and Conduction Disturbances,** 131
Simon Chakko, Agustin Castellanos, Kenneth M. Kessler,
and Robert J. Myerburg

19 **Congestive Heart Failure,** 156
Gary S. Francis

20 **Hypotension and Cardiogenic Shock,** 175
Mrinal Sharma and Richard C. Becker

21 **Sudden Cardiac Death,** 187
James L. Gilman and Gerald V. Naccarelli

IV   SPECIFIC DISEASE ENTITIES

22 **Ischemic Heart Disease,** 192
Kanu Chatterjee

23 **Acute Myocardial Infarction,** 209
Guy S. Reeder and Bernard J. Gersh

24 **Infective Endocarditis,** 225
Frederick A. Masoudi and Merle A. Sande

25 **Valvular Heart Disease,** 235
Shahbudin H. Rahimtoola

26 **Cardiomyopathies,** 262
Pravin M. Shah

27 **Pericardial Disease and Pericardial Heart Disease,** 271
Brian D. Hoit

28 **Congenital Heart Disease,** 280
Robert C. Schlant

29 **Pulmonary Hypertensive Heart Disease,** 293
Richard S. Irwin, Joseph S. Alpert, and James E. Dalen

30 **Diseases of the Aorta,** 299
Miguel Zabalgoitia and Robert A. O'Rourke

31 **Diseases of the Peripheral Arteries and Veins,** 304
Peter C. Spitell and John A. Spittell, Jr

32 **Arterial Hypertension,** 312
Norman M. Kaplan

33 **Cardiac Tumors; Cardiac Manifestations of Endocrine,
Collagen Vascular, and HIV Disease; and Traumatic
Injury of the Heart,** 329
John S. MacGregor and Melvin D. Cheitlin

34 **Cardiac Transplantation,** 335
Lynne Warner Stevenson

PART THREE
PULMONARY AND CRITICAL CARE MEDICINE

I   BASIC PHYSIOLOGY

35 Respiratory Pathophysiology, 346
Walter J. Daly and Jacob S.O. Loke

36 Abnormalities of the Control of Breathing, 352
Neil S. Cherniack

37 Respiratory Muscles and Respiratory Muscle Failure, 357
Dudley F. Rochester

38 Pulmonary Blood Flow, 360
J.T. Sylvester and Roy G. Brower

39 Host Defense Mechanisms in the Respiratory Tract, 364
Herbert Y. Reynolds

40 Mechanisms of Lung Injury and Repair, 370
Jamson S. Lwebuga-Mukasa

II   LABORATORY AND DIAGNOSTIC TESTS

41 Pulmonary Function Testing, 375
Jacob S.O. Loke

42 Invasive Diagnostic Techniques, 380
John A. Rankin

43 Pulmonary Diagnostic Imaging, 386
Robert D. Tarver, Lynn S. Broderick, and Dewey J. Conces, Jr.

44 Intensive Care Monitoring and Mechanical Ventilation, 390
Herbert P. Wiedemann

III   CLINICAL SYNDROMES AND THERAPEUTIC MODALITIES

45 Approach to the Patient with Respiratory System Disease, 400
John L. Stauffer and Herbert Y. Reynolds

46 Acute Respiratory Failure, 412
Leonard D. Hudson

47 Multiple Organ Dysfunction in the Context of ARDS, 421
Jean E. Rinaldo and Melissa Clark

48 Pulmonary Edema, 423
Arthur P. Wheeler, Gordon R. Bernard, and Kenneth L. Brigham

49 Respiratory Therapy and Monitoring, 428
David H. Ingbar and Linda Nici

50 Pulmonary Rehabilitation, 432
Barry J. Make

IV   SPECIFIC DISEASE ENTITIES

51 Chronic Obstructive Pulmonary Disease, 437
Gordon L. Snider

52 Interstitial Lung Disease, 448
Jack D. Fulmer† and K. Randall Young, Jr.

53 Sarcoidosis, 456
Geoffrey McLennan and Gary W. Hunninghake

54 Hypersensitivity Pneumonitis, 460
Herbert Y. Reynolds and Timothy J. Craig

55 Langerhans' Cell Granulomatosis (Histiocytosis X, Eosinophilic Granuloma), 463
Allan J. Hance, Abdellatif Tazi, and Francoise Basset

56 Primary Granulomatous Pulmonary Vasculitis, 465
Stephen B. Sulavik and Nav T. Singh

57 Occupational Lung Diseases, 471
Akshay Sood, J. Bernard Gee, and William S. Beckett

58 Adverse Pulmonary Reactions to Drugs and Other Therapeutic Modalities, 476
J. Allen Cooper, Jr.

59 Cystic Fibrosis and Bronchiectasis, 479
Pamela B. Davis and Michael D. Infeld

60 Neoplasms of the Lung, 486
Michael C. Iannuzzi and Galen B. Toews

61 Solitary Pulmonary Tumor, 493
Thomas Y. Sullivan

62 Pulmonary Hypertension: Primary and Secondary Causes, 497
Lewis J. Rubin and Barbara J. Kircher

63 Pulmonary Thromboembolism, 499
Charles K. Chan and Richard A. Matthay

64 Pleural Diseases, 505
Ian R.G. Dowdeswell

65 Diseases of the Mediastinum, 510
Ian R.G. Dowdeswell

66 Pulmonary Transplantation, 514
James H. Dauber, Penny A. Williams, and David R. Nunley

67 Sleep-Related Respiratory Disorders, 524
Laurel Wiegand

PART FOUR
HEMATOLOGY AND ONCOLOGY

I   BASIC PRINCIPLES

68 Molecular and Cellular Biology of Hematopoiesis, 530
David A. Williams

69 Hemostasis and Fibrinolysis, 534
James N. George

70 The Genetics of Cancer, 540
Joanna Groden

71 Principles of Cancer Treatment, 550
Beverly S. Mitchell

†Deceased.

II LABORATORY TESTS

72 **Evaluation of Peripheral Blood and Bone Marrow Cells,** 555
John C. Winkelmann

73 **Molecular Diagnostics,** 559
Harold R. Schumacher

74 **Evaluation of Monoclonal Proteins in Serum and Urine,** 564
Robert A. Kyle

75 **Evaluation of Hemostasis and Thrombosis,** 568
James N. George

III SPECIAL TOPICS

76 **Blood Transfusion,** 572
Jay E. Menitove

77 **Hematopoietic Stem Cell Transplantation,** 576
Frederick R. Appelbaum

78 **Complications of Cancer and Cancer Therapy,** 579
Sara L. Zaknoen

IV CLINICAL SYNDROMES

79 **Abnormal Hematocrit,** 586
Emmanuel N. Dessypris

80 **Abnormal Nucleated Blood Cell Counts,** 590
David H. Boldt

81 **Lymphadenopathy and Splenomegaly,** 596
David H. Boldt

82 **Excessive Bleeding and Clotting,** 602
James N. George

V SPECIFIC DISEASES

83 **Thrombocytopenia and Disorders of Platelet Function,** 610
Andrew I. Schafer

84 **Disorders of Blood Coagulation,** 617
Gilbert C. White II

85 **Thrombosis and Anticoagulation,** 630
Russell D. Hull, Graham F. Pineo, and Gary E. Raskob

86 **Iron Deficiency Anemia, Anemia of Chronic Disease, Sideroblastic Anemia, and Iron Overload,** 641
Robert T. Means, Jr.

87 **Megaloblastic Anemia,** 646
Robert T. Means, Jr.

88 **Hemoglobinopathies and Thalassemias,** 650
Martin H. Steinberg

89 **Hemolytic Anemia,** 661
John C. Winkelmann

90 **Bone Marrow Failure and Myelodysplasia,** 671
Frederick R. Appelbaum

91 **Abnormalities of Phagocytes, Eosinophils, and Basophils,** 678
David H. Boldt

92 **The Leukemias and Polycythemia Vera,** 682
John J. Hutton

93 **Hodgkin's Disease and Non-Hodgkin's Lymphoma,** 691
Thomas P. Miller and Thomas M. Grogan

94 **Multiple Myeloma and the Dysproteinemias,** 700
Robert A. Kyle

95 **Breast Cancer,** 706
C. Kent Osborne

96 **Gynecologic Cancers,** 713
Vicki V. Baker

97 **Cancer of the Prostate and Testis,** 717
Geoffrey R. Weiss

98 **Head and Neck Cancer,** 722
Jack L. Gluckman and Michael Farrell

99 **Lung Cancer,** 724
Manuel Valdivieso

100 **Cancer of Unknown Primary Site,** 729
Stephen C. Schwartz, Jared Klein, and William P. Peters

PART FIVE
RENAL AND ELECTROLYTE DISORDERS

I BASIC PHYSIOLOGY

101 **Principles of Renal Physiology,** 736
Jay H. Stein and George L. Bakris

II LABORATORY TESTS AND DIAGNOSTIC METHODS

102 **Urinalysis and Renal Function Tests,** 742
Charles R. Nolan, T. Dwight McKinney, and Marvin Forland

103 **Imaging of Renal Disorders,** 748
Abraham A. Ghiatas

III BASIC CLINICAL SYNDROMES

104 **Hematuria,** 756
B.S. Kasinath

105 **Proteinuria,** 758
B.S. Kasinath and Manjeri A. Venkatachalam

106 **Dysuria,** 762
Marvin Forland

107 **Acute Nephritic Syndrome,** 763
B.S. Kasinath

108 **Nephrotic Syndrome,** 765
B.S. Kasinath

109 **Acute Renal Failure,** 768
Satish Kumar and Jay H. Stein

110 **Chronic Renal Failure,** 776
Robert G. Luke, Charles E. Sanders, Jr., and John J. Curtis

111 **Nephrolithiasis,** 796
Stanley Goldfarb

IV   DISORDERS OF ELECTROLYTE AND ACID-BASE
      BALANCE

112 **Disorders of Water Balance,** 805
Robert G. Narins, Mark D. Faber, and G. Gopal Krishna

113 **Disorders of Sodium Balance,** 816
Murray Epstein

114 **Disorders of Potassium Balance,** 825
Richard H. Sterns and Robert G. Narins

115 **Disorders of Acid-Base Balance,** 834
Susan R. DiGiovanni and George M. Feldman

116 **Glomerular Diseases,** 841
William G. Couser

117 **Diabetic Nephropathy,** 859
Fuad N. Ziyadeh and Stanley Goldfarb

118 **Renal Manifestations of Dysproteinemias,** 862
Paul W. Sanders

119 **Drug- and Chemical-Induced Nephropathy,** 866
William M. Bennett and William F. Finn

120 **Cystic Diseases of the Kidney,** 871
Jared J. Grantham

121 **Glomerular and Interstitial Hereditary
     Nephropathies,** 876
Gerald F. DiBona

122 **Disorders of Renal Transport,** 878
Sidney Kobrin and Stanley Goldfarb

123 **Obstructive Uropathy,** 884
Saulo Klahr

124 **Tubulointerstitial Renal Diseases,** 888
Shreeram Aradhye, Shelley Albert, and Eric G. Neilson

125 **Renovascular Diseases,** 893
George L. Bakris and S. Luke Kusmirek

126 **Renal Cell Carcinoma,** 898
T. Dwight McKinney

PART SIX
NEUROLOGIC DISORDERS

I   CLINICAL AND LABORATORY EVALUATION
     OF THE NERVOUS SYSTEM

127 **Neurologic History and Examination,** 902
Jock Murray

128 **Psychologic Testing,** 903
William E.M. Pryse-Phillips

129 **Spinal Fluid Examination,** 904
Martin A. Samuels

130 **Electroencephalography and Evoked Responses,** 905
Rodney D. Bell and R. Mañon-Espaillat

131 **Electromyography,** 914
Allen B. Gruber and Richard J. Barohn

132 **Neuroradiologic Studies,** 917
Ashwani Kapila

133 **Autonomic Nervous System,** 930
Roy Freeman

II   CLINICAL SYNDROMES

134 **Sleep and Sleep Disorders,** 939
Jean K. Matheson

135 **Coma and Related Disorders,** 947
Martin A. Samuels

136 **Faintness and Syncope,** 952
Sumanth D. Prabhu, Robert A. O'Rourke, and J. Donald Easton

137 **Headache and Facial Pain,** 957
John Edmeads

138 **Neck and Back Pain,** 963
Kenneth K. Nakano

139 **Otoneurology,** 971
Stephen W. Parker

140 **Disorders of Speech and Language,** 975
Daniel B. Hier

III   NEUROLOGIC DISEASES

141 **Epilepsy,** 978
John Davenport

142 **Cognitive Failure Dementia,** 985
Thomas M. Walshe III

143 **Parkinsonism and Movement Disorders,** 989
Lewis Sudarsky

144 **Cerebrovascular Disease (Stroke),** 997
Louis R. Caplan

145 **Demyelinating Diseases,** 1007
David M. Dawson

146 **Myelopathies,** 1011
Frisso A. Potts

147 **Diseases of Peripheral Nerve and Motor Neurons,** 1014
Eric L. Logigian

148 **Diseases of the Neuromuscular Junction,** 1020
Marjorie E. Seybold

149 **Muscle Disease,** 1024
Robert H. Brown, Jr.

IV   NEUROLOGY OF BEHAVIOR

150 **Behavioral Neurology,** 1030
Roy Freeman

151 **Anxiety,** 1034
Barry S. Fogel

152 **Mood Disorders,** 1035
Barry S. Fogel

153 **Personality Disorders, Maladaptive Illness Behavior, and Somatization,** 1038
Barry S. Fogel

154 **Thought Disorders,** 1041
Barry S. Fogel

V NEUROLOGY IN GENERAL MEDICINE AND SURGERY

155 **Head Trauma,** 1043
Peter M. Black

156 **Spinal Cord Injury,** 1045
Paul A. Gutierrez and Robert R. Young

157 **Principles of Neurorehabilitation,** 1053
Bhagwan T. Shahani

158 **Ocular Manifestations of Neurologic Disorders,** 1056
John E. Carter

159 **Neurology of the Lower Urinary Tract,** 1065
Frances M. Dyro

160 **Neurooncology,** 1067
Amy A. Pruitt

161 **Neuroendocrinology,** 1075
David Borsook and Steven E. Hyman

162 **Metabolic and Toxic Disorders,** 1078
Stephen M. Sagar

163 **Principles of Coma and Neurologic Emergencies,** 1081
Allan H. Ropper

164 **Neurocardiology,** 1086
Martin A. Samuels

165 **Neurorheumatology,** 1091
Kenneth K. Nakano

166 **Neuropulmonology,** 1095
Frank W. Drislane and Martin A. Samuels

167 **Neurogastroenterology,** 1100
Martin A. Samuels

168 **Neurohepatology,** 1102
Martin A. Samuels

169 **Neurohematology,** 1103
Martin A. Samuels

170 **Neuronephrology,** 1105
Martin A. Samuels

PART SEVEN
CLINICAL IMMUNOLOGY, RHEUMATOLOGY, AND DERMATOLOGY

I PRINCIPLES OF IMMUNOLOGY

171 **Human Immune Response,** 1108
Robert R. Rich

172 **Human Leukocyte Antigen Complex,** 1115
Benjamin D. Schwartz

173 **Antibodies: Structure and Genetics,** 1121
Roger M. Perlmutter

174 **Cellular Immunity, Cytokines, and Immunoregulation,** 1126
John J. O'Shea and Thomas B. Nutman

175 **Complement System and Immune Complex Diseases,** 1132
Robert H. Carter

176 **Immediate Hypersensitivity,** 1139
Stephen I. Wasserman

177 **Tolerance and Autoimmunity,** 1142
Alfred D. Steinberg

II LABORATORY AND DIAGNOSTIC TESTS

178 **Complement Measurements,** 1147
Robert H. Carter, M. Kathryn Liszewski, and John P. Atkinson

179 **Evaluation of Cellular Immune Function,** 1150
John J. O'Shea

180 **Laboratory Methods in Immediate Hypersensitivity,** 1153
Stephen I. Wasserman

181 **Autoantibodies,** 1155
Liam Martin and Marvin J. Fritzler

182 **Rheumatoid Factors,** 1160
Dennis A. Carson

183 **Synovial Fluid Analysis,** 1161
Nathan J. Zvaifler

184 **Imaging Evaluation of Patients with Arthritis,** 1164
Donald Resnick, David R. Marcantonio, and David J. Sartoris

III CLINICAL IMMUNOLOGY

185 **The Primary Immunodeficiency Disorders,** 1174
David L. Nelson

186 **Inherited Complement Deficiencies,** 1178
Robert H. Carter, M. Kathryn Liszewski, and John P. Atkinson

187 **Rhinitis,** 1180
Robert S. Zeiger and Michael Schatz

188 **Asthma,** 1185
Timothy D. Bigby and Stephen I. Wasserman

189 **Anaphylaxis,** 1193
Diana L. Marquardt

190 **Periarticular Rheumatic Complaints,** 1195
Harry G. Bluestein

191 **Evaluation of Joint Complaints,** 1198
Nathan J. Zvaifler

192 **Rheumatoid Arthritis,** 1200
Nathan J. Zvaifler

193 **Sjögren's Syndrome,** 1209
Robert I. Fox

194 **Systemic Lupus Erythematosus,** 1212
John H. Klippel

195 **Vasculitic Syndromes,** 1218
Leonard H. Calabrese and George F. Duna

196 **Raynaud's Phenomenon,** 1226
Richard M. Silver

197 **Systemic Sclerosis,** 1228
Thomas A. Medsger, Jr.

198 **Diffuse Fasciitis With Eosinophilia,** 1233
Richard M. Silver

199 **Inflammatory Myopathies,** 1234
Paul H. Plotz

200 **Spondyloarthropathies,** 1237
Robert Inman

201 **Uncommon Arthropathies,** 1242
John H. Klippel and Nathan J. Zvaifler

202 **Cryoglobulinemia,** 1248
Peter D. Gorevic

203 **Infections of the Joints,** 1250
James S. Louie, Adolf W. Karchmer, and Michael H. Weisman

204 **Rheumatic Fever,** 1256
Angelo Taranta

205 **Antirheumatic Drugs,** 1258
Joseph M. Cash

IV JOINT DISEASES

206 **Osteoarthritis,** 1264
Kenneth D. Brandt

207 **Gout and Hyperuricemia,** 1268
Robert A. Terkeltaub

208 **Arthritis Associated With Calcium-Containing Crystals,** 1276
Lawrence M. Ryan and Daniel J. McCarty

209 **Ochronosis and Alkaptonuria,** 1280
J. Edwin Seegmiller

210 **Amyloidoses,** 1282
Merrill D. Benson

211 **Heritable and Developmental Disorders of Connective Tissue,** 1286
Stephen M. Krane

V DERMATOLOGY

212 **Cutaneous Manifestations of Connective Tissue Diseases,** 1290
Thomas T. Provost, Wendy Lynch, and Eva Simmons-O'Brien

213 **Bullous Diseases,** 1293
Hossein C. Nousari and Grant J. Anhalt

214 **Cutaneous Malignancies: Basal Cell Carcinoma and Squamous Cell Carcinoma,** 1297
Margaret O'Neill and Stanley Miller

215 **Melanoma,** 1298
Susan E. Koch

216 **Psoriasis,** 1300
Frederick G. Wenzel and Warwick L. Morison

217 **Dermatitis,** 1302
S. Elizabeth Whitmore

218 **Acne Vulgaris,** 1304
Charlotte E. Modly

219 **Photodermatoses,** 1306
Frederick G. Wenzel and Warwick L. Morison

220 **Superficial Fungal Infections,** 1307
Constantino Costarangos and Bernard Cohen

221 **Cutaneous Manifestations of Drug Reactions,** 1312
Antoinette F. Hood

222 **Cutaneous Manifestations of Internal Malignancy,** 1316
Terri Dunn and Susan D. Laman

223 **Cutaneous Manifestations of Gastrointestinal Disease,** 1320
Van Ha and Susan D. Laman

224 **Cutaneous Manifestations of Endocrine Disorders,** 1322
Diane Orlinsky and Susan E. Koch

225 **Cutaneous Manifestations of Sarcoidosis,** 1324
Steven R. Feldman

226 **Cutaneous Manifestations of Human Immunodeficiency Virus Infection,** 1325
Thomas D. Horn and Ciro R. Martins

227 **Kaposi's Sarcoma,** 1330
Kathryn A. O'Connell

228 **Mycosis Fungoides and Sézary's Syndrome,** 1331
Stanford I. Lamberg

PART EIGHT
INFECTIOUS DISEASES

I BASIC PRINCIPLES

229 **Basic Principles of Infectious Disease,** 1334
Peter Densen and Merle A. Sande

230 **Host Defense Against Infection: The Roles of Antibody, Complement, and Phagocytic Cells,** 1336
Peter Densen, David L. Weinbaum, and Gerald L. Mandell

231 **Principles of Antiinfective Therapy,** 1343
Robert C. Moellering, Jr. and George M. Eliopoulos

232 **Hospital Infection Control,** 1361
R. Michael Massanari and Richard P. Wenzel

II LABORATORY TESTS

233 **Use of Laboratory Tests in Infectious Diseases,** 1366
Thomas A. Drake

III CLINICAL SYNDROMES

234 **Fever of Unknown Origin,** 1375
Martin G. Täuber

235 **Fever and Rash,** 1380
Peter K. Lindenauer and Merle A. Sande

236 **Fever in the Compromised Host,** 1386
Lowell S. Young

237 **Respiratory Tract Infections,** 1390
Birgit Winther and Jack M. Gwaltney, Jr.

238 **Intraabdominal Infections,** 1396
Matthew E. Levinson

239 **Acute Meningitis,** 1402
Allan R. Tunkel and W. Michael Scheld

240 **Brain Abscess and Perimeningeal Infections,** 1413
Michael R. Chicoine and Ralph G. Dacey, Jr.

241 **Skin and Subcutaneous Infections,** 1419
Richard E. Bryant

242 **Gastrointestinal Tract Infections,** 1425
Herbert L. DuPont

243 **Osteomyelitis,** 1433
Jon T. Mader

244 **Sexually Transmitted Diseases (Urethritis, Vaginitis, Cervicitis, Proctitis, Genital Lesions),** 1437
Michael F. Rein

245 **Gram-Negative Bacteremia and the Sepsis Syndrome,** 1445
Lisa Istorico Sanders and C. Glenn Cobbs

246 **Urinary Tract Infections,** 1455
Donald Kaye, Allan R. Tunkel, and George R. Fournier, Jr.

247 **Infections in Travelers,** 1464
Philip J. Rosenthal

248 **Acquired Immunodeficiency Syndrome,** 1470
Julie Louise Gerberding and Merle A. Sande

249 **Fever in the Hospitalized Patient,** 1479
Rafael Jurado and John E. McGowan, Jr.

IV ORGANISMS INFECTIVE TO HUMANS

Viral Diseases

250 **Common Viral Infections, Picornavirus, and Orthomyxovirus Infections (Rhinovirus, Enterovirus, and Influenza),** 1483
R. Gordon Douglas, Jr.

251 **Paramyxovirus (Parainfluenza, Mumps, Measles, and Respiratory Syncytial Virus), Rubella Virus, Coronavirus, and Adenovirus Infections,** 1494
Eurico Arruda and Frederick G. Hayden

252 **Rabies,** 1505
Steven L. Chuck

253 **Unusual Viral Infections: Arenavirus, Colorado Tick Fever Virus, Parvovirus, Bunyavirus, and Togavirus (Ebola),** 1508
Charles J. Schleupner

254 **Rotavirus and Norwalk-Like Virus Infections,** 1519
Suzanne M. Matsui

255 **Herpesvirus Infections (Herpes Simplex Virus, Varicella-Zoster Virus, Cytomegalovirus, and Epstein-Barr Virus),** 1522
David A. Katzenstein and M. Colin Jordan

256 **Human Retrovirus Infections,** 1531
Jay A. Levy

CHLAMYDIAL AND MYCOPLASMAL DISEASES
Chlamydial Diseases

257 **Chlamydial Infections,** 1534
Julius Schachter

258 **Mycoplasmal Infections,** 1538
John Mills

Rickettsial Diseases

259 **Rickettsial Infections,** 1541
David T. Durack and David H. Walker

Bacterial Diseases

260 **Staphylococcal Infections,** 1546
John N. Sheagren

261 **_Streptococcus pyogenes_ Infections** 1553
Dennis L. Stevens

Enterococci

262 **Enterococcal and Other Non–Group A Streptococcal Infections,** 1560
Larry J. Strausbaugh

263 **Gram-Positive Bacillary Infections and Clostridial Infections,** 1565
Ronald Dworkin and James Leggett

264 **_Neisseria meningitidis_ Infections,** 1578
James A. Reinarz

265 **_Neisseria gonorrhoeae_ Infections,** 1581
Edward W. Hook III

266 **Infections Caused by _Haemophilus_ Species,** 1585
David T. Durack and John R. Perfect

267 **Infections Caused by _Campylobacter_ and _Helicobacter_ Species,** 1590
Jean-Paul Butzler

268 Infections Caused by *Vibrio* Species, 1593
Mary E. Wilson, Aldo A.M. Lima, and Richard L. Guerrant

269 Infections Caused by *Salmonella* and *Shigella* Species, 1598
David Bangsberg and Merle A. Sande

270 Infections Caused by *Brucella, Francisella tularensis, Pasteurella, Yersinia* Species, and *Bordetella pertussis* (Whooping Cough), 1604
Nancy K. Henry, Walter R. Wilson, and J. Owen Hendley

271 Infections Caused by *Bacteroides* and Other Mixed Nonsporulating Anaerobes, 1613
Anthony W. Chow

272 Infections Caused by Legionellae, 1621
Washington C. Winn, Jr. and Christopher J. Grace

273 Tuberculosis and Nontuberculous Mycobacterial Infections, 1625
Julie R. Brahmer and Merle A. Sande

274 Infections Caused by Spirochetes, 1640
David Bangsberg and Michael F. Rein

275 Infections With *Mycobacterium leprae* (Leprosy), 1648
Reuben Granich and Jonathan H. Mermin

Fungal Diseases
276 Infections Caused by Common Fungi, 1651
Thomas F. Patterson and John R. Graybill

277 Infections Caused by *Candida, Actinomyces,* and *Nocardia* Species, 1660
John E. Edwards, Jr.

278 *Cryptococcus neoformans* Infections, 1667
Thomas F. Patterson

Protozoal Diseases
279 Infections Caused by Protozoa, 1671
Carolyn Petersen

280 *Pneumocystis carinii* Infections, 1692
Sharon Safrin

Helminthic Diseases
281 Infections Caused by Helminths, 1696
G. Richard Olds

PART NINE
ENDOCRINOLOGY, METABOLISM, AND GENETICS

I   BASIC PHYSIOLOGY

282 Principles of Endocrine Physiology, 1708
Richard M. Jordan and Peter O. Kohler

283 Physiology of Bone and Mineral Homeostasis, 1714
Gregory R. Mundy and Charles A. Reasner II

284 Principles of Genetic Disorders, 1721
Robb E. Moses and R. Ellen Magenis

II   LABORATORY TESTS

285 Laboratory Diagnosis in Endocrinology, 1732
Richard M. Jordan and Peter O. Kohler

286 Diagnostic Approach to Bone and Mineral Disorders, 1744
Gregory R. Mundy and Charles A. Reasner II

III   CLINICAL SYNDROMES

287 Weight Loss, 1748
Richard M. Jordan and Peter O. Kohler

288 Obesity, 1750
Edward S. Horton

289 Weakness, 1753
David L. Vesely

290 Hirsutism, 1755
D. Lynn Loriaux

291 Amenorrhea, 1757
William F. Crowley, Jr.

292 Impotence and Altered Libido, 1760
John C. Marshall

293 Gynecomastia, 1764
John C. Marshall

294 Disorders of Adolescent Growth and Development, 1766
H. Verdain Barnes

IV   DISORDERS OF THE ENDOCRINE GLANDS

SPECIFIC ENDOCRINE, METABOLIC, AND GENETIC DISORDERS

295 Disorders of the Hypothalamus and Anterior Pituitary, 1773
Shlomo Melmed and Glenn D. Braunstein

296 Disorders of the Posterior Pituitary, 1788
Gary L. Robertson

297 Disorders of the Thyroid, 1797
Gerald S. Levey and Irwin Klein

298 Disorders of the Adrenal Cortex, 1817
John Kendall and D. Lynn Loriaux

299 Disorders of the Adrenal Medulla, 1826
Alan Goldfien

300 Disorders of the Ovary, 1832
William F. Crowley, Jr.

301 Disorders of the Testis, 1838
Richard J. Santen

302 Benign Breast Disease, 1846
Richard J. Santen and Joann Pinkerton

303 Diabetes Mellitus, 1850
Alan J. Garber

304 **Hypoglycemia,** 1874
William E. Clutter and Phillip E. Cryer

305 **Heritable Disorders of Carbohydrate Metabolism,** 1879
Alan J. Garber

306 **Disorders of Lipids and Lipoproteins,** 1883
Scott M. Grundy

307 **Lipodystrophies,** 1899
M. Joycelyn Elders

V **METABOLIC DISORDERS IN ADULTS**

308 **Disorders of Amino Acid Metabolism,** 1903
Jess G. Thoene

309 **Lysosomal Storage Diseases,** 1911
Alan J. Garber

310 **Phakomatoses,** 1920
Thomas D. Gelehrter

311 **Disorders of Porphyrin Metabolism,** 1923
Joseph R. Bloomer

312 **Hypercalcemia,** 1927
John P. Bilezikian

313 **Hypocalcemia,** 1930
John P. Bilezikian

314 **Disorders of Phosphate Homeostasis,** 1934
Fuad N. Ziyadeh and Stanley Goldfarb

315 **Disorders of Magnesium Homeostasis,** 1939
Sidney Kobrin and Stanley Goldfarb

316 **Osteoporosis,** 1944
Lawrence G. Raisz

317 **Osteomalacia and Disorders of Vitamin D Metabolism,** 1949
L. Lyndon Key, Jr. and Norman H. Bell

318 **Paget's Disease of Bone,** 1955
Frederick R. Singer

319 **Osteopetrosis,** 1958
Gregory R. Mundy and Charles A. Reasner II

320 **Fibrous Dysplasia,** 1960
Gregory R. Mundy

321 **Renal Bone Disease,** 1961
Hartmut H. Malluche and Marie-Claude Monier-Faugere

322 **Primary Hyperparathyroidism,** 1965
John P. Bilezikian

323 **Malignant Disease and the Skeleton,** 1971
Gregory R. Mundy and Charles A. Reasner II

PART TEN
ALIMENTARY TRACT, LIVER, BILIARY TREE, AND PANCREAS

I **PHYSIOLOGIC, BIOCHEMICAL, AND IMMUNOLOGIC PRINCIPLES**

ALIMENTARY TRACT

324 **Alimentary Tract Motor Function,** 1976
Raj K. Goyal

325 **Gastric Secretion,** 1980
Jean-Pierre Raufman

326 **Intestinal Absorption,** 1985
Jerry S. Trier

327 **Intestinal Immunity,** 1989
Martin F. Kagnoff

II **DIAGNOSTIC PROCEDURES AND TESTS**

328 **Gastrointestinal Endoscopy,** 1993
Bret T. Petersen

329 **Evaluation of Esophageal Disease,** 1998
Konrad S. Schulze-Delrieu and Robert W. Summers

330 **Evaluation of Gastroduodenal Diseases,** 2002
Walter L. Peterson

331 **Evaluation of Intestinal Disease,** 2004
Nicholas O. Davidson

III **CLINICAL SYNDROMES AND SPECIFIC DISEASE ENTITIES**

332 **Gastrointestinal Bleeding,** 2008
Gregory L. Eastwood

333 **Esophageal Diseases,** 2014
Robert W. Summers and Konrad S. Schulze-Delrieu

334 **Nausea, Vomiting, and Anorexia,** 2025
Irfan Soykan and Richard W. McCallum

335 **Abdominal Pain,** 2030
T. Edward Bynum

336 **Peptic Ulcer Disease,** 2035
Juan-R. Malagelada

337 **Gastritis and Other Gastric Diseases,** 2041
Gregory L. Eastwood

338 **Tumors of the Stomach,** 2045
Robert C. Kurtz

339 **Diarrhea, Constipation, and Irritable Bowel Syndrome,** 2050
Robin D. Rothstein

340 **Diseases of Small Bowel Absorption,** 2056
Michael R. Charlton and Edward V. Loftus, Jr.

341 **Idiopathic Inflammatory Bowel Disease,** 2068
Stephen B. Hanauer

342 **Intestinal Obstruction and Peritonitis,** 2077
T. Edward Bynum

343 **Tumors of the Small and Large Intestines,** 2080
Charles J. Lightdale

344 **Vascular Diseases of the Intestine,** 2086
T. Edward Bynum

345 **Diverticular and Other Intestinal Diseases,** 2089
Michael D. Apstein

346 **Gastrointestinal Manifestations of HIV Infection and AIDS,** 2094
Donald P. Kotler

347 **Nutrition and Internal Medicine,** 2099
Elliot Weser and Eleanor A. Young

LIVER, BILIARY TREE, AND PANCREAS

I   PHYSIOLOGIC, BIOCHEMICAL, AND IMMUNOLOGIC PRINCIPLES

348 **Hepatic Metabolism,** 2118
Seymour M. Sabesin

349 **Bile Production and Secretion,** 2123
James M. Crawford and Martin C. Carey

350 **Pancreatic Secretion,** 2129
Laurence J. Miller

II   DIAGNOSTIC PROCEDURES AND TESTS

351 **Evaluation of Hepatobiliary Diseases,** 2134
Albert J. Czaja

352 **Evaluation of Pancreatic Diseases,** 2144
C.S. Pitchumoni

III   CLINICAL SYNDROMES AND SPECIFIC DISEASE ENTITIES

353 **Jaundice and Disorders of Bilirubin Metabolism,** 2147
J. Donald Ostrow, Ronald P.J. Oude Elferink, and Piter J. Bosma

354 **Principal Complications of Liver Failure,** 2159
Steven Schenker and Anastacio M. Hoyumpa

355 **Acute and Chronic Viral Hepatitis,** 2172
Rakesh Vinayek and Jorge Rakela

356 **Drug- and Toxin-Induced Liver Disease,** 2184
Hyman J. Zimmerman

357 **Alcoholic Liver Diseases and Nonalcoholic Steatohepatitis,** 2194
David W. Crabb and Mats Estonius

358 **Primary Biliary Cirrhosis, Primary Sclerosing Cholangitis, and Other Cholangiopathies,** 2199
Adil E. Bharucha and Keith D. Lindor

359 **Hemochromatosis, Wilson's Disease, and Other Genetic Liver Diseases Affecting the Adult,** 2203
Kris V. Kowdley and Anthony S. Tavill

360 **Hepatic Veno-Occlusive Diseases,** 2207
Stephen C. Hauser

361 **Liver Abscesses and Cysts,** 2209
David R. Lichtenstein

362 **Hepatic Tumors,** 2212
Gregory J. Gores

363 **Liver Transplantation,** 2217
Michael F. Sorrell and Jeremiah P. Donovan

364 **Biliary Tract Stones and Associated Diseases,** 2220
Michael D. Apstein

365 **Other Diseases of the Gallbladder and Biliary Tree,** 2231
Stephen C. Hauser

366 **Pancreatic Diseases,** 2233
C.S. Pitchumoni

367 **Diseases of the Peritoneum, Mesentery, and Omentum,** 2247
James M. McGill

PART ELEVEN
SPECIAL TOPICS IN INTERNAL MEDICINE

368 **Periodic Health Examination,** 2254
Suzanne W. Fletcher

369 **Preoperative Evaluation,** 2256
Jane Appleby, C. Jeffrey Griffin, and Valerie A. Lawrence

370 **Prevention and Control of Injuries,** 2264
Arthur L. Kellerman

371 **Women's Health,** 2267
Jeane Ann Grisso, Michelle Berlin, Margo J. Krasnoff, and Anne W. Moulton

372 **Medical Disorders During Pregnancy,** 2272
Andrea J. Singer

373 **Gerontology and Geriatric Medicine,** 2282
Michael S. Katz and Meghan B. Gerety

374 **Substance Abuse,** 2293
Booker T. Bush

375 **Chronic Fatigue Syndrome,** 2298
Daniel J. Clauw

376 **Common Eye Problems,** 2300
William G. Tsiaras and Ananth V. Mudgill

377 **Common Ear, Nose, and Throat Problems,** 2306
Earl H. Harley

378 **Drug Interactions and Adverse Effects,** 2310
David A. Flockhart

APPENDIX
Immunization Schedule for Adults, 2315

COLOR PLATES

PART II
DISEASES OF THE HEART AND BLOOD VESSELS

Plate II-1 Color flow velocities in diastole.

Plate II-2 Color flow velocities in systole.

Plate II-3 Color Doppler image—aortic regurgitation.

Plate II-4 Color Doppler image—mitral regurgitation.

PART IV
HEMATOLOGY AND ONCOLOGY

Plate IV-1 Normal bone marrow.

Plate IV-2 Colony-forming unit grown from human bone marrow.

Plate IV-3 Maturing erythroid precursors in bone marrow.

Plate IV-4 Erythrocyte morphology in peripheral blood.

Plate IV-5 Lymphocyte morphology in peripheral blood.

Plate IV-6 Granulocyte morphology in peripheral blood.

Plate IV-7 Bone marrow of a patient with B_{12} deficiency.

Plate IV-8 Plasma cells in myeloma.

Plate IV-9 Iron in normal bone marrow.

Plate IV-10 Petechiae and hemorrhagic bullae in acute idiopathic thrombocytopenic purpura.

Plate IV-11 Ringed sideroblasts in sideroblastic anemia.

Plate IV-12 Leukoplakia of the lateral tongue.

Plate IV-13 Erythroplakia of the soft palate.

Plate IV-14 Deep infiltrating squamous cell carcinoma of the tongue.

PART VII
CLINICAL IMMUNOLOGY, RHEUMATOLOGY, AND DERMATOLOGY

Plate VII-1 Gram-stained expectorated sputum or transtracheal aspirate in aspiration anaerobic pneumonia.

Plate VII-2 Lupus erythematosus.

Plate VII-3 Dermatomyositis (Gottron's papules).

Plate VII-4 Dermatitis herpetiformis.

Plate VII-5 Basal cell carcinoma.

Plate VII-6 Squamous cell carcinoma.

Plate VII-7 A 45-year-old man with atypical mole syndrome and a history of two primary melanomas.

Plate VII-8 Superficial spreading malignant melanoma.

Plate VII-9 Psoriasis.

Plate VII-10 Porphyria cutanea tarda.

Plate VII-11 Stevens-Johnson syndrome.

Plate VII-12 Erythema nodosum.

Plate VII-13 Exanthematous eruption after administration of trimethoprim-sulfamethoxazole.

Plate VII-14 Addison's disease.

Plate VII-15 Toxic epidermal necrolysis.

Plate VII-16 Necrobiosis lipoidica diabeticorum.

Plate VII-17 Acanthosis nigricans.

Plate VII-18 Eruptive xanthomas.

Plate VII-19 Xanthelasma.

Plate VII-20 Papular lesions of sarcoidosis.

Plate VII-21 The lesions of lupus pernio at the nasal orifice.

Plate VII-22 Kaposi's sarcoma.

PART VIII
INFECTIOUS DISEASES

Plate VIII-1 Mature oocyst of *Isospora belli* in unstained fecal smear.

Plate VIII-2 *Treponema pallidum* by dark-field microscopy.

Plate VIII-3 Quellung reaction with pneumococcal omni serum.

Plate VIII-4 Staphylococci.

Plate VIII-5 *Haemophilus influenzae.*

Plate VIII-6 Gram-negative rods in *Klebsiella pneumoniae* or others caused by Enterobacteriaceae or *Pseudomonas.*

Plate VIII-7 Gram-stained expectorated sputum or transtracheal aspirate in aspiration anaerobic pneumonia.

Plate VIII-8 Gram stain of spun cerebrospinal fluid in *Haemophilus influenzae* type B meningitis.

Plate VIII-9 Gram stain of centrifuged cerebrospinal fluid in meningococcal meningitis.

Plate VIII-10 Giemsa stain of bronchial washings demonstrating *Pneumocystis carinii* cysts.

Plate VIII-11 Giemsa stain of conjunctiva scraping showing typical cytoplasmic inclusion of *Chlamydia trachomatis.*

Plate VIII-12 *Leishmania* amastigotes in cutaneous leishmaniasis.

Plate VIII-13 Photomicrographic scraping from base of a herpes blister demonstrating multinuclear giant cells.

Plate VIII-14 Giemsa-stained blood smear in *Plasmodium falciparum* malaria.

Plate VIII-15 Giemsa-stained blood smear in *Plasmodium vivax* malaria.

Plate VIII-16 Trypomastigotes of *Trypanosoma brucei rhodesiense* in a Giemsa-stained thick blood smear.

Plate VIII-17 Trypomastigote of *Trypanosoma cruzi* in a Giemsa-stained blood smear.

Plate VIII-18 Petechial and purpuric skin lesions in a severe case of Rocky Mountain spotted fever.

Plate VIII-19 Rocky Mountain spotted fever.

Plate VIII-20 Desquamation following toxic shock syndrome.

Plate VIII-21 Cutaneous lesions in meningococcemia.

Plate VIII-22   Cutaneous lesion in disseminated gonococcal infection.

Plate VIII-23   Cutaneous lesion in a leukemic patient with overwhelming *Pseudomonas aeruginosa* septicemia.

Plate VIII-24   Cutaneous sporotrichosis.

Plate VIII-25   Erysipelas.

Plate VIII-26   Periorbital *Haemophilus influenzae* cellulitis.

Plate VIII-27   Elephantiasis nostras.

Plate VIII-28   Hot tub folliculitis.

Plate VIII-29   Staphylococcal scalded skin syndrome.

Plate VIII-30   Acute gangrene of arm.

Plate VIII-31   *Mycobacterium marinum.*

Plate VIII-32   Modified Kinyoun stain of stool specimen demonstrating cryptosporidia.

Plate VIII-33   Oocysts of *Cryptosporidium.*

Plate VIII-34   Chancre of the penis.

Plate VIII-35   Hematoxylin and eosin preparation from peripheral lymph node.

Plate VIII-36   Lymph node biopsy with red-staining *Mycobacterium avium-intracellulare* organisms.

Plate VIII-37   Transbronchial biopsy specimen in cytomegalovirus pneumonitis.

Plate VIII-38   Cutaneous Kaposi's sarcoma lesions.

Plate VIII-39   Kaposi's sarcoma lesion in colonic mucosa.

Plate VIII-40   Typical lesion of bacillary angiomatosis.

Plate VIII-41   Retinochoroiditis caused by cytomegalovirus infection.

Plate VIII-42   Oral hairy cell leukoplakia.

Plate VIII-43   Negri bodies in human patient with rabies.

Plate VIII-44   Typical focus of rickettsial vasculitis in an arteriole.

Plate VIII-45   Small intradermal hemorrhage at a focus of vasculitis.

Plate VIII-46   Secondary syphilis.

Plate VIII-47   Palmar lesions of secondary syphilis.

Plate VIII-48   Ulcerative skin lesions of blastomycosis.

Plate VIII-49   Lymphangitic spread of sporotrichosis.

Plate VIII-50   Cerebrospinal fluid shows *Cryptococcus neoformans.*

Plate VIII-51   Severe papilledema in cryptococcal meningitis.

Plate VIII-52   *Entamoeba histolytica* in fecal specimen.

Plate VIII-53   *Giardia lamblia* trophozoite and cyst.

PART IX
ENDOCRINOLOGY, METABOLISM, AND GENETICS

Plate IX-1   Interstitial microdeletion of chromosome band 22q11.

Plate IX-2   Background diabetic retinopathy.

Plate IX-3   Exudative diabetic retinopathy.

Plate IX-4   Proliferative diabetic retinopathy.

Plate IX-5   Biopsies of iliac crest showing tetracycline labeling at the mineralization front in a normal subject and a patient with osteomalacia.

PART X
ALIMENTARY TRACT, LIVER, BILIARY TREE, AND PANCREAS

Plate X-1   Reflux esophagitis.

Plate X-2   Lower esophageal ring.

Plate X-3   Carcinoma of the stomach.

Plate X-4   Crohn's disease.

Plate X-5   Perianal manifestations of Crohn's disease.

Plate X-6   Endoscopic photographs of Crohn's disease.

Plate X-7   Histologic features of ulcerative colitis.

Plate X-8   Endoscopic features of ulcerative colitis.

Plate X-9   Pyoderma gangrenosum.

Plate X-10   Oral aphthous ulcer in a patient with Crohn's disease.

Plate X-11   Mulberry-shaped solitary cholesterol gallstone.

Plate X-12   Close-packed faceted cholesterol gallstones.

Plate X-13   Round solitary cholesterol gallstone.

Plate X-14   Black polymer pigment gallstones.

Plate X-15   Polarized light microscopy of bile-rich duodenal fluid.

PART XI
SPECIAL TOPICS IN INTERNAL MEDICINE

Plate XI-1   Drusen in age-related macular degeneration.

Plate XI-2   Optic nerve disc edema with peripapillary flame-shaped hemorrhages in malignant hypertension.

Plate XI-3   Arteriovenous nicking in hypertension.

Plate XI-4   Multiple areas of cotton-wool spots. Also visible are copper wiring and arteriovenous nicking.

Plate XI-5   Macular star: deposition of hard exudate in the center of the macula.

Plate XI-6   Silver wiring.

Plate XI-7   Intraretinal microvascular abnormalities and venous beading in diabetic retinopathy.

Plate XI-8   Neovascularization of the optic nerve and vitreous hemorrhage in diabetic retinopathy.

Plate XI-9   Branch retinal vein occlusion.

Plate XI-10   Central retinal vein occlusion.

Plate XI-11   Cytomegalovirus retinitis.

Color Plates

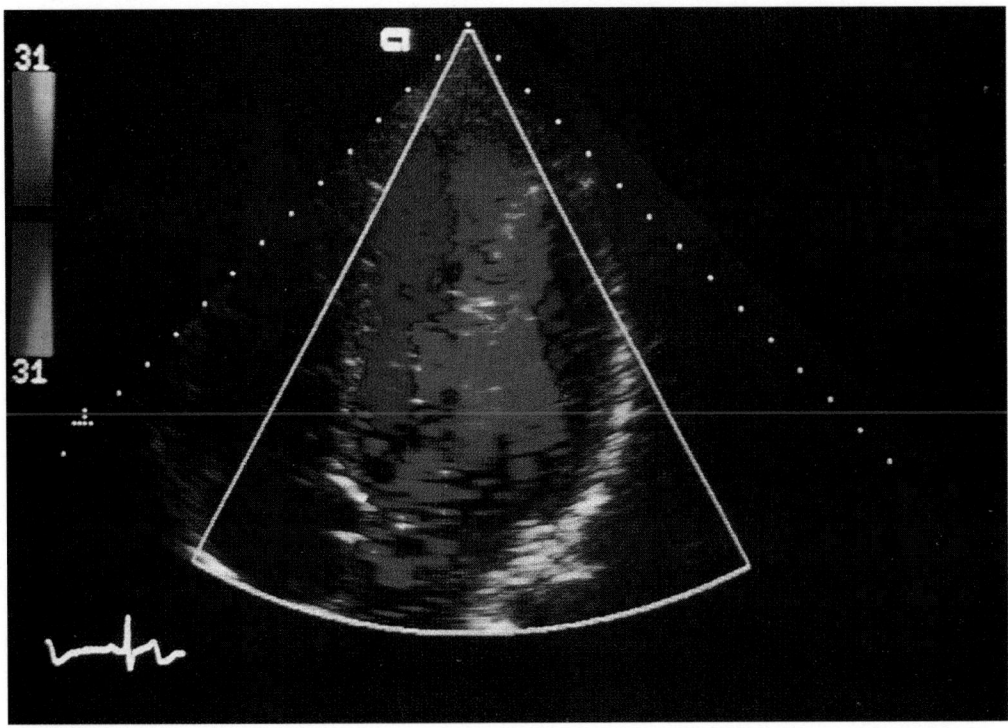

PLATE II-1   Flow velocities in diastole (shown in red) coming toward the transducer, which is located over the apex.

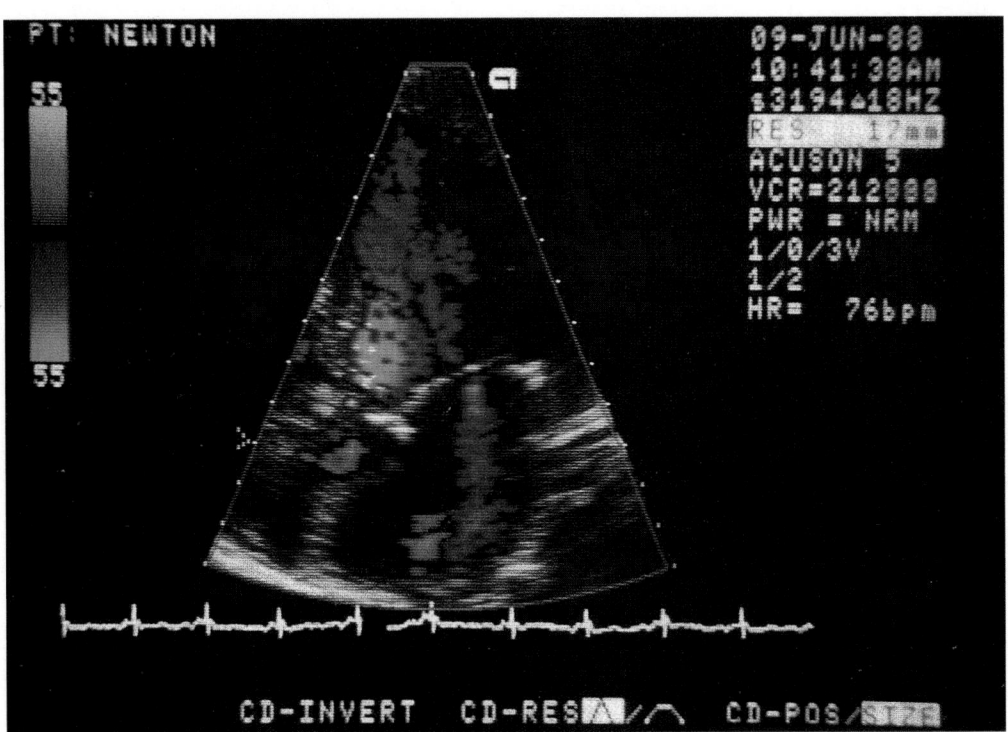

PLATE II-2   Flow velocities in systole (shown in blue) moving away from the transducer, which is located over the apex.

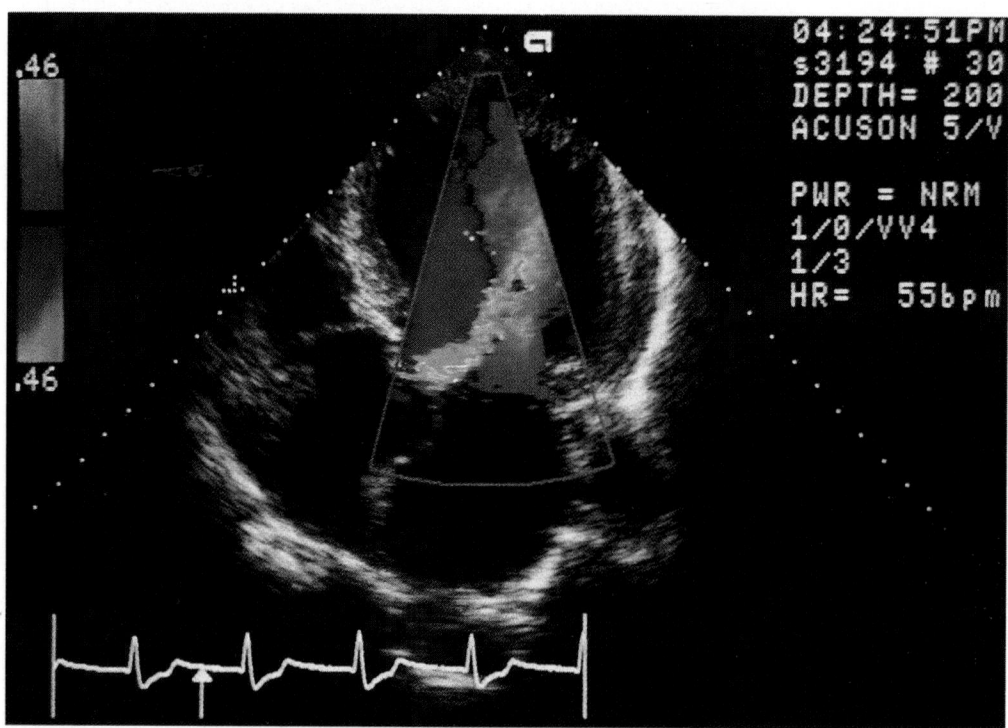

PLATE II-3 Doppler image from a patient with aortic regurgitation. This diastolic image showing the aortic regurgitant jet directed into the left ventricular cavity was acquired using transthoracic echocardiography.

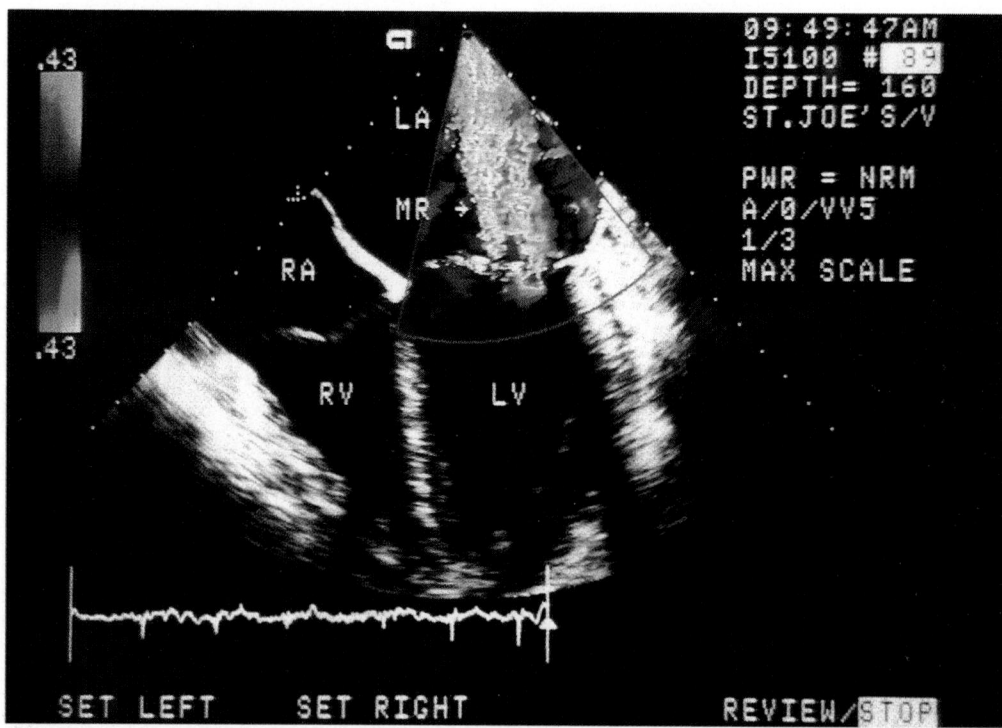

PLATE II-4 Doppler image from a patient with mitral regurgitation. This systolic image showing the mitral regurgitant jet directed into the left atrium was acquired using transesophageal echocardiography.

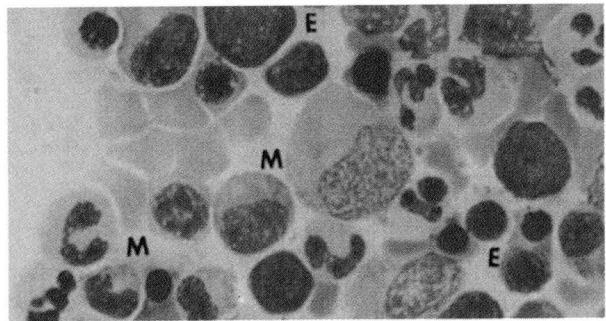

PLATE IV-1   Normal bone marrow. *M,* Myeloid precursor; *E,* erythroid precursor (× 600).

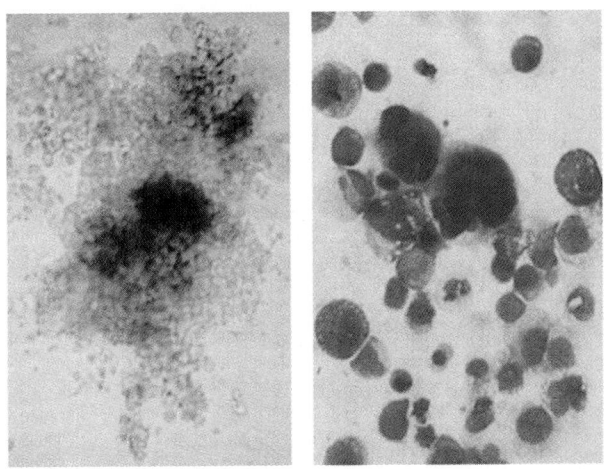

PLATE IV-2   Colony-forming unit grown from human bone marrow. **A,** CFU-GEMM colony derived from a pluripotent stem cell grown in methylcellulose. The colony contains granulocytes, erythrocytes, macrophages, and megacaryocytes. **B,** A Wright-stained smear of a single colony (CFU-GEMM) containing granulocytes, erythrocytes, and megakaryocytes.   *(Courtesy H.A. Messner.)*

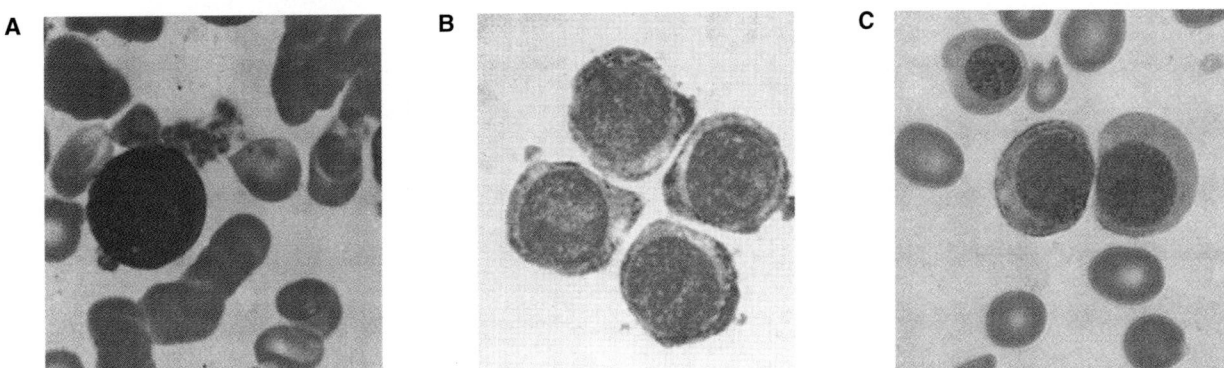

PLATE IV-3   Maturing erythroid precursors in bone marrow. **A,** Pronormoblast. **B,** Basophilic normoblasts. **C,** Polychromatophilic and orthochromatophilic normoblasts with a megaloblastic appearance.

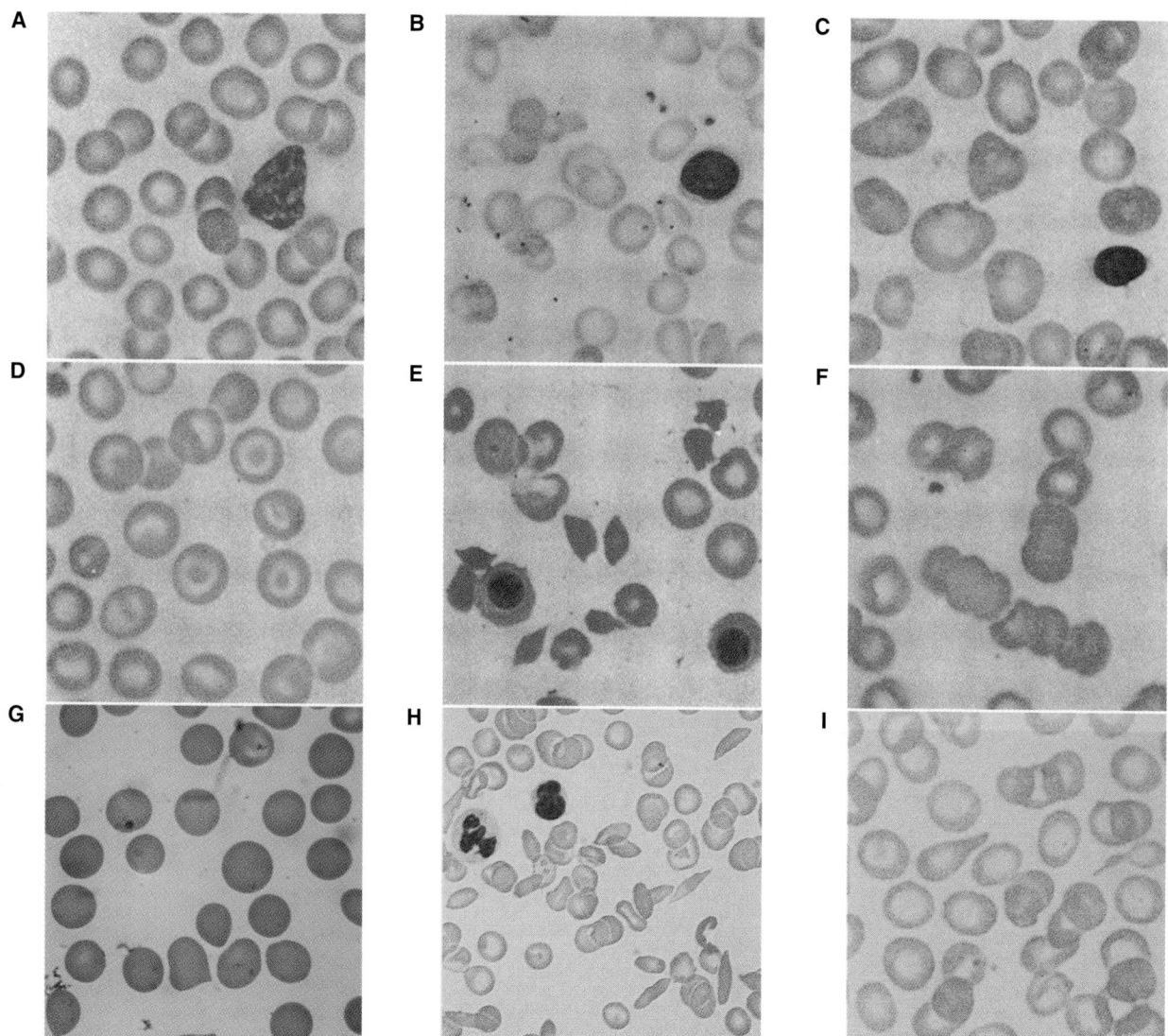

PLATE IV-4   Erythrocyte morphology in peripheral blood. Wright's stain (× 1000). **A,** Normal red cells. **B,** Microcytic hypochromic cells typical of iron deficiency. **C,** Macrocytosis typically seen in megaloblastic anemia. **D,** Target cells. **E,** Schistocytes and nucleated red cells. **F,** Rouleau formation. **G,** Normal red cells and microspherocytes in hereditary spherocytosis. **H,** Sickle cell anemia, showing sickled cells, a Howell-Jolly body, target cells, and polychromatophilia. **I,** Teardrop poikilocytes. **J,** Reticulocytes (special stain). **K,** Howell-Jolly body (nuclear remnant). **L,** Homozygous beta-thalassemia, showing microcytic and hypochromic erythrocytes, anisocytosis, poikilocytosis, basophilic stippling, a Howell-Jolly body, tar-get cells, and polychromatophilia. **M,** Heterozygous beta-thalassemia, showing hypochromia and microcytosis. **N,** Hemoglobin sickle cell disease, showing an HbC crystal, target cells, a folded taco-shaped cell, polychromatophilia, and Pappenheimer bodies. **O,** Eccentrocytes (blister cells) with a lop-sided distribution of hemoglobin. Typically seen during a hemolytic episode in G6PD deficiency. **P,** Heinz bodies (supravital stain). **Q,** HbS-beta^0-thalassemia, showing a nucleated erythrocyte, Howell-Jolly and Pappenheimer bodies, a sickle cell, target cells, polychromatophilia, hypochromia, and microcytosis. **R,** Elliptocytes.

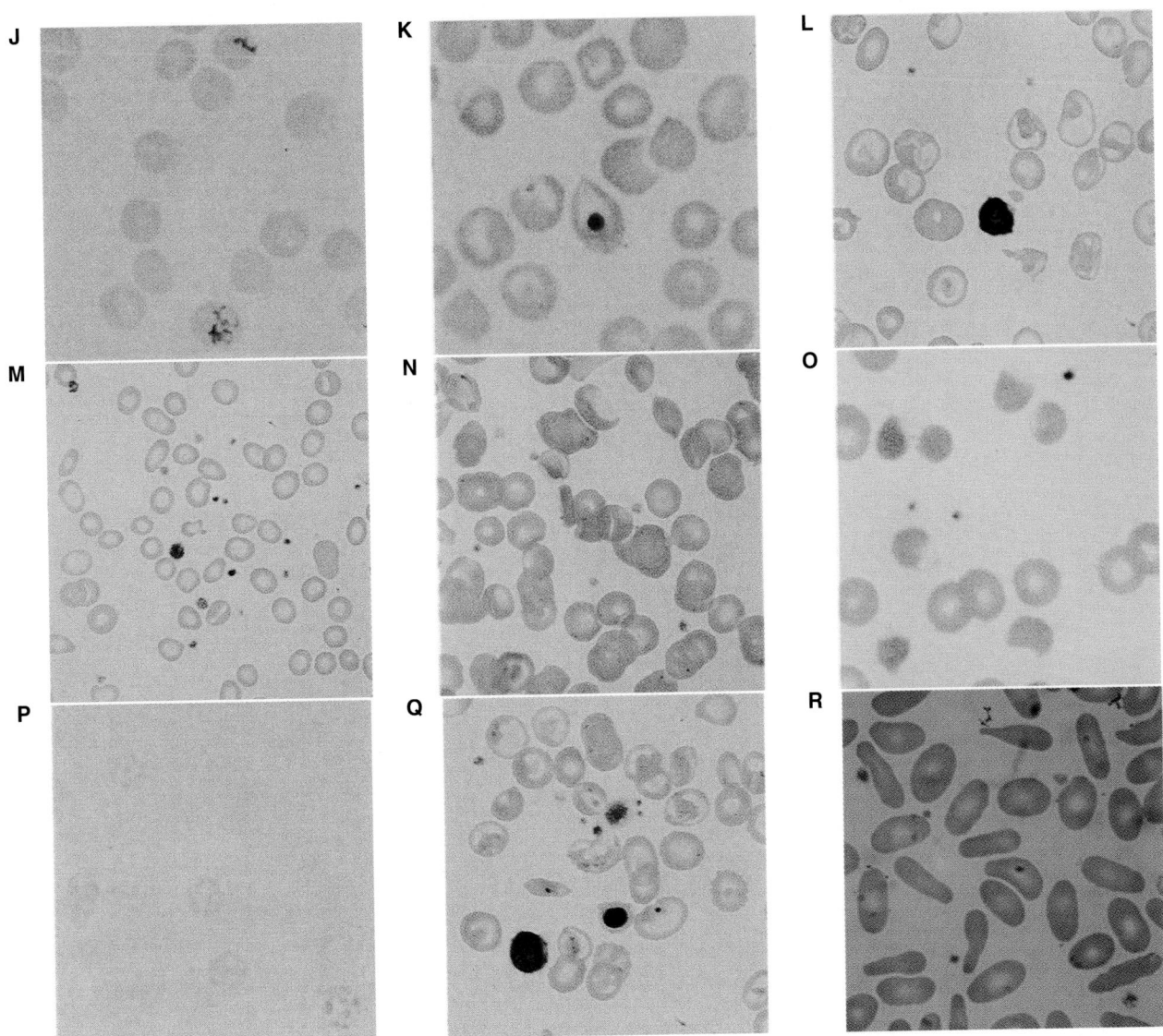

PLATE IV-4   For legend see opposite page.

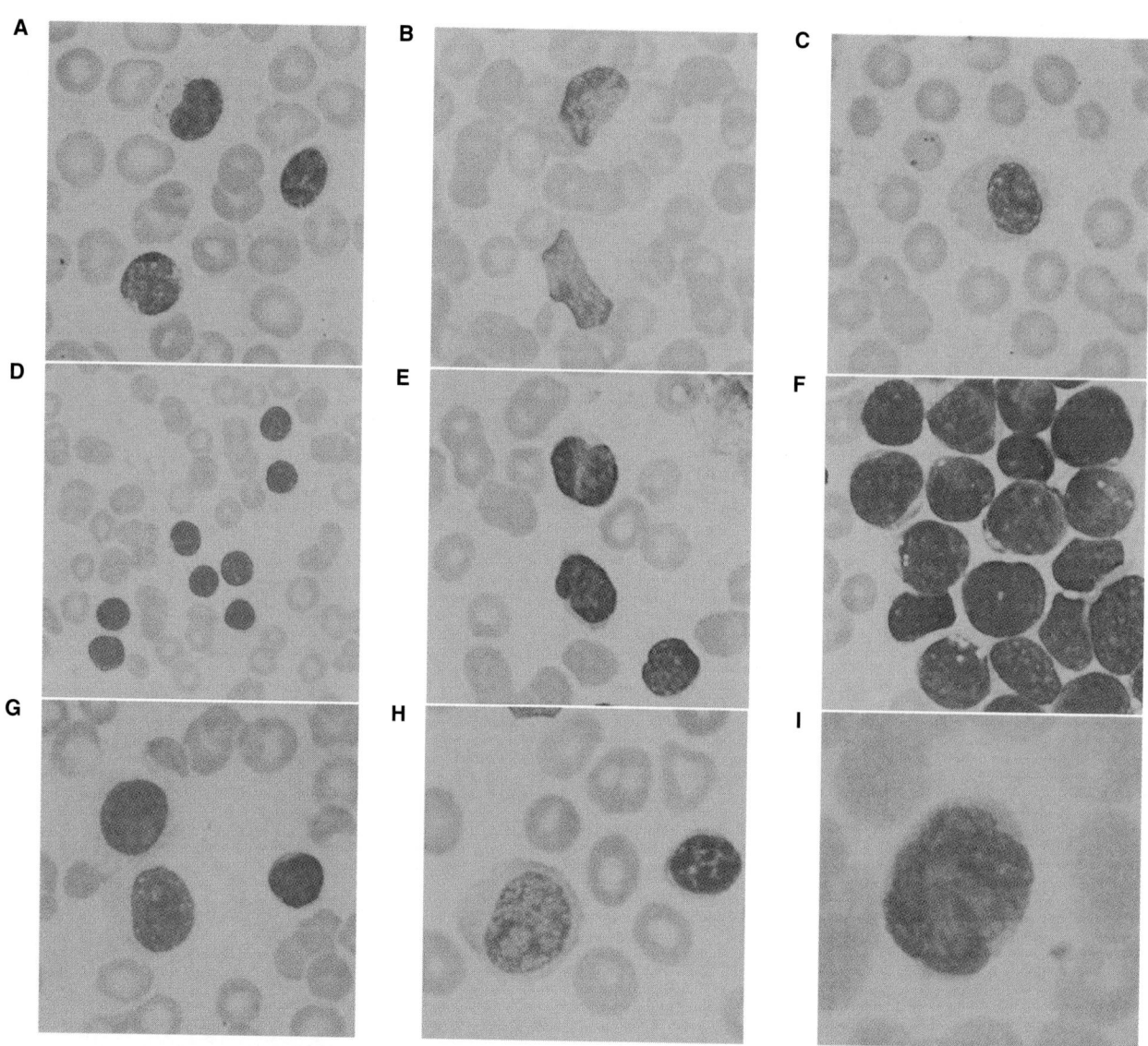

PLATE IV-5   Lymphocyte morphology in peripheral blood. Wright's stain ($\times$ 1000). **A,** Normal lymphocytes. **B,** Atypical lymphocytes (infectious mononucleosis). **C,** Plasmacytoid lymphocyte. **D,** Chronic lymphocytic leukemia ($\times$ 600). **E,** Lymphosarcoma "buttock" cells. **F,** Acute lymphoblastic leukemia. **G,** Hairy cells. **H,** The large cell is a prolymphocyte; the small cell is a normal, mature lymphocyte. **I,** Sézary cell with a lobulated, convoluted nucleus ($\times$ 2000).

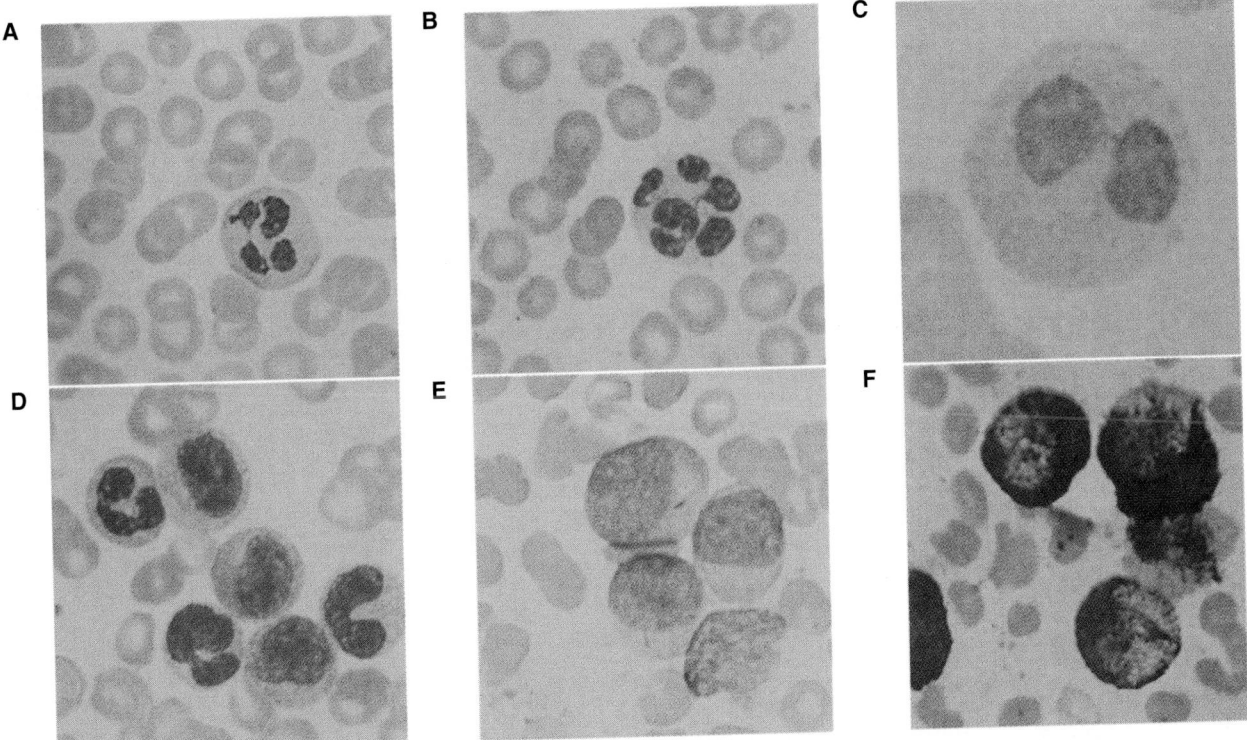

PLATE IV-6   Granulocyte morphology in peripheral blood. Wright's stain ($\times$ 1000). **A,** Normal neutrophil. **B,** Hypersegmented neutrophil. **C,** Pelger-Huët anomaly (bilobed neutrophil, magnified). **D,** Chronic myelogenous leukemia showing granulocytes at several stages of differentiation. **E,** Leukemic myeloblasts with Auer rods in the cytoplasm. **F,** Leukemic blasts that stain with Sudan black B.

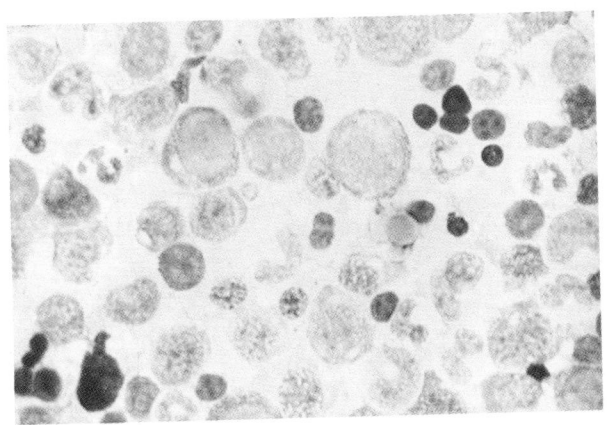

PLATE IV-7   Bone marrow of a patient with B$_{12}$ deficiency (Wright-Giemsa stain).   *(Courtesy Robert T. Means, Jr.)*

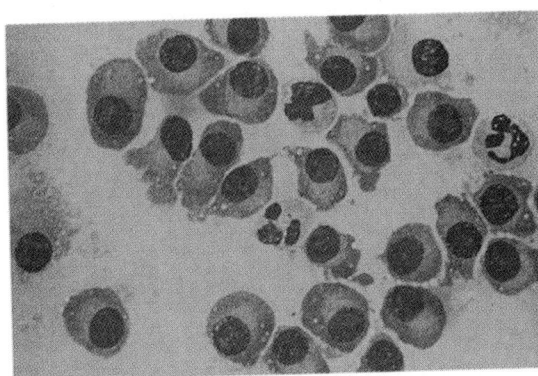

PLATE IV-8   Plasma cells in the bone marrow of a patient with myeloma.

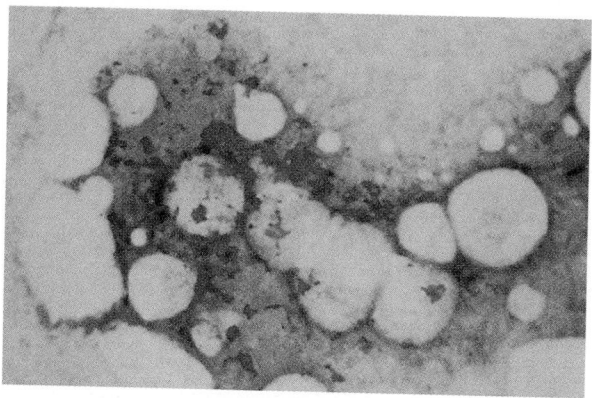

PLATE IV-9   Iron in normal bone marrow stained with Prussian blue (× 100).

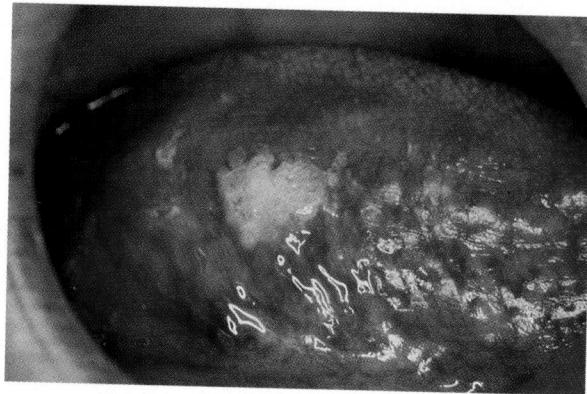

PLATE IV-12   Leukoplakia of the lateral tongue.

A 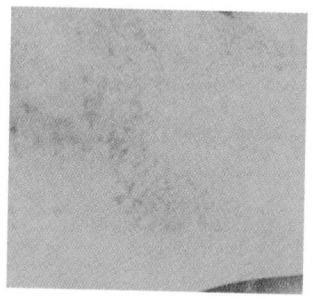 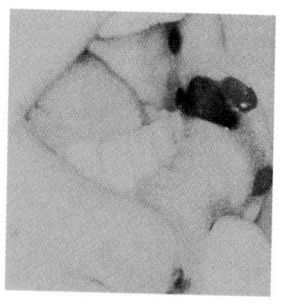 B

PLATE IV-10   Petechiae and hemorrhagic bullae in a patient with acute idiopathic thrombocytopenic purpura. These photographs were taken on the first day of illness in a previously healthy 25-year-old man. **A,** Petechiae over the lateral surface, right ankle, and foot. **B,** Hemorrhagic bullae in the oral mucous membranes.

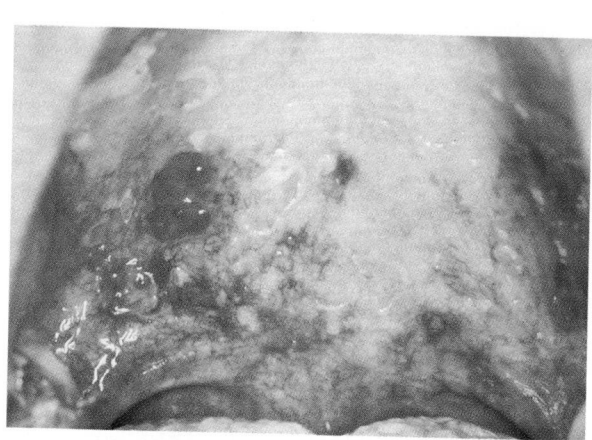

PLATE IV-13   Erythroplakia of the soft palate.

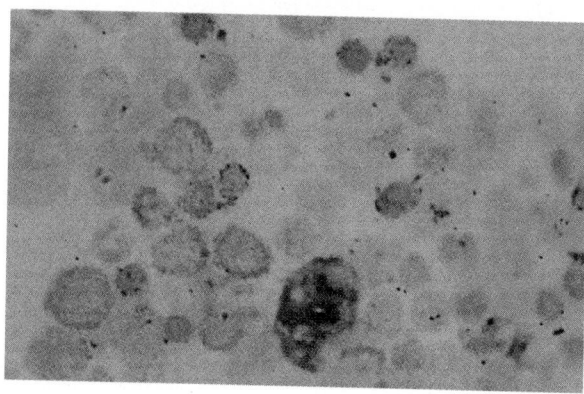

PLATE IV-11   Ringed sideroblasts in the bone marrow from a patient with sideroblastic anemia; Prussian blue stain (× 1000).

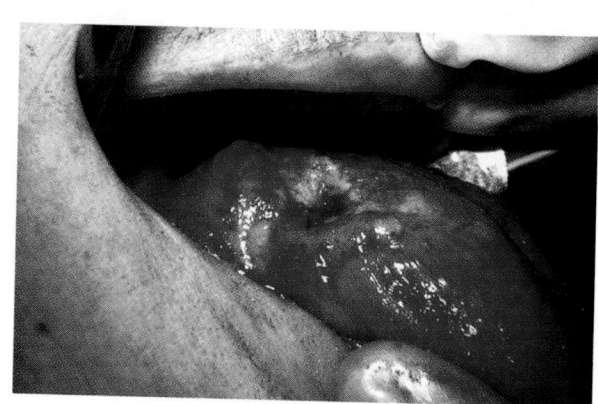

PLATE IV-14   Deep infiltrating squamous cell carcinoma of the tongue.

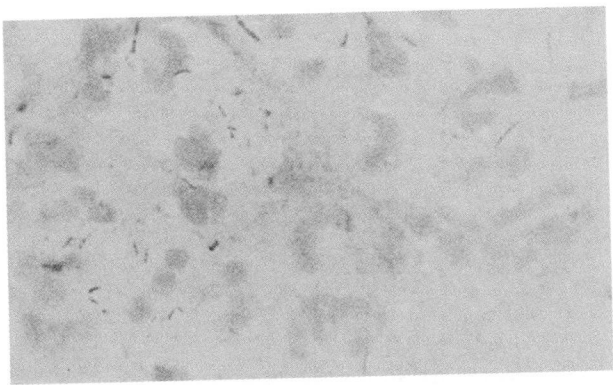

PLATE VII-1 Gram-stained expectorated sputum or transtracheal aspirate from patients with aspiration anaerobic pneumonia typically shows a mixture of gram-positive cocci rods with bizarre morphologic forms.

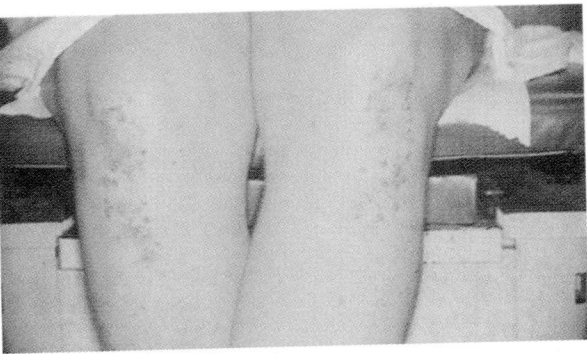

PLATE VII-4 Dermatitis herpetiformis.

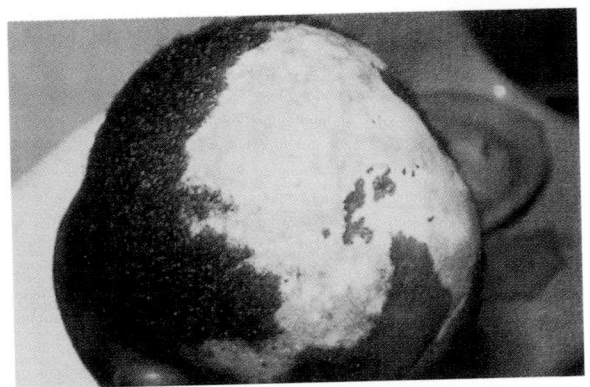

PLATE VII-2 Lupus erythematosus.

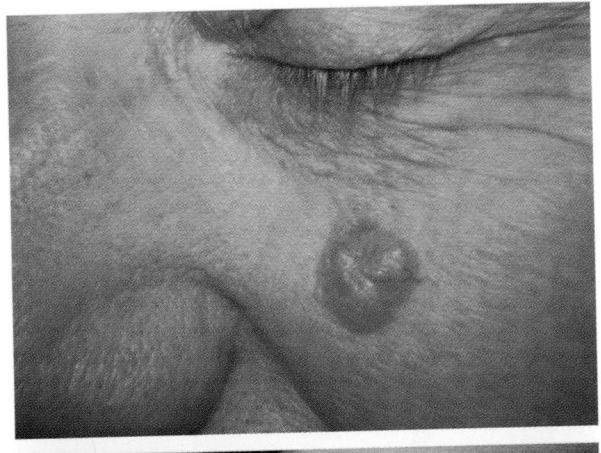

A

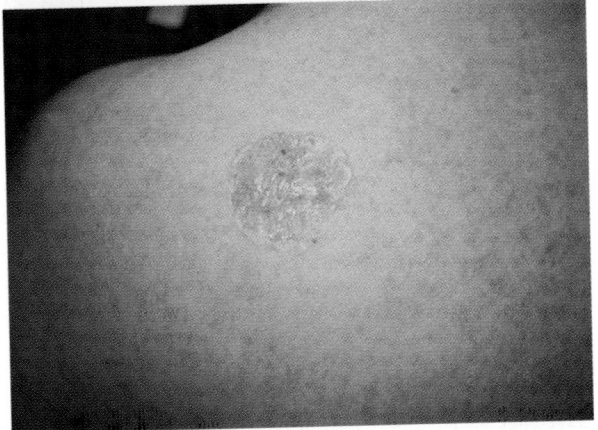

B

PLATE VII-5 Basal cell carcinoma.

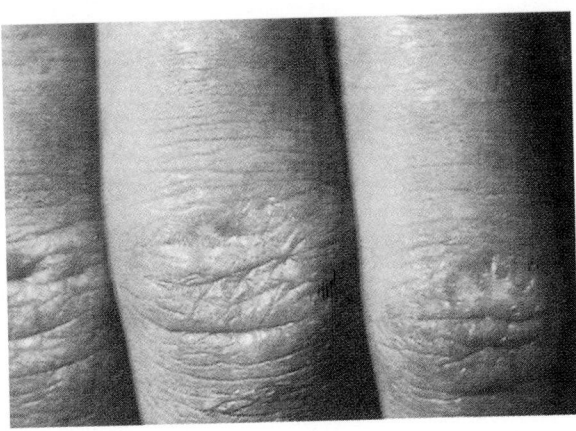

PLATE VII-3 Dermatomyositis (Gottron's papules).

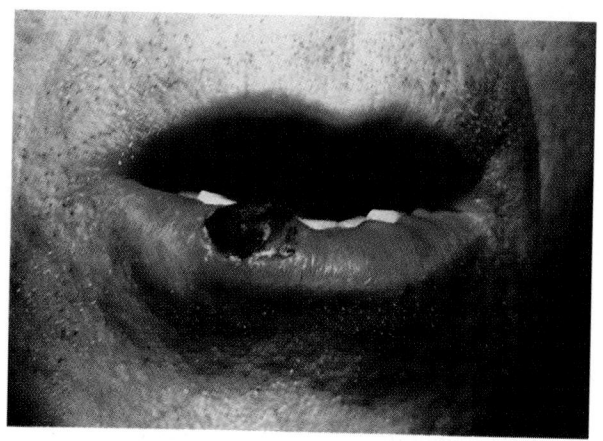

PLATE VII-6   Squamous cell carcinoma.

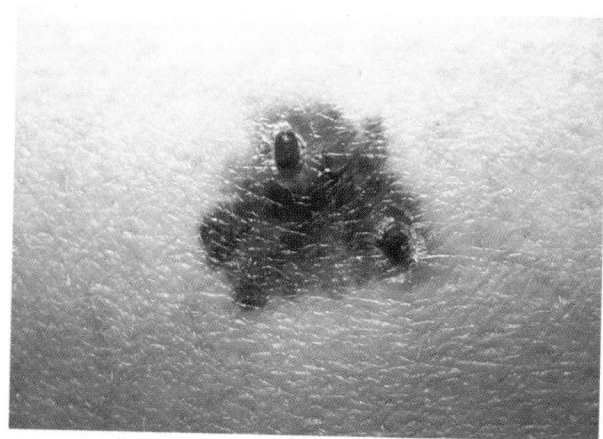

PLATE VII-8   Superficial spreading malignant melanoma.

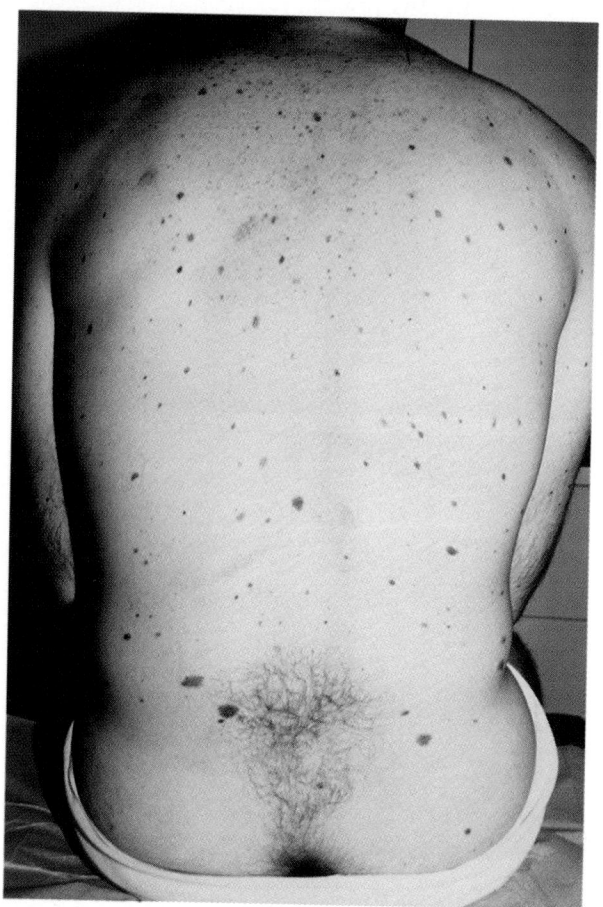

PLATE VII-7   A 45-year-old man with atypical mole syndrome and a history of two primary melanomas.

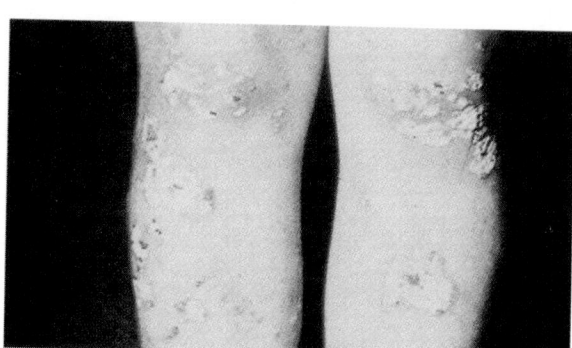

PLATE VII-9   Psoriasis.

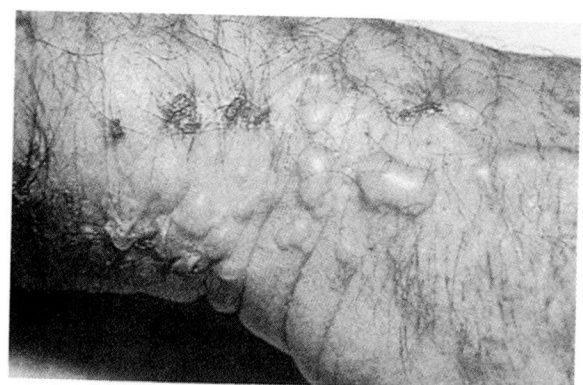

PLATE VII-10   Porphyria cutanea tarda.

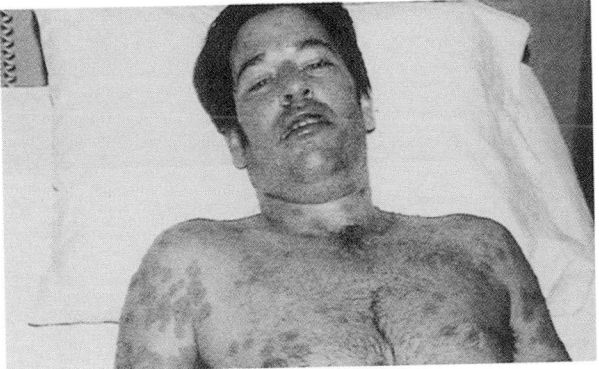

PLATE VII-11   Stevens-Johnson syndrome.

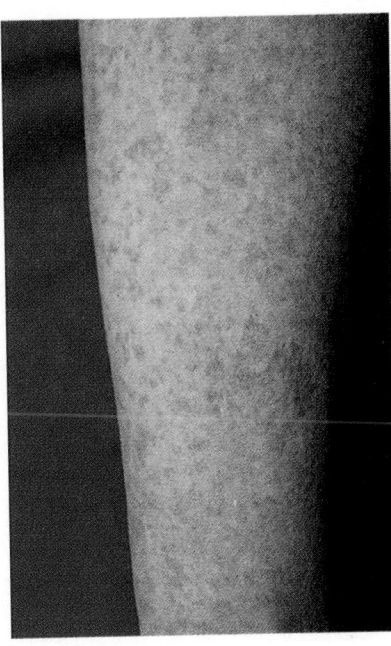

PLATE VII-13   Exanthematous eruption developing after the administration of trimethoprim-sulfamethoxazole.

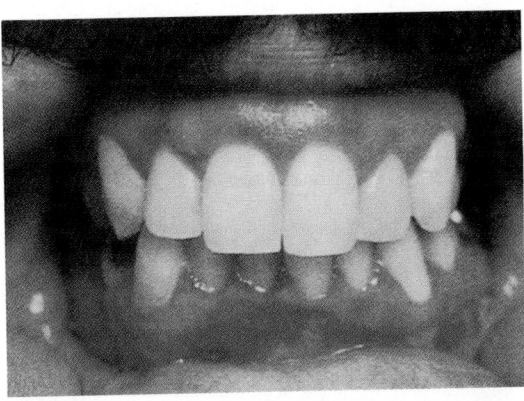

PLATE VII-14   Addison's disease: hyperpigmentation of the gums along the dentate margins.

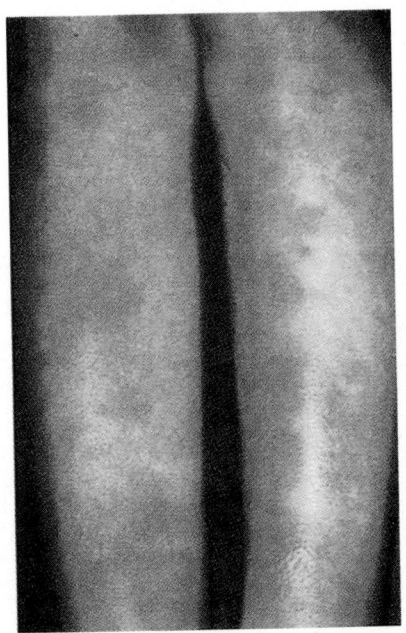

PLATE VII-12   Erythema nodosum.

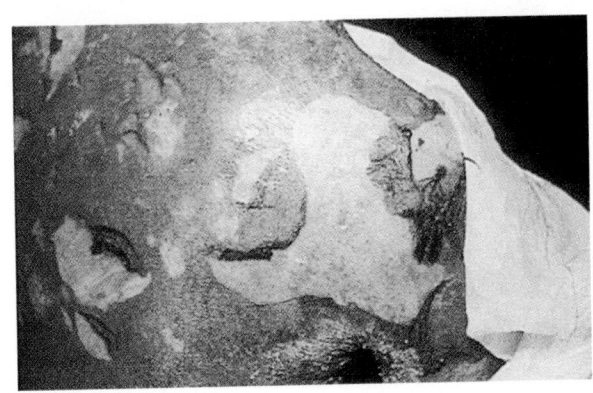

PLATE VII-15   Toxic epidermal necrolysis.

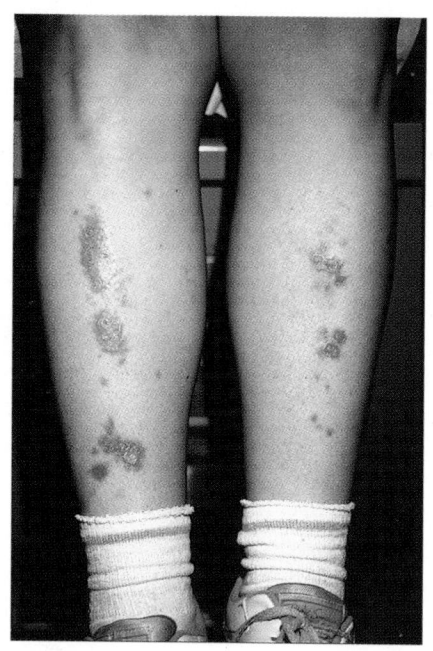

PLATE VII-16   Necrobiosis lipoidica diabeticorum.

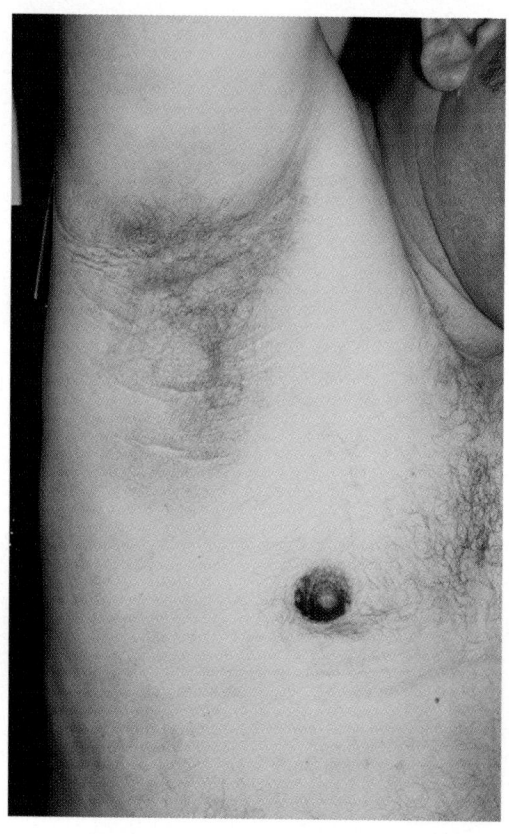

PLATE VII-17   Acanthosis nigricans.

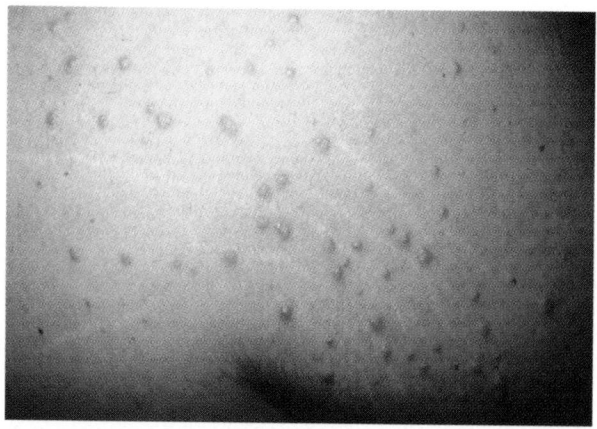

PLATE VII-18   Eruptive xanthomas.

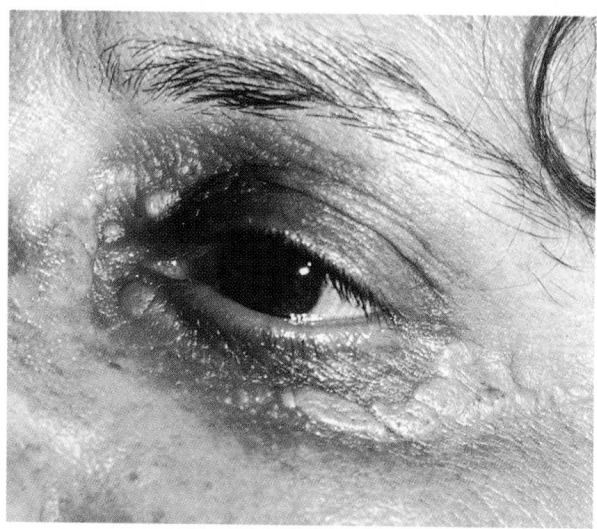

PLATE VII-19   Xanthelasma.

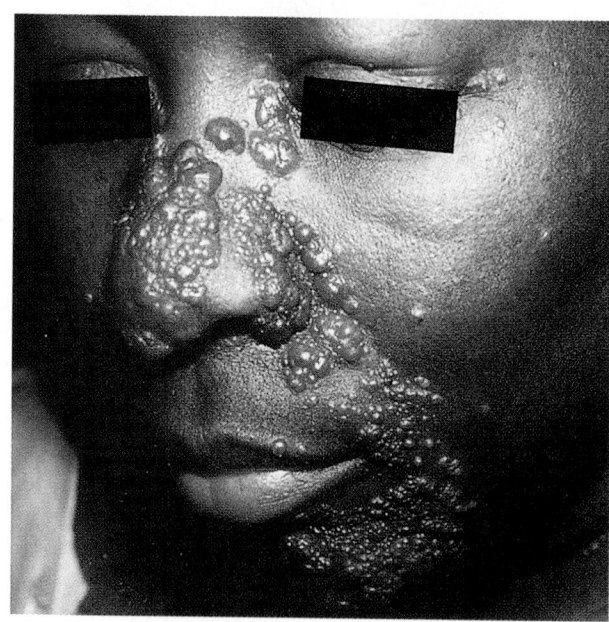

PLATE VII-20   The papular lesions of sarcoidosis often manifest as a symmetric eruption on the central face.

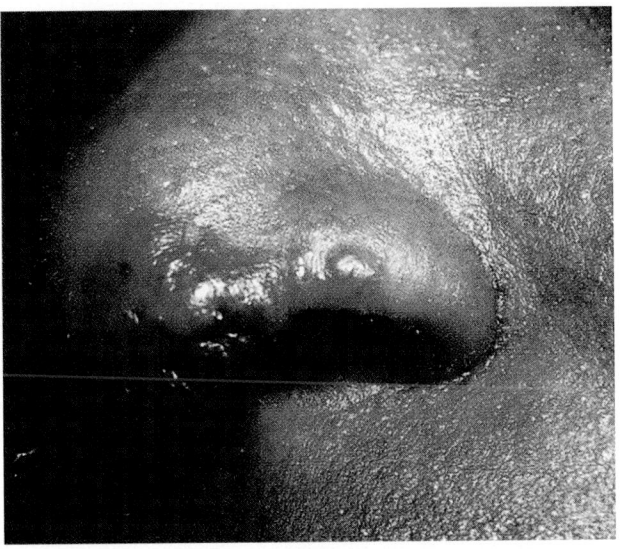

PLATE VII-21   The lesions of lupus pernio seen at the nasal orifice may be evidence of involvement of the upper respiratory tract.

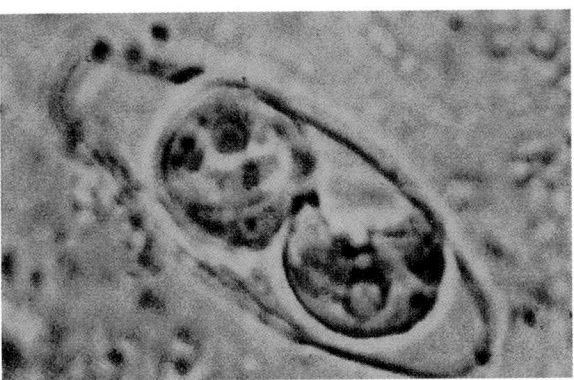

PLATE VIII-1   Mature oocyst of *Isospora belli* in unstained fecal smear. The oocyst is typically elongated, measures 20-33 μm by 10-19 μm, and has a wall consisting of two layers. Two sporocysts may be seen within the oocyst (× 2000).   *(Courtesy Dr. Keith Hadley, San Francisco General Hospital.)*

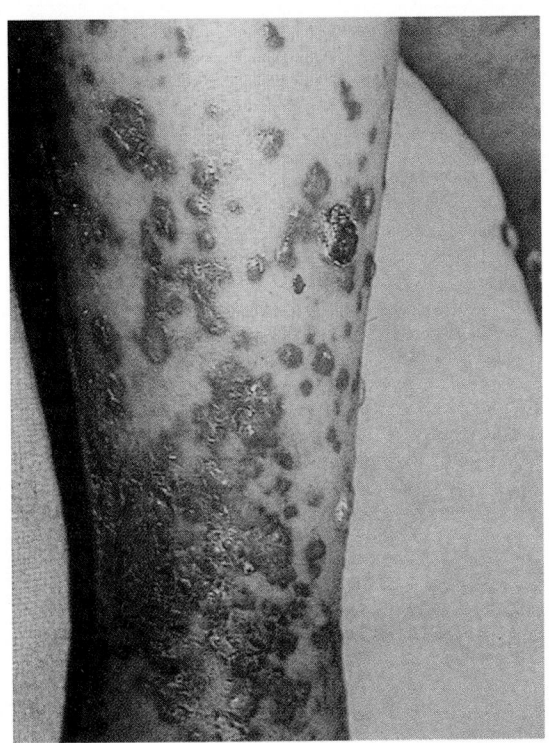

PLATE VII-22   Kaposi's sarcoma.

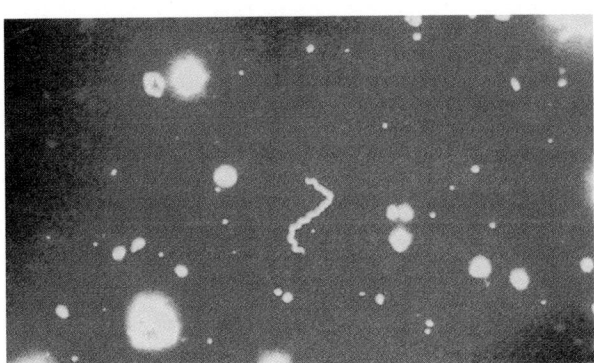

PLATE VIII-2   *Treponema pallidum* by dark-field microscopy (× 1000). Note the distinct spirals and characteristic bending. *(Courtesy Centers for Disease Control and Prevention.)*

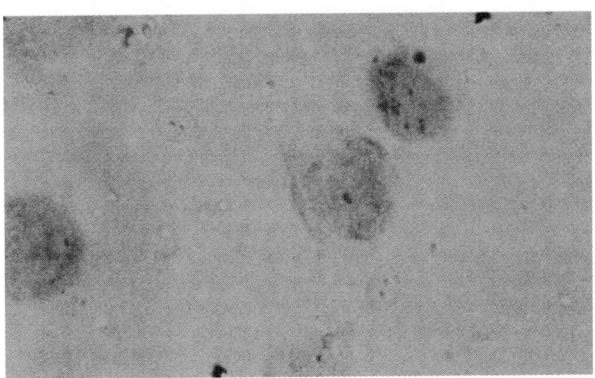

PLATE VIII-3   Inspection for a quellung reaction with pneumococcal omni serum improves the correlation of the Gram stain with the culture by nearly 90%, chiefly by reducing the number of false-positive smears caused by the otherwise indistinguishable oral alpha-hemolytic streptococcus.

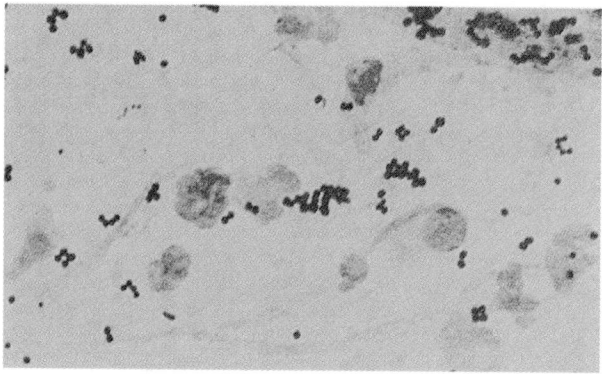

PLATE VIII-4   Staphylococci can be identified by the typical clustering (like grapes on a stem) of gram-positive cocci.

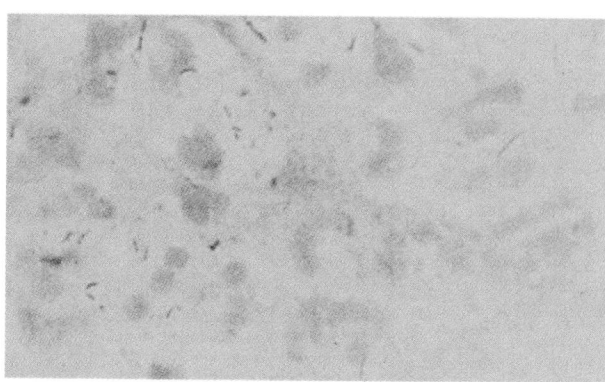

PLATE VIII-7   Gram-stained expectorated sputum or transtracheal aspirate from a patient with aspiration pneumonia.

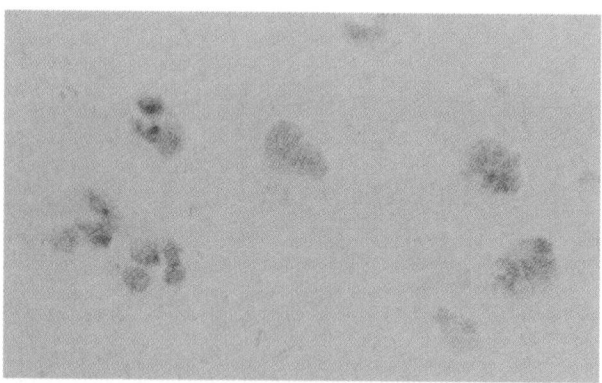

PLATE VIII-5   *Haemophilus influenzae* is often difficult to see because the gram-negative coccobacillary forms may be poorly stained and may blend with the red background.

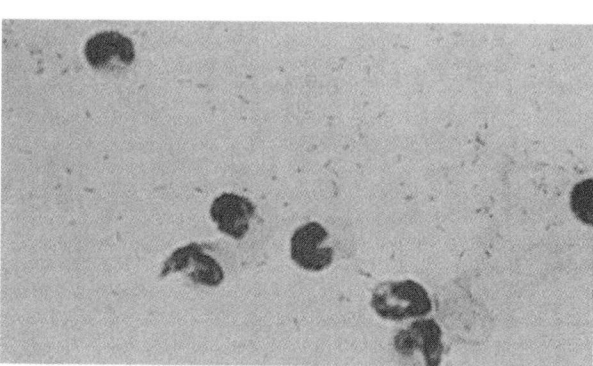

PLATE VIII-8   Gram stain of spun cerebrospinal fluid from a patient with *Haemophilus influenzae* type B meningitis. Note the presence of coccobacillary organisms in conjunction with polymorphonuclear leukocytes.

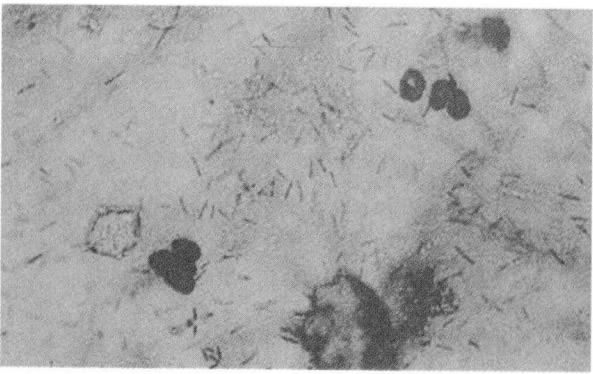

PLATE VIII-6   The large gram-negative rods predominate the field in *Klebsiella pneumoniae* or other infections caused by the Enterobacteriaceae or *Pseudomonas*.

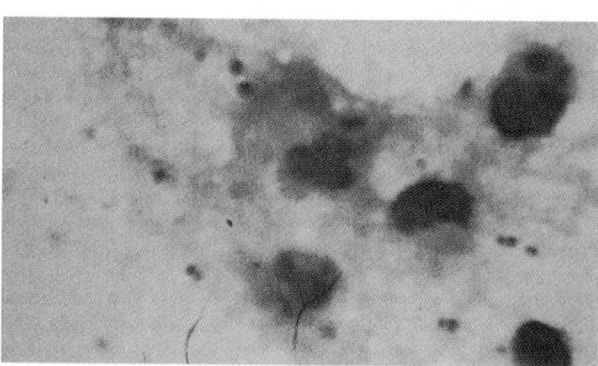

PLATE VIII-9   Gram stain of centrifuged cerebrospinal fluid from a patient with meningococcal meningitis. Note the presence of gram-negative cocci in pairs associated with polymorphonuclear leukocytes.

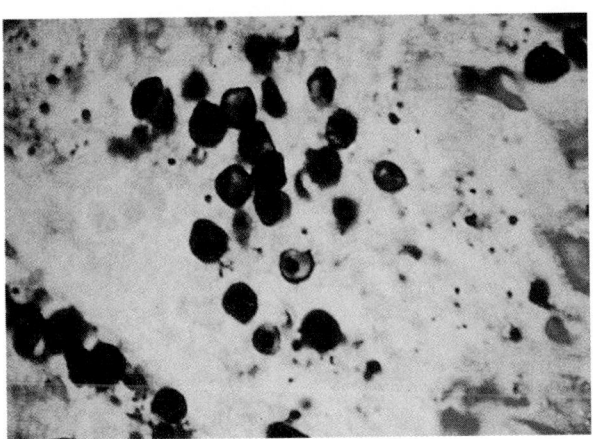

PLATE VIII-10   Giemsa stain of bronchial washings demonstrating *Pneumocystis carinii* cysts.

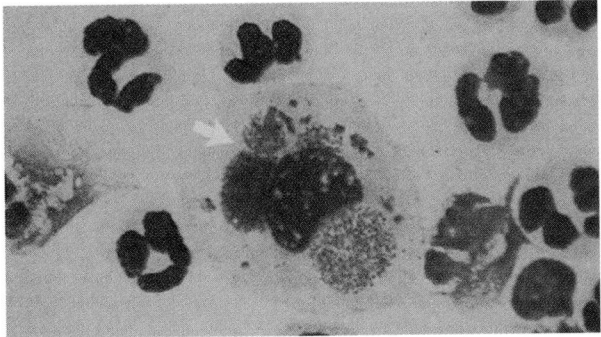

PLATE VIII-11   Giemsa stain of conjunctiva scraping showing typical cytoplasmic inclusion of *Chlamydia trachomatis*.

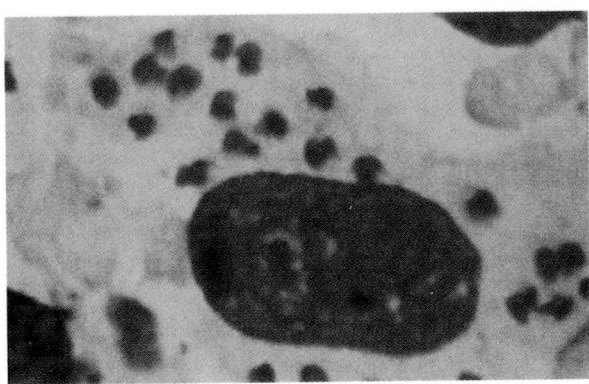

PLATE VIII-12   *Leishmania* amastigotes within an impression smear of a patient with cutaneous leishmaniasis. Giemsa stain (× 2000). *(Courtesy Dr. Keith Hadley, San Francisco General Hospital.)*

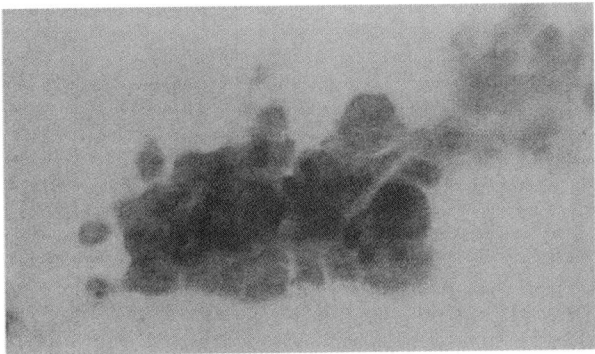

PLATE VIII-13   Photomicrographic scraping from the base of a herpes blister demonstrating multinuclear giant cells.

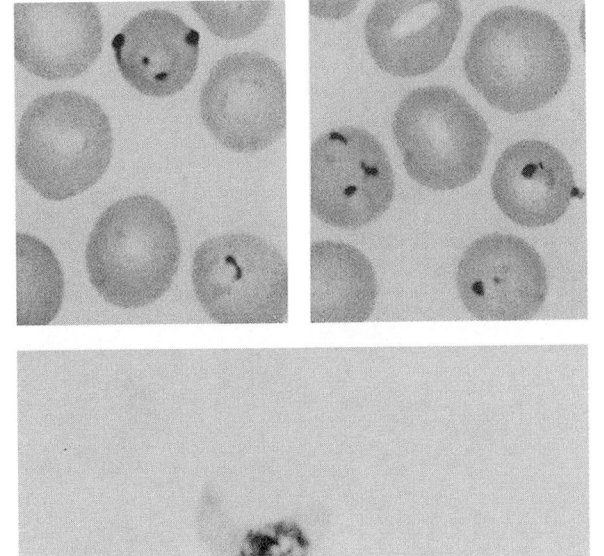

A

B

C

PLATE VIII-14   Giemsa-stained blood smear in *Plasmodium falciparum* malaria. **A** and **B,** Asexual parasites; note that ring forms predominate, some erythrocytes contain multiple parasites, and some parasites contain double nuclei (× 2000). **C,** Gametocyte has pathognomonic crescent shape (× 2000).

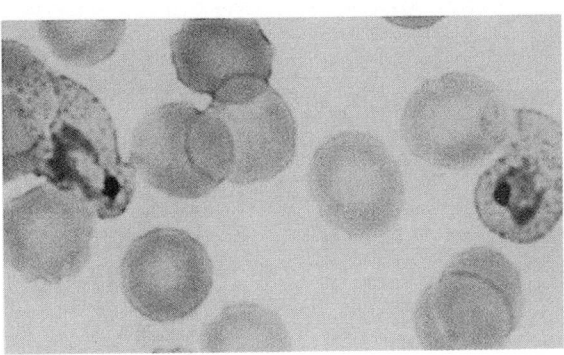

PLATE VIII-15   Giemsa-stained blood smear in *Plasmodium vivax* malaria. Asexual parasites. Note that the parasites are large and ameboid, the infected erythrocytes are the largest cells in the field (because they are reticulocytes), and the erythrocytes contain numerous pink dots (Schüffner's dots) (× 2000).

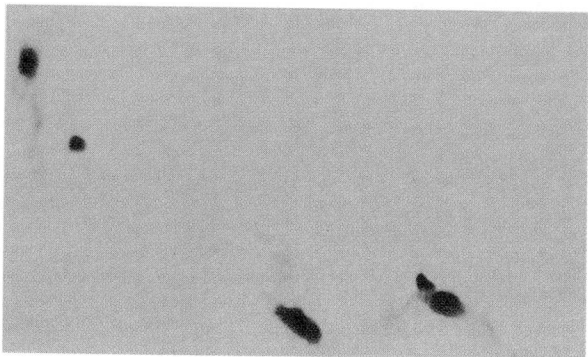

PLATE VIII-16 Trypomastigotes of *Trypanosoma brucei rhodesiense* in a Giemsa-stained thick blood smear. The central reddish nucleus is evident, but the kinetoplast cannot be distinguished (× 2000). *(Courtesy Dr. Keith Hadley, San Francisco General Hospital.)*

PLATE VIII-19 In Rocky Mountain spotted fever, the rickettsiae invade the vasculature of the integument as well as other organs and can be demonstrated in vessel walls by immunofluorescence.

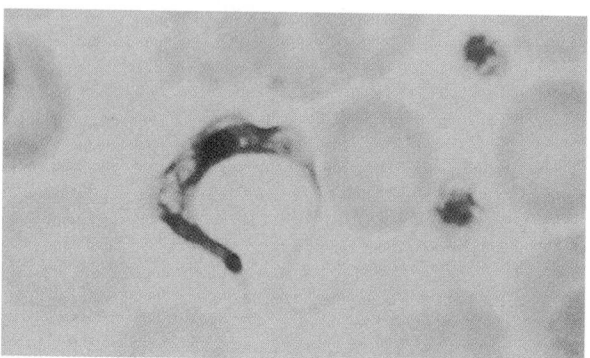

PLATE VIII-17 Trypomastigote of *Trypanosoma cruzi* in a Giemsa-stained blood smear. A central nucleus, flagellum, and posterior kinetoplast can be seen (× 2000). *(Courtesy Dr. Keith Hadley, San Francisco General Hospital.)*

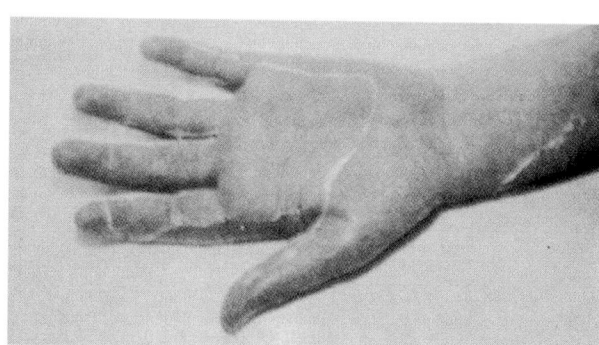

PLATE VIII-20 Desquamation following toxic shock syndrome.

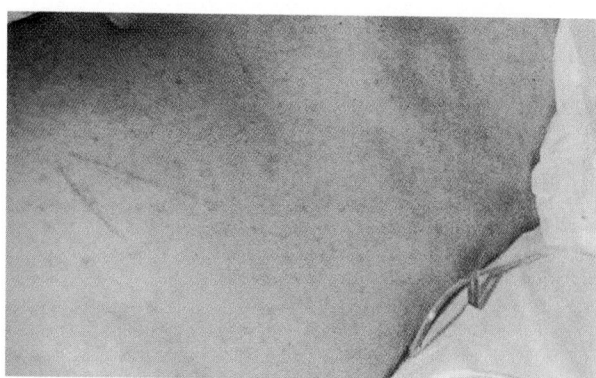

PLATE VIII-18 Petechial and purpuric skin lesions in a severe case of Rocky Mountain spotted fever, 7 days after the onset of symptoms.

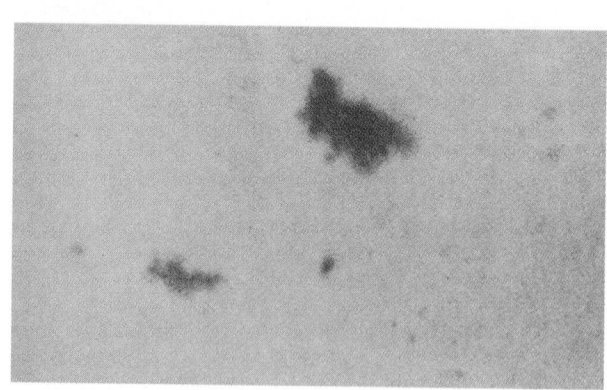

PLATE VIII-21 Cutaneous lesions in a patient with meningococcemia.

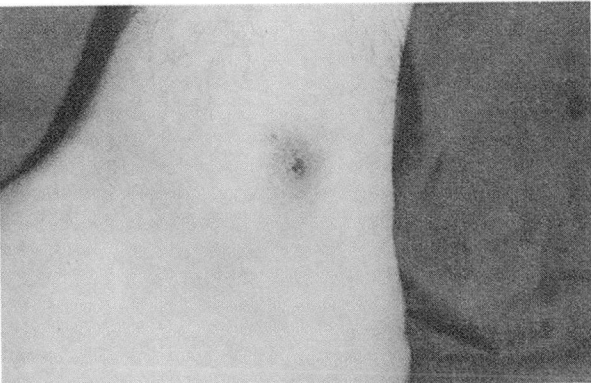

PLATE VIII-22 Cutaneous lesion from a patient with disseminated gonococcal infection. Note the characteristic appearance of the gray necrotic ulcer on an erythematous base in the typical location on the ankles.

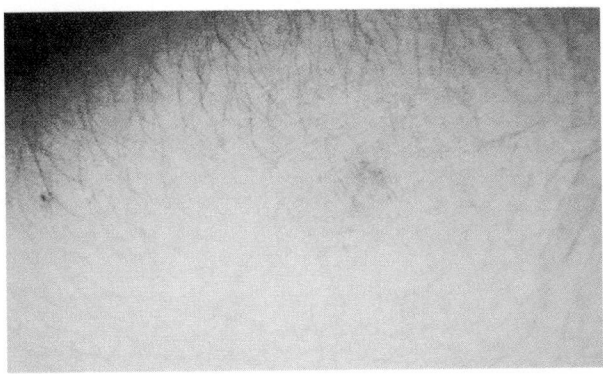

PLATE VIII-23 Cutaneous lesion in a leukemic patient with overwhelming *Pseudomonas aeruginosa* septicemia. The lesion is called *ecthyma gangrenosum*. Note the characteristics of the bluish central discoloration.

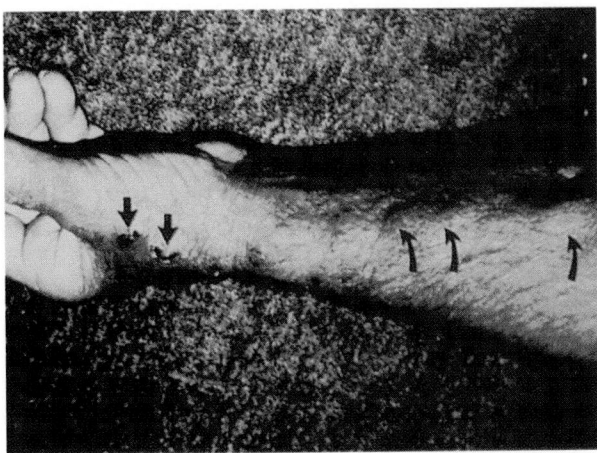

PLATE VIII-24 Cutaneous sporotrichosis, with peripheral ulcerative lesions *(large arrow)* and proximal satellite nodules *(small arrows)*.

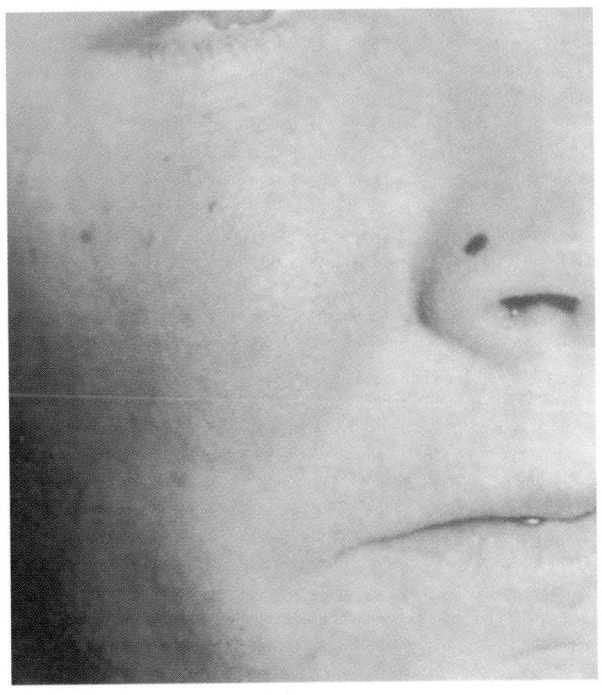

PLATE VIII-25 Erysipelas.

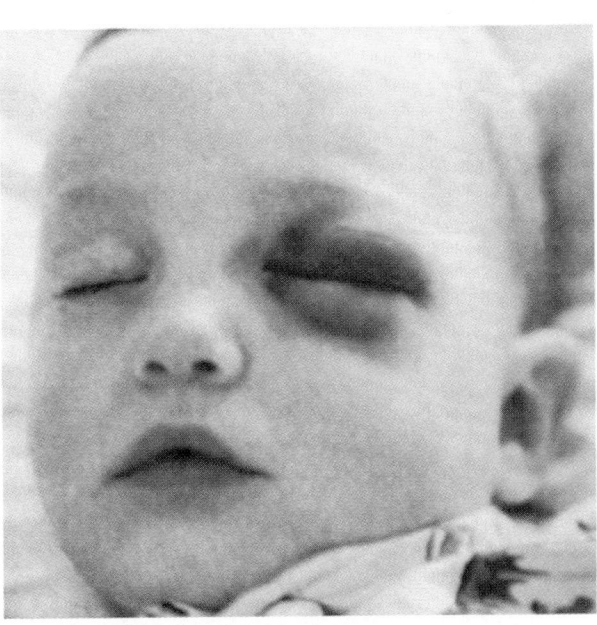

PLATE VIII-26 Periorbital *Haemophilus influenzae* cellulitis.

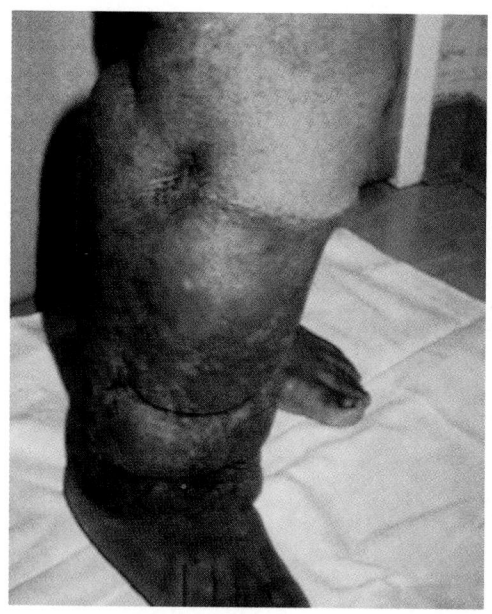

PLATE VIII-27   Elephantiasis nostras.

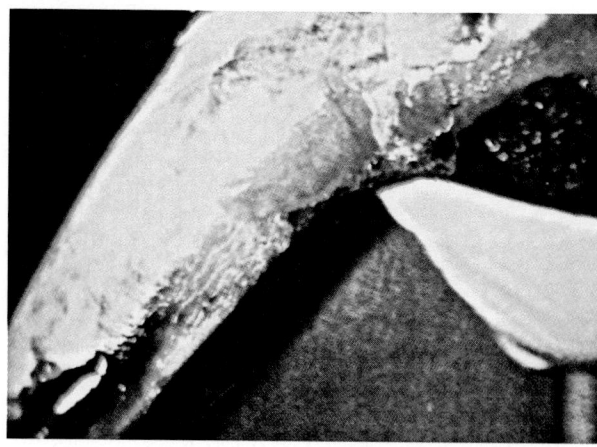

PLATE VIII-30   Acute gangrene of the arm caused by *Streptococcus pyogenes,* group A, type 12. (*From* Arch Intern Med *112:937, 1963.*)

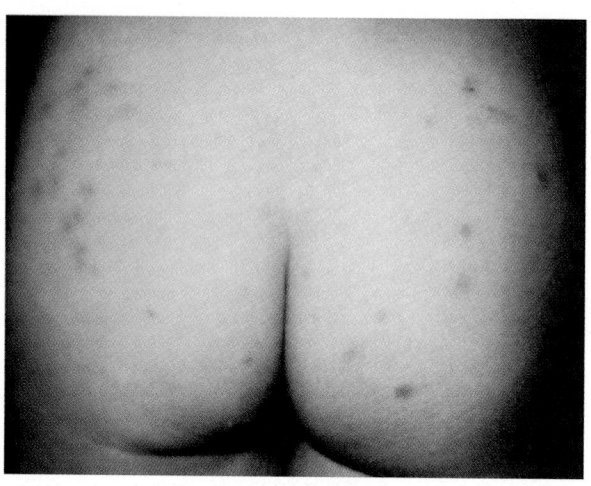

PLATE VIII-28   Hot tub folliculitis.

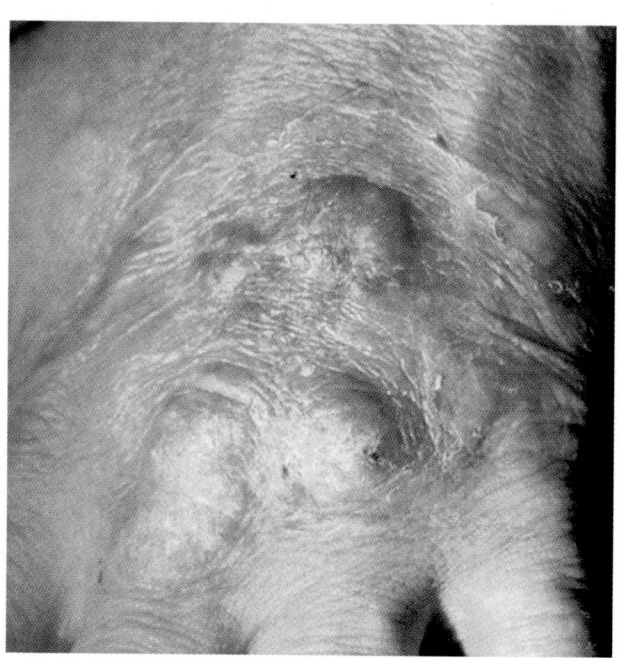

PLATE VIII-31   *Mycobacterium marinum.*

PLATE VIII-29   Staphylococcal scalded skin syndrome.

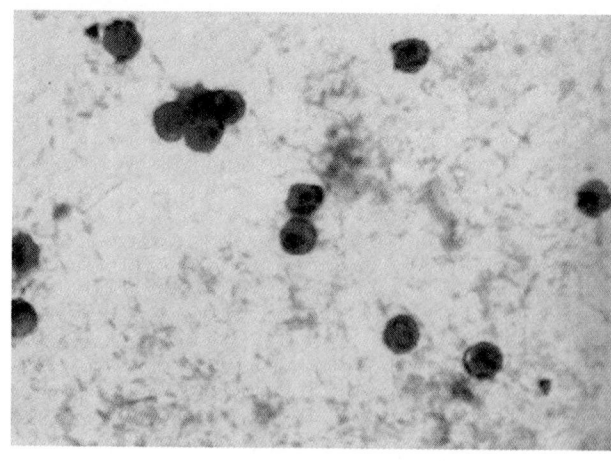

PLATE VIII-32   Modified Kinyoun stain of stool specimen demonstrating the numerous oval, red cryptosporidia.

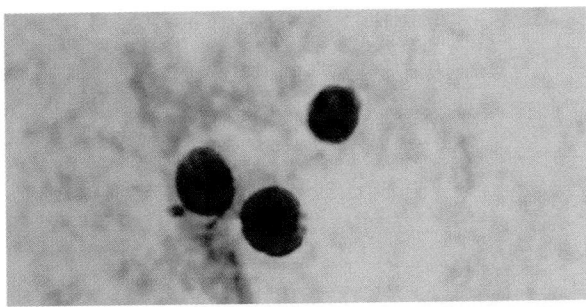

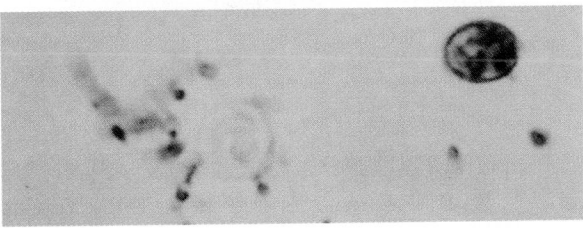

PLATE VIII-33 Oocysts of *Cryptosporidium*. **A,** Oocysts are acid fast and can be stained with modified Kinyoun stain or Ziehl-Neelsen stain (× 2000). **B,** Periodic acid Schiff (PAS) stain can assist in differentiating *Cryptosporidium* from yeast. Yeast stains with PAS; *Cryptosporidium* does not. (× 2000). *(Courtesy Dr. Keith Hadley, San Francisco General Hospital.)*

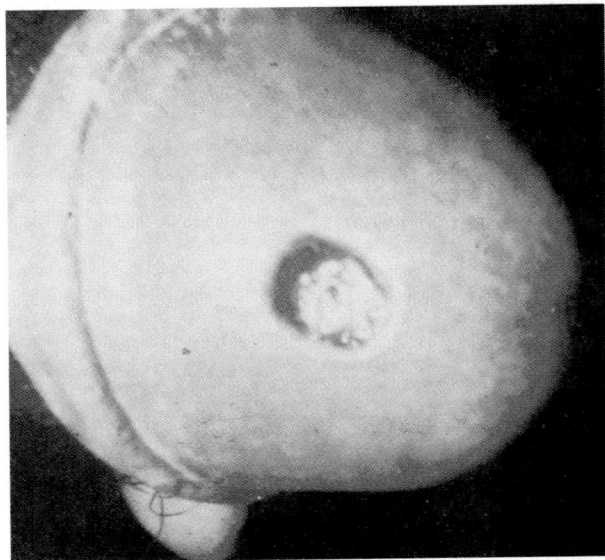

PLATE VIII-34 Chancre of the penis in a patient with primary syphilis. *(Courtesy Centers for Disease Control and Prevention.)*

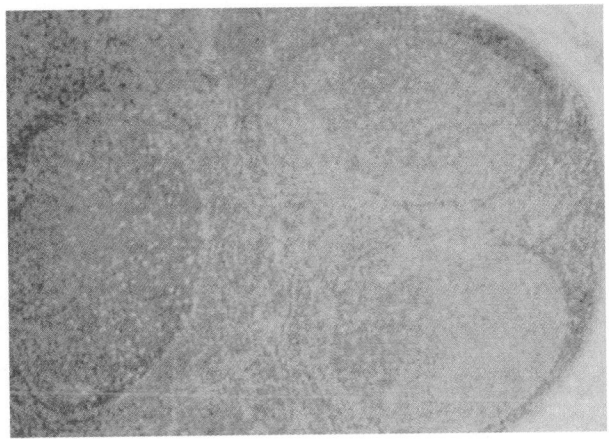

PLATE VIII-35 Hematoxylin and eosin preparation of biopsy specimen from a peripheral lymph node demonstrating reactive hyperplasia.

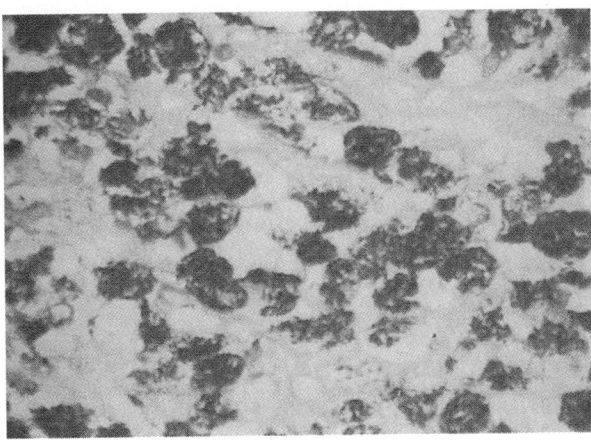

PLATE VIII-36 Acid-fast stain of a lymph node biopsy specimen demonstrating macrophages filled with numerous red-staining *Mycobacterium avium-intracellulare* organisms.

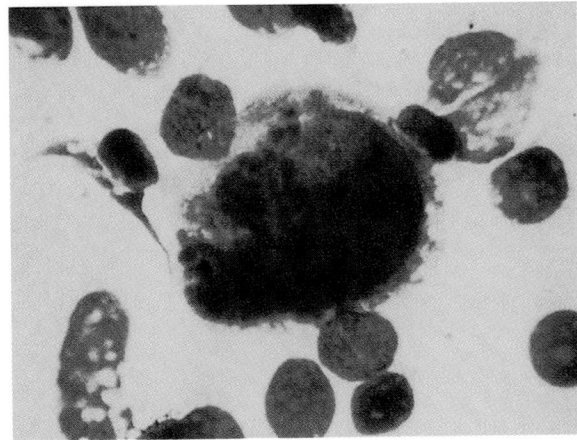

PLATE VIII-37 Transbronchial biopsy specimen from a patient with cytomegalovirus pneumonitis demonstrating a multinucleated cell with intranuclear and cytoplasmic inclusions.

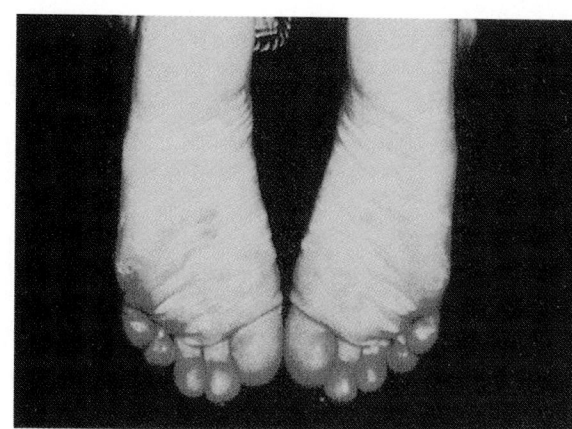

A

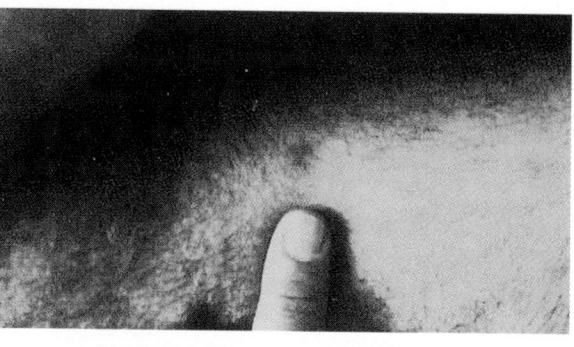

B

PLATE VIII-38 Cutaneous Kaposi's sarcoma lesions.

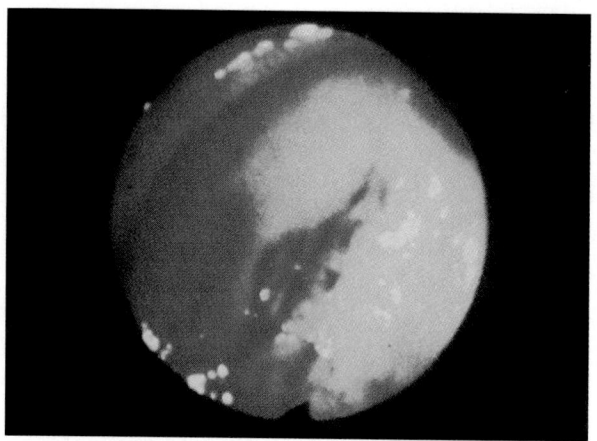

PLATE VIII-39 Kaposi's sarcoma lesion in colonic mucosa.

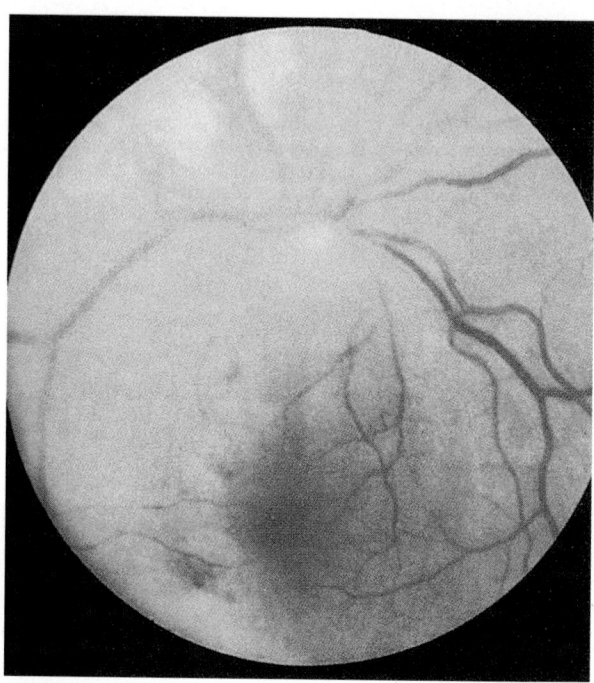

PLATE VIII-41 Retinochoroiditis caused by cytomegalovirus infection.

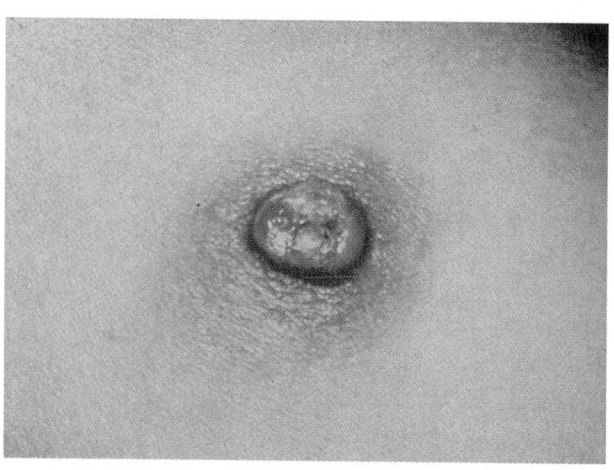

PLATE VIII-40 Typical lesion of bacillary angiomatosis.

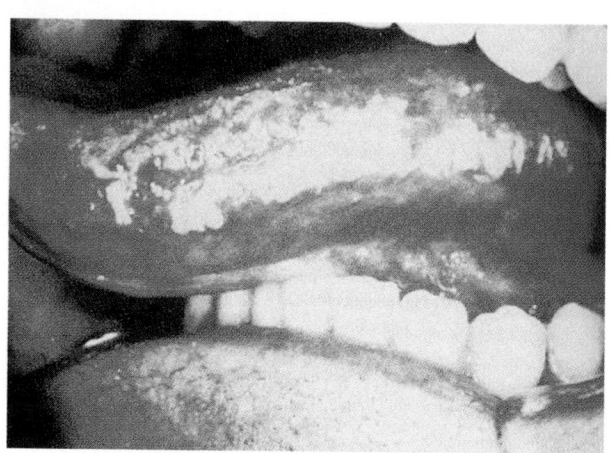

PLATE VIII-42 Oral hairy cell leukoplakia.

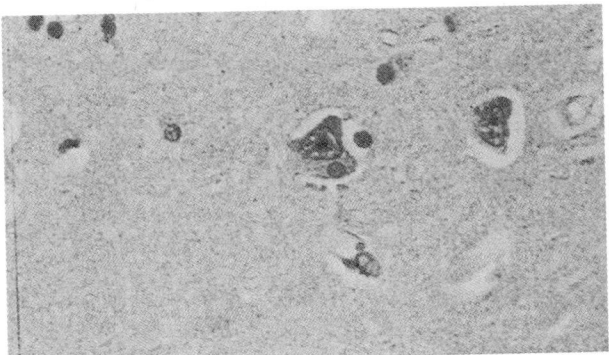

PLATE VIII-43 Negri bodies in human patient with rabies. In the center is a well-defined cell with a nucleus and a cytoplasmic Negri body. Hematoxylin-eosin stain (× 200). *(Courtesy Dr. Jerry Winkler, Centers for Disease Control and Prevention.)*

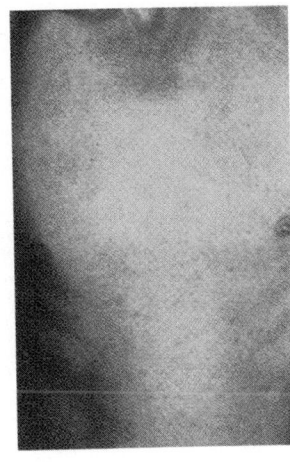

PLATE VIII-46 Secondary syphilis. *(Courtesy Dr. Charles J. Schleupner.)*

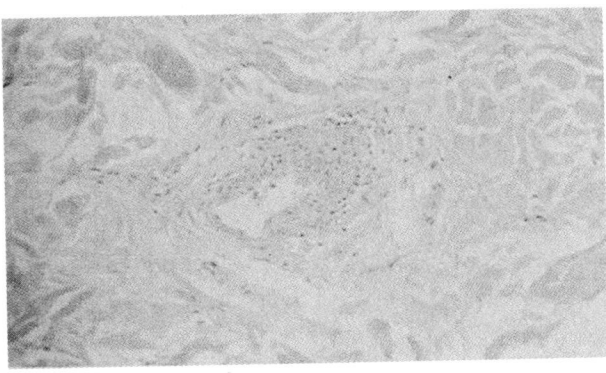

PLATE VIII-44 Typical focus of rickettsial vasculitis in an arteriole, with mononuclear inflammatory infiltrate and a small, nonocclusive thrombus.

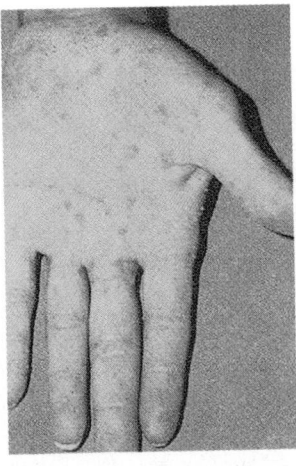

PLATE VIII-47 Palmar lesions of secondary syphilis. *(Courtesy Dr. Charles J. Schleupner.)*

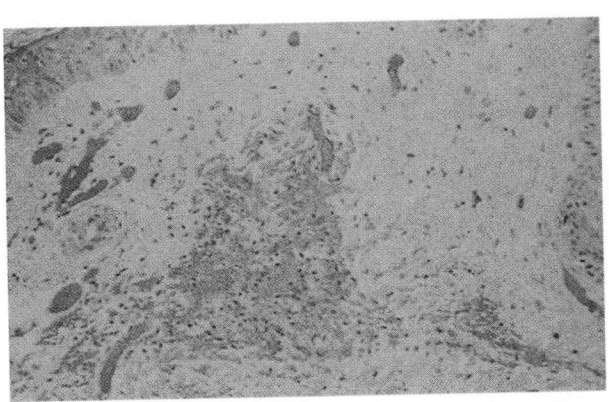

PLATE VIII-45 Small intradermal hemorrhage at a focus of vasculitis. This causes the palpable, petechial rash that does not blanch on pressure.

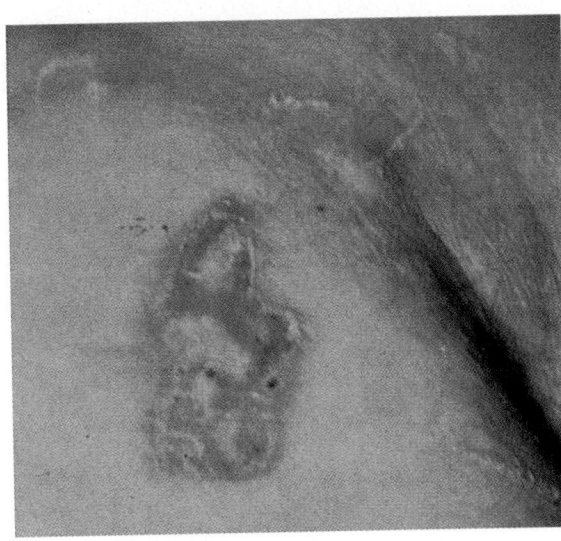

PLATE VIII-48 Ulcerative skin lesions of blastomycosis.

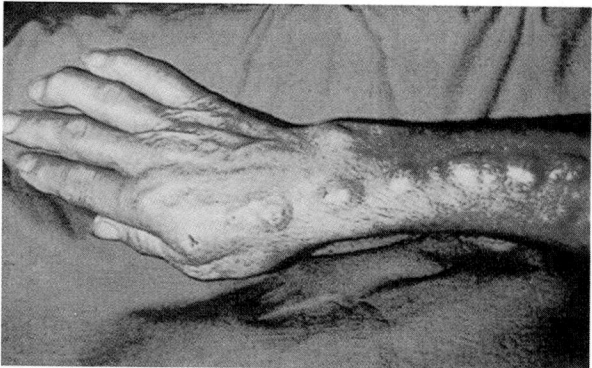

PLATE VIII-49   Lymphangitic spread of sporotrichosis.

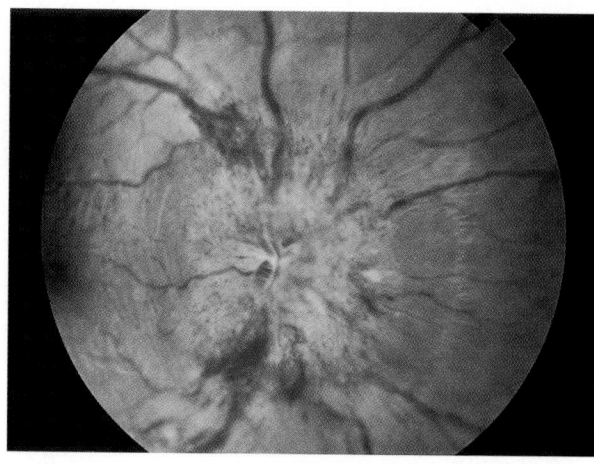

PLATE VIII-51   Funduscopic view of severe papilledema in a patient with cryptococcal meningitis and persistently elevated cerebrospinal fluid pressures.

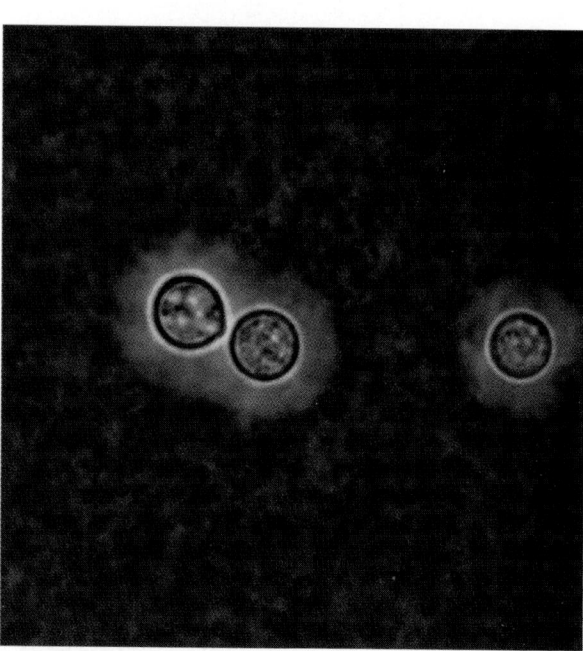

PLATE VIII-50   India ink preparation of cerebrospinal fluid shows cryptococcus neoformans with characteristic single budding and large polysaccharide capsules (× 1000).

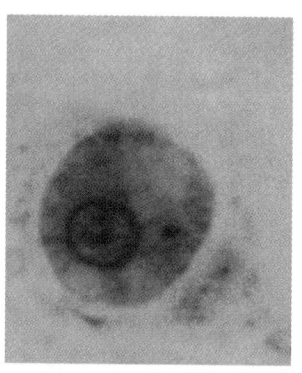

A
B

PLATE VIII-52   *Entamoeba histolytica* in fecal specimen (trichrome stain). **A,** A trophozoite or a very early cyst. Trophozoites measure 10-60 μm in diameter and may contain phagocytized erythrocytes. **B,** A cyst containing a chromatoidal bar and a single nucleus. Mature cysts are 10-20 μm in diameter and most often contain four nuclei (× 2000). *(Courtesy Dr. Keith Hadley, San Francisco General Hospital.)*

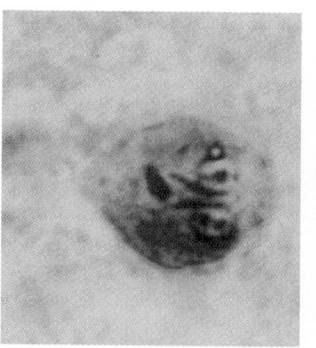
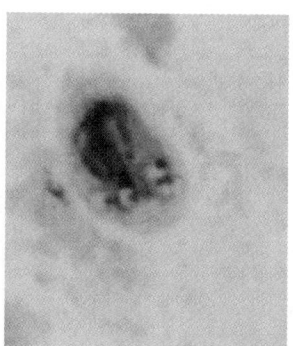

A
B

PLATE VIII-53   **A,** *Giardia lamblia* trophozoite and **B,** cyst. The trophozoite contains two nuclei and a flagellum. The cyst contains four nuclei (× 2000).   *(Courtesy Dr. Keith Hadley, San Francisco General Hospital.)*

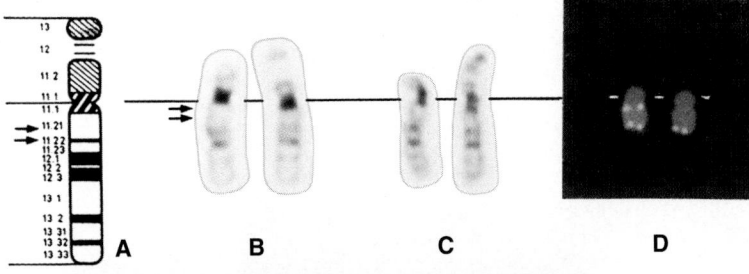

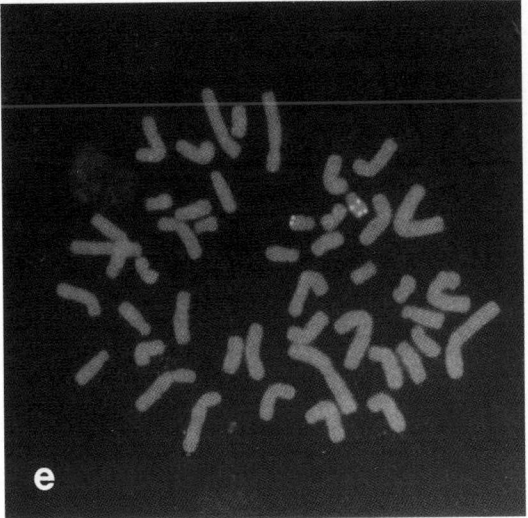

PLATE IX-1 Interstitial microdeletion of chromosome band 22q11. **A,** ISCN 1995 ideogram of chromosome 22. Arrows point to region deleted. **B,** G-banded chromosome 22 homologs from a patient with velocardiofacial syndrome. The chromosome 22 on the right is visibly deleted. Arrows on the normal homolog point out the region deleted. **C,** Apparently normal G-banded chromosomes 22 from a patient with velocardiofacial syndrome. **D,** Chromosomes 22 from the same patient as in C after fluorescent in situ hybridization (FISH) with biotin-labeled Oncor probe D22S75 together with distal 22 identifier probe D22S39. The deleted chromosome 22 on the right exhibits signal only from the identifier probe. **E,** Hybridized chromosome spread from which the chromosomes 22 in *D* were prepared.

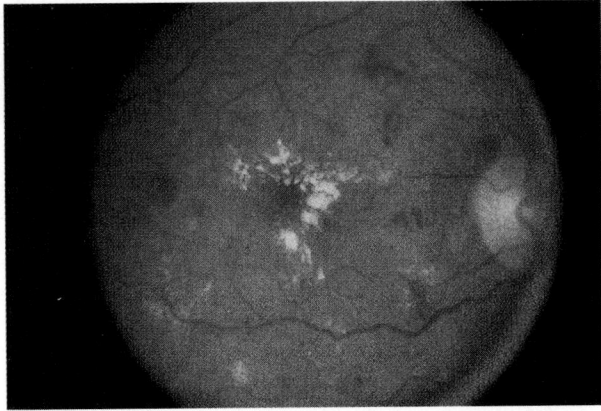

PLATE IX-3 Exudative diabetic retinopathy. Hard exudates, composed of lipid, carbohydrate, and protein, which are left in the retina after long-standing capillary endothelial leakage of serum, may take a variety of shapes. Rings of exudates suggest that microangiopathy in the center of the ring is leaking. Almost always, other evidence of nonproliferative retinopathy is present.

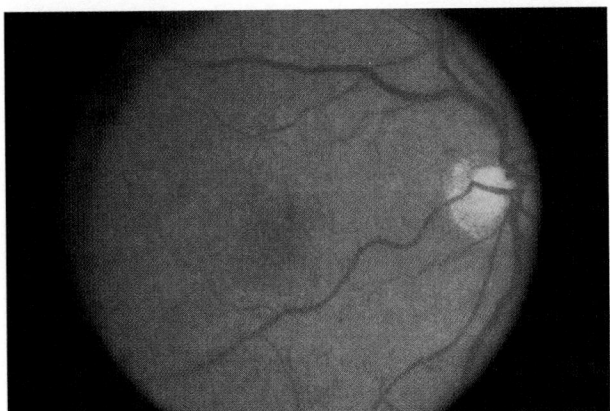

PLATE IX-2 Nonproliferative or background diabetic retinopathy. The characteristic features of nonproliferative retinopathy include microaneurysms, dot hemorrhages, slightly larger and irregular blot hemorrhages, and occasionally cotton-wool patches. Flame-shaped hemorrhages in the nerve fiber layer of the retina may also occur.

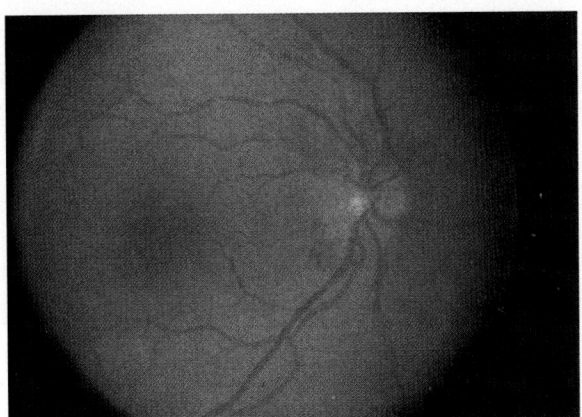

PLATE IX-4 Proliferative diabetic retinopathy. At a more advanced stage of diabetic retinopathy, new blood vessels form and grow from previously existing normal vessels. They are larger than normal caliber, and their unusual lacelike arrangement that follows no anatomic patterns and elevation above the retinal plane as they evolve distinguish them from alterations of preexisting normal retinal vessels.

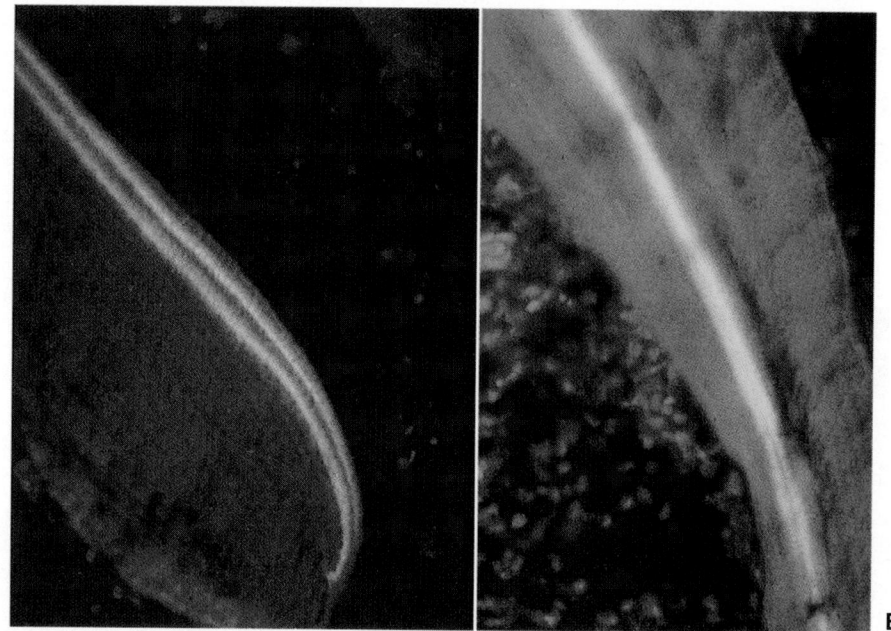

PLATE IX-5   Biopsies of iliac crest showing tetracycline labeling at the mineralization front in a normal subject **(A)** and a patient with osteomalacia **(B).** Note the two separate bands of fluorescence in the normal subject and the coalescence of the two bands in the affected patient.   *(Courtesy Dr. Robert Weinstein.)*

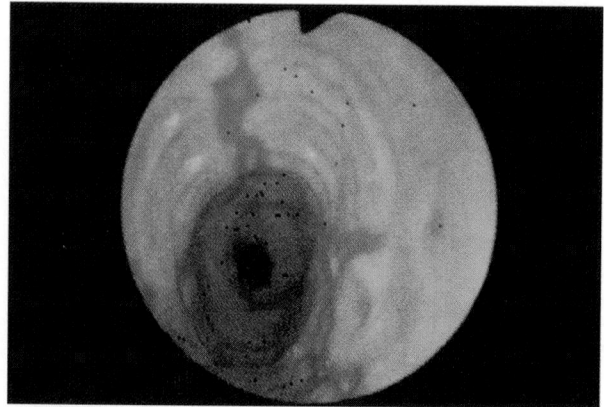

PLATE X-1   Reflux esophagitis.

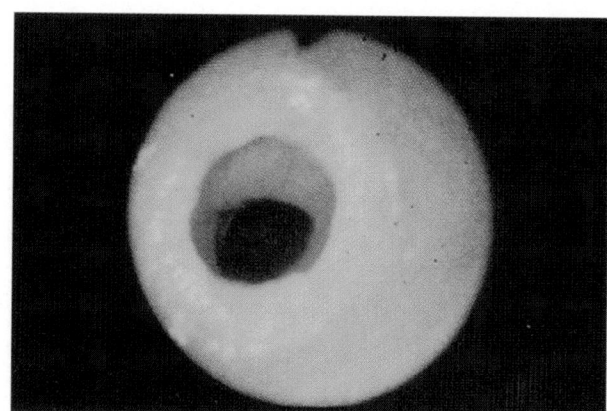

PLATE X-2   Lower esophageal ring.

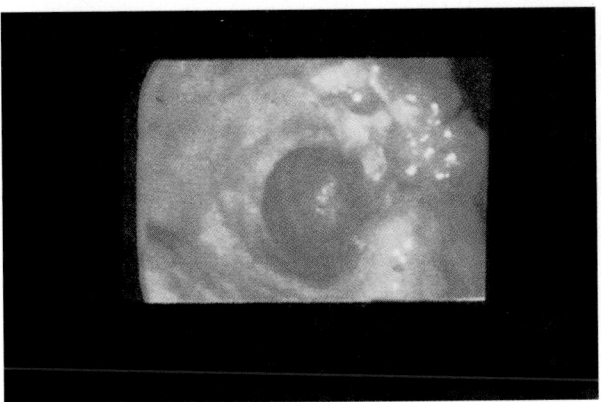

PLATE X-3 Carcinoma of the stomach.

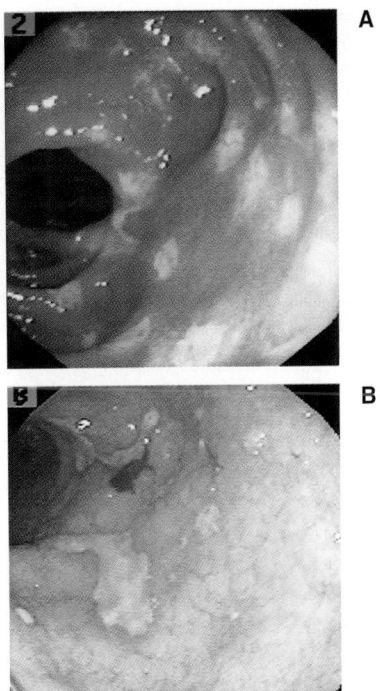

PLATE X-6 Endoscopic photographs of Crohn's disease. **A,** Aphthous ulcerations extending into the terminal ileum. **B,** Linear ulcerations with spared (normal) intervening mucosa.

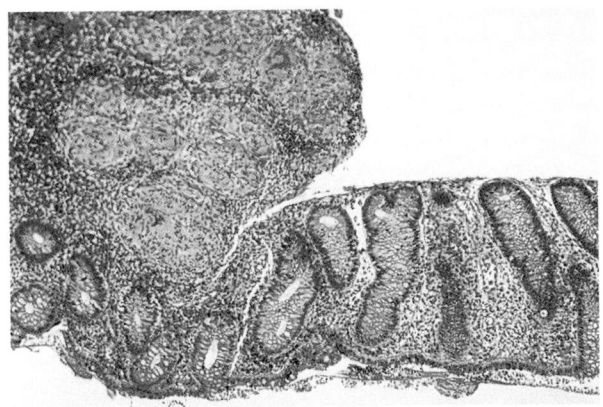

PLATE X-4 Crohn's disease. Fissuring ulceration with adjacent glandular structures and granuloma formation typical of the focal nature of Crohn's disease. The deeper, fissured ulcer may penetrate transmurally and result in fistulization.

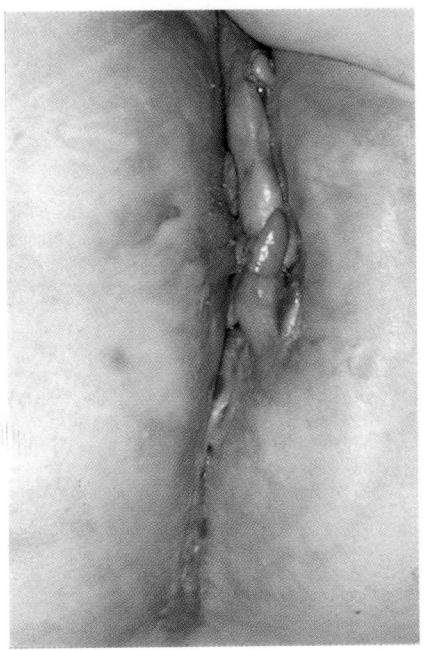

PLATE X-5 Perianal manifestations of Crohn's disease with hypertrophied skin tags, fissure, and fistula openings.

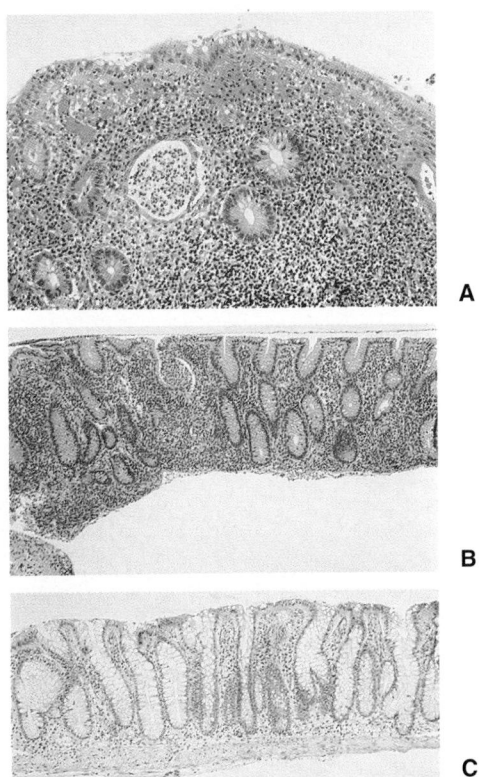

PLATE X-7 Histologic features of ulcerative colitis. **A,** Crypt abscess with neutrophil infiltrations into colonic epithelial glands. **B,** Diffuse, continuous superficial inflammation with glandular distortion and expansion of the lamina propria by neutrophils, eosinophils, and lymphocytes accompanying superficial ulceration. **C,** Chronic ulcerative colitis with absent acute (neutrophil) inflammation but distortion of the normal glandular architecture.

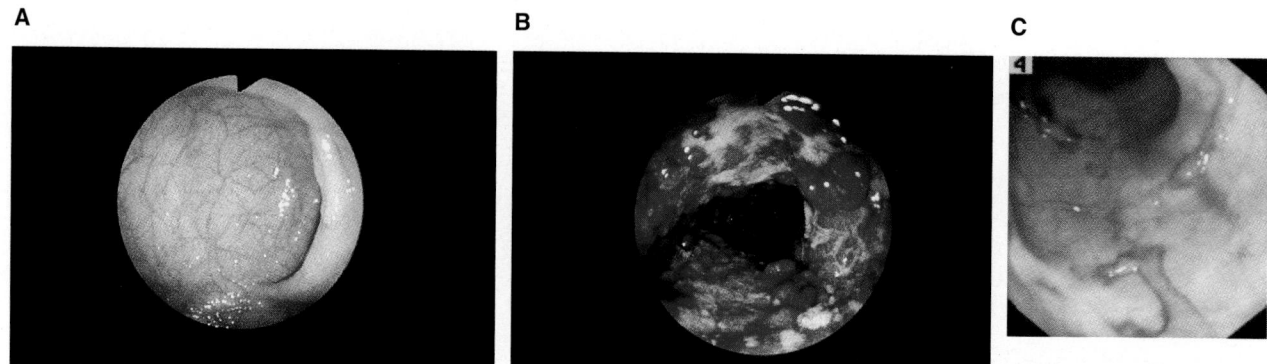

PLATE X-8   Endoscopic features of ulcerative colitis. **A,** Normal appearing colon with intact, glistening mucosa and preserved mucosal vascular pattern. **B,** Severe ulcerative colitis with contiguous ulceration, spontaneous hemorrhage, and exudation of mucopus. **C,** Chronic, quiescent ulcerative colitis with intact mucosa but distorted vascular pattern and filamentous postinflammatory pseudopolyps.

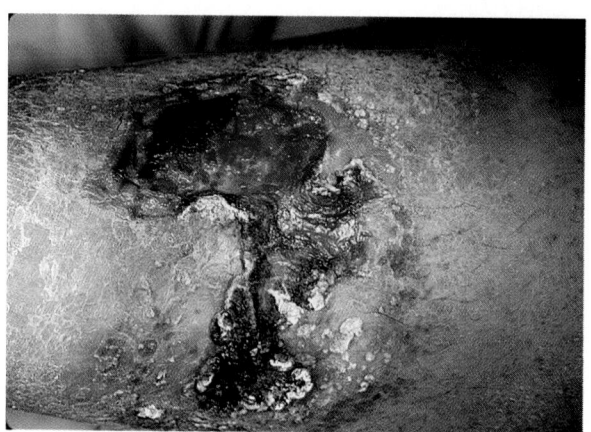

PLATE X-9   Pyoderma gangrenosum.

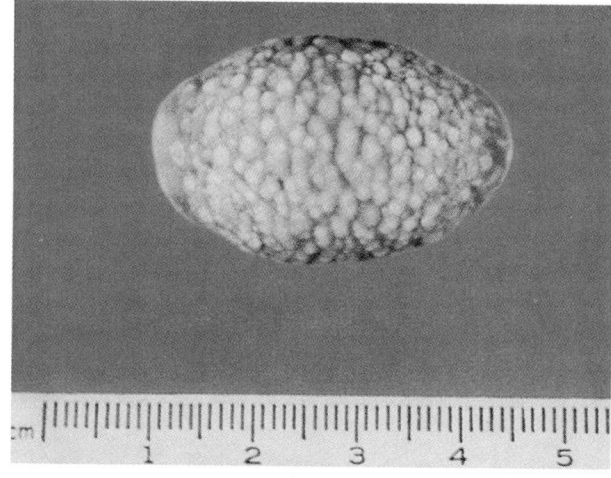

PLATE X-11   Mulberry-shaped solitary cholesterol gallstone (3.5 cm × 2.0 cm).   *(Courtesy David E. Cohen, Boston.)*

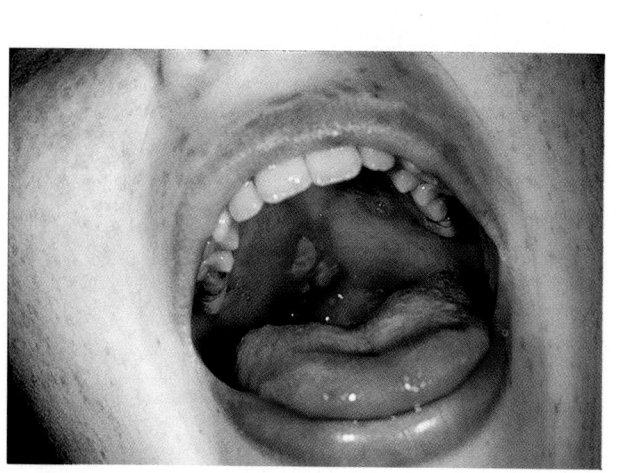

PLATE X-10   Oral aphthous ulcer in a patient with Crohn's disease.

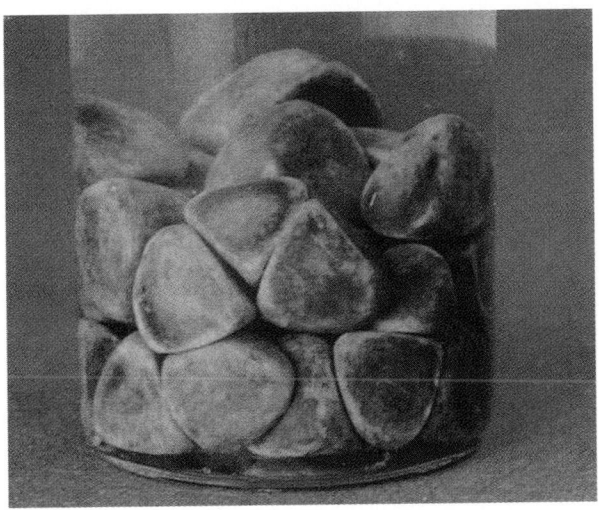

PLATE X-12 Close-packed faceted cholesterol gallstones conforming to the shape of a cylindric vessel.

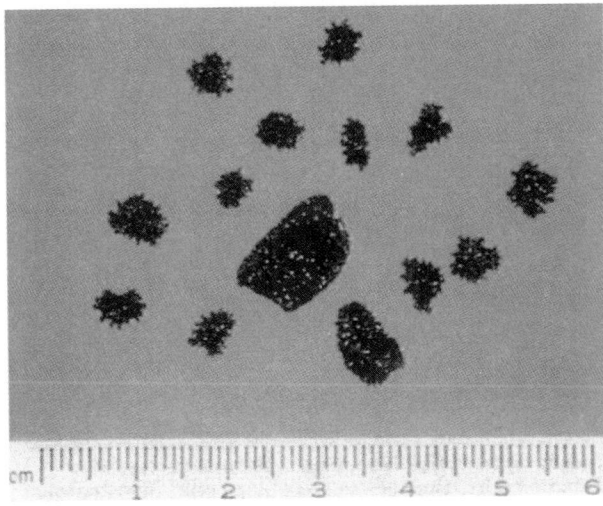

PLATE X-14 Black polymer pigment gallstones formed in a gallbladder. Most are small and spiculated; one is large and flat.

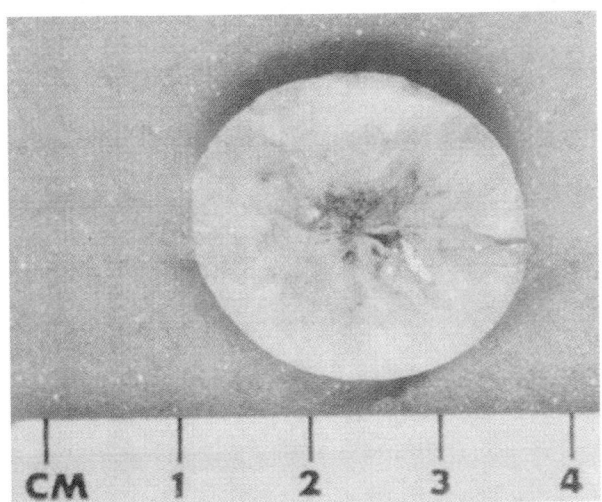

PLATE X-13 Round solitary cholesterol gallstone with cut surface displaying a pigmented nucleus composed of the acid salt of calcium bilirubinate.

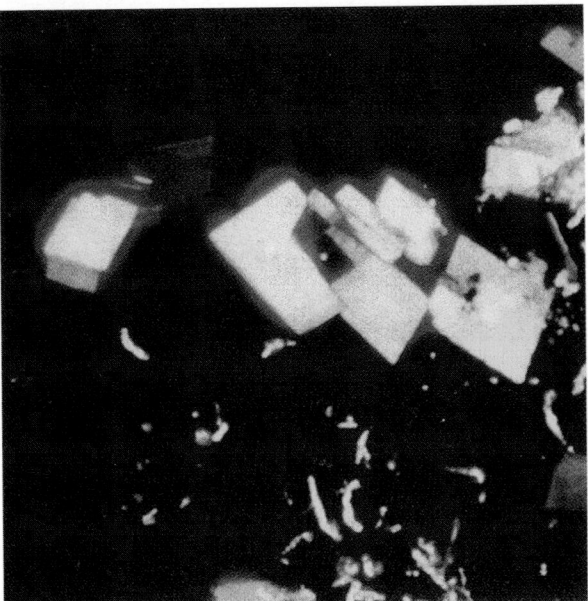

PLATE X-15 Polarized light microscopy of bile-rich duodenal fluid showing rhombohedral cholesterol monohydrate crystals and amorphous golden-yellow bilirubin precipitates ($\times$ 40).

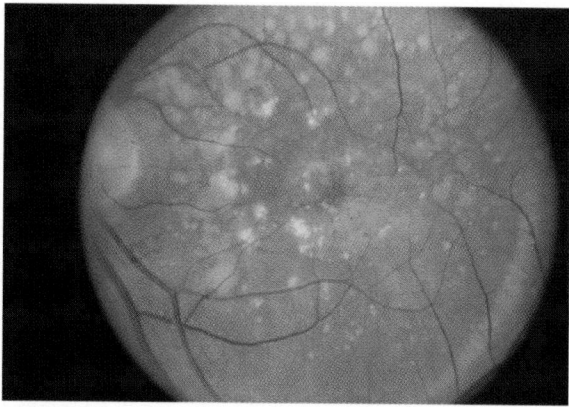

PLATE XI-1   Drusen in a patient with age-related macular degeneration.

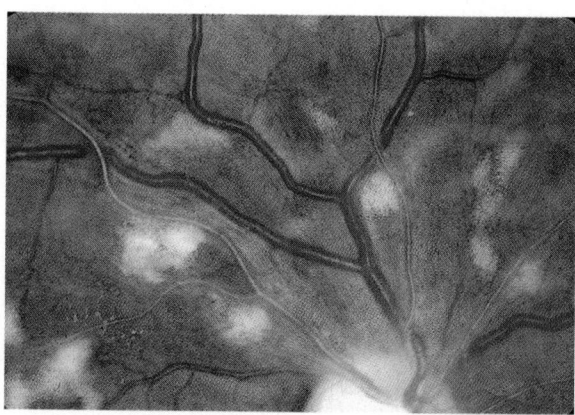

PLATE XI-4   Multiple areas of cotton-wool spots. Also visible are copper wiring and arteriovenous nicking.

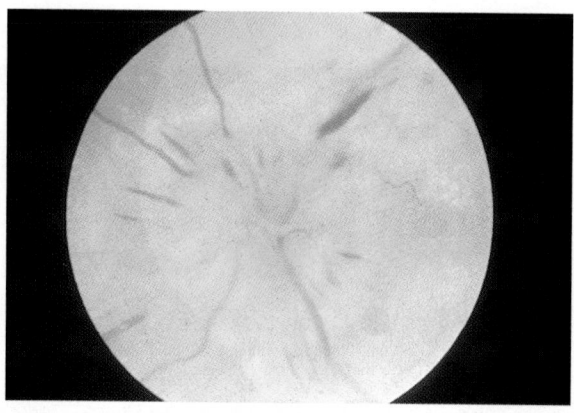

PLATE XI-2   Optic nerve disc edema with peripapillary flame-shaped hemorrhages in a patient with malignant hypertension.

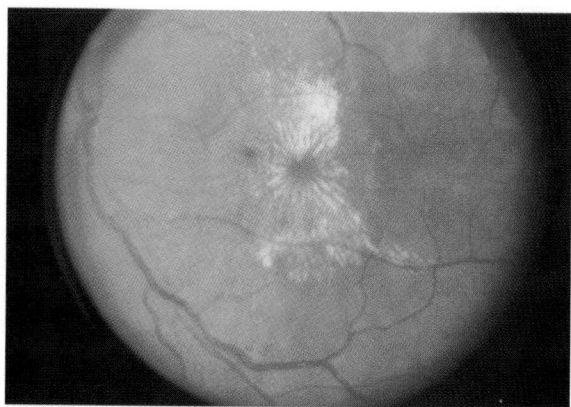

PLATE XI-5   Macular star: deposition of hard exudate in the center of the macula.

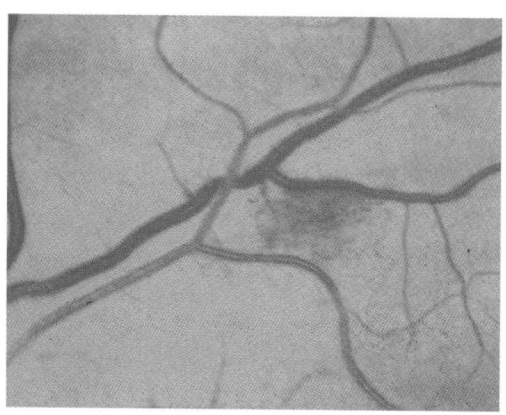

PLATE XI-3   Arteriovenous nicking in a patient with hypertension.

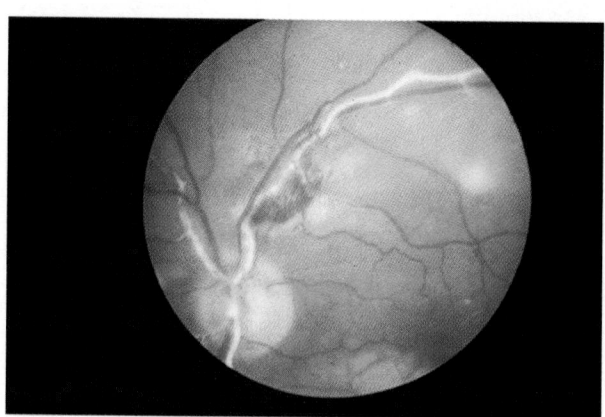

PLATE XI-6   Silver wiring.

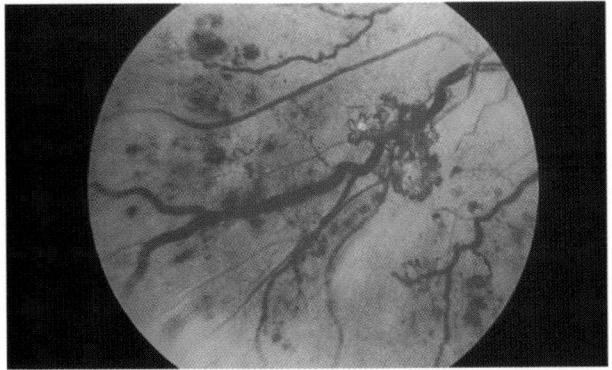

PLATE XI-7   Intraretinal microvascular abnormalities and venous beading in a patient with diabetic retinopathy.

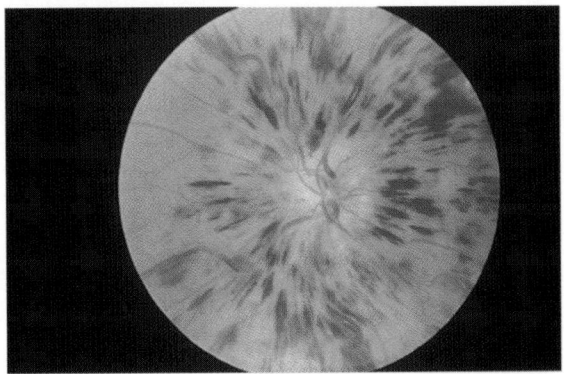

PLATE XI-10   Central retinal vein occlusion.

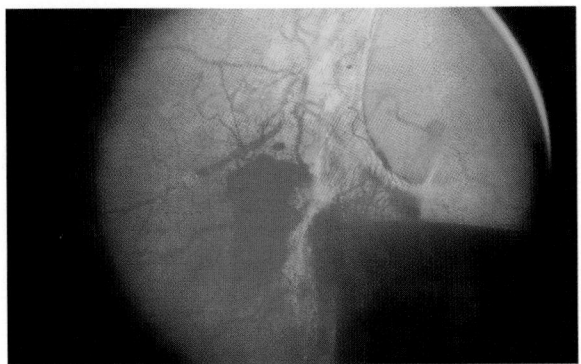

PLATE XI-8   Neovascularization of the optic nerve and vitreous hemorrhage in a patient with diabetic retinopathy.

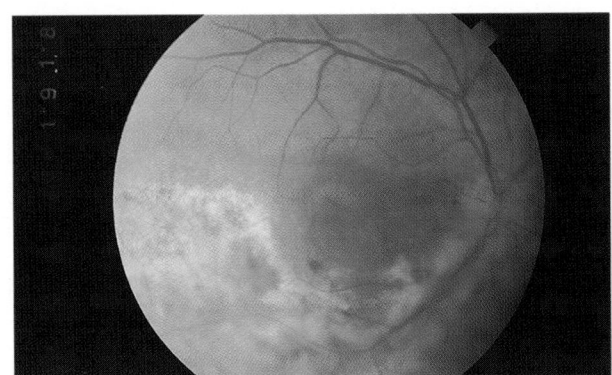

PLATE XI-11   Cytomegalovirus retinitis.

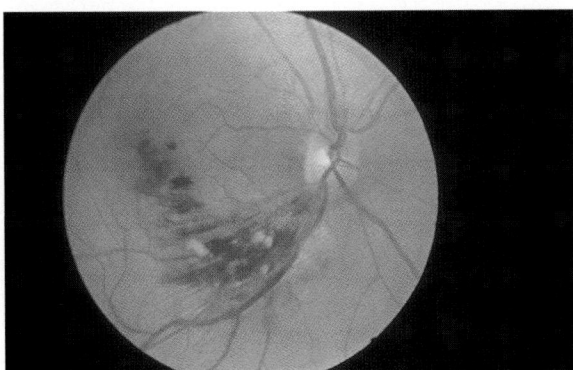

PLATE XI-9   Branch retinal vein occlusion with flame-shaped hemorrhages and cotton-wool spots along the distribution of the occluded vein.

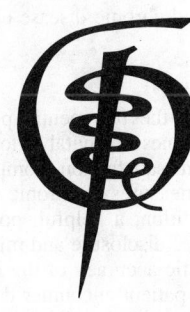

Introduction to Modern Medical Practice

1 Physician-Patient Encounter

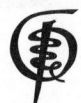

Jack Ende

Even as the focus of health care broadens and begins to address the quality of care provided to populations, the very basis of that care remains the physician-patient encounter. This encounter develops from the interview and the physical examination. Both are rooted in the traditions of internal medicine, yet both have evolved considerably since most practicing physicians received training.

The interview, or medical history, now is conceptualized as having three functions: data gathering, relationship building, and patient education and counseling. Through the interview the clinician comes to understand the patient's complaints, screens for additional problems, forges a therapeutic alliance, addresses emotional issues, and teaches the patient about his or her illness now and how illnesses might be prevented in the future. All this occurs in a brief span of time—in outpatient settings usually less than 15 minutes. The physical examination functions as a series of diagnostic tests—each maneuver with its own operating characteristics—that collectively are useful in confirming the history, identifying new problems, and completing the database.

MEDICAL INTERVIEW: A THREE-FUNCTION MODEL
Data Gathering

In inpatient and outpatient settings clinicians generally know something about the patient even before the encounter begins. Obviously this is true for patients already encountered, but it also may be true for patients who are new. Hospital or outpatient records can be reviewed; in office settings many clinicians use screening questionnaires that patients complete before the interview.

Clinical studies suggest that the data-gathering function of the interview yields 60% to 80% of the information required for diagnosis. This information comes through observation, inquiry, and analysis and through verbal and nonverbal channels. After an initial greeting, clinicians turn their attention to the patient's concerns. The traditional notion of the chief complaint often does not apply to office settings, where studies show that (1) patients typically have more than a single chief complaint and (2) the first complaint mentioned is not necessarily the most important. Accordingly, as the interview begins, physicians might do well to hold their interruptions to a minimum and encourage patients to relate all their major concerns before any particular one is explored. Studies show that facilitation (rather than interruption and questioning) during the early part of the encounter reduces patients' concerns that emerge later in the visit.

Multiple concerns identified at the beginning of the interview may require prioritization. When time is short and the patient's concerns are several and unrelated to a single diagnosis, patients can be encouraged to identify those they regard as most pressing and reassured that the rest will be addressed later or during subsequent visits. Then patients can be encouraged to tell the "story" of their illness. Open-ended questions and facilitative comments work best at this stage; more narrow questions are used later, to clarify and focus the patient's comments as the clinician mentally sorts through the possible diagnoses. Interview techniques and examples of comments useful during the critical early phase of the interview are shown in Table 1-1.

The review of systems, long the bane of first- and second-year medical students clutching lists of questions they hardly understand, is another matter entirely for experienced clinicians. In the hands of experienced clinicians the review of systems functions as a useful and time-efficient screening tool. It can be introduced with a general question, "Is there anything else you are concerned about?" Patients may find this reassuring, and it allows clinicians to then move more ex-

peditiously through a series of screening questions. How the questions are selected determines the thrust of the interview. Clinical outcomes data suggest that the greatest benefit is likely to come from asking about life-style, habits, and behavior, and from inquiry about specific symptoms that herald prevalent and important diseases. Based on disease prevalence, efficiency of inquiry, and benefit from early detection, the U.S. Preventive Services Task Force (USPSTF) has identified issues appropriate for routine screening in the context of the periodic health examination (Chapter 368). The periodic health examination represents an opportunity for delivering preventive services, but so do other forms of physician-patient encounters, including encounters for acute illness and chronic disease checkups.

Relationship Building

Recent studies have substantiated the therapeutic potential of the physician-patient encounter. Outcomes attributable to successful interactions include improved patient satisfaction, compliance, quality of life, and physiologic outcome measures of chronic illness, such as hypertension and diabetes. In addition, a helpful, positive relationship, particularly one that facilitates disclosure and minimizes defensiveness, can enhance the diagnostic accuracy of the interview.

The therapeutic aspects of the patient encounter derive from two of its most important aspects: relationship building or rapport and patient education and empowerment. The physician-patient relationship depends on a series of skills. It requires attention to the patient's comfort and ability to make patients feel at ease. This is done verbally with a sincere greeting and nonverbally as well, with attention to eye contact and seating arrangement, thoughtful gestures and, when appropriate, touching. Verbal techniques associated with patient comfort include facilitative comments that encourage patients to continue their story; echoing and summarizing, which reassure patients that they have been heard; and silence, perhaps the most potent technique, which encourages patients to express their feelings and thoughts.

Several barriers challenge the physician-patient relationship. These fall in the realm of the cognitive, cultural, physical, and emotional. Emotion handling is an essential skill for interviewing; fortunately, it can be learned. When emotion arises during the interview, it should be *recognized*, not ignored, and acknowledged. This often is as simple as naming the emotion, using empathic comments like, "you seem upset." Patients then should be encouraged to continue. Their feelings can be *legitimized* with comments such as, "I understand. Anyone would feel that way," and they should be *supported*, a promise conveyed by assurances that the physician is interested and will be available to help. Empathic interviewing strengthens the physician-patient relationship and adds to its therapeutic value. Additional suggestions for managing this aspect of the interview are found in Table 1-1.

Educating and Counseling

The educational function of the interview addresses problems of adherence (compliance) while empowering patients with knowledge of their disease and treatment. In several clinical situations patient education programs have been associated with measurable benefit in health outcomes. However, studies have called attention to how little information patients retain in the course of routine physician encounters. Patient education cannot be taken for granted. Successful approaches to patient education include the following: (1) initial elicitation of the patient's concept of either the disease or its therapy, (2) clear explanations that address misconceptions and provide measured amounts of information in terms that patients understand, (3) use of aids including instructional videos, and (4) repetition, review, and solicitation of questions. Studies suggest that efforts at patient education are beneficial, but it takes time. Many physicians use ancillary personnel to augment their efforts in patient education. Table 1-1 provides a model for patient education adapted from the recommendations of the USPSTF.

INTERVIEWING IN PROBLEMATIC AREAS

Patients with psychological, social, and behavioral problems are identified from the interview, including the screening review of systems;

Table 1-1 A three-function model for the medical interview*

FUNCTION	OBJECTIVE	EXAMPLE
Gathering data needed for diagnosis, prognosis, treatment, or counseling, or all of these functions	Identify major concerns	"Please tell me how I can help."
	Elicit other concerns	"What else?"
	Prioritize concerns	"What's most important? Where should we begin?"
	Develop the patient's narrative	"Tell me about that."
	Encourage a complete recounting	"Please go on. You're doing fine."
	Summarize and check	"I see. So if I understand correctly, first you noticed . . . and then . . ."
	Focus the history	"Be more specific. Did the pain start suddenly or gradually?"
	Make transition to the review of systems	"I have several other questions for you, but first, is there anything else?"
	Completing the database: the family history, past medical history, health maintenance history, and review of systems	(Specific questions based on patient's age and risk factors are used here; preinterview questionnaires often help)
Building a therapeutic relationship	Ensure the patient's comfort	"Are you comfortable? May we begin?"
	Project professionalism	(Attention to one's own demeanor, appearance, and surroundings)
	Address barriers to communication	
	1. Cognitive	"I want to be sure you understand. Let me say it another way."
	2. Cultural and personal	"Please tell me how you see this problem. What do we need to do?"
	3. Emotional	
	a. Showing empathy	"You seem sad."
	b. Legitimizing	"It's understandable that you feel that way. Anyone would."
	c. Showing support	"I'm here to help. Maybe we can work something out."
	Incorporating the patient's perspective	"That's what I think. How does that sound to you?"
Providing education and counseling†	Incorporate the patient's beliefs and concerns	"How do you feel about exercise?"
	Inform patients about purposes and effects of recommended behavioral change	"Exercise can lower your blood pressure, but it won't happen right away and you'll have to stick to it."
	Suggest changes that are small, not large	"Let's start slowly; I'd like for you to begin walking on a regular basis."
	Be specific	"Five minutes a day, every other day, is how you should begin for the first week."
	Adding new behaviors is easier than eliminating established ones	"We'll get to work on a diet soon. Let's get the exercise program going first."
	Link new behaviors to behaviors that are established or habitual	"Think about walking during your lunch hour for five minutes before you eat."
	Exploit the power of the profession	"I understand, but I do want you to begin exercising."
	Obtain the patient's commitment	"How will you make this happen? When will you start?"
	Employ multiple strategies; consider referral	"There are exercise classes I'd like for you to check out, and this pamphlet may be helpful."
	Monitor progress through regular follow-up	"I'm going to ask my nurse to call you next week to see how this is going, and let me see you in one month. Okay?"

*Developed by the American Academy on Physician and Patient. From Lipkin M, Putnam SM, Lazare A, editors: *The medical interview,* New York, 1995, Springer.
†Modified from U.S. Preventive Services Task Force: *Guide to clinical preventive services,* ed 2, Baltimore, 1996, Williams & Wilkins.

from other sources of information such as family and friends, past medical encounters, and past medical history (trauma, auto accidents, emergency room visits); or from the physical examination. Other channels of information, such as the patient's appearance and behavior—both verbal and nonverbal—may heighten the clinician's concern about psychologic and social issues. Of these, the most important for general internal medicine practice are alcoholism, violence, and issues related to sexuality.

Alcoholism

The medical encounter provides an opportunity to screen for and detect alcoholism, a common disease with an enormous health impact, which is responsive to treatment, particularly if diagnosed in early stages. As an entry point for screening for alcoholism, clinicians can ask, "How often do you drink?" and whether the patient and mem-

bers of his or her family have had alcohol problems in the past. "How often?" is a more helpful initial question than "Do you drink?", since the latter may be perceived as confrontational or judgmental. Asking about past or family problems with alcohol is consistent with alcoholism's chronic and inherited patterns. Responses to these questions that either are positive or are negative but obfuscated or embellished by comments signaling denial should be followed by more reliable screening questions such as the four CAGE questions (Box 1-1). Patients who answer positively to three or four questions have a high likelihood of alcoholism. Positive responses to any of the questions should be pursued with more extensive inquiry into the parameters of alcoholism including quantity, problems with control, tolerance, dependence, and impact, both physical and social. At times, family and friends must be interviewed. The questions contained in the Alcohol Use Disorders Identification Tool (AUDIT) (Box 1-1) are useful in following up on positive responses to the CAGE questions, or when

---

BOX 1-1

Screening questions for problematic use of alcohol

CAGE questions

Have you ever felt you ought to *C*ut down on drinking?
Have people *A*nnoyed you by criticizing your drinking?
Have you ever felt bad or *G*uilty about your drinking?
Have you ever had a drink first thing in the morning to steady your nerves or get rid of a hangover? (*E*ye opener)

AUDIT questions*

How often do you have a drink containing alcohol?
How many drinks do you have on a typical day when you are drinking?
How often do you have six or more drinks on one occasion?
How often during the last year have you found that you were unable to stop drinking once you had started?
How often in the last year have you failed to do what was normally expected from you because of drinking?
How often during the last year have you needed a first drink in the morning to get yourself going after a heavy drinking session?
How often during the last year have you had a feeling of guilt or remorse after drinking?
How often during the last year have you been unable to remember what happened the night before because you had been drinking?
Have you or someone else been injured as a result of your drinking?
Has a relative, doctor, or other health care worker been concerned about your drinking or suggested you cut down?

For scoring system see Saunders JB, Aasland OG, Babor TF et al: *Addiction* 88:791-804, 1993.

BOX 1-2

SAFE questions for domestic violence

Stress and Safety

What stress do you experience in your relationship?
Do you feel safe in your relationship?
Should I be concerned for your safety?

Afraid and Abused

Has your partner ever threatened or abused you or your children?
Have you been physically hurt by your partner?
People in relationships often fight; what happens when you and your partner disagree?

Friend and Family

Are your friends aware that you have been hurt?
Do your parents or siblings know about this?
Do you think you could tell them, and do you think they would be able to help you?

Emergency Plan

Do you have a safe place to go and the resources you need in an emergency?

BOX 1-3

Screening for sexual problems

For all patients (modified by patients' situations)

Are you sexually active?
Have you noticed any changes or problems in your sexual functioning lately?
(For men) Do you have any problems developing or maintaining an erection?
(For women) Do you have pain during intercourse?
Have you had any difficulty with lubrication (for women) or with orgasm (for men and women)?
Has your health affected your sexual functioning?
What is your sexual orientation? Do you have sex with men, women, or both?
Do you have any questions or concerns about sex?

For patients who may be at risk for sexually transmitted illness

What is your pattern of sexual activity (number of partners, frequency, casual partners, etc.)
Do you have sex with people who might be in high-risk groups (including partners of indeterminate risk)
Do you use condoms?
Do you have any concerns about getting a sexual disease or human immunodeficiency virus (HIV)?

Adapted from Ende J, Rockwell S, Glasgow M: *Arch Intern Med* 144:558-561, 1984; Lipkin M, Putnam SM, Lazare A, editors: *The medical interview*, New York, 1995, Springer.

---

suspicion of alcoholism or problematic drinking arises for other reasons. The AUDIT can be scored, or clinicians may use the items less formally, to gain an impression of the patient's relationship to alcohol and the likelihood that alcohol use has reached the stage at which it should be considered problematic.

Violence

Violence causes an enormous burden of suffering. Homicide and suicide are its most serious manifestations. Furthermore, its physical and psychologic morbidity extends beyond its immediate victims and makes violence one of the nation's leading health problems. Persons at greatest risk are young males of minority background, persons with a history of delinquent or criminal behavior, past victims, and persons living in impoverished urban environments. "Secondary" victims include persons, particularly elderly individuals, whose lives are affected by the threat of violent crime and assault. Possession of firearms, particularly handguns, places patients and family members at risk for violent acts and mishaps. Clinicians may be able to reduce this risk by including questions about guns at home in the routine database and then urging safety measures or removal.

Domestic violence, referring to harm induced by intimate partners, also exacts a large toll of suffering nationwide. Its victims are mostly women, particularly women who are pregnant, who have been victims before, or whose partners are affected by drug or alcohol abuse problems. Recent data have associated irritable bowel syndrome and somatoform disorders with past history of sexual abuse and violence. Twenty percent of women have experienced violence at some point in their lives; 2% to 3% report being kicked, bitten, or hit in the past year. Bruises, lacerations, and musculoskeletal injuries, particularly about the face, are the most common forms of injury. Suspicion of domestic violence and forced sexual activity or rape should prompt specific inquiry. The SAFE questions (Box 1-2) remind clinicians about the important issues to cover when caring for women at risk for violence and abuse.

Elderly persons are particularly prone to abuse, which can extend from psychologic neglect to physical violence. Risk factors associated with vulnerability among elderly persons include poor health, cognitive impairment, and lack of family, financial, or community support. Abusers most often are spouses or close relatives who themselves are affected by substance abuse or mental illness. Clinicians should not hesitate to ask elderly patients about exposure to violence or abuse. To date, no specific instrument or battery of questions has been tested or shown to be more helpful than routine inquiry in detecting elder abuse.

Sexual Functioning

Sexual functioning is part of general health. Inquiry into sexual health should be included in the review of systems. Studies show that inquiry about sexual functioning yields significant information about problems that are important to the patient, yet often omitted. Box 1-3 provides general questions that can be used in office settings. For pa-

BOX 1-4
Organization and sequence
of the physical examination

1. Before the examination begins
General appearance and hygiene
Overall state of health
Mobility, gait, and posture

2. With the (gowned) patient sitting upright, examiner in front
Hands: Nails, joints, peripheral circulation
Wrists: Radial pulses, joints
Elbows: Range of motion, nodes
Axillae: Nodes
Supraclavicular: Boney structure, nodes
Neck: Soft tissue, nodes
Head: Symmetry, cranial nerves V and VII
Eyes: Inspection; pupillary responses; conjunctivae; cranial nerves
   III, IV, and VI; funduscopic examination
Ears: Hearing, canals, tympanic membranes
Nose: Turbinates
Mouth and pharynx: Inspection of teeth, gums and buccal mucosa,
   oropharynx

3. Examiner moves behind seated patient
Thyroid: Palpation during swallowing
Lungs: Inspection, percussion, auscultation
Spine: Inspection, palpation for tenderness
Costovertebral space: Palpate for tenderness

4. Examiner moves to front
Breast examination (in women): inspection with arms down, then
   raised

5. Patient reclines
Breast examination: Palpation
Jugular veins: Inspection for level (changing angle of examining
   table may be needed)
Cardiac: Percussion, palpation, auscultation
Abdomen: Inspection, palpation, percussion, and auscultation of all
   quadrants
Genitourinary (in men): Inspection, palpation of testicles, genitalia,
   and inguinal regions
Lower extremities (from feet) advancing upward: Inspection for vas-
   cular sufficiency; palpation of pulses and for edema; joints (espe-
   cially knees and hips); deep tendon reflexes; plantar responses;
   motor, sensory, and cerebellar testing
Upper extremities: Motor, sensory, and cerebellar testing

6. Additional examination (as indicated)
General examination for skin lesions
Focal musculoskeletal examination
Gait and station
Mental status examination

7. Rectal, pelvic examination (properly positioned)
Rectal (for men): Palpation of prostate, rectum
Pelvic examination (for women)

Physical examination continues to play an essential role in confirming the history, completing the database, and uncovering important new findings, while symbolizing the healing powers of the physician with the laying on of hands. The well-performed physical examination remains the trademark of the respected internist. Its importance should not be minimized.

Novice clinicians may have difficulty arranging the components of the examination. The complete screening examination should be just that, complete, but it should not be tiring, either for the examiner or the patient. It should require the patient to change positions no more than twice; it should flow easily and be completed in no more than 20 minutes.

For office patients a prologue to the physical examination is afforded by observations of the patient as he or she enters the examination room. General appearance, demeanor, dress, and hygiene all come into view and provide useful information. In the office the examination itself begins with the gowned patient in a sitting position, providing an opportunity to take vital signs (if not already done) and to examine the head, eyes, ears, nose, and throat; the neck; the chest and back; and breasts. It continues with a patient lying back. The breast examination for women is completed with the patient supine. This is followed for women and men by the cardiovascular, abdominal, musculoskeletal, and neurologic examinations and, in men, genitourinary examination, As needed, additional dermatologic, musculoskeletal, and neurologic examinations can be carried out, including formal testing of gait, station, and mental status. Rectal examination in men and pelvic and rectal examinations in women usually are performed last. Patients can then dress in privacy, and the encounter is brought to a close with a final summary and opportunity for questions. Box 1-4 provides an organizational framework for the full physical examination.

BIBLIOGRAPHY

Albert EJ: Violence in intimate relationships and the practicing internist: new "disease" or new agenda? *Ann Intern Med* 123:224-281, 1995.
Asher ML: Asking about domestic violence: SAFE questions, *JAMA* 269(18):2367, 1993.
Buchsbaum DG et al: Screening for alcohol abuse using CAGE scores and likelihood ratios, *Ann Intern Med* 115:774-777, 1991.
Kaplan SH, Greenfield S, Ware JJ: Assessing the effects of physician-patient interactions on the outcomes of chronic disease, *Medical Care* 27(3 suppl):S110-127, 1989.
Lipkin M, Putnam SM, Lazare A, editors: *The medical interview,* New York, 1985, Springer.
Novack DH: Therapeutic aspects of the clinical encounter, *J Gen Intern Med* 2:346-355, 1987.
Sackett DL: The science of the art of the clinical examination, *JAMA* 267:2650-2652, 1992. (Series follows this introductory editorial.)
Schneiderman H: *Bedside diagnosis: an annotated bibliography of literature on physical examination and interviewing,* ed 2, Philadelphia, 1992, American College of Physicians.
U.S. Preventive Services Task Force: *Guide to clinical preventive services,* ed 2, Baltimore, 1996, Williams & Wilkins.

tients at risk for sexually transmitted illnesses or who have specific concerns about their sexual functioning or sexual orientation, additional questions should be added. Patients with chronic illness should be asked about sexual problems that may have arisen as a result of their underlying problems.

PHYSICAL EXAMINATION

Recent studies have called into question the value of the routine screening examination and the reliability of some physical examination maneuvers. At the same time, a renewed interest and a more scientific approach to the physical examination have substantiated the importance of physical examination findings in several clinical situations and even their superiority to more costly diagnostic procedures.

2 Principles of Diagnostic Testing

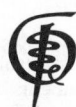

John M. Eisenberg

An essential skill of the excellent clinician is the ability to interpret diagnostic tests. These tests are sometimes used to screen large populations to determine the risk of disease and at other times to decide whether the probability of a patient having a disease is high enough to justify initiating specific therapy. In either case the clinician must be able to understand what test results mean. Diseases are rarely really "ruled in" or "ruled out." Instead, clinicians have to make patient care decisions based on the likelihood of one disease versus another and the likelihood of disease versus health.

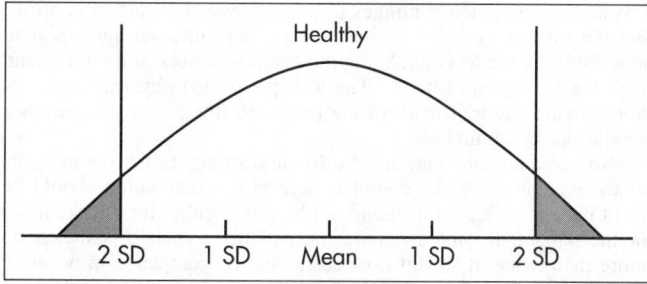

FIGURE 2-1   By convention, upper and lower limits of normal are set 2 standard deviations (2 SD) above and below the mean result in a healthy population. By this definition, 2.25% of healthy patients would be labeled as having too high a result and 2.25% of healthy patients would be labeled as having too low a result. *2 SD,* Abnormal.

WHAT IS ABNORMAL?

The first step in interpreting diagnostic tests is to decide on the definition of an abnormal test result. For some tests too high a result is abnormal (e.g., alkaline phosphatase level). For other tests too low a result is abnormal (e.g., albumin level). For still others an abnormal result may be too high or too low (e.g., serum sodium, hemoglobin, or thyroxine level).

Figure 2-1 demonstrates the distribution of test results for a population of healthy individuals (e.g., serum calcium level). Test results for a healthy group of people are likely to characterize a "normal" or gaussian distribution, with most results bunched around an average (or "mean") and with decreasing numbers of people having results farther away from the mean result. Of a representative population of typical, healthy people, about two thirds will have results lying within 1 standard deviation of the mean, and 95.5% of results are within 2 standard deviations. Thus 2.25% of healthy individuals have a test result more than 2 standard deviations above the mean. Similarly, 2.25% of results are more than 2 standard deviations below the mean. When an upper limit of normal is chosen for most laboratory tests, it is generally set at this level—2 standard deviations above the mean—recognizing that a small proportion of healthy people (2.25%) will be labeled incorrectly as having an abnormally high result and thus as being diseased. Similarly, the lower limit of normal is generally set (by convention) at a level 2 standard deviations below the mean; therefore 2.25% of healthy people will be incorrectly labeled as having an abnormally low result and thus as being diseased.

Although the upper and lower limits of normal may not always be set so that 2.25% of healthy people have too high or too low a result, there will be healthy individuals who are incorrectly labeled as diseased, or *false-positive results,* no matter where the upper limit is set. The only exception—at least theoretically—is when the cutoff point can be set high (or low) enough that the results of no one who is actually healthy fall outside the limits of normal. Healthy individuals whose test results are below the upper limit of normal (or above the lower limit of normal), and whose tests thus accurately reflect the absence of disease, have *true-negative results.*

DISEASED PATIENTS

Patients who have the disease in which the diagnostic test result is abnormal have a different distribution of test results than patients who are healthy. For example, men with prostate cancer have a different distribution of results on prostate-specific antigen (PSA) testing than do healthy men. If the test is one for which presence of disease results in abnormally high test values, the curve describing the results for the diseased patients will be shifted to the right (Fig. 2-2). Thus a larger proportion of these diseased patients have a test result above the upper limit of normal than do healthy patients. Generally, not all of the diseased patients have a result above the upper limit of normal. The diseased patients whose elevated test results accurately reflect the presence of disease have *true-positive results.* Those whose test results are below the upper limit of normal, despite the presence of disease, have *false-negative results.*

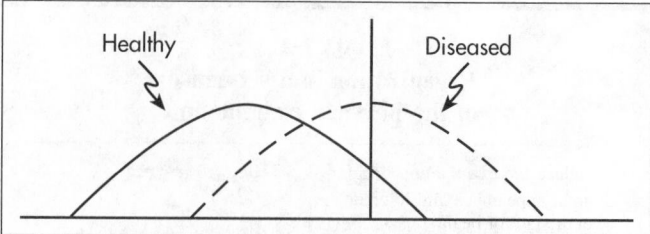

FIGURE 2-2   Setting an upper limit of normal. The test results for a group of patients with disease are different from the results for a healthy population. For a test result that is elevated in disease, the test results will be shifted to the right.

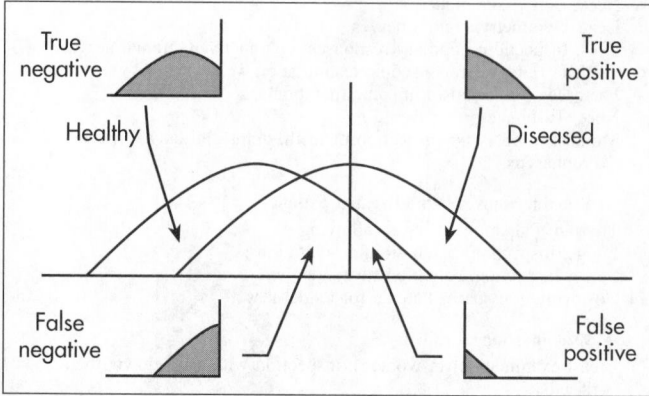

FIGURE 2-3   Four types of test results. The separation of healthy and diseased populations' test results into true-positive, true-negative, false-positive, and false-negative results.

Table 2-1   Characteristics of diagnostic test results

TEST RESULTS	DISEASE PRESENT	NO DISEASE	TOTAL
Abnormal	True positive (TP)	False positive (FP)	All abnormal results (TP + FP)
Normal	False negative (FN)	True negative (TN)	All normal results (TN + FN)
Totals	All with disease (TP + FN)	All without disease (TN + FP)	All patients

Figure 2-3 depicts how the overlapping test results of healthy and diseased populations are divided by the upper limit of normal into the four possible types of test results. Table 2-1 represents the four types of results on a 2 × 2 table, with two columns representing the presence or absence of disease and two rows representing abnormal or normal test results.

SENSITIVITY AND SPECIFICITY

Sensitivity and specificity are two fundamental characteristics of diagnostic tests. *Sensitivity* describes the ability of a test to detect persons with disease out of a population with the disease being considered, that is, to correctly identify diseased persons. This can be remembered as "positive in disease" (PID). Persons with disease have either an abnormal test result (true-positive result) or a misleading normal result (false-negative result). A test's sensitivity is the proportion of patients with true-positive results divided by the number of patients with disease (which includes both true-positive and false-negative results).

Specificity describes the ability of a test to detect normal persons out of a population without disease, that is, to correctly identify

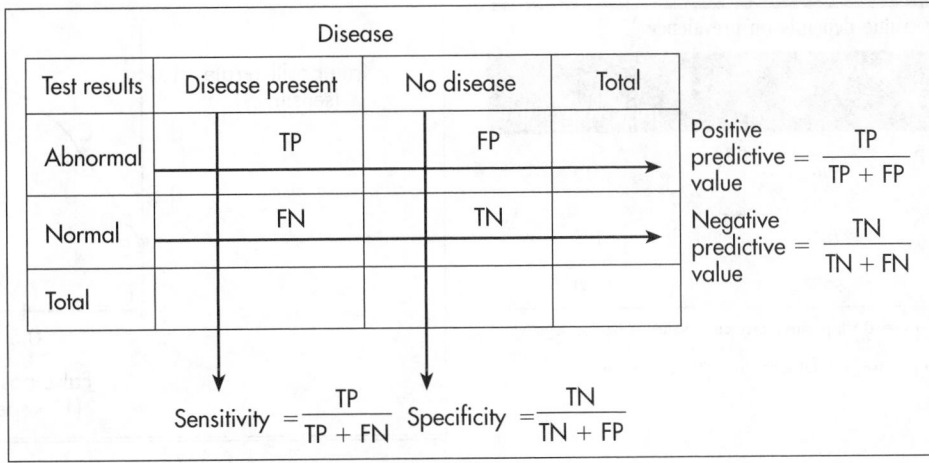

FIGURE 2-4   Characteristics of diagnostic tests. *TP,* True positive; *FP,* false positive; *TN,* true negative; *FN,* false negative.

Table 2-2   Predictive value depends on prevalence

	DISEASE		
	+	−	TOTAL (INDIVIDUALS)
+	TP 160	FP 160	320
−	FN 40	TN 640	680
Total	200*	800*	1000

Sensitivity = 0.80; specificity = 0.80; positive predictive value = 0.50; negative predictive value = 0.94.
TP, True positive; *FP,* false positive; *FN,* false negative; *TN,* true negative.
*20% Prevalence.

healthy individuals. This can be remembered as "normal in health" (NIH). Persons who are free of disease have either a normal test result (true-negative result) or a misleading abnormal result (false-positive result). A test's specificity is the proportion of true-negative results divided by the number of patients free of disease, which is the total of true-negative and false-positive results.

A 2 × 2 table (e.g., Table 2-1 and Fig. 2-4) facilitates the calculation of sensitivity and specificity when the distribution of test results into true-positive, false-positive, true-negative, and false-negative results is known. The 2 × 2 table also facilitates determining how many patients will be in these categories, when sensitivity, specificity, and the prevalence of disease in the population are known. Figure 2-4 shows how sensitivity is the test characteristic defined by the first column of the 2 × 2 table, that is, the proportion of patients who have disease and whose results are labeled true positive by their test results. Specificity is the test characteristic defined by the second column, that is, the proportion of patients who are free of disease and whose results are labeled true negative. For example, Table 2-2 shows a working 2 × 2 table. If a population of 1000 patients includes 20% with disease and a test is used with 80% sensitivity and 80% specificity, 160 patients will have true-positive results; 40, false-negative; 640, true-negative; and 160, false-positive.

PREDICTIVE VALUE

Sensitivity and specificity are useful statistics in understanding how effective a test will be in discriminating healthy and diseased individuals out of a large population of individuals undergoing testing. However, these statistics are less useful in interpreting test results for individual patients. With an individual patient the physician generally has an abnormal or a normal test result, and the challenge is to

interpret the test results for the patient who asks, "How likely is it that I have disease?" or "How likely is it that I am free of disease?" For these more clinical questions, predictive value is of more value.

Positive predictive value describes the probability that a patient who has an abnormal test result actually has disease. Thus positive predictive value is the proportion of true-positive results to all abnormal results (true-positive plus false-positive results) (Fig. 2-4). Conversely, negative predictive value represents the probability that a patient who has a normal test result is actually free of disease; this is represented by the proportion of true-negative results to all normal results (true-negative plus false-negative results). Therefore positive predictive value reveals the proportion of patients with an abnormal test result (false-positive and true-positive results) who have both the abnormal test result and the disease in question. As Fig. 2-4 shows, this proportion is represented by the fraction TP/(TP + FN). This probability tells a patient with an abnormal test result how likely it is that he or she has the disease. Similarly, negative predictive value shows the proportion of patients with a normal result (true-negative and false-positive results) who are actually free of the disease in question. As Fig. 2-4 shows, this proportion is represented by the fraction TN/(TN + FP). This probability tells a patient with a normal result how confident he or she can be that disease is absent. Thus whereas the first column of the 2 × 2 table provides information about sensitivity and the second column provides information about specificity, the first row describes positive predictive value and the second row describes negative predictive value. For example, in Table 2-2, among the 320 individuals with an abnormal test result, half (160) have disease and thus have true-positive results. Thus the positive predictive value is 0.50. Among the 680 patients with negative results, 640 are free of disease, so the negative predictive value is 0.94.

The positive and negative predictive values of a test depend on the prevalence of disease in the population being tested because they are calculated by using results in patients both with *and* without disease. In contrast, sensitivity and specificity describe the results of a test within groups of patients with *or* without disease and are thus independent of the prevalence of disease (assuming a constant spectrum of disease). If a disease is rare, the number of patients with true-positive results will probably be small compared with those who have false-positive results, even if the test has high levels of sensitivity and specificity. This is because of the large number of patients who are free of disease, some of whom have false-positive results.

The dependence of predictive value on prevalence is demonstrated by the following exercise.

If the 20% prevalence of disease shown in Table 2-2 is lower, for example, 2% (as in Table 2-3), there will be 20 individuals with disease, of whom 16 will have abnormal test results (TP) and 4 will have negative results (FN). Of the 980 patients who are free of disease among 1000 men with a 2% prevalence of disease, 80% (784) will have a normal result and 20% (196) will have an abnormal result. Thus positive predictive value will be (16) ÷ (16 + 196) =

Table 2-3 Predictive value depends on prevalence

	DISEASE			
	+		−	TOTAL (INDIVIDUALS)
+	16 TP		196 FP	212
−	4 FN		784 TN	788
Total	20*		980*	1000

Sensitivity = 0.80; specificity = 0.80; positive predictive value = 0.075; negative predictive value = 0.995.
TP, True positive; *FP*, false positive; *FN*, false negative; *TN*, true negative.
*2% Prevalence.

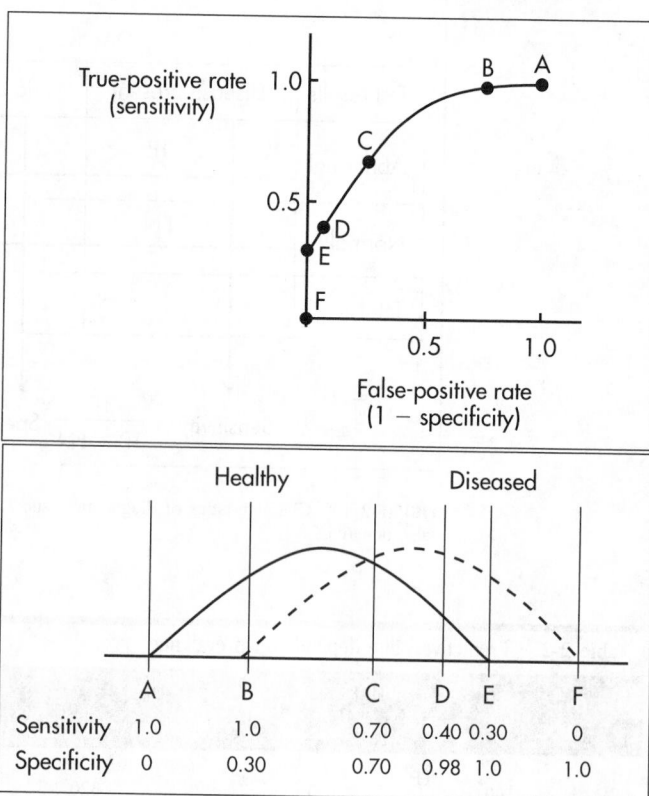

7.5%, and negative predictive value be (784) ÷ (784 + 4) = 99.5%. In this example, when a patient with lower prevalence of disease is tested, positive predictive value is lower but negative predictive value is higher.

Therefore the general principle is that positive predictive value is higher for populations with higher prevalence of disease, and negative predictive value is higher for populations with less frequent disease. Thus in screening populations for disease ("ruling out"), a low-prevalence population can be used to obtain high negative predictive values. Patients with negative results can be reassured with reasonable confidence that they are free of disease. The disease is not really "ruled out," but it is shown to be quite unlikely by the negative test result.

In choosing treatment options (especially, risky interventions), a high positive predictive value is preferred; therefore a high-prevalence population favors identification of patients who ought to get the diagnostic test if the treatment is effective and the test's operating characteristics are acceptable. Patients with an abnormal test result are likely to have disease, but often a more definitive test is needed until doctors and patients are comfortable that the likelihood of disease is high enough to justify initiating definitive treatment.

Patients who have symptoms of a disease are more likely to have that disease than the general population, and the prevalence of disease in this population is accordingly higher. Thus the positive predictive value of an abnormal result in a patient with symptoms is likely to be higher than among asymptomatic patients.

Sensitivity and specificity are often thought to be fixed characteristics of a test and, in contrast to predictive value, not a function of the population being tested. This is an oversimplification because the spectrum of disease in people with disease influences sensitivity and specificity. For example, patients with advanced lung cancer are likely to have larger lesions, and the sensitivity of chest radiography is likely to be higher than for patients with early-stage disease and smaller lesions. This effect is often described as "spectrum bias."

CHOOSING A CUT-OFF POINT

The traditional method of determining the upper limit of normal for a test result has been to use the point 2 standard deviations above the mean (or for choosing the lower limit of normal for a test result that may be too low in disease, the point defined by 2 standard deviations below the mean). However, this statistical determination may have little to do with the actual distribution of results in normal and abnormal patients. Often physicians (and laboratories) choose upper (and lower) limits of normal that are based more on traditional statistics than on clinical characteristics and clinical judgment.

When physicians decide on the test results that will define an abnormal result, one principle is paramount: the upper (or lower) limit of normal can be modified, but increased sensitivity will be offset by decreases in specificity, and vice versa. The only way in which both sensitivity and specificity can be improved simultaneously is to improve the test's performance or find a better test.

This principle is demonstrated best by a graph known as a receiver operating characteristic curve (ROC curve). The term *receiver* emphasizes the role that physicians play in interpreting diagnostic tests—

FIGURE 2-5 **A,** Receiver operating characteristic curve (ROC). Sensitivity and specificity vary as the upper limit of normal is changed. **B,** Different cut-off points. ROC curve demonstrates the relationship between the false-positive rate (specificity) and true-positive rate (sensitivity) as the upper limit of normal is varied.

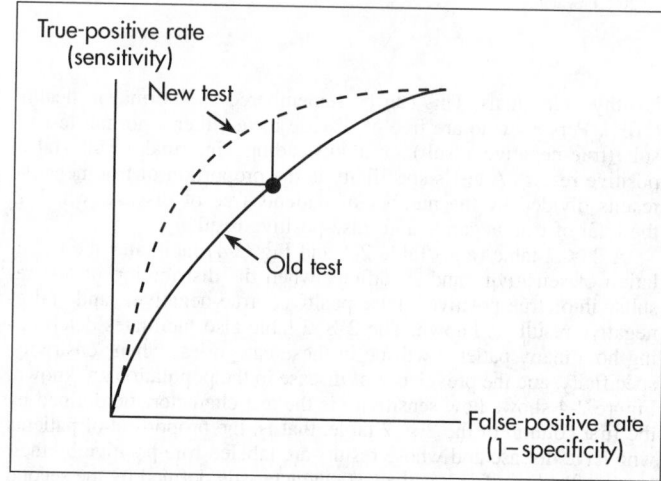

FIGURE 2-6 Comparing receiver operating curves of two tests. A superior test is "northwest" of an inferior one. Holding specificity constant, sensitivity is improved, and holding sensitivity constant, specificity is improved.

receiving information about their patients and interpreting these signals about whether the patient is well or sick. The term *receiver* also reflects the origin of the name *ROC curve*. This type of analysis is said to have been born of operations researchers' efforts during World War II to decide how sensitive radar equipment should be set. Too sensitive, and defending planes and forces would be mobilized unnecessarily (e.g., if a flock of birds flew over the English Channel and were mistaken for the German Luftwaffe)—a false-positive interpretation. Not sensitive enough, however, and enemy planes would

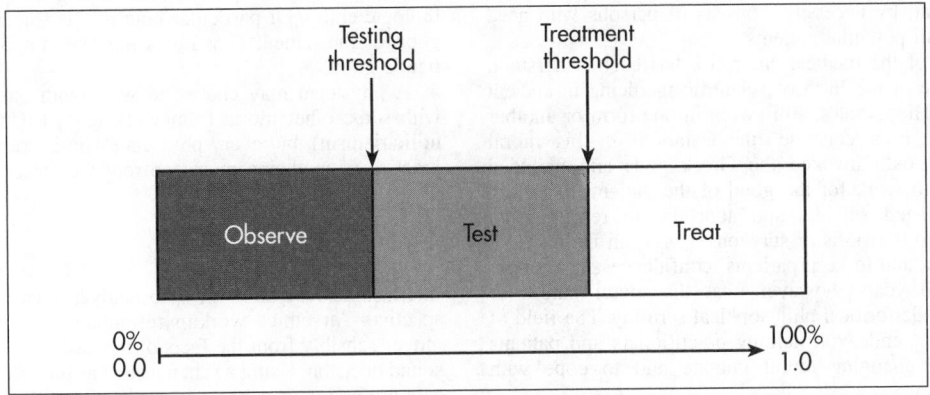

FIGURE 2-7   The threshold model for decision making.

not be detected by radar—a false-negative interpretation. In selecting and interpreting tests, physicians should define the limits of normal results in a way that balances the benefits of true-positive results with the disadvantages of false-positive test results.

Figure 2-5 demonstrates how an ROC curve can guide the selection of the upper (or lower) limit of normal for a diagnostic test. In Fig. 2-5, *A,* point A could be chosen as the upper limit of normal for a test result, and all test results would be above this point and would be interpreted as abnormal. Thus sensitivity would be 1.00 with 100% true-positive results among those with disease. However, specificity would be 0.00, with 100% false-positive results among those free of disease. Conversely, point F would characterize an upper limit of normal with no false-positive results but also no true-positive results. Sensitivity would be 0.0 and specificity 100.0. Point B would describe the upper limit of normal whereby sensitivity would be 1.00 but specificity about 0.30 with 70% false-positive results among healthy individuals. On the other hand, an upper limit of normal at point E would include only about 30% of those with disease as having true-positive results but would produce no false-positive results. Point D is the upper limit of normal that would be selected by the conventional method of choosing a point 2 standard deviations above the upper limit of normal, thus by definition including 2.25% of healthy people as having false-positive results. In this example, point D would result in sensitivity of about 0.40. Point C, an alternative upper limit of normal, would result in the test having sensitivity of about 0.70 and specificity of about 0.70.

Thus the upper (or lower) limit of normal for a test result is not fixed but can be selected depending on the decision maker's judgment about the inescapable trade-off between sensitivity and specificity. Both sensitivity and specificity can be improved simultaneously only if the test can be genuinely improved. For example, Fig. 2-6 shows the ROC curve for a new, improved test compared with an older test. A cut-off point can be selected for the new test whereby sensitivity is better than for the old test, even though specificity is maintained. Similarly, specificity can be improved (fewer false-positive results), even though sensitivity is maintained. Therefore a superior test has an ROC curve above and to the left of the ROC curve for an inferior diagnostic test.

SELECTING A THRESHOLD FOR DECISION MAKING

The results of diagnostic tests help clinicians determine the likelihood of disease in their patients. Positive predictive value describes the probability of disease based on test characteristics and the prevalence of disease in patients having positive test results. Conversely, negative predictive value describes the probability of disease in patients having negative test results.

In making decisions about patient care, clinicians have levels of likelihood that a disease is present at which they order definitive diagnostic evaluation and other levels of likelihood at which they start

therapy. For any probability of disease above the treatment threshold, treatment is started (Fig. 2-7). For any probability below the test threshold, no further diagnostic tests and no treatment are used. Between these two thresholds the patient's probability of disease resides in the testing region.

When the probability of disease is in the testing region—between the test threshold and treatment threshold—valuable information may be obtained from a test, the results of which can increase or decrease the probability of disease. In interpreting the implications of the new test results, the probability of disease before testing is the "prior probability" and the probability after testing is the "posterior probability." If the test result is abnormal, the posterior probability of disease is greater than before the test. If the test result is normal, the posterior probability is lower than before the test. If the posterior probability transcends a threshold compared with the prior probability, the probability of disease has become high enough to initiate treatment or low enough to stop testing and observe. If the posterior probability remains in the testing region, another test, if available, is performed. The threshold is a function of the risks and benefits of testing, as shown in the following equation.

(EQ. 1)

$$T = \frac{1}{\left(1 + \dfrac{B}{C}\right)}$$

T, Threshold; *B,* benefits; *C,* cost

The greater the benefit and smaller the cost, the larger the fraction (B/C) is. This increases the denominator (1 + B/C) and causes the threshold to be lower. Conversely, the higher the costs and lower the benefits, the higher the threshold for action.

3   **Clinical Bioethics**

Daniel P. Sulmasy

Medicine is an inherently moral enterprise. Illness and injury inevitably limit the patient's freedom, alter the patient's self-image, and render the patient extremely vulnerable. Physicians, through their public acts of profession, swear to put their knowledge and skills at the service of patients. But the striking imbalance in knowledge, power, and freedom between patients and physicians requires that physicians be entrusted with enormous responsibility—responsibility to the individual patients who present themselves, asking for help, and to the society that, by necessity, consists of persons who need one another and are all potential patients.

The moral nature of the medical enterprise has been understood since at least the time of the birth of scientific medicine in ancient Greece. The Oath of Hippocrates, still sworn in one form or another by physicians today, is a concrete manifestation of this moral content. The original oath invoked the Greek gods and included injunctions to teach, to work for the good of the patient, to refrain from euthanasia, assisted suicide, and abortion, to refrain from surgery in deference to the skills of surgeons, to refrain from sexual relations with patients, and to keep patients' confidences. It has only been for the last 30 years, however, that the moral nature of medicine has come under critical philosophical scrutiny. The field of bioethics is thus a new endeavor, helping practitioners and patients to make sense of a changing moral climate and to cope with advances in technology.

LAW AND MORALITY

It is important to recognize that law and morality are not equivalent, even in a democratic, pluralistic society. Not everything that is legal is moral, and not everything that is moral is legal. Clinical bioethics helps physicians and patients to locate their moral compasses in our litigious society. Physicians who carefully cultivate respectful, communicative relationships with their patients and always strive to do what they think is morally correct are substantially less likely than other physicians to be sued, and will be able to muster a formidable defense if suit is ever brought. But the central question of clinical bioethics is not, "How do I avoid lawsuits?" Rather, it is, "What is the right and good healing act for this patient in these circumstances?"

MORAL FRAMEWORKS

Anyone who thinks seriously about an ethical issue must do so from some basic moral position, regardless of whether he or she can articulate it. Several contemporary approaches help frame these moral positions in clinical bioethics. These frameworks are not necessarily mutually exclusive, but they may prove useful in analyzing morally troubling cases.

Principlism

One very popular framework is known as principlism. Beauchamp and Childress have argued that no matter what one's fundamental moral beliefs, there are four principles of bioethics that almost everyone can agree are important. These are (1) *respect for patient autonomy,* or the physician's duty to respect patient dignity and self-determination; (2) *beneficence,* or the physician's duty to do good for patients; (3) *nonmaleficence,* or the physician's duty not to harm patients; and (4) *justice,* or the physician's duties to other parties and to society in general. These principles are described as *prima facie,* or "first face," since it is inevitable that one or more of these principles will clash. Situations in which one can only act by violating one or another of these principles are called *dilemmas.* Principlists argue that dilemmas are resolved only through intuition.

Beneficence-in-Trust

As an alternative to principlism, Pellegrino and Thomasma have argued that since physicians pledge themselves to act for the good of their patients, this can be the central organizing principle of clinical bioethics. The virtuous physician is the one who habitually serves the good of the patient. They argue that there is a fourfold meaning of the patient's good, arranged in a hierarchy of importance, not in a merely *prima facie* manner. These meanings are (1) *the patient's ultimate good,* referring to the most fundamental values of the patient as the patient defines them; (2) *the good of the patient as a person,* referring to the intrinsic value of the individual as a human being, bearing an indelible dignity; (3) *the particular good of the patient's choice,* referring to the good the patient perceives in a given situation, such as the patient's perception of the quality of life associated

with the possible outcomes of various treatments; and (4) *the biomedical good of the patient,* concerning the patient's function as a biologic entity. Of particular note in this framework, the biomedical good of the patient constitutes the least important level of the patient's good.

A physician may choose to work with one or both of these, or with some other moral framework (e.g., Buddhism, Christianity, or utilitarianism), but every physician who is concerned with the moral practice of medicine must confront the issues raised by the frameworks presented.

"ETHICS WORKUP"

Internists should know how to analyze a case from an ethical perspective. An ethics workup resembles all clinical reasoning. One moves sensibly from the facts of the case to a medically and morally sound decision. Using a schema such as the one presented here, health care professionals holding a variety of philosophical and religious positions regarding ethics can share the following basic framework for thinking about and discussing morally troubling cases:

1. **What are the facts?** Good ethics begins with good data. These data are both medical and social. For example, both an estimate of prognosis and an understanding of the patient's home situation are often relevant to an ethical decision.
2. **What is the issue?** One must identify the specific ethical issue in the case. It may turn out, on reflection, that the problem is actually not an ethical problem, but a diagnostic problem or a communication problem. As the philosopher G.E. Moore has observed, "in Ethics . . . the difficulties and disagreements . . . are mainly due to a very simple cause: namely, to the attempt to answer questions, without first discovering precisely *what* question it is which you desire to answer."*
3. **Frame the issue.** Using one or several of the frameworks presented earlier, or an alternative framework, one should attempt to understand the important moral dimensions of the issue. For example, it may be the case that a patient with idiopathic thrombocytopenic purpura demands splenectomy as her first-line treatment. If the physician believes that splenectomy is very dangerous compared with prednisone therapy, respect for the patient's autonomy would seem to clash with a commitment to the principle of nonmaleficence and perhaps with the principle of justice. Or, a patient with a very treatable malignancy such as Hodgkin's disease may be refusing treatment. The physician's commitment to serving the patient's biomedical good would have to be examined in light of the patient's own choices, his good as a person, and the patient's own beliefs about the ultimate good.
4. **Situate the issue.** It is helpful to situate the case in relation to one's personal experience and that of the profession. This case-based method of analysis is called "casuistry." Is the case at hand analogous to any others where a broad moral consensus has been reached? How well does this case fit those paradigmatic cases? For example, in discussing whether it is permissible to remove a feeding tube from a young woman in permanent coma (such as Nancy Cruzan), it is useful to ask how closely this case approximates a case where there is substantial moral and legal consensus (such as the case of Karen Ann Quinlan).
5. **Reason.** It is important to weigh all the facts of the case in light of one's ethical framework and clinical experience in order to reason one's way to a judgment. Before deciding to act, the physician ought to play "devil's advocate" with his or her own position. He or she should also seek input from colleagues if time permits. A call to an ethics committee or an ethics consult service may be useful. Once resolved, a retrospective critique of the reasoning employed in the case can be helpful in preparing for the next time such a situation arises.
6. **Decide.** In medical ethics, as in all other aspects of medicine, a decision must be made. Taking all of the aforesaid into account, choices must be made in the midst of uncertainty. There

---

*Moore GE: *Principia Ethica,* Cambridge, 1986, Cambridge University, p vii.

is no simple formula here. The answer will require clinical judgment, practical wisdom, and common sense. In the final analysis the decision rests with the physician's moral judgment.

MORAL AGENTS: WHO DECIDES?

A critical issue in clinical bioethics is the identification of the morally appropriate decision maker. There are many individuals who are concerned about the patient's condition: the patient, the patient's family, friends, hospital administrators, lawyers, third-party payers, politicians, and, of course, the health care team. Ordinarily the patient is the primary decision maker. Perhaps the most salient contribution of contemporary bioethics to the practice of medicine has been the understanding that the patient has an enormous role to play in deciding what should be done in clinical practice. Out of respect for autonomy, quality-of-life judgments are generally thought to be the prerogative of the patient and family, not the physician. *Paternalism* refers to clinical practice that, while rooted in beneficence, fails to pay due regard to patient autonomy. Without seeking patient input a physician can only know the biomedical good of the patient and will fail to treat the patient as a whole person.

If a patient has lost decision-making capacity, respect for autonomy does not end. The physician should look for other indications of the patient's wishes. Generally the last statement made by the patient before becoming incapacitated takes precedence. For example, a patient with a living will stating that she did not want ventilator treatment might tell a nurse of her recent decision to give ventilator support a try, and then lose consciousness. This last decision would override the living will.

If there is no last "competent" decision, the team should ascertain whether the patient has an advance directive (e.g., a living will) and abide by the provisions of this document. If there is no advance directive, the physician should ask relatives or close friends what they think the patient would have wanted in such a situation. If no one is located who knows the patient, the physician should consult a hospital ethics committee. As a last resort it may be necessary to seek a court-appointed guardian. A schematic representation of this hierarchy of decision makers is depicted in Fig. 3-1.

DECISION-MAKING CAPACITY

An important skill for the internist is to determine whether a patient has lost decision-making capacity. Technically the term *competence* refers to a judge's decision that an individual has lost all capacity to make decisions. The internist, however, is concerned with a more narrow question: Is this patient capable of making a decision about *this* clinical option in these particular clinical circumstances? The threshold varies according to the gravity of the decision. For example, a suicidally depressed patient might be allowed to refuse blood drawing but would not be allowed to sign out of the hospital against medical advice. The assistance of a psychiatric consultant is often important, but ultimately the determination of decision-making capacity is the responsibility of the attending physician. In circumstances of obtundation or disorientation the answer is easy, but in many other cases the physician must make a clinical judgment based on the following clinical data:

1. Does the patient have intact judgment? That is, is the patient free of impulsiveness, able to correctly assess the seriousness of situations, able to set goals and make plans, and able to appreciate the connections between acts and consequences?

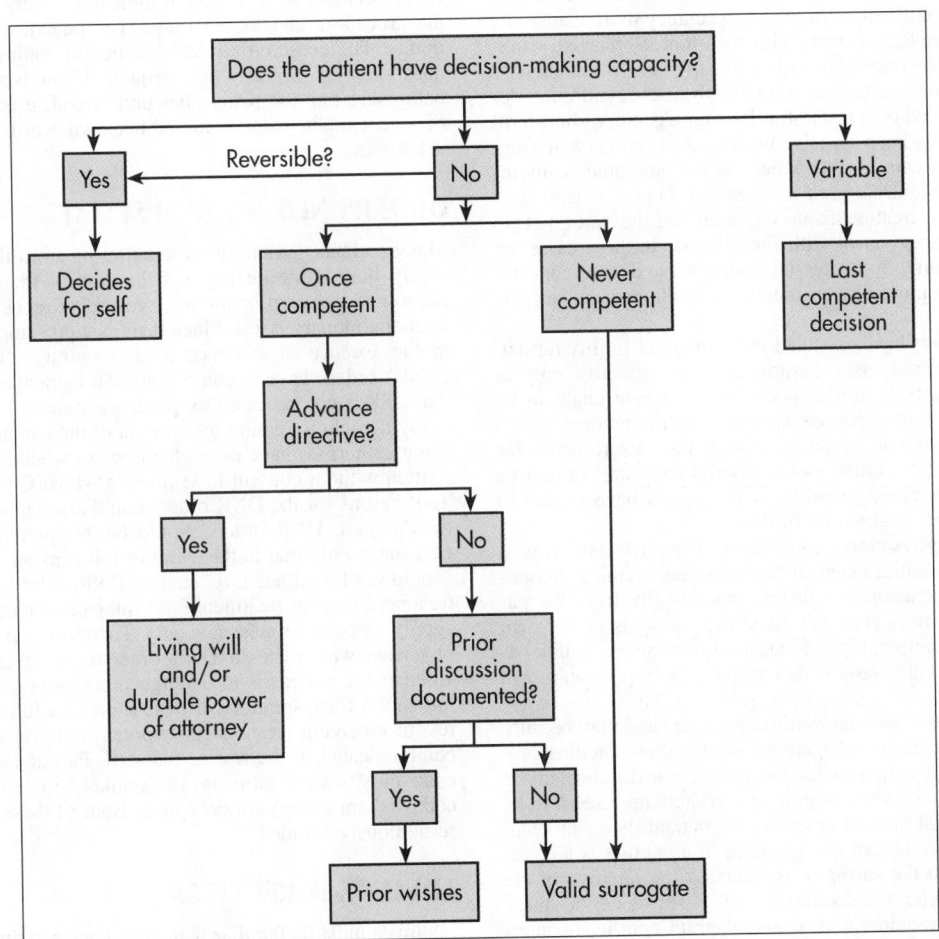

FIGURE 3-1   Flow diagram for ethically identifying the primary decision maker in patient care settings. (Modified from Sulmassy DP, FitzGerald D, Jaffin JH: *Crit Care Clin* 9:775–789, 1993. After Pellegrimo.)

2. Does the patient understand the nature of the procedure under consideration, its risks and benefits, and the consequences of deciding either to accept or to forgo the procedure?
3. Can the patient communicate a decision? A patient who cannot reach a decision of any sort may have impaired decision-making capacity.
4. Can the patient explain the reasons for a decision in a way that is consistent with his or her life history and previously held values?
5. Does the patient's decision remain relatively stable over time? Patients must certainly be free to change their minds, but a patient whose decision vacillates minute to minute may not have intact decision-making capacity.

Once it has been judged that a patient's decision-making capacity is impaired, the medical care team should next decide whether decision-making capacity can be restored through medical intervention and whether time will permit this approach. If the patient cannot participate in the decision-making process and it is unlikely that the patient's capacity can be restored in an appropriate time frame, one should then follow the procedures described in Fig. 3-1.

MORAL LIMITS TO PATIENT AUTONOMY

Internists should know that there are important limits to patient autonomy. The following are exceptions to the general rule that the physician should follow the wishes of the patient or surrogate:

Harm to specific, identifiable third party(ies). An example of such harm is the disturbed patient who expresses the intent, means, and method to kill another individual. It would be morally irresponsible to allow that individual to carry out such a threat.

Biomedical futility. Sometimes a request is made by a patient with a terminal illness or his or her family for interventions that are biomedically ineffective in reversing or arresting the disease process or in substantially improving life expectancy more than hours to days. For example, a patient with recurrent esophageal carcinoma refractory to surgery, radiation therapy, and chemotherapy may come to medical attention with Boerhaave's syndrome, demanding to be placed on a respirator. Barring a genuine short-term benefit (e.g., "Try to keep me alive until my son can get here from Guam"), ventilator care for this patient would be biomedically ineffective and not required, even if requested. Often, patients who demand ineffective treatments are experiencing the natural stage of denial in coming to terms with fatal illness. In these cases the denial should be directly addressed with compassionate concern, not necessarily supported by acquiescence in the request for ineffective therapy.

Some bioethicists have extended the concept of futility further, judging that in certain cases therapy might be effective only in maintaining a quality of life so poor that such care ought to be declared futile. A more cautious approach seems prudent. Judgments of futility have an objective basis if they are reserved for ineffective treatments. Quality-of-life judgments are subjective and ought to be reserved to patients. The courts have tended to support the cautious position on futility.

Violations of the physician's conscience. The physician, as well as the patient, is a moral agent. If the physician's ethical reasoning leads to a conclusion that differs dramatically from the patient's wishes, the physician may need to follow his or her own conscience. For example, a physician need not comply with a patient's request for euthanasia if this violates the physician's own moral beliefs.

Conflicts of interest. Sometimes it can become clear that, because of a conflict of interest, a surrogate decision maker is neither providing a substituted judgment for the patient nor deciding in the patient's best interests. For example, a surrogate may seem to be driven by a financial interest in seeing the patient die or in keeping the patient alive. The simple presence of a conflict is not sufficient to judge that the surrogate is violating the interests of the patient. To challenge the legitimacy of a surrogate on these grounds generally requires a clear and flagrant conflict of interest.

Therapeutic privilege. A very controversial exception, therapeutic privilege refers to the decision to override patient wishes or to withhold specific information on the grounds that one would otherwise endanger the patient's well-being. Such a decision should be made with great care in order to avoid inappropriate paternalism. It is extremely rare to encounter circumstances in which it is morally legitimate to invoke therapeutic privilege.

INFORMED CONSENT

Every internist must be able to obtain a morally adequate informed consent. This is not synonymous with obtaining a signature on a piece of paper. Informed consent is a process. It is one of the fundamental ways in which the physician shows respect for the autonomy of patients.

There are four basic elements in informed consent. First, the decision by the patient must represent an *autonomous* authorization. It must be free from coercion or even subtle manipulation by the physician or by others. Information must be presented in a fair and balanced fashion. This does not imply total neutrality, nor does it imply that the physician cannot make a recommendation or even try to persuade a patient, if the physician thinks the patient is making a mistake. But a physician ought not, for instance, purposefully distort the facts or threaten to sever the physician-patient relationship if the patient does not do as the physician requests.

The second element is that the patient must have *decision-making capacity.* The rudiments of how to make judgments about the patient's decision-making capacity have been described earlier.

The third element is that relevant information must be *disclosed* to the patient. The content to be disclosed is generally considered to include the nature of the procedure, its potential benefits and risks, and the alternatives to the procedure, including not having any procedure done.

The fourth element of informed consent, but certainly not the least, is *comprehension*. The patient must not merely have been told about the procedure and its outcomes. The patient must understand these things. The common clinical practice of asking, "Do you have any questions?" is probably not adequate. If one is seriously interested in being sure that the patient has understood, it is better to ask the patient to explain back in his or her own words the information just disclosed.

ORDERS NOT TO RESUSCITATE

Many patients, generally those suffering from illnesses that have severely limited the quality and duration of their lives, would prefer not to undergo cardiopulmonary resuscitation (CPR) in the event of a cardiopulmonary arrest. Since there is a presumption in favor of CPR in the absence of evidence to the contrary, "Do Not Resuscitate" (DNR) orders have become a standard practice for communicating that CPR is not indicated for particular patients. DNR orders are generally thought to require the consent of the patient or family, although some authorities have raised the issue of whether DNR orders can be written without consent in settings in which CPR is deemed "futile." The reasons for the DNR order should always be recorded in the patient's chart. DNR orders should be interpreted narrowly. Such orders mean only that in the event of full cardiopulmonary arrest, CPR should not be initiated. As such, a DNR order is compatible with all treatment short of treatment for a full cardiopulmonary arrest, or with supplying comfort measures only. Therefore it is incumbent upon the physician who writes a DNR order to make clear decisions about whether the patient is to undergo other sorts of treatments (such as intubation for respiratory distress short of a full cardiopulmonary arrest or receiving pressors for hypotension). These decisions must be communicated to the rest of the staff. Partial codes (e.g., "chemical code only") are confusing and unlikely to be successful. "Show" codes (sham codes) are deceptive. Both of these practices should be scrupulously avoided.

ADVANCE DIRECTIVES

Internists must be familiar with state laws pertaining to the two basic kinds of advance directives: living wills and durable powers of attorney for health care (DPAHC). Living wills specify treatments that the patient would or would not wish to receive in the event of terminal illness and the loss of decision-making capacity. These documents have the disadvantage that they apply only to terminal illness and may be vague or inflexible. DPAHCs are documents that specify a surrogate decision maker in the event that the patient loses decision-making capacity. They are flexible but are only as good as the surrogate's understanding of the patient's wishes. If the patient's living will appears to be contradicted by the decision maker specified in the DPAHC, one generally defers to the individual specified in the DPAHC to interpret the living will.

Sometimes conflicts occur among family members or other surrogates. If the patient has named an individual in a DPAHC, it is this person's judgments that should guide clinical decision making. If there is no DPAHC and surrogates cannot agree, one should attempt to ascertain who knows the patient best. Sometimes it is useful to ask the family to appoint a spokesperson. In all these cases of conflict one must be prepared to challenge the validity of the surrogate decision. Ethics consultation can be invaluable in helping to resolve these conflict situations.

WITHHOLDING AND WITHDRAWING CARE

Sometimes treatments are initiated with a hope of success that later proves quite limited. For instance, a patient may have intubation for pneumonia and respiratory distress but wind up several weeks later comatose and ventilator dependent with little hope of weaning or survival. Just as one ought to respect the valid wishes of a patient to refuse treatment, one ought to respect the valid wishes of a patient who would like treatment discontinued. However, one must recognize that it is psychologically more difficult to discontinue treatment once started. In addition, several religious groups allow the withholding but not the withdrawing of life support, and one should never justify the nonvoluntary withdrawal of treatment from one patient in favor of another patient with a better prognosis merely on the grounds that "there is no difference between withholding and withdrawing care." However, if one is relatively sure that a patient would not want treatment continued, respect for the patient generally requires that the treatment be withdrawn.

PAIN MANAGEMENT AND THE PRINCIPLE OF DOUBLE EFFECT

It is incontrovertible that there is a moral mandate to treat pain, particularly if the patient is terminally ill. Sometimes, however, physicians hesitate to do so because there is a risk that this might hasten the death of the patient. The centuries-old principle of double effect may be invoked in such cases. According to this rule, a physician completely opposed to euthanasia can act with clear conscience in administering a drug like morphine to a dying patient if several conditions are met. First, the physician must sincerely intend pain relief, not the death of the patient. Second, the dose must be consistent with a plan to relieve pain through the analgesic effects of morphine, not through causing respiratory arrest and death as the means of relieving pain. Third, the need for pain relief must be great compared with the risk of respiratory arrest and death in that patient. For example, if a patient is dying of metastatic breast cancer and is in severe pain, the potential benefit of intravenous morphine would seem overwhelming compared with the risk that morphine might contribute to hastening an already imminent death. If these conditions are fulfilled, a physician should be able to respond to the pain control needs of patients with a clear conscience, even knowing that death may unintentionally be hastened as a side effect.

At present, there is significant controversy about whether physicians should be authorized to *intentionally* hasten the death of the patient through euthanasia or assisted suicide, actions not permitted by Western medicine since the Hippocratic ethic became dominant many centuries ago. Legal bans on these practices are being challenged through legislative initiatives and civil suits.

ETHICS AND COST CONTROL

In an increasingly cost-constrained environment many ethical issues arise regarding the role of the individual practitioner in cost control.

Certainly, the internist should be a wise steward of medical resources. Contemporary medical care is expensive. Medical care is also associated with iatrogenic burdens. Therefore it is in the interest of the patient that the physician should strive to use only those tests and treatments that are truly necessary to help the patient. In a fee-for-service environment physicians who order more tests or treatments than are medically indicated (primarily to increase personal income) violate their moral duty to work for the patient's good. Likewise, in a capitated environment or under other conditions of financial reward for providing care less expensively, physicians who order fewer tests or treatments than are medically indicated (primarily to increase personal income) also violate their duty to work for the patient's good.

Physicians should not attempt to "ration" care at the bedside of individual patients. Such attempts, however nobly inspired, are fraught with moral difficulties. First, it would appear to be an act of hubris for an individual physician to decide unilaterally *that* rationing take place, *what* care should be rationed, and *from whom* care should be withheld. Second, it is formally unjust to withhold treatment from a patient simply because the patient happens to be seeing a particularly frugal physician, while a similar patient is receiving that same treatment elsewhere. Third, in an open system of care such as that in the United States it is nearly impossible to demonstrate empirically that the cost savings achieved by failing to treat one patient would be redirected to the treatment of the patients one might hope would be helped.

The proper role of physicians in cost control, then, is twofold. The first aspect is to practice carefully and to be wise in the use of medical resources. The second is to participate as an informed and involved citizen in the great debates about health care financing that are now affecting our society. Should cost control be achieved through market forces? Is it morally acceptable that almost 40 million Americans are without any form of health insurance at some time during a given year? Should the United States adopt a system of national health insurance? Are financial incentives to provide less care for patients the proper antidote to the incentives for overtreatment for personal gain under fee-for-service? The present turmoil in the financing of health care engenders these and many other new questions in medical ethics that physicians ignore at the peril of the profession and the peril of their patients.

CONCLUSION

Clinical bioethics is a new, growing field of investigation in medicine that helps to bridge the gap between the science and the art of practice. An understanding of the basic elements of bioethics is now a necessary competency for the internist. As the science of medicine has become increasingly powerful, questions arise about the proper use of health care technology. The fact that one can perform a test or treatment does not imply that one ought to do so. In addition, as the moral climate of the Western world changes, it is necessary for practitioners of the science and art of medicine to understand their own moral positions and how these moral positions will affect their practice. In the face of tremendous pluralism, much agreement about medical morality can be achieved by understanding the mission of medicine as an inherently moral enterprise in which competent, compassionate men and women undergo a long, serious period of training and dedicate themselves to working for the good of patients, whom they respect as whole persons.

BIBLIOGRAPHY

Annas G: The health care proxy and the living will, *N Engl J Med* 324:1210-1213, 1991.
Appelbaum PS, Grisso T: Assessing patients' capacities to consent to treatment, *N Engl J Med* 319:1635-1638, 1988.
Beauchamp TL, Childress JF: *Principles of biomedical ethics,* ed 4, New York, 1994, Oxford University Press.
Council on Ethical and Judicial Affairs, American Medical Association: Guidelines for the appropriate use of do-not-resuscitate orders, *JAMA* 265:1868-1871, 1991.
Pellegrino ED: Altruism, self-interest, and medical ethics, *JAMA* 258:1939-1940, 1987.
Pellegrino ED, Thomasma DC: *For the patient's good,* New York, 1988, Oxford University.

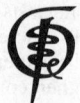

4 Costs and Outcomes

Kevin Schulman

Until recently, clinicians practiced medicine without consideration or knowledge of the costs of providing care to patients. In fact, in the United States, common reference sources for physicians omit information about the costs of medical services and pharmaceutical products. However, the rising costs of health care in the United States have created pressure on clinicians to understand the cost of providing care to patients.

These cost pressures have motivated the development of new ways of organizing clinical practice to control the cost of care for patients. This has led to a need for clinicians to understand both the costs and benefits of new therapies and procedures in order to assess the value of the therapies they provide to their patients. Moreover, hospitals and physicians have in recent years been held more directly accountable for the outcomes of the care they provide. These issues are now being addressed by investigators in the field of clinical economics.

HEALTH CARE EXPENDITURE

Medical care consumed 14.2% of the U.S. gross national product in 1995—an estimated $1 trillion. The cost of medical care grew at a rate faster than that of inflation in the general economy for almost the entire period from 1970 to 1994, reaching a peak rate of growth of 11.6% in the early 1990s. The cost of health care in the United States, expressed as a portion of the gross national product devoted to health care, is higher than that in any other developed nation. Canada has the second highest health care expenditure level, with 9.3% of its 1990 gross national product devoted to health care. France devoted 8.8%; Germany, 8.1%; Japan, 6.5%; and Great Britain, 6.2% of their gross national products in health care expenditures.

Increasing costs in the health care sector are generally thought to stem from several factors, including increasing costs in the overall economy, rising costs of medical technology, increasing age and size of the population, larger numbers of visits to doctors each year, and a greater intensity of services offered by physicians. Because the federal government provides Medicare medical insurance to people over 65 years of age in the United States, the aging of the population is one of the main factors behind the tremendous growth of annual Medicare spending (Medicare outlays were $180 billion in 1995 and were expected to grow at 8% annual rate for 1996) and of health expenditure in general.

The high cost of health care has led investigators to examine the effect of insurance on the use of medical resources in the United States. In a pivotal experiment investigators from the Rand Corporation determined that patients with insurance for all medical costs use more health care resources than patients who are required to pay a portion of their health care costs. A more recent study demonstrated a decline of about 15% in the use of emergency room services among members of health maintenance organizations (HMOs) who were required to make a small copayment for such services.

Several investigators have shown that, at least for elderly populations, a large proportion of the cost of medical services is consumed in a patient's last year of life. In 1991, about $34 billion, the equivalent of 28% of Medicare's budget, was spent on people in their last year of life. Other investigators have demonstrated substantial variation in clinical practice at the regional level. Physicians recommend elective surgeries for procedures such as hysterectomy with rates up to seven times greater than average in some geographic areas. This has led to the study of small-area variation, in which investigators explore the variation in treatment across geographic areas to better understand clinical practice and to make treatment decisions based on "best practices" for specific clinical services. It has also led to increased interest in evaluating the costs, effectiveness, and benefits of medical care.

Economic assessment includes the evaluation of both costs and benefits (outcomes) of a service or program. With knowledge of either costs or benefits alone, it is not possible to make a rational spending decision.

Costs of Care

There are four types of medical care costs: (1) direct medical costs, including the costs of medical services such as physician and hospital fees; (2) direct nonmedical costs, defined as the costs that accompany receiving medical care, such as the cost of transportation to physician offices or specialized treatment centers; (3) indirect medical costs, such as disability or lost productivity attributable to illness; and (4) intangible costs, which are the costs of pain and suffering related to the illness. Although each of these categories affects patients, families, and the health care system, direct medical costs are most often used to enumerate the costs of medical care to the nation as a whole, regardless of who pays. Projected direct medical costs in the United States for fiscal year 1995 included $441.1 billion for hospital costs, $206.1 billion for physician costs, $84.1 billion for pharmaceutical costs, and $92.9 billion for nursing home costs.

Researchers have recently begun to pay greater attention to the indirect costs of medical care. Because individuals have the highest value of future earnings when they are young, indirect costs are greatest for diseases that impact younger populations, such as those in their 20s and 30s. Indirect medical costs can also be substantial. The indirect costs of human immunodeficiency virus (HIV) disease, which generally strikes younger populations, are estimated to be at least six times greater that the direct costs of care for the disease.

Economic assessments of medical care may involve any or all of the four cost categories just discussed. Managed care organizations may be interested in the direct costs of hospital services, while employers may be most interested in the indirect costs of care stemming from employees' lost work days. Patients, on the other hand, are likely to be most interested in either direct out-of-pocket medical costs—such as copayments—or the intangible costs related to pain and suffering caused by disease and treatment.

Outcomes Research

Variation in the costs of medical care has led to new efforts to understand the outcomes of medical care and to assess the value of specific clinical services. These efforts form the core of what is described as "outcomes research." Traditionally physicians have evaluated specific clinical measures and end-points for either clinical or epidemiologic studies. These measures can assess morbidity (e.g., peak flow rates for lung function) or mortality (survival). Until the development of outcomes research, little information was collected on the effect of treatments and diseases on patients' quality of life and health state preferences. Outcomes research allows investigators to better measure the impact of medical therapies on patients' lives.

In addition to traditional clinical parameters such as survival and test results, outcomes of care can be measured using two very different measures: health status and patient preference (Table 4-1). Health status instruments are used to quantify patients' activities across a range of functional areas related to health. These areas, or "domains," typically include physical, emotional, and social parameters. Health status instruments are used in comparisons of patients' standardized levels of functioning, which can then be quantified into a quality-of-life score across each of the domains. For example, a health status instrument reports results for each patient by domain. These results are usually scaled from 0 to 100—with 0 representing the worst score for the domain. Thus an individual patient may receive a score of 90 in the physical function domain and a score of 80 in the emotional function domain.

Health status instruments can be general and unrelated to specific medical conditions, or they can be disease specific. Disease-specific measures of health status tend to be more sensitive than general measures to changes in a patient's condition. However, disease-specific measures do not always assess systemic side effects of treatments. Therefore many trials include both types of measures.

In contrast to health status assessment, which evaluates patient health status according to a standardized level of functioning, patient preference assessments measure patients' perceptions of their health states. The analysis requires patients or society to assign a weighted *utility*, or value, to overall treatment outcomes. For example, on a scale of 0 to 1—in which 0 is the worst imaginable health state and 1 represents perfect health—a patient with mild asthma may report her health state as 0.95. The outcome measure, known as a quality-adjusted life year (QALY), is calculated using both survival and patient preference information. Investigators are currently exploring the use of patient preference assessment in clinical trials.

Economic Assessment of Medical Technologies and Therapies

Economic analysis involves a series of analytic tools designed to compare the costs and outcomes of medical care. Several types of economic analysis are reported in the medical literature (Fig. 4-1).

Cost-benefit analysis compares the cost of a medical intervention with its benefit. Both costs and benefits are measured in the same (usually monetary) units. One of the potential difficulties of cost-benefit analysis is that it requires researchers to associate money values with morbidity and years of life. Outcomes (treatment benefits) may be difficult to measure in monetary terms, and many ethical problems arise in any such attempt. Economists believe that cost-benefit analysis is the most appropriate type of analysis for determining new health care investments. However, cost-benefit analysis is rarely conducted because of the measurement and ethical issues surrounding the method.

Cost-effectiveness analysis, the most common analytic approach reported in the medical literature, compares costs in monetary terms with effectiveness in clinical units. For example, one might measure clinical outcomes in terms of lives saved or toxicities prevented. As an alternative, health outcomes can be reported in terms of change in an intermediate clinical outcome, such as percentage of change in blood cholesterol level or percentage of lowering of blood pressure. Results of cost-effectiveness analysis are typically reported as a ratio of costs to clinical benefits (e.g., dollars per year of life saved). Examples of results of these analyses appear in Table 4-2.

Table 4-1   Outcome Measures

INSTRUMENT	NUMBER OF ITEMS	TIME TO COMPLETE (MINUTES)	SELF-ADMINISTERED
General measures			
Short form 36	36	15	Yes
Short form 12	12	5-10	Yes
Medical Outcomes Study HIV form	30	15	Yes
Sickness Impact Profile form	136	45	Yes
Nottingham Health Profile form	45	15	Yes
Disease-specific measures			
Asthma Quality of Life Questionnaire (Juniper)	32	10	Yes
Asthma Quality of Life questionnaire (Marks)	20	5	Yes
LHQ			
Diabetes Quality of Life Measure	46		Yes
Functional Living Index–Cancer (FLIC)	26	15	Partially
Cancer Rehabilitation Evaluation System (CARES)	139	30	Yes
Functional Assessment of Cancer Therapy (FACT-G)	29	15	Yes
Arthritis Impact Measurement Scales (AIMS)	48	15-20	Yes
Patient preference measures			
EuroQol	7	5	Yes
Time Trade-off	NA	10-15	Potentially
Standard Gamble	NA	10-15	No
Quality of Well-Being Scale	25	15	Yes
Health Utilities Index	15	15	Yes

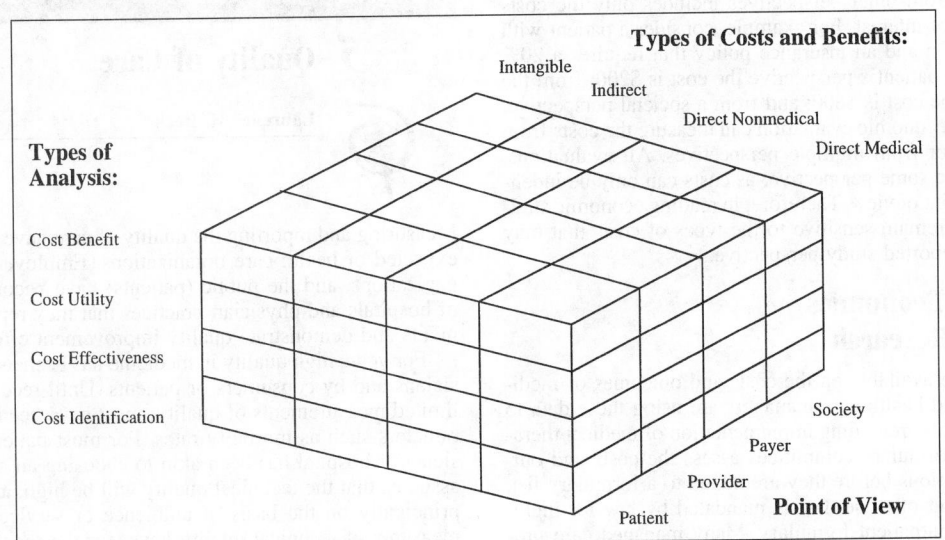

FIGURE 4-1   Clinical economic analysis.
Modified from Bombardier C, Eisenberg JM: *J Rheumatol* 12:201-204, 1985.

Table 4-2   Cost-utilities for various heart disease interventions

INTERVENTION	YOLS	$/YOLS	$QALY
ACE inhibitors for symptomatic heart failure			
SOLVD Treatment Trial lifetime projection	0.40	100	100
Screening asymptomatic adults for hypertension			
Men (40 years of age)	0.03	NA	18,050
Men (60 years of age)	0.05	NA	9,300
Beta-adrenergic antagonists after acute MI			
Low risk (55 years of age)	0.10	16,700	NA
High risk (55 years of age)	0.47	3,000	NA
Cardiac rehabilitation after MI	0.02	22,950	NA
Coronary revascularization			
PTCA, 1-vessel disease, ↓ LVF, mild angina	0.10	NA	103,000
PTCA, 1-vessel disease, ↓ LVF, severe angina	0.20	NA	7,350
CABG, 3-vessel disease, ↓ LVF, severe angina	1.40	NA	19,100
Thrombolysis			
t-PA incremental to streptokinase	0.14	32,700	NA

From Glick H, Cook J, Kinosian B et al: *J Cardiac Failure* 1:371-380, 1995.
All figures expressed in United States dollars adjusted to 1992 and rounded to the nearest $50.
ACE, Angiotensin-converting enzyme; *CABG,* coronary artery bypass graft; *LVF,* left ventricular function; *MI,* myocardial infarction; *NA,* not available; *PTCA,* percutaneous trans-luminal coronary angioplasty; *QALY,* quality-adjusted life year; *SOLVD,* Studies of Left Ventricular dysfunction; *t-PA,* tissue-type plasminogen activator; *YOLS,* years of life saved.

Cost-utility analysis, a subset of cost-effectiveness analysis, measures costs in monetary units and outcomes in terms of the value patients gain from medical treatment (patient utility). The results of a cost-utility analysis are expressed as the cost per quality-adjusted life year gained from treatment (Table 4-2).

Cost-identification analysis enumerates the costs involved in medical care, ignoring the resulting outcomes. By performing cost-identification analysis, researchers can determine the costs of alternative means of providing a service. Results are expressed in terms of cost per unit of service provided. For example, a cost-identification study might measure the cost of a course of a specific antibiotic regimen or the cost of an outpatient surgical treatment program. It would not, however, calculate the clinical outcomes associated with treatment (cost-effectiveness analysis) or the value of the outcomes of the treatment in units of currency (cost-benefit analysis). Cost-identification studies, which include comparisons between different treatments based on their costs alone, are appropriate only if treatment outcomes or benefits are equivalent for the therapies being evaluated.

Economic evaluation is unique in that costs may be different for different actors in the health care system. Costs can be calculated from different perspectives or points of view. Costs can be calculated from the viewpoint of the patient, caregiver, payer, or society. The calculation of societal costs represents the total cost of a transaction. The calculation of costs from other perspectives includes only the costs relevant to the party of interest. For example, consider a patient with a $1000 hospitalization and an insurance policy that requires a 20% copayment. From the patient's perspective the cost is $200; from the payer's perspective the cost is $800; and from a societal perspective, the cost is $1000. An economic evaluation can measure the costs from a single perspective or from multiple perspectives. All evaluations, however, must assume some perspective, as costs can only be identified from a given point of view. Therefore, in reading economic studies it is important to remain sensitive to the types of costs that may be excluded by the reported study perspective.

Use of Clinical Economics and Outcomes Research

As more data become available on the costs and outcomes of medical care, clinicians and health care managers are using these data to improve decision making regarding implementation of medical therapies. Many hospital formulary committees assess the costs and outcomes of new medications before they are added to a formulary list. In Australia assessment of these data is mandated by law for inclusion on the national outpatient formulary. Many managed care programs use cost-effectiveness analysis to improve the clinical treatment process for patients. Employers and employees are now demanding that managed care programs report information on the outcomes of care as part of their program assessment. At the national level the

Health Care Financing Administration is considering the use of cost-effectiveness analysis in deciding which services to offer as covered services under the Medicare program.

BIBLIOGRAPHY

Bodenheimer TS, Grumbach K: *Understanding health policy: a clinical approach,* Norwalk, Conn, 1995, Appleton & Lange.

Drummond MF, Stoddart GL, Torrance GW: *Methods for the economic evaluation of health care programmes,* New York, 1987, Oxford University.

Eisenberg JM: Clinical economics: a guide to the economic analysis of clinical practices, *JAMA,* 262:2879-2886, 1989.

Gold MR, Siegel JE, Russell LB, Weinstein MC: *Cost-effectiveness in health and medicine,* New York, 1996, Oxford University.

Selby JV, Fireman BH, Swain BE: Effect of copayment on use of emergency department in a health maintenance organization, *N Engl J Med,* 334:635-641, 1996.

Spilker B, editor: *Quality of life and pharmacoeconomics in clinical trials,* ed 2, Philadelphia, 1996, Lippincott-Raven.

Torrance GW, Feeny D: Utilities and quality-adjusted life years, *Int J Technol Assess Health Care* 5:559-575, 1989.

Wennberg JE: Future directions for small-area variations. *Med Care* 31:YS75-80, 1993.

CHAPTER

5   Quality of Care

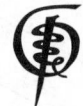

Laurence H. Beck

Measuring and reporting the quality of care have become increasingly expected of health care organizations. Employers, managed care organizations, and the public (patients) have become more demanding of hospitals and physician practices that they report quality measurements and demonstrate quality improvement efforts.

For years high quality in medicine has been assumed, both by physicians and by consumers or patients. Until recently there have been limited measurements of quality; most have been relatively crude parameters such as mortality rates. For most patients, choosing a physician or hospital has been akin to choosing an airline: the consumer assumes that the technical quality will be high, and choices are made principally on the basis of ambience or service quality. Legitimate measures of technical quality have, for the most part, been unavailable to the public.

Individual case review, both formal and informal, has been the principal mode of assessing quality, usually through peer review by physicians. Although a valid approach, review of individual cases may

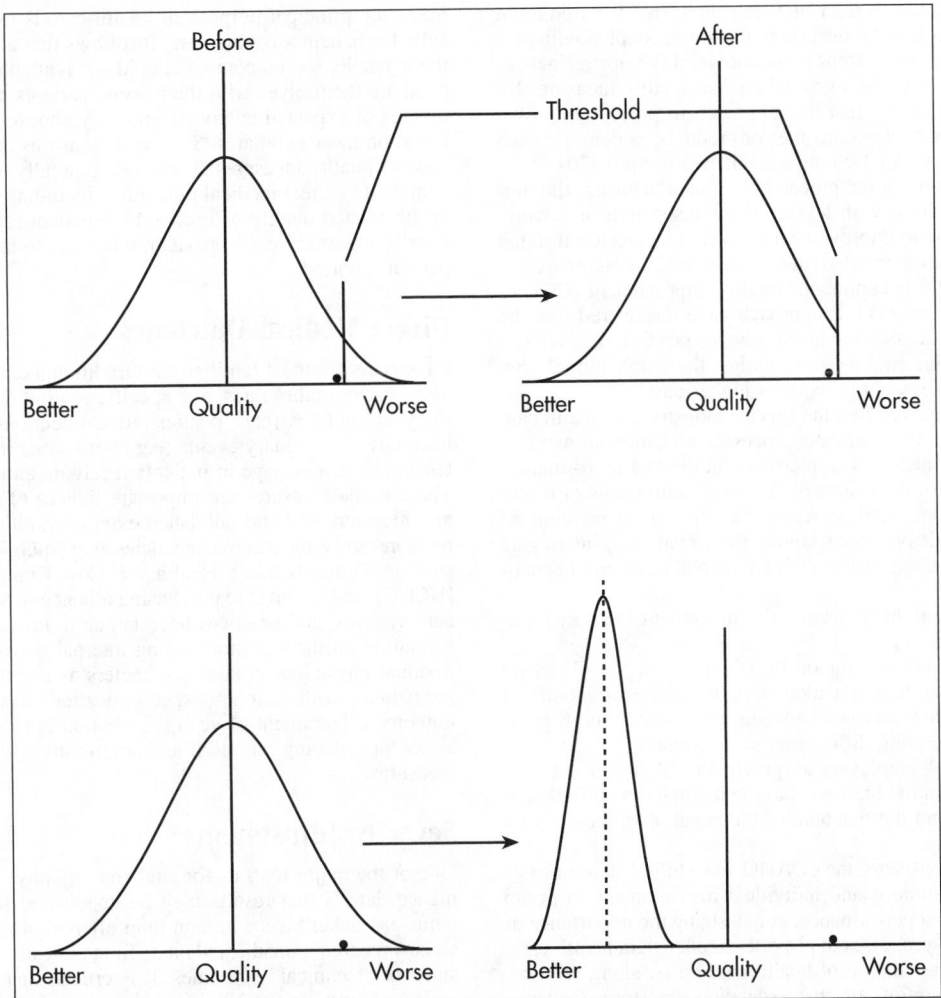

FIGURE 5-1 Comparison of the principles of, **A,** quality assurance (QA) with, **B,** quality improvement (QI). In QA the emphasis is on looking for and eliminating the few cases (or individuals) that fail to meet a minimal standard. The result is a minimal change in overall quality. In QI the emphasis is on improving the performance of the entire group by reducing case-to-case variation and by changing the processes of care so that the mean level of quality can improve dramatically.

From James BC: *Quality management for health care delivery,* Chicago, 1989, The Hospital Research and Educational Trust.

ignore patterns of care or outcomes that are more readily apparent when results of many patients or providers are aggregated.

For many years the stimulus for assessing quality has principally been driven by external accrediting organizations such as the Joint Commission on Accreditation of Healthcare Organizations (JCAHO). The primary basis for review has been quality assurance, which is a system of inspection. Quality assurance usually has involved the setting of minimum standards and then, by either external case review or peer review, identifying organizations that do not meet the standards. Organizations were considered to have good quality as long as they met or exceeded these minimal standards. The philosophy underlying this form of quality assurance assumes that *individuals* are responsible for result or outcomes. If there is a bad outcome, it can probably be traced to the actions of one or more *individuals*. This "bad apples" approach has tended to minimize evaluation of group or organizational performance.

Another feature of quality assurance is that it has principally been hospital based until recently. When outcomes have been measured, the parameters have been important but crude: mortality, complication rate, readmission rate to hospital. Only in the last decade have quality measures begun to be applied systematically to physicians' outpatient practices. Physicians rarely received meaningful feedback on their own practice or performance unless they happened to fall into the "bad apples" group.

The foundations of current quality improvement efforts in health care derive from the 1920s with the work of Walter Shewhart and, more recently, in the 1970s through the teaching of W. Edwards Deming. Deming studied variation in the output of industrial processes, showing that consistency in outcome, whether that outcome was a product or a service, depended on reducing the variation in the processes used to produce that outcome. Deming described two kinds of variation: *common* cause (or random) variation, which is the "wobble" inherent in any process, and *special* cause variation, which could be attributed to some special factor, either individual based or environment based, which is not part of the process and can be identified and eliminated.

Deming and others repeatedly emphasized that quality should be defined by the customer and that its measurement should assess how well the product or service meets the needs of the customer.

Deming demonstrated that 85% to 90% of defects in quality or of variation in outcomes were due to the processes of production and only 10% were due to the performance of individuals. Therefore the way to improve quality is to focus on processes, to make them consistent, thereby reducing variation, and then to study those processes intensively, attempting to make them more efficient by removing complexity, rework, and redundancy.

These concepts are demonstrated in Fig. 5-1, which compares traditional quality assurance with quality improvement. In the former, removal of those not meeting standards results in a minimal improvement in quality because those who are not cited have no incentive to change, but only to make certain they remain above the minimum threshold. On the other hand, reduction in variation, coupled with process improvement—the basic steps in modern quality improvement—can have a large effect on the mean or median quality measure. Industry has repeatedly shown that this approach to process improvement is effective in improving outcomes or products, as demonstrated by Japanese industry (under Deming's guidance) in the 1970s.

By reducing variation in the processes of manufacturing, the output is made more uniform with less need for inspection or rework. More important, dramatic improvement can often be created through fundamental changes in the underlying processes. Consistently, companies who have used this continuous quality improvement (CQI) or total quality management (TQM) approach have discovered that the new manufacturing processes produced a *better* product at a *reduced* cost of production. This finding goes against the conventional wisdom that high quality invariably requires higher cost.

As CQI gradually moved into the service industry and health care during the late 1980s, the focus on processes and measurement of outcomes resulted in much less emphasis on individual performance. Instead, measurement of the results of groups of individuals or of entire systems has predominated, in recognition that more meaningful measurement of overall processes comes from evaluating aggregate results and comparing those results with an internal or external benchmark.

The following factors have abetted the movement to quality improvement in health care:

1. The classic studies of variation by Wennberg in New England demonstrated that there is marked variation in the provision and use of health care services between communities or regions without corresponding differences in outcome.
2. The influence of employers as purchasers of health care for large groups of individuals has put great emphasis on the quality of services and the outcome of the health care received by their employees.
3. Over the last few years the JCAHO has shifted its emphasis from quality assurance and individual measurement to group and organizational performance, emphasizing the importance of interdisciplinary processes to provide excellence in health care.
4. The continuing escalation of health care costs, along with recent severe constraints on that escalation, has forced intense scrutiny on the appropriateness of use of health care services, as well as their cost and efficiency.

All of these changes have caused a shift of thinking for the individual physician, who must consider not only, "How can I achieve the best outcome for this patient in my office?" but also, "How can I improve the average outcome for all my patients?"

Although much of the recent emphasis has been on the reduction of costs in health care, quality is becoming increasingly important. Coalitions of large employers and health insurance organizations, believing that much of the excess cost has been driven out of health care, are now insisting on measures of quality, both in individual procedures and in overall outcomes for populations of patients. "Report cards" comparing performance of individual physicians in terms of patient satisfaction, use of resources, and population health outcomes have become increasingly prevalent, particularly for physicians working within large health maintenance organizations (HMOs) and integrated health care systems.

MEASURING QUALITY AND OUTCOMES

The definition of quality in health care has varied depending on the point of view of the individual defining it. Physicians have traditionally looked at the technical aspects of medical care in defining quality. Patients, on the other hand, have often been more concerned with service quality—the way in which the technical aspects of care are delivered. Measurement of patient satisfaction has become an important component of the definition. Most recently, with the emphasis on cost containment, the quest in quality improvement, particularly for purchasers of health care, has been for increased *value,* where

(EQ. 1)

$$ \text{Value} = \frac{\text{Quality}}{\text{Cost}} = \frac{\text{Medical outcomes} + \text{Service quality}}{\text{Resources used}} $$

Since the principal purpose of health care is to facilitate optimal results for patients seeking care, it follows that a valid measurement of these results (or outcomes) should be available. Physicians want to compare themselves with their peers; patients must have realistic estimates of expected outcomes and may choose their provider of care based on those estimates. Several dimensions of outcomes have been used as quality measures. These fall generally into the following categories: (1) direct medical outcomes (including functional status), (2) health-related quality of life, and (3) patient satisfaction. The first is usually reported by the provider, whereas the latter two are generally patient reported.

Direct Medical Outcomes

Physicians are most familiar with traditional outcome measures, such as 5-year mortality rates, and specific morbidities. These may be primary morbidities (e.g., postoperative infections, readmission to the hospital) or secondary events (e.g., stroke rate in patients with hypertension or hemorrhage in patients receiving anticoagulation therapy). These crude measures are important indices of quality of care. They are often reported and published externally, either by the provider or more recently by external agencies (e.g., public watchdog agencies such as Pennsylvania's Healthcare Cost Containment Commission [HCCC], and health care purchasing alliances). Many hospitals, health care systems, and practices have begun to measure and distribute information on the variation among internal departments or among individual physicians in such parameters as length of stay (LOS), cost per patient, readmission rates, complication rates, and numerous other outcomes. The intent of such distribution is to stimulate discussions aimed at reducing variation and improving overall quality outcome measures.

Severity Adjustment

One of the major reasons for challenge by physicians of such performance data is that results may be unadjusted for severity. "My patients are sicker" is a common (and often legitimate) concern of physicians receiving unadjusted data. To make valid comparisons of measures of "technical" outcomes, it is crucial that the data be defined, collected, and reported in a consistent manner and that the data be severity adjusted. For example, it is inappropriate to compare the mortality rate or re-stenosis rate of coronary artery bypass graft (CABG) operations between two surgeons if one surgeon primarily performs elective surgery on patients in stable condition with one- or two-vessel disease and another surgeon performs a high proportion of emergency operations on desperately ill patients who are transferred from other hospitals.

Numerous severity-adjustment systems have been developed, and each has its own strengths and weaknesses. Many are based on administratively reported patient data (e.g., from hospital discharge billing data), and the validity of these clinical data may be appropriately questioned or challenged by clinicians. Severity adjustment should usually be based on conditions present at the onset of a specific management process, but many systems in use include complications that may have resulted from the management. Therefore, when reporting or comparing medical outcome results, it is important for physicians to ascertain whether the comparison groups were similar and, if not, were appropriately adjusted for severity.

Functional Status Measures

Use of measurement of functional status to assess the quality of care has increased. Since for many medical conditions cure or long-term survival is not the primary goal, optimization of functional status is a more valid measure than survival or mortality. Many functional status measures are provider reported (e.g., New York Heart Association Functional Class, the active joint score in rheumatoid arthritis) and can be used as severity adjusters as well as outcome measures. Increasingly, patient-reported functional and health status measures are used, including scales such as the Katz activities of daily living (ADL) scale or disease-specific questionnaires such as those developed by InterStudy (Excelsior, Minn) (TyPE instruments).

More comprehensive patient-derived quality-of-life measures are most useful when comparing populations of patients receiving alter-

---

BOX 5-1
Examples of population-based health care measures

Health Plan Employer Data and Information Set (HEDIS) 3.0*†
Domain: Effectiveness of care
Childhood immunization status
Adolescent immunization status
Flu shots for high-risk adults
Breast cancer screening
Cervical cancer screening
Prenatal care in the first trimester
Low-birth weight babies
Domain: Use of services
Well-child visits in the first 15 months of life
Well-child visits in the third, fourth, fifth, and sixth year of life
Adolescent well-care visit
Frequency of selected procedures
Inpatient utilization: General hospital/acute care
Inpatient utilization: Nonacute care
Discharge and average length of stay for females in maternity care
Cesarean section and vaginal birth after cesarean rate (VBAC rate)
Ambulatory care

Checkups after delivery
Treating children's ear infections
Beta-blocker treatment after a heart attack
Eye examinations for people with diabetes
Follow-up after hospitalization for mental illness
Advising smokers to quit
Flu shots for older adults

Births and average length of stay, newborns
Mental health utilization: Inpatient discharges and average length of stay
Mental health utilization: Percentage of members receiving inpatient, day/night care and ambulatory services
Readmission for specified mental health disorders
Chemical dependency utilization: Percentage of members receiving inpatient, day/night care and ambulatory services
Readmission for chemical dependency
Outpatient drug utilization
Frequency of ongoing prenatal care
Chemical dependency utilization–inpatient discharges and average length of stay

Healthy People 2000

1. Reduce coronary heart disease deaths to no more than 100 per 100,000 people.
2. Reduce maternal mortality rate to no more than 3.3 per 100,000 live births.
3. Reduce the mean serum cholesterol level in adults to no more than 200 mg/dl.
4. Increase to at least 85% women aged 18 years and older with a uterine cervix who received a Pap test in the preceding 1 to 3 years.

---

*HEDIS is a registered trademark of the National Committee for Quality Assurance.
†HEDIS 3.0 Reporting Set Measures, 1997.

native treatments for well-defined conditions. One of the most frequently used, the Short Form 36 (SF-36 [from the Medical Outcomes Study]) contains 36 questions addressing several domains (physical, cognitive, and emotional function; social and role function; symptoms; and general well-being). These measures are not highly sensitive for detecting small changes in health in an individual but can be used to show rates of change (improvement or deterioration), particularly with groups of patients.

Patient Satisfaction

Patient satisfaction is a crucial and increasingly used measure of quality of care. Patients may have great faith in the technical quality of their care, but they usually make choices based on the degree to which their service needs are met. Therefore service measures such as accessibility, ease of making appointments, treatment by support staff, waiting time, and ambience of the practice setting are highly correlated with patients' overall satisfaction with care.

Patient satisfaction is frequently measured by health care providers but often in a nonscientific manner. The most common method, using voluntary questionnaires available to patients in waiting rooms or hospital hallways, selects a biased sample that cannot be readily compared with any other population. To be valid and comparable, a random (or total) sample of patients should be presented with a standardized satisfaction questionnaire, either written or by telephone interview. This methodology is being used more often by insurance companies and employers to compare the service quality of multiple providers. Patient satisfaction scores are appropriately used by individual practices or institutions to target areas for improvement and to demonstrate, through repeated measurements over time, that effective changes have been made. Standardized patient satisfaction instruments are available, and organizations are using them both to look for internal variation and to compare themselves with peer organizations using the same instrument.

Population Health Outcomes

As health care expenditures continue to increase and approach the limit that the public (and government) are willing to spend, it has become strategically important to measure the effectiveness of those expenditures in improving the health of the nation (or of populations within a given health care system).

Many large health care systems and HMOs have begun measuring such parameters as use of preventive health service, general health status, and use of health service in selected subpopulations (e.g., patients with asthma). A number of the parameters being measured derive from two documents: *Healthy People 2000* and *Health Plan and Employer Data and Information Set (HEDIS)*.

Healthy People 2000, a product of the U.S. Public Health Service, sets goals for the U.S. population for a large number of preventive services, mortality rates, and health status (Box 5-1).

HEDIS includes a comprehensive set of quality measures that are being used by employers to choose physician practices for their employees and by the National Committee for Quality Assurance (NCQA) to evaluate the performance of HMOs. Examples are shown in Box 5-1. As hospitals and health care systems develop integrated clinical information systems, they should include the capability to measure these population outcomes and report them internally and externally.

METHODS OF QUALITY IMPROVEMENT
Clinical Practice Guidelines

The literature is replete with practice guidelines developed over the last several years. As defined by the Institute of Medicine, practice guidelines are "systematically developed statements to assist practitioners and patients in making decisions about appropriate health care for specific clinical circumstances." The principles underlying practice guidelines are that, for a given clinical situation there is a best current practice; that this practice can be defined by a set of statements or, more commonly, by a branching algorithm; and that the use of the guideline should lead to more uniform and improved clinical outcomes with either reduction or less variation in resource use.

Guidelines have been developed and published by professional specialty organizations, by individual physicians and groups, by insurance companies, and in the largest coordinated effort to date, by the Agency for Health Care Policy and Research. One such guideline is shown in Fig. 5-2. Although many guidelines are developed by a consensus panel of experts, the more compelling and rigorous guidelines have been developed through an evidence-based approach. Guidelines have most commonly been developed for hospital-based situations, but an increasing number span the continuum between ambulatory care and appropriate hospital care.

Although hundreds of guidelines are now in the literature, successful implementation coupled with rigorous evaluation of their outcomes, has been scanty. Many guidelines have been developed an d reportedly put into place, with the authors describing improvements in care such as increased patient satisfaction, decreased length of stay, and decreased resource use. Most of these reports are uncontrolled, and it is difficult or impossible to separate the effects of the guideline implementation from other secular trends in the delivery of health care. However, when practice guidelines that fit rigorous criteria have been critically reviewed, most have demonstrated an improvement in the process of care or use of the guideline, although only a small proportion of these studies have measured and reported actual outcomes of care.

Critical Pathways

The most common hospital-based approach to CQI has been the development and deployment of critical pathway techniques. The majority of institutions have begun this activity (also known as care maps or clinical pathways) within the last several years.

A critical pathway is developed through a multidisciplinary team-involving representatives from the key professional disciplines that are involved in the care of a specific medical condition or procedure. The team develops a "best current approach" for the evaluation and management of the usual patient with that condition. The pathway reflects a combination of literature-based evidence, local practices, and the particular resources available in the institution developing the instrument. The usual product of this process is a matrix chart in which the various tasks to be completed are arrayed against time (usually segregated by the responsible discipline); time is measured in hospital days (Table 5-1).

Although most patients are expected to progress according to the timeline in the pathway, the determinant of when they pass from one stage to the next should be a measured clinical result or outcome. Certain steps in these pathways may activate standard order sets, a set of orders that are "automatically" activated if certain criteria are met. These protocol orders are carried out unless actively changed by the ordering physician.

In many institutions the critical pathway has been developed into a documentation tool that becomes part of the patient record; completion of the tasks is documented directly on the matrix. Variations are noted, and an explanation is required for divergence from the pathway. The variations are analyzed to determine ways of improving or altering the pathway. Many institutions plan to include

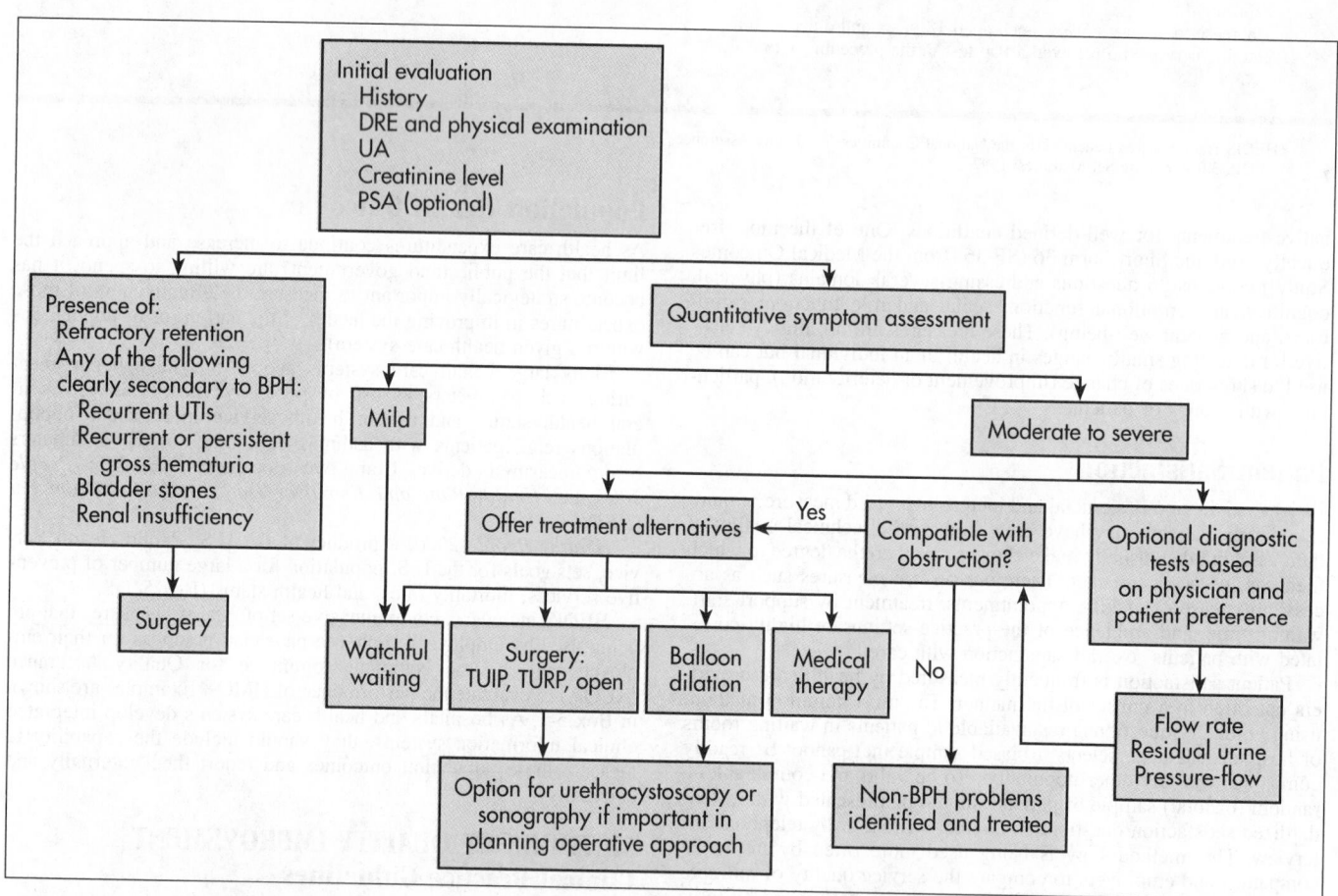

FIGURE 5-2 Clinical guideline for management of benign prostatic hyperplasia (BPH). *DRE,* Digital rectal examination; *PSA,* prostate-specific antigen; *TUIP,* transurethral incision of the prostate; *TURP,* transurethral prostatectomy; *UA,* urinalysis; *UTI,* urinary tract infection.

Modified from Agency for Health Care Policy and Research (AHCPR) Clinical Practice Guidelines for benign prostatic hypertrophy (Pub. no. 94-0582), Rockville, Md, 1994, The Agency.

Table 5-1 Critical pathway for management of lower-extremity deep venous thrombosis

DAY 1	DAY 2	DAY 3	DAY 4	DAY 5
Tests				
Standard admitting labs Screen for cancer: physical examination, CXR, urinalysis, and stool for occult blood Defer testing for hypercoagulable state to outpatient setting PTT q 4-6 hours until two consecutive results within 60-80 sec PT/INR qd with target INR of 2.0-3.0	CBC, platelets QOD PTT qd if stable at 60-80 sec	Arrange for inpatient or outpatient mammogram if woman >40 without recent mammogram		
Activity				
Bed or chair, depending on pain and need to control edema	Ambulate when pain allows after 24 hours of therapeutic heparin			
Treatment				
Local heat	Fit for graduated compressin stockings			
Medications				
In emergency department Heparin bolus and drip: use weight-based nomogram* Alternately, give 7,500 U bolus and 1,250 U/h drip Call research nurse re: DVT eligibility ***On floor*** Adjust heparin by nomogram* Pain relief medications prn Begin warfarin qAM or qPM as soon as PTT ≥60 sec. Initial dosage: 7.5 mg qd × 2d Stool softener	Heparin Adjust per nomogram* Warfarin Stool softener prn	Heparin Adjust per nomogram* Warfarin Stool softener prn	Heparin Adjust per nomogram* Warfarin Stool softener prn	Consider discharge for uncomplicated patients after 5 days of heparin and when INR = 2-3† Warfarin Stool softener prn
Diet				
No limits	No limits	No limits	No limits	No limits
Patient and family education				
1. Risks and complications of DVT (including symptoms of pulmonary embolism) 2. Risks and complications of heparin treatment 3. Need for regulation of heparin 4. Explain activity level	1. Rationale for warfarin 2. Need for daily labs 3. Explain INR target range 4. Explain INR versus PT 5. Teach how to use stockings	1. Provide patient with written instructions (e.g., warfarin teaching book) 2. Warfarin video 3. Review risk factor reduction strategies (e.g., smoking cessation)	1. Reinforce warning symptoms and signs of DVT complications	1. Arrange for next INR within 1-3 days 2. Identify the primary MD who will be responsible for follow-up care 3. Specify how patient will communicate with the primary MD 4. Phone or fax inpatient PT/INRs and warfarin dosages to primary MD

From Pearson SD et al: *Am J Med* 100:283-289, 1996.
Critical pathway for treatment of proximal lower-extremity deep vein thrombosis (DVT). Patient eligible for critical pathway unless: suspected of pulmonary embolism; is a pregnant woman; is a participant in a study protocol; or an inferior vena cava (IVC) filter is indicated for bleeding complications, current use of warfarin, acute major cerebrovascular accident, allergy to heparin, or compliance problems with warfarin treatment.
*Heparin weight-based nomogram.[1] Initial dose = 80 U/kg bolus, 18 U/kg/h. On repeat PTT: PTT <40 sec—rebolus with 80 U/kg, increase drip by 4 U/kg/h; PTT 40-60 sec—rebolus with 40 U/kg, increase drip by 2 U/kg/h; PTT 60-80 sec—no change; PTT 80-100 sec—decrease drip by 2 U/kg/h; PTT >100—hold drip for 1 hour, then decrease drip by 3 U/kg/h.
†Insufficient data to specify how many hours of heparin = 5 days. Some patients (e.g., iliofemoral DVT) likely require more days of heparin. *CXR,* Chest roentgenogram; *PTT,* partial thromboplastin time; *PT,* prothrombin time; *INR,* international normalized ratio; *CBC,* complete blood cell count; *prn,* as needed.

critical pathways and the accompanying order sets in their clinical information systems so that they will be readily available to ordering physicians.

Despite the widespread development and use of these pathways, formal evaluation of their effects on quality have, as for guidelines, been few.

Feedback of Physician Performance Data

Many institutions and, increasingly, many health care payers are collecting data on a wide variety of performance criteria and feeding that information back to individuals or groups, usually with a comparison to an appropriate peer group. The measured parameters include patient satisfaction scores, medical outcomes (e.g., cesarean section rates), performance of preventive practices (rate of Pap smears in women at risk), and resource use. In some cases these data, sometimes known as practice profiles, are returned to clinicians without further intervention with the assumption that physicians, like most professionals, want to be among the best and will consciously or unconsciously change their practice style to come closer to the benchmark. Review of effective practice profile feedback in the literature demonstrates that such feedback can improve performance, more so with individual or peer comparison feedback than with aggregate or grouped feedback. However, it also appears to be more successful when other interventions such as incentives, opinion leader reinforcement, or individual education are used in combination.

PHYSICIANS' RESPONSE TO QUALITY IMPROVEMENT

One of the obstacles to the successful implementation of clinical guidelines, critical pathways, or performance information feedback has been physician attitude. For most of their training, physicians have been taught to be individualists, to make independent decisions, and to value highly their autonomy in clinical decision making. For example, physician response to clinical guidelines is often that they represent "cookbook medicine" and that they are inappropriate for use because "my patients are different." This is often the response when physicians are first presented with clinical performance data; the data are challenged as being either incorrect or irrelevant to the patients cared for by a particular physician or group of physicians. Physicians usually consider their patients' conditions to be more complex than those of the comparison group.

Although there may be validity in some cases in these objections, more commonly when appropriate severity or case-mix adjustment is used, the trends shown by the data persist. For the previously discussed reasons it is crucial that if these efforts are to succeed, they must be supported by clinical leadership. Key clinicians should be champions of clinical guidelines and critical pathways, and physicians should scrutinize performance data carefully before releasing the information to peers. In the development of guidelines or pathways or in the adaptation for local use of published guidelines it is crucial for local "opinion leaders" to be involved in the process in order to modify the guidelines appropriately for the local environment and to prevent the "not invented here" syndrome in which physicians object to guidelines or pathways developed at other institutions.

Physician behavior can and often does change in the desired direction but variably so, depending on the methods used to induce change. Factors that have been used successfully include the following: (1) education, particularly when reinforced by opinion leaders; (2) feedback of information about practice or outcome, usually in comparison with an external standard ("benchmark") or with a peer group; (3) physician participation and leadership in developing standards or guidelines; (4) administrative interventions (e.g., restrictions on expensive drugs or changing order forms to reduce test options); (5) financial incentives or penalties (e.g., fixed reimbursements for hospital stay according to diagnosis-related group) resulting in more careful resource use. Use of each method has been reported to be successful in changing physician practice, but the combination of two or more methods is more likely to effect change.

The internist can and should be a champion of quality measurement and improvement. Internists have traditionally been "data driven" in their clinical decision making. They also frequently possess the epidemiologic, statistical, and analytic skills to evaluate aggregate data from their own or others' practices. By understanding the processes of care and by recognizing that variation in process or outcome often results from differences in practice style rather than from individual patient characteristics, the internist is ideally situated to work with colleagues to standardize and improve those processes, using explicit measurement of outcome to evaluate the results of the improvement.

What other skills are necessary for effective quality management? First, the internist must be able to work in teams, both in clinical care and in analysis of processes. Second, all clinical work must be understood as a process or series of processes. The internist must be able to collect, display, and analyze data on the *processes* and *out-*

comes of care. He or she must be able to analyze the processes of care and find opportunities to simplify and improve those processes. The internist must have the ability to define the service characteristics that lead to patient satisfaction, to measure them, and to respond by changing his or her practice when possible to meet those service requirements.

What does high quality look like in an internists' practice? An example might be illustrative. A five-physician general internal medicine practice was asked by an insurance-owned HMO to report the percentage of women over 50 years of age in their practice who received an annual mammogram. Through chart review, referral forms, and billing data, the physicians measured the group and individual physician rates, finding the group rate to be 73% but the individual rates varying among physicians from 51% to 86%. They recognized that they had five different practice styles for encouraging women to have mammograms. Because the external standard should approach 100%, they were determined to develop a system within the practice that could move them closer to that goal. Building on methods used by the physician with the 86% rate as a benchmark, they developed a standardized preventive screening matrix for every patient's chart and had the triage nurse check it and update it at each woman's visit. The nurse was authorized to order the mammogram if it was indicated. A system of follow-up calls by the secretary was begun for patients for whom a mammogram report had not been received within 4 weeks of the order.

When the physicians measured their performance 18 months after initiating this system, the group percentage had risen to 87% and the variation by individual was small, ranging from 83% to 92%. They were pleased to report this quality improvement to the HMO and at the same time began evaluating the reasons that the remaining 13% of their women patients did not receive a mammogram.

In approaching a clinical condition or evaluating care for quality it is tempting to measure multiple intermediate and final outcomes. Unless one is carrying out a robust outcomes research project, it usually suffices to choose only a few key quality outcomes that are the most important quality indicators. These should be readily available, measured in a standard way, and, ideally, collected into a clinical database from which the information can be subsequently searched and analyzed. Because such measures will increasingly be demanded by external organizations (which often do their own measurement through administrative data and patient questionnaires), it is imperative that physicians be proactive in evaluating their own performance, looking for variation in quality, and vigorously pursuing quality improvement opportunities.

BIBLIOGRAPHY

Greco P, Eisenberg JM: Changing physicians' practices, *N Engl J Med* 329:1271-1274, 1993.

Handley MR, Stuart ME: An evidence-based approach to evaluating and improving clinical practice, *HMO Practice* 8:10-19, 75-82, 1994.

Iezzoni LI et al: Predicting who dies depends on how severity is measured: implications for evaluating patient outcomes, *Ann Intern Med* 123:763-770, 1995.

Laffel G, Blumenthal D: The case for using industrial quality management science in health care organizations, *JAMA* 262:2869-2873, 1989.

Localio AR, Hamory BH: A report card for report cards, *Ann Intern Med* 123:802-803, 1995.

Salem-Schatz S et al: The case for case-mix adjustment in practice profiling: when good apples look bad, *JAMA* 272:871-874, 1994.

Schoenbaum SC: Feedback of clinical performance information, *HMO Practice* 7:5-11, 1993.

Walton M: The Deming management method, New York, 1986, Putnam Group.

Wennberg JE et al: Hospital use and mortality among medicare beneficiaries in Boston and New Haven, *N Engl J Med* 321:1168-1173, 1989.

Woolf SH: Practice guidelines: a new reality in medicine, *Arch Intern Med* 150:1811-1817, 1990.

CHAPTER

6 Implementing Clinical Practice Guidelines

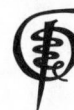

Scott Weingarten and Stephen Deutsch

During the past decade the practice of medicine has been undergoing rapid transformation as a result of economic pressures and market forces. The buyers and consumers of health care are demanding more accountability from health care plans and physicians. With health care cost containment being promoted by employer groups and governmental organizations, physicians and other health care providers are seeking new methods of improving care while maintaining or reducing health care costs. These strategies often include systematic approaches to clinical decision making. In the past, physicians and other health care providers would prescribe a diagnostic and therapeutic plan for patients based on the uniqueness of each clinical situation and the physician-patient interaction. This approach was guided by the physician's experience and understanding of the medical literature and ultimately by the patient's personal preferences regarding treatments. Clinical decisions were made in deference to clinical freedom and autonomy. Not surprisingly, medical care delivered in this manner was associated with great variability. The care that patients received depended in part on the geographic location where the care was received, as well as the particular hospital, physician organization, and physician responsible for providing that care.

Increasingly, questions are being asked regarding the cause of these variations in care. One possible explanation is that many clinical decisions cannot be supported by scientific evidence but rather are determined by an individual physician's experience and training, along with the "art of medicine." Of those clinical decisions that are based on scientific evidence, the scientific knowledge is at times inconsistent and difficult for physicians and other health care providers to access in real time while they are caring for patients. Moreover, it has been said that more than 100,000 medically related articles are published each month, and individual physicians can be expected to read and retain only a relatively small fraction of the published medical literature. Variations in care may be further accentuated by differences in preferences from patient to patient, since patients may choose different options when informed about alternative treatments. The provision of health care services is influenced by many factors, only some of which relate to the patient's medical condition.

Health services researchers have discovered a significant rate of inappropriate care, including the use of invasive procedures. Inappropriate care is defined as care in which the risks of treatment are judged by experts to exceed the potential benefits. Furthermore, it is believed that the provision of inappropriate care may contribute to rising health care costs without providing commensurate benefit to patients as demonstrated through improved patient outcomes.

Additional research has disclosed a significant gap between optimal medical care (care that would lead to the best patient outcomes) and care that is being provided on a widespread basis. Whether examining influenza immunization of elderly patients, the performance of mammograms, or the provision of the most protective forms of deep venous thrombosis prophylaxis therapy for patients undergoing total hip replacement, studies consistently demonstrate opportunities to improve the quality of patient care. Furthermore, the lack of a systematic approach to clinical decisions may at times compromise patient care. In addition, long gaps have been documented between the time that therapies are proven to be effective and their widespread adoption into clinical practice. For example, the published literature demonstrated that thrombolytic therapy was associated with a reduction in mortality long before it was widely recommended for clinical practice for patients who came to medical attention with acute myocardial infarction. Similar delays have been documented after a therapy was shown to be ineffective and before it was abandoned as a mainstay of treatment.

PRACTICE GUIDELINES

The health services research studies left a trail of observations regarding the delivery of medical care services, including unexplainable variations in medical care, the provision of inappropriate medical care, and gaps between optimal medical practice and widespread clinical practice. To address these issues, physicians and others involved in health care delivery promoted the idea that practice guidelines may remedy this situation. Medical practice guidelines, otherwise known as practice parameters or protocols, are a means of providing organized medical knowledge to clinicians that could potentially influence the care delivered to individual patients. Practice guidelines have been defined as "systematically developed statements to assist practitioner decisions about appropriate health care for specific clinical circumstances." The guidelines are often derived from systematic reviews of the scientific evidence, and the information condensed into documents to assist physicians and other clinicians. The guidelines consolidate available scientific knowledge about the best and most appropriate treatments for patients with common diseases and conditions.

Proponents of clinical guidelines believe that they will inform clinical decision making and thereby decrease undesirable variations in medical care, improve quality of care, and decrease health care costs. Practice guidelines, when used in this manner, could be applied to populations of patients as well as individual patients. However, in some circles, enthusiasm for guidelines is tempered by concerns that guidelines oversimplify the practice of medicine, devalue the "art of medicine," and infringe on physician autonomy and clinical freedom. There is also a concern that they may be used in a punitive manner or by plaintiff's attorneys against physicians and other health care providers in medical malpractice cases.

A number of organizations are either producing or sponsoring the development of practice guidelines. Those organizations include organizations associated with the United States Federal Government (United States Preventive Services Task Force [USPSTF], the Agency for Health Care Policy and Research), specialty societies (American College of Cardiology, American College of Physicians), academic medical centers, health plans, and commercial organizations. Attesting to the number of organizations producing practice guidelines, the American Medical Association's Directory of Practice Parameters lists and catalogues more than 2000 different guidelines. These guidelines, however, are of variable quality, ranging from rigorous scholarly syntheses of the available scientific evidence (e.g., American College of Physicians, Agency for Health Care Policy and Research) to guidelines that are less rigorous and comprehensive.

Although many different guidelines are in circulation, the impact of many of these guidelines on patient care is relatively unknown. Furthermore, the acceptability, credibility, and quality of individual guidelines vary. Recent studies have demonstrated that professional society guidelines receive a higher level of confidence from some physicians than guidelines produced by other sources.

With the large number of guidelines in existence it may be a daunting task for clinicians to decide which guidelines are most appropriate for their patients, and which guidelines offer the greatest opportunity to improve medical care. Guidelines vary widely in the method used to create them, the rigor with which the scientific evidence is reviewed and organized, the background of those individuals interpreting the evidence and translating the information into practice guidelines, and the resources devoted toward their development.

For many conditions there are multiple guidelines available on the same topic. Given the variability in the process used to create guidelines, it is not surprising that conflicts have been identified between different guidelines on the same topic. These conflicts can create confusion among physicians contemplating using them to assist in the care of their patients.

DEVELOPING GUIDELINES

There are different methods of developing practice guidelines. These methods include the following:

Informal consensus is a time-honored method of guideline development in which expert opinion is used as the basis for guideline development.

Formal consensus is a more systematic approach to codifying expert opinion. Multiple experts are convened, and the medical literature may be reviewed to inform the guideline decision makers.

Using the *explicit approach* to developing guidelines, developers specify the potential benefits, harms, and costs of potential interventions and derive explicit estimates of the probability of each outcome. This is an analytic approach for deriving quantitative estimates of the effects of interventions on health outcomes. This method can use both direct and indirect evidence to link interventions to patient outcomes.

Evidence-based guidelines produce recommendations that are linked to scientific evidence. Rules of evidence are emphasized over expert opinion alone.

Some physicians may inherently find evidence-based guidelines preferable to guidelines that are developed without careful review of the available scientific evidence. As the literature is reviewed, the scientific evidence can become a neutral arbiter in the consensus-building process that leads to guideline development, rather than reliance on differences in expert opinion that may not always be based on up-to-date scientific evidence. Since physicians and nurses are trained in using the scientific method, this approach to guideline development may hold significant appeal.

Creation of evidence-based guidelines requires the ability to search the medical literature for relevant medical research articles. After the published studies have been gathered, their validity is determined and the articles are critically appraised. Critical appraisal skills and techniques may be helpful for alerting guideline developers and potential users of the guidelines about the potential biases and limitations of guidelines. The Evidence-Based Working Group at McMaster University (Hamilton, Ontario, Canada) developed an explicit, structured approach for critically appraising research articles. Grading the evidence alerts users to the strength of the medical evidence and the potential biases that may confound interpretation of the study results. For example, one grading scheme yields a high grade of evidence (grade A) to information ascertained from large, double-blind, randomized, controlled clinical trials. A lower grade of evidence (grade C) is assigned when the study results are subject to greater bias (a study that is not randomized). In studies subject to greater bias the interpretation of the results and the guidelines based on these results should occur with greater caution.

Desirable attributes of practice guidelines include the following:
1. The purpose of the guideline should be clearly expressed.
2. The content must be frequently reviewed and updated regularly.
3. The guidelines must be flexible enough to account for the nuances of clinical medicine.
4. Guidelines should be easy to follow.
5. They should be applicable in a variety of geographic and health care settings.
6. They should be linked to patient outcomes, which may include morbidity, mortality, health status, quality of life, patient satisfaction, and cost of care, especially when scientific support for the recommendations is uncertain.

Evidence-based guidelines are intrinsically appealing to many clinicians, since much of medical training is predicated on the application of the scientific method. However, there are also limitations to the use of an evidence-based approach for this application. These limitations include a paucity of scientific evidence to support many common clinical practices. In other cases the evidence, when available, may be incomplete, contradictory, or of insufficient quality or credibility to be used to develop a guideline.

IMPROVING CLINICAL PRACTICE

Despite the explosive growth in the number of medical practice guidelines, until recently there has been relatively limited evidence that they have had an impact on medical care. There has been a disproportionate amount of time spent on development as compared with time spent on implementation and evaluation. However, a systematic review of the published literature on practice guidelines demonstrated that guidelines had significant potential to improve patient care. Of 59 published studies on practice guidelines, 55 demonstrated at least one significant change in care associated with the introduction of a guideline. The magnitude of the effects was variable. Moreover, of the 11

BOX 6-1

Implementation strategies for guidelines

1. Traditional education
2. Retrospective feedback
3. Concurrent feedback (reminders)
4. Incentives
5. Administrative solutions
6. "Academic detailing"
7. Opinion leaders
8. Patient education
9. Application of information technology
10. Physician (clinician) involvement in the development and implementation process

---

studies that examined patient outcomes, 9 demonstrated beneficial changes in patient care.

If a guideline is not adopted into practice, it will have relatively little impact on patient care. Many studies have demonstrated that dissemination of guidelines alone fails to produce widespread adoption, including guidelines published by prestigious scientific organizations such as the National Institutes of Health. Many barriers to physician adoption of guidelines must be overcome for guidelines to have the opportunity to improve patient care. The literature has convincingly demonstrated that a carefully crafted implementation plan is requisite for the adoption of guidelines; otherwise, there may be no sustained change in clinical practice.

Physician attitudes and beliefs about practice guidelines may influence their adoption. A recent survey of physician attitudes showed that a majority of physicians believed guidelines would be used for disciplinary actions and a significant number believed guidelines will increase health care costs, although their development was motivated by a desire to reduce costs. Less favorable attitudes were held by internists in private practice, those paid "fee-for-service," physicians in full-time practice, and those who had been practicing medicine for a longer time. While physicians' general attitudes about guidelines may not correlate with their adoption into practice, physician attitudes about specific guidelines have been shown to correlate with their adoption of those guidelines.

Many different implementation strategies have been employed to encourage clinician adoption of guidelines (Box 6-1). For example, any one of these strategies, or several of them, could be employed to implement the USPSTF guidelines on performing mammography.

The USPSTF guidelines for mammography are an excellent example of evidence-based guidelines; several levels of evidence are used to offer clinical recommendations ranging from an "A" recommendation ("there is good evidence to support the recommendation") to a "C" recommendation ("there is insufficient evidence to recommend for or against the condition in a periodic health examination, but recommendations may be made on other grounds"). Lower-level grades ("D" and "E") suggest that there is fair or good evidence for excluding the condition from the periodic examination. The recommendation of the 1996 USPSTF guideline is shown in Box 6-2.

Among the implementation strategies are the following:
1. *Traditional education.* Published studies have demonstrated that traditional continuing medical education programs fail to produce sustained changes in clinical practice. Although educational programs may appear to be a cost-effective method of gaining widespread acceptance of guidelines, available information on the effectiveness of education as a dissemination strategy suggests that expectations should be low, except when education is used in conjunction with other implementation strategies. A grand rounds or continuing medical education program could be used to inform clinicians about the USPSTF guidelines on mammography.
2. *Retrospective feedback.* Results are mixed regarding the effects of retrospective feedback and physician profiling on physician practice. Although changes in patient care have been demonstrated in studies employing retrospective feedback and profiling, the magnitude of the effect is often small. Therefore enthu-

BOX 6-2

**U.S. Preventive Services Task Force 1996 Guideline
for Screening Mammography**

Screening for breast cancer every 1 to 2 years, with mammography alone or mammography and annual clinical breast examination (CBE), is recommended for women ages 50 to 69 ("A" recommendation). Clinicians should refer patients to mammographers who use low-dose equipment and adhere to high standards of quality control. Such standards have recently been established by the Mammography Quality Standards Act, a federal law mandating that all mammography sites in the United States be accredited through a process approved by the Department of Health and Human Services. There is insufficient evidence to recommend annual CBE alone for women ages 50 to 69 ("C" recommendation). For women ages 40 to 49, there is conflicting evidence of fair to good quality regarding clinical benefit from mammography with or without CBE, and insufficient evidence regarding benefit from CBE alone; therefore, recommendations for or against routine mammography or CBE cannot be made based on the current evidence ("C" recommendation). There is no evidence specifically evaluating mammography or CBE in high-risk women younger than age 50; recommendations for screening such women may be made on other grounds, including patient preference, high burden of suffering, and the higher positive predictive value (PPV) of screening, which would lead to fewer false positives than are likely to occur from screening women of average risk in this age-group. There is limited and conflicting evidence regarding clinical benefit of mammography or CBE for women ages 70 to 74 and no evidence regarding benefit for women older than age 75; however, recommendations for screening women ages 70 and older who have a reasonable life expectancy may be made based on other grounds, such as the high burden of suffering in this age-group and the lack of evidence of differences in mammogram test characteristics in older women versus those ages 50 to 69 ("C" recommendation). There is insufficient evidence to recommend for or against teaching breast self-examination (BSE) in the periodic health examination ("C" recommendation).

siasm for physician profiling and retrospective feedback may not always be supported by proven changes in patient care.

Retrospective feedback could be used to provide clinicians with feedback about their mammography rates (e.g., 75% compliance with USPSTF mammography guidelines). Also, each clinician could compare his or her mammography rate with that of peers.

3. *Concurrent feedback (reminders).* Studies have demonstrated that real-time feedback of guideline information to physicians while they are caring for patients can be associated with significant increases in their adoption of the guidelines. Reminders enable physicians to decide whether a particular guideline is appropriate for their individual patient at the time when they are providing care. However, some studies have shown that the effects of the guidelines on clinical practice diminish when the reminders are discontinued.

To encourage adherence to USPSTF mammography guidelines, checklists, written reminders, or cues could be used to prompt physicians to perform mammograms in appropriate patients at the time of the visit (also see no. 9).

4. *Incentives.* Many studies have shown that incentives, monetary and otherwise, may significantly influence physician decision making. It stands to reason that incentives, or removal of disincentives, may promote physician adoption of practice guidelines. Linking physician reimbursement to adoption of USPSTF mammography guidelines would be considered a method of providing physicians with incentives to follow the guidelines.

5. *Administrative solutions.* In general, administrative rules have been shown to produce changes in physician practice. Therefore administrative mandates may be used to enforce adoption of guidelines, although the safety of this approach is largely unproved and the impact of this approach on physician satisfaction is unknown. An administrative solution to promote the adop-

tion of guidelines could best be illustrated by the exclusion of a particular drug from a formulary. An administrative fiat might be less appropriate for increasing adoption of USPSTF mammography guidelines.

6. *"Academic detailing."* "Academic detailing," a method involving one-on-one brief educational interactions, has been shown to change physician behavior. Face-to-face sessions may prove to be successful when the message is brief and repetitive. During these encounters the educator attempts to understand each physician's approach to a particular clinical situation. The "detailer" then explains the guideline, and the physician has the opportunity to raise questions and concerns about the potential impact of the guideline on patient care. Although this approach has been proven effective, it can be costly and labor intensive. Using the "academic detailing" model, the educator might schedule a meeting or series of meetings with each clinician to better understand their beliefs and attitudes about the USPSTF mammography guidelines. Using that information as background, the "detailer" could explain the potential benefits of following the USPSTF mammography guidelines using repetitive and brief messages.

7. *Opinion leaders.* Studies have shown that the visible support of practice guidelines by "opinion leaders" may promote adoption of the guidelines. Using a "social influence" model of changing physician behavior, local peer pressure and influence may affect practice patterns. Therefore recruiting local and influential "physician champions" to promote guidelines may prove to be effective. Respected opinion leaders could promote the USPSTF mammography guidelines.

8. *Patient education.* Patient educational programs and outreach programs can be used to promote patient understanding of the rationale behind guidelines. Patients may initiate questions with their physician that lead to adoption of the guideline (e.g., patient asks the physician whether a mammogram should be performed, since it has been more than 2 years since her last mammogram). Patient education could be used to directly inform women about the potential benefits of mammography with the hope that women who are overdue for a mammogram would contact their physician and request one.

9. *Application of information technology.* Recent technologic advances in clinical information systems have been accompanied by studies examining the use of computerized reminders to implement practice guidelines. Several of these studies have shown that real-time computer reminders lead to increased adoption of guidelines. The desire to implement multiple practice guidelines and the application of guidelines to patients with multiple conditions and comorbid illnesses will increase the potential benefits of using computerized reminders as an implementation strategy. When physicians interact with practice guidelines on a dynamic basis (such as with computerized order entry systems), computer technology may prove to be a cost-effective method of implementing several guidelines at the same time. Information technology may enable the performance of cost-effective outcomes studies and, eventually, an understanding of how systematically changing care affects patient outcomes.

Busy physicians and clinicians may be less likely to seek out guidelines if they either detract from the patient encounter or reduce time with patients. Time constraints may limit the adoption of paper-based guidelines, especially if they require a physician to search out guidelines while the patient waits in the office or the examining room. In the future, practice guidelines and other clinical decision support tools may be embedded in clinical decision support software housed in an electronic medical record. The key decision points and the guidelines to support the most appropriate clinical decisions may be linked to diagnoses, diagnostic tests, treatments, symptoms, or signs. The widespread deployment of this type of system may significantly advance attempts to implement complicated guidelines and allow for the capture of patient outcomes data and the use of this information to improve medical care. With each patient encounter computers could be used to process the age, gender, date of last mammogram (if appropriate), breast cancer risk factors (if appropriate and available), and the date of the visit to determine whether the patient is overdue for a mammogram. If the patient is overdue, the physician would be prompted to consider performing a mammogram.

10. *Physician (clinician) participation.* Social influence models suggest that the involvement of key individuals in the development of guidelines, especially those individuals involved with patient care, may encourage the eventual adoption of guidelines. Therefore many health care organizations encourage the involvement of diverse groups of health care practitioners to develop, adapt, and update guidelines. A multidisciplinary team might be assembled to review and adopt the USPSTF mammography guideline and to discuss possible strategies for effectively implementing the guideline.

The most effective guideline implementation efforts often involve several different approaches to implementation; the use of a single strategy may prove to be less effective. However, studies have shown that guidelines are imperfect and may not be relevant to many patients. In fact, a recent study demonstrated that preserving each physician's ability to override guidelines is important for maintaining the quality of patient care. Therefore, with very few exceptions, guidelines should be used to complement rather than substitute for physician decision making. Coercive implementation strategies, such as tying compliance with guidelines to physician incentives, may become problematic when the scientific evidence supporting a guideline is uncertain.

IMPACT ON PATIENT CARE

"Disease management," also known as "health care management," is a concept that has been promoted to address the comprehensive management of patients across the continuum of care. Disease management programs reduce the emphasis on treating acute episodes of illness while seeking a more comprehensive approach to the total care of a patient. The approach emphasizes preventive care and care that prevents or delays complications. Practice guidelines and clinical decision support aids are often developed to identify the primary determinants of both the quality and cost of care for patients enrolled in the disease management program. Therefore practice guidelines codify the desired diagnostic and therapeutic approach to populations of patients.

After a guideline has been implemented, especially guidelines based on uncertain scientific evidence, the effects on patient care, both intended and actual, should be evaluated. Considering the large number of guidelines that have been disseminated, relatively few have been evaluated. Measured effects could include the acceptance of the guidelines by physicians, the impact on clinical outcomes (e.g., mortality, morbidity), the effect on patient-centered outcomes (e.g., patient health status, patient satisfaction, return to work), and economic outcomes (e.g., cost of outpatient and inpatient care). There is a definable cost associated with developing, updating, implementing, and evaluating guidelines. The true economic impact of any guideline is the cost savings, if any, minus the program costs.

Practice guidelines and other systematic approaches to clinical decision making are being promoted to reduce undesirable variations in care, to reduce health care costs, and to improve quality of medical care. There is early evidence to suggest that guidelines based on available scientific evidence and implemented in an effective manner may improve patient care. However, some dissemination and implementation strategies may prove to be effective, while others may incur cost without benefit. Given the current enthusiasm for guidelines and the resources devoted to their development, the promise of guidelines may best be realized through careful attention to their implementation and evaluation in clinical practice. In this new era of physician accountability for clinical decisions and greater attention to improving the health of populations of patients, systematic approaches to clinical decision making, including the use of practice guidelines, are likely to continue to play an important role in the practice of medicine.

BIBLIOGRAPHY

Balas EA, Austin Boren S, Brown GD et al: Effect of physician profiling on utilization: meta-analysis of randomized clinical trials, *J Gen Intern Med* 11:584-590, 1996.
Brook RH: Practice guidelines and practicing medicine: are they compatible? *JAMA* 262:3027-3030, 1989.
Cook DJ, Guatt GH, Laupacis A, Sackett DL: Rules of evidence and clinical recommendations on the use of antithrombotic agents, *Chest* 102(suppl):305S-311S, 1992.
Davis DA, Thomson MA, Oxman AD et al: Changing physician performance: a systematic review of the effect of continuing medical education strategies, *JAMA* 274:700, 1995.
Eisenberg JM: *Doctors' decisions and the cost of medical care*, Ann Arbor, Mich, 1986, Health Administration Press.
Greco PJ, Eisenberg JM: Changing physicians' practices, *N Engl J Med* 329:1271-1273, 1993.
Grimshaw JM, Russell IT: Effect of clinical guidelines in medical practice: a systematic review of rigorous evaluations, *Lancet* 342:1317-1322, 1993.
Kosecoff J, Kanouse DE, Rogers WH et al: Effects of the National Institutes of Health Consensus Development Program on physician practice, *JAMA* 258:2708-2713, 1987.
Mugford M, Banfield P, O'Hanlon M: Effects of feedback of information on clinical practice: a review, *Br Med J* 303:398-402, 1991.
Pestotnik SL, Classen DC, Evans RS et al: Implementing antibiotic practice guidelines through computer-assisted decision support: clinical and financial outcomes, *Ann Intern Med* 124:884-890, 1996.
Soumerai SB, Avorn J: Principles of educational outreach ("academic detailing") to improve clinical decision making, *JAMA* 263:549-556, 1990.
Tunis SR, Hayward RSA, Wilson MC et al: Internists' attitudes about clinical practice guidelines, *Ann Intern Med* 120:956-963, 1994.
U.S. Preventive Services Task Force: *Guide to clinical preventive services*, ed 2, Baltimore, 1996, Williams & Wilkins.
Wennberg J, Gittelsohn A: Small-area variations in health care delivery, *Science* 182:1102-1108, 1973.

CHAPTER

7 Medical Informatics

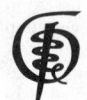

Mark E. Frisse

The availability of current, reliable medical information has always been central to the practice of internal medicine. More than a hundred years ago Osler wrote that the physician who cannot access and use current medical knowledge "flounders along in an aimless fashion, never able to gain any accurate conception of disease, practicing a sort of popgun pharmacy, hitting now the malady and again the patient, he himself not knowing which."

What Osler identified a century ago remains true today, but the context in which medicine is practiced has changed dramatically. In past eras medical care was often provided by one internist who saw the patient only episodically when acute illness arose and during prolonged periods of hospitalization. In these settings acute illness generally precipitated the office visit and, when in the hospital, the pace of patient recovery defined the use of hospital resources and the length of hospitalization. More recently internists serve as coordinators of an extensive array of health care providers and resources distributed throughout a community. Emphasizing lifetime patient care and prevention, the challenges of prevention and management of chronic illness have been added to the still daunting demands of episodic medical care. In the modern setting coordination of health promotion within a community and over the lifetime of the patient dominates the concern of the ambulatory care practitioner and, when hospitalization is indicated, financial exigencies require the internist to coordinate inpatient care and care after discharge from the hospital in a manner that maximizes patient benefit while considering the cost of this care. To meet these challenges, the internist requires access to "best practices" and a vast array of information at the point of medical care delivery.

Means by which internists obtain and communicate information are many (Table 7-1). The telephone, the textbook, and the paper-based medical record remain the dominant forms of medical communication, but they are often inadequate to meet the information needs of physicians. The rapid evolution of computer and communications technology holds the potential to be of invaluable support to the management of the patient in the modern medical care setting. Widespread availability of relatively inexpensive computers and network-based communication technologies promises secure, ubiquitous access to all types of information relative to patient care, health care administration, and professional education. Currently these technologies and information resources are at different stages of maturity and are not

Table 7-1   How new technologies are changing activities of the internist

CURRENT METHOD	EMERGING METHODS	POSSIBLE FUTURE METHODS
Hallway conversation Telephony	Telemedicine consults Electronic mail, beepers with text-messaging capabilities	Interactive "desktop" telemedicine systems Structured electronic mail and wireless communications devices integrated with clinical information systems
Prescription ordering	Internet-based prescription-writing systems	Medication-ordering systems integrated with patient profiles and effective adverse drug interaction advisors
Paper-based medical records	Limited computer-based medical records that are site specific and nonstandardized	Comprehensive computer-based medical record systems based on open standards and systems for ensuring confidentiality and privacy
Libraries, books, and journals	Analogous digital libraries delivered via CD-ROM or via the Internet	Intelligent agents designed to bring relevant information into clinical situations when it is needed
Continuing medical education	PC-based, interactive continuing medical education programs	Network-based continuing medical education programs based on educational objectives and integrated into clinical practice settings

well integrated, and the practice of internal medicine finds itself in a period of great transition from an era characterized solely by paper, voice, and telephony to a new era in which these methods of communication are enhanced or supplanted by digital communications. Information technology has the potential to change every aspect of medical communication, from the traditional "curbside" medical consult to the provision of continuing medical education. In some areas of medical practice systems are already in place in many clinical settings. In other areas prototypes are only beginning to demonstrate the potential of new information technology. In this period of transition one can only identify general themes underlying the use of information technology in medicine and outline how these concepts are being realized in two areas of most current interest to the internist—the computer-based medical record and Internet-based digital medical libraries.

COMPUTER-BASED MEDICAL RECORD

The record of the medical care of the patient has traditionally been kept separate from the record of its financial consequences. In the hospital setting most information systems concerned themselves more with the business processes of the hospital than with the clinical care of the patient. As a result, clinical information systems usually were composed of simple patient management issues like scheduling, laboratory reports, and radiographic study summaries. These systems were more concerned with the notion of medical care as a manipulation of objects (e.g., patients, blood samples, x-rays) and less concerned with the notion of medical care as the manipulation of medical knowledge (e.g., diagnostic aids, therapeutic recommendations, clinical monitoring, evidence-based medical practice).

In the early 1980s the nature of hospital-based medical practice changed dramatically with the introduction of a legislatively mandated system for Medicare payment based on diagnosis-related groups (DRGs). Under this system most hospital reimbursement would be based on the active problems leading to hospitalization rather than on the amount of services delivered in treating these problems. These problems would be identified by using discharge diagnoses encoded in the International Classification of Diseases (ICD) terminology. For the first time, those responsible for the financial aspects of hospitalization had to take a much greater interest not just in the care delivered, but also in the extent to which this care represented the optimal balance between the needs of the patient and the resource constraints on the institution. In the ensuing years emphasis on capitation-based health care financing has been extended to encompass professional services for Medicare patients and, increasingly, a number of different health maintenance and "managed care" schemes, all directed more toward the goal of cost-effective lifetime medical care and away from earlier methods emphasizing physician autonomy.

The coupling of health care financing with medical practice provides strong incentives for the development of systems that enhance the consistency and quality of medical care for individuals while also providing better data for the cost-effective management of the health care of large populations. Although most current hospital and practice-based systems do not completely meet either the clinical needs of physicians or the administrative needs of managers, there is increasing

evidence that systems that are of benefit to clinicians and patients can also benefit those concerned with medical costs. Much evidence in support of this claim comes from recent medical informatics research. For example, clinical reminder systems based on computer-based medical records can increase adherence to preventive medicine guidelines; physician-based computer order writing has been shown to significantly lower patient charges and hospital costs.

The characteristics of the computer-based patient record required by the practitioner depend on a number of core infrastructure elements (Table 7-2). Central to an effective system is a clinical database that can integrate diverse collections of information. At first glance, the creation of a clinical database may seem to be a straightforward application of a microcomputer program: it is not. Although simple microcomputer databases can be useful for clinical trials and extremely limited practice settings, most of the breadth of a general medical practice requires a complex database that may take months or years to construct. Clinical vocabularies are also a core component of a medical information system. These vocabularies relate the terms used by the practitioner with the codes necessary for billing and medical nomenclature. Often, different hospital and ambulatory care systems use slightly different codes to represent the same medical concept. For this reason, communication of data between different medical information systems can be difficult. A secure network connection is also a core element of any clinical information system. Measures taken to ensure easy access by qualified individuals while preventing unauthorized access are extremely important in the maintenance of trust between practitioner and patient. An easy-to-use computer-human interface is essential for regular clinical use. Increasingly, these interfaces are being created using World Wide Web browser technology, handheld personal computers, and in some instances even voice recognition. Although the type of instrument used to access clinical data may differ from setting to setting, its uniformity and ease of use are necessary for acceptance.

The way in which these core elements are combined to create an information system will vary. For example, some systems are extremely useful in the ambulatory care setting. These systems often simplify management of information within a medical practice, but often their ease of use is offset by difficulties in importing clinical information resident in hospital information systems or other databases. Other systems are better suited for large-scale health care enterprises but are less flexible and adaptable to the preferences of individual practitioners. Herein lies the major dilemma for the practitioner. Systems that are optimized for the practice of an individual or small group often cannot be easily integrated with systems from other groups or larger organizations. Systems suitable for larger organizations often impose on the individual practitioner a manner of clinical data management that is not the best fit with his or her practice preferences. Recently vendors of health care information systems are adopting common standards for data representation and communication. This should enable clinicians to use systems that are both optimal for practice and easily integrated with larger enterprises.

The same tension between the ease of use of smaller systems and the comprehensive nature of larger systems is seen in other information management needs. Scheduling software—a critical aspect of effective, coordinated medical practice—must be powerful enough to

Table 7-2 Components of the computer-based patient record

COMPONENT	CURRENT EXAMPLE	POSSIBLE FUTURE EXAMPLES
Network infrastructure	High-speed hospital networks, the Internet, dial-up access	Networks capable of delivering full-motion video and teleconferencing in the office and in the home
Security software	Public-key encryption systems, patient identification cards	Access based on encryption and identification from voice, retinal scan, or fingerprint
Databases	Distributed databases, each holding a portion of the medical record	Integrated databases capable of delivering a comprehensive medical record; "smart cards" capable of holding important personal medical information
Clinical lexicons	Coding systems used for diagnosis and billing (e.g., CPT, SNOP, ICD), specialized thesauri	Comprehensive, integrated links between codes used for diagnosis, treatment, and other aspects of health care delivery
Computer-human interface	Windows, mice, pen-based systems	Voice recognition; small, portable computers specialized for home health care, hospital rounds, and other tasks
Scheduling software	Isolated scheduling systems that do not communicate well with systems from other groups	Open standards systems that facilitate scheduling within and between health care delivery systems
Clinical reminder systems	Computer-based reminders based on generic risk stratification and delivery patterns	Customized reminders based on the unique attributes of patients and their health care delivery system
Adverse drug interaction systems	Comprehensive compendia of adverse drug reactions; some automated reminders based on limited dosage and clinical information	Highly "intelligent" software capable of discerning specific aspects of the clinical context and delivering reminders only when indicated
Clinical pathways, critical pathways, and patient care guidelines	Flow charts and other task-based systems for routine and relatively uncomplicated clinical problems	Sophisticated systems that will allow for effective management of complex problems and will be capable of handling exceptional cases in an effective way
Electronic mail	E-mail based on the sender and the time a message is sent	Work flow, "groupware" systems in which e-mail priorities are based on the acuity of a medical problem and the degree of urgency required
Reference works	CD-ROM or Internet-based compendia of traditional published materials	Patient care materials and data specifically produced for management of patients within a large, comprehensive health care system

optimize the allocation of resources to meet patient demands, yet flexible enough to accommodate the invariably unsuspected events that complicate the scheduling of patients across a complex set of procedures and office visits. Clinical reminder systems and adverse drug interaction systems, if properly linked to clinical data, may be able to enhance the reliability of routine screening health maintenance procedures and possibly dangerous drug interactions but these systems will require much work to ensure that their "advice" is sound across a wide range of clinical contexts. Clinical pathway software can evolve to serve as a map for all aspects of the care of a patient, regardless of the impact of specific actions on outcomes. Critical pathways software—a subset of clinical pathway systems—defines the rate-limiting steps to delivery of high-quality, cost-effective medical care. Initially focusing only on routine, high-volume procedures in which the course of events can be clearly delineated, over time clinical and critical pathway systems may evolve to systems that support a comfortable "buffer zone" capable of ensuring both physician judgment and care monitoring across a wide variety of medical problems.

Electronic mail (e-mail) is currently an adjunct to clinical care but promises to become a vital component of clinical practice support. Increasingly, e-mail will be used to solicit advice from health care professionals and to facilitate communication between parties engaged in the care of a common patient population. Medical discussions, clinical problem solving, adherence to guidelines, perusal of the medical literature, and medical communication all merge into a seamless set of human interactions facilitated—but not controlled—by the computer.

The embodiment of the medical record in digital form—the computer-based patient record (CPR)—holds both great promise and great peril for the internist. The promise lies in the ability to record and have available all information relevant to the care of the patient, to have automated assistance in monitoring treatment and appropriate drug dosage, to integrate active clinical problems with recent relevant medical literature, to link community health care information with appropriate public health agencies, and to provide adequate lifelong medical care for patients and populations. However, the perils associated with the CPR are equally significant. As information systems become more ubiquitous, they will be vulnerable to abuse and privacy violations if not created and managed correctly. In its finest form CPR is both the embodiment of the highest standards of medical practice

and the means by which the profession can learn more about improving these processes and enhancing the quality of patient care.

INTERNET-BASED MEDICAL INFORMATION

The Internet and related technologies will play an increasingly important role in the practice of medical care. Just as the distributed CPR will allow for near-instantaneous updating of clinical information and the availability of a comprehensive clinical record for those involved in patient care, the Internet promises to make available documents and current information to the medical practitioner (Table 7-3). Never has the need for such technologies been more acute. For example, conventional paper-based publishing processes require long delays between the authoring of a document and its receipt by interested readers. Because ideas must be communicated through physical objects (journals and books), the process requires literally tons of paper and enormous resources to move these printed resources from the writer to the reader. The Internet allows for the creation of an entirely different marketplace for medical information; publications become digital entities rather than paper, and they can be copied an infinite number of times and rapidly transmitted almost anywhere at a fraction of the cost of paper-based publications.

Like the CPR, Internet-based medical resources offer both promise and peril. The promise lies in the ability to update information rapidly and at low cost. For the writer the Internet offers an instantaneous readership for ideas; for the reader, a vast array of writings heretofore not available. But in this immediacy lies some of the peril of Internet-based publishing. In this environment the quality of publication may suffer: the degree of peer review is seldom known, the validity of information is often questionable, the credibility of the author is often not apparent, and the degree of consensus on published assertions is hard to know. Copyright laws may also change the financial aspects of information access and lead to increased charges for libraries and other groups. Increasingly, when seeking medical information on the Internet, one is flooded with information and is in essence trying to "drink from a fire hose." The din of thousands of ephemeral documents on a topic may drown out the truly relevant work valuable to the immediate needs of patient care.

For the reasons just mentioned it seems clear that the primary means by which clinicians will seek out Internet-based information

Table 7-3 Internet-based medical information resources

TYPE OF SERVICE	CHARACTERISTICS
The National Library of Medicine and related resources	Provide inexpensive access to MEDLINE and other citation databases; provide Agency for Health Care Policy and Research clinical guideline data. Numerous specialty resources available through the National Cancer Institute and other agencies
Local and regional medical libraries	Provide search services and resources catered to the needs of an individual institution or region; helpful in identifying the most cost-effective way of obtaining published clinical information
General-purpose Internet providers	Provide inexpensive access to services for individuals, families, and professionals; ample consumer health information resources and some biomedical literature resources
Professional societies	Provide access to Internet-based resources tailored to the needs of a specialty group; emerging as the dominant form of communication between professional societies and their members.
Individual medical journals	Provide immediate access to published journals and late-breaking medical news
Publishing consortia	Provide access to collections of journals and textbooks; recently published information may not appear in these resources as quickly as it appears in the sites of individual journals
Specialized services for health care institutions	Resellers for a wide range of citation databases and full-text journal collections obtained from the National Library of Medicine and publishers; generally marketed through medical libraries and offered to all members of a medical school, hospital, state, or health care provider
Specialized services for physicians	Offer many of the same services provided by other on-line literature providers and add to these collections a number of other services of value to the individual practitioner; sold to individuals or groups; services offered at no charge generally receive their revenue through advertising or coupling reader profiles with pharmaceutical marketing
Consumer information resources	Provide individuals with information concerning health care plans, costs, and services; provide members, when enrolled in a health care plan, with consumer health information and plan-specific guidelines for medical care

will be through some credible intermediary. In some instances this intermediary may be the professional librarian, whose job will change from managing a physical collection to managing a list of relevant links between the needs of the clinical community and the publications available in digital form. In other instances the intermediaries may be the on-line resources of the professional society, the professional journal, the commercial publishing firm, or the health care system in which one is employed. In each case the sustained excellence of an Internet resource will be ensured only if there is sufficient financial support. For this reason one must be wary of "free" services. In some instances services offering Medline searching at no cost to registered users may maintain a record of searches performed by a practitioner, in order to develop more effective marketing strategies for pharmaceuticals and other medical services. One must always remember that while one is learning about Internet-based resources, these products and services may be very busy characterizing the user; the feeling of privacy one has when using an on-line system may be an illusion.

The ability to distribute a message across the world in only a few seconds leads to powerful and sometimes disruptive changes in society. Although physicians are well trained not to discuss the affairs of their patients when in elevators or other public places, new communication technologies allow these same individuals to discuss confidential matters over discussion forums, e-mail, or newsgroups. Often the authors of sensitive documents write impulsively without giving thought to the damage that may result if a message to a colleague is intentionally or unintentionally distributed to a wider audience. Although the technology is changing rapidly, in most current computer systems one cannot guarantee that any personal message will be delivered in a secure form only to the intended recipients. As many e-mail users have discovered, one cannot generally "retract" a message that has already been sent, and the potential damage of an electronically disseminated regrettable utterance is far more substantive than if the same utterance was made in a hallway or an office. Similarly, all messages sent over the Internet must be assumed to be permanent, and the long-term implications of a recorded message must be considered. Messages that may seem appropriate within the context of an acute problem may appear very different when read at a later date in a different context. Although the legal status of e-mail in the medical setting remains a matter of debate, potential legal implications must be considered along with other ethical issues.

CONCLUSION

The practice of internal medicine will always center on the relationship between a patient and his or her physician working together with a wide array of other health care professionals. Information technol-

ogy promises to change both the manner in which physicians manage patient information and the way in which physicians communicate. Increasingly, the CPR will be the only repository for medical information on the care of the patient. This comprehensive nature of the emerging CPR requires that the internist be sure the record is accurate, comprehensive, and made available in the right context of privacy and confidentiality. Similarly, the increasing availability of educational information over the Internet holds the promise of creating new communities of practitioners and patients. Issues of reliability, credibility, and social convention must be pondered increasingly as these resources become more prevalent. As in the case of medical practice, the acquisition and effective use of information are best achieved in partnership with colleagues and trained information professionals.

BIBLIOGRAPHY

Covell DG, Uman GC, Manning PR: Information needs in office practice: are they being met? *Ann Intern Med* 103(3):569-599, 1985.

Dick R, Steen EB, editors: *The computer-based patient record: an essential technology for health care,* Washington, DC, 1991, National Academy Press.

Kiley R: *Medical information on the Internet: a guide for health professionals,* New York, 1996, Churchill Livingstone.

Osheroff JA: *Computers in clinical practice: managing patients, information, and communication,* Philadelphia, 1995, American College of Physicians.

Shortliffe EH et al: *Medical informatics: computer applications in health care,* Reading, Mass, 1990, Addison-Wesley.

Sittig DF, Stead WW: Computer-based physician order entry: the state of the art, *J Am Med Informatics Assoc* 2:108-123, 1994.

Tierney WM et al: Physician inpatient order writing on computer workstations: effects on resource utilization, *JAMA* 269(3):379-383, 1993.

Van Bemmel JH, Musen M, editors: *Handbook of medical informatics,* Houten, Netherlands, 1997, Bohn Stafleu Van Loghum.

CHAPTER

8 Managed Care

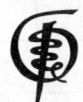

Andrew B. Bindman

Managed care in the United States began more than 60 years ago. It was not until the 1990s, however, that the majority of the overall population began receiving its health care through this type of insurance plan. In large part fueled by concerns about runaway health care costs, managed care is rapidly becoming the predominant health care delivery model in the United States. Managed care was credited with lowering health care costs to large employers in 1994 for the first time in more than two decades. Between 1985 and 1995 the number of people enrolled in health maintenance organizations (HMOs) increased by 300% (Fig. 8-1). In California, where organizational changes are among the fastest in the country, virtually the entire privately insured population is enrolled in some form of managed care. Nationwide, more than 75% of physicians are involved in some type of a managed care contract; such contracts result in an estimated 34% of their total revenues.

Managed care describes an integrated relationship between a health insurance plan and the providers who care for that plan's patients. In managed care a health insurance plan forms contracts with physicians and hospitals to provide for the comprehensive health care needs of the plan's enrollees. These contracts typically specify a fixed amount of money that will be paid for the care of the patient population and often place providers at some financial risk. Retrospective and prospective reviews are used to reduce the chance that limits on payments to providers will decrease the quality of care.

In traditional indemnity-based insurance a physician is paid on a fee-for-service basis for patient care. There is little oversight of the physician's decision making beyond the limits a plan sets on what services it covers. Indemnity-based insurance does not create any financial or other barriers that prevent a physician from advocating on a patient's behalf for any medical services that are perceived to be necessary. If anything, indemnity-based insurance creates an incentive for physicians to provide excessive care, since all services, independent of their appropriateness, are reimbursed. Health plans are more actively involved in physicians' practice decisions in managed care than they are in indemnity-based insurance plans.

It is becoming increasingly difficult to classify managed care plans (Table 8-1). The competition among plans for patients is forcing them to borrow and adapt strategies for controlling costs and maintaining

quality that are acceptable to the target enrollee population. In broad terms, most managed care plans can be described as either preferred provider organizations (PPOs) or HMOs. The PPO model is more similar to traditional indemnity insurance than is the HMO model. In a PPO a health insurance plan negotiates a reduced fee-for-service rate from physicians in exchange for the contracted physicians having an exclusive opportunity to provide care to the patients who sign up with that plan. In traditional PPOs, plans will not cover the cost of patients seeing physicians who are not under contract with the PPO. Point of service (POS) plans are a variant of PPOs in which patients are given a financial incentive to see the physicians who are under contract with the plan, but the plan will also pay some of the cost of seeing physicians who are outside the plan. The patients of a particular PPO or POS plan tend to form only a portion of a provider's overall practice.

There are two main types of HMOs: independent practice associations (IPAs) and group or staff model HMOs. Independent practice associations are loose networks of providers who typically remain in their office-based locations and who may or may not have a previous affiliation with one another. Similar to a PPO, a particular IPA's patients tend to form only a portion of an IPA provider's practice. In an IPA, however, providers often agree to accept at least part of the financial risk of caring for patients. In group model HMOs (e.g., Kaiser) physicians organize themselves into one or more groups of multispecialty practices that contract with a health plan to provide patient services, and their entire practice tends to be derived from the HMO. In staff model HMOs physicians are employees of the health plan. In HMO models, patients are covered only for care delivered by the HMO and providers are usually paid a fixed amount for their services. The fixed amount can be in the form of salary or as capitated payments. Capitated payments are predetermined monthly (or, rarely, yearly) dollar amounts for each managed care patient assigned to a provider. Plans and providers can agree to use the same capitation payment for all of the plan's enrollees but, more commonly, a

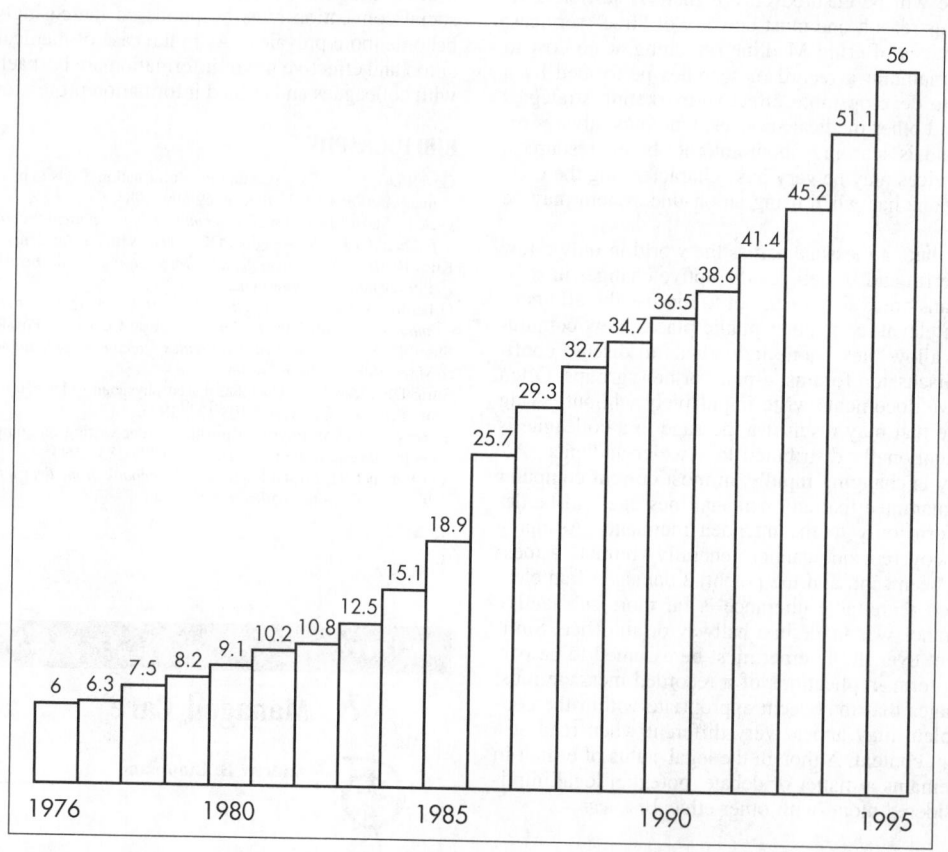

FIGURE 8-1 Number of people receiving their care in health maintenance organizations: 1976 to 1995 (millions).

From 1995 National Directory of HMOs, Group Health Association of America.

few different capitation amounts are used based on patient characteristics such as age and gender.

Managed care plans are in different stages of development throughout the country, but several trends are apparent. Health plans and providers are consolidating their services. Whereas the number of enrollees in managed care continues to climb, the total number of managed care plans is declining. Between 1977 and 1987 the number of HMOs in the United States grew from 165 to a peak of 650 plans. In the 1990s there have never been more than 600 plans. The greatest growth is among IPA plans and for-profit plans. Similarly, physicians are moving from solo and small-group practices to group and network arrangements. Between 1965 and 1991 the percentage of physicians in group practice grew from 10% to 33%. During the same time period the average number of physicians per group increased from 6 to 12.

Much of the private health insurance market has moved to managed care, and public health insurance programs are rapidly making this transition as well. Both the Medicaid and Medicare programs are expanding their use of managed care (Fig. 8-2). In 1995, more than 11 million Medicaid recipients and almost 4 million Medicare enrollees received their health care through managed care.

In most states Medicaid programs are sometimes using voluntary and, increasingly, mandatory approaches to shift their populations to managed care. In some cases this transition is accompanied by an expansion of the populations eligible to receive Medicaid-sponsored services. The stated purposes of expanding Medicaid's use of managed care are to lower health care costs and to improve access to providers who have refused to participate in fee-for-service–based state Medicaid programs. The pace at which Medicaid programs are changing health care delivery for their low-income, disabled, and el-

Table 8-1   Organization of health care delivery

INTENSITY OF MANAGED CARE	ORGANIZATION FORM	DEFINITION
Least managed	Indemnity plan with fee-for-service (FFS)	Complete freedom of choice to patients; insurer reimburses physicians on an FFS basis
	Managed indemnity plan (MIP)	Free choice and FFS, but insurer exercises some degree of utilization control to manage costs
	Preferred provider organization (PPO)	Insurer channels patients to "preferred" physicians who are usually paid discounted FFS; the insurer, not the physician, usually accepts financial risk for performance
	Point of service (POS) plan	Insurer uses financial incentives to channel patients to contracted physicians, but patients have some insurance coverage for providers outside the plan
	Independent practice association (IPA)	Insurer channels patients to physicians, usually solo or in small groups, who have agreed to some financial risk for performance; payment may be either capitation or FFS with financial incentives based on performance
	Network IPA	Similar to IPA but consists of a network of larger group practices; payment is usually capitation to each group, which then pays the physicians
	Staff/group health maintenance organization (HMO)	The classic prepaid, large multispecialty, group practice; patients are covered only for care delivered by the HMO; the doctors are usually salaried and work either for the plan (staff model HMO), or for a physician group practice (group model HMO) that has an exclusive contract with the plan
Most managed		

From the Council on Graduate Medical Education: Sixth report: managed health care—implications for the physician workforce and medical education, Washington, DC, 1995, US Department of Health and Human Services.

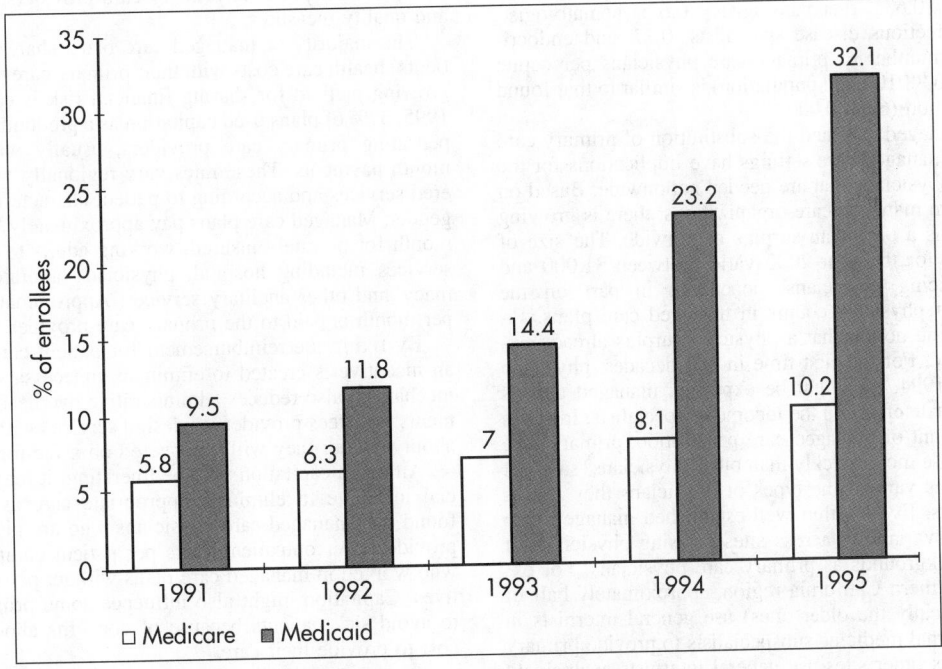

FIGURE 8-2   Managed care as a percentage of total Medicaid and Medicare.
From Group Health Association of America, Washington, DC, 1995, National Directory of HMOs database.

derly populations has raised concern about whether adequate safeguards are in place to ensure that Medicaid managed care does not erode the access to and quality of health care for these target populations. Evaluation of Medicaid managed care has been limited, and because of variation in how states structure their programs, the results are quite mixed.

Medicare's expansion into managed care is occurring almost exclusively through enrollees volunteering to receive their health care through managed care organizations. It is unlikely that Medicare will mandate managed care for its enrollees, since such a policy would not be acceptable in the near term for the constituency, predominantly elderly individuals, covered by this entitlement program. Typically, Medicare enrollees are provided with incentives such as the elimination of copayments or the expansion of covered services such as eyeglasses as a means to induce them to elect managed care over indemnity-based insurance plans. Unlike Medicaid managed care, which is prevalent throughout the country, most of the growth of Medicare managed care has been in particular markets such as the West (California and Arizona) and the South (Florida).

MANAGED CARE WORKFORCE

The constellation of physicians in managed care plans is different from that found in the general population. Managed care plans use fewer physicians than indemnity insurance plans to care for their patient populations. In 1992, estimates of the number of physicians per 100,000 population ranged from 77 to 119 among several surveyed HMOs, whereas the estimate was 180 for the general U.S. population overall. Furthermore, in group and staff model HMOs a higher percentage of generalist physicians is used to care for the population than is used in indemnity-based insurance plans. In HMOs the ratio of primary care physicians to subspecialty physicians is approximately 50:50, whereas the United States as a whole has approximately one third of practicing physicians identifying themselves as primary care physicians. The 50:50 ratio of primary care and specialty physicians found in group and staff model HMOs is similar to that found nationwide in most other industrialized countries. When one compares the physician staffing patterns available in the national physician supply pool with that of a typical group model HMO, there is an apparent excess of physicians nationwide in all of the internal medicine subspecialties. The ratio of the number of subspecialists per capita in a group model HMO to the number per capita in the U.S. population is less than 1.0. The ratios for subspecialists are as follows: cardiologists, 0.50; gastroenterologists, 0.53; pulmonologists, 0.59; nephrologists, 0.63; rheumatologists, 0.67; hematologist-oncologists, 0.67; infectious disease specialists, 0.77; and endocrinologists, 0.77. The number of primary care physicians per capita found in HMOs (54 to 88/100,000 population) is similar to that found in the general population (63/100,000).

The growth of managed care and the substitution of primary care for specialty care in managed care settings have implications for the number and type of physicians that are needed nationwide. Based on estimates derived from managed care organizations, there is growing consensus that there is a physician surplus nationwide. The size of the surplus projected for the year 2000 varies between 31,000 and 165,000 extra practicing physicians, depending in part on the suspected accuracy of physician counts in managed care plans. Financial data support the notion that a physician surplus already exists in the marketplace. For the first time in two decades, physician incomes dropped in 1994. As might be expected, managed care is having a disproportionate effect on the income of specialists. In states with the greatest amount of managed care penetration, primary care physicians' salaries rose more quickly than other physicians' salaries.

Managed care plans vary in the types of physicians they use as primary care providers. Even within well-established managed care organizations there is variability across sites in using physicians of different specialty backgrounds as primary care physicians. For example, in Kaiser's northern California region, approximately half of the clinical sites (typically the older ones) use general internists in combination with internal medicine subspecialists to provide primary care to adults, whereas other sites use general internists exclusively with family practitioners, with no internal medicine subspecialists serving as primary care physicians. In several states, including California, "direct-access" laws require managed care organizations to allow women to also choose obstetrician-gynecologists as primary care providers.

MANAGED CARE GATEKEEPER

The emphasis on the primary care provider is incorporated into more than 90% of HMOs by extending these physicians' roles into that of gatekeepers. As gatekeepers, physicians not only are responsible for the primary care functions, but also are the fulcrum for curtailing costs by matching patients' needs and preferences with the appropriate use of medical services. Some physicians object to the term "gatekeeper" because it implies that they are agents for an insurance plan rather than advocates for their patients. Those who view it more positively perceive the gatekeeping role as an opportunity to protect patients from unnecessary care. Managed care plans that use gatekeepers typically require patients to obtain the prior approval of their primary care provider to make use of emergency department, specialty, hospital, and other high-cost services. Without the approval of the primary care provider the patient may be at risk for these service charges.

While managed care plans have rapidly embraced primary care providers and their gatekeeper role, there has been little study of the independent contribution of primary care gatekeepers to cost savings and quality in managed care plans. Martin and others (1989) conducted a randomized trial within a managed care plan examining whether a primary care gatekeeper was associated with additional cost savings. Patients who were assigned a primary care gatekeeper had a greater proportion of their ambulatory visits with a primary care physician than with a specialist physician. This resulted in significantly lower ambulatory care charges ($21 per person per year) for patients assigned a primary care gatekeeper; however, hospital and total health care costs were not significantly different between the two groups.

MANAGING THE GATEKEEPER

To maximize the potential benefits of primary care physicians, managed care plans are, increasingly, attempting to manage the behavior of their gatekeepers. Managed care plans are exercising their influence over their primary care gatekeepers by (1) sharing financial risk with the primary care providers, usually through capitated payments; (2) developing exclusive contracting relationships; (3) scrutinizing primary care providers' decision making with utilization management tools; and (4) profiling primary care providers' performance on cost and quality measures.

The majority of managed care plans share financial risk for patients' health care costs with their primary care providers. The fastest-growing method for sharing financial risk is capitated payments. In 1995, 37% of plans used capitation as a predominant method for compensating primary care providers, usually with per-member, per-month payments. These rates vary regionally with the range of covered services and according to patient characteristics such as age and gender. Managed care plans pay approximately $100 per member per month for privately insured, working adults to receive medical care services including hospital, physician, laboratory, radiology, pharmacy, and other ancillary services. Approximately $10 per member per month is paid to the primary care provider.

By fixing the reimbursement for patient care through capitation, an incentive is created to eliminate unnecessary care. This payment mechanism also reduces administrative overhead in determining payments and frees providers to design services without being concerned about whether they will be covered on a fee-for-service basis.

Although capitation may be liberating, it may also create a financial incentive to eliminate appropriate care as well. Research has found that managed care physicians who are placed at financial risk provide fewer outpatient visits per patient compared with providers who worked in managed care plans without personal financial incentives. Capitation might also influence some primary care physicians to avoid sick patients because of concerns about how much it will cost to provide their care.

A growing trend in some IPA managed care plans is to capitate payments for specialists as well as primary care physicians. This removes the financial risk on primary care physicians for referring patients to specialists. Furthermore, it creates an incentive for specialists to decrease the intensity of services they provide patients and to quickly refer patients back to primary care providers.

A second mechanism by which managed care plans attempt to control providers is through exclusive contracts. Whereas it is typical for physicians in group and staff model HMOs to care exclusively for patients in their plan, this is not generally the case for PPO and IPA models. A recent General Accounting Office report found that fewer than 15% of primary care physicians received more than 30% of their patients from a single IPA. However, in a number of plans physicians are being offered financial incentives to sign exclusive contracting agreements because plans believe this will enhance their ability to influence physician practice behaviors. Concerned that exclusive contracting relationships could have a negative impact on competition, some states have passed laws making them illegal except for group and staff model HMOs.

Even with shared financial risk and exclusive contracts, 95% of managed care plans use health care utilization management tools to control primary care practices. IPA model HMOs tend to implement utilization review controls to a greater degree than in the staff or group model HMOs. Utilization review enables the managed care organization to alter the clinical plan developed between a physician and patient, and the utilization review controls have not been liked by patients or providers. Typically these strategies require primary care providers to obtain authorization from a nurse or another health care professional working on behalf of the plan before ordering expensive diagnostic tests, therapeutic procedures, or hospitalizations. The most visible challenge to utilization review was the condemnation by patients and providers of forcing new mothers to be discharged from the hospital less than 48 hours after delivery. Recently, federal legislation was passed preventing this practice. Utilization review approaches lead to a global decrease in service use. It has not been demonstrated, however, that utilization review accurately identifies and eliminates unnecessary care.

In addition to utilization review, managed care plans are using physician profiles to make decisions about whether they will contract with a particular physician or group. Most managed care plans obtain at least a qualitative description of a primary care provider's practice style before establishing a contract. Once primary care physicians are in a plan, decisions about retaining them are in part based on physician profiles generated by monitoring several aspects of practice, including number of visits per patient, rates of specialty referral, use of laboratory and expensive diagnostic tests, and hospitalization rates. Presently, few of the quality of care data are monitored, and monitoring tends to focus on immunization and cancer screening rates rather than on patients' health outcomes. There are no published reports demonstrating the validity of any cost or quality indicator used for physician profiling.

In many cases physicians are not aware of what aspects of their care is being monitored. They may first learn of their results in conjunction with being informed that their contract with a plan is ending (decertification) based on their performance. Physicians confronted with poor performance evaluations raise the argument that their performance might have appeared better had their patients complied with all of their recommendations. The majority of managed care plans, including those run by physicians, do not statistically correct physician profiles for differences in their patient populations (risk adjustment). The legality of either not offering or terminating contracts with physicians on the basis of these profiles has been challenged by individual physicians and at least two state medical societies, who argue that the profiling methodology is often cryptic and flawed. In addition, several states have enacted "any willing provider" laws that require health plans to contract with any physician who is willing to accept the terms of the plan. Managed care plans object to such legislation, asserting that controlling the choice of providers is essential for addressing health care costs.

PHYSICIAN AND PATIENT RELATIONSHIPS

The growth of managed care is leading to an evolution not only in the relationship between physicians and health plans, but also in the relationship between physicians and patients. Increasing numbers of patients are enrolling in managed care plans; however, in many cases

enrollment is due to an employer's rather than the patients' choice. Therefore the increased choice of managed care plans cannot be construed as an indicator that patients are more satisfied with these plans. In fact, patients in indemnity-based insurance plans tend to rate their satisfaction with care higher than those in managed care plans. Studies suggest that patients' interpersonal relationships with their primary care physicians do not differ dramatically across health plan settings, but patients tend to believe that physician visits are more rushed in managed care settings than in fee-for-service practices.

The increased use of capitation for primary care providers in managed care settings has the potential to create a perception that physicians are being paid to provide less than optimal care. Primary care physicians in managed care are required to balance the concerns of the patient, other patients in the plan, and their own financial risk in deciding how to ration access to specialists and diagnostic tests. Practice guidelines may provide physicians with some help in determining the appropriate choices to make with a particular patient; however, data deficiencies are likely to result in some inconsistent decisions that can undermine the public's confidence.

The public's trust in their personal physician may be further undermined by the revelation that some physicians have signed agreements ("gag clauses") with managed care plans that prohibit them from informing patients about a plan's use of financial incentives with providers or perceived deficiencies in the type or quality of health plan services.

MANAGED CARE QUALITY

Although financial incentives at the plan and provider level create the potential for undermining the quality of care delivered, several studies suggest that the process and outcomes of care in managed care plans are as good as if not better than in indemnity-based insurance plans. The limited number of studies on managed care plan quality does not allow comparisons among the different types of managed care plan models. Furthermore, the speed with which managed care plans are forming and changing may limit the generalizability of the research. However, there are reasons to suspect that integrated managed care practices are better equipped than solo practitioners to share rapidly changing information and technical expertise that is required to provide high-quality care.

Compared with indemnity-based plans, HMO plans have lower hospital admission rates and shorter lengths of hospital stays. HMO plan enrollees receive more health promotion activities, preventive tests, procedures, and examinations than do enrollees in indemnity-based plans. Predominantly by means of chart review and patient self-report data, patients with a variety of chronic conditions have been found to have similar outcomes in HMO and indemnity-based plans. Most of the study designs have been observational rather than randomized and are confounded by the fact that healthier patients disproportionately select managed care rather than indemnity-based insurance plans. Researchers performing the Medical Outcomes Study undertook one of the most ambitious attempts to date to examine health outcomes over time, adjusting for differences in patient severity between managed care and indemnity-based insurance plans. They followed hypertensive and diabetic patients who were cared for in staff model HMOs, IPAs, and indemnity-based insurance plans over a 4-year period and found no significant differences in physiologic and self-rated health associated with the type of insurance plan.

A few studies raise questions about the ability of managed care plans to provide high-quality care to certain vulnerable populations. Some patients may have more difficulty negotiating the managed care bureaucracy. Low-income, elderly, and mentally ill patients have been found in some studies to have worse self-reported outcomes in managed care versus indemnity-based insurance plans.

Although the results of studies of quality in managed care plans are generally good, the public remains skeptical about whether these plans can truly deliver more for less. Purchasers of health care, in particular, large employers, have catalyzed a movement to publicly disseminate information on the quality of managed care plans to help consumers make informed choices. Although there continues to be a lack of uniformity in what quality of care data should be reported, organizations such as the National Committee on Quality Assurance (NCQA) have proposed approaches to collecting and disseminating similar data across managed care plans. NCQA's Health Plan Employer Data and Information Set (HEDIS) is rapidly becoming one of the industry standards for measuring the performance of managed care plans. The HEDIS "report card" measures the degree to which the enrollee population receives preventive services such as childhood immunization, mammograms, and Pap smears; adequate prenatal care; and management of certain chronic conditions such as asthma and diabetes. Nonetheless, questions remain about whether the HEDIS indicators or indicators proposed by other organizations sufficiently measure quality, whether the indicators can be adequately risk adjusted, and whether the present system of having managed care plans voluntarily report their data can adequately protect the public from the potential harms of rationing resources within managed care.

FUTURE OF PRIMARY AND MANAGED CARE

A health care delivery revolution is under way in the United States. For a variety of reasons managed care is becoming the preferred health care delivery model, and this in turn is stimulating a demand for primary care providers. As managed care shifts the power of clinical decision making away from specialists and onto primary care providers, a new form of managed care plan is beginning to emerge in markets that have more experience with managed care. For example, in California, rather than serving as regulated employees in staff model HMOs, primary care physicians are, increasingly, forming their own IPAs that accept the full financial risk for their patients. To accept the full financial risk and administrative responsibilities for patient populations, these groups must become large enough to hire additional staff and to absorb the effects of high-cost patients. Specialty and hospital services are purchased through contracts with the primary care IPA. In many cases these IPAs are able to contract for specialty and hospital services at a lower rate than staff and group model HMOs pay to own these services because the penetration of managed care in the health care market has created an apparent excess of specialty and hospital services.

It is too early to determine which model of managed care will ultimately dominate the marketplace. Much of the recent growth of managed care plans has been stimulated by a focus on lowering costs. Many health care analysts believe that over the long term managed care plans must demonstrate not only an ability to lower costs, but also to improve quality, if they are to remain viable and convince some increasingly vocal patients and providers that health care is not just a business but a service that can improve the quality of life of individuals and the general population.

BIBLIOGRAPHY

American Medical Association: Ethical issues in managed care, *JAMA* 273:330-335, 1995.

Bodenheimer TS, Grumbach K: Capitation or decapitation: keeping your head in changing times, *JAMA* 276:1025-1031, 1996.

Council on Graduate Medical Education: Sixth report: managed health care—implications for the physician workforce and medical education, Washington, DC, 1995, US Department of Health and Human Services.

Franks P, Clancy CM, Nutting PA. Gatekeeping revisited: protecting patients from overtreatment, *JAMA* 327:424-429, 1992.

Gold M, Hurley R, Lake T, Ensor T, Berenson R: A national survey of the arrangements managed-care plans make with physicians, *N Engl J Med* 333:1678-1683, 1995.

Greenfield S, Rogers W, Mangotich M, Carney M, Tarlov A: Outcomes of patients with hypertension and non-insulin-dependent diabetes mellitus treated by different systems and specialties, *JAMA* 274:1436-1444, 1995.

Iglehart JK: Physicians and growth of managed care, *N Engl J Med* 331:1167-1171, 1994.

Martin D, Diehr P, Price K, Richardson W: Effect of a gatekeeper plan on health services use and charges: a randomized trial, *Am J Public Health* 79:1628-1632, 1989.

Miller R, Luft H: Managed care plan performance since 1980: a literature review, *JAMA* 271:1512-1519, 1994.

Ware JE Jr, Bayliss MS, Rogers WH et al: Differences in 4-year health outcomes for elderly and poor, chronically ill patients treated in HMO and fee-for-service systems: results from the Medical Outcomes Study, *JAMA* 276:1039-1047, 1996.

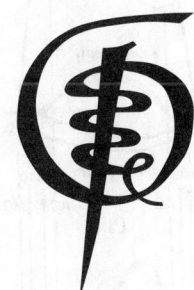

Diseases of the Heart and Blood Vessels

9 Cardiovascular Physiology

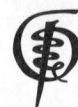

Martin M. LeWinter, Louis A. Mulieri, and George Osol

The function of the cardiovascular system is to deliver oxygen, nutrients, and other essential molecules to the tissues of the body and carry waste products (carbon dioxide, metabolic end-products) to the organs responsible for their elimination (lungs, liver, kidneys). To accomplish this, nature has designed a system with two separate circulations. The pulmonary circulation is a low-resistance, high-capacitance vascular bed specialized for gas exchange with the environment. The systemic circulation is composed of multiple relatively high-resistance beds specialized for tissue delivery of oxygen and nutrients and extraction of carbon dioxide and metabolic waste products. Blood, a solvent that dissolves and transports the substances required for and produced by metabolism, travels sequentially through both circulations and is pumped by two highly adapted pumps in series combined in one single organ, the heart, which is under coordinated local and neurohumoral control. This system must function under an extraordinary variety of demands, for example, the stress of exercise, in which cardiac output may increase four-fold or more, extremes of temperature during which the circulation must function to maximize either heat loss or conservation, and beat-to-beat variations in loading imposed by routine functions such as respiration. Moreover, the system has little room for error. For example, the slightest sustained mismatch in left and right heart output would result in a catastrophe. This chapter reviews cardiac function and the peripheral and coronary circulations and considers integrated function of the entire system in response to the stress of exercise.

CARDIAC FUNCTION
The Cardiac Cycle

As a frame of reference, we begin with a description of organ level events during the cardiac cycle (Fig. 9-1). Mechanical activity begins with electrical signaling provided by specialized conduction tissue. This tissue is a component of the cardiac excitation system that controls heart rate by responding to a variety of modulating influences; provides a normal sequence of activation, which in turn assists maximally efficient contraction and filling; and, at the cellular level, initiates the biochemical processes that underlie myocyte contraction. At the body surface, the activity of the excitation system is recognized by recording the electrocardiogram (ECG), which reflects electrical potential differences generated by the heart. At the cellular level, electrical excitation consists of transmission of a membrane-based depolarizing and then repolarizing current called the *action potential* (described in detail in a later section). Transmission occurs first through the aforementioned tissue specialized for its generation and spread, and then to atrial and ventricular myocytes, where the action potential is the signaling event that initiates contraction. Initiation and spread of excitation begin in the right atrium in the sinus node region of the specialized conduction tissue and continue through specialized intraatrial pathways that converge in the atrioventricular region of the conduction system. This region consists of the atrioventricular node and His bundle. Spread of excitation then continues through large intraventricular fascicles (the left and right bundle branches), ultimately reaching the smallest branches of the specialized conduction tissue, the Purkinje fibers. From the latter, electrical

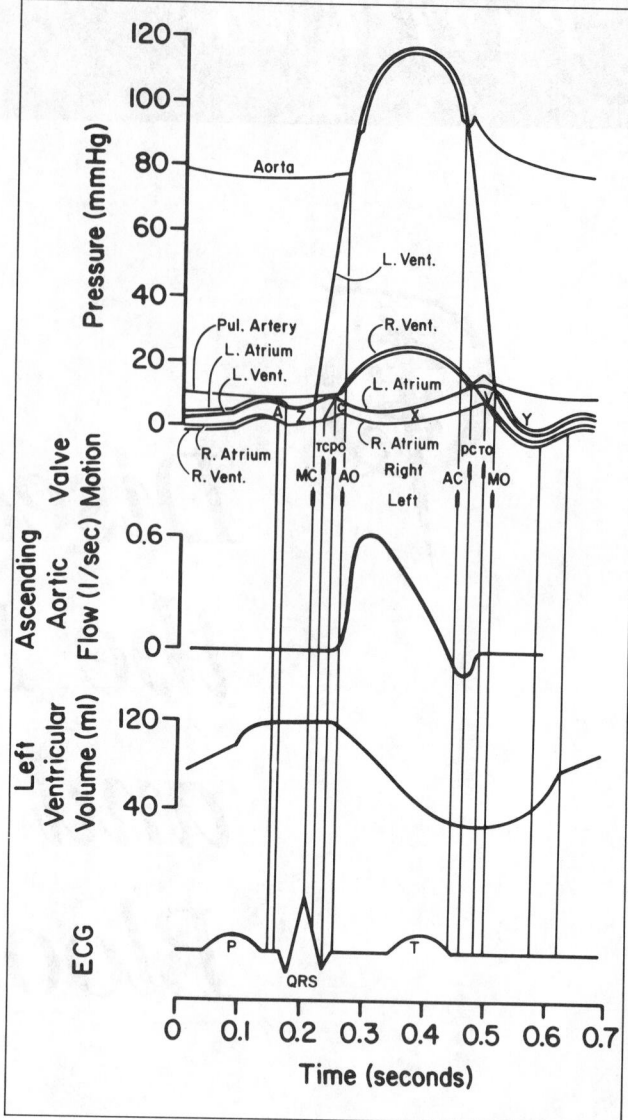

FIGURE 9-1 Electrical and mechanical events during the cardiac cycle. *MC* and *TC*, Mitral and tricuspid valve closure; *PO* and *AO*, pulmonic and aortic valve opening; *AC* and *PC*, aortic and pulmonic valve closure; *TO* and *MO*, tricuspid and mitral valve opening; *L*, left; *R*, right; *Vent*, ventricle; *Pul*, pulmonary.

(Modified from Hurst JW, editor: *The heart*, ed 5, New York, 1982, McGraw-Hill.)

excitation reaches the ventricular myocardium. The electrical signal spreads rapidly through most of the specialized conduction system. The atrioventricular node, however, delays the spread of the impulse, which maximizes efficiency of atrial booster pump function and protects the ventricles from excessively rapid stimulation when the atrial rate is abnormally high. Within the myocardium, the action potential spreads from myocyte to myocyte through specialized structures called intercalated disks, which contain low-resistance gap junctions across which current preferentially flows. The left ventricle, the most massive of the cardiac chambers, is the largest source of electrical potentials. Electrical activation of the left ventricle begins first in the interventricular septum, spreads toward the anteroapical region, and reaches the posterobasal portion last. The normal body surface ECG consists of the P wave, reflecting depolarization of right and then left atrium; the isoelectric PR interval (atrial repolarization and atrioventricular node delay); the QRS complex, reflecting ventricular depolarization; the isoelectric ST segment; and the T wave, the surface representation of ventricular repolarization (see Chapter 12).

Electrical activation causes a coordinated sequence of contraction and relaxation of the cardiac chambers that, with normal valve function, results in efficient ejection of blood by the ventricles, followed by relaxation and filling. The cardiac mechanical cycle may be considered to begin at ventricular end-diastole, the instant just before the ventricles begin to generate active tension signaled by a sudden rise in pressure at the onset of contraction. Because of the normal sequence of electrical activation, the left ventricle develops pressure slightly before the right. The mitral and tricuspid valves close when ventricular pressure just exceeds atrial pressure. Both ventricles then increase pressure rapidly until pressure in the aorta or pulmonary artery is exceeded, resulting in opening of the aortic and pulmonic valves and ejection of blood into the systemic and pulmonary circulations. The period during which ventricular pressure rises with constant volume is termed *isovolumic contraction.* The succeeding ejection phase continues until ventricular pressure peaks and then falls below aortic or pulmonary arterial pressure, resulting in closure of aortic and pulmonic valves. In the left ventricle, a period follows during which ventricular pressure drops rapidly and aortic and mitral valves are closed; this is called *isovolumic relaxation.* Normally, the right ventricular–pulmonary artery pressure crossover is so low that right ventricular isovolumic relaxation is virtually nonexistent. When ventricular pressure crosses atrial pressure, the mitral and tricuspid valves open, resulting in the onset of the filling phase of ventricular diastole.* The rapid inrush of blood shortly after mitral and tricuspid valve opening is caused by an atrioventricular pressure gradient of several millimeters of mercury (mm Hg). Subsequently, filling slows and may come to a complete halt (true diastasis) as the pressure gradient disappears. The last phase of ventricular filling, atrial contraction, results in transfer of a further bolus of blood into the ventricle. Ventricular contraction begins once again during atrial relaxation.

Ventricular volume patterns are similar in both chambers except for the virtual absence of isovolumic relaxation in the right ventricle. Systolic pressure waveforms differ, mainly because the left ventricle is thicker walled and generates a much higher pressure, reflecting the high-resistance nature of the systemic arterial bed. During ventricular filling, pressure waveforms in both ventricles are similar, but the pressure is slightly higher on the left side. Left and right atrial pressure waveforms are also similar. The positive wave during atrial contraction (a wave) is followed by atrial relaxation, which begins with or extends into ventricular systole. The decline of atrial pressure early during ventricular systole is termed the *x descent.* Once atrial relaxation is complete, atrial pressure rises once again during ventricular systole (v wave), as continuous venous inflow passively fills the atria. The v wave reaches its peak at the time of ventricular-atrial pressure crossover, signaling the onset of ventricular filling. The second descent of atrial pressure, beginning with the onset of ventricular filling, is the y descent. Paralleling ventricular diastolic pressure, right atrial pressure is normally lower than left atrial pressure. Normal inspiration results in (1) a substantial increase in venous return to the right heart as intrathoracic pressure decreases and (2) pooling of blood in the pulmonary circulation, which results in a small decrease in venous return to the left heart. During inspiration, right ventricular stroke volume increases in relation to left ventricular stroke volume. This prolongs right ventricular ejection time and delays the time of pulmonic valve closure, resulting in normal, increased splitting of the second heart sound on inspiration (see Chapter 11).

Cellular Basis of Cardiac Contraction

Cardiac myocytes may be considered to consist of three linked systems: (1) a plasmalemmal *excitation system,* which participates in spread of the action potential and functions as a switch that initiates the intracellular events, which give rise to contraction, and (2) an intracellular *excitation-contraction coupling system,* which amplifies and converts the electrical excitation signal to a chemical signal, which in turn directly results in activation of the (3) *contractile system,* a molecular motor using adenosine triphosphate (ATP) as its energy source (Fig. 9-2).

*We use the term *diastole* to refer to the sequence of ventricular relaxation and filling.

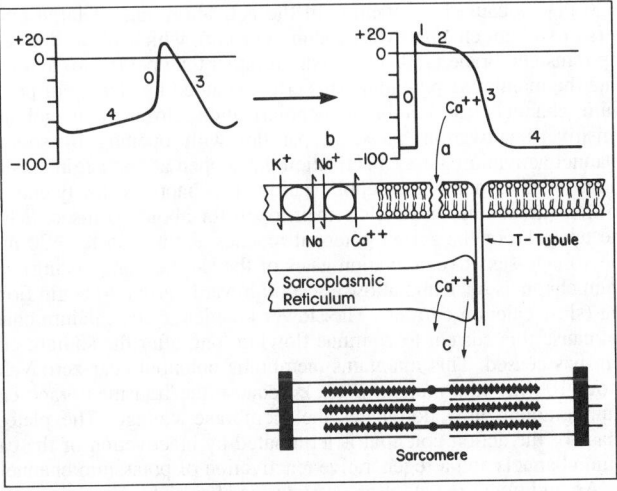

FIGURE 9-2 Schematic drawing of a myocardial cell showing the plasmalemmal excitation system with the principal channels responsible for the action potential, the excitation-contraction coupling system with T-tubule and sarcoplasmic reticulum, and the contractile system with the sarcomere building block. On the top are shown two action potentials, on the left from a sinus node cell displaying spontaneous diastolic depolarization, and on the right from a myocardial cell. *a,* Entry of calcium into cell via the slow calcium channel; *b,* sodium-calcium exchange; *c,* release of calcium from the sarcoplasmic reticulum.

Excitation System. Each myocyte is encased in a sarcolemma composed of the lipid sheet plasmalemma (cell membrane) and a covering of lamellar and collagen fiber layers. The electrical insulation afforded by the lipid layer allows the plasmalemma to support a charge separation, resulting in a transmembrane voltage gradient, the *resting potential* (normally −87 mV, inside negative). This charge separation, in combination with specialized plasmalemmal proteins, enables myocytes to generate a transient collapse (and slight reversal) of the resting potential, the *action potential.* The local current flow accompanying the collapse enables myocytes to signal their own intracellular organelles as well as propagate action potentials to neighboring myocytes.

The resting potential is established by a transmembrane protein, the *sodium pump,* which uses energy from ATP hydrolysis to pump sodium ions out of the myoplasm. Sodium pumping maintains intracellular sodium concentration at about one fifteenth the extracellular value. In contrast, potassium ions are freely permeable in the resting state, and their transmembrane concentration gradient therefore is in equilibrium with the negative transmembrane voltage.

The energy stored in the sodium gradient can be discharged periodically in an "avalanche" mode to generate a brief (0.02 sec) but powerful electrical force (110 mV). The mechanism resides in the voltage sensitivity of proteins lining conductance *channels* that pierce the plasmalemma. The avalanche occurs when a change in transmembrane voltage opens the channels and results in an increasing transmembrane flow of ions that markedly enhances the original voltage change. The latter is most prominent in sodium channels. The proteins lining each type of channel are specialized to select specific ions for entry. An ion cannot pass through its specific channel unless a specialized portion of the channel protein, the *activation gate,* ceases to obstruct the channel. A second portion, the *inactivation gate,* moves into an obstructing position to terminate ion flow. With both gates open, selected ions flow through the channel under the influence of their concentration and/or voltage gradient. Channels are either fully open or closed. The rate of ion flow is varied by changing the ratio of open time to closed time. In a *voltage-operated gate* the probability of being open depends mainly on the strength of the transmembrane electric field. Typically, in a resting myocyte, a 10% change in transmembrane voltage is sufficient to modify the shape of the positively charged "voltage sensor" portion of ion channel proteins, resulting in opening.

The upstroke of the action potential from −87 mV to its peak of

+20 mV is caused by opening of the activation gate of large numbers of sodium channels (fast sodium current), which allows the resting transmembrane gradient of sodium rather than potassium to dominate the membrane potential. This effect is aided by closing of potassium channels as membrane depolarization closes their voltage-sensitive inactivation gates. In parallel with opening of sodium channel activation gates, inactivation gates open at rest begin closing in response to membrane depolarization. This happens slowly enough so that the sodium channels remain open for about 20 msec. When the upstroke of the action potential reaches about −35 to −20 mV, the voltage-sensitive activation gates of the L-type (long lasting) calcium channels open and allow a second inward current to begin flowing (slow calcium current). The slower kinetics of the calcium channel cause this current to continue flowing long after the sodium current has ceased. This maintains membrane potential near zero V for about 100 ms (the *plateau phase*), because the transmembrane calcium gradient now dominates the membrane voltage. The plateau phase of the action potential is terminated by inactivation of the calcium channels and a regenerative reactivation of potassium channels.

An additional recovery process ensues after sodium, calcium, and potassium channels are returned to their resting states. The sequential flow of sodium, calcium, and potassium currents during the action potential results in an intracellular gain of sodium and calcium ions and a loss of potassium ions. Excess calcium ions are extruded mainly by the plasmalemmal *sodium-calcium exchanger pump*. The exchanger is a shuttle that moves one calcium ion out of the cell against its concentration gradient and uses energy from the sodium gradient to move one sodium ion into the cell.

In specialized conduction system tissue, the slow inward calcium current normally flows between beats in conjunction with a smaller diastolic transmembrane voltage gradient than is present in the myocyte (Fig. 9-2). This causes spontaneous diastolic depolarization and pacemaker activity when the transmembrane voltage achieves threshold for a propagated action potential.

Spread of the action potential within a myocyte or throughout the myocardium is an inherent result of the ion gradients that drive the membrane action potential itself. Sodium ions (or calcium ions) that have moved through the membrane via open channels (vice versa for potassium) create a local increased charge concentration that dissipates by electrostatic interaction with ions along the adjacent membrane whose channels have not yet opened. This spreading of depolarization outside the region of open channels, *electrotonic* flow, acts to open the voltage-sensitive activation gates of nearby regions. This results in self-sustaining propagation of the *action potential* over the whole membrane and then to adjacent cells by virtue of easy flow of ions through the intercalated disks between cells.

Excitation-Contraction Coupling System. The ability of the action potential to switch on and control the activity of the contractile proteins is enhanced by a system of intracellular membranes, the *sarcotubular system* (Fig. 9-3), which creates electrochemical couplings between the sarcolemma and intracellular organelles. Signals are communicated between these organelles more rapidly than possible by simple diffusion. The sarcotubular system consists of *transverse tubules* (T-tubules) and *sarcoplasmic reticulum* (SR). T-tubules are tubular invaginations of the sarcolemma. The SR is a longitudinally oriented system of intracellular membranous tubules and sacs in the form of a collar that encircles and divides contractile filaments into 1 to 2 μm diameter bundles, the *myofibrils,* and forms repeating, closed compartments that extend along the length of each myofibril from cross-striation to cross-striation. At each end of the collar is a bulge *(cistern)* that abuts a T-tubule, creating a *dyad* structure *(triad* if cisternae of adjacent collars bracket the T-tubule) held together by specialized junctional contacts *(feet)* between the adjacent membranes. The SR compartments contain an enormous intracellular store of bound calcium ions that can be released into the myoplasm in a controlled way to act as messengers for initiation and control of contraction in nearby myofilaments.

The membranes of the SR are spanned by *SR calcium-pump* proteins (SERCA2a) that use energy from ATP to rapidly (<½ sec) move calcium ions from the sarcoplasm to be stored in the interior of the SR against a large concentration gradient. Stored calcium can be released from the cisternae by opening special calcium-release chan-

nels *(ryanodine receptors)* that bridge the cisternal membrane near the foot proteins of the dyad. The opposite side of the foot proteins is near a different kind of calcium release channel (the *DHP receptor*), which spans the T-tubule membrane. Opening of the DHP receptor allows calcium ions to enter the cell from the extracellular fluid contained in the T-tubule lumen.

Arrival of a membrane action potential at the mouth of a T-tubule causes depolarization of the contiguous membrane and spread of the depolarization toward the center of the cell. As the depolarization spreads, it activates the voltage-sensitive calcium gates of the DHP receptor, causing both physical movement of the gate proteins and flow of calcium ions from the T-tubule lumen into the dyad gap. This opens the calcium gates of the nearby ryanodine receptors and allows calcium ions to flow from the SR-cisternal lumen into the myoplasm. Because the calcium channels of the ryanodine receptor are activated by a rise in calcium concentration, the initial release causes an avalanche of further release of calcium from the cisternae, giving rise to the twitch-inducing, myoplasmic *calcium spike*. Although only a small portion of the cisternal store of calcium is released, the amount is sufficient to raise the intracellular concentration from its diastolic value of 0.1 μm to 1 to 10 μm. The concentration increase is transient because free calcium ions are rapidly removed from the cytoplasm by binding to the contractile proteins, sodium-calcium exchange, and calcium pump uptake.

For the heart to remain in steady state, calcium entering the myoplasm by influx through the plasma membrane and SR release must

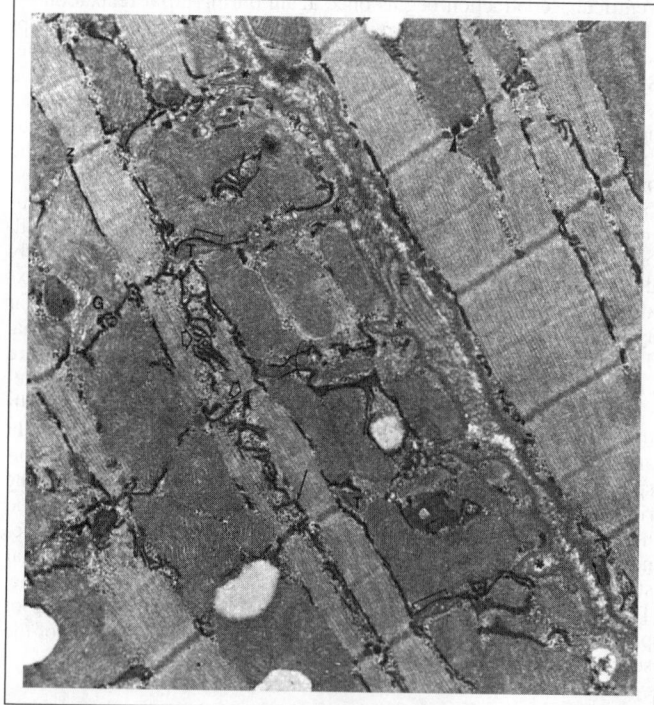

FIGURE 9-3 Longitudinal electron micrographic section through two cardiac myocytes with the sarcoplasmic reticulum stained in black contrast. Extracellular space *(E)* contains bundles of collagen. Asterisks indicate grooves from which transverse tubules *(T)* enter the interior of the cells. The laminar coat of the plasmalemma can be seen extending into the transverse tubule. The SR forms a tubular network around the sarcomere structure composed of free SR and networks termed M and Z retes *(open arrows)*. Z rete is often represented only by a single Z tubule (z). Interior couplings *(brackets)* composed of junctional SR and plasmalemma form dyads *(brackets)* or triads *(curved brackets)* with transverse tubules and peripheral couplings subjacent to plasmalemma *(brace)*. In areas where transverse tubules are sparse, SR structure is termed corbular SR *(arrowhead)*. Dark transverse lines are Z lines (see Fig. 9-4). Mitochondria are prominent, with nearby glycogen granules and lipid droplets. *G* indicates Golgi zones.

(Modified from Sommer JR, Johnson EA: Ultrastructure of cardiac muscle. In Berne RM, editor: *Handbook of physiology,* Bethesda, 1979, American Physiological Society.)

be removed by the end of diastole in order for the myocyte to relax. Plasma membrane influx is small and adequately extruded by sarcolemmal sodium-calcium exchange. The bulk of the released calcium is removed in approximately 0.2 sec by SERCA2a, which has high calcium affinity and effectively competes with the calcium-binding sites on the contractile proteins. Its pumping rate is intrinsically self-regulated because it speeds up when free calcium concentration rises.

Contractile System. Heart muscle is organized in *sarcomere* building blocks that allow structural modification according to the type of mechanical work performed (Fig. 9-4). Addition of sarcomeres in parallel increases force-producing capacity without changing shortening. Addition of sarcomeres in series increases shortening capacity (and velocity) without changing force production. Each sarcomere is composed of two bundles of longitudinally oriented filaments. *Thick filaments*, 1.6 μm long, are composed of myosin molecules in a trigonal array at the center of the sarcomere's length. At each end of this array, a set of 1 μm long *thin filaments* composed of actin molecules interdigitates with the thick filaments. The other ends of the thin filaments extend to the ends of the sarcomere where they are anchored to a transverse structure, the *Z-disk.* At a sarcomere length (distance between Z-disks) of 2.2 μm, the central end of each thin filament overlaps 0.7 μm of the distal ends of the thick filaments (the *overlap zone*). The 0.3 μm length of nonoverlapped thin filaments extending to the Z-disk and the neighbors of the Z-disk in the adjacent sarcomere constitute the *I-band.* The centrally positioned thick filaments constitute the *A-band.* Alternating A and I bands give rise to the *striated* appearance of cardiac muscle. The thick filaments are joined at the *M-line,* in the middle of the sarcomere.

A portion of each myosin molecule is oriented along the length of the sarcomere to form the thick filament. The remainder protrudes from the filament surface and is free to move in the space between thick and thin filaments (Fig. 9-4). This protruding portion, the *cross-bridge,* is the molecular structure responsible for conversion of chemical energy to directed, mechanical energy. The cross-bridge head contains the site of myosin's ATPase activity and a separate site that allows myosin to bind strongly to actin molecules in the nearby thin filament. The head also has auxiliary proteins *(light chains)* adsorbed to its surface that maintain structural requirements for effective mechanical function *(essential light chains)* and allow fine control of force and motion *(regulatory light chains).*

A group of proteins (the *tropomyosin-troponin complex)* adsorbed to actin at regular intervals allows for control of the myosin-actin interaction according to the presence or absence of calcium ions *(activator calcium)* (Fig. 9-5). The tropomyosin-troponin complex is anchored to the actin backbone by tropomyosin. An inhibitory protein, *troponin-I,* is adsorbed to tropomyosin in a position that allows it to prevent cross-bridges from binding to the underlying actin molecules. The ability to switch on cross-bridge binding to actin is conferred by two more adsorbed proteins, *troponin-T* and *troponin-C.* Binding of activator calcium to troponin-C reverses the inhibitory effect of troponin-I and allows actin-myosin interaction to occur. With this arrangement, cross-bridges interact with actin, hydrolyze ATP, and produce force and shortening in accord with the time course of calcium release from the SR as governed by the sarcolemmal action potential.

The energy released from hydrolysis of one ATP high-energy phosphate bond by myosin is stored in the form of a molecular conformational change in the head of the cross-bridge. While the myosin head is bound to an activated actin filament, the conformational energy is released, causing the myosin head to rotate slightly as would the oar of a rower seated on the actin filament (Fig. 9-6). This motion generates a force that propels the actin filament along the thick filament toward the center of the sarcomere. This process occurs repeatedly and randomly at millions of different actin-myosin cross-bridges in both halves of the sarcomere, causing large-scale force and/or motion generation.

If no external restraining force is applied to the muscle, the cross-bridges propel the filaments at the maximum speed their chemomechanical reactions permit. If muscle shortening is opposed by an external load, as during physiologic contraction, cross-bridge motion is

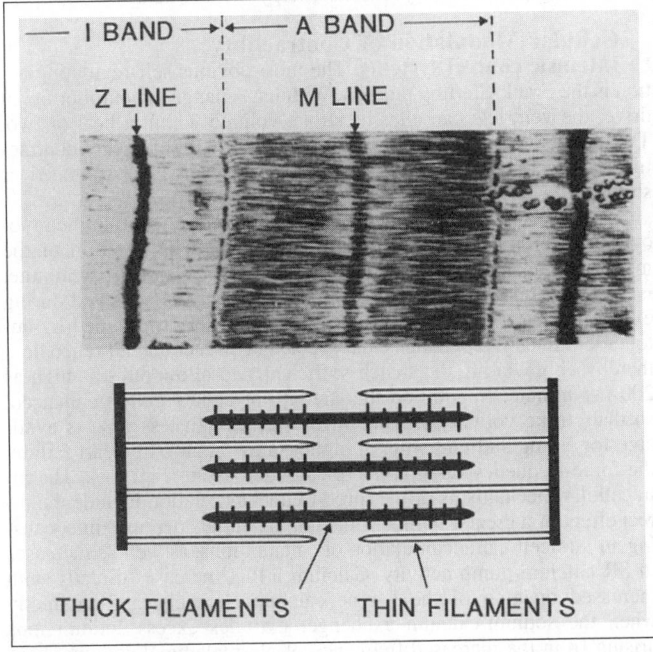

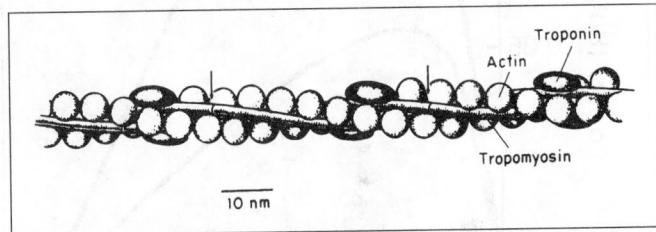

FIGURE 9-5 Schematic representation of the tropomyosin-troponin complex adsorbed to the actin filament (see text).

(Modified from Woledge RC, Curtin NA, Homsher E: *Energetic aspects of muscle contraction,* San Diego, 1985, Academic Press.)

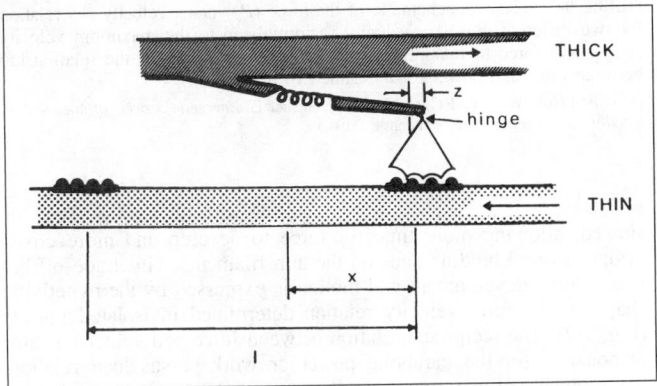

FIGURE 9-6 Schematic of the mechanical interaction between the thick myosin filaments and the thin actin filaments. The triangular structure in contact with the thin filament is the myosin head. Letter z denotes the distance moved by the thick filament as a result of rotation of the head region.

(From Woledge RC, Curtin NA, Homsher E: *Energetic aspects of muscle contraction,* San Diego, 1985, Academic Press.)

FIGURE 9-4 *Top,* electron micrograph of a sarcomere; *bottom,* schematic representation (see text).

(From Woledge RC, Curtin NA, Homsher E: *Energetic aspects of muscle contraction,* San Diego, 1985, Academic Press.)

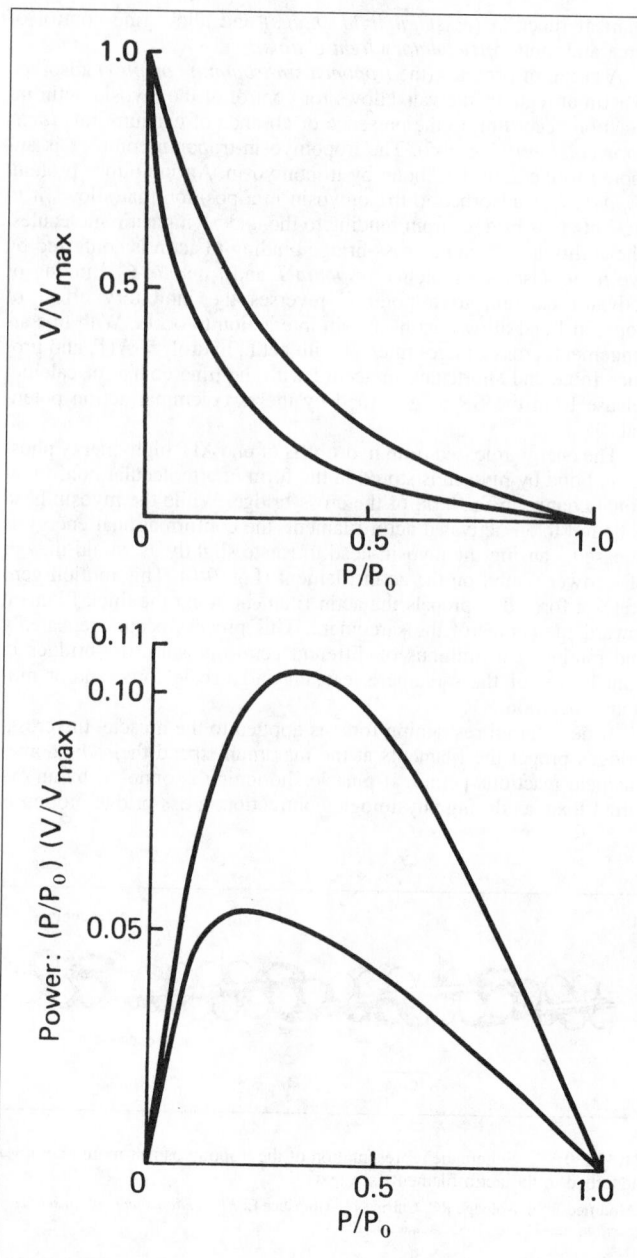

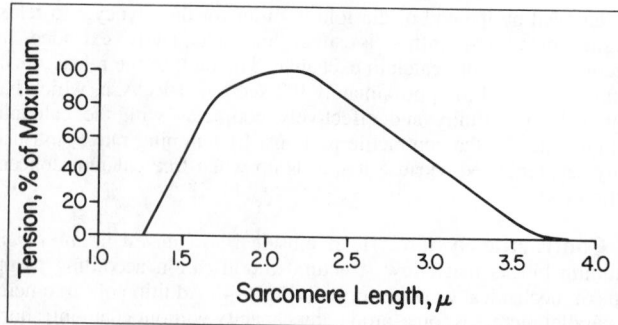

FIGURE 9-8 Schematic of the sarcomere length-tension (or force) relationship, showing marked diminution of tension development at sarcomeres below about 2.0 μm. At very long sarcomere lengths, overlap of thin and thick filaments is progressively reduced, resulting in the descending limb of the length-tension relationship.

(Modified from Braunwald E, Ross J Jr, Sonnenblick EH, editors: *Mechanisms of contraction of the normal and failing heart,* Boston, 1976, Little, Brown.)

FIGURE 9-7 *Above,* schematic of the force *(P)* versus velocity *(V)* relation for two different muscles. Velocity is normalized to the maximum velocity (V_{max}) and force to maximum isometric force (P_o). *Below,* the relationship between force and power for the same two muscles.

(Modified from Woledge RC, Curtin NA, Homsher E: *Energetic aspects of muscle contraction,* San Diego, 1985, Academic Press.)

actin and myosin filaments move farther apart at shorter sarcomere length. This changes the geometry of the myosin-actin bond during activation and results in a reduction in the effective degree of activation at any concentration of activator calcium (i.e., fewer cross-bridge connections are made). This gives rise to the tension-length relation of the sarcomere or isolated muscle strips, and is also the main cause of the Frank-Starling relation in the intact ventricle.

Myocardial Energy Metabolism. In view of the large amounts of energy used by the heart, it is not surprising that myocytes are richly endowed with mitochondria (see Fig. 9-3) and heavily dependent on oxidative metabolism. Under basal conditions, myocytes preferentially take up and oxidize fatty acids to generate ATP. During stress conditions, however, glucose uptake and anaerobic glycolysis become increasingly important. Certain ion pumps, for instance SERCA2a, may be especially dependent on ATP produced from glycolysis. Furthermore, the heart is an insulin-sensitive organ, and insulin lack causes a cardiomyopathy. Thus glucose utilization, although not as important as fatty acid oxidation, is nonetheless a significant component of myocardial energy metabolism.

Cellular Modulation of Contractility

Intrinsic control systems. The most obvious self-regulating action is the Frank-Starling relation. Without a change in neurohormonal drive, the ventricle can alter its stroke volume within a beat or two. This results directly from greater or lesser sensitivity of the contractile proteins to activator calcium when sarcomeres are stretched or shortened.

Another self-regulatory response residing entirely within the myocyte is the *force-frequency* relation (Fig. 9-9). The duration of the myocardial isometric twitch contraction, at a rate of 60 per minute, is such that relaxation would be incomplete at rates achieved during exercise and cause impaired diastolic filling. This is avoided by automatic intracellular changes that speed up contraction and relaxation, thereby abbreviating the twitch sufficiently to allow rates as high as 200 per minute. In addition the strength of contraction is enhanced, so that stroke volume is maintained even though less time is available for filling and emptying at higher rates. In chronic heart failure, the force-frequency relation is typically depressed (Fig. 9-9). The intracellular mechanisms of the force-frequency relation include the direct effect of a greater number of action potentials per unit time, causing an intracellular accumulation of calcium ions, as well as increases in SR calcium-pump activity. Calcium influx increases directly with increased opening of the L-type calcium channels, and indirectly when the sodium-calcium exchanger extrudes excess sodium ions arising from the increased frequency of plasmalemmal sodium channel opening. Although these factors support increased twitch force generation, in isolation they may risk elevation of diastolic calcium and force. This is avoided by an accompanying increase in speed of the SR calcium-pump, which increases relaxation rate and abbreviates the contraction. Activity of the SR calcium pump is partly con-

slowed, allowing more time for force to develop and more cross-bridges to find binding sites on the thin filaments. This trade-off between force development and motion is expressed by the hyperbolic shape of the force-velocity relation determined in isolated muscle (Fig. 9-7). The reciprocal relation between force and velocity is also responsible for the parabolic power or work versus load relation. Since power is force times velocity, power output is zero at both zero velocity and zero force (maximum velocity) and reaches its maximum at about 25% to 40% of maximum force.

The force produced by an activated sarcomere also depends on the length of the sarcomere, diminishing quite steeply below 2 μm (Fig. 9-8) because the degree of activation of cross-bridges depends on sarcomere length. The main reason for this appears to be related to the fact that because the sarcomere maintains a constant volume,

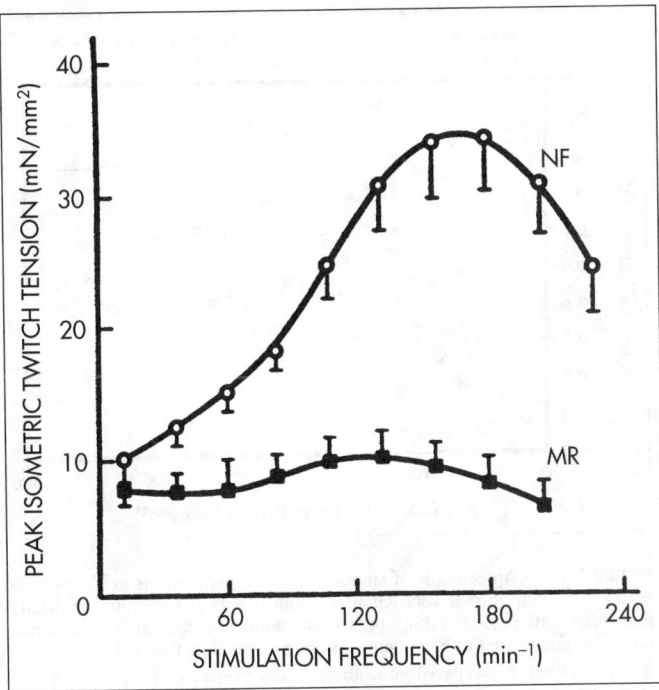

FIGURE 9-9   Examples of the force-frequency relationship obtained in non-failing *(NF)* and failing myocardial strips from patients with heart failure caused by mitral regurgitation *(MR),* with peak tension plotted against stimulation frequency. This relationship is characteristically depressed in heart failure.

(From Mulieri LA et al: Myocardial force-frequency defect in mitral regurgitation heart failure is reversed by forskolin, *Circulation* 88:2702, 1993. Reprinted by permission, American Heart Association.)

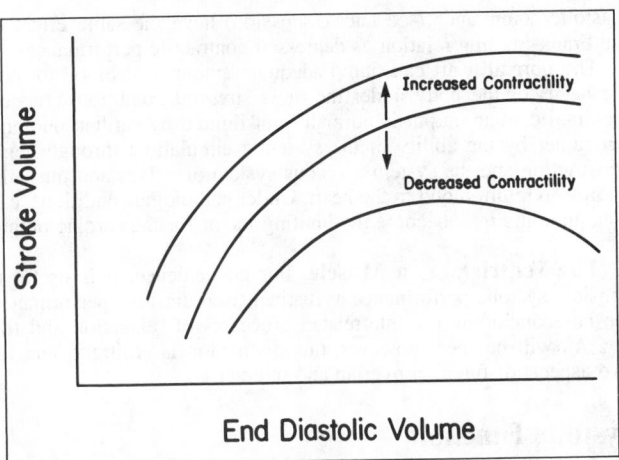

FIGURE 9-10   The ventricular Frank-Starling relationship, expressed as end-diastolic volume versus stroke volume (see text).

trolled by an associated protein, *calcium-activated calmodulin kinase,* or *CaM-K.* This kinase, which increases SERCA2a activity in response to increased calcium ion concentration, has a built-in frequency sensitivity. Slight, transient increases in calcium ions, even if insufficient to activate the kinase directly, are held in their binding sites long enough so that repeated increases are summated. This averaging process results in calcium pump speed being increased by the average as well as the instantaneous intracellular calcium ion concentration.

Extrinsic control systems. Similar changes in intracellular calcium handling are brought about by neurohormonal control systems via specialized receptor proteins that span the sarcolemmal membrane. Modulation of contractility by adrenergic and cholinergic neural discharge and circulating catecholamines is mediated by agonist binding to specific receptors that liberate second and third messengers intracellularly. β-adrenergic receptor binding ultimately results in changes in intracellular *cyclic adenosine monophosphate* (cAMP) concentration. In the case of norepinephrine, binding to surface membrane β-receptors stimulates interaction between G-protein and guanosine triphosphate within the membrane. The guanosine triphosphate combines with active subunit G_s, which activates enzymatic conversion of ATP to c-AMP by *adenylate cyclase* on the cytoplasmic side of the receptor complex. Calcium fluxes and concentrations are increased by increased cAMP because cAMP activates protein kinase A, which catalyzes phosphorylation of several calcium-handling proteins throughout the myocyte. Thus sarcolemmal calcium channel opening is enhanced by cAMP-induced phosphorylation of its subunit, and phosphorylation of the SR calcium-pump control protein *phospholamban* releases its inhibitory action on SERCA2a. Phosphorylation of troponin-I reduces contractile protein calcium sensitivity, which facilitates β-receptor mediated increases in relaxation rate.

Structure and Function of the Ventricles

Architecture. The left ventricle is a thick-walled (about 1.0 to 1.1 cm) chamber with a truncated ellipsoid shape composed of spi-

raling, sheetlike layers of myocyte bundles. The orientation of the bundles changes from subepicardium to subendocardium, progressing from a relatively longitudinal orientation (in relation to the long axis of the ellipsoid) to circumferentially oriented fibers that occupy roughly the middle two thirds of the wall, to longitudinally oriented fibers once again in the subendocardium. Contraction is associated with a wringing of the ventricle characterized by a counterclockwise rotation that is most prominent toward the apex. The wringing action is important for the ventricle to eject blood normally and is inherent in the normal spread of excitation and connections between fiber bundles. This complex architecture results in conversion of shortening of individual myocytes and fibers to thickening of the wall of the chamber, which is ultimately responsible for ejection of blood. The interventricular septum functions mainly as a part of the left ventricle. Reflecting the low-impedance/low-resistance nature of the pulmonary vascular bed, the right ventricle is thinner walled than the left. In cross section, it appears crescentic, and its contraction has been likened to a bellows. A significant portion of the mechanical output of the right ventricle appears to be related to energy transfer from the left ventricle through the interventricular septum (systolic ventricular interaction). This concept is supported by the observation that destruction of much of the free wall of the right ventricle is well tolerated.

The ventricles also have a well-developed connective tissue network. Cardiac collagen is characterized by a weave of fibers that forms a netlike structure around groups of six or more myocytes (visible as myofibers), connecting fibers that link adjacent myofibers, and strutlike projections that connect to adjacent blood vessels and may help maintain vessel patency during contraction. The collagen network of the ventricles appears to be largely responsible for their passive filling properties (see later discussion). The last major component of the ventricles from an anatomic standpoint is the vascular bed, described later in more detail.

The Ventricle as a Pump. Normal pumping requires delivery of appropriate amounts of blood to the tissues at acceptably low levels of filling pressure. Thus the most important means of assessing pump function clinically is the relationship between filling pressure or volume and output (stroke volume or work, minute output, power output). The ventricles display the Frank-Starling effect, the curvilinear relationship between filling pressure (classically mean atrial pressure, but more properly ventricular end-diastolic pressure) and output (Fig. 9-10). As discussed earlier, the Frank-Starling relation is due to increased contractile protein calcium sensitivity at longer sarcomere lengths. Increases or decreases in intrinsic contractile performance result in upward or downward shifts of the Frank-Starling relation. Since the Frank-Starling effect is related to sarcomere length, a more direct representation is the relation between output and end-diastolic volume (rather than pressure). In many clinical situations, however, filling pressure is more readily measurable than volume. Characterization of ventricular performance in terms of filling *pressure* and output is a "black box" approach in that abnormalities of diastolic compliance (see later discussion) have the same effect on the Frank-Starling relation as depressed contractile performance.

The normal heart can pump adequate amounts of blood to meet the needs of the body under the most stressful conditions. Indeed, maximal cardiac output is normally not limited by cardiac pumping but rather by the ability of the systemic circulation, through venoconstriction and the systemic venous system of valves and muscular pumps, to return blood to the heart. Under pathologic conditions, cardiac pumping may become the limiting factor for the cardiac output.

The Ventricle as a Muscle. For convenience, it is useful to consider systolic performance as distinct from diastolic performance, the latter including the interrelated processes of relaxation and filling. As will be seen, however, this distinction is arbitrary, and the two aspects of function overlap and interact.

Systolic Function

The systolic performance of the ventricle may be characterized in relation to loading conditions (preload, afterload) and changes in contractility. Although used frequently, contractility is difficult to define. We use the term here to indicate the intrinsic level of contractile performance (or change in contractile performance) independent of loading conditions or change in loading conditions. Thus one way to define a change in contractility is a change in contractile performance when loading conditions are unchanged or can be accounted for, for example, increased shortening despite increased afterload. Unfortunately, this is often impossible in the intact heart. Furthermore, contractility is not truly independent of loading conditions. Load-induced changes in fiber length directly influence intrinsic performance by modulating contractile protein calcium sensitivity. Thus the goal of defining "load-independent" contractility indexes is, in a sense, unrealistic.

Loading Conditions and Contractile Performance. In classic isolated muscle mechanics experiments, a force in the form of a weight is applied to a quiescent linear muscle specimen. This force is the preload, which stretches the muscle to an initial length. The muscle is then stimulated electrically to contract and lift an additional weight, the afterload. Once stimulated, the force in the muscle increases until it just meets the opposing force of the afterload, at which time shortening commences (i.e., the muscle lifts the weight). The sum of preload and afterload is the total load. As specified earlier, both preload and afterload influence myocardial contractile performance.

In isolated muscle, load is often expressed as *stress,* or force normalized to cross-sectional area. This normalization enables comparison of muscles of different size. It is useful to translate the concept of stress as a measure of load on the myofibers to the entire ventricle. To estimate wall stress in the left ventricle, the Laplace relation is used. For a spherical chamber, the Laplace relation states that average wall stress is equal to the product of pressure and internal radius divided by twice the wall thickness. Variants of this relation have been developed to account for the actual shape of the ventricle, fiber orientation, and other features. These equations allow an estimate of the stress "seen" by the myofibers as the ventricle fills and then contracts against an afterload. In diastole, the stress applied to the myofibers is their preload and determines their initial length. During contraction the stress resulting from both the preload and the systolic load (total load) determines velocity and extent of ejection. The total systolic load presented to the ventricle by the vascular system has two components, a resistive load determined at the level of small systemic arteries and arterioles by microvascular tone, and a less important capacitive load determined by the properties of the large arteries, which absorb a certain amount of blood pumped via expansion of their walls. A component of vascular load is caused by reflection of pressure waves back to the heart from the periphery.

Analogous to isolated muscle, in the intact ventricle one way of evaluating afterload (more precisely, instantaneous total load) is to estimate systolic wall stress. This has led to a useful approach for assessing ventricular function, estimation of stress-shortening or stress-shortening–velocity relationships (Fig. 9-11) in which a measure of wall stress (e.g., the end-systolic or peak value) is related to a

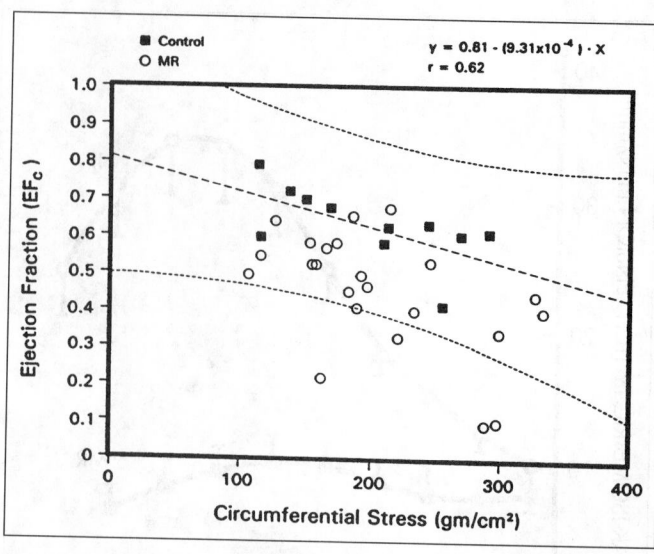

FIGURE 9-11   An example of stress-shortening relationships in a population of subjects with normal ventricular function *(Control)* and mitral regurgitation *(MR)*. MR patients falling below the confidence intervals of the normal range are considered to have depressed intrinsic contractile performance.

(From Starling M et al: Impaired left ventricular contractile function in patients with long-term mitral regurgitation and normal ejection fraction, *J Am Coll Cardiol* 22:243, 1993. Reprinted by permission, Elsevier Science.)

measure of shortening or shortening velocity (e.g., ejection fraction [stroke volume ÷ end-diastolic volume] or mean velocity of fiber shortening [V_{cf}; see later discussion below]). As seen in Fig. 9-11, the ventricle behaves in a similar fashion as isolated muscle (i.e., afterload is reciprocally related to shortening). With this approach a normal population can be characterized with single data points obtained with noninvasive techniques such as echocardiography and cuff sphygmomanometry. If the value in a patient is above or below the normal range, this may indicate an alteration in intrinsic contractile performance. Thus afterload is accounted for in attempting to understand variations in contractile performance.

The most common clinical index of ventricular function is the ejection fraction (determined by angiography, echocardiography, or radionuclide ventriculography). Although easily measurable, ejection fraction is sensitive to preload and afterload. Thus a normal ejection fraction can be considered to indicate normal intrinsic contractile function only if loading conditions are normal.

Elastance Concepts in the Assessment of Ventricular Function. As an alternative to characterizing the ventricle in terms of stress and shortening, Suga and Sagawa proposed ventricular elastance in the 1970s. This approach is based on the empirical observation that the ventricle behaves as a time-varying elastance. That is, during contraction the ventricle can be likened to a spring that progressively increases its stiffness (elastance) over time during contraction (Fig. 9-12). The elastance of a spring is the linear relationship between its stiffness and its length normalized to its unstressed or resting length. By analogy, in the ventricle, calculation of elastance requires knowledge of the "equivalent" of stiffness (pressure/volume ratio) and unstressed length (so-called dead volume, V_0). Elastance at any time during contraction can be estimated by varying loading conditions and generating a series of pressure-volume loops. (In their original studies, Suga and Sagawa used isolated perfused canine ventricles with controlled loading conditions and volume.) Using this approach, it was found that at any time t (for example, 100 msec after the start of contraction) during each of the above variably loaded contractions, the pressure/volume ratio was linear and reached a maximal value (maximal elastance) at time t_{max}, termed end-systole. Then, elastance progressively decreased as the ventricle relaxed. The slope (E_{max}) of the apparently linear end-systolic pressure-volume relation (ESPVR) changed predictably with acute interventions such as positive and negative inotropic drugs that alter intrinsic contractile per-

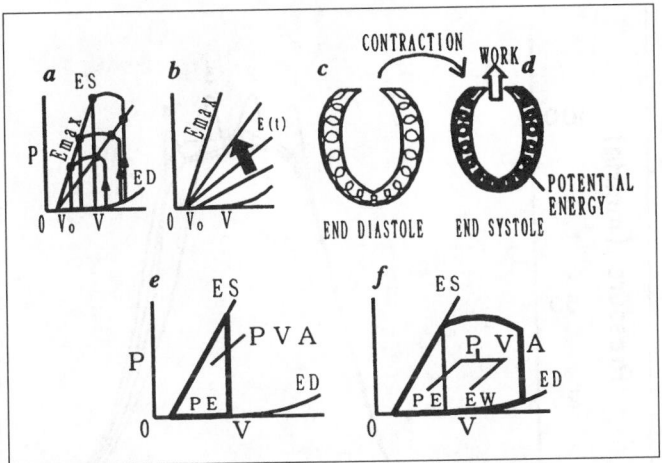

FIGURE 9-12   Schematic of the concept of ventricular elastance and its relationship to pressure-volume area (see text). In panel a, a series of pressure volume loops are displayed with varying end-diastolic *(ED)* and end-systolic *(ES)* volumes but constant contractility. Straight lines connecting points during the pressure-volume loops and intersecting at V_0 indicate an identical time (e.g., 100 msec) during each contraction. E_{max} represents slope of line connecting loops at time t_{max}, when maximum pressure/volume ratio occurs. Note that as afterload increases (higher pressure, *P*), *ES* volume increases. In panel b, elastance has been plotted as a function of time [E(t)] at four different times during contraction for the preceding pressure-volume loops. Elastance progressively increases until t_{max} when it is at its maximal value. Panels c and d schematize the concept of total mechanical energy being composed of external work and potential energy, which is stored in a "spring" at end-systole (i.e., the spring is stiffest at end-systole). In panel e, the same concept is expressed in terms of pressure-volume area *(PVA)* for an isovolumic contraction, in which pressure rises to an end-systolic value and then decreases, all at the same volume. Therefore all chemical energy is converted to potential energy *(PE)* by the contractile machinery. In panel f, an ejecting beat is shown. *PVA* consists of external work *(EW)*, the area within the pressure-volume loop, and *PE*, the area under the E_{max} line and to the left of the intersection of the pressure-volume loop and the end-systolic pressure-volume relationship.

(From LeWinter MM, Sugatt, Watkins MW, editors: *Cardiac energetics: from E_{max} to pressure-volume area,* Boston, 1995, Kluwer.)

formance. Specifically, E_{max} increased without a change in V_0 with increased contractility. The reverse occurred with decreased contractility. Thus E_{max} offered the possibility of an index of contractility that was "load independent." Although E_{max} remains a practically useful index of contractile performance, these initial observations have been modified. The ESPVR is often significantly curvilinear, especially in the intact heart and circulation. Furthermore, the ESPVR may be sensitive to the way in which afterload is varied (resistive versus capacitive load) and to preload. Systolic ventricular interaction also influences the ESPVR independent of changes in intrinsic performance. Last, it is problematic to use these concepts to compare different hearts because of difficulties in normalizing end-systolic relationships for size and the aforementioned curvilinearity. To overcome this problem, end-systolic relationships have been further modified by calculating end-systolic stiffness based on wall stress estimates.

Two extensions of elastance concepts have proved useful. In the first, elastance theory has been applied to ventricular energetics. The main determinants of myocardial energy demand are heart rate, afterload, and contractility; however, accurate quantification of afterload and contractility remains problematic. As an alternative, a pressure-volume or elastance-based approach to energetics predicts that total mechanical energy generated per beat can be considered to consist of two components (Fig. 9-12). One is external work, the area enclosed within the pressure-volume loop of a contraction. The second is potential energy, ultimately dissipated as heat during relaxation. (To understand potential energy, consider a fully isovolumic contraction, which can be produced experimentally. The contraction generates mechanical energy, but none is converted to external work; i.e., all mechanical energy is in the form of potential energy stored at end-systole.) The novelty of the elastance approach is that it provides

a basis for quantifying potential energy. In elastance theory, potential energy of a beat is the area under the ESPVR between its end-systolic point and V_0. The sum of external work and potential energy is the total mechanical energy of contraction and is termed *pressure-volume area* (PVA). PVA has been linearly correlated with myocardial oxygen consumption (VO_2). The linear VO_2-PVA relation has a positive VO_2 axis intercept, the unloaded VO_2, or oxygen consumption at zero PVA, when no mechanical energy is produced. Unloaded VO_2 is mainly accounted for by basal metabolism and excitation-contraction coupling.

Based on this analysis, it can be understood how changes in afterload and contractility and, to a modest extent, preload increase myocardial energy demands (Fig. 9-12). Increased contractility increases E_{max}, increasing external work at any preload. Most inotropic interventions also increase energy costs of excitation-contraction coupling by SERCA2a activity, resulting in increased unloaded VO_2. Increased afterload increases the level of pressure at which the pressure-volume loop intersects the ESPVR, thus increasing potential energy with variable effects on external work, but increased overall PVA. In the whole ventricle, increases in preload only modestly increase external work and therefore PVA, because the left ventricle does not markedly increase its diastolic volume acutely.

A second application of elastance theory is the concept of ventricular-vascular coupling. Just as the ventricle has an elastance relationship, the systemic arteries can also be considered in terms of an elastance relationship (which is not time varying). Arterial elastance is largely a function of the properties of the large arteries. There is an optimal relationship between ventricular and arterial elastance such that energy transfer is most efficient; that is, the largest possible proportion of total mechanical energy (PVA) generated by the ventricle is converted to usable external work. The normal heart and vascular system seem to operate at nearly optimal ventricular-vascular coupling. Various drugs can alter ventricular-vascular coupling. Moreover, in heart failure (Chapter 19) coupling between the ventricle and the vascular system is adversely affected, resulting in inefficient transfer of energy from the heart to the vascular system.

Other Approaches to the Assessment of Systolic Performance. A number of other indexes have been used to assess systolic function. Maximal rate of pressure rise (dP/dt) is highly sensitive to changes in intrinsic contractile performance, but also to afterload and, modestly, preload. V_{cf} is left ventricular internal minor axis (of the ellipsoid) shortening divided by ejection time and normalized to end-diastolic minor axis dimension; it can be derived from echocardiographic images. It is sensitive to changes in afterload, but it is a useful measure of intrinsic contractile performance if afterload is normal or can be accounted for. Measurement of ventricular power output has the attraction of being related to mechanical performance in a way that is highly physiologic, because power considers both the force generated by the ventricle and the time over which it is generated. Other empirical indexes have been developed that appear to be relatively load insensitive. One is preload recruitable stroke work, which relates end-diastolic volume to stroke work. This is obviously a form of the Frank-Starling relation. The other is the relation between end-diastolic volume and peak positive dP/dt. As with E_{max}, estimation of these indexes requires manipulation of loading conditions.

Diastolic Function

In addition to meeting demands for blood flow, the heart must function at levels of diastolic pressure that do not result in circulatory congestion. This requires a normal sequence of ventricular relaxation and filling. Ventricular relaxation begins at end-systole (defined as maximal elastance), slightly before aortic valve closure (end-ejection), continues through isovolumic relaxation, and does not reach completion until after mitral valve opening. Before filling commences, several factors combine to determine relaxation rate, or isovolumic ventricular pressure decline (Fig. 9-13). After filling begins, but before relaxation is complete, several other factors related specifically to the level of ventricular volume and/or the fact that the ventricle is changing its volume also influence the relation between pressure and volume. Certain of the latter features then dominate the diastolic pressure-volume relationship once relaxation is complete.

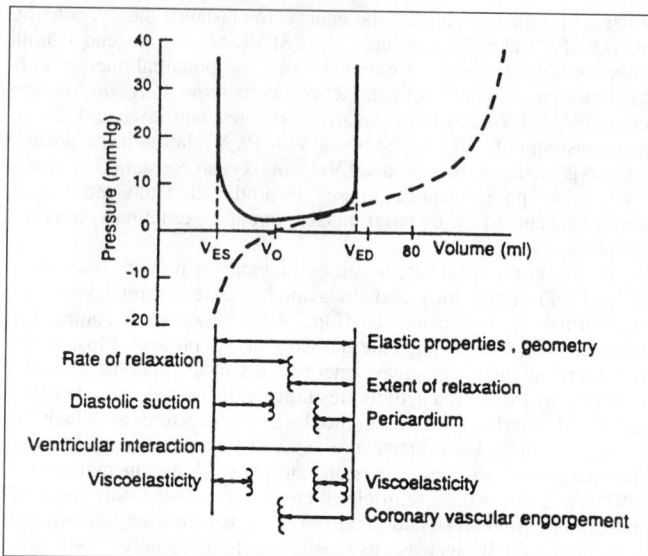

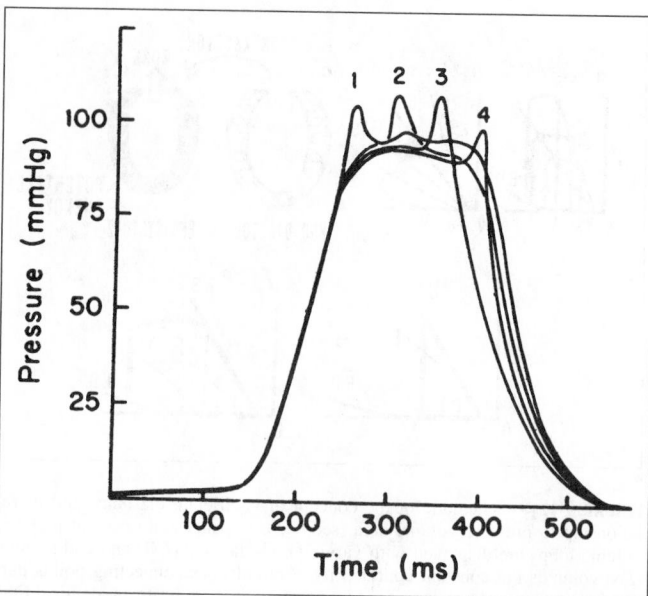

FIGURE 9-13 Schematic of the determinants of pressure and volume during isovolumic relaxation and filling. *Solid line* = actual pressure and volume. *Dashed line* = passive (fully relaxed) pressure-volume relationship. V_{ES} = end-systolic volume; V_{ED} = end-diastolic volume, V_0 = zero pressure intercept of passive pressure-volume relationship (which is not the same as dead volume of the ESPVR).

(From Gilbert JC, Glantz SA: *Circ Res* 64:828, 1989, Reprinted by permission, American Heart Association.)

FIGURE 9-14 Application of increased afterload at varying times during contraction. At time 1, relaxation is delayed. At times 3 and 4, the reverse occurs.

(From Ariel Y et al: Load-dependent relaxation with late systolic volume steps: servopump studies in the intact canine heart, *Circulation* 75:1290, 1987. Reprinted by permission, American Heart Association.)

During isovolumic relaxation, pressure falls exponentially. The determinants of isovolumic pressure fall are as follows. First, the underlying myocyte relaxation rate is determined by the balance between the avidity of the contractile proteins for calcium and the rate at which the sarcoplasmic reticulum and other uptake and extrusion mechanisms can remove calcium from the contractile proteins and restore intracellular calcium concentration to normal diastolic levels. In some pathologic situations, diastolic calcium concentration cannot be restored to normal, resulting in increased tension because of diastolic cross-bridge formation or incomplete relaxation. Relaxation rate is also modulated by the load on the myofibers. Increased afterload beginning early in systole results in delayed relaxation (Fig. 9-14). Changes in load occurring late during systole cause opposite effects. Although perturbations in load near end-systole might be considered to be of theoretical interest, this is not necessarily the case. Reflected waves typically return to the ventricle near end-systole and may function to accelerate relaxation. With noncompliant arteries, however, reflected waves return earlier and may result in an opposite effect. This may partly underlie delayed and/or slowed relaxation in elderly subjects. Last, temporal and spatial inhomogeneities of contraction and relaxation slow relaxation, as with regional ischemia.

Once ventricular pressure falls below atrial pressure, filling commences (see Fig. 9-1) and is related to variations in the pressure gradient between atrium and ventricle. Immediately after mitral opening, rapid filling occurs in association with a several millimeters of mercury (mm Hg) gradient, and an initial fall followed by a progressive increase in left ventricular pressure during the rest of diastole. As filling proceeds, the gradient markedly decreases, signaling the end of rapid filling. At slow heart rates, the gradient eventually virtually disappears, and filling may cease until atrial contraction increases the gradient once again and injects an additional volume of blood just before ventricular systole commences.

As indicated earlier, during early filling, ventricular relaxation is not yet complete. Therefore the same factors that influence isovolumic pressure fall continue to operate and influence ventricular pressure. The relationship between ventricular pressure and volume during diastolic filling is also influenced by the atrium. The passive filling characteristics of the atrium as it fills during ventricular systole partly determine the atrioventricular gradient present immediately after mitral valve opening. The less compliant the left atrium, the larger

the gradient and the more rapid the transfer of blood from atrium to ventricle. Indeed, as long as the atrioventricular valve is open, diastolic ventricular pressure, although dominated by the filling characteristics of the ventricle, is also partly determined by the properties of the atrium and even the pulmonary venous system.

In addition to the relaxation rate, other ventricular properties influence filling (see Fig. 9-13). One is generation of restoring forces during contraction. When ventricular filling is prevented experimentally, the ventricle can fully relax at its end-systolic volume. The fully relaxed pressure under these conditions can be negative (see Fig. 9-13), indicating that the chamber is under compression because of the generation of restoring or recoil forces during contraction, which result from stretching of functional springs in the myocardium. Restoring forces cause suction of blood into the ventricle, which lowers pressure during early filling. Restoring forces are inversely related to end-systolic volume (see Fig. 9-13). Thus suction is particularly important when the end-systolic volume is small, for example, during hypovolemia or increased contractility. Another ventricular property that is theoretically operative during early, rapid filling is a viscous effect that results because cardiac muscle resists stretch more at rapid lengthening rates.

Relaxation and the generation of restoring forces are dynamic aspects of filling whose influence varies markedly with time. Underlying these time-dependent properties is the so-called passive, or end-diastolic ventricular pressure-volume relation (Fig. 9-15), which is the relation between pressure and volume when the ventricle is in its fully relaxed, end-diastolic state, with either no or minimal levels of cross-bridge formation. Since this relation is exponential, passive compliance, the ratio of change in diastolic volume to change in pressure, is inversely related to volume. The passive pressure-volume relation is determined by the geometry of the ventricle (mainly wall thickness) and the stiffness of the myocardial tissue itself (ratio of change in stress to change in strain or extension of the tissue). Thus a thicker wall requires a larger pressure to fill the ventricle (i.e., it is less compliant at any volume). Similarly, if myocardial tissue is stiffer, for instance, because of increased connective tissue, this also results in decreased compliance. Throughout all of relaxation and filling, a portion of the pressure in the ventricle is dictated by its position on the passive pressure-volume relationship. The passive filling relationship is modified by external constraints (see Fig. 9-13). One constraint is the pericardium, which normally has a relatively small reserve vol-

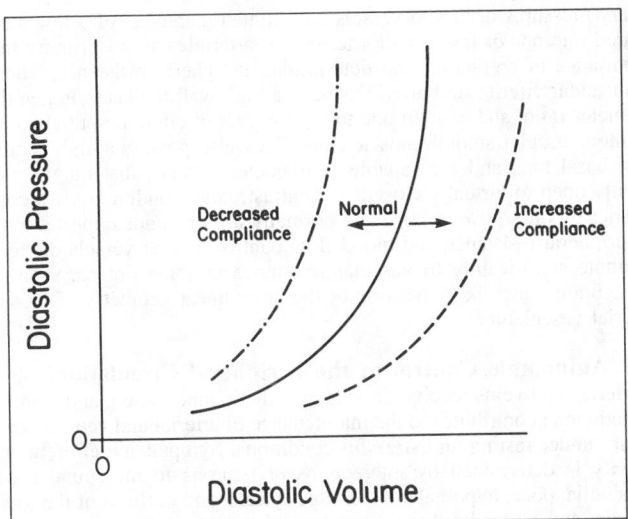

FIGURE 9-15 Schematic of the relation between pressure and volume in the passive ventricle (see text).

ume. Once this reserve volume is exceeded, the pericardium markedly resists further stretch and reduces ventricular compliance. For the left ventricle, this effect is likely very modest at physiologic volumes, but for the right ventricle it is an important determinant of diastolic pressure over the physiologic range of volume. The contribution of the pericardium to ventricular diastolic compliance can be important when the heart dilates rapidly. An additional constraint to filling of the left ventricle is the diastolic pressure in the right ventricle (and vice versa). Thus a portion of the right ventricular diastolic pressure is transmitted to the left ventricle, a phenomenon termed *diastolic ventricular interaction*. Diastolic interaction is likely a cause of elevated left ventricular diastolic pressure and decreased compliance observed with elevated right ventricular diastolic pressure, for example as a result of pulmonary hypertension.

One additional factor that influences diastolic filling is the amount of blood contained within the walls of the ventricle, or myocardial turgor. A significant component of the passive ventricular pressure-volume relation is accounted for by this effect. Changes in left ventricular compliance probably related to vascular turgor are observed soon after acute coronary occlusion, when there is often an increase in compliance.

Once relaxation is complete and recoil forces (if present) have dissipated, the passive pressure-volume relationship (modified by external constraints and turgor) is the chief determinant of the relationship between pressure and volume. During atrial contraction, ventricular pressure and volume usually track the passive pressure-volume relationship until end-diastole.

Echocardiography and Doppler flow velocity profiles are used clinically to delineate diastolic function (see Chapter 13). Transmitral velocity profiles are divided into E and A waves, corresponding to early inflow and atrial contraction, and filling characterized by their ratio and by filling rates. Abnormalities of relaxation and filling typically decrease the E/A ratio. The rate of deceleration of mitral inflow following the E wave peak is an index of passive left ventricular chamber compliance, and pulmonary venous inflow demonstrates consistent patterns when left atrial pressure is elevated. Using echocardiography, isovolumic relaxation time can be calculated from recordings of aortic and mitral valve motion, and left ventricular diastolic volume, wall thickness, and geometry can be estimated.

Short-Term Modulation of Ventricular Function

Heart rate. Heart rate is an important means of modulating ventricular function independent of changes in neurohumoral stimulation. Like the myocyte, the ventricle displays a positive "staircase" in response to increasing stimulation frequency (i.e., intrinsic contractile performance increases until an optimal rate is attained). Changes in contraction frequency also influence relaxation and filling. With in-

creased heart rate, diastole is shortened much more than systole, especially the slow filling phase between rapid filling and atrial contraction.

Paracrine modulation of ventricular function. A number of substances released locally and associated with vascular endothelium affect ventricular function, although their physiologic and pathophysiologic significance have not yet been clearly established. Nitric oxide itself and endothelium-dependent vasodilators cause modest depression in systolic performance and an earlier onset of left ventricular relaxation in association with an apparent increase in end-diastolic compliance. Although contractile performance assessed in terms of end-systolic indexes is depressed, peak positive dP/dt is unaltered. The mechanism(s) of these effects is uncertain. In contrast, under certain circumstances locally released vasoconstrictors such as endothelin and angiotensin II can have more or less opposite effects on ventricular function, causing delayed relaxation and decreased compliance.

Neurohumoral modulation of ventricular function. The most important short-term neurohumoral modulation occurs as a result of variations in sympathetic and parasympathetic stimulation caused by both cardiac neural activity and circulating catecholamines. Stimulation of β-receptors results in increased heart rate and contractility and more rapid relaxation. These effects are due to the influence of adrenergic stimulation on the sinus node and specialized conduction system and, within the myocyte, on the level of c-AMP and independent effects related to the force-frequency relationship. Other myocyte receptors include α-adrenergic, dopaminergic, angiotensin II, and histaminergic. Their importance in short-term modulation of ventricular function in the heart is uncertain. Some receptor-mediated responses are signals for cardiac hypertrophy (e.g., α-adrenergic agonism and angiotensin II). These agonists and endothelin appear to exert their effects via the inositol triphosphate second messenger system. This system causes increased intracellular calcium concentration but appears to be most important in relation to growth responses. Vagal stimulation has modest negative effects on contractility as well as profound heart rate lowering effects. Correspondingly, vagal withdrawal is important in the heart rate response to stress.

The heart participates in a number of reflex responses that also modulate short-term function and are integrated with the neurohumoral modulation described earlier. Thus the heart is an important part of the efferent limb of arterial baroreceptors and chemoreceptors. Similarly, pulmonary stretch receptors influence heart rate and play a role in sinus arrhythmia. Stretch receptors located in the atria may also modulate heart rate, especially tachycardia during increases in intravascular volume. Ventricular mechanoreceptors that respond to deformation rather than stretch per se are activated at small ventricular volumes. Discharge of these receptors results in vagally mediated bradycardia and hypotension and is likely involved in vasovagal syncope. Chemoreceptors located on the ventricular epicardial surface also connect to vagal efferents and may function physiologically in response to prostaglandins produced in the pericardial space.

Ventricular interaction. Another aspect of beat to beat control is interaction between the cardiac chambers. Interaction can be demonstrated among all of the chambers, but the most important are ventricle-ventricle interactions. Ventricular interaction is partly responsible for fine tuning of left and right heart output responses to frequent and rapid changes in loading conditions and heart rate (e.g., during changes in position and respiratory phase). Diastolic interaction across the septum has been mentioned earlier. The ventricles also interact during systole. Thus, for example, an abrupt increase in pulmonary artery pressure results in modest increases in left ventricular contractile performance.

Coronary perfusion. Changes in coronary perfusion pressure and/or flow per se influence ventricular function. In general, increases in perfusion pressure/flow augment systolic performance and most likely cause some decrease in passive compliance. Decreases in perfusion pressure/flow likely have opposite effects independent of myocardial ischemia, which occurs if perfusion is reduced to a sufficiently low level. A component of the influence of coronary perfusion on ventricular function is probably related to tissue turgor. Increased turgor caused by increased perfusion may stretch myocardial tissue, resulting in increased Frank-Starling effects and improved systolic performance. In addition, stretch-activated calcium channels may open as turgor increases. These effects may also be mediated by the afore-mentioned paracrine modulators of ventricular function. Subischemic decreases in perfusion pressure/flow underlie the clinical phenomenon of "hibernating" myocardium, in which systolic function is depressed but returns to normal with restoration of normal perfusion.

Long-term modulation of ventricular function. At the level of the whole ventricle, chronic stress is accompanied by various types of hypertrophy and remodeling of the myocardium. Patterns of remodeling are individualized, depending on the nature of the stress. Chronic pressure overload (aortic stenosis, hypertension) results in concentric hypertrophy (addition of new sarcomeres in parallel) in which wall thickness is increased with little change in chamber volume. This normalizes mean stress across the wall and improves systolic performance. In contrast, physiologic hypertrophy seen in endurance athletes or pure volume overload, for example as a result of mitral regurgitation, results in dilation of the left ventricle with little or no increase in wall thickness (addition of new sarcomeres in series). Often, chronic stress may encompass a combination of volume and pressure overload (e.g., aortic regurgitation) (see Chapter 25).

PERIPHERAL CIRCULATION
Distribution of Cardiac Output and Systemic Hemodynamics

The peripheral circulation distributes cardiac output throughout the various organs of the body. The elasticity of large arteries absorbs the highly pulsatile and discontinuous flow from the heart, such that the amplitude of pressure pulsations is diminished in small arteries and virtually absent in the venous circulation. Intravascular pressure also decreases from a mean value of 90 to 95 mm Hg in large arteries to about 30 mm Hg in capillaries and <20 mm Hg in veins.

The above values apply to resting conditions. Normally, the peripheral circulation must adapt rapidly to changes in arterial pressure and significant variations in end-organ metabolic demands. Even routine activities such as standing challenge the cardiovascular system profoundly. Because of gravitational forces, cerebral perfusion pressure and venous return are suddenly reduced. At the same time, capillary pressures in the ankles may exceed 90 to 100 mm Hg. The metabolic demands of exercise require redistribution of cardiac output to increase perfusion of coronary, pulmonary, and skeletal muscle circulations; diminish splanchnic flow; and maintain cerebral flow. Vascular regulatory mechanisms therefore must be bidirectional (i.e., blood flow can either increase or decrease on demand). For this to occur, the venous circulation must adjust its capacitance and modulate venous return (a major determinant of cardiac output), and the arterial vasculature must be in a position to modulate flow by constriction or dilation. Because it is impossible to dilate a vessel that is already fully relaxed, some portion of the arterial circulation must operate in a state of partial constriction or tone.

Arterial Diameter, Vascular Resistance, and Flow. Pressure, flow, and resistance are most often related through Poiseuille's equation, which predicts that flow is proportional to the fourth power of vessel radius and inversely proportional to the fourth power of resistance:

$$Q \propto r^4, \text{ or } Q \propto 1/R^4, \text{ where } r = \text{radius and } R = \text{resistance}$$

Thus given the same initial pressure, doubling inner radius results in a sixteen-fold increase in flow (2^4). Estimates from intact vascular networks suggest this may be an overestimation and that a third power equation may be more accurate. In any case, relatively minor changes in arterial caliber can produce large changes in resistance and flow, which are related through a simple equation analogous to Ohm's law: flow = perfusion pressure/resistance. Although resistance is also affected by fluid viscosity and vessel length, these parameters are normally relatively invariant in the cardiovascular system. Therefore lumen diameter is the most powerful determinant of vascular resistance (and therefore blood flow) under physiologic conditions. Because most of the >60 mm Hg drop between systemic arterial and capil-lary pressures occurs in vessels with lumen diameters of a few hundred microns or less, small arteries and arterioles are of primary importance in regulating and determining peripheral resistance. These muscular arteries and arterioles have a high wall thickness/lumen diameter ratio, and contain one to three layers of circumferentially oriented vascular smooth muscle cells. They also possess a high degree of basal tone and are capable of diameter changes that range from fully open to virtually closed. In contrast, large conduit arteries constrict by only 10% to 20% and normally are of minor importance to peripheral resistance and blood flow control. Larger vessels do contribute significantly to vascular resistance in some organs, such as the brain, most likely because of the more linear geometry of the arterial vasculature.

Autonomic Control of the Peripheral Circulation. Most arteries and veins receive direct sympathetic innervation, and sympathetic tone contributes to the maintenance of arterial and venous pressure under resting and stressful conditions. Sympathetic efferent activity is determined by interactions of neurons in the spinal cord, medulla, pons, hypothalamus, limbic system, and portions of the forebrain, and by feedback signals arising from cardiovascular mechanoreceptors and chemoreceptors that are localized in discrete baroreceptor centers in the carotid sinuses, aortic arch, and heart. The two central areas that appear to be of principal importance in regulating sympathetic outflow are the nucleus tractus solitarius (NTS) and the rostral ventral lateral medulla (RVLM). The influence of the NTS on the RVLM is inhibitory. In animals, bilateral lesions lead to malignant hypertension.

Sympathetic denervation produces varying effects on organ blood flow. The cerebral circulation is virtually unaffected, most likely because of autoregulatory mechanisms, whereas denervation of the skin increases flow as much as ten-fold. During intense sympathetic activation, large amounts of epinephrine (and, to a lesser extent, norepinephrine) are released from the adrenal medulla in response to activation of sympathetic preganglionic afferents. Blood pressure increases markedly, and a significant redistribution of cardiac output occurs, including increased perfusion of working skeletal muscle and decreased splanchnic flow. Stimulation of the venous circulation increases venous return, thereby augmenting cardiac output. The parasympathetic system, via the vagus nerve, generally produces effects opposite those of the sympathetic division (i.e., decreased cardiac rate and output and vascular relaxation) but is of secondary importance in vascular as opposed to cardiac tissues.

Integration of Control Mechanisms in the Peripheral Circulation. Minute-to-minute control of the peripheral circulation involves a complex interplay between several mechanisms, neural, myogenic, and endothelial. Metabolites released from adjacent tissues also impinge on the vascular wall (metabolic regulation). Under resting conditions skeletal muscle arteries and arterioles operate in a highly constricted state, and skeletal muscle perfusion is relatively low. Physical activity can result in manyfold increases in skeletal muscle blood flow because of increased cardiac output and arterial dilation, so that the proportion of cardiac output directed to skeletal muscles increases from 20% to >70%, and total blood flow is increased by a factor of ten (Table 9-1). Interestingly, some studies show that an increase in skeletal muscle blood flow can be detected before exercise actually begins, suggesting a neurally mediated anticipatory effect.

During exercise, dilation of skeletal muscle arteries and arterioles occurs because of metabolic factors such as adenosine, potassium, and hydrogen ions that diffuse from the adjacent myocytes into the vascular wall and induce hyperpolarization and relaxation of vascular smooth muscle either directly or indirectly, by stimulating the release of endothelial factors such as nitric oxide and prostacyclin. Increased flow itself serves as a stimulus for further vasodilation, presumably through a shear stress–induced release of vasoactive substances from the endothelium.

Blood Flow Autoregulation. Autoregulation is defined as the ability of an organ to maintain a relatively constant blood flow despite changes in arterial pressure. Although most organs autoregulate blood flow to some degree, this phenomenon is particularly well de-

Table 9-1 Distribution of cardiac output in normal human subjects at rest and after 10 minutes of strenuous exercise

	BLOOD FLOW (ML/MIN, % OF TOTAL)			
VASCULAR BED	REST		EXERCISE	
Skeletal muscle	1200	(21%)	12,500	(71%)
Splanchnic	1400	(24%)	600	(3%)
Renal	1100	(19%)	600	(3%)
Cerebral	750	(13%)	750	(5%)
Coronary	250	(4%)	750	(5%)
Skin	500	(9%)	1900	(11%)
Other organs	600	(10%)	400	(2%)
Cardiac output	5800	(100%)	17,500	(100%)

From Milnor WR: *Cardiovascular physiology,* Oxford, 1990, Oxford University Press.

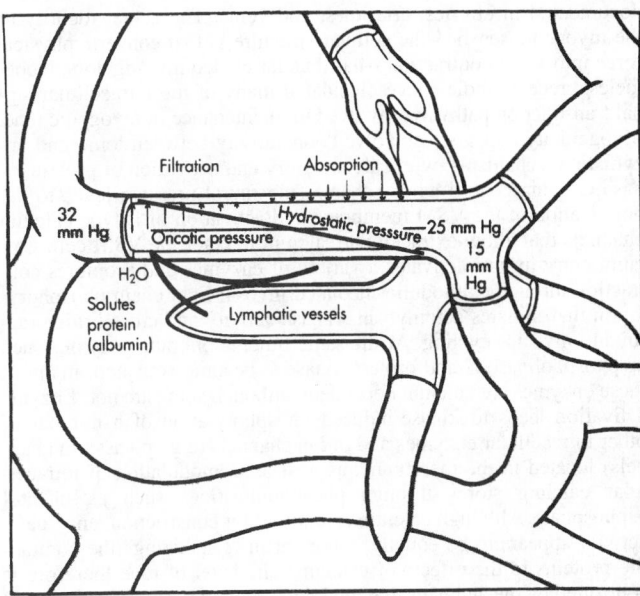

FIGURE 9-16 Schematic representation of the factors responsible for filtration and absorption across the capillary wall and the formation of lymph. (From Berne RM, Levy MN: *Cardiovascular physiology,* St Louis, 1992, Mosby.)

veloped in the cerebral, coronary, and renal circulations and is principally effected by adjustments in the caliber of smaller arteries and arterioles. Autoregulatory effectiveness is defined by the ability of the arteries to constrict to increased pressure and dilate in response to decreased pressure to keep total blood flow relatively constant. Autoregulation involves several mechanisms, most notably myogenic and metabolic. The process has upper and lower pressure limits. If perfusion pressure falls below a certain point (lower limit of autoregulation), tissue hypoperfusion ensues. Transmural pressures above the upper limit of autoregulation result in a breakthrough phenomenon in which forced dilation of arteries occurs, leading to loss of arterial and arteriolar tone. Large increases in organ blood flow, transmission of high intravascular pressures to capillaries and veins, and vessel leakage and rupture may occur.

Finally, the ability to autoregulate blood flow must be reserved for some but not all organs. If increased blood pressure stimulated arterial constriction throughout the body, total peripheral resistance would increase, raising pressure further via a positive feedback mechanism that could have dire consequences. An equally dangerous situation would occur in response to a fall in blood pressure and would lead to vascular collapse. Hence, simultaneous and opposite changes in arterial and arteriolar tone and/or adjustments in venous capacitance and plasma volume (driven by the nervous and endocrine systems) must occur normally to prevent hypertension or hypotension.

Principles of Capillary Exchange and Microcirculatory Control Mechanisms

Capillaries are the only segment of the vasculature capable of nutrient and gaseous exchange, and of hormonal delivery to target tissues. The underlying biophysical principles were defined in 1896 by Starling, who proposed that fluid exchange in the capillary resulted from an interplay between two opposing but balanced forces (Fig. 9-16). At the proximal end of a capillary, intravascular pressure slightly exceeds tissue pressure and results in hydraulic ultrafiltration—movement of fluid through the capillary wall and into the extracellular space. The capillary acts as a selective filter, and the degree of selectivity varies with the physical properties of the endothelium and cells associated with its outer edge, such as pericytes. The passage of relatively large molecules such as proteins is largely impeded, although some leakage occurs with subsequent reabsorption into lymphatic vessels and a return to the circulation. Consequently, plasma osmolarity increases along the length of a capillary, and the associated force (oncotic pressure) tends to pull extracellular fluid back into the capillary lumen through a process of reabsorption. The subtle, bidirectional percolation of fluid is modulated by the biophysical and biochemical properties of endothelial cells, along with specialized cells associated with the outside of a capillary (pericytes or astrocytes). These functions are in turn modulated by humoral and endocrine factors. An imbalance between the opposing forces can lead to edema if filtration exceeds reabsorption. If reabsorption exceeds filtration, plasma volume expands (primarily on the venous side) and cellular/extracellular volume decreases.

Elevations in hydrostatic pressure need not be strictly arterial to have adverse consequences. Increased venous pressure may cause a back pressure that increases capillary filtration and impedes reabsorption. Edema in patients with right-sided heart failure and elevated venous pressure is a clinical example of the way in which capillary forces are altered secondary to changes in venous hemodynamics. Under normal conditions, it is essential for the arterial tree to regulate resistance so as to maintain capillary pressure at levels at which normal fluid exchange may occur. The following section is devoted to reviewing the mechanisms by which the cells of the arterial wall regulate arterial tone and, hence, vascular resistance and capillary pressure.

In general, the amount of tone increases with decreasing arterial size and is greatest in smaller arteries and arterioles that play a major role in determining peripheral resistance and regulating regional blood flow. The level of tone at any time reflects an integration of multiple excitatory and inhibitory pathways that converge upon the ultimate effector, vascular smooth muscle (VSM), to "set" the level of tone. Changes in the physical forces impinging on the vascular wall (shear stress, transmural pressure), in neurotransmitter release from nerves (most often at the medial-adventitial junction), or in the concentration of metabolites released from surrounding tissues all modulate the set point to either increase or decrease arterial tone.

The endothelium, the interface between blood and VSM, is also an important modulator of tone via release of vasoactive factors having inhibitory (e.g., nitric oxide, prostacyclin) or excitatory (e.g., endothelin, thromboxane) effects on VSM. Moreover, in many arteries the endothelium is coupled to VSM through numerous myoendothelial junctions. The nature of the contact may vary but sometimes occurs through low-resistance gap junctions that allow bidirectional transfer of information and propagation of dilation or constriction. Finally, VSM itself is capable of constricting in response to pressure or stretch. Because this phenomenon occurs in isolated arterial segments denuded of endothelium and in the absence of metabolic or neural factors, it appears to be truly endogenous to VSM and therefore is termed *myogenic tone.* A discussion of myogenic tone and reactivity lends itself to an understanding of signal transduction by vascular smooth muscle and the way in which other exogenous (endothelial, neural, metabolic) inputs are integrated to produce a system that is responsive, bidirectional, and subject to a high degree of local control.

Arterial constriction to increased perfusion pressure was first described by Bayliss in 1902. Since then, myogenic responses have been documented in arteries, arterioles, and veins. The actual identity of the myogenic sensor—the cellular structure(s) that converts physical force into VSM contraction—has thus far eluded investigators. Nonetheless, recent studies have elucidated many of the intracellular signal transduction pathways involved in maintenance of myogenic tone. Myogenicity appears to involve cooperativity between ionic and enzymatic mechanisms, with calcium entry and activation of protein kinase C being central among them. Transmural pressure leads to depolarization of the VSM membrane and activation of L-type calcium channels that allow extracellular calcium to enter the VSM cell. Calcium entry in turn activates a variety of enzymes and promotes contraction through calmodulin-mediated myosin light chain phosphorylation that initiates actomyosin ATPase activity and cross-bridge (actin and myosin) cycling. At the same time, membrane enzymes such as phospholipase C and protein kinase C become activated; many of these enzymes are calcium dependent, although some are not. Enzyme activation leads to kinase-induced phosphorylation of a number of other intracellular enzymes and of ion channels (e.g., potassium channels) located in the membrane, as well as to modulation of intracellular calcium stores through phosphoinositides such as inositol triphosphate. Although calcium is required for constriction, enzymatic activity appears to be equally important in "sensitizing" the contractile proteins to the effects of calcium. The level of tone therefore is controlled by mechanisms that modulate calcium entry and efflux, and by enzymatic modulation of its effect on the contractile proteins. Feedback mechanisms are poorly understood but may involve calcium-induced activation of potassium channels whose opening facilitates potassium efflux and membrane hyperpolarization.

The importance of the endothelium in modulation of arterial tone was recognized in the early 1980s, when Furchgott and colleagues reported that this cell type was obligatory for the relaxation response to acetylcholine. They found that endothelial denudation abolished relaxation to acetylcholine and hypothesized that cholinergic stimulation led to release of a then-unidentified substance that relaxed VSM. This substance, initially called endothelium-derived relaxing factor (EDRF), was subsequently (1988) shown to be nitric oxide (NO). NO is produced during conversion of the amino acid L-arginine into L-citrulline by the enzyme nitric oxide synthase. In addition to its vasodilatory actions, NO is now known to be a cytotoxic molecule utilized by the immune system, a neurotransmitter, and a modulator of cell division. It is now clear that the endothelium performs a variety of chemotransduction and mechanotransduction functions and releases a host of vasoactive molecules in response to both physical and chemical stimulation. Foremost, in addition to NO, are the peptide endothelin and dilator and constrictor prostaglandins (such as prostacyclin and thromboxane, respectively). There is also experimental evidence for a non-NO factor that hyperpolarizes smooth muscle. This substance has not yet been identified and is simply called EDHF (endothelium-derived hyperpolarizing factor).

Endothelial secretions diffuse to adjacent VSM to activate a variety of signal transduction mechanisms that alter intracellular concentrations of cAMP (prostaglandins), cGMP (nitric oxide), phospholipase C (endothelin), and membrane potential (EDHF). Release of endothelium-derived vasoactive molecules is controlled by a variety of factors. Shear is thought to be an important stimulus for a number of endothelial events, including hyperpolarization (opening of potassium channels), calcium influx, up-regulation and down-regulation of mRNA for many different proteins (e.g., tPA, heat shock proteins), induction of G proteins and a number of kinases (protein kinase C, MAP kinase), cytoskeletal rearrangement, and release of cytokines and growth factors. Shear stress can also modulate arterial growth and remodeling through an endothelium-dependent mechanism. Aberrations in small artery endothelial function (most often diminished release of or paradoxical reactions to vasodilator substances) have been reported in several diseases, such as hypertension and diabetes. In larger arteries, abnormal flow patterns (turbulence, eddy currents, particularly at bifurcations) associated with lower than normal shear stress may lead to metabolic derangements in endothelial function and accelerate atherosclerosis.

The Coronary Circulation

The main coronary arteries (right and left) arise at the root of the aorta and provide the blood supply to the myocardium. The right coro-

nary artery normally supplies the inferior surface of the left ventricle and the right ventricle and atrium, whereas the left coronary artery divides into circumflex and anterior descending branches that perfuse the bulk of the left ventricular myocardium and the left atrium. Branches from the main arteries ramify and penetrate the myocardium, forming dense capillary beds. By some estimates, as much as 30% of the heart, by weight, consists of vascular cells. Venous blood returns to the right atrium through the coronary sinus. There is also some communication between the chambers of the heart and the myocardium via arteriosinusoidal channels that anastomose with other sinuses and capillaries (arteriosinusoidal and arterioluminal arteries and thebesian veins), and interconnect with cardiac veins.

Coronary blood flow is complicated by the myocardium, which compresses intramyocardial vessels during systole, sometimes to a degree sufficient to induce retrograde flow in epicardial arteries. As a result, the bulk of coronary flow occurs during diastole. This renders the subendocardial layer of the myocardium more susceptible to hypoperfusion because ventricular diastolic pressure opposes the driving pressure for flow. There has been some uncertainty about the actual driving pressure for coronary flow, in particular whether the downstream pressure should be considered equivalent to right atrial/coronary sinus pressure or a larger value related to tissue forces that cause collapse of the microcirculation (i.e., a critical closing pressure). Nonetheless, regulatory mechanisms similar to those already described function to modulate coronary flow (Fig. 9-17). The coronary circulation autoregulates in response to changes in perfusion pressure, although the level of flow is most closely linked to metabolic demand. Sympathetic stimulation of the heart, unlike in many other vascular beds, elicits a marked increase in coronary flow associated with acceleration of the cardiac rhythm and increased contractility. Under conditions of β-receptor blockade (thus preventing the chronotropic and inotropic effects of sympathetic stimulation on the myocardium), reflex activation of sympathetic nerves increases coronary resistance, demonstrating that the direct action of norepinephrine on coronary resistance vessels is constriction. The effect of norepinephrine on the coronary circulation is modulated by a combination of α- and β-receptors that mediate constriction and relaxation, respectively. The distribution of receptor subtypes on vascular smooth muscle and endothelium varies with type of vessel and may change with age.

Because myocardial oxygen extraction is near maximal even under basal conditions, the principal mechanism by which the heart increases its oxygen supply with increased demand is an autoregulatory decrease in coronary resistance with a concomitant increase in flow. Metabolites released from myocytes, most importantly adenosine and potassium, dilate the arterial circulation and augment myocardial perfusion during increased demand. The coronary circulation of a healthy individual possesses considerable reserve, and flow can increase by 400% during strenuous exercise. As expected, there is close parallelism between myocardial oxygen consumption and coro-

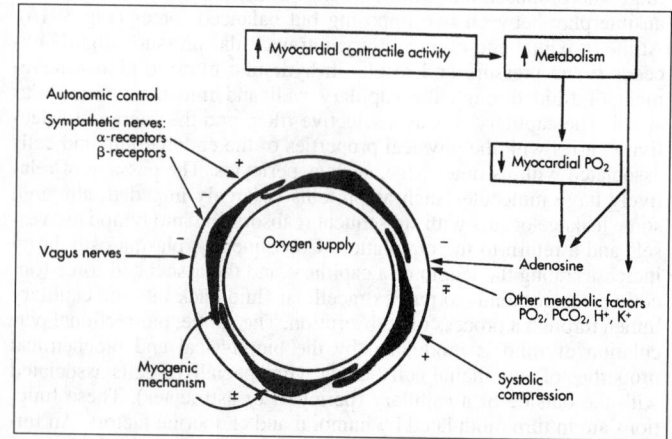

FIGURE 9-17 Schematic representative of factors that increase (+) or decrease (−) coronary vascular resistance. The intravascular pressure (arterial blood pressure) stretches the vessel wall.

(From Berne RM, Levy MN: *Cardiovascular physiology,* St Louis, 1992, Mosby.)

nary blood flow, which is required to avoid underperfusion and ischemia.

INTEGRATION OF THE CARDIOVASCULAR SYSTEM: THE CARDIOVASCULAR RESPONSE TO DYNAMIC EXERCISE

Isotonic exercise, consisting of endurance activities such as walking, running, swimming, and cycling with repetitive shortening against relatively low loads, causes a coordinated response that maximizes delivery of blood to working skeletal muscle and the heart (see Table 9-1). In the peripheral circulation, local vasodilatory influences reduce resistance in working muscle vascular beds. To facilitate heat transfer, cutaneous vascular beds dilate. In contrast, neurohumorally mediated responses cause vasoconstriction in nonworking skeletal muscle and other organs such as the abdominal viscera. With isotonic exercise in which large muscle groups are used, there is usually a decrease in total systemic vascular resistance. Coronary flow is augmented because of autoregulatory vasodilation in response to increased metabolic demands. As indicated earlier, in the normal circulation the ability to return blood to the heart is the limiting factor for increases in cardiac output during exercise. Accordingly, systemic venoconstriction, pumping of venous blood by working muscles, and the valves in the systemic veins are important in exercise responses. In addition, increased respiratory rate causes the intrathoracic pressure to be negative more often, which further assists venous return to the right heart. In the heart itself, adrenergic stimulation caused by the coordinated effects of increased central nervous outflow and circulating catecholamines, along with parasympathetic withdrawal, results in increased heart rate, accelerated atrioventricular conduction, and enhanced contractility. During upright exercise in normal subjects, ventricular end-diastolic volume remains fairly constant. Reflecting increased contractility, end-systolic volume decreases and therefore stroke volume and ejection fraction increase. The increased heart rate per se improves contractile performance as a result of the force-frequency relationship. Because the increase in heart rate is greater than the increase in stroke volume, increased rate is the most important factor accounting for increased cardiac output. The combination of increased heart rate and stroke volume with marked shortening of diastole means that ventricular filling must occur much more rapidly than under resting conditions. A likely important mechanism of the increase in rate of ventricular filling during exercise is increased generation of restoring forces resulting from the decrease in end-systolic volume. Thus the enhanced force of contraction is linked to increased suction, which, along with a more rapid relaxation rate, allows increased filling to occur without a rise in ventricular diastolic pressure. Systolic arterial pressure rises in parallel with heart rate, whereas diastolic blood pressure decreases. The increase in systolic pressure is related to the increase in stroke volume, whereas the decrease in diastolic pressure is related to the net decrease in systemic vascular resistance. Last, there is evidence that during exercise, changes in both ventricular and vascular elastance optimize ventricular-vascular coupling.

BIBLIOGRAPHY

Abboud FM, Thames MD: Interaction of cardiovascular reflexes in circulatory control. In Berne R, Sperelakis N, editors: *Handbook of physiology: the cardiovascular system*, vol 3, Bethesda, 1983, American Physiological Society.

Braunwald E, Sobel BE: Coronary blood flow and myocardial ischemia. In Braunwald E, editor: *Heart disease: a textbook of cardiovascular medicine*, ed 4, Philadelphia, 1992, WB Saunders.

Brown AM: Cardiac reflexes. In Berne R, Sperelakis N, editors: *Handbook of physiology*, vol 1, Bethesda, 1983, American Physiological Society.

Feigl EO: Coronary physiology, *Physiol Rev* 63:1-205, 1983.

Gaasch WH, Le Winter MM, editors: *Left ventricular diastolic dysfunction and heart failure*, Philadelphia, 1994, Lea & Febiger.

Gibbons WR, Zygmunt AC: Excitation-contraction coupling in the heart. In Fozzard et al, editors: *The heart and cardiovascular system*, vol 2, New York, 1991, Raven Press.

Guyton AC: The circulation. In Guyton AC, editor: *Textbook of medical physiology*, ed 7, Philadelphia, 1986, WB Saunders.

Hathaway DR et al: Vascular smooth muscle: a review of the molecular basis of contractility, *Circulation* 83:382-390, 1991.

Shroff SG et al: Mechanical and energetic behavior of the intact left ventricle. In Fozzard HA et al, editors: *The heart and cardiovascular system*, vol 1, New York, 1991, Raven Press.

Woledge RC, Curtin NA, Homsher E: *Energetic aspects of muscle contraction*, London, 1985, Academic Press.

Yellin EL, Nikolic S, Frater RWM: Left ventricular filling dynamics and diastolic function, *Prog Cardiovasc Dis* 32:247-271, 1990.

CHAPTER

10 Molecular Biology of the Cardiovascular System

Roger D. Bies and Robert Roberts

The study of the mechanisms controlling cardiovascular function has recently undergone a dramatic evolution from the traditional physiologic and anatomic paradigms that have dominated the field for many years to an intense interest in the cascade of molecular interactions responsible for cardiac and vascular development, growth, hypertrophy, adaptation to physiologic stress, cholesterol metabolism, thrombosis, and hormonal and autonomic effects in the myocardium. Molecular biology offers a unique technology that allows one to study the molecular diversity within the heart. Rare molecules difficult to detect at the protein level because of their low concentrations can now be analyzed. The specific gene product, as well as the regulatory mechanisms that control when a protein is expressed, and in what cell or tissue, to perform a programmed biologic function, can now be explored. This can be accomplished either in isolated cells or in the intact organism using recombinant deoxyribonucleic acid (DNA) technology, such as in a transgenic animal. Unique molecular control and expression of genes to generate specific proteins are important in the development and function of the myocardium, the valvular apparatus, the conduction system, and the vascular system. Recombinant DNA technology promises to provide not only an understanding of the basic mechanisms of cardiovascular science but also a therapeutic benefit. This chapter is an introduction to basic molecular biology, common molecular laboratory technology, and the recent advances made in molecular cardiology and cardiovascular genetics.

THE DNA CODE

The human chromosome, the largest molecule in the human body, comprises a long double-stranded helical molecule of DNA associated with different nuclear proteins. Each strand consists of a chain of deoxyribose sugars missing a hydroxyl group on the second carbon atom of the sugar ring. The deoxyribose sugar chain is linked by phosphodiester bonds between the fifth ($5'$) carbon atom on one sugar to the third ($3'$) carbon in the ring on the preceding sugar molecule. The first carbon of the sugar ring is linked to one of the four nucleotide bases found in all DNA molecules. Thus, by convention, DNA is arranged in a $5'$ to $3'$ direction through its phosphodiester linkages. *Genes* are discrete regions of DNA arranged sequentially along the molecule. Each gene contains a specific DNA code that directs the synthesis of a unique messenger ribonucleic acid (mRNA), a mirror image of the code contained on the DNA. The mRNA is processed and transported from the nucleus to the cellular cytoplasm. In the cytoplasm, the genetic code is "read" by a large molecule called a *ribosome*. It translates the language encoded by the linear sequence of the nucleotides (bases) in the mRNA into a language written in linear sequence of amino acids from which a unique polypeptide is synthesized to perform a specific cell function. Some genes, the so-called housekeeping genes, are turned on all of the time and provide the common proteins for cell structure, cellular organelles, and metabolic enzymes that perform basic cell function. In the heart and vascular system, as in other organs, some genes are specifically turned on or off to give these cells their tissue-specific characteristics to perform the unique function typical of that organ.

The specificity of the DNA code is spelled out by a simple four-letter code designated by the nucleotide bases. These letters A, C, G, and T refer to adenine, cytosine, guanine, and thymine, respectively. The information is stored in the DNA molecule and passed on to each generation through the variation in the linear sequence of these four letters. The variation in the linear sequence is also what provides the specificity of any DNA fragment. Each gene has a unique sequence (genotype), which codes for a unique protein that imparts a unique feature (phenotype) to the individual or its offspring. The two DNA strands are held together by hydrogen bonds between exclusive nucleotide base pairs such that each strand has a complementary strand that perfectly matches its mate (Fig. 10-1). Adenine binds only to thymine with two hydrogen bonds (A→T), and guanine binds only to cytosine with three hydrogen bonds (G→C). The uniqueness of the sequence of a particular stretch of nucleotides and the highly specific complementary hydrogen bond base pairing account for the specificity of the DNA code and serve as the basis for the sensitive and specific techniques currently used in molecular biology.

The mRNA is initially in the nucleus, where it is synthesized as a mirror image from the DNA template of a particular active gene. The mRNA found in a particular cell represents the activity of only those specific genes required for that particular cell's function. mRNA is a single-stranded molecule very similar to DNA in that it is composed of a long chain of ribose sugars, each linked to a phosphate group and a nucleotide base. The mRNA code is identical to the DNA code from which it is made, except that the nucleotide base thymine is not found in RNA and is replaced by the nucleotide base uracil (U). As with thymine, uracil associates only with adenine. mRNA is a processed form of nuclear RNA that is transported to the cell's cytoplasm, where the unique coding sequence is translated into a polypeptide. A group of three nucleotide bases is called a *codon,* and a unique combination of the A, U, G, and C bases encodes for each of the 20 common amino acids found in protein molecules.

The amino acid content and sequence for a particular protein are encoded by the mRNA molecule, which is synthesized from a chromosomal gene. Therefore the isolation and identification of the sequence of an individual mRNA provide unique information. One drawback to the study of mRNA is that it is an easily degraded, single-stranded molecule. One "trick" used in molecular biology to produce a stable copy of the information contained in mRNA is to use the enzyme reverse transcriptase to synthesize a complementary DNA molecule (cDNA) from the RNA template. cDNA is a stable copy of the mRNA that can then be manipulated for cloning, sequencing, or producing recombinant proteins in vivo.

GENE EXPRESSION AND ITS REGULATION

Gene expression refers to the processes whereby a gene gives rise to its end product, namely, its unique polypeptide. This implies transcription, processing of the mRNA, transport of the mRNA to the cytoplasm, and then translation into protein and subsequent postranscriptional modification. Normal and abnormal molecular responses to biologic or pharmacologic stress include changes in contractile protein isoforms in cardiac hypertrophy and failure, activation of endogenous injury and repair mechanisms in myocardial necrosis, changes in sodium channel properties during prolonged therapy with antiarrhythmic drugs, or regulation of cardiac β-receptor density with cardiac β-blocker therapy. Regulation of these processes occurs at multiple levels, from the gene in the cardiac cell to modification or phosphorylation of the resultant protein.

Gene transcription is the process of activation of a particular gene and the synthesis of that gene's specific RNA message. The regulation and selectivity of gene expression by a particular cell are the bases for cell differentiation and are what, for example, make cardiac muscle different from skeletal muscle or smooth muscle. Before transcription can occur, the DNA at the site of the gene of interest must unravel and expose its sequence to an enzyme that can synthesize an RNA copy of the gene. DNA is normally compacted around a class of well-characterized proteins called *histones,* which may act to regulate the availability of a particular segment of DNA for gene activity. Histones bind with the DNA, and changes in histone DNA binding may allow a conformational configuration in the DNA helix such that RNA polymerase can bind and begin synthesis of an RNA molecule. At the start site of a particular gene, the presence or absence of methyl (CH$_3$) groups in the dinucleotide sequence, —C—G—, has also been shown to be an important factor as to whether the gene is active in a particular cell. Gene activation involves the binding of RNA polymerase to a specific segment of the gene called the *promoter.* Once this binding occurs, RNA polymerase moves down the DNA molecule, reading and synthesizing an RNA copy of the gene until the end of the gene is reached and the RNA polymerase falls off. Several complex factors regulate the rate and frequency of RNA polymerase binding. Other unique elements at the start site of a gene include *enhancer* sequences, which interact with the promoter and regulate RNA polymerase binding, whereas other elements inhibit transcription and are referred to as *silencers* (Fig. 10-2).

Transcription factors are a heterogeneous group of proteins that bind to promoter, enhancer, and silencer sequences and further modulate RNA polymerase binding. They are nuclear proteins that can regulate the tissue-specific and physiologic activation of certain genes. There are at least three well-known classes of transcriptional factors referred to as zinc fingers, leucine zippers, and helix-loop-helix molecules. The zinc fingers represent a distinct class of specific DNA binding proteins that contain what is termed *zinc finger* motif: a fingerlike loop is stabilized at the base by a single zinc ion to form a common DNA binding structure. One familiar group of transcription factors belonging to the zinc finger family are the glucocorticoid and thyroid receptor proteins. Thyroid hormone, which binds to its cell surface receptor on cardiac myocytes, is transported as a receptor complex to the nucleus, where it is shown to be a prominent regulator of myosin heavy chain (MHC) gene expression. *Leucine zipper proteins* form a second category of transcription factors that regulate cardiac gene expression. Two well-studied proteins in the heart include c-*jun* and c-*fos*. These proteins generally form dimers held together by the interaction of four or five leucine residues, spaced seven residues apart in the sequence of each protein. These leucine residues interdigitate in a zipperlike dimer and are referred to as the *leucine zipper* motif, which is used to describe this class of transcrip-

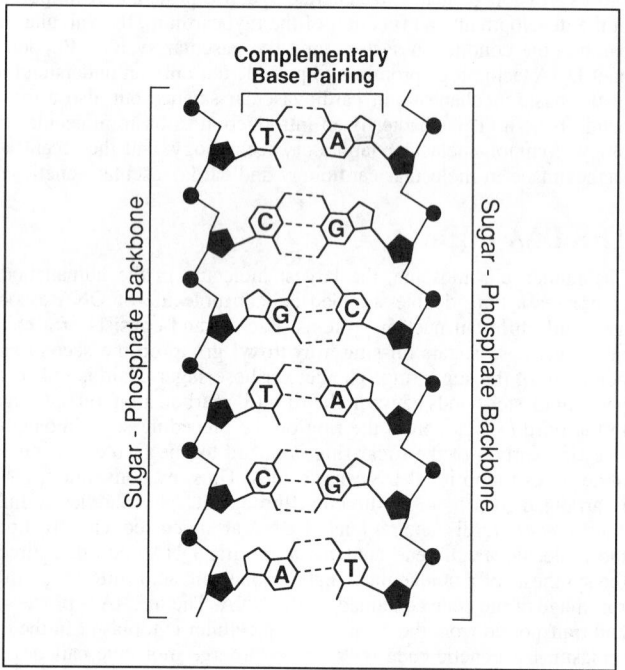

FIGURE 10-1   Specificity of deoxyribonucleic acid (DNA) base pairing. The two strands of DNA are bound together by hydrogen bonds between the nucleotide bases on each strand. The bonds are formed by strict pairing between two complementary bases, A—T or C—G, such that each strand reflects the exact sequence of the opposite strand. *A,* Adenine, *T,* thymine; *G,* guanine; *C,* cytosine. The sugar *(dark pentamer)* and phosphate *(dark circle)* linkages form the backbone of the DNA strand.

(From Roberts R et al: *A primer of molecular biology,* New York, 1992, Elsevier.)

tion factor proteins. The promoter region of some genes involved in cardiac hypertrophy contain a conserved DNA sequence (e.g., the AP1 site) that binds leucine zipper–type proteins. Pressure and volume overload of cardiac tissue induce the expression of oncogene proteins, which may then regulate the genes involved in compensatory hypertrophy or structural remodeling of the ventricular wall.

Some transcription factors are able to activate the genes that determine the tissue characteristics of a specific cell. For example, a transcription factor protein called *myo-D* is capable of turning on the gene programs that induce a cell to be skeletal muscle. This protein's influence is so strong that if the myo-D protein is introduced into a nonmuscle cell such as a fibroblast, it can transform that cell into a skeletal muscle by imposing its regulatory properties. Myo-D is a nuclear protein in the class of molecules called *helix-loop-helix* proteins, which describe a common structural conformation for this class of transcription factor proteins.

The next step in the regulation of gene expression is the process of *posttranscriptional regulation,* the cell's ability to modify or process the RNA transcript once it has been produced. One important mechanism of posttranscriptional regulation is the process of alternative mRNA splicing. This occurs in the nucleus before export of the mature RNA into the cytoplasm. Alternative splicing is a mechanism whereby a single RNA code from a single gene can be "edited" by the cell by splicing out or inserting some of the coding sequences, which ultimately results in a change in a portion of the protein's peptide sequence produced by that gene. In this way, multiple *isoforms* of a protein can be produced from a single gene. Various cardiac proteins, including the contractile elements troponin T and tropomyosin, as well as dystrophin, a cytoskeletal protein in the heart, are expressed as tissue-specific and developmentally specific isoforms that may confer variations in molecular function tailored for the cell's specific needs.

Further regulatory steps that modulate the ultimate quantity and activity of a particular protein product from an activated gene occur in the cell cytoplasm and relate to translation and posttranslational changes. For example, the stability of the mRNA can determine the quantity of protein produced at the level of the ribosome. Many protein modifications occur after translation, including proteolysis, which can cleave off a peptide fragment to form an active molecule; glyco-

sylation; phosphorylation, the formation of sulfhydryl bonds; or the coupling of fatty acids, which may affect the protein's destination within the cell. All these steps are potential targets for pharmacologic or genetic therapies.

INHERENT PROPERTIES OF DNA FUNDAMENTAL TO RECOMBINANT DNA TECHNIQUES

The DNA molecule possesses three inherent features that are essential and fundamental to recombinant techniques: (1) DNA consists of two strands held together by hydrogen bonding; (2) denaturation, such as by increasing the temperature from 50° C to 95° C, breaks the hydrogen bonds so that the strands fall apart; but on cooling to 50° C, the two strands through complementary base pairing reanneal (hybridize) to their previous identical structure; and (3) the phosphage group of each nucleotide imparts a negative charge so that molecules of different size can be separated by electrophoresis.

Several applications of recombinant DNA techniques are unique:
1. In vivo structure function analysis
2. Molecular genetics
3. Exploring the molecular basis of the growth response
4. Genetically engineered site-specific drugs

ISOLATION AND DIGESTION OF DNA

Molecular techniques using DNA have proved useful in the development of diagnostic tools to analyze cardiovascular diseases and have provided a unique approach to structure/function analysis of molecular interactions in the heart. DNA can be isolated from any human tissue, including blood. The white cells provide an easily accessible source of DNA and can be extracted manually or with an automatic DNA extraction device. About 200 μg of DNA can be obtained from 10 to 20 ml of blood, which can be stored almost indefinitely at subzero temperatures. The lymphocytes can be transformed with Epstein-Barr virus to propagate indefinitely in cell culture as immortal cell lines to provide a renewable source of DNA. In performing molecular genetic studies, researchers routinely use lymphocytes because a renewable source of DNA precludes the necessity of obtaining further blood from the family.

DNA is present in extremely large molecules because each chromosome is essentially a single, long DNA molecule. The smallest chromosome (chromosome 21) has about 50 million base pairs (bp), whereas the largest chromosome (chromosome 1) has more than 250 million bp. The techniques for identification and analysis of DNA became feasible and readily accessible with the discovery of restriction endonuclease enzymes found in bacteria. These particular enzymes made it possible to cut DNA into smaller fragments of specific sizes, a process usually referred to as *digestion.* They have specific recognition sites that vary from 2 to 8 bp in length. These enzymes cut only at these specific recognition sites, and thus the number of fragments generated for a particular DNA molecule remain consistent with the number of recognition sites and provide predictable patterns after separation by electrophoresis.

SEPARATION AND IDENTIFICATION OF DNA BY ELECTROPHORESIS

Separation of the DNA fragments after digestion is simplified by exploiting the observation that DNA is negatively charged. The phosphate groups have a net negative charge; thus the universal technique for separation of DNA fragments is electrophoresis, in which the fragments migrate in the gel in proportion to their length. The longer fragments migrate more slowly relative to the shorter fragments and give rise to a particular pattern of size-separated DNA. The electrophoresis is usually performed using either agarose or polyacrylamide gel, after which the fragments are stained with ethidium bromide and visualized in ultraviolet light as "bands" on the gel. Electrophoresis is used universally and routinely in the separation and detection of DNA fragments. The use of ethidium bromide staining provides for visualization of all DNA fragments but does not always give the desired resolution. Resolution is improved, however, by the use of a radiolabeled probe, which specifically hybridizes only with the fragment of interest. After hybridization the gel is exposed to x-ray film, and only

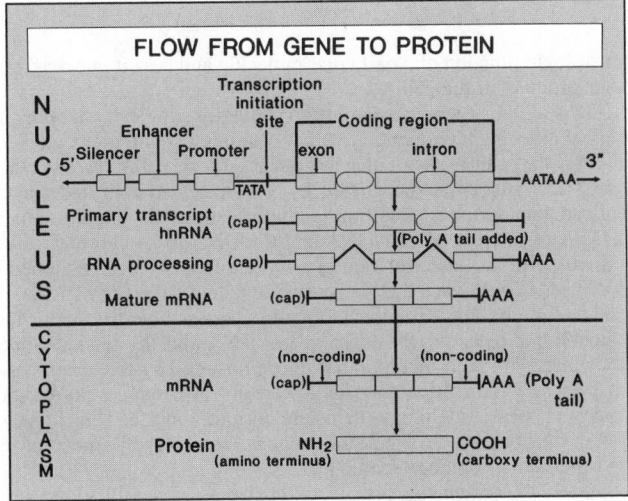

FIGURE 10-2   Regulation of gene activation. Schematic diagram of the components of gene structure that contribute to gene activation and protein synthesis. Ribonucleic acid (RNA) polymerase binds to a site at the beginning of a gene (promoter region), which often contains a TATA box. Other gene elements (enhancers) may regulate this process. A heteronuclear RNA copy of the gene (hnRNA) is produced, which contains protein-coding (exons) and noncoding (introns) sequences. The noncoding introns are spliced out, and the RNA is "capped" at the 5′ end and polyadenylated at the 3′ end (Poly A tail) to form a mature messenger RNA (mRNA). The mRNA is used to synthesize the protein encoded by this gene in the cell cytoplasm.

(From Roberts R et al: *A primer of molecular biology,* New York, 1992, Elsevier.)

the fragments of interest emit radioactivity and are visualized on the autoradiograph. A further modification of this technique is the transfer of the DNA fragments by diffusion from the gel to a nylon filter developed by E.M. Southern and discussed in the next section.

The size of the fragments of double-stranded DNA is indicated by their length in base pairs (nucleotides). For example, a 200 bp fragment is a piece of double-stranded DNA, with each complementary strand being 200 nucleotide bases long. A 1000 bp fragment is 1 kilobase (kb) long, and a 1 million bp fragment is 1 megabase (Mb) long. Many DNA endonucleases are now commercially available, each of which is specific for a particular DNA sequence. Each enzyme has only one recognition site, which may be a 4, 5, 6, or 8 bp sequence and will cut only a section of DNA that contains that particular sequence.

SOUTHERN, NORTHERN, AND WESTERN AND SOUTHWESTERN BLOTTING

The analysis of a few hundred bp of DNA in the region of interest may be difficult when the DNA from all the human chromosomes (which amounts to 3 billion nucleotide bp) is cut and separated on the same gel. This dilemma is resolved by using a DNA probe tagged with an easily recognizable marker such as a radionuclide. The technique has been further modified, with the DNA fragments transferred by osmotic diffusion from the gel to a solid support consisting of either nitrocellulose or nylon.

The method developed by Southern involves digestion of DNA and separation by electrophoresis, as described previously. Smaller fragments of DNA move more rapidly in the gel, whereas larger fragments move more slowly, each fragment moving a characteristic distance proportional to its size. The DNA is then transferred to a "hard copy" nitrocellulose or nylon membrane. The pattern of DNA separated and transferred onto the membrane is identical to the pattern of DNA separated on the agarose gel. This membrane can then be dried and used to detect DNA fragments of interest. To do this, a DNA probe is used. A probe is a fragment of DNA that contains a nucleotide sequence specific for the gene or DNA fragment of interest. The detection method requires that the probe be labeled with some identifiable tag, usually radioactive phosphorus-32 (^{32}P), and then denatured into a single DNA strand. The DNA on the membrane is denatured into single strands and the radioactive strand added in a solution to the membrane. Conditions are changed so that reannealing or hybridization occurs such that the probe can bind to its specific complementary fragments on the membrane. The binding of a foreign DNA probe to DNA fragments containing complementary sequences is called *hybridization* rather than *reannealling* (the latter term is used when the two original strands bind together). The membrane can then be washed and exposed to an x-ray film in a process called *autoradiography*. Only those fragments that have bound to the probe and contain the DNA of interest will be exposed on the film, and their sizes and pattern can be determined (Fig. 10-3).

If the material being isolated and identified is DNA, the procedure is referred to as Southern blotting; if the material is RNA, it is called Northern blotting. Correspondingly, the separation and membrane transfer of protein for detection are referred to as Western blotting. The probe used for Southern or Northern blotting is usually a radionuclide-labeled DNA fragment, whereas Western blotting usually uses a chemically tagged antibody. The procedures used to identify proteins that bind to DNA (transcriptional factors), where both DNA and protein are used, are referred to as Southwestern.

DNA CLONING

DNA cloning is a method of isolating and producing multiple copies of a DNA fragment of interest. These cloned fragments can then be used as DNA probes or organized to analyze the specific sequences of the cloned fragment. Cloned fragments representing a complete gene can be used for pharmaceutical purposes by producing vast amounts of a purified (recombinant) protein such as rtPA, now used daily in the treatment of myocardial infarction (Chapter 23). Cloned genes also can be used to express a particular protein in vivo in a transgenic animal. This type of experiment is useful in studying the

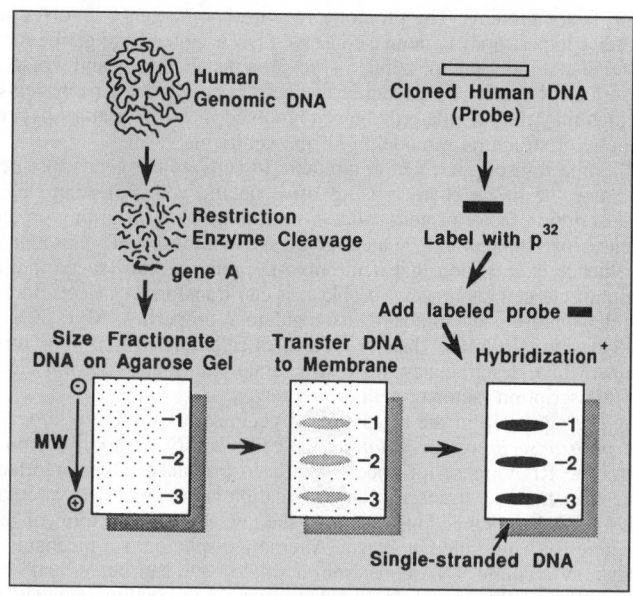

FIGURE 10-3   Southern blotting technique. Human DNA is isolated and digested with a restriction enzyme, creating small fragments that are then size separated on an agarose gel using electrophoresis. In this case, gene *A* is analyzed and is found to contain restriction enzymes sites cleaving it into three different-sized fragments labeled *1, 2,* and *3*. The largest fragment, *1,* moves most slowly through the gel, and *3,* the smallest fragment, moves farthest in the electric field. The complex DNA mixture is denatured into single-stranded molecules and then transferred to a solid-support nylon membrane for further manipulation and detection. Detection is accomplished by labeling a cloned complementary DNA probe containing the transcribed sequences from gene *A* with radioactive phosphorus-32 (^{32}P). The labeled probe is then capable of binding to (hybridizing) the complementary sequences of DNA that have been size separated. The filter is washed and exposed to x-ray film, and only fragments *1, 2,* and *3,* which have hybridized with the probe, are detected at the size position they have migrated to from the gel. Different individuals may vary by containing a different number of restriction enzyme sites within a particular gene, leading to different fragment patterns on the Southern blot autoradiogram.

(From Roberts R et al: *A primer of molecular biology,* New York, 1992, Elsevier.)

physiologic function of a particular molecule and how it interacts with other proteins in the cell.

DNA cloning techniques are fundamentally similar in that they all involve inserting a segment of the DNA of interest into a second piece of DNA that can replicate the desired fragment, called *vector DNA.* Vector DNA is DNA recognized by a host cell system and can be replicated many times, resulting in amplification of a single fragment of DNA of interest. Vector DNA and the DNA to be cloned are first both cut with the same restriction enzyme. The DNA to be cloned is then inserted into vector DNA, and an enzyme called *DNA ligase* is used to link the DNA fragments together to assemble the vector into a functioning piece of DNA. The vector DNA plus the desired cloned DNA insert are then incorporated into a host cell system that propagates them within the cell as if it were its own native DNA. Four general classes of cloning systems are currently in use. The choice of system depends on the DNA fragment's size and the purpose of using a particular cloning technique.

1. Small DNA fragments 5 to 15 kb in size are generally cloned into a piece of circular DNA vector called a *plasmid,* which is incorporated into bacterial cells and replicated many times. Plasmids are extrachromosomal DNA present in bacteria that contain an origin of DNA replication and also often contain sequences for a drug-resistance gene (Fig. 10-4).
2. *Phage* cloning systems can handle DNA pieces up to 20 kb in size, which are incorporated into a bacteriophage that invades and multiplies in a bacterial host. Phage refers to viruses that infect bacteria.
3. A combination vector system called a *cosmid* can accommodate DNA pieces up to 50 kb in size.

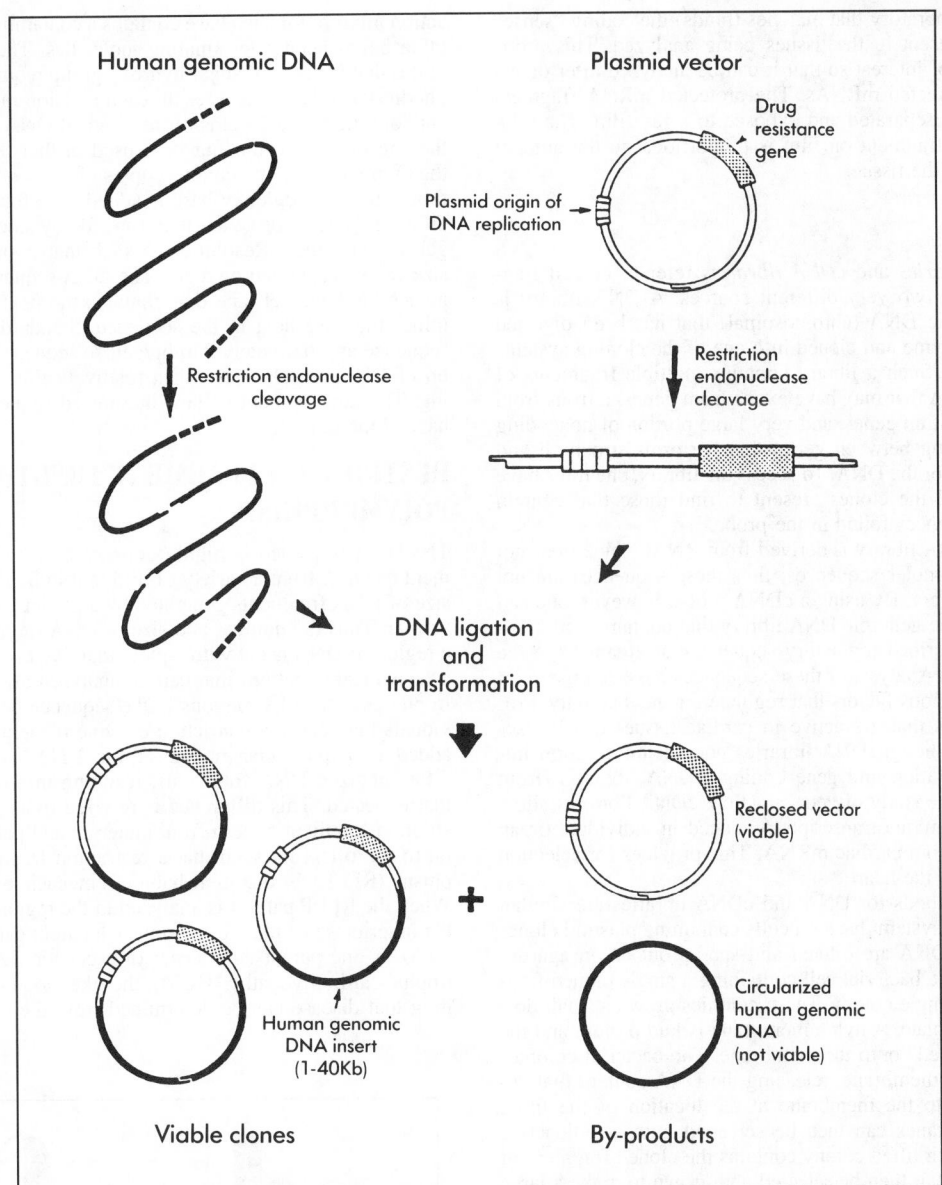

Human genomic DNA

Plasmid vector

Drug resistance gene

Plasmid origin of DNA replication

Restriction endonuclease cleavage

Restriction endonuclease cleavage

DNA ligation and transformation

Reclosed vector (viable)

Human genomic DNA insert (1-40Kb)

Circularized human genomic DNA (not viable)

Viable clones

By-products

FIGURE 10-4   Cloning of a DNA fragment using a plasmid as the vector. Initially the human genomic DNA is cleaved with a restriction enzyme and then inserted into the plasmid vector that contains a means of replication and a selectable marker, such as a drug-resistance gene. Various by-products of the procedure (i.e., closed vector, circularized human DNA) are also represented.

(From Roberts R et al: *A primer of molecular biology,* New York, 1992, Elsevier.)

4. A new system using yeast rather than bacteria can accommodate insertions of over 1 Mb (1 million bp) of human DNA fragments.

RNA ANALYSIS

It is estimated that only 12% of DNA is transcribed, and less than 5% of chromosomal DNA actually represents genes that encode for proteins. Therefore routine analysis of DNA is complicated by many noncoding sequences, the significance of which is still under investigation. mRNA, on the other hand, represents only DNA sequences that have been transcribed to perform a cell function; these sequences encode for the estimated 67,000 proteins needed for a human. Although the DNA content of different cells is the same, mRNA isolated from cardiac tissue varies significantly from mRNA isolated from another organ, such as the liver. The translated proteins from the mRNAs in these two organs are very different and perform quite different functions. Therefore the mRNA sequences provide unique information about tissue-specific proteins produced in a particular or-

gan and can define tissue-specific proteins that may differentially regulate function in these different tissues. From the sequence of the nucleotides in the mRNAs, one can derive the amino acid sequence of the polypeptide product. The mRNA sequence can also be used as a probe to analyze DNA fragments and find the gene that produces a particular polypeptide. mRNA is single stranded and a relatively unstable molecule that is often converted in the laboratory to a more stable cDNA copy of the sequence.

Because full-length mRNA transcripts can directly encode for a desired protein, it is often preferred to clone the mRNA sequence into an "expression vector" to allow one to make the recombinant protein and study its function. Northern blotting, one method of analyzing RNA, is performed similar to the Southern blot technique described earlier except that instead of using DNA, the RNA is used and separated electrophoretically, then blotted onto a membrane and probed with a radioactive probe. Ribonuclease protection assay (RPA) is another way of quantifying the cellular content of a specific mRNA. This procedure uses a radioactive complementary "antisense" probe synthesized in the laboratory that matches (binds) the coding "sense" strand of mRNA present in the tissues being analyzed. This probe protects the mRNA of interest so that it can be analyzed after digestion of all the unprotected mRNAs. The protected mRNA fragment is electrophoretically separated and exposed to x-ray film. The relative intensity of the fragment on film is proportional to the amount of mRNA present in the tissue.

DNA LIBRARIES

The terms *DNA libraries* and *cDNA libraries* refer to cloned fragments of DNA from two very different sources. A DNA library is derived from genomic DNA (chromosomal) that has been digested with a restriction enzyme and cloned into one of the cloning systems described previously. Such a library contains multiple fragments of different sizes of DNA that may have exons from genes, introns from noncoding regions within genes, and very large portion of noncoding genomic DNA existing between genes that performs structural and regulatory functions for the DNA. To access the library, one must have a probe to *screen* all the clones present to find those that contain complementary sequences found in the probe.

In contrast, a cDNA library is derived from RNA, which does not contain intron or promoter sequences; thus these sequences are not found in a cDNA library. By using a cDNA probe, however, one can select a clone from the genomic DNA library that contains both transcribed and nontranscribed regulatory sequences upstream from the gene's coding region. Analysis of these sequences has been useful in demonstrating the various factors that regulate a gene's activity. Promoters and enhancers that are active in cardiac tissues can be isolated in this way. Although DNA libraries contain information important in gene regulation and gene coding, cDNA libraries (from RNA) are useful in the study of gene function. cDNA libraries allow one to focus on the unique transcripts produced in individual organ types and are made from cardiac mRNA. This provides for selection of genes expressed in the heart.

The screening methods for DNA and cDNA libraries are similar. In a bacterial cloning system, bacteria cells containing plasmid clones of human DNA or cDNA are diluted and spread out on an agarose plate such that a single bacterial cell containing a single cloned fragment can grow as a single colony. These colonies grow as small dots on top of the culture plate. A nylon membrane is laid on top, and the colonies are then "lifted" onto the membrane. The bacterial colonies are then lysed on the membrane, releasing the DNA content that denatures and adheres to the membrane at the location of the lifted colony. These membranes can then be screened with a radioactive probe to identify which lifted colony contains the cloned fragment of interest. This colony can then be selected and grown to make a large preparation of a single cloned fragment of DNA or cDNA.

The expression, regulation, and function of a particular gene and its protein can be studied by manipulating and piecing together different cloned fragments of DNA from different sources. For example, cloned promoters and enhancers, which initiate gene function, can be ligated to a cDNA clone encoding for a particular protein. Recombinant human proteins such as rtPA are produced by ligating the human cDNA clone to the gene regulatory sequences active in bacteria. In this way a human protein can be artificially produced in a bacterial system in large quantities. The properties that control regulation of promoter and enhancer sequences in a human cardiac gene can be studied by ligating the regulating sequences to what is called a *reporter* gene. Reporter genes synthesize a product that is not normally found in human tissues and thus is easily quantifiable as a measure of gene activity.

SEQUENCING

DNA sequencing is an essential aspect of molecular biology. The nucleotide sequence of DNA, cDNA, or RNA is used to derive the amino acid sequence of a protein, find a particular endonuclease restriction enzyme site for molecular analysis, or detect mutations in a gene that produce human disease through deletions, insertions, or substitutions within the genetic code.

The Sanger technique involves the use of DNA polymerase to copy a cloned piece of DNA. Four separate reactions are performed for each of the four nucleotides, A, T, C, and G. The DNA synthesis re-

action mixture for each base contains a contaminating source of nucleotide base–specific terminating molecules. These are dideoxynucleotides that lack the 3′ sugar hydroxy group required for the next phosphodiester linkage. As a result, each reaction mixture contains different copy fragment lengths of the original DNA that are terminated at the site of the terminating base used in that reaction. For example, the thymine reaction contains copies of the sequence terminated each time a thymine dideoxy base is added. The four reactions, each specific for A, T, G, or C, are then run side by side on a polyacrylamide gel in four lanes. Resolution is such that a single bp difference in size can be separated on a gel. The DNA sequence is read so that the nucleotide base gel lane that contains the next longest strand determines the base next in the sequence. Standard sequencing gels can sequence approximately 250 bp/gel, so sequencing of a few thousand bp of DNA or cDNA is still a relatively time-consuming undertaking. The development of new automated sequencers has greatly enhanced the output.

RESTRICTION FRAGMENT LENGTH POLYMORPHISM

The DNA sequence is highly conserved, so when a particular segment of DNA from a variety of different individuals is compared, the size of DNA fragments generated by a particular enzyme generally is similar. Thus the number and size of DNA fragments produced when a region of DNA is cut with a particular *DNA restriction enzyme* form a recognizable pattern that can be analyzed after separation by electrophoresis. Small variations in the sequence between unrelated individuals may cause a restriction enzyme recognition site to be lost or added to a particular region of the DNA, which would produce different-sized DNA fragments, resulting in a different pattern from that expected. This difference is referred to as *polymorphic.* The restriction fragment pattern from maternal and paternal DNA is passed on to the offspring such that a restriction fragment length polymorphism (RFLP) is distinguishable from each parental chromosome. When the RFLP pattern is analyzed in the region of a particular gene, the inheritance of that gene from each parent can be determined (Fig. 10-5). If one parent is a carrier of a genetic disease, such as hypertrophic cardiomyopathy (HCM), the likelihood of an offspring inheriting that disease can be determined from the offspring's RFLP pat-

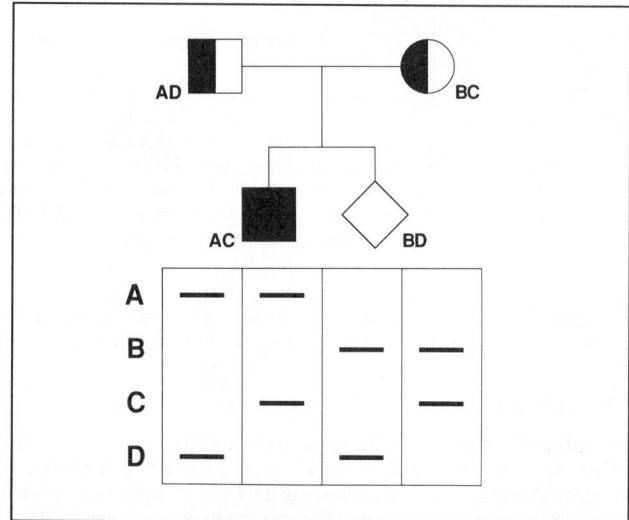

FIGURE 10-5 Restriction fragment length polymorphism (RFLP) detection of autosomal recessive disease transmission. Restriction fragment bands *A, B, C,* and *D* detected on Southern blot using a disease-linked probe. A small family pedigree is shown above. On the basis of the affected child's inheritance *(solid square below),* the father's diseased allele cosegregates with band *A,* and the mother's diseased allele cosegregates with band *C.* The normal offspring *(open diamond)* inherited the father's *B* and the mother's *D* bands, both of which are linked to the normal gene. A child containing only one diseased allele from either parent *(not shown)* would be a carrier for the disease.

(From Roberts R et al: *A primer of molecular biology,* New York, 1992, Elsevier.)

tern by a comparison with the RFLP pattern from the affected parent. If the RFLP from the disease-carrying region of the affected parent's DNA matches the son's or daughter's pattern, the likelihood of inheriting the disease is significant. With HCM, various families have been identified who have inherited mutations in the β-MHC gene, which cause the disease.

POLYMERASE CHAIN REACTION

The polymerase chain reaction (PCR) technique provides for rapid isolation and purification of a desired fragment of DNA by selective logarithmic amplification. The desired piece of DNA can be amplified from a complex mixture of very diluted DNA or a single copy of the target fragment within a few hours without the need for cloning and purification. The technique requires some knowledge of the DNA sequences in the region to be amplified. First, small specific oligonucleotide molecules approximately 25 bases long must be synthesized to act as "primers" for the reaction. The DNA to be copied is denatured with heat, causing the strands to separate and then cool so that the small, short, sequence-specific oligonucleotide primers can bind to the desired region of the DNA. The heat-stable *Taq* polymerase enzyme is used to initiate synthesis at the precise region of DNA bound by primer. This process is called *primer extension*. By selecting oligonucleotide primers flanking the region of interest and oriented inward toward each other, the intermediate sequence is amplified by doubling the amount of DNA copy in that particular region with each cycle. The DNA is repeatedly denatured and copied in this one region. Repeated cycles can synthesize approximately 1 million copies of the piece of DNA of interest in about 3 hours (Fig. 10-6). The PCR method is most efficient for pieces of DNA less than 1000 bp in size, although fragments up to 5000 to 7000 bp have been produced. The technique is so rapid and simple that it has quickly gained wide popularity in both diagnostic and research laboratories.

GENE TRANSFER

Numerous methods have now been developed to transfer foreign DNA into mammalian cells. This may be performed in cells in culture or in the intact animal. The gene may be transferred into somatic cells or into germline cells. Expression of a mutant myosin heavy chain gene in feline cardiac myocytes induced fiber disarray identical to that in the human disease, hypertrophic cardiomyopathy. Each method has its own advantages and pitfalls in terms of efficacy and utility of gene transfer. Transgenic animals provide a useful source for studying the impact of gene expression or gene mutations in the intact animal. Determination of a particular protein's or enzyme's function and its effect on the pathophysiology of disease may be best accomplished by this method. A foreign DNA vector designed to express a particular protein under the control of a selected promoter and enhancer system is introduced by injection into a fertilized ovum. The genetically altered ovum is then implanted into the uterus of a surrogate maternal animal, and the offspring's phenotypic effects are studied. Recently the effect of the intracellular calcium modulator *calmodulin* on cardiac growth has been studied in transgenic mice. Calmodulin was expressed specifically in the heart under the control of the promoter for atrial natriuretic factor. This expression vector overexpressed calmodulin in the atria of the offspring mouse hearts, causing myocyte growth and hypertrophy and often early death. Overexpression of G protein (Gα) in transgenic mice appears to result in development of fibrosis and cardiomyopathy similar to the changes seen in human heart failure and may be useful in analyzing the pathophysiology of hyperadrenergic states.

Gene transfer in the cardiovascular system is a developing field, and several interesting systems have already been developed. Using either tissue culture or intact animals, one can now induce cardiac myocytes, vascular smooth muscle cells, and endothelial cells to incorporate exogenous DNA into their cells by a variety of methods. Cellular uptake of exogenous DNA can be enhanced with the use of calcium phosphate, DEAE-dextran, liposomes (lipofection), electroporation, retrovirus transfection, adenovirus transfection, and direct injection. Another successful technique is to transplant genetically modified cells from tissue culture into an intact animal. Human gene therapy studies to promote angiogenesis in subjects with peripheral vascular disease are under way.

CARDIAC GROWTH AND HYPERTROPHY

Although the human heart exhibits remarkable physiologic reserve, the nondividing cardiac myocyte is limited in its ability to preserve function in response to disease or injury. The sustained compensatory response to ischemia, infarction, hypertension, and/or heart failure is cellular hypertrophy and chamber dilation. Cell division in heart tissue terminates during fetal development. However, some genes continue to show developmental differences in gene expression, such as the slow cardiac calcium adenosine triphosphatase (Ca-ATPase), which is dramatically increased in the adult human ventricle. In contrast, atrial natriuretic factor, which is expressed in the embryonic ventricle, is turned off as the heart matures into the adult stage. Differences in the cardiac myocyte's ability to divide or express different proteins or protein isoforms are regulated by transcription factors that determine cardiac gene expression during development and disease. Various physiologic stressors (e.g., pressure overload) can cause induction and reexpression of fetal genes, which may provide insight into the adaptive cellular response seen in patients with cardiac hypertrophy. For example, in patients with cardiac failure the atrial natriuretic gene is reexpressed in the diseased ventricular muscle, whereas in persons with healthy ventricles this gene is quiescent.

The observation that crude extracts from hypertrophied hearts induce hypertrophy when infused in vitro provides evidence that locally produced trophic substances are important as initiating signals for hypertrophy and altered gene expression. The factors responsible for hypertrophy are inherent in the myocyte and through paracrine, autocrine, or intracrine mechanisms stimulate the cells to hypertrophy. The signaling mechanisms that induce changes in the cascade of proteins affecting differential function in cardiac hypertrophy and failure have broad potential in the treatment of heart disease (Fig. 10-7). Several initiating signals have been identified that alter cardiac gene expression. Norepinephrine has been shown to alter β-MHC gene expression and skeletal α-actin expression in cultured cardiac cells. Mechanical stretch of isolated ventricular myocytes on distensible membranes has also been shown to induce RNA synthesis, β-MHC expression, and expression of the skeletal α-actin and atrial myosin light chain. The general pathway consists of a receptor→receptor coupled proteins→signalling proteins→transcriptional factor→gene expression. The acidic and basic fibroblast growth factors and transforming growth factor β (TGF-β) are some of the peptide growth factors that have been studied most extensively. These growth factors partially recapitulate the fetal cardiac phenotype by increasing production of atrial natriuretic factor and decreasing production of Ca-ATPase in ventricular myocardium. Although these growth factors have been identified in myocardial cells, some have suggested that fibroblasts may play the major role in the production of distinct trophic substances during injury or stress. Release of these growth factors has been demonstrated in ischemic myocardium and in the surviving myocardium surrounding infarcted cardiac muscle.

The nuclear oncogene proteins c-*myc,* c-*fos,* and c-*jun* have received considerable attention in the context of cardiac growth and hypertrophy. In the normal adult ventricle, relatively little expression of c-*myc* and c-*fos* occurs. During physiologic stress, however, these proteins increase dramatically in the cell nucleus. As previously discussed, these proteins are transcription factors that bind to the regulatory regions of genes and direct their activity. For example, a *fos/jun* heterodimer binds to the regulatory regions of the atrial natriuretic gene, which is activated in ventricular muscle during pressure overload hypertrophy. Serum growth factors and norepinephrine have both been shown to induce c-*myc* expression in cultured ventricular cells. C-*fos* is induced by both acidic and basic fibroblast growth factors, passive stretch, angiotensin, and endothelin. Depending on the initiating signal, a variety of receptors, coupling proteins, and signaling proteins transmit the extracellular stress to the nucleus, where nuclear transcription factors act to alter cell function.

The renin-angiotensin system appears to play a major role in cardiac growth and hypertrophy. This system mediates sodium retention and vasoconstriction, resulting in elevation of preload and afterload. Stimulation of mechanoreceptors in the heart can initiate the growth cascade described. In addition, angiotensin II exerts load-independent effects on cardiac myocyte growth. Angiotensin II stimulates DNA and protein synthesis, which appears to be mediated by activation of tyrosine kinase and mitogen-activated protein (MAP) kinases, independent of c-*fos* and c-*jun* protooncogene induction. The mechanism

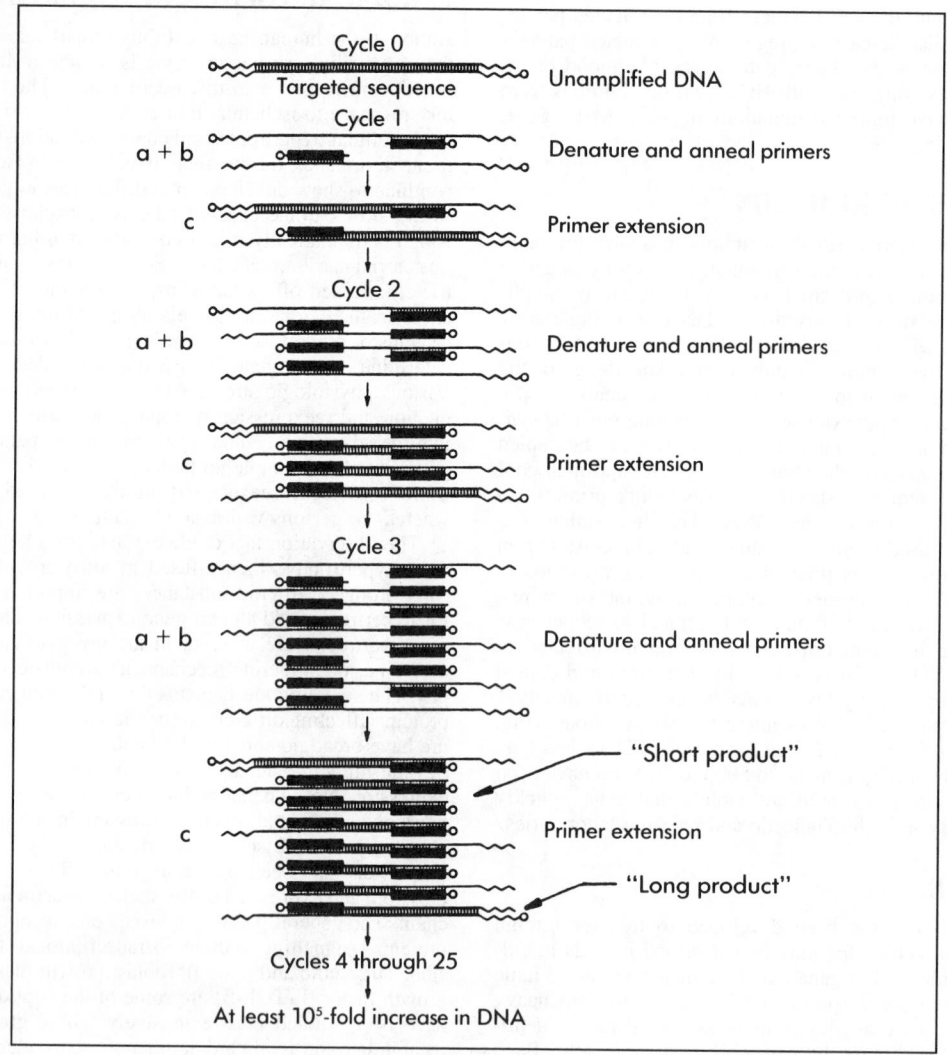

FIGURE 10-6   Polymerase chain reaction (PCR). Amplification of a selected region is accomplished by separating the two strands of DNA with heat denaturation and subsequent annealing of short oligonucleotide primers complementary to and flanking the region to be amplified (steps *a* and *b*). In step *c* the enzyme *Taq* polymerase is used to extend synthesis from the primer, creating double-stranded DNA in the selected region for amplification. A second cycle of denaturation and annealing of primers followed by primer extension again doubles the amount of double-stranded DNA in the region of interest, with some copies terminating at the site of the downstream primer. These "short products" eventually dominate the reaction, creating a single-size DNA fragment selected by the separation distance of the two primers used in the reaction. The PCR product is often visualized by agarose gel electrophoresis and ethidium bromide staining of the DNA *(not shown).*
(From Roberts R et al: *A primer of molecular biology,* New York, 1992, Elsevier.)

whereby angiotensin-converting enzyme (ACE) inhibitors prolong survival of patients with cardiac failure is through modulation of cardiac growth.

ADRENERGIC RECEPTORS AND G PROTEINS

Autonomic tone plays a pivotal role in the regulation of cardiac contractile function, heart rate, and conduction through the atrioventricular node. Muscarinic receptors in the heart interact with the neurotransmitter *acetylcholine,* which is released by the parasympathetic division of the autonomic nervous system via the vagus nerve. Alpha- and β-receptors in the heart interact with the neurotransmitter *norepinephrine,* released from sympathetic nerve terminals, and *epinephrine,* released from the adrenal cortex. Pharmacologic stimulation or inhibition of these receptors has proved useful in cardiovascular therapies for patients with congestive heart failure, hypertension, acute myocardial infarction, and bradyarrhythmias. Maladaptive responses to chronic stimulation of these receptors also occur, such as the induction of tachyarrhythmias and the alteration in gene expression and

cellular proteins demonstrated in congestive heart failure. Multiple isoforms of each receptor class have now been purified and cloned, allowing their study in both in vitro and in vivo experimental systems. At present, at least three subtypes of the α_1-adrenergic receptor (α_{1a}, α_{1b}, and α_{1c}), three subtypes of the α_2-adrenergic receptor (α_{2a}, α_{2b}, and α_{2c}), and three subtypes of the β-adrenergic receptor (β_1, β_2, and β_3) have been identified. Five different muscarinic receptors have also been cloned (M_1, M_2, M_3, M_4, and M_5). These receptors are all membrane proteins that share general features, including up to seven stretches of hydrophobic amino acids, each long enough to span the lipid bilayer. The amino terminus of the receptor proteins is usually extracellular, and the carboxy terminus is in the cytoplasm. Each receptor contains glycosylation sites, as well as amino acids, that serve as substrates for protein kinases. Protein kinases can phosphorylate the receptor and influence its activity.

The general mechanism for signal transduction for these receptor proteins involves *G proteins.* G proteins are so named because of their ability to bind guanosine triphosphate (GTP). This high-energy phosphate complex activates adenyl cyclase, which catalyzes the conver-

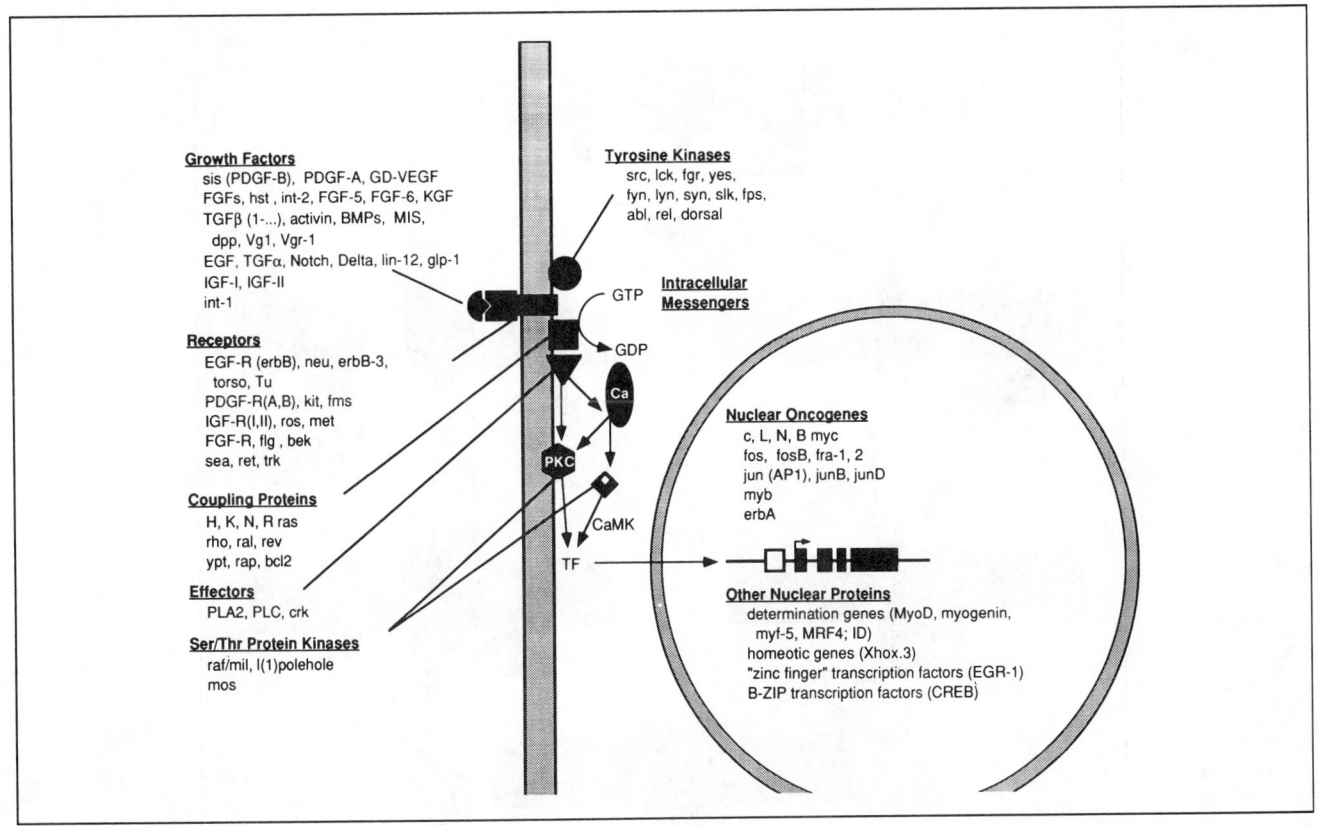

FIGURE 10-7   Oncogene proteins and cardiac growth and hypertrophy. Cellular oncogenes encode several proteins that may be involved in cardiac growth. The stimulus for cardiac gene regulation involves extracellular forces (i.e., pressure), neurotransmitters, hormones, or growth factors that stimulate membrane receptors and regulate cardiac gene transcription through various coupling proteins, tyrosine kinases, and intracellular messengers. These cellular mechanisms appear to regulate production of nuclear oncogenes, which encode transcription factors, leading to cardiac gene regulation.

sion of ATP to adenosine $3',5'$-cyclic monophosphate (cAMP). The β_1, β_2, and β_3 receptors are coupled to a G protein called G_s, which stimulates adenyl cyclase. The α_{2a} and α_{2b} receptors and the M_2 and M_4 receptors are coupled to a G protein called G_i, which inhibits adenyl cyclase. With the M_2 receptor the G-protein coupling may also directly activate the cardiac potassium channel. Not all these receptors work through adenyl cyclase. The α_1 receptor and M_1, M_3, and M_5 receptors appear to couple to a G_q member of the G protein family that activates phospholipase C. Both cAMP and phospholipase C can modulate a variety of cellular processes, including cardiac growth metabolism and ion channel activity. cAMP positively regulates the activity of protein kinase A (PKA), which can have several effects. Cardiac calcium channels are regulated by PKA-mediated phosphorylation of the channel protein. Overstimulation of the β receptors appears to cause PKA-modulated desensitization of β-receptor activity. The decrease in the capacity of the β receptor to activate the G_s protein results from a feedback loop in which PKA phosphorylates the β_2 receptor. The promoter regions of the β_1 and β_2 adrenergic receptors have also been sequenced and analyzed. PKA mediates active removal of the receptors from the membrane by downregulation and has also been shown to decrease synthesis and perhaps stability of β_2-receptor mRNA.

The activation of phospholipase C through the α_1-adrenergic receptor and several muscarinic receptors stimulates two separate pathways of cell regulation. Phospholipase C cleaves membrane phospholipids to produce both inositol phosphates and diacylglycerol. Diacylglycerol activates protein kinase C (PKC), whereas inositol phosphates regulate intracellular calcium. Although PKC cannot be stimulated by activation of the β receptor, several sites for PKC phosphorylation exist on the β_2 receptor. Therefore stimulation of α and muscarinic receptors may affect β-receptor function.

G proteins consist of a three-subunit G protein complex that associates with a signal-transducing cell surface receptor. Alpha, beta, and gamma (α, β, γ) subunits, and many isoforms of each have been identified. Initially, all three subunits are in contact with the receptor. When the β-adrenergic receptor is stimulated by hormone (i.e., epinephrine), the α subunit releases bound guanosine diphosphate (GDP), and the receptor undergoes a structural change, increasing its affinity for hormone. The empty α subunit can then bind GTP, which causes a release of the α subunit from the receptor (β/γ subunit) complex. The GTP-activated α subunit binds to and activates adenylyl cyclase, converting ATP to cAMP (Fig. 10-8). Some G proteins, such as G_k (activated by a muscarinic receptor), can directly modify the activity of the cardiac potassium channel without acting through a protein kinase. Molecular techniques have allowed modifications of cDNAs that express these various receptors and G proteins in an in vitro system in which the receptor's mutation has allowed identification of ligand binding sites and sequences that interact with the G proteins.

An important β-receptor regulator called β-*adrenergic receptor kinase* (BARK) has been cloned and purified and shown to be capable of phosphorylating the β receptor, but only in the presence of an agonist. The action of BARK is mediated by a second protein called β *arrestin*. The sequence of receptor deactivation requires binding of an agonist to the receptor, followed by the receptor's phosphorylation by BARK near the G protein binding site. This phosphorylated site is recognized by β arrestin, which binds to the receptor and prevents its binding to the G_s protein. Because receptor occupancy is required for BARK activity, BARK probably plays a physiologic role when receptors are exposed to high concentrations of agonists, such as in synaptic clefts. BARK may also play a role in β-receptor desensitization in patients with high catecholamine states, such as end-

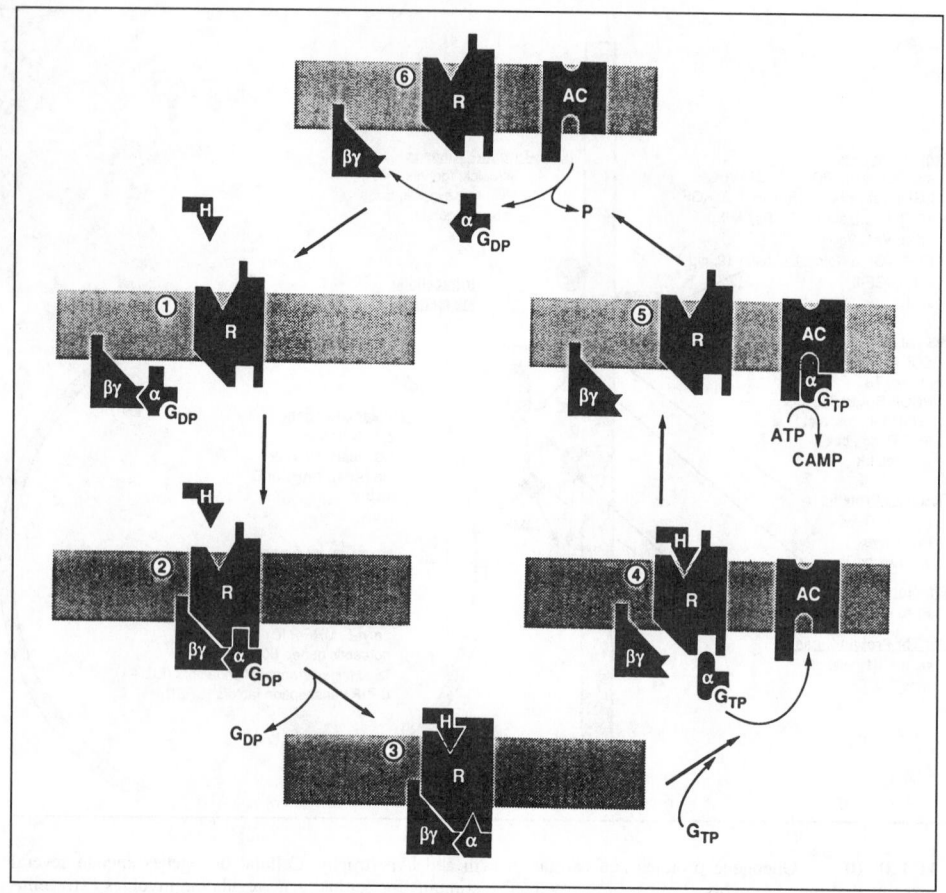

FIGURE 10-8   Outline of a cycle of signal transduction for the β_2-adrenergic receptor. The components include the hormone *(H)* epinephrine, the β_2 receptor *(R)*, the subunits of G$_s$ (α, β/γ), and adenylyl cyclase *(AC)*. See text for discussion.

stage congestive heart failure (interestingly, BARK expression is up-regulated in heart failure). BARK-mediated β-receptor desensitization contrasts greatly with the model for desensitization mediated by PKA.

ION CHANNELS

Membrane depolarization and excitation-contraction coupling are mediated by an important class of transmembrane proteins known as ion channels. These proteins are important pharmacologic targets that regulate the flow of sodium, calcium, and potassium currents across the cardiac myocyte plasma membrane and sarcoplasmic reticulum. The gating of ion channels generally falls into two categories: voltage dependent and receptor mediated. Many voltage-dependent channels are highly regulated by receptor-mediated modulation of voltage sensitivity. Advances in molecular genetics have demonstrated that mutations in ion channels are the cause of several human diseases.

Calcium Channels

Three cation pump enzymes catalyze the movement of calcium against its concentration gradient: (1) the ryanodine receptor, the calcium ATPase of the sarcoplasmic reticulum (SRCA); (2) the dihydropyridine receptor, the calcium ATPase of the plasma membrane (PMCA); and (3) the sodium/calcium exchanger powered by the sodium gradient created by the sodium/potassium ATPase (NKA), which secondarily moves calcium out of the cell. NKA has an α-catalytic subunit, which is stabilized by a β subunit that can be glycosylated. Both PMCA and SRCA contain an α-catalytic subunit, which can act as the functional unit. ATP hydrolysis converts the catalytic subunit into a high-affinity protein conformation to activate the channel. Mutations in the α_1 subunit of the dihydropyridine receptor (PMCA) cause a muscle disease called hypokalemic periodic paralysis

(hypoPP). HypoPP muscle has reduced calcium current amplitude and delayed channel inactivation. Cardiac defects resulting from calcium channel mutations have not yet been described.

PMCA, SRCA, and NKA are each encoded by tissue-specific, developmentally regulated gene families. Many of these mRNA gene products are alternatively spliced for multiple isoforms of the channel, encoded by a single gene. The functional significance of these isoforms is currently under investigation.

Alternate mechanisms for inducing cardiac hypertrophy clearly cause differential effects on expression of SRCA. For example, in cardiac hypertrophy induced by hyperthyroidism, thyroid hormone receptor appears to bind to the promoter region of SRCA to enhance expression and enzymatic activity. In contrast, pressure overload hypertrophy induces up to a 50% decrease in SRCA levels. Expression of NKA is also enhanced by both thyroid hormone and glucocorticoid induction.

SRCA is modulated by other intracellular proteins, including phospholamban, which reduces the enzyme's affinity for calcium. Phospholamban can be dissociated from the SRCA by phosphorylation through cAMP-dependent protein kinase and calmodulin-dependent protein kinase, both of which can be activated by cell surface receptors. PMCA is also activated by intracellular proteins, with calmodulin-dependent protein kinase and direct activation by calmodulin being the most important.

SRCA has been extensively studied as a recombinant molecule expressed in tissue culture cell systems. Site-directed mutagenesis of various regions of the protein has identified the ion binding sites and the ATP binding site for the protein. These homologous regions contained within both PMCA and NKA suggest that these sequences are partially conserved motifs.

Beta-adrenergic stimulation causes a five-fold increase in calcium currents through G protein stimulation of adenyl cyclase and PKA.

Acetylcholine decreases cardiac calcium currents only after they have been stimulated by β-adrenergic agonists, a process mediated by an inhibitory G protein mechanism. PKC phosphorylation has a biphasic effect, with initial calcium current stimulation followed by inhibition.

Sodium Channels

The voltage-dependent cardiac sodium channel has been cloned and studied electrophysiologically in the cell system of the *Xenopus laevis* (frog) oocyte. Initial rapid membrane depolarization is achieved via fast changes in sodium permeability through a voltage-activated gate. Cardiac sodium channel activation has a fast phase opening and closing, followed by a slow component characterized by "burst" openings that last several milliseconds. This burst component of the cardiac channel characterizes the late sodium current plateau typical of cardiac sodium channels.

The cardiac sodium channel is susceptible to gating modification by β-adrenergic stimulation. The G_s protein appears to be responsible for modulating cardiac sodium currents through cAMP-dependent phosphorylation or direct interaction of G_s with the channel. Adrenergic stimulation depresses the sodium current and slows conduction, which may produce a substrate for reentrant arrhythmias or ventricular fibrillation. A decrease in action potential threshold may also be mediated by angiotensin II, which stimulates PKC-mediated modulation of the cardiac sodium channel. Angiotensin-converting enzyme inhibitor drugs may have an antiarrhythmic effect by blocking cardiac angiotensin II effects on sodium currents. Antiarrhythmic agents such as lidocaine exert their effect through binding to open depolarized inactivated sodium channels, which slows their recovery from inactivation (Chapter 17). The effect is to prevent impulse generation from the damaged depolarized tissue. A subset of patients with congenital long QT syndrome have mutations in the α-subunit of the cardiac sodium channel gene (SN5A) on chromosome 3(p21). Studies of mutant channels in *Xenopus* oocytes have demonstrated a sustained inward current, which explains the prolongation of cardiac action potentials in this disease. Three hereditary muscle diseases, hyperkalemic periodic paralysis, paramyotonia congenita, and potassium aggrevated myotonia, are caused by mutations in the α subunit of the muscle sodium channel on chromosome 17q.

Potassium Channels

A potassium channel inhibited by intracellular ATP was first described in cardiac muscle, and is also found in skeletal muscle, arteriolar smooth muscle, and pancreatic β cells. Sulfonylureas are highly specific for this channel and block its activity. Ischemia causes these channels to open and shorten action potential duration, causing decreased contractile force. Cardiac hypertrophy has been associated with reduced ATP inhibition of this potassium channel, which may have a protective function.

Acetylcholine stimulation of the muscarinic M_2 receptor appears to cause an unidentified G protein to interact directly with the cardiac potassium channel. The possibility of comediated PKC activation of the channel has not been excluded. Another pathway for G protein–mediated modulation of the cardiac potassium channel may be via the cardiac adenosine receptor. These receptors may be particularly important for activating potassium channels in ischemic cardiac muscle.

Mutations in a putative potassium channel gene (HERG) on chromosome 7(q35) have been linked to a subset of patients with congenital long QT syndrome. It is hypothesized that delayed myocellular repolarization in these patients causes a secondary reactivation of the dihydropyridine receptor L-type calcium channel (PMCA), and causes secondary repolarization, the etiology for torsades de pointes arrhythmia in this disease.

CONTRACTILE AND CYTOSKELETAL PROTEINS

The observation that the contractile and cytoskeletal proteins undergo isoform transitions both in cardiac hypertrophy and in cardiomyopathy has led to an intense investigation regarding the pathophysiology of these diseases and the fundamental cellular defects. The cardiac sarcomere is composed of thick and thin filaments (Chapter 9). Thick filaments are composed of approximately 400 molecules of MHCs. Each MHC molecule consists of two α helixes wound together with two attached myosin light chains (MLCs). MHCs are encoded by both an α-MHC gene and a β-MHC gene, which allow the formation of three possible MHC combinations: α/α, α/β, or β/β. Alpha/alpha-MHC has a four-fold to five-fold greater ATPase activity than the β/β-MHC combination. The predominant form in the adult ventricle is β-MHC, whereas the α form appears to be present primarily in the adult atrium. In patients with cardiac hypertrophy, β-MHC expression increases. Mutations in β-MHC have been described in families with the inherited form of hypertrophic cardiomyopathy.

Changes in MLC expression have also been described, and several MLC isoforms exist. Absent or significantly reduced MLC 2 (the regulatory MLC, which can be phosphorylated) has been found in patients with idiopathic dilated cardiomyopathy. Dramatically reduced or absent MLC 2 may alter ATPase activity and result in generalized destabilization of the sarcomere's lattice geometry.

Each thick filament of myosin is associated with six thin-filament protein complexes. The thin filament contains two chains of globular actin associated with the dimeric superhelix tropomyosin molecule and three different troponin molecules. Troponin C binds calcium, troponin I binds to actin and inhibits contraction, and troponin T stabilizes the complex and binds it to tropomyosin. Both troponin T and I can also be phosphorylated and may induce changes in the activity of these molecules during contraction. Phosphorylation of troponin I appears to decrease the sensitivity for calcium and may account for the lusitropic effect of β-adrenergic agonists on cardiac relaxation. The tropomyosin genes encode both α and β subunits and are capable of alternative splicing to produce a variety of tropomyosin isoform proteins. Similarly, the α-actin protein is present in three different isoforms produced by separate genes: the skeletal, cardiac, and smooth muscle α actins. Although the smooth muscle α actin has been found in embryonic myocardium, only the skeletal and cardiac α actins are present in the adult ventricle. No consistent differences in α actin have yet been observed in human cardiac disease.

Several intermediate and accessory proteins are associated with the contractile proteins and are involved in their assembly, stability, and organization. *Desmin* is an intermediate filament found in muscle cells that appears to tie the edges of the Z disks (lines) together. Intermediate filament assembly is controlled through phosphorylation by protein kinases. Interestingly, alterations in desmin and other cytoskeletal proteins have been described in patients with cardiomyopathy. Thick filaments of myosin are linked to the Z disk via a large 2500 kd (kilodalton) protein called *titin*, whereas actin filaments within the sarcomere are linked to the Z disk via an elongated 600 kd protein called *nebulin*. Alpha actinin is another Z disk–associated protein, which acts within the sarcomere to bundle actin molecules and link these filaments together near their attachment to the Z disk. Spectrin is a 280 kd protein localized to the cytoplasmic surface of the cardiocyte membrane. Spectrin forms a complex with the protein ankyrin and binds to a number of important molecules, including the voltage-dependent sodium channel, sodium ATPase, and the acetylcholine receptor. In cardiac pressure overload, volume overload, hypercontractile states, and failure, the forces exerted on the heart's cytoskeletal contractile elements may cause pathophysiologic responses in the organization and relative content of these various filaments.

Microtubules are long rodlike structures formed in the cytoplasm of the cardiocyte via polymerization of α-tubulin and β-tubulin. The microtubules are involved in a variety of cellular processes including cell division, cell shape and movement, vesicular transport, and regulation and adenylyl cyclase activity. Pressure overload hypertrophy induces an increase in microtubule formation (a resistive force), which appears to be partially responsible for the contractile defect in hypertrophic cardiocytes. Depolymerization of microtubules with colchicine is capable of reversing this defect in an animal model.

Mutations in the gene that encodes the cytoskeletal protein *dystrophin* cause the skeletal and cardiac disease seen in Duchenne and Becker muscular dystrophies. Dystrophin is localized to the cell membrane's cytoplasmic surface, where it is associated with a large, transmembrane glycoprotein complex that binds the extracellular matrix protein laminin. Skeletal muscle and cardiac cells deficient in dystrophin develop necrosis presumably related to membrane instability and elevation of intracellular calcium. The cardiomyopathy and conduction defects seen in Duchenne and Becker muscular dystrophies are directly related to the defective expression of dystrophin in the heart.

LIPOPROTEINS, APOLIPOPROTEINS, AND ATHEROSCLEROSIS

Atherosclerosis and accelerated atherogenesis remain the most recognized and most treatable forms of cardiac disease (Chapter 171). Diagnosis and treatment of the major dyslipoproteinemias have been advanced mainly by molecular techniques that have elucidated the various mechanisms for this heterogeneous group of disorders. Premature cardiovascular disease is caused either by defects in lipoprotein receptors or by the associated apolipoproteins that modulate their metabolism. Elevated levels of low-density lipoprotein (LDL), β–very-low-density lipoprotein (β-VLDL), and lipoprotein a (LPa) and diminished levels of high-density lipoprotein (HDL) all increase the risk of early atherosclerotic ischemic heart disease (Chapter 171).

Plasma lipids are important substrates for energy metabolism, membrane integrity, and steroid synthesis. They are transported as lipoproteins and are separated into five major classes by the content of triglycerides, cholesterol, cholesterol esters, phospholipids, and apolipoproteins. Intestinally absorbed lipids are transported to the liver as large, hydrated lipoproteins called *chylomicrons*. The intestines, liver, and capillary endothelium modify these particles by the addition of lipoproteins and by interactions with the enzyme hepatic lipase in the liver and lipoprotein lipase in the capillary endothelium. Lechithin-cholesterol acetyltransferase (LCAT) catalyzes the esterification of plasma cholesterol to cholesterol esters. Triglyceride-rich VLDL secreted by the liver is converted to the cholesterol-rich LDL by the combined action of these lipolipases (Chapter 297).

The pathologic mechanisms for the accumulation of plasma lipids within macrophages with subsequent foam cell formation, and the formation of an occlusive atherosclerogenic plaque, are now largely understood (Chapter 171). The dyslipoproteinemias result in increased transport and transudation of lipoproteins into the intima of the coronary vessels, where blood-derived macrophages also migrate. Oxidative modification of LDL enhances uptake by macrophages and foam cell formation. Cytokinins liberated by macrophages stimulate additional migration of bloodborne macrophages and migration and proliferation of smooth muscle cells into the intima, which ultimately progress into a complex atherosclerotic lesion.

The structural similarity of LPa to plasminogen has led to a proposal that this lipoprotein particle may enhance thrombosis formation by binding tissue plasminogen activator and deactivating it, resulting in diminished steady-state thrombolysis and enhanced thrombogenesis. HDLs have been proposed to play a pivotal role in retarding foam cell formation by removing excess cholesterol from peripheral cells and transporting the cholesterol back to the liver, where it is secreted as free cholesterol or bile acids. Diminished HDL levels alter the equilibrium of cholesterol deposition by reducing cholesterol removal and transport back to the liver, which promotes lipid accumulation in peripheral cells.

The apolipoproteins associated with these various lipid particles are responsible for their receptor recognition, enzyme activation, secretion, and cellular uptake. For example, apolipoprotein B100 and E interact with the LDL receptor to initiate endocytosis and cellular uptake of LDL. Apolipoprotein A1 on HDL is believed to interact with an HDL receptor to facilitate the removal of cholesterol from peripheral cells.

Genetic diseases that alter expression of the LDL receptor or one of the apolipoprotein molecules can severely affect cholesterol metabolism. The LDL receptor gene is located on chromosome 19, where the genes for apolipoproteins E, C2, and C1 are also located. The genes for apolipoproteins A1, C3, and A4 are found on chromosome 11. The apolipoprotein B isoproteins are synthesized from a single gene on chromosome 2, and LPa is a polymorphic apolipoprotein with multiple genetic alleles present at a single locus on chromosome 6.

Familial hypercholesterolemia established the importance of LDL levels in atherogenesis and has now been characterized by four classes of mutations in the LDL receptor gene. Patients who are heterozygous for the disease have LDL cholesterol levels of 250 to 500 mg/

dl, and homozygous patients have concentrations of 600 to more than 1200 mg/dl. The dramatic coronary disease in these patients may appear as early as age 2 years to as late as the mid-20s. Class I mutations result from failure of LDL receptor biosynthesis. Class II mutations are characterized by an LDL receptor that cannot be transported to the cell surface from the endoplasmic reticulum. Class III mutations produce an LDL receptor that is present at the cell surface but cannot bind LDL normally. Class IV mutations lead to receptors that bind LDL at the cell membrane but that cannot be normally internalized and metabolized by the cell. Triple drug therapy is often required to treat patients with familial hypercholesterolemia. Liver transplantation is the most effective, although the most costly, treatment. Gene therapy using recombinant LDL receptor has shown promise in the LDL-deficient Watanabe rabbit.

Type III lipoproteinemia (dys-β-lipoproteinemia) is characterized by a structural or functional defect in apolipoprotein E. The genetic defects in this disease cause either an apolipoprotein E deficiency or the production of a functionally defective apolipoprotein E. The altered E variants have a decreased affinity for the LDL receptor, producing delayed catabolism and accumulation of remnant lipoprotein particles. Although these patients develop premature cardiovascular disease, in contrast to those with LDL receptor disorders, they respond well to diet and medical therapy (Chapter 297).

Patients with low HDL levels have been characterized by several genetic defects in apolipoprotein A1. Several families have been described who have increased catabolism of A1, whereas other families have an A1 deficiency from structural mutations in the gene. Patients with combined deficiency of A1, C3, and A4 often have reduced levels of HDL and VLDL, with relatively normal LDL levels.

Increased LPa levels have also been shown to increase five-fold the relative risk of premature vascular disease. The genetic mechanism for increased plasma levels of LPa has not yet been defined. Elevated LPa levels are not effectively reduced by diet, and the only medication shown to reduce LPa levels consistently is niacin (Chapter 297).

The disorder designated *familial combined hyperlipidemia* (FCH) is probably a heterogeneous disease and is the most common of all the dyslipoproteinemias. The gene frequency of this codominantly inherited disease has been estimated as 1 in 300 in the U.S. population. The lipid and lipoprotein profile of these patients varies, and elevations in cholesterol, triglycerides, or both may be observed in the plasma. Patients with FCH often have an abnormal cholesterol/apolipoprotein B ratio, and plasma HDL levels are frequently reduced. They generally respond to diet and medical therapy for control of their hyperlipidemia.

APPLICATION OF MEDICAL GENETICS TO THE CARDIOMYOPATHIES

Several advances have been made in recent years that have accelerated the identification of genes responsible for disease. To identify the responsible gene, one must first map the region (locus) on the chromosome where the gene resides, referred to as *chromosomal mapping*. This is now possible by the technique of genetic linkage analysis, which affords the opportunity to map the locus without knowing the protein defect. Several thousand markers of known chromosomal location distributed throughout each of the 46 chromosomes are now available. While genes are inherited independently of each other when a DNA marker and a disease-related gene are in close physical proximity on the same chromosome, they tend to be coinherited more often than by chance (>50%) and are said to be genetically linked. Because there are markers of known location every one million base pairs, the chances of a particular diseased gene and one of these markers being coinherited are high, which provides the opportunity to map the location of practically any disease-related gene, provided one has a family of two generations with seven or more living affected individuals. The DNA markers used initially were RFLPs detected by Southern blotting, which requires 7 to 10 days to perform. The markers today are short tandem repeat polymorphisms (STRP), which are analyzed by PCR, often requiring only 2 to 3 days and offering much greater resolution and information. Once the locus of the gene has been mapped, the gene must be identified. Techniques for isolation and identification of genes recently developed have also accelerated this process. The two strategies consist of positional candidate and positional cloning techniques. One first attempts to determine whether genes known to be mapped to the chromosomal locus are responsible for the disease; if they are not, one often has to clone the region relative to the position of the markers (positional cloning) and subsequently identify the DNA sequences that make up the gene. The identification of the causal gene depends on finding a gene expressed in cardiac tissue exhibiting the disease and demonstrating a causal relationship between the mutation and the disease.

Major advances have been made in uncovering the molecular basis for cardiomyopathy in patients who have inherited genetic diseases that influence their cardiac function. This group of diseases dramatically illustrates the important interplay of many different cellular elements and the way in which defects in many different aspects of cellular physiology can produce a cardiomyopathic phenotype. Defects in the sarcomere proteins, such as mutations in the β-MHC, have been shown to induce hypertrophic cardiomyopathy. Defective expression of the cytoskeletal protein dystrophin is responsible for the cardiomyopathy and conduction defect seen in patients with Duchenne and Becker muscular dystrophies, as well as X-linked cardiomyopathies. The cardiomyopathy seen in patients with myotonic dystrophy is probably caused by the altered expression of a protein kinase in cardiac tissues. Maternally inherited mitochondrial defects have also been described in patients with cardiomyopathy, in whom impaired oxidative phosphorylation may cause both conduction defects and cardiac failure.

Congenital long-QT syndrome has been mapped to three separate loci on chromosomes 3, 7, and 11; X-linked cardiomyopathy to the short arm of the X chromosome; and a form of complete atrial standstill and muscle weakness called Emery-Dreyfuss muscular dystrophy, to the distal long arm of the X chromosome. Myotonic dystrophy associated with a dilated cardiomyopathy has been mapped to chromosome 19q13.2, and the responsible gene appears to be a myotonin protein kinase. A family with a conduction defect and dilated cardiomyopathy has been mapped to chromosome 1, but the gene has not yet been identified. Most recently, two loci responsible for idiopathic dilated cardiomyopathy have been mapped to chromosome 1q32 and 9q13-q22, but no gene has yet been identified.

FAMILIAL HYPERTROPHIC CARDIOMYOPATHY

Familial hypertrophic cardiomyopathy (FHCM) has long been an interesting disease for the cardiologist because its clinical, hemodynamic, and morphologic profile may be used as a paradigm of many other cardiac diseases (Chapter 26). The disease is said to be the most common cause of sudden death in the young and is by far the most common cause of death in athletes. The disease is known to have an autosomal dominant pattern of inheritance and was the first primary cardiac disorder for which the causative gene was isolated. The first gene was localized to the long arm of chromosome 14 and the gene was identified to be β-MHC. Three other genes have now been identified, α-tropomyosin on chromosome 15, troponin T on chromosome 1, and myosin-binding protein on chromosome 11p. It is estimated that these four genes account for 50% of FHCM. Several other families have been identified whose disease is not due to any of these genes and has yet to be mapped to its chromosomal locations. Recently, a family with FHCM and Wolff-Parkinson-White syndrome was mapped to chromosome 9q, but the gene has not yet been identified. There have been more than forty mutations identified in the β-MHC, three in α-tropomyosin, and six in troponin T. The mutations in the first three genes were missense mutations, meaning a single nucleotide is substituted, resulting in the substitution of a single amino acid. There is one exception for β-MHC in a family shown to have a 2000 bp deletion. In the recently identified myosin-binding protein, however, the three mutations have been identified: a deletion, a six-amino acid duplication, and a missense mutation.

The clinical manifestations with respect to hypertrophy appear to be similar for all of the genes. De novo mutations have been identified in the β-MHC and α-tropomyosin genes and documented to be transmitted to subsequent generations, clearly establishing that these mutations are responsible for FHCM. Experimental studies have shown that the mutant β-MHC protein exhibits defective contractility as determined from an in vitro motility assay. Thus the hypothesis that the hypertrophy is compensatory is widely accepted as a most plausible mechanism. Studies in feline species using gene transfer of the mutant β-MHC resulted in myocyte and sarcomere disarray similar to that of HCM seen in humans. Other studies have shown that the extent of hypertrophy and the frequency of sudden death may result, in part, from the interaction of the primary mutant gene with that of other genes. Patients with FHCM resulting from β-MHC mutations who also have the ACE DD genotype exhibit more extensive hypertrophy and a much higher incidence of sudden death. This may have profound therapeutic implications, particularly in individuals with DD genotypes in whom an ACE inhibitor may prevent the hypertrophy. Despite having the same mutation present in the same family, individuals affected with FHCM often exhibit marked variation in the extent of hypertrophy, as well as other clinical features such as sudden death.

Based on genetic screening for the mutations identified so far, genotype-phenotype correlations suggest that risk stratification may be possible on the basis of specific mutations. This feature is illustrated in Fig. 10-9, where it is seen that one mutation has essentially a normal life span and the other has a shortened life span of only 33 years. Studies have indicated that at least three mutations in the β-MHC gene ($Arg^{403}Gln$, $Arg^{453}Cys$, and $Arg^{719}Trp$) have a very malignant course with a very high incidence of sudden death, whereas another three mutations ($Val^{606}Met$, $Phe^{513}Cys$, and $Leu^{908}Val$) have a far more benign course.

Familial Idiopathic Dilated Cardiomyopathy

Dilated cardiomyopathy (DCM) is the more common of the two responses of the heart to injury such as hypertension, ischemic heart disease, and volume overload. DCM is also the most common cause for cardiac transplantation, which costs more than $200 million per year. The incidence of familial DCM (FDCM) is unknown but is estimated to account for 20% to 30% of all cases of idiopathic DCM. The etiology of DCM is so diverse, including myocarditis in childhood, that it is often difficult to determine the cause and not infrequently to determine whether it is familial or acquired. The first loci for DCM were mapped in 1995 to chromosomes 1 and 9. Neither of the genes has yet been identified, and another form of FDCM occurring in association with a conduction disorder was mapped to chromosome 7. FDCM is a lethal disease with a high incidence of sud-

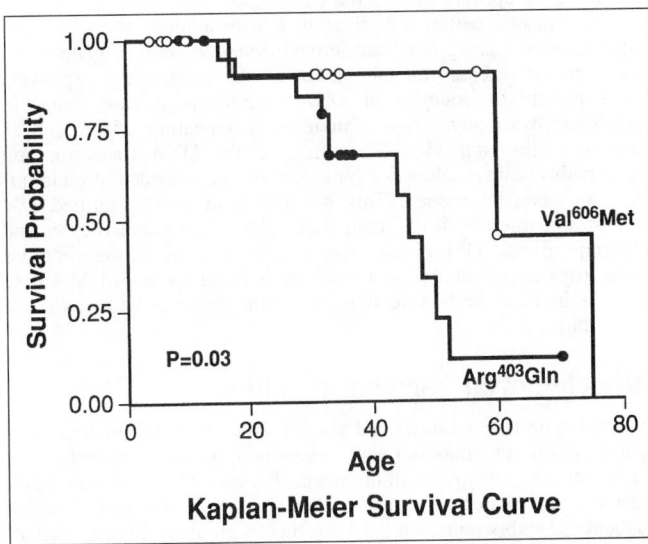

FIGURE 10-9 Kaplan-Meier survival curve comparing families having the malignant $Arg^{403}Gln$ mutation with another family having the more benign $Val^{606}Met$ mutation.

(From Marian AJ, Roberts R: *Circulation* 92:1336, 1995.)

den death occurring in the teenage years. Until the first gene is identified, the nature of this disease, whether it be familial or acquired, remains an enigma.

Cardiomyopathy of Duchenne and Becker Muscular Dystrophy

Duchenne and Becker muscular dystrophies are allelic X-linked recessive disorders caused by mutations in the gene encoding the cytoskeletal protein dystrophin. These diseases affect approximately 1 in 3500 newborn males and are the most common and devastating of the human muscular dystrophies. Phenotypic effects of dystrophin gene mutations are primarily manifested in limb skeletal muscle, although patients usually die from respiratory failure, congestive heart failure, or cardiac conduction abnormalities. Patients who have a milder form of Becker dystrophy often express detectable amounts of a truncated form of dystrophin protein of intragenic deletions that presumably occur in noncritical regions of the molecule. In contrast, patients with Duchenne dystrophy have been characterized by low levels or complete absence of dystrophin in skeletal muscle. *X-linked cardiomyopathy* is a term used to describe families who have low or absent dystrophin in the heart and preserved dystrophin expression in skeletal muscle. These patients present with cardiomyopathy but no skeletal myopathy. The diagnosis can be made in patients with cardiomyopathy and unexplained elevation of serum creatine kinase by Southern blot of lymphocyte DNA, or demonstration of low cardiac dystrophin by immunochemical analysis of an endomyocardial biopsy specimen. Dystrophin is a cytoskeletal protein localized to the sarcolemma, although it appears to lack a transmembrane domain. Dystrophin is associated with an integral membrane glycoprotein complex that links the cytoskeleton to the extracellular molecule laminin. When dystrophin is absent from dystrophic muscle, the integral membrane glycoproteins are destabilized at the membrane surface.

Myotonic Muscular Dystrophy

Myotonic muscular dystrophy (Steinert disease) is a systemic disease that has many nonmyopathic features, including frontal baldness, cataracts, and muscle atrophy with a characteristic long face and slightly nasal voice (Chapter 125). As many as 80% of patients have interventricular conduction defects, which may culminate in fatal Stokes-Adams episodes unless anticipated and treated by pacemaker insertion. The gene responsible for this disease has been localized to the long arm of chromosome 19, and sequence homology has shown that the gene appears to be a protein kinase.

The unusual pattern of inheritance with a more severe phenotype in the offspring has been termed *anticipation.* The genetics of this type of disease mutation involves the progressive expansion of a repetitive sequence of DNA within the disease gene. In myotonic dystrophy, amplification of a repeating triplet (GCT) occurs in the noncoding $3'$ region of the DNA transcript and presumably causes altered expression of the encoded protein kinase in diseased tissues. This novel protein kinase, termed *DM kinase,* is expressed at the intercalated disk of cardiac myocytes and Purkinje fibers. DM kinase may play a role in normal impulse transmission in the heart, and there are reduced levels of DM kinase protein in heart and skeletal muscle from patients with myotonic dystrophy.

Mitochondrial Cardiomyopathies

Several reports have described abnormalities in mitochondrial morphology and mitochondrial gene deletions in patients with either isolated cardiomyopathy or multisystem diseases who primarily manifest cardiac conduction defects. The mitochondrial defects in these patients probably represent a heterogeneous group of diseases that affect mitochondrial function. One family with an apparent X-linked recessive inheritance pattern for disease was characterized by the deaths of four related male infants from dilated cardiomyopathy and heart failure. Morphologic studies revealed mitochondria that were greatly enlarged, with irregular shape and increased crista, and that

contained unidentified dense granules. The incidence of these mitochondrial changes was noted four times more frequently in cardiac tissues than in skeletal muscle and the diaphragm at autopsy. Electron microscopy of a biopsy sample from a mother of the proband revealed no abnormalities. The genetic defect in this disorder has not yet been identified but illustrates the potential importance of mitochondrial dysfunction in a subgroup of patients with cardiomyopathy.

Kearns-Sayre syndrome is a well-described myopathy characterized by external ophthalmoplegia, pigmentary retinopathy, and heart block. The morphologic changes in skeletal muscle observed using a trichrome stain involve the identification of so-called ragged red fibers. Cardiac involvement appears almost exclusively to affect the specialized conduction system rather than the myocardium. Patients with this disorder have deletions in the genes encoded by the mitochondrial genome. Kearns-Sayre syndrome is transmitted by maternal inheritance because all the mitochondria in the ovum during the zygote's formation are from the mother. As a result, the affected mother passes the disease to all children, but only her daughters can transmit the mitochondrial abnormality to subsequent generations. The relative proportion of mitochondrial genomes affected varies from 30% to 85% in different patients. Biochemical analysis of the mitochondrial enzymes from muscle extracts shows widely scattered values. Most patients, however, have reduced activity of four enzymes in the respiratory chain: cytochrome *c* oxidase, cytochrome *c* oxoreductase, rotenone-sensitive NADH–cytochrome *c* reductase, and NADH dehydrogenase (cytochrome *c* reductase).

Congenital Long Q-T Syndrome

Several disorders have been shown to target the cardiac conduction system through mechanisms that prolong the Q-T interval (Chapter 18). These patients have a high incidence of sudden death from episodic ventricular arrhythmias and also have Stokes-Adams attacks, characterized by fainting spells and usually precipitated by exertion or emotional stress. Antiarrhythmic drugs that modulate the activity of ion channels can prolong the Q-T interval, prompting early speculation that these disorders involve gene defects in proteins involved in membrane repolarization.

The *Romano-Ward syndrome* is predominantly a childhood illness associated with QT prolongation on the electrocardiogram. Onset of symptoms is usually before age 3 years, although some patients do not show clinical signs until age 30. Affected individuals may appear healthy except for episodes of palpitations, chest pain, and sudden loss of consciousness or sudden death. Romano-Ward syndrome is inherited as an autosomal dominant trait, and this heterogeneous disease has been linked to three distinct genetic loci on chromosome 11 (LQT1), chromosome 7 (LQT2), and chromosome 3 (LQT3). The genetic probe used to show linkage to chromosome 11 is the gene encoding the Harvey-*ras* oncogene (H-*ras*-1). No mutations have yet been identified in the coding sequence of the H-*ras*-1 gene in patients with long QT syndrome; therefore this gene cannot be implicated as a causative gene in the disease. In families with linkage to chromosome 7 (LQT2), mutations have been found in the HERG gene. The HERG gene product is believed to be a calcium-dependent potassium channel; this may be responsible for the observed repolarization abnormality. The chromosome 3–related variant of long QT (LQT3) is caused by mutations in the cardiac sodium channel SCN5A. The mutant channel displays a persistent inward sodium current, which explains prolongation of cardiac action potentials in this form of congenital long QT syndrome.

Jervell and Lange-Nielsen syndrome is an autosomal recessive inherited disease associated with a cardiac abnormality similar to that seen in Romano-Ward syndrome; however, it is also characterized by bilateral high-tone perceptive deafness. The incidence is about 1 in 300,000 persons in the general population and about 1 in 100 among all deaf children. Histologic abnormalities in the artery to the sinus and atrioventricular nodes have been demonstrated, and the administration of digitalis can reduce the Q-T interval and diminish the frequency of syncopal attacks. The chromosomal location and molecular defect in these individuals remain undefined.

BIBLIOGRAPHY

Bennet P et al: Molecular mechanisms for an inherited cardiac arrhythmia, *Nature* 376:683-685 (letter), 1995.

Bies RD et al: Expression and localization of dystrophin in human cardiac Purkinje fibers, *Circulation* 86:147-153, 1992.

Caforio ALP et al: Identification of α- and β-cardiac myosin heavy chain isoforms as major autoantigens in dilated cardiomyopathy, *Circulation* 85:1734-1742, 1992.

Curran M et al: A molecular basis for cardiac arrhythmia: *HERG* mutations cause long QT syndrome, *Cell* 80:795-803, 1995.

Hoffman E et al: Overexcited or inactive: ion channels in muscle disease, *Cell* 80:681, 1995.

Kelly DP, Strauss AW: Mechanisms of disease: inherited cardiomyopathies, *N Engl J Med* 330:913-919, 1994.

Maeda M et al: Identification, tissue specific expression, and subcellular localization of the 80- and 71-kDa forms of myotonic dystrophy kinase protein, *J Biol Chem* 270:20246-20249, 1995.

Mares A et al: Molecular biology for the cardiologist, *Curr Probl Cardiol* 17:1-72, 1992.

Marian AJ et al: Sudden cardiac death in hypertrophic cardiomyopathy: variability in phenotypic expression of β-myosin heavy chain mutations, *Eur Heart J* 16:368-376, 1995.

Marian AJ et al: Angiotensin converting enzyme polymorphism in hypertrophic cardiomyopathy and sudden cardiac death, *Lancet* 342:1085-1086, 1993.

Marian AJ, Roberts R: Recent advances in the molecular genetics of hypertrophic cardiomyopathy, *Circulation* 92:1336-1347, 1995.

Melacini P et al: Correlation between cardiac involvement and CTG trinucleotide repeat length in myotonic dystrophy, *J Am Coll Cardiol* 25:239, 1995.

Muntoni F et al: A mutation in the dystrophin gene selectively affecting dystrophin expression in the heart, *J Clin Invest* 96:693, 1995.

Perryman MB et al: Expression of a missense mutation in the mRNA for β-myosin heavy chain in myocardial tissue in hypertrophic cardiomyopathy, *J Clin Invest* 90:271, 1990.

Roberts R, editor: *Molecular basis of cardiology,* Hamden, CT, 1992, Blackwell Scientific Publications.

Theifelder L et al: α-tropomyosin and cardiac troponin T mutations cause familial hypertrophic cardiomyopathy: a disease of the sarcomere, *Cell* 77:701, 1994.

Vikstrom KL: The molecular genetic basis of familial hypertrophic cardiomyopathy, *Heart Failure* 11:5, 1995.

Watkins H et al: Characteristics and prognostic inplications of myosin missense mutations in familial hypertrophic cardiomyopathy, *N Engl J Med* 326:1108, 1992.

II LABORATORY TESTS AND DIAGNOSTIC METHODS

CHAPTER

11 Physical Examination of the Cardiovascular System

James A. Shaver

The physical examination of the cardiovascular system, together with a history, is the foundation on which the evaluation of a cardiac patient is based. The synthesis of information obtained by these two exercises allows the clinician to order the most appropriate and cost-effective additional tests necessary to confirm the diagnosis and treat the patient. The accuracy of these physical signs is based on firm anatomic and physiologic principles, thereby permitting precise pathophysiologic inferences to be drawn from them. Although the student of medicine can easily acquire the theory and mechanics of the cardiovascular examination, it is only by the careful examination of a large number of patients with normal and abnormal physical findings and correlation of these findings with the anatomic and physiologic gold standards that the art and science of this discipline can be mastered.

Proper assessment of the heart and circulation includes evaluation of the patient's physical appearance, determination of blood pressure, examination of the arterial and jugular venous pulses, inspection and palpation of the precordial movements, and cardiac auscultation.

GENERAL APPEARANCE

The physical examination begins when the physician first meets the patient. The patient's general appearance often provides important clues to a primary cardiac condition. The apprehensive, diaphoretic patient with a clenched fist attesting to the severity of the chest pain is a classic presentation of acute myocardial infarction. The cachectic patient with edematous lower extremities, a distended abdomen full of ascites, and peripheral cyanosis may be suffering from the ravages of long-standing congestive heart failure. Acute left heart failure with pulmonary edema is manifested by a frightened, apprehensive, and diaphoretic patient with labored respirations; the patient is often sitting upright and coughing up pink frothy sputum. Likewise, the individual leaning forward and splinting the chest with a pillow is probably suffering from acute pericardial disease. In each of these conditions, the astute clinician will immediately focus the physical examination to confirm the suspected diagnosis.

Many congenital anomalies have typical physical appearances that are associated with cardiac disease. Although their review is beyond the scope of this chapter, a few are highlighted. The cardiac manifestations of Marfan's syndrome include aortic root disease, which may be evidenced by an acute dissection, as well as myxomatous degeneration of the mitral valve and mitral annular ectasia. Down's syndrome is easily recognized and predicts the presence of an endocardial cushion defect. Coarctation of the aorta and a bicuspid valve are often associated with Turner's syndrome, found in the female with short stature, webbing of the neck, and sexual infantilism. When the general appearance suggests a congenital anomaly in a patient with cardiovascular symptoms, a possible associated cardiac anomaly should be suspected.

The morbidly obese patient with peripheral edema often presents with typical left heart failure or, more rarely, is observed to have the pickwickian syndrome of hypersomnolence and pulmonary hypertension secondary to alveolar hypoventilation. The patient with severe chronic obstructive lung disease has dyspnea at rest, uses accessory muscles to aid respiration, and may have coexisting right heart failure secondary to cor pulmonale. Puffiness of the face and periorbital edema, especially on arising in the morning, may be due to marked increase in the central venous pressure, as commonly seen in constrictive pericarditis, severe tricuspid regurgitation, and tricuspid stenosis. Cardiac problems are commonly associated with collagen vascular disease (Chapter 33). Other systemic diseases such as sarcoidosis, amyloidosis, and hemochromatosis should always raise the suspicion that the heart may be one of the target organs of the underlying illness.

Central cyanosis of the head and neck is readily observed at the bedside when the O_2 saturation is less than 80% and more easily appreciated when associated with polycythemia. Right-to-left intracardiac shunting at the atrial or ventricular level should always be suspected, whereas cyanosis and clubbing of the toes with sparing of the fingers are diagnostic of a reversed patent ductus arteriosus that joins the aorta distal to the left subclavian artery. Peripheral cyanosis is a manifestation of low cardiac output and wide arterial venous difference and is much more obvious in the distal extremities. It is frequently observed in patients with severe right heart failure secondary to advanced mitral stenosis or chronic constrictive pericarditis. In such patients, mild icterus of the sclera secondary to the hepatic congestion is often present.

Both advanced hypothyroidism and hyperthyroidism have typical clinical appearances (Chapter 33). The myxedematous patient has a hoarse, raspy voice with a dull, expressionless face, periorbital puffiness, a large tongue, dry skin, and sparse hair. The thyrotoxic patient is often hyperkinetic, with warm, salmon-colored skin, excessive perspiration, exophthalmos, and a fine tremor. Advanced acromegaly is easily recognized and is associated with accelerated coronary atherosclerosis and myocardial hypertrophy, whereas the truncal obesity of Cushing's syndrome with thin extremities and abdominal striae is often associated with severe systemic hypertension.

More subtle findings on the general examination can be of equal diagnostic importance. Such is the case in infective endocarditis (Chapter 24), in which splinter hemorrhages on the nail beds, Osler's nodes, clubbing of the fingers, and conjunctival hemorrhages are apparent on more detailed examination. Mucocutaneous telangiectasia on the face, lips, and oral mucous membranes may be associated with pulmonary or hepatic arteriovenous fistulas (Osler-Weber-Rendu disease). Corneal arcus and earlobe creases, particularly when present in the younger patient, should raise the suspicion of possible coronary artery disease; xanthomas on the dorsum of the hand, extensor surfaces of the elbows, and Achilles tendon should alert the clinician to lipid abnormalities associated with atherosclerosis.

The importance of the general appearance of the patient cannot be overemphasized and will often alert the clinician to search for additional physical signs in order to arrive at a definitive cardiac diagnosis.

MEASUREMENT OF BLOOD PRESSURE

Brachial artery blood pressure should routinely be determined in both arms. The patient should be seated or lying comfortably, and the arm should be slightly flexed and at the level of the heart. Proper technique is important for obtaining accurate measurements of blood pressure by the indirect method. The sphygmomanometer compression cuff, the hand-operated rubber ball for inflation, and the adjustable valve for cuff deflation should be in perfect working order. The inflatable rubber bag must be contained completely within the sealed inelastic cuff, so that the cuff evenly compresses the area to which it is applied. The width of the cuff should be 20% greater than the limb diameter, and the length should be adequate to compress two thirds of the limb. It should be applied snugly around the arm. The diaphragm of the stethoscope should be placed close to or under the edge of the cuff. The cuff is then quickly inflated to approximately 20 to 30 mm Hg above the systolic pressure as indicated by obliteration of the pulse. The auscultatory pressure is determined by noting the onset of the Korotkoff sounds as the cuff is deflated at a rate of approximately 3 mm Hg/sec. These sounds are produced by flow of blood through the brachial artery as the blood pressure cuff is gradually released; they consist of five phases. Phase 1 is the first appearance of a clear, tapping sound representing peak systolic pressure. This is replaced by soft murmurs during phase 2 and louder murmurs during phase 3, as the volume of blood flowing through the constricted artery increases. They suddenly become muffled in phase 4, as arterial diastolic pressure is approached. Korotkoff sounds disappear at phase 5, usually approximately 10 mm Hg lower than phase 4. Systolic pressure should be recorded at the point at which the first tapping sounds occur for two consecutive beats (phase 1). The diastolic pressure should be recorded in adults when sounds become inaudible. When the pulse pressure is wide, diastolic pressure should be recorded when muffling of the sounds occurs (onset of phase 4). When the difference between muffling and disappearance of the Korotkoff sounds is considerable, both pressures should be recorded.

If the cuff is deflated too slowly or is immediately reinflated for repeat blood pressure determination, the resultant venous congestion elevates diastolic pressure and decreases the intensity of Korotkoff sounds such that the systolic pressure is underestimated and the diastolic pressure is overestimated. When Korotkoff sounds are difficult to auscultate, their amplitude may be increased by having the patient open and close the hand vigorously five or six times. An erroneously low systolic pressure may also result from a failure to detect the presence of an auscultatory gap, a silent interval occasionally present just below the systolic blood pressure. This may be avoided by inflating the cuff to 20 to 30 mm Hg above the level necessary to obliterate the pulse. Systolic blood pressure may also be estimated by palpation alone, by inflating the cuff to 20 to 30 mm Hg greater than that necessary to obliterate the pulse and then slowly deflating it until the pulse returns. The first palpable pulse is recorded as the systolic blood pressure and is approximately 5 to 10 mm Hg lower than that obtained by auscultation.

Blood pressure also can be measured in the lower extremity by applying a cuff of the appropriate size and fit to the thigh, with auscultation of Korotkoff sounds in the popliteal fossa. Blood pressure in the lower extremity also may be obtained by applying a standard arm cuff to the lower half of the calf and auscultating either the dorsalis pedis or posterior tibial pulse. Blood pressure in the lower extremity is measured in the supine position and normally is up to 20 mm Hg higher than that in the arm; however, the diastolic pressures are nearly identical. In coarctation of the aorta, the blood pressure in the lower extremity is decreased relative to the upper extremity and should be measured in all patients (particularly younger) with hypertension.

When the regular-sized cuff is applied to a large upper arm or a normal adult thigh, arterial pressure may be overestimated, a common problem in obese patients. Likewise, when it is applied to a small arm, the pressure may be underestimated. The arterial pressure also may be underestimated if the cuff is deflated too rapidly, particularly when bradycardia or irregular rhythms are present.

In the adult population, systolic pressure greater than 140 mm Hg and diastolic pressure greater than 90 mm Hg are considered elevated. A single blood pressure measurement should never be used in the diagnosis of hypertension (Chapter 32).

ARTERIAL PULSES

Arterial pulses that can easily be palpated during the cardiovascular examination include the carotid, subclavian, brachial, radial, abdominal aorta, femoral, popliteal, posterior tibial, and dorsalis pedis pulses. The radial or brachial artery is most commonly palpated for the evaluation of heart rate and rhythm, whereas the carotid pulse gives the most accurate representation of the central aortic pressure. Whether the artery is palpated with the thumb or the pads of the fingertip depends on the preference of the examiner. When two pulses are compared (right and left, or upper and lower extremity), both arteries should be palpated simultaneously or in rapid succession, the latter being more appropriate for palpation of the carotid arteries. Auscultation over both the carotid arteries and subclavian arteries is an important aspect of their evaluation and may reveal bruits, indicating either local arterial obstruction or the transmitted murmur of left ventricular outflow obstruction. Healthy children and young adults may have easily heard innocent supraclavicular systolic murmurs that can be attenuated or vanish with hyperextension of the shoulders.

The volume and contour of the arterial pulses are determined by a complex interplay of factors, including left ventricular stroke volume and its rate of ejection, the compliance and capacity of the arterial tree, and the pressure wave that results from antegrade flow of blood, as well as the reflection of a pulse wave returning from the periphery. For practical purposes at the bedside, the amplitude of the pulse correlates well with the arterial pulse pressure, which in turn is primarily determined by the ratio of the stroke volume to the compliance of the vessel. The amplitude of the arterial pulse can conveniently be graded 0 to +3, with 0 designating an absent pulse, +1 a reduced pulse, +2 a normal pulse, and +3 an exaggerated pulse.

Differences in peripheral pulses are most commonly caused by localized obstructive arteriosclerotic vascular disease (Chapter 31), particularly in the carotid and femoral vessels. Obstruction also can be caused by arterial emboli, thrombosis in situ, arteritis, dissecting aortic aneurysms, and prior surgical vascular procedures. Unequal pulses in the upper extremity can be caused by a cervical rib or the scalenus anticus syndrome, and a selected decrease in the pulse in the right arm is seen in patients with supravalvular aortic stenosis.

Femoral pulses may be decreased or absent with localized arteriosclerosis of the external or common iliac arteries. Unilateral or bilateral impairment is common with dissecting aneurysms, and absent femoral pulses may be found with thrombotic occlusion or saddle embolus to the aortic bifurcation. In the child or young adult, if both femoral pulses are equally weakened or delayed, coarctation of the aorta is a likely possibility, particularly if hypertension exists in the upper extremities. Bilateral absence of both the dorsalis pedis and posterior tibial pulse or unilateral absence of either usually indicates atherosclerotic vascular disease. Neither of these pulses should be considered absent unless palpated in the dependent position.

A recording of the normal carotid pulse is shown in Fig. 11-1. As the pulse wave travels distally, the upstroke becomes steeper, with a higher systolic peak, and the dicrotic incisura is replaced by a smoother, later dicrotic notch. With aging, as well as in patients with arteriosclerosis, the tidal wave may become higher than the percussion wave, with the pulse reaching its peak in late systole.

Abnormal pulses may be due to alterations in the physiologic state or a disease process or both (Fig. 11-2). A hyperkinetic pulse is seen in high-output states, having a rapid upstroke, an increased amplitude and pulse pressure, and a large stroke volume (Fig. 11-2, *A*). In

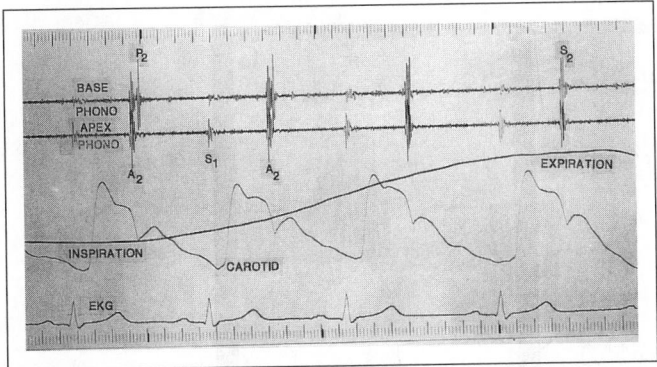

FIGURE 11-1 The indirect carotid pulse is recorded simultaneously with the base and apex phonocardiogram in a normal subject. The normal carotid pulse has a brisk upstroke, terminating in an initial higher percussion wave followed by a lower second wave, the tidal wave. The systolic portion of the pulse is terminated by the sharp incisura related to aortic valve closure, which normally follows A_2 by 20 to 40 msec. A small dicrotic notch is present, followed by a gradual decline of the pulse during the remainder of diastole. Normal physiologic splitting of S_2 is present during inspiration. A_2 and P_2 are clearly separated into two distinctly audible sounds. During expiration, the splitting narrows and A_2 and P_2 are separated by less than 30 msec and are appreciated as a single sound. Note the absence of P_2 at the apex.

(From Shaver JA, Salerni R: Auscultation of the heart. In Hurst JW, Schlant RC, editors: *The heart,* ed 7, New York, 1990, McGraw-Hill.)

contrast, a hypokinetic pulse is a weak pulse of small volume and pulse pressure and is usually a reflection of low stroke volume and low blood pressure. Pulsus bisferiens is a pulse having a double systolic peak and is most commonly observed in combined aortic stenosis and regurgitation, severe aortic regurgitation without stenosis, and hypertrophic cardiomyopathy (Fig. 11-2, *B, C*). In severe chronic aortic regurgitation, there is an extremely rapid upstroke with a large volume pulse and wide pulse pressure (Corrigan or Waterhammer pulse). Pistol shot sounds are also heard over the brachial and femoral arteries (Traube's sign), and a to-fro murmur may also be heard over the femoral artery when compressed by the bell of the stethoscope (Duroziez's sign). A classic pulsus parvus et tardus pulse of severe aortic stenosis is shown in Fig. 11-2, *D*. Severe aortic stenosis in the elderly may have a near-normal pulse contour because of the decreased distensibility of the carotid vessels; however, a transmitted systolic murmur is almost always present (Chapter 25). A dicrotic pulse is a double-peaked pulse, with one peak in systole and the second in early diastole, because of an accentuated dicrotic wave following S_2. It is observed in two disparate conditions: (1) severe left ventricular failure in young or middle-aged patients associated with a low stroke volume and high peripheral vascular resistance (Fig. 11-2, *E*), and (2) young patients having a high cardiac output with low peripheral vascular resistance, such as with high fever. A quick-rising pulse with a rapid fall-off and shortened ejection time is observed in severe mitral regurgitation (Fig. 11-2, *F*).

Pulsus alternans is usually a sign of severe left ventricular dysfunction (Fig. 11-3, *A*). The cardiac rhythm must be regular since varying cycle lengths will normally alter the pulse amplitude. It is commonly precipitated by a premature contraction and may be exaggerated by having the patient abruptly assume the upright posture. Pulsus paradoxus is an exaggeration of the normal respiratory variation in the pulse amplitude and is a classic finding in cardiac tamponade (Fig. 11-3, *B*). When severe tamponade is present, this can be appreciated by palpation of the brachial or radial artery. During quiet respiration, when a decrease in pulse amplitude during inspiration can be appreciated, the maximum difference in systolic pressure is usually 20 mm Hg or greater between expiration and inspiration. When less severe tamponade is present, the extent of the pulse pressure difference can be quantitated by cuff sphygmomanometry. After the cuff has been inflated above systolic pressure, it is deflated at a rate of 2 to 3 mm Hg per heartbeat, and a pulsus is defined as the pressure difference between the first discernible Korotkoff sound on expiration and the pressure level at which Korotkoff sounds are heard

during all phases of quiet respiration. A difference of 10 mm Hg or more is considered abnormal.

The normal response of pulse amplitude following a premature beat in a patient with fixed left ventricular outflow obstruction is shown in Fig. 11-4, *A*. A similar increase in pulse pressure is also present in the normal subject following a premature beat, both being due to the increased stroke volume following a long diastolic filling period. In Fig. 11-4, *B*, a decrease in the pulse pressure is shown following a premature beat, a finding pathognomonic for hypertrophic obstructive cardiomyopathy. When normal sinus rhythm with AV dissociation is present with complete heart block, paced ventricular rhythms, and ventricular tachycardia, there will be a random beat-to-beat variation in the pulse amplitude depending on the appropriate or inappropriate timing of the atrial contribution to ventricular filling.

JUGULAR VENOUS PULSE

The right jugular venous pulse (JVP) is a direct "pipeline" into the right atrium, and its careful inspection gives valuable information regarding both the level of right atrial pressure as well as its waveform. The left internal jugular and the two external jugular veins are less reliable for estimating right atrial pressure because of the presence of valves and the fact that the left innominate vein transverses the mediastinum and may be compressed or kinked by a variety of normal or diseased mediastinal structures. During inspiration, venous return to the right heart increases, whereas mean right atrial pressures and the JVP fall, closely paralleling the decline in intrathoracic pressure.

In Fig. 11-5, the right JVP is recorded in a normal subject and has a similar waveform to the normal right atrial pressure. The A wave of the JVP results from venous distention because of right atrial systole, whereas the first part of the X descent is due to active right atrial relaxation. The C wave, which can be recorded in the right atrial pressure trace, is a vibration resulting from the sudden tensing of the retrograde bulging tricuspid valve when its elastic limits are met and may be reflected retrograde into the JVP with a lesser amplitude. At times the C wave in the JVP may be an artifact produced by the carotid pulse, which occurs almost simultaneously with tricuspid closure. It is followed by the X^1 descent, caused by the pulling down of the floor of the atrium (descent of the base) by ventricular contraction. The subsequent V wave is due to passive flow into the right atrium during systole, when the tricuspid valve is closed. The rapid descent of the V wave (Y descent) is due to the fall in the right atrial pressure during the rapid phase of right ventricular filling. Following the nadir of the Y descent (Y trough), a diastasis or H wave may be produced during the slow phase of ventricular filling before the subsequent A wave.

Although all of these events usually can be recorded by pressure transducers in the right atrium or applied directly over the right JVP, they are not easily identified on inspection. The downward collapsing movement of the jugular veins, that is, the X^1 and Y descents, is more easily appreciated by the eye than are the ascents, because they produce large, rapid excursions. The predominate X^1 jugular venous descent occurs just before S_2, whereas Y descent follows S_2 (Fig. 11-5). In the normal subject, the A wave has the most prominent ascent, occurring just before S_1 or the carotid pulse, whereas the V wave is less conspicuous, occurring close to S_2, just after the carotid pulse. With elevation of central venous pressure, the V wave becomes higher and the Y collapse more prominent.

The technique of estimating central venous pressure is shown in Fig. 11-5. The patient's upper thorax is positioned such that the column of blood in the internal jugular vein is visible in the neck by using an examining table that breaks in the middle, allowing the entire thorax to be raised and lowered. This can also be accomplished by slowly raising the head of an electric bed until the oscillating meniscus of the JVP can be seen in the column of blood. The center of the right atrium is approximately 5 cm from the sternal angle of Louis, and this relationship is maintained in every position between supine and sitting upright. The vertical height of the column in the neck can be measured from the sternal angle, and the estimated right atrial pressures (centimeters of blood) can be obtained by adding 5 cm (Fig. 11-5). Additional information can be gained by observing the response to gradual, sustained abdominal compression (abdominal jugular or

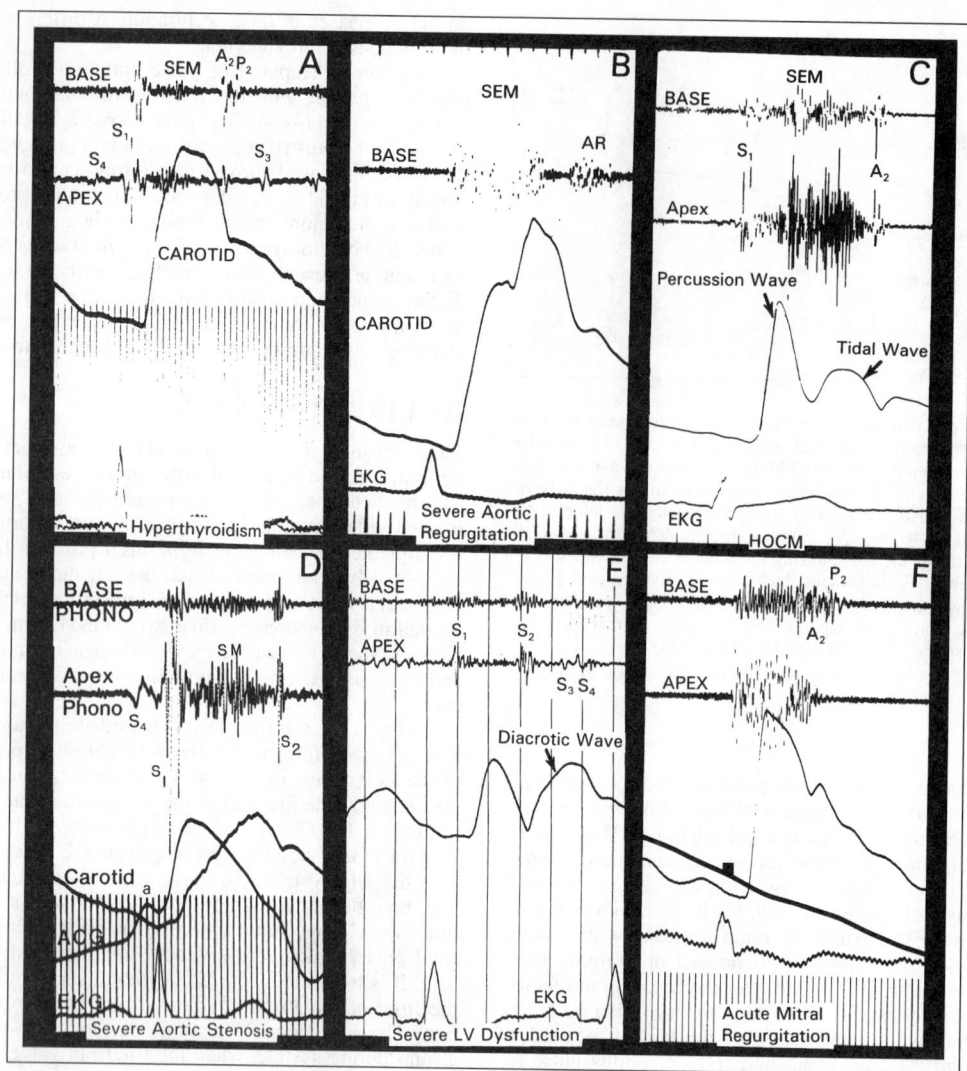

FIGURE 11-2   Abnormalities of the carotid pulse are recorded with the base and/or apex phonocardiogram. **A,** In hyperthyroidism, a hyperkinetic carotid pulse is associated with a prominent systolic ejection murmur (SEM) and audible S_3 and S_4 gallops. **B,** The classic Corrigan pulse of severe aortic regurgitation is associated with a grade V SEM followed by a pandiastolic murmur of aortic regurgitation *(AR)*. **C,** The classic bisferiens pulse of hypertrophic obstructive cardiomyopathy (HOCM) is associated with an SEM recorded at the base and apex. Note the late accentuation of the murmur at the apex, consistent with concomitant mitral regurgitation. Marked prolongation of left ventricular ejection time causes reversed splitting of S_2. **D,** The classic slow-rising anacrotic pulse of calcific aortic stenosis is associated with a grade V SEM, recorded at both the base and apex. A very prominent presystolic pulsation *(a)* is recorded on the apex-cardiogram (ACG), coincident with a loud S_4 at the apex. The systolic pulsation of the ACG is prominent and sustained. **E,** A patient with severe left ventricular dysfunction. The carotid pulse is of small amplitude and short duration associated with an extremely large dicrotic wave, equal in height to the systolic wave. An incomplete summation gallop (S_3, S_4) is recorded on the apex phonocardiogram. **F,** The quick-rising pulse with rapid fall-off and a short ejection time, typical of severe mitral regurgitation, is associated with wide splitting of S_2.

hepatojugular reflux) for approximately 30 seconds. The normal response to this increase in venous return is a transient increase in the prominence of the external jugular veins and the crests and troughs of the internal jugular veins for a few beats, which is promptly followed by a fall to control levels as abdominal compression continues. In patients with right ventricular failure, the initial rise in JVP is not followed by a prompt fall, but instead falls gradually or is maintained during the entire compression period. The evaluation of the individual waves of the JVP can be greatly facilitated by directing a light source tangentially across the neck to highlight their ascents and descents.

Elevations of the JVP and abnormalities of its waveform occur with right-sided congestive failure, obstruction to right ventricular inflow or reduction of right ventricular compliance, pericardial disease and restrictive cardiomyopathy, volume overload, obstruction to the

superior vena cava, and both atrial and ventricular arrhythmias. Prominent A waves are associated with increased impedance to right ventricular filling, as shown in Fig. 11-6, *A-C*. In patients with large atrial septal defects, the A wave is prominent and equal in height to the V wave, because the JVP is reflecting left atrial pressure as the large communication equilibrates pressure in the two chambers. With atrial fibrillation, the a wave disappears, but the X^1 descent remains. In complete heart block, when a contraction occurs against the closed tricuspid valve, giant A waves (Cannon waves) are produced. In slow or rapid junctional rhythms, a waves occur synchronously with the carotid pulse.

The classic M- or W-shaped contour of the central venous pressure in chronic constrictive pericarditis is shown in Fig. 11-6, *E* (see Chapter 27). Prominent X^1 and Y descents are present, which increase in excursion with inspiration. With progressively more severe tricus-

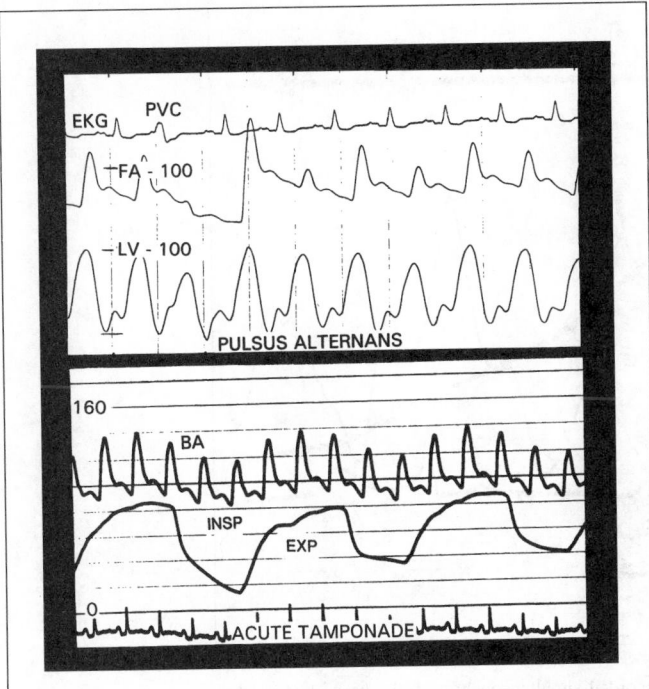

FIGURE 11-3   A, femoral arterial and left ventricular pressures are recorded in a patient with severe left ventricular dysfunction. Following a premature ventricular contraction *(PVC),* classic pulsus alternans is initiated with alternations in the amplitude, pulse pressure, and duration of the femoral artery pulse on a beat-to-beat basis. **B,** Brachial artery pressure is recorded in a patient with acute cardiac tamponade demonstrating pulsus paradoxus. Note the 20 mm Hg decrease in arterial pressure during quiet inspiration.

(**B** From Reddy PS: Hemodynamics of cardiac tamponade in man. In Reddy PS, Leon DF, Shaver JA, editors: *Pericardial disease,* New York, 1982, Raven Press.)

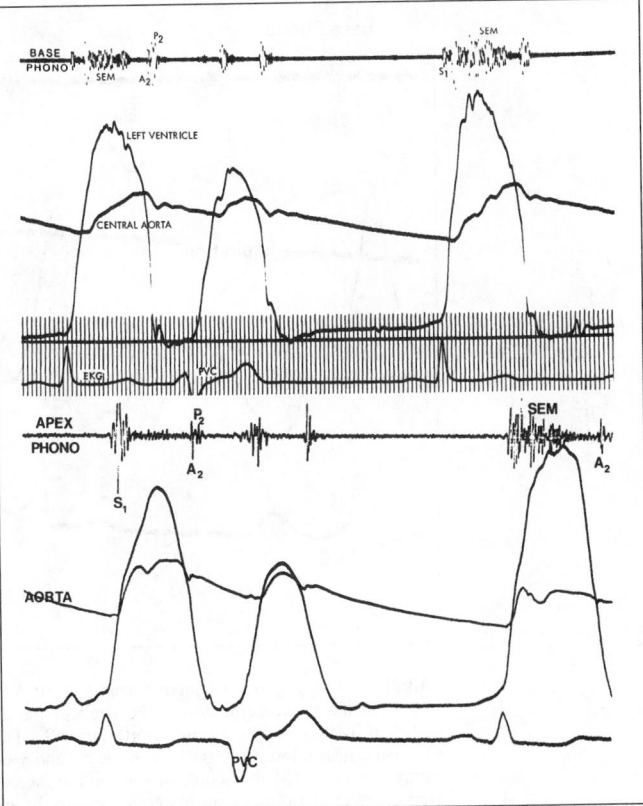

FIGURE 11-4   A, Simultaneous left ventricular and central aortic pressures are recorded with the phonocardiogram in a patient with fixed orifice valvular aortic stenosis and **(B),** hypertrophic obstructive cardiomyopathy. In fixed orifice aortic stenosis, there is an increase in the pulse amplitude and pulse pressure following the long diastolic pause after a premature beat. In contrast, in HOCM, there is a decrease in the pulse amplitude and pulse pressure following a premature beat, which is pathognomonic of this condition. Note that in both conditions there is a significant increase in the intensity of the murmur following the premature beat.

(**A** From Reddy PS, Shaver JA, Leonard JJ: Cardiac systolic murmurs: pathophysiology and differential diagnosis, *Prog Cardiovasc Dis* 14:10, 1971.)

pid regurgitation, the V wave becomes early and higher with a very rapid Y descent, and the duration of the X^1 prime descent is progressively abbreviated. With severe tricuspid regurgitation, the X^1 descent is absent and the JVP is said to be ventricularized with a large V wave (Fig. 11-6, *D*). Severe tricuspid regurgitation also may be associated with pulsations of the earlobe, liver, and, occasionally, pulsation of the veins of the temple. In patients with marked increase in central venous pressure, observation of the JVP may be facilitated by having the patient in the sitting, or even standing, position. Also, in such patients, a paradoxical rise in the height of the JVP may occur during inspiration (Kussmaul's sign).

INSPECTION AND PALPATION

Inspection of the chest wall and bony thorax should be carried out before palpation. Frequently, cardiac abnormalities may be associated with abnormalities of the bony thorax, such as the straight back syndrome, pectus excavatum, pectus carinatum, ankylosing spondylitis, and kyphoscoliosis. In young patients with congenital heart disease, asymmetric prominence of the anterior chest wall may be present, reflecting enlargement of the underlying cardiac structures involved in the congenital anomaly. Prominent parasternal or apical pulsations may be observed in patients with volume or pressure overloading of the right and left ventricle, respectively. A late systolic bulge, either at the apex or in an ectopic area, also may be observed in patients having large dyskinetic left ventricular aneurysms. On occasion, prominent presystolic or early diastolic pulsations are visually evident at the apex in patients having an exaggerated atrial contribution to ventricular filling or excessively rapid early diastolic filling. Abnormal pulsations in the third left intercostal space may be observed with enlargement of the pulmonary artery, whereas enlargement of the aorta, as seen with aortic aneurysms, may result in abnormal pulsation in the second right intercostal space. Careful

examination of the skin may reveal scars from prior cardiac or thoracic surgery.

After inspection, palpation of the anterior chest wall should be carried out. In patients having chest pain suggesting a musculoskeletal origin, palpation of these areas may reproduce the exact pain that the patient is experiencing, thereby ruling out a cardiac cause. Both inspection and palpation of the chest are best performed with the patient in the supine position or with the upper trunk elevated to 30 degrees, with the examiner on the right side of the patient. In general, outward movements are best evaluated by palpation, whereas inward movements are usually more easily seen than felt. Parasternal impulses arising from the right ventricle, pulmonary artery, or ascending aorta are best appreciated during exhalation and better examined when the patient is supine. Apical movements, however, are best evaluated with the patient in the left lateral decubitus position, rotated 45 to 90 degrees. The precordial movements should be evaluated with the flat portion of the fingers, then with the fingertips, and finally, as precisely as possible, with the tip of the first or second finger. Light pressure of the fingertips is the best technique for eliciting the faint pulsations, such as a palpable S_3 or S_4 or a bifid apical impulse. Timing of the impulses can be accomplished by simultaneous palpation of the right carotid artery or auscultation of the heart.

In addition to palpating the systolic and diastolic motion of the ventricles, it is frequently possible to feel heart sounds and heart murmurs (thrills). The vibrations of a loud S_1 and the opening snap of mitral stenosis may be palpated at the apex, whereas the loud A_2 and

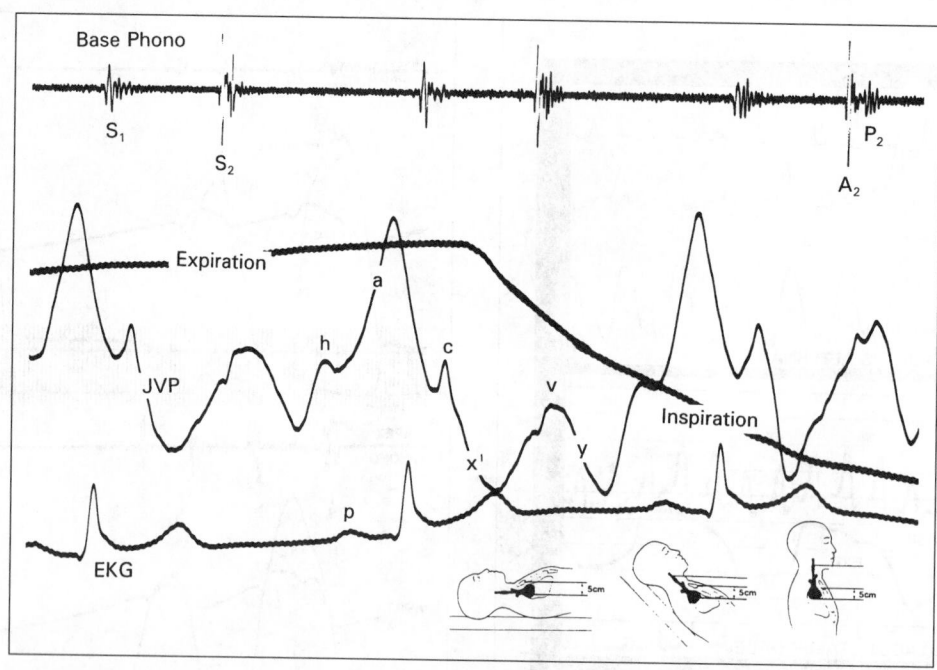

FIGURE 11-5   The normal jugular vein pulse (JVP) is recorded simultaneously with the base phonocardiogram and the electrocardiogram. The peak of the a wave slightly precedes S_1, and the peak of the v wave followed by its y descent occurs shortly after S_2. The trough of the x^1 descent is the lowest point on the JVP. On visual inspection of the JVP, both the x^1 and y descents are the more prominent waves, and the c wave is rarely observed. The method of measuring the mean jugular venous pressure as the vertical distance above the sternal angle of Louis (5 cm above the mid-right atrium, regardless of trunk elevation) is shown in the right lower corner of the illustration (see text for details).

(Insert From Crawford MH: *Examination of the heart.* Part 2: *Inspection and palpation of venous and arterial pulses,* Dallas, 1990, American Heart Association.)

P_2 of systemic and pulmonary hypertension may be palpated at the base. Prominent valvular ejection clicks and pericardial knocks also can be palpated. Prominent presystolic pulsations, as well as early diastolic pulsations, can often be palpated when their auscultatory counterpart, the S_4 and the S_3 cannot be heard. Thrills are palpable vibrations from murmurs and are associated with murmurs grade IV/VI or louder. These vibrations are best felt with the fingertips or firm pressure from either the proximal heel or distal palm of the hand. Seven areas of the anterior chest should be examined for abnormal cardiovascular pulsations by inspection and palpation. Common abnormalities observed in each of these areas are tabulated in Box 11-1.

The normal apical impulse in the adult is usually located at or within the left midclavicular line in the fifth intercostal space. This impulse is less than 2 cm in diameter and in most instances is considerably smaller. It is normally located within the midclavicular line. The normal apical impulse, as recorded by the apex cardiogram, is shown in Fig. 11-7, *A*. The rapid upstroke of the apex cardiogram is caused by the early systolic outward movement of the apical area, which is produced by isovolumic contraction of the left ventricle and the counterclockwise rotation and anterior motion of the heart. It begins at about the time of S_1, just before the upstroke of the carotid pulse. The peak outward motion normally occurs with or just after the stroke volume is being ejected into the aorta. Following that, the apex normally moves inward. Although a presystolic wave is recorded by the apexcardiogram, it is rarely palpated in the normal individual unless the patient has a very thin, ascetic body habitus. In children and young adults, however, the normal early rapid diastolic filling wave can be felt. Common clinical conditions that can produce abnormal apical pulsations are illustrated in Fig. 11-7, *B-F,* and Fig. 11-2, *D*.

AUSCULTATION

For cardiac auscultation to be optimal, it should be carried out in a quiet, well-lit room, with an examining table large enough to allow the patient to lie flat, sit up, or roll to either side with ease. The clinician should choose a stethoscope that fits the ears comfortably, has a short segment of flexible tubing, and is equipped with both a diaphragm and a bell. When the diaphragm is pressed firmly against the skin, it will accentuate high-pitched sounds and murmurs. The bell of the stethoscope accentuates low-frequency sounds and filters out high-pitched sounds. With very light pressure, low-pitched sounds, such as diastolic filling sounds and rumbling murmurs, are accentuated. With firm pressure, the skin itself becomes a tense diaphragm and the rumbling, low-pitched murmurs and sounds are pressed out and attention then can be directed to the high-frequency components.

The four primary areas of auscultation are (1) the primary aortic area in the second right interspace and the secondary aortic area in the third left interspace adjacent to the sternum, (2) the pulmonary area in the second left interspace, (3) the tricuspid area in the fourth and fifth interspaces adjacent to the left sternal border, and (4) the mitral area at the cardiac apex. Although auscultatory events arising from each valve are usually heard best in their respective areas, this is not always the case. The murmur of aortic stenosis in elderly persons is frequently heard best at the apex, whereas the regurgitant murmur of a flail posterior mitral leaflet may radiate to the base, simulating the murmur of aortic stenosis. Furthermore, cardiac auscultation should not be restricted to just these four areas. In some patients the murmur of aortic regurgitation secondary to abnormalities of the aortic root may be heard best to the right of the sternum. The continuous murmur of a patent ductus arteriosus is best heard just below the left clavicle, whereas the murmur of large bronchial collaterals may be most prominent in the posterior thorax. In each of these conditions, the patient's overall clinical presentation will usually guide the experienced clinician to the appropriate area to auscultate.

While auscultating, one listens both specifically and selectively for heart sounds and murmurs. The physician should adopt a systematic way of listening. One method is to start at the apex, then move to the lower left sternal border and progress along the sternal border to the base of the heart. In each area, the physician listens specifically for S_1,

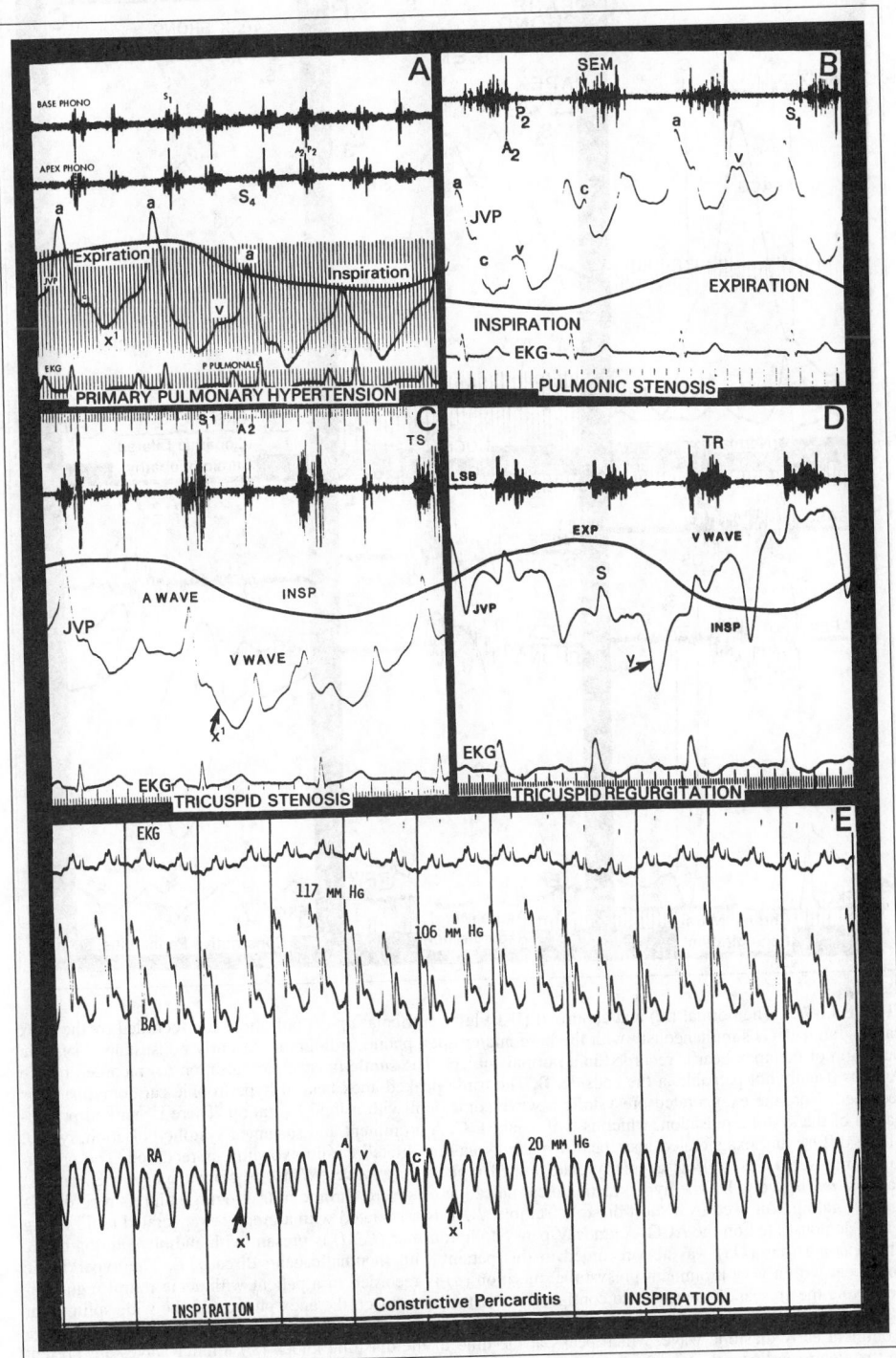

FIGURE 11-6   **A-D,** Abnormalities of the JVP are recorded simultaneously with the base and/or apex phonocardiogram. **A-C,** Prominent a waves associated with increased resistance to right ventricular filling are demonstrated in primary pulmonary hypertension, valvular pulmonic stenosis, and tricuspid stenosis. In tricuspid stenosis (TS), note the crescendo-decrescendo presystolic murmur of *TS* is coincident with the rapid rise and decline of the a wave. **D,** The murmur of severe tricuspid regurgitation *(TR)* increases in intensity with inspiration and is associated with a very prominent v wave, having a rapid y descent. The onset of the v wave in severe tricuspid regurgitation is early, as shown by a prominent systolic *(S)* wave. **E,** The right atrial and brachial artery pressures are recorded in a patient with severe chronic constrictive pericarditis. Although not commonly present in this condition, pulsus paradoxus is observed in this patient. There is marked elevation of right atrial pressure with a classic M or W configuration of its contour caused by the very rapid x¹ and y descents, following the a and v waves, respectively. Note the increase in both the peaks and the valleys of the waveforms during inspiration.

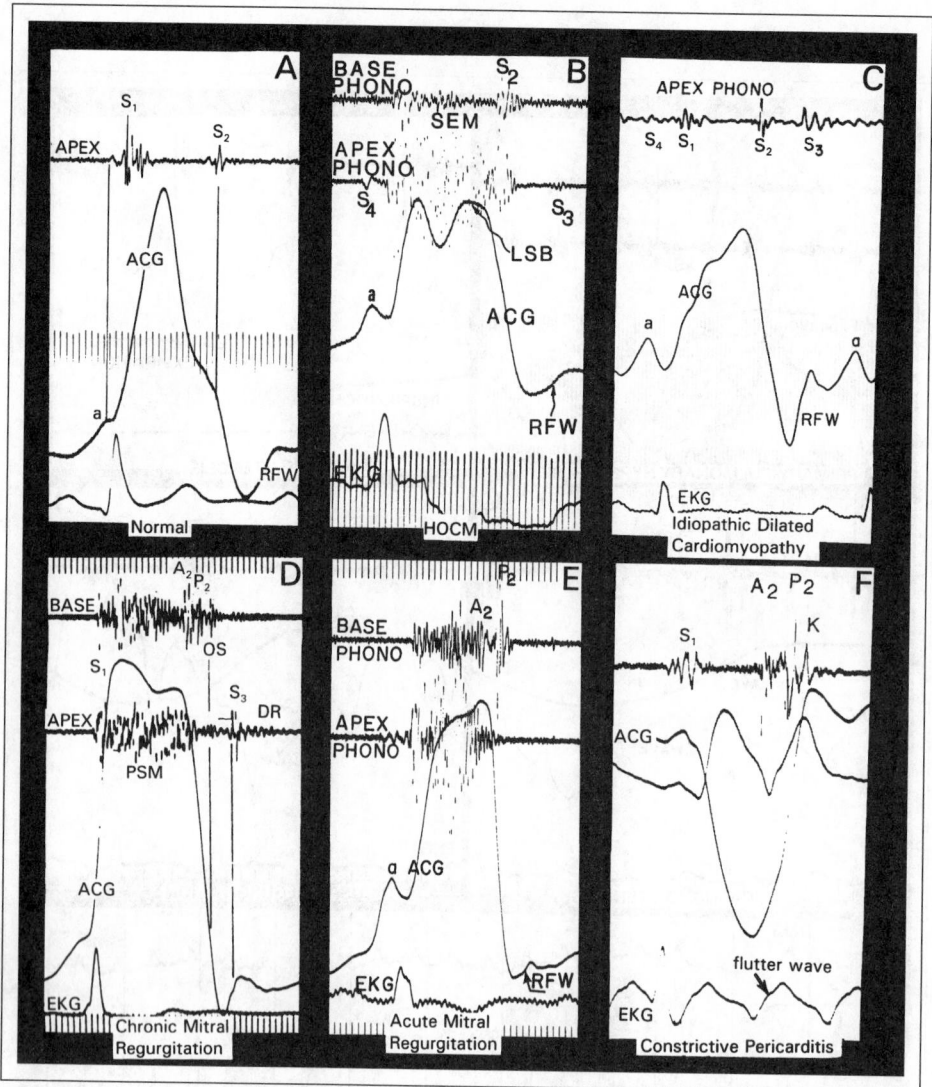

FIGURE 11-7 The normal **(A)** and abnormal **(B-F)** left ventricular apical pulsations are recorded by the apex cardiogram *(ACG)* simultaneously with the base and/or apex phonocardiogram. **A,** Early nonsustained systolic pulsation of the apex beat is recorded in a normal subject. The subtle presystolic pulsation *(a)* recorded by the ACG is usually not palpable at the bedside. **B,** The triple-peaked apex beat of hypertrophic cardiomyopathy is recorded. Note the exaggerated presystolic a wave coincident with a loud S_4 gallop. There is marked prolongation of the systolic pulsation, which is twin peaked. **C,** A prominent and sustained systolic pulsation, typical of the diffuse and exaggerated apex beat of patients having dilated cardiomyopathy, is recorded. The presystolic impulse *(a)*, as well as a greatly exaggerated rapid filling wave *(RFW)*, is coincident with S_4 and S_3 gallops, respectively. **D,** The hyperkinetic apical pulsation of severe chronic mitral regurgitation is recorded. A loud S_3 gallop, followed by a short diastolic rumble *(DR)*, is associated with a greatly exaggerated rapid filling wave, demonstrated on the ACG. A grade V pansystolic murmur *(PSM)* is present with audible splitting of S_2. The opening snap *(OS)* was also recorded in this patient having rheumatic heart disease. **E,** The hyperkinetic apex beat with a very prominent presystolic pulsation *(a)* is recorded in a patient with acute mitral regurgitation. Note the crescendo-decrescendo configuration of the murmur on the apex phono and the wide splitting of S_2. **F,** Recorded in a patient with constrictive pericarditis. The ACG demonstrates systolic retraction and a prominent early diastolic wave, which peaks at the time of the diastolic knock *(K)*. Flutter waves are present on the electrocardiogram.

noting its intensity, constancy, presence of splitting, and variation with respiration. This is followed by selective listening to the S_2, noting again the same characteristics. Subsequently, extra sounds are carefully listened for, first in systole, then in diastole, with special attention to their timing, pitch, and other characteristics that may identify them as ejection sounds, gallop sounds, or opening snaps. Murmurs are then listened for, first in systole and then diastole. After this general survey, the physician listens selectively for certain sounds and murmurs. With the bell applied lightly at the apex, the patient is instructed to roll onto the left side and the clinician concentrates on dias-

tole, searching for diastolic filling sounds or rumbles arising from the atrioventricular valves.

Auscultation is continued with the patient in the sitting position. With the patient leaning forward, the aortic and pulmonic areas are examined, with the diaphragm pressed firmly against the chest wall, first during quiet respiration and then with the breath held in forced expiration. The examiner focuses on the high frequency auscultatory range to detect a faint, blowing diastolic murmur of semilunar valve regurgitation or the presence of a pericardial friction rub.

Cardiac auscultation should be considered a dynamic exercise and

---

BOX 11-1
Areas to be examined for abnormal cardiovascular pulsation, palpable heart sounds, and thrills

A. Sternoclavicular Area
  1. Abnormal pulsations—tortuous great vessels, dilated aorta (aortic dissection, atherosclerotic or luetic aneurysm, aortic regurgitation), right-sided aortic arch (tetralogy of Fallot)
B. Aortic
  1. Abnormal pulsation—aortic aneurysm, dilated ascending aorta secondary to aortic regurgitation
  2. Palpable A_2—arterial hypertension
  3. Palpable thrill—aortic stenosis and regurgitation
C. Pulmonic
  1. Abnormal pulsation—dilated pulmonary artery
    a. Slow, sustained and forceful—pulmonary hypertension
    b. Hyperkinetic, vigorous, less sustained—atrial septal defect, hyperkinetic state
  2. Palpable P_2—pulmonary hypertension
  3. Palpable thrill—valvular pulmonic stenosis
D. Left parasternal—right ventricle and tricuspid
  1. Abnormal right ventricular systolic pulsation
    a. Pressure load—sustained—primary pulmonary hypertension, pulmonic stenosis, cor pulmonale, mitral stenosis, Eisenmenger's reaction
    b. Volume load—hyperkinetic—atrial septal defect, ventricular septal defect
    c. Late systolic—severe mitral regurgitation secondary to expanding left atrium
  2. Abnormal diastolic pulsation (increases with inspiration)
    a. Presystolic impulse—decreased right ventricular compliance
    b. Rapid early diastolic filling—severe tricuspid regurgitation, atrial septal defect, right ventricular failure, pericardial knock
  3. Palpable thrill—ventricular septal defect

E. Apical
  1. Abnormal left ventricular systolic pulsation
    a. Pressure load—exaggerated and sustained—aortic stenosis, hypertrophic cardiomyopathy, systemic hypertension
    b. Volume overload—hyperkinetic—mitral regurgitation, aortic regurgitation, hyperkinetic circulation (fever, exertion, hyperthyroidism)
    c. Left ventricular systolic dysfunction with cardiac enlargement, forceful, diffuse and sustained
  2. Palpable M_1, OS, midsystolic click, tumor "plop"—mitral stenosis, mitral valve prolapse, left atrial myxoma
  3. Palpable thrill—mitral regurgitation, mitral stenosis, hypertrophic obstructive cardiomyopathy
  4. Abnormal diastolic pulsation
    a. Presystolic impulse—abnormal left ventricular compliance, aortic stenosis, hypertrophic cardiomyopathy, ventricular aneurysm, dilated cardiomyopathy
    b. Rapid early diastolic filling—mitral regurgitation, left ventricular failure, pericardial knock
  5. Systolic retraction—constrictive pericarditis and severe organic tricuspid regurgitation
F. Epigastric
  1. Abnormal pulsation
    a. Abdominal aortic—hyperkinetic circulation, aortic regurgitation, abdominal aneurysm
    b. Hepatic—tricuspid regurgitation, tricuspid stenosis, right ventricular enlargement
    c. Right ventricular—cor pulmonale secondary to emphysema
G. Ectopic—between pulmonary and apical area
  1. Paradoxical left ventricular pulsation secondary to left ventricular aneurysm, acute myocardial infarction, dilated cardiomyopathy

---

should be performed with the patient in the left lateral decubitus position, standing, and squatting, and during the Valsalva maneuver and after its release. This dynamic examination changes the preloading and afterloading conditions of the heart and may yield diagnostic information because of the typical response of heart sounds and murmurs to these maneuvers. Because every patient cannot be examined in such depth, information obtained from the history and clues from the examination of the arterial, venous, and precordial pulsations should guide the clinician to the appropriate maneuvers and interventions during dynamic auscultation.

Cardiac Cycle

The left-sided cardiac cycle is depicted in Fig. 11-8. The isometric contraction period is the interval from the onset of ventricular pressure rise until ventricular pressure exceeds the diastolic pressure in the aorta and the aortic valve opens (Chapter 9). During isometric contraction, the rapidly rising ventricular pressure causes a sudden retrograde surge of blood toward the mitral valve, which is abruptly decelerated when the elastic limits of the leaflets of the closed mitral valve are reached. This sudden deceleration of blood sets the entire cardiohemic system into vibration, producing the C-wave on the left atrial pressure tracing. The higher frequency components of this pressure phenomenon are recorded as M_1 and are appreciated at the bedside as the major component of S_1. The left ventricular ejection period is the interval from the onset of pressure rise in the central aorta to the aortic incisura. During the first 75% to 80% of ventricular ejection, the ventricular pressure exceeds the pressure in the central aorta and is responsible for acceleration of blood into the aorta. In the latter part of systole, the ventricle begins its relaxation phase and ventricular pressure rapidly declines. However, forward flow in the aorta continues for a brief period despite a negative pressure gradient resulting from the inertia of the stroke volume.

As a positive pressure gradient rapidly develops between the aorta and the rapidly declining left ventricular pressure, the column of blood

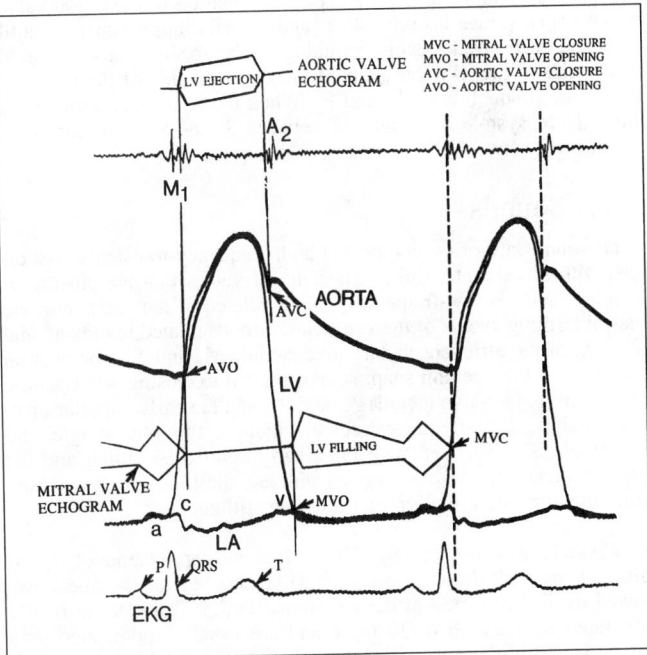

FIGURE 11-8 The normal cardiac cycle is recorded by catheter-tipped micromanometer in the left atrium, left ventricle, and central aorta simultaneously with the electrocardiogram and phonocardiogram. The aortic and mitral valve echocardiograms have been added to indicate the duration of left ventricular ejection and the left ventricular filling period, respectively. (See text for details.)

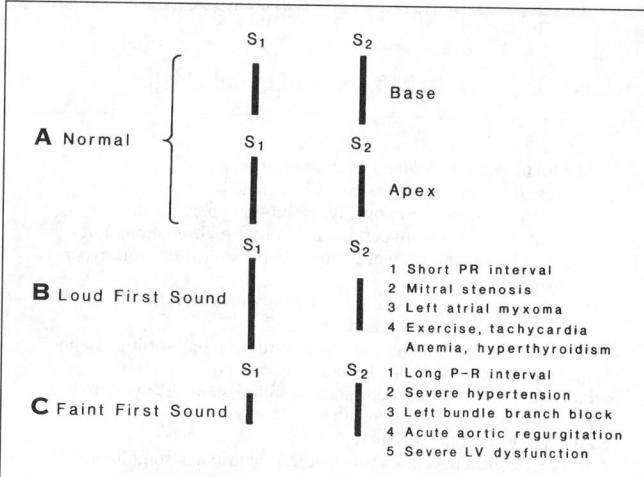

FIGURE 11-9   The first heart sound. **A,** S_2 is characteristically louder than S_1 at the base. Although S_1 is usually more prominent than S_2 at the apex, this relationship is less constant and less reliable for timing purposes. Conditions causing loud, **B,** and faint, **C,** S_1 sounds are listed above.

(From Shaver JA, Leonard JJ, Leon DF: *Examination of the heart.* Part 4: Auscultation of the heart, Dallas, 1990, American Heart Association.)

in the aorta is reversed and the retrograde flow is abruptly checked by the tensed closed aortic valve. At this time, the incisura on the central aortic pressure is inscribed and its higher frequency components are recorded and heard as A_2. The left ventricular pressure continues to fall rapidly during the isovolumic relaxation phase, while both aortic and mitral valves are closed (Chapter 9). During systole, when the mitral valve is closed, blood returns from the pulmonary veins into the left atrium, generating a passive V wave. When the pressure in the left atrium exceeds rapidly declining left ventricular pressure, the mitral valve opens, and the rapid phase of early left ventricular filling begins. Following this, the slow phase of ventricular filling occurs and the anterior and posterior leaflets of the mitral valve slowly float toward each other and remain approximated until reopened with atrial systole, resulting in the second phase of rapid ventricular filling. Similar events from the right side of the heart result in the production of T_1 and P_2. When the heart is auscultated at the bedside, systole is the interval between S_1 and S_2, and diastole is the interval between the S_2 and the subsequent S_1.

Heart Sounds

Heart sounds are of two types: (1) high-frequency transients, associated with the abrupt terminal checking of valves that are closing or opening, and (2) low-frequency sounds related to the early and late diastolic filling events of the ventricles. Sounds related to closing and opening of the atrioventricular valve include M_1 and T_1, nonejection sounds, and the opening snap; sounds related to closing and opening of the semilunar valve include A_2 and P_2, and the early valvular ejection sounds. Low-frequency sounds include the physiologic and pathologic S_3 associated with rapid early ventricular filling and the presystolic atrial, or S_4, associated with late diastolic filling resulting from the atrial contribution of ventricular filling.

First Heart Sound (S_1). The two major components of S_1 audible at the bedside are the louder M_1 heard best at the apex, followed by T_1 heard best at the left sternal border. They are normally separated by only 20 to 30 msec and are usually appreciated as a single sound in the normal subject. The intensity of S_1 depends primarily on three factors: (1) the rate of pressure rise and tension development in the ventricle, (2) the degree of separation of the atrioventricular valve leaflets at the onset of ventricular pressure rise, and (3) the structure of the valve leaflets themselves (normal or scarred). Common conditions producing a loud or soft first heart sound are displayed in Fig. 11-9.

Because T_1 is quite faint, only the louder M_1 that occurs earlier or almost simultaneously usually is heard. Although T_1 becomes louder as a result of pulmonary hypertension, this sound is still difficult to distinguish from M_1 unless the splitting interval widens. This commonly occurs in right bundle branch block where the onset of right ventricular systole is delayed, and T_1 may be sufficiently late to be easily appreciated as a distinct sound following M_1. Wide splitting of S_1 is also present in left ventricular pacing, left ventricular ectopic beats, and idioventricular rhythms originating from the left ventricle. In a similar fashion, pacing from the right ventricle and ectopic beats and idioventricular rhythms originating from the right ventricle will produce reversed splitting of S_1 (T_1, M_1). Although the sequencing of valve closure may be reversed in left bundle branch block and/or severe left ventricular function, splitting of S_1 usually cannot be appreciated at the bedside.

Second Heart Sound (S_2). The relationship of A_2 and P_2 to the hemodynamic events of the cardiac cycle is shown in Fig. 11-10. Right ventricular ejection begins before left ventricular ejection, has a longer duration, and terminates after left ventricular ejection; as a result, P_2 normally occurs after A_2. Right and left ventricular systole are nearly equal in duration and the pulmonary artery incisura is delayed relative to the aortic incisura, primarily because of a larger interval separating the pulmonary incisura from the right ventricular pressure compared with the same left-sided event. This interval has been called the "hangout" interval, and its duration is thought to be a reflection of the impedance of a vascular bed into which the blood is being received. In the low resistant, highly capacitant pulmonary bed, this interval is normally much greater than on the left and contributes significantly to the duration of right ventricular ejection. Awareness of this interval is essential for proper understanding of normal physiologic splitting and for the abnormal splitting seen in conditions where significant alterations in pulmonary vascular impedance have occurred.

The intensity of S_2 is directly proportional to the pressure gradient that develops across the valve (i.e., the driving force accelerating the blood in a retrograde fashion into the base of the great vessels). This gradient is primarily determined by the level of the diastolic pressure in the great vessel and is consistent with the clinical observation of a loud A_2 or P_2 in systemic or pulmonary hypertension. Both A_2 and P_2 may be decreased by disease processes that decrease the mobility of the leaflets (calcific fixation) or would destroy the leaflets (endocarditis) such that adequate coaptation cannot occur.

During normal respiration, A_2 and P_2 are separated by less than 30 msec during expiration and are appreciated as a single sound (see Fig. 11-1). During inspiration, both components become distinctly audible as the splitting interval widens, primarily because of a delayed P_2, although an earlier A_2 contributes to a lesser degree. Splitting is heard best at the second left intercostal space. Normally, P_2 is softer than A_2 and is rarely heard at the apex unless either significant pulmonary hypertension is present or the apex is occupied by an enlarged right ventricle (e.g., atrial septal defect). The width of the splitting interval varies with age and the depth of respiration. In younger patients, maximal splitting during inspiration averages 40 to 50 msec, and its value decreases with aging; a single second heart sound during both phases of respiration may be normal in patients older than 40 years of age.

All conditions in which abnormal splitting exists can be identified at the bedside by the presence of audible expiratory splitting. The three causes of audible expiratory splitting are diagrammed in Fig. 11-11. In Fig. 11-10, the common causes of wide physiologic splitting and reversed splitting of S_2 are classified according to the abnormality of the cardiac cycle responsible for the altered timing of A_2 and P_2. Narrow physiologic splitting is a common finding in severe pulmonary hypertension in which both A_2 and P_2 are easily heard during expiration, even though the splitting interval is less than 30 msec (see Fig. 11-11). Wide splitting of S_2 with an increase in P_2 may also be heard in severe pulmonary hypertension, usually a sign of compromised right ventricular function. Cardiac conditions that delay A_2 may produce a single S_2 when the splitting interval becomes less than 30 msec. Conditions in which one component of S_2 is either absent or inaudible will also produce a single S_2 (severe tetralogy of Fallot and severe calcific aortic stenosis). The most common

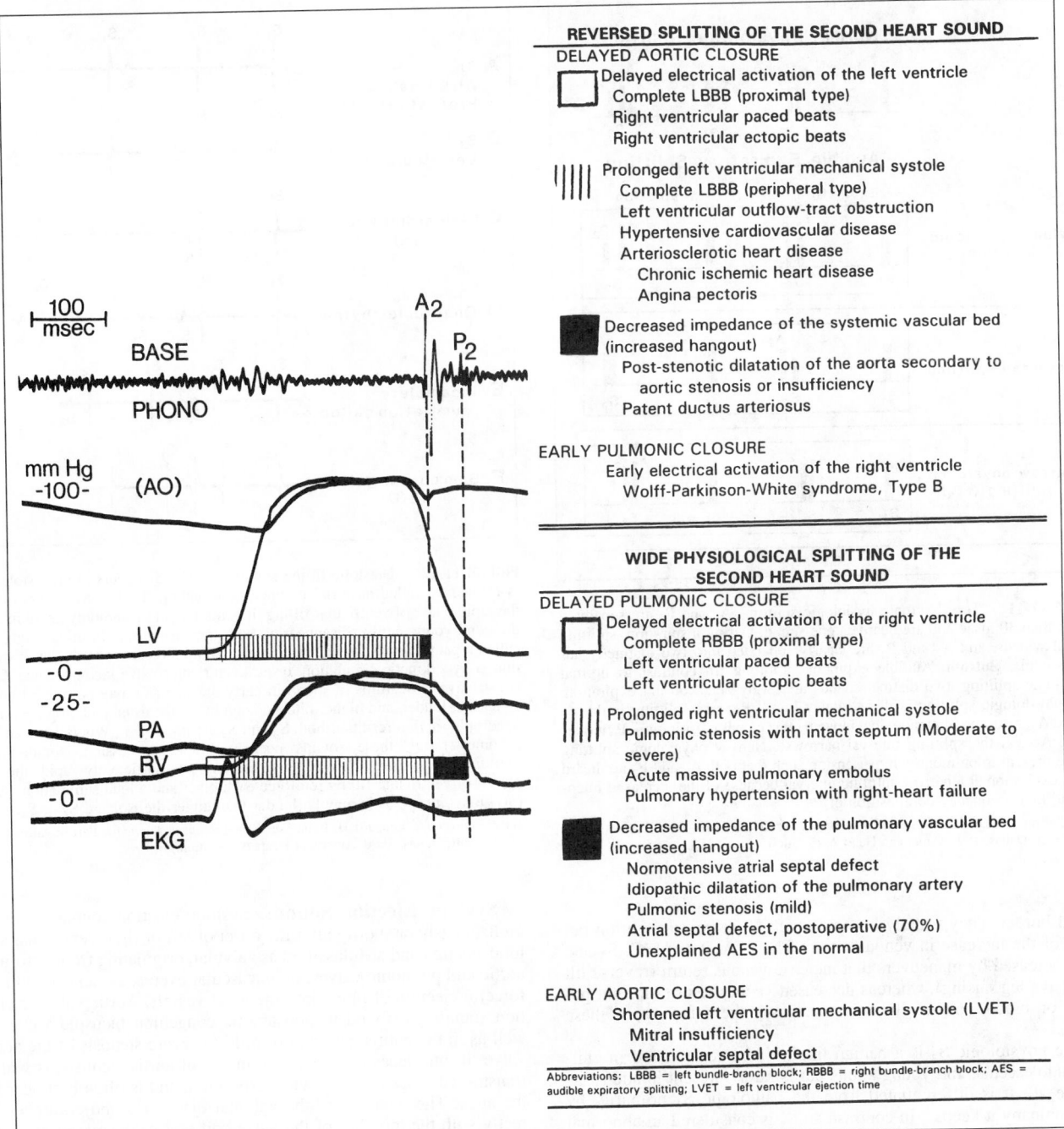

FIGURE 11-10   Simultaneous left ventricular, central aortic, right ventricular, and pulmonary artery pressures are recorded by catheter-tipped micromanometer simultaneously with the electrocardiogram and the base phonocardiogram. A_2 and P_2 are coincident with the incisura of the respective arterial traces. Left and right ventricular mechanical systoles are nearly equal in duration, and the right ventricular systolic ejection period terminates after left ventricular ejection because of an increased right-sided "hangout" interval. Abnormalities of splitting of S_2 are classified according to the abnormality of the cardiac cycle responsible for the alteration in timing of A_2 and P_2. (See text for details.)

(Modified from Shaver JA, O'Toole JD: The second heart sound: newer concepts. Part 1: Normal and wide physiological splitting, and part 2: Paradoxical splitting and narrow physiological splitting, *Mod Concepts Cardiovasc Dis* 46:7213, 1977.)

cause of an apparently single S_2 is inability to hear the fainter of the two components of the sound (usually P_2) because of emphysema, obesity, or respiratory noise.

Third (S_3) and Fourth (S_4) Heart Sounds. S_3 and S_4 are low-frequency sounds related to early and late diastolic filling of the ventricles (Fig. 11-12). They are called *gallops* in pathologic conditions, and their presence alerts the clinician to abnormalities of ven-

tricular function, compliance, or both. Box 11-2 lists the common conditions in which S_3 and S_4 are heard.

Physiologic and pathologic S_3, as well as the S_4 originating from the left heart, are heard best at the apex with the patient in the left lateral position, listening with the bell of the stethoscope pressed lightly against the chest wall. Frequently the S_4 is associated with a presystolic impulse palpated in the left lateral position. Right-sided S_3 and S_4 gallops are heard best near the xiphoid or the left lower

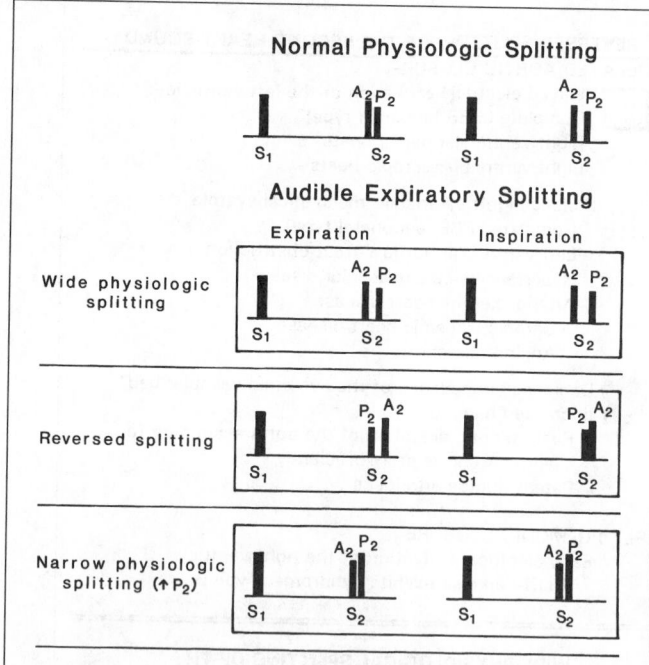

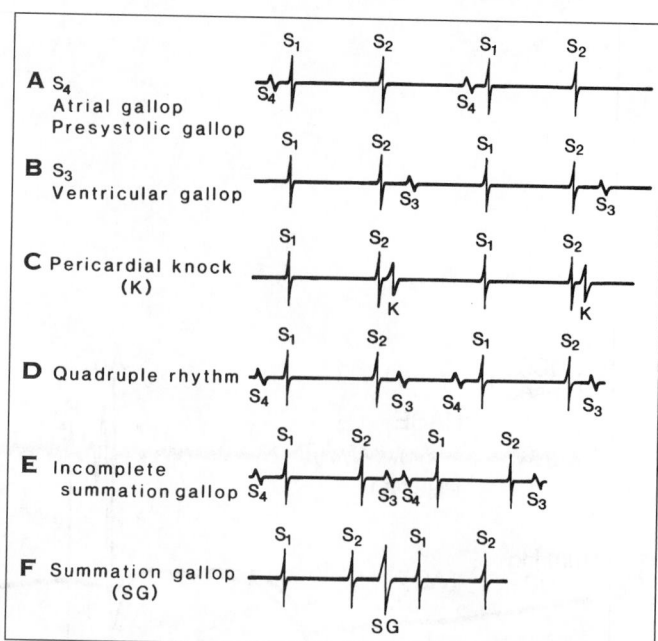

FIGURE 11-11 **Top,** Normal physiologic splitting. A_2 and P_2 are separated by less than 30 msec and are heard as one sound. During inspiration, splitting interval widens, and A_2 and P_2 are clearly separated into two distinctly audible sounds. **Bottom,** Audible expiratory splitting. In contrast to normal physiologic splitting, two distinct sounds are easily heard during expiration. Wide physiologic splitting is due to delay in P_2. Reverse splitting is due to delayed A_2, resulting in paradoxical movement (i.e., with inspiration, P_2 moves toward A_2 and the splitting interval narrows). Narrow physiologic splitting may be present in pulmonary hypertension such that both A_2 and P_2 are heard during expiration at a narrow splitting interval because of the increased intensity and high frequency composition of P_2.

(From Shaver JA, Leonard JJ, Leon DF: *Examination of the heart.* Part 4: Auscultation of the heart, Dallas, 1990, American Heart Association.)

FIGURE 11-12 Diastolic filling sounds. **A,** The S_4 occurs in presystole and is frequently called an atrial or presystolic gallop. **B,** The S_3 occurs during the rapid phase of ventricular filling. It is normal and commonly heard in children and young adults, disappearing with increasing age. In middle age, it is called a pathologic S_3 or ventricular gallop and indicates ventricular dysfunction, a hyperkinetic circulation, or atrioventricular valve incompetence. **C,** In constrictive pericarditis, a sound in early diastole *(K)* may be present and is an earlier, louder, and higher pitched sound than the usual pathologic S_3. **D,** A quadruple rhythm results if both S_3 and S_4 are present. **E,** When the heart rate becomes faster, these sounds occur in rapid succession, simulating a mid-diastolic rumble. **F,** When the heart rate is sufficiently rapid, the two phases of ventricular filling reinforce each other and a loud summation gallop *(SG)* may appear. This may be louder than either the isolated S_3 or S_4.

(From Shaver JA, Leonard JJ, Leon DF: *Examination of the heart.* Part 4: Auscultation of the heart, Dallas, 1990, American Heart Association.)

sternal border. They usually become much louder on inspiration because of the increase in venous return. The intensity of both S_3 and S_4 is increased by maneuvers that increase venous return (reverse tilt or passive leg raising), whereas decreased venous return (upright position or blood volume diuresis) decreases the intensity of these sounds.

The physiologic S_3 is a benign finding commonly heard in children, adolescents, and young adults but is rarely present in adults after age 40. It is differentiated from the pathologic S_3 primarily by "the company it keeps." In contrast, an S_4 is considered an abnormal finding in a younger patient. In some elderly patients, an S_4 may be a normal finding. Because atrial contraction is essential for the production of an S_4, this sound is absent in atrial fibrillation.

The classic gallop rhythm associated with poor systolic pump function, congestive heart failure, and tachycardia is usually a summation gallop because of the fusion to both the S_3 and S_4. The S_3 associated with hyperkinetic states and atrioventricular valve regurgitation does not necessarily imply heart failure; such patients may maintain normal ventricular function for years after the S_3 is detected. Pathologic S_3 is also heard in both restrictive and hypertrophic cardiomyopathy, occurring somewhat earlier in diastole, and may have after-vibrations, which simulate a short diastolic rumble.

Another prominent early diastolic sound, the pericardial knock, is an important physical finding in chronic constrictive pericarditis (Chapter 27), and is sometimes confused with the opening snap of mitral stenosis or an S_3. The pericardial sound appears earlier than the pathologic S_3, is of higher frequency, and is more widely transmitted. It usually increases in intensity with inspiration and occurs near the nadir of the Y descent of the JVP.

Systolic Ejection Sounds. Systolic ejection sounds occur simultaneously or shortly after the onset of left or right ventricular systolic ejection and are classified as valvular, originating from deformed aortic and pulmonic valves, or as vascular events, associated with the forceful ejection of blood into the great vessels. Aortic valvular ejection sounds are found in nonstenotic congenital bicuspid valves as well as in the entire spectrum of mild to severe stenosis of the aortic valve. It introduces the ejection murmur of aortic stenosis, is widely transmitted, does not vary with respiration, and is often best heard at the apex. The intensity of the valvular ejection sound correlates directly with the mobility of the valve and will be decreased or absent with progressive valve calcification. A similar sound arises from the stenotic pulmonary valve; however, there is a significant decrease in the intensity of this sound with inspiration, and it is heard well only at the base.

Aortic ejection sounds also originate from the aortic root and are common in systemic hypertension, aneurysms of the ascending aorta, and nonvalvular aortic regurgitation secondary to abnormalities of the aortic root. This sound is likely the result of sudden tensing of the dilated aortic root with the onset of forceful ventricular ejection. These root sounds tend to be poorly transmitted from the aortic area and are not well heard at the apex.

Vascular or root ejection sounds also may originate from the pulmonary artery where the common denominator is dilation of the pulmonary artery, idiopathic or secondary to severe pulmonary hypertension. These sounds are heard best at the second and third left intercostal spaces.

Opening Snaps. Opening of the normal atrioventricular valve is a silent event. However, with thickening and deformity of the valve (usually rheumatic in origin), a sound is generated in early diastole

BOX 11-2
Common conditions in which S₃ and S₄ are heard

Third heart sound (S₃), ventricular diastolic gallop, protodiastolic gallop, and pericardial knock
Physiologic S₃—children and young adults
Decreased prevalence with increasing age
Pathologic S₃
Ventricular dysfunction—poor systolic function, increased end-diastolic and end-systolic volume, decreased ejection fraction, and high filling pressures
  Idiopathic dilated cardiomyopathy
  Ischemic heart disease
  Valvular heart disease
  Congenital heart disease
  Systemic and pulmonary hypertension
Excessively rapid early diastolic ventricular filling
  Hyperkinetic states
    Anemia
    Thyrotoxicosis
    Arteriovenous fistula
  Atrioventricular valve incompetence
  Left to right shunts
Restrictive myocardial or pericardial disease
  Constrictive pericarditis (pericardial knock)
  Restrictive cardiomyopathy
  Hypertrophic cardiomyopathy

Fourth heart sound (S₄), atrial diastolic gallop, and presystolic gallop
Physiologic S₄—recordable, rarely audible
Pathologic S₄
Decreased ventricular compliance
  Ventricular hypertrophy
    Left or right ventricular outflow obstruction
    Systemic or pulmonary hypertension
    Hypertrophic cardiomyopathy
  Ischemic heart disease
    Angina pectoris
    Acute myocardial infarction
    Old myocardial infarction
    Ventricular aneurysm
  Idiopathic dilated cardiomyopathy
Excessively rapid late diastolic filling secondary to vigorous atrial systole
  Hyperkinetic states
    Anemia
    Thyrotoxicosis
    Arteriovenous fistula
  Acute atrioventricular valve incompetence
Arrhythmias
  Heart block

(From Shaver JA, Salerni R: Auscultation of the heart. In Hurst JW, Schlant RC, editors: *The heart*, ed 7, New York, 1990, McGraw-Hill.)

similar to the valvular ejection sounds originating from deformed semilunar valves. As with valvular ejection sounds, this sound is produced by the sudden checking of the early diastolic descent of the funnel-shaped stenotic valve when its elastic limits are met. The opening snap is a crisp, sharp sound usually heard best from the left sternal border to just inside the apex. Its intensity does not vary with respiration and correlates well with the mobility of the valve. A loud sound is heard in mobile stenotic valves, and a soft or absent sound is present with calcific fixation of the valve. The opening snap of mitral stenosis follows A₂ by 30 to 150 msec, and there is an inverse relationship between the duration of this interval and the severity of mitral stenosis.

A similar sound, the tricuspid opening snap, may also arise from a deformed stenotic tricuspid valve. This sound tends to be heard closer to the left sternal border and, unlike the mitral opening snap, increases with inspiration. It usually follows the mitral opening snap. An early diastolic sound can also be caused by a right or a left atrial myxoma, with the tumor "plop" occurring at the maximal diastolic descent of the myxoma.

Nonejection Systolic Sounds. Nonejection systolic sounds (clicks) are caused by prolapse of the A-V valves, often associated with the murmur of mitral or tricuspid regurgitation. Like other high-frequency cardiac sounds, systolic nonejection sounds are produced by vibrations when the elastic limit of the prolapsed valve is suddenly reached. The presence of a nonejection click on examination in and of itself is sufficient for the diagnosis of mitral valve prolapse. The sound has a sharp, high-frequency clicking quality and, although it is often confined to the apex, it can be transmitted widely over the precordium. It may be an isolated finding occurring in mid or late systole, or there may be multiple clicks, presumably as a result of different areas of large redundant scalloped mitral leaflets that prolapse at different times.

Variability of the auscultatory findings from examination to examination is typical of mitral valve prolapse. These variations in the timing of the click can be most easily understood by considering mitral valve prolapse a condition in which the valve is too big for the ventricle. This valvular-ventricular disproportion is manifested at a given volume and geometric configuration during left ventricular emptying (Fig. 11-13). Situations that decrease end-diastolic volume, decrease vascular impedance, or increase contractility allow the heart

to reach this size earlier in systole, resulting in earlier onset of the click and a longer murmur. Increased heart size and peripheral vascular impedance and decreased contractility will have the opposite effect. These dynamic changes can best be heard at the bedside by examining the patient in the supine, left lateral, sitting, and standing positions and during prompt squatting.

Extra Cardiac Sounds. Pericardial friction rubs may be produced by inflammation of the pericardial sac, with or without fluid. These sounds are typically high-pitched, leathery, scratchy in nature, and appear close to the ear. They are auscultated best with the patient leaning forward or in the knee-chest position. The components of the rub occur during the three intervals of the cardiac cycle when the heart has its greatest excursion within the pericardial sac, during atrial systole, ventricular systole, and rapid early diastolic filling. The usual friction rub occurs during the first two intervals, although three-component rubs may be heard in uremic pericarditis where a hyperkinetic hypertrophied ventricle is frequently present. A scratchy sound should not be considered a friction rub unless both systolic and diastolic components are heard.

A mediastinal crunch, or Hamman's sign, may occur when air is in the mediastinum. In this condition, a series of crunching sounds is heard from time to time, occurring most frequently during ventricular systole in a random fashion. Mediastinal emphysema may be confirmed by crepitation in the neck secondary to subcutaneous air. Often the patient may be aware of the sound and may describe the position or respiratory phase in which it occurs. Both pericardial friction rubs and mediastinal crunching sounds are common after cardiac surgery.

Pacemaker sounds are high-frequency sounds of brief duration that are occasionally present in patients with transvenous pacemakers located in the right ventricular apex. They occur nearly coincident with the pacemaker spike and are due to stimulation of the intercostal nerves next to the endocardial electrode, which results in contractions of the intercostal muscles.

Heart Murmurs

A cardiac murmur is defined as a relatively prolonged series of auditory vibrations of varying intensity (loudness), frequency (pitch), quality, configuration, and duration. Most authorities now agree that

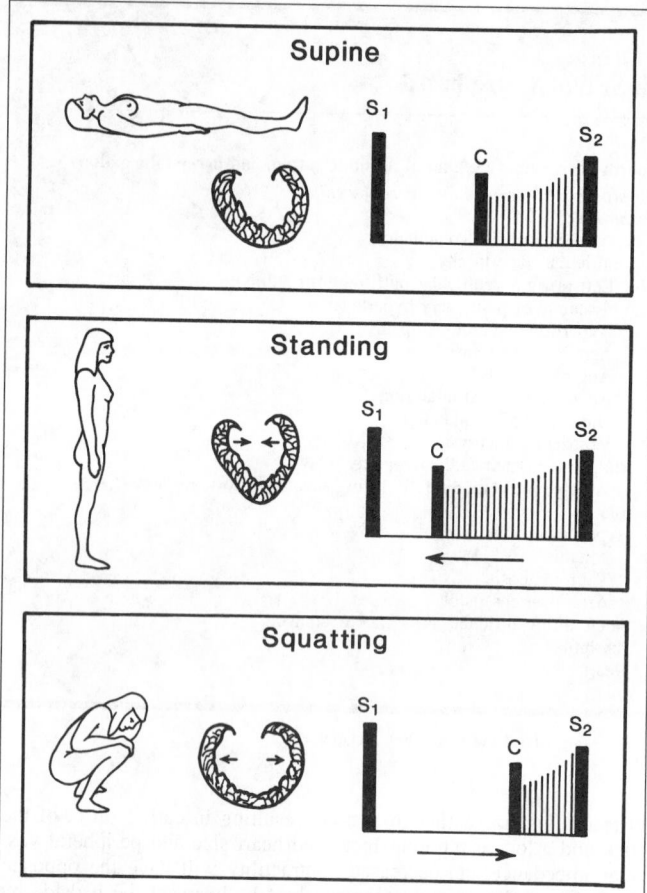

FIGURE 11-13 A mid-systolic nonejection sound *(C)* occurs in mitral valve prolapse and is followed by a late systolic murmur that crescendos to S₂. The upright posture decreases venous return and the heart becomes smaller, and the C moves closer to S₁, with an earlier onset of the mitral regurgitation murmur. With prompt squatting venous return increases, the heart becomes larger, the click moves toward S₂, and the duration of the regurgitant murmur shortens.

(From Shaver JA, Leonard JJ, Leon DF: *Examination of the heart.* Part 4: Auscultation of the heart, Dallas, 1990, American Heart Association.)

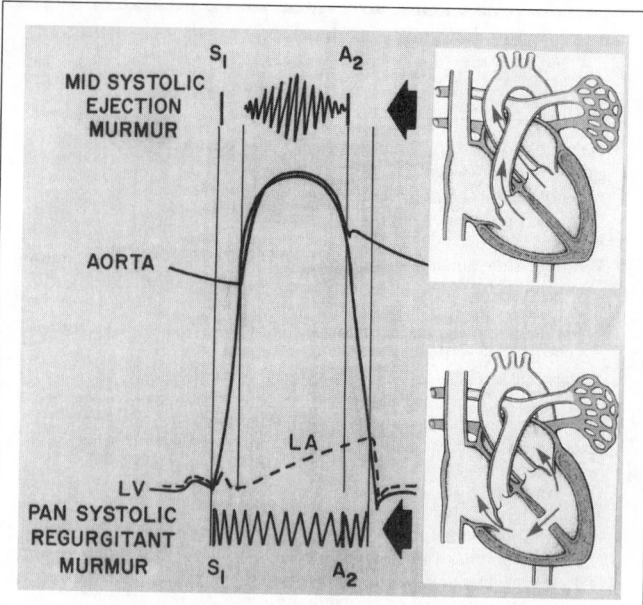

FIGURE 11-14 *Right,* Flow diagram. Mid-systolic ejection murmurs are caused by forward flow across the left or right ventricular outflow tract, whereas pansystolic regurgitant murmurs are caused by retrograde flow from a high-pressure cardiac chamber to a low-pressure one. *Left,* Diagrammatic representation of the mid-systolic ejection murmur and the pansystolic regurgitant murmur, as related to left ventricular *(LV)*, aortic, and left atrial *(LA)* pressures. The systolic ejection murmur occurs during the period of LV ejection; the onset of the murmur is separated from S₁ by the period of isovolumic contraction, and the crescendo-decrescendo murmur terminates before A₂. The pansystolic regurgitant murmur begins with, or may replace, S₁, and the murmur continues up to and through A₂ as left ventricular pressure exceeds left atrial pressure during the period of isovolumic relaxation. The murmur has a plateau configuration and varies little with respiration.

(From Shaver JA: Systolic murmurs, *Heart Dis Stroke* 2:9-17, 1993.)

turbulence is the prime factor responsible for most murmurs; it occurs when blood velocity becomes critically high.

The clinician's description of a murmur should include its timing (systolic, diastolic, or continuous), location, radiation, and intensity. It is also important to note the effect of respiration on the murmur, as well as maneuvers or pharmacologic interventions that affect the preloading and afterloading conditions of the ventricle. There is seldom any difficulty distinguishing between systole and diastole because systole is considerably shorter at normal heart rates. With tachycardia, however, the duration of systole and diastole may approach each other. In this situation, the clinician can usually rely on the fact that S₂ is the louder sound auscultated at the base. Once S₂ is identified, murmurs can be properly located in the cardiac cycle as systolic or diastolic. If the murmur is at the apex, the proper timing can be ensured by "inching." This technique consists of slowly moving the stethoscope down from the base to the apex while repeatedly fixing the cardiac cycle in one's mind, using S₂ as a reference point. Simultaneous palpation of the carotid artery will also readily identify systole coincident with the upstroke of the pulse.

The location and radiation of a murmur are multifactorially determined by the site of origin, intensity, and direction of blood flow. The intensity of the murmur as heard at the chest wall is determined by the transmission characteristics of the tissue intervening between the source of the murmur and the stethoscope. Obesity, emphysema,

and significant pleural or pericardial effusions will decrease the intensity of the murmur, whereas a thin, ascetic body type will often accentuate it.

Systolic murmurs are graded from 1 to 6. A grade 1 murmur is audible only after the listener has tuned in. Grade 2 is the faintest systolic murmur audible immediately after placing the stethoscope on the chest. Grade 5 is a loud murmur that cannot be heard with the stethoscope removed from the chest wall but can be heard with just the edge of the stethoscope touching the skin. A grade 6 murmur is audible with the stethoscope removed from the chest wall. Grade 3 and 4 are intermediate. Systolic murmurs of grade 3 or more in intensity are usually hemodynamically significant. Systolic thrills are usually associated with grade 4 or louder murmurs. A murmur's intensity varies directly with the velocity of blood flow, which in turn is directly related to the pressure head that propels the blood across the murmur-producing area. High velocity through a small ventricular defect produces a loud murmur, whereas high flow at low velocity through an atrial septal defect produces no murmur. The frequency composition of a murmur is also directly related to the velocity of blood flow. Low velocity resulting from a small pressure head across a stenotic mitral valve produces a low-pitch rumbling murmur, whereas a large diastolic pressure gradient across a regurgitant semilunar aortic valve results in high-velocity retrograde flow and the typical high-pitched murmur of aortic regurgitation.

Systolic Murmurs. Systolic murmurs may be classified as systolic ejection or pansystolic regurgitant. Systolic ejection murmurs (SEM) are caused by forward flow across the left or right ventricular outflow tract, whereas pansystolic regurgitant murmurs are caused by retrograde flow from a high-pressure chamber into a lower-pressure chamber (Fig. 11-14). A more detailed breakdown of this classifica-

---

BOX 11-3
Physiologic classification of systolic murmurs

A. Systolic ejection murmurs—forward flow across the left or right ventricular outflow tract
   1. Normal flow across the anatomically normal left or right ventricular outflow tract (innocent murmurs)
   2. High flow across the anatomically normal left or right ventricular outflow tract (functional murmurs of anemia, thyrotoxicosis, exercise, fever, atrial septal defect, complete heart block, etc.)
   3. High flow across an incompetent semilunar valve without significant stenosis (aortic or pulmonic regurgitation)
   4. Forward flow into a dilated great vessel (dilated aortic root, dilation of the pulmonary artery, idiopathic or secondary to pulmonary hypertension)
   5. Forward flow across a stenosed area in the left or right ventricular outflow tract (subvalvular, valvular, and supravalvular aortic or pulmonic stenosis)
   6. Combinations of 2 through 5
B. Systolic regurgitant murmurs—regurgitant flow from a high-pressure chamber to a lower-pressure chamber
   1. Pansystolic regurgitant murmurs (mitral and tricuspid regurgitation, ventricular septal defect, left ventricle to right atrial defect)
   2. Early systolic regurgitant murmurs (acute mitral regurgitation, tricuspid regurgitation secondary to isolated disease of the valve, small ventricular septal defect)
   3. Mid and late systolic regurgitant murmurs (papillary muscle dysfunction, mitral and tricuspid valve prolapse)

(From Shaver JA, Salerni R: Auscultation of the heart. In Hurst JW, Schlant RC, editors: *The heart,* ed 7, New York, 1990, McGraw-Hill.)

tion based on the physiologic mechanisms of production of these murmurs is shown in Box 11-3.

Systolic ejection murmur. The midsystolic ejection murmur begins shortly after the left or right ventricular pressure exceeds aortic or pulmonary diastolic pressure sufficiently to open the aortic or pulmonic valve (see Fig. 11-14). The contour of the time-intensity pattern, or murmur envelope, parallels the contour of flow velocity, and the murmur is heard when the sound produced by the peak turbulence exceeds the audible threshold. The intensity of SEMs is related directly to peak flow velocity during ventricular ejection. Any condition that increases forward flow, such as exercise, anxiety, or the increased stroke volume associated with a long diastolic pause following a premature beat (see Fig. 11-4), will increase the intensity of the murmur. Likewise, conditions that decrease stroke volume or its rate of ejection (congestive heart failure or negative inotropic drugs) will decrease the intensity of the murmur.

Innocent murmurs are systolic ejection in nature and are found in patients without evidence of physiologic or structural abnormalities of the cardiovascular system. This definition excludes murmurs produced by minor structural abnormalities such as a prolapsing mitral valve, even if such murmurs are hemodynamically insignificant. Although systolic murmurs produced by high cardiac output are functional, physiologic, and flow related, they are excluded from this definition because of the associated altered physiologic state. Innocent murmurs are less than grade 3 in intensity and vary considerably with body position and level of activity, and from one examination to another. They are found in approximately 30% to 50% of all children and are common in adolescents and young adults. In elderly persons, innocent murmurs caused by flow across the left ventricular outflow tract may have a musical quality and are frequently heard best at the apex.

Because both innocent murmurs and systolic ejection murmurs associated with physiologic or structural abnormalities of the cardiovascular system have the same mechanism of production, it is not the nature of the murmur itself that allows the differential diagnosis, but rather the associated cardiac findings. Therefore the "company

the murmur keeps" establishes the proper diagnosis; the innocent murmur must be found in the setting of an otherwise normal cardiovascular examination (Fig. 11-15).

A prominent systolic ejection murmur is almost always present with obstruction to right or left ventricular outflow, which may be located at the valvular, supravalvular, or subvalvular level. These murmurs are crescendo-decrescendo in nature, and their murmur envelope closely parallels the instantaneous ventricular–great vessel pressure gradient. As long as the cardiac output is maintained, the intensity and duration of the murmur increase as the stenotic lesion progressively narrows. When cardiac output decreases, the intensity of the murmur decreases, although careful auscultation will usually reveal that the murmur still has a prolonged duration. In the elderly patient, the murmur of aortic stenosis often is heard best at the apex, having a musical quality, and may be confused with the pansystolic murmur of mitral regurgitation. However, careful inching of the stethoscope from the base to the apex with attention to the crescendo-decrescendo quality of the murmur will usually allow proper identification of the apical murmur (see Fig. 11-2, *D*).

Pansystolic regurgitant murmurs. Pansystolic regurgitant murmurs are produced by retrograde flow from a chamber of high pressure to one of low pressure (see Fig. 11-14). Because there is usually a large pressure differential between the two chambers throughout systole, the murmurs are holosystolic in duration, high-pitched and blowing in quality, and plateaulike in configuration. In contrast to systolic ejection murmurs, these murmurs vary little with changes in forward cardiac output or beat-to-beat changes in stroke volume. Their intensity, however, is closely related to the pressure gradient causing the regurgitant flow from the ventricular chamber into the recipient chamber. Interventions that increase left ventricular pressure, such as hand grip, the squatting position, and vasoconstrictor drugs, increase the intensity of the regurgitant murmur, whereas measures that decrease the left ventricular pressure (inhalation of amyl nitrite) decrease the intensity of these murmurs.

The pansystolic murmur of mitral regurgitation is blowing in character and heard best at the apex radiating well into the axilla. There is a good correlation between the intensity of the murmur and the degree of mitral regurgitation. Severe mitral regurgitation is usually accompanied by a hyperdynamic apical impulse, and frequently a systolic thrill is palpable; a hyperkinetic S_3 is present, often followed by a short diastolic flow rumble (see Fig. 11-7, *D*). The classic pansystolic murmur of tricuspid regurgitation is heard best at the lower left sternal border; however, when a large right ventricle occupies the apex, it may be heard well lateral to the midclavicular line. It is usually easily identified by its typical augmentation in intensity with inspiration. Simultaneous observation of the JVP while listening to this murmur will help define its right-sided origin, revealing prominent v waves with rapid y descents that augment with inspiration (see Fig. 11-6, *D*). When tricuspid regurgitation is severe, a right-sided S_3 gallop followed by a short flow rumble that increases in intensity with inspiration is present. The murmur of a ventricular septal defect is heard at the parasternal border of the fourth, fifth, and sixth intercostal spaces, frequently accompanied by a systolic thrill. In contrast to mitral regurgitation, the murmur does not radiate well to the axilla, and its intensity does not correlate well with the degree of left to right shunting, nor does it have the respiratory variation characteristic of tricuspid regurgitation.

Not all regurgitant murmurs are pansystolic. Common variants of regurgitant murmurs are illustrated in Fig. 11-16, and the typical response of the late systolic murmur of mitral prolapse to postural changes is shown in Fig. 11-13. Another systolic murmur, associated with a ballooning mitral valve, is the systolic "whoop" or "honk." Such murmurs are loud, high-pitched, musical, and frequently intermittent, being heard best at the apex in mid or late systole. They are often associated with nonejection sounds and may vary markedly with respiration, from beat to beat, and from examination to examination. Occasionally, they are readily audible to both the clinician and the patient without the aid of a stethoscope. Similar whooping or honking noises may originate from the tricuspid valve and are occasionally caused by transvenous catheters positioned across the valve.

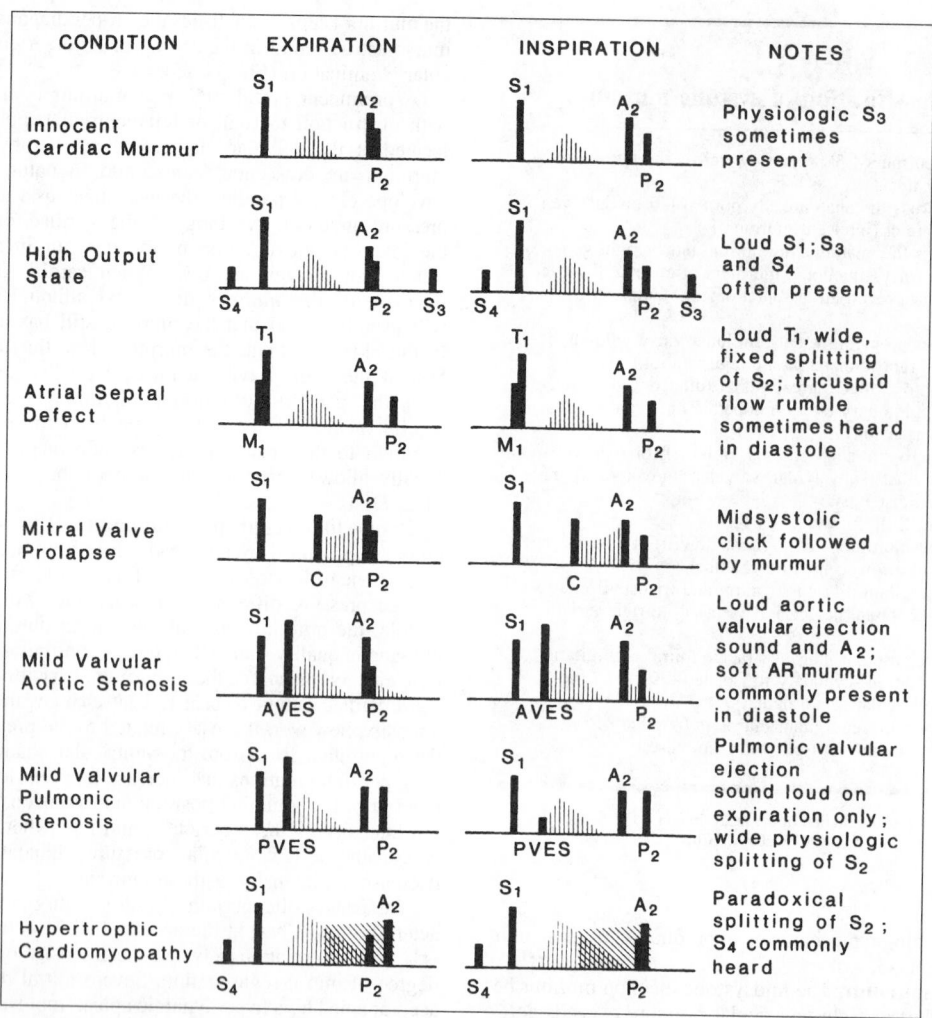

FIGURE 11-15   The differential diagnosis of the innocent murmur versus the systolic murmur associated with physiologic or anatomic abnormalities of the cardiovascular system is made by the company the murmur keeps. Innocent murmurs must be found in an otherwise normal cardiovascular examination. *C*, Mid-systolic ejection sound; *AVES*, aortic valvular ejection sound; *PVES*, pulmonary valvular ejection sound; *AR*, aortic regurgitation.

(From Shaver JA, Leonard JJ, Leon DF: *Examination of the heart.* Part 4: Auscultation of the heart, Dallas, 1990, American Heart Association.)

Diastolic Murmurs. Diastolic murmurs are caused by either structural abnormalities of the atrioventricular and semilunar valves, or increased flow across anatomically normal atrioventricular valves. In contrast to some systolic ejection murmurs that are innocent, diastolic murmurs should never be considered innocent. They have two basic mechanisms of production. Diastolic filling murmurs or rumbles are due to forward flow across the atrioventricular valves, whereas diastolic regurgitant murmurs are due to retrograde flow across an incompetent semilunar valve (Fig. 11-17). A further breakdown of this classification based on the mechanism of production of each murmur is shown on Box 11-4.

Diastolic filling murmurs (rumbles). Diastolic rumbles are caused by forward flow across the atrioventricular valves, and their onset is delayed from their respective semilunar closure sound by the isovolumic relaxation period (see Fig. 11-17). When the atrial pressure exceeds the declining ventricular pressure, the atrioventricular valves open and filling begins. There are two phases of rapid ventricular filling, early diastole and presystole, the time at which these murmurs tend to be most prominent.

The diastolic rumble of the stenotic mitral valve is heard best at the apex. As long as the stenotic valve has mobility, the murmur is introduced by an opening snap and is most prominent during the two phases of rapid ventricular filling (Fig. 11-18). The duration of the

mitral rumble correlates well with the duration of the diastolic gradient across the mitral valve, whereas its intensity is related to both the severity of the obstruction and the forward flow across the stenotic valve. When atrial fibrillation is present, the persistence of the rumble throughout a long diastolic filling period indicates that there is a diastolic gradient throughout the long cycle and that the obstruction is significant. In normal sinus rhythm, the presystolic murmur crescendos up to S_1 (see Fig. 11-18). A left atrial myxoma also may produce obstruction of the mitral orifice, and the diastolic rumble is similar to that produced by mitral stenosis and is introduced by a loud tumor "plop" (Chapter 33). A presystolic crescendo murmur occurs as the tumor mass protrudes through the mitral orifice into the left atrium during early systole. The diastolic rumble of the stenotic tricuspid valve is usually heard in the xiphoid area just off the left sternal border. In contrast to the presystolic murmur of mitral stenosis, which crescendos up to the loud S_1, the earlier onset of right atrial systole relative to left atrial systole results in a presystolic tricuspid murmur with a crescendo-decrescendo configuration, which ends before S_1 and increases with inspiration (see Fig. 11-6, *C*).

Short mid-diastolic flow rumbles, often introduced by S_3, are also produced by high flow across the normal or regurgitant atrioventricular valve (see Box 11-4). A rumbling diastolic murmur (Austin Flint murmur) associated with hemodynamically significant

BOX 11-4
Physiologic classification of diastolic murmurs

A. Diastolic filling murmurs (rumbles)—forward flow across the atrioventricular valves
1. Forward flow across a stenosed or obstructed atrioventricular valve (mitral or tricuspid stenosis, left or right atrial myxoma)
2. High flow across a normal atrioventricular valve (mitral flow rumble of a ventricular septal defect or patent ductus arteriosus, tricuspid flow rumble of an atrial septal defect, hyperkinetic states, complete heart block)
3. High flow across an incompetent atrioventricular valve without significant stenosis (flow rumble of mitral and tricuspid regurgitation)
4. Forward flow across a partially closed atrioventricular valve (presystolic murmur of mitral stenosis, Austin Flint murmur secondary to severe aortic or pulmonary regurgitation)
5. Combinations of 1 through 4
B. Diastolic regurgitant murmurs—regurgitant flow across an incompetent semilunar valve
1. Pandiastolic regurgitant murmurs (aortic regurgitation and pulmonic regurgitation secondary to pulmonary hypertension)
2. Abbreviated diastolic regurgitant murmurs (acute aortic regurgitation, minimal aortic regurgitation)
3. Delayed diastolic regurgitant murmur (organic pulmonic regurgitation)

(From Shaver JA, Salerni R: Auscultation of the heart. In Hurst JW, Schlant RC, editors: *The heart*, ed 7, New York, 1990, McGraw-Hill.)

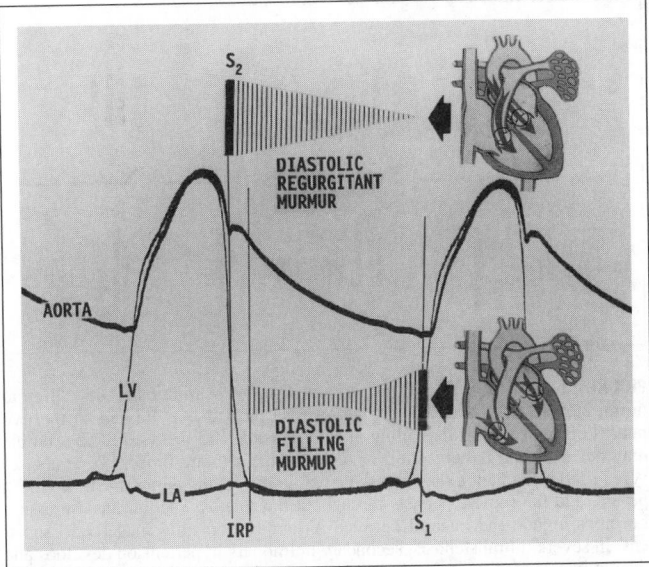

FIGURE 11-17 **Left,** Diagrammatic representation of the diastolic filling murmur and the diastolic regurgitant murmur as related to left ventricular *(LV)*, aortic, and left atrial *(LA)* pressures. The diastolic filling murmur occurs during the diastolic filling period and is separated from S_2 by the isovolumic relaxation period. The rumbling murmur is most prominent during rapid, early ventricular filling and presystole, terminating with S_1. The diastolic regurgitant murmur begins immediately after S_2 and continues in a decrescendo fashion up to S_1, closely paralleling the aortic left ventricular diastolic pressure gradient. **Right,** Flow diagram. Diastolic filling murmurs or rumbles are caused by forward flow across the atrioventricular valves, whereas diastolic regurgitant murmurs are caused by retrograde flow across incompetent semilunar valves.

(From Shaver JA: Diastolic murmurs. *Heart Dis Stroke* 2:98-103, 1993.)

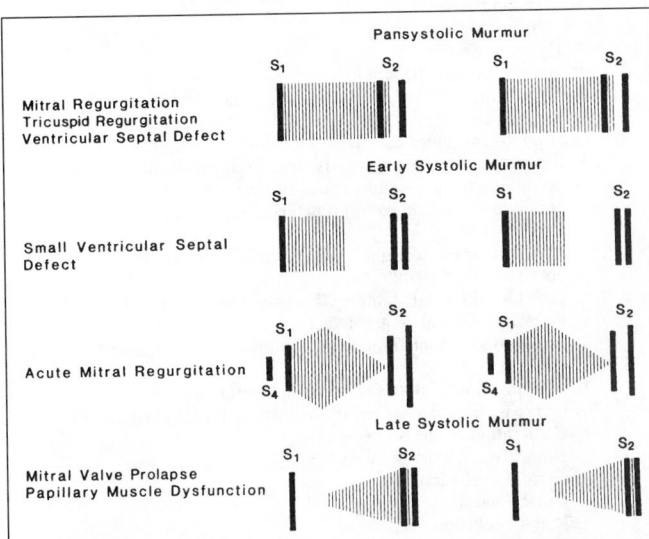

FIGURE 11-16 Variations of regurgitant murmurs that exist in addition to the classic pansystolic regurgitant murmurs heard in mitral regurgitation, tricuspid regurgitation, and ventricular septal defect (VSD). In patients with small VSDs, the murmur that starts with S_1 may suddenly stop during early or mid systole because, as the ventricular volume decreases and the septum thickens during ejection, the defect seals and the murmur ceases. In acute mitral regurgitation, the murmur may end well before A_2 as a result of an extremely high left atrial v wave, which abolishes the left ventricular–left atrial pressure gradient during late systole. S_1 may be soft if a flailed mitral leaflet is present and it is preceded by a prominent S_4. Audible expiratory splitting with an accentuated P_2 is present. Mid to late systolic murmurs may be caused by papillary muscle dysfunction and prolapse of the mitral or tricuspid valve. In the latter condition, the valve is competent in earlier systole, but as the ventricular volume decreases, the leaflets become incompetent and the murmur begins building in late systole, becoming maximal at the time of S_2.

(From Shaver JA, Leonard JJ, Leon DF: *Examination of the heart*. Part 4: Auscultation of the heart, Dallas, 1990, American Heart Association.)

aortic regurgitation is often heard at the apex, having many of the qualities of the murmur of mitral stenosis (Fig. 11-19). In contrast to mitral stenosis, the Austin Flint murmur is introduced by an S_3 rather than an opening snap, and the S_1 is of normal or decreased amplitude. When the aortic regurgitation is acute, marked elevation of the left ventricular end-diastolic pressure occurs, resulting in a reverse pressure gradient between the left ventricle and the left atrium in late diastole, causing premature closure of the mitral valve, and the presystolic component of the Austin Flint murmur disappears (see Fig. 11-19).

Pandiastolic aortic regurgitant murmurs. When the aortic valve becomes incompetent, a blowing high-pitched decrescendo diastolic murmur develops (see Fig. 11-17). The murmur of aortic regurgitation resulting from deformity of the aortic valve is usually best heard in the third and fourth left parasternal areas. When the murmur is heard best to the right of the sternum (Harvey's sign), however, the clinician should be alerted to a possible aortic root etiology for the regurgitation. The murmur of mild aortic regurgitation is frequently quite faint and may be overlooked if the examiner does not listen with the patient sitting up and leaning forward, with the diaphragm of the stethoscope pressed firmly against the chest wall during held forced expiration. Pharmacologic agents or maneuvers that increase or decrease the diastolic aortic left ventricular pressure gradient will increase or decrease the intensity of the regurgitant murmur. For example, prompt squatting or hand grip often elicits a faint aortic regurgitant murmur at the bedside, whereas inhalation of amyl nitrite will markedly decrease an easily heard aortic regurgitant murmur.

In many patients, combined aortic stenosis and regurgitation are present when the deformed aortic valve is both obstructive and incompetent. In this situation, the classic to-fro murmur of aortic stenosis and regurgitation is present (Fig. 11-20). Unlike a continuous murmur that reaches its peak intensity at about the time of S_2, the to-fro murmur has two separate components that can be clearly distinguished by the presence of a silent period before the onset of the regurgitant component.

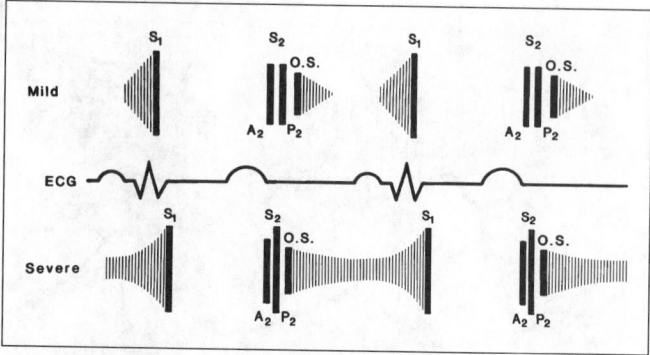

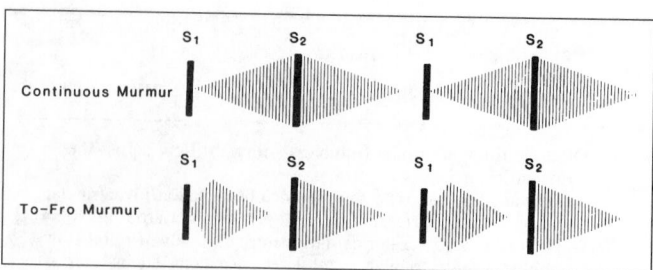

FIGURE 11-18 Diastolic filling murmur (rumble of mitral stenosis). In mild mitral stenosis, the diastolic gradient across the valve is limited to the two phases of rapid ventricular filling in early diastole and presystole. The rumble may occur during either period or both. As the stenotic process becomes severe, a large gradient exists across the valve during the entire diastolic filling period, and the rumble persists throughout diastole. As the left atrial pressure becomes higher, the interval between A_2 and the opening snap *(O.S.)* shortens. In severe mitral stenosis, secondary pulmonary hypertension develops and results in a louder P_2, and the splitting interval usually narrows.

(From Shaver JA, Leonard JJ, Leon DF: *Examination of the heart*. Part 4: Auscultation of the heart, Dallas, 1990, American Heart Association.)

FIGURE 11-20 The continuous murmur versus the to-fro murmur. The to-fro murmur is a combination of a systolic ejection murmur and a diastolic regurgitant murmur. The classic example of a to-fro murmur is aortic stenosis and regurgitation. At times, this type of murmur may be confused with a continuous murmur, such as a patent ductus arteriosus, in which there is an abnormal communication between the high-pressure aorta and the low-pressure pulmonary artery. This results in a large pressure gradient throughout the cardiac cycle, producing a continuous murmur. Note that the continuous murmur builds to a crescendo around S_2, where the to-fro murmur has two components. The mid-systolic ejection component decrescendos and disappears as it approaches S_2, leaving a silent period before the onset of the regurgitant murmur.

(From Shaver JA, Leonard JJ, Leon DF: *Examination of the heart*. Part 4: Auscultation of the heart, Dallas, 1990, American Heart Association.)

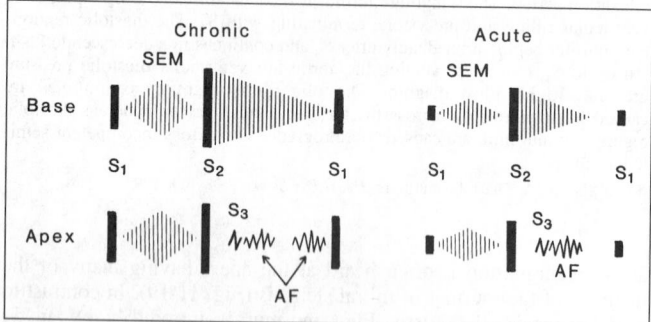

FIGURE 11-19 Auscultatory findings in chronic and acute aortic regurgitation. In chronic aortic regurgitation, a prominent systolic ejection murmur *(SEM)* resulting from the large forward stroke volume is heard at the base and apex and ends well before S_2. The aortic diastolic regurgitant murmur begins with S_2 and continues in a decrescendo fashion, terminating before S_1. At the apex, the early diastolic component of the Austin Flint murmur *(AF)* is introduced by a prominent S_3. A presystolic component of the AF is also heard. In acute aortic regurgitation, there is a significant decrease in the intensity of the SEM compared with chronic aortic regurgitation because of the decreased forward stroke volume. S_1 is markedly decreased in intensity because of preclosure of the mitral valve, and at the apex the presystolic component of the AF murmur is absent. The early diastolic murmur at the base ends well before S_1 because of the equilibration of the left ventricular and aortic end-diastolic pressure. Significant tachycardia is usually present.

(From Shaver JA: Diastolic murmurs, *Heart Dis Stroke* 2:98-103, 1993.)

Pulmonary regurgitation is most commonly found when severe pulmonary hypertension is present with dilation of the pulmonary artery. This type of pulmonary regurgitant murmur (Graham Steell's murmur) is identical in contour and pitch to that of aortic regurgitation, both murmurs being produced by similar hemodynamics. Although these murmurs cannot be differentiated by their acoustic qualities, the Graham Steell's murmur is almost always accompanied by physical findings of severe pulmonary hypertension.

Continuous murmurs. A continuous murmur is defined as one that begins in systole and extends through S_2 into part or all of diastole. It does not necessarily have to occupy the entire cardiac cycle; thus a systolic murmur that extends into diastole without stopping at S_2 is considered to be continuous, even if it fades away before the subsequent S_1. Continuous murmurs can be congenital or acquired. Although it is beyond the scope of this chapter to detail

---

BOX 11-5
Physiologic classifications of continuous murmurs

A. Continuous murmurs caused by rapid blood flow
   1. Venous hum
   2. Mammary souffle
   3. Hemiangioma
   4. Hyperthyroidism
   5. Acute alcoholic hepatitis
   6. Hyperemia of neoplasm (hepatoma renal cell carcinoma, Paget's disease)
B. Continuous murmurs caused by high-to-low pressure shunts
   1. Systemic artery to pulmonary artery (patent ductus arteriosus, aortopulmonary window, truncus arteriosus, pulmonary atresia, anomalous left coronary, bronchiectasis, sequestration of the lung)
   2. Systemic artery to right heart (ruptured sinus of Valsalva, coronary artery fistula)
   3. Left-to-right atrial shunting (Lutembacher's syndrome, mitral atresia plus atrial septal defect)
   4. Venovenous shunts (anomalous pulmonary veins, portosystemic shunts)
   5. Arteriovenous fistula (systemic or pulmonic)
C. Continuous murmurs secondary to localized arterial obstruction
   1. Coarctation of the aorta
   2. Branch pulmonary stenosis
   3. Carotid occlusion
   4. Ciliac mesenteric occlusion
   5. Renal occlusion
   6. Femoral occlusion
   7. Coronary occlusion

(From Myers JD: The mechanisms and significances of continuous murmurs. In Leon DF, Shaver JA, editors: *Physiologic principles of heart sounds and murmurs*. Monograph 46, New York, 1975, American Heart Association.)

the many conditions that may cause a continuous murmur, a few of the more common clinical conditions are reviewed. A more complete physiologic classification of continuous murmurs is provided in Box 11-5.

The differential diagnosis of a continuous murmur should include the benign cervical venous hum heard commonly in children, in nearly all pregnant women, and in persons with high cardiac output. This murmur is usually poorly heard in the supine position, and its presence in an adult in this position strongly suggests a hyperdynamic circulatory state. Its peak intensity is in the supraclavicular fossa just lateral to the sternocleidomastoid muscle and is usually more prominent on the right side, peaking in early diastole. A cervical venous hum can be terminated easily by digital compression of the JVP. Another benign continuous murmur is a mammary souffle, which occurs in 10% to 15% of pregnant women during the second and third trimesters and in early postpartum lactation. This murmur may be obliterated by firm pressure on the stethoscope or by digital pressure lateral to the site of auscultation.

A patent ductus arteriosus is a classic example of a cardiovascular congenital anomaly in which there is shunting from a high-pressure systemic to the low-pressure pulmonary circulation, resulting in a large pressure gradient between the two circulations throughout the cardiac cycle. This murmur is heard best in the left infraclavicular area and the second left intercostal space, and peaks in intensity at the time of S_2. Sinus of Valsalva aneurysms may cause a continuous murmur when they rupture into the right heart, which is heard maximally at the lower sternal border or xiphoid over the area corresponding to the fistulous tract. An important sign in differentiating a ruptured sinus from a patent ductus arteriosus is diastolic accentuation of the murmur.

Arteriovenous fistulas between peripheral vessels produce a classic continuous murmur with systolic accentuation caused by the shunting of blood at high flow rates from a high-pressure artery into a low-pressure vein. This condition should always be considered as a potential cause for heart failure. These murmurs are best heard at the site of the fistula and local compression on the venous side decreases its intensity. Complete obliteration of the fistula abruptly terminates the murmur; if the shunt is large, a baroreceptor-mediated reflex bradycardia (Branham's sign) occurs. Upon release of the obstruction, a reflex tachycardia also occurs.

Continuous murmurs in adults are also caused by severe localized arterial obstructions. Although partially occluded arteries usually have only a delayed systolic murmur, this murmur may be continuous if the obstruction is critical, and adequate collateral flow is not available. Such murmurs are commonly heard directly over the carotid, subclavian, and femoral arteries. Continuous murmurs caused by obstruction of the renal or mesenteric arteries can also be heard by careful auscultation over the back or abdomen, respectively. In addition to critical obstruction of the systemic arteries, a continuous murmur may arise from branch pulmonary artery stenosis or partial obstruction of a major pulmonary artery occluded by a massive pulmonary embolus.

BIBLIOGRAPHY

Abrams J: *Essentials of cardiac physical diagnosis,* Philadelphia, 1987, Lea & Febiger.

Braunwald E: The physical examination. In Braunwald E, editor: *Heart disease: a textbook of cardiovascular medicine,* ed 4, Philadelphia, 1992, WB Saunders.

Constant J: *Bedside cardiology,* ed 3, Boston/Toronto, 1985, Little, Brown.

Crawford MH: *Examination of the heart,* Part 2: Inspection and palpation of venous and arterial pulses, Dallas, 1990, American Heart Association.

Fowler NO: *Cardiac diagnosis and treatment,* ed 3, Hagerstown, 1980, Harper & Row.

Leon DF, Shaver JA, editors: *Physiologic principles of heart sounds and murmurs.* Monograph 46, New York, 1975, American Heart Association.

O'Rourke RA, Shaver JA, Salerni R et al: The history, physical examination, and cardiac auscultation. In Alexander RW, Schlant RC, Fuster V, editors: *The heart,* ed 9, New York, 1998, McGraw-Hill.

Perloff JK: Physical examination of cardiovascular system. In Stein JH, editor: *Internal medicine,* ed 4, St Louis, 1994, Mosby.

Reddy PS: Hemodynamics of cardiac tamponade in man. In Reddy PS, Leon DF, Shaver JA, editors: *Pericardial disease,* New York, 1982, Raven Press.

Reddy PS, Shaver JA, Leonard JJ: Cardiac systolic murmurs: pathophysiology and differential diagnosis, *Prog Cardiovasc Dis* 14:10, 1971.

Schlant RC, Hurst JW: *Examination of the heart.* Part 3: Examination of the precordium: inspection and palpation, Dallas, 1990, American Heart Association.

Shaver JA: Cardiac auscultation: a cost-effective diagnostic skill. In O'Rourke RA, editor: *Current problems in cardiology,* St Louis, 1995, Mosby.

Shaver JA: Diastolic murmurs, *Heart Dis Stroke* 2:98-103, 1993.

Shaver JA. Heart murmurs: innocent or pathologic? Part I. Hosp *Med* 18:6 13-31, 1982.

Shaver JA: Systolic murmurs, *Heart Dis Stroke* 2:9-17, 1993.

Shaver JA: Heart murmurs: innocent or pathologic? Part II. *Hosp Med* 18:7 13-22, 1982.

Shaver JA, Leonard JJ, Leon DF: *Examination of the heart.* Part 4: Auscultation of the heart, Dallas, 1990, American Heart Association.

Shaver JA, Salerni R: Auscultation of the heart. In Schlant RC, Alexander RW, editors: *The heart,* ed 8, New York, 1994, McGraw-Hill.

Tavel ME: *Clinical phonocardiography and external pulse recording,* ed 4, Chicago, 1985, Year Book.

12 Electrocardiography

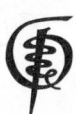

Frederick A. Masoudi and Nora Goldschlager

Since the introduction of the string galvanometer by Einthoven in the early 1900s, electrocardiography has been one of the most widely used diagnostic tools in all of clinical medicine. This technique, which records the electrical potentials produced by cardiac tissue, is useful in the evaluation of certain cardiac conditions, including abnormalities of conduction of cardiac electrical impulses, myocardial ischemia and infarction, pericarditis, cardiac chamber enlargement and hypertrophy, arrhythmias, and electronic pacemaker function. Electrocardiography can also be useful in evaluating patients with systemic diseases and metabolic states and drugs that affect the heart.

CARDIAC ELECTRICAL ACTIVITY AND THE ELECTROCARDIOGRAM

The heart is characterized by both the capacity to generate electrical impulses—automaticity—and to propagate these impulses—conductivity. The electrical impulses are translated into mechanical energy, allowing the heart to perform its function as a pump. Each cardiac cycle begins with the formation of an impulse in an area of the heart capable of spontaneous electrical activation (generally the sinoatrial node); the impulse is propagated through the conducting system of the heart (Fig. 12-1) and finally to the cardiac myocytes, which are capable of transmission of the impulse to other myocytes. After activation is completed, the cardiac tissue repolarizes, allowing it to undergo a subsequent depolarization (Chapter 9). The electrocardiogram (ECG) provides an assessment of these cycles of impulse formation and conduction and myocardial depolarization and repolarization.

The ECG is a graphic representation, from a number of different perspectives, of the changes in electrical potential of the heart during the cardiac cycle. The electrical potential of the heart during the car-

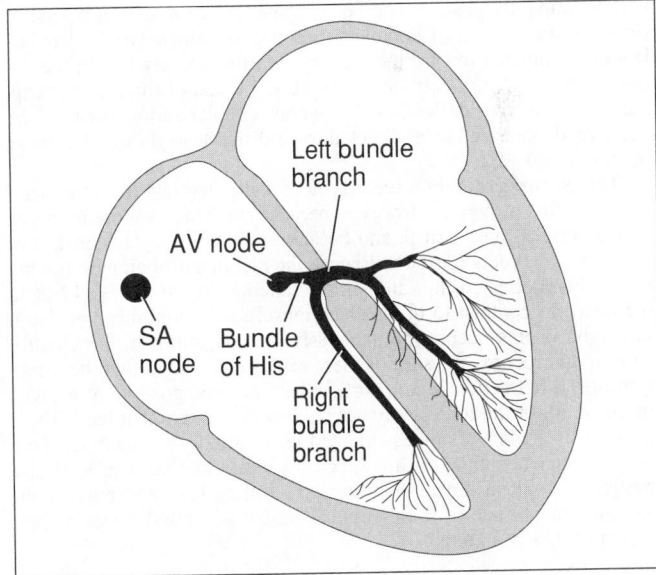

FIGURE 12-1 Schema of the cardiac conduction system. Normally, the sinoatrial *(SA)* node serves as the site where cardiac electrical activity is generated. The impulse spreads throughout the atrial myocardium and reaches the AV node. From the AV node, the electrical impulse is transmitted to the bundle of His and continues to the bundle branches, finally entering the ventricular myocardium through the Purkinje fibers, which are the numerous terminal branches of the bundle branches. The intraventricular septum is depolarized by the impulse propagated through septal Purkinje fibers of the left bundle branch.

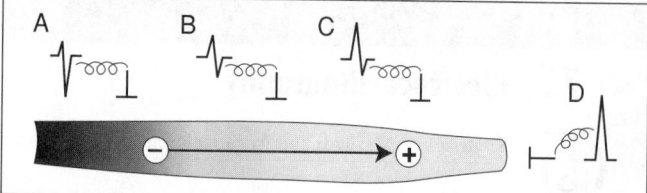

FIGURE 12-2 Schematic representation of a muscle strip undergoing depolarization. As the wave of depolarization passes from left to right, it is recorded by a number of electrodes (leads) placed on the muscle surface. A surface electrode records a positive deflection as the depolarization travels toward it and a negative deflection as the depolarization travels away from it.

diac cycle can be conceived of as a vector having a particular direction and magnitude that is changing over time. As electrical current flows through the heart, the characteristics of this vector of electrical potential change. As a result, the projections of these vectors on the different electrocardiographic leads change. The electrocardiographic tracing displays the projections of the vectors of this changing electrical potential on the external body surface lead axes.

Fig. 12-2 depicts a muscle strip with a number of external recording electrodes, or leads. These electrodes record the electrical activity in this muscle strip as a wave of depolarization passes from left to right. By convention, current flows from a negative to a positive direction. Any recording from a surface electrode will result in a positive deflection as current flows toward it and a negative deflection as current flows away from it. For example, the depolarization wave in Fig. 12-2 is directed toward electrode A on the left side of the muscle strip for a small portion of the depolarization and is subsequently directed away from electrode A for the remainder of depolarization. Thus the recording from this electrode is positive for a short time at the beginning of the depolarization but is negative for the majority of the depolarization. Electrode B is placed in the middle of the muscle strip. For the first half of depolarization, the impulse travels toward this electrode; then it passes under it midway through the depolarization and subsequently heads away from it. Therefore the recording from electrode B is positive for the first half of the depolarization and is negative for an equivalent amount of time in the second half of the depolarization. Electrode C records a deflection that is predominantly positive and becomes negative for a short period of time toward the end of depolarization because the wave of depolarization is directed toward the electrode until relatively late in the depolarization cycle. Electrode D, on the right side of the muscle strip, records a positive deflection throughout depolarization because the wave of depolarization is directed toward this lead during the entire process.

The electrocardiogram records electrical potentials from the heart based on this principle. However, because the heart is more complex than a simple muscle strip, and because the cardiac cycle consists of a number of events (described later), the electrocardiographic tracing is more complicated than the simple schema shown in Fig. 12-2. In the heart, in contrast to the isolated muscle strip, a number of depolarization events occur simultaneously. At any moment, the electrocardiogram records the sum of these events. Thus although the direction of the deflection in any surface lead may be positive at a given moment, all of the forces may not be directed toward that lead. There may be a number of forces oriented in a variety of directions, both positive and negative, with respect to a particular surface lead at a particular point in time. Any surface recording lead will register the summed magnitude of these simultaneously generated forces as projected on that lead axis.

STANDARD ELECTROCARDIOGRAPHIC LEADS

Before the electrocardiogram can be recorded, electrodes are applied to the patient. The limb electrodes are applied to each of the four limbs. The precordial electrodes are applied to the anterior chest wall. Conventional electrocardiography uses a set of 12 different perspectives, called *external* or *body surface leads,* which provide different views of the vector of the heart's electrical activity throughout the cardiac cycle.

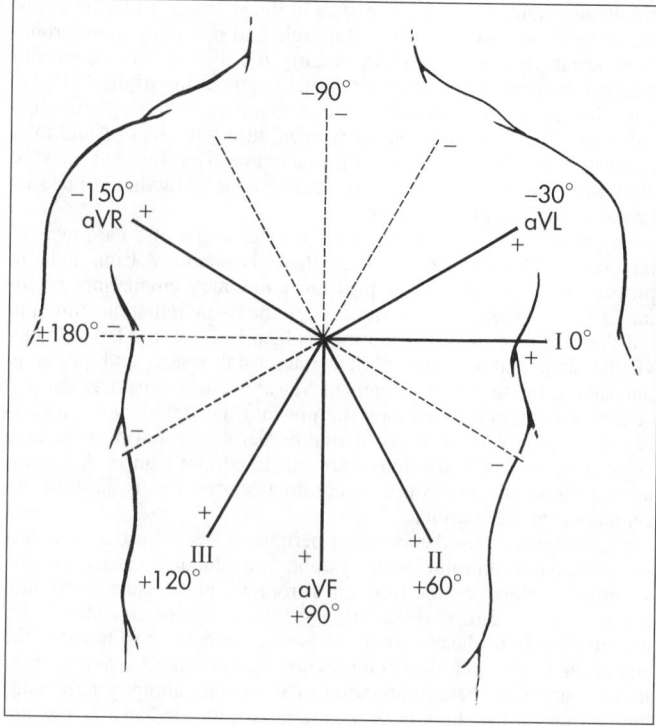

FIGURE 12-3 The axes of the limb leads in the frontal plane.

The standard electrocardiographic leads are schematized in Figs. 12-3 through 12-5. Fig. 12-3 depicts the six standard limb leads that detect the electrical activity of the heart in the frontal plane. One group of these leads records the potential difference between different limb electrodes. These bipolar limb leads are designated I, II, and III. By convention, lead I is a horizontally oriented dipole with the negative pole at the right arm and the positive pole at the left arm. Thus, forces directed from right to left are inscribed as positive deflections in lead I, and likewise, forces directed rightward are inscribed as negative deflections in this lead. Any forces that are directed superiorly or inferiorly, that is, perpendicular to lead I, will have a magnitude of zero in lead I. By convention, the plane of lead I is designated as 0 degrees in the frontal plane. The angle of any other lead is determined by the deviation of the direction of the lead in question from the axis of lead I; clockwise deviation is designated as positive and counterclockwise deviation is designated as negative. Lead II records the potential difference between the right arm (negative) and the left leg (positive) with an axis that is 60 degrees clockwise from lead I. By the convention, the axis of lead II is thus designated as +60 degrees. The final bipolar limb lead is lead III, which records the potential difference between the left arm (negative) and left leg (positive). The axis of this lead is 120 degrees clockwise from lead I and is designated as +120 degrees.

The remaining limb leads are unipolar leads with a common central ground and a single limb electrode as the positive pole. These unipolar leads, called the augmented limb leads, are named aV_R (*R*ight arm), aV_L (*L*eft arm), and aV_F (left *F*oot). The axes of these leads, as shown in Fig. 12-3, are −120 degrees, −30 degrees, and +90 degrees, respectively. The electrical axes of aV_R and aV_L are designated negative because this is the deviation of these leads from lead I in a counterclockwise direction.

Another set of unipolar leads records electrical potential in a horizontal plane (see Figs. 12-4 and 12-5). These leads, also known as precordial leads, are designated V_1 to V_6. They record the cardiac electrical activity from positions on the chest wall from the right fourth intercostal space to the left midaxillary line. The precise placement of these leads (see Fig. 12-4) is important. Incorrect lead placement makes comparisons with previously recorded electrocardiograms difficult. Leads V_1 through V_6 complete the group of 12 leads

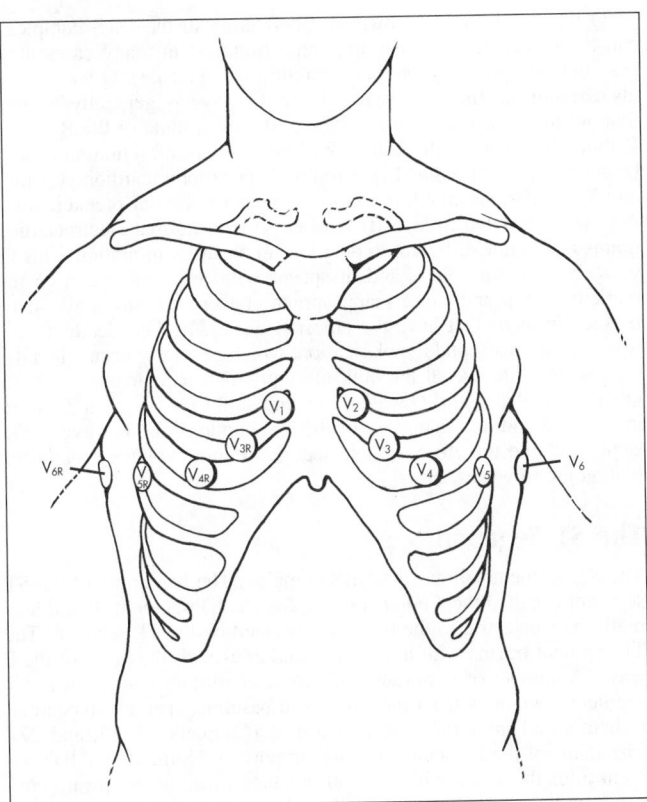

FIGURE 12-4 Schema of the locations of the precordial leads on the chest wall.

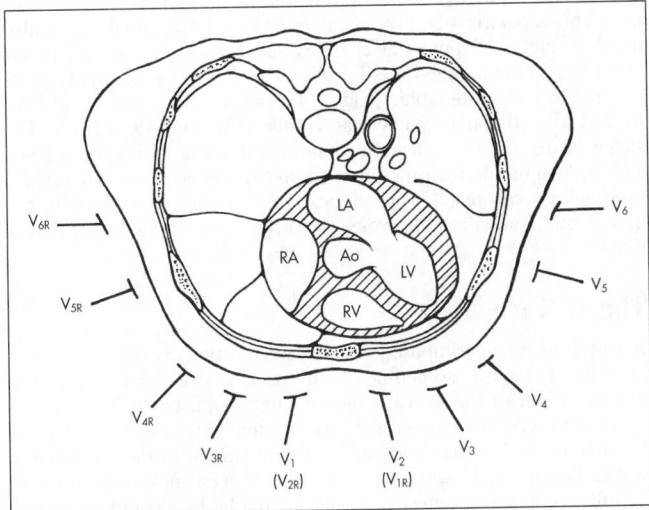

FIGURE 12-5 The precordial leads in cross section. Leads V_1-V_6 are the most widely used precordial leads. Leads V_{1R}-V_{6R} are the right-sided precordial leads.

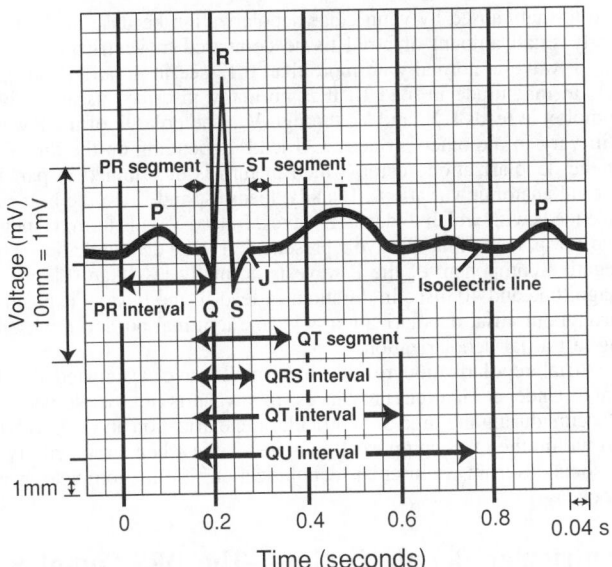

FIGURE 12-6 Normal electrocardiographic waveforms and intervals on a standard electrocardiographic grid.

(From Goldschlager N, Goldman M: *Principles of clinical electrocardiography,* ed 13, East Norwalk, CT, 1989, Appleton & Lange.)

used in the standard electrocardiogram. In certain circumstances, the use of nonstandard leads is helpful. The right precordial leads, which are designated $V1_R$ through $V6_R$ (Fig. 12-5), can be particularly useful in the diagnosis of acute right ventricular myocardial infarction (Chapter 23). The precordial leads V_7 through V_{10} are occasionally used to provide a better representation of the electrical activity of the posterior wall of the heart in conditions such as suspected posterior myocardial infarction.

The different surface electrocardiographic leads are often considered in groups because they are aligned in similar direction. These groupings can be particularly useful in the evaluation of ischemia and infarction (see later section), in which they are used to describe an electrocardiographic "territory" where the pathologic process is taking place. Leads II, III, and aV_F are designated as *inferior* leads because their axes are aligned such that inferiorly directed forces are recorded as positive deflections (Fig. 12-3). Leads I and aV_L are called *lateral* leads; leads V_5 and V_6 are called *apical* leads; and leads V_1 through V_4 are called *anterior* leads. These general designations are useful to communicate information about the electrocardiogram but do not necessarily correspond to a particular anatomic territory. Variations in body habitus and chest wall deformities may make these designations anatomically invalid in particular patients.

THE NORMAL ELECTROCARDIOGRAM

A normal cardiac cycle inscribed on standard electrocardiogram paper is shown in Fig. 12-6. The horizontal axis represents time, with each small box representing 0.04 sec (40 msec) and each large box representing 0.2 sec (200 msec) at standard recording speed (25 mm/sec). The vertical axis represents the magnitude of electrical potential, with each small box representing 0.1 mV and each large box representing 0.5 mV using the most common standardization of 1 mV/10 mm. Because these values hold only for these standard recording speeds and sensitivities, it is important to evaluate each electrocardiogram for voltage calibration and documentation of recording speed in order to calculate rates and to evaluate chamber enlargement.

Atrial Depolarization—The P Wave

All cardiac tissue is capable of automatic impulse formation, but under normal conditions, the sinoatrial node is the site where the electrical activity of the cardiac cycle originates. The impulse, formed in the sinus node at the junction of the superior vena cava and the right atrium, spreads through the atrial myocardium and results in the depolarization of the atria. The right atrium is normally depolarized slightly before the left; thus the early part of atrial electrical activity consists of right atrial depolarization, and the latter part represents left atrial depolarization. The electrical vector of normal atrial depolarization is directed inferiorly and leftward in the frontal plane, causing a positive deflection in surface leads I and II. The vector is directed anteriorly and leftward in the horizontal plane, leading to a positive deflection in leads V_3 through V_6. Atrial depolarization results in a deflection called the P wave. This deflection is small relative to that caused by ventricular depolarization because of the relatively small amount of atrial tissue compared to ventricular tissue. The P wave is normally no more than 0.12 sec in duration and 0.25 mV in magnitude in lead II. It is normally inscribed as an upright complex in leads I, II, and V_3 through V_6. The polarity of the P wave will vary in the other surface ECG leads depending on the direction of the depolarization vector, which in turn is determined in part by normal anatomic variations. Usually, leads V_1 and II are the best surface leads with which to detect P waves. In lead V_1, the terminal negative component of the P wave represents left atrial depolarization. This negative component of the P wave is normally less than 0.1 mV in magnitude and 40 msec in duration. In lead II, the P wave is positive throughout atrial depolarization, with the terminal portion representing left atrial depolarization.

Atrial repolarization results in a small wave designated the Ta wave. Under normal circumstances, this wave is not visible because it occurs during the time of ventricular depolarization and is thus buried within the QRS complex. It may be visible when atrial activity is dissociated from ventricular depolarization, as in complete heart block.

Ventricular Depolarization—The QRS Complex

After the atria have depolarized, the impulse reaches the atrioventricular (AV) node and passes to the His bundle and subsequently to the bundle branches (see Fig. 12-1). During this time (the PR segment), there is no detectable electrical activity on the surface electrocardiogram. The impulse then spreads from the bundle branches throughout the Purkinje network to the ventricular myocardium. Ventricular depolarization is inscribed on the electrocardiogram as the QRS complex.

Ventricular depolarization normally begins with interventricular septal depolarization. Normally, the electrical impulse is transmitted from the His bundle to the septum via centroseptal fibers of the left bundle branch, and septal depolarization proceeds from the left to the right portion of the septum. As a result, normal septal depolarization forces are inscribed as initial negative deflections in the leftward leads (I and V_6), and as positive deflections in the rightward leads (lead V_1), although some variability exists because of the position of the heart within the chest cage. Normal septal depolarization is completed in less than 0.03 sec.

Because the bulk of ventricular myocardium is contained in the left ventricle, the later portion of the QRS complex is predominantly the result of depolarization of this chamber. Under normal conditions, the net vector of left ventricular depolarization is directed leftward and inferiorly, resulting in a positive deflection in leads I, II, V_5, and V_6, and a predominantly negative deflection in the rightward leads (leads V_1 and aV_R). The QRS complex is significantly larger than the P wave because of the greater mass of the ventricles compared to the atria. Thus the magnitude of the vector of depolarization is larger. The duration of the QRS wave is normally less than 0.12 sec.

Because of the relatively large mass of ventricular myocardium, the QRS complex is usually the largest complex in the cardiac cycle. There can be variation in QRS voltage among normal individuals. Conditions that lead to an abnormally large ventricular mass such as long-standing hypertension or aortic valvular disease can cause an abnormal increase in the magnitude of the QRS forces. In contrast, an abnormally low QRS voltage of less than 0.5 mV in all of the limb leads occurs in conditions that cause diffuse myocardial injury, such as coronary disease and cardiac failure, or infiltrative diseases such as sarcoidosis, amyloidosis, and hemochromatosis. Low voltage can also be seen in conditions in which high impedance exists between the heart muscle and the body surface recording electrodes, such as pericardial effusion, obesity, chronic obstructive pulmonary disease, and anasarca.

If the first deflection of the QRS complex is negative, the deflection is called a Q wave. The first positive deflection of the QRS complex, no matter how small and regardless of what precedes it, is called an R wave. A negative deflection that follows an R wave is called an S wave. A second discrete positive deflection is called an R′ (R-prime) wave, and a subsequent negative deflection is called an S′ (S-prime) wave. Because the QRS complex morphology is different in each lead, the labeling of the complex may also be different in each lead.

Q waves (the initial downward deflection in the QRS complex) can be important electrocardiographic findings; in many cases they may indicate prior myocardial infarction (Chapter 23). Q waves can also be normal findings. A pathologic Q wave is generally greater than 40 msec in duration or ≥25% of the magnitude of the R wave. Pathologic Q waves, the hallmark of myocardial infarction, may also be seen with ventricular hypertrophy, hypertrophic cardiomyopathy, and Wolff-Parkinson-White syndrome with ventricular preexcitation. A Q wave isolated to lead III is often seen in normal electrocardiograms and is not sufficient to diagnose myocardial infarction. This Q wave, which can appear and disappear with respiration, can be remarkably deep and cause inappropriate concern. Q waves also may be seen in leads that have the tallest R waves. In these leads, the Q wave represents septal depolarization, which generally occurs in a direction opposite that of the bulk of ventricular depolarization. These Q waves, called *septal Q* waves, are almost always less than 30 msec in duration and less than 25% of the magnitude of the R wave in the same lead and therefore do not meet duration or voltage criteria for pathologic Q waves.

The ST Segment

The ST segment follows the QRS complex. The beginning of the ST segment is called the *J point* (Fig. 12-6). The ST segment should normally be isoelectric to the baseline provided by the TP segment. The TP segment begins with the T wave and ends with the onset of the P wave. A number of important pathologic conditions can result in ST segment deviations from the isoelectric baseline, such as myocardial ischemia and infarction and pericarditis (Chapters 22, 23, and 27). The shape of the ST segment is also important. Normally the ST segment joins the T wave in a smooth manner, forming an upward concavity with a smooth contour.

The T Wave

After ventricular depolarization and a short pause, indicated by the QRS wave and the ST segment, the ventricular myocardium repolarizes. This repolarization process, like the depolarization process, also involves electrical potential changes and forms a deflection in the electrocardiogram called the T wave. The T wave is normally positive in electrocardiographic leads I, II, and V_3 to V_6 and is negative in lead aV_R. Its polarity may vary in the remaining ECG leads. The shape of the T wave is usually smooth and asymmetric, and it has a smaller magnitude than the QRS complex. Abnormalities in T wave morphology can result from myocardial ischemia or infarction, hyperkalemia, and central nervous system disease, among other conditions.

The U Wave

A small wave superimposed on the later portions of the T wave or after the T wave is sometimes seen and is called the U wave. The precise origin of the U wave remains unproved, but it has been attributed to repolarization of the His-Purkinje network. Normally, the U wave is smaller than and has a polarity similar to the preceding T wave. Prominent U waves are most often seen in association with hypokalemia, hypomagnesemia, left ventricular hypertrophy, and bradycardia. U wave inversion can be seen with coronary artery disease involving the left anterior descending vessel and left ventricular hypertrophy. In general, isolated abnormalities of the U wave are unreliable means of making specific diagnoses.

APPROACH TO THE ELECTROCARDIOGRAM

The importance of a systematic approach to interpreting the electrocardiogram cannot be overemphasized. Failure to evaluate every electrocardiogram with respect to all of the components listed here may result in the oversight of critical findings. Although a number of sophisticated algorithms have been developed to provide a means by which computers can "read" electrocardiograms, these systems are not perfect, and errors commonly occur. Reliance on computer-generated ECG interpretations without independent and systematic overreading by the physician can result in incorrect diagnoses, occasionally with devastating clinical consequences. Perhaps the best first step in the interpretation of any electrocardiogram is to ignore the computer-generated reading until an independent interpretation has been made.

An appropriate approach to the electrocardiogram should involve evaluation of all of the following:

1. The rate of both the P waves and the QRS complexes and their relationships to each other.
2. The rhythm (see Chapter 18).
3. The mean electrical axis of the P wave and QRS complex in the frontal plane.
4. The PR interval, the QRS duration, and the QT interval.
5. The waveforms; for evidence of injury or ischemia, chamber enlargement, intraventricular conduction delays, drug and electrolyte effects, and repolarization abnormalities associated with conduction delays or ventricular hypertrophy.

Determination of Rate

The ventricular rate can be approximated by a variety of methods, of which the following are the most useful. If the QRS complexes occur with regularity, the rate can be calculated by dividing the number of large (0.2 sec) boxes between two consecutive QRS complexes into 300. For example, if the QRS complexes are separated by four large boxes (0.8 sec), the ventricular rate is 300/4 or 75/min. This method is useful only when the QRS complexes occur at regular intervals. In the case of irregular QRS rhythms, the number of QRS complexes occurring in 6 sec is multiplied by 10 to calculate the average ventricular rate per minute. On the bottom margin of most standard electrocardiographic recording paper, marks spaced at 3-sec intervals allow for an easy assessment of the rate using this method. This latter method is accurate regardless of the rhythm.

Determination of Axis

Although the axis of any of the electrocardiographic complexes can be determined, the most clinically relevant is that of the QRS complex in the frontal plane. To determine the mean frontal QRS axis, it is necessary to evaluate the net area under the QRS complexes in each of the limb leads. If the net area under the QRS complex is zero, the net QRS vector must be perpendicular to that lead. If the net area under the QRS complex is positive, the net vector must lie within that half of the frontal plane defined by the positive pole of that lead. The reverse is true if the net area is negative. Thus if the area under the QRS complex is positive in lead I, the net QRS vector must fall somewhere in the range of −90 degrees to +90 degrees. If the net QRS area is negative in lead II, the QRS axis must fall between −30 degrees and +120 degrees.

The normal mean frontal plane QRS axis lies between −30 degrees and +90 degrees. In order for the QRS axis to fall within these normal limits, the net area under the QRS complexes must be positive in leads I and II (Fig. 12-7). If the net QRS area is positive in lead I and negative in II, the QRS axis lies between −30 degrees and −90 degrees, and is designated *left axis deviation*. If the area under the QRS complexes is negative in lead I and positive in lead II, the axis lies between +90 degrees and +150 degrees and is designated *right axis deviation*. If the net QRS area is negative in both leads I and II, the axis lies between −90 degrees and +150 degrees and is designated *extreme axis deviation*. Deviations in the mean frontal plane QRS axis may indicate the existence of specific cardiac abnormalities or delays in the intraventricular conduction system (Box 12-1).

The mean frontal plane axis of the P wave is measured in a similar manner. An unusual P wave axis may indicate right or left atrial abnormality or that the site of formation of the impulse that depolarizes the atrium does not originate in the SA node.

Measurement of Intervals

The important intervals that should be measured on every tracing include the PR interval, the QRS duration, and the QT interval (Fig. 12-6). The PR interval is the interval from the beginning of the P wave to the beginning of the QRS complex and is normally between 0.12 and 0.20 sec. Shorter PR intervals can be normal or seen in patients with accessory pathways, in which the electrical impulse bypasses the AV node and depolarizes a portion of the ventricle earlier

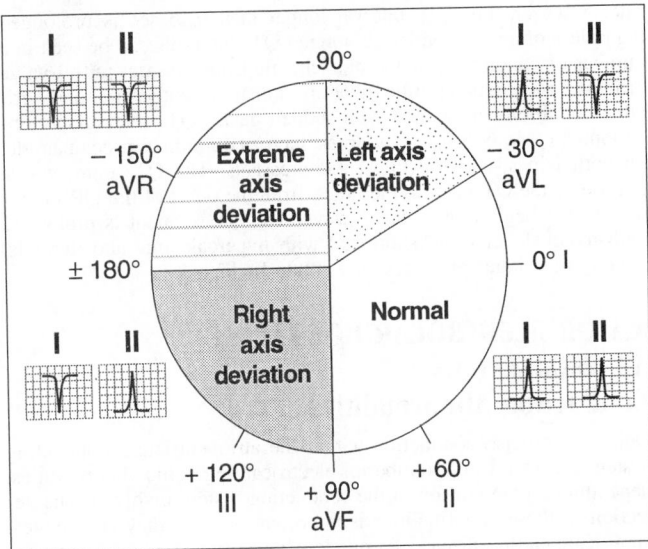

FIGURE 12-7 The determination of the QRS axis in the frontal plane. An analysis of the QRS complexes in leads I and II provides the information for a qualitative assessment of the axis.

BOX 12-1
Causes of Axis Deviations

A. Left axis deviation (−30 degrees to −90 degrees)
 1. Left anterior fascicular block (LAFB)
 2. Inferior wall myocardial infarction
 3. Some Wolff-Parkinson-White patterns
 4. Chronic obstructive lung disease
 5. Severe hyperkalemia (levels >7 mEq/L)
 6. Some congenital heart diseases (e.g., ostium primum atrial septal defect)

B. Right axis deviation (+90 degrees to +180 degrees)
 1. Right ventricular hypertrophy
 2. Lateral wall myocardial infarction
 3. Some Wolff-Parkinson-White patterns
 4. Left posterior fascicular block (LPFB)
 5. Chronic obstructive lung disease
 6. Acute pulmonary embolus
 7. Left pneumothorax

---

than normal. A prolonged PR interval implies impairment of conduction within the atrium, AV node, or the His bundle.

The QRS duration is measured from the onset of the QRS complex to its end. This interval is usually between 0.05 and 0.10 sec, and prolongation greater than 0.12 seconds is considered abnormal. Prolongation of the QRS complex occurs as the result of any process or condition that impairs conduction within the bundle branches or myocardium, or in situations in which ventricular depolarization originates in the ventricle itself (as seen with a premature ventricular depolarization or with an implanted ventricular pacing electrode).

The QT interval is measured from the onset of the QRS complex to the termination of the T wave. Where the T wave merges with the U wave, the end of the T wave can be extrapolated from its peak to the baseline to measure the interval. The QT interval depends on age and gender, as well as on heart rate and variations in autonomic tone. The QT interval is longer on average in younger patients, in women, and at slow heart rates. The measured QT interval can be corrected for heart rate (*QTc*) by dividing the measured QT interval in seconds by the square root of the RR cycle length in seconds:

$$QT(sec)/[RR(sec)]^{1/2}$$

The clinical value of QTc is controversial as the formula corrects for only one of the many sources of QT interval variability. As a general rule, however, any QTc interval longer than 0.46 sec is prolonged regardless of age or gender. Prolonged QTc intervals can be seen in a number of conditions, including ischemic heart disease, mitral valve prolapse, rheumatic carditis, hypothyroidism, hypothermia, and heritable conditions associated with sudden death. QTc interval prolongation can also be caused by drugs such as quinidine, procainamide, phenothiazines, and tricyclic antidepressants. The QT segment is a portion of the QT interva. measured from the onset of the QRS complex to the beginning of the T wave. The QT segment is prolonged with hypocalcemia and shortened with hypercalcemia and digitalis, although the latter produces only subtle findings.

MAJOR ELECTROCARDIOGRAPHIC ABNORMALITIES
Conduction Abnormalities

Delay of impulse conduction within the atrioventricular conducting system can result in a number of electrocardiographic abnormalities, depending on the portion of the conducting system involved. The detection of these abnormalities is important because they can suggest significant cardiac disease. As previously mentioned, normal ventricular depolarization begins with interventricular septal depolarization from left to right by septal fibers of the left bundle branch. Subsequently, as the impulse is propagated through the right and left bundle branches, the right and left ventricles are depolarized. During normal conduction, because of the orderly transmission of the electrical impulse through the bundle branches to the ventricular myocardium, the QRS complex is inscribed in less than 0.12 seconds. If either of the bundle branches is diseased, the normal ventricular depolarization sequence is altered, leading to an alteration in the QRS complex morphology. The impulse travels through the His bundle and through the normally conducting bundle branch, and the corresponding ventricle depolarizes normally. The other ventricle will not depolarize normally because of the conduction delay in the bundle branch that normally activates it. Instead, the wave of depolarization will reach this ventricle through myocyte-to-myocyte transmission of the impulse from the normally activated ventricle. This route of myocyte-to-myocyte transmission of the wave of depolarization is relatively slow when compared to the normal process. Thus in intraventricular conduction abnormalities, the directions and magnitudes of the vector of depolarization will be altered, and the time required for complete depolarization of the ventricle will be prolonged. The resulting QRS complex will have an abnormal morphology and prolonged duration. Bundle branch "blocks" do not cause QRS axis deviation. If the frontal plane QRS axis is abnormal in the presence of bundle branch block, another cause of this deviation should be sought (see Box 12-1).

Right Bundle Branch Block

Right bundle branch block (RBBB) is a common electrocardiographic abnormality seen in conditions affecting the conducting system, as well as in up to 2.5% of normal subjects. As an isolated finding, it has little prognostic significance. In conjunction with other electrocardiographic findings or in specific situations, however, the pattern may be more important. RBBB is more common than left bundle branch block, possibly because the right bundle branch is smaller and follows a longer course than the left bundle, thereby making it more prone to damage from infiltration or fibrosis. It is not uncommon to see RBBB in association with trauma, either external (such as after chest trauma) or internal (during the placement of a pulmonary artery catheter). It can also be present in more serious conditions such as pulmonary hypertension and idiopathic fibrosis of the conduction system (Lenegre's disease).

Delay in or failure of conduction in the right bundle branch results in a delay in activation of the right ventricle while left ventricular depolarization remains normal. The initial portion of ventricular depolarization (septal depolarization by fibers of the left bundle branch) is normal, whereas the terminal portion, which consists in part of muscle-to-muscle conduction of the impulse within the right ventricle, results in a prolonged QRS complex with terminal forces that are directed rightward. The criteria for the diagnosis of RBBB

BOX 12-2
Diagnostic Criteria for Conduction Abnormalities

A. Right bundle branch block (RBBB)
  1. QRS duration of 0.12 sec or more
  2. An rsr′, rsR′, or rSR′ pattern in leads V_1 or V_2
  3. Wide (>40 msec) S waves in leads I and V_6
  4. Time to R wave peak in lead V_1 >0.05 sec and normal in leads V_5 and V_6
B. Left bundle branch block (LBBB)
  1. QRS duration of 0.12 sec or more
  2. Broad and notched or slurred R waves in leads I, aV_L, V_5, and V_6
  3. Absent Q waves in leads I, V_5, and V_6
  4. Time to R wave peak in leads V_5 and V_6 >0.06 seconds and normal in leads V_1 and V_2
  5. Small initial R waves in leads V_1 and V_2
C. Left anterior fascicular block (LAFB)*
  1. Left axis deviation of −45 degrees to −90 degrees
  2. A qR pattern in lead aV_L
  3. Time to R wave peak in aV_L greater than 0.045 sec
  4. QRS duration less than 0.12 sec
D. Left posterior fascicular block (LPFB)
  1. Right axis deviation of +90 degrees to +180 degrees
  2. An rS configuration in leads I and aV_L and Q waves in leads III and aV_F
  3. QRS duration of less than 0.12 sec

Modified from Willems JL et al: Criteria for intraventricular conduction disturbances and pre-excitation, *J Am Coll Cardiol* 5:1261, 1985.
*Warner et al. have proposed a simple means of determining the presence of LAFB, which involves an analysis of the time at which the peak of the R wave occurs in simultaneously recorded tracings of leads aV_R and aV_L. During normal ventricular depolarization, the R wave peak in aV_R should occur before the peak in lead aV_L. This study showed that in LAFB, the R wave peak in lead aV_L occurred before the peak in lead aV_R. This method was found to be more sensitive and specific than the traditional criteria. The method, which has not been widely used, requires simultaneous recordings of leads aV_L and aV_R.

---

are shown in Box 12-2, and the QRS morphology is demonstrated in Fig. 12-8. Because ventricular depolarization is abnormal, ventricular repolarization is altered, typically resulting in ST-T segment depression and T wave inversion in leads V_1 and V_2, and occasionally in lead V_3. These changes can obscure the electrocardiographic manifestations of ischemia or infarction.

Left Bundle Branch Block

In contrast to RBBB, left bundle branch block (LBBB) is usually associated with organic heart disease and is only occasionally seen in normal subjects. It is commonly seen in association with longstanding hypertension, coronary disease, dilated cardiomyopathies, degenerative conduction system disease, and calcific aortic valvular disease.

Delay in or failure of conduction in the left bundle branch changes the sequence of ventricular depolarization beginning with altered septal depolarization, resulting in significantly altered QRS morphology. Ventricular depolarization begins in the right ventricle and subsequently proceeds in part by slow muscle-to-muscle conduction in a leftward direction. The criteria for LBBB are shown in Box 12-2, and representative QRS morphology is shown in Fig. 12-8. With LBBB ventricular repolarization is altered such that the ST segments are isoelectric or depressed and the T waves inverted in leads I, aV_L, V_5, and V_6. Because of these abnormalities of repolarization, the diagnosis of myocardial ischemia or infarction is obscured and cannot be made with certainty.

Fascicular Blocks

The left bundle branch consists of two major divisions, an anterosuperior and an inferoposterior fascicle. Conditions that affect the left bundle branch before the bifurcation or that affect both fascicles lead to an LBBB pattern. Isolated delay in or block of conduction in the anterosuperior division of the left bundle branch—left anterior fascicular block (LAFB)—is generally associated with structural heart

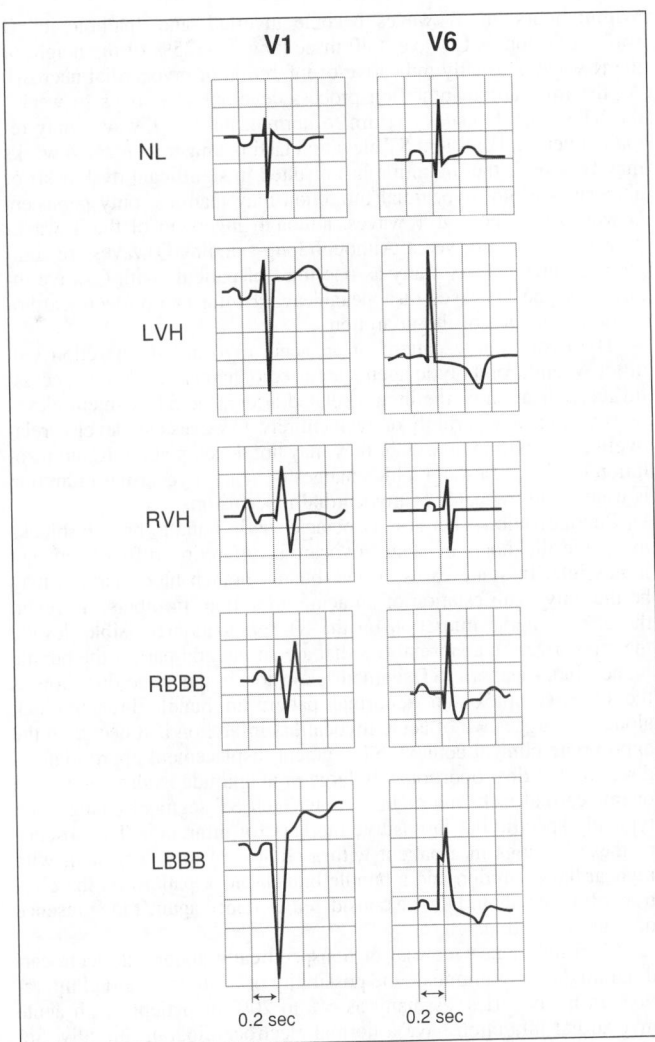

V1   V6

NL

LVH

RVH

RBBB

LBBB

0.2 sec   0.2 sec

FIGURE 12-8 The morphology of right bundle branch block *(RBBB)*, left bundle branch block *(LBBB)*, left ventricular hypertrophy *(LVH)*, and right ventricular hypertrophy *(RVH)* in leads V_1 and V_6 compared to normal *(NL)*.

disease, usually hypertensive heart disease or coronary artery disease. In LAFB, ventricular depolarization occurs via the right bundle branch and the posterior fascicle of the left bundle branch. As a result, the anterior and lateral walls of the left ventricle are depolarized last. The mean QRS vector in the frontal plane is thereby deviated to the left. The criteria for LAFB are shown in Box 12-2.

Left posterior fascicular block (LPFB) is rarer than LAFB and is often associated with RBBB. In LPFB, ventricular depolarization occurs via the right bundle branch and the anterior fascicle of the left bundle branch. Thus the inferoposterior wall of the left ventricle is depolarized last, deviating the mean frontal plane QRS vector to the right. Criteria for the diagnosis of LPFB are shown in Box 12-2. The diagnosis of LPFB should be confirmed on clinical grounds, and other causes of right axis deviation, particularly right ventricular hypertrophy, should be excluded.

Other Conduction Abnormalities

Often, the morphology of LBBB or RBBB is present, but the QRS duration is less than 0.12 sec, leaving an important criterion for the diagnosis of these conditions unfulfilled. *Incomplete LBBB* or *incomplete RBBB* are terms used when all of the criteria for bundle branch block exist except QRS duration prolongation. Incomplete bundle branch block patterns are often associated with ventricular hypertrophy.

When the diagnostic criteria for RBBB exist together with the criteria for either LAFB or LPFB, bifascicular block is said to exist.

Chamber Enlargement and Hypertrophy

The electrocardiogram can be useful in detecting the presence of chamber enlargement and hypertrophy. Typically, electrocardiographic signs of chamber enlargement are specific, but relatively insensitive, meaning that their presence indicates that the presence of chamber enlargement is highly likely, but their absence does not eliminate the possibility that chamber enlargement exists.

Left Ventricular Hypertrophy

The diagnosis of left ventricular hypertrophy (LVH) is important for several reasons. First, LVH may be a manifestation of end-organ damage, most commonly resulting from long-standing arterial hypertension, but also from aortic stenosis and dilated and hypertrophic cardiomyopathy. Second, the electrocardiographic pattern of LVH with associated repolarization abnormality has been correlated with a significant increase in cardiovascular mortality. Finally, LVH is a common cause of alterations in the ST segments and T waves and can confound the diagnosis of myocardial ischemia and infarction.

The electrocardiographic pattern of LVH results from an increase in left ventricular mass. As a result, the wave of depolarization takes longer to traverse the ventricle and creates a depolarization vector of greater magnitude. The result is a QRS complex that is taller in the leftward leads, more prominently negative in the right-sided leads, and slightly wider. LVH thus causes an exaggeration of the normal QRS pattern.

A number of criteria have been developed that indicate the presence of LVH. When compared to autopsy or echocardiogram, these criteria are generally insensitive but highly specific for the presence of an increased left ventricular mass. The sensitivities of the most commonly used criteria range from 15% to 40% (that is, an increased left ventricular mass is difficult to rule out based on the absence of any of these findings). On the other hand, the specificities range from 93% to 98% (that is, an increased left ventricular mass is highly likely in the presence of the findings when the criteria are applied to the appropriate patient populations). The criteria that perform best with respect to sensitivity and specificity for the diagnosis of LVH are the Cornell voltage criteria (approximate sensitivity of 40% and specificity of 95%): if the sum of the magnitude of the R wave in lead aV_L plus the magnitude of the S wave in V_3 exceeds 28 mm in men or 20 mm in women (assuming a normal standard of 0.1 mV/mm), LVH is present. The Sokolow-Lyon criteria, with a sensitivity of 25% and specificity of 97%, require that the height of the R wave in lead aV_L is greater than 11 mm (or 13 mm if left axis deviation is present), or the height of the R wave in V_5 or V_6 exceeds 25 mm, or the sum of the depth of the S wave in lead V_1 plus the height of the R wave in V_5 or V_6 exceeds 35 mm. The Romhilt-Estes score involves assigning points on the basis of not only increased QRS amplitudes, but also the presence of characteristic ST segment abnormalities, left atrial enlargement, and left axis deviation.

ST segment and T wave abnormalities are common in LVH. These are often referred to as a *strain* pattern, although there is no physiologic reason to support the use of this term, and its use should be discouraged. Typically, the ST segments and T waves in LVH are oriented opposite to the main deflection of the QRS complex. Thus in the left-sided leads (leads I, aV_L, V_5 and V_6), in which the QRS complex is largely positive, the ST segment will be depressed and the T wave inverted. Similarly, in leads V_1 and V_2, in which the QRS complex is largely negative, the ST segments will be elevated and the T waves upright (see Fig. 12-8).

Right Ventricular Hypertrophy (RVH)

Right ventricular hypertrophy (RVH) can result from a number of conditions, including some forms of congenital heart disease, long-standing mitral stenosis, and pulmonary disease. The diagnosis of RVH, similar to that of LVH, is based on relatively insensitive criteria. RVH should be considered whenever the mean QRS axis in the frontal plane is deviated to the right. In addition to right axis deviation, other criteria for the diagnosis of RVH include an R/S ratio in precordial lead V_1 >1 without other evidence of posterior wall myocardial infarction, an R wave in lead V_1 greater than 7 mm in height, or an S wave >7 mm in precordial leads V_5 or V_6. A right intraventricular conduction delay also may be present. All of these findings might be expected in the context of an enlarged or hypertrophied right

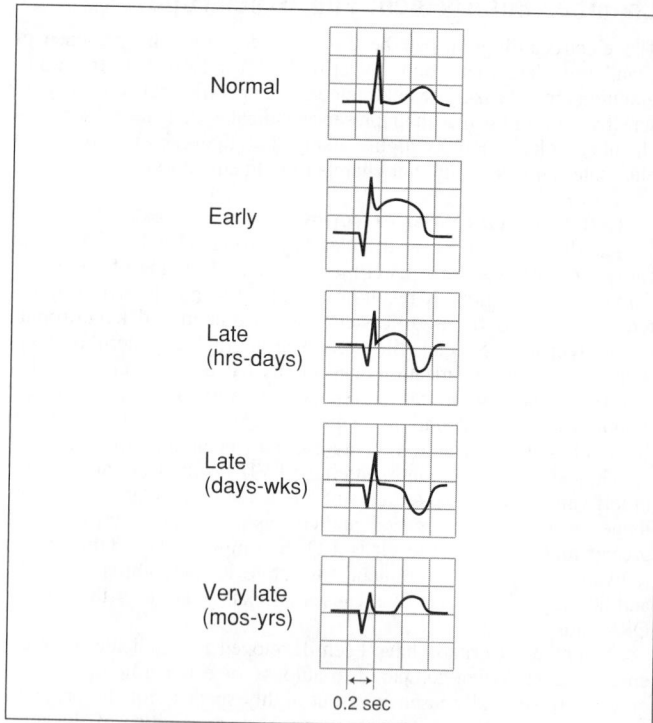

Normal

Early

Late
(hrs-days)

Late
(days-wks)

Very late
(mos-yrs)

0.2 sec

FIGURE 12-9 Schema of the evolution of a myocardial infarction.

ventricle, where the QRS, which under normal circumstances mainly reflects left ventricular depolarization, is overshadowed by right ventricular forces (see Fig. 12-8).

Atrial Abnormalities

Left atrial abnormality refers to a pattern that can occur with left atrial hypertrophy or dilation or with any process such as atrial fibrosis in which atrial conduction and depolarization are delayed. It is misleading therefore to use the term *atrial enlargement,* a commonly used phrase.

The initial component of the P wave is caused predominantly by right atrial depolarization and its latter part predominantly by left atrial depolarization. In left atrial abnormality, the latter (left atrial) part of the P wave is exaggerated. The criteria for left atrial abnormality are a biphasic P wave in lead V_1 with a negative terminal component larger than 1 mm (0.04 sec) in duration and 1 mm (0.01 mV) in height. A broad, notched P wave of more than 0.12 sec in duration in lead II is also highly suggestive of left atrial abnormality.

The electrocardiographic diagnosis of right atrial abnormality is suggested by a P wave greater than 2.5 mm in height in lead II or more than 1.5 mm in height in precordial leads V_1 or V_2. Because of the strong correlation between right atrial hypertrophy and right ventricular hypertrophy, the mean QRS axis in the frontal plane is often deviated rightward.

Ischemic Heart Disease

Acute Myocardial Infarction

Electrocardiography is a mainstay in the diagnosis of acute myocardial infarction, along with clinical history and assays for serum enzyme levels (Chapter 23). The electrocardiographic diagnosis of acute myocardial infarction requires that the characteristic findings develop over time, and thus serial electrocardiograms are required in the acute setting. The classic electrocardiographic changes during acute myocardial infarction are schematized in Fig. 12-9. In the earliest stages of infarction, the T waves become tall and peaked, indicative of acute myocardial ischemia. If ischemia persists for more than a few minutes, a pattern of injury develops. This pattern consists of elevation of the ST segments, typically with an upward convexity. Although this pattern of ST segment elevation indicates transmural ischemic injury, it is not indicative of myocardial necrosis.

Within hours, the T waves become inverted, and "pathologic" Q waves develop. A Q wave >40 msec long or ≥25% of the height of the R wave is usually indicative of infarction or myocardial necrosis. As the myocardial infarction process develops over days to weeks, the ST segments usually return to normal, but the T waves may remain inverted. Persistent ST elevation lasting longer than 2 to 4 weeks may be seen if the infarction has resulted in significant dyskinesis or akinesis. An old myocardial infarction may manifest only persistent Q waves with normal T waves, although inversion of the T waves may also persist for years. Although long-standing Q waves are common, occurring in as many as one third of patients with Q-wave infarctions, the Q waves disappear, leaving little or no electrocardiographic evidence of the infarction.

The evolutionary pattern of an acute myocardial infarction will differ when thrombolytic agents are used (Chapter 23). With successful recanalization of the infarct-related artery, the ST segment elevations will resolve partially or even entirely. Q waves can develop relatively early (within hours), or they may not develop at all. Rapid resolution of electrocardiographic changes of acute myocardial infarction is used as an indicator of myocardial reperfusion.

Repolarization changes associated with bundle branch blocks make the diagnosis of acute myocardial infarction difficult but not impossible. In some cases, a new bundle branch block pattern may be the only manifestation of an acute infarction. In others, however, the effects of the infarction on the ST segments are visible despite the repolarization abnormalities that are an integral part of the bundle branch block pattern. ST segment elevation in the same direction as the QRS complex—an abnormal pattern in bundle branch block alone—is suggestive of acute myocardial infarction if it occurs in the appropriate clinical context. ST segment displacement appropriate in direction but disproportionately large in magnitude is also suggestive of myocardial ischemia or infarction. Such ST segment changes are typically specific but insensitive markers for infarction. The absence of these findings in a patient with a clinical history consistent with myocardial infarction and a bundle branch block pattern on the electrocardiogram should not be considered evidence against the presence of acute infarction.

A normal or near normal or nonspecifically abnormal electrocardiogram does not eliminate the possibility of acute myocardial infarction. In many series, as many as 6% to 20% of patients with acute myocardial infarction have a normal electrocardiogram initially. Serial tracings, however, often confirm the diagnosis, and abnormalities are seen at some point in the majority of patients.

The electrocardiographic findings in acute myocardial infarction occur generally in leads that correspond, albeit not precisely, to the location of the infarction. The distribution of the electrocardiographic changes and the number of leads involved may provide important prognostic information. For instance, anterior wall myocardial infarctions are associated with a worse prognosis than are inferior wall infarctions, and the prognosis in anterior infarction worsens with an increasing number of leads involved.

The electrocardiographic abnormalities recorded during acute myocardial infarction will occur in the leads facing the area of injury and infarction. Thus if the anterior wall of the left ventricle is involved, the electrocardiographic changes occur in leads V_1 through V_6. Abnormalities occurring only in leads V_1 and V_2 are designated as septal infarction; those involving leads V_1 through V_4 are designated as anteroseptal infarction; those involving only leads V_5 and V_6 are designated as apical infarction. Involvement of leads I and aV_L occurs in an anterolateral infarction, and these changes are frequently accompanied by apical involvement. The correlation of the infarction site with the electrocardiographic leads involved, however, is not high and depends in part on body habitus and heart size.

Acute infarction patterns involving leads II, III, and aV_F are seen during acute inferior wall infarction. When these are present, it is important to look carefully for involvement in "contiguous" areas of the electrocardiogram, because prognosis is affected by the extent of the infarction. These areas include the right ventricle and the apex, posterior wall, and septum of the left ventricle. Right ventricular infarction is diagnosed by recording right-sided precordial leads V_{1R} through V_{6R} (see Fig. 12-4); ST elevation in these leads confirms the diagnosis. The finding with the highest sensitivity and specificity for right ventricular infarction is ST elevation exceeding 1 mm in lead

V_{4R}. In all cases of suspected or documented inferior wall infarction, right-sided precordial leads should be recorded. Apical injury is indicated by ST segment elevations in leads V_5 and V_6. Posterior wall infarction is suggested if there is ST depression with tall R waves in leads V_1 and V_2, which are the leads that face away from the posterior wall. These abnormalities are the mirror image of the ST segment elevations and deep Q waves typically seen in transmural infarction. ST elevation and Q waves can be seen in leads placed on the patient's back, which face the posterior wall of the left ventricle.

During acute myocardial infarction it is not uncommon to see ST depressions in leads opposite the area of ST segment elevation. These ST segment depressions are called *reciprocal changes*. They can be seen in leads III and aV_F when there is primary ST elevation in leads I and aV_L, and in leads I and aV_L when there is ST elevation in leads II, III, and aV_F. ST segment depression in leads V_1 and V_2 and occasionally in leads V_3 and V_4 in the context of an acute inferior wall myocardial infarction are reciprocal changes indicative of posterior wall infarction. Reciprocal changes, which will occur only in the context of myocardial injury, can be helpful in the differential diagnosis of ST segment elevation, as such changes should not occur with other causes of ST segment abnormalities such as pericarditis. ST depression in leads that are remote from the acute myocardial infarction pattern may also represent myocardial ischemia in a territory separate from the infarction.

A patient often will have an acute myocardial infarction by clinical history accompanied by electrocardiographic abnormalities but will not develop Q waves. In the past, infarction accompanied by Q waves was considered to result from transmural infarction, whereas an infarction not accompanied by Q waves was thought to result from subendocardial, nontransmural infarction. Correlation between Q waves and transmural necrosis has not been confirmed by pathologic evaluation. There are differences, however, in outcome between patients with Q wave and non–Q wave infarction. Patients with Q wave infarction tend to have a higher early mortality from their infarction, whereas patients with non–Q wave infarction have a lower in-hospital mortality but a higher late mortality (Chapter 23). One year after infarction, both groups have a similar risk of death, with the majority of the deaths in the Q wave group occurring in the acute phase (within the first month). These differences in outcome have been significantly altered by the advent of new therapies for myocardial infarction.

Chronic Ischemic Heart Disease

Aside from the presence of Q waves in the context of an old myocardial infarction, the electrocardiographic findings in ischemic heart disease are nonspecific. Nonspecific ST-T changes are common and include ST segment depression and flat or inverted T waves (Chapter 22).

Acute Pericarditis

The diagnosis of acute pericarditis can be difficult because, similar to myocardial ischemia and infarction, it causes chest pain and is accompanied by ST segment and T wave abnormalities on the electrocardiogram (Chapter 27). There are some important differences between the electrocardiographic manifestations of pericarditis and those of ischemia and infarction. In the early stage of pericarditis, there is elevation of the J point and the ST segments. In contrast to infarction, however, in which the ST segment elevations are typically located in a set of contiguous leads and in which reciprocal ST depressions may be seen, the ST segments in pericarditis are often diffusely elevated, and ST depressions do not occur (except in lead aV_R). The ST segments in pericarditis are usually flat or concave upward, in contrast to those seen in myocardial infarction (Fig. 12-10, *A*). Abnormalities of the PR segments are frequently seen in pericarditis. Most often, the PR segments are depressed in precordial leads V_2 through V_6, but PR segment depression also can be seen in the limb leads. PR segment elevation also can be seen in lead aV_R; however, PR segment abnormalities are not specific for pericarditis. Although they are rare in myocardial infarction, they can be seen in the relatively rare case of atrial infarction. Over the ensuing 2 weeks, the diffusely elevated ST segments normalize. Finally, T wave inversions occur. Although T wave inversions may persist indefinitely, the electrocardiogram usually returns to normal.

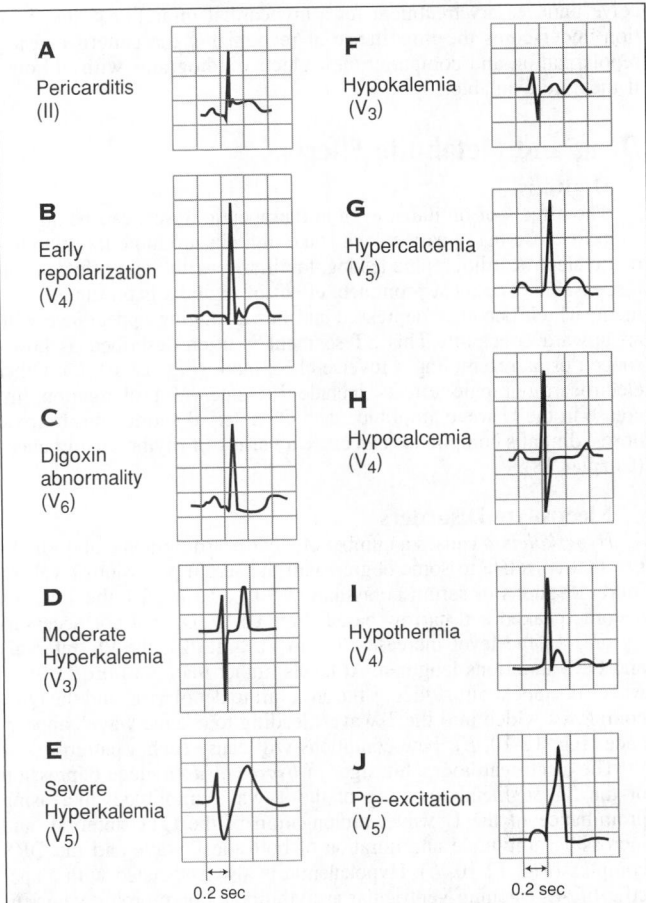

FIGURE 12-10   Other electrocardiographic abnormalities shown in leads where the abnormalities are often most prominent: **A**, early acute pericarditis; **B**, "early repolarization"; **C**, digitalis effect; **D**, moderate hyperkalemia; **E**, severe hyperkalemia; **F**, hypokalemia; **G**, hypercalcemia; **H**, hypocalcemia; **I**, hypothermia; **J**, Wolff-Parkinson-White pattern.

Other electrocardiographic features are helpful in distinguishing pericarditis from acute myocardial infarction; Q waves are absent, in the former, and frequently evolve in the latter. Also, the electrocardiographic resolution of pericarditis typically occurs within weeks, whereas that of acute myocardial infarction may take months. Because these last two features are apparent only after the passage of time, they are of no use in the acute setting.

The pathologic process causing the pericardial inflammation may result in the accumulation of a significant amount of fluid in the pericardial space. Several electrocardiographic findings have been attributed to pericardial effusion (Chapter 27): decreased QRS voltage, variations in the QRS and T wave magnitudes from one complex to the next ("electrical alternans"), flattening of the T wave, and notching of the P waves. In practice, however, the electrocardiographic findings of pericardial effusion are too insensitive and nonspecific to be of clinical use.

Early Repolarization

This electrocardiographic finding, characterized by J point elevation, is a variant of normal, usually seen in young men. The ST segment itself has a normal configuration. Early repolarization may be confused with myocardial injury or pericarditis. The pattern is best seen in leads V_2 through V_5, and rarely in lead V_6. It is generally not seen in the limb leads. In early repolarization, the downstroke of the R wave is notched at the point where it merges with the ST segment. This J point and the takeoff of the ST segment are elevated. An upward concavity characterizes the ST segment. Reciprocal changes in other leads do not occur (Fig. 12-10, *B*). On occasion, a patient with this normal variant finding will complain of chest pain and will receive unnecessary treatment for a myocardial infarction. This situation underscores the importance of recognizing the pattern of early repolarization and comparing new electrocardiograms with old ones if they are available.

Drug and Metabolic Effects

Digitalis

The effects of digitalis, even in therapeutic doses, can be significant. Because many patients who take digitalis are more likely to undergo electrocardiographic testing, familiarity with these effects is indispensable. The most prominent effect of digitalis is on the ST segment, which becomes depressed and has a sagging appearance with an upward concavity. This ST segment is often described as bowl-shaped or as resembling a reverse checkmark (Fig. 12-10, *C*). Other electrocardiographic effects include PR interval prolongation, increase in the U wave amplitude, and QT interval shortening. In toxic doses, digitalis compounds can cause a variety of rhythm disturbances (Chapter 18).

Electrolyte Disorders

Hyperkalemia causes a number of electrocardiographic abnormalities that correlate to some degree with the serum potassium level. At mild elevations of serum potassium (5.5 to 6.5 mEq/L), the T waves become peaked and narrow based (Fig. 12-10, *D*), but not necessarily tall. As the level increases (6.5 to 7.5 mEq/L), the PR intervals and QRS durations lengthen. At levels higher than 7.5 mEq/L, the P waves disappear altogether as the atria fail to depolarize, and the QRS complexes widen into the T waves, leading to a "sine wave" appearance (Fig. 12-10, *E*). Few conditions will cause such a pattern.

The electrocardiographic signs of *hypokalemia* include depression of the ST segment, lowering of the T wave amplitude, increasing prominence of the U wave, prolongation of the QTU interval, and increasing amplitude and duration of both the P wave and the QRS complex (Fig. 12-10, *F*). Hypokalemia is also associated with a specific life-threatening ventricular arrhythmia, a polymorphic ventricular tachycardia known as torsades de pointes (Chapter 18).

Hypercalcemia causes shortening of the QT interval. In addition, the T waves characteristically have an abrupt upslope and a gradual downslope (Fig. 12-10, *G*). PR interval prolongation and J waves also may be seen. *Hypocalcemia* will produce QT interval prolongation through lengthening of the Q-T segment. The QRS and T wave durations themselves remain normal (Fig. 12-10, *H*).

Hypothermia

At body temperatures less than 34° C, the electrocardiogram may manifest characteristic changes of hypothermia. These changes include bradycardia, lengthening of the PR, QRS, and QT intervals, and the development of J waves. The J wave is found in the terminal part of the QRS complex (Fig. 12-10, *I*), and is usually best seen in leads V_3 and V_4.

Myxedema

Myxedema produces a "low and slow" electrocardiographic picture. The T waves are of low amplitude or inverted, the QRS voltage is low, and the rate is slow. This constellation of findings should prompt an investigation of thyroid function.

Accessory Pathways

Accessory pathways (Fig. 12-10, *J*) are abnormal connections between portions of the atrial and ventricular tissue. In the presence of some accessory pathways, the wave of depolarization from the atria can depolarize the ventricles directly, bypassing the normal route of depolarization, including the AV node to varying degrees. In many, but not all, cases of these "extranodal" accessory pathways, because the AV node is bypassed, the PR interval is shortened. Accessory pathways occur in a number of locations, some involving the AV node and His bundle, and others entirely removed from these structures. In cases where the accessory pathway is extranodal and the ventricle is preexcited through the pathway, ventricular depolarization may be sufficiently disordered to cause abnormalities in the QRS complex. The classic pattern of such a pathway, the Wolff-Parkinson-White

(WPW) pattern, consists of a short PR interval and a slurring of the initial portion of the QRS complex. This slurring, called the *delta wave,* represents preexcitation of the ventricular myocardium and intramyocardial conduction of the depolarization impulse that has entered the ventricles via the accessory pathway. The remainder of the QRS complex represents the net contribution of two separate waves of depolarization: one originating from the accessory pathway and the other from the normal route of conduction through the AV node, His bundle, and Purkinje system. Depending on the location of the accessory pathway, the mean QRS axis in the frontal plane may also be abnormal (see Box 12-1). Because the WPW pattern may have features that mimic myocardial infarction, LVH, and RVH, these diagnoses cannot be established in the presence of an electrocardiographically evident extranodal accessory pathway.

Electronic Pacemakers

The effects of cardiac pacemakers on the electrocardiogram depend on which chambers are paced and in which chambers sensing of the intracardiac electrical signal occurs. The right atrium, right ventricle, or both can be stimulated by implanted transvenous pacemaker leads. The electrical stimulus generated by the pacemaker occurs over a very short period of time (1 msec or less). As a result, the pacemaker stimuli are recorded on the electrocardiogram as sharp artifacts of variable amplitude that are too brief to be mistaken for native cardiac electrical activity. They may be of too low a magnitude in some surface leads to be appreciated, and simultaneous recording of multiple ECG leads is mandatory for an accurate interpretation of pacemaker activity.

If the atrium is paced, a pacemaker stimulus artifact will precede the P wave. The P wave morphology and axis will depend on the location of the pacemaker lead in the atrial endocardium and the consequent atrial depolarization pathway. If the ventricle is paced, a pacemaker stimulus artifact will precede the QRS complex. The QRS complex itself will be wide because the wave of depolarization depends on relatively slow muscle-to-muscle propagation of the impulse. The most common site for a ventricular pacing lead is the right ventricular endocardium at the apex, although on occasion, the lead is positioned along the interventricular septum. The right ventricle is depolarized first, and the depolarization wavefront passes slowly throughout the ventricles until the left ventricle depolarizes, creating a pattern resembling left bundle branch block. The abnormal pattern of depolarization, and therefore repolarization, which results from ventricular pacing, makes meaningful interpretation of ST segment and T wave abnormalities impossible.

BIBLIOGRAPHY

Castellanos A, Myerburg RJ: Electrocardiography. In Schlant RC, Alexander RW, Lipton MJ (editors): *Atlas of the heart,* New York, 1996, McGraw-Hill.

Flowers NC: Left bundle branch block: a continuously evolving concept, *J Am Coll Cardiol* 9:684, 1987.

Gold BS et al: The utility of preoperative electrocardiograms in the ambulatory surgical patient, *Arch Intern Med* 152:301, 1992.

Goldschlager N, Goldman MJ: *Principles of clinical electrocardiography,* ed 13, East Norwalk, Conn, 1989, Appleton & Lange.

Haisty WK et al: Recognition of electrocardiographic electrode misplacements involving the ground (right leg) electrode, *Am J Cardiol* 71:1490, 1993.

Hands ME et al: Electrocardiographic diagnosis of myocardial infarction in the presence of complete left bundle branch block, *Am Heart J* 116:23, 1988.

Hazen MS, Marwick TH, Underwood DA: Diagnostic accuracy of the resting electrocardiogram in detection and estimation of left atrial enlargement: an echocardiographic correlation in 551 patients, *Am Heart J* 122:823, 1991.

Levy D et al: Determinants of sensitivity and specificity of electrocardiographic criteria for left ventricular hypertrophy, *Circulation* 81:815, 1990.

Meyers DG, Bagin RG, Levene JF: Electrocardiographic changes in pericardial effusion, *Chest* 104:1422, 1993.

Rouan GW et al: Clinical characteristics and outcome of acute myocardial infarction in patients with initially normal or nonspecific electrocardiograms (a report from the Multicenter Chest Pain Study), *Am J Cardiol* 64:1087, 1989.

Schlant RC et al: Guidelines for electrocardiography: a report of the American College of Cardiology/American Heart Association task force on assessment of diagnostic and therapeutic cardiovascular procedures, *J Am Coll Cardiol* 19:473, 1992.

Sgarbossa EB et al: Electrocardiographic diagnosis of evolving acute myocardial infarction in the presence of left bundle-branch block, *N Engl J Med* 334:481, 1996.

Spodick DH: Differential characteristics of the electrocardiogram in early polarization and acute pericarditis, *N Engl J Med* 295:523, 1976.

Tan HL et al: Electrophysiologic mechanisms of the long QT interval syndromes and torsade de pointes, *Ann Intern Med* 122:701, 1995.

Vandenberg BF, Romhilt DW: Electrocardiographic diagnosis of left ventricular hypertrophy in the presence of bundle branch block, *Am Heart J* 122:818, 1991.

Warner RA et al: Improved electrocardiographic criteria for the diagnosis of left anterior hemiblock, *Am J Cardiol* 51:723, 1983.

Willems JL et al: Criteria for intraventricular conduction disturbances and pre-excitation, *J Am Coll Cardiol* 5:1261, 1985.

Wong ND, Levy D, Kannel WB: Prognostic significance of the electrocardiogram after Q wave myocardial infarction: the Framingham study, *Circulation* 81:780, 1990.

Zehender M et al: Right ventricular infarction as an independent predictor of prognosis after acute inferior myocardial infarction, *N Engl J Med* 328:981, 1993.

CHAPTER

13 Cardiac Noninvasive Techniques

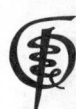

George A. Beller and Sanjiv Kaul

Cardiac noninvasive techniques refer to those diagnostic procedures that do not necessitate the placement of intravascular or intracardiac catheters. This chapter includes information on all frequently used noninvasive cardiac diagnostic methods except standard electrocardiography (Chapter 12). In ordering noninvasive tests, the physician should reflect on the quality of the available laboratory for performing the test(s), the accuracy and cost of the test(s) compared with alternative diagnostic methods, and the influence of test results on subsequent clinical decision making.

CHEST RADIOGRAPH

Before the advent of echocardiography, the chest radiograph was the only means of estimating cardiac size and status of the pulmonary vasculature. The radiograph is still useful in determining associated pulmonary pathology in patients with cardiac disorders and in determining the presence of pulmonary edema, particularly when other pulmonary conditions (e.g., pneumonia) coexist. Mediastinal widening on the chest radiograph may be the first indication of aortic pathology (e.g., dissection, aneurysm).

Figure 13-1 illustrates the cardiac structures that can be seen in different views on the chest radiograph. Because the cardiac silhouette represents a "summation" planar image, it is difficult to determine the exact cause of increased heart size, which can occur from enlargement of any chamber or the presence of pericardial effusion. Images from different views (Fig. 13-1, *A* to *D*) sometimes can assist in this purpose. Certain characteristic features on the cardiac silhouette and pulmonary vasculature are noted in specific cardiac conditions such as mitral stenosis (Chapter 25) and left-to-right cardiac shunts (Chapter 28). A rough estimate of the severity of these conditions can be derived from the chest radiograph. Echocardiography (with Doppler), however, provides more accurate assessments of these conditions and generally has replaced the radiograph for this purpose.

The findings of pulmonary venous congestion, such as prominent superior pulmonary veins, interstitial or alveolar edema, Kerley B lines, and the presence of fluid in the interlobar fissures, are usually noted with left atrial pressures greater than 20 mm Hg (Chapter 19). When these findings are present on the radiograph, they are usually also evident on physical examination. Sometimes, however, coexisting pulmonary disease may make it difficult to separate these from other findings.

Calcification of the aorta or coronary arteries indicates atherosclerosis of these structures. Calcification may also be noted in the mitral annulus, mitral valve, aortic valve, left ventricular (LV) mural thrombus, LV aneurysm, or left atrial or LV tumors. The presence and type of prosthetic valve can also be seen, and correct placement of a pacemaker lead can be confirmed on the chest radiograph.

The presence of dextrocardia, with or without situs inversus, may assist in the echocardiographic examination, particularly in the identification of abnormally placed structures. Classic radiographic patterns, such as a "boot-shaped" heart (Chapter 28), are usually associated with tetralogy of Fallot and may narrow the differential diagnosis in a child with central cyanosis. An anomalous pulmonary vein draining into the inferior vena cava may lead to the "scimitar" sign. Similarly, increased pulmonary vasculature may indicate the presence of undetected left-to-right cardiac shunts, and lack of pulmonary vasculature may indicate pulmonic or subpulmonic stenosis (Chapter 28).

In summary, the chest radiograph has had an important historical role in the evaluation of patients with cardiac disorders and is still useful, particularly in determining coexisting pulmonary pathology.

EXERCISE ELECTROCARDIOGRAPHIC TESTING

Electrocardiographic (ECG) stress testing is a clinically valuable technique that provides important diagnostic and prognostic information in patients with suspected or known coronary artery disease. The two major types of muscular exercise that can be used to stress the cardiovascular system are isometric (static) and isotonic (dynamic). Exercise is considered *isometric* when sustained muscular contraction occurs without motion (e.g., with handgrip), whereas isotonic exercise is defined as muscular contraction that results in some motion (e.g., running). Isometric exercise, which primarily presents a pressure load to the left ventricle, is rarely used for diagnostic ECG stress testing but can be used as an adjunct to pharmacologic stress, as with intravenous (IV) dipyridamole or adenosine infusion. *Isotonic* exercise, which imposes a volume load to the left ventricle, is the preferred mode of exercise used for stress testing, and the cardiovascular response to isotonic exercise is proportional to the intensity of the exercise.

Physiology

When a subject exercises maximally, the cardiac output may increase from 5 to 25 L/min, which results in increased systemic arterial pressure despite vasodilation in the skeletal muscles, which assists the increase in flow. The increase in stroke volume during exercise varies and depends on the intensity of exercise and the posture in which exercise is performed. Although stroke volume usually increases, the primary mechanism for the rise in cardiac output is augmented heart rate. The increase in heart rate with exercise is attributed to a diminished vagal tone, followed by an increase in sympathetic neural outflow to the heart and blood vessels. Maximum heart rate decreases with age; it usually can be calculated by subtracting the subject's age from 220.

When isotonic exercise commences at a certain intensity, oxygen (O_2) uptake by the lung increases, then remains stable at a steady state after 2 minutes. At this steady state, heart rate, cardiac output, arterial blood pressure, and pulmonary ventilation are maintained at relatively constant levels. The *maximum oxygen uptake* (Vo_{2max}) is the maximum O_2 a person consumes when performing isotonic exercise involving a large part of total muscle mass. For exercise stress testing, the *metabolic equivalent* (MET) is used as a surrogate for Vo_{2max} and is expressed in multiples of resting requirements. One MET is equal to 3.5 ml O_2/kg of body weight/min. A person walking on a level surface at 4 miles/hr would exercise at a workload of 4 METs. Vo_{2max} is also equal to the maximum cardiac output times the maximum arteriovenous O_2 difference. The Vo_{2max} decreases progressively with age. Because cardiac output is equal to the product of stroke volume and heart rate, Vo_2 is directly proportional to heart rate.

Myocardial Vo_2 is the product of heart rate and systolic blood pressure, often referred to as the *double product* or *rate-pressure product*. The major determinants of myocardial Vo_2 include myocardial wall tension, myocardial contractility, and heart rate (Chapter 9). The increase in myocardial O_2 demand during exercise is met by an increase in myocardial blood flow. Regional myocardial ischemia develops during exercise when a patient with a coronary artery stenosis cannot produce enough blood flow to supply the myocardium's increased metabolic needs (Chapter 22). In a patient with symptomatic coronary artery disease, angina pectoris usually occurs at the same double product regardless of the activity.

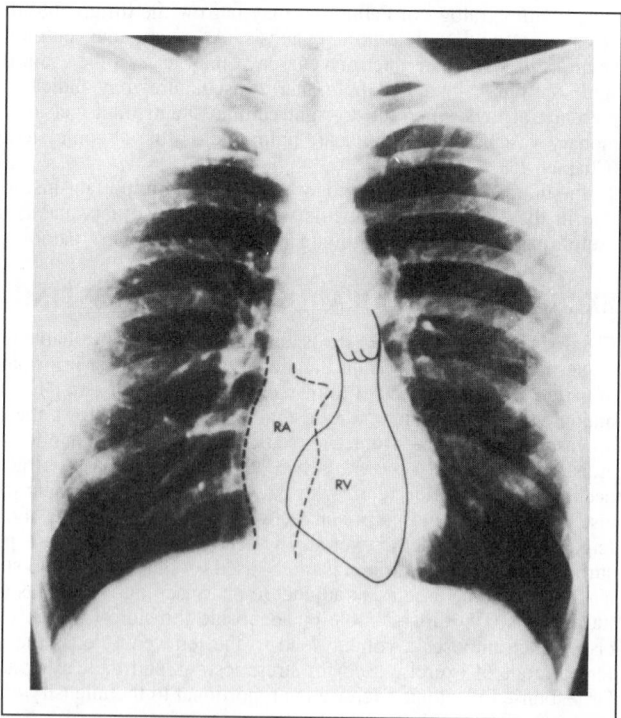

A

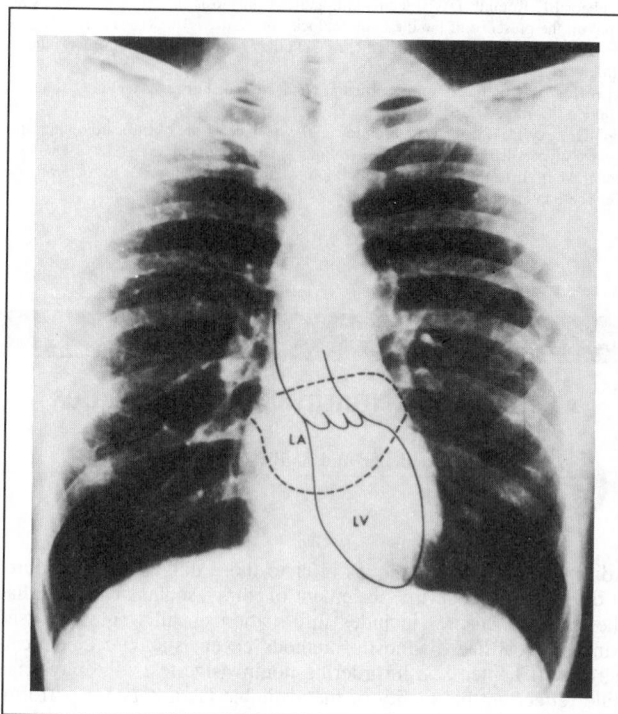

B

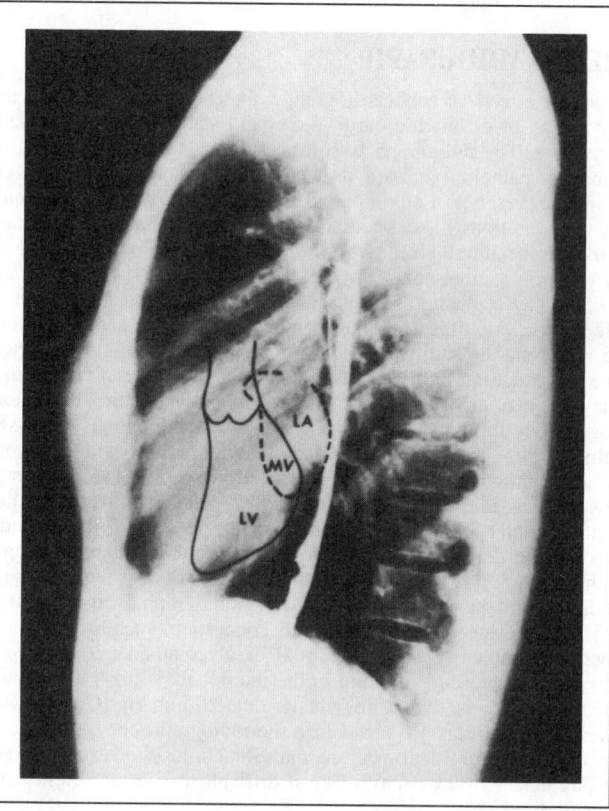

C

D

FIGURE 13-1   Posterior anterior and lateral views of the normal heart showing major structures, including cardiac chambers. **A** and **C,** Right-sided heart chambers; **B** and **D,** left-sided heart chambers. *RA,* Right atrium; *RV,* right ventricle; *TV,* tricuspid valve; *LA,* left atrium; *LV,* left ventricle; *MV,* mitral valve.

(From Dinsmore RE: Chest roentgenography. In Pohost GM, O'Rourke RA, editors: *Principles and practice of cardiovascular imaging,* Boston, 1991, Little, Brown.)

Procedures

Exercise testing should be conducted solely by well-trained personnel with basic knowledge of exercise physiology who are trained to provide cardiopulmonary resuscitation (CPR). Testing should be performed under the supervision of a physician familiar with general indications and contraindications to the test and familiar with normal and abnormal responses. Competency standards for performance of exercise testing have been defined by a joint statement from the American College of Physicians, American College of Cardiology, and American Heart Association Task Force on Clinical Privileges in Cardiology. The physician or physician's assistant responsible for supervising an exercise test must first ask pertinent questions about the patient's medical history, should perform a brief physical examination, and must review a standard 12-lead ECG acquired immediately before testing.

General contraindications to exercise testing for myocardial ischemia include very recent acute myocardial infarction (within 3 to 5 days); active endocarditis; active unstable angina with rest pain; potentially life-threatening arrhythmias; acute pericarditis; severe aortic stenosis; hypertrophic cardiomyopathy; marked elevation of arterial blood pressure (>200 mm Hg systolic or >120 mm Hg diastolic); severe symptomatic LV dysfunction; acute pulmonary embolus or infarction; acute or serious noncardiac disorder; acute thrombophlebitis or deep venous thrombosis; neurologic, musculoskeletal, or arthritic condition precluding adequate exercise; and inability or lack of motivation to perform the test.

Technical Aspects

The ECG recording electrodes are placed on the trunk and should mimic the standard 12-lead conventional system. A recorder designed to capture high-quality ECG data during exercise is mandatory, and microprocessors are useful for generating average waveforms and for making certain ECG measurements. The exercise test can be performed on a treadmill or a mechanically or electrically braked cycle. A treadmill should have both variable-speed and variable-grade capability and must be accurately calibrated. The treadmill should have front and side rails for patients to steady themselves; patients should not tightly grasp siderails because this decreases Vo_2, increases exercise time, and enhances muscle artifact. Bicycle ergometers are most often used to evaluate the functional capacity and response to therapy with cardiovascular drugs in patients with coronary artery disease or heart failure.

Before commencing the exercise test protocol, a 12-lead ECG tracing should be obtained in the standing position when performing treadmill exercise and after voluntary hyperventilation. The latter may induce ST-T wave changes that must be taken into account when interpreting exercise-induced alterations. Clinical testing consists of an initial warm-up load, progressive uninterrupted exercise with an adequate duration at each level, and a recovery period. The 12-lead ECG is recorded each minute, with frequent three-lead recordings taken according to clinical circumstances. Blood pressure determinations are made frequently, and the patient is observed closely for limiting endpoints or complications. The exercise workload is usually changed every 3 minutes, and testing for detection of coronary artery disease is conducted to symptom-limited end-points. The Bruce protocol is the most popular one used in the United States, and its advantages include a seventh or final stage that cannot be completed by most individuals. The optimum protocol should last 6 to 12 minutes and should be individualized to the patient. Submaximum testing is most often conducted during the predischarge phase after recovery from an uncomplicated acute myocardial infarction.

Indications for terminating an exercise test include a drop in systolic blood pressure to below baseline levels despite an increase in exercise workload, new-onset or increasing anginal chest pain, central nervous system symptoms, signs of poor peripheral perfusion, high-grade ventricular arrhythmias, technical difficulties monitoring the ECG or systolic blood pressure, and the patient's request to cease. Frequently a test is terminated when marked (>4.0 mm) ischemic S-T segment depression is observed or new S-T segment elevation appears in leads without Q waves. This latter finding reflects transmural ischemia, which may result from exercise-induced vasospasm or rarely from sudden occlusion of a coronary vessel. Similarly, a less serious arrhythmia (e.g., supraventricular tachycardia) may result in premature termination of the test.

Because abnormal responses may occur only during recovery after exercise, patients should be continuously monitored in the supine position during the postexercise periods for at least 5 minutes.

Clinical Applications

The main indication for exercise testing is to assist in the diagnosis of coronary artery disease in patients with chest pain (Chapter 22). A second major indication is to evaluate functional capacity and aid in assessing the prognosis of patients with known coronary artery disease. When exercise stress is sufficient to produce a mismatch between myocardial O_2 supply and demand, myocardial ischemia will develop and often is identified by certain alterations in the S-T segment of the ECG. Although anginal chest pain induced by the test is strongly predictive of coronary artery disease, 1.0 mm of horizontal or downsloping S-T segment depression is considered a positive endpoint for ischemia (Chapter 12). The S-T depression must persist for 80 msec or longer and must be recognized in at least three consecutive beats with a steady ECG baseline. Slow upsloping S-T segment depression in which the S-T segment is still depressed by 1.0 mm at 0.08 seconds has a 50% predictive value for diagnosing coronary artery disease. Increasing S-T segment elevation often can be seen in leads demonstrating pathologic Q waves at rest in patients with prior myocardial infarction. These changes are predominantly observed in patients with a depressed ejection fraction and severe regional myocardial asynergy.

A review of published studies shows that the sensitivity of exercise ECG stress tests averaged 68%, with average specificity of 77% for detection of coronary artery disease. The extent of coronary artery disease may affect the test's sensitivity. An ischemic ECG response occurs in 85% or more of patients with three-vessel disease, but in only 45% to 50% of patients with single-vessel disease. The administration of antianginal drugs may influence exercise stress test results. Beta-adrenergic blockers, calcium antagonists, and nitrates may prevent the appearance of abnormal S-T segment changes. Beta blockers may prevent the patient from attaining the desired heart rate–blood pressure product at which ischemic S-T segment depression would appear.

An ECG stress test is considered to be "diagnostic" when 85% or more of the maximum predicted heart rate adjusted for age is attained. Sensitivity is reduced if the test is terminated at suboptimum heart rates in the absence of limiting symptoms.

In certain situations, horizontal or downsloping S-T segment depression can appear in the absence of significant coronary artery disease. Causes of false-positive S-T segment responses include ST-T wave abnormalities on the resting ECG caused by digitalis administration, LV hypertrophy, mitral valve prolapse syndrome, hyperventilation, electrolyte abnormalities such as hypokalemia, bundle branch block, Wolff-Parkinson-White syndrome, pericardial disease, systemic hypertension, and noncardiac disorders such as nonischemic cardiomyopathy.

Although sensitivity and specificity values define a test's essential accuracy, the interpretation of any patient's test results depends on the pretest likelihood of coronary artery disease in that individual or in the overall population being tested. Bayes' theorem expresses the posttest likelihood of disease as a function of the test's sensitivity and specificity and the disease's prevalence in the population being tested. A diagnostic test such as exercise electrocardiography is of greatest value with an intermediate probability of disease in the range of 50%, where uncertainty is greatest. In a population with a high prevalence of coronary artery disease, a positive test merely confirms the presence of disease, but a negative test does not exclude disease. In a low-prevalence population, a negative test merely confirms the absence of disease, but a positive test result does not establish disease presence because such a response may represent a false-positive test result.

Conversely, although ECG exercise testing does not add substantially to the diagnosis of coronary artery disease in male patients with typical angina pectoris, the test may be useful for prognostication. Several high-risk exercise test variables are associated with an increased cardiac event rate and a high incidence of left main or three-

---

BOX 13-1

Exercise ECG and thallium-201 (^{201}Tl) imaging variables associated with high-risk coronary artery disease

---

Exercise ECG stress testing

Impairment of exercise tolerance

Ischemic S-T segment depression and/or angina at 4 METs or less

2 mm or more of horizontal or downsloping S-T depression

Ischemic S-T depression lasting longer than 5 minutes into recovery period

S-T depression observed in five or more ECG leads

Decrease in systolic blood pressure of 10 mm Hg or greater with exercise

Exercise ^{201}Tl scintigraphy

Multiple perfusion defects, particularly of the redistribution type, in more than one coronary supply region

Increased lung ^{201}Tl uptake

Transient left ventricular cavity dilation observed on exercise images

---

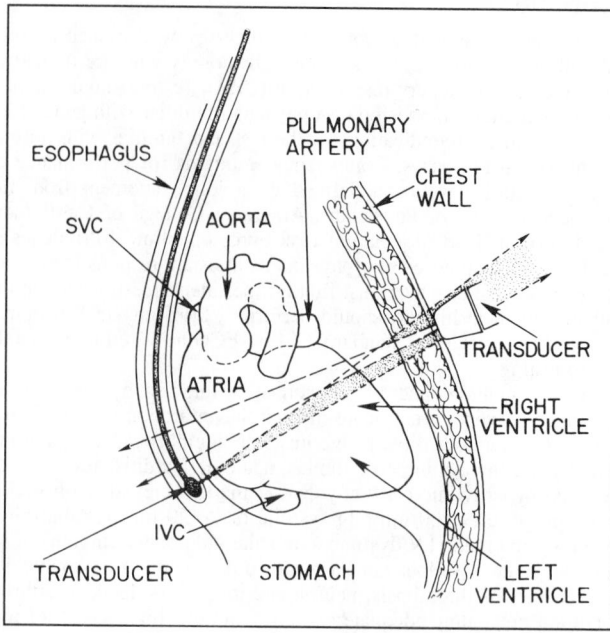

FIGURE 13-2   Methods of acquiring images of the heart using echocardiography. The transducer placed on the chest wall can be used to acquire most images. Because of its proximity to these structures, however, the transducer placed in the esophagus can acquire better images of the posterior cardiac structures and the great vessels.

vessel coronary artery disease (Box 13-1). Patients with 2.0 mm or more of S-T segment depression, particularly when manifested at a low exercise heart rate or workload, have a higher incidence of high-risk anatomic disease compared with patients with lesser degrees of S-T segment depression. Patients failing to progress further than stage 1 of the Bruce protocol or to achieve a workload of at least 4 METs are at higher risk for subsequent ischemic cardiac events compared with patients with better exercise capacity. Peak heart rate alone on exercise testing is related to survival. Patients achieving a heart rate of only 120 beats/min or less on exercise testing have a significantly worse survival compared with patients whose heart rate exceeds 120 beats/min. Patients who attain exercise heart rates greater than 160 beats/min have a much lower subsequent cardiac event rate even with S-T segment depression. Normally the systolic blood pressure increases with exercise because of the increased cardiac output with maintenance of stroke volume. Exercise-induced mechanical dysfunction resulting in impaired systolic contraction from ischemia often causes a failure to increase the systolic blood pressure by 10 mm Hg or more or may result in exercise-induced hypotension. A decrease in systolic blood pressure of 10 mm Hg or more during exercise has been shown to predict left main or three-vessel coronary artery disease. The ratio of the systolic blood pressure measured 3 minutes after exercise to the systolic blood pressure at peak exercise is predictive of the extent of inducible ischemia. The higher the value, the greater the extent of ischemia. Finally, the demonstration of complex ventricular ectopy at peak exercise is associated with increased risk of an adverse outcome.

CONTINUOUS AMBULATORY ELECTROCARDIOGRAPHIC RECORDING

The initial objective of ambulatory ECG was to detect arrhythmias in ambulatory patients with symptoms such as dizziness, palpitations, and syncope, and this still remains its major role. Three or four ECG leads are placed on the chest wall and connected to a small tape recorder, which the patient clips to a belt. Usually the ECG is continuously recorded on tape for 24 hours; however, the recordings may last up to 72 hours. A diary is usually provided so the patient can record symptoms and the time when these occurred. In some patients an *event monitor* is used. This unit is attached to the patient for up to a month at a time, and several seconds to minutes of the most recent ECG recordings are retained within the device's computer memory. When patients experience a symptom, they can trigger the device and play back the recordings to an analysis system via the telephone.

The data on the recording devices are played back on an automated analysis system that scans the data extremely rapidly. Abnormalities are detected and printed out, along with the time at which

they occurred. Such data as slowest and fastest heart rates, total premature atrial and ventricular beats, and abnormal pauses are all noted. The physician then can correlate these with the patient's symptoms.

Another use of ambulatory ECGs is the detection of ischemic S-T segment changes when symptoms are or are not present. The entity of *silent myocardial-ischemia* (Chapter 22) was first described when painless S-T elevation was first documented on the ambulatory ECG in patients with coronary artery disease. Ambulatory ECG monitoring for identifying periods of ischemic S-T segment depression has excellent prognostic value in patients with chronic coronary artery disease and in patients with a recent myocardial infarction. Exercise testing with cardiac imaging (radionuclide, echocardiographic) is more accurate for detecting myocardial ischemia and provides more prognostic information than does ambulatory electrocardiography.

Patients with variant angina (Chapter 22) are more likely to show ECG ST-T wave changes during normal activity than during exercise testing. Ambulatory electrocardiography may be useful in such patients, particularly for monitoring the results of therapy. The results of therapy can also be assessed by this technique in patients with arrhythmias (Chapter 18).

ECHOCARDIOGRAPHY

Echocardiography is used to image cardiac structures and function and also flow direction and velocities within cardiac chambers and vessels. Usually these images are obtained from several positions on the chest wall and abdomen using a hand-held transducer (Fig. 13-2); this technique is referred to as *transthoracic* echocardiography. In some circumstances a specially designed transducer is inserted into the esophagus and stomach to obtain images from behind the heart; this technique is referred to as *transesophageal* echocardiography (Fig. 13-2). Although traditionally considered noninvasive, echocardiography is now often used in the operating room, where either transesophageal echocardiography is used or the transducer is hand held directly over the heart's surface. In the cardiac catheterization laboratory, miniature transducer-tipped catheters are inserted directly into coronary arteries to obtain cross-sectional images of the arterial lumen and wall or into the cardiac chambers to visualize cardiac structures.

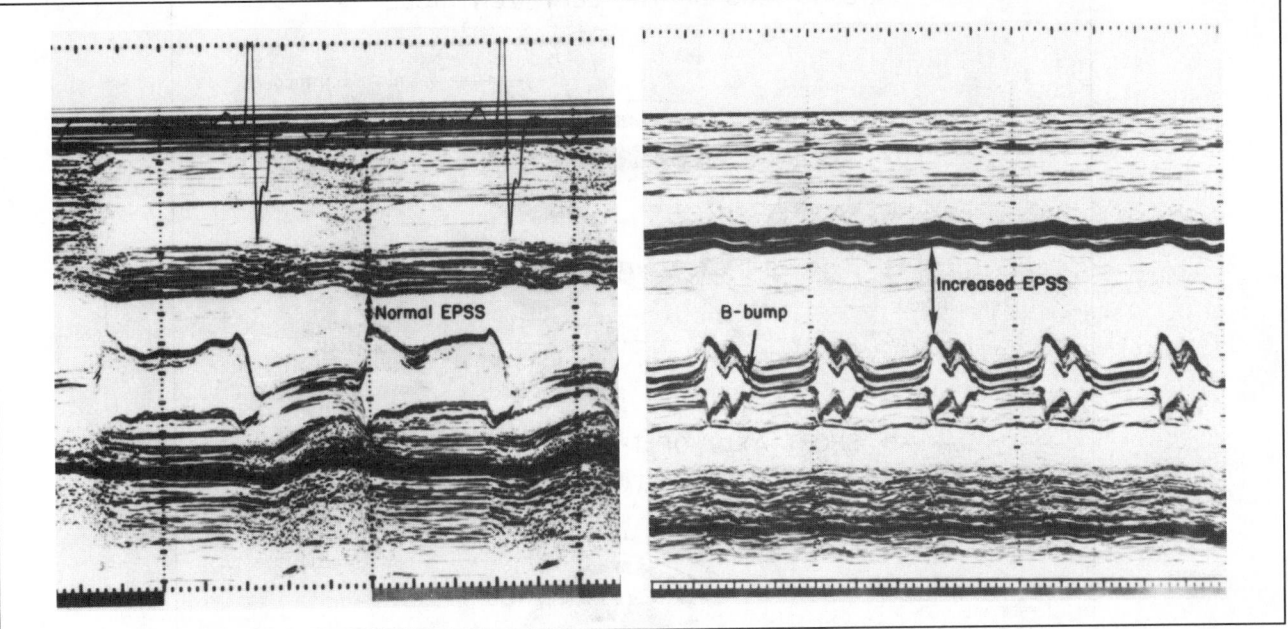

FIGURE 13-3   M-mode echocardiogram through the left ventricle at the mitral valve level in a normal subject *(left)* and in a subject with dilated ischemic cardiomyopathy *(right)*. *EPSS,* E-point septal separation, indicates the distance between the anterior mitral leaflet and the interventricular septum in diastole.

Imaging Cardiac Structures and Function

Echocardiography uses ultrasound to image the heart. Ultrasound is emitted by piezoelectric crystals housed within a transducer. When the shape of the crystals is changed electronically, the crystals emit ultrasound waves that travel within tissue at 1540 cm/sec and are reflected back from tissues and tissue-blood interfaces. The returning sound waves distort the piezoelectric crystals within the transducer, and the energy is transformed into an electric signal, which is converted to a video signal for display on a screen. Within a certain range, the video signal's intensity is roughly proportional to that of the reflected sound wave, and the signal's location on the screen indicates the time for the sound wave to return from the tissue. Because the time for the sound wave to return from a structure within the heart is inversely related to the structure's distance from the transducer, cardiac structures are displayed on the video screen in their true anatomic orientation.

When a beam created by a single crystal is directed through the heart, it interrogates the heart as an "ice pick." This method is called *M-mode* echocardiography and provides excellent axial and temporal resolution. Fig. 13-3 depicts an M-mode image through the heart at the mitral valve level in a normal subject and in a patient with dilated cardiomyopathy. Because the tracing represents an ice pick view, cardiac structures are not represented in a tomographic format and only a very limited view of the cardiac chambers is provided.

To image more of the heart at the same time, several individual beams can be emitted from many piezoelectric crystals housed within the same transducer, creating a wide beam capable of imaging the heart in an entire plane. This beam can be created either mechanically, in which the crystals are moved within the transducer using a motor, or electronically, in which the crystals are stimulated one after the other to produce a wide-angled beam. The beam can be of any size and contains several imaging lines. Because the speed of sound in tissue is constant, the rate at which each sector is created depends on the number of lines to be formed and their length. For a 90-degree sector with a depth of 20 cm, the frame rate is 30/sec for a conventional system.

This imaging method is termed *two-dimensional* (2D) echocardiography and is the standard format used for imaging the heart. The same transducer can also be used to obtain M-mode data, which are more valuable when the M-mode beam is guided from the 2D image,

because the exact orientation of the beam is known (Fig. 13-4). Using the transthoracic approach, 2D images are acquired from four standard locations: parasternal, apical, subcostal, and suprasternal. The parasternal approach provides long-axis and short-axis images of the LV (Fig. 13-4) and right ventricular (RV) inflow. The apical approach provides two-chamber, four-chamber (Fig. 13-5), and long-axis views of the LV. The subcostal and suprasternal approaches often are not needed if the parasternal and apical images are adequate; however, in some patients in whom these images are inadequate, subcostal views provide useful information. Also, the subcostal four-chamber view provides the best approach for imaging the interatrial septum, whereas the suprasternal view is valuable for imaging the great vessels.

By using several planes, the heart can be imaged comprehensively in real time using 2D echocardiography. Cardiac chamber dimensions and wall thickness can be measured and valve structure and motion assessed. In addition, proximal portions of the great vessels can be imaged and any echo-free space within the pericardial cavity noted. Classic patterns can be used to define disease entities, as shown in Fig. 13-3, which compares images from a normal subject and a patient with dilated cardiomyopathy. Compared with the normal image, the other shows a dilated LV cavity and an increased distance between the mitral valve and the interventricular septum, which indicates low ejection fraction. A "B bump" is also noted on the anterior mitral leaflet, which indicates a high LV end-diastolic pressure. The end-systolic four-chamber view of the same patient (Fig. 13-5, *C*) also shows incomplete mitral leaflet closure, indicating mitral regurgitation, as well as a thrombus in the LV apex.

Because the echo beam traverses tissue and is reflected back from intervening structures, it becomes weaker when it reaches structures located farthest from the transducer. The echo beam can be artificially strengthened at greater depth, a technique called *time-gain compensation*. Despite this modification, however, structures located farthest from the transducer may not be imaged as clearly as those nearest to the transducer, particularly when structures are imaged using the lateral resolution of ultrasound. For instance, structures such as the left atrial appendage, the pulmonary veins, and the aorta are not imaged well using the transthoracic approach.

Because the esophagus is close to both the atria and the great vessels, a transducer positioned in it (see Fig. 13-2) provides a more com-

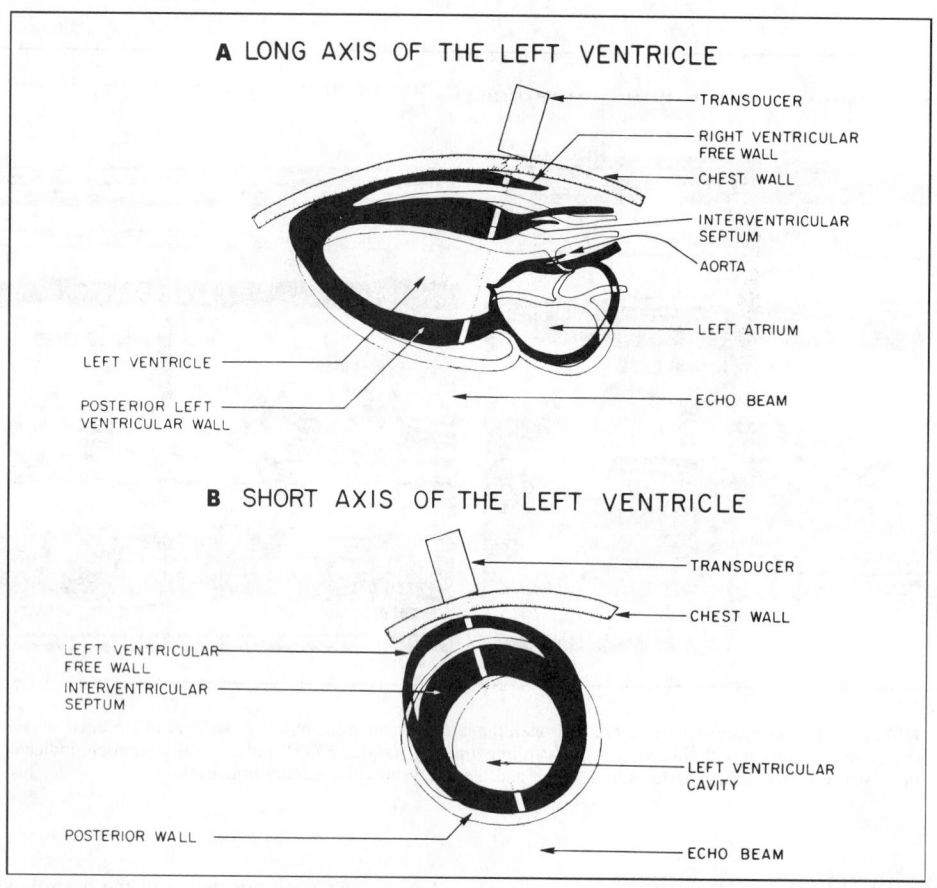

FIGURE 13-4 Parasternal long-axis **(A)** and short-axis **(B)** views on two-dimensional (2D) echocardiography obtained in end-diastole *(white)* and end-systole *(black)*. The M-mode beam can be guided using the 2D image. (From Kaul S: *Am Heart J* 112:568, 1986.)

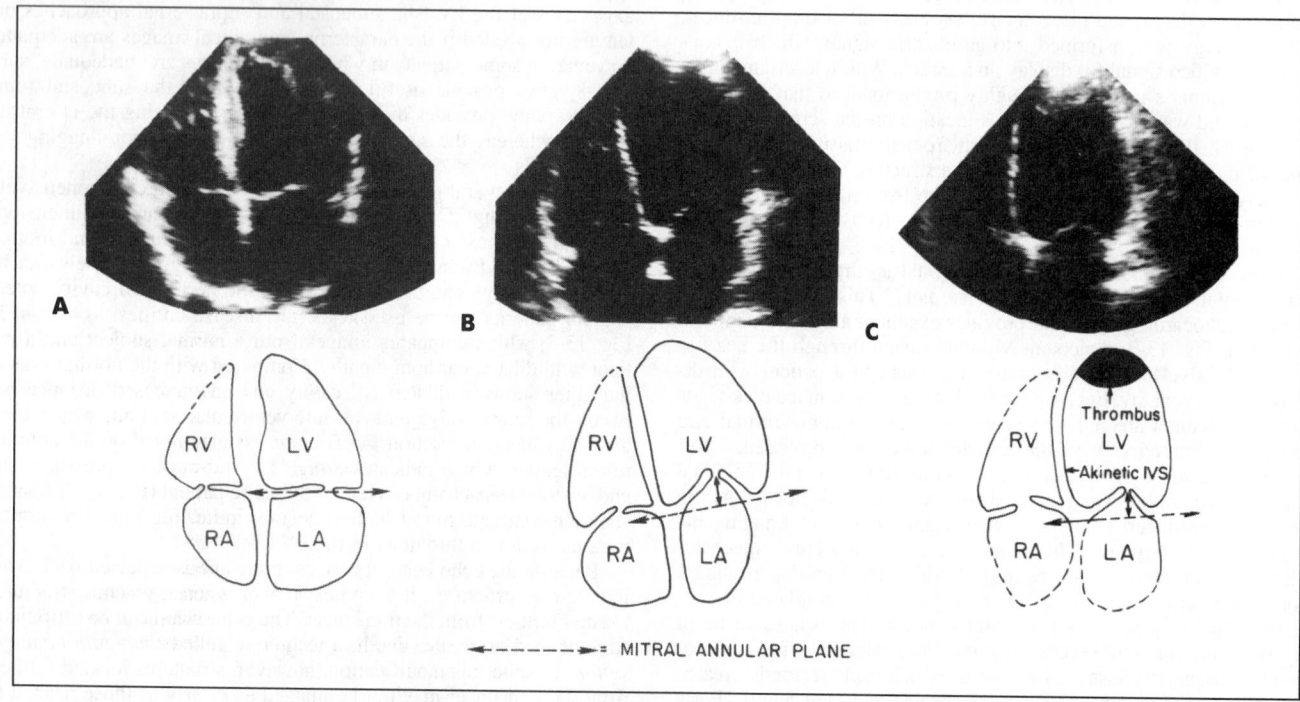

FIGURE 13-5 Four-chamber views from three different subjects. **A,** Normal subject with normal left ventricular size and normal end-systolic position of the mitral leaflets in relation to the mitral annulus. **B,** Patient with dilated cardiomyopathy and incomplete mitral leaflet closure, in which the leaflets hang up in the left ventricle in end-systole and result in mitral regurgitation. **C,** Patient with dilated cardiomyopathy similar to the one in **B,** with the additional finding of a thrombus in the left ventricular apex. The interventricular septum (IVS) is also akinetic. This patient's M-mode echocardiogram is depicted in the right panel in Fig. 13-3. (From Kaul S: *Am Heart J* 118:963, 1989.)

prehensive view of these structures. Fig. 13-6 is an example of dissection of the thoracic aorta noted on transesophageal echocardiography. Fig. 13-7 illustrates a thrombus in a mechanical prosthetic mitral valve that could not be visualized from the transthoracic approach because of "shadowing" created by the prosthesis. The thrombus was clearly seen on transesophageal echocardiography (Fig. 13-7, *A*), however, and its position was confirmed when the prosthetic valve was surgically removed (Fig. 13-7, *B*). Moreover, because there is no intervening lung and the imaging depth from the transesophageal approach is less, requiring less tissue penetration, higher-frequency transducers can be used, resulting in even better resolution.

Despite the definitely superior image quality obtained with transesophageal echocardiography, the procedure is uncomfortable for the awake patient, who requires sedation and a local anesthetic to the pharynx. The procedure is also more time consuming and resource consuming; a nurse is required to assist, and a trained physician is required to perform it. This differs from transthoracic echocardiography, which can be performed by a trained sonographer. As a consequence, the transesophageal procedure should be performed only when the information required cannot be obtained by other less involved methods.

Imaging Flow Velocities and Direction

When a moving source of light is interrogated from a stationary object, the frequency of light emitted from the moving source changes, becoming higher as it moves toward the stationary object (white to red) and lower as it moves away (white to blue). The direction of shift in frequency therefore indicates the moving source's direction of motion and has been termed the *Doppler effect* after the Austrian physicist who described this phenomenon. This same phenomenon is noted when ultrasound is emitted from a stationary transducer and the reflected waves from the red blood cells (RBCs) within cardiac chambers and great vessels are received by the same or another stationary transducer. The direction of shift in ultrasound frequency is used to determine the direction of flow of the RBCs in relation to the transducer. This direction of flow can be displayed as a spectral velocity profile, with the profile oriented toward the transducer for blood coming toward it or oriented away from the transducer for blood flowing away.

Fig. 13-8 illustrates the spectral display of signals from the LV outflow tract using a continuous-wave Doppler transducer positioned at the heart's apex, with the ultrasound beam directed from the LV apex to the aortic root. The flow signals directed upward are oriented toward the transducer, and those directed downward are oriented away from the transducer. These signals indicate that the patient has aortic regurgitation because in diastole, flow is directed toward the transducer (toward the LV apex). The flow directed downward indicates the maximum peak velocity in systole is along the line of interrogation. This *velocity* is normal (almost 1 m/sec), indicating the absence of any obstruction in the LV outflow tract.

The direction of flow can also be depicted by using color coding of velocity shifts within the cardiac chambers. Red depicts blood directed toward the transducer (see Color Plate II-1), and blue depicts blood moving away from the transducer (see Color Plate II-2). Not only can the direction of RBC flow be assessed, but the RBC velocity can be measured as well. Unlike imaging cardiac structures, in which the best resolution is obtained when the structure is imaged with the echo beam perpendicular to it, accurate measurement of RBC velocity is obtained by having the beam as parallel to the cells as possible. The degree of shift in the frequency of ultrasound after it strikes the RBCs reflects the velocity at which the RBCs are moving. The faster they move, the greater the frequency shift. As long as the RBCs are sampled along their direction of flow (± 15 degrees), the Doppler shift produced by them provides an accurate assessment of RBC velocity. This velocity information can be used to quantify flow and to measure pressures within cardiac chambers. Because flow equals mean velocity times area, if the aortic root area (2D imaging of the heart) and the mean flow velocity across the aortic valve are known, the stroke volume can be calculated. When multiplied by heart rate, the stroke volume can provide the cardiac output. The same principle can be used to measure valve area, using the continuity equation, which is based on energy proximal to a stenosis being the same as distal to it. Because mean velocity times area equals flow, this flow should be the same downstream as upstream from a stenosed aortic valve. If the aortic root area just proximal to the valve (from 2D imaging) and the mean velocity at this plane are known, aortic valve area can be calculated by dividing the product of these two by the mean velocity across the stenotic aortic valve.

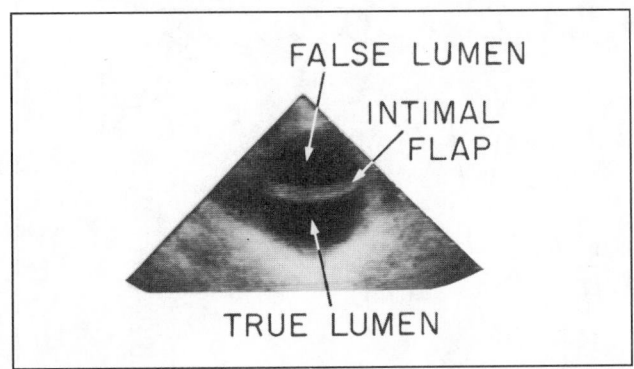

FIGURE 13-6   Dissection of the thoracic aorta noted on transesophageal echocardiography.

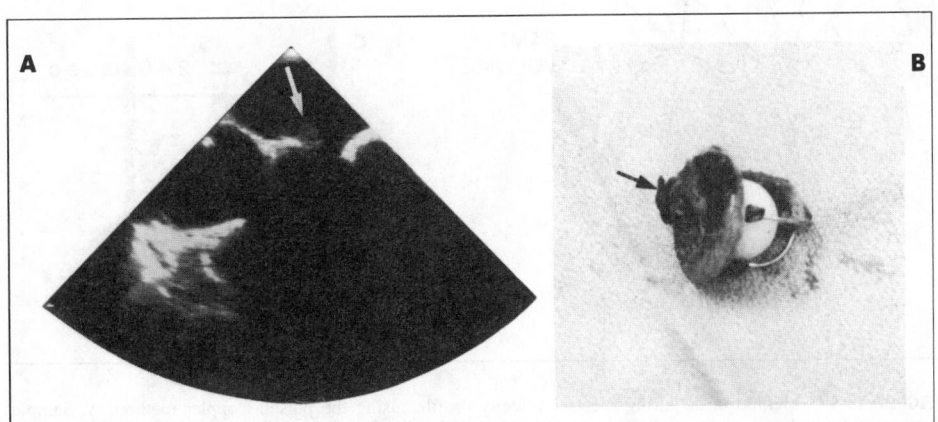

FIGURE 13-7   **A,** Thrombus on the left atrial aspect of the prosthetic mitral valve noted on transesophageal echocardiography. **B,** Presence of the thrombus was confirmed with inspection of the valve after it was surgically removed.

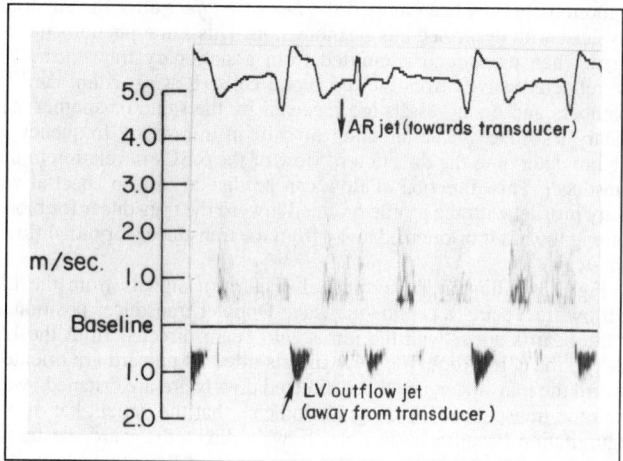

FIGURE 13-8 Continuous-wave Doppler recordings obtained from a line of interrogation extending from the left ventricular *(LV)* apex to the LV outflow tract. It depicts abnormal diastolic flow oriented toward the transducer, indicating aortic regurgitation *(AR),* and normal systolic velocity, indicating absence of any obstruction in the entire outflow tract.

In practice, measurement of velocities is performed using either the pulsed-Doppler or the continuous-wave Doppler technique. For the pulsed technique, a sample volume is placed over a region where the velocity has to be measured, such as at the mitral leaflet tips (Fig. 13-9, *A*). As the ultrasound signals return from the heart, all except those returning from this sample volume will be rejected. The signals from the sample volume are then depicted as a spectral display, with time on the *x* axis. Fig. 13-9, *B* illustrates pulsed-Doppler signals from a normal mitral valve, whereas Fig. 13-9, *C* illustrates those from a patient with mitral stenosis. This technique is excellent for quantification of velocities at a discrete site; however, it is limited by the maximum velocity it can measure and is not used for the quantification of velocities greater than 2 m/sec.

Unlike pulsed Doppler, in which the transducer emits ultrasound and then goes into the "receive mode" to acquire the returning waves, continuous-wave Doppler uses two transducers: one to emit ultrasound and the other to receive it. Although this technique cannot localize the exact region within the beam length producing the greatest Doppler shift, it can measure very high velocities, such as those created by valvular stenosis and regurgitation and intracardiac shunts.

Using the modified Bernoulli equation ($P = 4V^2$), the peak instantaneous velocity across a region (*V*) can be converted to the peak instantaneous pressure gradient (*P*) across it. For instance, if *V* across a stenotic aortic valve is 5 m/sec, *P* across it is 100 mm Hg. *V* can be converted to mean gradient by integrating the velocity profile. Similarly, as shown in Fig. 13-10, if *V* measured from a regurgitant jet across the tricuspid valve during systole is 4.8 m/sec, the gradient across the tricuspid valve in systole is 92 mm Hg. If, based on the

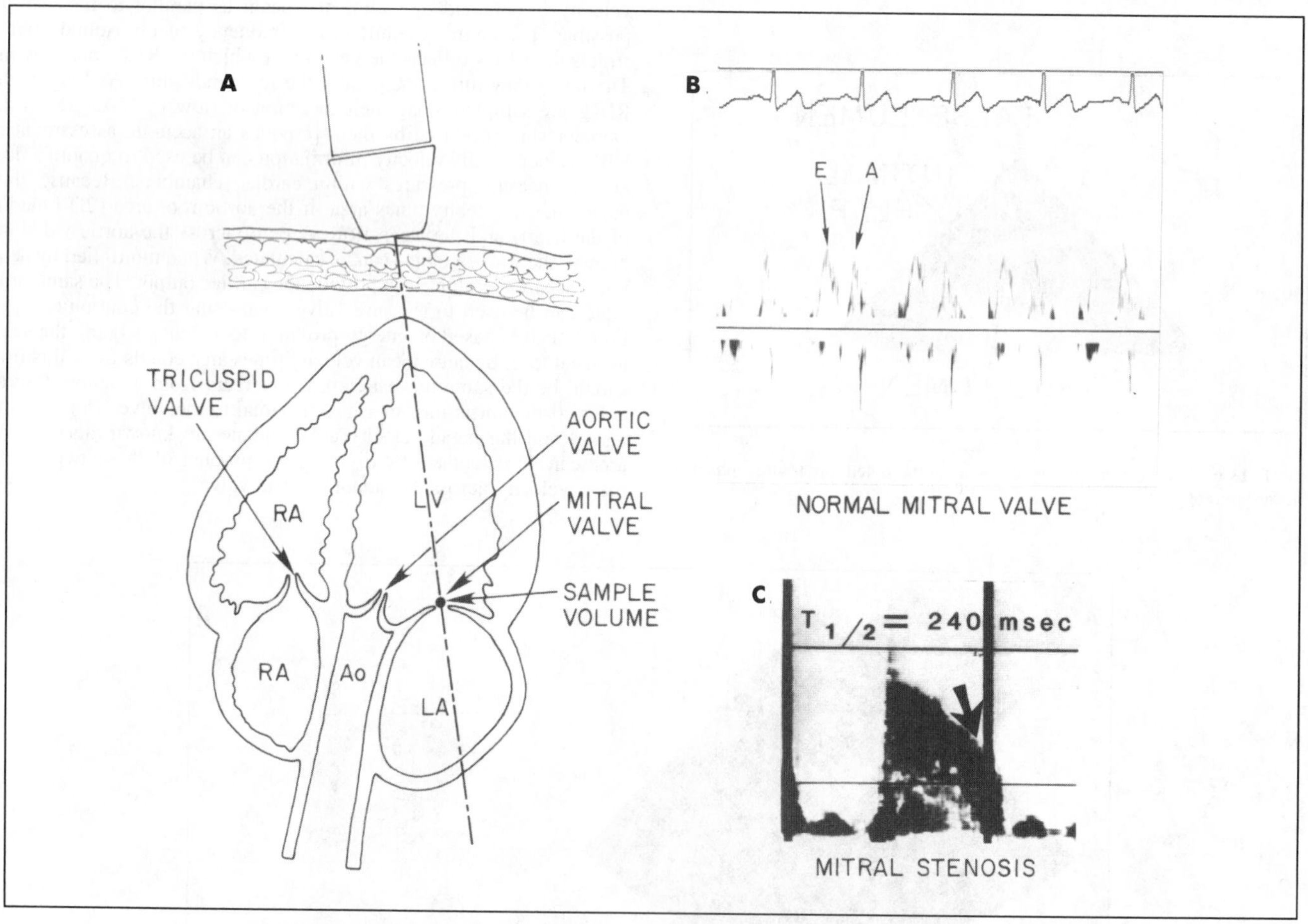

FIGURE 13-9 Method of acquiring spectral velocity profiles using the pulsed-Doppler method. **A,** Sample volume is located at the mitral valve tips, resulting in a spectral velocity profile oriented toward the transducer (**B** and **C**). **B,** Normal mitral velocity profile in which the E wave results from early LV filling and the A wave from LV filling caused by left atrial contraction. **C,** Velocity profile from a patient with severe mitral stenosis in which the pressure half-time is 240 msec. No A wave exists because the patient is experiencing atrial fibrillation.

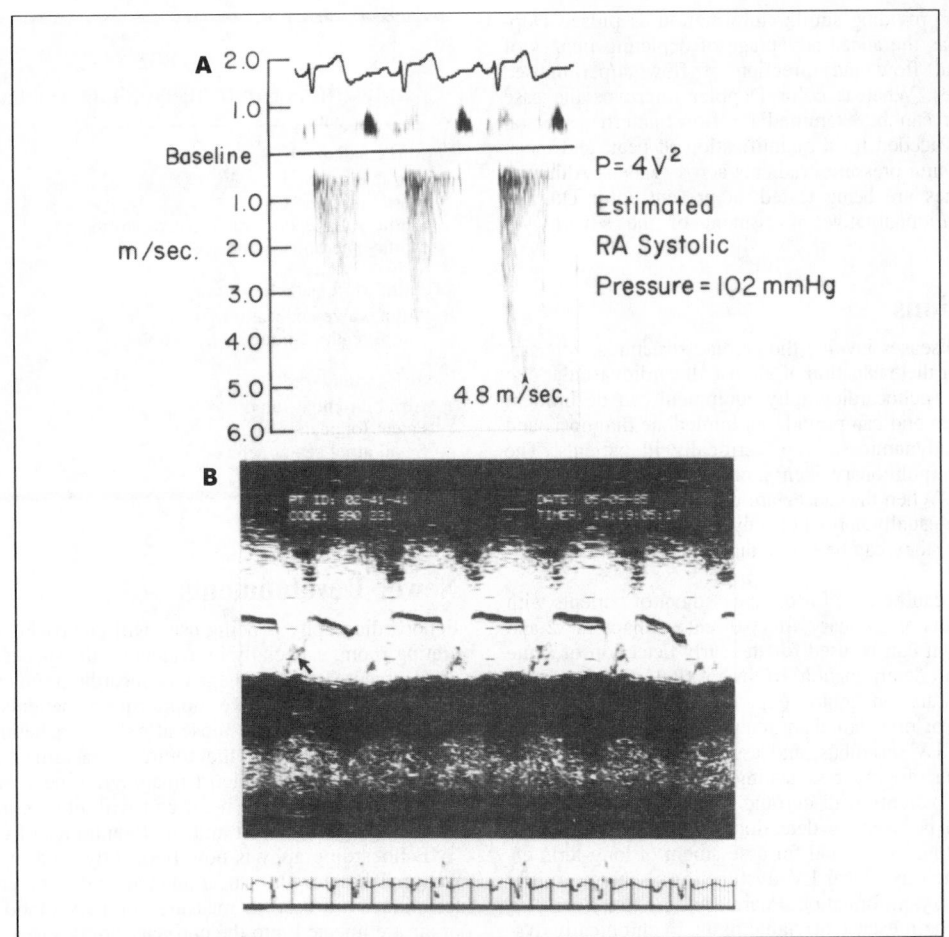

A   P= 4V²
Estimated
RA Systolic
Pressure = 102 mmHg

4.8 m/sec.

FIGURE 13-10   Continuous-wave Doppler **(A)** and M-mode tracings **(B)** from a patient with pulmonary hypertension (see text for details).

jugular venous pressure, the mean right atrial pressure is estimated to be 10 mm Hg, the peak ventricular systolic (and hence the pulmonary artery systolic pressure, unless pulmonic stenosis is present) pressure is 102 mm Hg. Pulmonic valve motion on M-mode images in the patient whose Doppler signal is depicted in Fig. 13-10, *A*, also shows the classic "flying W" pattern for pulmonary hypertension, as depicted in Fig. 13-10, *B*.

The rate of pressure gradient decline across a stenotic mitral valve provides an estimate of the severity of stenosis. The time required during diastole to go from peak pressure gradient to half that value provides a direct assessment of mitral stenosis; the longer this interval, the more severe the mitral stenosis. The simultaneous left atrial and LV pressure recordings in a patient with mitral stenosis (Fig. 13-11) indicate a 260 msec interval (normal, 20 to 60 msec) for the maximum pressure gradient to reach half its original value and severe mitral stenosis. Fig. 13-9, *C*, illustrates a Doppler signal from the same patient. The pressure half-time of 240 msec derived from pulsed Doppler was very close to the 260 msec obtained at cardiac catheterization.

The information available from pulsed-Doppler echocardiography in terms of mean velocities and turbulent flow can also be obtained by simultaneously color-coding velocities in different regions of the cardiac cavities and great vessels. Different-colored maps can be used, and higher velocities of blood are coded brighter. When turbulence is present, the range of velocities within a region is large. The variance from the mean velocity, therefore, is great compared with the situation when flow is laminar. This variance is color coded as a mosaic pattern. For instance, aortic regurgitation causes a mosaic pattern in the LV outflow tract in diastole on a transthoracic image (see Color Plate II-3), and a mosaic pattern is noted in the mitral regurgitant jet in the left atrium in systole on a transesophageal image (see Color

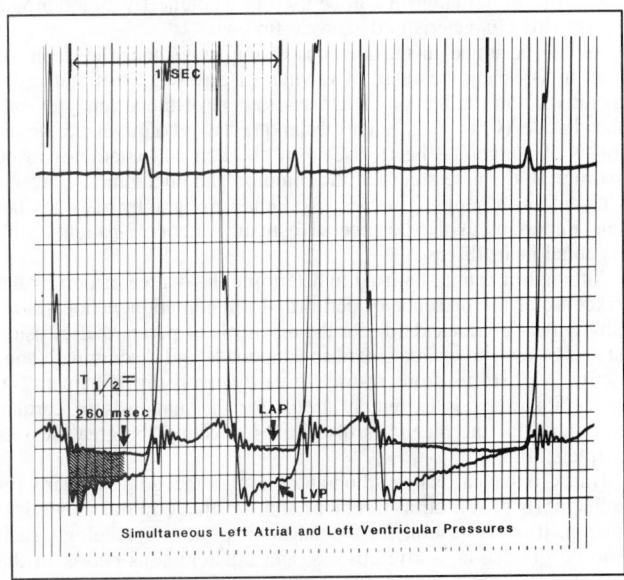

FIGURE 13-11   Simultaneous left atrial and left ventricular pressure tracings from a patient with mitral stenosis to illustrate the principle of *pressure half-time*. It takes 260 msec for the maximum pressure gradient between the left atrium *(LAP)* and left ventricle *(LVP)* in diastole to reach half that value. This patient had a pressure half-time of 240 msec with the pulsed-Doppler method.

Plate II-4). Although providing similar information as pulsed Doppler, color Doppler has the added advantage of depicting images of normal and abnormal flow and direction of flow superimposed on routine 2D images. Whereas color Doppler improves the ease with which the heart can be examined for flow patterns, spectral Doppler displays are needed for a quantification of peak and mean velocities when assessing pressure gradients across valves. Although quantitative approaches are being tested, at present color Doppler provides only a semiquantitative assessment of the severity of regurgitation.

Clinical Indications

Because most heart diseases involve the cardiac structures, echocardiography is useful for the evaluation of almost all cardiovascular diseases. Being portable, echocardiography equipment can be brought to the patient's bedside and can provide an immediate diagnosis and measure of the hemodynamic status of critically ill patients. The causes of hypotension, pulmonary edema, or both can be determined (Chapters 19 and 20). When the causes are noncardiac, cardiac function and structures are usually normal or only mildly abnormal. When the causes are cardiac, they can be easily diagnosed on echocardiography.

Echocardiography can be used for the assessment of patients with acute and chronic forms of coronary artery disease (Chapters 22 and 23). In these patients, it can be used for the early detection of acute myocardial infarction, determination of in-hospital prognosis and complications after infarction (infarct expansion, ventricular remodeling), demonstration of myocardial "stunning," diagnosis of RV infarction, detection of LV thrombus, and assessment of viable myocardium using pharmacologic stress testing or myocardial contrast echocardiography. In patients with chronic coronary artery disease, echocardiography can be used for detection of disease using either exercise or pharmacologic stress and for assessment of long-term effects of infarction, such as global LV dysfunction, ischemic mitral regurgitation, and aneurysm formation. Pharmacologic stress can also be used to assess for the presence of viable tissue in chronically dysfunctional myocardium with or without a previous history of infarction.

Echocardiography is excellent for evaluating patients with primary myocardial disorders such as ventricular hypertrophy (obstructive or nonobstructive) and restrictive and dilated cardiomyopathies (Chapter 26). In the former, it can define the distribution of hypertrophy and estimate the severity of outflow tract obstruction and mitral regurgitation; in the latter, it can be used to examine LV function and may provide characteristic diagnostic findings.

As can be noted in the previous examples, echocardiography is useful in assessing the cause of valvular disease (e.g., rheumatic, degenerative) and the hemodynamic assessment of the severity of valvular disease (Chapter 25). This technique has revolutionized the diagnosis of congenital heart disease in children and continues to be important in the assessment of the common and uncommon congenital disorders in adults (Chapter 28). Echocardiography also has become important in the postoperative management of patients with congenital heart disease.

Although it cannot be used to determine the degree of pericardial thickening or the presence of pericardial inflammation, echocardiography is the "gold standard" for the diagnosis of pericardial effusion and can be used to evaluate cardiac tamponade and discriminate constrictive pericarditis from restrictive cardiomyopathy (Chapter 27). Echocardiography is extremely useful for the diagnosis of cardiac masses and for the diagnosis of diseases affecting the great vessels (Chapters 30 and 33).

Transesophageal echocardiography is also the gold standard for the diagnosis of left atrial thrombus and prosthetic mitral valve dysfunction. It is also useful for the diagnosis of aortic pathology, such as aortic dissection, aortic abscess, and atheromatous debris in the aorta. Transesophageal echocardiography can also detect a thrombus in the main or left or right pulmonary artery in patients with pulmonary embolus and can visualize the proximal portions of the coronary arteries. The indications for transesophageal echocardiography are listed in Box 13-2.

BOX 13-2
Indications for transesophageal echocardiography

Aortic pathology
Aortic dissection
Aortic root abscess
Aortic valve endocarditis (native/prosthetic)
Aortic atheromatous debris

Mitral valve pathology
Mitral valve endocarditis (native/prosthetic)
Mitral regurgitation (unclear etiology)

Atrial pathology
Atrial thrombus/tumor
Patent foramen ovale
Small atrial septal defect

Newer Developments

Echocardiography is being used with increasing frequency in the operating room, especially in evaluating the success of valve repair and replacement. Transesophageal echocardiography is also being used for the on-line intraoperative monitoring of patients undergoing noncardiac surgery, especially those at risk for ischemic events during aortic cross-clamping. In the future, intracardiac catheters likely will have transducers capable of imaging the heart, which can be placed in the right side of the heart and will allow continuous on-line cardiac imaging of the left and right ventricles of critically ill patients.

Echocardiography is now frequently used in the cardiac catheterization laboratory as an adjunct to coronary angiography. Doppler techniques are used to measure coronary blood flow. Microbubbles of air are injected into the coronary arteries to assess myocardial perfusion, a technique termed *myocardial contrast echocardiography.* This technique can be used to assess myocardial viability after infarction by determining the spatial extent of collateral blood flow and the extent of no-reflow. This technique can now be used to assess myocardial perfusion after IV injection of bubbles capable of transpulmonary transit. Newer forms of data acquisition, such as harmonic imaging, make the detection of bubbles in the myocardium more feasible. In the future, it is anticipated that myocardial contrast echocardiography will be used in the outpatient laboratory to diagnose coronary artery disease and in the emergency department to better diagnose acute myocardial infarction.

Catheter-tipped transducers are introduced into coronary arteries to obtain cross-sectional images, particularly after intervention procedures, and have the potential for quantification of residual atheroma. Three-dimensional (3D) echocardiography has also become a feasible clinical tool. Its implications in the clinical assessment of patients, however, need to be defined.

NUCLEAR CARDIOLOGY TECHNIQUES

Significant advances in the ability to image the heart under stress and resting conditions in patients with suspected or known coronary artery disease have been made using radionuclide imaging agents. After the IV administration of various radiolabeled agents, either the myocardium or the cardiac blood pools and great vessels can be imaged with the patient at rest or during exercise or under pharmacologic stress by using planar or single photon emission tomography (SPECT), scintigraphy, or positron imaging and appropriate computer processing. Many diagnostic and prognostic applications of nuclear cardiology techniques are based on the principle that physiologic and functional information, rather than just structural or anatomic information, is the ultimate value of this noninvasive methodology. Myocardial perfusion imaging or radionuclide angiography performed in conjunction with exercise electrocardiography can provide clinically relevant data about the presence and extent of ischemia. This may be more prognostically important than the mere classification of the number of diseased vessels by angiography.

With the emergence of coronary angioplasty and thrombolytic therapy as highly effective interventions for patients with acute ischemic syndromes, nuclear cardiology tests have been used frequently for the noninvasive determination of the efficacy of revascularization or reperfusion with these therapeutic approaches. Finally, significant advances have been made in the application of nuclear cardiology techniques for assessing myocardial viability in patients with LV dysfunction. Quantitative SPECT imaging of thallium-201 (^{201}Tl) uptake at rest and positron emission tomographic imaging of myocardial blood flow and metabolism are gaining increased attention as noninvasive approaches for evaluating myocardial viability in patients with chronic ischemic heart disease or acute myocardial infarction.

Myocardial Perfusion Imaging

Myocardial perfusion imaging is most often performed with exercise ECG testing for detecting coronary artery disease and determining prognosis. ^{201}Tl is the perfusion agent most often used, but the new agents, technetium-99m (^{99m}Tc) sestamibi and ^{99m}Tc tetrofosmin are gaining increased clinical use, particularly with SPECT imaging.

Thallium-201 Imaging

Thallium, a metallic element in group IIIA of the periodic table, is transported intracellularly by both passive and active mechanisms. Early myocardial uptake of IV ^{201}Tl is directly proportional to regional myocardial blood flow and the extraction fraction of ^{201}Tl by the myocardium. After the initial phase of myocardial uptake, there is continuous exchange of myocardial ^{201}Tl and ^{201}Tl from the extracardiac compartments. ^{201}Tl is continually washing out of normally perfused myocardium and replaced by recirculating ^{201}Tl from residual activity in the blood pool compartment. This process of continuous exchange forms the basis of the phenomenon of ^{201}Tl redistribution that is observed when the tracer is administered during transient underperfusion of the myocardium, as induced by exercise in patients with significant coronary artery disease. In clinical imaging studies, ^{201}Tl redistribution is defined as the total or partial resolution of initial postexercise defects when assessed by repeat imaging 2½ to 4 hours after tracer administration. The ^{201}Tl perfusion scan is most often performed with conventional treadmill exercise testing. A dose of 2.5 to 3.0 mCi of ^{201}Tl is administered through a freely flowing IV cannula during symptom-limited end-points such as angina pectoris, shortness of breath, fatigue, lower extremity claudication, or hypotension. The patient then exercises for another 30 to 45 seconds to ensure that the initial myocardial uptake phase will reflect the perfusion pattern present at peak exercise. Within 5 minutes after cessation of exercise, the patient is positioned under the collimator of a gamma camera to obtain anterior and multiple oblique projection images for the planar approach and for multiple-angle images acquired using the SPECT technique, with rotation of the camera around the patient.

Areas of diminished ^{201}Tl uptake on the images obtained immediately after exercise represent either zones of stress-induced transient ischemia or myocardial scar. To differentiate the two, delayed images are obtained to look for redistribution. Redistribution or reversible defects imply stress-induced ischemia, whereas persistent or fixed defects on serial images suggest myocardial scar. Approximately 30% of persistent defects actually represent severe ischemia rather than scar. Reinjection of a second dose of ^{201}Tl, with the patient at rest after acquisition of the redistribution images, has shown further reversibility in approximately 30% of defects that appear fixed at 2½ to 4 hours.

Most nuclear cardiology laboratories perform SPECT, rather than planar, imaging because SPECT yields images of slices of the heart without interference of activity from noncardiac or overlapping myocardial regions. The tomographic approach yields better defect contrast than planar imaging, permitting enhanced detection of small zones of hypoperfusion. Three-headed SPECT cameras permit more rapid acquisition of image data, thereby reducing the chance of artifacts caused by patient motion. Planar or SPECT ^{201}Tl scintigraphy performed with symptom-limited exercise stress testing has enhanced

both sensitivity and specificity of detecting coronary artery disease. Sensitivity and normalcy rate of SPECT ^{201}Tl scintigraphy using planar imaging technology are about 92% and 84%, respectively. Sensitivity rate is 83% for detection of single-vessel disease as compared to 93% and 95% for detection of two-vessel and three-vessel disease, respectively. SPECT perfusion defect size increases with increasing severity of stenosis. Defect size is quantitated from polar maps or "bull's-eye plots."

Several factors increase or decrease sensitivity of ^{201}Tl scintigraphy for detecting coronary artery disease. With both planar and SPECT imaging lesions of the left circumflex coronary artery are more difficult to resolve. A proximal stenosis in the left anterior descending artery produces a perfusion defect approximately twice as large as that produced by a proximal right coronary artery lesion. Also, branch stenoses of the major coronary arteries are more difficult to resolve than when more proximal narrowings are present. Stenoses that are >70% narrowed are more likely to be detected by SPECT imaging than 50% to 70% stenoses. Quantitative SPECT ^{201}Tl imaging can correctly predict multivessel disease in 65% of patients with two or more stenoses. The level of exercise achieved during stress testing influences the exercise ECG more than the ^{201}Tl scintigram. Throughout the range of exercise workloads or peak heart rates achieved, the frequency of ^{201}Tl scan abnormalities is more prevalent than exercise S-T segment depression. Long-acting nitrates administered just before testing may reduce defect size on exercise ^{201}Tl scintigrams.

The specificity of SPECT ^{201}Tl scintigraphy may vary tremendously among laboratories and depends on the ability of the interpreter to differentiate artifacts from true myocardial perfusion abnormalities. Attenuation artifacts in women resulting from overlying breast tissue are most often localized in the anteroseptal region. A high diaphragm can cause attenuation artifacts in the inferior wall. Artifacts can occur if a patient moves as the gamma camera is being rotated around the torso. New techniques for correcting for attenuation are being validated.

Exercise ^{201}Tl imaging is useful for the noninvasive assessment of prognosis in patients with chest pain syndromes or known coronary artery disease. Box 13-1 summarizes the high-risk ^{201}Tl scan variables. On initial postexercise images, high-risk scan findings include multiple ^{201}Tl defects in one or more coronary supply regions, increased ^{201}Tl uptake in the lung that can be quantitated using the lung/heart ratio, and exercise-induced transient LV cavity dilation. Presence of redistribution compared with solely persistent defects indicates a higher risk for subsequent cardiac events. The extent of stress-induced hypoperfusion, as reflected by the total number of defects identified or total defect size, is one of the best prognostic predictors of subsequent death and reinfarction in patients with coronary artery disease. This is particularly true when extensive hypoperfusion is observed at low exercise heart rates and workloads and is accompanied by ischemic S-T segment depression. Fig. 13-12 shows the survival rate for patients stratified by total extent of exercise ^{201}Tl SPECT defects, represented as percent of LV area, from the study of Marie et al (1995). Several studies have shown that extent of hypoperfusion on SPECT ^{201}Tl images provides supplementary prognostic information to clinical variables and the resting left ventricular ejection fraction (LVEF). Patients with chest pain and completely normal myocardial ^{201}Tl perfusion scans have an excellent prognosis, with less than a 1% per year death or infarction rate. Increased lung uptake of ^{201}Tl reflects ischemia-induced LV diastolic dysfunction with development of pulmonary edema. A portion of the ^{201}Tl dose equilibrates with this pulmonary interstitial edema fluid, giving the appearance of increased ^{201}Tl activity in the lung on the anterior view. Some observers have reported that an increased lung/heart ^{201}Tl ratio is even a better predictor of prognosis than the number of perfusion defects identified. Fig. 13-13 shows serial postexercise images in a patient with inferior and anteroseptal defects reflecting multivessel coronary artery disease.

^{201}Tl imaging can be performed solely in the resting state to identify residual myocardial viability in regions of severe wall motion abnormalities. Patients with chronic coronary artery disease and LV dysfunction caused by "hibernation" demonstrate preservation of ^{201}Tl uptake at rest (Chapter 22). With this technique, IV ^{201}Tl is admin-

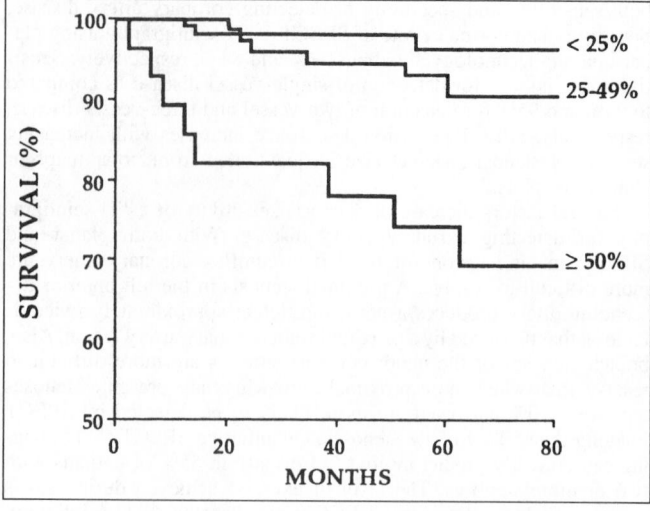

FIGURE 13-12 Survival related to total extent of ^{201}Tl SPECT defects on exercise imaging. Values represent percent of left ventricular area.

(From Marie P-Y et al: Long-term prediction of major ischemic events by exercise thallium-201 single-photon emission computed tomography. Incremental prognostic value compared with clinical, exercise testing, catheterization and radionuclide angiographic data, *J Am Coll Cardiol* 26:879, 1995.)

istered, and initial and delayed rest images are acquired at 15 minutes and 4 hours after tracer injection. Areas of resting hypoperfusion that are viable will demonstrate initial defects that show a late filling or redistribution or mild irreversible defects. Zones of myocardial asynergy showing >50% [201]Tl uptake, compared to peak uptake, exhibit improved regional systolic function after revascularization. This technique is now used clinically to assist in the selection of patients with coronary artery disease and severely depressed LVEF who will benefit most from revascularization. Patients undergoing revascularization with LV dysfunction primarily resulting from hibernation have a better short- and long-term prognosis than patients with comparable reductions in LV function but relatively more nonviable myocardial regions as assessed by ^{201}Tl scintigraphy.

Technetium-99m Sestamibi Imaging

[99m]Tc sestamibi is a lipophilic cationic ^{99m}Tc complex that, as with ^{201}Tl, is taken up in myocardial tissue in proportion to regional myocardial blood flow. The 140 keV photon energy peak of ^{99m}Tc is ideal for gamma camera imaging and can produce higher-quality images than those produced by [201]Tl. The relatively short half-life (6 hours) of ^{99m}Tc provides favorable patient dosimetry and permits administration of 10 to 15 times larger doses than with ^{201}Tl, yielding better images in a shorter period.

Because ^{99m}Tc sestamibi does not redistribute over time after IV administration, separate injections of the radionuclide must be administered during stress and resting states to differentiate between transient ischemia and myocardial scar. The most common protocol using this radionuclide is to perform the resting study in the morning using a dose of 8 to 10 mCi and the exercise portion of the study 3 to 4 hours later using a dose of 24 to 30 mCi. Acquisition of the images is performed 30 to 45 minutes after ^{99m}Tc sestamibi injection, allowing for clearance of radioactivity from the lungs and liver. Ideally, a "2-day" protocol is preferable because 24 to 30 mCi can be administered for both the rest and exercise portions of the imaging procedure. Another protocol is called a *dual-isotope rest ^{201}Tl/exercise ^{99m}Tc sestamibi study* in which ^{201}Tl imaging is performed first, followed immediately by exercise imaging using ^{99m}Tc sestamibi. Defect reversibility is determined by comparing the two sets of images. This protocol markedly shortens the total time for an imaging study.

Sensitivity detection of coronary artery disease with ^{99m}Tc sestamibi is comparable to that cited for ^{201}Tl, whereas specificity is higher, particularly in women. The higher photon energy and enhanced count rate with somewhat decreased attenuation and scatter make ^{99m}Tc sestamibi a better radionuclide for SPECT imaging com-

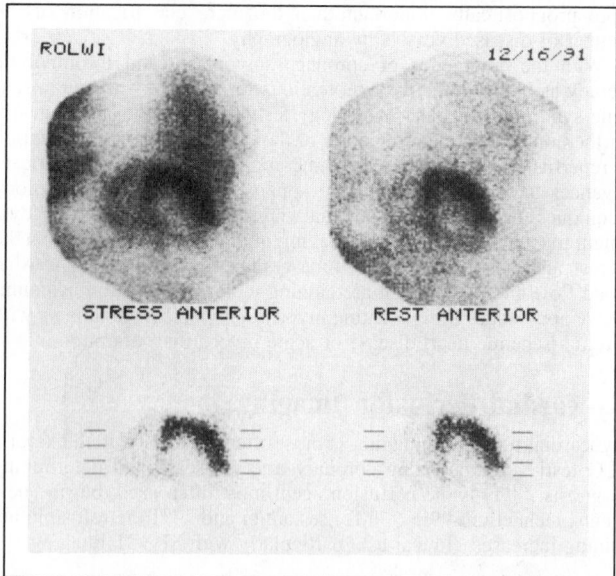

A

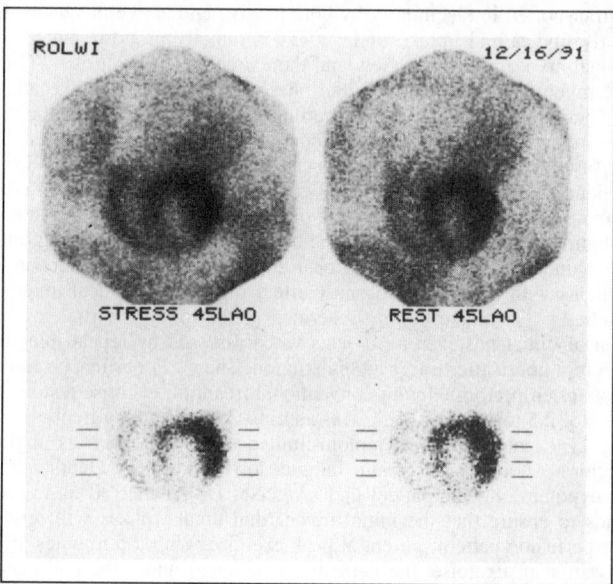

B

FIGURE 13-13 **A,** Postexercise and delayed (after rest) anterior view, planar, thallium-201 (^{201}Tl) images obtained 10 minutes and 2½ hours after ^{201}Tl injection, respectively. Note increased ^{201}Tl uptake in the lung and an extensive inferior wall defect that is predominantly persistent. The background-subtracted images are shown below the processed images. **B,** Postexercise and delayed 45-degree left anterior oblique (LAO) images in the same patient showing an anteroseptal defect with partial delayed redistribution.

pared with [201]Tl. This is why specificity is enhanced. Image quality is superior, and there are fewer image artifacts. Fig. 13-14 shows stress and rest short-axis ^{99m}Tc sestamibi tomograms in a normal patient and stress and rest short-axis tomograms in a patient with a reversible inferior defect.

There are two other potential advantages of ^{99m}Tc sestamibi imaging. First, this procedure has the ability to gate the perfusion images with the ECG to assess regional wall thickening. Assessment of regional systolic function and perfusion simultaneously may assist in the noninvasive detection of viability and in distinguishing attenuation artifacts from scar. LVEF can also be calculated from the gated SPECT tomograms. Second, first-pass radionuclide ventriculography can be undertaken with the IV bolus injection of ^{99m}Tc sestamibi before acquisition of myocardial perfusion scans. The LVEF can be mea-

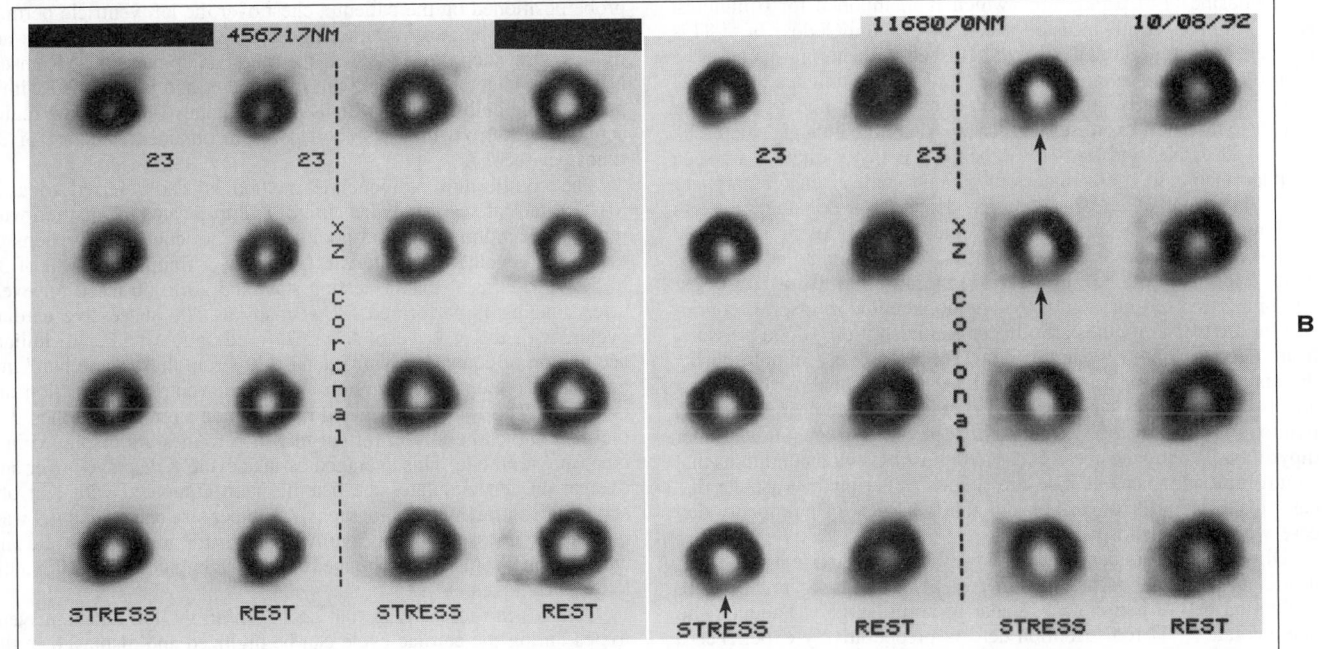

FIGURE 13-14   **A,** Normal stress and rest short-axis ^{99m}Tc sestamibi tomograms showing uniform tracer uptake in all myocardial regions. The sequence is from the apical slices *(upper left)* to basilar slices *(lower right)*. **B,** Short-axis ^{99m}Tc sestamibi tomograms in a patient with an inferior defect on stress images, which show reversibility on rest images *(arrow)*.

sured both at rest and during exercise as is undertaken with conventional radionuclide angiography. The ability to measure LVEF and regional myocardial perfusion simultaneously with a single IV injection of ^{99m}Tc sestamibi may significantly enhance the prognostic value of this agent.

As with ^{201}Tl scintigraphy, exercise ^{99m}Tc sestamibi SPECT imaging provides additional prognostic value to clinical and exercise stress test variables. Mortality rate is <0.5% per year in patients with a normal exercise ^{99m}Tc sestamibi scan. ^{99m}Tc-labeled agents such as sestamibi are preferable to ^{201}Tl for risk stratification in women.

Some limitations to ^{99m}Tc sestamibi imaging deserve mention. First, because the agent does not redistribute over time, it may not be as useful for assessing myocardial viability in the resting state in patients with coronary artery disease and LV dysfunction. Nevertheless, several recent studies have shown that resting ^{99m}Tc sestamibi uptake is comparable to resting ^{201}Tl uptake when both tracers were administered to the same patients with resting regional wall motion abnormalities. ^{99m}Tc sestamibi uptake in the lung has not been validated as a prognostic variable and thus may somewhat diminish the agent's prognostic usefulness.

Other Technetium-99m Perfusion Agents

^{99m}Tc teboroxime is a boronic acid adduct of technetium dioxime (BATO) compound that is a neutral lipophilic agent with high initial myocardial extraction and rapid myocardial clearance. Because of its rapid myocardial clearance, all imaging protocols must be performed rapidly; ideally, no more than 1 minute should pass between ^{99m}Tc teboroxime injection and the onset of imaging. SPECT acquisition is difficult using this radionuclide perfusion agent because of the short imaging time needed to acquire high-quality scintigrams. Another drawback of this agent is the substantially high level of liver activity that is seen in some patients, causing difficulty in assessing the heart's inferior wall. Nevertheless, despite these limitations, sensitivity and specificity of exercise ^{99m}Tc teboroxime imaging have been in the 85% to 90% range.

^{99m}Tc tetrofosmin is a compound of the diphosphene group that is rapidly cleared from the blood pool after intravenous injection and, like ^{99m}Tc sestamibi, is taken up by the myocardium in proportion to blood flow. This agent does not redistribute over time, and separate in

jections are required for rest and exercise SPECT imaging. Sensitivity and specificity for coronary artery disease detection with exercise stress are comparable to ^{201}Tl imaging, although defects are somewhat less severe with ^{99m}Tc tetrofosmin. ^{99m}Tc bis(N-ethoxy N-ethyldithiocarbanate) nitrido technetium (NOET) is a new neutral lipophilic myocardial imaging agent that does "redistribute" over time after a single intravenous injection. Preliminary studies in patients show high concordancy with ^{201}Tl uptake patterns in the same patient.

Pharmacologic Stress Imaging

Pharmacologic stress is an appropriate substitute for exercise stress imaging for detecting significant coronary artery stenoses and separating high-risk and low-risk subgroups of patients with coronary artery disease. When either IV dipyridamole, adenosine, or dobutamine is administered in a patient with a critical coronary stenosis, flow reserve is impaired in the stenotic region. Also, the degree of vasodilation is significantly less relative to the increase in flow in response to these agents in normally perfused zones. When ^{201}Tl or ^{99m}Tc sestamibi is administered during peak pharmacologic effect in the patient with significant coronary narrowing, diminished uptake of the radionuclide is observed in the stenosis zone, producing an initial defect. Ischemic defects are most often reversible on resting images, whereas areas of scar correlate with nonreversible defects.

The sensitivity and specificity of dipyridamole, adenosine, and dobutamine ^{201}Tl imaging for detection of coronary artery disease are comparable to those of exercise scintigraphy. Dipyridamole ^{201}Tl stress scintigraphy is performed in the following manner. First, no caffeinated beverages are permitted for 12 hours before imaging. Patients receiving theophylline compounds are not eligible for testing unless these drugs have been discontinued. After baseline hemodynamic values are obtained, 0.56 mg/kg of dipyridamole is infused over 4 minutes. A dose of 2.0 to 3.0 mCi of ^{201}Tl is injected at 9 minutes, and initial images are obtained 5 minutes later. As with exercise scintigraphy, delayed images are obtained 2½ to 4 hours later. Vital signs and serial 12-lead ECGs are obtained every minute during dipyridamole infusion and for at least 5 minutes thereafter. Aminophylline (50 to 100 mg IV) can be administered to reverse dipyridamole-associated side effects, such as systemic hypertension, chest pain, wheezing, and nausea. The adenosine protocol involves infusion of

IV adenosine (140 µg/kg/min), which is maintained for 6 minutes. After 3 minutes at this infusion rate, a 2.0 to 3.0 mCi dose of ^{201}Tl is injected in a contralateral vein and flushed with normal saline. The adenosine infusion is maintained for 3 additional minutes after ^{201}Tl administration. Early and delayed images are acquired in a manner similar to that after exercise stress or dipyridamole imaging. Increased lung ^{201}Tl uptake and transient ischemic LV cavity dilation are seen on pharmacologic stress images in patients with extensive coronary artery disease and ischemic perfusion defects. For dobutamine stress imaging, the drug is infused at incremental doses of 5, 10, 20, 30 and 40 µg/kg/min at 3-minute intervals. After 1 minute at the maximally tolerated dose, 3.0 mCi of ^{201}Tl or 24 to 30 mCi of ^{99m}Tc sestamibi are injected intravenously. The dobutamine infusion is continued for another 2 minutes after tracer administration. Blood pressure, heart rate, and the 12-lead ECG are recorded every minute during the test. Dobutamine is most often used instead of dipyridamole or adenosine in patients with a history of bronchospasm or in those with pulmonary disease receiving oral theophylline compounds. Either dipyridamole or adenosine is indicated in patients with conditions that would limit adequate exercise stress, such as peripheral vascular disease, disabling arthritis, orthopedic abnormalities, or pulmonary disease without bronchospasm.

Dipyridamole or adenosine ^{201}Tl imaging can provide useful prognostic information, particularly in patients undergoing preoperative evaluation before peripheral vascular or aortic surgery. Patients who demonstrate ^{201}Tl redistribution defects preoperatively experience a seven-fold higher perioperative ischemic cardiac event rate compared with patients not demonstrating such scan abnormalities. Patients who benefit most from preoperative risk assessment with pharmacologic stress imaging are those with more than two clinical risk factors known to be associated with increased risk of perioperative ischemic events (e.g., diabetes, advanced age, history of angina, poor functional capacity). Dipyridamole or adenosine ^{201}Tl scintigraphy can be performed early after uncomplicated acute myocardial infarction for separation of high-risk and low-risk subgroups. Pharmacologic stress imaging is safe when performed as early as 4 days after onset of infarction in patients who remain asymptomatic after the early acute phase of hospitalization. Patients with recurrent angina at rest should not be considered for pharmacologic stress imaging. Vasodilator stress imaging is superior to exercise imaging for detection of coronary artery disease in patients with baseline left bundle branch block. Fewer false-positive defects in the septum for detection of left anterior descending coronary stenoses occur with vasodilator stress in these patients.

Side effects of either dipyridamole or adenosine imaging are predominantly minor, with chest pain and S-T segment depression occurring more frequently after adenosine infusion than after dipyridamole administration. Third-degree atrioventricular block is occasionally observed with adenosine administration. Chest pain occurs with vasodilator stress, even in the absence of underlying coronary artery disease. S-T segment depression after infusion of dipyridamole occurs in approximately 10% to 15% of patients. Side effects related to dobutamine infusion are frequent, and ischemic chest pain occurs in 30% of patients. Palpitations are common and can be quite bothersome. Arbutamine, a mixed β_1- and β_2-adrenoreceptor agonist and a mild α-receptor stimulant, is an alternative agent to dobutamine for stress imaging and is used with a closed-loop delivery system that uses the patient's heart rate response to modulate the rate of drug administration.

Radionuclide Angiography

Imaging of ventricular function differs significantly from myocardial perfusion imaging in that the radioactive tracer remains in the blood pool during scintigraphy and cardiac dynamics are assessed in a manner similar to that used in contrast ventriculography. An in vivo labeling technique with ^{99m}Tc radiopharmaceuticals is the approach most often used. With this technique, unlabeled IV stannous pyrophosphate reconstituted in normal saline is injected 15 to 20 minutes before injection of 15 to 30 mCi of [99m]Tc. Radionuclide angiography implies the dynamic imaging of the LV and RV blood pools using ECG gating. Two approaches to gated radionuclide angiography have emerged: the first-pass and the equilibrium methods. A nonimaging

probe positioned on the patient's chest over the left ventricle permits continuous ambulatory monitoring of LVEF during ambulatory activities. One such device, called the VEST (Capintec, Inc., Ramsey, NJ), has a detector that is 5.5 cm in diameter and is equipped with a parallel-hole collimator. It weighs approximately 0.75 kg. The radioactive counts from the LV blood pool are obtained at a rate of 32 times per second.

The equilibrium radionuclide method is also referred to as a MUGA nuclear scan study because of *mu*ltiple-*g*ated *a*cquisition with repetitive sampling of blood pool counts from equal subdivisions of the cardiac cycle's R-R interval. Generally, a framing interval of 30 to 50 msec is used for the resting state and 20 to 30 msec for exercise. Imaging is performed for as many as 200 successive cardiac cycles, with the R wave of the ECG used as the marker to initiate acquisition of count data with each cycle. From these "resultant" images, both regional wall motion and global ventricular function are evaluated. The equilibrium-gated radionuclide angiogram is then displayed in an endless-loop format in which frames are displayed in a ciné (movie) mode. This averaged cardiac cycle is displayed over and over again and simulates the beating heart compared with that observed in contrast ventriculography. Chamber size and segmental wall motion are assessed visually, and ventricular EF and end-systolic and end-diastolic volumes can be measured by computer-assisted quantitation techniques.

Changes in radioactivity that occur within the left and right ventricles during the cardiac cycle can be digitized and displayed in the form of a relative volume curve (Fig. 13-15). This curve is based on the principle that a change in radioactivity is proportional to the change in blood volume. When corrections for background have been performed, the LV time-activity curve represents the average change in blood volume when all the cardiac cycles have been integrated to form a composite cycle.

To assess regional ventricular function, multiple imaging views are obtained. They include the anterior, 45-degree left anterior oblique (LAO), and steep 70-degree LAO projections.

Perhaps the most useful parameter derived from the radionuclide angiogram is the LVEF. The method for calculating the LVEF is called the *area-counts technique*. The supposition for this technique is that proportionality exists between ^{99m}Tc counts and the LV blood pool and actual blood volume. The end-diastolic counts are proportional to the end-diastolic volume, and the end-systolic counts are proportional to the end-systolic volume. The change in radioactivity in the LV blood pool between end-diastole and end-systole is proportional to stroke volume, and this change is referred to as *stroke counts*. The ejection fraction is computed as the end-diastolic counts minus the end-systolic counts divided by the end-diastolic counts after adjusting for background radioactivity. The area-counts technique for calculation of ejection fractions correlates well with ejection fractions assessed from contrast ventriculography (Fig. 13-15).

Other indices that can be obtained from the radionuclide angiogram include peak systolic ejection rate, ejection time, RVEF, regurgitant fraction, and diastolic filling time. Left-to-right intracardiac shunts can also be quantitated using radionuclide angiographic methods. A semiquantitative assessment of valvular regurgitation can be assessed by measuring the ratio of the LV stroke volume to the RV stroke volume.

With the first-pass radionuclide method, a single bolus of ^{99m}Tc is injected rapidly through the IV route, and analysis is limited to the initial transit of radioactivity through the central circulation. A multicrystal scintillation camera is preferable to the single-crystal Anger camera for first-pass radionuclide angiography, since high count rates of up to 400,000 counts/sec are obtained with the multicrystal device.

Clinical Uses

In most patients the etiology of congestive heart failure can be ascertained by the history, physical findings, chest radiographic manifestations, and ECG patterns (Chapter 19). In certain patients, however, the cause of heart failure is not evident. In such patients a gated radionuclide angiogram at rest may be useful in distinguishing between ischemic cardiomyopathy and primary idiopathic dilated cardiomyopathy. Patients with ischemic cardiomyopathy have multiple segmental wall motion abnormalities, whereas patients with primary myocardial disease usually have diffuse hypokinesis.

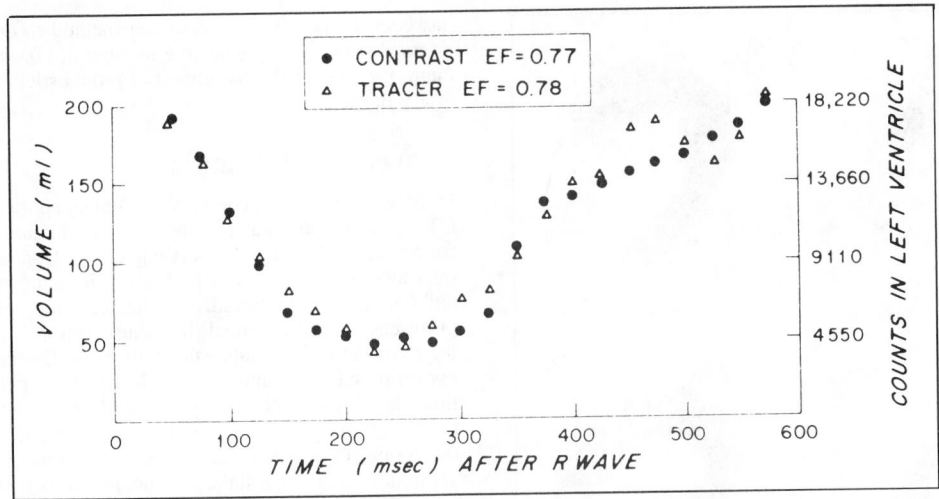

FIGURE 13-15 Technetium-99m (^{99m}Tc) activity represented by "counts" in the LV region of interest versus time curve and the LV volume from contrast angiography versus time curve plotted on the same axes. The ejection fraction *(EF)* is almost identical for the two techniques.

(From Burow RD et al: *Circulation* 56:1024, 1977.)

Resting radionuclide angiography can be valuable in the evaluation of patients with chronic ischemic heart disease and those with recent myocardial infarction. The LVEF is one of the most useful prognostic variables that can be obtained. As with echocardiography, radionuclide angiography can be used for assessing myocardial viability. Preservation of systolic wall motion after infarction or in patients with chronic coronary artery disease and heart failure implies residual viability. Such patients may benefit from revascularization, with improvement in function coincident with amelioration of symptoms. The resting radionuclide angiogram is also well suited for recognition of aneurysmal LV dilation, which can be distinguished from pseudoaneurysms and thinned myocardial segments that are unsuitable for surgery.

Radionuclide angiography has been used successfully in cancer patients to evaluate cardiotoxicity of doxorubicin by serial assessment of LVEF. Imaging RV size and contraction pattern is particularly useful in the evaluation of patients who have inferior wall infarction and signs of low cardiac output. Patients with hemodynamically significant RV infarction show a depressed RVEF and RV dilation, although the LVEF may be normal or only mildly reduced. Radionuclide angiography can be performed with supine bicycle exercise to detect coronary artery disease and determine prognosis (Chapters 21 and 22). Coronary artery disease is detected by demonstrating an exercise-induced decrease or a failure to increase LVEF from rest to exercise. Inducible ischemia with exercise stress is manifested by a new regional wall motion abnormality when compared with the resting assessment. The lower the exercise LVEF, the worse the prognosis in patients with coronary artery disease.

Other Gamma Camera Imaging Agents

Imaging of acute myocardial necrosis can be accomplished with intravenous injection of either ^{99m}Tc pyrophosphate or indium-111 (^{111}In) antimyosin Fab fragments. These radiopharmaceuticals are preferentially sequestered in necrotic myocardial tissue. They produce "hot spots" of radioactive uptake on scintigraphy. The size of the hot spot correlates with infarct size. Imaging with these agents is rarely performed in clinical practice because the diagnosis of acute myocardial infarction can be made readily by clinical history, typical ECG changes, and measurement of serum markers of myocardial imaging, such as creatine kinase and its MB fraction, troponin I, and troponin T (Chapter 23).

Iodine-123 (^{123}I) radiolabeled metaiodobenzylguanidine (MIBG), an analog of norepinephrine, concentrates in adrenergic neurons and can be used for scintigraphic assessment of regional cardiac adrenergic innervation. ^{123}I-MIBG uptake is decreased before deterioration of LVEF in patients receiving doxorubicin, suggesting that damage to cardiac neurons is a consequence of doxorubicin therapy for malignancies. The heart/mediastinum activity ratio of ^{123}I-MIBG has prognostic value in patients with congestive heart failure. Survival rate is worse for patients with a heart/mediastinum ratio of <120%, compared to those with a ratio of >120%.

^{123}I-labeled fatty acids can be used for imaging myocardial metabolism with a SPECT camera. ^{123}I-phenylpentadecanoic acid (IPPA) has proven to be the most clinically applicable for patient studies. Myocardial regions with reduced systolic function but preserved viability demonstrate significantly higher uptake of the tracer at rest as compared with nonviable regions. In one study, 80% of asynergic segments shown to be viable by ^{123}I-IPPA imaging exhibited improved regional systolic function after revascularization.

Positron Emission Tomography

Positron emission tomography (PET) provides the capability for quantitative noninvasive imaging of regional concentration of positron-emitting radioisotopes. PET is undertaken after the IV administration of short-lived positron emitters such as carbon-11 (^{11}C), nitrogen-13 (^{13}N), oxygen-15 (^{15}O), fluorine-18 (^{18}F), and rubidium-82 (^{82}Rb). ^{82}Rb is generator produced and has a half-life of 75 seconds. The myocardial uptake of ^{82}Rb is proportional to regional blood flow, and this agent is given during peak vasodilator stress after dipyridamole or adenosine administration. Sensitivity and specificity for detection of coronary artery disease with ^{82}Rb PET are about 90%. Clinical imaging studies use approximately 20 mCi of ^{13}N ammonia. ^{15}O-labeled water, another positron-emitting flow tracer, has a first-pass extraction fraction approaching 100% and an ultrashort half-life of 2 minutes, which requires administration of high doses of tracer activity.

Perhaps the most interesting and potentially useful application of PET is the noninvasive assessment of myocardial metabolism. ^{18}F, 2-fluoro-2-deoxyglucose (FDG), is a glucose analog used with PET imaging to assess regional glucose metabolism in the myocardium. The magnitude of FDG activity reflects the magnitude of glucose consumption. Under conditions of severe ischemia, increased FDG uptake reflects substrate utilization in the glycolytic pathway. Increased FDG activity on PET images in areas of diminished perfusion (mismatch pattern) is characteristic of "hibernating myocardium" and reflects preservation of myocardial viability. Areas showing FDG/blood flow mismatch usually demonstrate improved regional function after coronary revascularization. Regions of myocardium that show both diminished perfusion and diminished FDG uptake (match pattern) are indicative of nonviability and lack of improvement in systolic func-

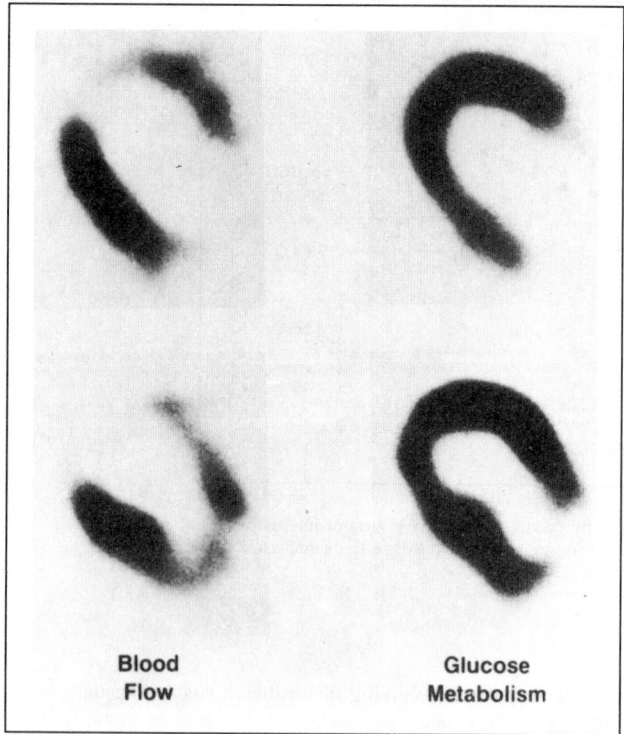

Blood Flow   **Glucose Metabolism**

FIGURE 13-16   Positron emission tomographic (PET) images of blood flow *(left)* and glucose metabolism *(right)* obtained at two levels of the heart's midportion. Note that the perfusion abnormalities on the nitrogen-13 (^{13}N) ammonia PET images of blood flow correspond to increased FDG uptake on the glucose metabolism images indicative of a mismatch pattern characteristic of preserved viability.

(From Brunken R: *J Am Coll Cardiol* 10(3):563, 1987.)

tion after bypass surgery or angioplasty. The positive predictive accuracy of a perfusion-metabolism mismatch for improvement of segmental function after coronary bypass surgery is in the range of 80%. The accuracy of a match pattern for predicting that function will not improve after revascularization is approximately 83%. Fig. 13-16 is an example of diminished myocardial perfusion, as evaluated by ^{13}N ammonia imaging, and increased FDG uptake indicative of viable myocardium in this region.

Carbon-11 (^{11}C) acetate with PET imaging is another approach for noninvasive assessment of viability. Uptake and clearance of ^{11}C acetate are quantified, and if oxidative metabolism is reduced, the clearance of the tracer is prolonged. Dysfunctional but hibernating myocardium exhibits oxidative metabolism equivalent to 74% of that of normal myocardium.

COMPUTED TOMOGRAPHY OF CARDIOVASCULAR SYSTEM
Electron Beam Computed Tomography

Electron beam computed tomography, formerly called ultrafast computed tomographic (CT) scanning, can acquire images faster and at multiple levels without scanner or patient movement when compared with conventional CT scanning. The resolution of most ultrafast CT devices is in the range of 0.7 to 1.5 mm, and the slice thickness can be varied from 3 to 10 mm. The scanner is operable in either a ciné, flow, or volume mode. Contrast enhancement is mandatory for CT to distinguish the blood pool from the myocardium. Clinical applications include the detection of coronary calcification in the proximal coronary vessels; quantitation of LV mass; measurement of LVEF and end-diastolic, end-systolic, and stroke volumes; evaluation of regional myocardial systolic contraction; and evaluation of myocardial perfusion after bolus injection of contrast medium. Quantification of coronary artery calcification using electron beam computed tomography

has been proposed as a screening method to detect occult coronary artery disease. The greater the number of coronary vessels with calcium, the greater the likelihood of prognostically important coronary artery disease.

Conventional Scanning

Perhaps the most frequently used clinical application of conventional CT for cardiovascular imaging is the evaluation of the thoracic aorta for presence of an aneurysm (Chapter 30). Conventional CT with contrast medium allows for a highly sensitive diagnosis of an aneurysm and can accurately measure its diameter and determine the presence or absence of intraluminal thrombus. Although aortography provides the most definitive diagnostic study for a dissecting aortic aneurysm, conventional CT demonstrates clearly the segment of aortic dissection, showing an intimal flap between the true and false lumina. Contrast medium is also injected for detection and localization of aortic dissection. Pericardial disease can also be well evaluated using conventional CT. Pericardial cysts, neoplastic pericardial infiltration, effusions, and constrictive pericarditis are well delineated by conventional CT.

MAGNETIC RESONANCE IMAGING

Magnetic resonance imaging (MRI) has revolutionized imaging of the brain and other body structures. It is a true 3D imaging modality because it acquires data from an entire volume of tissue, which can then be depicted in tomographic slices. MRI involves placing the body region to be imaged within a large-bore superconducting magnet, which for most imaging requires a field strength of 1 to 2 Tesla. Because the heart moves as a result of both cardiac contraction and respiration, the best-quality images are obtained by ECG and respiratory gating.

The theory of MRI and physics of image construction are beyond the scope of this chapter. In brief, however, MRI depends on the absorption and reemission of radiofrequency (RF) energy from certain nuclei when these are placed within a magnetic field. To create cardiac images, the hydrogen nuclei are used most often because these are abundant in the body. When placed in a magnetic field, these nuclei align themselves parallel to the field. If the proper RF pulse is then applied, the alignment of the nuclei changes in relation to the magnetic field, and this change depends on the RF signal's strength and duration. The signal generated by the movement of the nuclei away from their aligned positions within the magnetic field can be detected by a receiver coil placed within the magnet.

After the RF pulse stops, the nuclei begin to realign themselves again parallel to the magnetic field of the external magnet, which can be measured by T1 and T2 relaxation times. These values vary for different tissues and are used to provide contrast in the images. The signals detected within the tissue are subjected to fast-Fourier transform, and the number of times the nuclei have to be perturbed to produce an image depends on the resolution required. This, coupled with the number of images required during the cardiac cycle and the heart and respiratory rates, will determine how long the patient needs to be within the magnet. Different pulse-generating sequences used to create different types of images also affect the imaging time.

The images produced by MRI are of excellent resolution, and because the data are acquired in three dimensions, measurements of cardiac mass and volume can be very precise. In addition, by using certain imaging sequences, flow through cardiac chambers can be measured. Newer imaging sequences allow for fast acquisition with greater temporal resolution, so images can be viewed in a ciné loop similar to radionuclide cineangiography. MRI contrast agents provide the potential for measuring myocardial blood flow. Development of ultrafast imaging techniques will allow for the application of echo-planar techniques for cardiac imaging. MR spectroscopy offers the capability for studying myocardial metabolism.

MR images are particularly useful in the diagnosis of aortic disease (e.g., dissection, aneurysm), constrictive pericarditis, anomalous pulmonary venous connections, and systolic pulmonary arterial shunts. MRI also is being used with increased frequency for detecting intracardiac masses, defining complex congenital heart disease, assessing myocardial infarction and viability, determining coronary

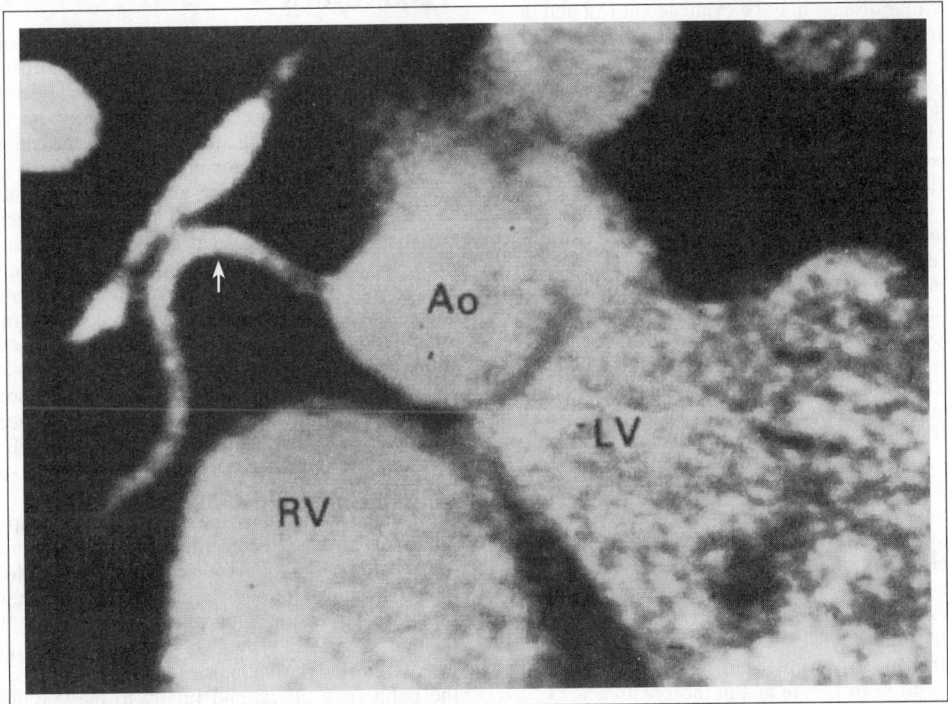

FIGURE 13-17   Oblique magnetic resonance image at the level of the origin of the right coronary artery *(arrow). Ao,* Aorta; *RV,* right ventricle; *LV,* left ventricle.

(From Manning WJ et al: *Circulation* 87:94, 1993.)

artery bypass graft patency, and delineating the course of anomalously originating coronary arteries. MRI angiography may permit visualization of the coronary arteries for noninvasive identification of stenoses in the left main or proximal portions of the three main coronary vessels. Fig. 13-17 is an MRI image at the level of the proximal right coronary artery. Myocardial perfusion and detecting regions of inducible ischemia with pharmacologic stress can also be accomplished with MRI techniques. MRI's clinical usefulness compared with other available noninvasive techniques (e.g., transthoracic and transesophageal echocardiography, nuclear imaging techniques, CT) remains to be clarified.

BIBLIOGRAPHY

Bansal RC, Shah PM: Transesophageal echocardiography, *Curr Probl Cardiol* 15:643-720, 1990.

Beller GA: *Clinical nuclear cardiology,* Philadelphia, 1995, WB Saunders.

Beller GA: Myocardial perfusion imaging with thallium-201, *J Nucl Med* 35:674, 1994.

Blackwell GG, Pohost GM: The usefulness of cardiovascular magnetic resonance imaging, *Curr Probl Cardiol* 19:117-175, 1994.

Cheitlin MD et al: ACC/AHA guidelines for clinical application of echocardiography, *J Am Coll Cardiol* 29:862-879, 1997.

Dinsmore RE: Chest roentgenography. In Pohost GM, O'Rourke RA, editors: *Principles and practice of cardiovascular imaging,* Boston, 1991, Little, Brown.

Feigenbaum H: *Echocardiography,* ed 4, Philadelphia, 1985, Lea & Febiger.

Fletcher GF et al: Exercise standards: a statement for health professionals from the American Heart Association, *Circulation* 91:580-615, 1995.

Hatle L, Angelsen B: *Doppler ultrasound in cardiology: physical principles and clinical applications,* ed 3, Baltimore, 1994, Williams & Wilkins.

Kajinami K et al: Noninvasive prediction of coronary atherosclerosis by quantification of coronary artery calcification using electron beam computed tomography: comparison with electrocardiographic and thallium exercise stress test results, *J Am Coll Cardiol* 26:1209, 1995.

Kaul S: Echocardiography in coronary artery disease, *Curr Probl Cardiol* 15:235, 1990.

Mangano DT, Goldman L: Preoperative assessment of patients with known or suspected coronary disease, *N Engl J Med* 333:1750, 1995.

Marie P-Y et al: Long-term prediction of major ischemic events by exercise thallium-201 single-photon emission computed tomography. Incremental prognostic value compared with clinical, exercise testing, catheterization and radionuclide angiographic data, *J Am Coll Cardiol* 26:879, 1995.

Ritchie JI et al: ACC/AHA guidelines for clinical use of cardiac radionuclide imaging, *J Am Coll Cardiol* 25:521-547, 1995.

Schelbert HR: Metabolic imaging to assess myocardial viability, *J Nucl Med* 35(suppl):85, 1994.

Weyman AE, editor: *Principles and practice of echocardiography,* ed 2, Philadelphia, 1994, Lea & Febiger.

Zaret BL et al: Nuclear cardiology, *N Engl J Med* 329:775-783; 855-863, 1993.

CHAPTER

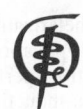

14 Cardiac Catheterization and Angiography

William H. Gaasch and Joseph P. Murgo

Catheterization of the heart provides hemodynamic, angiographic, and other information that describes the anatomy and physiology of a variety of disease states. These data include valuable prognostic information and are often necessary to evaluate potential candidates for surgical or other forms of therapy. In addition to this diagnostic function of the cardiac catheterization laboratory, several important therapeutic procedures are now available for the management of patients with coronary, valvular, and congenital heart disease (Chapter 15). Thus it is important to understand the indications and risks as well as the capabilities and limitations of the procedure.

INDICATIONS

Patients with known or suspected coronary artery disease may require cardiac catheterization to assess the presence or extent of disease. Fixed atherosclerotic lesions, intimal disruption, thrombus, and coronary artery spasm may be visualized and ventricular function assessed.

The severity of valvular disease may be evaluated at rest and during exercise or other hemodynamic stress. Ventricular function is assessed, and associated conditions such as coronary artery disease and pulmonary hypertension are evaluated.

Hemodynamic and angiographic studies are necessary to define the type and complexity of congenital heart disease and assess the possibility of associated coronary or other abnormalities.

Diseases of the pericardium, myocardium, or endocardium require extensive diagnostic evaluation that often includes catheterization. It is particularly important to identify patients with treatable disorders, especially pericardial disease.

In patients with congestive heart failure, catheterization is used to assess and evaluate ventricular function and to rule out intracardiac shunts and valvular, coronary, and other associated or contributory abnormalities.

Postoperative catheterization may provide diagnostic information in patients who have undergone coronary bypass surgery, valve replacement, repair of congenital defects, or other surgical procedures.

Pulmonary hypertension and its severity can be assessed, and the potential causes (e.g., intracardiac shunts, pulmonary embolic disease, pulmonary venous hypertension) can be identified.

Right heart catheterization, often performed with a balloon flotation catheter in the intensive care unit, provides diagnostic information and allows an assessment of the response to therapy. Although complete right and left heart catheterization with angiography may eventually be necessary, an early right heart catheterization can be invaluable in patients with heart failure and in those with acute coronary syndromes, especially those with the mechanical complications of myocardial infarction (i.e., mitral regurgitation and ventricular septal defect).

An endomyocardial biopsy can provide diagnostic information in patients with heart failure. It is typically used to identify rejection after cardiac transplantation, but it can also be useful in patients with myocardial dysfunction of unknown cause. Electrophysiologic studies can provide a specific diagnosis as well as an evaluation of therapeutic interventions (Chapter 18).

Percutaneous transluminal coronary angioplasty is the most common therapeutic procedure performed in the cardiac catheterization laboratory, but coronary atherectomy and coronary stents are increasingly used (Chapter 15). Balloon catheter valvotomy of stenotic mitral or aortic valves also can be effective in selected patients with valvular heart disease (Chapter 25). Therapeutic procedures (e.g., balloon septostomy or dilatation of aortic coarctation) may be especially valuable in children with congenital heart disease (Chapter 28).

RISKS

The mortality rate associated with diagnostic cardiac catheterization is approximately 0.1%, but the frequency of nonfatal complications is greater. These complications include myocardial infarction, perforation of the heart or great vessels, ventricular fibrillation, induction of atrial arrhythmias or atrioventricular block, thromboembolic complications such as cerebrovascular accident (stroke) or peripheral embolization, bleeding, infection, and hypersensitivity reactions to angiographic contrast materials.

The complications of therapeutic procedures such as coronary angioplasty or balloon valvuloplasty are considerably greater than those of diagnostic cardiac catheterization. For example, abrupt closure occurs in 1% to 3% of patients undergoing coronary angioplasty; some of these patients require urgent bypass surgery. These are relatively new procedures, and the complication rate will continue to decline as experience grows and the techniques evolve.

The risks of cardiac catheterization can be minimized if relative contraindications are considered. These include uncontrolled arrhythmias as well as hypokalemia and digitalis intoxication, uncontrolled hypertension or heart failure, allergy to radiographic contrast agents, and intercurrent febrile or other illness. Heparin is usually substituted for oral anticoagulants before catheterization. Special arrangements must be made for patients with severe renal insufficiency.

TECHNIQUES

Many techniques allow specially designed catheters to be introduced into peripheral blood vessels and (with fluoroscopic and/or pressure monitoring) selectively advanced into the various cardiac chambers or great vessels. Once in place, catheters are used for a variety of purposes, such as pressure and flow measurements, angiography, blood sampling, indicator injection and sampling, recording of electrophysiologic data, biopsy, and therapeutic procedures.

Right heart catheterization has classically been performed with the patient under local anesthesia by direct exposure of an antecubital vein; the catheter is introduced through a small venotomy and is guided into the heart. A percutaneous approach through the femoral, jugular, or subclavian veins may also be used; this technique involves cannulation of the vessel with a needle through which a guidewire is introduced. When the wire is satisfactorily positioned, the needle is removed, and the catheter is guided over the wire into the vessel. The wire is then removed, and the catheter is advanced into the heart. Alternatively, a vein dilator with sheath may be advanced over the wire. The wire is then removed, and a catheter is inserted through the sheath. As the catheter is advanced through the right side of the heart, pressure measurements are made, blood samples are obtained for blood gas analysis, and cardiac output can be measured.

A balloon flotation catheter may be introduced directly into an exposed vein or through a sheath. The catheter is advanced while monitoring pressure, and when it approaches the right atrium, the balloon is inflated. Blood flow through the right side of the heart usually carries the balloon catheter through the right ventricle, into the pulmonary artery, and finally to the "pulmonary artery wedge" position, where pulmonary venous pressure is measured. This technique may be used without fluoroscopic assistance, but it is essential to monitor pressure continuously and to avoid excessive balloon inflations.

Left heart catheterization may be performed by introducing the catheter into an exposed artery by a percutaneous approach similar to that just described. The use of vascular sheaths for catheter insertion and exchange has greatly reduced the potential for trauma to the artery. The catheter is advanced under fluoroscopic guidance from the brachial or femoral arteries to the ascending aorta and then retrograde across the aortic valve into the left ventricle. Pressures are measured, blood samples are obtained for blood gas analysis, and angiography is performed. It is difficult to enter the left atrium using the retrograde approach, and thus the pulmonary artery wedge pressure is used as a close approximation of left atrial pressure.

The transseptal approach to the left atrium and left ventricle may be used. This method is especially useful in the presence of severe aortic stenosis or a prosthetic aortic valve. The technique uses a unique catheter through which a specially designed needle and stylet can be advanced from the femoral vein and inferior vena cava through the interatrial septum into the left atrium.

Coronary arteriography is performed with specially designed catheters, inserted via brachial or femoral arteries, that allow selective injection of contrast material in the right and left coronary arteries (Figs. 14-1 and 14-2). This procedure may be accompanied by transluminal angioplasty (Chapter 15).

PRESSURE MEASUREMENT

Intracardiac pressures are measured with specially designed catheters and transducers. These instruments allow the pressure pulse to displace or deform a mechanical device such as a membrane or diaphragm; mechanical displacement is transformed into an electrical signal by *pressure transducers*. The electrical signals produced by the transducers are subsequently amplified and displayed or recorded. By convention, cardiovascular pressures are measured relative to middle right atrial position and atmospheric pressure.

The fidelity with which a transducer electrically represents a pulsatile pressure wave depends on the frequency response of the catheter and transducer system. Conventional fluid-filled catheter transducer systems provide a limited frequency response. Therefore proper care is necessary to eliminate or minimize the factors that limit frequency response (e.g., excessively long tubing, presence of air bubbles). For more accurate measurements, miniaturized transducers have been mounted on cardiac catheters so that pressure signals are

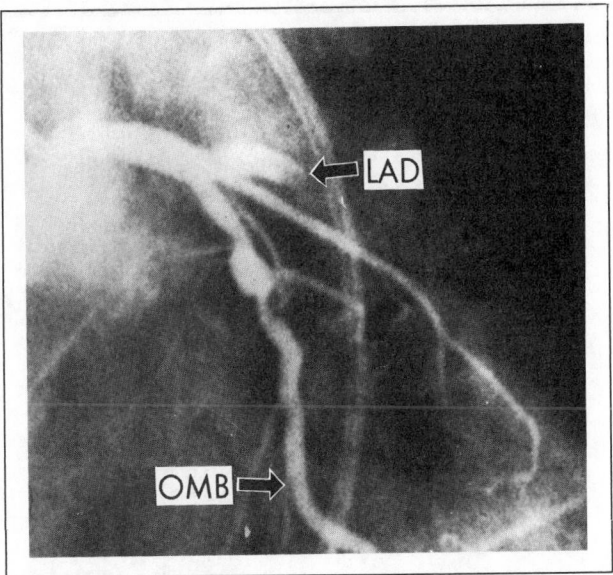

A

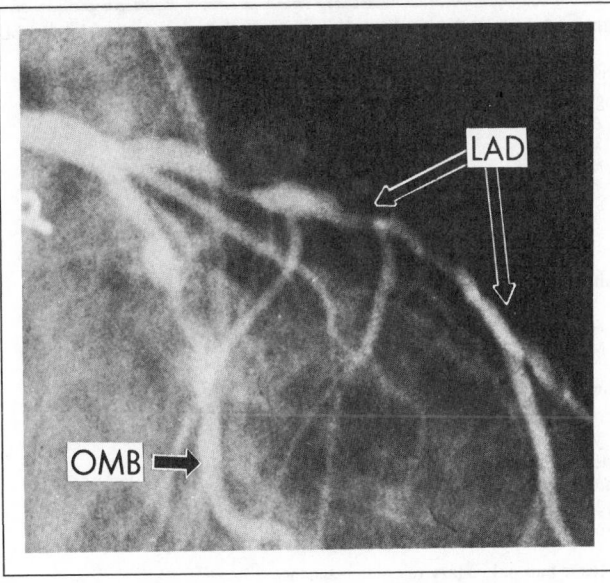

B

FIGURE 14-1 **A,** Arteriogram of left coronary artery (right anterior oblique projection) in a patient 2 hours after onset of myocardial infarction. The arrow indicates site of total occlusion of left anterior descending artery *(LAD)*. **B,** Same coronary artery after 60 minutes of intracoronary streptokinase administration; antegrade flow in the LAD has been restored. *OMB,* Obtuse marginal branch.

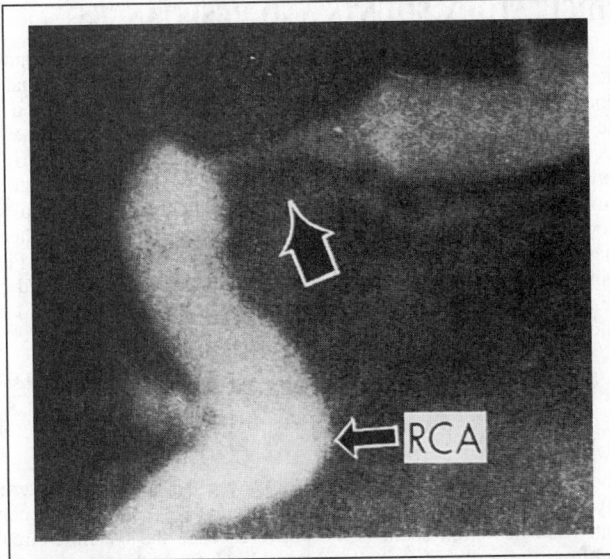

FIGURE 14-2 Arteriogram of proximal right coronary artery *(RCA)* in the 60-degree left anterior oblique projection showing a segment of high-grade obstruction before angioplasty.

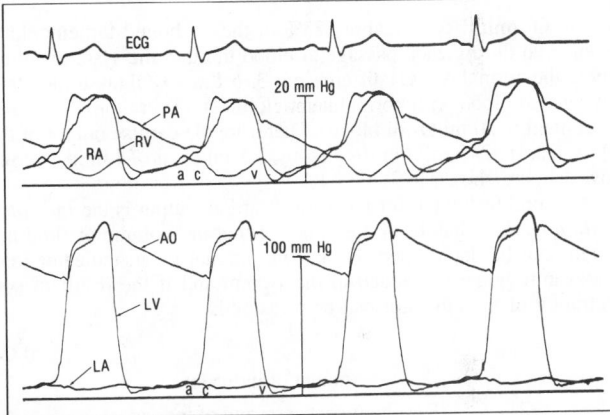

FIGURE 14-3 Normal pressure recordings from the great arteries and cardiac chambers. Simultaneous high-fidelity tracings were obtained with special catheters on which multiple micromanometers were mounted. *ECG,* electrocardiogram; *PA,* pulmonary artery; *RV,* right ventricle; *RA,* right atrium; *AO,* aorta; *LV,* left ventricle; *LA,* left atrium. The *a, c,* and *v* refer to right and left atrial pressure waveform.

converted to electrical signals at the site of interest in the cardiovascular system.

The normal pressure relationships of the chambers of the human heart and great vessels are shown in Fig. 14-3. Small physiologic flow-related pressure gradients between the ventricle and great vessels persist until midsystole; the flow of blood continues until the arterial dicrotic notch (incisura). Normal pressure values are listed in Table 14-1.

CARDIAC OUTPUT

During catheterization the cardiac output can be measured by methods based on the Fick principle, indicator-dilution techniques, or angiography. The *Fick principle* states that the uptake or release of a substance by an organ equals the product of blood flowing through the organ and the arteriovenous (A-V) difference of the substance. By measuring the oxygen (O_2) content of pulmonary arterial (mixed-venous) and pulmonary venous (or systemic arterial) blood, the pulmonary blood flow is measured. In the absence of intracardiac shunts (see following discussion), the pulmonary blood flow is assumed to be equal to the systemic blood flow. The formula for measurement of cardiac output (CO, L/min) by the Fick principle for O_2 is as follows:

(EQ.1)

$$CO = \frac{\dot{V}O_2}{\text{Arterial } O_2 \text{ content} - \text{Mixed-venous } O_2 \text{ content}}$$

where $\dot{V}O_2$ is oxygen uptake (ml/min), arterial O_2 content is systemic arterial oxygen content (ml/L), and mixed venous O_2 content is pulmonary arterial oxygen content (ml/L).

O_2 consumption has been classically determined by spirometry and chemical analysis of the expired gas. In the resting subject, $\dot{V}O_2$ is approximately 3.5 ml O_2/kg/min, or in a 70 kg man, approximately

Table 14-1   Hemodynamic data in normal humans at rest (± 1 SD)

Pressure data

Right atrium	
A wave	5 ± 3 mm Hg
V wave	4 ± 3 mm Hg
Mean	4 ± 2 mm Hg
Right ventricle	
Systolic	21 ± 3 mm Hg
End diastolic	6 ± 2 mm Hg
Pulmonary artery	
Systolic	19 ± 2 mm Hg
Diastolic	8 ± 2 mm Hg
Mean	12 ± 2 mm Hg
Pulmonary capillary wedge	
A wave	8 ± 3 mm Hg
V wave	8 ± 3 mm Hg
Mean	7 ± 2 mm Hg
Left ventricle	
Systolic	115 ± 11 mm Hg
End diastolic	8 ± 3 mm Hg
dP/dt_{max}	1600 ± 360 mm Hg/sec
Aorta	
Systolic	115 ± 11 mm Hg
Diastolic	74 ± 8 mm Hg
Mean	93 ± 8 mm Hg

Flow data

Hemoglobin (Hb) oxygen-carrying capacity	1.36 ml/g Hb
Oxygen consumption	126 ± 24 ml/min/m^2
Arteriovenous oxygen difference	3.6 ± 0.5 vol/dl
Cardiac index	3.6 ± 0.5 L/min/m^2
Stroke index	48.0 ± 9 ml/beat/m^2
Stroke work index	0.54 ± 0.12 joules/m^2

Systemic and pulmonary vascular resistance

Total pulmonary resistance	144 ± 33 dynes-cm-sec^{-5}
Pulmonary arteriolar resistance	62 ± 29 dynes-cm-sec^{-5}
Systemic vascular resistance	1086 ± 270 dynes-cm-sec^{-5}

dP/dt$_{max}$, Maximum rate of rise of ventricular pressure.

245 ml O_2/min. Because about 25% of the O_2 bound to hemoglobin is removed during each passage of blood through the systemic circulation, the normal A-VO_2 difference is 3 to 4 ml O_2/dl (assuming fully oxygenated blood with normal hemoglobin concentration, the arterial O_2 content is 20 ml O_2/dl blood). Therefore the cardiac output of this 70 kg man is 245 ml/min divided by 3.5 ml/dl, or 7 L/min. Normal flow data are shown in Table 14-1.

A second technique for measuring cardiac output is the *indicator-dilution method*, based on the principle that the volume of fluid in a system can be determined if a known amount of an indicator (e.g., indocyanine green) is added to the system and if the resultant concentration of the indicator can be measured:

(EQ.2)

$$\text{Vol} = \frac{\text{Amount of indicator}}{\text{Resultant concentration of indicator}}$$

where vol is volume (ml), amount of indicator is indocyanine green (mg) added to the venous system, and resultant concentration is concentration (mg/ml) in the arterial blood. This concentration is determined by sampling arterial blood and measuring the concentration with a densitometer over time and thus measuring volume as a function of time or cardiac output in milliliters per minute. Assumptions about mixing and sampling are necessary, but the indocyanine green method is acceptable for determining the cardiac output. The *thermodilution* (i.e., cold saline) *method* is somewhat easier to use because no arterial puncture is required and no blood need be withdrawn. Use of a cold fluid as the indicator uses the same principle, but the site of injection must be close to the site of observation. Special adaption of the balloon-tipped, flow-directed catheter allows the indicator (5 to 10 ml of cold saline) to be injected rapidly in the right atrium and sensed by a thermistor located 25 to 30 cm away (at the catheter tip in the main pulmonary artery). Substituting temperature for concentration of indicator in equation 2, a bedside computer determines the cardiac output. Properly performed, the indicator-dilution methods have an error of only 5% to 10%. They are most accurate in normal or high cardiac output states and are much less accurate in the presence of valvular regurgitation or low output states, when Fick cardiac outputs are more reliable.

Stroke volume (ml/beat) is the cardiac output (ml/min) divided by the heart rate (beats/min). The cardiac index (L/min/m^2) is the cardiac output (L/min) divided by the body surface area (m^2).

CIRCULATORY SHUNTS AND RESISTANCES

A special use of blood flow measurements is to detect and quantitate intracardiac shunts. Left-to-right shunts mix fully oxygenated blood from the left side of the heart with the desaturated blood in the right side of the heart. For example, a left-to-right shunt will occur in the patient with an atrial septal defect when right ventricular diastolic stiffness is lower than left ventricular diastolic stiffness. The shunt may be detected and an increase or "step up" in blood O_2 content noted as blood is sampled in the right heart chambers. A left-to-right shunt may be quantitated by using the Fick principle. First, flow through the pulmonary circuit is calculated by using equation 1. Next, systemic blood flow (SBF, L/min) is calculated as follows:

(EQ.3)

$$\text{SBF} = \frac{\dot{V}O_2}{\text{Arterial } O_2 \text{ content} - \text{Mixed-venous } O_2 \text{ content}}$$

where $\dot{V}O_2$ is oxygen uptake, arterial O_2 content is systemic arterial oxygen content, and mixed-venous O_2 content is venae cavae content. The calculation of the A-VO_2 difference for the systemic circuit requires a sample of mixed-venous blood from the venae cavae (proximal to the shunt); the calculation for the pulmonary circuit requires blood from the pulmonary artery (distal to the shunt). Thus the magnitude of a left-to-right intracardiac shunt (L/min) is calculated as follows:

(EQ.4)

$$\text{Shunt} = \text{PBF} - \text{SBF}$$

where PBF is pulmonary blood flow (L/min) and SBF is systemic blood flow (L/min). In the case of an atrial septal defect, a pulmonary/systemic flow ratio exceeding 1.5 indicates a significant shunt. Smaller shunts cannot be detected reliably with the oxymetry method.

Right-to-left intracardiac shunts cause a mixture of desaturated blood from the right side of the heart with oxygenated blood returning from the pulmonary circuit. Detection and localization of the shunt are accomplished by noting a decrease in O_2 content as blood is sampled in the left heart chambers and aorta. Application of the methods outlined earlier permits quantitation of a right-to-left shunt. Bidirectional shunting also may occur, but a discussion of methods for estimating the severity of complex intracardiac shunts is beyond the scope of this chapter.

Indicators other than O_2, such as indocyanine green dye or ascorbic acid, are often used in the detection of intracardiac shunts. Other agents, such as hydrogen or krypton-85, may be introduced at the pulmonary capillary level by inhalation and detected in the right side of the heart by special techniques that permit the detection of very small left-to-right shunts. Angiographic methods also permit detection and precise localization of intracardiac shunts. Flow data are summarized in Table 14-1.

The principle for calculating systemic and pulmonary vascular resistances is that resistance is directly proportional to the pressure drop across the vascular bed and inversely proportional to the flow through the bed. Thus systemic vascular resistance (SVR, Wood units) is calculated as follows:

(EQ.5)

$$SVR = \frac{AOP - RAP}{SBF}$$

where AOP is mean aortic pressure (mm Hg), RAP is mean right atrial pressure (mm Hg), and SBF is systemic blood flow (L/min). Similarly, pulmonary arteriolar resistance (PAR, Wood units) is calculated as follows:

(EQ.6)

$$PAR = \frac{PAP - LAP}{PBF}$$

where PAP is mean pulmonary artery pressure (mm Hg), LAP is mean left atrial (or pulmonary artery wedge) pressure (mm Hg), and PBF is pulmonary blood flow (L/min). These formulas give resistances in arbitrary (Wood) units; multiplication of these units by a factor of 80 produces metric units of dynes-cm-sec^{-5}.

An increase in flow results in an increase in pressure if downstream vascular resistance remains constant; if vasoconstriction produces an increase in resistance, maintenance of normal flow requires a ventricle to generate increased pressure. These principles form the basis for vasodilator therapy in patients with congestive heart failure (Chapter 19).

VALVE ORIFICE SIZE

A special case of resistance to blood flow is that produced by stenotic valves. As valve orifice area decreases, an exponential increase in the pressure gradient across the stenotic valve is generated for any given flow. Conversely, a minor increase in flow, as occurs during exercise, is associated with large increases in the pressure gradient. These predictions are based on the hydraulic orifice-area formulas developed by Gorlin and Gorlin. The effective orifice areas (cm^2) of stenotic aortic and mitral valves may be calculated as follows:

(EQ.7)

$$Aortic\ valve\ area = \frac{Flow/SEP}{44.5\sqrt{\Delta P}}$$

(EQ.8)

$$Mitral\ valve\ area = \frac{Flow/DFP}{38\sqrt{\Delta P}}$$

where flow is flow across the orifice (ml/beat), SEP is systolic ejection period (sec/beat), DFP is diastolic filling period (sec/beat), and ΔP is the mean pressure gradient across the orifice. Thus the pressure gradient across a stenotic orifice provides a reasonable estimate of the orifice area when the cardiac output is normal but not when heart failure is present. These orifice equations are not valid in the presence of significant valvular regurgitation if systemic blood flow (Fick or indicator dilution) is used in the equations; because only effective stroke volume is considered by this method, the orifice size will be underestimated. If, however, the total stroke volume is determined, the orifice formulas may be used in patients with mixed stenotic and regurgitant lesions.

ANGIOGRAPHY

Angiography permits assessment of cardiac volume and morphology and allows analysis of cardiac motion. To create and record a visual image of cardiovascular structures, a radiopaque material is injected into the chamber or vessel of interest. Various x-ray techniques then record the silhouette created by the contrast material. Most often, recording is done on 35 mm film at imaging speeds of 30 to 60 frames/sec, producing a cineangiogram that allows study of the chamber or vessel in real-time, slow-motion, and single-frame modes.

With the newer technique of digital angiography, the x-ray image is detected by a high-resolution television camera rather than on film. The analog signal output from the camera is digitized and sent to a central processing unit for storage, display, and processing. Subsequent computer processing of the images obtained by digital angiography allows better quantitative assessment of parameters such as coronary stenosis and ventricular volumes. Computerized assessment and quantification of video densitometry from coronary arteriography can provide estimates of myocardial perfusion and coronary blood flow. Most importantly, the increased contrast enhancement allows for a significant reduction in the amount of contrast material required for injection.

Angiography of the *right side of the heart* is useful in evaluating congenital abnormalities as well as acquired disorders such as tricuspid regurgitation or constrictive pericarditis. Injection of radiopaque material in the pulmonary arteries provides images for detecting pulmonary thromboemboli and congenital abnormalities of the pulmonary vasculature and, after passage through the lungs, for determining left heart size and morphology.

Angiography of the *left side of the heart* is used to assess mitral and aortic valves and the size and function of the left heart chambers and the ascending aorta. Selective left ventriculography may be used to diagnose and assess the severity of mitral regurgitation and to define abnormalities of the mitral leaflets and subvalvular structures. Ventriculography is also used to assess the ventricular outflow tract, the presence of mural thrombi, the aortic valve, and left-to-right shunts at the ventricular level.

Global and regional function of the left ventricle can be assessed by analyzing the ventriculogram, most often using the right arterior oblique projection alone. However, the accuracy is improved substantially if a left arterior oblique projection is also obtained. Thus it is possible to detect and assess quantitatively wall motion abnormalities (ventricular asynergy). Fig. 14-4 shows examples of regional wall motion abnormalities: reduced motion (hypokinesis), absent motion (akinesis), and paradoxical systolic expansion (dyskinesis).

By modeling the left ventricle as an ellipsoid and determining a radiographic magnification factor, its end-diastolic and end-systolic volumes can be calculated. Thus total stroke volume can be determined. If the effective stroke volume (Fick or indicator-dilution technique) is known, the regurgitant volume can be measured in patients with mitral or aortic regurgitation. This is accomplished by subtracting the effective stroke volume from the total stroke volume.

Angiography of the ascending aorta is performed to assess the severity of aortic regurgitation and to define aortic root anatomy of congenital or acquired disorders, including aortic dissection.

Selective coronary arteriography provides detailed visualization of the coronary arteries. Atherosclerotic and congenital lesions and collateral vessels can be assessed, coronary spasm or thrombus diagnosed, and coronary bypass graft patency confirmed. Finally, coronary arteriography is an essential part of therapeutic procedures such as transluminal angioplasty and during or after the administration of thrombolytic agents.

LEFT VENTRICULAR FUNCTION

The evaluation of left ventricular (LV) function and myocardial contractility has been extensively investigated. Various indices derived from the pre-ejection and ejection phases of the cardiac cycle have been devised to assess and evaluate systolic function. Similarly, diastolic function (i.e., heart's ability to fill without a compensatory increase in diastolic pressure) has been studied by measuring relaxation and filling parameters as well as the myocardium's passive elastic properties. Systolic and diastolic dysfunction often coexist, but it is well established that elevated filling pressures (diastolic dysfunction) may be present in the absence of systolic dysfunction.

END-DIASTOLE   END-SYSTOLE

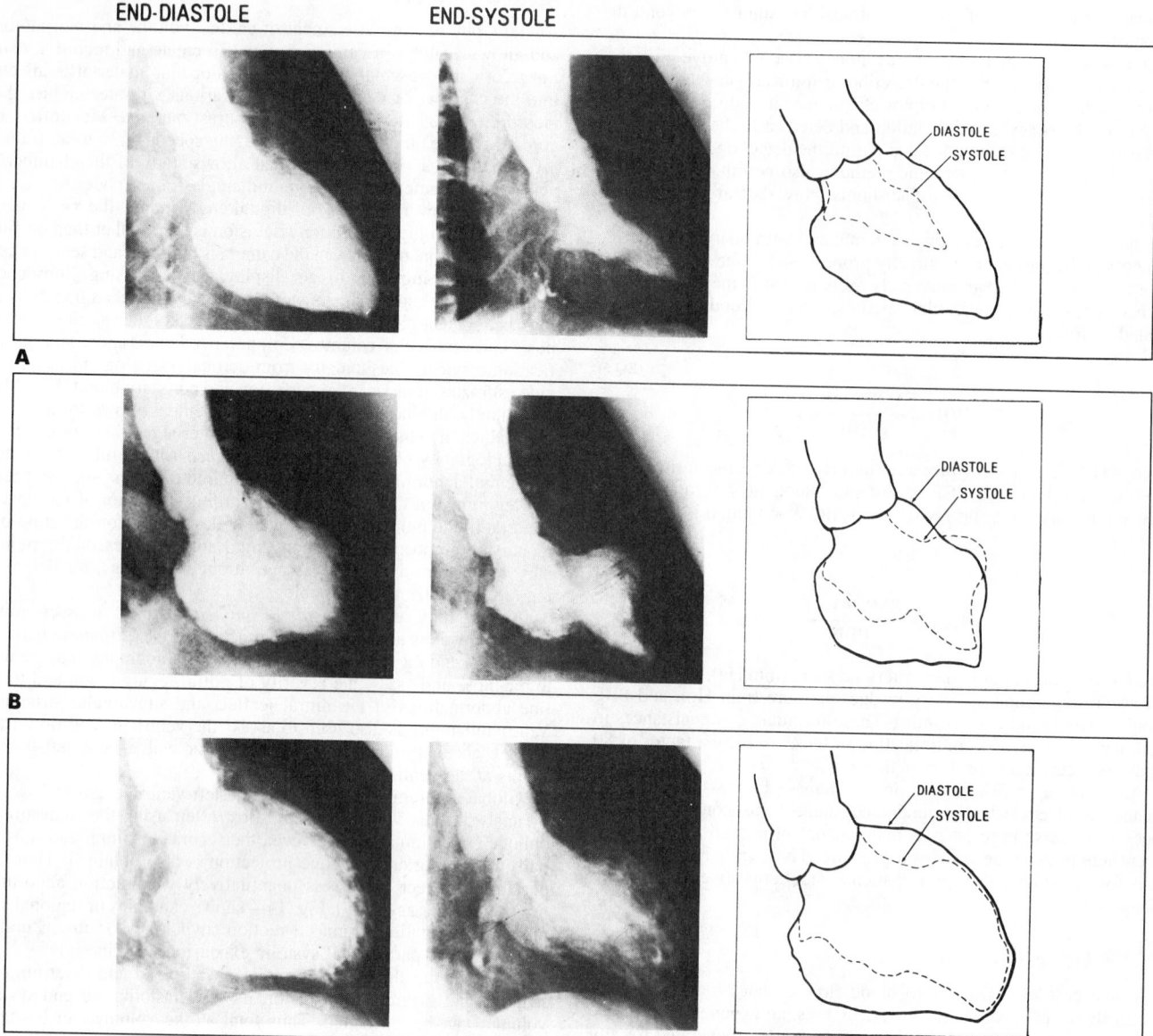

FIGURE 14-4   End-diastolic and end-systolic frames from the left ventricular cineangiograms (right anterior oblique projection) of three different patients. Superimposed silhouette outlines are shown in the panels on the right. **A,** Normal left ventriculogram showing symmetric left ventricular contraction. **B,** Ventriculogram from a patient who had multiple myocardial infarctions, showing dyskinesis of the anterior ventricular wall and hypokinesis of the inferior wall. **C,** Ventriculogram from a patient with extensive anterior infarction; akinesis of the anterior and apical portions of the left ventricle is demonstrated.

Of the preejection or isovolumic indices of contractility, the first derivative of LV pressure with respect to time, the rate of rise of ventricular pressure (*dP/dt*, mm Hg/sec), is the simplest to obtain and interpret. If LV end-diastolic pressure and volume remain relatively constant, changes in the maximum rate of rise of pressure *(dP/dt$_{max}$)* reflect changes in contractility. Calculations of contractile element velocity and other derived indices can reflect acute changes in contractility, but they are of very limited use in the assessment of basal contractile state in diseased hearts (Chapter 9).

The ejection phase indices of contractility or systolic function can be derived from an analysis of the LV cineangiogram. The *ejection fraction* (EF, %), defined as the ratio of stroke volume to end-diastolic volume, is calculated as follows:

(EQ.9)

$$EF = \frac{\text{Stroke volume}}{\text{End-diastolic volume}}$$

where the stroke volume is end-diastolic volume minus end-systolic volume. A major advantage of this parameter is that absolute ventricular volume calculations are not necessary. Moreover, because the EF is a normalized parameter, interpatient comparisons may be made without considering body size. Since cineangiographic techniques permit description of the time course of volume change, special techniques may be applied to calculate the rate of change of ventricular dimensions or volume. When coupled with pressure measurements, ventriculographic dimension and wall thickness data may be used to calculate LV wall tension or stress and thus to construct LV stress–dimension–shortening plots, which may be used to assess ventricular function and contractility. These analyses are based on the well-known inverse relation between afterload (systolic stress) and shortening (Chapter 9).

The stroke work (SW, joules) performed by the left ventricle may be calculated as follows:

(EQ.10)

$$SW = (LVSP - LVEDP) \cdot SV \cdot 0.136$$

where LVSP is LV systolic pressure (mm Hg), LVEDP is end-diastolic pressure (mm Hg), SV is stroke volume (ml), and 0.136 is a conversion factor of mm Hg to metric units (joules). Comparing values for SW among patients of different size requires normalization of the SV for body surface area. By plotting the SW index (joules/m²) against LVEDP in different physiologic states (e.g., rest, exercise, drug administration), a modified "Starling" ventricular function curve can be generated (Chapter 9).

Diastolic pressure-volume and stress-strain data are used to assess LV passive elastic stiffness. Stiffness may be increased in hypertrophied and fibrotic hearts, in the presence of infiltrative disease, and in chronic constrictive pericarditis.

Abnormalities of LV diastolic relaxation may be assessed by measuring the rate of isovolumetric pressure decline and/or the rate and time course of ventricular filling. These relaxation parameters, which are determined in part by active energy-requiring processes, may be abnormal in chronic disease states (e.g., hypertrophy, cardiomyopathy) and during acute or transient disorders (e.g., angina pectoris). Relaxation abnormalities often precede impaired systolic function (Chapters 9 and 22).

CATHETERIZATION DATA IN VARIOUS DISEASES
Ischemic Heart Disease

An imbalance between myocardial blood supply and demand underlies the manifestations of ischemic heart disease. Coronary arteriography is used to determine the cause of inadequate myocardial blood supply and its severity; the technique allows identification of fixed coronary obstruction caused by atherosclerosis, obstructions caused by coronary artery spasm or thrombus, and congenital or traumatic coronary abnormalities.

An abnormal left coronary arteriogram is shown in Fig. 14-1. The left anterior descending artery is completely occluded, and there is moderate disease in the obtuse marginal branch. After the administration of intracoronary streptokinase, flow is restored, but a severe fixed obstruction persists. Complete coronary arteriography requires multiple contrast injections and filming in multiple radiographic projections. Such information is important in planning myocardial revascularization and provides valuable prognostic information.

Coronary artery spasm causes or contributes to myocardial ischemia in Prinzmetal's variant angina and in a variety of other ischemic syndromes (Chapter 22). The intravenous (IV) administration of ergonovine maleate during coronary arteriography may permit the detection of coronary artery spasm in patients with atypical clinical presentations. The angiographic demonstration of coronary spasm provides the clinician with important information about the cause of the myocardial ischemia and aids in planning therapy.

The evaluation of ventricular function in the patient with coronary artery disease is very important. Of the many variables by which ventricular function may be assessed, measurement of ventricular filling pressure and cardiac output and angiographic determination of LV size, wall motion, and EF are the most frequently used.

Examples of information obtained from left ventriculography in patients with coronary artery disease are shown in Fig. 14-4. Three ventriculograms are presented. Drawings of the end-diastolic and end-systolic silhouettes are also provided to aid in the interpretation of the systolic contraction pattern. Fig. 14-4, *A*, depicts a normal left ventricle, and Fig. 14-4, *B*, illustrates a ventricle damaged by infarction. During systole the anterior wall of the damaged ventricle bulges outward (i.e., dyskinesis). The remainder of the ventricular silhouette is irregular in the systolic frame. The apex of the chamber demonstrates decreased inward motion (i.e., hypokinesis). Fig. 14-4, *C*, demonstrates akinesis. The anterior and apical portions of this patient's left ventricle show absent motion during systole. The end-diastolic ventricular dimension is enlarged because of the ventricle's diminished pumping capacity.

By combining angiographic and hemodynamic data, cardiac catheterization should provide information regarding the cause of myocardial ischemia, a description of the heart's functional state, and a determination of the damage already produced by the disease.

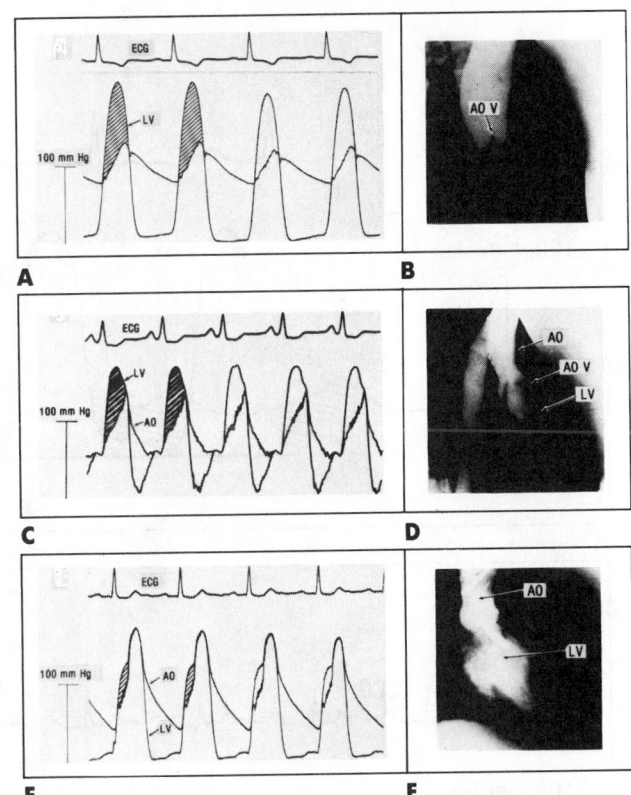

FIGURE 14-5   Pressure and angiographic data from patients with aortic valve disease. **A,** Simultaneous micromanometer recordings of left ventricular *(LV)* and aortic *(AO)* pressure from a patient with severe aortic stenosis showing a pressure gradient *(shaded area)* between the left ventricle and the aorta. **B** and **F,** Aortic root and LV angiograms, respectively, showing thickening and doming of the aortic valve *(AO V)*, poststenotic dilation of the aortic root, and concentric hypertrophy of the left ventricle. **C** and **E,** LV and AO pressure tracings from patients with acute and chronic aortic regurgitation, respectively. **D,** Aortic root angiogram from a patient with aortic regurgitation reveals reflux of radiopaque material across the aortic valve into the left ventricle.

Aortic Stenosis

As aortic stenosis develops, an abnormal pressure difference or gradient is generated across the valve. This results in an increase in LV pressure and high flow velocities in the narrowed orifice. The resultant turbulent flow is associated with the characteristic murmur of aortic stenosis (Chapter 25). Catheterization data in aortic stenosis are illustrated in Fig. 14-5, *A.* Simultaneous LV and aortic pressure curves illustrate the high LV pressure and the pressure gradient across the stenotic valve.

Fig. 14-5, *B,* is a representative aortic root angiogram in a patient with significant aortic stenosis. A prominent bulge in the aortic root is the site of poststenotic dilation of the vessel, an abnormality that arises in response to the turbulent blood flow across the narrowed, thickened, and irregular aortic valve. The left ventriculogram, shown in Fig. 14-5, *F,* demonstrates the greatly thickened aortic valve that is prevented from opening fully during systole. The valve appears domelike, and the narrowed orifice is easily seen. The LV systolic dimensions are small as a result of concentric hypertrophy.

Aortic Regurgitation

Examples of the different pressure waveforms obtained from patients with acute and chronic aortic regurgitation are shown in Fig. 14-5, *C* and *E.* A major difference between acute and chronic aortic regurgitation is the relatively normal LV chamber size and high diastolic pressures in the acute form in contrast to ventricular dilation and increased chamber compliance in the chronic form.

In acute aortic regurgitation a substantial elevation in LV diastolic pressure may be seen; in some patients it may increase to such an

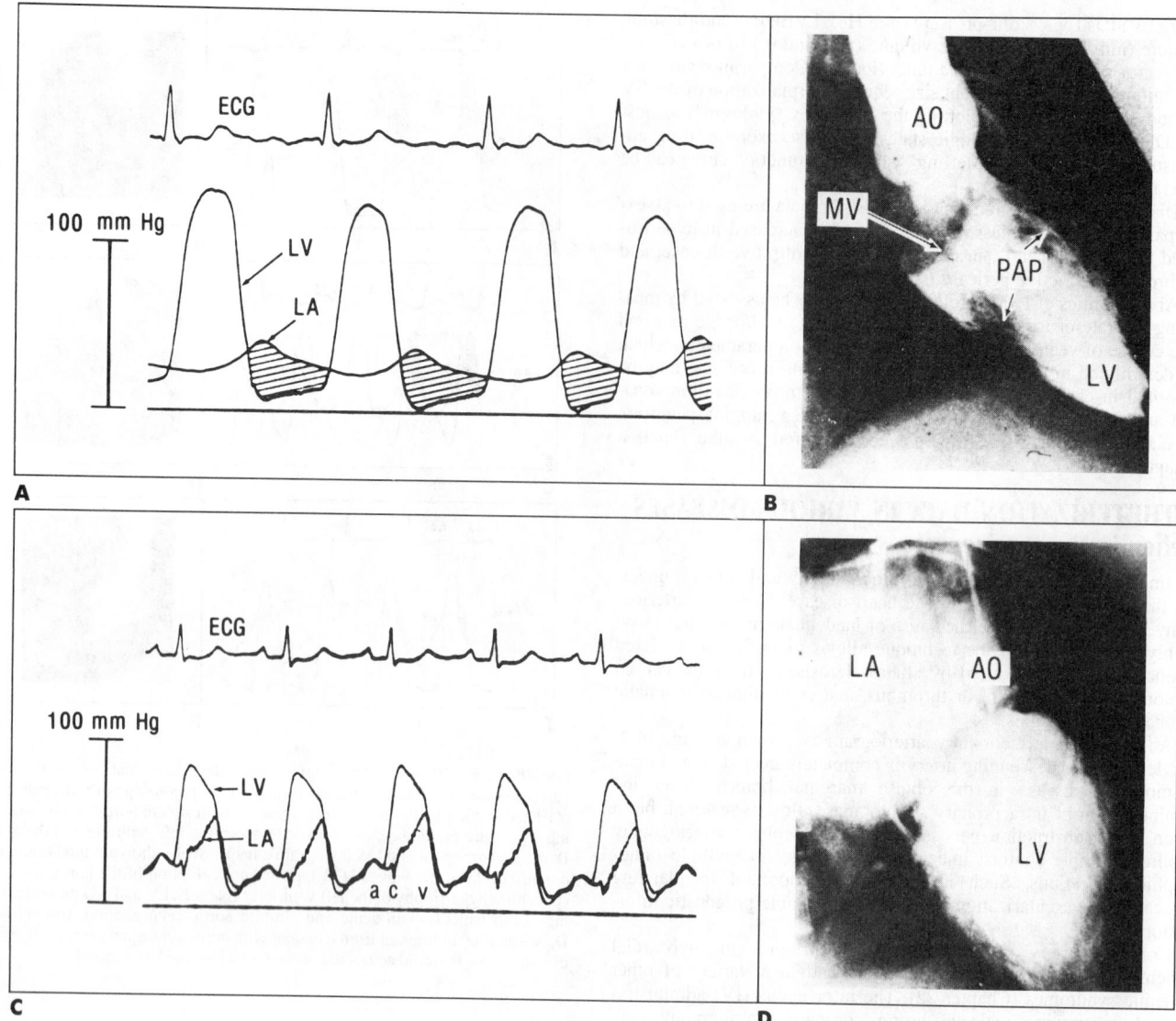

FIGURE 14-6   Pressure and angiographic data from patients with mitral valve disease. **A,** Simultaneous left ventricular *(LV)* and left atrial *(LA)* pressure recordings from a patient with mitral stenosis. The "left atrial" pressure was recorded indirectly through the pulmonary wedge position. This example illustrates a pandiastolic pressure gradient *(shaded area)* across the mitral valve. **B,** LV angiogram from the same patient shows a thickened mitral valve *(MV)*, prominent papillary muscle and a small LV cavity. *AO,* Aorta. **C,** LV and LA pressure tracings from a patient with acute mitral regurgitation showing a prominent regurgitant wave *(v)* in the left atrium. The *a* and *c* also refer to LA pressure waves. **D,** Left ventriculogram from a patient with chronic mitral regurgitation showing an enlarged LV cavity and a massively enlarged left atrium.

extent that equilibration with aortic pressure occurs before the end of diastole (Fig. 14-5, *C*). A considerable systolic pressure gradient may be observed between the left ventricle and the aorta. Such gradients may result from ejection dynamics of increased blood flow associated with a large volume load and do not necessarily imply associated valvular stenosis.

LV and aortic pressure tracings from a patient with chronic aortic regurgitation are shown in Fig. 14-5, *E*. This ventricle is compliant and accepts the large diastolic volume without major changes in diastolic pressure. The physical characteristics of the ascending aorta also change with chronic aortic regurgitation so that flow-related systolic gradients are generated across the aortic valve but are extremely different in magnitude and duration when compared with the hemodynamics of acute aortic regurgitation.

An aortic root angiogram performed in a patient with aortic regurgitation is shown in Fig. 14-5, *D*. The early diastolic frame reveals regurgitation of opacified blood across the aortic valve into the left ventricle.

Mitral Stenosis

As mitral stenosis develops, a progressive rise in left atrial (LA) pressure is required to maintain adequate flow across the valve. As shown in Fig. 14-6, *A*, the elevated LA pressure and the diastolic pressure gradient across the mitral valve are present throughout diastole, but the presence of atrial fibrillation causes a beat-to-beat variation in the diastolic pressure gradient. When the diastolic filling period is shortest, the end-diastolic LA pressure (and the pressure gradient) is highest.

In patients whose heart rates are well controlled, long diastolic filling periods may allow adequate decompression of the left atrium, resulting in surprisingly low filling pressures during rest or when cardiac output demands are at a minimum. Thus an adequate evaluation of the severity of mitral stenosis is achieved by increasing heart rate and cardiac output by exercise. If the valve orifice area is significantly decreased, substantial increases in pressure will occur in the left atrium, pulmonary capillary bed, and the pulmonary artery. Pressure information and valve gradient measurements alone do not pro-

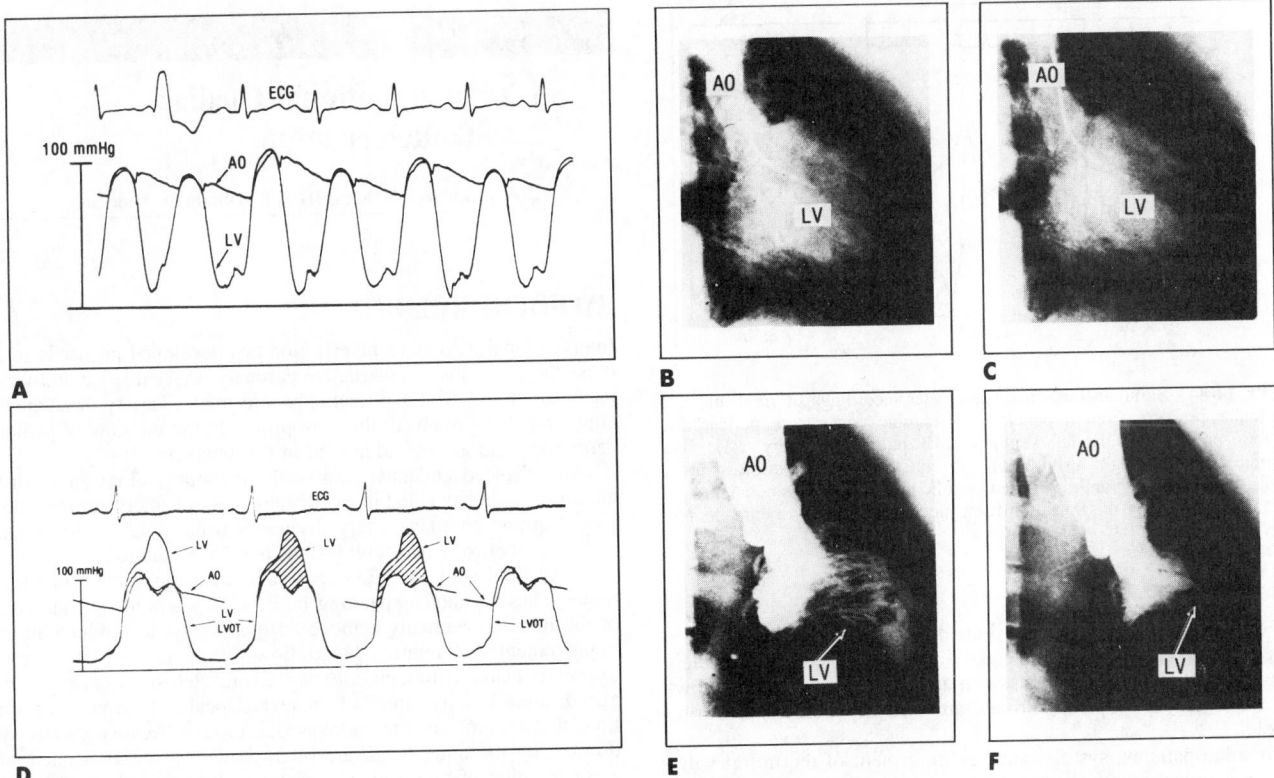

FIGURE 14-7   Pressure and angiographic data from patients with cardiomyopathy. **A,** Left ventricular *(LV)* and aortic *(AO)* pressure tracings from a patient with congestive (dilated) cardiomyopathy demonstrating elevated LV diastolic pressure and LV alternans after a ventricular ectopic beat. **B** and **C,** End-diastolic and end-systolic frames from the left ventriculogram of a patient with congestive cardiomyopathy. The left ventricle is dilated and the ejection fraction is greatly reduced. **D,** Simultaneous high-fidelity pressure tracings from a patient with hypertrophic obstructive cardiomyopathy demonstrating the characteristic pressure gradient *(shaded area)* between the LV body and outflow tract *(LVOT)*. In the first cardiac cycle, pressures are recorded in the LV cavity, LVOT, and ascending aorta by three micromanometers mounted on a single catheter. In the second cycle the ascending aortic pressure tracing has been eliminated, revealing a systolic pressure gradient between the LV body and LVOT. In the third cycle the LVOT pressure has been eliminated, revealing a pressure gradient between the LV body and the aorta. In the fourth cycle the pressure tracing from the LV body has been removed; no abnormal pressure gradient exists across the aortic valve. **E** and **F,** End-diastolic and end-systolic frames, respectively, from the LV cineangiogram of the same patient shown in **D.** The LV cavity is small in diastole and almost obliterated in systole.

vide an adequate characterization of the degree of stenosis. Blood flow rates and a calculation of valve orifice area should be a part of the evaluation of all stenotic valves.

The typical angiographic appearance of the mitral valve and left ventricle in a patient with rheumatic mitral stenosis is shown in Fig. 14-6, *B.* A diastolic frame is shown. The limited excursion of the thickened mitral valve produces a sharp line of demarcation between the nonopacified blood in the left atrium and the contrast medium in the small left ventricle. Since the rheumatic process involves the entire mitral apparatus, the angiographic appearance of the ventricle also reveals prominent papillary muscles, with their tips positioned close to the mitral annulus as a result of chordal fusion and shortening.

Mitral Regurgitation

As with aortic regurgitation, substantial hemodynamic differences exist between acute and chronic mitral regurgitation (Chapter 25). In patients with acute mitral regurgitation the left atrium remains small and noncompliant, and a sudden regurgitant volume into a small left atrium produces a marked rise in LA pressure, with a large regurgitant v wave in the LA pressure pulse (Fig. 14-6, *C*). In chronic mitral regurgitation, progressive LA dilation with an associated increase in LA compliance allows large regurgitant volumes of blood without significant increases in LA pressure. The left ventriculogram in Fig. 14-6, *D*, demonstrates the marked LA dilation that accompanies significant chronic mitral regurgitation. Because progressive, insidious damage to LV myocardium may occur in the disease's more advanced stages,

an accurate evaluation of LV function is especially important in these patients.

Cardiomyopathies

Two clinical examples illustrate the most common disorders of cardiac muscle: congestive (dilated) and hypertrophic cardiomyopathies (Chapter 26).

Dilated cardiomyopathies are primarily characterized by the heart's reduced ability to eject blood. The end-diastolic and end-systolic frames from an LV cineangiogram are shown in Fig. 14-7, *B* and *C*. There is diffuse hypokinesis of the left ventricle, a reduced EF, and a low cardiac output. The LV and aortic pressure tracings are shown in Fig. 14-7, *A*. In addition to the elevated LV end-diastolic pressure, LV alternans is present in the beats after a premature ventricular contraction. In patients with congestive cardiomyopathy the purposes of cardiac catheterization are to identify the cause when possible, determine the degree of functional impairment, and assess responses to pharmacologic interventions, such as afterload reduction or positive inotropic agents.

Hypertrophic cardiomyopathies are characterized by an asymmetric myocardial hypertrophy, small LV cavities, and hypercontractile systolic function (Chapter 26). Abnormalities of diastolic function, often caused by the extraordinary hypertrophy that accompanies this disorder, result in marked reductions of LV diastolic compliance.

The typical angiographic appearance of the left ventricle in a patient with hypertrophic cardiomyopathy is shown in Fig. 14-7, *E*

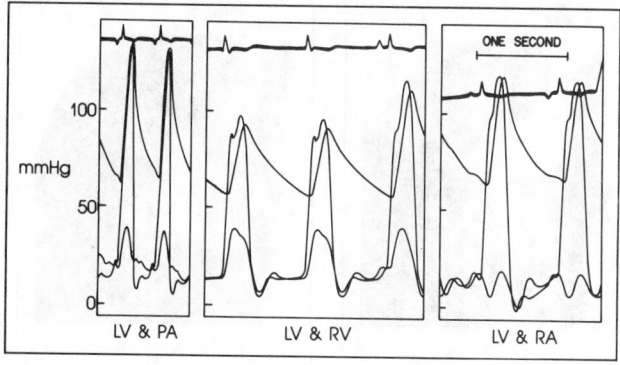

FIGURE 14-8 Simultaneous micromanometer recordings of right and left ventricular pressure from a patient with chronic constrictive pericarditis. Diastolic pressures in the left ventricle *(LV)*, pulmonary artery *(PA)*, right ventricle *(RV)*, and right atrium *(RA)* are equal. The contribution of atrial systole to end-diastolic and developed systolic pressures in this noncompliant heart is illustrated by the transition from junctional to atrial rhythm *(middle panel)*.

and *F*. In the diastolic frame (Fig. 14-7, *E*), a distorted, highly trabeculated ventricular chamber is illustrated. The left ventricle's hypercontractile quality is illustrated in Fig. 14-7, *F*, which shows that the chamber's apical portions are virtually obliterated during systole.

In some patients, systolic anterior movement of the mitral valve may be associated with the presence of intraventricular pressure gradients (Fig. 14-7, *D*). Not all patients with hypertrophic cardiomyopathy demonstrate such gradients, and various interventions, such as the production of a premature ventricular contraction, inhalation of amyl nitrite, or an infusion of isoproterenol, may be employed to produce such gradients during cardiac catheterization. Some investigators interpret the presence of such a gradient as indicating an obstruction to LV outflow. Others, who believe that ejection is not impeded, interpret a gradient as the result of combined hyperdynamic ejection and geometric factors. The interpretation and significance of these intraventricular gradients remain controversial.

Chronic Constrictive Pericarditis

When scarring and fibrosis affect the pericardium, diastolic filling is impaired, whereas systolic function is preserved (Chapter 27). The insidious progression of chronic constrictive pericarditis eventually results in systemic and pulmonary venous hypertension and the signs and symptoms of congestive heart failure (Fig. 14-8). Thus the diagnosis of constrictive pericarditis should be considered in all patients with heart failure. Complete right-sided and left-sided heart catheterization is performed to exclude the diagnosis of restrictive cardiomyopathy, confirm the diagnosis of pericardial constriction, and evaluate the presence of other disease.

BIBLIOGRAPHY

Abrams HL, editor: *Abrams angiography: vascular and interventional radiology,* ed 3, Boston, 1983, Little, Brown.

Gaasch WH, LeWinter MM, editors: *Left ventricular diastolic dysfunction and heart failure,* Philadelphia, 1994, Lea & Febiger.

Grossman W: *Cardiac catheterization and angiography,* ed 4, Philadelphia, 1991, Lea & Febiger.

Grossman W, Baim DS: *Coronary arteriography, angiography, and intervention,* ed 5, Baltimore, 1995, Williams & Wilkins.

King SB, Douglas JS: *Coronary arteriography and angioplasty,* New York, 1985, McGraw-Hill.

Kruger RA, Riederer SJ: *Basic concepts of digital subtraction angiography,* Boston, 1984, GK Hall.

Levine HJ, Gaasch WH, editors: *The ventricle: basic and clinical aspects,* Boston, 1985, Martinus Nijhoff.

Pepine CJ, Hill JA, Lambert CR, editors: *Diagnostic and therapeutic cardiac catheterization,* Baltimore, 1994, Williams & Wilkins.

Yang SS et al: *From cardiac catheterization data to hemodynamic parameters,* ed 3, Philadelphia, 1988, Davis.

15   Interventional Cardiac Catheterization

Spencer B. King III and William D. Anderson

PATHOPHYSIOLOGY

Interventional cardiac catheterization has developed primarily to address the problems of obstructive coronary artery disease and valvular obstructions. Although techniques to treat a variety of congenital conditions have evolved, they are primarily the purview of pediatric cardiology and are not addressed in this chapter.

An enhanced understanding of the pathophysiology of coronary atherosclerosis has aided in the development of interventional strategies. Chronic coronary artery disease is usually the result of longstanding atherosclerosis with lesions that have matured and are composed of lipid core, calcific deposits, and a large amount of fibrous tissue. These lesions, expanding both radially and toward the center of the lumen, eventually achieve adequate mass to produce luminal impingement that reduces blood flow during periods of increased oxygen demand. Although coronary atherosclerosis is usually generalized, these lesions can result in severe localized coronary obstructions that are amenable to endovascular therapy. Acute coronary syndromes, on the other hand, are often thought to be associated with a combination of mural plaque, platelet fibrin thrombus, and sometimes arterial spasm. The lesions may have a superficial accumulation of lipid-rich material covered by a thin fibrous cap with altered endothelial function on which platelets can adhere, become activated, and aggregate. Activated platelets release a number of vasoactive substances that may promote constriction of the smooth muscle cells of the arterial media. Acute myocardial infarction is often associated with fracture of the plaque or the thin fibrous cap at the junction of plaque and less involved media, resulting in exposure of highly thrombogenic tissue components leading to complete thrombotic occlusion of the artery. These unstable syndromes may also be amenable to catheter-based interventions, and knowledge of the underlying pathophysiology may aid in planning therapeutic approaches.

BACKGROUND

Coronary angioplasty, developed by Andreas Gruentzig as a less invasive approach to myocardial revascularization, was built on the foundation of coronary arteriography, first introduced by Mason Sones, and peripheral vascular angioplasty, introduced by Charles Dotter. Since the first coronary angioplasty performed in 1977 by Gruentzig, the procedure has continued to expand in popularity, with more than 400,000 procedures performed annually in the United States alone and a resultant moderation in the growth of bypass surgery. At present, angioplasty is used both as a less invasive alternative to bypass surgery and as an adjunct to medical therapy. We will discuss the selection of patients for angioplasty, some of the techniques of performing the procedure, complications and how to avoid them, and the data relative to long-term outcome. Also, new devices that have evolved in the 1990s, including directional atherectomy, extraction atherectomy, rotary ablation, laser therapy and, most importantly, stenting, are examined. The role of angioplasty in acute myocardial infarction and its relationship to thrombolytic therapy and finally the most refractory problem in angioplasty, that of restenosis, are discussed.

Revascularization of obstructed coronary arteries was first accomplished by surgical means. The value of coronary artery bypass surgery when compared to medical therapy was established for many subsets of the disease in studies carried out in the 1970s. Patients with left main disease, triple vessel disease, and all forms of disease involving the proximal left anterior descending coronary artery were shown to have improved survival when compared to medically treated patients in a recent *meta-analysis* of prior studies. Surgery had an even greater advantage in those patients with left ventricular dysfunction.

Angioplasty of the coronary arteries was developed in the late 1970s as a less invasive method for treating coronary obstructive disease. It was first applied in patients with a single culprit lesion, severe symptoms, and ischemia usually documented by stress testing. In the earliest Zurich series, the patients were relatively young, and most were heavy smokers. They have now been followed 10 years with an overall survival rate of 90%; and 95% for those with single-vessel disease. Of interest, most no longer smoke. Patients treated at Emory in 1981 had predominantly single-vessel disease (88%). The 10-year survival rate has been 91%.

A registry of angioplasty patients was established with the support of the National Heart, Lung, and Blood Institute (NHLBI) in the late 1970s, and a second registry was collected in the mid 1980s. Although angioplasty was in its infancy during the first registry, by 1985 the second registry contained 52% multivessel disease patients and the success rate was 82%. Five-year survival rate was 93% in patients with single-vessel disease and 87% for patients with multivessel disease.

RANDOMIZED TRIALS

A randomized trial comparing percutaneous transluminal coronary angioplasty (PTCA) and medical therapy was conducted in eight VA hospitals (angioplasty compared to medicine [ACME] trial). A total of 212 patients with single-vessel disease with abnormal stress tests received either angioplasty or medical therapy. The differences found at 6 months were a greater freedom from angina in the angioplasty group (64% vs. 46%) and a greater improvement in treadmill time (2.1 vs. 0.5 minutes) in the angioplasty group. There was no difference in death or myocardial infarction rates.

Nine trials comparing angioplasty and coronary bypass surgery have now been performed, including more than 5200 randomized patients. Two of these trials were sponsored by the NHLBI and performed in the United States. The first, the Emory Angioplasty vs. Surgery Trial (EAST) was a single-center study, and the largest, the Bypass Angioplasty Revascularization Investigation (BARI) was a multicenter study. There are many similarities in the baseline features of these two studies. The average age was 61 to 62 years, the percentage of patients with three-vessel disease was 40% to 42%, and the ejection fraction averaged 57% to 60%. Many other similarities existed (Table 15-1). Likewise, outcomes were similar. The hospital mortality rate (approximately 1%) did not differ between surgery and PTCA randomized patients, and 5-year survival rate, ranging between 87% and 91%, did not differ based on the group assignment.

There was more heterogeneity among the other trials conducted in Europe and South America (Table 15-2). The trials also varied in the participation of patients with one-, two-, or three-vessel disease. A recent meta-analysis of all the trials except BARI reported on 1-year outcomes. There was no difference in mortality or myocardial infarction at 1 year between angioplasty-assigned and surgery-assigned patients, but overall 18% of the angioplasty group had bypass surgery performed by the end of the first year (see Table 15-2). Longer term follow-up in BARI and EAST showed that more than 25% of the angioplasty-assigned patients had surgery by the end of 5 years and more than 50% had either surgery or angioplasty. Although angioplasty had a significant cost advantage during the initial hospitalization, much of that was lost during follow-up because of excess repeat procedures in the angioplasty group. A 3-year analysis of the cost in EAST showed that angioplasty had been 95% as costly as surgery by that time. Similar cost relationships were also found in a substudy of the BARI trial.

Limitations of Randomized Trials

Entry into trials had to be limited to patients who were suitable for either procedure; therefore those eligible represent less than 20% of the multivessel population. The consistent finding of no difference in mortality between surgery and angioplasty is in contrast to more variation in the need for further intervention in the angioplasty-assigned patients. This later parameter relates to the percentage of patients with two- and three-vessel disease and by the restudy strategy in the vari-

Table 15-1 Percutaneous transluminal coronary angioplasty versus coronary artery bypass grafting in multivessel coronary artery disease

	EAST		BARI	
	CABG	PTCA	CABG	PTCA
Patient population				
Age (years)	61	62	61	62
LVEF	62	61	58	57
Prior MI	41	41	55	54
CHF	4	3	9	9
No. of diseased vessels				
Two	60	60	58	57
Three	40	40	41	41
In-hospital outcome				
Death	1	1	1.3	1.2
MI	10.3	3	4.6	2.1
Further revascularization				
PTCA	0	0	0	2.2
CABG	—	10.1	0.1	6.3
Five-year outcome				
Death	8.8	12.1	10.7	13.7

EAST, Emory Angioplasty Surgery Trial; *BARI*, Bypass Angioplasty Revascularization Investigation; *LVEF*, left ventricular ejection fraction; *MI*, myocardial infarction; *CHF*, congestive heart failure; *CABG*, coronary artery bypass grafting; *PTCA*, percutaneous transluminal coronary angioplasty.

ous studies. The striking increased need for repeat revascularization in the angioplasty patients is primarily driven by the restenosis phenomenon. These studies were carried out in an era before the wide availability of new devices. Whether application of new technologies, especially stents, might decrease the need for repeat revascularization remains speculative but interesting. Stenting has also allowed more procedures to be completed in one step rather than multiple stages. This change in procedure may influence cost for patients undergoing angioplasty.

Subgroup Analysis

Most of the studies have been small and have not shown significant differences in subgroups, such as three-vessel disease, older age, and women. BARI, however, found that diabetic patients receiving therapy (insulin or oral agents) had a significantly worse 5-year mortality rate when treated with angioplasty (35%) compared with surgery (19%) (Frye personal communication). The explanation for this is not completely clear, but the diabetic patients did have more diffuse coronary artery disease. The BARI findings raised questions about the safety of multivessel angioplasty in treated diabetics and about long-term management of this population that may have blunted warning symptoms of ischemia.

NEW DEVICES

The first of the currently used devices was the directional atherectomy catheter developed by John Simpson. It is composed of a catheter with a metal cylinder on the end (Fig. 15-1, *A*). One side is open in the configuration of a dugout canoe. When the device is placed into a lesion, the plaque prolapses into the cannister. The cutting cylinder, located within the cannister, spins at 2500 revolutions per minute and by advancing the drive shaft can be moved through the cylinder in order to slice off the plaque. A balloon mounted on the side of the cannister opposite the opening can be inflated to push the device against the plaque.

This was the first device to undergo extensive objective testing in a comparison to balloon angioplasty. These trials, CAVEAT, CCAT, and CAVEAT II, did not show a major advantage of atherectomy over balloon angioplasty in a population of patients with lesions suitable

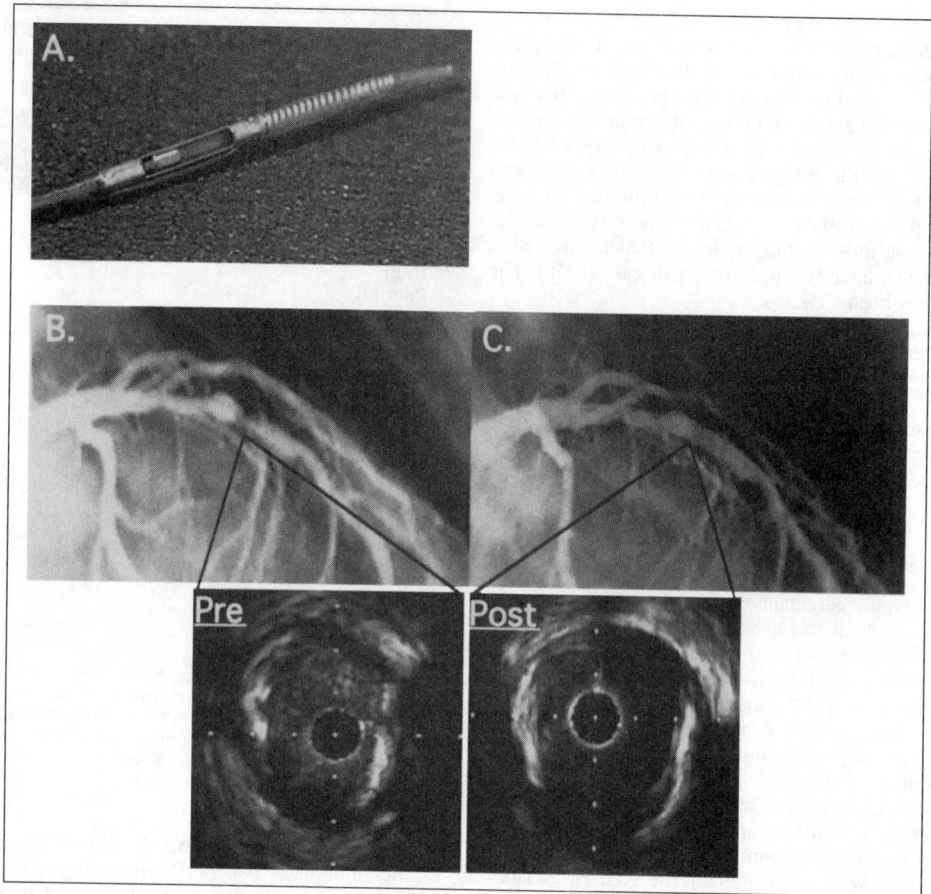

FIGURE 15-1   Directional atherectomy device. **A,** No. 7 French atherocath shown with open window (housing cutting cylinder) and nose cone for removal of excised atheromatous tissue. **B,** RAO angiogram and intravascular ultrasound (IVUS) image of severe mid LAD lesion before intervention. **C,** RAO angiogram following directional atherectomy and adjuvant balloon angioplasty demonstrating significant improvement in stenosis while accompanying IVUS image confirms removal of soft plaque from mid left anterior descending artery.

Table 15-2   Percutaneous transluminal coronary angioplasty versus coronary artery bypass grafting

TRIAL	SINGLE VS. MULTIVESSEL	NUMBER OF PATIENTS	CARDIAC DEATH OR MI		ANGINA (CCS II-IV)		ADDITIONAL PTCA		ADDITIONAL CABG	
			CABG	PTCA	CABG	PTCA	CABG	PTCA	CABG	PTCA
CABRI	Multi	1054	5.7	7.9	11	15.6	2.1	20.1	0.8	15.7
RITA	Both	1011	6.2	6.7	10.6	20.6	3.2	18.2	1.6	18.8
EAST	Multi	392	18.4	13.7	9	18.5	4.1	33.8	0	18.2
GABI	Multi	359	10.2	5.5	25.2	28.4	—	—	1.1	17.6
Toulouse	Multi	152	7.9	7.9	—	—	—	—	1.3	9.2
MASS	Single	142	1.4	6.9	—	—	—	—	0	13.9
Lausanne	Single	134	3	6.8	4.9	8.3	3	11.8	1.5	13.2
ERACI	Multi	127	10.9	12.7	—	—	—	14.5	0	17.5
TOTAL/MEAN		3371	8.0	8.5	12.1	18.3	3.1	19.7	1.0	17.8

MI, Myocardial infarction; *CABG,* coronary artery bypass grafting; *PTCA,* percutaneous transluminal coronary angioplasty; *CCS,* Canadian Cardiovascular Society Angina Class. (All data presented are percentages unless otherwise specified.)
Follow-up data on additional PTCA or CABG obtained from 1-year follow-up except RITA (30 months) and Lausanne (24 months).

for either procedure. Directional atherectomy has found its greatest use in bulky lesions and in bifurcation lesions (Fig. 15-1, *B* and *C*). Recently, the popularity of stenting has significantly affected the use of the atherectomy device. A study of atherectomy, BOAT (Balloon vs. Optimal Atherectomy Trial), using techniques to accomplish optimal opening of the vessels has been completed. If the restenosis rate is significantly reduced without excess complications, a resurgence of atherectomy use may occur.

Another atherectomy device is the transluminal extraction catheter (TEC). This device consists of a rotating conical cutting head behind which is a large-bore catheter with suction potential that can aspirate the cut material and clot from arteries and vein grafts. Heavily thrombotic vein grafts have been the primary target for this device.

The rotational ablation device is an olive-shaped burr coated with diamond microchips (Fig. 15-2, *A*). Spinning at 150,000 to 200,000 revolutions per minute produces a differential cutting effect on the least compliant tissue, especially calcified tissue (Fig. 15-2, *B* and *C*). This device has been valuable in extremely firm stenoses that cannot be opened easily with a balloon. Studies comparing restenosis rates with this device have so far not demonstrated an advantage.

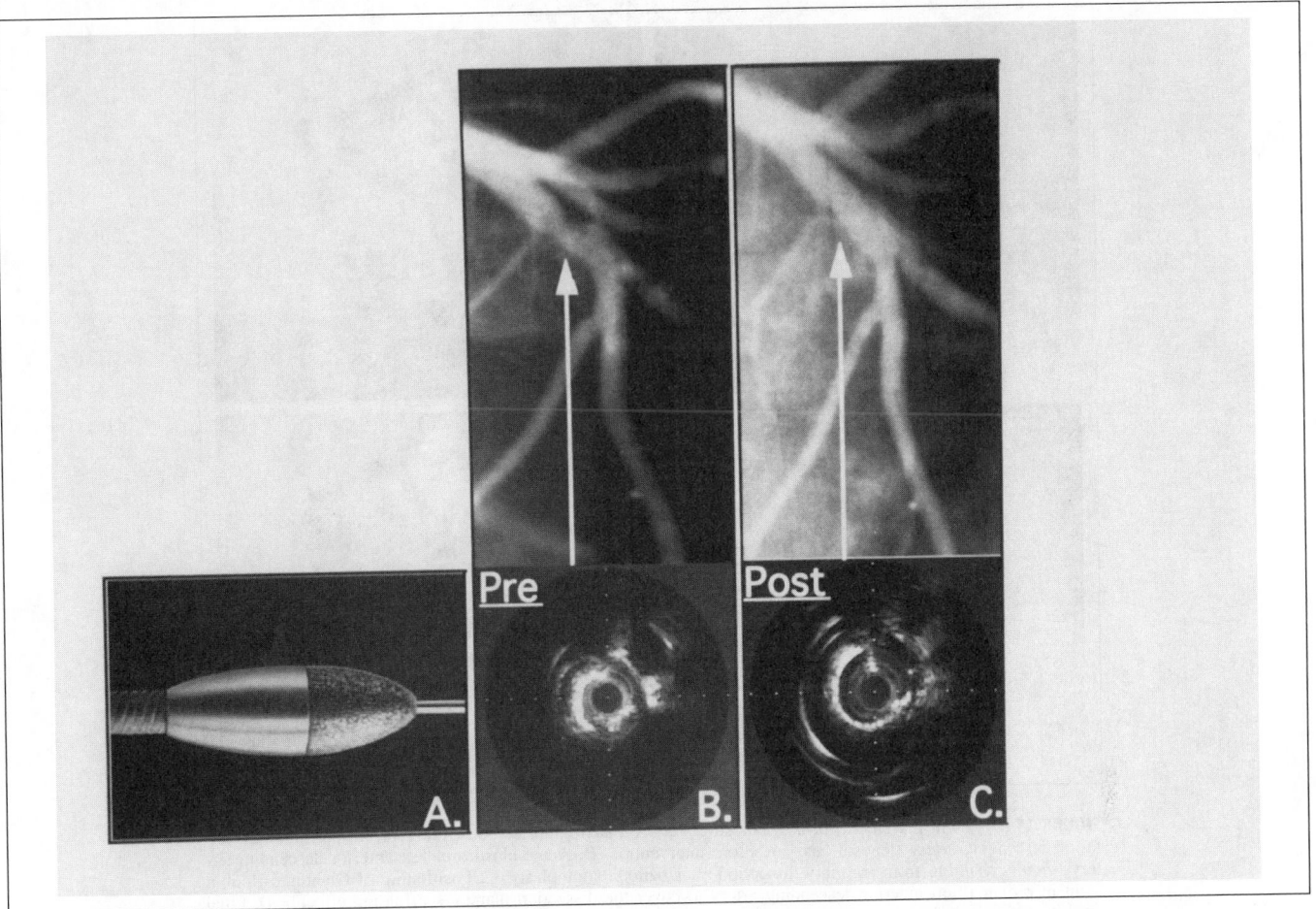

FIGURE 15-2   Rotational atherectomy device. **A,** Magnified view of rotablator burr, demonstrating rotating cable on left and head of oval burr (impregnated with abrasive diamond chips) on right. **B,** RAO angiogram and IVUS image confirming severe stenosis and heavy calcification of proximal left anterior descending artery before intervention. **C,** RAO angiogram and IVUS image after rotational atherectomy and adjuvant balloon angioplasty demonstrating a small residual stenosis <15%.

Laser angioplasty has had a relatively uneven course in coronary interventions. Currently two types of laser systems are in clinical use, the homium YAG and the excimer laser. The catheters deliver the laser energy by a fiberoptic bundle system that transports the light to the end of the catheter. These systems work over a central or eccentric guidewire lumen. When the laser is activated with the catheter tip against the plaque, tissue ablation occurs, which is accompanied by vaporization and bubble formation and by shock waves. All these forces are involved in opening the obstructions. Limited trials have not shown any benefit of laser in restenosis prevention. The niche for laser has been limited, and only a few institutions are currently using the device.

Stents are endoprosthetic devices designed to provide radial support to enlarge the vessel lumen, displace intraluminal tissue, seal dissections, create a smoother final channel, and resist forces that lead to arterial constriction. The initial use of stents was to treat arteries that occluded after angioplasty (Fig. 15-3). Later stents were applied in an attempt to reduce restenosis. Although more than 15 stent designs have been tested clinically worldwide, only two stents are approved for clinical use in the United States. The Gianturco-Roubin stent is a single-strand stainless steel wire bent in a redundant loop spiral shape and expanded by a balloon. This stent has been approved by the Food and Drug Administration (FDA) for treatment of acute vessel closure including severe dissection and other outcomes thought to cause acute closure. The main impact of stent use for acute closure is a reduced incidence of acute myocardial infarction (MI) and a diminished need for emergency surgery in this setting. Problems of stenting have been occasional difficulty in placement, throm-

botic occlusion, and bleeding complications of prolonged anticoagulation.

One stent has been approved by the FDA for restenosis reduction. The Palmaz-Schatz stent is a stainless steel slotted tube that opens to a diamond-shaped mesh when expanded with a balloon. FDA approval was granted after the completion of two randomized studies that showed a reduction in restenosis rates with the stent. Included in these trials were patients undergoing single-lesion angioplasty in vessels ranging from 3 to 4 mm to treat lesions ≤15 mm long. Both studies were positive, with a reduction in the restenosis rate from 42% to 32% in the STRESS (STent REStenosis Study) trial and 32% to 22% in the BENESTENT (balloon-expandable stent implantation with balloon angioplasty) trial. The differences in restenosis rates between the European and American studies may have been partially influenced by the different quantitative measurement systems used (Fig. 15-4). Adverse effects in stent patients were a higher thrombosis rate at the treatment site and an excess of bleeding complications that resulted from the use of heparin and coumadin in these trials. Although this reduction in restenosis rates has created a high degree of enthusiasm for the application of stents, several points must be borne in mind. A recent observation in the BENESTENT trial showed that patients who underwent balloon angioplasty with excellent results had a restenosis rate not significantly different from patients who were stented (Patrick Serruys, personal communication, 1996). This raises the question of whether lesions should be stented primarily or only after observing a less than satisfactory outcome with balloon angioplasty. Another consideration is that studies so far have been with a specific type of lesion, and randomized trials of longer lesions,

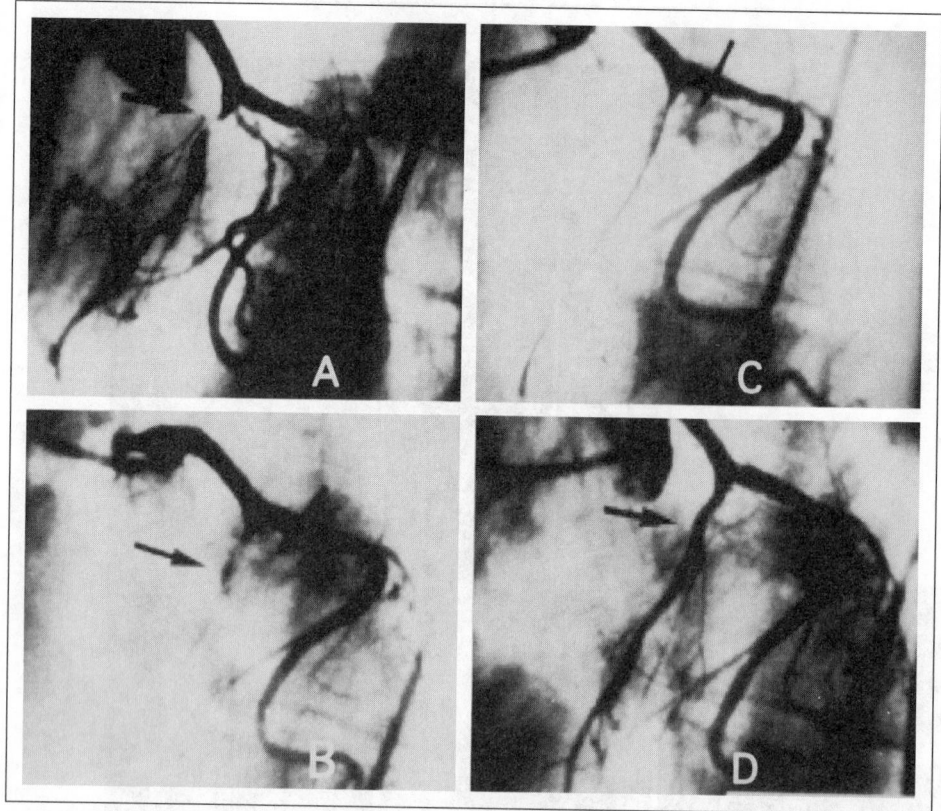

FIGURE 15-3   Stent placement for acute closure. **A,** LAO angiogram demonstrating severe proximal left anterior descending artery stenosis *(arrow)* before intervention. **B,** Acute closure of left anterior descending artery *(arrow)* resulting from coronary dissection after balloon angioplasty. **C,** Positioning of Gianturco-Roubin stent in proximal left anterior descending artery to cover the dissection plane ("scaffolding effect"). **D,** Final angiographic result demonstrating minimal residual stenosis.

smaller vessels, bifurcation and ostial lesions, vein grafts, or patients who require multiple stents have not been conducted. Although there are observational data in all these conditions, the value of stenting in such circumstances has not been firmly established. One randomized trial comparing stenting to balloon angioplasty in vein grafts has shown a moderate advantage for stenting in the final lumen diameter at follow-up (SAVED trial).

The most important development in stenting has been the observation that complete deployment of the stent can result in a lower acute thrombosis rate and in most cases obviate the need for systemic anticoagulation. Such complete deployment can usually be obtained through the use of high-pressure balloon inflation in the range of 14 to 20 atmospheres. Using a high-pressure stent deployment strategy, many operators have recently abandoned the use of warfarin and have substituted the antiplatelet therapy of aspirin and ticlopidine; observational studies have shown this practice to be associated with a low thrombosis rate, decreased bleeding complications, and earlier hospital discharge. Recently, antithrombotic coatings have been applied to stents. A heparin bonding process was used with Palmaz-Schatz stents in the BENESTENT II pilot study. There was no early stent thrombosis in that experience, and the restenosis rate was remarkably low at 13%. A larger trial with heparin-coated stents utilizing only aspirin and ticlopidine is currently under way. Several other trials (RAVES, STARS, STRESS III) are being carried out to objectively evaluate this reduced anticoagulation regimen.

A number of new stent designs are currently undergoing evaluation. The Wallstent, a self-expanding device, has been designed in long lengths and has been used in Europe primarily in vein graft disease. A number of single-wire stents are also undergoing testing, including the tantalum Wiktor stent and Cordis stent. The Gianturco-Roubin stent, approved in the United States for bailout, has been modified and a new version with denser wire frequency and flat rather than round wires is undergoing initial clinical testing. The Johnson & Johnson Interventional Systems (JJIS) stent has undergone modification, and new systems are being tested with coatings and a helical articulation. Other stents are in early testing.

APPROACH TO SPECIFIC LESIONS

A number of lesions remain problematic for angioplasty. They are chronic total occlusions, long diffuse lesions, lesions located in the ostium or bifurcations, lesions containing thrombi or hard calcified lesions, and diffusely diseased vein grafts.

The leading angiographic finding that is a contraindication for balloon angioplasty is chronic total occlusion. Most series that have attempted chronic total occlusions report success rates in the 60% to 70% range. Balloon angioplasty remains the primary approach to chronic total occlusions, although as with new technology, the key element is the ability to cross the total occlusion with a guidewire. In this regard, stiff or standard guidewires have been most consistently successful, with important successes recently reported with ultralubricious hydrophilic wires.

Long, diffusely diseased arterial segments have a higher propensity for dissection, and the opportunity to achieve excellent angioplasty results is somewhat limited. Debulking of these long and often calcified lesions has been performed using the rotablator and also the excimer laser. Also helpful for long diffuse disease is the development of long balloons. Currently most manufacturers have balloons 30 and 40 mm long and some longer. By crossing all of the diseased segment, these balloons may be less prone to creating dissection planes. It is not yet clear which approach is superior.

Lesions at the ostium of the coronary arteries or vein grafts or at the bifurcation of coronary arteries pose a special problem. Dilating in a straight segment gives the possibility for plaque displacement, not only radially but longitudinally. It also ensures that the force can be applied equally in the circumference of the vessel. When ostial or

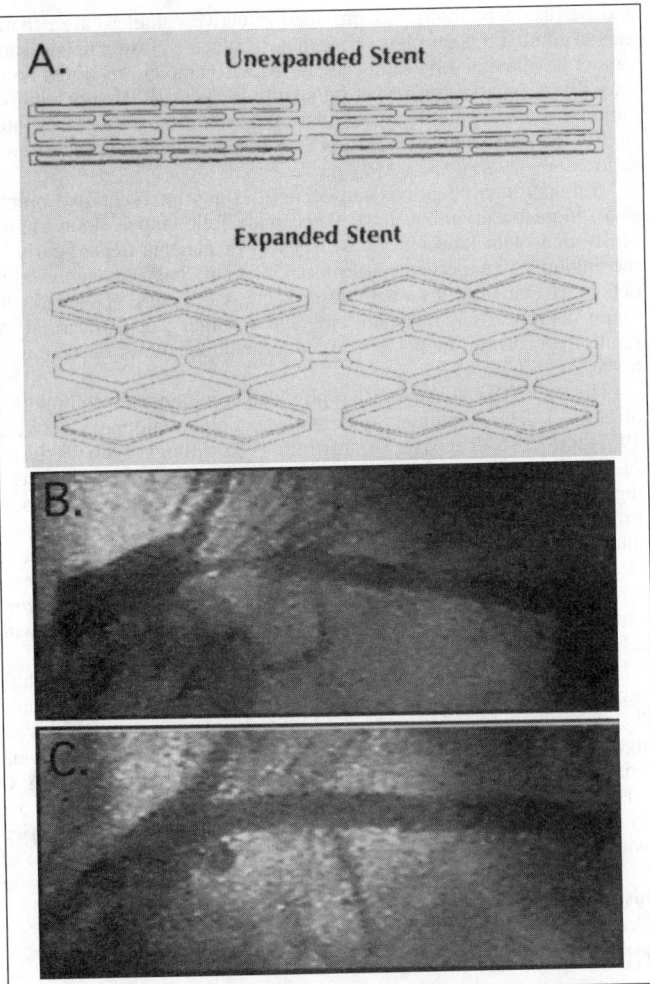

FIGURE 15-4   Palmaz-Schatz stent. **A,** Diagram demonstrating slotted tube design of Palmaz-Schatz stent in unexpanded and expanded states. **B,** LAO angiogram of ostial left circumflex lesion before intervention. **C,** LAO angiogram of same lesion after implantation of a 3.0 mm Palmaz-Schatz stent (followed by high-pressure balloon inflations at 20 atmospheres) demonstrating a residual stenosis of 5% to 10%.

bifurcation lesions are approached, there is often nothing to push against; therefore elastic recoil is much more common than in lesions located in straight segments. Debulking devices, especially the rotablator and directional atherectomy, have found a niche in these types of lesions. Laser has been helpful for aortic ostial lesions. In large bifurcation lesions, directional atherectomy has the potential to remove a significant amount of tissue, thereby decreasing the effect of elastic recoil. Stenting in these lesions also has been performed and is often successful in ostial vein graft disease and sometimes in ostial right coronary disease. In bifurcation lesions, stenting becomes technically challenging because multiple stents must be placed and the possibility of occluding or "jailing" the side branch sometimes diminishes the enthusiasm for stenting in such lesions.

Lesions containing thrombus have previously been found to have a higher risk of acute closure after angioplasty. Two developments have made thrombus-containing lesions easier to approach. The first is the development of stenting. If the thrombus is associated with a severe flow disruption and a rheology favorable toward rethrombosis, then improvement of that lumen by stenting and reestablishment of a laminar flow pattern can often solve the problem. The second powerful tool has been the development of IIb/IIIa platelet receptor blockers. In the EPIC trial, patients who were judged at high risk of having thrombus, such as those who were unstable or were in the early postmyocardial infarction period, were randomized to receive the IIb/IIIa receptor blocking antibody (C7E3) or placebo. The treat-

ment group had a 35% reduction in the end-point of death, nonfatal infarction, surgery, angioplasty, stent implantation, or insertion of an intraaortic balloon pump for refractory ischemia. Though bleeding complications were increased in the C7E3 group study, a subsequent trial (EPILOG) using a weight-adjusted heparin dose (and actually withholding heparin after the procedure in most cases) resulted in no increase in bleeding complications and a sustained improvement in the clinical event rate.

The hard calcified plaque that cannot be opened with a balloon has been uniquely suited for rotablator therapy. Lesions that resist balloon inflation, even up to high pressures, can be dilated with balloons when treated with rotablator burrs, indicating a release from highly constrictive unyielding lesions. Strategies continue to be developed regarding the technique of rotary ablation and how much enlargement of the vessel should be obtained with the rotablator burr to achieve optimal benefit.

Vein graft disease poses a major problem at this time with so many patients presenting who have had bypass surgery 8 to 15 years previously. These degenerative vein grafts have shown very high restenosis rates when treated with balloon angioplasty. Many of the other techniques have been tried without dramatic success. Directional atherectomy also resulted in a high restenosis rate and perhaps an increased embolic rate. The rotary ablation approach has generally been contraindicated in vein grafts, and laser has been used with mixed success. The TEC atherectomy catheter has been used more than any other device in diffusely diseased vein grafts. Intracoronary stenting seems rational for fairly discrete stenoses and with longer stents perhaps for more diffuse disease. The potential for stenting the entire course of vein grafts with a single stent may improve long-term results. Adjuncts such as prolonged urokinase infusion have been helpful in opening some vein grafts, although in other patients they have resulted in embolization of thrombotic debris. The IIb/IIIa antagonist is just beginning to be used for this indication, and initial observations are encouraging, although none of these techniques has been able to produce good long-term patency in diffusely diseased grafts.

CORONARY ANGIOPLASTY FOR ACUTE MYOCARDIAL INFARCTION

Angioplasty is helpful in three situations after myocardial infarction: (1) as an elective procedure to relieve the remaining stenosis after myocardial infarction (with or without prior thrombolytic therapy), (2) as a "rescue" procedure for those patients who have undergone thrombolytic therapy but continue to manifest signs or symptoms of ongoing injury suggesting reocclusion or a lack of reperfusion, and (3) as a primary procedure in the place of thrombolytic therapy (Chapter 23).

Several trials have evaluated the use of angioplasty as an adjunct after thrombolytic therapy. The rationale was that if the artery were opened but a high-grade stenosis remained, then further improvement in perfusion could be achieved with angioplasty. Three trials testing this approach failed to show an advantage of early intervention after thrombolysis with tPA. It should be pointed out that in the TIMI trial, patients were undergoing early angioplasty only if the artery had opened with thrombolysis but still retained a high-grade lesion. In arteries that were totally occluded, angioplasty was not attempted. Based on these trials, elective angioplasty immediately after thrombolytic therapy was largely abandoned. The reason for this outcome could have been further stimulation of platelet activation in the presence of a thrombolytic agent or the increased hemorrhage at the site of angioplasty. A strategy of deferring angioplasty was tested by the TIMI investigators who investigated 3262 patients randomized within 18 to 48 hours after infarction to elective catheterization and angioplasty versus a conservative strategy of angioplasty only for recurrent ischemia. Angioplasty was performed in 54% of the invasive strategy group and 13% of the conservative strategy group. There was no difference in the primary end-point of death or reinfarction at 6 weeks (averaging 7%) and no difference in left ventricular function. Late survival was also equal between the groups, although more rehospitalizations occurred in the conservative strategy group. Another trial, SWIFT (Should We Intervene Following Thrombolysis), using anistreplase also found no advantage to the aggressive strategy. Although these trials have not established that elective angioplasty after thrombolysis in asymptomatic patients is essential, it continues to be a common practice, and further studies to evaluate the long-term economic impact of an in-hospital catheterization would seem appropriate.

RESCUE CORONARY ANGIOPLASTY

Reperfusion after thrombolytic therapy is not complete and occurs in 55% to 85% of patients. The mortality rate in those patients whose arteries do not achieve patency is high, and therefore opening those arteries would seem to be intuitively correct. The TAMI V (Thrombolysis in Acute Myocardial Infarction V) trial tested the strategy of immediate catheterization and subsequent rescue angioplasty, if needed, after thrombolytic therapy against a strategy of catheterization and angioplasty, if needed, at the time of discharge. The early intervention group achieved a higher degree of patency (94% vs. 90%) and improved wall motion and fewer adverse outcomes than the late intervention group. A recent study, The Randomized Evaluation of Salvage angioplasty with Combined Utilization of Endpoints (RESCUE), compared rescue angioplasty with conservative therapy. That trial showed a significant benefit to rescue angioplasty.

The decision to perform early catheterization and potential rescue angioplasty is complicated by present limitations in determining reperfusion after the administration of thrombolytic agents (Chapter 23). Among the indices of patency are the complete resolution of ST segments and the complete alleviation of chest pain. These signs are frequently absent even in the situations in which flow has been restored. Arrhythmias during thrombolytic administration have not been shown to be predictive of reperfusion. The creatine kinase release curve is sensitive and specific for patency but is attainable only after the fact.

PRIMARY CORONARY ANGIOPLASTY

Primary angioplasty without the use of thrombolytic agents has become popular in recent years. Three investigations recently reported comparisons of primary angioplasty with thrombolytic therapy (Table 15-3). The largest of these was the Primary Angioplasty in Myocardial Infarction (PAMI) trial. A total of 395 patients who were within 12 hours of the onset of pain were randomized to angioplasty or thrombolytic therapy using tPA. Patients had to be eligible for thrombolytic therapy as well as primary angioplasty and therefore were not the highest risk group with infarction. Total occlusion with no antegrade flow was seen in 78% of the patients. There was a strong trend toward decreased mortality in the angioplasty group (2.6%) compared to the thrombolytic group (6.5%, $P = 0.06$). Features putting the patients in a high-risk group, such as the occurrence of anterior infarction, older age, and female gender, all were associated with an even greater benefit from primary angioplasty over thrombolysis.

Two other trials, one at the Mayo Clinic and one from the Netherlands, showed a significantly decreased need for subsequent revascularization in the angioplasty group. In the Mayo study, no difference was detectable in death or left ventricular function at 6 weeks; however, the angioplasty patients had fewer readmissions for ischemia (Table 15-4).

It is difficult to extrapolate the results of these trials to the broad population of patients undergoing primary angioplasty. The hospitals involved in these studies were committed to the process of primary angioplasty, and the patient population was not the highest risk group. Nonetheless, primary angioplasty seems to be a valuable and viable method for treating acute myocardial infarction, and larger prospective studies are planned.

COMPLICATIONS

Patients undergoing angioplasty are subject to a variety of complications, including coronary dissection, vessel perforation, thrombus formation, and coronary spasm, as well as those complications associated with diagnostic catheterization such as hematomas at vascular access sites and occasional strokes. Some of these complications, particularly coronary dissection and thrombus formation, may lead to abrupt coronary closure in approximately 5% to 7% of patients within 24 hours of the initial procedure. The evolution of intracoronary stents

and perfusion balloons has provided effective catheter-based therapies to combat this problem. Nonetheless, if acute closure persists and cannot be alleviated by such catheter-based therapies, emergent coronary artery bypass grafting is frequently performed. With or without surgery, some degree of myocardial infarction often ensues, accounting for the significant mortality (4% to 10%) associated with this condition.

Although complications can occur after any interventional procedure, more observations have been made following balloon angioplasty than with newer devices. A series of patients treated early in the angioplasty experience at Emory University has been analyzed in detail. At that time the angioplasty success rate was 91%, with the major complications of death, emergency surgery, or myocardial infarction occurring in 4.1% and minor complications occurring in 6.9%.

The NHLBI PTCA Registry provided a multicenter compilation of clinical data on patients undergoing balloon angioplasty between 1977 and 1981 (Registry 1) and from 1985 through 1986 (Registry 2). Death (<1%) and MI (4.6%) rates were similar between the two registries despite more extensive coronary disease in the latter group. Procedural success was similarly improved and the need for surgical intervention significantly reduced in the Registry 2 population, due largely to technical advances in catheter technology. The most recent reports of balloon angioplasty populations have demonstrated a continued increase in procedural success rates (usually above 93%) with a leveling of complication rates in the range of 1% to 3%.

An evaluation of the safety and efficacy of newer devices, including stents, atherectomy catheters, and laser devices was recently published by the NACI (New Approach to Coronary Intervention) investigators. Of 2835 patients undergoing percutaneous coronary interventions with these devices, major complications (consisting of death, Q wave MI, or performance of emergency CABG) ranged from 2.6% to 7.1%, depending on the device chosen. Procedural success varied widely (from 78% to 95%) between devices, with an overall value of 91%. Many of the lesions represented in this cohort of patients were historically recalcitrant to balloon angioplasty.

RESTENOSIS

Following interventional procedures, the coronary arteries undergo a healing process during which renarrowing of the artery frequently occurs. This renarrowing of the lumen has been arbitrarily defined as restenosis when the lumen diameter is reduced to 50% or less than the diameter of the adjacent reference segment. There are many other definitions of restenosis, but this one has become standard. The process of restenosis usually runs its course within the first 6 months and if systematic angiograms are obtained, the average rate of this degree of renarrowing has been approximately 35% to 40%.

The pathobiology of this process consists of three major components. First is the elastic recoil that occurs after most interventions. Inherent to angioplasty is the stretching of the entire vessel, and if one waits a few minutes after the procedure, some immediate loss of lumen diameter occurs. This has been observed to result in a 40% to 50% reduction in luminal cross-sectional area compared to that of the fully inflated balloon. Second is the process of neointimal formation. This process is most akin to the proliferative phase of wound healing in which cells multiply, migrate to the site of injury, and produce extracellular matrix, forming a new and significantly thickened intima, especially in the zones where the most severe vascular damage has occurred. The third process, observed only recently, is the reduction in arterial size produced by a shrinking of the entire artery or "remodelling." This term, *remodelling,* commonly used for adaptive expansion of the artery to compensate for atherosclerosis, may not be the most appropriate term for a process that seems more akin to wound contracture in the latter phases of wound healing. In any case, the result of this process is a decreased circumference of the external elastic lamina compared to the early postangioplasty condition. The relative contributions of these three phenomena must vary widely, but it has been estimated that the late contributions to luminal narrowing from neointimal formation and arterial contracture may be approximately equal.

Animal models of restenosis have been targeted primarily at understanding the neointimal proliferative response. Although a num-

Table 15-3   Primary angioplasty versus thrombolytic therapy in acute myocardial infarction

TRIAL	NUMBER OF PATIENTS		DEATH		REINFARCTION		DEATH/NONFATAL REINFARCTION		LEFT VENTRICULAR EJECTION FRACTION		RECURRENT ISCHEMIA		STROKE	
	PTCA	TPA OR SK	PTCA	TPA OR SK	PTCA	TPA OR SK	PTCA	TPA OR SK	PTCA	TPA OR SK	PTCA	TPA OR SK	PTCA	TPA OR SK
PAMI	195	200	3	7	3	7	5	12	53	53	3	7	0	2
Netherlands Study	70	72	0	6	0	9	0	15	51	45	9	38	0	3
Mayo Clinic Study	47	56	4	4	—	—	—	—	53	50	15	36	—	—
Total/Mean	312	328	2	6	1	8	3	14	52	49	9	27	0	3

PAMI, Primary Angioplasty in Myocardial Infarction; *PTCA*, percutaneous transluminal coronary angioplasty; *tPA*, tissue plasminogen activator; *SK*, streptokinase.
All data presented are percentages unless otherwise specified.
Left ventricular ejection fraction at 6 weeks for PAMI and Mayo Clinic Study; before hospital discharge for Netherlands study.

✔ *WHEN TO REFER*

The American College of Cardiology and the American Heart Association have published guidelines for indications for coronary angioplasty. Several considerations should precede selection for angioplasty: Will angioplasty have a reasonable chance of solving the clinical problem at hand? Is there a high chance of procedural success? What is the risk of acute complications with angioplasty? What is the chance of serious complications, including death or myocardial infarction, should the procedure fail? What is the long-term chance that the result will be sustained? What results would be expected from alternative therapy such as medical treatment or surgery? These questions should be asked any time an interventional cardiology procedure is contemplated.

Patients most suitable for angioplasty include those who have lesions amenable to angioplasty, plus ischemia on medical therapy or angina unresponsive to therapy, or patients intolerant to the side effects of therapy who have a moderate to high chance of angioplasty success with a low to moderate risk of serious complications (Chapter 22). When considering referral of patients with mild symptoms or no symptoms, one should insist on more severe ischemia on laboratory testing or patients who are rescued from cardiac arrest or those with threatening coronary lesions who are in need of high-risk noncardiac surgery.

Angioplasty has become the treatment of choice in patients who are referred for revascularization with single-vessel disease. One possible exception is those patients with involvement of the origin of the anterior descending coronary artery or the circumflex artery in a way that might affect the left main artery. These lesions also may have a higher restenosis rate, and a case for surgical intervention is sometimes made. Patients with multivessel disease are increasingly sent for angioplasty, and results of the randomized trials mentioned earlier show that this is a viable technique, although not superior to surgery. Most cases of multivessel coronary disease do not fit within the entry criteria of those trials; therefore selection of patients, particularly those with prior bypass surgery, significant left ventricular dysfunction, and other conditions must depend on the answer to the questions posed in the beginning of this section. As with any technique, referral for an interventional coronary procedure should be to experts with extensive experience. Recent efforts by the American Board of Internal Medicine to establish a certificate of added qualification in interventional cardiology should help identify experts in the field who can serve as consultants to those cardiologists not performing interventions.

ber of approaches at controlling restenosis have been successful in small animals, the most appropriate model so far seems to be the porcine coronary artery overstretch model.

Although there has been some success with drug therapy in these models, there has not been a convincing reduction in restenosis rates in human trials. Some of the agents that have been tested include aspirin, coumadin, ticlopidine, ciprostene, trapidil (a PDGF inhibitor), heparin, steroids, angiotensin-converting enzyme inhibitors, angiopeptin (a growth hormone inhibitor), ketanserin (a serotonin inhibitor), lovastatin, and omega-3 fatty acids. Despite mixed results from these trials, no drug has yet been approved or is generally used for restenosis prevention. It has been recently observed in the EPIC trial (Evaluation of 7E3 for the Prevention of Ischemic Complications) that an improvement in acute complications was also associated with an improvement in late clinical events, especially repeat revascularization. This has been interpreted as possibly being due to a reduction in restenosis rates using the IIb/IIIa antiplatelet antibody. Confirmation of this finding awaits angiographic documentation of the mechanism of these improved results.

The search for a method for preventing restenosis has also extended to the use of new devices. Trials such as CAVEAT I and C-CAT unfortunately showed no advantage for directional atherectomy in this regard. A new trial, BOAT, is testing the possibility that more vigorous atherectomy may indeed improve that rate. Definitive trials with other devices, such as rotational ablation and laser, have not been carried out, and trials that have been performed have not

Table 15-4   Success and complication rates of percutaneous interventions

	NHLBI REGISTRY 1 (1977-81)	NHLBI REGISTRY 2 (1985-86)	NACI REGISTRY (1994)
Procedural success	58	82	91
Major complications			
Death	1.0	0.8	1.6
MI	4.9	4.4	1.3
Emergency CABG	6.1	3.7	1.7

All data are presented as percentages.
NHLBI, National Heart, Lung, and Blood Institute; *NACI,* New Approaches to Coronary Intervention; *MI,* myocardial infarction; *CABG,* coronary artery bypass grafting.

shown any reduction in restenosis. Encouraging results with stents from STRESS and BENESTENT, however, have led the way to a proliferation of new trials using stenting to further improve the restenosis rate. Most encouraging in this regard is the BENESTENT II pilot trial, which showed a restenosis rate as low as 13%.

Experimental efforts to control restenosis have recently concentrated on local drug delivery devices ranging from porous balloons to ionophoresis methods. These methods of applying drug either in the artery or against the wall of the artery with polymeric drug alluding systems have as yet produced no reduction in restenosis rates and have not been applied in patients.

A recent approach of applying low-dose endovascular radiation has been effective in blocking the neointima formation in the porcine coronary model. This approach has now been used in the first patient studies, and the results are anxiously awaited.

In summary, restenosis is a multifactorial process common to all interventional cardiology techniques. Coronary stenting blocks the chronic constriction phase of restenosis but exaggerates the proliferative response. An attractive combination seems to be the application of stents plus a method to reduce the proliferative response. On the other hand, if methods such as endovascular radiation or local drug delivery can blunt the neointimal response, these may be themselves be satisfactory for retaining an adequate lumen.

BIBLIOGRAPHY

Baim DS, Kent KM, King SB III et al: Evaluating new devices: acute (in hospital) results from the New Approaches to Coronary Intervention Registry, *Circulation* 89:471-481, 1994.
Califf RM, Topol EJ, Stack RS et al: Evaluation of combination thrombolytic therapy and timing of cardiac catheterization in acute myocardial infarction: results of Thrombolysis and Angioplasty in Myocardial Infarction—phase 5 randomized trial, *Circulation* 83:1543-1556, 1991.
Detre K, Yeh W, Kelsey S et al: Has improvement in PTCA intervention affected long-term prognosis? The NHLBI PTCA Registry experience, *Circulation* 91:2868-2875, 1995.
Frye RL, King SB III, Sopko G, Detre KM: A symposium: multivessel PTCA versus CABG: baseline data from the bypass angioplasty revascularization investigation (BARI) and the Emory angioplasty surgery trial (EAST), *Am J Cardiol* 75:1C-59C, 1995.
Grines CL, Browne KF, Marco J et al: A comparison of immediate angioplasty with thrombolytic therapy for acute myocardial infarction, *N Engl J Med* 328:673-679, 1993.
Gruentzig AR, King SB, Schlumpf M, Siegenthaler W: Long term followup after percutaneous transluminal coronary angioplasty: the early Zurich experience, *N Engl J Med* 316:1127-1132, 1987.
Ivanhoe RJ, Weintraub WS, Douglas JS et al: Percutaneous transluminal coronary angioplasty of chronic total occlusions: primary success, restenosis and long term clinical followup, *Circulation* 85:1214-1216, 1992.
King SB III, Lembo NJ, Weintraub WS et al: A randomized trial comparing coronary angioplasty with coronary bypass surgery, *N Engl J Med* 331:1044-1050, 1994.
King SB III, Schlumpf M: Ten-year completed follow-up of percutaneous transluminal coronary angioplasty: the early Zurich experience, *J Am Coll Cardiol* 22:353-360, 1993.
Parisi AF, Folland ED, Hartigan P: A comparison of angioplasty with medical therapy in the treatment of single-vessel coronary artery disease, *N Engl J Med* 326:10-16, 1992.
Pocock SJ, Henderson RA, Rickards AF et al: Meta-analysis of randomised trials comparing coronary angioplasty with bypass surgery, *Lancet* 346:1184-89, 1995.
Ryan TJ, Bauman WB, Kennedy WJ, et al: Guidelines for percutaneous transluminal coronary angioplasty: a report of the American Heart Association/American College of Cardiology Task Force on Assessment of Diagnostic and Therapeutic Cardiovascular Procedures (Committee on Percutaneous Transluminal Coronary Angioplasty), *Circulation* 88:2987-3007, 1993.

Serruys PW, de Jaegere P, Kiemeneij F et al: A comparison of balloon-expandable stent implantation with balloon angioplasty in patients with coronary artery disease, *N Engl J Med* 331:489-495, 1994.

SWIFT (Should We Intervene Following Thrombolysis?) Trial Study Group: SWIFT trial of delayed elective intervention vs conservative treatment after thrombolysis with antistreplase in acute myocardial infarction, *Br Med J* 302:555-560, 1991.

The EPIC Investigators: Use of a monoclonal antibody directed against the platelet glycoprotein IIb/IIIa receptor in high-risk coronary angioplasty, *N Engl J Med* 330:956-961, 1994.

TIMI Research Group: Immediate vs delayed catheterization and angioplasty following thrombolytic therapy for acute myocardial infarction: TIMI II A results, *JAMA* 260:2849-2858, 1988.

TIMI Study Group: Comparison of invasive and conservative strategies after treatment with intravenous tissue plasminogen activator in acute myocardial infarction: results of the Thrombolysis in Myocardial Infarction (TIMI) phase II trial, *N Engl J Med* 320:618-627, 1989.

Topol EJ, Leya F, Pinkerton CA et al: A comparison of directional coronary atherectomy with coronary angioplasty in patients with coronary artery disease, *N Engl J Med* 329:221-227, 1993.

Weintraub WS, Mauldin PD, Becker E et al: A comparison of the costs of and quality of life after coronary angioplasty or coronary surgery for multivessel coronary artery disease: results from the Emory Angioplasty versus Surgery Trial (EAST), *Circulation* 92:2831-2840, 1995.

Yusuf S, Zucker D, Peduzzi P et al: Effect of coronary artery bypass graft surgery on survival: overview of 10-year results from randomised trials by the Coronary Artery Bypass Graft Surgery Trialists Collaboration, *Lancet* 344:563-570, 1994.

III CLINICAL SYNDROMES

CHAPTER

16 Chest Pain

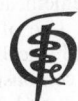

Louis J. Dell'Italia and Douglas J. Pearce

Chest pain, often referred to as "chest discomfort," is a frequent complaint of patients seeking medical evaluation. An accurate assessment of the cause and significance of the various types of chest discomfort is important and in some instances life-saving. Etiologies of chest pain can be separated into two major categories, cardiac and noncardiac (Box 16-1).

CARDIAC CAUSES OF CHEST PAIN
Ischemic Causes

Although no uniform presenting symptom exists for ischemic heart disease, chest pain or discomfort represents the most common reason for seeing a physician. William Heberden is credited with the original description of his own angina in 1768:

> But there is a disorder of the breast marked with strong and peculiar symptoms, considerable for the kind of danger belonging to it, and not extremely rare, which deserves to be mentioned more at length. The seat of it and sense of strangling and anxiety with it is attended, make it not improperly called angina pectoris.
>
> They who are afflicted with it are seized while they are walking (more especially if it be up a hill and soon after eating) with a painful and most disagreeable sensation in the breast, which seems as if it would extinguish life if it were to increase or to continue; but the moment they stand still, all this uneasiness vanishes.

Angina pectoris is defined as chest pain or discomfort of cardiac origin that results from a temporary imbalance between myocardial oxygen (O_2) supply and demand (Chapter 22). A patient's description of ischemic chest pain may take many forms, including burning, viselike tightness, squeezing, choking, heaviness, knifelike, and suffocating. These various descriptions may be further modified by the pa-

---

BOX 16-1
Differential diagnosis of chest pain

Cardiovascular
Ischemic in origin
   Coronary atherosclerosis
   Aortic stenosis
   Hypertrophic cardiomyopathy
   Severe systemic hypertension
   Severe right ventricular hypertension
   Aortic regurgitation
   Severe anemia/hypoxia
Nonischemic in origin
   Aortic dissection
   Pericarditis
   Mitral valve prolapse/autonomic dysfunction

Gastrointestinal
Esophageal reflux
Esophageal spasm
Esophageal rupture

Pulmonary
Pulmonary embolus
Pneumothorax
Pneumonia

Neuromusculoskeletal
Thoracic outlet syndrome
Degenerative joint disease of cervical/thoracic spine
Costochondritis (Tietze's syndrome)
Herpes zoster

Psychogenic
Anxiety
Depression
Cardiac psychosis
Self-gain

---

tient's intelligence, education, and sociocultural background. However, the patient is usually able to describe a deep rather than a superficial origin of the pain. Although the etiology of the different forms of discomfort is complex and not fully understood, an adequate anatomic explanation exists for the many patterns of referred pain that can be manifested in the neck, jaw, left shoulder, and left arm. It is likely that nonmedullated, small sympathetic nerve fibers that parallel the coronary arteries provide the afferent sensory pathway for angina and enter the spinal cord in the lowest cervical and upper thoracic segments (C8-T4). Here these sympathetic afferent impulses converge with impulses from somatic thoracic structures onto the same ascending spinal neurons. Thus impulses reaching visceral afferent neurons may stimulate nearby intermediate neurons that are receptors for somatic impulses and subsequently may produce a sensation of discomfort in the various referred areas in the chest, neck, or arms. Because the quality or character of the chest discomfort can be difficult to interpret, the location, radiation, duration, precipitating factors, and means of relief are very important in the systematic assessment of the patient with chest pain (Box 16-2).

Localization of the site of discomfort may help determine its cause. Although the deep, visceral character of ischemic chest pain often defies localization, anginal pain usually begins in the midsternum or slightly to the left of the midline. Pain localized to a discrete area of the chest by pointing a finger to the inframammary region or cardiac apex usually is not angina pectoris. However, one or two clenched fists held by the patient over the upper sternum (Levine's sign) when describing the discomfort strongly suggests angina. Pain that originates entirely outside the thorax or epigastrium and subsequently radiates to the chest is not caused by myocardial ischemia. However, ischemic pain may be felt only in the arm or may start in the arm and radiate to the chest. As discussed, the patterns of *radiation* can vary because of the convergence of visceral and somatic impulses. In

---

BOX 16-2
Characteristics of angina pectoris

Quality
Pressure of heavy weight on the chest
Burning
Tightness
Constriction about the throat
Visceral quality (deep, heavy, squeezing, aching)
Gradual increase in intensity followed by gradual fading

Location
Over sternum or very near to it
Anywhere between epigastrium and pharynx
Occasionally limited to left shoulder and left arm
Rarely limited to right arm
Limited to lower jaw
Lower cervical or upper thoracic spine
Left interscapular or suprascapular area

Radiation
Medial aspect of left arm
Left shoulder
Jaw
Occasionally right arm

Duration
30 seconds to 30 minutes

Precipitating factors
Relationship to exercise
Effort that involves use of arms above the head
Cold environment
Walking against the wind
Walking after a large meal
Emotional factors involved with physical exercise
Fright, anger, anxiety
Coitus

Nitroglycerin relief
Relief of pain occurring within 45 seconds to 5 minutes after taking
  nitroglycerin

Associated symptoms
Shortness of breath
Dizziness, lightheadedness, syncope
Palpitations
Weakness

---

ventricle as opposed to the normal-sized ventricle because of differences in wall stress. Nevertheless, myocardial O_2 supply depends greatly on the ability to increase coronary blood flow. Therefore the extent of physical activity (double product) that precipitates angina is related to the degree of fixed coronary artery stenosis but is not necessarily related to the number of coronary arteries with obstructive lesions. However, many episodes of angina, especially variant and unstable angina, are probably caused by coronary vasoconstriction or thrombosis without an increase in myocardial O_2 demand.

Typical angina pectoris usually comes on gradually and reaches its maximum intensity over 2 to 5 minutes. If pain is related to exertion, *relief* should occur within 2 to 5 minutes after cessation of exercise or with administration of sublingual nitroglycerin (Chapter 22). Nitroglycerin dilates the coronary vessels, thereby increasing blood flow and O_2 delivery through the diseased vessel and by way of collateral vessels. Nitroglycerin also decreases both preload and afterload through its venous and arterial vasodilating properties, thereby decreasing both diastolic and systolic wall stress. However, nitroglycerin's effect on arterial vasodilation may not be apparent by a simple cuff sphygmomanometer pressure recording. Recent data have demonstrated that nitroglycerin's effect on arterial afterload reduction is accomplished by decreasing wave reflection in the arterial circulation (Fig. 16-1). Delayed relief at 10 to 15 minutes after nitroglycerin administration is not compatible with ischemic chest pain and may be caused by a placebo effect. Pain that occurs after exercise or at the end of a stressful day is not usually due to ischemic chest pain. Occasionally, patients experience dissipation of angina during continuation of exercise (walk-through phenomenon) or absence of chest pain during a subsequent exercise effort (warm-up phenomenon) that previously elicited angina. These phenomena have been attributed to opening of important collaterals during the initial episode of ischemia.

Other precipitating factors unrelated to physical activity can increase myocardial O_2 demand (double product) through reflex discharge of catecholamines. When the patient is carefully questioned, the physician may find that episodes of *chest pain at rest* may be associated with emotional lability such as occurs during anger, fright, or uncomfortable situations. Exposure to cold air causes an increase in systemic arterial pressure and heart rate, whereas extreme heat results in an augmented cardiac output from vasodilation. Use of tobacco may elicit chest pain at rest or at a lower level of physical activity by two mechanisms. Carbon monoxide, which is a combustion product in cigarette smoke, may combine with hemoglobin and shift the hemoglobin-oxygen dissociation curve to the left, thereby reducing tissue O_2 delivery. The absorption of nicotine through the lungs increases myocardial O_2 demand by increasing heart rate, systolic arterial pressure, and contractility through the release of endogenous catecholamines.

Some patients with exertional angina pectoris experience *angina at rest* as a result of progression of disease severity or as an isolated clinical event. Coronary vasomotor tone is an important determinant of coronary blood flow and is influenced by several factors, including autonomic activity, metabolic products, and circulatory neurohumoral substances (Chapter 22). One or a combination of these factors is presumably responsible for an acute decrease in myocardial O_2 supply in patients with fixed coronary disease and in those with otherwise normal coronary arteries. This added feature may produce variable clinical manifestations of angina, ranging from angina at rest on certain days to pain that can be elicited only with maximum physical exertion at other times. Another cause of an acute decrease in myocardial O_2 supply includes coronary thrombosis superimposed on coronary atherosclerosis with spontaneous thrombolysis or coronary artery embolism. Angina at rest also may be caused by intermittent tachyarrhythmias that increase myocardial O_2 demand while decreasing diastolic filling time for coronary perfusion. Alternatively, labile hypertension acutely increases myocardial wall stress, resulting in rest angina. Another mechanism of rest angina may occur just before sleep, soon after the patient reclines. This occurs because of an increase in LV wall stress caused by the increased LV volume resulting from an augmentation in venous return in the supine position. Angina that occurs in the early morning hours, however, usually results from increased coronary vasomotor tone, which is common during this time of the day.

It is apparent that many potential causes of ischemic rest pain are unrelated to the number of diseased coronary arteries. Therefore de-

---

general, however, angina does not radiate to the upper jaw, the lower back, or below the umbilicus.

The assessment of chest pain is not complete without an evaluation of *precipitating factors* that elicit chest discomfort. This information is not only of diagnostic value but also provides an index of the severity of narrowing in the coronary arteries. Chest discomfort usually is induced by exercise, cold environment, or emotion or after eating a large meal. All these activities increase the O_2 demand of cardiac muscle by increasing heart rate, blood pressure, and myocardial contractility mediated through sympathetic stimulation. Increased O_2 demand must be balanced by an augmentation in coronary blood flow because the coronary circulation is not capable of increasing its O_2 extraction, since oxygen extraction is near maximal at baseline.

The *double product* (heart rate times blood pressure) has been used as a bedside index of the heart's myocardial O_2 demand. Although it does not include contractility, the double product demonstrates a high correlation with directly measured O_2 consumption in the normal left ventricle (LV). An increase in heart rate decreases diastolic filling time when most blood flow to LV endocardium occurs. An augmentation in pressure increases the tension developed in the ventricular wall (Laplace's law = Pressure $\times$ Radius/wall thickness), and in the normal ventricle a higher pressure indicates greater contractility. However, larger increments in myocardial O_2 demand can occur for a comparatively lower heart rate times pressure product in the dilated

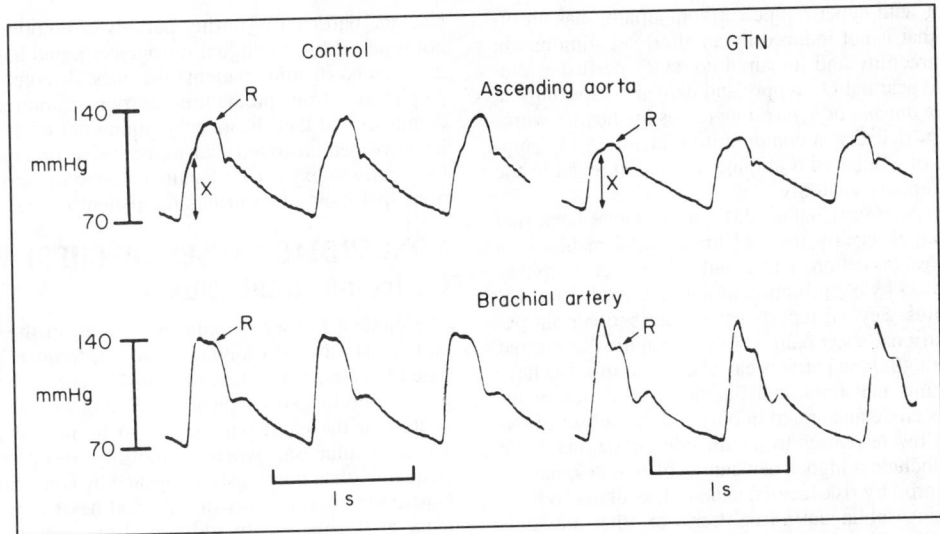

FIG. 16-1   High-fidelity pressure waveforms in the same patient from the brachial artery and ascending aorta at control valves and after nitroglycerin glyceryl trinitrate *(GTN)* administration. Reduction in amplitude of the reflected wave *(R)* by GTN is responsible for a change in contour of ascending aortic and brachial arterial waveforms. Because R constitutes a large part of the aortic pressure waveform, GTN produces a fall in the central systolic pressure.

(From Kelly RP et al: *Eur Heart J* 11:138, 1990.)

BOX 16-3
The Canadian Cardiovascular Society's classification of angina pectoris

1. Ordinary physical activity, such as walking and climbing stairs, does not cause angina. Angina with strenuous or rapid or prolonged exertion at work or recreation.
2. Slight limitations of ordinary activity. Walking or climbing stairs rapidly, walking uphill, walking or stair climbing after meals, or in cold, or in wind, or under emotional stress, or only during the few hours after awakening. Walking more than two blocks on the level and climbing more than one flight of ordinary stairs at a normal pace and in normal conditions.
3. Marked limitation of ordinary physical activity. Walking one to two blocks on the level and climbing one flight of stairs in normal conditions and at normal pace.
4. Inability to carry on any physical activity without discomfort—anginal syndrome may be present at rest.

From Campeau L: Letter to the editor. *Circulation* 54:522, 1976.

---

spite the more malignant natural history observed in many patients with angina at rest, the predictive value of the history alone is not as accurate as with exertional angina, which can be related to O_2 demand by the double product. The number of diseased arteries and amount of myocardium at risk, however, are directly related to prognosis, and the likely severity often can be estimated from a careful history. A classification of the functional severity of angina pectoris is detailed in Box 16-3. Episodes of angina pectoris can be *associated with symptoms* that result from ischemic LV dysfunction or life-threatening arrhythmias. Severe ischemia may produce an increase in diastolic filling pressures or papillary muscle dysfunction, resulting in pulmonary venous congestion and symptoms of shortness of breath. This may also be the only manifestation of ischemia, or "anginal equivalent," in the absence of chest discomfort, particularly in diabetic patients. Low cardiac output may produce other associated symptoms of fatigue, weakness, or dizziness resulting from arrhythmias or ischemic LV dysfunction. Prolonged, severe pain associated with shortness of breath results from elevated LV diastolic pressures caused by ischemia involving a large amount of myocardium. These patients are clearly at increased risk. In addition, prolonged, severe pain at rest associated with nausea, vomiting, and diaphoresis sug-

gests myocardial infarction. Furthermore, myocardial infarction is more frequently associated with signs of LV dysfunction (dyspnea, orthopnea) and autonomic nervous system hyperactivity (tachycardia, diaphoresis, bradycardia). However, up to 30% of patients may have no pain or may have atypical symptoms, particularly elderly and diabetic patients.

An evaluation of the patient who complains of chest pain is not complete without an assessment of the risk factors for coronary artery disease. Increased age, hypertension, diabetes, hypercholesterolemia, and cigarette smoking are established independent risk factors for coronary artery disease. Other important risk factors include a family history of premature coronary artery disease, obesity, sedentary lifestyle, type A personality, hypertriglyceridemia, and hyperuricemia. This information, coupled with a detailed history of the chest pain (see Box 16-2), should permit the physician to categorize the patient as being at low, intermediate, or high risk for coronary artery disease. This interview process is extremely important not only in determining whether an exercise test is necessary, but also in interpreting exercise test results to rule out the diagnosis of coronary artery disease, especially in the patient with a low pretest likelihood of disease. More important, a careful history may alert the physician to an unstable pattern. For example, an older patient with multiple risk factors complaining of frequent painful episodes relieved by two or three nitroglycerin tablets, the recent onset of rest angina, angina with minimal exertion, or angina with associated symptoms may be at increased risk during exercise. In this patient, it may be more appropriate to proceed directly to cardiac catheterization. This underscores the importance of a physician-patient interaction that results in a comprehensive chest pain history based on the known physiology of the coronary circulation and the bedside hemodynamic determinants (double product) of myocardial O_2 demand. Taken in this manner, this history classifies the patient as low risk versus high risk and stable versus unstable, thereby providing important supplemental information to noninvasive and invasive testing (Chapter 22).

It is important to emphasize that angina is a symptom and not solely a manifestation of coronary atherosclerosis. For example, classic symptoms of exertional angina may occur in the patient with *aortic stenosis* (Chapter 25), in whom increased resistance to LV ejection occurs with each heartbeat. This imbalance in myocardial O_2 demand results from increased systolic tension, a prolonged ejection period relative to the diastolic filling period (when most coronary flow occurs), and decreased coronary perfusion to the subendocardium caused by a thicker muscle mass and high diastolic filling pressures. Chronic elevation of afterload produces a similar physiologic mechanism for exertional angina in patients with *systemic hypertension* and *pulmonary hypertension* resulting from primary or secondary causes.

In contrast, the patient with hypertrophic cardiomyopathy has an increased muscle mass that is not induced by an afterload stimulus. In this patient, hypercontractility and impaired coronary perfusion create an imbalance of myocardial O_2 supply and demand, especially at high heart rates. Severe *anemia* or *hypoxia* increases the heart's workload at a time when O_2 delivery is compromised, resulting in symptoms of angina at rest or angina with minimum exertion, even in the patient with normal coronary anatomy.

Severe *aortic regurgitation* (Chapter 25) may produce nocturnal angina during sleep when vagally induced bradycardia results in a longer diastole, more regurgitation, and greatly decreased coronary perfusion pressure caused by equilibration of aortic diastolic and LV diastolic filling pressures. Several reports have described certain patients with typical exertional chest pain and angiographically normal coronary arteries. Although these patients have been classified as having microvascular angina, metabolic and functional evidence of inducible ischemia has been demonstrated in only a small subset of patients having limited flow responses to pharmacologic or metabolic stress. These patients include a higher percentage of females, have a decreased number of coronary risk factors, and are less likely to have relief of pain after taking sublingual nitroglycerin or other antianginal drugs that are usually effective in patients with myocardial ischemia caused by obstructive coronary artery disease. At this time, the underlying cause of this chest pain syndrome is highly speculative; however, these patients' life expectancies appear no different from those of an age-matched and sex-matched population without chest discomfort.

Nonischemic Causes

Pericarditis is a common cause of nonischemic cardiac pain (Chapter 27). The chest pain of pericarditis is usually sharp and penetrating. In contrast to ischemic cardiac chest pain, this pain comes on suddenly and lasts for hours to days. In addition, pericardial pain is worsened by deep inspiration and by lying in a flat, recumbent position. The pain is relieved by nonsteroidal antiinflammatory agents and by sitting upright and leaning forward. Radiation of the discomfort may involve the shoulders, upper back, and neck. This pattern of radiation can be explained by the innervation of the pericardium. The visceral pericardium is virtually insensitive to pain, whereas pain fibers originating in the parietal pericardium innervate only the diaphragmatic surface. Consequently, radiation of the discomfort of pericarditis may involve the shoulders, upper back, and neck because of irritation of the diaphragmatic pleura, which is innervated through the phrenic nerve by fibers originating in the cervical sympathetic ganglia (C3-C5). On occasion, the pain of acute pericarditis may mimic that observed in acute myocardial infarction, possibly because of periadventitial coronary artery nerve stimulation. In addition, because the pain is sharp, it must be differentiated from that of acute aortic dissection.

As mentioned earlier, the pain of *acute aortic dissection* must be differentiated from that of acute myocardial infarction and acute pericarditis (Chapter 30). The pain of aortic dissection is sudden in onset, in contrast to the pain of acute myocardial infarction, which increases in intensity with time. The pain is usually sharp and may radiate into the neck, back, flanks, and legs. The pattern of radiation depends on the location of the arterial dissection. Patients frequently characterize the pain as "tearing" in quality and the most excruciating pain that they have ever experienced. Manifestations of arterial occlusion may occur, including syncope and other neurologic symptoms when dissection involves the carotid and cerebral arteries and vascular insufficiency of the limbs when dissection extends to the subclavian and femoral arteries. In general, most patients have a long-standing history of systemic arterial hypertension, except patients with Marfan syndrome or idiopathic cystic medial necrosis.

Chest pain is a frequent complaint of patients with *mitral valve prolapse* (Chapter 25). The pain may be substernal but is more often perceived in the left anterior thorax. The pain is described in many ways, including a sharp or sticking pain or less frequently a dull ache. In addition, the duration of the pain is highly variable, often being characterized as momentary or lancinating, but it may also last several minutes to several hours. In contrast to ischemic chest pain, the chest pain of mitral valve prolapse is usually nonradiating. In addition, the pain is usually not related to exercise and tends to occur in clusters, particularly during periods of emotional stress. The pain is not relieved by sublingual nitroglycerin and has no consistent relieving factors. In some patients the chest discomfort actually represents palpitations from premature ventricular contractions. Many patients complain that their heart is "jumping out of their chest." Many studies have demonstrated that mitral valve prolapse and panic disorder frequently coexist. Chest pain is the symptom in both these conditions that most often brings the patient to seek medical attention.

NONCARDIAC CAUSES OF CHEST PAIN
Gastrointestinal Causes

The clinical history of pain originating in the gastrointestinal tract, particularly that of esophageal origin, frequently cannot be differentiated from ischemic cardiac pain. Recent studies of *reflux esophagitis* with prolonged esophageal pH and pressure monitoring demonstrate that the chest pain seems to be related primarily to an acid-sensitive mucosa, whereas motility disorders occur much less frequently than previously suggested by conventional laboratory tests. Gastroesophageal reflux disease and heart disease increase in prevalence as people age. In addition, drugs used to treat coronary artery disease, such as nitrates, β-blockers, and calcium entry blockers, may decrease lower esophageal sphincter pressure and contraction amplitude, thereby aggravating or predisposing to gastroesophageal reflux. Therefore reflux-induced chest pain occurs frequently in patients with obstructive coronary artery disease.

Gastroesophageal reflux pain is usually described as burning and is located in the epigastric or retrosternal area. The pain is frequently precipitated by assuming the recumbent position or by bending over. However, gastroesophageal reflux pain may be triggered by exercise. Symptoms suggesting an esophageal origin of chest pain include pain that continues for hours, retrosternal pain without lateral radiation, pain that occurs after meals or interrupts sleep, and pain that is relieved with antacids. Other esophageal symptoms can often be elicited, including regurgitation, dysphagia, and odynophagia.

Esophageal spasm results from a neuromuscular disorder of the esophagus that produces pain frequently confused with ischemic chest pain. This condition may occur in any age-group but most often affects those between ages 50 and 60 years. As with ischemic chest pain, pain from esophageal spasm is located in the retrosternal area and often radiates to the back, arms, and jaw. The pain may be described as a burning, squeezing, or aching sensation. Features that may distinguish it from ischemic chest pain include associated symptoms of dysphagia, regurgitation of gastric contents, and pain during or after ingestion of extremely hot or cold drinks. Patients may have pain precipitated by exercise; this pain can be relieved with sublingual nitroglycerin, which relaxes esophageal smooth muscle. The definitive diagnosis is made by demonstrating abnormal esophageal motility on ciné esophagrams or by performing esophageal manometry.

Acute esophageal rupture may occur after a prolonged bout of vomiting or retching or after esophageal instrumentation. The event is characterized by severe retrosternal pain resulting from the chemical mediastinitis produced by acidic gastric contents. The pain of peptic ulcer disease and biliary colic may be confused with ischemic chest pain because both conditions may be associated with a burning sensation in the epigastrium.

Pulmonary Causes

The acute substernal chest pain of *pulmonary embolus* (Chapter 29) often occurs in a specific clinical setting, such as during the postoperative period, during long trips, in patients with congestive heart failure, and in patients with deep vein thrombophlebitis. The chest pain is usually sharp and may be located in the right or left thorax, depending on the location of the embolus. Frequently, the chest pain is also aggravated by inspiration. Although the clinical findings of acute pulmonary embolus may be quite variable, massive embolus is often associated with dyspnea, tachypnea, and cyanosis. The physical examination may also reveal an elevated jugular venous pressure, tricuspid regurgitation, and other signs of acute right-sided heart failure.

Acute spontaneous pneumothorax may also be associated with chest pain. However, this condition may be readily differentiated from ischemic chest pain because it usually occurs in young, otherwise healthy men in the third and fourth decades of life. The clinical presentation is typically marked by the sudden onset of agonizing, unilateral, pleuritic chest pain accompanied by severe shortness of breath. The plain or expiratory chest radiograph provides the definitive diagnosis. The chest pain of *pneumonia* results from pleural irritation, which manifests as a sharp, pleuritic pain frequently accompanied by decreased inspiratory efforts. This condition is usually associated with fever, chills, and increased sputum production.

Neuromuscuoskeletal Causes

The various *thoracic outlet syndromes* may produce symptoms that are sometimes confused with cardiac chest pain. Compression of the neurovascular bundle by a cervical rib or the scalenus anterior muscle may cause discomfort radiating to the chest, neck, and ulnar surface of either arm. The prominence of associated paresthesias, the lack of clear relation of the pain to physical exercise, and its aggravation by certain body positions are helpful differential features.

Tietze's syndrome, or *idiopathic costochondritis,* is an occasional cause of anterior chest wall pain that is aggravated by movement and deep breathing. The reproduction of the chest pain syndrome by direct pressure over the involved costochondral junction and the relief of pain after local infiltration with lidocaine are helpful diagnostic maneuvers. Degenerative arthritis of the cervical and thoracic vertebrae may cause bandlike pain confined to the chest, neck, or back, which often radiates to the arms. Radiologic evidence of degenerative changes involving the cervical and thoracic vertebrae is often found in asymptomatic elderly patients. The production or exacerbation of pain by various postures, movement, sneezing, or coughing is more useful in the diagnosis of chest discomfort caused by vertebral disease.

The prevesicular phase of *herpes zoster* may be characterized by bandlike chest pain in a dermatomal distribution. The patient's advanced age, the presence of hyperesthesia on physical examination, and the eventual eruption of typical lesions 3 or 4 days after the onset of symptoms resolve any diagnostic difficulties.

Psychogenic Causes

Chest pain of emotional origin may be difficult to distinguish from chest pain resulting from angina pectoris because both may be precipitated by anxiety. However, a careful history (see Box 16-2) will document that chest pain of emotional origin is frequently sharp, left inframammary in location, and usually very well circumscribed. Psychogenic chest pain may be described as stabbing or lightninglike episodes of pain lasting less than 1 minute and not precipitated by any activity. Alternatively, the patient may complain of a substernal ache that lasts for hours or days and is unrelieved by nitroglycerin. These symptoms of chest discomfort are very dissimilar from those resulting from myocardial ischemia. Patients may complain of atypical symptoms such as air hunger, palpitations, giddiness, circumoral paresthesias, and other multiple somatic complaints that may suggest a neurasthenic personality. The patient often admits to having mild episodes of discomfort during the history and physical examination. During this time, nonverbal communication, such as a flat or worried facial expression, retarded motor activity, and hand wringing, may indicate underlying depression. As stated previously, many studies have demonstrated that mitral valve prolapse and psychogenic chest pain may frequently coexist. Recent studies of patients with mitral valve prolapse syndrome have demonstrated that faulty autonomic regulation can easily lead to inappropriate tachycardia or bradycardia, orthostatic hypotension, dyspnea, reduced effort tolerance and fatigability, chest pain, and rhythm disturbances. The similarity between these symptoms and the somatic expressions of anxiety just described may be related to autonomic dysfunction rather than a collection of neurotic complaints. Therefore appropriate tests of the autonomic nervous system may be indicated in some patients.

LIMITATIONS OF CHEST PAIN HISTORY

Although a complete history as outlined earlier provides a framework for further diagnostic workup in the patient with chest pain, the history may be misleading because of several factors. The physician's inability to interview the patient systematically results in incomplete data. This may result from different physicians' variable skills in obtaining a correct history or from the patient's failure to describe accurately the symptom complex because of sociocultural or educational reasons. Furthermore, many patients may withhold symptoms from the physician to maintain job security. In contrast, other patients may fabricate symptoms to obtain disability benefits.

Finally, it must be emphasized that a typical history of angina pectoris does not necessarily coincide with the extent of coronary atherosclerosis. In addition, the physician must be alert to the existence of obstructive coronary artery disease in the absence of chest pain, especially in the diabetic patient. In these situations a high index of suspicion should lead the physician to appropriate diagnostic tests to rule out the presence of significant obstructive coronary artery disease.

CHEST PAIN CENTERS

Chest pain centers have proliferated in this country during the first half of this decade. There are now an estimated 700 to 1000 chest pain centers in the United States. Chest pain centers are usually located adjacent to the emergency department. A fully developed chest pain center consists of (1) a chest pain evaluation unit to promptly diagnose and treat acute cardiac ischemia, (2) an observation unit to rule out ischemia in patients with chest pain of intermediate likelihood of cardiovascular disease, (3) appropriate cardiovascular monitoring equipment including continuous 12-lead ST segment monitoring, (4) specially trained nurses and physicians, (5) a community outreach education program, and (6) a continuous quality improvement program.

Chest pain centers have decreased the time to reperfusion therapy for acute coronary thrombosis by more than 50%, often to less than 30 minutes (Chapter 23). Chest pain centers have also been shown to reduce the costs of ruling out ischemia. Ischemic heart disease is excluded in 40% to 70% of patients hospitalized with chest pain, at an estimated expense of 1.6 million unnecessary inpatient days annually. Protocol-driven assessment in a short-stay observation unit can safely risk-stratify patients with intermediate likelihood of ischemic heart disease and at half the cost of hospitalization. Patients are typically observed over 12 to 24 hours with continuous ST segment monitoring and frequent assessment of serum markers of cardiac injury (Chapter 23). If these remain negative, some form of provocative testing for inducible ischemia is subsequently performed before discharge. Finally, as part of the mission to optimize care of the cardiac patient, most chest pain centers participate in community programs aimed at increasing cardiac awareness and access to the medical system. In summary, changing medical reimbursement and marketing have spawned much of the growth in chest pain centers, but improved patient care has been demonstrated in clinical studies.

BIBLIOGRAPHY

Alpert MA et al: Mitral valve prolapse, panic disorder and chest pain, *Med Clin North Am* 75:1119, 1991.

Berman DS, Rozanski A, Knowbel SB: The detection of silent ischemia: cautions and precautions, *Circulation* 75:101, 1987.

Cannon RO: Microvascular angina: cardiovascular investigations regarding pathophysiology and management, *Med Clin North Am* 75:1097, 1991.

Coghlan HC: Autonomic dysfunction in the mitral valve prolapse syndrome: the brain-heart connection and interaction. In Boudoulas H, Wooly CF, editors: *Mitral valve prolapse and mitral valve prolapse syndrome*, Mount Kisco, NY, 1988, Futura.

Dell'Italia LJ, O'Rourke RA, Pohost GM: Evaluation of the patient with signs and symptoms of ischemic heart disease. In Chatterjee K, Parmley WW, editors: *Cardiology*, Philadelphia, 1998, JB Lippincott.

Gibler WB, Runyon JP, Levy RC et al: A rapid diagnostic and treatment center for patients with chest pain in the emergency department, *Ann Emerg Med* 25:108, 1995.

Jesse RL, Kontos MC, Tatum JL: Evaluation of chest pain in the emergency department, *Curr Prob Cardiol* 22:149-236, 1997.

Kerns JR, Shaub TF, Fontanarosa PB: Emergency cardiac stress testing in the evaluation of emergency department patients with atypical chest pain, *Ann Emerg Med* 22:794-798, 1993.

Richter JE: Gastroesophageal reflux disease as a cause of chest pain, *Med Clin North Am* 75:1065, 1991.

Uhl GS, Froelicher V: Screening for asymptomatic coronary artery disease, *J Am Coll Cardiol* 1:946, 1983.

Weiner DA et al: Correlations among history of angina, ST-segment response, and prevalence of coronary artery disease in the coronary artery surgery study (CASS), *N Engl J Med* 301:230, 1979.

17 Palpitations

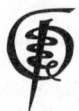

Sumanth D. Prabhu and Robert A. O'Rourke

The term *palpitation* denotes an unpleasant awareness of the heartbeat that may result from alterations in cardiac rate, rhythm, stroke volume, and/or contractility. This common symptom is nonspecific and often reflects a functional rather than organic problem. Palpitations may be the only manifestation of important cardiac arrhythmias or they may be benign and unrelated to structural heart disease, requiring no treatment. Conversely, some patients with definite heart disease may be unaware of significant rhythm disturbances. Patients with various anxiety states may describe palpitations resulting from normal heart action. Such individuals may be convinced that palpitations result from underlying heart disease and indicate impending death. These concerns cause apprehension, increase autonomic nervous system activity, and often eventuate in a vicious cycle that results in complete emotional disability and cardiac neurosis. Thus whether palpitations are a manifestation of incapacitating anxiety requiring empathy and reassurance or a result of cardiac arrhythmias necessitating further diagnostic testing and treatment, they deserve careful assessment.

PATHOPHYSIOLOGY

A patient's awareness of the heartbeat may result from several mechanisms. Normal persons exposed to physiologic stressors experience forceful sensations of cardiac motion because of increased circulating catecholamines and attendant augmentation of heart rate and contractility. Pathologic stressors, such as fever, hyperthyroidism, anemia, and pheochromocytoma, may cause palpitations on a similar basis. Anxiety and emotional stressors often sensitize individuals to normal cardiac motion within the thoracic cavity. Thus sympathetic nervous system activity often determines whether the patient complains of palpitations.

Forceful, regular palpitations may be described by patients with abnormally increased stroke volume, such as occurs with aortic and mitral regurgitation or ventricular septal defect and a variety of hyperkinetic circulatory states (e.g., anemia, thyrotoxicosis, arteriovenous fistula). These patients frequently complain of palpitations at night while lying on the left side, when the heart most closely approximates the chest wall.

Intermittent tachyarrhythmias, bradyarrhythmias, or isolated premature contractions may cause palpitations by sporadic, irregular alterations in heart motion. Palpitations are most often perceived during the onset or at the termination of the arrhythmia. During premature contractions, patients most commonly feel the postextrasystolic beat, which is associated with an increased stroke volume, rather than the ectopic beat per se. Patients with atrioventricular nodal reentrant tachycardia may also experience a rapid pounding sensation in the neck as a result of simultaneous atrial and ventricular contraction, elevated right atrial pressure, and reversal of flow in the great veins.

DIAGNOSTIC EVALUATION

The evaluation of the patient presenting with palpitations includes defining symptom severity, determining the underlying pathophysiologic mechanism, defining the presence or absence of structural heart disease, and establishing whether the symptoms correlate with cardiac rhythm disturbances. The initial evaluation comprises the history, physical examination, basic laboratory evaluation, and 12-lead electrocardiogram (ECG). Further diagnostic testing is directed by the information derived from this initial assessment. If symptoms are mild and there is no evidence of associated cardiac or noncardiac disorders, further workup is generally not necessary. Patients who have findings suggestive of underlying heart disease or who have severe symptoms usually require additional evaluation. This can include

Table 17-1   Value of the history in detecting the cause of palpitations

DESCRIPTION OF PALPITATIONS	DEFINING LIKELY CAUSE
Occasional "flip-flops," "skipped beats"	Premature beats
Sudden onset, rapid, regular	Supraventricular tachycardia
Sudden onset, rapid, irregular	Paroxysmal atrial fibrillation
Gradual onset, regular with exercise	Sinus tachycardia
Associated with drugs	Tobacco, coffee, tea, catecholamines, xanthines, thyroid hormone
Associated with atypical chest pain and hyperventilation symptoms	Anxiety state, mitral valve prolapse syndrome

echocardiography to define the extent of structural heart disease, ambulatory ECG monitoring or transtelephonic ECG transmission to correlate cardiac rhythm and symptoms, and treadmill testing to evaluate for exercise-induced arrhythmias and underlying coronary artery disease. Based on the results of noninvasive studies, selected patients may require invasive assessment with cardiac catheterization or electrophysiologic study.

DIFFERENTIAL DIAGNOSIS
Cardiac Arrhythmias

Important clues can be obtained from the history in determining the cause of palpitations (Table 17-1). The nature of onset, pulse rate, and pulse regularity should be specifically sought. Many patients have taken their pulse during the palpitations or can characterize the rhythm by tapping out a representative episode.

The gradual onset and cessation of palpitations associated with stress or exercise suggest sinus tachycardia. This rhythm can be associated with anxiety, stimulant drugs, and hyperkinetic circulatory states. The sudden onset of rapid, regular palpitations not associated with stress or exercise suggests the diagnosis of supraventricular tachycardia. A rate of 100 to 140 beats/min suggests sinoatrial reentry or atrial tachycardia, a regular rate of 150 beats/min suggests atrial flutter, and a regular rate exceeding 160 beats/min suggests paroxysmal supraventricular tachycardia (SVT), especially if the episode is terminated by vagal maneuvers (Chapter 18). Paroxysmal SVT often occurs in young patients who are otherwise healthy. Ventricular tachycardia (VT) is not usually associated with palpitations, perhaps because of the reduced cardiac output. However, prominent cerebral symptoms often occur. Patients with VT tend to be older with underlying structural heart disease. The sudden onset of rapid, irregular palpitations suggests atrial fibrillation or chaotic atrial tachycardia.

Episodic second- or third-degree atrioventricular block may be accompanied by slow, forceful palpitations, often associated with varying degrees of light-headedness or frank syncope. Palpitations described as "flip-flops" or "skipped beats" suggest premature and postectopic beats. The postextrasystolic pause may be perceived as an actual cessation of heartbeat ("my heart stopped"), in contrast to the complete lack of awareness of similar pauses during atrial fibrillation. Premature ectopic beats occur commonly both in the presence and absence of structural heart disease. When premature beats are frequent, clinical differentiation from atrial fibrillation may be aided by physical exercise. Exercise-induced sinus tachycardia may abolish premature beats, whereas ventricular contractions remain irregular in atrial fibrillation.

The physical examination is usually performed between attacks rather than during an episode of palpitations. This examination may uncover evidence of underlying heart disease or may be entirely unremarkable. Examination during a symptomatic episode may yield additional information. Patients with VT display varying intensity of the first heart sound and often have episodic cannon A waves in the jugular venous pulse because of atrioventricular (AV) dissociation and asynchronous atrial and ventricular contraction. Patients with SVT resulting from AV nodal reentry typically display prominent jugular venous pulsations matching the rate of the tachycardia that results from simultaneous atrial and ventricular contraction, along with constant intensity of the first heart sound.

The precise characterization of the basis for palpitations depends on the correlation of symptoms with ECG evidence of arrhythmias. Although the baseline ECG may reveal evidence for underlying heart disease or conduction abnormalities, it is often entirely normal. Ambulatory ECG recording often fails to disclose irregularities of heart rhythm in patients complaining of palpitations. In patients with infrequent episodes, long-term ambulatory ECG recordings may have to be performed on multiple occasions to detect the rhythm during symptoms (Chapters 13 and 18). An alternative approach is ECG telephone transmission during symptoms or the use of a patient-activated recording system with a 30-second memory loop. This approach is probably more cost effective than long-term ambulatory ECG monitoring in such patients.

Psychiatric Disorders

The symptom of palpitation is commonly described by patients with psychiatric illnesses such as panic disorders, anxiety reaction, depression, and somatization and is among the diagnostic criteria for some of these syndromes. Indeed, nearly half of medical outpatients referred for ambulatory ECG recording for palpitations have a psychiatric disorder. These patients are more likely to report symptoms during the ECG recording period, with symptoms less likely to be secondary to demonstrable arrhythmias.

Many patients with anxiety disorders are distressed by the awareness of normal heart action during daily exercise, such as walking up stairs or doing housework. A history of the gradual onset and offset of this sensation before and after intense physical activity usually suggests sinus tachycardia as the underlying mechanism. Alternatively, symptoms may be noted during introspective moments and at night rather than during periods of marked physical activity. In addition to increased awareness of normal heart action, anxious patients may be more sensitive to the presence of premature beats. Both atrial and ventricular premature depolarizations have been documented frequently by ambulatory ECG recordings in otherwise healthy adults, particularly during periods of emotional stress and fatigue.

Palpitations may be part of a chronic anxiety neurosis that is manifested by protracted autonomic nervous system overactivity. This condition has been variously termed *neurocirculatory asthenia, soldier's heart, Da Costa's syndrome, cardiac neurosis,* and *functional cardiovascular disease.* These patients often have physical findings of a hyperkinetic circulatory state manifested by resting sinus tachycardia, excessive perspiration, widened arterial pulse pressure, and a functional systolic murmur in the absence of other physical findings or laboratory data that suggest hyperthyroidism (Chapter 288). The common association of nonspecific ST-T wave changes on the ECG with the patient at rest, together with the frequent complaints of chest pain (Chapter 16), may lead to the mistaken diagnosis of coronary artery disease. Diagnostic error may be compounded by stress ECG testing because hyperventilation alone may provoke S-T segment depression in some patients.

A subgroup of patients with the mitral valve prolapse syndrome has been recognized as having a psychologic profile and signs of autonomic dysfunction similar to patients with neurocirculatory asthenia (Chapter 25). These observations, when combined with atrial or ventricular arrhythmias and/or false-positive ECG exercise test results, often complicate evaluation of the patient with mitral prolapse who has anxiety, atypical chest pain, and palpitations. Symptoms suggestive of hyperventilation (giddiness, circumoral/distal paresthesias) associated with transient or extremely prolonged and well-circumscribed "stabbing" chest pain in the region of the cardiac apex suggest a functional etiology rather than organic heart disease.

MANAGEMENT

The management of patients with palpitations depends on the underlying cause and severity of symptoms. If the symptoms are determined to be secondary to a specific arrhythmia, an underlying cardiac disease in the absence of arrhythmia, or a noncardiac systemic disorder, treatment is directed toward that particular condition with further referral as appropriate. Successful treatment of palpitations resulting from a chronic anxiety state may simply require reassurance and behavioral modification. Stimulant drugs, caffeine, and alcohol should be avoided or limited, and the patient should be advised to stop smoking. Patients with more severe symptoms may require long-term counseling and psychotherapy, along with appropriate use of sedatives and tranquilizers. Beta blockade with propranolol in doses ranging from 80 to 320 mg/day may be useful in treating refractory patients with palpitations associated with sinus tachycardia or some patients with the mitral valve prolapse syndrome.

BIBLIOGRAPHY

Alexander RW, Schlant RC, Fuster V, editors: *Hurst's the heart: arteries and veins,* ed 9, New York, 1998, McGraw-Hill.

Barsky AJ, Cleary PD, Coeytaux RR, Ruskin JN: Psychiatric disorders in medical outpatients complaining of palpitations, *J Gen Intern Med* 9:306-313, 1994.

Barsky AJ, Cleary PD, Sarnie MK, Ruskin JN: Panic disorder, palpitations, and the awareness of cardiac activity, *J Nerv Ment Dis* 182:63-71, 1994.

Braunwald EB, editor: *Heart disease: a textbook of cardiovascular medicine,* ed 4, Philadelphia, 1992, WB Saunders.

Gürsoy S, Steurer G, Brugada J et al: Brief report: the hemodynamic mechanism of pounding in the neck in atrioventricular nodal reentrant tachycardia, *N Engl J Med* 327:772-774, 1992.

Knudson MP: The natural history of palpitations in a family practice, *J Fam Pract* 24:357-360, 1989.

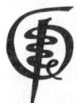

CHAPTER

18 Cardiac Arrhythmias and Conduction Disturbances

Simon Chakko, Agustin Castellanos, Kenneth M. Kessler, and Robert J. Myerburg

Cardiac arrhythmias are caused by abnormal impulse generation, abnormal impulse conduction, or a combination of both. Management of arrhythmias is based on three interacting considerations:

1. Accurate diagnosis of the arrhythmia. Electrocardiography (ECG) is the cornerstone of diagnosis, but clinical signs are often helpful and electrophysiologic studies may be occasionally necessary.
2. Evaluation of the clinical setting. Arrhythmias may occur in the presence or absence of structural heart disease. Clinical settings that lead to arrhythmias may be *acute or transient* abnormalities such as myocardial infarction, electrolyte disturbances, or *chronic* abnormalities such as cardiomyopathies, which cause *persistent or recurrent* arrhythmias.
3. Decision to treat an arrhythmia depends on the presence and type of symptoms and the potential for morbidity and mortality. Some arrhythmias may produce bothersome symptoms but may not affect the long-term prognosis, whereas other arrhythmias that cause few or no symptoms may predict a poor outcome.

In this chapter, the general principles of diagnosing and treating arrhythmias are discussed first, followed by specific arrhythmias.

PATHOPHYSIOLOGY OF ARRHYTHMIAS

The specialized conduction system of the heart that initiates and conducts the cardiac impulse consists of three major parts: (1) sinoatrial (SA) node, (2) atrioventricular (AV) junctional area including the AV node and bundle of His, and (3) bundle branches and Purkinje network (Chapter 12). The SA node is located at the lateral junction of the right atrium and superior vena cava. The sinus node artery, which supplies the SA node, arises from the right coronary artery in 60% of cases and from the left circumflex artery in 40%. Three internodal tracts connecting the SA and AV nodes have been reported, but their functional significance is controversial. The AV node is a compact ovoid structure located anterior to the ostium of the coronary sinus above the insertion of the septal leaflet of the tricuspid valve. It is

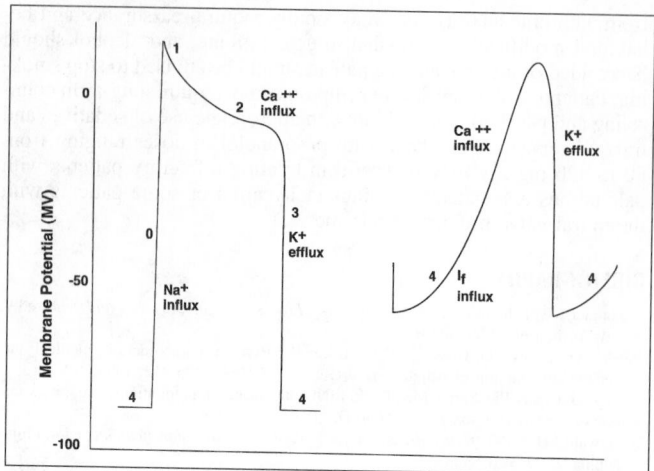

FIGURE 18-1   Mechanism of automaticity. Action potential of a Purkinje fiber cell *(left)* is compared to a pacemaker cell *(right)*. In the pacemaker cell, note the spontaneous rise in resting potential to threshold potential. I_f, pacemaker current.

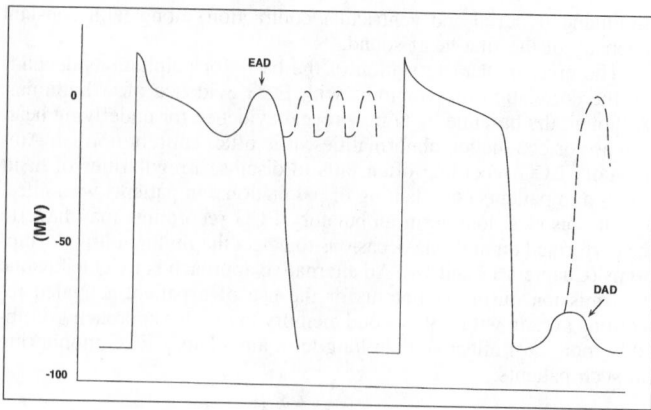

FIGURE 18-2   Triggered activity. Action potential is followed by oscillations of membrane voltage called afterdepolarizations. Early afterdepolarizations *(EADs)* occur before the cell fully repolarizes and repetitive EADs *(dashed line)* may cause tachyarrhythmia. Delayed afterdepolarizations *(DADs)* occur shortly after repolarization, and if the threshold voltage is reached, an action potential may follow *(dashed line)*.

supplied by the AV nodal artery, which originates from the right coronary artery in 90% of cases and left circumflex artery in 10%. The bundle of His originates from the distal portion of the AV node and penetrates the central fibrous body of the heart and bifurcates into left and right bundle branches. The left bundle in turn bifurcates into left anterior and posterior fascicles.

Cardiac impulse originates in the sinus node and activates both atria, and the atrial depolarization results in the P wave on the surface electrocardiogram (ECG). Normally conduction from atria to ventricles takes place only through the AV node and His bundle. The impulse is physiologically delayed in the AV node, which is responsible for most of the duration of the P-R interval. The long refractory period of the AV node protects the ventricles from being depolarized at dangerously rapid rates during some supraventricular tachycardias. Occasionally, abnormal accessory pathways of specialized conduction tissue connect the atria and ventricles, bypassing the AV node, which can lead to arrhythmias. After the AV node, the impulse travels down the bundle of His, bundle branches, and the Purkinje system and activates both ventricles, which results in the QRS complex. Normally, activation of both ventricles is rapid and orderly and lasts less than 0.10 sec. When there is a block in one of the bundle branches, activation is delayed, and the QRS complex becomes widened. Such widening of the QRS complex is described as aberrant conduction. Widening of the QRS complex is also seen if cardiac activation originates in the ventricle and does not use the specialized conduction system (e.g., premature ventricular complex). Determining whether a wide QRS complex is due to aberrant conduction or ectopic origin is a common problem in the diagnosis of arrhythmias. Cardiac arrhythmias result from abnormalities of impulse formation and impulse conduction.

Abnormalities of Impulse Formation

Specialized cardiac conducting system cells have intrinsic automaticity, which is the ability to depolarize themselves to the threshold potential and generate an action potential. The action potential of a pacemaker cell is different from other cells of the heart (Fig. 18-1). These cells have a higher resting potential. The upstroke is more gradual because the Ca^{2+} channels that provide the inward current are slow. Efflux of K^+ causes repolarization. Automaticity is explained by the net gain in intracellular positive charges during diastolic depolarization, which is caused by a decrease in the outward K^+ current and an inward pacemaker current (I_f) of Na^+ and K^+. When the threshold potential of approximately -40 mV is reached, voltage gated Ca^{++} channels open, providing an inward current that causes the upstroke of the action potential. Rate of discharge of an automatic cell is determined by the rate of diastolic depolarization and resting and

threshold potentials. Because the sinus node discharges more rapidly, it is the dominant pacemaker. If the sinus node fails, other latent pacemakers become dominant. The dominant pacemaker also suppresses other pacemakers by a mechanism called overdrive suppression; the depolarization of subsidiary pacemaker cells increases the activity of their Na^+/K^+ pump, which results in hyperpolarization and counteracts the pacemaker activity.

Sympathetic stimulation increases automaticity by altering the action potential threshold and by increasing the I_f. Increased automaticity of the sinus node may result in sinus tachycardia. Sympathetic stimulation and tissue injury can increase the automaticity of latent pacemakers, resulting in ectopic rhythms. Examples of arrhythmias caused by increased automaticity of latent pacemakers include atrial tachycardia, junctional tachycardia, and accelerated idioventricular rhythm. Parasympathetic (vagal) stimulation leads to decreased automaticity by raising the threshold potential, reducing I_f, and increasing the efflux of K^+. The SA and AV nodes are most sensitive to vagal stimulation and sinus bradycardia and AV block may result. Tissue injury and degeneration may lead to decreased automaticity. When a latent pacemaker discharges because of failure of SA node, it is described as an *escape beat* or *escape rhythm*. Examples include junctional escape rhythm and idioventricular escape rhythm.

Triggered Activity

Triggered activity (which is a form of automatic activity different from normal or enhanced automaticity) is another mechanism of arrhythmia formation. Under certain conditions, an action potential may be followed by oscillations of the membrane voltage known as afterdepolarizations (Fig. 18-2). Triggered activity is single or repetitive firing of a cell or group of cells initiated by afterdepolarizations. Early afterdepolarizations (EADs) occur before the cell fully repolarizes and delayed afterdepolarizations (DADs) occur shortly after the completion of repolarization. EADs are seen in conditions that prolong repolarization (e.g., hypokalemia, prolonged QT interval, and bradycardia). The torsade de pointes type of ventricular tachycardia is caused by EAD. DADs are usually too small to reach threshold voltage, but their amplitude increases with rapid pacing, increased catecholamine concentrations, and digitalis toxicity. When the amplitude of DAD reaches threshold voltage, triggered activity may be provoked. DAD is the probable mechanism of many arrhythmias caused by digitalis toxicity.

Reentry

The most common mechanism of arrhythmogenesis is reentry. A reentrant loop is an electrical circuit that can self-sustain depolarizations continuously. The mechanism of reentry is illustrated in Fig.

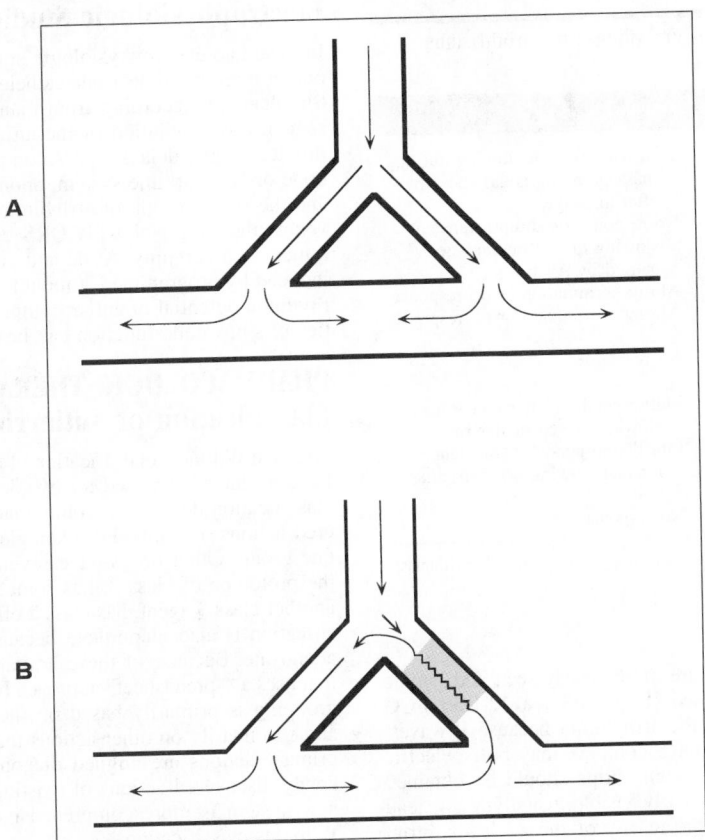

FIGURE 18-3 Reentry. Normally an impulse travels down both branches of the conduction system and cannot conduct retrograde because of refractoriness **(A).** In a reentrant circuit **(B),** presence of unidirectional block and delayed conduction in one branch *(stippled area)* make repeated reentry possible.

18-3. When an action potential reaches a division of conduction system, it travels down both branches simultaneously. The impulse that traveled down one branch cannot return through the other branch because of refractoriness to conduction. If unidirectional block and delayed conduction are present in one branch, the impulse is able to conduct antegrade via one division and then retrograde through the other. Because retrograde conduction is delayed, the other branch has recovered from its refractoriness when the impulse reaches it again. Thus a reentrant circuit is set up. It then repeatedly reenters the same pathway to generate reentrant rhythms. Reentrant circuits may be located anywhere in the heart. They may be well defined anatomically or may be functional in which cellular electrophysiologic properties determine the reentrant circuit. An example of an anatomically defined reentrant circuit is the AV node, which comprises a slow pathway (with slow conduction and shorter refractory period) and a fast pathway (with fast conduction and longer refractory period). These differences in conduction properties may lead to reentrant tachycardias, which are described further under AV nodal reentrant tachycardias. Other examples of reentrant tachycardias include atrial flutter, most monomorphic ventricular tachycardias, and AV reciprocating tachycardias. Functional reentrant circuits may change their size and location and lead to random reentry. Examples of such random reentry are atrial and ventricular fibrillation.

History and Physical Examination

History and physical examination are helpful in evaluating patients with arrhythmias (Chapter 11). Knowledge of the underlying heart disease is helpful in the diagnosis and guiding the therapy of arrhythmias. For example, ventricular tachycardia is uncommon in the absence of myocardial disease. A tachyarrhythmia is likely to be supraventricular in a young man with a structurally normal heart, ventricular in a patient with previous myocardial infarction (MI) and syncope, or atrial fibrillation in a patient with severe mitral stenosis. The

history must include an inquiry into conditions that may precipitate or aggravate arrhythmias. Caffeine, alcohol, prescription drugs (e.g., tricyclic antidepressants), sympathomimetic agents in nonprescription drugs, and illicit drugs such as cocaine and amphetamines may trigger arrhythmias. Thyrotoxicosis, mitral valve prolapse, pericarditis, and hypokalemia are states conducive to the genesis of arrhythmias. Failure to recognize these conditions will result in inappropriate and often futile therapy. Although familial disorders leading to arrhythmias are uncommon, it is important to recognize them, since treatment of these arrhythmias may be unique. Examples include β-adrenergic blocker therapy for ventricular tachycardia secondary to congenital long Q-T syndromes and prophylactic pacemaker placement in myotonic dystrophy.

History must include specific questions about symptoms such as palpitations, syncope, and dizziness. Angina and heart failure may be worsened by arrhythmias. Some patients may not feel palpitations in the presence of recurrent arrhythmias, and others may complain of palpitations when no arrhythmias are present (Chapter 17).

Physical examination should include a search for heart failure and valvular heart disease (Chapter 11). An irregularly irregular rhythm and pulse deficit (all auscultated heart beats do not result in peripheral pulses) suggest atrial fibrillation. A-V dissociation results in intermittent large A waves in the jugular venous pulse (cannon A waves) when the atrium contracts against the closed tricuspid valve. Among patients with wide QRS complex tachycardia of unknown origin, presence of cannon A wave is suggestive of ventricular tachycardia. In the presence of slow heart rate, cannon A waves indicate that AV block is present.

Electrocardiography

The definitive diagnosis of the type of arrhythmia can be made by ECG in most cases (Chapter 12). For continuous monitoring, MCL$_1$ (positive lead in V$_1$ position and negative at the left shoulder) is pref-

Table 18-1 Response of various arrhythmias to carotid sinus massage or intravenous adenosine

TYPE OF ARRHYTHMIA	RESPONSE
Sinus tachycardia	Transient, gradual slowing during massage and gradual speeding after massage
Atrial tachycardia	No response or abrupt, transient slowing of ventricular rate caused by AV block
AV nodal reentry tachycardia	Abrupt termination or no response
Accessory pathway reentry tachycardia	Abrupt termination or no response
Nonparoxysmal junctional tachycardia	No response
Atrial flutter	Flutter persists. Transient stepwise slowing of ventricular rate
Atrial fibrillation	Fibrillation persists. Transient gradual slowing of ventricular rate
Ventricular tachycardia	No response

(From Chakko S, Kessler KM: Recognition and management of cardiac arrhythmias, *Curr Prob Cardiol* 20:53-120, 1995.)

erable to lead II, because P waves are more clearly seen and bundle branch patterns are easily diagnosed. If possible, a 12-lead ECG should always be obtained during the arrhythmia because P waves, flutter waves, and portions of the QRS complex may be isoelectric and not visible in a single lead. Rhythm strips should be obtained using leads in which P waves are clearly visible, usually V_1 or lead II. If P waves are not clearly visible in any of the 12 leads, atrial activity can be demonstrated by placing the right and left arm leads in various positions on the chest (Lewis leads) or by using esophageal leads. Carotid sinus massage triggers a reflex increase in vagal activity and sympathetic withdrawal and is very helpful in the diagnosis of arrhythmias. It should not be performed in patients with cerebrovascular disease or carotid bruits. It is preferable to limit the duration to 5 seconds. Simultaneous bilateral massage should never be done. Response of various arrhythmias to carotid sinus massage is shown in Table 18-1. Similar responses are seen with intravenous injection of adenosine (Fig. 18-4).

Ambulatory ECG (Holter) monitoring is used to detect intermittent arrhythmias, but the yield is low because many such arrhythmias may not occur on a daily basis. It is also useful for monitoring response to drug therapy and to detect proarrhythmia. Continuous loop recorders or event recorders are useful in the diagnosis of infrequent symptomatic arrhythmias and to document that symptoms are related to arrhythmias. These small devices can be used to monitor the ECG of patients for periods of weeks to months. The ECG is continuously digitized and placed into a temporary memory. Because the memory is limited, at any given point in time only the data from the previous few minutes are retained, and older data are continuously discarded. The patient activates the device when symptoms are felt, and the device places the digitized ECG data from the previous and subsequent few minutes into a permanent memory that can be printed out later or transmitted immediately via telephone (Fig. 18-5).

Signal Averaged ECG

Low-amplitude, high-frequency waveforms in the terminal portion of the QRS complex are often present in patients vulnerable to sustained ventricular tachycardia. These waveforms are called *late potentials*. They correlate with delayed and fragmented activation of the ventricles and indicate that a substrate for reentry is present. Late potentials can be detected from magnified QRS complexes obtained from surface ECG. Random artifacts and skeletal muscle noise are eliminated by averaging 300 to 400 QRS complexes. The signal-averaged ECG is useful for risk stratification after MI. Ventricular tachycardia is unlikely in the absence of late potentials among patients recovering from an MI; however, the positive predictive value is low.

Electrophysiologic Studies

Intracardiac electrophysiologic studies are performed by positioning one or more multielectrode catheters in various positions in the heart. Simultaneous recording from many sites allows the mapping of the sequence of excitation of the atria, AV junction, and ventricles. By this technique, delays in AV conduction can be localized to the AV node or His-Purkinje system, anomalous pathways can be identified, and the site of origin of arrhythmias determined. Supraventricular or ventricular origin of wide QRS complex tachycardia can be determined with certainty. Atrial and ventricular tachyarrhythmias can be induced by programmed stimulation, and the effectiveness and proarrhythmic potential of antiarrhythmic drugs can be tested. Abnormalities of sinus node function can be documented.

PHARMACOLOGIC THERAPY OF ARRHYTHMIAS
Classification of Antiarrhythmic Drugs

Vaughan Williams classification of antiarrhythmic drugs and its modifications have been used for two decades (Table 18-2). However, this classification does not accommodate newer drugs and newly discovered actions of drugs. For example, moricizine does not fit into any one group. Other drugs have several classes of action. Amiodarone, the prototype of class 3, has some class 1, 2, and 4 effects. Sotalol, another class 3 agent, has class 2 effects. The Vaughan Williams classification is also incomplete because it does not include digoxin or adenosine. Because of these limitations, a new classification system that uses a "spreadsheet" approach has been proposed (Fig. 18-6). The grouping is primarily based on the predominant action of the drug and secondarily on other actions that may be clinically relevant. The primary actions are aligned diagonally. Newly discovered drugs or newly discovered actions of existing drugs can easily be added. The new system is more comprehensive and flexible than the Vaughan Williams classification.

The CAST Study

The use of antiarrhythmic drugs has been dramatically altered by the findings of the Cardiac Arrhythmia Suppression Trial (CAST). The fundamental premise underlying the design and implementation of CAST was the "PVC hypothesis," which had guided thoughts on antiarrhythmic therapy for many years. The PVC hypothesis proposed the PVC (premature ventricular contraction) as the primary triggering factor for initiation of ventricular tachycardia or ventricular fibrillation and assumed that PVC suppression by an antiarrhythmic drug would protect against sudden cardiac death by eliminating the trigger. CAST was implemented to test the PVC suppression hypothesis, using a study design in which suppression of PVCs by a specific agent as compared to placebo was a requirement for randomization to that agent. It was a multicenter, double-blind, placebo-controlled study to evaluate the effects of antiarrhythmic therapy with encainide, flecainide, or moricizine in patients with myocardial infarction in the recent past and asymptomatic or mildly symptomatic ventricular arrhythmias. Groups receiving the antiarrhythmic drugs had greater mortality rates than those receiving placebo. The common practice of treating asymptomatic PVCs to prevent lethal arrhythmias was determined to be not beneficial and potentially harmful. CAST also demonstrated that an early favorable response of PVCs to antiarrhythmic drugs does not exclude an adverse outcome later. Also, meta-analysis of data of randomized trials has suggested a net adverse effect of antiarrhythmic drugs used to suppress PVCs after myocardial infarction. Furthermore, in the SPAF (Stroke Prevention in Atrial Fibrillation) study designed to evaluate the efficacy of warfarin and aspirin in prevention of strokes among patients with atrial fibrillation, patients with heart failure who were receiving class 1A or 1C antiarrhythmic drugs had a higher incidence of arrhythmic death when compared to those not taking antiarrhythmic drugs.

Proarrhythmia

Drug-induced arrhythmia or drug-aggravated arrhythmia is a serious problem. Proarrhythmic events, when defined as the initiation of sustained ventricular tachycardia in a patient in whom only nonsustained ventricular tachycardia was induced at baseline, have been reported

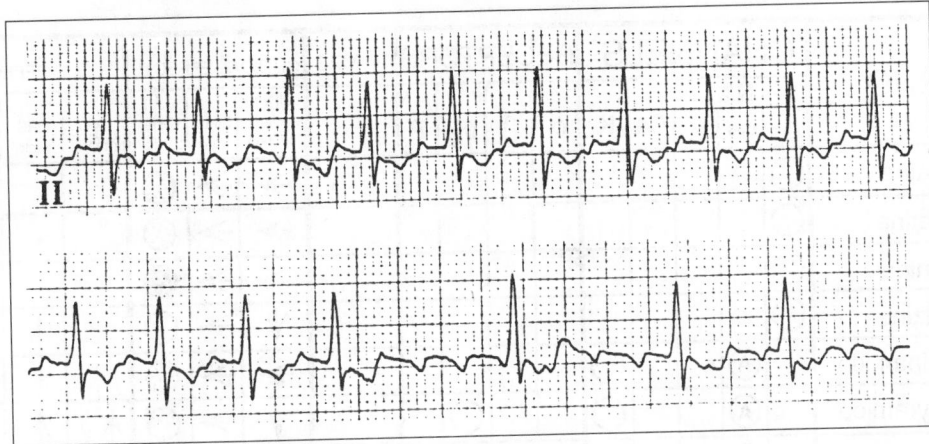

FIGURE 18-4   In a patient with supraventricular tachycardia *(top)*, carotid sinus pressure decreases the AV conduction, and flutter waves become clearly visible *(bottom)*.

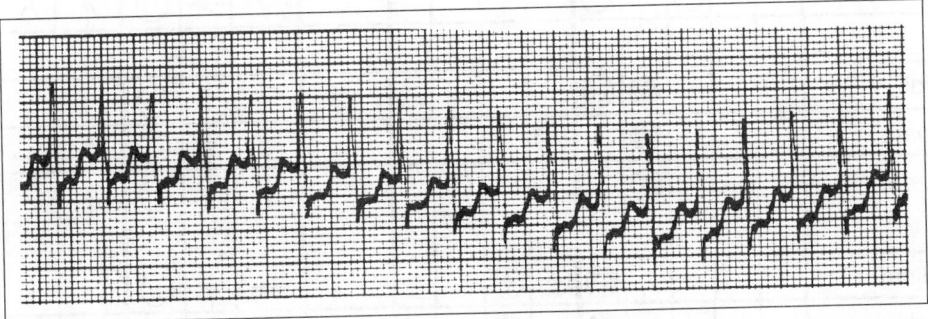

FIGURE 18-5   Supraventricular tachycardia recorded and transmitted through the telephone by a patient who had isolated episodes of palpitations and dizziness. He had been asymptomatic during repeated Holter recordings.

Table 18-2   Vaughan Williams classification of antiarrhythmic drugs

CLASS	ACTION	DRUGS
Class 1	Sodium channel blockade	Moricizine
1A	Moderate phase—0 depression and slow conduction, prolong repolarization	Quinidine, procainamide, disopyramide
1B	Minimal phase—0 depression and slow conduction, shorten repolarization	Lidocaine, tocainide, mexiletine
1C	Marked phase—0 depression and slow conduction, little effect on repolarization	Encainide, flecainide, propafenone
Class 2	β-adrenergic blockade	Propranolol, acebutolol, others
Class 3	Prolong repolarization	Amiodarone, bretylium, sotalol
Class 4	Calcium-channel blockade	Verapamil, diltiazem

in 18% of drug trials using electrophysiologic testing. Patients with left ventricular dysfunction, concomitant therapy with digitalis and diuretics, or prolonged QT interval are at increased risk for proarrhythmia. Significant suppression of PVCs by an antiarrhythmic drug does not exclude possible proarrhythmia. The classic drug-induced proarrhythmia is torsades de pointes, a polymorphic ventricular tachycardia associated with long QT interval that is seen more commonly with class 1A agents and amiodarone. In addition, incessant ventricular tachycardia is seen with either class 1A or class 1C agents; a clinical, paroxysmal ventricular tachycardia becomes incessant and may

be interrupted for only one or two sinus complexes before the tachycardia reinstates itself. A third type of proarrhythmia is a wide sinewave-like tachycardia, which is more common with type 1C drugs and is often fatal; the drug level is often high.

The definition of proarrhythmia has been expanded. Aggravation of an existing arrhythmia, appearance of a new asymptomatic arrhythmia, or a change in inducibility may now be considered as proarrhythmic events. Another category referred to as *transient proarrhythmic risk* identifies a response in which the drug itself is not prone to generate a proarrhythmic response until a third factor—such as transient ischemia, changes in hemodynamics, or alterations in autonomic tone—changes the relationship between drug and patient from benign to potentially fatal. Because all antiarrhythmic drugs have some potential for proarrhythmia, therapy should be initiated under ECG monitoring in most cases, especially when organic heart disease is present or malignant ventricular arrhythmias are being treated.

Selected Antiarrhythmic Drugs

Detailed description of all antiarrhythmic drugs is beyond the scope this chapter. The reader should consult standard sources and have a full understanding of pharmacokinetics, dosage, drug interactions, and toxicity before prescribing these drugs. Fig. 18-6 shows the mechanism of action and some of the clinical and electrocardiographic effects of antiarrhythmic drugs. Pharmacokinetics and some common drug interactions are shown in Table 18-3. Drug interactions are often difficult to evaluate. Studies in normal volunteers may not predict responses in cardiac patients; observations from animal studies and isolated case reports are of limited clinical significance. Some interactions are obvious: combining two antiarrhythmic drug with β-adrenergic blocking activity or negative inotropic effect will have additive effect. Cimetidine inhibits the hepatic cytochrome P_{450} and

DRUG	CHANNELS: NA Fast	CHANNELS: NA Mod.	CHANNELS: NA Slow	CHANNELS: Ca	CHANNELS: K	RECEPTORS: α	RECEPTORS: β	RECEPTORS: M_2	RECEPTORS: P	PUMPS: Na-K ATPase	CLINICAL EFFECTS: Left ventricular function	CLINICAL EFFECTS: Sinus rate	CLINICAL EFFECTS: Extracardiac	ECG EFFECTS: PR interval	ECG EFFECTS: QRS width	ECG EFFECTS: JT interval
Lidocaine	Low										→	→	Moderate			↓
Mexiletine	Low										→	→	Moderate			↓
Tocainide	Low										→	→	High			↓
Moricizine	Low (I)										↓	→	Low		↑	
Procainamide		Low (A)			Moderate						→	→	Moderate	↑	↑	↑
Disopyramide		Low (A)			Moderate			Low			↓	→	Moderate	↑↓	↑	↑
Quinidine		Low (A)			Moderate	Low		Low			→	↑	Moderate	↑↓	↑	↑
Propafenone		Low (A)					Moderate				↓	↓	Low	↑	↑	
Flecainide			Low (A)		Low						↓	→	Low	↑	↑	
Bepridil	Low			High	Moderate						?	↓	Low			↑
Verapamil	Low			High		Moderate					↓	↓	Low	↑		
Diltiazem				Moderate							↓	↓	Low	↑		
Bretylium					High	Agonist/Antagonist	Agonist/Antagonist				→	↓	Low			↑
Sotalol					High		High				↓	↓	Moderate	↑		↑
Amiodarone	Low			Low	High	Moderate	Moderate				→	↓	High	↑		↑
Propranolol	Low						High				↓	↓	Moderate	↑		
Atropine								High			→	↑	Moderate	↓		
Adenosine									Agonist		?	↓	Low	↑		
Digoxin								Agonist		High	↑	↓	Moderate	↑		↓

Relative potency of block / severity of effects:

○ Low ◎ Moderate ● High

= Agonist = Agonist/Antagonist

A = Activated state blocker

I = Inactivated state blocker

FIGURE 18-6 New classification of antiarrhythmic drugs, which uses a spreadsheet approach. (Modified from American Heart Association: *Circulation* 84:1848, 1991; and Smeets JLRM: Advances in arrhythmology, *Impulse* 1992.)

reduces hepatic blood flow, resulting in decreased clearance of many antiarrhythmic drugs. It is preferable to use one of the newer H_2-receptor antagonists in patients receiving antiarrhythmic agents. Drugs that induce the hepatic cytochrome P_{450} (e.g., phenobarbital, phenytoin, and rifampin) may accelerate the clearance of antiarrhythmic drugs metabolized in the liver. Erythromycin increases serum digoxin levels by destroying enteric flora that break down digoxin. It is also an inhibitor of hepatic microenzymes. Approximately 10% of the population is congenitally deficient in cytochrome P_{450} microenzymes. Thus serum levels of antiarrhythmic drugs should be moni-

Table 18-3 Pharmacokinetics of selected antiarrhythmic drugs.

CLASS	DRUG	HALF-LIFE (HRS)	PLASMA PROTEIN BINDING (%)	MAJOR ROUTE OF EXCRETION	THERAPEUTIC SERUM LEVELS (μg/ml)	INTERACTIONS
	Moricizine	1.5-3.5*	95	H	n/a	Cimetidine
I A	Quinidine	6-7	80-90	H/R	2-5	Digoxin, warfarin, cimetidine
	Procainamide	2.5-5	14-23	H/R	4-8	
	Disopyramide	4-10	20-60†	H/R	2-5	
B	Lidocaine (IV)	1-2	40-80	H	1.5-6	Cimetidine, propranalol
	Tocainide	11-15	10-20	H/R	4-10	
	Mexiletine	10-12	50-60	H	0.5-2	
C	Flecainide	12-27‡	40	H/R	0.2-1	Cimetidine, propranalol
	Propafenone	2-10	97	H	—	Warfarin, propranolol
II	Propranolol	2-3	90-95	H	0.05-0.1	Cimetidine
	Esmolol (IV)	0.15	55	H	—	
	Acebutolol	3-4	26	H/R		
III	Bretylium (IV)	5-10	0-8	R	0.5-1.5	
	Amiodarone	50 days	96	H	1-2.5	Digoxin, warfarin, phenytoin
	Sotalol	12	0	R	—	
IV	Verapamil	3-7	90	H	0.5-2 ng/ml	Amiodarone, quinidine, erythromycin, verapamil
—	Digoxin	30-40	20-25	R	n/a	Dipyridamole, theophylline
—	Adenosine (IV)	10sec	—	—		

n/a, not applicable; *H*, Hepatic; *R*, Renal.
*Half-life may be shortened in patients after multiple dosing.
†Protein binding is concentration-dependent.
‡Half-life increases with increasing dosage.

tored whenever possible. Two antiarrhythmic drugs should be combined cautiously.

Quinidine

Quinidine is used in the prevention and treatment of ventricular and many supraventricular arrhythmias. Although it can cause AV block, more often its vagolytic effect enhances AV conduction. Thus patients with atrial flutter or atrial fibrillation should first receive drugs that control the ventricular rate by decreasing AV conduction (e.g., digoxin, β-adrenergic blockers, or verapamil) before quinidine is used. The α-adrenergic blocking effect of quinidine may lead to hypotension. Long-acting preparations of quinidine are preferred, and the usual dose is 300 to 600 mg three times a day, with monitoring of serum levels. Marked prolongation of QT interval (>500 msec) warrants discontinuation of quinidine. Proarrhythmia (worsening ventricular arrhythmias or torsades de pointes ventricular tachycardia) may also occur in the absence of marked QT prolongation and at therapeutic serum levels. Gastrointestinal adverse effects such as diarrhea and nausea are common. Idiosyncratic reactions include fever, rash, thrombocytopenia, and hemolytic anemia.

Procainamide (Procan, Pronestyl)

Indications and proarrhythmic effects of procainamide are similar to those of quinidine. Procainamide is acetylated to *N*-acetyl procainamide (NAPA) in the liver. NAPA has its own antiarrhythmic effects and is excreted by the kidney. Long-acting preparations at a dose of 500 to 1000 mg three or four times a day with monitoring of serum procainamide and NAPA levels is recommended. Intravenous preparation of procainamide is used in the intensive care unit setting to achieve serum levels rapidly and to treat ventricular arrhythmias resistant to lidocaine and at times for supraventricular tachycardias. The intravenous form is preferred for atrial fibrillation with very rapid ventricular response in the presence of Wolff-Parkinson-White (WPW) syndrome. The loading dose is 50 mg infused over 2 minutes, every 5 minutes, up to a total dose of 800 mg with ECG monitoring of QRS duration and QT interval; the maintainance dose is 2 to 4 mg/kg/min. Procainamide has fewer gastrointestinal side effects than quinidine. However, immune-mediated fever, agranulocytosis, and lupuslike syndrome may develop. A lupuslike syndrome is noted in 15% to 20% of patients receiving procainamide and is character-

ized by the insidious onset of fever, arthritis, malar rash, pleural and/or pericardial effusions, and antinuclear antibodies with a "smooth" or "diffuse" pattern. Although most patients treated chronically develop antinuclear antibodies, only 15% to 20% develop the lupuslike syndrome. Cimetidine decreases the renal clearance of procainamide and *N*-acetylprocainamide.

Disopyramide (Norpace)

Indications and electrophysiologic and proarrhythmic effects of disopyramide are similar to quinidine and procainamide. Disopyramide has a negative inotropic effect and should be avoided in the presence of left ventricular dysfunction, especially if there is a history of congestive heart failure. Its anticholinergic actions cause dry mouth, constipation, blurred vision, and urinary obstruction. It is poorly tolerated when prostatism or glaucoma is present. Disopyramide is available in an oral form, and the usual dose is 100 to 200 mg every 6 hours.

Moricizine (Ethmozine)

Moricizine has class 1A, 1B, and 1C properties. It is a well-tolerated drug that is moderately effective in suppressing ventricular ectopy. In the CAST study, however, increased mortality was noted during the initial 14-day period of moricizine therapy, and no survival benefit was noted during long-term therapy. Thus use of moricizine has been limited to life-threatening ventricular arrhythmias, and it does not appear to be more effective than other class 1 drugs. Usual dosage is 600 to 900 mg/day in three divided doses.

Lidocaine (Xylocaine)

Lidocaine is usually the drug of choice for acute suppression of ventricular arrhythmias. Disposition of intravenous lidocaine is represented by the two-compartment pharmacokinetic model. Thus to achieve and maintain serum therapeutic levels quickly, multiple loading doses and simultaneous initiation of a maintainance infusion are necessary. Recommended dose is an initial IV bolus of 1 mg/kg, followed by 0.5 mg/kg IV bolus injections every 8 to 10 minutes, if necessary, to a total of 3 mg/kg. Maintenance infusion is at 2 to 4 mg/kg. The dose should be adjusted by measuring serum levels. Lower doses should be used in the elderly and in the presence of heart failure, hypotension, or hepatic dysfunction. Abrupt termination of infusion will result in a gradual decline of serum levels over the next 8 to 10 hours. Adverse reactions include confusion, stupor, convulsions, and rarely coma. Sinus node dysfunction and suppression of escape rhythms may occur.

Mexiletine (Mexitil) and Tocainide (Tonocard)

These two oral drugs are similar to lidocaine in their electrophysiologic properties and adverse effects. They are used in the treatment of symptomatic ventricular arrhythmias and may be appropriate when the QT interval is prolonged; however, they are not very potent in suppressing ventricular tachycardias. Use of tocainide is declining because of the high incidence of adverse effects, which include tremor, dizziness, and other central nervous system effects similar to those of lidocaine as well as the rare occurrence of lupuslike syndrome, pulmonary fibrosis, and agranulocytosis. Mexiletine has similar central nervous system adverse effects but is better tolerated. The usual dose of mexiletine is 150 to 250 mg every 8 hours, taken with meals.

Propafenone (Rhythmol)

Propafenone has class 1C antiarrhythmic properties and moderate β-adrenergic antagonism. It is used primarily in the treatment of life-threatening ventricular arrhythmias. Seven percent of the population, deficient in cytochrome P_{450} microenzymes, fail to convert propafenone into 5-hydroxypropafenone and accumulate high concentrations of propafenone, which causes significant β-adrenergic blockade. This metabolic phenotype, however, does not affect the antiarrhythmic actions or dosage because both propafenone and 5-hydroxypropafenone have similar antiarrhythmic properties. The usual oral dose is 150 to 300 mg every 8 hours.

Flecainide (Tambocor)

Flecainide is effective in suppressing premature ventricular contractions and moderately effective in the treatment of life-threatening ventricular arrhythmias. Because of the findings of the CAST study, its use is limited to life-threatening ventricular tachycardias. The risk of flecainide-induced proarrhythmia, however, is low in the absence of structural heart disease. Thus flecainide is approved for the prevention of supraventricular tachycardias, paroxysmal atrial flutter, and fibrillation in the absence of structural heart disease. Among older patients, it is preferable to exclude coronary artery disease using non-invasive testing (Chapter 13) before initiating flecainide therapy. It has a negative inotropic effect and should be avoided in the presence of severe left ventricular dysfunction. Slow elimination makes twice-a-day dosing possible. The usual oral dose is 100 to 150 mg every 12 hours.

Beta-adrenergic Blockers

The properties and role of β-blockers in the treatment of hypertension and ischemic heart disease are described in Chapters 22 and 32. In addition to β-adrenergic blockade, propranolol and acebutolol have membrane-stabilizing effects caused by sodium channel blockade. Propranolol is effective in controlling arrhythmias precipitated by adrenergic stimulation during emotional stress or exercise. It is the drug of choice for ventricular arrhythmias in mitral valve prolapse and congenital QT prolongation syndromes. All β-blockers are effective in controlling the ventricular rate in atrial fibrillation or flutter. Esmolol, an ultra–short acting intravenous β-blocker is useful in the intensive care settings. Many β-blockers have been shown to reduce mortality and incidence of sudden death after myocardial infarction (Chapter 23). Beta-blockers with intrinsic sympathomimetic activity (pindolol, acebutolol) should be avoided in ischemic heart disease.

Amiodarone (Cordarone)

Amiodarone is classified as a class 3 drug, but it has class 1, 2, and 3 effects. It is the most potent antiarrhythmic drug available. Although it is effective in the treatment of many supraventricular arrhythmias including those associated with WPW syndrome, its use is limited to life-threatening ventricular arrhythmias because of potential toxicity. It is the drug of choice for survivors of cardiac arrest who are not candidates for an automatic implantable cardioverter defibrillator. Adverse effects include bradyarrhythmias, photosensitivity, liver function abnormalities, and hypothyroidism or hyperthyroidism. Pneumonitis and pulmonary fibrosis, an idiosyncratic but dose-related adverse effect, can be fatal; it usually occurs after 3 to 12 months of therapy and may be minimized by using the lowest possible maintenance dose. Usual oral loading dose is 800 to 1600 mg/day for 7 to 10 days, and the maintenance dose is 200 to 400 mg/day.

Sotalol (Betapace)

Sotalol is a class 3 antiarrhythmic agent with strong β-adrenergic blocking properties. It is commonly used in the prevention of sustained ventricular tachycardia but is also effective in many supraventricular tachycardias. In the ESVEM (Electrophysiologic Study Versus Electrocardiographic Monitoring) study sotalol was noted to be superior to mexiletine, procainamide, propafenone, or quinidine in preventing the recurrence of ventricular tachyarrhythmias. Adverse reactions are those caused by β-adrenergic blockade and proarrhythmia. Risk of developing torsades de pointes increases with higher dosage, bradycardia, and hypokalemia. The usual oral dose is 80 to 160 mg twice a day.

Calcium Channel Blockers

Not all calcium channel blockers have antiarrhythmic properties. Verapamil and diltiazem block the calcium-dependent slow current in the SA node and AV node. Intravenous verapamil (10 mg over 1 to 2 minutes) is effective in terminating reentrant supraventricular tachycardias. Intravenous infusion of diltiazem is effective in controlling the ventricular rate in atrial flutter and fibrillation. Oral forms of both drugs are useful in the prevention of reentrant supraventricular tachycardias and for control of ventricular rate in atrial flutter and fibrillation. Adverse effects include bradyarrhythmias, AV block, and negative inotropy. Bepridil (Vascor), used in the treatment of angina, has class 1 antiarrhythmic properties and can cause prolongation of QT and torsades de pointes ventricular tachycardia.

Digitalis

Digitalis slows AV conduction by increasing the vagal tone and by a direct effect. It is used in the treatment of supraventricular tachycardias and to control the ventricular rate when atrial flutter or fibrillation is present. The role of digoxin in preventing and converting atrial fibrillation is controversial. Digoxin, the most commonly used preparation, requires an oral loading dose of 1 mg in divided doses and a maintenance dose of 0.125 to 0.5 mg. Serum digoxin levels must be used to guide dosing. Reduction in dosage is necessary in the elderly and in renal insufficiency. Digitalis toxicity may cause gastrointestinal, neurologic, or visual disturbances; cardiac toxicity can be potentially lethal. Premature ventricular contractions are commonly seen, but are nonspecific. The following arrhythmias are suggestive of digitalis toxicity: atrial tachycardia with block, nonparoxysmal junctional tachycardia, bidirectional ventricular tachycardia, sinus bradycardia, sinus arrest, Mobitz-1 or third-degree AV block, and AV dissociation caused by acceleration of a subsidiary pacemaker. Many digitalis-induced arrhythmias may be treated by stopping the drug. Hypokalemia should be corrected. Potassium is effective in suppressing digitalis-induced ventricular arrhythmias. However, potassium may worsen conduction disturbances and AV block. Lidocaine and phenytoin are used to treat digitalis-induced ventricular arrhythmias. If possible, cardioversion should be avoided in the presence of digitalis toxicity because ventricular fibrillation may be precipitated. Antidigoxin antibodies in the form of Fab fragments can rapidly reverse digitalis toxicity by binding to digoxin and forming an antibody-digoxin complex, which is then excreted by the kidneys. Cost limits its use to life-threatening arrhythmias or arrhythmias that require prolonged monitoring in the intensive care unit.

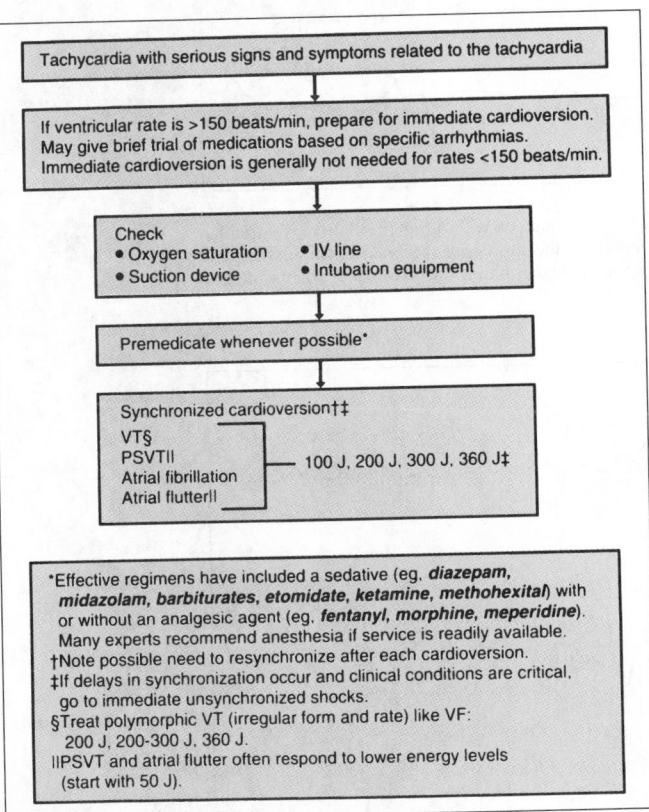

FIGURE 18-7   Algorithm for emergency cardioversion recommended by the Emergency Cardiac Care Commitee.
(From *JAMA*, 268:2221, 1992.)

Adenosine

Adenosine is an endogenous nucleoside that slows sinus node discharge and depresses AV nodal conduction, often with transient AV block. It has a very short half-life of 10 seconds. It is better tolerated than verapamil in the presence of ventricular dysfunction and hypotension and is the drug of choice for termination of supraventricular tachycardias. Unlike verapamil, it can be used to treat wide QRS complex tachycardias. The usual dose is 6 to 12 mg injected as a rapid intravenous bolus. Adverse effects include flushing and the sensation of chest pressure, which are transient. Dipyridamole enhances and theophylline or caffeine inhibits the action of adenosine.

NONPHARMACOLOGIC THERAPY
Cardioversion

The use of direct electrical current for elective or emergency conversion of arrhythmias has become standard therapy. The algorithm for emergency cardioversion recommended by the Emergency Cardiac Care Committee is shown in Fig. 18-7. If time permits, electrolyte abnormalities and digoxin toxicity should be excluded. The discharge to the tallest R wave must be synchronized to prevent triggering of ventricular fibrillation; exceptions include ventricular fibrillation and ventricular tachycardias with wide QRS complex when synchronization may not be possible and in tachyarrhythmias causing circulatory collapse with no time for synchronization. Recommended initial energy levels for cardioversion are 50 J for atrial flutter and supraventricular tachycardia, 100 J for atrial fibrillation and monomorphic ventricular tachycardia, and 200 J for polymorphic ventricular tachycardia and ventricular fibrillation. Stepwise increases in energy are used if the initial shock fails. Complications are rare. Transient creatine kinase elevation is usually from the skeletal muscle. If severe conduction system disease is suspected, a temporary pacemaker should be inserted before cardioversion. When ventricular fibrillation occurs,

it is usually attributed to improper synchronization or digitalis toxicity. The risk of systemic embolization is discussed later under atrial fibrillation.

Pacemakers

Temporary pacemakers are used for the immediate treatment of severe and most often symptomatic bradyarrhythmias or when the potential for severe bradyarrhythmia is high (e.g., acute anterior wall infarction with bifascicular block). The pacer wire is inserted percutaneously into a central vein and is positioned in the right ventricular apex under ECG or fluoroscopic guidance; the generator remains outside. Temporary pacing is also used for overdrive suppression of ventricular tachycardia, including torsade de pointes, and the prevention of ventricular tachycardias associated with a long QT interval. Atrial pacing techniques are used to terminate some supraventricular tachycardias. Transcutaneous pacemaker accomplishes pacing using two large-patch electrodes applied to the chest wall. Although it is noninvasive and very useful in emergencies, transcutaneous pacing causes considerable discomfort to the patient, and it is usually used as a stopgap measure.

Permanent pacing means that the generator is implanted under the skin. In general, permanent pacing is recommended for symptomatic irreversible bradyarrhythmias, Mobitz type II AV block, and complete AV block. A variety of permanent pacemakers are available. They are programmable, permitting adjustment of sensing and pacing functions noninvasively. Pacemakers are categorized by a five-letter identification code: the first letter indicates the chamber paced (A, atrium; V, ventricle; D, dual; and O, none), the second letter indicates the chamber sensed (A, V, D and O), and the third letter indicates response to sensing (I, inhibited by sensed signal; T, triggered by sensed signal; and D, inhibited or triggered). The fourth and fifth letters indicate programmability and antitachycardia features. The letter *R* in the fourth position indicates rate modulation (i.e., ability to change rate in response to body motion, respirations, etc.). Most pacemakers used in clinical practice are either VVI or DDD; if rate-responsive features are also available, they are called VVIR or DDDR.

The VVI pacemaker is a single-chamber pacemaker that senses and paces only in the ventricle; it is inhibited when an R wave is sensed. For example, a VVI pacer programmed at 60 beats/min will pace every second if there is no intrinsic R wave. Presence of an R wave will inhibit the pacer for the next 1 second (Fig. 18-8). VVI pacers are simple to evaluate; however, because only the ventricles are paced, AV synchrony is lost. Loss of the atrial contribution may lead to symptomatic hypotension during pacing in some patients. This phenomenon is described as *pacemaker syndrome*. Uncontrolled studies suggest that there may be a higher incidence of atrial fibrillation and strokes with VVI pacing than with DDD pacemakers. DDD pacemakers maintain AV synchrony and are preferred but are somewhat more difficult to evaluate and program. They sense and pace both in the atria and ventricle. Various DDD functions are shown in Fig. 18-9. DDD pacemakers should be avoided in the presence of atrial fibrillation or flutter. Occasionally, DDD pacemakers may function at rapid rates when ventricular pacing causes retrograde P waves, which in turn trigger pacing in the ventricles. Such a tachyarrhythmia is called *pacemaker-mediated tachycardia* and can be prevented by appropriate programming. All patients with pacemakers require periodic surveillance for impending battery depletion, including telephonic or bedside ECG assessment of pacing rate, which slows as battery power depletes. Pacemaker programming devices can noninvasively assess more sophisticated measurements of pacemaker function and power reserve. For details regarding the indications for and the selection of appropriate pacemakers, see the guidelines compiled by a joint task force of the American College of Cardiology and the American Heart Association.

Automatic Implantable Cardioverter Defibrillator

The automatic implantable cardioverter defibrillation (AICD) comprises two components: the pulse generator and a lead system for detection of arrhythmias and for the delivery of shock. Current systems use heart rate as a primary arrhythmia-sensing parameter. When heart

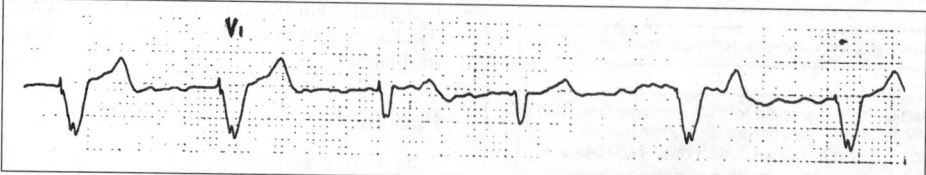

FIGURE 18-8   VVI pacemaker programmed at 60 beats/min in a patient with atrial fibrillation. Ventricular pacing resulting in wide QRS complex is noted every second. In the third beat, pacemaker stimulation and intrinsic QRS complex occur simultaneously. Intrinsic QRS complexes inhibit the pacemaker for the next 1 second.

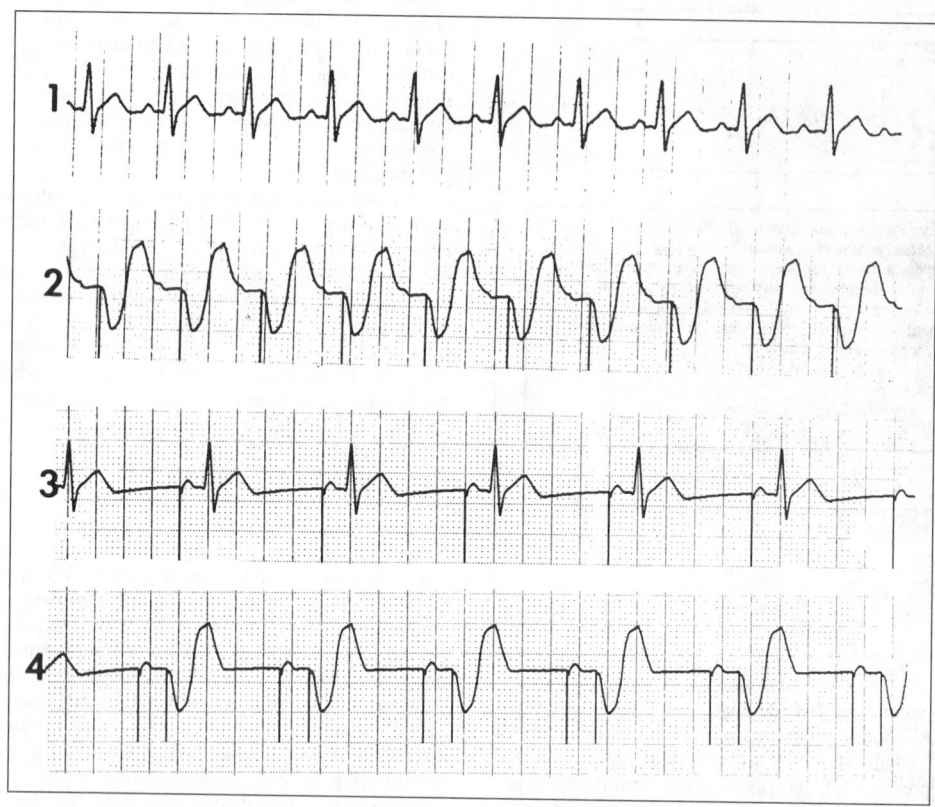

FIGURE 18-9   Various functions of a DDD pacemaker. Tracing 1: Normal atrial and ventricular activity inhibits the pacemaker. Tracing 2: Atrial rhythm is sinus tachycardia; pacemaker senses the atrial activity and paces the ventricle because no intrinsic ventricular activity is sensed during the programmed AV interval. Tracing 3: Because heart rate is lower than the programmed minimum rate, pacemaker paces the atria at the programmed minimum rate. Normal ventricular activity is sensed and ventricular pacing is inhibited. Tracing 4: After atrial pacing, no intrinsic ventricular activity is sensed during the programmed AV interval and ventricular pacing occurs.

rate exceeds a preset value and the arrhythmia detection algorithm is satisfied, shock is delivered. If the shock is unsuccessful, the AICD will recycle and deliver four additional shocks. Although the AICD is remarkably effective in preventing sudden arrhythmic deaths, older systems have some limitations. Newer AICDs have better arrhythmia detection algorithms, antitachycardia pacing, and stand-by pacing capabilities. Another major initial limitation was the need for thoracotomy to place the epicardial patch electrodes. Nonthoracotomy lead systems that use subcutaneous and/or transvenous electrodes are now available. Currently accepted indications for AICD placement include drug-resistant sustained ventricular tachycardia and survivors of cardiac arrest caused by ventricular tachycardia or fibrillation, in whom the arrhythmia is not inducible in the laboratory or is drug refractory. AICD placement is not indicated for ventricular tachycardia or ventricular fibrillation occurring in the first 2 days after acute myocardial infarction or if it is secondary to a remediable cause (e.g., hypokalemia, ischemia).

Catheter-ablative procedures using radiofrequency energy are now available at many centers. Arrhythmias caused by accessory pathways that were previously treated medically or by surgical interruption can now be ablated with a catheter. Drug-refractory atrial arrhythmias can be controlled by ablating the AV node and inserting a pacemaker. Within the AV node are two pathways, fast and slow conducting. Selective ablation of one of these pathways is called modification of the AV junction, which results in control of AV nodal reentrant tachycardia while preserving AV nodal conduction, obviating the need for a pacemaker. Catheter ablation is also useful in the treatment of ventricular tachycardias, especially the bundle branch reentry and right ventricular outflow tract varieties. Radiofrequency catheter techniques have replaced surgery for AV node modification and accessory pathway interruption. Aneurysmectomy and endocardial resection procedures are useful in the removal of the arrhythmogenic focus of ventricular tachycardia, usually seen in ischemic cardiomyopathy. Because many of these patients have left ventricular dysfunction, operative mortality associated with these procedures is high, and implantation of AICD has become the preferred treatment.

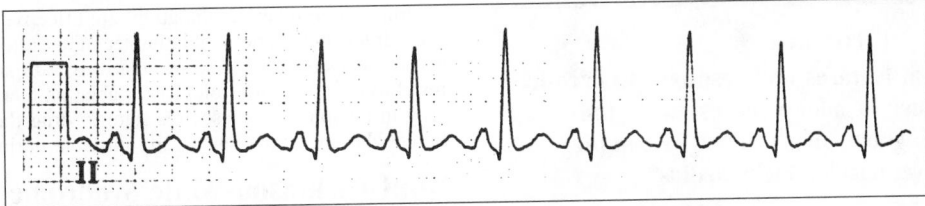

FIGURE 18-10 Sinus tachycardia. P wave is upright in lead II, indicating normal P wave vector.

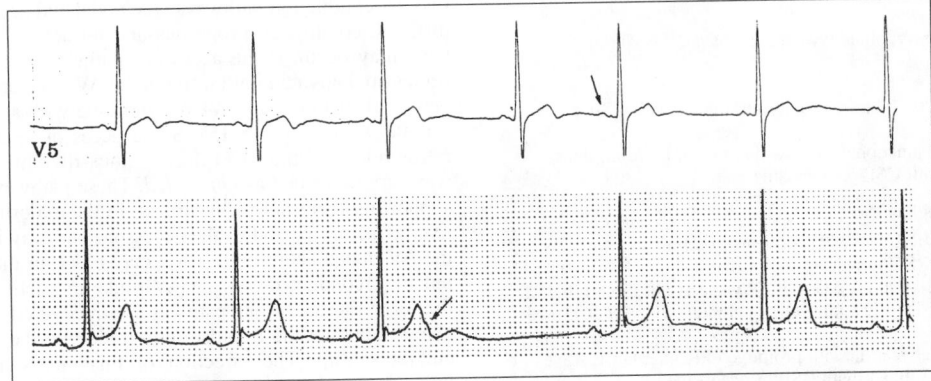

FIGURE 18-11 Premature atrial contraction (PAC). In both strips, PAC resets the sinus node, and a less than fully compensatory pause results. In the bottom strip, the PAC is not conducted. A nonconducted PAC is a common cause of sinus pause.

SUPRAVENTRICULAR TACHYCARDIAS
Sinus Tachycardia

Sinus rhythm at a rate above 100 beats/min is defined as sinus tachycardia. Sinus tachycardia is normal in infants and children and in adults during physical or emotional stress. Sympathomimetic drugs, anticholinergic drugs, nicotine, alcohol, caffeine, and pathologic conditions such as fever, anemia, hypotension, thyrotoxicosis, and hypoxemia may cause sinus tachycardia. A normal P wave vector (upright P in lead II) and normal relationship between P and R waves are necessary to diagnose sinus tachycardia (Fig. 18-10). Management almost always depends on the control of these triggering factors. Specific therapy is rarely needed.

Premature Atrial Contractions

Premature atrial contractions (PACs) are common and may occur in normal individuals. Conditions that cause sinus tachycardia may initiate and increase PACs. ECG characteristics include a premature P wave, which has a different vector and a less than fully compensatory pause (Fig. 18-11, *top*). Occasionally, the P wave is superimposed on the preceding T wave and can be recognized by a change in the shape of the T wave. A PAC may not conduct to the ventricle if it is early and the conduction system is still refractory (Fig. 18-11, *bottom*). Alternatively, the PAC may conduct aberrantly, and right bundle branch morphology is most common. PACs usually do not require treatment. Occasionally, PACs trigger sustained arrhythmias, and therapy is aimed at the prevention of the sustained arrhythmias. If PACs cause annoying palpitations, treatment may be necessary. Reassurance and removal of triggering factors should be tried first. Digitalis and β-adrenergic blockers are often used, but their efficacy has not been clearly documented.

Supraventricular Tachyarrhythmias

The term *supraventricular tachyarrhythmia* (SVT) includes all tachyarrhythmias originating above the bifurcation of the bundle of His with an atrial rate above 100 beats/min. On examination, atrial fibrillation and multifocal atrial tachycardia produce an irregularly ir-regular pulse, and atrial flutter may be regular or irregular dpending on the pattern of AV block. Others SVTs are usually regular. SVTs are caused by reentry or increased automaticity of an ectopic focus. The reentrant tachycardias can be disrupted with carotid sinus pressure or drugs that decrease AV nodal conduction (see Table 18-1). Presence of AV block during the tachycardia excludes the diagnosis of AV nodal reentry and AV reciprocating tachycardia, because these arrhythmias include the AV node in their reentry circuit, and AV block will usually terminate them. A physiologic degree of AV block (not all atrial impulses are conducted to the ventricle) is typical of atrial flutter and fibrillation and may be seen in ectopic atrial tachycardia and sinus node reentry tachycardia. Automatic tachycardias are not terminated by carotid sinus pressure or drugs that decrease AV nodal conduction, but AV block may increase, resulting in a decrease in the ventricular rate. Arrhythmias that are sudden in onset and termination and are transient are described as paroxysmal. For the differential diagnosis of SVTs, a 12-lead ECG with a rhythm strip of the lead in which the P wave is clearly visible should be obtained. Determine whether the P wave follows (RP < PR) or precedes (RP > PR) the QRS complex. Response to carotid sinus pressure and adenosine should be documented. Using clinical and electrocardiographic criteria, a definite diagnosis of the type of SVT can be made in most cases (Box 18-1). QRS complexes are usually narrow in SVTs, but a widened QRS may be seen if aberrant conduction is present. The treatment algorithm proposed by the Emergency Cardiac Care Committee of the American Heart Association for the management of tachyarrhythmias is shown in Fig. 18-12.

Atrioventricular Nodal Reentrant Tachycardia (AVNRT)

Atrioventricular nodal reentrant tachycardia (AVNRT) is the most common type of paroxysmal supraventricular tachycardia. The AV node has two types of conduction pathways: one with faster conduction and a longer refractory period and the other with slower conduction and a shorter refractory period. A PAC may be blocked in the faster pathway because of the longer refractory period but is conducted in the slower pathway. As antegrade conduction occurs, the faster pathway recovers its excitability, and the impulse can now

> **BOX 18-1**
>
> **Electrocardiogram features and response to carotid sinus pressure or adenosine useful in the differential diagnosis of narrow QRS complex supraventricular tachycardias***
>
> 1. *AV block is present at baseline or with CSP or adenosine*
>   a. Atrial flutter: flutter waves, regular at ≥240/min
>   b. Atrial fibrillation: irregular, atrial rate =350/min
>   c. Ectopic atrial tachycardia: abnormal P wave, atrial rate <240/min
>   d. Sinus nodal reentry: sinus P waves, atrial rate ≤150/min
>
> 2. *No discernible P waves*
>   a. AVNRT: rate 120-200/min, usually terminates with CSP or Adenosine
>   b. Nonparoxysmal junctional tachycardia: rate <130/min, does not terminate with CSP or adenosine
>
> 3. *P following QRS (PR > RP)*
>   a. Orthodromic AVRT: 160-240/min, usually terminates with CSP or adenosine. QRS alternans is suggestive
>   b. AVNRT: rate 120-200/min. Usually P wave is not discernible, but may be inscribed just after QRS complex with RP <95 ms (see 2a)
>   c. Ectopic atrial tachycardia with prolonged PR interval: P waves are abnormal, AV block with CSP or adenosine
>   d. Nonparoxysmal junctional tachycardia: Rate <130/min, P inscribed just after the QRS. Does not terminate with CSP or adenosine
>
> 4. *P precedes QRS (PR < RP)*
>   a. Sinus nodal reentry tachycardia: sinus P waves, atrial rate <150/min, AV block with CSP or adenosine
>   b. Ectopic atrial tachycardia with normal PR interval: abnormal P waves, AV block with CSP or adenosine
>   c. Atypical AVNRT: abnormal P wave, rate 120-200/min, usually terminates with CSP or adenosine
>   d. Nonparoxysmal junctional tachycardia: rate <130/min, P inscribed just before the QRS. Does not terminate with CSP or adenosine
>
> 5. *AV dissociation is present*
>   Nonparoxysmal junctional tachycardia: ventricular rate <130/min
>
> *12-lead ECG or leads II, V_1, and V_5 are necessary to evaluate P waves.
> *AVNRT*, AV nodal reentry tachycardia; *AVRT*, AV reciprocating tachycardia; *CSP*, carotid sinus pressure.

propagate in the retrograde direction in the faster pathway. Thus a reentry circuit is set up (Fig. 18-13, *A*). The ventricles are activated normally through the His-Purkinje system, and the atria are activated in a retrograde fashion. Because the retrograde conduction is fast, the atria and ventricles are activated simultaneously, and the P wave is inscribed in the QRS complex and is not visible (Fig. 18-14, *top*). If the retrograde conduction is slower than usual, the P wave may occur just after the QRS complex. AVNRT is typically a narrow QRS complex tachycardia with no visible P waves and has an abrupt onset and offset. In the atypical type of AVNRT, antegrade conduction occurs through the fast pathway and retrograde conduction through the slow pathway (Fig. 18-13, *B*). Because atria are activated after the ventricular activation, a retrograde P wave with RP > PR is seen (Fig. 18-14, *middle*).

AVNRT is usually a benign condition and is well tolerated. Palpitations are common; occasionally, the rate is rapid enough to cause additional symptoms. Rest, sedation, and vagotonic maneuvers are useful in terminating AVNRT. Currently adenosine, 6 mg IV followed by 12 mg IV bolus, is the treatment of choice. IV verapamil is also effective. Most AVNRTs can be terminated with one of these drugs. If the patient is hemodynamically unstable, DC cardioversion (25 to 50 J) should be used. Infrequent well-tolerated attacks of AVNRT do not require chronic therapy. Digoxin, β-adrenergic blockers, and ve-

rapamil, alone or in combination, are effective preventive measures. Radiofrequency catheter ablation techniques that modify the AV node without causing AV block are relatively safe and very effective. Referral to an electrophysiologist for ablation therapy should be considered in symptomatic cases resistant to drug therapy, or in those patients who are hemodynamically unstable during the arrhythmia.

Wolff-Parkinson-White Syndrome and Atrioventricular Reciprocating Tachycardias

AV reciprocating tachycardias (AVRT) use the abnormal accessory pathways that connect the atria and the ventricles. Because there are two AV conduction pathways (AV nodal and accessory pathway) with different conduction properties and refractory periods, reentrant circuits may occur. If the accessory pathway conducts antegrade, ventricles are activated both through the AV node and the accessory pathway, and ECG reveals WPW syndrome with a short PR interval and a delta wave (Fig. 18-15). Some accessory pathways conduct only retrograde, and the ECG during sinus rhythm is normal; such pathways are described as *concealed*. These pathways are still capable of supporting reentrant tachycardias. In the majority of cases, the effective refractory period of the accessory pathway is greater than that of the AV node. Therefore a PAC may block in the accessory pathway, but may conduct down the AV node and activate the ventricle. By this time the accessory pathway has recovered its excitability and is able to conduct the impulse retrograde into the atria. A reentrant circuit is set up. The direction of this circus movement, antegrade through the AV node and retrograde through the accessory pathway, is described as *orthodromic* and is the common variety (Fig. 18-13, *C*). With concealed accessory pathways, only orthodromic tachycardias are possible. Because ventricular activation occurs normally through the conduction system in orthodromic tachycardias, the QRS complex is normal and narrow. Uncommonly, the accessory pathway has a shorter refractory period than the AV node, and the circus movement will be in the opposite direction (i.e., antegrade through the accessory pathway and retrograde through the AV node, which is called an antidromic tachycardia) (Fig. 18-13, *D*). Because ventricular activation during an antidromic tachycardia is through the accessory pathway, the QRS complex will be wide. Differentiation between antidromic tachycardia and ventricular tachycardia is often difficult. Orthodromic tachycardia may resemble AV nodal reentry tachycardia, but the former has a faster rate (>200/min), and retrograde P wave occurs after rather than within the QRS complex (Fig. 18-14, *bottom*). Electrical alternans of the QRS complex is more common in AVRT. When the refractory period of the accessory pathway is short, potential exists for very rapid ventricular rates (>250/min) during atrial fibrillation and atrial flutter (Fig. 18-16). Such rapid rates may lead to fatal ventricular fibrillation. AVRT may also degenerate into atrial fibrillation. Thus when prescribing therapy for AVRT, the possibility that the patient may develop atrial fibrillation with very rapid ventricular response should be kept in mind.

The risk of sudden death is increased in WPW syndrome, but the magnitude of risk is unknown. No intervention is necessary in asymptomatic patients. A short refractory period of the accessory pathway, presence of multiple bypass tracts, and family history of premature sudden death are associated with an increased risk for sudden death. Acute treatment to terminate AVRT and AVNRT is similar. Chronic therapy to prevent AVRT, however, is more complex because many antiarrhythmic drugs have variable effects on the AV node and accessory pathway, and the possibility that the patient will develop atrial fibrillation with very rapid ventricular rates is a concern. Propranolol, verapamil, digoxin, and adenosine reduce conduction across the AV node but not across the accessory pathway. Digoxin also reduces the refractory period of the accessory pathway and is particularly dangerous because it may accelerate the ventricular rate during atrial flutter or fibrillation. Type 1A drugs (see Table 18-2) reduce conduction across the accessory pathway and may be beneficial in interrupting or preventing AVRT, but they are not effective in reducing AV nodal conduction. Amiodarone and type 1C drugs reduce both AV nodal and accessory pathway conduction and are useful in the long-term management of selected patients.

AVRT may be terminated safely with carotid sinus pressure or vagomimetic drugs. Drugs that depress conduction in the AV node or

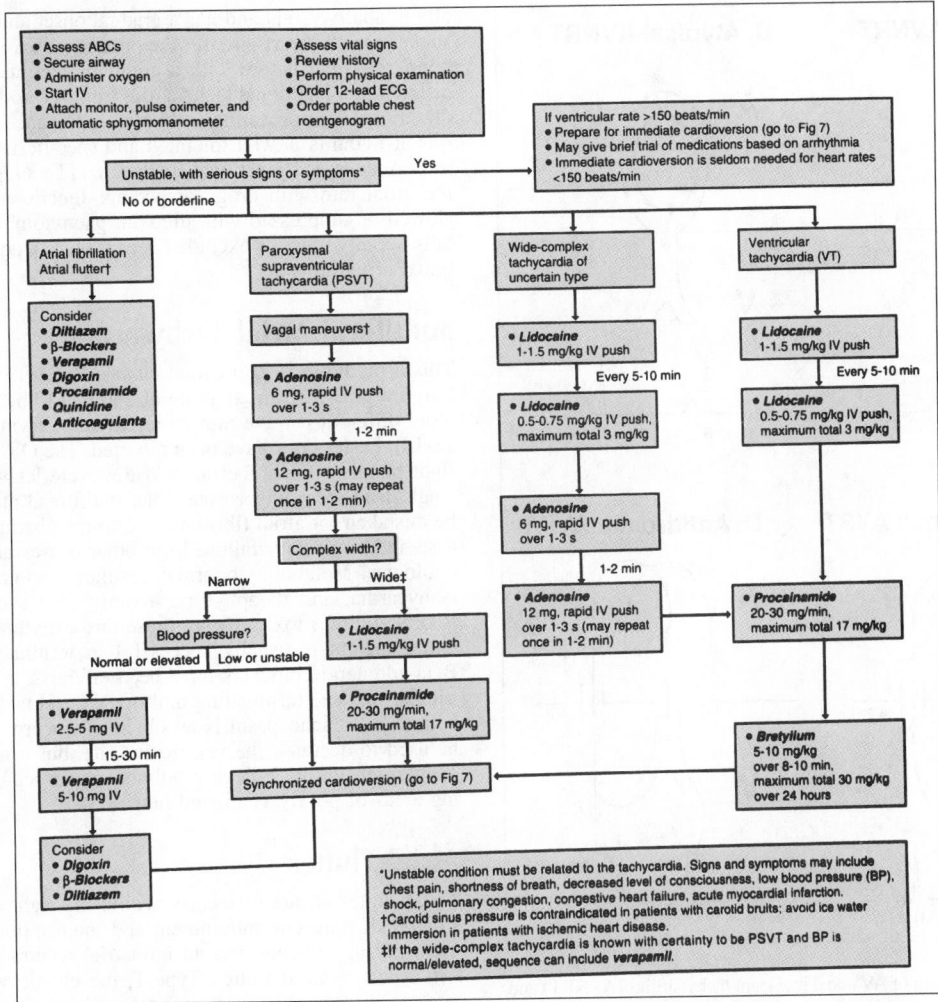

FIGURE 18-12   Algorithm for the treatment for tachycardias recommended by the Emergency Cardiac Care Committee.

(From *JAMA* 268:2223, 1992.)

accessory pathway may be effective in terminating AVRT. If atrial fibrillation develops, however, ventricular rate will be dangerously rapid if the accessory pathway is not blocked (see Fig. 18-16). Digoxin must be avoided because it shortens the refractory period of the accessory pathway. It is preferable to limit the therapy to drugs that will depress the conduction in the accessory pathway (e.g., procainamide) or to drugs such as adenosine that have no effect on the accessory pathway. Patients who do not have life-threatening arrhythmias and respond well to drugs may be managed medically. Type 1A drugs, 1C drugs, and amiodarone are usually effective for chronic therapy. Ablation of the accessory pathway using radiofrequency energy is now performed at many centers and is cost effective because it is curative. Asymptomatic patients with WPW syndrome do not require therapy; patients with recurrent arrhythmias, those prone to develop atrial flutter or fibrillation, and those with a family history of sudden cardiac death should be referred for possible ablation therapy.

Ectopic Atrial Tachycardias

There are two types of ectopic atrial tachycardias: automatic atrial tachycardia and paroxysmal atrial tachycardia. The pathophysiologic mechanism appears to be increased automaticity. Certain ECG features are helpful in differentiating automatic from reentrant supraventricular tachycardias. In automatic tachycardias, the first P wave occurs late and has the same morphology and similar PR interval as the rest of the P waves during tachycardia. In reentrant tachycardias, the first P wave is premature, has a longer PR interval, and has a differ-

ent morphology from the rest of the P waves of the tachycardia. This difference is due to the fact that, unlike automatic tachycardias, in reentrant tachycardias, a PAC is delayed in one limb of the reentrant circuit (leading to long PR); and the subsequent P waves are from retrograde activation of the atria. In automatic atrial tachycardias, the P waves always precede the QRS complex, and the rate gradually speeds at the beginning of the tachycardia *(warm-up phenomenon)*. Vagotonic measures are ineffective. Automatic tachycardias cannot be initiated or terminated by pacing or programmed stimulation.

Automatic atrial tachycardia is rare in adults and more common in children; the electrophysiologic mechanism has not been studied extensively. It is persistent and lasts for weeks, months, and sometimes years. In children it is commonly associated with cardiomyopathy, which may be a complication of persistent tachyarrhythmia. In the few adults reported to have automatic atrial tachycardia, no consistent history of heart disease is present. Antiarrhythmic drugs are not effective in its termination. Propranolol and verapamil may decrease the rate. Recent studies suggest that radiofrequency ablation may successfully terminate many cases of ectopic atrial tachycardia with a low incidence of recurrence.

Paroxysmal atrial tachycardia is usually seen among patients with severe heart disease and/or digitalis toxicity. The clinical electrophysiology of this arrhythmia is not well understood. The atrial rate is usually between 120 and 250 beats/minute, and 2:1 AV block is common (Fig. 18-17). As the name implies, it is transient and resolves when the underlying condition improves. Hemodynamic compromise is rare because the ventricular rate is usually not very rapid. Cardio-

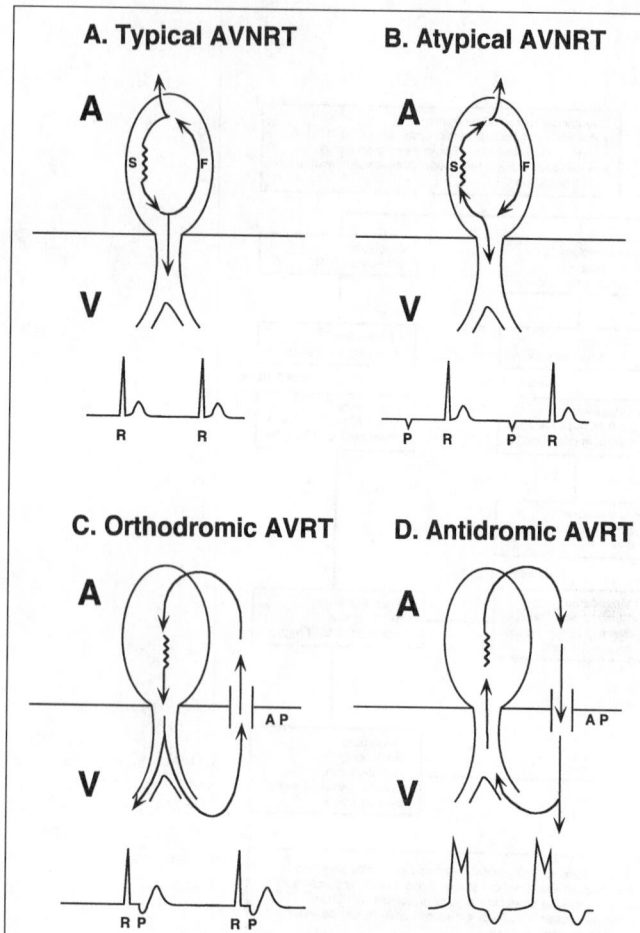

FIGURE 18-13 Mechanism of AV nodal reentrant tachycardias (AVNRT) and AV reciprocating tachycardias (AVRT). See text for details. *A*, atria; *AP*, accessory pathway; *F*, fast pathway; *S*, slow pathway; *V*, ventricles.

version may be effective, but digitalis toxicity should be excluded first. In the absence of digitalis toxicity, this arrhythmia will respond to digitalis and control of heart failure.

Accelerated Atrioventricular Junctional Rhythm and Junctional Tachycardia

AV junctional premature beats, accelerated junctional rhythm, and junctional tachycardia are arrhythmias that originate in the AV junction. They are more likely to arise in tissues adjacent to the node rather than within the node itself. The AV junction includes the approaches to the AV node, the AV node itself, and the bundle of His. The AV junctional tachycardias may be automatic or reentrant. Tachycardias caused by AV nodal reentry and reciprocating tachycardias that incorporate AV node in their macroreentry circuit were described earlier. The inherent rate of the AV junctional pacemaker is 40 to 60 beats/min. Junctional escape rhythm during sinus bradycardia and AV block is a normal physiologic phenomenon.

Accelerated junctional rhythm is caused by enhanced automaticity and has a rate of 60 to 100 beats/min. AV junctional tachycardia is diagnosed when the rate of the junctional rhythm exceeds 100 beats/min. Like other automatic rhythms, these arrhythmias cannot be induced or terminated by programmed stimulation, and cardioversion is not effective. Digitalis toxicity, myocardial infarction, cardiac surgery, and rheumatic fever are the common etiologies. The QRS complex is usually normal. The P wave is inscribed in the QRS complex or just before or after it, depending on the rapidity of retrograde conduction. AV dissociation is commonly present, with atrial and ventricular rates being close to each other. Junctional tachycardia is usu-

ally nonparoxysmal and has a gradual onset and termination. The association with heart disease, the presence of AV dissociation, and the nonparoxysmal nature with a gradual onset and termination help to differentiate junctional tachycardia from AV nodal reentrant tachycardia and AV reciprocating tachycardia. Because the rate is not rapid, this arrhythmia is well tolerated and specific treatment is not necessary. Accelerated junctional rhythms can be suppressed by increasing the atrial rate with drugs or pacing. Junctional tachycardia can be slowed or suppressed with digoxin, phenytoin, or propranolol. Digitalis toxicity must be excluded because it is a common cause of junctional arrhythmias.

Multifocal Atrial Tachycardia

This arrhythmia is also called *chaotic atrial rhythm*. It is an irregularly irregular rhythm at a rate of 100 to 140 beats/min, with three or more different P wave morphologies and varying P-R intervals (Fig. 18-18). Faster rates have been reported. The QRS complex may show right bundle branch aberrancy if the cycle length is short. If only a single lead recording is available, multifocal atrial tachycardia may be mistaken for atrial fibrillation. Chronic obstructive pulmonary disease and respiratory failure from other causes are the most common etiologies. Metabolic abnormalities may also cause multifocal atrial tachycardia, and theophylline toxicity may cause or exacerbate it. Rarely, digitalis toxicity may cause this arrhythmia. Correction of inciting factors is usually successful in terminating the arrhythmia. Beta-adrenergic blockers have been effective in decreasing the ventricular rate and terminating multifocal atrial tachycardia, but exacerbation of bronchospasm is an obvious concern. Verapamil may also be used to decrease the ventricular rate, but it may decrease arterial oxygen tension by relieving pulmonary vasoconstriction and perfusing areas of poorly ventilated lung.

Atrial Flutter

Atrial flutter is due to reentry within the right atrium. The demonstration of transient entrainment and interruption of atrial flutter by atrial pacing indicate it is an intraatrial reentrant rhythm. There are two types of atrial flutter. Type 1, the classic variety, has an atrial rate of 240 to 340 beats/min and can always be interrupted by rapid atrial pacing. Type 2 has an atrial rate of 350 to 450 beats/min and cannot be interrupted by rapid atrial pacing. There is some overlap between the upper rate of type 1 and the lower rate of type 2 atrial flutter. The ventricular rate is usually regular with 2:1 or 4:1 AV conduction. Irregularity or grouped beating may occur and is due to two levels of block in the AV junction.

Atrial flutter may be paroxysmal, persistent, or chronic. Chronic atrial flutter often converts to atrial fibrillation. Atrial flutter is rare in the absence of heart disease. It is noted in patients with chronic obstructive lung disease, or with atrial enlargement from any cause, after cardiac surgery, and in patients who have undergone corrective surgery for congenital heart disease. The ECG reveals a typical sawtooth pattern in leads II, III, and aV$_F$ (Fig. 18-19); discrete flutter waves with isoelectric baseline is common in lead V$_1$. The ventricular rate, which depends on the AV conduction, is usually around 150 beats/min (2:1 AV block) or 75 beats/min (4:1 AV block). Atrial flutter should be considered in the differential diagnosis of narrow QRS complex tachycardia at a rate of 150 beats/min. Carotid sinus massage or adenosine is helpful in transiently increasing the AV block and unmasking the occult flutter waves (see Table 18-1 and Fig. 18-1).

Patients with myocardial dysfunction, advanced coronary artery disease, and mitral stenosis may not tolerate atrial flutter well if the ventricular rate is rapid. Ventricular rate may be slowed with digitalis, β-adrenergic blockers, verapamil, or diltiazem. Intravenous β-adrenergic blockers, verapamil, or diltiazem is preferred for acute therapy because they are effective and act quickly. When the arrhythmia is poorly tolerated, immediate conversion by electrical cardioversion or rapid atrial pacing is the treatment of choice. Anticoagulation is not necessary before or after conversion of pure atrial flutter. Antiarrhythmic drugs may be used to convert atrial flutter, but their effectiveness is unpredictable. Quinidine is traditionally used, but other class 1A and 1C drugs may also be used for conversion.

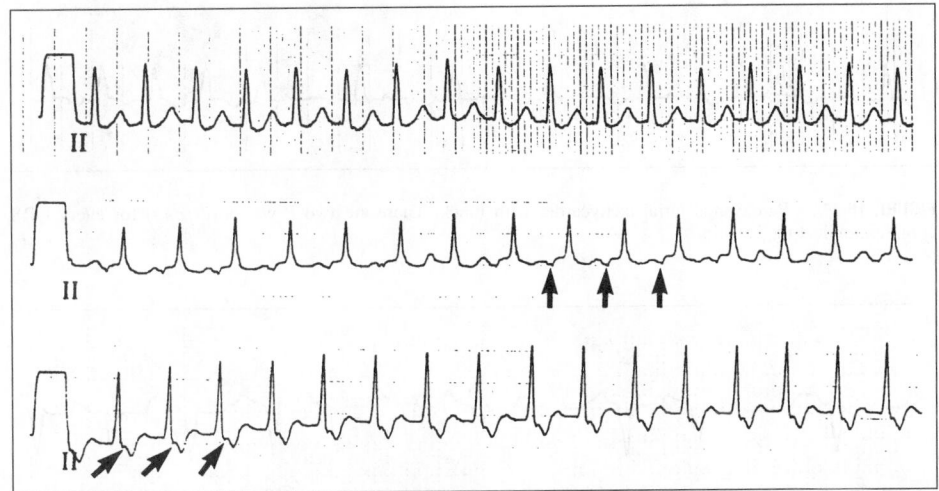

FIGURE 18-14   Typical *(top)* and atypical *(middle)* forms of AV nodal reentrant tachycardia. *Bottom*, orthodromic AV reciprocating tachycardia. Arrows denote P waves. (See text for details.)

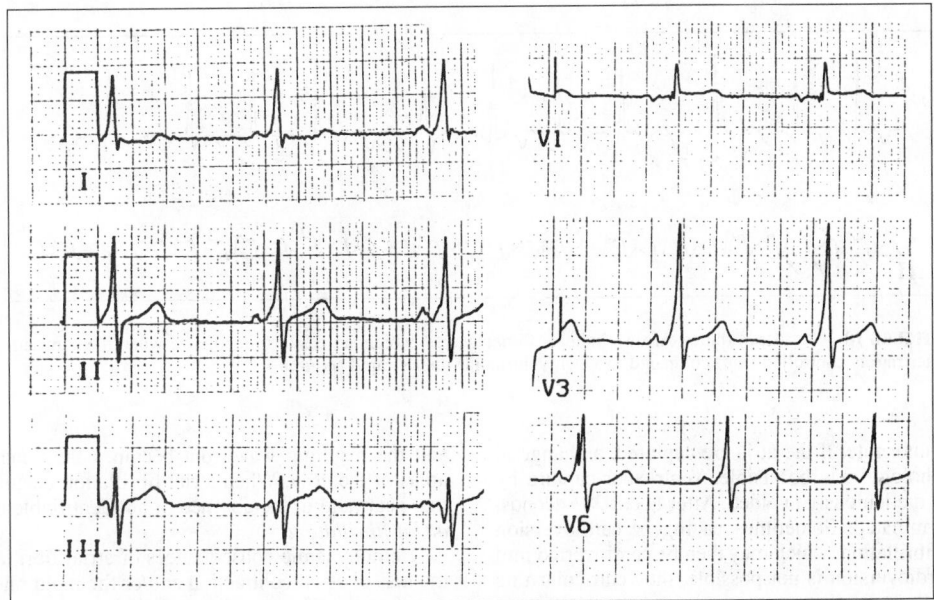

FIGURE 18-15   WPW syndrome. Selected leads show short PR interval and delta wave.

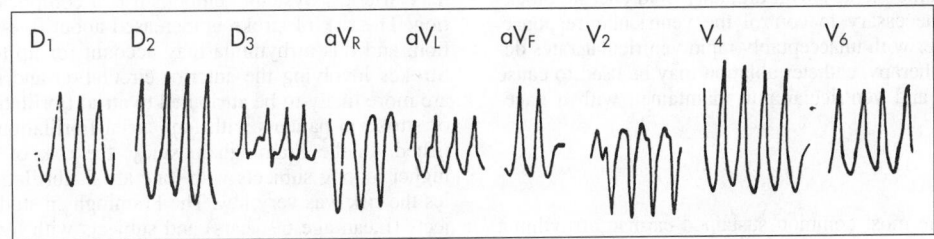

FIGURE 18-16   Atrial fibrillation with very rapid ventricular response in a patient with WPW syndrome.

These drugs may decrease the rate of the atrial flutter and may result in 1:1 AV conduction with a potentially dangerous increase in the ventricular rate to 220 to 240 beats/min. To prevent this complication, AV conduction should be first suppressed with digitalis, β-adrenergic blockers, verapamil, or diltiazem. The major problem with chronic drug therapy for rate control is that the changes in ven-

tricular rate are not smooth because ventricular conduction may change from 4:1 to 2:1 AV conduction. Thus conversion by electrical cardioversion or rapid atrial pacing is the treatment of choice for atrial flutter. Synchronized cardioversion at 25 to 100 J converts most patients with atrial flutter to sinus rhythm. Bipolar atrial pacing is performed from the high right atrium at a rate that is about 50 beats

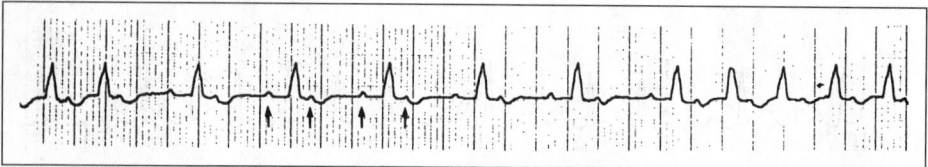

FIGURE 18-17   Paroxysmal atrial tachycardia with block. There are two P waves *(arrows)* for every QRS complex, indicating 2:1 block.

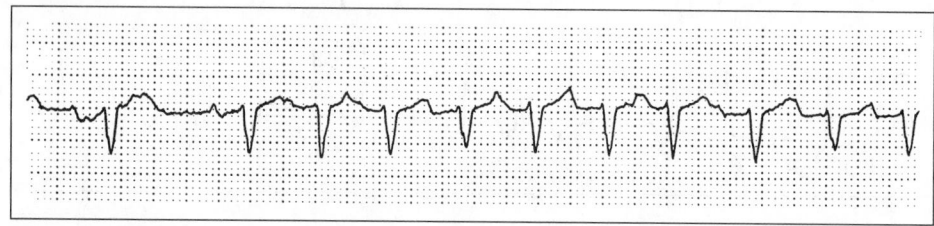

FIGURE 18-18   Multifocal atrial tachycardia. Irregularly irregular rhythm with varying morphologies of P waves.

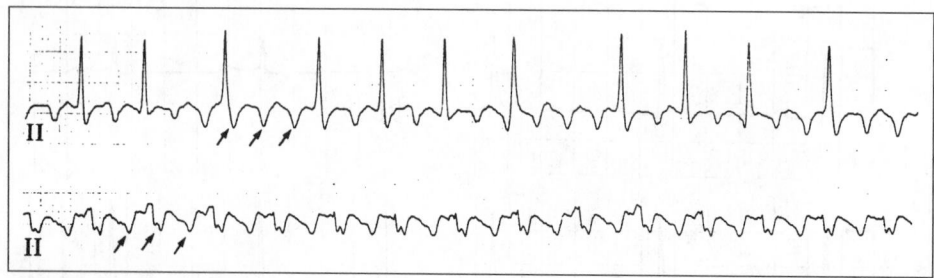

FIGURE 18-19   Atrial flutter. Arrows indicate flutter waves, which are easier to recognize when the ventricular rate is controlled *(top)* compared to when ventricular rate is rapid *(bottom.)*

faster than the atrial flutter rate. If the atria are captured, a change in the flutter wave morphology may be visible. Ventricular capture by the atrial lead must be meticulously avoided. After about 30 seconds, pacing is abruptly terminated. Sometimes pacing or cardioversion may precipitate atrial fibrillation, which may then be cardioverted into sinus rhythm, or if cardioversion is not possible, the ventricular rate is then easier to control medically.

For control of recurrent episodes of paroxysmal atrial flutter, class 1A drugs, especially quinidine, are commonly used. Class 1C and class 3 drugs are also effective. Occasionally, atrial flutter cannot be terminated and chronic therapy with digitalis, β-adrenergic blockers, or verapamil is necessary to control the ventricular response. For chronic atrial flutter with unacceptably rapid ventricular rates despite aggressive drug therapy, catheter ablation may be used to cause complete heart block and ventricular rate maintained with a pacemaker.

Atrial Fibrillation

Atrial fibrillation is the most common sustained cardiac arrhythmia encountered in clinical practice. Its prevalence increases with age. In epidemiologic studies, age, valvular disease, congestive heart failure, hypertension, and diabetes are independent risk factors. It is common after cardiac surgery. Hyperthyroidism, alcohol intoxication, coronary artery disease, cardiomyopathy, atrial septal defect, pulmonary embolism, and pericarditis may lead to atrial fibrillation. Echocardiographic left ventricular hypertrophy, left atrial enlargement, and left ventricular dysfunction are often associated with atrial fibrillation. The most widely accepted proposed mechanism of atrial fibrillation is the so-called multiple reentrant wavelet mechanism. It is believed that orderly progression of depolarization wavefront is not possible,

and the resulting wavefront becomes fractionated around refractory areas of the atria. When atrial fibrillation occurs in an otherwise normal heart and in the absence of an identifiable cause, it is called *lone atrial fibrillation.*

Hemodynamic consequences of atrial fibrillation are secondary to the loss of atrial contraction and/or the rapid rate. Loss of atrial transport function is not well tolerated by patients with poorly compliant ventricles (e.g., left ventricular hypertrophy caused by aortic stenosis) or in the presence of systolic dysfunction. The rapid ventricular rate decreases the diastolic filling time for the ventricles and coronary arteries. Systemic embolism is a complication of atrial fibrillation. The risk of stroke is increased about five-fold by atrial fibrillation, and this arrhythmia may account for up to 15% of all strokes. Strokes involving the anterior circulation and strokes in the elderly are more likely to be attributed to atrial fibrillation. An increased risk of stroke in patients with lone atrial fibrillation is not clearly established. In the Framingham study, the risk of stroke was four-fold higher among subjects with lone atrial fibrillation, but in other studies the risk was very low. The Framingham study included older subjects (mean age 69 years) and subjects with hypertension; also transient ischemic attacks were included as an end-point. Paroxysmal atrial fibrillation is associated with a lower stroke risk than chronic atrial fibrillation. The risk of embolic events tends to be higher during the first few months after the onset of chronic atrial fibrillation. There is a 1% to 2% risk of systemic embolism during the first few days after conversion to sinus rhythm.

Atrial fibrillation is diagnosed at the bedside by irregularly irregular pulse; pulse deficit is due to a low stroke volume during the more rapid beats, which fail to generate a peripheral pulse. The ECG is characterized by grossly irregular atrial electrical activity. Atrial fibrillatory waves are best seen in lead V_1, as well as II, III, and aV_F.

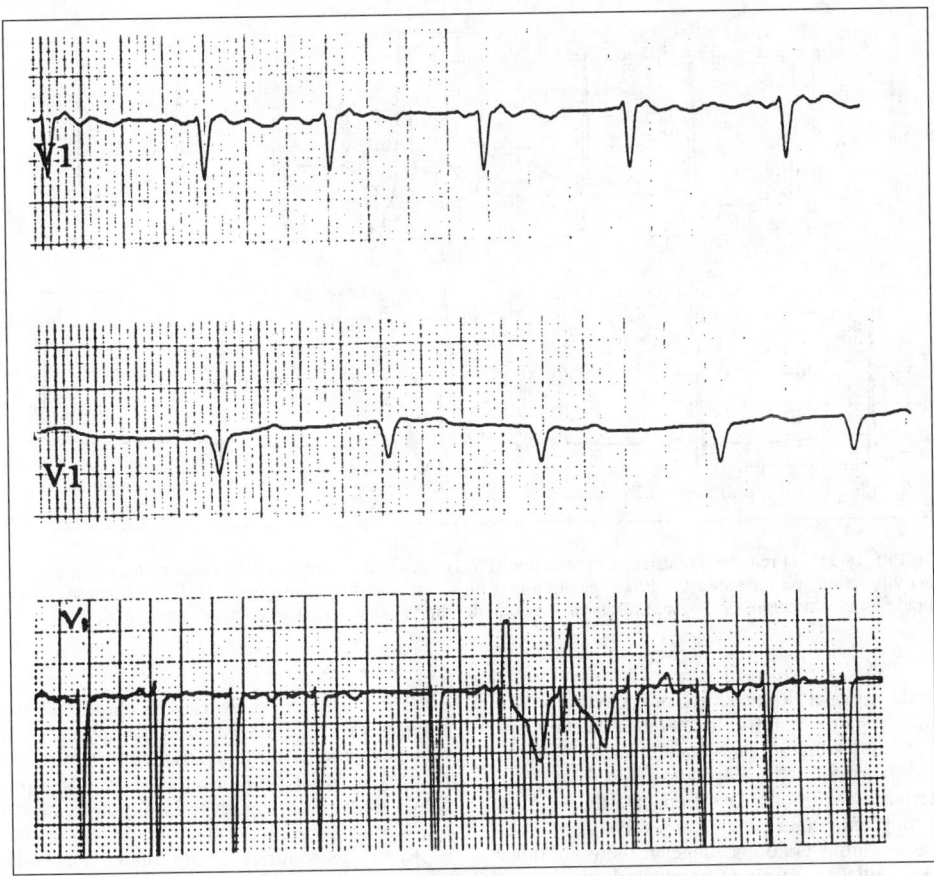

FIGURE 18-20 *Top,* Coarse atrial fibrillation with clearly visible fibrillatory waves. *Middle,* Fine atrial fibrillation with invisible fibrillatory waves. *Bottom,* Ashman phenomenon: right bundle branch type of aberrancy occurs when a long RR interval is followed by short RR interval.

They may be clearly visible or almost imperceptible (Fig. 18-20). The ventricular rate is usually 120 to 160 beats/min. Ventricular rates below 100 beats/min, in the absence of drug therapy, indicate significant conduction system disease; drugs that will depress AV nodal conduction further should be used with caution in these patients. Aberrant ventricular conduction is not uncommon, and the aberrant QRS complexes may be difficult to distinguish from ventricular ectopic beats. Because the refractory period of a depolarization is determined by the previous RR interval, aberrancy tends to occur when a long ventricular cycle is followed by short cycle; the short cycle terminates with an aberrantly conducted beat. This is referred to as the Ashman phenomenon (Fig. 18-20, *bottom*). A series of short cycles may generate a run of aberrantly conducted beats that mimics ventricular tachycardia. An initial QRS vector similar to that of the narrow QRS complex, a right bundle branch block pattern, and the long-short cycle sequence strongly favor aberrancy. Ventricular rates above 200 beats/min with a wide QRS complex is suggestive of the WPW syndrome with antegrade conduction through the accessory pathway (Fig. 18-16). Slow, regular ventricular response in the presence of atrial fibrillation is usually due to an accelerated junctional rhythm with AV block as a result of digitalis toxicity.

Management of atrial fibrillation depends on whether it is new onset, paroxysmal, or chronic. Investigation to determine the etiology of new onset atrial fibrillation is especially important. An echocardiogram is mandatory to evaluate left ventricular function, left atrial size, and valvular and pericardial disease. Exercise testing to assess the presence of important coronary artery disease may be necessary in selected patients. Pulmonary embolism, thyrotoxicosis, and alcohol abuse should be considered. It is difficult to determine the best treatment for new onset atrial fibrillation, since about half the patients will revert to sinus rhythm spontaneously within 24 to 48 hours. In some cases the reversion is due to improvement of the underlying condition. New onset atrial fibrillation often terminates with antiarrhythmic therapy, but the reversion rate is low after 3 days.

Our approach to new onset atrial fibrillation is to first control the ventricular rate with intravenous digoxin. Intravenous verapamil, diltiazem, or β-adrenergic blockers may be used if more rapid rate control is necessary; these drugs have negative inotropic effects and should be used cautiously in patients with heart failure. Immediate DC cardioversion is used for patients with significant hemodynamic compromise. Studies to determine the etiology of atrial fibrillation are then undertaken. Cardioversion can be performed without preceding anticoagulation for up to 48 hours after the onset of atrial fibrillation; anticoagulation is recommended for 4 weeks after cardioversion because atrial contractile function does not recover immediately and the risk of embolism remains. Quinidine is occasionally administered before cardioversion in the hope of enhancing the success rate of DC cardioversion; quinidine alone may restore sinus rhythm in 10% of patients. When atrial fibrillation lasts longer than 2 days or is of uncertain duration, the current recommendation is to administer warfarin therapy to an INR of 2.0 to 3.0 for 3 weeks before attempting reversion to prevent embolic events. In emergency cardioversion, heparin therapy with simultaneous initiation of warfarin therapy is recommended. In patients who are poor candidates for anticoagulation, transesophageal echocardiography may be performed to exclude atrial appendage thrombi before cardioversion; however, atrial function does not recover immediately after cardioversion. Stroke may occur in nonanticoagulated patients despite screening by transesophageal echocardiography because of de novo thrombus formation after cardioversion. Attempts at reversion should be deferred if chances of spontaneous reversion are high or correction of an underlying abnormality is necessary; examples include atrial fibrillation after cardiac surgery or during hyperthyroidism. Reversion may be attempted with

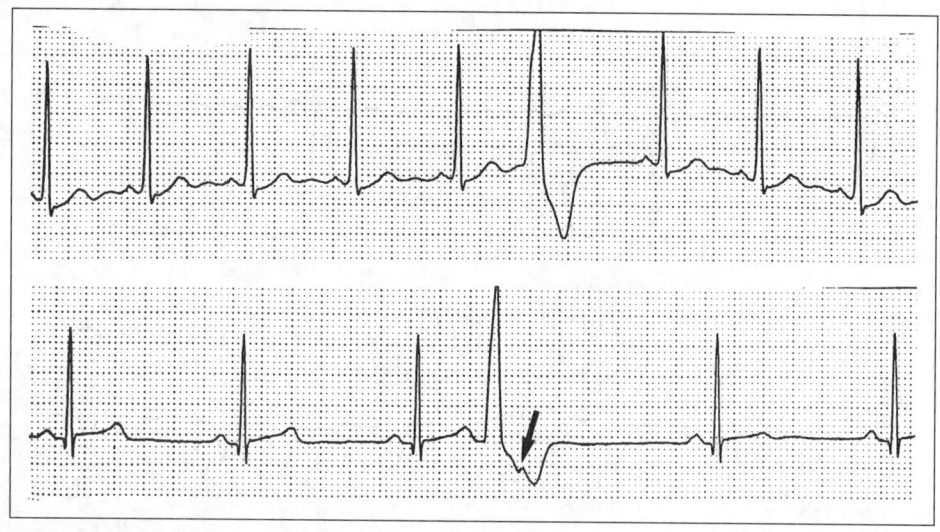

FIGURE 18-21   Premature ventricular contraction (PVC) usually does not reset the sinus node, and the sinus activity returns on time after the PVC, resulting in a fully compensatory pause *(top)*. If the PVC causes retrograde atrial activation *(arrow)* and resets the sinus node, the pause is less than compensatory *(bottom)*.

quinidine or procainamide in usual dosages, but proarrhythmia is a risk. Synchronized cardioversion using 100 to 200 J is the best approach. Success rate of cardioversion and maintenance of sinus rhythm depend on the duration of atrial fibrillation, atrial size, the patient's age, and underlying conditions. Duration of atrial fibrillation appears to be the most important predictor. Anticoagulation is continued for 4 weeks after cardioversion or longer if there are other indications for continuing anticoagulation. Once sinus rhythm is established, the question arises of antiarrhythmic therapy to prevent recurrence. A clinical assessment of the risk for recurrent atrial fibrillation should be made. Risk of antiarrhythmic therapy must be balanced against the benefits of maintaining sinus rhythm. Patients with only mild structural heart disease and those who tolerate atrial fibrillation well may be observed without antiarrhythmic therapy. Antiarrhythmic therapy should be avoided unless there are frequent recurrences or atrial fibrillation is poorly tolerated, because an excess mortality has been suggested.

Patients with WPW syndrome may develop a very rapid ventricular rate (>250 beats/min) if conduction occurs through the accessory pathway. The QRS complex is wide and the rhythm is irregularly irregular (see Fig. 18-16). Drugs such as digoxin and verapamil should be avoided because they may increase the ventricular rate and increase the risk for secondary ventricular fibrillation. Intravenous procainamide and electrical cardioversion are the best treatments.

Brief paroxysms of atrial fibrillation may be treated conservatively in the absence of heart disease. If the paroxysms are longer in duration or result in hemodynamic compromise, drug therapy is needed. Digoxin, β-adrenergic blockers, or verapamil may be used to control the ventricular response. It has been suggested that digoxin may increase the risk for recurrence in paroxysmal atrial fibrillation. Class 1A drugs are commonly used to prevent episodes of atrial fibrillation; class 1C or III antiarrhythmic drugs are also effective. As mentioned above, proarrhythmic effect of these drugs is a concern. In chronic atrial fibrillation, control of ventricular rate and prevention of systemic emboli are the main aims of treatment. Digoxin is commonly used to control the ventricular rate. In some patients, addition of a second drug, diltiazem, verapamil, or a β-adrenergic blocker, is necessary to control the ventricular rate. Although digoxin is effective in controlling the ventricular rate at rest, it is not as effective during exercise because its electrophysiologic effects are mediated through increased vagal tone. Beta-adrenergic blockers and calcium channel blockers alone or in combination with digoxin may provide better control of the ventricular rate during exercise.

Results of five randomized trials have consistently shown that moderate anticoagulation to an INR of 1.5 to 3 reduces the risk of stroke by two thirds or more in patients with nonrheumatic atrial fi-

brillation. Thus all patients with chronic atrial fibrillation should receive warfarin anticoagulation therapy unless there are contraindications; exceptions are lone atrial fibrillation and brief and isolated paroxysms of atrial fibrillation. The role of aspirin is not clear. In the SPAF study, both aspirin (325 mg/day) and warfarin were effective, but warfarin was more effective in reducing the incidence of strokes.

Rarely, the ventricular rate cannot be adequately controlled despite correction of underlying conditions and pharmacologic therapy. In such cases, complete AV block is produced by ablating the AV junction, and a VVIR pacemaker is implanted. The obvious drawback of this approach is the need for a pacemaker. Recently, attempts have been made to selectively ablate the area of the AV node responsible for conducting rapid rates. Control of the ventricular rate without the need for a pacemaker can be achieved by this technique. Patients whose ventricular rates are difficult to control despite aggressive medical therapy may be referred for these techniques.

VENTRICULAR ARRHYTHMIAS
Premature Ventricular Contractions

Premature ventricular contractions (PVCs) are characterized by their prematurity, wide QRS complex, change in QRS vector, fixed coupling interval, and a fully compensatory pause that follows (Fig. 18-21, *top*). None of these characteristics is totally sensitive or specific. The QRS complex of a PVC may appear narrow, especially in single-lead monitor systems. Premature atrial contraction may cause a wide QRS complex if aberrant conduction is present. The QRS vector may be normal depending on the site of origin of PVCs. The sinus cycle is usually unaffected by PVCs, and a fully compensatory pause results. However, the pause will be less than compensatory if the PVC results in retrograde atrial activation and depolarization of the sinus node (Fig. 18-21, *bottom*). Rarely, no compensatory pause occurs, and the PVC is termed an interpolated PVC. The coupling interval may change with PVCs; if this is noted, the possibility of ventricular parasystole—an automatic ectopic rhythm that is independent of the normal electrical activity of the heart—should be considered. PVCs may be classified by their morphology (uniform or multiform) and their relationship to the dominant rhythm (bigeminy, trigeminy). Two consecutive PVCs are described as a couplet or pair (Fig. 18-22, *top*).

Clinical significance of PVCs is determined by evaluating the patient for the presence of heart disease and other ventricular arrhythmias. Echocardiography and exercise testing may be necessary to exclude coronary, valvular, and myocardial disease and to estimate left ventricular ejection fraction. Ambulatory ECG monitoring will provide an estimate of the frequency of PVCs and other ventricular arrhythmias. PVCs seen among patients without heart disease are be-

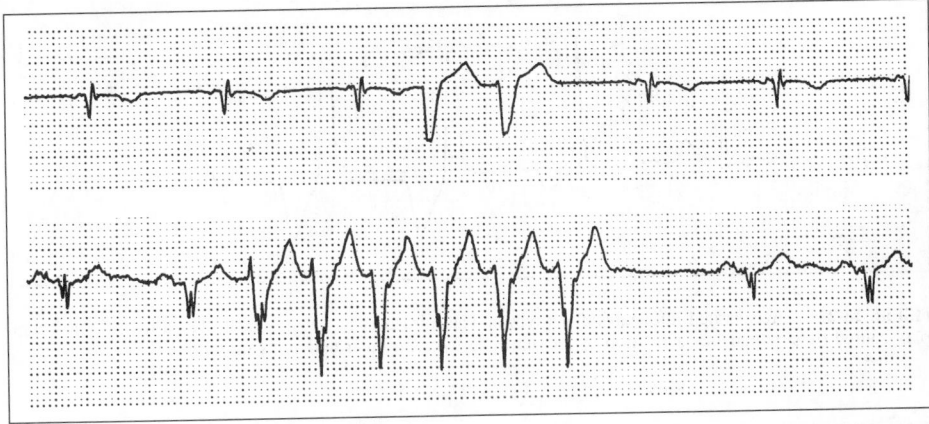

FIGURE 18-22 *Top,* Paired premature ventricular contractions. *Bottom,* Nonsustained ventricular tachycardia.

nign and require no intervention. Physicians may feel obligated to treat PVCs that are accompanied by higher grades of ventricular arrhythmias (e.g., paired PVCs and unsustained ventricular tachycardia). Follow-up of asymptomatic healthy subjects with frequent and complex ventricular ectopy for as long as 10 years revealed that the survival of the study cohort was similar to that of the healthy U.S. population. It should be noted, however, that patients with complex ventricular ectopy usually have organic heart disease.

Sometimes the physician is forced to treat benign PVCs to control palpitations that are bothersome to the patient. Reassurance and avoidance of aggravating factors (e.g., caffeine, tobacco, and stress) should be tried first. Although proarrhythmia is uncommon in patients without heart disease, every effort should be made to avoid antiarrhythmic drugs. Beta-adrenergic blockers are often effective in low doses and are the drugs of choice, especially in patients with mitral valve prolapse. Prevalence of PVCs is increased in hypertension with left ventricular hypertrophy, dilated cardiomyopathy, congestive heart failure, hypertrophic cardiomyopathy, and mitral valve prolapse, as well as after a myocardial infarction. Although there is an increased incidence of sudden death in these disease states, there is no evidence that suppression of PVCs using antiarrhythmic drugs (other than β-adrenergic blockers after myocardial infarction) is beneficial.

PVCs are common in acute myocardial infarction, but the threshold for treatment remains unsettled. The prophylactic administration of lidocaine to all patients with suspected myocardial infarction appears to increase mortality, despite reducing the risk for ventricular fibrillation, and is no longer recommended. Administration of lidocaine to patients with myocardial infarction and "warning arrhythmias" (frequent PVCs, multiform PVCs, pairs, salvos, and R-on-T phenomenon) has been practiced for many years but is controversial.

Nonsustained Ventricular Tachycardia

Nonsustained VT is defined as three or more consecutive ventricular impulses lasting ≤30 sec (Fig. 18-22, *bottom*). Some investigators define three to five impulses as salvos and six or more impulses lasting ≤30 sec as nonsustained VT. In general, nonsustained VT is considered to be a marker for sustained VT and ventricular fibrillation. However, patients with no organic heart disease are not at increased risk. Polymorphic varieties with a rapid rate may have a worse prognosis. Conceptually, nonsustained VT may be viewed as a self-terminating VT or as an intense triggering event in a susceptible myocardium. Treatment is generally similar to that outlined for other patterns of PVCs. In patients with heart failure secondary to idiopathic or ischemic cardiomyopathy, nonsustained VT is a marker for sudden death, but in a recent VA cooperative study, amiodarone therapy did not improve survival. Among patients recovering from myocardial infarction, the presence of nonsustained VT and a depressed left ventricular ejection fraction (≤30%) increases the risk for arrhythmic death to 25% per year. The risk for arrhythmic death is low if left ventricular function is preserved and ventricular aneurysm is not present. Patients with depressed ejection fraction and nonsustained VT may be further risk stratified using signal-averaged ECG (SAECG). Because the negative predictive value of SAECG is high, electrophysiologic studies or antiarrhythmic therapy other than β-adrenergic blockers is unnecessary if late potentials are not detected. The presence of late potentials is moderately predictive of inducible VT, and electrophysiologic studies are recommended. Inducible sustained monomorphic VT indicates higher risk, and it is suggested, although not certain, that antiarrhythmic therapy guided by electrophysiologic testing is beneficial.

Accelerated Idioventricular Rhythm

Accelerated idioventricular rhythm (AIVR) is sometimes described as *slow VT.* The mechanism of AIVR is abnormal automaticity. The ventricular rate is usually between 60 and 110 beats/min and is close to the sinus rate. Fusion beats are commonly present at the origin and termination (Fig. 18-23). AIVR is usually short lived and terminates spontaneously; precipitation of more rapid ventricular rhythm is rare. It is seen in myocardial infarction, especially when reperfusion occurs. Cardiomyopathy and digitalis toxicity are other etiologies. Suppressive therapy is not necessary because the rate is slow. Rarely, hemodynamic compromise may occur from loss of atrioventricular synchrony; increasing the sinus rate with atropine is usually effective or as an alternative, AV sequential pacing may be initiated.

Sustained Ventricular Tachycardia and Wide QRS Complex Tachycardia

Ventricular tachycardia (VT) may be classified according to its morphology: monomorphic, polymorphic, bidirectional, and torsades de pointes. Sustained VT is defined as consecutive ventricular complexes lasting more than 30 seconds or resulting in hemodynamic collapse. The usual rate of VT is 120 beats/min or more. It is important to recognize that both duration and ECG pattern of VT are useful in determining its etiology, prognosis, and treatment. Before diagnosing VT, supraventricular tachycardia with a wide QRS complex should be excluded. Sometimes treatment must be initiated before a definitive diagnosis can be made (Fig. 18-12).

Wide QRS complex tachycardias may be caused by VT or supraventricular tachycardia with aberrant conduction secondary to a functional bundle branch block, a preexisting bundle branch block, or antegrade conduction over an accessory atrioventricular pathway. A correct diagnosis can be made from clinical and surface ECG criteria in most patients. Most patients with VT have structural heart disease, most commonly myocardial infarction. Hemodynamic stability or instability is not useful in the differential diagnosis. History of undiagnosed tachycardia for more than 3 years makes VT very unlikely. Cycle length of the tachycardia is not helpful in diagnosis. AV dissociation, a reliable criterion for diagnosing ventricular tachycardia, may be recognized by the presence of cannon A waves on physi-

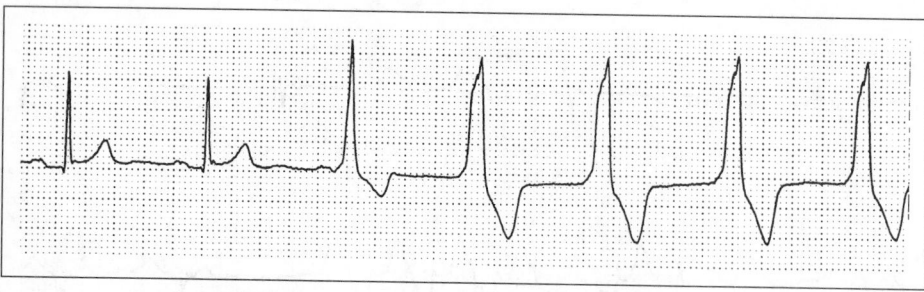

FIGURE 18-23   Accelerated idioventricular rhythm. The third beat is a fusion beat (i.e., a hybrid QRS complex caused by simultaneous activation of the ventricle by ventricular and sinus impulses).

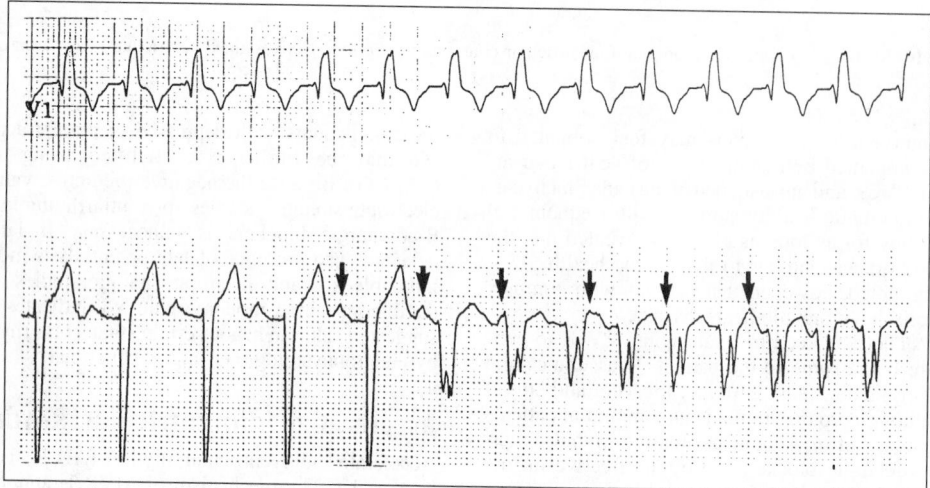

FIGURE 18-24   *Top,* Wide QRS complex tachycardia recorded on lead V₁. Triphasic rSR′ pattern strongly favors supraventricular tachycardia with aberrant conduction. *Bottom,* Wide QRS tachycardia is of ventricular origin because AV dissociation is present. Note P waves *(arrows)* that are unrelated to the QRS complexes.

cal examination or by ECG. A single-lead recording is diagnostic of VT if P waves are distinguishable and AV dissociation is present (Fig. 18-24, *bottom*). Look for fusion beat, which is a hybrid QRS complex caused by the simultaneous activation of the ventricle by a ventricular and sinus impulse (Fig. 18-23), and capture beat, which is a normal QRS complex during wide QRS tachycardia caused by a fortuitously timed sinus discharge that captures the ventricle. Fusion beats and capture beats have high specificity in diagnosing ventricular tachycardia. Polymorphic tachyarrhythmias are almost always ventricular in origin.

If time permits, 12-lead ECG should be performed because the likelihood of visualizing P waves is better. AV dissociation is the most reliable criterion for diagnosing VT. Obtaining a previous ECG for comparison is extremely helpful. If the previous ECG reveals a Q-wave infarction, assume the tachycardia is VT. If preexisting bundle branch block with morphology similar to the present tachycardia is noted, the diagnosis is supraventricular tachycardia with aberrancy. QRS duration and morphology are helpful in diagnosing the etiology of wide QRS tachycardia. VT is highly likely if the QRS duration is greater than 140 msec with a right bundle branch block pattern and greater than 160 msec with a left bundle branch block pattern, especially when the QRS duration was normal during sinus rhythm. Abnormal QRS axis beyond −30 degrees is more common in VT; QRS axis between −90 degrees and ±180 degrees is a reliable marker of VT. Left bundle branch configuration in the precordial leads with right axis deviation is almost exclusively ventricular in origin.

The QRS configuration is also helpful. Generally, concordantly positive or negative QRS complexes across the precordium strongly favor VT (Fig. 18-25). In lead V₁ a right bundle branch configuration that is monophasic (R) or biphasic (qR) suggests VT, but a tripha-

sic pattern (rSR′) strongly favors aberrant conduction (Fig. 18-24, *top*). A correct diagnosis of VT can be made in most but not all cases when the reported criteria are collectively applied (Box 18-2).

Definitive diagnosis can be made in all cases by intracardiac electrograms, but treatment often must be initiated before a definitive diagnosis can be made. Response to pharmacologic agents also may have diagnostic value. However, unless a definitive diagnosis of supraventricular tachycardia can be made, the use of verapamil should be avoided. Administration of verapamil to patients with VT often results in hemodynamic deterioration, acceleration of the tachycardia, or degeneration into ventricular fibrillation. Adenosine appears to be better tolerated because of the very short half-life of the drug. Adenosine terminates most of the supraventricular tachycardias secondary to reentry but has no effect on VT. Only VT responds to lidocaine. Regardless of the origin of the wide QRS complex tachycardia, patients with hemodynamic compromise should be promptly cardioverted. The treatment algorithm for wide QRS complex tachycardia recommended by the Emergency Cardiac Care Committee is shown in Fig. 18-12.

Sustained Monomorphic Ventricular Tachycardia

Sustained monomorphic VT occurs at a rate greater than 120 beats/min, has uniform QRS morphology, and lasts 30 sec or more. A common misconception is that VT will always result in hemodynamic collapse. Although the majority of patients with VT have accompanying dizziness, syncope, or clinical cardiac arrest, some patients tolerate sustained monomorphic VT remarkable well. The etiology of VT determines the clinical presentation. In patients with prior myocardial infarction or ventricular aneurysm, the VT is monomorphic and occurs at a rate of 150 to 180 beats/min and may be well tolerated.

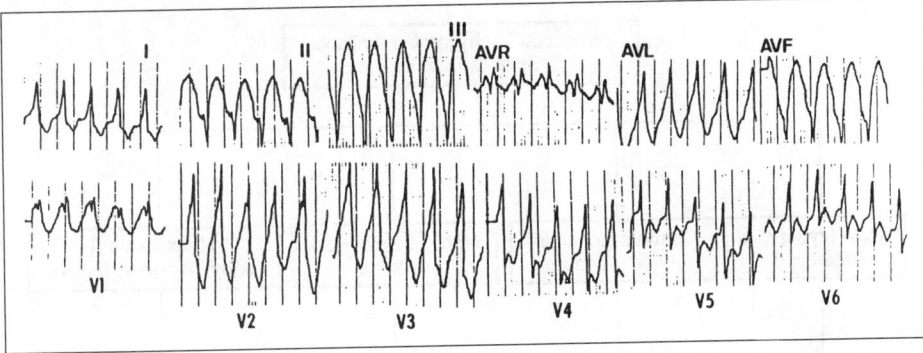

FIGURE 18-25   Twelve-lead ECG of ventricular tachycardia. Left axis deviation and concordantly positive QRS complexes across the precordium.

BOX 18-2

Wide QRS complex tachycardia: highly reliable criteria for the diagnosis of ventricular tachycardia

1. Preexisting bundle branch block in a previous ECG and a different QRS morphology during tachycardia
2. Q wave myocardial infarction in previous ECG
3. Atrioventricular dissociation
4. QRS duration >140 msec with a RBBB morphology and >160 msec with LBBB morphology. Specificity of these criteria is even higher in the absence of preexisting BBB or antiarrhythmic drugs
5. QRS axis between −90 degrees and ±180 degrees
6. Polymorphic tachycardia
7. LBBB pattern in precordial leads with right axis deviation
8. Concordantly positive or negative QRS complex across the precordium

(From Chakko S, Kessler KM: Recognition and management of cardiac arrhythmias, *Curr Probl Cardiol* 20:53-120, 1995.)

Patients with acute ischemia have polymorphic VT at rates in excess of 250 beats/min, which results in hemodynamic collapse. Most patients with sustained VT have organic heart disease, with ischemic heart disease and cardiomyopathies being the most common. Reduced ejection fraction, slowed ventricular conduction, ventricular aneurysm, prior myocardial infarction, and myocarditis are often noted.

In acute myocardial infarction, sustained VT occurs most often during the first 24 hours and often degenerates into ventricular fibrillation (Chapter 23). If the hemodynamic status is stable, intravenous lidocaine or procainamide may be tried. If VT persists, synchronized cardioversion starting at low energies (25 to 50 J) should be used. Very rapid VT, ventricular flutter, or VT accompanied by hemodynamic collapse is treated with immediate unsynchronized cardioversion using 200 to 400 J. Sustained VT during the acute phase of myocardial infarction is due to transient factor and does not predict future arrhythmic events after hospital discharge.

Treatment to terminate VT in conditions other than acute myocardial infarction is the same (Fig. 18-12). However, the risk of recurrence is high and the approach to prevent recurrence is complex and controversial. Our approach to managing these patients is guided by programmed electrical stimulation (PES), and the recommended algorithm is shown in Fig. 18-26. The first step is to determine the etiology of VT. Patients with VT secondary to acute myocardial infarction (<72 hours), correctable heart disease (e.g., severe aortic stenosis), or reversible precipitating factors (e.g., hypokalemia, proarrhythmic drug effect) do not require PES. If transient myocardial ischemia is thought to be the cause of VT, it should be corrected by appropriate medical, interventional, or surgical therapy. In some clinical situations, prevention of VT is not ensured by the correction of such precipitating causes, and PES may still be necessary. For example, a patient with severe coronary artery disease and VT undergoes revascu-

larization followed by PES to ensure that that the arrhythmia has been controlled. Management of patients in whom reversible causes are not identified is based on the results of PES. The subgroup of patients whose VT is noninducible often receives an automatic implantable cardioverter defibrillator (AICD) because risk of recurrent VT is still high and effectiveness of pharmacologic therapy cannot be evaluated in the absence of inducible VT. If a patient's clinical condition precludes invasive procedures, medical therapy with amiodarone is preferred. Otherwise serial drug testing guided by PES is done until an antiarrhythmic drug is identified that makes the VT noninducible or stable and well tolerated. Patients in whom VT is resistant to drug therapy usually undergo AICD implantation. If anatomy is suitable (e.g., ventricular aneurysm), antiarrhythmic surgery is an option. PES is performed postoperatively on all patients who undergo arrhythmia surgery or AICD implantation to ensure that the arrhythmia has been eradicated or can be terminated if it recurs.

PES-guided management is not universally accepted, and therapy guided by ambulatory ECG (Holter) monitoring and empiric therapy have also been recommended. Some investigators believe that if a patient with sustained VT also has 10 or more PVCs per hour, serial testing for antiarrhythmic drug efficacy may be performed by Holter monitoring. Effectiveness of antiarrhythmic drugs and proarrhythmia are evaluated by changes in arrhythmia frequency and appearance of new ventricular arrhythmias. In the ESVEM study, survival and arrhythmia recurrence was similar regardless of whether Holter monitoring or EPS was used to select an antiarrhythmic drug. However, many patients with sustained VT do not have PVCs during monitoring. Empiric amiodarone therapy has also been effective in some studies.

Polymorphic Ventricular Tachycardia Including Torsades de Pointes

VT with a continuously varying QRS morphology is called polymorphic VT. Torsades de pointes, a French phrase that means "twisting of the points," is a polymorphic VT characterized by QRS peaks that seem to twist around the baseline (Fig. 18-27). There are three types of polymorphic VT: (1) polymorphic VT associated with a normal QT interval, (2) torsades de pointes that is bradycardia dependent and associated with a prolonged QT interval, and (3) torsades de pointes that is adrenergic dependent and associated with a prolonged QT interval. Management of polymorphic VT associated with a normal QT interval is similar to monomorphic VT, which is described earlier. Polymorphic VT is usually associated with acute ischemia and is due to very rapid rates (>250 beats/min); hemodynamic collapse is common, and serial EPS is not possible.

The second type, bradycardia-dependent torsades de pointes, is usually considered to be part of a syndrome that includes a prolonged QT interval plus a predisposing factor that may have caused the QT prolongation. The common predisposing factors are antiarrhythmic drugs (classically type IA, but also class III and bepridil), psychotropic drugs (phenothiazines, tricyclic antidepressants), hypokalemia, hypomagnesemia, and rarely antimicrobials (erythromycin, trimethoprim-sulfamethoxazole, pentamidine). This arrhythmia often

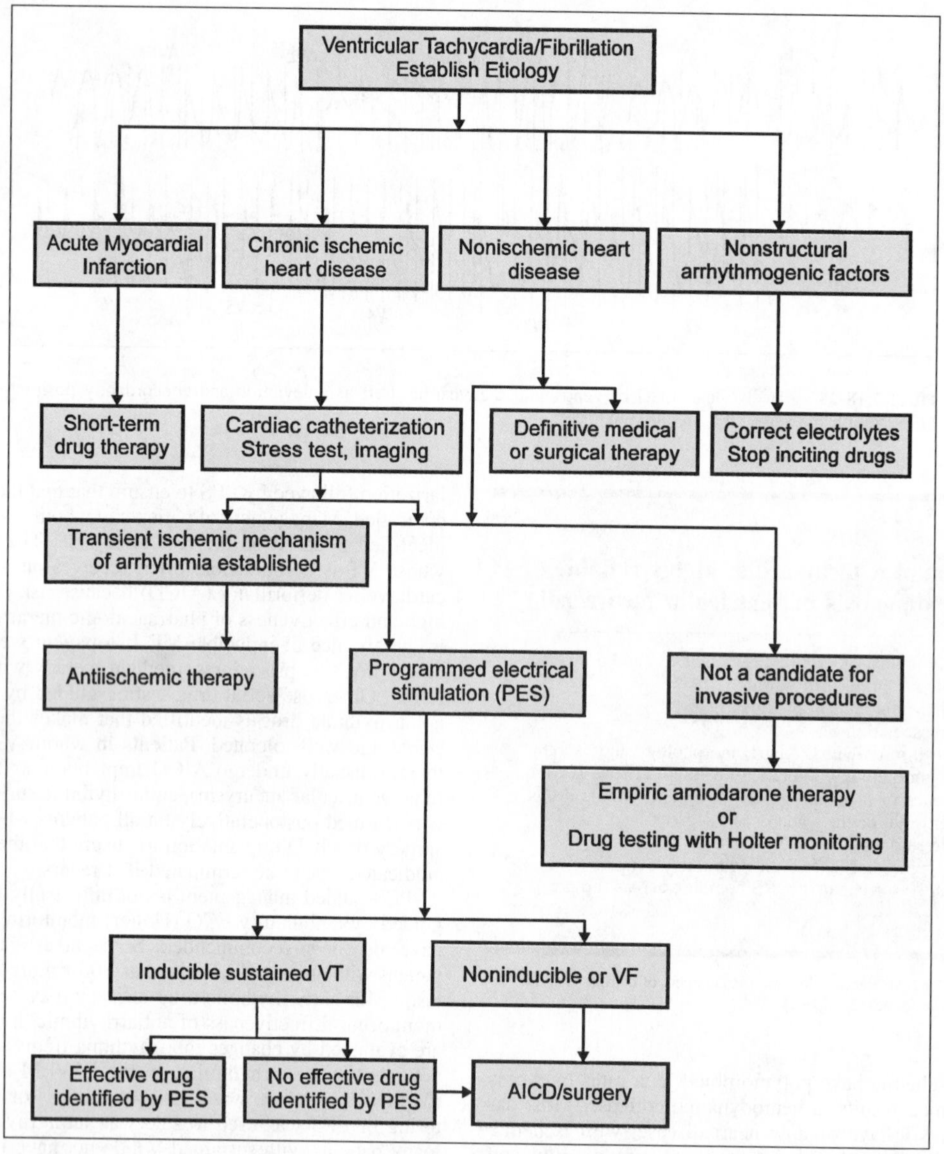

```
                  ┌─────────────────────────────┐
                  │ Ventricular Tachycardia/Fibrillation │
                  │        Establish Etiology         │
                  └─────────────────────────────┘
```

Ventricular Tachycardia/Fibrillation Establish Etiology

- Acute Myocardial Infarction
- Chronic ischemic heart disease
- Nonischemic heart disease
- Nonstructural arrhythmogenic factors

- Short-term drug therapy
- Cardiac catheterization Stress test, imaging
- Definitive medical or surgical therapy
- Correct electrolytes Stop inciting drugs

- Transient ischemic mechanism of arrhythmia established

- Antiischemic therapy
- Programmed electrical stimulation (PES)
- Not a candidate for invasive procedures

- Empiric amiodarone therapy or Drug testing with Holter monitoring

- Inducible sustained VT
- Noninducible or VF

- Effective drug identified by PES
- No effective drug identified by PES
- AICD/surgery

FIGURE 18-26   Recommended approach to preventing recurrence of ventricular tachycardia (VT) or ventricular fibrillation (VF).

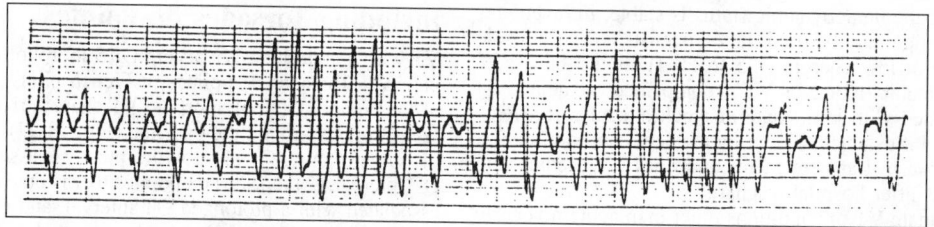

FIGURE 18-27   Torsades de pointes ventricular tachycardia.

begins during bradycardia or during a pause that follows a premature beat. A normal QT interval does not exclude the diagnosis of torsades de pointes because it may occur in the absence of a prolonged QT interval, and QT prolongation may be intermittent. Polymorphic VT noted in the presence of a prolonged QT interval and a known predisposing factor may not have the typical torsades de pointes pattern. Thus clinical correlation is often necessary to diagnose torsades de pointes. Treatment includes correction of electrolyte abnormalities and withdrawal of drugs that may have caused the arrhythmia. Even

in the absence of hypomagnesemia, intravenous infusion of magnesium sulfate is reported to be effective. Increasing the heart rate with isoproterenol or pacing are effective preventive measures; the latter is preferred when ischemic heart disease cannot be excluded. Cardioversion should be avoided because this arrhythmia is episodic and recurrent.

The third type, adrenergic-dependent torsades de pointes, is typically seen in patients with congenital long QT syndromes. Two varieties have been reported: those with autosomal recessive inheritance

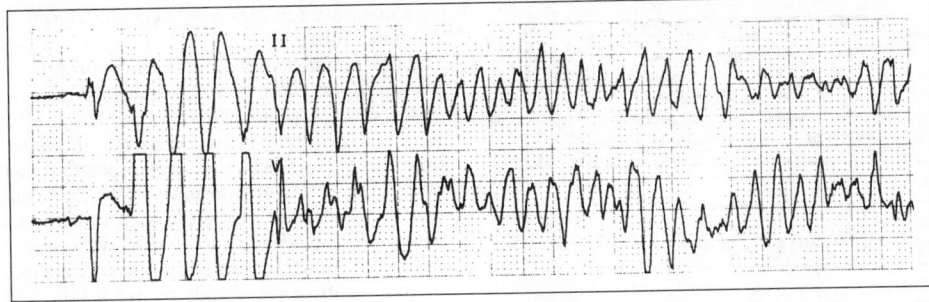

FIGURE 18-28   Rapid ventricular tachycardia degenerates in to ventricular fibrillation.

and associated deafness, the Jervell and Lange-Nielsen syndrome; and those without deafness, the Romano-Ward syndrome. VT often occurs during exertion, sudden awakening, and emotional stress. These patients are younger and the QT interval is prolonged; a history of syncope is often present among family members. Beta-adrenergic blockade reduces mortality. If drug therapy fails, high thoracic left sympathectomy should be recommended.

Uncommon Types of Sustained Ventricular Tachycardia

Right ventricular dysplasia, a condition in which right ventricular musculature is replaced by fatty and fibrous tissue, has been reported to cause sustained VT. Right ventricular enlargement can usually be demonstrated by any of the imaging modalities. T wave inversion is present in the right precordial leads. During VT, the QRS complex has a left bundle branch morphology. Amiodarone and class 1 drugs are reported to be effective. The prognosis is good, especially in patients who tolerate VT well. Right ventricular tachycardia mediated by exercise or catecholamines has been reported in young or middle-aged subjects without any evidence for heart disease. The VT originates in the right ventricular outflow tract and has a left bundle branch morphology with inferior axis; it can be induced by the administration of catecholamines and responds well to β-adrenergic blockers, verapamil, and adenosine. VT originating in the left ventricle in young patients without evidence for heart disease has also been reported. This form of VT has right bundle branch morphology with left axis deviation and responds well to verapamil.

Bundle branch reentry VT is a macroreentry tachycardia seen in dilated cardiomyopathies. One of the bundle branches functions as the antegrade limb. The impulse then crosses the septum and uses the other bundle as a retrograde limb. The VT usually has left bundle branch morphology. Catheter ablation of the right bundle is very effective.

Ventricular Fibrillation

Ventricular fibrillation (VF) is the most frequently identified arrhythmia associated with sudden death. It occurs commonly in the setting of acute ischemic events or unpredictably in chronic ischemic heart disease. It is also the mode of death in 25% to 50% of fatalities in cardiomyopathies. Occasionally, VF occurs in the absence of cardiac abnormalities. The ECG reveals a continuous undulating pattern without discrete P, QRS, or T waves (Fig. 18-28). Fine fibrillation is diagnosed when the waveforms are less than 0.2 mV in amplitude. Coarse fibrillation can be more easily defibrillated and has a better prognosis.

The first goal of therapy is immediate resuscitation. Basic life support with cardiopulmonary resuscitation is performed only until defibrillation can be carried out. In acute myocardial infarction, early VF is associated with increased hospital mortality but does not affect posthospital mortality, and long-term antiarrhythmic therapy is not warranted. Automatic implantable cardioverter defibrillators are reliable and effective and are becoming the preferred treatment. A defibrillator is recommended for survivors of VF who do not have inducible sustained ventricular arrhythmia or inducible VF during EPS.

Our approach to prevention of VF is shown in Fig. 18-26 and is discussed in detail under sustained ventricular tachycardia.

BRADYARRHYTHMIAS AND AV BLOCKS

Bradyarrhythmias are caused by depression of impulse formation or decreased AV conduction. Symptoms are the result of hypoperfusion caused by the slow heart rate. However, the rate at which symptoms appear is highly variable. Sinus bradycardia at a rate less than 40 beats/min may cause no symptoms in some individuals and is normal in well-trained athletes and during sleep, but the same rate may cause dizziness or syncope in others. Because dizziness and syncope may be caused by many conditions other than bradyarrhythmia, it is important to document the relationship between the rhythm and symptoms. Holter monitoring for 24 to 48 hours is commonly used for this purpose, but the yield is low because the arrhythmias and symptoms are often infrequent. Event recorders are more useful. Bradyarrhythmias are exacerbated by drugs, increased vagal tone, hypothyroidism, hypothermia, and hyperkalemia. If the patient is symptomatic, the first step is to increase the heart rate with parasympatholytic drugs (atropine) or, less frequently, sympathomimetic drugs (isoproterenol); the latter is not well tolerated by patients with coronary disease. Small doses of atropine (<0.3 mg) may cause paradoxical worsening of the bradyarrhythmia and are avoided. A temporary transvenous pacemaker is necessary for bradyarrhythmias unresponsive to drug therapy or if it is likely that the bradyarrhythmia may worsen (e.g., Mobitz type II AV block). Transcutaneous pacemakers are very useful because pacing can be initiated immediately without the need for an invasive procedure. Many patients, however, find it very uncomfortable, and it is often used to maintain adequate rhythm while inserting a transvenous pacemaker or as a standby when the potential for severe bradyarrhythmia exists but is low. Algorithm for the treatment of symptomatic bradyarrhythmias recommended by the Emergency Cardiac Care Committee is shown in Fig. 18-29.

Sinus Bradycardia and Sinoatrial Block

Sinus bradycardia may be physiologic or pathologic as a result of sinus node dysfunction. Increased vagal tone, which causes sinus bradycardia, may be physiologic (e.g., athletes) or pathologic (e.g., inferior myocardial infarction). Sinus rate less than 60 beats/min is defined as sinus bradycardia, but it is rarely considered to be pathologic until it is less than 50 beats/min. Unexpected absence of sinus node activity is described as sinus arrest (Fig. 18-30, *top*). Sinoatrial (SA) block refers to abnormal conduction from the sinus node to atrial muscle. There are three degrees of SA block similar to the three degrees of AV block. Since sinus node discharge is not visible on the surface ECG, SA block can be recognized only by the unexpected absence of a P wave and subsequent QRS complex. First-degree and third-degree SA block cannot be diagnosed from a surface ECG. SA Wenckebach block is recognized by the progressive shortening of the P-P intervals followed by a dropped P-QRS complex. It is often mistaken for sinus arrhythmia. Type II second-degree SA block can be diagnosed only if it is intermittent; an abrupt decrease in sinus rate to half the baseline rate is very suggestive (Fig. 18-30, *middle*). SA block may be caused by digitalis, ischemia, or vagal stimulation.

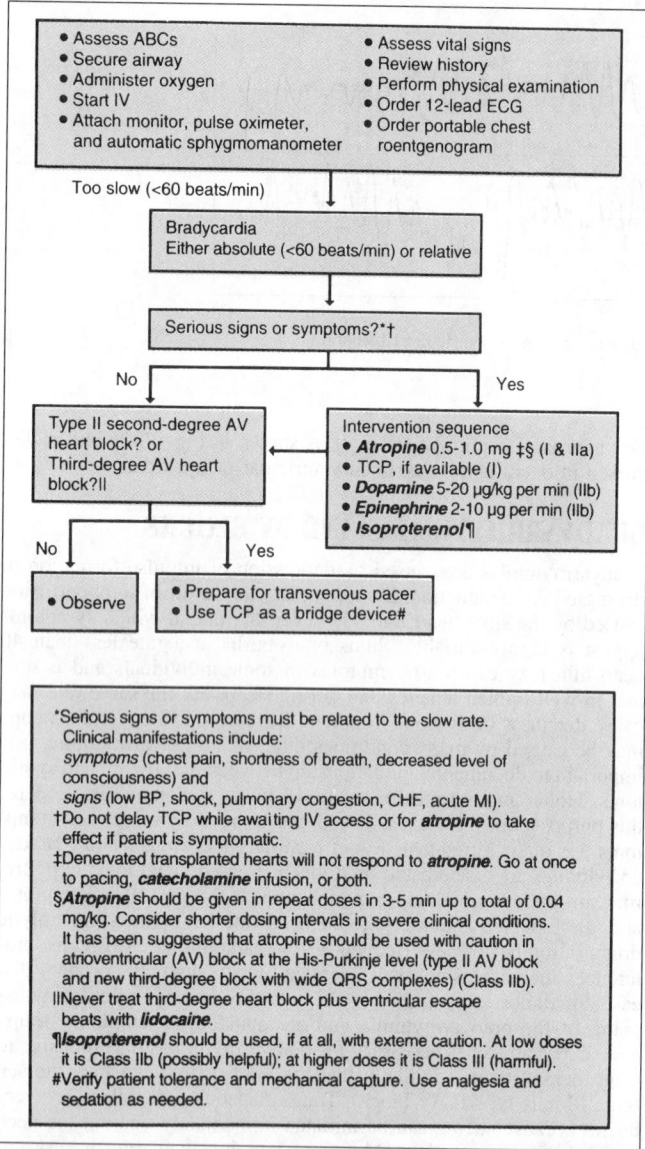

- Assess ABCs
- Secure airway
- Administer oxygen
- Start IV
- Attach monitor, pulse oximeter, and automatic sphygmomanometer
- Assess vital signs
- Review history
- Perform physical examination
- Order 12-lead ECG
- Order portable chest roentgenogram

Too slow (<60 beats/min)

Bradycardia
Either absolute (<60 beats/min) or relative

Serious signs or symptoms?*†

No — Yes

Type II second-degree AV heart block? or Third-degree AV heart block?‖

Intervention sequence
- *Atropine* 0.5-1.0 mg ‡§ (I & IIa)
- TCP, if available (I)
- *Dopamine* 5-20 μg/kg per min (IIb)
- *Epinephrine* 2-10 μg per min (IIb)
- *Isoproterenol*¶

No — Yes

- Observe
- Prepare for transvenous pacer
- Use TCP as a bridge device#

*Serious signs or symptoms must be related to the slow rate. Clinical manifestations include:
  symptoms (chest pain, shortness of breath, decreased level of consciousness) and
  signs (low BP, shock, pulmonary congestion, CHF, acute MI).
†Do not delay TCP while awaiting IV access or for *atropine* to take effect if patient is symptomatic.
‡Denervated transplanted hearts will not respond to *atropine*. Go at once to pacing, *catecholamine* infusion, or both.
§*Atropine* should be given in repeat doses in 3-5 min up to total of 0.04 mg/kg. Consider shorter dosing intervals in severe clinical conditions. It has been suggested that atropine should be used with caution in atrioventricular (AV) block at the His-Purkinje level (type II AV block and new third-degree block with wide QRS complexes) (Class IIb).
‖Never treat third-degree heart block plus ventricular escape beats with *lidocaine*.
¶*Isoproterenol* should be used, if at all, with extreme caution. At low doses it is Class IIb (possibly helpful); at higher doses it is Class III (harmful).
#Verify patient tolerance and mechanical capture. Use analgesia and sedation as needed.

FIGURE 18-29 Algorithm for the treatment of symptomatic bradyarrhythmias recommended by Emergency Cardiac Care Committee. *TCP*, Transcutaneous pacemaker.
(From *JAMA* 268:2221, 1992.)

Treatment of sinus bradycardia, sinus arrest, and SA block is similar to that of sinus node dysfunction and is discussed in the next section.

Sick Sinus Syndrome

Sick sinus syndrome is a generalized abnormality of cardiac impulse formation and intraatrial and AV nodal conduction that is manifested by a wide range of combinations of bradyarrhythmias and tachyarrhythmias. It may be caused by conditions that result in fibrosis in the sinus node region, such as aging, atherosclerosis, hypertension, myocarditis, trauma, and cardiomyopathies. The sinoatrial dysfunction may be exacerbated by drugs such as digitalis, β-adrenergic blockers, calcium channel blockers, antiarrhythmic agents, and lithium carbonate. Sinus bradycardia, sinus arrest, and sinoatrial block may be present. As a consequence, there is insufficient suppression of excitable atrial foci resulting in atrial tachycardias. These abnormal atrial tachycardias may suppress the sinus node, further producing long posttachycardia pauses. This phenomenon is described as tachycardia-bradycardia syndrome (Fig. 18-30, *bottom*). Drug therapy for tachycardias will also worsen the bradyarrhythmia. These arrhyth-

mias may result in dizziness, syncope, dyspnea, fatigue, lethargy, and systemic embolism.

ECG manifestations include inappropriate sinus bradycardia, sinus arrest, sinoatrial block, and atrial fibrillation with slow ventricular response. A prolonged asystolic period after spontaneous or electrical conversion of tachycardias may be seen. Atrial flutter, ectopic atrial tachycardia, and sinus node reentrant tachycardia may be seen. Ambulatory ECG monitoring may be necessary when these arrhythmias are transient. Often these transient arrhythmias occur as isolated events, and prolonged monitoring with an event recorder is necessary for documentation. During invasive electrophysiologic testing, measurements of sinus node recovery time and sinoatrial conduction time are used to diagnose sinus node dysfunction. Invasive electrophysiologic studies have many drawbacks and are not necessary for diagnosis in most cases. Abnormalities of sinus node function are detected only variably in patients with symptomatic sinus node disease, and prognostic implications of abnormalities of sinus node function in asymptomatic patients are unknown. Thus documentation of bradyarrhythmia during symptoms is the cornerstone to diagnosis.

Since both bradyarrhythmias and tachyarrhythmias occur in sick sinus syndrome, drug therapy to control tachyarrhythmia may worsen bradyarrhythmia. Pacemaker implantation may be necessary before drug therapy or cardioversion for tachyarrhythmia. Pacemakers are extremely effective in controlling symptoms caused by bradyarrhythmias. In the past, the majority of patients with sick sinus syndromes were treated with VVI pacemakers. However, VVI pacemakers result in loss of AV synchrony and may result in higher incidence of atrial fibrillation, systemic embolism, and heart failure. DDD pacemakers are probably superior. Single-chamber atrial pacemakers are usually avoided in sick sinus syndrome because associated AV nodal abnormality may be present. If AV nodal conduction is found to be normal on electrophysiologic study, however, an atrial pacemaker with rate adaptive features (AAIR) is also an appropriate choice.

AV Conduction Abnormalities

AV block refers to conduction abnormalities between the atria and ventricles that may be pathologic or physiologic because of increased vagal tone. Management depends on the degree of block, associated symptoms, and clinical setting. AV blocks are classified into three degrees. In first-degree AV block, all sinus impulses are conducted, but the PR interval is >200 msec (Fig. 18-31, *A*). The site of delayed conduction may be at the AV node or the infranodal conduction system and cannot be localized by surface ECG. Drugs such as digoxin and calcium-channel blocker drugs that decrease AV nodal conduction may cause first-degree AV block. Isolated first-degree AV block does not cause symptoms, and no treatment is necessary.

In second-degree AV block, there is intermittent failure of conduction from the atria to ventricles; it is subdivided into Mobitz type I (Wenckebach phenomenon) and type II. In type I second-degree AV block, there is progressive lengthening of the PR interval, with an eventual nonconducted P wave resulting in a dropped QRS complex (Fig. 18-31, *B*). The degree of PR lengthening diminishes with subsequent beats, and thus the RR intervals get shorter; however, such shortening of the RR interval is not always present. This pattern recurs in a regular fashion, leading to grouped beating. Finding grouped beating should always raise the possibility of Wenckebach phenomenon. Location of the conduction abnormality is almost always in the AV node, and the QRS complex is usually narrow. Wenckebach phenomenon may be secondary to vagal tone and is not uncommon among athletes; digitalis toxicity and inferior wall infarction are other common causes. It is usually asymptomatic and does not progress to higher degrees of AV block; prognosis is related to the severity of underlying heart disease. It may be abolished by atropine; pacing is usually not necessary. Rarely in inferior wall infarction, the ventricular rate is slow enough to cause symptoms, and temporary pacing may be necessary.

In Mobitz type II block, there is intermittent failure of P waves to conduct, but the pattern of PR prolongation is absent. The location of the block is infranodal and usually infrahisian, and the QRS complex is usually widened (Fig. 18-31, *D*). Sometimes the AV block is 2:1 and because only a single PR interval is present before the nonconducted P wave, the presence or absence of lengthening of the PR interval cannot be evaluated. In these instances, a narrow QRS com-

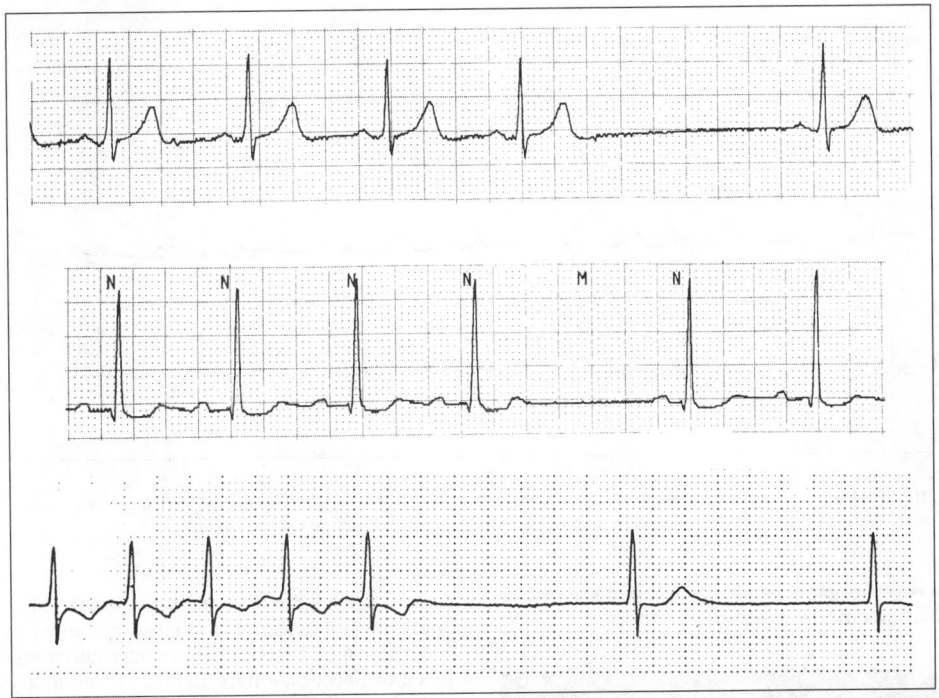

FIGURE 18-30   *Top,* Sinus arrest; unexpected prolonged absence of sinus activity. *Middle,* Type 2, second-degree SA block; abrupt decrease in sinus rate with the duration of the pause *(M)* double of baseline sinus rate (N-N). *Bottom,* Tachycardia-bradycardia syndrome; supraventricular tachycardia is followed by sinus arrest and junctional escape rhythm.

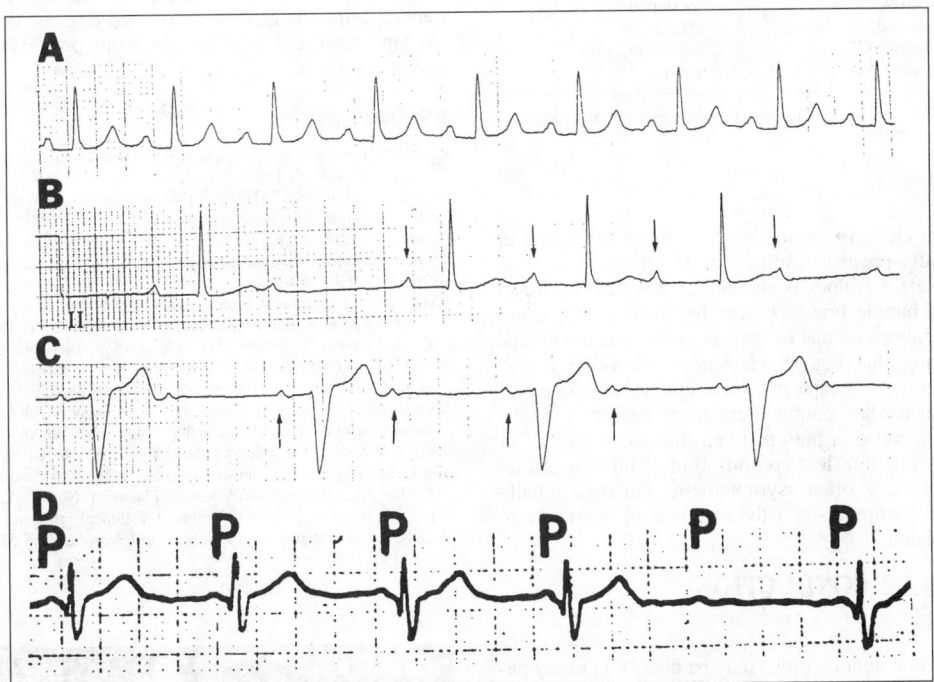

FIGURE 18-31   **A,** Sinus rhythm with first-degree AV block; PR interval is prolonged. **B,** Mobitz type I AV block (Wenckebach phenomenon). P waves *(arrows)* are regular with progressive prolongation of the PR interval and a nonconducted P wave. **C,** 2:1 AV block. Widened QRS complex suggests Mobitz II AV block. **D,** Mobitz type II AV block. P waves are regular, with normal PR interval with a nonconducted P wave.

plex favors type I block and a widened QRS complex favors type II block (Fig. 18-31, *C*). High conduction ratios such as 3:1 are described as high-degree AV block (Fig. 18-32, *top*). Type II AV block is always pathologic, and the risk of progression to complete heart block is high. When complete heart block develops, escape rhythms

are idioventricular and therefore slow. Permanent pacing is recommended to prevent syncope, but it may not improve survival. The differences in type II AV blocks between inferior and anterior wall infarctions are shown in Table 18-4.

In third-degree AV block, there is complete absence of conduc-

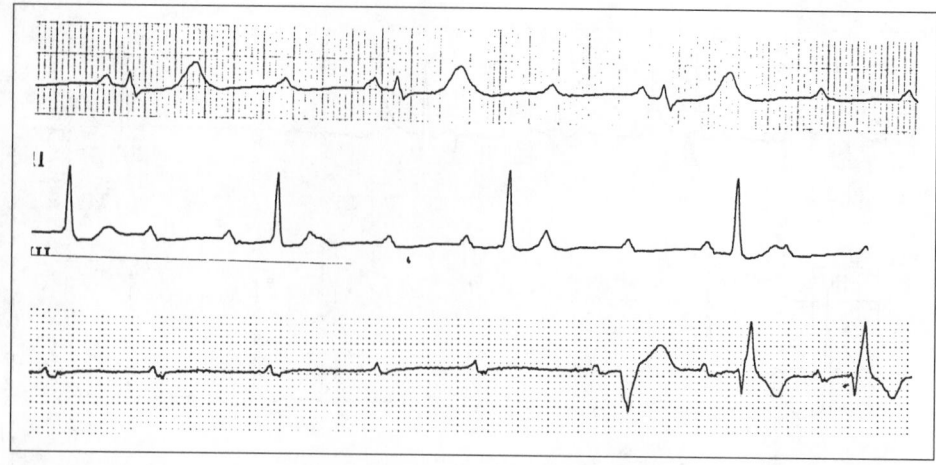

FIGURE 18-32   *Top,* High-degree AV block with 3:1 conduction. *Middle,* Complete heart block with junctional escape rhythm. *Bottom,* Episode of complete heart block without an escape rhythm.

Table 18-4   Type II atrioventricular block in myocardial infarction

	AV BLOCK	
	INFERIOR MYOCARDIAL INFARCTION	ANTERIOR MYOCARDIAL INFARCTION
Site	AV nodal	Infrahisian
Mechanism	Vagal tone, ischemia	Extensive necrosis
Type, degree	Mobitz I, third degree	Mobitz II, third degree
QRS complex	Narrow	Widened
Progression	Gradual	Abrupt
Escape rhythm	Junctional	Idioventricular
Prognosis	Good	Poor

(From Chakko S, Kessler KM: Recognition and management of cardiac arrhythmias, *Curr Probl Cardiol* 20:53-120, 1995.)

tion from atria to ventricles. An escape rhythm, either junctional or idioventricular, is usually present, resulting in AV dissociation (Fig. 18-32, *middle*). Complete AV block is sometimes preceded by lower grades of AV block or bundle branch blocks for many years. Complete heart block may cause syncope or cardiac collapse if the escape rhythm is slow idioventricular (Fig. 18-32, *bottom*). However, it may be an incidental finding if the escape rhythm is junctional with a sufficient rate to maintain cardiac output. Permanent pacing is necessary unless a reversible cause is present (e.g., digitalis toxicity), or the complete AV block is a transient complication of inferior infarction. Congenital AV block is often asymptomatic, but occasionally pacing will be needed. Symptoms and the response of heart rate to exercise guide the decision.

INTRAVENTRICULAR CONDUCTION ABNORMALITIES

Intraventricular conduction abnormalities may be present in many patients before the development of complete heart block. The surface ECG may reveal bifascicular or trifascicular blocks. Intracardiac recordings may show a prolonged H-V interval resulting from delayed conduction from the His bundle to the ventricles. Prospective studies, however, have shown that prophylactic pacing does not improve survival in patients with intraventricular conduction abnormalities or prolonged H-V intervals. In acute anterior wall infarction, appearance of new left bundle branch block or bifascicular block (right bundle branch block with left anterior or posterior hemiblock) indicates a 40% to 50% chance of complete heart block (Chapter 23). Prophylactic pacemaker insertion is usually recommended in these situations. Pacing is not necessary if the bundle branch block was present be-

fore the acute infarction, but if the duration of the bundle branch block is unknown it is assumed to be new. Temporary pacemakers are useful in management because in acute anterior infarction, complete heart block can occur abruptly and may result in asystole or severe bradyarrhythmia. Survival is not improved, however, because the high mortality rate that accompanies these conduction disturbances is the result of extensive myocardial necrosis. The availability of external pacing devices has reduced the urgency for transvenous pacemaker placement in these situations. Permanent pacing is usually not necessary in patients with inferior infarction and transient high-degree AV block. Survivors of anterior infarction with bundle branch block who experienced transient Mobitz II or third-degree AV block are at risk for sudden death and may benefit from prophylactic permanent pacemaker insertion.

REFERENCES

Chakko S, Kessler KM: Recognition and management of cardiac arrhythmias, *Curr Probl Cardiol* 20:53-120, 1995.

Dreifus LS et al: ACC/AHA guidelines for implementation of cardiac pacemakers and antiarrhythmic devices, *J Am Coll Cardiol* 18:1-3, 1991.

Emergency Cardiac Care Committee and Subcommittees, American Heart Association: Guidelines for cardiopulmonary resuscitation and emergency cardiac care, *JAMA* 268:2171-2302, 1992.

Guidelines for permanent cardiac pacemaker implantation: a report of the Joint American College of Cardiology/American Heart Association Task Force on Assessment of Cardiovascular Procedures, *J Am Coll Cardiol* 14:1827, 1989.

Myerburg RJ, Castellanos A: Cardiac arrest and sudden cardiac death. In Braunwald E, editor: *Heart disease*, Philadelphia, 1992, WB Saunders.

Myerburg RJ, Kessler KM, Castellanos A: Recognition, clinical assessment and management of arrhythmias and conduction disturbances. In Alexander RW, Schlant RC, Fuster V, editors: *The heart*, ed 9, New York, 1998, McGraw-Hill.

Waldo AL, Wit AL: Mechanism of cardiac arrhythmias and conduction disturbances. In Schlant RC, Alexander RW, editors: *The heart*, New York, 1994, McGraw-Hill.

Zipes DP et al: ACC/AHA guidelines for clinical intracardiac electrophysiological and catheter ablation procedures, *J Am Coll Cardiol* 26:555-573, 1995.

CHAPTER

19   Congestive Heart Failure

Gary S. Francis

Heart failure is a complex clinical syndrome that defies simple definition. It is clinically characterized by breathlessness and fatigue and can occur as a consequence of virtually any form of heart disease. The performance of the myocardium is inadequate to pump blood sufficient for the needs of the body. However, this simple definition fails to take into account many nuances of the syndrome such as pure diastolic heart failure or restrictive cardiomyopathy, whereby ejection phase or pumping indexes are normally retained, but abnormalities of relaxation or left ventricular (LV) filling may lead to extreme dyspnea, a syndrome that can be every bit as disabling as heart failure resulting from markedly reduced systolic function. How then, from a conceptual standpoint, should one think about heart failure? The following points should be considered:

- *Heart failure* is a term that may be preferred to *congestive heart failure,* because today many patients lack congestion, and pulmonary capillary wedge pressure bears little relation to breathlessness in the chronic stages of the syndrome.

- Heart failure is a syndrome, like fever or renal failure, and cannot stand alone as a diagnosis. It is always due to some etiologic factor (e.g., idiopathic dilated cardiomyopathy). Any form of heart disease can lead to heart failure.

- There is no single laboratory test for heart failure. It is always a clinical diagnosis made by taking a careful history and doing a careful physical examination. Even conventional hemodynamic measurements such as cardiac output or LV filling pressure may be normal in patients with a very low ejection fraction (EF). On the other hand, ejection fraction may be normal in patients with diastolic heart failure who have extremely elevated LV filling pressures.

- Knowledge of LV function is critical to understanding the mechanism of heart failure. Because therapy is predicated on the mechanism of the symptoms, an understanding of how the symptoms are occurring is vital to management of the patient. An echocardiogram should be done in every patient in whom the diagnosis of heart failure is a consideration. For example, the approach to critical aortic stenosis is very different than the approach to severely dilated cardiomyopathy, and therefore the mechanisms of the syndrome must always be sought out.

One reason that heart failure is so difficult to define is that there is no consistent or unique distinguishing feature in terms of how the syndrome is characterized. In many congenital heart or valvular lesions, LV function may be normal. In hypertrophic cardiomyopathy, systolic function may be hypercontractile, whereas diastolic filling is markedly impaired. In heart failure resulting from critical aortic stenosis, mitral stenosis, aortic regurgitation, mitral regurgitation, and flagrant hyperthyroidism, LV performance may remain intact or even hyperkinetic, thereby excluding LV dysfunction as a defining factor. Moreover, patients with severe cardiomyopathy from coronary artery disease or idiopathic dilated cardiomyopathy may have none of the cardinal features of edema, rales, S3 gallop, jugular venous distention, or murmur of mitral regurgitation, especially in the modern era when compensation occurs from the use of powerful loop diuretics and angiotensin converting enzyme (ACE) inhibitors. Nevertheless, such patients may be very symptomatic with breathlessness and fatigue, and can be said to have "heart failure." Young patients with astonishingly low EF (i.e., <15%) may occasionally be completely without symptoms, and may even retain near-normal exercise tolerance despite severe LV dysfunction. Do such patients have heart failure, or are they better classified as LV dysfunction without heart failure? Perhaps they have New York Heart Association (NYHA) Class I heart failure. However one classifies them, all such patients are part of the large syndrome of heart failure and if left untreated, most go on to develop all of the features well known to experienced physicians including edema, rales, jugular venous distention, ascites, a gallop rhythm, and a murmur of mitral insufficiency accompanied by dyspnea and fatigue. It is important to bring these various examples to the attention of the reader to underscore the idea that heart failure is a complex clinical syndrome with a seemingly endless list of causes, but unfortunately it has no consistent clinical or laboratory feature that allows for a simple definition. The heart must be involved in heart failure in some fashion to distinguish it from circulatory congestion, a condition of pure volume overload such as might occur in acute renal failure where there is no inherent myocardial abnormality. Despite all the problems in defining heart failure, the diagnosis of the syndrome and determination of the cause are usually rather straightforward. In virtually every case, knowledge of valvular function and myocardial shape and function must be sought, and the echocardiogram has clearly emerged as the cornerstone of diagnosis. The

---

BOX 19-1
Classification of cardiac failure

I. Mechanical abnormalities
   A. Increased resistance to forward outflow (pressure overload)
   B. Increased ventricular inflow (volume overload): valvular regurgitation, shunts, increased blood volume
      1. Primary
      2. Secondary (valvular regurgitation from ventricular dilation)
   C. Pericardial disease (constriction and tamponade)
   D. Restrictive heart disease (endocardial or myocardial)
   E. Ventricular aneurysm
II. Myocardial failure
   A. Primary
      1. Cardiomyopathy
      2. Myocarditis
      3. Metabolically induced muscle dysfunction (hypothyroidism)
      4. Reduction in muscle mass (myocardial infarction)
   B. Secondary
      1. Dysdynamic heart failure (long-standing volume or pressure overload)
      2. Drug induced
      3. Cardiac involvement in systemic disease
III. Electrical disorders
   A. Asystole
   B. Ventricular fibrillation
   C. Heart block
   D. Ventricular tachycardia

---

combination of a careful history, physical examination, chest radiograph, electrocardiogram, and an echocardiogram allows one to classify heart failure (Box 19-1).

EPIDEMIOLOGIC CONSIDERATIONS AND PROGNOSIS

Although age-adjusted death rates for heart disease in general and coronary artery heart disease in particular have been decreasing steadily since 1968, the incidence of heart failure continues to increase, particularly in those over age 65 years (Fig. 19-1). Heart failure is the only cardiovascular diagnosis that is increasing in incidence and is the leading Diagnosis Related Group (DRG) for inpatients older than age 65. The prevalence probably approaches 10% in people older than 75 years. There has been a four-fold increase in hospital admissions for heart failure since 1971. In 1989, the National Heart, Lung, and Blood Institute estimated the annual health care costs of heart failure in the United States to be just under $9 billion, with indirect costs of another $1.4 billion. About $6.4 billion of this was spent on hospital care, $500 million on professional services, $1.7 billion on nursing home care, and $200 million on pharmaceuticals. In 1991 more money was spent on heart failure than cancer or acute myocardial infarction (Fig. 19-2). Far and away, most of these patients are cared for by family physicians and general internists, with only 17% being cared for by a cardiologist in 1991 (Fig. 19-3).

In addition to gender differences, there are important racial differences in the epidemiology of heart failure. Blacks and whites had striking differences in etiology of heart failure in the SOLVD (Studies of Left Ventricular Dysfunction) registry of 6273 consecutive unselected patients with heart failure or LV dysfunction. Whites were far more likely than blacks to have ischemic etiology of heart failure (73% vs. 36%), whereas blacks were far more likely than whites to have a hypertensive etiology (32% vs. 4%). There were no overall differences in mortality, but hospital admissions for heart failure were more frequent in blacks. For men, African-American race appeared not to be a risk factor to develop heart failure after adjusting for hypertension, diabetes mellitus, left ventricular hypertrophy, and body mass index. Among younger African-American women, however, ad-

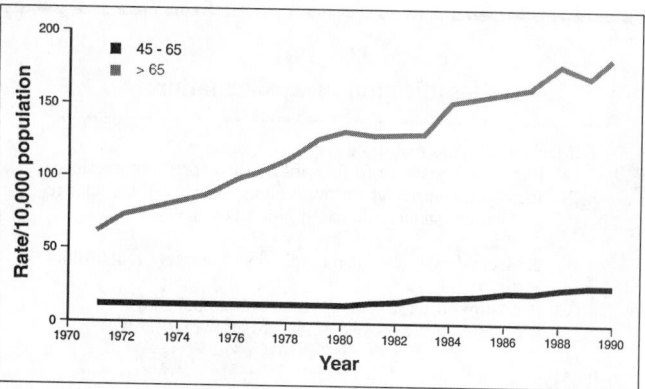

FIGURE 19-1   Rates of admission to hospital for heart failure according to age in the United States, 1971-1990.

(From Kannel WB, Ho K, Thom T: *Br Heart J* 72:S3, 1994.)

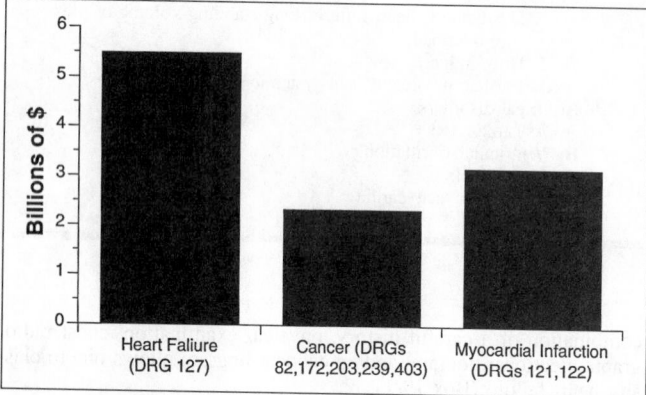

FIGURE 19-2   Comparison of Health Care Financial Administration (HCFA) expenditures on heart failure compared with cancer and myocardial infarction according to the medicare program.

(Modified from O'Connell J, Bristow M: *J Heart Lung Transplant* 13:S107, 1993.)

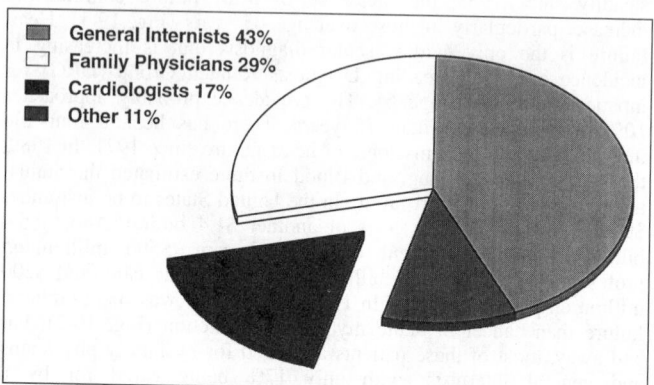

FIGURE 19-3   Physicians responsible for the care of patients with heart failure.

(Modified from O'Connell J, Bristow M: *J Heart Lung Transplant* 13:S107, 1993.)

justment of these variables does not reduce the risk of developing heart failure. These findings highlight the role of hypertension and diabetes in the development of heart failure among blacks.

The median survival in the Framingham Heart Study after the onset of heart failure was 1.7 years in men and 3.2 years in women. Overall 1-year and 5-year survival rates were 57% and 25% for men and 64% and 38% in women, respectively. Mortality increases with

advancing age in both genders, although women probably have a somewhat lower mortality rate. In the Framingham study, the advances in the treatment of hypertension, myocardial ischemia and valvular heart disease during 40 years of observation have not translated into an appreciable improvement in overall survival. It is as if all we do with treatment is forestall the onset of heart failure to a later date, thereby pushing the prevalence onto the older population. These observations emphasize that ACE inhibitors, although powerful new therapeutic tools, usually prolong life only 9 to 18 months. Clearly, there is still a need to develop improved techniques to prevent heart failure.

Despite the data from the Framingham study demonstrating no real decline in mortality rate from vasodilators, data from the Mayo Clinic, UCLA, and the Brigham and Women's Hospital show marked improvement in survival in patients with idiopathic dilated cardiomyopathy, underscoring the effects of referral bias and secular trend, as well as improved diagnostic criteria. Also, in the SOLVD, the mortality rate for patients developing new onset heart failure was only 30% at 2 years, which is substantially lower than the Framingham study data. The Framingham investigators used criteria developed in the 1940s, which clearly lack sensitivity and specificity. In all likelihood, the prognosis of patients with heart failure has improved with vasodilator therapy.

Despite some uncertainties regarding the influence of modern therapy on survival, it seems clear that prevention of heart failure holds the key to reducing the huge economic burden. Preliminary data suggest that in Glasgow almost 8% of the population have LV dysfunction, and 40% of these have no symptoms of heart failure. Likewise, a preliminary population-based study from Sweden suggests that the prevalence of asymptomatic LV dysfunction may be just as high as that of heart failure. If these findings are substantiated, there may be a very large base of patients with asymptomatic LV dysfunction who are candidates for treatment with ACE inhibitors to prevent heart failure. It is also possible that information from the recent postmyocardial infarction ACE inhibitor trials will lead to a reduction in cases of overt heart failure.

PATHOGENESIS

The pathogenesis of heart failure depends on the etiology. In the overly nourished Western world, coronary artery disease is the most common cause of heart failure. Often, but not always, such patients have loss of substantial myocardial tissue because of recurrent myocardial infarction and replacement fibrosis. Eventually LV filling pressure rises and cardiac output begins to fall. These characteristic findings also occur in idiopathic dilated cardiomyopathy, severe myocarditis, aortic regurgitation and mitral regurgitation, and during the end stages of severe aortic stenosis. Toxic cardiomyopathy from adriamycin and cytoxan also shares these features. The failing myocardium shares two important principles: (1) There is an inability to raise stroke volume and cardiac output sufficiently as LV filling pressure rises (Fig. 19-4), and (2) the failing myocardium is exquisitely sensitive to afterload. As afterload increases, there is a more pronounced depression of LV performance (Fig. 19-5).

The preload of the heart is the end-diastolic myocardial fiber length. At the turn of the nineteenth century, Starling pointed out that the force of contraction is related to the end-diastolic fiber length. Obviously this is something that cannot be measured at the bedside. Therefore, the end-diastolic volume or end-diastolic pressure (i.e., pulmonary capillary wedge pressure) is often substituted for preload. Measurement of LV filling pressure is not equivalent to preload, as it is influenced by diastolic properties of the heart, such as chamber stiffness. Nevertheless, it is a reasonable bedside substitute for preload measurement. Unlike normal subjects, patients with heart failure simply fail to demonstrate a brisk increase in stroke volume with an increase in filling pressure. The curve is flattened (Fig. 19-4), but does not actually descend.

Afterload is circumferential LV wall stress during ejection, an important component of total impedance to ejection that also includes compliance of the peripheral vasculature, arteriolar resistance, and viscosity of the blood. Impedance is tedious to measure, but it is conceptually very important. There is an inverse relation between circumferential wall stress (afterload) and both ejection fraction and ve-

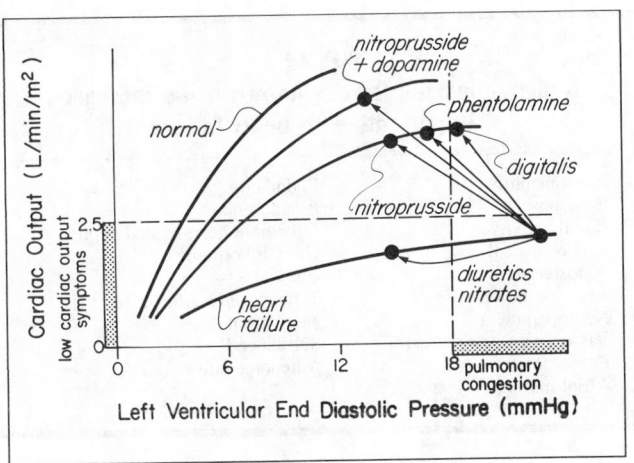

FIGURE 19-4   Ventricular function curve in congestive heart failure (CHF) compared with normal curve. At any level of left atrial pressure, cardiac output is decreased in the failing heart. The dotted area indicates the level of cardiac output and filling pressure at which symptoms develop.

(Modified from Mason DT, editor: *Congestive heart failure,* New York, 1976, Yorke Medical Books.)

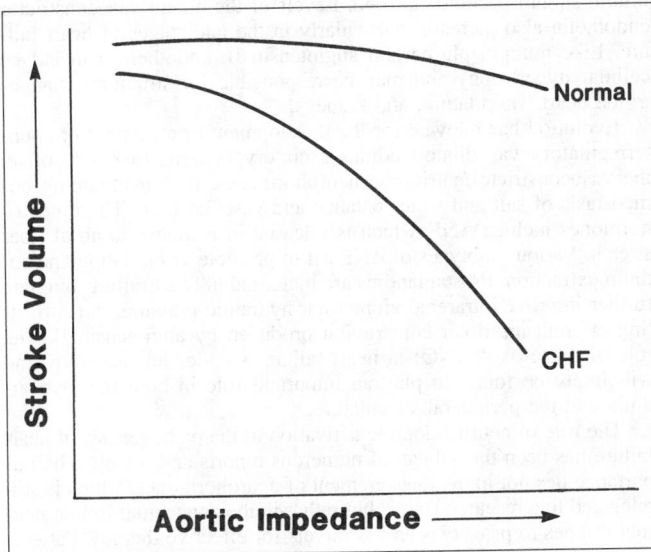

FIGURE 19-5   Patients with heart failure are exquisitely sensitive to an afterload stress. Compared with normal subjects, an increment in aortic impedance in patients with heart failure is accompanied by a profound reduction in stroke volume.

locity of fiber shortening, which is magnified in the failing heart. Afterload or wall stress is defined by the Laplace relationship:

(EQ.1)

$$\sigma = \frac{P x r}{2h}$$

Where σ is wall stress, P is chamber pressure, r is chamber radius, and h is chamber thickness. This implies that LV wall thickness is a critical determinant of ventricular performance. Poor cardiac performance in patients with heart failure can be secondary to inadequate hypertrophy leading to increased wall stress (afterload), which is responsible for inadequate muscle shortening. It is important not to equate afterload with systemic vascular resistance (SVR), as the latter is a calculated ratio of flow and pressure and does not serve as an adequate surrogate for afterload. Rather, afterload is an integration of

pressure, chamber size, and wall thickness and may bear little relation to SVR.

THE DIFFERENCE BETWEEN CONTRACTILITY AND PERFORMANCE OF THE HEART

It is important when considering heart failure to remember the primary determinants of cardiac output:

Heart rate → cardiac output ← stroke volume ←
{preload, afterload, contractility}

The stroke volume is a product of (1) preload, (2) afterload, and (3) the inherent "contractility" of the heart. Contractility of the heart, which cannot be measured in the intact circulation, is the force of contraction *independent* of loading conditions (preload and afterload) and heart rate. Although not usually directly measurable, contractility is profoundly altered by certain drugs in either a positive (e.g., dobutamine, digitalis) or negative (e.g., first-generation Ca^{++} channel blockers, β-adrenergic blockers) direction. From a clinician's perspective, it is best to separate contractility from performance. The cardiac output and ejection fractions reflect the *performance* of the LV, which is the sum total of contractility, heart rate, and loading conditions. Performance therefore is a more precise term when characterizing LV function. The term *ejection fraction* is end-diastolic volume − end systolic volume/end diastolic volume and is normally 62%±12%. It is the clinical index most commonly used to characterize LV performance. LV performance may be reduced when contractility is reduced, but it incorporates loading conditions and heart rate and is therefore a more comprehensive term than *contractility*. It is possible for contractility to be normal in the face of reduced LV performance, such as might occur in severe aortic stenosis or cardiac tamponade. For the clinician, it is the performance of the heart that is inadequate in heart failure, and often clinical improvement is forthcoming when measures to optimize loading conditions are used pharmacologically.

COMPENSATORY MECHANISMS

For purposes of discussion, we will assume that heart failure is due to a poorly functioning LV with reduced contractility (loss of sarcomeres) and therefore reduced performance (i.e., a low ejection fraction). In this setting, as in any situation in which an excessive hemodynamic burden is placed on the left ventricle, the heart depends on three principal compensatory mechanisms for maintenance of its pumping function: (1) the Frank-Starling mechanism, in which there is an increased preload (i.e., increased length of the sarcomeres from 2.0 to 2.2 μm); (2) increased release of catecholamines, mainly norepinephrine from adrenergic cardiac nerves, which augments contractility; and (3) myocardial hypertrophy, with or without cardiac chamber dilation, which augments the number of sarcomeres. Frequently, these changes are accompanied by an increase in muscle and chamber stiffness, which contributes to a higher LV filling pressure for any given chamber volume. Although these compensatory mechanisms may enhance myocardial performance in a temporary fashion, they are limited and ultimately may play an important role in the pathogenesis of the syndrome. Hence they have become important therapeutic targets.

CELLULAR ABNORMALITIES OF MYOCARDIAL FAILURE

Various cellular abnormalities have been described in the myocardium, both from human patients and from experimental animals with heart failure. Among the earliest was the demonstration that cardiac norepinephrine stores were depleted in patients with severe heart failure, a finding that appears to be specific for the failing myocardium. A more interesting and consistent biochemical change in the failing myocardium is a decrease in myosin adenosine triphosphatase (ATPase) activity. This change appears to be caused by a change in the individual isoenzymes of myosin, resulting in a preponderance of the slow over the fast component. Diminished myosin ATPase activity results in a decrease in cross-bridge interaction between actin and myosin, which in turn results in a reduced velocity of muscle short-ening. Although this observation represents an interesting correlation between biochemistry and muscle mechanics, its significance is un-clear. As with many other biochemical changes in the myocardium, this may represent an adaptive response designed as an energy-sparing process to minimize ATP utilization. Our better understanding of mo-lecular biology (Chapter 10) is making it increasingly clear that this, similar to other adaptive responses, represents an alteration in gene-specific expression.

Other studies have demonstrated a decrease in calcium (Ca^{++}) transport by the sarcoplasmic reticulum (SR). This finding, together with ATP depletion, could influence diastolic as well as systolic pa-rameters of myocardial function. It has been clearly demonstrated in experimental animals and in tissue obtained from human hearts at bi-opsy that a decrease occurs in the activity of the Ca^{++} ATPase sys-tem responsible for SR Ca^{++} transport. Most recently, samples from human biopsies have shown a decrease in the expression of messen-ger ribonucleic acid (mRNA) for the Ca^{++} ATPase of the SR. Other studies have demonstrated abnormalities of mitochondrial function and a decrease in high-energy phosphate production. Nevertheless, a causal relationship between decreased ATP levels and diminished contractile activity of the failing myocardium has not been estab-lished.

Despite these observations of significant biochemical dysfunction, the relationship between these biochemical changes and the contrac-tile properties of the failing myocardium has yet to be established. They may well represent a secondary phenomenon but equally well may represent primary and basic underlying abnormalities that could precipitate, or at least perpetuate, the heart failure state.

HIGH-OUTPUT FAILURE

High-output failure is a form of heart failure in which cardiac output is elevated compared with values for the normal resting state in hu-mans. Many symptoms and physical findings, however, are identical to those of low-output failure. The primary physiologic abnormality in high output failure is either circulatory shunting or greatly increased peripheral demands for blood. Examples of high-output fail-ure include arteriovenous (AV) fistula, anemia, thyrotoxicosis, Paget's disease (multiple AV fistulas in bone), and beriberi. Although actual cardiac index is high (>3.6 L/min/m^2), the "effective" cardiac output arriving at the peripheral tissues is low for any given atrial pressure. This is true in an absolute sense with AV shunting and in a relative sense with anemia. The effective cardiac output versus atrial pressure curve is depressed downward and to the right. In high-output states, however, myocardial performance may remain normal or even be aug-mented. Thus absolute cardiac output for any given end-diastolic *vol-ume* may be normal or increased. As a consequence, treatment in these conditions should be directed primarily toward relieving the defect that renders stroke volume inadequate rather than toward improving myocardial performance.

NEUROENDOCRINE ACTIVATION

As LV performance is diminished, a host of biologic factors are re-leased (Box 19-2). It is now clear that plasma norepinephrine (PNE) and atrial natriuretic factor (ANF) are increased even before the overt expression of the full syndrome of heart failure (Fig. 19-6). Arginine vasopressin (AVP) and plasma renin activity (PRA) may also be in-creased very early, but this finding is less consistent. The mechanisms whereby neuroendocrine activation occurs, especially the sympathetic nervous system, remain incompletely understood. Norepinephrine re-lease probably evolved as a mechanism to protect blood pressure and to maintain flow to exercising muscle, particularly during short-term stress. The sympathetic nervous system is a quickly acting vasocon-strictor and chronotropic system primarily designed to act "on com-mand" to restore blood pressure and cardiac output. The renin-angiotensin system (RAS) is a slower acting system with both a cir-culating and a tissue component. Its major component, angiotensin II, has a vast array of biologic properties (Fig. 19-7). In addition to its vasoconstrictor properties, angiotensin II has important salt and water retaining activity, both directly on the renal tubules and indi-

---

BOX 19-2

Neuroendocrine factors known to be increased in patients with heart failure

Norepinephrine	Endothelin
Epinephrine	β-endorphins
Renin activity	Calcitonin gene-related peptide
Angiotensin II	Growth hormone
Aldosterone	Cortisol
Arginine vasopressin	Tumor necrosis factor-α
Neuropeptide Y	Neurokinin A
Vasoactive intestinal peptide	Substance P
Prostaglandins	Adrenomedullin
Atrial natriuretic factor	

---

rectly by stimulating the release of aldosterone from the adrenal cor-tex. The tissue RAS has important influences on myocardial and vas-cular hypertrophy, leading to structural changes in the myocardium and peripheral vessels. AVP is released during the course of heart fail-ure, causing a reduction in free water clearance and regional vaso-constriction. Its importance in the pathogenesis of heart failure is less clear, but as specific AVP antagonists are developed, its role in heart failure should become clarified. Levels of the potent vasoconstrictor endothelin also increase, particularly in the late stages of heart fail-ure. Like norepinephrine and angiotensin II, endothelin can induce cellular hypertrophy and may be responsible for structural changes in the heart, vasculature, and kidneys.

Evolution has allowed for the development of a number of coun-terregulatory vasodilator/sodium excretory systems that may offset the vasoconstrictor/natriuretic neurohormones, thus maintaining ho-meostasis of salt and water balance and vascular tone. These neuro-hormones include ANF, which is released in response to atrial fiber stretch. Various subtypes of ANF act to promote vasodilation and so-dium extraction. Prostaglandins are increased in heart failure and may further improve intrarenal glomerular hydraulic pressure, thus offset-ting efferent arteriolar constriction produced by angiotensin II. The role of nitric oxide (NO) in heart failure is under intense study and will likely be found to play an important role in both the myocar-dium and the peripheral vasculature.

The role of neuroendocrine activation in the pathogenesis of heart failure has been the subject of numerous reports and reviews. Its im-portance lies not in the measurement of neurohormones, which is still relegated to a research status, but rather in the conceptual link of neu-rohormones to prognosis and as targets for effective therapy. Patients with high levels of plasma norepinephrine clearly have a worse prog-nosis. The so-called neurohormone hypothesis would suggest that drugs that inhibit various neuroendocrine systems are far more effec-tive in the chronic therapy of heart failure than drugs designed to stimulate the inotropic state of the heart. The ACE inhibitors have now become the cornerstone of therapy, underscoring the importance of the RAS in the pathophysiology of heart failure. There is now great interest in β-adrenergic blocking agents for the treatment of heart fail-ure, and preliminary data suggest such treatment may prolong sur-vival. The success of ACE inhibitors and the promising new data on β-blockers are consistent with the view that neuroendocrine compen-satory mechanisms may actually produce an overadjustment; that is, excessive renin activity, sympathetic drive, and other neurohormones may be detrimental to the myocardium and peripheral circulation by leading to left ventricular remodeling, adverse myocardial structural changes, and hemodynamically adverse peripheral vasoconstriction and salt and water retention (Fig. 19-8). A more penetrating under-standing of various neuroendocrine abnormalities is now a primary focus in the development of new drug therapy for heart failure. How-ever, the sympathetic and renin-angiotensin-aldosterone systems re-main pivotal in the pathogenesis of heart failure (Fig. 19-9), and their interruption by β-blockers and ACE inhibitors has been a major thera-peutic step forward.

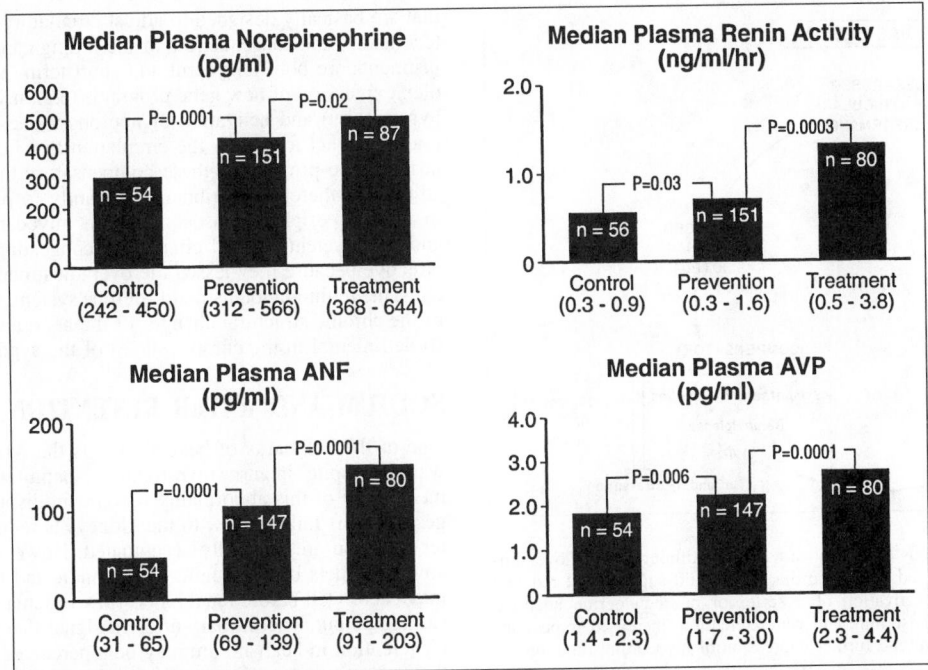

FIGURE 19-6   Bar grafts of incremental increase in plasma norepinephrine, plasma renin activity, plasma arginine vasopressin (AVP), and plasma atrial natriuretic factor (ANF) in control subjects, prevention patients, and treatment patients. These are baseline data collected from patients entering the SOLVD Trial. Prevention refers to patients with asymptomatic or minimally symptomatic left ventricular dysfunction, whereas Treatment represents a group of patients with overt congestive heart failure. The data are median values and interquartile ranges, 25% to 75%.

(From Francis GS et al: *Circulation* 82:1724, 1990.)

THE NEUROHORMONAL HYPOTHESIS

The symptoms of heart failure have traditionally been blamed on the weakened heart's inability to pump blood. Although there is an inexorable decline of pump function over time, the mechanism of this decline is poorly understood. New findings suggest a progressive loss of myocardial cells. The hemodynamic theory fails to explain how these cells die. Drugs that simply improve the inotropic state have failed to improve long-term survival and may in some cases accelerate mortality, whereas drugs that reduce neurohormonal influences, such as ACE inhibitors and β-adrenergic blockers, seem to improve survival. Endogenously released agents that may promote cell death include norepinephrine, angiotensin II, vasopressin, endothelin, and tumor necrosis factor (TNF)-α. Cytokines such as TNF-α mediate myocardial depression in septic shock, and appear to be overexpressed in chronic heart failure. Monocytes and macrophages in underperfused tissue may release TNF-α, and adult mammalian cardiac myocytes may also produce the cytokine. It is possible that progressive dilation of the LV may be the trigger for TNF-α synthesis. There is also the possibility that TNF-α may stimulate apoptosis, or programmed cell death of cardiac myocytes. Undoubtedly the role of neurohormones and cytokines is very complex, and no single factor will account for the derangements characterized in heart failure. Nevertheless, the neurohormonal hypothesis has stimulated much new thinking regarding the pathophysiology of heart failure and opened the door for potentially exciting new therapies designed to block or attenuate neurohormones and cytokines.

PERIPHERAL VASCULAR AND REFLEX CONTROL ABNORMALITIES

Functional and structural changes in the arterial circulation appear to be critical factors in the development of heart failure. The failing myocardium cannot cope with the increasing impedance to ejection. Resistance to ejection is predominantly at the arteriolar level, but the

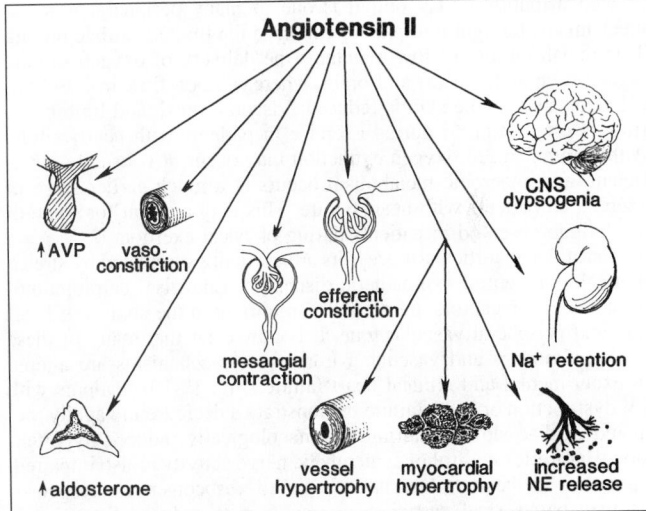

FIGURE 19-7   Angiotensin II has multiple biologic functions. In heart failure, it likely contributes to enhancement of AVP release, arteriolar vasoconstriction, increased secretion of aldosterone, mesangial contraction (which reduces glomerular filtration rate), efferent arteriole constriction (which maintains glomerular filtration rate), vascular and myocardial hypertrophy, enhanced release of norepinephrine (NE) from sympathetic nerve endings, a direct effect of sodium reabsorption, and an increased sensation of thirst. The net result of these activities is increased systemic vascular resistance, heightened sympathetic activity, peripheral edema, and hyponatremia—all hallmarks of advanced heart failure.

(Modified from Francis GS. In Antonaccio MJ, editor: *Cardiovascular pharmacology,* ed 3, New York, 1990, Raven Press.)

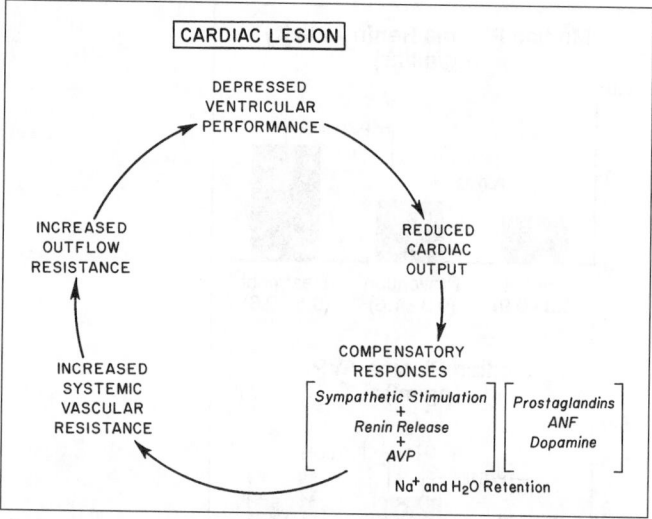

FIGURE 19-8   The vicious cycle of heart failure. Although vastly oversimplified, this commonly used schematic diagram would suggest that reduced cardiac output leads to activation of a series of neuroendocrine adaptive mechanisms. The result is sodium and water retention, increased impedance to left ventricular ejection, and further depression of myocardial function. (Modified from Francis GS. In Antonaccio MJ, editor: *Cardiovascular pharmacology,* ed 3, New York, 1990, Raven Press.)

compliance of the conduit vessels is also reduced. Both structural and functional changes in the vasculature may account for the alteration in impedance. Vascular smooth muscle may remodel, and the release of NO from the endothelium is blunted in response to various stimuli, thereby narrowing the vascular lumen and decreasing vascular distensibility.

Redistribution of LV output is one of many peripheral vascular mechanisms brought into play to conserve the limited cardiac output. This redistribution of flow maintains the delivery of oxygen to vital organs such as the heart and brain, whereas blood flow to less critical areas such as the skin is reduced. Visceral, renal, and limb blood flow is often reduced during exercise in patients with heart failure. Although enhanced oxygen extraction may occur, it is usually insufficient, and anaerobic metabolism occurs at a much earlier stage of exercise in patients with heart failure. This may account for some of the fatigue observed in patients during physical exertion.

Carotid and aortic baroreceptors are normally stimulated by stretch that inhibits central sympathetic discharge. Likewise, cardiopulmonary mechanoreceptors are normally important in the control of heart rate and peripheral vascular tone. It is now clear that many of these cardiopulmonary and vascular baroreceptor mechanisms are altered in experimental and clinical heart failure (Fig. 19-10). Patients with LV dysfunction or heart failure demonstrate a decrease in vagally mediated cardiac slowing during pharmacologically induced hypertension. Baroreflex control of sympathetic nerve activity is also impaired. Patients with heart failure have impaired vasoconstrictor responses or even paradoxical vasodilatory responses to reduced filling pressure. Neurohumoral responses to upright tilt or orthostatic stress are also blunted. Baroreceptor sensitivity is reduced in heart failure, but it remains unclear how much these reflex control abnormalities actually contribute to the development of the neurohumoral excitatory state. Experimentally, arterial baroreflex sensitivity in heart failure is preserved until late in the course of developing heart failure. Nevertheless, reflex control abnormalities may contribute to activation of the sympathetic nervous system by failing to inhibit central sympathetic drive to the periphery in response to day-to-day physiologic adjustments such as an expanding cardiac volume.

Abnormalities of neuroendocrine activation, altered reflex control mechanisms, and structural changes in the myocardium and peripheral vasculature are extremely complex and our understanding of them continues to evolve. A very simplified manner of thinking about heart failure is that nature has evolved a large number of redundant steps

that are basically designed to adjust circulatory homeostasis and protect against the consequences of the falling cardiac output. These adjustments are both long-term and short-term, and they include complex expression of new gene programs (e.g., myocardial and vascular hypertrophy) and activation of neurohormones that are highly integrated and act to protect the circulation and flow to vital organs. As heart failure progresses, these compensatory mechanisms may overadjust and thereby contribute importantly to pathogenesis, resulting in intense peripheral vasoconstriction, myocardial remodeling, salt and water retention, and circulatory congestion. ACE inhibitors are effective because they lessen the overadjustment of one of these systems, the renin-angiotensin-aldosterone system, thus forestalling some of the chronic structural changes of the heart and vasculature that are so detrimental in the chronic stages of the syndrome.

SODIUM AND WATER RETENTION

One of the hallmarks of heart failure is the retention of sodium and water. Despite intense investigation spanning many decades, the mechanism of this abnormality remains in dispute. In advanced congestive heart failure, flow to the kidneys is reduced and salt and water retention are markedly accentuated. However, studies of various animal models of heart failure have indicated that sodium retention may occur well before renal blood flow is actually diminished by low cardiac output. The primary afferent signal that initiates salt and water retention in heart failure may be a perceived reduction in a hypothetical entity referred to as *effective blood volume.* Unfortunately, effective blood volume is poorly defined and cannot be measured. Moreover, even though total blood volume is increased in heart failure, proponents of the concept of effective blood volume would suggest that the fullness of the arterial compartment is actually reduced. The inability to measure effective blood volume has obfuscated our understanding of how the kidney senses a perceived reduction in circulatory volume.

Whatever the signal, the kidney responds in heart failure in a way that is similar to blood loss or dehydration. There is an increase in sympathetic nervous system activity, which in turn activates the renin-angiotensin-aldosterone system. Renin release is also stimulated in heart failure by diminished pressure/volume activity in the renal artery, by hyponatremic perfusate to the macula densa as a direct result of sympathetic stimulation and diuretic use. Superimposed on these renin release mechanisms, release of arginine vasopressin (AVP) is also enhanced, which further favors sodium and water retention. The result is an expansion of the extracellular volume, which in a teleologic sense may protect against a perceived fall in blood pressure or flow. The expanded blood volume increases intracardiac pressure causing atrial distention, which in turn releases atrial natriuretic peptide (ANP). Multiple peptides may be released from the heart that have both natriuretic and vasodilator properties. However, the natriuretic and vasodilator effects of ANP are overwhelmed by peripheral vasoconstrictor and sodium retentive influences so that the overall effect is one of salt and water retention.

Patients with untreated heart failure may have a marked reduction in effective renal plasma flow even when cardiac output is not decreased, implying some renal artery vasoconstriction. Glomerular filtration rate is reduced to a lesser extent than renal blood flow, so the filtration fraction may be increased. These findings suggest a disproportionate increase in glomerular efferent arteriolar tone compared with afferent arteriolar tone. We now know that increased levels of angiotensin II are responsible for much of the heightened efferent arteriolar tone that occurs in heart failure, and this efferent arteriolar constriction is useful in maintaining intraglomerular hydraulic pressure. ACE inhibitors, which reduce angiotensin II formation, may consequently reduce intraglomerular hydraulic pressure by lessening efferent arteriolar tone. The net result may be manifested by a rise in blood urea nitrogen (BUN) and serum creatinine. High levels of circulating angiotensin II also stimulate the adrenal cortex to release aldosterone, which further acts on the renal tubules to promote salt and water retention. In addition to its direct vasoconstrictor effects, angiotensin II sensitizes the vasculature to norepinephrine and acts directly to release norepinephrine from sympathetic neurons via a presynaptic receptor mechanism. Angiotensin II also stimulates thirst through a central nervous system mechanism (Fig. 19-7).

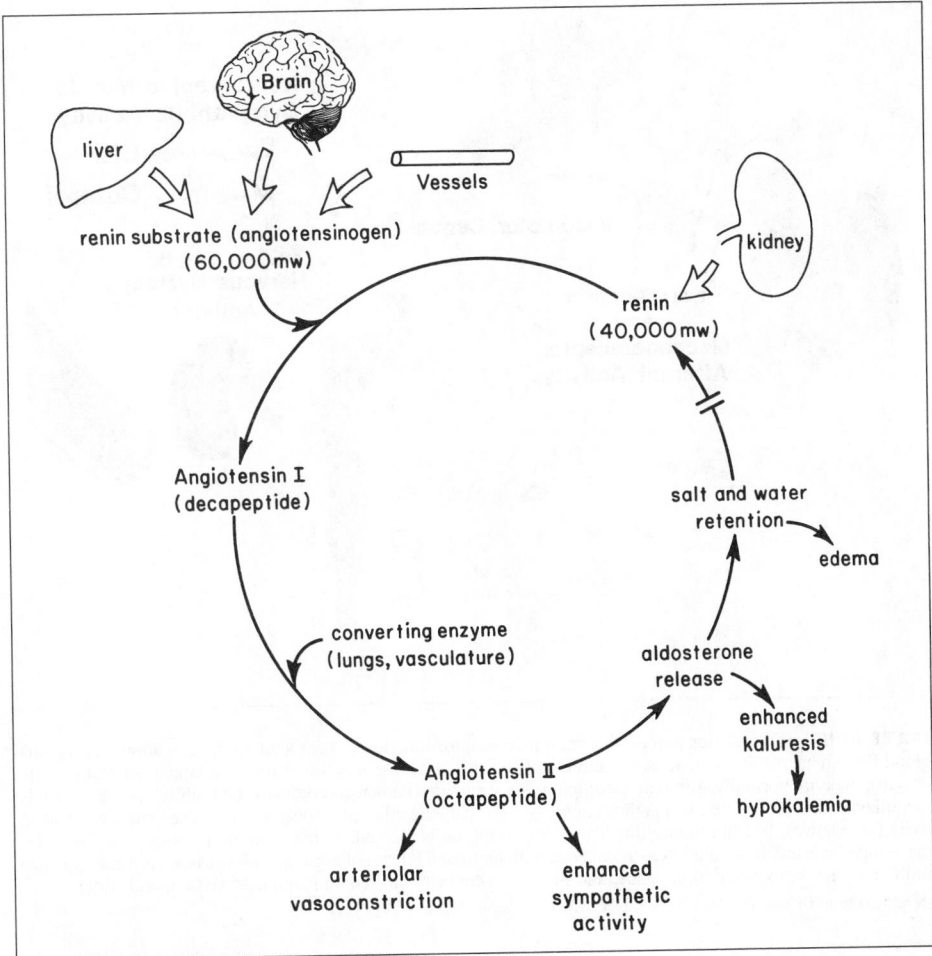

FIGURE 19-9   The renin-angiotensin-aldosterone system. Arterial vasoconstriction, salt and water retention, hypokalemia, and increased sympathetic nervous system activity can result from increased renin and angiotensin II.

(Modified from Francis GS. In Engelmeier RS, O'Connell JB, editors: *Drug therapy and dilated cardiomyopathy and myocarditis,* New York, 1988, Marcel Dekker.)

The mechanism of salt and water retention in heart failure is extraordinarily complex and still poorly understood. As extracellular volume increases, there may be a secondary reduction in plasma renin activity. Yet episodes of clinical decompensation are usually accompanied by marked stimulation of the renin-angiotensin-aldosterone system. Ultimately, patients develop circulatory congestion, peripheral edema, ascites, and all of the manifestations of severe congestive heart failure. Although powerful loop diuretics and ACE inhibitors are particularly useful in this regard, dietary sodium restriction is critically important. Many patients with advanced heart failure will become resistant to diuretic therapy unless sodium is markedly restricted. On the other hand, restriction of fluids or water is rarely necessary in patients with heart failure unless there is attendant hyponatremia.

CLINICAL MANIFESTATIONS
Symptoms

The cardinal symptom of heart failure is the sensation of breathlessness (dyspnea) or shortness of breath. Dyspnea is the consciousness of the necessity for increased respiratory effort or the sensation of difficult, labored, uncomfortable breathing. Despite being the central symptom of heart failure, the mechanism of dyspnea is complex and surprisingly poorly understood. It is unclear whether dyspnea serves any useful purpose, although it may deter patients from imposing an excessive strain on the cardiovascular system. In acute heart failure, such as occurs in acute pulmonary edema, pulmonary vascular congestion and consequent hypoxemia clearly lead to dyspnea, which can

be promptly relieved by diuresis. However, the mechanism of shortness of breath in chronic heart failure is much less clear. Many studies now demonstrate that there is no direct relationship between pulmonary capillary wedge pressure and dyspnea or exercise tolerance. Likewise, there is no simple relationship between dyspnea and the level of ventilation or of dead space ventilation in patients with chronic heart failure. Pulmonary venous congestion probably plays some role, and the apparent lack of correlation may simply be a matter of inadequacy of measurements. There may also be individual variation in the perceptual threshold for dyspnea. Diuretics reduce pulmonary vascular congestion and remain a mainstay of therapy. It is important to realize, however, that multiple mechanisms may be operative, including increased physiologic dead space, decreased pulmonary compliance, increased small airway resistance, respiratory muscle fatigue, and as yet unspecified signals from pulmonary J-receptors and respiratory muscles.

Additional disturbances of respiration include orthopnea, which is shortness of breath that is more pronounced on assuming a recumbent position. Patients with severe heart failure prefer to sleep more upright, even assuming the sitting posture. In paroxysmal nocturnal dyspnea (PND), patients awake from sleep with breathlessness and often sit at the side of the bed for relief. These symptoms are thought to be due to increased positional dependence of pulmonary congestion resulting from the recumbent position. A dry, nonproductive cough may occur, which can be indistinguishable from an ACE inhibitor–induced cough. Wheezing and Cheyne-Stokes respirations may also occur.

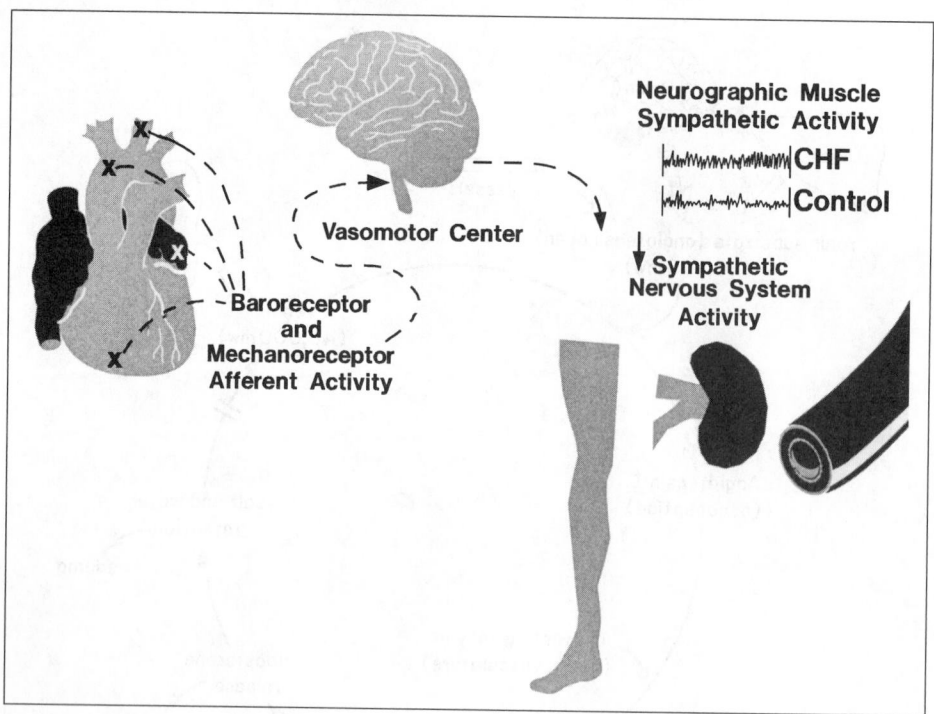

FIGURE 19-10   The relationship of abnormal baroreceptor function to neuroendocrine activation and regional blood flow in heart failure. Increases in atrial and ventricular filling pressure or increased mean arterial pressure or pulse pressure normally stimulate cardiopulmonary and arterial baroreceptors to send inhibitory signals to the medullary vasomotor center, which then suppresses sympathetic efferent activity and increased vagal efferent activity (not shown). In heart failure this baroreflex inhibition is blunted, with a resultant increase in activation of the sympathetic and renin-angiotensin systems, with increased release of arginine vasopressin. As a consequence, limb and renal vasoconstriction ensue, and there is accompanying renal retention of sodium and water. (Modified from Hirsch AT, Dzau VJ, Creager MA: *Circulation* 75[suppl IV]:IV-36, 1987.)

In the most advanced stages of heart failure, sleeping may become impossible and this may be the chief complaint. Patients fall asleep, but soon awaken, not due to PND, and are unable to return to sleep. Inability to sleep soundly and loss of appetite are more often symptoms of very severe heart failure and are frequently resistant to therapy.

Patients with heart failure complain of fatigue. The sensation of fatigue is nonspecific and, like dyspnea, is complex and not well understood. In the past fatigue has been regarded as a function of low cardiac output, and this likely is an important mechanism in severe, end-stage heart failure. In more mild forms of chronic, ambulatory heart failure, however, there is little evidence of reduced skeletal muscle blood flow at rest or during exercise. Drugs that acutely and chronically improve blood flow do not consistently improve exercise capacity or reduce fatigue. However, oxygen supply to exercising muscles is limited, and the vasodilatory reserve to large muscle groups is impaired. Chronic severe heart failure reduces lean body mass, and skeletal muscle mitochondrial oxidative enzymes are decreased. Abnormalities of muscle histology, ultrastructure, and biochemistry are similar to those observed in deconditioning. Psychologic factors can be important, and a mild state of situational depression may contribute to physical inactivity. It is possible that limited physical activity simply leads to a state of deconditioning, which then further retards muscle activity. Disuse atrophy may eventually play a major role in the fatigue experienced by patients with heart failure. While exhibiting significant atrophy, however, patients with heart failure usually have relatively well-preserved strength. At least some skeletal muscle abnormalities appear not to be characteristic of disuse alone. Patients with heart failure can become better conditioned with exercise training programs, and ambulatory patients should be encouraged to stay as active as possible.

Right upper quadrant pain, abdominal fullness, and even nausea and vomiting may occur as a consequence of fluid accumulation in the peritoneal cavity and bowel, but these are relatively late symptoms or occur during acute decompensation.

Physical Findings

Particular attention should be directed at the jugular veins, the lungs, the heart, the abdomen, and the lower extremities. Today, in an era when loop diuretics and ACE inhibitors are in common use, it is rare to see a patient who has not received some prior treatment. The cardinal features such as jugular venous distention, rales, an S3 gallop, and edema may be absent in compensated heart failure. Of course, pedal edema is very nonspecific and may be from Ca^{++} channel blocker treatment or previous coronary artery bypass surgery, but it is often the first abnormal physical finding noted by the patient.

In untreated or undertreated heart failure, elevated jugular venous pressure is present either at rest or during provocative maneuvers. Patients with heart disease are examined most effectively in the 45 degree position. The internal jugular vein is deep and is not normally visible as a discrete structure; however, it is visible when there is severe venous hypertension such as in uncompensated heart failure. Its pulsations are transmitted and usually are visible. Careful visual inspection of the neck is required to identify the level above which the venous pulsation is absent. The upper limit of normal is 4 cm above the sternal angle. Because the right atrium is approximately 5 cm below the sternal angle, the upper limit of normal venous pressure corresponds to a central venous pressure of approximately 8 cm H_2O (Chapter 11).

Simple maneuvers can be used to test right ventricular response to a volume challenge. Applying firm pressure to the periumbilical region for 10 to 30 seconds with the patient breathing quietly will normally raise venous pressure less than 3 cm H_2O, and this occurs only transiently. Heart failure causes a sustained increase in jugular venous pressure, which remains elevated until the abdominal pressure is withdrawn. Positive abdominal-jugular reflux may occur in heart failure, even when resting jugular pressure is normal. Passive leg raising and exercise can also increase jugular venous pressure in patients with heart failure.

In chronic heart failure, considerable dyspnea may exist in the absence of rales. Characteristically, however, an elevated pulmonary capillary wedge pressure is associated with fine rales over the lung bases. The threshold at which extravasation of interstitial lung fluid occurs and rales appear is highly variable and dependent on the chronicity of the increased filling pressure. Pleural effusions may reflect more chronic elevation of cardiac filling pressure. Unilateral pleural effusions in heart failure are more often on the right side. Small airways may be compromised, leading to wheezing and bronchospasm. In acute pulmonary edema, rales and rhonchi are usually heard throughout the lung fields.

The cardiac examination should be carried out in both the supine and left lateral decubitus position. In heart failure, when there is cardiomegaly, the apex impulse is often sustained and displaced and may occupy two interspaces. A palpable A wave (S4) and S3 gallop are frequently present. Auscultation for heart sounds, gallops, clicks, and murmurs is standard. An S3 is usually audible most clearly at the apex with the patient in the left lateral decubitus position. A murmur of mitral regurgitation radiating to the axilla is frequently present in heart failure. Tricuspid regurgitation, although present on echocardiography, is sometimes inaudible (Chapter 11).

Palpation of the carotid, brachial, and femoral arteries to evaluate the contour of the arterial pulse wave is also performed. The abdomen should be carefully palpated. Often the liver is enlarged in patients with heart failure and may be quite tender when acute passive congestion is present. The spleen is less commonly palpable. Ascites may be present and for some patients is the dominant location for fluid collection. Not uncommonly patients will sense an increase in abdominal girth in the absence of obvious ascites. Gross ascites, as seen in end-stage liver disease, can occur in heart failure but is uncommon in this era of modern treatment. Peripheral edema is highly variable, with some patients never manifesting any trace of leg edema despite severe heart failure whereas others demonstrate pedal edema as one of the earliest signs of heart failure.

LABORATORY AND OTHER DIAGNOSTIC TESTS
Chest Radiograph

A standard posteroanterior (PA) and lateral chest film should be performed in every patient suspected of having heart failure. Cardiac chamber enlargement and plethoric pulmonary vasculature may help establish the diagnosis (Fig. 19-11). The chest radiograph, however, may occasionally be normal in patients with heart failure, such as those with pure diastolic dysfunction, and is therefore not sensitive enough to exclude the diagnosis. Moreover, the range of normal cardiac silhouette size is quite wide, so that apparent cardiomegaly on chest radiograph may be absent on echocardiography. Cardiomegaly is said to be present on chest radiograph when the cardiac silhouette in the posteroanterior projection is greater than half the total thoracic diameter. Enlargement of the cardiac silhouette can be due to right, left, or biventricular enlargement. With heart failure one can see perihilar engorgement of the pulmonary vasculature, cephalization of pulmonary vascular markings, and sometimes haziness at the bases, suggesting a pleural effusion, which occurs more often on the right. Fluid in the interlobar septa in the lung periphery may be demonstrated as 1-cm horizontal markings at the edge of the lung fields (Kerley B lines). When pulmonary edema ensues, alveolar fluid is present with perihilar confluent infiltrates in a "butterfly" pattern. There is a very weak relation between cardiothoracic ratio and left ventricular ejection fraction, although both variables have important prognostic implications.

Echocardiography and Radionuclide Ventriculography

Every patient with heart failure should have an echocardiogram performed to assess LV size and function, as well as valvular morphology and function. This form of imaging is necessary to distinguish systolic from diastolic dysfunction, which have major therapeutic and prognostic differences. Echo will also indicate whether valvular stenosis or insufficiency is present, which may be silent or difficult to diagnose by conventional bedside techniques. Pericardial effusion, myxoma, hypertrophic cardiomyopathy, regional wall motion abnormalities, and unsuspected severe aortic stenosis or mitral insufficiency can be diagnosed by Doppler echocardiography (Chapter 13). It remains the cornerstone of diagnostic tests. Other imaging techniques

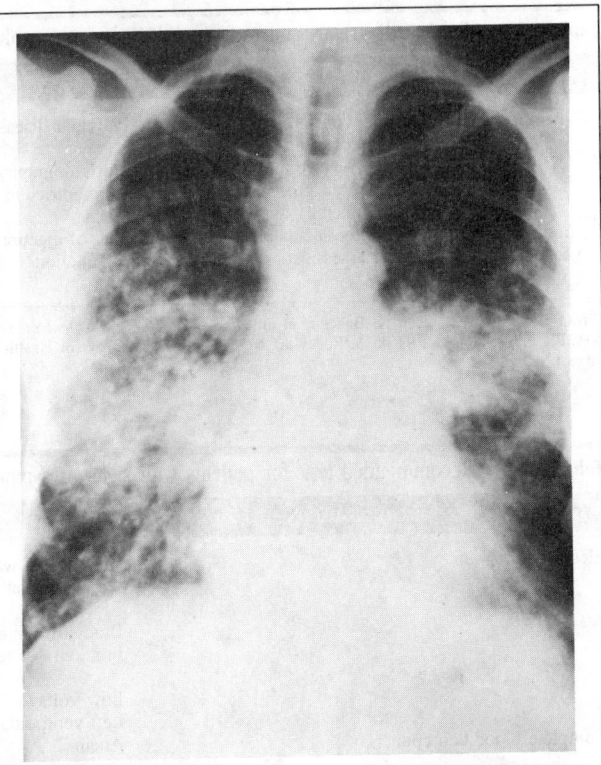

A

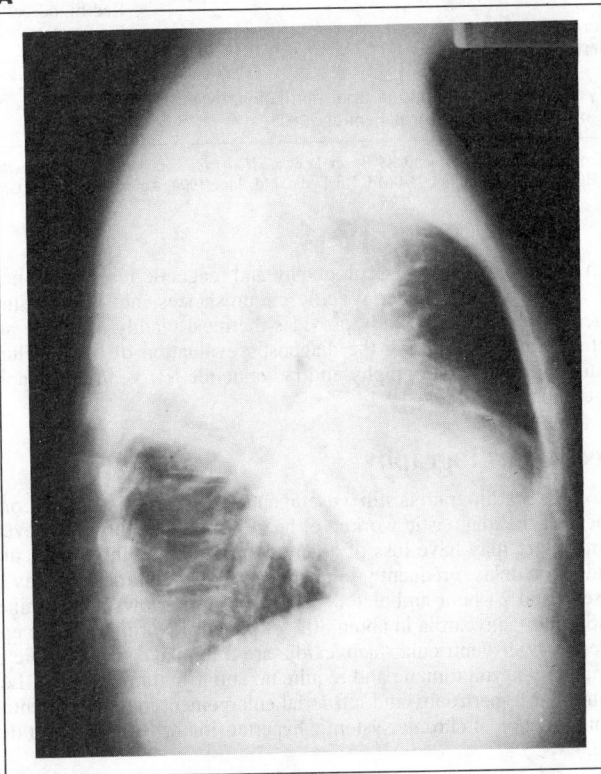

B

FIGURE 19-11   **A,** Posterior and **B,** lateral chest radiographs of a patient in heart failure. There is cardiac enlargement, which is seen on the lateral projection as primarily left ventricular. Lung fields demonstrate the typical butterfly pattern of pulmonary edema.

Table 19-1   Echocardiography and radionuclide ventriculography compared in evaluation of left-ventricular performance

TEST	ADVANTAGES	DISADVANTAGES
Echocardiogram	Permits concomitant assessment of valvular disease, left ventricular hypertrophy, and left atrial size Less expensive than radionuclide ventriculography in most areas Able to detect pericardial effusion and ventricular thrombus More generally available	Difficult to perform in patients with lung disease Usually only semiquantitative estimate of ejection fraction provided Technically inadequate in up to 18% of patients under optimal circumstances
Radionuclide ventriculogram	More precise and reliable measurement of ejection fraction Better assessment of right ventricular function	Requires venipuncture and radiation exposure Limited assessment of valvular heart disease and left ventricular hypertrophy

(From Konstam M, Dracup K, Baker D et al: *Heart failure: management of patients with left-ventricular systolic dysfunction.* Quick Reference Guide for Clinicians No. 11. AHCPR Publication No. 94-0613. Rockville, Md, June 1994, Agency for Health Care Policy and Research, Public Health Service, U.S. Department of Health and Human Services.)

Table 19-2   Recommended tests for patients with signs or symptoms of heart failure

TEST RECOMMENDATION	FINDING	SUSPECTED DIAGNOSIS
Electrocardiogram	Acute ST-T wave changes	Myocardial ischemia
	Atrial fibrillation, other tachyarrhythmia	Thyroid disease or heart failure from rapid ventricular rate
	Bradyarrhythmias	Heart failure from low heart rate
	Previous MI (e.g., Q waves)	Heart failure from reduced left-ventricular performance
	Low voltage	Pericardial effusion
	Left ventricular hypertrophy	Diastolic dysfunction
Complete blood cell count	Anemia	Heart failure due to or aggravated by decreased oxygen-carrying capacity
Urinalysis	Proteinuria	Nephrotic syndrome
	Red blood cells or cellular casts	Glomerulonephritis
Serum creatinine	Elevated	Volume overload from renal failure
Serum albumin	Decreased	Increased extravascular volume due to hypoalbuminemia
T_4 and TSH (obtain only if atrial fibrillation, evidence of thyroid disease, or patient age >65)	Abnormal T_4 or TSH	Heart failure caused by or aggravated by hypothyroidism or hyperthyroidism

(From Konstam M, Dracup K, Baker D et al. *Heart failure: management of patients with left-ventricular systolic dysfunction.* Quick Reference Guide for Clinicians No. 11. AHCPR Publication No. 94-0613. Rockville, Md, June 1994, Agency for Health Care Policy and Research, Public Health Service, US Department of Health and Human Services.)

such as radionuclide ventriculography and magnetic resonance imaging may be helpful under specific circumstances, but the transthoracic Doppler echo probably provides the most readily available and useful information during the diagnostic evaluation of heart failure. Features of echocardiography and radionuclide left ventriculography are compared in Table 19-1.

Electrocardiography

The electrocardiogram is still a useful and relatively inexpensive component of the diagnostic workup of heart failure. Patients with severe heart failure may have loss of anterior forces and an intraventricular conduction delay. Frequent premature ventricular contractions may be present, and 24-hour ambulatory ECG recording shows nonsustained ventricular tachycardia in about 30% of patients. Normally, these episodes of brief ventricular tachycardia are minimally symptomatic or completely asymptomatic and require no antiarrhythmic therapy. Left ventricular hypertrophy and left atrial enlargement may be present as a consequence of chronic systemic hypertension or valvular heart disease.

Routine Laboratory Tests

There are no blood tests specific for the diagnosis of heart failure. Routine laboratory work usually ordered during the evaluation of a new patient with chronic heart failure should include the following:
1. Complete blood cell count (CBC) and urinalysis
2. Blood serum: electrolytes, BUN, creatinine, glucose, phosphorus, magnesium, calcium, and albumin levels
3. Thyroid-stimulating hormone (TSH) level in patients with atrial fibrillation and unexplained heart failure

Recommended routine tests are outlined in Table 19-2.

Plasma norepinephrine levels and plasma atrial natriuretic factor are almost always elevated in patients with heart failure and may have important pathophysiologic and prognostic implications. The sympathetic nervous system is activated early in the syndrome, and the renin-angiotensin-aldosterone system appears to be activated later in the disease process. Measurement of these neurohormone levels is not routine and is not part of the standard diagnostic workup for heart failure, although it remains an area of intense research interest.

Exercise Testing

It should be recognized that today many patients have heart failure in the absence of pulmonary rales or pedal edema. So-called noncongestive heart failure requires a very careful history and objective physical examination, coupled with a Doppler-echo examination to verify LV dysfunction. Assessment of exercise tolerance can be very difficult and cannot be assumed by knowledge of LV function. There is only a very weak relation between LV function and exercise tolerance in patients with heart failure (Fig. 19-12). Yet knowledge of functional capacity is crucial because it has a major impact on patient well-being and quality of life. Functional capacity is also an important predictor of mortality in patients with heart failure and may help guide therapy, including potential surgical approaches. Exercise testing with gas analysis to determine maximal oxygen consumption ($VO_{2\ max}$) is the preferred format for determining functional capacity and is necessary when considering patients as potential candidates for heart transplantation. Patients with heart failure should undergo a bicycle or treadmill exercise test using a gradually incremental workload such as the Naughton or modified Naughton protocol. Normal individuals under the age of 60 should be able to achieve a $VO_{2\ max}$ of at least 25 ml/kg/min, whereas over the age of 60, a $VO_{2\ max}$ of

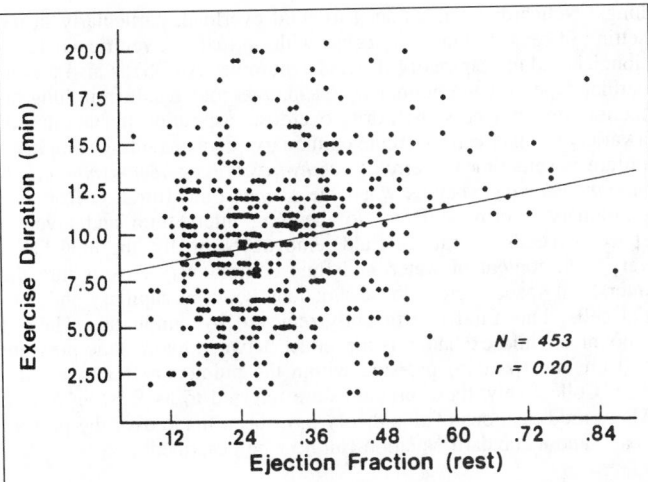

FIGURE 19-12 V-HeFT-I data indicating the relationship between baseline resting ejection fraction and exercise duration by bicycle ergometry in patients with heart failure. The weak relation between exercise capacity and resting left ventricular function has been repeatedly demonstrated in patients with heart failure.

(Modified from Francis GS. In Shaver JA, editor: *Cardiomyopathies: clinical presentation, differential diagnosis, and management,* Philadelphia, 1988, FA Davis.)

greater than 20ml/kg/min should be anticipated. Values below this are consistent with the diagnosis of heart failure.

PATIENT AND FAMILY COUNSELING; NEED FOR HOSPITALIZATION

Patients with heart failure should be informed about their diagnosis, including what to do if symptoms worsen (Box 19-3). Prognosis, activity level, diet, medications, and compliance need to be discussed in some detail. Heart failure is a lethal syndrome with a prognosis worse than that for many types of cancer. Many heart failure centers specialize in treating such patients and have extensive ancillary resources for patients to draw on. Some patients may need hospitalization when first seen or when seen for follow-up, especially if the following findings are present:

- Clinical or ECG evidence of acute ischemia
- Pulmonary edema or respiratory distress, oxygen saturation <90%
- Complicating other medical illness (e.g., pneumonia, renal failure)
- Anasarca
- Symptomatic hypotension or syncope
- Symptoms refractory to outpatient therapy
- Inadequate social support for safe outpatient management

CARDIAC CATHETERIZATION

In some cases cardiac catheterization and coronary angiography are necessary. There is still not uniform agreement as to which patients benefit most from such invasive studies. It is of some importance to know if coronary artery disease is present, as revascularization may benefit selected patients. Patients with angina should undergo cardiac catheterization and coronary angiography if they are otherwise candidates for interventional procedures. Patients with advanced heart failure frequently have severe coronary artery disease but no angina pectoris. Dyspnea on exertion, however, may be an anginal equivalent. It may be impossible to know by simple clinical assessment in many cases whether underlying coronary artery disease is present, thus prompting diagnostic coronary angiography. If severe coronary artery disease coexists with heart failure, further imaging studies with isotope perfusion scanning (e.g., thallium 201) or dobutamine echocardiography may be necessary to determine whether hypokinetic heart muscle is hibernating but will respond to revascularization.

Patients with severe end-stage heart failure refractory to outpatient therapy are frequently admitted to the intensive care unit for hemo-

BOX 19-3
Suggested topics for patient, family, and caregiver education and counseling

General counseling
Explanation of heart failure and the reason for symptoms
Cause or probable cause of heart failure
Expected symptoms
Symptoms of worsening heart failure
What to do if symptoms worsen
Self-monitoring with daily weights
Explanation of treatment/care plan
Clarification of patient's responsibilities
Importance of cessation of tobacco use
Role of family members or other caregivers in the treatment/care plan
Availability and value of qualified local support group
Importance of obtaining vaccinations against influenza and pneumococcal disease
Prognosis
　Life expectancy
　Advance directives
　Advice for family members in the event of sudden death
Activity Recommendations
　Recreation, leisure, and work activity
　Exercise
　Sex, sexual difficulties, and coping strategies
Dietary Recommendations
　Sodium restriction
　Avoidance of excessive fluid intake
　Fluid restriction (if required)
　Alcohol restriction
Medications
　Effects of medications on quality of life and survival
　Dosing
　Likely side effects and what to do if they occur
　Coping mechanisms for complicated medical regimens
　Availability of lower cost medications or financial assistance
Importance of Compliance with the Treatment/Care Plan

(From Konstam M, Dracup K, Baker D et al. *Heart failure: management of patients with left-ventricular systolic dysfunction.* Quick Reference Guide for Clinicians No. 11. AHCPR Publication No. 94-0613. Rockville, Md, June 1994, Agency for Health Care Policy and Research, Public Health Service, U.S. Department of Health and Human Services.)

dynamic monitoring and to assess therapy. Insertion of a Swan-Ganz catheter is extremely useful in such patients in guiding acute therapy. In general, these are patients with severe symptoms refractory to diuretics who are failing outpatient therapy. Hemodynamic monitoring has proven to be indispensable in the care of these critically ill patients. Short-term use of dobutamine, milrinone, and nitroprusside may be helpful. Such patients are often referred to a Heart Failure Center experienced in the care of the severely ill heart failure patient.

DIASTOLIC HEART FAILURE

The majority of patients with heart failure have an enlarged heart and severe systolic dysfunction, but a large segment of patients with heart failure, perhaps as many as 30%, have the syndrome of pure *diastolic heart failure.* Nearly all patients with systolic heart failure have some element of diastolic dysfunction. Part of the enigma of pure diastolic heart failure lies in the lack of clear definition. There is no uniformly agreed on definition, and diastolic heart failure therefore is a clinical diagnosis of exclusion made when the patient has all of the hallmarks of heart failure but has normal systolic function. Often times patients with pure diastolic dysfunction are elderly, hypertensive women with normal or small hearts and a normal ejection fraction. Not infrequently, severe mitral regurgitation is present and causally related to the heart failure. Because the management of patients with pure diastolic heart failure is very different than that of systolic heart failure, it is critical to make the distinction.

Diastolic dysfunction impairs ventricular filling by diminishing relaxation or reducing compliance of the left ventricle, or both. The hemodynamic consequences include elevation of left ventricular filling pressure and pulmonary venous and pulmonary capillary wedge pressure engorgement. Causes of pure diastolic heart failure include myocardial ischemia, left ventricular hypertrophy of any etiology, and occasionally infiltrative processes of the heart such as amyloid deposition. Patients with diastolic heart failure may have coronary artery disease, systemic hypertension, diabetes mellitus, aortic stenosis, hypertrophic cardiomyopathy, or infiltrative cardiomyopathy. It is likely that a decrease in ventricular compliance also occurs as part of a normal aging process.

Doppler echocardiography and radionuclide imaging are of value in assessing systolic function and detecting diastolic dysfunction. Cardiac catheterization may be useful and is particularly of value when noninvasive studies are nondiagnostic.

The treatment of diastolic heart failure remains controversial, and there is no uniform agreement regarding therapy. If the patient is hypertensive, control of blood pressure is essential. ACE inhibitors and calcium channel blockers may be useful in this regard. β-adrenergic blocking agents tend to slow the heart rate and improve left ventricular filling characteristics. In general, the prognosis of patients with pure diastolic heart failure is better than that of patients with systolic heart failure, but the treatment may be difficult.

DIFFERENTIAL DIAGNOSIS

The differential diagnosis of heart failure is expansive and includes chronic obstructive lung disease, asthma, pulmonary embolus, constrictive pericarditis, or virtually any other clinical condition producing breathlessness and/or fatigue. The primary goal of the clinician is to determine whether the heart is making a major contribution to the symptoms. Because heart failure is such a common syndrome, it may coexist with other diagnoses known to cause shortness of breath, such as chronic obstructive lung disease. In addition to a careful history and physical examination, the echocardiogram with Doppler interrogation of the heart should be performed. In patients who have severe, chronic, breathlessness, obstructive airway disease and heart failure both may contribute to dyspnea and fatigue. In such cases, a cardiopulmonary exercise test with gas exchange and pulmonary function tests are useful in determining which entity is dominantly affecting the patient. Patients with severe obstructive lung disease generally fail to reach an anaerobic threshold during exercise, whereas patients with heart failure usually achieve anaerobic threshold, albeit at an earlier point in the exercise test than normal subjects. VO_{2max} is typically reduced in heart failure. The combination of Doppler echocardiography, cardiopulmonary exercise testing with gas analysis, and pulmonary function tests are usually sufficient to distinguish severe lung disease from congestive heart failure. Pulmonary function tests alone, however, may be insufficient because patients with heart failure frequently demonstrate abnormalities of pulmonary function such as restrictive defects and small airway obstruction.

THE TREATMENT OF CONGESTIVE HEART FAILURE
Acute Pulmonary Edema

Few disorders in medicine are as common as pulmonary edema. The high incidence stems in part from the high prevalence of heart failure and its tendency to produce severe pulmonary venous hypertension. Moreover, acute pulmonary edema is a true cardiac emergency and needs to be treated promptly. The mortality rate associated with acute pulmonary edema remains about 10%. The fundamental problem is a disturbance of fluid transport across capillary endothelium within the lungs, resulting in an abnormal accumulation of fluid. It occurs as the result of a variety of clinical settings and has many causes. Like heart failure, pulmonary edema should be considered a clinical syndrome rather than a specific etiologic entity.

As with chronic heart failure, the treatment of acute pulmonary edema is predicated on an understanding of the pathogenesis of the syndrome. Management will vary greatly depending on the underlying mechanism of the abnormal accumulation of fluid within the lungs. Noncardiac causes such as fluid overload, particularly in the setting of renal failure, may occur with normal left ventricular function. The adult respiratory distress syndrome (ARDS) is also a noncardiac type of acute pulmonary edema that may result from lung infection, generalized sepsis, drug overdose, aspiration pneumonia, or a variety of other causes. Acute pulmonary edema resulting from heart failure is sometimes referred to as *hydrostatic* or *hemodynamic pulmonary edema*. It begins when the rate of fluid filtration from the pulmonary microvasculature to the lung interstitium and alveolar spaces exceeds the rate of fluid removal. Normally, the lung has a very high content of water, and fluid continuously crosses into the interstitial spaces across loose junctions between capillary endothelial cells. This fluid is efficiently removed by lymphatics. The net amount of fluid exchange is a product between hydrostatic pressure and oncotic (protein) pressure within the pulmonary microvasculature. Collectively, these pressures are referred to as *Starling forces*. Many modifications of this theory have been made over the past 90 years, and a standard equation can now be described:

$$\text{(EQ.2)}$$
$$Q_F = K[(P_{cap} - P_{is}) - \sigma(\P_{pl} - \P_{is})]$$

where Q_F = net fluid exchange, K = membrane filtration coefficient, P_{cap} = capillary hydrostatic pressure, P_{is} = interstitial hydrostatic pressure, σ = reflection coefficient, $\P_{pl}$ = plasma oncotic pressure, and $\P_{is}$ = interstitial oncotic pressure.

Oncotic pressure opposes hydrostatic pressure. Capillary osmotic pressure (about 25 mm Hg) is normally greater than capillary hydrostatic pressure (approximately 10 mm Hg), although there is no flow of fluid into the vascular space. On the contrary, under normal conditions there is a net movement of fluid from the intervascular to the interstitial space. This is possible because the interstitial hydrostatic pressure is negative and the interstitial oncotic pressure is close to the capillary oncotic pressure, resulting in a net Starling force from vascular to interstitial space.

The most common cause of increased capillary hydrostatic pressure leading to acute pulmonary edema is left ventricular heart failure. Specific causes include acute myocardial infarction, severe and uncontrolled systemic hypertension, acute and chronic valvular heart disease, and decompensation of a previously stable cardiomyopathic condition. Virtually any form of heart disease can lead to heart failure, and therefore acute pulmonary edema is potential from many etiologies.

Patients with pulmonary edema are often severely breathless and are unable to give a clear and detailed history. They appear pale and diaphoretic and are nearly always tachypneic. Fine rales are often heard throughout all lung fields. The chest radiograph is normally confirmatory, and right heart catheterization is not usually necessary. It is important to recognize that patients with chronic heart failure may tolerate increased pulmonary capillary wedge pressure for long periods of time. For example, patients with chronic mitral stenosis are notorious for tolerating very high pulmonary capillary wedge pressure, often exceeding values that under normal conditions would produce acute pulmonary edema.

In my experience the usual precipitating causes of acute pulmonary edema include the sudden onset of rapid atrial arrhythmias, acute myocardial ischemia with mitral regurgitation, dietary indiscretion, noncompliance with medications, and the use of nonsteroidal antiinflammatory drugs. In many cases, however, undertreated chronic heart failure may simply progress to acute pulmonary edema in a slow and insidious fashion.

Management of Acute Pulmonary Edema

The most important treatment for acute pulmonary edema is to lower the hydrostatic pulmonary microvasculature pressure. The usual first-line treatment is intravenous loop diuretics such as furosemide or bumetanide. Noncardiac causes of pulmonary edema should always be excluded. Although the treatment of acute pulmonary edema usually occurs in the emergency room or accident ward, without exception all patients require hospital admission.

It is important to quickly exclude causes of acute heart failure that can be treated by special therapeutic approaches. An electrocardiogram should be promptly performed to exclude acute myocardial infarction or injury, a high degree of atrial-ventricular (AV) block, or ventricular tachycardia. Pericardial tamponade and acute pulmonary embolism should be considered and excluded when appropriate. A secure intravenous catheter should be placed, and blood should be obtained for essential laboratory studies. Patients should be placed on oxygen therapy. Sublingual nitroglycerin, 0.4 to 0.6 mg, should be given every 5 to 10 minutes as needed, provided that the patient is not severely hypotensive. If systemic blood pressure is acceptable (i.e., >90 mm Hg systolic), nitroglycerin can be administered intravenously with a starting dose of 0.3 to 0.5 μg/kg/min. Patients who are hypertensive should have sodium nitroprusside begun at a dose of 0.1 μg/kg/min. Nitroprusside, which has balanced arteriolar and venodilator effects, is also particularly useful when pulmonary edema is attributable to severe mitral or aortic valve regurgitation. It can be quickly titrated over 20 to 30 minutes to target a fall in blood pressure to 85 to 100 mm Hg systolic. If a balloon pulmonary artery catheter is in place, the wedge pressure should be lowered to 15 mm Hg, provided the blood pressure remains adequate.

The initial dose of furosemide is sometimes difficult to determine, but probably 20 to 80 mg should be given intravenously as soon as the diagnosis of acute pulmonary edema is suspected. Patients with chronic renal insufficiency may require a higher dose of loop diuretic. A Foley catheter is frequently helpful to accurately assess urine output. Morphine sulfate, 3 to 5 mg intravenously, is effective in ameliorating many of the symptoms of acute pulmonary edema (e.g., anxiety, breathlessness, diaphoresis) but must be used with caution in patients who have concomitant chronic obstructive lung disease with respiratory or metabolic acidosis. If chronic airway disease is suspected, arterial blood gases should be analyzed. Intubation and mechanical ventilation are a value in selected patients with severe hypoxemia or respiratory acidosis that does not respond readily to therapy.

In most cases, patients with acute pulmonary edema can be stabilized in the emergency room or ward and then transported to the intensive care unit for further treatment. Placement of a pulmonary artery balloon catheter should be considered if the patient is hypotensive and/or deteriorating or requires dopamine to augment systemic blood pressure. If there is uncertainty regarding the diagnosis of hydrostatic acute pulmonary edema, a pulmonary artery balloon catheter may be highly instructive.

After the patient is comfortably stabilized, a transthoracic Doppler echocardiogram should be performed unless the patient's status has recently been adequately evaluated. Depending on the urgency for confirming or establishing the diagnosis, echocardiography should be performed as soon as possible after initial stabilization. In some cases, transesophageal echocardiography may be required to diagnose and define certain types of lesions such as aortic dissection, ruptured chordae tendineae, or acute bacterial endocarditis. Conditions such as acute pericardial tamponade, massive pulmonary embolism, ruptured chordae tendineae or papillary muscles, ruptured intraventricular septum, critical aortic stenosis, acute aortic regurgitation, and aortic dissection can all be diagnosed by echocardiography. As with chronic heart failure, the echocardiogram remains the cornerstone of diagnosis.

The successful treatment of acute pulmonary edema is very gratifying, and patients often manifest prompt alleviation of their severe symptoms. Follow-up care is largely predicated on the precipitating cause of the acute problem. Most patients typically remain in the intensive care unit for 24 to 48 hours followed by several days of convalescence in the hospital. Recurrent, *flash* pulmonary edema is a severe form of acute heart failure that often requires diagnostic cardiac catheterization and coronary angiography. The prognosis of patients with recurrent flash pulmonary edema is very poor.

Treatment of the Ambulatory Patient with Chronic Heart Failure

Once the diagnosis of heart failure is secure, it is the physician's responsibility to determine the primary goals of therapy and quickly move to relieve symptoms and improve the quality of life. Heart failure is an exceedingly common and lethal clinical condition, and it is important to gain the patient's confidence early and spend considerable time counseling the patient and the family (see Box 19-3). Non-

pharmacologic, pharmacologic, and surgical approaches to management should all be considered. Nonpharmacologic treatment includes restriction of sodium to <2 g/day, weight loss (if there is excessive weight), and dietary supplementation of potassium. Regular dynamic exercise should be encouraged. It is now well known that patients with heart failure can safely undergo physical conditioning programs and may actually demonstrate modest improvement in left ventricular function. However, the primary goal of having the patient exercise on a regular basis is to maintain adequate skeletal muscle mass and to condition the skeletal muscles. Isometric exercise (work against gravity) should be discouraged, since it places an acute afterload stress on the left ventricle and is usually poorly tolerated. Patients should be discouraged from any sort of heavy lifting or working with their arms held above their heads. Depression is a common manifestation of chronic heart failure and should be recognized and treated.

Diuretics

Although not all patients exhibit congestion or edema, eventually signs and symptoms of circulatory congestion do develop, and at that point diuretic therapy becomes mandatory. The need for diuretic therapy should be determined by observing elevated jugular venous pressure and/or truncal or pedal edema. Pulmonary rales or chest radiograph evidence of lung congestion is also an indication for diuretic therapy. Loop diuretics are traditionally prescribed, and thiazides may be ineffective if glomerular filtration is markedly reduced. Nearly all patients will require supplemental potassium chloride, usually in the range of 20 to 60 mEq/day. In some cases, potassium-sparing agents may be used in lieu of potassium chloride (Table 19-3). In advanced heart failure, diuretics may not be very well absorbed, and intravenous loop diuretics may be necessary on a temporary basis. Typically furosemide is prescribed at 10 to 40 mg once or twice a day (see Table 19-3). If large doses of diuretics become necessary, patients should be queried about their salt intake. The most common cause of diuretic resistance is excessive salt intake.

It is often appropriate to augment the loop diuretic with a second diuretic that has an alternative mechanism of action. Metolazone administered in a dose of 2.5 or 5 mg 30 minutes to 1 hour before the oral administration of furosemide can sometimes greatly augment the diuresis in patients who are resistant to furosemide alone; however, severe hypokalemia and volume depletion may occur with this strategy. It is prudent therefore to use supplemental metolazone on an intermittent rather than on a regular basis. One strategy is to have patients weigh themselves daily. If they gain 3 or more pounds or feel particularly congested, supplemental metolazone might be added for 1 to 3 days and then stopped. Patients should be cautioned that a profound diuresis may occur, necessitating the intake of additional potassium chloride. Home measurements of daily morning weight can provide a useful guide to the need for altering the diuretic dosage. If the patient is being sequentially followed in the clinic, careful evaluation of the jugular venous pressure is perhaps the most sensitive guide toward alteration in diuretic dose.

Patients who become volume depleted on diuretics often develop prerenal azotemia. A small increase in BUN may occur when diuretic therapy is increased, which is often an acceptable consequence of heightened diuretic dosage. Signs of more severe volume depletion may require a reduction in diuretic dose. Usually such patients need to be seen frequently in clinic.

Angiotensin-Converting Enzyme Inhibitors

Perhaps the most exciting development in the treatment of heart failure the last two decades has been the emergence of angiotensin-converting (ACE) inhibitors. More than any other therapy, these drugs have proved to be safe and effective and have the potential to prolong survival. The only contraindications to a trial of ACE inhibitors include shock, angioneurotic edema, or significant hyperkalemia. Mild asymptomatic hypotension is not a contraindication to ACE inhibitor therapy, since many patients with advanced heart failure have systolic blood pressures in the range of 70 to 90 mm Hg. Nevertheless, clinical judgment must always govern such therapeutic decisions. In general, low doses should be started, and the ACE inhibitor should be gradually titrated to the maximal doses used in the various large clinical trials. This titration should take place over several weeks. Numerous randomized, placebo-controlled, multicenter studies have been performed over the last two decades in support of this strategy (Table 19-4) (V-HeFT II, CONSENSUS I, SOLVD). Even patients who are New York Heart Association (NYHA) functional Class I may benefit from the use of ACE inhibitors, which delay the onset of heart failure and thus reduce the need for hospitalization (SOLVD–Prevention Trial). In the SOLVD–Prevention Trial, enalapril significantly reduced the incidence of heart failure and the rate of related hospital admissions compared with placebo. However, survival was not improved in this minimally symptomatic group (Fig. 19-13). The target dose of enalapril that showed survival benefit in the SOLVD–Treat-

ment Trial was 10 mg twice a day (Fig. 19-14). It is unclear whether smaller doses of ACE inhibitors are effective, and physicians are encouraged to titrate the patients up to maximal doses used in the large trials when the drug is well tolerated. A trial of ACE inhibitors is indicated in all patients with congestive heart failure, unless contraindicated.

Patients with more advanced heart failure (New York Heart Association Functional Class III and IV) benefit the most from ACE inhibitors, although all functional classes derive some benefit. ACE inhibitors likely all share the same mechanism of action, but the majority of the data have been derived from the use of enalapril and captopril. Lisinopril (5 to 20 mg/day), quinapril (5 to 20 mg twice a

Table 19-3   Oral medications commonly used for heart failure

DRUG	INITIAL DOSE (mg)	TARGET DOSE (mg)	RECOMMENDED MAXIMAL DOSE (mg)	MAJOR ADVERSE REACTIONS
Thiazide diuretics				
Hydrochlorothiazide	25 qd	As needed	50 qd	Postural hypotension, hypokalemia, hyperglycemia, hyperuricemia, rash. Rare severe reaction includes pancreatitis, bone marrow suppression, and anaphylaxis.
Chlorthalidone	25 qd	As needed	50 qd	
Loop diuretics				
Furosemide	10-40 qd	As needed	240 bid	Same as thiazide diuretics.
Bumetanide	0.5-1.0 qd	As needed	10 qd	
Ethacrynic acid	50 qd	As needed	200 bid	Ototoxicity.
Torsemide	5-20 qd	As needed	20 qd	
Thiazide-related diuretic				
Metolazone	2.5*	As needed	10 qd	Same as thiazide diuretics.
Potassium-sparing diuretics				
Spironolactone	25 qd	As needed	100 bid	Hyperkalemia, especially if administered with ACE inhibitor; rash; gynecomastia (spironolactone only).
Triamterene	50 qd	As needed	100 bid	
Amiloride	5 qd	As needed	40 qd	
ACE inhibitors				
Enalapril	2.5 bid	10 bid	20 bid	Hypotension, hyperkalemia, renal insufficiency, cough, skin rash, angioedema, neutropenia.
Captopril	6.25-12.5 tid	50 tid	100 tid	
Lisinopril	5 qd	20 qd	40 qd	
Quinapril	5 bid	20 bid	20 bid	
Fosinopril	10 qd	20-40 qd	40 qd	
Digoxin	0.125 qd	As needed	As needed	Cardiotoxicity, confusion, nausea, anorexia, visual disturbances.
Hydralazine	10-25 tid	75 tid	100 tid	Headache, nausea, dizziness, tachycardia, lupuslike syndrome.
Isosorbide dinitrate	10 tid	40 tid	80 tid	Headache, hypotension, flushing.

ACE, angiotensin-converting enzyme; *BID*, twice a day; *QD*, once a day; *TID*, three times a day.
*Given as a single test dose initially.

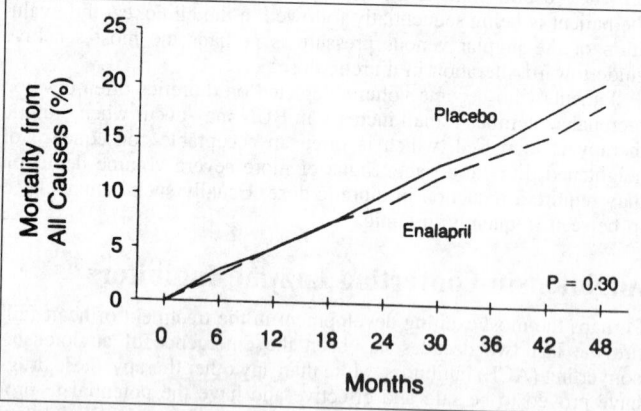

FIGURE 19-13   Total mortality in the SOLVD Prevention Trial. There is no significant difference in mortality between patients randomly assigned to placebo or enalapril. This study included patients with left ventricular dysfunction but no or very minimal symptoms.

(From SOLVD Investigators: *N Engl J Med* 327:685, 1992.)

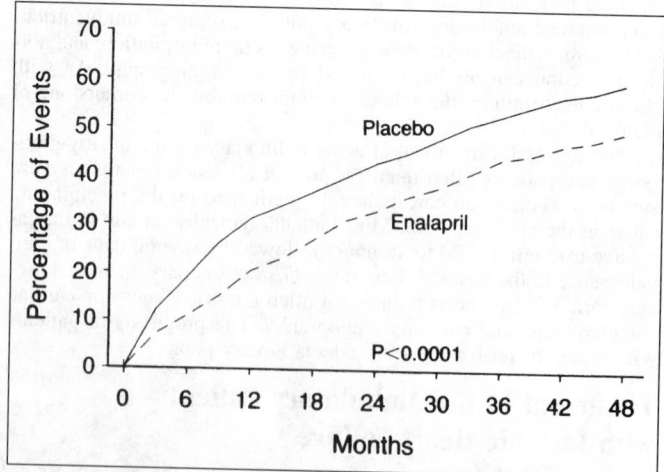

FIGURE 19-14   Mortality curves from the SOLVD Treatment Trial demonstrating the placebo and enalapril groups. There is a statistically significant reduction in mortality in patients randomly assigned to enalapril. The SOLVD Treatment Trial included only patients with symptomatic or overt heart failure.

(From SOLVD Investigators: *N Engl J Med* 325:293, 1991.)

Table 19-4 Randomized, controlled, multicenter survival trials in heart failure

ACRONYM	FULL TITLE	STUDY DRUGS	NYHA CLASS	OUTCOME	PUBLICATION
V-HeFT I	Vasodilator Heart Failure Trial I	Placebo vs. hydralazine and isosorbide dinitrate vs. placebo Background therapy—digitalis and diuretics	II, III	Hydralazine (75 mg qid) and Isosorbide Dinitrate 40 mg qid improved survival	Published: *N Engl J Med* 314:1547-1552, 1986
CONSENSUS I	Cooperative New Scandinavian Enalapril Survival Study	Placebo vs. enalapril 10 mg bid Background therapy—digitalis, diuretics, some vasodilators	IV	Enalapril improved survival (average dose 18.4 mg/day)	Published: *N Engl J Med* 316:1429-1435, 1987
V-HeFT II	Vasodilator Heart Failure Trial II	Enalapril vs. hydralazine and isosorbide dinitrate Background therapy—digitalis, diuretics	II, III	Enalapril 20 mg/day improved survival more than Hyd-Iso. Exercise and EF were improved more by Hyd-Iso	Published: *N Engl J Med* 325:303-310, 1991
SOLVD– Treatment	Studies of Left Ventricular Dysfunction–Treatment	Enalapril 10 mg bid vs. placebo in patients with symptomatic heart failure. Background—digitalis and diuretics	II, III	Enalapril improved survival	Treatment trial published: *N Engl J Med* 325:293-302, 1991
SOLVD– Prevention	Studies of Left Ventricular Dysfunction - Prevention	Enalapril 10 mg bid vs. placebo in asymptomatic patients with EF ≤ 35%	I	Enalapril delayed progression of heart failure, but did not improve survival	Prevention trial published: *N Engl J Med* 327:685-691, 1991
PROMISE	Prospective Randomized Milrinone Survival Evaluation	Milrinone 10 mg qid vs. placebo Background—Digitalis, Diuretics, ACE inhibitors	III, IV	Milrinone increase mortality	Published: *N Engl J Med* 325:1468-1475, 1991
Vesnarinone (OPC–8212)	Vesnarinone (OPC–8212)	Vesnarinone 60 mg/day and 120 mg/day vs. placebo Background—Digoxin, Diuretics, ACE inhibitors	III, IV	Vesnarinone 60 mg/day improved survival, while 160 mg/day increased mortality	Published: *N Engl J Med* 329:149-155, 1993
VEST	Vesnarinone Survival Trial	Vesnarinone 60 mg or 30 mg/day vs. placebo 3500 pts., EF ≤ 30%	III, IV	Vesnarinone increased mortality	Preliminary results reported
PROFILE	Prospective Randomized Flosequinan Longevity Evaluation	Flosequinan 100 mg/day vs. placebo Background—Digoxin, Diuretics, ACE inhibitor	III, IV	Terminated May 1993 from excess mortality with flosequinan	Preliminary results reported
MDC	Metoprolol in Dilated Cardiomyopathy	Metoprolol vs. placebo Dose of metoprolol 100-150 mg daily following slow titration	II, III, IV	Trend for improved survival plus reduced need for heart transplant in patients treated with metoprolol	Published: *Lancet* 342:1441-1446, 1993
BEST	Beta-blocker Evaluation Survival Trial	Bucindolol 6.25 to 200 mg bid vs. placebo; E.F≤35%	III, IV	In progress	
PRAISE	Prospective Randomized Amlodipine Survival Evaluation	Amlodipine (Dihydropyridine) 10 mg/day vs. placebo Background therapy—Digoxin, Diuretics, ACE inhibitors	III, IV	No overall difference in survival vs. placebo; trend for "nonischemic" cardiomyopathy patients to have improved survival	Preliminary results reported
PRAISE II	Prospective Randomized Amlodipine Survival Evaluation II	Amlodipine vs. placebo in patients with nonischemic cardiomyopathy	III, IV	In progress	
CHF–STAT	Congestive Heart Failure Survival Trial of Anti-Arrhythmic Therapy	Amiodarone vs placebo in patients with heart failure and >10 PVCs per hour	I, II, III, IV	No overall difference in survival vs. placebo; trend for patients with nonischemic cardiomyopathy to have improved survival and improved EF	Published: *N Engl J Med* 333:77-82, 1995
GESICA	Group Study of Heart Failure in Argentina	Nonrandomized, placebo-controlled trial of amiodarone (300 mg/day)	II, III, IV	Mortality and hospital admission rate reduced by low-dose amiodarone independent of complex ventricular arrhythmias	Published: *Lancet* 344:493-498, 1994
PRECISE/ MOCHA	Prospective Randomized Evaluation of Carvedilol on Symptoms and Exercise/Multicenter Oral Carvedilol Heart Failure Assessment	Carvedilol vs. placebo	II, III, IV	Significant improvement in survival with carvedilol; pending FDA approval for heart failure	Published: *Circulation* 94:2793-2799, 1996; *Circulation* 94:2807-2816, 1996
FIRST	Flolan International Randomized Survival Trial	IV epoprostenal vs. conventional therapy	IV	Terminated in June 1993 due to increased mortality and clinical deterioration in the epoprostenal group	Preliminary results reported
DIG	Digitalis Investigators Group	Digoxin vs. placebo in stable heart failure. Background therapy—Diuretics and ACE inhibitors; 7788 patients	II, III	No overall effect on mortality; fewer hospitalizations and pump failure deaths with digitalis; trend for more arrhythmic deaths with digitalis	Published: *N Engl J Med* 336:525-533, 1997
ATLAS	Assessment of Treatment With Lisinopril and Survival	Survival study of high vs. low dose lisinopril in moderate to severe CHF	II, III, IV	Completion in 1997	
RALES	Randomized Aldactone Evaluation Study	Placebo vs. spironolactone in patients on triple therapy with digoxin, diuretics, ACE inhibitors	II, III, IV	In progress	

Hyd, hydralazine; *Iso,* isosorbide dinitrate; *CHF,* congestive heart failure.

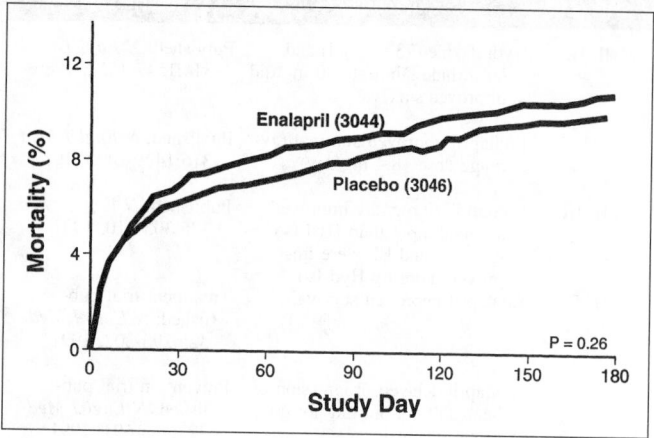

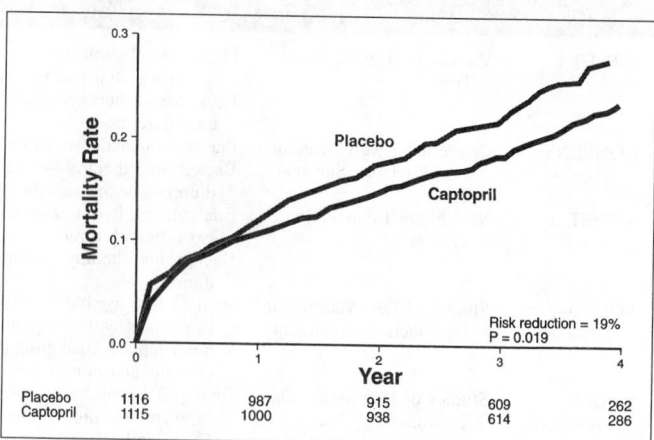

FIGURE 19-15   Kaplan-Meier Life-Table mortality curves for the placebo and enalapril groups in CONSENSUS II. Patients were randomly allocated to either intravenous enalaprilat followed by enalapril or placebo as treatment for acute myocardial infarction. There was no statistically significant difference in mortality between the two therapies.

(From CONSENSUS Trial Study Group: *N Engl J Med* 327:678, 1992.)

FIGURE 19-16   Cumulative mortality from all-cause in the SAVE Trial. Patients were randomly allocated to either placebo or captopril. Entry into the trial required reduced left ventricular function as a complication of acute myocardial infarction. Captopril significantly reduced mortality.

(From Pfeffer MA et al: *N Engl J Med* 327:669, 1992.)

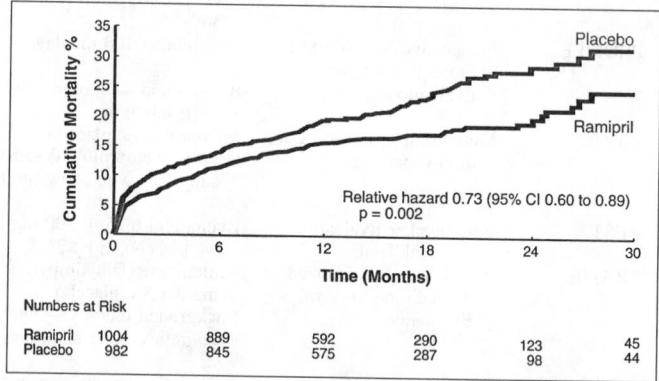

FIGURE 19-17   Mortality curves illustrating the primary endpoint of all-cause mortality analyzed by intention to treat in the AIRE study. Ramipril significantly reduced mortality when compared to placebo in patients with acute myocardial infarction and clinical evidence of heart failure.

(From Acute Infarction Ramipril Efficacy [AIRE] Study Investigators: *Lancet* 342:821, 1993.)

day) and fosinopril (20 to 40 mg/day) have now also been approved for the treatment of heart failure. Although there is far less experience with these last three drugs. It is possible that fosinopril will offer some advantage when there is associated renal dysfunction, since it is partially excreted by the biliary system.

Patients who are severely ill with advanced heart failure and who have modest hypotension should probably have ACE inhibitors initiated in the hospital. If symptomatic hypotension occurs, the legs should be raised and in some cases intravenous fluids may be necessary. Patients with hyponatremia are often markedly hyperreninemic, often as a result of antecedent aggressive diuretic therapy, and are at greater risk to develop hypotension from ACE inhibitors.

Occasionally, dangerous hyperkalemia can occur when using ACE inhibitors, particularly when they are used in combination with potassium-sparing agents or with nonsteroidal antiinflammatory drugs. Likewise, patients with bilateral renal artery stenosis or relative volume depletion may develop abrupt renal insufficiency following the institution of ACE inhibitors. Therefore it is prudent to monitor the volume status, serum potassium, and renal function when instituting such therapy. Although drugs such as spironolactone, triamterene, and amiloride can be used in combination with ACE inhibitors (see Table 19-3), serious hyperkalemia can occasionally occur with these combinations. The medications and their commonly used dosages for the treatment of heart failure are outlined in Table 19-3.

The Use of ACE Inhibitors in Patients with Acute Myocardial Infarction

Several studies have recently been published supporting the use of ACE inhibitor therapy in patients following acute myocardial infarction. The first study, CONSENSUS II, compared intravenous enalaprilat followed by oral enalapril with placebo in patients with acute myocardial infarction. It had a relatively short follow-up period. No statistically significant difference was demonstrated between these two therapies during the brief follow-up period (Fig. 19-15). Subsequently, the SAVE (Survival and Ventricular Enlargement) study trial indicated that captopril given to patients with acute myocardial infarction with an ejection fraction of 40% or less improved survival when compared with placebo (Fig. 19-16). In the SAVE study, captopril was begun an average of 11 days after the onset of acute infarction when patients were clinically stable, and the dose was gradually titrated from 6.25 mg three times a day to 50 mg three times a day over several weeks. Patients with overt heart failure were excluded from SAVE. In the AIRE (Acute Infarction Ramipril Efficacy) study, ramipril 2.5 mg twice a day titrated to 5 mg twice a day or placebo was given to patients 5 to 6 days after the onset of the

infarction with acute myocardial infarction and clinical evidence of heart failure. As in the SAVE study, there was a statistically significant improvement in survival in patients randomly assigned to ramipril (Fig. 19-17). More recently, the ISIS IV (Fourth International Study of Infarct Survival) study and the GISSI III study also indicated improvement in survival in patients randomly assigned to lisinopril after the onset of acute myocardial infarction, and these findings were confirmed in the Chinese Cardiac Study with captopril and with zofenopril and trandolapril in similar large, post-MI trials. There now seems to be no question that selected patients with acute myocardial infarction benefit from the use of an ACE inhibitor. Questions still remain regarding the timing of when the ACE inhibitor should be instituted, and what the duration of therapy should be. In general, it is probably safest to institute therapy after the patient is clinically stable, perhaps on day two or three after myocardial infarction. Treatment should be started with a relatively small dose of ACE inhibitor, and then the dose should be gradually titrated up over several weeks' time.

Positive Oral Inotropic Agents

Digitalis.   Digitalis has been in use for more than 200 years, but some controversy persists regarding its use for patients with congestive heart failure. There seems to be an emerging realization that digitalis is an effective and safe orally available positive inotropic agent. In fact, digitalis is the only positive inotropic agent available for long-term oral use. The controversy is regarding the influence of digitalis on long-term mortality in patients with heart failure. This uncertainty is about to be resolved with the publication of the Digitalis Investigators Group (DIG) study. In this multicenter, randomized, placebo-controlled survival trial, 7788 patients were randomly allocated to either digoxin or placebo. The treatment has been superimposed on diuretics and ACE inhibitors. The results demonstrated no overall effect of digoxin on mortality. However, there were fewer hospitalizations and deaths from pump failure in patients treated with digoxin. There was also a disturbing trend for more presumed arrhythmic deaths in patients treated with digoxin. On balance, digoxin had a favorable effect on the prevention of worsening heart failure.

The mechanism of enhanced contractility mediated by digitalis is still not entirely clear, although inhibition of the sodium-potassium-ATPase pump is thought to play a major role. Inhibition of this membrane pump allows for increases in intracellular sodium, which in turn activates the calcium/sodium exchange mechanism, leading to heightened intracellular calcium. In theory, more intracellular calcium is then available for operation of contractile proteins.

Digoxin is most useful in patients with moderate to severe congestive heart failure when there is a baseline tachycardia, third heart sound (S_3), and other signs of excessive sympathetic nervous system activity. Recent studies have suggested that digoxin can modulate neurohormonal compensatory mechanisms, leading to a reduction in sympathetic muscle nerve activity. Whether this neuroendocrine modulation contributes significantly to the beneficial effects of digitalis is still not entirely clear.

Digoxin is approximately 60% to 85% absorbed by the GI tract. Its onset of action is usually within 30 minutes, but the peak effect is at 1.5 to 5 hours. The average half-life for digoxin is rather long, approximately 36 to 42 hours. It is primarily excreted by the kidneys, although there is some GI excretion. Intravenous digoxin is usually not necessary for the treatment of heart failure. The usual maintenance dose is 0.125 to 0.5 mg/day, depending on renal function, how the patient responds, and the serum digoxin level. The therapeutic level of digoxin is considered to be between 0.9 and 2.0 ng/ml. Serum digoxin levels should be checked at least 6 hours after the previous dose to ensure that a steady pharmacokinetic state has been established.

Vesnarinone. Several new positive oral inotropic agents have recently been the subject of clinical trials. One such drug is vesnarinone, which has been shown to reduce mortality in patients with heart failure when used at a dose of 60 mg/day. Unfortunately, a higher dose of 120 mg/day increased the mortality rate. Vesnarinone has now been studied in a large multicenter trial to determine its role in the treatment of patients with heart failure. The drug increased mortality. The mechanism of action of vesnarinone remains obscure, but it appears to increase cyclic AMP by inhibition of a specific isoform of phosphodiesterase. Vesnarinone also increases intracellular sodium, increases calcium channel open frequency, and prolongs the cardiac cell action potential by inhibiting the outward potassium channel. In animal models vesnarinone can inhibit natural killer cell activity and attenuates TNF-α. In rare cases vesnarinone can impair marrow function, and the white blood cell (WBC) count must be monitored carefully. In view of increased mortality with vesnarinone, it can no longer be considered as treatment for heart failure.

Intravenous Inotropic Agents and Nitroprusside

Patients with severe or unstable heart failure require hospitalization and aggressive medical therapy. Factors leading to acute decompensation should be corrected when possible. Such factors may include rapid atrial fibrillation, pneumonia, acute myocardial ischemia, dietary indiscretion, and inappropriate or inadequate drug therapy. Drugs that are known to aggravate congestive heart failure include nonsteroidal antiinflammatory agents, the first-generation calcium-channel blockers, β-adrenergic blocking agents, and certain chemotherapy regimens including Adriamycin and Cytoxan.

In most circumstances it is prudent to admit patients with unstable or severe heart failure to the intensive care unit for hemodynamic

monitoring. When blood pressure is elevated in the setting of severe heart failure, the vasodilator nitroprusside is the preferred treatment of choice. Most patients presenting with severe unstable heart failure, however, are modestly hypotensive, with blood pressures in the range of 70 to 100 mm Hg systolic. In such cases, it may be preferable to begin therapy with dobutamine at 2 to 3 μg/kg/min. There are important differences between nitroprusside and dobutamine. Nitroprusside is energetically neutral and does not usually precipitate myocardial ischemia. It can be quickly titrated with the starting dose of 5 to 15 μg/min up to 300 μg/min in an attempt to reduce pulmonary capillary wedge pressure to 15 mm Hg. The primary goal should be reduction in pulmonary capillary wedge pressure rather than an increase in cardiac output. With nitroprusside, filling pressure is consistently diminished and cardiac output tends to improve. The limiting factor with nitroprusside is the systemic blood pressure. In general, it is imprudent to allow the *mean* blood pressure to fall to less than 65 mm Hg, which usually corresponds to a systolic blood pressure of 70 to 85 mm Hg.

If there is modest hypotension, or if nitroprusside tends to reduce blood pressure to an undesirable extent, dobutamine can either be added to nitroprusside or used in lieu of nitroprusside. As with nitroprusside, dobutamine should be titrated to reduce pulmonary capillary wedge pressure to 15 mm Hg. Unfortunately, reduction in filling pressure with dobutamine is not nearly as consistent as with nitroprusside. Moreover, dobutamine can increase myocardial oxygen demand by increasing heart rate and inotropy, thereby having the potential to precipitate myocardial ischemia. Dobutamine, like all catecholamines, can also be arrhythmogenic. For most patients a combination of nitroprusside and low-dose dobutamine (less than 5 μg/kg/min) will suffice in reducing pulmonary capillary wedge pressure and improving cardiac output.

Milrinone is a selective cardiac phosphodiesterase III inhibitor that increases intracellular cyclic AMP. It thereby increases the inotropic state of the heart through phosphorylation of membrane-bound calcium channels. As with dobutamine, prolonged use of milrinone can lead to tolerance. There are explicit pharmacologic differences between dobutamine and milrinone. Dobutamine has a half-life of only a few minutes. Milrinone has a relatively long half-life that requires that it be given as an intravenous loading dose of 50 μg/kg over 10 min followed by an infusion rate of 0.37 to 0.50 μg/kg/min. Because milrinone is cleared by the kidneys, the dose may have to be adjusted downward in patients with a marked reduction in creatinine clearance. The half-life of milrinone in patients with NYHA Class III and IV heart failure varies from 50 minutes to 1.7 hours. Compared with dobutamine, there is less incremental change in heart rate with milrinone. Moreover, milrinone tends to reduce blood pressure slightly, usually in the range of 5% to 10%. Dobutamine, on the other hand, tends to slightly increase mean arterial blood pressure. Because there is less increase in the heart rate–blood pressure product with milrinone compared with dobutamine, there appears to be less increase in myocardial oxygen demand for any given increase in cardiac output. These findings would suggest that milrinone may be preferable in patients with severe coronary artery disease.

There is no role for dopamine in the treatment of patients with severe congestive heart failure unless restoration of blood pressure is the primary goal. Dopamine should be reserved for patients with more advanced hypotension. The ability of low-dose dopamine to increase sodium excretion and improve renal blood flow has recently come under question. In general, its role in the treatment of patients with severe advanced heart failure is limited. The pharmacologic effects of these potent intravenous agents are summarized in Fig. 19-18.

Direct-Acting Oral Vasodilator Therapy

Although diuretics, digitalis, and ACE inhibitors remain conventional therapy for most patients with heart failure, selected patients may benefit from direct-acting vasodilators such as long-acting nitrates and hydralazine. The V-HeFT investigators in the mid 1980s established the efficacy of hydralazine 75 mg four times a day and isosorbide dinitrate 40 mg four times a day in patients with NYHA functional class II and III heart failure. These same investigators later reported a small but statistically significant further improvement in survival with enalapril 10 mg twice a day compared with the combination of

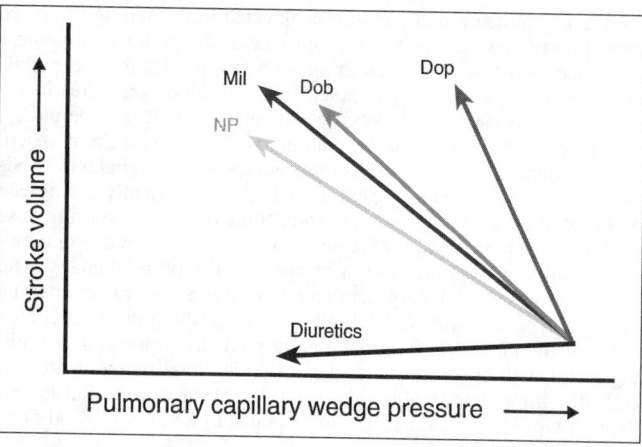

FIGURE 19-18   The hypothetical hemodynamic effects of nitroprusside and intravenous inotropic agents in patients with severe heart failure. *NP*, nitroprusside; *Mil*, milrinone; *Dob*, dobutamine; *Dop*, dopamine.

hydralazine and isosorbide dinitrate. Recent information suggests that nitrate tolerance is attenuated by hydralazine, thus rendering further support for the combination of hydralazine and long-acting nitrates. However, many patients do not tolerate large doses of hydralazine and nitrates, and in the first V-HeFT trial a substantial proportion of patients either had to have the dosages reduced or have the drugs stopped altogether. Nevertheless, for patients who are not responding to conventional *triple therapy,* the addition of hydralazine and isosorbide dinitrate should be considered. If ACE inhibitors are not tolerated because of symptomatic hypotension, azotemia, recurrent hyperkalemia, cough, rash, or angioneurotic edema, the combination of isosorbide dinitrate or some other long-acting nitrate plus hydralazine should be considered. The usual starting dose for isosorbide dinitrate is 5 to 10 mg three times a day, and for hydralazine the starting dose should be 10 mg four times a day. If tolerated, hydralazine should be gradually titrated to a dose of 75 mg four times a day and isosorbide dinitrate to 40 mg three times a day. It is appropriate for patients to have a 10-hour nitrate-free period for each 24-hour time frame to help avoid nitrate tolerance. The role of angiotensin II receptor antagonists such as losartan in the treatment of heart failure is currently under study. Until more data are available, these interesting new agents should be considered investigational.

Calcium Channel Blockers

Patients with reduced LV function and concurrent ischemic heart disease, angina pectoris, or high blood pressure may be suitable candidates for calcium channel blockers. However, physicians should not consider calcium channel blockers as *primary* agents in the treatment of heart failure. The first-generation calcium channel blockers have the distinct potential to aggravate congestive heart failure. The newer dihydropyridines may be somewhat safer in this regard. The recently completed PRAISE I Trial (see Table 19-4) suggests that patients with nonischemic cardiomyopathy may even have a survival advantage when treated with amlodipine 10 mg/day used in conjunction with conventional therapy. This hypothesis is now being tested in the recently launched PRAISE II study. Nevertheless, it appears that the newer dihydropyridines amlodipine and felodipine are tolerated in patients with congestive heart failure. More clinical experience is required before calcium channel blockers can be considered as *primary* therapy for heart failure.

Beta-Adrenergic Blockers

Considerable interest continues in the use of β-adrenergic blocking agents for the treatment of chronic congestive heart failure. Recently a series of small studies has been completed with carvedilol, a potent β₁-selective blocking agent with α₁-receptor blocking properties. It appears that when carvedilol is begun at very low doses (3.125 mg orally twice a day) and is then gradually titrated up on a weekly basis to 50 mg twice a day, left ventricular performance improves and survival is enhanced. Carvedilol is now approved by the FDA for the treatment of heart failure.

The carvedilol studies, as well as a broader experience with other β-adrenergic blockers for the treatment of heart failure, would suggest that patients may have some worsening of heart failure when β-blockers are being titrated up to the maximal dosage. Therefore, patients should be carefully monitored for worsening heart failure, and adjustments of diuretics and other therapies may be necessary. It is possible that the α-blocking moiety of carvedilol will offset the potential of the drug to worsen heart failure during its initiation. Drugs such as carvedilol have the potential to cause a complete adrenergic blockade and thereby reduce the detrimental effect of excessive catecholamine activity, a hallmark of severe heart failure. It is likely that the nonadrenergic blockade properties of carvedilol are also operative, including a very potent antioxidant activity. It will be important for physicians to familiarize themselves with the pharmacology and potential adverse effects of β-blockers before considering their use in patients with heart failure. β-blockers are still considered investigational for the treatment of heart failure, but the results of preliminary studies are quite promising.

Antiarrhythmic Therapy in Heart Failure

Ventricular arrhythmias are nearly omnipresent in patients with heart failure. Asymptomatic ventricular arrhythmias causing mild palpitations and brief nonsustained ventricular tachycardia should not be treated because currently no data support this strategy. It is well known that antiarrhythmic drugs can worsen ventricular arrhythmias and produce negative inotropic effects in patients with advanced heart failure. Routine Holter monitoring and signal averaged electrocardiography are not indicated as a primary screening tool but might be useful in selected patients with symptoms suggestive of sustained arrhythmias. When patients have symptomatic ventricular arrhythmias and heart failure, including bradyarrhythmias and syncope, they should be referred to cardiac specialists for further evaluation. Patients who sustain a cardiac arrest should also be referred for specialized diagnostic studies and therapy. In many cases, an implantable cardioverter defibrillator (ICD) will be indicated. In some cases, amiodarone may be added, primarily to diminish the spontaneous initiation of symptomatic ventricular arrhythmias and/or to reduce the rate of the sustained ventricular tachycardia.

The results of two large studies would suggest that the empiric use of amiodarone for patients with heart failure is still not clear. A reexamination of the data from the CHF-STAT trial and the GESICA trial (see Table 19-4) would suggest that amiodarone might be more beneficial in patients with nonischemic cardiomyopathy, but further investigation of this hypothesis will be necessary.

Patients with symptomatic supraventricular tachycardia, atrial fibrillation, and/or atrial flutter who have severe heart failure should be referred to a cardiac specialist for further evaluation. In some cases, low-dose amiodarone can reverse even long-standing atrial fibrillation and prevent its recurrence. Patients with chronic, severe supraventricular tachycardia may be candidates for radiofrequency (RF) ablation.

Anticoagulation

Selected patients with heart failure should be considered candidates for long-term anticoagulation with warfarin. This would include patients with chronic atrial fibrillation, patients with a previous history of systemic emboli, and patients with a large left atrium and mitral stenosis. Overall, the incidence of systemic emboli in patients with heart failure remains relatively low, with only 46 clinical embolic events in 804 patients followed for an average of 2.6 years in V-HeFT II. In the SOLVD trial, only 5.3% of patients experienced a clinical embolism during 39.2 months of follow-up. Looking at all of the major studies, the incidence of arterial thromboembolism ranges from 0.9 to 5.5 events per 100 patient years, with the largest studies reporting an incidence of 2% and 2.4% per 100 patient years. It seems clear that clinical embolic complications are linked to a low ejection fraction, and many physicians prefer to institute chronic anticoagulation with warfarin in patients with an ejection fraction of less than 20%. In addition, many physicians administer anticoagulation to pa-

infarction ISIS-4 (Fourth International Study of Infarct Survival) collaborative group, *Lancet* 345:669-685, 1995.

Krum H et al: Double-blind, placebo-controlled study of the long-term efficacy of carvedilol in patients with severe chronic heart failure, *Circulation* 92:1499-1506, 1995.

Metra M et al: Effects of short and long-term carvedilol administration on rest and exercise hemodynamic variables, exercise capacity and clinical conditions in patients with idiopathic dilated cardiomyopathy, *J Am Coll Cardiol* 24:1678-1687, 1994.

Packer M et al: Double-blind, placebo-controlled study of the effects of carvedilol in patients with moderate to severe heart failure: The PRECISE Trial, *Circulation* 94:2793-2799, 1996.

Pfeffer MA: Effect of captopril on mortality and morbidity in patients with left ventricular dysfunction after myocardial infarction: results of the Survival and Ventricular Enlargement trial, *N Engl J Med* 327:669-677, 1992.

Singh SN et al: Amiodarone in patients with congestive heart failure and asymptomatic ventricular arrhythmia. Survival Trial of Antiarrhythmic Therapy in Congestive Heart Failure, *N Engl J Med* 333:77-82, 1995.

The SOLVD Investigators: Effect of enalapril on mortality and the development of heart failure in asymptomatic patients with reduced left ventricular ejection fractions, *N Engl J Med* 327:685-691, 1992.

SOLVD Investigators: Effect of enalapril on survival in patients with reduced left ventricular ejection fractions and congestive heart failure, *N Engl J Med* 325:293-302, 1991.

Swedberg K et al: Effect of the early administration of enalapril on mortality in patients with acute myocardial infarction: results of the Cooperative New Scandinavian Enalapril Survival Study II (CONSENSUS II), *N Engl J Med* 327:678-684, 1992.

Williams JF et al: ACC/AHA guidelines for the evaluation and management of heart failure, *Circulation* 92:2764-2784, 1995.

tients with a low ejection fraction and an associated intracardiac thrombus.

If the decision is made to institute chronic anticoagulation with warfarin, the target range of international normalized ratio (INR) is 2.0 to 3.0. The optimal range of anticoagulation for patients with a documented embolism is perhaps somewhat higher at 2.0 to 3.5. There are no controlled trials demonstrating the efficacy of routine anticoagulation in other patients with heart failure and normal sinus rhythm, and the routine use of chronic warfarin therapy for patients with heart failure cannot be recommended based on our current database. It is likely, however, that selected patients, such as those with atrial fibrillation, previous embolic events, or ultra-low ejection fraction, will benefit the most.

BIBLIOGRAPHY

Acute Infarction Ramipril Efficacy (AIRE) Study Investigators: Effect of ramipril on mortality and morbidity of survivors of acute myocardial infarction with clinical evidence of heart failure, *Lancet* 342:821-828, 1993.

Baker DW, Wright RF: Management of heart failure. IV. Anticoagulation for patients with heart failure due to left ventricular systolic dysfunction, *JAMA* 272:1614-1618, 1994.

Chatterjee K: Heart failure in evolution, *Circulation* 94:2689-2693, 1996.

Cody RJ, Kubo SH, Pickworth KK: Diuretic treatment for the sodium retention of congestive heart failure, *Arch Intern Med* 154:1905-1914, 1994.

Cohn JN et al: A comparison of enalapril with hydralazine-isosorbide dinitrate in the treatment of chronic congestive heart failure, *N Engl J Med* 325:303-310, 1991.

CONSENSUS Trial Study Group: Effects of enalapril on mortality in severe congestive heart failure: results of the Cooperative North Scandinavian Enalapril Survival Study (CONSENSUS), *N Engl J Med* 316:1429-1435, 1987.

Digitalis Investigation Group: The effect of digoxin on mortality and morbidity in patients with heart failure, *N Engl J Med* 336:525-533, 1997.

Doval HC et al: Randomised trial of low-dose amiodarone in severe congestive heart failure: Groupo de Estudio de la Sobrevida en la Insuficiencia Cardiaca en Argentina (GESICA), *Lancet* 344:493-498, 1994.

Ferguson DW et al: Sympathoinhibitory responses to digitalis glycoside in heart failure patients. Direct evidence from sympathetic neural recordings, *Circulation* 80:65-77, 1989.

Francis GS: Calcium channel blockers and congestive heart failure, *Circulation* 83:336, 1991.

GISSI-3: Effects of lisinopril and transdermal glyceryl trinitrate singly and together on 6-week mortality and ventricular function after acute myocardial infarction: Gruppo Italiano per lo Studio della Sopravivenza nell"infarto Miocardico, *Lancet* 343:1115-1122, 1994.

Goldsmith SR, Dick C: Differentiating systolic from diastolic heart failure: pathophysiologic and therapeutic considerations, *Am J Med* 95:645-655, 1993.

ISIS-4: A randomized factorial trial assessing early oral captopril, oral mononitrate, and intravenous magnesium sulphate in 58,050 patients with suspected acute myocardial

20 Hypotension and Cardiogenic Shock

Mrinal Sharma and Richard C. Becker

Shock is one of the most feared medical conditions, and although potentially reversible, a majority of patients will not survive the event unless a prompt diagnosis is made and treatment initiated. Most patients with shock are hypotensive; however, hypotension in and of itself does not secure a diagnosis of shock. In general, hypotension is defined as a systolic blood pressure less than 90 mm Hg or a decrease in mean blood pressure of ≥30 mm Hg below baseline.

DEFINITION

Shock is a systemic clinical syndrome characterized by hypotension and hypoperfusion. Hypoperfusion at the tissue level causes cellular dysfunction. An inability to generate high-energy phosphate, which is required for adequate cellular function, ultimately leads to cellular injury and necrosis. Hypoperfusion can be determined clinically by the presence of several clinical variables: (1) altered mental status, (2) reduced urine output (<20 ml/hr), and (3) cool clammy skin. The absence of these clinical markers despite a systolic blood pressure of 90 mm Hg or less, or a mean blood pressure 30 mm Hg below baseline constitutes hypotension but not overt shock. Thus tissue hypoperfusion is the key element securing a diagnosis of shock.

Inherent to an understanding of shock (as a systemic syndrome) is an appreciation that flow (at the cellular level) can diminish to a point that cell viability is not possible; however, blood pressure can still be maintained by an increase in systemic vascular resistance. Accordingly, if arterial blood pressure is increased by simply increasing vascular resistance, blood flow and tissue perfusion may decrease. In the setting of hypotension, the desired therapeutic goal is to raise blood pressure; in overt shock the goal is to both raise blood pressure and improve tissue perfusion.

DIFFERENTIAL DIAGNOSIS AND ETIOLOGY OF SHOCK

Although tissue and cellular hypoperfusion remain the hallmarks of shock, a variety of mechanisms can lead to the same clinical endpoint. The causes of shock are outlined in Box 20-1.

EPIDEMIOLOGY OF CARDIOGENIC SHOCK

Cardiogenic shock develops in 5% to 15% of patients with acute myocardial infarction. The in-hospital mortality remains in excess of 80%. The 5-year mortality rate for those who survive the initial insult is 60%.

PATHOPHYSIOLOGY
Hemodynamic Alterations

In cardiogenic shock, the decrease in the cardiac output is accompanied by an increase in sympathetic/autonomic output, which leads to postcapillary venule and arteriolar vasoconstriction. The adrenergic-mediated venule constriction overrides the arteriolar constriction with a resultant increase in capillary hydrostatic pressure. The net result of this change is an egress of fluid from the intravascular to the interstitial space. This process is detailed in Fig. 20-1. Intravascular volume depletion, acting through the Bainbridge reflex and ventricular baroreceptor activation, causes a further increase in sympathetic output. In turn, increased sympathetic drive in the presence of decreased intravascular volume leads to renal hypoperfusion and activation of the renin-angiotensin-aldosterone cascade. Angiotensin II stimulates the release of vasopressin and endothelin; both are potent vasoconstrictors.

Myocardial Function

Peripheral vasoconstriction increases aortic diastolic pressure. This minimizes the decrease in coronary perfusion that accompanies systolic hypotension. However, coronary perfusion is not maintained unless the mean arterial pressure is greater than 65 mm Hg. Accordingly, there is a reduction in left ventricular ejection fraction and an increase in left ventricular diastolic dimension. In later stages of shock there is myocardial fluid retention causing a decrease in both left ventricular end-diastolic volume and ventricular compliance. Therefore shock states are characterized by both systolic and diastolic myocardial dysfunction. Lefer and colleagues identified a peptide produced by lysosomal hydrolase in sections of an ischemic pancreas as the culprit myocardial depressant in shock states. Others believe that L-leucine is the major circulating myocardial depressant factor, whereas other investigators have suggested that tumor necrosis factor is the major circulating myocardial depressant substance.

Elevation of Serum Lactate and Anaerobic Metabolism

Hypoperfusion limits the delivery of oxygen to cellular mitochondria. The aerobic oxidation of carbohydrates takes place within mitochondria when pyruvate enters the Krebs cycle. During the oxidation process, electron transfer occurs via pyridine nucleotides to oxygen, which serves as the final recipient of electrons and ultimately is converted to water. In the absence of oxygen however, pyruvate is converted to lactate without entering the Krebs cycle. This results in formation of two adenosine triphosphate (ATP) molecules as opposed to the 36 that normally would be generated by the citric acid cycle. Clearly circulatory shock leads to overproduction of lactate with limited generation of ATP (Fig. 20-2). A cell devoid of an adequate supply of energy fails to maintain its structural integrity and cellular death rapidly ensues. The oxygen deficit incurred during glycolytic cellular metabolism and the generation of serum lactate both portend a poor prognosis in circulatory shock.

Other Abnormalities in Shock States

Histamine and bradykinin release are increased in shock states. Activation of the arachidonic acid pathway generates prostaglandin (PGE_2) and prostacyclin (PGI_2), both of which have vasodilating properties. In the setting of gram-negative septicemia, lipid A endotoxin causes a profound cellular insult through lipid peroxidation of cell membranes and activation of the complement system. This leads to thrombocytopenia and disseminated intravascular coagulation. In severe cases purpura fulminans with extensive tissue necrosis and gangrene ensue. In addition to decreased concentrations of factors V and VIII, there can also be depletion of antithrombin III and α_2-macroglobulin. Injury to type 2 pneumocytes, activation of T lymphocyte killer cells, and macrophage-induced neutrophil sequestration with oxygen-derived radical generation set the stage for adult respiratory distress syndrome (ARDS). Its development adds further oxy-

---

BOX 20-1
Causes of Shock

Hypovolemic shock

I. Inadequate circulating blood volume
  A. Acute hemorrhage (e.g., trauma, gastrointestinal bleeding, retroperitoneal bleeding, hemoptysis, hemothorax, ruptured aortic aneurysm)
  B. Plasma volume loss
    1. Intestinal obstruction
    2. Peritonitis, pancreatitis, rapid accumulation of ascites
    3. Splanchnic ischemia
    4. Extensive burns or exudative skin disease
    5. Increased capillary permeability (prolonged hypoxia and ischemia, extensive tissue injury, anaphylaxis)
  C. Excessive water and electrolyte losses
    1. Inadequate fluid and salt intake
    2. Excessive sweating
    3. Severe vomiting or diarrhea
    4. Excessive urinary losses (e.g., diabetes mellitus, diabetes insipidus, nephrotic syndrome, salt-losing nephropathy, postobstructive uropathy, diuretic phase of acute renal failure, excessive diuretic use)
    5. Acute adrenocortical insufficiency

Septic shock

Gram-negative septicemia

Cardiogenic shock

I. *Impaired contractility/excessive preload*
  A. Acute myocardial infarction
  B. Dilated cardiomyopathy
  C. Mitral insufficiency (subacute, chronic)
  D. Aortic insufficiency (subacute, chronic)
  E. Ventricular septal rupture
  F. Tachyarrhythmias/bradyarrhythmias
II. *Decreased preload*
  A. Right ventricular infarction
  B. Pericardial tamponade
  C. Pulmonary embolism
  D. Hypovolemia resulting from blood loss (e.g., ruptured aneurysm)
  E. Cardiac myxoma
  F. Tension pneumothorax
  G. Mitral stenosis
III. *Excessive afterload*
  A. Malignant hypertension
  B. Coarctation of the aorta
  C. Aortic stenosis
  D. Hypertrophic cardiomyopathy (Preload may also be reduced)

Neurogenic shock (loss of vasomotor tone)

I. Spinal anesthesia
II. Spinal cord or brain damage
III. Drugs (ganglionic or adrenergic blocking agents)
IV. Anaphylaxis
V. Addisonian crisis

gen deficit to already hypoperfused and oxygen-deprived cells. The deficit is further augmented as erythrocyte 2,3-diphosphoglycerate (DPG) declines because of lactic acidosis with increased affinity of hemoglobin for oxygen. As a result there is less oxygen delivery at the tissue level.

If hypotension and hypoperfusion persist, there is a progressive loss of peripheral vascular compensation. Box 20-2 illustrates the physiologic compensatory responses to the shock state. Box 20-3 outlines the pathologic mechanisms culminating in the final loss of vascular tone. Fig. 20-3 provides a detailed pathophysiologic scheme for the shock syndrome.

Clinical Presentation of the Shock Syndrome

Hypotension and hypoperfusion represent the cardinal manifestations of the shock syndrome. An altered mental status, obtundation, restlessness, agitation, cool and clammy skin, and reduced urine output (<20 ml/hr) suggest reduced end-organ tissue perfusion. The presence of jugular venous distention, rales on lung examination, a loud S3 gallop, and systolic heart murmur are common findings in cardiogenic shock, whereas a history of hematemesis, melena, or diarrhea in the presence of reduced or normal jugular venous pressure supports a diagnosis of hypovolemic shock. The presence of high spiking fevers or hypothermia with a prodrome or history of a productive cough, urinary tract infection, or persistent diarrhea may suggest an infectious etiology. Physical findings, including costovertebral angle tenderness, dullness to percussion, bronchial breathing, and rhonchi, assist in localizing the site of infection. Spastic paralysis of the lower extremities accompanied by complete sensory loss and hyperreflexia are observed in transection of the spinal cord, which is a recognized cause of neurogenic shock.

A variety of causative mechanisms are associated with the development of cardiogenic shock in the setting of acute myocardial infarction (MI) (Chapter 23). Several mechanisms are discussed here.

Left Ventricular Dysfunction. Approximately 7.0% of patients with acute MI experience injury to 40% or more of the left ventricle. Physical examination typically reveals signs of hypoperfusion accompanied by pulmonary rales and either an S3 gallop or a summation (S3, S4 gallop).

Mechanical Complications. Although uncommon, the mechanical complications of acute myocardial infarction are potentially treatable if recognized early. In contrast to patients with primary myocardial pump failure and those with intractable arrhythmias, patients with mechanical complications may experience relatively small (but strategically placed) infarctions.

Acute mitral regurgitation often presents as acute "flash" pulmonary edema 2 to 7 days after an inferoposterior MI. The posterior papillary muscle is particularly vulnerable to injury because of its single blood supply, most often from the right coronary artery. Overall, papillary muscle rupture accounts for nearly half of all acute MI-related deaths.

Ventricular septal rupture accounts for 5% of all acute MI-related deaths, with an incidence of 1% to 3% during the initial 2 to 7 days. An anterior site of infarction typically causes rupture of the anterior septum, whereas defects in the posterior basal septum occur with inferoposterior infarctions.

Myocardial rupture (free wall) causes between 10% and 15% of all MI-related deaths. In approximately 50% of cases, rupture occurs within the initial 5 days. Risk factors for cardiac rupture include advanced age, female gender, a history of hypertension, and recent steroid or nonsteroidal antiinflammatory drug use. A sudden worsening or return of chest pain accompanied by hypotension or electromechanical dissociation supports the diagnosis. Thrombolytic therapy has changed our perspective on cardiac rupture. Although the overall incidence of rupture has not changed in the thrombolytic era, a greater proportion of early deaths (within 24 to 48 hours) can be attributed to this nearly always fatal event.

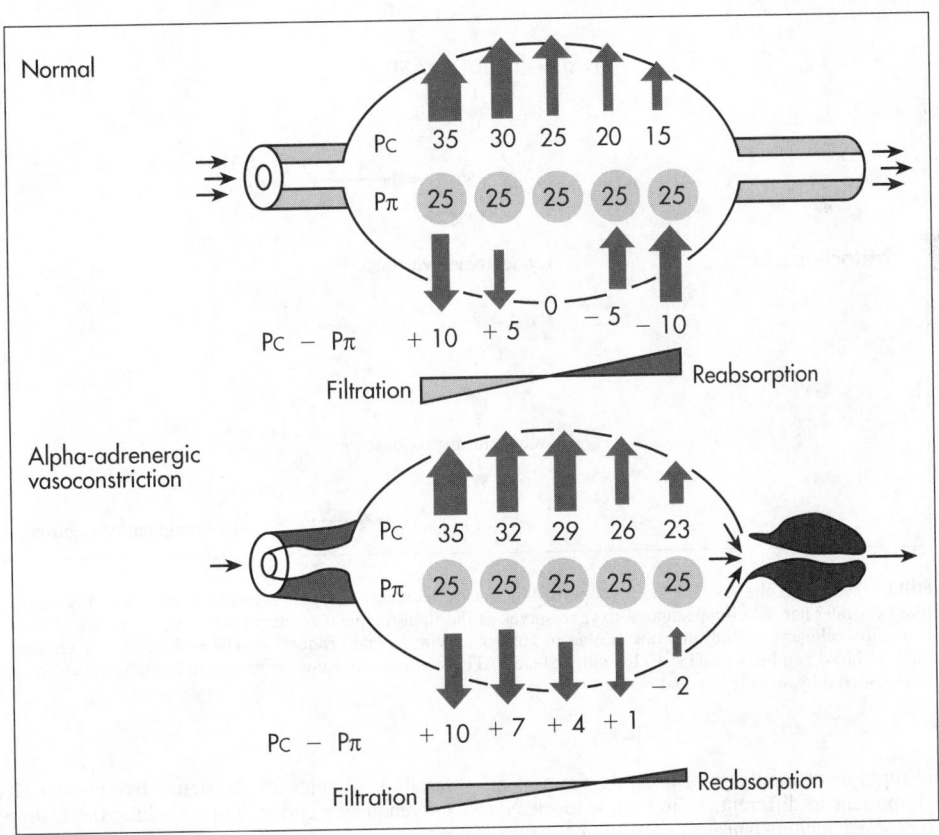

FIGURE 20-1   With circulatory shock adrenergic vasoconstriction causes an increase in capillary hydrostatic pressure (Pc), while oncotic pressure $(P\pi)$ remains unchanged. Since vasoconstriction on the venular side overrides arteriolar vasoconstriction, a net egress of fluid occurs into the interstitial space.

(From Weil HM, Planta VM, Rackow E: Acute circulatory failure. In Braunwald E, editor: *Heart disease: a textbook of cardiovascular medicine*, ed 4, Philadelphia, 1992, Saunders.

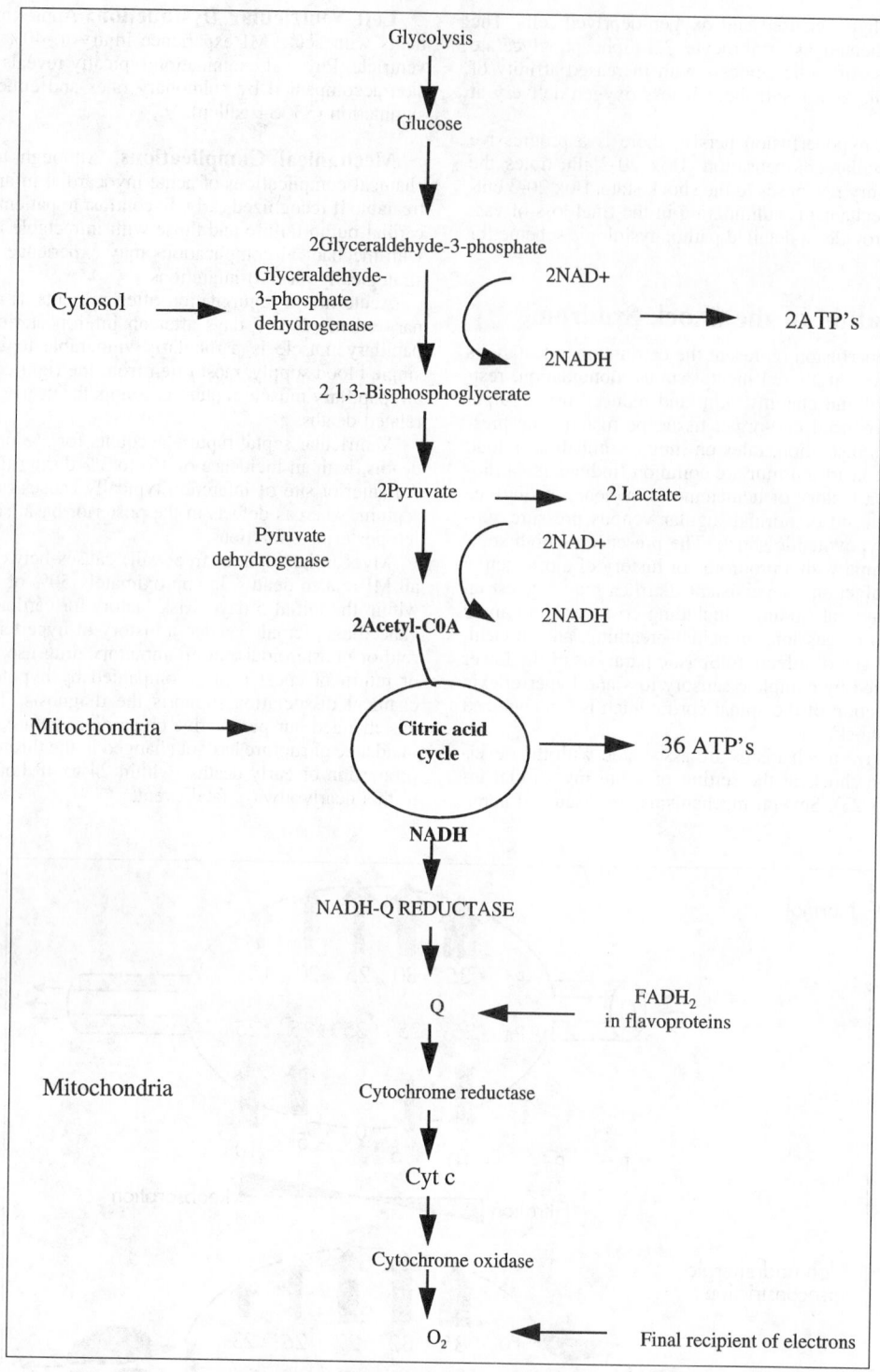

FIGURE 20-2   In the shock state, hypoperfusion causes decreased oxygen delivery to metabolically active tissues. Under normal circumstances, oxygen serves as the final recipient of electrons; however, a lack of oxygen shifts cellular metabolism from aerobic to anaerobic with lactate production. The end result is a substantially reduced number of ATPs. Cells with reduced ATP generation are unable to maintain integrity and over time undergo hypoxic injury and death.

Subacute myocardial rupture commonly presents in the form of a pseudoaneurysm. It is important to differentiate it from a localized pericardial effusion. The former requires surgical correction because of the possibility of enlargement and overt rupture into the pericardial space, causing sudden tamponade.

Right Ventricular Infarction. Right ventricular infarction occurs in one third of all patients with an acute inferior myocardial in-

farction (Chapter 23). Systemic hypotension, Kussmaul's sign, jugular venous distention, and clear lung fields support the diagnosis. The surface electrocardiogram reveals ST-segment elevation in leads V_{3R} and V_{4R}. Intravenous volume expansion is the treatment of choice. If an improvement in blood pressure is not observed, several possibilities should be considered. Right ventricular volume loading in the setting of pericardial constraint and increased right ventricular pressure can cause left ventricular diastolic dysfunction. Furthermore, a

BOX 20-2
Compensatory mechanisms in shock states

Increased sympathetic tone
Decreased parasympathetic tone
  Enhanced myocardial contractility
  Increased heart rate
  Arteriolar constriction
  Peripheral venoconstriction
  Decreased capillary hydrostatic pressure
  Increased central blood volume

(From Grella DR, Becker RC: Cardiogenic shock complicating coronary artery disease: diagnosis, treatment and management, *Curr Probl Cardiol* 19(12):701, 1994.)

BOX 20-3
Contraregulatory mechanisms in shock states

Factors associated with a loss of peripheral vascular tone

Acidemia
Decreased central sympathetic nervous system activity resulting from cerebral ischemia
Catecholamine depletion from vascular smooth muscle nerve endings
Antiadrenergic actions of increased endorphin concentrations
Release of nitric oxide and vasodilating prostaglandins

Factors associated with decreased cardiac performance

Acidemia
Inappropriate bradycardia
Circulating myocardial depressant factors
Decreased coronary arterial perfusion

(From Grella DR, Becker, RC: Cardiogenic shock complicating coronary artery disease: diagnosis, treatment and management, *Curr Probl Cardiol* 19(12):702, 1994.)

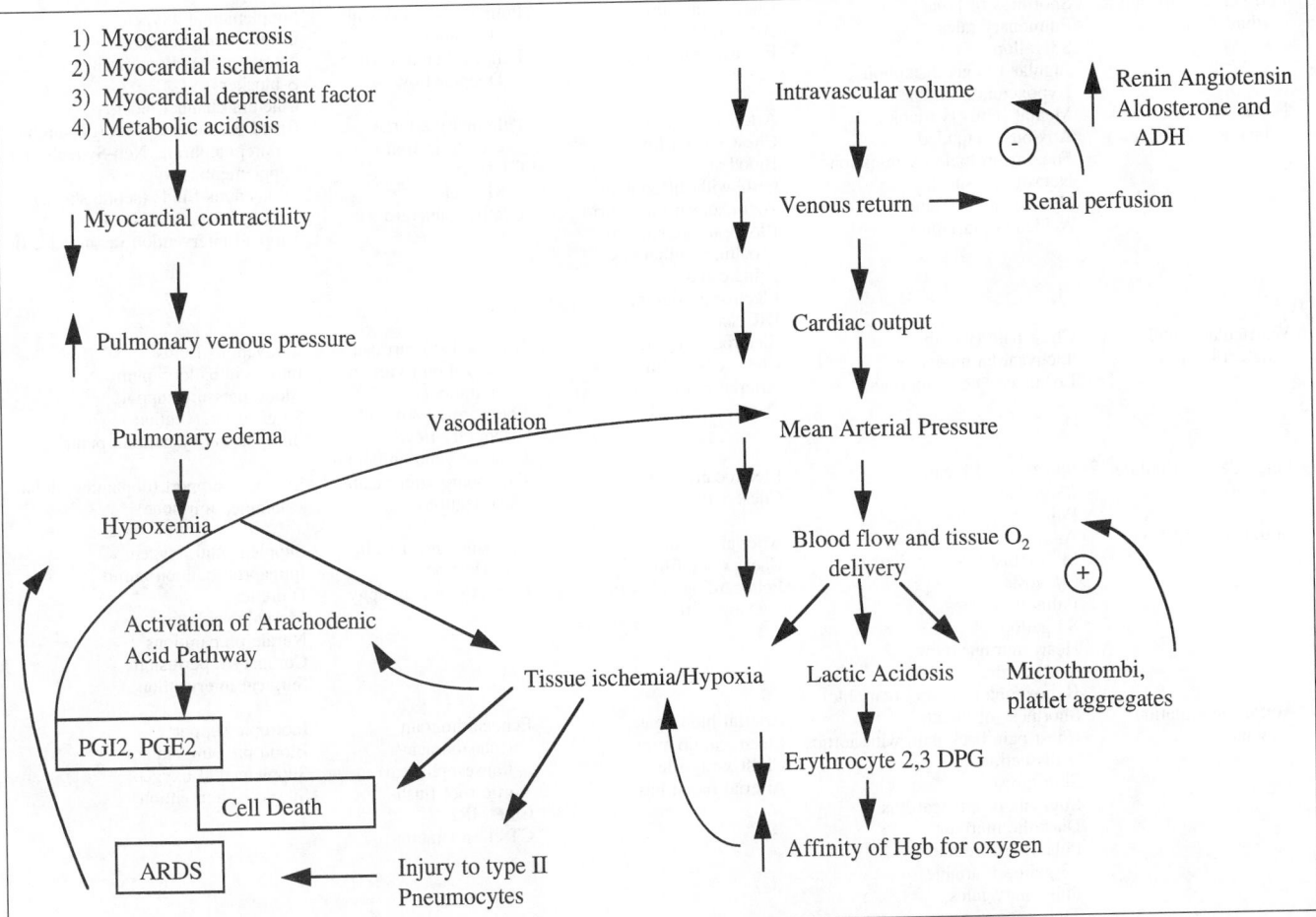

FIGURE 20-3 Pathophysiology of the shock syndrome. Various factors that can contribute to reduced myocardial contractility are shown. Reduced contractility causes pulmonary edema with resultant hypoxemia. Hypoxemia in turn causes tissue ischemia and ultimately cell death, activation of the arachidonic acid pathway, and injury to type II pneumocytes with onset of ARDS (adult respiratory distress syndrome). ARDS typically causes further hypoxemia, while PGI$_2$ and PGE$_2$ (metabolites of arachidonic acid) serve as vasodilators, lowering mean arterial pressure, and decreasing tissue perfusion. A depletion of intravascular volume activates the renin-angiotensin system. This system tends to increase the intravascular volume but also causes vasoconstriction. A reduced cardiac output ultimately leads to reduced blood flow and oxygen delivery (hypoperfusion). Microthrombi and platelet aggregation can develop in small vessels, further compromising tissue perfusion. Lactic acidosis and an increased oxygen affinity for hemoglobin further exacerbate the hypoxic insult. These various mechanisms ultimately lead to tissue ischemia/hypoxia with resultant cellular death. ↓ = Decreased, ↑ = increased, ⊖ = inhibition and ⊕ = stimulation.

right-to-left shunt can develop as increased right atrial pressure causes opening of the foramen ovale. In some circumstances biventricular failure with marked desaturation necessitates early endotracheal intubation and inotropic/vasopressor support.

Complete Heart Block. Complete heart block develops in 7% of patients with an acute MI (Chapter 23). Hemodynamic instability is more common among patients with an anterior site of infarction. This may be a reflection of the overall size of infarction. However, patients with inferior infarctions, particularly in the presence of right ventricular involvement, can experience profound hemodynamic deterioration with the loss of an atrial kick. These patients may require temporary atrial ventricular (AV) pacing. Although patients with inferior MI in the presence of complete heart block and hemodynamic stability can be observed, the patient with anterior wall myocardial infarction requires temporary transvenous pacemaker irrespective of hemodynamic stability.

Ventricular Tachycardia. Ventricular tachycardia develops in as many as 15% of patients with acute MI (Chapter 23). Patients with large infarctions are particularly prone to early hemodynamically significant ventricular tachyarrhythmias. Although myocardial injury in and of itself can serve as a focus for life-threatening arrhythmias, it is important to consider ischemia/ongoing infarction as well.

Table 20-1　Keys to differential diagnosis of circulatory shock

PATIENT CLASSIFICATION	HISTORICAL FEATURES AND PHYSICAL FINDINGS	DIAGNOSTID SCREENING TOOLS	DEFINITIVE DIAGNOSTIC STUDIES	TREATMENT CONSIDERATION
Volume overload	Shortness of breath Tachycardia (variable) S3 gallop Pulmonary rales Jugular venous distention Hypoxemia (variable)	Chest x-ray film Arterial blood gas Electrocardiogram Echocardiogram Hematocrit Serum electrolytes	Pulmonary artery catheterization	Supplemental oxygen Inotropic support Diuretics Morphine sulfate Nitrate preparations
Left-sided heart failure (diastolic)	Shortness of breath Pulmonary rales S3 gallop Jugular venous distention Hypoxemia (variable)	Chest x-ray film Arterial blood gas Electrocardiogram	Pulmonary artery catheterization Echocardiogram with Doppler flow	Supplemental oxygen Control arrhythmias Nitrate preparations (ischemia) β-blockers Calcium channel blockers
Noncardiogenic shock (septic, neurogenic)	Mental status (variable) Anxious, obtunded Focal neurologic examination Neurogenic shock Hypoxemia (variable) Acidemia (variable)	Arterial blood gas Chest x-ray film Blood sugar CBC with differential Toxin screen blood urine Blood, urine, sputum cultures, others as indicated Electrocardiogram DIC screen	Pulmonary arterial catheterization CT scan MRI scan Lumbar puncture	Blood pressure support (dopamine, norepinephrine, Neo-Synephrine) Supplemental oxygen Intravenous fluids (septic shock) Antibiotics (septic shock) Surgical intervention (as indicated)
Ventricular septal defect (acute)	Chest pain (variable) Tachycardia moderate Localized "new" murmur	Electrocardiogram Chest x-ray film Arterial blood gas	Right-sided heart catheterization (with saturations) Echocardiogram with Doppler flow Contrast ventriculogram	Intravenous fluids Intraaoric balloon pump Blood pressure support Surgical intervention Intrapulmonary balloon pump
Left-side heart failure (systolic)	Shortness of breath S3 gallop Pulmonary rales	Electrocardiogram Chest x-ray film	Pulmonary artery catheterization	Inotropic support (dopamine, dobutamine, amrinone)
Mitral regurgitation	Anxious Skin moist livedo reticularis Cyanosis Pulmonary rales S3 gallop Heart murmur (new) Tachycardia Hypoxemia acidemia (variable)	Arterial blood gas Chest x-ray film Echocardiogram with Doppler flow	Left-sided heart catheterization Coronary angiography	Supplemental oxygen Intraaortic balloon pump Diuretics Morphine sulfate Nitrate preparations Coronary reperfusion Surgical intervention
Aortic regurgitation (acute)	Shortness of breath Chest pain back pain with aortic dissection Skin moist Stigmata of endocarditis Diastolic murmur Pulse pressure narrow S3 gallop (variable) Pulmonary rales Tachycardia Hypoxemia	Arterial blood gas Electrocardiogram Chest x-ray film Arterial blood gas	Echocardiogram (transthoracic/transesophageal) Aortic root flush Ciné MRI CT chest (trauma)	Inotropic support Blood pressure support Supplemental oxygen Surgical intervention
Critical aortic stenosis	Shortness of breath Pulmonary rales Jugular venous distention Tachycardia (variable) Late-peaking systolic murmur Diminished carolid upstroke Hypoxemia	Electrocardiogram Chest x-ray film Arterial blood gas	Echocardiogram with Doppler flow Pulmonary artery catheterization Left heart catheterization Pulmonary artery catheterization	Inotropic support Supplemental oxygen Control arrhythmias Surgical intervention Balloon valvuloplasty Surgical intervention

CBC, complete blood cell count; *DIC*, disseminated intravascular coagulation; *CT*, computed tomography; *MRI*, magnetic resonance imaging.
(From Grella DR, Becker, RC: Cardiogenic shock complicating coronary artery disease: diagnosis, treatment and management, *Curr Probl Cardiol* 19(12):708-712, 1994.)

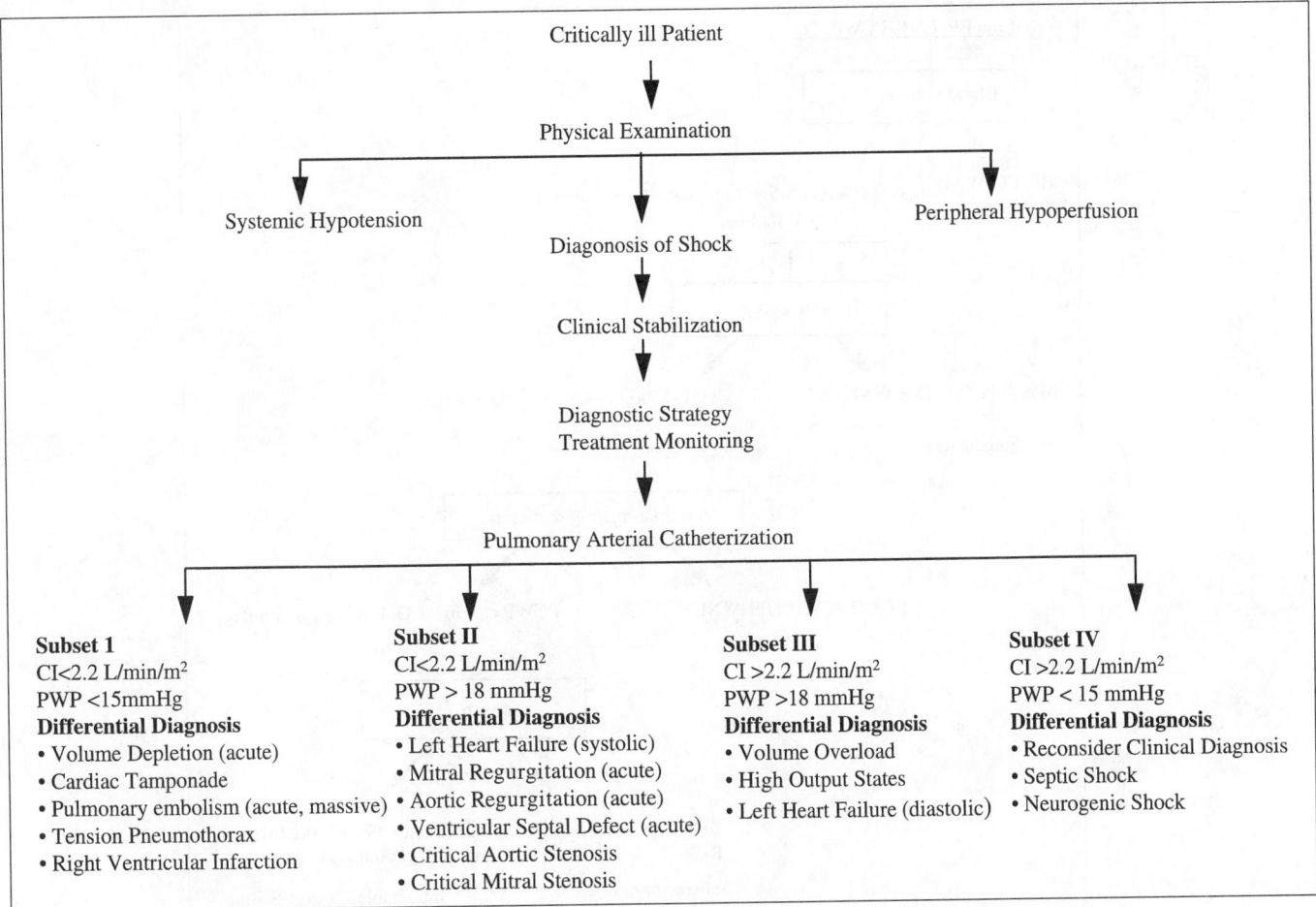

FIGURE 20-4 Patients with a clinical diagnosis of shock can be further characterized using hemodynamic information provided by pulmonary arterial catheterization. Depending on the cardiac index (CI) and pulmonary wedge pressure (PWP), patients can be divided into four different subsets. A diagnosis can be secured with pertinent history and physical examination along with additional testing (e.g., echocardiogram, cardiac catheterization).

(From Grella DR, Becker RC: Cardiogenic shock complicating coronary artery disease: diagnosis, treatment and management, *Curr Probl Cardiol* 19(12):707, 1994.)

Evaluation and Treatment of Patients With Cardiogenic Shock

The key to definitive treatment is establishing a prompt diagnosis. A brief medical and surgical history followed by physical examination and carefully selected diagnostic tests will foster a diagnosis in a majority of patients. A transthoracic or transesophageal echocardiogram may provide important information in the evaluation of mechanical defects stemming from acute MI or in the diagnosis of aortic dissection. Ventilation/perfusion (V/Q) scanning, a lower extremity duplex scan, or pulmonary angiography should be performed if there is a high clinical suspicion for pulmonary embolism.

A stepwise approach to patients with circulatory shock and its differential diagnosis is outlined in Table 20-1.

1. *Initial clinical stabilization* follows the basic ABC (Airway, Breathing, and Circulation) approach to life-threatening illnesses. In patients with obtundation and a moderate to severe degree of hypoxemia, we advocate early endotracheal intubation. Because some patients with shock require aggressive volume repletion, large-gauge venous access should be secured. Central line placement is also advocated when vasopressor support is likely to be required.
2. *Hemodynamic monitoring:* Many patients with a full-blown shock syndrome develop multisystem organ failure. Accordingly, early hemodynamic monitoring permits a tailored approach to treatment (Fig. 20-4).

Pharmacologic Therapy

Persistent systemic hypotension and end-organ hypoperfusion often dictate the need for inotropic/vasopressor support.

Dobutamine has two enantiomeric forms. The (+) enantiomer has α_1-receptor activity and is also 10 times more potent than (−) enantiomer in its ability to stimulate β-receptors. Dobutamine has β_1 activity that is much greater than β_2. However, the presence of β_2 activity does override α_1-mediated vasoconstriction in the periphery. An initial increase in cardiac output may cause baroreceptor-mediated vasodilation with a resultant decrease in systolic blood pressure; however, increasing the dobutamine dose often solves the problem. The half-life of this agent is 2 to 3 minutes.

Dopamine is a naturally occurring precursor of norepinephrine. In low doses (2 to 5 μg/kg/min), it produces nonadrenergic vasodilation of the renal and mesenteric vascular beds. At higher doses it produces predominately α-mediated vasoconstrictive effects.

Norepinepherine has a predominantly vasoconstrictive effect with some β_1 activity. This mediator is released by postganglionic adrenergic terminals and remains the agent of choice in profound hypotension (particularly in the setting of septic shock).

Isoproterenol is "pure" β-agonist that is utilized in the presence of symptomatic bradyarrhythmias unresponsive to atropine while the arrangements for a temporary transvenous pacemaker are being made. It may also be useful in the treatment of torsades de pointes.

Epinephrine has equal α- and β-receptor activity and remains the

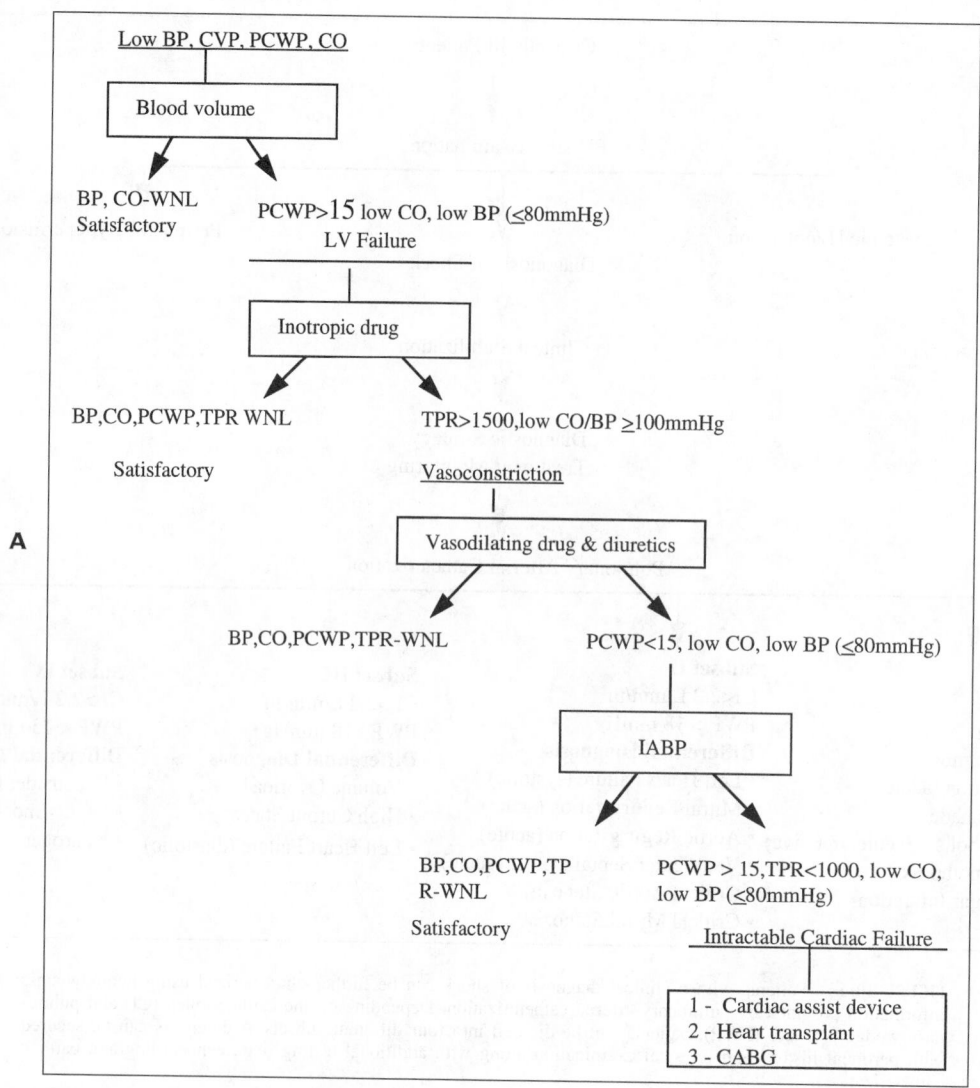

FIGURE 20-5   **A,** A stepwise approach to the treatment of circulatory shock is outlined.

Continued.

treatment of choice in anaphylaxis and anaphylactic shock. It is also used commonly during cardiopulmonary resuscitation, refractory asthma, and as a racemic mixture in the treatment of postextubation glottic edema.

Amrinone exhibits inotropic and vasodilatory effects by inhibiting phosphodiestrase, an enzyme required for the breakdown of cAMP. Increased concentrations of cAMP activate protein kinase, which phosphorylates the calcium channel. The phosphorylated calcium channel allows an influx of calcium, which at the level of sarcolemma promotes increased inotropy by combining with troponin C and allowing actin-myosin interactions. Amrinone is the agent of choice when cardiogenic shock is complicated by recurrent coronary vasospasm. A combination of amrinone and dobutamine increases the stroke volume index and decreases the left ventricular end diastolic volume more than does either agent alone.

Digitalis is useful when rapid atrial fibrillation complicates the shock picture. However, in acute shock secondary to myocardial failure, digoxin as an inotrope has a limited role.

Nitroprusside is a potent vasodilator with a half-life of 1 to 3 minutes. The degradation of this agent produces cyanide, which is converted to thiocyanate in the liver (with subsequent renal excretion). This agent should be considered when cardiogenic shock occurs in the presence of severe mitral regurgitation or ventricular septal defects. Unfortunately, many of these patients are profoundly hypotensive, precluding use of vasodilating agents. Toxic levels of thiocyanate (>10 mg/dl) may be seen in the circulatory shock as a result of

renal hypoperfusion and renal failure. The symptoms produced include nausea, mental status changes, seizures, and abdominal pain; however, these may be difficult to discern in critically ill patients. Therefore a high degree of clinical suspicion is required. Fig. 20-5 details various pharmacologic strategies used in the treatment of cardiogenic shock.

Reperfusion Therapy in Cardiogenic Shock

Cardiogenic shock accompanying anterior wall MI carries a mortality rate of greater than 80%. Occlusion of the infarct-related artery contributes to this high rate. Although some authors have reported encouraging results with thrombolytic therapy, a number of large clinical trials have failed to show a benefit. This lack of benefit is likely due to inability of the thrombolytic to reach the occluding thrombus because of low coronary perfusion pressure. The problem is further compounded by metabolic acidosis, as it increases the Michaelis-Menton constant and hence lowers the catalytic rate of plasminogen to plasmin conversion.

Although only 3% of the patients are found to be in cardiogenic shock on initial presentation, an additional 3% to 4% develop this complication at a later stage, suggesting a role for extension, recurrent ischemia or infarct extension, or recurrent ischemia or infarct expansion. There is a direct correlation between the mortality and the Killip class at initial presentation. Table 20-2 shows the mortality data for different clinical trials. Unfortunately, the mortality rate remains

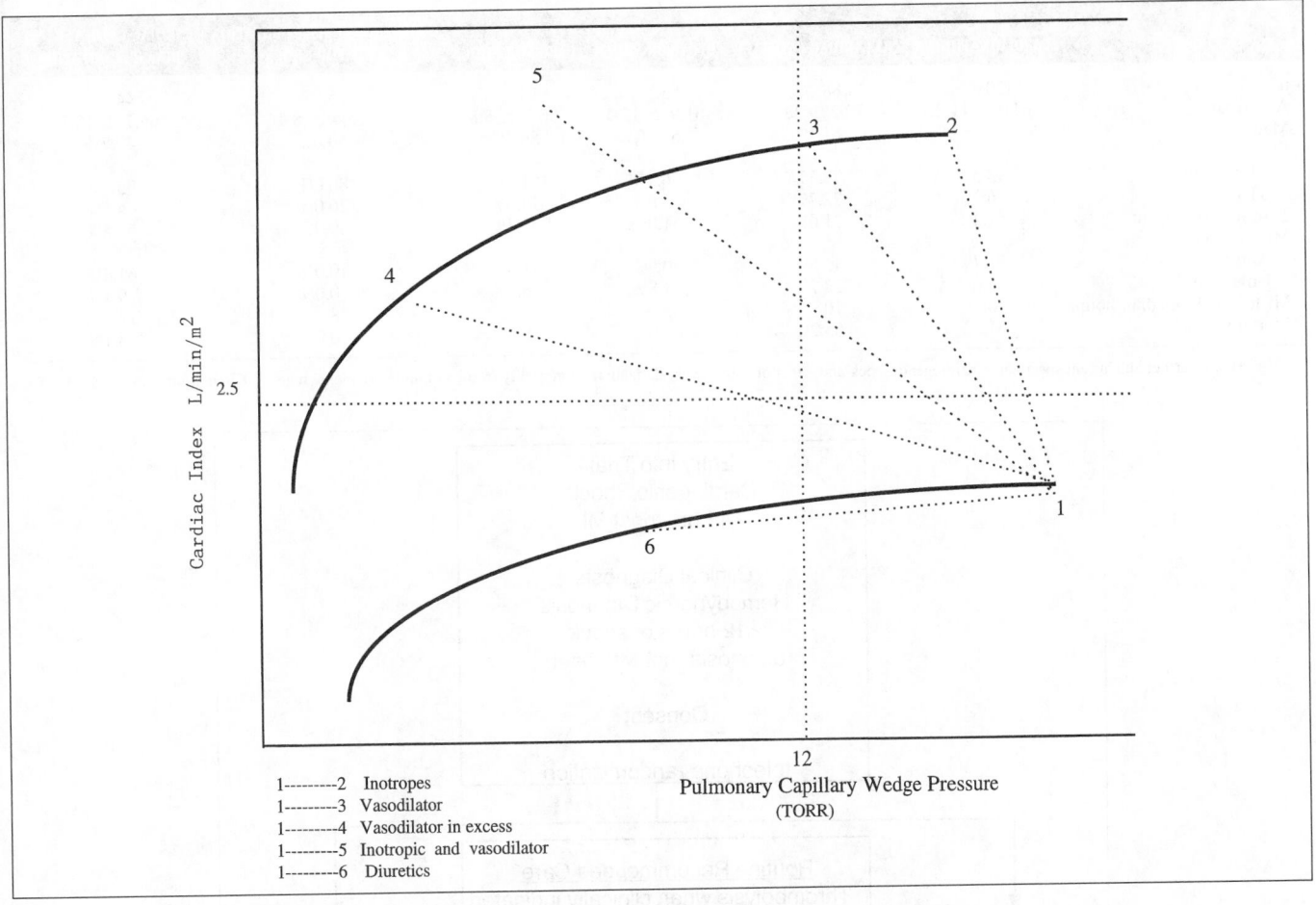

1--------2 Inotropes
1--------3 Vasodilator
1--------4 Vasodilator in excess
1--------5 Inotropic and vasodilator
1--------6 Diuretics

FIGURE 20-5, cont'd.   B, The effect of different pharmacologic interventions on the cardiac index and capillary wedge pressure. Treatment with an inotropic agent increases the cardiac index, with little change in the wedge pressure (1→2). However, the combined administration of inotropic agents and diuretics causes a decrease in the capillary wedge pressure and an increase in the cardiac index (1→5). Vasodilators cause an increase in the cardiac index and a small decrease in the capillary wedge pressure (1→3). However, vasodilators given in excess may cause a marked decrease in filling pressure (preload) (1→4). Diuretics decrease capillary wedge pressure without a significant increase in cardiac index (1→6). *BP,* Blood pressure; *CO,* cardiac output; *TPR,* total peripheral resistance; *PCWP,* pulmonary capillary wedge pressure; *IABP,* intraaortic balloon pump; *WNL,* within normal limits; *CABG,* coronary artery bypass graft.

in excess of 50% with cardiogenic shock (Killip class IV) irrespective of thrombolytic use.

Coronary Angioplasty

Although randomized clinical trial results are not available, there is sufficient evidence that PTCA of the infarct-related coronary artery leads to a significant reduction in in-hospital mortality. Some retrospective studies suggest a long-term mortality benefit, especially when single-vessel coronary artery disease presents as cardiogenic shock. Patients with cardiogenic shock from ischemic mitral regurgitation and patients with a prior history of coronary artery bypass grafting (CABG) may also experience a significant reduction in in-hospital mortality.

A follow-up of 200 patients with cardiogenic shock from the Duke Data Base showed patency of the infarct-related coronary artery as the most important prediction of in-hospital mortality. Various investigators have reported markedly improved survival after successful PTCA of infarct-related artery compared to unsuccessful coronary angioplasty. Recent clinical experience clearly shows an improved in-hospital survival in patients with cardiogenic shock who underwent PTCA compared to traditional mortality in excess of 80%. Thus it appears that PTCA of infarct-related artery, in the setting of cardiogenic shock, has a survival benefit, although this is not proven in the randomized controlled trials.

Table 20-2   Thrombolytic therapy clinical experience: mortality subdivided by Killip classification

	MORTALITY (%)			
	KILLIP I	KILLIP II	KILLIP III	KILLIP IV
GISSI-1				
SK	5.9	16.1	33	69.9
Placebo	7.3	19.9	39	70.1
International study				
SK/aspirin	5.1	17.8	33.3	64.9
tPA/aspirin	4.1	17.7	29.9	78.1
GUSTO-1				
tPA	4.4	13.0	23.3	63.4
SK (subcutaneous heparin)	5.2	15.0	31.0	58.0
SK (intravenous heparin)	4.4	13.0	23.0	63.0
tPA plus SK	5.3	13.8	37.0	56.0

SK, streptokinase; *tPA,* tissue plasminogen activator.
(From Grella DR, Becker, RC: Cardiogenic shock complicating coronary artery disease: diagnosis, treatment and management, *Curr Probl Cardiol* 19(12):715, 1994.)

Table 20-3 Characteristics and outcome of patients selected for cardiac catheterization and revascularization

	CARDIAC CATHETER	NO CARDIAC CATHETER	PTCA FOR SHOCK	CABG FOR SHOCK	VERY LATE REVASCULARIZATION NOT FOR SHOCK	CARDIAC CATHETER, NO REVASCULARIZATION
n	120	88	55	16	5	44
Age, years	64.0 ± 11.2	70.2 ± 11.7	61.9 ± 12.4	66.3 ± 8.8	65.4 ± 8.4	65.7 ± 10.3
Male	56.7%	61.4%	63.6%	56.3%	60.0%	47.7%
ECG						
ST elevation	93.3%	77.3%	96.4%	81.2%	80.0%	95.5%
ST depression	6.7%	22.7%	3.6%	18.8%	20.0%	4.5%
Thrombolytic agent	51.4%	31.0%	51.0%	33.3%	40.0%	59.5%
MI location						
Anterior	51.7%	45.5%	50.9%	31.3%	40.0%	61.4%
Unknown	5.0%	22.7%	1.8%	6.3%	0.0%	9.1%
MI to shock, median hours	6	10	5	18	8	12
Mortality	51.3%	85.2%	60.0%	18.8%	0.0%	58.1%

(From Hochman J et al: Current spectrum of cardiogenic shock and effect of early revascularization on mortality: results of an international registry, *Circulation* 91:873-881, 1995.)

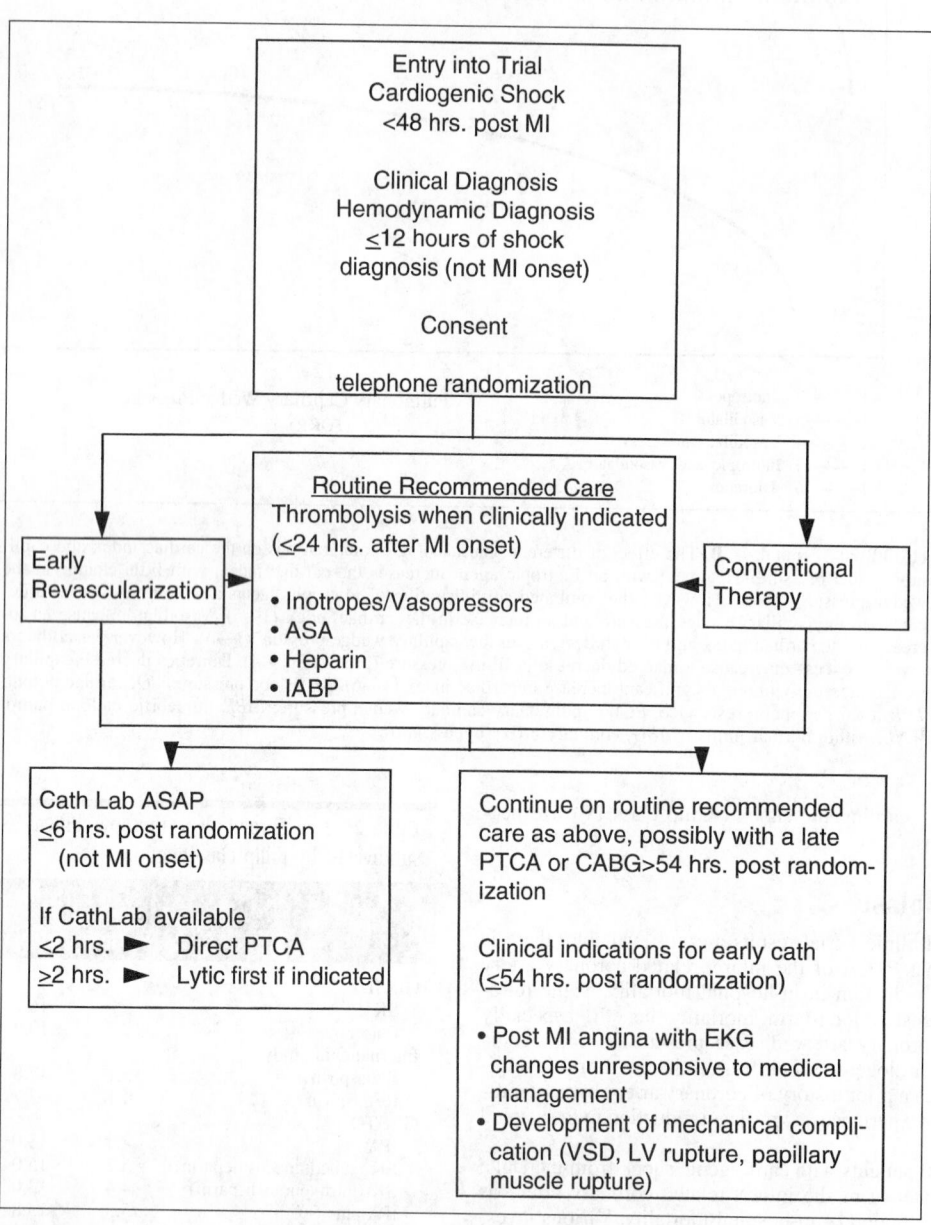

FIGURE 20-6 Shock trial algorithm. Patients who within 48 hours of an acute MI and ≤12 hours from the onset of shock are to be randomized to conventional therapy (e.g., inotropes/vasopressors), ASA (aspirin), IABP (intraaortic balloon pump) heparin, early revascularization with PTCA (percutaneous transluminal coronary angioplasty), or CABG (coronary artery bypass grafting). Patients randomized to early revascularization can receive conventional therapy, including thrombolytic therapy, if immediate access to the cardiac catheterization laboratory is not possible. Patients undergoing cardiac catheterization more than 54 hours after randomization will not be considered part of early revascularization group. The primary endpoint of the study is all-cause mortality at hospital discharge.

(From Grella DR, Becker RC: Cardiogenic shock complicating coronary artery disease: diagnosis, treatment and management, *Curr Probl Cardiol* 19(12):727, 1994.)

Coronary Artery Bypass Grafting

Dewood and co-workers found that when revascularization is performed within 16 hours of onset of acute MI there is a mortality rate of 25%; however, the rate increases to 72% if revascularization is delayed for more than 18 hours. Furthermore, there is a 62.5% mortality rate with anterior wall myocardial infarction compared to 20% with inferior wall myocardial infarction.

Although the available literature shows significant survival benefit as with PTCA, there is lack of randomized clinical trials supporting the use of CABG as a treatment for cardiogenic shock.

Clinical Trials in Cardiogenic Shock

The ideal treatment approach to cardiogenic shock remains an open-ended question; however, several points merit discussion.

Thrombolysis Versus No Thrombolysis. Although the GISSI-I trial, which used streptokinase (without aspirin or heparin), found no benefit, Kennedy et al. found intracoronary streptokinase resulted in similar mortality as with successful PTCA. In addition, GUSTO investigators showed that 6-week mortality with recombinant tPA use was 51%, similar to the mortality rate with PTCA. It should be emphasized, however, that these trials were not randomized.

PTCA Versus CABG. Recently, Hockman et al. reported the results of an international registry for cardiogenic shock. In this study 251 patients with cardiogenic shock were enrolled to assess the impact of early revascularization on mortality. The characteristics and outcomes of patients who underwent cardiac catheterization and revascularization are summarized in the Table 20-3.

As shown in the table, patients with cardiogenic shock had much lower mortality rate with CABG than with PTCA. Further investigations are needed to assess whether this difference reflects a selection bias or an ability to perform complete revascularization with CABG. In any event, randomized clinical trials are needed to further analyze this question.

Randomized Clinical Trial of Cardiogenic Shock. An NIH-sponsored multicenter clinical trial is currently under way to determine whether revascularization (PTCA or CABG) offers a survival

advantage over conventional therapy using aspirin, heparin, thrombolytic agents, vasopressors, and intraaortic balloon counterpulsation. The treatment algorithm is shown in the Fig. 20-6.

Mechanical Intervention

Intraaortic balloon counterpulsation should be used when hemodynamic instability persists despite adequate medical therapy. Patients with mechanical complications of MI and those with profound global ischemia are particularly likely to benefit. Hemodynamic effects of intraaortic balloon pump are outlined in Table 20-4.

In femorofemoral extracorporeal bypass venous blood is removed from the vena cava and then passed through the membrane oxygenator. The oxygenated blood is then pumped into the femoral artery.

BOX 20-4
Hemodynamic criteria for mechanical circulatory support

A. Cardiac index <1.8 L/m^2/min
B. Systolic arterial pressure <90 mm Hg
C. Left and/or right atrial pressure >20 mm Hg
D. Urine output <20 ml/hr (adult)
E. Systemic vascular resistance >2100 dynes/sec/cm^{-5}
F. Metabolic acidosis
G. The existence of (A-F) despite adequate preload, maximal pharmacologic support, and intraaortic balloon pumping.

(From Pennington G, Swartz M: Assisted circulation and mechanical hearts In Braunwald, *Heart disease: a textbook of cardiovascular medicine*, ed 4, Philadelphia, 1992, Saunders.)

Table 20-4 Effects of intraaortic balloon pumping (IABP) in 35 patients with cardiogenic shock

	BEFORE	IABP	CHANGE (%)
Pulmonary artery occlusive pressure mm Hg	24	19	−21
Aortic systolic/diastolic mm Hg	78/55	68/95	−13/+73
Cardiac index L/min/M^2	1.7	2.4	+41

(From Weil MH, von Planta M, Rackow EC: Acute circulatory failure (shock). In Braunwald, *Heart disease: a textbook of cardiovascular medicine*, ed 4, Philadelphia, 1992, Saunders.) (Modified from Resenekov L: Cardiogenic shock, *Chest* 83:893, 1983.)

Table 20-5 Effects of nonsynchronized mechanical circulatory assist devices on cardiac physiology

	LEFT VENTRICLE		RIGHT VENTRICLE	
	PRELOAD	AFTERLOAD	PRELOAD	AFTERLOAD
LVAD	↓	↑	↑	↓
RVAD	↑	−	↓↑	↑↓
BVAD	↓↑	↑	↓↑	↓↑
ECMO	↓	↑	↓	↓

LVAD, left ventricular assist device; *RVAD*, right ventricular assist device; *BVAD*, biventricular assist device; *ECMO*, extracorporeal membrane oxygenation.
(From Pennington G, Swartz M: Assisted circulation and mechanical hearts. In Braunwald, *Heart disease: a textbook of cardiovascular medicine*, ed 4, Philadelphia, 1992, Saunders.)

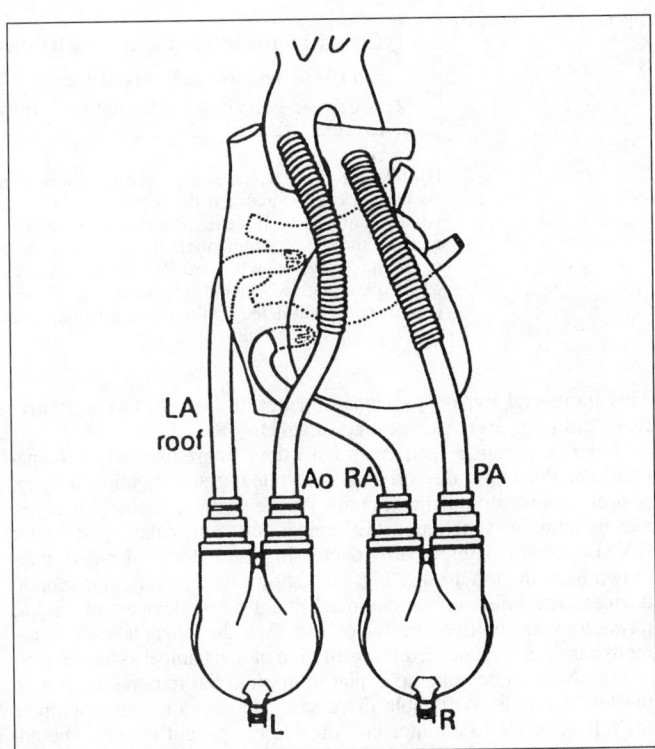

FIGURE 20-7 Biventricular assist device (BVAD). Blood is taken from the left atrium *(LA)* and is pumped into the aorta *(AO)*, thus bypassing the left ventricle. Blood is taken from the right atrium *(RA)* and is pumped to the pulmonary artery *(PA)*, thus bypassing the right ventricle.

(From Grella DR, Becker RC. Cardiogenic shock complicating coronary artery disease: diagnosis, treatment and management, *Curr Probl Cardiol* 19(12):723, 1994.)

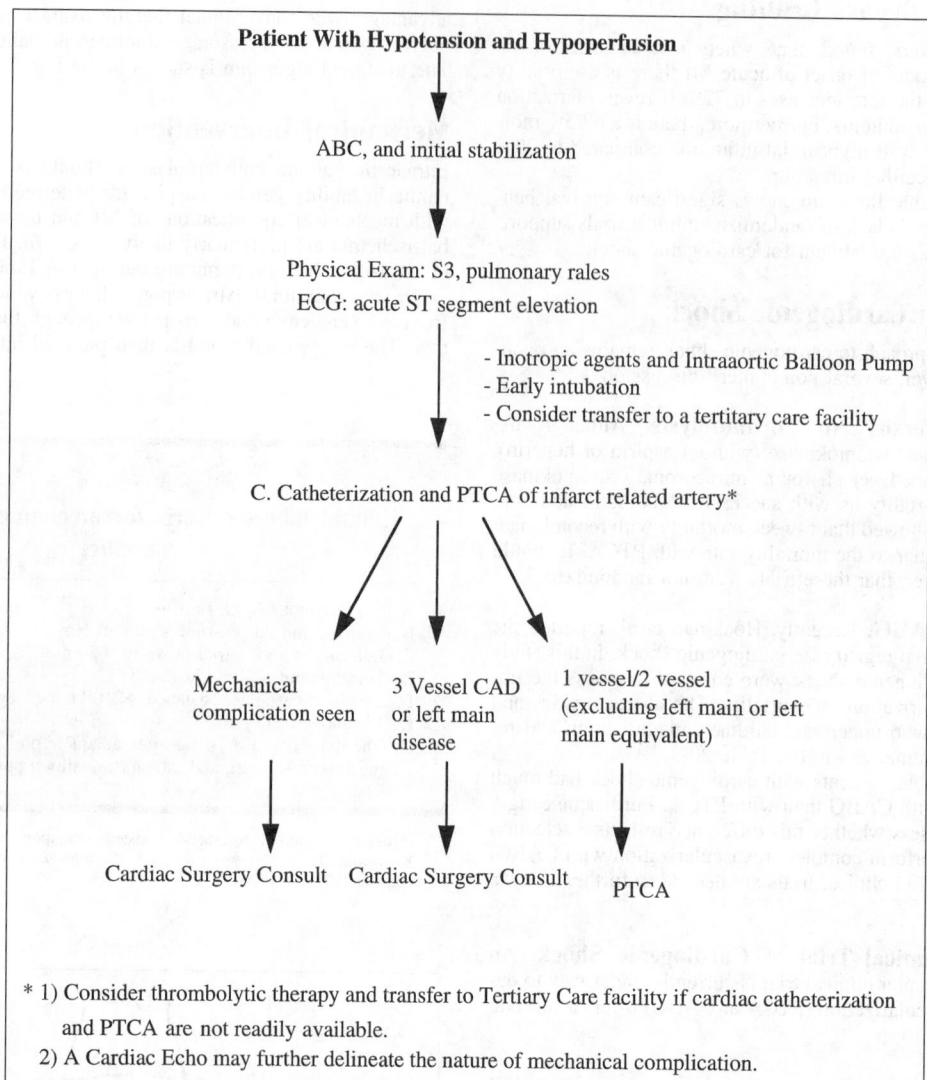

Patient With Hypotension and Hypoperfusion

↓

ABC, and initial stabilization

↓

Physical Exam: S3, pulmonary rales
ECG: acute ST segment elevation

- Inotropic agents and Intraaortic Balloon Pump
- Early intubation
- Consider transfer to a tertiary care facility

↓

C. Catheterization and PTCA of infarct related artery*

Mechanical complication seen → Cardiac Surgery Consult

3 Vessel CAD or left main disease → Cardiac Surgery Consult

1 vessel/2 vessel (excluding left main or left main equivalent) → PTCA

* 1) Consider thrombolytic therapy and transfer to Tertiary Care facility if cardiac catheterization and PTCA are not readily available.

2) A Cardiac Echo may further delineate the nature of mechanical complication.

FIGURE 20-8   A suggested approach to treatment of patients with cardiogenic shock. Once a clinical diagnosis of shock is secured and the patient is stabilized, an attempt should be made to transfer the patient to a tertiary care facility. If the transfer cannot be done in a timely fashion, however, strong consideration should be given to the use of thrombolytic therapy. Once the patient is in the tertiary care facility, prompt cardiac catheterization with a view toward PTCA (percutaneous transluminal coronary angioplasty)/CABG (coronary artery bypass grafting) should be undertaken. If cardiogenic shock is due to complications of MI (e.g., VSD [ventricular septal defect], mitral regurgitation) an early echocardiogram may be a useful diagnostic test.

This peripheral bypass provides a bridge toward a more definitive treatment (e.g., PTCA or cardiac surgery).

External pulsatile ventricular assist devices are used when the patient is unable to be taken off bypass despite revascularization and support of an intraaortic balloon pump. As the stunned ventricle recuperates its pumping function, a TEE-guided left ventricular assist device (LVAD) wean is attempted by decreasing the volume of blood withdrawn from the left atrium. Fig. 20-7 shows the biventricular support devices. The effect of various mechanical assist devices on cardiac physiology are outlined in Table 20-5. Box 20-4 details various hemodynamic criteria needed for institution of mechanical assist devices.

The Nimbus hemopump is placed through the femoral artery into the left ventricle. A flexible drive shaft couples this hemopump in the left ventricle to a motor unit outside the patient's body. The advantage of this system is that it obviates the need for sternotomy, which is a must if a ventricular assist device is used.

Novacor left ventricular assist system, Thermocardiac left ventricular assist system, and Symbion Jarvik-7 are mechanical support devices used to provide permanent support. However, they are rarely used in patients with acute MI and cardiogenic shock. These devices

provide only temporary support while definitive treatment of cardiogenic shock is undertaken.

SUMMARY

Circulatory shock remains a medical emergency requiring immediate supportive therapy while attempts are made to address the underlying etiology. MI can present as a cardiogenic shock either due to massive infarction itself or due to complications arising from MI. In any event, after initial stabilization a prompt transfer to a tertiary care facility should be initiated. Although no randomized trials are done to determine the best treatment approach, based on the available literature, the treatment algorithm in Fig. 20-8 is suggested.

BIBLIOGRAPHY

Becker RC, Charlesworth A, Wilcox R et al. for the LATE investigators: Cardiac rupture associated with thrombolytic therapy: impact of time to treatment in the LATE study, *J Am Coll Cardiol* 25:1063-1068, 1995.

Bengtson JR, Kaplan AJ, Pieper KS et al: Prognosis in cardiogenic shock after acute myocardial infarction in the interventional era, *J Am Coll Cardiol* 20:1482-1489, 1992.

Bolooki H: Emergency cardiac procedures in patients in cardiogenic shock due to complications of coronary artery disease, *Circulation* 79(suppl I):137-148, 1989.

Brodie BR, Wientraub RA, Stuckey TD et al: Outcomes of direct coronary angioplasty for acute myocardial infarction in candidates and noncandidates for thrombolytic therapy, *Am J Cardiol* 67:7-12, 1991.

DeWood MA, Notske RN, Hensley GR et al: Intra-aortic balloon counterpulsation with and without reperfusion for myocardial infarction shock, *Circulation* 61:1105-1112, 1980.

Gacioch GM, Ellis SG, Lee L et al: Cardiogenic shock complicating acute myocardial infarction: the use of coronary angioplasty and the integration of the new support devices into patient management, *J Am Coll Cardiol* 19:647-653, 1992.

Goldberg RJ, Gore JM, Alpert JS et al: Cardiogenic shock resulting from acute myocardial infarction: a fourteen year community-wide perspective, *N Engl J Med* 325:1117-1122, 1991.

Grella RD, Becker R: Cardiogenic shock complicating coronary artery disease: diagnosis, treatment and management, *Curr Probl Cardiol* 19:693-744, 1994.

Guyton RA, Arcidi JM Jr, Langford DA et al: Emergency coronary bypass for cardiogenic shock, *Circulation* 76(suppl V):22-27, 1987.

Hibbard MD, Holmes DR Jr, Bailey KR et al: Percutaneous transluminal coronary angioplasty in patients with cardiogenic shock, *J Am Coll Cardiol* 19:639-646, 1992.

Hochman J, Boland, Sleeper L et al: Current spectrum of cardiogenic shock and effect of early revascularization on mortality: results of an international registry, *Circulation* 91:873-881, 1995.

Kennedy JW, Gensini GG, Timmis GC, Maynard C: Acute myocardial infarction treated with intracoronary streptokinase: a report of the Society for Cardiac Angiography, *Am J Cardiol* 55:871-877, 1985.

Laks H, Rosenkranz E, Buckberg GD: Surgical treatment of cardiogenic shock after myocardial infarcion, *Circulation* 74(suppl III):11-16, 1986.

Lee L, Bates ER, Pitt B et al: Percutaneous transluminal coronary angioplasty improves survival in acute myocardial infarction complicated by cardiogenic shock, *Circulation* 78:1345-1351, 1988.

Lee L, Erbel R, Brown TM et al: Multicenter registry of angioplasty therapy of cardiogenic shock: initial and long term survival, *J Am Coll Cardiol* 17:599-603, 1991.

Lefer AM: Pharmacologic and surgical modulation of myocardial depressant factor formation and action during shock, *Prog Clin Biol Res* 111:111, 1993.

McCall D, O'Rourke RA: Hypotension and cardiogenic shock. In Stein JH, editor: *Internal medicine,* Boston, 1990, Little, Brown.

Moosvi AR, Khaja F, Villanueva L et al: Early revascularization improves survival in cardiogenic shock complicating acute myocardial infarction, *J Am Coll Cardiol* 19:907-914, 1992.

Weil M, Von Planta M, Rackow E: Acute circulatory failure (shock). In Braunwald E, editor: *Heart disease: a textbook of cardiovascular medicine,* Philadelphia, 1992, Saunders.

CHAPTER

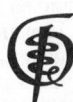

21 Sudden Cardiac Death

James L. Gilman and Gerald V. Naccarelli

Sudden cardiac death is an enigma. Although it is the most common mode of death in most Western societies and occurs approximately one thousand times each day in the United States alone, understanding of the basic mechanisms responsible for sudden cardiac death remains rudimentary. Furthermore, treatment strategies for the primary and secondary prevention of sudden cardiac death have proliferated although conclusive proof for the efficacy of these strategies remains ethereal.

Sudden cardiac death is best viewed not as a separate clinical syndrome but as a final common pathway for a wide spectrum of cardiac pathology (Box 21-1). The best clinical definition of sudden death is an operational one: Sudden cardiac death is characterized by unexpected and abrupt cardiovascular collapse not associated with trauma. The syndrome may occur in patients without *previously diagnosed* cardiac disease; however, some form of chronic cardiac pathology is the norm. In the patient with known heart disease, sudden cardiac death implies that the underlying cardiac disorder is symptomatically stable and that symptoms of congestive heart failure and ischemia are controlled before the event.

BOX 21-1

Cardiac substrates predisposing to sudden cardiac death

1. Ischemic heart disease
   a. Acute myocardial infarction (MI)
   b. Post-MI (especially in patients with left ventricular dysfunction)
   c. Chronic ischemic cardiomyopathy
2. Dilated cardiomyopathy
   a. Idiopathic
   b. End-stage valvular heart disease
3. Diseases characterized by hypertrophy
   a. Hypertrophic cardiomyopathy
   b. Hypertensive cardiomyopathy
   c. Marked hypertrophy caused by valvular disease
4. Primary electrical disorders
   a. Wolff-Parkinson-White syndrome
   b. Long QT syndromes
   c. Idiopathic ventricular fibrillation

RELEVANT PHYSIOLOGY AND PATHOPHYSIOLOGY

Monitoring of in-hospital episodes of sudden death in early coronary care units revealed that most sudden cardiac deaths were due to ventricular tachyarrhythmias. Ambulatory electrocardiography (Holter monitoring) confirmed this finding in outpatients. A frequent finding from recordings in both settings was the presence of monomorphic or polymorphic ventricular tachycardia at the onset of the event, with subsequent deterioration to ventricular fibrillation. Ventricular tachyarrhythmias account for nearly 80% of sudden cardiac deaths. The rest of sudden arrhythmic deaths are due to bradyarrhythmias. However, not all sudden death is arrhythmic. Myocardial rupture, aortic dissection, and papillary muscle rupture may produce the clinical appearance of sudden arrhythmic death. Similarly, massive pulmonary emboli and central nervous sytem vascular catastrophes should be included in the differential diagnosis (Box 21-2).

Reentry is thought to be the mechanism responsible for most sustained monomorphic ventricular tachycardias. Reentry is made possible by critical pathologic relationships between conduction velocity and refractoriness in an anatomic circuit of conductive tissue. The mechanisms responsible for ventricular fibrillation and polymorphic ventricular tachycardia are less well elucidated. Multiple circulating wavefronts of depolarization form the basis of one hypothesis. Collision, cancellation, and summation of these wavefronts account for the chaotically changing morphology.

Clinical pathophysiologic schemae emphasize three factors that are requisite for sustained ventricular arrhythmias and sudden cardiac death. The first factor is the anatomic substrate. Primary electrical disorders of the heart can and do occasionally occur. However, most patients who have survived an episode of sudden cardiac death and patients who are at high risk for one of these events have underlying structural pathology. In general, the associated disease processes are characterized by fibrosis and scar formation. The substrate for reentry is easiest to conceptualize in the case of a large area of infarcted myocardium adjacent to and interdigitated with normal myocardium. Processes characterized by more diffuse fibrosis and scarring and dilated cardiomyopathy and hypertensive cardiovascular disease are also associated with the propensity for sudden cardiac death. Hypertrophic cardiomyopathy is another important associated clinical entity. In contrast to ischemic heart disease and dilated cardiomyopathy, the risk for sudden death in hypertrophic cardiomyopathy is not associated with left ventricular dysfunction (Chapter 26).

In the processes of fibrosis and scar formation, the second factor necessary for sudden cardiac death evolves: the electrical substrate necessary to sustain a lethal arrhythmia. Assuming that reentry is the basic mechanism for these arrhythmias, a circuit capable of conduction at a rate rapid enough to produce hemodynamic compromise is

---

BOX 21-2
Differential diagnosis of sudden cardiac death

1. Syncope
   a. Syncope caused by bradyarrhythmia
   b. Syncope caused by tachyarrhythmia
   c. Nonarrhythmic syncope (including neurocardiogenic syncope)
2. Seizure
3. Hemodynamic causes of abrupt cardiovascular collapse
   a. Myocardial rupture after myocardial infarction
   b. Papillary muscle rupture
   c. Massive pulmonary emboli
   d. Acute aortic dissection
4. Arrhythmia
   a. Tachycardias
      (i) Ventricular tachycardia/ventricular fibrillation
      (ii) Rapid supraventricular arrhythmias (e.g., atrial fibrillation in Wolff-Parkinson-White syndrome)
   b. Bradycardias
      (i) Atrioventricular block
      (ii) Sick sinus syndrome
5. CNS vascular catastrophes
   a. Massive stroke
   b. Hemorrhage

---

required. The tachycardia rate necessary to produce hemodynamic collapse varies among patients; younger patients without severe heart disease often tolerate rapid rates for substantial periods. Elderly patients with cerebrovascular disease and severe ventricular dysfunction may suffer collapse with relatively slow tachycardias. Even in a single patient, hemodynamic collapse may occur during some episodes and not during others. Patient position, volume status, and intercurrent illness are among the factors that affect the hemodynamic consequences of the arrhythmia.

Even in patients with the appropriate anatomic and electrical substrates, ventricular arrhythmias are seldom incessant. Some perturbation of the usual milieu is necessary for the arrhythmia to be initiated. This third factor is often referred to as the trigger factor. Known triggers include electrolyte imbalance, especially hypokalemia and hypomagnesemia, ischemia, activity of the sympathetic nervous system, and, all too frequently, antiarrhythmic drugs. Some triggers, such as electrolyte abnormalities, are relatively easy to assess and quantify. The means to assess ischemia are also in widespread clinical use. However, the effects of the autonomic nervous system are more difficult to quantify. The means to assess the brain-heart interactions and the effects of circulating catecholamines are still in the developmental stages.

LABORATORY AND OTHER DIAGNOSTIC TESTS

Evaluation of the patient who has survived an episode of out-of-hospital sudden cardiac death is fairly standard. The first step is to determine whether the epsiode of sudden death occurred in association with an acute myocardial infarction. Patients experiencing malignant arrhythmias early (within 48 hours of the onset of an acute myocardial infarction) are at no higher risk for a recurrence than if these early arrhythmias had not occurred. The in-hospital evaluation of these patients is directed at their underlying coronary artery disease, with little attention directed to their risk of arrhythmias. However, patients experiencing ventricular tachycardia or ventricular fibrillation unassociated with acute infarction have a risk of recurrence of 10% to 30% per year. These patients require a full characterization of their anatomic and electrical substrates.

Initial evaluation begins with a complete history and physical examination. A thorough description of the episode of presumed sudden death is mandatory. Because patients often have little recall of their behavior just before and during one of these events, information should be gathered from any available witnesses, as well as from the emergency medical response personnel who first cared for the pa-

tient. Earliest rhythm recorded by the initial responders must be documented. Response to all therapies delivered, including cardiopulmonary resuscitation, should also be carefully recorded. No amount of subsequent testing can compensate for a mistaken diagnosis of aborted sudden cardiac death.

The second step in the evaluation of the sudden death survivor is the complete characterization of the underlying cardiac substrate. The baseline chest radiograph and electrocardiogram should be assessed. Chest radiograph may indicate the presence of cardiac enlargement or congestive heart failure. The electrocardiogram is of obvious importance in the exclusion of an acute infarction, as well as indicating the presence of an old infarction, ventricular hypertrophy, conduction system disease, and heart block. The first specialized cardiac test used is an echocardiogram. The presence of ventricular dysfunction, regional wall motion abnormalities, valvular pathology, pericardial disease, intracardiac tumors, and ventricular hypertrophy can all be determined quickly and reliably by echocardiography (Chapter 13). Echocardiography can be used very early in the hospital course while the patient is still in the coronary care unit; the results are used to guide the remainder of the diagnostic evaluation. Radionuclide ventriculography is performed to assess global and regional ventricular function when a diagnostic-quality echocardiogram is not possible. Because coronary artery disease is the most common substrate for sudden cardiac death, almost every sudden death survivor undergoes cardiac catheterization and coronary arteriography. The presence or absence of significant coronary disease and the need for revascularization affect management plans significantly. Ancillary tests not routinely used but invaluable in the appropriate clinical settings include treadmill testing with or without myocardial perfusion imaging.

The third step in the evaluation of the sudden death survivor is the assessment of the electrical substrate. Twenty-four-hour ambulatory ECG recording is used routinely. The primary means used to assess the heart's electrical function, however, is an electrophysiology (EP) study. Placement of electrode catheters in the right atrium (near the sinus node), the right ventricle, and in the region of the atrioventricular node to record His bundle activation allows measurement of normal cardiac conduction intervals. Furthermore, the responses to various pacing protocols (programmed electrical stimulation) can also be documented. The ability to induce the patient's clinical arrhythmia reproducibly by common pacing techniques indicates a higher propensity for recurrence than if the patient's arrhythmia is not inducible by these techniques. In EP testing, the distinction between diagnostic testing and testing used to guide treatment becomes blurred. Although there is diagnostic and prognostic information in a baseline EP study, the greater role for this technique is in its use to guide therapy (vide infra).

Noninvasive tests predictive of arrhythmia occurrence and sudden death risks have been developed. These tests have been studied best in the postmyocardial infarction patient population and in patients with chronic coronary disease and less extensively in patients with hypertensive heart disease, dilated cardiomyopathy, and hypertrophic cardiomyopathy. These tests include signal-averaged electrocardiography, measurement of T wave alternans, baroreceptor sensitivity, and measurement of heart rate variability. The former two tests are assessments of the cardiac electrical substrate, and the latter two are assessments of the autonomic milieu in which the diseased heart functions. In various reports, the results of each of these tests appear to be independently predictive of the risk for sudden death after an episode of myocardial infarction, especially if the infarction produces significant ventricular dysfunction; however, the tests have been shown only to have prognostic significance thus far. Use of the tests as an indication for treatment or as a means to guide treatment is not yet justified. Furthermore, the risk stratification function of these tests is of greatest value in patients without symptomatic arrhythmias. They have little role at this time in the routine evaluation of the sudden death survivor.

DIFFERENTIAL DIAGNOSIS

Sudden cardiac death resulting from a ventricular arrhythmia can be easily confused with syncope or a seizure. In patients with syncope

---

BOX 21-3

General cardiac care of the sudden death survivor

1. Control ischemia
   a. Medical therapy—β-blockers, calcium channel antagonists, nitrates
   b. Revascularization
      (i) Angioplasty
      (ii) Bypass surgery
2. Treat congestive heart failure and left ventricular dysfunction
   a. Angiotensin-converting enzyme (ACE) inhibitors
   b. Hydralazine and nitrates in patients unable to take ACE inhibitors
   c. Digitalis and diuretics in patients unable to tolerate ACE inhibitors
3. Eliminate as many triggers as possible
   a. Supplemental potassium if medical regimen results in hypokalemia
   b. Magnesium supplements for patients receiving large doses of diuretics

---

BOX 21-4

Treatment approaches useful in preventing sudden cardiac death

1. Coronary revascularization
2. Empiric antiarrhythmic therapy
   a. Beta-blockers
   b. Amiodarone
3. Holter or electrophysiology-guided antiarrhythmic therapy
4. Catheter or surgical ablation of ventricular tachycardia
5. Implantable cardioverter defibrillators

BOX 21-5

Vaughn Williams classification of antiarrhythmic drugs

1. Class I
   Ia—Quinidine, procainamide, disopyramide
   Ib—Mexiletene, tocainide, lidocaine
   Ic—Propafenone, flecainide
2. Class II—β-adrenergic receptor antagonists: metoprolol, propranolol, acebutolol
3. Class III—Bretylium, sotalol, amiodarone
4. Class IV—Calcium channel antagonists: diltiazem, verapamil, nifedipine

---

resulting from a ventricular arrhythmia, differentiation is moot because these patients are managed in much the same manner as patients who have survived sustained tachyarrhythmias. However, ventricular tachyarrhythmias account for only a small percentage of patients with syncope, regardless of etiology, and seizures are, by definition, self-limited, whereas termination of a malignant ventricular tachyarrhythmia requires intervention. Careful documentation of pulselessness and all cardiac rhythms at the time of the event are obviously crucial. Rhythm strips are requisite for excluding a bradyarrhythmia as a cause of cardiovascular collapse. Unfortunately, the necessary haste in initiating treatment and transporting the patient to the hospital often preclude optimal documentation. Rhythm strips often are not recorded or are of poor quality. Strips are often not maintained for later analysis. Poor quality data may preclude the correct diagnosis and result in mismanagement.

The cardiac mechanical events that produce rapid cardiovascular collapse and may be confused with arrhythmic sudden death are best assessed by echocardiography in the coronary care unit. Echocardiography is the preferred initial procedure of choice for the postmyocardial infarction patient who collapses suddenly. Transthoracic echocardiography may indicate evidence of myocardial rupture or papillary muscle rupture. The echocardiogram may also provide diagnostic evidence in cases of massive pulmonary emboli. "Emboli in transit" may be detected in the right heart chambers, or acute right heart dilation and failure may be evident. A transthoracic echocardiogram is sometimes helpful in the diagnosis of aortic dissection. However, a transesophageal echocardiogram is the preferred technique when dissection is clinically suspected. Transesophageal echocardiography is also a useful technique in the evaluation of acute mitral valve dysfunction.

MANAGEMENT

Just as evaluation of the sudden death survivor requires delineation of the underlying cardiac disease as well as the characteristics of the electrical substrate, treatment is aimed at the underlying pathology, not just at the arrhythmia (Box 21-3). Ischemia and heart failure symptoms should be controlled. Ventricular function in patients with cardiomyopathy should be optimized by the use of afterload-reducing agents and digitalis. Revascularization for patients with significant demonstrable ischemia is often beneficial. In those patients in whom symptomatic ischemia immediately preceded the presenting arrhythmia, revascularization alone may be sufficient therapy to prevent a recurrence. Medical regimens should be tailored to avoid electrolyte disturbances that trigger a lethal arrhythmia. Once treatment has optimized the underlying cardiac disease, arrhythmia-specific treatment can be chosen.

Considerable controversy continues regarding the optimal antiarrhythmic therapy for survivors of sudden cardiac death. Survivors can be treated medically, surgically, or with the aid of an implantable device (Box 21-4). Medical therapy may be empiric (unguided), guided by ambulatory ECG recording, or guided by electrophysiologic study.

Early attempts to prevent recurrence of sudden cardiac death using antiarrhythmic drugs relied on these agents in an unguided fashion. The agents used in these early trials, Vaughn Williams Class Ia drugs (Box 21-5), were relatively weak antiarrhythmic agents by current standards. These agents were ineffective in the prevention of sudden death recurrence. Class Ic drugs are more potent antiarrhythmics, but the efficacy in patients with sustained arrhythmias remains sufficiently low to preclude routine empiric use. Empiric use of Class III drugs, amiodarone and sotalol, has been under consideration most recently. In a study performed in Seattle, empiric amiodarone compared favorably with electrophysiologically guided treatment strategies, although the arrhythmia recurrence rate in both treatment groups was high. In the ESVEM (Electrophysiology Study Versus Electrocardiographic Monitoring) clinical trial, patients treated with sotalol fared better than patients on other agents, regardless of how treatment was guided. In postmyocardial infarction patients, propranolol, metoprolol, timolol, and acebutolol have all been demonstrated to improve survival. In an uncontrolled study of survivors of cardiac arrest, β-blockers improved patient survival as compared with patients not taking β-blockers.

Patients with frequent ventricular premature beats or nonsustained ventricular tachycardia are candidates for Holter recording–guided antiarrhythmic therapy. After a baseline Holter study is performed in the drug-free state, the patient receives an antiarrhythmic drug, and another Holter recording is obtained after the drug reaches a steady state level. Suppression of ventricular premature beats and nonsustained ventricular tachycardia is the requirement for efficacy. Because the occurrence of spontaneous arrhythmias can vary greatly from one day to the next, suppression of at least 80% of the baseline premature beats is required before therapeutic effect is ensured. Patients with infrequent spontaneous ectopy and arrhythmias are not candidates for this approach.

EP-guided therapy relies on similar principles to Holter ECG recording–guided therapy. A baseline EP study is performed in the drug-free state in an attempt to induce the patient's presenting arrhythmia. The patient is then prescribed an antiarrhythmic drug or drug regimen and the EP study is repeated. The endpoint of EP-guided treatment is the inability to induce sustained arrhythmia. Persistent inducibility of a slower, hemodynamically tolerated arrhythmia is also an acceptable partial efficacy endpoint. Several electropharmacologic trials may be necessary before one of these endpoints is reached. In fact, no EP-effective regimen is found in a significant number of cases. This is one major drawback of EP-guided treatment along with the expense and discomfort of multiple EP studies. Another major pitfall is that approximately one third of sudden death survivors do not have inducible arrhythmias at baseline EP study.

Direct comparison of Holter monitoring–guided treatment and EP-guided therapy was performed in the ESVEM trial. Patients presenting with sudden death were included but the study also included patients with hemodynamically better tolerated arrhythmias. Sudden death survivors actually made up only a small portion of the study population. Patients included in this study had easily inducible arrhythmias at baseline EP study, as well as frequent ectopy on Holter monitoring. Assignment to Holter-guided or EP-tailored therapy was random. The study found no differences in survival between patients randomized to Holter-guided therapy and those in whom treatment was based on serial electropharmacologic trials. Holter-guided therapy was less expensive, and suitable endpoints were achieved more often in those treated by Holter-guided therapy. Sometimes lost in the debate over the results of this important trial is the fact that arrhythmia recurrence rates in both arms were quite high; nearly 60% of patients experienced arrhythmia recurrence in the first 2 years of study. Rather than conclusively demonstrating the benefits of one treatment strategy over another, the results of ESVEM are viewed by many as an indictment of pharmacologic treatment strategies in general.

The only therapeutic modality that has the potential for patient cure in the traditional sense is surgical resection. This technique is used to good advantage in a few specialized centers in the United States. To be a candidate for surgical resection, the patient must have an inducible arrhythmia and a discrete aneurysm. The technique is also limited by severe preoperative ventricular dysfunction; surgical resection almost invariably causes an additional decrement in ventricular performance. The arrhythmia is mapped intraoperatively, and resection of the region responsible for arrhythmia initiation is then performed. Multiple tachycardia morphologies and origin of the tachycardia near the mitral valve apparatus add further technical difficulty. In experienced centers, elimination of inducible arrhythmia can be accomplished more than 90% of the time. However, the mortality rate of map-guided ventricular resection is 10% to 15% in most centers even when patients are selected carefully. This risk is seldom justified unless the patient requires concomitant surgery for revascularization or valve replacement.

Catheter ablation has high cure rates in specific ventricular tachycardia syndromes, including bundle-branch reentry, right ventricular outflow, or left ventricular septal ventricular tachycardia. This technique has had limited success in curing ventricular tachycardia in patients with coronary artery disease.

Automatic implantable defibrillators were first implanted in 1980, and automatic implantable cardioverter-defibrillators (ICDs) were approved for commercial release by the Food and Drug Administration (FDA) in 1985. Since their release, their use has grown rapidly and device-based therapies are preferred for most sudden death survivors by most cardiac electrophysiologists. Unlike medical or surgical therapies, ICD-based treatment does not prevent life-threatening arrhythmias. The device monitors heart rate much as a pacemaker does. A life-threatening arrhythmia is detected as an abrupt increase in rate. Once programmable detection criteria are met, antitachycardia therapy is delivered. The earliest devices had few programmable features. Current devices have more sophisticated, programmmable detection criteria and can provide backup bradycardia pacing as well as antitachycardia therapies. Tiered therapy devices may be programmed to pace terminate tachycardias in lower rate ranges, deliver a low-energy shock at an intermediate rate or if pacing fails, and deliver a high-energy shock for very rapid rates or if all other treatments fail.

Implantation of an ICD is a relatively simple procedure, especially when compared with the complexities of map-guided surgical resection for treatment of an arrhythmia. Current devices are much smaller and can be implanted in the pectoral region much like a pacemaker. Current lead systems incorporate the rate-sensing electrodes and defibrillation electrodes in a single lead that can be placed by the transvenous route. A procedure that once required a thoracotomy and a fairly lengthy hospital stay can now be performed during an overnight hospital stay. Once lead positioning is accomplished, testing is performed to ensure that the ICD will detect and terminate a lethal arrhythmia. Ventricular fibrillation is induced repeatedly, and the amount of energy necessary to reliably defibrillate the heart—the *defibrillation threshold* (DFT)—is determined. The implanted device should be able to deliver at least 10 J of energy more than the DFT before device implantation is accomplished.

ICD use offers many advantages over medical therapy. Patient compliance is not an issue with an ICD. Medication toxicity also is less of a problem. Although most patients receiving ICDs also receive some form of antiarrhythmic medication, the intensity of medical therapy is less than in patients treated with medicines alone. Also, breakthrough arrhythmias are unlikely to be fatal. ICD therapy does not require that arrhythmias be inducible at baseline EP study. The primary reason that ICD therapy has become so popular, however, is its success in preventing mortality as a result of recurrence of sudden cardiac death. Sudden death mortality as low as 1% per year has been reported in large uncontrolled series. Most patients with ICDs also have significant ventricular dysfunction and noncardiac comorbid conditions. A significant impact of ICDs on total mortality has yet to be demonstrated. The results of ongoing clinical studies will determine the lasting impact of ICDs on the treatment strategies for sudden death survivors.

ICD therapy should not be used for every sudden death survivor. Some patients are psychologically intolerant of therapy that rescues them with a painful shock when the arrhythmia occurs. Patients with a history of frequent arrhythmias that would result in very frequent shocks should not have an ICD implanted without extensive counseling and consideration of all alternatives. ICD therapy is expensive but compares favorably to serial electropharmacologic trials requiring a prolonged hospital course.

Although the last two decades have witnessed the development of several treatment strategies for sudden death survivors, this development has had little effect on the public health problem of sudden cardiac death. Unfortunately and immutably, most patients do not survive the first episode of sudden cardiac death. Sudden death mortality can be addressed in a major way only by efforts to prevent heart disease and the initial episode of sudden death in patients with known heart disease. This latter issue has been studied extensively. These studies have focused particularly on patients with ischemic heart disease who have survived an episode of myocardial infarction.

Large-scale, carefully controlled, randomized studies in the United States and abroad indicate that β-blocker use after myocardial infarction affects subsequent sudden death mortality, as well as overall mortality. Subgroup analysis indicates that β-blocker use is most valuable in high-risk cases, that is, patients with left ventricular dysfunction and complex or frequent ventricular ectopy on Holter monitoring. In patients with left ventricular dysfunction after myocardial infarction, as well as in patients with left ventricular dysfunction of other etiologies, angiotensin-converting enzyme (ACE) inhibitors have a favorable effect on mortality. The large studies addressing this issue are concordant with regard to the improvement in total mortality but discordant with regard to the impact of ACE inhibitors on sudden death mortality. ACE inhibitors should be used routinely in patients with left ventricular dysfunction who are at risk for sudden death because of their favorable impact on symptoms and overall survival.

Although the use of β-blockers and ACE inhibitors after myocardial infarction is well substantiated by scientific evidence, the data indicate that the routine use of antiarrhythmic agents after myocardial infarction is deleterious. This was best demonstrated in CAST (Cardiac Arrhythmia Suppression Trial). This study targeted postmyocardial infarction patients at increased risk for sudden cardiac death. Study drugs included encainide, flecainide, and moricizine. Long-term therapy was chosen for the patients based on demonstrated sup-

✔ *WHEN TO REFER*

Care of the sudden death survivor is a complex, multifaceted process (Box 21-6). An organized team approach is required for many patients. In many instances, the patient's primary cardiac disorder may be managed effectively by a primary care physician or general cardiologist. Management of postresuscitation complications may require the services of an intensivist. Arrhythmia management often requires consultation with a cardiologist experienced in the management of arrhythmias or a specially trained cardiac electrophysiologist. The physician responsible for managing the arrhythmia should have experience in the techniques of EP testing, as well as ICD implantation. ICD implantation may require the services of a thoracic surgeon, although implantation by cardiologists in cardiac catheterization laboratories has become a standard practice in many centers. Map-guided surgery should be considered in selective cases and in centers experienced in these specialized techniques. Open communication between the primary care physician and the physician(s) responsible for arrhythmia management is requisite for optimal outcomes.

Patients experiencing sudden cardiac death within the first 48 hours of a well-documented acute myocardial infarction do not require referral (Chapter 23). Arrhythmias in the acute setting should be treated conventionally with lidocaine, procainamide, and bretylium. Once the acute arrhythmias have been controlled, antiarrhythmics should be discontinued and the patient observed closely for recurrences. In the absence of recurrent symptomatic arrhythmias, no further antiarrhythmic therapies are warranted. Patients experiencing sudden death in the late in-hospital phase of an acute infarction or soon after discharge are among the most difficult patients to evaluate. Although the risk of recurrent life-threatening arrhythmias in these patients is significant, the scar from the episode of infarction is not fully formed and the mature postmyocardial infarction electrical substrate has not fully developed. The hazards of selecting long-term therapy during a time when the electrical substrate is changing are apparent. The management of patients experiencing late acute phase (more than 48 hours but less than 4 to 6 weeks) arrhythmias should probably involve an arrhythmia specialist.

Another special circumstance is the patient who experiences sudden cardiac death as a complication of treatment with an antiarrhythmic drug. In many cases, the antiarrhythmic agent was prescribed for atrial fibrillation. These patients do not require referral. Discontinuation of the offending drug, reconsideration of the need for antiarrhythmic therapy, and, if a drug is required, use of an agent with a lower risk of proarrhythmia (e.g., amiodarone) represent one appropriate course of action.

The issue of patients at increased risk for lethal ventricular arrhythmias but who have yet to experience a symptomatic episode is also problematic, and management of these patients remains controversial. Examples in this group include patients with ischemic cardiomyopathy and late potentials on signal-averaged electrocardiograms or frequent nonsustained ventricular tachycardia on Holter monitoring, patients with dilated cardiomyopathy and frequent spontaneous arrhythmias, and patients with hypertrophic cardiomyopathy and syncope or a family history of sudden death. There is no consensus regarding the management of these cases. Although selective cases may warrant aggressive intervention, sudden death prophylaxis in these settings deserves further study, and patients treated prophylactically should be treated in a research environment where the merit of the treatment can be rigorously assessed.

✔ *WHEN TO REFER*

1. Patients experiencing sudden cardiac death unassociated with an acute myocardial infarction
2. Patients experiencing symptomatic arrhythmias after myocardial infarction
   a. Late acute phase (2 days to 6 weeks)
   b. Chronic phase
3. High-risk patients yet to experience a symptomatic episode of arrhythmia (more controversial)
   a. Dilated cardiomyopathy and frequent ectopy
   b. Hypertrophic cardiomyopathy
      (i) Family history of sudden death
      (ii) Syncope
   c. Left ventricular dysfunction and syncope

patients at increased risk for sudden death is currently under investigation. The strategy of prophylactic ICD implantation in patients at increased risk for sudden death is also under study in several trials.

BIBLIOGRAPHY

Cardiac Arrhythmia Suppression Trial (CAST) Investigators: Preliminary report: effect of encainide and flecainide on mortality in a randomized trial of arrhythmia suppression after myocardial infarction, *N Engl J Med* 321:406-412, 1989.

Cardiac Arrhythmia Suppression Trial (CAST) II Investigators: Effect of the antiarrhythmic agent moricizine on survival after myocardial infarction, *N Engl J Med* 327:227-233, 1992.

Cascade Investigators: Cardiac arrest in Seattle: conventional versus amiodarone drug evaluation, *Am J Cardiol* 67:578-584, 1991.

Cascade Investigators: Randomized antiarrhythmic drug therapy in survivors of cardiac arrest, *Am J Cardiol* 72:280-287, 1993.

Cox JL: Patient selection criteria and results of surgery for refractory ischemic ventricular tachycardia, *Circulation* 79(suppl I):I163-I177, 1989.

DiMarco JP, Haines DE: Sudden cardiac death, *Curr Probl Cardiol* 15:187-232, 1990.

Engelstein E, Zipes D: Sudden cardiac death. In Alexander RW, Schlant RC, Fuster V, editors: *The heart,* New York, 1998, McGraw-Hill.

ESVEM Investigators: Electrophysiologic study versus electrocardiographic monitoring for selection of antiarrhythmic therapy for ventricular arrhythmias, *Circulation* 79:1354-1360, 1989.

ESVEM Investigators: Determinants of predicted efficacy of antiarrhythmic drugs in the electrophysiologic study versus electrocardiographic monitoring trial, *Circulation* 87:323-329, 1993.

Gillum RF: Sudden coronary death in the United States 1980-1985, *Circulation* 79:756-765, 1989.

Gilman JK, Jalal S, Naccarelli GV: Predicting and preventing sudden death from cardiac causes, *Circulation* 90:1083-1092, 1994.

Gilman JK, Naccarelli GV: Sudden cardiac death, *Curr Probl Cardiol* 17:699-778, 1992.

Greene HL: The CASCADE study: randomized antiarrhythmic drug therapy in survivors of cardiac arrest in Seattle, *Am J Cardiol* 72(suppl F):70F-74F, 1993.

Kelly P et al: Surgical coronary revascularization in survivors of prehospital cardiac arrest: its effect on inducible ventricular arrhythmias and long-term survival, *J Am Coll Cardiol* 15:267-274, 1990.

Kleman JM et al: Nonthoracotomy versus thoracotomy implantable defibrillators: intention-to-treat comparison of clinical outcomes, *Circulation* 90:2833-2842, 1994.

Kupperman M et al: An analysis of the cost-effectiveness of the inplantable cardioverter defibrillator, *Circulation* 90:91-100, 1990.

Libertson RR: Sudden death from cardiac causes in children and young adults, *N Engl J Med* 334:1039-1044, 1996.

Mason JW: A comparison of electrophysiologic testing with Holter monitoring to predict antiarrhythmic drug efficacy for ventricular arrhythmias, *N Engl J Med* 329:445-451, 1993.

Mason JW: A comparison of seven antiarrhythmic drugs in patients with ventricular tachyarrhythmias, *N Engl J Med* 329:452-458, 1993.

O'Donoghue S et al: Automatic implantable cardioverter defibrillator: is early implantation cost-effective? *J Am Coll Cardiol* 16:1258-1263, 1990.

Wilber DJ et al: Out-of-hospital cardiac arrest: use of electrophysiologic testing in the prediction of long-term outcome, *N Engl J Med* 318:19-24, 1988.

Winkle RA et al: Long-term outcome with the automatic implantable cardioverter-defibrillator, *J Am Coll Cardiol* 13:1353-1361, 1989.

pression of ventricular ectopy on Holter monitoring. Despite the demonstrated efficacy of antiarrhythmic agents, more deaths and more cardiac arrests occurred in patients receiving these drugs than in patients receiving placebo. CAST graphically illustrated that antiarrhythmic agents can be proarrhythmic or can make arrhythmias worse instead of better. Every antiarrhythmic drug is associated with proarrhythmia to some degree. Class Ia and Ic drugs have the greatest incidence of proarrhythmia. Amiodarone is a potent antiarrhythmic with a low incidence of proarrhythmia. The routine use of amiodarone in

IV SPECIFIC DISEASE ENTITIES

CHAPTER

22 Ischemic Heart Disease

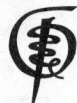

Kanu Chatterjee

The manifestations and pathophysiologic consequences of ischemic heart disease are protean. Ischemic heart disease may be totally silent or may manifest in angina, arrhythmias, and heart failure. Myocardial ischemia stems from the imbalance between myocardial oxygen (O_2) requirements and O_2 supply. Myocardial O_2 supply (arterial O_2 content times coronary blood flow) primarily depends on coronary blood flow; in most patients, arterial O_2 saturation and content are normal. An imbalance between myocardial O_2 supply and demand can occur from a primary decrease in coronary blood flow or from a disproportionate increase in myocardial O_2 requirements or their combination. In some clinical syndromes of ischemic heart disease, the capacity to increase coronary blood flow for the increment in myocardial O_2 demand is limited, and myocardial ischemia results whenever this reserve for myocardial perfusion is exceeded. Impaired myocardial perfusion, caused by primary decrease in coronary blood flow resulting from fixed or dynamic increase in the coronary arterial resistance and/or abnormalities of the coronary vascular autoregulatory mechanisms, appears to be the principal cause for myocardial ischemia in other clinical syndromes. Conceivably the mechanisms for myocardial ischemia may vary in the same individuals in different circumstances, and, as a result, the clinical manifestations may also change. Considerable advances have been made in the last few years in the understanding of the pathophysiologic mechanisms of myocardial ischemia in the different clinical syndromes of chronic ischemic heart disease.

ETIOLOGY

Obstructive coronary artery disease caused by atherosclerosis is the most common cause of chronic ischemic heart disease. In addition, manifestations of chronic and episodic myocardial ischemia can occur from nonatherosclerotic coronary artery disease and in the absence of any coronary artery disease.

Debate over the precise mechanism by which atherosclerotic lesions of the coronary arteries develop in patients with chronic ischemic heart disease continues (Chapter 306). Nevertheless, it is generally believed that the intimal layer is principally involved in atherosclerosis, and three different types of lesions can be identified: the fatty streak, the fibrous plaque, and the complicated lesion. Current evidence suggests that intimal endothelial injury is important in initiating the atherosclerotic process. Experimental studies suggest that the endothelial barrier, broken by mechanical or chemical injury, is associated with a tissue response that includes local platelet adhesion and aggregation. Various factors, including hypertension and hyperlipidemia, can injure the arterial endothelium and trigger this tissue response. The disruption of endothelium exposes the subendothelial connective tissue to platelets, as well as to circulating lipids. With repeated or continuous endothelial injury, deposition of intracellular and extracellular lipids and proliferation of arterial smooth muscle then contribute to the formation of obliterative atherosclerotic lesions. Cellular necrosis, hemorrhage, lipid deposition, and smooth muscle proliferation then lead to complicated lesions that contain newly formed connective tissue and lipids that may eventually calcify.

Alternative hypotheses have also been promulgated to explain human coronary artery atherosclerosis. Cellular mechanisms for lipid deposition might be involved in the development of the atherosclerotic process. Continued, enhanced synthesis of cholesterol, deficient high-density (alpha) lipoproteins (HDLs), and a defective lysosomal lipoprotein transport mechanism have been proposed as potential contributory mechanisms in the pathogenesis of coronary artery atherosclerosis.

Precisely how well-recognized, important risk factors such as hypertension, smoking, diabetes mellitus, increased low-density lipoproteins (LDLs), and decreased HDL levels contribute to the development of atherosclerotic coronary artery lesions has not been established. Hypertension is regarded as an important contributing factor for the entrance of lipids. The ingredients of cigarette smoke that are thought to promote atherosclerosis are carbon monoxide and nicotine, but the mechanisms remain unclear. Diabetic patients have been reported to have circulating substances that promote muscle proliferation, as well as an increased propensity to bind lipoproteins.

High levels of total cholesterol and increased levels of LDL fraction, decreased total HDL, and its subfractions HDL_2 and HDL_3, particularly HDL_2, have been found to be important risk factors for coronary artery disease. Insulin resistance, which may be associated with impaired glucose tolerance, hyperinsulinemia, elevated plasma triglyceride levels, and decreased HDL cholesterol, has been identified as a risk factor for atherosclerotic coronary artery disease.

Hyperlipidemia may be secondary (mainly dietary) or primary (from familial defects in cellular LDL receptors). The mechanism of the "protective" effects of HDLs needs clarification. Nevertheless, recent studies suggest that modification is feasible in clinical practice and may be associated with halting the progression and even with regression of atherosclerosis. Thus modification of risk factors is important in the management of chronic ischemic heart disease.

Although atherosclerotic obstructive coronary artery disease is the most common cause of chronic myocardial ischemia, myocardial ischemia can result from nonatherosclerotic coronary artery disease, as well as appear in the absence of coronary artery lesions (Box 22-1). Congenital anomalies of the coronary arteries (e.g., anomalous origin of the left coronary artery from the pulmonary artery) can precipitate myocardial ischemia and infarction. Hereditary metabolic disorders are infrequently associated with nonatherosclerotic coronary artery lesions. Systemic collagen vascular disease, irradiation, chest trauma, and extrinsic compression of the coronary arteries by tumors can infrequently cause obstructive lesions and myocardial ischemia.

When myocardial ischemia occurs in the presence of normal coronary arteries, several pathologic conditions should be considered. If coronary artery spasm is demonstrated, variant angina (Prinzmetal's angina) is most likely the diagnosis. Although acute episodes of myocardial ischemia can result from coronary artery embolism, chronic myocardial ischemia is a rare sequela.

Increase in myocardial O_2 requirements and impaired myocardial perfusion may precipitate myocardial ischemia in patients with valvular heart disease and hypertrophic cardiomyopathy. In dilated nonischemic cardiomyopathy, myocardial O_2 demand may also increase disproportionately because of a marked increase in left ventricular wall stress. Decreased transmyocardial pressure gradient caused by elevated left ventricular diastolic pressure and impaired coronary vasodilatory reserve may also compromise myocardial perfusion and induce myocardial ischemia.

PATHOPHYSIOLOGY
Determinants of Myocardial Oxygen Demand

The major determinants of myocardial oxygen demand ($M\dot{V}O_2$) and perfusion are shown in Box 22-2 (Chapter 9). Even under conditions of no increased stress, the myocardium extracts approximately 75% of the available O_2. This O_2 is used to provide energy by oxidative metabolism, and the rate of myocardial O_2 consumption parallels the cardiac energy requirements.

Heart rate is a major determinant of $M\dot{V}O_2$, which increases as heart rate increases. Tachycardia also produces deleterious effects on myocardial perfusion because of the decreased duration of diastole, during which left ventricular perfusion occurs. Reduction of heart rate

---

BOX 22-1

Causes of myocardial ischemia in presence and absence of coronary artery disease

---

I. Atherosclerotic obstructive coronary artery disease
II. Nonatherosclerotic coronary artery disease
  A. Coronary artery spasm
  B. Congenital coronary artery anomalies
    1. Anomalous origin of coronary artery from pulmonary artery
    2. Aberrant origin of coronary artery from aorta or another coronary artery
    3. Coronary arteriovenous fistula
    4. Coronary artery aneurysm
III. Acquired disorders of coronary arteries
  A. Coronary artery embolism
  B. Dissection
    1. Surgical
    2. During percutaneous coronary angioplasty
    3. Aortic dissection
    4. Spontaneous, e.g., during pregnancy
  C. Extrinsic compression
    1. Tumors
    2. Granulomas
    3. Amyloidosis
  D. Collagen vascular disease
    1. Polyarteritis nodosa
    2. Temporal arteritis
    3. Rheumatoid arthritis
    4. Systemic lupus erythematosus
    5. Scleroderma
  E. Miscellaneous disorders
    1. Irradiation
    2. Trauma
    3. Kawasaki disease
  F. Syphilis
IV. Hereditary disorders
  A. Pseudoxanthoma elasticum
  B. Gargoylism
  C. Progeria
  D. Homocystinuria
  E. Primary oxaluria
V. "Functional" causes of myocardial ischemia in absence of anatomic coronary artery disease
  A. Syndrome X
  B. Hypertrophic cardiomyopathy
  C. Dilated cardiomyopathy
  D. Muscle bridge
  E. Hypertensive heart disease
  F. Pulmonary hypertension
  G. Valvular heart disease; aortic stenosis, aortic regurgitation

---

BOX 22-2

Major determinants of myocardial oxygen consumption and coronary blood flow

---

I. Myocardial oxygen consumption
  A. Heart rate
  B. Contractility
  C. Wall stress
    1. Intraventricular pressure
    2. Ventricular volume
    3. Wall thickness
II. Myocardial perfusion
  A. Perfusion pressure (arterial diastolic pressure)
  B. Epicardial coronary artery resistance, including resistance at the site of stenosis
  C. Coronary arteriolar resistance
  D. Extravascular resistance
  E. Left ventricular diastolic pressure and coronary sinus venous pressure

---

Determinants of Coronary Blood Flow and Myocardial Oxygen Supply

Myocardial O_2 supply is a function of O_2 delivery and extraction. Arterial O_2 content cannot be significantly increased under normal atmospheric conditions, and myocardial O_2 extraction is nearly maximum at rest. Thus augmenting coronary blood flow remains the principal means of providing increased O_2 supply.

Coronary blood flow is directly related to the perfusion pressure (aortic diastolic pressure) and the duration of diastole and is inversely proportional to coronary vascular bed resistance, the latter being determined by a number of factors (Chapter 9). The degree of epicardial coronary artery stenosis is a major determinant of coronary blood flow in patients with atherosclerotic ischemic heart disease. In addition the autonomic activity, circulating neurohumoral substances, and local vasoactive components modulate the epicardial coronary arterial tone. Alpha-adrenergic stimulation is associated with decreased caliber and increased tone of the epicardial coronary arteries. The role of local and circulating vasoactive substances (prostacyclin, thromboxane, endothelial-derived relaxing factor, endothelin, serotonin, histamine, angiotensin) in the regulation of the coronary vascular tone, either in normal or in pathologic conditions, has not been clearly delineated. It has been suggested, however, that the dynamic variations in the caliber of both the normal and the stenosed coronary artery segments may occur in response to these vasoactive stimuli.

The extravascular mechanical compression of the intramyocardial coronary arteries offers resistance to coronary blood flow during systole. The resistance offered by arteriolar vessels, the site of autoregulation, modulates coronary vascular resistance and plays a major role in regulating myocardial perfusion with or without coronary artery disease. The arteriolar tone is influenced by autonomic activity, metabolic products, circulating neurohumoral substances, and various pharmacologic agents. During increased myocardial metabolic demand, such as during exercise, arteriolar resistance declines, which augments blood flow (autoregulatory reserve). With increasing severity of epicardial coronary artery stenosis, the autoregulatory reserve is progressively diminished, and with very severe coronary artery stenosis, the distal coronary vascular bed resistance may reach minimum levels. In such circumstances, myocardial perfusion depends primarily on perfusion pressure, and a reduction in arterial diastolic pressure may precipitate myocardial ischemia.

Left ventricular diastolic pressure and coronary sinus venous pressure also serve to resist myocardial perfusion, particularly to the subendocardium. A decrease in left ventricular diastolic pressure, without a concomitant reduction in arterial diastolic pressure, increases the transmyocardial pressure gradient and thereby improves subendocardial perfusion.

is therefore associated with decreased MVO_2 and improved left ventricular myocardial perfusion. Intraventricular systolic pressure (same as systemic arterial pressure in the absence of left ventricular outflow obstruction), ventricular volume, and wall thickness are the major determinants of left ventricular wall stress. Increased ventricular volume and/or pressure increase wall stress; increased wall thickness (hypertrophy) decreases wall stress. The rationale for reducing arterial pressure and/or left ventricular volume in order to decrease MVO_2 is apparent. Enhanced contractility increases MVO_2. Therefore reduction of contractility is another potential method of decreasing O_2 requirements.

In clinical practice, the most frequently used index of MVO_2 is the product of peak systolic pressure and heart rate (*double product*). This index, however, does not incorporate changes in contractility or ventricular volume. The tension-time index (*triple product*) includes the area under the systolic portion of the arterial pressure curve, left ventricular ejection time, and heart rate but excludes left ventricular volume and contractility. Little difference exists between the double product and the triple product as indices of MVO_2.

Angina of Effort (Classic Angina). By far the most common cause of *exertional angina* is atherosclerotic narrowing of the large epicardial coronary arteries. The resulting intraluminal resistance is added to the autoregulatory resistance of the arterioles and contributes significantly to the total coronary arterial resistance to blood flow.

In patients with effort angina, resting coronary blood flow is adequate and proportional to MVO_2 at rest, indicating that stenotic resistance and the resistance of the distal coronary vascular bed are below the critical level required to limit flow at rest. During exercise, there is a two-fold to four-fold decrease in resistance of the distal coronary vascular bed mediated by local metabolites that promote coronary blood flow to meet the increased MVO_2. Although such vasodilation always increases flow to the potentially ischemic myocardial zones, the increment in flow for a given increase in demand becomes progressively curtailed as the degree of stenosis increases, resulting in relative myocardial ischemia. The principal mechanism for the increased MVO_2 is increased heart rate and arterial pressure, as well as a reflex increase in contractility. A relative increase in left ventricular diastolic volume and pressure and decreased diastolic perfusion time might also be contributory in some patients. The mechanism for the efficacy of pharmacologic agents that decrease MVO_2 in effort angina is apparent.

Absolute reduction of coronary blood flow to the potentially ischemic myocardial zones can also occur during increased myocardial stress and during exercise. This reduction in flow may result from a decrease in the perfusion pressure distal to the stenosis associated with increased flow velocity through the stenosis and/or diversion of flow from the subendocardium toward the epicardium. Thus exertional angina may result from either an excessive increase in myocardial O_2 requirements, causing an imbalance of O_2 demand and supply, or an absolute reduction of flow, producing true myocardial ischemia. An increase in the coronary arterial tone, either at the site of stenosis or at the nonatherosclerotic segments, may occur during exercise and may contribute to decreased coronary blood flow.

Variant Angina (Prinzmetal's Angina). Variant angina is characterized by cyclically recurrent angina at rest, usually unrelated to effort. It is often associated with S-T segment elevation on the electrocardiogram (ECG) during angina.

The primary mechanism of variant angina is a spontaneous decrease in coronary blood flow unrelated to changes in MVO_2. Arteriographic studies have documented transient complete or incomplete, localized or diffuse narrowing of the epicardial coronary arteries (coronary artery spasm), causing interruptions of flow to the ischemic myocardium during spontaneous angina. Coronary artery spasm can also be provoked by intravenous (IV) injection of vasoconstrictors such as ergonovine or by hyperventilation. Such spasm is usually accompanied by symptoms and ECG changes similar to those associated with the patient's spontaneous angina attacks. The mechanism for the focal or diffuse spasm of the coronary arteries still remains speculative. Activation of histamine or serotonin receptors, an imbalance between the beta- and alpha-adrenoreceptor activity, an imbalance between vasodilator prostacyclin and vasoconstrictive thromboxane activity, and decreased production of endothelial-derived relaxing factors in the presence of atherosclerosis have been regarded as potential mechanisms. It must be emphasized that both the precise mechanism for coronary artery spasm and the precise triggering mechanism in individual patients remain unclear.

Most patients with variant angina also have fixed obstructive coronary artery lesions of varying severity. Only a few have completely normal coronary arteries. The sites of coronary artery spasm may vary, although they most frequently occur at, or in the vicinity of, atherosclerotic lesions. However, in the same patient, single or multiple coronary arteries, different coronary arteries, or different locations in the same artery may demonstrate coronary artery spasm during anginal attacks. This variability should be considered in the management of patients with variant angina.

Silent Myocardial Ischemia. Myocardial ischemia can occur without any symptoms referable to ischemia. The existence of *silent ischemia* has been documented by arteriographic, scintigraphic, metabolic, ECG, and hemodynamic studies. Reversible wall motion abnormalities, and myocardial thallium perfusion defects, transient de-

crease in myocardial rubidium-82 uptake, and S-T segment shifts in the ECG, occurring during stress or spontaneously without angina provide evidence for silent ischemia. Abnormal myocardial lactate metabolism and regional and global ventricular systolic and diastolic dysfunction during induced ischemia, in the absence of angina are further indicators of silent ischemia.

The mechanism for silent asymptomatic ischemia during exercise appears to be similar to that for exercise-induced angina, that is, increased myocardial O_2 requirements producing imbalance between O_2 demand and supply. Continuous ambulatory ECG and blood pressure monitoring in patients with chronic stable angina reveals that both heart rate and blood pressure increase frequently during a few minutes preceding the onset of ischemic S-T segment changes, suggesting that increased myocardial O_2 demand may, in part, be a potential mechanism for silent ischemia in these patients. Decreased heart rate or lack of increase in heart rate with beta-adrenergic blocking agents associated with reduction in the frequency and duration of silent ischemia also provides evidence for increased MVO_2 as a contributory mechanism for silent ischemia. Spontaneous episodes of silent ischemia, however, may occur without any increase in the MVO_2. Heart rate preceding or during the episodes of ischemia is often lower than that during exercise-induced angina. During the episodes of unprovoked ischemic S-T segment depression without angina, there is decreased myocardial uptake of rubidium-82. This suggests that a primary decrease in coronary blood flow may be the mechanism for spontaneous episodes of silent myocardial ischemia. The mechanisms for the primary decrease or an inadequate increase in coronary blood flow when there is an increment in MVO_2 may be different in the different anginal syndromes. It is likely that in patients with variant angina, the mechanisms that precipitate symptomatic myocardial ischemia also induce silent myocardial ischemia.

In patients with unstable ischemic syndromes (unstable angina, postinfarction angina), spontaneous episodes of silent ischemia probably result from formation of labile nonocclusive thrombi at the site of ruptured or fissured atheromatous plaques, causing transient interruption of blood flow. Coronary arterial vasoconstriction mediated by vasoactive substances released because of platelet and endothelial dysfunction may further decrease coronary blood flow and compromise myocardial perfusion. Increased coronary vascular tone resulting from heightened sympathetic activity and/or platelet aggregation, release of vasoactive substances such as thromboxane, and a reduced vasodilating regulatory effect of endothelial-derived relaxing factors are other potential mechanisms for spontaneous silent myocardial ischemia. Until the mechanism for silent ischemia can be determined, the therapy, when indicated, will remain empirical, utilizing nonspecific coronary vasodilators or reperfusion therapy.

Mixed Angina. Patients with mixed angina are those whose clinical profiles are not typical of either classic angina or variant angina. Since the exercise threshold is variable, alterations in coronary vascular tone and spontaneous changes in coronary blood flow have been implicated as causes of ischemia. Variable responsiveness of the coronary vascular bed to adrenergic stimulation might explain the changes in coronary vasculature resistance. A simultaneous increase in MVO_2 also contributes to mixed angina. Although these patients have variable exercise thresholds, the rate-pressure product at the onset of angina or S-T segment depression during exercise remains unchanged.

Postprandial Angina. The mechanism of postprandial angina also needs further clarification. The hypothesis that the diversion of blood flow from the myocardium to the gastrointestinal system precipitates postprandial angina has not been substantiated. The hemodynamic changes associated with ingestion are characterized by increased heart rate and blood pressure caused by reflex sympathetic stimulation. Thus increased MVO_2 provides a possible explanation, particularly when angina occurs during exercise after meals. In these patients, significant obstructive atherosclerotic lesions are likely to be present. However, it is also possible that an inappropriate increase in coronary vascular tone resulting from sympathetic stimulation causes a primary reduction in coronary blood flow, causing postprandial angina. Despite increased heart rate and blood pressure, which increase MVO_2, coronary blood flow is not proportionally increased and may even fall. Thus both a "vasoactive mechanism" and increased $M\dot{V}O_2$ likely contribute to postprandial angina.

Walk Through Angina. In this syndrome, angina is experienced at the beginning of physical activity, for example, walking, and angina is relieved later despite continuing the same physical activity. An inappropriate increase in coronary resistance resulting in an inadequate increase or decrease in coronary blood flow at the beginning of the exercise has been thought to be the mechanism. Walk through angina usually indicates the presence of coronary artery disease. In the majority of patients with obstructive atherosclerotic coronary artery disease, however, the intensity of angina increases with continued physical activity.

Linked Angina. In this syndrome, typical angina occurs during visceral stimulation (e.g., during drinking cold liquids or during esophageal reflux) associated with evidence of myocardial ischemia such as S-T segment depression in the ECG. Linked angina can occur in the presence or absence of atherosclerotic coronary artery disease. Primary decrease in coronary blood flow due to centrally mediated increase in coronary resistance resulting from visceral stimulation appears to be the mechanism of linked angina.

Unstable Angina. The syndrome of unstable angina is clinically characterized by angina of changing character, duration, and intensity in patients with either a relatively long history of stable angina or a recent onset of angina. Discrete, single, or multiple episodes of prolonged rest angina are important features of the clinical profile.

Patients with stable angina may become "unstable" because of the development of concurrent illness such as severe anemia, hyperthyroidism, and aortic stenosis (secondary unstable angina). However, in most patients such secondary causes are absent, and a primary change in the pathoanatomy of the coronary artery lesions appears to precipitate unstable angina syndrome. The distribution of coronary artery lesions is similar in patients with stable and unstable angina, but the type of lesions in patients with unstable angina may be different from those in patients with stable angina. In unstable angina an eccentric atheromatous plaque with irregular surface protruding into the lumen of the coronary artery (type IIb) is the most frequent type of lesion identified angiographically. In patients with stable angina, smooth concentric (type I), smooth eccentric (type IIa), or diffuse lesions (type III) are more frequent. The lesions' irregular surface probably represents fissuring or ulceration of the plaques, which may initiate platelet aggregation and adhesion and formation of labile nonocclusive thrombi at the site or vicinity of the atheromatous plaque.

Increased platelet aggregability and increased production of vasoconstrictor thromboxane A_2 appear to occur more frequently in patients with unstable angina than in patients with stable angina or acute myocardial infarction. Furthermore, intraoperative angioscopic studies have demonstrated thrombus at the site of the atheromatous plaque, causing partial or total occlusion of the offending coronary artery. The increased serum concentrations of fibrin-related antigen, D dimer, the principal breakdown fragment of fibrin and of fibrin monomer, an intermediate product of fibrin formation, in the serum of patients with unstable angina compared with that of control subjects and patients with chronic stable angina provides indirect evidence for the presence of an active thrombotic process in patients with unstable angina. Fibrinopeptide A concentration is also higher in patients with unstable angina. Coronary arteriographic studies have demonstrated the presence of atherosclerotic coronary artery lesions in most patients with unstable angina and the presence of thrombus in the artery supplying the area of ischemia.

Autopsy studies indicate that in patients with acute ischemic syndromes, vulnerable plaques with tear, ulceration, and disintegration of their fibrous cap with deep injury of the atheroma lie beneath approximately 75% of intraluminal thrombi. The vulnerable plaques are usually less obstructive and have larger atheromatous and less sclerotic components with more cholesterol esters than crystalline cholesterol and thinner rather than thicker fibrous caps. Plaque disruption tends to occur more frequently at the shoulder regions, that is, at the junctions of the plaque and the normal arterial wall. The thinner plaque cap is friable and relatively avascular with decreased smooth muscle cells and collagen. Decreased synthesis and/or increased degradation of collagen, mediated by infiltrating activated inflammatory cells (macrophages, T-lymphocytes, mast cells), and activation of the programmed death (apoptosis) of vascular smooth muscle cells are a few of the proposed mechanisms of "cap thinning" of the vulnerable plaques. The triggering mechanisms of plaque disruption are not known but are likely multifactorial. Increased tension on the fibrous cap resulting from increased coronary artery luminal pressure (hypertension) and diameter, increased intraplaque pressure, compression of the cap and plaque, vasospasm, and abnormal bending deformation of the plaque-containing arterial wall—all may contribute to plaque disruption. Whatever the mechanisms of plaque disruption may be, associated platelet dysfunction, exposure of plaque thrombogenic material to flowing blood, and thrombotic-thrombolytic disequilibrium contribute to the formation of nonocclusive thrombi—the principal mechanism of interruption of coronary blood flow in primary unstable angina. Phasic vasoconstriction of the plaque-containing epicardial coronary arteries mediated by released vasoconstrictive substances such as thromboxane, serotonin, and endothelin may also cause phasic reduction in coronary blood flow.

Patients with recent catheter-based myocardial revascularization (e.g., percutaneous transluminal coronary angioplasty [PTCA]) or surgical myocardial revascularization (coronary artery bypass [CABG]) may have a clinical profile similar to those with primary unstable angina. The pathophysiologic mechanisms of unstable angina in these patients, however, are different. Restenosis in patients with prior PTCA and graft stenosis in patients with prior CABG surgery are more frequent mechanisms in these patients than the disruption of a vulnerable plaque as in patients with primary unstable angina. In patients with progressively worsening exertional angina (accelerated angina), progression of coronary artery stenosis is more likely the mechanism.

Nocturnal Angina. The mechanism for angina that occurs after a patient has retired to bed is unlikely to be similar in all patients. Two distinct types of nocturnal angina are recognized: (1) pain that affects the patient soon after retiring or lying down, even before going to sleep, and (2) pain that wakes the patient after several hours of resting, usually in the early morning.

Nocturnal angina occurring soon after going to bed is most likely caused by an increase in $M\dot{V}O_2$ associated with increased left ventricular volume and as a result of an increment in left ventricular wall tension.

Nocturnal angina occurring in the early morning hours may be related to increased coronary vascular tone, although the precise triggering mechanism remains unclear.

Syndrome X. Typical exertional or stress-induced angina occurring in the absence of angiographically documented epicardial coronary artery disease is defined as *syndrome X*. Secondary causes of angina in patients with normal coronary arteries, such as aortic and mitral valvular disease, pulmonary hypertension, and muscle bridge, need to be excluded before the diagnosis of syndrome X can be considered. During treadmill exercise tests, patients develop typical angina associated with ischemic changes in the stress ECG. In some patients, focal impairment of myocardial perfusion, as evident from reversible myocardial thallium defects and transient reduction of blood flow to vascular territory, may be observed. The mechanism for myocardial ischemia in syndrome X remains unclear; abnormality of vasodilation of coronary microvasculature, regional or global, is the proposed explanation of stress-induced angina, which is also the reason for another term for syndrome X, *microvascular angina*. The prognosis of patients with this syndrome generally is excellent. Calcium channel blockers and nitrates are effective in controlling angina.

CLINICAL MANIFESTATIONS

Several syndromes resulting from ischemic heart disease are recognized clinically, although myocardial ischemia can be entirely asymptomatic. Acute myocardial infarction may be the first evidence of ischemic heart disease (Chapter 23). Infrequently, arrhythmias and congestive heart failure can be the predominant consequence of ischemic heart disease. However, angina pectoris is by far the most common

Table 22-1   The clinical presentations of angina syndromes with potential mechanisms of myocardial ischemia

TYPE	DESCRIPTION
Exertional angina	Angina during predictable level of physical activity or during emotional stress (demand ischemia)
Mixed angina	Variable exercise threshold (demand and supply ischemia)
Vasospastic angina	Spontaneous angina at rest, usually not provoked by exercise (supply ischemia)
Walk through angina	Angina at the onset of exercise, relieved during continued exercise (supply ischemia)
Linked angina	Angina precipitated by stimulation of other viscera (supply ischemia)
Nocturnal angina	Occurs soon after retiring, assuming recumbent position (demand ischemia), or occurs many hours after retiring (supply ischemia)
Syndrome X	Exertional angina (abnormal coronary vasodilation during exercise)
Postprandial angina	Angina during or soon after eating meals (supply and demand ischemia)
Primary unstable angina	Progressively worsening angina with rest angina (supply ischemia due to formation of nonocclusive coronary thrombi following disruption of a vulnerable atheromatous plaque)

clinical manifestation. The principal clinical presentations along with the proposed mechanisms of myocardial ischemia are summarized in Table 22-1.

Angina

The term *angina,* first used by Dr. William Heberden in 1768, was intended to indicate a sense of strangling associated with anxiety and frequently accompanied by a sense of death *(angor animi).* However, this classic description of precordial discomfort is not uniformly expressed by patients with angina pectoris, whose distress can otherwise be described as "viselike," "constricting," "suffocating," "crushing," "a heaviness," "a tightening," "pressure," or even "indigestion." Some patients complain of a burning sensation in the chest; others of the chest "expanding or bursting" (Chapter 16).

The location of chest discomfort is most frequently retrosternal but can be left pectoral or epigastric. Infrequently the discomfort can be located only in the interscapular or epigastric regions.

Radiation is common and usually occurs down the medial aspect of the left arm. Radiation can also occur to both arms, the throat, lower jaw, back, and epigastrium. Rarely the discomfort may start distally, in the arms, elbows, and wrists, and radiate centrally toward the chest. The absence of radiation does not exclude a diagnosis of angina pectoris.

The duration of chest discomfort may vary in the different anginal syndromes. However, discomfort of a fleeting, stabbing, or shock-like nature that lasts for only 2 to 3 seconds is not caused by myocardial ischemia; similarly, discomfort that lasts for several hours or days without any remission is unlikely to be angina.

Precipitating factors should be evaluated for a diagnosis of angina. Classic angina is most frequently experienced during exercise. In patients with chronic stable angina, the level of exercise that precipitates angina is usually reproducible and predictable. The extent of physical activity that precipitates angina appears to be inversely related to the severity (but not necessarily to the extent) of coronary artery lesions.

Angina pectoris may develop after less effort than usual in the morning, in a cold environment, walking against the wind, and walking after a large meal. Emotional states (e.g., anger, anxiety), isometric exercises, and sexual intercourse can also induce angina.

Analysis of the mode of relief of chest discomfort is helpful in diagnosing angina pectoris. Typical angina dissipates gradually over a period of minutes, usually as a result of cessation of the activity that precipitated it. Angina pectoris also begins gradually and reaches its maximum intensity over a period of minutes (Chapter 16). Relief

of chest discomfort in response to nitroglycerin is also a helpful diagnostic clue. Relief of angina typically occurs within 45 seconds to 5 minutes after the sublingual administration of nitroglycerin. However, chest pains associated with esophageal spasm are also relieved by nitroglycerin; thus response to nitroglycerin is not specific for angina pectoris. In some patients, carotid sinus massage can cause relief of angina by decreasing heart rate and blood pressure.

The character, location, and radiation of angina are similar in the different clinical syndromes. However, the duration, precipitating factors, and clinical presentations are different. In patients with classic angina the duration is usually brief, precipitated by physical activity, and relieved by the cessation of activity. The intensity of the discomfort is extremely variable. Emotional stress, various forms of isometric exercise, and activity after meals may precipitate angina. When nocturnal angina is experienced by patients with classic angina, it usually occurs soon after retiring or after lying down and is usually relieved promptly by sitting up.

In patients with variant angina, repeated episodes of angina occur at rest, usually without a history of predictable effort-induced angina. The duration can be considerably longer (30 to 40 minutes), and the angina dissipates either spontaneously or in response to nitroglycerin. ECGs obtained during prolonged episodes of angina often reveal reversible S-T segment elevation, indicating transmural myocardial ischemia. Cyclic occurrence (i.e., angina recurring more or less at the same time of the day or night in the same patient) is also observed. Nocturnal angina is usually experienced long after retiring to bed, frequently in the early morning hours, and is not relieved by assuming an upright position. An increased prevalence of migraine headache and Raynaud's phenomenon has been noted in patients with variant angina, suggesting a general propensity to vasoreactivity.

The typical clinical presentation, however, may be lacking in variant angina. In addition to rest angina, some patients may experience angina during physical activity, although the level of physical activity that induces angina is unpredictable. The cyclic occurrence and nocturnal angina might be absent, and an ECG might demonstrate S-T segment depression (subendocardial ischemia) instead of S-T segment elevation.

The clinical characteristics of angina in patients with unstable angina depend on the definition used to distinguish this syndrome. Presently, *unstable angina* is most frequently defined according to criteria used in the National Institutes of Health (NIH)–sponsored National Cooperative Study. The diagnosis depends on the presence of one or more of the following history features: (1) angina pectoris of new onset (usually within 2 months and brought on by minimal exertion); (2) development of more severe, prolonged, or frequent (crescendo) angina superimposed on a preexisting pattern of relatively stable, effort-related angina pectoris; or (3) angina pectoris at rest as well as with minimal exertion.

Because rest angina is an important criterion, variant angina is sometimes diagnosed as unstable angina; however, variant angina should be distinguished from unstable angina.

The duration of this discomfort is usually longer (up to 40 minutes), and the intensity may be more severe. Relief of angina in response to nitroglycerin is frequently incomplete. In patients with a history of stable angina, a sudden reduction in the level of physical activity that induces angina or an increase in frequency, severity, and duration of angina should be suspected of heralding the onset of unstable angina. A new site of radiation or the onset of new symptoms, such as dyspnea, palpitations, and diaphoresis, along with angina, may also suggest unstable angina.

The incidence of the unstable angina syndrome in patients with new onset of angina remains unclear. Different studies have reported that between 25% and 88% of patients with unstable angina give a history of new onset of angina.

Dyspnea

Dyspnea without associated angina is an infrequent clinical manifestation of myocardial ischemia. However, concomitant with angina, many patients with classic angina experience "a sensation of being unable to take a deep breath." In patients with variant or unstable angina, severe dyspnea may accompany prolonged episodes of angina caused by marked increase in pulmonary venous pressures.

Symptoms and signs of low cardiac output may also be seen in these patients. Nocturnal dyspnea soon after retiring indicates myocardial ischemia in some patients; the dyspnea is relieved by assuming an upright posture and also by nitroglycerin.

Dizziness, Palpitations, and Syncope

Palpitations alone are infrequent in patients with chronic ischemic heart disease (Chapter 17) but can be experienced along with angina. They result most frequently from premature ventricular beats. Dizziness and syncope caused by ventricular tachycardia or fibrillation during myocardial ischemia rarely occur without being preceded by angina. These complications may be precipitated by physical activity (e.g., treadmill exercise). In patients with variant or unstable angina, dizziness or syncope during prolonged episodes of angina may result from ventricular tachyarrhythmias or atrioventricular conduction disturbances.

Syncope caused by hypotension is an infrequent clinical manifestation of myocardial ischemia. However, its occurrence indicates severe ischemia involving large segments of myocardium, results in severe pump failure, and carries an ominous prognosis.

Several cardiac and noncardiac disorders can cause chest discomfort that mimics angina pectoris (Chapter 16). With a careful clinical history, physical examination, and appropriate laboratory tests, these disorders can usually be distinguished from angina.

PHYSICAL EXAMINATION

The physical examination may yield entirely normal findings or may reveal manifestations of risk factors for coronary artery disease. Tendon xanthomas, xanthelasma, and corneal arcus, particularly in younger subjects, may suggest lipid abnormalities. A diagonal ear lobe crease may be more prevalent in patients with ischemic heart disease.

Cardiovascular examination should include determination of blood pressure, examination of peripheral pulses, and funduscopic examination (Chapter 11). Detection of hypertension or its manifestations and peripheral vascular disease is important because there is a higher prevalence of atherosclerotic coronary artery disease in these patients. In young patients, coarctation of the aorta and supravalvular aortic stenosis should be excluded because these conditions are associated with premature atherosclerosis.

Cardiac examination may reveal manifestations and sequelae of ischemic heart disease, as well as the causes of angina other than coronary artery disease. In patients with chronic ischemic cardiomyopathy, particularly those with overt heart failure, physical examination may reveal signs of left-sided and right-sided heart failure (Chapter 11). However, these physical findings are not specific for ischemic cardiomyopathy and are present in patients with dilated congestive cardiomyopathy of any etiology.

Certain physical findings may provide information regarding the presence and severity of ischemic heart disease. Third and fourth heart sounds (gallops) are palpable in some patients with coronary artery disease. During hand-grip exercise, which may induce myocardial ischemia, palpable or audible gallops may appear transiently. During exercise-induced angina or spontaneous angina, these physical findings are frequently present. Fourth heart sounds are detected during auscultation in most patients with symptomatic coronary artery disease, and third heart sounds are also common, but neither is specific for ischemic heart disease (Chapter 11).

Abnormalities of the outward movement of the apical impulse can be detected in some patients. A sustained apical impulse often indicates the presence of dyskinetic myocardial segments and/or a depressed left ventricular ejection fraction. This abnormal finding is most frequently appreciated in patients with a previous myocardial infarction and chronic left ventricular aneurysms. However, it can appear transiently during either spontaneous or hand-grip exercise–induced ischemia.

Paradoxical (reversed) splitting of the second heart sound can occur transiently during an anginal attack. Transient depression of left ventricular function and a prolonged ejection time appear to be the mechanisms. The murmur of mitral regurgitation can be detected in some patients; papillary muscle dysfunction is the most frequent cause, but left ventricular dilation may also be contributory. A rela-

tively high-frequency diastolic murmur or a continuous murmur along the left parasternal area, associated with proximal coronary artery stenosis, usually of the left anterior descending coronary artery, occurs infrequently.

LABORATORY STUDIES
Electrocardiography

ECG evaluation is an important tool in the diagnosis of ischemic heart disease (Chapter 12). A normal resting ECG is found in 50% of patients with chronic stable angina without a history of previous myocardial infarction and does not exclude significant coronary artery disease. Q waves, diagnostic of anterior or inferior myocardial infarctions, are highly specific indicators of left ventricular wall motion abnormalities related to previous myocardial infarction and also indicate atherosclerotic obstructive coronary artery disease in a vast majority of patients. Other ECG abnormalities may be observed in patients with ischemic heart disease, but they are not specific; they are minor ST-T changes, conduction disturbances, including left bundle branch block and left anterior hemiblock, and ventricular arrhythmias.

The resting ECG, when recorded during an episode of variant or unstable angina, may reveal a variety of abnormalities indicative of myocardial ischemia (Chapter 12). Reversible S-T segment elevation suggests transmural myocardial ischemia, whereas S-T segment depressions suggest subendocardial ischemia. S-T segment alternans, occasionally seen during acute ischemic episodes, is usually associated with later development of ventricular tachyarrhythmias or advanced conduction disturbances. Transient Q waves have been observed infrequently in patients with severe myocardial ischemia without infarction. T wave inversions, the appearance of "U" waves or negative "U" waves, normalization of preexisting T wave changes, transient prolongation of the Q-T interval, and appearance of arrhythmias may indicate myocardial ischemia; however, the predictive value of these changes for the diagnosis of myocardial ischemia remains undetermined. Nevertheless, an ECG obtained during an episode of chest pain that does not show changes in the S-T segments or T waves is strong evidence against myocardial ischemia as the cause of chest pain. When the resting ECG shows left ventricular hypertrophy or a conduction defect, the reliability of any ECG change as a predictor of myocardial ischemia is reduced. In patients with unstable or variant angina, ECG changes are transient and normalize partially or completely with relief of myocardial ischemia.

A resting ECG is useful for the diagnosis of previous myocardial infarction. In patients with variant or unstable angina, the ECG should be obtained during chest pain, both to detect myocardial ischemia and to define the likely ischemic myocardial region.

The exercise ECG is more useful than the resting ECG in detecting myocardial ischemia (Chapter 13). Downsloping S-T segments are highly specific for coronary artery disease; most patients with this response have double- or triple-vessel involvement. Horizontal or slowly upsloping S-T segments are much less specific indicators of coronary artery disease. Marked S-T segment depression (0.2 mV or more) in symptomatic patients is associated with a high incidence of multivessel coronary artery disease and left main artery disease. Earlier onset of S-T segment depression and greater persistence of S-T segment changes after the cessation of exercise strengthen the diagnosis of coronary artery disease. S-T segment changes occurring in the early stages of exercise and persisting for 8 minutes or longer after exercise are strongly associated with extensive coronary artery disease.

The value of exercise ECG findings for the diagnosis of coronary artery disease is related to the prevalence of coronary artery disease in the patient population being evaluated (Bayes theorem) (Chapter 13). An abnormal resting ECG caused by left ventricular hypertrophy, intraventricular conduction abnormalities, or electrolyte disturbances or by drug therapy (e.g., digitalis) decreases the predictive value of stress electrocardiography for the diagnosis of coronary artery disease. On the other hand, hemodynamic abnormalities observed during exercise in association with an abnormal stress ECG improve the predictive value. A fall in systolic blood pressure, the lack of significant increase in heart rate, a low heart rate–blood pressure product at the onset of S-T segment changes, and significant dyspnea during exercise all increase the probability of extensive coronary artery disease (Chapter 13).

Ambulatory ECG recordings may reveal evidence of transient myocardial ischemia (S-T segment shifts) in patients with ischemic heart disease (Chapter 13). Angina may not accompany the S-T segment changes. Ambulatory ECG recording has been recommended for the diagnosis of variant angina. The ambulatory ECG is frequently employed to detect episodes of silent myocardial ischemia. A flat or downsloping S-T segment depression of at least 1.0 mm or more below an isoelectric baseline and lasting for at least 1 minute is regarded as evidence for myocardial ischemia in patients with known coronary artery disease. Such ECG changes correlate well with other markers of myocardial ischemia, such as changes in myocardial thallium-201 or rubidium-82 uptake. Characteristic S-T depression occurs less frequently in totally asymptomatic patients without any other evidence of coronary artery disease. J point depression with upsloping S-T segments, however, occurs frequently, in as many as 36% of normal individuals. It must be emphasized that although characteristic S-T segment changes in the absence of angina often indicate silent myocardial ischemia in patients with known coronary artery disease, caution must be used in interpreting such changes in asymptomatic persons. The ECG changes must be supported by other evidence for myocardial ischemia.

Radiologic Investigations

Plain chest radiographs usually do not reveal any diagnostic information in patients with ischemic heart disease. Intracardiac linear calcification involving the apical portion of the cardiac silhouette may indicate chronic left ventricular aneurysm and, indirectly, the presence of ischemic heart disease, since previous myocardial infarction resulting from atherosclerotic coronary heart disease is the most frequent cause. Coronary artery calcification of more than one major coronary artery branch is frequently associated with significant coronary artery disease. However, this is an infrequent finding on standard chest films; fluoroscopy is more sensitive in detecting intracardiac calcification. Cardiac fluoroscopy, along with an exercise treadmill test, has a higher predictive value for the diagnosis of significant coronary artery disease. Fast computed cardiac tomography (cardiac CT) is useful to detect coronary artery calcification and can be of value for diagnosis of coronary atherosclerotic disease. When coronary artery calcification is detected in an individual with a positive exercise test, significant obstructive coronary artery disease is almost always present. In patients with prolonged episodes of chest pain, radiographic findings of pulmonary venous hypertension are strong evidence for myocardial ischemia. Unusual causes of ischemic heart disease, such as calcific aortic stenosis, coarctation of aorta, pseudoxanthoma elasticum, and coronary artery aneurysm, occasionally are suggested by standard chest films.

Standard Laboratory Tests

Hyperlipidemia and carbohydrate intolerance are established risk factors for coronary artery disease. Therefore assessment of lipid profile and carbohydrate tolerance should be considered in patients with ischemic heart disease. Among relatively young patients (i.e., under the age of 50 years) with arteriographically proved coronary artery disease, the incidence of carbohydrate intolerance or type II or I hyperlipoproteinemia may be as high as 90%.

Noninvasive Imaging Studies

In the diagnosis of ischemic heart disease and its severity, myocardial perfusion scintigraphy, gated blood pool scintigraphy, and echocardiography are of value in appropriate subsets of patients (Chapter 13). These studies aid in establishing the diagnosis of ischemic heart disease, as well as in localizing and quantitating the ischemic myocardial segments. Box 22-3 lists their potential clinical applications.

Myocardial Perfusion Scintigraphy. Thallium-201 myocardial perfusion scintigraphy is often employed in the diagnosis of ischemic heart disease. Images made at the peak of dynamic exercise, the time of maximum blood flow and therefore of isotope distribu-

---

BOX 22-3
Noninvasive studies in anginal syndromes

1. Classic angina
   a. History, physical examination, and resting ECG
   b. Normal resting ECG: stress electrocardiography to detect high-risk patients or to assess response to therapy
   c. Abnormal resting ECG (uninterpretable): stress thallium myocardial perfusion scan to detect high-risk patients
   d. In patients with poor exercise tolerance: dipyridamole-thallium myocardial perfusion scan to detect severity of coronary artery disease
   e. In patients in whom concurrent assessment of left ventricular function is indicated: resting and exercise gated blood pool scintigraphy or two-dimensional (2D) echocardiography
   f. In patients with previous myocardial infarction and stable angina: stress thallium myocardial perfusion scan (in patients with adequate exercise tolerance) or dipyridamole-thallium myocardial perfusion scan or exercise ventriculography to assess the severity of coronary artery disease and to localize the new vascular territory involved with atherosclerosis
2. Atypical chest pain syndrome
   a. Normal resting ECG: stress electrocardiography
   b. Abnormal resting ECG: stress thallium myocardial perfusion scintigraphy or stress ventriculography (in the absence of other detectable heart disease)
   c. Mitral valve prolapse, chest pain, and abnormal resting ECG: echocardiography and stress thallium myocardial perfusion scintigraphy
   d. Suspected valvular heart disease: 2D echocardiography
3. Variant and unstable angina
   a. History
   b. ECG during chest pain
   c. In patients with prolonged chest pain and uninterpretable ECG: 2D echocardiography; thallium myocardial perfusion scintigraphy and/or gated blood pool scintigraphy

---

tion, are compared with resting images made later (Chapter 13). Perfusion abnormalities related to reversible myocardial ischemia are transient and normalize when the ischemia is relieved. In contrast, image abnormalities caused by myocardial infarction or scar tissue are persistent. The appearance of perfusion defects during stress-induced myocardial ischemia and subsequent normalization of the defects on relief of the ischemia form the basis for stress thallium myocardial perfusion scintigraphy. Thallium images may be planar or tomographic (single photon emission computed tomography) and at present tomographic images are used more frequently to assess the presence and extent of ischemic myocardium. Exercise treadmill thallium myocardial scintigraphy has a sensitivity and specificity of over 80% for detecting coronary artery disease.

IV dipyridamole-thallium myocardial perfusion scintigraphy is an alternative technique to exercise thallium perfusion scintigraphy, and its sensitivity, specificity, and predictive value in the diagnosis of significant coronary artery disease appear to be very similar to those of exercise thallium scintigraphy (Chapter 13). Dipyridamole blocks adenosine deaminase and prevents adenosine reuptake by red blood cells, increasing local concentration of adenosine. Adenosine, being a potent coronary vasodilator, decreases coronary vascular resistance and increases coronary blood flow. However, the magnitude of reduction of coronary vascular resistance and therefore the magnitude of increase in coronary blood flow is related to the severity of coronary artery stenosis. After dipyridamole administration in patients with varying degrees of coronary artery stenosis in the different vascular territories, heterogeneity of flow distribution and thus of thallium uptake occurs, which allows the diagnosis of coronary artery disease. Dipyridamole-thallium perfusion scintigraphy is safe and is indicated in patients who cannot perform adequate exercise (e.g., with peripheral vascular disease) or when exercise testing is contraindicated. Adenosine thallium scintigraphy has diagnostic accuracy, sensitivity, and specificity similar to those of dipyridamole-thallium perfusion scintigraphy and can be used for similar indications. Both dipyridamole and adenosine stress tests show close agreement with thallium exercise scintigraphy in terms of sensitivity, specificity, and predictive values.

Technetium-99m, a calcium analog with a higher photon energy and a shorter half-life than thallium chloride, can be linked to a variety of agents and used as a marker of myocardial perfusion. Sestamibi is an isonitrile compound that is taken up by the myocardium proportional to blood flow but does not undergo redistribution. Tomographic images with sestamibi provide better resolution and are being more frequently used for assessment of myocardial perfusion. The physical properties of technetium-99m also allow images to be acquired on the first pass through the ventricle, therefore allowing assessment of ventricular ejection fraction.

Dobutamine, a β-adrenergic agonist positive inotropic agent, is also frequently used for pharmacologic stress perfusion scintigraphy. The hemodynamic effects of dobutamine when given in larger doses increase heart rate and contractility, causing an increase in myocardial oxygen demand and a decrease in arterial pressure and perfusion time, which compromise myocardial perfusion. Thus an imbalance between myocardial oxygen supply and demand is induced that precipitates myocardial ischemia, which can be detected by myocardial perfusion scintigraphy. Dobutamine has also been used in conjunction with simultaneous wall motion imaging by radionuclide ventriculography, echocardiography, ultrafast computer tomography, and magnetic resonance imaging. The sensitivity and specificity to detect coronary artery disease by dobutamine stress tests may both exceed 80%.

Positron emission tomography (PET) to assess coronary blood flow and its reserve with the use of rubidium-82, or ammonia (NH_3) as the radionuclide tracer, and to assess myocardial metabolism with the use of labeled carbohydrates such as fludeoxyglucose F-18 is being increasingly used to detect presence and extent of chronically ischemic but viable myocardium (hibernating myocardium). Although sensitivity and specificity for the detection of coronary artery disease may exceed 90%, PET is a very expensive test and its use is limited in clinical practice. Many studies have demonstrated the improved sensitivity of the perfusion scintigraphic technique compared with stress electrocardiography in the diagnosis of coronary artery disease, particularly in the identification of single- and double-vessel disease. Thus an exercise myocardial perfusion scan is useful for excluding significant coronary artery disease in patients who have atypical chest pains and for establishing presence of high-risk coronary artery disease (left main coronary artery or triple-vessel involvement), and in patients in whom stress electrocardiography shows an equivocal response or cannot be interpreted because of baseline repolarization abnormalities, ST-T changes from drugs, left ventricular hypertrophy, or conduction disturbances. Stress myocardial perfusion scintigraphy also provides information regarding the distribution and extent of myocardial ischemia.

Clinical use of radioisotopic imaging in the diagnosis of unstable and variant angina is limited by logistic problems. Diagnosis should be made primarily by the history and the ECG evidence of myocardial ischemia. Myocardial scintigraphy may aid in the diagnosis of rest angina by demonstrating decreased segmental myocardial perfusion defects during prolonged episodes of chest pain or soon after the ischemic episode (Chapter 13).

Gated Blood Pool Scintigraphy. Global and regional left ventricular wall motion abnormalities during exercise or pharmacologic stress detected by radionuclide ventriculography using technetium-99m–labeled erythrocytes may indicate the presence and extent of myocardial ischemia and therefore indirectly the presence and severity of coronary artery disease. Although high sensitivity and specificity (up to 90%) have been observed for detecting coronary artery disease, impaired ejection fraction and regional wall motion abnormalities at rest or during exercise can be observed in hypertensive heart disease, valvular heart disease, and in cardiomyopathies in the absence of coronary artery disease. Radionuclide ventriculography combined with myocardial perfusion scintigraphy, however, is a useful technique to detect hibernating myocardium.

Echocardiography. Echocardiography is most commonly used to assess global and regional left ventricular systolic and diastolic functions that are frequently abnormal in ischemic heart disease. Up-

right treadmill and supine bicycle exercise, pacing, and pharmacologic stress, using dobutamine, dipyridamole, or adenosine in conjunction with 2D echocardiography, can be used to detect stress-induced regional and global wall motion abnormalities including changes in wall thickening that result from induced ischemia and correlate with the severity and extent of coronary artery disease. For detecting coronary artery disease, exercise echocardiography and high-dose (up to 50 g/kg/min) dobutamine stress echocardiography have been reported to have sensitivities and specificities exceeding 90%. Low-dose dobutamine stress echocardiography can also be used to assess response of "stunned" and "hibernating" myocardium. Administration of contrast agents such as albumen microbubbles can enhance ultrasonic signals reflected from the myocardium, and contrast echocardiography can be used to detect abnormalities of myocardial perfusion. Transesophageal echocardiography during transesophageal pacing is another potential technique to detect stress-induced wall motion abnormalities resulting from coronary artery disease (Chapter 13).

Coronary Arteriography

The definitive diagnosis of coronary artery disease and its anatomic extent can be made only by coronary angiography. Techniques are described in Chapter 14. The discussion in this section is confined to indications for the technique and interpretation of the information gained.

Indications for Coronary Arteriography
1. In patients with classic angina, coronary arteriography is not required for the diagnosis of coronary artery disease.
2. In patients with stable angina in whom a stress ECG or a thallium myocardial perfusion scan suggests high-risk coronary artery disease (e.g., left main coronary artery stenosis), coronary arteriography is indicated.
3. In patients with stable angina, when revascularization surgery or angioplasty is contemplated, coronary arteriography must be performed.
4. In occasional patients with atypical chest pain (e.g., patients admitted to a coronary care unit several times to rule out myocardial infarction), when other diagnostic tests have failed to clarify the diagnosis, coronary arteriography may be required to exclude coronary artery disease.
5. In patients with angina and valvular heart disease, coronary arteriography is required to delineate the coronary anatomy and establish the mechanism of angina.
6. In most patients with unstable angina, coronary arteriography is indicated. Timing of coronary arteriography, however, is variable, largely depending on the response to medical therapy. In patients who have partial or no relief of angina with medical therapy, coronary arteriography should be done promptly.
7. In patients with variant angina who have S-T elevation or depression during angina, coronary arteriography is indicated to determine whether the coronary arteries are normal or if fixed coronary artery stenosis is present.
8. When a diagnosis of variant angina is strongly suspected but cannot be documented by noninvasive studies, coronary arteriography with ergonovine provocation is indicated.
9. The diagnosis of syndrome X requires documentation of the absence of atherosclerotic coronary artery disease.

Interpretation of Arteriographic Findings. In patients with stable angina the incidence of single-, double-, and triple-vessel coronary artery disease is approximately the same. Abnormalities of left ventricular wall motion can be detected by contrast ventriculography in approximately 60% of patients with chronic ischemic heart disease. Asynergy is usually caused by scar tissue and reflects previous myocardial infarction. However, abnormal segmental wall motion and decreased global ejection fraction may also result from reversible myocardial ischemia (hibernating myocardium). In the catheterization laboratory, intervention ventriculography can be performed (with nitroglycerin or postextrasystolic potentiation) to differentiate between scar tissue and reversible ischemic myocardial segments. Reversible hypokinetic myocardial segments often demonstrate improved systolic motion after ingestion of nitroglycerin or with postextrasystolic potentiation. Contrast left ventriculogram also reveals mitral regurgitation when present.

In patients with unstable angina, single-, double-, and triple-vessel disease also occurs with approximately equal frequency. However, the following exceptions or qualifications may be noted. The incidence of single-vessel disease is higher in patients with recent-onset of angina. Left main coronary artery stenosis is also more frequent in patients with unstable angina. The left anterior descending coronary artery is the most frequently affected vessel. Less developed collateral circulation has been observed in patients with unstable angina than in those with chronic stable angina. In approximately 10% of patients diagnosed with unstable angina, coronary arteriography does not reveal hemodynamically significant coronary artery stenosis. Coronary artery spasm is considered to be the mechanism for rest angina in these patients. Type IIb coronary artery lesions are more frequently encountered, and in patients with an abnormal resting ECG, thrombus at the site of coronary artery stenosis is also discovered more frequently.

As described earlier, hemodynamic abnormalities are variable in patients with unstable angina. In some patients, severe depression of cardiac function may be observed during ischemic episodes, whereas the hemodynamics may be normal between episodes of angina.

In patients with variant angina, coronary arteriography reveals atherosclerotic lesions of varying severity involving at least one major coronary artery in most patients (Chapter 14), although in some patients, arteriographically detectable lesions are absent. Coronary artery spasm as the mechanism for variant angina has been well documented. In some patients with suspected variant angina, provocation of coronary artery spasm is required to confirm the diagnosis (Chapter 14). Ergonovine, methacholine, and hyperventilation have been used to provoke coronary artery spasm; IV injection of ergonovine (0.05 to 0.4 mg) appears to be the method most likely to provoke coronary artery spasm. Demonstration of coronary artery spasm alone, however, does not confirm a diagnosis of variant angina. Unless the provoked coronary artery spasm is accompanied by the patient's usual chest pain, along with ECG changes indicating myocardial ischemia, the diagnosis of variant angina is not established. In patients with severe fixed coronary artery stenosis, an ergonovine provocation test should be avoided because of the risk of precipitating a myocardial infarction.

At catheterization, atrial pacing is occasionally used to induce myocardial ischemia by increasing heart rate; however, it is considerably less sensitive and specific for diagnosing coronary artery disease than is treadmill exercise testing.

MEDICAL MANAGEMENT

Management of a patient with ischemic heart disease should incorporate modification of risk factors for coronary atherosclerosis along with interventions to prevent adverse consequences of myocardial ischemia. Thus treatment of hypertension, hyperlipidemia, obesity, and diabetes and cessation of smoking should be part of the routine management of such patients. That tobacco smoking is associated with increased risk of coronary artery disease is well established. Angina can be precipitated by inhalation of tobacco smoke, which can increase heart rate and blood pressure and myocardial oxygen demand. Inhalation of tobacco smoke can increase coronary vascular resistance and impair myocardial perfusion. Tobacco smoking can also interfere with the efficacy of antianginal drugs. Thus all patients should be advised to discontinue smoking.

Hypertension is not only a risk factor for coronary artery disease but also a major hemodynamic determinant for increase in myocardial oxygen demand. Thus adequate control of blood pressure, which should include weight reduction and avoidance of excess sodium intake, should be considered as a part of the therapeutic strategies for management of ischemic heart disease.

Treatment of hyperlipidemia is essential if not imperative for optimal management of patients with documented coronary artery disease. Partial ileal bypass, a surgical approach to control hyperlipidemia, is effective in decreasing total and low-density lipoprotein (LDL) cholesterol and reducing the risk of death and adverse cardiac events. In patients with established ischemic heart disease and with moderate hyperlipidemia, HMG coenzyme reductase inhibitor sim-

vastatin has the potential to decrease the total and cardiovascular mortality by 34% and 40%, respectively. In postinfarction patients with mild hyperlipidemia, pravastatin, another HMG-CoA reductase inhibitor, decreases the risk of total and cardiovascular mortality almost by similar magnitudes, along with reduction in total and LDL cholesterol. In patients with manifest chronic coronary artery disease and hyperlipidemia, pravastatin has been reported to reduce the risk of fatal and nonfatal myocardial infarction by 62%. These beneficial effects were observed in younger and older patients, men and women, and in patients with and without histories of hypertension and prior myocardial infarction. A substantial reduction (30% to 62%) in the risk of fatal and nonfatal cerebrovascular events has also been observed with the use of statins in hyperlipidemic patients with atherosclerotic ischemic heart disease and peripheral vascular disease. Although the risk of coronary events may also decrease with the rigid dietary treatment of hyperlipidemia or with the use of other lipid-lowering agents, vigorous exercise, and stress reduction, the magnitude of reduction in the risk of total mortality, cardiovascular mortality, adverse coronary events, and fatal and nonfatal cerebrovascular events with the use of statins seem much larger. Thus if tolerated, statins are preferable with established ischemic heart disease. Lipid-lowering therapies may be associated with regression of atherosclerotic lesions, which at best is modest and not adequate to explain the magnitude of reduction of cardiovascular mortality and acute coronary events. Plaque stabilization associated with decreased atheroma is a potential mechanism.

Physical exercise has been advocated for patients with ischemic heart disease to decrease the complications of coronary artery disease. The relationship between physical activity and the development of coronary artery disease is unclear, but physical training clearly produces beneficial effects on cardiac performance. Furthermore, physical activity provides patients with a sense of well-being. Thus regular physical exercise is recommended for patients with chronic stable angina.

Patients with exertional angina should be discouraged from performing very strenuous, vigorous exercise that can trigger acute ischemic syndromes and encouraged to engage in regular moderate exercise, which appears to provide beneficial effects. Exercise programs preferably should be based on the results of treadmill exercise tolerance testing; it is desirable not to exceed 75% of the ischemia heart rate. Arm exercise, which is associated with earlier onset of angina threshold, and exercising in cold weather, which brings on angina more frequently, should be avoided. Mean maximal heart rate during sexual intercourse usually does not exceed 70% of the maximal predicted heart rate and thus, patients who can achieve a heart rate up to 120 beats per minute during an exercise tolerance test can engage in sexual activity safely.

Although aspirin provides substantial benefit in acute ischemic syndromes, its efficacy in chronic ischemic heart disease has not been firmly established. Nevertheless, if there is no contraindication, it is advisable to use low-dose aspirin (75 to 325 mg once a day).

Diabetes and obesity are independent risk factors for coronary heart disease, but the impact of rigid control of diabetes and treatment of obesity on the prognosis of patients with ischemic heart disease remains unclear. However, since insulin resistance has been implicated not only in the pathogenesis of atherosclerosis but also as a contributing factor in unstable plaque syndrome, adequate control of diabetes is desirable. Similarly, weight reduction and treatment of obesity are also desirable because they facilitate control of hypertension and angina.

The treatment of angina and other manifestations of myocardial ischemia is based on a reduction of MVO_2 and an increase in coronary blood flow to the potentially ischemic myocardium. Pharmacologic agents, in general, decrease MVO_2, although some agents have the potential to enhance myocardial perfusion. Revascularization surgery and transluminal coronary angioplasty, on the other hand, increase coronary blood flow and O_2 delivery to the myocardium.

Pharmacologic Agents: Nitroglycerin and Nitrates

Nitroglycerin and nitrates are direct-acting endothelium-independent smooth muscle relaxants that cause vasodilation of the peripheral vas-

Table 22-2 Potential beneficial and deleterious effects of nitroglycerin and other nitrates in management of angina

EFFECTS	RESULTS
Beneficial	
Decreased ventricular volume	
Decreased arterial pressure	Decreased MVO$_2$
Decreased ejection time	
Decreased left ventricular diastolic pressure	Improved subendocardial perfusion
Increased collateral flow	Improved perfusion to ischemic myocardium
Vasodilation of epicardial coronary arteries	Relief of coronary artery spasm
Improved ventriculoaortic coupling	Decreased MVO$_2$
Deleterious	
Reflex tachycardia	Increased MVO$_2$
Reflex increase in contractility	
Decreased diastolic perfusion time because of tachycardia	Decreased myocardial perfusion

From Chatterjee K, Rouleau J-L, Parmley WW: *JAMA* 252:1173, 1984.

cular bed. It is generally accepted that "the nitrate receptors," which contain sulfhydryl (SH) groups, are probably located on the myocytes rather than on the vascular endothelium. After receptor binding, nitrates are converted by enzymatic mechanism to nitric oxide, which stimulates guanylate cyclase to produce cyclic guanosine monophosphate (GMP) in the smooth muscles. The mechanism of cyclic GMP–mediated vasodilation is unclear but may be related to decreased calcium entry to the cell or increased calcium uptake by the sarcoplasmic reticulum. The SH groups, required for the stimulation of guanylate cyclase, are oxidized by excess exposure to nitrates. The depletion of SH groups is one of the proposed mechanisms for nitrate tolerance, and this hypothesis is supported by the observations that SH donor *N*-acetylcysteine at least partially reverses nitrate tolerance. It has been suggested that the augmented cyclic adenosine monophosphate (c-AMP) production in response to prostaglandins contributes to nitrate-induced vasodilation.

Nitroglycerin and nitrates produce more pronounced vasodilation of the venous capacitance bed than the arteriolar resistance bed. The hemodynamic effects of nitroglycerin are characterized by decreased ventricular diastolic volumes associated with decreased systemic and pulmonary venous pressures. Arterial pressure tends to decrease, and heart rate and contractility may increase. Decreased arterial pressure and left ventricular volume are associated with decreased wall tension and a resulting decreased MVO$_2$. In rare instances a paradoxical increase in MVO$_2$ may occur because of excessive reflex tachycardia and increased contractility. Nitroglycerin and nitrates improve compliance of the conduit arteries including aorta and enhance ventriculoaortic coupling, which is associated with decreased left ventricular ejection resistance and myocardial oxygen demand. Myocardial oxygen demand also diminishes due to decreased central aortic pressure that may not be always reflected in peripheral pulses.

Nitroglycerin also dilates the large epicardial conductance coronary arteries. Coronary arteriolar resistance tends to decrease, although to a much lesser extent. Since collateral coronary arteries tend to respond in the same way as larger arteries, nitroglycerin can potentially increase collateral blood flow.

The potential beneficial and deleterious effects of nitroglycerin and nitrates in the treatment of angina are summarized in Table 22-2. In patients with stable angina associated with fixed obstructive coronary artery disease, nitroglycerin exerts its beneficial effects primarily by decreasing MVO$_2$.

Relaxation of the smooth muscles of the epicardial coronary arteries and relief of coronary artery spasm are the mechanisms of beneficial effects in patients with variant angina. Increases in regional coronary blood flow and myocardial perfusion are associated with the relief of angina. For maintenance therapy, long-acting nitrates or nitroglycerin administered transcutaneously are frequently effective. In

general, relatively larger doses of these agents are needed compared with those used for the treatment of stable angina.

Nitroglycerin and nitrates are effective in decreasing the frequency and duration of episodes of spontaneous S-T segment shifts without angina in patients with stable angina and with vasospastic angina. Enhanced left ventricular regional wall motion provides additional evidence for their effectiveness in ameliorating silent myocardial ischemia.

Nitroglycerin and nitrates are also useful in the treatment of unstable angina, although the precise mechanism is not clear. Both decreased MVO$_2$ and increased myocardial perfusion associated with decreased coronary vascular tone might be contributory. Nitroglycerin also decreases platelet aggregation, which may also contribute to its beneficial effects in primary unstable angina. In patients with repeated episodes of rest angina, administration of nitroglycerin by the IV route is preferable because it permits easier control of angina.

Some of the forms of nitroglycerin and nitrates used in the treatment of angina are listed in Table 22-3. The onset of action of sublingual nitroglycerin is rapid (1 to 3 minutes), which is why it is the most frequently used agent for the immediate treatment of angina pectoris. Because of its shorter duration of action (not exceeding 20 to 30 minutes), it is not a suitable agent for maintenance therapy. The onset of action of IV nitroglycerin is also rapid (5 minutes), but its hemodynamic effects are quickly reversed on discontinuation of its infusion. Its clinical application is therefore restricted to the treatment of recurrent rest angina. However, tolerance to the hemodynamic effects of nitroglycerin certainly occurs both in patients with angina and with heart failure. It has been suggested that an 8- to 12-hour nitroglycerin-free period avoids the development of tolerance. Cross-tolerance to isosorbide dinitrate has been documented; thus substitution of isosorbide dinitrate for nitroglycerin is not effective. Improvement in exercise tolerance of patients with stable angina is more apparent when nitroglycerin is given three times rather than four times daily, presumably because an 8-hour nitrate-free period is required to prevent tolerance. Buccal and oral preparations and several transdermal forms of nitroglycerin are also available. It is claimed that these formulations provide effective blood concentrations for long periods, but their effectiveness in the maintenance therapy of angina remains uncertain. Treadmill exercise tests have demonstrated that the beneficial effects of nitroglycerin patches do not last more than 6 to 8 hours.

The onset of action of sublingual or chewable isosorbide dinitrate, pentaerythrityl tetranitrate, and erythrityl tetranitrate is rapid (2 to 3 minutes), but their duration of action is relatively short (1½ to 3 hours). Isosorbide 5-mononitrate does not undergo liver metabolism and is fully bioavailable after oral administration. Its elimination half-life is 4 to 6 hours and duration of action about 8 hours.

The most common undesirable effect of nitrate therapy is a throbbing headache, which tends to decrease with continued therapy. Postural dizziness and weakness also occur, but frank syncope is rare. Because of the potential for withdrawal symptoms, nitrate therapy should be tapered rather than abruptly stopped.

Methemoglobinemia is virtually never seen in the clinical management of angina and has been observed only when very large (nonpharmacologic) doses of nitrates have been used. Nitrates do not worsen glaucoma, once thought to be a contraindication, and nitrates can be used safely in the presence of increased intraocular pressure. However, nitrates are contraindicated if intracranial pressure is elevated.

Beta-Adrenergic Blocking Agents

The beneficial effects of β-blocking agents are primarily related to their potential to decrease MVO$_2$. In general, β-blocking drugs decrease heart rate, blood pressure, and contractility, which in turn decrease MVO$_2$. Exercise-induced increases in heart rate and blood pressure are also blunted by β-blocker therapy. Decreased heart rate is associated with a larger left ventricular end-diastolic volume, which increases MVO$_2$, but the net effect in most patients is reduction of MVO$_2$.

Some β-blocking drugs have the potential to enhance myocardial perfusion because of their differential effects on coronary vascular resistance in the relatively ischemic and nonischemic myocardial segments. Myocardial perfusion also may improve because of increased

Table 22-3   Nitroglycerin and nitrates in angina

COMPOUND	ROUTE	DOSAGE	DURATION OF EFFECTS
Nitroglycerin	Sublingual tablets	0.3-0.6 mg up to 1.5 mg	1½-7 minutes
	Spray	0.4 mg, as needed	Similar to sublingual tablets
	Ointment	2% 6×6 in	Up to 7 hours
		15×15 cm	
		7.5-40 mg	
	Transdermal patches	0.2-0.8 mg/h every 12 hours	8-12 hours during intermittent therapy
	Oral–sustained release	2.5-13 mg 1-2 tabs 3 times daily	4-8 hours
	Buccal	1-3 mg 3 times daily	3-5 hours
	Intravenous	5-200 g/min	Tolerance in 7-8 hours
Isosorbide dinitrate	Sublingual	2.5-15 mg	Up to 60 minutes
	Oral	5-80 mg 2-3 times daily	Up to 8 hours
	Spray	1.25 mg	2-3 minutes
	Chewable	5 mg	2-2½ hours
	Oral–slow release	40 mg 1-2 daily	Up to 8 hours
	Intravenous	1.25-5.0 mg/h	Tolerance in 7-8 hours
	Ointment	100 mg/24 h	Not effective
Isosorbide mononitrate	Oral	10-20 mg twice daily	12-24 hours
		60-240 mg once daily	
Pentaerythritol tetranitrate	Sublingual	10 mg as needed	Not known
Erythritol tetranitrate	Sublingual	5-10 mg as needed	Not known
	Oral	10-30 mg, 3 times daily	Not known

Modified from Thadani U, Opie LH: Nitrates. In Opie LH, editor: *Drugs for the heart,* ed 4, Philadelphia, 1995, Saunders.

Table 22-4   Effects of β-adrenergic blocking drugs, nitrates, and combined β blocker–nitrate therapy in patients with angina pectoris

	BETA BLOCKERS	NITRATES	COMBINED NITRATES AND BETA BLOCKERS
Heart rate	Decrease	Reflex increase	Decrease
Atrial pressure	Decrease	Decrease	Decrease
End-diastolic volume	Increase	Decrease	None or decrease
Contractility	Decrease	Reflex increase	None
Ejection time	Increase	Decrease	None
Diastolic perfusion time	Increase	Decrease	Increase

From Katzung BG, Chatterjee K: *Basic and clinical pharmacology,* Los Altos, Calif, 1983, Lange.

diastolic perfusion time associated with decreased heart rate. It has been suggested that β-blocking agents cause a rightward shift of the oxyhemoglobin dissociation curve, which increases O_2 delivery. However, decreased MVO_2 seems to be the most important mechanism for the relief of myocardial ischemia.

Beta-blocker therapy enhances exercise tolerance and delays the onset of angina and S-T segment depression during exercise in patients with effort angina. The magnitude of S-T segment depression may also decrease. Although exercise tolerance improves, the heart rate–blood pressure product at the onset of myocardial ischemia remains unchanged.

The increase in end-diastolic volume that results from relative bradycardia is an undesirable effect of β-blocking drugs. Furthermore, a significant reduction in contractile function, if it occurs, may also increase left ventricular end-systolic and end-diastolic volumes and end-diastolic pressure. These potential deleterious effects can be overcome by the concomitant use of nitrates. Beta-blocking drugs and nitrates tend to offset each other's deleterious effects on MVO_2 (Table 22-4), and the net result is a decrease in MVO_2. An additive effect of the two agents in improving exercise tolerance has been observed, although it may not occur in all patients with chronic stable angina. The differences in the important properties of the different β-blocking agents are summarized in Table 22-5.

No conclusive evidence proves that any particular β-blocking drug is superior to any other for the management of stable angina. Relatively cardioselective β blockers are competitive antagonists to $β_1$ receptors, and nonselective β blockers are antagonists to both $β_1$ and

$β_2$ receptors. Nonselective β blockers therefore may have the potential to increase coronary vascular tone because of unopposed α-adrenergic activity. Worsening leg claudication and Raynaud's phenomenon are observed more frequently with nonselective than with cardioselective β blockers. $Beta_2$ receptor inhibition is associated with increased serum potassium levels. Correction of hypokalemia therefore is more likely to occur with nonselective β blockers than with cardioselective β blockers. Beta-blocking agents with intrinsic sympathetic stimulating activity attenuate the exercise-induced increase in heart rate and blood pressure without causing a significant decrease in resting heart rate or blood pressure. In clinical circumstances in which reduction of resting heart rate or blood pressure is not required or undesirable, β-blocking agents with intrinsic sympathetic activity may provide some advantage.

The side effects profile of different β-blocking drugs may differ and should be considered in the selection of a particular β-blocking agent in the long-term management of patients with angina pectoris. Bronchospasm is more likely to occur with nonselective β blockers. Intensification of insulin-induced hypoglycemia is more common with nonselective β-blocking drugs. Depression of cardiac function and precipitation of overt congestive heart failure may complicate β-blocker therapy, particularly in patients with already compromised left ventricular function. Beta-blocking agents with intrinsic sympathetic-stimulating activity theoretically are less likely to precipitate heart failure. Central nervous system side effects (e.g., fatigue, depression, lack of concentration) have been reported less frequently with β-blocking drugs that do not substantially cross the blood-brain barrier (lipophilic β blockers). Gastrointestinal side effects and sexual dysfunction are common with all β-blocking agents. Beta-adrenergic blocking agents may increase blood sugar and impair insulin sensitivity, particularly when used concurrently with diuretics. In patients with insulin-dependent diabetes β blockers may decrease reaction to hypoglycemia. Beta blockers may have unfavorable effects on the blood lipid profile, with an increase in triglycerides and decrease in HDL cholesterol. The clinical significance of these potential adverse metabolic changes with β blockers remains unclear and should not be deterrent to their use when indicated.

The effective dose of any β-blocking drug varies considerably from patient to patient; dose titration in individual patients against both resting and exercise heart rates is desirable, along with monitoring of changes in blood pressure and cardiac function. In patients with severe effort angina, considerable reduction in resting heart rate (50 to 60 beats/min) and maximum heart rate during exercise (100 to 120 beats/min) may be required to control angina effectively.

For maintenance therapy of stable angina, β-blocking drugs with a relatively long half-life are preferred because of improved patient

Table 22-5   Properties of various β-adrenergic blocking agents

AGENT	SELECTIVITY	INTRINSIC SYMPATHETIC ACTIVITY	LIPID SOLUBILITY	PLASMA HALF-LIFE (HOURS)	USUAL DOSE FOR ANGINA
Propranolol	−	−	+++	1-6	60-320 mg/day
Metoprolol	+	−	+	3	100-200 mg/day
Nadolol	−	−	0	16-24	80-240 mg/day
Timolol	−	−	+	4-5	15-45 mg/day
Atenolol	+	−	0	6-9	50-100 mg/day
Pindolol	−	+++	+	4	5-20 mg/day
Acebutolol	+	++	0	8-12	600-1200 mg/day
Labetolol (combined β- or α-blocking effects)	−	−	+++	3-4	300-600 mg/day
Betaxolol	+	−	+	19-22	10-20 mg/day
Bisoprolol	+	−	+	9-12	10 mg/day
Cartelol	−	+	+	6	2.5-10 mg/day
Celiprolol	+	+ (β₂)	−	4-5	400 mg/day
Sotalol	+	−	+	12	240-480 mg/day
Esmolol (intravenous)	+	−	+	10 minutes	50-300 μg/kg/min

−, Absent; +, Present; ++, moderate; +++, marked.

Table 22-6   Calcium channel blocking agents potentially useful in management of angina syndromes

AGENT	USUAL DOSE	ABSOLUTE OR RELATIVE CONTRAINDICATIONS
Dihydropyridines		
Nifedipine	Oral: 30-120 mg/day Sublingual: 10 mg q4-6h	Hypotension
Nitrendipine	20-40 mg/day	Hypotension
Felodipine (potent vasodilator)	15-30 mg/day	Hypotension
Nimodipine (useful in cerebral ischemia)	0-35 mg/kg, 4 hourly	Hypotension
Nisoldipine	30-60 mg/day	Hypotension
Nicardipine	15-90 mg/day	Hypotension
Verapamil	IV bolus: 5-10 mg in 10 min IV infusion: 1 mg/min to total of 10 mg Oral: 120-480 mg/day	Sick sinus syndrome, A-V conduction defects, sinus bradycardia, digitalis toxicity, overt heart failure, hypotension
Diltiazem	IV: 0.15-0.25 mg/kg over 2 min Oral: 90-230 mg/day	As for verapamil
Mixed agents		
Tiapamil (as with verapamil, also a sodium blocker)	1500 mg/day	As for verapamil
Bepridil (mixed sodium blocker)	200-400 mg/day	Prolonged Q-T interval

compliance. The potential disadvantage of the long-acting β blockers, however, is the longer persistence of hemodynamic effects and untoward effects when, in certain clinical circumstances, withdrawal of β-blocker therapy becomes necessary. It must be emphasized that sudden withdrawal of effective β-blocker therapy in ambulatory patients may result in worsening of angina and precipitation of acute ischemic episodes, including myocardial infarction. During elective withdrawal of β-blocker therapy, patients should be instructed to reduce their physical activity, and withdrawal should be gradual. Beta-blocker therapy is effective in controlling symptoms in patients with mixed, postprandial, and walk through angina. Beta-adrenergic blocking agents also decrease silent ischemic episodes in patients with atherosclerotic coronary artery disease, supporting the hypothesis that increase in myocardial oxygen demand contributes to the occurrence of silent ischemia.

Despite the potential for the β-blocking drugs to increase coronary vascular tone (unopposed alpha-adrenergic effect), in clinical practice, many patients (50% to 85%) with primary unstable angina become free of anginal attacks on a regimen of combined β-blocker and nitrate therapy. For patients who have not been on β-blocker therapy, relatively short-acting β-blocking drugs should be administered to decrease resting heart rate to between 50 and 60 beats/min and systolic blood pressure to 100 to 110 mm Hg without precipitating heart failure or compromising organ perfusion. In some patients, therapy may be initiated with IV propranolol (0.1 to 0.2 mg/kg), metoprolol (5 to 10 mg), or the short-acting β blocker esmolol. In patients already receiving β-blocker therapy, the dose of β-blocking drugs should be increased to achieve the desired hemodynamic ef-

fects. In patients with unstable angina, β blockers should be used in conjunction with nitrates.

In patients with variant angina, β blockers do not appear to be effective; coronary vasodilators remain the primary therapy.

Calcium Channel Blocking Agents

Drugs that block the slow inward current of a propagated cardiac impulse, frequently called calcium channel blocking agents, have emerged as additional pharmacotherapy of anginal syndromes (Table 22-6). Calcium channel blocking drugs have the potential to decrease MVO₂ as well as to increase coronary blood flow.

All calcium channel blocking drugs possess a negative inotropic effect: they decrease myocardial contractile force because of decreased availability of calcium to the contractile elements. These agents also inhibit calcium entry to the smooth muscles of the peripheral vascular bed and cause peripheral vasodilation. Arterial and intraventricular pressures decrease because of the decreased systemic vascular resistance. Heart rate may also decrease with the use of some calcium channel blocking agents. These hemodynamic effects (decreased contractility, heart rate, and arterial pressure) decrease MVO₂.

Calcium channel blocking agents may increase coronary blood flow and myocardial perfusion by several mechanisms. All calcium channel blocking agents can cause dilation of the epicardial coronary arteries and thus relieve and prevent vasospasm of the large coronary arteries. Arterial dilation results partly from the direct effect on smooth muscles and partly from inhibition of the vasoconstrictive ef-

Table 22-7   Properties of calcium-channel blocking drugs in clinical use

DRUGS	VASCULAR SELECTIVITY*	USUAL DOSE	PLASMA HALF-LIFE	SIDE EFFECTS
Dihydropyridines				
Nifedipine	3.1	Immediate release: 20-40 mg 3 times a day orally Slow release: 30-180 mg orally	4 hours	Hypotension, dizziness, flushing, nausea, constipation, edema
Amlodipine	++	5-10 mg once daily	30-50 hours	Headache, edema
Felodipine	5.4	5-10 mg once daily	11-16 hours	Headache, dizziness
Isradipine	7.4	2.5-10 mg twice daily	8 hours	Headache, fatigue
Nicardipine	17.0	20-40 mg three times a day	2-4 hours	Headache, dizziness, flushing, edema
Nisoldipine	++	20-40 mg once daily	2-6 hours	Similar to nifedipine
Nitrendipine	14.4	20 mg once or twice daily	5-12 hours	Similar to nifedipine
Miscellaneous				
Bepridil	–	200-400 mg once daily	24-40 hours	Arrhythmias, dizziness, nausea
Diltiazem	0.3	Immediate release: 30-80 mg 4 times a day Slow release: 120-320 mg once daily	3-4 hours	Hypotension, dizziness, flushing bradycardia
Verapamil	1.3	Immediate release: 80-160 mg three times a day Slow release: 120-480 mg once daily		Hypotension, myocardial depression, heart failure, edema

Modified from Katzung BG, Chatterjee K: Vasodilators and the treatment of angina. In Katzung BG, editor: *Clinical Pharmacology,* Norwalk, Conn, 1994, Appleton & Lange.
*=Numeric data give the ratio of vascular potency to cardiac potency; higher numbers indicate greater vascular, less cardiac potency.
−=Myocardial depression greater than vasodilation.
++=Significant degree of vasodilation greater than myocardial depression.

fect of the α receptors. Evidence also shows that calcium channel blocking agents have the potential to promote coronary collateral blood flow.

Other physiologic effects of calcium channel blocking agents, such as improved left ventricular diastolic function and myocardial relaxation and decreased myocardial injury in the presence of ischemia from decreased myocardial calcium overload, have been observed. However, the significance of these effects in the treatment of ischemic heart disease remains undetermined.

Several calcium channel blocking drugs are available for clinical use (Table 22-7). Tiapamil and bepridil appear to possess sodium channel blocking effects in addition to calcium channel blocking properties. Nifedipine, verapamil, and diltiazem are structurally different, and there are also differences in their cardiovascular effects. Sinoatrial and atrioventricular nodal tissues, which are mainly composed of slow-response cells, are affected by verapamil and diltiazem but not by nifedipine. Thus verapamil and diltiazem decrease atrioventricular conduction and are effective for the treatment of supraventricular tachycardia and for decreasing ventricular responses in atrial fibrillation or flutter. In patients with a history of supraventricular tachycardia or atrial fibrillation and flutter, diltiazem or verapamil provides advantages over nifedipine. However, in patients with sinoatrial or atrioventricular nodal disease, nifedipine is preferable. All three agents decrease arterial pressure; however, nifedipine seems to be a more potent arteriolar dilator, and the hypotensive response to nifedipine is usually more pronounced. Negative inotropic effects, least likely with diltiazem, can cause a depression in left ventricular pump function. Reduction of systemic vascular resistance and a decrease in left ventricular afterload usually compensate for the potential deleterious consequences of their negative inotropic effects on cardiac performance. Thus overall left ventricular pump function may remain unchanged. However, verapamil is not well tolerated by patients with significantly depressed left ventricular function.

Concomitant use of β blockers should also be avoided in patients with depressed left ventricular function because of the risk of precipitating overt heart failure from the combined negative inotropic effects of both classes of agents.

It has been demonstrated that both nonspecific sympathetic antagonism and α-adrenergic antagonism can occur with some calcium channel blocking agents. Nonspecific sympathetic antagonism is most marked with diltiazem and much less with verapamil. Nifedipine does not seem to have this effect. Thus reflex tachycardia, in response to

hypotension, occurs most intensely with immediate release nifedipine and less so with verapamil. With diltiazem, heart rate may even decrease despite a fall in arterial pressure. As a consequence, in patients with bradycardia in whom further reduction in heart rate is not desired, nifedipine is preferable to verapamil or diltiazem. Conversely, when reduction in heart rate is desired, verapamil or diltiazem is more likely to produce this effect than nifedipine.

Drug interaction, such as with digitalis, is a practical clinical problem with the use of some calcium channel blocking agents. Serum digoxin levels consistently increase with verapamil, and digitalis toxicity can occur. Both decreased distribution volume and impaired clearance of digoxin appear to contribute to increased serum digoxin levels. Serum digoxin levels have rarely been found to increase after nifedipine or diltiazem therapy.

The short-acting immediate release calcium channel blocking agents such as nifedipine may activate the adrenergic system in response to acute and rapid decrease in arterial pressure, which has been thought to be the potential mechanism for the observed dose-related increase in morbidity and mortality in hypertensive patients. Slow-release nifedipine, however, may not increase the risk of adverse cardiac events and decrease the frequency of manifest and silent ischemic episodes in patients with chronic ischemic heart disease. The safety and potential benefits of longer-acting dihydropyridines and calcium-channel blockers, such as amlodipine, felodipine, and nisoldipine, have been observed. Thus longer-acting or slow-release calcium channel blockers can be used when indicated and are preferable to short-acting and immediate-release agents. Shorter-acting diltiazem or verapamil may also increase the risk of adverse cardiac events in patients with clinical heart failure and reduced left ventricular ejection fraction. In contrast, in patients with preserved left ventricular systolic function, these agents are well tolerated and in patients with angina, there is no difference in morbidity and mortality with these agents compared to β blockers.

In the management of effort angina, calcium channel blockers, preferably slow-release or long-acting agents, should be added to nitrates and β blockers when nitrate–β blocker therapy is inadequate for relief of symptoms. Heart rate–lowering calcium channel blockers such as diltiazem or verapamil may be useful in patients intolerant to β blockers or when β blocker therapy is contraindicated (bronchospastic disease). For the management of unstable angina, calcium channel blockers, particularly the immediate release short-acting agents such as nifedipine should not be used alone because of the enhanced risk of myocardial ischemia and adverse cardiac events. Similarly, in patients with overt heart failure or reduced ejection fraction, calcium channel blockers should be avoided. Diltiazem, however, has been found effective in decreasing the incidence of silent and symptomatic myocardial ischemia as well as of acute cardiac events in patients with non–Q wave myocardial infarction, the pathophysiologic mechanism of which appears to be similar to that of primary unstable angina.

Calcium channel blockers are effective in preventing a recurrence of anginal episodes in patients with variant angina. In approximately 70% of patients, anginal attacks are completely abolished; in another 20% a marked reduction in frequency can be expected. The prevention of coronary artery spasm is the principal mechanism for this beneficial effect. Nifedipine, administered sublingually, can cause prompt relief of angina.

Although nitroglycerin and nitrates are also effective in the management of variant angina, the incidence of undesirable side effects with nitrates compared with calcium-entry blocking agents is higher. Furthermore, beneficial effects of calcium channel blocking agents have been documented in patients refractory to nitrate therapy.

Calcium channel blocking agents decrease the frequency and duration of the silent episodes of ischemia. A decrease in coronary vascular tone and improved myocardial perfusion are the likely mechanisms.

The side effects of the different calcium channel blocking agents differ to some extent. Symptoms related to hypotension (e.g., dizziness) can occur with any of these agents but are more frequent with nifedipine. Headaches, flushing, gastrointestinal symptoms (e.g., nausea, constipation), and dependent edema are common to all the agents. Nonspecific central nervous system symptoms are observed infrequently after administration of calcium channel blocking drugs. Frank psychosis (mania) has been reported after the use of diltiazem, although this complication is extremely rare. Bradyarrhythmias occur more frequently with verapamil than with diltiazem. As described earlier, overt heart failure and elevation of serum digoxin levels are more likely to occur with verapamil than with nifedipine and diltiazem.

Other Antianginal Therapies

Long-term anticoagulant therapy with coumadin derivatives does not appear to have any role in the management of chronic ischemic heart disease. Aspirin decreases the incidence of acute cardiac events (infarction, sudden death, need for coronary artery bypass surgery) by almost 50% in patients with unstable angina. IV heparin has been found more effective than aspirin in controlling angina and decreasing the incidence of adverse cardiac events in patients with unstable angina. However, it is preferable to use both aspirin and heparin concurrently despite a higher risk of bleeding complications. To avoid heparin rebound when heparin therapy needs to be discontinued, low-molecular weight heparin may be of benefit in unstable angina but its superiority to standard heparin has not been firmly established. Newer antithrombotic (hirudin, hirulog) and antiplatelet agents (glycoprotein IIb/IIa antagonists) are undergoing clinical trials, and their use in the management of unstable angina remains to be determined. Thrombolytic therapy (e.g., rt-PA, streptokinase) not only is ineffective in controlling recurrence of ischemia but also has the potential to enhance the risk of adverse cardiac events.

Ticlopidine, another antiplatelet agent with different mechanisms of action than aspirin, is also effective in reducing the incidence of ischemia and infarction in patients with unstable angina. Ticlopidine, at a dose of 250 mg twice daily given for 6 months, may reduce the incidence of mortality and of myocardial infarction by 50%. Ticlopidine primarily inhibits the adenosine diphosphate pathway of platelet aggregation but, unlike aspirin, does not inhibit the cyclooxygenase pathway; it does not prevent the production of thromboxane by platelets or the production of prostacyclin by endothelial cells. Ticlopidine can be used when aspirin is contraindicated; its gastrointestinal and bleeding complications are similar to those of aspirin.

IV prostacyclin, although it increases coronary blood flow, does not improve the angina threshold in patients with effort angina. Similarly, it does not provide any advantage, compared with conventional therapy, in patients with unstable angina.

Beneficial effects were anticipated in the treatment of vasospastic angina with α-adrenergic blocking agents; however, controlled studies have failed to demonstrate the efficacy of α-blocking agents, such as prazosin, in variant angina. Low-dose amiodarone along with nitrates and calcium channel blockers is occasionally effective in patients with refractory vasospastic angina. Cardiac denervation, although it has been attempted, is seldom necessary for control of vasospastic angina.

Intraaortic balloon counterpulsation is effective in controlling episodes of rest angina in patients with unstable angina. "Systolic unloading" decreases MVO_2, and diastolic augmentation has the potential to enhance myocardial perfusion. Patients with preserved left ventricular function and stable hemodynamics usually do not require intraaortic balloon counterpulsation. In patients with significantly depressed left ventricular function and unstable hemodynamics, intraaortic balloon counterpulsation is useful for stabilization. In patients with chronic refractory angina, intermittent enhanced external counterpulsation (EECP), transthoracic spinal nerve stimulation, and carotid artery stimulation have been attempted but their efficacy for treatment of refractory angina remains to be established. Transmyocardial laser revascularization surgery has also been used for treatment of chronic angina, but its role also is uncertain in the management of refractory angina.

CORONARY ANGIOPLASTY AND MYOCARDIAL REVASCULARIZATION SURGERY
Coronary Angioplasty

Percutaneous transluminal coronary balloon angioplasty, directional atherectomy, combined angioplasty and stenting, and laser angioplasty are several nonsurgical techniques for myocardial revascularization. The details of these procedures are described in Chapter 15.

Catheter-based revascularization therapy relieves myocardial ischemia and improves symptoms, quality of life, and cardiac function in patients with obstructive coronary artery disease. The relative efficacies of medical therapy, balloon angioplasty, or coronary artery bypass surgery in decreasing mortality and myocardial infarction rate in patients with stable angina are often uncertain, even in patients with proximal stenosis of the left anterior descending coronary artery. With normal left ventricular ejection fraction, long-term survival is similar in patients treated medically or with bypass surgery or angioplasty. The need for repeat revascularization procedures is significantly lower in patients undergoing coronary artery bypass surgery compared to those having angioplasty or medical therapy. Both catheter-based revascularization therapy and coronary artery bypass surgery result in greater symptomatic relief and a lower incidence of ischemia on treadmill exercise tests compared to medical therapy. In patients with multivessel coronary artery disease and stable angina, the overall mortality rate and incidence of myocardial infarction are similar in patients undergoing coronary artery bypass surgery and coronary angioplasty. A second revascularization procedure, predominantly coronary angioplasty, is needed significantly more often in patients originally treated with coronary angioplasty. Although the immediate cost of performing coronary artery bypass surgery is higher than that for catheter-based myocardial revascularization procedures, the long-term cost is similar.

The major advantage of the catheter-based myocardial revascularization therapy compared to coronary artery bypass surgery is that the short-term morbidity associated with surgery can be avoided. Furthermore, the option for surgery at some future date remains available to patients who have undergone successful angioplasty.

The major disadvantage of coronary angioplasty is restenosis, which occurs at a rate of 30% to 40%. The use of stents following balloon angioplasty may decrease the incidence of restenosis to about 20%. Various antiplatelet and antithrombolic agents, lipid-lowering agents, angiotensin-converting enzyme inhibitors, and drugs that can potentially attenuate *smooth* muscle and fibroblast growth have been used to reduce the incidence of restenosis without success. The inhibitors of glycoprotein IIb/IIIa that impair platelet function decrease the incidence of acute reocclusion following angioplasty of complex coronary artery lesions. It should be appreciated that not all types of coronary artery lesions are amenable to catheter-based revascularization. Both initial success rate, which may exceed 90%, and long-term results also depend on knowledge, skill, and experience of the interventionalists.

Patients with stable angina refractory to medical therapy are the ideal candidates for catheter-based revascularization. Patients with mild symptoms but with a large amount of myocardium at ischemic risk may also be considered for such therapy. The role of angioplasty for the management of silent ischemia has not been established.

Patients with primary unstable angina should not be considered for immediate angioplasty because of the increased risk of acute reocclusion and adverse cardiac events. Elective angioplasty following heparin therapy for 3 to 5 days may decrease the risk of adverse complications, hospital stay, and recurrence of ischemic symptoms.

Coronary Artery Bypass Surgery

Surgical creation of a bypass shunt from the aorta to a diseased coronary artery beyond the area of fixed obstruction is now an established therapy for ischemic heart disease. Most often, a saphenous vein is used for the shunt material, although other veins may also be used. The internal mammary artery is being used with increasing frequency and in most patients is the vessel of choice for left anterior descending coronary artery lesions because of its higher long-term patency rate.

Perioperative mortality in patients with normal or slightly depressed left ventricular function is presently quite low at 1.0% to 2.5%. In patients with depressed left ventricular function, operative mortality is considerably higher and the operative risk increases with the increasing severity of depressed cardiac function. Left main coronary artery stenosis, incomplete revascularization, a combined surgical procedure (bypass grafts along with aneurysmectomy or valve replacement), and female gender appear to influence operative risk adversely. Operative mortality is higher in patients older than 65 years and in the presence of other organ dysfunction (e.g., renal failure, peripheral vascular disease, COPD).

The incidence of perioperative myocardial infarction has also declined with the availability of better myocardial protection techniques (cold cardioplegia). The incidence of clinically significant perioperative infarction is presently 5% or less.

The early graft patency rate (within 6 months) exceeds 80%. Early graft occlusion usually results from thrombosis. The saphenous vein graft patency rate after 6 to 10 months is 70% to 86%, and the graft closure rate decreases significantly after the first year. After the first year the graft attrition rate is approximately 2% per year. However, at 10 to 15 years, only 50% to 30% of the vein grafts are expected to remain patent and functioning. The patency rate of the internal mammary artery grafts is higher than that of saphenous vein grafts. Fibrous intimal, medial, and adventitial proliferation and atherosclerotic involvement of the bypass grafts are the principal causes of late graft occlusion. The risk for late graft occlusion is significantly higher in patients with higher LDL and lower HDL cholesterol. Thus control of hyperlipidemia should be considered as an important part of management after bypass surgery. Aspirin therapy during the immediate preoperative period also decreases the rate of graft occlusion, which is the rationale for aspirin therapy in patients undergoing coronary artery bypass surgery.

Between 70% and 95% of patients with stable or unstable angina report either complete or marked relief of anginal symptoms. Improved exercise tolerance and improved quality of life are expected for most patients. Improvements in regional and global myocardial mechanical and metabolic function also occur (Fig. 22-1). Coronary artery bypass surgery also decreases the frequency and duration of the silent episodes of spontaneous S-T segment depression. The benefits of bypass surgery in relieving symptoms and improving quality of life decline with time, and at 10 years postsurgery the incidence of recurrence of anginal symptoms and of decreased exercise tolerance is similar to those of medically treated patients.

Coronary artery bypass surgery also provides survival benefits in certain subsets of patients with stable angina. Improved survival with surgical therapy compared to medical therapy has been documented in patients with left main coronary artery disease. Patients without left main coronary artery disease but in the high-risk subgroups are also likely to derive survival benefit with surgery. The high-risk subgroups are defined angiographically and clinically and include

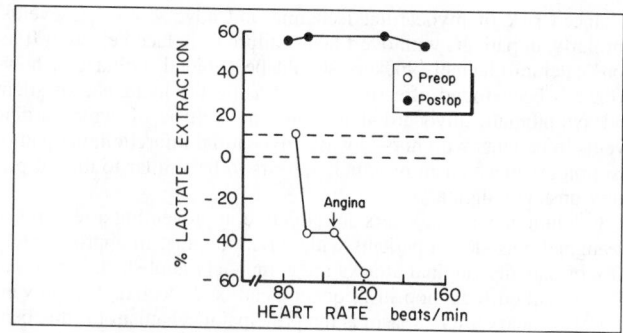

FIG. 22-1   Changes in myocardial lactate extraction during atrial pacing before and after coronary artery bypass surgery. Positive values indicate lactate extraction by the myocardium and thus adequate O_2 supply. Negative values indicate lactate production and myocardial ischemia. Preoperatively with increased heart rate and at the onset of angina, myocardial lactate production rather than extraction occurred. Postoperatively, despite a higher pacing rate, lactate extraction was normal and angina did not develop. These findings suggest that revascularization surgery can improve angina threshold and prevent myocardial ischemia.

(From Katzung BG, Chatterjee K: *Basic clinical pharmacology,* Los Altos, Calif, 1983, Lange.)

patients with three-vessel disease and impaired left ventricular ejection fraction, resting S-T segment depression, and a history of previous myocardial infarction or a history of previous hypertension. In these high-risk patients survival benefit with surgery tends to decrease beyond 7 years, probably related to increased frequency of late graft occlusion. Survival with surgery appears to be better compared to that with medical therapy in patients with three-vessel disease and in patients with two-vessel disease in which one of these vessels is the proximal segment of the left anterior descending coronary artery. In patients with one-vessel disease and in those with two-vessel disease without involvement of the proximal left anterior descending coronary artery, surgical myocardial revascularization is not associated with improved survival compared to that with medical therapy. Also, in patients with mild angina and preserved left ventricular ejection fraction, surgical therapy may not decrease mortality and myocardial infarction rates but may improve quality of life.

Long-term survival following bypass surgery appears to have improved due to better surgical techniques and more frequent uses of arterial conduits. The 10-year and 15-year survival rates, even after saphenous vein bypass graft surgery, are approximately 74% and 55%, respectively. The long-term survival following bypass surgery is influenced by a number of factors such as gender, age, and the state of left ventricular function before surgery. The long-term survival is better in males than in females; in patients with normal ejection fraction and in younger patients the 10-year survival in those with normal left ventricular ejection fraction exceeds 80%, whereas it is approximately 65% in patients with reduced ejection fraction. In patients older than 75 years, 10-year survival is approximately 40%, whereas it exceeds 80% in patients younger than 45 years. During postsurgery follow-up, the incidence of myocardial infarction and need for reoperation progressively increase with time and at 15 years, rates of myocardial infarction and reoperation are 26% and 33%, respectively, after saphenous vein bypass graft surgery. Nevertheless, surgical revascularization therapy provides substantial benefit in relieving symptoms and improving quality of life and survival in clearly identifiable subsets of patients with stable angina.

Indications for and timing of revascularization surgery in patients with unstable angina remain controversial. The NIH National Cooperative Study compared medical and surgical therapy; improvement in survival following surgical therapy was not demonstrated. It appears established, however, that emergency revascularization surgery is rarely required and that most patients can be "cooled off" with aggressive medical therapy as outlined previously. Thus coronary arteriography and the decision regarding revascularization surgery can be made electively following the cooling-off period in most patients, usually during the same hospitalization. Some patients who develop angina with limited physical activity or who continue to experience rest

---

BOX 22-4
Therapeutic approach for stable angina

I. General medical therapy—modification of risk factors such as cessation of smoking, control of hypertension, diabetes, and hyperlipidemia. Regular exercise and reduction of weight. Use of aspirin if not contraindicated.

II. Medical therapy in patients with stable angina in the absence of significant triple-vessel coronary artery disease or left main coronary artery stenosis—β blockers and then add nitrates. For those who become refractory to β blocker and nitrate therapy, add calcium channel blockers. For those who become refractory to triple therapy, consider revascularization therapy (catheter-based revascularization or surgical revascularization procedure depends on the anatomic considerations).

III. Indication for revascularization therapy
   A. Significant left main coronary artery restenosis → coronary artery bypass surgery.
   B. Significant triple-vessel coronary artery disease with or without associated left main coronary artery stenosis and with or without normal left ventricular ejection fraction → coronary artery bypass surgery, including internal mammary artery as conduit.
   C. Single- or double-vessel coronary artery stenosis, including proximal left anterior descending coronary artery stenosis and refractory angina → catheter-based revascularization or coronary artery bypass surgery.
   D. Single vessel coronary artery stenosis and refractory angina → initially catheter-based revascularization followed by surgical revascularization, if necessary.

IV. Intolerance to pharmacologic agents because of side effects or if quality of life with medical therapy unacceptable → catheter-based revascularization or surgical revascularization based on the anatomy.

V. In patients with moderately to severely depressed left ventricular ejection fraction with angina or angina equivalent with or without signs of heart failure → surgical revascularization if feasible.

BOX 22-5
Therapeutic approach for primary unstable angina

1. High-risk patients: Admission in the monitored cardiac care unit
   Prolonged rest angina
   Rest angina with S-T changes
   Early postinfarction rest angina
   Angina with hemodynamic compromise
   • Left ventricular failure
   • Hypotension
   • Mitral regurgitation
   Previous myocardial infarction
   Postcoronary angioplasty
   Postcoronary bypass surgery
2. Intravenous continuous heparin infusion
3. Aspirin
4. IV nitroglycerin for 24 hours, followed by nonparenteral nitrates
5. Beta blockers (IV esmolol or other β blockers) followed by nonparenteral β blockers
6. Intractable to 2-5, add slow-release or long-acting calcium channel blockers
7. Intractable to 2-6 → intraaortic balloon counterpulsation in presence of hemodynamic compromise → catheter-based or surgical myocardial revascularization
8. Intractable to 2-6, no hemodynamic compromise → cardiac catheterization → catheter-based or surgical myocardial revascularization
9. Responsive to 2-6 and stress-induced myocardial ischemia → elective cardiac catheterization → elective catheter-based or myocardial revascularization
10. Responsive to 2-6 and no stress-induced myocardial ischemia → continue medical therapy including aspirin, lipid-lowering agents, antiischemic therapy, and angiotensin-converting enzyme inhibitors in selected patients
11. Postangioplasty and postcoronary artery bypass surgery patients: IV heparin and aspirin and antiischemic drugs → cardiac catheterization → catheter-based or surgical myocardial revascularization

---

angina require early coronary arteriography for consideration of semiemergent reperfusion therapy. Patients who remain asymptomatic with medical therapy and tolerate medical therapy well can undertake an elective stress test. If evidence of myocardial ischemia is detected during the early stage of exercise despite medical therapy, coronary arteriography and reperfusion therapy are recommended. If myocardial ischemia does not appear during the stress test, medical therapy can be continued and surgery deferred.

When a vasospastic mechanism for unstable angina is suspected based on the clinical profile, coronary arteriography must be performed during the same hospitalization to delineate the coronary anatomy. If fixed coronary artery lesions are revealed, decisions regarding medical and surgical therapy can then be made in the same way as in patients with a history of effort angina. Patients with normal coronary arteries or with hemodynamically insignificant coronary artery stenosis should be regarded as having variant angina, and aggressive medical therapy should be continued.

The benefits of revascularization surgery in patients with variant angina have been unimpressive, even when significant fixed obstructive lesions are present. Episodes of coronary artery spasm may continue despite revascularization surgery. Therefore surgery is recommended only when aggressive medical therapy has failed and only in patients with associated severe fixed coronary artery stenosis. It has been suggested that cardiac sympathectomy along with coronary artery bypass surgery may provide better results than coronary artery bypass surgery alone.

SUGGESTED THERAPEUTIC APPROACHES

In patients with chronic stable angina, once the diagnosis is established, pharmacotherapy is initiated usually with nitrates, and then β-adrenergic blocking agents and/or calcium channel blocking agents are added to control angina. Reperfusion therapy with angioplasty or coronary artery bypass surgery is considered in patients who become refractory to pharmacotherapy or cannot tolerate pharmacotherapy because of either the drug's side effects or poor acceptance of the quality of life during pharmacotherapy. Coronary artery bypass surgery should also be considered in patients with hemodynamically significant left main coronary artery stenosis or triple-vessel coronary artery disease with a large extent of myocardium at risk. Modification of the risk factors including reduction in serum lipids should be considered in all patients (Box 22-4).

In patients with variant angina, with normal or hemodynamically insignificant coronary artery stenosis, nitrates and/or calcium channel blocking agents are effective in the vast majority of patients. In patients with significant coronary artery stenosis and those who continue to be symptomatic despite adequate medical therapy, reperfusion therapy by angioplasty or coronary artery bypass surgery is frequently required. These patients, however, require continued coronary vasodilator therapy after angioplasty or bypass surgery. In patients refractory to combination therapy with nitrates and calcium channel blockers, the addition of amiodarone is sometimes effective in controlling variant angina.

Patients with unstable angina (Box 22-5), a history of recurrent rest angina, and ischemic ECG changes should be admitted to the intensive care unit for better monitoring. Continuous IV infusion of heparin (5000 U bolus and 1000 U/hr) rather than intermittent heparin therapy should be instituted. In those patients already taking aspirin, aspirin (75 to 325 mg/day) should be continued. Aspirin should be continued indefinitely if conservative therapy is indicated. IV nitroglycerin is preferable to nonparenteral nitrates for 48 hours, although continuous infusion of nitroglycerin may produce tolerance. IV esmolol has been shown to be effective in reducing the frequency of ischemic episodes and thus is preferable to other β-blocking agents for initial management. For maintenance therapy, nonparenteral β-blocking drugs are titrated according to the changes in heart rate and blood pressure. Nifedipine and probably other dihydropyridines alone should be avoided for treatment of unstable angina because of increased risk of infarction; these agents, however, can be used in combination with nitrates and β blockers. Presently available data suggest that thrombolytic agents (e.g., rt-PA) are not more effective than heparin in reducing the frequency of ischemic episodes in unstable angina; thus thrombolytic agents are not indicated. Patients refractory to aspirin, heparin, and antianginal drugs require coronary arteriography with a view to revascularization. Patients with hemodynamic instability and severely depressed left ventricular function may benefit from prophylactic intraaortic balloon counterpulsation therapy before coronary arteriography.

Silent myocardial ischemia occurs frequently in patients who had manifestations and/or complications of coronary artery disease previously. In patients with documented prior myocardial infarction, chronic stable angina, unstable angina, and variant angina, more than half the episodes of ischemia occur without angina. The incidence of coronary artery disease in patients who never had manifestations of coronary artery disease but exhibit evidence of silent myocardial ischemia is relatively small at approximately 4%.

Frequent episodes of silent myocardial ischemia in patients with unstable angina and acute myocardial infarction appear to indicate a worse prognosis. The prognosis of patients with chronic stable angina or variant angina and episodes of silent ischemia has not been adequately assessed. It also remains uncertain whether pharmacotherapy or reperfusion therapy influences the ultimate prognosis. Nevertheless, until such evidence is available, it is reasonable to assess for silent myocardial ischemia in certain high-risk groups. In these specific subsets of patients, pharmacotherapy should be considered initially, followed by even more aggressive therapy such as angioplasty or coronary artery bypass surgery later. However, in the low-risk group or in patients without prior evidence of coronary artery disease, any therapeutic intervention for the prevention of silent myocardial ischemia is unnecessary and unjustified.

PROGNOSIS

Manifest ischemia such as angina is associated in the United States with an annual mortality of approximately 4%. In the Framingham Study the annual mortality of those who had a nonfatal myocardial infarction was 5%. However, recurrent myocardial infarctions are associated with a higher mortality. Hypertension, cigarette smoking, an abnormal ECG, ventricular arrhythmias, and ischemic S-T segment changes during exercise all are adverse prognostic indicators in patients with ischemic heart disease.

The extent and severity of coronary artery disease and the state of left ventricular function appear to be the most important prognostic factors for all patients with ischemic heart disease. With significant stenosis of only one of the major coronary arteries, the annual mortality rate is approximately 2%. With two-vessel disease, the annual mortality rate is about 7%. In patients with significant triple-vessel disease, it is 11%. Left main coronary artery stenosis carries an ominous prognosis: the 5-year mortality has been reported to be as high as 57%.

Evidence of heart failure from left ventricular dysfunction is associated with a mortality almost three times as high as the mortality in patients without heart failure who have a similar extent of coronary artery disease. The degree of depression of left ventricular function appears to bear a direct relation to mortality. In patients with three-vessel coronary artery disease and with normal ejection fraction, the 2-year mortality is approximately 12%; with an ejection fraction less than 50%, 2-year mortality increases to 36%. In patients with diffuse left ventricular dysfunction (usually an ejection fraction of 25% or less) and with triple–coronary artery disease, a 5-year mortality rate of 90% has been reported.

Current medical therapy, particularly with β blockers, appears to influence the long-term prognosis of patients with stable angina. The Coronary Artery Surgery Study (CASS) reported an annual mortality of 1.6% in patients with mild to moderate angina and preserved left ventricular function. Even in patients with decreased ejection fraction, the prognosis is better than expected.

The prognosis for patients with unstable angina has been evaluated by both retrospective and prospective studies. Early studies had reported an early mortality ranging from 10% to 60%, with an incidence of myocardial infarction of 20% to 80%. More recent studies

have suggested, however, that the early mortality rate (within 1 month of hospitalization) is 1% to 2% and that the infarction rate is approximately 10%. The NIH National Cooperative Study reported an in-hospital mortality of 3% and late mortality of 7% during follow-up (average 30 months). In patients with progressively worsening effort angina or rest angina, a very unfavorable long-term prognosis has been reported. Five-year and 10-year mortality rates of 39% and 52%, respectively, have been observed. In patients whose angina is not relieved within 48 hours of bed rest, 1-year mortality may be as high as 57%. Spontaneous S-T segment depression unaccompanied by angina, particularly lasting for 1 hour or longer per 24 hours of ECG monitoring, is also associated with worse prognosis in patients with unstable angina. The mortality of patients with unstable angina treated medically is lower than that of acute myocardial infarction but higher than that of patients with stable angina. The majority of deaths occur within the first month of presentation. History of recurrent episodes of rest angina, ischemic changes in the electrocardiogram, hemodynamic compromise (hypotension, mitral regurgitation, left ventricular failure), and previous myocardial infarction are the adverse risk factors.

The prognosis of patients with variant angina remains undetermined. However, sudden death has been reported in approximately 15% of patients with severe variant angina, usually within 3 months of the onset of symptoms. Patients with variant angina and with normal coronary arteries appear to have a better prognosis than do those with fixed obstructive coronary artery lesions. Prognosis of patients with syndrome X is excellent and mortality or myocardial infarction is not expected.

BIBLIOGRAPHY

Ambrose JA et al: Angiographic morphology and the pathogenesis of unstable angina pectoris, *J Am Coll Cardiol* 5:609-616, 1985.

Berman DS et al: Incremental value of prognostic testing in patients with known or suspected ischemic heart disease: a basis for optimal utilization of exercise technetium-99m sestamibi myocardial perfusion single-photon emission computed tomography, *J Am Coll Cardiol* 26:639-647, 1995.

Braunwald E et al: Diagnosing and managing unstable angina, *Circulation* 90:613-620, 1994.

Byington RP et al: Reduction in cardiovascular events during pravastatin therapy: pooled analysis of clinical events of the pravastatin atherosclerosis intervention program, *Circulation* 92:2419-2425, 1995.

Cameron A et al: Coronary bypass surgery with internal thoracic artery grafts: effects on survival over a 15-year period, *N Engl J Med* 334:263-265, 1996.

Chatterjee K: The history. In Parmley WW, Chatterjee K, editors: *Cardiology,* Philadelphia, 1988, Lippincott.

Furberg CD, Patsy BM, Meyer JV: Nifedipine: dose-related increase in mortality in patients with coronary heart disease, *Circulation* 92:1326-1331, 1995.

Hoffman BB: Adrenoreceptor-blocking drugs. In Katzung BG, editor: *Clinical pharmacology,* Norwalk, Conn, 1994, Appleton & Lange.

Hueb WA et al: The medicine, angioplasty or surgery study (MASS): a prospective, randomized trial of medical therapy, balloon angioplasty or bypass surgery for single proximal left anterior descending artery stenosis, *J Am Coll Cardiol* 26:1600-1605, 1995.

Katzung BG, Chatterjee K: Vasodilators and the treatment of angina pectoris. In Katzung BG, editor: *Clinical pharmacology,* Norwalk, Conn, 1994, Appleton & Lange.

Kirklin JW et al: ACC/AHA guidelines and indications for coronary artery bypass graft surgery, *Circulation* 83:1125-1173, 1991.

Maseri A: Medical therapy of chronic stable angina pectoris, *Circulation* 82:2258-2262, 1990.

Mertes H et al: Symptoms, adverse effects, and complications associated with dobutamine stress echocardiography: experience in 1118 patients, *Circulation* 88:15-19, 1993.

Messerli FH: Case-control study, meta-analysis, and bouillabaisse: putting the calcium antagonist scare into context, *Ann Intern Med* 123:888-889, 1995.

Opie LH, Messerli FH: Nifedipine and mortality: grave defects in the dossier, *Circulation* 92:1068-1073, 1995 (editorial).

Rahimtoola SH et al: Survival 15 to 20 years after coronary bypass surgery for angina, *J Am Coll Cardiol* 21:151-157, 1993.

Riberio PA, Shah PM: Unstable angina: new insights into pathophysiological characteristics, prognosis, and management strategies, *Curr Probl Cardiol* 21:669-732, 1996.

Rodriquez A et al: Argentine randomized trial of coronary angioplasty percutaneous transluminal versus coronary artery bypass surgery in multiple vessel disease (ERACI): in-hospital results and 1-year follow-up, *J Am Coll Cardiol* 22:1060-1067, 1993.

Rosen SD et al: Central nervous system pathways mediating angina pectoris, *Lancet* 344:147-150, 1994.

Scandinavian Simvastatin Survival Study Group: Randomized trial of cholesterol lowering in 4,444 patients with coronary heart disease: the Scandinavian simvastatin survival study (4S), *Lancet* 344:1383-1389, 1994.

Thadani U, Opie LH: Nitrates. In Opie LH, editor: *Drugs for the heart,* ed 4, Philadelphia, 1995, Saunders.

Younis LT, Chaitman BR: Management of stable angina pectoris, *Cardiology* (special edition) 1(2):61, 1995.

23 Acute Myocardial Infarction

Guy S. Reeder and Bernard J. Gersh

INCIDENCE

Despite the approximate 40% decline in cardiovascular deaths during the last three decades, atherosclerotic cardiovascular disease still represents the most frequent cause of death in the United States. There are approximately 700,000 coronary artery–related deaths per year and more than 1 million myocardial infarctions (MIs), with early death in 10% to 15% and a subsequent 1-year mortality of 10% to 15%. The decreasing individual mortality from MI, possibly accounted for by earlier detection, widespread use of coronary care units, advances in drug therapy, and reperfusion with thrombolytic agents or balloon angioplasty, may be offset by the general aging of the population. These older patients at risk for atherosclerotic heart disease make up a group in whom the case-fatality rate for acute MI remains high.

PATHOPHYSIOLOGY

Acute MI occurs when profound and prolonged ischemia leads to irreversible myocardial cell damage and necrosis. In most patients, this results from thrombotic coronary occlusion. Infrequently, MI may occur with prolonged or severe coronary spasm in the absence of underlying coronary artery disease; this mechanism is implicated in cases related to cocaine use, ergot therapy, and severe emotional stress. Rare causes of MI include spontaneous coronary artery dissection, nitroglycerin withdrawal, serum sickness and various allergic conditions, profound hypoxemia, sickle cell crisis, carbon monoxide poisoning, and acquired hypercoagulable states. Epidemiologic studies demonstrate an increase in MI event rates in the early morning hours, probably related to circadian variation in coronary vascular tone, catecholamines, and coagulability (Fig. 23-1). This phenomenon is blunted by beta-adrenergic receptor blockade.

Recently, much investigation has centered on complex atherosclerotic plaque as a precursor of MI and unstable angina. Postmortem studies demonstrated that the nidus for intracoronary thrombus formation is usually disruption of a lipid-rich atherosclerotic plaque with exposure of thrombogenic plaque material to the bloodstream (Fig. 23-2). Serial angiographic studies demonstrated that plaque rupture and thrombosis in mild stenoses more often lead to MI than similar processes involving tight lesions, presumably as a result of better distal collateralization in the latter.

The sequence of events leading to plaque rupture is not fully understood, but it is known that lipid-rich plaques have an increased risk of rupture. Such plaques usually have an eccentrically located lipid pool separated from the vessel lumen by only a thin, fibrous cap. Plaque rupture usually occurs at the junction between the fibrous cap and the normal vessel wall, probably from increased stress at this area. Whether increased shear forces caused by the stenosis, repeated oscillatory stress resulting from contraction of the heart, or changes in coronary tone related to circulating catecholamines act singly or in concert to potentiate plaque rupture remains conjectural. Once rupture occurs, platelets adhere to the exposed collagen and lipid matrix, and the thrombotic cascade is initiated.

Totally occlusive thrombus in patients with inadequate distal collateralization most often results in Q wave MI. Transiently occluding thrombus, with spontaneous lysis, or distal collateralization may yield lesser degrees of necrosis and produce non–Q wave MI. Patients with intermittent or subtotal occlusive thrombi, adequate collateralization, or both may have the syndrome of unstable or prolonged angina in the absence of myocardial necrosis. Thus a common underlying process (i.e., plaque rupture and superimposed thrombus) is responsible for unstable angina, non–Q wave MI, Q wave MI, and probably sudden death in many patients. Extent of MI relates to the size of the territory supplied by the infarct-related vessel, the presence and ad-

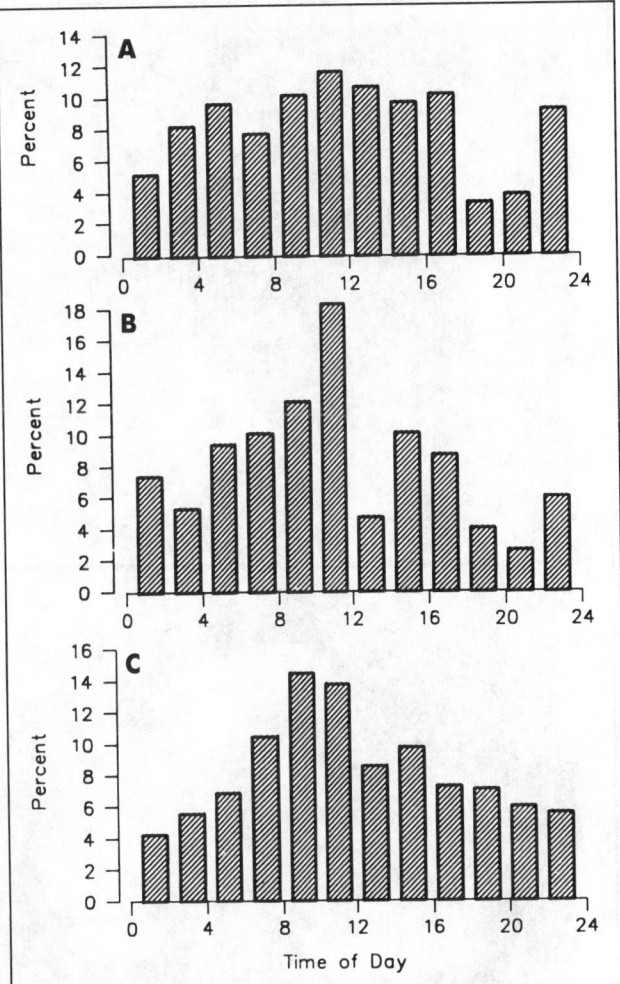

FIGURE 23-1   Diurnal variation in myocardial infarction (MI). **A,** Incidence of MI in 206 patients receiving beta-adrenergic receptor blocker therapy before their MI. Morning incidence of MI did not increase. Percent of MIs per 2-hour interval is indicated on *y* axis, and time of day is indicated on *x* axis (military time). **B,** Incidence of MI in 147 patients receiving calcium antagonists before their MI. Morning incidence of MI increased ($P < 0.01$) similar to that observed in total study population. **C,** Incidence of MI in 1473 patients who did not receive beta-adrenergic receptor blocker therapy. Morning incidence of MI is increased ($P < 0.001$).

(From Willich SN et al: *Circulation* 80:853, 1989.)

equacy of distal collateralization, and the metabolic needs of the jeopardized myocardium. In the majority of nonreperfused Q wave infarcts, most of the jeopardized myocardium becomes necrotic, whereas in non–Q wave infarcts and unstable angina, a substantial amount of residual jeopardized (ischemic) myocardium has not yet become necrotic.

Myocardial necrosis leads to an inflammatory response with infiltration of neutrophils and monocytes. Necrotic myocardium is gradually replaced by the deposition of collagen fibers and scar tissue. This healing process is complete within 4 to 6 weeks after necrosis.

CLINICAL PRESENTATIONS

The classic symptom of acute MI is discomfort in the central area of the chest that may radiate to the neck, back, or arms. It is persistent (unrelieved by nitrates) and is frequently associated with diaphoresis, nausea, weakness, and fear of impending death. The discomfort gradually builds to maximum intensity over several minutes, and this feature may help to differentiate MI from other conditions, such as aortic dissection or perforated peptic ulcer, in which maximum pain is usually instantaneous. In patients with preexisting angina pectoris the pain of MI is usually similar but persistent.

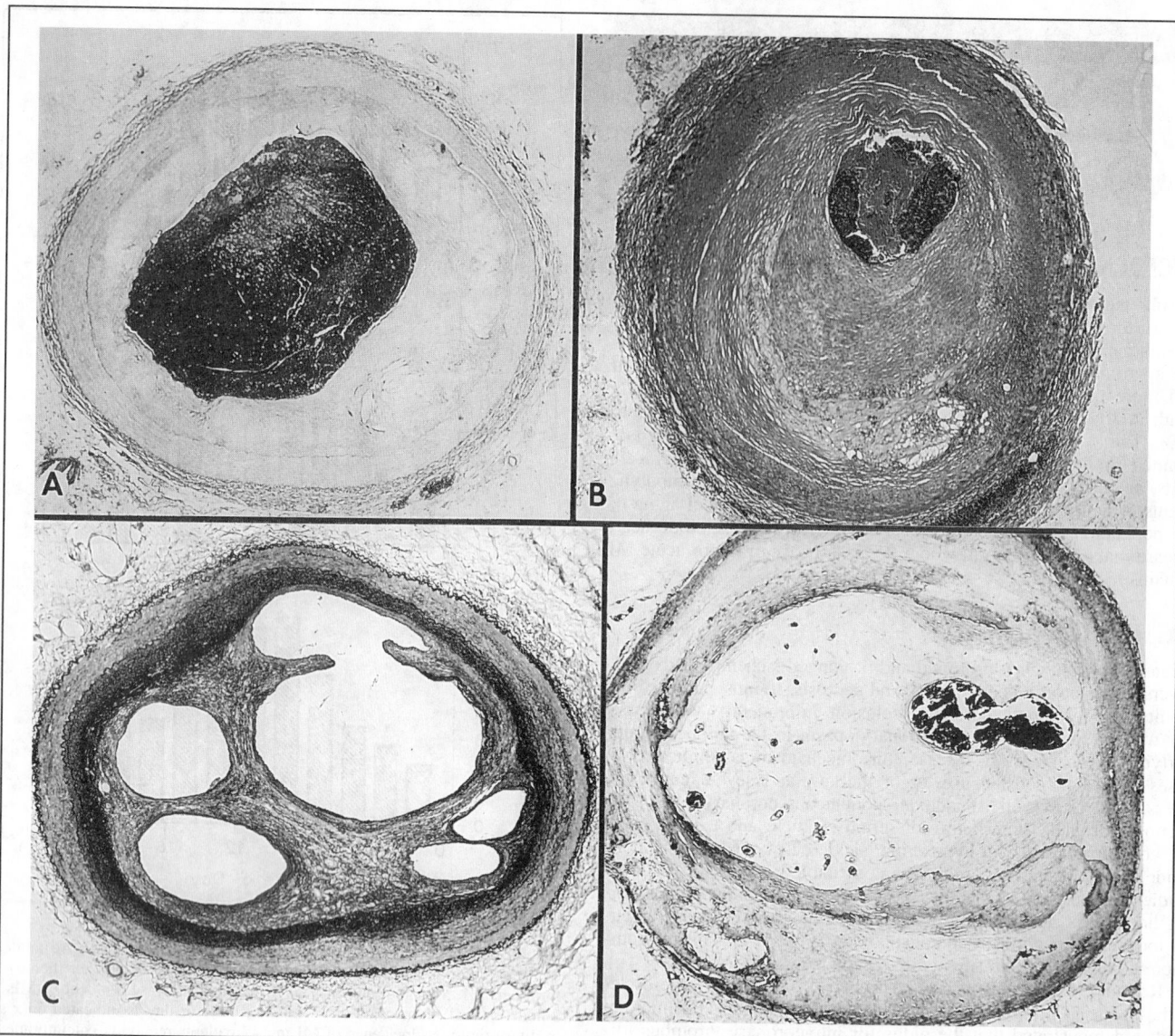

FIGURE 23-2   Coronary thrombosis and its consequences. Occlusive thrombi involving grade 2 plaque **(A)** and grade 4 plaque **(B).** Organization and fibrosis of thrombus with **(C)** and without **(D)** appreciable lysis and recanalization.

(From Edwards WD: In Gersh BJ, Rahimtoola SH, editors: *Current topics in cardiology: acute myocardial infarction,* New York, 1991, Elsevier.)

At least one fifth of MIs are clinically unrecognized because of atypical symptoms, especially in elderly patients (Table 23-1), or absence of chest discomfort. Painless MI is known to occur in elderly persons, in patients with diabetes mellitus, and in postoperative patients, especially those receiving analgesics. If the pain of myocardial ischemia is perceived in the epigastrium, back, or in one arm only, the diagnosis may not be considered by the patient and sometimes not by the physician (Chapter 16). Occasionally, MI may be recognized in retrospect only by the clinical occurrence of a complication, such as peripheral embolization of mural thrombus, development or worsening of congestive heart failure, new mitral regurgitation, or syncope caused by arrhythmia.

The physical examination may be entirely normal in patients with uncomplicated MI, although a fourth heart sound is typical. A minority of patients may demonstrate findings that suggest hyperlipidemia, including corneal arcus, xanthelasma, or tendon xanthomas. Patients with substantial left ventricular dysfunction at presentation may demonstrate tachycardia, pulmonary rales, tachypnea, and a third heart sound. A mitral regurgitant murmur should suggest papillary muscle dysfunction or partial papillary muscle rupture; however, the latter is

unlikely at presentation. An aortic regurgitant murmur occurs infrequently and should suggest the possibility of aortic dissection, as should asymmetry in blood pressure or pulse amplitude in the upper extremities.

In patients with right ventricular involvement, increased jugular venous pressure, Kussmaul's sign, and a right ventricular third heart sound may be present. Such patients virtually always have inferior MIs and may demonstrate exquisite blood pressure sensitivity to nitrates. In patients with massive left ventricular dysfunction, shock is indicated by hypotension, diaphoresis, cool skin and extremities, pallor, oliguria, and possible confusion. These patients have a high mortality. Some estimation of prognosis at presentation is possible with the use of the Killip classification (Table 23-2). However, more accurate stratification of risk of early mortality can be obtained by the use of hemodynamic subsets, as described later.

The differential diagnosis of the patient with acute MI should include aortic dissection, pericarditis, acute pulmonary embolism, intercostal neuralgia, costochondritis, and abdominal visceral disorders such as peptic ulcer disease, pancreatitis, and biliary colic. The physical examination alone often allows accurate differentiation of MI from

Table 23-1   Atypical symptoms of myocardial infarction (MI) in elderly patients

	PATIENTS (%)		
SYMPTOMS	65-74 YEARS	75-84 YEARS	≥85 YEARS
Chest pain	78	60	38
Dyspnea	41	44	43
Sweating	34	23	14
Syncope	3	18	18
Confusion	3	8	19
Stroke	2	7	7

Modified from Bayer AJ et al: *J Am Geriatr Soc* 34:263, 1986.

Table 23-2   Killip class and hospital mortality

KILLIP CLASS		HOSPITAL MORTALITY (%)
I	No CHF	6
II	Mild CHF, rales, S3 heart sound, congestion on chest radiograph	17
III	Pulmonary edema	38
IV	Cardiogenic shock	81

Modified from Killip TK III, Kimball JT: *Am J Cardiol* 20:457, 1967. *CHF,* Congestive heart failure.

many of these other disorders, as do the electrocardiogram (ECG) and other laboratory tests.

ELECTROCARDIOGRAPHIC MANIFESTATIONS

The ECG remains the most useful test for making the diagnosis of MI (Chapter 12). In Q wave MI the initial ECG manifestation involves an increase in the amplitude of the T wave (peaking) followed within minutes by ST segment elevation (Fig. 23-3). The R wave may initially increase in height but soon decreases as Q waves form. If the jeopardized myocardium is reperfused, the ST segment may promptly revert to normal, although T waves usually remain inverted and Q waves may or may not regress. In the absence of reperfusion the ST segment gradually returns to baseline in several hours to days, and T waves are symmetrically inverted. These changes describe anterior and inferior transmural MI. Posterior transmural MI is an exception to these rules because there generally is ST depression in leads V_1 to V_3 at presentation, and MI may therefore be mistaken for an anterior non–Q wave MI. Conduction disturbances are common with inferior MI and may include first-, second-, or third-degree atrioventricular block or, less often, sinus bradycardia (Chapter 12).

Patients with non–Q wave MI may demonstrate various nonspecific ST segment and T wave abnormalities but most often demonstrate ST depression with or without T wave inversion; Q waves do not evolve.

"Reciprocal" ST segment depression may occur in leads remote from those with ST segment elevation. The presence of reciprocal depression denotes a patient at higher risk for later complications. In some patients a large MI may produce reciprocal depression simply because of electrical phenomena. In other patients, the presence of remote depressions indicates "ischemia at a distance" and the presence of multivessel disease or compromised collateralization. Finally, ST depression in leads V_1 to V_3 may represent posterior injury rather than anterior ischemia (Chapter 12). Failure of the T wave to invert within 24 to 36 hours or renormalization of previously inverted T waves in the infarct zone should suggest regional pericarditis, which in some patients has been a precursor to cardiac rupture.

OTHER LABORATORY TESTS

Measurement of the serum level of creatine kinase (CK) is useful for confirmation of MI. The MB isoenzyme of CK (CK-MB) is present in largest concentration in myocardium, although small amounts (1%

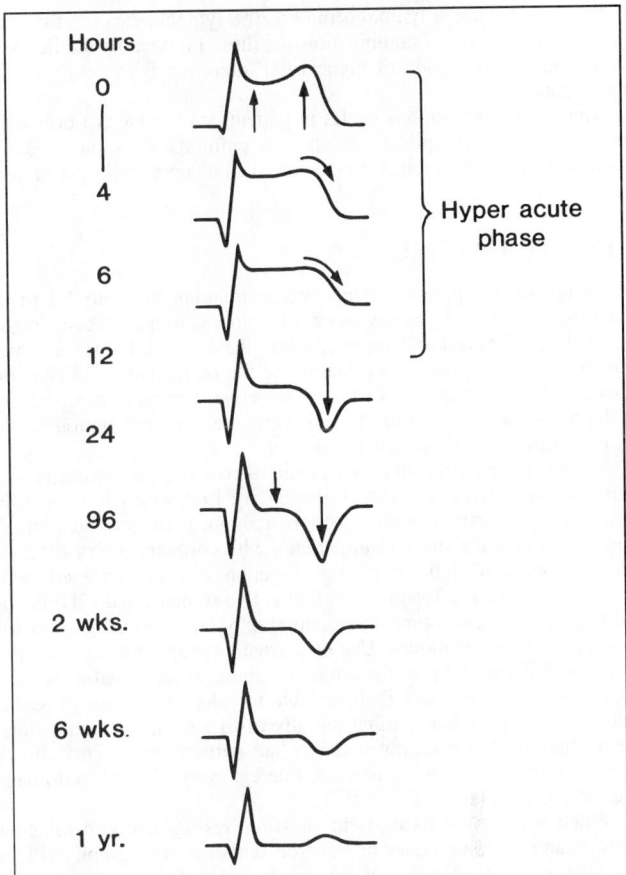

FIGURE 23-3   Evolution of electrocardiographic changes in MI. Serial, morphologic, typical QRST changes with time after transmural MI are depicted. (From Gau GT: In Brandenburg RO et al, editors: *Cardiology: fundamentals and practice,* vol 1, Chicago, 1987, Mosby–Year Book.)

to 2%) can be found in skeletal muscle, especially the tongue, small intestine, and diaphragm. CK-MB appears in serum within approximately 3 hours of MI onset, reaches peak levels at 12 to 24 hours, and has a mean duration of activity of 1 to 3 days. Because of the short time for release of this enzyme, phlebotomy for CK-MB analysis should be performed at admission, 12 to 18 hours later, at 24 to 30 hours, and possibly at 36 to 48 hours. False-positive cardiac increases in CK-MB levels can occur after cardioversion, cardiac surgery, myopericarditis, percutaneous transluminal coronary angioplasty, and occasionally after rapid tachycardia. Noncardiac causes of false-positive increases in CK-MB levels may occur with extensive skeletal muscle trauma, rhabdomyolysis, hypothyroidism, the muscular dystrophies, and some other neuromuscular disorders. Rarely, some patients may have low and constant elevations of serum levels of CK-MB for no known cause.

In patients who are first seen more than 24 hours after symptom onset, MB-CK activity may be decreasing or normal, and in selected patients it may be useful to measure serum levels of aspartate aminotransferase (AST) or lactic dehydrogenase (LDH). Although these enzymes have a longer duration of increased levels in the bloodstream, they are not specific for myocardium, and therefore their routine measurement is not justified. Moreover, in a patient with an infarct confirmed on the basis of creatine phosphokinase analyses, the AST level provides little additional information and is expensive to measure.

Occasionally the concentration of CK-MB isoenzyme may be increased in patients with normal total levels of CK enzyme. This finding usually indicates a small amount of myocardial necrosis in a patient whose baseline total CK enzyme level is at the low-normal end of the range, a not unusual finding in the elderly patient. Newer markers of myocardial infarction include MB-CK isoforms, myoglobin, troponin, and relative lymphopenia ($<20\%$ lymphocytes on differential count). The use of combinations of these markers for earlier and more sensitive detection of myocardial infarction is currently under investigation.

The chest radiograph is useful in patients with acute MI primarily for exclusion of complications, such as pulmonary edema, or other conditions in the differential diagnosis, such as pneumothorax or aortic dissection.

CARDIAC IMAGING

There are many applications of cardiac imaging in acute MI (e.g., diagnosis, prognosis, management of complications, assessment of underlying diseases) (Chapter 13) but the current focus on cost-effectiveness warrants a reevaluation of the *incremental* information provided by the imaging technique. Selective coronary arteriography is the most common method for assessing the coronary anatomy, and its indications in MI are presented later.

Various imaging techniques are used to visualize the cardiac chambers, cardiac valves, or both (Chapter 13). Left ventricular systolic function, as measured by the ejection fraction, is the strongest prognostic indicator for survival in patients with coronary artery disease. Measurements of left ventricular function can be obtained with contrast-enhanced left ventriculography, two-dimensional (2D) echocardiography, radioisotope ventriculography, and fast computed tomography (CT) techniques. Use of perfusion imaging to indicate the extent of MI may help to determine response to reperfusion; helpful techniques include either thallium scintigraphy or the use of sestamibi, a technetium isotope that initially distributes in a manner similar to thallium but does not undergo late redistribution. This allows demonstration of the initial perfusion defect even with delayed imaging, unlike with thallium.

When viability of tissue is in question, resting thallium imaging with 4- and 24-hour views or positron emission tomography (PET) has been used. Application of PET is limited to the few centers that have this technology.

When mechanical complications of MI are suspected, 2D and transesophageal echocardiography are the methods of choice for detecting left ventricular mural thrombus, right ventricular MI, papillary muscle and valve pathology, pericardial effusion and tamponade, and cardiac rupture. Left ventricular wall motion analysis and quantitation of valvular regurgitation can also be performed with contrast-enhanced ventriculography. In many institutions, however, patients are initially evaluated with 2D echocardiography and color-flow Doppler imaging because of the low cost, absence of risk, and convenience of this technology, which can be used at the patient's bedside.

Routine application of any imaging modality in every patient with MI cannot be justified from either an intellectual or a financial standpoint. The quality and availability of each technique at an institution are crucial to the use of a particular imaging modality. Before performing any imaging technique on the patient who has had an MI, the physician must have firmly in mind the clinical question to be answered as well as the likelihood that the test results will affect clinical decision making.

APPROACH TO THE PATIENT

There are four immediate goals in the management of the patient with acute MI: (1) relief of ischemic pain, (2) stabilization of hemodynamics, (3) reduction of myocardial oxygen demand ($M\dot{V}O_2$), and (4) maintenance or increase of myocardial perfusion. As much as possible, these goals should be achieved simultaneously.
1. Pain relief is best achieved with O_2, nitroglycerin, and intravenously (IV) administered morphine sulfate.
2. Estimation of the patient's volume status and the presence of left ventricular failure can be established to some extent by the results of the physical examination. If the patient is hypertensive, the careful IV administration of nitroglycerin and beta-adrenergic receptor blockers can be beneficial. If the patient is hypotensive without pulmonary congestion or rales, cautious fluid administration can be performed, perhaps with 2D echocardiographic imaging of left and right ventricular function. Pulmonary artery catheterization and measurement of pulmonary artery wedge pressure remain

---

BOX 23-1
Thrombolytic therapy for patients with MI

Indications

Ongoing Q wave MI longer than 30 minutes and less than 12 hours manifested by ST segment elevation of 1 mV or greater in two or more ECG leads
Chest pain and ST depression in anterior precordial leads coupled with imaging test demonstrating posterior left ventricular wall motion abnormality
Patient consent
Absence of absolute contraindications

Contraindications

Absolute
  Active bleeding
  Recent (<6 weeks) major surgical procedure or arterial puncture in noncompressible area or recent major trauma
  Symptomatic cerebrovascular disease or intracranial pathologic condition
Relative
  History of gastrointestinal bleeding or active ulcer disease
  Recent (6 months) administration of streptokinase or allergy to this drug (applies only to streptokinase)
  History of bleeding diathesis
  Remote history of cerebrovascular disease
  Prolonged cardiopulmonary resuscitation

---

the most accurate method of determining proper left ventricular filling pressure.
3. Reduction of $M\dot{V}O_2$ is achieved with sedation, pain relief, reduction of the heart rate (if tolerated) to 70 beats/min or less with IV administration of beta-adrenergic receptor blockers, and IV administration of nitroglycerin as long as a mean arterial pressure of 80 mm Hg is preserved. In patients in whom concern exists regarding precipitation of left ventricular failure, a short-acting beta-adrenergic receptor blocker such as esmolol is useful.
4. To maintain myocardial perfusion, aspirin (325 mg chewable) and IV administered heparin (5000 to 10,000 U boluses) are used for antiplatelet and anticoagulant effect. Although these measures provide some relief of pain and partial resolution of ST segment deviation in many patients, the cornerstone of modern therapy for MI is early reperfusion, with either thrombolytic therapy or emergent angioplasty. Therefore patients must be assessed rapidly as candidates for one of these interventions.

Thrombolytic Therapy

The rationale of thrombolytic therapy is largely based on laboratory investigations of experimental acute MI. The appreciation that myocardial necrosis occurs in a progressive wavefront from the endocardium to the epicardium and that this progression could be halted with prompt reperfusion led to the concept of myocardial salvage by lysis of intracoronary thrombi, using IV thrombolytic agents. General indications and contraindications for IV thrombolytic therapy are shown in Box 23-1. Patients with evidence of Q wave MI who are not judged to be at increased risk for bleeding complications may be considered for thrombolysis. Active menstruation is not considered to be a contraindication to thrombolysis.

Table 23-3 illustrates features of the currently available thrombolytic agents. These vary with respect to fibrin selectivity, antigenicity, side effects, and cost.

The fibrin-selective agents, such as tissue plasminogen activator (t-PA), have been shown conclusively to produce higher 90-minute patency rates compared with nonselective agents (i.e., streptokinase), but the clinical results in terms of mortality and left ventricular function are remarkably similar.

Fig. 23-4 shows pooled mortality data from five trials involving more than 28,000 patients treated within 6 hours of symptom onset

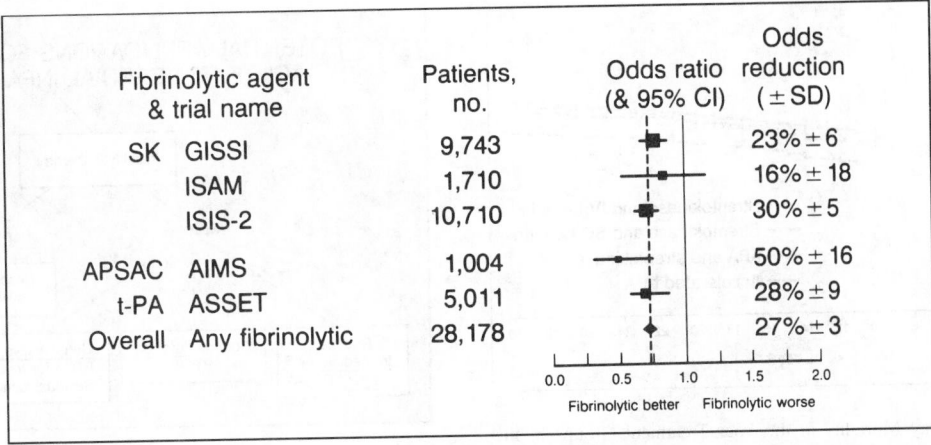

Fibrinolytic agent & trial name		Patients, no.	Odds ratio (& 95% CI)	Odds reduction (±SD)
SK	GISSI	9,743		23% ± 6
	ISAM	1,710		16% ± 18
	ISIS-2	10,710		30% ± 5
APSAC	AIMS	1,004		50% ± 16
t-PA	ASSET	5,011		28% ± 9
Overall	Any fibrinolytic	28,178		27% ± 3

0.0   0.5   1.0   1.5   2.0
Fibrinolytic better   Fibrinolytic worse

FIGURE 23-4   Mortality reduction in five large randomized trials of thrombolysis versus placebo for MI. Trial size is represented by size of square; relative mortality reduction is shown by position of square in relation to vertical line; confidence limits *(CI)* are demonstrated by horizontal line. Diamond shows pooled results of trials, with an average 27% mortality reduction. *SD,* Standard deviation; *SK,* streptokinase; *t-PA,* tissue plasminogen activator; *APSAC,* activated plasminogen streptokinase activator complex.

(Modified from Topol EJ, editor: *Textbook of interventional cardiology,* Philadelphia, 1990, Saunders.)

Table 23-3   Features of thrombolytic agents

AGENT	FIBRIN SELECTIVITY	ANTIGENICITY	HYPOTENSION	COST ($)*	USUAL DOSAGE
Streptokinase	−	+	+	206	1.5 million U/3 hr
Urokinase†	−	−	−	3192	3 million U/3 hr
scu-PA	+	−	−	NA	NA
t-PA	+	−	−	2244	100 mg/3 hr
APSAC	−	+	+	1665	30 Unit bolus

*Pharmacy cost at one institution in 1992 dollars.
†Not approved for this use.
scu-PA, Single-chain urokinase-type plasminogen activator; *t-PA,* tissue plasminogen activator; *APSAC,* activated plasminogen streptokinase activator complex; *NA,* not applicable.

and demonstrates an average mortality reduction of approximately 27% ± 3% compared with those receiving placebo.

Subsequently, a meta-analysis of nine placebo-controlled thrombolytic trials including 58,600 patients demonstrated an absolute mortality reduction of 30 lives per 1000 for patients presenting within 0 to 6 hours of symptom onset, 20 lives per 1000 for presentation between 7 to 12 hours, and no statistically significant benefit of thrombolytic therapy for those presenting beyond 12 hours. There was an excess of one disabling stroke per 1000 patients treated versus control. Patients with ST segment elevation or bundle branch block achieved the most benefit; those with ST depression achieved no benefit from thrombolytics.

Three large trials directly compared different thrombolytic agents with each other, as opposed to placebo. In GISSI-2 and its international arm, 20,000 patients were randomized to t-PA (100 mg) or streptokinase (1.5 million U), with a second randomization to heparin (12,500 U given subcutaneously two times a day) or placebo. All received aspirin, and 36% received beta-adrenergic receptor blocking agents. The mortality in the streptokinase arm was 8.5% and in the t-PA arm, 8.9%. In the Third International Study of Infarct Survival (ISIS-3) involving 46,000 patients randomized to streptokinase, activated plasminogen streptokinase activator complex (APSAC), or t-PA, the 5-week mortalities were 10.5%, 10.6%, and 10.3%, respectively. The rate of hemorrhagic stroke was slightly higher in the t-PA (0.7%) and APSAC (0.6%) groups compared with the streptokinase group (0.3%). Despite the known higher patency afforded by t-PA, neither of these trials demonstrated a clinical benefit of this more expensive agent.

The GUSTO trial succeeded in demonstrating an advantage of t-PA over streptokinase (Fig. 23-5). In this multicenter trial of 41,021 patients, an "accelerated" dosing regimen of t-PA was compared to two streptokinase arms (differing with respect to IV vs. SC heparin)

and a t-PA/streptokinase combination arm. Intravenous heparin was used with t-PA and the combination strategy. Thirty-day mortality was 6.3% for accelerated t-PA, 7.3% for the averaged streptokinase arms, and 7.0% for the combination treatment. The rate of hemorrhagic stroke was 0.49% and 0.54% for the two streptokinase arms and 0.72% for accelerated t-PA.

In the GUSTO angiographic substudy, 2431 patients were randomly selected to undergo angiography at 90 minutes, 180 minutes, 24 hours, and 5 to 7 days after thrombolysis. Normal flow in the infarct artery was present at 90 minutes in 54% of patients treated with t-PA but only 30% of those treated with streptokinase. Mortality was strongly and inversely related to infarct artery flow rate: 4.4% at 30 days for those with normal flow regardless of thrombolytic used versus 7.4% to 8.9% for lesser rates of flow. This study demonstrated the importance of restoring normal infarct artery flow rates as the mechanism for reduced mortality of reperfusion therapy.

The effects of thrombolytic therapy on left ventricular ejection fraction, as a surrogate of myocardial salvage, have been moderate. Pooled data from trials of thrombolytic therapy demonstrate an average change in ejection fraction of only 9% between treatment and control groups. More recent imaging techniques using technetium sestamibi, however, do document unequivocally that successful reperfusion results in significant salvage (approximately 40% to 50% of the area at risk). The substantial improvement in survival with thrombolytic therapy is probably not totally explainable by myocardial salvage alone. Repeated observations that survival is better with an open infarct-related rather than a closed infarct-related artery led to the so-called open artery hypothesis (which implies a benefit of thrombolysis independent of myocardial salvage).

Potential explanations for a survival benefit included improved tissue healing, less cavity dilation, and a source for collaterals if another artery becomes jeopardized in the future. Additionally, electri-

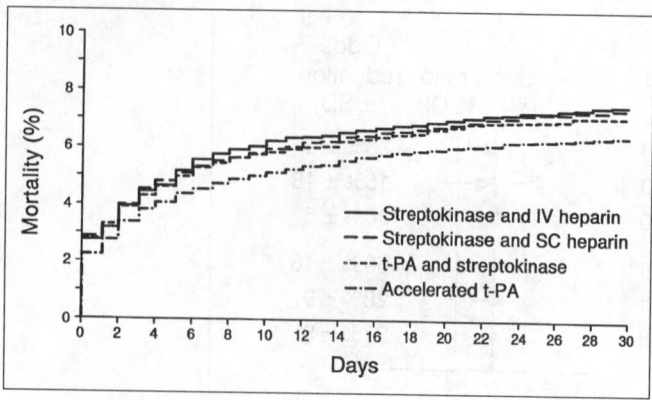

FIGURE 23-5   Thirty-Day Mortality in the Four Treatment Groups of the GUSTO Trial. The group receiving accelerated treatment with t-PA had lower mortality than the two streptokinase groups ($P = 0.001$) and than each individual treatment group: streptokinase and subcutaneous (SC) heparin ($P = 0.009$), streptokinase and intravenous (IV) heparin ($P = 0.003$), and t-PA and streptokinase combined with IV heparin ($P = 0.04$).

(Redrawn from GUSTO investigators: *N Engl J Med* 329:673, 1993.

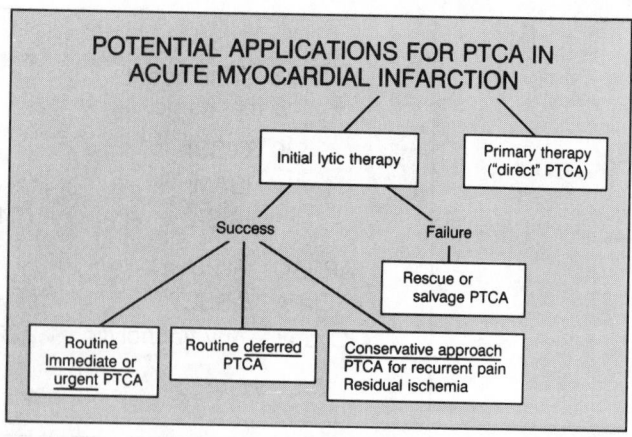

FIGURE 23-6   Potential application of percutaneous transluminal coronary angioplasty *(PTCA)* during acute myocardial infarction.

(From Holmes DR Jr, Gersh BJ: In Gersh BJ, Rahimtoola SH, editors: *Current topics in cardiology: acute myocardial infarction,* New York, 1991, Elsevier.)

cal instability of the myocardium may be decreased in the presence of an open infarct-related artery.

The general acceptance of the efficacy of thrombolytic therapy in Q wave MI and the enhanced benefits of early treatment led to investigational use of prehospital administration of thrombolytic agents. Prehospital thrombolysis is justified only when transportation to the hospital is prolonged (greater than 1 hour).

Those likely to gain the most benefit from thrombolysis include patients with large MIs, bundle branch block, continued pain at presentation, and collaterals to the infarct-related vessel and patients who are at high risk due to other factors.

At present, controversy exists about the application of thrombolytic therapy to certain patient subsets.

Elderly. There has been reluctance to apply thrombolysis to elderly patients because of an increased risk of bleeding. However, because these patients have a highly increased risk of death with MI, the potential for gain is increased, and in general, thrombolytic therapy in elderly patients has been underused. No upper age limit exists for thrombolysis; however, the older the patient, the more rigorous should be the search for contraindications.

Late Presentation. The use of thrombolytic therapy in patients who first appear late after the onset of symptoms (≥ 6 hours) is an important issue that applies to a substantial number of patients. The benefits clearly diminish with time, as does the potential for myocardial salvage; the risk of rupture may increase with time as well.

However, both the LATE trial and the FTT meta-analysis demonstrated definite benefit in treatment with thrombolytics up to 12 hours after symptom onset but not beyond, with a relative mortality reduction of approximately 26% and an absolute mortality reduction of 20 lives per 1000 patients treated. In selected patients with continued pain beyond 12 hours' duration, it may still be reasonable to offer thrombolysis if clinically high risk.

ST Segment Depression. The bulk of evidence suggests that thrombolytic therapy has little value in patients with non–Q wave infarction. Although most of these patients have persistent chest pain and ST segment depression, a subset of these patients (i.e., those with ST depression in leads V_1 to V_3) may have posterior Q wave MI (in the area of the circumflex coronary artery), and such patients may benefit from thrombolytic therapy.

New Bundle Branch Block. The presence of new bundle branch block is a marker for extensive MI. Although the conduction abnormality may mask the diagnosis of Q wave MI, several trials

demonstrated a benefit of thrombolytic therapy in this group, and such patients should be considered candidates unless contraindications to thrombolysis exist.

Reocclusion. Reocclusion of the infarct-related vessel occurs in 6% to 20% of patients and is silent in half of these. Causes of vessel reocclusion are probably multifactorial but relate to persistence of thrombus, the underlying thrombogenic lesion, and activation of the clotting system by lytic therapy itself.

With t-PA, the use of intravenous heparin is mandatory to preserve patency and in GUSTO, this strategy resulted in a low reocclusion rate of 6%. With streptokinase, the need for heparin is less well established and delayed SC heparin is acceptable. Newer agents include the direct antithrombin, hirudin, which unlike heparin, is able to bind with and inactivate clot-bound thrombin, and a group of agents that inhibit the glycoprotein 2B-3A platelet receptor responsible for platelet aggregation. Further experience in the use of these agents may decrease reocclusion after successful thrombolytic therapy.

Angioplasty

Percutaneous transluminal coronary angioplasty has assumed an important role in treatment of patients with acute MI (Fig. 23-6) (Chapter 15).

Direct angioplasty implies the use of this technique instead of thrombolytic therapy early in acute MI. Patency rates of 80% to 95% (higher than that achievable with thrombolytic therapy) are possible with reocclusion rates and in-hospital mortality similar to that reported in trials of thrombolysis. Advantages of this approach include the avoidance of thrombolytic therapy with its small but important risk of intracranial hemorrhage and the production of wide patency in the infarct-related vessel. However, this approach is limited by the lack of universal availability of catheterization facilities and the resultant delays for many patients located far from available centers.

Several randomized trials comparing results of direct angioplasty to thrombolytic therapy have been reported. Results in 103 patients in one trial from the Mayo Clinic demonstrated no significant difference in myocardial salvage between these two initial treatment strategies, with approximately half of myocardium at risk salvaged in each group. Complications, overall mortality, and aggregate cost were also similar. In the largest single trial (The Primary Angioplasty in Myocardial Infarction [PAMI] trial), 395 patients with ST segment elevation myocardial infarction within 12 hours of symptom onset were randomized to acute angioplasty versus thrombolysis with t-PA. The combined endpoint of death or reinfarction occurred in 5.1% of the angioplasty group versus 12.0% of the thrombolytic group. Recurrent ischemia (10.3% versus 28.0%) and stroke (0% versus 3.5%) were also significantly different between the groups. These results

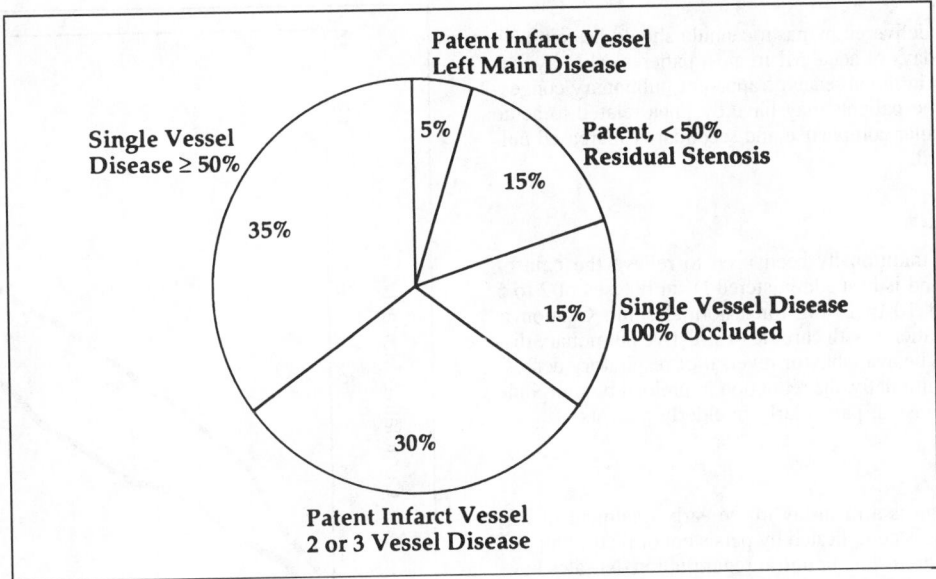

FIGURE 23-7 Proportion of patients in each of five anatomic subsets distinguished after thrombolytic therapy. (From Topol EJ, Holmes DR, Rogers WJ: *Ann Intern Med* 114:877, 1991.)

await confirmation by the GUSTO II trial, in which a subgroup of 1200 patients with ST segment elevation infarction will be randomized between angioplasty and accelerated t-PA.

For most of the U.S. population, however, direct angioplasty is limited by logistic constraints, and it is reassuring to see that thrombolytic drugs are equally effective in achieving myocardial salvage. Nonetheless, an important role exists for direct angioplasty in institutions with the available resources. Furthermore, direct angioplasty should be strongly considered (1) when a contraindication to thrombolytic therapy exists or (2) when the diagnosis of MI is uncertain by ECG criteria. Also, several uncontrolled series of patients with cardiogenic shock demonstrated an apparent marked decrease in mortality compared with historical control subjects and with results of trials of thrombolysis for patients in whom little or no benefit was apparent. Therefore it is reasonable to offer direct angioplasty to patients who have cardiogenic shock for whom mortality otherwise may reach 80% to 90%.

Angioplasty performed after thrombolytic therapy can be subdivided into three clinical situations: routine, rescue, and late elective angioplasty (see Fig. 23-6). *Routine* angioplasty implies early use of the technique after thrombolytic therapy, despite the presence of an open infarct-related artery. Three large-scale randomized trials investigated this approach (TIMI, TAMI, European Cooperative Study Group). Each trial demonstrated a higher mortality, increased bleeding complications, no decrease of reocclusion, and a higher rate of emergency coronary bypass surgery in the early angioplasty group. Early routine angioplasty in asymptomatic patients after thrombolytic therapy therefore cannot be recommended and is contraindicated.

Rescue angioplasty implies the early use of angioplasty in patients whose arteries failed to recanalize after thrombolytic therapy. Both TAMI-5 and the RESCUE trial prospectively examined the strategy of rescue angioplasty. In the former, there was a trend toward higher predischarge vessel patency (94% vs. 90%, $P = 0.065$) and better regional left ventricular function. In RESCUE, the occurrence of death or CHF tended to be lower in the treatment group (6.5% vs. 16.4%, $P = 0.055$). Mortality rates and vessel reocclusion are higher than for patients undergoing direct angioplasty or thrombolysis.

The current inability to assess noninvasively the patency of an infarct-related artery is a major limitation to the more widespread use of rescue angioplasty and to the conduct of a trial. Currently it is reasonable for patients who have continued pain and ST segment elevation after thrombolytic therapy to undergo cardiac catheterization for determination of infarct vessel patency and to undergo angioplasty if the vessel remains occluded or has suboptimal flow.

Late elective angioplasty implies the selective use of angioplasty in the convalescent stage of myocardial infarction. Both the TIMI-2 trial and the SWIFT trial compared a conservative strategy of angioplasty for patients with spontaneous or exercise-induced ischemia after MI versus an early invasive strategy of routine catheterization and angioplasty at 18 to 48 hours. At follow-up the number of deaths and repeat infarctions and the measurements of ejection fraction were similar in the conservative and routine catheterization groups, demonstrating no definite advantage for the latter.

The findings from these large multicenter trials are consistent and emphasize that a conservative policy of watchful waiting accompanied by angiography for these patients with spontaneous or exercise-induced ischemia is not only safe but the correct and most cost-effective approach for those with a stable clinical course after thrombolytic therapy.

Whereas the role of angioplasty after thrombolytic therapy has been clarified, an issue of continued debate is the role of routine predismissal angiography in stable postthrombolytic patients, as opposed to exercise or pharmacologic stress testing.

Fig. 23-7 shows the proportion of patients in various anatomic subgroups found at angiography after thrombolytic therapy. Some patients, those with left main coronary artery disease or three-vessel disease, might be selected for early surgical revascularization on the basis of findings from routine postinfarction angioplasty. However, identification of high-risk patients is also likely from clinical features such as presence of pulmonary congestion or overt congestive heart failure, recurrent angina, hypotension, or ejection fraction less than 40% on noninvasive testing.

The major argument against routine angiography after MI is "reperfusion momentum": the temptation to intervene with angioplasty for an anatomically severe lesion that may or may not be clinically important. At present, one may recommend either routine, post-MI angiography or a more conservative approach of selective angiography on the basis of spontaneous or exercise-induced ischemia. If routine angiography is elected, subsequent revascularization must be limited to patients with high-risk coronary anatomy, demonstrable ischemia, or both.

ADJUNCTIVE THERAPY

Pharmacologic therapy for patients with acute MI retains an important role in patient management, with or without the use of reperfusion techniques.

Oxygen

Low-flow O_2 therapy delivered by nasal cannula should be routinely given during the first days of acute MI in most patients. Mild hypoxemia may occur, even in the absence of apparent pulmonary congestion. Additionally, some patients may have dyspnea related to acute changes in left ventricular compliance and secondarily increased pulmonary interstitial fluid.

Morphine Sulfate

Morphine sulfate has traditionally been used to relieve the pain of myocardial ischemia and is best administered IV in boluses of 2 to 5 mg, to a maximum of 10 to 15 mg for a normal adult. Caution is necessary in treating patients with chronic obstructive pulmonary disease. Naloxone should be available for reversal of respiratory depression if this occurs. Additionally, the reduction in preload by morphine may exacerbate hypotension, particularly in elderly patients.

Nitrates

The use of nitroglycerin is a mainstay in the early treatment of MI, particularly in those cases complicated by persistent or recurrent pain, congestive failure, hypertension, or mitral regurgitation. Nitrates have several salutary effects, including dilation of venous capacitance vessels, arterial resistance vessels, and coronary arteries, and possibly redistribution of flow to ischemic areas. Animal experiments demonstrated reduction in infarct size when nitroglycerin was administered IV within the first 4 to 6 hours after coronary occlusion, and several clinical studies in certain subgroups of patients support these findings.

IV nitroglycerin, starting at a dose of 5 to 10 μg/min, can be used in most patients early in the course of MI and is often useful as initial treatment for relief of pain. In normotensive patients the usual goal is to decrease systolic blood pressure by 10%; in hypertensive patients a 30% decrease is allowable, but adequate perfusion pressure must be maintained because infarct size can actually increase if mean blood pressure decreases below 80 mm Hg. IV nitroglycerin is usually administered for 24 to 48 hours, depending on the patient's clinical condition and the use of nitrates given orally or of other afterload-reducing agents. Approximately 10% of patients demonstrate a sensitivity to nitroglycerin manifested by a profound decrease in blood pressure after administration of even a small dose. This vagally mediated reflex is especially prominent in patients with inferior wall MI and those with substantial right ventricular involvement. Nitroglycerin therapy is best avoided in this subgroup of patients. Additionally, nitrate tolerance may occur, even within the first 24 hours of continuous IV infusion. The routine use of oral nitrates in patients without symptomatic ischemia has been questioned by the GISSI-3 and ISIS-4 trials, which found no benefit in this subgroup of myocardial infarction survivors.

Beta-Adrenergic Receptor Blockers

The use of β-adrenergic receptor blockade in patients with acute MI is logical, and the theoretic advantages have been supported by much data from clinical trials. Nonetheless, it appears that these agents are still underused, particularly in the United States.

Mechanisms whereby β-adrenergic receptor blockers may be beneficial include (1) a reduction in myocardial O_2 consumption, which by slowing the rate of necrosis can increase the time available for myocardial salvage and decrease the risk of recurrent ischemia; (2) antagonism of arrhythmogenic and toxic biochemical effects of catecholamines; and (3) a possible direct effect on myocardial ventricular fibrillation threshold. Also, in ISIS-1, a trial of IV atenolol, a reduction in mortality was achieved by a highly significant decrease in the frequency of cardiac rupture compared with placebo treatment.

The results of clinical trials document an impressive decrease in early and late mortality despite minimum change in left ventricular function. In pooled data from 28 trials of β-adrenergic receptor blockers, the average mortality decrease was 28% at 1 week, with most benefit obtained in the first 48 hours. An average 18% reduction in reinfarction and 15% reduction in cardiac arrest were also documented. The long-term effects of β-adrenergic receptor blockade by agents without intrinsic sympathetic activity in secondary prevention

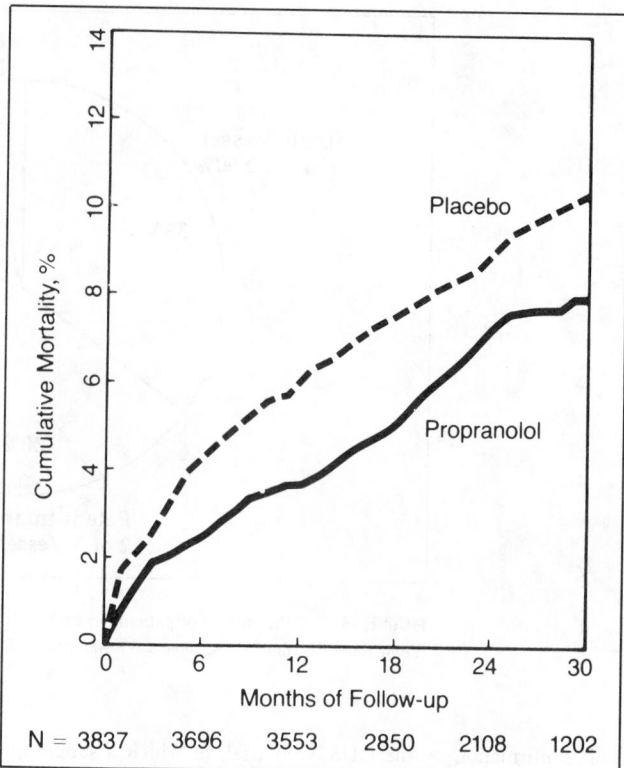

FIGURE 23-8   Survival after acute MI: the BHAT trial. Life table cumulative mortality curves for propranolol hydrochloride and placebo groups. *N* denotes total number of patients followed up through each time point.

(From Friedman L et al: *JAMA* 246:2073, 1981.)

of death after MI were established by large-scale randomized trials (Fig. 23-8). Although most of the benefit of β-adrenergic receptor blockade was demonstrated within the first week of infarction and occurred in patients at increased risk, continuing benefit in terms of decreased mortality was documented up to 3 years later.

Many experts recommend the early IV administration of β-adrenergic receptor blockers followed by beta blockers given orally for most patients with MI who do not demonstrate overt congestive heart failure or shock at admission. Major left ventricular dysfunction is not necessarily a contraindication; when concern exists regarding this, IV administration of a short-acting β-blocker, such as esmolol, can be used, with rapid termination of its effects if hypotension or increased pulmonary congestion occurs.

The studies demonstrating mortality reduction due to β-blockers were performed predominantly in nonthrombolysed patients. The use of β-blockers in patients receiving thrombolysis is a logical extension of these data but remains formally untested.

Calcium-Channel Blockers

Studies of the calcium-channel blockers failed to demonstrate a consistent benefit in patients with Q wave MI. In a meta-analysis of 22 trials, no improvement in mortality, reduction of infarct size, or reduction in the incidence of reinfarction was documented (Fig. 23-9). The lack of benefit probably relates to the negative inotropic action of the calcium-channel blockers, with an adverse effect in patients with left ventricular failure and the potential for nifedipine reflexly to increase heart rate and myocardial O_2 consumption. In patients with non–Q wave MI, two trials (Diltiazem Reinfarction Study, Multicenter Diltiazem Postinfarction Trial) demonstrated a decreased incidence of reinfarction and post-MI angina in patients treated with diltiazem compared with placebo. Further analysis in one of these trials demonstrated that patients with left ventricular failure, manifested by pulmonary congestion, actually had an adverse response to diltiazem, with benefit limited to those without pulmonary congestion.

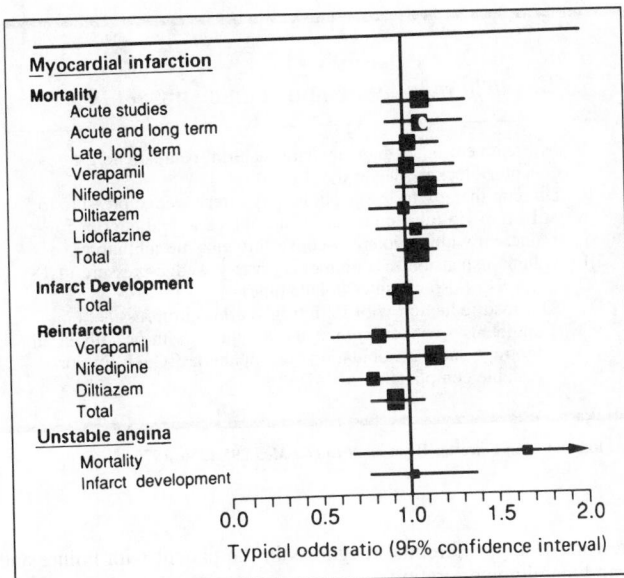

FIGURE 23-9   Published studies of calcium-channel blockers in patients with acute MI. Typical odds of death, infarct development, and reinfarction according to disease, types of trials, and drug used. Area of squares proportional to number of patients. Bars indicate 95% confidence intervals. Portions to left of vertical line (corresponding to odds ratio <1) indicate reduced risk with treatment; portions to right of vertical line indicate increased risk with treatment. Upper 95% confidence limit for effect on mortality in unstable angina, 6.2. Note that treatment does not seem to reduce risk of any event.

(From Held PH, Yusuf S, Furberg CD: *Br Med J* 299:1187, 1989.)

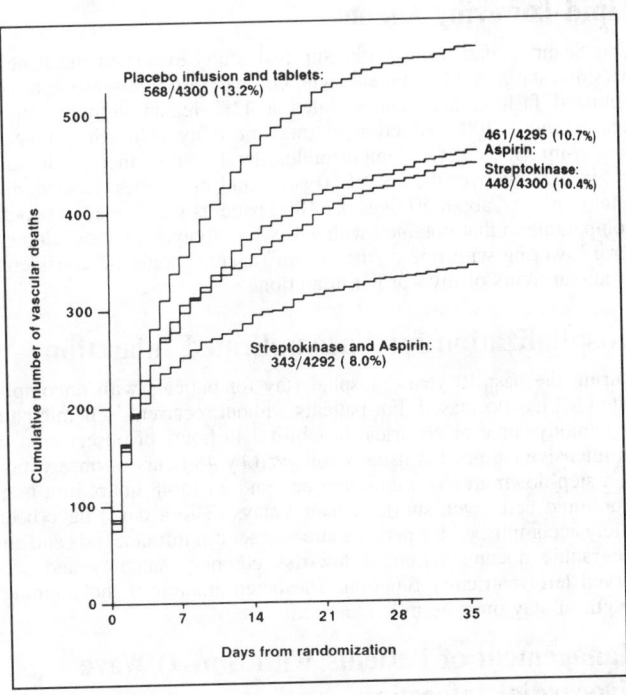

FIGURE 23-10   Effect of aspirin, streptokinase, both, or neither on 35-day vascular mortality in the ISIS-2 study.

(From ISIS-2 [Second International Study of Infarct Survival] Collaborative Group: *Lancet* 2:349, 1988.)

Although it is reasonable to treat a subgroup of patients who have non–Q wave MI with diltiazem, most such patients undergo invasive study and prompt revascularization.

Aspirin

Aspirin decreases mortality in patients with MI, undoubtedly through its antiplatelet effects. This was perhaps best illustrated in the ISIS-2 study (Fig. 23-10), in which patients were randomized to treatment with aspirin, streptokinase, or placebo, with later heparin therapy. The decrease in the death rate with aspirin and heparin was 23% compared with 25% for streptokinase and heparin and 41% for the combination of all three agents. Thus the effect of aspirin was nearly as great as that of streptokinase in this study, and the benefits of each were partially additive. At the present time, 325 mg of chewable aspirin usually is administered when the patient with acute MI is first seen.

Prophylactic Use of Lidocaine

Prophylactic use of lidocaine can decrease the risk of primary ventricular fibrillation but also appears to increase the risk of fatal asystolic events. In a recent meta-analysis of six trials of prophylactic use of lidocaine in patients with acute MI, the mortality was slightly higher in the lidocaine group. Currently, prophylactic use of lidocaine is not recommended for patients with acute MI.

Heparin

Heparin is a key adjunctive agent for treatment of patients with acute MI receiving thrombolysis with t-PA. Heparin acts to inhibit the thrombotic cascade by its potentiation of antithrombin III and by a direct antithrombin effect. It has recently become clear that thrombosis occurs simultaneously with thrombolysis and may even be potentiated by thrombolytic agents such as streptokinase or t-PA. Additionally, thrombin is a strong inducer of platelet aggregation, and these factors undoubtedly account in part for the propensity toward reocclusion after successful artery recanalization.

The major benefit of heparin in patients receiving thrombolytic therapy appears to be in decreasing reocclusion rather than in enhancing initial salvage. However, controversy surrounds the timing and administration of heparin. Probably the best method for administration of heparin is bolus IV administration followed by a continuous drip with titration to an activated partial thromboplastin time of 55 to 85 seconds. Although heparin can be administered before, during, or after the conclusion of thrombolytic therapy, we usually elect to administer it at the onset of treatment.

Angiotensin-Converting Enzyme Inhibitors

The administration of angiotensin-converting enzyme inhibitors (ACE) after myocardial infarction has clearly been shown to reduce postinfarction mortality. Two megatrials, GISSI 3 and ISIS-4, involving approximately 77,000 patients, demonstrated that the nonselective early oral administration of captopril or enalapril resulted in four or five lives saved per 1000 patients treated. Smaller trials using selective administration (low ejection fraction, congestive heart failure, or anterior wall infarction) have shown 40 to 70 lives saved per 1000 patients treated. ACE inhibitors can be administered on the first or second hospital day, orally, in low dosage, and gradually increased as long as hypotension is avoided. Duration of therapy is not established, though patients with ejection fraction <45% are usually treated indefinitely.

Magnesium Sulfate

The use of intravenous magnesium sulfate remains controversial. Animal studies and early human trials showed a relative mortality reduction of approximately 25% but these salutary effects were not confirmed by the ISIS-4 megatrial, which showed no benefit of this agent. However, the relatively late administration of magnesium in this trial, as well as subsequent experimental data demonstrating myocardial salvage when magnesium was administered prior to or at the time of reperfusion, casts the ISIS-4 results in some doubt. This agent is undergoing further trial testing; in the meantime, because of the low cost and low toxicity, magnesium can be considered in high-risk patients pending further data. Renal impairment and second degree heart block are relative contraindications.

Lipid-Lowering Agents

The Scandinavian Simvastatin Survival Study evaluated the benefit of Simvastatin in 4444 patients with coronary artery disease in a randomized fashion and demonstrated a 42% reduction in coronary deaths and a 30% reduction in total mortality at mean 5.4 years follow-up. Benefit was demonstrable after 1 year of therapy, including in patients over the age of 60 years and in females. Considering total mortality, about 50 lives per 1000 patients were saved, a benefit comparable to that obtained with early thrombolytic therapy. Cholesterol lowering with one of the "statin" agents should be considered in all survivors of myocardial infarction.

Hospitalization for Uncomplicated Infarction

During the past 10 years, hospital stay for patients with uncomplicated MI has decreased. For patients without recurrent ischemic pain or hemodynamic or electrical instability, 48 hours of observation in an intensive care bed is usually followed by 48 hours of observation in a step-down area or monitored bed and 24 to 48 hours in a non-monitored bed. Even shorter hospital stays (3 to 4 days) have been safely accomplished for patients after successful thrombolysis and angiographic documentation of low-risk coronary anatomy and preserved left ventricular function. The determination of the optimum length of stay must be individualized.

Management of Patients With Non–Q Wave Myocardial Infarction

The differentiation between Q wave and non–Q wave MIs is useful because the management, clinical course, and late prognosis differ between the two entities. Pathologic studies of non–Q wave MIs demonstrate an incomplete MI in relation to the myocardial territory at risk. Even though the incidence of severe coronary artery disease is roughly similar in Q wave and non–Q wave MIs, patients with non–Q wave MIs are two to four times more likely to have a patent infarct-related artery at presentation, with residual severe stenosis or prominent collateralization. Because of the smaller amount of infarcted tissue, the risk of congestive heart failure and significant arrhythmia is lower than with Q wave MI, as is in-hospital mortality. However, in the 6 to 12 months after non–Q wave MI, the cumulative mortality reaches or exceeds that for patients dismissed from the hospital after Q wave MI because of a higher incidence of reinfarction.

Patients presenting with non–Q wave myocardial infarction are a heterogeneous group with regard to myocardial territory at risk, extent of damage, and clinical outcome. Risk factors for further events in patients with non–Q wave MI include anterior location, persistent ST segment depression at dismissal, occurrence or progression of ST depression with angina, and inability to perform a low-level stress test. On the other hand, patients with non–Q wave MI who have no ST segment depression are in a lower-risk group.

The immediate treatment of patients with non–Q wave MI should consist of aspirin, β blockers, IV heparin, and perhaps treatment with diltiazem, depending on the presence or absence of pulmonary congestion. In general, at our institution, patients with non–Q wave MI, particularly if the extent of enzyme release is small, are treated similarly to patients with angina at rest. Thrombolytic therapy is of no proven value and may be harmful. The initial step is stabilization of the symptoms and hemodynamics, followed by coronary angiography. Thereafter, therapy is individualized on the basis of the coronary anatomy, left ventricular function, age, and other clinical variables. An alternative approach after stabilization is for the patient to begin mobilization under observation. In the absence of recurrent symptoms, angiography may be limited to patients with documented ischemia during stress testing.

COMPLICATIONS

Because of the ubiquity of cardiac rhythm monitoring, most patients who die in the hospital from acute MI do so because of either extensive myocardial damage with pump failure or mechanical complication of MI, such as severe mitral regurgitation or cardiac rupture. The mechanical complications are potentially curable and should be in the

---

BOX 23-2
Therapy by hemodynamic subset

I　No treatment other than standard (aspirin, beta-adrenergic receptor blockers, heparin)

II　Diuretic therapy to lower pulmonary artery wedge pressure to 18 mm Hg (also consider IV nitroglycerin and afterload reduction with angiotensin-converting enzyme inhibitors)

III　Volume expansion to a pulmonary artery wedge pressure of 18 mm Hg (also consider dobutamine)

IV　Afterload reduction with IV nitroglycerin, nitroprusside, or angiotensin-converting enzyme inhibitors with or without an inotrope such as dobutamine or dopamine (search for correctable complication of MI)

Modified from Forrester JH et al: *N Engl J Med* 295:1356, 1976.

---

forefront of any differential diagnosis in the patient with failure and hemodynamic deterioration.

Left Ventricular Failure

More than 20 years ago, Killip and Kimball (see Table 23-2) described the outcome of patients without or with various degrees of left ventricular failure occurring during hospitalization for acute MI. In patients with mild congestive heart failure characterized by rales covering less than 50% of the lung fields or an S3 gallop, mortality was 17%, whereas those with pulmonary edema had a doubling of mortality to approximately 38%. Treatment of the patient with mild congestive heart failure in the absence of ongoing ischemia may require no more than usual methods, such as sodium restriction, digitalis, afterload reduction, and diuretics. Most patients with adequate peripheral perfusion and urine output do not require invasive hemodynamic monitoring.

In patients with more than mild pulmonary congestion but no evidence of ongoing ischemia, invasive hemodynamic monitoring using a balloon-tipped pulmonary artery catheter allows immediate access to valuable hemodynamic information and guides therapy. The management of such patients has been described on the basis of hemodynamic subsets related to pulmonary artery wedge pressure and cardiac output (see Box 23-2 and Fig. 23-11). The basic goals of this approach include adjustment of volume status to bring pulmonary artery capillary wedge pressure to 18 to 20 mm Hg, optimization of cardiac output with inotropic agents or vasodilators, or both. In hypotensive patients, dopamine is the preferred inotropic agent because of its peripheral constricting properties with preservation of renal perfusion. Nitroglycerin is the preferred vasodilator and may be added cautiously once an acceptable systemic pressure has been obtained. Nitroprusside is less desired because of its potential coronary steal effect. For normotensive patients with low cardiac output, dobutamine, which has mixed inotropic and vasodilatory properties, may be preferable.

Severe left ventricular dysfunction (pump failure) may present as florid pulmonary edema or cardiogenic shock with hypotension, cool underperfused extremities, oliguria, and evidence of cerebral and visceral hypoperfusion (Chapters 19 and 20). Such patients constitute a high-risk subset, occurring in approximately 7% of myocardial infarctions and carrying historical mortality of about 80%. The goals for management of these patients are two-fold: (1) immediate hemodynamic stabilization, including adequate oxygenation and correction of acid-base and tissue perfusion abnormalities, including the use of intraaortic balloon pumping or ventricular assist devices, and (2) nearly simultaneous urgent investigation for ongoing ischemia and possible mechanical complications of myocardial infarction. In a prospective international registry of cardiogenic shock and effect of early revascularization on mortality, 19 centers in the United States and Europe prospectively registered 251 patients. The overall in-hospital mortality was 66%, and patients clinically selected to undergo cardiac catheterization had a lower mortality (51% vs. 85%, $P < 0.0001$) than

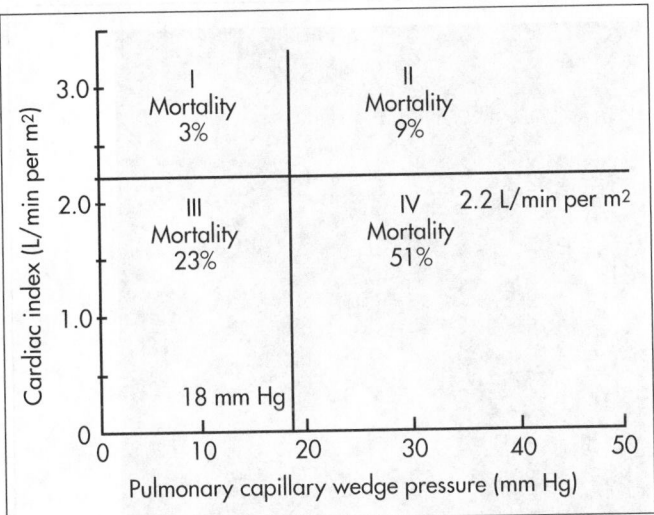

FIGURE 23-11   Hemodynamic subsets and hospital mortality in myocardial infarction.
(Modified from Forrester JS, Diamond G, Chatterjee K et al: *N Engl J Med* 295:1356, 1976.)

those not selected, even if no revascularization was performed (mortality 58%). Patients selected for early revascularization tended to be younger, had an earlier presentation of shock, and had a lower mortality than those not selected for revascularization (62% vs. 73%, $P = 0.077$). The mortality for patients undergoing urgent percutaneous transluminal coronary angioplasty was 60%, slightly higher than those undergoing selection for catheterization, suggesting that much of the benefit attributed to early revascularization may be due to patient selection. A randomized trial of revascularization strategies in patients presenting with cardiogenic shock is currently undergoing enrollment and will help settle this issue. For the present, however, urgent angiography and revascularization, if possible, are recommended for all patients presenting with cardiogenic shock.

Mechanical Complications

The mechanical complications of acute MI occur infrequently but are important because they are potentially reversible. Moreover, among patients who die of mechanical complications, infarct size is considerably smaller than in patients dying of arrhythmias or primary pump failure. Thus the mechanical complication per se is the major cause of death and not left ventricular dysfunction.

The mechanical complications of MI include myocardial free wall rupture, ventricular septal defect, acute ischemic disruption of the mitral valve with severe regurgitation, and right ventricular infarction. Infarction expansion or extension and left ventricular aneurysm formation are also mechanical complications, but these do not generally result in major acute deterioration of hemodynamics.

Although use of the balloon-tipped pulmonary artery flotation catheter provides useful diagnostic information and is helpful in monitoring therapy, the most efficient method for diagnosing the mechanical complications is bedside 2D echocardiography, including the use of the transesophageal approach when necessary. With these two modalities, virtually every patient who has experienced a mechanical complication can be rapidly diagnosed and plans for corrective therapy instituted.

Acute Mitral Regurgitation

Although the presence of transient mitral regurgitation caused by papillary muscle dysfunction is common in patients with MI, severe mitral regurgitation from papillary muscle rupture (Fig. 23-12) is a life-threatening, eminently correctable complication. Papillary muscle rupture accounts for approximately 5% of deaths in patients with acute MI, as determined by autopsy studies. Rupture of the entire pap-

illary muscle is rapidly fatal because of the torrential mitral regurgitation that results. Usually, survivors have had partial tearing of one or more heads of the papillary muscle, with severe regurgitation caused by a flail mitral segment. Papillary muscle rupture usually involves the posterior medial papillary muscle, presumably because its blood supply is derived only from the posterior descending artery, whereas the anterolateral papillary muscle has a dual blood supply from both left anterior descending and circumflex branches.

The clinical presentation of papillary muscle rupture is the acute onset of pulmonary edema, usually within 2 to 7 days after inferior MI. The characteristics of the murmur vary; no murmur may be audible as a result of a rapid increase of pressure in the left atrium. Therefore a high degree of suspicion, especially in the patient with inferior wall infarction, is necessary for diagnosis. 2D echocardiographic examination demonstrates the severed papillary muscle head and a flail segment of the mitral valve. Left ventricular function is hyperdynamic as a result of the severe regurgitation into the low-impedance left atrium; this finding alone should suggest the diagnosis.

The cornerstone of successful therapy is prompt diagnosis and emergency surgery. Surgical correction requires mitral valve replacement or repair. The current approach of emergency surgery accrues an overall operative mortality of approximately 25%, but this appears to be decreasing, and the late results of this approach are excellent.

Myocardial Rupture

Rupture of the free wall of the left ventricle accounts for approximately 10% of deaths in patients with acute MI. The characteristics of patients with free wall rupture are similar to those with rupture of the papillary muscle or ventricular septum. Rupture of the free wall of the left ventricle typically occurs in small infarcts (Fig. 23-13), often in patients with single-vessel disease and poor collaterals and typically in elderly females with first MIs. Although any wall may be involved, rupture of the lateral wall probably occurs most often. Rupture occurs within the first 5 days of infarction in 50% of patients and within 14 days in 87%. The area of rupture always occurs within the MI area but usually is eccentrically located near the junction with normal myocardium.

The clinical presentation is usually sudden electromechanical dissociation. The great majority of patients die even when rapid resuscitative measures, including pericardiocentesis, balloon pumping, and urgent rush to cardiac surgery, are attempted. Occasionally, rupture may be subacute, with periodic small amounts of blood leaking into the pericardial space. Pericardial pain and failure of the T wave to undergo usual inversion may be a manifestation of this phenomenon, and the subsequent inflammatory process may wall off the area of pericardial leakage from the remaining pericardial space. In this way a false aneurysm or pseudoaneurysm of the left ventricle may form. The entity is easily and reliably detected by 2D echocardiography and mandates early surgical intervention because of the risk of further expansion of the false aneurysm or release of its contents into the remaining pericardial space, producing tamponade and death. The major impediment to surgical correction of acute free wall rupture is logistic, but among the few patients who can undergo surgery early enough, immediate surgery can be performed with gratifying results.

Ventricular Septal Rupture

Rupture of the ventricular septum occurs in 1% to 3% of patients with acute MIs and causes approximately 5% of periinfarction deaths. The substrate is quite similar to that of free wall rupture in terms of number of vessels diseased and infarct size. Typically, ventricular septal rupture associated with anterior MI is located in the apical septum, and that associated with inferior MI is located in the basal inferior septum. Incidence in anterior and inferior MIs is approximately equal, unlike papillary muscle rupture.

The diagnosis should be suspected clinically when a new pansystolic murmur is present. Once again, echocardiography, including the transesophageal approach, can diagnose this condition. Additionally, withdrawal of venous samples from the pulmonary artery catheter and an arterial line, as well as measurement of O_2 consumption, allow calculation of the percentage of shunt. As with other cardiac ruptures,

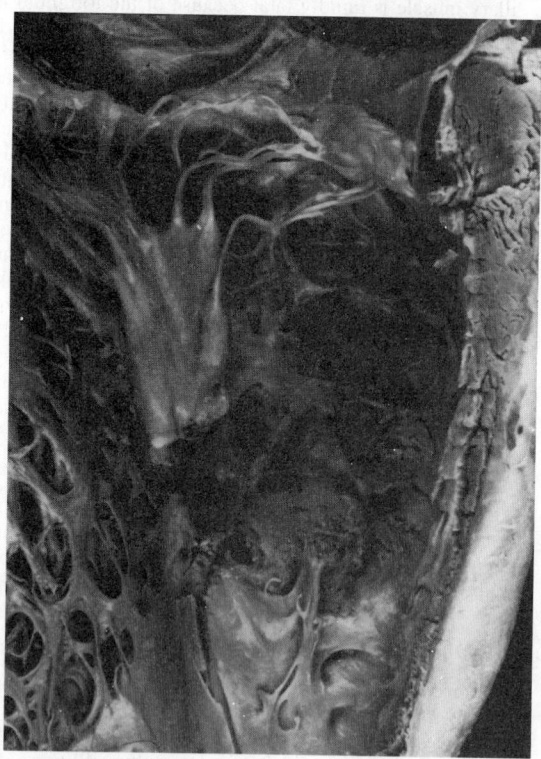
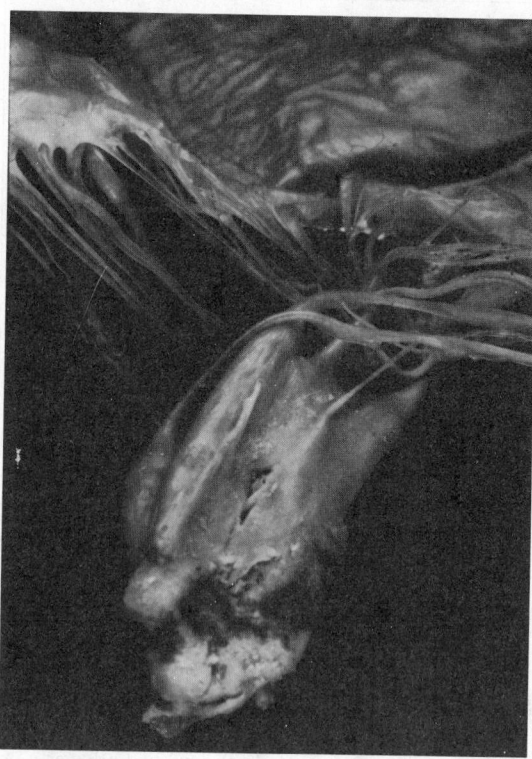

FIGURE 23-12 Pathologic specimen demonstrates complete transection of papillary muscle *(left)* and close-up view *(right)* caused by MI. Severe mitral regurgitation and death resulted.
(Courtesy William D. Edwards, MD.)

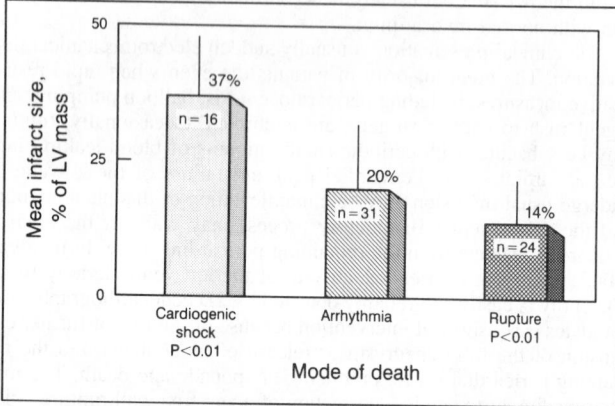

FIGURE 23-13 Mean infarct size as percentage of left ventricular mass in patients dying of cardiogenic shock, arrhythmia, and cardiac free wall rupture. *LV,* Left ventricular.

(Data from Saffitz JE, Fredrickson RC, Roberts WC: *Am J Cardiol* 57:1249, 1986.)

aggressive and early angiography and surgical management are advocated, although the outcome in these patients is not as gratifying as in those with acute mitral regurgitation because the extent of myocardial necrosis is generally larger.

Right Ventricular Infarction

Involvement of the right ventricle (Fig. 23-14) is a common sequela of acute inferior MI. However, *hemodynamically significant* right ventricular dysfunction occurs in relatively few patients with right ventricular infarction.

The diagnosis of hemodynamically significant right ventricular infarction rests on the clinical triad of hypotension, increased jugular venous pressure, and clear lung fields in a patient with acute inferior wall MI. A more sensitive finding suggestive of right ventricular involvement is a positive Kussmaul's sign. Additional diagnostic techniques that can document right ventricular involvement include ECG ST segment elevation in right-sided chest leads (V_{3R} or V_{4R}), visualization of right ventricular wall motion abnormalities, and right ventricular dilation on radionuclide angiography or echocardiography.

From a management standpoint, it is crucial to identify the patient in whom the abnormal hemodynamic profile is predominantly the result of right ventricular involvement, that is, dominant right ventricular infarction. Documentation that right ventricular function rapidly improves in a few days and the usually favorable response of the hemodynamic abnormality to fluid loading with or without inotropic support emphasize the importance of correctly identifying this problem. In patients with normal hemodynamics, the need to diagnose right ventricular infarction is debatable. If it is suspected, avoidance of preload reduction is sufficient.

Pulmonary artery balloon-tipped flotation catheter measurements in patients with significant right ventricular infarction demonstrate elevation of the right atrial pressure, usually greater than 10 mm Hg, and often show a right atrial pressure/pulmonary artery wedge pressure ratio of 0.8 or greater. However, in patients with significant left ventricular dysfunction and elevation of the wedge pressure, this ratio may be lower and does not exclude the presence of significant right ventricular involvement. The incidence of high-grade atrioventricular (AV) block is also increased in patients with right ventricular infarction.

Treatment of patients with right ventricular infarction typically involves volume loading with normal saline to achieve a pulmonary artery wedge pressure of 18 to 20 mm Hg. In some patients, this alone is sufficient to improve cardiac output and systemic pressure. How-

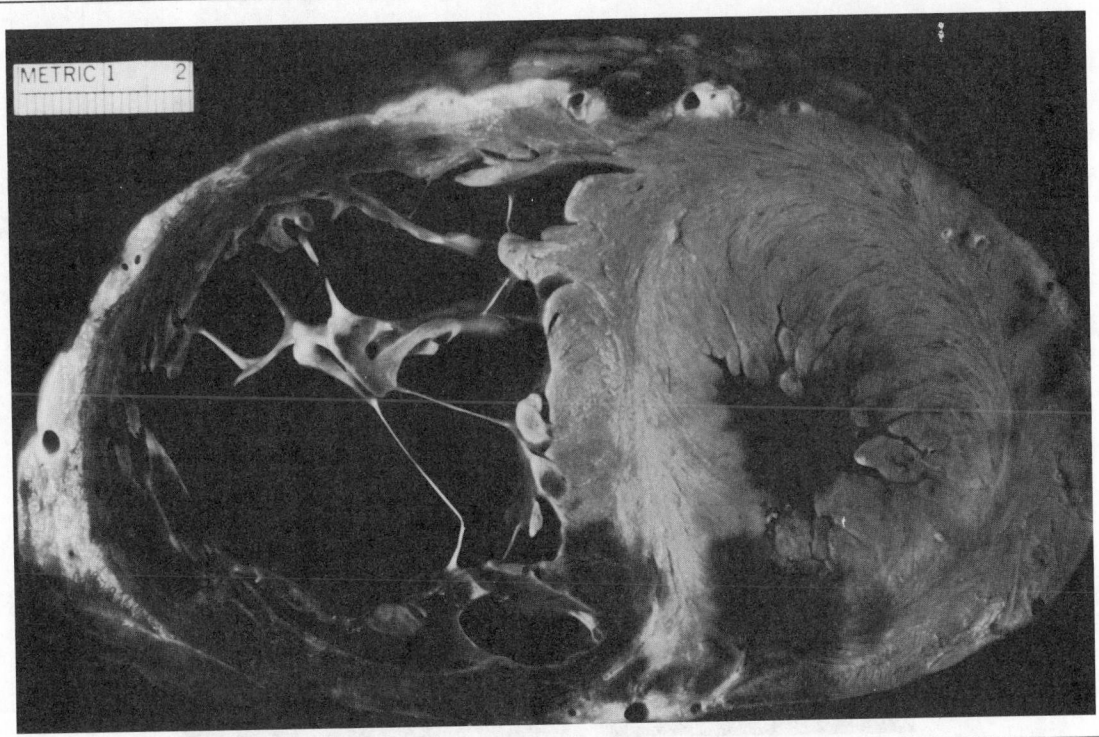

FIGURE 23-14   Extensive right ventricular MI associated with inferior wall infarction. Severe right ventricular failure resulted in patient's death.
(Courtesy William D. Edwards, MD.)

ever, some patients will not respond to fluid-loading alone. Recent investigations suggest that this may be the result of marked right ventricular enlargement within a relatively noncompliant pericardium, which may result in functional left ventricular compression caused by ventricular interaction. When volume loading alone does not suffice, the use of an inotropic agent, such as dobutamine, has been advocated and has demonstrated limited success. Cautious use of agents such as nitroprusside may occasionally be warranted.

Most patients, even those with substantial right ventricular dysfunction, spontaneously improve in 48 to 72 hours after the acute event. Patients in shock may benefit from attempted angioplasty of the occluded right coronary artery or even possibly the temporary use of a right ventricular assist device; however, many of these patients have associated significant left ventricular dysfunction complicating the picture. The overall balance between the extent of right ventricular and left ventricular dysfunction is a major determinant of long-term outcome.

Infarct Expansion and Left Ventricular Aneurysm

Infarct expansion refers to thinning and dilation of the infarct segment, usually without clinical manifestations of myocardial enzyme release. This is in contradistinction to infarct extension, in which recurrent pain and another increase in the CK-MB values are generally observed. Infarct expansion has been described primarily in sequential echocardiographic studies and is a precursor of aneurysm formation and myocardial rupture in a minority of patients.

The formation of a left ventricular true aneurysm occurs in the days and weeks after MI, probably beginning with infarct expansion, necrosis and removal of dead cellular elements, and replacement with fibrous scar tissue. Patients at increased risk for aneurysm formation include those with large infarcts, those with uncontrolled hypertension, and those receiving corticosteroids or nonsteroidal antiinflammatory agents. The early development of apical dyskinesis or aneurysm formation predisposes to mural thrombus and embolization dur-

ing the first 3 to 6 months after MI. Furthermore, it appears likely that early infarct expansion, by altering regional wall stress, predisposes to ventricular remodeling, with dilation of the noninfarct portion of the left ventricle and ultimately late congestive heart failure and death.

Left Ventricular Thrombus

Left ventricular thrombus (Fig. 23-15) can be observed in 10% to 40% of anterior wall infarcts and rarely in inferior wall infarcts. Thrombus is usually located within hypokinetic or dyskinetic segments, that is, in areas of relative stasis of blood flow, usually the left ventricular apex. Large or mobile thrombi, as observed on echocardiographic examination, have a relatively high risk of embolization. We usually provide 3 to 6 months of anticoagulant therapy in patients with (1) large anterior MI, (2) congestive heart failure, (3) documented mural thrombus, or (4) large apical aneurysmal or dyskinetic segments.

The incidence of left ventricular thrombus formation probably is decreased by the early use of thrombolytic therapy because extent of MI and degree of wall motion abnormality may be decreased and because of a direct effect against thrombus formation.

Pericarditis

Pericarditis frequently occurs early in the course of transmural MI. It may manifest as a pericardial rub, pleuritic chest pain, or pericardial effusion seen on 2D echocardiography, or it may be clinically silent (Chapter 27). Late pericardial inflammation (2 weeks to 3 months after MI) has been termed *Dressler's syndrome* and is probably related to an autoimmune mechanism. It is becoming increasingly infrequent for reasons unknown. Treatment with salicylates, nonsteroidal antiinflammatory agents, or colchicine is preferred to the use of corticosteroids because of the high frequency of relapse when corticosteroid therapy is discontinued. Echocardiography in patients with pericardi-

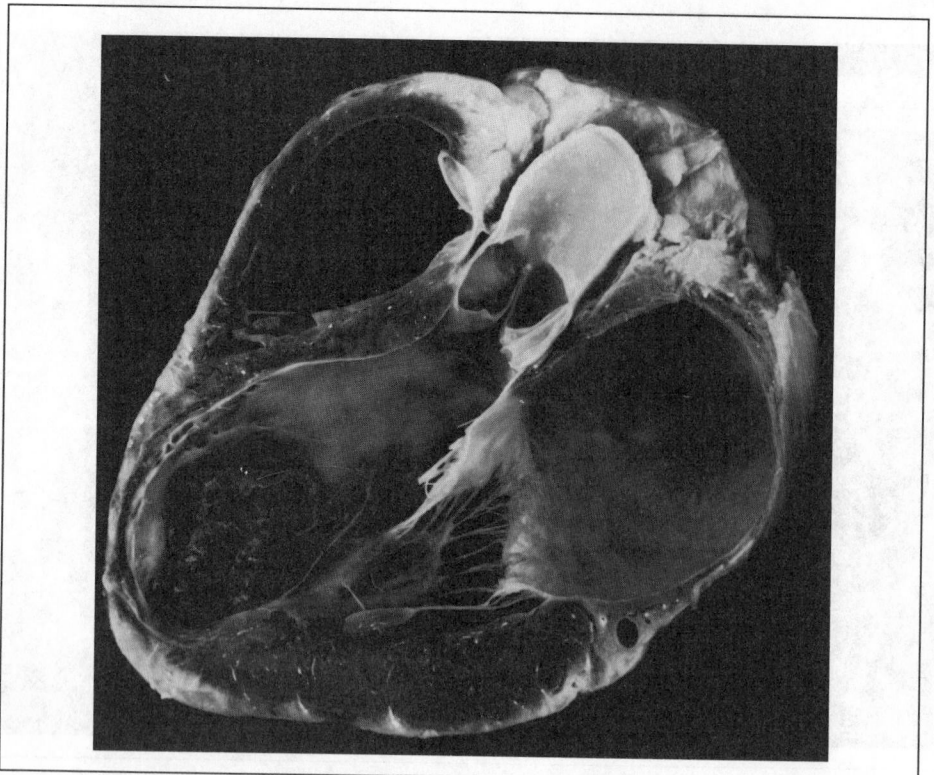

FIGURE 23-15 Left ventricular thrombus. Extensive anterior and apical MI with apical thrombus. Systemic embolization occurred before death.

(From Edwards WD: In Gersh BJ, Rahimtoola SH, editors: *Current topics in cardiology: acute myocardial infarction,* New York, 1991, Elsevier.)

tis is useful to determine the extent of effusion and to exclude the possibility of partial rupture or pseudoaneurysm.

Electrical Complications

Conduction Disturbances. Conduction disturbances in patients with acute MI generally result from two mechanisms: ischemic injury to the conduction system or surrounding myocardium and abnormal reflexes that are usually vagally mediated and precipitated by MI. The blood supply (Fig. 23-16) to the sinus node arises from the proximal right coronary artery in 55% of patients and from the proximal left circumflex in 45%. The blood supply to the AV node arises from the distal branches of the right coronary artery in 90% of patients and from the distal portions of the left circumflex artery in 10%. There is usually a dual blood supply to the AV node and bundle of His, which accounts for the lack of necrosis of these structures even with extensive MI. The right bundle branch is supplied primarily by the septal perforator vessels originating from the left anterior descending artery, as is the distal portion of the anterior left bundle branch. The main left bundle branch has a dual supply from both distal branches of the right coronary and proximal circumflex vessels, and the posterior division of the left bundle branch is supplied from branches of the circumflex coronary artery.

In general, all conduction disturbances associated with inferoposterior MI are related largely to enhanced vagal activity, tend to be more transient, are often responsive to atropine, and imply a more benign outcome than those involved in anterior MI. Conversely, major conduction disturbances associated with anterior MI usually imply extensive septal necrosis and more significant reduction in left ventricular function.

Sinus bradycardia. Sinus bradycardia and sinus pauses occurring in either anterior or inferior MI are usually benign and are generally observed unless prolonged asystole or symptoms are present. First-degree AV block occurs in 4% to 13% of patients with MI. Ob-

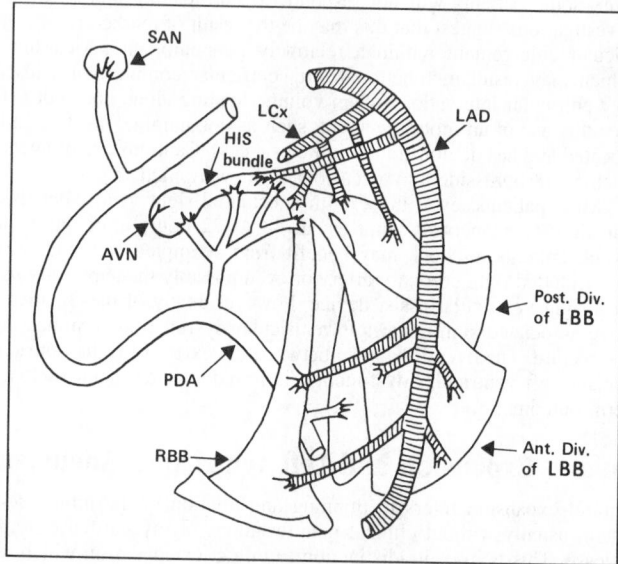

FIGURE 23-16 The conduction system and its blood supply. *AVN,* Atrioventricular node; *LAD,* left anterior descending; *LCx,* left circumflex; *LBB,* left bundle branch; *PDA,* posterior descending artery; *RBB,* right bundle branch; *SAN,* sinoatrial node.

(From DeGuzman M, Rahimtoola SH: *Cardiovasc Clin* 13:191, 1983.)

servation and avoidance of any medications that might prolong AV conduction are all that is required.

Second-degree atrioventricular block. This usually develops within the first 24 hours of MI in 3% to 10% of individuals. With type I second-degree AV block, progressive prolongation of the PR interval is observed; this usually occurs with inferoposterior MI and may often respond to atropine. A narrow QRS complex is usually present, and careful observation is the rule unless the ventricular rate decreases below 45 beats/min or symptoms of ischemia or impaired perfusion develop. Type II second-degree AV block is identified by intermittent dropped beats in the absence of progressive PR prolongation and implies extensive infranodal conduction system injury. Often the QRS complex is wide, indicating associated bundle branch block (BBB), and progression to complete heart block occurs in approximately one third of these patients. Most patients with anterior MI and type II second-degree AV block receive temporary transvenous pacing because of the unpredictable risk of complete heart block.

Complete heart block. This occurs in 3% to 7% of patients with acute MIs. In general, patients with inferoposterior MI progress to third-degree heart block after a period of second-degree block and again may demonstrate some responsiveness to atropine. Often a reliable junctional escape rhythm is present, and recovery tends to occur within 3 to 7 days, although occasionally it can be delayed. Many of these patients can be observed; in some with standby, temporary, transcutaneous pacing patches in place. Complete heart block in patients with anterior MI usually indicates an extensive area of myocardial necrosis, may occur unpredictably, and carries a poor prognosis. Most patients require temporary transvenous pacing, and some physicians advocate permanent transvenous pacing. Late mortality in these patients is usually caused by pump failure or ventricular fibrillation rather than persistent, high-grade AV block.

The occurrence of any new BBB with acute MI also identifies patients with extensive infarction who are at higher risk for later complications. Unifascicular block, especially left anterior hemiblock, occurs in approximately 5% of patients and has a relatively benign prognosis. Complete right or left BBB occurs in 10% to 15% of patients and most often involves the right bundle branch. In the past, the new occurrence of left or right BBB has been a generally accepted indication for temporary transvenous pacing. However, mortality in these patients is related primarily to pump failure or ventricular fibrillation.

The indications for temporary transvenous pacing were a source of discussion and interest in the 1970s. The indications still apply, but the availability of transcutaneous pacing (if capture can be documented in advance) simplifies the management in patients with marginal indications or in whom venous access is limited.

Late Postinfarction Bradyarrhythmias. Permanent transvenous pacing is indicated in patients with persistent complete or high-grade AV block or persistent, type II second-degree AV block after MI and in patients with a new BBB and transient but resolved complete heart block during the acute course of MI. However, this indication remains controversial, and no proved benefit of pacing exists in this subgroup of patients. Occasionally, patients may require electrophysiologic study to determine the site of AV block and to aid in the decision of whether permanent pacing is indicated. Permanent pacing may also be indicated in the rare patient with profound sinus node dysfunction.

Tachyarrhythmias. The genesis of tachyarrhythmias in patients with MI is multifactorial. Decreased blood flow leads to anaerobic metabolism, and decreased venous outflow allows accumulation of by-products of this process, resulting in acidosis, increased extracellular potassium concentration, and increased intracellular calcium concentration. In addition, there may be alterations in sympathetic and vagal tone and increased concentrations of circulating catecholamines. The electrophysiologic correlates of these cellular abnormalities include slowing of conduction and prolongation of refractoriness, and the inhomogeneous nature of the MI process produces an ideal situation for the occurrence of reentrant arrhythmias (Chapter 18). The presence of injury currents may directly enhance phase IV depolarization of Purkinje cells, resulting in increased automaticity. Fiber stretch, resulting from increased atrial and ventricular end-diastolic pressures, is also arrhythmogenic. Finally, reperfusion, possibly from intracellular calcium overload or production of free O_2 radicals, may generate reperfusion arrhythmias, which may be either automatic or reentrant.

Supraventricular Arrhythmias. Sinus tachycardia occurs in up to 25% of patients with acute MI and often results from pain, anxiety, and sometimes hypovolemia. Persistent sinus tachycardia, related to increased circulating catecholamines, may be a marker of severe left ventricular dysfunction and is a poor prognostic sign. Whatever the cause, sinus tachycardia is undesired because of increased O_2 demand. After relief of pain and assessment for the presence of pulmonary congestion, it is desirable to decrease the heart rate below 70 beats/min by IV administration of beta-adrenergic receptor blockers. A short-acting beta-adrenergic receptor blocker, such as esmolol, may be appropriate for patients in whom the extent of left ventricular dysfunction is of particular concern.

Atrial premature beats typically occur in patients with acute MI and may represent increased left atrial pressure. They may also be a harbinger of other atrial tachyarrhythmias. However, when they occur in isolation, observation alone suffices.

Atrial fibrillation occurs in 10% to 15% of patients with acute MI. Its presence early signifies atrial ischemia; later it may also represent atrial stretch from increasing filling pressures. Immediate cardioversion is the best treatment for patients with symptomatic rapid atrial fibrillation or in whom the rapid ventricular response produces ischemia. If the ventricular response is only moderate and the patient is asymptomatic, IV diltiazem or esmolol is useful for control of heart rate, along with digoxin given orally; the latter may take 4 to 8 hours for full effect. Recurrent episodes of atrial fibrillation should be suppressed with an antiarrhythmic agent such as procainamide or quinidine. The treatment of atrial flutter is similar to that of atrial fibrillation except that drug treatment is less effective in producing an easily controlled ventricular response. Occasionally, atrial overdrive pacing may be used to terminate atrial flutter without resorting to cardioversion.

AV nodal reentrant tachycardia (supraventricular tachycardia) occurs infrequently in patients with acute MI, probably relates to underlying dual AV nodal pathways, and may respond to adenosine or digitalis, among other agents. Accelerated junctional rhythm is a benign disorder that may be observed.

Ventricular Tachyarrhythmias. Although many patients with MI may have ventricular premature beats, few develop more advanced arrhythmias. Conversely, ventricular fibrillation or tachycardia may develop without warning. Suppression of ventricular premature beats can be accomplished if they are symptomatic, are frequent (more than 5/min), or occur in runs of bigeminy. Otherwise, they may be observed.

The ubiquity of early ventricular ectopy and primary ventricular arrhythmias is well established in patients seen within the first few hours of MI. These rhythms remain a major indication for the prompt initiation of ECG monitoring during the treatment of acute MI, and they typically decrease in frequency during the first 24 to 36 hours of infarction. In contrast, ventricular arrhythmias occurring late after the completion of MI are usually a manifestation of underlying left ventricular dysfunction and thus have been termed *secondary* ventricular arrhythmias. Such rhythms portend a less benign prognosis, not only because of the electrical disturbance per se, but also because this indicates significant systolic dysfunction.

Accelerated idioventricular rhythm may occur in up to 40% of continuously monitored patients and may signify reperfusion in some. Although this rhythm disturbance is generally considered benign and is usually untreated, idioventricular rhythms that accelerate to 110 to 120 beats/min may then be more appropriately considered automatic ventricular tachycardias with a less benign prognosis, and these more rapid rhythms should be suppressed with lidocaine.

Ventricular tachycardia occurs in up to 15% of patients during acute MI. The ventricular rate is usually 140 to 200 beats/min, and this rhythm disturbance may degenerate to ventricular fibrillation. The rhythm disturbance usually responds to IV lidocaine. However, procainamide, bretylium, cardioversion, ventricular overdrive pacing, or amiodarone may all be required in the acute stages for resistant cases (Chapter 18). The use of lidocaine prophylactically for prevention of ventricular tachycardia is contraindicated.

Ventricular fibrillation is seen in approximately 8% of patients surviving to hospitalization for acute MI. It is more frequent in large Q wave infarcts and may occur with or without warning arrhythmias.

The occurrence of ventricular fibrillation within the first 24 hours of hospitalization was thought not to confer any long-term risk to patients successfully resuscitated. However, recent studies indicate poorer outcome for patients with ventricular fibrillation at any time during their hospital course. Ventricular fibrillation or tachycardia occurring late in the hospital course may result from pump failure, severe electrolyte imbalance, effects of antiarrhythmic medications, or other metabolic derangements. However, it is usually associated with decreased left ventricular systolic function and portends a poor prognosis. *Sustained monomorphic* ventricular tachycardia, occurring early or late during the hospital course, occurs infrequently but implies an arrhythmogenic substrate and a propensity for recurrence after discharge. An invasive electrophysiologic study can be justified in these patients before dismissal.

Treatment of ventricular fibrillation in the early phase of MI involves immediate cardioversion and lidocaine given IV for 24 to 36 hours as prophylaxis for a recurrent episode. Late-phase ventricular fibrillation should prompt a search for severe residual ischemia or reinfarction and consideration of implantable cardioverter-defibrillator (ICD) therapy.

The treatment of patients with asymptomatic, late-phase, nonsustained ventricular tachycardia remains problematic and is the current focus of several randomized trials. Nonsustained ventricular tachycardia is an independent predictor of mortality and sudden death after MI. Decreased left ventricular systolic function and late potentials on signal-averaged ECGs are also independent additional predictors of mortality.

Electrophysiologic testing was proposed as a procedure to assess asymptomatic patients at increased risk for ventricular fibrillation and sudden death, but the results have been disappointing; although quite sensitive, the test is nonspecific. At present such testing remains investigational. A second problem in treatment of such patients relates to antiarrhythmic drugs (Chapter 17). The bulk of available data indicates that antiarrhythmic therapy for asymptomatic, nonsustained ventricular tachycardia in patients after MI worsens survival.

The only pharmacologic treatments that have been shown to improve survival in the patient after MI include beta-adrenergic receptor blockade, thrombolytic therapy, and aspirin, and these agents should be used whenever possible. Additionally, patients with late-phase, nonsustained ventricular tachycardia should have a thorough search for residual myocardial ischemia, which, in conjunction with left ventricular dysfunction and ventricular arrhythmias, identifies a subgroup at high risk for sudden cardiac death in whom coronary revascularization may be of benefit.

LATE MANAGEMENT

Late management of patients with MI includes risk stratification, rehabilitation, and preventive cardiology.

Risk Stratification

Reasonable estimates of survival and morbidity after MI can be established by using clinical and noninvasive laboratory parameters. The history and physical examination can identify factors such as advanced age, prior MI, presence of New York Heart Association (NYHA) class II to IV congestive heart failure, postinfarction angina, mechanical complications of MI, and non–Q wave MI, all of which identify patients at higher risk for reinfarction and death in the first 6 months after MI. As stated previously, decreased ejection fraction, complex ventricular ectopy, and late potentials on the signal-averaged ECG also identify individuals at increased risk for continued problems. The absence of these clinical and noninvasively determined risk factors identifies a population at low risk for reinfarction and death in the months immediately after MI.

Exercise testing, with or without the use of radioisotopes, has been used for detecting patients at relatively higher or lower risk for a poor outcome. In patients who do not manifest pump failure or severe ischemia, have negative results of a predischarge exercise test, have an ejection fraction greater than 40%, and have negative results of a symptom-limited outpatient exercise test at 6 weeks, a 1-year mortality of 5% or less can be expected.

Virtually all the studies examining prognosis after MI were performed in the prethrombolysis era. As a group, such patients might typically have a 1-year post-MI mortality of up to 30%, and these risk stratification algorithms remain useful in patients not receiving thrombolytic or reperfusion therapy. However, the increasingly aggressive use of reperfusion strategies (thrombolysis, acute angioplasty, myocardial revascularization) and the selection process for thrombolytic therapy resulted in 1-year postdischarge cumulative mortality rates of 2% to 5% in some studies. The previously established criteria for risk stratification in the prethrombolysis era may not apply to most patients treated with thrombolytic drugs or mechanical reperfusion. For example, in the GISSI-2 trial, patients with EF >40% and uncomplicated hospital course had a 6-month mortality of less than 1%, regardless of whether a postinfarction exercise test was positive or negative.

Rehabilitation and Preventive Cardiology

The goals of cardiac rehabilitation are to enhance quality of life, facilitate return to normal activities, and provide secondary prevention to correct risk factors for further ischemic events. At our institution a four-phase program is instituted for patients after uncomplicated MI. An interdisciplinary approach involving members of the medical and nursing staff, social and vocational rehabilitation counselors, occupational therapists, dietitians, and an exercise physiologist allows an integrated strategy of patient education, modification of risk factors, vocational adjustment, and improvement in quality of life.

The phase I program begins when the patient is hemodynamically and electrically stable in the coronary care unit and continues until discharge. It begins with passive range-of-motion exercises and progresses to sitting in a chair twice daily, minimum self-care exercises, then ambulating with physical therapists, having bathroom privileges, showering in a wheelchair, and gradually increasing levels of supervised activities. Initially an upper limit heart rate of 20 beats/min above the standing rate is used, but by the end of phase I, the patient can generally walk at a pace of 1 to 2 miles/hr for up to 10 minutes three times a day. At this stage a predismissal or an early postdismissal rehabilitation treadmill exercise test is performed, usually using the Naughton protocol with a target of either symptoms or achievement of 5 metabolic equivalents (METs) of activity. A positive result on such a test or intercurrent symptoms are usually an indication for an invasive study.

Phase II begins at patient discharge and generally continues for 1 to 3 months. Objectives include continued patient education, modification of risk factors, preparation for gradual return to occupational and avocational activities, and improvement of cardiovascular fitness by aerobic exercise. In general a standard program includes three visits weekly for supervised exercise sessions as well as unsupervised and regular home exercise sessions, sometimes including telephone ECG transmission for monitoring of ischemia or arrhythmia. A symptom-limited treadmill exercise test is performed at the beginning and end of phase II to establish a safe upper-limit heart rate during exercise and to assess aerobic improvement during the program's course.

After successful completion of phase II, the phase III program is initiated with the goal of continued improvement in cardiorespiratory fitness, usually with group exercise and education sessions at a community exercise facility or a strictly home exercise program without direct supervision. Exercise to 50% to 70% of functional aerobic capacity is usually prescribed as long as no ischemia is present during treadmill testing to this level. The duration of phase III is 6 months to 1 year, and patients are released from this program when their functional capacity can be sustained at 8 METs with a stable rest and exercise ECG and without symptoms of angina or dyspnea at normal activity levels.

Finally, patients may enter a phase IV program, designed to maintain the exercise capacity achieved in phase III, and the length of this program is indefinite.

A mandatory aspect of the rehabilitation program is modification of risk factors. Smoking cessation is the most important, in addition to blood pressure control and treatment of hyperlipidemia and diabetes mellitus. Periodic reinforcement and regular follow-up are essential.

BIBLIOGRAPHY

Cardiac Arrhythmia Suppression Trial (CAST) investigators: Preliminary report: effect of encainide and flecainide on mortality in a randomized trial of arrhythmia suppression after myocardial infarction, *N Engl J Med* 321:406, 1989.

Chesebro JH et al: Thrombolysis in Myocardial Infarction (TIMI) Trial, Phase I: a comparison between intravenous tissue plasminogen activator and intravenous streptokinase: clinical findings through hospital discharge, *Circulation* 76:142, 1987.

Ellis SG et al: Coronary angioplasty as primary therapy for acute myocardial infarction 6 to 48 hours after symptom onset: report of an initial experience, *J Am Coll Cardiol* 13:1122, 1989.

Fibrinolytic Therapy Trialists' (FTT) Collaborative Group: Indications for fibrinolytic therapy in suspected acute myocardial infarction: collaborative overview of early mortality and major morbidity results from all randomised trials of more than 1000 patients, *Lancet* 343:311, 1994.

Gersh BJ, Rahimtoola SH, editors: *Current topics in cardiology: acute myocardial infarction,* New York, 1991, Elsevier.

Gomes JA et al: The prognostic significance of quantitative signal-averaged variables relative to clinical variables, site of myocardial infarction, ejection fraction and ventricular premature beats: a prospective study, *J Am Coll Cardiol* 13:377, 1989.

Grines CL, Browne KF, Marco J et al: A comparison of immediate angioplasty with thrombolytic therapy for acute myocardial infarction, *N Engl J Med* 326:673, 1993.

Gruppo Italiano per lo Studio della Sopravvivenza nell'Infarto Miocardico: GISSI-2: a factorial randomised trial of alteplase versus streptokinase and heparin versus no heparin among 12,490 patients with acute myocardial infarction, *Lancet* 336:65, 1990.

Gruppo Italiano per lo Studio della Sopravvivenza nell'Infarto Miocardico: GISSI-3: effects of lisinopril and transdermal glyceryl trinitrate singly and together on 6-week mortality and ventricular function after acute myocardial infarction, *Lancet* 343:1115, 1994.

GUSTO Investigators: An international randomized trial comparing four thrombolytic strategies for acute myocardial infarction, *N Engl J Med* 329:673, 1993.

Hochman J, Boland J, Sleeper LA et al: Current spectrum of cardiogenic shock and effect of early revascularization on mortality: results of an international registry, *Circulation* 91:873, 1995.

ISIS-1 (First International Study of Infarct Survival) Collaborative Group: Mechanisms for the early mortality reduction produced by beta-blockade started early in acute myocardial infarction: ISIS-1, *Lancet* 1:921, 1988.

ISIS-2 (Second International Study of Infarct Survival) Collaborative Group: Randomised trial of intravenous streptokinase, oral aspirin, both, or neither among 17,187 cases of suspected acute myocardial infarction: ISIS-2, *Lancet* 2:349, 1988.

ISIS-3 (Third International Study of Infarct Survival) Collaborative Group: ISIS-3: a randomised comparison of streptokinase *vs* tissue plasminogen activator *vs* anistreplase and of aspirin plus heparin *vs* aspirin alone among 41,299 cases of suspected acute myocardial infarction, *Lancet* 339:753, 1992.

ISIS-4 (Fourth International Study of Infarct Survival) Collaborative Group: ISIS-4: A randomised factorial trial assessing early oral captopril, oral mononitrate, and intravenous magnesium sulphate in 58,050 patients with suspected acute myocardial infarction, *Lancet* 345:669, 1995.

LATE Study Group: Late Assessment of Thrombolytic Efficacy (LATE) study with alteplase 6-24 hours after onset of acute myocardial infarction, *Lancet* 342:759, 1993.

MacMahon S et al: Effects of prophylactic lidocaine in suspected myocardial infarction: an overview of results from randomized, controlled trials, *JAMA* 260:1910, 1988.

Ryan T et al: ACC/AHA guidelines for the management of patients with acute myocardial infarction (special report), *J Am Coll Cardiol* 1328–1428, 1996.

Scandinavian Simvastatin Survival Study Group: Randomised trial of cholesterol lowering in 4444 patients with coronary heart disease: the Scandinavian Simvastatin Survival Study (4S), *Lancet* 344:1383, 1994.

Stone GW, Grines CL, Browne KF et al: Predictors of in-hospital and 6-month outcome after acute myocardial infarction in the reperfusion era: the primary angioplasty in myocardial infarction (PAMI) trial, *J Am Coll Cardiol* 25:370, 1995.

TIMI Study Group: Comparison of invasive and conservative strategies after treatment with intravenous tissue plasminogen activator in acute myocardial infarction: results of the Thrombolysis in Myocardial Infarction (TIMI) Phase II Trial, *N Engl J Med* 320:618, 1989.

CHAPTER

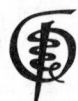

24 Infective Endocarditis

Frederick A. Masoudi and Merle A. Sande

Infective endocarditis is a localized infection consisting of fibrin, platelets, and microorganisms that adhere to the cardiac valves or other endothelial surfaces. The clinical manifestations are protean and systemic, including fever, cardiac murmurs, anemia, splenomegaly, petechiae, pyuria, and peripheral emboli. Without appropriate treat-

ment, the mortality approaches 100%, though its pace varies from a subtle, indolent, wasting condition to fulminant, overwhelming sepsis. Endocarditis must be considered early in the differential diagnosis of a wide variety of conditions; prompt diagnosis and aggressive appropriate antibiotic therapy are critical. Successful therapy requires close cooperation between the internist and the surgeon since emergency cardiac surgery has become a critical therapeutic intervention in some patients.

PATHOPHYSIOLOGY

Normal native cardiac valves are remarkably resistant to attachment of bacteria and subsequent infection; intravenous injection of very high titers of pyogenic bacteria into experimental animals fails to produce endocarditis. Damage to the endothelial surface either by scarring (as from rheumatic heart disease) or direct trauma (as from turbulent blood flow or jet streams produced by intracardiac shunts) renders the tissue susceptible to colonization of circulating microorganisms. The critical predisposing lesion seems to be a deposit of platelets and fibrin on the endothelium—so-called nonbacterial thrombotic endocarditis. Studies in animals have shown that these clotting elements are the receptive surface for adhesion of circulating microorganisms and subsequent infection (Fig. 24-1). Preexisting structural cardiac diseases that result in scarring or lead to turbulent blood flow can be identified in more than half of all patients with endocarditis. Most of the others probably have clinically undetectable abnormalities.

Recently the epidemiology of conditions predisposing to infective endocarditis has changed, primarily for three reasons: decreasing incidence of rheumatic heart disease, increasing recognition and diagnosis (because of widespread use of echocardiography) of mitral valve prolapse, and the aging of the population, which has increased the prevalence of degenerative heart disease. In previous series, rheumatic heart disease accounted for 40% to 60% of recognized preexisting diseases; in more recent series, it accounts for less than 25% of native valve endocarditis (Table 24-1). Stenosis and/or regurgitation of the mitral (85%), aortic (50%), and tricuspid (less than 10%) valves are the predisposing valve lesions.

In many centers mitral valve prolapse has surpassed rheumatic heart disease as the most common predisposing condition for infective endocarditis (Chapter 25). The prevalence of mitral valve prolapse is 4% in unselected populations, and the risk for infective endocarditis is three to eight times higher in persons with mitral valve prolapse than in the general population. However, this increased risk is greater in the subset of patients with mitral valve prolapse associated with a systolic murmur of mitral regurgitation. In addition, patients with mitral valve prolapse and diffusely thickened redundant leaflets on echocardiogram (with or without mitral regurgitation) have a higher risk of endocarditis than patients without this condition (Chapter 25). Although the risk of endocarditis is relatively low among persons with mitral valve prolapse, this condition is common in the general population, which accounts for the increased proportion of cases of endocarditis. In most recent series, mitral valve prolapse accounts for 20% to 25% of the cases of endocarditis. Therefore mitral valve prolapse with mitral regurgitation and/or myxomatous proliferation (leaflet thickening and redundancy) may account for a majority of cases of endocarditis.

Congenital heart disease accounts for approximately 20% of identifiable lesions. These include all high-pressure shunts, such as ventricular septal defects, tetralogy of Fallot, and patent ductus arteriosus, as well as stenotic lesions, including coarctation of the aorta and congenital valvular and subvalvular lesions of the pulmonic and aortic valves. In hypertrophic obstructive cardiomyopathy, the infection is usually found on either the mitral or aortic valve. Endocarditis is rare in patients with isolated secundum atrial septal defects, probably because of the low-pressure shunt with little turbulence. It is also rare in patients with surgically repaired intracardiac lesions without significant residual hemodynamic abnormality more than 6 months after the corrective procedure.

Degenerative heart diseases, including Marfan syndrome, syphilitic aortitis, calcification of the mitral annulus, and calcific nodular lesions resulting from arteriosclerosis, account for the largest proportion of cases without demonstrable underlying valvular disease.

Many iatrogenic conditions render the host susceptible to endo-

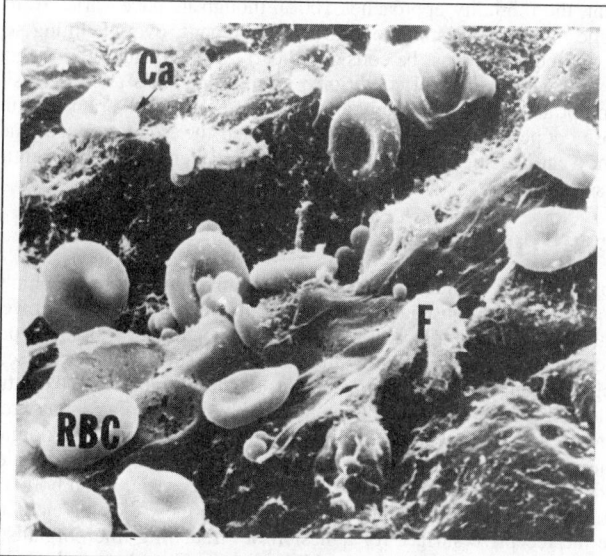

FIG. 24-1   Traumatized heart valve endothelium showing adherent erythrocyte *(RBC)* and fibrin *(F)*. Note the erythrocyte covered by fibrin. Yeast cells *(Ca)* are also present on the developing vegetation.

Table 24-1   Approximate distribution of predisposing conditions to native valve endocarditis*

PREDISPOSING CONDITION	PERCENTAGE
Mitral valve prolapse	20-25
Rheumatic heart disease	15-20
Congenital heart disease	20
Degenerative heart disease	20
None	20

*Distribution may vary markedly depending on geographic location, hospital, and patient population.

Table 24-2   Approximate distribution of organisms causing endocarditis

ORGANISM	NATIVE VALVE (PERCENTAGE)	PROSTHETIC VALVE* <2 MO (PERCENTAGE)	PROSTHETIC VALVE* >2 MO (PERCENTAGE)
Viridans and other streptococci	60	10	30
Staphylococcus aureus	25	20	15
Enterococci	10	5	10
Coagulase-negative staphylococci	<1	30	20
Gram-negatives†	5	15	10
Candida species	<1	10	5
Other	<1	10	10

*Time after valve implantation.
†HACEK organisms for native valve endocarditis and other gram-negative aerobic bacilli for prosthetic valve endocarditis.

carditis and endarteritis. They include arterio-arterial fistulas, hemodialysis shunts or fistulas, and peritoneovenous shunts. Hospitalized patients who are immunocompromised or who undergo invasive intravascular access procedures, including pulmonary artery or central venous pressure monitoring and the insertion of hyperalimentation lines, are particularly susceptible. Endocarditis also complicates implanted prosthetic cardiac valves in 0.5% to 2.0% of cases. These infections frequently result from intraoperative contamination, but the presence of the foreign body and the turbulence created by the prosthesis also render these valves susceptible to colonization by circulating microorganisms. The risk in patients with permanent transvenous cardiac pacemakers is not increased, however. Intravenous drug abusers have a high incidence of infective endocarditis, and in two thirds of such patients there are no known predisposing cardiac lesions. At least 75% of these patients have tricuspid valve involvement, a preponderance that remains unexplained.

The infection is usually localized along the line of closure of the damaged valve leaflet on the atrial side of the atrioventricular valves and on the ventricular surface of the semilunar valves, distal to the stenosis of a coarctation of the aorta; on the low-pressure side of an intracardiac shunt; or at the jet stream impact area on the ventricular wall of a ventricular septal defect. These are the areas where fibrin-platelet thrombi are deposited and where turbulent flow and eddy currents are present, providing a receptive surface for attachment of circulating microorganisms.

Bacteria that cause endocarditis reach the heart through the bloodstream; in general, the organisms that produce disease are those that most commonly produce transient bacteremia (i.e., streptococci and staphylococci) (Table 24-2). Bacteremia is extremely common in humans and seems to occur whenever a heavily colonized mucous membrane or infected area is traumatized. Procedures in or manipulations of the oral cavity and genitourinary and gastrointestinal tracts commonly produce transient bacteremia.

The level of bacteremia (i.e., titers of circulating organisms) probably depends on the degree of trauma and the number of microorganisms colonizing or infecting the traumatized site. In one study, 10% of patients with severe gingival disease had detectable bacteremia even before undergoing any dental procedure, and in a recent study more than 60% had positive blood cultures 5 minutes after simple dental cleaning. Experiments in animals with damaged cardiac valves have demonstrated that a critical level of bacteremia is required to produce endocarditis and that this level is species-specific and even strain-specific. Interestingly, the infectious dose for gram-negative rods such as *Escherichia coli* is nearly 100 times higher than for gram-positive cocci such as *Staphylococcus aureus* and viridans streptococci. This difference in median infective dose (ID_{50}) correlates with the relative frequency with which these organisms produce disease in humans.

Organisms that rarely produce other common infections (e.g., oral streptococci, diphtheroids, and *Staphylococcus epidermidis*) are important pathogens in infective endocarditis, suggesting that classic virulence factors (such as are found in *S. aureus* and gram-negative bacilli) may be less important in the pathogenesis of this disease. The ability of bacteria to adhere firmly to fibrin and platelets, however, seems to be a critical characteristic. For example, species of viridans streptococci that produce extracellular dextran from sucrose strongly adhere to dental enamel and produce dental plaque. These same dextran-producing strains are responsible for the majority of cases of streptococcal endocarditis, even though non–dextran-producing strains are more commonly isolated from the bloodstream after dental procedures. In animal models, dextran formation by *Streptococcus sanguis* has been shown to increase its ability to produce endocarditis (lower ID_{50}). The presence of fibronectin, a glycoprotein produced by endothelial cells, also appears to markedly increase adherence of streptococci and staphylococci but not *E. coli*. Thus as the bacteria are rapidly swept past the damaged valve, the strains that can most strongly adhere to the receptive surface of fibrin and platelets are the organisms that are most likely to produce disease.

After adherence and multiplication of the organism, further deposition of platelets and fibrin occurs, leading to the development of the mature vegetation. This lesion consists of a friable mass of bacteria in very high titers (10^8 to 10^{10} bacteria per gram) tightly encased in the fibrin platelet mesh. Few phagocytic cells are present in the deep recesses of the vegetation; thus the organisms appear protected from the host's major defenses. Vegetation propagation (platelet and fibrin deposition) continues until the organisms are eradicated by antimicrobial agents or surgery. Vegetations caused by the more indolent streptococcal strains usually grow slowly but may reach a large size. Fungi (*Candida* and *Aspergillus*) tend to produce very large friable vegetations that frequently embolize.

Cardiac complications of endocarditis result from invasion or destruction of the valves or adjacent structures by pathogens. In some instances, especially when disease is caused by *S. aureus*, the infection may extend into the valve ring, producing an abscess or an aneurysm of the sinus of Valsalva; through the interventricular septum to involve the conduction system, producing arrhythmias; or out to the pericardium, producing purulent pericarditis or cardiac rupture. Cardiac valves may be quickly destroyed by the more virulent organisms (*S. aureus* and *Streptococcus pneumoniae*). Involvement of the chordae tendineae or papillary muscles may lead to rupture and acute valvular regurgitation or to outflow obstruction, which result in acute congestive heart failure. Progressive scarring of the valve after successful treatment may also eventually lead to hemodynamically significant regurgitation.

The extracardiac manifestations of the disease are usually the result of arterial embolization of pieces of the friable vegetation. Embolization to the vasa vasorum of major arteries or contiguous spread from a septic arterial embolus may produce a mycotic aneurysm. These commonly occur at the bifurcation of medium-sized arteries. The brain is involved in 50% of cases, the thorax and abdomen in 40%, and the extremities in 10%. Embolization to all major arteries may occur. When the coronary vessels are involved, myocardial infarction may result. Cerebral embolization may produce temporary vascular insufficiency or stroke. Metastatic abscess formation is common in the spleen, kidney, or other vital organs when the disease is caused by *Streptococcus aureus* and, occasionally, viridans streptococci (*Streptococcus anginosus*, also called *Streptococcus milleri* group). Many of the unique peripheral manifestations of the disease (Janeway lesions, cutaneous infarcts, Osler nodes) are thought also to be the result of small-vessel embolization.

Immune-complex deposition also appears to play a role in the pathophysiology of extracardiac manifestations of endocarditis, especially those in the kidney. Abnormalities in renal architecture can be found in nearly all cases of infective endocarditis. In the preantibiotic era the incidence of glomerulonephritis was greater than 75% in subacute endocarditis but less than 40% in acute endocarditis, suggesting that infections with less virulent organisms and a more prolonged antigenic challenge produce high levels of circulating immune complexes and concomitant glomerulonephritis. Glomerulonephritis has been reported in 2% to 60% of patients treated with antibiotics for endocarditis, but the true incidence has not been established. *S. aureus* endocarditis is frequently associated with glomerulonephritis, particularly in parenteral drug users, regardless of the duration of the illness. Glomerular lesions may be focal or diffuse, and crescents may be present. Interstitial involvement may produce tubular damage, endarteritis, and arteriosclerosis. Embolization is common, and septic renal infarcts occur in nearly all patients with fatal *S. aureus* endocarditis. Since this disease is associated with a constant intravascular antigenic challenge, it is not surprising that high titers of antibodies of several classes are found. Circulating immune complexes can be identified in more than 90% of patients with infective endocarditis of long duration and fall when appropriate antibiotic therapy is administered. Some of the peripheral manifestations of endocarditis (Roth spots, Osler nodes, petechiae, and some diffuse purpuric lesions) may be due in part to immune complex deposition.

CLINICAL SYNDROME

The clinical presentation of infective endocarditis is primarily that of unexplained fever and cardiac murmur. However, the disease may manifest in a wide variety of ways. The symptoms and signs may be protean, and essentially any organ system can be involved. Four pathophysiologic processes contribute to the clinical picture: (1) the infectious process on the valve, (2) arterial embolization of vegetation, (3) bacteremia with metastatic infection, and (4) immunopathologic phenomena.

The clinical presentation is to a large extent determined by the nature of the infective organism. With pyogenic bacteria such as *S. aureus* and, less commonly, *S. pneumoniae* and *Neisseria gonorrhoeae*, the disease may be acute and fulminant, with high fever, multiple metastatic abscesses and peripheral embolic phenomena, rapid valve destruction, and a high mortality. About one third of patients with staphylococcal endocarditis have a history of a preceding staphylococcal infection, and symptoms generally start within 2 weeks of the initial infection. This form of acute bacterial endocarditis may involve a normal valve, in contrast to the subacute infection, which al-

---

BOX 24-1
Clinical presentations of endocarditis

Fever and heart murmur
Sepsis
Fever of unknown origin
Transient ischemic attacks or stroke
Meningitis
Subarachnoid hemorrhage
Peripheral arterial embolization
Myocardial infarction
Unexplained congestive heart failure
Pulmonary infarction, necrotizing pneumonia
Constitutional symptoms suggestive of
- Neoplasm
- Hematologic malignancy
- Collagen vascular disease
Musculoskeletal complaints suggestive of
- Polymyalgia rheumatica
- Acute rheumatic fever
- Rheumatoid arthritis
Anemia
Renal failure

---

most always occurs on a damaged valve. All age-groups are involved, but mortality is particularly high in patients older than 50 years of age. *S. aureus* endocarditis has a particular predilection for developing in parenteral drug users, although the disease may be less fulminant than in a nonaddict population. Staphylococcal endocarditis may be confused with other severe acute infectious diseases, such as gram-negative sepsis with endotoxemia or meningococcemia, and occasionally with an acute vasculitis such as systemic lupus erythematosus. Of patients with staphylococcal bacteremia, 60% in older autopsy series and 10% in recent reports show evidence of endocarditis.

The subacute form of infective endocarditis accounts for approximately two thirds of cases and is usually caused by either viridans streptococci or enterococci. A history of dental procedures is found in 15% to 20% of patients with viridans streptococcal endocarditis, and about 50% of patients with enterococcal disease have had a preceding genital or urologic procedure. In the vast majority of cases, symptoms begin within the 2-week period after the procedure, but because of the protean nature of the disease, the diagnosis is not made for an average of 5 weeks. Eighty percent of these patients have a previous history of cardiac disease. Symptoms usually begin insidiously with anorexia, weakness, weight loss, fatigue, feverishness with night sweats, and arthralgias. The nonspecific presentation often leads to incorrect diagnoses, such as malignancy, collagen vascular disease, tuberculosis, fever or anemia of unknown origin, glomerulonephritis of unknown origin, or other chronic diseases. Although the distinction between acute and subacute forms of the disease is clinically important, they represent the two extremes of a continuum, and there is considerable overlap between the clinical syndromes produced by the individual organisms. The various clinical presentations of endocarditis are listed in Box 24-1.

The physical findings in infective endocarditis can provide important diagnostic clues. Almost all patients have fever, but elderly patients and those with renal failure, severe disability, or congestive heart failure may not. The fever is usually remittent and rarely exceeds 39.5° C (103° F) except in acute endocarditis. Heart murmurs are present in more than 85% of patients but may not be detected in patients with tricuspid or pulmonic disease. The detection of a changing murmur or appearance of a new murmur during the course of disease is an important diagnostic clue, but such a change is found in only 3% to 10% of patients.

Cutaneous manifestations are found in approximately 50% of patients. Petechiae are the most common and usually appear in the conjunctiva, palate, buccal mucosa, and extremities. They occur most frequently in patients with prolonged illness. They occur as small, nonblanching lesions in crops but discolor and disappear within 2 to 3 days. Osler nodes are small, painful nodular lesions, usually in the pads of the fingers or toes or occasionally on the thenar eminence. They range in size from 2 to 15 mm, may be multiple, and disappear in hours to days. They are most common in patients with subacute endocarditis but may also be found in those with systemic lupus erythematosus or marantic endocarditis, hemolytic anemias, and gonococcal infections, and in extremities with cannulated radial arteries. Janeway lesions are hemorrhagic, macular, flat, painless plaques with a predilection for the palms and the soles. They are most commonly found in patients with acute staphylococcal endocarditis and are frequently multiple. Roth spots are pale, oval retinal lesions with a peripheral area of hemorrhage; they are usually found near the optic disc. They are rare (<5% of cases) and can also be identified in patients with anemia, leukemia, or connective tissue disorders (systemic lupus erythematosus). Splinter hemorrhages are subungual, linear, reddish-brown streaks found in the fingernails or toenails. They are most suggestive of endocarditis when located proximal in the nail bed. Distal splinter hemorrhages are also seen in patients with occupational trauma to the nails. Clubbing of the nail beds has been found and is especially common when the disease is of long duration.

Splenomegaly is reported in as many as 60% of patients, and its incidence correlates with the duration of disease. Musculoskeletal complaints are common, occurring in as many as 44% of patients. They usually appear early in the disease and may be the only initial complaint; they include arthralgias, arthritis, low back pain, and diffuse myalgias. Neurologic manifestations occur in 30% to 40% of patients and may dominate the clinical picture. Neurologic manifestations are more common in staphylococcal endocarditis than in streptococcal infections. A sudden neurologic event in a young person should always suggest the possibility of infectious endocarditis. Major cerebral emboli are found in 10% to 30% of patients and may produce transient or permanent neurologic defects. Mycotic aneurysms of the cerebral vessels occur in up to 10% of patients and are usually clinically silent but may present as an expanding mass lesion of the brain or, with rupture, as a subarachnoid hemorrhage, resulting in a severe headache, stiff neck, and fever. Other neurologic features include seizures, visual changes, choreoathetoid movement, mononeuropathy, cranial nerve palsies, and toxic encephalopathy.

Major embolic episodes occur in approximately one third of patients with endocarditis, often early in the disease or after therapy has been completed. The incidence appears to be highest in those with large vegetations as determined by echocardiogram (Chapter 13). Splenic infarctions are common and may present as left upper quadrant pain radiating to the left shoulder, accompanied by a splenic or pleural friction rub and a left pleural effusion. An embolus lodging in a mesenteric artery may precipitate signs and symptoms of an acute abdominal process. Emboli to large peripheral arteries, which are particularly common in fungal endocarditis, may produce acute limb ischemia. Pulmonary emboli may arise from right-sided (tricuspid) infection and are a common feature in endocarditis associated with parenteral drug use. Coronary artery emboli usually arise from the aortic valve and may produce acute myocardial infarction.

Congestive heart failure may predominate in the presentation and may result from valvular dysfunction, associated myocarditis that commonly complicates endocarditis early in the course of the disease, or myocardial infarction. The signs of uremia, once a common presenting feature of bacterial endocarditis, are now rarely observed. However, 10% to 15% of patients with endocarditis also have immune-complex glomerulonephritis, and signs of azotemia are occasionally present.

LABORATORY FINDINGS

The laboratory manifestations of endocarditis are summarized in Table 24-3. Most patients with endocarditis have the anemia characteristic of chronic inflammation, with normochromic, normocytic indices, low serum iron, and low iron-binding capacity. The anemia progressively worsens with the duration of the illness. Leukocytosis is found primarily in patients with acute endocarditis, whereas leukopenia may be found in subacute disease and is usually associated with splenomegaly. Large histiocytes (mononuclear cells) can be detected in peripheral blood. The presence of these cells is not diagnostic of endocarditis; they may also be seen in patients with malaria, typhoid

Table 24-3 Laboratory manifestations of endocarditis

LABORATORY FINDING	INCIDENCE (PERCENTAGE)
Hematologic	
Anemia	70-90
Thrombocytopenia	5-15
Leukocytosis*	20-30
Leukopenia	5-15
Histiocytosis	25
Elevated ESR	90-100
Serologic	
Hypergammaglobulinemia	20-30
Rheumatoid factor	40-50
Hypocomplementemia	5-15
Immune complexes	90-100
Mixed cryoglobulins	80-95
Urine	
Proteinuria	50-65
Microscopic hematuria	30-50
RBC casts	10-12
Bacteremia	
Positive blood cultures	95
Intraleukocytic bacteria	50

*Primarily in acute endocarditis.

fever, and tuberculosis. The erythrocyte sedimentation rate (ESR) is nearly always elevated; however, it may be normal in patients with renal failure, congestive heart failure, or disseminated intravascular coagulation. Rheumatoid factor can be detected in the majority of patients who have had symptoms of endocarditis for at least 6 weeks.

Detection of bacteremia with blood culture is the single most important diagnostic test. Bacteremia is usually continuous and low grade (less than 100 bacteria/ml of blood) in the subacute form of the disease but may be high grade in acute staphylococcal endocarditis. In patients who eventually have positive blood cultures, 80% of the first set of blood cultures drawn are positive, as are 89% of the first two sets and 99% of the first three sets. Therefore, if subacute bacterial endocarditis is suspected, three cultures (each consisting of 5 to 10 ml of blood obtained from separate venipuncture sites) should be collected over a 24-hour period and cultured with both aerobic and anaerobic techniques. In acute situations, several cultures may be drawn at approximately 20-minute intervals before starting empiric therapy.

Modern blood-culturing techniques fail to identify the etiologic agents of endocarditis in about 5% of cases. If initial cultures are negative at 48 to 72 hours, additional cultures should be obtained and all should be held for 2 to 3 weeks with periodic Gram stains and subculturing. If gram-positive cocci are grown initially but fail to grow in subculture, a nutritionally deficient variant streptococci should be suspected, which may require broth supplemented with pyridoxal hydrochloride or cysteine. Possible causes of culture-negative endocarditis are extensive and include antimicrobial therapy before obtaining cultures; fastidious organisms (anaerobic bacteria, nutritionally variant streptococci, HACEK-group and other fastidious organisms, *Brucella* species); *Chlamydia psittaci* (psittacosis); *Rickettsia* such as *Coxiella burnetti* (Q fever); fungi (e.g., *Candida, Aspergillus*); chronic endocarditis; marantic endocarditis; atrial myxoma; Libman-Sacks endocarditis; and incorrect diagnosis. When endocarditis cultures are negative, a careful history should be taken and more extensive evaluation for unusual causes should be initiated. Cultures may be negative in patients who were treated with antibiotics either by a physician or by themselves before the cultures were drawn. Patients with endocarditis caused by fungi frequently have negative blood cultures, but large vegetations are usually detected by echocardiogram, and embolic complications are common.

Serologic detection of antigen or antibodies is useful in diagnosing some forms of endocarditis. Serologies are becoming increasingly important in the diagnosis of *Candida* and *Aspergillus* endocarditis. Serologic evidence of infection with *C. psittaci* and the causative agent of Q fever would be diagnostic of endocarditis in some clinical situations.

Table 24-4 Comparison of test characteristics of transesophageal echocardiography (TEE) and transthoracic echocardiography (TTE) in endocarditis

	TTE		TEE	
	SENS (%)	SPEC (%)	SENS (%)	SPEC (%)
Valvular vegetations*	60†	>95	90	>95
Abscesses‡	28	97	87	95

*Estimate based on various studies.
†The sensitivity of TTE is probably higher for right-sided vegetations and is significantly lower for prosthetic valve abnormalities.
‡Data from Daniel WG et al: Improvement in the diagnosis of abscesses associated with endocarditis by transesophageal echocardiography, *N Engl J Med* 324:795, 1991. Surgery or autopsy results used as "gold standard" to calculate test characteristics in a severely ill study population (n = 118).

Echocardiography has become a valuable tool for evaluating patients suspected of having endocarditis (Chapter 13). The evaluation of endocarditis has benefited dramatically from developments in non-invasive cardiology, particularly with regard to 2D transthoracic echocardiography (TTE), Doppler echocardiography, and transesophageal echocardiography (TEE). The TEE procedure is very safe, usually lasts about 10 to 15 minutes, and is well tolerated by patients (Chapter 13). Transesophageal echocardiography has improved visualization of the cardiac structures by taking advantage of the anatomic relationship of the esophagus to the heart; structures of 1 to 2 mm can be visualized. Valvular morphology and valve structures, chordae, and attachments are better defined by TEE than TTE. Major advantages of TEE over TTE include improved image quality; superior visualization of valve ring abscesses, mycotic aneurysms, prosthetic valve abnormalities, and small vegetations; improved hemodynamic assessment of prosthetic valve dysfunction; intraoperative assessment of cardiac hemodynamics and structures; and clarification of abnormal but nondiagnostic TTE studies. The disadvantages of TEE are that the procedure is more invasive and more labor intensive and carries a potential risk of bacteremic seeding of abnormal valves. Although both TTE and TEE have high specificity, TEE is much more sensitive than TTE in detecting vegetations and abscesses involving left-sided structures of the heart (Table 24-4). TTE may be as sensitive as TEE in imaging right heart structures, and in some studies, the sensitivity of TTE for right-sided vegetations is equivalent to the sensitivity of TEE. This remains a subject of some debate, however. TEE is clearly superior in evaluating any suspected prosthetic valve infection. In endocarditis, TEE should be performed when the site, extent of infection, and effect on cardiac function have not been clearly defined by TTE, when persistent fever, bacteremia, or other evidence suggests ongoing infection and possible abscess formation, or when a prosthetic heart valve may limit the accuracy of TTE. Transesophageal echocardiography should not replace TTE, but should complement it when TTE is nondiagnostic or if additional data will influence therapy, management, or surgical approach (Chapter 13). Doppler echocardiography uses sound waves to identify and quantitate flow through intracardiac and extracardiac vascular structures; it can be used to measure a variety of hemodynamic parameters. For evaluation of endocarditis, Doppler echocardiography enables the severity of valvular regurgitation to be estimated and is an integral part of TTE and TEE. In evaluating mitral valve dysfunction and mitral regurgitation, the Doppler TEE is far superior to the standard TTE approaches.

The echocardiogram provides important prognostic information as well, since patients with vegetative lesions visualized by echocardiography have a higher incidence of congestive failure, embolization, need for surgery, and death than those lacking detectable vegetations. Vegetations that are large (1 cm), multiple, left-sided, or that increase in size during appropriate antibiotic therapy indicate a particularly high-risk subpopulation. The echocardiogram may also image local complications such as valve ring abscesses, myocardial abscesses, or pericardial effusions. It is also useful to assess left ventricular function in patients with aortic regurgitation (Chapter 25).

DIFFERENTIAL DIAGNOSIS

Although the diagnosis of endocarditis may be obvious in patients with underlying cardiac valvular disease who present with fever and peripheral embolic phenomena, these classic findings are frequently absent. Up to 50% of patients do not exhibit peripheral manifestations, and the murmur may be absent or subtle; this is particularly common in parenteral drug users with right-sided endocarditis. In the elderly there may be no fever, and patients may present with no more than confusion, wasting, anorexia, and lethargy (see Box 24-1).

The classic manifestations of endocarditis may mimic those of other diseases. Fever, petechiae, splenomegaly, microscopic hematuria, and anemia with a cardiac murmur may resemble acute rheumatic fever with carditis, collagen vascular diseases such as systemic lupus erythematosus with cardiac involvement, or neoplasia such as atrial myxomas. The clinical picture may be dominated by the manifestations of arterial embolization mimicking acute myocardial infarction, transient cerebral ischemic attacks, stroke, sudden occlusion of a major artery, or splenic or renal infarction.

SPECIAL CONSIDERATIONS
Infection in Parenteral Drug Users

Parenteral drug users have a unique predilection for developing infective endocarditis and in some large metropolitan hospitals account for the majority of cases. The bacteremia in parenteral drug users occurs with injection and probably arises from bacterial colonization of their skin and nares. The disease tends to differ from conventional forms in location and microbiology. In over 70% the tricuspid valve is involved, followed in frequency by the aortic (and mitral) valves. Approximately three fourths of the cases are caused by *S. aureus*. There is an appreciable incidence of community-acquired methicillin resistance in the *S. aureus* isolated in Detroit, Michigan, and this organism is becoming more prevalent in other areas. *Pseudomonas aeruginosa, Pseudomonas cepacia,* and other gram-negative aerobic bacilli account for an additional 15%, *Candida albicans* and various streptococci for about 10%. The latter two organisms affect the aortic and mitral valves more commonly than the tricuspid valve. These figures are approximate, and the microbiology of endocarditis as well as the distribution of the valves involved in this patient population can vary significantly by region. The effect of an increasing prevalence of human immunodeficiency virus (HIV) disease on the epidemiology and clinical management of endocarditis in this group remains to be seen.

A diagnosis of endocarditis must be considered in all febrile parenteral drug users since fever may be the only manifestation. As many as 15% of febrile parenteral drug users who present without a clear cause of their fever will have endocarditis. Prospective studies of the emergency room evaluation of such patients have shown that neither signs, symptoms, laboratory tests, nor clinical judgment can be used to accurately predict which patients have endocarditis, which provides the rationale for admitting all febrile parenteral drug users to the hospital. For reasons that are unclear, the majority of endocarditis in this patient population involves the right side of the heart, specifically the tricuspid valve. Pulmonic valvular involvement is very rare. When the tricuspid valve is involved, the clinical presentation frequently reflects septic pulmonary involvement, including fever, chills, pleurisy, cough, and hemoptysis. Signs of tricuspid regurgitation, such as a short or pansystolic murmur that increases with inspiration or ventricularization of the jugular venous wave, may also be present. A murmur is frequently absent in tricuspid valve endocarditis, however. A significant minority of parenteral drug users with tricuspid endocarditis will not have a characteristic murmur at the time of presentation. The chest radiograph may demonstrate multiple poorly defined peripheral infiltrates, which may cavitate, reflecting septic pulmonary infiltrates. Peripheral embolization and metastatic infection are indicative of left-sided valvular involvement or of the presence of a right-to-left intracardiac shunt such as a patent foramen ovale. Such findings are rare in isolated right-sided disease.

Therapy with appropriate antimicrobial drugs is usually successful in curing this disease in patients without prosthetic valves. Traditional therapy consists of 4 weeks of intravenous antibiotics, but recent trials have shown comparable results with a 2-week combination of nafcillin and an aminoglycoside in selected drug users who have isolated, uncomplicated right-sided *S. aureus* endocarditis. Other studies have shown that a 4-week course of oral therapy with cipro-floxacin and rifampin is also effective in carefully selected patients.

The mortality from native valve staphylococcal endocarditis in this patient population is relatively low (less than 10%), compared with 30% to 40% in the nonaddict population. The reasons for these differences are not clear but in part reflect the high incidence of right-sided disease and the youthful population involved. Therapy of highly resistant microbes, such as *P. cepacia,* may require surgical excision of the tricuspid valve. Once infection has occurred, these patients are highly susceptible to recurrent episodes of endocarditis.

Prosthetic Valve Endocarditis

Infective endocarditis is a relatively common (0.5% to 2.0% incidence) and devastating complication of prosthetic cardiac valve or tissue graft valve replacement. With the increasing use of valve replacement, the prevalence of this disease has continued to rise, and in some major hospitals accounts for up to 30% of all cases of infective endocarditis. The disease has been separated for convenience into two forms: early (within the first 2 months after surgery; one third of the patients) and late (more than 2 months after valve replacement; two thirds of the patients).

In early disease the organism is probably introduced at the time of surgery or stems from infectious complications of the procedure, such as wound infections, urinary tract infections, and intravenous catheter infections. This is reflected in the causative organisms in early prosthetic valve endocarditis. Half of the cases are caused by staphylococcal species (*S. epidermidis,* approximately 30%; *S. aureus,* 20%). *Pseudomonas* and Enterobacteriaceae account for 15% to 20%, and fungi, particularly *Candida* and *Aspergillus* species, account for an additional 15%. Streptococci occur in less than 10% of cases. Early endocarditis is frequently fulminant and rapidly progressive. The aortic valve is more commonly affected than the mitral valve. Initial clinical manifestations include fever, a regurgitant murmur associated with perivalvular leak, or a systolic murmur suggestive of outflow obstruction. The opening and closing prosthetic valve sounds may be muted by vegetation invasion of the cage. Peripheral manifestations are unusual except for petechiae, which occur in about 50% of patients. However, emboli to major organs are common; large emboli can be especially common in patients with *Aspergillus* or *Candida* prosthesis infection. A traumatic (impact) hemolytic anemia may occur as a result of perivalvular leak. The incidence of early prosthetic valve endocarditis appears to have decreased in the last decade, probably because of perioperative antibiotic prophylaxis and improved surgical care. Mortality, however, remains high (approaching 80% in some series), reflecting the virulence of the etiologic agents.

Late prosthetic valve endocarditis is similar to natural valve endocarditis. Predisposing factors include oral-dental and genitourinary procedures. Streptococci account for approximately 40% of cases, *S. epidermidis* for 25%, and *S. aureus* for 15%. Gram-negative organisms, particularly fastidious organisms such as *Haemophilus aphrophilus,* other *Haemophilus* species, and *Actinobacillus,* and fungi are uncommon, occurring in less than 10% of patients. The clinical manifestations of late prosthetic valve endocarditis are similar to those found in natural valve disease and are, again, dictated by the virulence of the infecting organism. Prognosis is somewhat better with late infection, and mortality is approximately 40%. Infection in both early and late prosthetic valve endocarditis is usually at suture lines and may result in ring abscess formation with dissection, fistula formation, rarely purulent pericarditis, valve dysfunction with dehiscence leading to instability of the prosthesis, or vegetation growth with valvular outflow obstruction.

When prosthetic valve endocarditis is suspected, cinefluoroscopy may detect alterations in the rocking motion of the valve. The ECG may reveal conduction disturbances, such as those commonly occurring with a ring abscess. Because of the multiple echoes caused by the prosthesis itself, the transesophageal echocardiogram is clearly superior to the transthoracic echocardiogram for the hemodynamic assessment of prosthetic valve dysfunction and the visualization of vegetations and ring abscesses. As in native valve endocarditis, the diagnosis is established by detecting bacteremia (or fungemia) by serial

blood culture techniques. All patients with bacteremia in the postoperative period do not have endocarditis. This is especially true with gram-negative rod infections, in which bacteremia may result from urinary tract infection from indwelling urinary catheters, septic phlebitis from intravenous catheters, or respirator-induced gram-negative pneumonic or sternal wound infections. However, when bacteremia persists after the local infection is eradicated or foreign bodies are removed, patients should be considered to have prosthetic valve endocarditis and treated accordingly.

The differential diagnosis of fever in the postoperative period involves considering a long list of conditions, including those that have been listed, as well as postcardiotomy syndrome, drug fever, thrombophlebitis, transfusion-induced hepatitis, cytomegalovirus infection, and mononucleosis. Repeated blood culturing is therefore critical in identifying cases of endocarditis and in instituting appropriate therapy.

Antimicrobial therapy of prosthetic endocarditis needs to be specifically tailored to the infecting organism (Table 24-5). Even with appropriate antimicrobials, surgical intervention is frequently required in patients with staphylococcal, fungal, or gram-negative infection or who develop hemodynamic compromise.

THERAPY FOR ENDOCARDITIS

Successful therapy for infective endocarditis entails administering rapidly bactericidal antimicrobial agents in high enough dosages and for long enough periods to sterilize the vegetations completely. This therapy should be coupled with aggressive surgical management of complications, including valve replacement and drainage of myocardial abscesses when clinically indicated.

Antimicrobial Therapy

Infective endocarditis is unique because the focus of infection is contained within the protective environment of the valvular vegetation. Few phagocytic cells are present within this tightly woven matrix of fibrin, platelets, and very high numbers of microorganisms. Host defenses appear to be relatively ineffective in eradicating the infective organisms. Thus, the antimicrobial regimen used must be bactericidal and given in high enough dosages to ensure adequate bactericidal activity. Bacteriostatic drugs should never be used. In addition, although there are numerous circumstances in which vancomycin is an indispensable component of the therapeutic regimen, it is generally preferable to use combinations that do not include vancomycin if possible. This is recommended for two reasons: vancomycin, although bactericidal, kills bacteria at a very slow rate in vitro; also, because of years of indiscriminant use of this antibiotic, alarming resistance patterns are emerging, particularly in enterococci. In any event, the antimicrobial regimen must be tailored to the infecting organism. Thus, isolation of the organism is vital to optimum management. Once the organism has been isolated and identified, its susceptibility to antimicrobial agents should be determined by serial tube dilution techniques in broth. The disk sensitivity method has little value in managing this disease.

Antibiotics should be administered parenterally and meticulous attention should be given to aminoglycoside levels to prevent toxicity. Specific recommendations are outlined in Table 24-5. There is no merit to routinely monitoring serum bactericidal levels since this test, even when performed in a standardized manner, has not been shown to provide clinically useful information in the majority of patients. Its utility in patients with infections caused by unusual organisms or who exhibit inadequate clinical responses to standard treatment regimens remains to be determined.

Highly penicillin-susceptible viridans streptococci and *S. bovis* are sensitive to penicillin with minimum inhibitory concentrations (MICs) less than or equal to 0.1 µg/ml. A regimen of 4 weeks of penicillin G alone has been successful in nearly 99% of patients treated. The addition of an aminoglycoside increases the rate of bacterial killing in vitro and has been shown in experimental animals to increase the rate at which organisms are eradicated from the vegetations in vivo. Four weeks of penicillin alone is preferred for patients likely to have side effects with an aminoglycoside. Combination therapy with 2 weeks of penicillin and gentamicin is as effective as 4 weeks of penicillin alone and is appropriate for uncomplicated infections. A combination

Table 24-5 Current recommendations for treatment of bacterial endocarditis

ANTIBIOTICS	DOSAGE[a]	ADMINISTRATION	DURATION	COMMENTS
Penicillin-susceptible viridans streptococci and *Streptococcus bovis* (MIC ≤ 0.1 µg/ml)				
1. Penicillin G	2 million units every 4 hr	IV	4 wk	Preferred in patients >65 years old and those with renal or eighth cranial nerve impairment, heart failure, or CNS complications. Effective for other penicillin-susceptible nonviridans streptococci.
2. Penicillin G	2 million units every 4 hr	IV	2 wk	Uncomplicated patient: age <65; no renal or eighth cranial nerve impairment; no CNS complication; no severe heart failure; viridans streptococci and *S. bovis* only.
& gentamicin[b]	1 mg/kg (not to exceed 80 mg) q8h	IV	2 wk	
3. Penicillin G	2 million units every 4 hr	IV	4 wk	Relapse; complications such as shock or extracardiac focus of infection.
& gentamicin[b]	1 mg/kg (not to exceed 80 mg) q8h	IV	2 wk	
4. Vancomycin[c]	15 mg/kg (not to exceed 1 g) q12h	IV	4 wk	Penicillin allergy.
5. Cefazolin[d]	1-2 g every 8 hr	IV	4 wk	Penicillin allergy.
6. Ceftriaxone[d]	2 g once daily	IV or IM	4 wk	Uncomplicated patient with viridans streptococci; candidate for outpatient therapy; penicillin allergy
7. Ceftriaxone	2 g once daily	IV	2 wk	This once-a-day combination regimen is becoming increasingly popular for home IV prescription for patients with penicillin-susceptible viridans *Streptococcus* and uncomplicated diseases.
& gentamicin	3 mg/kg once daily	IV	2 wk	
Strains of vifidans streptococci & *S. bovis* relatively resistant to penicillin G (0.1 µg/ml < MIC < 0.5 µg/ml)				
1. Penicillin G	2 million units every 4 hr	IV	4 wk	For MIC >0.5 µg/ml or prosthetic valve infection, treat same as enterococci.
& gentamicin	1 mg/kg (not to exceed 80 mg) q8h	IV	2 wk	
2. Vancomycin[c]	15 mg/kg (not to exceed 1 g) q12h	IV	4 wk	Penicillin allergy; avoidance of gentamicin.
3. Cefazolin[d]	1-2 g every 8 hr	IV	4 wk	Penicillin allergy; avoidance of gentamicin.
Enterococci (*Enterococcus faecalis*)[e] (or viridans streptococci with MIC ≥0.5 µg/ml, nutritionally deficient viridans streptococci, or prosthetic valve infection caused by viridans streptococci or *S. bovis*)				
1. Penicillin G	4 million units every 4 hr	IV	4-6 wk	Increase to 6-8 wk for symptoms longer than 3 months, complicated course, or prosthetic valve infection. Some would use ampicillin, but no evidence of superiority available.
& gentamicin[b]	1 mg/kg (not to exceed 80 mg) q8h	IV	4-6 wk	
2. Vancomycin[c]	15 mg/kg (not to exceed 1 g) q12h	IV	4-6 wk	Penicillin allergy. Cephalosporins may be useful substitutes in streptococcal infections but should not be used for enterococcal infections.
& gentamicin[b]	1 mg/kg (not to exceed 80 mg) q8h	IV	4-6 wk	
S. aureus				
1. Nafcillin	2 g every 4 hr	IV	4 wk	Methicillin-susceptible strain; increase duration to 6 wk for complicated infection; omit gentamicin for significant renal impairment. Some recommend gentamicin for 5-7 days.
& gentamicin	1 mg/kg (not to exceed 80 mg) q8h	IV	3-5 days	
2. Vancomycin[c]	15 mg/kg (not to exceed 1 g) q12h	IV	4-6 wk	Penicillin allergy or methicillin-resistant strain; increase duration to 6 wk or longer for complicated infection. Higher relapse rate when compared to β-lactam regimens.
3. Cefazolin[d]	2 g every 8 hr	IV	4-6 wk	Penicillin allergy; increase duration to 6 wk for complicated infection.
& gentamicin[b]	1 mg/kg (not to exceed 80 mg) q8h	IV	3-5 days	
4. Nafcillin	2 g every 4 hr	IV	2 wk	Methicillin-susceptible strain; **intravenous drug user, tricuspid valve infection only,** no extrapulmonary infection, no renal impairment.
& gentamicin[b]	1 mg/kg (not to exceed 80 mg) q8h	IV	2 wk	
5. Nafcillin	2 g every 4 hr	IV	6-8 wk	Prosthetic valve infected with methicillin-susceptible strain; for methicillin-resistant strain substitute vancomycin for nafcillin.
& rifampin[f]	300 mg every 12 hr	PO or IV	6 wk	
& gentamicin[b]	1 mg/kg (not to exceed 80 mg) q8h	IV	2 wk	
Coagulase-negative staphylococci or prosthetic valve infection				
1. Nafcillin	2 g every 4 hr	IV	6-8 wk	Methicillin-susceptible strain; vancomycin recommended in case of uncertain methicillin susceptibility.
& rifampin[f]	300 mg every 12 hr	PO or IV	6-8 wk	
& gentamicin	1 mg/kg (not to exceed 80 mg) q8h	IV	2 wk	

[a]Dosages are for patients with normal renal function.
[b]Streptomycin 500 mg every 12 hr intramuscularly may be used instead of gentamicin. Gentamicin doses should be adjusted to achieve a peak serum concentration of 3 µg/ml, and streptomycin a peak serum concentration of 20 µg/ml.
[c]Vancomycin peak serum concentrations 1 hour after infusion should be in the range of 30 to 45 µg/ml.
[d]Cephalosporins should be avoided in patients with an immediate-type hypersensitivity reaction to penicillin.
[e]All enterococci should be tested for resistance to penicillin, vancomycin, and aminoglycosides.
[f]This use of rifampin is not listed in the manufacturer's official directive. Rifampin increases dose of warfarin needed for antithrombotic therapy.

Continued

Table 24-5   Current recommendations for treatment of bacterial endocarditis—cont'd

ANTIBIOTICS	DOSAGE[A]	ADMINISTRATION	DURATION	COMMENTS
Coagulase-negative staphylococci or prosthetic valve infection—cont'd				
2. Vancomycin[c]	15 mg/kg (not to exceed 1 g) q12h	IV	6-8 wk	Methicillin-resistant strain; penicillin allergy.
& rifampin[f]	300 mg every 12 hr	PO or IV	6-8 wk	
& gentamicin	1 mg/kg (not to exceed 80 mg) q8h	IV	2 wk	
HACEK group[g]				
1. Ampicillin	2 g every 4 hr	IV	4 wk	Definitive regimen determined by in vitro susceptibilities.
& gentamicin[b]	1 mg/kg (not to exceed 80 mg) q8h	IV	4 wk	
2. Ceftriaxone[d]	2 g once daily	IV or IM	6 wk	Penicillin allergy.

[g]*Haemophilus* species, *Actinobacillus actinomycetemcomitans, Cardiobacterium hominis, Eikenella corrodens, Kingella kingii.*
MIC = minimum inhibitory concentration.

of ceftriaxone and gentamicin given once a day for 2 weeks has also been shown to be effective and lends itself to home therapy in uncomplicated cases. For complicated infections, 4 weeks of penicillin plus 2 weeks of gentamicin is recommended. For prosthetic valve infection, appropriate therapy is 6 weeks of penicillin plus 2 weeks of gentamicin. For penicillin-allergic patients with a history of a rash, cefazolin, vancomycin, and ceftriaxone are acceptable alternatives. However, ceftriaxone is reserved for patients who have uncomplicated infections caused by viridans streptococci and are candidates for outpatient therapy. Patients should be carefully evaluated and stabilized in the hospital before management as outpatients is considered. Cephalosporin antibiotics should be avoided in patients with immediate-type hypersensitivity reactions to penicillin.

Relatively penicillin-resistant viridans streptococci (and *S. bovis*) have MICs between 0.1 and 0.5 µg/ml. The recommended therapy is 4 weeks of penicillin plus 2 weeks of gentamicin. For penicillin-allergic patients with a history of a rash, 4 weeks of cefazolin alone is an appropriate alternative. For patients with an immediate-type hypersensitivity reaction to penicillin, 4 weeks of vancomycin is recommended. Infection caused by viridans streptococci with an MIC greater than 5 µg/ml or nutritionally deficient variant strains should be treated with the same regimen used for infections caused by enterococci.

Enterococci are unique because of their relative resistance to penicillin and their universal resistance to cephalosporins. Therapy with these drugs alone is frequently ineffective; the synergistic combination of penicillin and gentamicin or streptomycin must be administered. For enterococci, or viridans streptococci with an MIC greater than 0.5 µg/ml, 4 weeks of penicillin plus 4 weeks of gentamicin is recommended. Duration of therapy should be extended to 6 weeks for prolonged disease (symptoms for 3 months or longer), a complicated course, or prosthetic valve infection. For penicillin-allergic patients, vancomycin should be substituted for penicillin. The degree of resistance to aminoglycosides is variable. Highly resistant enterococci (MIC greater than or equal to 2000 µg/ml) are not synergistically killed by an aminoglycoside combined with penicillin or vancomycin in vitro or in experimental models. Susceptibility of the enterococci should guide final selection of the appropriate aminoglycoside, but tobramycin is not recommended because *Enterococcus faecium* is highly resistant to it. Prolonged use of aminoglycosides, particularly gentamicin, in patients with renal insufficiency may be associated with auditory and vestibular toxicity; serum levels in these patients should be monitored carefully during therapy. Irreversible vestibular toxicity is reported in 20% of patients who receive streptomycin for 4 weeks. The incidence of nephrotoxicity (rise in serum creatinine of greater than 5 mg/dl) with gentamicin ranges from 20% (doses of 3 mg/kg or less) to 100% (doses greater than 3 mg/kg), although the drug-associated nephrotoxicity can be reversible. Antibiotic susceptibility, the nature of the toxicity associated with each agent, and the ease of monitoring therapy should be weighed in choosing the most appropriate antibiotic regimen.

Enterococci have developed drug resistance in increasing and alarming numbers. In certain geographic areas, vancomycin resistance and high level aminoglycoside resistance are common. For this reason, all isolates of *Enterococcus* should be tested for resistance to vancomycin as well as both gentamicin and streptomycin. Any infection with a resistant strain should prompt an immediate specialty consultation.

Staphylococcal endocarditis is caused by *S. aureus* or coagulase-negative staphylococci (e.g., *S. epidermidis*). For methicillin-susceptible *S. aureus,* 4 weeks of nafcillin plus 3 to 5 days of gentamicin is recommended. Experimental and clinical data suggest that the addition of gentamicin for the first several days increases the rate of both clinical response and clearance of the bacteremia. Recent studies have demonstrated that vancomycin may not be as effective as nafcillin for therapy of *S. aureus* endocarditis; vancomycin should be reserved only for patients infected with methicillin-resistant *S. aureus* (4 weeks of vancomycin is recommended) or for those who are penicillin-allergic (4 weeks of either vancomycin or cefazolin can be used). For complicated *S. aureus* endocarditis, therapy is extended for 6 weeks or longer. *S. aureus* prosthetic valve infection with methicillin-susceptible strains requires 6 weeks of nafcillin plus 6 weeks of rifampin plus 2 weeks of gentamicin therapy. With a methicillin-resistant strain, vancomycin is substituted for nafcillin. Unless unequivocal in vitro tests show it to be methicillin-susceptible, coagulase-negative staphylococcal native or prosthetic valve endocarditis should be treated with 6 weeks of vancomycin plus 6 weeks of rifampin plus 2 weeks of gentamicin.

Fastidious gram-negative coccobacilli such as the HACEK group (*Haemophilus, Actinobacillus, Cardiobacterium, Eikenella,* and *Kingella* species) occasionally cause native valve endocarditis. In vitro they are susceptible to ampicillin, cephalosporins, aminoglycosides, and penicillin-aminoglycoside combinations. Ampicillin plus gentamicin for 4 weeks is recommended; ceftriaxone is highly active in vitro and may be a suitable alternative. In prosthetic valve infections with these organisms, a 6-week regimen with these drugs is recommended.

The mainstay of therapy for fungal endocarditis is surgery combined with antifungal treatment. Amphotericin B up to 1 mg/kg/day intravenously is given to a minimum total dose of 40 to 50 mg/kg (2.5 to 3.5 g). Flucytosine 150 mg/kg/day in four divided doses orally is usually added. To avoid bone marrow suppression, 2-hour postdose flucytosine levels should be between 50 to 100 µg/ml.

Antimicrobial therapy for other organisms, including anaerobes, gram-negative cocci, and gram-negative bacilli, should be tailored according to the in vitro sensitivities of the organisms. Empiric therapy in patients suspected of having endocarditis should be instituted after appropriate blood cultures have been obtained. For acute native valve endocarditis, empiric therapy should include antibiotics that are bactericidal against streptococci, staphylococci, and enterococci. The three-drug combination of nafcillin plus penicillin plus gentamicin can be used. Nafcillin can be omitted if *S. aureus* is not suspected, such as in subacute endocarditis. For penicillin-allergic patients, vancomycin can be substituted for both nafcillin and penicillin. Empiric therapy for endocarditis in parenteral drug users must be active against *S. aureus;* for example, a nafcillin-gentamicin combination.

BOX 24-2

Common cardiac conditions at risk for endocarditis

Endocarditis prophylaxis recommended
Prosthetic cardiac valves
Previous bacterial endocarditis
Most congenital cardiac malformations
Rheumatic and other acquired valvular dysfunction
Hypertrophic cardiomyopathy
Mitral valve prolapse with valvular regurgitation*

Endocarditis prophylaxis not recommended
Isolated secundum atrial septal defect
Surgical repair without residua beyond 6 mo. of secundum ASD, VSD, or PDA
Previous coronary artery bypass surgery
Mitral valve prolapse without mitral regurgitation*
Physiologic, functional, or innocent heart murmurs
Previous Kawasaki disease without valvular dysfunction
Previous rheumatic fever without valvular dysfunction
Cardiac pacemakers and implanted defibrillators

Modified from Dajani AS et al: Prevention of bacterial endocarditis: recommendations by the American Heart Association, *JAMA* 264:2919, 1990.
*Prophylaxis is recommended for patients with MVP with a holosystolic murmur of mitral regurgitation or leaflet redundancy (myxomatous degeneration) on echocardiography. Prophylaxis is optional in patients with late systolic murmur or echocardiographic mitral regurgitation that is nonaudible on physical examination.
ASD, atrial septal defect; *VSD,* ventricular septal defect; *PDA,* patent ductus arteriosis.

✔ *WHEN TO REFER*

Uncomplicated endocarditis with usual organisms without significant drug resistance can be managed appropriately by the primary internist. Other cases can be more challenging to the physician and life-threatening to the patient, however, and judicious use of specialists in infectious disease, cardiology, and/or cardiothoracic surgery is often appropriate.

Infectious diseases specialists can be useful in a number of circumstances. Endocarditis caused by unusual organisms such as the HACEK group or fungi; infections with highly resistant organisms such as vancomycin-resistant enterococci, nutritionally deficient streptococci or methicillin-resistant staphylococci; or infections that have relatively low cure rates such as all cases of enterococcal or prosthetic valve endocarditis are conditions where such consultation should be sought early.

Patients who are persistently febrile (i.e., for more than 5 to 7 days) in spite of seemingly adequate therapy should be evaluated by an infectious diseases specialist. Although some of these patients will have a drug fever, as many as 45% of such patients in one series had a cardiac complication such as a myocardial abscess. Other causes of persistent fever include iatrogenic infections in another site, such as a catheter-associated urinary tract infection.

Patients with evidence of cardiac complications manifested as conduction abnormalities or congestive heart failure should be evaluated immediately by a cardiologist and a cardiothoracic surgeon. Emergent transesophageal echocardiography is often required, and many such patients require prompt surgical intervention. In addition, those patients who are at high risk for such complications, particularly patients with aortic valve disease, should also be evaluated early. A patient with recurrent clinically significant embolic events should be evaluated for possible surgery. Although such events may not represent a failure of antibiotic therapy per se, surgery should be considered, lest further embolic events lead to incapacitation or death of the patient.

BOX 24-3

Dental or surgical procedures at higher risk to cause bacteremia that results in endocarditis

Endocarditis prophylaxis recommended
Dental procedures known to induce gingival or mucosal bleeding, including professional cleaning
Tonsillectomy and/or adenoidectomy
Surgical operations that involve intestinal or respiratory mucosa
Bronchoscopy with a rigid bronchoscope
Sclerotherapy for esophageal varices
Esophageal dilatation
Gallbladder surgery
Cystoscopy
Urethral dilatation
Urethral catheterization if urinary tract infection is present*
Prostatic surgery
Incision and drainage of infected tissue*
Vaginal hysterectomy
Vaginal delivery in the presence of infection*

Endocarditis prophylaxis not recommended†
Dental procedure not likely to induce gingival bleeding
Injection of local intraoral anesthesia (except intraligamentary)
Shedding of primary teeth
Tympanostomy tube insertion
Endotracheal intubation
Bronchoscopy with a flexible bronchoscope with or without biopsy
Cardiac catheterization
Gastrointestinal endoscopy with or without biopsy
Cesarean section
In the absence of infection for urethral catheterization, dilatation and curettage, uncomplicated vaginal delivery, therapeutic abortion, sterilization procedures, or insertion or removal of intrauterine devices

---

Modified from Dajani AS et al: Prevention of bacterial endocarditis: recommendations by the American Heart Association, *JAMA,* 264:2919, 1990. This table is not meant to be all-inclusive.
*In addition to the prophylactic regimen for genitourinary procedures, antibiotic therapy should be directed against the most likely bacterial pathogen.
†In patients at high risk for endocarditis (those with prosthetic valves or history of endocarditis), physicians may choose to administer prophylactic antibiotics even for low-risk procedures.

In some communities, unusual organisms (e.g., methicillin-resistant *S. aureus* or *Pseudomonas*) may be more prevalent, and empiric therapy should be modified appropriately. In patients with prosthetic valves, agents should be active against staphylococci, both *S. aureus* and coagulase-negative and gram-negative organisms. Vancomycin, gentamicin, and rifampin are recommended. Culture-negative endocarditis should be evaluated for fastidious or slow-growing organisms and other unusual causes; empiric therapy should be directed against enterococci and viridans streptococci. Four weeks of penicillin (or vancomycin for the penicillin-allergic patient) plus gentamicin is recommended. With right-sided endocarditis, an acute clinical course, a history of parenteral drug use, or lack of response to penicillin plus aminoglycoside, *S. aureus* should be suspected and nafcillin added or vancomycin substituted for penicillin. For culture-negative prosthetic valve endocarditis, vancomycin plus rifampin plus gentamicin should be used to cover against coagulase-negative staphylococci.

The exact role of cardiac surgery in infective endocarditis is controversial, and decisions regarding surgical intervention are best made on an individual basis in consultation with an experienced surgeon. In general, surgery should be considered for patients who, despite appropriate medical therapy, develop deep-seated myocardial abscesses (frequently manifested by emerging conduction defects), persistent bacteremia, or fungal endocarditis, or who have infected prosthetic valves. Aortic insufficiency resulting in shock requires emergent cardiac valve replacement. Patients with valvular insufficiency with congestive heart failure should be treated aggressively with diuretics and afterload reduction; surgery is indicated if they do not improve within 24 hours. Patients with hemodynamically stable valvular insufficiency

Table 24-6   Recommended prophylactic antibiotic regimens for patients at risk having dental, oral, upper respiratory tract, genitourinary, or gastrointestinal procedures

PROCEDURE	RISK FACTOR	DOSING REGIMEN*	COMMENTS
Dental, oral, or upper respiratory tract	Standard risk† with native valve	**Amoxicillin** 3 g orally 1 hr before procedure, then 1.5 g after initial dose.	Standard oral regimen.
		Erythromycin 1 g orally 2 hr before procedure, then 0.5 g 6 hr after initial dose.	Amoxicillin/penicillin allergy.
		Clindamycin 300 mg orally 1 hr before procedure, then 150 mg 6 hr after initial dose.	Amoxicillin/penicillin allergy or unable to tolerate erythromycin.
		Ampicillin 2 g IV or IM 30 min before procedure, then 1 g IV or IM 6 hr after initial dose.	Unable to take oral medications.
		Clindamycin 300 mg IV 30 min before procedure, then 150 mg 6 hr after initial dose.	Unable to take oral medications; amoxicillin/ ampicillin/penicillin allergy.
	High risk† (prosthetic valve or history of endocarditis)	**Ampicillin** 2 g IV or IM plus **gentamicin** 1.5 mg/kg (not to exceed 80 mg) IV or IM 30 min before procedure, then amoxicillin 1.5 g orally 6 hr after initial dose.	Alternatively, instead of oral amoxicillin the IV regimen can be repeated 8 h after initial dose.
		Vancomycin 1 g IV starting 1 hr before procedure.	Amoxicillin/ampicillin/penicillin allergy; no repeat dose necessary.
Genitourinary or gastrointestinal	Standard or high risk	**Ampicillin** 2 g IV or IM plus **gentamicin** 1.5 mg/kg (not to exceed 80 mg) IV or IM 30 min before procedure, then amoxicillin 1.5 g orally 6 hr after initial dose.	Alternatively instead of oral amoxicillin the IV regimen can be repeated 8 hr after initial dose.
		Vancomycin 1 g IV plus **gentamicin** 1.5 mg/kg (not to exceed 80 mg) IV or IM starting 1 hr before procedure. May repeat gentamicin 8 hr after initial dose.	Amoxicillin/ampicillin/penicillin allergy; no repeat dose necessary for vancomycin.
	Low risk (minor procedures)‡	**Amoxicillin** 3 g orally 1 hr before procedure, then 1.5 g after initial dose.	Not for amoxicillin/penicillin-allergic patients.

Modified from Dajani AS et al: Prevention of bacterial endocarditis: recommendations by the American Heart Association, *JAMA* 264:2919, 1990. Reader should refer to article for more detailed discussion of this topic.
*In patients with impaired renal function it may be necessary to omit second dose of gentamicin.
†Standard oral regimens can be used in higher risk patients as per AHA recommendations; however, clinicians may choose parenteral regimens.
‡Patients without prosthetic valve and no history of endocarditis and no urinary tract infection undergoing minor procedures.

should be treated with a full course of antibiotics before being evaluated for cardiac surgery. The presence of active infection is not a contraindication to surgical intervention (Chapter 25). Surgery followed by a full course of antimicrobial therapy is often curative. Remarkably, the incidence of recurrent infection in patients who undergo surgery with active disease does not greatly exceed the risk of infection in patients who receive a prosthetic valve for other reasons.

ENDOCARDITIS PROPHYLAXIS

The use of chemoprophylaxis to prevent bacterial endocarditis in high-risk patients has become accepted practice. Although its value has never been proved in humans, administration of bactericidal antibiotics has been shown to prevent endocarditis in experimental animals. Current recommendations are based on these animal studies as well as on clinical, epidemiologic, and bacteriologic data. Patients at risk are those with cardiac or vascular disease known to be associated with endocarditis (Box 24-2). Penicillin-sensitive oral streptococci (various species of viridans streptococci) are likely to be isolated from the bloodstream in patients undergoing dental, oral, or respiratory tract procedures; enterococci, which are more resistant to penicillin, are seeded in patients undergoing genitourinary or gastrointestinal procedures (Box 24-3). Drug selection is based on the sensitivity of the endocarditis-producing organisms likely to disseminate during a given procedure, and current recommendations are set forth in the 1990 American Heart Association guidelines (Table 24-6). These recommendations emphasize the use of oral over parenteral regimens, of amoxicillin over penicillin V as the standard oral regimen, and of prophylaxis for patients with mitral valve prolapse when mitral regurgitation is present (Chapter 25). Amoxicillin is as active as penicillin V against oral streptococci, but plasma levels and half-life are increased. The oral regimen is also recommended for high-risk patients (e.g., patients with prosthetic valves) undergoing dental, oral, or respiratory tract procedures; however, some authorities would still select the parenteral regimens provided. When used in other countries for high-risk

patients, oral amoxicillin therapy has been associated with better compliance and few failures. For penicillin-allergic patients, clindamycin and erythromycin are recommended. Because patients taking oral penicillins for secondary prevention of rheumatic fever or for other purposes may harbor oral streptococci relatively resistant to the penicillins, erythromycin or clindamycin should be used for prophylaxis. The main prophylactic regimens recommended for genitourinary or gastrointestinal procedures are still parenteral for standard- or high-risk patients. However, for standard-risk patients undergoing minor (low-risk) procedures, an oral amoxicillin regimen is optional. When infected tissue is manipulated, antibiotic selection should be based on the sensitivities of the most likely infecting organism. Antibiotic prophylaxis should start 30 to 60 minutes before the procedure and, unless indicated clinically, should not be continued beyond the recommended postprocedure dose. Maximum protective benefit is probably derived within the first 6 to 8 hours, and prolonged antibiotic administration predictably leads to the emergence of resistant strains.

In patients with mitral valve prolapse, the AHA recommends antibiotic prophylaxis only for those with mitral regurgitation. However, exactly how mitral regurgitation should be defined in this setting (by physical examination or echocardiography) has not been clarified. In addition, a recent echocardiographic study defined a subset of patients with mitral valve prolapse with thickened mitral valve leaflets and redundancy who are at high risk for endocarditis. Based on current knowledge, prophylaxis is recommended for patients with mitral valve prolapse with a holosystolic murmur of mitral regurgitation or with leaflet thickening and redundancy (myxomatous proliferation) on echocardiography. Prophylaxis is optional in patients with a late systolic murmur or with echocardiographic mitral regurgitation that is inaudible on physical examination (Chapter 25). Antibiotic prophylaxis is recommended perioperatively in patients undergoing open heart surgery, valve replacement, or placement of intracardiac materials. The antibiotic chosen should be directed against *S. aureus* and coagulase-negative staphylococci and tailored to the pathogens most commonly isolated in the particular institution. Prophylaxis should be given in the years after most heart or valvular surgery in patients undergoing high-risk dental, oral, respiratory tract, genitourinary, gastrointestinal, or other procedures. This is not recommended for patients who have undergone coronary artery bypass graft surgery. All patients at risk for endocarditis should establish and maintain the best possible oral health and dental hygiene to reduce potential sources of bacterial seeding, and should receive regular dental care.

BIBLIOGRAPHY

Bayer AS, Theofilopoulos AN: Immunopathogenetic aspects of infective endocarditis, *Chest* 97:204, 1990.

Chambers HF, Miller T, Newman M: Two-week therapy of *Staphylococcus aureus* right-sided endocarditis and bacteremia in intravenous drug users, *Ann Intern Med* 109:619, 1988.

Dajani AS et al: Prevention of bacterial endocarditis. Recommendations by the American Heart Association, *JAMA* 264:2919, 1990.

Daniel WG et al: Improvement in the diagnosis of abscesses associated with endocarditis by transesophageal echocardiography, *N Engl J Med* 324:795, 1991.

Dinubile MJ: Surgery in active endocarditis, *Ann Intern Med* 96:650, 1982.

Freedman LR, Valone J Jr: Experimental infective endocarditis, *Prog Cardiovasc Dis* 23:169, 1979.

Kanter MC, Hart RG: Neurologic complications of infective endocarditis, *Neurology* 41:1015, 1991.

Marks AR et al: Identification of high-risk and low-risk subgroups of patients with mitral-valve prolapse, *N Engl J Med* 320:1031, 1989.

Mathew J et al: Clinical features, site of involvement, bacteriologic findings, and outcome of infective endocarditis in intravenous drug users, *Arch Intern Med* 155:1641, 1995.

McKinsey DW et al: Underlying cardiac lesions in adults with infective endocarditis. The changing spectrum, *Am J Med* 82:681, 1987.

Pelletier LL Jr, Petersdorf RG: Infective endocarditis: review of 125 cases from the University of Washington Hospitals, 1963-1972, *Medicine* (Baltimore) 56:287, 1977.

Sande MA, Kaye D, Root RK, editors: Endocarditis, vol 2, *Contemporary issues in infectious diseases,* New York, 1984, Churchill Livingstone.

Sande MA, Scheld WM: Combination antibiotic therapy of bacterial endocarditis, *Ann Intern Med* 92:390, 1980.

Scheld WM, Sande MA: Endocarditis and intravascular infections. In Mandell GL, Douglas RG Jr, Bennett JE, editors: *Principles and practice of infectious diseases,* ed 4, New York, 1995, Churchill Livingstone.

Shapiro SM et al: Transesophageal echocardiography in the diagnosis of infective endocarditis, *Chest* 105:377, 1994.

Shively BK et al: Diagnostic value of transesophageal compared with transthoracic echocardiography in infective endocarditis, *J Am Coll Cardiol* 18:391, 1991.

Small PM, Chambers HF: Vancomycin for *Staphylococcus aureus* endocarditis in intravenous drug users, *Antimicrob Agents Chemother* 34:1227, 1990.

Van Scoy RE: Culture-negative endocarditis, *Mayo Clin Proc* 57:149, 1982.

Wilson WR et al: Antibiotic treatment of adults with infective endocarditis due to streptococci, enterococci, staphylococci, and HACEK microorganisms, *JAMA* 274:1706, 1995.

CHAPTER

25 Valvular Heart Disease

Shahbudin H. Rahimtoola

The clinical assessment and management of valvular heart disease have undergone many changes in the last three decades. The incidence of acute rheumatic fever has declined, and as a result rheumatic heart disease is not the most important cause of valve disease. Prolapse of the mitral valve and congenital aortic valve disease are now the most common valvular lesions. Valve surgery has been the major therapeutic advance in treating severe valve disease; in fact, most patients with severe valve disease are now considered candidates for operation. Doppler echocardiography (Chapter 13) has an important role in the diagnosis and follow-up of these patients. Catheter balloon valvuloplasty is a useful technique for the treatment of some stenotic cardiac valves.

AORTIC STENOSIS
Etiology

Aortic stenosis is obstruction to outflow of blood from the left ventricle to the aorta. The obstruction may be at the valve, above the valve (supravalvular), or below the valve (subvalvular). Supravalvular aortic stenosis is a congenital lesion. Subvalvular aortic stenosis results either from a discrete fibromuscular obstruction, which is a congenital lesion, or from a muscular obstruction (hypertrophic cardiomyopathy).

Congenital abnormalities of the aortic valve account for most cases of isolated aortic valve stenosis. Recent data indicate that calcific aortic stenosis in the older patient (often called degenerative) may represent an autoimmune reaction to antigens present in the valve. The most common cause of acquired aortic stenosis is rheumatic heart disease; patients with this disease usually have additional mitral valve disease. Rare disorders that produce aortic valve stenosis include rheumatoid disease and atherosclerosis associated with severe hypercholesterolemia.

Pathology

In congenital aortic valve stenosis, the valve may be unicuspid, bicuspid, or tricuspid, depending on the patient's age. In the first two decades of life, over 90% of stenotic valves are either unicuspid or bicuspid, whereas in patients 65 years of age or over, 90% of the valves are tricuspid. Unicuspid valves produce severe obstruction in infancy and are the most frequent malformation found in fatal valvular aortic stenosis in children under the age of 1 year (Chapter 28). Congenital bicuspid valves are capable of producing severe obstruction to left ventricular outflow after the first few years of life. The valvular abnormality produces turbulent flow, which traumatizes the leaflets and eventually leads to fibrosis, rigidity, and calcification of the valve. In a congenitally abnormal tricuspid aortic valve, the cusps are of unequal size and have some degree of commissural fusion; the third cusp may be diminutive. Eventually, the abnormal structure leads to changes similar to those seen in a bicuspid valve, and significant left ventricular outflow obstruction often results.

Rheumatic aortic stenosis results from adhesions and fusion of the commissures and cusps. The leaflets and the valve ring become vascularized, which leads to retraction and stiffening of the cusps. Calcification occurs, and the aortic valve orifice is reduced to a small triangular or round opening, which is frequently regurgitant as well as stenotic. Importantly, the heart exhibits other evidence of rheumatic heart disease, namely, involvement of the mitral valve and presence of Aschoff's nodules in the myocardium. Rheumatoid aortic stenosis is extremely rare and results from nodular thickening of the valve leaflets and the involvement of the proximal part of the aorta. In severe forms of hypercholesterolemia, lipid deposits occur not only in the aortic wall but also in the aortic valve and occasionally produce valvular stenosis.

The left ventricle is concentrically hypertrophied. The hypertrophied cardiac muscle cells are increased in size, with their transverse diameters ranging from 15 to 70 μm (normal, 10 to 15 μm). There is a variable amount of fibrous tissue (collagen fibrils) in the interstitial tissue. Usually, the cardiac muscle cells do not degenerate in patients with aortic valve stenosis.

Subclinical calcific emboli are commonly found if diligently sought.

Abnormal Physiology

With reduction in the aortic valve area, energy is dissipated during the transport of blood from the left ventricle to the aorta. The aortic valve area has to be reduced by 50% of normal before a measurable gradient can be demonstrated in humans. When a pressure gradient develops between the left ventricle and the ascending aorta, left ventricular pressure rises; aortic pressure remains within the normal range until end-stage heart failure occurs. The relationship of the valve area to cardiac output and pressure gradient is discussed in the section on mitral stenosis. As left ventricular pressure rises, ventricular wall stress increases, which leads to impaired left ventricular function.

Therefore, the heart normalizes wall stress by becoming hypertrophic (Chapter 9). Since aortic stenosis develops slowly over the years in humans, hypertrophy develops in proportion to increased intraventricular pressure, and myocardial stress remains normal. Thus, the major compensatory mechanism by which the heart copes with left ventricular outflow obstruction is ventricular hypertrophy. Left ventricular mass in patients with severe aortic stenosis undergoing valve replacement averages 229 g per square meter (normal, 105 g/m²); at autopsy, left ventricles weighing as much as 1000 g have been reported. However, left ventricular volume is within the normal range. Therefore, there is a considerable thickening of the left ventricular wall.

The diastolic properties of the left ventricle are affected in aortic stenosis. There is a resistance to left ventricular filling, because the hypertrophied left ventricle per se offers increased resistance to filling, the stiffness of the left ventricle is increased, or both. As a result, left ventricular end diastolic pressure is elevated, but this cannot be used as a measure of left ventricular failure. Powerful atrial contraction produces the required left ventricular filling and results in an elevated left ventricular end diastolic pressure (atrial booster pump function). The necessary left ventricular filling and fiber length are achieved by atrial systole, which occupies only a small part of the cardiac cycle. Therefore, there is a transient increase in left atrial pressure due to the large A wave, but mean left atrial pressure remains in the normal range or is only minimally increased.

Left atrial contraction is therefore of considerable benefit to these patients. Loss of effective atrial contraction, either because of atrial fibrillation or because of an inappropriately timed atrial contraction (e.g., that associated with first-degree heart block or with atrioventricular [AV] dissociation), results in elevations of mean left atrial pressure, reduction of cardiac output, or both, and may precipitate heart failure.

Patients with severe left ventricular hypertrophy may exhibit left ventricular diastolic dysfunction. This may produce the syndrome of clinical heart failure (paroxysmal nocturnal dyspnea, orthopnea, and even pulmonary edema) even if left ventricular systolic pump function is normal. In patients 60 years of age or older, a higher percentage of women (41%) compared to men (14%) have "excessive" hypertrophy, that is, greater amounts of hypertrophy in spite of similar degrees of severity of aortic stenosis. They have supernormal left ventricular systolic pump function and a small thick-walled chamber with lower end-systolic wall stress.

Left ventricular systolic pump function is determined by myocardial (muscle) function and by a combination of left ventricular afterload and preload (Chapter 9). Thus, impaired left ventricular systolic pump function (as measured by ejection fraction) may be the result of impaired myocardial function, afterload-preload mismatch, or both. Left ventricular systolic pump function is normal in most patients with severe aortic stenosis. When the left ventricular hypertrophy alone is not adequate to overcome the outflow obstruction, the left ventricle uses the Frank-Starling mechanism (preload reserve) to maintain systolic pump function. When the preload reserve is no longer adequate, a reduction of left ventricular systolic pump function occurs (Fig. 25-1). In aortic stenosis, use of the preload reserve is not a good compensatory mechanism. Even small increases in left ventricular volume result in major increases in left ventricular end-diastolic pressure, because the left ventricle is on the very steep portion of its diastolic pressure-volume curve, and the corresponding increase in mean left atrial pressures produces pulmonary edema. Eventually, pulmonary artery, right ventricular, and right atrial pressures are elevated. Peripheral edema results from increases in systemic venous pressure and salt and water retention.

In most patients with aortic valve stenosis, cardiac output is in the normal range and initially increases normally with exercise. Later, as the severity of aortic stenosis increases progressively, the cardiac output remains within the normal range at rest, but, on exercise, it no longer increases in proportion to the amount of exercise undertaken or does not increase at all (fixed cardiac output). With the development of congestive heart failure, there is a reduction in the resting cardiac output and a tachycardia. As a result, stroke volume may be so lowered that it results in a small gradient across the left ventricular outflow tract in spite of severe aortic stenosis.

In severe aortic stenosis, myocardial oxygen needs are increased because of an increased muscle mass (hypertrophy), elevations in ventricular pressures, and prolongation of the systolic ejection time. Blood flow to the myocardium, particularly flow to the subendocardium, is inadequate, because the abnormally elevated pressure compresses the coronary arteries as they traverse the myocardium to supply the subendocardium, and the elevated left ventricular end-diastolic pressure lowers the diastolic aortic–left ventricular pressure (coronary perfusion pressure) gradient. Associated obstructive coronary artery disease from atherosclerosis further increases the imbalance between myocardial oxygen needs and supply.

Clinical Manifestations

History. Patients with congenital valve stenosis may give a history of a murmur since childhood or infancy; those with rheumatic stenosis may have a history of rheumatic fever. Most patients with valvular aortic stenosis, including a few with severe valve stenosis, are asymptomatic. The symptoms of aortic stenosis are angina pectoris, syncope, exertional presyncope, and the symptoms of heart failure. It must be emphasized that once symptoms occur in a patient with severe aortic stenosis, the life span of the patient is very short without surgical treatment. Sudden cardiac death occurs in 5% of patients with aortic stenosis. It occurs only in those with severe valve stenosis, most of whom have had some cardiac symptoms before the fatal episode. Typical angina pectoris occurs with or without associated coronary artery disease and results from an imbalance between myocardial oxygen demand and supply, as previously discussed.

Syncope is the result of reduced cerebral perfusion. Syncope occurring on effort is caused by either systemic vasodilatation in the presence of a fixed or inadequate cardiac output, an arrhythmia, or both. Syncope at rest is usually due to a transient ventricular tachyarrhythmia, from which the patient recovers spontaneously. Other possible causes of syncope include transient atrial fibrillation or transient AV block during which the ventricle is deprived of the powerful atrial booster pump function and/or the ventricular rate is slow.

Dyspnea on exertion, orthopnea, paroxysmal nocturnal dyspnea, and pulmonary edema result from varying degrees of pulmonary venous hypertension. Systemic venous congestion with enlargement of the liver and peripheral edema results from increased systemic venous pressure and salt and water retention. There is an increased incidence of gastrointestinal arteriovenous malformations. As a result, these patients are susceptible to gastrointestinal hemorrhage and anemia. Calcific systemic embolism may occur.

Physical Findings. The arterial pulse rises slowly, taking a longer time than normal to reach peak pressure, and the peak is reduced; the pulse pressure may be narrowed. The anacrotic notch on the upstroke is best appreciated in the carotid arteries. The more severe the valve stenosis, the lower the anacrotic notch on the arterial pulse. A systolic thrill may be felt in the carotid arteries. The jugular venous pulse is normal unless the patient is in congestive heart failure. In the absence of heart failure, the heart size is normal. The cardiac impulse is heaving and sustained in character, and there may be a palpable fourth heart sound (S₄). An aortic systolic thrill often is present at the base of the heart. In 80% to 90% of adult patients with severe aortic stenosis, there is an S₄ gallop sound, a midsystolic ejection murmur that peaks late in systole, the second heart sound (S₂) is single, and there is a faint early diastolic murmur of minimal aortic regurgitation. In the young patient with valvular aortic stenosis, a systolic ejection sound initiates the systolic murmur but later tends to disappear as aortic stenosis becomes severe. The S₂ may be paradoxically split, and there may be no early diastolic murmur. In many patients, particularly the elderly, the systolic ejection murmur is atypical, may be soft or cooing, and may be heard only at the apex of the heart. In the presence of congestive heart failure, the jugular venous pressure often is increased, the left ventricle is dilated, there is a third heart sound, and the systolic murmur may be very soft or absent. Thus, the clinical features on physical examination resemble those of heart failure from a variety of causes such as cardiomyopathy, rather than aortic stenosis.

Severe valvular aortic stenosis is common in patients 60 years of age or older. The clinical features in many of these patients tend to be somewhat different from those typical of younger patients. Systemic hypertension is common, occurring in about 20% of the pa-

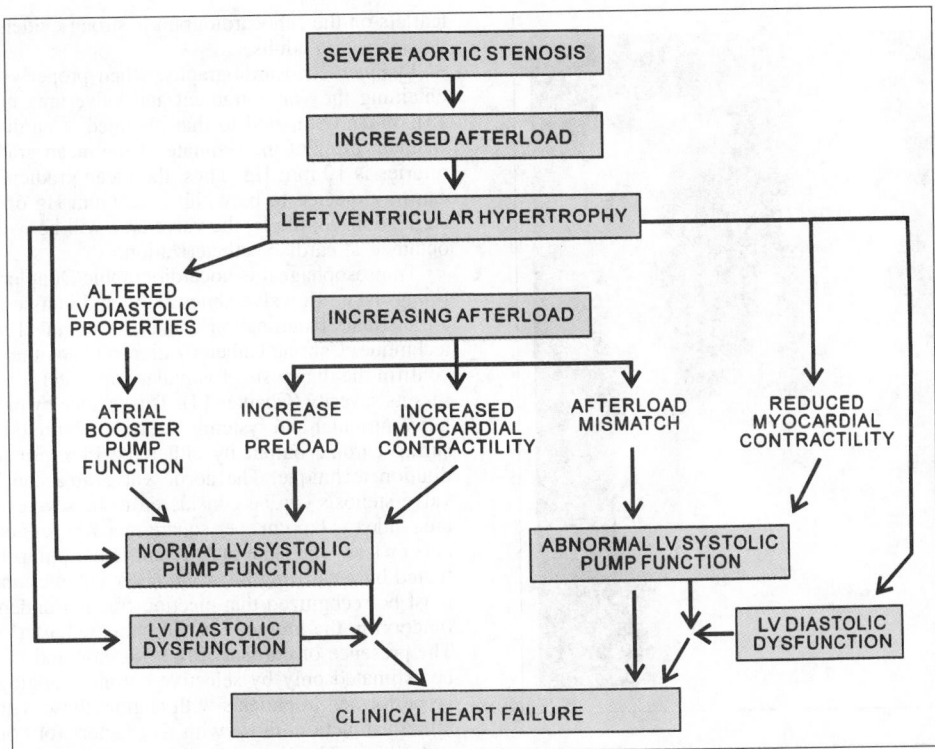

FIGURE 25-1   Some aspects of the pathophysiology in severe aortic stenosis. The heart responds to aortic stenosis by hypertrophy, and left ventricular systolic pump function remains normal. Left ventricular hypertrophy may alter the left ventricular diastolic properties and there is increased resistance to left ventricular filling. As a result, left ventricular end-diastolic pressure is elevated, but powerful atrial contraction produces the required left ventricular filling and fiber length (atrial booster pump function). Because atrial systole occupies only a small part of the cardiac cycle, there is only a transient increase in left atrial pressure; therefore, mean left atrial pressure remains in the normal range or is only minimally increased. As left ventricular afterload continues to increase, the left ventricle uses two additional compensatory mechanisms, namely, increase of preload and increase of myocardial contractility. Both of these help maintain normal left ventricular systolic pump function. When the limit of the preload reserve has been reached (afterload mismatch) or myocardial contractility is reduced, left ventricular systolic pump function becomes abnormal. Clinical heart failure is usually a result of abnormal left ventricular systolic pump function; diastolic dysfunction may also be present in some patients. Clinical heart failure in those with normal left ventricular systolic pump function is a result of left ventricular diastolic dysfunction.

From Rahimtoola SH: Aortic valve stenosis. In Rahimtoola SH, editor: Valvular heart disease and endocarditis. In Braunwald E, editor-in-chief: *Atlas of the heart,* Philadelphia, Current Medicine, 1997.

tients, half of whom have moderate or severe systolic and diastolic hypertension. A fifth of the patients first present in congestive heart failure. The male/female ratio is 2:1. Because of thickening of the arterial wall and its associated lack of distensibility, the arterial pulse rises normally or even rapidly, and the pulse pressure is wide. The S_2 is either absent or single.

Chest Radiograph. The characteristic finding is a normal-sized heart with a dilated ascending aorta (Fig. 25-2). Calcium in the aortic valve can be seen on the lateral film but is best appreciated by fluoroscopy with image intensification. Calcium in the aortic valve is the hallmark of aortic stenosis in adults 40 to 45 years of age. In patients aged 45 years or above, the diagnosis of aortic valve stenosis of any severity is not tenable if calcium in the aortic valve is not present. However, the presence of calcium does not necessarily denote that the aortic stenosis is severe. In patients with heart failure, the cardiac size is increased because of dilatation of the left ventricle and left atrium; the lung fields show pulmonary edema and pulmonary venous congestion with redistribution of blood flow. In the presence of congestive heart failure, the right ventricle and the right atrium may be dilated.

Electrocardiogram. The ECG in severe aortic stenosis shows left ventricular hypertrophy with or without secondary ST-T wave changes (Chapter 12). However, it is important to recognize that in

about 10% to 15% of patients with severe aortic stenosis, left ventricular hypertrophy cannot be appreciated on the ECG. In fact, the ECG may be entirely normal in some of these patients. The P wave abnormalities of left atrial enlargement and hypertrophy or conduction delay are usually present. The ECG may show left bundle branch block, right bundle branch block with left or right axis deviation, or, occasionally, isolated right bundle branch block. In some of the patients the conduction abnormality results from aortic valve calcification extending into the specialized conducting tissue. The patients are usually in sinus rhythm. The presence of atrial fibrillation indicates the presence of either associated mitral valve disease, coronary artery disease, or heart failure secondary to aortic valve disease.

Special Laboratory Studies. On the echocardiogram, the aortic valve leaflets normally are barely visible in systole, and the normal range of aortic valve opening is 1.6 to 2.6 cm (Chapter 13). In the presence of a bicuspid aortic valve, eccentric valve leaflets may be seen. The aortic valve leaflets may appear to be thickened as a result of calcification and/or fibrosis; however, the older patient without valve stenosis may also have thickened cusps. The aortic valve may have a reduced opening, but this also occurs in other conditions in which the cardiac output is reduced. The left ventricular hypertrophy often results in thickening of both the interventricular septum and the posterior left ventricular wall. The left ventricular size is normal.

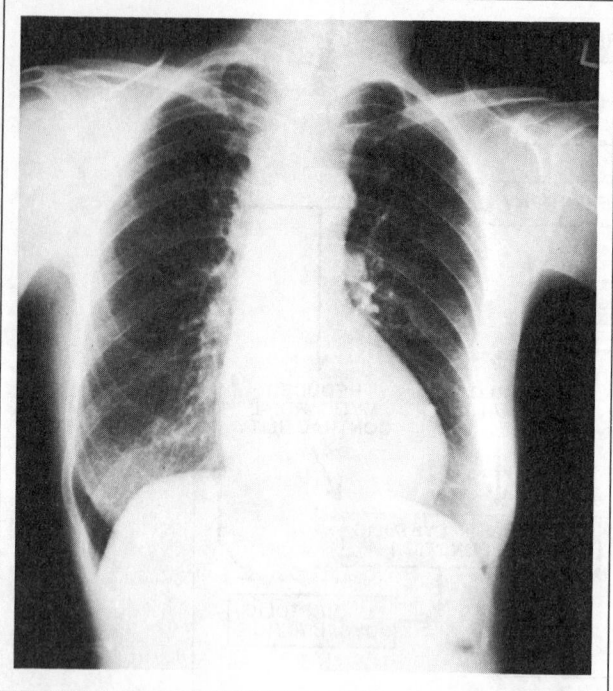

A

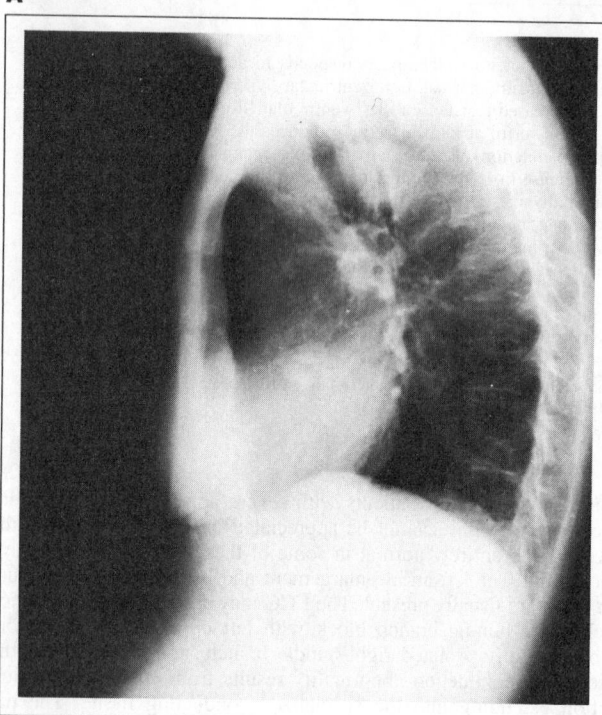

B

FIGURE 25-2   Chest radiograph in the frontal **(A)** and left lateral **(B)** projection in a patient with severe aortic stenosis. The aortic valve is heavily calcified, a finding best appreciated on the lateral projection **(B)** or with fluoroscopy.

All these abnormalities are better appreciated on two-dimensional (2D) echocardiography. When left ventricular function is impaired, the left ventricle and left atrium are dilated and the percentage of dimensional shortening (Chapter 13) is reduced.

In many patients the severity of aortic valve stenosis is incorrectly estimated by M-mode or 2D echocardiography. Neither is a completely reliable technique for assessing the severity of valvular aortic stenosis. However, the presence of normal movement of thin aortic leaflets on the echocardiogram is strong evidence against severe aortic stenosis in adults.

Doppler echocardiography, when properly applied, is useful for obtaining the valve gradient and valve area noninvasively (Chapter 13). When compared to that obtained at cardiac catheterization, the standard error of the estimate of the mean gradient in the best laboratories is 10 mm Hg. Thus, the mean gradient obtained by Doppler can be expected to be within ± 20 mm Hg of that obtained at catheterization. Similarly, the valve area will be within ± 0.3 cm² of that obtained at cardiac catheterization.

Transesophageal echocardiographic/Doppler is very useful in defining the aortic valve abnormality and in assessing its severity when an adequate examination cannot be obtained with the transthoracic technique. Cardiac catheterization remains the standard technique to confirm the diagnosis of valvular aortic stenosis and to accurately assess its severity (Chapter 14). This is done by measuring simultaneous left ventricular and systemic arterial pressure (see Fig. 14-3) and measuring cardiac output by either the Fick principle or the indicator-dilution technique. The aortic valve area can be calculated. Aortic valve stenosis can be considered to be severe when the aortic valve area index is 0.6 cm² per square meter or less or the valve area is 1.0 cm² or less. The state of left ventricular pump function can be quantitated by measuring left ventricular volumes and ejection fraction. It must be recognized that ejection fraction underestimates myocardial function in the presence of the increased afterload of aortic stenosis. The presence of coronary artery disease and its site and severity can be estimated only by selective coronary angiography, which should be performed in patients with angina, those with left ventricular systolic dysfunction, those with risk factors for coronary artery disease, and all patients 35 years of age or older being considered for aortic valve surgery. The incidence of associated coronary artery disease is related to the prevalence of coronary artery disease in the population. In general, in persons 50 years of age or older it is about 50%.

Gated blood pool radionuclide scans provide information on ventricular function similar to that provided by left ventricular cineangiography (Chapter 13). These studies are of particular value in the occasional patient in whom left ventricular cineangiography is unsuccessful and echocardiographic studies are suboptimal.

It is recommended that exercise tests of any kind not be undertaken in patients with severe aortic stenosis unless there is a specific reason for such studies. Exercise tests in these patients may precipitate ventricular tachyarrhythmias and ventricular fibrillation. If there is doubt about the severity of aortic stenosis and concern that the patient's symptoms may not be caused by aortic stenosis, then it is usually wise to document the absence of severe aortic stenosis before performing an exercise test.

Ambulatory ECG recording may be needed in an occasional patient suspected of having an arrhythmia, since symptoms occur only during arrhythmias in some patients with mild or moderate aortic stenosis.

Natural History and Prognosis

Valvular aortic stenosis is frequently a progressive disease, the severity increasing over time. The factors that control this progression and the time it takes for severe outflow obstruction to develop are unknown. In a recent study in patients with "mild" stenosis (aortic valve area > 1.5 cm²), the rate of progression to moderate or severe stenosis was 12% in 10 years and 62% in 25 years. The duration of the asymptomatic period after the development of severe aortic valve stenosis is also unknown; some recent data suggest it may be less than 2 years. The overwhelming majority of adults with severe aortic stenosis who are seen by cardiologists have symptoms. Severe disease in adults is lethal, particularly if the patient is symptomatic, with a prognosis that is worse than for many forms of neoplastic disease. The 3-year mortality is approximately 36% to 52%. The 5-year mortality is about 52% to 80% and the 10-year mortality is 80% to 90%. A recent study of elderly patients (average age 77 years) showed 1-year and 3-year mortalities were 44% and 75%, respectively. With the onset of severe symptoms (angina, syncope, or heart failure) the average life expectancy is 3 years. A combination of symptoms is much more ominous, a sign of a greatly reduced survival. Sudden death, like syncope, occurs in the presence of severe aortic stenosis.

Its exact incidence is difficult to determine but is probably about 5%. Most, but not all, of these patients have had some cardiac symptoms before the fatal episode; at times, the only symptom has been exertional presyncope.

Management

All patients with aortic stenosis need antibiotic prophylaxis against infective endocarditis (Chapter 24). Those in whom the valve lesion is of rheumatic origin need additional rheumatic fever prophylaxis (Chapter 204). Patients with mild or moderate stenosis rarely have symptoms or complications and do not need any specific medical therapy. In mild stenosis, the patient should be encouraged to lead a normal life. Those with moderate valve stenosis should avoid moderate to severe physical exertion and competitive sports. In patients with mild or moderate disease, if atrial fibrillation should occur, it should be reverted rapidly to sinus rhythm. In severe stenosis, reversion to sinus rhythm often becomes a matter of some urgency.

Operation should be advised if the patient has severe aortic valve stenosis. In young patients, if the valve is pliable and mobile, simple commissurotomy may be feasible, and it will relieve outflow obstruction to a major degree; overly enthusiastic commissurotomy with production of significant aortic regurgitation should be avoided. This is probably a palliative procedure that puts off valve replacement for many years. Older patients and even young patients with calcified, rigid valves need valve replacement. In view of the natural history of severe aortic valve stenosis, that is, a 10-year mortality of 80% to 90%, it is reasonable to recommend surgery even to the asymptomatic patient. Asymptomatic adults with severe aortic stenosis are uncommon.

The operative mortality of valve replacement is about 5% or less. In those without associated coronary artery disease or heart failure, it may be 1% to 2%. Patients with associated coronary artery disease should have coronary bypass surgery at the same time as valve surgery. Left ventricular function remains normal postoperatively if perioperative myocardial damage has not occurred. Left ventricular hypertrophy regresses toward normal; after 2 years, the regression continues at a slower rate up to 8 to 10 years after valve replacement. In those with very excessive ventricular hypertrophy preoperatively, the hypertrophy may regress slowly or not at all. These patients may then have severe left ventricular diastolic dysfunction, which may be a difficult clinical problem both in the early postoperative period and after hospital discharge. Surviving patients are functionally improved. The 10-year survival is 60% or better; 15-year survival is 45% or better.

Patients who present with heart failure should be hospitalized and treated with digitalis and diuretics and should undergo surgery as soon as possible. If heart failure does not respond satisfactorily and rapidly to medical therapy, surgery becomes a matter of considerable urgency. Catheter balloon valvuloplasty is an important bridge procedure that usually greatly improves the patients' hemodynamics and makes them better candidates for valve replacement. Valve replacement in patients with aortic stenosis and heart failure can be performed at an operative mortality of 10% or less. Although this is higher than in patients not in heart failure, the risk is justified, because late survival in those who live through the operation is excellent and is far superior to that which can be expected with medical therapy. The 7-year survival of patients who survive operation is 84%. The impaired left ventricular function improves in *all* such patients provided there has been no perioperative myocardial damage and becomes normal in two thirds of the patients. In addition, the operative survivors are functionally much improved. Left ventricular hypertrophy and dilatation (if present preoperatively) regress toward normal.

Despite the excellent results of valve replacements in patients with severe aortic stenosis who are in heart failure, it is important to recognize that surgery should *not* be delayed until heart failure develops.

The role of catheter balloon valvuloplasty in the older patient has now been clarified. In calcific aortic stenosis after catheter balloon valvuloplasty, the average increase in valve area is 0.3 cm^2 and the final aortic valve area usually averages 0.8 cm^2; thus, many patients continue to have severe aortic stenosis. The 30-day, 1-year, and 3-year mortalities average 14%, 35%, and 71%, respectively, in the older

patient with calcific aortic stenosis, a mortality rate that may be similar to the natural history of this lesion. This technique is indicated in those who have an expected limited short life span, as a bridge procedure in those who need emergent noncardiac surgery and in those who are in heart failure, or in cardiogenic shock, when operative risks are considered to be prohibitively high, and in those who refuse surgery. When performed as a bridge procedure, valve surgery should not be unduly delayed. It is the procedure of choice in young patients who have pliable, noncalcified valves with commissural fusion.

CHRONIC AORTIC REGURGITATION
Etiology

In North America, the most common cause of isolated severe aortic regurgitation is aortic root/annular dilatation that is presumably the result of medial disease. Other common causes include a congenital (bicuspid) valve, previous infective endocarditis, and rheumatic disease. Chronic aortic regurgitation also occurs in association with a variety of other diseases, such as

1. Congenital lesions, for example, supravalvular and discrete subvalvular aortic stenosis, ventricular septal defect, and aneurysm of the sinus of Valsalva.
2. Connective tissue diseases, for example, Marfan's syndrome, osteogenesis imperfecta, and Ehlers-Danlos syndrome.
3. Autoimmune diseases, for example, ankylosing spondylitis, rheumatoid arthritis, and systemic lupus erythematosus.
4. Various forms of aortitis and arteritis, for example, giant-cell arteritis and Takayasu's disease.
5. Syphilis.

Forty percent to 60% of the surgically removed valves from patients with isolated severe aortic regurgitation are classified as idiopathic. Half of these (or 20% to 30% of all the valves removed) showed histologic criteria of myxomatous degeneration.

Pathology

Depending on the cause, the valve cusps show thickening, shortening, commissural lesions, and calcification. Regardless of the cause, the left ventricle is dilated and hypertrophied; some of the largest ventricles have been described in association with chronic severe aortic regurgitation. Little pockets may be seen in the left ventricular outflow tract. These are pouches out of the endocardial lining formed by the regurgitant jet's striking the left ventricle.

The myocardium is hypertrophied, with replication of sarcomeres in series, elongation of fibers, and wall thickening. The wall is not as thickened as in patients with aortic stenosis. Ultrastructural changes in the myocardial cells are similar to those seen in aortic stenosis; an important difference, however, is the frequent presence of degenerated cardiac muscle cells in patients with severe aortic regurgitation. Cardiac muscle cells with mild degeneration show focal myofibrillar lysis, with preferential loss of thick myofilament and focal proliferation of tubules of the sarcoplasmic reticulum. Moderately degenerated muscle cells show a marked decrease in the number of myofibrils and T-tubules and proliferation of sarcoplasmic reticulum, mitochondria, or both. Severely degenerated muscle cells usually are present in areas of marked fibrosis; they are often atrophic, have thickened basement membranes, and have lost their intercellular connections. These degenerated cardiac muscle cells may represent the ultrastructural basis for impaired left ventricular function, which is seen more commonly in severe aortic regurgitation than in severe aortic stenosis.

In patients with rheumatoid arthritis and ankylosing spondylitis, nodules on the outer surface of the anterior leaflet of the mitral valve have been described.

Abnormal Physiology

The left ventricle responds to chronic aortic regurgitation by an increase in left ventricular diastolic volume, the increment in end diastolic volume being proportional to the amount of regurgitation. The left ventricle hypertrophies to normalize stress (Chapter 9). The left ventricular wall is not as thickened as in aortic stenosis; however, the

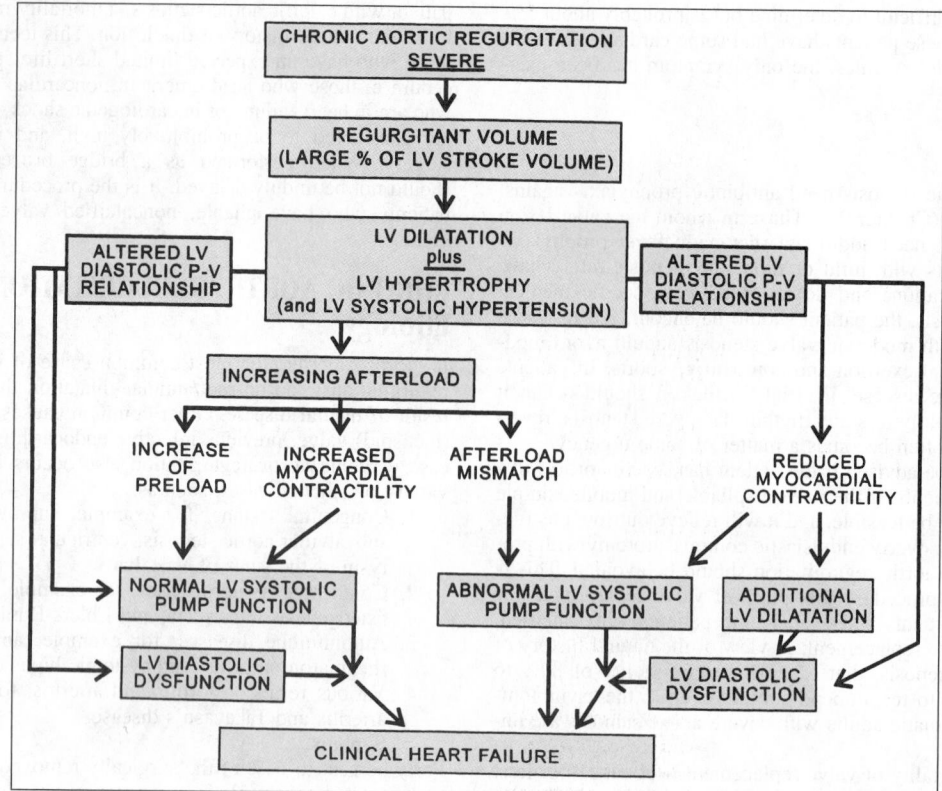

FIGURE 25-3 Some aspects of the pathophysiology of severe chronic aortic regurgitation. Severe chronic aortic regurgitation results in a large regurgitant volume (a large percentage of left ventricular stroke volume). The left ventricle responds by dilating in proportion to the amount of the regurgitant volume. The subsequent large left ventricular stroke volume results in left ventricular systolic hypertension. Both of these increase left ventricular wall stress (afterload), which could result in an impairment of left ventricular function. The heart responds by hypertrophy, myocardial stress remains normal, and left ventricular systolic pump function remains normal. There is an alteration of the left ventricular diastolic pressure-volume relationship. However, some patients with normal left ventricular systolic pump function become symptomatic because of the abnormal left ventricular diastolic function. As left ventricular afterload (a result of left ventricular dilatation, hypertrophy, and systolic hypertension) continues to increase, the left ventricle uses two additional compensatory mechanisms, namely, increase of preload and increase of myocardial contractility. Both of these help maintain normal left ventricular systolic pump function. When the limit of preload reserve has been reached (afterload mismatch) or myocardial contractility is reduced, left ventricular systolic pump function becomes abnormal. The additional left ventricular dilatation also results in further alteration of the left ventricular diastolic pressure-volume relationship.

Clinical heart failure is usually a result of the abnormal left ventricular systolic pump function; diastolic dysfunction may also be present in some patients. Clinical heart failure in those with normal left ventricular systolic pump function is a result of left ventricular diastolic dysfunction.

From Rahimtoola SH: Aortic valve stenosis. In Rahimtoola SH, editor: *Valvular heart disease and endocarditis.* In Braunwald E, editor-in-chief: *Atlas of the heart,* Philadelphia, Current Medicine, 1997.

total left ventricular mass is greatly increased, and the wall is usually thicker than normal.

Because of the leak of blood from the ascending aorta to the left ventricle in diastole, the aortic diastolic pressure is reduced and is frequently below 50 mm Hg. The large left ventricular stroke volume (a combination of forward stroke volume and regurgitant volume) results in elevation of the aortic systolic pressure, and thus the pulse pressure is considerably increased. Reduction or normalization of aortic systolic pressure is suggestive of left ventricular systolic dysfunction in these patients. The left ventricular end-diastolic pressure is increased because the regurgitant volume increases ventricular end-diastolic volume. However, the relation between left ventricular end-diastolic volume and end-diastolic pressure is not linear (Chapter 9), and in any group of patients there is a considerable scatter between the two measurements. In fact, many patients have a normal ventricular end-diastolic pressure in spite of severe aortic regurgitation and large left ventricles, indicating a shift of the ventricular pressure-volume curve to the right.

The increased left ventricular end-diastolic volume is associated with a normal ejection fraction, and, as a result, left ventricular stroke volume is large. The left ventricle in aortic regurgitation is ejecting against systemic resistance, and the myocardial tension that is developed to open the aortic valve and eject the huge stroke volume is great. This contrasts with another volume-overload lesion, mitral regurgitation, in which there is a low-resistance chamber into which the left ventricle is also emptying (the left atrium). Thus, for the same degree of regurgitant volume, myocardial tension or afterload is higher in aortic regurgitation. As the regurgitation increases, the left ventricle adapts by increasing end-diastolic volume (Frank-Starling mechanism) and/or by increasing myocardial contractility. When these two mechanisms are inadequate, left ventricular systolic function declines (afterload mismatch). At this stage, correction of aortic regurgitation will result in a normalization or marked improvement in left ventricular systolic function (Fig. 25-3).

Left ventricular stroke volume in aortic regurgitation consists of the forward stroke volume (blood delivered to the body tissues and the heart), which, multiplied by heart rate, makes up the forward cardiac output and the regurgitant volume (the volume of blood that regurgitates back to the left ventricle). In the early stages, even in severe aortic regurgitation, the forward cardiac output and left ventricular ejection fraction are normal at rest. During exercise, end-diastolic volume is reduced and ejection fraction is increased. As in normal subjects, the systemic vascular resistance is decreased, and the heart rate is increased, which reduces the length of diastole. Both these factors reduce the regurgitant volume, and forward stroke volume and cardiac output are increased during exercise.

A certain number of patients who are symptomatic have normal left ventricular systolic function. In these patients the symptoms of elevated left atrial pressure are a result of altered left ventricular diastolic function.

Progressive impairment of left ventricular systolic function in aortic regurgitation produces the following changes: at first, left ventricular ejection fraction fails to increase normally or actually diminishes during exercise, with the resulting increment in cardiac output with exercise being inadequate. An abnormal response of the left ventricular ejection fraction (failure to increase) on exercise is also related to lack of an adequate fall in systemic vascular resistance during exercise. Thus, a decline in ejection fraction on exercise cannot be used as a specific marker of left ventricular function in these patients. However, an ejection fraction on exercise of less than 0.50 has been shown to correlate with increased left atrial pressure during exercise and an abnormal left ventricular contractile state at rest. Further impairment of left ventricular function produces demonstrable abnormalities at rest; there is a further increase in left ventricular end-diastolic volume, which helps to maintain forward stroke volume. The resting left ventricular ejection fraction is reduced, and mean left atrial pressure begins to increase. Even at this stage, the forward cardiac output may be maintained in the normal range. The increases in left atrial pressure may produce various grades of pulmonary edema. Finally, in the state of severe heart failure, ejection fraction may be low, left ventricular end-diastolic volume is large, and end-diastolic pressure is greatly increased and is associated with increases in left atrial, pulmonary, right ventricular, and right atrial pressures. Cardiac output is no longer normal. An increase in systemic venous pressure in association with salt and water retention produces engorgement of systemic organs (e.g., the liver) as well as peripheral edema.

Because of the increase in left ventricular mass, myocardial oxygen needs are increased. Coronary blood flow is inadequate with stress because of the reduction in the aortic diastolic pressure and increased diastolic ventricular pressure. The inadequate coronary blood flow jeopardizes the subendocardium, which may become ischemic. Associated obstructive coronary artery disease exacerbates the reduction in coronary blood flow.

Clinical Manifestations

History. Patients with mild to moderate aortic regurgitation usually do not have symptoms that can be attributed to the heart. Even patients with severe aortic regurgitation may be asymptomatic. They may complain of pounding of the head or palpitations, which result from their awareness of the beating of a dilated left ventricle that undergoes a large volume change in systole, during either sinus beats or postectopic beats. The main symptoms of severe aortic regurgitation result from elevated pulmonary venous pressures and include dyspnea on exertion, orthopnea, and paroxysmal nocturnal dyspnea. When congestive heart failure occurs, patients complain of fatigue and weakness. Angina pectoris occurs in 20% of such patients and may be present even if the coronary arteries are normal. Angina associated with syphilitic aortic regurgitation may be due to associated ostial stenosis of the coronary arteries. In such patients, angina often occurs at rest and is difficult to control.

Physical Findings. A variety of interesting but not very useful signs may be present in patients with chronic severe aortic regurgitation. These include de Musset's sign (bobbing of the head with each heartbeat), Traube's sign (pistol-shot sound heard over the femoral artery), Duroziez's sign (systolic murmur over the femoral artery when it is compressed proximally and diastolic murmur when it is compressed distally), and Quincke's pulse (capillary pulsations that can be detected by pressing a glass slide on the patient's lip or transmitting a light through the patient's fingertips).

The arterial pulse is very characteristic and consists of an abrupt distention with a rapid rise and a quick collapse (Corrigan's pulse).

The arterial pulse may be bisferiens, a double impulse during systole that signifies severe aortic regurgitation (Chapter 11). The systolic arterial pressure is increased, the diastolic pressure is reduced, and the Korotkoff's sounds persist down to 0 mm Hg. Even in such instances, however, the recorded intraarterial pressure rarely falls below 30 mm Hg. The vasoconstriction that occurs in the presence of severe heart failure may result in some elevation of the arterial diastolic pressure. The jugular venous pressure is normal except in heart failure and in instances in which the greatly dilated ascending aorta obstructs the superior vena cava.

On inspection, the chest may rock and the cardiac impulse may be visible. The cardiac impulse is hyperdynamic. There may be a systolic thrill at the base of the heart, over the carotids, and in the suprasternal notch. This results from a large left ventricular stroke volume across a diseased aortic valve. A diastolic thrill signifies severe aortic regurgitation. The first heart sound is usually soft, because the mitral valve leaflets are close to each other at the onset of systole, or, if valve closure is premature, the valve is closed. This is exaggerated if the P-R interval is prolonged. The S_2 is usually single because the aortic valve does not close properly, or because the left ventricular ejection time is prolonged, and the P_2 may not be heard. Often, a systolic ejection murmur that is sometimes very loud is present. The clinical sine qua non of aortic regurgitation is an early or immediate decrescendo, blowing diastolic murmur beginning after the S_2. It is best heard with the diaphragm of the stethoscope at the left sternal border, or, in difficult instances, by having the patient sit up and lean forward and by auscultating in held respiration at the end of a deep expiration. In severe aortic regurgitation, the murmur may be holodiastolic. When it is soft, its intensity can be increased by doing isometric exercise, for example, a handgrip, which increases aortic diastolic pressure. At times, this murmur is better heard along the right sternal border, which should draw attention to the possibility that the cause of the aortic regurgitation is aortic root disease. Classically, rupture of the sinus of Valsalva into the right heart chambers produces a continuous murmur.

In many patients with severe aortic regurgitation, an Austin Flint murmur is present in presystole and/or middiastole (Chapter 11). Two inferences can be drawn from the presence of an Austin Flint murmur: (1) It signifies that the aortic regurgitation is severe, and (2) it requires that associated mitral stenosis be excluded. The most helpful sign at the bedside is the response of the murmur to the inhalation of amyl nitrite. The vasodilatation produced by amyl nitrite increases forward flow, reduces the regurgitant volume, and results in the Austin Flint murmur becoming much softer or disappearing. On the other hand, the increased cardiac output and the tachycardia accentuate or increase the murmur of mitral stenosis. Alternatively, echocardiography can easily demonstrate the presence of organic mitral stenosis.

Chest Radiograph. The left ventricle is increased in size, and this can be appreciated on the chest x-ray by an increase in the cardiothoracic ratio (Fig. 25-4). Since the upper limit of normal of the cardiothoracic ratio is 0.49, many patients with increased left ventricular size have an enlarged ventricular volume and still have a cardiothoracic ratio within the normal range. The ascending aorta is dilated, and there may be calcium in the aortic valve. There might be evidence of an enlarged left atrium and an increased left atrial and pulmonary venous pressure, which are manifested in the pulmonary vascular shadows by a redistribution of blood flow, pulmonary congestion, and pulmonary edema.

Electrocardiogram. The ECG shows left ventricular hypertrophy with or without associated secondary ST-T wave changes. In a small percentage of patients, ECG evidence of left ventricular hypertrophy is absent in spite of severe aortic regurgitation. Conduction abnormalities, such as left bundle branch block or right bundle branch block with or without axis deviation, may be present. The P-R interval may be prolonged, particularly in patients with ankylosing spondylitis. The rhythm is usually sinus. The presence of atrial fibrillation should make one suspect the presence of associated mitral valve disease or heart failure.

Special Laboratory Studies. The sign of aortic regurgitation on echocardiography is diastolic fluttering of the anterior leaflet of

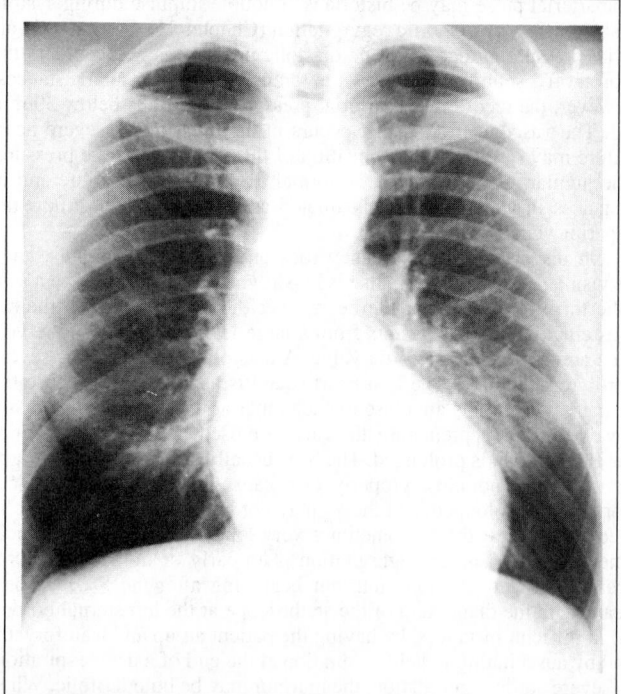

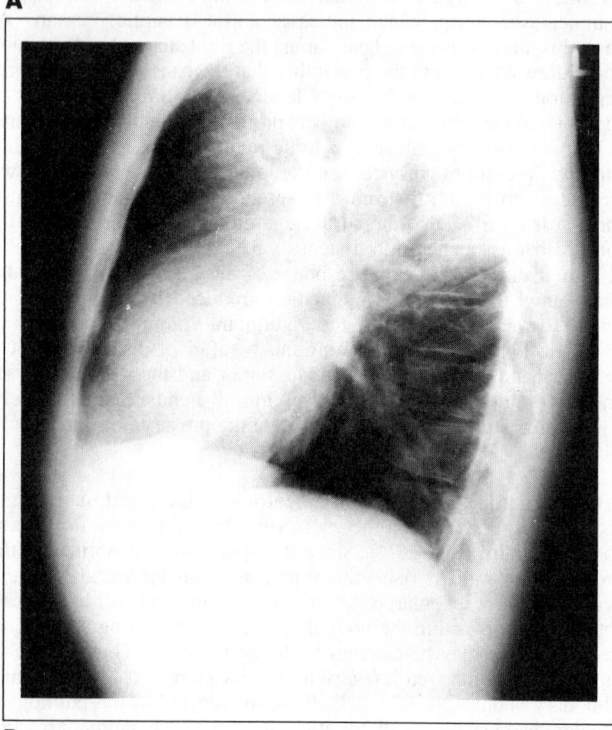

FIGURE 25-4   Chest radiograph in the frontal **(A)** and left lateral **(B)** projection in a patient with severe aortic regurgitation. The ascending aorta and left ventricle are enlarged.

the mitral valve (Chapter 13). Echocardiography is of particular value for excluding the presence of associated mitral stenosis in patients with an Austin Flint diastolic murmur. Left ventricular dimensions are increased, and if ventricular function is normal, the percentage of dimensional shortening is normal. Because of the increase in left ventricular dimensions caused by the volume overload, there is separation between the open anterior leaflet of the mitral valve and the endocardial surface of the interventricular septum (septal–E point separation), but this does not necessarily indicate impaired left ventricu-

lar function when aortic regurgitation is present. In aortic regurgitation, as in other volume-overloaded lesions, the response in mild volume overload is an elongation of the heart. Since M-mode echocardiography takes a pencil look at the short axis of the heart, left ventricular dimensions by M-mode echocardiography may appear to be normal. 2D echocardiography (Chapter 13) is much superior to the M-mode technique for assessing left ventricular volumes and systolic function in such patients. A dilated ascending aorta can be detected on echocardiography and so can an enlarged left atrium. Aortic valve vegetations suggest infective endocarditis. Some unusual conditions can easily be detected by echocardiography, for example, prolapse of the aortic leaflet into the left ventricle in diastole. Doppler echocardiography (Chapter 13) is useful for diagnosing and assessing the severity of aortic regurgitation. There is a significant incidence of false positives in the mild grade. There is also an overlap between the various grades of severity of assessment of aortic regurgitation by Doppler when compared to angiography. Transesophageal echocardiography is a useful technique when a transthoracic echocardiogram is unsatisfactory and in certain instances to identify the anatomy of the valve leaflets, aortic root, and annulus. Echocardiography/Doppler ultrasound is also very useful to assess disease of other valves.

Cardiac catheterization allows the measurement of intracardiac and intravascular pressures and cardiac output both at rest and on exercise and demonstrates the changes described under Abnormal Physiology. In addition, other valvular diseases, for example mitral stenosis, aortic stenosis, and mitral regurgitation, can be excluded. Left ventricular angiography demonstrates enlarged left ventricular volumes and allows the calculation of ejection fraction. Angiography performed with injection of contrast medium in the ascending aorta demonstrates aortic regurgitation and allows a semiquantitative assessment of the degree of aortic regurgitation (Chapter 14). In addition, the angiogram demonstrates the dimension of the aortic root and the state of the ascending aorta. Selective coronary angiography allows assessment of the site, severity, and extent of associated obstructive coronary artery disease and should be performed in patients with angina, those with left ventricular systolic dysfunction, those with risk factors for coronary artery disease, and those 35 years of age or older who are being considered for surgery.

Gated blood pool radionuclide scans also allow the measurement of left ventricular volumes and ejection fraction. In addition, with this technique it is now possible to quantify the amount of aortic regurgitation. However, these scans assess regurgitation present at both the aortic and mitral valves. Thus, if both valves are incompetent, the total amount of regurgitation present at both valves will be evaluated. This technique also allows measurement of left ventricular ejection fraction on exercise and on serial studies.

A treadmill exercise test provides an objective assessment of the degree of functional impairment and documentation of arrhythmias related to exertion.

Ambulatory ECG recording may be needed in an occasional patient suspected of having an arrhythmia.

Natural History and Prognosis

Patients with mild aortic regurgitation that does not progress should have a normal life expectancy. Their major risk is the development of infective endocarditis and further valve destruction. Patients with moderate aortic regurgitation, if their disease does not progress, would be expected to have a life expectancy that is reasonably close to the normal range. However, the disease does progress, and mortality at the end of 10 years appears to be about 15%.

Patients with severe aortic regurgitation are known to have a long asymptomatic period before the condition is discovered. In asymptomatic patients with normal left ventricular function at rest, symptoms and/or left ventricular dysfunction and/or sudden death developed at the rate of 3% to 6% per year. The predictor of development of symptoms is left ventricular systolic dysfunction at rest. In those with normal left ventricular systolic function at rest, the predictors are an increased left ventricular size (left ventricular dimension at end-diastole of ≥ 70 mm, at end-systole of ≥ 50 mm, and left ventricular end-diastolic volume index of ≥ 150 ml/m^2) and abnormal left-ventricular ejection fraction on exercise of <0.50. Sudden death in asymptomatic patients appears to occur only in those with a massively dilated left ventricle (left ventricular end-diastolic dimension of ≥ 80 mm). It is likely that left ventricular dysfunction first appears on exercise and later also at rest; eventually, heart failure ensues. However, severe symptoms may occur even when left ventricular systolic pump function is normal at rest. The 5-year mortality of symptomatic patients with severe aortic regurgitation is about 25% and the 10-year mortality averages 50%. Once symptoms occur in patients with aortic regurgitation, it is likely that the rate of deterioration will be rapid. Most patients with angina are dead within 4 years. The 2- to 3-year mortality of those in heart failure is 50% to 70%. The overall 5-year and 10-year mortalities after appearance of mild to moderate symptoms without overt heart failure are approximately 30% and 50%, respectively.

Management. All patients with aortic regurgitation need antibiotic prophylaxis to prevent infective endocarditis (Chapter 24). Patients with aortic regurgitation of a rheumatic origin need antibiotic prophylaxis to prevent recurrences of rheumatic carditis (Chapter 204). Patients with syphilitic aortic regurgitation need a course of antibiotics to treat syphilis.

Patients with mild aortic regurgitation need no specific therapy. They do not need to restrict their activities and can lead a normal life. Patients with moderate aortic regurgitation also usually need no specific therapy. However, these patients should avoid heavy physical exertion, competitive sports, and isometric exercise.

Patients with severe aortic regurgitation need medical treatment and eventually surgical treatment, which usually consists of valve replacement. Medical treatment consists of the administration of digitalis, diuretics, and vasodilators. Digitalis acts by increasing myocardial contractility, often reducing end-diastolic volume while increasing the ejection fraction and also the cardiac output if it is reduced in the resting state. Digitalis is clearly indicated in patients with symptoms. The need for and benefits of this therapy in asymptomatic patients have not been well documented. Diuretics are of value when the left atrial pressure is elevated and in the presence of congestive heart failure.

Vasodilators are either arterial, venous, or both. Vasodilators act by reducing the peripheral arterial resistance, which favors forward cardiac output and reduces regurgitant volume; initially, the total left ventricular stroke volume remains unchanged. If the left atrial pressure is elevated and left ventricular ejection fraction reduced, vasodilators frequently result in an improvement in both.

The value of long-term vasodilators in asymptomatic patients has been evaluated in placebo-controlled randomized trials. Hydralazine produced modest reduction of end-diastolic volume and increase in ejection fraction; however, because of side effects, long-term compliance (1 to 2 years) was poor. A calcium-channel blocking agent, nifedipine, produced significant reduction in blood pressure and left ventricular end-diastolic volume and mass, and major increases in left ventricular ejection fraction. Almost all patients completed the 1-year trial. Recently, a prospective randomized trial in *asymptomatic* patients with *normal* left ventricular systolic function showed that at the end of 6 years, 34 ± 6% of patients treated with digoxin developed left ventricular systolic dysfunction and/or symptoms and thus needed valve replacement compared with 15 ± 3% of patients treated with long-acting nifedipine ($P < 0.001$) (Fig. 25-5). All asymptomatic patients with severe aortic regurgitation and normal left ventricular systolic function should be treated with a vasodilator (calcium-channel blocking agent, long-acting nifedipine) unless there is a contraindication to its use. Long-term hydralazine therapy in symptomatic patients results in significant benefit in 20% to 35% of patients. Vasodilators are indicated in patients who refuse surgery or are not operative candidates for any reason. It is also indicated for short-term therapy in patients awaiting valve replacement to optimize their hemodynamics (reduce filling pressures and increase cardiac output) and thus reduce their operative risks.

Vasodilators are of considerable short-term benefit in patients in functional classes III and IV but ideally should be started after the institution of hemodynamic monitoring, that is, measurement of pulmonary artery wedge pressure and cardiac output with the use of balloon flotation catheters. Hemodynamic monitoring identifies patients who need the therapy, whereas clinical judgments can be wrong. It

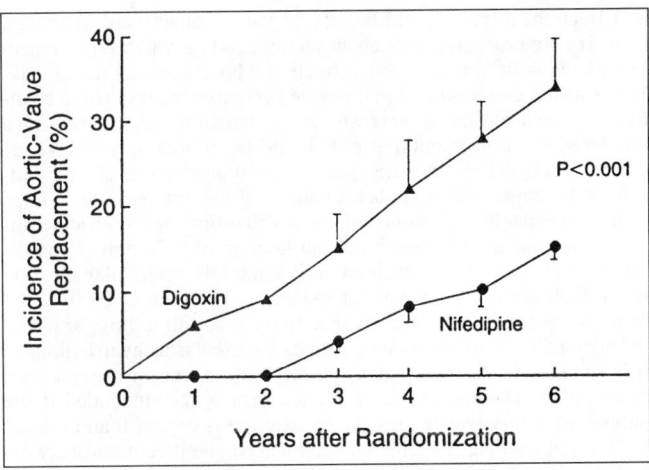

FIGURE 25-5 Cumulative actuarial incidence of progression to aortic replacement in the patients assigned to digoxin and to nifedipine therapies. Data from a prospective randomized trial in asymptomatic patients with normal left ventricular systolic function who had chronic, severe aortic regurgitation.

From Scognamiglio R et al: *N Engl J Med* 331:689, 1994.

establishes whether arterial dilators alone will suffice or additional venodilators are needed. Finally, it provides information on the optimum dosage of vasodilator therapy. After the initial hemodynamic measurements are made, arterial dilators are given in progressively increasing dosage until an optimum effect on cardiac output has been obtained. If cardiac output does not show any further increase but left atrial pressure is still very high, additional venodilator therapy should be given. If the patient is very ill or the hemodynamic abnormalities are marked, intravenous therapy (e.g., sodium nitroprusside) may be the vasodilator of first choice. Small doses of hydralazine (≤50 mg) are without therapeutic effect and larger doses (≥150 mg) need to be given only twice daily. The twice-daily regimen reduces the incidence of side effects and can be expected to improve patient compliance. Alternatively, patients can be given angiotensin-converting enzyme inhibitors; however, benefit of such therapy except for treatment of associated left ventricular dysfunction has not been documented.

Patients with severe chronic aortic regurgitation need valve replacement. The correct timing of surgical therapy has not been fully clarified. Valve replacement should be performed before irreversible left ventricular dysfunction occurs. However, the major problem is identifying the precise point at which left ventricular dysfunction will occur. Here, two major difficulties are encountered: (1) Patients may already have impaired left ventricular systolic pump function at rest when they first present or at the time of the first symptom; and (2) patients with severe symptoms may have normal left ventricular systolic pump function. Patients may be in functional class III (symptoms with less than ordinary activity), with a normal left ventricular ejection fraction, or they may be in functional class I (asymptomatic), with a reduced left ventricular ejection fraction. A reduced ejection fraction by 2D echocardiography and/or radionuclide ventriculography are the best noninvasive indicators of depressed systolic ventricular function (Chapter 13).

Decisions about surgery in aortic regurgitation should be based on the functional class and on the left ventricular ejection fraction at rest. Patients with chronic severe aortic regurgitation who are in functional class III or IV (symptoms at rest) need valve replacement. Benefit from valve replacement has been demonstrated even when the left ventricular ejection fraction is 0.25 or less. As opposed to aortic stenosis, in which no lower level of ejection fraction indicates inoperability, it is likely that some patients with aortic regurgitation and a low ejection fraction will become inoperable. This level has not been precisely defined but may be about 0.15 or less. Patients who are in functional class II (symptoms with ordinary activity) and those who have impaired left ventricular systolic pump function (reduced ejection fraction) at rest should be offered valve replacement. Although there is some disagreement about recommending valve replacement to patients with normal ejection fraction who are in functional class II, we would do so. Although the issue is controversial in some countries, we believe that patients who are in functional class I and have a reduced ejection fraction at rest should be offered aortic valve replacement. If the ejection fraction is normal at rest, one should consider valve replacement in class I patients if the left ventricle is huge (left ventricular end-diastolic volume $\geq$150 ml/m^2, left ventricular internal dimension on M-mode echocardiogram of $\geq$70 mm at end diastole, $\geq$50 mm at end systole) and/or the left ventricular ejection fraction shows a new, persistent reduction to $\leq$0.54 to 0.60, if the patients have reduced exercise capacity on treadmill testing, or if ambulatory ECG monitoring demonstrates ventricular tachyarrhythmias. It is suggested that such patients undergo an exercise test with right heart catheterization, and valve replacement is recommended if the pulmonary artery wedge pressure on exercise is greater than or equal to 20 to 24 mm Hg. Patients with associated significant coronary artery disease should have coronary bypass surgery performed at the time of valvular surgery.

Aortic valve replacement, with or without associated coronary bypass surgery for obstructive coronary disease, can be performed at many surgical centers with an operative mortality of 5% or less. In those without associated coronary artery disease or reduced left ventricular systolic function, the operative mortality may be in the 1% to 2% range. If aortic valve replacement is successful and uncomplicated, left ventricular volume and hypertrophy regress but do not return to normal. Impaired left ventricular systolic pump function improves postoperatively in 50% or more of the patients; recent data show improvement is more likely to occur if left ventricular dysfunction was present preoperatively for 12 to 14 months or less. Even if left ventricular systolic pump function does not improve, there is a reduction in end-diastolic volume and hypertrophy; from a cardiac point of view, this is advantageous to the patient. The 5-year survival of patients undergoing aortic valve replacement in severe aortic regurgitation is 85% (includes operative and late cardiac deaths). The 5-year survival of patients with a left ventricular ejection fraction of 0.45 or greater is 87% versus 54% in patients with an ejection fraction less than 0.45. Late survival after valve replacement for chronic severe aortic regurgitation is best predicted by variables indicative of left ventricular systolic pump function.

New techniques of aortic valve repair are being developed and evaluated. Eventually, it is possible that some patients may need to have valve repair rather than valve replacement for aortic regurgitation.

ACUTE AORTIC REGURGITATION
Etiology

Infective endocarditis is the usual etiology of acute aortic regurgitation. It may also be caused by aortic dissection and trauma to the heart. Severe systemic hypertension is often associated with transient aortic regurgitation, which disappears as the blood pressure is brought under control.

Abnormal Physiology

The major difference between acute and chronic severe aortic regurgitation is the extent of left ventricular enlargement. The left ventricle is large in chronic aortic regurgitation but is only somewhat dilated in patients with acute aortic regurgitation. However, there is a limit to how much the left ventricle can increase its volume acutely (probably no more than 20% to 30%) and the left ventricle often appears normal both on physical examination and on the chest x-ray. Nevertheless, the increase in left ventricular volume is inadequate for the amount of regurgitation. Since the left ventricle is only slightly increased in size, the increase in left ventricular stroke volume is limited even if the ejection fraction is increased. Most of the left ventricular stroke volume is regurgitated back into the left ventricle; as a result, the forward stroke volume to the body and the cardiac output may be severely compromised in spite of a marked compensatory sinus tachycardia. An acute increase in left ventricular end-diastolic volume results in a marked increase in left ventricular end-diastolic pres-

sure, because the left ventricle is operating on the steep portion of the diastolic pressure-volume curve. If, in addition, the left atrial pressure is normal or mildly increased, the mitral valve may close prematurely. If the left atrial pressure rises considerably, pulmonary edema and passive pulmonary hypertension commonly occur. Compensatory tachycardia is the rule; it helps to shorten diastole, hence the time available for aortic regurgitation to occur, and attempts to maintain the cardiac output. The left ventricular and aortic systolic pressures remain normal. The aortic diastolic pressure cannot fall below the elevated left ventricular end-diastolic pressure, and thus the arterial pulse pressure may be in the normal range. It is important to recognize that left ventricular systolic pump function is frequently normal in these patients at least in the initial stages.

Clinical Manifestations

The patient may have a history of trauma and exhibit the clinical features of infective endocarditis. Usually, however, the symptoms of heart failure are predominant.

On physical examination, these patients have tachycardia. The peripheral pulse shows a rapid rate of rise in arterial pressure, but the systolic pressure is normal. The diastolic pressure is normal or even reduced, and the pulse pressure is often normal. Thus, although the classic peripheral signs of chronic severe aortic regurgitation are often absent, an important diagnostic clue is the rapid rate of rise of arterial pressure. If there is frank congestive heart failure, the usual clinical manifestations of heart failure are present. The left ventricle is often hyperkinetic. The S_1 is soft; the S_2 is soft and often single. There is usually a loud diastolic gallop (S_3). An aortic systolic murmur is often present, and the classic early or immediate diastolic murmur of aortic regurgitation is present. An Austin Flint murmur may be heard.

The ECG often shows nonspecific ST-T wave changes and a sinus tachycardia. However, the ECG may be normal. The chest radiograph shows that the cardiothoracic ratio may be within the normal range. The aorta is not dilated unless aortic root disease or dissection of the aorta is the cause of the acute regurgitation. The lung fields show the signs of increased pulmonary venous pressure and of pulmonary edema.

One must be aware of the typical clinical picture of patients with gross acute aortic regurgitation in severe heart failure to recognize it. These patients are often intravenous drug abusers and have marked sinus tachycardia and pulmonary edema. However, an aortic diastolic murmur may be absent or difficult to appreciate, which often causes the diagnosis to be missed. The chest x-ray shows a "normal" heart size with pulmonary edema. The important diagnostic clues include (1) a peripheral arterial pulse that has a rapid rate of rise and fall, even though the pulse pressure is small; (2) the telltale signs of intravenous drug abuse; and (3) "normal" heart size with pulmonary edema on chest x-ray.

Echocardiography shows the diastolic flutter of the anterior leaflet of the mitral valve. In addition, the echocardiogram may show vegetations on the aortic valve, prolapse of an aortic valve leaflet into the left ventricle in diastole, and premature mitral valve closure. The mitral valve may be seen to open for only a short time because the stroke volume is limited. Occasionally, the aortic valve leaflets have been totally destroyed, and none is seen on the echocardiogram. Doppler ultrasound can easily demonstrate the aortic regurgitation and provide an estimate of its severity. For detection of dissection of the aorta, infective endocarditis, and in acutely ill patients, transesophageal echocardiography/Doppler ultrasound is overall probably the best of the noninvasive tests for most patients (Chapter 30). Magnetic resonance imaging has a very high specificity for diagnosis of dissection of the aorta and may be used in stable patients if the diagnosis has not already been made. Cardiac catheterization and angiography show the abnormal physiology described, and aortography shows gross aortic regurgitation. A radionuclide gated blood pool scan may be helpful in demonstrating normal left ventricular ejection fraction and a mild increase in left ventricular volume.

The natural history of this condition is variable. If the aortic regurgitation is mild to moderate in severity, these patients are likely to do well with medical therapy. Eventually, the changes of chronic aortic regurgitation will be seen. In patients with severe aortic regurgitation, the natural history depends on whether they have heart failure. If heart failure is present, which is common, the prognosis is very poor without valve surgery.

Management

The underlying cause of the regurgitation must be treated, which often is difficult. In patients with infective endocarditis, the appropriate antibiotic therapy has to be given. If the aortic regurgitation is mild, no other specific therapy may be needed. If aortic regurgitation is moderate, digitalis therapy and vasodilators may be beneficial. Aortic regurgitation caused by dissection of the aorta is an indication for surgery regardless of the degree of regurgitation.

For patients with severe aortic regurgitation, the choices of medical therapy include digitalis, diuretics, and vasodilators. Patients with heart failure should be given digitalis, diuretics, and vasodilators. In patients with moderate or severe heart failure, despite medical therapy, aortic valve replacement is indicated. If the patient responds dramatically to digitalis, diuretics, and vasodilators, surgical therapy often can be delayed until heart failure and the infection (when caused by endocarditis) are controlled, and the patient is in a more stable condition. If the patient does not respond immediately and dramatically to therapy, valve replacement should not be delayed, even if the infection is uncontrolled or the patient has had little antibiotic therapy.

MITRAL STENOSIS
Etiology

Mitral stenosis is an obstruction to blood flow between the left atrium and the left ventricle caused by abnormal mitral valve function. Congenital mitral stenosis is uncommon. It is usually caused by a "parachute" deformity of the valve in which shortened chordae tendineae insert in a large, single papillary muscle. In virtually all adult patients, the cause of mitral stenosis is previous rheumatic carditis. However, about 60% of patients with rheumatic mitral valve disease do not give a history of rheumatic fever or chorea, and about 50% of patients with acute rheumatic carditis do not eventually have clinical valvular heart disease. Mitral stenosis, usually rheumatic, in association with atrial septal defect is called *Lutembacher's syndrome*. A rare cause of mitral stenosis is massive mitral valve anular calcification. This process occurs most frequently in elderly women and produces mitral stenosis by limiting leaflet motion. The degree of stenosis, when present, is usually mild. Other causes of obstruction to left atrial outflow include a left atrial myxoma, massive left atrial ball thrombus, and cor triatriatum, in which a congenital membrane is present in the left atrium.

Pathology

In temperate climates and developed countries, there is usually a long interval (an average of 20 years) between an episode of rheumatic carditis and the clinical presentation of symptomatic mitral stenosis. In tropical and subtropical climates and in less developed countries, the latent period is often shorter, and mitral stenosis may occur during childhood or adolescence. The pathologic hallmark of rheumatic carditis is Aschoff's nodule. The most common lesion of acute rheumatic endocarditis is mitral valvulitis. The mitral valve has vegetations along the line of closure and chordae tendineae. Mitral regurgitation may be present during the acute episode.

Mitral stenosis is usually the result of repeated episodes of carditis alternating with healing and is characterized by the deposition of fibrous tissue. Ultimately, the deformed valve is subject to nonspecific fibrosis and calcification. Lesions along the line of closure result in fusion of the commissures and contracture and thickening of the valve leaflets. The chordal lesions are manifested as shortening and fusion of these structures. The combination of commissural fusion, valve leaflet contracture, and chordae tendineae fusion results in a narrow, funnel-shaped orifice, which restricts the flow of blood from the left atrium to the left ventricle. The rapidity with which patients become symptomatic with this lesion may depend on the number and severity of repeated bouts of rheumatic valvulitis. Frequently, the rheumatic episodes are not clinically apparent.

In pure mitral stenosis, the left ventricle is usually normal, but there may be evidence of previous carditis with deposition of fibrous tissue. The left atrium is enlarged and hypertrophied as a consequence of left atrial hypertension. Mural thrombi are often found in the left atrium, particularly if atrial fibrillation has been present. Calcification of the mitral valve frequently also involves the mitral anulus.

Abnormal Physiology

The pathophysiologic features of mitral stenosis all result from obstruction of the flow of blood between the left atrium and the left ventricle. With reduction in valve area, energy is lost to friction during the transport of blood from the left atrium to the left ventricle. Accordingly, a pressure gradient is present across the stenotic valve. The relationship between valve area, cardiac output, flow period, and average diastolic gradient between the left atrium and the left ventricle is defined by the formula of Gorlin and Gorlin (Chapter 14).

It is readily apparent that maintaining cardiac output when the valve area is small requires a large gradient and thus elevated left atrial pressure. Similarly, an increased demand for cardiac output, such as occurs during exercise or in pregnancy, results in an increase in gradient and high left atrial pressures. More subtle is the effect of the length of the diastolic flow period on the relationship between output and gradient. The time available for diastole is that part of the cardiac cycle not taken up by isovolumetric contraction and relaxation or by ejection. As the heart rate increases, the total amount of time spent during systole increases despite a reduction in the systolic time per beat. Thus, time available for diastole decreases as the heart rate increases. Because blood can flow through the mitral valve only during diastole, the flow rate is inversely proportional to the flow period at a constant cardiac output. Of course, a higher flow rate results in a greater loss of energy to friction and requires a larger gradient and higher left atrial pressures.

The pressure gradient between the left atrium and the left ventricle, which increases markedly with increased heart rate or cardiac output, is responsible for left atrial hypertension. The left atrium gradually enlarges and hypertrophies. Pulmonary venous pressure rises with left atrial pressure and is passively associated with an increase in pulmonary arterial pressure (Fig. 25-6). In up to 20% of patients, the pulmonary vascular resistance is also elevated, which further increases pulmonary artery pressure. Pulmonary arterial hypertension results in right ventricular hypertrophy and right ventricular enlargement. The changes in right ventricular function eventually result in right atrial hypertension and enlargement, in systemic congestion, and frequently in tricuspid regurgitation also.

Pulmonary venous hypertension alters lung function in several ways. Distribution of blood flow in the lung is altered, with a relative increase in flow to the upper lobes and therefore in physiologic dead space. Pulmonary compliance generally decreases with increasing pulmonary capillary pressure, adding to the work of breathing, particularly during exercise. Chronic changes in the pulmonary capillaries and pulmonary arteries include fibrosis and thickening. These changes protect the lungs from transudation of fluid into the alveoli (pulmonary edema). Indeed, it is not uncommon to find patients with severe mitral stenosis whose resting pulmonary artery wedge pressure (indirect left atrial pressure) exceeds 30 mm Hg. However, capillary and alveolar thickening further add to the abnormalities of ventilation and perfusion. Pulmonary vascular changes result in increasingly elevated pulmonary vascular resistance.

In some patients with high pulmonary vascular resistance and right ventricular dysfunction, cardiac output may be low. The body maintains oxygen consumption by extracting more oxygen from the arterial blood, and mixed venous oxygen content falls. The hemoglobin oxygen dissociation curve is shifted to the right, facilitating the unloading of oxygen from hemoglobin to the tissues. The reduced cardiac output results in surprisingly small gradients across the mitral valve despite severe stenosis. Although pulmonary congestion may be less striking in these patients, the cardiac output does not increase normally with exercise, and, typically, the patients are severely limited by fatigue.

Long-standing mitral stenosis with severe pulmonary hypertension and resultant right ventricular dysfunction may be accompanied by chronic systemic venous hypertension. Tricuspid regurgitation is fre-

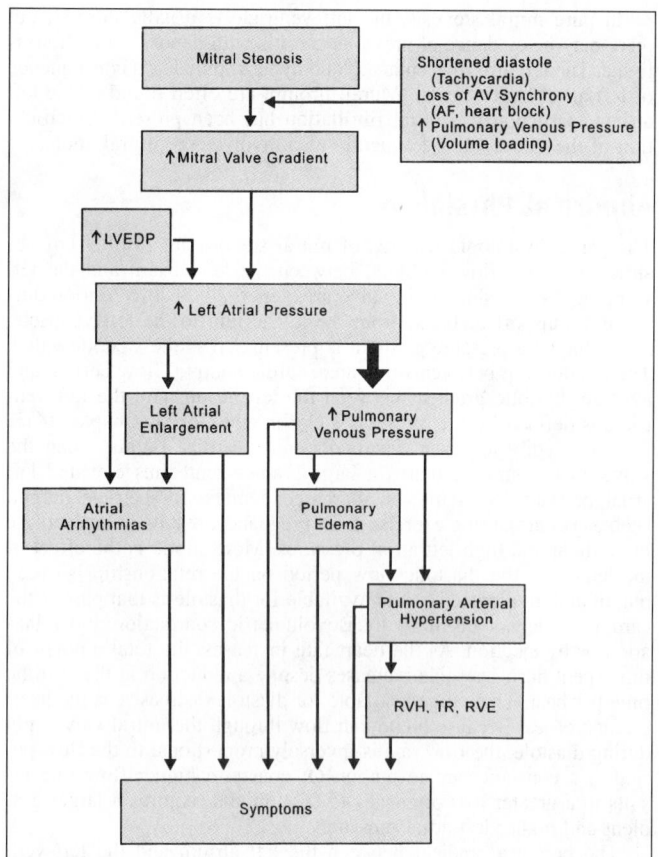

FIGURE 25-6   Some aspects of the pathophysiology in mitral stenosis. Mitral stenosis results in a diastolic pressure gradient from the left atrium to the left ventricle. The actual gradient is dependent on the mitral valve area and the mitral valve *flow per diastolic second.* As a result, there is an elevation of left atrial pressure and, therefore, also of pulmonary venous pressure. Physiologic and pathologic changes, such as tachycardia and atrial fibrillation (which shorten diastole and may also result in loss of effective atrial contraction) or pregnancy, volume loading, and left-to-right shunts (at ventricular and aortopulmonary levels), which increase pulmonary venous flow, will increase the mitral valve gradient, left atrial, and pulmonary venous pressures. An increased left ventricular diastolic pressure will also result in further increase of left atrial pressure.

An elevated left atrial pressure has several important effects; these include enlargement of the left atrium, atrial arrhythmias, and an increase of pulmonary venous pressure. Pulmonary venous hypertension may result in pulmonary edema and pulmonary arterial hypertension. Pulmonary arterial hypertension and right ventricular hypertension result in right ventricular hypertrophy, and may result in tricuspid regurgitation and right ventricular enlargement. All of these changes contribute to producing symptoms. In addition, a fixed or even reduced cardiac output will also contribute to the symptomatic state of the patient.

From Kawanishi DT, Rahimtoola SH: Mitral valve stenosis. In Rahimtoola SH, editor: Valvular heart disease and endocarditis. In Braunwald E, editor-in-chief: *Atlas of the heart,* Philadelphia, Current Medicine, 1997.

quently present, even in the absence of intrinsic disease of this valve. Functional pulmonic regurgitation may also be present. Dependent edema formation and visceral congestion directly reflect elevated venous pressure and salt and water retention. Chronic passive congestion in the liver leads to central lobular necrosis and eventually cirrhosis.

Clinical Manifestations

History. An asymptomatic interval is usually present between the initiating event of acute rheumatic fever and the presentation of symptomatic mitral stenosis. During this interval, the patient feels well. Initially, there is little or no gradient at rest, but with increased cardiac output, left atrial pressure rises, and exertional dyspnea devel-

ops. As mitral valve obstruction increases, dyspnea occurs at lower work levels. The progression of disability is so subtle and so protracted that many patients adapt by circumscribing their lifestyles. It becomes imperative, then, to document what activities the patient can perform without symptoms, and at what activity level symptoms begin; failure to do this often results in an underestimation of disability.

As obstruction progresses, the patients note orthopnea and nocturnal dyspnea that apparently results from redistribution of blood to the thorax on assuming the supine position. With severe mitral stenosis and elevated pulmonary vascular resistance, fatigue rather than dyspnea may be the predominant symptom. Dependent edema, nausea, anorexia, and right upper quadrant pain reflect systemic venous congestion resulting from right heart failure.

Palpitations are a frequent complaint in mitral stenosis and may represent frequent premature atrial contractions or paroxysmal atrial fibrillation. Of patients with severe symptomatic mitral stenosis, 50% or more have chronic atrial fibrillation. Paroxysmal atrial fibrillation may produce pulmonary edema in some patients with mitral stenosis. The acute increase in left atrial pressure that produces pulmonary edema results both from a decrease in the diastolic flow period caused by increased heart rate and from a loss of atrial transport function.

Systemic embolism, a frequent complication of mitral stenosis, may result in stroke, occlusion of extremity arterial supply, occlusion of the aortic bifurcation, or visceral or myocardial infarction. Atrial fibrillation, increasing age of the patient, increasing left atrial size, and a previous history of embolism are associated with an increased incidence of systemic embolism. Hemoptysis may result from increased pulmonary venous pressure. Blood streaking of pulmonary edema fluid may result, or hemoptysis may be severe and, rarely, life-threatening. Pulmonary embolism, which is more common in patients with heart failure, also may cause hemoptysis.

Exertional chest pain, typical of angina pectoris, may be present in some patients with severe mitral stenosis but normal coronary arteries. Severe pulmonary hypertension has been postulated as a cause. Infective endocarditis is an uncommon complication of pure mitral stenosis.

Progression of symptoms in mitral stenosis is generally slow but relentless. Thus, a sudden change in symptoms rarely reflects a change in valve obstruction. Rather, there usually is a noncardiac precipitating event or paroxysmal atrial fibrillation. Fever, pregnancy, and noncardiac surgery, all of which increase cardiac output, can precipitate decompensation in patients with moderate to severe obstruction.

Physical Findings. During the latent, presymptomatic interval, incidental physical findings may be normal or may provide evidence of mild mitral stenosis. Frequently, the only characteristic finding noted at rest will be a loud S_1 and a presystolic murmur. A short diastolic decrescendo rumble may be heard only with exercise. In patients with symptomatic mitral stenosis, the findings are more obvious, and careful physical examination usually leads to the correct diagnosis.

The general appearance of the patient in mitral stenosis is usually normal. The mitral stenosis facies, characterized by malar flush, is uncommon and is caused by peripheral cyanosis, which is usually associated with a low cardiac output and severe pulmonary hypertension. Tachypnea may be present if left atrial pressure is high. The jugular venous pressure may be normal or may show evidence of elevated right ventricular end-diastolic pressure or tricuspid regurgitation (Chapter 11). Atrial fibrillation produces an irregular venous pulse with absent A waves. The arterial pulse is normal except for irregularity in atrial fibrillation and low volume when cardiac output is reduced. All peripheral pulses should be carefully examined because of the frequency of systemic embolism. The chest findings may be normal or may reveal signs of pulmonary congestion with rales or pleural fluid (dullness and absent breath sounds). Marked left atrial enlargement may produce egophony at the tip of the left scapula.

The precordium is usually unremarkable on inspection. On palpation, the apical impulse should feel normal. An abnormal left ventricular impulse suggests disease other than pure mitral stenosis. A diastolic thrill usually is appreciated only when the patient is examined in the left lateral decubitus position. When pulmonary hypertension is present, a sustained right ventricular lift along the left sternal border and pulmonic valve closure may be palpable. On auscultation in the supine position, the only abnormality appreciated may be the accentuated S_1. Failure to examine the patient in the left lateral decubitus position accounts for most of the misdiagnoses of symptomatic mitral stenosis. The diastolic rumble is heard best with the bell of the stethoscope applied at the apical impulse. Nevertheless, the murmur may be localized, and the region around the apical impulse also should be auscultated. The opening snap is heard best with the diaphragm and is often most easily appreciated midway between the apex and the left sternal border. In this intermediate region, the S_1, the pulmonary component of the second heart sound (P_2), and the opening snap can be identified.

The opening snap occurs after the left ventricular pressure falls below left atrial pressure in early diastole. When left atrial pressure is high, as in severe mitral stenosis, the snap occurs early in diastole. The converse is true with mild mitral stenosis. The interval between the A_2 and the opening snap varies from 40 to 120 ms. Although the opening snap is present in most cases of mitral stenosis, it is absent in patients with stiff, fibrotic, or calcified leaflets. Thus, absence of the opening snap in severe mitral stenosis indicates that mitral valve replacement rather than commissurotomy may be necessary.

The diastolic rumble follows the opening snap. In some patients with low cardiac output or mild mitral stenosis, brief exercise, such as sit-ups or walking, is adequate to increase flow and bring out the murmur. The murmur is low pitched, rumbling, and decrescendo. In general, the more severe the mitral stenosis, the longer the murmur. Presystolic accentuation of the murmur occurs in sinus rhythm and has been reported even in atrial fibrillation. A diastolic rumble is not diagnostic of mitral stenosis (Chapter 11).

Systolic murmurs also may be heard in association with the murmur of mitral stenosis. A blowing holosystolic murmur at the apex suggests associated mitral regurgitation, whereas a systolic blowing murmur heard best at the lower left sternal border that increases with inspiration usually signifies tricuspid regurgitation. The Graham Steell murmur is a high-pitched diastolic decrescendo murmur of pulmonic regurgitation caused by pulmonary hypertension. In most patients with mitral stenosis, such a murmur usually indicates aortic regurgitation. In general, a left-sided third heart sound (S_3) is not compatible with important mitral stenosis, with the possible exception of concomitant severe aortic regurgitation and significant left ventricular systolic dysfunction. If an S_3 and a rumble are present, mitral regurgitation is usually the predominant lesion.

Chest Radiograph. The posteroanterior and lateral chest films are often so typical that experienced clinicians can make the tentative diagnosis from the film before the history and physical examination are complete (Fig. 25-7). The thoracic cage is normal. The lung fields show evidence of elevated pulmonary venous pressure. Blood flow is redistributed to the upper lobes, resulting in prominence of upper lobe vascularity. Increased pulmonary venous pressure results in transudation of fluid into the interstitium. Accumulation of fluid in the interlobular septa produces linear streaks in the bases, which extend to the pleura (Kerley B lines). Interstitial fluid may also be seen as perivascular or peribronchial cuffing. With transudation of fluid into the alveolar spaces, pulmonary edema is seen. Chronic hemosiderin deposition results in an interstitial radiodensity that does not resolve after the relief of stenosis. Pulmonary hypertension results in enlargement of the main pulmonary trunk and right and left main pulmonary arteries. These changes are not specific for mitral stenosis but represent long-standing elevated left atrial pressure.

The cardiac silhouette usually does not show generalized cardiomegaly, but the left atrium is invariably enlarged. This is manifested in the posteroanterior film by a density behind the right atrial border (double atrial shadow), prominence of the left atrial appendage on the left heart border between the main pulmonary artery and left ventricular apex, and elevation of the left main bronchus. The lateral film shows the left atrium bulging posteriorly. The left ventricular silhouette is normal. The right ventricle may be enlarged if pulmonary hypertension has been present. Right ventricular enlargement is usually noted by filling of the retrosternal space but is an unreliable sign in adults. The combination of a normal-sized left ventricle, enlarged left atrium, and pulmonary congestion should immediately raise the possibility of mitral stenosis. Mitral valve calcification is occasionally seen on the plain chest film.

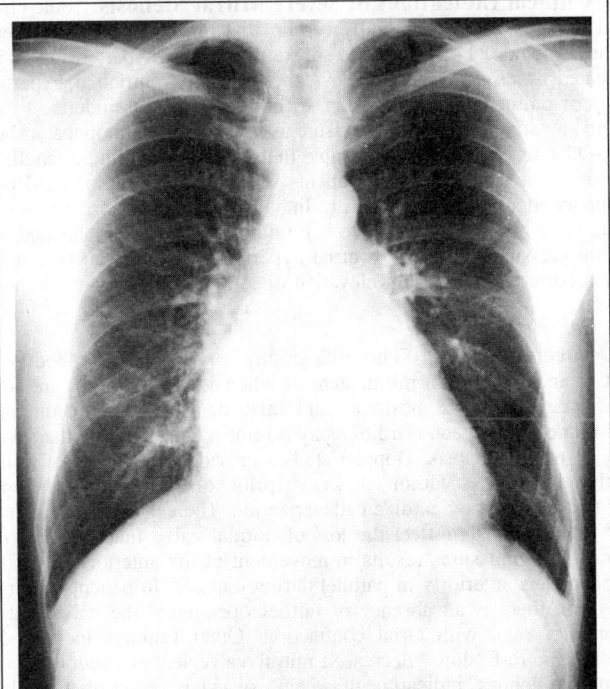

A

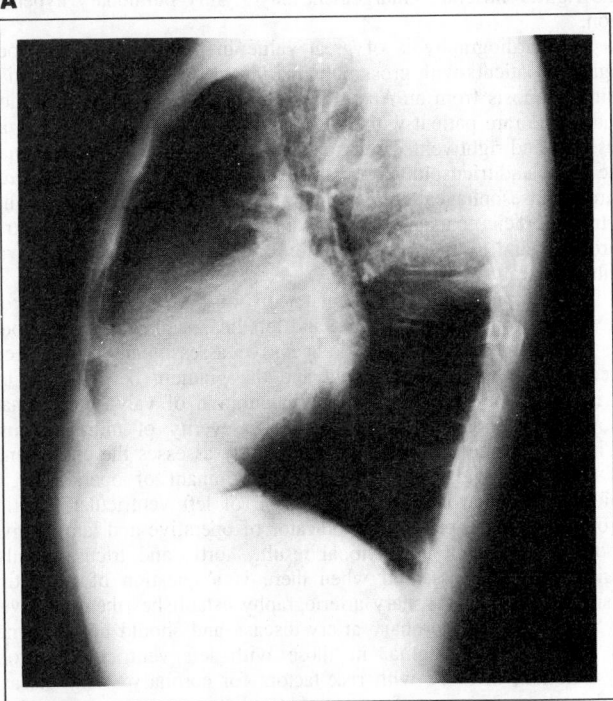

B

FIGURE 25-7 Chest radiograph in the frontal **(A)** and left lateral **(B)** projection in a patient with severe mitral stenosis. Marked left atrial enlargement and pulmonary vascular engorgement are present in the absence of left ventricular enlargement.

Electrocardiogram. The ECG is not usually as helpful as the chest x-ray. For patients in sinus rhythm, the widened P wave is caused by interatrial conduction delay and/or prolonged left atrial depolarization (Chapter 12). The P wave is broad and notched in lead II and biphasic in lead V_1, and measures 0.12 s or more. Atrial fibrillation is common. Left ventricular hypertrophy is almost never present unless there are associated lesions. Right ventricular hypertrophy may be present if pulmonary hypertension is marked.

Clinical Indications of Severe Mitral Stenosis. Some clinical features make it virtually certain that mitral stenosis is severe. These include (1) moderate to severe pulmonary hypertension as indicated by clinical and ECG evidence of right ventricular hypertrophy or pulmonary hypertension, or both, and/or (2) moderate to severe elevation of left atrial pressure as indicated by orthopnea, a short P_2-OS interval, a diastolic rumble that occupies the whole length of a long diastolic interval in patients with atrial fibrillation, and pulmonary edema on the chest x-ray. In both these clinical circumstances, one must be certain that there is no other cause for the elevated left atrial pressure and that left atrial hypertension is not caused mainly by a correctable transient elevation of left ventricular diastolic pressure.

Special Studies. Echocardiography has proved to be both sensitive and specific for mitral stenosis when adequate studies are done (Chapter 13). False positives and false negatives are uncommon. M-mode and 2D echocardiography do not reliably predict the severity of mitral stenosis. Doppler studies provide an estimate of mitral valve area that is within ± 0.4 cm^2 (prior to interventional therapy) of that obtained by cardiac catheterization. The echographic findings of mitral stenosis reflect the loss of normal valve function. The fusion of commissures results in movement of the anterior and posterior leaflets anteriorly in parallel during diastole. In patients in sinus rhythm, there is an absence of further opening of the valve that is normally seen with atrial contraction. Other findings include decreased E-to-F slope, decreased mitral valve leaflet excursion, and multiple echoes, indicating thickening or calcification of the valve. Left atrial enlargement is seen. Abnormal pulmonary valve motion and right ventricular enlargement may signify pulmonary hypertension.

Echocardiography is of great value in patients with equivocal signs, in patients with gross pulmonary hypertension, to differentiate mitral stenosis from an Austin Flint murmur of aortic regurgitation, and in the rare patient with "silent" mitral stenosis. It is used to assess left and right ventricular and atrial size and function, to evaluate the aortic and tricuspid valves, and to estimate pulmonary artery pressure. Transesophageal echocardiography is a useful technique when a transthoracic echocardiogram is unsatisfactory to assess left atrial thrombus and to assess the anatomy of the mitral valve and subvalvular apparatus.

In the majority of patients with disabling symptoms from presumed mitral stenosis, right and left heart catheterization should be performed as part of a preoperative assessment. Simultaneous measurement of cardiac output and the gradient between the left atrium and the left ventricle and calculation of valve area remain the "gold standard" for assessing the severity of mitral stenosis (Chapter 14). Left ventricular angiography assesses the competence of the mitral valve, an important determinant of operability for mitral commissurotomy. Quantification of left ventricular function provides a useful prognostic indicator of operative and late survival and of the expected functional result. Aortic and tricuspid valve function can be assessed when there is a question of coexisting lesions. Selective coronary arteriography establishes the site, severity, and extent of coronary artery disease and should be performed in patients with angina, in those with left ventricular systolic dysfunction, in those with risk factors for coronary artery disease, and in those 35 years of age or older who are being considered for surgery.

Natural History

The population presenting with mitral stenosis is changing because of the sharp decline in the incidence of acute rheumatic fever in the past 40 years. Native-born American citizens with symptomatic mitral stenosis are presenting at an older age. Young adults in the third and fourth decades with symptomatic mitral stenosis are more likely to come from low socioeconomic backgrounds and from the inner city or be immigrants, particularly from Latin America, the Middle East, Southeast Asia, or the Orient. Therefore, the latent period between acute rheumatic fever and symptomatic mitral stenosis is variable and appears to be related to the presence of repeated streptococcal infection. Females with mitral stenosis outnumber males by almost 2:1. The most important feature of the asymptomatic interval,

then, is the susceptibility to repeated bouts of both rheumatic valvulitis and streptococcal infection. The mechanism for the progression from no symptoms to mild to severe symptoms is progressive stenosis of the mitral valve.

With the onset of exertional dyspnea and fatigue, the valve area is usually reduced to one half to one third its normal size. Further small reductions in valve area markedly obstruct flow and result in symptoms with minimal exertion. The interval from initial mild symptoms to disabling symptoms may be 10 years. During this time, the patient is at little risk of death, permanent injury, or irreversible cardiac damage, except from atrial fibrillation with rapid ventricular rate resulting in pulmonary edema and from systemic embolus. Unfortunately, it is not possible to predict who is at risk of embolism. When functional class III symptoms are present, the valve area is usually 1.0 cm^2 or less, and both rest and exercise hemodynamics are deranged. Further small reductions in valve area result in symptoms at rest. The survival of patients with functional class III symptoms treated nonsurgically is markedly reduced, and fewer than 50% can be expected to survive 10 years and almost none with class IV symptoms will survive 10 years.

Management

Mitral stenosis can be prevented through two approaches. First, all streptococcal infections should be diagnosed and correctly treated. This prevents most initial episodes of acute rheumatic fever. Second, all patients with known previous acute rheumatic fever should receive appropriate antibiotic prophylaxis (Chapter 204).

Although the incidence of infective endocarditis is low, in isolated mitral stenosis, all patients exposed to bacteremia should receive appropriate prophylaxis against infective endocarditis (Chapter 24). Family and vocational planning should be considered. Women with this disease should consider bearing children before symptoms occur, since pregnancy is usually well tolerated with mild mitral stenosis. Occupations that require strenuous exertion in middle age and later should probably be avoided if possible. When patients reach the symptomatic threshold, medical treatment may be of some benefit. Digitalis offers no improvement for the patient with normal sinus rhythm and normal left ventricular function. When atrial fibrillation is present, however, digitalis plays a critical role in controlling ventricular rate. In selected patients beta-adrenergic blocking agents, diltiazem, or amiodarone may be added to reduce exercise-induced severe tachycardia. Beta-adrenergic blocking agents should be used with great caution or not at all in patients with impaired left ventricular function or associated significant aortic stenosis. In my view, digoxin and diltiazem are probably the best combined therapy. Diuretics reduce pulmonary congestion and peripheral edema and allow most patients freedom from salt restriction. For the patient with mild symptoms, maintenance of sinus rhythm is desirable. Cardioversion of atrial fibrillation and maintenance of antiarrhythmic therapy with digitalis and quinidine or digitalis and amiodarone should be offered to these patients. Anticoagulation is usually begun about 3 weeks in advance of cardioversion and is continued for 4 weeks after cardioversion. Patients with chronic atrial fibrillation and those with a previous history of embolism should receive anticoagulation unless there is a specific contraindication.

Unless there is a contraindication, surgery should be recommended to a mitral stenosis patient with functional class III or IV symptoms. For younger patients with a pliable valve and without important mitral regurgitation, this means commissurotomy. Because of the low morbidity and mortality of mitral commissurotomy, surgery is also offered to these patients when functional class II symptoms are present. The results of successful commissurotomy are excellent, and surgical mortality is less than 1%. Late mortality at 10 years is less than 5%, the thromboembolism rate is 2% per year or less, and the reoperation rate ranges from 0.5% to 4.5% per year. The return of symptoms after commissurotomy usually is the result of an incomplete operation, other valvular lesions, or deterioration of myocardial function. In less-developed countries, excellent results have been reported in a very high percentage of patients for up to 25 years.

For the older patient with a stiff or calcified valve, or when moderate mitral regurgitation is present, mitral valve replacement is usually performed. Valve replacement carries a higher operative mortality than does commissurotomy (approximately 5%) and the morbid-

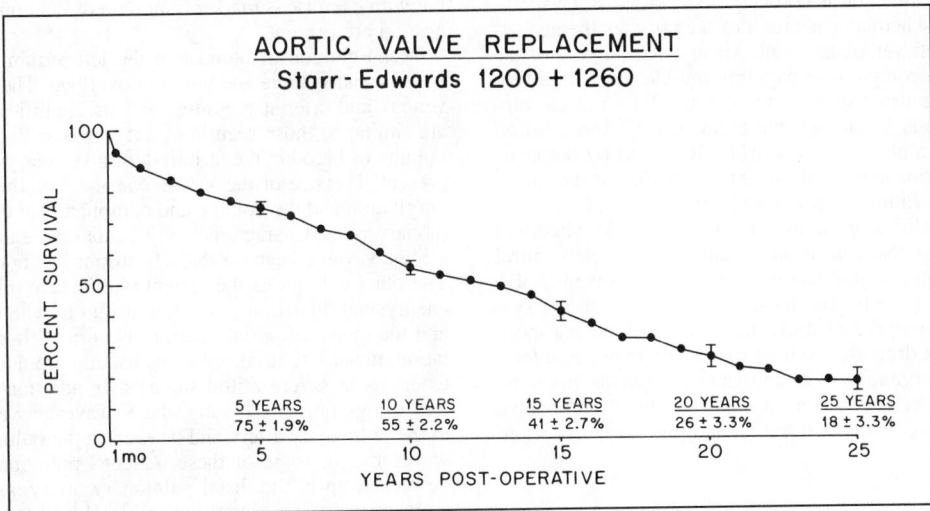

A

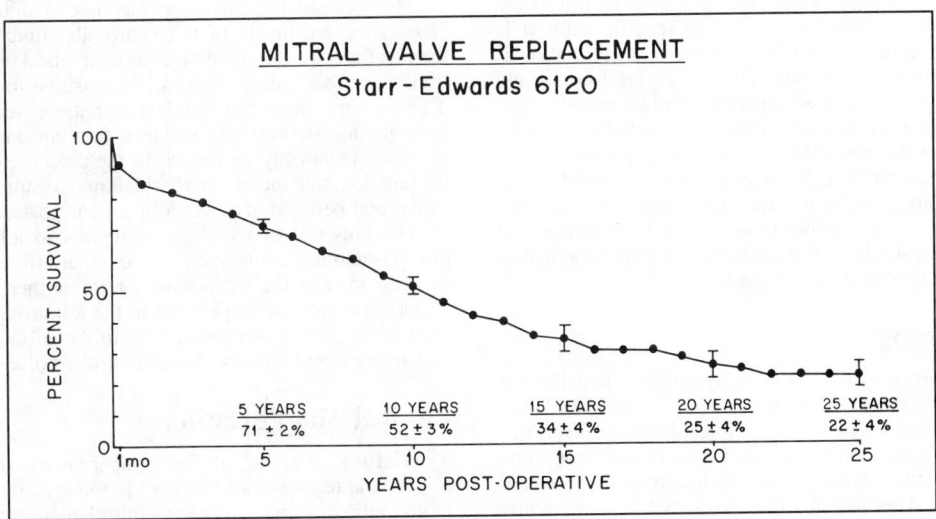

B

FIGURE 25-8   Survival after aortic **(A)** or mitral **(B)** valve replacement with a non–cloth-covered, caged Si-lastic ball prosthesis. The numbers indicate percentages of survival with one standard error.

Data from Albert Starr, MD.

ity that is associated with prostheses (see Prosthetic Valves). Survival at 10 years after mitral valve replacement for functional class III and IV patients is better than 60% (Fig. 25-8).

Catheter balloon commissurotomy with use of the double balloon technique or the Inoue balloon produces immediate and 3-month hemodynamic and clinical results comparable to those obtained by surgical commissurotomy. The results of catheter balloon commissurotomy are greatly influenced by the characteristics of the valve and its supporting apparatus, which are best determined by 2D echocardiography (transthoracic and/or transesophageal). In one study, the 7-year survival was 95 ± 1% and the event-free survival was 65 ± 6%. The 7-year event-free survival ranged from 13% to 90% in various subgroups. In the appropriate patient, in centers with skilled and experienced staff, catheter balloon commissurotomy is the procedure of first choice for relief of severe mitral stenosis.

MITRAL REGURGITATION
Etiology

Competent mitral valve function requires functioning of individual mitral leaflets, chordae tendineae, anulus, left atrium, papillary muscles, and supporting left ventricular segments. Disruption of the function of any of these elements can cause mitral valve regurgita-tion. The abnormalities causing mitral regurgitation reflect the multiple elements necessary for normal function. The valve leaflets are the most delicate components of this system, and disruption of leaflet substance invariably leads to important mitral regurgitation. For this reason, rheumatic fever, which most commonly attacks the mitral leaflets, has been a leading cause of mitral regurgitation. With the sharp decline in primary and secondary cases of rheumatic fever in this country, isolated mitral regurgitation caused by rheumatic disease requiring surgery is now less common.

Mitral valve prolapse (see Mitral Valve Prolapse) is now one of the commonest causes of isolated mitral regurgitation requiring surgery. Rupture of chordae tendineae may occur in both rheumatic and prolapsing mitral valves and may result from trauma or endocarditis. In a substantial number of patients, however, the cause remains unknown. Mitral valve anular dilatation, which occurs in marked left ventricular and left atrial enlargement and in Marfan's syndrome, prevents normal coaptation of the leaflets, leading to mitral regurgitation. Idiopathic mitral anular calcification prevents the anulus from contracting normally during systole, again promoting regurgitation. There is a known association between mitral valve prolapse, anular calcification, and chordal rupture with or without Marfan's syndrome.

Left ventricular enlargement also impairs normal papillary muscle function by displacing the muscles laterally. The most common cause of papillary muscle dysfunction is coronary artery disease. Dysfunction may result from ischemia or necrosis of the muscles themselves or of the underlying left ventricular wall. Aneurysmal bulging of the left ventricle may also compromise papillary muscle function. Myocardial infarction is the usual setting in which papillary muscle rupture occurs and it results in catastrophic mitral regurgitation. Mitral regurgitation in hypertrophic cardiomyopathy is caused by the characteristic systolic anterior motion of the anterior leaflet of the mitral valve, which results in failure of adequate leaflet coaptation.

Congenital abnormalities of the mitral valve caused by abnormal development of the endocardial cushions and resultant cleft mitral valve may result in mitral regurgitation. Systemic illnesses may also affect the mitral valve leaflets. The most common of these are systemic lupus erythematosus, rheumatoid arthritis, and ankylosing spondylitis. Methysergide, a drug used to treat headaches, may cause leaflet thickening and regurgitation; the regurgitation may disappear on cessation of therapy. Infective endocarditis may also involve the valve leaflet primarily, causing leaflet perforation and mitral regurgitation.

Pathology

The pathology of mitral regurgitation is as varied as the causes. The changes caused by rheumatic fever and mitral valvulitis were reviewed in the section on mitral stenosis. The specific pathologic feature of rheumatic valvulitis that results in mitral regurgitation is loss of leaflet area through contracture. There is severe fibrosis and rigidity of the whole of the valvular apparatus. Unlike mitral stenosis, mitral regurgitation may be present from the initial episode of acute rheumatic fever. Commissural fusion is an unimportant feature of rheumatic mitral regurgitation. When it is present, mixed mitral stenosis and mitral regurgitation result. The regurgitation of blood into the left atrium during systole results in left atrial enlargement and hypertrophy. The left ventricle is also enlarged and hypertrophied to maintain the large left ventricular stroke volume.

Abnormal Physiology

The fundamental abnormality of mitral regurgitation is that the left ventricle simultaneously ejects blood through two orifices, the aorta and the incompetent mitral valve. There are three direct results of this abnormality. First, the volume of blood that moves through the aortic valve, that is, the effective cardiac output, is less than the left ventricular stroke volume. This requires that the actual left ventricular end-diastolic and stroke volumes be increased to supply the normal circulatory demands. Second, the regurgitation of blood back into the left atrium during systole increases the volume, and therefore the pressure, of the left atrium. Third, the total impedance (left atrium and aorta) against which the left ventricle ejects is reduced. The reduction of impedance enhances left ventricular systolic pump function by allowing the ventricle to empty more rapidly early in systole and thereby decreases left ventricular radius and therefore wall stress. The reduction in stress permits greater shortening and, accordingly, stroke volume is increased for a given preload, aortic resistance, and myocardial contractility.

To compensate for the fraction of stroke volume lost to the left atrium, left ventricular stroke volume must be increased. As previously described, the reduction in impedance to ejection increases stroke volume. However, additional mechanisms are necessary. With acute valvular regurgitation, preload (sarcomere length) is increased. This mechanism, however, is sharply limited by the diastolic pressure-volume curve of the ventricle and pericardium. Thus, acute severe mitral regurgitation frequently results in high filling pressure and pulmonary edema. The chronic adaptation to volume overload uses increased numbers of sarcomeres in an enlarged circumference operating at their optimum length. Left ventricle volume and mass are increased, and the pressure-volume curve is shifted to the right. Long-standing, severe volume overload often leads to myocardial dysfunction, the cause of which is not understood. Continued left ventricular enlargement is used to compensate for decreased left ventricular function. Left ventricular and left atrial enlargement further impair mitral valve function, increasing mitral valve regurgitation. Left ventricular end-diastolic pressure and left atrial pressure eventually rise, whereas cardiac output falls. The ability to increase cardiac output with exercise is markedly impaired. Pulmonary and systemic congestion are present.

Regurgitation of blood into the left atrium during systole results in left atrial volume and pressure overload. The effects on pulmonary venous and arterial pressures and the significance of these changes are similar to those seen in mitral stenosis. Because of the increased volume of blood in the atrium during systole, a large V wave may be present. The size of the V wave depends on the amount of mitral regurgitation and the volume and compliance of the left atrium and pulmonary veins. Characteristically, acute severe mitral regurgitation has a high V wave because the left atrium has not had time to enlarge. The other extreme is the patient with severe mitral regurgitation and aneurysmal dilatation of the left atrium in whom the V wave is small and the mean left atrial pressure is normal. In severe mitral regurgitation, mean left atrial pressures usually are not elevated to the same extent as in severe mitral stenosis. In addition to the pulmonary artery wedge pressure tracing, the V wave may also be reflected back to the pulmonary artery and be seen in the pulmonary artery pressure waveform. In some of these patients, pulmonary venous blood can be picked up in the distal pulmonary artery, as demonstrated by an increase in oxygen saturation of blood in the distal pulmonary arteries.

The reduced impedance to ejection in mitral regurgitation may cause an overestimate of left ventricular function. This stems from the fact that ejection fraction, commonly used in determining left ventricular systolic pump function, is sensitive to changes in afterload. This becomes important in selecting patients for surgery. After mitral regurgitation is surgically stopped, the impedance to left ventricular ejection is suddenly increased. In the presence of poor left ventricular function, this increased afterload may result in cardiac decompensation and perioperative death or a poor postsurgical result.

The presence of parallel impedances to left ventricular ejection also has another implication. Factors that affect the impedance in either the aorta or the left atrium determine their relative flows. Thus, factors that increase impedance in the left atrium or decrease impedance in the aorta favor blood flow to the aorta and decrease regurgitant fraction and increase forward stroke volume.

Clinical Manifestations

History. Because of the compensatory mechanisms available, mild mitral regurgitation does not produce cardiac symptoms, and patients with moderate to severe mitral regurgitation may have long asymptomatic intervals. In contrast, acute severe mitral regurgitation is usually associated with congestive heart failure.

The predominant symptoms relate to pulmonary and systemic venous congestion and impaired rest and exercise cardiac output. As a consequence, patients are most frequently limited by exertional dyspnea and fatigue. Orthopnea and paroxysmal nocturnal dyspnea may result from redistribution of blood volume in the supine position. Acute episodes of pulmonary edema are less common than with mitral stenosis unless an acute change in mitral valve function occurs with chordae tendineae or papillary muscle rupture, or valve perforation with endocarditis. Long-standing pulmonary hypertension results in tricuspid regurgitation and systemic venous congestion, manifested by peripheral edema, abdominal pain, and swelling. Systemic embolism and hemoptysis are less common than with mitral stenosis. Patients with anular calcification may have calcific systemic emboli. Chest pain typical of angina pectoris usually indicates coexisting coronary artery disease. As with many volume-overload lesions, patients frequently complain of palpitations, which often represent an awareness of the large left ventricle contracting to expel the large stroke volume. Irregular palpitations indicate ectopic beats or atrial fibrillation, which may be present in up to 75% of these patients. Infective endocarditis may occur on damaged leaflets, further compromising mitral valve function.

Physical Findings. The general appearance shows no features characteristic of mitral regurgitation, but tachypnea, peripheral cyanosis, and edema may be readily apparent in patients with end-stage mitral regurgitation and severe heart failure. The jugular venous pressure is elevated when pulmonary hypertension has been long-standing. A prominent A wave reflects increased filling pressure, and a large V wave may represent tricuspid insufficiency. Only a CV wave is present in patients with atrial fibrillation. The carotid pulse is normal or shows a brisk upstroke, except with severe reduction in cardiac output, which results in a small-volume pulse. The precordium is hyperactive. The left ventricular impulse is laterally and caudally displaced and larger than usual. An apical systolic thrill is not infrequent. A right ventricular impulse and pulmonary valve closure may also be felt along the left sternal border when pulmonary hypertension is present. An impulse along the left sternal border may represent sustained left atrial filling during systole. This expansile pulsation of the left atrium may displace the right ventricle and has to be distinguished from a right ventricular heave.

The sine qua non of clinical diagnosis of mitral regurgitation is the mitral systolic murmur; therefore, careful auscultation is important. A typical murmur may be notably absent in severe prosthetic perivalvular leak and in some patients may be very localized and heard in only one spot on the precordium. When mitral regurgitation is caused by leaflet damage, such as with rheumatic heart disease or endocarditis, the murmur is holosystolic. The exception to this rule is acute severe mitral regurgitation due to chordal rupture or leaflet perforation. In this setting, the left atrium is small and noncompliant. The V wave in the left atrium may approach left ventricular pressure toward the end of systole, reducing regurgitant flow and causing the murmur to be early and midsystolic in timing. As the lesion becomes less acute, the murmur becomes holosystolic. Murmurs not caused by leaflet damage may vary in intensity and duration during systole.

The murmur of mitral regurgitation is typically high frequency and blowing in quality. It is heard best with the diaphragm of the stethoscope placed firmly over the left ventricular impulse. The murmur often radiates well to the axilla. The exception to this rule is acute chordal rupture of the posterior leaflet, which produces a loud murmur that radiates to the left sternal border. The murmur is thus frequently confused with ventricular septal defect and aortic stenosis. With anterior leaflet involvement, the murmur radiates to the back and the spine and can be conducted to the top of the head. A characteristic of mitral regurgitation murmurs caused by leaflet damage is the constancy of the murmur at different cycle lengths. This helps to differentiate this murmur from that of hypertrophic cardiomyopathy and aortic stenosis. Thus, the careful listener can use the natural variation of cycle length in atrial fibrillation or fortuitous extrasystoles to help confirm the presence of mitral regurgitation and its cause. The S_1 is reduced in intensity and may be obscured by the murmur. An S_4 is uncommon except in acute mitral regurgitation. A third heart sound, or S_3, often is present with severe mitral regurgitation. In some patients with severe mitral regurgitation, a diastolic rumble is present because of increased diastolic flow. The pulmonary component of S_2 is increased when pulmonary arterial hypertension is present.

Chest Radiograph. The thoracic cage is normal except in patients with mitral valve prolapse or Marfan's syndrome, who have a higher incidence of scoliosis, pectus excavatum, and thin chest with decreased anteroposterior diameter. The lung fields show evidence of elevated pulmonary venous pressure, and the findings are similar to, but less marked than, those seen in mitral stenosis. The pulmonary arteries are enlarged in long-standing pulmonary hypertension. The cardiac silhouette usually shows overall enlargement; left ventricular and left atrial enlargement constitutes most of this increase. The left atrium reaches larger dimensions than in any other cardiac disease in long-standing severe mitral regurgitation, and in some patients the left atrium is aneurysmal. Right ventricular and right atrial enlargement reflect elevated pulmonary pressures. Calcification of the anulus of the mitral valve may be present, but leaflet calcification is uncommon in pure mitral regurgitation. Left ventricular aneurysm may be present when coronary artery disease is the cause of mitral regurgitation.

Electrocardiogram. Atrial fibrillation is present in up to 75% of patients with chronic severe mitral regurgitation. Signs of left atrial enlargement or increased pressure or interatrial conduction delay are manifested in patients with sinus rhythm by broad-notched P waves in lead II and biphasic P waves in V_1. Signs of left ventricular hypertrophy are frequently present in chronic severe mitral regurgitation. Biventricular hypertrophy and biatrial enlargement may also be

demonstrated when pulmonary artery pressure is elevated. In acute severe mitral regurgitation, the ECG may be entirely normal.

Special Studies. Unlike the echocardiogram in mitral stenosis, the echocardiogram of mitral regurgitation may not be diagnostic of mitral valve dysfunction. Occasionally, ruptured chordae tendineae, or flail leaflets, are seen with severe acute mitral regurgitation. Multiple or thick echoes on the leaflets suggest fibrosis or calcification and are typically seen with rheumatic heart disease. Vegetations may be seen on the valve in infective endocarditis. The left atrium and left ventricle are enlarged, reflecting the severity of the mitral regurgitation. More important, echocardiography can be used serially to assess left ventricular dimensions and function. Doppler echocardiography (Chapter 13) is useful for diagnosing and assessing the severity of mitral regurgitation. There is a significant incidence of false positives in the mild grade, and the lesion may be erroneously judged to be severe in the presence of significant aortic stenosis. There is also an overlap between the various grades of severity of assessment of mitral regurgitation by Doppler when compared to angiography. Transesophageal echocardiography is of considerable value in defining mitral valve morphology and assessing the severity of mitral regurgitation (Chapter 13). It is particularly helpful in determining whether the valve can be repaired and the type of repair operation that will need to be performed.

Radionuclide-derived ejection fractions can be used to assess left ventricular function reliably. Comparison of simultaneous right and left ventricular stroke counts may be used to assess the severity of left-sided regurgitant lesions; this technique does not distinguish between aortic and mitral regurgitations. The effect of exercise on left ventricular systolic function can be obtained with this technique (with the limitations mentioned under Chronic Aortic Regurgitation), as can serial evaluations.

Right and left heart catheterization remains the cornerstone of evaluation of patients with symptomatic mitral regurgitation. Left ventricular cineangiography is used to assess quantitatively left ventricular volume and function, as well as the degree of valvular regurgitation. Pulmonary vascular resistance and cardiac output are measured. The effect of exercise on hemodynamics and cardiac function can be evaluated. Coexisting lesions of the aortic and tricuspid valves are assessed. Coronary arteriography determines the presence, site, and severity of coronary arterial obstruction and should be performed in patients with angina, in those with risk factors for coronary artery disease, in those with left ventricular systolic dysfunction, and in those 35 years of age or older who are being considered for cardiac surgery.

Natural History

The course of mitral regurgitation is determined by the cause and the interplay between the severity of the regurgitation and the ability of the left ventricle to compensate. Chronic mild mitral regurgitation is rarely responsible for symptoms because of adequate compensation; the major risk in such patients is infective endocarditis. With moderate to severe mitral regurgitation, there may be a long asymptomatic interval, and, when symptoms occur, they may progress slowly. However, functional capacity with severe mitral regurgitation may decline because of deterioration of left ventricular function rather than worsening of valve function. Or worsening of function may be caused by chordal rupture. Survival of symptomatic patients with important mitral regurgitation is about 60% at 10 years, but additional studies are needed to determine the natural history of severe mitral regurgitation.

Management

As with mitral stenosis, primary or secondary rheumatic fever prophylaxis reduces the incidence of rheumatic mitral regurgitation. Prevention of myocardial infarction reduces the incidence of mitral regurgitation caused by coronary artery disease.

Infective endocarditis prophylaxis is essential for all patients with mitral regurgitation, including the patient with trivial or mild valvular regurgitation (Chapter 24). Patients with rheumatic mitral regurgitation need antibiotic prophylaxis to prevent recurrence of rheumatic carditis (Chapter 204).

The patient with mild mitral regurgitation needs no specific therapy. The symptomatic patient can be helped by medical treatment through several approaches. Symptoms of systemic and pulmonary congestion are improved with diuretics. Digitalis reduces symptoms by improving left ventricular systolic pump function and controlling ventricular rate in patients with atrial fibrillation. Reduction of aortic impedance by decreasing systemic vascular resistance also helps relieve symptoms of mitral regurgitation and improve hemodynamic abnormalities. Afterload and preload reductions are helpful, but the effect of chronic vasodilator therapy on the natural history of mitral regurgitation is unknown; preliminary results are disappointing. It is recognized that any treatment that tends to reduce left ventricular size may reduce mitral regurgitation by improving the function of the mitral apparatus. Thus, the combination of decreased activity, diuresis, digitalis, and vasodilators reduces symptoms and improves hemodynamics in most patients. Maintenance of sinus rhythm is not as important for patients with mitral regurgitation as for those with mitral stenosis; however, at least one attempt should be made to convert the patient to sinus rhythm. Unless there is a clear reduction in function after the onset of atrial fibrillation, most patients with severe mitral regurgitation should probably be left in atrial fibrillation, with the rate controlled by digitalis; others may need small doses of beta-blocking agents, diltiazem, or amiodarone to control ventricular rate adequately.

The optimum timing of operation for the patient with chronic severe mitral regurgitation has not been determined. The problem of timing of valve replacement in chronic mitral regurgitation arises from the observation that disabling symptoms may be the result of irreversible left ventricular dysfunction. Thus, the best time to intervene in chronic mitral regurgitation is just before irreversible left ventricular dysfunction occurs. It is clear that this point cannot be determined from the symptoms. Furthermore, ejection phase indices commonly used to assess left ventricular function are elevated by the reduced impedance to ejection in mitral regurgitation. It is generally agreed that as the left ventricle enlarges and function decreases, a point is reached when mitral valve replacement is not beneficial. It may not be possible to determine this point prospectively in each patient. However, a study suggests that when the end-diastolic dimension is greater than 7 cm and the fractional shortening is reduced or low normal, a reduction in left ventricular volume and mass does not occur after mitral valve replacement, and ventricular function may actually deteriorate. Clinical use of this information should be tempered by knowledge of the difficulties intrinsic to M-mode echocardiography, including reproducibility of measurements and effects of volume overload on geometry. More recent data show that significantly better results, both with regard to lower operative mortality and better 10-year survival, are obtained in patients less than 75 years of age who are in functional class I or II and whose left ventricular ejection fraction is 0.60 or greater. These patients are ideal candidates for valve repair. For these reasons, our current practice is to recommend mitral valve replacement to patients with severe mitral regurgitation and evidence of borderline or reduced left ventricular function even if symptoms are mild or absent.

For patients whose valves are suitable for repair, left ventricular ejection fraction that is less than 0.60 should be considered as reduced left ventricular function. It is uncertain at this time if this is also true for patients who would need valve replacement. Factors that favor the balance toward surgery include a valve that is suitable for repair, a rheumatic or prolapse etiology, potential for major hemodynamic benefit, potential for correction of a large area of myocardial ischemia, and a dramatic response to medical treatment. Patients with symptoms and good left ventricular function are ideal candidates for valve replacement. Because of the increased operative mortality and poor postoperative results, we are reluctant to routinely recommend surgery in patients with ejection fractions of 0.30 or less. Pending new data, these patients should be treated vigorously with digitalis, diuretics, and vasodilators. If there is good improvement with this therapy, they should be reevaluated for surgery.

The expected results of mitral valve replacement for rheumatic mitral regurgitation are similar to those for mitral stenosis. In patients with mitral regurgitation caused by coronary artery disease, the results are poorer. Patients with significant associated coronary artery disease should also have coronary bypass surgery at the time of valve replacement. Preservation of chordae at the time of valve replacement results in better postoperative left ventricular systolic function. Patients who postoperatively have a left ventricular ejection fraction of greater than or equal to 0.50 have much better long-term survival than those with a left ventricular ejection fraction of less than 0.50. Preoperative predictors of postoperative left ventricular ejection fraction of 0.50 or more are left ventricular ejection fraction of at least 0.50, left ventricular end-systolic volume index of no more than 50 ml/m^2, and absence of pulmonary hypertension.

The current practice is to perform mitral valve repair, rather than replacement, when feasible. When successful, the results of valve repair are similar to those of valve replacement and left ventricular function may be better with valve repair. Moreover, the incidence of many of the complications of prosthetic heart valves and especially of systemic emboli is much lower with valve repair. It is uncertain whether valve repair results in better survival compared with valve replacement in patients with identical preoperative clinical left ventricular function and comorbid conditions.

ACUTE MITRAL REGURGITATION
Etiology

Acute mitral regurgitation usually results from infective endocarditis or trauma, both of which may result in rupture or perforation of the valve leaflets and chordae tendineae. Chordal rupture also occurs in rheumatic and prolapsing mitral valves, but in many patients the cause is unknown. Spontaneous chordal rupture is more common in men and in patients with systemic hypertension, acute left ventricular dilatation from any cause, or fibrosis of the papillary muscles. Papillary muscle dysfunction from ischemia, infarction, or fibrosis of the papillary muscle, the underlying left ventricular muscle, or both often causes acute mitral regurgitation. The most common cause of papillary muscle dysfunction is coronary artery disease. Rupture of a papillary muscle from myocardial infarction or trauma usually causes acute, catastrophic mitral regurgitation, particularly when the belly rather than an apical head of a papillary muscle is affected.

Abnormal Physiology

The major difference between acute and chronic severe mitral regurgitation is the extent of left ventricular and left atrial enlargement and the magnitude of left atrial (and pulmonary venous) hypertension. The left ventricle is large in chronic mitral regurgitation but is only somewhat dilated in acute mitral regurgitation. To compensate for the left ventricular stroke volume lost to the left atrium, total left ventricular stroke volume has to increase. This is achieved by an "increase" of ejection fraction and an increase of left ventricular end-diastolic volume and sarcomere length. However, this compensatory mechanism is limited by the characteristic sarcomere length-tension curve and the diastolic pressure-volume relationships of the left ventricle and the pericardium. The left ventricle can increase acutely probably by no more than 20% to 30%, which accounts for its "normal size" on both physical examination and chest x-ray. This increased size is usually inadequate to maintain forward stroke volume; the compensatory tachycardia is often inadequate to maintain a normal forward cardiac output. The regurgitant volume increases left atrial volume. However, increases of left atrial size are limited by the left atrial pressure-volume curve and, as a result, left atrial pressure rises precipitously, producing pulmonary edema. Pulmonary hypertension is common. The regurgitant volume frequently cannot be accommodated in the left atrium and is transmitted into the pulmonary veins. In the absence of myocardial infarction, left ventricular systolic pump function frequently is normal in these patients; indeed, measured indicators of left ventricular systolic function may yield increased values because of the reduced impedance to left ventricular emptying.

Clinical Manifestations

The patient may have a history of trauma or myocardial infarction, and the patient may exhibit the clinical features of infective endocarditis. Usually the symptoms of heart failure are predominant.

On physical examination, these patients have tachycardia; they may also be orthopneic. The usual clinical manifestations of heart failure often are present. As opposed to patients with chronic mitral regurgitation, of whom 75% are in atrial fibrillation, patients with acute mitral regurgitation are usually in sinus rhythm. The left ventricle is hyperkinetic. The S_1 is soft, and a loud S_3 is the rule. In contrast to patients with a chronic lesion, patients with acute mitral regurgitation usually have a presystolic gallop (fourth heart sound). They have a mitral systolic murmuring that may be holosystolic, late systolic, or crescendo-decrescendo. There may be a diastolic mitral flow murmur. The P_2 is increased in intensity.

The electrocardiogram often shows nonspecific ST-T wave changes and a sinus tachycardia. However, the ECG may be normal or may demonstrate the findings of a myocardial infarct. On the chest radiograph the cardiothoracic ratio may be within the normal range. The lung fields show signs of increased pulmonary venous pressure and of pulmonary edema.

Echocardiography (M-mode, 2D, or transesophageal) may show a variety of abnormalities, which include vegetations, prolapse of the mitral valve, flail leaflets, mitral valve aneurysm, mitral anular calcification, and the changes of a myocardial infarction. Two-dimensional echocardiography is also of value in determining left ventricular size and function, left atrial size, and presence of other cardiac lesions. Doppler echocardiography (Chapter 13) is useful in demonstrating mitral regurgitation, especially in those rare instances when there is no characteristic murmur (also see Mitral Regurgitation). A radionuclide gated blood pool scan may help demonstrate normal left ventricular ejection fraction and an increase in left ventricular volumes.

The natural history of this condition is variable. If the mitral regurgitation is mild to moderate in severity, patients are likely to do well with medical therapy. Eventually, the changes of chronic mitral regurgitation occur. In patients with severe mitral regurgitation, the natural history depends on whether they have heart failure, coronary artery disease, papillary muscle rupture, or a combination. If heart failure is present, which is common, the prognosis is very poor. If coronary artery disease is the cause, the prognosis is that of the coronary artery disease and its complications. If papillary muscle rupture is present, 95% or more of patients die within 48 hours. In those with a flail leaflet, the annual mortality is high (6.3%).

Management

The underlying cause of regurgitation must be treated, which often is difficult. In patients with infective endocarditis, the appropriate antibiotic therapy must be given. If the mitral regurgitation is mild, no other specific therapy may be needed. If mitral regurgitation is moderate, digitalis, diuretics, and vasodilators may be advisable.

For patients with severe mitral valve regurgitation, the choices of medical therapy include digitalis, diuretics, and vasodilators. Patients with heart failure should be given digitalis, diuretics, and vasodilators. In patients with mild, moderate, or severe heart failure that persists despite medical therapy, surgery is indicated. If the patient responds dramatically to digitalis, diuretics, and vasodilators, surgical therapy often can be delayed until heart failure and the infective endocarditis are controlled so that the operation is performed when the patient is in a more stable condition. If the patient does not respond immediately and dramatically to medical therapy, surgery should not be delayed, even if the infection is uncontrolled or the patient has had little antibiotic therapy. Surgery usually involves mitral valve replacement, but if the valve is suitable for repair, valvuloplasty is the procedure of choice. Associated or causative coronary artery disease requires coronary artery bypass surgery if it is technically feasible. Valve rupture, if diagnosed, is an indication for immediate valve surgery. Valve surgery is relatively urgent for severe regurgitation due to a flail leaflet.

MITRAL VALVE PROLAPSE
Etiology

Mitral valve prolapse occurs in the presence of redundant mitral valve leaflets, elongated chordae tendineae, enlarged mitral anulus, and abnormally contracting left ventricular wall segments. Mitral valve prolapse is associated with the physical findings of one or more systolic clicks and a late systolic murmur. Echocardiographic and angio-

graphic studies reveal protrusion of the mitral leaflet or leaflets beyond the plane of the mitral anulus and into the left atrium, with associated mitral regurgitation. The cause of mitral valve prolapse is at present unknown. Our inability to determine the cause probably means that the clinical features have heterogeneous origins.

The syndrome has been noted in all ages but is most common (5%) in women of childbearing age. Autosomal dominant inheritance has been demonstrated both with, and in the absence of, muscular dystrophy. Many patients with Marfan's syndrome have mitral valve prolapse. Mitral valve prolapse associated with segmental wall motion abnormalities develops in some patients with coronary artery disease. Mitral valve prolapse has been demonstrated in up to 37% of patients with ostium secundum atrial septal defect. Myxomatous proliferation of the mitral leaflet tissue is often found in patients with mitral valve prolapse who require valve surgery or are studied at autopsy. The incidence of myxomatous proliferation of the mitral valve in patients with incidental findings of prolapse is unknown and may be small.

Thus, the clinical syndrome that we know as mitral valve prolapse does not have a single cause. It may occur as an autosomal dominant heritable disorder, as part of a generalized connective tissue abnormality, or sporadically in otherwise normal people. Our imprecise knowledge of the natural history, complications, and treatment of this disorder naturally follows from our inability to characterize its etiology or the significance of the click-murmur syndrome or isolated echocardiographic findings of mitral valve prolapse in individual patients. It is possible that mitral valve prolapse is being significantly overdiagnosed.

Pathology

The presumed normal life span of most patients with mitral valve prolapse has limited the pathologic examination of the heart and the mitral valve to a small subset of patients who have severe mitral regurgitation or who die suddenly or accidentally. Pathologic findings most commonly include redundant mitral leaflet tissue involving predominantly the posterior leaflet. The chordae tendineae may be elongated. In the absence of coronary artery disease, the papillary muscles underlying the left ventricular myocardium are normal. The mitral anulus of patients with mitral valve prolapse and severe mitral regurgitation may be strikingly enlarged. Histologic examination shows myxomatous infiltration of the valve leaflets, with increased acid mucopolysaccharides. The normal collagenous and elastic elements are disrupted. These changes, however, are not specific for this syndrome. There is great variability in the amount of myxomatous tissue (spongiosa portion of leaflet) present in otherwise normal valves, but in the mitral valve prolapse syndrome, the spongiosa portion of the mitral leaflet actually invades and disrupts the fibrosa portion (elastin and collagen tissue). There is an increased incidence of associated mitral anular calcification and ruptured chordae tendineae, particularly in elderly patients with mitral valve prolapse.

Abnormal Physiology

Except for the mitral valve, the cardiovascular system functions normally in most persons with mitral valve prolapse. The major pathophysiologic event is mitral regurgitation. Mitral regurgitation may be absent, trivial, slowly progressive, or sudden and severe in onset, with chordae tendineae rupture. When mitral regurgitation is hemodynamically important, pathophysiologic changes of left ventricular volume overload and regurgitation into the left atrium are present and are identical to those previously discussed under Mitral Regurgitation. The systolic click and murmur of mitral valve prolapse result from abnormal valve function. Early in systole, the valve is competent. However, as the ventricle contracts and becomes smaller, the redundant mitral leaflets and/or chordae tendineae allow the affected leaflet to fall back into the left atrium, disrupting leaflet coaptation and allowing mitral regurgitation. At the moment of maximum prolapse, the chordae tendineae and leaflets tense, producing the click or multiple clicks. Events that alter left ventricular size, contractility, and/or aortic impedance affect the timing of maximum prolapse and thus the systolic click and murmur. A reduction of ventricular volume (by standing up), an increase in myocardial contractility (exercise), or a decrease in arterial resistance (amyl nitrite) often accentuates a systolic click or murmur and causes this auscultatory finding to occur earlier in systole.

Autonomic dysfunction has been demonstrated in women with mitral valve prolapse and is characterized by decreased parasympathetic and increased alpha-adrenergic tone. Arrhythmias, including supraventricular and ventricular tachycardia, are common in patients with this syndrome (the mechanism is unknown), and the rare occurrence of sudden death is presumed to be on this arrhythmic basis. Abnormal electrophysiologic function has not otherwise been documented in mitral valve prolapse. Shortened platelet survival time has been noted in some patients with mitral valve prolapse, and there is an increased incidence of mitral valve prolapse in young persons with cerebrovascular accidents. This is probably caused by fibrin emboli from the abnormal mitral leaflet tissue, as several postmortem studies suggest.

Clinical Manifestations

Most patients with mitral valve prolapse are asymptomatic and therefore are diagnosed only because the characteristic click and murmur are heard incidentally during a physical examination or on echocardiographic/Doppler study performed for some other indication. Occasionally, the patient hears a loud whoop on standing up and seeks medical help. In others, the diagnosis is actively pursued because of atypical chest pain, palpitations, cerebrovascular episodes, or history of heart murmur.

History. There is no symptom complex diagnostic of mitral valve prolapse. In instances of severe mitral regurgitation, the previously described symptoms of shortness of breath, fatigue, weakness, orthopnea, and paroxysmal nocturnal dyspnea predominate. Some patients with mitral valve prolapse seek medical attention because of atypical (for angina) chest pain, unusual shortness of breath, easy fatigability, syncope, and palpitations. These complaints are not specific for mitral valve prolapse and frequently occur in patients without cardiac or other organic disease.

Chest pain in mitral valve prolapse is usually not related to exertion. It may last for hours and yet may allow continued activity. The pain responds poorly to nitroglycerin. Since both mitral valve prolapse and coronary artery disease are common, some patients with coronary artery disease also have mitral valve prolapse. Shortness of breath and fatigue may be only subjective or may be demonstrable on a graded exercise test. Palpitations are a frequent subjective complaint and may or may not correlate with arrhythmias documented by ambulatory ECG recording. Occasional patients report frank syncopal episodes in addition to lightheadedness and dizzy spells. These may or may not correlate with arrhythmias. There is an association between mitral valve prolapse and transient cerebral or retinal ischemic events or stroke.

Physical Findings. The diagnosis of mitral valve prolapse is most frequently made by physical examination. Although the patient's general appearance may be normal, the incidence of thoracic skeletal abnormalities is high and warrants careful inspection. Loss of the normal dorsal thoracic kyphosis (straight back), scoliosis, pectus excavatum, and decreased anteroposterior/transverse diameter ratio are present singly or in combination in over half of the affected patients. Diseases with a high incidence of mitral valve prolapse (e.g., Marfan's syndrome, myotonic dystrophy, atrial septal defect) have their own characteristic findings.

In the absence of hemodynamically important mitral regurgitation, most physical findings are restricted to auscultation of the heart. The precordial examination may reveal a sharp midsystolic tap, coincident with the click. The auscultatory phenomena are diagnostic of mitral valve prolapse. These include a nonejection click or multiple clicks heralding a midsystolic or late systolic murmur. The clicks and murmur are best heard at the apex, and the murmur is typically soft and blowing, sometimes with radiation to the axilla, consistent with mitral regurgitation. Occasionally, a loud whoop or honk is heard. It is important to note that the click(s) and murmur are variable and may be heard only intermittently; at times, only the click or the murmur is heard. When present, the click and murmur behave in the following manner: Maneuvers that decrease left ventricular size move

the click and murmur closer to or simultaneous with the S_1. With standing up from a supine position or amyl nitrite inhalation, therefore, the click moves closer to S_1 and the duration of the murmur lengthens. In some, a holosystolic murmur follows these manipulations. Maneuvers that increase left ventricular size cause the click and the onset of the murmur to occur later in systole. Squatting, passive leg lifting in the supine position, or sustained hand grip exercise thus move the click and the murmur to later in systole and may even abolish one or both. In patients with suggestive symptoms and normal auscultatory findings, the physical examination is incomplete without a provocative maneuver to bring on the click and/or murmur. In some patients, the murmur is holosystolic.

Chest Radiograph. The abnormalities of the thoracic skeleton previously described are readily recognized on the chest x-ray (scoliosis, straight back, pectus excavatum). The lungs and cardiac silhouette are normal unless hemodynamically important mitral regurgitation is present; these changes are described under Mitral Regurgitation.

Electrocardiogram. The scalar ECG may show flat or inverted T waves in the inferior leads (II, III, aV_F) in about one third of patients with mitral valve prolapse. These abnormalities may fluctuate with time and may be readily confused with myocardial ischemia. The Q-T interval may be prolonged. Most often the ECG is entirely normal.

Special Laboratory Studies

Echocardiography. After the physical examination, the test most commonly used to diagnose mitral valve prolapse is echocardiography. The specific findings on M-mode echocardiography are abrupt late systolic or, occasionally, pansystolic movement of the closed mitral valve toward the left atrium. Caudal angulation (Chapter 13) of the transducer must be avoided because it may produce an artifact resembling pansystolic prolapse. As with auscultation, maneuvers that change left ventricular volume change the echocardiographic timing of prolapse, and the diagnostic sensitivity may be enhanced. Two-dimensional echocardiography also demonstrates prolapse and is probably the more sensitive of the two techniques. The combination of M-mode and 2D echocardiography is superior to either alone (Chapter 13). However, the absence of the classic findings of prolapse on the echocardiogram does not exclude the diagnosis of mitral valve prolapse, since false-negative results may be obtained in up to 10% of patients.

Cardiac catheterization and angiography. Hemodynamic and angiographic procedures are not indicated to make the diagnosis of mitral valve prolapse. These invasive tests may be useful in evaluating the occasional patient with hemodynamically important mitral regurgitation. Coronary arteriography may be necessary in some patients with anginal pain to establish whether coronary obstructive disease is present. The left ventriculogram shows posterior displacement of the mitral leaflets across the plane of the mitral anulus and into the left atrium during systole. Both 30-degree right anterior oblique and 60-degree left anterior oblique views are necessary to assess the mitral apparatus for prolapse accurately by left ventriculography.

Radionuclide studies. Myocardial perfusion scintigraphy in association with a graded exercise test may be used successfully to differentiate patients with mitral valve prolapse and anginal pain from those with and without associated obstructive coronary artery disease. Blood pool scans are not as effective for the diagnosis of prolapse.

Exercise testing. Exercise testing may induce frequent and complex ventricular extrasystoles, particularly during the recovery period. The high incidence of false-positive S-T segment depression in patients with mitral valve prolapse during exercise testing diminishes the importance of this finding. Exercise testing also enables one to evaluate objectively the degree of functional impairment.

Ambulatory ECG recordings. Ambulatory ECG recordings reveal premature atrial contractions or premature ventricular contractions in half the patients studied. Supraventricular or ventricular tachycardias have been observed in 6% of patients who have been evaluated by ambulatory ECG recording. However, these recorded arrhythmias often do not correspond in time to symptoms such as palpitations.

Natural History

Mitral valve prolapse is found at all ages in both sexes but is most prevalent in women of childbearing age. Consequently, most of those who reach the physician's office for evaluation of a heart murmur or symptoms subsequently found to be related to mitral valve prolapse are young women. Most patients with mitral valve prolapse are asymptomatic, and the diagnosis of prolapse is usually made in these patients during routine physical examination or from an echocardiographic examination performed for some other purpose.

Complications of mitral valve prolapse are infrequent but important. Chest pain is not common and is usually atypical for angina pectoris. Since prolapse and coronary artery disease are both common disorders, it is not surprising that some patients have severe associated atherosclerotic obstructive coronary artery disease. Endocarditis may occur in patients with prolapse, even in the absence of previously documented mitral regurgitation; mitral regurgitation often is intermittent. Progressive mitral regurgitation may occur because of increasing mitral dilatation, lack of leaflet coaptation, or chordae tendineae rupture. Acute severe mitral regurgitation may follow chordal rupture involving a large segment of leaflet. There is a known association between mitral valve prolapse and mitral anular calcification. These patients are also likely to have supraventricular and ventricular tachyarrhythmias. Some patients have associated preexcitation, and in most the accessory pathway appears to be on the left side of the heart. Sudden death is rare in prolapse and is probably caused by ventricular fibrillation or tachycardia; it occurs usually in those with symptomatic ventricular tachyarrhythmias. There is a relationship between mitral valve prolapse and cerebral and retinal ischemic events. Platelet survival is known to be shortened in some patients with mitral valve prolapse. Two-dimensional echocardiography of the mitral valve and the left atrium in some patients with mitral valve prolapse, stroke, and normal cerebral angiograms has shown densities consistent with thrombus on the mitral valve or in the left atrium, in the groove between the prolapsing valve and the left atrial wall. Transesophageal echocardiography may be of particular value in demonstrating thrombus in the left atrium when it is not seen on transthoracic echocardiography. Data show that patients with mitral valve prolapse who also have a thickened mitral valve on 2D echocardiography have a higher incidence of associated cardiovascular abnormalities and of complications of mitral valve prolapse.

Management

Because of the good prognosis in most patients with prolapse, management should be supportive. For patients who are incidentally found to have mitral valve prolapse on physical examination, echocardiographic examination with a brief explanation of the problem, a recommendation for infective endocarditis prophylaxis (Chapter 24), and reassurance seem most appropriate. If the physical findings are not classic for prolapse, the echocardiogram can be used to substantiate the diagnosis. Left ventricular cineangiography is unwarranted for diagnosis alone in most patients. Patients with mitral valve prolapse (whether they have a mitral systolic murmur, midsystolic click, or both) need antibiotics to prevent infective endocarditis.

For patients who have symptoms, with chest pain, palpitations, dyspnea, or possibly cerebral or retinal emboli, a more extensive evaluation may be indicated. Echocardiography can aid in supporting the clinical diagnosis of prolapse, in evaluating left ventricular function and volume overload (if significant mitral regurgitation is present), and in showing ruptured chordae. If the patient has had cerebrovascular episodes, anticoagulant and/or antiplatelet therapy is reasonable. Patients with recurrent tachyarrhythmias or syncope or who aborted sudden death should undergo electrophysiologic study with provocative stimulation to determine whether they have abnormal conduction function or an accessory pathway and to guide drug therapy. Mitral regurgitation is managed as described previously.

In the absence of coronary artery disease, hemodynamically important mitral regurgitation, or a symptomatic arrhythmia, most patients with mild symptoms can be treated with reassurance. For those with refractory chest pain or palpitations, beta-adrenergic blocking agents may be effective. These agents also may be effective for the treatment of supraventricular tachyarrhythmias or premature ventricular contractions. Except for the management of important mitral regurgitation, significant obstructive coronary artery disease, or life-threatening arrhythmias in association with an accessory pathway, surgical therapy is not recommended. In the appropriate patient, catheter ablation therapy or implantation of a cardioverter defibrillator with or without a pacemaker may be indicated.

TRICUSPID STENOSIS
Etiology

Tricuspid stenosis is almost always rheumatic in origin. It rarely occurs as an isolated lesion and is associated with mitral valve disease (often stenosis) and with aortic stenosis. Tricuspid stenosis in the cardinoid syndrome is usually accompanied by tricuspid regurgitation. Obstruction of right atrial outflow occurs with a right atrial myxoma and, rarely, with a particular form of constrictive pericarditis.

Pathology

The valvular abnormalities in tricuspid stenosis are similar to the findings in rheumatic mitral valve disease; calcification of the valve, however, is rare. The normal area of the tricuspid valve is 7 cm^2; in severe tricuspid stenosis, the area is less than 1.5 cm^2. Although tricuspid stenosis is diagnosed in 3% to 4% of patients with multivalvular disease, it has been detected at autopsy and by 2D echocardiography in 10% or more of these patients.

Abnormal Physiology

Stenosis of the tricuspid valve prevents adequate filling of the right ventricle and may lower cardiac output. The right atrium is enlarged and its pressure elevated, whereas the right ventricle is of normal size. Severe tricuspid stenosis may prevent or ease the pulmonary congestion resulting from associated severe mitral stenosis. In severe tricuspid stenosis, the altered hemodynamics are similar to those in mitral stenosis with two exceptions: (1) Instead of pulmonary congestion and pulmonary edema, these patients have systemic congestion and systemic edema; and (2) since the right ventricle is much more compliant than the left, right ventricular, and therefore right atrial, pressures are lower than the left atrial pressures that are seen in mitral stenosis.

Clinical Manifestations

History. The age and sex ratios are the same as in mitral stenosis. The symptoms are dominated by the left-sided valvular disease, but effort intolerance and easy fatigability may be caused in part by tricuspid stenosis. If increased jugular venous pressure and liver enlargement are present, they may be caused mainly by tricuspid stenosis. The lack of pulmonary congestion in patients with severe mitral stenosis may be caused by severe tricuspid stenosis. If there is no pulmonary venous hypertension, hemoptysis, pulmonary edema, orthopnea, and paroxysmal nocturnal dyspnea are also usually absent.

Physical Findings. The arterial pulse is normal. When sinus rhythm is present, giant A waves are present in the jugular pulse (Chapter 11). In such patients, if a right ventricular heave is absent, the diagnosis of right atrial obstruction is nearly certain. In atrial fibrillation, large V waves with a *slow* Y descent are the characteristic finding in this condition. A diastolic murmur and, if the patient is in sinus rhythm, a presystolic murmur are audible at the left sternal edge. It may be difficult to distinguish these murmurs from those caused by mitral stenosis, but an increase in intensity of the murmur(s) during inspiration suggests tricuspid stenosis. An opening snap is rarely heard or is difficult to distinguish from the mitral opening snap; when it is heard, it is present after the mitral opening snap. Since tricuspid stenosis may be associated with regurgitation, a holosystolic murmur that increases during inspiration may also be heard in the same area.

Chest Radiograph. The right atrium may be enlarged. Calcification of the tricuspid valve is rare. Signs of associated mitral stenosis are often present.

Electrocardiogram. If sinus rhythm is present, tall, pointed P waves indicating right atrial enlargement and/or hypertension may be identified. Atrial fibrillation is common.

Echocardiography. An echocardiogram of the tricuspid valve shows a pattern similar to that in mitral stenosis. Findings on 2D echocardiography, namely, doming of the tricuspid valve, are more specific than those of M-mode echocardiography. In patients with suspected tricuspid stenosis, careful 2D echocardiographic and Doppler study of the tricuspid valve must be performed. Evidence of mitral and aortic valve disease may be seen.

Cardiac Catheterization. Simultaneous recording of right ventricular and right atrial pressures is the way to demonstrate a gradient across the tricuspid valve. The gradient is often small and can be difficult to detect, especially when atrial fibrillation or a low cardiac output is present. The gradient can be increased with exercise. Normally, there is less than a 1 mm Hg diastolic gradient across the tricuspid valve. A gradient greater than 3 mm Hg suggests moderate stenosis, whereas a gradient greater than 5 mm Hg is associated with severe stenosis. If sinus rhythm is present, tall A waves can be seen in the right atrial pressure tracing.

Natural History

Tricuspid stenosis is never a primary lesion. The mitral and aortic valvular abnormalities usually dominate and determine the clinical course. Diuretics should be used with some caution in moderate to severe tricuspid stenosis, because when venous pressure is lowered, right ventricular filling and output are reduced. As a consequence, left ventricular filling and output may be compromised. Tricuspid commissurotomy is the usual treatment if severe stenosis is present. Valve replacement may be indicated if significant regurgitation through the valve is also present.

TRICUSPID REGURGITATION
Etiology

Tricuspid regurgitation most commonly results from right ventricular dilatation caused by left ventricular failure, mitral stenosis, pulmonary hypertension, pulmonary stenosis, or atrial septal defect. It may resolve after correction of the primary abnormality, but tricuspid regurgitation associated with rheumatic disease is usually permanent. Causes not associated with right ventricular dysfunction are infective endocarditis, carcinoid, and trauma. Thus, the patients most likely to have tricuspid regurgitation are those with severe heart failure or with severe mitral valve disease and intravenous drug abusers with infective endocarditis. Prolapse of the tricuspid valve usually occurs with mitral valve prolapse. Rarely, tricuspid regurgitation has been associated with a protein-losing enteropathy, lymphocytopenia, and immunologic deficiency. Congenital lesions, such as Ebstein's anomaly and endocardial cushion defect, also cause tricuspid regurgitation (Chapter 28).

Abnormal Physiology

The physiologic effects of tricuspid regurgitation are analogous to those of mitral regurgitation, except that the right atrium is more compliant than the left atrium, and right ventricular systolic pressure is lower than that present in the left ventricle. Thus, in tricuspid regurgitation, the right ventricle is delivering blood into a more compliant atrium at a lower driving pressure than in mitral regurgitation. Forward flow may be decreased, and right ventricular volume is increased.

Clinical Manifestations

History. Symptoms are usually dominated by the underlying disease. Symptoms that may be primarily related to tricuspid regurgitation are fatigue and dyspnea on exertion, a throbbing in the neck or abdomen, epigastric distention, nausea, loss of appetite, and peripheral edema.

Physical Findings. Large V waves with a rapid Y descent are noted in the jugular venous pulse. The neck vein findings are often not prominent because the right atrium is very compliant. Atrial fibrillation is present in 80% of patients. The right ventricle feels hyperdynamic. A holosystolic murmur that increases with inspiration (Carvallo's sign) is heard best at the xiphoid area and adjacent to the left sternal edge.

Chest Radiograph. The chest x-ray may reveal evidence of right atrial enlargement. If the tricuspid regurgitation is related to other problems, the overall heart size is usually increased.

Electrocardiogram. The rhythm is usually atrial fibrillation. Evidence of right atrial and ventricular enlargement may be present.

Echocardiogram. The M-mode echocardiogram provides only indirect evidence of tricuspid valve regurgitation. Diminished or paradoxical interventricular septal motion reflecting volume and/or pressure overload of the right ventricle may be present. Intravenous injection of indocyanine green or microscopic air bubbles allows detection of tricuspid regurgitation on 2D echocardiography. Vegetations may be seen on the tricuspid valve, as may a right-sided myxoma. Flail leaflet, Ebstein's anomaly, and endocardial cushion defects may be seen, as may tricuspid valve prolapse. Doppler studies are of particular value in diagnosing and assessing the severity of tricuspid regurgitation. However, there is an incidence of false-positive for the mild lesion.

Cardiac Catheterization. It is difficult to quantitate the degree of tricuspid regurgitation by catheterization. Right ventricular angiography and indicator-dilution curves show tricuspid regurgitation and provide semiquantification, but there is a high incidence of false-positive findings as a result of technical problems, for example, a catheter across the valve or atrial fibrillation. Demonstration of a systolic murmur in the right atrium by intracardiac phonocardiography may be necessary to establish the diagnosis but is usually not clinically necessary.

Natural History and Management

The hemodynamic burden of tricuspid incompetence is usually well tolerated. An exception is the acute type that results from rupture of the valve or its supporting structure.

Mild to moderate tricuspid regurgitation usually requires no specific therapy. Severe regurgitation can be treated by digitalis and diuretics. As in tricuspid stenosis, overenthusiastic use of diuretics entails some danger. In all forms of tricuspid regurgitation, therapy is directed to the primary lesion or to associated left-sided valvular lesions. If the regurgitation is secondary to another problem, and at operation for that problem the tricuspid valve appears normal, correcting the primary cause is usually sufficient. In some patients, tricuspid valvuloplasty corrects the severe regurgitation. However, valve replacement may be necessary for regurgitation that is part of multivalve rheumatic disease. Some intravenous drug abusers with severe tricuspid insufficiency and no right ventricular systolic hypertension may be treated temporarily by valve resection alone.

PULMONIC STENOSIS

Pulmonic valve stenosis is usually a congenital lesion and is considered in detail in Chapter 28. It may be produced in rare instances by carcinoid, rheumatic disease, myxoma, and myxosarcoma of the pulmonary valve. Extrinsic compression from tumors and aneurysm of the aorta or sinus of Valsalva and a particular kind of constrictive pericarditis may produce right ventricular outflow obstruction. The abnormal hemodynamics, history, and physical findings are dependent on the degree of obstruction and are similar to those seen in congenital valve stenosis. Diagnosis is usually made by cardiac catheterization and angiography. Treatment, if needed, is usually directed to the primary cause. Resection of the tumor and valve replacement may be necessary.

PULMONIC REGURGITATION
Etiology

Pulmonic regurgitation can occur as a primary or secondary lesion. Primary regurgitation associated with normal pulmonary artery pressure is caused by congenital absence or deformity of the valve, infective endocarditis, or dilatation of the pulmonary artery from any cause, including the idiopathic variety or, perhaps most commonly, pulmonary-valve surgery. However, most cases of pulmonic regurgitation are secondary and are associated with elevated pulmonary artery pressure (>80 mm Hg) caused by mitral stenosis, primary pulmonary hypertension, cor pulmonale, and other sources of pulmonary hypertension. Rare causes include rheumatic disease, carcinoid, trauma, and syphilis.

Abnormal Physiology

Since there is normally only a 5 mm Hg gradient in diastole across the pulmonary valve, pulmonic regurgitation with normal pulmonary artery pressure is usually of no hemodynamic consequence. As pulmonary artery pressure and diastolic gradient increase, so does the hemodynamic significance of the lesion. Occasionally, right ventricular enlargement and failure result.

Clinical Manifestations

History. In patients with normal pulmonary artery pressure, symptoms are absent. In patients with high pulmonary artery pressure, symptoms are usually related to the underlying lesion but may be aggravated by the pulmonic regurgitation.

Physical Findings. Pulmonic regurgitation is usually diagnosed only by auscultation. With normal pulmonary artery pressures, the heart sounds are normal; P_2 is followed by a short pause, then by a short, rough, low-pitched decrescendo murmur that ends well before the S_1. It is best heard in the second or third left intercostal space. If pulmonary hypertension is present, the murmur occurs immediately after a P_2, which is usually louder than normal. It is a higher-pitched, blowing, decrescendo diastolic murmur (Graham Steell murmur).

Chest Radiograph and Electrocardiogram. The chest x-ray and ECG are usually normal. If the pulmonic regurgitation is secondary to another lesion, both reflect the original lesion.

Cardiac Catheterization. With severe pulmonic valve regurgitation, the pulmonary artery diastolic pressure approaches right ventricular diastolic pressure and its pressure tracing is similar to the right ventricular tracing. Injection of a contrast agent into the pulmonary artery demonstrates pulmonic regurgitation.

Natural History and Prognosis

Although large series are not available, it appears that patients with pulmonic regurgitation without pulmonary hypertension do reasonably well for long periods of time. Surgical removal or destruction of the valve does not produce heart failure unless pulmonary hypertension is present. However, some of these patients are now presenting 10 to 20 years later with severe right ventricular dilatation and impaired cardiac performance. Thus, pulmonic regurgitation with low pulmonary artery pressure may not be totally benign. In patients with high pulmonary pressure, symptoms and complications are usually related to the primary lesion.

Management

Pulmonic regurgitation with normal pulmonary artery pressure requires no special treatment. Valve replacement can be performed if the regurgitation causes major hemodynamic and cardiac problems. When it is secondary to another lesion, treatment is directed toward the primary cause.

MULTIVALVULAR DISEASE

Multivalvular disease occurs frequently. Common forms of this disease include stenosis and regurgitation at one valve, for example, mitral stenosis and mitral regurgitation, aortic stenosis and aortic regurgitation. Also very common are various combinations of stenosis and regurgitation of the aortic, mitral, and tricuspid valves. Many combinations are possible.

BOX 25-1
Major complications of valve replacement

1. Operative mortality
2. Perioperative myocardial infarction
3. Prosthetic endocarditis
4. Prosthetic dehiscence
5. Prosthetic dysfunction
   a. Obstruction: usually thrombotic, occasionally due to item 3, 4, or 8
   b. Regurgitation
   c. Hemolysis
   d. Structural failure
6. Thromboemboli
7. Hemorrhage with anticoagulant therapy
8. Valve prosthesis–patient mismatch
9. Prosthetic replacement often caused by item 3, 4, or 5; occasionally caused by item 6, 7, or 8
10. Late mortality, including sudden, unexplained death

The abnormal physiology, history, and physical and other findings depend on the combination of valves affected, the degree of stenosis and regurgitation, and associated factors such as pulmonary hypertension and coronary artery disease.

PROSTHETIC VALVES

Intracardiac prosthetic heart valves have been in use for 36 years. Because of the success of valve replacement in improving symptoms and offering some patients prolonged survival (see Fig. 25-8), hundreds of thousands of patients now have prosthetic heart valves. These patients are not cured but still have serious heart disease. They have exchanged native valve disease for prosthetic valve disease (Box 25-1) and must be followed with the same care as patients with native valvular disease. The clinical course of patients with prosthetic heart valves is influenced by several factors.

Ventricular Dysfunction

Despite relief of valvular obstruction or regurgitation, some patients fail to improve or even deteriorate after valve replacement because of impaired myocardial function. The cause of dysfunction may be carditis associated with rheumatic disease, myocardial degeneration and fibrosis from long-standing pressure or volume overload, ischemic damage at the time of valve replacement, coronary artery disease, or other associated diseases such as congestive (dilated) cardiomyopathy. Perioperative myocardial damage is an important cause of postoperative ventricular dysfunction. The importance of myocardial protection at the time of valve surgery is now recognized, and current operative techniques reduce myocardial oxygen consumption by hypothermic, potassium-arrest cardioplegia and use a variety of means for maintaining adequate myocardial perfusion and protection.

Other Cardiac Lesions

Cardiac diseases affecting primarily one valve often affect other valves, the conduction system, coronary arteries, and pulmonary vasculature. With the exception of pulmonary hypertension and functional tricuspid regurgitation, these disorders do not improve after isolated valve replacement. Rheumatic disease typically affects both mitral and aortic valves but not necessarily with the same severity at the same time. Therefore, patients who have mitral valve replacement may subsequently require aortic valve replacement years later, or vice versa. Calcification of the aortic and mitral valve anuli accompanying disease of these valves may extend to the conduction system. High-degree or complete atrioventricular block may occur at the time of surgery or during the late postoperative period, requiring pacemaker implantation. Coronary artery disease is very common in the age range of patients requiring valve replacement. We recommend that coronary arteriography be performed preoperatively in all patients with myocardial ischemic pain, in those with left ventricular systolic dysfunction, in those with risk factors for coronary artery disease, and in those 35 years of age or older. Coronary bypass surgery of technically suitable vessels is performed at the time of valve replacement.

Prosthesis-Related Problems

As stated, the patient with a heart valve prosthesis has traded native valvular disease for prosthetic valvular disease.

Operative mortality for valve replacement averages 5% (range 2% to 10%) for aortic valve replacement and averages 8% (range 5% to 12%) for mitral valve replacement. Operative mortality is related to older age of patient, functional classes III to IV, increased left ventricular size, left ventricular dysfunction, heart failure, pulmonary hypertension, low cardiac output, and presence of associated diseases such as systemic hypertension, diabetes, and renal and hepatic failure. Coronary bypass surgery performed at the same time as valve replacement increases the operative mortality modestly, but associated coronary artery disease if not bypassed increases the operative and late mortality significantly. Other very important factors include the occurrence of perioperative myocardial infarction, the duration of the operation, aortic cross-clamp time, and whether the patient needed reoperation within 1 to 2 weeks after the initial operation, and on an elective or emergency basis.

The risk of prosthetic endocarditis is about 3% in the first year and 0.5% in subsequent years. Despite therapy, infections in the early postoperative period (up to 2 to 12 months) are the result of hospital-based organisms. They are difficult to cure and have a high mortality (about 77%); early reoperation is usually recommended. Mortality from late (2 to 12 months or later) postoperative infection is approximately 40%. About half the patients can be treated successfully with medication alone. The infected valve should be replaced in patients who do not respond to medical treatment or who have evidence of heart failure, anular invasion, embolism, prosthetic dysfunction, unstable prosthesis, or gram-negative, staphylococcal, or fungal infection. The importance of adequate antibiotic prophylaxis for the prevention of endocarditis cannot be overemphasized (Chapter 24).

Prosthetic dehiscence is the result of sutures pulling out of the cardiac tissues. It may result from infection, inadequate surgical technique, or diseased cardiac tissue (e.g., edema, necrosis, calcification).

Because of the continued proliferation of new types and models of prostheses and their relatively brief history of clinical use, the natural history of prosthetic failure is incompletely determined. Although some mechanical prostheses had initial problems with component failure, the most common cause for dysfunction of mechanical prosthetic valves is thrombotic obstruction. The incidence of thrombotic obstruction with the Björk-Shiley spherical occluder valve is higher than that seen with the Starr-Edwards or St. Jude valves, particularly in the mitral position. Failure of tissue valves is more common than failure of mechanical prostheses because of leaflet deterioration or calcification; progressive prosthetic regurgitation is the rule. Bioprosthesis failure is greater in younger patients and in the mitral position. In patients over 50 years old, failure of mitral prosthesis usually starts at 7 to 8 years and of aortic prosthesis at 8 to 10 years. It is unlikely that the tissue valves currently in use will be able to provide the long-term performance demonstrated by the ball valve mechanical prosthesis.

Red cells are fractured by turbulence and contact with foreign surfaces. Some degree of hemolysis is present with all mechanical prostheses but not with bioprostheses. However, important hemolysis may occur with a perivalvular leak or severe prosthetic obstruction regardless of prosthesis type. Serum lactic dehydrogenase (LDH) is usually the simplest and most reliable index of hemolysis to follow in patients with prosthetic valves. A sudden increase in LDH may indicate prosthesis dysfunction, perivalvular leak, or cloth tear. Iron and folate therapy usually correct anemia. Valve re-replacement may be required for severe, refractory hemolytic anemia.

Important systemic embolization is an unfortunate complication of prosthetic valve replacement. Anticoagulation is recommended for all patients with mechanical prostheses. Despite long-term anticoagulation, patients with mechanical prostheses face a 1% to 2% or less

per year embolic rate for aortic prostheses and a 3% to 4% or less per year rate for mitral prostheses. If patients experience an embolism, aspirin is added to the anticoagulant therapy if they are not already receiving aspirin. Tissue prostheses in the aortic position have a similar embolic rate *without* anticoagulation. Tissue mitral prostheses do not have a lower incidence of emboli than do mechanical prostheses when atrial fibrillation is present. Therefore, long-term anticoagulation is recommended in patients with this rhythm. Cessation of anticoagulation in patients with mechanical prostheses should be avoided because it carries a 20% to 25% incidence of systemic embolism in the first year. If it is necessary to discontinue anticoagulation temporarily, it is recommended that it be slowly tapered.

Long-term anticoagulant therapy is associated with bleeding episodes. The incidence of minor bleeding is about 2% to 4% per year or less. The incidence of major bleeding is about 1% to 2% per year or less, with a mortality of about 0.5% per year or less. The incidence of these complications is lower in patients who take their medications reliably and in those in whom smooth long-term anticoagulation can be achieved. With oral anticoagulants, low-dose or mid-dose warfarin therapy is combined with low-dose aspirin. Higher degrees of anticoagulation increase the incidence of bleeding without reducing the incidence of thromboembolism.

When using oral anticoagulants (warfarin), international normalized ratio (INR) should be ≤3.5 to 4.0 and prothrombin time (PT) ratio should be ≤2.0. With low-dose warfarin INR should average 2.5 (range 2.0 to 3.0) and PT ratio should average 1.5 (range 1.3 to 1.7). With mid-dose warfarin, INR should average 3.0 (range 2.5 to 3.5) and PT ratio should average 1.8 (range 1.6 to 2.0). For the first 2 to 3 months after valve replacement, mid-dose warfarin therapy is combined with low-dose aspirin (81 mg in the United States). Subsequently, for mechanical prostheses, patients with aortic valve replacement in sinus rhythm should receive low-dose warfarin; those with aortic replacement in atrial fibrillation and patients with mitral valve replacement should receive mid-dose warfarin. Subsequently for bioprostheses, patients with aortic valve replacement in atrial fibrillation and mitral valve replacement in sinus rhythm should receive low-dose warfarin; those with mitral valve replacement in atrial fibrillation should receive mid-dose warfarin. All patients should receive low-dose aspirin after valve replacement with mechanical or biologic valves.

No prosthesis currently employed has an effective orifice as large as that of the native valve, and valve prosthesis–patient mismatch may occur. All patients with prosthetic heart valves have mild to moderate stenosis. Patients with aortic valve prostheses have obstruction to left ventricular outflow (aortic stenosis), and patients with mitral valve prostheses have obstruction to left atrial emptying (mitral stenosis). This is most important with the large patient in whom a small prosthesis must be placed for technical reasons. The resulting patient-prosthesis mismatch contributes to incomplete relief of symptoms. The long-term effect of intrinsic prosthetic stenosis on survival and ventricular dysfunction is unknown. The presence of intrinsic prosthetic stenosis must be considered when advising patients with prosthetic heart valves concerning activity.

Reoperation to replace a prosthetic heart valve is a serious complication. It is usually required for moderate to severe prosthetic dysfunction and dehiscence, for prosthetic endocarditis, and occasionally for recurrent thromboembolism, severe recurrent bleeding from anticoagulant therapy, and valve prosthesis–patient mismatch.

Late cardiac death may result from ventricular dysfunction, other cardiac lesions, or prosthesis-related causes. Late, sudden death is not uncommon. It may result from a bradyarrhythmia, a tachyarrhythmia that is often associated with ventricular dysfunction, prosthetic dysfunction or mismatch, coronary artery disease, or a combination of these.

Management

All patients with prosthetic valves need appropriate antibiotics for prophylaxis against infective endocarditis (Chapter 24). Patients with rheumatic heart disease continue to need antibiotics as prophylaxis against the recurrence of rheumatic carditis. Adequate anticoagulation is needed for appropriate patients (see above).

Table 25-1   Normal auscultatory findings in patients with prosthetic heart valves

| TYPE OF PROSTHETIC VALVE | AUSCULTATORY FINDING* | |
	AORTIC	MITRAL
Starr-Edwards ball valve	Sharp opening sound after S₁	Sharp opening sound after S₂, 0.07–0.15 s
	Sharp closing sound at S₂	Sharp closing sound at S₁
	Ball "rattles" during systole	Ball "rattles" during diastole
	SEM	SEM
Björk-Shiley spherical occluder	Soft opening sound after S₁	Soft opening sound after S₂, 0.07–0.15 s
	Sharp closing sound at S₂	Sharp closing sound at S₁
	SEM	SEM
Xenograft	SEM	Diastolic rumble†
		SEM

*Absence of opening or closing sounds with mechanical prostheses usually signifies severe prosthetic dysfunction.
†Indicates bioprosthetic obstruction or prosthesis-patient mismatch.
SEM, Systolic ejection murmur.

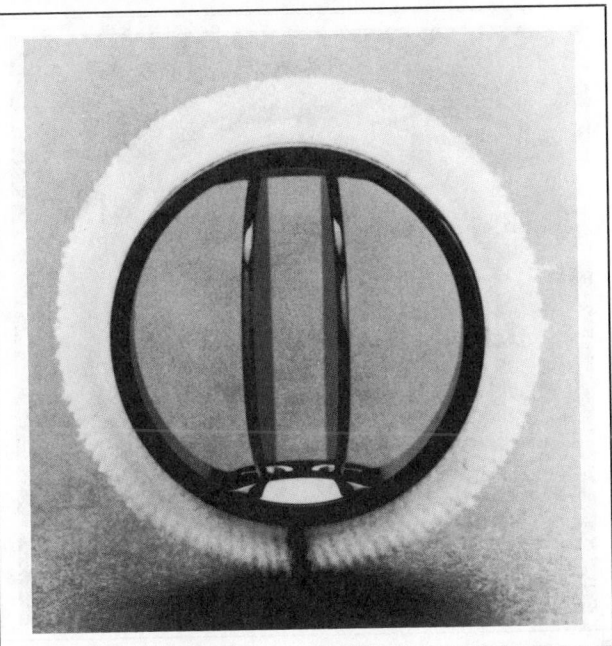

FIGURE 25-9   St. Jude valve.

During the first 4 to 6 weeks after surgery, the physician and surgeon jointly manage the patient, directing their attention toward relieving postoperative discomfort, readjusting cardiac medications, and instituting anticoagulation if not contraindicated. A graduated plan of activity is started that, in most cases, enables the patient to return to full activity in 4 to 6 weeks.

Several syndromes are peculiar to the postoperative period. The postperfusion syndrome, which occurs in up to 5% of patients, usually appears in the third or fourth postoperative week. Characterized by fever, splenomegaly, and atypical lymphocytes, it is benign and self-limited. Another effect of surgery, the postpericardiotomy syndrome, occurs in up to 25% of the patients and is characterized by fever and pleuropericarditis. It usually develops in the second or third postoperative week but can appear as late as 1 year after surgery and sometimes recurs. Although this syndrome is usually self-limited, most patients benefit from taking antiinflammatory drugs, such as aspirin or indomethacin, and a short course of corticosteroids is also occasionally required.

Even though the pericardium is left open at the end of surgery, cardiac tamponade has been known to occur during the first 6 weeks. The critically ill patient improves promptly with pericardial drainage, which underscores the need to consider this uncommon postoperative complication. Usually, anticoagulants have been given and the fluid is hemorrhagic.

The 4- to 6-week postoperative visit is critical, because by this time the patient's physical capabilities and expected improvement in functional capacity can usually be assessed. At this time, the physician should assemble essential records and data for the subsequent office follow-up, including preoperative history, physical examination, chest x-ray, ECG and indication for surgery, the preoperative echocardiographic/Doppler ultrasound and cardiac catheterization/angiographic reports, surgeon's operative report, and hospital discharge summary. The prosthesis model, serial number, and size should of course be recorded.

The workup on this visit should include an interval or complete initial history and physical examination, ECG, chest x-ray, echocardiography/Doppler studies, complete blood count, electrolytes, LDH, and INR/prothrombin time, if indicated. The examination's main focus is on physical signs that relate to functioning of the prosthesis or suggest the presence of a myocardial, conduction, or valvular disorder. The auscultatory sounds to expect with some normally functioning prostheses are listed in Table 25-1. Severe perivalvular mitral regurgitation may be inaudible on physical examination, a fact to remember when considering possible causes of functional deterioration in a patient.

The interval between routine follow-up visits depends on the patient's needs. Anticoagulant regulation does not require office physician visits.

Multiple noninvasive tests have emerged for assessing valvular and ventricular function. Fluoroscopy can reveal abnormal rocking of a dehiscing prosthesis or limitation of the occluder if the latter is opaque. Phonocardiography can detect variant poppets if "normal" sounds were previously established. Radionuclide angiography is useful to determine whether functional deterioration is the result of reduced ventricular function. M-mode echocardiography has proved unreliable in assessing ventricular and prosthetic function, but 2D echocardiography with Doppler velocity recordings yields useful information about both.

"Heart failure" after valve replacement may be the result of (1) preoperative left ventricular dysfunction that improved partially or not at all, (2) perioperative myocardial damage, (3) other valve disease that has progressed, (4) complications of prosthetic heart valves, and (5) associated heart disease, such as coronary artery disease and systemic hypertension.

Any patient with a prosthetic heart valve who does not improve after the surgery or who later shows deterioration of functional capacity should undergo appropriate testing, including cardiac catheterization and angiography to determine the cause. Such studies are also necessary for patients who require reoperation for endocarditis or repeated embolism, to determine the hemodynamics and anatomy for the surgeon.

The indications for reoperating on a patient with prosthetic valve endocarditis have already been discussed. The patient in stable condition, without prosthetic valve endocarditis, can probably undergo reoperation with slightly greater risk than that accompanying the initial surgery. For the patient with catastrophic dysfunction, surgery is clearly indicated and urgent. The patient without endocarditis or severe dysfunction requires careful hemodynamic evaluation, and the decision about reoperation should then be based on the hemodynamic abnormalities, the symptoms, ventricular function, and current knowledge of the natural history of the particular prosthesis.

Choice of Prosthesis

In the United States, two main kinds of prosthetic heart valves are presently being implanted: mechanical prostheses and biologic valves. The three main types of mechanical valves that are being used are a bileaflet (St. Jude) valve (Fig. 25-9), a ball and cage (Starr-Edwards)

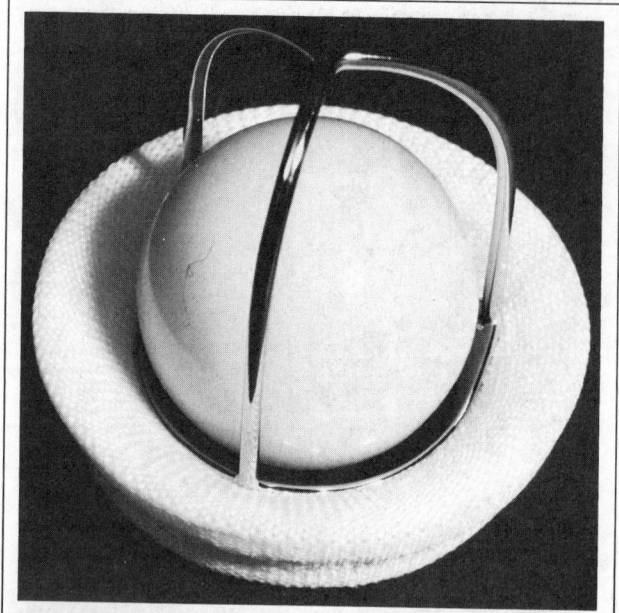

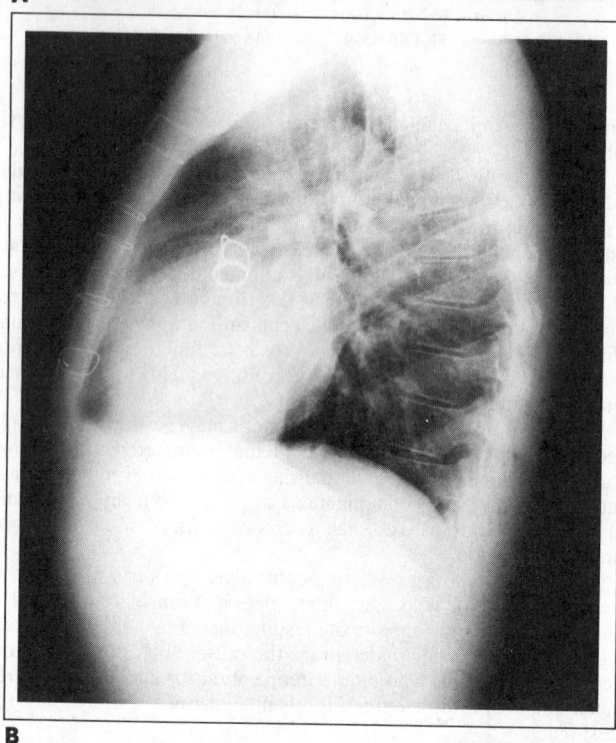

FIGURE 25-10   **A,** Starr-Edwards model 1260 aortic prosthesis. **B,** The radiolucent Silastic poppet is not seen on the chest radiograph.

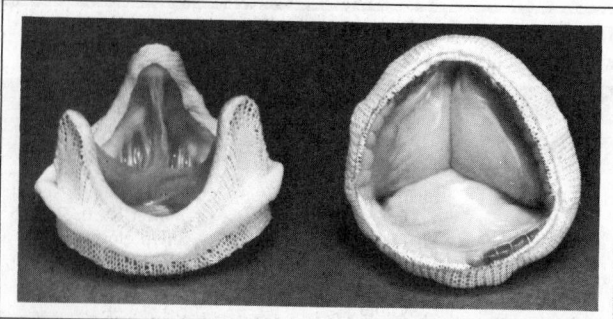

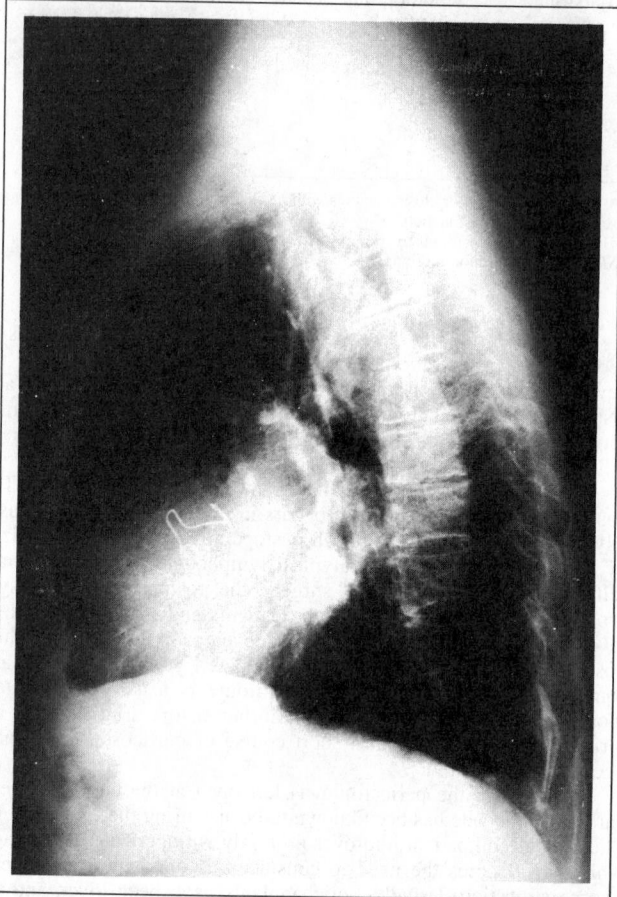

FIGURE 25-11   **A,** Carpentier-Edwards aortic prosthesis. **B,** Only the wire stent of this bioprosthesis is visualized on the chest roentgenogram.

valve (Fig. 25-10), and the Medtronic Hall valve; the tilting disk valve (e.g., the Björk-Shiley spherical occluder valve) is no longer being used in the United States. The biologic valves are porcine heterografts or xenograft (e.g., Hancock and Carpentier-Edwards) (Fig. 25-11) and bovine pericardial heterograft valves (e.g., Carpentier-Edwards).

The main advantages of the mechanical prostheses are their *proved* durability (Starr-Edwards valves last for up to 36 years; the Björk-Shiley spherical occluder valve, for up to 15 to 20 years) and the accumulated knowledge of their complications, including rate of occurrence. The later model Björk-Shiley 60-degree convexoconcave prosthesis has a high incidence of strut fracture and is no longer avail-

able for clinical use. Follow-up on the St. Jude valve is available for 10 to 15 years. The main advantage of porcine heterografts is that anticoagulant therapy is not required for patients in sinus rhythm. Since mechanical valves with anticoagulation and heterografts without anticoagulation have demonstrated similar thromboembolism rates, the main disadvantage of mechanical valves is the need for anticoagulant therapy and its associated morbidity and mortality. The main disadvantage of heterografts is their limited durability (Table 25-2). At present, structural valve deterioration of heterografts (degeneration and obstruction) occurs at an average rate of ≤5% at 5 years, 10% to 20% at 10 years, and 40% to 65% at 15 years; the incidence is lower in aortic prostheses and in the older patient. The incidence is very high in young patients. The Carpentier-Edwards bovine pericardial valve (available for aortic valve replacement) has as good or lower complication rate (including structural valve failure rate) than the porcine heterograft up to 10 years after valve replacement.

Table 25-2 Probability of death from any cause, any valve-related complication, and individual valve-related complications 11 years after randomization, according to type and location of replacement valve.*

EVENT	AORTIC VALVE			MITRAL VALVE		
	MECHANICAL PROSTHESIS (N = 198)	BIOPROSTHESIS (N = 196)	P VALUE	MECHANICAL PROSTHESIS (N = 88)	BIOPROSTHESIS (N = 93)	P VALUE
Death from any cause	0.53 ± 0.04	0.59 ± 0.04	0.26	0.64 ± 0.05	0.67 ± 0.05	0.41
Any valve-related complication	0.62 ± 0.04	0.64 ± 0.04	0.64	0.71 ± 0.05	0.79 ± 0.06	0.34
Systemic embolism	0.16 ± 0.04	0.15 ± 0.03	0.49	0.18 ± 0.05	0.15 ± 0.04	0.61
Bleeding	0.43 ± 0.04	0.24 ± 0.04	<0.001	0.41 ± 0.06	0.28 ± 0.07	0.02
Endocarditis	0.07 ± 0.02	0.08 ± 0.02	0.79	0.11 ± 0.04	0.17 ± 0.05	0.37
Valve thrombosis	0.02 ± 0.01	0.01 ± 0.01	0.33	0.01 ± 0.01	0.01 ± 0.01	0.95
Perivalvular regurgitation	0.04 ± 0.02	0.02 ± 0.01	0.28	0.17 ± 0.05	0.09 ± 0.06	0.05
Reoperation	0.07 ± 0.02	0.16 ± 0.04	0.07	0.21 ± 0.05	0.47 ± 0.09	0.23
Structural valve failure	0.00 ± 0.00	0.15 ± 0.04	<0.001	0.00 ± 0.00	0.36 ± 0.08	<0.001

From Hammermeister KE et al: Comparison of outcome in men 11 years after heart-valve replacement with a mechanical valve or bioprosthesis, *N Engl J Med* 328:1289, 1993.
*Plus–minus values are means ±SE. P values are for the difference in the probability of event-free survival between patients with a mechanical prosthesis and those with a bioprosthesis.

BOX 25-2
Valve selection criteria*†

Reasons for preferring mechanical valve
Quality of life as perceived by the patient
Age <40 years
Renal failure
Long expected lifetime
Composite graft
Patient needs anticoagulants, for example, for other mechanical valve, atrial fibrillation, previous stroke(s)
Coronary bypass using internal mammary artery
Previous dysfunctional tissue valve
Double valve replacement

Reasons for preferring bioprosthesis
Quality of life as perceived by the patient
Anticoagulant intolerance
Unreliable anticoagulant risk
Age ≥60 to 65 years
Short expected lifetime
Pregnancy anticipated
Previous thrombosed mechanical valve

---

*Criteria set in *italics* are more compelling.
†Please see text. This box refers only to mechanical and bioprosthetic valves. It does not consider the impact on valve selection of the appropriate use of homograft valves (i.e., endocarditis) or the pulmonary autografts (i.e., children). The indications for these procedures are still evolving, and these procedures are not universally available options.

Antibiotic-sterilized homograft valves have a low incidence of many complications, in particular of prosthetic endocarditis. However, they are more difficult to insert and the failure rate averages 19% at 10 years, 54% at 14 years, and 88% at 20 years. Viable cryopreserved homografts may have a very low failure rate. An autograft is a valve that has been translocated within the same individual. For example, with the Ross procedure the patient's pulmonary valve is inserted in the aortic position and a porcine valve is inserted in the pulmonary position. This procedure is more difficult to perform but has good results in young patients, especially if they cannot take anticoagulants.

The prosthetic valve should be chosen after a careful consideration of all factors. Guidelines for selection of a mechanical or heterograft are listed in Box 25-2. It needs to be emphasized that the choice of operative procedure and selection of valve replacement device has to be *individualized* for each patient after a careful consideration of all factors.

Section Editor's Note The association of valvular heart disease with the use of the anorectic agents fenfluramine and dexfenflura-

---

✔ WHEN TO REFER

Patients with valvular heart disease should be referred to an appropriate cardiologist according to the following guidelines:
1. When there is uncertainty about the diagnosis of the valve lesion(s) or the assessment of their severity.
2. When there is uncertainty whether the symptoms are due to the valve disease.
3. All asymptomatic patients considered to have moderate or severe valve disease.
4. For follow-up of asymptomatic patients when:
   a. Valve disease is mild, every 2 to 5 years if necessary.
   b. Valve disease is moderate, every 1 to 2 years.
   c. Valve disease is severe, every 6 to 12 months.
   d. Patients develop symptoms due to valve disease, early or immediate.
5. When the valve lesion is acute.
6. All patients with valve disease who are symptomatic from, or have any limitation because of, their valve disease.
7. Relief of symptoms or response to therapy is inadequate, or is inappropriate, or is not to the patient's and/or family's satisfaction.
8. Every 6 to 12 months for follow-up of symptomatic patients or as often as is necessary for any specific reason.
9. For follow-up after valve surgery:
   a. At 4 to 6 weeks after surgery for first postoperative visit.
   b. Asymptomatic patients at annual intervals.
   c. Symptomatic patients every 6 to 12 months.
   d. Response to therapy is inadequate, or is inappropriate, and/or symptoms persist.
   e. Early or immediately if patients develop new symptoms due to valve disease.
   f. Early or immediately if a complication occurs.
10. For advice about anticoagulant regimen if there is unsatisfactory, inappropriate, or inadequate control of their anticoagulant regimen, or if there is a complication of anticoagulant therapy.

It needs to be reemphasized that the above are suggested guidelines; care of a patient should be *individualized*, taking into consideration many factors.

---

mine, particularly when either was combined with phentermine, was reported in the summer of 1997. All 24 patients had aortic regurgitation and/or mitral regurgitation; 8 had associated pulmonary hypertension, and in 5, the histopathologic findings of the excised valves demonstrated plaque-like encasement of the leaflets and chordal structures with intact architecture. The incidence of valvular pathology in asymptomatic patients receiving these drugs is not known at this time.

The drugs fenfluramine and dexfenfluramine have been withdrawn from the market. Controversy exists regarding some cardiologists' recommendations concerning patients who have used these drugs. Most agree that all such patients should undergo a careful cardiovascular physical examination, followed by echocardiogram if heart murmur is detected and that patients with clinical and echocardiographic evidence of valvular heart disease should then undergo appropriate treatment and/or further testing. Recommendations that all exposed patients undergo echocardiography would be an expensive approach for patients who have no heart murmurs or cardiac symptoms.

BIBLIOGRAPHY

Connolly HM, Crary JL, McGoon MD et al: Valvular heart disease associated with fenfluramine-phentermine, *N Engl J Med* 337:581-588, 1997.

Grunkemeier GL et al: Replacement heart valves. In O'Rourke RA, editor: *Hurst's the heart, update I*, New York, 1996, McGraw Hill.

Hammermeister KE et al: Comparison of outcome in men 11 years after heart-valve replacement with a mechanical valve or bioprosthesis, *N Engl J Med* 328:1289-1296, 1993.

Kawanishi DT, Rahimtoola SH: Catheter balloon commissurotomy for mitral stenosis: complications and results, *J Am Coll Cardiol* 19:192, 1992.

Rahimtoola SH: Catheter balloon valvuloplasty for severe calcific aortic stenosis: a limited role, *J Am Coll Cardiol* 23:1076-1078, 1994.

Rahimtoola SH (editor): Valvular heart disease and endocarditis. In Braunwald (editor): *Atlas of the heart*, Philadelphia, 1997, Current Medicine.

Scognamiglio R et al: Nifedipine in asymptomatic patients with severe regurgitation and normal left ventricular function, *N Engl J Med* 331:689-694, 1994.

26   Cardiomyopathies

Pravin M. Shah

CARDIOMYOPATHY: GENERAL CONSIDERATIONS

Cardiomyopathy is best defined as diffuse myocardial disorder attributable neither to pressure or volume overload nor to segmental loss of muscle function secondary to ischemic damage. This definition does not exclude the coexistence of valvular, hypertensive, or coronary artery disease; it merely requires that these be judged not responsible for the myocardial dysfunction. Hence, the diagnosis of cardiomyopathy involves identifying concomitants and excluding other causes.

The current definition used by the World Health Organization/International Society of Cardiology Task Force on Cardiomyopathies specifically describes these as "heart muscle disease or diseases of unknown cause or causes." The previous use of etiologic classification into primary and secondary types is therefore redundant. However, it is important to consider etiologies that may result in cardiac involvement simulating cardiomyopathies (Box 26-1).

It is generally unnecessary to subject every patient to laboratory investigation for each possible cause, since clinical clues to the probable cause are often present. The potentially correctable conditions—hemochromatosis, hypophosphatemia, and, rarely, beriberi and endocrine states without other end-organ features—should be carefully considered. Similarly, it may be necessary to examine the possible role of toxic agents such as alcohol, since these may add to myocardial dysfunction even when not causing the disease.

The pathophysiologic classification (Box 26-2) offers an excellent opportunity to characterize the underlying myocardial dysfunction and thus approach therapy more physiologically. Although there is some overlap, the dilated cardiomyopathies are characterized by abnormal systolic pump function; the hypertrophic cardiomyopathies, by disordered diastolic function from reduced distensibility; and the restrictive cardiomyopathies, by elements of both. In addition, myocarditis will be considered in this discussion as it is often indistinguishable from dilated cardiomyopathy.

MYOCARDITIS

Myocarditis is inflammation of the myocardium that is commonly caused by infectious agents, particularly viruses. It may occur in an

acute, subacute, or chronic form, and the inflammation may involve the myocardial cell, interstitium, and/or vascular elements. Any infectious agent may produce cardiac inflammation by direct invasion of the myocardium, by production of a myocardial toxin, or by autoimmunity. The viral etiologies include echovirus, poliovirus, and coxsackie A and B viruses, with coxsackie B being the most frequent. Myocarditis may also be caused by pharmacologic agents, chemicals, metabolic disorders, radiation, or other physical agents. In some patients, myocarditis presents as acute congestive heart failure; in others, it results in chronic insidious congestive cardiomyopathy. In most patients with acute myocarditis, the inflammatory process is transient and subclinical, and no evidence of persistent cardiac disease exists.

The clinical manifestations are highly variable and may fall into one of the following categories: (1) Asymptomatic patients generally have focal myocarditis, diagnosed as an incidental finding at autopsy, with a reported incidence varying between 1% and 7%. (2) Symptomatic patients may have a predominantly systemic illness with few or no signs of cardiac involvement except for subtle clues such as persistent tachycardia or electrocardiographic changes. (3) Cardiac presentation includes chest pain of myopericarditis or symptoms of heart failure. (4) Uncommonly, focal myocarditis with features of acute myocardial infarction is noted. (5) Similarly, presentation with arrhythmia conduction disturbance and occasionally with sudden death has been described. (6) Some patients may present with pulmonary or systemic emboli.

Myocarditis may result in nonspecific symptoms, including fatigue, dyspnea, palpitations, and precordial discomfort. Chest pain is usually caused by associated pericarditis but may suggest myocardial ischemia.

Physical examination commonly reveals tachycardia. The first heart sound (S_1) is often soft; third or fourth heart sounds (S_3, S_4) are frequent, and a soft apical systolic murmur (mitral regurgitation) may be present. Diastolic murmurs are rare. A friction rub is often heard in patients who have associated pericarditis.

Clinical evidence of congestive heart failure is present in the more severe cases. The heart size is usually normal in asymptomatic pa-

---

BOX 26-1

Conditions that may simulate cardiomyopathies

Infective (e.g., viral, rickettsial, protozoal, bacterial, Chagas' disease)
Metabolic and infiltrative (e.g., hemochromatosis, amyloidosis, glycogen storage disease)
Toxic (e.g., alcohol, anticancer agents, amphetamines, cobalt)
Radiation
Endocrine (e.g., hyperthyroidism, hypothyroidism, acromegaly, Cushing's disease)
Deficiency (e.g., beriberi, hypophosphatemia)
Ischemic (e.g., diffuse nonsegmental ischemic dysfunction)
Collagen disease (e.g., periarteritis nodosa, rheumatic fever, rheumatoid arthritis)
Immunologic (transplant rejection, peripartum)
Neuromuscular (Duchenne's muscular dystrophy, myotonic dystrophy, Erb's limb-girdle dstrophy, Friedreich's ataxia)

BOX 26-2

Pathophysiologic classification of cardiomyopathies

I. Dilated (congestive) cardiomyopathy
II. Hypertrophic cardiomyopathy
   A. Asymmetrical
      1. Dynamic outflow obstruction
      2. Absence of resting or provoked outflow obstruction
   B. Concentric: dynamic outflow obstruction is uncommon
III. Restrictive cardiomyopathy

tients but may be enlarged in patients with heart failure or pericardial effusion. Pulmonary and systemic embolism may occur.

The most common electrocardiogram abnormalities involve the S-T segment and the T wave, but atrial and ventricular arrhythmias and atrioventricular (AV) conduction defects may result. Pathologic Q waves are rare. Complete AV block is usually transient but occasionally results in sudden death. Chest x-rays may reveal a normal or enlarged heart, with or without signs of pulmonary venous hypertension.

The diagnosis is often based on determining the associated systemic illness and its characteristics. Methods for identifying the responsible infectious agents are described in Chapter 233. In experienced hands, transvenous endomyocardial biopsy is a safe method of establishing the diagnosis and assessing the results of therapy in severe cases of myocarditis. Although the biopsy does not usually identify the responsible infectious agent, a diagnosis of active myocarditis may be made on the basis of inflammatory infiltrate accompanied by necrosis of adjacent myocytes. Although the histologic appearance of acute myocarditis is often characteristic, the criteria for diagnosis of chronic, indolent, resolving "myocarditis" are often subtle and subject to considerable interobserver variability. Furthermore, the inflammatory changes may be spotty, requiring several biopsy specimens from different regions to provide diagnostic information. Noninvasive techniques, such as echocardiography and radionuclide angiography (Chapter 13), may be useful for detecting impaired left ventricular performance or pericardial effusion during the systemic illness. Continuous ambulatory ECG recordings have been used to document atrial and ventricular arrhythmias in various infectious diseases. Positive gallium scans, although not specific for myocarditis, have been reported in a subgroup of patients responsive to immunosuppressive therapy.

Treatment is often supportive and includes rest and adequate oxygenation. Congestive heart failure is treated in the usual manner with digitalis, diuretics, and vasodilators, with particular attention to the possibility of digitalis toxicity. Important arrhythmias should be treated with the usual antiarrhythmic agents. The use of corticosteroids in acute viral myocarditis is controversial; it is generally believed to be contraindicated, since in vitro studies indicate that the use of corticosteroids during the acute viral illness may actually exacerbate the infectious process. A recent prospective multicenter trial of immunosuppressive agents and of steroid therapy in histologically proven myocarditis failed to confirm substantial benefits over placebo. Currently, most authorities recommend that immunosuppressive therapy be used in acute viral myocarditis only as a last resort.

DILATED (CONGESTIVE) CARDIOMYOPATHY

As the term implies, the most frequent underlying anatomic change in dilated (congestive) cardiomyopathy is chamber (ventricular) dilation, generally accompanied by an alteration in systolic pump function that results in the clinical syndrome of congestive heart failure. Although most patients in the past came under observation only after symptoms of heart failure developed, current widespread use of echocardiography permits recognition of the disorder at an early stage. Occasionally, a development of new bundle branch block may predate an early stage of cardiomyopathy even prior to any signs of chamber dilation or pump dysfunction.

Pathology

Postmortem examination reveals enlargement and dilation of all four cardiac chambers. The cardiac valves are intrinsically normal, as are the coronary arteries. However, cardiomyopathy may coexist in a patient with associated valvular or coronary artery disease. Mural thrombi are often noted in the ventricles or the atria.

Histologic examination reveals myocardial cell degeneration and areas of necrosis and fibrosis; cellular infiltration is generally not pronounced except in patients with an acute inflammatory process.

Needle biopsy was introduced as a technique for evaluating myocardial damage caused by specific conditions. However, the usefulness of needle biopsy has so far been limited to occasional conditions such as amyloid disease, hemochromatosis, and sarcoidosis.

Pathophysiology

Diffuse myocardial damage leading to dilated cardiomyopathy predominantly affects systolic pump function. In the early phases, the only objective evidence may be signs of circulatory insufficiency occurring with imposed stress, such as physical exercise. Progressive impairment of cardiac function subsequently develops. Chamber dilation is the result of increased residual volume caused by reduced ejection fraction, but in turn may provide a partial compensation on the basis of the Frank-Starling mechanism. Eventually, however, hypertrophy results, with an increase in muscle mass. All patients with dilated cardiomyopathy, except those with the most acutely fulminant disease (i.e., acute myocarditis), have cardiac hypertrophy (i.e., increased muscle mass) although wall thicknesses are generally normal (i.e., so-called eccentric hypertrophy).

The symptomatic phase of dilated cardiomyopathy is generally the result of elevated filling pressures and resulting venous congestion, although reduced cardiac output may contribute by decreasing glomerular filtration rate and increasing sodium reabsorption. In addition, a prominent symptom of generalized fatigue results from subnormal resting cardiac output. The symptom complex in dilated cardiomyopathy may differ from that in congestive heart failure from other causes, in which primary involvement of the left heart chambers with pulmonary congestion, edema, and pulmonary arterial hypertension precedes the development of right heart failure. Most patients with dilated cardiomyopathy have simultaneous involvement of both left and right heart chambers. Thus the sequence of progressive symptomatology is different and involves systemic venous congestion in the early phases. Isolated left or right ventricular cardiomyopathy may be present in less than 10% of cases.

Clinical and Laboratory Manifestations

Dyspnea is a common early symptom. Effort intolerance is often a rapidly progressive symptom. In advanced disease, orthopnea develops with superimposed episodes of paroxysmal nocturnal dyspnea. Episodic coughing with frothy expectoration may accompany dyspnea. Some patients can comfortably lie flat despite pulmonary edema, especially when it is chronic or is associated with right ventricular failure.

Palpitation may represent sinus tachycardia with minimum exertion or commonly occurring arrhythmias. Easy fatigability is often due to low cardiac output and may replace dyspnea as a prominent presenting symptom.

Dependent edema is secondary to systemic venous congestion and constitutes evidence of right ventricular failure, whereas right upper quadrant abdominal pain with tenderness indicates hepatic congestion. Generally, weight loss and anorexia are late features, although apparent weight gain from water retention may mask muscle wasting.

The physical examination may provide important diagnostic clues in the more advanced phase, but is generally not helpful in the early phase of minimum or no symptoms.

Signs of systemic venous congestion may include jugular venous distention, hepatomegaly, dependent edema, ascites, and, in advanced cases, mild jaundice and cachexia. Signs of pulmonary venous congestion include pulmonary rales and pleural effusions.

There is lateral and caudal displacement of a sustained left ventricular apical impulse, and the diastolic rapid-filling phase (S_3) and presystolic (S_4) phase of the left ventricle are often palpable. A prominent pulmonic component of S_2 is heard in patients with severe pulmonary hypertension. The presence of an apical S_3 is related to an increased left atrial (filling) pressure, dilated chamber, and reduced cardiac output. An apical S_4 is related to diminished left ventricular compliance and strong atrial contraction and is often absent in advanced cases. The presence of both S_3 and S_4 results in a quadruple rhythm and, in the presence of tachycardia, may simulate a middiastolic rumble. When S_3 and S_4 are superimposed during tachycardia, a loud summation gallop sound may be heard. Not infrequently, the S_3 or summation gallop sound may be the loudest sound appreciated over the apex. Similar gallop sounds originating in the right heart are generally best heard over the lower left sternal edge and subxiphoid areas (Chapter 11).

An apical systolic murmur of mitral regurgitation may be heard as a high-pitched, blowing murmur of variable duration and intensity. A similar murmur at the lower left sternal edge may represent tricuspid regurgitation. A diastolic rumble suggests a more severe degree of mitral regurgitation.

Pulsus alternans is often noted as evidence of ventricular dysfunction (Chapter 11). It is generally accentuated by upright posture and other maneuvers resulting in decreased ventricular volume.

On the chest x-ray, cardiomegaly with enlargement of all chambers is generally noted in symptomatic patients. The lung fields show signs of pulmonary venous congestion and edema.

On the ECG, sinus tachycardia, intraventricular conduction disturbances, signs of left ventricular or biventricular enlargement, signs of left or biatrial enlargement, and low voltage are noted, singly or in combination. Although first- or second-degree AV block may be observed, higher degrees of heart block are uncommon.

Echocardiography is extremely useful to confirm diagnosis and to quantitatively assess ventricular function. The left ventricular internal dimension is increased, often in excess of 7 cm; its percentage of dimensional shortening is markedly reduced (Chapter 13). The ventricular septum and posterior left ventricular walls are of normal thickness. The percentage of thickening and excursions of both walls during systole are reduced. The degree of left ventricular dilation is variable and some symptomatic patients may have a normal-sized left ventricle despite marked reduction of contractile function. A striking appearance of the mitral leaflets in the middle of the left ventricular cavity may draw attention to the diagnosis. The diastole opening E point of the anterior mitral leaflet is further removed from the left side of the interventricular septum, denoted as E point–septal separation. This distance may be well in excess of 1 cm and reflects reduced ejection fraction. Reduced ejection fraction is generally associated with a diffuse reduction in contractility; however, occasionally regional dysfunction may be present, mimicking an ischemic etiology. The valves are structurally normal in the absence of coexisting organic valvular heart disease. The left atrium and the right ventricle are often enlarged. The reported prognostic study of echocardiography revealed that the ratio of left ventricular dimension to wall thickness ejection fraction and the E point–septal separation are highly predictive of long-term survival.

Doppler echocardiography commonly demonstrates moderate regurgitation across the mitral and tricuspid valves even in the absence of murmurs. Mitral inflow velocity pattern may show tall, peaked E wave with rapid deceleration suggesting elevated left atrial pressure. Right ventricular and pulmonary artery pressures can be estimated by the use of continuous-wave Doppler signal of tricuspid regurgitation. Cardiac output can be accurately assessed by Doppler methods.

Radionuclide angiography also allows accurate assessment of ejection fraction, as well as semiquantitative evaluation of regional wall motion abnormalities, and may be used when echocardiography is technically not feasible.

A diagnosis of dilated cardiomyopathy may be made in most patients from the clinical and echocardiographic studies. Cardiac catheterization may be indicated (1) to assess the severity of coexisting valvular heart disease, (2) to assess the presence of associated coronary artery disease, and (3) to evaluate the acute effects of therapeutic interventions.

Extensive multivessel coronary artery disease may coexist without symptomatic ischemic events. The term *ischemic cardiomyopathy* is often used to describe patients with global dysfunction secondary to chronic global ischemia (hibernating myocardium) without clinically evident myocardial infarction. Those with truly ischemic cardiomyopathy may benefit from myocardial revascularization (e.g., coronary bypass surgery), in the presence of substantial segments with myocardial viability (e.g., by dobutamine echocardiography or by positron emission tomography).

Management

Since the underlying cause in most cases of dilated cardiomyopathy is unknown or no longer relevant, the principles of management are largely symptomatic or supportive. These may best be considered under (1) reduction in cardiac work, (2) supportive measures, (3) measures directed toward specific causes, and (4) radical therapy.

Although it appears to make intuitive sense to restrict physical ac-

tivity in order to reduce cardiac work, the salutary effects of moderate activity (such as walking) are well demonstrated for most patients in classes I to III. More strict bed rest is indicated for class IV patients until the functional class is improved with aggressive medical treatment.

The introduction of vasodilator therapy in the treatment of acute or chronic congestive failure with or without acute myocardial infarction is a major therapeutic advance (Chapter 19). Patients with dilated or congestive cardiomyopathy are often managed effectively with the use of these agents. The usefulness of vasodilators is well established in the presence of moderate or severe heart failure in addition to digitalis and diuretic therapy. Reductions of both preload and afterload by vasodilator therapy are desirable endpoints in the setting of increased filling pressures and result in decreased ventricular volume, reduced wall tension, decreased oxygen and metabolic demands, and often an increase in cardiac output. Vasodilator agents currently in use include intravenous sodium nitroprusside, sublingual and oral nitrates, intravenous and oral hydralazine, and converting enzyme inhibitors such as captopril or enalapril (Chapter 19).

The agents captopril and enalapril inhibit conversion of angiotensin I to angiotensin II and the degradation of bradykinin. They cause a reduction in systemic vascular resistance and ventricular filling pressures, with an increase in cardiac output and no change in heart rate.

The use of vasodilators is shown to improve survival. This beneficial effect was seen in patients with mild symptoms (class II), as well as with more advanced symptoms (classes III or IV).

The oral administration of digitalis has long-established effectiveness in treating chronic congestive heart failure (Chapter 19). The drug is generally used along with the vasodilators. The basic therapeutic use of digitalis in patients with dilated cardiomyopathy is similar to that for congestive heart failure from any cause. It is especially indicated in the presence of resting sinus tachycardia and supraventricular arrhythmias, including atrial fibrillation.

Among the catecholamines and other sympathomimetic amines, the agents with the most therapeutically potent beta-adrenergic effects on the myocardium are dopamine and dobutamine (Chapters 19 and 20). The role of these agents in dilated cardiomyopathy with congestive heart failure is restricted to advanced refractory heart failure. They favorably influence circulatory and metabolic balance. Intravenous infusions of these agents for 5 to 10 days may be attempted with appropriate monitoring in an intensive care unit setting. Intraarterial pressures may also be monitored. These agents may be less effective and possibly detrimental in the absence of high filling pressure (wedge pressure < 15 mm Hg). Newer inotropic agents, for example, amrinone and milrinone, are often beneficial when administered acutely; however, a deleterious effect on survival with their chronic use is reported (Chapter 19).

Long-term oral anticoagulant therapy may be considered in patients on prolonged bed rest, since the likelihood of venous thromboembolic disease is increased in the setting of low cardiac output. Similarly, patients with chronic or frequent atrial fibrillation, echocardiographically demonstrated intracardiac clots, or evidence of systemic or pulmonary thromboembolism are candidates for anticoagulant therapy. A routine use of anticoagulants in all patients is controversial because there are no prospective studies showing improved risk-benefit ratio. Chronic hepatic congestion and previous alcohol-induced hepatic damage may complicate successful anticoagulant therapy.

Since the beta-adrenergic blocking drugs tend to depress myocardial function, their use in heart failure was felt to be contraindicated. However, several recent trials report favorable long-term effect in a substantial number of patients. A new class of beta blocker, carvediol, has recently shown impressive survival benefit over placebo, when added to digitalis, diuretics, and angiotensin-converting enzyme (ACE) inhibitors.

Antiarrhythmic drugs may be required in patients with dilated cardiomyopathy who have documented arrhythmias. Both supraventricular and ventricular arrhythmias are frequent, and the latter probably explains many of the sudden deaths observed in these patients. It remains to be demonstrated if the use of antiarrhythmic agents improves survival in this subset of patients. Indeed, increased proarrhythmia with class I agents may produce an adverse outcome.

Cardiac transplantation (Chapter 34) may be considered for

younger patients with advanced myocardial damage refractory to medical therapy who show no evidence of severe pulmonary hypertension or other organ involvement. This procedure is carried out at selected centers. The 1-year patient survival rate is in excess of 80%, which is comparable to the survival rate with cadaver kidney transplants. With improved understanding of the immunologic aspects of rejection, as well as improved availability of donor organs, transplantation may offer considerable promise for patients with advanced dilated cardiomyopathy.

A large body of evidence incriminates heavy alcohol intake in dilated cardiomyopathy. In early cases, total abstinence may produce dramatic recovery. The cardiac depressant effects of alcohol make it an undesirable substance for such patients, even when no definite causal connection appears likely.

Severe hypophosphatemia in burn patients, prolonged respiratory alkalosis, chronic phosphate-binding antacid use, and treatment of diabetic ketoacidosis resulting in serum phosphate levels below 1.0 mg/dl may lead to dilated cardiomyopathy and congestive heart failure. Replenishment of phosphate rapidly leads to complete recovery.

Lithium carbonate used in manic-depressive disorders may result in toxic damage to the myocardium, with cardiac dilation, ventricular arrhythmias, and sudden death. High doses of cyclophosphamide have been associated with congestive heart failure and death from hemorrhagic myocarditis with cardiac dilation.

Doxorubicin therapy is associated with progressive cardiomegaly and depression of cardiac function. The toxicity is dose related and is observed in about 2% of patients so treated. Ingestion of a toxic dose is fatal in more than half the patients. Its occurrence may be prevented if a cumulative dose of less than 500 mg/m^2 is given. Daunorubicin shows a greater propensity than doxorubicin for cardiac toxicity in the doses used. Patients receiving these agents should be followed up with periodic echocardiograms to reveal early evidence of cardiac involvement.

Beriberi heart disease, although rare in Western countries, may cause high-output congestive heart failure with cardiomegaly in nutritionally deprived parts of the world. It is rapidly reversible with replacement of thiamine.

HYPERTROPHIC CARDIOMYOPATHIES

Hypertrophic cardiomyopathy (HCM) is a form of primary myocardial disease with a characteristic clinical and pathologic expression. Several terms have been used for the disorder: *idiopathic hypertrophic subaortic stenosis* (IHSS) in the United States, *muscular subaortic stenosis* in Canada, and *hypertrophic obstructive cardiomyopathy* (HOCM) in Europe.

A term that includes "subaortic stenosis" is unfortunate, since the disorder may be expressed without left ventricular outflow obstruction, and patients with isolated infundibular subpulmonic stenosis have been described. It is more accurate and potentially less confusing to refer to the disorder as *hypertrophic cardiomyopathy* and add the word *obstructive* if either left or right ventricular outflow obstruction can be demonstrated.

Etiology

Despite considerable progress in understanding the clinical hemodynamic, pathologic, and functional aspects of HCM, the underlying cause and pathogenesis of this disease are largely unknown. The asymmetric type of HCM is commonly a genetically transmitted disorder, but sporadic cases are also recognized.

Familial hypertrophic cardiomyopathy is inherited as an autosomal dominant disease. The exact incidence of the familial form is difficult to determine owing to the variable phenotypic expression. Several molecular genetic studies have reported mutations of β cardiac myosin heavy chains as being responsible for familial hypertrophic cardiomyopathy (Chapter 10). The chromosome loci identified in genetic mapping include 14q11, 1q3, 15q2 and 11p13-q13. Thus the genetic basis is heterogenous despite the common phenotype, hypertrophic cardiomyopathy.

The relative frequency of sporadic cases suggests that spontaneous mutations in the gene loci for this disease occur commonly and are responsible for sporadic forms of hypertrophic cardiomyopathy.

Pathology

The pathologic findings are remarkably uniform and include massive and often asymmetric hypertrophy. Thickening of the walls involves both the atria and the ventricles, although the most characteristic findings involve the left ventricle. The interventricular septum is generally much more massively hypertrophied than the free wall. This peculiar asymmetric septal hypertrophy may provide the necessary hemodynamic conditions that produce a dynamic outflow obstruction. Localization of such hypertrophy in the midlateral wall may result in midventricular obstruction and its distribution in the right ventricular infundibulum in subpulmonic stenosis.

In a subgroup of patients defined by 2D echocardiographic, cineangiographic, and/or postmortem examination, the hypertrophy involved primarily the apical portion of the left ventricle rather than the outflow tract. This is termed *asymmetric apical hypertrophy,* and such patients have none of the clinical features of intraventricular obstruction.

Striking pathologic features common to most patients with outflow obstruction include fibrous thickening of the anterior mitral leaflet and plaques in the upper interventricular septum constituting the left ventricular outflow tract. The former is thought to represent the result of frequent contacts of the anterior mitral leaflet against the interventricular septum. The endocardial plaques in the septum may be the result of jet lesions distal to the obstruction. The aortic valve is generally normal, and the coronary arteries are large and patent in the absence of coexisting disease.

On microscopy, a bizarre and disorderly array of muscle fibers is a striking feature and is associated with increased connective tissue that interrupts and crisscrosses muscle bundles. Myofibril disarray is not pathognomonic for this disease and is often spotty in distribution, but the disarray is quantitatively more severe in this condition than in others. Additional features include deep clefts in the septum, abnormal narrowing of small intramural coronary arteries, and sclerosis of the sinus node.

Pathophysiology

The functional end results of the abnormal anatomy are characteristic. They include changes in both systolic and diastolic left ventricular function, with profound effects on pressures and flow.

The integrity of overall systolic function is rather well preserved until the end stage; indeed, hyperkinetic function is a hallmark of the disorder. The cardiac output is generally normal or even increased; the ejection fraction is often supernormal. Although global function is well preserved, regional abnormalities occur; for example, the upper interventricular septum is often hypodynamic and shows reduced thickening during systole. The free walls are generally hypercontractile.

Left ventricular outflow obstruction is dynamic and variable. The variability can be observed within the same cardiac cycle, from one beat to the next and from one physiologic state to another. When present, outflow obstruction begins after the onset of early uninterrupted ejection. Present evidence suggests that the obstruction is caused by a sharp systolic anterior motion (SAM) of the mitral leaflet, which obliterates the outflow space. The actual mechanism of SAM is not clear, although it is likely to be the result of a Venturi effect from the rapid ejection of a jet of blood through an anatomically narrowed outflow space. The degree of left ventricular outflow obstruction can be accentuated by factors that reduce preload (end-diastolic volume), diminish afterload (arterial pressure), or increase contractility or heart rate. Echocardiographic recordings have demonstrated that SAM of the mitral valve is both exacerbated and prolonged by interventions that accentuate the outflow obstruction, and vice versa. Some investigators attribute the intraventricular pressure gradients to cavity obliteration. Recent echocardiographic and Doppler techniques have elucidated differences between true gradients resulting from obstruction and those caused by cavity obliteration.

Mitral regurgitation is demonstrated by color-flow Doppler echocardiography in about 90% of obstructive patients and its severity is related to the severity of outflow obstruction. Thus when outflow obstruction is accentuated with a more persistent and prominent SAM, mitral regurgitation is more severe. The factors that decrease outflow obstruction tend to reduce the degree of mitral regurgitation.

Severe right ventricular infundibular stenosis is rare and may occur either independently or concurrently with left ventricular outflow obstruction. The mechanism of right ventricular outflow obstruction is different from that on the left side, since the infundibulum is circumferentially bound by muscle. Excessive muscle contraction in this disorder results in outflow obstruction, and the factors resulting in increased contractility tend to accentuate obstruction. The tricuspid valve does not play a role in the right-sided outflow obstruction.

Distensibility and compliance of the hypertrophied ventricles are reduced, with resulting elevation in end-diastolic pressure without an increase in volume. The abnormalities of early diastolic relaxation coupled with reduced distensibility tend to influence the pattern of diastolic filling. Thus, early, rapid, passive filling is notably impaired, necessitating a stronger atrial contraction to deliver diastolic inflow into a relatively nondistensible left ventricle. This dependence on atrial contraction to maintain efficient flow is exemplified by a sudden drop in cardiac output when atrial fibrillation supervenes. Although this abnormality of diastolic compliance has important hemodynamic consequences, namely, elevations of left atrial and pulmonary venous pressures with resultant pulmonary congestion and edema, actual obstruction to inflow is rare.

Clinical Features

Effort dyspnea and paroxysmal nocturnal dyspnea constitute the most common symptoms and represent evidence of pulmonary congestion. Because elevations in pulmonary venous and left atrial pressures occur in the presence of a hyperdynamic left ventricle, they are attributed to increased stiffness of the hypertrophic ventricles. In some patients, especially those with volume overload, frank pulmonary edema may be noted.

Syncope and dizziness short of loss of consciousness (presyncope) are common. These may be effort-related, although they are not predictably so. The frequency of the episodes is highly variable. The exact mechanism is obscure; however, it is probably related to reflex vasodilation and hypotension induced by stretching the left ventricular baroreceptors. As an alternative, arrhythmia may play a role by producing a decrease in cardiac output.

Typical effort angina simulating symptomatic coronary artery disease is frequent, although episodes of chest pain may be prolonged and may occur spontaneously at rest. Typically, sublingual nitroglycerin fails to provide prompt relief, although this is not a universal finding. In the presence of large, patent coronary arteries, ischemia is probably caused by intramyocardial compression of coronary arteries and increased myocardial tension and muscle mass, with oxygen requirements outstripping oxygen delivery.

Palpitations may merely represent awareness of forcible heartbeats, especially in the left lateral decubitus position. More commonly, atrial and ventricular arrhythmias are responsible. Tachyarrhythmias are poorly tolerated and are often associated with symptoms of low output and hypotension. Isolated or short runs of ventricular and supraventricular premature depolarizations often occur without symptoms.

The physical signs also tend to vary considerably from minimal or nonspecific to highly characteristic. The characteristic signs include evidence of left ventricular hypertrophy and obstruction of left ventricular outflow, left ventricular inflow, and right ventricular outflow.

A powerful systolic thrust of the left ventricle on palpation indicates an increase in muscle mass, and, although less frequent, the characteristic bifid apex in systole is virtually diagnostic of this condition. A prominent atrial contraction imparts a strong presystolic impulse that is palpable at the apex. A trifid impulse composed of a prominent A wave and bifid systolic peaks is sometimes palpable and often recordable on apex cardiogram. Such a finding is highly characteristic of this disease. S_4 is present in virtually every patient in sinus rhythm.

A jerky arterial pulse with sharp upstroke is typical, although not diagnostic. Occasionally, a bifid (bisferiens) pulse may be felt, especially in the carotid artery (Chapter 11). A bifid arterial pulse in association with a normal pulse pressure is highly characteristic of HOCM (Fig. 26-1). The pulse contour in HOCM is influenced by the presence and severity of outflow obstruction. In the absence of resting obstruction, the arterial pulse is essentially normal.

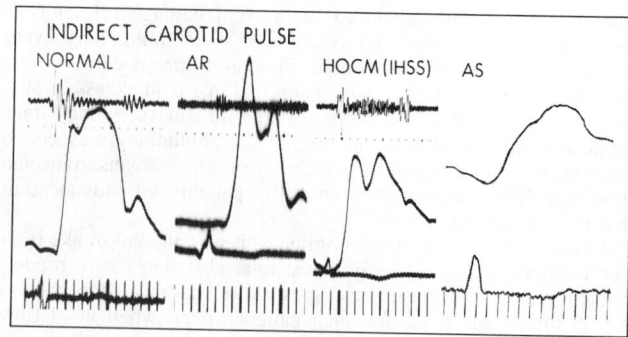

FIGURE 26-1   Contour of indirect carotid pulse in hypertrophic obstructive cardiomyopathy, HOCM (IHSS), compared with normal, aortic regurgitation *(AR)*, and aortic stenosis *(AS)*. Note the bifid systolic pulse in *AR* and *HOCM*, although the former is associated with wide pulse pressure and the latter with normal pulse pressure.

Table 26-1   Effects of physiologic and pharmacologic maneuvers in hypertrophic obstructive cardiomyopathy

INTERVENTION	LEFT VENTRICULAR OUTFLOW OBSTRUCTION	MURMUR
Valsalva		
Phase 2-3	Increased	Increased
Phase 4	Decreased	Decreased
Squatting	Decreased	Decreased
Upright posture	Increased	Increased
Exercise	Increased	Increased
Amyl nitrite inhalation	Increased	Increased
Methoxamine	Decreased	Decreased
Isoproterenol	Increased	Increased
Propranolol	Decreased or unchanged	Decreased or unchanged

A systolic murmur of variable intensity is present along the left sternal border and apex. It is poorly transmitted to the aortic area and neck vessels. It is medium pitched or high pitched, with onset after the S_1. The murmur resembles a long ejection murmur along the left sternal border and attains a regurgitant quality (high pitched, blowing) toward the apex. The apical murmur may be well transmitted to the axilla. The S_2 is clearly audible, and both components are well preserved. Reverse splitting with a delayed aortic component is diagnostic of severe outflow obstruction in the absence of left bundle branch block. The signs of outflow obstruction, including intensity of the systolic murmur, are accentuated by maneuvers that augment the severity of obstruction (Table 26-1 and Fig. 26-2).

The blowing apical murmur of mitral regurgitation also generally varies in intensity with dynamic outflow obstruction. In some instances mitral valve regurgitation may be independent of outflow obstruction. This can be detected by raising the blood pressure with methoxamine or angiotensin, which, while relieving outflow obstruction, does not diminish murmur intensity. These patients may require mitral valve surgery; hence this differentiation is clinically important.

Whereas a prominent atrial sound (S_4) is a constant feature of a noncompliant hypertrophied left ventricle, a mitral diastolic murmur simulating mitral stenosis may occasionally lead to consideration of rheumatic mitral disease. The absence of an opening snap and the presence of severe, unexplained left ventricular hypertrophy should point to a correct diagnosis.

The systolic murmur of infundibular pulmonic stenosis is similar to that noted in congenital infundibular pulmonic stenosis. The murmur is not prominent at the lower left sternal edge. The ejection sound is absent, and the pulmonary closure sound is delayed. When infundibular obstruction accompanies left ventricular outflow obstruction, the clinical signs of the latter dominate. However, isolated right ventricular outflow obstruction may be difficult to differentiate from con-

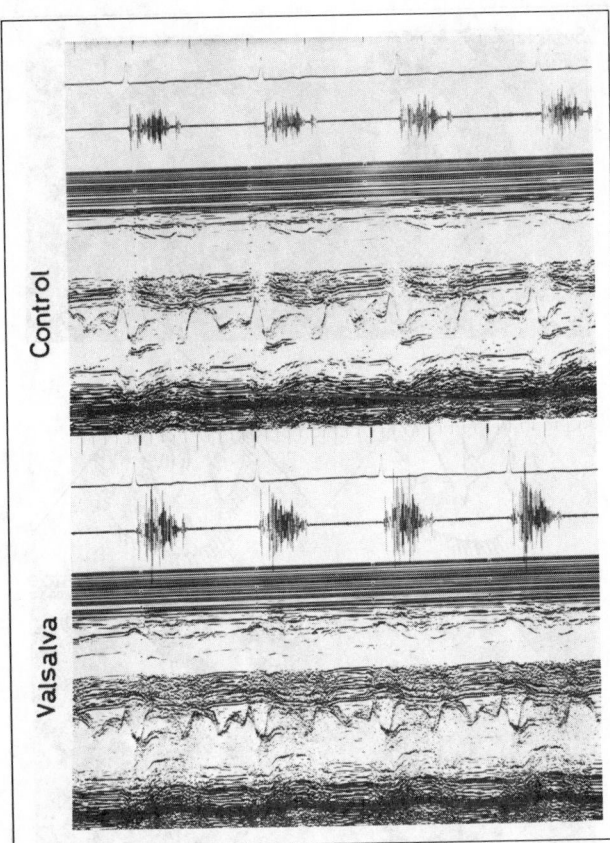

FIGURE 26-2 Effects of Valsalva maneuver on the murmur intensity and SAM of the mitral valve are shown in the control *(upper panel)* and during Valsalva strain *(lower panel)*. Note the increase in amplitude of the murmur along with more prominent systolic motion.

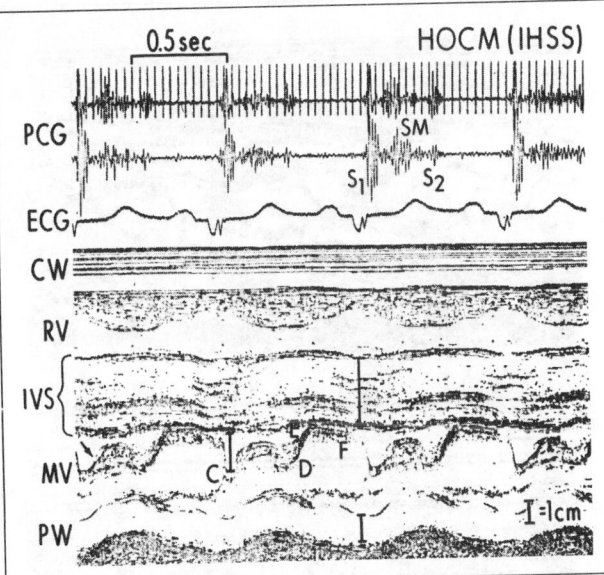

FIGURE 26-3 M-mode echocardiogram in a patient with HOCM. The interventricular septum *(IVS)* is markedly thickened (2 cm) and is more than 1.5 times the thickness of the posterior wall *(PW)*. The mitral valve *(MV)* echo shows systolic anterior motion *(arrow)*, which starts after closure point *C* and returns to baseline before diastolic opening point *D*. The open valve in early diastole at point *E* comes in contact with the *IVS*, and the diastolic slope *(E-F)* is attenuated. *PCG,* Phonocardiogram.

genital infundibular pulmonic stenosis until evidence for unexplained left ventricular hypertrophy is sought.

The common conditions to be considered in the differential diagnosis include other forms of left ventricular outflow obstruction, mitral regurgitation, and coronary artery disease.

Laboratory Diagnosis

A routine 12-lead ECG often discloses evidence of left ventricular hypertrophy with increased QRS voltage or ST-T wave changes in the lateral precordial leads (V_4 to V_6). All signs of left ventricular hypertrophy are absent in about 10% of patients despite the massive increase in cardiac muscle mass. Hence a normal ECG does not exclude the diagnosis of HCM. On occasion, large, abnormal Q waves simulating myocardial infarction are noted, representing septal depolarization.

Other features include a short P-R interval, Wolff-Parkinson-White syndrome, left-axis deviation caused by left anterior hemiblock, and complete left or right bundle branch block. Atrial and ventricular premature depolarizations are common but may be detected only with ambulatory ECG recording. Complete heart block is rare.

Posteroanterior and lateral chest x-rays are often reported to be normal. Evidence of left ventricular enlargement may be subtle, since the cavity size is not increased. Left atrial size shows a mild enlargement, except in a stage of advanced decompensation or severe mitral regurgitation. Pulmonary venous engorgement may be seen, but frank pulmonary edema and signs of pulmonary arterial hypertension are infrequent.

Echocardiography (Chapter 13) is an important method of diagnosing HCM (Fig. 26-3). This technique is useful for evaluating the thickness of the interventricular septum and left ventricular posterior wall; their movements in systole; the end-diastolic and end-systolic

dimensions of the left ventricular cavity along its minor axis; the left ventricular outflow size, defined as the space between the anterior mitral leaflet and interventricular septum; and the functional aspects of mitral and aortic valve motion. It also permits differentiation of concentric from asymmetric hypertrophy. In the former, the interventricular septum/left ventricular posterior wall ratio is close to unity; in the latter, the ratio exceeds 1.5 : 1.0.

Dynamic left ventricular outflow obstruction is diagnosed by analyzing the systolic motion of the mitral valve. Abnormal SAM of the anterior mitral leaflet with its apposition against the interventricular septum localizes the outflow obstruction in HOCM. The SAM begins sometime after onset of early ejection and is terminated in endsystole before the S_2.

The dynamic nature of obstruction may be interpreted from variations in the extent of SAM with different maneuvers designed to alter the dynamic obstruction. Patients without resting obstruction usually have small and incomplete SAM, whereas those with high resting gradients tend to have complete SAM touching the septum. Since SAM of the anterior mitral leaflet is probably caused by a Venturi effect from rapid, early ejection across the left ventricular outflow space, its occurrence in other conditions may be predicted. It has been noted in hyperkinetic circulatory states, in aortic regurgitation, and during infusion of dopamine in a patient in shock. Echocardiographic simulation of SAM may be observed in mitral valve prolapse and in pericardial effusion, but the differentiation is generally easy. As a result of the dynamic midsystolic obstruction to outflow, the aortic valve cusps may show premature closure with late systolic reopening. Diastolic movement of the mitral valve is impaired, with a flat E to F slope (Chapter 13).

A combination of narrow left ventricular outflow space, thickened interventricular septum, and the typical SAM of the anterior mitral leaflet is virtually diagnostic of HOCM. When the interventricular septal wall/posterior wall ratio exceeds 1.5 : 1.0, asymmetric hypertrophy can be diagnosed confidently. With rare exceptions, patients with HCM demonstrate asymmetric septal hypertrophy, although the latter is not specific for HCM. Two-dimensional echocardiography may reveal the asymmetric hypertrophy to involve the lateral free wall, the apex, the distal septum, and rarely the posteroinferior wall. Additional findings include midsystolic preclosure of one or more aortic valve cusps (Fig. 26-4), a hypodynamic interventricular septum

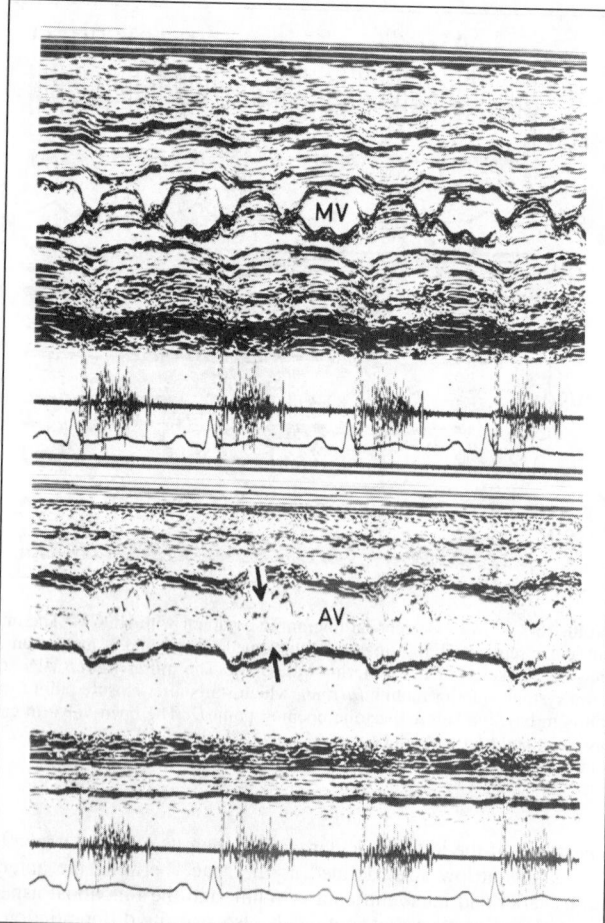

FIGURE 26-4   M-mode echocardiogram at the levels of the mitral valve *(MV)* *(upper panel)* and aortic valve *(AV)* *(lower panel)*, in a patient with HOCM. Note the systolic anterior motion of the mitral valve and midsystolic aortic valve closure *(arrow)*. Simultaneous ECG and phonocardiograms are shown in both panels. Note the phonocardiogram showing a late-onset murmur that ends before the S_2.

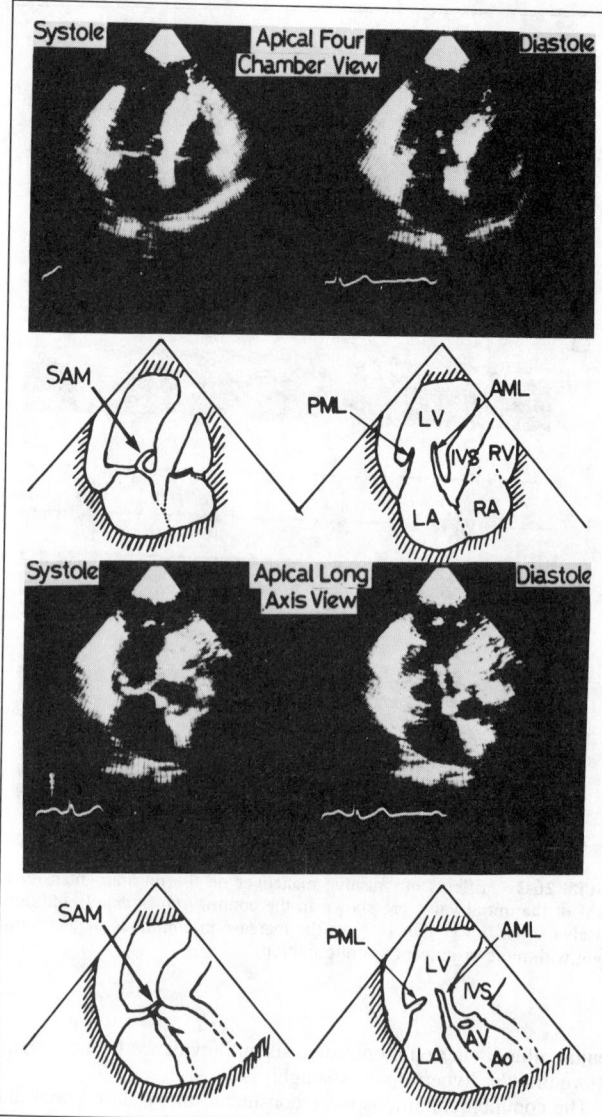

FIGURE 26-5   Two-dimensional echocardiograms with the apical four-chamber view *(upper panel)* and apical chamber view *(lower panel)* in a patient with HOCM. Midsystolic frames are shown on the left and middiastolic to late diastolic on the right. Note the anterior *(AML)* and posterior *(PML)* mitral leaflets in diastole and systole. The systolic coaptation is abnormal, with the distal AML bending toward the interventricular septum *(IVS)* and causing systolic anterior motion *(SAM)*.

with diminished systolic motion, and reduced diastolic slope of the anterior mitral leaflet. When SAM is absent at rest and following provocative maneuvers (i.e., Valsalva maneuver or amyl nitrite inhalation), it may be inferred that HCM is of the nonobstructive type. A confirmed diagnosis can be made from the echocardiographic evaluation alone.

The advent of Doppler methods has demonstrated (1) mitral regurgitation, (2) localization of outflow obstruction with increased velocity, and (3) quantitation of outflow gradients using continuous-wave Doppler method. The 2D echocardiography technique (Fig. 26-5) generally permits differentiation of SAM involving the mitral leaflet from that involving the chordae tendineae. The leaflet SAM is more characteristically associated with outflow obstruction, whereas the chordal SAM is nondiagnostic and represents passive buckling of the chordae tendineae in a rapidly emptying left ventricle. With the advent of Doppler echocardiography, it is possible to obtain information on flow and pressure dynamics using pulsed- and continuous-wave modes. The pulsed-wave Doppler method can localize the site of obstruction by showing aliasing or turbulence below the aortic valve when obstruction is localized in the left ventricular outflow tract; the measurement of high velocities by the continuous-wave Doppler method can be used to measure the pressure drop across the subvalvular obstruction on the basis of simplified Bernoulli equation. The contour of the outflow tract velocity profile mirrors the profile of the pressure drop from the left ventricular cavity to the outflow tract and assumes a characteristic dagger shape. As ventricular ejection begins, the early velocity is around 1.5 m/sec, commensurate with

the rapid early ejection. Subsequently, the Doppler velocity increases progressively to reach a peak in mid to late systole and returns to baseline at the end of ejection. This profile differs sharply from that seen in fixed obstruction, such as valvular aortic stenosis, where a smooth contour of increasing velocity is observed, even when it peaks in midsystole (Fig. 26-6). In addition, the presence and severity of mitral regurgitation can be assessed. A similar approach can be used to evaluate right ventricular infundibular obstruction.

Until the advent of echocardiography, final confirmation of diagnosis rested with cardiac catheterization and selective cardiac angiography (Chapter 14). A key diagnostic feature is the demonstration of dynamic left ventricular outflow obstruction. Special care must be taken, however, to avoid recording an artifactual gradient from entrapment of the catheter. Analysis of the recorded arterial pressure and pressure gradient during a postectopic beat often provides an important clue. Typically, the arterial pulse pressure is narrower in the postectopic beat than the sinus beat, in contrast to the normal and the fixed forms of left ventricular outflow obstruction (e.g., valvular aortic stenosis), when the

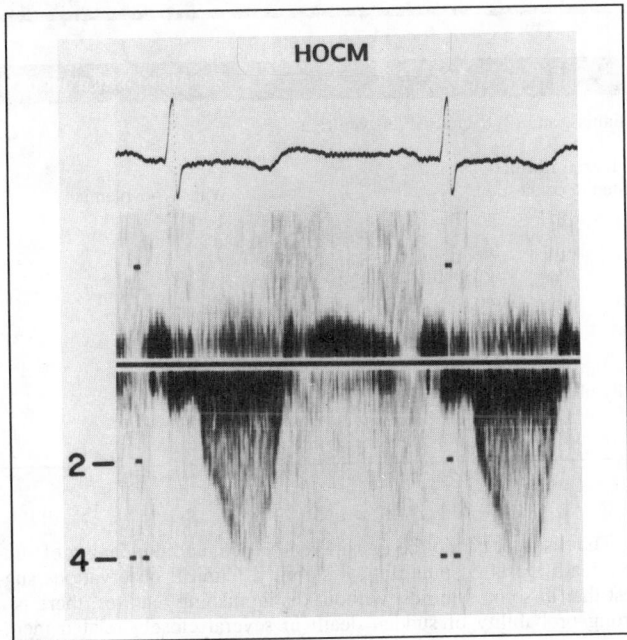

A

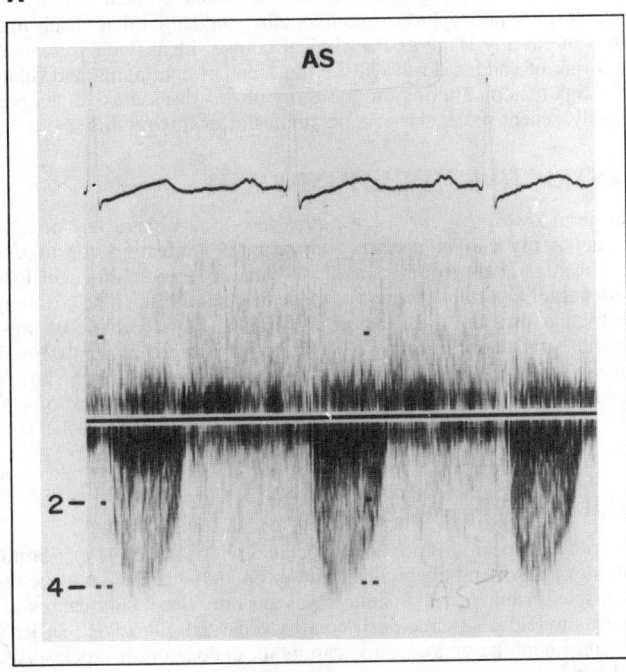

B

FIGURE 26-6   The continuous-wave Doppler spectral display of velocity profile of outflow obstruction in hypertrophic obstructive cardiomyopathy *(HOCM)* **(A)** shows a characteristic dagger shape. The peak velocity is reached in mid to late systole of 4.0 m/sec, consistent with peak systolic gradient of 64 mm Hg $(\Delta P = 4.V^2)$. In contrast, the velocity profile in aortic valve stenosis *(AS)* **(B)** shows a smooth progressive rise to a peak. The striking difference in the shapes of the velocity profiles by continuous-wave Doppler provides an important clue of dynamic *(HOCM)* versus fixed *(AS)* outflow obstruction.

pulse pressure is wider in the postectopic beat. Accentuation of outflow gradient with the Valsalva maneuver, amyl nitrite inhalation, or isoproterenol infusion provides added confirmation.

Selective left ventricular cineangiography demonstrates the characteristic anatomic and functional features (Chapter 14). Ventricular geometry is altered, the cavity assuming a sausage shape in the right anterior oblique projection. In a few patients, simultaneous left and right ventricular angiograms have been reported to demonstrate a

massively thickened interventricular septum, especially in its midportion. Since echocardiography provides a reliable means of diagnosing HCM and defining its anatomic and functional aspects, catheterization-angiography studies are reserved for selected patients and on rare occasions. The invasive diagnostic confirmation is unnecessary in most cases and should be avoided.

Management

Both medical and surgical management are at present palliative. The major objectives of therapy are to improve symptoms, ameliorate outflow obstruction, improve left ventricular compliance, suppress arrhythmias, and prevent and treat major complications, that is, bacterial endocarditis and thromboembolism.

Sudden severe physical activities such as competitive sports should be avoided owing to the risk of sudden death.

Medical Management. The cardiac drugs commonly used for symptomatic relief of dyspnea or angina in other cardiac disorders are either contraindicated or must be used with caution (Table 26-2). Thus digitalis must be avoided except to treat rapid atrial fibrillation when beta-adrenergic blockade and calcium channel blockers are unsuccessful or poorly tolerated. Nitrates are generally contraindicated and are often ineffective in relieving angina. Diuretics must be used with caution so as not to produce hypovolemia.

Beta-adrenergic blocking agents have been used extensively. Slowing the heart rate is generally beneficial. Although amelioration of obstruction induced by exercise and beta-adrenergic stimulation has been demonstrated, resting gradients are reduced only in some patients with labile obstruction. Symptomatic improvement is striking in some patients and may last several years, although increasing doses may be needed; others fail to experience sustained improvement. A daily dose in excess of 480 mg may be required for some patients. These agents have not been shown to decrease the incidence of ventricular arrhythmias or sudden death. The dose of propranolol should be increased gradually and the effects monitored, especially in those without a major component of outflow obstruction.

A beneficial effect of the calcium channel–blocking drugs verapamil and long-acting nifedipine has been reported. Symptomatic amelioration is frequently observed; however, worsening of heart failure may result. In some patients with undue hypotensive effect, severe deterioration or even death may ensue. The use of these agents should be carefully monitored. Disopyramide has been used for its negative inotropism to provide symptomatic improvement in some patients with hypertrophic obstructive cardiomyopathy. A combination therapy may be cautiously considered in refractory cases.

The use of antiarrhythmic agents may be considered since sudden cardiac death is overwhelmingly the most common mode of demise, probably from arrhythmias. Atrial and ventricular arrhythmias occur in the majority of patients with HCM regardless of the symptomatic or hemodynamic state. Although supraventricular tachycardias may worsen symptoms, they are not commonly associated with sudden death. Ventricular tachycardia and other high-grade ventricular arrhythmias have been demonstrated in at least 30% of patients monitored by 72-hour ambulatory ECG recordings. Asymptomatic family members screened and found to have HCM also have a high incidence of asymptomatic ventricular arrhythmias. Treatment of ventricular tachycardia in all patients with HCM regardless of the presence of obstruction or symptoms is currently recommended. Unfortunately, ventricular arrhythmias generally have been found to be refractory to conventional agents alone or in combination with beta-adrenergic blockade. Amiodarone, a class III antiarrhythmic agent (Chapter 18), has been shown to suppress the majority of atrial and ventricular arrhythmias and is reported in an uncontrolled clinical trial to prevent sudden cardiac death in this disorder. Sotalol with combined class III antiarrhythmic and beta blocking effects may prove beneficial. However, the experience with this agent is limited.

Bacterial endocarditis is a well-known complication, and the use of prophylactic antibiotics at times of risk is recommended. Thromboembolism is observed, especially in the presence of intermittent or sustained atrial fibrillation. Anticoagulation is advised in this clinical setting, particularly if an embolic episode has been diagnosed.

The use of an AV sequential (DDD) pacemaker with appropriately

Table 26-2   Drugs used in hypertrophic cardiomyopathy

CARDIOVASCULAR DRUGS	INDICATIONS FOR USE	GENERALLY CONTRAINDICATED
Propranolol and other beta blockers	Obstruction, arrhythmias, and (?) decreased left ventricular compliance	
Digitalis	Rapid, uncontrolled atrial fibrillations	Yes
Diuretics	Pulmonary and systemic congestion	With hypovolemia
Antianginal agents—nitrates and other vasodilators		Yes
Inotropic agents—isoproterenol, dopamine, epinephrine, bitartrate		Yes
Vasopressors—angiotensin, methoxamine	Hypotension	
Atropine sulfate	Extreme bradycardia	
Antiarrhythmic agents—procainamide, quinidine sulfate, quinidine gluconate, amiodarone	Arrhythmias	Yes
Oral anticoagulants	Atrial fibrillation or thromboembolism	
Calcium channel blockers—verapamil, nifedipine	Symptoms caused by obstruction or decreased left ventricular compliance	
Disopyramide	Symptoms caused by outflow obstruction	

programmed A-V interval may ameliorate the outflow obstruction and has been recommended as a therapeutic option. Its long-term role in management remains to be elucidated. For the present, pacemaker therapy should be restricted to a setting of clinical trials in patients refractory to medical therapy.

Surgical Management. Considerable experience has been reported with transaortic ventriculomyotomy or ventriculomyectomy in patients with HOCM. Although the amount of muscle removed is small, several echocardiographic and cardiac catheterization studies have reported postoperative relief of outflow obstruction. Symptomatic improvement is often dramatic, along with reduction or abolition of the systolic murmur and other features of left ventricular outflow obstruction. The surgical approach of replacing the mitral valve to relieve outflow obstruction should be avoided, except in a few patients with severe, independent mitral regurgitation.

Surgical relief of right ventricular outflow obstruction can be carried out successfully, as in infundibular pulmonary stenosis. The current surgical approach to myectomy is considerably aided by intraoperative echocardiography. Epicardial echo accurately localizes hypertrophy and permits visualization of resected muscle in the shape of a tunnel in the outflow tract. Transesophageal echo is useful to demonstrate normalization of SAM and improvement or abolition of mitral regurgitation. This operation, to achieve consistent and optimal results, requires a team effort by an operating surgeon and cardiologist-echocardiographer. The present-day operative risk should not exceed 5%, and relief of obstruction should be realized in more than 95% of cases.

Natural History

Longitudinal studies on the course of HCM are limited in length of follow-up, but future long-term studies with additional anatomic and functional observations using echocardiography and ambulatory ECG recordings should provide useful data on its natural course.

Sudden cardiac death is the most common cause of death in patients with HCM regardless of symptomatic or hemodynamic states. Sudden death is statistically increased in patients who have a family history of sudden death and does not seem to be altered by treatment with beta-adrenergic blockers, calcium channel blockers, or surgical myotomy-myectomy, although patients surviving surgery are reported to have a lower incidence of sudden death in some series. Studies currently in progress suggest that ventricular tachycardia as documented by ambulatory ECG recordings is associated with sudden death, but a significant causal relationship has not yet been established. Furthermore, prevention of sudden death by the use of antiarrhythmic drugs remains to be demonstrated.

Progressive congestive heart failure with visceral congestion was rare, although this outcome may be more common during the end-stage disease with a longer follow-up. Twelve percent of patients had atrial arrhythmias, and almost half of those patients had established atrial fibrillation. Overall attrition rate is approximately 3.4% per year.

The disorder cannot be considered benign, and the danger of sudden death exists despite clinical stability. Clinical observations suggest that in some families, without distinguishing features, there is a strong probability of sudden death in several closely related members.

Although slow progression of the disease and clinical stability are the rule in hypertrophic cardiomyopathy, sudden cardiac death may intervene at any stage of the clinical course. Identifying patients at high risk of sudden death will be the focus of continuing and future investigations on altering the mortality of this disease. As noted previously, recent molecular-genetic studies offer this promise.

RESTRICTIVE CARDIOMYOPATHY

The term *restrictive cardiomyopathy* describes a characteristic syndrome of myocardial disease with features simulating constrictive pericarditis. The predominant hemodynamic abnormalities include evidence of diastolic restriction of ventricular filling. The resulting ventricular pressure pulse recording shows a rapid decline of pressure in early diastole, followed by a brisk rise to a plateau (termed the *square root sign*). The venous or atrial pressure pulses show a rapid Y descent and often a rapid X descent. Some evidence of systolic dysfunction may also be evident, especially on noninvasive testing.

Etiology

A variety of specific processes associated with infiltrative or fibrotic pathology involving the myocardium or endomyocardium may be responsible. Primary or idiopathic cases are rare. Secondary causes include amyloidosis, sarcoidosis, endomyocardial fibrosis, Loeffler's hypereosinophilic endocarditis, carcinoid, endocardial fibroelastosis, and hemochromatosis.

Pathology

The conspicuous features are infiltration and fibrosis involving to a varying degree the myocardium and endocardium. The ventricular size is often normal or mildly enlarged. The muscle is often stiff and thickened. The endocardium may be scarred and thickened. The atria may be conspicuously dilated. The valves are generally spared except in endomyocardial fibrosis, in which the AV valves are predominantly involved. The etiologic diagnosis rests on histologic identification of the specific infiltration. Needle biopsy may be especially useful in this regard and may assist in therapy in some instances, for example, hemochromatosis or sarcoidosis.

Pathophysiology

The diastolic restriction of ventricular filling common to this syndrome results in elevations of atrial and venous pressures. Sinus tachycardia is a compensatory feature and helps to maintain cardiac output, since the stroke volume may be relatively fixed by diastolic restriction. The venous congestion may be evident in both the lungs and the systemic organs, depending on the relative severity of involvement of the two ventricles. The ventricular pressure pulse shows a dip and plateau (square root sign). The resulting atrial pressure pulse finding is a rapid Y descent. In addition, the X descent may be prominent in some cases.

Clinical Manifestations

The clinical features are predominantly those of pulmonary and systemic venous congestion, as in dilated cardiomyopathy. Clinical evidence of cardiomegaly usually is conspicuous by its absence. The symptoms and signs of left and right heart failure are often present (Chapter 19).

On the chest x-ray, marked atrial enlargement with mild ventricular enlargement and pulmonary venous congestion, pulmonary edema, and pleural effusions are commonly present. On the ECG, sinus tachycardia with low voltage and diffuse ST-T changes are noted. Atrial fibrillation is frequently present.

The characteristic features of the echocardiogram include thickened walls with a normal or slightly enlarged ventricular cavity and moderate to marked dilation of the atria. The systolic function, as measured by fractional shortening, may be reduced. The echo appearance of the ventricular walls in amyloidosis shows a typical granular or sparkling appearance. The Doppler findings include evidence of impaired diastolic filling detected by the mitral inflow pattern. As filling pressures increase, the early filling wave becomes more pronounced and has a more rapid deceleration. This latter pattern is associated with worse prognosis. Mitral and tricuspid regurgitation are also commonly present.

The pressure waveforms and intracardiac pressures obtained during cardiac catheterization are highly suggestive of constrictive pericarditis (Chapter 27). However, differences in end-diastolic pressures in the two ventricles, with exercise, volume loading, or catecholamine infusion, are seen more often with restrictive cardiomyopathy. Right ventricular end-diastolic pressure is frequently more than one third of the peak systolic pressure in constrictive pericarditis, but is less commonly so in restrictive cardiomyopathy.

Differentiation from constrictive pericarditis may not be possible despite all the invasive and noninvasive testing and may require thoracotomy for confirmation. Such a radical approach may be needed, since constrictive pericarditis is a surgically remediable lesion.

Treatment

The basic principles of treatment are similar to those in dilated or congestive cardiomyopathy, with the following differences. First, it may be neither practical nor desirable to reduce venous pressure markedly toward normal, because a sharp reduction in cardiac output and a drop in blood pressure may result. Second, moderate tachycardia is beneficial in maintaining cardiac output, since the stroke volume is limited by diastolic restriction of filling. Third, digitalis therapy may have no beneficial effect in the absence of left ventricular enlargement, and the resulting bradycardia may reduce cardiac output. Finally, a beneficial role of vasodilator drugs has not been demonstrated.

Clinical Course and Prognosis

Most of the conditions causing restrictive cardiomyopathy have a poor prognosis and frequently a rapidly deteriorating course. Some patients with hemochromatosis may be improved by phlebotomy, and valve replacement may be indicated in those with carcinoid heart disease. Surgical resection of fibrotic endocardium has been undertaken with some success in patients with endomyocardial fibrosis in endemic areas. Treatment of the other associated infiltrative disorders is not satisfactory.

BIBLIOGRAPHY

Anderson JL et al: A randomized trial of low-dose beta-blockage therapy for idiopathic dilated cardiomyopathy, *Am J Cardiol* 55:471, 1985.

Cohn JN, Johnson G, Ziesche S et al: A comparison of enalapril with hydralazine-isosorbide dinitrate in the treatment of chronic congestive heart failure, *N Engl J Med* 325:303-310, 1991.
Dec GW, Fuster V: Idiopathic dilated cardiomyopathy, *N Engl J Med* 331:1564, 1994.
Dec GW et al: Active myocarditis in the spectrum of acute dilated cardiomyopathies: clinical features, histologic correlates and clinical outcome, *N Engl J Med* 312:885, 1985.
Kelly DP, Strauss AW: Inherited cardiomyopathies, *N Engl J Med* 330:913, 1994.
Kowey PR, Eisenberg R, Engel TR: Sustained arrhythmias in hypertrophic obstructive cardiomyopathy, *N Engl J Med* 310:1566, 1984.
Maron BJ: Hypertrophic cardiomyopathy, *Curr Probl Cardiol* 18:639, 1993.
O'Connell JB: Dilated cardiomyopathy: emerging role of endomyocardial biopsy, *Curr Probl Cardiol* 11:450, 1986.
O'Connell JB: Immunosuppression for dilated cardiomyopathy, *N Engl J Med* 321:1119, 1989.
The SOLVD Investigators: Effect of enalapril on survival in patients with reduced left ventricular ejection fraction and congestive heart failure, *N Engl J Med* 325:293, 302, 1991.
Symanski JD, Nishimura RA: The use of pacemakers in the treatment of cardiomyopathies, *Curr Probl Cardiol* 21:385-444, 1996.

CHAPTER

27 Pericardial Disease and Pericardial Heart Disease

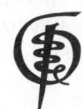

Brian D. Hoit

The pericardium is a two-layered sac consisting of a mesothelial monolayer that adheres firmly to the epicardium (visceral pericardium), reflects over the origin of the great vessels, and continues as the inner surface of a tough outer fibrous layer (parietal pericardium); between the two is a "potential" space containing a small amount (about 20 cc) of fluid. Reflections of the pericardium around the great vessels result in the formation of two recesses, the oblique and transverse sinuses. Ligamentous attachments to the sternum and diaphragm limit displacement of the pericardium and its contents within the chest. Pericardial chemoreceptors and mechanoreceptors with sympathetic afferents are described and may be related to the transmission of pericardial pain.

Although the pericardium is not essential for life, it serves many important, albeit subtle, functions. The pericardium is less compliant than, and limits distention of, the cardiac chambers, facilitating ventricular (and atrial) interaction and coupling. The latter refers to the manner in which changes in pressure and volume on one side of the heart influence pressure and volume on the other side. The pericardium also has complex effects on ventricular filling, with both qualitative and quantitative differences in restraint of right versus left ventricular filling. Although the magnitude and importance of pericardial restraint of ventricular filling at physiologic cardiac volumes remains controversial, there is general agreement that pericardial reserve volume, that is, the difference in unstressed pericardial versus cardiac volume, is relatively small, and that pericardial influences become significant when reserve volume is exceeded, as in hypervolemia and in disease states characterized by rapid increases in heart size (e.g., acute mitral and tricuspid regurgitation, pulmonary embolism, and right ventricular infarction). Moreover, the limitation of cardiac filling volumes by the pericardium may limit cardiac output and oxygen delivery during exercise. The pericardium also prevents excessive torsion and displacement of the heart, minimizes friction with surrounding structures, and is an anatomic barrier to the spread of infection from contiguous structures. In addition to its function as a lubricant, pericardial fluid may equalize gravitational, inertial, and hydrostatic forces. Finally, epicardial mesothelial cells may modulate myocyte structure, function, and gene expression.

Much of our understanding of pericardial physiology is based on pericardial pressures measured with fluid-filled catheters. However, pericardial restraint is best considered as a contact force, defined as fluid pressure plus deformational force. Pericardial contact pressure measured with flat balloons is considerably higher than liquid pressure measured with fluid-filled catheters (which is subatmospheric), and varies regionally. Although the implications are not completely understood, pericardial contact pressure is likely to be pertinent in conditions characterized by altered ventricular loading, such as pulmonary hypertension, aortic stenosis, and congestive heart failure.

Pericardial heart disease comprises pericarditis and its complications, tamponade and constriction, and congenital lesions (cysts and complete and partial absence of the pericardium). The prevalence of pericarditis has increased in recent years, owing largely to the greater use of cardiovascular surgery, hemodialysis, and immunosuppressive therapy, and to the longer survival of many cancer patients. In the last several years, acquired immunodeficiency syndrome (AIDS) has become an important cause of pericardial heart disease. In addition to its increasing prevalence, recent advances in diagnosis and therapy of pericarditis and its complications have resulted in a resurgence of interest in pericardial heart disease.

ETIOLOGY OF PERICARDIAL HEART DISEASE

Pericarditis may arise as an isolated phenomenon or may complicate a variety of systemic disorders or the use of certain drugs. It often remains clinically silent, detected only by electrocardiography (ECG) or echocardiography performed in the pursuit of unrelated complaints. In many instances, the cause of pericardial heart disease is never identified. The major definable causes of pericardial disease are infectious, neoplastic, immune/inflammatory, metabolic, iatrogenic, traumatic, and congenital (Box 27-1). Although this classification scheme is ad-

---

BOX 27-1
Causes of pericardial heart disease

Idiopathic
Infectious
  Viral
  Bacterial
  Mycobacterial
  Fungal
  Protozoal
  AIDS
Neoplastic
  Primary (mesothelioma—rare)
  Secondary (breast, lung, melanoma, lymphoma, leukemia)
Immune/inflammatory
  Connective tissue diseases
  Myocardial infarction (MI)
  Dressler's (post MI) syndrome
  Postcardiotomy
  Posttraumatic
Metabolic
  Uremia
  Dialysis-associated
  Myxedema
  Amyloidosis
Iatrogenic
  Radiation injury
  Cardiac perforation (catheters)
  Automated implantable cardioverter defibrillator placement
  Drugs (hydralazine, procainamide, isoniazide anticoagulants, minoxidil, methysergide)
Traumatic
  Blunt trauma
  Penetrating trauma
  Chylopericardium
Congenital
  Pericardial cysts
  Congenital absence of pericardium
  Mulibrey nanism
Other
  Dissecting aortic aneurysm
  Whipple's disease
  Sarcoidosis
  Familial Mediterranean fever

---

mittedly arbitrary and contains considerable overlap, it serves as a useful framework for differential diagnosis.

Infectious Pericarditis

Viral pericarditis is the most common infectious type, and along with idiopathic pericarditis, accounts for the majority of cases encountered in the outpatient setting. Agents most often implicated include coxsackie, echovirus, adenovirus, influenza, mumps, varicella-zoster, and Epstein-Barr viruses. Although definitive diagnosis is made by acute and convalescent (3 weeks) viral neutralizing antibodies, these studies are generally not helpful in sporadic cases of pericarditis.

The most common causative agents of bacterial pericarditis are streptococci, staphylococci, and gram-negative rods; *Haemophilus influenzae* is an important cause in children. Bacterial pericarditis is often mistaken for aseptic pericarditis after cardiac surgery or hemodialysis. In addition, pericardial involvement may be unrecognized when it complicates systemic infection. Children and immunosuppressed patients of all ages are most vulnerable, and unusually high fever and white cell counts are helpful clues to the presence of bacterial pericarditis. The characteristic features of acute pericarditis are frequently absent. The course is often fulminant and commonly eventuates in cardiac tamponade. Adhesive and constrictive pericarditis are common sequelae in survivors and may develop suddenly and early. Tuberculosis is an uncommon cause of pericarditis in the United States but remains a major cause of pericarditis in nonindustrialized countries. Tuberculous pericarditis results from hematogenous spread of primary tuberculosis or from breakdown of infected mediastinal lymph nodes. Therefore affected individuals generally lack typical symptoms and signs of pulmonary tuberculosis. Mycobacteria are difficult to culture from pericardial fluid, which is diagnostic in only one third of cases. Presumptive diagnosis generally requires a history of contact and/or purified protein derivative (PPD) conversion.

Although pericarditis due to histoplasmosis often resembles tuberculous pericarditis, the former seldom leads to pericardial calcification and constriction. Serologic testing is diagnostic; skin tests are useless in endemic areas such as the Ohio River valley. In contrast to histoplasmosis, other fungal infections (e.g., blastomycosis, coccidioidomycosis, aspergillosis, and candidiasis) are notably indolent, do not remit spontaneously, and if untreated, frequently result in pericardial constriction.

There is a high incidence and prevalence (11%/yr and 5%, respectively) of pericardial effusion in AIDS patients (Chapter 33). Although effusions are typically small in outpatients, large effusions and tamponade are common in hospitalized patients. The pericarditis may be due to associated malignancies (e.g., lymphoma and Kaposi's sarcoma), viruses (including human immunodeficiency virus [HIV]) and opportunistic infections (e.g., mycobacteria, cytomegalovirus, *Nocardia,* and *Cryptococcus*). However, the etiology is often unclear. An asymptomatic pericardial effusion may signal end-stage HIV disease, independent of CD4 count and albumin level.

Neoplastic Pericarditis

Metastatic neoplasia remains the leading cause of pericardial disease in hospitalized patients, most often in patients with lung or breast cancer, melanoma, lymphoma, and acute leukemia. Many cases are asymptomatic and found only incidentally at autopsy, but others cause symptoms and may progress to cardiac tamponade. Primary mesothelioma of the pericardium is rare. The presence of pericarditis in cancer patients does not imply imminent death; indeed, more than 50% of pericardial effusions in these patients are due to causes other than metastatic disease, such as infections, radiation, and drug therapy.

Immune and Inflammatory Pericarditis

Pericarditis may accompany virtually any connective tissue disease. Nearly one third of patients with rheumatoid arthritis develop pericarditis; although tamponade and effusive-constrictive disease are recognized complications, most cases are subclinical. Pericarditis does not correlate with the duration of rheumatoid arthritis and may occur more frequently when the arthritis is inactive and in patients with nodular disease. Serologic tests almost always yield positive results, and the pericardial fluid has characteristically low glucose and complement concentrations. Pericarditis may be the only manifestation of juvenile arthritis. The majority of patients with either primary or drug-induced lupus erythematosus (LE) (as may occur with procainamide and hydralazine) develop pericarditis. Although effusions, which contain LE cells, commonly occur, tamponade is unusual. Pericarditis is also a complication of acute rheumatic fever, scleroderma, Wegener's granulomatosis, polyarteritis nodosa, dermatomyositis, ankylosing spondylitis, Reiter's syndrome, Behçet's disease, and familial Mediterranean fever.

Pericarditis is common in the first few days after myocardial infarction but is clinically apparent in only 10% to 15% of cases. Cardiac tamponade seldom occurs, except in patients who receive systemic anticoagulants or suffer cardiac rupture. Pericarditis that begins more than 10 days to 2 weeks after a myocardial infarction probably represents Dressler's syndrome, which is rarely complicated by cardiac tamponade or pericardial constriction (Chapter 23).

Metabolic Pericarditis

Pericarditis affects about one third of patients with uremia and has a high associated mortality. Patients with dialysis-associated pericarditis often have neither pain nor a friction rub. Cardiac tamponade may develop, but constriction is rare. The cause of pericardial disease in this setting is unknown; nondialyzable "middle molecules," immunologic abnormalities, and infection have all been implicated. Pericarditis with effusion (sometimes containing cholesterol) occurs in about one third of patients with myxedema. This typically remains asymptomatic and regresses when the patient becomes euthyroid; cardiac tamponade is a rare complication. Pericardial effusions are common in amyloidosis but are generally small and asymptomatic.

Iatrogenic Pericardial Disease

Iatrogenic pericardial disease results from both the calculated complications and the unanticipated effects of diagnostic and therapeutic procedures. Radiation injury to the pericardium, following exposure in excess of 4000 rads, frequently occurs within 1 year after completing intensive therapy to the mediastinum; however, chronic effusions or pericardial constriction may become manifest only after many years. Postcardiotomy syndrome, which complicates 5% to 30% of cardiac operations, usually appears in the second or third week to 2 months after cardiac surgery; affected patients frequently have high titers of antiheart and antiviral antibodies and may suffer cardiac tamponade. Cardiac perforation complicating diagnostic cardiac catheterization and pacemaker insertion, complications of endoscopic sclerotherapy of esophageal varices, automatic defibrillator electrode placement, and drugs (anticoagulants, thrombolytics, drugs causing a lupuslike syndrome, minoxidil, methysergide) are other causes of iatrogenic pericardial disease.

Traumatic Pericardial Disease

Blunt and penetrating trauma are important causes of pericarditis, particularly among young males. Although traumatic pericarditis is often overshadowed by associated injuries and usually resolves uneventfully, cardiac tamponade and pericardial constriction occur occasionally. As a result, presentation may be delayed weeks or years after the chest injury. Chylous pericardial effusions generally follow traumatic or surgical injury to the thoracic duct but may be idiopathic.

Congenital Pericardial Disease

Pericardial cysts usually become evident as a prominent, round, sharply demarcated opacity seen on chest radiography (most often in the right cardiophrenic border) in an asymptomatic patient. Congenital absence of the pericardium is an uncommon anomaly that involves either a portion of, or more commonly the entire, left parietal pericardium. Right-sided defects and bilateral complete absence of the pericardium are extremely rare. Pericardial defects are usually asymptomatic; rarely, herniation and strangulation of the left atrial appendage through a partial defect occurs.

ACUTE PERICARDITIS
History and Physical Examination

Acute pericarditis typically produces sharp retrosternal pain that radiates to the trapezius ridge (especially the left) and is aggravated by lying down and relieved by sitting up. However, the quality, severity, and location of pain vary greatly. Pericardial pain may radiate down the left arm and suggest cardiac ischemia or may be localized to the epigastrium and mimic an acute condition in the abdomen. The pain of pericarditis is often worse with inspiration and is difficult to distinguish from that of pleurisy; its onset is frequently heralded by a prodrome of fever, malaise, and myalgia. Chest pain may be absent in acute pericarditis, especially in early pericarditis complicating myocardial infarction or cardiac surgery and in uremic pericarditis. Patients with acute pericarditis complain of dyspnea, particularly when there is concomitant fever, splinting, or significant pericardial effusion. Other uncommon symptoms include cough, dysphagia, and singultus.

The hallmark of acute pericarditis is the pericardial friction rub. Superficial and scratchy (often likened to the sound of walking on dry snow), the pericardial rub may be confined to ventricular systole but most often includes a component during atrial systole, and occasionally during ventricular diastole, resulting in biphasic and triphasic rubs, respectively. The evanescent nature of the rub necessitates frequent examination. The stethoscope diaphragm should be placed firmly on the chest wall, usually between the lower left sternal border and the cardiac apex, and the patient examined in both the supine and sitting positions. Pleural rubs are associated with the respiratory, not cardiac cycle, but may coexist with pericardial rubs. Pericardial rubs are confused with cardiac murmurs, sounds due to pneumodiastinum, ejection sounds and valve clicks, and, most commonly, with artifacts produced by skin rubbing against a loosely placed stethoscope head. Proper examination technique and experience should minimize such confusion. Although pericardial effusion may silence a rub, the presence of a rub does not exclude even a large pericardial effusion.

In uncomplicated pericarditis, the jugular venous pressure usually remains normal. Cardiac gallops indicate coexisting myocardial disease. The history and physical examination are also helpful in identifying underlying diseases associated with pericarditis.

Electrocardiography

The electrocardiogram (Fig. 27-1) may either confirm the clinical suspicion or first alert the clinician to the presence of pericarditis. Serial tracings are frequently needed to distinguish the ST segment elevations due to acute pericarditis from those due to acute myocardial infarction and early repolarization (Chapter 12). In the former, the ECGs reveal a different sequence of ST-T wave changes; in the latter, the ECG pattern does not evolve. A ratio of ST junction to T wave amplitudes greater than 0.25, especially in lead V_6, also distinguishes pericarditis from early repolarization.

ST-T wave changes are diffuse and have a characteristic evolution in acute pericarditis. In the first stage, ST segment elevations, which differ from ischemic ST elevations by their upward concavity, and which seldom exceed 5 mm in height, typically occur within a few hours of the onset of chest pain and persist for hours or days. Depression of the PR segment is also seen in this stage. In the second stage, the ST segments return to baseline; at this point, the T waves may appear normal or exhibit loss of amplitude. In the third stage, tracings show inversion of T waves; these changes are known to persist indefinitely, particularly with tuberculous, uremic, or neoplastic pericarditis. In the variably present fourth stage, the ECG normalizes. In a "typical" case of acute pericarditis, the approximate time frame for these ECG changes is 2 weeks. However, only about half of patients with acute pericarditis display all four ECG stages, and variations are very common. Atrial arrhythmias complicate 5% to 10% of cases of acute pericarditis.

Imaging Studies

The chest radiograph may reveal an enlarged cardiac silhouette because of a moderate or large pericardial effusion and may detect evidence of tuberculosis, fungal disease, pneumonia, or neoplasm.

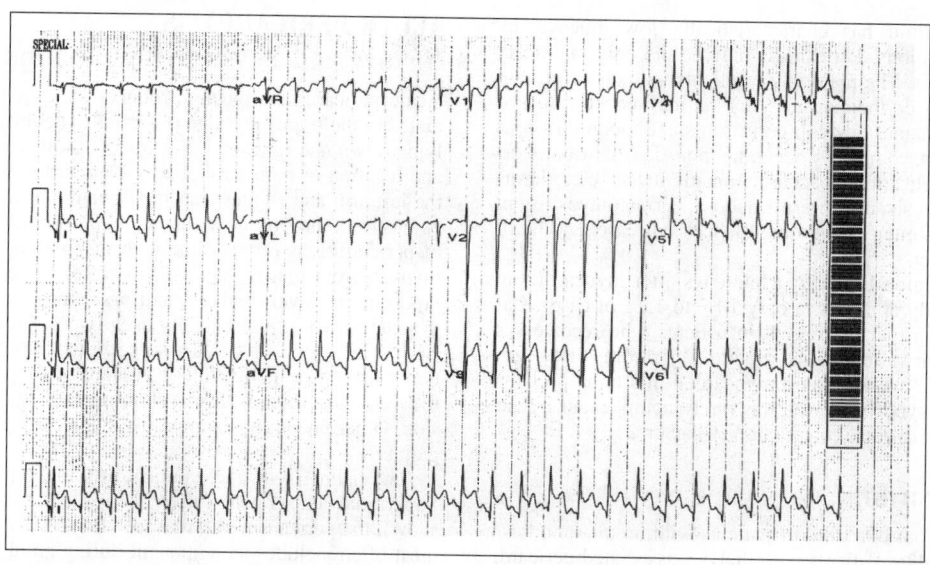

FIGURE 27-1   A 12-lead electrocardiogram of a patient with acute pericarditis. The ST segments are elevated in leads II, III, aV_F and V_3 to V_6 and depressed in aV_R and V_1. Depression of the PR segment is also evident in many leads.

Echocardiographic identification of pericardial effusion confirms the clinical diagnosis of acute pericarditis (Chapter 13). Echocardiography also proves valuable in estimating the volume of pericardial fluid and identifying cardiac tamponade, in suggesting the basis of pericarditis, and in documenting associated acute myocarditis with congestive heart failure. However, it should be recognized that the patient with purely fibrinous acute pericarditis often has a normal echocardiogram.

Although technetium-99 pyrophosphate scans may be positive in patients with pericarditis associated with epicarditis, and gallium scans have proven useful in displaying characteristics of purulent pericarditis, these tests are rarely used to diagnose acute pericarditis.

Laboratory Studies

Nonspecific blood markers of inflammation, such as the erythrocyte sedimentation rate (ESR) and the white blood cell (WBC) count, usually rise in cases of acute pericarditis. Patients with extensive epicarditis occasionally have elevations of serum cardiac isoenzymes suggestive of acute myocardial infarction.

Clinical Course

As a rule, acute idiopathic pericarditis is a benign, self-limited disease lasting 2 to 6 weeks. The most common complication, recurrence, occurs in about one quarter of cases and occasionally proves resistant to therapy. Small pericardial effusions commonly occur, but cardiac tamponade is unusual. Other unusual complications include heart failure due to associated myocarditis and late constrictive pericarditis. These complications can usually be detected by clinical evaluation and echocardiography. The clinical course and prognosis of individuals with pericarditis otherwise vary largely with the presence and nature of the underlying disease.

PERICARDIAL EFFUSION

Accumulation of transudate, exudate, or blood in the pericardial sac is a frequent complication of pericardial disease and should be considered in all patients with acute pericarditis. An unexplained increase in heart size on the chest radiogram remains one of the most common clues to pericardial disease. Pericardial effusions are very common after cardiac surgery. They are frequently loculated and usually resolve without sequelae within the first postoperative month. Pericardial effusions in cardiac transplant patients are associated with an increased incidence of acute rejection. Chronic effusive pericarditis

is an entity of unknown etiology that may be associated with large, asymptomatic effusions. Many conditions causing pericarditis (e.g., uremia, tuberculosis, neoplasia, connective tissue disease, heart failure) produce chronic pericardial effusions.

History and Physical Examination

Effusions that do not elevate pericardial and venous pressures (either because of their size or the rapidity of their development) are usually asymptomatic. The physical examination frequently is not helpful. A large effusion may increase the area of cardiac dullness and compress the lower lobe of the left lung, causing atelectatic rales or bronchial breath sounds and egophony (Ewart's sign) over the left lung base.

Laboratory Studies

Other than culture and cytology, characteristics of the pericardial fluid are usually too nonspecific to be of diagnostic value. Transudative effusions (hydropericardium) occur in heart failure and other states associated with chronic salt and water retention (including pregnancy), and exudative effusions occur in the large number of infectious and inflammatory causes of pericarditis. Although frank hemorrhagic effusions suggest recent intrapericardial bleeding, sanguineous and serosanguineous effusions occur in many infectious and inflammatory disorders. In certain disorders, the nature of the pericardial fluid has greater diagnostic value. For example, chylous pericarditis implies injury or obstruction to the thoracic duct, and cholesterol pericarditis is either idiopathic or associated with hypothyroidism, rheumatoid arthritis, or tuberculosis.

Diagnostic Studies

Flask-shaped enlargement of the cardiac silhouette on chest radiograph occurs with moderate or large pericardial effusion, but differentiation of large effusions from cardiac dilation is often difficult; pulmonary congestion suggests cardiac dilation. Small effusions (less than a few hundred milliliters) are associated with a normal cardiothoracic ratio. Low voltage on the ECG is typical when the effusion is large.

Echocardiography (Fig. 27-2) is the procedure of choice for the diagnosis of pericardial effusion. Attention to technical detail results in excellent sensitivity and specificity. The diagnostic feature on M-mode echocardiography is the persistence of an echo-free space between parietal and visceral pericardium throughout the cardiac cycle. Separations that are observed only in systole represent clini-

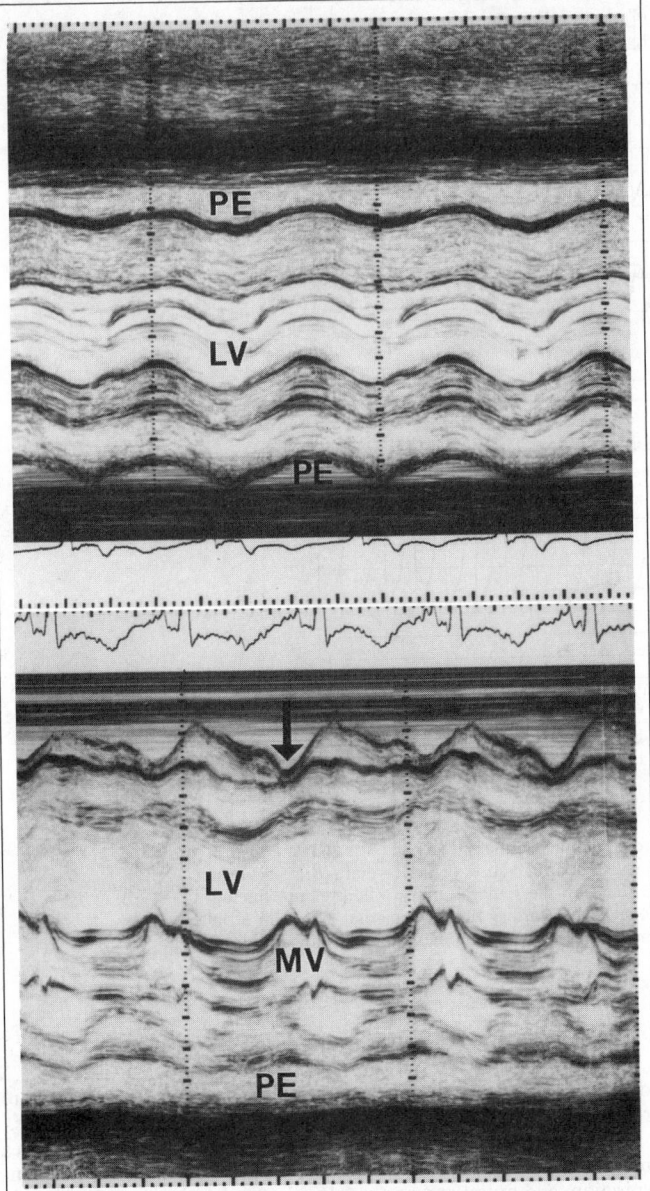

FIGURE 27-2 M-mode echocardiograms of pericardial effusion. The effusion *(PE)* appears as an echo-free space surrounding the heart. The effusion on the left does not cause cardiac compression. The effusion on the right demonstrates right ventricular diastolic collapse *(arrow)*, evident as abnormal motion of the anterior free wall of the right ventricle that occurs after the mitral valve *(MV)* opens. *LV*, Left ventricle.

cally insignificant accumulations. The superior spatial orientation of two-dimensional (2D) echocardiography enables delineation of the size and distribution of pericardial effusion, as well as detection of loculated fluid. As the amount of pericardial fluid increases, fluid distributes from the posterobasilar left ventricle apically and anteriorly, and then laterally and posteriorly to the left atrium. Fluid adjacent to the right atrium is an early sign of pericardial effusion. Echocardiographic signs of large effusions and tamponade are discussed later.

Echocardiography readily identifies chamber enlargement and characterizes ventricular function. Thus the relative contributions of cardiac enlargement and pericardial effusion to overall cardiac enlargement and the relative roles of tamponade and myocardial dysfunction to altered hemodynamics can also be evaluated.

Pericardial effusions are easily detected by computed tomography (CT); size, geometry, and distribution of pericardial effusions are readily determined by this technique. In addition, the attenuation co-

efficients for blood, exudate, chyle, and serous fluid may be sufficiently characteristic to permit their identification.

Magnetic resonance imaging (MRI) effectively detects loculated pericardial effusion and pericardial thickening. Inflamed pericardium and adhesions have a high signal intensity relative to pericardial fluid and myocardium, providing a potential means of identifying the nature of the effusion.

Radionuclide techniques are used infrequently to seek out pericardial disease, but pericardial effusion may be detected as an incidental finding.

CARDIAC TAMPONADE

Cardiac tamponade is a hemodynamic condition characterized by equal elevation of atrial and pericardial pressures, an exaggerated inspiratory decrease in arterial systolic pressure (pulsus paradoxus), and arterial hypotension. The latter is generally a late sign in chronic effusions, and occasionally, a heightened sympathoadrenal state produces systemic hypertension. As intrapericardial pressure rises, venous pressures increase to maintain cardiac filling and prevent collapse of the cardiac chambers. Although the absolute intracardiac pressures are elevated, the transmural (distending) pressures, that is, cavitary diastolic minus pericardial pressures, are practically zero or even negative. The greatly reduced preload is responsible for the fall in cardiac output, and when compensatory mechanisms are exhausted, a decrease in arterial pressure.

History and Physical Examination

Cardiac tamponade is best viewed as a continuum, ranging from mild, sometimes unsuspected tamponade (pericardial pressure less than 10 mm Hg), to severe (pericardial pressure greater than 15 to 20 mm Hg). Mild cardiac tamponade is frequently asymptomatic, whereas moderate, and especially severe tamponade produces precordial discomfort and dyspnea. In extreme cases, patients are often incapable of reporting symptoms. After cardiac surgery, dyspnea and fatigue should raise the suspicion of tamponade; in these instances the effusion is often loculated, and echocardiographic and hemodynamic findings may be unreliable.

Physical findings are dictated similarly by the severity of cardiac tamponade. Venous pressure may not be frankly elevated in early tamponade, whereas extreme elevations of venous pressure may go unrecognized in the recumbent or semirecumbent patient in whom the top of the pulsatile jugular venous waveform is above the angle of jaw. Compression of the heart by pericardial fluid results in a characteristic loss of the atrial Y descent. Owing to the decrease in intrapericardial pressure that occurs during ventricular ejection, the systolic atrial filling wave and the X descent are preserved. Thus careful inspection of the jugular venous pulse waveform is essential for the diagnosis. Kussmaul's sign, a failure of venous pressure to decrease during inspiration, is not seen in cardiac tamponade.

An inspiratory decline of systolic arterial pressure exceeding 10 mm Hg defines pulsus paradoxus. Pulsus paradoxus may be detected by palpation of an arterial pulse (generally over a large artery). In milder cases of tamponade, the pulse decreases with inspiration, whereas in more severe cases, the pulse disappears with inspiration. Pulsus paradoxus is quantitated using sphygmomanometry by subtracting the pressure at which Korotkoff's sounds are heard during expiration only from the pressure at which sounds are heard throughout the respiratory cycle.

The paradoxical pulse is complex and multifactorial in origin. Inspiratory filling of the right heart is necessary for its development; increased right heart volume results in both a leftward shift of the interventricular septum (reducing left ventricle [LV] filling and compliance) and increased pericardial pressure (reducing the gradient for left atrial filling). It should be recognized that pulsus paradoxus is neither sensitive nor specific for cardiac tamponade. A paradoxical pulse may be absent in tamponade associated with LV dysfunction and elevated LV diastolic pressures, atrial septal defect, aortic regurgitation, and regional tamponade (as occurs in the postoperative patient). Conversely, pulsus paradoxus is seen occasionally in cases of constrictive pericarditis, obstructive pulmonary disease, pulmonary embolus, right ventricular infarction, and large bilateral pleural effu-

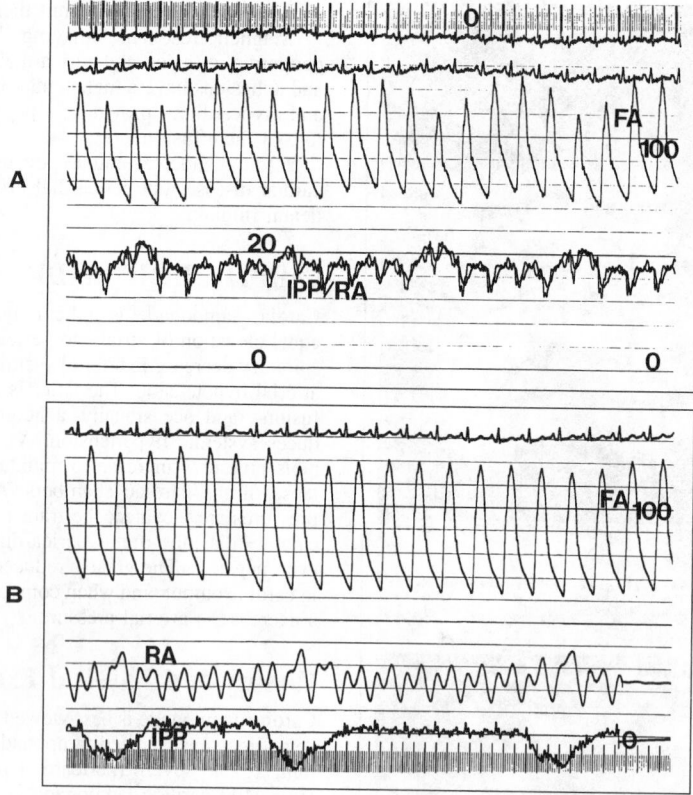

FIGURE 27-3   Hemodynamic record of a patient with cardiac tamponade before **(A)** and after **(B)** removal of 480 ml of pericardial fluid. Before pericardiocentesis, there is equal elevation of pericardial *(IPP)* and right atrial *(RA)* pressures. Pulsus paradoxus (15 mm Hg) is evident on the femoral artery *(FA)* pressure tracing. Note the absent Y descent on the RA tracing. After removal of pericardial fluid, pericardial and right atrial pressures decrease and the pulsus paradoxus disappears. Pericardial pressure becomes subatmospheric with inspiration.

(Courtesy Noble O. Fowler, MD.)

sions. Nevertheless, in the appropriate clinical setting, pulsus paradoxus is a key finding signifying cardiac tamponade, and its presence should be sought with diligence.

Diagnostic Studies

Low voltage on the ECG and electrical alternans, particularly when P, QRS, and T waves are involved, should raise the suspicion of cardiac tamponade. However, this finding is insensitive, occurring in only about 20% of instances. When effusion is massive, the heart swings freely within the pericardial sac and acquires a pendular, rotary motion that is associated with electrical alternans. This sign is very specific but insensitive for cardiac tamponade.

Unless the situation is life threatening, an echocardiogram should be obtained. During inspiration, a greater than normal increase in right ventricular dimension and decrease in left ventricular dimension occur in many cases of tamponade. These respiratory changes also occur in other conditions associated with pulsus paradoxus, such as chronic obstructive lung disease and pulmonary embolism. Diastolic collapse of the right ventricle, an abnormal posterior motion of the anterior right ventricular wall during diastole (see Fig. 27-2), signifies that pericardial pressure exceeds early diastolic right ventricular pressure (i.e., negative transmural pressure). Although this sign is a relatively sensitive and specific marker for tamponade, right ventricular diastolic collapse is sensitive to alterations in ventricular loading conditions and may not be seen in the presence of right ventricular hypertrophy. Late diastolic right atrial collapse is virtually 100% sensitive for tamponade, but is less specific. For example, small effusions produce right atrial collapse in the presence of left ventricular

dysfunction. Posteriorly loculated effusions after cardiac surgery are reported to produce left atrial and left ventricular diastolic collapse.

During cardiac tamponade, tricuspid and pulmonic flow velocities measured by Doppler echocardiography increase markedly with inspiration, and mitral and aortic valve flow velocities decrease significantly compared with normal control patients and patients with asymptomatic effusions. Changes in the pattern of venous flow (reflecting the predominance of systolic flow) and exaggerated respiratory variations of venous flow velocities are also seen in cardiac tamponade.

The diagnosis of cardiac tamponade is confirmed by right heart catheterization (Fig. 27-3). The right atrial, pulmonary capillary wedge, and pulmonary artery diastolic pressures are elevated and equal within 4 mm Hg; neither Kussmaul's sign nor the early ventricular diastolic dip and plateau (square root sign) characteristic of pericardial constriction are seen in tamponade. Pericardial pressure is elevated and equal to right atrial pressure; the degree of elevation is related to both the severity of tamponade and the patient's intravascular volume status. The right atrial and wedge pressure tracings reveal an attenuated or absent Y descent. Cardiac output is reduced and systemic vascular resistance is elevated. Equal elevation of diastolic pressures may also be seen with dilated cardiomyopathy and right ventricular infarction.

Owing to the steep pericardial pressure-volume relation, removal of small amounts of pericardial fluid (about 50 ml) produces considerable symptomatic and hemodynamic improvement. Unless there is concomitant cardiac disease or coexisting constriction (effusive-constrictive pericarditis, see later discussion), removal of all of the pericardial fluid normalizes pericardial, atrial, ventricular diastolic and arterial pressures, and cardiac output.

CONSTRICTIVE PERICARDITIS

Constrictive pericarditis is a condition in which a thickened, scarred, and often calcified pericardium limits diastolic filling of the ventricles. Unlike cardiac tamponade, early diastolic filling is unrestrained, and only at the end of the first third of diastole does the unyielding, stiff pericardium abruptly restrict ventricular filling. As a result, ventricular pressure falls rapidly in early diastole and subsequently rises abruptly to an elevated level, where it remains until the next ventricular systole. End-diastolic ventricular pressures and mean atrial pressures are elevated and nearly equal (within 5 mm Hg), and end-diastolic volumes and, consequently, stroke volume and cardiac output are reduced. These pathophysiologic changes are responsible for the characteristic hemodynamic and physical findings described later.

Although acute pericarditis from most causes may eventuate in constrictive pericarditis, the most common antecedents are idiopathic, tuberculosis (particularly common in nonindustrialized countries) and other infectious diseases, neoplasm (particularly lung and breast), radiation therapy, renal failure, connective tissue diseases, and following cardiac trauma and surgery. Rare causes include Dressler's syndrome, sarcoidosis, Whipple's disease, amyloidosis, and dermatomyositis. Mulibrey nanism is a hereditary form of constrictive pericarditis that is associated with abnormalities of the *mu*scle, *li*ver, *br*ain, and *ey*es.

History and Physical Examination

Constrictive pericarditis resembles congestive heart failure due to myocardial disease and chronic liver disease. The history is useful in making these critical distinctions and in identifying an antecedent cause of constrictive pericarditis. Patients generally complain of fatigue, dyspnea, weight gain, abdominal discomfort, nausea, increased abdominal girth, and edema. Although symptoms usually develop over years, symptoms progress over a period of months in patients with subacute constrictive pericarditis after trauma, cardiac surgery, and mediastinal irradiation.

Striking features on physical examination include ascites, hepatosplenomegaly, edema, and in long-standing cases, severe wasting. This general appearance often leads to a misdiagnosis of hepatic cirrhosis. However, confusion is readily circumvented by a careful examination of the neck veins. The venous pressure is elevated and displays deep Y, and often deep X descents. The venous pressure fails to decrease with inspiration (Kussmaul's sign), but frank inspiratory swelling of the neck veins is uncommon. It should be remembered that Kussmaul's sign is seen also in cases of restrictive cardiomyopathy, right ventricular failure and infarction, and tricuspid stenosis. The heart is often normal sized and when not, enlargement is rarely extreme. A pericardial knock, similar in timing to the third heart sound (but 0.06 to 0.08 sec earlier), signifies the end of rapid ventricular diastolic filling; in several series, this characteristic finding occurred infrequently. Systolic retractions of the chest may be evident. The arterial blood pressure is normal except in severe cases. Pulsus paradoxus is an inconsistent finding, most often found in subacute constrictive pericarditis with associated pericardial effusion (effusive-constrictive pericarditis).

Diagnostic Studies

Serum chemistries suggest hepatic insufficiency. Protein-losing enteropathy and proteinuria further reduce plasma proteins.

The electrocardiographic findings are nonspecific. Low QRS voltage, nonspecific T wave changes, and an intraatrial conduction defect (P mitrale) are common. Atrial fibrillation is seen in approximately one third of cases, and atrial flutter is less common. Unusual ECG findings include right ventricular hypertrophy due to a fibrous band constricting the right ventricular outflow tract, and Q waves that are thought to be due to myocardial penetration by the pericardial scar.

The cardiac silhouette may be normal or enlarged. Pericardial calcification is present in less than half of cases seen in the United States and Europe. Pericardial calcification is seen in the absence of constriction, but then it is usually less dense and has a more patchy distribution. Pericardial thickness can be estimated angiographically

from the thickness and contour of the right atrial free wall and the depth of the epicardial coronary arteries.

Pericardial thickening and calcification and abnormal ventricular filling produce characteristic changes on the M-mode echocardiogram. Increased pericardial thickness is suggested by parallel motion of the epicardium and parietal pericardium, which are separated by a relatively echo-free space at least 1 mm thick. Only in the presence of pericardial and pleural effusions can the pericardial thickness be measured directly. Echocardiographic correlates of the hemodynamic abnormalities of constrictive pericarditis include flattening of the left ventricular posterior wall endocardium, abnormal septal motion, and occasionally premature opening of the pulmonic valve. These findings, which reflect abnormal filling of the ventricles, are insensitive and subtle, and they lack the specificity to be clinically useful. Although no sign or combination of signs on M-mode echocardiograms is diagnostic of constrictive pericarditis, a normal study virtually rules out the diagnosis.

Two-dimensional echocardiography frequently assists in the evaluation of suspected constrictive pericarditis. Atrial enlargement, inferior vena caval and hepatic venous dilation, hypermobile atrioventricular valves, a sharp halt in ventricular diastolic filling, and an apical shell of pericardium are echocardiographic findings that should be sought. Ventricular systolic function often is normal or only slightly reduced except in far-advanced cases in which fibrotic scar has deeply invaded the myocardium.

The clinically crucial distinction between constrictive pericarditis and restrictive cardiomyopathy may be aided by differences in ventricular filling provided by quantitative M-mode and 2D echocardiography and Doppler echocardiography (Chapter 13). Patients with constrictive pericarditis show marked respiratory variation in diastolic transmitral and tricuspid valve flow velocities and isovolumic relaxation time, whereas patients with restrictive cardiomyopathy show inspiratory shortening of tricuspid deceleration time and diastolic atrioventricular valve regurgitation. The sensitivity and specificity of these signs remain to be elucidated.

Computed tomography is a highly accurate method of evaluating pericardial thickness and therefore plays a pivotal role in diagnosis and management of constrictive disease. The normal pericardium is identified as a 1- to 2-mm curvilinear line of soft tissue density, whereas, in constrictive pericarditis, the parietal pericardium is 4 to 20 mm thick. Failure to visualize the posterolateral left ventricular wall on dynamic CT suggests myocardial fibrosis or atrophy and is associated with a poor surgical outcome. Because of the close physiologic similarities of constrictive pericarditis and restrictive cardiomyopathy, increased pericardial thickness detected by tomographic scanning is the most reliable means of distinguishing between the two disorders, as normal pericardial thickness excludes most cases of constrictive pericarditis. The CT scan is also useful in planning pericardiectomy because of its ability to define the distribution of pericardial thickening.

Accurate definition of pericardial thickness and its distribution is also possible with MRI (Fig. 27-4). Unlike CT, electrocardiographic gating is necessary for adequate visualization, resolution is not quite as good, and calcification is difficult to distinguish from fibrosis.

Hemodynamics

Cardiac catheterization is used to confirm the clinical impression, uncover occult constriction, diagnose effusive-constrictive disease, and identify associated coronary and valvular disease. Endomyocardial biopsy is sometimes necessary to exclude restrictive cardiomyopathy, which shares many hemodynamic abnormalities with constrictive pericarditis. Characteristic hemodynamic findings of constrictive pericarditis include equal (i.e., less than 5 mm Hg difference) elevation of right and left ventricular diastolic and atrial pressures, prominent X and Y descents on the right atrial and PA wedge pressure tracings (resulting in an M shape), an early diastolic dip and plateau (square root sign) on the ventricular pressure waveforms, and lack of an inspiratory decrease in right atrial pressure (Fig. 27-5). The pulmonary arterial systolic pressure is usually normal or only slightly elevated (usually no greater than 50 mm Hg) and the right ventricular (RV) diastolic pressure exceeds one third of the RV systolic pressure. Stroke volume and cardiac output are reduced, although in early constrictive

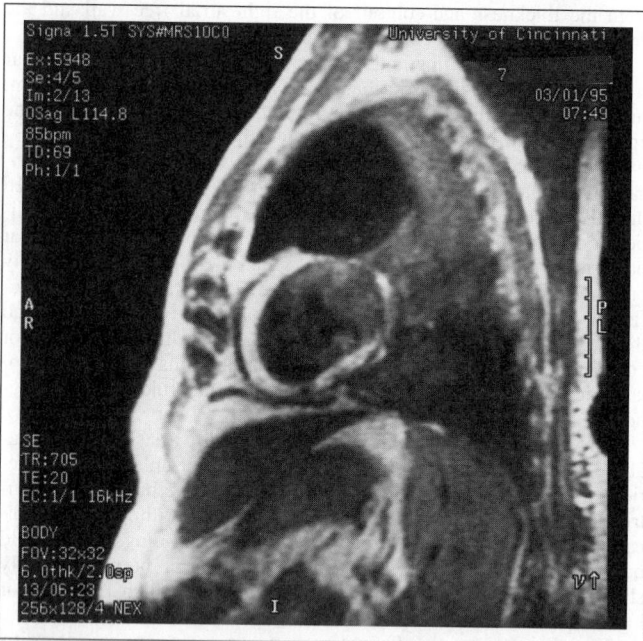

FIGURE 27-4   MRI scan (spin echo image) of a patient with surgically proven constrictive pericarditis. The pericardium is viewed as a line of low signal intensity (black) sandwiched between higher intensity epicardial and pericardial fat (white). Note the regional variation of pericardial thickness, which is normally 1 to 2 mm.

pericarditis (occult constriction) they are often normal. Rarely, localized constriction by fibrous bands produces hemodynamic characteristics of right ventricular outflow tract obstruction, and mitral and tricuspid stenosis.

Occult constrictive pericarditis is diagnosed when the characteristic hemodynamic findings of constriction appear after a rapid infusion of saline (e.g., 1 L over 6 to 8 min).

Effusive-constrictive pericarditis occurs when pericardial fluid accumulates between the thickened, fibrotic parietal and visceral pericardium. Neoplasia, chest irradiation, infection, idiopathic pericarditis, and connective tissue diseases are common antecedents. The hemodynamic features are those of cardiac tamponade before, and constrictive pericarditis after pericardiocentesis. Thus removal of pericardial fluid fails to lower atrial and ventricular diastolic pressures, but the attenuated or absent Y descent becomes prominent.

Restrictive cardiomyopathy impairs ventricular filling and increases ventricular diastolic pressures. Features favoring the diagnosis of restrictive cardiomyopathy include an RV systolic pressure greater than 50 mm Hg, RV diastolic pressure less than one third of the RV systolic pressure, and a greater than 5 mm Hg difference between right and left ventricular diastolic pressures. Although endomyocardial biopsy is useful in distinguishing between constrictive pericarditis and restrictive cardiomyopathy due to myocardial infiltration (e.g., amyloid), neoplasia, radiation therapy, and connective tissue disease may cause both pericardial and myocardial disease.

MANAGEMENT OF PERICARDIAL HEART DISEASE
Acute Pericarditis

Acute pericarditis usually responds to oral nonsteroidal antiinflammatory agents (e.g., acetylsalicylic acid ASA 650 mg q 3-4h, ibuprofen 600-800 mg q 6 h, or indomethacin 25-75 mg qid); however, narcotics may be required for severe pain. Some cases necessitate steroid therapy (prednisone 60-80 mg/day) for a week to control pain, with the dosage tapered rapidly thereafter. Steroids are also useful in acute pericarditis associated with uremic pericarditis and connective tissue diseases. Tuberculous and pyogenic pericarditis should be excluded before steroid therapy is initiated.

Painful recurrences of pericarditis tend to respond to the same therapeutic agents that successfully treated the initial episode, but some patients require steroids; in these cases, the risks of long-term steroids should be minimized by using either the lowest possible dose, alternate day therapy, or combinations with nonsteroidal drugs. Recurrent pericarditis may respond dramatically to colchicine, 1 mg/day, although the experience with this microtubular inhibitor is relatively limited. Although recurrences of pericarditis generally respond to medical therapy, rare cases require pericardiectomy to control painful recurrences. Left stellate ganglionectomy has also been employed successfully in selected instances.

Pericardiocentesis usually proves unnecessary unless either a suspected diagnosis (e.g., purulent pericarditis suggested by continued fever, high white blood cell [WBC] count, associated septicemia, immunosuppression) demands fluid analysis or cardiac tamponade supervenes. Occasionally pericardiocentesis is needed to establish the etiology of a pericardial effusion. Persistent or progressive effusion, particularly when the cause is uncertain, also warrants pericardiocentesis. Anticoagulants should be temporarily discontinued if possible, in order to reduce the risk of cardiac tamponade; patients who must continue taking anticoagulants should be switched to heparin, the effect of which can be reversed rapidly.

Dialysis-associated effusive pericarditis usually responds to an intensification of dialysis and regional heparinization, or by changing to peritoneal dialysis; a minority of patients require pericardial drainage. Pericardial instillation of triamcinolone may be beneficial.

Finally, patients in whom pericarditis represents one manifestation of systemic illness, such as connective tissue disease, uremia, infection, or neoplasia, should also receive therapy directed toward the primary disorder.

Pericardial Effusion and Cardiac Tamponade

Unless the situation is immediately life threatening, pericardiocentesis should be performed by experienced staff in a catheterization laboratory or a facility similarly equipped for hemodynamic monitoring. The ability to perform careful hemodynamic measurements, and simple logistic and personnel requirements are advantages of needle pericardiocentesis. Moreover, 2D echo is helpful in guiding the needle and has increased the safety of the procedure. A catheter can be advanced over a guidewire into the pericardial space and can remain for several days. Sclerosing agents, steroids, and specific chemotherapeutic agents may then be given through the catheter.

Open surgical drainage offers several advantages, including complete drainage, access to pericardial tissue for histopathologic and microbiologic diagnoses, the ability to drain loculated effusions, and the absence of traumatic injury due to blind placement of a needle into the pericardial sac. Although the choice between needle pericardiocentesis and surgical drainage depends on institutional resources and physician experience, needle pericardiocentesis is often the best option when the etiology is known and/or the diagnosis of tamponade is in question, and surgical drainage is optimal when the etiology is unclear but the presence of tamponade is certain. Irrespective of the method of retrieval, pericardial fluid should be sent for smear, culture, and cytology. Adenosine deaminase activity and carcinoembryonic antigen level are useful diagnostic adjuncts; values are higher in malignant and tuberculous effusions than in benign effusions.

Recurrent effusions are treated by repeat pericardiocentesis, sclerotherapy with tetracycline, surgical creation of a pericardial window, or pericardiectomy. A pericardial window is usually performed in patients with malignant effusions, and pericardiectomy may be required for recurrent effusions in dialysis patients. In critically ill patients, a pericardial window may be created percutaneously with a balloon catheter.

Patients with cardiac tamponade awaiting pericardial drainage should receive fluids to expand the intravascular volume. Dobutamine or nitroprusside may be used after the blood volume has been expanded, but only as a temporizing measure.

Constrictive Pericarditis

Pericardiectomy is the definitive treatment for constrictive pericarditis, but is not indicated in very early constriction (occult and

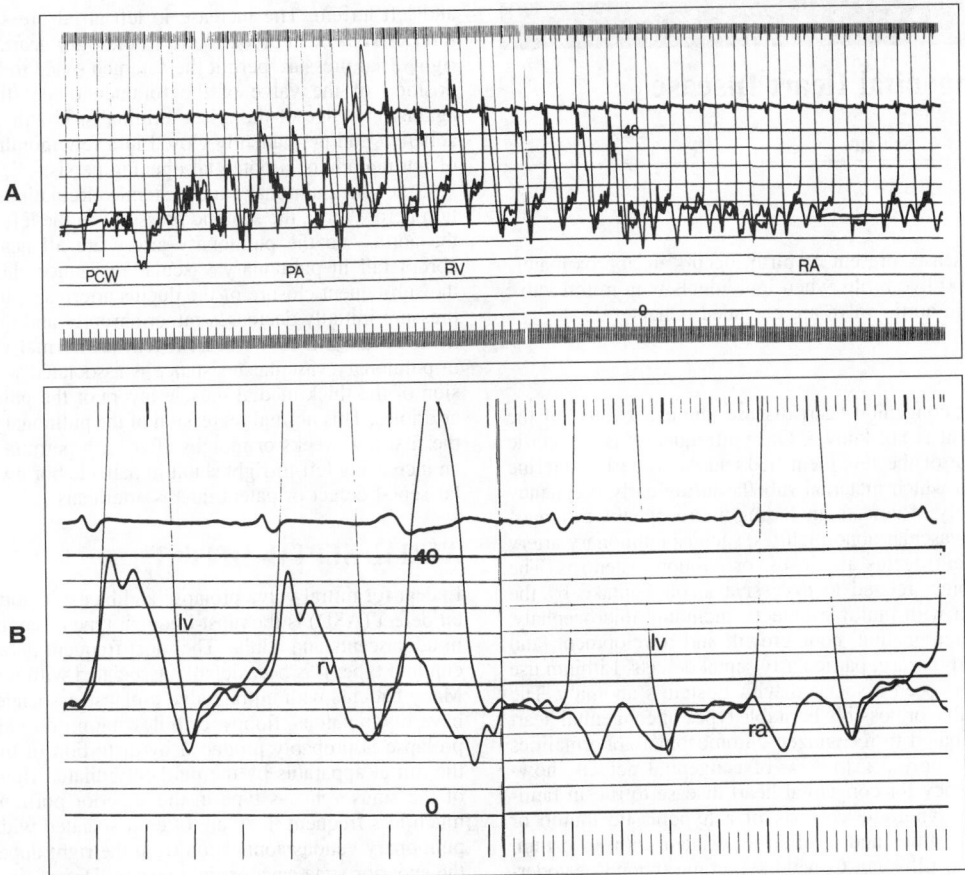

FIGURE 27-5   Hemodynamic record of a patient with surgically proven constrictive pericarditis. **A,** Slow paper speed recording of high gain left ventricular *(LV)* pressure and simultaneous right heart pullback from pulmonary capillary wedge *(PCW)* to pulmonary artery *(PA)*, right ventricle *(RV)*, and right atrium *(RA)*. **B,** Fast paper speed recording of LV and simultaneous RV and RA pressure tracings. Note the elevated and equal atrial and diastolic pressures, the prominent X and Y descents on the RA tracing, and the dip and plateau on the RV and LV tracings during longer diastoles.

(Courtesy of Peter J. Engel, MD.)

✔ *WHEN TO REFER*

Hospitalization is warranted for most patients with an initial episode of acute pericarditis to rule out myocardial infarction and to observe for the development of cardiac tamponade. Establishing the exact cause of acute pericarditis is an important part of management, but considerable judgment must be exercised when deciding whether (and how) to investigate the possibility of concomitant systemic disease. PPD skin tests, blood cultures, fungal serology, ASO titers, cold agglutinin tests, heterophil antibody assay, thyroid function tests, renal function profiles, ANA and RF assays, extractable nuclear antigen test, and complement assays may be indicated in various combinations, depending on the clinical setting.

An extensive evaluation is generally unnecessary in a young, previously healthy adult who presents with a viral syndrome, typical pericardial chest pain, and a pericardial friction rub. Depending on the history and symptoms at presentation, trauma, myocarditis, SLE, and/or purulent pericarditis require consideration in younger patients. In older adults, myocardial infarction, tuberculosis (TB), and neoplastic disease should be considered. Differentiating viral from idiopathic pericarditis is difficult, expensive, and of little practical importance.

Patients with suspected pericardial disease should have an echocardiogram, and those with complicated pericarditis (recurrent pericarditis, large, nonresolving, or progressive effusion, suspected cardiac tamponade or constrictive pericarditis) should be referred to a cardiologist.

functional class I) or in severe, advanced disease (functional class IV) when the risk of surgery is excessive and the benefits are diminished. Involvement of the visceral pericardium also increases the surgical risk. Symptomatic relief and normalization of cardiac pressures may take several months following pericardiectomy. In some patients, constrictive pericarditis resolves either spontaneously or in response to various combinations of nonsteroidal antiinflammatory agents, steroids, and antibiotics. Diuretics and digoxin (in the presence of atrial fibrillation) are useful in patients who are not candidates for pericardiectomy because of their high surgical risk.

BIBLIOGRAPHY

Fowler NO: Recurrent pericarditis, *Cardiol Clin* 8:621, 1990.

Fowler NO: Constrictive pericarditis: its history and current status. *Clin Cardiol* 18:341, 1995.

Hoit BD: Imaging the pericardium, *Cardiol Clin* 8:587, 1990.

Hoit BD, Lew WY, LeWinter M: Regional variation in pericardial contact pressure in the canine ventricle. *Am J Physiol* 255:H1370, 1988.

Oh JK, Hatle Lk, Seward JB, et al: Diagnostic role of Doppler echocardiography in constrictive pericarditis, *J Am Coll Cardiol* 23:154, 1994.

Shabetai R: The pericardium: an essay on some recent developments, *Am J Cardiol* 42:1036, 1978.

Shabetai R, Fowler NO: Diseases of the pericardium. In Alexander RW, Schlaut RC, Fuster V, editors: *The heart,* ed 9, New York, 1998, McGraw-Hill.

Spodick DH: The normal and diseased pericardium: current concepts of pericardial physiology, diagnosis and treatment, *J Am Coll Cardiol* 1:240, 1983.

28 Congenital Heart Disease

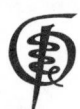

Robert C. Schlant

Congenital heart disease, present at birth, occurs in approximately eight infants per 1000 live births when individuals with mitral valve prolapse and bicuspid aortic valve are excluded (Chapter 25).

ETIOLOGY

In most instances of congenital heart disease, the exact cause of the defect in development is not known. Only infrequently is a specific cause identified. One of the few identified causes is the intrauterine rubella syndrome, in which maternal rubella during early pregnancy may result in a variety of defects, including microcephaly, cataracts, deafness, and cardiovascular abnormalities, such as pulmonary artery branch stenosis, patent ductus arteriosus, or pulmonic stenosis. The fetal alcohol syndrome, related to excessive alcohol intake by the mother, is associated with multiple defects, including microcephaly, microophthalmia, micrognathia, poor growth and development, and often congenital heart disease, particularly septal defects. Lithium use during pregnancy has been associated with Ebstein's anomaly. The many forms of heritable or possibly heritable types of congenital heart disease that are attributed to recognized chromosomal abnormalities probably account for only 5% to 10% of congenital defects; however, there is a tendency for congenital heart disease to run in families. The Holt-Oram syndrome consists of a hypoplastic thumb or other skeletal abnormalities and is often associated with an ostium secundum defect. The Ellis-van Creveld syndrome (chondroectodermal dysplasia) is an autosomal recessive defect consisting of dwarfism, polydactyly of the hands and occasionally the feet, and a common atrium. Down's syndrome is associated with trisomy 21 and in about 20% with endocardial cushion defect. Patent ductus arteriosus is more common in infants born at high altitudes (above 1500 m) and, like ventricular septal defect, in infants born prematurely. Bicuspid aortic valve, aortic atresia, and complete transposition of the great arteries occur more commonly in male infants, whereas ostium secundum atrial septal defect, partial endocardial cushion defects, and patent ductus arteriosus are found more frequently in females.

FETAL CIRCULATION AND CHANGES ASSOCIATED WITH BIRTH

The fetus obtains all of its nutrition and oxygen from the placental circulation. The fetal circulation is characterized by three special vascular channels, all of which normally disappear after birth: (1) the foramen ovale in the atrial septum, through which blood passes from the right atrium to the left atrium; (2) the ductus arteriosus, through which most of the blood reaching the pulmonary artery reaches the aorta; and (3) the ductus venosus, which shunts about half of the blood returning from the placenta through the liver to the inferior vena cava, where much of it preferentially streams to the heart and across the foramen ovale and into the left atrium and systemic circulation. Blood from the superior vena cava, on the other hand, preferentially streams across the tricuspid valve into the right ventricle. Because of the right-to-left shunts through the foramen ovale and the ductus arteriosus, the output of the fetal right ventricle is twice that of the left ventricle and relatively little blood (about 8% of the total cardiac output) reaches the uninflated lungs. Soon after birth there is an eight-fold to ten-fold increase in pulmonary blood flow in association with a marked decrease in the resistance to blood flow in the lungs; this is related to the inflation of the previously collapsed lungs and to a decrease in pulmonary arterial vasoconstriction produced by changes in pulmonary arterial oxygen tension, prostaglandin PGI_2, and leukotrienes. The increased systemic vascular resistance produced by vasoconstriction or by tying of the umbilical cord and umbilical arteries is associated with an increase in the pressures in the left ventricle

and left atrium. The increase in left atrial pressure, the decrease in inferior vena cava blood return to the right heart, and the decrease in right atrial pressure permit the foramen ovale to be closed by the opposition of the valve of the foramen ovale (the septum primum) against the edge of the crista terminalis. Usually, the valve becomes adherent and permanently closed in a few months, but in about 35% of normal adults, a potential opening persists.

Since the pulmonary and systemic circulations are in communication before birth, the systolic pressures in the left and right ventricles, the aorta, and the pulmonary artery are all nearly equal. With the abrupt fall in pulmonary vascular resistance shortly after birth and the subsequent closure of the ductus arteriosus, the pulmonary artery pressure initially decreases rather abruptly and then more slowly until, after about 2 to 6 weeks, it reaches normal values. The decrease in pulmonary vascular resistance is associated with a marked regression of the thick medial muscle layers of the pulmonary arteries and arterioles. This normal regression of the pulmonary vasculature within the first few weeks or months after birth permits the development of an increasing left-to-right shunt in patients born with a large ventricular septal defect or patent ductus arteriosus.

ATRIAL SEPTAL DEFECT

Except for mitral valve prolapse and bicuspid aortic valve, atrial septal defect (ASD) is the most frequent type of congenital heart disease in adolescents and adults. The most frequent defect is the ostium secundum type; it is occasionally associated with mitral valve prolapse. Many patients with mitral valve prolapse associated with ASD do not have myxomatous, floppy, or billowing mitral valve leaflets, and the prolapse is probably produced by distortion of the left ventricle and the mitral apparatus by the markedly dilated right ventricle. Defects of the sinus venosus type in the superior portion of the septum are much less frequent; they are often associated with partial anomalous pulmonary venous connection from the right upper or middle lobe to the superior vena cava or right atrium. Defects in the ostium primum involve the inferior portion of the atrial septum and are grouped as endocardial cushion defect or common atrioventricular canal defects (see discussion of Common Atrioventricular Canal Defects [Endocardial Cushion Defect]). After birth, the foramen ovale usually closes, although patency to a probe persists permanently in about 35% of adults. Very rarely, such patients may acquire a functional atrial septal defect ("blown-open foramen ovale") if the left atrial pressure increases markedly as a result of mitral valve disease, stretching the atrial septum and permitting a left-to-right shunt to develop. Conversely, if the right atrial pressure increases markedly, as in acute pulmonary embolus, a right-to-left shunt may develop or a paradoxical embolus may occur. ASD often occurs in association with other lesions. The combination of ostium secundum ASD and mitral stenosis is known as Lutembacher's syndrome.

The relative magnitude of the left-to-right (L-R) or right-to-left (R-L) shunt depends on the size of the ASD, the relative compliance of the two atria, the resistance to flow across the tricuspid and mitral valves, and especially the relative distensibility of the right and left ventricles. At birth, the two ventricles have similar diastolic filling characteristics, since they function at nearly the same systolic pressures in utero. As a result, there is little or no L-R shunting until the normal regression of the fetal pulmonary vasculature occurs and the normal growth hypertrophy of the left ventricle causes it to become thicker and less compliant than the right ventricle. With medium or large atrial septal defects, there is no significant pressure difference between the two atria, and the direction and amount of shunting are determined primarily by the relative compliance of the right and left ventricles. Some atrial defects present at birth may spontaneously close over the ensuing 5 years. Because of the tremendous reserve of the pulmonary circulation, the pressure in the pulmonary artery may not be elevated in some patients even with a pulmonary flow three times greater than the systemic flow. After at least 20 years, however, a minority of patients (perhaps 15%) develop progressively more severe pulmonary vascular disease, which eventually may markedly increase pulmonary vascular resistance and, consequently, pulmonary artery and right ventricular pressure. The compliance of the hypertrophied right ventricle may decrease, causing the L-R shunt to decrease and, eventually, to reverse. When there is sufficient R-L shunt to produce significant arterial oxygen unsaturation and clinical cyanosis, the patient is said to have Eisenmenger's reaction. In general, this syndrome develops much later (usually between 20 and 40 years of age), and less often in patients with ASD than in patients with either a large ventricular septal defect or a patent ductus arteriosus. Patients with Eisenmenger's reaction may have exertional syncope, hemoptysis, angina, and polycythemia. Patients who develop Eisenmenger's reaction have a high operative mortality for closure of the defect, and a high percentage of such patients do not have a decrease in the pulmonary artery or right ventricular pressure after surgery. On the other hand, children who have surgical correction of their ASD at a young age may be dramatically improved and may be capable of normal physical activities.

Children with ASD tend to be thin, asthenic, and relatively gracile in habitus. ASD occurs twice as often in girls as in boys. A history of frequent upper respiratory tract infections and slight effort intolerance or dyspnea is frequently noted, but many patients reach adolescence or young adulthood with only mild or no symptoms. As these patients get older, however, they have a progressively increasing prevalence of cardiac symptoms, primarily fatigue and dyspnea on exertion. In patients over age 40, congestive heart failure may develop, often in association with supraventricular arrhythmias, especially atrial fibrillation.

The pathophysiology of heart failure in ASD is frequently complex and multifactorial. In patients with a medium- or large-sized ASD, the right and left atrial pressures and therefore the filling pressures of both ventricles are essentially equal. When this pressure becomes elevated, there are symptoms and signs of increased venous pressure in both the pulmonary and the systemic circulation. In many patients it is not possible to determine whether the failure was caused primarily by dysfunction of the left or the right ventricle.

In general, a decrease in left ventricular diastolic distensibility increases the left-to-right shunt and right ventricular (RV) stroke volume, whereas a decrease in right ventricular distensibility decreases the left-to-right shunt and RV stroke volume and may even produce a right-to-left shunt across the ASD. The causes of changes in left ventricular (LV) distensibility in patients with ASD include the following: age-related changes in LV distensibility, coronary artery disease, systemic arterial hypertension, mitral regurgitation, idiopathic myocardial dysfunction, and right ventricular dysfunction. Changes in the right ventricular distensibility may be produced by several mechanisms including the chronic volume load from the ASD; the pressure load from pulmonary hypertension, particularly when marked; right ventricular ischemia; and left ventricular dysfunction. In patients with a chronically overloaded RV whose right ventricles remain abnormal after surgery, the right ventricle may transmit the diastolic pressure abnormalities to the left ventricle. Patients with ASD and heart failure frequently have atrial fibrillation, which may be either a contributing factor or a worsening consequence.

The physical findings vary considerably with the size of the L-R shunt and the pulmonary vascular resistance. The jugular venous pulse tends to have equal A and V waves or more prominent A waves if there is pulmonary hypertension. Since the pressures in the left and right atria are essentially equal with a large defect, the jugular venous pressure directly reflects the filling pressure of both ventricles. In patients with a significant shunt, right ventricular dilation and hypertrophy may be manifest as a hyperdynamic right ventricular lift along the left parasternal border and a palpable pulmonary trunk and pulmonary component of the second heart sound (P_2). The first sound is usually loud and prominently split. The two components (A_2) and (P_2) of the second heart sound are classically widely split, and during expiration the interval between the two sounds is fixed or does not decrease or disappear in the normal fashion (Chapter 11). A systolic murmur of grade III or less in the second or third left intercostal space is usually present, sometimes in association with an early ejection sound. Patients with a large L-R shunt may have a low-pitched diastolic murmur along the lower left sternal border produced by high flow across the tricuspid valve. This may disappear if the L-R shunt decreases as a result of Eisenmenger's reaction or marked RV hypertrophy. Some patients have evidence of mitral valve prolapse (Chapter 25). Mitral regurgitation caused by thickening of the anterior mitral valve leaflet, perhaps related to improper mitral leaflet coaptation produced by the dilated RV, occurs in about 15%

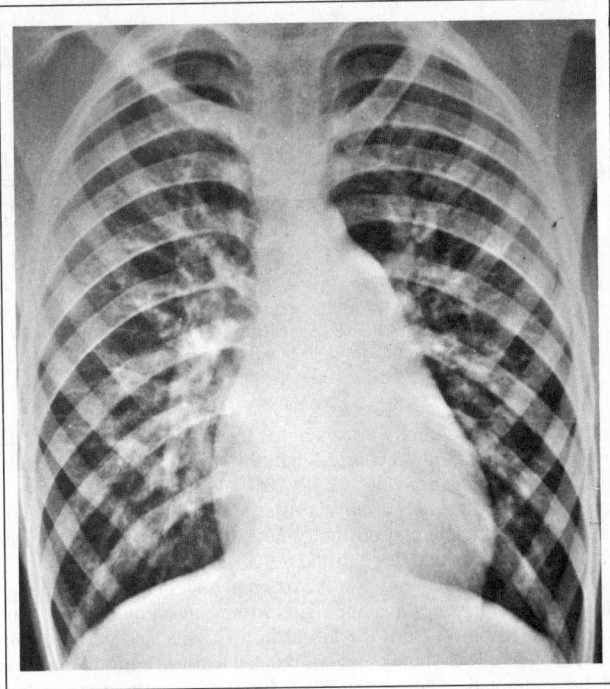

FIGURE 28-1   Chest film of a 12-year-old patient with ostium secundum ASD showing mild cardiomegaly and increased pulmonary blood flow through enlarged main and peripheral pulmonary vessels.

(Courtesy Dr. Wade H. Shuford, Professor of Radiology, Emory University School of Medicine.)

of patients over age 50 and may increase in frequency and severity with age. Rarely, high flow in the pulmonary vessels may produce systolic murmurs that can be heard over the posterior lung fields and that may extend past the second heart sound. Also in rare cases, a decrescendo, blowing diastolic murmur of pulmonary regurgitation from pulmonary hypertension is heard along the upper left sternal border. Patients with severe right ventricular hypertension and dilation may develop tricuspid regurgitation. Cyanosis and clubbing may be present in individuals in whom Eisenmenger's reaction develops.

The chest radiograph characteristically shows slight or moderate cardiomegaly with prominence of the pulmonary outflow tract and increased pulmonary vascular markings when the pulmonary flow is at least twice as great as systemic flow (Fig. 28-1). Dilation of the right ventricle may occasionally be evident on the lateral view; right atrium (RA) and RV dilation produce marked cardiomegaly. Calcification can be seen in pulmonary vessels with severe hypertension. In patients with severe pulmonary vascular disease, the pulmonary vasculature has a "pruned-tree" appearance, with prominent central vessels but decreased small, distal vasculature. The left atrium is usually enlarged only in adults with congestive heart failure and atrial fibrillation.

The electrocardiogram (ECG) classically shows right axis deviation and incomplete right bundle branch block (Fig. 28-2). The rhythm is usually sinus until age 20, after which there is a progressive increase in supraventricular arrhythmias, including atrial fibrillation, atrial flutter, and atrial tachycardia. The development of right ventricular hypertrophy may be reflected in further widening of the QRS complex and in increased amplitude of the R' wave in lead V_1. The PR interval is prolonged in about 20% of patients. The P axis is usually nearly vertical in ostium secundum defects but tends to be horizontal in sinus venosus defects.

Two-dimensional (2D) transthoracic (TTE) or transesophageal (TEE) echocardiography can directly image the atrial septal defect, in addition to demonstrating dilation of the right ventricle and paradoxical motion of the ventricular septum. The diagnosis is often aided by color Doppler or contrast echocardiography. Pulmonary hypertension may be reflected in abnormal motion of the pulmonic valves.

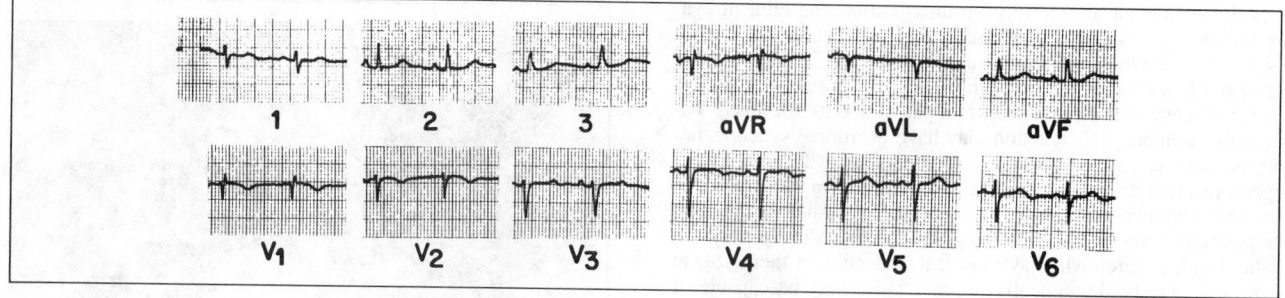

FIGURE 28-2   Electrocardiogram of a patient with ostium secundum ASD with right axis deviation and incomplete right bundle branch block.

Doppler echocardiography (Chapter 13) may provide evidence of the L-R shunt. Clinical and echocardiographic evidence of mitral valve prolapse is present in about 10% to 20% of patients with an ostium secundum ASD but may disappear after surgical correction of ASD.

At cardiac catheterization the catheter may pass freely from the right to the left atrium through the defect, and blood samples demonstrate an abnormal step-up in the oxygen content of blood sampled from the superior vena cava and right atrium caused by the L-R shunt of oxygenated blood from the left atrium (Chapter 14). The quantities of L-R and R-L shunts and pulmonary and systemic blood flows can be estimated. The presence of anomalous pulmonary venous drainage may be detected. The pressures in the pulmonary artery and right ventricle can be directly measured and the pulmonary vascular resistance calculated by dividing the pulmonary pressure by the pulmonary flow. It is important to distinguish patients with a high pulmonary artery pressure in association with a high flow (and therefore normal or low pulmonary vascular resistance) from patients with high pulmonary artery pressure with a low flow (and high pulmonary vascular resistance). In the presence of a large L-R shunt, there may be a functional peak pressure gradient across the pulmonary valve, which is usually only 5 to 20 mm Hg but can be 50 to 60 mm Hg.

Most individuals with ASD and a pulmonary flow more than 1.7 times systemic flow should have the defect repaired, preferably between the ages of 3 and 6 years, to prevent the subsequent development of pulmonary vascular disease and/or heart failure. Surgical repair can also be successfully performed in adults, including those over the age of 60. Individuals with pulmonary flow that is calculated to be 1.5 to 1.7 times systemic flow are in a borderline zone, although many probably should undergo surgery. Individuals with normal pressures and calculated pulmonary flow less than 1.5 times systemic flow usually do not require repair. Surgical closure is less clearly indicated in older patients, adult patients with sinus venosus defects with coronary flow less than 1.8 times systemic flow, and patients with severe pulmonary vascular disease or mitral regurgitation. A few patients with severe pulmonary vascular disease have had transplantation of one lung, although it is probable that severe pulmonary vascular disease will eventually develop in this lung. In contrast to most other forms of congenital heart disease, patients with isolated ostium secundum ASD rarely acquire infective endocarditis. Patients with chronic atrial fibrillation should be maintained on low-dose warfarin. Closure of an ASD with a double-umbrella device introduced by a catheter is feasible if the defect is circular and less than 2 cm in diameter and has a well-defined rim. These necessary conditions for this investigational technique are often not present in adult patients.

After successful closure of an ASD before the age of 20, the heart size usually returns to normal and the pulmonary vasculature on chest radiograph returns to normal. The electrocardiographic evidence of incomplete right bundle branch block and the abnormal splitting of the second heart sound often persist, although the splitting may vary with respiration if the conduction disturbance regresses.

After surgical repair of an atrial septal defect, a small percentage of patients may have a small residual L-R shunt of no hemodynamic consequence. Years after successful repair of an ASD, a small percentage of patients develop atrial arrhythmias such as sinus bradycardia, atrial fibrillation, or atrial flutter. Patients who have their ASD closed with a patch of synthetic material and who subsequently develop mitral regurgitation can have intravascular hemolysis from a jet of regurgitant blood striking the patch. In a very small percentage of patients, the patch may become detached and the left-right shunt can return.

Most women who have had an ASD repaired tolerate pregnancy well but have a risk of about 6% of having a child with the same defect. The risk is about 1.5% if only the father has had an ASD.

PARTIAL TRANSPOSITION OF THE PULMONARY VEINS (PARTIAL ANOMALOUS PULMONARY VENOUS CONNECTION)

In this condition, one or more of the four pulmonary veins is connected to the right atrium or a systemic vein. The most frequent type is abnormal connection of the veins from the right upper and middle lobes to the superior vena cava or right atrium in patients with a sinus venosus type of ASD. The defect can readily be repaired at the time of repair of the ASD. When isolated transposition of the pulmonary veins occurs, it has the physiologic effects of a small ASD with L-R shunt. Occasionally, the abnormal right pulmonary vein appears on the chest radiograph as a crescentlike shadow (scimitar syndrome) in the right lung field before it enters the inferior vena cava either just above or just below the diaphragm. There are often associated abnormalities and hypoplasia of the lung segments connected to the anomalous vein, hypoplasia of the right pulmonary artery, and a shift of the heart to the right side of the chest. Other cardiac defects are common.

COMMON ATRIOVENTRICULAR CANAL DEFECTS (ENDOCARDIAL CUSHION DEFECT)

This group of anomalies encompasses a variety of abnormalities, including ostium primum defects of the inferior atrial septum, with or without defects of the high ventricular septum, and defects or clefts in the mitral and/or tricuspid valves that result in mitral and/or tricuspid regurgitation. In some patients only one atrioventricular valve is present. Ostium primum defects are common in patients with Down's syndrome.

The combination of L-R shunt and atrioventricular valve regurgitation is usually associated with earlier and more severe symptoms and disability than is ostium secundum ASD. In childhood, upper respiratory infections are common and weight gain tends to be retarded, as in patients with ostium secundum defects. If significant mitral regurgitation is present, there may be dyspnea and fatigue on exertion or even pulmonary edema. In general, elevation of pulmonary artery pressure and the development of pulmonary vascular disease tend to occur earlier than in ostium secundum defects. Adults may develop atrial fibrillation, complete heart block, and heart failure.

The findings on physical examination are similar to those of a patient with ostium secundum ASD plus possible evidence of mitral or, less frequently, tricuspid regurgitation (Chapter 11). The chest radiograph is similar to that of an ostium secundum ASD except for dilation and hypertrophy of the left ventricle if there is significant mitral regurgitation. In contrast to patients with other types of chronic mitral regurgitation, the left atrium is usually only mildly enlarged, if at all.

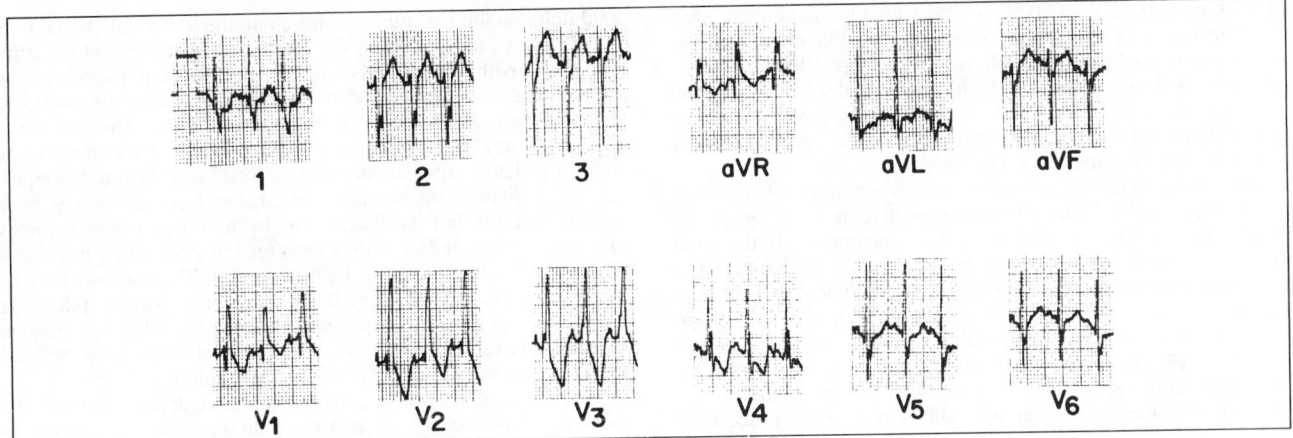

FIGURE 28-3   Electrocardiogram of a patient with ostium primum ASD, showing incomplete right bundle branch block and marked left axis deviation.

The ECG is often the first clue to the presence of an ostium primum type of endocardial cushion defect rather than an ostium secundum ASD. The characteristic findings are the combination of incomplete right bundle branch block with an rSr′ in lead V$_1$ in combination with a QRS axis between 0 and −150 degrees (Fig. 28-3). If there is significant mitral regurgitation, there may also be increased R wave voltage in the left precordial leads. The PR interval is usually prolonged.

The transthoracic (TTE) or transesophageal (TEE) echocardiogram may demonstrate the low atrial septal defect as well as abnormal motion of the mitral or tricuspid valve leaflets or even complete absence of the tissues formed at the middle of the heart from the endocardial cushion. Dilation of both ventricles may be present. Doppler echocardiography provides an estimate of the severity of the regurgitation.

Cardiac catheterization provides evidence of an ASD with an increase in oxygen content in blood samples from the right atrium compared with those in the superior vena cava. It may be possible to pass the catheter across the defect into the left atrium and ventricle. Left ventricular angiography may demonstrate a characteristic "gooseneck" deformity of the left ventricular outflow tract in the presence of a cleft anterior mitral valve leaflet. It may also demonstrate the L-R shunt, at times directly from the left ventricle to the right atrium, or mitral regurgitation.

Patients with an endocardial cushion defect require antibiotic prophylaxis against endocarditis during any dental procedure or surgical procedure likely to be associated with bacteremia. When only an ostium primum defect is present, surgical repair of an endocardial cushion defect is very similar to that of an ostium secundum defect; however, clefts in the mitral or tricuspid valves are much more difficult to repair satisfactorily without residual regurgitation. Some patients require repair or pulmonary artery banding in the first year of life. Occasionally, the valve cannot be repaired and must be replaced with a prosthetic valve.

A woman with an endocardial cushion defect has about a 14% likelihood of having a child with the same defect. The risk is 1% if only the father is affected.

VENTRICULAR SEPTAL DEFECT

In infants ventricular septal defect (VSD) is the most common recognized congenital heart defect after mitral valve prolapse or bicuspid aortic valve. About 10% of adolescents and adults with congenital heart disease have an isolated VSD. It is unusual in adults older than age 50 since the majority of infants who are born with a VSD experience spontaneous closure of the defect. Such closure is most likely to occur in the first 10 years and with small defects, but closure can occur later, and even large defects may close. The defects may be small or large, single or multiple. Defects are located usually in the superior, membranous portion of the ventricular septum (in-

fracristal defect) and less frequently in the subpulmonic (supracristal) area or in the inferior muscular portion.

The clinical course and natural history of VSD vary markedly with the size of the defect(s). Small defects (less than 0.5 cm^2/m^2) produce a loud holosystolic murmur and thrill along the lower left sternal edge but only a small L-R shunt of no hemodynamic consequence. Such a defect, however, does predispose the patient to infective endocarditis. This type of defect, maladie de Roger, is very likely to close spontaneously. Intermediate-size defects (0.5 to 1.0 cm^2/m^2) permit a moderate to large L-R shunt and produce moderate to large elevation of right ventricular and pulmonary artery pressures. In patients with large defects (more than 1.0 cm^2/m^2), who usually have equal pressures in both ventricles and the hemodynamics of a single ventricle, the direction and amount of shunt between the two ventricles depend on the compliance of the two ventricles and the relative impedance to the ejection of blood out the aorta and out the pulmonary artery. Patients with a large VSD have both increased pulmonary blood flow and increased pulmonary artery pressure. Thus they are likely to develop Eisenmenger's reaction much earlier and more severely than patients with an ostium secundum ASD.

Infants with a large VSD may have little L-R shunt at birth when the pulmonary vasculature is still markedly hypertrophied and the pulmonary vascular resistance is high. As hypertrophy of the media in the pulmonary vessels regresses over the first 3 to 12 weeks in full-term infants at sea level, the pulmonary vascular resistance decreases, allowing a much greater L-R shunt and exposing the pulmonary capillaries to relatively high pressures. Also, the increasing L-R shunt imposes a volume load on the left ventricle, which may cause an elevation of the diastolic pressures in the left ventricle, left atrium, and pulmonary veins, further contributing to the development of pulmonary edema. In many, perhaps most, children a secondary increase in the pulmonary vascular resistance begins after a few days or weeks. This increase in resistance tends to decrease the L-R shunt, to "protect" the pulmonary capillaries from the high pulmonary artery pressure, and to decrease the volume load on the left ventricle. In patients with a large VSD the pulmonary vascular resistance often increases excessively after a variable period of time, usually 3 to 20 years, with the development of severe pulmonary vascular disease and Eisenmenger's reaction. At that stage the pulmonary vascular resistance, which is usually more than 600 dynes/sec/cm^{-5}, or about 7 R units per square meter, is so high relative to the systemic vascular resistance that the L-R shunt decreases or even disappears completely, together with the murmur from the shunt across the VSD. Surgical correction is usually prohibitive in adults when the pulmonary vascular resistance is more than 800 dynes/sec/cm^{-5}, or 11 R units per square meter. Such patients often have dyspnea on exertion, chest pain, hemoptysis, and syncope. A R-L shunt may develop, together with a marked right ventricular left parasternal lift, arterial unsaturation, cyanosis, clubbing, and polycythemia. At this stage, the pulmonary vascular disease is largely irreversible; surgical repair of the defect is of limited benefit and is associated with a high operative mortality. Pregnancy and oral contraceptives are prohibited for such patients. In a few adolescents or adults with a large VSD, a marked infundibular stenosis develops, which decreases the L-R shunt and can also produce a R-L shunt and cyanosis. Therapy with combined cardiac and pulmonary transplantation is a potential form of therapy for patients with Eisenmenger's syndrome.

Patients with small VSDs usually have no symptoms. Those with medium or large defects may develop congestive heart failure at 3 to 12 weeks, which may be misdiagnosed as pneumonia. If the child survives this period, he or she may then show only mild symptoms, with exertional dyspnea, failure to thrive, and fatigue, but with relatively poor growth until the subsequent development of Eisenmenger's reaction, with cyanosis, clubbing, dyspnea, and weakness. Eventually, such patients may die suddenly, or may develop biventricular heart failure and/or pulmonary emboli and thrombi.

At birth there may be no murmurs, although usually a moderately

loud holosystolic murmur is heard along the lower left sternal border at a few days of age. Often the murmur is accompanied by a thrill. In patients with a small defect and small L-R shunt, there is no parasternal lift or accentuated P_2, but usually there is a holosystolic murmur and thrill along the lower left sternal border. The murmur and L-R shunt may end in midsystole if the defect is in the muscular septum. In patients with a small VSD the ECG and chest radiograph are normal. Patients with moderate or large defects and shunts have a similar murmur, but the apical impulse may be sustained, forceful, and displaced, together with a forceful left parasternal impulse, reflecting the volume load on both ventricles. The components of the second heart sound are normally or moderately widely split, usually with a loud pulmonic component. An early diastolic, low-frequency murmur and third heart sound may be heard at the apex, reflecting the increased flow across the mitral valve into the LV.

The chest radiograph of patients with large defects shows enlargement of all four chambers and the pulmonary artery, together with pulmonary plethora. Patients with Eisenmenger's reaction may have a pruned-tree appearance on radiograph with normal or decreased pulmonary blood flow (Fig. 28-4). The ECG may show biatrial and left ventricular or biventricular hypertrophy (Fig. 28-5). Patients with VSD and Eisenmenger's reaction may be inoperable when they have lost the ECG evidence of left or combined ventricular hypertrophy and have only right ventricular hypertrophy. The transthoracic or transesophageal echocardiogram may demonstrate the VSD directly in addition to dilation of both ventricles and evidence of pulmonary hypertension. Doppler echocardiography provides evidence of the magnitude and direction of ventricular shunt.

Cardiac catheterization (Chapter 14) permits measurements of pressures in the cardiac chambers and blood sampling to estimate the direction and magnitude of intracardiac shunts and to estimate pulmonary vascular resistance. Left ventricular angiography may demonstrate the shunt to the right ventricle. Coronary arteriography is usually performed in adults, especially those with risk factors for coronary artery disease. The VSD and the size of both ventricles can also be demonstrated by magnetic resonance imaging (MRI).

Patients with small VSDs, a small L-R shunt, and a pulmonary to systemic flow ratio less than 1.5 : 1.0 require only prophylaxis for bacterial endocarditis (Chapter 24). Most of these small defects close spontaneously, and those that remain open do not require surgery. If pulmonary edema develops in an infant with a large VSD and does not respond to therapy with digitalis and diuretics, the patient may require primary closure of the defect or, less frequently, pulmonary artery banding to decrease the pulmonary artery flow. Patients with a persistent large defect who survive infancy with medical therapy or with pulmonary artery banding should have complete repair at about 12 to 24 months of age. In patients in whom Eisenmenger's reaction develops, there is a much higher operative mortality and only a slight chance of a significant decrease in the pulmonary vascular resistance or pressure. Patients who develop infundibular stenosis with an R-L

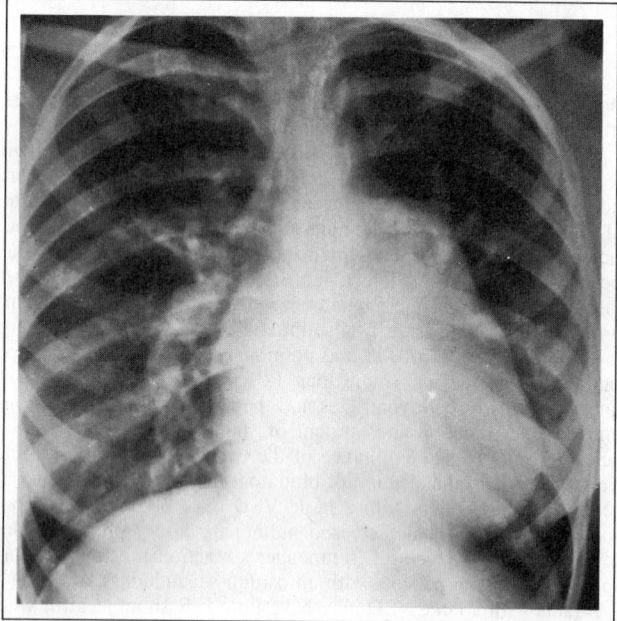

FIGURE 28-4   Chest film of a patient with a large VSD and Eisenmenger's reaction. The film shows moderate cardiomegaly, enlarged main and central arteries, and a pruned-tree appearance of the distal pulmonary arteries.

(Courtesy Dr. Wade H. Shuford, Professor of Radiology, Emory University School of Medicine.)

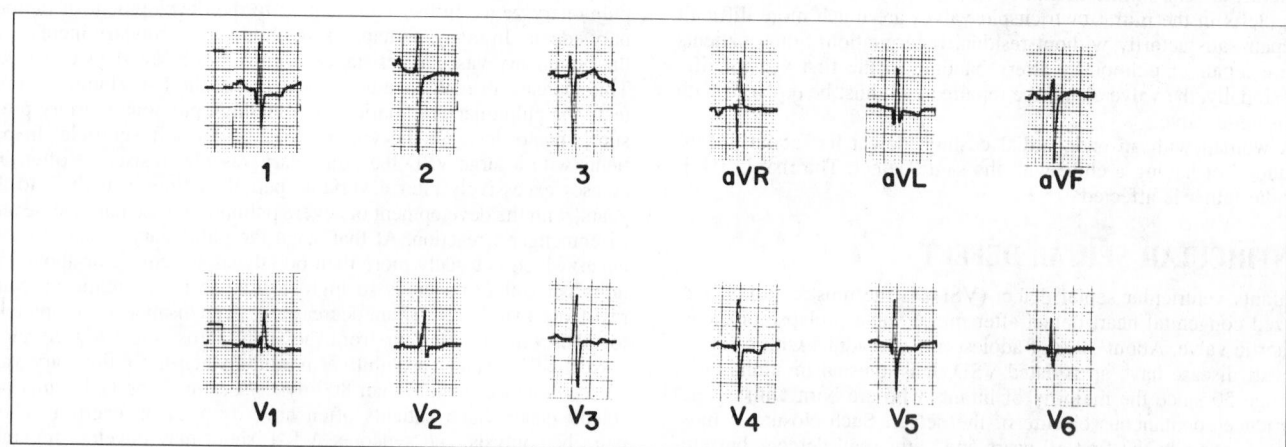

FIGURE 28-5   Electrocardiogram of patient with VSD and biventricular hypertrophy. Tracing also shows incomplete right bundle branch block but no definite left atrial abnormality.

shunt may develop secondary polycythemia. In patients with hyperviscosity symptoms the hematocrit can be lowered to below 65% by phlebotomy with fluid replacement to decrease the likelihood of thrombosis. Repeated phlebotomy may require iron therapy to avoid iron deficiency. Some of these patients can have corrective surgery with good results. In adults without severe pulmonary vascular disease, surgical correction of a VSD is usually indicated if the pulmonary blood flow is more than 1.4 times systemic flow.

A woman who has a VSD has about a 9.5% likelihood of having a child with the same defect, whereas the likelihood is only 2.5% if the father has had a VSD.

VENTRICULAR SEPTAL DEFECT WITH AORTIC REGURGITATION

There is usually a large defect in the superior, supracristal portion of the membranous ventricular septum just under the right coronary cusp of the aortic valve. In most patients the support for the aortic valve is adequate until early childhood, when the diastolic murmur of aortic regurgitation first is heard. The clinical course of such patients is usually more problematic than is that of patients with an isolated VSD. Often the aortic regurgitation becomes progressively more severe and may require valve replacement. Occasionally, the VSD closes spontaneously, leaving only moderate to severe aortic regurgitation. The aortic regurgitation may be directly demonstrated by aortography, which may also demonstrate the VSD. Echocardiography may demonstrate the VSD and may show diastolic fluttering of the anterior mitral valve leaflet produced by the aortic regurgitation. Doppler echocardiography provides an estimate of both the regurgitation and the L-R shunt.

The VSD should be repaired if there is moderate pulmonary artery hypertension with a significant L-R shunt. At times, repair of the VSD can correct the support of the aortic valve and decrease or eliminate the aortic regurgitation; more often, however, it is necessary to replace the aortic valve.

PATENT DUCTUS ARTERIOSUS

Patent ductus arteriosus (PDA) is common in infants and children but accounts for only about 2% of congenital heart defects in adults. It tends to occur with higher frequency in siblings and can result from maternal rubella in the first trimester of pregnancy. Persistence of PDA is more frequent in females, in premature infants, and in infants born at high altitudes.

The ductus arteriosus is normally patent during fetal life, when it provides a shunt from the pulmonary artery to the aorta. After birth, the ductus normally closes functionally over the first 24 to 48 hours of life and anatomically over the first 3 months; closure at a later age can occur but is infrequent. PDA may occur with many other defects, especially coarctation of the aorta and VSD.

The hemodynamic consequences and physiologic changes produced by a PDA are related to the vascular resistance through the ductus and to the pulmonary vascular resistance. In infants with high-resistance PDA, there may be only a very small L-R shunt and little hemodynamic consequence other than increased susceptibility to infective endarteritis. Infants with large, low-resistance PDA and large L-R shunts may develop left ventricular failure and pulmonary edema at 3 to 12 weeks, when the fetal vasculature undergoes its normal regression of early infancy. Usually, the left ventricle is able to compensate for the increased L-R shunt by dilation and hypertrophy and the pulmonary vasculature increases its resistance. Although the PDA closes spontaneously in many children within 3 months, a large ductus may persist and can eventually result in Eisenmenger's reaction with pulmonary vascular resistance equal to or greater than systemic resistance and an R-L shunt through the PDA with differential cyanosis of the lower extremities. This can occur at any age beyond 3 years.

Individuals with a small PDA may have no symptoms. Infants with a large PDA may develop pulmonary edema with severe dyspnea, cyanosis, and tachypnea at about 6 to 12 weeks of age. The heart failure and respiratory distress tend to occur in the first week in premature infants and in the second or third month in nonpremature infants. Children who survive this period may be relatively asymptomatic except

for mild exertional fatigue and dyspnea. Some patients with medium or large defects and a chronic volume load on the left ventricle develop left ventricular failure after the age of 20. Right ventricular failure caused by the chronic pressure load may also occur.

The classic finding of PDA is a thrill and continuous "machinery" murmur with a late systolic accentuation that is loudest in the first to third left parasternal intercostal spaces (Chapter 11). Some patients have only a systolic murmur. The murmur is often not present immediately after birth in full-term infants. The arterial pulse pressure tends to be increased, reflecting the large diastolic runoff into the pulmonary circuit. In patients with a large L-R shunt the apical impulse is displaced leftward and sustained. Patients with a large L-R shunt through the PDA may have a middiastolic murmur and a third heart sound at the apex related to the large flow across the mitral valve into the left ventricle. Patients who develop Eisenmenger's reaction with severe pulmonary vascular obstructive disease and an R-L shunt may have a right ventricular lift and a loud pulmonic component of the second heart sound, no ductus thrill or murmur, but differential cyanosis with cyanosis of the toes and intermediate cyanosis of the left fingers, but no cyanosis of the right fingers.

The chest radiograph may be normal in patients with a very small PDA, whereas patients with a large PDA may have pulmonary plethora together with enlargement of the ascending aorta and aortic knob, left ventricle and atrium, and pulmonary artery (Fig. 28-6). Patients who develop severe pulmonary vascular disease may have a normal left ventricle and atrium but a pruned-tree appearance of the peripheral pulmonary vasculature. Older patients occasionally have calcification of the PDA. The ECG in patients with a significant L-R shunt usually shows evidence of left ventricular hypertrophy and left atrial abnormality. Right ventricular hypertrophy may be present in patients with pulmonary hypertension. Echocardiography may demonstrate the ductus, dilation and hyperfunction of the left ventricle, and occasionally left atrial enlargement. Doppler echocardiography

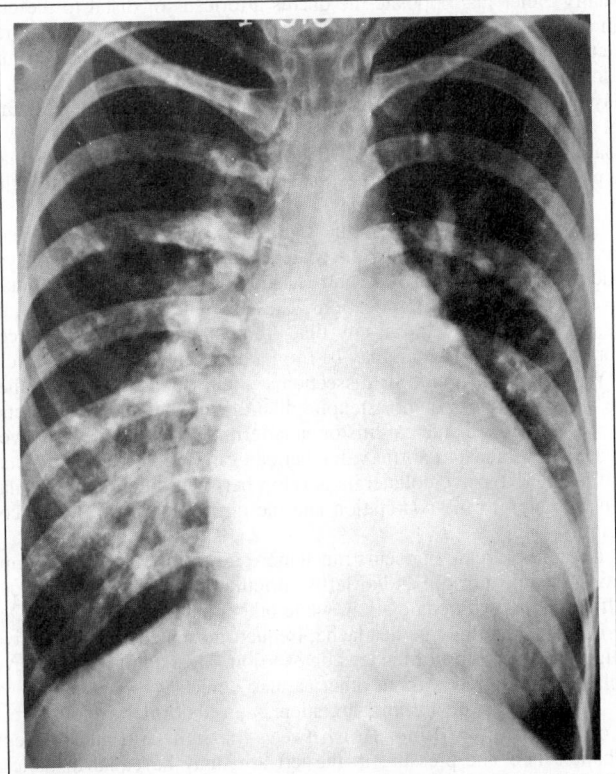

FIGURE 28-6 Chest film of a patient with a PDA showing moderate cardiomegaly and very prominent peripheral pulmonary vessels. In this film the aorta is not enlarged.

(Courtesy Dr. Wade H. Shuford, Professor of Radiology, Emory University School of Medicine.)

may be used to diagnose and quantify the shunt. Cardiac catheterization permits direct measurement of cardiac pressures and estimation of any L-R or R-L shunts. Aortography demonstrates the PDA, as does MRI.

Infants with PDA in whom congestive heart failure develops may be treated with indomethacin (which inhibits synthesis of prostaglandins) in an attempt to induce closure of the ductus, but most full-term infants eventually require elective surgical closure at 1 to 2 years of age. A patent ductus in premature infants is more likely to close either spontaneously or with indomethacin, although some require surgical closure. All patients should receive prophylaxis against infective endarteritis of the ductus. In general, any child or adult discovered to have a PDA should have it surgically corrected unless the patient either has already developed Eisenmenger's reaction or is elderly.

A mother who has a PDA has a 4% likelihood of having a child with the same defect. The likelihood is 2% if only the father has had a PDA.

AORTOPULMONARY SEPTAL DEFECT

This relatively rare defect consists of a communication, or "window," which is often relatively large, between the ascending aorta and the main pulmonary artery. A large aortopulmonary artery communication permits equalization of their pressures and, in most instances, a large L-R shunt until the development of severe pulmonary vascular disease and Eisenmenger's reaction. Patients with this defect clinically resemble those with a large, low-resistance PDA, and the two lesions can coexist. The distinction is usually made by passage of a catheter across the defect or by TTE or TEE, left ventricular angiography, aortography, or MRI. Early surgical repair is necessary to prevent progressive pulmonary vascular disease.

COARCTATION OF THE AORTA

There is a discrete, congenital narrowing of all layers of the aorta, usually either just opposite the ductus arteriosus or distal to the origin of the left subclavian artery just above the ductus arteriosus (preductal coarctation). In adolescents or adults, it is often located just below the ligamentum arteriosum (postductal coarctation). Rarely, it may be proximal to the left common carotid artery or in the abdominal aorta. About 25% to 46% of patients have a bicuspid aortic valve. Coarctation may be associated with other defects and in females may be part of Turner's syndrome (short stature, webbed neck, small chin, and other skeletal abnormalities).

The basic abnormality is the significant obstruction to left ventricular outflow produced by the coarctation. As a consequence of systolic hypertension in the left ventricle and upper body, the patient may develop a number of complications. These include left ventricular failure, which may develop at any time from infancy to adulthood; cerebral hemorrhage, which may be from a berry aneurysm in the circle of Willis; aortic rupture or dissection, which usually involves either the ascending aorta or poststenotic dilation just beyond the coarctation; and infective endocarditis or endarteritis, which usually involves a coexisting bicuspid aortic valve but can rarely involve the coarctation itself. Extensive collaterals develop between the arterial circulation proximal to the coarctation and the circulation distal to the coarctation.

Isolated coarctation occurs much more frequently in males. Symptoms and signs of right and/or left ventricular failure develop in about half of infants with coarctation, while others have no symptoms. Occasionally, there may be headache, frequent nosebleeds, or excessive fatigue or discomfort of the legs on exertion. Most adult patients have isolated coarctation without other cardiac defects.

The hallmark of aortic coarctation is an abnormal systolic pressure difference ($\geq$30 mm Hg) between the right arm and the legs (Chapter 11). The pressure in the left arm may be equal to or less than that in the right arm, depending on the site of coarctation. The diastolic pressure below the coarctation is often normal or nearly normal. In some patients the pressure difference between the right arm and the legs is relatively mild at rest but increases dramatically during exercise. The carotid pulses are often very forceful while the pulses in the leg are delayed, weak, or impalpable. The legs are oc-

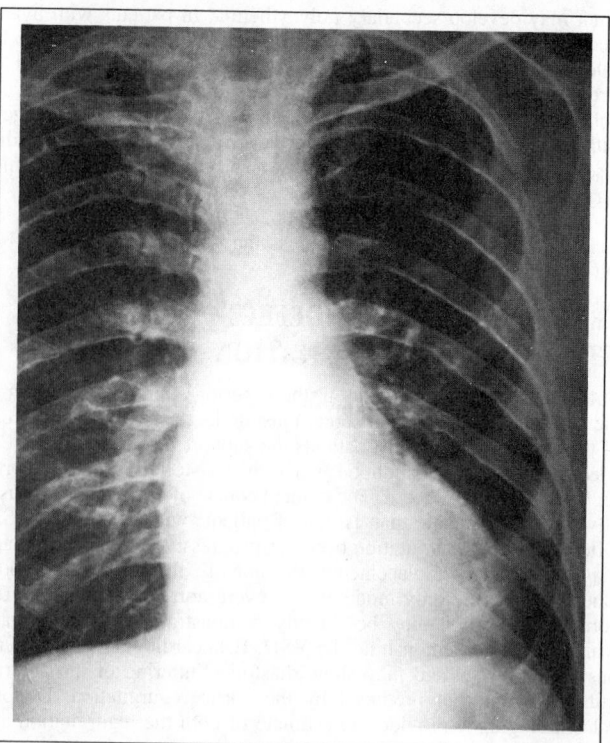

FIGURE 28-7   Chest film of a patient with coarctation of the aorta showing mild cardiomegaly and notching on the undersurfaces of the posterior ribs. (Courtesy Dr. Wade H. Shuford, Professor of Radiology, Emory University School of Medicine.)

casionally poorly developed relative to the chest and arms. The apical impulse is sustained, forceful, and displaced leftward and inferiorly. Patients with a biscuspid aortic valve may have a harsh midsystolic murmur and thrill along the second right intercostal space and an early systolic ejection click at the apex. In addition, there may be a blowing, decrescendo diastolic murmur of aortic regurgitation along the left sternal border. A midsystolic blowing murmur from the flow across the coarctation may often be heard faintly along the left sternal border or louder posteriorly in the left interscapular space. At times, this murmur extends into early diastole. Collateral vessels produce systolic murmurs that may continue into or throughout diastole and are commonly heard over the posterior chest wall beyond childhood. At times, these collateral intercostal vessels are palpable, particularly over the posterior chest.

The chest radiograph may show prominence of the ascending aorta and enlargement of the left ventricle and left atrium. The poststenotic dilation of the aorta and the dilated proximal left subclavian artery and aorta may produce a "figure 3" sign along the left side of the upper descending thoracic aorta. Classically, notching on the undersurfaces of the posterior ribs bilaterally is present after the age of 7 or 8 years (Fig. 28-7). If the coarctation is proximal to the origin of the left subclavian artery, however, notching may occur only on the right side, whereas patients with coarctation of the abdominal aorta may have no notching of the upper ribs.

The usual ECG findings are those of left ventricular hypertrophy and left atrial abnormality (Chapter 12). Infants may have ventricular or combined ventricular hypertrophy, often in association with an interatrial L-R shunt. Aortography proximal to the suspected site demonstrates the character of the coarctation and the collateral vessels and may also demonstrate aortic regurgitation or a biscuspid aortic valve. Two-dimensional echocardiography, especially transesophageal, and MRI can also demonstrate the coarctation. Upper- and lower-extremity blood pressure measurements during exercise are useful in assessing the significance of systolic pressure differences that are only mild at rest.

Most young patients with significant coarctation should undergo cardiac catheterization to assess possible associated lesions. Children with isolated coarctation should have elective surgical repair at age 4 to 6 years to decrease the likelihood of heart failure, aortic dissection or rupture, and cerebral hemorrhage. Balloon dilation has been used with reasonably good success in children and a few adults although recurrence is possible. Older children and young adults should have surgical repair as soon as feasible. In patients older than age 50 without evidence of a complication, the indication for surgery is less definite. After surgical repair, some patients with coarctation have a post-coarctation syndrome of acute abdominal pain, ileus, and even necrotizing mesenteric vasculitis that appears to be related to suddenly exposing the abdominal vessels to a higher than usual blood pressure. This can usually be prevented or satisfactorily controlled by careful blood pressure control with sodium nitroprusside and beta blockers; in very rare cases it may require emergency surgery. Patients should be followed consistently after repair of the coarctation, since many have an associated bicuspid aortic valve and many redevelop systemic hypertension for which they will require therapy. A small percentage of patients operated on in childhood develop evidence of recurrence of the stenosis at the site of coarctation. Such patients can usually be managed with balloon dilation or medication to control their hypertension; only rarely do they require repeat surgery.

A woman with coarctation of the aorta has about a 4% chance of having a child with the same defect. The likelihood is about 2.5% if only the father has had a coarctation.

CONGENITAL AORTIC STENOSIS*

The obstruction may be either supravalvular, valvular, or subvalvular. Supravalvular stenosis is usually produced by a fibrous band or ring just above the aortic valve. Valvular stenosis in infants or children is usually produced by cuspal fusion of a bicuspid valve, or by a unicuspid (unicommissural) or noncommissural valve. It is four times as frequent in males. Congenital subvalvular stenosis is usually produced by a discrete fibromembranous or fibromuscular band or ring that extends from the anterior leaflet of the mitral valve to the ventricular septum just below the aortic valve. In older children or adults, subvalvular obstruction is most often produced by hypertrophic obstructive cardiomyopathy (Chapter 26).

Infants and children may die suddenly without significant symptoms. Others have symptoms of dyspnea or distress on feeding or on exertion, fatigue, exertional angina, or syncopal or near-syncopal episodes. In occasional infants, the stenosis is critical at birth or in the first 6 months and requires prompt surgical correction to prevent congestive heart failure. More often, the symptoms of congestive heart failure or of distress while eating, which are equivalent to angina pectoris in an older patient, occur after several years or during the rapid growth phase of childhood. Valvular aortic stenosis is usually associated with an ejection click, which is often loudest at the apex. Half the patients with subvalvular aortic stenosis have the murmur of aortic regurgitation caused by fibrosis and retraction of the aortic valve leaflets from the jet of blood through the subvalvular obstruction. When the regurgitation is moderate or severe, it may require repair or replacement of the aortic valve.

Some patients with supravalvular aortic stenosis have Williams' syndrome, with a particular elfin appearance, mental retardation, retarded growth, small chin, and malformed teeth. Peripheral pulmonary artery stenosis is frequently an associated condition. Hypercalcemia has occasionally been noted in infancy. Usually the blood pressure is higher in the right arm than in the left, and there is no ejection click. The midsystolic murmur is usually loudest in the first right intercostal space and radiates to both carotids. A fourth heart sound may be heard at the apex in this and all other types of moderate to severe aortic stenosis.

The examination of patients with valvular aortic stenosis is similar except that the murmur is usually loudest in the second right intercostal space, frequently with a systolic thrill. An ejection click is heard either in this area or at the apex, and occasionally the murmur of aortic regurgitation is heard along the left sternal border. In infants or children with valvular aortic stenosis, the carotid pulse may

be normal and the aortic component of the second heart sound may be well preserved. The presence of paradoxical splitting of the second heart sound is rare and implies severe obstruction (Chapter 11). A fourth heart sound is frequently heard with moderate or severe obstruction.

The chest radiograph may show slight convexity of the left ventricle. Prominence of the ascending aorta is usual in valvular stenosis, but is unusual in supravalvular stenosis, and is only occasionally found in subvalvular stenosis. Calcification is usually seen only in valvular stenosis after age 20. Evidence of pulmonary edema may be present.

All forms of aortic stenosis usually have electrocardiographic evidence of left ventricular hypertrophy and left atrial enlargement when the obstruction is significant. Doppler echocardiography demonstrates the location and provides a good estimate of the severity of the obstruction. MRI can also demonstrate the location of the obstruction, while cardiac catheterization and left ventricular angiography permit estimation of the effective orifice of the obstruction and evaluation of left ventricular function in addition to outlining the obstruction. Coronary arteriography is performed on all patients with angina and most adult patients. In patients with low peak or mean gradients across the aortic valve, it is important to calculate the valve area since a decreased stroke volume can result in existence of only a mild pressure gradient across a severely stenotic valve. Some patients have a dramatic, progressive increase in the severity of obstruction over 3 to 5 years.

Surgery is generally indicated in children or adolescents with a peak pressure difference between the left ventricle and the aorta of 75 mm Hg or greater or a valve area less than 0.5 cm^2/m^3. Surgery may also be indicated with less severe obstruction in patients with symptoms, cardiomegaly, or ECG changes (Chapter 25).

A woman with congenital AS has about an 18% chance of having offspring with the same defect, whereas the likelihood is only 5% if only the father has had congenital AS.

BICUSPID AORTIC VALVE

This lesion, which may be the most common type of congenital heart disease other than mitral valve prolapse, occurs more frequently in males, with an incidence of 1% to 2%. In most instances one leaflet is larger than the other. It often occurs in association with PDA, coarctation of the aorta, or interruption of the aortic arch.

A bicuspid aortic valve is the most frequent cause of significant valvular aortic stenosis in infancy and childhood, of congenital aortic regurgitation, and of isolated calcific stenosis before the age of 65. While some bicuspid aortic valves are fully competent at birth, the abnormal structure of the valve produces abnormal stresses on the valve that eventually result in premature fibrosis and calcification after 30 to 60 years. A minority of patients have aortic regurgitation from early life. Infective endocarditis is a constant threat to any patient with a bicuspid aortic valve. Whereas the majority of patients with a bicuspid aortic valve eventually develop valvular fibrosis and calcification with calcific aortic stenosis (Chapter 25), a rare patient over the age of 70 is found at autopsy to have only mild fibrosis with no significant stenosis. There is a suggestion that calcification and stenosis occur earlier in patients with systemic hypertension or hypercholesterolemia.

Patients with a functionally normal bicuspid aortic valve have no symptoms. Patients who have significant congenital stenosis or regurgitation, however, may develop symptoms of congestive heart failure, angina, or syncope in infancy or childhood (Chapter 25). The presence of a bicuspid aortic valve can be suggested in a young patient who is found to have a midsystolic murmur loudest in the second right intercostal space together with an ejection click, which is often heard loudest at the apex. An early diastolic blowing murmur of aortic regurgitation may occasionally be heard along the left sternal border. The diagnosis and management of patients with significant aortic stenosis or regurgitation are described in Chapter 25. For most of their lives, the main danger is infective endocarditis. With the development of any one of the classic triad of symptoms—congestive heart failure, angina, or syncope—patients are candidates for prompt surgery because of the high risk of sudden death without such therapy (Chapter 25).

---

*See also acquired aortic stenosis, Chapter 25.

VALVULAR PULMONIC STENOSIS WITH INTACT VENTRICULAR SEPTUM

There is usually a dome-shaped stenosis of the pulmonic valve with fused commissures, often associated with poststenotic dilation of the main pulmonary artery. The severe obstruction is associated with marked hypertrophy of the right ventricle, which at times is associated with secondary muscular infundibular stenosis of the outflow tract. Maternal rubella may be associated with pulmonic stenosis, although patent ductus arteriosus and pulmonary artery branch stenosis are more frequent.

Many patients have no symptoms even with severe stenosis. When present, the most frequent symptoms are easy fatigability and dyspnea on exertion. Angina pectoris on exertion and syncope can also occur, especially with severe stenosis.

In patients with moderate or severe pulmonic stenosis there is usually a prominent A wave in the jugular venous pulse; a palpable, sustained right ventricular lift along the left sternal border; a widely split second heart sound with delayed or usually faint or inaudible pulmonic component; a moderately loud and long, harsh, spindle-shaped midsystolic murmur, often with a thrill that is loudest in the second left intercostal space and tends to radiate to the left infraclavicular area and the neck; and a right-ventricular fourth heart sound along the left sternal border. In patients with mild to moderate pulmonic stenosis, a pulmonic ejection sound may be heard at the base or upper left sternal edge (Chapter 25). Patients with severe pulmonic stenosis and elevation of right atrial pressure may have arterial oxygen unsaturation and cyanosis from an R-L shunt through a patent foramen ovale.

The chest radiograph may show varying degrees of prominence of the right atrium and right ventricle, occasionally producing marked enlargement of the heart. There is often prominence of the main and/or left pulmonary artery produced by poststenotic dilation; however, the pulmonary blood flow appears normal or diminished (Fig. 28-8, *A*). In adults, the pulmonic valve may be calcified.

There is a reasonably good correlation between the severity of stenosis and the relative ECG evidence for right ventricular hypertrophy in lead V_1. In addition, there is usually right axis deviation and right atrial enlargement. Doppler echocardiography provides a good estimate of the severity of pulmonic stenosis and of right ventricular function. Contrast echocardiography may document an R-L shunt at the atrial level. Cardiac catheterization permits direct measurements of the pressure difference across the stenotic valve and right ventricular pressures and permits calculation of the effective valve orifice. Right ventricular angiography visualizes the dome-shaped stenosis and poststenotic dilation of the pulmonary artery (Fig. 28-8, *B*).

Patients with pulmonic stenosis are susceptible to infective endocarditis, for which they should receive appropriate antibiotic prophylaxis (Chapter 24). Balloon valvuloplasty (valvotomy) is the treatment of choice for most patients with isolated congenital pulmonic stenosis. In general, valvotomy is indicated, preferably in childhood, if the peak systolic pressure difference between the right ventricle and the pulmonary artery is 80 mm Hg or more and is indicated for many, but not all, patients with a resting pressure difference of 50 to 79 mm Hg. Occasionally, balloon valvotomy is indicated in symptomatic patients with pressure differences of 25 to 49 mm Hg at rest, but only very rarely is it indicated with lower pressure differences. If catheter balloon valvuloplasty is not successful, surgical valvotomy may be performed. Surgery should include infundibular resection if hypertrophy of this region is thought to contribute significantly to the obstruction.

In contrast to valvular aortic stenosis, patients over the age of 12 with pulmonic stenosis who have serial cardiac catheterizations usually show no increase in a pressure difference of less than 50 mm Hg across the valve. Most children and many adults do very well after balloon valvuloplasty or surgical valvotomy, whereas some adults occasionally do not, perhaps because of right ventricular fibrosis and persistent hypertrophy. Some patients may develop significant infundibular obstruction. Many patients have mild pulmonary regurgitation after pulmonary valvotomy; occasionally this regurgitation is severe and leads to right ventricular volume overload and tricuspid regurgitation. Rarely, pulmonic stenosis can recur after valvotomy.

A woman with pulmonary stenosis has a 6.5% chance of having a

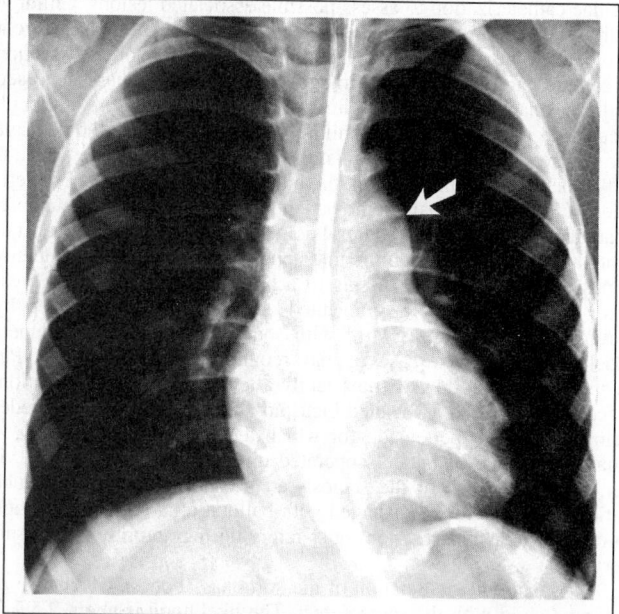

A

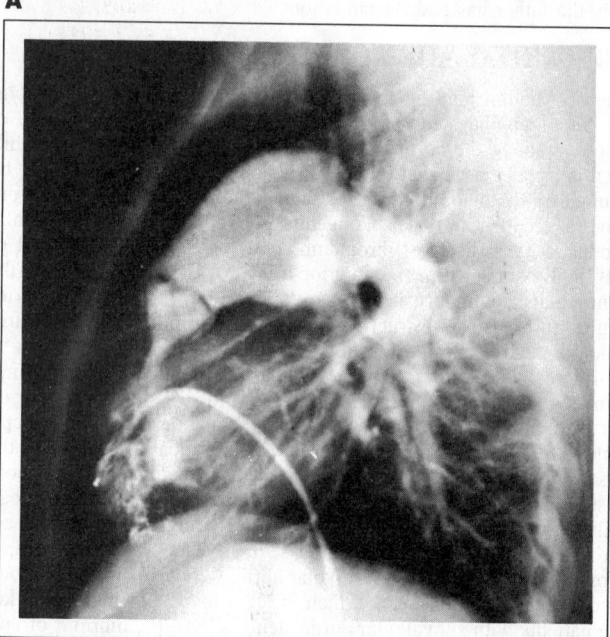

B

FIGURE 28-8   Chest film **(A)** and right ventricular angiogram **(B)** in a patient with isolated pulmonic stenosis. The chest film shows a slight prominence of the main pulmonary artery *(arrow)* and diminished pulmonary blood flow. The angiogram shows dome-shaped stenosis of the pulmonary valve with poststenotic dilation of the main pulmonary artery.

(Courtesy Dr. Wade H. Shuford, Professor of Radiology, Emory University School of Medicine.)

child with the same defect, whereas the likelihood is 2% if only the father is affected.

TETRALOGY OF FALLOT

Tetralogy of Fallot is the most common type of cyanotic congenital heart disease in older children and adults. The four features of the syndrome are a large VSD, pulmonic stenosis of varying severity but usually predominantly infundibular, overriding of the aorta over the VSD, and right ventricular hypertrophy. Other cardiac lesions are frequently present, including a right aortic arch in about 30% of patients. There is great variation in the pathology and pathophysiology, de-

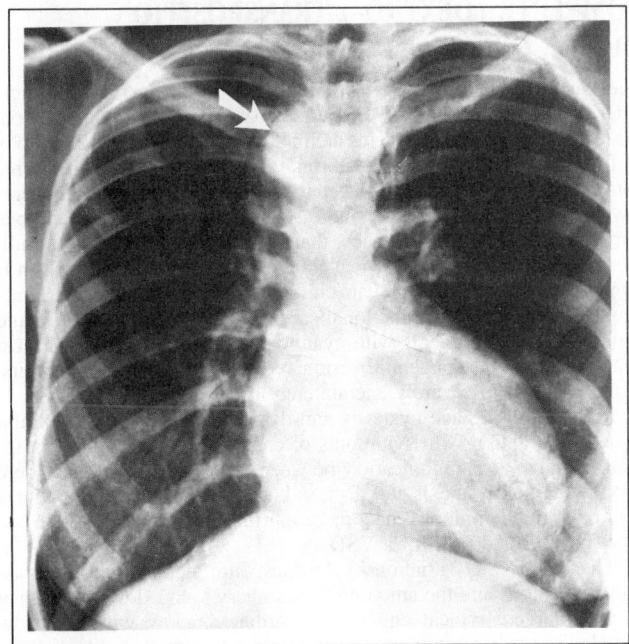

FIGURE 28-9   Chest film of a patient with tetralogy of Fallot showing mild cardiomegaly, uplifting of the cardiac apex, decreased pulmonary blood flow, and a right aortic arch *(arrow)*.

(Courtesy Dr. Wade H. Shuford, Professor of Radiology, Emory University School of Medicine.)

pending on the severity of pulmonic stenosis and the size of the VSD. Thus some patients initially have only mild infundibular stenosis and have an L-R shunt from the large VSD. Subsequently, they may develop marked infundibular stenosis and an R-L shunt and cyanosis. The level of systemic vascular resistance also influences the amount of pulmonary blood flow and, therefore, of cyanosis.

Cyanosis is usually noted shortly after birth in patients with severe pulmonic stenosis. A systolic murmur along the left sternal border may also be noted shortly after birth if there is moderate obstruction to pulmonary flow, but the murmur may be faint or absent if there is very severe pulmonic stenosis or pulmonary atresia. Episodic loss of consciousness or hypercyanotic episodes may occur in association with severe stenosis, often after exertion or crying, and are often caused by transient worsening of infundibular stenosis. Classically, infants or children with tetralogy assume the knee-chest position or squat to obtain relief from exertional cyanosis. These maneuvers compress the femoral arteries and increase systemic resistance, producing an increase in pulmonary blood flow and increasing arterial oxygen saturation; they also increase venous return.

Growth and development often are below average. Some patients have no detectable cyanosis, whereas others have marked generalized cyanosis with clubbing of the fingers and toes. In most cyanotic patients there is a faint right ventricular impulse felt along the lower left sternal edge and a midsystolic murmur that is loudest in the third intercostal space near the sternum and is often associated with a thrill. In most patients with cyanosis and tetralogy of Fallot the pulmonic component of the second heart sound is not heard; only a loud, single aortic component is heard. In patients who have mild pulmonic stenosis and so-called acyanotic tetralogy or pink tetralogy, the findings are similar to those of patients with a large VSD, including a widely split second heart sound.

The classic chest film of patients with cyanosis shows a boot-shaped heart produced by right ventricular hypertrophy, small pulmonary artery, and small left ventricle, in association with relatively clear lung fields. In patients with acyanotic tetralogy of Fallot, the pulmonic stenosis is mild, and there may even be an L-R shunt across the VSD with increased pulmonary vascular markings. The aortic arch is on the right side in about 30% of patients (Fig. 28-9).

The ECG in cyanotic patients usually shows right-axis deviation, right ventricular hypertrophy, absent Q waves over the left pericar-

dium, and often right atrial abnormality. In patients with mild pulmonic stenosis, the ECG shows Q waves and higher R waves in the left precordial leads.

Both 2D echocardiography and MRI usually provide an accurate picture of the anatomy and permit a reasonable evaluation of ventricular function. Cardiac catheterization and angiography provide an accurate assessment of the severity of the pulmonic stenosis, the amount of R-L shunting, the character of the ventricular septal defect, and the presence of associated lesions, including coronary artery anomalies.

Medical management consists primarily of trying to prevent brain abscess, cerebrovascular accidents, and infective endocarditis. Infants and children rarely have congestive heart failure, which does occasionally occur in adult patients. In some patients, the cyanosis is associated with marked polycythemia, which can produce headaches, fullheadedness, or rarely, cerebral venous thrombosis. Repeated phlebotomy may be necessary for such hyperviscosity symptoms, which usually do not occur unless the hematocrit is more than 65%. Repeated phlebotomy can produce iron deficiency anemia unless iron supplementation is provided. Propranolol is often useful in preventing hypoxic spells.

Surgery should usually be offered to patients with tetralogy of Fallot who have more than mild cyanosis. Preferably, elective total correction is performed at age 4 or 5 years, or, if necessary, in infancy. In some instances, especially in some very small infants, it is necessary to perform a palliative shunt procedure such as a Blalock-Taussig procedure, in which a subclavian artery from the opposite side of the aortic arch is anastomosed to a pulmonary artery. Most patients have complete right bundle branch block after total repair.

Complications of the Blalock-Taussig procedure include outgrowing the size of the anastomosis or, rarely, the development of severe pulmonary vascular obstructive disease (PVOD). PVOD is more likely to occur in adults who have had a Potts procedure, which is a side-to-side anastomosis of the descending aorta to the left pulmonary artery, or a Waterston-Cooley anastomosis, in which the ascending aorta is anastomosed to the right pulmonary artery. Patients who have had a palliative procedure in childhood should usually have total correction at an early age before they either outgrow the shunt or develop severe PVOD.

Patients with uncorrected tetralogy have an increased morbidity and mortality during pregnancy. Patients who have had a palliative procedure continue to be at risk for brain abscess and infective endocarditis.

Overall, the most common cause of death in patients with tetralogy after surgical repair is sudden death caused by ventricular arrhythmias. Patients should be followed regularly after repair to detect ventricular arrhythmias on routine ECG, as well as on periodic ambulatory ECG and/or 24-hour ambulatory ECG. Ventricular arrhythmias detected should be treated aggressively. Other causes of death include congestive heart failure related to residual ventricular septal defect and severe PVOD after a palliative procedure.

A woman with tetralogy of Fallot has a 2.5% chance of producing a child with the same defect. The likelihood is 1.5% if only the father is affected.

EBSTEIN'S ANOMALY OF THE TRICUSPID VALVE

In this defect there is downward displacement of the septal and posterior leaflets of the tricuspid valve, which are broadly attached to the wall of the right ventricle below the true anulus of the valve and have poorly developed papillary muscles and chordae tendineae. Usually the anterior leaflet is attached normally to the anulus. The wall of the "atrialized" portion of the right ventricle above the valve is abnormally thin. The markedly reduced pumping ability of the small functional right ventricle is further hindered by the bulging of the anterior leaflet into the right atrium during systole. The tricuspid valve is usually regurgitant, although it can also be stenotic. There is usually an ASD or a patent foramen ovale, through which a large R-L shunt develops. A significant number of patients have the Wolff-Parkinson-White (WPW) syndrome (Chapter 12) and have recurrent supraventricular tachycardias. In a few patients there is evidence that the maternal use of lithium may have been a factor in the development of Ebstein's anomaly.

A few patients are acyanotic, although there may be a history of cyanosis at birth that subsequently decreased or of chronic cyanosis together with episodes of tachycardia in association with fatigue and breathlessness. At times, chest pain occurs. Ebstein's anomaly is relatively rare beyond the fourth decade, although survival to age 85 has been reported.

Although there is usually an R-L shunt, many patients are not clinically cyanotic. There may be systolic pulsations of the jugular veins with large V waves and an early to midsystolic murmur of tricuspid regurgitation along the left sternal border. The murmur may increase with inspiration (Carvallo's sign) and may be associated with a thrill. Occasionally, there is a low-pitched murmur of tricuspid stenosis along the left sternal border. There is usually no parasternal lift or right ventricular hypertrophy. In most cases there is wide splitting of both the first and second heart sounds, which, together with loud right ventricular third and fourth heart sounds, can produce a loud cacophony of sounds.

The chest radiograph characteristically shows a large heart without enlargement of the right ventricle or main pulmonary artery. The pulmonary vasculature is normal or diminished. In about 10% of patients, the ECG shows a short PR interval and evidence of type B WPW syndrome (Chapter 12). Other ECG findings in patients with Ebstein's anomaly include prominent right atrial P waves, a prolonged PR interval, and complete or incomplete right bundle branch block. Right ventricular hypertrophy is absent.

Echocardiography shows that closure of the tricuspid valve occurs more than 65 msec later than mitral valve closure in association with abnormally increased motion of the tricuspid leaflet. The abnormal displacement of the tricuspid valve into the right ventricle is well shown by echocardiography, and the location of the R-L shunt can be identified by contrast and Doppler echocardiography. MRI also shows the essential anatomic features. Cardiac catheterization permits the recording of right ventricular electrocardiograms from the lower portion of the "right atrium" that is formed by the atrialized portion of the right ventricle. Cardiac catheterization and right ventricular angiography also permit estimation of the severity of tricuspid regurgitation, evaluation of right ventricular function, identification of any associated abnormalities, and localization of the site of R-L shunting.

Management varies greatly, as do the many abnormalities that may be encountered in mild to severe cases. Most patients die before the age of 25 from either congestive heart failure or sudden death. In general, surgery should be considered in any patient with progressive cyanosis, heart failure, or effort intolerance. The most encouraging surgical results have been from anuloplasty with plication of the atrialized portion of the right ventricle, although the results have been only fair. Patients with recurrent supraventricular tachycardia and type B WPW syndrome can usually be controlled medically, but intracardiac mapping and ablation (Chapter 18) of the anomalous pathway may be necessary.

TRUNCUS ARTERIOSUS (COMMON AORTOPULMONARY TRUNK)

In this condition a single large vessel leaves the base of the heart, usually above a ventricular septal defect. There is a single semilunar valve at the base of the truncus, which gives rise to the coronary arteries, the pulmonary arteries, the aorta, and all systemic arteries. There is moderate variation in the origins of the pulmonary arteries, which occasionally are partially stenotic near their origins. Such stenosis tends to decrease the pulmonary flow and to protect the pulmonary arteries from systemic arterial pressure.

Most children with this condition have mild to moderate cyanosis from birth and a large L-R shunt, develop PVOD, and die in childhood. A rare patient with stenosis near the origin of the pulmonary arteries may live to young adulthood without surgery.

Echocardiography and MRI can usually establish the diagnosis. The complete study of the condition requires cardiac catheterization, right ventricular angiography, and aortography. Both medical and surgical management are unsatisfactory. Surgery can be attempted with construction of a conduit containing a prosthetic valve from the right ventricle to the pulmonary arteries. Both the conduit tubing and the prosthetic heart valve should be carefully monitored for dysfunction.

COMPLETE (DEXTRO-) TRANSPOSITION OF THE GREAT ARTERIES

The basic defect is the origin of the aorta from the right ventricle anterior and to the right of the pulmonary artery, which arises from the left ventricle. The ventricles are in the normal position ("D-loop"), and the atria and ventricles are normally related. To sustain life, some communication must exist between the two circulations. Most patients have a patent foramen ovale, about two thirds have a PDA, and one third have a VSD. Other defects that may be present include a rudimentary right ventricle and tricuspid atresia or stenosis. The lesion is more frequent in males and in children of diabetic mothers. It accounts for about 4% of functional cardiac malformations at birth and about 10% of all patients with cyanotic heart disease. It is the most common cyanotic congenital lesion requiring treatment in the first weeks of life and is rarely encountered in adults.

Most children have cyanosis and dyspnea from birth and exhibit growth retardation with symptoms of congestive heart failure. In infants without a communication between the two circulations, there may be marked cyanosis and distress but no murmurs. Other patients may have the continuous machinery murmur of PDA or the holosystolic murmur and thrill of a VSD.

There is a great variation in the chest film, depending on the associated lesions and the amount of pulmonary blood flow. There may be an enlarged, typical egg-shaped cardiac shadow with a narrow pedicle. There is often evidence of increased pulmonary blood flow. The ECG is normal for age, with right ventricular predominance. Doppler echocardiography and MRI can usually provide the diagnosis and define the associated defects, although cardiac catheterization and angiography may be necessary.

Infants in acute distress should have emergency cardiac catheterization and balloon atrial septostomy to allow communication between the two circulations and thus survival until a more definitive procedure can be attempted. Survival depends on the associated lesions and the rate of development of PVOD.

CONGENITALLY CORRECTED TRANSPOSITION OF THE GREAT ARTERIES

The two basic defects are transposition of the aorta and the pulmonary artery and inversion of the ventricles ("L-loop"). Thus there is functional correction with systemic venous blood passing through the morphologic right atrium to a bicuspid mitral valve into a right-sided morphologic left ventricle and into the pulmonary artery, while pulmonary venous blood passes through a morphologic left atrium and a tricuspid valve into a left-sided morphologic right ventricle and into the aorta, which is anterior to the pulmonary artery. There may be no symptoms unless there is an associated defect, for example, Ebstein's anomaly of the tricuspid valve, VSD, obstruction to outflow of the venous ventricle, mitral regurgitation, pulmonic stenosis, congenital heart block, or variations in the pattern of coronary arteries. Most patients have an associated defect. There may be no abnormalities on physical examination, but one fourth of the patients have a loud single second sound that is loudest in the second left intercostal space and is produced by aortic valve closure. An apical holosystolic murmur is heard in about half the patients.

In some patients the chest film is essentially normal. The normal shadow of the main pulmonary artery may be absent, and there may be a convexity, or "shoulder," on the left middle cardiac border produced by the displaced anterior aorta. The ECG may show a prolonged PR interval, and there may be small Q waves over the right precordium but not in the lateral chest leads. Supraventricular arrhythmias, including paroxysmal atrial tachycardia, atrial fibrillation, and atrial flutter, may occur. The abnormal location of the aorta, pulmonary artery, and atrioventricular valves can be demonstrated by echocardiography, MRI, or cardiac catheterization and selective angiography. Palliative surgery may be necessary for associated defects.

TOTAL ANOMALOUS PULMONARY VENOUS CONNECTION

In this syndrome, the four pulmonary veins return oxygenated blood from the lungs to the right atrium or to one of its tributaries. In the right atrium some blood is shunted to the left atrium through an atrial septal defect and produces systemic cyanosis, which may be mild or marked. Physiologically, there is a large L-R shunt and a smaller R-L shunt. Most infants with this condition have cyanosis with increased fatigue on exertion and develop congestive heart failure and die by the age of 1 year. The chest radiograph shows increased pulmonary blood flow, and the heart may have a figure-of-eight or "snowman" appearance if the pulmonary venous blood enters a vertical vein in the upper chest and a dilated superior vena cava is in the right upper chest. The ECG usually shows evidence of right axis deviation, right ventricular hypertrophy, and right atrial enlargement. Echocardiography and MRI can visualize the dilated right atrium and right ventricle and, in many cases, the anomalous pulmonary veins joining the right atrium or a tributary. Doppler echocardiography provides an estimate of the location, magnitude, and direction of shunts. Cardiac catheterization and selective pulmonary angiography are used for precise delineation of the anatomic defects and for confirmation of the R-L and L-R shunts.

Emergency balloon atrial septostomy may provide temporary relief if the atrial defect is too small, but most patients require complete surgical correction with connection of the pulmonary venous return to the left atrium and closure of the ASD to prevent death from congestive failure in the first year of life.

TRICUSPID ATRESIA

The rare syndrome of atresia of the tricuspid valve is always associated with an interatrial communication and often with hypoplasia of the right ventricle. The systemic blood returns to the right atrium, where it passes into the left atrium. Pulmonary blood flow, which is usually markedly decreased, is achieved by a patent ductus arteriosus or a VSD. There is usually marked cyanosis, a single heart sound, and left axis deviation on the ECG. If the interatrial communication is inadequate in size, balloon septostomy can be utilized to increase pulmonary blood flow, along with other palliative procedures, such as the creation of a systemic arterial-pulmonary artery shunt. More nearly complete correction of the defect involves the anastomosis of the right atrium to the right ventricle or creation of a conduit between the right atrium and the pulmonary artery in combination with closure of the interatrial communication. Very few children with this defect live to adulthood.

CORONARY SINUS ANEURYSM (SINUS OF VALSALVA FISTULA)

In this condition, which is more common in males, there is a congenital defect between the anulus fibrosus of the aortic valve and the media of the aorta. Over a period of three to four decades, the aortic pressure causes progressive dilation and aneurysm formation at the area of weakness. Eventually, the aneurysm ruptures, most often into the right ventricle, less frequently into the right atrium, and, rarely, into the left ventricle, left atrium, or pericardium. Occasionally, bacterial endocarditis is responsible for the rupture.

There are no symptoms until the aneurysm ruptures. There may be the abrupt onset of severe, tearing chest pain and symptoms of acute heart failure. There may be a wide pulse pressure with bounding arterial pulses. Classically, there is a very loud continuous precordial murmur with thrill; occasionally, the murmur can be heard from the foot of the bed.

The diagnosis of the aneurysm and the location of the fistula and the chamber into which it ruptures can be confirmed by aortography, transthoracic Doppler echocardiography, transesophageal echocardiography, or MRI (Chapter 13). It is possible to diagnose an asymptomatic aortic sinus aneurysm before rupture if one of these procedures happens to be performed for some other reason.

Surgical repair is indicated for virtually all individuals in whom a fistula develops from an aortic sinus aneurysm. On the other hand, if an aneurysm is incidentally discovered before it ruptures to form a fistula, surgery is probably not indicated, since it is difficult to know exactly the location and extent of the congenital defect until it ruptures.

COR TRIATRIATUM

A relatively rare syndrome, cor triatriatum is produced by a congenital fibromuscular band that divides the left atrium into a superior and posterior chamber and an inferior and anterior chamber and produces obstruction to the flow of the pulmonary venous blood through the left atrium into the left ventricle. The symptoms resemble those of mitral stenosis with progressive dyspnea and pulmonary congestion (Chapter 25). There may be evidence of pulmonary artery hypertension and right ventricular hypertrophy, but a loud snapping S_1, opening snap, and diastolic rumble are absent. The condition can be demonstrated by transthoracic or, preferably, transesophageal echocardiography, MRI, or pulmonary angiography. The abnormal diaphragm can be surgically excised with excellent results.

ABERRANT RIGHT SUBCLAVIAN ARTERY

The aberrant right subclavian artery arises from the aorta distal to the origin of the left subclavian artery and passes behind the esophagus to the right arm. It may occur as an isolated lesion or together with other lesions, particularly right aortic arch, tetralogy of Fallot, or coarctation of the aorta. In the presence of aortic coarctation, the pressure in the right arm can be lower than that in the left arm if the aberrant artery originates distal to the coarctation. The anomaly rarely produces symptoms, although formerly it was thought to produce dysphagia. The diagnosis can usually be confirmed by barium swallow. No treatment is necessary.

MALPOSITIONS OF THE HEART

Situs inversus refers to a condition in which the arrangement of organs is the reverse of normal. In complete situs inversus the heart and cardiac apex and abdominal organs are located on the opposite side of normal (mirror-image dextrocardia), and the heart is usually normal. On the other hand, when there is situs inversus of the viscera but the heart is in the left side of the chest (isolated levocardia), a serious cardiac malformation is usually present. *Dextroversion* refers to the condition in which the viscera, atria, and aortic arch are in their normal position but the cardiac apex is on the right. Congenital heart disease is usually present, particularly corrected transposition of the great arteries, pulmonic stenosis, or VSD. In patients in whom the visceral situs is indeterminate, complex heart disease is usually present, together with asplenia or polysplenia.

CONGENITAL ABNORMALITIES OF THE CORONARY ARTERIES

The three congenital anomalies of the coronary arteries encountered most frequently in adult patients are an ectopic origin of a coronary artery from the aorta, an anomalous origin of a coronary artery from the pulmonary artery, and coronary arteriovenous fistula.

Ectopic origin of a coronary artery from the aorta is an isolated finding in approximately 0.6% of individuals undergoing coronary arteriography. Of the numerous variations, two are especially likely to produce clinical symptoms: either an ectopic left coronary artery arising from the right sinus of Valsalva or an ectopic right coronary artery arising from the left sinus of Valsalva. Both ectopic arteries may pass between the aorta and the pulmonary artery. The coronary circulation can be compromised by hypoplasia either of the coronary ostia or of the proximal coronary artery or, less frequently, by compression between the aorta and pulmonary artery or by extreme angulation of the proximal coronary artery. It is likely that only a minority of patients with this condition have myocardial ischemia from the anomaly. Clinical manifestations may include angina pectoris, myocardial infarction, ventricular tachycardia, and sudden death. Symptoms may occur in adolescence or young adult life, depending on the degree of proximal narrowing, mass of muscle supplied, and collateral circulation. Echocardiography, especially transesophageal, can often provide the diagnosis, but coronary arteriography is necessary for proper definition of the abnormality.

Patients with significant objective evidence of myocardial ischemia should be treated by coronary artery bypass graft surgery. An ectopic right coronary artery incidentally discovered at coronary arteriography requires no specific therapy. Many other varieties of ectopic origin and unusual course of the coronary arteries occur; they seldom produce symptoms and are usually discovered incidentally. Knowledge of aberrant coronary arteries before surgery for congenital heart disease is important if the surgery involves ventriculotomy, in which an aberrant coronary artery might be damaged. This damage is especially likely to occur in patients with tetralogy of Fallot. Knowledge of the presence of an aberrant coronary artery is also important in patients undergoing intraoperative myocardial perfusion by coronary cannulation.

In anomalous origin of the left coronary artery from the pulmonary artery, the left main coronary artery originates from a sinus just above the pulmonic valve, whereas the right coronary artery originates from its normal aortic sinus. In utero, the pressures in the pulmonary artery and aorta are nearly equal, and myocardial perfusion is reasonably normal. After birth, however, pressure in the pulmonary artery rapidly declines and the perfusion pressure in the pulmonary artery and the left coronary artery is no longer high enough to perfuse the left ventricle, which has a much higher intramyocardial systolic pressure. As a consequence, the heart is perfused by the right coronary artery originating from the right aortic sinus, while collateral vessels carry some blood from the right coronary artery to the anomalous left coronary artery and to the pulmonary artery. The infant or child usually develops myocardial ischemia or infarction, often within the first 6 months of life. Mitral regurgitation frequently results from the myocardial infarction.

Some infants have no symptoms preceding sudden death, while others have great distress, which probably represents angina pectoris, while feeding. Most children die before the age of 12, usually from sudden death or chronic left ventricular failure from myocardial scarring and mitral regurgitation. Some patients, however, may survive until adulthood. Often, there is no clear history of chest pain, since the infarction occurs in infancy before the child can describe symptoms. There may be evidence of a left ventricular aneurysm, left ventricular hypertrophy, and an apical holosystolic murmur from mitral regurgitation. Occasionally, there is a continuous murmur produced by the intercoronary anastomoses.

The chest radiograph usually shows evidence of left ventricular hypertrophy and often pulmonary congestion. The ECG often shows evidence of an extensive anterolateral myocardial infarction. Coronary arteriography and aortic root aortography demonstrate the right coronary artery originating normally from the aorta and connecting by collaterals to the left coronary artery, which drains into the pulmonary artery. Left ventricular angiography or echocardiography can demonstrate the area of myocardial infarction and dyskinesia and may also demonstrate mitral regurgitation. Transesophageal echocardiography can also demonstrate the abnormal origin of a coronary artery.

If the extent of myocardial infarction is not excessive, the left coronary artery can be anastomosed to either the aorta or the subclavian artery. Heart transplantation should be considered in some patients. Otherwise, management is purely supportive for symptoms of myocardial ischemia and heart failure. Patients with a large ventricular aneurysm and diminished left ventricular function should be considered for chronic anticoagulation with warfarin (INR = 2 − 3).

In congenital coronary arteriovenous fistula, the right and left coronary arteries originate normally from the aorta, but one or more branches form a fistula with a cardiac chamber or the pulmonary artery. Most fistulas originate from a branch of the right coronary artery and communicate with the right ventricle, right atrium, or coronary sinus. The fistula functions as an L-R shunt but usually does not seriously interfere with myocardial oxygenation, so angina and myocardial infarction usually do not occur. On the other hand, the shunt can be so large that it imposes a volume load on the left ventricle and whatever right-sided chambers the shunt involves.

Many patients have no symptoms. Others may have retarded growth, mild exertional fatigue, and dyspnea. The fistula can also become the site of infective endarteritis, with symptoms similar to those of infective endocarditis (Chapter 24). If the fistula enters the right atrium, right ventricle, or coronary sinus, there may be evidence of biventricular enlargement with both a parasternal impulse and a displaced and sustained apical impulse. The hallmark is a continuous murmur, which often is less loud than the murmurs of PDA and usually is located in a lower position on the chest. At times it is maximal to the right of the sternum. The systolic murmur is often loudest during systole if the fistula enters the right atrium, loudest during either systole or diastole if it enters the right ventricle, and loudest about the second heart sound if it enters the pulmonary artery.

If the fistula is large, the chest radiograph usually shows left ventricular, right ventricular, and pulmonary artery dilation, except for the small number of cases in which the fistula enters the pulmonary artery, producing only dilation of the left ventricle and pulmonary artery. The pulmonary vasculature is often increased because of the large L-R shunt and increased pulmonary flow. Occasionally, the cardiac border is slightly irregular as a result of the aneurysmal dilation of the involved coronary artery.

There may be ECG evidence of left or combined ventricular hypertrophy. Coronary arteriography or aortography delineates the size and course of the involved coronary artery and the site of entry into the right heart or pulmonary artery. MRI and echocardiography, especially transesophageal, can also delineate the involved coronary artery when it is markedly dilated. Coronary arteriovenous fistulas should usually be surgically corrected to decrease the risk of infective endarteritis, abolish the L-R shunt, and perhaps improve the coronary blood flow reserve.

CONGENITAL PERICARDIAL DEFECTS

Congenital defects may involve any portion of the parietal pericardium, although the left side is more frequent. Most patients are asymptomatic, but partial defects can rarely cause chest pain, which can resemble angina pectoris. Herniation and strangulation, particularly of the left atrial appendage through a partial pericardial defect, can occur and produce sudden death. The presence of partial left defect may be suggested on a chest film by a prominence in the area of the pulmonary artery produced by herniation of the left atrial appendage. Echocardiography, particularly transesophageal, and MRI usually provide a proper diagnosis. Partial defects should usually be surgically corrected by closure to prevent herniation and strangulation of the left atrium or ventricle. Complete pericardial absence or large defects do not require therapy.

DISTURBANCES OF CONDUCTION

The Wolff-Parkinson-White syndrome, the Romano-Ward syndrome (prolonged QT interval with deafness), and the Jervell and Lange-Nielsen syndrome (prolonged QT interval with deafness) are discussed in Chapter 18.

BIBLIOGRAPHY

Adams FH, Emmanouilides GC, Riemenschneider TA, editors: *Moss' heart disease in infants, children and adolescents*, ed 5, Baltimore, 1995, Williams & Wilkins.

Dearfield JE, Warnes CA, Gersh BJ: Congenital heart disease in adults. In Alexander RW, Schlant RC, Fuster V, editors: *The heart*, ed 9, New York, 1998, McGraw-Hill.

Garson A Jr et al: Prevention of sudden death after repair of tetralogy of Fallot: treatment of ventricular arrhythmias, *J Am Coll Cardiol* 6:221, 1985.

Graham TP Jr: Ventricular performance in congenital heart disease, *Circulation* 84:2259, 1991.

McNamara DG: The adult with congenital heart disease, *Curr Probl Cardiol* 14:57, 1989.

Nora JJ, Berg K, Nora AH: *Cardiovascular diseases: genetics, epidemiology, and prevention*, New York, 1991, Oxford University Press.

Nugent EW et al: The pathology, pathophysiology, recognition, and treatment of congenital heart disease. In Schlant RC et al, editors: *Hurst's the heart*, ed 8, New York, 1994, McGraw-Hill.

Perloff JK: Congenital heart disease in adults. In Braunwald E, editor: *Heart disease*, ed 4, Philadelphia, 1992, Saunders.

Perloff JK, Child JS, editors: *Congenital heart disease in adults*, Philadelphia, 1991, Saunders.

Perloff JK et al: Adults with cyanotic congenital heart disease: hematologic management, *Ann Intern Med* 109:406, 1988.

Perloff PK: *The clinical recognition of congenital heart disease*, ed 4, Philadelphia, 1994, Saunders.

Perloff PK et al: Bethesda Conference: Congenital heart disease after childhood: an expanding patient population, *J Am Coll Cardiol* 18:311, 1991.

Roberts WC: *Adult congenital heart disease*, Philadelphia, 1987, FA Davis.

CHAPTER

29 **Pulmonary Hypertensive
Heart Disease**

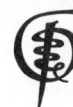

Richard S. Irwin, Joseph S. Alpert, and James E. Dalen

The resistance to pulmonary blood flow is only one twelfth the resistance across the systemic bed in normal individuals. The mean pulmonary artery (PA) pressure is only 12 ± 2 mm Hg and the mean left atrial pressure is only 6 ± 2 mm Hg in normals. Thus the left pressure gradient across the normal pulmonary circulation is only 6 ± 2 mm Hg. A normal cardiac output of 5 to 6 liters per minute flows from the right ventricle to the left atrium with a pressure drop of only 6 mm Hg, as opposed to a pressure drop of about 90 mm Hg in the systemic circulation between the left ventricle and right atrium. The resistance of the pulmonary vascular bed is much lower than that of the systemic circulation because the media of the precapillary pulmonary arterioles are thin compared with the more muscular media of the systemic arterioles. The low resistance of the pulmonary circulation accounts for a right ventricle that is less than half as thick as the left ventricle.

Pulmonary hypertension occurs if resistance to flow across the pulmonary bed increases. Such an increase occurs as a result of a variety of diseases that affect the pulmonary circulation. Pulmonary hypertension is present when mean PA pressure exceeds 20 mm Hg, and in the vast majority of cases, it is secondary to cardiac or pulmonary diseases. Pulmonary hypertension can be subdivided into three categories based on its pathophysiology: precapillary, passive, and reactive. In precapillary pulmonary hypertension the abnormality that leads to elevated pulmonary pressures is located in the pulmonary arteries or arterioles. Individuals with passive pulmonary hypertension have diseases that lead to increased pulmonary venous pressure that, in turn, produces secondary elevations in pulmonary arterial pressure, for example, mitral stenosis. Patients with reactive pulmonary hypertension have long-standing elevated pulmonary venous pressure complicated by pulmonary arteriolar vasoconstriction (Table 29-1). The only "pure" form is the rare entity primary pulmonary hypertension. Examination of this entity will allow elucidation of the clinical manifestations of pulmonary hypertension from any cause. In most patients with secondary pulmonary hypertension, the clinical manifestations are overshadowed by the underlying cardiac or pulmonary disease. The natural history, prognosis, and management also depend on the underlying disease.

An approach to the differential diagnosis of pulmonary hypertension is shown in Table 29-1.

PRECAPILLARY PULMONARY HYPERTENSION
Pathophysiology

In patients with precapillary pulmonary hypertension, the disease involves the pulmonary circulation proximal to the pulmonary capillaries, that is, the PAs or arterioles. Pressure in the PA is increased (mean PA pressure >20 mm Hg), but wedge pressure and left atrial pressure remain normal (<12 mm Hg). As a result, the mean PA to left atrial pressure gradient is increased and exceeds 12 mm Hg.

Patients with precapillary pulmonary hypertension have dyspnea, but because their pulmonary venous pressure is normal, they do not experience orthopnea, paroxysmal nocturnal dyspnea, or pulmonary edema. On physical examination such patients are often observed to have tachypnea, but the auscultatory findings in the lungs are usually normal. The chest x-ray may show evidence of right ventricular enlargement and prominent pulmonary arteries, but the left ventricle is normal. Pulmonary venous redistribution and Kerley B lines do not occur. The electrocardiogram (ECG) usually demonstrates right ventricular hypertrophy or right axis deviation.

Causes of Precapillary Pulmonary Hypertension

The causes of precapillary pulmonary hypertension are listed in Box 29-1.

Primary Pulmonary Hypertension. Primary pulmonary hypertension is the rarest cause of pulmonary hypertension, but it is described here in detail because it illustrates the clinical manifestations of pulmonary hypertension not accompanied by other cardiac or pulmonary disease.

Primary pulmonary hypertension is a disease of unknown origin, characterized by diffuse pathologic changes in the pulmonary vasculature. Patients with primary pulmonary hypertension do not have intrinsic pulmonary or cardiac disease or extrinsic causes of pulmonary vascular obstruction.

Several theories have been advanced concerning the cause of primary pulmonary hypertension. Some authorities argue that it is the result of recurrent episodes of asymptomatic pulmonary embolism. Supporting this theory is the common autopsy finding of clinically unrecognized, organizing, or recanalized pulmonary emboli in patients with primary pulmonary hypertension. An alternative explanation for the development of primary pulmonary hypertension is thrombosis in situ of small pulmonary arteries, with resultant widespread pulmonary vascular obstruction. Various abnormalities of coagulation, including abnormal platelet function and defective fibrinolysis, have been demonstrated in patients with primary pulmonary hypertension. Arrayed against recurrent pulmonary thromboembolism or in situ arterial thrombosis as the cause are the findings of several pathologic studies that demonstrate clear morphologic differences between patients with thromboembolic or thrombotic pulmonary hypertension and those with primary pulmonary hypertension. However, veno-occlusive disease affecting the majority of small pulmonary venules has been observed in a number of patients with primary pulmonary hypertension (see Reactive Pulmonary Hypertension).

Drug hypersensitivity has also been suggested as a cause of pri-

---

BOX 29-1
Causes of pulmonary hypertension

Precapillary pulmonary hypertension
  Primary pulmonary hypertension
  Disorders of ventilation
  Congenital heart disease with pulmonary vascular disease
  Pulmonary embolism
  Schistosomiasis
  Collagen vascular diseases
  Pulmonary vasculitis
  Sickle hemoglobinopathies
  Portal hypertension
  Ingestion of drugs and herbal remedies
Passive pulmonary hypertension
  Left ventricular failure
  Mitral valve disease
  Cor triatriatum
  Obstruction of major pulmonary veins
  Congenital pulmonary vein stenosis
  Left atrial myxoma or thrombus
Reactive pulmonary hypertension
  Some patients with mitral valve disease
  Rarely, other causes of pulmonary venous hypertension, including
    pulmonary veno-occlusive disease

Table 29-1 Differential diagnosis of pulmonary hypertension

PRESSURE VARIABLE	PRECAPILLARY	PASSIVE	REACTIVE
PA mean pressure	↑/↑↑	↑	↑↑
Left atrial pressure	Normal	↑	↑
PA left atrial pressure gradient	>12 mm Hg	<12 mm Hg	>12 mm Hg

mary pulmonary hypertension, although allergic vasculitis would be unlikely to affect only the pulmonary vasculature. Some type of immunologic process may play a role in the development of primary pulmonary hypertension, but the nature and extent of such a process remain unknown.

Increased pulmonary vascular reactivity and pulmonary vasoconstriction have been demonstrated in patients with primary pulmonary hypertension, leading to the conclusion that a marked vasospastic or vasoconstrictive tendency underlies the development of primary pulmonary hypertension in predisposed persons. Heightened autonomic nervous system activity is considered by some to be a factor in the development of primary pulmonary hypertension. Primary pulmonary hypertension is more common at high altitudes than at sea level, suggesting that hypoxic pulmonary vasoconstriction predisposes to this condition. Patients with primary pulmonary hypertension appear to have increased pulmonary vasomotor tone early during their illness. However, as the disease progresses, functional changes progress to fixed, anatomic pulmonary vascular lesions.

A number of pathologic findings are common to almost all patients with primary pulmonary hypertension: (1) intimal thickening and fibrosis in small pulmonary arteries and arterioles, producing a characteristic "onion-skin" configuration; (2) increased medial thickness of small muscular pulmonary arteries and arterioles; (3) dilated, thin-walled side branches of muscular pulmonary arteries known as *plexiform lesions;* and (4) necrotizing arteritis and fibrinoid necrosis in the walls of muscular pulmonary arteries.

Most patients with primary pulmonary hypertension come to the attention of a physician late in the course of the disease, or when symptoms of right ventricular failure develop. Women with primary pulmonary hypertension outnumber men 3:1 or 4:1. The disease occurs sporadically or with a familial pattern suggestive of autosomal dominant inheritance with variable penetrance.

Patients with primary pulmonary hypertension usually complain of exertional dyspnea without orthopnea, as well as effort syncope, anginal chest pain, and weakness. Late in the disease, dyspnea occurs at rest. Palpitations are commonly reported and may be related to the sudden death of some patients. Occasionally, patients complain of cough and/or hemoptysis.

Physical examination of patients with primary pulmonary hypertension discloses findings consistent with pulmonary hypertension and right ventricular pressure overload: a large A wave in the jugular venous pulse; left parasternal (right ventricular) heave; pulmonic ejection sound and flow murmur; prominent pulmonic component of the second heart sound; right ventricular fourth heart sound; and signs of right ventricular failure (hepatomegaly, peripheral edema, and even ascites). Patients with severe pulmonary hypertension may also have a prominent V wave in the jugular venous pulse, a right ventricular third heart sound, and murmurs of tricuspid and/or pulmonic regurgitation. The lungs are clear, but the respiratory rate is increased, even at rest.

The results of routine laboratory tests are usually normal in patients with primary pulmonary hypertension. Abnormal platelet function, defects in fibrinolysis, and other abnormalities of coagulation are occasionally noted in such patients. The ECG demonstrates right ventricular hypertrophy and right atrial enlargement (P pulmonale). Chest radiography in patients with primary pulmonary hypertension demonstrates enlargement of the main pulmonary artery and its major branches, with marked tapering of peripheral arteries (Fig. 29-1). The lung fields are strikingly lucent. The right ventricle and atrium are often enlarged.

The results of pulmonary function tests are usually normal. Arterial blood gas analysis usually reveals evidence of hyperventilation, with a low Pco_2 and elevated pH. The arterial Po_2 may be normal or reduced. Echocardiography demonstrates enlarged right ventricular dimensions, small or normal left ventricular dimensions, and a thickened interventricular septum. Right ventricular systolic and diastolic dysfunction may be present. Doppler echocardiographic examination usually demonstrates tricuspid and pulmonic regurgitation. Perfusion lung scans in patients with primary pulmonary hypertension are usually normal or demonstrate small, nonspecific defects. Lung scanning may be hazardous late in the course of the disease, because the macroaggregated albumin particles used in scanning may significantly reduce the cross-sectional area of the already critically limited pulmonary vascular bed.

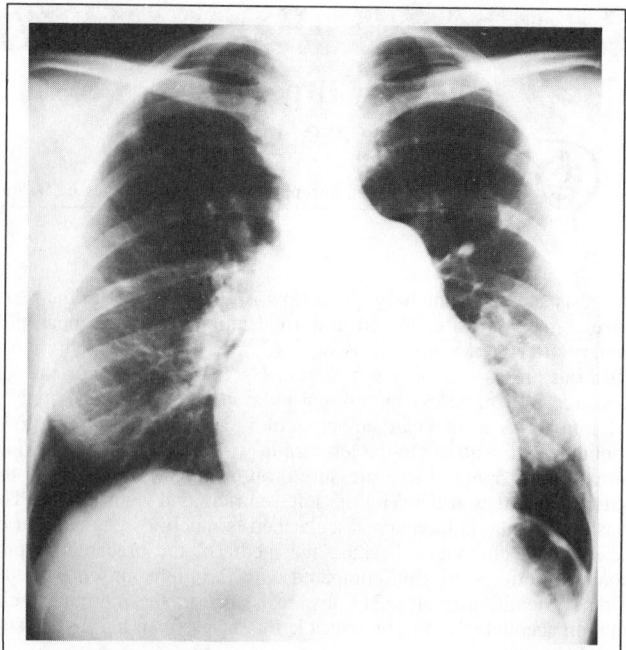

A

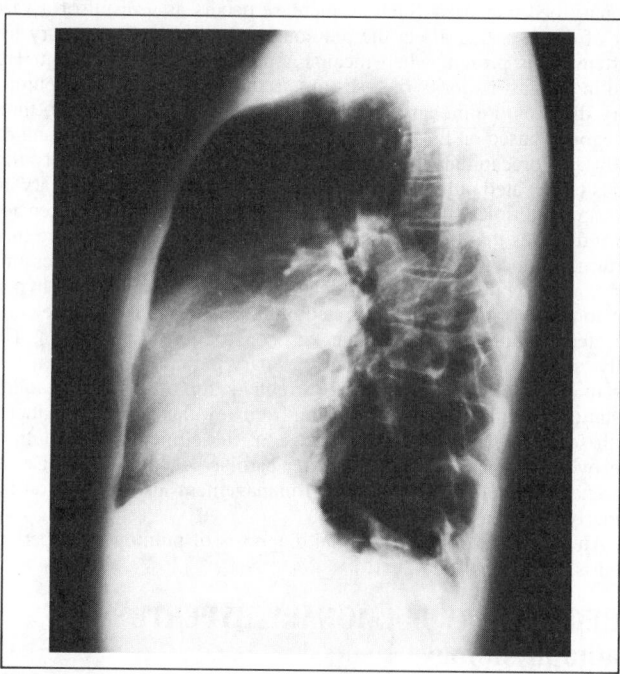

B

FIGURE 29-1 Posteroanterior **(A)** and lateral **(B)** chest radiograph of a patient with primary pulmonary hypertension. Note the large central pulmonary arteries, with tapering of the distal arteries. A very large right ventricle is evident on the lateral film.

The diagnosis of primary pulmonary hypertension cannot be confirmed without cardiac catheterization and lung scan or pulmonary angiography to exclude other cardiac or pulmonary causes of pulmonary hypertension. Some patients are too ill for one or both these procedures, and, in such patients, the diagnosis remains tentative. Right heart catheterization reveals markedly elevated pulmonary arterial and right ventricular pressures. Right atrial pressure is increased if right ventricular failure is present. Left ventricular, left atrial, and pulmonary capillary wedge pressures are low or normal. Pulmonary angiography demonstrates large central pulmonary arteries, with marked pe-

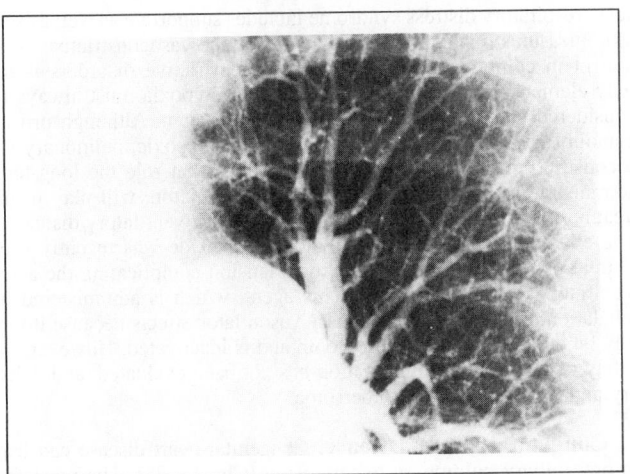

FIGURE 29-2   Pulmonary angiogram in a patient with primary pulmonary hypertension (same patient as in Figure 29-1). The contrast medium was injected into the left upper pulmonary artery. Note the large central pulmonary arteries, with marked tapering of the distal branches.

ripheral tapering (Fig. 29-2). It should be noted that pulmonary angiography presents a potential risk of death to the patient with primary pulmonary hypertension; subselective injections are usually employed rather than injection into the main pulmonary artery.

The differential diagnosis of primary pulmonary hypertension entails ruling out many causes of secondary pulmonary hypertension. Entities that must be excluded before a clinical diagnosis of primary pulmonary hypertension can be entertained include mitral stenosis, congenital cardiac defects with Eisenmenger's reaction, recurrent pulmonary embolism, sickle cell disease, collagen vascular disease, and such rare entities as cor triatriatum and pulmonary venous obstruction.

Rarely, primary pulmonary hypertension may spontaneously regress and may respond to vasoactive agents. However, there is no uniformly effective medical therapy for the majority of these patients. Mortality is largely determined by the severity of pulmonary artery pressure elevation and the state of function of the right ventricle.

Although vasoactive drug therapy is not consistently effective in primary pulmonary hypertension, it is the only hope at present for reversing elevated pulmonary vascular resistance. Recent reports on the use of oxygen, prostacyclin, prostaglandin E_1, and chronic oral medications such as the calcium-channel blocking agents nifedipine and diltiazem have shown that these agents as well as others can improve hemodynamics in certain patients. However, since all of these agents can produce serious adverse reactions, they should not be given empirically. Careful monitoring and initial evaluation with a Swan-Ganz catheter in place are necessary to determine which patients will benefit from initial and continued therapy. When assessing the response to vasodilators, the overall effects of a drug on pulmonary and systemic hemodynamics, gas exchange, and oxygen transport must be considered. The goal of a decrease in pulmonary artery pressure accompanied by an increase in cardiac output with little or no change in systemic pressure or gas exchange occurs in approximately 25% to 30% of patients. A decrease in pulmonary vascular resistance greater than 20% is considered by some to represent a favorable response as long as gas exchange and systemic blood pressure are not adversely affected. Since (1) prostacyclin and prostaglandin E_1 are powerful pulmonary vasodilators with very short half-lives (minutes) when given intravenously, (2) substantial data show that they can be given safely to patients with primary pulmonary hypertension, and (3) the acute response to these agents has predictive value for subsequent oral vasodilator therapy, these agents may become an integral part of the routine management of patients with primary pulmonary hypertension as test drugs. In addition, continuous intravenous infusion of prostacyclin has been used in some patients for periods ranging from months to years. If vasoactive agent therapy is ineffective, symptomatic treatment consisting of salt restriction, oxygen, and diuretics is usually prescribed. Oral anticoagulant therapy with coumarin derivatives is also commonly undertaken and may prolong sur-

---

BOX 29-2

Disorders of ventilation that can cause precapillary pulmonary hypertension

I. Vasoconstriction of the precapillary and capillary vascular bed
   A. With structurally normal pulmonary parenchyma and vascular bed
      1. High-altitude pulmonary hypertension (residence at or above 3000 m)
      2. Primary central hypoventilation
      3. Peripheral, obstructive sleep apnea
      4. Obesity-hypoventilation syndrome
      5. Paralytic poliomyelitis
      6. Myasthenia gravis
   B. With pulmonary parenchymal disease
      1. Chronic obstructive pulmonary disease
      2. Cystic fibrosis
II. Anatomic restriction of the pulmonary capillary vascular bed
   A. Diffuse lung disease*
      1. Sarcoidosis
      2. Progressive systemic sclerosis
      3. Idiopathic interstitial fibrosis
      4. Acute respiratory distress syndrome
   B. Extensive lung resection
   C. Extensive fibrothorax
III. Vasoconstriction plus anatomic restriction of the pulmonary vascular bed
   A. Kyphoscoliosis
   B. Chronic fibrotic tuberculosis

*Any disease that leads to diffuse interstitial fibrosis may be complicated by pulmonary hypertension.

vival. Lung or combined heart-lung transplantation should be considered in patients who are unresponsive to vasodilators and who have low cardiac output.

Disorders of Ventilation. The ventilatory respiratory diseases that can cause precapillary pulmonary hypertension include vasoconstriction of the pulmonary vascular bed, anatomic restriction of the pulmonary vascular bed, or a combination of both, as shown in Box 29-2.

Pulmonary vasoconstriction occurs in response to a number of different stimuli. The most potent, clinically important, and best documented is alveolar hypoxia. The mechanism of hypoxic vasoconstriction is not well understood. Alveolar hypoxia occurs in a number of different pulmonary diseases as a consequence of alveolar hypoventilation or ventilation-perfusion inequalities (Chapter 35). Increases in plasma hydrogen ion concentration (acidemia), particularly when produced by hypercapnia, not only cause pulmonary vasoconstriction directly but also augment the effect of alveolar hypoxia. Although these two stimulants may produce only modest increases in pressure in normal subjects at sea level, the vasoconstrictive effects may become greatly magnified and sustained in various clinical situations.

High-altitude pulmonary hypertension is caused by the hypoxic vasoconstrictive effects of chronic alveolar hypoxia and occurs in humans born and raised at high altitude. As long as these persons reside at altitudes above 3000 m, pulmonary hypertension is sustained because of persistent pulmonary vasoconstriction. However, it can be reversed on return to sea level, since alveolar hypoxia is no longer present.

Pulmonary hypertension may occur in a wide variety of extrapulmonary respiratory diseases solely on the basis of alveolar hypoventilation, even with a structurally normal pulmonary parenchyma and vascular bed, for example, peripheral, obstructive sleep apnea.

The main determinants of pulmonary hypertension in patients with the chronic obstructive pulmonary diseases (COPD), chronic bronchitis, and emphysema are alveolar hypoxia and acidemia (Chapter 51). Pulmonary hypertension occurs in many patients with COPD and cystic fibrosis when Pa_{O_2} is less than 50 mm Hg and Pa_{CO_2} is greater than 45 mm Hg. These degrees of hypoxemia and hypercapnia become predictable in COPD patients when the absolute value of FEV_1 is less than 1 L. Although respiratory acidosis and other factors, such as anatomic restriction of the pulmonary vascular bed, increased cardiac output, polycythemia, and an expanded lung volume may contribute, all these influences are secondary to alveolar hypoxia in the pathogenesis of the pulmonary hypertension of COPD.

Anatomic restriction of the pulmonary vascular bed may also cause pulmonary hypertension. The cross-sectional area of the pulmonary vascular bed can be reduced in several ways. In diffuse interstitial lung diseases, parenchymal disease probably compresses and gradually obliterates the small pulmonary arteries, causing increased resistance to blood flow, with resultant pulmonary hypertension. Since hypoxic vasoconstriction does not appear to contribute significantly to the resistance to blood flow in these diseases, other pulmonary function tests can be useful in predicting the presence of pulmonary hypertension. When the vital capacity is 50% of the predicted value in sarcoidosis or idiopathic interstitial fibrosis, pulmonary hypertension may well be present at rest; when it is between 50% and 80% of predicted, pulmonary hypertension may develop with exercise. In progressive systemic sclerosis, a diffusing capacity of less than 43% of predicted is a better predictor of pulmonary hypertension than is a vital capacity of less than 50% of predicted; in this disease, diffusing capacity has a sensitivity of 67% in predicting definite pulmonary hypertension.

A combination of vasoconstriction plus anatomic restriction of the pulmonary vascular bed is involved in the pathogenesis of pulmonary hypertension in diseases such as kyphoscoliosis and long-standing fibrotic tuberculosis complicated by fibrothorax, thoracoplasty, and/or an acute respiratory infection (Chapters 35 and 62).

Although idiopathic kyphoscoliosis affects 2% to 3% of the population of the United States, a deformity of the thoracic spine severe enough to produce pulmonary hypertension is found in a relatively small number of these patients. Pulmonary hypertension at rest in this disease should not be anticipated unless the vital capacity is less than 60% of predicted.

The clinical manifestations of pulmonary hypertension fall into two categories: those resulting from the primary ventilatory disorder and those resulting from abnormal cardiac function. Against the background of the primary ventilatory clinical manifestations are the signs and symptoms of pulmonary hypertension and cor pulmonale (see Primary Pulmonary Hypertension).

In addition to the pulmonary function studies that help predict the presence of pulmonary hypertension and often determine its cause, chest radiographs frequently are useful for determining the type of pulmonary disease.

The diagnostic value of the ECG in pulmonary hypertension and cor pulmonale depends on the underlying ventilatory disorder. Although the ECG is reliable in demonstrating right ventricular hypertrophy in diseases that anatomically restrict the vascular bed, it is less reliable in vasoconstrictive diseases, since the levels of pulmonary hypertension are generally less. Perhaps because of the hyperinflated lungs, episodic hypoxemia, and respiratory acidosis that occur in COPD patients, ECG evidence of right ventricular hypertrophy is uncommon. Serial changes are the ones most likely to occur. When arterial PO_2 falls below 50 mm Hg in COPD patients with pulmonary hypertension, one or more of the following ECG changes should be seen: a rightward shift of the mean QRS axis, T wave abnormalities in right precordial leads, S-T depressions in leads II, III, and aV_F, and transient right bundle branch block. With improvement in gas exchange, all these changes should subside.

Pulmonary hypertension caused by ventilatory disorders may be treated in a variety of ways. For primary central hypoventilation, a respiratory center stimulant such as progesterone may suffice. For the morbidly obese hypoventilator, weight reduction is the primary mode of therapy. For peripheral obstructive sleep apnea, nasal continuous positive airway pressure (CPAP) is often helpful and a permanent tracheostomy may be curative. While cessation of cigarette smoking and a Milwaukee brace prevent pulmonary hypertension from occurring in many patients with minimal COPD and kyphoscoliosis, respectively, continuous oxygen therapy may be helpful late in the course of both diseases (Chapter 51). Decortication may be curative in pulmonary hypertension caused by fibrothorax, as may corticosteroids in idiopathic interstitial fibrosis and sarcoidosis. Treatment of the

acute respiratory distress syndrome includes supportive as well as specific measures (Chapter 46). Finally, since the vasoconstrictive component in combined anatomic and vasoconstrictive disorders is the only element that can be reversed, alveolar hypoxia must always be considered and treated with supplemental oxygen. Although prostaglandin E_1 and nifedipine can acutely inhibit hypoxic, pulmonary vasoconstriction, it is not known at this time what role the long-term administration of these agents or other vasodilators will play in the treatment of pulmonary hypertension caused by ventilatory disorders. The endothelium-derived vasodilator nitric oxide was recently used to treat patients with pulmonary hypertension complicating the acute respiratory distress syndrome. This agent, which is administered by inhalation, has selective pulmonary vasodilator effects because it rapidly binds to circulating hemoglobin and is inactivated. However, the safety of long-term administration has not been evaluated, and delivery and monitoring are cumbersome.

Congenital Heart Disease. Congenital heart disease can lead to precapillary pulmonary hypertension (Chapter 28). The most frequent congenital lesions leading to pulmonary hypertension in adults are those characterized by a left-to-right shunt: ventricular septal defect, patent ductus arteriosus, and ostium secundum atrial septal defect (ASD). As the pulmonary vascular resistance increases, the magnitude of the left-to-right shunt decreases. Late in the course, the patient may be cyanotic as a result of right-to-left shunting. The development of severe pulmonary hypertension in patients with these cardiac defects is termed Eisenmenger's reaction. The clinical findings and/or symptoms of ventricular septal defect and patent ductus arteriosus usually lead to their detection in childhood. However, the clinical manifestations of ASD are subtle, and therefore this lesion can remain undetected until adult life.

The primary symptom of ASD is decreased exercise tolerance. Such patients are not disabled but often avoid strenuous athletic activities and adjust their lifestyle to their modest limitation. On physical examination, there is a systolic pulmonic murmur and usually fixed splitting of the second heart sound (Chapter 28). The ECG usually indicates a right ventricular volume overload, and the chest radiograph often shows increased pulmonary vascular markings, an enlarged right ventricle, and a small aortic knob.

An echocardiogram usually confirms the clinical diagnosis by demonstrating right ventricular volume overload. Doppler echocardiographic examination or first-pass radionuclide angiography demonstrates the left-to-right shunt and yields an estimate of its size. Cardiac catheterization quantifies the magnitude of the left-to-right shunt and determines whether the lesion is complicated by pulmonary hypertension.

Pulmonary hypertension in patients with ASD may be modest and associated with increased pulmonary blood flow. This condition is termed *hyperkinetic pulmonary hypertension.* In this circumstance, the pulmonary hypertension is reversible if the left-to-right shunt is eliminated by closure of the ASD. However, PA pressure may reach systemic levels and be associated with a minimal left-to-right shunt or even a net right-to-left shunt. When ASD is complicated by pulmonary hypertension, patients note dyspnea; with severe pulmonary hypertension, they may experience chest pain, hemoptysis, and syncope. The ECG demonstrates right ventricular hypertrophy, and the chest x-ray shows very prominent proximal pulmonary arteries with tapered distal arteries. The outlook is poor when ASD is complicated by precapillary pulmonary hypertension. Death occurs within 10 years in at least half of such patients.

The cause of pulmonary hypertension in patients with ASD is unclear. Although some patients survive to advanced age without the development of pulmonary hypertension, it occurs in about 30% of adults with ASD. Pulmonary hypertension is a response of the pulmonary arterioles to the large pulmonary blood flow associated with ASD. The media of the arterioles hypertrophy, thereby increasing resistance to flow and increasing PA pressure. Intimal proliferation may occur, with a resultant further increase in resistance and pressure. Why this process develops in some patients with ASD and not others is unknown. The size of the defect does not determine in which patients pulmonary hypertension develops as long as the ASD is greater than 1 cm in diameter.

In patients with ASD living at sea level, pulmonary hypertension rarely occurs before age 20, but it may do so in ASD patients living at modest altitudes (>1220 m). This earlier incidence in patients with ASD living at higher altitudes has been attributed to the effects of mild alveolar hypoxia.

Serial cardiac catheterizations have demonstrated the development of pulmonary hypertension in patients with ASD whose PA pressure was normal at the first study. However, patients age 50 or older with ASD and normal pulmonary artery pressures rarely develop subsequent pulmonary hypertension.

The inability to predict which patients with ASD will develop pulmonary hypertension and the poor prognosis once severe pulmonary hypertension develops are facts favoring the surgical closure of ASD when first detected, especially in patients under age 50. The operative risk of closing an uncomplicated ASD is less than 1% (Chapter 28).

Pulmonary Embolism. Pulmonary embolism is the commonest cause of acute pulmonary hypertension. There are two mechanisms by which pulmonary hypertension occurs in patients with acute pulmonary embolism: embolic obstruction of the pulmonary circulation and vasoconstriction.

The major factor causing pulmonary hypertension in pulmonary embolism is the embolic obstruction of the pulmonary vascular bed. Significant pulmonary hypertension does not occur unless more than 50% of the pulmonary bed is obstructed. It should be noted that in patients without previous heart or lung disease, pulmonary embolism, even when massive, does not cause severe pulmonary hypertension. In response to acute increases in afterload, the normal right ventricle can only generate 40 to 50 mm Hg pressure, at which point it dilates and fails.

Mild pulmonary hypertension is found in patients with minor pulmonary embolism (obstruction of less than 25% of the pulmonary circulation). Pulmonary hypertension in this case cannot be explained on a mechanical basis. It is very probably caused by pulmonary vasoconstriction, secondary to hypoxemia.

In general, pulmonary hypertension secondary to pulmonary embolism is reversible with anticoagulation or thrombolytic agents. As the degree of pulmonary embolic obstruction and the hypoxemia decrease, the PA pressure returns to normal levels.

Chronic pulmonary hypertension is rare when acute pulmonary embolism is treated with anticoagulation or venous interruption. Patients with chronic pulmonary hypertension secondary to pulmonary embolism usually have had multiple symptomatic episodes of pulmonary embolism that were not treated.

Pulmonary hypertension caused by repeated attacks of silent pulmonary embolism is a very rare syndrome. Clinically, it is difficult to distinguish such patients from those with the equally rare syndrome of primary pulmonary hypertension. Ventilation-perfusion lung scans and a search for deep venous thrombosis are essential to distinguish between these two entities. Patients with pulmonary emboli will have multiple unmatched segmental or lobar perfusion defects. Patients with unresolved proximal vessel obstruction should be referred to a center experienced in performing pulmonary thromboendarterectomy.

Schistosomiasis. Although schistosomiasis is not endemic in the United States, it is a worldwide problem that affects 200 million people in 71 countries. It is the leading cause of chronic pulmonary hypertension in the world. The infection occurs when individuals are exposed to water infested by snails that serve as hosts for the blood flukes *Schistosoma mansoni* and *Schistosoma japonicum*. Cercariae penetrate the skin and are carried by the blood to the liver, where they mature into adult parasites (Chapter 281). If ova enter the venous circulation, they lodge in pulmonary arterioles, where they produce an inflammatory lesion and granulomas. The obstruction of pulmonary arterioles results in pulmonary hypertension. With extensive involvement of the arterioles, PA pressure reaches systemic levels. The main pulmonary arteries may become aneurysmal. Death occurs secondary to chronic pulmonary hypertension with right ventricular failure.

The most effective treatment for pulmonary hypertension due to schistosomiasis is preventive: avoiding wading and swimming in water contaminated with the snail host. Once pulmonary hypertension occurs, medical treatment will not reverse the process. However, ad-

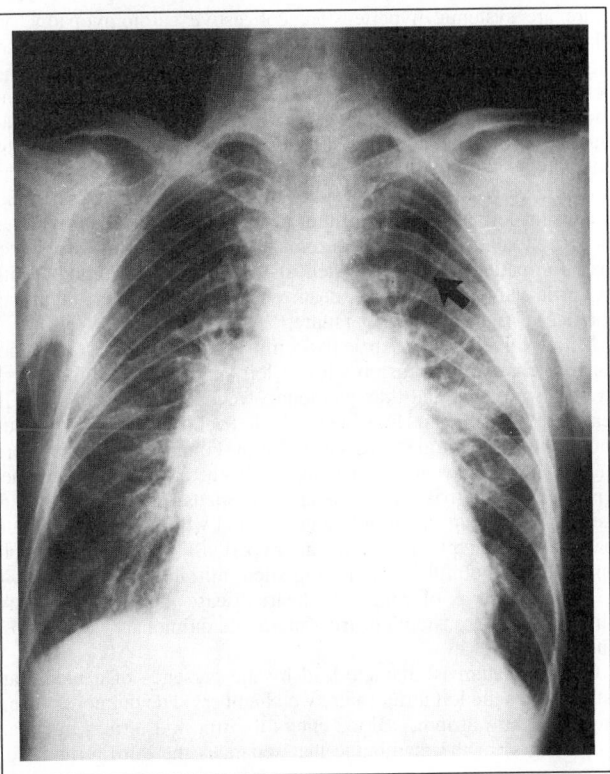

FIGURE 29-3   Chest radiograph from a patient with severe mitral stenosis and pulmonary venous hypertension. Note pulmonary vascular redistribution *(arrow)*, fluid in the major fissure of the left lung, and hazy infiltrates of interstitial edema bilaterally.

ditional damage caused by additional egg emboli can be prevented with praziquantel, an effective, relatively nontoxic drug.

PASSIVE PULMONARY HYPERTENSION
Pathophysiology

A variety of diseases result in elevation of pulmonary venous pressure (see Box 29-1). As pulmonary venous pressure increases, PA pressure must rise if pulmonary blood flow is to continue. This mandatory increase in PA pressure in response to increased pulmonary venous pressure is termed *passive pulmonary hypertension*. The gradient across the pulmonary bed remains normal, that is, less than 12 mm Hg. Since pulmonary venous pressure is rarely sustained above 25 to 30 mm Hg, mean PA pressure in patients with passive pulmonary hypertension rarely exceeds 35 to 40 mm Hg. The increased PA pressure places a burden on the right ventricle and may eventually lead to right ventricular failure.

In evaluating patients with pulmonary hypertension, a first step is to distinguish between passive and precapillary pulmonary hypertension. The primary clue to the diagnosis of passive pulmonary hypertension is the presence of pulmonary venous hypertension, which is recognized by the following symptoms: dyspnea, orthopnea, and paroxysmal nocturnal dyspnea. Radiographic signs of pulmonary venous hypertension include prominence of the upper lobe pulmonary veins, increased density of the central lung fields (Fig. 29-3), and Kerley B lines. Kerley B lines are particularly useful in detecting chronic pulmonary venous hypertension and are caused by interstitial edema or fibrosis in the interlobular septa. They appear as fine, dense, horizontal linear densities in the lateral lower lobes, just above the diaphragm.

Causes of Passive Pulmonary Hypertension

Any disease that causes left ventricular failure results in increased pulmonary venous pressure and thereby leads to passive pulmonary hypertension (Chapter 19). The commonest causes of left ventricular failure are systemic hypertension, congestive cardiomyopathy, and ischemic heart disease. In all of these conditions symptoms of left ventricular failure, including dyspnea, orthopnea, and paroxysmal nocturnal dyspnea, occur before signs of passive PA hypertension appear. Signs of right ventricular failure do not appear until pulmonary venous hypertension has been sufficiently sustained to lead to PA hypertension.

Aortic valve disease may lead to passive pulmonary hypertension by causing left ventricular failure and pulmonary venous hypertension. Right ventricular failure secondary to passive pulmonary hypertension in patients with aortic stenosis is particularly ominous. Without aortic valve replacement, death occurs within a year of the appearance of right ventricular failure.

Mitral valve disease, particularly mitral stenosis, may lead to pulmonary venous hypertension without left ventricular failure. That is, left atrial pressure, and thus pulmonary venous pressure, may be increased to 20 to 30 mm Hg, whereas the left ventricular filling pressure remains normal. Mitral stenosis is one of the commonest causes of prolonged pulmonary venous hypertension, hence one of the commonest causes of chronic passive pulmonary hypertension. Since mitral stenosis may be silent, it should be considered whenever one evaluates a patient with unexplained pulmonary hypertension. Echocardiography is particularly helpful in diagnosing silent mitral stenosis.

Two rare forms of congenital heart disease may lead to passive pulmonary hypertension: cor triatriatum and pulmonary vein stenosis (Chapter 28).

Cor triatriatum is characterized by the presence of a membrane that separates the left atrium into two chambers. The pulmonary veins enter the "third atrium." Blood enters the true left atrium by means of opening(s) in the membrane that separates the third atrium from the true atrium.

Pulmonary vein stenosis is most likely to occur at the junction of the pulmonary veins with the left atrium. If the lesion affects multiple veins, pulmonary hypertension occurs.

The diagnosis of these two rare causes of pulmonary hypertension is made by echocardiography and cardiac catheterization. Pulmonary artery and pulmonary wedge pressures are increased, whereas pressure in the true left atrium is normal.

Patients with these two rare forms of congenital heart disease usually present with symptoms of pulmonary venous hypertension very early in life.

The signs of passive PA hypertension are usually masked by the underlying cause of pulmonary venous hypertension. However, pulmonary hypertension should be suspected whenever the chest radiograph shows enlargement of the pulmonary arteries or right ventricle, or when the ECG shows biventricular hypertrophy in a patient expected to have left ventricular hypertrophy.

Treatment

Passive pulmonary hypertension is clearly reversible if the underlying cause of pulmonary venous hypertension is corrected. Treatment of systemic hypertension or correction of valvular disease lowers pulmonary venous pressure and thereby also relieves passive pulmonary hypertension.

REACTIVE PULMONARY HYPERTENSION

In certain patients with long-standing pulmonary venous hypertension, PA pressure may rise out of proportion to the increased pulmonary venous pressure. The pressure gradient from the PA to the left atrium increases, and PA pressure may reach systemic levels. This reaction to pulmonary venous hypertension is most likely to occur in patients with mitral valve disease, particularly mitral stenosis. It is uncommon in patients with left ventricular failure secondary to aortic valve disease, coronary heart disease, or systemic hypertension; individuals with the latter two conditions usually succumb before reactive pulmonary hypertension can develop. When the gradient is more than 12 mm Hg in patients with these diseases, one should suspect associated mitral valve disease or some superimposed cause of precapillary pulmonary hypertension, such as pulmonary embolism or chronic lung disease.

The cause of this inordinate increase in PA pressure and pulmo-

nary vascular resistance in patients with reactive pulmonary hypertension resides in the precapillary pulmonary arterioles. These arterioles demonstrate medial hypertrophy and possibly intimal proliferation—findings similar to those noted in patients with severe precapillary pulmonary hypertension secondary to congenital heart disease.

Reactive pulmonary hypertension greatly increases the patient's disability. Right ventricular hypertrophy develops, and right ventricular failure may follow. Cardiac output and exercise tolerance decrease markedly.

The ECG shows right ventricular hypertrophy, and the chest radiograph demonstrates right ventricular enlargement with very prominent central pulmonary arteries. On physical examination, a systolic parasternal heave is present, and the pulmonic component of the second heart sound is loud. The stigmata of right ventricular failure (distended neck veins, hepatomegaly, peripheral edema) may be present.

Even though the pathologic findings are similar to those in patients with severe precapillary pulmonary hypertension secondary to congenital heart disease, reactive pulmonary hypertension is reversible if pulmonary venous pressure is returned to normal. When patients with mitral stenosis complicated by passive and reactive pulmonary hypertension have mitral valve replacement, passive pulmonary hypertension resolves immediately after surgery, although the PA to left atrial pressure gradient may persist. Follow-up catheterizations months to years after mitral valve replacement demonstrate a progressive decrease in the gradient and a return of PA pressure to near-normal levels.

An additional cause of reactive pulmonary hypertension is pulmonary veno-occlusive disease. This disease is characterized by diffuse, patchy involvement of small pulmonary veins and venules. The affected veins show fibrous narrowing or obliteration of the intima. Some observers believe that these lesions represent organized or recanalized thromboses of pulmonary veins. The disease affects children and young adults and is usually fatal within 2 years. It leads to severe pulmonary hypertension resembling that seen in primary pulmonary hypertension.

Pulmonary hypertension resulting from pulmonary veno-occlusive disease is differentiated from primary pulmonary hypertension by the presence of pulmonary venous hypertension in the former. Therefore, patients with veno-occlusive disease often have orthopnea and paroxysmal nocturnal dyspnea, and their chest radiographs usually show Kerley B lines.

It is difficult to measure wedge pressure accurately in this disease. It may be elevated, normal, or "zero." Left atrial pressure is normal. The cause of veno-occlusive disease is unknown, and no treatment is available except for combined heart/lung or single lung transplantation.

BIBLIOGRAPHY

Bergofsky EH: Respiratory failure in disorders of the thoracic cage, *Am Rev Respir Dis* 119:643, 1979.

D'Alonzo GE et al: Survival in patients with primary pulmonary hypertension—results from a National Prospective Registry, *Ann Intern Med* 115:343, 1991.

Frishman AP: Pulmonary hypertension. In Alexander RW, Schlant RC, Fuster V, editors: *The heart*, ed 9, New York, 1998, McGraw Hill.

Harvey RM, Enson Y, Ferrer MI: A reconsideration of the origins of pulmonary hypertension, *Chest* 59:82, 1971.

Moser KM, Spragg RG, Utley J et al: Chronic thrombotic obstruction of major pulmonary arteries: results of thromboendarterectomy in 15 patients, *Ann Intern Med* 99:299, 1983.

Nocturnal Oxygen Therapy Trial Group: Continuous or nocturnal oxygen therapy in hypoxemic chronic obstructive lung disease: a clinical trial, *Ann Intern Med* 93:391, 1980.

Packer M, Medina N, Yushak M: Adverse hemodynamic and clinical effects of calcium channel blockade in pulmonary hypertension secondary to obliterative pulmonary vascular disease, *J Am Coll Cardiol* 4:890, 1984.

Pietra GG et al: Histopathology of primary pulmonary hypertension—a qualitative and quantitative study of pulmonary blood vessels from 58 patients in the National Heart, Lung, and Blood Institute Primary Pulmonary Hypertension Registry, *Circulation* 80:1198, 1989.

Rich S, Brundage BH: High-dose calcium channel-blocking therapy for primary pulmonary hypertension: evidence for long-term reduction in pulmonary arterial pressure and regression of right ventricular hypertrophy, *Circulation* 76:135, 1987.

Round S, Hill NS: Pulmonary hypertensive diseases, *Chest* 85:397, 1984.

Rubin LJ: ACCP consensus statement on primary pulmonary hypertension, *Chest* 104:236, 1993.

Rubin LJ, Mendoza J, Hood M et al: Treatment of primary pulmonary hypertension with continuous intravenous prostacyclin (epoprostenol), *Ann Intern Med* 112:485, 1990.

Thadani U et al: Pulmonary veno-occlusive disease, *Q J Med* 44:133, 1975.

Voelkel NF: Mechanisms of hypoxic pulmonary vasoconstriction, *Am Rev Respir Dis* 133:1186, 1986.

Wagenvoort CA, Wagenvoort N: *Pathology of pulmonary hypertension,* ed 2, New York, 1977, Wiley.

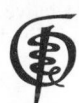

CHAPTER

30 Diseases of the Aorta

Miguel Zabalgoitia and Robert A. O'Rourke

Anatomically, the aorta is divided into four segments: ascending, arch, descending, and abdominal. In the normal adult, the ascending aorta extends from the base of the heart up to 5 to 6 cm cephalad. It continues as the arch, from where the three brachiocephalic arteries (innominate, left common carotid, and left subclavian) branch off. The descending thoracic aorta is the continuation beyond the arch. It courses in front of the spine and behind the esophagus, measures approximately 20 cm long, and ends at the level of the diaphragm. The aortic isthmus is the junction between the arch and the descending thoracic aorta where coarctations are usually located. The abdominal aorta extends from the diaphragm to its bifurcation (at the level of the umbilicus) into the common iliac arteries.

The aortic wall is composed of a thin intima lined by endothelium, a thick media containing elastic tissue arranged in a spiral, and a thin adventitia, composed mainly of collagen, containing the vasa vasorum and lymphatics. The great tensile strength of the aorta lies in its elastic medium, which serves as an expansible reservoir and accommodates each stroke volume ejected by the left ventricle during early systole. It then recoils during late systole and diastole, propelling the column of blood distal to the arterial bed. This converts the pulsatile inflow into a continuous outflow.

In addition to its conductance and pumping functions, the aorta plays a role in the control of systemic vascular resistance and heart rate. Baroreceptors analogous to those in the carotid sinus lie in the ascending aorta and the aortic arch and send afferent signals to the vasomotor center in the brain stem by way of the vagus nerves (Chapter 9). Raising the aortic pressure causes reflex bradycardia and reduction of systemic vascular resistance, whereas lowering the blood pressure increases the heart rate and systemic resistance.

The systolic aortic pressure is a function of the *volume* of blood ejected, the *compliance* of the aorta, and the *resistance* to blood flow (Chapter 9). The aorta and its branches tend to stiffen with age, which accounts for the increase in systolic blood pressure with advancing age. Specific disease entities that affect the aorta deserve a brief description.

ATHEROSCLEROSIS

Atherosclerosis is the most common cause of aortic aneurysms in adults older than 50 years of age. Atherosclerosis starts during early adult life in the abdominal aorta, and from there extends in both cephalad and caudal directions. On pathologic examination, the atherosclerotic process is frequently seen to extend from the intima into the media, destroying its elastic and muscular supports. A combination of atherosclerotic plaque and thrombus is common in aneurysms. Distal arterial embolization of cholesterol crystals and small thrombi may produce catastrophic consequences.

MARFAN SYNDROME

Histologically, Marfan syndrome (cystic medial necrosis) consists of multiple clefts of mucoid material within the aortic media. The nature of the process responsible for the degeneration of elastic and collagen fibers is unknown, but the development of the lesion seems to be accelerated by hypertension and pregnancy. The typical lesion is a fusiform aneurysm affecting the ascending aorta and the sinuses of Valsalva. Aortic regurgitation may be present as a result of dilation of the aortic ring. This condition is particularly prevalent in patients with Marfan syndrome. However, careful examination of patients with anuloaortic ectasia and cystic medial necrosis reveals that about 25% to 50% of these patients may have some, but not all, of the clinical features of the Marfan syndrome, indicating that many patients represent a forme fruste of this disorder.

The physical examination in patients with Marfan syndrome may reveal abnormal pulsation of the dilated ascending aorta over the second and third right intercostal spaces. As with other cases of aortic regurgitation secondary to dilation of the ascending aorta, the intensity of the diastolic murmur is greater to the *right* of the sternum, whereas in patients with aortic regurgitation secondary to primary valvular abnormality, the murmur is best heard along the *left* sternal border (Chapter 11).

The chest radiograph shows a markedly dilated ascending aorta and left ventricular dilation proportional to the severity of aortic regurgitation. Calcification of the ascending aorta and aortic valve is uncommon. Two-dimensional (2D) echocardiographic findings include widened aortic root, aneurysmal dilation of the sinuses of Valsalva, and incomplete coaptation of the aortic cusps during diastole (Chapter 13).

Complications of aneurysms of the ascending aorta account for more than 90% of deaths from Marfan syndrome. Elective composite graft repair of the aorta is recommended when the aortic root diameter reaches 6.0 cm, even if the patient is asymptomatic. Surgical correction is also advised when aortic regurgitation is severe, causing symptoms of congestive heart failure. The risks of failure of aortic valve replacement and aneurysm resection in this group of patients are between 10% and 15%. Recently, a 90% postsurgical survival at 8 years has been reported for ascending aortic aneurysms in patients with Marfan syndrome.

MYCOTIC ANEURYSMS

The so-called mycotic aneurysms of the aorta are of bacterial, not fungal, origin. Because the intact endothelium is quite resistant to bacterial invasion, a previously damaged area almost always provides the site for infection. Bacterial endocarditis is the usual setting in which mycotic aneurysms occur, but they may also develop during sepsis or by direct spread of infection from surrounding tissues. Direct invasion of the aortic wall adjacent to an aortic valve endocarditis may result in a ring abscess or in sinus of Valsalva rupture. Mycotic aneurysms tend to be saccular in appearance. Staphylococci, streptococci, and salmonellae are the usual infectious agents. Treatment includes parenteral antibiotics followed by surgical excision.

Diseases of the aorta are primarily the result of degenerative changes in the aortic wall. Among the factors that lead to this degeneration are aging and hypertension. Diseases of the aorta can be classified into the categories outlined in Box 30-1.

AORTIC ANEURYSMS

An aneurysm of the aorta is a pathologic dilation of any of its anatomic segments. A *true aneurysm* includes all three layers of the wall, as opposed to a *pseudoaneurysm,* in which disruption of the intima and media layers has occurred, and the wall is composed of the adventitia and thrombus. According to their macroscopic appearance, aneurysms may be described as *fusiform,* when the entire circumference is affected resulting in a diffusely dilated lesion, or *saccular,* when only a portion of the circumference is affected resulting in a diverticular formation. In most cases, aneurysms result from weakening of the media from defects in collagen and elastin. Once dilation starts, it tends to progress because wall stress at constant arterial pressure increases proportionally to chamber diameter (Laplace's law). Hypertension (particularly diastolic) promotes further dilation.

The most common cause of death in patients with thoracic or abdominal aneurysms is rupture. Thoracic aneurysms tend to rupture into the left pleural space, whereas abdominal aneurysms tend to rupture into the retroperitoneal space.

BOX 30-1
Classification of diseases of the aorta

Aneurysm
  Thoracic
    Ascending
    Arch
    Descending
  Abdominal
    Suprarenal
    Infrarenal
Dissection
  Type I
  Type II   }Type A
  Type III }Type B
Aortitis
  Syphilitic
  Rheumatic diseases
    Rheumatoid arthritis
    Ankylosing spondylitis
    Psoriatic arthritis
    Reiter's syndrome
    Relapsing polychondritis
    Enteropathic arthropathies
  Takayasu's arteritis
  Giant-cell arteritis
Occlusive disease
  Atherosclerotic
  Thrombotic
  Embolic
Trauma
Coarctation (Chapter 28)

Thoracic Aortic Aneurysms

In the normal adult, the diameter of the ascending aorta is 3.5 cm or less, the aortic arch is between 2.8 and 3.5 cm, and the thoracic descending aorta is between 2.2 and 3.0 cm. The signs and symptoms of a thoracic aortic aneurysm depend on its size and location. Most thoracic aneurysms are asymptomatic, being recognized on routine chest radiograph as a mediastinal widening. Thus an aortic aneurysm should be considered in the differential diagnosis of any mediastinal mass. Further investigation should include noninvasive methods such as computed tomography (CT) scanning, magnetic resonance imaging (MRI), or transesophageal echocardiography (TEE). If surgical repair is indicated, contrast aortography may be needed. Because progressive layering of thrombus frequently occurs within the aneurysmal sac and because an arteriogram shows only the intraluminal dimensions, the true size of the aneurysm may be underestimated. The exact dimensions of the aneurysm, including the thickness of the thrombus, can be better measured by CT, MRI, or TEE (Chapter 13).

Chronic chest pain, arising from compression of adjacent structures, may radiate into the neck, shoulders, or back. Severe chest pain in patients with a thoracic aneurysm may represent sudden expansion, rupture, or dissection. Compression of the left mainstem bronchus or the trachea may produce respiratory symptoms. Compression of the left recurrent laryngeal nerve may produce hoarseness, and esophageal compression may result in dysphagia. Aortic regurgitation is unusual in arteriosclerotic ascending aortic aneurysms but common with anuloaortic ectasia or dissections. Laminated thrombus is frequently present inside of the aneurysm, which may embolize to the distal arterial circulation, including the brain.

Management depends on the size and location of the aneurysm, the clinical presentation, and the relative risks of rupture versus operation. Rupture is the most serious complication of an aneurysm. It has an exceedingly high mortality rate, whereas elective repair in a low-risk patient can be performed safely with less than 10% mortality. A direct relationship exists between aneurysmal size and risk of rupture. Aneurysms larger than 6 cm in patients with low operative risk should be considered for elective repair. On the other hand, asymptomatic patients with stable aneurysms less than 6 cm, asymp-

tomatic patients with Marfan syndrome with an aneurysm less than 5 cm, and high-risk patients with large thoracic aneurysms should undergo CT, MRI, or TEE at 6- or 12-month intervals to assess aneurysmal growth. In the presence of signs and symptoms of expansion suggesting impending rupture (pain, compression of adjacent structures, new diastolic murmur, and objective evidence of aneurysmal growth), urgent surgical intervention is needed.

Aneurysms are repaired by replacing the dilated segment of the aorta with a Dacron graft. If the aortic valve and the fibrous ring are involved, resulting in aortic regurgitation, replacement of the aortic valve with reimplantation of the coronary arteries is required. Serious complications after repair include myocardial infarction, stroke, and respiratory and renal failure. Therefore complete preoperative assessment is mandatory to establish the operative risk on an individual basis.

Abdominal Aortic Aneurysms

Because atherosclerosis is most common in the abdominal aorta, 75% of atherosclerotic aneurysms are found in the distal abdominal aorta below the renal arteries. An abdominal aneurysm commonly produces no symptoms and is usually detected on routine examination as a palpable, pulsatile, and nontender mass or as an incidental finding on abdominal radiograph or abdominal ultrasound obtained for other reasons. Some patients may complain of pulsations in the abdomen, others of low back pain. During periods of rapid expansion, abdominal aneurysms produce pain in the low back, abdomen, or groin; the pulsatile mass frequently becomes tender and appears more fixed than in the asymptomatic patient. Acute abdominal or low back pain and hypotension occur with rupture of the aneurysm, requiring emergent surgery.

An abdominal aneurysm should be suspected when physical examination reveals a pulsatile, expansible, and occasionally tender mass between the xiphoid process and the umbilicus. The diagnosis is confirmed by abdominal ultrasound, which delineates the size, location, and characteristics of the aneurysmal sac contents. A mural thrombus is present in almost all cases. Serial ultrasound studies are extremely useful for documenting aneurysm expansion. Computed tomography and magnetic resonance imaging have also been used for this purpose. Contrast aortography is essential in the preoperative evaluation to document the extent of atherosclerosis in adjacent vascular territories. However, since the mural thrombus reduces the intraluminal size, aortography may underestimate the size of the aneurysm.

The risk of rupture increases with size. The mortality rate of patients with abdominal aneurysms exceeding 6 cm in diameter is 50% in 1 year, 75% in 2 years, and 90% in 3 years; in those with lesions between 4 and 6 cm, it is 25% in 1 year, 28% in 2 years, and 30% in 3 years. Thus operative resection of the aneurysm is indicated in symptomatic patients, in those with evidence of rapidly expanding aneurysms regardless of their size, and in patients with aneurysms larger than 5 cm in diameter, regardless of their symptoms. For aneurysms less than 5 cm in diameter, follow-up with serial ultrasound studies is mandatory.

The prognosis depends on the extent, location, and severity of atherosclerosis in vessels supplying vital organs. Frequently, the severity of accompanying coronary artery and cerebrovascular disease determines the long-term prognosis. Thus careful preoperative cardiac and general medical evaluation is essential. Operative mortality rate for a "triple A" (abdominal aortic aneurysm) resection ranges between 1% and 5% in most centers. After acute rupture, however, the mortality rate of an emergent operation is generally greater than 50%.

DISSECTION OF THE AORTA

Aortic dissection is usually initiated by an intimal tear that allows blood driven by arterial pressure to dissect through the aortic media, separating the intima from the adventitia and creating a double-lumen vessel. Because most dissections occur in the outer half of the media, the false lumen wall is exceedingly thin and prone to rupture. Occasionally, the false lumen reenters the true lumen in a more distal location through a spontaneous fenestration of the intimal flap.

Most aortic dissections occur in men (ratio of men to women is

3:1) between the ages of 40 and 60 years. Predisposing factors include systemic hypertension, coarctation of the aorta, atherosclerosis, pregnancy, cystic medial necrosis, and trauma. The elevated incidence noted in patients with systemic hypertension and coarctation is probably related to abnormally high wall stress. In elderly patients with extensive atherosclerosis, dissection may originate from perforation of an atheromatous plaque, the so-called *penetrating aortic ulcer.* The increased incidence of dissection in females in the third trimester of pregnancy may be the result of changes in connective tissue that occur late in pregnancy.

The two widely accepted classifications of aortic dissections are those of DeBakey and Stanford. DeBakey classifies dissections into type I (60%), which originates in the ascending aorta and extends into the descending aorta; type II (10%), which affects only the ascending aorta; and type III (30%), which originates at the upper descending aorta and extends distally. Stanford's classification separates dissections into type A (proximal) and type B (distal).

Severe chest pain occurs in more than 90% of patients. It is frequently described as a sudden, tearing pain associated with diaphoresis. The pain is so severe that it tends to persist despite the use of narcotics. The location may be useful in determining the site and extent of the dissection. As a general rule, pain in the chest, neck, and jaw suggests dissection involving the ascending aorta, whereas pain in the back suggests involvement of the descending aorta.

Other clinical features of acute onset of aortic dissection are manifestations of its four major complications: (1) compression of adjacent structures such as superior cervical ganglia (Horner's syndrome), superior vena cava (superior vena cava syndrome), left laryngeal nerve (hoarseness), bronchus (dyspnea), and esophagus (dysphagia); (2) occlusion of major branch vessels; (3) retrograde extension into the aortic valve (regurgitation); and (4) rupture (shock). Myocardial ischemia or infarction may occur as a result of coronary artery involvement. Because most type A dissections extend along the greater aortic curvature, the right coronary artery is more commonly affected than the left. Proximal aortic dissection may rupture into the pericardial sac, creating hemopericardium and cardiac tamponade. Neurologic ischemic symptoms may occur as a result of occlusion of cerebral or spinal arteries. Ischemic signs and symptoms affecting the upper and lower extremities may result from involvement of the subclavian or iliac arteries. Splanchnic vascular occlusion can result in bowel infarction and renal failure. Severe hypertension should suggest renal artery involvement.

Although half the patients with aortic dissection present with hypertension, others present with normal or low blood pressure. If significant hypotension is present, aortic rupture into the left pleural or pericardial space should be suspected. Examination of the jugular veins is helpful in distinguishing between cardiac tamponade and hypovolemia (Chapter 27). An emergent echocardiogram is mandatory to confirm this diagnosis.

Physical examination reveals an acutely distressed patient. Neurologic deficit or a pulse discrepancy between the arms may indicate compromise of the aortic arch vessels. Similarly, acute abdominal pain or diminished femoral pulses may suggest splanchnic or iliofemoral vessel involvement. Aortic regurgitation in a patient with aortic dissection strongly suggests that the dissecting process involves the aortic ring.

The electrocardiogram usually excludes acute myocardial ischemia unless there is coronary artery involvement or cardiac tamponade. As seen in Fig. 30-1, the chest radiograph may be helpful in suggesting the presence of aortic dissection. The unusually widened mediastinum may be present in either type A or type B dissection. Although a nonspecific finding, a widened mediastinum should lead to more specific diagnostic procedures. Precordial echocardiography can reveal dilation and double lumen of the aortic root. However, dissections involving the upper part of the ascending aorta or the aortic arch are more difficult to diagnose through this approach. Thus a negative precordial echocardiographic study should not exclude the possibility of a dissecting aortic arch.

The method of choice for diagnosing aortic dissection is transesophageal echocardiography (Chapter 13). Other imaging modalities such as MRI and CT with contrast have also been shown to be highly accurate in detecting aortic dissection. However, TEE has the following advantages over MRI and CT scanning: (1) It can be performed

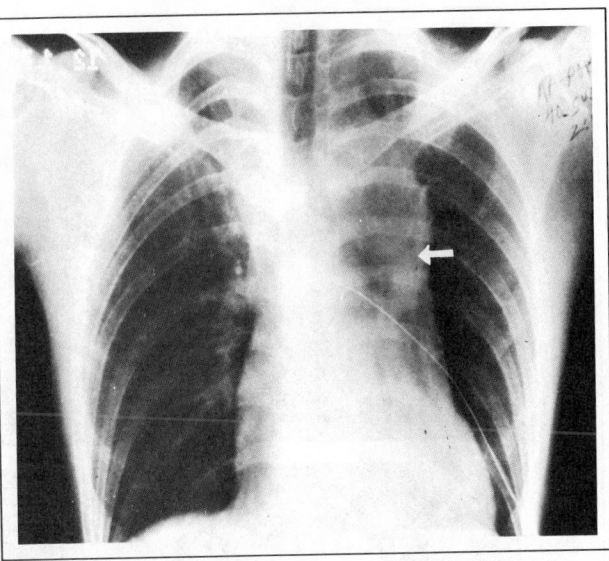

FIGURE 30-1   Posteroanterior chest radiograph of a patient with acute aortic dissection caused by anuloaortic ectasia associated with Marfan syndrome. Note the wide mediastinal shadow.
(From Walsh RA, O'Rourke RA: The diagnosis and management of acute left-sided valvular regurgitation, *Curr Probl Cardiol* 4(9):1-34, Dec, 1979.)

as a bedside procedure in the emergency room or in the intensive care area; (2) it requires less than 20 minutes; and (3) it does not require contrast media. Figure 30-2 illustrates a patient with type I aortic dissection. The separation between the true lumen and the false lumen by the intimal flap is clearly identified. A moderate amount of anterior pericardial effusion is also evident. Contrast aortography may be needed to determine the status of the coronary and aortic arch arteries (Fig. 30-3).

The prognosis for survival in untreated patients with aortic dissection is extremely poor. In one series of 505 patients, one third died within 48 hours of presentation; three fourths were dead within 2 weeks; nine out of ten did not survive 1 year. Thus transesophageal echocardiography should be performed as soon as possible in all patients in whom aortic dissection is suspected.

Medical therapy should be initiated as soon as possible. Unless hypotension is present, therapy should be aimed at reducing cardiac contractility and systemic arterial pressure, and thereby shear stress. Systolic blood pressure should be maintained between 100 and 120 mm Hg. A β-adrenergic blocker (labetelol) should be immediately administered simultaneously with sodium nitroprusside infusion. Direct vasodilators, such as diazoxide and hydralazine, are contraindicated, since these agents can increase hydraulic shear and may propagate dissection.

Definitive therapy is dictated by the type of dissection and by the complications noted on presentation. Ascending aortic dissections (type A) are unstable and pose the threat of retrograde dissection, rupture, acute severe aortic regurgitation, or fatal pericardial tamponade; thus surgical intervention is the preferred treatment. The goals of surgery are to correct complications and to limit the dissecting process. The intimal tear is either excised or oversewn; the false lumen is obliterated by oversewing the aorta. In proximal dissections (type A) and severe aortic regurgitation, a composite Dacron conduit with a prosthetic valve and reimplantation of the coronary arteries is the preferred therapy. The distal dissection plane, which may extend into the descending thoracic or abdominal aorta, often becomes obliterated. The major causes of perioperative mortality and morbidity include myocardial infarction, paraplegia, renal failure, tamponade, hemorrhage, and sepsis.

For patients with descending aorta dissection (type B) who are stable without vascular complications, medical therapy is the preferred mode of treatment. Transesophageal echocardiography may be useful in the decision-making process in patients with type B dissections. If the upper and lower margins of the dissection can be identi-

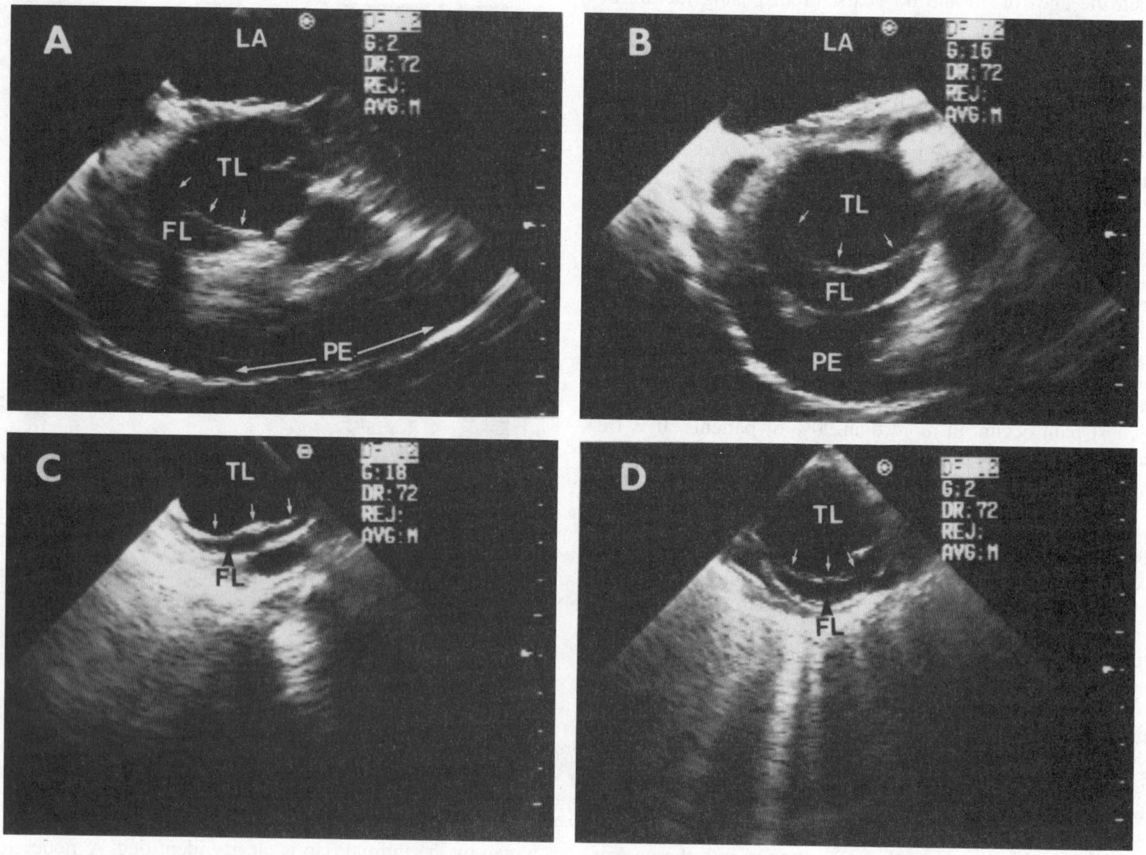

FIGURE 30-2 Transesophageal echocardiography in a patient with type I acute aortic dissection. The true lumen *(TL)* and the false lumen *(FL)* are clearly separated by an intimal flap *(arrows).* A moderate amount of anterior pericardial effusion *(PE)* is also noted. **A,** Image at the level of the aortic valve and aortic root. **B,** Image at the level of the ascending aorta. **C,** Image at the level of the aortic arch. **D,** Image at the level of the middescending thoracic aorta.

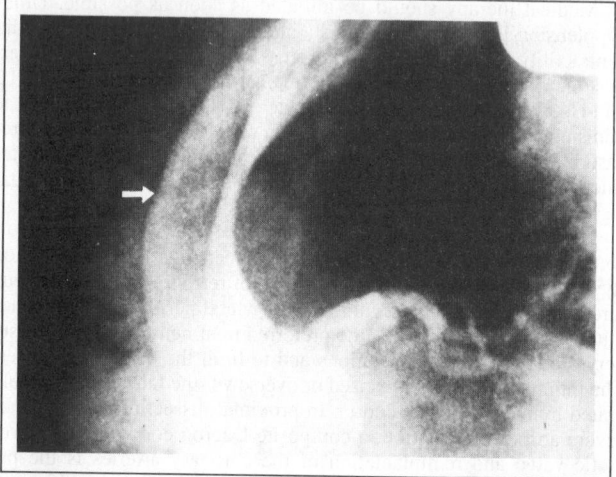

FIGURE 30-3 Angiogram of a patient with acute aortic dissection of the ascending aorta. Contrast material fills the true lumen; the false lumen is to the left.

(From Walsh RA, O'Rourke RA: The diagnosis and management of acute left-sided valvular regurgitation, *Curr Probl Cardiol* 4(9):1-34, Dec, 1979.)

fied and are limited to the thoracic descending aorta, if the false lumen is completely or almost completely occupied by thrombus, and if active circulation between the true lumen and the false lumen is not evident by color-flow Doppler, the decision for medical management alone is well supported. However, if the distal end of the dissection cannot be identified because it extends into the abdominal aorta, if the false lumen is not obliterated by thrombus, and if there is evidence of blood flow between the true and the false lumens, emergent thoracoabdominal contrast aortography is recommended to detect splanchnic vessels and lower limb involvement. The decision for an emergent operation should be based on these angiographic results. Figure 30-4 illustrates serial TEE images in a patient with type B dissection.

Long-term management of patients with aortic dissection treated either medically or surgically should include careful control of blood pressure with the use of long-acting β-adrenergic blockers and serial noninvasive follow-up by means of CT, MRI, or TEE.

AORTITIS

Although the causes of aortitis are diverse, the pathologic consequences are similar: aneurysm formation or stenosis of aortic branch vessels. Syphilis, ankylosing spondylitis, and rheumatoid arthritis result in inflammation, scarring, and weakening of the aortic media. Involvement of the aortic ring and cusps often results in aortic regurgitation. In contrast, Takayasu's arteritis and giant-cell arteritis produce ischemic symptoms related to occlusive disease of the branches of the aorta.

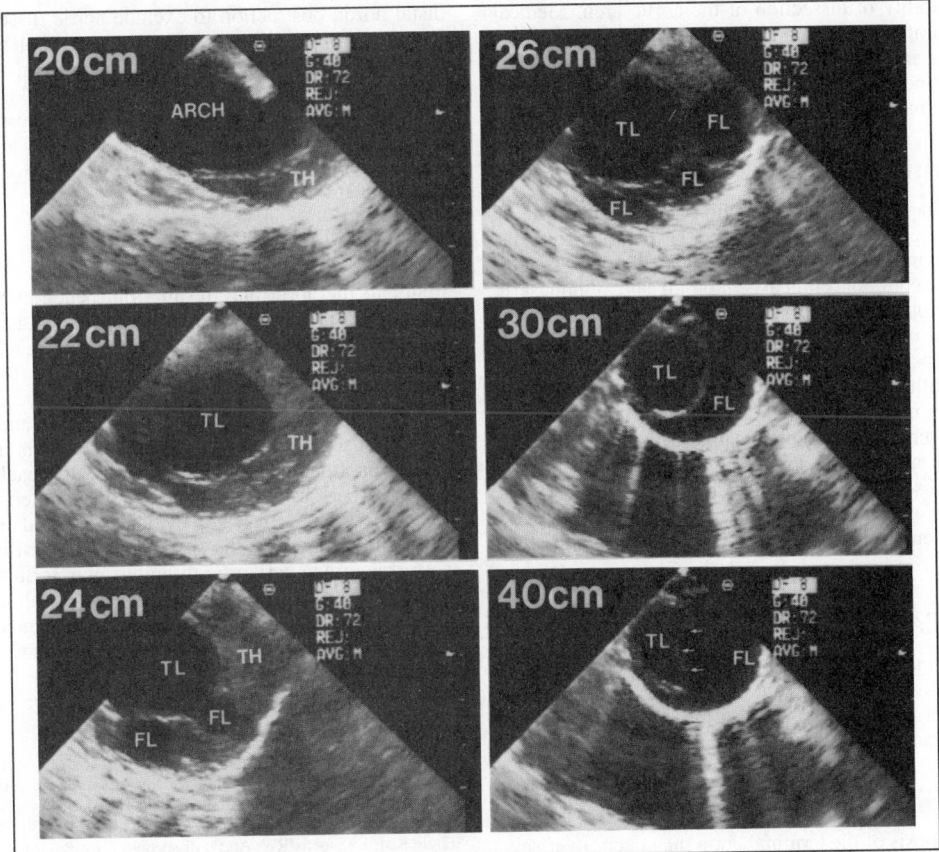

FIGURE 30-4   Transesophageal echocardiography in a patient with type III acute aortic dissection. The proximal end of the dissection can be clearly identified at 20 cm, where the true lumen at the level of the aortic arch can be separated from the false lumen, which is obliterated by thrombus *(TH)* formation. At 22 cm, the centrally located true lumen is being surrounded by the thrombus-obliterated false lumen; at 24 and 26 cm, the false lumen is partially obliterated by the thrombus; at 30 cm, the false lumen is thrombus-free, suggesting free-flow circulation between the true lumen and the false lumen. At 40 cm, the dimensions of the false lumen are now larger than the true lumen, and external compression of the intimal flap can be clearly appreciated *(arrows),* which is indicative of a hypertensive false lumen. At this latter level, the transesophageal transducer is beyond the diaphragm, that is, at the uppermost portion of the abdominal aorta. More distal imaging of the abdominal aorta is not possible because the aorta and the esophagus are no longer in contact.

SYPHILIS

Treponema pallidum affects the aorta by direct invasion of the adventitia. The spirochetes spread through the lymphatics into the media and produce an obliterative endarteritis of the vasa vasorum. Inflammation leads to destruction of elastic tissue and eventually to scar and calcification along the ascending aorta. The characteristic radiographic appearance of dilation and calcification of the ascending aorta (not the aortic knob) should suggest syphilitic aortitis. Other clinically important manifestations of tertiary syphilis of the aorta include aortic regurgitation and coronary ostial stenosis. Positive serologic tests support the diagnosis. Penicillin therapy as recommended for tertiary syphilis is necessary (Chapter 274).

Chronic Rheumatoid Diseases

Aortitis involving predominantly the ascending aorta has been documented in patients with rheumatoid arthritis (Chapter 192), ankylosing spondylitis (Chapter 200), psoriatic arthritis (Chapter 200), Reiter's syndrome (Chapter 200), relapsing polychondritis (Chapter 191), and enteropathic arthropathies (Chapter 191). The aortitis in each of these conditions may result in aortic dilation and consequently in aortic regurgitation.

Cardiovascular symptoms occur in 3% to 10% of patients with ankylosing spondylitis and may be present before manifestations of arthritis are evident. Aortic regurgitation is the predominant cardiac manifestation of ankylosing spondylitis. Mitral regurgitation may be present but is rarely isolated or severe. Conduction abnormalities are usually not clinically important, but complete heart block has been reported.

Takayasu's Arteritis

Takayasu's arteritis (Chapter 195) is a type of vasculitis that characteristically results in inflammation and obstruction of the aorta and its major branches. Panarteritis occurs during the active phase of the disease and is replaced by intimal proliferation. Wall scarring and intravascular thrombosis are late manifestations of the disease. The term *pulseless disease* is applied because of frequent severe obstruction of the innominate, left common carotid, and left subclavian arteries. Involvement of the abdominal branches of the aorta may produce gastrointestinal symptoms or renovascular hypertension. Obstruction of the iliofemoral arteries is rare.

The syndrome should be suspected in young females (particularly those of Asian origin) whose symptoms suggest proximal obstruction of upper extremity and head arteries. Examination reveals diminished or absent upper extremity and carotid pulses, with good preservation of lower extremity pulses. Bruits are frequently present. Contrast aortography may help determine the extent and severity of obstruction and exclude the possibility of dissection of the aortic arch. Medical therapy includes antiinflammatory and immunosuppressive agents during the acute phase and anticoagulants during the late stage of the disease. Surgical treatment may be needed for relief of ischemia resulting from critically narrowed arteries.

Giant-Cell Arteritis

Giant-cell arteritis (Chapter 195) is a vasculitis that is a subacute or chronic inflammatory process with local and systemic manifestations. It occurs predominantly in women over the age of 55. Headache is the most common clinical symptom, and blindness is the most dreaded complication. Symptoms may range from fatigue, morning stiffness, and myalgia noted in polymyalgia rheumatica to those resulting from obstruction of medium-sized arteries, especially the temporal and ophthalmic arteries. On laboratory examination, the erythrocyte sedimentation rate is markedly elevated and mild anemia may be present, but serum creatine kinase is normal. Diagnosis is typically made by biopsy of the superficial temporal artery. Although the disease is self-limited, it can result in arterial obstruction and infarction. Corticosteroid therapy is usually effective in controlling symptoms and progression of the inflammatory process.

OCCLUSIVE DISEASE

Occlusion of the terminal aorta may occur gradually, as a result of progressive atherosclerosis, or suddenly, secondary to arterial embolism. Symptoms and prognosis are related to the underlying disease and to the amount of collateral circulation.

Chronic Aortic Obstruction

Slowly progressive stenosis of the terminal aorta may occur over several years. Exercise-induced pain characteristically involves the low back, buttocks, and thighs and may progress to pain at rest as the severity of stenosis increases. Inability to maintain penile erection is common. Absence of pulses in both femoral arteries and more distal locations are characteristic. Bruits are usually audible over the abdomen near the umbilicus and over both femoral arteries. Loss of lower extremity hair, atrophy of the skin and subcutaneous tissue, and loss of leg muscle mass are common in such patients; gangrene is a late manifestation of the disease.

Acute Aortic Obstruction

Systemic emboli are the primary cause of acute aortic obstruction. A cardiac source should be strongly considered. The presence of atrial fibrillation, mitral stenosis, cardiomyopathy, valve prostheses, or recent myocardial infarction makes emboli of cardiac origin more likely.

The severity of reduced arterial circulation to the lower extremities depends on the level of the occlusion, the competence of collateral circulation, the severity of acute arterial spasm, and the extent of thrombus propagation. Clinically, the patient notes the sudden onset of ischemic pain at the level of the occlusion. If collateral circulation is inadequate, cutaneous sensation and muscle strength are lost within the first hour. Severe muscle contractures may occur at 6 hours. Muscle swelling and skin discoloration signify prolonged ischemia. Initial improvement in symptoms may be followed by increased evidence of ischemia caused by proximal propagation of the arterial thrombus. On examination, the legs are cool and the lower extremity pulses, including those of the femoral arteries, are absent. Muscle strength and cutaneous sensation are diminished. Muscle fasciculations and/or contractures may be present. Edema is a late finding. Similar clinical findings may occur in patients with dissection of the descending aorta. These patients are usually identified by the presence of severe back pain and asymmetric extremity pulses.

Acute aortic obstruction is an emergency condition. The patient's life and the viability of both lower extremities depend on rapidly establishing the correct diagnosis and promptly instituting appropriate therapy. Doppler ultrasonographic measurement of lower extremity arterial pressures is useful in establishing the presence, severity, and site of arterial occlusion. Contrast aortography is necessary in acute distal aortic obstruction to exclude aortic dissection and to establish the site of obstruction and the amount of collateral circulation.

Prompt institution of intravenous heparin therapy is essential as soon as aortic dissection is excluded. Surgical embolectomy or thrombectomy should be performed as soon as possible. Heparin therapy should be continued after surgery. Lifetime anticoagulation therapy is indicated in the majority of patients to prevent recurrent embolism or propagation of arterial thrombus.

AORTIC TRAUMA

Injury to the aorta may result from penetrating wounds or nonpenetrating chest trauma. During motor vehicle accidents, the aorta may be completely or incompletely transected. Under such acceleration-deceleration injuries, the most common site (80%) of tear or rupture is the aortic isthmus located just distal to the origin of the left subclavian artery where the mobile (ascending and arch) and fixed (descending) segments of the aorta join. Patients may be in shock from exsanguination. The presence of chest and back pain, upper extremity hypertension with lower extremity hypotension, decreased or absent pulses in the legs, or evidence of fluid in the left side of the chest should increase the suspicion of aortic rupture. In survivors of aortic rupture, a periaortic thrombus may form, the aortic lumen may recanalize, and a pseudoaneurysm may develop just distal to the left subclavian artery. Because of the high incidence of spontaneous rupture of such aneurysms, surgical resection and repair should be performed immediately.

BIBLIOGRAPHY

Bergstein EF, Chan EL: Abdominal aortic aneurysm in high risk patients. Outcome of selective management based on size and expansion rate, *Ann Surg* 200:255, 1984.

Boucek RJ, Noble NL, Gunja-Smith Z et al: The Marfan syndrome: a deficiency in chemically stable collagen cross-links, *N Engl J Med* 305:988-991, 1981.

Eagle KM, DeSanctis RW: Aortic dissection, *Curr Probl Cardiol* 14:227, 1989.

Erbel R et al: Echocardiography in diagnosis of aortic dissection, *Lancet* 1:457, 1989.

Gott VL et al: Surgical treatment of aneurysms of the ascending aorta in the Marfan syndrome, *N Engl J Med* 314:1070, 1986.

Griepp RB, Ergin MA, Lansman SL et al: The natural history of thoracic aortic aneurysms. *Semin Thorac Cariovasc Surg* 3:258-265, 1991.

Hall S et al: Takayasu arteritis. A review of 32 North American patients, *Medicine (Baltimore)* 64:89, 1985.

Hirata K, Kyushima M, Asato H: Electrocardiographic abnormalities in patients with acute aortic dissection, *Am J Cardiol* 76:1207-1212, 1995.

Ishikawa K: Patterns of symptoms and prognosis in occlusive thromboaortopathy (Takayasu's disease), *J Am Coll Cardiol* 8:1041, 1986.

Kato M, Bai H, Sato K et al: Determining surgical indications for acute type B dissection based on enlargement or aortic diameter during the chronic phase, *Circulation* 92(suppl II):II107-II112, 1995.

Lynch DR, Dawson TM, Raps EC et al: Risk factors for the neurologic complications associated with aortic aneurysms, *Arch Neurol* 49:284-288, 1992.

Nienaber CA, von Kodolitsch Y, Nicolas V et al: The diagnosis of thoracic aortic dissection by noninvasive imaging procedures, *N Engl J Med* 328:1-9, 1993.

Perruquet JL, Davis DE, Harrington TM: Aortic arch arteritis in the elderly. An important manifestation of giant cell arteritis, *Arch Intern Med* 146:289, 1986.

Stanson AW, Kazmier FJ, Hollier LH et al: Penetrating atherosclerotic ulcers of the thoracic aorta: natural history and clinicopathologic correlations, *Ann Vasc Surg* 1:15-23, 1986.

Sterpnetti AV et al: Abdominal aortic aneurysms in elderly patients. Selective management based on clinical status and aneurysmal expansion rate, *Am J Surg* 150:772, 1979.

CHAPTER

31 Diseases of the Peripheral Arteries and Veins

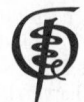

Peter C. Spittell and John A. Spittell, Jr.

The competent clinician should be familiar with peripheral vascular disorders, confident in making an accurate diagnosis, and knowledgeable regarding the available therapeutic options. Peripheral vascular disorders occur commonly, present important therapeutic opportuni-

Table 31-1 Grading of elevation pallor*

GRADE OF PALLOR	DURATION OF ELEVATION
0	No pallor in 60 sec
1	Definite pallor in 60 sec
2	Definite pallor in less than 60 sec
3	Definite pallor in less than 30 sec
4	Pallor on the level

From Spittell JA Jr: Recognition and management of chronic atherosclerotic occlusive peripheral arterial disease, *Mod Concepts Cardiovasc Dis* 50:19, 1981.
*Elevation of extremity at angle of 60 degrees above the level.

Table 31-2 Color return and venous filling times

	COLOR RETURN (SEC)	VENOUS FILLING TIME (SEC)
Normal	10	15
Moderate ischemia	15-20	20-30
Severe ischemia	40+	40+

From Spittell JA Jr: Recognition and management of chronic atherosclerotic occlusive peripheral arterial disease, *Mod Concepts Cardiovasc Dis* 50:19, 1981.

ties, and often serve as valuable diagnostic clues to other significant conditions. Accordingly, a systematic and careful evaluation of the arterial and venous circulation should be included in the history and physical examination of every patient.

In this chapter the clinical aspects and management of acute and chronic occlusive peripheral arterial disease, arterial aneurysms, vasospastic disorders, arteritides, varicose veins, venous thrombosis, and chronic venous insufficiency are presented.

DISEASES OF THE PERIPHERAL ARTERIES

Peripheral arterial disease can be caused by one or more etiologic factors—aging, atherosclerosis, hypertension, infection, inflammatory disorders, degenerative disease, iatrogenic, and trauma. Atherosclerosis is by far the most common cause of peripheral arterial disease, including both occlusive and aneurysmal disease; however, the less common types of occlusive arterial disease must also be considered since they often present important diagnostic and/or therapeutic opportunities. In addition to atherosclerotic occlusive disease and aneurysms, the peripheral arteries may be affected by vasospastic disorders, inflammation, and trauma.

Peripheral arterial disease, whether occlusive, aneurysmal, or vasospastic, is not difficult to diagnose since the peripheral arteries are easy to examine, and symptoms of peripheral arterial disease, when present, are fairly distinctive.

Examination of the upper extremity arteries (subclavian, brachial, radial, and ulnar), the abdominal aorta, and the lower extremity arteries (femoral, popliteal, posterior tibial, and dorsalis pedis) should be a part of every general medical evaluation. Auscultation over the major arteries for bruits is an additional important method for detecting proximal occlusive disease. The degree of any ischemia can be estimated at the bedside or in the office by the observation of elevation pallor (Table 31-1) and the time required for return of color and filling of the veins with dependency after elevation (Table 31-2). Active pedal plantar flexion is also a useful method to assess the degree of ischemia in the office. While the patient stands with only fingertip support for balance, the feet are extended fully and then returned to a baseline stance, with feet flat on the floor. This symptom-limited test is repeated for up to 50 repetitions. Ankle systolic pressure measurements before and after the test are obtained; a decrease in absolute ankle systolic pressure of greater than 20 mm Hg or a decrease in ankle brachial systolic pressure index of greater than 20% constitutes an abnormal test.

The Allen test (Fig. 31-1, *A, B*) for assessing the adequacy of circulation in the hand is useful when there are symptoms or signs of peripheral arterial disease in the upper extremities, and routinely applying it before and after radial artery puncture is good practice. An-

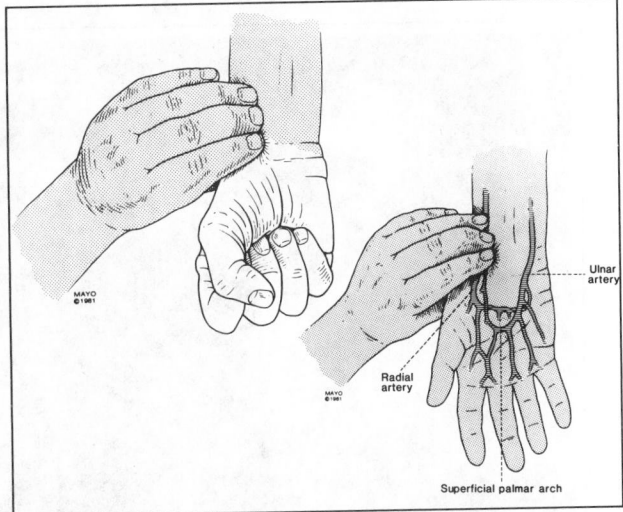

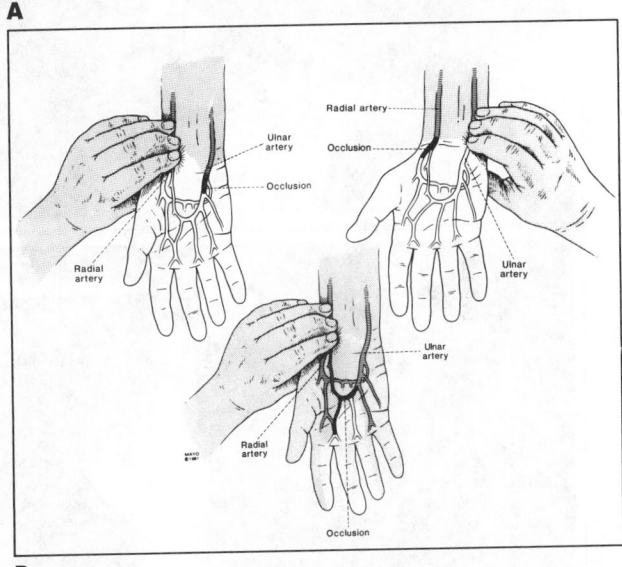

FIGURE 31-1 The Allen test. **A,** Normal (negative) result indicating patency of ulnar artery and superficial palmar arch. **B,** Abnormal (positive) results caused by occlusion of ulnar artery *(left)*, radial artery *(right)*, and superficial palmar arch *(center)*.

(From Spittell JA Jr: Occlusive peripheral arterial disease: guidelines for office management, *Postgrad Med* 71:137, 1982.)

other useful maneuver is palpation of the two radial arteries simultaneously; a delay in the pulsation of one may be noted when narrowing of the origin of the ipsilateral subclavian artery (not uncommon) occurs with consequent reversal of flow in the ipsilateral vertebral artery. In addition, compression of the subclavian artery in the thoracic outlet should be evaluated by the thoracic outlet maneuvers (Fig. 31-2, *A, B*).

Objectivity in the diagnosis of peripheral arterial disease has been aided by the development of noninvasive methods, which are useful for detecting occlusive arterial disease, aneurysmal disease, and vasospastic disorders.

Occlusive arterial disease in the lower extremities may be further evaluated by obtaining supine systolic brachial and ankle blood pressures, using a hand-held Doppler velocity transducer and a standard arm blood pressure cuff. Normally, the systolic pressure at the ankle equals or exceeds that at the brachial level; in the case of occlusive arterial disease in the lower extremity, the systolic pressure at the ankle is reduced. Determination of systolic brachial and ankle blood pressures before and after standard exercise is a more sensitive means of detecting occlusive arterial disease, providing an estimate of the degree of disability imposed by any

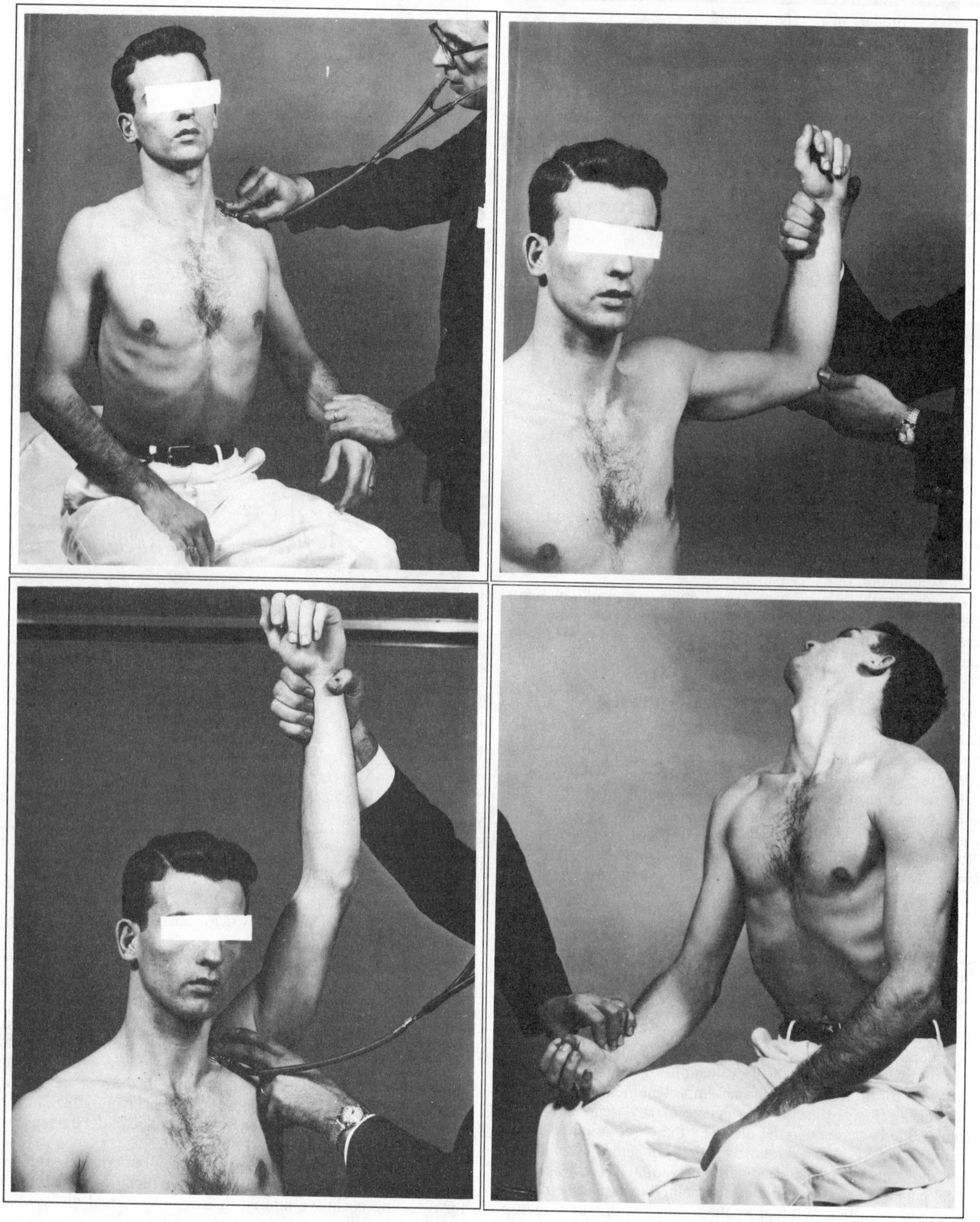

FIGURE 31-2   **A,** Costoclavicular maneuver, active. Auscultation over subclavian artery, above or below midportion of clavicle, may reveal systolic bruit as artery is being compressed. Radial pulse and bruit over subclavian artery disappear when complete compression of subclavian artery occurs. **B,** Costoclavicular maneuver, passive. **C,** Hyperabduction maneuver. Axillary artery may be completely or incompletely compressed by maneuver. In latter case, bruit may be heard above or below clavicle or, on occasion, deep in axilla. **D,** Scalene or Adson's maneuver. This test is used in both cervical rib or anomalous first thoracic rib syndrome and scalenus anticus syndrome. Auscultation over subclavian artery being tested may reveal bruit when artery is partially compressed.

(From Fairbairn JF, Campbell JK, Payne WS: Neurovascular compression syndromes of the thoracic outlet. In Juergens JL, Spittell JA, Fairbairn JF, editors: *Peripheral vascular diseases,* ed 5, Philadelphia, 1980, WB Saunders.)

BOX 31-1
Classification of occlusive arterial disease

I. Acute arterial occlusion
  A. Thrombotic arterial occlusion secondary to
    1. Atherosclerosis
      a. Arteriosclerosis obliterans
      b. Atherosclerotic aneurysm
    2. Thromboangiitis obliterans (Buerger's disease)
    3. Arteritis resulting from
      a. Connective tissue diseases
      b. Giant-cell (temporal or cranial) arteritis
      c. Takayasu's arteritis
    4. Myeloproliferative disease
      a. Polycythemia vera
      b. Thrombocytosis
    5. Hypercoagulable states
      a. Complicating neoplastic disease
      b. Complicating ulcerative bowel disease
      c. Idiopathic ("simple") arterial thrombosis
    6. Trauma
      a. Arterial puncture and arteriotomy
      b. Secondary to fractures and bone dislocations
      c. Arterial entrapment
        (1) Lower extremity
          (a) Adductor tendon compression of superficial femoral artery
          (b) Popliteal artery entrapment
        (2) Upper extremity
          (a) Thoracic outlet compression
          (b) "Crutch" thrombosis
      d. Frostbite
  B. Embolic arterial occlusion (arising from thrombi of)
    1. Cardiac origin
      a. Valvular heart disease, including valvular prostheses
      b. Acute myocardial infarction
      c. Myocardial aneurysm
      d. Atrial fibrillation
      e. Cardiomyopathy
      f. Infective endocarditis
      g. Left-sided myxoma
    2. Proximal atherosclerotic plaques or arterial narrowing
    3. Proximal arterial aneurysms
      a. Atherosclerotic
      b. Poststenotic dilatation
      c. Fibromuscular dysplasia
  C. Miscellaneous causes
    1. Arterial spasm, secondary to
      a. Ergotism
      b. Trauma of blunt or penetrating type
      c. Intraarterial injections
    2. Aortic dissection
      a. Luminal compression (by extension of the dissection into branch[es] of the aorta)
      b. Occlusion at site of reentry of dissection
    3. Foreign bodies
      a. Bullet embolism
      b. Guidewires and catheters
II. Chronic arterial occlusive disease
  A. Arteriosclerosis obliterans
  B. Thromboangiitis obliterans (Buerger's disease)
  C. Arteritis
    1. Connective tissue disorders
    2. Giant-cell (temporal or cranial) arteritis
    3. Takayasu's disease
  D. Trauma
    1. Blunt trauma
      a. Chronic occupational arterial occlusion in the hand
    2. Arterial entrapment
      a. Superficial femoral artery
      b. Popliteal artery
  E. Congenital arterial narrowing

From Spittell JA Jr: Office and bedside diagnosis of occlusive arterial disease, *Curr Probl Cardiol* 8:1, 1983.

intermittent claudication. Duplex ultrasonography, combining two-dimensional, pulsed-wave and color-flow Doppler, can reliably identify the degree of stenosis in the extracranial carotid and vertebral arteries, the upper and lower extremity arteries, as well as the aortoiliac region. Two-dimensional ultrasonography is also the noninvasive diagnostic method of choice for aneurysmal disease in the aorta and iliofemoral and lower extremity arteries. Magnetic resonance angiography is another noninvasive method to assess arterial occlusive disease in the same territories as described for duplex ultrasonography.

Although arteriography remains the best procedure for demonstrating the location and extent of occlusive arterial disease and the character of the arterial circulation proximally and distally, it is usually reserved for patients for whom restoration of pulsatile flow is being considered or when the etiology of the occlusive arterial disease is uncertain.

Raynaud's phenomenon can be confirmed by measuring the skin temperature of the digits before and after their immersion in ice water for 30 seconds. Normally, digital skin temperatures return to preimmersion levels in 3 to 10 minutes, whereas in patients with a vasospastic disorder, the time required to reach preimmersion temperatures exceeds 10 minutes.

OCCLUSIVE PERIPHERAL ARTERIAL DISEASE

Occlusive peripheral arterial disease (OPAD), whether acute or chronic, results in ischemia to the affected limb(s) or digit(s) supplied by the affected artery. The symptoms and signs depend on the location and extent of the occlusion and the adequacy of the collateral circulation.

Acute Occlusive Arterial Disease

The etiologies of acute arterial occlusion are enumerated in Box 31-1. Acute peripheral arterial occlusion can be the initial or dominant manifestation of cardiac or systemic disease, as well as acute aortic dissection. The degree of ischemia depends on the size of the occluded artery and the adequacy of the collateral circulation. Associated arterial spasm, hypotension, and fragmentation of an occluding embolus also influence the impact of an acute arterial occlusion.

The clinical presentation of an acute arterial occlusion is variable and may include any or all of the "five P's"—pain, pallor, paresthesia, pulselessness, and paralysis. Occasionally, abrupt shortening of the distance necessary to elicit claudication may be the presenting complaint of an acute arterial occlusion in the person with preexisting occlusive arterial disease.

A thorough peripheral vascular examination usually allows one to localize the site of an acute occlusion when the larger- or medium-sized arteries are involved. With arteriolar occlusions, livedo reticularis and cyanotic digits are the manifestations; when there is associated renal insufficiency and hypertension, atheroembolism from proximal atherosclerotic plaques or an aortic aneurysm should be suspected.

The diagnosis of acute arterial occlusion is usually readily apparent after a careful history taking and physical examination. Initial management includes protection of the extremity from trauma, plus pain relief, heparin anticoagulation, and immediate hospitalization. Arteriography and appropriate surgical therapy (thrombectomy or embolectomy) on an emergent basis are indicated to restore adequate circulation to the affected limb.

Embolic arterial occlusions can usually be relieved by embolectomy using a Fogarty catheter. It is important to identify the source

BOX 31-2

Clinical features suggesting uncommon types of occlusive arterial disease

Person younger than age 40
Acute ischemia in the absence of prior evidence of occlusive arterial disease
Occlusive arterial disease confined to the upper extremity
Digital occlusive arterial disease, particularly if accompanied by systemic symptoms

From Spittell JA Jr, Spittell PC: Diseases of the aorta and peripheral arteries. In Parmley W, Chatterjee K, editors: *Cardiology,* Philadelphia, 1987, JB Lippincott.

BOX 31-3

Clinical features of thromboangiitis obliterans

More common in young (less than 30 years of age) males
Activity of disease correlates with tobacco use
Small arteries and veins of upper and lower extremities involved, producing
   Migratory superficial thrombophlebitis
   Claudication of arch and/or calf

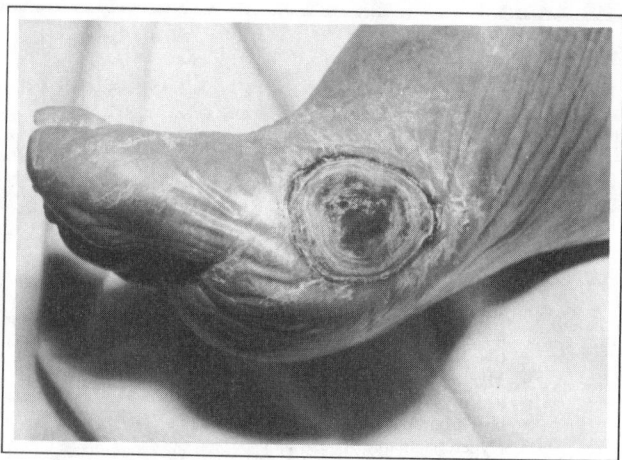

FIGURE 31-3   Ischemic ulceration of the foot.

of the emboli (most often the heart, less often a proximal arterial aneurysm), then to correct it, if possible, or to institute oral anticoagulant therapy to prevent recurrent embolic arterial occlusion.

Thrombotic arterial occlusion may be managed in several ways, depending on the size of the involved artery, the duration of the arterial occlusion, and the associated underlying disease. Thrombectomy, thrombolysis (often followed by balloon angioplasty [PTA]), and arterial bypass surgery are the available therapeutic options.

In the patient with atheroembolism (cholesterol embolization), surgical resection of the source of the atheromatous debris (aneurysm or atherosclerotic artery) is the only effective therapy; antiplatelet and anticoagulant therapy have not been effective in atheroembolism and at times may even precipitate atheroembolism.

Chronic Occlusive Arterial Disease

Chronic occlusive peripheral arterial disease, most commonly caused by atherosclerosis, results in luminal narrowing of large and medium-sized arteries, especially of the lower extremities. Clinical recognition of chronic occlusive arterial disease, even in its early stages, is important since much of the limb loss that occurs results from preventable trauma to the ischemic limb.

Less common causes of chronic occlusive arterial disease such as thromboangiitis obliterans (TAO, Buerger's disease), trauma, arteritis, and extrinsic compression of arteries (e.g., popliteal artery entrapment) can be suspected at the time of initial evaluation of the patient (see Box 31-2). Thromboangiitis obliterans has distinct clinical features (see Box 31-3) and deserves special mention because of its consistent relationship to tobacco use. If the patient with TAO abstains from using tobacco, the activity of the disease stops, but it recurs just as surely if tobacco use is resumed.

Differentiation of TAO and occlusive arterial disease of the hand caused by repetitive blunt trauma is also important and can present a diagnostic challenge in a person who smokes. Features suggestive of occlusive arterial disease of the hand caused by repetitive blunt trauma include unilateral symptoms and signs of digital ischemia and/or infarction, most commonly involving the dominant hand in a person whose occupation or leisure activity involves repetitive blunt palmar trauma. Arteriography is usually necessary to establish the diagnosis, and connective tissue disease and diabetes mellitus should

be excluded. Treatment of occlusive arterial disease of the hand resulting from repetitive blunt trauma depends on both the severity of the clinical manifestations and arteriographic findings. Conservative treatment includes protection of the hands from mechanical and thermal trauma, the use of padded gloves, and tobacco cessation. Calcium-channel blockers and α-1 adrenergic receptor blockers (prazosin, doxazosin) can alleviate episodic digital vasospasm but are of no benefit in treating fixed obstructive arterial disease. For severe cases and those that are refractory to medical therapy, surgical sympathectomy and/or direct revascularization using microvascular techniques are indicated.

The clinical manifestations of chronic occlusive arterial disease are a direct result of ischemia of the tissues of the extremity supplied by the affected arteries. In milder cases there may be no symptoms, and the peripheral arterial examination may be nearly normal. The hallmark of symptomatic occlusive peripheral disease, intermittent claudication, is as typical in its occurrence with walking and its relief with standing still as angina pectoris is with exertion or stress. A careful history and physical examination usually allow differentiation of intermittent claudication from neurologic or musculoskeletal conditions. Pseudoclaudication, resulting from lumbar spinal stenosis, differs from true intermittent claudication in several respects. The patient with pseudoclaudication usually develops symptoms with long standing as well as with walking and gets relief only by sitting down or leaning over some object. Importantly, standing still will not relieve pseudoclaudication, although it does relieve true intermittent claudication.

When ischemia becomes more severe, the patient may develop pain at rest; this usually involves the toes and/or foot, is aggravated by cool temperatures, is often worse at night, and is relieved temporarily by dependency. Ischemic ulceration, commonly resulting from trauma, occurs most often on the toes, heel, or foot. An ischemic ulcer (Fig. 31-3) is painful and on examination has a discrete edge, a pale base, or is covered by an eschar.

All persons with occlusive peripheral arterial disease should be instructed in conservative measures. Avoidance of vasoconstrictive influences such as cold and certain pharmacologic agents (β-blocking agents, ergot preparations, clonidine) and the complete cessation of tobacco use should be stressed. The need for tobacco cessation is of paramount importance for the patient with intermittent claudication. Epidemiologic studies have demonstrated that 5-year mortality, major amputation rate, and the need for revascularization are all significantly increased in persons who continue to smoke compared to those who stop smoking (27% versus 12%, 11% versus 0%, and 31% versus 8%, respectively).

The risk factors for atherosclerosis such as obesity, diabetes mellitus, hyperlipidemia, and hypertension should also be modified. When intermittent claudication is the major complaint, a program of walking to the point of claudication, several times a day, may improve walking distance. Vasodilators are of no benefit in the symp-

---

BOX 31-4

Elective restoration of pulsatile flow to limb in chronic atherosclerotic occlusive arterial disease with intermittent claudication

1. It does not affect longevity or ameliorate coronary or cerebrovascular disease.
2. The incidence of severe ischemia is relatively low.
3. Runoff should be adequate.
4. Complications of the procedure, though infrequent, do occur.
5. Reocclusion may occur.

From Spittell JA Jr: Peripheral vascular disease: advances in diagnosis and management, *Baylor Cardiology Series* 7:1, 1984.

BOX 31-5

Restoration of pulsatile flow in chronic atherosclerotic occlusive arterial disease with rest pain or ischemic ulceration

1. The incidence of limb loss is relatively high without treatment.
2. It may permit a lower level of amputation.
3. The risks of the procedure are less than the risk of amputation

From Spittell JA Jr: Peripheral vascular disease: advances in diagnosis and management, *Baylor Cardiology Series* 7:1, 1984.

BOX 31-6

Vasospastic disorders

Raynaud's phenomenon
  Primary (Raynaud's disease)
  Secondary
Livedo reticularis
  Primary
  Secondary
Acrocyanosis
Reflex sympathetic dystrophy
Chronic pernio

From Spittell JA Jr, Spittell PC: Diseases of the aorta and peripheral arteries. In Parmley W, Chatterjee K, editors: *Cardiology*, Philadelphia, 1987, JB Lippincott.

---

tomatic treatment of intermittent claudication. Pentoxifylline (a methylxanthine), which is reported to lower blood viscosity and decrease erythrocyte rigidity, may improve the walking distance of some patients with intermittent claudication. The likelihood of successful treatment with pentoxifylline is increased in a "target" population consisting of persons with a history of intermittent claudication for more than 1 year and an ankle/brachial index of 0.8 or less. Propionyl-L-carnitine, by improving energy metabolism in ischemic skeletal muscle, may also improve walking distance in patients with intermittent claudication.

Reconstructive arterial surgery for chronic occlusive arterial disease has specific indications. These include the relief of disabling claudication (Box 31-4), improved prognosis for limb survival in the diabetic patient (Box 31-5), as well as the need to relieve rest pain and to heal ischemic ulcerations. Percutaneous balloon angioplasty (PTA) provides a means of restoring pulsatile arterial blood flow with reduced morbidity, mortality, and cost when compared to arterial surgery. The indications for PTA are the same as for reconstructive arterial surgery except that PTA is most successful for focal lesions (less than 10 cm long) in the iliac, femoral, and popliteal arteries. Surgical sympathectomy is reserved for the patient in whom restoration of pulsatile blood flow is not possible, as an aid to the healing of ischemic ulceration.

PERIPHERAL ARTERIAL ANEURYSMS

Peripheral arterial aneurysms are most commonly caused by atherosclerosis; thus they are more common in males over 50 years of age. Less common causes of aneurysmal disease include familial tendency, inherited elastic tissue defects (Marfan, Ehlers-Danlos, and fragile X syndromes), infections, arteritides, congenital defects, and trauma. Regardless of etiology, aneurysmal disease is related to weakening of the media of the artery. Hypertension often coexists and directly or indirectly contributes to weakening of the arterial wall and expansion of the aneurysm.

Once initiated, aneurysmal dilation tends to be progressive. Progressive enlargement of the aneurysm and slowing of flow contribute to the formation of laminated mural thrombus, which may progress to complete thrombosis of the lumen or be the source of emboli in the distal arterial circulation; as an aneurysm enlarges, it may exert pressure on surrounding structures and/or rupture.

When uncomplicated, aneurysms produce no symptoms or findings other than a pulsatile mass. Compression of surrounding structures, such as veins, may produce symptoms and signs of chronic venous obstruction. Rupture of an aneurysm presents acutely, usually with evidence of pain and bleeding. Less commonly, when rupture is into a companion vein, the acute development of signs of an arteriovenous fistula is the mode of presentation.

Ultrasound is currently the preferred method to detect and determine the size and extent of an abdominal aortic aneurysm. Computed tomography scanning with intravenous contrast is also an excellent, but more expensive, method of diagnosis. Aortography is usually reserved for patients in whom there is associated peripheral, renal, or mesenteric occlusive arterial disease.

The risk of rupture of an abdominal aortic aneurysm smaller than 4 cm is small but increases progressively as an aneurysm reaches 5 cm in diameter. Elective surgical resection is indicated in most patients with aneurysm diameter exceeding 4.5 cm, in the absence of other significant medical problems. Other indications for surgical intervention include a symptomatic (painful) aneurysm or an aneurysm enlarging under observation. Percutaneous repair of an abdominal aortic aneurysm using advanced endovascular techniques may be indicated in highly selected patients at increased surgical risk.

In the extremities, atherosclerotic aneurysms are most commonly found in the femoral and popliteal arteries. The aneurysm is bilateral in over half of the patients; more than 40% of patients with popliteal artery aneurysm have aneurysmal disease involving the abdominal aorta, femoral, or popliteal arteries. The most common complication of femoropopliteal aneurysms is thromboembolic. Surgical resection produces the best results when carried out before complications occur.

Atheroembolism occasionally complicates abdominal aortic aneurysms, producing a distinctive clinical picture of livedo reticularis, blue toes, hypertension, and renal insufficiency. Prompt recognition of this symptom complex is important because resection of the aneurysm is the only effective treatment. Unilateral atheroembolism—livedo reticularis and blue toes—may occur with femoropopliteal aneurysm; again, resection of the aneurysm is the only effective therapy.

Aneurysms involving the upper extremity arteries are usually the result of blunt or penetrating trauma; in the subclavian artery they result from compression of the artery between the uppermost rib and clavicle. Thromboembolism from mural thrombus to the distal arterial circulation may be the first manifestation of aneurysms in the upper extremity.

VASOSPASTIC DISORDERS

The vasospastic disorders (Box 31-6)—Raynaud's phenomenon, livedo reticularis, acrocyanosis, chronic pernio, and reflex sympathetic dystrophy—involve the small arteries and arterioles in the digits and

Table 31-3 Differential diagnosis of vasospastic and occlusive arterial disease

	VASOSPASTIC DISORDERS	OCCLUSIVE ARTERIAL DISEASE
Arteries involved	Small	All
Color changes	+	±
Claudication	−	+
Absent pulses	−	+
Ischemic ulceration	±	±
Major gangrene	−	±

From Spittell JA Jr: The vasospastic disorders, *Curr Probl Cardiol* 8:1, 1984.

BOX 31-7

Conditions that may cause secondary Raynaud's phenomenon

A. After trauma
  1. Related to occupation
    a. Pneumatic hammer disease
    b. Occupational occlusive arterial disease of the hand
    c. Occupational acroosteolysis
    d. Vasospasm of typists and pianists
  2. Following injury or operation
B. Neurologic conditions
  1. Thoracic outlet syndrome
  2. Carpal tunnel syndrome
  3. Other neurologic diseases
C. Occlusive arterial disease
  1. Arteriosclerosis obliterans
  2. Thromboangiitis obliterans
  3. Postembolic or postthrombotic arterial occlusion
D. Miscellaneous conditions
  1. Scleroderma
  2. Lupus erythematosus
  3. Rheumatoid arthritis
  4. Dermatomyositis
  5. Fabry's disease
  6. Paroxysmal hemoglobinuria
  7. Cold agglutinins or cryoglobulinemia
  8. Primary pulmonary hypertension
  9. Myxedema
  10. Associated with certain neoplasms
  11. Associated with hepatitis B antigenemia
  12. Pheochromocytoma
  13. Ergotism
  14. After combination chemotherapy for testicular cancer

Adapted from Spittell JA Jr: Vasospastic disorders: recognition and management, *Cardiovasc Clin* 10:279, 1980.

BOX 31-8

Procedures to evaluate recent Raynaud's phenomenon

History (include drugs)
Exam
  Thoracic outlet maneuvers
  Allen's test
Lab
  Blood count
  Sedimentation rate
  Protein electrophoresis
  Antinuclear antibody
  Cold agglutinins
  Cryoglobulin
  Urinalysis
  Other "indicated" by history or physical findings

From Spittell JA Jr, Spittell PC: Diseases of the aorta and peripheral arteries. In Parmley W, Chatterjee K, editors: *Cardiology,* Philadelphia, 1987, JB Lippincott.

BOX 31-9

Classification of livedo reticularis

Primary (idiopathic) livedo reticularis
Secondary livedo reticularis
  Connective tissue diseases
  Vasculitis
  Myeloproliferative disorders
  Dysproteinemias
  Atheroembolism (cholesterol embolization)
  After cold injury
  Use of amantadine hydrochloride (Symmetrel)
  Reflex sympathetic dystrophy

From Spittell JA Jr: Vasospastic disorders, *Cardiovasc Clin* 13:75, 1983.

---

skin, producing changes in skin color and temperature. The vasospastic disorders are transient, reversible, and precipitated by exposure to cold, emotional stress, or other vasoconstrictive influences (Table 31-3).

Raynaud's phenomenon, the most common vasospastic disorder, is defined as brief and intermittent color changes (usually triphasic—pallor, cyanosis, rubor) involving the digits and precipitated by exposure to cold or stress. Raynaud's disease (primary Raynaud's phenomenon) is a benign disorder; secondary Raynaud's phenomenon occurs with a broad spectrum of underlying disorders, and at times the Raynaud's phenomenon is the initial clue to the underlying disorder (Box 31-7). An evaluation of the patient with Raynaud's phenomenon should consider the causes listed in Box 31-8. If the initial evaluation is negative, the patient should be observed for a period of 2 years before a diagnosis of Raynaud's disease can be made. Management of all patients includes protection from cold and avoidance of causes of vasoconstriction (tobacco, trauma, and drugs). In addition, a trial of an α-1 adrenergic blocker such as doxazosin (1 to 2 mg QHS) or of a calcium-channel blocker such as nifedipine (30 mg QD

[extended release]) may be useful in reducing vasospastic episodes. Biofeedback is useful in younger patients and in those whose occupation precludes pharmacologic therapy. Sympathectomy is generally reserved for patients with Raynaud's disease who are refractory to the above therapies. In secondary Raynaud's phenomenon, results of sympathectomy are unfortunately less beneficial.

Livedo reticularis is a bluish-purple mottling of the skin of the extremities caused by spasm of dermal arterioles. Like Raynaud's phenomenon, it is classified into primary and secondary forms. The differentiation of primary and secondary livedo reticularis is based on clinical and laboratory features (Box 31-9). The management of idiopathic livedo reticularis includes protection from cold and reassurance; for more symptomatic patients, a trial of doxazosin or nifedipine may be beneficial. Lumbar sympathectomy is reserved for ischemic ulceration not controlled by medication.

Chronic pernio is a vasospastic disorder of the toes seen most commonly in women with a prior history of cold injury. With the onset of cold weather each year, erythematous, cyanotic, and hemorrhagic vesiculation and/or ulcerative lesions of the toes occur. These resolve spontaneously in the spring with warmer weather. Small doses of doxazosin (1 mg daily) are extremely effective in preventing and treating symptomatic chronic pernio.

Acrocyanosis is a benign disorder resulting in almost constant coldness and bluish discoloration of the hands and fingers and occasionally the feet and toes. It is important not to confuse this disorder with the cyanotic phase of Raynaud's phenomenon. A right-to-left shunt and methemoglobinemia should be excluded. Reassurance that it is a benign condition is all that most patients need.

Although reflex sympathetic dystrophy is basically a neurologic disorder, vasospastic phenomena—coldness and cyanosis—are present and can be relieved by doxazosin (1 mg daily), which aids in the rehabilitation process.

ARTERITIS

The arteritides known to involve the extremity arteries include scleroderma, systemic lupus erythematosus, periarteritis nodosa, giant-cell arteritis, and Takayasu's arteritis. Except for the last two, arteriography is of little value in this group of disorders.

Takayasu's arteritis, or pulseless disease, is a chronic focal arteritis of the aorta and large elastic arteries seen predominantly in women less than 40 years of age. Aortic valve regurgitation is often present (Chapter 25). It involves the outer media and adventitia of the aorta and larger elastic arteries. Early in the disease nonspecific systemic manifestations such as malaise, low-grade fever, arthralgia, and weight loss are seen. Later, the symptoms of arterial insufficiency develop depending on the degree of arterial occlusion. Laboratory findings at the onset of the disease include an elevated erythrocyte sedimentation rate, mild anemia, and leukocytosis; later characteristic findings of occlusive arterial disease develop. Arteriography shows focal, segmental stenosis with smooth, tapered walls.

Management in the acute phase of Takayasu's arteritis includes adequate doses of corticosteroids; immunosuppressive agents have been used with success in some cases. In the late inactive phase general measures for occlusive arterial disease are used, and arterial bypass grafting or balloon angioplasty can be used to relieve significant residual ischemia when the activity of the disease is suppressed. The overall prognosis is variable and depends on the arteries involved and the promptness and adequacy of treatment.

Giant-cell arteritis (cranial arteritis, temporal arteritis) is a granulomatous arteritis that affects segments of major arteries and the aorta, particularly branches of the carotid system, in persons more than 60 years of age. Although the most common symptoms of giant-cell arteritis are throbbing headaches and scalp tenderness and the major complication is loss of vision, involvement of other large arteries is being recognized with increasing frequency. Patients may develop intermittent claudication of the upper and/or lower extremities, and this may be a dominant feature. Arteriography is useful when there is peripheral arterial involvement; it shows smooth, tapering segmental stenosis in otherwise normal-appearing arteries. Definitive diagnosis is made by biopsy of a temporal or occipital artery and is recommended since corticosteroid therapy must sometimes be prolonged to control the arteritis. With steroid therapy the activity of giant-cell arteritis subsides; peripheral arterial involvement and resultant symptoms may require a prolonged course of corticosteroid therapy for control. Untreated, giant-cell arteritis is usually self-limited, lasting 1 to 5 years. A rare complication of giant-cell arteritis is aortic dissection.

DISEASES OF THE VEINS

Varicose veins are the most common peripheral vascular disorder affecting the lower extremity. Primary varicose veins are caused by a hereditary weakness of the vein wall and valves, whereas secondary varicose veins result from deep venous obstruction. Obesity, orthostatism, pregnancy, ascites, and right heart failure favor the formation of varicose veins. Symptoms vary from none to complaints of aching, heaviness, and swelling of the lower extremities. On examination dilated tortuous veins are seen with the patient standing, and there may be stasis changes of the skin of the medial aspect of the distal leg. The patient with primary varicose veins will usually describe disease that progresses distally from the upper thigh, whereas secondary varicose veins usually spread proximally from the lower leg. Nonspecific treatment of varicose veins includes adequate elastic support stockings. Sclerotherapy and surgical stripping of varicose veins are indicated for those who fail more conservative therapy or those with recurrent superficial thrombophlebitis or cosmetic problems caused by large varicosities.

Venous thrombosis complicates many types of surgical and medical illnesses and is a common cause of morbidity and mortality despite increased attention to early and accurate diagnosis. An increased incidence of venous thrombosis occurs in patients in the postoperative state and with trauma, congestive heart failure, malignant disease, myeloproliferative disease, obesity, oral contraceptives, tamoxifen, and inherited coagulopathies such as antithrombin III deficiency,

protein C deficiency, protein S deficiency, and activated protein C resistance.

Recurrent venous (and arterial) thrombosis is also associated with the presence of antiphospholipid antibodies, a heterogeneous group of autoantibodies to anionic phospholipids. Primary (idiopathic) and secondary (connective tissue and autoimmune diseases) antiphospholipid syndromes have both been associated with recurrent large- and small-vessel arterial and venous thrombosis, recurrent fetal loss, transient ischemic attack, cerebrovascular accident, cerebral venous thrombosis, thrombocytopenia, and livedo reticularis. Of note is the association of mitral and aortic valvular lesions, especially in persons with recurrent arterial thrombosis. The presence of antiphospholipid antibodies should be suspected in persons with unexplained recurrent venous and arterial thrombosis and in persons with an underlying connective tissue or autoimmune disease. Anticardiolipin antibodies can be readily identified using an enzyme-linked immunosorbent assay (ELISA). Therapy consists of treatment of the underlying disorder, if present, and long-term anticoagulation with warfarin in all patients with venous or arterial thrombosis associated with the presence of antiphospholipid antibodies. Subcutaneous heparin therapy may be an alternative in women of child-bearing age and during pregnancy.

Superficial thrombophlebitis presents as a firm, red, tender cord or nodule and is readily recognized on examination. It must be differentiated from acute lymphangitis, cellulitis, and inflammatory nodular conditions such as erythema nodosum or vasculitis. The management of superficial thrombophlebitis includes warm, moist packs for pain relief and aspirin to decrease associated inflammation. For recurrent disease oral anticoagulant therapy may be used prophylactically.

The clinical presentation of deep venous thrombosis is highly variable and often necessitates the use of noninvasive and invasive diagnostic techniques for confirmation. Noninvasive diagnosis can be accomplished using Doppler flow-velocity studies and impedance plethysmography; these will confirm most deep venous thrombosis proximal to the calf veins. Duplex Doppler imaging can now reliably examine the deep venous system of the leg from the level of the common femoral vein to the distal popliteal vein and has become the noninvasive screening examination of choice for patients suspected of having deep venous thrombosis. The reported sensitivity of duplex Doppler imaging for detecting deep venous thrombosis in the femoral and popliteal veins is 89% to 100%, and the specificity is 97% to 100%. Limitations of duplex Doppler imaging for suspected deep venous thrombosis include poor visualization of the inferior vena cava and iliac veins as well as incomplete visualization of the numerous branches of the deep venous system of the calf. When results are equivocal, contrast venography remains the accepted standard in diagnosis. Pulmonary embolism remains the most serious complication and is seen most commonly with popliteal and thigh vein thrombosis, the latter posing a significantly higher risk.

Management of deep venous thrombosis begins with identification of patients with predisposing factors. Once they are identified, prophylaxis is accomplished by early ambulation, anticoagulant therapy, or intermittent calf compression in the patient at risk. Small-dose subcutaneous heparin (5000 units q8-12h) has proved effective in preventing deep venous thrombosis in general medical and surgical patients.

Once thrombosis has occurred, anticoagulant therapy is the treatment of choice, if no contraindications exist. Initial anticoagulation with intravenous heparin is followed by oral anticoagulant therapy, which is continued for 3 to 6 months. Thrombolytic therapy, with streptokinase or urokinase, followed by heparin and then oral anticoagulant therapy to prevent recurrent thrombosis, is the preferred treatment in extensive deep venous thrombosis (which is more likely to progress to chronic venous insufficiency if heparin therapy is used alone). As with anticoagulant therapy, the main contraindications to thrombolytic therapy relate to bleeding. Additional measures include bed rest with elevation of the involved extremity, along with the application of local warm packs. Surgical treatment of deep venous thrombosis is largely limited to inferior vena cava interruption in patients with a contraindication to anticoagulant or thrombolytic therapy, or in those who have recurrent pulmonary emboli despite adequate anticoagulant therapy.

Chronic venous insufficiency usually results from postphlebitic valvular incompetence or varicose veins with underlying dysfunction of venous valves. The clinical presentation of patients with chronic venous insufficiency is similar to that described for varicose veins, although the manifestations of venous stasis are usually more pronounced. Characteristic findings include dependent edema, cutaneous venous breakdown, and stasis changes (pigmentation, dermatitis, and ulceration). Therapy of chronic venous insufficiency includes adequate elastic support to prevent complications. Stasis dermatitis and stasis ulceration are both treated with bed rest, elevation of the foot of the bed, and intermittent moist dressings of normal saline; skin grafting is desirable for larger ulcers that require more than 2 or 3 weeks to heal. Additional measures include weight reduction in obese patients, low-sodium diets to help prevent leg edema, and adequate elastic support after healing. The overall outlook with chronic venous insufficiency is good with the regular use of adequate elastic support. The topical application of growth factors derived from homologous platelets has been shown to improve the healing rate of venous ulceration. Outpatient treatment with platelet-derived growth factors, applied topically to a wound twice a day for 8 weeks, can be accomplished using approximately 6 ounces of the patient's peripheral blood.

BIBLIOGRAPHY

Atri SC et al: Use of homologous platelet factors in achieving total healing of recalcitrant skin ulcers, *Surgery* 108:508, 1990.

Brevetti G, Perna S, Sabba C et al: Propionyl-L-carnitine in intermittent claudication: double-blind, placebo-controlled, dose titration, multicenter study, *J Am Coll Cardiol* 26:1411-1416, 1995.

Carter SA: Arterial auscultation in peripheral vascular disease, *JAMA* 246:1682, 1981.

Doubilet P, Abrams HL: The cost of underutilization. Percutaneous transluminal angioplasty for peripheral vascular disease, *N Engl J Med* 310:96, 1984.

Evans JM, O'Fallon WM, Hunder GG: Increased incidence of aortic aneurysm and dissection in giant cell (temporal) arteritis: a population-based study, *Ann Intern Med* 122:502-507, 1995.

Harris LM, Koerner NA, Curl GR et al: Active pedal plantar flexion: a hemodynamic measurement of claudication, *J Vasc Technol* 19:115-118, 1995.

Hirsh J: The optimal duration of anticoagulant therapy for venous thrombosis, *N Engl J Med* 332:1710-1711, 1995.

Langsfeld M et al: The use of deep duplex scanning to predict hemodynamically significant aortoiliac stenoses, *J Vasc Surg* 7:395, 1988.

Lensing AWA et al: Detection of deep-vein thrombosis by real-time B-mode ultrasonography, *N Engl J Med* 320:342, 1989.

Lindgarde F et al: Conservative drug treatment in patients with moderately severe chronic occlusive peripheral arterial disease, *Circulation* 80:1549, 1989.

Love PE et al: Antiphospholipid antibodies: anticardiolipin and the lupus anticoagulant in systemic lupus erythematosus (SLE) and in non-SLE disorders, *Ann Intern Med* 112:682, 1990.

McDaniel MD, Cronenwett JL: Basic data related to the natural history of intermittent claudication, *Ann Vasc Surg* 3:273, 1989.

Pairolero PC et al: Subclavian-axillary artery aneurysms, *Surgery* 90:757, 1981.

Pederson OM et al: Compression ultrasonography in hospitalized patients with suspected deep venous thrombosis, *Arch Intern Med* 151:2217, 1991.

Rooke TW et al: Percutaneous transluminal angioplasty in the lower extremities: a 5 year experience, *Mayo Clin Proc* 62:85, 1987.

Rosenfield K, Schainfeld R, Eisner JM: Percutaneous revascularization in peripheral arterial disease, *Curr Prob Cardiol* 21:1-96, 1996.

Spittell JA Jr: Hypertension and arterial aneurysm, *J Am Coll Cardiol* 1:523, 1983.

Spittell JA Jr: Pentoxifylline and intermittent claudication, *Ann Intern Med* 102:126, 1985.

Spittell JA Jr: Some uncommon types of occlusive arterial disease, *Curr Probl Cardiol* 8:3, 1983.

Spittell JA Jr: Vasospastic disorders, *Curr Probl Cardiol* 8:1, 1984.

Spittell PC, Spittell JA: Occlusive arterial disease of the hand due to repetitive blunt trauma: a review with illustrative cases, *Int J Cardiol* 38:281-292, 1993.

CHAPTER

32 Arterial Hypertension

 Norman M. Kaplan

Hypertension remains the most common indication for visits to physicians in the United States. Nonetheless, data from the 1988 to 1991 National Health and Nutrition Examination Survey (NHANES III)

shows that fewer than 25% of hypertensive Americans have their disease well controlled, defined as a blood pressure below 140/90. Comparisons between previous NHANES surveys document continued improvement in the percentages of Americans whose hypertension has been diagnosed (now 69%) and is under treatment (now 53%). Regardless, we and all other societies continue to suffer the consequences of uncontrolled hypertension, in part because of inadequacies in the delivery of health care but mainly because of the nature of hypertension—a chronic disease that is usually asymptomatic but whose treatment imposes numerous burdens.

On the other hand, the NHANES III survey found that about 13 million American adults who had been previously diagnosed as hypertensive were normotensive while receiving no antihypertensive drug therapy. Many of these people may have lowered their blood pressure by lifestyle modifications, but most probably had been misdiagnosed on the basis of too few blood pressure recordings.

We remain in an unsettled situation. More people need to be diagnosed and treated, but many people are being falsely diagnosed and unnecessarily treated. There is a need, then, to consider the evidence about the true frequency of hypertension, the risks of the untreated disease, and the rationale and practices of therapy in hopes of maximizing the benefits while minimizing the risks of treatment.

FREQUENCY OF HYPERTENSION

The frequency of hypertension rises progressively with the age of the population. The data in Fig. 32-1 were obtained in the 1988 to 1991 NHANES III survey of almost 10,000 persons carefully chosen to be a representative sample of the American population. The criterion for the presence of hypertension was a systolic blood pressure of at least 140 mm Hg or a diastolic blood pressure of at least 90 mm Hg.

The rise in systolic blood pressure that is common in older persons is responsible for the progressive increase in the prevalence of hypertension after age 55. Among the general population, diastolic pressures tend to rise little after age 45, reflecting the usual appearance of primary (essential) hypertension by that time. Pure or predominant systolic hypertension should be considered separately from the combined systolic and diastolic elevations seen with primary hypertension. Although they share many risks, they are different in pathogenesis and management.

Another problem with survey data such as those summarized in Fig. 32-1 is their reliance on only a few measurements in the face of a tendency for initial blood pressure readings to be higher than subsequent readings. For example, in the screening program for the Hypertension Detection and Follow-up Program (HDFP), among the white men whose second reading at the initial home visit was over 95 mm Hg diastolic, 44% were below 90 mm Hg at the second examination. Part of this tendency for repeated blood pressures to be lower reflects the regression toward the mean observed with repeated measurements of all biologic variables: outlying values, either high or low, tend to come toward the mean when repeated measurements are taken. A larger part of the tendency probably reflects the relief from some of the anxiety associated with initial examinations. Even after repeated visits, readings taken by a physician are usually higher than those obtained by a nurse and higher to an even greater degree than those obtained by the patient at home. The prevalence of "office" or "white-coat" hypertension is around 20% so that, if at all possible, out-of-the-office readings should be obtained in both diagnosing and monitoring hypertension.

Beyond the tendency for office readings to be higher, the blood pressure is markedly variable under ordinary conditions. This variability has been increasingly apparent with the wider use of ambulatory measurements over periods of 24 hours or longer. As seen in Fig. 32-2, readings vary a good deal during the day, mainly in relation to physical activity, and fall during sleep, only to rise abruptly upon arising. The early morning increase in sudden death, heart attacks, and strokes reflects, at least in part, this abrupt rise in blood pressure.

Precautions in Measuring Blood Pressure

To minimize errors caused by variability, three readings should be taken each time and the average recorded. Additional precautions are given in Box 32-1. Particular emphasis should be given to ensuring

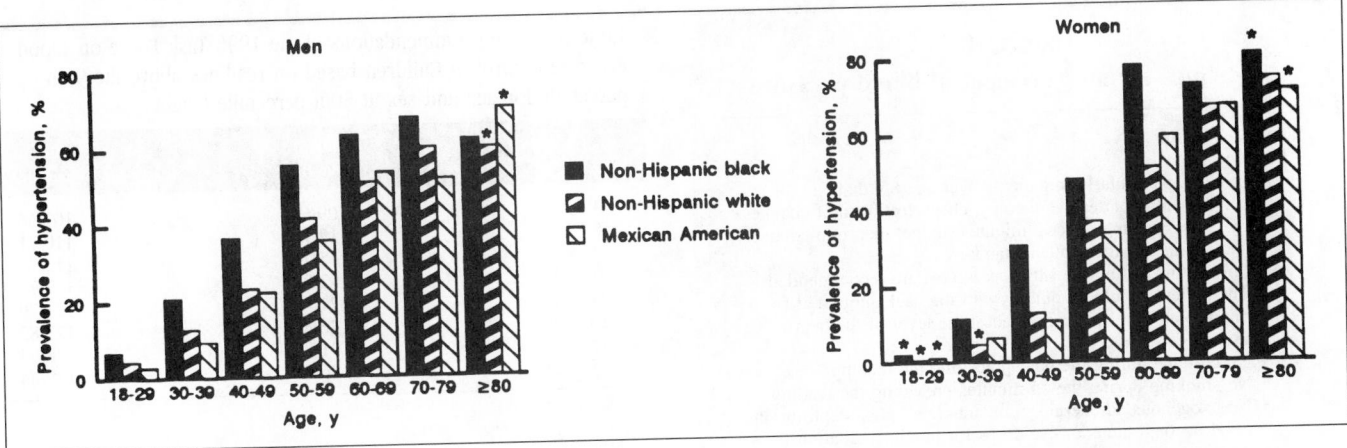

FIGURE 32-1   Prevalence of high blood pressure by age and race/ethnicity for men and women, US population 18 years of age and older. *Estimate based on sample size not meeting minimum requirements of the National Health and Nutrition Examination Survey III design or relative SEM greater than 30%.

(From Burt VL et al: Trends in the prevalence, awareness, treatment, and control of hypertension in the adult US population, *Hypertension* 26:60-69, 1995.)

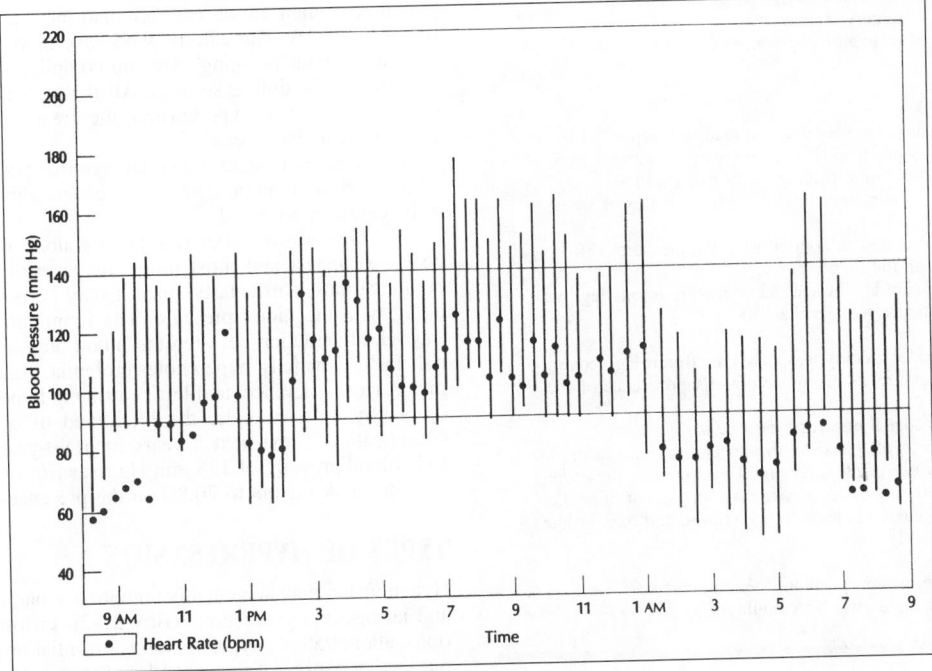

FIGURE 32-2   Computer printout of blood pressures obtained by ambulatory blood pressure monitoring over 24 hours beginning at 9 AM in a 50-year-old man with hypertension receiving no therapy. The patient slept from midnight until 6 AM. •, Heart rate.

(From Zachariah PK, Sheps SG, Smith RL: Defining the roles of home and ambulatory monitoring, *Diagnosis* 10:39-50, 1988.)

that the patient is as near basal level as possible, avoiding cigarettes, coffee, physical exertion, and anxiety-inducing activities. Attention should be paid to the use of properly functioning gauges and appropriately sized cuffs.

In the absence of automatic ambulatory recordings, multiple readings taken by the patient outside the physician's office may be used to establish the usual range of the blood pressure. The average of the readings taken under various circumstances may be taken since there is increasing evidence that the risks of hypertension are most closely predicted by the average of multiple out-of-the-office readings.

In the study by Verdecchia et al. of more than 1200 patients who had a 24-hour ambulatory recording and who were then followed for up to 7 years, there was no increase in cardiovascular events among the 228 patients with "white-coat" hypertension compared to the nor-

motensives. On the other hand, those with hypertension suffered more than a threefold increase in cardiovascular morbidity, which increased another threefold in those whose pressures did not fall by more than 10% during sleep, referred to as *nondippers*.

Definition of Hypertension

Regardless of the problems in defining the usual or average blood pressure, there is a need for standard criteria to diagnose and categorize patients by. Despite the arbitrariness of the division, the upper limit of normal blood pressure is usually taken as 140/90 mm Hg in the office setting and as 160/95 mm Hg in community screening.

In view of the expected variability, a practical approach is to consider initial readings greater than 140/90 mm Hg as "suspicious" and

BOX 32-1

Guidelines for measurement of blood pressure

Patient conditions
  Posture
  • Initially, particularly in patients over age 65, diabetic, or receiving antihypertensive therapy, check for postural changes by taking readings after 5 minutes supine, then immediately and 2 minutes after patient stands.
  • For routine follow-up, sitting pressures are recommended. The patient should sit quietly with the back supported for 5 minutes and the arm supported at the level of the heart.
  Circumstances
  • No caffeine during the hour preceding the reading.
  • No smoking during the 15 minutes preceding the reading.
  • No exogenous adrenergic stimulants (e.g., phenylephrine in nasal decongestants or eye drops for pupillary dilation).
  • A quiet, warm setting.
  • Home readings taken under varying circumstances and 24-hour ambulatory recordings may be preferable and more accurate in predicting subsequent cardiovascular disease.
Equipment
  • Cuff size: The bladder should encircle and cover two thirds of the length of the arm; if it does not, place the bladder over the brachial artery. If bladder is too small, high readings may result.
  • Manometer: Aneroid gauges should be calibrated every 6 months against a mercury manometer.
  • For infants, use ultrasound equipment (e.g., the Doppler method).
Technique
  Number of readings
  • On each occasion, take at least two readings, separated by as much time as is practical. If readings vary by more than 5 mm Hg, take additional readings until two are close.
  • For diagnosis, obtain three sets of readings at least 1 week apart.
  • Initially, take pressure in both arms; if the pressures differ, use the arm with the higher pressure.
  • If the arm pressure is elevated, take pressure in one leg, particularly in patients younger than 30.
  Performance
  • Inflate the bladder quickly to a pressure 20 mm Hg above the the systolic pressure, as recognized by disappearance of the radial pulse.
  • Deflate the bladder 3 mm Hg every second.
  • Record the Korotkoff phase V (disappearance), except in children, in whom use of phase IV (muffling) may be preferable.
  • If the Korotkoff sounds are weak, have the patient raise the arm, open and close the hand 5 to 10 times, and then inflate the bladder quickly.
  Recordings
  Note the pressure, patient position, the arm, cuff size (e.g., 140/90, seated, right arm, large adult cuff).

From Kaplan NM: *Clinical hypertension,* ed 6, Baltimore, 1994, Williams & Wilkins.

Table 32-1　Recommendations of the 1996 Task Force on Blood Pressure Control in Children based on readings above the 95th percentile for age and sex at 50th percentile height

AGE (YR)	BOYS (mm Hg)	GIRLS (mm Hg)
3	109/65	107/66
5	112/71	110/71
7	115/76	113/74
9	117/79	117/77
11	121/80	121/79
13	126/82	125/82
15	131/83	128/83
17	136/87	129/84

ing associated with a greater overall risk for both stroke and coronary heart disease (Fig. 32-3). In the Framingham study, the systolic blood pressure was more closely correlated with risk than was the diastolic.

A number of other factors are also responsible for the development of the cardiovascular complications of hypertension. The patient's demographic features play a role. At any given level of blood pressure, women are at less risk than men, and blacks are at higher risk than whites. The elderly, who have more underlying atherosclerosis as a result of aging, develop complications more quickly than the younger in similar settings. All things being equal, however, the earlier the onset of hypertension, the greater the eventual likelihood of cardiovascular disease.

The degree of target organ damage that occurs in response to any given level of blood pressure varies considerably and obviously needs to be carefully assessed.

The presence of other risk factors along with hypertension may be the strongest and most important determinant of cardiovascular complications, particularly since it may be possible to modify them along with the blood pressure. The Framingham study clearly portrays the interaction between the blood pressure and the other major risk factors, namely hypercholesterolemia, cigarette smoking, abnormal glucose tolerance, and left ventricular hypertrophy on electrocardiography. For example, the likelihood of a major cardiovascular complication in the next 8 years for a 40-year-old man with a systolic blood pressure of 195 mm Hg rises from 4.6% in the absence of the other risk factors to 70.8% in the presence of all four of them.

TYPES OF HYPERTENSION

Hypertension may accompany numerous renal, hormonal, neurologic, and iatrogenic dysfunctions (Box 32-2). In truly unselected populations, about 95% of hypertension is essential or primary, that is, without known cause. Of the secondary forms, excluding those related to alcohol, oral contraceptives, and other drugs, renal parenchymal disease is most common, responsible for 2% to 3%. Renovascular disease is the only other mechanism responsible for as much as 1% of hypertension. Among younger women, oral contraceptive use is the most common mechanism for secondary hypertension. The various adrenal hyperfunctions, medullary (i.e., pheochromocytoma) and cortical (i.e., Cushing's syndrome or primary aldosteronism), are involved in less than 0.5% of all hypertension.

PATHOPHYSIOLOGY

The cause of primary (essential) hypertension is unknown. All the various factors known to affect the blood pressure have been implicated, and it is likely that many of these are involved, because if only one were responsible, the counterregulatory actions of the others should work to return the pressure to normal. In the search for causes, multiple hypotheses have been proposed, linking various factors directly or indirectly to the hemodynamic fault of established hypertension, namely an increased peripheral vascular resistance (Fig. 32-4).

The most widely held views implicate a renal defect in sodium

to diagnose "hypertension" only if the average of readings at a third office visit is higher than 140/90 mm Hg. The term *labile* should be discarded. Patients with only occasional high readings may be called *borderline* and advised to keep close check on their blood pressure while also modifying their lifestyles to prevent a further rise. Since the systolic blood pressure tends to rise with the progressive large-vessel atherosclerosis that usually accompanies aging, a level of 160 mm Hg after age 60 seems to be an appropriate upper limit of normal.

For children, the recommendations of the 1996 Task Force on Blood Pressure Control in Children are based on readings persistently above the 95th percentile for age and sex (Table 32-1).

Risks of Hypertension

The level of the blood pressure remains the most direct risk factor for premature cardiovascular disease, every increment of pressure be-

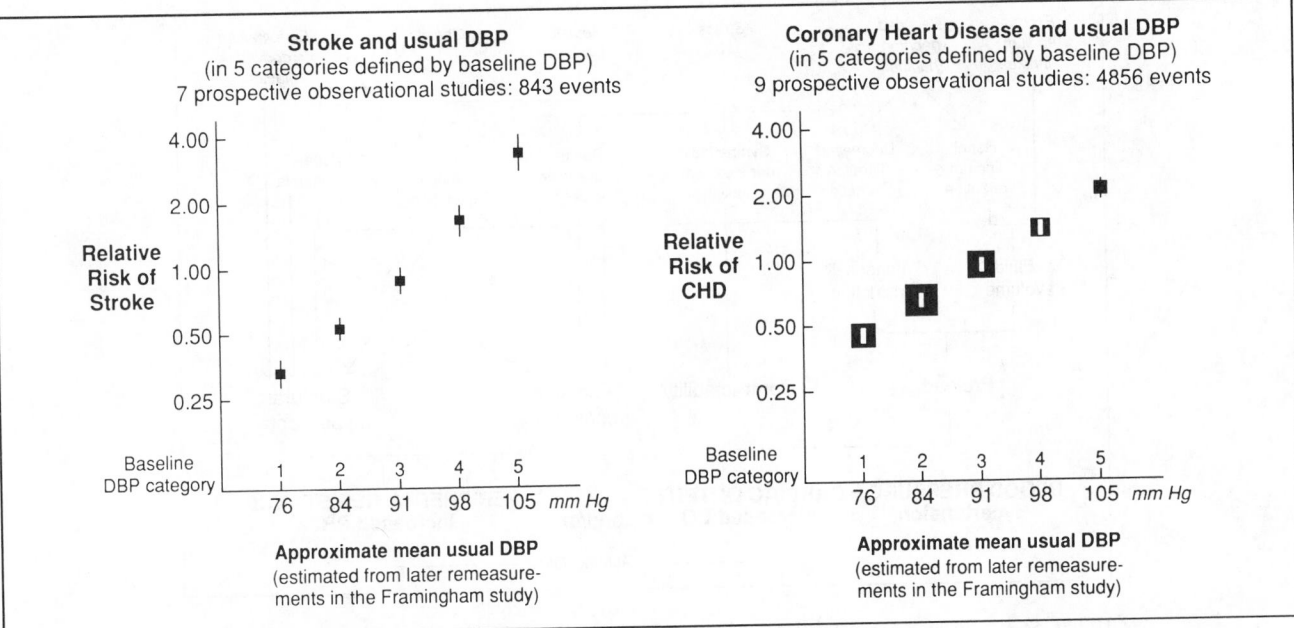

FIGURE 32-3 The relative risks of stroke and of coronary heart disease, estimated from the combined results of the prospective observational studies, for each of five categories of diastolic blood pressure. The solid squares represent disease risks in each category relative to risk in the whole study population; the sizes of the squares are proportional to the number of events in each DBP category, and 95% confidence intervals for the estimates of relative risk are denoted by vertical lines.

(From MacMahon S et al: *Lancet* 335:765, 1990.)

BOX 32-2
Types of hypertension

I. Systolic and diastolic hypertension
  A. Primary, essential, or idiopathic
  B. Secondary
    1. Renal
      a. Renal parenchymal disease
        (1) Acute glomerulonephritis
        (2) Chronic nephritis
        (3) Polycystic disease
        (4) Connective tissue diseases
        (5) Diabetic nephropathy
        (6) Hydronephrosis
      b. Renovascular
      c. Renin-producing tumors
      d. Renoprival
      e. Primary sodium retention (Liddle's syndrome, Gordon's syndrome)
    2. Endocrine
      a. Acromegaly
      b. Hypothyroidism
      c. Hyperthyroidism
      d. Hypercalcemia (hyperparathyroidism)
      e. Adrenal
        (1) Cortical
          (a) Cushing's syndrome
          (b) Primary aldosteronism
          (c) Congenital adrenal hyperplasia
        (2) Medullary: pheochromocytoma
      f. Extraadrenal chromaffin tumors
      g. Carcinoid
      h. Exogenous hormones
        (1) Estrogen
        (2) Glucocorticoids
        (3) Mineralocorticoids: licorice
        (4) Sympathomimetics
        (5) Tyramine-containing foods and monoamine oxidase inhibitors

    3. Coarctation of the aorta
    4. Pregnancy-induced hypertension
    5. Neurologic disorders
      a. Increased intracranial pressure
        (1) Brain tumor
        (2) Encephalitis
        (3) Respiratory acidosis
      b. Sleep apnea
      c. Quadriplegia
      d. Acute porphyria
      e. Familial dysautonomia
      f. Lead poisoning
      g. Guillain-Barré syndrome
    6. Acute stress, including surgery
      a. Psychogenic hyperventilation
      b. Hypoglycemia
      c. Burns
      d. Pancreatitis
      e. Alcohol withdrawal
      f. Sickle cell crisis
      g. Postresuscitation
      h. Postoperative
    7. Increased intravascular volume
    8. Alcohol, drugs, etc.
II. Systolic hypertension
  A. Increased cardiac output
    1. Aortic valvular regurgitation
    2. Arteriovenous fistula, patent ductus
    3. Thyrotoxicosis
    4. Paget's disease of bone
    5. Beriberi
    6. Hyperkinetic circulation
  B. Rigidity of aorta

From Kaplan NM: *Clinical hypertension,* ed 6, Baltimore, 1994, Williams & Wilkins.

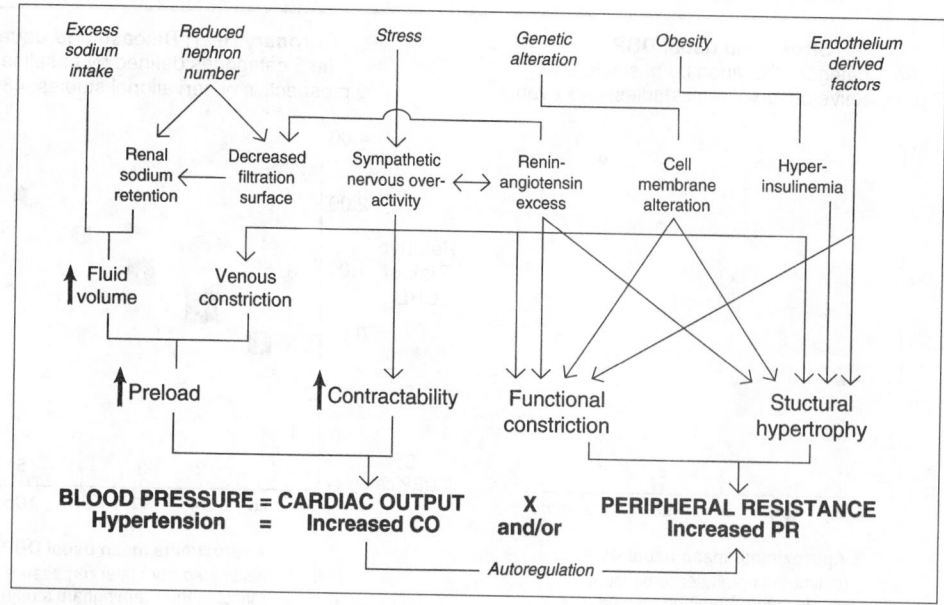

FIGURE 32-4   Some of the factors involved in the control of blood pressure that affect the basic equation: Blood pressure = cardiac output × peripheral resistance.
(From Kaplan NM: *Clinical hypertension,* ed 6, Baltimore, 1994, Williams & Wilkins.)

excretion, often caused by a congenital deficiency of nephrons seen in infants of low birth weight, along with a certain threshold level of sodium intake. Some believe that stress by itself is sufficient. More recently, an inherited or acquired defect in sodium transport across cell membranes has been postulated. We will review the evidence for these mechanisms, with the awareness that, whatever else is responsible, heredity must be in the background. As much as half of the variability of blood pressure in the population can be ascribed to heredity, and the blood pressure tends to be similar in first-degree relatives. Inheritance appears to be polygenic.

Increased Peripheral Resistance

Once initiated, the elevated pressure is maintained by an increased peripheral vascular resistance. Most of this resistance arises in small arteries and arterioles, whose proportionately large amount of smooth muscle provides a high wall/lumen ratio. When these smooth muscle cells contract or hypertrophy, relatively small decreases in luminal diameter induce marked increases in resistance. Folkow has postulated that those who are genetically predisposed have an exaggerated or reinforced pressor response to stress, which, by inducing an increase in perfusion pressure, leads to an immediate protective functional vasoconstriction to normalize tissue blood flow via the myogenic reflex mechanism, autoregulation. Soon thereafter, smooth muscle hypertrophy and the deposition of collagen and interstitial material lead to persistent structural thickening of resistance vessels.

Folkow's original hypothesis has been expanded to include the possible role of one or more trophic mechanisms that may cause hypertrophy directly (Fig. 32-5). Insulin is a likely candidate to be one of the trophic mechanisms in primary hypertension, particularly since high plasma insulin levels and resistance to insulin have been described in nonobese hypertensive patients as well as those who are obese.

In addition to various mechanisms that lead to increased contraction and hypertrophy, other forces are involved in relaxation of blood vessels (Fig. 32-6). One, an endothelium-derived relaxing factor (EDRF) that is now known to be nitric oxide (NO), may be deficient, whereas endothelin, a potent vasoconstrictor, may be increased. The role of these and a number of other endothelium-derived relaxing and contracting factors may turn out to be important, but their place in the pathogenesis of hypertension remains uncertain.

Stress and the Sympathetic Nervous System

As shown in Figs. 32-3 and 32-4, stress-induced activation of the sympathetic nervous system may lead to hypertension. Additional evidence for a direct mechanism is presented first. Then the evidence for an indirect path involving renal sodium retention is reviewed.

Persons under high levels of stress may develop more hypertension. Perhaps the best demonstration was by Cobb and Rose, who showed that highly stressed air traffic controllers had 5.6 times the annual incidence of hypertension of less-stressed weekend pilots who started with similar blood pressures and other characteristics. Less direct evidence indicates a higher prevalence of hypertension among American blacks and less-educated whites.

Stress may increase the release of epinephrine from the adrenal medulla and norepinephrine from adrenergic neurons activated by central nervous system (CNS) stimulation. High levels of circulating epinephrine mediate α-adrenergic effects including increases in heart rate and cardiac output. Epinephrine may also be taken up by β₂ receptors on the presynaptic neuronal membrane and may enhance release of norepinephrine from storage granules. Thereby the transient epinephrine surge may produce considerably more prolonged vasoconstriction.

Higher levels of circulating epinephrine and norepinephrine have been found in hypertensives in the majority of carefully performed comparisons of matched normotensive and hypertensive persons. Moreover, the normotensive offspring of hypertensive parents have been shown to display an exaggerated pressor response to the stress of complex arithmetic problems compared with the similarly normotensive children of normotensive parents. Therefore all the ingredients suggested by Folkow are in place: increased stress, increased levels of circulating catechols, and increased pressor reactivity to stress. Whether these can directly lead to sustained hypertension by inducing structural hypertrophy of resistance vessels remains to be seen.

Renal Sodium Retention

The stress-induced activation of the sympathetic nervous system could also lead to hypertension via an indirect route, involving stimulation of renal sodium retention. One way or another, the renal retention of part of the daily sodium intake—at an absolute rate too small to measure—may be an essential part of the initiation of hyperten-

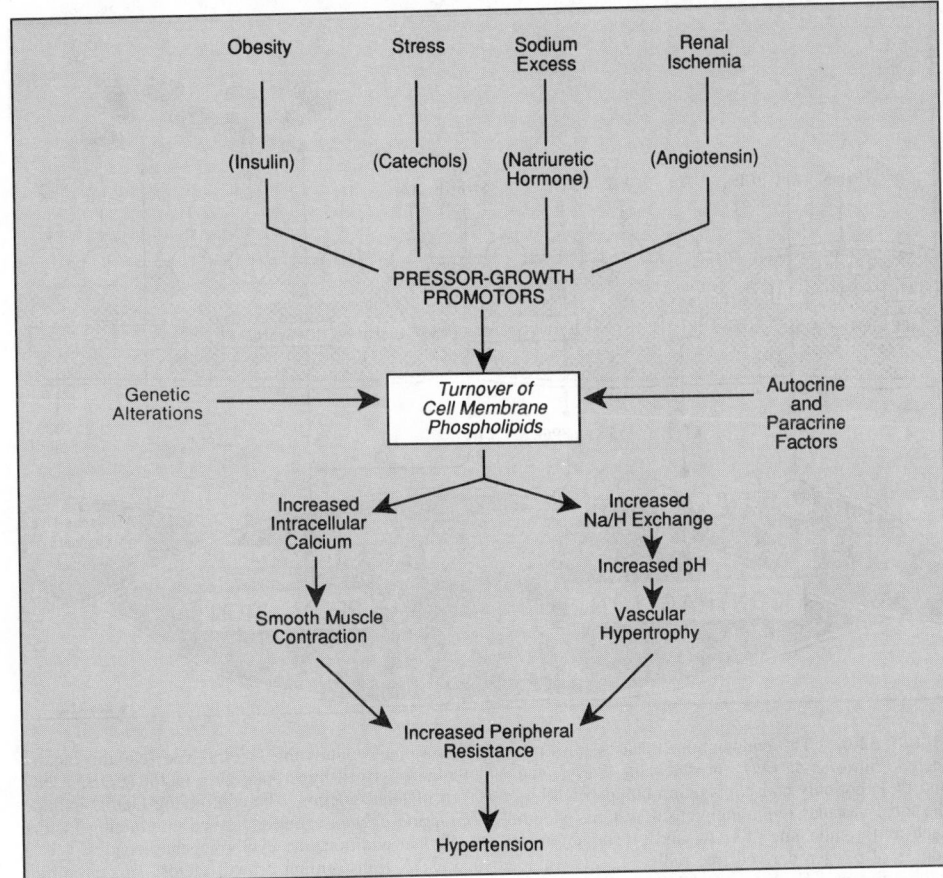

FIGURE 32-5   Scheme for the induction of hypertension by numerous pressor hormones that act as vascular growth promotors.
(From Kaplan NM: *Clinical hypertension,* ed 6, Baltimore, 1994, Williams & Wilkins.)

sion. Guyton has long argued that the kidneys have to reset their normal pressure-natriuresis relationship for hypertension to develop. Otherwise, whenever pressure might rise for whatever reason, the prompt natriuresis that normally occurs in the face of higher pressure would promptly return the pressure exactly to normal. This resetting could be explained by a greater constriction of the renal efferent arterioles, decreasing renal blood flow more than glomerular filtration and thereby increasing filtration fraction and eventually increasing sodium retention.

To explain renal sodium retention, Brenner and co-workers have postulated a congenital deficit in the number of nephrons as a result of intrauterine growth retardation seen in low-birth-weight infants (Fig. 32-7). Barker has documented an increase in the subsequent development of both hypertension and cardiovascular disease during adult life in those with low birth weight compared to those of normal birth weight.

The renal retention of sodium and water, however it arises, would expand body fluid volume, if not in absolute values at least in relative excess for the level of blood pressure and the volume of the circulatory bed.

This higher-than-expected blood volume for the level of pressure could increase cardiac output, which according to the concept of autoregulation, would lead to an increased peripheral resistance. Such a pattern of high output changing over to high resistance has been documented by Lund-Johansen in a small number of hypertensives left untreated for 20 years. Whether this is the usual hemodynamic pattern for most patients is uncertain.

Some believe it is unnecessary to invoke an initially high cardiac output but rather hold to the view that peripheral resistance is primarily increased. Such an increase could come about very simply by an increase in the sodium and water content of vascular tissue, which

could be a passive consequence of an expanded plasma volume. But in recent years, more active ways to explain an increase in intracellular sodium within vascular tissue have been proposed along with other explanations for the hypertension-inducing effect of the increased intracellular sodium.

Increased Intracellular Sodium and Calcium

At least two distinct mechanisms have been proposed to explain the origin of increased intracellular sodium in hypertension. Both postulate a defect in the normal movement of sodium across the cell membrane, a process that preserves the usual sodium concentration within cells at around 10 mmol/L with plasma at a concentration of 140 mmol/L. One hypothesis proposes an acquired inhibitor of the $(Na^+ + K^+)$-ATPase pump, the major physiologic regulator of sodium transport; the other proposes an inherited defect in one or more of the multiple sodium transport systems.

Acquired Pump Inhibitor. This hypothesis begins with the renal retention of sodium and water, which expands the total extracellular fluid volume or some portion of it, so that the secretion of a natriuretic hormone is activated in an attempt to shrink the expanded volume back to normal. In animal models, the source of this natriuretic hormone appears to be the AV3V region of the hypothalamus. After more than 30 years of active search in numerous laboratories, this putative hormone has only recently been identified as ouabain. In the meantime, another natriuretic factor arising from cardiac atrial tissue has been identified and synthesized. This atrial natriuretic factor dilates the renal vascular bed while increasing sodium excretion but does not inhibit the $(Na^+ + K^+)$-ATPase pump nor affect sodium efflux from cells.

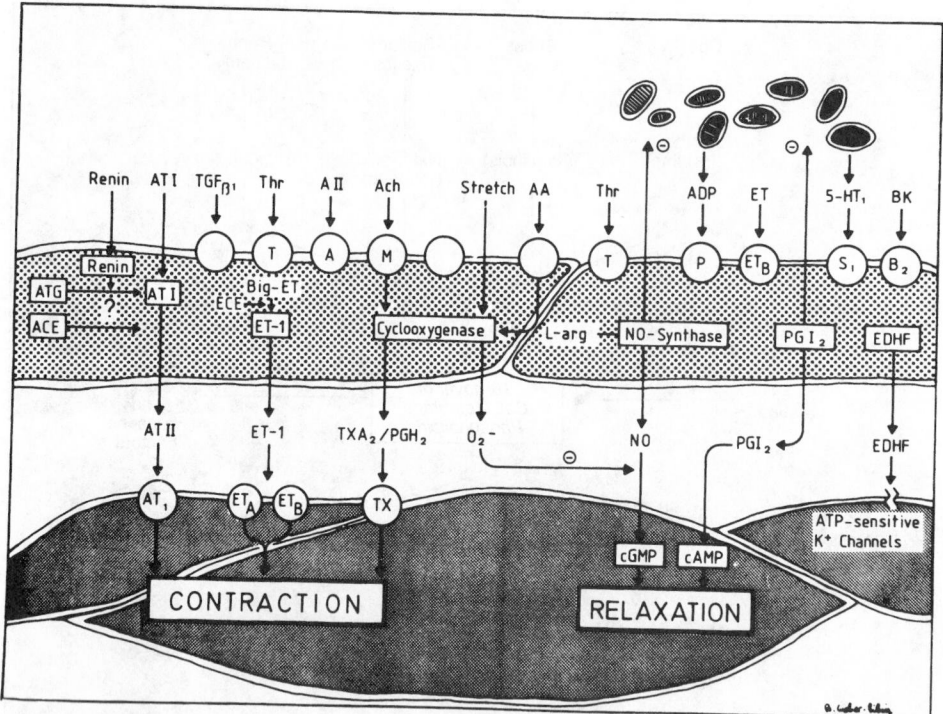

FIGURE 32-6 The endothelium releases both relaxing factors and contracting factors. The relaxing factors include nitric oxide *(NO)*, prostacyclin *(PGI$_2$)*, and endothelium-derived hyperpolarizing factor *(EDHF)*. NO and PGI$_2$ not only cause relaxation but also inhibition (O) of platelet function. The contracting factors include the local vascular renin-angiotensin system, endothelin *(ET)*, and cyclooxygenase-derived contracting factors such as thromboxane *(TX)* A$_2$ and prostaglandin H$_2$ *(PGH$_2$)*. In addition, the cyclooxygenase pathway is a source of oxygen-derived free radicals. *ATI*, Angiotensin I; *TGF*, transforming growth factor; *Thr*, thrombin; *AII*, angiotensin II; *Ach*, acetylcholine; *AA*, arachidonic acid; *5-HT$_1$*, 5-hydroxytryptamine-1; *BK*, bradykinin; *T*, thrombin receptor; *A*, angiotensin receptor; *M*, muscarinic receptor; *P*, purinic receptor; *S$_1$*, serotonin receptor; *B$_2$*, bradykinin receptor; *ATG*, angiotensinogen; *ACE*, angiotensin converting enzyme; *ECE*, endothelin converting enzyme; *L-arg*, L-arginine; *cAMP*, cyclic AMP; *cGMP*, cyclic GMP.

(From Lüscher TF: The endothelium in hypertension, *J Hypertens* 12(suppl 10):S105-116, 1994.)

The inhibitory action of the ouabain natriuretic hormone on $(Na^+ + K^+)$-ATPase pump activity in the kidney would induce a natriuresis, thereby countering the retention of sodium and returning the extracellular fluid to normal. At the same time, however, the inhibition of the pump in vascular smooth muscle would reduce sodium efflux, increasing intracellular sodium concentration. As postulated by Blaustein and Hamlyn, this would immediately increase the concentration of free calcium within these cells, causing an increase in tone and reactivity in response to any pressor stimulus. Thereby peripheral resistance is increased and hypertension induced.

Inherited Defect in Transport. Alterations in other membrane transport mechanisms for sodium have been measured in red and white blood cells both of patients with primary hypertension and of the normotensive children of hypertensive parents. Most investigators find an increased rate of Na^+, Li^+-countertransport, which may be a marker for Na^+-H^+ exchange. The field is confused with multiple assays, mostly involving highly artificial conditions, usually showing some alteration in most hypertensives. Beyond the confusion as to the type and frequency of alterations in sodium flux mechanisms, there remains the much more fundamental issue of their pathogenetic role in hypertension. None of these alterations have been measured in human vascular smooth muscle cells, so the role of this mechanism remains uncertain.

Increased concentrations of free intracellular calcium could also arise more directly from defective binding of calcium to the cell membrane, as shown by the Russian workers Postnov and Orlov.

Increased Sodium Intake

Any theory about the pathogenesis of hypertension should account for the observation that the intake of increased amounts of dietary

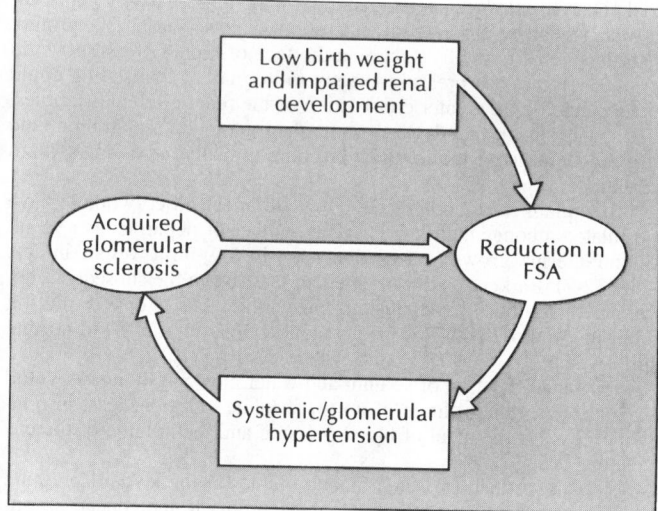

FIGURE 32-7 Hypothesis: the risks of developing essential hypertension and progressive renal injury in adult life are increased as a result of congenital oligonephropathy, an inborn deficit of filtration surface area *(FSA)* caused by impaired renal development. Low birth weight, caused by intrauterine growth retardation and/or prematurity, contributes to this oligonephropathy. Systemic and glomerular hypertension in later life results in progressive glomerular sclerosis, further reducing FSA and thereby perpetuating a vicious cycle, leading, in the extreme, to end-stage renal failure.

(From Brenner BM, Chertow GM: *Am J Kidney Dis* 23:171-175, 1994.)

sodium is necessary but not sufficient in itself. The evidence for the involvement of sodium, although it remains circumstantial, is impressive. It includes the following:

1. Animal models in which hypertension develops in those genetically susceptible when they are given large sodium loads. The most impressive of these animal studies is that of Denton et al., who induced hypertension in a group of previously normotensive chimpanzees by adding progressively more sodium to their diet over 20 months, up to a high-normal level for humans. The average blood pressure rose 33/10 mm Hg, only to promptly fall to normotensive levels when the extra sodium was removed from the diet.

2. Multiple epidemiologic surveys correlating sodium intake and hypertension: those ingesting less than 50 to 75 mmol of sodium per day have little or no hypertension; those ingesting more than the threshold level of 100 to 150 mmol per day have a certain incidence of hypertension that is increased little if at all by higher levels of sodium intake.

3. Evidence that when groups of persons introduce more sodium into their diets, their mean blood pressures tend to rise.

4. Conversely, there is usually a 5 to 10 mm Hg fall in blood pressure when dietary sodium intake is reduced in patients with hypertension.

5. The induction of hypertension by the retention of sodium by exogenous mineralocorticoids or by the loss of renal function.

6. The demonstration that normotensive children of hypertensive parents tend to increase their blood pressure when given sodium loads and retain sodium during periods of emotional stress.

To these may be added the previously noted increased concentration of sodium within blood cells and the vascular smooth muscle tissue of patients with hypertension. All this evidence strongly supports a role for sodium, at least in the half of hypertensives who are sodium sensitive (i.e., whose pressures rise when given a sodium load). Modern humans have been ingesting a high-sodium diet only in very recent times. Our ancestors consumed a naturally low-sodium, high-potassium diet. Much of what is attributed to the "unnatural" sodium load may be equally attributable to the "unnatural" reduction in potassium intake that has followed the substitution of processed foods for natural ones.

Other Environmental Mechanisms

Beyond too much sodium or too little potassium, a lower level of calcium intake, an excess of calories, and the ingestion of ethanol have also been found to be associated with hypertension. The data concerning calcium intake remain fragmentary and conflicting. Furthermore, no logical explanation as to how a reduced calcium intake could evoke a rise in blood pressure has been provided. Since increased concentrations of calcium in the blood or within cells raise the blood pressure, and since drugs that antagonize the entry or actions of calcium lower the blood pressure, skepticism remains appropriate.

The evidence for a connection between obesity and hypertension is much more solid. Although the specific mechanism is unknown, increased levels of plasma insulin may provide a common bond, particularly in those with predominately upper body obesity, the typical pattern in middle-aged males (Fig. 32-8). In addition to hypertension, dyslipidemias and type II diabetes often accompany the hyperinsulinemia of upper body obesity.

Of even greater interest, hyperinsulinemia secondary to resistance to insulin-mediated glucose utilization in peripheral muscles has been documented in about half of *nonobese* hypertensives. The role of insulin resistance and resultant hyperinsulinemia remains under intensive study. As will be noted later in this chapter, both nondrug and drug therapies may alter insulin sensitivity and these effects may prove to be important in the overall impact of therapy on cardiovascular risk.

Ethanol, in excess amounts, exerts a pressor action. Those who consume an average of 2 or more ounces a day, as found in four to five bottles of beer, glasses of wine, or potions of 80-proof distilled spirits, may thereby develop considerable hypertension. In view of the large number of persons who consume that much or more, ethanol abuse is probably the most common form of rapidly reversible

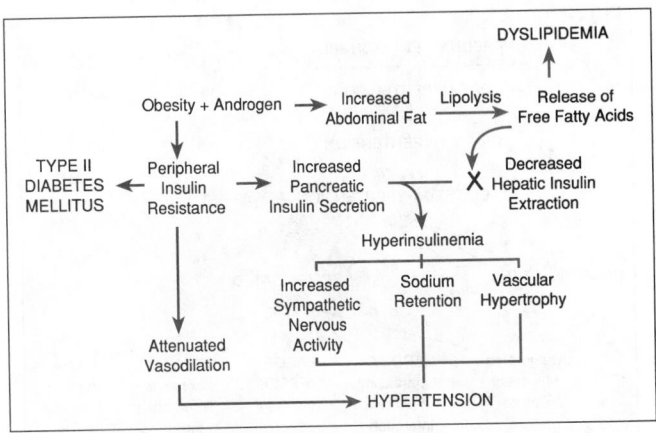

FIGURE 32-8 Overall scheme for the mechanism by which upper body obesity could promote glucose intolerance, hypertriglyceridemia, and hypertension via hyperinsulinemia.

(From Kaplan NM: *Clinical hypertension*, ed 6, Baltimore, 1994, Williams & Wilkins.)

hypertension. On the other hand, ingestion of one to two drinks per day has been associated with less coronary disease.

Other Postulated Mechanisms

Hypertension may arise from either excessive pressor or deficient depressor mechanisms. As shown in Fig. 32-4, the renin-angiotensin system may be activated by stress along with the sympathetic nervous system. Laragh has long argued for a primary role of renin in the pathogenesis of primary hypertension. At the least, it is probably involved in those with high renin levels, since an elevated blood pressure would be expected to inhibit the release of renin through the juxtaglomerular baroreceptors so that low renin levels would be expected.

As noted previously, a host of endothelium-derived vasoactive substances have been identified, and they may play an important role in the pathogenesis of hypertension (see Fig. 32-6). Too much vasoconstricting by endothelin or other constricting factors or too little vasodilation by nitric oxide, the major endothelium-derived relaxing factor, may be critical.

We are left with a mass of disparate data that may never fit together logically. However, while the search for the mechanisms continues, hints suggest preventive actions, including avoidance of obesity, regular physical activity, moderate restriction of dietary sodium and increase in dietary potassium, and moderation of alcohol intake.

In view of the known difficulties in controlling the disease, the intrinsic wisdom of applying these probably effective measures to the entire population seems logical, even if it is not certain that they will prevent hypertension but certain that they pose no danger, even to those not predisposed.

NATURAL HISTORY OF ESSENTIAL HYPERTENSION

If left untreated, patients may proceed along the course shown in Fig. 32-9. Fewer are now proceeding into an accelerated malignant course, and the mortality, and probably the morbidity, from both coronary and cerebral vascular disease has been declining steadily in the United States since the late 1960s. We are uncertain, however, about the contribution of the greater recognition and treatment of hypertension to these improvements. Most analyses of the evidence suggest that there has been a fall in the incidence of coronary and cerebral vascular disease in addition to improved survival of patients after the complication develops.

Nonetheless, hypertension remains both common and poorly managed in much of the population. The problem is particularly prevalent among blacks, who have a higher incidence of hypertension and a higher mortality rate at every level of blood pressure than do whites.

Part of the problem among all populations is the asymptomatic

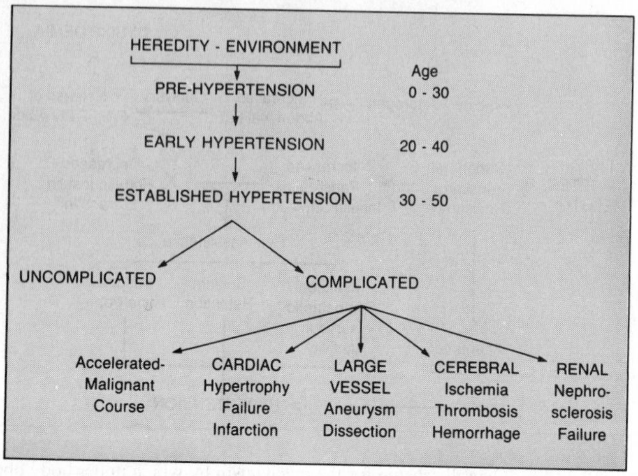

FIGURE 32-9   A representation of the natural history of untreated essential hypertension.

(From Kaplan NM: *Clinical hypertension,* ed 6, Baltimore, 1994, Williams & Wilkins.)

Table 32-2   Overall guide to workup of hypertension

DIAGNOSIS	DIAGNOSTIC PROCEDURE	
	INITIAL	ADDITIONAL
Chronic renal disease	Urinalysis, BUN or creatinine, sonography	Renin assay, renal biopsy, IVP
Renovascular disease	Bruit, duplex sonography, isotopic renography and plasma renin before and 1 hr after 50 mg captopril	Aortogram, renal vein renins
Coarctation	Blood pressure in legs	Aortogram
Primary aldosteronism	Plasma potassium Plasma renin:aldosterone ratio	Urinary potassium; plasma aldosterone after saline
Cushing's syndrome	AM plasma cortisol after 1 mg dexamethasone at bedtime	Urinary cortisol after variable doses of dexamethasone
Pheochromocytoma	Spot urine for metanephrine	Urinary VMA and catechols; plasma catechols, basal, and after 0.3 mg clonidine

From Kaplan NM: *Clinical hypertension,* ed 6, Baltimore, 1994, Williams & Wilkins. *BUN,* Blood urea nitrogen; *IVP,* intravenous pyelogram; *VMA,* vanillylmandelic acid.

BOX 32-3
Features of "inappropriate" hypertension

1. Onset before age 20 or after age 50
2. Markedly elevated pressures, particularly with grade III or IV funduscopic changes
3. Organ damage
   a. Funduscopic findings of grade II or higher
   b. Serum creatinine >1.5 mg/dl
   c. Cardiomegaly (on radiograph or echocardiogram) or left ventricular hypertrophy (on ECG)
4. Features suggesting secondary causes
   a. Unprovoked hypokalemia
   b. Abdominal diastolic bruit
   c. Variable pressures with tachycardia, sweating, tremor
   d. Family history of renal or endocrine disease
   e. Hematuria, palpable kidneys
   f. Decreased femoral pulses
5. Poor response to therapy that is usually effective

---

nature of the disease for the first 10 to 20 years, while it is provoking cardiac and vascular damage. With use of more sensitive diagnostic procedures such as echocardiography, such damage is being recognized to be even more common than previously realized. Although some left ventricular hypertrophy may be either primary to the development of hypertension or essential for the maintenance of cardiac output in the face of an increased afterload, left ventricular hypertrophy has been observed by echocardiography in as many as half of young patients with asymptomatic, uncomplicated, mild hypertension.

Diagnostic Tests

For most patients, only a hematocrit, urinalysis, automated blood chemistry study (electrolytes, glucose, creatinine, and cholesterol), and an electrocardiogram (ECG) are needed. More testing should be done on those with features that suggest secondary hypertension (Box 32-3). Selectivity in the performance of screening tests is needed, since more false positives than true positives would be uncovered if procedures such as an intravenous pyelogram (IVP) or assay of plasma renin activity (PRA) were performed on all hypertensives.

Those found to have one or more features suggestive of a secondary form of hypertension during the initial screening by the history, physical examination, and routine laboratory work should have the additional confirmatory studies shown in Table 32-2 for the most com-

mon secondary causes. The choice and sequence of confirmatory tests will vary with the type of patient and circumstances. As an example, a young woman with the sudden onset of severe hypertension and an abdominal bruit should probably immediately have a selective renal arteriogram, in view of the high likelihood of renovascular hypertension. On the other hand, an older man with moderate hypertension of recent onset who has an abdominal bruit may be appropriately evaluated by a less hazardous procedure, the response of PRA or an isotopic renogram to a single dose of captopril or duplex sonography. In such a patient, a negative screening study excludes the less likely diagnosis of renovascular hypertension with virtual certainty.

Although the various secondary forms are present in no more than 5% of the hypertensive population, that segment may comprise some 2 million persons in the United States alone.

Differential Diagnosis

Oral Contraceptive–Induced Hypertension. Most young women who take oral contraceptives have a rise in blood pressure of 2 to 4 mm Hg. In a survey of 23,000 pill users by the British Royal College of General Practitioners, the overall incidence of hypertension in 5 years was 5%, a figure 2.6 times that noted among 23,000 non–pill users. Although usually mild, the hypertension may on rare occasions be severe with resultant irreversible renal damage. The mechanism is uncertain. All women taking estrogens have an increase in renin substrate with increased levels of angiotensin II and aldosterone. Why hypertension develops only in some instances and whether this is hypertension produced de novo or simply uncovered at an earlier time remains unknown.

It should be possible to prevent serious problems from oral contraceptive–induced hypertension by these maneuvers:
1. Recheck the blood pressure every 3 to 6 months, with no refill of prescriptions permitted so that patients must return for observation.
2. Restrict estrogen use in women who are over 35, obese, smokers, or already hypertensive.
3. If hypertension develops, recommend other forms of contraception.

It should be noted that low-dose postmenopausal estrogen use is not a cause of hypertension.

Renal Parenchymal Disease. The diagnosis is simple, based on the presence of renal insufficiency and hypertension. Most patients start with primary hypertension that causes progressive renal damage. Among whites, hypertension is responsible for perhaps 20% of end-stage renal disease; in blacks, it is responsible for about 50%.

BOX 32-4
Diagnosis of renovascular hypertension

Suggestive clinical features
1. Abdominal diastolic bruit
2. Hypertension of recent onset and rapid progression, particularly in young women and older men
3. Rapidly deteriorating renal function, particularly after angiotensin-converting enzyme (ACE) inhibitor therapy
4. Hypertension difficult to control medically

Screening studies
1. Renal Duplex Sonography
2. Evidence of renal ischemia
   a. IVP (rapid sequence)
   b. Isotopic renogram: 1 hr after 50 mg captopril
3. Demonstration of renin excess
   a. PRA in peripheral blood
   b. Response to captopril: 1 hr after 50 mg

Confirmatory studies
1. Visualization of renal arteries by angiography
2. Renal vein PRA from stenotic side increased more than 1.5 to 2.0 times; no increase from contralateral side above vena cava blood

---

Bilateral renovascular disease may be the underlying problem in a significant number of patients with refractory hypertension and azotemia; 39 of 106 such patients were reported in one series by Ying and colleagues.

Diabetics are particularly vulnerable to renal damage when hypertensive. Effective control of hypertension has been shown to slow the progression of their renal damage. Therefore the diabetic hypertensive patient should be carefully monitored with measurements of urine protein excretion and serum creatinine and have even minimal hypertension treated vigorously, probably to a diastolic blood pressure level of less than 80 mm Hg (Chapter 117).

Recent advances in medical therapy of chronic renal disease may engender more hypertension: cyclosporine, erythropoietin, and perhaps extracorporeal shock wave lithotripsy.

Renovascular Hypertension (also see Chapter 125). Many patients have renal artery lesions that are not functionally significant, the degree of stenosis being less than that required to activate renin release. It is therefore necessary to ensure the functional significance of a lesion before surgery and, to a lesser degree, before angioplasty. Among the usual clinical and laboratory features, only the presence of an abdominal bruit was of differential diagnostic value in the Cooperative Study on Renovascular Hypertension, being heard in 46% of those with renovascular hypertension and 9% of those with essential hypertension. The diagnosis can be made by the sequence of steps shown in Box 32-4.

Particular attention should be given to any patient with severe hypertension as reflected in funduscopic changes of accelerated-malignant hypertension or refractoriness to potent therapy. A high frequency of renovascular hypertension among such patients, well beyond the 1% or less seen in the overall hypertensive population, has been documented. Most of them should have a renal arteriogram. Of the other procedures in Box 32-3, the "captopril challenge test" measuring the rise of PRA and renal blood flow or glomerular filtration rate (GFR) by isotopic renography 1 hour after a single 50 mg dose of captopril has been found to be a useful screening test to exclude the disease in those less likely to have renovascular hypertension. When performed by experienced technicians, renal duplex sonography has been found to accurately reflect arteriographic findings.

The increasing availability of transluminal balloon angioplasty has made the search for functional renovascular disease even more attractive, since elderly and other persons who are poor risks for surgery probably can be successfully managed by that procedure. However, the place of angioplasty remains uncertain. Despite its low risk, it may not provide prolonged relief, particularly among those with atherosclerotic renovascular disease, who are by far the majority of patients. For now, reparative surgery is probably the best choice for those with proved renovascular hypertension, but angioplasty at the same time as renal arteriography may be used. Despite better antihypertensive efficacy with ACE inhibitors, chronic use of these agents is generally not favored because of the distinct possibility of progressive loss of function in the ischemic kidney by removal of the support to perfusion provided by high levels of angiotensin II.

Renin-Secreting Tumors. Only a few dozen of these hemangiopericytomas of the juxtaglomerular cells have been reported. Most have been in young patients who have severe hypertension and markedly high renin levels with secondary aldosteronism manifested by hypokalemia and metabolic alkalosis. A similar but milder process may occur more commonly among patients with Wilms' tumor and other malignancies of the kidney.

Primary Aldosteronism (also see Chapter 289). Aldosterone hypersecretion induces hypertension and renal potassium wastage, but hypokalemia may not always be present, making its recognition more difficult. In a series of 80 patients with primary aldosteronism seen at the Cleveland Clinic, although 75 had a history of hypokalemia, 22 were normokalemic when admitted to the clinic, and 10 remained normokalemic even when given sodium loads to increase potassium wastage.

Conversely, adrenal masses are being found incidentally when abdominal computed tomography (CT) is performed for various reasons. Since as many as 8% of normotensive persons and 15% of hypertensives may have a nonfunctioning tumor, usually a lipoma, of the adrenal at autopsy, there is an obvious need to exclude the few functioning tumors that may require surgery from the larger number of nonfunctioning ones that should be left alone. The initial screening studies for the adrenal disorders shown in Table 32-2 should be performed on patients found by CT scan to have an adrenal mass. Surgery should only be done if hormone hypersecretion is proved.

In patients with aldosterone-producing adenomas, the hypertension may be of any degree of severity. In the Medical Research Council (MRC) series of 136 patients, the mean blood pressure was 205/123 mm Hg, and 31 had experienced either stroke or myocardial infarction. The diagnosis of primary aldosteronism can be best begun by measuring aldosterone and PRA in a single blood sample obtained whenever unexplained hypokalemia is observed.

The plasma aldosterone (PA) must be increased above 20 (ng/dl); the PRA must be suppressed below 0.5 (ng/ml/hr) so that the PA/PRA ratio should be well above 40:1. A very low PRA with a normal PA, as often seen in patients with essential hypertension, will give a high ratio; therefore, the PA level must also be elevated. Most patients who have secondary aldosteronism (induced by diuretics, for example) have higher PRA and a ratio below 20:1. The diagnosis may be confirmed by finding more than 30 mmol of potassium per 24-hour urine collection *in the presence of hypokalemia*. The finding of less than 30 mmol suggests gastrointestinal losses or earlier use of diuretics, the more likely explanation in most hypokalemic hypertensive patients.

Once an elevated blood aldosterone and suppressed PRA are found along with renal wastage of potassium, the nature of the adrenal pathology must be determined by CT scan of the adrenals. Aldosterone-producing adenomas are usually small, but most can be differentiated from bilateral adrenal hyperplasia. The hyperplasia, usually causes milder degrees of the usual features. It must be recognized to avoid unnecessary surgery. Patients with hyperplasia should be treated with spironolactone; those with a tumor should have surgery. The rare familial form of glucocorticoid-remediable aldosteronism (GRA) has been shown to arise from a mutation of the 11β-hydroxylase and aldosterone synthase genes, producing a chimeric gene that catalyzes the formation of 18-hydroxylated steroids outside the zona glomerulosa. Increased levels of 18-hydroxycortisol characterize the syndrome.

The glycyrrhizic acid in licorice inhibits the 11β-OH-dehydrogenase enzyme responsible for conversion of cortisol, which exerts potent mineralocorticoid action in the kidney, to cortisone, which is much less potent, thereby inducing "apparent" mineralocorticoid excess.

Cushing's Syndrome (see Chapter 289). Hypertension may also be induced by the mineralocorticoid activity of high levels of

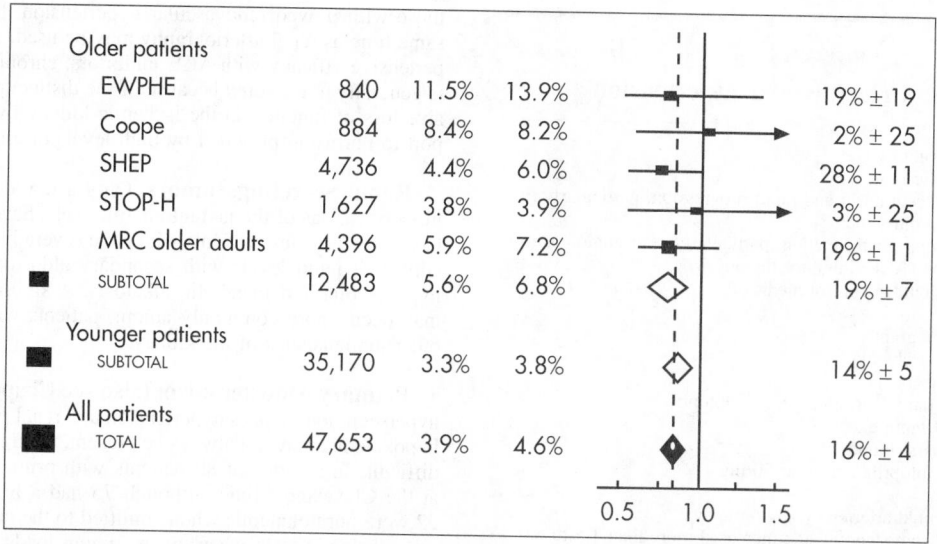

Older patients				
EWPHE	840	11.5%	13.9%	19% ± 19
Coope	884	8.4%	8.2%	2% ± 25
SHEP	4,736	4.4%	6.0%	28% ± 11
STOP-H	1,627	3.8%	3.9%	3% ± 25
MRC older adults	4,396	5.9%	7.2%	19% ± 11
SUBTOTAL	12,483	5.6%	6.8%	19% ± 7
Younger patients				
SUBTOTAL	35,170	3.3%	3.8%	14% ± 5
All patients				
TOTAL	47,653	3.9%	4.6%	16% ± 4

FIGURE 32-10　Effects of blood pressure reduction on coronary heart disease incidence in 12 randomized controlled trials of younger patients (most under age 60) and 5 trials in older patients (all over age 60). Box size is proportional to number of events recorded. Horizontal lines denote 99% confidence intervals of odds ratios from individual trial results and diamonds denote 95% confidence intervals for odds ratios for combined trial results.

(From MacMahon S, Rodgers A: The effects of blood pressure reduction in older patients: an overview of five randomized controlled trials in elderly hypertensives, *Clin Exp Hypertens* 15:967-978, 1993.)

cortisol. Hypokalemia is usually less prominent than with primary aldosteronism except in those with very high cortisol levels, as with ectopic adrenocorticotropic hormone (ACTH)-producing tumors. In the more common pituitary ACTH-induced bilateral adrenal hyperplasia, hypertension may be prominent and, if left untreated, may lead to serious cardiac damage.

Pheochromocytoma (see Chapter 290). The hypertension may be wildly episodic or fairly constant but is almost always accompanied by peculiar spells of profuse sweating, tremor, palpitations, headache, and various other symptoms. Although most recurrent spells are caused by anxiety-induced hyperventilation, menopause, or a number of other catecholamine-induced syndromes, the possibility of a pheochromocytoma can be easily excluded by the measurement of metanephrine in a single voided urine specimen. If the spot urine contains more than 1.2 μg of metanephrine/mg of creatinine, 24-hour urine catecholamine levels should be determined. Plasma catechols may also be measured before and after an attempt to suppress them with the sympathetic inhibitor clonidine. Those with a pheochromocytoma have high plasma levels that cannot be suppressed by more than 50% or to a level of less than 400 pg/ml in the 3 hours after oral intake of 0.3 mg of clonidine.

Once the clinical signs have been confirmed by the biochemical assays, the pathology should be elucidated by abdominal CT scanning. Most pheochromocytomas—about 90%—are solitary and in an adrenal gland. About 10% are extraadrenal, most along the abdominal sympathetic chain. About 10% are malignant, as ascertained by the finding of metastases. A few are associated with the type 2 multiple endocrine neoplasia syndrome or multiple neurofibromatosis.

After adequate α-adrenergic blockade, surgery is almost always indicated, with caution to avoid severe hypertension during induction of anesthesia and manipulation of the tumor.

Miscellaneous Causes. As shown by the long list of secondary types of hypertension in Box 32-2, numerous other mechanisms can induce hypertension. A variety of drugs and chemical agents may be responsible. Many of these, such as nasal decongestants and diet pills containing the sympathetic agonist phenylpropanolamine, are readily available and widely used. Nonsteroidal antiinflammatory drugs (NSAIDs) have been found to interfere with the efficacy of numerous antihypertensive drugs. The potential of various drugs and chemical agents to induce or aggravate hypertension should be recognized in the evaluation of all patients.

MANAGEMENT

Many practitioners treat all persons with a diastolic pressure above 90 mm Hg and most with a systolic above 140 mm Hg. The reasons for this approach include the recognition that hypertension is common and, if left untreated, is a major risk factor for premature cardiovascular disease. After the benefits of antihypertensive drug therapy for the more severe degrees of hypertension were demonstrated in the late 1960s, the logical assumption was made that the millions with relatively milder degrees of hypertension should also be treated, particularly since medications became available that could be taken once or twice a day and seemed to be largely free of bothersome side effects. Therefore, more and more of the 80% of the hypertensive population who have mild hypertension (defined as a diastolic blood pressure between 90 and 104 mm Hg) have been begun on drug therapy; these include a large share of the 40% with diastolic blood pressure between 90 and 94 mm Hg. However, the extension of treatment to these less hypertensive patients began without proof that it was beneficial.

Results of Clinical Trials

Clinical trials of the therapy of mild hypertension were begun in the early 1970s. The results of initial trials provided confirmatory evidence for the benefits of therapy in regard to the prevention of stroke and congestive heart failure. The results of three more recent studies in elderly hypertensives have strengthened the evidence for protection against coronary disease, perhaps because they used lower doses of diuretics than used in earlier trials (Fig. 32-10).

Analyses of the results of the multiple trials have clearly demonstrated significant overall protection from cardiovascular complications by the treatment of mild-moderate hypertension, averaging a 38% reduction in the relative risk from stroke and a 16% reduction for coronary disease. As shown by Lever and Ramsay in their analysis of the six trials involving elderly patients and one other of similar design involving middle-aged patients, the relative or proportionate benefit from the incidence of stroke was fairly uniform across the entire range of risk seen in the placebo groups (Fig. 32-11). When

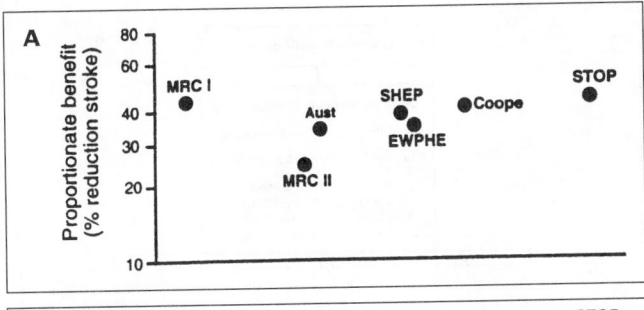

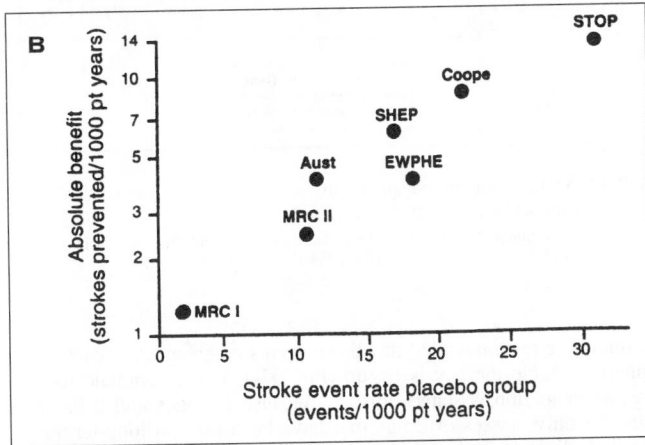

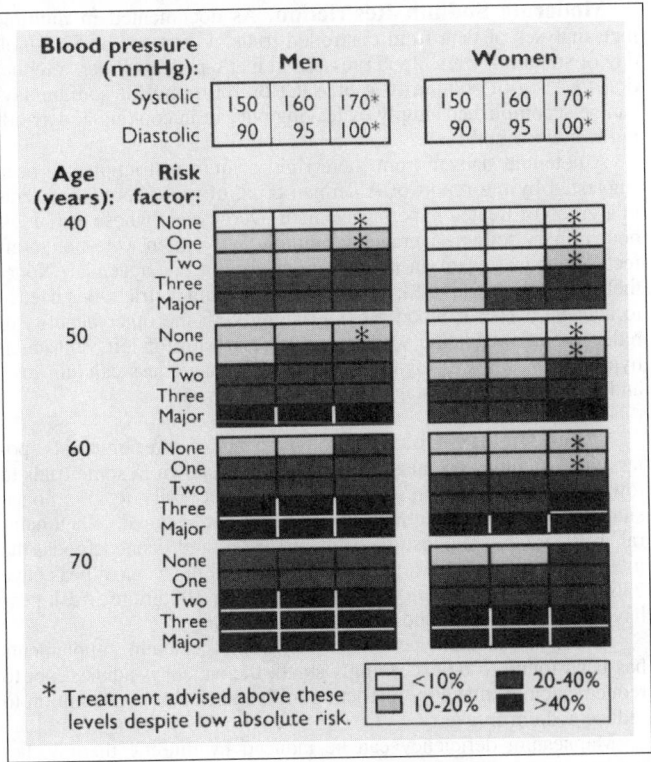

FIGURE 32-11   Comparison of **(A)** proportionate (relative) and **(B)** absolute benefit from reduction in the incidence of stroke in the six trials in the elderly and in one other with similar design, but in which the absolute risk of stroke was much lower. Event rates are for fatal and nonfatal stroke combined. *MRC I,* Medical Research Council (MRC) trial I; *MRC II,* MRC trial II; *Aust,* Australian study; *SHEP,* Systolic Hypertension in the Elderly Program; *EWPHE,* European Working Party on High Blood Pressure in the Elderly trial; *Coope,* Coope and Warrender; *STOP,* Swedish Trial in Old Patients with Hypertension.

(From Lever AF, Ramsay LE: Treatment of hypertension in the elderly, *J Hypertens* 13:571-579, 1995.)

FIGURE 32-12   Absolute risk (%) of having a cardiovascular event in 10 years according to age, blood pressure, and other risk factors.

(From Jackson R et al: Management of raised blood pressure in New Zealand: a discussion document, *Br Med J* 307:107-110, 1993.)

the actual number of strokes prevented is shown, however, the absolute benefit clearly varies with the level of risk in the placebo groups. As the authors state: "When contemplating lifelong treatment of asymptomatic condition, a 33% reduction of risk from fatal stroke is of no importance to someone whose risk of stroke is almost zero. The same 33% reduction is of considerable interest to someone at high and imminent risk of stroke."

Recognition of the minimal if any protection provided by treatment of low-risk patients has prompted a call for consideration of the entire risk status rather than just the level of blood pressure when determining the need for therapy. Jackson and co-workers from New Zealand have formulated a nomogram including levels of blood pressure, age, and gender, along with the number of other major risk factors (Fig. 32-12). They recommend institution of drug therapy only if the absolute risk of having a cardiovascular event (based on the Framingham Heart Study data) in 10 years is 20% or higher. Most U.S. practitioners would likely find these recommendations too conservative and would treat most patients at lesser overall risk. Nonetheless, I believe the concept is valid, and perhaps a compromise of starting drug treatment in patients above a 10% absolute risk is most appropriate.

Whatever level of blood pressure is used to decide upon the need for therapy, it is essential to adequately monitor the pressure for a few months, preferably by home measurements to recognize the 20% or more with only "white-coat" hypertension. The wisdom of this approach is shown by the results of the Australian trial: 48% of those who entered the trial with diastolic blood pressure between 95 and 109 mm Hg on the second set of readings had a fall to less than 95 mm Hg that persisted during the subsequent 4 years while they received no active drug (or nondrug) therapy. Most of this fall occurred in the first 4 months of observation.

Part of the hesitation in starting drug therapy reflects the increasing awareness of the potential for any drug therapy to produce various side effects that may diminish the quality of life. In addition, the high cost of medications, particularly the newer ACE inhibitors and calcium blockers, has prompted many to either withhold therapy or substitute less-expensive generic forms for others that may be preferable.

Nondrug Therapies

One way to minimize or delay the need for drug therapy is by the use of various nondrug modalities, better called "lifestyle modifications." Although these, too, may interfere somewhat with the quality of life, they should have no bothersome side effects. These therapies should be continued and offered to all hypertensives whether or not they also need medication. The hope is that these lifestyle modifications will lower blood pressure to levels wherein drugs are not required or, failing that, will reduce the amounts of medication needed. There is hope, but certainly no proof, that their widespread use could prevent the development of hypertension.

There is also no proof that these lifestyle modifications protect against cardiovascular complications or that they will be accepted by or effective in lowering the blood pressure for most hypertensives. But they do no harm, and they may do some good not only by lowering blood pressure but also by reducing other risk factors for cardiovascular disease. If the modifications are offered in a reasonable manner, as a gentle recommendation for gradual change rather than as a massive attack against current habits, most patients should be willing to at least try them.

Weight Reduction.   Weight gain clearly tends to raise blood pressure, and weight loss usually lowers blood pressure. The effect of reduced caloric intake is probably independent of concomitant sodium restriction. A 1- to 2-mm Hg fall in blood pressure usually accompanies each kg of weight loss.

Moderate Sodium Restriction. As documented in multiple metaanalyses of data from controlled trials, a decrease of 50 mmol/day of sodium lowers blood pressure in many patients. Such a reduction to 2.4 g of sodium (6 g of NaCl or 100 mmol of sodium/day) can be accomplished simply by leaving out salt in cooking and avoiding heavily salted foods.

A potential danger from more rigid sodium restriction has been suggested by the report of Alderman et al. of more coronary events in a group of treated hypertensive men over 4 years whose initial 24-hour urinary sodium averaged 65 mmol/day. Women were not so affected, nor was there an increase in strokes in either gender. Nonetheless, caution is advised: only moderate sodium restriction is needed to achieve a fall in blood pressure along with the other benefits of reduced sodium intake, which include regression of left ventricular hypertrophy, slower progression of renal damage, less calcium loss, and less potassium wastage if diuretics are given.

Other Dietary Changes. Supplements of three minerals, potassium, calcium, and magnesium, have been shown in some trials to lower the blood pressure. It should not be necessary to give potassium supplements if a lower sodium intake is consumed. When natural, fresh foods are substituted for processed and canned foods, the intake of potassium rises markedly. As an example, canned peas have 236 mg of sodium and 96 mg of potassium per 100 grams; fresh peas have 2 mg of sodium and 316 mg of potassium.

Although the antihypertensive efficacy of calcium supplements has been found to be exceedingly small, the patient is advised not to reduce calcium intake by restricting milk and cheese consumption to reduce sodium intake.

Magnesium deficiency can be induced by diuretic therapy, but magnesium supplements have not been shown to lower blood pressure.

A few clinical studies have shown a lowering of the blood pressure by ingestion of a lacto-ovovegetarian diet, a low-saturated, high-polyunsaturated fat diet, or 2 to 3 g/day of omega-3 fatty acids. Such diets may reduce the blood pressure by increasing levels of vasodilatory prostaglandins.

Moderate Alcohol Consumption. Too little or too much alcohol may be harmful—too little by increasing the risks for coronary heart disease presumably through a lowering of high-density lipoprotein (HDL) cholesterol, too much by raising the blood pressure and, when carried further, by the ravages of alcohol abuse. Beyond 2 ounces/day, ethanol may raise the blood pressure and, in larger amounts, it is probably by far the most common cause of reversible, curable hypertension.

Exercise. Regular isotonic exercise may lower the blood pressure, perhaps through reduction of sympathetic nerve activity. Isometric exercise probably does no good for cardiovascular fitness and causes a reflex rise in blood pressure, so it should be avoided.

Relaxation. Various techniques to relieve tension and induce relaxation have been shown to lower the blood pressure, but in the majority of controlled studies, the effect is no greater than seen with placebo.

Drug Therapy

Even if all of these lifestyle modifications are used, most hypertensives need antihypertensive drugs. As noted, the treatment of hypertension constitutes the largest single indication for drug use in the United States.

Almost any of the drugs shown in Table 32-3 may be chosen for initial therapy with the expectation that about half of patients will have a 10% or greater fall in blood pressure, which will bring the diastolic blood pressure of most of those who start with fairly mild hypertension below 90 mm Hg, the usual goal of therapy. Drugs that tend to reduce renin-aldosterone activity such as β-blockers, ACE inhibitors, and calcium entry blockers may work particularly well in the absence of a diuretic.

Despite the progressive decline in the use of diuretics and β-blockers over the last 5 years, the report of the fifth Joint National

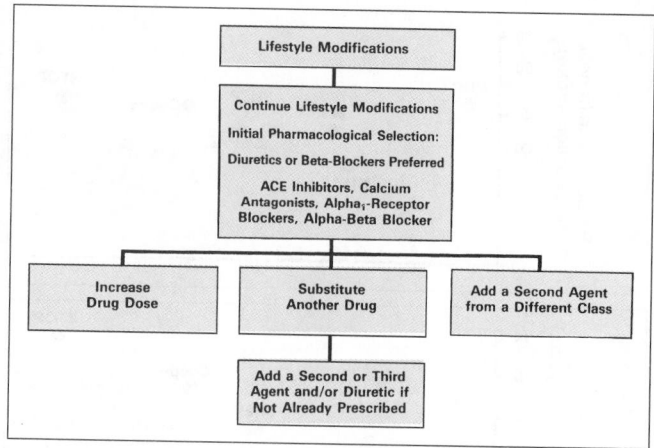

FIGURE 32-13 Simplified algorithm for treatment of hypertension. *ACE,* Angiotensin-converting enzyme.

(From Joint National Committee on Detection, Evaluation, and Treatment of High Blood Pressure, *Arch Intern Med* 153:154-183, 1983.)

Committee recommended that these agents be given preference when pharmacologic therapy is begun (Fig. 32-13). The rationale for this recommendation is stated thusly: "Because diuretics and β-blockers are the only classes of drugs that have been used in long-term controlled clinical trials and shown to reduce morbidity and mortality, they are recommended as first-choice agents unless they are contraindicated or unacceptable, or unless there are special indications for other agents."

This recommendation, which counters the choices being made by most U.S. practitioners in recent years, has been criticized as a "backward step." However, the last two phrases of the statement indicate that the other choices listed as acceptable (ACE inhibitors, calcium antagonists, α-blockers, and α-β-blockers) can be used when diuretics or β-blockers are unacceptable or when indications for the newer drugs are present. The last phrase is most important: "The presence of a number of concomitant conditions or demographic features should be used to make the choice most appropriate for each individual patient" (Table 32-4). If the initial choice is ineffectual or causes bothersome side effects, that drug should be discontinued and one from another class substituted.

Subsequent Drug Therapy. If the first choice is well tolerated but only partially effective, either increase the dose or add a second drug from another class. The wisdom of adding a second drug or of starting therapy with very low doses of two drugs is becoming increasingly obvious. Thereby additive effects are achieved, whereas drug-specific side effects are kept minimal. In about 10% of hypertensives, a third drug, usually a vasodilator, is needed. In the past, hydralazine was the usual choice, with minoxidil reserved for resistant cases. Calcium entry blockers will probably be used increasingly, since they are effective vasodilators of the systemic arteries as well as of the coronary arteries.

Other Guidelines

The goal of therapy should be to reduce the diastolic pressure to below 90 mm Hg, but caution is needed in reducing it below 85 mm Hg since that may induce myocardial ischemia, particularly in patients with preexisting coronary disease. The progressive fall in coronary mortality seen with progressive lowering of pressure is aborted at diastolic levels below 85 mm Hg and coronary mortality then begins to rise, producing a J-curve relationship. Some deny the presence of a J-curve for coronary mortality and the results of a controlled study (the HOT trial) are eagerly awaited. No such J-curve has been seen for stroke, and increasing evidence documents the need for a much lower blood pressure to preserve renal function in those with proteinuria or other evidences of renal damage.

In the elderly with predominantly systolic hypertension, the sys-

Table 32-3   Oral antihypertensive drugs

DRUG	TRADE NAME	DOSE RANGE (MG/DAY) (FREQUENCY)	SIDE EFFECTS
Diuretics (partial list)			
Hydrochlorothiazide	Hydrodiuril Esidrix	12.5-50	Biochemical abnormalities: ↓ potassium, ↑ cholesterol, ↑ glucose Rare: blood dyscrasias, photosensitivity, pancreatitis
Chlorthalidone	Hygroton	12.5-50	
Metolazone	Microx, Diulo	0.5-10	Less if any hypercholesterolemia
Indapamide	Lozol	2.5	Short duration of action
Furosemide	Lasix	40-240	Longer duration of action
Torasemide	Demadex	5-40	
Potassium-sparing agents (plus thiazide)			
Spironolactone	Aldactazide	25-100	Hyperkalemia, gynecomastia
Dyrenium	Dyazide, Maxzide	25-100	Hyperkalemia
Amiloride	Moduretic	5-10	Hyperkalemia
Adrenergic inhibitors			
Peripheral:			
Reserpine	Serpasil	0.05-0.25(1)	Sedation, depression
Guanethidine	Ismelin	10-150	Orthostatic hypotension, diarrhea
Guanadrel	Hylorel	10-75	
Central α-agonists:			
Methyldopa	Aldomet	500-3000(2)	Hepatic and autoimmune disorders
Clonidine	Catapres	0.2-1.2(2)	Sedation, dry mouth, "withdrawal"
Guanabenz	Wytensin	8-32(2)	Sedation, dry mouth, "withdrawal"
Guanafacine	Tenex	1-3(1)	Sedation, dry mouth
α-blockers:			
Doxazosin	Cardura	1-20(1)	
Prazosin	Minipress	2-20(2)	Postural hypotension (mainly with first dose), lassitude
Terazosin	Hytrin	1-20(1)	
β-blockers:			
Acebutolol	Sectral	200-800(1)	
Atenolol	Tenormin	25-100(1-2)	Serious: bronchospasm, congestive heart failure, masking of insulin-induced hypokalemia, depression
Betaxolol	Kerlone	5-20(1)	
Bisoprolol	Zebeta	2.5-10(1)	
Carteolol	Cartrol	2.5-10(1)	
Metoprolol	Lopressor, Toprol XL	50-300(1-2)	Less serious: poor peripheral circulation, insomnia, fatigue, decreased exercise tolerance, hypertriglyceridemia, decreased HDL (except with ISA-agents)
Nadolol	Corgard	40-320(1)	
Penbutolol	Levatol	10-20(1)	
Pindolol	Visken	10-60(2)	
Propranolol	Inderal	40-480(2)	
Timolol	Blocadren	20-60(2)	
Combined α- and β-blocker			
Labetalol	Normodyne, Trandate	200-1200(2)	Postural hypotension, β-blocking side effects
Carvedilol	Coreg	12.5-50(2)	
Direct vasodilators			
Hydralazine	Apresoline	50-400(2)	Headaches, tachycardia, lupus syndrome
Minoxidil	Loniten	5-100(1)	Headaches, fluid retention, hirsutism
Calcium entry blockers			
Verapamil (SR)	Isoptin, Calan, Verelan	90-480(1-2)	Constipation, conduction defects
Diltiazem (SR & CD)	Cardizem, Dilacor	120-240(1-2)	Nausea, headache, conduction defects
Dihydropyridines			
Amlodipine	Norvasc	2.5-10(1)	Flush, headache, local ankle edema
Felodipine	Plendil	5-20(1)	(All same as amlodipine)
Isradipine	DynaCirc	5-20(2)	
Nicardipine	Cardene	60-90(2-3)	
Nifedipine (XL)	Procardia, Adalat	30-120(1)	
Nisoldipine	Sular	20-60(1)	
Converting enzyme inhibitors			
Benazepril	Lotensin	5-40(1)	Cough, rash, loss of taste
Captopril	Capoten	25-150(2)	Rare: Leukopenia, proteinuria
Enalapril	Vasotec	5-40(1-2)	(All same as captopril)
Fosinopril	Monopril	10-40(1)	
Lisinopril	Prinivil, Zestril	5-40(1)	
Moexipril	Univasc	2.5-10(1)	
Quinapril	Accupril	5-80(1)	
Ramipril	Altace	1.25-20(1)	
Trendolapril	Maxik	1-4(1)	
Angiotensin-receptor blockers			
Losartan	Cozaar	50-100(1-2)	No cough, but angioedema occurs

Table 32-4   Recommended choices of antihypertensive drugs for various coexisting conditions

COEXISTING CONDITION	DIURETIC	β-BLOCKER	α-BLOCKER	CALCIUM BLOCKER	ACE INHIBITOR
Older age	++	+/−	+	+	+
Black race	++	+/−	+	+	+
Angina	+	++	+	++	+/−
Postmyocardial infarction	+	++	+	+/−*	+
Congestive heart failure	++	+/−	+	+/−	++
Cerebrovascular	+	+	+/−	+/−	++
Renal insufficiency	++	+/−	+	+	+
Diabetes	+/−	−	++	++	++†
Dyslipidemia	−	−	++	+	++
Prostatism	+	+	++	+	+

++, Preferred; +, suitable; +/−, usually not preferred; −, usually contraindicated.
*Short-acting dihydropyridines contraindicated.
†Caution if renovascular disease not ruled out.

tolic pressure should be gently lowered toward 145 mm Hg. The failure of cerebral autoregulation may cause postural symptoms to appear in the elderly even with small falls in blood pressure.

In view of the significantly greater occurrence of cardiovascular catastrophes in the morning hours after arising from sleep, a time when blood pressure abruptly increases, it is vital to ensure that the antihypertensive effects of therapy be maintained at this time, preferably by having patients check their pressures soon after arising with home devices. Some agents approved for once-a-day dosing may not provide 24-hour control, so twice-a-day dosing may be needed or other longer-acting agents may be used once daily.

If the goal blood pressure has been reached on two or more drugs, the substitution of comparable combination tablets should be attempted. If the goal has been maintained for at least 1 year, the doses of drugs should be slowly reduced and, rarely, discontinued under careful surveillance.

Specific Drugs

Diuretics. The most commonly used diuretics are listed in Table 32-3. The most appropriate choice for most patients is hydrochlorothiazide, with its 12- to 16-hour duration of action and mild, smooth effect, although the longer-lasting chlorthalidone may provide better efficacy. Patients on direct vasodilators or with renal insufficiency (i.e., serum creatinine above 2.5 mg/dl) may need more potent diuretics, either two or three doses per day of a loop diuretic, such as furosemide, or one dose a day of torsemide or metolazone. Indapamide may have additional vasodilatory effects.

The side effects of large doses of diuretics largely reflect their pharmacologic actions (Fig. 32-14). Three of these metabolic changes may increase cardiovascular risk: the rise in serum cholesterol, up to 20 mg/dl; the fall in serum potassium, which averages 0.7 mmol/L; and the worsening of glucose tolerance, which reflects greater insulin resistance. Efforts should be made to prevent hypokalemia by use of the smallest effective dose of diuretic, concomitant reduction in sodium intake, and generous use of potassium-sparing agents or supplemental potassium. Although microencapsulated potassium chloride tablets may be safely used, a level teaspoonful of a potassium chloride–containing salt substitute provides 40 mmol of potassium at less cost. Prudence suggests that a fall of serum potassium of more than 0.5 mmol/L be reversed by the same measures.

The rise in serum uric acid and calcium levels shown in Fig. 32-14 need not be corrected unless the patient has concomitant gout or hyperparathyroidism. Although impotence has been considered unusual with diuretics, it was reported in 22% of men in the British MRC trial taking 10 mg/day of bendrofluazide, compared with 10% of those on a placebo and 13% on propranolol.

All diuretic side effects are lessened when usually effective smaller doses (12.5 mg hydrochlorothiazide [HCTZ] a day) are used. In combinations, as little as 6.25 mg HCTZ may be enough.

Adrenergic Inhibitors. All of the agents shown in Table 32-3 lower the blood pressure about 10% and, if used with a diuretic, bring

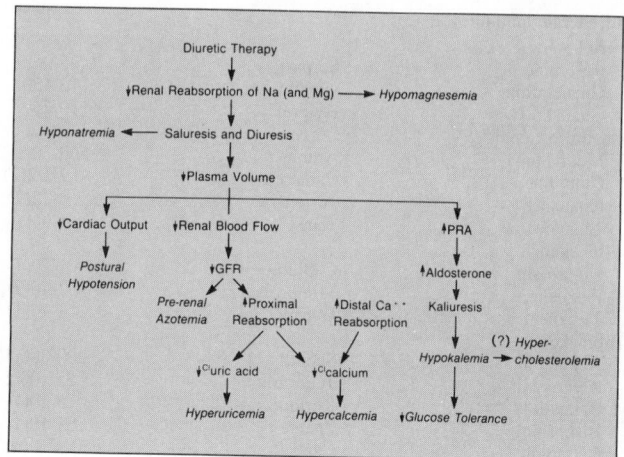

FIGURE 32-14   The mechanisms by which chronic diuretic therapy may lead to various complications. The mechanisms for hypercholesterolemia remains in question, although it is shown as arising via hypokalemia.
(From Kaplan NM: *Clinical hypertension,* ed 6, Baltimore, 1994, Williams & Wilkins.)

at least 80% of hypertensives to the goal of a diastolic blood pressure below 90 mm Hg. The choice between these drugs should be based on their propensity to induce metabolic mischief or bothersome side effects, although prescribing habits, in fact, largely determine the choice.

Peripheral Inhibitors. Reserpine remains an effective, inexpensive, and generally well-tolerated drug. It can be effective in even smaller doses, 0.05 mg/day, than usually prescribed. Guanethidine is now reserved for resistant patients as a step 4 drug. Guanadrel is a shorter-lasting guanethidine-like agent, which seems to cause fewer side effects when used twice a day.

Central Inhibitors. Clonidine, guanabenz, guanfacine, and methyldopa act in a similar manner to decrease sympathetic drive from the CNS. Other than for a variety of autoimmune syndromes with methyldopa, their side effects are similar, mainly sedation and dry mouth. Guanabenz has been approved for monotherapy since it appears to induce less fluid retention.

Alpha Blockers. Three are now available—prazosin, terazosin, and doxazosin—which act selectively on the postsynaptic α_1 receptor on the vascular smooth muscle. The most widely perceived side effect, first-dose hypotension, is seen infrequently, is seldom severe, and can be minimized by discontinuation of diuretic therapy for the day before and the day after start of the drug. Among this class of drug's advantages are the beneficial effects on plasma lipid levels and insulin resistance, the lack of interference with the ability to perform physical activity, and relief of the symptoms of prostatism.

Beta Blockers. Of those now available, equivalent doses probably exert similar antihypertensive effects. If one does not work, it is unlikely that another will, but if one causes side effects, it may be worth trying another with different pharmacologic properties.

β-Blockers differ in three major ways:

1. *Relative β-₁ selectivity.* In the fairly large doses used to treat hypertension, the relatively greater β_1 selectivity of atenolol, bisoprolol, and metoprolol may not be enough to prevent β_2-mediated side effects such as bronchospasm.
2. *Intrinsic sympathomimetic activity* (ISA). The greater ISA of pindolol and acebutolol may translate into less bradycardia, vasoconstriction, and alterations in lipid levels than are seen with the other beta blockers.
3. *Lipid solubility.* The lesser lipid solubility of atenolol and nadolol enables them to remain in the blood longer and they are slowly excreted, largely unchanged, through the kidneys.

The major side effects of β-blockers are largely a magnification of their pharmacologic β_1- and β_2-receptor blockade: decrease in cardiac output limiting exercise ability and, very rarely, inciting heart failure; bronchospasm; and the masking of the symptoms (except for sweating) while prolonging the duration of insulin-induced hypoglycemia. In addition, they may induce considerable fatigue, depression, and insomnia; these side effects may be less common with the lipid-insoluble beta blockers atenolol and nadolol, which do not enter the brain as much. All but pindolol and acebutolol may so constrict the peripheral circulation as to cause cold extremities and diminish the conversion of triglycerides into HDL cholesterol, raising the level of triglycerides and lowering the level of HDL cholesterol.

Combined α- and β-Blockers. These agents have both α- and β-blocking effects, which results in even greater antihypertensive potency than an α- or β-blocker alone, with little reduction in cardiac output. Labetaolo, available for both oral and intravenous use, has been used especially for severe hypertension. The most bothersome side effect is postural hypotension. Carvedilol has been found to be especially beneficial in the treatment of congestive heart failure.

Vasodilators. A direct-acting vasodilator has usually been the third drug added for the 10% of patients who do not respond adequately to two. When added to a diuretic and an adrenergic inhibitor, the antihypertensive effect of all three is fully developed, and their side effects are minimized. Hydralazine is the usual choice and need be given only twice daily. Beyond the expected side effects of direct-acting vasodilators of tachycardia, flushing, and headache, hydralazine may cause a febrile lupuslike reaction that is almost always totally reversible. Patients who inactivate the drug more slowly via acetylation may develop the reaction with total doses of less than 200 mg/day; fast acetylators rarely develop it with less than 400 mg/day.

Minoxidil, more potent than hydralazine, is usually reserved for those with renal insufficiency, near the end of their course. But, if given in small doses, it may provide excellent antihypertensive action on a once-daily schedule and not cause much hirsutism, the most common side effect. Significant fluid retention usually accompanies its antihypertensive action, often requiring the addition of potent diuretics.

Calcium Entry Blockers. These vasodilators may be used as first, second, or third drug. Of those now available, the dihydropyridines are the most potent peripheral vasodilators, but all lower blood pressure. The availability of verapamil, diltiazem, and some of the dihydropyridines in slow-release forms that provide once-a-day dosage adds to their attractiveness. Some find that calcium entry blockers are especially effective in the elderly hypertensive population.

Nifedipine as a liquid in a capsule has been useful for semiemergency situations in which very high blood pressure must be lowered within 20 to 30 minutes. However, this short- and rapid-acting formulation has been found, in large doses, to increase mortality in the postmyocardial infarction period. A case-control study by Psaty et al. showed an increase in the use of various short-acting calcium entry blockers in patients who had had a myocardial infarction compared to controls who had not. The inability of such retrospective analyses to ensure comparability of cases and controls makes them frequently wrong, as shown for claims in 1974 that reserpine increased the risk for breast cancer and a claim in 1995 that β-blockers increased the risk for sudden death.

Regardless of the potential hazards of short-acting calcium entry blockers, the long-acting formulations have been tested and found to be effective and safe for both hypertension and angina so their appropriate use should not be restricted.

Angiotensin-Converting Enzyme Inhibitors. ACE inhibitors also act as vasodilators. By their inhibition of the enzyme that converts the inactive angiotensin I to the potent vasoconstrictor angiotensin II, the drugs are particularly effective in high renin-angiotensin forms of hypertension. They probably also work in other ways, so most patients with primary hypertension have some benefit from them. They work particularly well when renin levels are raised by concomitant diuretic therapy or sodium restriction.

ACE inhibitors have been found to provide excellent protection from progression of renal insufficiency in diabetics with nephropathy, presumably by their ability to selectively dilate renal efferent arterioles, reducing intraglomerular pressure. Whether this protection is greater than obtainable from other antihypertensive agents, however, is uncertain.

By removing angiotensin II–mediated systemic vasoconstriction, ACE inhibitors have proved to be particularly valuable in reducing after demands on a heart that has failed from prolonged hypertension. These drugs are generally free of the CNS- and cardiac-mediated side effects such as sedation, fatigue, and exercise limitation often seen with adrenergic inhibitors. However, these drugs may cause side effects, such as cough, loss of taste, and rash, that are irritating, as well as some rare but serious problems such as angioneurotic edema. Rarely, they induce renal failure when given to patients dependent on high levels of renin-angiotensin II to maintain renal perfusion. This dependence has been noted primarily in patients with stenoses in both renal arteries or in the one artery to a solitary kidney. When their renin support is removed by an ACE inhibitor, renal blood flow may fall precipitously, far below the level expected from the fall in systemic blood pressure.

A-II-Receptor Blockers. Losartan is the first of this new class of agents that inhibit the renin-angiotensin system at the receptors for A-II on the vascular wall. Since kinins do not simultaneously increase as they do with ACE inhibitors, kinin-induced cough does not occur, but, surprisingly, reports of angioedema have appeared with the use of losartan. Whether these agents provide better or equal effectiveness as ACE inhibitors in nephropathy and congestive heart failure remains to be seen.

Some Special Problems

Systolic Hypertension in the Elderly. Elderly persons often have isolated systolic hypertension caused by loss of elasticity in large arteries from atherosclerosis. They are at high risk for stroke and other cardiovascular catastrophes and, with publication of the results of the Systolic Hypertension in the Elderly Program (SHEP), antihypertensive drug treatment has been found to reduce these risks. Therefore, such patients should be treated in the same general way as described for systolic and diastolic hypertension in preceding portions of this chapter, but in a slower, more gentle manner toward a goal of a systolic blood pressure of 145 mm Hg.

All of the drugs listed in Table 32-3 may be used in the elderly; a low dose of the diuretic chlorthalidone, 12.5 mg, was the initial drug in the SHEP trial, and a low dose of the beta blocker atenolol, 25 mg, was the second. Special precautions are needed:

1. Diuretics may cause more volume depletion and hypokalemia.
2. Adrenergic inhibitors may cause more postural hypotension since the baroreceptor reflexes are less active. This sluggish baroreceptor response may allow for the use of hydralazine without an adrenergic inhibitor.
3. Any drug that effectively lowers the blood pressure may cause a fall in perfusion to the brain. Those that also cause sedation may lead to dementia in the elderly.
4. The widespread use of antidepressants and NSAIDs may block some of the expected effects of antihypertensive agents.

Table 32-5   Parenteral drugs for treatment of hypertensive emergency (in order of rapidity of action)

DRUG	DOSAGE	ONSET OF ACTION	ADVERSE EFFECTS
Vasodilators			
Nitroprusside (Nipride, Nitropress)	0.25-10 µg/kg/min as IV infusion	Instantaneous	Nausea, vomiting, muscle twitching, sweating, thiocyanate intoxication
Nitroglycerin	5-100 µg/min as IV infusion	2-5 min	Tachycardia, flushing, headache, vomiting, methemoglobinemia
Diazoxide (Hyperstat)	50-100 mg/IV bolus repeated, or 15-30 mg/min by IV infusion	2-4 min	Nausea, hypotension, flushing, tachycardia, chest pain
Hydralazine (Apresoline)	10-20 mg IV / 10-50 mg IM	10-20 min / 20-30 min	Tachycardia, flushing, headache, vomiting, aggravation of angina
Enalapril (Vasotec IV)	1.25-5 mg q 6 hr	15 min	Precipitous fall in BP in high renin states; response variable
Nicardipine (Cardene)	5-10 mg/hr IV	10 min	Tachycardia, headache, flushing, local phlebitis
Adrenergic inhibitors			
Phentolamine (Regitine)	5-15 mg IV	1-2 min	Tachycardia, flushing
Trimethaphan (Arfonad)	0.5-5 mg/min as IV infusion	1-5 min	Paresis of bowel and bladder, orthostatic hypotension, blurred vision, dry mouth
Esmolol (Brevibloc)	500 µg/kg/min for 4 min, then 150-300 µg/kg/min IV	1-2 min	Hypotension
Propranolol (Inderal)	1-10 mg load; 3 ng/hr	1-2 min	Beta-blocker side effects, e.g., bronchospasm, decreased cardiac output
Labetalol (Normodyne, Trandate)	20-80 mg IV bolus every 10 min / 2 mg/min IV infusion	5-10 min	Vomiting, scalp tingling, burning in throat, postural hypotension, dizziness, nausea

Hypertension in Children. The 1996 update of the 1987 report of the Second Task Force on Blood Pressure Control in Children confirmed that

Nonpharmacological intervention strategies can be introduced as initial treatment and tailored to meet the needs of the individual patient. Traditional forms of antihypertensive drug therapy should be reserved for use in patients with severe hypertension or when BP remains markedly elevated after several weeks to months of nonpharmacological therapy. . . . Major questions still remain with regard to the long-term effects of drug treatment on children and adolescents. In particular, drugs altering peripheral or central adrenergic activity may adversely affect physical performance or cognitive function. Also, the recognized adverse effects of diuretics on glucose metabolism and of diuretics and beta-adrenergic blocking agents on lipid metabolism are of equal concern. Thus a definite need for treatment must be established before therapy with any of these agents is introduced during the first or second decade of life with the possibility of 50 to 60 years (or more) of continuous antihypertensive therapy.

Patients Who Need Special Care. Patients at higher risk from their hypertension need even more protection by effective antihypertensive therapy. This includes diabetics, blacks, and hypertensive patients with target organ damage affecting their brain, heart, or kidneys.

Of these patients, hypertensive diabetics are particularly vulnerable to rapidly progressive renal damage. They should be followed with frequent measurements of urine protein and creatinine clearance. If either is abnormal, intensive therapy to prevent hyperperfusion of remaining glomeruli by either hypertension or hyperglycemia may protect them from progressive sclerosis and thereby delay, if not stop, the hitherto inexorable progression to renal failure.

Hypertensive Crises. Several clinical circumstances require rapid reduction of the blood pressure. These circumstances include hypertensive encephalopathy, severe hypertension in the presence of rapidly developing target organ damage, and accelerated malignant hypertension.

In most hypertensive crises, the diastolic blood pressure is greater than 140 mm Hg. Funduscopic findings may include hemorrhages, exudates, and papilledema. The manifestations of encephalopathy include headache, confusion, somnolence, stupor, visual loss, focal defects, seizures, or coma. Cardiac findings include a hyperdynamic sustained left ventricular impulse, cardiac enlargement, and pulmonary venous hypertension. Oliguria and azotemia are usually present, as are symptoms of nausea and vomiting.

The drugs listed in Table 32-5 should provide as rapid and complete a reduction in markedly elevated pressures as needed. Oral agents with rapid onset of action work very well for those not needing parenteral therapy who have only a hypertensive urgency, that is, severe hypertension but no immediate danger to vital organs. Intravenous nitroprusside is surely the most effective and certain way to lower dangerously high blood pressure, but it requires constant surveillance and blood pressure monitoring. Intravenous nicardipine or labetalol is easier to use.

Maintaining Adherence to Therapy

Most patients for whom drug therapy is prescribed take the drug assiduously at first. But with the onset of either bothersome side effects or the natural tendency to lose motivation and forget, as many as half are not adhering to therapy a year later. The following practices should be helpful in improving patients' adherence to therapy:

1. Inform patients of their blood pressure and overall cardiovascular risk status by use of Framingham predictive data available from the American Heart Association's *Coronary Risk Handbook* or pharmaceutical companies' hand calculators.
2. Be gentle in trying to change unhealthy lifestyles, but insist on the need to do so.
3. Repeatedly emphasize the need to stop smoking, and to reduce calories, sodium, and saturated fat and to increase isotonic exercise, perhaps not all at one time but eventually.
4. Prescribe medications in the fewest number and lowest doses possible, slowly building up to required levels.
5. Go slow with medications to avoid symptoms of cerebral hypoperfusion, allowing the system to readjust by autoregulation to a lower blood pressure level. With the initial fall in blood pressure, even if not to "hypotensive" levels, cerebral blood flow may decrease. The range of blood pressure over which autoregulation maintains a normal cerebral blood flow is shifted to the right in chronic hypertensives; when blood pressure is lowered below the lower end of this range, but still at a level above 140/90 mm Hg, cerebral blood flow may fall, leading to postural dizziness, weakness, and fatigue.
6. Involve the patient (and, if acceptable, the spouse) in the process as a willing partner, not as a passive recipient. Use home blood pressure measurements, medication diaries, and self-determined behavioral goals. The currently available home blood pressure units with microphone detectors and digital readouts can be easily used by virtually every patient, and their relatively low cost makes them accessible to most. Their use will provide a better idea of the usual range of the blood pressure, helping to establish the diagnosis and to make the decision to start treatment. Once patients are on therapy, it is particularly important to ensure dampening of the abrupt rise in pressure upon awakening that is responsible for the increased incidence of heart attacks and strokes in the early

✔ *WHEN TO REFER*

Few patients need referral for either the diagnosis or treatment of their hypertension if primary care practitioners follow appropriate guidelines and are reasonably patient. Referral may be needed for these reasons: (1) to establish the presence of hypertension by ambulatory monitoring if the diagnosis cannot be made by multiple home measurements, (2) to ascertain a secondary form of hypertension in those with inappropriate features such as rapidly progressive renal insufficiency or abnormal findings on screening studies, (3) to control those who are truly resistant despite the use of adequate diuretics and multiple antihypertensives in full doses, and (4) to manage the few with accelerated malignant hypertension with or without hypertensive encephalopathy. Often patients who are symptomatic with virtually any and all medications need only to have their anxiety dealt with or restarted on very low doses of medication to overcome falls in cerebral perfusion.

morning. If these postawakening pressures are not lowered, longer-acting medications or twice-a-day dosing may be needed.

7. Use nonphysician personnel for follow-up and psychological support. As physician extenders, they can be particularly effective in monitoring and encouraging the use of nondrug regimens.

The application of these maneuvers to improve adherence to treatment and the judicious use of both nondrug and drug therapies should make it possible to bring the blood pressure down to safe levels in virtually all patients with hypertension.

BIBLIOGRAPHY

Alderman MH, Madhavan S, Cohen H et al: Low urinary sodium is associated with greater risk of myocardial infarction among treated hypertensive men, *Hypertension* 25:1144-1152, 1995.

Brenner BM, Chertow GM: Congenital oligonephropathy and the etiology of adult hypertension and progressive renal injury, *Am J Kidney Dis* 23:171-175, 1994.

Burt VL et al: Trends in the prevalence, awareness, treatment, and control of hypertension in the adult US population. Data from the Health Examination Surveys, 1960 to 1991, *Hypertension* 26:60-69, 1995.

Burt VL et al: Prevalence of hypertension in the US adult population. Results from the Third National Health Nutrition Examination Survey, 1988-1991, *Hypertension* 25:305-313, 1995.

Cruickshank JM: Coronary flow reserve and the J curve relation between diastolic blood pressure and myocardial infarction, *Br Med J* 297:1227, 1988.

Folkow B: Psychosocial and central nervous influences in primary hypertension, *Circulation* 76(suppl I):I, 1987.

Guyton AC: Kidneys and fluids in pressure regulation. Small volume but large pressure changes, *Hypertension* 19(suppl I):I, 1992.

Hallett JW Jr et al: Advanced renovascular hypertension and renal insufficiency: trends in medical comorbidity and surgical approach from 1970 to 1993, *J Vasc Surg* 21:750-760, 1995.

Harper R, Ennis CN, Sheridan B et al: Effects of low dose versus conventional dose thiazide diuretic on insulin action in essential hypertension, *Br Med J* 309:226-230, 1994.

Hoes AW, Grobbee DE, Lubsen J: Does drug treatment improve survival? Reconciling the trials in mild-to-moderate hypertension, *J Hypertens* 13:805-811, 1995.

Horan MJ, Sinaiko AR: Synopsis of the report of the Second Task Force on Blood Pressure Control in Children, *Hypertension* 10:115, 1987.

Joint National Committee on Detection, Evaluation, and Treatment of High Blood Pressure: The Fifth Report of the Joint National Committee on Detection, Evaluation, and Treatment of High Blood Pressure (JNC V), *Arch Intern Med* 153:154-183, 1993.

Kaplan NM: *Clinical hypertension*, ed 6, Baltimore, 1994, Williams & Wilkins.

Kaplan NM: Management of hypertensive emergencies, *Lancet* 344:1335-1338, 1994.

Kaplan NM: Do calcium antagonists cause myocardial infarction? *Am J Cardiol* 77:81-82, 1996.

Lever AF: Slow pressor mechanisms in hypertension: a role for hypertrophy of resistance vessels? *J Hypertens* 4:515, 1986.

Lever AF, Ramsay LE: Treatment of hypertension in the elderly, *J Hypertens* 13:571-579, 1995.

Lithell HOL: Effect of antihypertensive drugs on insulin, glucose, and lipid metabolism, *Diabetes Care* 14:203, 1991.

Lund-Johansen P: Central haemodynamics in essential hypertension at rest and during exercise: a 20-year follow-up study. *J Hypertens* 7(suppl 6):S52, 1989.

Lüscher TF: The endothelium in hypertension: bystander, target or mediator? *J Hypertens* 12(suppl 10):S105-S116, 1994.

National High Blood Pressure Education Program: Update on the 1977 Task Force report on high blood pressure in children and adolescents, *Pediatrics* 98:649-658, 1996.

Neaton JD, Wentworth D: Serum cholesterol, blood pressure, cigarette smoking, and death from coronary heart disease. Overall findings and differences by age for 316,099 white men, *Arch Intern Med* 152:56, 1992.

Olin JW et al: The utility of duplex ultrasound scanning of the renal arteries for diagnosing significant renal artery stenosis, *Ann Intern Med* 122:833-838, 1995.

Perloff D, Sokolow M, Cowan R: The prognostic value of ambulatory blood pressures, *JAMA* 249:2792, 1983.

Peterson JC et al: Blood pressure control, proteinuria, and the progression of renal disease, *Ann Intern Med* 123:754-762, 1995.

Pickering TG: Blood pressure measurement and detection of hypertension, *Lancet* 344:31, 1994.

SHEP Cooperative Research Group: Prevention of stroke by antihypertensive drug treatment in older persons with isolated systolic hypertension. Final results of the Systolic Hypertension in the Elderly Program (SHEP), *JAMA* 265:3255, 1991.

Verdecchia P et al: Ambulatory blood pressure. An independent predictor of prognosis in essential hypertension, *Hypertension* 24:793-801, 1994.

Yanagisawa M et al: A novel potent vasoconstrictor peptide produced by vascular endothelial cells, *Nature* 332:411, 1988.

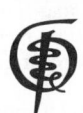

CHAPTER

33 Cardiac Tumors; Cardiac Manifestations of Endocrine, Collagen Vascular, and HIV Disease; and Traumatic Injury of the Heart

John S. MacGregor and Melvin D. Cheitlin

CARDIAC TUMORS

Primary tumors of the heart are relatively rare, but correct and timely diagnosis is important because surgical cure is often possible. Seventy-five percent of primary cardiac tumors are benign histologically; however, because of their location, they frequently produce life-threatening complications. Protean clinical manifestations, which are in part determined by the size and location of the tumor, have been described. They include chest pain, dyspnea, syncope, arrhythmias, murmurs, systemic and central nervous system emboli, and coronary artery and pulmonary artery emboli, as well as pericardial effusion, cardiac tamponade, fever, weight loss, and edema. The diagnosis most often is made by two-dimensional echocardiography and/or angiography. More recently it has been established with increasing frequency by computer tomography or magnetic resonance imaging. The relative incidence of primary cardiac tumors is shown on Table 33-1.

Table 33-1   Incidence of primary cardiac tumors

	PERCENTAGE OF PRIMARY CARDIAC TUMORS
Benign	
Myxoma	30.5
Lipoma	10.5
Papillary fibroelastoma	9.9
Rhabdomyoma	8.5
Fibroma	4.0
Hemangioma	3.5
Teratoma	3.3
AV node mesothelioma	2.8
Other benign tumors	2.1
TOTAL BENIGN TUMORS	75.1
Malignant	
Angiosarcoma	9.2
Rhabdomyosarcoma	6.1
Fibrosarcoma	3.2
Lymphoma	1.6
Other malignant tumors	4.8
TOTAL MALIGNANT TUMORS	24.9

Modified from McAllister HA, Fenoglio JJ: *Atlas of tumor pathology.* Washington, DC, 1978, Armed Forces Institute of Pathology.

MYXOMA

Myxomas account for about one third of primary cardiac tumors. They are much more common in adults, with the greatest incidence between the third and sixth decades. Most cases are sporadic, but familial autosomal dominant transmission has been reported. Rare cases have been associated with a syndrome that includes multiple pigmented skin lesions, myxomatous mammary fibroadenomas, and adrenocortical disease. The left atrium is the most common location for myxomas, accounting for about 80% of cases. Fifteen percent are located in the right atrium, with most of the remainder arising in the right ventricle. Left ventricular myxomas are exceedingly rare. Atrial myxomas are usually attached to the interatrial septum in the region of the limbus of the fossa ovalis. Less often they are attached to the posterior or anterior atrial walls or to the atrial appendage. Cardiac myxomas arise from multipotential mesenchymal cells present in subendocardial tissue. At the time of excision, they are usually 5 to 6 cm in diameter and project into a cardiac chamber on a short, broad-based fibrovascular stalk, which is in communication with the subendocardium. Characteristically, they have a polypoid and pedunculated appearance.

Although cardiac myxomas are generally considered to be benign histologically, several reports have suggested that they may rarely possess a malignant potential. These include reports of distant metastasis with independent growth, local invasion, and local recurrence after excision.

Clinical manifestations fall into three major categories: hemodynamic compromise, embolization, and constitutional symptoms. The nature of the hemodynamic manifestations depends on the size and location of the tumor. Left atrial myxomas commonly mimic mitral valve disease, especially mitral stenosis, in their clinical presentation. Symptoms are those of left-sided heart failure, including dyspnea and occasionally chest pain. Intermittent obstruction of the mitral outflow tract by a large mobile myxoma can lead to syncope or sudden death. Physical findings with left atrial myxoma may include a low-pitched, early to middiastolic sound known as a "tumor plop," and a diastolic murmur resembling that of mitral stenosis. Mitral valve disease can sometimes be distinguished from atrial myxoma on physical examination by identifying marked positional variation of the physical findings. The systolic murmur of mitral regurgitation may result from injury to the mitral valve caused by the tumor.

Right atrial myxomas produce hemodynamic symptoms, either by intermittently obstructing the tricuspid valve and mimicking tricuspid stenosis, or by damaging the valve and producing tricuspid regurgitation. Hemodynamic manifestations of right atrial myxoma include dyspnea, edema, hepatosplenomegaly, and elevated jugular venous pressure. These findings may be confused with cor pulmonale, constrictive pericarditis, and Ebstein's anomaly.

About 50% of patients with myxoma have embolic manifestations, including emboli to the central nervous system, coronary arteries, peripheral organs and viscera, and in the case of right atrial myxoma, to the lungs. Constitutional symptoms are common in patients with myxoma, and in some cases may dominate the presentation. Constitutional manifestations of myxoma include fever, fatigue, malaise, weight loss, arthralgias, myalgias, rash, Raynaud's phenomenon, leukocytosis, elevated erythrocyte sedimentation rate, abnormal serum proteins, and hypergammaglobulinemia. These symptoms result from an immunologic reaction to a "foreign" antigen. Typically, these systemic signs resolve after excision of the myxoma.

The diagnosis of myxoma is confirmed by either transthoracic or transesophageal two-dimensional echocardiography, which usually demonstrates the size and site of attachment of a myxoma (Chapter 13). Magnetic resonance imaging has been used to verify or exclude the presence of intracardiac tumors in cases where the echocardiographic diagnosis is equivocal. In most cases cardiac catheterization and cineangiography are not necessary to make this diagnosis. It may be necessary, however, to diagnose coexistent cardiac or coronary artery disease before surgery. When catheterization is required, direct catheterization of the chamber from which the tumor arises should be avoided, because it can lead to tumor dislodgement and embolization. Surgical excision including the portion of the atrium from which the tumor arises is usually curative, although local recurrence occasionally occurs. Operative mortality and morbidity are low, and the prognosis after excision is generally excellent, usually with total resolution of preoperative symptoms.

OTHER BENIGN CARDIAC TUMORS

Lipomas and papillary fibroelastomas each account for about 15% of benign cardiac tumors. Lipomas most often occur in the interatrial septum, where they grow as a nonencapsulated mass of adipose tissue, which bulges in the subendocardium into the right atrium. Lipomas develop by hypertrophy of adipose tissue, which is in continuity with epicardial fat, and are not true neoplasms. They are most commonly asymptomatic and are usually incidental findings at autopsy. Supraventricular arrhythmias, conduction disturbances, and hemodynamic compromise may be seen.

Papillary fibroelastomas arise from cardiac valves or adjacent endothelium. They are usually asymptomatic and, like lipomas, are usually incidental findings on postmortem examination. They occasionally cause symptoms either by embolization or by interference with valve function. Rarely they lodge in the ostium of one of the coronary arteries, resulting in sudden death. Rhabdomyomas are the most common benign cardiac tumor in children, 90% of cases occurring before age 15. Rhabdomyomas are thought to be hamartomatous growths derived from fetal cardiac myoblasts. They are multicentric in up to 90% of cases. They are found most commonly in the ventricles, but up to 30% involve the atria. This tumor usually grows deep within the myocardium but can also have intracavitary extension. There is a strong association between rhabdomyomas and tuberous sclerosis, a condition characterized by mental retardation and convulsions (Chapter 310). Clinical manifestations include tachyarrhythmias and heart failure. Surgical resection can be difficult because of multicentric growth, lack of encapsulation, and intramyocardial location; but it should be considered to relieve symptoms in suitable individuals.

Fibromas occur in both pediatric and adult patients but are more common in children. They are solitary and usually involve the ventricular septum. Symptoms relate to conduction system involvement and often include arrhythmias and sudden death. Surgical therapies have included tumor resection, and in the case of unresectable tumors, cardiac transplantation. Mesotheliomas are intramyocardial tumors that most commonly occur near the atrioventricular node. They can cause conduction disturbances including complete heart block and sudden death. Antiarrhythmic agents and pacemaker implantation in selected patients with fibromas and mesotheliomas may be useful.

MALIGNANT PRIMARY CARDIAC TUMORS

Malignant tumors comprise about 25% of all cardiac tumors. Sarcomas account for almost all of the malignant tumors, with angiosarcomas and rhabdomyosarcomas being the most common histologic types. These tumors may arise in any cardiac chamber, but right-sided involvement is more common. Symptoms at presentation include rapidly progressive heart failure, arrhythmias, and hemopericardium with tamponade. At the time of diagnosis, advanced regional extension and distant metastasis are often present, precluding curative surgical excision. Surgery may be needed, however, to establish a tissue diagnosis to guide chemotherapy and radiation therapy, which may slow progression in some cases. The prognosis is poor, with most patients dying within 1 year of the diagnosis. Figure 33-1, *A* shows a two-dimensional echocardiogram with a large mass that extends from the right atrium, across the tricuspid valve, into the right ventricle. The patient reported a brief illness that included abdominal swelling, lower extremity edema, near-syncope, and profound fatigue. Physical findings included marked jugular venous distention, hepatomegaly, ascites, and lower extremity edema. The lung fields were clear and no murmur was heard. The clinical presentation outlined here is the result of near-total obstruction of the tricuspid valve by the tumor resulting in decreased cardiac output. The mass was surgically resected and light microscopy demonstrated a high-grade angiosarcoma (Fig. 33-1 *B, C*).

METASTATIC TUMORS INVOLVING THE HEART

Metastasis of noncardiac tumors to the heart is a much more common cause of neoplastic heart disease than primary cardiac tumors. In a large autopsy series, up to 20% of patients dying of a malignancy had cardiac or pericardial metastases. Like metastasis elsewhere in the body, mechanisms of metastasis to the heart include direct tumor extension and lymphatic and hematogenous spread. The

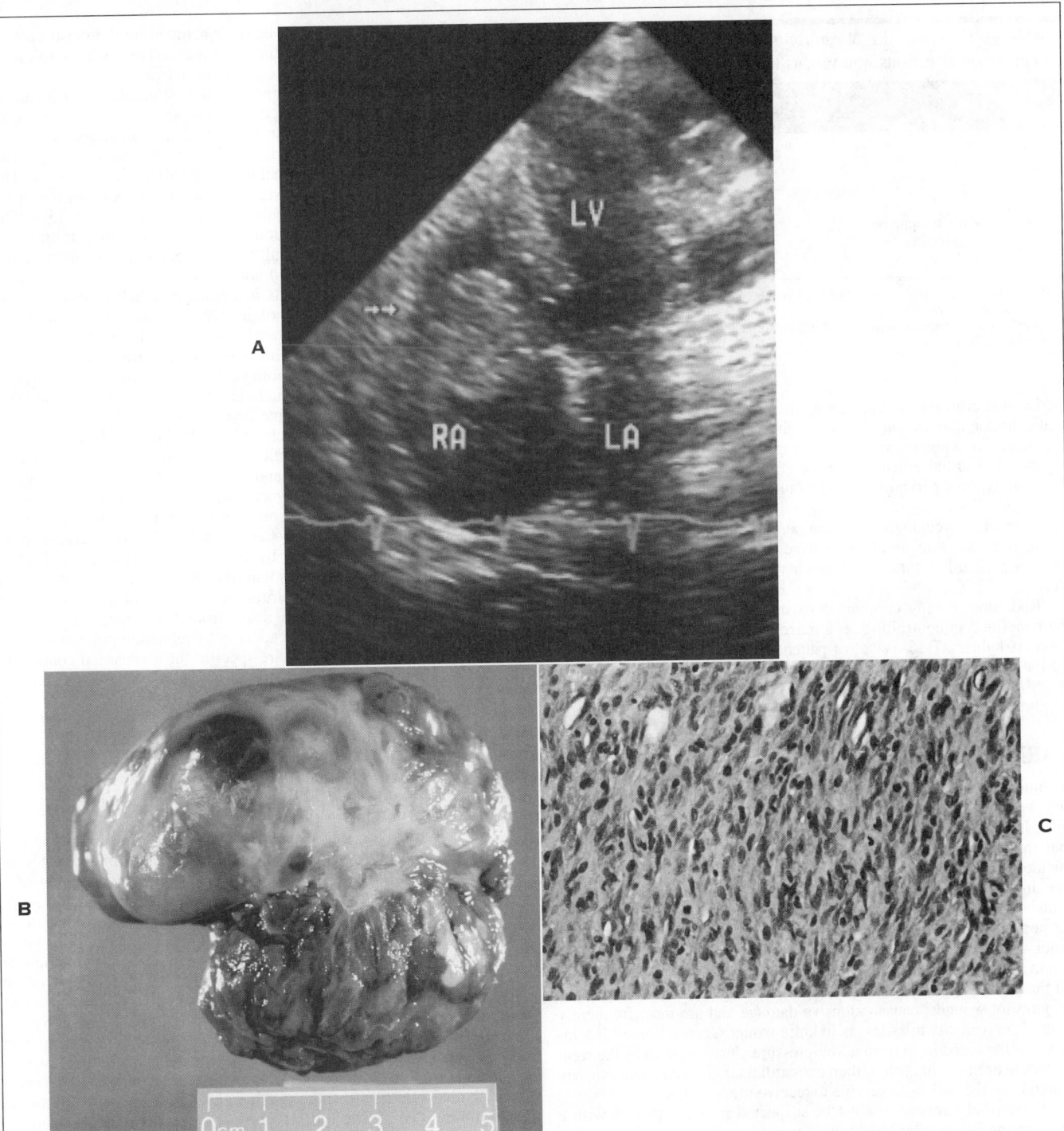

FIGURE 33-1   A, Two-dimensional echocardiogram showing a large tumor extending from the right atrium across the tricuspid valve into the right ventricle. **B,** Gross pathology specimen of tumor, which measured over 8 cm in its largest dimension. **C,** Light microscopy of mass after hematoxylin and eosin stain, showing a highly malignant angiosarcoma.

pericardium, myocardium, and endocardium may all be involved. The gross appearance of the metastatic tumor may be either diffuse and infiltrative or nodular.

The prevalence of cardiac involvement with several specific noncardiac primary tumors is shown in Table 33-2. Melanoma and leukemia commonly involve the heart, with a 45% and 33% incidence of cardiac metastasis diagnosed at autopsy, respectively. Lung and breast cancers account for the largest absolute number of cardiac metastases, accounting for 28% and 12% of all cardiac metastases, respectively. If cardiac involvement is present, widespread metastatic disease is usually present. With the advent of the adult immunodefi-

ciency syndrome resulting from HIV infection, Kaposi's sarcoma and non-Hodgkin's lymphoma have become important tumors involving the heart. Cardiac symptoms attributable to metastases are present in only about 10% of the patients with metastatic tumors to the heart. Symptoms, when present, typically relate to heart failure, pericarditis, pericardial tamponade, and vena caval obstruction. The latter is seen frequently in tumors that can grow up from the kidney into the inferior vena cava and the right side of the heart.

A chest roentenogram showing an enlarged cardiac silhouette or evidence of mediastinal tumor may suggest the diagnosis of tumor metastasis to the heart. Echocardiography is useful for identifying

Table 33-2   Prevalence of cardiac metastasis at postmortem examination in patients with various tumors

TUMOR	PERCENTAGE WITH CARDIAC METASTASES*
Melanoma	45 (433)
Leukemia	33 (1345)
Lung	23 (3523)
Breast	21 (1639)
Non-Hodgkin's lymphoma	20 (953)
Hodgkin's lymphoma	8 (562)
Renal	10 (501)

Pooled data from 19 studies, modified from Weinberg BA, Conces DJ Jr, Waller BF: *Clin Cardiol* 12:289-296, 1989.
*Numbers in parentheses indicate total number of autopsy examinations performed in each tumor category.

pericardial effusion and confirming the presence of tamponade. Metastatic tumor masses may be seen with echocardiography, magnetic resonance imaging, or computed tomography. Large symptomatic malignant pericardial effusions can be effectively treated with drainage by a subxyphoid pericardial window under local anesthesia with minimal morbidity.

Recently, percutaneous balloon pericardiotomy has been found to be an effective, safe, and less invasive technique than surgery for creating a pericardial window in patients with malignant pericardial effusions.

Radiation therapy or treatment with a local sclerosing agent can be beneficial in controlling recurrence of malignant pericardial effusions (Chapter 27). Survival of patients with metastatic involvement of the heart depends on the extent and rate of progression of the primary disease. In one series, up to 50% of patients treated with a subxyphoid pericardiectomy were dead within 3 months.

CARDIOVASCULAR TRAUMA

Trauma to the myocardium, septum, valves, coronary arteries, aorta, and veins can occur with both penetrating and nonpenetrating injuries. In most instances of nonpenetrating cardiovascular trauma, the patient has multiple injuries, and the cardiovascular trauma may be incidental and overlooked. This is especially true with nonpenetrating injuries, such as compression injuries in automobile accidents causing myocardial contusion. When a cardiac chamber is lacerated in nonpenetrating injury, the laceration is usually extensive and the injury fatal.

In penetrating trauma the amount of damage is related to the mass of the penetrating object and to its velocity. High-velocity missiles, as in gunshot wounds, cause extensive damage and are most frequently fatal. Low-velocity missiles, as in knife wounds, cause limited lacerations; if the bleeding is from a low-pressure chamber, such as the right ventricle or the right atrium, then pericardial tamponade occurs slowly enough for the patient to survive to receive medical care.

Pericardial tamponade must be suspected in every patient with a penetrating injury who has hypotension. If the intravascular volume is normal and tamponade occurs gradually, the patient may have the usual clinical picture of pericardial tamponade including tachycardia, increased central venous pressure, and hypotension. However, in trauma patients with hypovolemia caused by hemorrhage, pericardial tamponade must be suspected when the penetrating injury could have involved the heart and when there is hypotension despite fluid and blood replacement, even if the central venous pressure is not elevated. If the patient is hemodynamically stable, pericardiocentesis can be attempted. If the bleeding is rapid, however, blood often clots in the pericardium and is impossible to extract through a needle. In this case thoracotomy is necessary with extraction of the pericardial blood and clot. If the patient is hemodynamically unstable, immediate thoracotomy with relief of the tamponade and repair of the laceration is lifesaving. Aside from the clinical picture, two-dimensional echocardiography is the fastest way to make a diagnosis of bleeding into the pericardium. The echocardiogram can demonstrate the amount of fluid and whether clots are present. Furthermore, the pathophysiol-

ogy of cardiac tamponade can be demonstrated by the presence of a distended inferior vena cava that does not collapse with inspiration and the diastolic collapse of the right and left atrium.

With nonpenetrating injury the commonest problem is myocardial contusion. This results from chest compression, as occurs with steering-wheel injuries, and also from sudden deceleration where the chest wall suddenly stops moving and the mediastinum crashes into the chest wall at the velocity that the vehicle had been traveling. The incidence of myocardial contusion at postmortem examination in fatal accidents involving thoracoabdominal trauma is about 15%. The incidence of myocardial contusion in survivors of nonpenetrating thoracoabdominal trauma is difficult to assess and depends on the criteria used to diagnose myocardial contusion.

Myocardial contusion results in intramyocardial hemorrhage and myocardial necrosis. Because of its location, the right ventricle is most frequently involved, followed in frequency by the left ventricle. The retrosternal right atrium and posterior left atrium are less commonly involved. Arrhythmias, both ventricular and atrial, are frequent; electrocardiographic changes, including ST-T wave changes and QRS changes, including those of acute myocardial infarction, are seen, as are varying degrees of AV block and bundle-branch block.

Myocardial contusion is difficult to diagnose. Pericardial friction rubs with pericardial effusion and congestive heart failure are good evidence for the presence of myocardial contusion. However, arrhythmias are less specific and can be seen with sympathetic stimulation and anxiety after injury. Electrocardiographic (ECG) changes can be either pre-existing or caused by hypoxia. Arrhythmias and ECG changes can be related to drugs that have been taken, such as alcohol or other therapeutic or illicit drugs involved in the precipitation of the accident. Hypotension can result from hemorrhage. Pulmonary edema on chest radiograph can actually be related to pulmonary contusion. None of these findings are specific for myocardial contusion. A rise in serum creatine kinase (CK) is usually caused by skeletal-muscle injury. A rise in CK-MB fraction is more specific for myocardial necrosis but also occurs with smooth-muscle injury and even with massive skeletal muscle necrosis. Imaging techniques such as radionuclide angiography or two-dimensional echocardiography can show areas of hypokinesia or even akinesia in myocardial contusions and thus indicate that the ECG changes seen are probably related to myocardial contusion.

All the complications seen after acute myocardial infarction can occur after myocardial contusion, including rupture of the left ventricular free wall, rupture of the septum with the development of a ventricular septal defect, mitral regurgitation, fatal arrhythmias, congestive heart failure, and false and true ventricular aneurysms. However, if the patient has a suspected, uncomplicated myocardial contusion without tamponade and without heart failure, serious complications from the contusion rarely occur either in the hospital or on follow-up. In the absence of symptomatic arrhythmias the patient can safely be observed on a nonmonitored ward before discharge. Symptomatic arrhythmias should be observed in a monitored ward and treated with lidocaine. Late complications of uncomplicated myocardial contusion are very unusual. After pericardial injury or myocardial contusion, a posttraumatic pericarditis can result probably on an autoimmune basis. The typical story is that of the development of chest discomfort, usually with a pleuritic component developing 1 week to several months after the trauma. The discomfort may be accompanied by a low-grade fever and other signs of an inflammatory reaction. Not infrequently, a pericardial friction rub is present. The treatment as long as tamponade has not occurred is that of idiopathic pericarditis with nonsteroidal antiinflammatory drugs. If there is no response, a short course of high-dose steroids is effective. In most cases, only one episode occurs. Occasionally, there are several episodes. Very infrequently, the pericarditis can be repetitively recurrent, requiring antimetabolite drugs; occasionally pericardiectomy is necessary to relieve the pain.

On rare occasions penetrating and nonpenetrating injuries can injure the interventricular septum and cause an interventricular septal defect, or can rupture an aortic, mitral, or tricuspid valve cusp, or even rupture a papillary muscle, all resulting in valvular regurgitation, varying in degree from severe acute valvular regurgitation requiring afterload reduction and immediate surgery to mild degrees of valvular regurgitation that do not require surgery.

Coronary arteries can be injured, especially with penetrating injuries, and tamponade can occur from a laceration of the coronary artery. Injury to a coronary artery and coronary vein can result in a coronary arteriovenous fistula. Occasionally, coronary-cameral fistulas result from injury. All these can best be evaluated by coronary arteriography.

Of the great vessel injuries, traumatic rupture of the aorta is the most serious. It occurs most frequently in deceleration injuries in automobile accidents. The most common site of rupture is in the proximal descending aorta, just after the take-off of the subclavian artery, and about 15% of patients with ruptured aorta survive long enough to reach medical care and be diagnosed clinically. The second most common site of rupture is in the ascending aorta, just above the aortic valve; because of the intrapericardial position of the ascending aorta this almost always results in death from tamponade. Aortic rupture should be suspected on the basis of chest roentgenograms showing a widened mediastinum. Other signs such as fluid capping the left lung, left pleural effusion, and obscuration of the descending aorta by bleeding in the mediastinum should all alert the physician to possible rupture of the aorta. When suspected, immediate aortography followed by immediate repair is indicated. In false aneurysms caused by remote injury, repair is still indicated because false aneurysms can rupture at any time. In some centers, computed tomography scans are recommended as a screening test for ruptured aorta in patients with widened mediastinum. Transesophageal echocardiography (TEE), especially using the Omniprobe, can visualize the ascending aorta, most of the aortic arch, and the entire thoracic descending aorta. Therefore a skilled echocardiographer using TEE can reliably and rapidly make a diagnosis of aortic rupture. Aortography used to be the preferred way of making the diagnosis. In many centers, computed tomography or TEE has become the dominant imaging technique.

Slow-velocity missiles can enter the heart muscle or cardiac chambers or vessels and lodge there. These missiles can cause infection and damage to the chambers. Moreover, if they lie in the lumen of veins, arteries, or cardiac chambers they can migrate forward, the venous missiles lodging finally in the right heart or pulmonary artery and left heart or arterial missiles migrating distally causing obstruction. Another complication is the development of thrombus and fibrin, which can then embolize. Foreign bodies, especially in the left chamber of the heart or arteries, should be removed. If the missile is small and intramyocardial and causes no mechanical dysfunction, the patient can be observed without surgical removal.

Finally, the fastest growing cause of traumatic cardiovascular injury is iatrogenic trauma resulting from the increase in invasive medical procedures being performed. This includes laceration of arteries and veins, perforation of the right ventricle with a catheter resulting in tamponade, and cutting off of intravascular lines. These lost catheters usually can be removed with snare catheters without surgery.

ACQUIRED IMMUNODEFICIENCY SYNDROME (AIDS)

Infection with the human immunodeficiency virus (HIV), a retrovirus that invades the nucleus of the host cell and incorporates a copy of its DNA in the host genetic material, was first recognized in 1981 (Chapter 248). After a latent period, the virus releases into the cytoplasm double-stranded DNA copies of the virus, eventually killing the cell and invading other immune cells, usually T-helper lymphocytes, eventually compromising the immune defense mechanism of the host. This makes the host susceptible to opportunistic infections and unusual cancers such as Kaposi's sarcoma and non-Hodgkin's lymphoma from which the patient eventually dies.

In the United States, the populations at high risk are homosexual men, IV-drug-abusing patients, prostitutes, and patients receiving blood products, such as hemophiliacs. Heterosexual transmission occurs in women who are IV drug abusers and/or have sexual intercourse with infected men (Chapter 248).

Cardiovascular involvement in AIDS is usually clinically of little consequence, possibly because the myocardial cell lacks the CD-4 receptor necessary for the virus to enter the cell. Cardiovascular involvement is seen with opportunistic infections such as toxoplasmosis, *Candida, Cryptococcus,* and cytomegalovirus. Rarely, the patient can have a severe, clinically important myocarditis with toxo-

plasmosis. Pericarditis with pericardial effusion and tamponade is the commonest clinical cardiovascular problem in our experience; about a third of the patients with pericardial fluid develop tamponade requiring pericardiocentesis. Most often an etiologic agent is not found on culture of the pericardial fluid or biopsy of the pericardium. However, involvement with lymphoma and with *Mycobacterium tuberculosis* and *avium* is not uncommon. The presence of a pericardial effusion in a patient with AIDS is a bad prognostic sign because such patients have a shorter survival than AIDS patints without pericardial effusion.

Patients with severe pulmonary hypertension, right ventricular dilatation, and even right ventricular failure have been reported. This usually occurs in patients with multiple episodes of *Pneumocystis carinii* infections. Patients with primary pulmonary hypertension have been reported with electron microscopic changes in the pulmonary vascular endothelium similar to those seen in lupus erythematosus. No evidence of HIV organism was found in the pulmonary endothelium by *in situ hybridization.* The postulated mechanism is the production of endothelial injury by paracrine cytokines releasing vasoactive substances or growth factors that result in increased pulmonary vascular resistance.

Other cardiovascular abnormalities in patients with HIV infection have included thrombotic noninfectious endocarditis (marantic endocarditis) and mitral valve prolapse. When infective endocarditis is seen, it is usually in IV drug abusers.

The most interesting cardiovascular involvement seen is the patient with decreased left ventricular function, with or without left ventricular dilation. This is not an uncommon echocardiographic finding, and wall motion abnormalities including hypokinesis are reported in 15% to 40% of patients with AIDS. At postmortem examination, focal collections of round cells in the myocardium—so-called focal myocarditis—can be seen in 20% to 40% of patients. Diffuse myocarditis, on the other hand, is rare. At autopsy, dilated cardiomyopathy is also rare as is dilated cardiomyopathy with clinical congestive heart failure. In one prospective echocardiographic survey of 296 HIV- infected adults conducted over 4 years, 13 (4%) were found to have dilated cardiomyopathy.

The etiology of cardiomyopathy is unknown, but there are probably multiple explanations. Myocarditis resulting from HIV infection is the most obvious explanation. Attempts have been made to demonstrate the HIV organism in the myocardium, with limited success. Calebrese reported culturing the HIV virus from a right ventricular myocardial biopsy from a patient with a normal left ventricular myocardium and no evidence of left ventricular disease. Lewis and colleagues have reported positive identification of portions of the HIV virion in the myocardium from people dying of AIDS by in situ hybridization techniques. These positive findings were infrequent and from this technique it is not clear that the identified nucleic acid sequences were derived from myocytes. They could have been from endothelial cells, circulating lymphocytes, or tissue macrophages. Furthermore, the hearts of these patients were all normal without clinical or microscopic evidence of cardiac abnormality.

Other explanations of poor systolic contractile function have been suggested. These patients often are taking a wide variety of drugs, some of which are known cardiac depressants capable of causing cardiomyopathy. Such drugs as adriamycin, interleukin II, and interferon-α have all been reported to cause cardiomyopathy, which is at times irreversible. The patients with hypokinesis and poor contractile function on echocardiography have been described as improving when azidothymidine (AZT) is withdrawn, and a "drug holiday" has been advised in such patients. Another possible explanation for hypokinesis is cytokine production, either systemically or locally in the myocardium, which could produce myocardial depression.

If the patient has a known pathogen as the cause of the myocarditis or pericarditis, obviously treatment specific for the organism is indicated. The value of myocardial biopsy is limited in such patients, since the finding of round cell infiltration is not likely to alter treatment.

DIABETES

Patients with diabetes have increased cardiovascular mortality and morbidity (Chapter 303). Diabetes is an independent risk factor for the development of coronary artery disease, which is frequently more diffuse and severe than in patients without diabetes. The concept that strict glycemic control can reduce both macrovascular and microvascular complications in diabetics is becoming increasingly accepted. Silent ischemia, or angina with atypical features, is more common in diabetics, probably resulting from autonomic and sensory neuropathies. Patients with insulin-dependent diabetes mellitus have an increased risk of developing congestive heart failure even in the absence of coronary artery disease, leading to the postulation of a diabetes-induced cardiomyopathy. Systolic and diastolic dysfunction have both been demonstrated in diabetics.

HYPERTHYROIDISM

Excess thyroid hormone stimulates the heart both through direct effects on cardiac muscle and by stimulating the sympathetic nervous system (Chapter 297). Cardiovascular manifestations of hyperthyroidism include palpitations, dyspnea, angina, heart failure, tachycardia, atrial fibrillation, hypertension, and increased cardiac output. Angina and congestive heart failure more commonly occur in patients with underlying heart disease, but they can occur in patients without coronary artery disease. In elderly patients, cardiovascular dysfunction, including atrial fibrillation and congestive heart failure, may be the only manifestations of hyperthyroidism. Therefore all elderly patients with these conditions should have laboratory determination of thyroid function. Findings on cardiac examination in hyperthyroid patients may include a wide pulse pressure, hyperdynamic precordium, accentuation of S_1 and S_2, and a pleuropericardial rub (Means-Lerman scratch) usually best heard in the second left intercostal space. Definitive therapy of hyperthyroidism is either surgical or pharmacologic ablation of the gland. Cardiac glycosides have been used to treat atrial arrhythmias; however, in hyperthyroidism there is frequently decreased sensitivity to conventional doses of these drugs. β-Adrenoceptor antagonists are useful in controlling rapid atrial arrhythmias and may also decrease other symptoms related to thyrotoxicosis. In the presence of severe heart failure they must be used cautiously.

HYPOTHYROIDISM

Hypothyroid patients may present with bradycardia, dyspnea, and easy fatigability (Chapter 297). Physical findings may include bradycardia, hypotension, distant heart sounds, edema, and rales. Cardiomegaly with global hypokinesis and four-chamber enlargement may be present in advanced cases. Pericardial and pleural effusion may be present, but pericardial tamponade is rare. Hypothyroidism is associated with hypercholesterolemia and hypertriglyceridemia, and patients are at increased risk for atherosclerotic vascular disease. Cardiac dysfunction related to hypothyroidism can be totally reversible with thyroid replacement therapy. Repletion of thyroid hormone should be done slowly, starting with a low dose, especially in the presence of coronary artery disease, to avoid precipitating episodes of unstable angina or myocardial infarction.

OBESITY

Increased cardiovascular mortality and morbidity in obese patients are in part related to increased rates of hypertension, atherosclerosis, and glucose intolerance (Chapter 288). Hemodynamic effects of obesity include increased left ventricular filling pressures, increased left ventricular end-diastolic volume, and increased cardiac output. Some obese patients develop an eccentric left ventricular hypertrophy with chamber dilation, which is associated with an increased incidence of ventricular ectopy and episodes of pulmonary edema. Weight reduction may have a salubrious effect on cardiac dysfunction related to obesity.

Some patients with extreme obesity hyperventilate causing hypoxia, hypercarbia, and respiratory acidosis, all powerful stimulators of pulmonary vasoconstriction. This causes severe pulmonary hypertension and cor pulmonale, the so-called Pickwickian syndrome (Chapter 36). The pulmonary hypertension is rapidly reversible with hyperventilation, and weight loss is the definitive treatment.

RHEUMATOID DISEASES

Cardiac manifestations of chronic rheumatoid diseases include pericardial effusion, pericarditis, myocarditis, arteritis, valvular abnormalities, conduction disturbances, heart failure, angina, and myocardial infarction. Systemic lupus erythematosus involves the heart in over 75% of patients; postmortem series demonstrate evidence of pericarditis in over two thirds of patients (Chapter 194). Pericardial tamponade and constrictive pericarditis are rare. Valvular pathology occurs in 30% to 50% of patients. Lesions include thickened valve leaflets with impaired function, which may lead to regurgitation or stenosis, and sterile Libman-Sacks vegetations. Myocarditis and coronary arteritis are sometimes seen. Accelerated or premature atherosclerosis may result in myocardial ischemia or infarction.

Necropsy series demonstrate cardiac involvement with rheumatoid arthritis in up to 50% of patients, pericarditis being the most common manifestation (Chapter 194). The clinical incidence of pericarditis is much lower than this, in the range of 5%, and is usually easily treated with steroids and antiinflammatory agents. Tamponade and constriction are rare. Coronary arteritis is present at autopsy in about 20% of patients with rheumatoid arthritis and may rarely lead to severe luminal narrowing with development of angina or myocardial infarction. Rheumatoid arthritis patients also have a higher incidence of atherosclerosis. Granulomatous inflammation of the cardiac valves can result in deformity and valvular insufficiency.

Progressive systemic sclerosis carries a poor prognosis when there is cardiac involvement (Chapter 197). Diffuse myocardial fibrosis with congestive heart failure occurs late in the course of this disease. Pericarditis and coronary arteritis are often also present in patients with progressive systemic sclerosis. Restrictive lung disease as a consequence of systemic sclerosis can result in cor pulmonale.

Polyarteritis nodosa results in a necrotizing vasculitis of the coronary arteries in up to 50% of cases, often with the formation of multiple areas of aneurysmal dilation (Chapter 195). Myocarditis and focal myocardial necrosis may follow the arteritis with subsequent development of congestive heart failure, a common cause of death in these patients. Valvular pathology is uncommon in patients with polyarteritis nodosa. Pericarditis is present in about 20% of these patients.

BIBLIOGRAPHY

Currie PF, Jacob AJ, Foreman AR et al: Heart muscle disease related to HIV infection: prognostic implications, *Br Med J* 309:1605-1607, 1994.

Doherty NE, Siegel RJ: Cardiovascular manifestations of systemic lupus erythematosus, *Am Heart J* 110:1257-1265, 1985.

Dubrow TJ, Mihalka J, Eisenhauer DM et al: Myocardial contusion in the stable patient: what level of care is appropriate? *Surgery* 106:267-273, 1989.

Follansbee WP, Curtiss EI, Medsger TA Jr et al: Physiologic abnormalities of cardiac function in progressive systemic sclerosis with diffuse scleroderma, *N Engl J Med* 310:142-148, 1984.

Forfar JC, Muir AL, Sawyers SA, Toft AD: Abnormal left ventricular function in hyperthyroidism: evidence for a possible reversible cardiomyopathy, *N Engl J Med* 307:1165-1170, 1982.

Heidenreich PA, Eisenberg MJ, Kee LL et al: Pericardial effusion in AIDS: incidence and survival, *Circulation* 92:3229-3234, 1995.

Hiatt JR, Yeatman LA Jr, Child JS: The value of echocardiography in blunt chest trauma, *J Trauma* 28:914-922, 1988.

Hossack KF, Moreno CA, Vanway CW, Burdick DC: Frequency of cardiac contusion in nonpenetrating chest injury, *Am J Cardiol* 61:391-394, 1988.

Khan AH, Spodick DH: Rheumatoid heart disease, *Semin Arthritis Rheum* 1:327-337, 1972.

Mette SA, Palevsky HI, Pietra GG et al: Primary pulmonary hypertension in association with human immunodeficiency virus infection: a possible viral etiology for some forms of hypertensive pulmonary arteriopathy, *Am Rev Respir Dis* 145:1196-1200, 1992.

Michaels AD, Lederman RJ, Mac Gregor JS, Cheitlin MD: Cardiovascular involvement in AIDS, *Curr Probl Cardiol* 22:109-148, 1997.

Nathan DM: Long-term complications of diabetes mellitus, *N Engl J Med* 328:1676-1685, 1993.

Nihoyannopoulos P, Gomez PM, Joshi J et al: Cardiac abnormalities in systemic lupus erythematosus, *Circulation* 82:369-375, 1990.

Potkin RT, Werner JA, Trobaugh GB et al: Evaluation of noninvasive tests of cardiac damage in suspected cardiac contusion, *Circulation* 66:627-631, 1982.

Reynen K: Cardiac myxomas, *N Engl J Med* 333:1610-1617, 1995.

Salcedo EE, Cohen GI, White RD, Davison MB: Cardiac tumors: diagnosis and management, *Curr Probl Cardiol* 17:73-137, 1992.

Schrader ML, Hochman JS, Bulkley BH: The heart in polyarteritis nodosa: a clinicopathologic study, *Curric Cardiol* 109:1353-1359, 1985.

Woeber KA: Thyrotoxicosis and the heart, *N Engl J Med* 327(2):94-98, 1992.

Ziskind AA, Pearce AC, Lemmon CC et al: Percutaneous balloon pericardiotomy for the treatment of cardiac tamponade and large pericardial effusions: description of technique and report of the first 50 cases, *J Am Coll Cardiol* 21(1):1-5, 1993.

34 Cardiac Transplantation

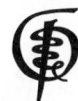

Lynne Warner Stevenson

CURRENT STATUS OF TRANSPLANTATION

Since the first cardiac transplantation was performed in 1967, more than 35,000 have been performed in the world. Survival has improved from 25% at 1 year in 1970 to 80% at 1 year in 1991, and is now 60% to 70% at 5 years for orthotopic transplantation (the new heart replaces the old, as opposed to heterotopic, where the new heart is attached "piggy-back" to the old heart, a procedure rarely done now). The improving results of transplantation have expanded the pool of potential candidates, both to patients with less critical compromise and to older patients with other systemic medical problems.

The increasing number of patients considered for transplantation contrasts with the relatively fixed supply of donor hearts: approximately 2500 hearts are available each year in the United States, and almost 1 million people have a history of severe symptoms of heart failure. Currently twice as many patients are listed than receive transplants each month. Paradoxically, the alternative medical therapy originally designed to stabilize patients before transplantation now frequently rivals transplantation for improving the quality of life and survival for many patients with heart failure. The major current challenges are (1) to identify those patients for whom transplantation offers the greatest benefit for quality and length of life, (2) to optimize the status of candidates until transplantation can be performed, (3) to maximize the use of suitable donor hearts, and (4) to prevent the accelerated coronary artery disease that limits extended survival of the transplanted heart.

REFERRAL FOR CARDIAC TRANSPLANTATION
Evaluation of Potential Candidates

At times in the past, cardiac transplantation and aggressive medical therapy for heart failure were not often offered in the same institutions. As medical therapy for advanced heart failure has improved and the supply of donor hearts has become more limiting, those institutions committed to either have developed expertise in both. The question no longer is when to refer for cardiac transplantation, but rather when to refer for advanced heart failure management, which may include transplantation, but only after consideration of other medical and surgical options. Referral of patients with advanced heart failure frequently leads to improved quality of life, exercise capacity, and reduced rehospitalizations for heart failure even when cardiac transplantation is not performed. All patients whose daily life remains limited by symptoms of heart failure after therapy with angiotensin-converting enzyme (ACE) inhibitors, diuretics, and digoxin should be considered for referral to a center with special expertise in heart failure. Although more than 95% of patients evaluated for transplantation have severe symptoms of heart failure, patients should also be evaluated when currently available therapy has not relieved daily limitation caused by angina or ventricular arrhythmias. Rare indications for transplantation include primary cardiac tumors or trauma.

Referral After Transplantation

The majority of hospitalizations after transplantation are triggered by rejection or infection. Any patient with unusual fatigue, dizziness, shortness of breath, or syncope merits immediate evaluation. New dysrhythmia or evidence of hemodynamic compromise that may represent rejection necessitates consultation with a transplant cardiologist. Hypotension may result from either rejection or infection, in addition to medications.

Patients take their temperatures daily and should in general be hospitalized for temperature above 100° Fahrenheit, except in occasional

BOX 34-1
Evaluation of heart failure patients for potentially reversible components

Patient factors
Extensive myocardial ischemia
Severe valvular lesions in the absence of irreversible myocardial decompensation
Recent viral infection
Excessive alcohol consumption
Frequent or incessant tachyarrhythmias
Hypertension
Anemia
Endocrine disorders
Electrolyte disturbances

Health care factors
Perception of "failure"
Incomplete adjustment of therapy
    Inadequate diuresis
    Vasodilator regimen adjusted to "standard" doses rather than optimal doses
    Transient stabilization on intravenous inotropic agents without revising oral regimen for discharge.
Lack of appropriate patient education
Excessive restriction of activity
Therapy with negatively inotropic agents during decompensation
Therapy with prostaglandin inhibitors

cases of obvious upper respiratory infections traversing a family. Determining the source of infection and the optimal antibiotic regimen requires consultation with a team experienced in the care of immunosuppressed patients.

Because of the multiple potential drug interactions, particularly with cyclosporine, the transplant specialist should be consulted for addition of any new medications or major change in medication dosages. Patients who are unable to absorb oral medications because of gastrointestinal illness or surgery will need to follow a parenteral immunosuppressive regimen until they can again establish adequate oral intake. The potential for adrenal suppression during medical or surgical stress should be recognized in all patients who have recently received glucocorticoid therapy.

EVALUATION AND MEDICAL THERAPY OF HEART FAILURE IN THE CANDIDATE
Etiology

During the evaluation of heart failure in a potential transplant candidate, it is important to establish the underlying cause if possible. Coronary artery disease accounts for approximately half of the heart failure in transplantation candidates. In 2% to 5% of these patients, revascularization of "hibernating" myocardium can lead to gradual improvement of ventricular function in the native heart, thus averting transplantation.

Dilated nonischemic cardiomyopathy is the other major cause of transplantation referral, whereas restrictive cardiomyopathy, valvular heart disease, and congenital heart disease together account for only 10% of primary transplantation recipients. The causative factors of most concern during an evaluation for transplantation are those with potential reversibility (Box 34-1) and those having a negative impact on posttransplantation outcome. Even after referral for transplantation, patients with symptoms lasting less than 6 months from nonischemic cardiomyopathy have almost a 30% chance of significant recovery of left ventricular function during the next 6 to 12 months, if transplantation can be avoided during that time. (Occasionally, young patients with total circulatory collapse associated with a recent viral infection may require mechanical circulatory support but recover virtually normal left ventricular function within 2 weeks.) Heart failure patients with a history of heavy alcohol consumption or

---

BOX 34-2

Tailored therapy for heart failure before cardiac transplantation

1. Measurement of baseline hemodynamics
2. Intravenous nitroprusside and diuretics tailored to hemodynamic goals:
   PCW ≤ 15 mm Hg   RA ≤ 8 mm Hg
   SVR ≤ 1200 dynes/sec/cm^{-5} SBP ≤ 80 mm Hg
3. Definition of optimal hemodynamics by 24 to 48 hours
4. Titration of high-dose oral vasodilators as nitroprusside weaned; captopril and isosorbide dinitrate with occasional addition of hydralazine
5. Monitored ambulation and diuretic adjustment for 24 to 48 hours
6. Maintenance digoxin levels 0.8 to 1.5 ng/dl if no contraindication
7. Detailed patient education including sodium restriction
8. Flexible outpatient diuretic regimen including intermittent metolazone based on daily weight
9. Progressive walking program
10. Vigilant follow-up through high-intensity heart failure clinic

---

PCW, pulmonary capillary wedge pressure; *RA*, right atrial pressure; *SBP*, systolic blood pressure; *SVR*, systemic vascular resistance.

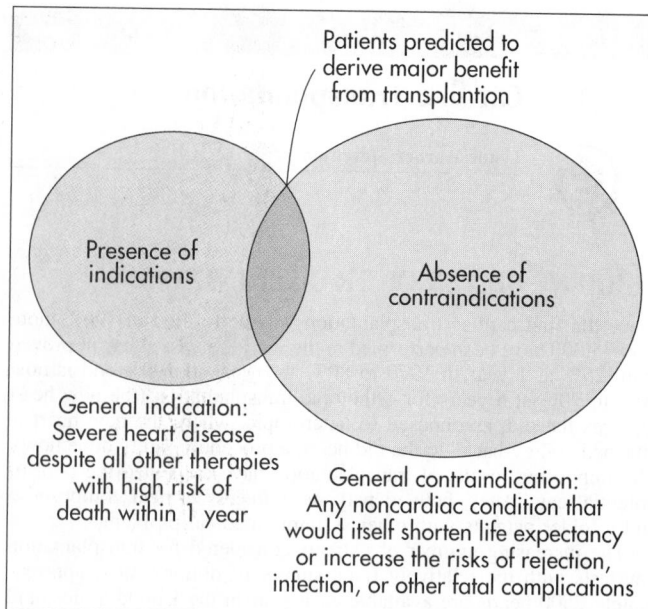

FIGURE 34-1   Venn diagram of small intersection between those people with sufficient severity of heart disease to warrant transplantation and those people without any contraindications to the procedure. Current practice in the patient at the time of referral is often to establish absence of contraindications and then to observe over time for evidence of progressive heart failure causing unacceptably limited quality and expected length of life without transplantation.

catecholamine-related drug addiction have a good chance of improvement to good clinical function with total abstention, but are at high risk of recurrent substance abuse after transplantation.

These and other factors can contribute to decompensation even if they did not originally cause the heart failure (see Box 34-1). Many physicians continue to perceive symptomatic heart failure as an untreatable disease terminated only by early death or transplantation. This perception is unfortuantely transmitted to patients, who often arrive at transplantation centers convinced that they will either die within a few months or resume normal life after transplantation, neither of which is generally true. Many patients with advanced heart failure can enjoy quality of life and survival similar to that achieved by transplantation, which brings its own burdens and risks.

Medical Therapy for Advanced Heart Failure

The majority of patients currently referred for transplantation have severe symptoms of congestion arising from elevated left-sided filling pressures (orthopnea, paroxysmal nocturnal dyspnea [PND] and immediate dyspnea on light exertion [IDLE]), right-sided filling pressures (anorexia, hepatoabdominal distention, and peripheral edema), or both. Repeated hospitalizations to relieve congestion have in most cases led to only brief symptomatic improvement, with longer-term stability hindered by poor diuretic response, hypotension, declining renal function, or other complicating cardiac conditions. The majority of these potential transplantation candidates can still be rendered free of congestion when further therapy with vasodilators and diuretics is tailored to hemodynamic goals of near-normal filling pressures and systemic vascular resistance (Box 34-2).

Before referral, many patients have been unable to comply with complicated medical regimens because of lack of education about their condition and their drugs. Patients must participate actively in their own care team to maintain normal volume status by watching their fluid and salt intake, and adjusting diuretic dosage in response to weight change. In addition, exercise capacity, well-being, and some of the physiologic abnormalities of heart failure can be improved through progressive exercise programs. It should be emphasized that the complexity of an optimal medical regimen for heart failure is often exceeded by the complexity of the regimen after transplantation.

SELECTION FOR TRANSPLANTATION
Indications for Transplantation

Selection for transplantation once focused on the enumeration of contraindications but has increasingly shifted to include specific indica-

---

BOX 34-3

Criteria for stability on medical therapy

Stable blood pressure (SBP ≥ 80 mm Hg)
Stable weight on flexible oral diuretic regimen
No congestive symptoms at rest
Ambulatory ≥ 1 city block
Stable creatinine and blood urea nitrogen (BUN ≤ 60 mg/dl)
Stable serum sodium (usually ≥ 132 mEq/L)
No angina
No recurrent sustained ventricular arrhythmias or syncope
No recurrent arterial emboli on anticoagulation
No serious drug side effects

---

tions describing the patients for whom transplantation offers a major benefit in quality of life and length of life compared to that expected without transplantation (Fig. 34-1). Patients who remain critical despite optimal medical therapies clearly have unacceptable quality of life and survival. They need to be further evaluated only for contraindications (see later discussion). Although their early postoperative mortality is approximately twice that in patients without urgent need, their 1-year survival rate is still approximately 80%, compared to virtually no chance of 1-year survival without transplantation. The overall expected benefit (difference between transplantation and no transplantation) is so large for the critically ill patients that they should continue to receive priority for the limited donor hearts. Although less than 30% of patients are initially listed urgently for transplantation, 60% to 70% of recent transplantations have been performed in candidates who have deteriorated to the point of requiring hospitalization until transplantation.

Patients who are unstable (Box 34-3) have disabling symptoms and a poor prognosis and may require frequent brief hospitalizations. Evaluation for contraindications is the focus of further evaluation for these patients. Although the immediate risk is not as great as for the critical patients, there is still an obvious major benefit of transplan-

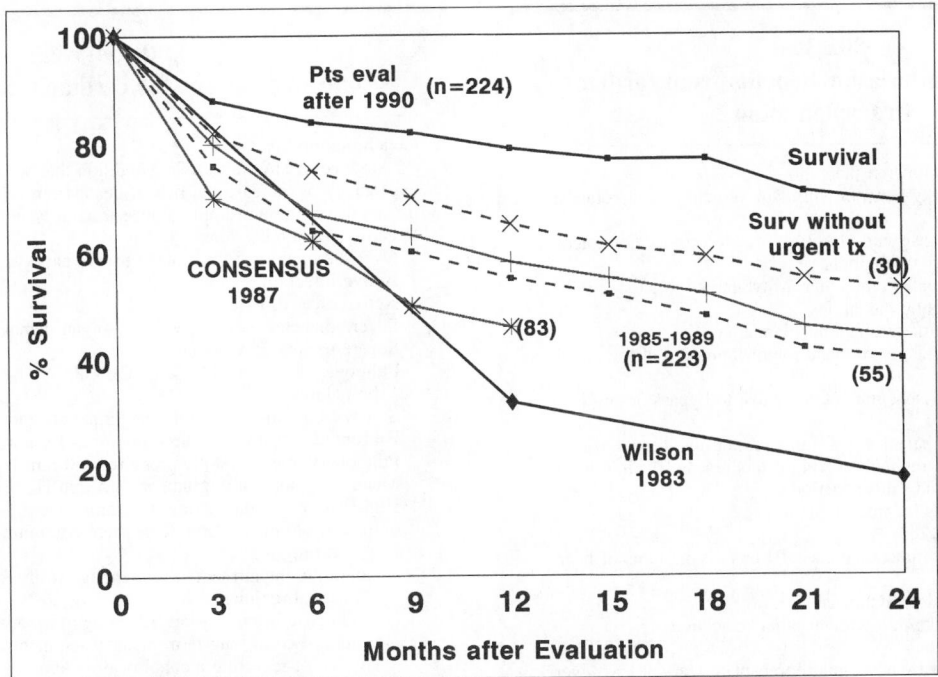

FIGURE 34-2 Kaplan Meier curves showing improving survival for 447 patients referred with New York Heart Association Class IV symptoms of heart failure. All 447 patients underwent therapy tailored to hemodynamic goals as described. Survival is compared to previously published survival for Class IV populations.

(From Wilson et al: *JACC* 2:403-410, 1983 and 1987 CONSENSUS *N Eng J Med* 316:1429-1435, 1987). The solid upper lines indicate survival with censoring at the time of transplant.

Table 34-1 Peak exercise oxygen consumption and expected benefit from transplantation

PEAK Vo₂ WITH HEART FAILURE	EXPECTED AFTER TRANSPLANTATION	ESTIMATED 1-YEAR SURVIVAL WITH HEART FAILURE	ESTIMATED 1-YEAR SURVIVAL AFTER TRANSPLANTATION	DECISION REGARDING TRANSPLANTATION
<10	<14-18	<50%	≤80% to 90%	Transplantation (if eligible)
10-14	14-18	60% to 75%	80% to 90%	Toward transplantation
14-18	14-18	75% to 85%	80% to 90%	Away from transplantation
>18	>14-18	85% to 95%	>80% to 90%	No transplantation (unless other indications)

(Data from Mancini DM et al: Value of peak exercise oxygen consumption for optimal timing of cardiac transplantation in ambulatory patients with heart failure, *Circulation* 83:778-786, 1991; Stevenson LW et al: Exercise capacity for survivors of cardiac transplantation or sustained medical therapy for stable heart failure. *Circulation* 81:78-85, 1990; and Stevenson LW et al: Improvement in exercise capacity of candidates awaiting heart transplantation, *J Am Coll Cardiol* 25:163-178, 1995.)

tation. As the waiting list grows longer, however, some patients will die before transplantation can be performed, whereas others will eventually achieve greater stability and should be reevaluated after 6 months for evidence of new "stability" (Box 34-3).

For most patients with left ventricular ejection fraction, less than 25% who fulfill the criteria for stability whether or not they have previously had a period of decompensation, the benefits of transplantation for functional capacity and survival are less clear. Many of these patients may have exercise performance similar to that achieved after transplantation. Survival for potential transplantation candidates discharged on aggressive medical therapy after evaluation with New York Heart Association Class IV symptoms of heart failure is considerably better than predicted from earlier eras (Fig. 34-2). Although transplantation still provides better survival, increasing experiences suggest that there are subpopulations of stable patients in whom transplantation can be deferred in favor of more critically ill recipients.

A major determinant of transplantation benefit for both functional capacity and survival in an ambulatory heart failure patient is the peak oxygen consumption achieved during exercise, which has become a yardstick by which candidate populations can be standardized between programs (Table 34-1 and Box 34-4). It should be noted that in current criteria for transplant candidacy, a low ejection fraction is neither necessary nor sufficient indication for transplantation. Severe

angina in a patient without targets for revascularization could confer a dismal prognosis and quality of life despite an ejection fraction greater than 25%. Patients with idiopathic restrictive disease or "burned out" hypertrophic cardiomyopathy with a left ventricular ejection fraction of 30% to 45% may require transplantation for refractory congestive symptoms without severely reduced ejection fraction. Not all candidates are listed primarily for congestive symptoms, however (Fig. 34-3); some candidates have very low functional capacity.

Contraindications to Cardiac Transplantation

Contraindications, listed in Box 34-5, were often considered "absolute" during the era when transplantation was an experiment, but many are now "relative" because the procedure is more widely available. Patients with heart failure resulting from chronic systemic illnesses such as scleroderma would be excluded. The benefit of transplantation for amyloidosis is questionable since the disease progresses after transplantation. Investigation continues regarding Chagas' disease, which frequently recurs after transplantation. Older patients have less rejection but more complications, and in the largest studies, survival is slightly but significantly worse in patients older than 60 to 65 years, in whom relative contraindications often become abso-

---

BOX 34-4

Selection criteria for benefits from cardiac transplantation

Accepted indications for transplantation
   Peak V_{O_2} ≤10 ml/kg per min with achievement of anaerobic metabolism
   Severe ischemia consistently limiting routine activity not amenable to bypass surgery or angioplasty
   Recurrent symptomatic ventricular arrhythmias refractory to all accepted therapeutic modalities
Probable indications for cardiac transplantation
   Peak V_{O_2} <14 ml/kg per min and major limitation of the patient's daily activities
   Recurrent unstable ischemia not amenable to bypass or angioplasty
   Instability of fluid balance/renal function not due to patient noncompliance with regimen of weight monitoring, flexible use of diuretic drugs, and salt restriction
Inadequate indications for transplantation
   Ejection fraction ≤20%
   History of previous functional class III or IV symptoms of heart failure
   Previous ventricular arrhythmias
   Peak V_{O_2} >15 ml/kg/min without other indications
Continuing evaluation
   Clinical assessment by heart failure/transplant team at least every 1 to 2 months to determine persistence of indications
   Reevaluation at 6-month intervals to include assessment of clinical stability and measurement of peak oxygen consumption

(Modified from Mudge GH, Goldstein S, Addonizio JL et al: *J Am Coll Cardiol* 22:21-31, 1993.)

BOX 34-5

Contraindications for cardiac transplantation

General eligibility
   Absence of any noncardiac condition that would itself shorten life expectancy or increase the risk of death from rejection or from complications of immunosuppression, particularly infection
Specific contraindications
   Over the upper age limit of 55 to 65 years (various programs)
   Active infection
   Active ulcer disease
   Severe diabetes mellitus with end-organ damage
   Severe peripheral vascular disease
   Pulmonary function (FEV_1, FVC) <60%* or history of chronic bronchitis
   Serum creatinine >2 mg/dl; creatinine clearance <50 ml/min*
   Bilirubin >2.5 mg/dl, transaminases >2× normal*
   Pulmonary artery systolic pressure >60 mm Hg*
   Mean transpulmonary gradient >15 mm Hg*
   High risk of life-threatening noncompliance
      Inability to make strong consistent commitment to transplantation program
      Cognitive impairment severe enough to limit comprehension of medical regimen
      Psychiatric instability severe enough to jeopardize incentive for adherence to long-term medical regimen
      History of recurring alcohol or drug abuse
      Failure to establish stable address or telephone number
      Previous demonstration of repeated noncompliance with medication or follow-up

*May need to provide optimal hemodynamics with nitroprusside and/or dobutamine for 72 hours to determine reversibility of organ dysfunction caused by heart failure.

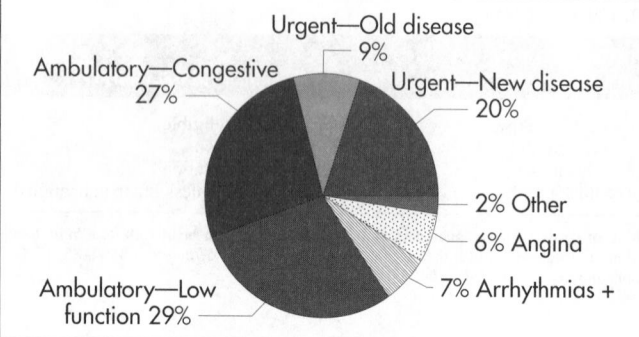

FIGURE 34-3   Clinical profile at the time of listing for transplantation for 1994-1995 at the Brigham and Women's Hospital. Patients may be listed urgently for transplantation during their initial hospitalization, often following an acute event such as myocardial infarction or postcardiotomy shock. Ambulatory patients listed for transplantation may be listed primarily for refractory symptoms of congestion, severe limitation of functional capacity determined by peak oxygen consumption in the absence of congestive symptoms, angina, uncontrollable symptomatic ventricular arrhythmias, or combinations of these factors.

lute. Diabetes mellitus was once an absolute contraindication but does not preclude transplantation if blood sugars are easily controlled, and there is no evidence of neuropathy, retinopathy, or distal vascular disease. Patients with a recent malignancy are excluded since immunosuppression may accelerate recurrence and progression.

All patients undergo measurement of pulmonary pressures and resistance, which can be elevated as a result of either chronic left heart failure or unrecognized pulmonary conditions. Pulmonary hypertension that cannot be reversed pharmacologically can cause immediate failure of the right ventricle of the transplanted heart. The majority of elevated pulmonary pressures will respond well to optimization of hemodynamics, including occasional use of nitric oxide.

Evaluation of other organ systems is complicated by the effects of the compromised circulation, and often patients are accepted with some degree of renal or hepatic impairment expected to reverse after normal hemodynamics are restored by transplantation. Active infection remains an absolute contraindication to either transplantation or the insertion of a mechanical support device to "bridge" the patient to transplantation.

A major cause of late deaths after transplantation is patient noncompliance. The psychologic and physical stresses after transplantation, combined with the emotional lability of steroid therapy, can precipitate fatal episodes of noncompliance. Evaluation by the psychiatrist and social worker includes consideration of previous noncompliance, substance abuse, and family support.

Most transplantation centers find approximately half of patients who undergo complete evaluation to be acceptable in terms of contraindications, although the indications for transplantation vary more widely. Candidacy for transplantation is increasingly considered to be a dynamic state (Fig. 34-4). Between 10% and 30% of listed outpatient candidates will deteriorate to require hospitalization until transplantation. These patients and those who cannot be discharged after their initial transplantation evaluation are increasingly considered for implantable left ventricular support devices to allow hemodynamic stability and physical rehabilitation before transplantation.

Selection of Donors for Transplantation

The heart must be harvested while still perfused after documentation of brain death. Criteria for brain death vary among states but generally include cessation of all brain function. Most states have adopted the "required request," which requires hospitals to offer the option of organ donation to the family.

Hemodynamic consequences of brain death include severe volume depletion from diabetes insipidus, sympathetic storm causing hypertension and tachycardia, and rapid depletion of triiodothyronine. The rapid volume loss resulting from diabetes insipidus often requires massive fluid replacement, which is critical to avoid the need for excessive intravenous inotropic support. Insertion of a central venous

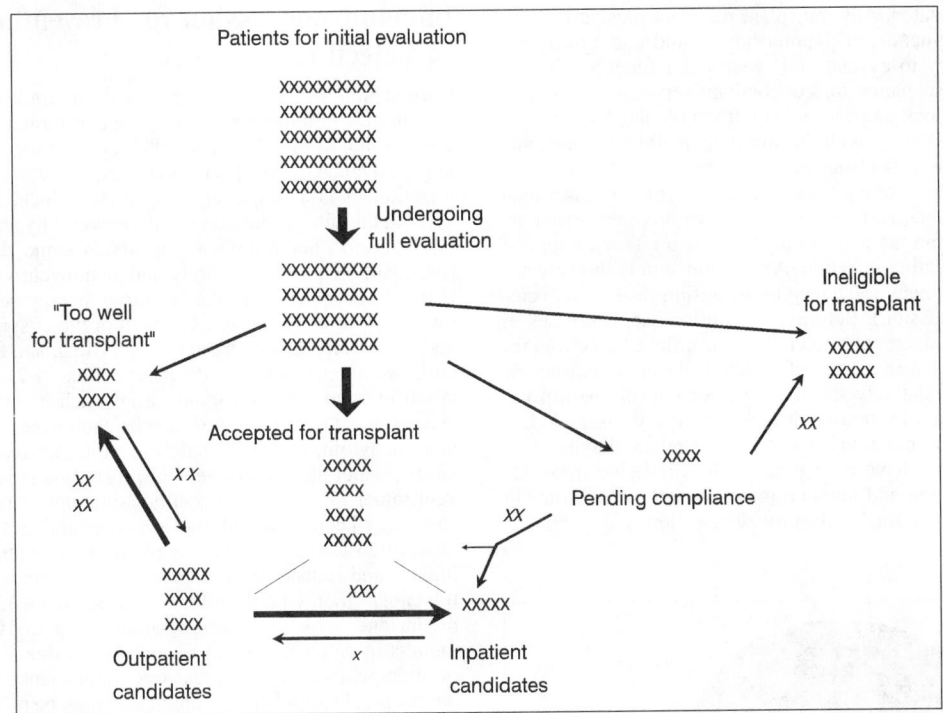

FIGURE 34-4   Flow chart indicating the dynamic nature of candidacy and priority for cardiac transplantation. Patients may improve or deteriorate following initial evaluation, developing new indications or contraindications for transplantation.

line or pulmonary artery catheter to optimize filling pressures may allow use of an otherwise "marginal" donor heart. Echocardiography is now widely used to assess ventricular function in donors. Coronary angiography is often performed in donors over 40 years old, whose hearts are being used more often than previously, often after coronary arteriography. Previous limits are also being extended for the ischemic time between harvest and implantation, but current data demonstrate decreased long-term graft survival when 5 hours are exceeded.

Donors are screened for evidence of human immunodeficiency virus (HIV) or hepatitis infections, which if present would exclude donation. Patients are matched to donors primarily on the basis of ABO blood group and body size. After potential recipients are screened for the presence of circulating antibodies to a random panel of antigens, those with elevated levels frequently do not undergo transplantation unless a specific cross-match to the donor blood is negative.

REJECTION AND IMMUNOSUPPRESSION
Rejection

Prevention, recognition, and therapy of rejection and of the consequences of immunosuppression constitute the major specific issues in the care of the transplantation recipient. Immune injury can be caused by cytotoxic T-lymphocytes, natural killer cells, monocyte-macrophages, cytokine effects, and multiple antibody-mediated mechanisms. Hyperacute rejection occurring within minutes after the recipient's blood fills the newly transplanted heart indicates the presence of preformed antibodies, which can usually be detected and avoided through pretransplantation screening of the recipient and donor. The other clinical syndromes of rejection probably reflect a concert of immunologic mechanisms (Box 34-6).

Rejection is the second greatest cause of total mortality (Fig. 34-5). The majority of patients will develop one episode of rejection in the first year after transplantation. The Cardiac Transplant Research Database, including 25 transplantation centers and the largest collected experience, describes a cumulative incidence of 0.8 episodes by the third month and 1.1 by the sixth month, with markedly decreasing new incidence thereafter. By 12 months, the average incidence is 1.3 episodes/patient, but this represents multiple episodes in

---

BOX 34-6
Presentations of rejection

Hyperacute rejection causing graft failure at implantation
Asymptomatic acute cellular rejection diagnosed on routine surveillance biopsy
Acute cellular rejection with hemodynamic compromise
"Vascular" rejection on biopsy with or without accompanying cellular infiltrate
Reversible graft dysfunction without cellular infiltrate
Chronic irreversible graft dysfunction without cellular infiltrate
Transplant coronary artery disease detected by angiography or autopsy

---

some patients, and no rejection at all in more than one third of patients during the first year. After the first year, the risk of rejection declines dramatically but was still 17% in patients who had already had an earlier episode of rejection. Risk factors for rejection include younger age and female gender, both associated with increased immune responses.

Most rejection episodes are diagnosed in asymptomatic patients by routine surveillance endomyocardial biopsies, performed using a bioptome inserted through the internal jugular or femoral vein initially at weekly intervals, then monthly by 6 months. After the first year, routine biopsies are performed with decreasing frequency and not at all in some centers. There are four histologic grades of biopsy based on the degree of lymphocyte infiltrate and myocyte necrosis. Grades I and II are often not treated, whereas grades III and IV (rarely seen) usually warrant intensification of immunosuppression (Fig. 34-6).

Of 918 episodes of rejection in the multicenter series, 16% were associated with clinical hemodynamic compromise. Interestingly, one third of these occurred without major cellular infiltrate, in which antibody-mediated injury to the myocardium and coronary vasculature ("humoral" or "vascular" rejection) or biopsy sampling error have sometimes been implicated. Any transplant recipient presenting with shortness of breath, syncope, or hypotension should undergo immediate echocardiography to evaluate left ventricular function. Unless there is high clinical suspicion for concomitant sepsis, patients with new hypotension or shock and decreased left ventricular function are usually treated immediately with intravenous methylprednisolone, even before biopsy tissue is obtained.

Other clinical evidence of rejection is rare, occurring in fewer than 20% of patients who receive therapy for positive biopsies. Atrial arrhythmias and vague fatigue may occur. Fever is a rare symptom of rejection, usually indicating infection. A common sign is the new apparent control of previously refractory hypertension related to cyclosporine (see later discussion). Before cyclosporine use, decreases in electrocardiographic voltage reflected intramyocardial edema from rejection. This is not a sensitive sign of rejection during cyclosporine therapy, but it is still relatively specific for rejection (or silent myocardial infarction caused by transplant coronary artery disease). Endomyocardial biopsy remains the major technique for diagnosis of rejection, although there have been multiple less invasive measurements of cardiac function and immune response with sensitivities in the range of 60% to 70% for biopsy-proven rejection.

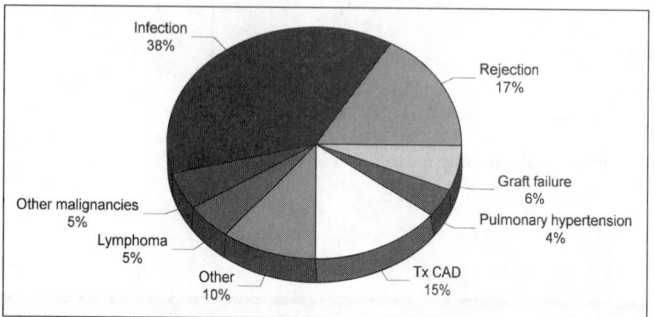

FIGURE 34-5 Causes of death after transplantation in the cyclosporine era, as described by Grattan et al. from the Stanford experience. *Tx CAD*, transplant coronary artery disease.

Immunosuppression for Prevention and Therapy of Rejection

Current immunosuppression is based on "triple therapy" with cyclosporine A, azathioprine, and varying corticosteroid doses. After introduction into clinical trials in 1982, cyclosporine A was heralded as a major advance, and indeed has decreased the severity of infection and rejection. It is a fungal endecapeptide, which, like the newer agent FK506, inhibits production of interleukin-2 by activated lymphocytes. Cyclosporine nephrotoxicity occurs to some degrees in almost all transplant recipients and rarely may require chronic hemodialysis. Hypertension requiring one- or two-drug therapy occurs in most patients on cyclosporine A, partly as a result of direct sympathetic stimulation and perhaps from endothelin release. Hirsutism, tremor, and hyperkalemia are other common side effects (Box 34-7). Cyclosporine A metabolism is affected by many drugs such as erythromycin, calcium channel blockers, cimetidine, and ketoconazole, which increase levels; and phenytoin, isoniazid, nafcillin, sulfamethoxazole, and cholestyramine, which decrease levels. Cyclosporine is primarily used to prevent rather than to treat rejection, although increased dosing has occasionally been used both intravenously and orally for mild rejection.

Corticosteroids inhibit cytokine transcription, stabilize membranes, and reduce local edema. Steroid therapy is initiated with intravenous methylprednisolone and subsequently maintained with prednisone, which is tapered rapidly to 5 to 10 mg/day by 3 to 6 months in patients without recurrent rejection. The vigor and timing of attempts to achieve steroid-free maintenance vary among centers, but eventual steroid-free maintenance may be possible in 50% to 80% of transplant recipients. The anticipated benefits of reduced weight, diabetes, hyperlipidemia, osteoporosis, and late infection may be in part offset by greater vulnerability to rejection, particularly in the setting of inadequate cyclosporine levels. Glucocorticoid administration, given either over 3 days as intravenous pulse therapy or as an "oral pulse" of 10 to 14 days, is successful as sole therapy for over 80% of rejection episodes.

Azathioprine is a purine antimetabolite converted hepatically to 6-mercaptopurine, which inhibits proliferation of lymphocytes. Addition of azathioprine adjusted to maintain white blood counts over 4000/cm^3 allows lower doses of both steroids and cyclosporine A. Methotrexate and cyclophosphamide have at times been used instead

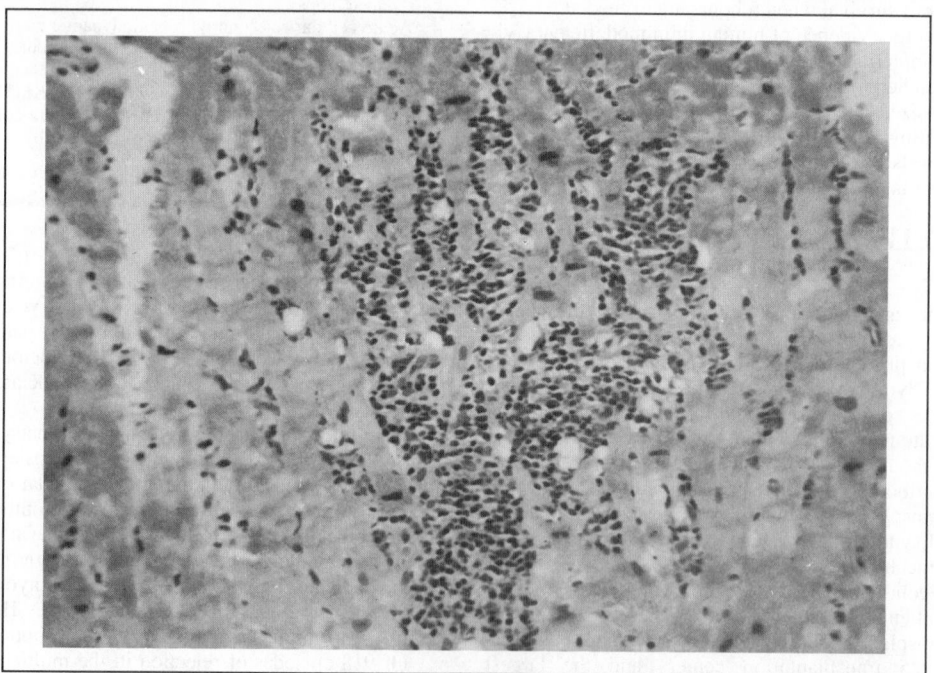

FIGURE 34-6 Severe cardiac rejection with heavy infiltrate of mononuclear cells with occasional neutrophils and myocyte necrosis with vacuolization and myofibrillar degeneration.

(From Stevenson LW, and Miller L: *Curr Probl Cardiol* 4:219, 1991.)

BOX 34-7
Potential adverse effects of triple-drug immunosuppression

Cyclosporine A
  Hypertension
  Renal dysfunction
  Hyperkalemia
  Hypomagnesemia
  Hyperuricemia
  Hepatic dysfunction
  Central nervous system
    Tremor
    Seizures
    Paresthesias
    Anxiety
    Insomnia
  Hirsutism
  Rhinorrhea
  Gingival hyperplasia
  Malignancy
Corticosteroids
  Cushingoid habitus
  Osteoporosis
  Diabetes exacerbation
  Obesity
  Labile emotions
  Sodium retention
  Hyperlipidemia
  Easy bruisability
  Peptic ulcers
  Cataracts
  Insomnia
  Avascular bone necrosis
  Corticosteroid myopathy
  Growth retardation in children
Azathioprine
  Leukopenia
  Thrombocytopenia
  Macrocytic anemia
  Pancreatitis
  Cholestatic jaundice
  Hepatitis
  Interstitial pneumonitis

Modified from Kobashigawa J: *J Critical Illness* 8:607-615, 1993.

of or in addition to azathioprine in patients with recurrent rejection. These drugs are not generally used as part of acute therapy for the rejection episode.

In some programs, antilymphocyte antibodies are used intravenously for 5 to 14 days to initiate immunosuppression, either with polyclonal antilymphocyte globulin or murine monoclonal antibody against the CD3 receptor on activated lymphocytes (OKT3). Many programs reserve their use in the peritransplant period for those patients at high risk for early renal failure if cyclosporine were to be initiated immediately. These antibodies are also used in 10- to 14-day courses in combination with glucocorticoids for therapy of refractory rejection. The first 2 or 3 days of antilymphocyte therapy are associated in some patients with acute pulmonary and hemodynamic compromise attributed to cytokine release. These antibodies are administered initially only after adequate pretreatment and with provisions for emergency respiratory and hemodynamic intervention.

Total lymphoid irradiation is also used as therapy for recurrent rejection. Because of the 5 to 10 weeks required for completion, it is not helpful during acute rejection. Plasmapheresis is occasionally used before transplantation to reduce preformed antibodies and after transplantation to reduce levels of circulating antibodies that may be contributing to severe hemodynamic compromise.

Attempts continue to increase the specificity of immunosuppression. Current agents under investigation include RS-61443, rapamycin, 15-deoxyspergualine, brequinar, other compounds inhibiting cytokine release or binding, and antibodies against adhesion molecules.

Accelerated Transplant Coronary Artery Disease

Although acute rejection syndromes occur primarily during the first 6 months after transplantation, subsequent graft function and survival are most threatened by accelerated coronary artery disease, which has also been called "chronic rejection." The first long-term heart transplant survivor died after 19 months from coronary artery disease in the new heart, although both recipient and donor were under 25 years old and previously free of coronary artery disease. Most transplant recipients develop diffuse intimal thickening of the coronary arteries, which is evident on angiography in 50% of patients by 5 years, seen earlier on intracoronary ultrasound. Compared to native atherosclerosis, transplant arteriosclerosis is more diffuse and characterized by greater cellular infiltration (both of mononuclear and smooth muscle cells) but less lipid accumulation.

Prolonged ischemic time and cytomegalovirus (CMV) infection are commonly considered to be risk factors. Hyperlipidemia, smoking, and obesity are implicated but appear to be permissive factors rather than dominant as they are in native atherosclerosis. Therapy with HMG-CoA reductase inhibitors, if carefully monitored for evidence of rhabdomyolysis, can be safe and effective for lowering cholesterol levels in this population. They appear to reduce the incidence of coronary vascular disease when begun early after transplantation and may decrease major rejection episodes. Diltiazem also may decrease the incidence of transplant coronary artery disease.

Because the transplanted heart remains essentially denervated, the majority of patients with transplant coronary artery disease have no symptoms until ventricular function is markedly impaired, although rare patients have reported chest pain during a positive exercise stress test. The distal and diffuse nature of the disease limits the reliability of noninvasive testing. Baseline and yearly coronary angiography are the current standard for diagnosis but are now complemented by intracoronary ultrasound for earlier detection.

Once graft coronary artery disease is diagnosed, risk of death is related to the number of vessels involved and left ventricular function. One-year survival with three-vessel disease and left ventricular ejection fraction <40% is less than 50%, with most deaths occurring suddenly as a result of ischemic arrhythmias. Percutaneous angioplasty or surgical bypass grafting is technically successful for "discrete" proximal lesions but the disease often progresses rapidly in other vessels. Retransplantation is the best therapy for severe transplant arteriosclerosis but is often excluded because of renal disease and other conditions. Even in the best candidates, retransplantation yields a 1-year survival rate of only 60%, compared to 80% to 90% for first transplants.

Infection

The immunosuppression currently necessary to allow graft acceptance predisposes the transplant recipient to infection, which led to the death of the first human heart transplant recipient from pneumonia within the first month. Infection has been the most common cause of death after transplantation (see Fig. 34-5). The incidence of major infection requiring intravenous therapy has declined to 0.62 episodes per patient during the first year, most occurring during the first 3 months. Multiple infections frequently occur in the same patient, particularly after CMV infection, so 67% of patients are actually free of major infection during that year. Death has occurred in 17% of overall episodes but in 36% of documented serious fungal infections.

The approach to fever in the transplant recipient includes careful history and physical examination, complete blood cell count, chest radiograph, and cultures of blood, sputum, and urine. The lung is the most common site, involved in 28% of treated infections (Fig. 34-7). Hypoxia or pulmonary infiltrates should be aggressively evaluated with bronchoscopy. Fever with gastrointestinal symptoms may indicate CMV, candidal infection, or atypical presentation of lymphomas. Fever with any neurologic symptoms merits computerized axial tomography and lumbar puncture. The sinuses should not be overlooked.

In the early posttransplantation period, bacterial infections are dominant, although cutaneous herpes can be troublesome. Systemic viral infections such as CMV often become apparent within the first 3 months. CMV accounts for 25% of all infections requiring therapy after transplantation. Treatment with ganciclovir, which inhibits viral-

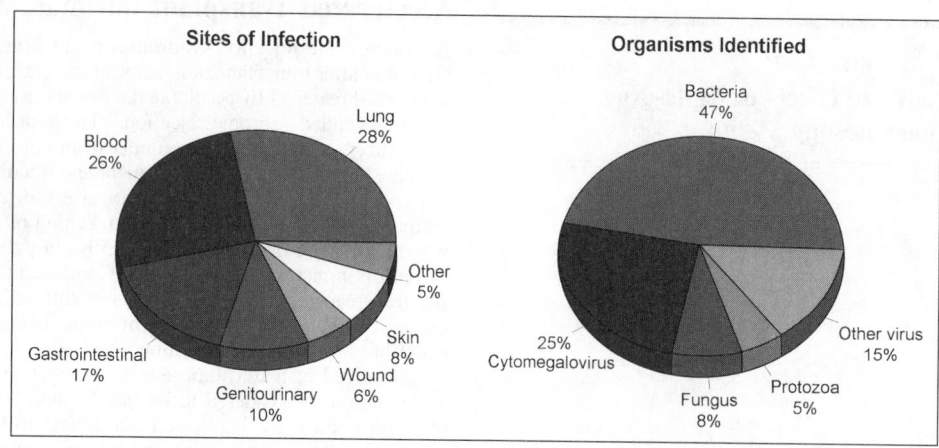

FIGURE 34-7　Pie chart depicting the sites and organisms implicated in 409 infectious episodes from the Cardiac Transplant Research Database, including patients from 25 major transplant centers. *CMV,* Cytomegalovirus.

(Modified from Miller LW, Naftel DC, Bourge RC et al: A multiinstitutional study, *J Heart Lung Transplant* 13:381-393, 1994.)

induced DNA polymerase, can be life saving. Infections occurring later after transplantation include fungal infections such as *Aspergillus* and *Pneumocystis.* Additional organisms often encountered are *Listeria, Legionella, Nocardia,* and *Toxoplasma.*

These patients do not have lymphopenia and are thus less vulnerable to opportunistic infections than patients with bone marrow transplants or acquired immunodeficiency syndrome. Community upper respiratory infections are usually well tolerated. Facemasks are recommended only for the first few weeks after transplantation, and during hospital visits. Patients are urged to avoid gardening or open construction areas. Prophylaxis with trimethoprim-sulfa is frequently given to prevent *Pneumocystis.* Prophylaxis against CMV may help decrease the severity of infections in high-risk patients.

Malignancy After Transplantation

The occurrence of malignancy is increased after transplantation to almost 100-fold that of age-matched controls, presumably caused by the impaired immune surveillance. Approximately 5% of transplant survivors develop malignancy, which accounts for 10% of all deaths (see Fig. 34-5). Cutaneous malignancy is most common, followed by those of the lung and intestinal tract. Lymphoma is particularly common and may be found in extranodal locations such as the gastrointestinal tract and central nervous system. The Epstein-Barr virus has frequently been implicated in these lymphomas, which may occur within the first year after transplantation. Therapy with acyclovir and reduced immunosuppression can occasionally cause dramatic resolution, but highly aggressive tumors may progress rapidly over a few days.

CARDIAC FUNCTION AFTER TRANSPLANTATION

Function of the transplanted heart is affected by denervation, acute rejection, arteriosclerosis, hypertension, and other side effects of immunosuppression (Box 34-8). Vagal reinnervation does not appear to occur in humans, so vagal stimulation by carotid sinus massage or digoxin will not slow atrioventricular conduction. Late sympathetic reinnervation has been demonstrated in some patients, but most hearts function "independently" of the central nervous system, responding instead to alterations in venous return and the effects of circulating catecholamines to increase heart rate and contractility.

The cardiac output is usually within normal limits at rest, with a higher heart rate and lower stroke volume that is the product of a normal left ventricular ejection fraction and slightly reduced left ventricular volume. With the classic anastomotic technique, the donor atria are anastomosed to the recipient atria, creating a snowman configuration (Fig. 34-8) and varying patterns of atrial contraction. The newer techniques of bicaval anastomoses leave the donor atria largely intact.

BOX 34-8

Factors affecting cardiac performance after transplantation

Before implantation
  Donor:
    Body size, gender, and cardiac function
    Age
    Adequacy of preservation
    Ischemic time
  Recipient:
    Irreversible pulmonary hypertension to cause new right heart failure
    Obesity
    Diabetes
    Hypertension
Denervation
  Afferent denervation
    Impaired reflex response of peripheral circulation
    Impaired neural regulation of fluid balance and renal function
    Absence of anginal symptoms during ischemia
  Efferent denervation
    Absent vagal tone
    Elevated resting heart rate
    Delayed heart rate response to increased demand
    Limited maximal heart rate response
    Possible impairment of relaxation
  Hypersensitivity to catecholamines, adenosine
Atrial anastomoses
  Atrial distortion and asynchronous contraction
  Mitral and tricuspid regurgitation
  Increased baseline atrial natriuretic factor
Effects of rejection
  Acute myocardial depression from cytokines
  Chronic fibrosis
  Nonspecific graft dysfunction
  Decreased coronary vascular reserve
  Epicardial coronary artery disease
Complications of hypertension
  Left ventricular hypertrophy
  Increased peripheral afterload
  Cardiodepressant effects of calcium channel blockers, β-blockers
Obesity

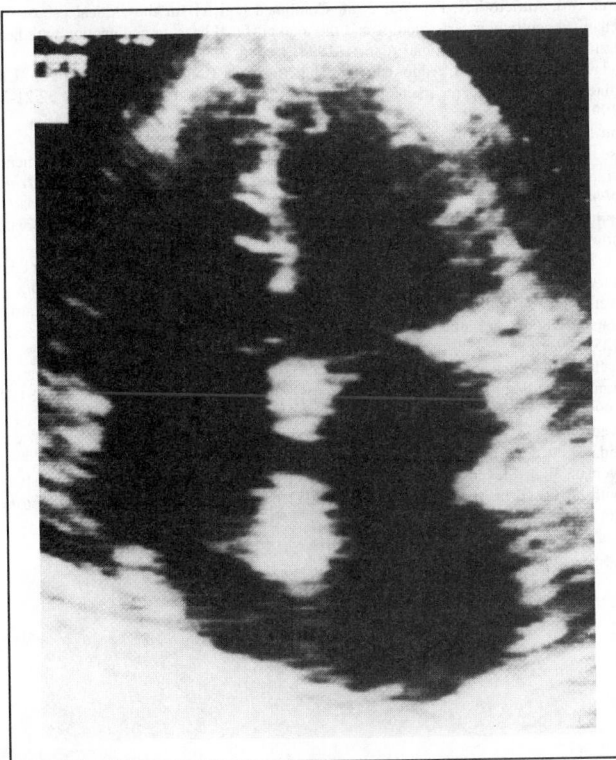

FIGURE 34-8   Four-chamber view of the transplanted heart using two-dimensional echocardiography, showing the "snowman" atria created by the anastomosis of donor and recipient atria during orthotopic cardiac transplantation. Atria are at the bottom of the picture.

(From Stevenson LW: *Am J Cardiol* 60:119-122, 1987.)

Table 34-2   Typical medical regimen six months after transplantation

DRUG	DOSE†
Cyclosporine	180 mg bid
Azathioprine	150 mg daily
Prednisone	5 mg daily*
Enalapril	10 mg bid
Furosemide	40 mg daily
Diltiazem slow release	60 mg bid
Pravastatin	40 mg daily
Trimethoprim-sulfasoxazole	0-4 times weekly
Antacids, H₂-blockers or sucralfate	Usually prescribed early after transplantation and after steroid pulses
Nystatin or clotrimazole	Used orally to prevent candidiasis during high-dose steroid therapy

*In absence of recent rejection. Patients with recent rejection would receive higher-dose prednisone. Some patients will undergo steroid weaning and be maintained on a steroid-free regimen.
†Actual doses will vary.

Maintenance of normal volume status frequently requires diuretic therapy, although at lower doses than before transplantation. The transplanted hearts do not provide the normal cardiorenal feedback for volume regulation. Fluid retention is also promoted by high steroid doses and some drugs used to treat the hypertension. The tendency to retain fluid occurs despite elevation of atrial natriuretic factor, which probably results from the abnormal geometry and stretch of the anastomosed atria. On appropriate therapy, resting ventricular filling pressures are frequently within normal limits in the absence of rejection. However, 10% to 20% of patients have persistently reduced compliance and elevated filling pressures despite adequate diuretic doses and normal systolic function. Many transplant recipients reveal mildly decreased ventricular compliance only during volume loading or exercise.

The response to exercise is delayed and blunted in the denervated heart. Heart rate does not increase until circulating catecholamines rise after 3 to 5 minutes of exercise and does not reach maximum levels predicted for the donor age. Although ejection fraction eventually increases as in normal hearts, compliance is reduced and the peak stroke volume is lower. Impaired right ventricular function may also be limiting. Transplant recipients generally perform at 50% to 70% of maximal levels predicted for age, with oxygen consumption equivalent to that of patients with stable heart failure. This limitation results both from limited cardiac reserve and from the musculoskeletal effects of glucocorticoid therapy and previous deconditioning (see Box 34-8). However, transplantation patients describe less limitation of routine activity than many heart failure patients, perhaps because of diminished exertional congestion.

LIFE AFTER TRANSPLANTATION

There are currently more than 20,000 patients alive after cardiac transplantation. The longest documented survival is 22 years after transplantation. Of patients undergoing transplantation, 90% to 95% survive to hospital discharge, 80% to 90% survive 1 year, 60% to 70% survive 5 years, and an estimated 30% to 40% survive 10 years, although there are few numbers for late survival. The first 3 months are dominated by the highest frequency of rejection and infection episodes, as described previously. Hypertension requires therapy in 70% of patients, usually with disproportionate diastolic elevation and loss of diurnal variation. The serum creatinine usually stabilizes to between 1.3 and 1.8 mg/dl by the end of the first year, although patients occasionally progress to dialysis. Obesity, defined as weight 25% above ideal, occurs in 20% to 40% of recipients. Symptomatic osteoporosis develops in up to 10% of recipients.

By 3 to 6 months, most patients are physically capable of returning to the level of employment or school before their cardiac disability, excepting heavy physical labor. Despite their good functional status, fewer than half of patients actually return to employment, in some cases because they have chosen early retirement but often because employers are reluctant to cover transplant recipients for health and liability. The National Transplantation Study of United States programs described 85% of transplant survivors to be physically active, although 66% continue to perceive themselves as limited in some way from performing their desired activities. Their lives continue to be shaped by the complicated medical regimen, including 15 to 20 biopsies during the first year, and daily drug schedules, including 10 to 16 daily doses of medicines (Table 34-2).

Patient education includes not only the medication schedule but warning signs of rejection or infection. Patients are instructed in low-calorie and low-fat diets to decrease obesity and accelerated coronary artery disease. Most patients need to follow a moderate restriction of salt intake. Physical activity and rehabilitation are strongly encouraged. The most effective education begins before transplantation. Patients' perceptions of the success of transplantation depend in large part on their expectations, which should not be of return to a completely normal life, but to a set of problems that is less limiting than those of their previous heart failure.

THE FUTURE OF TRANSPLANTATION

Results of transplantation will continue to improve as the immune response can be better regulated, particularly to prevent coronary artery disease. Transplantation of the approximately 2500 hearts available yearly can have little impact, however, on the total heart failure population of 3 million in the United States, many of whom will do well without transplantation. Some patients may eventually be maintained at home on mechanical assist devices. The excitement and glamor of transplantation and other newer surgical techniques should not divert attention from the more fundamental challenges of managing left ventricular dysfunction. Refinement of neurohumoral and hemodynamic modulation of the circulation along with improved techniques for preventing sudden death will allow quality and length of life to be improved despite impairment of native heart function. Ultimately, elucidation of the myocardial responses to injury may allow us to interrupt the progression to heart failure and limit the population for whom transplantation need ever be considered.

BIBLIOGRAPHY

Bourge RC, Naftel DC, Constanza-Nordin MR, Transplant Cardiology Research Group: Risk factors for death after cardiac transplantation, *J Heart Lung Transplant* 11:191, 1992.

Corcos T, Tamburino C, Leger P et al: Early and late hemodynamic evaluation after cardiac transplantation: a study of 28 cases, *J Am Coll Cardiol* 11:264-269, 1988.

Erickson KW, Costanzo-Nordin MR, O'Sullivan F et al: Influence of pre-operative transpulmonary gradient on late mortality after orthotopic heart transplantation, *J Heart Transplant* 9:526-537, 1990.

Gao SZ, Schroeder JS, Alderman EL et al: Prevalence of accelerated coronary artery disease in heart transplant survivors. Comparison of cyclosporine and azathioprine regimens, *Circulation* 80:III100-105, 1989.

Grattan MT, Moreno-Cabral CE, Starnes VA et al: Eight-year results of cyclosporine-treated patients with cardiac transplants, *J Thorac Cardiovasc Surg* 99:500-509, 1990.

Kahan BD: Cyclosporine, *N Engl J Med* 321:1725-1738, 1989.

Kavanagh T, Yacoub MH, Mertner DJ et al: Cardiorespiratory responses to exercise training after orthotopic cardiac transplantation, *Circulation* 77:162-171, 1988.

Mancini DM, Eisen H, Kussmaul W et al: Value of peak exercise oxygen consumption for optimal timing of cardiac transplantation in ambulatory patients with heart failure, *Circulation* 83:778-783, 1991.

Mehta SM, Aufiero TX, Pae WE et al: Combined registry for the clinical use of mechanical ventricular assist pumps and the total artificial heart in conjunction with heart transplantation: Sixth official report—1994. 14:585-593, 1995.

Mudge GH, Goldstein S, Addonizio LJ et al: Bethesda Conference Task Force 3: Cardiac transplantation: recipient guidelines/prioritization, *J Am Coll Cardiol* 22:21-31, 1993.

Penn I: Cancers following cyclosporine therapy, *Transplantation* 43:32-35, 1987.

Rose AG, Novitsky D, Cooper DKC. Pathophysiology of brain death in the experimental animal: extracranial aspects/myocardial and pulmonary histopathologic changes, *Transplant Proc* 20(5-S7):29-32, 1988.

Salomon RN, Hughes CW, Schoen FJ et al: Human coronary transplantation-associated arteriosclerosis, *Am J Pathol* 138:791-798, 1991.

Shao-Zhou G, Hunt SA, Schroeder JS et al: Early development of accellerated graft coronary artery disease: risk factors and course, *J Am Coll Cardiol* 28:673-679, 1996.

Stevenson LW, Hamilton MA, Tillisch JH et al: Decreasing survival benefit from cardiac transplantation for outpatients as the waiting list lengthens, *J Am Coll Cardiol* 18:919-925, 1991.

Stevenson LW, Sietsema K, Tillisch JH et al: Exercise capacity for survivors of cardiac transplantation or sustained medical therapy for stable heart failure, *Circulation* 81:78, 1990.

Stevenson LW, Steimle AE, Fonarow G et al: Improvement in exercise capacity of candidates awaiting heart transplantation, *J Am Coll Cardiol* 25:163-170, 1995.

Stevenson WG, Stevenson LW, Middlekauff HR et al: Improving survival for patients with advanced heart failure: a study of 737 consecutive patients, *J Am Coll Cardiol* 26:1417-1423, 1995.

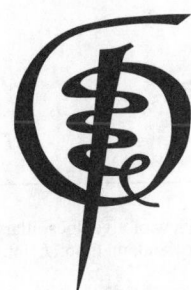

Pulmonary and Critical Care Medicine

CHAPTER

35 Respiratory Pathophysiology

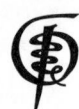

Walter J. Daly and Jacob S.O. Loke

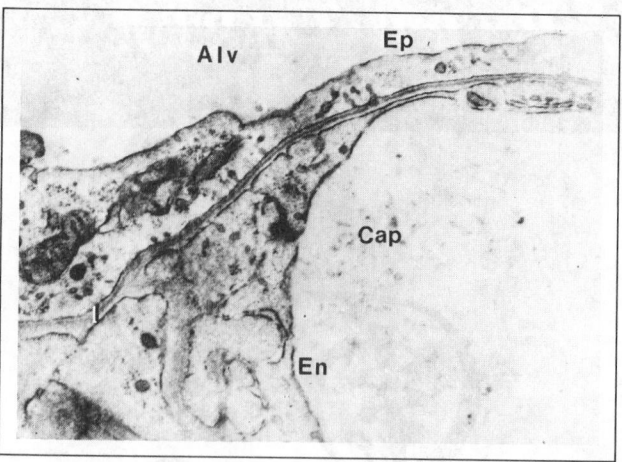

FIGURE 35-1   Electron microscopic view of alveolocapillary membrane. *Alv,* Alveolus; *Cap,* capillary; *En,* capillary endothelium; *I,* interstitium; *Ep,* alveolar epithelium.

The major components of the respiratory system include (1) a neural control mechanism, (2) a ventilatory "pump", (3) gas exchange, and (4) the pulmonary circulation. Impairment of one or more of these components due to a disease process can lead to dysfunction and the corresponding development of symptoms, especially dyspnea.

NONRESPIRATORY FUNCTIONS OF THE LUNG
Filtering

The lung serves a vital filtering function. It protects the systemic circulation against constant threat of focal ischemia and even infarction by filtering embolic material of various types, that is, fibrin clumps, clots, and other material that may be endogenous or exogenous in origin.

Metabolic Functions

The lung has an important set of metabolic functions. Because the entire cardiac output flows through the lung during a single circulation, a large fraction of the circulating blood is in contact with respiratory endothelial cells two or more times each minute. This finding suggests that the lung is uniquely situated to perform metabolic changes on the blood. In some instances, the lung seems to act like a metabolic filter, removing certain locally important vasoactive substances such as serotonin, bradykinin, norepinephrine, and certain prostaglandins (PGs). Substances important to systemic regulation such as epinephrine, prostacycline, and PGI_2 pass unaffected. Angiotensin I is specifically converted to angiotensin II by angiotensin-converting enzyme (ACE). These important activities are performed by the pulmonary endothelial cells. Disorders that impair endothelial cell function also affect amine-processing efficiency. Best studied of these disorders is oxygen toxicity.

Lung Defenses

See Chapter 39 for a discussion on defense functions of the lungs.

Microvascular Fluid Exchanges

The principal forces active in transcapillary fluid movement in the lung are the capillary hydrostatic pressure and the plasma oncotic pressure. The balance of these pressures favors reabsorption of fluid from the interstitium and thus provides for a "dry" alveolocapillary membrane and effective gas exchange. Fig. 35-1 depicts an electron microscopic view of the alveolocapillary relationship. Fig. 35-2 diagrams the forces of the capillary membrane. In everyday life, transient increases in capillary pressure during exercise must exceed the oncotic pressure; fluid transudation occurs particularly at the lung bases. Fluid is readily drained from the interstitium into the lymphatics, and lung water increases only a little. As long as interstitial oncotic pressure remains low and plasma protein concentration remains relatively normal, capillary hydrostatic pressure is usually not sufficiently high to cause edema. Factors that increase hydrostatic pressure or lower plasma oncotic pressure can be expected to produce interstitial edema. If the draining capacity of the lymphatics is ex-

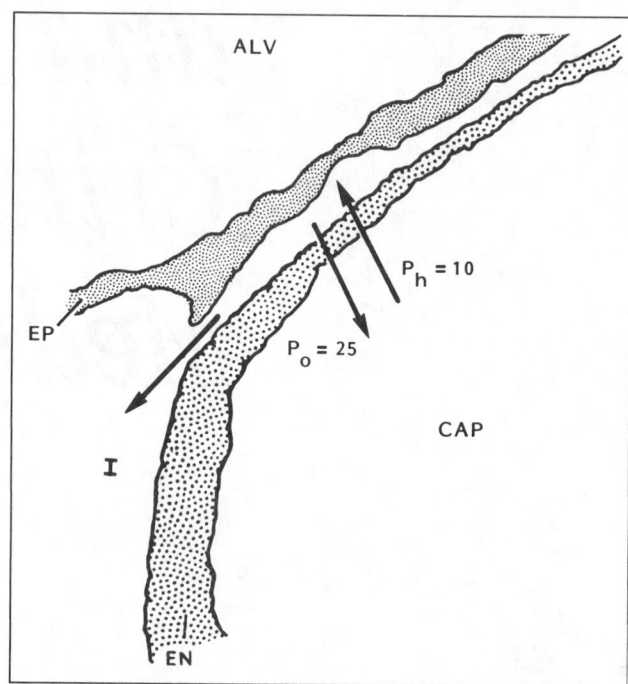

FIGURE 35-2   Diagram of forces acting at alveolocapillary membrane. *Alv,* Alveolus; *Cap,* capillary; *Ep,* alveolar epithelium; *En,* capillary endothelium; P_h, hydrostatic pressure; P_o, plasma oncotic pressure; *I,* interstitium.

ceeded, water accumulates in the interstitium, the lung stiffens, and alveolar flooding may occur. Fluid leaving the capillary bed under these circumstances is characteristically low in protein concentration. If capillary pressure exceeds about 20 mm Hg, protein leakage occurs and edema formation is enhanced by decreasing the transendothelial oncotic gradient.

Other conditions may increase the permeability of the capillary membrane directly, leading to a permeability edema. In this event, the membrane leaks protein as well as water at lower capillary pressures, the osmotic gradient is lessened, and fluid movement may occur at less elevated or even more normal capillary pressures. When permeability is increased, lymph protein concentration increases. This change in lymph protein clearly differentiates lung fluid accumulation caused by permeability from that caused by hydrostatic pressures, except when pressure is very high and effective pore size increases.

As fluid accumulates in the interstitium, it finds its way to the lymphatics, which first appear at the level of the respiratory bronchioles. When the interstitium is fluid-filled and the draining capacity of the lymphatics has been exceeded, alveolar flooding occurs and clinical pulmonary edema is evident. Dyspnea, hypoxemia, and early radiographic changes may appear before alveolar flooding.

RESPIRATORY FUNCTION

The lung is efficient for gas exchange so that up to 6 liters of oxygen can move into the blood each minute as comparable quantities of carbon dioxide can be expired. Thus about 7×10^{23} molecules of oxygen individually diffuse across a surface of 90 m^2 into an instantaneous capillary volume of about 100 ml, which is changed 400 times each minute during extremes of exercise. During rest, transfer is appropriately reduced to the level of 200 to 400 ml of oxygen each minute.

The forces driving this remarkable movement of gas between alveolus and capillary are entirely those that drive diffusion of gas from places of higher to lower partial pressures. No active processes requiring metabolic energy are required.

Simply, the function of the lung as a gas exchanger has three components: delivery of gas to and from the alveolus, diffusion across the membrane, and movement of blood to and from contact with the membrane.

Mechanical Properties

Briefly stated, the mechanical properties of the lung important to understanding clinical disorders are compliance and airway resistance. The forces applied to the surface of the lung are transmitted by the chest wall and diaphragm acting as a ventilatory "pump."

Ventilatory "Pump." The forces driving the lung during ventilation are the muscles of the chest wall and diaphragm. These muscles are coordinated and cycled in response to metabolic and neurologic drive. The lung is ventilated as a passive response to contraction of the inspiratory muscles as modified by compliance and resistance. With muscle weakness or paralysis caused by a variety of disorders, for example, poliomyelitis, muscular dystrophy, paraplegia, or phrenic nerve injury, hypoventilation may occur. Also, decreased deformability of the thorax (e.g., kyphoscoliosis, obesity, or ascites) may impair respiratory muscle function. In any case, the volume of air moved during a tidal volume depends on the force of inspiratory muscle activity and the mechanical impediments to movement. Respiratory muscle dysfunction or fatigue can lead to ventilatory failure.

Compliance. Compliance is an expression of the elastic properties of the lung. It is measured as the change in volume divided by the change in transpulmonary pressure and is expressed as liters per centimeter of water. Customarily, the transpulmonary pressure is measured as the difference between airway and esophageal pressure. In actual practice, static compliance is measured as the slope of a curve relating lung volume and transpulmonary pressure—measured during periods of no air flow. This relationship is outlined in Fig. 35-3. The normal lung compliance is about 0.2 L/cm H$_2$O. The fibrotic lung and the congested lung are stiffer; that is, they have lower compliance. In emphysema, the lung contains less tissue per unit volume of air and has a higher compliance.

Total compliance (C$_T$) is the compliance of lung and chest wall measured together. If C$_C$ = compliance of the chest wall 1/C$_T$ = 1/C$_L$ + 1/C$_C$. Normal C$_T$ = 0.1 L/cm H$_2$O. The compliance usually measured in patients connected to ventilators is total compliance. In such measurements, the condition of no airflow must be met, but chest wall relaxation or paralysis is crucial.

Since C$_L$ is a measure of the force required to stretch the lung, the lower the C$_L$, the greater the force required for a given tidal volume. Thus, when C$_L$ is low, the respiratory pattern is low tidal volumes and increased frequency.

Dynamic Compliance. The pressure-volume relationship measured without allowing for complete cessation of airflow is called *dynamic compliance*. In normal individuals, static compliance and dynamic compliance approximate each other. If the internal mechanical properties of the lung are unevenly distributed, each breath is also unevenly distributed, and without the time that a period of no airflow allows for redistribution, volumes are unevenly distributed, and each part of the lung may be on a different portion of its pressure-volume curve. Thus when mechanical heterogeneity exists, dynamic compliance is less than static compliance and becomes still less as breathing frequency increases.

Airway Resistance. Airway resistance expresses the force required to move air from alveolus to mouth. Normally the resistance of the upper airway is about 50% of the total. Resistance of airways less than 2 mm in diameter is only about 20%. However, diseases involving the small airways may have an important impact on distribution of ventilation, ventilation-perfusion matching, and arterial Po$_2$.

Since resistance measurements are made during airflow and really measure the force required to move air through the resistance of the airway, the force required is highly dependent on the rate of flow. For a given resistance (R$_L$), rapid breathing requires more effort than slow, deeper breathing.

Work. The overall resistance (R$_L$) and compliance (C$_L$) account for the work required to ventilate the lung. Normally the process is so efficient that little added effort is necessary to increase ventilation within clinical ranges. However, when resistance is high or the lung is stiff, increased ventilation is accomplished only with vigorous effort of the respiratory muscles. When the inspiratory effort is high to achieve a desired flow and/or volume, neuroventilatory dissociation develops and leads to the sensation of breathlessness.

Surfactant. Type II alveolar epithelial cells produce a unique phospholipid, dipalmitoyl-lecithin, which lines alveolar surfaces. This material is capable of changing its surface tension so that the surface tension of small alveoli is less than that of large alveoli. If such material were not present, small alveoli would be expected to empty into large alveoli and collapse.

Surfactant has been extracted from the lung, its surface-active properties have been measured, its composition has been analyzed, and its presence at the alveolar surface has been demonstrated by special electron microscopic techniques. Surfactant is an "antiatelectasis" factor that tends to prevent alveolar closure at small volumes. In vivo or excised lungs seem to decrease their surfactant activity and compliance as their volume of expansion decreases. In other words, both compliance and surfactant activity are affected by the volume history of the lung. This change is partially explained by alveolar closure at small volumes, but may also be caused by extracellular changes in surfactant molecules; that is, surfactant molecules may aggregate or disaggregate as volume changes. Large-volume sighs at 4- to 5-minute intervals seem sufficient to maintain surfactant activity and prevent alveolar collapse.

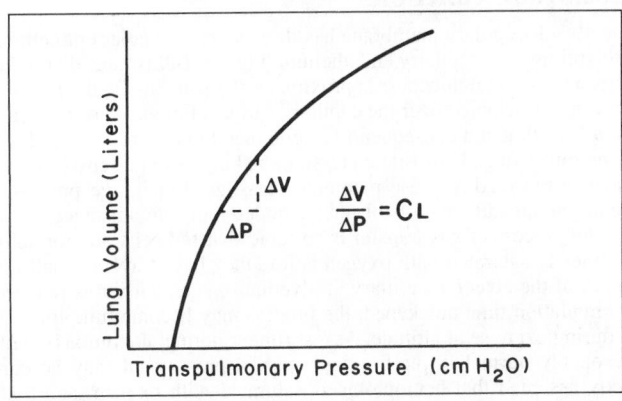

FIGURE 35-3   Measurement of the static compliance (C$_L$) of the lung. The change in lung volume (ΔV) is plotted against the change in transpulmonary pressure (ΔP) (the pressure required for lung inflation) during periods of no airflow.

Membrane Functions

The alveolocapillary membrane has three layers: alveolar epithelium, interstitium, and capillary endothelium. Fig. 35-1 illustrates their relationship. The total thickness approximates 0.3 μm, but the thickness is unevenly distributed over the capillary surface. For gas to diffuse easily, a very thin and consequently fragile membrane is required. Membrane forces (e.g., hydrostatic pressure) and injury (e.g., sepsis, shock, pancreatitis) readily cause membrane leakage. Reparative processes are important and are probably active under many circumstances.

The process of gas transfer is so rapid that red cells are normally completely saturated with oxygen before they have traversed half the length of the alveolar capillary. If alveolar oxygen tension is reduced or circulation time quickened, the process may become time-limited, as during exercise at altitude. At rest (under normal conditions), with reasonably normal inspired oxygen partial pressure, it may be correctly assumed that hemoglobin is saturated with oxygen, and both carbon dioxide and oxygen in a given alveolus are in equilibrium with gas concentrations in the adjacent capillary by the time alveolar capillary transit is completed. Calculations show and physiologic observations confirm that oxygen transfer across the membrane is not limited by membrane thickness; that is, oxygenation is not diffusion-limited except during exercise in patients with interstitial lung disease. Although gas transfer is conceptualized as occurring from a single alveolus across a single alveolocapillary membrane to a single capillary containing a single red blood cell, it is readily apparent that these processes take place in several million sets of alveoli and capillaries simultaneously. As shown in Fig. 35-4, each alveolus is liberally supplied with a network of capillaries.

It is possible to measure this aggregate transfer of oxygen as an oxygen-diffusing capacity, but the measurement is too cumbersome for clinical use. Rather, trace carbon monoxide concentrations are used as a test gas, and the calculations become simpler because hemoglobin removes carbon monoxide from the plasma so rapidly that plasma PCO opposing diffusion across the membrane can be assumed to be zero. A low value for the diffusing capacity for carbon monoxide (DLCO) is characteristic of a number of diseases, including interstitial lung disease, emphysema, and pulmonary vascular disease. DLCO may also be decreased in anemia, as the capillary mass of hemoglobin available to bind carbon monoxide is decreased.

Alveolar Gas and Dead Space

At the end of an expiration, conducting airways are filled with expired gas. As inspiration begins, this gas is the first to reenter the alveoli. At the end of inspiration, those same nonexchanging parts are filled with inspired air that never reaches the alveoli. This space is called the *dead space*. Furthermore, regions of alveoli that are not perfused or are "underperfused" function as dead space because they do not contribute to oxygenation or carbon dioxide elimination. The gas contained in this dead space is called the *dead space volume* (VD).

The volume of gas remaining in the lung at the end of a normal expiration is the functional residual capacity (FRC). Thus functioning alveoli are not empty at end-expiration but contain a volume of gas that is diluted as inspiration occurs. This residual gas serves to buffer against wide swings in gas tension during the respiratory cycle.

The forces acting on the lung to drive ventilation are not directly applied to each alveolus, so given alveoli are ventilated according to the ease with which air flows into them; the inspired air flows to alveoli that are most easily opened, through bronchi with the least resistance. Because normally there is uneven distribution of ventilation, some unevenness of alveolar ventilation and of individual alveolar gas tensions occurs. However, in any single alveolus, given reasonable inspired oxygen concentrations and circulation time that is not excessively rapid, P_{O_2} and P_{CO_2} in the alveolus and end-capillary blood may be assumed to be nearly identical.

Selection of reasonable values of P_{O_2} and P_{CO_2} to represent the sum of all alveolar P_{O_2}s and P_{CO_2}s is a more complex consideration. The rapidity of carbon dioxide movement and the shape of the blood-carbon dioxide dissociation curve (Fig. 35-5) have led to the theoretical demonstration that arterial P_{CO_2} (Pa_{CO_2}) can be taken as equal to alveolar P_{CO_2} (PA_{CO_2}). The different dissociation relationship for blood and oxygen does not permit a similar assumption, and PA_{O_2} must be calculated. A simplified calculation is

(EQ. 1)

$$PA_{O_2} = PI_{O_2} - 1.25\ (Pa_{CO_2})$$

PI_{O_2} is the partial pressure of oxygen inspired. A respiratory quotient (RQ) of 0.8 is assumed.

Unevenness of Ventilation

Because the forces applied to the surface of the lung by the ventilatory "pump" are not evenly distributed and because the individual resistances and compliances within the lung are not evenly distributed, some alveoli are normally better ventilated than others. Unevenness may be diffusely distributed as in the diffuse diseases of the lung, regionally distributed as with a local partial bronchial obstruction, or distributed according to vertical pressure gradients. This heterogeneity of ventilation may be exaggerated by irregular stiffening of the lung with scattered foci of edema, inflammation, or fibrosis, or with irregularly distributed areas of increased airway resistance due to obstructive airway diseases. Furthermore, resistances are constantly changing with clearing of mucous plugs, coughing, deep breathing, or local perfusion changes. It is well established that local bronchial constriction occurs in response to local decreases in alveolar P_{CO_2} caused by redistribution of perfusion to other areas. Local factors also cause frequency-dependent unevenness. Given irregularly scattered areas

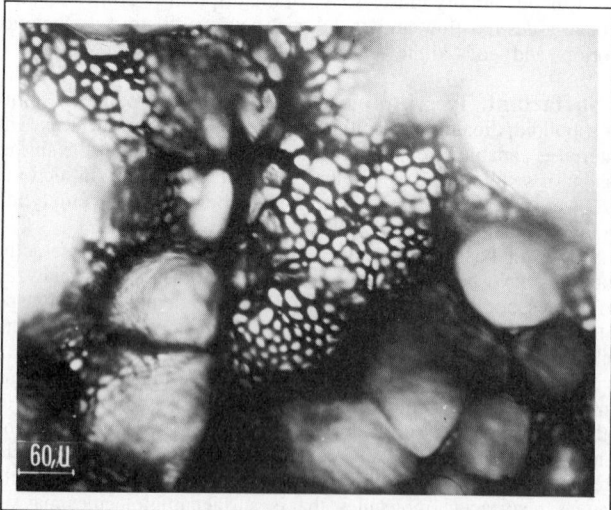

FIGURE 35-4 Microscopic view of the capillary network at the alveolar surface viewed on face. This preparation was from a thick cut of an India ink–perfused, fume-fixed lung.

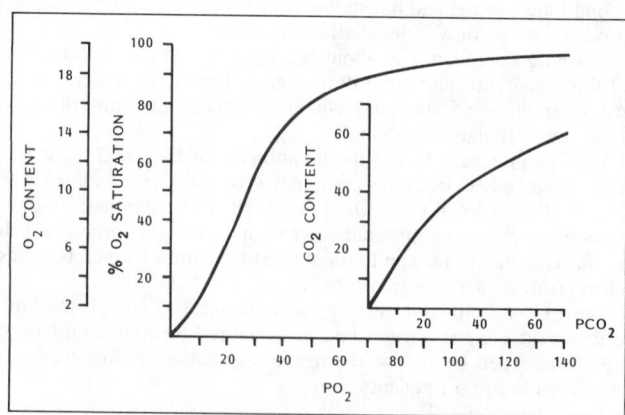

FIGURE 35-5 Dissociation curves of O_2 and CO_2 with blood. These curves are represented as normal curves. Hemoglobin concentration = 15 g/dl. Content = ml gas/dl blood.

difficult to ventilate, increased respiratory frequency can redistribute ventilation away from the difficult areas to the areas of easier access. With diseases such as asthma, chronic obstructive pulmonary disease (COPD), or interstitial lung disease, that unevenness is exaggerated.

In normal individuals, regionally determined gradients of ventilation are more important than differences caused by local resistance changes. Such gradients are dependent on the structure of the chest and of the lung and on regional pressure-volume relationships. The net result is a gradient of ventilation such that the lower zones of the vertical lung receive the largest fraction of ventilation. At low lung volumes, there is even a tendency for lower zone airway closure, which accounts for some hypoxemia found at low lung volumes. Obesity may contribute to airway closure in lower lung zones.

Capillary Blood Gas

Once oxygen enters the plasma, it rapidly diffuses along concentration gradients into the red cell and loosely associates with hemoglobin according to the relationship known as the *oxygen-hemoglobin dissociation curve*. The shape of this curve (Fig. 35-5) and the factors affecting it are important. Carbon dioxide leaves the blood, even more rapidly than oxygen enters, and diffuses freely into the alveolus. The carbon dioxide dissociation curve describes the carbon dioxide partial pressure–volume relationship (Fig. 35-5).

In normal gas environments, the principal alveolar gases are oxygen, carbon dioxide, nitrogen, and water. Water vapor remains as a constant pH_2O, dependent on body temperature and barometric pressure. Oxygen enters the alveolus as alveolar gas is partially exchanged during ventilation, and, with each breath, carbon dioxide is removed. Carbon dioxide diffuses into the alveolus from the capillary blood, having been delivered to the lung from peripheral production sites. Thus, there is a reciprocal relationship between $PACO_2$ and PAO_2. In fact, if PAN_2 remained constant, the sum of $PACO_2$ and PAO_2 would be a constant fraction of barometric pressure during air breathing.

It is evident that decreased ventilation of a given alveolus decreases end-capillary PO_2 and increases PCO_2 with resultant change in capillary blood oxygen and carbon dioxide content. When ventilation is increased above normal, however, alveolar PO_2 and end-capillary PO_2 move toward the level of inspired PO_2 and alveolar end-capillary PCO_2 decreases.

Perfusion

Just as alveolar ventilation is unevenly distributed, so is capillary perfusion. Unevenness of perfusion is dependent on gravity, local structural change, and local alveolar PO_2. In the normally low-pressure pulmonary circulation, the effect of gravity is large, increasing the perfusion of dependent areas and leaving apical portions of the lung unperfused. With increases in pulmonary vascular pressure, perfusion is "redistributed" toward the apices, a radiographic sign of increased pulmonary venous pressure. With local fibrosis, embolic obstruction of the pulmonary artery, or loss of vasculature caused by emphysema, there are foci of absent or decreased perfusion. Perfusion distribution is singularly sensitive to local alveolar PO_2, so that areas of focal alveolar hypoxia cause local arterial constriction and perfusion unevenness.

Relationship of Ventilation to Perfusion

When, for whatever reason, local ventilation and perfusion are not ideally matched, blood gas abnormalities occur in end-capillary blood. Arterial blood sampled peripherally for PCO_2 and PO_2 measurement represents the aggregate of end-capillary contributions together with admixture from venous blood totally bypassing alveolar exchange. When foci of alveolar underventilation with respect to perfusion occur (low $\dot{V}/\dot{Q}$), end-capillary blood has low PO_2 and high PCO_2. When such blood is mixed with blood from areas of normal $\dot{V}/\dot{Q}$, the consequence is reduced arterial PO_2 and increased PCO_2. Increased PCO_2 stimulates increased ventilation, which is chiefly distributed to the areas of normal or high $\dot{V}/\dot{Q}$ ratios, reducing the PCO_2 and increasing the PO_2 in the blood from those areas. But the result of mixing this blood with blood from areas of low $\dot{V}/\dot{Q}$ is only correction of the PCO_2 levels, not PO_2. The slope of oxygen- and carbon dioxide–blood dissociation curves determines this difference. Thus, hyperventilation

of some areas may remove sufficient carbon dioxide to compensate for carbon dioxide retained in foci of reduced ventilation, whereas the hyperventilated areas do not add sufficient oxygen to correct for the hypoxemia. This important phenomenon is illustrated in Fig. 35-6. In this example, hyperventilation sufficient to reduce $PaCO_2$ to 33 mm Hg failed to raise PaO_2 above 59 mm Hg.

Mismatching of ventilation and perfusion is the most common cause of hypoxemia. A representative list of other causes of hypoxemia is presented in Box 35-1.

Hyperventilation and Hypoventilation

Overall increases or decreases in alveolar ventilation have profound effects on alveolar and arterial blood gas levels. These effects are predictable from consideration of the oxygen- and carbon dioxide–blood dissociation curves (Fig. 35-5). The rate of carbon dioxide production is also an important determinant of $PACO_2$. The relationship is expressed as

$$PACO_2 = 0.863\ (\dot{V}CO_2/\dot{V}A)$$

0.863 being a conversion constant; $\dot{V}CO_2$, an expression of CO_2 production; and $\dot{V}A$, alveolar ventilation. From this equation an increase in $\dot{V}CO_2$ requires an increase in alveolar ventilation if $PACO_2$ is to remain stable.

As total alveolar ventilation increases without a change in $\dot{V}CO_2$, alveolar PCO_2 is reduced and alveolar PO_2 approaches inspired PO_2. Examination of the dissociation curves shows that this change profoundly affects blood carbon dioxide content with little change in oxy-

---

BOX 35-1
Causes of hypoxemia

Anatomic shunting of venous to arterial shunt
  Pulmonary arteriovenous fistula
  Patent ductus arteriosus with reversal flow
  Intracardiac septal defect with severe pulmonary hypertension, pulmonic stenosis, tricuspid atresia, single ventricle
Physiologic derangements
  Hypoventilation
  Ventilation-perfusion mismatching
Altitude
  Low PIO_2

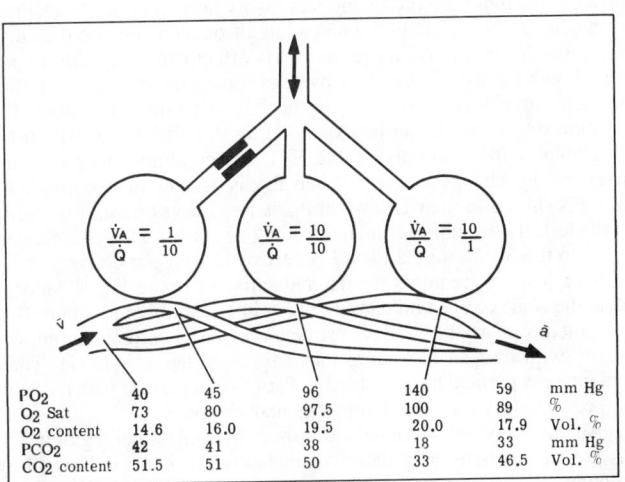

PO2	40	45	96	140	59	mm Hg
O2 Sat	73	80	97.5	100	89	%
O2 content	14.6	16.0	19.5	20.0	17.9	Vol. %
PCO2	42	41	38	18	33	mm Hg
CO2 content	51.5	51	50	33	46.5	Vol. %

FIGURE 35-6 Ventilation-perfusion mismatching. Three alveoli (A) with different V/Q are illustrated. $\dot{V}$, Ventilation (volume/time); $\dot{Q}$, blood flow (volume/time). Mixed venous ($\bar{v}$) values are tabulated in the first column. Values have been calculated and listed for each end capillary. Mixed arterial values ($\bar{a}$) are listed in the last column. Hemoglobin concentration = 15 g/dl.

gen content. Conversely, decreases in overall alveolar ventilation increase alveolar PCO_2 and decrease alveolar PO_2, affecting both arterial PO_2 and oxygen content as well as arterial PCO_2 and carbon dioxide content.

Because $PaCO_2$ is taken as a measure of overall $PACO_2$, increased $PaCO_2$ occurs when alveolar ventilation is decreased, and decreased $PaCO_2$ reflects increased alveolar ventilation. In clinical practice, increases in $PaCO_2$ do not occur unless there is alveolar hypoventilation. If the lungs are normal and central hypoventilation occurs, $PaCO_2$ rises. If the lungs are abnormal and ventilation-perfusion mismatching is present, $PaCO_2$ does not rise unless the neural control does not respond appropriately to increased $PaCO_2$, restoring it to normal. Thus, for clinical purposes, even with mismatching, $PaCO_2$ does not rise without absolute or relative "hypoventilation."

Oxygen Transport

Oxygen transport is the volume of oxygen moved through the circulation in a unit of time. Thus, O_2 transport (ml/min) = O_2 content (ml/dl) × blood flow (dl/min). Cardiac output or blood flow to a specific site is important to oxygen transport and tissue delivery. Blood oxygen content depends on the pulmonary capillary PO_2 produced by gas exchange, the amount of hemoglobin present, and the slope of the oxygen-hemoglobin dissociation curve (Fig. 35-5). If the curve is normal, PaO_2 above 80 mmHg adds little more than dissolved oxygen to the blood. Because only 0.003 ml of oxygen/mm Hg PO_2/ml blood is carried as dissolved oxygen, oxygen in solution is not important to oxygen transport except during hyperbaric conditions. Given the shape of the dissociation curve, when PaO_2 is less than 60 mm Hg, the availability of oxygen changes greatly with small changes in PaO_2. Thus addition of small concentrations of inspired oxygen adds substantial amounts of oxygen when PaO_2 is less than 60 mm Hg. Often attention is focused only at the upper end of the curve where the relationships determining loading of oxygen in the lung are described. The unloading of oxygen in the systemic capillaries also has great importance and is described by the same curve. Systemic capillary PO_2 varies widely from time to time and from place to place, depending on metabolic activity and local blood flow. The oxygen-hemoglobin relationship is sensitive to a number of factors that "shift the curve" to right or left, reflecting changing hemoglobin affinity for oxygen. These shifts have important implications for oxygen unloading.

DISORDERS OF OXYGEN TRANSPORT
Oxygen-Hemoglobin Curve

The right or left displacement of the oxygen-hemoglobin dissociation curve expresses a relationship that is an important determinant of oxygen transport. Fig. 35-7 illustrates abnormal variations in the curve. If the lungs are producing reasonably normal PaO_2, the changes in the curve chiefly affect the unloading of oxygen because the curve is steeper in the unloading region. This effect can be readily appreciated with the use of Fig. 35-7 by determining the percent saturation of each curve for a given PO_2 in the 20- to 40-mm Hg range. The position of the curve can be expressed as P_{50}, the PO_2 at which hemoglobin is 50% saturated. Table 35-1 lists conditions that are characterized by changes in P_{50}. When P_{50} is greater than normal, the curve is shifted to the right; when P_{50} is less than normal, it is shifted to the left. If one supposes that unloading oxygen in the systemic capillary to the 30% saturated level is needed for oxygen delivery, a left shift or low P_{50} requires greater reduction in tissue PO_2 to accomplish the same oxygen unloading. In regional circulations, where flow is limited by partial vascular obstruction or fixed cardiac output, difficulty with oxygen unloading may aggravate tissue hypoxia. These patients are particularly troubled if PaO_2 is decreased, which should be prevented by the use of supplemental oxygen.

Anemia may reduce oxygen transport, but unless hemoglobin levels are substantially low, there is an adaptive increase in blood flow to compensate.

Carbon Monoxide

Carbon monoxide poisoning produces important derangements in oxygen transport, mainly by occupying the oxygen-binding sites in

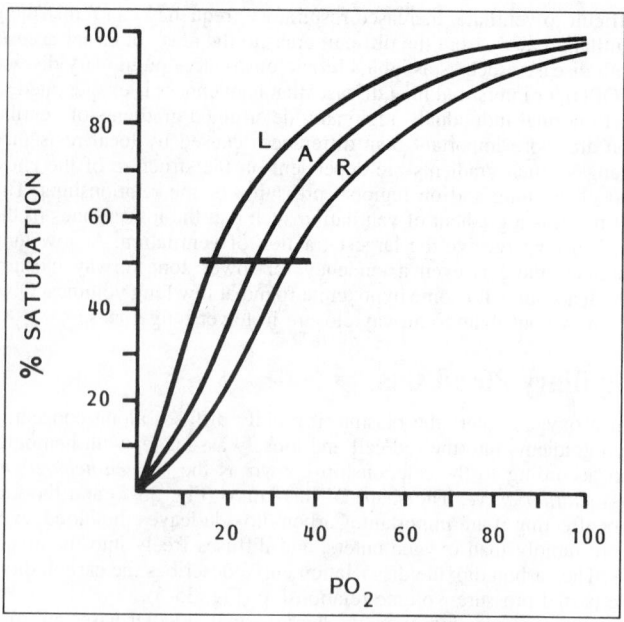

FIGURE 35-7   Shifts in oxygen-hemoglobin affinity curve. Curve A depicts the normal relationship. *L* represents a left-shifted curve (increased affinity). *R* represents a right-shifted curve (decreased affinity). Curve L: P_{50} = 17 mm Hg. Curve A: P_{50} = 26 mm Hg. Curve R: P_{50} = 34 mm Hg.

Table 35-1   Factors affecting oxygen-hemoglobin affinity

LOW P_{50}*	HIGH P_{50}
LEFT SHIFT OF CURVE (INCREASED AFFINITY)	**RIGHT SHIFT OF CURVE (DECREASED AFFINITY)**
High pH (alkalosis)	Low pH (acidosis)
Low temperature	High temperature
Low 2,3-DPG	High 2,3-DPG
Stored blood	Anemia
Phosphorus deficiency	Altitude acclimatization
Carbon monoxide poisoning	Rare hemoglobinopathies (Kansas, Beth Israel)
Hemoglobinopathies (e.g., Kempsey, Yakima)	

2,3-DPG, 2,3-diphosphoglycerate.
*Normal P_{50} = 27 mm Hg.

the hemoglobin molecule. Because the carbon monoxide–hemoglobin affinity is 200 times greater than the oxygen-hemoglobin affinity, small concentrations of carbon monoxide can convert large quantities of hemoglobin to carboxyhemoglobin. The carbon monoxide–hemoglobin affinity further complicates oxygen transport by causing a left shift in the oxygen-hemoglobin curve (low P_{50}). Thus what oxygen is transported is released with difficulty at the capillary level, driving tissue PO_2 even lower. Moreover, because carbon monoxide binds to myoglobin avidly, intracellular oxygen transport in active muscles—both skeletal and myocardial—is further impaired. The overall effect on oxygen transport of small quantities of carbon monoxide is greater than the loss of comparable quantities of oxygen capacity through anemia.

Abnormal Hemoglobins

Rarely, congenital hemoglobinopathies (e.g., Kansas, Beth Israel) shift the oxygen-hemoglobin curves so far to the right that hemoglobin is barely saturated with the PO_2 available during air breathing. If oxygen-hemoglobin affinity is reduced sufficiently, oxygen unloading occurs so readily that adequate amounts of reduced hemoglobin may be present in peripheral vessels to produce cyanosis without low tissue PO_2 or difficulty with oxygen transport. Conversely, other hemoglobinopathies can have increased oxygen-hemoglobin affinity that tissue P_{O_2} may be lowered to the point that erythropoietin is increased and erythrocytosis occurs. Often patients in this situation are detected through evaluation of polycythemia and demonstration of P_{50} that is abnormally low.

Other abnormalities of oxygen-hemoglobin affinity include sulfhemoglobinemia and methemoglobinemia. Sulfhemoglobin occurs as the consequence of binding of hydrogen sulfide to hemoglobin and, like carboxyhemoglobin, loses sites in the molecule usually available for oxygen binding. Sulfhemoglobin occurs after industrial or accidental exposure to hydrogen sulfide, in users of certain medications, and even as a consequence of environmental exposure to polluted air. In contrast to the left shift of the oxygen dissociation curve found in carboxyhemoglobin, the curve is shifted to the right when sulfhemoglobin is present. Thus the sulfhemoglobin effect on oxygen transport seems less than that predicted by estimating the fraction of sulfhemoglobin present, whereas the carbon monoxide effect is greater than predicted by carbon monoxide–hemoglobin levels.

Methemoglobinemia occurs as a congenital defect in hemoglobin metabolism or as a result of exposure to various toxic or medicinal substances such as nitrites, sulfonamides, and primaquine. The basic defect is conversion of the ferrous iron to the ferric form in the hemoglobin molecule, destroying its oxygen-carrying capacity. Methemoglobinemia, when present in sufficient concentrations (1.5 to 2.0 g/dl), produces brown discoloration of the skin. In acute situations, intravenous methylene blue (1 to 2 mg/kg) ordinarily causes rapid reversal. As with carbon monoxide–hemoglobin, methemoglobin causes a left shift of the dissociation curve, increasing oxygen affinity for hemoglobin and impeding oxygen unloading.

Acid-Base Regulation by the Lung

The prime determinant of acid-base balance and arterial pH is the buffer ratio of carbon dioxide to bicarbonate. The concentration of gaseous carbon dioxide is rapidly changed by ventilation, whereas bicarbonate is more slowly regulated by the renal tubule. Abrupt changes in alveolar ventilation increase or decrease Pa_{CO_2} and produce a set of pH levels dependent on the bicarbonate concentration. Chronic deviations in Pa_{CO_2} are accommodated partially by tubular retention or excretion of bicarbonate to produce a different set of carbon dioxide–bicarbonate relationships. Thus it is important to recognize both acute and chronic P_{CO_2}-pH curves. Ordinarily, renal compensation for a given acute P_{CO_2} change is not complete for many hours. When carbon dioxide retention is produced, Pa_{CO_2} increases, but respiratory acidemia may be severe or slight, depending on whether it is acute or chronic.

Given this relationship, it is possible to construct a series of curves to fit P_{CO_2}-pH pairs characterizing acute or chronic respiratory aci-

demia or alkalemia (Fig. 35-8). Understanding of this difference between acute and chronic P_{CO_2}-pH curves is important (1) to the diagnosis and management of respiratory acidosis and differentiation from metabolic acidosis, and (2) to the recognition of mixed states (i.e., combined respiratory and metabolic acidosis).

Alveolar-Arterial Difference—Oxygen

It can be assumed that blood leaving alveolar capillaries has nearly the same P_{O_2} as the alveoli they perfused, providing reasonably slow circulation time and normal or high alveolar P_{O_2} (PA_{O_2}). Furthermore, if ventilation to all alveoli is equal, PA_{O_2} is uniform throughout the lung. The ideal lung should have only such perfectly matched ventilation and perfusion relationships. If the ideal lung existed, there would be virtually no alveolar-arterial oxygen difference. PA_{O_2} can be calculated by Equation 1.

Even in normal lungs, a small alveolar-arterial oxygen difference exists because of ventilation-perfusion mismatch. This difference, $P(A-a)_{O_2}$, is normally about 6 mm Hg at ages less than 30 and about 15 mm Hg in normal persons older than 60 years of age. The effect of age on $P(A-a)_{O_2}$ is depicted in Fig. 35-9. The $P(A-a)_{O_2}$ is a rather sensitive index of oxygenation and is easily calculated. Arterial P_{O_2} (Pa_{O_2}) is a less sensitive measure; it provides information about the adequacy of blood oxygenation but incomplete information about lung function. For example, a young asthmatic may have a Pa_{O_2} of 80 mm Hg, indicating satisfactory oxygenation, but if Pa_{CO_2} is 20 mm Hg during air breathing ($FI_{O_2} = 0.21$), it follows that $P(A-a)_{O_2}$ is 44 mm Hg, an abnormal value, demonstrating impaired oxygenation, presumably due to ventilation-perfusion mismatch.

$$
\begin{aligned}
\text{Calculations: Barometric pressure} &= 760 \text{ mm Hg}\\
\text{Water vapor pressure} &= \underline{47 \text{ mm Hg}}\\
&\;713 \text{ mm Hg}
\end{aligned}
$$

$$
\begin{aligned}
FI_{O_2} \times (PB - 47) &= PI_{O_2}\\
0.21 \times (760 - 47) &= 149 \text{ mm Hg}\\
PA_{O_2} &= PI_{O_2} - 1.25\, Pa_{CO_2}\\
&= 149 - 1.25\,(20)\\
&= 124\\
P(A-a)_{O_2} &= PA_{O_2} - Pa_{O_2}\\
&= 124 - 80\\
&= 44 \text{ mm Hg}
\end{aligned}
$$

If alveolar ventilation is depressed in a patient with normal lungs (e.g., narcotic overdose), Pa_{O_2} decreases and Pa_{CO_2} increases without changing $P((A-a)_{O_2}$. If, however, a patient has increased Pa_{CO_2}, it is useful to calculate $P(A-a)_{O_2}$ to determine whether Pa_{O_2} is appropriately decreased or whether there is impaired oxygenation.

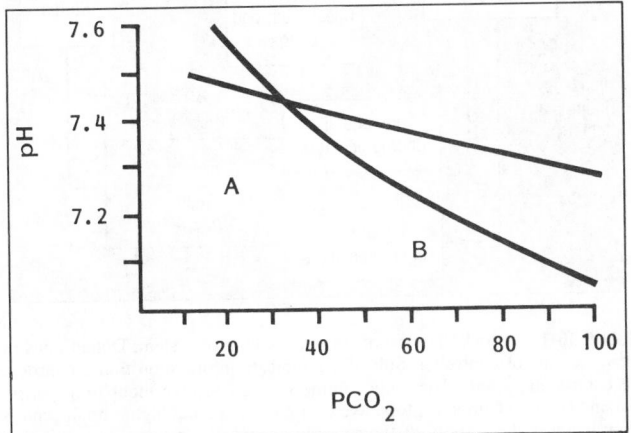

FIGURE 35-8 P_{CO_2}-pH curve. The steep curve outlines the P_{CO_2}-pH relationship during acute changes in P_{CO_2}. The flat curve represents changes during chronic P_{CO_2} deviations. Zone A is the area containing the P_{CO_2}-pH pairs found during metabolic acidosis. Zone B contains a mixed area observed with combined respiratory and metabolic acidosis.

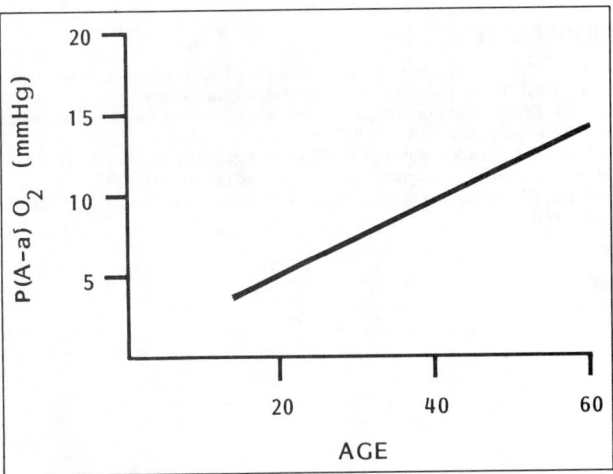

FIGURE 35-9   Effect of age on alveolar-arterial oxygen difference.

Venous Admixture

Though the most common cause of hypoxemia at rest (at sea level) is ventilation-perfusion mismatch, some "nonventilated" blood enters the left heart, having passed through thebesian cardiac veins, bronchial veins, or anatomic arteriovenous (A-V) shunts in the lung. In clinical situations, large right-to-left shunts may exist in pulmonary A-V fistulas or right-to-left intracardiac shunts. Furthermore, perfused but nonventilated or grossly underventilated alveoli contribute to this nonventilated circulation, which is collectively called *venous admixture*. Venous admixture is usually expressed as percentage of cardiac output (QS/QT). In general, QS/QT is greater than 20% if Pa_{O_2} is less than 100 mm Hg during 100% oxygen breathing.

Effects of Oxygen Breathing on Blood Gases

Air is 21% oxygen. If one assumes barometric pressure to be 760 mm Hg, the combined gas pressure at the alveolus is 760 mm Hg. At body temperature, water vapor has a pressure of 47 mm Hg, so this pressure contributes to the 760 mm Hg, leaving 713 mm Hg for the sum of P_{N_2}, P_{O_2}, and P_{CO_2}. The highest that P_{O_2} could be if no CO_2 were present would be $0.21 \times 713 = 149$ mm Hg. If all metabolism converted oxygen only to CO_2 and all CO_2 were excreted, $P_{CO_2} + P_{O_2}$ could then not exceed this ideal value of 149 mm Hg. If the lung were "ideal," $Pa_{CO_2} + Pa_{O_2}$ would also equal 149 mm Hg, but this situation never occurs because there is always a difference between PA_{O_2} and Pa_{O_2}. The degree to which Pa_{CO_2} and Pa_{O_2} departs from 149 mm Hg (during air breathing) is another measure of the extent of ventilation-perfusion mismatch and/or venous admixture.

In clinical settings, $Pa_{CO_2} + Pa_{O_2}$ often exceeds 149 mm Hg. This excess can happen only if there has been oxygen breathing or if the blood gas determinations are in error.

Each 1% of oxygen added to the inspired mixture adds 7 mm Hg P_{O_2} at the alveolar level. Given the shape of the oxygen-hemoglobin dissociation curve (Fig. 35-5), it is evident that small increases in inspired oxygen concentration have large effects on oxygen transport unless substantial fractions of blood totally bypass alveoli and enter the arterial circulation as unoxygenated venous blood (venous admixture).

An interesting and important therapeutic issue is the use of supplemental oxygen in patients with severe lung disease and chronic hypercapnia. When excessive oxygen is administered to such patients, Pa_{CO_2} may rise and can reach potentially high levels. Although the standard explanation for this observation is that oxygen suppresses hypoxic ventilatory drive, the mechanism appears more complex. Rather, increased ventilation-perfusion mismatching can occur with oxygen therapy; this can cause an increase in dead space and a resultant decrease in alveolar ventilation. Fortunately, the clinical implications of CO_2 retention with oxygen therapy are minimal with judicious use of supplemental oxygen. The target oxygen saturation of 90% is quite safe in the majority of patients with COPD and respiratory failure.

BIBLIOGRAPHY

Handbook of physiology: the respiratory system, vol 1, Circulation and non-respiratory functions, Bethesda, Md, 1985, American Physiological Society.

O'Donnell DE: Breathlessness in patients with chronic airflow limitation: mechanisms and management, *Chest* 106:904-912, 1994.

Sassoon CSH, Hassell KT, Mahutte CK: Hyperoxic-induced hypercapnia in stable chronic obstructive pulmonary disease, *Am Rev Respir Dis* 135:907-911, 1987.

Weinberger SE, Schwartzstein RM, Weiss JW: Hypercapnia, *N Engl J Med* 321:1223-1231, 1989.

CHAPTER

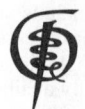

36   Abnormalities of the Control of Breathing

Neil S. Cherniack

The constancy of blood gases (arterial P_{CO_2}, P_{O_2}, and pH) seen in healthy persons is achieved by a complex interplay of control systems that rely on signals from chemoreceptors and mechanoreceptors in the body. These systems govern the rate and depth of breathing so that blood gases are maintained within a narrow range despite a variety of conditions that might otherwise cause unfavorable changes.

When respiratory function is severely impaired, these control systems may be unable to maintain arterial blood gases at normal levels. Indeed pulmonary disorders are the usual cause of persistent hypoxemia, hypercapnia, or hypocapnia, but frequently abnormalities are caused by a combination of impaired pulmonary performance and control system inadequacies. More rarely defects in the control system alone cause abnormal blood gases.

The respiratory control system itself is subject to two broad classes of disorders. The first affects the regularity of breathing and causes fluctuations in blood gas tensions. Acutely these fluctuations can be sufficiently great so as to be life threatening. The second kind of abnormality affects the mean level of alveolar ventilation so that arterial P_{CO_2} is excessively low or high, but breathing remains regular.

CHEMICAL CONTROL

Changes in blood gas tensions or in blood or brain pH cause compensatory changes in ventilation that tend to restore gas tension and pH toward their usual levels. Fig. 36-1 schematically diagrams the system responsible.

A reduction in ventilation, for example, decreases arterial P_{O_2}, exciting peripheral chemoreceptors in the carotid bifurcation and aortic

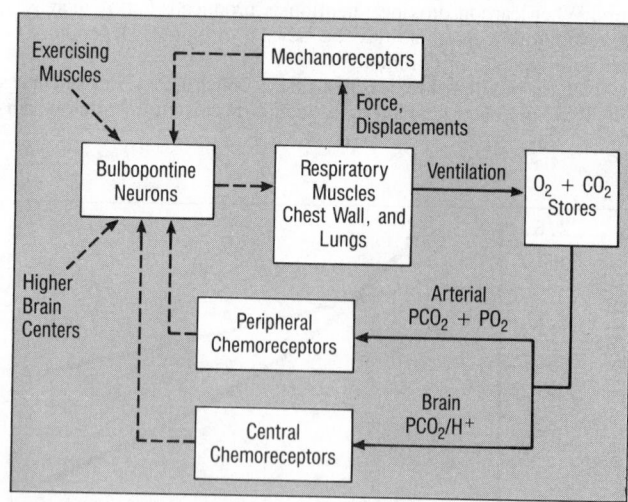

FIGURE 36-1   Block diagram of respiratory control system. Dotted lines indicate actions of controller. Solid lines indicate information transfer through the controlled system. The bulbopontine neurons receive input from peripheral and central chemoreceptors, exercising muscles, and higher brain centers. They increase the activity of the respiratory muscles to augment ventilation. Ventilation changes the amount of O_2 and CO_2 stored in chemical combination and physically dissolved in the tissues alters the P_{CO_2}, P_{O_2}, and H^+ concentrations in the arterial blood and brain, and thus affects chemoreceptor activity. Movements of the chest wall, lungs, and respiratory muscles alter mechanoreceptor activity.

arch (the carotid and aortic bodies) that sample the level of P_{O_2} and increase their signal to respiratory neurons in the medulla according to the degree of the hypoxemia. The greater signal in turn augments the activity of respiratory neurons and the motor discharge to the inspiratory muscles. This is a feedback control system because information concerning the effect of ventilation on arterial blood gases (in this case arterial P_{O_2}) is transferred (fed back) to the respiratory neurons through the chemoreceptors so that corrective action can be taken.

The level of peripheral chemoreceptor discharge is influenced by an intricate interplay of neurotransmitters released by hypoxia. For example, acetylcholine, neurokinin A and SP enchance the peripheral chemoreceptor signal, whereas nitric oxide and endorphin formation inhibits it.

The peripheral chemoreceptors are exclusively responsible for the increased ventilation in response to hypoxia. With a progressive reduction in arterial P_{O_2}, chemoreceptor discharge increases hyperbolically. A decrease in arterial P_{O_2} from 50 to 40 mm Hg produces a greater change in chemoreceptor activity and ventilation than does a change from 100 to 90 mm Hg, as shown in Fig. 36-2. Unlike its effects on the peripheral chemoreceptors, hypoxia is believed to have a depressant effect on brain respiratory neurons. This seems to be caused by the release by brain cells of depressant neurotransmitters and neuromodulators such as γ-aminobutyric acid (GABA), enkephalins, and adenosine. The exact level of arterial P_{O_2} at which depression of central respiratory neurons occurs probably depends on the rate of oxygen delivery by the cerebral circulation and ultimately on the ability of the cerebral blood vessels to dilate and brain blood flow to increase with hypoxia. An increase in arterial P_{CO_2} also stimulates peripheral chemoreceptors. But in normal individuals, the increase accounts for only 15% to 30% of the total ventilatory response to carbon dioxide.

Medullary chemoreceptors, which seem to respond directly to changes in brain interstitial or intracellular fluid pH and only indirectly to changes in arterial pH, are responsible for most of the augmentation of breathing seen with increases in P_{CO_2}. The relationship between arterial P_{CO_2} and ventilation is linear, unlike the hyperbolic relationship of arterial P_{O_2} and ventilation.

Figure 36-2 also shows the usual interactive effects of hypoxia and hypercapnia on ventilation in normal humans. Hypoxia increases the slope of the ventilatory response to carbon dioxide. This multiplying effect of hypoxia on the carbon dioxide response takes place mainly at the arterial chemoreceptors. Administration of oxygen to hypoxemic patients removes this hypoxia-driven augmentation, suppresses hypoxic drive, and sometimes causes considerable carbon dioxide retention.

Changes in arterial pH caused by metabolic disorders shift the position of the carbon dioxide response line. Metabolic alkalosis shifts the response line to the right so that resting P_{CO_2} is increased and ventilation is decreased, whereas acidosis causes a leftward shift so that resting P_{CO_2} is decreased and ventilation is greater. In addition, severe alkalosis seems to depress the effect of P_{CO_2} changes on ventilation, decreasing the slope of the ventilatory–carbon dioxide response line; acidosis has the opposite effect.

NEURAL FACTORS IN THE CONTROL OF VENTILATION

The rhythmic cycle of inspiration and expiration depends on the interaction among groups of neurons located in the medulla. The time spent in each phase of respiration is modified by signals from mechanoreceptors in the lungs and muscles of the chest wall. The mechanoreceptors in the lung are supplied to the vagus and can be classified into three broad categories: (1) receptors in the airways, which are stretched as the lungs expand and are responsible for the classic Hering-Breuer reflex in which lung inflation inhibits inspiratory and excites expiratory activity; (2) irritant receptors located in the epithelial layer of the airways, which are excited by dust, noxious gases, and mechanical stimuli; and (3) J receptors located in the alveolar wall, which are activated by congestion of the lung interstitium.

Stimulation of the receptors may be an important factor in the hyperventilation seen in asthmatic attacks. Irritant receptors in large airways are responsible for the cough reflex.

Three types of receptors in the chest wall innervated by spinal nerves—joint, tendon, and spindle—signal changes in the force exerted by the respiratory muscles and movement of the chest wall. Although these receptors are not believed to be important in normal breathing, they affect breathing patterns in diseases of the lung and chest wall and help compensate when there are impediments to breathing. Adjustment of the relationships among tidal volume, inspiratory time, and expiratory time by chest wall and pulmonary mechanoreceptors may be important in minimizing the work of breathing and the energy expenditure of the respiratory muscles and so can affect the endurance characteristics of the respiratory muscles. Fatigue of these muscles occurs more quickly when the ratio of inspiratory time to total breath duration is greater; endurance is prolonged by smaller ratios.

Higher brain centers also affect breathing. In awake subjects, voluntary hyperventilation with oxygen even to extremely low levels of P_{CO_2} is rarely followed by apnea. This is not true in anesthetized or in sleeping subjects who stop breathing when overhyperventilated. This difference in the effect of hyperventilation in conscious and unconscious humans has been attributed to a "wakefulness drive" arising in the reticular formation of the brain, which preserves ventilation even in the absence of chemical stimulation. This drive may be caused by the impingement of random stimuli from the external environment on the brain, which maintains respiratory neuron activity. After discharge is a possibly related phenomen in which breathing continues for several seconds after the termination of respiratory stimulation. It is of interest that after discharge does not occur in hypoxia.

Ventilation can be controlled consciously as well as involuntarily, that is, automatically influenced. Indeed, separate neural pathways for the voluntary and automatic control of the respiratory muscles have been described. Multiple inputs also allow the respiratory muscles to be sufficiently versatile so that ventilation can be adjusted to satisfy needs for chemical homeostasis and also to be used in communication and emotional expression. Higher brain centers may also play a key role in breathing, allowing adequate ventilation to be achieved with a minimum expenditure of work and with least discomfort.

IRREGULAR BREATHING

It has been known for many years that patients with congestive heart failure (particularly those with arteriosclerotic cardiac disease) as well as patients with brain disorders, such as tumors or cerebrovascular disease, sometimes breathe with a crescendo-decrescendo pattern of ventilation, with each swing of ventilation terminating in apnea. This kind of breathing, called *Cheyne-Stokes respiration,* has been considered an ominous prognostic sign. However, a similar breathing pattern has been observed in apparently normal individuals during sleep and even during wakefulness in sojourners at altitude. A Cheyne-Stokes-like pattern of breathing is also common in metabolic alkalosis, in premature infants, and in adults with the sleep apnea syndrome (Box 36-1).

Oscillations in several physiologic systems can be observed during Cheyne-Stokes breathing. Together with swings in ventilation, cyclic changes occur in blood pressure, heart rate, and cerebral blood

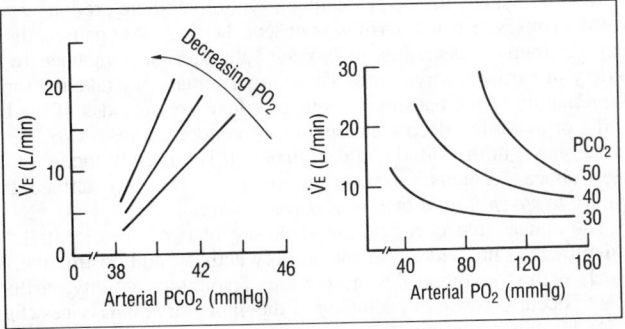

FIGURE 36-2   *Left,* Ventilatory response to CO_2. The slope of the response line increases with hypoxia. *Right,* Ventilatory response to hypoxia. Note how hypercapnia increases the curvature of the ventilatory response to hypoxia.

flow. Upper airway resistance decreases during the periods of increased ventilation. There may also be striking fluctuations in alertness. Signs of depression occur during the apneic phase: The pupils are often constricted, and the patient may be motionless. With hyperventilation, the pupils dilate; there may be thrashing of the extremities and electroencephalogram (EEG) evidence of arousal.

When measured simultaneously, arterial blood and alveolar gas tension swings have been shown to be out of phase. During hyperventilation, alveolar P_{CO_2} tends to be low and alveolar P_{O_2} high; the reverse occurs during the apneic phase (Fig. 36-3). These alveolar changes are the expected effects of ventilation changes on lung gas tensions. On the other hand, arterial gas tensions seem to change in the opposite way so that arterial P_{O_2} is lower and arterial P_{CO_2} is higher during hyperventilation than during apnea. This difference between arterial and alveolar gas tensions is believed to reflect the time required (circulation time) to transport blood from pulmonary capillaries to the systemic arteries. In general, the cycle length of Cheyne-Stokes respiration (the time required for a complete cycle of hyperventilation and apnea) is proportional to the circulation time; the time of hyperventilation and apnea increases as circulation time is prolonged (as in congestive heart failure).

It was previously thought that during the period of apparent apnea (as indicated by the absence of discernible airflow), all respira-

tory movements ceased, but in some patients respiratory activity seems to continue, and airflow is absent because of upper airway obstruction.

Many believe that Cheyne-Stokes respiration is a manifestation of instability in the feedback control of breathing similar to instabilities observed in manufactured control systems that regulate temperature or the output of machines. In these physical control systems, delays in information transfer from the controller to the controlled system (corresponding to lengthening in circulation time in the respiratory system), increases in controller gain (analogous to heightened ventilatory responses to changes in P_{CO_2} and P_{O_2}), or changes in set point (corresponding to increases in the level of P_{CO_2} and P_{O_2} needed to initiate breathing) cause the output of these systems to be oscillatory. Whether these analogies are correct is still controversial.

In patients with Cheyne-Stokes breathing and heart disease or some brain abnormality, treatment ought to be directed at reversing cardiac failure, increasing cerebral blood flow, or alleviating the central nervous system dysfunction. Occasionally, the intermittent decreases in P_{O_2} that occur during apnea are sufficiently great as to warrant treatment. Oxygen inhalation is helpful in these patients and may abolish the breathing irregularity. Sometimes Cheyne-Stokes breathing can be made to disappear by theophylline administration. Breathing carbon dioxide–enriched gas mixtures also frequently eliminates Cheyne-Stokes respiration. Respiratory depressants, which increase resting P_{CO_2} levels and cause hypoxemia, frequently produce Cheyne-Stokes breathing in predisposed patients.

BREATHING DURING SLEEP AND THE SLEEP APNEA SYNDROME

Normally during sleep, ventilation decreases along with metabolic rate, but because the fall in ventilation is greater than the decrease in metabolism, P_{CO_2} rises slightly and arterial P_{O_2} decreases a bit.

The changes in blood gas tension probably reflect the loss of stimuli from the surroundings, such as light and sound, which normally excite breathing. Even though in most normal patients these blood gas changes are minimal, sometimes changes in arterial P_{O_2} are clinically significant, particularly in patients with lung disease or neuromuscular disorders if hypoxemia is present during wakefulness. Because of the shape of the oxyhemoglobin dissociation curve, the oxygen saturation of arterial blood can fall to dangerous levels even with small P_{O_2} changes once patients are on the steep slope of the curve. The hypoxia and hypercapnia occurring during sleep in these patients can contribute to the cardiovascular consequences of lung disease and may accelerate bicarbonate retention, leading to even more pronounced alveolar hypoventilation when awake. The changes in gas tensions resulting from altered controller properties during sleep are probably aggravated by other changes that accompany sleep, such as the fall in functional residual capacity (FRC), which may increase ventilation-perfusion mismatching, and the increase in upper airway resistance, which tends to reduce ventilation.

In addition to changes in blood gas tensions, normal subjects may experience brief periods of apnea during sleep. Usually these apneas are less than 10 seconds and occur sporadically less than 10 times a night, especially in early slow-wave sleep (stages I and II) and in rapid eye movement (REM) sleep.

In individuals with the sleep apnea syndrome, there are longer repetitive pauses in which airflow is absent. During these pauses, there may be dramatic decreases in oxygen saturation accompanied by a variety of cardiac arrhythmias. These arrhythmias may take the form of premature beats, but more frequently there are episodes of bradycardia or asystole. Sleep apnea is more frequent in those who snore, in the obese, in the elderly, and in males. It is currently thought that sleep apnea accounts for most of the cases formerly termed the *obesity-hypoventilation* or *pickwickian syndrome*.

The apneas that occur during sleep are of two types: central, in which there is no evidence of respiratory activity, and obstructive, in which airflow is absent despite obvious respiratory activity; airflow fails to occur because of occlusion of the upper airway passages (Fig. 36-4). Usually obstructive apneas are more frequent than central ones, last longer, and hence are of greater clinical significance. Sometimes apneas occur irregularly, but frequently both central and obstructive apneas and electroencephalographic (EEG) evidence of arousal dur-

---

BOX 36-1
Causes of irregular breathing

Congestive heart failure (particularly arteriosclerotic disease)
Disease of the central nervous system (particularly cerebrovascular disease, meningitis, encephalitis, and brain tumors)
Sleep-disordered breathing (central and obstructive apneas)
Metabolic alkalosis
Prematurity

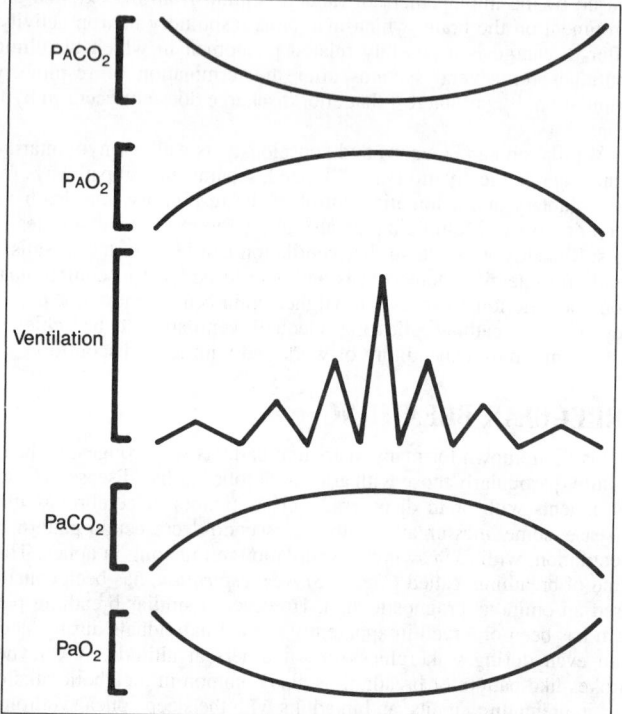

FIGURE 36-3 Changes in alveolar and arterial blood gas tensions during Cheyne-Stokes breathing. Arterial P_{O_2} is lowest and arterial P_{CO_2} is highest during the hyperventilation phase.

ing the hyperventilation phase are associated with a Cheyne-Stokes pattern of breathing.

The same mechanisms that have been used to explain Cheyne-Stokes respiration may also account for central apneas during sleep. On one hand, shifts in the operating point of the control system (elevated P_{CO_2} during sleep) may cause unstable respiratory control; it is also possible that depressed drives to breathing caused by inherently low chemosensitivity or large reductions in metabolic rate during sleep may be instrumental.

Cephalometric measurements and computed tomography (CT) scans reveal anatomic narrowing of the upper airway in some patients with obstructive sleep apnea. Nasal obstruction, for example, has been found to increase the number of sleep apneas. Many obese patients with obstructive sleep apnea seem to have narrower upper airway passages, which increase resistance to airflow.

The upper airway passages are formed by semirigid structures. The cross section of the upper airway can be actively narrowed or dilated by contraction of muscles in the nasal and oral cavities, the hypopharynx, and the larynx. During inspiration when the chest wall muscles contract, a negative pressure is produced in the pharynx that not only draws in air to inflate the lungs but also tends to collapse the upper airway. This can cause occlusion unless the muscles that dilate the upper airway can respond appropriately to withstand this collapsing force. It is believed that abnormalities in the control and coordination of the upper airway muscles may contribute to episodes of obstructive apnea during sleep.

The cranial nerves that innervate the upper airway muscles frequently display respiratory-related changes in their activity. In the case of the muscles that help widen the upper airway, such as the alae nasi (nostril flarer), the genioglossus (which protrudes the tongue), and the posterior cricoarytenoid (which abducts the vocal cords), activity is greater during inspiration than expiration. In addition, this respiratory-related activity increases with many of the same stimuli that excite breathing, for example, hypercapnia, hypoxia, and low blood pressure. The upper airway muscles may respond differently in patients with obstructive apnea than in normal patients. Arousal induced by hypoxia and hypercapnia occurs frequently in association with the termination of apnea.

Negative pressure in the upper airways has been shown to stimulate activity of the upper airway muscles. The large intrapharyngeal negative pressures that develop during obstructive breathing during sleep may also help terminate the episodes of obstruction.

Respiratory stimulants are not effective in terminating sleep apnea. However, continuous positive airway pressure (CPAP) applied through a mask eliminates obstructive sleep apnea in most patients. When CPAP has not been successful or not well tolerated, a prosthesis or an operation that widens the upper airways, uvulopalatopharyngoplasty, has benefited some patients.

HYPOCAPNIA AND HYPERVENTILATION

Box 36-2 lists some causes of persistent hyperventilation. Diseases that decrease lung compliance, such as fibrosis or pulmonary edema, are often associated with constant and regular hyperventilation. Although these patients frequently have mild to moderate hypoxemia, the hyperventilation is disproportionate to the severity of the hypoxemia and persists even when hypoxemia is relieved by the administration of 100% oxygen. It has been postulated that increased activity of vagally mediated reflexes contributes to the hyperventilation.

Acidosis of the arterial blood or the brain extracellular fluid is sometimes the explanation for hyperventilation. Diabetes may produce a severe metabolic acidosis associated with hyperventilation (Kussmaul's breathing). In subjects returning to sea level after a stay at altitude, hyperventilation often occurs and continues for several days even though arterial pH is normal or even alkaline. In some, persistent acidity of the cerebrospinal fluid is associated with the phenomenon. A reduction in brain extracellular fluid bicarbonate usually occurs during a sojourn at altitude, which is only gradually restored to normal levels with return to sea level. Hyperventilation may be maintained until cerebrospinal fluid acidity is also reversed. Acidosis also seems to account for the hyperventilation observed in uremia. This hyperventilation, which remains for a time even after dialysis restores arterial pH to normal levels, may also be caused by a persistent acidosis of brain extracellular fluid.

The cause of the hyperventilation seen in hepatic failure is still not clear. The hypoxia sometimes seen in patients with this disease caused by venous to arterial shunting seems insufficient to explain the hyperventilation that may be caused by elevated levels of brain ammonia.

The most severe instances of respiratory alkalosis occur in the presence of central nervous system disorders such as meningitis. Pontine lesions are a well-known cause of hyperventilation. At times, though, pontine hemorrhage produces the prolonged inspiratory pauses of apneustic breathing rather than increased breathing.

Fever is known to produce a shortening of inspiratory time and an increase in respiratory frequency in humans and even in vagotomized animals. The increase in frequency seems to be a direct effect of temperature on the discharge of bulbopontine neurons.

Hyperventilation is a common sign of salicylate intoxication. Salicylates increase metabolic rate but also seem to have a direct respiratory-stimulating effect on the brain.

Occasionally, hyperventilation is intermittent and associated with changes in position. The tachypnea associated with orthopnea probably arises from pulmonary congestion and airway closure in the supine position, which produces hypoxia and J-receptor stimulation. In rare cases, tachypnea and hyperventilation are observed only when patients are placed in an upright position (so-called platypnea). The explanation for this is uncertain but may be caused by poor perfusion of the lung when the patient is in the upright position, which improves when pulmonary artery pressure is increased by placing the patient supine.

Anxiety in some patients produces panic attacks in which episodes of hyperventilation lead to numbness and tingling of the extremities or even syncope. The hyperventilation may also produce cardiac arrhythmias or chest pain symptoms that mimic those of organic heart disease. Specific phobias in some patients (e.g., fear of heights, crowds) elicit panic attacks. Patients with panic attacks usually re-

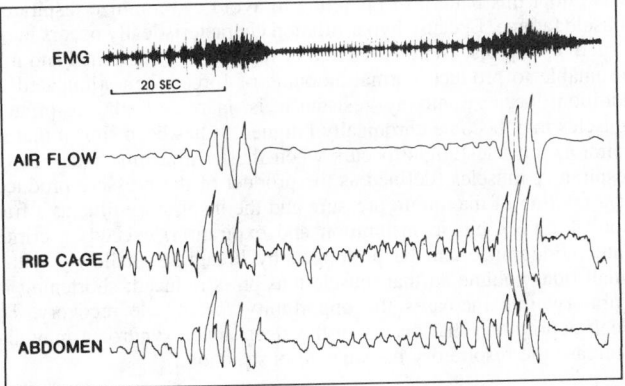

FIGURE 36-4 Tracing of electromyogram (EMG) measured from a chin surface electrode, airflow, and rib cage and abdominal movement in a patient with sleep apnea. Note that the airflow pattern resembles that seen in Cheyne-Stokes respiration. Associated with the waxing and waning of airflow are swings in the chin EMG (reflecting change in the activity of upper airway muscles). Note that chest wall movements persist even in the absence of airflow; the apnea is obstructive in type.

BOX 36-2
Causes of persistent hyperventilation

Fibrotic lung disease
Metabolic acidosis (e.g., diabetes, uremia)
CNS disorders (midbrain and pontine lesions)
Hepatic coma
Salicylate intoxication
Fever
Psychogenic (e.g., panic disorders)

quire a broad treatment approach that includes treatment of the phobia as well as education in controlled breathing techniques; the latter may reduce hyperventilation in these patients.

The deleterious effects of hyperventilation alkalosis are primarily cardiovascular (e.g., arrhythmias, reductions in cardiac output, hypotension) and nervous (e.g., decreases in cerebral blood flow, obtundation, tetany, seizures).

Treatment of acute hyperventilation should aim at reversal of the process inciting the disturbance (e.g., treatment of meningitis, sepsis). However, when the pH rises to 7.55 or above, special measures should be considered to raise the arterial PCO_2 and lower the pH. In subjects in whom an airway is in place, this can be achieved by artificially increasing respiratory dead space. Sedative drugs, which may be tried only if hypoxemia is not present, are usually ineffective because the doses required to depress the medullary respiratory neurons also depress the vasomotor center and produce hypotension.

HYPOVENTILATION AND HYPERCAPNIA IN SUBJECTS WITH NORMAL LUNGS

Increased levels of arterial PCO_2 are generally a consequence of obstructive pulmonary disease but can also occur in patients with normal lungs in certain circumstances, as shown in Box 36-3. Hypercapnia in patients without lung or chest wall disease sometimes results from an abnormality in the medullary respiratory neurons caused either by infection or cerebrovascular disease. The response to both hypercapnia and hypoxia may be depressed, and minute ventilation is decreased. The rate and depth of breathing tend to be less regular than in normal persons, and breath-holding time is frequently prolonged. Although hypoxia and hypercapnia are present at rest, the hypoxia can be explained entirely by the hypoventilation, and the gradient between alveolar and arterial PO_2 is within normal limits. Arterial blood gases can be restored to normal limits by voluntary hyperventilation.

Progesterone stimulates respiration in some of these patients, and oral administration of this drug may produce a significant reduction in the $PaCO_2$. Phrenic nerve stimulation has been used successfully in these patients to restore normal blood gas tensions and pH.

Occasionally, extreme elevations in $PaCO_2$, hypoxia, and cor pulmonale occur in patients with severe metabolic alkalosis. In contrast, other patients with equally great blood bicarbonate elevations show little if any carbon dioxide retention. This discrepancy is not explained by differences in brain interstitial fluid pH but may reflect altered intracellular pH.

In part, the hypoventilation observed in myxedema is a direct effect of the disease on the lung and respiratory muscles. The vital capacity may be reduced by muscular weakness, and a decrease in diffusing capacity has been observed. Myxedema may also produce abnormal EEG results, and it has been suspected that respiratory neuron depression contributes to the hypoventilation, which is relieved by thyroid hormone replacement. Hyperventilation is not observed in

hyperthyroid patients, and carbon dioxide sensitivity is within normal limits. It should also be noted that patients with sleep apnea may also have persistent hypercapnia while awake.

Although depression of hypercapnic and hypoxic sensitivity usually occur together, in some subjects a selective blunting of hypoxic drive occurs. For example, hypoxic response is depressed, but the response to hypercapnia may be normal in patients with surgically resected carotid bodies in a now-discarded treatment for asthma or in patients in whom inadvertent injury to the carotid body has been produced (by carotid endarterectomy, for example).

Birth at altitude or long-term exposure to altitude depresses hypoxic response but has little effect on the response to hypercapnia. Children with congenital cyanotic heart disease who in effect also have had prolonged exposure to hypoxia, like altitude dwellers, also display a blunted hypoxic response.

These patients with isolated defects in hypoxic response are able to maintain normal blood gas tensions during rest and exercise. However, anesthesia and the resulting depression of carbon dioxide sensitivity may produce hypoventilation and a progressive and life-endangering hypoxia.

Diseases that severely restrict movements of the chest wall, such as kyphoscoliosis and ankylosing spondylitis, may cause hypoventilation and retention of carbon dioxide.

Neuromuscular disorders, such as myasthenia gravis, the Guillain-Barré syndrome, amyotrophic lateral sclerosis, acid maltase disease, or muscular dystrophy, often terminate in respiratory failure with carbon dioxide elevation and depressed oxygen saturation. Bilateral paralysis of the diaphragm, the major muscle of inspiration, may cause carbon dioxide retention particularly when the patient is supine. This is associated with inward movement of the diaphragm during inspiration and outward movement of the rib cage. As in the patients with primary alveolar hypoventilation, in these patients, carbon dioxide retention occurs mainly because minute ventilation is reduced.

HYPERCAPNIA IN PATIENTS WITH OBSTRUCTIVE LUNG DISEASE

Chronic obstructive pulmonary disease (emphysema and bronchitis) is the most common cause of hypercapnia. An inborn decrease in chemosensitivity may contribute to the hypoventilation in some patients. In others, metabolic alkalosis or the use of sedatives or opiate drugs causes a depressed response to carbon dioxide and to hypoxia and further reduces ventilation. Some patients have a decreased minute ventilation, but in many patients with chronic obstructive pulmonary disease, the level of minute ventilation is even greater than normal. In these patients, hypercapnia is associated with shallow, rapid breathing in which each breath has a reduced inspiratory time. The hypercapnia is caused by an increase in physiologic dead space ventilated with each breath. This kind of respiratory pattern may be caused by reflex stimulation of breathing by inflamed airways, but some patients may adopt this pattern of breathing to avoid or minimize respiratory muscle fatigue. Because hyperinflation characteristically occurs in obstructive lung disease, the respiratory muscles are shortened and may be unable to produce normal amounts of force when stimulated. In addition, because airway resistance is increased, the respiratory muscles may become chronically fatigued. It has been shown that respiratory muscle fatigue occurs when the tension time index of the respiratory muscles (defined as the product of the pressure produced as a fraction of maximum pressure and the inspiratory time as a fraction of time spent in inspiration and expiration) exceeds a critical value. Endurance can be prolonged by breathing shallowly with a small tidal volume so that muscle tension is reduced; shortening inspiratory time increases the opportunity for muscle recovery. The sleep deprivation that occurs in the sleep apnea syndrome may also decrease the respiratory response to obstruction.

BEHAVIORAL CONTROL OF BREATHING AND ITS RELATION TO DYSPNEA

In addition to being regulated automatically (through chemoreceptor and mechanoreceptor reflexes), breathing can be altered volitionally. Obvious examples of this are voluntary breath-holding and the mild

---

BOX 36-3
Causes of persistent hypercapnia

1. With normal lungs:
   a. CNS disturbances (e.g., cerebrovascular disease, Parkinson's disease, encephalitis)
   b. Metabolic alkalosis
   c. Myxedema
   d. Primary alveolar hypoventilation (Ondine's curse)
   e. Spinal cord lesions
2. Diseases of the chest wall (e.g., kyphoscoliosis, ankylosing spondylitis)
3. Neuromuscular disorders (e.g., myasthenia gravis, Guillain-Barré syndrome, amyotrophic lateral sclerosis, acid maltase disease, muscular dystrophy, poliomyelitis)
4. Chronic obstructive pulmonary disease

hyperventilation that occurs with speech. Anxiety and depression may have more long-lasting effects on ventilatory patterns. Emotional factors may also explain the irregular breathing observed at times in normal individuals.

Volitional factors may be more important clinically when dyspnea (a sensation of difficult or labored breathing) is present. Although normal breathing occurs effortlessly without conscious awareness, the dyspneic patient is cognizant of every breath. Dyspnea is one of the more common presenting symptoms in patients with lung disease. Sometimes dyspnea is the major cause of disability and appears to be disproportionate to the severity of the lung disease.

To study dyspnea, standard psychophysical methods that relate the physical intensity of a stimulus to the sensation experienced have been used. These studies show that the sensations produced by changes in tidal volume increase as they do in response to other stimuli (e.g., light and sound) as a power function of the physical intensity of the stimulus. This power relationship also applies to the sensations produced by changes in respiratory muscle contraction. The sensory effects that occur with respiratory muscle contraction and the degree of dyspnea experienced increase with the pressure produced and length of time the pressure is maintained. Of the two effects, pressure changes seem more potent than time changes. Some evidence shows that some patients breathe more shallowly and rapidly to relieve dyspnea. Although this would decrease the sensation produced by breathing, it worsens gas exchange.

Hypercapnia and hypoxia are respiratory stimulants that increase the force generated by the respiratory muscles. Relief of hypoxia and hypercapnia is an effective way of diminishing dyspnea. Nonetheless, a clear relationship between respiratory sensitivity to hypoxia or hypercapnia and the dyspnea experienced by patients with lung disease has not yet been demonstrated. Sedative drugs have been used to diminish sensitivity to hypoxia and hypercapnia with the expectation that this would also reduce dyspnea. Although lifestyle has been improved in a few patients by this kind of treatment, in many patients significant adverse effects on gas exchange have been demonstrated.

ASSESSMENT OF RESPIRATORY CONTROL

Usually chemosensitivity has been evaluated by plotting the relationship between ventilation and arterial P_{CO_2} and P_{O_2} after steady-state inhalation of different inspired gas mixtures. These tests were long and tedious for both the patient and the examiner. Recently much more rapid single-breath and rebreathing methods of assessing ventilatory responses to hypoxia and hypercapnia have been developed.

Ventilation may not be an adequate measure of the response to chemical stimuli in patients with disease of the lungs or chest wall who have impaired respiratory mechanics. Methods of assessing efferent activity, which measures inspiratory pressures generated during airway occlusion or diaphragm electrical activity, have allowed respiratory regulation to be studied, even in the presence of significant lung disease.

Difficulties still remain; for example, methods of assessing the neural control of breathing are still in the developmental stage. However, there is now sufficient experience so that most patients with suspected abnormalities in respiratory control can be assessed and a diagnosis made.

Evaluation begins with the history, physical examination, and chest radiograph, which determine whether symptoms or signs of pulmonary or neuromuscular diseases are present. Tests that measure airway caliber and the strength of the respiratory muscles are particularly useful because obstructive lung disease and respiratory muscle weakness are the functional abnormalities most often associated with carbon dioxide retention.

Patients with obstructive lung disease rarely develop carbon dioxide retention if the forced expiratory volume at 1 second (FEV_1) is greater than 1.5 liters, although the ventilatory response to carbon dioxide will be reduced in patients with even modest reductions in FEV_1. Significant carbon dioxide retention with less reduction in FEV_1 should lead one to suspect concomitant respiratory controller dysfunction. If carbon dioxide retention is caused entirely by respiratory controller dysfunction, the A-a gradient is normal or nearly so, and breath-holding time will be unaffected by changes in P_{CO_2}. Also,

voluntary hyperventilation will return the arterial P_{CO_2} to normal values.

When lung function tests are normal, controller performance can be more directly evaluated by determining the ventilatory response to hypoxia and hypercapnia. When lung function is abnormal, measurements of occlusion pressure or the electromyogram (EMG) of the diaphragm can be used to evaluate whether there is any response to chemical stimuli. Polysomnography is essential in determining whether carbon dioxide retention is caused by disordered breathing during sleep.

BIBLIOGRAPHY

Cherniack NS: Sleep apnea and its causes, *J Clin Invest* 73:1501, 1984.
Cherniack NS, Nochomovitz ML, Altose MD: Disorders of respiratory control. In Simmons DH, editor: *Pulmonology*, vol 4, New York, 1982, Wiley.
Dowell AR et al: Cheyne-Stokes respiration: a review of clinical manifestations and critique of physiological mechanisms, *Arch Intern Med* 127:712, 1971.
Longobardo GS, Cherniack NS: Abnormalities in respiratory rhythm. In Cherniack NS, Widdicombe JG, editors: *The handbook of physiology*, sect. 3, vol 2, Washington, DC, 1986, American Physiological Society.
Neubauer JA, Melton JE, Edelman NH: Modulation of respiration during brain hypoxia, *J Appl Physiol* 68:441-451, 1990.
Oku Y, Saidel GM, Altose MD, Cherniack NS: Perceptual contributions to optimization of breathing, *Ann Biomed Eng* 21:509-515, 1993.
Prabhakar NR, Kumar GK, Chang CH et al: Nitric oxide in the sensory function of the carotid body, *Brain Res* 625:16-22, 1993.
Strohl KP, Cherniack NS, Gothe B: Physiologic basis of therapy for sleep apnea, *Am Rev Respir Dis* 134:791, 1986.
van Lunteren E, Strohl KP: The muscles of the upper airways, *Clin Chest Med* 7:171, 1986.

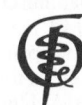

CHAPTER

37 Respiratory Muscles and Respiratory Muscle Failure

Dudley F. Rochester

The respiratory muscles are striated skeletal muscles under neural control. Their vital function, driven automatically, is to generate the inspired breath (tidal volume) at a size and rate appropriate to the prevailing metabolic needs. In effect, the respiratory muscles represent the "air pump" of the body, just as the heart is the blood pump. The respiratory muscles also participate in speech, breath-holding, pulmonary function tests, and other activities under voluntary control.

The principal inspiratory muscles are the diaphragm, the parasternal intercostal muscles, and the scalene muscles in the neck. The principal expiratory muscles are the external and internal oblique and transversus abdominis muscles of the abdomen, and the triangularis sterni muscles in the thorax. The lateral intercostal and sternomastoid muscles contribute to breathing, but these muscles also have nonventilatory postural functions.

RESPIRATORY MUSCLE CONTRACTILE PROPERTIES

The contractile force of skeletal muscles is affected by the degree of electrical or neural excitation. The physiologic range of phrenic nerve discharge rates lies between 5 and 40 impulses per second. Diaphragmatic contractile force and shortening vary approximately fivefold over this range, so increasing stimulation frequency is an important mechanism for regulating respiratory muscle force output and the size of the tidal volume.

Another factor that bears on contractile force is the resting length of the muscle. Diaphragm muscle length changes with lung volume. At the normal breathing position (functional residual capacity, FRC), the diaphragm is at or near its optimal resting length, whereas at full inspiration (total lung capacity, TLC), the diaphragm is 40% shorter. Diaphragmatic force and volume displacing capacity are highest near FRC and are reduced by half at TLC.

The velocity at which the muscle shortens during contraction also affects its force output. During quiet breathing, the diaphragm shortens slowly by 5% to 10% per breath, but during maximal voluntary or exercise ventilation, it shortens by approximately 20% per breath in a much shorter time. The velocity of shortening increases almost tenfold from quiet breathing to maximal ventilation, so at peak exercise the maximal inspiratory muscle dynamic force is only 65% of the maximal static force measured at rest.

RESPIRATORY MUSCLE NEURAL CONTROL AND INTERACTIONS

The integrated neuromuscular apparatus has the flexibility to maintain breathing even when the respiratory system is subjected to a variety of loads consequent to posture and physical activity. Fortunately, diaphragmatic contraction can expand the lungs, especially the lower lobes, in several ways. When the dome of the diaphragm descends, pressure in the abdomen increases and displaces the anterior abdominal wall outward. In addition, abdominal pressure exerts a lateral force on the lower rib cage in the area where the diaphragm is apposed to the rib cage. The diaphragm also expands the lower rib cage by pulling up on it. In the supine position, the outward excursion of the abdomen predominates and there is little rib cage motion. In the upright posture the actions of the diaphragm on the lower rib cage predominate, so the abdominal excursion is smaller and the rib cage excursion is larger.

Because contraction of the diaphragm lowers the pressure inside the thorax, it tends to cave in the upper chest. Contraction of inspiratory muscles in the upper rib cage and neck not only prevents chest distortion, but also contributes to the inspired volume, especially in the upper lobes.

During quiet breathing in the supine position, inspiration results from active contraction of the diaphragm and the parasternal muscles. The subsequent expiration is driven by the passive recoil of the respiratory system back to FRC. Merely assuming an upright position causes inspiratory recruitment of the scalene muscles as well as tonic and phasic expiratory recruitment of the abdominal muscles. At higher levels of physical activity, activation of these muscles increases and additional inspiratory and expiratory muscles are recruited.

With increased airway resistance and air trapping, lung volume increases. Diaphragmatic shortening capacity is impaired, and at very high lung volumes the diaphragm becomes flattened so it cannot effectively convert its contractile force into the pressure needed to inflate the lungs. The diaphragm no longer expands the lower rib cage, and the flat diaphragm may even draw the lower rib cage inward during inspiration (Hoover's sign). The compensatory mechanisms for breathing against high airway resistance or at very high lung volumes involve recruitment of the lateral intercostal and sternomastoid inspiratory muscles and the abdominal expiratory muscles.

The abdominal muscles have an important role in assisting inspiration. Their expiratory contraction increases abdominal pressure and pushes the diaphragm to a more cranial position. This lengthens the diaphragm and improves its mechanical advantage for the next inspiration. In addition, the sudden relaxation of the abdominal muscles at the end of expiration facilitates the onset of inspiratory airflow even before the diaphragm contracts.

RESPIRATORY MUSCLE STRENGTH

The strength of the respiratory muscles can be assessed by measuring the pressure generated by maximal inspiratory and expiratory efforts against a closed airway (PI_{max}, PE_{max}). PI_{max} is highest at full expiration (residual volume, RV) and PE_{max} is highest at TLC. Typically, PI_{max} and PE_{max} in adult males are -120 and $+250$ cm H_2O, respectively. Values in women are about 70% of those in men, and in both sexes PI_{max} and PE_{max} are substantially lower in old age.

One can also measure the strength of the diaphragm. Esophageal pressure (P_{es}) and gastric pressure (P_{ga}) reflect pleural and abdominal pressures, respectively. The difference between P_{ga} and P_{es} is re-

ferred to as *transdiaphragmatic pressure* (P_{di}). During maximal inspiratory efforts against a closed airway, P_{di} is similar in magnitude to P_{es} and PI_{max}. However, maximal P_{di} is twice as high during respiratory maneuvers that also increase abdominal pressure. The P_{es} during a sniff is similar to PI_{max}, and P_{es} during a cough is similar to PE_{max}. Because sniffing and coughing are natural actions, they are useful to test patients who have trouble performing the PI_{max} and PE_{max} maneuvers correctly, or in cases of suspected malingering.

RESPIRATORY MUSCLE ENDURANCE AND FATIGUE

Breathing is an endurance activity that requires repetitive contraction of the respiratory muscles for life. Normal breathing requires very little energy expenditure, and the perceived effort of breathing is minimal. Perhaps the most remarkable aspect of the respiratory muscle and neuromotor control system is its versatility. The respiratory muscles can support speech and singing, swimming the crawl and chopping wood, walking, cycling, and a host of other activities, all largely hidden from consciousness.

Two factors that bear on endurance are muscle fiber type and blood supply. About 75% of the fibers in respiratory muscles have good to excellent intrinsic endurance characteristics, and respiratory muscle blood supply is bountiful. Respiratory muscle endurance also depends on respiratory muscle strength and the force and duration of contraction with each breath.

The force and duration of inspiratory muscle contraction are assessed from the pressure required to inspire the tidal volume (P_{breath}), and the duration of inspiration (T_i). Both P_{breath} and T_i are expressed as fractions of their maximal values, PI_{max}, and T_{tot} (T_{tot} is the duration of one whole breath). Combining these variables yields a pressure-time index (PTI): $PTI = (P_{breath}/PI_{max}) \times (T_i/T_{tot})$.

In normal subjects breathing quietly, P_{breath}/PI_{max} is typically 0.05, T_i/T_{tot} is 0.4, and PTI is 0.02. Any combination of P_{breath}/PI_{max} or T_i/T_{tot} that causes P_{breath}/PI_{max} to exceed 0.5 or PTI to exceed 0.15 leads to fatigue. The time to onset of overt fatigue is 90 minutes when PTI is 0.15, but only 3 minutes when PTI is 0.40. Thus the respiratory muscles may be in a fatiguing pattern of contraction without having developed overt contractile failure. When overt fatigue of the diaphragm does occur, it may persist for 24 hours or more.

There are several mechanisms of respiratory muscle fatigue. Central fatigue represents inhibition of neural drive, perhaps owing to inhibitory influences from the overstressed muscle, or to a sense of excessive effort required to breathe. Transmission fatigue is failure at the level of the nerve or neuromuscular junction. Muscle cell fatigue is associated with production of free radicals and impairment of the mechanism that couples excitation to contraction.

Physicians should know and heed clinical manifestations of severe stress on the respiratory muscles, signs that reflect both their weakness and the recruitment of additional respiratory muscle groups. Increasing dyspnea with tachypnea and flaring of the alae nasi are detected by observation. Contraction of neck inspiratory and abdominal muscles can be assessed by palpation. The smooth outward inspiratory excursion of the chest and abdomen is replaced by abrupt, jerky movements in which the chest and abdomen are out of phase with each other (chest-abdomen asynchrony). Diaphragmatic paralysis is associated with paradoxical inward movement of the abdomen during inspiration.

An increase in P_{breath}/PI_{max} or inspiratory PTI, slowing of inspiratory muscle relaxation rate, and a shift in the power in the electromyogram (EMG) from higher to lower frequency (fall in the high/low ratio) all indicate that the respiratory muscles are in a fatiguing pattern of contraction, but are not necessarily evidence of overt fatigue. Electromyographic evidence of impending fatigue has been observed in chronic obstructive pulmonary disease (COPD) during exhaustive exercise and in trials of weaning from mechanical ventilation.

The best test for respiratory muscle fatigue is to detect a reduction in the P_{di} twitch response to stimulation of the phrenic nerves, while the amplitude of the EMG is preserved. This technique has been used to show that overt diaphragmatic fatigue occurs after exhausting exercise in normal subjects and to demonstrate the absence of overt diaphragmatic fatigue after exercise in patients with COPD.

RESPIRATORY MUSCLE WEAKNESS

Respiratory muscle weakness is a major factor in the pathogenesis of dyspnea, exercise limitation, nocturnal arterial oxyhemoglobin desaturation, and ventilatory failure. Other consequences of respiratory muscle weakness are impaired coughing and sighing, atelectasis, and pneumonia.

Respiratory muscle weakness related to malnutrition or other metabolic abnormalities is characteristic of COPD and other pulmonary or chest wall diseases (Box 37-1). Respiratory muscle weakness is common in acute, critical illness and occurs in many chronic non-pulmonary diseases (Box 37-2).

Another leading cause of inspiratory muscle weakness is mechanical disadvantage to the diaphragm. This stems from hyperinflation of the lung in obstructive lung diseases such as asthma, chronic bronchitis, and emphysema. Conversely, in severe obesity and ascites, the diaphragm may lose force because it is overstretched, especially when the patient is supine.

The respiratory muscles are usually involved in neuromuscular diseases. The clinical manifestations depend on the nature of the disease and the site of the lesion (Box 37-3). In spinal cord injury, expiratory muscle paralysis exceeds inspiratory paralysis because the diaphragm and scalene muscles are innervated above the C6 level. Diseases such as myasthenia gravis, dystrophies, and myopathies tend to involve inspiratory and expiratory muscles about equally.

Paralysis of the diaphragm usually occurs without other respiratory muscle weakness. Diaphragmatic paralysis is a complication of open-heart surgery, as a result either of cold injury to the phrenic nerves or damage to phrenic nerve blood supply. Diaphragmatic contractility is reflexly inhibited for about a week after upper abdominal surgery, and expiratory strength is reduced for approximately a week after thoracic surgery.

A definitive diagnosis of respiratory muscle weakness is made by measuring PI_{max} and PE_{max}, or by measuring the P_{di} twitch response to stimulation of the phrenic nerves. Other valuable clues are unexplained reductions in vital capacity and maximal voluntary ventilation, as well as unexplained increases in RV and Pa_{CO_2}. One should suspect respiratory muscle weakness in any patient with ventilatory failure, especially when the severity of underlying lung disease does not appear to account for CO_2 retention.

BOX 37-1

Principal pulmonary and chest wall causes of respiratory muscle weakness

Pulmonary
Acute hypoxic respiratory failure
Acute ventilatory failure
Chronic obstructive pulmonary disease (COPD)
Cystic fibrosis
Interstitial lung diseases (pulmonary fibrosis, sarcoidosis)

Chest wall
Kyphoscoliosis
Obesity hypoventilation syndrome (OHS)

BOX 37-2

General medical causes of respiratory muscle weakness

Age greater than 70 years
Congestive heart failure
Chronic renal failure
Collagen vascular diseases (rheumatoid arthritis, systemic lupus erythematosus, scleroderma, dermatomyositis)
Endocrine disorders (diabetes mellitus, hyperthyroidism, hypothyroidism)
Electrolyte imbalance (low K, P)
Infection (acute and chronic)
Malnutrition
Myopathies (alcohol, steroids)
Neoplasm (cachexia and paraneoplastic syndromes)
Shock (circulatory and septic)

BOX 37-3

Neuromuscular diseases associated with respiratory muscle weakness

Anterior horn cell diseases (amyotrophic lateral sclerosis, poliomyelitis)
Diaphragmatic paralysis
Diseases of neuromuscular junction (myasthenia gravis, Lambert-Eaton, organophosphate poisoning, botulism)
Dystrophies (Duchenne, Steinert)
Myopathies (congenital, inflammatory)
Neuropathies (alcoholic, diabetic, Guillain-Barré)
Spinal cord injury

RESPIRATORY MUSCLE FAILURE, DYSPNEA, AND VENTILATORY FAILURE

Significant ventilatory failure (Pa_{CO_2} greater than 50 mm Hg) does not occur with muscle weakness alone until inspiratory muscle strength (PI_{max}) falls below approximately 25% of normal. However, when the work of breathing is increased, as in COPD, kyphoscoliosis, and morbid obesity, ventilatory failure occurs when PI_{max} falls below 50% of normal.

In diseases that predispose to ventilatory failure, mechanical abnormalities of lungs, airways, and chest wall increase P_{breath}, and respiratory muscle weakness reduces PI_{max}. In COPD the combined effects are such that P_{breath}/PI_{max} and PTI approach the fatigue threshold. The increase in P_{breath}/PI_{max} contributes to dyspnea, respiratory distress, and rapid, shallow breathing.

This breathing pattern is associated with an increase in the neural drive to breathe. It also reflects the respiratory center response to respiratory distress, in that with increasing severity of disease, both tidal volume and T_i/T_{tot} fall. Smaller, shorter breaths reduce P_{breath}, minimize dyspnea, and lower the risk for overt respiratory muscle fatigue. The increase in respiratory rate maintains minute ventilation at normal levels, but the small tidal volume leads to CO_2 retention, especially when the efficiency of gas exchange is severely compromised by lung disease.

TREATMENT OF RESPIRATORY MUSCLE FAILURE

The immediate treatment of respiratory muscle failure is the treatment of acute ventilatory failure, that is, provide oxygen and initiate mechanical ventilation to normalize blood gas composition. It is also necessary to remove adverse influences on the muscles by correcting electrolyte balance, treating shock and abnormal fluid volume status, controlling infection, and relieving bronchospasm.

When patients in ventilatory failure receive adequate mechanical ventilation, their spontaneous breathing efforts cease and they lose their dyspnea. During trials of weaning from mechanical ventilation, development of dyspnea, tachypnea, and chest-abdomen asynchrony signifies that significant respiratory muscle failure persists and that the trial is likely to fail.

Dyspnea and tachypnea also occur with complications such as inflammation of the airways, pneumonia, pulmonary embolism, pulmonary edema, atelectasis, pleural effusion, and pneumothorax. The persistence or reappearance of dyspnea and tachypnea despite adequate oxygenation and ventilation should serve as a warning to look for such complications in patients who are being ventilated mechanically.

Patients with severely limited ventilatory endurance may need mechanical ventilator support several hours each day. The benefits include improved blood gas composition, better respiratory muscle function, relief of dyspnea, and prevention of nocturnal hypoventilation. Prolonged, intermittent mechanical ventilation can be provided using negative pressure body ventilators, or positive pressure ventilation via nose mask or lip seal devices. Patients with severe muscle weakness alone may be ventilated with the rocking bed or an inflatable abdominal belt.

Several classes of pharmacologic agents have been used in an attempt to improve respiratory muscle contractility. Although methylxanthines (theophylline, caffeine), β-adrenergic agonists, and digitalis glycosides enhance diaphragmatic contractility in vitro, the results in the clinical arena have been disappointing.

Measures designed to restore the contractile apparatus are more successful. Nutritional repletion increases respiratory muscle strength and endurance, provided caloric intake is approximately 1.5 times resting energy expenditure. The limitations are that it does not work unless underlying catabolic processes can be controlled, excessive repletion of critically ill patients may lead to difficulty in weaning owing to excessive CO_2 production, and patients with COPD find it hard to manage the diet.

Inspiratory muscles can be trained using voluntary hyperventilation to enhance ventilatory endurance, inspiratory resistive loads to increase respiratory muscle endurance, and/or maximal static efforts to increase strength. Inspiratory flow-resistive training in COPD increases inspiratory muscle strength and endurance but has modest effects on dyspnea and almost none on capacity for activities of daily living. Regimens that combine inspiratory muscle and walking training are better in this regard. Training that involves all three forms of inspiratory muscle training improves exercise capacity in patients with congestive heart failure.

SUMMARY

Normal respiratory muscles have excellent endurance and use little energy. The extraordinary versatility of the respiratory musculature stems from a sophisticated control mechanism that can adapt the pattern of breathing to a wide variety of physical activities.

Respiratory muscle dysfunction contributes to exercise limitation, dyspnea, tachypnea, and the development of acute and chronic ventilatory failure. Respiratory muscle fatigue sometimes occurs in acute ventilatory failure, but the rapid, shallow pattern of breathing usually forestalls development of overt fatigue. Weakness of respiratory muscles is associated with many pulmonary and nonpulmonary diseases. Mechanisms include mechanical disadvantage, catabolic effects of infection or malnutrition, metabolic disarray, hypoxemia, and respiratory acidosis.

Respiratory muscle function can be improved by treating hypoxia, acidosis, electrolyte imbalance, infection, and shock, reducing the work of breathing, and ameliorating the underlying disease when possible. Improvement of respiratory muscle contractility by nutritional repletion and training is often the key to enhancing capacity for physical exercise and reversing ventilatory failure.

In any patient with respiratory distress, it is appropriate to test respiratory muscle strength and to look for pulmonary, chest wall, neurologic, and general medical conditions that are associated with significant respiratory muscle weakness (see Boxes 37-1 to 37-3). It may be appropriate to refer the patient to a neurologist, and when respiratory muscle weakness is severe, the patient should be referred to a pulmonary or critical care physician skilled in the management of ventilatory failure.

BIBLIOGRAPHY

Babcock MA et al: Contribution of diaphragmatic power output to exercise-induced diaphragmatic fatigue, *J Appl Physiol* 78:1710, 1995.

Begin P, Grassino A: Inspiratory muscle dysfunction a nd chronic hypercapnia in chronic obstructive pulmonary disease, *Am Rev Respir Dis* 143:905, 1991.

Dekhuijzen PN, Folgering HT, van Herwaarden CL: Target-flow inspiratory muscle training during pulmonary rehabilitation in patients with COPD, *Chest* 99:128, 1991.

Efthimiou J et al: The effect of supplementary oral nutrition in poorly nourished patients with chronic obstructive pulmonary disease, *Am Rev Respir Dis* 137:1075, 1988.

Laghi F et al: Pattern of recovery from diaphragmatic fatigue over 24 hours, *J Appl Physiol* 79:539, 1995.

Leblanc P et al: Breathlessness and exercise in patients with cardiorespiratory disease, *Am Rev Respir Dis* 133:21, 1986.

Leblanc P et al: Inspiratory muscles during exercise: a problem of supply and demand, *J Appl Physiol* 64:2482, 1988.

Mancini DM et al: Benefit of selective respiratory muscle training on exercise capacity in patients with congestive heart failure, *Circulation* 91:320, 1995.

Polkey MI et al: Exhaustive treadmill exercise does not reduce twitch transdiaphragmatic pressure in patients with COPD, *Am J Respir Crit Care Med* 152:959, 1995.

Rochester DF: Respiratory muscles and ventilatory failure: 1993 perspective, *Am J Med Sci* 305:394, 1993.

Rochester DF, Braun NMT: Determinants of maximal inspiratory pressure in chronic obstructive pulmonary disease, *Am Rev Respir Dis* 132:42, 1985.

Tobin MJ et al: Konno-Mead analysis of ribcage-abdominal action during successful and unsuccessful trials of weaning from mechanical ventilation, *Am Rev Respir Dis* 135:1320, 1987.

Tolep K et al: Comparison of diaphragm strength between healthy adult elderly and young men, *Am J Respir Crit Care Med* 152:677, 1995.

White JES et al: Respiratory muscle activity and oxygenation during sleep in patients with muscle weakness, *Eur Respir J* 8:807, 1995.

Zakynthynos SG, Vassilakopoulos T, Roussos C: The load of inspiratory muscles in patients needing mechanical ventilation, *Am J Respir Crit Care Med* 152:1248, 1995.

CHAPTER

38 Pulmonary Blood Flow

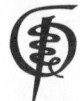

J. T. Sylvester and Roy G. Brower

The major function of the pulmonary vasculature is to bring blood into sufficiently intimate contact with ventilated air to allow adequate uptake of oxygen and elimination of carbon dioxide. In addition, this circuit provides the reservoir that fills the left ventricle during diastole and the mechanical filter that prevents air, thrombi, and other particulate material from reaching the systemic circulation, where embolic infarction or ischemia could have disastrous consequences. Finally, the pulmonary endothelium, with a large surface area of about 130 m², performs important metabolic functions, such as production and inactivation of certain vasoactive hormones.

STRUCTURE

The pulmonary arteries accompany the airways in bronchovascular bundles and branch asymmetrically as they travel peripherally. Arterial diameters, which approximate those of the accompanying airways, decrease from about 20 mm in the main pulmonary artery to about 20 to 50 μm in precapillary arterioles. Despite this, the increased number of branches causes the total cross-sectional area of the arterial vasculature to increase peripherally. At the central part of the acinus, the arterial end branches connect to a dense alveolar capillary network. This network is interconnected throughout the acinus, providing numerous pathways for blood to flow from the center of the acinus to the postcapillary venules at its periphery. The venules converge to form progressively larger veins, which follow an independent course toward the left atrium approximately midway between pairs of bronchovascular bundles.

Vascular smooth muscle allows active control of the flow through pulmonary vessels. The larger extraparenchymal pulmonary arteries contain several elastic lamini and a paucity of smooth muscle. Intraparenchymally, muscularity progressively increases until arteries about 2 mm in diameter are reached and then decreases so that virtually no arteries less than 30 μm in diameter have smooth muscle. At any given external diameter, pulmonary veins have thinner walls than arteries. In addition, the transitions from nonmuscular to muscular veins occur in larger vessels. Although they have no smooth muscle themselves, capillaries may nevertheless be subject to active control by interstitial myofibroblasts extending from the endothelial to the epithelial basement membrane. Contraction of these cells may cause capillary compression.

RESISTANCE

Although the entire cardiac output (CO) flows through the lung, the pressure gradient from the main pulmonary artery to the left atrium is usually no greater than 10 mm Hg, whereas about 100 mm Hg is normally required to drive the same CO through the systemic vasculature. Thus, in comparison to the systemic vasculature, the pulmonary vasculature is a low-resistance circuit. Under normal conditions, resistance in the pulmonary vasculature is approximately equally divided among arteries, capillaries, and veins. This contrasts with the systemic circulation, where most of the resistance is found in arterial vessels.

The flow-resistive properties of the pulmonary circuit are described by the relationship between mean pulmonary artery pressure (Ppa) and CO (Fig. 38-1). Two features of this pressure-flow relationship are noteworthy. First, the pressure axis intercept is the backpressure to flow, or the pressure that pulmonary artery pressure must exceed before blood can flow through the lung. The backpressure may vary in different parts of the lung because of gravity. This variation serves as the basis for dividing the lung into three zones. In zone 3, normally found in the basilar, dependent parts of the lung, both pulmonary arterial and left atrial pressures exceed alveolar pressure, and left atrial pressure is the backpressure to flow. In zone 2, normally found in the middle regions of the lung, gravity causes left atrial pressure to become less than alveolar pressure, but pulmonary artery pressure remains greater than alveolar pressure. The thin-walled capillaries are surrounded by alveolar pressure and do not resist collapse when left atrial pressure (and therefore intravascular capillary pressure) falls below alveolar pressure. For blood to flow through this region, pulmonary artery pressure must exceed alveolar pressure, which therefore acts as the backpressure. In zone 1, normally found at the apices of the lung, gravity causes both pulmonary arterial and left atrial pressure to become less than alveolar pressure. Thus, in this lung region, no blood flows through the collapsed alveolar capillaries.

The second noteworthy feature of this pressure-flow relationship is its curvilinearity: as Ppa increases, the change in pressure required to generate a given change in flow decreases. This occurs because at higher pressures perfused vessels distend and nonperfused vessels, such as those in zone 1, open and become perfused. The latter is termed *recruitment*. Both distention and recruitment increase the cross-sectional area of the vasculature and thereby lower its resistance.

Resistance can be measured as the inverse of the slope of the pressure-flow relationship (ΔPpa/ΔCO); but, this is impractical in patients because the pressure-flow curve is unknown and difficult to determine. In patients with thermodilution pulmonary artery catheters, resistance can be quantified as the difference between mean pulmonary artery and wedge pressures divided by CO. This ratio, known as *pulmonary vascular resistance* (PVR), has a normal value of less than or equal to 4 mm Hg · L^{-1} · min.

Increases in PVR are usually interpreted to indicate an increase in the flow-resistive properties of the vasculature, and vice versa. This interpretation is unambiguous if the change in PVR occurs with either Ppa or CO remaining constant or with P$_{pa}$ and CO changing in opposite directions; however, if P$_{pa}$ and CO change in the same direction, changes in PVR can occur without any change in the pulmonary artery pressure-flow relationship, as shown in Fig. 38-2. Pulmonary vascular resistance is the inverse of the chord slope connecting two points on the pressure-flow relationship: mean P$_{pa}$ at the measured CO and pulmonary capillary wedge pressure (P$_{pcw}$) at a CO of zero. Increases in CO along an unchanged pressure-flow relationship decrease PVR, and decreases in CO increase PVR because of the curvilinearity of the relationship. Furthermore, as illustrated in Fig. 38-3, changes in the pressure-flow relationship can occur without any change in PVR. If the pressure-flow curve were shifted to higher pressures, as would occur with vasoconstriction, and CO increased appropriately, the new P$_{pa}$-CO point could lie on the old PVR line. The result would be no change in PVR despite the vasoconstriction-induced change in the pressure-flow relationship. The same result could be obtained if the P$_{pa}$-CO relationship were shifted to lower pressures (vasodilation) and CO were appropriately decreased.

One way to deal with these ambiguities is illustrated in Fig. 38-4. Draw a straight line through the control Ppcw and P$_{pa}$-CO points on a set of pressure-flow coordinates. Draw a second straight line parallel to the flow axis through the control P$_{pa}$-CO point. Shade the area between the two lines. If a new P$_{pa}$-CO point falls to the right or left of the shaded area, then pulmonary vasoconstriction or vasodilation has occurred, respectively. If the new P$_{pa}$-CO point falls within the

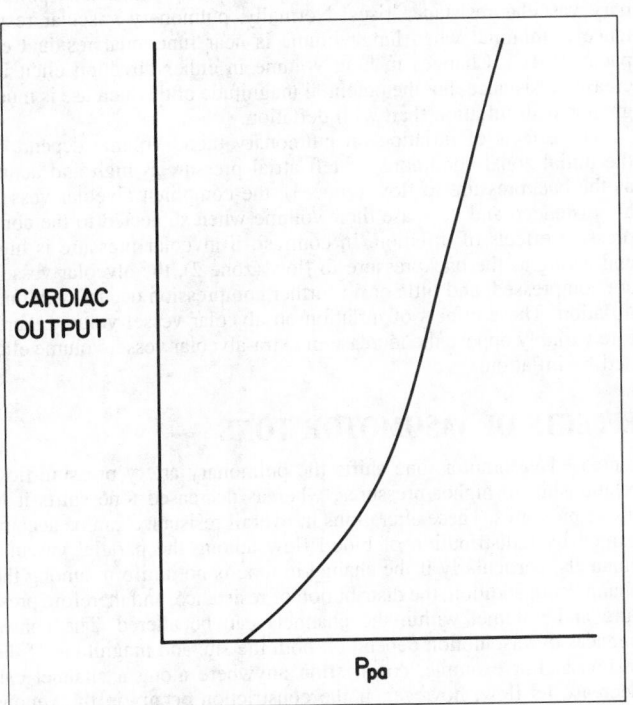

FIGURE 38-1   Pulmonary artery pressure-flow relationship. *P$_{pa}$*, Mean pulmonary arterial pressure.

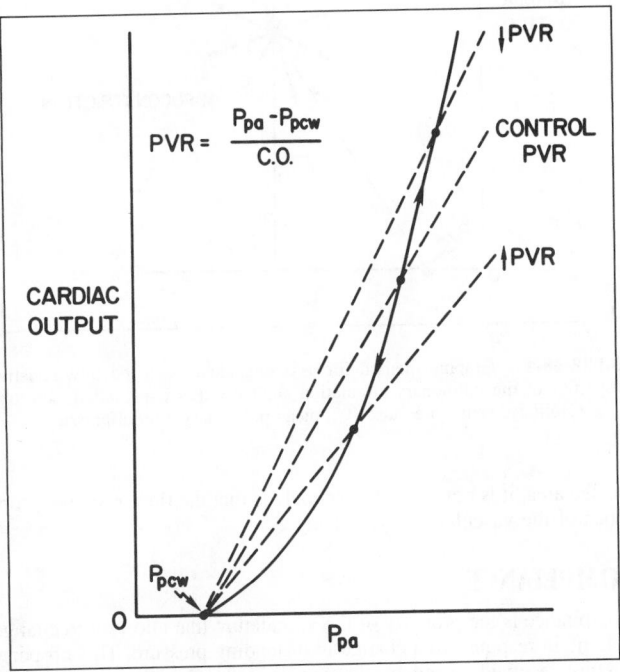

FIGURE 38-2   Change in pulmonary vascular resistance *(PVR)*, calculated as the difference between mean pulmonary arterial *(P$_{pa}$)* and capillary wedge pressures *(P$_{pcw}$)* divided by cardiac output *(CO)*, can occur without a change in the pulmonary artery pressure-flow curve.

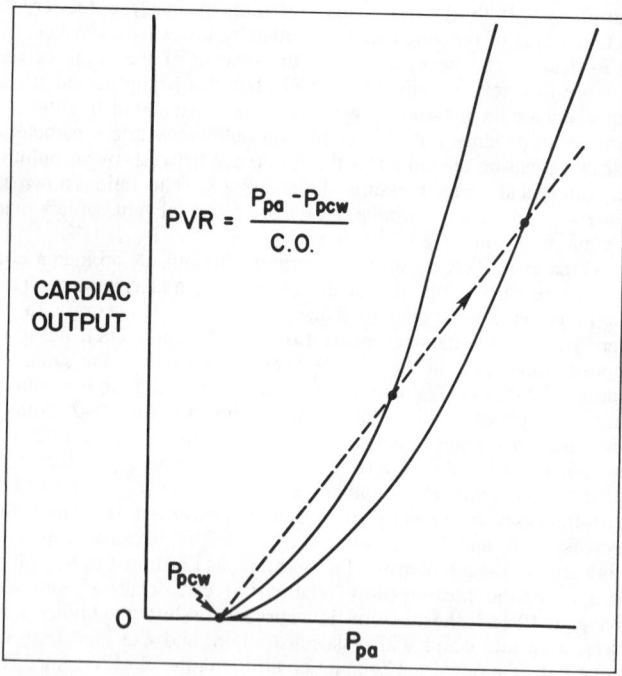

FIGURE 38-3   A change in the pulmonary artery pressure-flow curve can occur without a change in pulmonary vascular resistance *(PVR)*. P_{pa}, Mean pulmonary arterial pressure; P_{pcw}, capillary wedge pressure; *CO*, cardiac output.

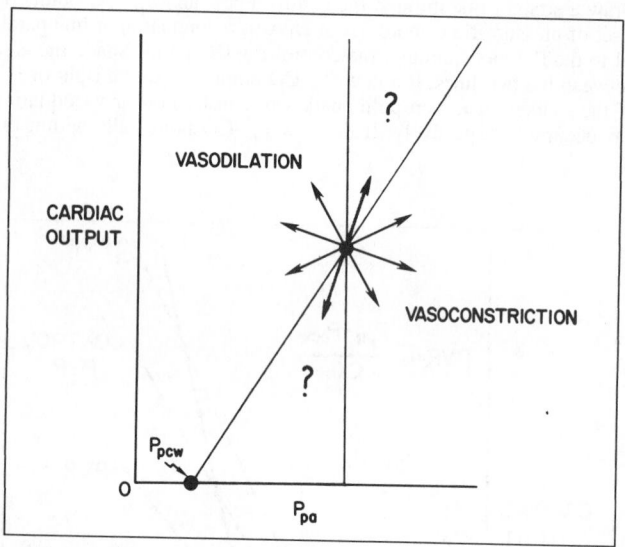

FIGURE 38-4   Graphic method for assessing changes in the flow-resistive properties of the pulmonary circulation clinically. For explanation, see text. P_{pcw}, Capillary wedge pressure; P_{pa}, mean pulmonary arterial pressure.

shaded area, it is not possible to conclude that the flow-resistive properties of the vasculature have changed.

COMPLIANCE

Compliance is the property of the vasculature that allows it to change volume in response to a change in distending pressure. This property has not received as much attention as resistance but is nonetheless essential to normal circulatory function. For example, during diastole, the aortic and pulmonary valves are closed, and the left ventricle must be filled from the pulmonary vasculature. This could not occur if the pulmonary circulation had no compliance.

Like resistance, the compliance of the pulmonary circulation is

less than that of the systemic circulation. For example, in animals pulmonary vascular compliance is about 0.25 ml · mm Hg^{-1} · kg^{-1}, whereas systemic vascular compliance is about 2.5 ml · mm Hg^{-1} · kg^{-1}. Because of its low compliance and intravascular pressure, the pulmonary circuit contains only about 10% of the total vascular volume. The distribution of this volume within the pulmonary circuit is not known with certainty, but recent studies suggest that the majority of pulmonary vascular compliance is located in the capillaries. This contrasts with the systemic circulation, where most of the compliance is thought to reside in small veins.

EFFECTS OF LUNG INFLATION

The lungs undergo cyclic changes in gas volume during the respiratory cycle, subjecting the pulmonary blood vessels to unique stresses. The effects of these stresses can be best understood by dividing the lung vessels into two functional categories. Alveolar vessels are surrounded by alveolar pressure, which rises relative to the pressure on the surface of the lung (pleural pressure) when the lung inflates. Thus alveolar vessels tend to be compressed by inflation. Alveolar vessels include not only capillaries but also arteries and veins, which lack effective attachments to the pulmonary parenchyma. Extra-alveolar vessels are surrounded by the sum of inward-acting alveolar pressure and outward-acting tissue pressure exerted by connections between the vessel and lung parenchyma. The distending effect of the tissue connections is predominant, causing extra-alveolar vessels to expand as the lung inflates. Extra-alveolar vessels include most arteries and veins and also the capillaries located at the junctions of alveolar septae, the so-called corner vessels. Thus the effect of inflation on the lung vasculature can be viewed as the net result of its opposing effects on alveolar and extra-alveolar vessels.

At residual lung volume, there is little tension in the parenchymal tissue, and extra-alveolar vessels may be narrowed, folded, or kinked. As lung volume increases, tissue tension increases, and the extra-alveolar vessels lengthen, expand, and unfold, decreasing their resistance. At low lung volumes, this decrease in extra-alveolar vessel resistance exceeds the simultaneous increase in alveolar vessel resistance caused by compression. Thus, total pulmonary vascular resistance falls. With further increases in lung volume, however, the increase in alveolar vessel resistance continues, while extra-alveolar vessels approach the limit of their distensibility. Thus, total pulmonary vascular resistance rises. Normally, pulmonary vascular resistance is minimal when lung volume is near functional residual capacity (FRC). Changes in lung volume in either direction elicit increased resistance, but the potential magnitude of the increase is much greater with inflation than with deflation.

The effects of inflation on pulmonary blood volume depend on the initial zonal conditions. If left atrial pressure is high and acting as the backpressure to flow (zone 3), the compliant alveolar vessels are distended and decrease their volume when subjected to the compressive effects of inflation. In contrast, if alveolar pressure is high and acting as the backpressure to flow (zone 2), the alveolar vessels are compressed, and little or no further compression occurs with lung inflation. These effects of inflation on alveolar vessel volume therefore variably oppose the increase in extra-alveolar vessel volume elicited by inflation.

EFFECTS OF VASOMOTOR TONE

Increased vasomotor tone shifts the pulmonary artery pressure-flow relationship to higher pressures, whereas decreased tone shifts it to lower pressures. These alterations in overall resistance can be accompanied by redistribution of blood flow among the parallel vascular channels, particularly if the change in tone is not uniform among the channels. In addition, the distribution of resistance, and therefore pressure and volume, within the channels can be altered. The consequences of vasomotion depend on both the site and magnitude of the response. For example, constriction anywhere along a channel can decrease its flow; however, if the constriction occurs in the venous part of the channel rather than the arterial, the volume of the channel and the amount of fluid filtered into the interstitium from its permeable region increases. Such effects could cause edema and deterioration of gas exchange.

Table 38-1 Substances with vasoactive effects on the pulmonary circulation

VASOCONSTRICTION	VASODILATION
Catecholamines (α-adrenergic)	Catecholamines (β-adrenergic)
Acetylcholine	Acetylcholine
Histamine	Histamine
Bradykinin	Bradykinin
Endothelin	Endothelin
Serotonin	Vasoactive intestinal polypeptide
Angiotensin II	Substance P
Vasopressin	Prostaglandin I_2
Leu-enkephalin	Prostaglandin E_1
Prostaglandin H_2	Adenosine
Prostaglandin $F_2 \alpha$	Adenosine triphosphate
Prostaglandin D_2	Carbon dioxide
Prostaglandin E_2	Hydrogen ion
Thromboxane A_2	Nitric oxide
Leukotriene C_4	
Leukotriene D_4	
Leukotriene E_4	
Platelet activating factor	
Adenosine triphosphate	
Carbon dioxide	
Hydrogen ion	
Potassium ion	

From McMurtry I: Humoral control. In Bergofsky EH, editor: *Abnormal pulmonary circulation,* New York, 1986, Churchill Livingstone.

Many substances are capable of changing pulmonary vasomotor tone (Table 38-1). Stimulation of the sympathetic nervous system and hypoxia cause pulmonary vasoconstriction. Nitric oxide, a highly diffusible endothelium-derived relaxing factor, causes pulmonary vasodilation. Several substances cause either constriction or dilation, depending on the initial state of tone, the presence of different receptor types, and other factors. For example, endothelin, a vasoactive peptide released from endothelium, causes vasoconstriction by stimulating receptors on vascular smooth muscle, and vasodilation by stimulating receptors on endothelium. The latter causes release of nitric oxide, which activates guanylate cyclase and increases intracellular cyclic guanosine monophosphate (cGMP) concentration in vascular smooth muscle. Nitric oxide release can be triggered by a wide variety of stimuli, including increased shear stress at the endothelial surface, which occurs when flow increases or vascular caliber decreases. With the exception of hypoxia, the significance of these responses is not well understood.

Hypoxic pulmonary vasoconstriction adjusts local pulmonary perfusion to match local ventilation. For example, when ventilation to a region of lung is impaired, as by a bronchial mucus plug or bronchoconstriction, the carbon dioxide tension of the region rises and the oxygen tension falls. If PO_2 falls below about 75 mm Hg, vasoconstriction occurs, resulting in a decrease in regional perfusion and readjustment of PCO_2 and PO_2 toward normal values. Thus the pulmonary vasoconstrictor response to hypoxia ameliorates the detrimental effects of regional hypoventilation on systemic arterial oxygen tension. The ability of the hypoxic response to maintain appropriate regional ventilation-perfusion relationships becomes limited as the size of the hypoxic region increases. If the entire lung were hypoxic, vasoconstriction would occur in all regions and no redistribution of perfusion would occur. This occurs in normal subjects at high altitude, in patients with weak respiratory muscles or depressed ventilatory drive, and in patients with diffuse parenchymal lung disease severe enough to cause generalized alveolar hypoxia. Under these conditions, hypoxic pulmonary vasoconstriction increases right ventricular afterload but does little to optimize gas exchange.

Administration of pulmonary vasodilators such as isoproterenol can cause hypoxemia, presumably as a result of abrogation of hypoxic vasoconstriction and secondary deterioration of ventilation-perfusion matching. In some cases, hypoxemia does not occur despite deterioration of ventilation-perfusion relationships because the vasodilator simultaneously increases CO through reduction of right and left ventricular afterload. The result is an increase in mixed venous oxygen tension, which nullifies the deleterious effects of poor ventilation-perfusion matching on arterial oxygen tension.

The mechanism of hypoxic pulmonary vasoconstriction remains unknown despite intensive investigation. Much of this work has focused on the identification of a unique humoral mediator released from hypoxic lung tissue, such as catecholamines, serotonin, histamine, prostaglandins, and leukotrienes. Alternatively, hypoxia may act directly on vascular smooth muscle. For example, recent evidence suggests that hypoxia may decrease the conductance of potassium channels located in the plasma membrane of pulmonary arterial smooth muscle cells, causing membrane depolarization, calcium influx through voltage-dependent calcium channels, and increased intracellular calcium concentration, and triggering of the cell's contractile machinery. The nature of the hypoxic stimulus remains unclear, but hypoxia-induced changes in both energy state and redox state have been considered. Similar uncertainty exists with respect to local hypoxic responses of systemic vessels, which dilate rather than constrict. Whatever the mechanisms, the opposite responses of pulmonary and systemic vessels to hypoxia act to maintain oxygen transport under conditions of hypoxic stress.

Pulmonary vasoconstriction preserves systemic arterial oxygen content by matching pulmonary perfusion to ventilation. Systemic vasodilation promotes distribution of oxygen-rich arterial blood to where it is most needed.

PATHOPHYSIOLOGY OF PULMONARY HYPERTENSION

Pulmonary hypertension (Chapters 29 and 62) can occur by three mechanisms: an increase in pulmonary vascular resistance, an increase in the backpressure to pulmonary blood flow, or an increase in flow.

Pulmonary vascular resistance can be increased by removal, obstruction, or obliteration of vascular channels. For example, with lung resection or pulmonary embolism, the number of patent parallel channels is reduced. Normally, the remaining vessels can distend or be recruited sufficiently to accommodate all of the CO without a large increase in pressure. If, however, the remaining vasculature is not capable of recruitment or distention, the increase in pulmonary artery pressure after obstruction or obliteration of vascular channels is more severe. Pulmonary vascular resistance also increases if individual channels become narrowed by vasospasm or by medial and endothelial hypertrophy, as occurs with chronic hypoxia and primary pulmonary hypertension. Again, this decreases the total cross-sectional area of the vasculature, necessitating an increase in pulmonary artery pressure to maintain a normal flow of blood.

If the backpressure to flow rises, pulmonary artery pressure must also rise to maintain an adequate pressure gradient for blood flow. This occurs when left atrial pressure is increased to high levels by mitral stenosis. With high levels of positive end-expiratory pressure (PEEP), alveolar pressure can be increased sufficiently to compress alveolar vessels and become the backpressure to flow. Further increases in PEEP then necessitate increases in pulmonary artery pressure to maintain cardiac output. Hyperinflation caused by asthma has the same effect. In this case, contraction of inspiratory muscles decreases pleural pressure to very negative values while alveolar pressure remains close to zero. Because pleural pressure surrounds the heart as well as the lungs, the decrease in pleural pressure causes left atrial pressure to decrease relative to alveolar pressure, and thus alveolar pressure becomes the backpressure to flow. Pulmonary artery pressure is also lowered by the reduction in pleural pressure, resulting in a decrease in the pressure gradient (pulmonary artery pressure–alveolar pressure) for flow. To restore this gradient, the right ventricle must raise pulmonary artery pressure relative to pleural pressure. This form of pulmonary hypertension would not be detected by the usual measurement of pulmonary artery pressure, which uses atmospheric pressure as a reference. It becomes apparent only if pulmonary artery pressure is referenced to pleural pressure. Thus, from its perspective in the chest the right ventricle sees an increase in pulmonary artery pressure during hyperinflation whether the hyperinflation is produced by raising alveolar pressure relative to atmospheric pressure (PEEP) or lowering pleural pressure relative to atmospheric pressure (asthma).

Increased CO can also lead to pulmonary hypertension. In patients with atrial or ventricular septal defects or with a patent ductus arteriosus, there is left-to-right shunting and an increase in pulmonary blood flow at rest. At first, the resulting increase in pulmonary artery pressure is mild because of the distensibility and recruitability of the pulmonary vessels. With time, however, anatomic changes occur in the vasculature that decrease its cross-sectional area, causing pulmonary hypertension. The mechanisms by which these anatomic changes occur are not well understood.

To understand the effects of pulmonary hypertension on the heart, it is useful to consider the relationship between right atrial pressure and CO (the Frank-Starling, or CO curve) and the relationship between right atrial pressure and venous return (the venous return curve). The CO curve demonstrates that the output of the heart progressively increases to a plateau as its filling pressure is increased. The curve is shifted downward (lower right ventricular output at a given right atrial pressure) by a decrease in cardiac contractility or an increase in afterload. The venous return curve demonstrates that the flow of blood to the right heart form the peripheral circulation is progressively decreased as the backpressure to venous return (the right atrial pressure) is increased. The venous return curve is shifted upward (higher venous return at a given right atrial pressure) by an increase in blood volume, a decrease in systemic vascular compliance, or a decrease in the resistance to venous return. In the steady state, venous return must equal CO. The intersection of the curves (Fig. 38-5) indicates what the steady state CO and right atrial pressure must be (point A).

If pulmonary artery pressure and therefore right ventricular afterload are increased, the CO curve shifts downward, intersecting the venous return curve at a lower CO and higher right atrial pressure (point B). Compensatory mechanisms such as constriction of peripheral vessels and renal retention of sodium and water are activated, shifting the venous return curve upward. The new intersection (point C) indicates a restoration of CO, albeit at an even higher right atrial pressure. If this situation persists, the right ventricle may hypertrophy, causing an upward shift of the CO curve and perhaps some return of the right atrial pressure toward normal. If, however, the pulmonary hypertension progresses, as is frequently the case, further increases in right atrial pressure as well as peripheral vascular pressure

and volume occur. At some point, the increase in peripheral vascular pressure results in edema. With time, the hypertrophied, dilated right ventricle weakens, particularly if hypoxemia and acidosis are present. This causes a further downward shift of the CO curve, leading eventually to lowered CO in the face of a markedly enlarged blood volume and massive peripheral edema (point D). This sequence of events can vary with the acuity of the insult. Under some circumstances, as in chronic bronchitis, the process may occur over a period of years and may be punctuated by numerous remissions and exacerbations. In contrast, when pulmonary hypertension is severe and occurs abruptly, as with pulmonary embolism, compensatory mechanisms may be inadequate or have insufficient time to develop fully. Under these conditions, CO may fall to severely low levels, resulting in shock and death.

The treatment and clinical causes of pulmonary hypertension are discussed in Chapters 29 and 62.

BIBLIOGRAPHY

Dawson CA: The role of pulmonary vasomotion in the physiology of the lung, *Physiol Rev* 4:2, 1984.

Fishman AP: Pulmonary circulation. In Fishman AP et al, editors: *The respiratory system: circulation and non-respiratory function,* Bethesda, Md, 1985, American Physiological Society.

Grover RF et al: Pulmonary circulation. In Shepherd JT, Abbored FM, editors: *The cardiovascular system: peripheral circulation and organ blood flow part 1,* Bethesda, Md, 1983, American Physiological Society.

Guyton AC, Jones CE, Coleman TG: *Circulatory physiology: cardiac output and its regulation,* Philadelphia, 1973, Saunders.

McMurtry IF: Humoral control. In Bergofsky EH, editor: *Abnormal pulmonary circulation,* New York, 1986, Churchill Livingstone.

Mitzner W: Resistance of the pulmonary circulation, *Clin Chest Med* 4:2, 1983.

Sylvester JT et al: Acute hypoxic responses. In Bergofsky EH, editor: *Abnormal pulmonary circulation,* New York, 1988, Churchill Livingstone.

Weibel ER: *The pathway for oxygen,* Cambridge, Mass, 1984, Harvard University Press.

Weir EK, Archer SL: The mechanism of acute hypoxic pulmonary vasoconstriction: the tale of two channels, *FASEB J* 9:183, 1995.

CHAPTER

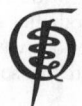

39   Host Defense Mechanisms in the Respiratory Tract

Herbert Y. Reynolds

A complex network of mechanical barriers and of immunologic and cellular mechanisms present in the nasooropharynx and along the trachea and conducting airways helps protect the respiratory mucosa from particles and microorganisms that are inhaled with ambient air or aspirated with oropharyngeal secretions. This local defense system also impedes the attachment and growth of microbes that inhabit the nose, throat, and central airways. The peripheral airways generally protect the alveolar surfaces, which normally are probably devoid of microbes. However, particles of small size (less than 3.0 μm in diameter) or with special aerodynamic properties (such as fragments of asbestos fibers) can reach the alveolar surface where mucociliary clearance and coughing mechanisms are not effective. Thus the air exchange surface has different mechanisms to cleanse itself. These include the scavenger activity of mobile alveolar macrophages, aided by nonimmune (surfactant and fibronectin) and immune (immunoglobulin [Ig] antibody) opsonins, or creation of an inflammatory reaction, which attracts polymorphonuclear (PMN) cells from adjacent capillaries and other components of systemic defense (complement factors) to the alveoli.

This chapter reviews normal components of the defense apparatus in the conducting airways and on the air exchange surface. Impairment of one or several of these host defenses can predispose to sinopulmonary and/or chronic lung infections; overactivity or a smoldering inflammatory reaction can cause bronchitis or an alveolitis,

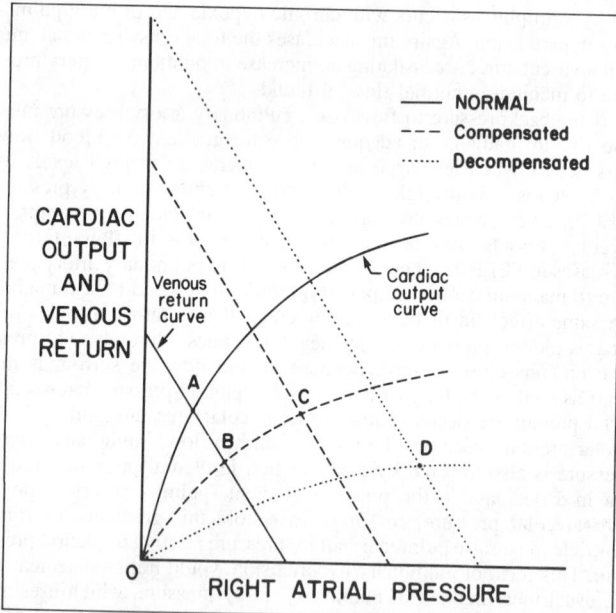

FIGURE 38-5   Graphic analysis of the regulation of cardiac output and right arterial pressure under normal conditions and compensated and decompensated pulmonary hypertension. **A,** Normal; **B,** pulmonary hypertension without peripheral vascular compensation; **C,** pulmonary hypertension with peripheral vascular compensation; **D,** decompensated pulmonary hypertension. For details, see text.

which stimulates fibroblasts to make collagen and can lead to interstitial fibrosis.

CONDUCTING AIRWAYS

A mucosal surface covers the airways (Fig. 39-1). In the nares and oropharynx, the surface is squamous epithelium; but over the nasal turbinates and from the trachea down to the respiratory bronchioles, it consists of a pseudostratified, columnar, ciliated, mucus-secreting epithelium. A turnover of mucosal cells occurs approximately every 7 days. This ciliated epithelium is interspersed with goblet cells and orifices leading from the submucosal bronchial glands. A tuft of possibly 100 to 200 cilia on each epithelial cell beats with amazing speed, approaching 300 times per minute, creating waves of coordinated ciliary motion over the airways' surface. Lymphocytes and plasma cells are distributed in the submucosa and lamina propria areas of the larger conducting airways and nasal passages. Some surface lymphocytes are found, perhaps extruded from bronchial-associated lymphoid aggregates. A few surface macrophages exist, either coming up from the alveoli, or perhaps they are dendritic macrophages, which have a special ability to process antigens that have been inhaled and have impacted on the surface. These cells might initiate immune responses in the airways. Joining all of these glandular and cellular networks together are nerves, exerting their control through neuropeptides and by adrenergic and cholinergic nerve fibers. A rich vascular supply also exists.

Autonomic nervous control regulates humidification of air and heat exchange on the mucosal surface, conserving fluid, especially in the nose and trachea. Interest is usually directed to the secretory potential of the mucosa, whereby mucus is produced by bronchial glands and goblet cells, serous and Clara cell secretions are added, local immunoglobulins are produced, and proteins transudate from the vascular space. However, absorption of fluid and debris from the mucosa and across the alveolar epithelial surface can be equally important. Several mechanisms accomplish this: lymphatic routes clear fluid and senescent cells or cell remnants after apoptosis has occurred, phospholipids can be ingested by surface macrophages, and brush cells with their apical border microvilli submerged in the periciliary sol fluid (microvillous cells) absorb fluid. The integrity of tight apical junctions between epithelial cells is also crucial in overall fluid balance and in preventing submucosal deposition or penetration of airway antigens. These junctions can be affected by irritation from airborne pollutants and by immediate allergic injury, which can occur with antigen-antibody reactions.

Accurate quantification of these various components in respiratory lining secretions remains limited in humans to date. General balance of fluid along the airways and the status of local irritation of the mucosal surface are important as variables in obtaining precise values. As for local secretion of proteins, the thickness of the stratified epithelial surface separating the lamina propria and basement membrane from the luminal surface of the airway might also be a significant factor. As an example, to facilitate secretion of dimeric IgA, epithelial cells have developed a receptor for secretory component. Mast cell or macrophage cytokines may alter local mucosal permeability. Bradykinin and neuropeptides can also have an effect, such that values for immune components measured on the mucosal surface can fluctuate along the surface; allowance must be made for this dynamic interplay.

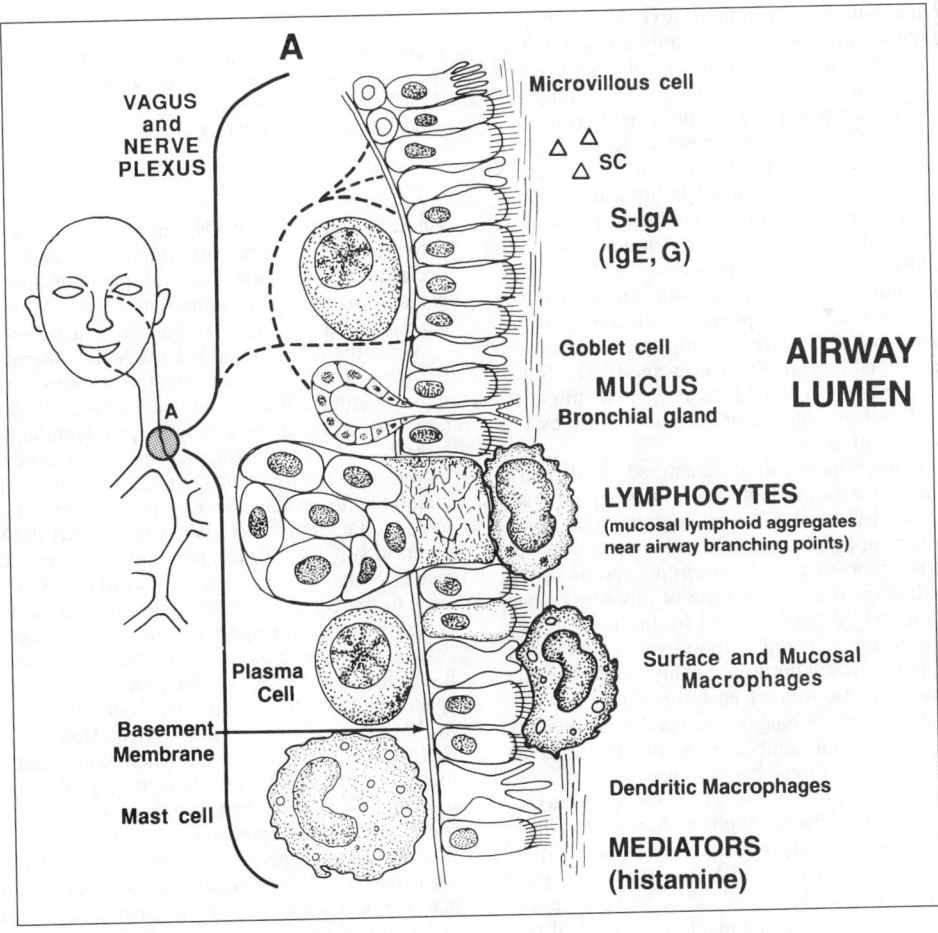

FIGURE 39-1   Enlarged portion *(A)* of the conducting airway surface depicting the mucosa and the major submucosal structures under the lamina propria. See text for details. *SC,* Secretory component, *S-IgA,* serum immunoglobulin A; *IgE, G,* immunoglobulin E and G.

(Modified from Reynolds HY: *Chest* 95:223S, 1989.)

DEFENSE MECHANISMS ON THE AIR EXCHANGE OR ALVEOLAR SURFACE

Toward the periphery of the airways, the epithelial layer gradually becomes thinner and less stratified; the cells become cuboidal in shape, and cilia are shorter. In the terminal air sacs and over the alveolar surface, the cell layer flattens and blends into a single layer of epithelium (type 1 pneumocytes) interspersed with type 2 pneumocytes distributed in the corners of alveoli. Goblet cells and mucous glands that were present in the conducting airways disappear (below the level of the respiratory bronchioles) as the alveolar surface is reached. This epithelial layer supports freely moving, detachable phagocytic cells and lymphocytes. In the transitional zone at the level of the respiratory bronchioles, other secretory cells (Clara cells) are present.

Particles or microbes of small dimensions in inspired air may elude trapping mechanisms in the conducting airways and reach the alveolar surface. As an example (Fig. 39-2), bacteria (B) can be of critical size, between 0.5 and 3 μm diameter including an envelope of moisture, so that they may escape aerodynamic filtration in the upper repiratory tract (URT) and proximal airways and descend to the alveoli. As mentioned, mucociliary clearance and coughing are not effective in removing particles from the alveolar surface, so other mechanisms have been developed. Based on experiments in rabbits and rodents exposed to aerosolized bacteria, bacteria deposited on the alveolar surface are rapidly captured by alveolar macrophages and ingested within a half hour or so. Because one macrophage services about three alveoli, these mobile cells must move quickly to cover a large area; shortcuts through the pores of Kohn facilitate this rapid coverage. What actually occurs following entry of a bacterium into an alveolus and before its final phagocytosis by a macrophage is speculation, but the following scenario could be envisioned.

Momentarily, the bacterium is free within the alveolus, but expansion and closure of the alveolus, a product of inspiration and expiration, probably forces the bacterium against the alveolar wall, where it becomes coated with several constituents of the alveolar lining material. These could be surfactant proteins, glycoproteins (fibronectin), humoral immune factors (IgG), and complement factor B. Two of these substances can be considered as nonimmune opsonins, surfactant and fragments of fibronectin; immunoglobulin with antibody specificity would be an immune opsonin. Complement, particularly C_3b, can promote receptor-mediator attachment to a macrophage or interact with an antibody to augment receptor binding. Also, a microbe might trigger activation of the alternate complement pathway and create directly a lytic situation. Complement activation may not occur readily, as minimal concentrations of complement factors are present as measured in normal bronchoalveolar lavage (BAL) fluids, and inhibitors of complement that would be needed to modulate complement activity and prevent indiscriminate tissue injury by this lytic system seem to be absent as well.

Immunoglobulin G is the principal opsonic antibody available in BAL fluid. Immunoglobulin A is available in limited amounts and has much less opsonic activity than IgG. Immunoglobulin M occurs in minimal amounts in normal persons. As IgM does not have prominent specific mu chain receptors on alveolar macrophages, its role as an opsonin is minor. Whatever the final mixture of opsonins, a bacterium so coated is more avidly phagocytosed by the macrophage. Macrophages can ingest inanimate particles (polystyrene balls) without prior opsonization, but they will not ingest many viable bacteria, especially gram-negative species, without an opsonic coating. Certainly, a specific opsonin increases phagocytic uptake appreciably. Therefore the availability of opsonic antibodies is important in clearing encapsulated bacteria such as *Streptococcus pneumoniae.*

Once inside the macrophage, the fate of the microbe in part reflects the condition (activation) of the macrophage. Moreover, a large inoculum of microbes, or an unusually virulent species or an initial exposure to a new species not encountered before (hence no prior chance for the host to have mounted any cellular or humoral immunity) could overwhelm the defense system and allow a microbial species to persist and create infection (pneumonia). Activation of the macrophage becomes another variable, and this requires coordination with T lymphocytes in the lung. Cytokines, interferon-γ and interleu-

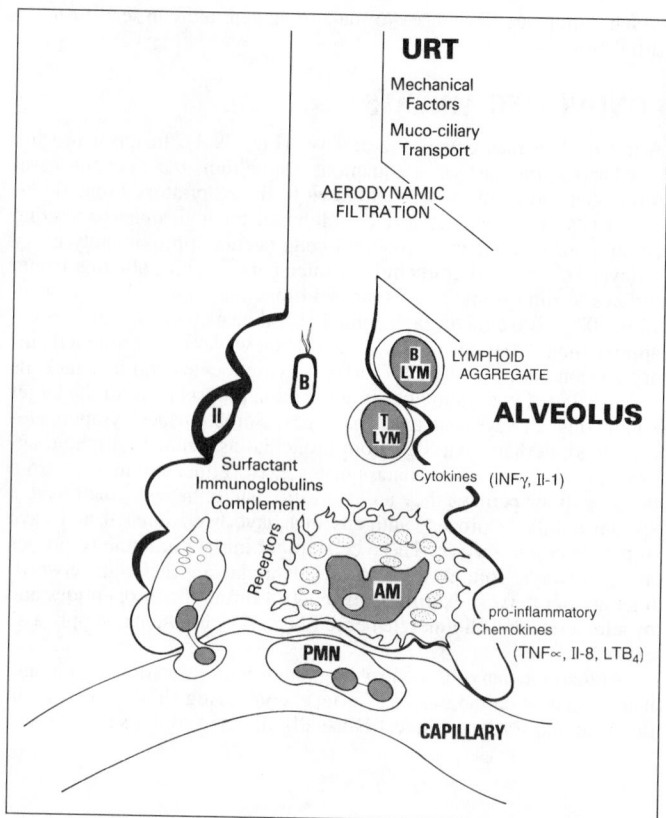

FIGURE 39-2   Enlargement of the alveolar unit illustrating components of the host defense system active on the alveolar surface. See text for details. *AM,* Alveolar macrophage.

(Modified from Reynolds HY: *Disease-a-Month* 31:13, 1985.)

kin 2, produced by the TH_1 subset of lymphocytes, can energize and activate macrophages, thus improving phagocytic and intracellular bactericidal capabilities. Several important species of intracellular organisms, including *Mycobacterium tuberculosis* and *Legionella pneumophila,* require that macrophages be activated to contain them.

Once the macrophage has ingested a microbe, the phagocyte may be able to kill or contain it, and the problem is resolved; cell-mediated immune stimulation may not be necessary to complete the action. Alternatively, conditions that favor proliferation of the microbe, that is, large inoculum and virulence, or virgin exposure of the host, may require that the macrophage recruit additional phagocytic help. One method is to produce several proinflammatory cytokines (i.e., chemotactic factors or chemokines that attract PMNs into the alveoli). A plentiful supply of PMNs exists as marginated cells in capillaries adjacent to alveoli that are readily available. PMNs roll along and then stick to the capillary endothelium by way of several adhesive glycoproteins found on respective cell surfaces, such as selectins or intercellular adhesion molecules (ICAMs), endothelial-leukocyte adhesion molecules (ELAMs), and integrins. In normal, uninflamed alveolar spaces, few PMNs are present. About 1% of airway cells recovered in BAL fluid (Table 39-1) are PMNs. However, human alveolar macrophages can produce several chemokines that initiate and direct the migration of granulocytes into the alveolar spaces. The major chemokines are interleukin 8, tumor necrosis factor (TNF-α) and leukotriene B_4 from the lipoxygenase pathway of arachidonic acid metabolism. Although PMNs are the prominent inflammatory cells responding to bacterial infection, other cells such as eosinophils, lymphocytes, and monocytes are involved in other kinds of inflammatory reactions as found in granulomatous (sarcoidosis) or eosinophilic lung diseases. Suppression of inflammation occurs when cytokines such as Il-10 and Il-13 inhibit macrophage production of chemokines and cause macrophages to engulf apoptotic PMNs.

Table 39-1 Profile of respiratory cells recovery in BAL fluid (for nonsmoker normals following 100- to 300-ml lavage)

		DIFFERENTIAL COUNT (%)			CYTOCENTRIFUGE CELL STAIN (%)		
CELL NUMBER TOTAL	VIABILITY	MACROPHAGES	PMN	EOSINOPHIL/BASOPHIL	LYMPHOCYTES	CILIATED CELLS	ERYTHROCYTES
15×10^6	<90%	85	1-2	<1	7-12	1-5	<5

IMMUNOGLOBULINS

In the analysis of proteins in BAL fluid recovered from normal subjects, albumin represents approximately one third of the total protein and accounts for the largest share.

Another group of proteins found in high concentration and easily detected in lavage fluid are the immunoglobulins. Immunoglobulin A constitutes approximately 5% of the total protein in BAL fluid. Serum IgA is principally a monomer, and little exists in polymeric form. In contrast, IgA in BAL fluid is a typical secretory IgA, as found in secretions from the breasts (colostrum), parotid glands, and gastrointestine, in that it contains bound secretory component glycoprotein as well as joining chain (J chain). Compared with values of about 2 mg/ml in serum, concentrated BAL fluid (about 25-fold concentration) contained about 150 μg/ml; differences between smokers and nonsmokers were not significant. Precipitin analysis of purified secretory IgA fractionated from BAL fluid has identified both α heavy chain subtypes. Delacroix and colleagues measured the relative proportions of IgA_1 and IgA_2 in serum and in a variety of external secretions. In general, excretory fluids contain mostly A_1 but relatively more A_2 than in comparison with serum. In bronchial secretions about 33% of the IgA was the A_2 variety.

Although IgA accounts for a sizable percentage of the total protein in BAL fluid, IgG is more abundant. Immunoglobulin G, expressed as a ratio of albumin, is present in concentrated BAL fluid obtained from nonsmokers in the same proportion as in serum (ratio about 0.25 to 0.3); for smokers, the lavage fluid contains slightly more IgG in proportion than does serum (ratio about 0.4), based on the finding that some 20% of normal smokers have elevated IgG in their lavage fluid. Because IgG in BAL approximates its serum value, most of it arrives by transudation from the plasma compartment. In addition, intraluminal secretion of IgG and IgA is possible by plasma cells or by release of cell membrane–bound immunoglobulin from lymphocytes and possibly macrophages in the alveolar space.

Immunoglobulin G in BAL fluid is composed of the four heavy chain subclasses of IgG, and these are quantitatively in almost the same proportions as found in serum. In BAL fluid, IgG_1 is most abundant (66%), IgG_2 is next (27%), and IgG_3 and IgG_4 are in small amounts accounting for 3% to 4% each of the total IgG. Immunoglobulin G_4 is in higher proportion in BAL fluid than in serum.

Immunoglobulin E is considered part of the mucosal secretory immune system because IgE plasma cells can be identified in the airway submucosa. However, its concentration of about 10 ng/ml of concentrated BAL fluid obtained from normal humans is very low in the nonallergic subject. Probably such measurements do not represent fairly the actual presence of IgE in the lungs because IgE is in part tissue bound, especially to submucosally located and intraluminal mast cells. Immunoglobulin E–secreting plasma cells are not plentiful in normal nonatopic subjects.

Immunoglobulin M, an approximately 900,000 daltons molecular weight protein, is detected in BAL fluid in very low concentrations, which are minuscule compared with those for IgA and IgG. Lactoferrin is present in BAL fluid. As it is quite similar in size to secretory IgA, it is a difficult contaminant to remove when purifying IgA from BAL fluid for biochemical analysis. Transport of these two proteins into the airways is considered to be linked. Lactoferrin and transferrin, which can also be identified in alveolar fluid, have antimicrobial activity because iron is a required nutrient for microbial growth.

Several proteins collected with the lavage technique have more relevance for the conducting airways than the alveolar spaces. Secretory component (SC) is a glycoprotein selectively produced by serous epithelial cells along various mucosal surfaces of the body and is of special interest in the airways because it is added to respiratory secretions selectively without an additional source from the intravascular fluid. Much of the SC supply is bound to secretory IgA, but a surprisingly large amount exists in pulmonary lavage fluid in a free or unattached state.

RESPIRATORY CELLS

Bronchoalveolar lavage fluid provides a sample of cells that are present on the surface of the terminal conducting airways and alveoli. As BAL requires successive aliquots of saline to be infused and aspirated from a sublobar segment of a lung, cells are detached and recovered in serial aspirates. If serial BAL fluid samples are assessed for their content of cells, some variation is found in that PMN cells are disproportionately high in the first aspirate and more lymphocytes appear in later ones; macrophages are plentiful in all samples. A representative population of intraluminal cells in BAL fluid is given in Table 39-1. From cigarette smokers without overt bronchitis or other respiratory disease, the recovery of cells in lavage is usually threefold to fivefold greater, reflecting primarily more alveolar macrophages. The population of alveolar macrophages is not homogeneous, and the variable size and morphology of these cells reinforce this. When alveolar macrophages are separated into subpopulations by cell surface markers or by size and density, different functions are evident. Moreover, macrophages should not be considered as just scavenger phagocytes for they have significant immune effector function as well and modulate immune responses on the alveolar surface. As macrophages undergo a transition and maturation from blood monocytes into differentiated alveolar macrophages in the interstitial compartment of the lung tissue, intermediate stages, or so-called interstitial macrophages, may have a special activity in forms of chronic lung injury and fibrosis.

As shown in Table 39-1, the usual cell recovery from a healthy nonsmoking volunteer is about 15 million cells, depending on the volume of lavage fluid used and recovered. The viability of the cells is about 95% and on a differential cell count (prepared from cytocentrifuged cell specimen and stained with Wright-Giemsa), most of the cells are macrophages. PMN cells are rare, as are erythrocytes; the amount of coughing induced by the bronchoscopy and lavage influences the number of ciliated epithelial cells found. These cells are often viable in a wet preparation mount of the BAL cells, and ciliary motion is visible.

Considerable interest has focused on the identification of lymphocytes, which may account for 10% or so of the total cells (Table 39-2). Aided by the use of T-cell-specific monoclonal antibody staining, most of the lymphocytes are T cells, and with further T-cell subset identification, about half of these are CD_4 helper cells, and a lesser percentage are of the CD_8 suppressor or cytotoxic variety. The ratio of T helper to suppressor cells is about 1.5 in the normal airways, and this is approximately the same ratio obtained for peripheral blood lymphocytes. Among the T-helper cells, a small percentage (about 7% in normal subjects) have an HLA-DR antigen; this subpopulation may increase when a lymphocytic alveolitis develops, as in active sarcoidosis, and is responsible for much of the interleukin-2 (IL-2) produced. TH_1 and TH_2 subsets produce different groups of cytokines, which can have differential effects on responder cells. For example, TH_1 lymphocytes produce interferon-γ and Il-2, which can activate macrophages, whereas TH_2 cells secrete Il-4, 5, 6 that can affect immunoglobulin production by B-lymphocytes and plasma cells. Approximately 7% of the airway T cells are killer cells, but these seem dormant in normal subjects. In addition, about 5% of the lymphocytes are B cells or plasma cells. These cells can release various class-specific immunoglobulins from their surface as already mentioned. Among normal T cells, a few have a γ/δ T-cell receptor; this subset can be increased in atopic asthma patients.

Disordered interaction between lymphocytes and macrophages is evident in the pathogenesis of several lung diseases. In Fig. 39-3, the complexity of these cellular functions, facilitated by locally produced soluble mediators (cytokines), is illustrated. Although the interaction between activated lung macrophages and lymphocytes is emphasized, especially subtype T helper/inducer (T_H) and T suppressor (T_S), similar connections are applicable for other immune cells, such as cytotoxic or killer lymphocytes, immunoglobulin-producing plasma cells, and B lymphocytes.

Alveolar macrophages, which originate from circulating blood monocyte precursors, undergo further maturation and differentiation in the interstitial spaces before emerging on the alveolar surface as potentially long lived, aerobically metabolizing phagocytes. Vitamin D metabolites are important in this developmental process. A major responsibility of these roving scavenger phagocytes is to clean debris from the alveolar surface. When activated, however, macrophages can secrete a large array of cellular mediators that affect the function of other cells (cytokines). As mentioned, macrophage proinflammatory

chemokines, which include leukotriene B_4, Il-8, and tumor necrosis factor α (TNFα), can attract other inflammatory cells to the alveoli, or macrophage fibroblast growth factors, such as platelet-derived growth factor, can stimulate fibroblast replication. Activated macrophages also can secrete interleukin-1 (IL-1), which may attract T lymphocytes into the alveoli. Other mediators such as tumor necrosis factor and plasminogen activator can have local alveolar effects (autocrine function) but may diffuse into the systemic circulation and produce remote effects as well. The list of enzymes, regulatory proteins, and inhibitors produced by macrophages continues to lengthen as more than 100 substances have been attributed to this heterogenous cell population.

The macrophage also serves as an antigen-presenting cell, which can process an antigen and display it on its cell membrane, where it is taken up by an appropriate T_H lymphocyte and matched with respect to class II major compatibility antigens. Antigen is received on the lymphocyte's membrane by a T-cell antigen receptor, which has an intricate structure composed of two β and α chains.

Within the lumen of the alveolar spaces, the majority of lymphocytes are T cells with the proportion of CD_4 T-helper cells greater than CD_8 suppressor cells; this ratio is approximately 1.5. The activated T_H cells can secrete a variety of cytokines, such as γ-interferon

Table 39-2   Lymphocyte subsets (%)

T CELLS (% OF TOTAL)	T HELPER/CD_4*,†	CD_8 CYTOTOXIC*	T KILLER‡,* LYMPHOCYTES	B LYMPHOCYTES (PLASMA CELLS)§	UNTYPABLE LYMPHOCYTES
70	50	30	7	5-10	5

*As percent of T cells, the T_H/T_S ratio is approximately 1.5:1.8.
†The T helper subset contains approximately 7% of cells with HLA DR$^+$ antigen, and these can preferentially produce interleukin-2.
‡Killer lymphocytes seem inactive when retrieved from a normal lung.
§Among plasma cells are immunoglobulin-releasing cells with the following frequency: IgG = IgA > IgE.

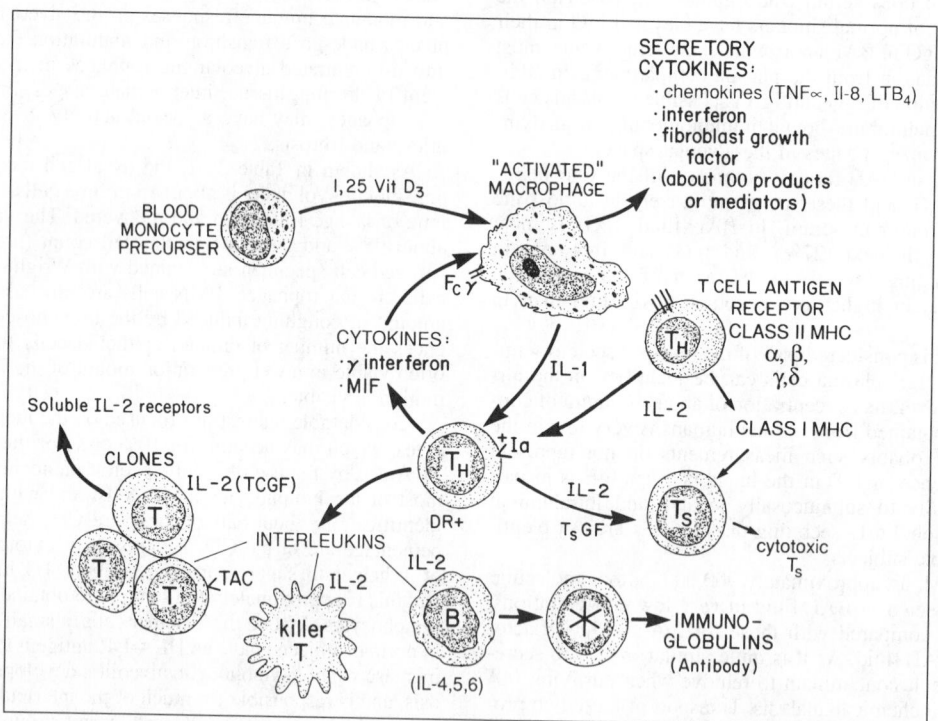

FIGURE 39-3   Immunologic interactions on the alveolar surface illustrated by various secretory functions of alveolar macrophages and lymphocytes. See text for details. Activated T-helper cells can produce cytokines that affect macrophage function, such as migration inhibition factor *(MIF)* and gamma (γ) interferon. *LTB₄,* Leukotriene B₄; *MHC,* major histocompatibility; *Tₛ,* subclass T suppressor cell; *TCGF,* T-cell growth factor; *Tₕ,* subclass T helper cell.

(Modified from Reynolds HY: *J Allergy Clin Immunol* 78:833, 1986.)

and migration inhibition factor (MIF), that modulate macrophage activity in turn; Gamma-interferon in particular can energize or activate the macrophage. Also T_H cells secrete cytokines that affect other lymphocytes. Interleukin-2 appears to be an important mediator in this respect, produced by a subset of T_H cells identified as DR-positive lymphocytes. It can stimulate T cells to replicate, thus expanding the clone and number of cells in the alveoli (formerly known as T cell growth factor [TCGF]), or it can activate natural killer lymphocytes that usually are dormant in normal lung. It is important to note that IL-2 in concert with other interleukins ($Il_{4,5,6}$ from TH_2 cells) can stimulate B lymphocytes to secrete immunoglobulin and may promote their differentiation into plasma cells. The effect of T suppressor cells is less well defined in terms of special mediators produced, but T cells may produce T suppressor growth factors. Natural inhibitors exist that may neutralize the effect of certain cytokines. For example, certain other cytokines, such as Il-10, Il-13, macrophage chemotactic inhibitor, and transforming growth factor B, will counteract others or down-regulate macrophages, suppressing activity through immunomodulation. Inhibition of IL-2 can be accomplished by immunosuppressive drugs such as corticosteroids and cyclosporine A. Thus the potential for cellular interactions within the air spaces are multiple and complicated, and derangements can cause or perpetuate respiratory illnesses.

POTENTIAL DEFECTS OR DYSFUNCTION IN HOST DEFENSES THAT COULD LEAD TO RESPIRATORY ILLNESS

The nasooropharynx and major conducting airways have an intricate network of barriers and movable mechanisms that prevents particles or microbes from adhering to or penetrating the mucosal surface and then sweeps them off. As reviewed, these include mucus coating of the surface, tight apical junctions between epithelial cells, beating cilia, angulation of the airways, and the cough reflex. Also present are immunologic components: secretory IgA and IgG, a few lymphocytes and macrophages that may initiate immune responses, various mediators such as histamine produced by mast cells, and an array of cytokines secreted by macrophages and epithelial cells. A very dynamic airway mucosal surface is equipped to react breath to breath with the many toxic substances inhaled with ambient air. At the level of the respiratory bronchioles where the airways change from serving as conduits for airflow to adapting for air exchange, host defenses are different. On the alveolar surface, clearance of particles and microbes is a combined function of phagocytic cells and various lipids, glycoprotein, and immunoglobulins that serve as opsonins (see Fig. 39-2).

Individual components or a combination of them may malfunction or be defective from a hereditary deficiency in structure and predispose the host to illness. Respiratory infections are usual, often recurrent ones that involve the upper airways and sinuses and the lungs. Other defects, such as a deficiency of the antiproteases α_1 antitrypsin, to inactivate proteolytic enzymes, may take longer to manifest and require additive effects from other injury, such as cigarette smoking, to accelerate illness and produce emphysema. If a patient has a propensity for sinopulmonary infections or a puzzling illness, it may be important to consider whether a defect, hereditary or acquired, in pulmonary host defense is contributory. In some situations an accurate diagnosis will permit replacement therapy of the absent component, or awareness of the specific problem can help put the illnesses into an overall health perspective for the patient and his or her family. Early on in infancy or childhood when recurrent infections occur, pediatricians are alerted quickly to the possibility of congenital illnesses such as cystic fibrosis. However, because children with acute respiratory infections are effectively treated with antibiotics, the appearance of cystic fibrosis and related problems may be delayed and not recognized until later in life—as a teenager or young adult. Therefore the internist may be confronted with a patient who has recurrent otitis media, sinusitis, and bronchitis, seemingly as independent problems; infertility concerns may be present also. At this juncture, a differential diagnosis that includes cystic fibrosis, structural defects in cilia leading to dyskinetic ciliary action, and immunoglobulin deficiencies, particularly of IgG subclasses IgG_2 and/or IgG_4, is appropriate to consider.

Another situation in which an acquired defect in pulmonary host defenses could be the cause of respiratory infection(s) would be the new onset of lower tract bacterial infections (at any age) or with particular opportunistic microorganisms. Several components of alveolar space defenses could be implicated and are illustrated with these examples. As the macrophage is centrally positioned in the defense of the alveolar surface, it must be responsive to a number of things. This scavenger phagocyte first intercepts the microbe and can either kill or contain it or must call in some other phagocytic cells for assistance, using chemokines to attract PMNs. Opsonic antibodies (IgG) plus other nonimmune opsonins discussed facilitate phagocytosis, but an absence of specific antibody may permit infection to develop with encapsulated bacteria such as *Streptococcus pneumoniae*. Insufficient bone marrow reserve of PMNs, reflecting effects of antineoplastic chemotherapy, may allow gram-negative bacilli and fungal organisms to flourish. Inability of immune T-helper lymphocytes to energize macrophages, through cytokines (interferon γ) that provide cell-mediated immunity and activation, makes containment of certain intracellular microbes difficult for these phagocytes (e.g., *Legionella pneumophila* or *Mycobacterium tuberculosis*). Similarly, concomitant infection of macrophages with viruses (e.g., human immunodeficiency virus, cytomegalovirus, or herpes viruses) plus an excessive number of CD_8 T-lymphocyte suppressor cells could influence macrophage function and containment of *Pneumocystis carinii* and common bacterial and fungal organisms. Patients with the acquired immunodeficiency syndrome are susceptible to infection from all of these microbes.

Identification of the precise lung host deficiency can make therapy more specific through immunization to develop special antibodies, replacement of certain immunoglobulins (IgG subclasses), or selective administration of cell mediators (γ interferon or interleukins). These ideas are expanded in several other chapters (see Chapters 229, 242, 261, 272, and 280) that examine the specific diseases or infections cited previously.

BIBLIOGRAPHY

Cox G et al: Macrophages' engulfment of apoptotic neutrophils contributes to the resolution of acute pulmonary inflammation in vivo, *Am J Respir Cell Mol Biol* 12:232, 1995.

Delacroix DL et al: IgA subclasses in various secretions and in serum, *Immunology* 44:383, 1982.

Downey GP et al: Neutrophil sequestration and migration in localized pulmonary inflammation, *Am Rev Respir Dis* 147:168, 1993.

Ley K, Tedder TF: Leukocyte interactions with vascular endothelium, *J Immunol* 155:525, 1995.

Liles WC, Van Voorhis WC: Review: nomenclature and biologic significance of cytokines involved in inflammation and the host immune response, *J Infect Dis* 172:1573, 1995.

Martin RJ et al: The effects of inhaled interferon gamma in normal human airways, *Am Rev Respir Dis* 148:1677, 1993.

Merrill WW et al: Immunoglobulin G subclass proteins in serum and lavage fluid of normal subjects: quantitation and comparison with immunoglobulins A and E, *Am Rev Respir Dis* 131:584, 1985.

Mosmann TR et al: Two types of murine helper T cell clone. I. Definition according to profiles of lymphokine activities and secreted proteins, *J Immunol* 136:2348, 1986.

Murray HW: Interferon-gamma and host antimicrobial defense: current and future clinical applications, *Am J Med* 97:459, 1994.

Pikaar JC et al: Opsonic activities of surfactant proteins A and D in phagocytosis of gram negative bacteria by alveolar macrophages, *J Infect Dis* 172:481, 1995.

Rankin JA et al: Human airway macrophages—a technique for their retrieval and descriptive comparison with alveolar macrophages, *Am Rev Respir Dis* 145:928, 1992.

Reynolds HY: Lung immunology and its contribution to the immunopathogenesis of certain respiratory diseases, *J Allergy Clin Immunol* 78:833, 1986.

Reynolds HY: Immunoglobulin G and its function in the human respiratory tract, *Mayo Clin Proc* 63:161, 1988.

Reynolds HY: Pulmonary host defenses—state of the art, *Chest* 95:223S, 1989.

Reynolds HY: Immunologic system in the respiratory tract, *Physiol Rev* 71:1117, 1991.

Reynolds HY: Cytokines: role in respiratory illnesses and potential control with immunomodulatory therapy *Focus and Opinion: Intern Med* 1(6):1, 1994.

Robinson BWS et al: Natural killer cells are present in the normal human lung but are functionally impotent, *J Clin Invest* 74:942, 1984.

Sibille Y, Reynolds HY: Macrophages and polymorphonuclear neutrophils in lung defense and injury, *Am Rev Respir Dis* 141:471, 1990.

Spinozzi F et al: Increased allergen-specific, steroid sensitive gamma/delta T cells in bronchoalveolar lavage fluid for patients with asthma, *Ann Intern Med* 124:223, 1996.

Strieter RM, Kunkel SL: Acute lung injury: the role of cytokines in the elicitation of neutrophils, *J Invest Med* 42:640, 1994.

CHAPTER

40 Mechanisms of Lung Injury and Repair

Jamson S. Lwebuga-Mukasa

Acute lung injury may occur as a result of insults originating in the lungs such as aspiration, toxic inhalation, or prolonged hyperoxia intraalveolar hemorrhage, or as a result of injury initiated in other parts of the body such as in the systemic inflammatory syndrome associated with sepsis, trauma, acute pancreatitis, and ischemic-reperfusion injury. Regardless of the initiating factor, the lung has a stereotypic response to acute injury. Acute injury to the alveolar-capillary barrier results in the exudation of vascular components into the alveoli, associated with type I epithelial cell necrosis, disruption and denudation of the alveolar basement membrane (BM), and formation of hyaline membranes. Inflammatory cells, cytokines, leukotrienes, and fibrinolytic and complement components amplify the injury. Subsequently, there is type II alveolar epithelial cell and myofibroblast proliferation and the remodeling of the extracellular matrix (ECM). Type II cells, the precursors of type I pneumocytes, migrate to cover the denuded BM and differentiate into type I cells, thus restoring a continuous epithelial lining. Severe initial lung injury, exaggerated inflammatory response, or repeated (chronic) injury results in a fibrotic response.

The cellular and molecular mechanisms mediating lung injury are beginning to be elucidated, and commonality of pathways may in part explain the stereotypic response. The key components in lung injury include cytokines, oxygen-derived free radicals, nitric oxide products, proteases, endotoxin, complement activation products, platelet activating factor (PAF), and coagulation products.

Cellular elements include alveolar macrophages (AMs), epithelial cells, interstitial cells, endothelial cells, polymorphonuclear leukocyte cells (PMNs) and peripheral blood mononuclear leukocytes. All cellular and ECM components participate in the amplification of the inflammatory reaction and in subsequent tissue repair. Repair processes require a coordinated, optimal replication of epithelial, fibroblast, and endothelial cell populations, with the restoration of normal tissue boundaries. These processes are mediated through cell-cell, cell-ECM, cytokine growth factor interactions, and hormonal factors.

Although common mechanisms may be involved in the initial injury and inflammatory response, the course of lung repair is more complex. It is influenced by (1) the nature and severity of the initial insult and inflammatory response; (2) superimposition of a second insult during the recovery period or chronicity of injury; (3) cell-to-cell and cell-to-ECM interactions; (4) effects of soluble growth factors from alveolar macrophages (AMs) and lymphocytes; (5) growth factors and cytokines bound to lung ECM, which may be released during inflammatory reactions; and (6) secretion of autocrine and paracrine factors by lung parenchymal cells. Growth factors secreted by lung parenchymal cells may also influence macrophage and lymphocyte functions. The variety of factors released during an inflammatory reaction and the ensuing repair probably reflects the interaction among the different factors and the target cells.

Inflammatory cytokines IL-1α, IL-1β TNF-α, IL-6, IL-8 and INF-γ, MIP-1α, MIP-1β, and MCP-1, along with toxic oxygen products and L-arginine metabolites nitrite (NO_2^-) and nitrate (NO_3^-) play critical roles in the mediation of the immediate inflammatory response. Monocytes express IL-1β, whereas tissue macrophages secrete IL-1α. As monocytes differentiate into tissue macrophages they switch their IL-1β expression to IL-1α. IL-1α, IL-1β, TNFα, in concert with the O_2 or NO metabolites are commonly induced in the various conditions that are associated with acute lung injury. In contrast, the expression of IL-4, IL-1 receptor antagonist (IL-1ra) is delayed over several hours in the course of an inflammatory response and serves to down-regulate the inflammatory response. Repair of damaged tissue requires coordinated proliferative and biosynthetic re-

sponse that is regulated by growth factors and cell-cell and cell-ECM interactions. Dysregulation of repair processes may result in a failure to restore normal alveolar cytoarchitecture.

Cell-to-cell adhesion is required for normal development, repair, and maintenance of continuous polarized alveolar, epithelial, and endothelial cell layers. Tight epithelial junctions are essential to the maintenance of fluid-free alveoli. Cell-to-cell interactions may be mediated by homologous cell adhesion molecules (CAMs), which are involved in cell recognition and tight-junction formation. Cell adhesion molecules permit sorting, migration, and reestablishment of continuous epithelial layers consequent to lung damage. A number of cell-cell adhesion molecules have been isolated and characterized. They include the cadherins (members of the integrin superfamily) and the platelet-endothelial cell adhesion molecule-1 (PECAM-1). They localize at sites of cell-cell contact. E-cadherins are a subfamily of epithelial cell CAMs that are found on lung epithelial cells. They are integral membrane glycoproteins that mediate Ca^{2+}-dependent homophilic cell-to-cell adhesion.

Cell interaction with ECM is a dynamic process in which the cells deposit and organize ECM components and the ECM in turn regulates cell function and differentiation during injury and repair. The major constituents of ECM are collagens, proteoglycans, and adhesive glycoproteins. Some proteoglycans have the capacity to bind other ECM molecules and growth factors. The cells synthesize ECM components, which assemble into complex three-dimensional structures. Both spatial organization and composition may be important for tissue-specific properties of the ECM. When ECM is damaged or modified, for example, after proteolysis during inflammatory reactions, solubilized fragments of ECM components may mediate many important biologic functions, such as chemotaxis and proliferation. The ECM, through cell-to-ECM receptors, is capable of regulating cellular functions and differentiation.

Integrins are a superfamily of cell surface receptors that anchor cells to ECM molecules. Integrins are heterodimeric glycoproteins that consist of an α(130 to 200 kilo-Dalton [kDa]) subunit and a β(90 to 130 kDa) subunit. Both subunits span the plasma membrane. When integrins bind to ECM ligands, the interaction is relayed into the cytoplasmic domains of the receptors, which results in activation of genes that control diverse cellular functions such as migration, proliferation, adhesion, cell shape changes, and cell differentiation. Integrin signaling has been recently reviewed by Clark and Brugge. Two complementary mechanisms are believed to be important for the signal transduction caused by integrins. In one mechanism the signal is transduced through the cytoplasmic domains to the cytoskeleton, which regulates cell shape. In another mechanism, the binding of the ligand to its integrin results in activation of phospholipase C and the tyrosine kinase cascade of the *src* family of oncogenes, which results in specific gene activation. The surface expression of the receptor as a consequence of posttranslational modification, or by differential splicing of ligands such as fibronectin or laminin. The expression of the ECM integrins is controlled by the ECM, growth factors, and cytokine networks. All known integrin functions require divalent cations. Nine β integrins, 16 α integrins, and at least 22 α/β combinations have thus far been identified. Alternative splicing of subunit mRNAs provides further diversity. In general, $β_1$ and $β_3$ integrins function as adhesive receptors for ECM, whereas $β_2$ integrins mediate cell-to-cell interactions of leukocytes and the immune system. A $β_4$ integrin is involved in lymphocyte adhesion. $α_v$ can associate with several different β subunits: $α_v β_5$, which binds vitronectin; $α_v β_6$, which is a fibronectin receptor; and $α_v β_8$, whose ligand has not yet been identified. $α_4$ can associate with $β_1$ and $β_7$ and functions as a receptor for fibronectin or for VCAM-1.

First, we review the structural and cellular components of the alveolar wall, using the adult respiratory distress syndrome (ARDS) to illustrate mechanisms of acute injury and the lung's defenses against them. Next, we discuss repair processes after acute lung injury.

COMPONENTS OF THE ALVEOLAR WALL

The alveolar wall consists of cellular and ECM components. Structural components of the alveolar wall provide a thin barrier across which gas exchange occurs. They also control the permeability of water solutes. In addition, cellular components of the lung perform many biochemical functions that are important for normal organ function and repair.

Cells of the Alveolar Epithelium

The alveolar epithelium is a mosaic consisting of type I and type II pneumocytes. Type I cells are extremely thin, flat cells that cover about 95% of the respiratory surface. They are the major barrier to diffusion of fluid and electrolytes into the alveoli and account for 60% of the resistance of fluid influx into alveoli. Because of their large surface area and their capacity for pinocytosis, they may contribute to the bulk transport of fluids across the alveolar septum. They may be capable of limited repair and of phagocytosis of particulate matter from the alveolar space. Little is known about their biosynthetic and metabolic functions.

Type II pneumocytes are cuboidal cells that are usually located at alveolar corners. They synthesize, store, secrete, and recycle surfactant. Type II cells synthesize, deposit, and remodel epithelial basement membrane. They regulate fluid and electrolyte transport. They are the precursors of adult type I cells during regeneration of the epithelium. In chronic hyperoxic states, type II cells adapt to oxygen injury by increasing cellular content of antioxidant enzymes. Along with Clara cells, type II cells are the major stem cells of the distal air spaces.

Type II alveolar epithelial cells participate in inflammatory reactions in several ways. They can be activated by the cytokine network in presence of TNFα and IL-1α to express MIP-1α and in presence of TGFβ to express IL-8, which may play important roles in recruitment of inflammatory cells. Type II cells can be induced to express nitric oxide synthase (iNOS) by IL-1α, TNFα, and INFγ, which results in production of NO_2^- and NO_3^- that can induce IL-1α or IL-β and TNFα, thus amplifying the inflammatory response. Type II cells also may play important roles in repair processes by production of growth factors that modulate fibroblast and endothelial cell proliferation and differentiation.

Cells of the Interstitial Space

The alveolar interstitial space contains fibroblasts, smooth muscle cells, and pericytes. Fibroblasts, of which there are several subpopulations, are the most commonly encountered cell type. They synthesize and secrete collagen, glycosaminoglycans, elastin, adhesive glycoproteins, and other components. Fibroblasts play important roles in pathologic conditions associated with abnormal deposition of ECM components. Their interactions with type II cells may be important for the maintenance of the type II pneumocyte–differentiated state. They also release enzymes that degrade the ECM such as collagenase and plasminogen activator (PA). The interstitial space at alveolar junctions contains lymphatics, which are important for removal of interstitial fluid and other metabolic products. Migration of fibroblasts in alveolar space may result in intraalveolar fibrosis.

Capillary Endothelium

The capillary endothelium provides a nonthrombogenic surface for gas exchange and accounts for 30% to 40% of the barrier to fluid efflux into the alveolus. Capillary cells are involved in receptor and bulk transport of macromolecules, metabolism of biogenic amines, and vasoactive peptides. Capillary endothelial cells also function as endocrine cells and participate in immunologic reactions. Endothelial cells secrete factors that may regulate alveolar epithelial cell functions. Endothelial cells are active participants in the initiation and amplification of inflammatory reactions of the lung. The endothelial surface nearest injury becomes more adhesive to leukocytes. In vitro IL-1, γ interferon (IFN-γ), and TNFα, all of which are macrophage products, induce expression of leukocyte adhesion molecules on cultured endothelial cells.

Vascular cells produce several members of cys-cys chemotactic cytokine family (chemokines). This family is characterized by the presence of tandem cysteine residues in the primary amino acid sequence. In contrast, IL-8 and gro-α, have the cysteine tandem interrupted by an extra amino acid residue. IL-8 and gro-α are chemoattractive to neutrophils, basophils, lymphocytes, and melanoma cells.

Recent studies using reconstructed vessels suggest that transmigration induced by IL-1α or TNFα was partially dependent on local production of IL-8. On exposure to inflammatory signals, endothelial cells produce monocyte chemotactic protein (MCP-1), a member of the cys-cys family. The regulation of MCP-1 expression by IL-1 and TNFα is at the gene transcription level. IL-8, MIP-1α and MCP in concert stimulate the expression of adhesion molecules on PMNs. IL-1α and TNFα also induce endothelial cell production of MIP-1α, MCP-1, and IL-8, which are chemoattractants of PMNs. Endothelial cells also synthesize PAF, prostaglandins, platelet-derived growth factor (PDGF), and class II major histocompatibility (MHC) antigens. Gamma interferon (INF-γ) causes organizational changes of endothelial cells, producing gaps between cells. IFN-γ induces endothelial cells to express class II MHC antigens and augments levels of class I MHC. It amplifies IL-1α production by LPS-stimulated endothelial cell and causes slow increase in ICAM-1. Its effects are synergistic with those of TNFα and IL-1α. Finally, endothelial cells may release enzymes that degrade the ECM.

Lung Extracellular Matrix

Current knowledge of the composition of the lung ECM is incomplete. Four broad classes of structural macromolecules have been identified: (1) collagens (of which 20 types have been identified); (2) noncollagenous adhesive glycoproteins such as laminin, fibronectin, cytotactin, entactin, and osteonectin (SPARC); (3) elastin; and (4) glycosaminoglycans. Review of this area is beyond the scope of this chapter. Each ECM component has the potential for isoform diversity that contributes to the unique properties of the ECM in different organs and tissues.

The ECM constitutes the three-dimensional mechanical framework that accounts for a significant component of the physical properties of the lung. The ECM, through ECM-to-cell receptors such as integrins, provides important functional cues that are necessary for the maintenance of normal cellular functions, response to injury, and restoration of tissue architecture during repair. Basement membranes separate the alveolar epithelium from the interstitium and thus provide boundaries along which orderly repair of the epithelium can occur. During repair the ECM provides a scaffold for attachment, proper orientation, support, shape determination, and migration of the cellular components of the alveolus. During wound repair, parenchymal cells have been shown to express differentially spliced isoforms of ECM components such as fibronectin and tenascin. In vitro, cytokines such as TGFβ have been shown to stimulate synthesis of ECM constituents and their receptors that may regulate repair processes. The ECM may function as a permissive substratum on which cells are responsive to soluble factors or as an inducer for the expression of new cellular functions in adherent cells during lung development and repair. Because of the net negative charge the alveolar epithelial basement membrane is believed to play an important role in the retention of cations. Intact or cleaved components of ECM may be important in chemoattraction of inflammatory cells into the alveolar space. Finally, ECM may function as a reservoir of growth factors such as basic fibroblast growth factor (bFGF) and transforming growth factor β (TGFβ), which may be released during lung remodeling.

MECHANISMS OF LUNG INJURY

Because of the large gaps in our understanding of the mechanisms of lung injury and repair, we borrow from observations made on nonpulmonary systems or on in vitro model systems and attempt to corroborate the observations with those in a clinical setting. It must be noted, however, that the involvement of specific cytokines or cells in repair processes of different tissues may differ; there is thus a need for confirming that processes observed in other systems also occur in the lung. Excessive lung parenchymal injury may result from inappropriately high secretion of inflammatory cytokines, proteolytic enzymes, and/or toxic O_2 or NO products. Some of the cellular and molecular mechanisms involved in acute lung injury are described here. The relative importance of the different mechanisms depends on the physiologic conditions in which the injury occurs.

Acute lung injury resulting in ARDS may be direct, as occurs with inhalation lung injury, or it may be secondary such as occurs in settings of sepsis, massive trauma, or massive blood transfusions. Sepsis and trauma are the most freuqent causes of acute lung injury leading to ARDS. The initiating injury mechanisms probably differ, depending on the clinical settings. Once initiated, however, lung damage may be amplified by recruitment and activation of PMNs, complement, fibrinolytic and lipoxygenase products, and local tissue factors. Generalized damage to the alveolar septum leads to leakage of fluid and protein into the interstitium. When the capacity of lung lymphatics to clear the fluid is overwhelmed, fluid exudes to the alveolar space, resulting in pulmonary edema. As a result, there is reduced lung compliance and functional residual capacity (FRC), a large right-to-left intrapulmonary shunt, and impaired gas transport. Decrease or dysfunction of surfactant occurs and may be caused in part by influx of inhibitory plasma factors. Some of the postulated mechanisms of acute lung injury are detailed later.

Cytokines and Lung Injury

Cytokines are soluble protein mediators that regulate functions of immune and nonimmune cells through binding to cell surface receptors. Cytokines play a key role in the initiation of lung injury, the inflammatory response, its maintenance, and resolution. They function as networks that influence each other's effects most frequently at gene transcription level. Although earlier clinical and histologic studies failed to demonstrate a causal relationship between the degree and duration of lung inflammation and a progression to fibrosis, recent studies have revealed elevated bronchoalveolar lavage (BAL) fluid and plasma cytokine levels in patients with severe lung injury and progression to fibrosis.

TNFα and IL-1α are well recognized early mediators of inflammation and are induced by a variety of injury agents. However, neither TNFα nor IL-1α is directly chemotactic for PMNs. Recruitment of PMNs is due to local synthesis of chemotactic proteins induced by IL-1α and TNFα. TNFα promotes adhesion of inflammatory cells to capillary endothelium at the sites of inflammation by induction of adhesion receptors for PMNs and stimulates peripheral blood monocytes to express IL-1α. Local mediators of inflammation include PAF; leukotriene B_4 (LTB$_4$); formylmethionine peptides; complement products C5a; macrophage/granulocyte inflammatory proteins MIP-1α, MIP-1β, and MCP-1; and IL-8. IL-1α and TNFα induce platelet-activating factor (PAF) synthesis. PAF (acetyl-glyceryl ether phosphoryl choline) is a potent platelet and leukocyte activator and a vasoconstrictor that also promotes leukocyte adhesion to endothelial cells. Normally the inflammatory reaction is transient. Sustained inflammatory response requires cytokines with chemotactic factors such as IL-8, MIP-1α, and MIP-1β; MCP-1 properties; and cytokines with proliferative, growth, and differentiation effects such as TGFβ, PDGF, insulin-like growth factor (IGF), bFGF, VEGF, TGFα, GMCSF, IL-6, and IL-10.

The interactions among the different cytokines, positive or negative, frequently occur at mRNA transcriptional level. The transcriptional factor nuclear factor-κB (NF-κB) plays an important role in modulation of cytokine-cytokine interactions. NF-κB is a pleiotropic regulator of many genes involved in immune and inflammatory responses including leukocyte adhesion molecules. This family of diverse transcription factor complex consists of a P_{50} (NF-κB1) and a p_{52} (NF-κB2), which are obtained from a nonlysosomal proteolytic products of precursor p_{105} and p_{100} proteins. NF-κB and its inhibitor, IκB-α, play a key role in regulating leukocyte adhesion and migration across the alveolar epithelium. NF-κB can be activated by inflammatory cytokines IL-1α, IL-1β, TNFα, LPS, and INF-γ and oxidative and mechanical stress. In a resting cell, NF-κB is complexed with inhibitory proteins, IκB-α and others. On activation of the cell, IκB-α is activated and degraded by a nonlysosomal mechanism, and NF-κB is translocated to the nucleus, where it binds to promoter elements in E-selectins, VCAM-1 and ICAM-1 genes, and presumably genes of inflammatory cytokines and induces their expression. NF-κB also increases expression of its inhibitor IκB-α. NF-κB mediates activation of IκB-α gene resulting in replenishment of cytoplasmic pool of the inhibitor and decreased NF-κB activation and expression of the NF-κB activated genes. Thus the effects of NF-κB is transient and the cell returns to a basal state. It has been proposed that once

translocated to the nucleus, NF-κB may be under additional regulatory control.

IL-1α and TNFα induce E-selectin and ICAM-1 and ICAM-2. Endothelial-leukocyte adhesion molecule-1 (ELAM-1) is a member of the E-selectin family induced by IL-1α and TNFα. Leukocytes contain preformed E-selectin, which can be immediately expressed on cell surface upon activation. E-selectin mRNA can also be induced in endothelial cells and is observed within the first 4 hours of an inflammatory response. VCAM-1 expression peaks in 6 hours and remains elevated for up to 72 hours. ICAM-1, ICAM-2, and VCAM-1 are members of the Ig superfamily. The ligand for VCAM-1 is $\alpha_4\beta_4$. PMNs bind ICAM-1 and ELAM-1 on endothelial cells. The ligands for ICAM-1 are β_2 integrins on leukocyte membranes. Natural killer lymphocytes adhere to vascular endothelium via ICAM-1 and VCAM-1. Endothelial cells possess receptors for GMCSF and respond to these cytokines with migration and proliferation.

Resolution of an inflammatory reaction requires down-regulation of the expression of inflammatory signals. A number of mechanisms have been described that decrease the expression of the effects of inflammatory cytokines. Prostaglandin E_2 (PGE$_2$), TGFβ, IL-4, and IL-10 have been shown to down-regulate expression of inflammatory cytokines. For example, IL-4 has been shown to decrease monocyte IL-1α and TNFα on endothelial cells. IL-4 and IL-10 decrease IL-1α and TNFα mRNA expression. IL-4, originally recognized as a growth and differentiation factor for lymphocyte, also has regulatory activities on nonimmune cells. IL-4 increases VCAM-1 expression but decreases ICAM-1 and ELAM-1 expression by endothelial cells. IL-4 has been shown to have inhibitory effect on monocyte adhesion to endothelial cells and down-regulates thrombomodulin anticoagulation pathway. Effects of inflammatory cytokines can be further antagonized by soluble factors that compete for the cell surface cytokine receptors. The most extensively studied system involves the IL-1 receptor antagonist (IL-1ra). IL-1ra is expressed late in the inflammatory response and blocks IL-1α, IL-1β, and TNFα mRNA expression.

Alveolar macrophages are the principal cells involved in the recruitment of PMNs in the air space; however, other cellular constituents of the alveolar wall participate in this process. Epithelial cells, fibroblasts, and endothelial cells have been shown to produce MIP-1α and MIP-1β, MCP-1, TNFα, O_2, NO, IL-8 in response to TNFα, and IL-1α. During inflammatory reactions, pulmonary endothelial cells express, on their surfaces, inducible adhesion molecules such as ELAM-1, ICAM-1, and VCAM-1. The adhesion molecules are important for PMN and platelet adhesion and thus serve to localize the PMN and platelet adhesion to sites of inflammation. Components of the lung ECM such as type IV collagen, fibronectin, and laminin in their native or cleaved states are PMN chemoattractants. Finally, arachidonic acid produced by pulmonary epithelial cells is metabolized to a potent chemoattractant, LTB$_4$, by pulmonary alveolar macrophages.

Inflammatory Cell Hypothesis

Both AMs and PMNs, which contain mechanisms for protease and oxidant lung injury, are believed to mediate lung damage. Macrophages contain lysosomal enzymes and neutral proteases that may damage the ECM. Activated AMs release substances (e.g., MIP-1α, MIP-1β, MCP, IL-1α, and IL-8) that are chemotactic to PMNs. The latter are frequently found at sites of alveolar and endothelial damage. PMN leukocytes and products of leukocytes are observed in BAL fluid of patients at risk of ARDS and those with ARDS. PMN leukocytes release oxygen radicals (superoxide anion O_2^- and the hydroxyl radical [$\cdot$OH]) as well as hydrogen peroxide (H_2O_2). Finally, substances capable of activating both PMNs and AMs are present in pulmonary microvasculature and BALF.

Polymorphonuclear leukocytes are normally absent from lung parenchyma. However, activated PMNs adhere to the surface of the pulmonary endothelium at the site of alveolar injury. They migrate through the endothelium, between cell junctions, and penetrate the basement membrane into the interstitium and finally into alveolar spaces. PMN leukocytes may degranulate at any stage of their migration, releasing factors that may amplify the initial damage to cellular and ECM components. However, PMNs are not the sole source of lung injury because neutropenia does not completely protect the lung from prolonged hyperoxia.

Oxidant Injury Hypothesis

Toxic O_2 Products. Both PMNs and AMs have mechanisms for release of toxic oxygen radicals, which damage cell membrane components and ECM. Superoxide dismutase, catalase, and ceruloplasmin are important protective mechanisms against oxidative damage to lungs. Oxygen radical scavengers, such as dimethyl thiourea (DMTU), protect alveolar cells from hyperoxic injury and resultant ARDS after phorbol myristate acetate–induced lung damage. Oxygen radicals may mediate their toxic effects by increasing pulmonary perfusion pressures and peroxidative damage to cell membranes and ECM. Thus papaverine, an inhibitor of smooth muscle contraction, prevents increased lung damage in isolated lung preparations.

Cell-free systems consisting of xanthine and xanthine oxidase mixtures have been used to generate O_2^- (superoxide) and hydrogen peroxide (H_2O_2). In the presence of iron, they react to form hydroxyl radical ($\cdot OH$). Hydroxyl radicals can be converted to water and oxygen by catalase. Superoxide anion O_2^- is converted to H_2O_2 by superoxide dismutase. The H_2O_2 or its derived product such as $\cdot OH$ probably causes the lung damage since superoxide dismutase does not protect from lung damage.

Products of Inducible Nitric Oxide Synthase (iNOS). Nitric oxide metabolites have emerged as important mediators of acute lung injury. Nitric oxide is generated from L-arginine in a nitric oxide synthase (NOS)-catalyzed reaction, which results in the formation of citrulline. There are two distinct classes of nitric oxide synthases, constitutive (cNOS) and inducible (iNOS) isoforms. Constitutive isoforms of NOS play important roles in neuronal transmission of some nonadrenergic, noncholinergic neurons, and in the modulation of vascular tone. Inducible forms of NOS are important in the modulation of inflammatory reactions and are expressed in phagocytic cells and a variety of other cell types including alveolar type II cells. The expression of iNOS can be induced by LPS, complement activation products, or cytokines. It has been shown that superoxide can react with nitric oxide to generate peroxynitrite ($ONOO^-$). Peroxynitrite decomposes to generate hydroxyl radical by the following mechanism:

$$NO + O_2^- \rightarrow ONOO^-$$
$$ONOO^- + H^+ \rightarrow ONOOH$$
$$ONOOH \rightarrow HO^\cdot + NO_2^\cdot$$

Protonation of peroxynitrite gives rise to a hydroxyl radical. Nitric oxide is on one hand potentially protective and on another hand cytotoxic. Low concentrations of NO protect against ARDS and inhibit adhesion to vascular walls and activation and mediate important tumoricidal and bacteriocidal effects of inflammatory cells. In contrast, excessive NO may cause cellular damage by deamination of deoxynucleotides and intact DNA. Peroxynitrite decomposition to hydroxyl radical may mediate cytotoxic damage when superoxide is present. Nitric oxide may also bind tyrosine residues of proteins producing nitrotyrosine and modify protein functions. The spectrum of oxidant species generated during phagocytic stimulation is variable and depends on the cell type, target cell, and extracellular environment. Although these systems have been studied most extensively in phagocytic cells, it is believed that similar processes also occur in other cells such as type II cells that express iNOS.

Protease Hypothesis

According to this hypothesis, inflammatory cells release proteases, elastases, collagenases, trypsin/chymotrypsin, and plasminogen activator–plasmin system, which damage both cells and ECM. In all cases the enzyme system has a corresponding inhibitor for regulation of its activity. The degree of proteolysis is determined by the granule content of PMNs, timing, location of proteases, substrates, and corresponding enzyme inhibitors.

Elastases. Leukocyte elastase is a serine protease that is released from PMN granules. It is bound by AM membrane and is secreted when the macrophage is activated. This enzyme can degrade a wide range of substrates including elastin, collagens, fibronectin, fibrinogen, factors VIII and XII, fibrin split products, and glycosaminoglycans. Alpha 1-antiprotease is the primary inhibitor of leukocyte elastase. This elastase is present in BAL fluid of patients with ARDS. Cathepsin L is a cysteine protease with elastolytic properties and an acid pH optimum that is also found in the leukocyte granule and macrophages.

Collagenases. The PMN granule also contains leukocyte collagenase, which is a metalloenzyme capable of degrading all collagen types and fibronectin.

Trypsin and Chymotrypsin. The trypsin activity can degrade type III collagen and cell surface glycoproteins. Leukocyte granules also contain chymotryptic activity, another serine protease, which degrades fibronectin and other glycoproteins. Elevated serum trypsin levels have been described in patients with severe acute pancreatitis and ARDS.

Plasmin-Plasminogen Activator-Inhibitor System. Plasminogen activators are involved in many cellular degradative processes and are distributed on many cell types. Plasminogen activators convert plasminogen to plasmin. Plasmin degrades fibrin and other proteins. There are two principal plasminogen activators: urokinase and tissue plasminogen activators.

Plasminogen activator is secreted as a 50,000-Dalton proenzyme. Many cell types possess surface receptors for proPA. Cells also synthesize several PA inhibitors. Type 1 is secreted by placenta, macrophages, and monocytes. Type 3 PA inhibitor is produced by fibroblasts. Types 1 and 2 are specific for PA. Type 3 also inhibits plasmin, thrombin, and trypsinlike proteases. It is believed that secreted PA binds to a plasma membrane receptor. After activation, PA triggers localized proteolysis of ECM, thus facilitating cell migration and lung remodeling. PA's binding receptor may protect the enzyme from its inhibitors. The AM contains a PA that is identical to urokinase and enhances elastolytic activity of AMs.

Products of the Fibrinolytic System

Diffuse intravascular coagulation with fibrinolysis often occurs during ARDS associated with trauma. It is associated with excessive formation of thrombin and plasmin in circulation. Platelet thrombi and microaggregates develop within lung microcirculation. Also during endotoxin-associated ARDS, activation of PMNs, AMs, and complement results in PMNs aggregation with release of PAF, endothelial cell injury, activation of blood-coagulating system and platelet microaggregation, and impaired clearance of activated blood products by the macrophage/monocyte system. Purified fibrinogen fragment D causes progressive complement depletion and pulmonary dysfunction, presumably via endothelial cell damage. Release of tissue factor at the site of injury may trigger the blood coagulation system in this form of ARDS. IL-1α and TNFα shift the fibrinolytic properties of endothelial cells by increasing plasminogen activator inhibitor-1 (PAI-1) production while leaving unchanged or decreasing tissue type plasminogen activator.

Factor XII is activated at the site of injury, and kallikrein is formed. Simultaneously, plasminogen is converted to plasmin, presumably by endothelial cell–derived PA. Alpha$_2$-macroglobulin and α_2-antiplasmin, which inhibit plasmin, are the protective mechanisms. When both inhibitors are overwhelmed, plasmin digests fibrinogen, fibrin, factor V, and factor VIII:C. Plasmin absorbed on fibrin surface is protected from both plasma inhibitors. Experimental data support possible toxic roles in the lung for fibrin(ogen) fragment D, fibrin peptide 6A, elastase or its fibrin(ogen) derivatives, kallikrein, and the platelet derivatives (thromboxane A$_2$ and lipoxygenase derivatives), and leukocyte-produced mediators (leukotrienes such as LTC$_4$ and LTD$_4$).

Tissue factor, which is an important initiator of the coagulation system, may play an important role in the formation of hyaline membranes. During severe ARDS intravascular and intraalveolar accumulation of fibrin and cellular debris occurs. Large amounts of tissue factor protein are present in normal lung parenchyma. During sepsis, expression of tissue factor protein and mRNA is enhanced. The majority of tissue factor positive cells are located at septal corners, suggesting that type II cells may be important for production of the tissue factor. LPS and inflammatory cytokine response elements have been demonstrated in promoter regions of tissue factor gene. LPS induction of tissue factor expression in human monocytes and endothelial cells is inhibited by immunosuppressive cytokines IL-4 and IL-10 by decreasing transcription of tissue factor.

Complement By-Products Hypothesis

Complement activation may play an important role in sepsis-induced lung damage. In septic shock and in an experimental model of sepsis, lung injury depends on complement activation and release of C5a, which is a chemotactic fragment. The C5a complement fragment may bind on surfaces of endothelial cells or on exposed endothelial cytoskeletal components, leading to further cellular and endothelial cell damage.

The C5, 6-9 complexes cause irreversible target cell membrane damage. Protective mechanisms against complement-mediated cell damage include C_1 inhibitors (C1-INH), (C4Bp)-C4 binding protein, and factor 1 (C4b-C3b inhibitors), which are regulators of the classic pathway. The C4a, 3a, and 5a anaphylatoxins cause smooth muscle contraction and increased production of factors H (B-H), P (properdin), and factor 1, which are regulators of the alternate pathway. The S protein and antithrombin III are modulators of the common pathway. In an experimental model of intraalveolar complement activation, complement activation was associated with induction of MIP-1α and NO_2/NO_3.

Platelets

Platelets play an important role in acute lung injury. Activated platelets express IL-1. Platelet-associated IL-1 induces endothelial cells to express leukocyte adhesion molecules and cytokines, with resultant amplification of the reaction.

Kininogen

Kinins cause marked permeability changes of the alveolar microvasculature. Proteases from human PMNs can generate kinins from kininogens. However, the exact enzyme responsible has not been established.

REPAIR MECHANISMS

Factors that determine the path of the repair process are only beginning to be elucidated. They include (1) severity and nature of the initial insult, (2) chronicity of the insult or superimposition of a second insult during the period of recovery from the initial injury, (3) cell-to-cell and cell-to-ECM interactions, (4) local effects caused by growth factors bound to ECM, (5) contributions of soluble growth factors secreted by inflammatory and parenchymal cells, (6) serum-derived growth factors, and (7) formation of cross-links of newly synthesized ECM components.

Normal Recovery From Acute Alveolar Injury

Repair of the lung epithelium requires remodeling of damaged basal lamina on which reorganization of cellular components and transformation of type II into type I cells occurs. Alveolar fluid is cleared by type II cells. Lung ECM provides a three-dimensional scaffold and boundaries along which reepithelialization occurs. Its constituents (e.g., glycosaminoglycans, collagens, laminin, fibronectin, and entactin) influence many cellular functions. Newly synthesized ECM components undergo normal cross-linking, thus forming stable structures. Structural microdomains, which exist beneath type I and II pneumocytes, are probably reestablished at this stage and may play a role in transformation of type II into type I cells.

Mesenchymal-epithelial interactions are important for normal lung development; their role during repair is speculative at present. Type II cells have basal processes with which they interact with interstitial cells. The processes are most frequent during periods of lung remodeling and rapid growth. Their role during repair is speculative at the present time. Current published evidence suggests that proliferative responses of alveolar epithelium and interstitium are interdependent. Their coordination results in normal repair, whereas their imbalance may result in a fibrotic response.

Alveolar macrophages phagocytize and break down cellular debris from sloughed epithelium. They synthesize and secrete numerous soluble growth factors, chemotactic factors, and cytokines that regulate cell proliferation and metabolic biosynthetic functions of lung cells. Cytokines secreted by mononuclear phagocytes attract inflammatory cells, mesenchymal, epithelial, and endothelial cells to injury sites and stimulate them to produce additional factors that may amplify the response. Responsiveness of the lung cells to the soluble factors is, in turn, regulated by the nature of the ECM that the cells are in contact with differentiation state and metabolic state of the cells. Monocyte phagocytes play a key role in repair responses as is demonstrated by the delayed wound healing that is observed in animal models with monocyte/macrophage depletion.

In vivo, IL-1, TGFβ, TNF, PDGF, and FGF are fibrogenic. In contrast, INFγ has a dual purpose: early in an inflammatory response it activates AMs, and later in the repair process it down-regulates collagen synthesis by transcriptional regulation of collagen mRNA.

Vascular Endothelial Growth Factor

Vascular endothelial growth factor (VEGF), a 46kDa protein related to PDGF, is mitogenic for vascular endothelium and has synergistic activity with TNFα in inducing procoagulant activity. In vitro, it promotes monocyte migration across endothelial monolayers. VEGF is believed to play an important role in regeneration of pulmonary capillary endothelium.

Pathologic Reparative Response to Lung Injury

Abnormal repair may occur when the lung's three-dimensional architecture is severely altered in the initial injury or ensuing response. Thus after oleic acid injury when lung basement membranes are preserved, normal healing occurs. When the basement membranes are damaged, however, lung repair results in scar formation. In bleomycin-induced lung injury, the intensity of chronic inflammation and fibrosis has been found to be directly related to the severity of acute lung injury.

The nature of injury is important. For example, intratracheal instillation of elastase results in emphysematous response, whereas instillation of collagenase does not heal with emphysema. Chronicity of the insult is also important. Thus while the same inflammatory mechanisms are believed to be involved in lung damage in ARDS that may not progress to fibrosis, chronic inflammatory responses are thought to result in the fibrotic reactions of idiopathic pulmonary fibrosis.

A second insult superimposed during the recovery phase may result in a fibrotic response. For example, after radiation-induced lung damage, administration of oxygen exacerbates the injury and may result in a fibrotic response. Similarly, patients with bleomycin-induced lung damage may worsen when they are concomitantly treated with oxygen, which presumably enhances oxidant damage.

Formation of cross-links of newly synthesized ECM is an important determinant of the course of repair. For example, intratracheal administration of cadmium chloride ($CdCl_2$) to Golden Syrian hamsters causes acute lung injury that results in fibrosis. However, when β-aminopropionitrile (BAPN), an inhibitor of lysyl oxidase, is simultaneously administered, bullous emphysema results. Lysyl oxidase is required for cross-linking of collagens and elastin during lung remodeling. Penicillamine similarly interferes with cross-linking of collagens and may prevent fibrotic lung reactions.

The exact molecular mechanisms that tip the balance toward normal, fibrotic, or emphysematous reparative responses in clinical settings are unknown at present; however, the general patterns tend to be (1) an initial inflammatory response and (2) a proliferative, migratory, and biosynthetic phase under the influence of ECM and soluble factors and cell-to-cell interactions. The transformation of the thickened alveolar epithelium into a normal respiratory surface occurs by differentiation of cuboidal type II cells into type I pneumocytes.

One of the mechanisms by which the inflammatory response and damage to ECM may influence repair is by recruitment of fibroblasts into the alveolar space. Fibroblast chemotaxis may be mediated by proteolytic products of ECM components such as collagens, tropoelastin, elastin, and fibronectin; peptides secreted by AMs, lymphocytes, and platelets; and LTB$_4$. Macrophages play key roles in repair processes of acute lung injury because they are capable of secreting factors that stimulate or inhibit proliferation of lung parenchymal cells (PDGF, TGFβ, PAF, IL-1α, and prostaglandin E$_2$ [PGE$_2$]). Macrophages may also regulate procoagulant activity of alveolar fluid and thus promote fibrin deposition in alveolar spaces. In chronic inflammatory states, the lymphocytes may produce factors that directly regulate lung parenchymal functions. Lung parenchymal cells may also produce factors that regulate immune responses or macrophage functions. For example, endothelial cells can secrete IL-1α, granulocyte monocyte colony—stimulating factor (GMCSF), and express MHC antigens.

The alveolar epithelial surface lining fluid is known to contain tissue factor and factor VII complexes and promotes coagulation of plasma. Thus exudation of plasma into the alveolar space, as occurs in ARDS, results in fibrin clot deposition in alveolar spaces. Crosslinking reactions mediated by factor XIIIa may also cross-link serum growth factors into fibrin clots, providing for their subsequent slow release during repair phases of the injury. For example, serum fibronectin can be cross-linked to fibrin by factor XIIIa and is a component of the "fibrin" clot. Fibronectin is an adhesive, chemoattractant, and proliferative factor for lung fibroblasts. It may stimulate fibroblasts to migrate from the lung interstitium through breaks in damaged alveolar basement membranes and enter into the alveolar spaces. The fibroblasts adhere and proliferate in the fibrin clots and, in severe cases, may obliterate the respiratory spaces. Thrombin, an enzyme that mediates conversion of fibrinogen to fibrin, is also a known mitogen. Potentially, thrombin may stimulate type II and other parenchymal cells to proliferate.

Although the initial response to acute lung injury is the same regardless of the nature of the insult, the outcome of the repair process may be either restoration of normal architecture, fibrotic reaction, or emphysema. Studies examining mechanisms of lung injury and repair at cellular and molecular levels may in the future permit the development of drug therapies targeting signal transduction mechanisms to minimize further lung damage and promote restoration of normal lung architecture and function.

BIBLIOGRAPHY

Bone RC et al: Adult respiratory distress syndrome: sequence and importance of development of multiple organ failure, *Chest* 101:320, 1992.

Clark EA, Brugge JS: Integrin and signal transduction pathways: the road taken, *Science* 268:233-239, 1995.

Crapo JD et al: Cell number and cell characteristics of normal human lung, *Am Rev Respir Dis* 125:740-745, 1982.

Kovacs E, DiPietro L: FIbrogenic-cytokines and connective tissue production, *FASEB J* 8:854-861, 1994.

Lwebuga-Mukasa JS: Matrix-driven pneumocyte differentiation, *Am Rev Respir Dis* 133:452, 1991.

Mackman N: Regulation of the tissue factor gene, *FASEB J* 9:883-889, 1995.

Meduri GU, Headley S, Tolley E et al: Plasma and BAL cytokine response to corticosteroid rescue treatment in late ARDS, *Chest* 108:1315-1325, 1995.

Meduri GU, Kohler G, Headley S et al: Inflammatory cytokines in the BAL of patients with ARDS. Persistent elevation over time predicts poor outcome, *Chest* 108:1303-1314, 1995.

Moncada S, Higgs A: The L-arginine-nitric oxide pathway, *N Engl J Med* 329:2002-2012, 1993.

Plow EF, Herren T, Redlitz A et al: The cell biology of the plasminogen system, *FASEB J* 9:939-945, 1995.

Raghow R: The role of extracellular matrix in post inflammatory wound healing and fibrosis, *FASEB J* 8:823-831, 1994.

Rosen GM, Pou S, Ramos CL et al: Free radicals and phagocytic cells, *FASEB J* 9:200-209, 1995.

Tomashefski JF Jr: Pulmonary pathology of the adult respiratory distress syndrome, *Clinic Chest Med* 11:593-619, 1990.

Ward PA: Oxygen radicals, cytokines, adhesion molecules and lung injury, *Environmental Health Perspectives* 102(suppl 10):13-16, 1994.

Wolpe SD, Cerami A: Macrophage inflammatory proteins 1 and 2: members of a novel superfamily of cytokines, *FASEB J* 3:2565, 1989.

II LABORATORY AND DIAGNOSTIC TESTS

CHAPTER

41 Pulmonary Function Testing

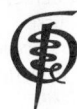

Jacob S.O. Loke

In the clinical evaluation of patients with cardiopulmonary disorders, pulmonary function tests can be used to separate patients with pulmonary abnormalities from those with cardiac diseases, noting that both cardiac and pulmonary diseases may coexist. The respiratory system consists of the respiratory center, the lung with its conducting system of the upper airway and the tracheobronchial tree (the gas-exchanging portion), and a ventilatory pump composed of the chest cage and the respiratory muscles. Malfunction of any part of the respiratory system can lead to pulmonary disease, and specific tests may be needed to detect these abnormalities.

Pulmonary function tests are used to objectively evaluate the patient with respiratory symptoms such as dyspnea. The patient may have psychosomatic complaints of dyspnea at rest and/or on exertion, and lung function tests are helpful in assessing whether the patient has obstructive or restrictive lung disease, or both, or normal lung function. This distinction is important because reassurance or anti-anxiety medication may be needed in those with a psychogenic respiratory disorder, whereas patients with a condition such as asthma may need bronchodilator therapy. In the latter, lung function tests are able to detect physiologic and abnormal changes in the respiratory system. In patients who use amiodarone for control of ventricular tachycardia or bleomycin for chemotherapy, lung function tests are able to detect pulmonary lung toxicity caused by these agents. Also, pulmonary function forms an integral part of the preoperative and functional assessment of the patient going for surgery. This is especially important in patients with significant bullous obstructive lung disease who will be undergoing bullectomy or lobectomy, or those undergoing pneumonectomy for lung cancer. In occupational lung disease and lung disability evaluation, lung function tests are useful for assessing decreased function and impairment. Finally, lung function tests have been used to evaluate the success of therapy, whether bronchodilator therapy in asthmatic patients or corticosteroid therapy in patients with sarcoidosis. It is important to note that the pulmonary abnormalities may not be present at rest but may be evident when lung function tests are performed during exercise and sleep. Patients may complain of dyspnea on exertion, and using the exercise test, exercise-induced asthma can be diagnosed. Similarly, in a patient who complains of hypersomnolence, sleep apnea, and cor pulmonale, obstructive or central sleep apnea may be demonstrated during the performance of a sleep study.

Pulmonary function tests that are available in a complete pulmonary function laboratory include the measurement of the following:

1. Nasal airway resistance to evaluate the patency of the nasal passages
2. Lung volumes to assess hyperinflation, air trapping, and restrictive ventilatory defect
3. Spirometry for assessing obstructive or restrictive processes
4. Single-breath diffusing capacity for obstructive and restrictive defects
5. Pulmonary mechanics (airway resistance, compliance—dynamic and static—maximal elastic recoil pressures, and pressure-volume curves) for obstructive and restrictive diseases
6. Maximal respiratory mouth pressures during expiration (PE$_{max}$), inspiration (PI$_{max}$), and transdiaphragmatic pressures (P$_{di}$) for assessing respiratory muscle function including the diaphragm

7. Spirometry before and after inhaled bronchodilator to assess reversibility of airway obstruction in patients with obstructive airway disease
8. Bronchoprovocation inhalation tests with nonspecific or specific agents to determine airway hyperreactivity and occupational asthma
9. Exercise testing to evaluate cardiopulmonary integrity and function
10. Arterial blood gases to assess the gas exchange properties of the lung (i.e., to detect hypoxia and/or hypoventilation and acid-base disturbances)
11. Ventilatory control studies such as ventilatory responses to hypoxia and hypercapnia to assess the respiratory control centers in patients with the pickwickian syndrome or Ondine's curse
12. Sleep studies to detect central or obstructive sleep apnea or sleep disturbance and to evaluate nocturnal oxygen therapy in patients with lung diseases.

SPIROMETRY

The lung has certain intrinsic properties, which include volume, elasticity, ventilatory ability, and gas exchange. Spirometry has been used to assess ventilatory ability. Also, one of the ways to detect airway obstruction is by measuring the forced expiratory volume in 1 second (FEV_1), the forced vital capacity (FVC), and the FEV_1/FVC ratio.

The FEV_1 and FVC can be determined with the patient exhaling into a water-sealed spirometer in which volume is measured against time (Fig. 41-1) or into a flow-volume device in which a pneumotachygraph with its associated circuits integrates flow into volume, and a flow-volume curve is generated (Fig. 41-2). The spirometer test requires a maximal effort during exhalation from total lung capacity. In obstructive airway disease, the FEV_1 is decreased more than the FVC so that the FEV_1/FVC ratio is less than 70%. The normal FEV_1/FVC ratio increases in children and young adults and decreases with age. Various criteria have been used to quantitate the severity of airway obstruction based on the predicted formula for FEV_1. When the FEV_1 is 65% to 79% of the predicted FEV_1, the airway obstruction is classified as mild; when it is 50% to 64% of predicted FEV_1, the airway obstruction is moderate, and when the FEV_1 is below 50% of predicted FEV_1, severe obstructive airway disease is present. These criteria are used when the FEV_1/FVC ratio is decreased and obstructive in nature. It should be noted, however, that in patients with asthma or lung disease who have significant coughing on exhalation, the FVC is underestimated or abruptly cut off because of coughing. Although the FEV_1 is decreased, the FEV_1/FVC may still be above 70%. A slow vital capacity (VC) maneuver should be performed, which may show an increase in slow VC compared with FVC, thus showing an abnormal FEV_1/FVC ratio. In addition, clinical correlation should be determined together with pulmonary function tests after inhaled bronchodilator therapy. Serial lung function tests may show an obstructive pattern later when the coughing episodes are resolved or diminished. The shape of the flow-volume curve is of value in assessing airway obstruction. The pattern of the airway obstruction can be caused by pressure limitation (Fig. 41-3, *A*) or volume-dependent limitation (Fig. 41-3, *B*). Expiratory wheeze caused by dynamic air compression can be heard during quiet or forced expiration on auscultation of the chest. For restrictive disease, FEV_1 and FVC decrease proportionally, but more so with the FVC such that the FEV_1/FVC is normal or increased.

From the spirometric studies, one can measure the flow rates at 25% to 75% ($FEF_{25\%-75\%}$) of the FVC. When the FEV_1, FVC, and FEV_1/FVC are normal, a decrease in forced expiratory flow at 25% to 75% of FVC (below 70% of predicted) indicates small airway disease, which is the earliest obstructive lung disease pattern seen in cigarette smokers. With the computer system available in most pulmonary function laboratories, the computer can digitize the flow at 50% of FVC from the spirometric tracing, enabling the flow rate at 50% of FVC ($\dot{V}_{max}$ 50) to be calculated without performing flow-volume curve studies. The decrease in $\dot{V}_{max}$ 50 below 70% of predicted in the presence of a normal FVC, FEV_1, and FEV_1/FVC ratio indicates mild obstructive lung disease of the small airways.

Other studies that have been used to assess small airway function include the closing volume, breathing air, and an 80% helium–20%

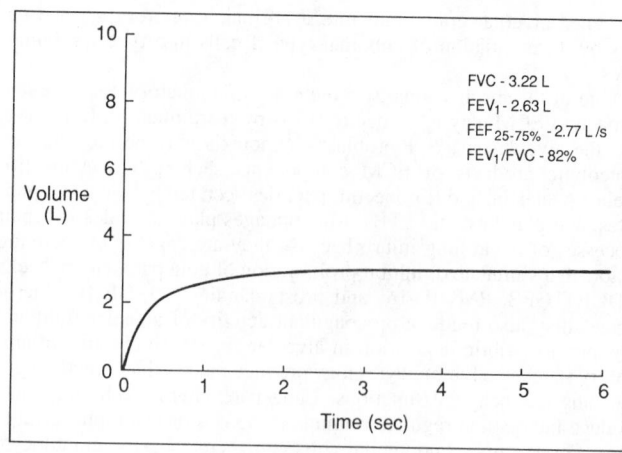

FIGURE 41-1   Normal spirogram in a 59-year-old white woman (154 cm in height). $FEF_{25\%-75\%}$, Forced midexpiratory flow (L/s) between 25% and 75% of the forced vital capacity (FVC); FEV_1, forced expiratory volume in 1 second.

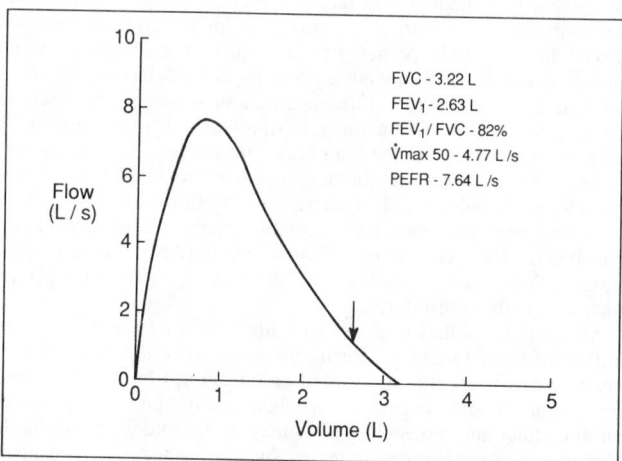

FIGURE 41-2   Normal maximal expiratory flow-volume curve study in a 59-year-old white woman (154 cm in height). *Small arrow,* Forced expiratory volume in 1 second (FEV_1) time marker; $\dot{V}_{MAX}$ 50, rate of air flow (L/s) at 50% of forced vital capacity (FVC); *PEFR,* peak expiratory flow rate in liters per second.

oxygen mixture for the flow-volume curve studies. These tests are generally investigational or research studies. The normal predictive range for pulmonary function test results, that is, spirometry, subdivisions of lung volume, single-breath diffusing capacity, is based on normal population studies. Generally, when the values are below 80% of predicted or above 120% of predicted (for total lung capacity [TLC] and residual volume [RV], the values are abnormal. However, the 95% confidence limits of a normal reference population may be a better way to assess the normal range. When one is evaluating results of pulmonary function tests, the predicted equations used in different pulmonary function laboratories should be considered. Also, predicted equations should be corrected for age, sex, and height, as well as for race because blacks and Asians have spirometry and lung volumes 15% lower than those of whites.

The maximal expiratory and inspiratory flow-volume curves are especially useful in detecting upper airway obstruction. Various types of upper airway obstruction can be elicited depending on the configuration of the flow-volume curves (Fig. 41-4). In fixed upper airway obstruction, the flow-volume curve shows a plateau in both the inspiratory and expiratory limb (Fig. 41-4, *A*). These upper airway obstructive lesions are caused by circumferential narrowings that are not influenced by intratracheal or extratracheal pressure changes. The constricted narrowed areas can be localized from the history or physi-

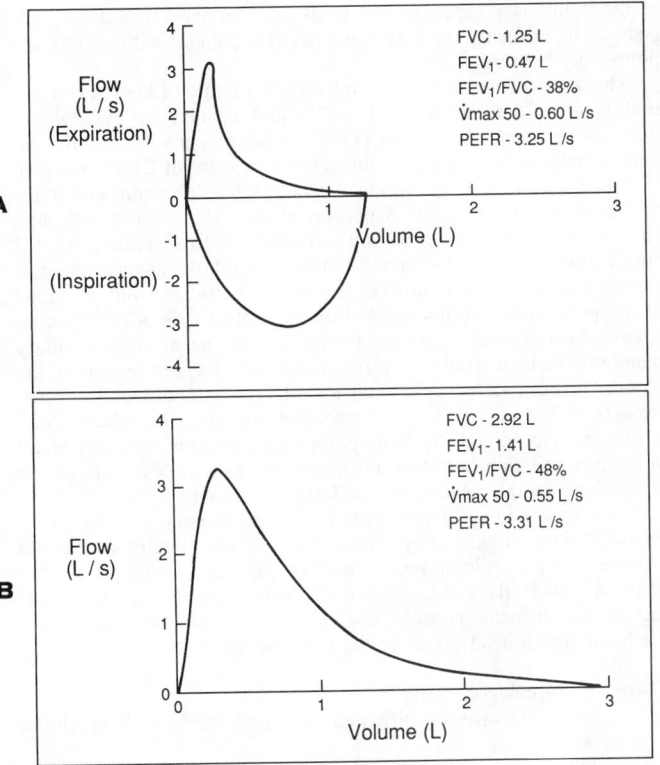

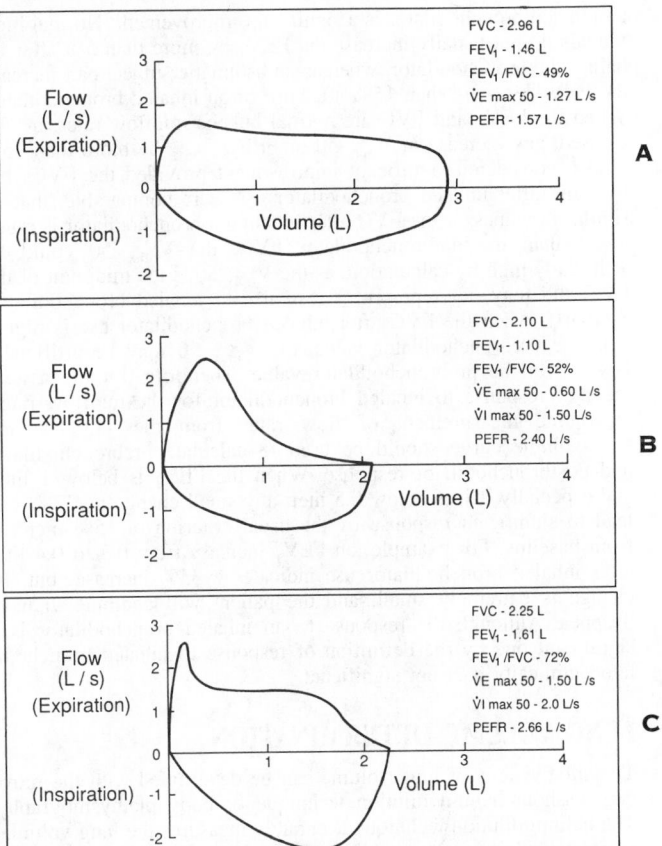

FIGURE 41-3   **A,** Pressure limitation maximal expiratory and inspiratory flow-volume curve study in a 65-year-old white man (173 cm in height) with severe obstructive airway disease. $\dot{V}_{MAX}$ *50,* Rate of air flow (L/s) at 50% of forced vital capacity (FVC); *PEFR,* peak expiratory flow rate in liters per second; *FEV₁,* forced expiratory volume in 1 second. **B,** Volume-dependent limitation maximal expiratory flow-volume curve study in a 62-year-old white man (161 cm in height) with moderate obstructive airway disease. $\dot{V}_{max}$ *50,* Rate of air flow (L/s) at 50% of forced vital capacity (FVC); *PEFR,* peak expiratory flow rate in liters per second; *FEV₁,* forced expiratory volume in 1 second.

FIGURE 41-4   **A,** Maximal expiratory and inspiratory flow-volume curve study in a 52-year-old black man who has obstructive airway disease in addition to fixed upper airway obstruction. $\dot{V}E_{max}$ *50,* Rate of air flow (L/s) at 50% of forced vital capacity (FVC) during expiration; *PEFR,* peak expiratory flow rate in liters per second; *FEV₁,* forced expiratory volume in 1 second. **B,** Maximal expiratory and inspiratory flow-volume curve study in a 77-year-old white man who has obstructive airway disease in addition to a variable extrathoracic upper airway obstruction caused by a thyroid carcinoma with tracheal compression. $\dot{V}E_{max}$ *50,* Air flow rate at 50% of forced vital capacity (FVC) during expiration; $\dot{V}I_{max}$ *50,* air flow rate at 50% of FVC during inspiration; *PEFR,* peak expiratory flow rate in liters per second; *FEV₁,* forced expiratory volume in 1 second. **C,** Maximal expiratory and inspiratory flow-volume curve study in a 69-year-old black woman who has a retrosternal goiter and a variable intrathoracic upper airway obstruction. $\dot{V}E_{max}$ *50,* Rate of air flow (L/s) at 50% of forced vital capacity (FVC) during expiration; $\dot{V}I_{max}$ *50,* rate of air flow (L/s) at 50% of FVC during inspiration; *PEFR,* peak expiratory flow rate in liters per second; *FEV₁* forced expiratory volume in 1 second.

cal examination or by performing a fiberoptic bronchoscopic examination. At times, the patient may present with stridor, and the flow-volume curve is still normal in configuration. A critical narrowing of the trachea has to be attained in some cases before the plateau pattern is evident on flow-volume curve.

Variable Extrathoracic Upper Airway Obstruction

The suprasternal notch is used to separate extrathoracic upper airway obstruction from intrathoracic upper airway obstruction. Any lesion (enlarged tonsils, goiter) that occurs in the upper airway and trachea above the suprasternal notch is extrathoracic in origin and may produce a plateau pattern on the inspiratory loop (Fig. 41-4, *B*). During inspiration the intratracheal pressure is less than the atmospheric pressure around the neck and leads to compression of the upper airway obstruction. During exhalation, the intratracheal pressures are greater than the atmospheric pressure, and, therefore, there is no limitation of airflow. The ratio of flow at 50% FVC during expiration ($\dot{V}E_{max}$ 50) and flow at 50% FVC during inspiration ($\dot{V}I_{max}$ 50), that is, $\dot{V}E_{max}$ 50/$\dot{V}I_{max}$ 50 is greater than 1.

Variable Intrathoracic Upper Airway Obstruction

Obstructive lesions in the tracheobronchial tree that are below the suprasternal notch give rise to a plateau pattern during expiration. During inspiration, the intrapleural pressure is negative relative to the tracheal lumen, and the caliber of the tracheal lumen increases. During forced exhalation, the positive intrapleural pressure is greater than the intratracheal pressure, leading to tracheal narrowing. The ratio of

$\dot{V}E_{max}$ 50/$\dot{V}I_{max}$ 50 is less than 1. During a routine spirometric test, variable intrathoracic upper airway obstruction or fixed upper airway obstruction can be suspected when the FEV₁, FVC, midflow rates, and FEV₁/FVC ratio are normal but there is a significant decrement in peak flow rate such that the FEV₁(ml)/peak flow (liters per minute) is greater than 10 (normal, <10). A flow-volume curve study during inspiration and expiration is requested to further document the variable or fixed pattern of upper airway obstruction.

INHALED BRONCHODILATOR STUDIES

Bronchial asthma, asthmatic bronchitis, viral upper respiratory tract infection, chronic obstructive pulmonary disease (COPD), occupational asthma, and psychogenic vocal cord dysfunction are some of the causes of reversible airway disease. To evaluate the reversibility of airway obstruction, one gives an inhaled bronchodilator—isoproterenol or metaproterenol (two puffs)—and assesses again the spirometric findings of FEV₁, FVC, and $\dot{V}_{max}$ 50 or FEF₂₅%₋₇₅%. The most reliable parameter for the response to inhaled bronchodilator is the FEV₁. A 15% increase in FEV₁ from the baseline value after use of an inhaled bronchodilator is a significant improvement. Normal individuals do not usually increase the FEV$_1$ by more than 5% after inhaling the bronchodilator, whereas an asthmatic subject can increase the FEV$_1$ by more than 15% after use of an inhaled bronchodilator. When the FEV$_1$ and FVC are normal but the midflow rates are decreased, any increase in $\dot{V}_{max}$ 50 or FEF$_{25\%-75\%}$ by more than 15% is also considered significant improvement provided the FVCs before and after inhaled bronchodilator use were comparable, that is, similar in values. If the FVC after inhaling a bronchodilator is much lower than the prebronchodilator FVC, the $\dot{V}_{max}$ 50 could be artificially high by calculation, as the $\dot{V}_{max}$ 50 is the midpoint of the FVC and may not represent a response to inhaled bronchodilator. Similarly, when the FVC after inhaled bronchodilator use is higher than the prebronchodilator value, the $\dot{V}_{max}$ 50 may be artificially lower than the prebronchodilator value. Therefore, for the assessment of response to inhaled bronchodilator for the midflow rates, isovolume measurement of flow rates from the TLC on the flow-volume curve should be used to calculate prebronchodilator and postbronchodilator response. When the FEV$_1$ is below 1 liter, and especially if it is below 0.5 liter, any small change in FEV$_1$ can lead to significant response by the usual criterion of 15% increase from baseline. For example, an FEV$_1$ increase from 0.3 to 0.4 liter after inhaled bronchodilator use indicates a 33% increase, but the change is extremely small, and the patient will continue to have dyspnea. Although the response to an inhaled bronchodilator is a significant one by the definition of response to inhaled bronchodilator, clinically it is not significant.

LUNG VOLUME DETERMINATION

The subdivisions of lung volume can be determined with the nitrogen washout–helium dilution technique or body plethysmography. The helium dilution technique accurately measures the lung volumes when there is no evidence of significant airway obstruction. In patients with obstructive lung disease, the helium dilution technique may underestimate lung volume because of poor mixing or inhomogeneity of gases in the lungs. However, the body plethysmograph determines intrathoracic lung volume whether or not the airways or alveoli are in communication with the other airways, and this is a more accurate way of determining the functional residual capacity. In patients with emphysema, there is usually hyperinflation and air trapping manifested by an increase (above 120% of predicted) in functional residual capacity (FRC) and RV, respectively. In contrast, for patients with restrictive ventilatory defect, TLC decreases and is classified as mild when TLC is between 66% and 81% of predicted, moderate when 51% to 65% of predicted, and severe when less than 51% of predicted value. In restrictive disease when the FEV$_1$/FVC is normal or increased, the increase in RV may be caused by muscle weakness and not to air trapping per se. In the presence of a normal TLC, FRC, RV, and FEV$_1$/FVC ratio, a decrease in FVC suggests also a restrictive process. The flow-volume curve shows a characteristic curve for restrictive process. Initially, the flow rates are increased with an increase in FEV$_1$/FVC ratio caused by an increase in elastic recoil in patients with interstitial lung disease or pulmonary fibrosis. Subsequently, with progressive increase in the restrictive process, the FEV$_1$, peak flow, and midflow rates are also decreased significantly, but the FEV$_1$/FVC ratio is normal or increased. When the TLC is decreased significantly together with a decrease in the FEV$_1$/FVC ratio, then both a restrictive and obstructive disease process exists.

It has also been shown that an isolated decrease in RV in the subdivisions of lung volume may indicate a restrictive intrathoracic process whether it is caused by lymphoma, cardiomegaly, or pleural disease.

SINGLE-BREATH DIFFUSING CAPACITY

The single-breath diffusing capacity is useful to assess occupational and interstitial lung disease, pulmonary vascular disease, and the effects of certain drugs (such as amiodarone and bleomycin) or after chemotherapeutic agents that can affect the interstitial portion of the lung. Also it is of value in emphysema with destruction of the pulmonary parenchyma and loss of the pulmonary capillary bed. Because diffusing capacity is related to the capillary blood volume, any loss

of the pulmonary capillary bed leads to a decrease in diffusing capacity. The diffusing capacity is increased in patients with asthma and pulmonary hemorrhage.

The test involves the patient inhaling a mixture of known concentration of air, carbon monoxide (CO), and an inert gas such as helium (He) or neon (Ne). After certain respiratory maneuvers, the patient exhales to RV and then inhales the mixture of 21.5% oxygen, 68.3% nitrogen, 0.295% carbon monoxide, 9.9% helium, and holds the breath for 10 seconds. A portion of the exhalation is collected, and concentrations of the carbon monoxide and the helium exhaled are measured. During the breath-holding period, the concentration of carbon monoxide in the lung decreases as it "diffuses" into the blood in the pulmonary capillaries. A diffusion defect was originally considered to assess an increase in thickness of the alveolar capillary membrane, which would lead to a decrease in oxygen tension in the blood. Diffusion defect is not considered to be a major factor in causing arterial hypoxemia. Other factors that can affect the values of diffusing capacity include the hemoglobin concentration, capillary blood volume, ventilation-perfusion mismatch, the ratio of alveolar volume to capillary blood volume, and carboxyhemoglobin.

An increase in diffusing capacity is seen in patients with an increase in hemoglobin concentration or an increase in pulmonary blood volume. The hemoglobin level should be determined with the test because anemia leads to a decrease in diffusing capacity. Before assuming that the diffusing capacity is abnormal, it should be corrected for the hemoglobin level given by the formula:

Corrected diffusing capacity =
$$\text{uncorrected diffusing capacity}/0.06965 \times \text{hemoglobin}$$

Smokers have higher carboxyhemoglobin levels in the blood than nonsmokers, and the single-breath diffusing capacity assumes that the carbon monoxide tension in pulmonary capillaries is zero. Therefore, without correcting for carboxyhemoglobin, the diffusing capacity may still be normal when it is above 70% of predicted, in contrast to the above 80% of predicted for nonsmokers. Our normal predicted equations for single-breath diffusing capacity include smokers and nonsmokers.

The diffusing capacity in patients with restrictive lung disease such as interstitial fibrosis is decreased. This decrease is associated with a decrease in TLC and vital capacity (VC) and a normal or increased FEV$_1$/FVC. In contrast, patients with restrictive disease caused by chest cage weakness or weakness of the respiratory muscles may have a decrease in TLC and VC and a normal or increased FEV$_1$/FVC ratio, but the diffusing capacity is normal.

The typical patterns of lung function tests in patients with restrictive or obstructive disease or both are shown in Table 41-1.

SPECIAL PULMONARY STUDIES
Ventilatory Control Studies

In a patient with pulmonary hypertension and heart failure or alveolar hypoventilation in the absence of lung disease, abnormalities in the respiratory control center should be suspected. Patients with primary alveolar hypoventilation (Ondine's curse) have no abnormalities in their lungs. Spirometry determinations of lung volumes and diffusing capacity in these patients are normal. However, one can detect the alveolar hypoventilation by performing an arterial blood gas analysis, which shows alveolar hypoventilation with a normal alveolar-arterial oxygen difference. Also, when one asks the patient to hyperventilate voluntarily, an increase in arterial oxygen tension (Pao$_2$) and a decrease in arterial carbon dioxide tension (Paco$_2$) occurs. Also, arterial oxygen saturation determined noninvasively with the pulse oximeter increases when the patient hyperventilates. When the patient inhales a 5% carbon dioxide and 95% oxygen mixture using a rebreathing technique for the ventilatory response to hypercapnia, the response of ventilation is blunted or absent, with progressive increase in end-tidal Pco$_2$. In normal individuals, there is a 2- to 3-liter increase in minute ventilation per 1 mm Hg change in end-tidal Pco$_2$. With regard to the ventilatory response to hypoxia, the patient breathes ambient air in a spirometer using the rebreathing technique. The rise in end-tidal Pco$_2$ is maintained at an isocapnic level of approximately 40 mm Hg by a carbon dioxide absorber. A pulse oximeter is used to assess oxygen saturation with progressive depletion of

Table 41-1 Patterns of pulmonary function abnormalities in various pulmonary diseases

PATTERNS OF ABNORMALITIES	VC	RV	TLC	FEV₁/FVC	D_LCO
Obstructive	N or ↓	N or ↑	N or ↑	↓	N or ↑
Asthma	N or ↓	N or ↑	N	↓	N
Chronic bronchitis	N or ↓	↑	↑	↓	↓
Emphysema	N or ↓	↑	↑	↓	↓
Restrictive	↓	↓	↓	N or ↑	↓
Pulmonary parenchyma	↓	↓	↓	N	N
Extrapulmonary	↓	↓	↓	↓	N or ↓
Restrictive and obstructive diseases	↓	N or ↓	↓		

VC, vital capacity; *RV*, residual volume; *TLC*, total lung capacity; *FEV₁*, forced expiratory volume in 1 second; *FVC*, forced vital capacity; *D_LCO*, diffusing capacity of carbon monoxide; *N*, normal; ↓, decreased; ↑, increased.

oxygen in the system as a result of the rebreathing maneuvers. When the ventilatory response is plotted against oxygen saturation, a linear relationship is found. Normally a 0.6 liter increase in minute ventilation occurs per 1% change in oxygen saturation. In patients with respiratory center abnormalities, the ventilatory response to hypoxia is blunted or absent. Subjects who have had removal of carotid bodies for treatment of asthma can also have a blunted ventilatory response to hypoxia.

The ventilatory response of breathing when there is a progressive decrease in arterial oxygen tension or hypoxia is a curvilinear one, but when oxygen saturation is plotted against ventilation, a linear relationship results. In patients with severe obstructive lung disease, the ventilatory response to hypercapnia and hypoxia may not be determined because of the mechanical abnormalities of the lung, which can produce a limitation in the ventilatory response. The occlusion pressure during the first 100 msec of inspiration has been used to assess the respiratory center output in these patients with lung disease.

Bronchoprovocation Inhalation Tests

The indications for bronchoprovocation inhalation tests are a clinical suspicion of hyperreactive airways, atypical presentation of asthma, and occupational asthma. Patients may have cough, dyspnea, and chest tightness and yet have normal pulmonary function tests at rest. Although abnormal lung function tests can be documented in the workplace, normal lung function tests may be found away from the working environment. The two types of bronchoprovocation inhalation tests are specific antigen challenge tests and nonspecific bronchial challenge tests. For the former, the particular agent that is producing the occupational asthma is given to the patient to inhale. With the specific challenge tests, the patient should be observed in a hospital environment for 24 hours because there may be an immediate reaction followed by a delayed reaction in the decrement of pulmonary function tests being monitored. The provocation dose is the dose of the agent that produces a decrease in FEV₁ by 20% or more from baseline. It is also known as PD₂₀(FEV₁).

In the nonspecific bronchial inhalation tests, methacholine or histamine is inhaled periodically at increasing concentrations, and the FEV₁ and FVC are monitored. In normal individuals, there is no decrease in FEV₁ below 20% of baseline values with the inhalation of the highest concentration of methacholine. In contrast, those patients with occupational asthma (symptomatic) or asthma usually react at a low concentration of methacholine. Because the methacholine test is a nonspecific bronchoprovocation test used to detect hyperreactivity of the airways, a negative test does not rule out a positive test with a specific antigen or agent to which the patient is allergic in the workplace.

Bronchodilator therapy, coffee or tea, and β-blockers should not be taken before the nonspecific bronchoprovocation tests to avoid false-negative or false-positive tests.

Clinical Exercise Tests

Exercise testing is useful in the evaluation of patients with dyspnea, with or without cardiopulmonary disease. Because of somatic complaints of dyspnea on exertion in an individual with a normal lung function test, an exercise test can be used to evaluate the cardiorespiratory responses to exercise. If one uses either a treadmill or bicycle ergometer for the exercise test, the blood pressure, heart rate (HR), electrocardiogram (ECG), ventilation, tidal volume, respiratory rate, carbon dioxide production, oxygen consumption, and oxygen saturation can be measured. The normal response of the cardiovascular system to progressive incremental exercise is an appropriate increase in HR and blood pressure reaching a targeted HR of close to 90% of the predicted maximal HR given by the formula $(210 - 0.65 \times \text{age})$. There should be no exertional hypotension or significant increase in diastolic blood pressure above 90 mm Hg or ECG changes suggestive of S-T segment depression or ischemia. The oxygen consumption at maximal exercise ($\dot{V}O_{2max}$) should be normal, and the slope of the $\dot{V}O_2/HR$ should be normal. $\dot{V}O_2/HR$ is also known as oxygen pulse. The $\dot{V}O_{2max}$ is increased in athletes and in fit individuals. It is decreased in unfit persons and decreased markedly in patients with significant cardiovascular disease or congestive heart failure. Also, the $\dot{V}O_{2max}$ is decreased in subjects with pulmonary disease. In a normal individual, the cardiovascular system and not the pulmonary system is the main limiting factor of exercise performance.

Associated with the gradual increase in HR during exercise in a normal individual is an appropriate increase in minute ventilation (i.e., tidal volume × respiratory rate). The maximal minute ventilation that can be achieved with maximal exercise is about 60% of the estimated maximal voluntary ventilation (MVV) (based on the FEV₁ × 35). Therefore for a person with an FEV₁ of 3 liters, the estimated MVV is approximately 105 liters. There should be no oxygen desaturation with exercise, and if the subject achieves a maximal minute ventilation, which is approximately 60% of the estimated MVV, then some ventilatory reserve for exercise exists. In an individual with a normal lung function test, an abnormal exercise test (in the absence of exercise-induced bronchospasm) may indicate cardiovascular abnormalities, especially if the $\dot{V}O_2$ is significantly decreased and associated with ischemic changes in ECG or exertional hypotension, and the ventilatory limitation was not reached.

In patients with obstructive lung disease, exercise tests may show that the targeted maximal HR is not attained but that the patient may reach maximal ventilation as shown by the maximal ventilation ($\dot{V}E_{max}$)–estimated MVV ratio, that is $\dot{V}E_{max}/\text{MVV} \times 100\%$ approaching or greater than 100%, and thus indicates ventilatory limitation. In patients with obstructive lung disease, the estimated MVV is given by the formula FEV₁ × 40. In COPD patients the anaerobic threshold is usually not reached, the $\dot{V}O_2$ is described as peak $\dot{V}O_2$ and not $\dot{V}O_{2max}$, and the peak $\dot{V}O_2$ is low. Also, oxygen desaturation can be seen if there is significant oxygen desaturation (below 90%) at a low exercise workload. This type of patient may need to receive supplemental nasal oxygen therapy with exercise.

In restrictive interstitial lung disease, exercise tests are useful to determine the work capacity and degree of oxygen desaturation. The patient can be ventilatory limited or may show significant oxygen desaturation before reaching ventilatory limitation. There is a decrease in the tidal volume response with the exercise because of the restrictive process, and this is associated with an inappropriate increase in respiratory rate to compensate for the blunted tidal volume response. Oxygen therapy is valuable in interstitial lung disease patients with significant oxygen desaturation to prevent the complications of pulmonary hypertension associated with hypoxia. Assessment can be done with serial exercise tests to determine the effect of corticosteroid or cyclophosphamide therapy.

The majority of patients with end-stage chronic obstructive lung disease may not be able to tolerate an exercise test on the treadmill or bicycle ergometer. Instead, a walking test of 2-, 6-, and 12-minute duration can be performed with monitoring of oxygen saturation with a portable pulse oximeter. If the patient shows significant oxygen desaturation below 85% while ambulating on a level surface for short distances, oxygen therapy is warranted, and the amount of oxygen therapy can be assessed by repeating the walking test to ensure an adequate oxygen saturation with the required nasal oxygen concentration.

Sleep Studies

Patients with COPD may have relatively normal Po_2 and Pco_2 at rest when the arterial blood gases are performed. During sleep, however, they may show significant oxygen desaturation. The oxygen desaturation is associated with pulmonary hypertension and can aggravate their COPD, leading them to seek medical help for their dyspnea. Thus sleep studies with monitoring of oxygen saturation provide us with the oxygenation status of patients with COPD. The use of oxygen therapy for prevention of oxygen desaturation or hypoxia has been shown in the nocturnal oxygen therapy trial studies in the United States and in the Medical Research Council studies in England to increase the survival of COPD patients with hypoxia.

The other major disease category for which sleep studies are indicated is the sleep apnea syndrome, whether central or obstructive sleep apnea (see Chapters 36 and 67).

A sleep study includes monitoring of stages of sleep, oral and nasal airflow, and ECG. By assessing the oral and nasal airflow and the rib cage and abdominal movements, obstructive or central types of sleep apnea syndrome can be diagnosed. Significant oxygen desaturation can occur with obstructive or central sleep apnea. Therapy can be directed at obstructive sleep apnea by using nasal continuous positive airway pressure (CPAP), thus improving the oxygen saturation as well as their sleep pattern or stages of sleep. Sleep studies can also be used to evaluate narcolepsy and myoclonus (see Chapters 36 and 166).

BIBLIOGRAPHY

American Thoracic Society: Evaluation of impairment/disability secondary to respiratory disorder, *Am Rev Respir Dis* 133:1205, 1986.

Bates DV: *Respiratory function in disease,* ed 3, Philadelphia, 1989, WB Saunders.

Clausen JL, editor: *Pulmonary function testing. Guidelines and controversies,* Orlando, 1984, Grune & Stratton.

Forster II RE et al: *The lung. Physiologic basis of pulmonary function tests,* ed 3, Chicago, 1986, Year Book.

Jones NL: *Clinical exercise testing,* ed 3, Philadelphia, 1988, WB Saunders.

Kryger MH, Roth T, Dement WC: *Principles and practice of sleep medicine,* Philadelphia, 1989, WB Saunders.

Miller A, editor: *Pulmonary function tests. A guide for the student and house officer,* Orlando, 1987, Grune & Stratton.

Morris AH et al: *Clinical pulmonary function testing. A manual of uniform laboratory procedures,* Salt Lake City, 1984, Intermountain Thoracic Society.

Wilson AF, editor: *Pulmonary function testing. Indications and interpretations,* Orlando, 1985, Grune & Stratton.

CHAPTER

42   Invasive Diagnostic Techniques

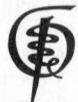

John A. Rankin

Clinicians have at their disposal several procedures for the diagnosis of pulmonary disease. They range from the essentially noninvasive analysis of expectorated sputum to the significantly invasive open lung biopsy via thoracotomy. A diagnostic evaluation/algorithm (Fig. 42-1) lists the separate techniques and the approximate order in which these procedures are performed in the evaluation of a patient with intrathoracic disease. Of course, every patient is unique and the art of medicine entails weighing the risks and benefits of a particular procedure with the likelihood of the procedure's yielding a diagnosis, when considering any or all of these procedures.

SPUTUM EXAMINATION

Examination of an expectorated sputum sample is one of the easiest and most cost-effective analyses to perform in evaluating suspected pulmonary disease. Although the retrieval and examination of expectorated sputum is not an invasive diagnostic technique, aspects of its examination not covered elsewhere in this text are discussed here. Either direct wet-mount examination of unstained sputum or the examination of a specimen stained with any of a variety of techniques (Chapter 233) can yield valuable and occasionally diagnostic information. For a wet-mount examination, a thin layer of freshly expectorated sputum is smeared on a slide, protected with a cover slip, and viewed under a microscope. The presence of large numbers of eosinophils (more than 20% to 30%) suggests atopic or parasitic disease. Some find it easier to identify eosinophils and perform a more accurate differential cell count on a Wright-Giemsa–stained specimen (Chapter 233). Additional findings supportive of asthma include the presence of Charcot-Leyden crystals, which are formed by the crystalization of eosinophil lysophospholipase; Curschmann's spirals, which are bronchiolar casts; and Creola bodies, which are composed of exfoliated epithelial cells.

The diagnosis of a specific bacterial pneumonia based on the presence or absence of bacteria and neutrophils in a Gram stain of a sputum specimen is subject to many pitfalls and consequently must be made with caution. The diagnosis of pneumonia caused by a specific etiologic agent can be made with certainty from a sputum sample only when the organism present in sputum is not part of the normal host oral flora and is not known to colonize the upper or lower respiratory tracts of subjects without pneumonia.

In some instances the induction of a sputum sample is helpful in establishing the etiology of suspected pulmonary pathology. This is especially true for patients who may have *Pneumocystis carinii* pneumonia complicating the acquired immunodeficiency syndrome (Chapters 248 and 280). A careful protocol has been worked out that has a sensitivity as high as 70%. Patients are allowed nothing by mouth for several hours and then prepped by brushing their teeth and gums and by washing their mouth several times with sterile saline or water. An ultrasonically generated mist of 3% saline is inhaled for approximately 10 to 15 minutes to induce cough and sputum production. The expectorated specimen then is liquefied using dithiothreitol and concentrated before making a slide to stain for the presence of *Pneumocystis* organisms.

Sputum also may be examined for the presence of malignant cells. If a sample cannot be delivered immediately for cytologic examination, it should be expectorated directly into a fixative solution. This procedure permits optimal preservation of cell morphology and helps maximize the positivity rate. As a general rule, the volume of sputum should not exceed the volume of fixative. If a patient is not spontaneously producing sputum, inhalation of an ultrasonically generated mist may induce cough and sputum production and thereby enhance the yield. It is important to note that the finding of malignant cells in sputum is not necessarily diagnostic of lung carcinoma, as their presence may be caused by malignancy in respiratory passages above the vocal cords. In general, sputum cytologic examination has a sensitivity of approximately 30% to 50% in patients with centrally located tumors. The yield of sputum examination from patients with lung lesions located in the peripheral airways is significantly less. Examination of three to five specimens appears to maximize the yield in all instances. In view of the ease with which sputum may be obtained and the relatively low cost, cytologic examination is still regarded as the first step in the evaluation of a patient with suspected lung malignancy.

Alveolar macrophages with large cytoplasmic vacuoles can be seen in patients with lipoid pneumonia resulting from aspirating oily substances such as mineral oil or oil-based nose drops. The presence of fat in the alveolar macrophage vacuoles can be confirmed by us-

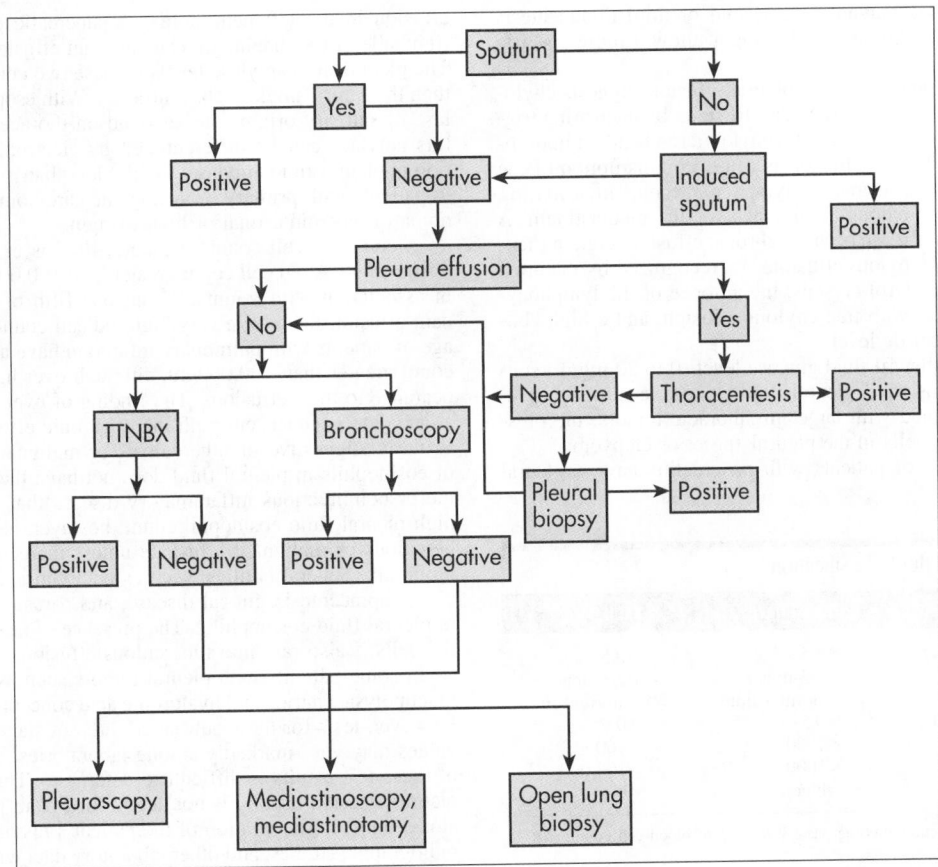

FIGURE 42-1   Diagnostic evaluation algorithm.

ing a Sudan stain. A positive Sudan stain, however, is not pathognomonic of lipoid pneumonia or of fat embolism, since sudanophilic cytoplasmic inclusions may be of endogenous origin.

THORACENTESIS

The space separating the visceral pleura and the parietal pleura normally contains several ml of fluid. The parietal pleura is perfused by systemic arterial vessels with a mean capillary pressure of 30 cm H_2O. The visceral pleura is perfused by vessels of the pulmonary circulation with a mean capillary pressure of 11 cm H_2O. The 19 cm difference in hydrostatic pressure normally causes fluid to enter the pleural space from the parietal pleura and to be reabsorbed by the visceral pleura. Cells and macromolecules return to the circulation via the lymphatics. A variety of disorders can disrupt the normal equilibrium of transudation and reabsorption and lead to accumulation of a pleural effusion. Alterations in hydrostatic pressures, obstruction of lymphatic drainage, reduction in osmotic pressure, or changes in capillary permeability from inflammation or tumor invasion can result in fluid accumulation. Thus pleural effusion can be a sign of either intrathoracic or extrathoracic disease. Thoracentesis, aspiration of pleural fluid for symptomatic relief and/or analysis, sometimes yields a specific diagnosis but often just narrows the diagnostic possibilities.

Conditions that alter the vascular and osmotic pressure without directly involving the pleura itself, such as heart failure, nephrotic syndrome, myxedema, and cirrhosis, cause a transudative fluid to accumulate.

Conditions associated with inflammation of the pleura such as tumor, connective tissue disease, trauma, and infection cause the accumulation of an exudative fluid. Criteria based on the pleural fluid protein concentration and pleural fluid lactic dehydrogenase concentration allow the differentiation of exudates and transudates (Table 42-1). In exudates the pleural fluid protein/serum protein concentration

ratio is greater than 0.5. The pleural fluid lactic dehydrogenase concentration to serum lactic dehydrogenase concentration ratio is greater than 0.6, and the absolute pleural fluid lactic dehydrogenase concentration is greater than two thirds of the upper limit of normal. Pleural fluid meeting any one of these three criteria qualifies as an exudate. White blood cell count (WBC), red blood cell count (RBC), and glucose determinations tend to be as shown in Table 42-1 but are not included in the separation of transudative and exudative effusions. Thoracentesis should be performed in any patient with a pleural effusion of unknown cause. The only major exception is a patient with clinical findings of congestive heart failure whose effusion decreases with appropriate therapy. With the initial diagnostic aspiration, no more than 1 liter should be removed. Acute pulmonary edema and hypotension have been reported after removal of larger quantities.

Information useful in the diagnosis of a pleural effusion is summarized in Box 42-1. Two findings on analysis of the effusion can yield a specific etiologic diagnosis. A positive smear and/or culture for bacteria, fungi, or mycobacteria has clinical importance since the pleural space is normally sterile. In a patient with a pneumonic process and a pleural effusion, culture of the effusion provides a reliable means of identifying the pathogen. Only one third of patients with a tuberculous pleural effusion have a positive culture of the fluid. Pleural biopsy for microscopic examination and culture increases the diagnostic yield to almost 70%.

A positive cytology is a second specific diagnostic aid from pleural fluid examination. For patients with malignant effusions, one third to two thirds have positive cytologic findings in their initial pleural fluid examination. The incidence of a positive cytology increases with the volume of fluid analyzed. Thus up to 90% of malignant effusions can be confirmed cytologically if three separate pleural fluid specimens are analyzed. Inflammation can cause bizarre mesothelial cell changes that can be confused with neoplastic changes. Also, in patients with large, long-standing neoplastic effusions, the free malignant cells in the effusion can degenerate in vivo with time and prevent definitive cytologic diagnosis. A second or third thoracentesis specimen containing freshly shed cells might allow a more specific diagnosis.

A milky or creamy appearance to pleural effusion suggests chylothorax, which can be confirmed by Sudan III stain, by measuring triglyceride levels, and by the presence of a chylomicron band on lipoprotein electrophoresis. Chylous effusion is caused by disruption of the thoracic duct resulting from trauma, lymphoma, tumor invasion, or, less commonly, granulomatous involvement of the mediastinum. A pseudochylous appearance can occur in chronic effusion (e.g., in rheumatoid disease). Pseudochylous effusions are recognized by the presence of rhomboid cholesterol crystals, the absence of the lymphocytosis seen in association with true chylous effusion, and a high cholesterol but low triglyceride level.

An extremely low pleural fluid glucose level (0 to 20 mg/dl) suggests a rheumatoid effusion. A pleural fluid glucose level of 20 to 40 mg/dl is commonly noted with large intrathoracic tumors, the presence of free malignant cells in the pleural space, or empyema.

Approximately 10% of patients with pancreatitis have a pleural

Table 42-1 Pleural fluid classification

	TRANSUDATE	EXUDATE
Pleural TP/Serum TP	<0.5	>0.5
LDH	<2/3 upper normal limit	>2/3 upper normal limit
Pleural LDH/Serum LDH	>0.6	>0.6
WBC	<1000	>1000
RBC	<1000	>100,000
Glucose	=blood	<blood

TP, Total protein; *LDH*, lactic dehydrogenase; *WBC*, white blood cell count; *RBC*, red blood cell count.

BOX 42-1
Information useful for the diagnosis of pleural effusions

I. Specific diagnostic aids
   A. Positive smear and/or culture for bacteria, mycobacteria, or fungi
   B. Positive cytology for primary or metastatic neoplasm or for lymphoma
   C. "True" chylous effusion-disruption or invasion of thoracic ducts
II. Potentially useful characteristics in differential diagnosis
   A. Elevated pleural fluid amylase/serum amylase ratio suggests
      1. Pancreatitis
      2. Pancreatic pseudocyst
      3. Ruptured esophagus (salivary amylase)
      4. Neoplasm
   B. Pleural fluid/serum glucose ratio <0.5 suggests tuberculosis, tumor, parapneumonic effusion, rheumatoid arthritis, or systemic lupus erythematosus
   C. Red blood count >100,000/mm³ associated most often with tumors, trauma, and embolus with infarction
   D. Lymphocytosis in exudate (>50% lymphocytes) seen in chronic effusions
   E. Pleural fluid eosinophilia rare in malignant and tuberculous effusions unless there is a coincident pneumothorax
   F. Greater than 1% mesothelial cells rare in tuberculous effusion
   G. Pseudochylous effusions (cholesterol crystals) seen with chronic effusion of rheumatoid disease, tuberculosis, and trapped lung
   H. Elevated acid mucopolysaccharide and hyaluronic acid levels usually associated with mesothelioma
   I. Lupus erythematosus cells: presence diagnostic of lupus pleuritis
   J. pH <7.1 in parapneumonic effusion suggests, but alone does not mandate, need for closed-tube thoracostomy
   K. Foul-smelling odor characteristic of anaerobic infection

effusion in the left hemithorax. A pancreatic pseudocyst under the right side of the diaphragm can cause an effusion in that hemithorax. The pleural fluid amylase levels in these two conditions can be higher than the serum amylase concentration. With esophageal rupture, amylase of salivary origin can be found on thoracentesis. The source of this amylase can be differentiated by electrophoresis. Slight elevation in pleural fluid amylase, usually less than 1000 units, can be seen in patients with primary bronchogenic carcinoma or metastatic carcinoma of gastrointestinal or breast origin.

A complete cell count on pleural fluid is of relatively little diagnostic value. A red cell count greater than 100,000/ml is usually found in association with trauma. About one fifth of patients with malignant effusions also have very high red cell counts. A smaller percentage of patients with pulmonary infarction have a pleural fluid red cell count greater than 100,000/ml, although over half have a bloody appearance to their effusions. The finding of over 50% lymphocytes in an exudate is consistent with many chronic effusions and is not particularly suggestive of tuberculosis or malignancy. A predominance of eosinophils in pleural fluid does not have the specificity for allergic or noninfectious inflammatory disease that it does in sputum. A high pleural fluid eosinophil count, however, is reputedly rare in tuberculous or malignant effusions unless there is a concurrent pneumothorax. Several entities, such as hemothorax, pneumothorax, previous thoracentesis, fungal disease, and parasitic disease, predispose to pleural fluid eosinophilia. The presence of more than 1% mesothelial cells is also rare in a tuberculous effusion.

In some patients with pleural tumors such as mesothelioma, acid mucopolysaccharide and hyaluronic acid concentrations are increased. However, tests for these substances are not standardized, and normal values may vary markedly among laboratories. Hence, the reliability of these test results is difficult to determine. The specific cause of a pleural effusion usually is not determined from pleural fluid analysis alone, but from integration of the patient's history, physical findings, radiographic studies, and other laboratory data with pleural fluid characteristics. The various biochemical assays should be ordered selectively for each patient. In spite of appropriate analyses, 20% of patients may not have a specific etiology determined at the time of their initial examination.

PLEURAL BIOPSY

Thoracentesis can be performed safely on small pleural effusions, especially if performed with ultrasound guidance. Because pleural biopsies are performed with a much larger needle (e.g., Abrams needle), a sufficiently large amount of fluid must be present to ensure that parietal and visceral pleura are separated widely and thus that an adequate sample of pleura can be obtained safely.

Percutaneous pleural biopsy can increase the diagnostic yield over thoracentesis alone when an exudate is documented and the etiology remains unclear. The complications of pleural biopsies should be little more than those of thoracentesis alone, if there is an adequate amount of pleural effusion. The procedure should not be uncomfortable for the patient if the skin, periosteum of the upper surface of the rib at the biopsy site, and parietal pleural are adequately anesthetized. Generally, biopsies are taken from tissue sites located at the 3, 4, 5, 6, 7, 8, and 9 o'clock positions relative to the entrance site of the needle. Samples are not taken at other positions to avoid the neurovascular bundle that runs along the inferior surface of the rib above the entrance site. Pleural biopsies are particularly helpful in diagnosing pleural effusions secondary to tuberculosis or malignancy. A recent review of more than 400 patients who had both thoracentesis and pleural biopsy showed that thoracentesis established a diagnosis of malignancy in 58% and pleural biopsy in 43%. The pleural biopsy was positive in 7% of patients with a tumor when thoracentesis cytology was negative. Because pleural biopsies remove parietal pleura that is supplied by arterioles under systemic pressure, the presence of a coagulopathy represents a relative contraindication to this procedure.

Typical granulomas may be seen on microscopic visualization, and occasionally organisms are revealed by special stain. Culture of the pleural tissue may grow mycobacteria, even if the histologic study does not show specific changes.

Primary pleural tumors, such as mesotheliomas, may be difficult to diagnose with certainty on the relatively small samples obtained from pleural biopsies. A variety of inflammatory processes can lead to bizarre changes in the mesothelial lining cells, which the pathologist may have difficulty in differentiating from neoplastic changes. The definitive diagnosis of mesothelioma often requires an open biopsy.

SWANN-GANZ CATHETERIZATION

Details of this technique are discussed in Chapter 14. In addition to providing assistance with hemodynamic monitoring, the simple aspiration of blood from the pulmonary vasculature via the distal port will provide a specimen that can be examined cytologically for tumor cells when tumor emboli are suspected or for fetal components when amniotic fluid emboli are suspected. No reliable studies have reported on the true positivity of this method, but patients with these diseases frequently develop respiratory failure and receive right heart catheterization for hemodynamic monitoring purposes. Positive cytology obviates the need for further diagnostic procedures in these patients who are already very ill.

BRONCHOSCOPY AND BIOPSIES

Table 42-2 summarizes the invasive techniques used to evaluate potential pulmonary disease. The introduction of the flexible fiberoptic bronchoscope in the late 1960s added a powerful tool for the diagnostic workup of many patients with bronchial or pulmonary parenchymal abnormalities. It has largely, though not completely, replaced the older rigid bronchoscope for examination of the tracheobronchial tree. The typical diagnostic fiberoptic bronchoscope has a 4 to 6 mm external diameter and contains a 2 mm biopsy and suction channel. Biopsy forceps, cytology brushes, and saline for lavage and washings can be introduced through the channel. The distal end can be flexed at least at an angle of 120 degrees for insertion into segmental and subsegmental bronchi. By contrast, the rigid bronchoscope can visualize directly only the trachea, the major bronchi, and the openings to some of the segmental bronchi. The fiberoptic bronchoscope, therefore, offers greatly increased visual and biopsy range with greater patient comfort.

Fiberoptic bronchoscopy is useful for the following:
1. For diagnosing lung masses or infiltrates of uncertain etiology
2. To evaluate hemoptysis or abnormal cytologic findings with normal chest radiograph
3. In preoperative evaluation of a patient with known chest malignancy
4. To evaluate the extent of an inhalational injury
5. To assess a potential etiology for cough, a localized wheeze, a pleural effusion, recurrent laryngeal nerve paralysis, or diaphragmatic paralysis
6. To perform laser therapy on an endobronchial tumor
7. To place a stent within an airway to alleviate an obstruction.

It is possible to perform biopsies or obtain aspirates for culture. In addition to having diagnostic functions, the fiberoptic bronchoscope is used therapeutically to remove retained secretions and to remove foreign bodies beyond the reach of the rigid bronchoscope.

The fiberoptic bronchoscope is used generally with only topical anesthesia while the patient is awake or slightly sedated. It is important that the patient be able to cooperate with the bronchoscopist. The bronchoscope can be introduced through either the nose or mouth, with or without an endotracheal tube. Diagnostic fiberoptic bronchoscopy is a very safe procedure. Fluoroscopic guidance can be helpful but is not always necessary when pulmonary parenchymal biopsies are to be obtained or when peripheral masses or nodules are to be sampled. About half of the primary chest neoplasms presenting as radiographic abnormalities can be visualized directly through the fiberoptic bronchoscope. Better than a 90% diagnostic yield is obtained for central endobronchial lesions. A greater than 70% diagnostic yield can be obtained form peripheral lesions when cytology brushes and biopsy forceps are guided successfully into the lesion under fluoroscopic control. Carcinoma metastatic to the lung also can be diagnosed by biopsy through the fiberoptic bronchoscope. With the exception of tumors of genitourinary tract origin, metastatic lesions to the lung tend to be peripheral and need to be subjected to biopsy under fluoroscopic control. The diagnostic yield for fiberoptic bronchoscopy decreases to about 20% for lesions less than 2 cm in diameter and for those located in the outer periphery of the lung field.

In addition to establishing the cell type of primary or metastatic

Table 42-2   Summary of diagnostic techniques

BIOPSY TECHNIQUE	APPROPRIATE APPLICATION	POTENTIAL COMPLICATIONS
Thoracentesis	Any pleural effusion of uncertain etiology Diagnostic and therapeutic reasons	Pneumothorax (R) Hemothorax (R) Infection (R)
Pleural biopsy	Exudate of uncertain etiology Increases diagnostic yield with malignancy and granulomatous disease	Pneumothorax (R) Hemothorax (R) Hypoxemia
Fiberoptic bronchoscopy with brush and biopsy	Central endobronchial lesion	Hemoptysis (R)
	Peripheral nodules or infiltrates—moderate yield; drops to low yield with lesion <2 cm	Pneumothorax Hemoptysis
	Diffuse interstitial disease—moderate yield	Pneumothorax Hemoptysis
	Evaluate extent of inhalational injury	
	Unexplained cough, localized wheeze, pleural effusion, diaphragm paralysis, laser therapy, stent placement	
	Search for bleeding with mild to moderate hemoptysis	Worsens hemoptysis (R)
	Preoperative staging for thoracotomy with neoplastic disease	
Bronchoalveolar lavage	Infiltrates (particularly in immunocompromised host)—high yield and very low morbidity. Particularly safe in patient at high risk for bleeding	Worsens hypoxia (C)
Rigid bronchoscopy	Massive hemoptysis Biopsy of upper airway obstructive lesion Foreign body removal	Worsens hemoptysis Further compromises upper airway
Needle aspiration	Peripheral nodules—high yield Pneumonic infiltrates (particularly in immunocompromised patients)—moderate yield	Pneumothorax (C) Hemoptysis Air embolus (R)
Thoracoscopy Mediastinoscopy Mediastinotomy Open biopsy	Pleural disease, peripheral lung mass, or interstitial lung disease Right paratracheal masses Left aortopulmonary masses In patient in whom other techniques have not yielded a specific diagnosis and clinical condition warrants surgery; in patient who is critically ill and does not have time to try serial procedures prior to starting therapy Bleeding diathesis or pulmonary hypertension	Pneumothorax (C) Pneumothorax (R) Infection (R) Pneumothorax (C)

R, Rare; *C*, common.

carcinomas of the lung, fiberoptic bronchoscopy is useful in preoperative staging. Blind biopsy of a normal-appearing main carina in patients with bronchogenic carcinoma has uncovered microscopic neoplastic invasion in as many as 10% of patients. This finding alters the therapeutic approach. In patients with positive cytologic findings and an abnormal chest radiograph, the tumor site has been localized to lobes other than the site of the apparent radiographic abnormality. In other patients tumors have been found bilaterally by bronchoscopy, although the involvement of only one side was apparent radiographically. In patients with hemoptysis or abnormal sputum cytologies but normal chest radiographs, the fiberoptic bronchoscope is the best diagnostic tool for locating the site of disease. Occult bronchogenic neoplasms can be found in a significant percentage of adult smokers presenting with hemoptysis and normal chest films. By including a thorough examination of the nasal and oral pharynx with the fiberoptic scope, one can uncover additional occult neoplasms. With the use of a transbronchial needle, subcarinal, right paratracheal, and, to a limited extent, left paratracheal nodes can be aspirated through the fiberoptic bronchoscope to aid in staging and diagnosis of carcinoma of the lung.

In patients with diffuse interstitial disease, transbronchial biopsy through the fiberoptic bronchoscope may provide adequate histologic material for specific diagnosis. Complications include a low (less than 5%) incidence of pneumothorax, fever, and hemoptysis of more than 10 ml of blood. Fluoroscopic control may be helpful in obtaining tissue. Multiple samples (six to eight) can be taken but are obtained generally from only one lung, as pneumothorax remains a risk even when the biopsy is done under fluoroscopic control.

Not all patients are candidates for fiberoptic bronchoscopy. Relative contraindications are (1) severe hypoxemia that cannot be readily corrected with supplemental oxygen, (2) acute hypercapnia, (3) bleeding diatheses that cannot be corrected for the performance of brush or forceps biopsies, (4) unstable cardiac conditions, and (5) untreated symptomatic patients with asthma. Patients in whom extra caution needs to be taken include those with treated bronchospastic disease such as asthma, pulmonary hypertension, superior vena cava obstruction, massive hemoptysis, and uremia. Unconscious patients and patients at risk for a serious complication or with one or more relative contraindications can be sedated and intubated. The procedure then can be performed with or without mechanical ventilation. With careful preprocedure evaluation, proper technique, and monitoring during the procedure, the incidence of complications is low. However, bleeding, pneumothorax, adverse reaction to an anesthetic agent, blood gas deterioration with associated arrhythmias, and death are all potential complications. The procedure should be carried out only by well-trained physicians with adequate support personnel and in facilities that can handle emergencies.

The rigid bronchoscope still has a clinical role. It is of value in pediatric patients and in patients with partial upper airway obstruction in which the solid fiberoptic bronchoscope would completely obstruct the upper airway. The rigid scope is also useful in patients with massive hemoptysis; for internal drainage of lung abscesses in which the small suction channel of the fiberoptic scope would be overwhelmed by large volumes of fluid, blood, or pus; and for the removal of foreign bodies not recoverable with the fiberoptic bronchoscope. The rigid scope generally is used in an operating suite with the patient under general anesthesia.

BRONCHOALVEOLAR LAVAGE

Bronchoalveolar lavage (BAL) is a relatively new tool for the clinician. This procedure is performed through a fiberoptic bronchoscope that is wedged in a segmental bronchus. Usually 20 to 50 ml of a physiologic solution such as sterile normal saline are infused sequentially with aspiration after each instillate. Instilled volumes totaling 100 to 300 ml are used most commonly. Bronchoalveolar lavage fluid can be analyzed for total cells, differential cell count, and the presence of parasites. It can also be stained and cultured for bacteria, viruses, and fungi. The isolation of almost any organism that does not normally colonize the upper or lower respiratory tract, such as *Legionella, Histoplasma, P. carinii,* or *Mycobacterium tuberculosis,* is diagnostic of infection. Recent data suggest that the isolation of commonly encountered gram-positive or gram-negative bacteria at greater

---

BOX 42-2
Diagnostic applications of bronchoalveolar lavage

Infectious pneumonias
  Pneumocystis carinii
  Cytomegalovirus
  Legionellosis
  Cryptococcosis
  Histoplasmosis
  Tuberculosis
  Aspergillosis
Other pulmonary disorders
  Malignancy
  Hemorrhage
  Alveolar proteinosis
  Eosinophilic granuloma
  Chronic eosinophilic pneumonia
  Drug-induced lung disease
  Berylliosis
  Hypersensitivity pneumonitis

---

than 10^5 colony-forming units/ml in a semiquantitative culture is very suggestive of pneumonia caused by the isolated organism(s). Swan-Ganz–like catheters now exist that can be inserted through the bronchoscope's channel. The balloon at the tip is inflated to sequester a portion of the lung, and a smaller volume lavage is performed through the catheter tip. Similar catheters can be passed into the lungs of intubated and mechanically ventilated patients without the aid of a bronchoscope. A small-volume lavage is then performed to sample the lung area of interest. A few relatively uncommon diseases such as eosinophilic pneumonia, alveolar proteinosis, and eosinophilic granuloma also can be diagnosed by findings in BAL fluid from patients with a clinical syndrome that is consistent with the preceding diseases. Additional diagnoses that can be made with the assistance of BAL include lung carcinoma, berylliosis, and pulmonary hemorrhage (Box 42-2).

Lung lavage initially was used as a method for the removal of inspissated airway secretions; later BAL was used to investigate immunopathogenic mechanisms relevant to numerous interstitial lung diseases or lung defense mechanisms in normal hosts. Some data suggest BAL cell differentials are useful in the initial evaluation of patients with undiagnosed interstitial lung disease. BAL fluid from patients with granulomatous lung diseases such as sarcoidosis or hypersensitivity pneumonitis frequently, but not always, has a preponderance of lymphocytes in the lavage fluid. By contrast, BAL fluid from patients with nongranulomatous lung diseases such as idiopathic pulmonary fibrosis frequently, but not always, has a preponderance of neutrophils and eosinophils. Thus the finding of one or the other of these cell profiles can tilt the diagnostic balance in favor of or against certain specific diagnoses. In addition, BAL cell differentials also may be helpful in the assessment of the activity of various lung diseases such as idiopathic pulmonary fibrosis. However, most pulmonologists agree that its usefulness as a clinical tool resides with the ease, safety, and sensitivity with which BAL can assist in the diagnosis of lung infections. A major advantage to BAL is that it can be performed with relative safety in patients with significant disturbances of their coagulation systems and on patients requiring mechanical ventilation. Potential major complications are similar to those for fiberoptic bronchoscopy except that pneumothorax and hemorrhage rarely occur. BAL should be distinguished from whole lung lavage, which is used only occasionally in the treatment of alveolar proteinosis.

PROTECTED BRUSH CATHETER

Samples of lower respiratory tract secretions can be retrieved with minimal contamination by upper respiratory tract organisms through the use of a protected brush catheter. This catheter has a brush within a double sheath that is sealed at the distal end with a soluble plug. After introduction through the fiberoptic bronchoscope and into the airway to be sampled, the plug is extruded, the brush is advanced into the airway or secretions to be sampled, the sample is obtained, and the brush is withdrawn within its sheath. Data on the value of this technique in the diagnosis of pneumonia are variable but appear promising, particularly when meticulous attention is paid to details of the procedure. The isolation of organisms at greater than 10^4 colony-forming units/ml suggests bacterial pneumonia.

TRANSTRACHEAL ASPIRATION

Transtracheal aspiration is another technique used to obtain lower respiratory tract secretions relatively free from contamination by upper respiratory tract flora. The procedure is performed under local anesthesia using a needle with an indwelling catheter that is advanced through the cricothyroid membrane. Aspirated secretions can be stained and cultured for pathogenic organisms. As with the protected brush catheter, data on the value of this technique vary. Interpretation of results is particularly difficult for patients with chronic bronchitis, many of whom have tracheal colonization with bacteria. When the procedure is performed by an experienced individual, the incidence of significant complications is low, and the results are helpful in diagnosing infectious pneumonias.

TRANSTHORACIC NEEDLE ASPIRATION

An alternative approach to fiberoptic bronchoscopy in the diagnosis of suspected lung pathology is transthoracic needle aspiration. A small-gauge spinal needle or a thin-walled 23- or 25-gauge needle made specifically for needle aspiration can be introduced with the patient under local anesthesia into lung nodules percutaneously with the assistance of computed tomography (CT) or fluoroscopy. The operator can often determine when the lesion has been entered by seeing it move and feeling a sense of resistance at the end of the needle. If attempts to aspirate fluid and cells from the lesion are unsuccessful initially, a few milliliters of saline can be injected into the lesion and the aspiration repeated. Material can be obtained for cytologic evaluation and culture. With malignant lesions, a greater than 90% diagnostic yield has been reported in some series.

The incidence of pneumothorax has been 20% to 30%. Many of these pneumothoraces are quite small, and therefore a smaller percentage of the patients have required a chest tube to reexpand the lung. A 10% to 20% incidence of hemoptysis has been reported, but this side effect is usually self-limited. In addition to evaluating solitary pulmonary nodules, needle aspiration can sample parenchymal or pleural masses and mediastinal or hilar lymph nodes.

Contraindications to needle aspiration are a bleeding diathesis, the presence of blebs or bullae in the immediate vicinity of the potential biopsy site, pulmonary hypertension, suspected vascular lesions such as arteriovenous malformations, and the inability of the patient to cooperate or to hold his or her breath for short periods. Aspiration with a thin, flexible needle also can prove useful in diagnosing pneumonia, particularly in the complex setting of the host who has undergone immunosuppression. Thus needle aspiration provides an alternative to BAL or brushing with a protected brush catheter.

THORACOSCOPY

Thoracoscopy (also referred to as *pleuroscopy*) is a procedure in which a fiberoptic thoracoscope is introduced into the pleural space through a small intercostal incision with the patient under either general or local anesthesia. Most often the procedure is carried out in an operating room. Thoracoscopy is potentially useful in the following situations: (1) the diagnosis of exudative pleural effusions of uncertain etiology, (2) decortication of complicated parapneumonic effusions, (3) pleurodesis of malignant pleural effusions, (4) biopsy of pleural or peripheral parenchymal lung lesions, and (5) blebectomy or bullectomy for pneumothoraces. One distinct advantage to thoracoscopy is that the pleura or lung can be inspected visually and biopsied under direct observation. Thus it can spare the patient the more invasive thoracotomy. Thoracoscopy has been used extensively in Europe and now is being used with an increasing frequency in the United States (Box 42-3). Complications associated with thoracoscopy are similar to those that result from thoracotomy. One important advan-

---

BOX 42-3
Diagnostic and therapeutic applications of thoracoscopy

Diagnosis
Exudative effusions of uncertain etiology
Pleural or peripheral parenchymal lung lesions

Therapy
Decortication
Pleurodesis
Blebectomy
Bullectomy

---

tage to thoracoscopy is that one or two small (1 to 2 cm) incisions are made in the chest wall rather than the much larger incision made for a full thoracotomy.

Video-assisted thoracoscopic surgery is an extension of thoracoscopy. This procedure is always performed in an operating room with the patient under general anesthesia. Resection of entire lung lobes and mediastinal dissection are possible with this procedure.

Because thoracoscopy and video-assisted thorascopic surgery are relatively new procedures, vigorous cost-benefit analyses for them have not been published. Their less invasive nature and their impressive low morbidity and mortality suggest they will find a place in algorithms for patient care as relates to the chest.

MEDIASTINOSCOPY AND MEDIASTINOTOMY

For mediastinoscopy a small incision is made at the suprasternal notch with the patient under general anesthesia. A mediastinoscope is inserted and advanced as tissue planes are dissected along the right side of the trachea. Right paratracheal lymph nodes or masses can be biopsied as far down as the main carina. A similar procedure cannot be performed on the left side of the trachea because of the presence of the great vessels. When it is necessary to biopsy selectively anterior left-sided masses or nodes situated near the aorta and pulmonary artery, a mediastinotomy is performed in which a small incision is made in the area of the second or third costal cartilages near the sternum with the patient under general anesthesia. This permits an extrapleural approach to left-sided lesions and can be performed quickly. These procedures are associated with a low morbidity and mortality. They are used almost exclusively in the diagnosis of potential lung tumors. They simultaneously provide a histologic diagnosis and an assessment of the spread of disease to mediastinal structures. The yield is high only when the nodes accessible with either procedure are enlarged on chest radiograph or CT scan. Because diagnoses are made most frequently by other procedures, these techniques are being used less often.

OPEN LUNG BIOPSY

The decision to proceed to open lung biopsy is predicated on several points, such as the diagnostic success or failure of less invasive tests and the speed with which a diagnosis is needed. This procedure requires general anesthesia and is the most invasive of diagnostic tests used to diagnose thoracic disease. Infectious and noninfectious lung diseases frequently alter lung architecture to a variable degree. Therefore small biopsies sometimes sample a relatively "normal" area of lung within a diseased lung zone and thus do not yield truly representative pathology. Larger quantities of lung parenchyma can be removed during an open lung biopsy than by other less invasive techniques, yielding a sample that is more representative of the true pathologic process. A significant advantage of open lung biopsy is that through a large chest wall incision, the surgeon gains access to one entire chest cavity. Furthermore, hilar and mediastinal lymph nodes can be sampled, which permits an assessment of the spread of a disease. Because the mortality rate of this procedure approximates 1%

and the morbidity rate is modest, ranging from 10% to 20%, the decision to proceed to open lung biopsy depends on the likelihood that the additional information gained will have a positive impact on patient outcome. Studies involving immunocompromised hosts do not suggest that patients on whom an open lung biopsy is performed actually fare better. Thus this procedure should be used selectively and only after considering carefully all the risks and benefits.

BIBLIOGRAPHY

Colt HG: Thoracoscopy: a prospective study of safety and outcome, *Chest* 108:324-329, 1995.

Goldstein RA et al: Clinical role of bronchoalveolar lavage in adults with pulmonary disease, *Am Rev Respir Dis* 142:481, 1990.

Ogirala RG, Agarwal V, Vizioli LD et al: Comparison of the Raja and Abrams pleural biopsy needles in patients with pleural effusion, *Am Rev Respir Dis* 147:1291, 1993.

Prakash UBS, Reiman HM: Comparison of needle biopsy with cytologic analysis for the evaluation of pleural effusion, *Mayo Clin Proc* 60:158, 1985.

Sahn SA: The pleura, *Am Rev Respir Dis* 138:184, 1988.

Salazar AM, Westcott JL: The role of transthoracic needle biopsy for the diagnosis and staging of lung cancer, *Clin Chest Med* 14:99-110, 1993.

Shellito J: Application of bronchoalveolar lavage to the diagnosis of pulmonary infection, *Clin Pulmonary Med* 1:144, 1995.

CHAPTER

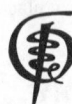

43 Pulmonary Diagnostic Imaging

Robert D. Tarver, Lynn S. Broderick, and Dewey J. Conces, Jr.

Pulmonary imaging methods vary from noninvasive to invasive. They are associated with varying degrees of discomfort, risk, and expense. In approximately 90% of instances, the plain chest radiograph is the only imaging study needed. Unfortunately, it can be normal or nonspecific in the presence of significant disease.

To make the plain radiograph and other modes of imaging most useful, the clinician should:

1. View all films independently.
2. Review all films with a radiologist. Do not depend solely on the written report.
3. Know that previous or old chest radiographs can be invaluable. Most adults have had one. Take the trouble to obtain it.
4. Be aware that anatomic abnormalities may reflect physiologic changes, for example, elevated diaphragms in noncompliant lungs and large upper lobe vessels in pulmonary venous hypertension.
5. Use the radiologist as a consultant in planning the patient's investigation.

The variety of specialized pulmonary imaging modalities presented in the discussion that follows has not lessened the importance of a competent clinician.

COMPUTED TOMOGRAPHY

Computed tomography (CT) makes use of a collimated x-ray beam of variable width (1.5 to 10.0 mm) to obtain information limited to that slice thickness. The anatomy is studied and displayed in cross section. The area of interest is studied with successive slices of predetermined thickness and spacing. Information for each slice is obtained in approximately 2 seconds. Density discrimination on CT is ten times that of conventional radiographs. Soft-tissue pulmonary nodules as small as 1 mm can be detected. Density graduations called Hounsfield units (HU) are based on a scale of -1000 for air to 0 for water. The ability to discriminate density differences allows the detection of tissue interphases such as fluid in cysts or lymph nodes surrounded by fat in the mediastinum. Fat can be recognized by its low density (-70 to -130 HU).

Contrast agents may be given intravenously to identify normal or abnormal vascular structures. The information can be displayed at different window widths of density and at different levels of density, allowing optimal demonstration of abnormalities.

CT is not a routine screening procedure. It should be used to help clarify specific problems and should always be preceded by a recent chest radiograph.

CT is indicated in the presence of a known extrapulmonary malignancy, for example, renal cell carcinoma, osteosarcoma, and melanoma, when the detection of pulmonary metastasis alters therapy. A significant number of nodules of less than 5 mm are benign, so the problem of a false-positive diagnosis of metastasis is always present.

The solitary pulmonary nodule is a common problem. No change in growth over 2 years and the unequivocal presence of central calcification are the only two reliable signs of benignancy. CT is able to identify calcium not visible on plain films. Phantoms that simulate specific anatomic locations and appropriate test objects are available to avoid the technical variables that are inherent in density determinations. In our department CT density determination using this phantom has been found to be very useful in evaluating the solitary nodule that does not contain calcium on a low-kV radiograph. Density measurements done without the phantom require special care. Accuracy of the equipment cannot be presumed but requires frequent calibration. Emphasis is placed on previous films, history of a prior malignancy, smoking history, associated disease, and age factors that might indicate the need for needle aspiration biopsy or other more definitive studies.

CT is also useful to establish or exclude a questionable lesion seen on the chest radiograph and to detect the presence of cavitation.

Evaluation of lung nodules with CT is not without its difficulties. Because information is obtained during suspended respiration, it is essential that each slice be obtained with the same lung volume; otherwise the nodule may move out of the field of interest. A cooperative, instructed patient is required.

Hila and Mediastinum

CT is useful in identifying hila adenopathy. When done with intravenous contrast (contrast enhancement), small nodes can be separated from confusing vessels. Magnetic resonance imaging (MRI) can also be used.

Computed tomography is clearly the superior method for examining the mediastinum, whether one is evaluating disease seen on the chest radiograph, looking for suspected abnormalities such as a thymoma in myesthesia gravis, or staging a known lung malignancy (Fig. 43-1). The low density of the normal fat of the mediastinum makes it possible to detect nodes as small as 5 mm regularly. Complete evaluation requires histologic study of these nodes. Location on CT determines the approach best for biopsy (mediasti-

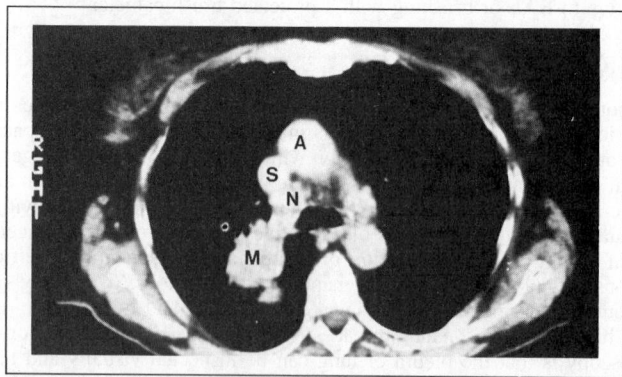

FIGURE 43-1   Transverse CT image with intravenous contrast at the level of the tracheal bifurcation. Biopsy of nodes by mediastinoscopy showed poorly differentiated adenocarcinoma. *M,* Right upper lobe mass; *S,* superior vena cava; *A,* ascending aorta; *N,* right paratracheal and retrocaval lymph nodes.

noscopy, transbronchial aspiration, percutaneous aspiration, parasternal thoracotomy).

Not only can the extent of mediastinal disease be evaluated with CT, but the appearance of certain lesions is relatively specific. Lipomas are low density, and cysts usually have a denser rim than their center. Contrast enhancement identifies normal vessels and vessel variants and demonstrates aneurysms.

Chest Wall and Pleura

The demonstration of anatomy in cross section makes CT an excellent method for evaluating the pleura and chest wall. Empyemas can be differentiated from lung abscesses. Lipomas are readily apparent. The localization and extent of pleural implants from metastasis or mesothelioma are well shown. The best site for biopsy is apparent, and follow-up comparison studies are easily carried out. Unless there is obvious rib destruction or tumor bulging externally, suspected chest wall invasion requires histologic verification. When confusion exists, CT may be used to distinguish benign pleural plaques from extrapleural fat.

High-Resolution CT

Compared to plain film radiography, CT has increased sensitivity for parenchymal disease. This is a result of the elimination of superimposition of structures and the increased ability of CT to discriminate parenchymal structures. Recently the technique of high-resolution CT (HRCT) has been developed. In this technique the slice thickness of 1.5 mm is used, which results in the images having much greater detail than conventional CT images.

HRCT has been found to be very useful in evaluating diffuse lung disease. It is useful in identifying parenchymal disease in patients who are symptomatic or with abnormal pulmonary function tests, but who have normal chest radiographs. Similarly, in febrile immune-compromised patients, infiltrates can be identified that are not visible on chest films. The HRCT findings can be used to characterize diffuse lung disease. The HRCT findings for sarcoidosis, lymphangitic spread of carcinoma, and bronchiectasis are fairly characteristic (Fig. 43-2). The activity of the lung disease can be assessed with HRCT because the presence of "ground glass densities" indicates active alveolitis. The response of the lung disease to therapy can be assessed with serial examinations. Finally, if biopsy is needed for diagnosis, HRCT can identify the best site for obtaining the biopsy.

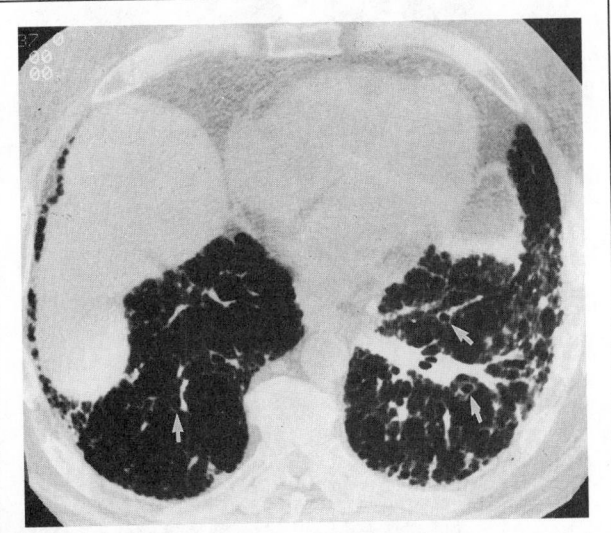

FIGURE 43-2 HRCT scan through the lung base of a patient with idiopathic pulmonary fibrosis. Subpleural reticular opacities and traction bronchiectasis *(arrows)* are demonstrated bilaterally.

LUNG SCANS

The major use of scintiscanning studies of the lung is in the diagnosis of pulmonary thromboembolism (PE). Small particles introduced intravenously distribute themselves in the pulmonary capillaries according to blood flow. If these particles are tagged with radioactive material, their distribution can be recorded with a gamma camera. At the present time the most frequently used particles are macroaggregated albumin (10 to 60 μ in diameter) labeled with technetium 99m. These particles are biodegradable, and their number is small in comparison to the total number of pulmonary arterioles providing a large margin of safety. Soon after perfusion (P) lung scans became an accepted clinical examination in the 1960s, it became apparent that although the study was highly sensitive in detecting abnormalities, it lacked specificity for thromboembolic disease. Almost any lung abnormality affects lung perfusion.

To improve specificity, ventilation (V) studies done with xenon-133 or xenon-127 were introduced. Their use was based on the fact that an area of diminished perfusion that maintains normal ventilation is most characteristic of vascular occlusion. Krypton-81m gas or DTPA technetium 99m as an aerosol may also be used. This is true in the absence of bronchoconstriction, congestive atelectasis, edema, hemorrhage, or infarction that may be produced by PE.

A normal V scan in an area of a P defect is a mismatch characteristic of vascular occlusion. The matched defect that is present when the V-P scans are both abnormal in the same area occurs in a wide spectrum of primary pulmonary diseases, as well as in the parenchymal changes that may occur secondary to a vascular occlusion. Not only can pulmonary emboli show matched defects, but less often other diseases can produce a V-P mismatch characteristic of an acute PE.

The evaluation of a patient with a suspected PE should include a chest radiograph to detect pulmonary infiltrates, pneumothorax, atelectasis, or other pulmonary diseases. Unless a contraindication exists, heparin may be started while the diagnostic evaluation is extended. Lung scans are then done within 12 to 24 hours; later scans are less diagnostic. For technical reasons related to photon energy, xenon-133 V scans are done before P scans. Both wash-in and wash-out ventilation should be evaluated, preferably both anteriorly and posteriorly. The labeled macroaggregated albumin for the P scan may be injected as a split dose in the vein of each foot to evaluate thrombi above the knees. The P scan should be imaged in multiple views. Ventilation done with xenon-127 is less available but has the advantage that it can be done after the P scan.

Abnormalities of ventilation are shown by failure of areas to fill during the wash-in phase and/or delayed clearing of xenon from areas during the wash-out phase. Perfusion is normal if radioactivity is uniformly present in all expected areas. An area of diminished or absent radioactivity indicates a perfusion abnormality.

Because V-P scans done for thromboembolism are an indirect demonstration of disease, they are interpreted as "normal," "high probability," or "indeterminate." This is based on the appearance of the chest radiograph together with the presence and size of perfusion abnormalities and whether associated ventilation abnormalities exist. The larger the area of V-P mismatch or the larger the P defect compared to the density on the chest radiograph, the more likely is the presence of PE. Nonthromboembolic occlusion of vessels produces similar findings.

A normal P scan excludes the diagnosis of a PE. Over 80% of V-P scans done for suspected PE show some abnormality. A high-probability scan, which is 85% to 90% accurate for a positive diagnosis, is present in fewer than half (41%) of patients who have a PE. The large number of nonspecific abnormal scans is where the major problems and controversies exist. Clinical evaluation is useful in deciding which abnormal scans should be further investigated with an angiogram. The patient with an indeterminate scan can be expected to have a PE more often than those with low-probability scans (33% vs 16%). In one series, however, 31% of patients with a low probability scan had angiographic PE. Most clinicians would agree that the majority of indeterminate scans should be evaluated with an angiogram. Because indeterminate scans are seen in at least 33% of patients with a suspected PE, this would result in a relatively large number of pulmonary angiograms—more than are now being done. It might be useful to think of V-P scans as "normal," "high probability," or "nondiagnostic."

Most PEs have their origin in the large veins of the lower extremities. When thrombi are present in these large veins, they are associated with a high incidence (50%) of PE. Impedance plethysmography and compression sonography are accurate methods for detecting and excluding large vein thrombi. Although the absence of vein clots does *not* exclude a PE, their presence would greatly facilitate the decision to use anticoagulants in patients with nondiagnostic lung scans. The role of these peripheral vein studies in patients with suspected PE is being evaluated.

V-P scintiscans can separate pulmonary hypertension secondary to old or recurrent PE from primary pulmonary hypertension. Unresolved emboli produce a high-probability scan; primary hypertension shows a low-probability or normal scintiscan.

V-P scans are useful in evaluating regional lung function. They may be especially helpful to evaluate the amount of lung resection that can be tolerated in a patient with lung cancer and in the evaluation of a patient with bullae being considered for resection.

Gallium-67 citrate has an affinity for inflammatory and neoplastic tissue. Scans done with this substance should be delayed at least 48 hours after the injection. The greatest value of gallium scans in the thorax is in evaluating the activity of diffuse pulmonary disease. Such applications include idiopathic fibrosis, sarcoidosis, and in patients receiving drugs with potential pulmonary toxicity such as amiodarone. Not only is the activity evaluated, but also the sensitivity of detecting diffuse abnormalities is often greater on gallium scans than on the chest radiograph.

PULMONARY ANGIOGRAM

Most pulmonary angiograms (PAs) are done to evaluate patients for suspected thromboemboli. A few angiograms are done to evaluate arteriovenous (AV) fistulas.

The decision to do a PA in a patient with a suspected PE is based on clinical circumstances and the findings of a prior V-P lung scan. A normal P lung scan excludes a significant pulmonary embolus and makes an angiogram unnecessary. Because the PA is the most definitive way of making the correct diagnosis, it should be used whenever the scan findings are inconclusive or at variance with the clinical evaluation. It is especially important to do a PA when the risk of therapy is so great as to make a correct diagnosis mandatory or when interventive therapy such as inferior vena cava occlusion or, more rarely, an embolectomy is considered. At most institutions 10% to 20% of patients with abnormal perfusion scans are evaluated with a PA. As with all imaging studies for pulmonary thromboemboli, the sooner an angiogram is done, the more reliable it is. Emboli begin to resolve within 24 hours and complete resolution may occur within 7 days. At times emboli do not resolve but organize and cause chronic pulmonary hypertension.

With few exceptions a PA done for suspected thromboembolic disease should be preceded by a V-P scan. An abnormal perfusion scan delineates those areas that must be well visualized on the angiogram. Using the lung scan and chest radiograph as a road map, the most probable areas of embolus can be studied first to shorten the study, decrease the contrast load, and allow more selective, detailed evaluation of abnormal areas.

Pulmonary angiograms are not easy studies. Considerable experience is required to ensure that examinations are satisfactory in patients whose ability to cooperate is often compromised by severe illness. The study is expensive and requires specialized equipment and an experienced team. Therefore the indications should be carefully considered and do vary among medical centers. The procedure is safely accomplished by experienced operators. Serious complications are more frequent in the presence of pulmonary hypertension and/or a failing right ventricle. Even in such circumstances the mortality rate has been 0.5% or less. In the evaluation of chronic thromboembolism and pulmonary hypertension for possible surgery, a PA is essential and should not be avoided. The use of supplemental oxygen and nonionic contrast agents, which alter physiology less than the older contrast agents, should make the procedure safer. In the presence of left bundle branch block, facilities for pacing must be immediately available because complete heart block may occur. Major arrhythmias, although uncommon (about 1%), need to be recognized and appropriately treated. Contrast reactions, usually minor, occur in about

1% of patients. The currently used catheters have eliminated perforation as a complication.

To diagnose a PE, the actual clot must be visualized as a filling defect or an abrupt termination of a vessel (Fig. 43-3). If these criteria are followed, a false-positive diagnosis is rare. A normal PA reliably indicates that therapy of pulmonary embolism is not needed. Follow-up of 311 such patients for periods up to 30 months showed no deaths from pulmonary embolism.

The actual diagnosis of a pulmonary AV fistula requires demonstrating an extracardiac right-to-left shunt with blood gas studies in the absence of pulmonary parenchymal disease. The number and location of these fistulas are best determined by PA. Treatment of these pulmonary AV fistulas can usually be accomplished with some form of transcatheter embolization.

Bronchial artery angiograms as a preliminary to embolization may be useful in hemoptysis. Massive (500 to 600 ml/day), life- threatening hemoptysis is the most clear indication, but chronic episodic hemoptysis in a patient with poor pulmonary drainage and function impairment (e.g., cystic fibrosis) are possible candidates as well. The bleeding site is best localized endoscopically first. In some patients with recurrent hemoptysis, however, it may be necessary to rely on the degree of hypervascularization seen to decide which vessel to embolize. Gelfoam or more permanent Ivalon particles are usually used. A skilled and experienced operator is essential because the anatomy of the feeding arteries is variable, and care must be taken to avoid injecting the vascular supply to the spinal cord. Paraplegia is the most feared complication. Some operators monitor somatosensory-evoked potentials during test injections into the vessel before embolization.

Bleeding stops immediately about 70% of the time. Recurrence of bleeding is seen in 20% of cases. The most frequent causes of hemoptysis that lend themselves to this form of therapy are cystic fi-

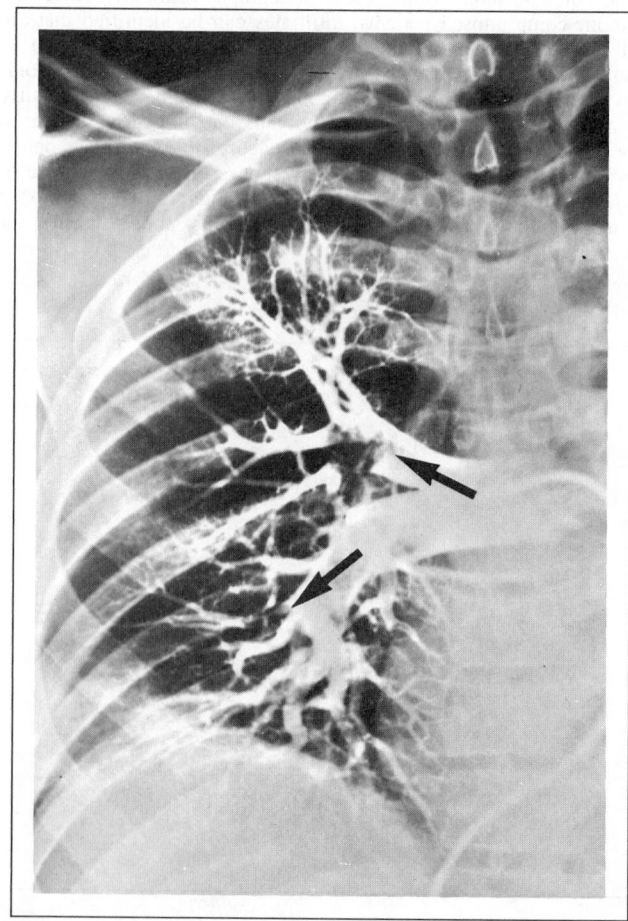

FIGURE 43-3   Right pulmonary angiogram. Clots are located within arteries *(arrows).*

brosis with bronchiectasis, aspergillosis (fungus ball), and occasionally tuberculosis, lung abscess, or lung cancer. The vast majority are high-risk patients for surgery.

PULMONARY ULTRASONOGRAPHY

Diagnostic ultrasonography depends on the reflections of sound waves from the interphase of tissues with different acoustic properties. These differences in acoustical impedance for soft tissues are relatively small. Much greater differences occur with air and bone, which do not permit enough sound to penetrate to evaluate deeper structures. Only those disease processes that can be approached without intervening air or bone can be studied. Therefore, except for the heart (echocardiography), ultrasound plays a relatively minor role in evaluating thoracic disease. Imaging is done through the intercostal spaces or from a subchondral or suprasternal approach.

The most valuable use of ultrasound is to detect and/or accurately localize fluid collections within the thorax or about the diaphragm. Fluid is recognized by an absence of internal echoes (Fig. 43-4). Each study contains its own acoustically determined ruler so that once fluid is localized, its depth can be accurately measured. This measurement allows a needle tip for aspiration to be precisely placed, avoiding penetration of lung, diaphragm, liver, or spleen. On occasion, a fluid-containing cavity may contain some internal echoes from blood clots or tissue debris, and at times solid structures such as lymphomas and neurofibromas may be so uniform acoustically as to appear cystic: because the needle tip can be so accurately placed, no harm comes from attempts at aspiration in either situation. In the case of solid tumors, aspirated cells for cytology may be diagnostic.

Most pleural effusions are readily diagnosed from chest radiographs, including lateral decubitus and oblique views. Ultrasound is used when small effusions are to be aspirated to obtain material for diagnostic purposes, when densities adjacent to the chest wall cannot be differentiated from fluid collections, or when there has been a prior unsuccessful attempt at fluid aspiration.

MAGNETIC RESONANCE IMAGING

The nuclei of atoms that have an odd number of neutrons plus protons have a magnetic moment. When these nuclei are placed in a magnetic field, they attempt to align themselves to this field. In doing so they rotate (precess) about the direction of the magnetic field at a specific frequency for a given nucleus. These precessing nuclei can absorb energy if they are exposed to a radio wave of the same frequency (resonance). After such a pulse, the nuclei release energy as they return to their ground state (relaxation). Longitudinal (T_1) and transverse (T_2) relaxation times may be measured and are thought to be specific for each substance. The recording of this energy release is the basis of MRI. Hydrogen nuclei are magnetic and, because of their abundance in living tissue, are the nuclei involved in imaging by most present-day devices.

All studies that use x-rays are limited in recording the differences in tissue based on photon absorption alone. Magnetic resonance imaging, however, can make use of a large variety of pulse sequences to enhance tissue discrimination. A further characteristic of MRI is that flowing blood usually gives no signal, allowing easy recognition of vascular structures from surrounding tissue. MRI has no known adverse biologic effects.

Tesla is the unit of strength of the magnet. Most newer scanners are 1.5 T, although excellent images can be obtained on lower field strengths of 0.3 T to 1.0 T. Cardiac gating is needed to image the chest and requires 4 to 6 minutes to scan 10 slices. Respiratory compensation, a form of respiratory gating, is also needed. MRI is not a routine study but should be used to solve specific problems.

MRI has a number of advantages over CT scanning in evaluating the heart and mediastinum. Moving blood can be made to have no signal or to have a bright signal without the addition of contrast material. This capability aids in the identification of masses and nodes in the hili or mediastinum and offers an alternative modality to CT in patients who are allergic to contrast. The ability to image the chest in saggital, coronal, and oblique planes is a significant advantage over CT. Cardiac gating allows improved visualization of intracardiac anatomy and pathology.

In the evaluation of lung cancer and mediastinal masses, CT and MRI offer similar results. However, MRI is better at evaluating invasion of the chest wall, brachial plexus, and subclavian vessels such as in superior sulcus tumors. Coronal imaging improves detection of subcarinal and AP window adenopathy. MRI is the imaging method of choice for evaluating posterior mediastinal neurogenic tumors that may involve the spinal canal. MRI cannot detect calcification, which is often important in chest imaging. MRI of the aorta is very good at evaluating acquired diseases such as aneurysms and dissections as well as congenital lesions such as vascular rings and coarctations. The ability to image the entire aorta on one oblique scan is a distinct advantage. MRI is the imaging modality of choice for imaging intracardiac tumors and masses and for evaluating the extent of cardiac involvement by paracardiac lesions (Fig. 43-5). MRI is also useful in

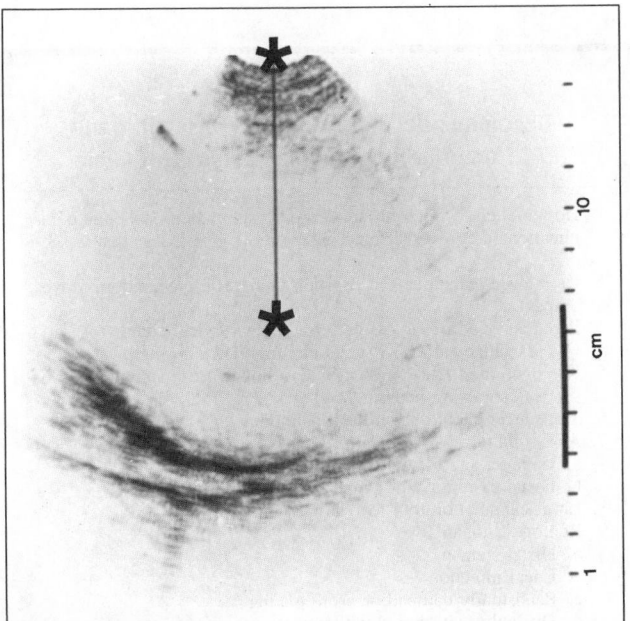

FIGURE 43-4   Ultrasound of a left lower posterior thoracic density. *Upper**, on skin surface, *lower**, within echo-free fluid. Depth indicated by 1 cm gradation marks at right. Needle aspiration at 6 cm depth revealed an empyema.

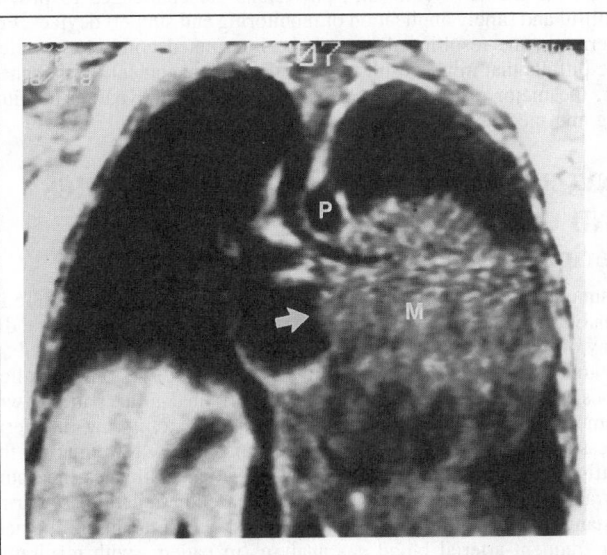

FIGURE 43-5   Coronal plane MRI in a patient with a lung mass *(M)* that has invaded the left atrium *(arrow)*. *P,* Pulmonary artery lateral to the trachea and superior to the left bronchus.

evaluating obstruction, compression, or thrombosis of the mediastinal veins.

Cardiac pacemakers, ferromagnetic vascular clips, implants or foreign bodies in critical areas (e.g., intracerebral, eye, cochlea), and the very early Starr-Edwards or other loosened heart valves are contraindications to MRI studies.

MRI of the chest is evolving rapidly as new imaging techniques are discovered. Imaging of the lung parenchyma and pulmonary arteries and more detailed cardiac imaging will be available in the near future.

BIBLIOGRAPHY

Kelley MA et al: Diagnosing pulmonary embolism: new facts and strategies, *Ann Intern Med* 114:300, 1991.

Naidich DP, Zerhouni EA, Siegelman SS: *Computed tomography and magnetic resonance of the thorax*, ed 2, New York, 1991, Raven.

Pinet F et al: Embolization of the systemic arteries of the lung, *J Thorac Imaging* 2:11, 1987.

Webb WR, Muller NL, Naidich DP: *High-resolution CT of the lung*, New York, 1992, Raven.

Webb WR, Sostman HD: MR imaging of thoracic disease: clinical uses, *Radiology* 182:621, 1992.

CHAPTER

44 Intensive Care Monitoring and Mechanical Ventilation

Herbert P. Wiedemann

Critically ill hospitalized patients are treated almost exclusively within specialized intensive care units. Two major developments during the last 30 years provided the impetus behind the flourishing of intensive care units. In the late 1960s, the value of volume-cycled ventilators and of delivering assisted ventilation in special centralized units was documented. The other major advance was the emergence of technologies that allowed the monitoring of important hemodynamic parameters. Most notable in this regard was the introduction of bedside pulmonary artery catheterization in the early 1970s.

In the intensive care unit, physicians are challenged to provide skillful and timely application of monitoring and support devices. Furthermore, the resulting data must be interpreted correctly, avoiding the pitfalls that might result in clinical mismanagement. In this chapter, the major procedures and techniques of hemodynamic monitoring and mechanical ventilation are discussed.

INVASIVE MONITORING OF HEMODYNAMICS AND GAS EXCHANGE
Peripheral Artery Catheterization

Cannulation of a peripheral artery is frequently performed in the intensive care unit, allowing (1) continuous monitoring and graphic display of the systemic arterial blood pressure, and (2) repeated analysis of arterial blood gases. Because of the low risk of serious complications, peripheral artery cannulation is warranted in all patients with hemodynamic instability in whom continuous monitoring of arterial pressures is important. Arterial catheters also improve accuracy in this setting, since sphygmomanometry usually underestimates the actual intraarterial pressure in patients with increased peripheral vascular resistance caused by hypovolemia or overt shock. In addition, the need for frequent arterial blood gas analyses in patients with respiratory failure is a relative indication for the use of an indwelling catheter to avoid the inconvenience and discomfort of frequent "single-stick" arterial samples. However, the advent of noninvasive techniques for monitoring arterial oxygen saturation (e.g., oximetry) and $Paco_2$ (e.g.,

capnography) is reducing the need for indwelling arterial catheters in hemodynamically stable patients being monitored solely for respiratory failure.

With proper technique (Box 44-1) peripheral artery cannulation is generally safe. The major complications are ischemia distal to the insertion site and infection. Ischemia may be secondary to either local thrombosis or distal embolization. Subclinical and reversible arterial occlusion are common, with up to one fourth of arteries remaining angiographically occluded 1 week after catheter removal. However, clinically significant ischemia (e.g., necrosis of fingers or toes) is rare (less than 0.2%). Hypotension, severe peripheral vascular disease, and the use of vasopressor drugs increase the risk of serious ischemic complications. The incidence of catheter-related septicemia can be reduced to less than 1% with proper precautions. Risk factors favoring infection include cannulation exceeding 4 days at one site and insertion by surgical cutdown rather than percutaneously.

Pulmonary Artery Catheterization

Routine bedside catheterization of the pulmonary artery became feasible with the introduction of the balloon-tipped catheter by Swan and colleagues in 1970. Since the inflatable balloon at the tip allows the catheter to be directed by blood flow, fluoroscopy usually is not necessary for proper placement. Several versions of the pulmonary artery catheter, commonly referred to as the *Swan-Ganz catheter,* are now available. One important modification of the original design is the placement of a thermistor near the distal tip, which allows for measurement of cardiac output by the thermodilution technique. Figure 44-1 depicts the most frequently used pulmonary artery catheter.

Pulmonary artery catheterization rapidly became an integral aspect in the management of many intensive care unit patients because the properly positioned catheter allows the direct acquisition of three important physiologic variables (Box 44-2): (1) cardiac output, (2) intravascular pressures (right heart chambers, pulmonary artery, and pulmonary artery occlusion or "wedge" pressure), and (3) mixed venous oxygenation. Additionally, a large number of calculated physiologic parameters can be derived from these primary measurements (Table 44-1).

Insertion and Normal Wave Forms. Venous access can be achieved via percutaneous insertion of the catheter through the subclavian, internal jugular, external jugular, femoral, or antecubital vein; cutdown may be necessary with the antecubital route. The catheter is

---

BOX 44-1

Recommended technique for inserting and maintaining systemic artery lines

1. Do an Allen test before radial artery cannulation. Ischemic complications are lowest if ulnar artery refill time is less than 5 seconds.
2. Use sterile technique for insertion (antiseptic preparation, gloves, drapes).
3. Percutaneous insertion is preferred over surgical cutdown.
4. Use 20-gauge catheter if wrist circumference is small.
5. Use continuous flush system with a nondextrose solution (normal saline) containing heparin.
6. Transducer should have disposable dome.
7. Assess daily
   a. Catheter site for evidence of inflammation
   b. Distal extremity for evidence of ischemia
8. Limit cannulation to 4 to 5 days at one site
9. Remove catheter for
   a. Distal ischemia
   b. Local infection
   c. Persistently damped pressure tracing
   d. Difficulty with blood withdrawal

Modified with permission from Matthay MA: Invasive hemodynamic monitoring in critically ill patients, *Clin Chest Med* 4:233, 1983.

advanced with continuous monitoring of the electrocardiogram (ECG) (for arrhythmia detection) and venous pressures recorded from the distal orifice. A sudden increase in the respiratory fluctuation of recorded pressures signals that the catheter tip has reached a central intrathoracic vein. The balloon is then inflated with air to the full recommended volume (1.5 ml for the 7 French catheter; 0.8 ml for the 5 French catheter) for flow-directed passage through the right atrium, right ventricle, and into the pulmonary artery. As a general guide, the right atrium should be reached about 10 cm from the subclavian vein, 10 to 15 cm from the jugular vein, 30 cm from a femoral vein insertion site, 40 cm from the right antecubital fossa, and 50 cm from the left antecubital fossa. Representative normal pressure tracings seen during passage of the catheter are shown in Fig. 44-2. The catheter is advanced until a pulmonary artery "wedge" tracing is obtained. This occurs when the balloon occludes the pulmonary artery segment; with absent flow, the pressure tracing from the distal orifice of the catheter reflects left atrial pressure. During flotation of the catheter, it is important to have the balloon fully inflated to prevent the catheter tip from protruding (Fig. 44-3). A catheter tip that is too distal and located in a small pulmonary artery may cause falsely high measurements of cardiac output and mixed venous PO2.

Because measurement of the pulmonary artery wedge pressure (PAWP) is a major use of the pulmonary artery catheter and provides the basis for important diagnostic and therapeutic decisions, it is essential to obtain a valid PAWP. Adherence to the following criteria helps ensure a valid PAWP:

1. A tracing characteristic of a left atrial wave form should be seen; a highly "damped" tracing devoid of oscillations except those resulting from ventilation-induced pressure changes is not acceptable. The PAWP wave form should disappear promptly with balloon deflation, yielding a pulmonary artery tracing, and return rapidly after balloon reinflation
2. The mean PAWP should be lower than or equal to the pulmonary artery diastolic pressure (the PAWP may transiently exceed pulmonary artery diastolic pressure in severe mitral regurgitation)
3. Catheter obstruction is ruled out by the ability of a saline flush solution to flow through the distal lumen.
4. Blood gas analysis of blood withdrawn from the distal port should reflect systemic arterial PO2 and PCO2 rather than that of mixed venous blood. Although this last criterion is usually not routinely tested, it may be of help in confusing situations. The validity of this criterion is supported by information that highly oxygenated blood is usually withdrawn from a true wedge position even in areas of radiographic infiltrates or in patients with large intrapulmonic shunts.

Although flow-directed passage of the catheter into the pulmonary artery usually presents little difficulty, a problem may occur in the presence of low cardiac output, tricuspid valve regurgitation, right ventricular dilation, or severe pulmonary hypertension. In such circumstances, a left-sided venous access route is advantageous, because the catheter has to loop in only one direction in going from the left subclavian vein to the right ventricular outflow. In some instances it may be necessary to advance the catheter with fluoroscopy to provide a direct visual assessment of catheter position.

Inability to obtain a valid PAWP tracing could be caused by a catheter tip that is not located in zone 3 of the lung (Fig. 44-4). If the catheter tip is located outside zone 3, the pulmonary artery tracing may appear normal until the balloon is inflated. Because alveolar pressure exceeds pulmonary capillary pressure in zone 2, the vessel distal to the inflated balloon then collapses, causing PAWP to reflect alveolar pressure rather than left atrial pressure. Because the vast ma-

---

BOX 44-2

Directly measured physiologic variables obtained with pulmonary artery catheterization

Cardiac output
Intravascular pressures
  Right atrial pressure
  Right ventricular pressure
  Pulmonary artery pressure
  Pulmonary artery "wedge" pressure
Mixed venous oxygenation

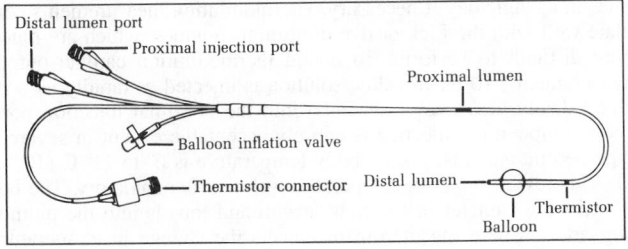

FIGURE 44-1 Typical triple-lumen pulmonary artery catheter. When the catheter is properly positioned and the balloon is deflated, the distal lumen records pulmonary artery pressure. When the balloon is inflated enough to occlude the segmental pulmonary artery, the distal lumen measures "wedge" pressure. The proximal lumen is 30 cm from the catheter tip and lies in the right atrium. A thermistor located just proximal to the balloon is used for cardiac output studies; the thermistor senses a temperature change shortly after a cold bolus of fluid exists from the proximal lumen.

(From Matthay MA: Invasive hemodynamic monitoring in acute respiratory failure, *J Respir Dis* 2:40, 1981.)

Table 44-1   Physiologic data derived from invasive monitoring

	NORMAL RANGE
Cardiac index (L/min/m²) $$CI = \frac{CO}{BSA}$$	2.4-4.4
Systemic vascular resistance (dynes · sec · cm⁻⁵) $$SVR = \frac{MAP - CVP}{CO} \times 79.9$$	900-1400
Pulmonary vascular resistance (dynes · sec · cm⁻⁵) $$PVR = \frac{MPAP - PAWP}{CO} \times 79.9$$	150-250
Stroke volume (ml) $$SV = \frac{CO}{HR}$$	
Stroke volume index (ml/m²) $$SVI = \frac{SV}{BSA} = \frac{CI}{HR}$$	30-65
Left ventricular stroke work index (g · m/m²) $$LVSWI = SVI \times (MAP - PAOP) \times 0.0136$$	43-61
Right ventricular stroke work index (g · m/m²) $$RVSWI = SVI \times (MPAP - CVP) \times 0.0136$$	7-12
Oxygen content (ml/dl blood) $$CaO_2 = Hgb \times \text{arterial O}_2 \text{ saturation} \times 1.36 + (Po_2 \times 0.003)$$	About 19.5
Arteriovenous oxygen content difference (ml/dl) $$avDO_2 = CaO_2 - CvO_2$$	3-5
Oxygen delivery (ml/min) $$\text{O}_2 \text{ delivery} = CO \times CaO_2 \times 10$$	800-1200
Oxygen consumption (ml/min) $$\dot{V}O_2 = CO \times (CaO_2 - CvO_2) \times 10$$	180-280
Pulmonary shunt (venoarterial admixture) (%) $$\frac{QS}{Qt} = \frac{CcO_2 - CaO_2}{CcO_2 - CvO_2}$$	<3-5%

Modified from Sprung CL, editor: *The pulmonary artery catheter: methodology and clinical applications*, Baltimore, 1983, University Park.
BSA, Body surface area; *CaO₂*, arterial oxygen content; *CcO₂*, pulmonary capillary oxygen content (assumed equal to alveolar Po₂); *CI*, cardiac index; *CO*, cardiac output; *CvO₂*, mixed venous oxygen content; *CVP*, central venous pressure; *Hgb*, hemoglobin concentration; *HR*, heart rate; *LVSWI*, left ventricular stroke work index; *MAP*, mean arterial pressure; *PAOP*, pulmonary artery occlusion pressure; *MPAP*, mean pulmonary artery pressure; *PAWP*, pulmonary artery wedge pressure; *PVR*, pulmonary vascular resistance; *Qs/Qt*, pulmonary shunt; *RVSWI*, right ventricular stroke work index; *SV*, stroke volume; *SVI*, stroke volume index; *SVR*, systemic vascular resistance.

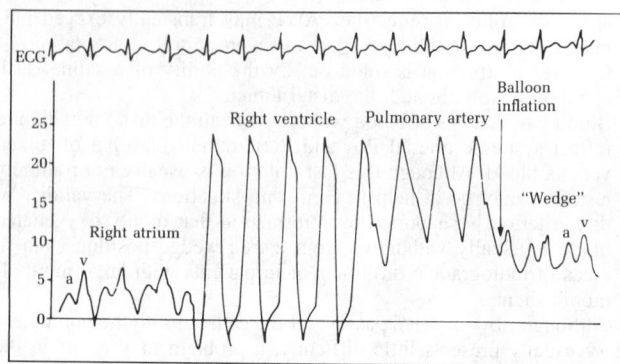

FIGURE 44-2   Representative recording of normal pressures and wave forms as a Swan-Ganz catheter is passed through the right side of the heart into the pulmonary artery. The first waveform is a right atrial tracing with characteristic a and v waves. The right ventricular, pulmonary artery, and pulmonary artery wedge tracings follow in sequence. Note that the wedge tracing shows a and v waves transmitted from the left atrium. In addition, the wedge pressure (mean) is less than pulmonary artery diastolic pressure. The wedge tracing is not always this distinct, but a very damped tracing or a mean wedge pressure greater than pulmonary artery diastolic pressure usually indicates some mechanical problem in the system (e.g., air bubble in the connecting tubing, catheter tip "overwedged," balloon inflated over distal orifice, or catheter tip in zone 1 or zone 2). In severe mitral regurgitation, the large transmitted left atrial v waves occasionally may cause the wedge tracing to resemble a pulmonary artery tracing. In such a case, careful analysis of the waveforms and attention to where the peak pressure occurs in relation to the ECG complex (top tracing) usually will avoid misinterpretation.

(From Matthay MA: Invasive hemodynamic monitoring in critically ill patients, *Clin Chest Med* 4:233, 1983.)

jority of pulmonary blood flows through zone 3, the flow-directed catheter usually migrates into this region during initial insertion. However, the size of the lung zones may change in response to physiologic alterations. For instance, diuresis or ventilation with high levels of positive end-expiratory pressure (PEEP) reduces the size of zone 3 because of a decrease in pulmonary venous pressure or an increase in alveolar pressure, respectively. Thus a catheter tip originally correctly positioned in zone 3 may subsequently be in zone 2. To obtain a valid wedge position, it may be necessary to refloat the catheter under these new physiologic conditions.

If a proper wedge tracing cannot be obtained, pulmonary artery diastolic pressure is sometimes used to estimate PAWP. In individuals with a normal heart rate and a normal pulmonary vascular bed, the relationship between these values is close. However, with tachycardia (especially heart rates above 120 per minute) or pulmonary hypertension, pulmonary artery diastolic pressure exceeds PAWP by large amounts. Thus in many situations requiring monitoring (e.g., adult respiratory distress syndrome, pulmonary embolism), estimation of PAWP from the pulmonary artery diastolic pressure is unreliable.

The normal waveforms depicted in Fig. 44-2 may be altered significantly by pathophysiologic conditions. For example, infarction of the right ventricle may reduce the pressure generated by this chamber to such a degree that right atrial, right ventricular, and pulmonary artery wave forms and pressures are nearly identical. Severe mitral valve insufficiency leads to a wedge tracing with a large left atrial "v" wave that may mimic the pulmonary artery waveform. These and other situations may cause significant confusion unless the clinician anticipates the possibility of aberrant waveforms through an understanding of the clinical setting.

Because intravascular pressure readings such as PAWP are calibrated relative to atmosphere, these measurements reflect transmural vascular pressures (pressure difference across the wall of the vessel or heart chamber) only if the pleural and atmospheric pressures are equal. (The importance of correctly assessing transmural pressure and the interpretation of PAWP during PEEP therapy are addressed more fully in the subsequent discussion of the relationship between PAWP and left ventricular preload.) Because pleural pressure most closely approximates atmospheric pressure at end expiration, vascular pressure readings should be obtained at this time (Fig. 44-5).

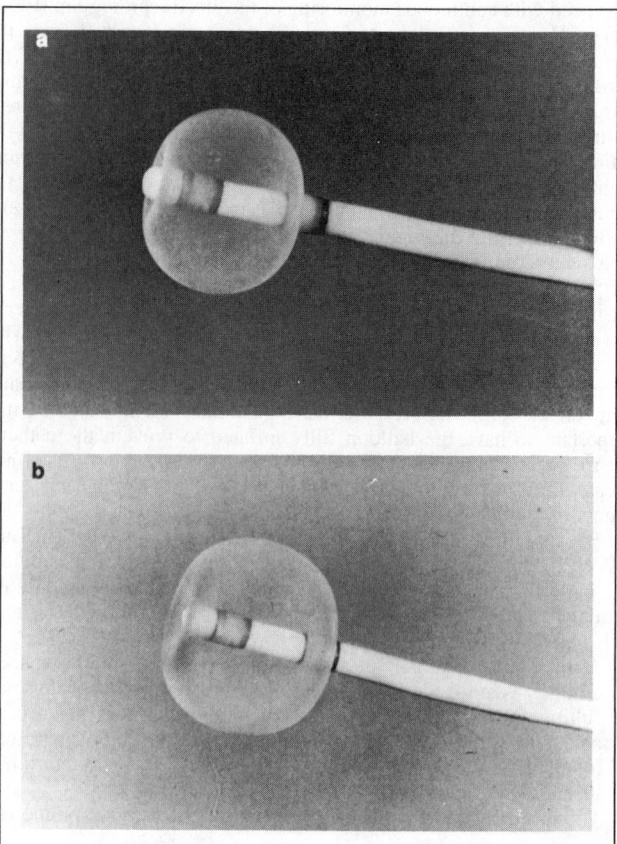

FIGURE 44-3   Photographs of a 7 French Swan-Ganz catheter balloon inflated with **A,** 1.0 ml, and **B,** 1.5 ml of air. Notice that the catheter tip protrudes beyond the inflated balloon if less than the full recommended volume is used. The exposed catheter tip may cause endocardial damage, induce ventricular arrhythmias, or damage the pulmonary artery. Also, using the recommended volume helps ensure a relatively proximal wedge position, which is important to lessen the risk of pulmonary infarction and to help maintain accuracy of thermodilution cardiac output and mixed venous PO_2 determinations. A catheter tip that is too distal and located in a small pulmonary artery may cause falsely high measurements of cardiac output and mixed venous PO_2.

(From Sprung CL: Complications of pulmonary artery catheterization. In Sprung CL, editor: *The pulmonary artery catheter: methodology and clinical applications,* Baltimore, 1983, University Park.)

Thermodilution Cardiac Output. (Also see Chapter 13.) With a thermistor-tipped pulmonary artery catheter and a commercially available bedside microprocessor, the measurement of cardiac output is an easy and rapid procedure that can be performed many times in a single day if necessary. Thermodilution measurements correlate well with the Fick or dye dilution techniques, which are much more difficult to perform. To obtain thermodilution cardiac output measurements, 10 ml of saline solution is injected as rapidly as possible (ideally, less than 4 seconds) into the proximal injection port. Room temperature injectate is entirely acceptable except in severely hypothermic patients; if core body temperature is 6° to 11° C (10° to 20° F) below normal, ice temperature solution is mandatory. The bolus exits the catheter in the right atrium and travels into the pulmonary artery where the thermistor detects the change in temperature over time. The bedside microprocessor quickly calculates and displays the cardiac output.

Phasic changes in intrathoracic pressure and venous return induced by spontaneous or mechanical ventilation may cause significant variability in single measurements. To reduce this problem, as well as other causes of variability, it is standard practice to average three consecutive measurements (about 1 minute apart), which are all obtained at end expiration, to constitute a single determination. Cardiac output determinations performed in this manner have an accuracy and reproducibility that are usually very acceptable for clinical use. How-

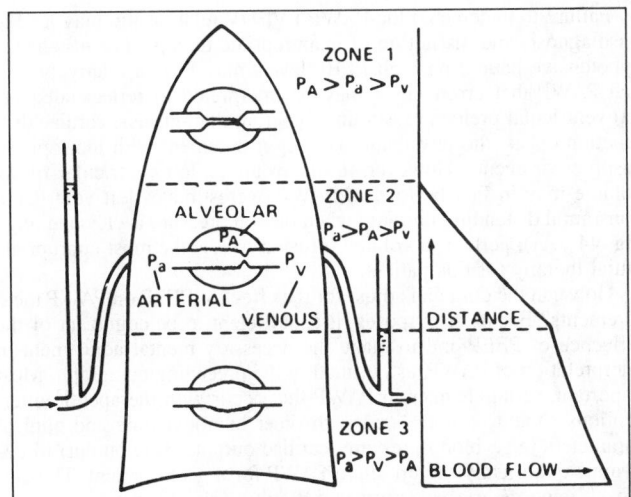

FIGURE 44-4   Zones of the lung, based on the relationship among pulmonary artery (P_a) pressure, alveolar pressure (P_A), and pulmonary venous pressure (P_V). The zones are not constant. For instance, a decrease in P_V (e.g., diuresis) or an increase in P_A (e.g., PEEP therapy) converts some zone 3 area into zone 2 or zone 1. The pulmonary wedge pressure reflects P_V (and thus left atrial pressure) only if the tip of the Swan-Ganz catheter lies in zone 3 before balloon inflation. If the balloon is inflated in zone 2, the occluded vessel collapses because P_A is greater than P_V. Without a continuous column of the blood between the catheter tip and the left atrium, the wedge pressure cannot reflect left atrial pressure.

(From West JB, Dollery CT, Naimark A: Distribution of blood flow in isolated lung: relation to vascular and alveolar pressure, *J Appl Physiol* 19:713, 1964.)

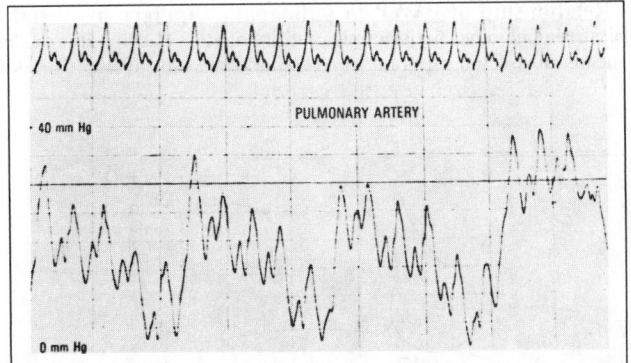

FIGURE 44-5   Example of how rapid, labored respiration can result in marked fluctuations of the pulmonary artery pressure tracing *(lower tracing)*. The upper tracing is the ECG. The patient's respiratory rate was 40, and the peak pulmonary artery pressure varied from 35 to 40 to 18 mm Hg. Because the pressures are recorded on calibrated strip chart paper, the pressures corresponding to the brief period of end expiration can be easily identified. A digital readout could be very misleading, as this value would be an electronic average of a 3- to 4-second scanning period.

(From Matthay MA: Invasive hemodynamic monitoring in critically ill patients, *Clin Chest Med* 4:233, 1983.)

ever, the thermodilution technique may not be accurate in the presence of significant tricuspid valve regurgitation (which causes a falsely low measurement), intracardiac shunts, or a too distally placed catheter (may be suspected when less than 1.0 ml of air in the balloon produces a wedge pressure).

Mixed Venous Oxygen Saturation.   Mixed venous blood is sampled through the distal orifice of the pulmonary artery catheter with the balloon deflated. (The 7 French catheter has a 2.5 ml dead space that must first be eliminated by discarding the initial sample.) In patients receiving mechanical ventilation and very high inspired oxygen concentration, a fast rate of blood withdrawal may lead to a falsely elevated mixed venous oxygen saturation caused by contamination of the sample with pulmonary capillary blood. A slow rate of blood withdrawal (less than 3 ml/minute) eliminates this possibility. Severe mitral valve regurgitation may also cause a falsely elevated mixed venous oxygen saturation as a result of retrograde pulmonary capillary blood flow.

Clinically, mixed venous oxygenation is used to monitor changes in cardiac output and assess tissue oxygenation. In normal individuals and many patients, as oxygen delivery (cardiac output × arterial oxygen content) decreases, increased extraction of oxygen from circulating blood allows tissue oxygen consumption to remain stable (oxygen consumption is independent of oxygen delivery until a critically low level of delivery) but causes the mixed venous oxygen content to decrease. Thus a decrease in cardiac output is reflected by a corresponding decline in mixed venous oxygen. Furthermore, as mixed venous Po$_2$ approaches 27 to 30 mm Hg (normal, 39 mm Hg), blood lactate levels usually increase, indicating that tissue oxygenation is reaching a critically low level. These interpretations of mixed venous oxygenation are most valid in patients with "simple" hemodynamic problems, such as isolated myocardial dysfunction. In more complex illnesses, including sepsis and the adult respiratory distress syndrome (ARDS), the interpretation of mixed venous oxygenation is much more complex. In sepsis, peripheral "shunting" of arterial blood past tissue beds may lead to maintenance of a high mixed venous oxygen level despite tissue oxygen deprivation indicated by high blood lactate levels. Furthermore, in some ARDS patients, oxygen consumption varies with oxygen delivery, even at normal or high cardiac outputs, suggesting an abnormal "supply dependency" of oxygen consumption. This phenomenon may be related in part to abnormalities in the systemic capillary circulation, which prevent normal tissue oxygen extraction. The result is that mixed venous oxygenation may remain high and relatively stable despite large, and presumably clinically important, decreases in cardiac output, oxygen delivery, and oxygen consumption. It is clear that solely monitoring mixed venous oxygenation in patients with sepsis or ARDS is inadequate. The clinician needs to monitor several other parameters, including cardiac output, arterial oxygen saturation, and lactate levels to be informed about changes in hemodynamic states of these patients.

Pulmonary artery catheters that provide a continuous measurement of the mixed oxygen saturation through use of fiberoptic reflectance oximetry are currently available. Although the continuous monitoring of mixed venous oxygenation may provide a helpful "early warning system" for detecting adverse hemodynamic trends, its value in this regard is limited by the factors outlined in the preceding discussion. Reliance on stable mixed venous oxygenation may provide a false sense of security in patients with illnesses such as ARDS or sepsis.

Left-to-right intracardiac shunts cause an elevated mixed venous oxygenation. This fact may be helpful in diagnosing atrial or ventricular septal defects; during passage of the catheter, blood samples show an abnormal "step-up" in oxygen saturation as the tip is passed into the right atrium or right ventricle. An example of how this maneuver may provide important diagnostic information is a patient with myocardial infarction who develops sudden hemodynamic instability and a systolic murmur. The major diagnoses to be considered are acute ventricular septal defect or acute mitral valve insufficiency. These possibilities can be easily distinguished through an assessment of oxygen saturation in the chambers of the right heart.

It is important to remember that mixed venous oxygenation has an important influence on arterial oxygenation saturation when there is a high degree of shunt through the lungs (e.g., ARDS) (Fig. 44-6). Although clinicians often reflexively attribute a decrease in Pao$_2$ to a worsening of lung function, such a decrease may in fact result from nonrespiratory factors that cause a reduction in mixed venous oxygenation (e.g., anemia, increased oxygen consumption, low cardiac output). If such factors are corrected, arterial oxygen saturation may improve even if lung disease does not improve.

Pulmonary Artery Wedge Pressure.   The measurement of the PAWP is a major use of the pulmonary artery catheter. The PAWP allows the clinician to make important assumptions regarding left ventricular preload and pulmonary capillary hydrostatic pressure.

Balloon occlusion of a branch of the pulmonary artery causes flow to cease between the catheter tip and the "junction point" at which pulmonary venous radicles served by the occluded artery join other radicles in which blood is still flowing toward the left atrium. Pulmonary artery wedge pressure reflects venous pressure at this junction point, which appears to be located in a pulmonary vein of about the same size as the occluded pulmonary artery. Thus the usual wedge pressure produced by balloon occlusion of a lobar artery correlates well with venous pressure at or near the left atrium. Because little pressure difference normally exists among the large pulmonary veins, left atrium, and left ventricle during end diastole, PAWP usually is a good approximation of intracavitary left ventricular end diastolic pressure (LVEDP). Under certain circumstances, however, normal pressure equilibration is prevented, and this relationship does not hold. For instance, obstruction of the large pulmonary veins (e.g., atrial myxoma, thoracic tumors, mediastinal fibrosis) may cause PAWP to exceed left atrial pressure. Similarly, mitral valve stenosis or insufficiency causes PAWP and left atrial pressure to exceed LVEDP. If left ventricular compliance is very reduced, left atrial contraction causes an increase in LVEDP such that it may exceed PAWP by 5 mm Hg or more. Although the clinician needs to be alert to these and related exceptions, PAWP usually provides a good estimate of LVEDP.

Relationship of PAWP to left ventricular preload. (See Chapter 14). According to the Frank-Starling principle, left ventricular preload determines the force of cardiac contraction for any given level of myocardial contractility. Therefore a measurement of left ventricular function (e.g., cardiac output) taken in conjunction with an assessment of left ventricular preload allows the clinician to make important conclusions regarding left ventricular contractility. Because PAWP is frequently used to assess left ventricular preload, it is important to understand the relationship between the two, which are sometimes incorrectly assumed to be identical.

Preload refers to stretch of myocardial fibers, and therefore is best assessed by left ventricular end diastolic *volume* (LVEDV). The LVEDV is determined by the transmural ventricular distending pressure (intracavitary pressure, or PAWP, minus juxtacardiac pressure) and ventricular compliance (pressure − volume relationship). The relationship between PAWP and left ventricular preload is shown in Fig. 44-7, which illustrates how a given PAWP may be associated with varying degrees of left ventricular filling in critically ill patients with altered juxtacardiac pressure (e.g., mechanical ventilation and PEEP) or ventricular compliance (e.g., myocardial ischemia, pericardial effusion).

Failure to understand the PAWP-LVEDV relationship may lead to misdiagnosis and institution of inappropriate therapy. For instance, a hypotensive patient on high PEEP levels may have a relatively normal PAWP that erroneously may be interpreted to reflect adequate left ventricular preload. Assuming therefore that intrinsic cardiac dysfunction exists, the physician may begin treatment with inotropic or vasopressor agents. However, in this example, left ventricular filling volume may in fact be low, as PAWP overestimates left ventricular transmural distending pressure when pleural pressure is elevated (e.g., Fig. 44-7, *A*); perhaps a volume infusion trial is the most appropriate initial therapy for this patient.

How can the clinician adjust for the effect of PEEP on PAWP measurements? For most purposes, it is sufficient to be cognizant of the influence of PEEP and to make the necessary mental adjustment in interpretation of PAWP, as outlined in the preceding paragraph. Most important, serial changes in PAWP that occur with therapeutic interventions should be correlated with other hemodynamic and clinical parameters (e.g., blood pressure, cardiac output, urine output) to determine empirically the optimum PAWP for a given patient. This approach is necessary because it is difficult to directly measure or calculate juxtacardiac pressure in patients. Pleural pressure at endexpiration cannot be assumed to be equal to PEEP, as lung and chest wall compliance affects the relationship between these pressures. In patients with poor lung compliance (e.g., ARDS), the change in pleural pressure is usually less than one half of the applied PEEP. Direct measurement of pleural pressure with an esophageal balloon is impractical in intensive care patients; furthermore, this measurement may underestimate the immediate juxtacardiac pressure in ventilated patients. Temporarily disconnecting PEEP to measure PAWP is discouraged. The resulting new measurement is of questionable value because hemodynamics are altered (e.g., an acute increase in venous return). In addition, abrupt removal of PEEP may cause dangerous hypoxemia, and this may not be fully and rapidly reversible with reinstitution of PEEP.

Relationship of PAWP to pulmonary capillary hydrostatic pressure. The other major clinical utility of PAWP is that it provides a means of assessing pulmonary capillary pressure, or the filtration

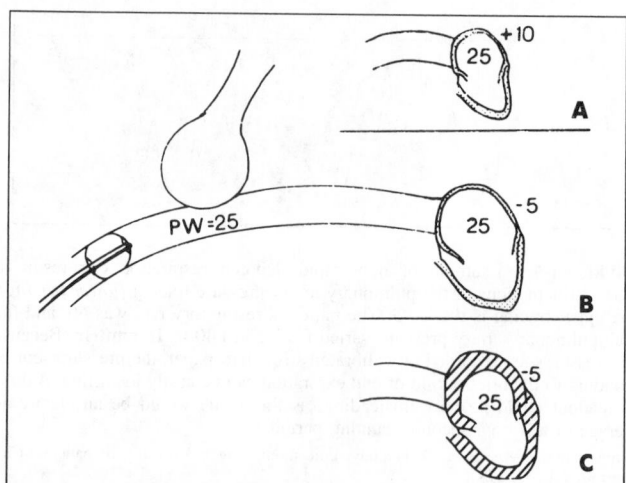

FIGURE 44-7   Relationship of pulmonary artery wedge pressure (PW) to left ventricular preload (left ventricular volume or "stretch") in three situations, illustrating the importance of considering pleural (juxtacardiac) pressure and ventricular compliance, along with PW, when making assumptions about left ventricular preload. The PW is elevated in each example and reflects the intracavitary left ventricular end diastolic pressure. **A,** The pleural pressure is increased, as might occur with PEEP therapy. Transmural left ventricular pressure is approximately normal, as is the preload. **B,** The pleural pressure is normal. Transmural left ventricular pressure is elevated, and preload is increased. **C,** The ventricle is stiff, as might occur with myocardial ischemia. Although PW and pleural pressure are identical to example **B,** the preload in this instance is normal.

(From O'Quin R, Marini JJ: Pulmonary artery occlusion pressure: clinical physiology, measurement, and interpretation, *Am Rev Respir Dis* 128:319, 1983.)

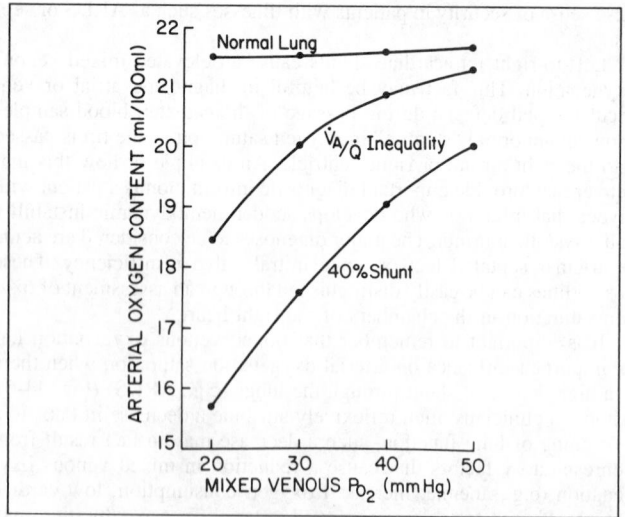

FIGURE 44-6   The effect of changing the mixed venous P_{O_2} on the arterial oxygen content in a patient with normal lungs, one with marked ventilation-perfusion inequality, and one with a large shunt. Each theoretical patient was assumed to be breathing 50% oxygen, and cardiac output and minute ventilation were held constant.

(From Dantzker DR: Gas exchange in the adult respiratory distress syndrome, *Clin Chest Med* 3:57, 1982.)

pressure favoring the development of pulmonary edema. This information often allows for the distinction between cardiogenic ("hydrostatic") and noncardiogenic ("leaky capillary") origins of lung edema fluid. Thus the presence of pulmonary edema with a normal PAWP suggests capillary injury (e.g., ARDS), whereas pulmonary edema with a high PAWP supports a cardiogenic cause such as congestive heart failure (but does not rule out coexisting lung injury). In most clinical settings, PAWP provides a reasonable assessment of pulmonary capillary pressure. However, these values are not equivalent, and the common practice of referring to PAWP as "pulmonary capillary wedge pressure" should be discouraged.

In fact, PAWP is less than true capillary pressure by a variable amount that depends on pulmonary venous resistance. Remembering that PAWP estimates pressure in the large veins near the left atrium, it is apparent that PAWP must be less than capillary pressure to maintain forward blood flow. The difference between these pressures depends on the magnitude of flow resistance between the pulmonary capillaries and left atrium. Usually about 40% of the total pressure drop from pulmonary artery to left atrium occurs on the pulmonary venous side of the capillaries. Because PAWP approximates left atrial pressure, pulmonary capillary pressure normally can be estimated as PAWP + 0.4 (mean pulmonary artery pressure − PAWP). However, influences such as hypoxia, sympathetic nervous system discharge, and vasoactive medications may significantly increase pulmonary venous resistance with the result that pulmonary capillary pressure may far exceed PAWP. A rare but prototypic example is pulmonary veno-occlusive disease, in which the PAWP is frequently normal but the chest roentgenogram exhibits pulmonary edema. Increased pulmonary venous resistance probably also sometimes contributes to pulmonary edema in more common problems such as central nervous system injury (neurogenic pulmonary edema), myocardial infarction, and ARDS. Further research is necessary, but it does appear that reliance on PAWP causes the physician to underestimate the role of hydrostatic forces in the development of pulmonary edema under some clinical circumstances. However, until more direct measurements of pulmonary capillary pressure become available, PAWP remains an extremely valuable, and often essential, measurement for the assessment and management of pulmonary edema.

Complications of Pulmonary Artery Catheterization.

The potential adverse effects of pulmonary artery catheterization are now well understood from over a decade of experience (Box 44-3). Ventricular arrhythmias occur frequently during insertion of the catheter but are usually self-limited. In critically ill patients, the incidence of ventricular tachycardia (three or more consecutive premature ventricular contractions [PVCs]) is reported to be 20% to 50%. However, sustained ventricular tachycardia requiring therapy occurs in only 1% to 2% of such patients. Risk factors for ventricular tachycardia include hypocalcemia, myocardial infarction or ischemia, hypotension, and hypokalemia. However, the two most significant risk factors are hypoxemia (Po_2 less than 60 mm Hg) and acidosis (pH less than 7.2). In such high-risk patients, the use of prophylactic lidocaine during catheter insertion should be considered.

During the initial years of Swan-Ganz catheter use, pulmonary infarction was one of the most common serious complications. The incidence of pulmonary infarction was found to be greater than 7% in the mid-1970s. However, more recent experience suggests that the incidence of pulmonary infarction is now at most 1%. The difference may result from better understanding of techniques that minimize this complication. For instance, the risk of thrombus developing on the catheter tip is now reduced by the use of continuous flush with heparin solutions. Equally important is the avoidance of persistent wedging of the catheter tip. Also, the balloon should never be inflated for longer than is necessary to obtain a wedge pressure reading (15 to 20 seconds).

The incidence of pulmonary artery rupture is about 0.2%. This is a serious complication with approximately a 50% mortality. The major risk factor for pulmonary artery rupture is pulmonary artery hypertension. Proper technique can minimize the risk of this serious complication. The balloon should always be inflated slowly and with continuous pressure monitoring; inflation should cease as soon as a wedge tracing is obtained. Hand flushing of the catheter while it is in a wedge position should be avoided.

Indications for Pulmonary Artery Catheterization.

Use of the pulmonary artery catheter should be reserved for those patients in whom the diagnosis or reasonable initial therapeutic plan remains unclear after a careful clinical and noninvasive assessment, or in patients who are so unstable that the proposed treatment requires invasive monitoring. Clinical settings in which pulmonary artery catheters are frequently used include complicated myocardial infarction or congestive heart failure, ARDS (especially if PEEP greater than 10 cm H_2O is required), septic shock, pulmonary embolism with hypotension, and during major cardiac or vascular surgery (Box 44-4).

The physician should maintain respect for the possibility of a serious complication, albeit uncommon, from the pulmonary artery catheter and avoid the overzealous use in patients in whom the information obtained is unlikely to change the diagnosis or therapy.

BOX 44-3

Complications of balloon flotation right heart catheterization

1. Arrhythmias
   a. Transient premature ventricular contractions (PVCs)
   b. Sustained ventricular tachycardia
   c. Ventricular fibrillation
   d. Atrial fibrillation
   e. Atrial flutter
2. Right bundle branch block
3. Pulmonary infarction
4. Pulmonary artery rupture
5. Catheter-related infections
6. Balloon rupture
7. Catheter knotting
8. Endocardial damage
   a. Valve cusps
   b. Chordae tendineae
   c. Papillary muscles
9. Complications at insertion site
   a. Pneumothorax
   b. Arterial puncture
   c. Venous thrombosis or phlebitis
   d. Air embolism

BOX 44-4

Some indications for pulmonary artery catheterization

1. Distinguish noncardiogenic and cardiogenic pulmonary edema
2. Adult respiratory distress syndrome: manage PEEP and volume therapy
3. Myocardial infarction complicated by
   a. hypotension unresponsive to volume challenge
   b. hemodynamic instability requiring vasoactive drugs or mechanical assist devices
   c. suspected cardiac tamponade (equalization of end diastolic pressures)
   d. suspected mitral regurgitation (giant "v" waves)
   e. suspected ruptured interventricular septum (step-up in right heart oxygen saturation)
4. Unresponsive congestive heart failure
5. Resolving doubts about volume and cardiovascular status in complex illnesses (e.g., sepsis, pulmonary embolism)
6. Diagnosis and monitoring of pulmonary hypertension
7. Major cardiac surgery

Modified from Goldenheim PD, Kazemi H: Cardiopulmonary monitoring of critically ill patients, *N Engl J Med* 331:717, 1984.

NONINVASIVE MONITORING OF GAS EXCHANGE
Pulse Oximetry

Pulse oximetry provides a simple, accurate, and noninvasive technique for the continuous monitoring of arterial oxygen saturation. This technology is gaining widespread application in intensive care units. Pulse oximetry operates on a spectrophotometric principle that exploits the different absorptive properties of oxygenated and deoxygenated hemoglobin. A small lightweight device attaches to the finger or toe and directs through the nailbed usually two wavelengths of light; a photodetector measures absorption. Arterial pulsation is used to gate the signal to the arterial component of blood contained within the nailbed.

Loss of adequate finger pulsation interferes with the instrument's ability to calculate arterial saturation. Inadequate finger pulsation may occur with (1) infusion of vasoconstrictive drugs, (2) hypotension (mean blood pressure less than 50 mm Hg), and (3) hypothermia. With most instruments, inadequate pulsation triggers a "low-perfusion" alarm, which should prevent the clinical application of inaccurate data. Dark skin pigmentation and jaundice do not significantly affect accuracy. However, many units have a tendency to overestimate true arterial saturation at very low values. Furthermore, the presence of elevated carboxyhemoglobin or methemoglobin produces falsely high oxyhemoglobin saturation measurements. This could have serious clinical consequences, as the physician may not recognize important decreases in arterial oxygen content. Direct measurement of an arterial blood sample with the traditional four-wavelength cooximeter (arterial blood gases) distinguishes oxyhemoglobin from carboxyhemoglobin and methemoglobin.

Transcutaneous Oxygen and Carbon Dioxide

Heated skin probes are able to measure the concentration of oxygen or carbon dioxide that diffuses from the capillaries through the skin. At relatively normal cardiac outputs, the transcutaneous P_{O_2} (Ptc_{O_2}) is a reliable trend monitor of the Pa_{O_2}, although the Ptc_{O_2} averages only about 80% of the Pa_{O_2} (a Ptc_{O_2} value of 80 mm Hg corresponds to a Pa_{O_2} of 100 mm Hg). However, at moderate levels of hypoperfusion (cardiac index between 1.5 and 2.2 L/min/m^2), even when not associated with frank hypotension, the Ptc_{O_2} averages only about 50% of the Pa_{O_2}. This represents an important limitation of transcutaneous monitoring because such patients may not be easily distinguished without invasive monitoring of the cardiac output. And finally, in cardiogenic shock (cardiac index less than 1.5 L/min/m^2), changes in Ptc_{O_2} actually reflect changes in the cardiac output (or tissue oxygen delivery), rather than the Pa_{O_2}. The physiologic interpretation of the Ptc_{O_2} value therefore is complex but relatively well established. In patients with normal cardiac output and cutaneous blood flow, the Ptc_{O_2} reflects Pa_{O_2}. However, in low-flow states, the Ptc_{O_2} diverges from Pa_{O_2} and reflects tissue oxygen delivery instead. This represents both a problem and an opportunity. The problem is that monitoring of the Ptc_{O_2} alone may be inadequate in many clinical situations since a decreasing Ptc_{O_2} may reflect either pulmonary decompensation (decreasing Pa_{O_2}) or hemodynamic failure (decreasing cardiac output). A separate, independent measurement of respiratory or cardiac function may be necessary to properly interpret the change in Ptc_{O_2}. On the other hand, Ptc_{O_2} can detect overall decreases in tissue oxygen delivery that are otherwise difficult to assess noninvasively.

Several practical considerations affect the use of transcutaneous monitors. The heated electrodes may produce mild erythema, need to be moved frequently, have a fairly long initial equilibration time (about 5 minutes), and take time to fully respond to subsequent changes (about 1 minute). Conjunctival monitors are available, which have much shorter equilibration and response times.

The transcutaneous P_{CO_2} is usually about 5 to 20 mm Hg higher than Pa_{CO_2}. The transcutaneous P_{CO_2} measurement is less sensitive to changes in hemodynamic status than Ptc_{O_2} and responds faster to changes in arterial gas tension.

Because of the practical and theoretical considerations, transcutaneous monitoring has not achieved widespread use as a noninvasive technique to monitor arterial blood gases in adult intensive care unit patients. However, as discussed, this technology does have immediate potential application in the noninvasive assessment of tissue oxygenation in patients with hypoperfusion.

End-Tidal Carbon Dioxide Monitoring

The carbon dioxide concentration of expired gas can be continuously monitored by mass spectroscopy or infrared absorption spectrophotometry. After anatomic dead space is cleared, the exhaled carbon dioxide tension tracks the mean alveolar value, which in turn closely approximates arterial carbon dioxide tension if pulmonary ventilation and perfusion are evenly distributed. However, in most critically ill patients, end-tidal carbon dioxide monitoring does not provide a reliable approximation of absolute arterial P_{CO_2}, as ventilation and perfusion are usually not optimally matched. Nevertheless, capnography has several potential roles in the intensive care setting, including the monitoring of patients after attempted intubation, during cardiopulmonary resuscitation, and during weaning from mechanical ventilation. Quick confirmation of appropriate endotracheal intubation is sometimes difficult. Capnography is a rapid and practical technique for detecting inadvertent esophageal intubation, which causes the CO_2 tension of the "expired" gas to quickly fall to very low levels. Cardiac arrest is associated with a marked drop in the end-trial CO_2, and the return of adequate cardiac output during successful cardiopulmonary resuscitation is associated with a dramatic rise in expired CO_2. Capnography therefore is one of the earliest and most reliable indicators of adequate resuscitation. During weaning from mechanical ventilation, capnography allows easy visualization of low total volume breaths or apneic periods.

MECHANICAL VENTILATION

In the 1950s, positive pressure ventilation supplanted negative pressure ventilation (e.g., iron lung) as the method of choice for providing respiratory support to critically ill patients. The major advantages of positive pressure ventilators include (1) the ability to ventilate adequately despite the presence of increased airway resistance or decreased pulmonary compliance, (2) better "control" of the airway through endotracheal intubation (e.g., suctioning of secretions), and (3) significantly improved access to the patient because the ventilator does not encase the patient.

The major adverse consequences of positive pressure ventilation (Box 44-5) are chiefly related to the altered physiology of inspiration. Instead of the normal bellows function of the chest wall and diaphragm, which creates negative pleural and airway pressure during spontaneous inspiration, positive pressure ventilation increases tracheal and pleural pressure during inspiration, altering normal interactions among lung, chest wall, and diaphragm. As a result, positive pressure ventilation may worsen ventilation-perfusion matching within the lung, leading to increased dead space ventilation and physiologic shunting. Usually, such inefficiency can be overcome by the increased ventilatory and oxygenation capacity of mechanical ventilation itself. Another physiologic consequence of positive pressure ventilation, decreased cardiac output, may present more of a clinical problem. This may be especially true when PEEP is also applied.

Initiating Mechanical Ventilation

Indications. The gas exchange function of the lung is twofold: (1) to provide oxygenation of arterial blood, and (2) to eliminate carbon dioxide and help regulate normal arterial acid-base balance. Inadequacy of either process such that there exists an immediate threat to life constitutes acute respiratory failure, which is the major indication for mechanical ventilation.

Hypoxemia severe enough to require mechanical ventilation is

BOX 44-5
Complications of mechanical ventilation

Barotrauma (e.g., pneumothorax, pneumomediastinum, subcutaneous emphysema)
Decreased cardiac output
Nosocomial pneumonia
Complications of endotracheal or tracheostomy tubes

usually caused by disorders of the lung parenchyma that produce marked ventilation-perfusion mismatch or intrapulmonary shunting, and such hypoxemia remains relatively unaffected by increases in minute ventilation. Hypoxemia therefore is often referred to as "gas exchange" failure. In contrast, hypercapnia requiring mechanical support of respiration is usually the result of inadequate alveolar ventilation, or "ventilatory" failure. Box 44-6 lists some disorders that may require mechanical ventilation for treatment of gas exchange or ventilatory failure.

Acute respiratory failure is assessed by measurement of the arterial blood gases, but there are no absolute threshold values of arterial Po_2, Pco_2, or pH at which mechanical ventilation should be instituted. Rather, it is necessary also to consider the underlying disease process, the patient's course and response to therapy, and other factors within the overall clinical context. As a general guide, acute hypercapnia resulting in a pH less than 7.30 should lead to consideration of beginning mechanical ventilation. Hypoxemia frequently can be initially treated with supplemental oxygen via nasal prongs or face mask without resorting to mechanical ventilation. If the arterial Po_2 cannot be maintained above about 60 mm Hg with such external devices, intubation and mechanical ventilation are necessary. In addition to ensuring controlled delivery of a high oxygen concentration to the lungs, mechanical ventilation may reduce the oxygen requirement in some patients by lessening shunt through the recruitment of previously collapsed alveolar units.

Initial Ventilator Settings. After intubation, most patients are initially placed on a conventional positive pressure–volume-controlled ventilator. The settings typically selected at the start of mechanical ventilation include a tidal volume of 10 to 12 ml/kg (ideal body weight), a respiratory frequency of 12 machine-delivered breaths per minute, an oxygen concentration of 100%, and an inspiratory flow rate of 40 to 60 liters/min (80 to 100 liters/min in patients with chronic obstructive lung disease to allow more expiratory time and improve ventilation-perfusion matching). The high-pressure alarm should be set at about 10 cm above the peak airway pressure observed on these settings.

Within 20 minutes of initiating mechanical ventilation, arterial blood gases should be obtained to document the adequacy of the initial ventilator settings and to guide subsequent adjustments. If possible, the inspired oxygen concentration should be lowered to nontoxic levels (less than 40% to 50%), while maintaining an adequate arterial concentration (Po_2 more than 60 mm Hg). The minute ventilation (tidal volume and respiratory rate) is adjusted to achieve an appropriate arterial Pco_2 and pH.

In some patients receiving mechanical ventilation, the goal of achieving normocapnia may require large tidal volumes and high minute ventilation, often resulting in high peak and plateau airway pressures (see subsequent discussion on monitoring ventilatory mechanics). This may lead to lung damage because of high pressures *(barotrauma)* and/or overdistention of normally compliant alveolar units that may be present *(volutrauma)*. To prevent these consequences, a strategy of *permissive hypercapnia* is now advocated by many authorities for the management of ventilated patients with conditions such as severe asthma or ARDS. In permissive hypercapnia, the $Paco_2$ is allowed to rise, if necessary, as tidal volumes are reduced to maintain pressures within certain putative thresholds (e.g., plateau pressure ≤30 cm H_2O in ARDS patients). Some authorities recommend using intravenous bicarbonate to maintain blood pH at greater than 7.15 to 7.20.

Modes of Mechanical Ventilation

Mechanical ventilation can be delivered via different modes and modifications thereof (Box 44-7). Although few data exist to support the overall superiority of one form of mechanical ventilation over the others, the purported advantages of certain modes have fostered their selective application in particular clinical circumstances.

Controlled Mechanical Ventilation. With this mode, a preset tidal volume is delivered at a predetermined frequency. The patient is unable to trigger additional ventilator breaths, frequently leading to patient discomfort. This mode of ventilation is now seldom used and is appropriate only for unconscious and apneic patients.

Assist/Control Ventilation. The assist/control mode, or assisted mechanical ventilation (AMV), allows the patient to trigger a ventilator-delivered breath (at the preselected tidal volume) by initiating a minimal inspiratory effort. If the patient does not make inspiratory efforts, the ventilator ensures a minimal minute ventilation at a frequency and tidal volume preselected by the physician. The major advantage of this system is that the patient is able to interact with the ventilator, thereby minimizing discomfort and allowing for an increase in minute ventilation in response to changes in physiologic demands. For these benefits to be realized, the sensitivity of the patient-triggering mechanism needs to be adjusted to avoid unintentional machine ventilation (leading to respiratory alkalosis) but should allow for patient-initiated breaths without excessive effort. Assist/control is the mode usually chosen for the initiation of mechanical ventilation.

Intermittent Mandatory Ventilation. Intermittent mandatory ventilation (IMV) delivers a preset tidal volume at a specified frequency, thereby guaranteeing a minimum ventilator-delivered minute ventilation, but additionally allows the patient to breathe spontaneously without triggering the ventilator. Respiration by the patient during IMV ventilation therefore mimics the physiology of normal spontaneous ventilation (e.g., full respiratory muscle effort throughout inspiration, negative pleural pressure during inspiration).

When compared to AMV, the putative advantages of IMV include (1) better patient synchrony with ventilator, (2) less tendency toward respiratory alkalosis, (3) maintenance of respiratory muscle function, (4) usefulness as a weaning technique, and (5) less reduction in cardiac output. Some evidence is available to support the contention that IMV is indeed helpful in patients who are "fighting" the ventilator in the assist/control mode or in patients whose cardiac output is depressed during positive pressure ventilation as a result of hypovolemia or the use of PEEP. A trial of IMV is warranted for these purposes. In contrast, no appropriately controlled studies indicate the superiority of IMV for enhancing respiratory muscle function or for expediting weaning. Two prospective investigations failed to find any

---

BOX 44-6
Some indications for mechanical ventilation

Gas exchange (oxygenation) failure
  Pneumonia
  Adult respiratory distress syndrome
  Pulmonary edema
Ventilatory failure
  Neuromuscular disease (e.g., Guillain-Barré syndrome, myasthenia gravis, poliomyelitis)
  Drug overdose
  Respiratory muscle fatigue or dysfunction
  Restrictive defects of the chest wall
  Depressed respiratory center drive
  Severe asthma
  Exacerbation of chronic obstructive pulmonary disease

BOX 44-7
Some modes of mechanical ventilation

Controlled mechanical ventilation (CMV)
Assist/control ventilation (AMV)
Intermittent mandatory ventilation (IMV)
Positive end-expiratory pressure (PEEP)
Pressure support ventilation (PSV)
High-frequency ventilation (HFV)
Inverse-ratio ventilation (IRV)

clinically significant difference in pH among patients ventilated with IMV or AMV. Although there was a slight trend toward a reduction in alkalosis with IMV, this occurred because of an increase in carbon dioxide production rather than a reduction in minute ventilation. This suggests that the small improvement in alkalosis occurs at the expense of increased breathing work.

The consequences of IMV are most appropriately discussed in the context of the frequency of ventilator-delivered breaths. If the IMV rate is low, the patient is receiving only partial ventilatory support because the ventilator does not provide an adequate minute ventilation. In such a case, the patient is required to supplement the difference. For unstable patients or patients with respiratory muscle fatigue, a low IMV rate clearly is inappropriate. In contrast, a low IMV setting may be of benefit in weaning a stable patient from mechanical ventilation. A high IMV rate provides full ventilatory support to the patient and obviates the need for additional spontaneous breaths. Used in this manner, IMV differs little from the traditional use of AMV.

Positive End-Expiratory Pressure. PEEP can be used with any of the modes of ventilation. It generally improves arterial oxygenation when applied to patients with diffuse lung edema and refractory hypoxemia caused by intrapulmonary shunting (e.g., ARDS). This is accomplished by preventing atelectasis in fluid-filled alveoli and terminal bronchioles, thereby improving ventilation-perfusion relationships. Frequently, the improvement in arterial PO_2 allows reduction of the inspired oxygen concentration to less toxic levels. Most evidence suggests that PEEP does not reduce total lung water, prevent ARDS when applied early to patients at risk, or hasten lung repair. Most clinicians therefore advocate the use of PEEP only when necessary to support oxygenation and only at the minimal level necessary to achieve this goal. Ideally, the arterial PO_2 should be maintained greater than or equal to 60 mm Hg (oxygen saturation greater than 90%) with an inspired oxygen concentration less than or equal to 50%.

The major adverse effect of PEEP is a depression of cardiac output. This is attributable chiefly to an increase in mean intrathoracic pressure and a consequent decrease in venous return to the thorax. No evidence shows that PEEP has a direct effect on myocardial contractility. A decrease in cardiac output is usually seen with PEEP levels greater than 10 cm H_2O, but this may occur at lower levels in patients with hypovolemia or cardiac disease. When cardiac output decreases significantly in a patient receiving PEEP, this may result in a net decrease in systemic oxygen delivery despite the improvement in PaO_2 and arterial oxygen saturation.

An empirical trial is necessary to determine the optimum level of PEEP under any given clinical circumstances. This usually involves gradually increasing the PEEP (e.g., 0, 5, 10 cm H_2O and so on) while monitoring arterial PO_2, lung compliance (compliance usually improves until excessive PEEP levels are reached), and the hemodynamic status. A pulmonary artery catheter should be placed to monitor hemodynamic variables if it is apparent that PEEP greater than 10 cm H_2O is required or if hemodynamic instability occurs at lower levels.

If PEEP is applied inappropriately to patients with *focal* lung consolidation (e.g., unilateral pneumonia), a paradoxical decrease in arterial PO_2 may occur. Alveolar expansion caused by PEEP preferentially occurs in the more compliant normal lung, increasing pulmonary vascular resistance in this area and thereby directing more pulmonary blood flow through the consolidated lung, aggravating the shunt.

Inverse Ratio Ventilation. Recent evidence suggests that conventional ventilatory support of ARDS patients with volume-cycled ventilation and PEEP (see preceding discussion) may perpetuate lung injury by overinflating. A strategy termed *inverse ratio ventilation* (IRV) may maintain or improve gas exchange at lower levels of PEEP and lower peak airway pressures, thereby theoretically reducing lung damage caused by mechanical ventilation. IRV can be achieved by two methods: (1) volume-cycled inspiratory flow rate, or (2) pressure-controlled ventilation, by utilizing a long inspiratory time. A limitation of IRV is the need to heavily sedate or paralyze most patients during its use. Clinicians appear to be using IRV with increasing fre-

quency, although no clinical trials have as yet compared the outcome in ARDS patients treated with IRV versus conventional ventilation.

Pressure Support Ventilation. A recent development in mechanical ventilation is pressure support ventilation (PSV), the augmentation of inspiratory efforts by a set amount of positive airway pressure. This pressure is sustained at a plateau level as long as a minimal inspiratory flow is occurring, providing the patient with significant control over the volume and duration of inspiration. Among different ventilators there is as yet no standard algorithm for maintaining and terminating pressure support during each breath; such pressure-flow specifications are dependent on the particular model used.

More clinical experience is necessary before conclusions about the role of PSV can be made. Pressure support ventilation may improve patient comfort and reduce pressure work during mechanical ventilation (e.g., spontaneous breaths during IMV) and may also be a valuable adjunct to weaning patients from mechanical ventilation.

High-Frequency Ventilation. High-frequency ventilation (HFV) is a generic term for mechanical ventilation with a frequency of greater than 60 cycles per minute. Three major types of ventilators are available: high-frequency positive pressure ventilators (HFPPV), high-frequency jet ventilators (HFJV), and high-frequency oscillators (HFO). Although each uses different mechanics and produces gas displacement in different ways, each is characterized by small tidal volumes that are less than or approximate to the anatomic dead space volume. Among other potential benefits, HFV provides adequate gas exchange at lower peak airway pressure than conventional positive pressure ventilation.

The HFPPV and HFJV are open systems that are effective without the use of a tight-fitting endotracheal tube. These systems are therefore useful when ventilatory support is required during upper airway surgery, laryngoscopy, or bronchoscopy. Except for these situations, HFV has not been documented to offer consistent benefits over conventional ventilation. A large prospective and randomized study comparing HFJV and conventional ventilation in intensive care unit patients with respiratory failure from a variety of causes (e.g., ARDS, pneumonia, aspiration) found no superiority for either technique. Conventional ventilation provided a higher PaO_2 at equivalent PEEP levels than HFJV, but alveolar ventilation was slightly better on HFJV. On HFJV, oxygenation and ventilation were maintained with lower peak inspiratory pressures than those with conventional volume-cycled ventilation. These differences were all small and not likely to be clinically significant. Similarly, no data are available indicating a reduction in the incidence of barotrauma with HFV or showing improved survival in patients with bronchopleural fistula, despite anecdotal reports that HFJV might be effective in ventilating patients with bronchopleural fistula.

Further clinical experience and investigation are necessary to define the role of HFV in the intensive care unit.

Monitoring Ventilatory Mechanics

Total thoracic (lung and chest wall) compliance characteristics can be assessed in the ventilated patient. The pressure dial on the ventilator indicates, for any given tidal volume, both peak pressure and a static pressure (assessed when there is no air flow just before the start of exhalation) (Fig. 44-8). Momentarily occluding the expiratory tubing immediately before exhalation may be necessary to reveal the brief plateau of the static pressure. Dividing the tidal volume by either peak or static pressure gives a measure of the thoracic dynamic characteristic or the thoracic static compliance, respectively. Static compliance reflects changes in the lung parenchyma, whereas the dynamic characteristic additionally reflects changes in airways resistance. It is valuable to evaluate respiratory compliance characteristics when taking care of the critically ill. Such monitoring provides means of assessing therapeutic interventions such as PEEP (static compliance usually increases during initial application of PEEP and may begin to decrease if the optimal PEEP level is exceeded) or assessing disease trends (a decreasing compliance signals worsening of lung parenchymal disease). Furthermore, an acute increase in peak airway pressure may be a valuable early indicator of problems such

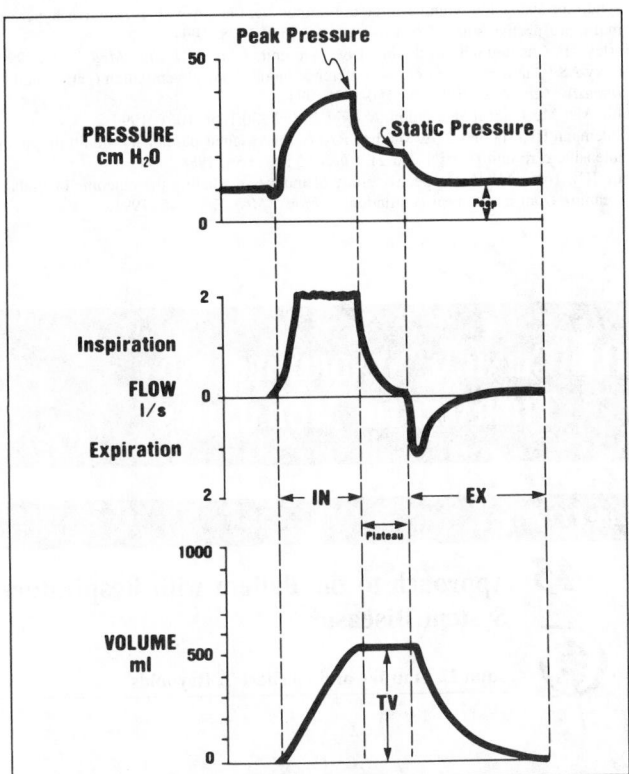

FIGURE 44-8 Relationship of tidal volume (TV), air flow rates, and ventilator dial reading in a patient receiving mechanical ventilation with 10 cm H_2O of PEEP. The static pressure is more apparent if expiratory retard or inspiratory hold is used, or if the expiratory tubing is momentarily occluded or pinched.

$$\text{Static compliance} = \frac{\text{Tidal volume}}{\text{Static pressure} - \text{PEEP}}$$

In this example, static compliance equals $500 \div (20 - 10) = 50$ ml/cm H_2O. The normal static compliance of the lung and chest wall in a mechanically ventilated patient is about 50 to 70 ml/cm H_2O. If lung and chest wall compliance is reduced (<25 ml/cm H_2O), the increased work of breathing will hinder weaning. If flow is also measured (requires a pneumotachograph), then airway resistance (R_{aw}) can be calculated:

$$R_{aw} = \frac{\text{Peak pressure} - \text{Static pressure}}{\text{Flow}}$$

In this example $(40 - 20) \div 2 = 10$ cm H_2O/liters per second (l/s). Normal R_{aw} is between 2 and 3 cm H_2O/liters per second. Increased airway resistance might be due to bronchospasm or secretions, for instance.

(From Bone RC: Monitoring ventilatory mechanics in acute respiratory failure, *Respir Care* 28:597-604, 1983.)

as pneumothorax, endotracheal tube sliding into the right mainstem bronchus, or endotracheal tube (or airways) becoming plugged with blood or secretions.

Endotracheal Intubation and Tracheotomy

Mechanical ventilation requires intubation of the trachea with either an endotracheal or a tracheotomy tube. In a patient with acute respiratory failure, endotracheal intubation can be performed much quicker and with fewer complications than tracheotomy, which requires surgical expertise and is associated with a twofold to fivefold increase in complication rate when performed on an emergency rather than elective basis. With current respiratory care techniques and soft-cuff endotracheal tubes, endotracheal intubation can usually be maintained for several days or even a few weeks without excessive complications. Nevertheless, the requirement for "prolonged" mechanical ventilation is an indication for elective tracheotomy. However, the timing of elective tracheotomy in mechanically ventilated patients remains a controversial topic.

Proponents of delayed tracheotomy cite studies demonstrating that the complications from tracheotomy are greater than those of 2 or 3 weeks of endotracheal intubation. However, these nonrandomized investigations (in which the tracheotomy groups were exposed to the tracheotomy procedure only after fairly prolonged translaryngeal intubation) may be biased against tracheotomy because prolonged translaryngeal intubation increases the risk for airway injury from a subsequent tracheotomy. Advocates of early tracheotomy also point to studies suggesting that laryngeal injuries from endotracheal intubation may be more severe and difficult to repair than tracheal injuries from tracheotomy.

A reasonable approach is to continue translaryngeal intubation in most mechanically ventilated patients for a week to 10 days and consider tracheotomy if weaning and extubation are not likely within the next week. Clinical judgment and individual patient factors may provide grounds for altering this approach. Specifically, the risks and advantages of each technique need to be considered in the particular clinical context.

Problems encountered with endotracheal intubation may include patient discomfort, difficulty in suctioning tracheobronchial secretions, patient self-extubation, and with nasotracheal intubation, sinusitis or otitis. Problems with tracheotomy include stomal infection, stomal hemorrhage, and subcutaneous emphysema.

A major advantage of tracheotomy is less interference with the pharyngeal area, allowing possibilities for speech and eating. Tracheotomy tubes also are more easily changed when necessary and have less resistance to air flow as compared with endotracheal tubes. These considerations account for the need for tracheotomy in virtually all patients undergoing a prolonged weaning process.

Weaning From Mechanical Ventilation

The process of returning a mechanically ventilated patient to normal spontaneous breathing is termed *weaning*. The clinician faces two major issues in the weaning process. First is the decision regarding when the patient is ready to begin the weaning process. Once the patient is deemed ready for weaning, an appropriate plan for accomplishing this goal must be devised. Prediction of weaning success and the weaning process itself are considerably more straightforward in the patient who has received short-term mechanical ventilation (less than 7 days). In contrast, patients who have received mechanical ventilation for longer than 1 month often require a fairly prolonged and complex weaning process.

Initiation of weaning should be considered when the patient has sufficiently recovered from the underlying processes that necessitated mechanical ventilation. The patient should also be hemodynamically stable, alert, cooperative, and without physical distress. At this point, gas exchange and spontaneous ventilatory parameters should be assessed. The criteria indicated in Box 44-8 are highly predictive of weaning success after short-term ventilatory support. In many of these

---

BOX 44-8
Criteria predictive of successful weaning from short-term mechanical ventilation

Arterial oxygen tension >60 mm Hg with inspired oxygen concentration ≤40%
Tidal volume >5 ml/kg
Vital capacity >10 ml/kg
Maximum inspiratory force <−25 cm H_2O
Spontaneous minute ventilation ≤10 liters/minute (and maintains acceptable $PaCO_2$)
Able to double spontaneous minute ventilation with maximal voluntary effort
Respiratory frequency/tidal volume ratio <100 breaths per minute/liter

---

BOX 44-9

Nonpulmonary factors to consider in the difficult-to-wean patient

Medications (e.g., sedatives, analgesics)
Malnutrition
Hypophosphatemia, hypomagnesemia, hypokalemia
Small-bore endotracheal tube (8 mm tube or larger is preferred)
Respiratory muscle dysfunction (e.g., diaphragm paralysis following open heart surgery)
Metabolic alkalosis (depresses respiratory drive)
Unstable medical status (e.g., uncontrolled infection)
Interference with chest wall (e.g., casts, bandages, chest tube, restraints)
Hypothyroidism

---

patients, it is reasonable to allow the patient to breathe spontaneously on a T-piece circuit with an inspired oxygen concentration of approximately 40%. Provided that the arterial blood gases obtained after 30 to 60 minutes are adequate, and the patient does not exhibit tachypnea, tachycardia, cardiac arrhythmias, or hemodynamic instability, the patient can usually be extubated.

Patients who have received long-term mechanical ventilation or who have significant unresolved underlying lung disease or other medical complications are usually not appropriate for the rapid T-piece weaning technique. In such patients, fulfilling the criteria of Box 44-8 does not necessarily predict quick success, and the weaning process is frequently prolonged over several days or even weeks.

Three methods used in this setting are the use of intermittent T-piece, IMV weaning, and pressure support weaning. The intermittent T-piece technique involves the use of progressively longer and more frequent periods of full spontaneous ventilation through the T-piece circuit, followed by periods of complete rest with full ventilatory support. The IMV method involves a gradual decrease in the IMV rate. In this method, the patient receives partial ventilatory support in a progressively decreasing manner, rather than intermittent periods of no ventilatory support as with the T-piece technique. Pressure support may provide a more physiologic workload to the ventilatory muscles than does IMV (with pressure support, the pressure-volume load on the muscles is more normal and the work is applied more regularly). In addition, because the patient has more control over the flow and volume of each breath, patient comfort might be expected to be improved with pressure support ventilation. At the start of weaning, levels of pressure support that produce tidal breaths equivalent to that supplied by conventional ventilation are provided. Subsequently, the level of pressure support is gradually reduced as tolerated. In all three methods, it is customary to return the patient to full ventilatory support during the night until the final stages of weaning are approached. No conclusive data exist that indicate the superiority of any single weaning method. Although further studies are necessary to define the relative merits of T-piece, IMV, and pressure support weaning, it is clear that each technique, when used appropriately, has been a successful weaning method. In the difficult-to-wean patient, it is worthwhile considering a number of nonrespiratory factors that may be contributing to the problem (Box 44-9), such as medications, metabolic alkalosis, or hypothyroidism.

BIBLIOGRAPHY

Brouchard L, Harf A, Lovino H et al: Comparison of three methods of gradual withdrawal from mechanical ventilation, *Am J Respir Crit Care Med* 150:896-903, 1994.

Clark JS et al: Noninvasive assessment of blood gases, *Am Rev Respir Dis* 145:220, 1992.

Darioli R, Perret C: Mechanical controlled hypoventilation in status asthmaticus, *Am Rev Respir Dis* 129:385-387, 1984.

Esteban A, Frutos F, Tobin MJ et al: A comparison of four methods of weaning patients from mechanical ventilation, *N Engl J Med* 332:345-350, 1995.

Falk JL, Rackow ED, Weil MH: End-tidal carbon dioxide concentration during cardiopulmonary resuscitation, *N Engl J Med* 318:607, 1988.

Hefner JE: Timing of tracheotomy in mechanically ventilated patients, *Am Rev Respir Dis* 147:768-771, 1993.

Hickling KG, Walsh J, Henderson S et al: Low mortality rate in adult respiratory distress syndrome using low-volume, pressure-limited ventilation with permissive hypercapnia: a prospective study, *Crit Care Med* 22:1568-1578, 1994.

Morley TF: Capnography in the intensive care unit, *J Intensive Care Med* 5:209, 1990.

Slutsky AS (Chairman): Consensus conference on mechanical ventilation (parts 1 and 2), *Intensive Care Med* 20:64-79, 150-162, 1994.

Tobin MJ: Mechanical ventilation, *N Engl J Med* 330:1056-1061, 1994.

Wiedemann HP, Matthay MA, Matthay RA: Cardiovascular-pulmonary monitoring in the intensive care unit (parts 1 and 2), *Chest* 85:537, 656, 1984.

Yang KL, Tobin MJ: A prospective study of indexes predicting the outcome of trials of weaning from mechanical ventilation, *N Engl J Med* 324:1445, 1991.

III   CLINICAL SYNDROMES AND THERAPEUTIC MODALITIES

CHAPTER

45   Approach to the Patient with Respiratory System Disease*

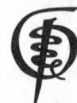

John L. Stauffer and Herbert Y. Reynolds

The diagnosis and treatment of patients with disorders and diseases of the respiratory system have changed substantially over the last two to three decades. Remarkable new advances in technology (diagnostic imaging, fiberoptic endoscopy, monitoring, and surgical techniques) and therapeutic modalities (pharmaceuticals, gene therapy, continuous positive airway pressure devices, life support systems, and ambulatory oxygen therapy), combined with an explosion in knowledge about respiratory biology and medicine, have revolutionized our approach to management of patients with respiratory system diseases.

Moreover, the spectrum of pulmonary disease continues to change. Cancer of the lung, especially in women, continues to increase. The "white plague" of tuberculosis is on the rise again, especially in patients with acquired immunodeficiency syndrome (AIDS) who are at risk for many kinds of infection from common encapsulated bacteria, *Pneumocystis carinii*, and fungal organisms. Chronic obstructive pulmonary disease (COPD) is increasing in the aging populations, and disorders of breathing during sleep such as obstructive sleep apnea are recognized much more often than in the past. Increasingly, lung transplantation is a reality for selected patients with pulmonary hypertension, interstitial fibrosis, COPD, and cystic fibrosis. Low-grade graft-versus-host disease causing mucositis and bronchiolitis obliterans is encountered in recipients of bone marrow transplants.

Advances in technology and new forms of pulmonary illness notwithstanding, the time-honored skills of taking a thorough medical history and performing a complete physical examination remain the cornerstones of diagnosis of respiratory system disease. This fundamental truth cannot be overemphasized. Selective supplemental tests may be ordered if needed to complement the history and physical examination. Skillful interpretation of these tests, combined with expertise in the medical history and physical examination, often precludes the need for expensive and invasive diagnostic studies such as fiberoptic bronchoscopy, computed tomography (CT) and surgical lung biopsy. A hierarchical organization of diagnostic modalities should be used in the evaluation of patients with respiratory system disease (Fig. 45-1). Simple diagnostic tests should precede the more invasive and expensive ones.

The purpose of this chapter is to remind the reader of the usefulness of what is old but tested and to present an approach to the respiratory patient by reviewing the history, the performance of the

---

*The authors appreciate the prior contributions of Dr. Richard E. Brashear.

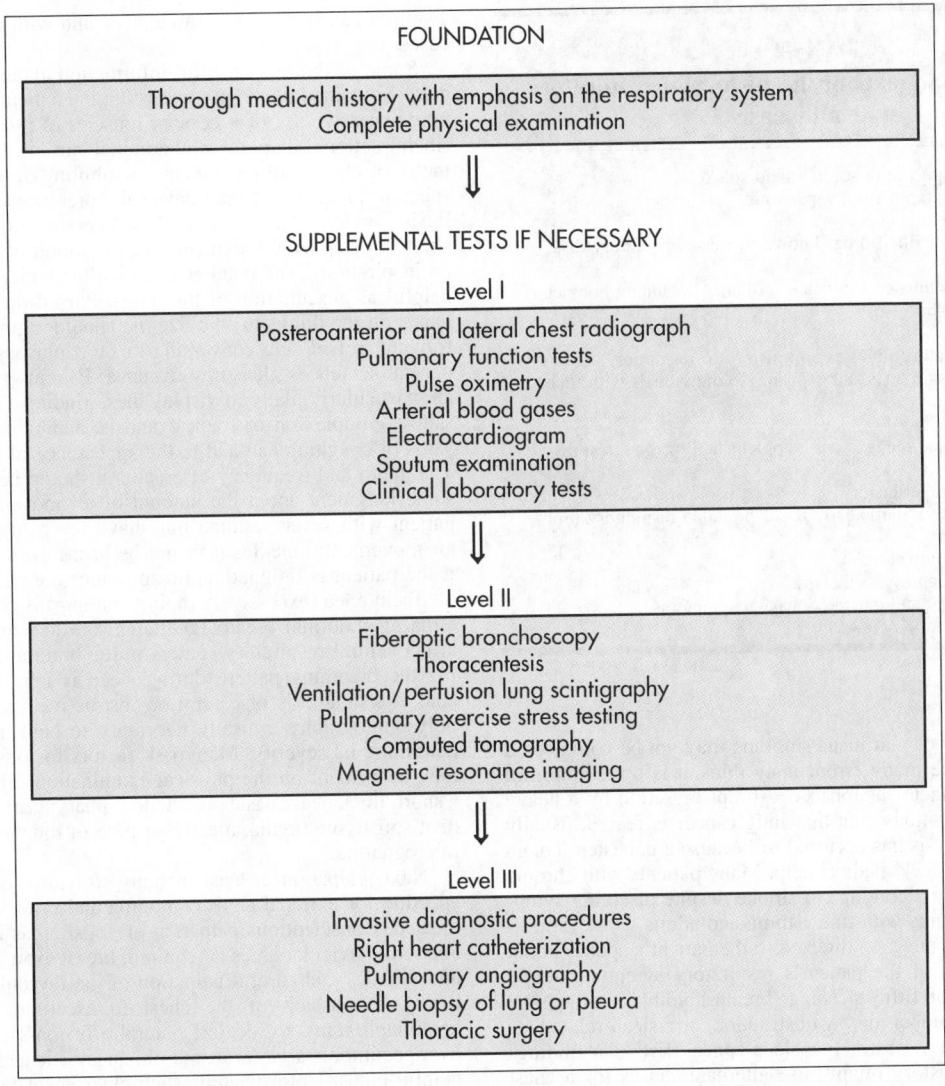

FIGURE 45-1 The medical history and physical examination are the foundation for the diagnosis of respiratory system disease. Diagnostic tests of increasing levels of complexity and invasiveness are performed if necessary to supplement the initial history and physical examination.

physical examination, and the main symptoms of some pulmonary diseases.

IMPORTANCE OF THE MEDICAL HISTORY

A thorough review of the patient's medical history, coupled with the presenting symptoms or circumstances of the acute illness, provides the background for the physician's initial diagnosis. The medical history must include identifying features of the patient, the chief complaint, history of the present illness, past medical history, family history, social history, and review of systems. These elements dictate how extensive a physical examination is needed and suggest what ancillary diagnostic studies are necessary to confirm or identify the disease process. Acute situations created by trauma or catastrophic illness obviously curtail history taking and by necessity direct medical attention to emergency care. It is possible that a busy house staff physician or hurried practitioner may not take the time to question and listen to the patient or may quickly scan a checklist history sheet and go straight for objective laboratory data and a chest radiograph. The physician may plan to fill in the details of the history later but, as can happen, may not get back to this as originally planned. Thus part of the patient's database may not be evaluated adequately. Sometimes only in retrospect do serious omissions in history taking become apparent.

Many unrelated things may have to be asked of the patient before a composite history is formed; the patient's occupational history is an example. Exposure to inhaled chemical fumes or organic dusts can cause asthmalike symptoms; the breathing of airborne particles from the grinding or cutting of heavy metal, or inhaling of sand or asbestos fibers can initiate forms of diffuse interstitial pulmonary fibrosis that produce chronic dyspnea. Usually, many years must elapse between the initial exposure to such materials and the development of respiratory symptoms, so that dating the exposure(s) or correctly identifying the work-related circumstances may be difficult. A detailed account of each job, including summer work during youth and assignments in military service, may be necessary to pinpoint a casual exposure to asbestos, for example. Exposure to inhaled mold spores and organic antigens that can cause hypersensitivity pneumonitis may be insidious, so unsuspected avocations or unusual hobbies need to be probed. Sometimes a visit to the patient's workplace or home is required to assess the environmental milieu. Other components of a relevant history in evaluating the patient with respiratory disease are listed in Box 45-1. The length of this list underscores the need for thoroughness in the medical history.

An accurate history of cigarette smoking is usually obtained, and some attempt to quantify the exposure by calculating "pack years" (average number of packs per day multiplied by the number of years of smoking) and noting if filtered or unfiltered cigarettes were smoked

---

BOX 45-1

Important components of the history of respiratory system disease

---

Smoking history; exposure to second-hand smoke
Previous chest radiographs for comparison
Complete occupational history
Use of medications or illicit drugs known to cause respiratory disease
Exposure to noxious inhaled substances at home (including hobbies), outdoors, and at work
Radiation exposure
Recent family respiratory illnesses and history of respiratory disease
Previous tuberculin skin tests and exposure to individuals with tuberculosis
Immunization history
Previous use of inhaled medications, supplemental oxygen, respiratory therapy, etc.
Recent and remote travel history
Interview of the spouse, particularly if sleep-related respiratory problems are suspected
Risk factors for HIV infection
History of immunosuppressive therapy
Upper respiratory tract and gastroesophageal symptoms

---

are of value. A history of marijuana smoking may not be volunteered by the patient, because many erroneously think it is not as harmful or as much of a risk factor as tobacco. Abrupt cessation by a heavy smoker is often an ominous sign that lung cancer is feared, usually because some hemoptysis has occurred or because a persistent cough prompts the patient to seek medical help. Many patients with chronic bronchitis or emphysema continue to smoke despite disabling symptoms. In contrast, patients with true asthma and adults with cystic fibrosis rarely smoke. A question directed to the patient's spouse about the latter's perception of the patient's respiratory symptoms could evoke the complaint of fitful sleeping, breath-holding, snoring that directs attention to an upper airway obstruction, or a sleep-related respiratory disorder such as obstructive sleep apnea. Particular findings in a patient's travel history might raise alternate causes for a chest mass or mediastinal calcification and redirect the diagnostic evaluation. Likewise, recurrent bacterial respiratory infections, perhaps also with sinus involvement in a young adult, could prompt the physician to consider pursuing one of several congenital diseases that affect the respiratory system, such as impaired ciliary movement (syndromes associated with an intrinsic structural defect in the dynein arms or radial spokes of cilia that alters rhythmic beating), acquired hypogammaglobulinemia, selective immunoglobulin G (IgG) subclass deficiency, or a subtle presentation of cystic fibrosis. A family history revealing affected siblings is of obvious importance. An association between recurrent sinopulmonary infections and infertility problems could be a clue for cystic fibrosis or a ciliary defect. Increasingly, drugs are implicated as a cause of hypersensitivity and interstitial pulmonary fibrosis, and a complete inventory of drug usage must be recorded. Antineoplastic chemotherapy agents and immunosuppressant drugs (such as cyclophosphamide, methotrexate, or bleomycin) are usually obvious, but gold or penicillamine therapy used for the patient with rheumatoid arthritis, an antibiotic prescribed for chronic suppression of a bladder infection (such as nitrofurantoin), or some other very common medication can all be culprits.

PHYSICAL EXAMINATION OF THE RESPIRATORY SYSTEM

Careful inspection of the nose and throat is necessary. Evidence of nasal obstruction from polyps or a deviated septum can explain postnasal secretions and coughing. Polyps can be associated with asthma, allergic rhinitis, and other diseases such as aspirin-induced asthma or cystic fibrosis. Nasal ulceration and sinusitis may suggest a vasculitis of the respiratory tract (Wegener's granulomatosis). Parotid gland

swelling can be found in sarcoidosis and with collagen vascular diseases.

Some of the most helpful information about breathing mechanics can be obtained by simply observing the patient. The careful eye will note excessive use of accessory muscles of respiration, nasal flaring, rib retractions, diaphragm-abdominal muscle incoordination, asymmetry of chest wall movement, or splinting of the thorax. Careful inspection of the chest may detect the presence of gynecomastia, scoliosis or kyphosis, increased anteroposterior dimension ("barrel chest"), or Hoover's sign (inward migration of the lower lateral ribs on inspiration). The manner in which the patient breathes is often as helpful as auscultation of the lungs. Pursed-lip breathing, fixing the hands on the thighs to stabilize the shoulder girdle, sitting or leaning forward in bed, and conversing in short phrases or words instead of normal sentences all betray dyspnea. Patients with advanced COPD are particularly likely to display these findings. Anxiety, restlessness, sallow complexion or frank cyanosis, audible wheezing, and paroxysms of coughing can add to the appearance of respiratory difficulty. The depth and frequency of breathing should be recorded, as well as some judgment about the amount of air movement. For example, a patient with severe asthma may have few wheezes because of poor air movement; crackles may not be heard even in pulmonary edema if the patient is fatigued and respirations are shallow.

Tachypnea (excessively rapid breathing) is obvious, but other patterns of abnormal breathing often relate to neurologic diseases that affect central respiratory centers in the brain and brainstem. Observing the breathing pattern during sleep is important because it may lead to a diagnosis of central or obstructive sleep apnea. Diagnostic polysomnography is usally necessary to confirm the diagnosis and determine its severity. Many risk factors for obstructive sleep apnea may be evident on the physical examination. These include obesity; a short, thick neck; nasal obstruction; pharyngeal narrowing by prominent soft tissue (uvula, tonsils, or base of tongue); macroglossia; and micrognathia.

Next, palpation at least of bony structures of the thorax and inspection for external signs of trauma and prior surgical scars are indicated. Conscientious palpation of nodal areas in the neck, axillary, and retroclavicular areas is required; breast examination in both males and females and careful palpation of the thyroid gland are also necessary. Percussion of the chest to ascertain movement of both hemidiaphragms, to localize pleural effusion(s), or to elicit dullness over pneumonic areas is an age-old diagnostic technique that can yield helpful clues. Unfortunately, such clues seem less important for the accuracy of diagnosis, because modern imaging procedures provide more objective data. However, auscultation of the lung fields remains useful because it provides unique information that the chest radiograph or CT scan cannot capture and helps the physician immediately to assess functioning of the airways. Crackles, wheezes, rhonchi, and diminished breath sounds can be distinguished. These findings can be correlated with those of chest inspection, palpation, and percussion, often leading to a specific diagnosis such as pneumonia, pleural effusion, or atelectasis with lobar bronchus obstruction. Auscultation of all lung fields should be performed. The topographic anatomy of the lungs should be recalled during auscultation (Fig. 45-2). Merely listening at the posterior bases of the lungs alone may not be sufficient; axillary and frontal projections of the lungs to the chest wall may yield pleural rubs or important clues to infection. Patients with a variety of diffuse interstitial pulmonary diseases that lead to fibrosis usually have dry, inspiratory crackles throughout much of the lung fields. Descriptive adjectives, such as *cellophane* and *Velcro* rales, have been given to these adventitious lung sounds. Examination of the heart must be considered as an extension of the lung examination, and a thorough assessment of left and right ventricular function must be made. Evidence of left heart failure, right heart failure, and pulmonary hypertension must be sought.

Obviously, an entire physical examination is required, and other sites removed from the chest can give important clues about lung function and the type of lung disease present. Needle puncture marks in the skin may identify an unsuspected intravenous drug user and provide a clue for the cause of multiple pulmonary abscesses and endocarditis. Acral cyanosis can reflect hypoxemia. Most collagen vascular diseases, particularly progressive systemic sclerosis, dermatomyositis, lupus erythematosus, and rheumatoid arthritis, involve the

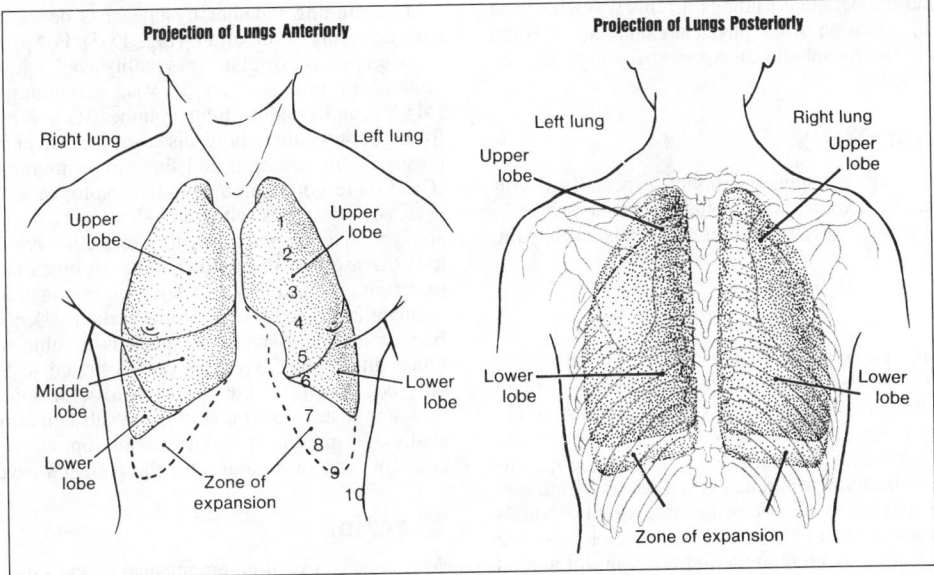

FIGURE 45-2 Projection of the lobes of the lung on the chest wall. Percussion and auscultation of the lungs reveal findings in specific lobes as projected.

(From Burnside JW, McGlynn TJ: *Physical diagnosis,* ed 17, Baltimore, 1987, Williams & Wilkins.)

BOX 45-2

Cardinal physical findings in normals and in selected common pulmonary disorders

Normal

Resonant percussion note over lung tissue
Vesicular sounds in lung periphery
Bronchovesicular sounds over large central bronchi
Inspiratory time to expiratory time ratio 2:3
No adventitious sounds

Asthma

Prolonged expiration
Wheezes
Crackles in some cases

Atelectasis

Dullness to percussion
Bronchophony, egophony, and/or whispered pectoriloquy in some cases
Variable effect on breath sounds
    Bronchus patent—bronchovesicular or bronchial sounds
    Bronchus obstructed—reduced or absent breath sounds

Bronchitis

Rhonchal fremitus
Rhonchi
Prolonged expiration in some cases

Consolidation

Dullness to percussion
Increased tactile fremitus in some cases
Bronchophony, egophony, and/or whispered pectoriloquy
Crackles in some cases

Variable effect on breath sounds
    Bronchus patent—bronchovesicular or bronchial sounds
    Bronchus obstructed—reduced or absent breath sounds

Emphysema

Chest hyperinflation
Hoover's sign (movement of the costal margins toward the midline on inspiration) in some cases
Hyperresonance
Distant, vesicular breath sounds
Prolonged expiration

Interstitial infiltrates

Physical examination may be normal
Intercostal retractions in some cases
Crackles in some cases
Digital clubbing in some cases

Pleural effusion

Dullness or flatness to percussion
Decreased tactile fremitus
Distant breath sounds
Pleural rub in some cases
Signs of consolidation if lung is compressed above effusion

Pneumothorax

Decreased tactile fremitus
Hyperresonance in some cases
Contralateral shift of mediastinal structures in tension pneumothorax
Distant breath sounds

---

skin, as well as having an appreciable incidence of interstitial pulmonary fibrosis. Clubbing of the digits always provokes an interesting differential diagnosis. Evidence of primary tumor in other organs can explain pulmonary metastases, and a tumor-associated hypercoagulable state may cause deep-vein thrombosis and result in pulmonary emboli. Because so many interrelationships exist among systemic and pulmonary diseases, it is useless to catalog even the most frequent

associations. The point for emphasis, however, is that a clear understanding of medical pulmonary disease requires a global view of the patient, and this requires a thorough physical examination. Normal chest findings and abnormal findings in common pulmonary disorders are summarized in Box 45-2.

If a chest radiograph is obtained, it is important that the physician performing the physical examination view the radiograph directly and correlate the clinical and radiographic findings. In this way, the chest radiograph is seen as an extension of the physical examination. If the chest radiograph reveals significant and unexpected findings, the patient should be reexamined.

RESPIRATORY SYMPTOMS

Certain respiratory symptoms are quite important, especially if volunteered by the patient. The cardinal ones include dyspnea or breathlessness, wheezing, coughing, expectoration of secretions, chest pain, and hemoptysis.

Dyspnea

Dyspnea may be an insidious symptom that is difficult for the patient to define or to pinpoint with regard to onset. *Dyspnea* means difficult or uncomfortable breathing and in aggregate is more than just an abnormal breathing pattern, for example, tachypnea, hyperventilation, and irregular or nonsynchronous breathing. Dyspnea can be quantitated. It is a subjective sensation that often is described as breathlessness, "air hunger," an awareness of not being able to catch one's breath, or having insufficient breath to perform a simple or mundane task (toweling off after bathing or climbing a flight of stairs). Labored breathing is expected with exertion and exercise, but the point at which one becomes aware of an unusual breathing pattern or perceives an excessive effort to breathe or to recover the breath is quite subjective. Breathlessness, which is an approximate synonym for dyspnea, can be quantitatively quite different from one person to the next, and, as a symptom of respiratory illness, it must be verified for each patient. For a conditioned athlete or jogger, breathlessness is associated only with vigorous exertion, whereas an active parent, supervising children and a household, may find breathlessness in the course of accustomed activity very debilitating. At times, dyspnea may not be a specific symptom of respiratory disease but a derivative symptom indicating congestive heart failure, anemia, thyrotoxicosis, anxiety, or myositis, and weak-muscle syndromes. Breathlessness commonly heralds a variety of interstitial lung diseases that produce less compliant lungs and restrictive patterns of pulmonary function. Finally, emotional illness (e.g., depression, hysteria) can produce various forms of dyspnea that are manifested as sighing, hyperventilation, rapid shallow breathing, or throat clearing and frequent coughing.

Because of its subjective nature, dyspnea may not correlate with various physiologic measurements such as pulmonary function tests; thus attempts have been made to quantitate it with various indices and scales. One such indexing method couples the patient's measured functional impairment with the magnitude of the task, the effort required, and the psychologic factors contributing. Thus a clinical rating of dyspnea may provide quantitative information that complements measurement of lung function.

The pathophysiologic mechanisms underlying the complaint of dyspnea are complex and poorly understood. Stimulation of various types of receptors in the upper airway, lung, and chest wall; inappropriate length-tension relationships in the respiratory muscles; and stimulation of peripheral and central chemoreceptors all appear to play some role, depending on the underlying disorder or disease process.

The complaint of dyspnea must always be taken seriously. It may be the first clue to the presence of one or more of a myriad of respiratory diseases. It may reflect defective respiratory drive or impaired respiratory muscles, or it may be a secondary symptom of cardiac or hematologic dysfunction. Orthopnea and paroxysmal nocturnal dyspnea strongly suggest the diagnosis of left ventricular dysfunction as the cause of dyspnea. The association of dyspnea with chronic productive cough points to the diagnosis of COPD or bronchiectasis. Evaluation of dyspnea is always carried out in sequential fashion, with the history and physical examination preceding relevant diagnostic studies. Interpretation of the chest radiograph, measurement of airflow by peak expiratory flow rate recording or spirometry, and assessment of oxyhemoglobin saturation by pulse oximetry or arterial blood gas analysis are the most useful tests to complement the history and physical examination. They should be obtained when necessary but preferably not as a routine, because the history and physical examination alone may often provide the correct diagnosis.

Determining whether dyspnea has developed acutely or is of a chronic nature is important (Fig. 45-3). For patients with COPD, dyspnea seems to correlate reasonably well with the forced expiratory volume in one second (FEV_1), maximum voluntary ventilation (MVV), and residual lung volume (RV). For patients with various forms of interstitial lung disease, the fall in arterial oxygen partial pressure with exertion and the carbon monoxide diffusion capacity ($DLCO$) are good parameters to monitor in assessing dyspnea. However, some patients with sarcoidosis may have normal lung spirometry yet have dyspnea, possibly reflecting endobronchial granulomatous disease and irritation. Finally, dyspnea may be a criterion used to determine disability in a legal or administrative sense that implies an inability to work or perform certain tasks; in other words, to define limitation. Because dyspnea is a subjective feeling and has a broad differential diagnosis (as illustrated in Fig. 45-3), it must not only be recognized but also judged with objectivity that requires a thorough history, examination, and substantiating pulmonary function studies. Its treatment should be appropriate for the underlying systemic or lung disease and for the patient's psychologic situation.

Wheezing

Wheezing is a continuous musical sound produced by turbulent airflow in narrowed bronchi or bronchioles. It may be both a symptom and an abnormal finding on physical examination. It is frequently accompanied by dyspnea and an unpleasant sensation of chest tightness. Often the patient with wheezing complains of inability to get a deep enough breath or to expel all the air after a deep inhalation. Wheezing, which is usually detected on expiration, must be distinguished from stridor, a crowing sound caused by upper airway obstruction.

Wheezing is most commonly associated with asthma; however, the adage that "all that wheezes in the chest is not caused by asthma" must be remembered. Indeed, the differential diagnosis of wheezing is broad (Box 45-3). Wheezing associated with bronchospasm may be an aftermath of viral or bacterial infection and is ascribed to hyperactive, irritated airways. Peribronchial fluid that accumulates from left heart failure can cause bronchoconstriction ("cardiac asthma") as well. Pulmonary thromboembolism may cause diffuse wheezing, usually of a transient nature. Isolated areas of unilateral wheezing in the chest carry a different connotation and may reflect localized obstruction by a neoplasm, mucus plug, or an aspirated particle. Many patients with asthma are never free of wheezing, and diffuse expiratory phase wheezing can be felt and also heard even when the subject is asymptomatic and under good medication control. Wheezing heard in both the inspiratory and expiratory phases of breathing denotes a more advanced stage of bronchospasm and often an acute attack. The silent chest in an asthmatic when little air is moving is a signal that airway obstruction is severe and vigorous therapy is needed.

Cough

Coughing is a normal mechanism for forcefully expelling secretions or inhaled particles from the airways, and it complements the mucociliary clearance system of the epithelial cell lining surface. Cough can be initiated voluntarily; however, it is most important as a protective reflex. This simple or reflexive coughing is infrequent and develops little force. However, deep or frequent coughing represents more than a nuisance and is an obvious sign of respiratory illness that demands attention and explanation.

The cough mechanism represents an interesting network of neurosensory-muscular coordination. The sensory arm of the cough reflex originates from afferent receptors in the epithelium of the airways. Excitation of the receptors by mechanical or chemical factors initiates impulses upward along the vagus nerve to integrative areas in the medulla oblongata and pons. Efferent impulses are transmitted to the diaphragm, the chest wall and abdominal muscles, and to the larynx.

Coughing has three phases. During the first, or inspiratory phase, the glottis opens wide and an initial inspiration increases static elastic recoil and lung volume. The compressive phase is initiated with closure of the glottis, continues with active contraction of the expiratory muscles, and ends with the sudden opening of the glottis. The expulsive phase begins with opening of glottis and the explosive re-

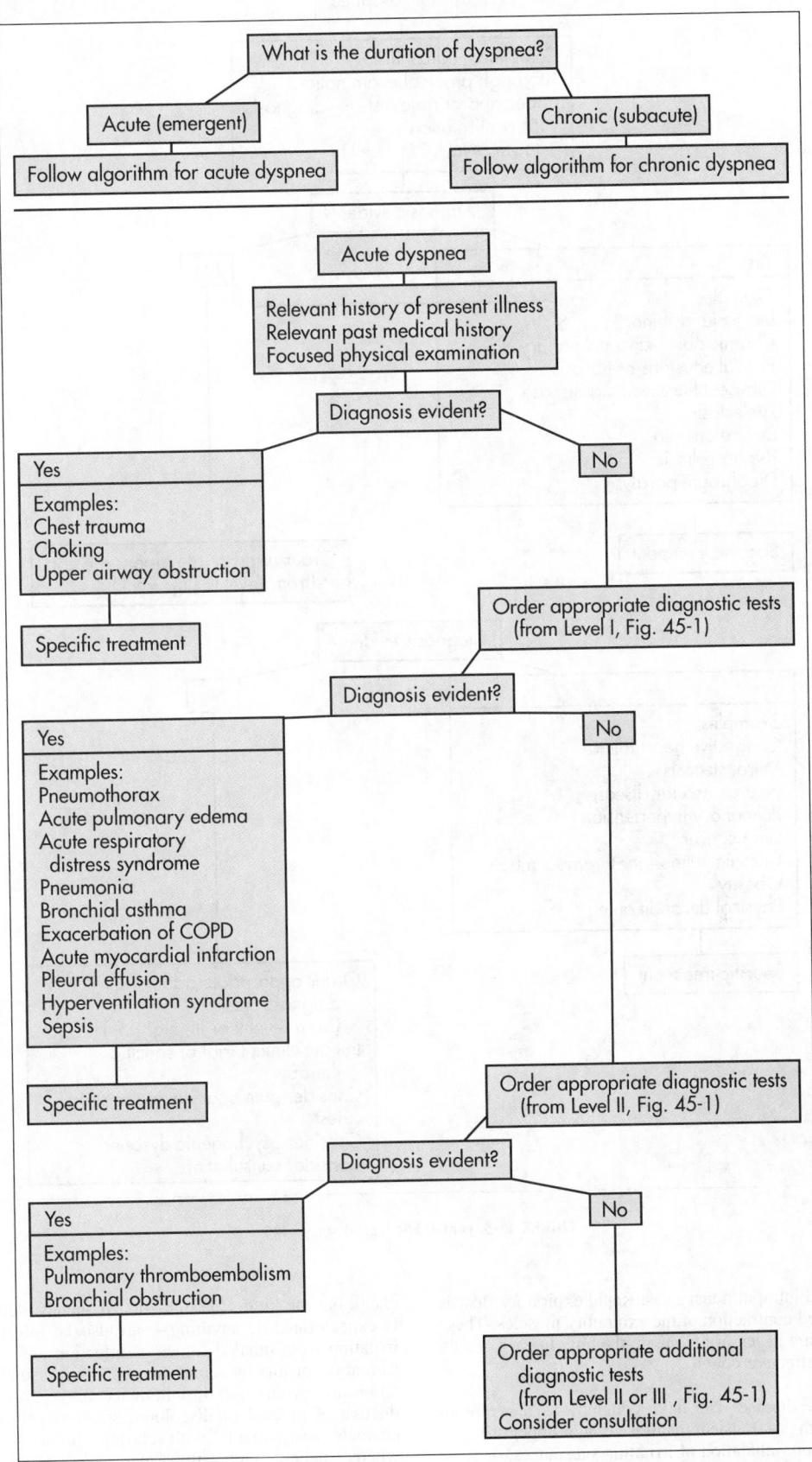

FIGURE 45-3   An algorithmic approach to evaluation of the patient with dyspnea.   *Continued.*

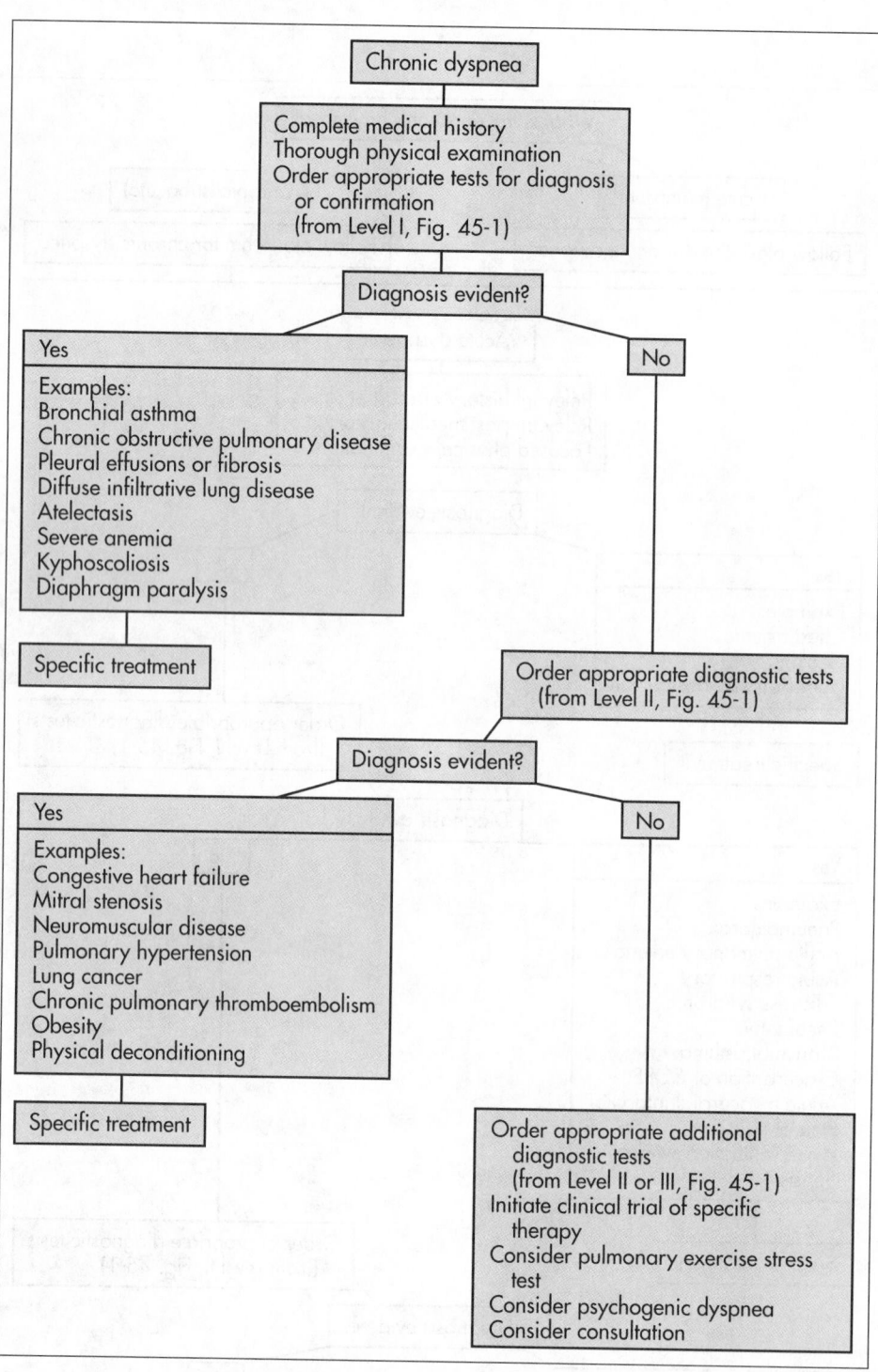

FIGURE 45-3, cont'd. For legend see p. 405.

lease of the pressurized intrapulmonary gas. Rapid expiratory flow is maintained by continued contraction of the expiratory muscles. These three phases of cough are necessary to create the high linear velocity of air required for an effective cough.

Evaluation. Many diseases can have coughing as a symptom (Box 45-4). Acute cough is a transient manifestation of upper or lower respiratory tract infection, inhalation of irritating substances, or aspiration. Not only is the anatomic location or the organ system involved helpful in determining why coughing is present (for example, postnasal secretions irritating the glottis, or an enlarged thyroid gland, an aortic aneurysm, or another mediastinal structure compressing the tra-

chea), but the kind of cough—its frequency, depth, sound, and what is expectorated, if anything—can also be informative. With airway irritation from inhaled fumes or infection and subsequent excessive formation of airway secretions, coughing usually becomes frequent and is an obvious sign of pulmonary disease. A raspy, wet cough productive of mucoid or discolored sputum (yellow, green, or brown) characterizes patients with chronic bronchitis or bronchiectasis, whereas patients with asthma may have a cough that produces scant, tenacious whitish sputum and mucus plugs.

Chronic cough, defined as cough that has persisted for more than 3 weeks, is a common disorder that is usually explained by a careful history and physical examination, often supplemented with pulmo-

---

BOX 45-3
The differential diagnosis of wheezing

Airway infection, inflammation, or edema
  Pharyngitis, epiglottitis
  Laryngitis, laryngeal edema
  Tracheitis
  Bronchitis, bronchiectasis
  Bronchiolitis
Allergic bronchopulmonary aspergillosis and other mycoses
Anaphylaxis
Bronchial asthma
  "Extrinsic" (allergic)
  "Intrinsic" (nonallergic)
  Exercise induced
  Drug induced (e.g., β-adrenergic blockers)
  Triad asthma (e.g., aspirin)
  Occupational (e.g., grain dust)
Chronic obstructive pulmonary disease
Congestive heart failure ("cardiac asthma")
Cystic fibrosis
Factitious asthma (a spectrum of disorders including laryngeal dyskinesia)
Inhalation lung injury
Parasitic diseases
Partial obstruction of central airways
  Foreign body aspiration
  Neoplasms
  Tracheal or bronchial stenosis
  Vascular lesions
Pulmonary thromboembolism
Pulmonary vasculitis

BOX 45-4
Selected important causes of cough

Acute cough
Aspiration of foreign body
Aspiration of upper airway or gastric secretions
Inhalation of noxious gases or dusts
Lower respiratory tract infection
  Laryngitis
  Tracheobronchitis
  Pneumonia
Postnasal drip
Upper respiratory tract infection
  Otitis
  Pharyngitis
  Rhinitis
  Sinusitis

Chronic cough (>3 weeks' duration)
Allergic bronchopulmonary aspergillosis (or mycosis)
Bronchial asthma
Bronchiectasis
Chronic bronchitis
Chronic inflammatory diseases involving the lower airways
  Vasculitis
  Sarcoidosis
Chronic rhinosinusitis with postnasal drip
Cigarette smoking
Congestive heart failure ("cardiac asthma")
Disorders of the auditory canals or tympanic membranes
Pharyngeal or laryngeal disease
Gastroesophageal reflux
Idiopathic pulmonary fibrosis
Recurrent aspiration
Primary or secondary lung cancer
Prolonged cough secondary to upper respiratory tract infection (including *Bordetella pertussis* and *Chlamydia pneumoniae*)
Psychogenic cough
Therapy with angiotensin-converting enzyme inhibitor

---

nary function tests and a chest radiograph. Asthma, COPD, cigarette smoking, and lingering effects of an upper respiratory tract infection are the most common causes of this symptom.

As postnasal drip can trigger coughing, a thorough examination of the nose, sinuses, pharynx, and larynx should be part of the evaluation of a patient with a chronic cough. A cough alone, without wheezing, can be the principal manifestation of asthma in some patients. In nonsmokers with a chronic persistent cough who have a normal chest radiograph, 25% or more may have unrecognized asthma—so-called cough-variant asthma, in which coughing instead of wheezing is the main symptom. A cough can also herald the development of more obvious heart failure and pulmonary edema. A nonproductive, short, shallow cough is a usual manifestation of diffuse interstitial fibrotic lung disease, because stiff, noncompliant airways do not distend readily with inspiration, and stretching them seems to precipitate reflex coughing. With airway irritation after infection, even shallow breaths may evoke coughing by stimulating abnormally sensitive irritant receptors in the bronchial walls. Coughing and clearing the throat can also be anxiety responses, and some patients with a history of chronic cough may actually not have airway disease but may just be manifesting self-consciousness and nervousness. In the wake of respiratory infection from viruses or microbes such as *Mycoplasma pneumoniae*, *Chlamydia pneumoniae*, and *Bordetella pertussis*, a persistent cough may linger for weeks. Such pathogens directly injure ciliated epithelial cells and can decrease the effectiveness of mucociliary clearance; thus coughing may be a compensating or adaptive host mechanism to ensure adequate clearance of stagnant secretions. A cough is a symptom that usually needs evaluation and a reasonable explanation for its occurrence.

For a cough of new onset to be worrisome enough to demand a thorough assessment, it should have been present for at least 6 to 8 weeks and not be just a residual effect of a prior mild respiratory infection. Occasionally, the physician will encounter patients with cough of such duration that cannot be readily explained. It is important to emphasize that these patients should be evaluated carefully and not just given antitussive medication or considered to have a psychosomatic disorder. The differential diagnosis of chronic cough is broad, and a thorough medical history and physical examination are

required; occasionally serious pulmonary or nonpulmonary diseases are detected. Nevertheless, in most cases, chronic "unexplained" cough represents a manifestation of one or more of the following: postnasal drip, occult bronchial asthma, or gastroesophageal reflux. Skilled clinical management for each of these common disorders is necessary for effective treatment of the cough. Long-term treatment is usually necessary, and recurrences are common on withdrawal of therapy.

A careful medication history may detect the current use of an angiotensin-converting enzyme (ACE) inhibitor for hypertension. Up to 20% of patients treated with ACE inhibitors develop chronic cough. A clinical trial of withdrawal of this medication allows the cough to disappear within a few days if the medication is responsible.

The cigarette smoking status of the patient is important, and an attempt to decrease smoking should be stressed. If the cough is productive, a sputum analysis of cells, a microbial culture, and a cytology study should be obtained initially. Thereafter, the evaluation is largely dictated by the patient's history, which provides the clues for the origin of the coughing. As mentioned, an ear-nose-throat examination with sinus radiographs or CT scan and perhaps an allergy workup, if upper airway infection or rhinitis is likely, may be required. Nocturnal "asthma" or glottic dysfunction from regurgitation would suggest the need for esophageal studies to document reflux from a hiatus hernia or esophageal dysmotility. Ambulatory monitoring of the esophageal pH for a 24-hour period is a useful test for the detection of gastroesophageal reflux.

Episodic coughing induced by exercise or athletics may warrant a methacholine inhalational challenge test to document hyperactive airways. Endobronchial obstruction can occur from a benign cause resulting from aspiration of a particle or a piece of vegetable matter into the airways, or may ominously suggest a neoplasm. Therefore diagnostic bronchoscopy may be required. The appearance of a normal chest film may not obviate the need for bronchoscopy in assessing early manifestations of obstruction or endobronchial disease. If coughing is part of a diffuse interstitial lung process, an etiologic evaluation often requires tissue biopsy. In systematically working through the differential diagnosis of a chronic, persistent cough and in deciding what tests and invasive procedures may be indicated, the problem of habitual or psychogenic cough should be placed purposely at the bottom of the differential list. These considerations are summarized in the algorithmic approach to cough shown in Fig. 45-4.

Treatment. Treatment of coughing requires therapy for the underlying problem that caused the cough. Cessation of cigarette smoking produces significant decreases in coughing. Within 4 to 6 weeks after stopping, a noticeable decrease in coughing may have occurred; however, the cough may linger and can persist for several years. A persistent cough in a smoker or exsmoker that cannot be attributed to chronic bronchitis raises the possibility of neoplasm and therefore the need for close observation.

Therapy includes aerosolized bronchodilators for asthma, cessation of smoking for chronic bronchitis, elevation of the head of the bed and no food or fluid before retiring for gastroesophageal reflux, and antibiotics and decongestants for sinusitis. Symptomatic (nonspecific) treatment is indicated only when the cause of the cough consistently eludes diagnosis so that specific or definitive therapy cannot be given. Cough suppressants are given for symptomatic relief rather than cure. Antitussive drugs act either on the afferent pathway of the reflex (peripherally) or centrally where the cough is coordinated. The drugs that appear to act on the afferent side of the cough reflex arc are local anesthetics. Central cough suppression is probably achieved by depressing the medullary integrative areas. The central cough suppressants include both narcotic and nonnarcotic agents. All narcotics are reasonably effective cough suppressants. The most commonly used is codeine phosphate. It is usually effective in oral doses of 10 to 20 mg, but as much as 30 mg is occasionally required. As an antitussive agent, dextromethorphan may be as effective as codeine. Expectorants and mucolytics do not function as cough suppressants. Guaifenesin (glycerol guaiacolate) has been demonstrated to have no antitussive effect in patients with the common cold.

Complications. *Cough syncope,* defined as a loss of consciousness preceded by a paroxysm of coughing, occurs most often in males. The patients are usually obese, well-muscled cigarette smokers, with underlying chronic obstructive disease. The more violent the cough, the more likely syncope is to occur. The duration of unconsciousness is brief, often only several seconds; rarely, a convulsion may occur.

Vigorous coughing may promote loss of urine and sometimes fecal incontinence. Coughing is a frequent prelude to hemoptysis, which has many causes and will be discussed. Rib fractures caused by very forceful cough are common. In patients with infections of the respiratory tract, the incidence of cough fractures is 5% or less. Cough fractures commonly involve the lateral aspect of one of the fifth through the tenth ribs; intense local pain and tenderness are found.

Pneumothorax, pneumomediastinum, splenic rupture, rupture of the rectus abdominis muscle, heart block, inguinal hernia, and rupture of anal, nasal, and subconjunctival veins are some of the more unusual complications of coughing.

Expectoration

Expectoration of sputum from the lower respiratory tract by coughing or "phlegm" from the pharynx by "hawking" and spitting is a commonly witnessed respiratory defense mechanism. Although patients often cannot be certain whether the mucus they expectorated originated in the chest or the nasopharynx, it is important to try to make this distinction. Secretions from the lower respiratory tract are cleared by deep, often raspy coughs and signal the presence of tracheobronchial or parenchymal lung disease, or occasionally aspiration of upper airway or gastric secretions. Secretions from the nasopharynx are often cleared by an inspiratory snorting maneuver, followed by throat clearing, or occasionally coughing; they are a manifestation of nasal or sinus disease. Conscious clearance of mucus from any level of the respiratory tract is not normal; it should always be considered a sign of acute, or possibly chronic, disease.

It is uncertain how much fluid normally is produced along the tracheobronchial surface because the humidification of inspired air and recovery of water from air during expiration are efficient mechanisms. The normal mucosal surface, viewed at bronchoscopy in normal persons, appears rather dry. Mucus does not uniformly cover the ciliated surface but is seen in patches. The pH of the mucosal surface of the trachea is 6.7. Ciliary clearance sweeps the surface secretions up the airways to the larynx where they are swallowed. It is important to emphasize that regular coughing and production of phlegm or sputum are indicative of airway irritation, which can be from many causes that may require medical investigation.

The patient's description or physician's inspection of an expectorated specimen has always had value in deciding what the abnormal process is—discoloration suggesting an exacerbation of infection in a person with chronic bronchitis, mucus plugs in a decompensating asthmatic, or blood mixed with sputum versus pure hemoptysis. Smelling the specimen (anaerobes sometimes give a foul odor), looking at the layering of sputum in a container, and quantitating the amount are recommended. How accurate these parameters are in judging the nature or severity of the lung process is debatable. Assessing sputum purulence as a gauge of infection is an imprecise measurement. Mucoid or whitish sputum may be expectorated routinely by a person with underlying airway irritation and hyperreactivity, for example, a cigarette smoker with bronchitis or a symptomatic asthmatic. When the sputum color changes abruptly to yellow or green and the sputum becomes sticky and more copious, an intercurrent microbial infection is suspected. Unfortunately, an analysis of inflammatory cells in sputum, ribonucleic acid value for polymorphonuclear content, and quantitative bacterial cultures do not correlate well with objective evidence of infection.

The texture of the sputum is often described by patients. Sticky phlegm in the trachea can be felt or perceived as a fullness and tickle when breathing and coughing, yet it might not be cleared; it remains adherent and does not come up and frustrates the patient. Hard flecks or strings of mucus can be interspersed in the sputum. Asthmatics often expectorate plugs of mucus variously described to be like rice particles, worms (bronchial casts), or pieces of spaghetti. Episodes of hard coughing that produce gelatinous, blood-colored plugs, perhaps as large as the tip of a small fifth finger, may be the clue for bronchiectasis and an allergic bronchopulmonary mycosis complicating asthma. The volume of expectorated fluid can be appreciable, roughly quantitated in quaint terms of tablespoons or portions of a cupful. A person with active bronchitis or with bronchiectasis as found with cystic fibrosis can produce several ounces a day or more of secretions. The purulent solid material may float on the watery secretions causing the specimen to layer, which is taken as evidence of bronchorrhea from bronchiectatic, infected airways, or rarely of drainage from a lung abscess.

Chest Pain

Chest pain(s) (Chapter 16) is a symptom that is readily communicated by the patient; however, identifying its cause or origin may require considerable effort and thought. The differential diagnosis of the complaint of chest pain is broad (Box 45-5). Pain, like hemoptysis, is not likely to be ignored by the patient unless it has a familiar and recurrent pattern, as in the case of the pain associated with angina or with esophageal irritation. Even under these circumstances, its appearance may cause considerable anxiety because of what it portends.

The origin of pain felt in the chest may be confusing. Pain originating in the biliary tract and in epigastric structures may radiate to the chest and cause dyspnea, and it may mimic the pain arising from mediastinal organs or the parietal pleura. Likewise, acute bacterial lobar pneumonia in a lower lung lobe may produce epigastric tenderness, directing attention to the abdomen as well as the lung. Atypical anginal chest pains can be difficult to differentiate from esophageal and gastric causes. Because postprandial heartburn can represent angina, exercise stress testing and often cardiac angiography may be needed to determine the precise cause of this pain. A rib injury or costochondritis can sometimes be a confusing cause of acute, severe chest wall pain, but the relationship of the pain to position or movement and the point tenderness elicited with examination usually resolve the issue. The complex description of pain is subjective but is

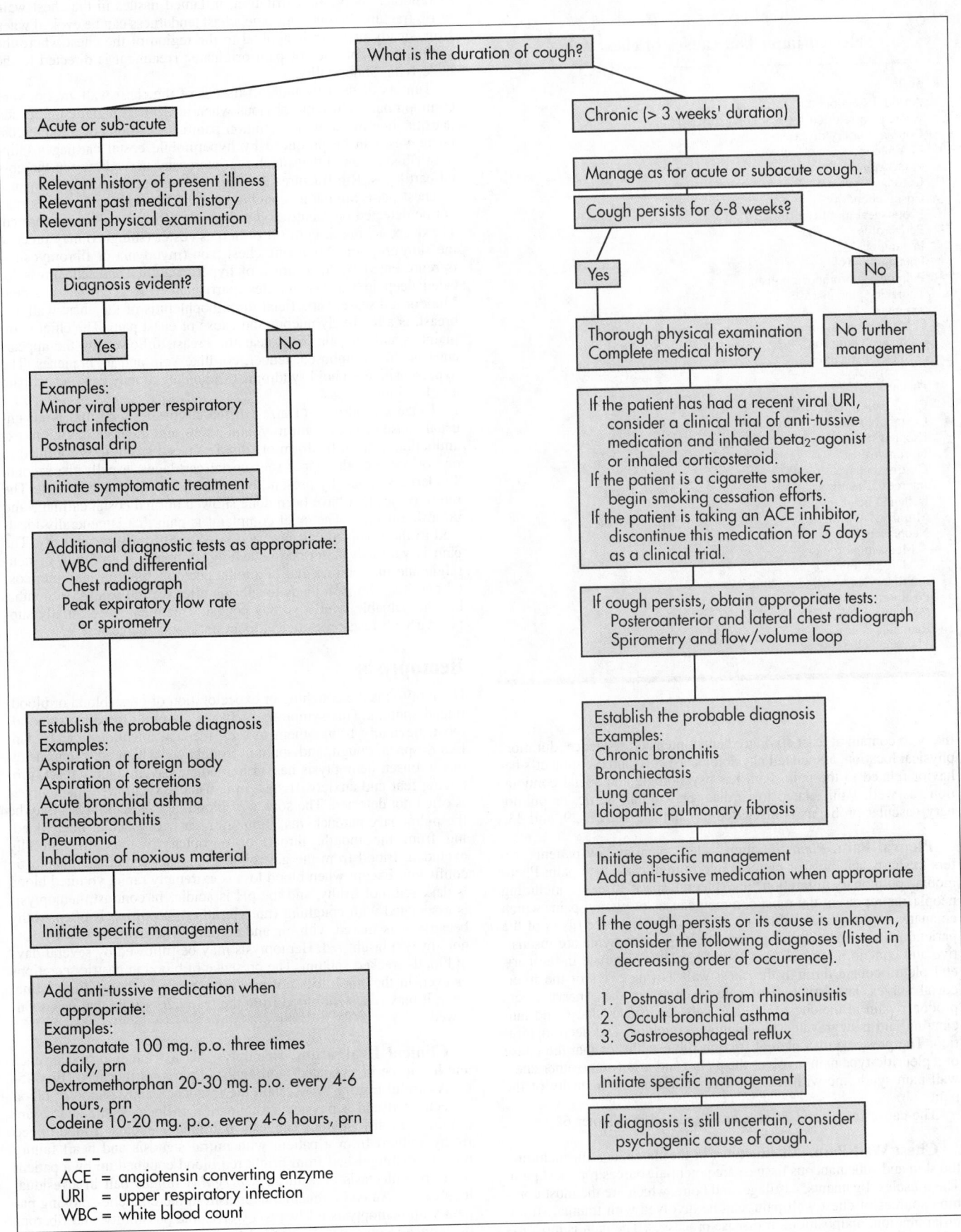

FIGURE 45-4   An algorithmic approach to evaluation and treatment of the patient with cough.

BOX 45-5
Selected important causes of chest pain

Acute

Aortic dissection
Chest pain referred from abdominal source
Coronary artery disease
    Acute myocardial infarction
    Ischemia
Coronary spasm
Costal chondritis
Esophageal motility disorders
Pericarditis
Pneumonia
Pneumothorax
Pulmonary thromboembolism
Thoracic spine disease
Trauma
    Mediastinal injury
    Muscle contusion
    Skeletal fractures

Chronic

Chest pain referred from abdominal source
Costal chondritis
Esophageal motility disorders
Fibromyositis
Gastroesophageal reflux
Intercostal neuritis
Ischemic heart disease
Mitral valve prolapse
Neoplasms
    Mediastinal tumors
    Mesothelioma
    Primary and secondary lung cancer
Postthoracotomy pain
Psychogenic pain
Radicular pain
Thoracic spine disease

---

likely to contain at least six ingredients: intensity, sequence, duration, physical location, associated physiologic aspects, and the subject's behavior related to the pain. Pain has psychologic and social connotations as well. Pain related to cardiac, pericardial, aortic, or pulmonary vascular problems is discussed in Chapters 16, 27, 29, and 33.

Pleural Pain. *Pleuritis,* often called "pleurisy" by patients, refers to sharp, stabbing, or piercing intermittent chest wall pain. Pneumonia, pulmonary infarction, and pleural space diseases including neoplasms represent the most common causes of pleural pain, which emanates from irritation of the endings of afferent nerve fibers of the parietal pleura. The visceral pleura and lung parenchyma are insensitive and contain no pain fibers. Pain fibers that originate in the parietal pleura course through the chest wall as fine twigs of the intercostal nerves, and irritation of pain receptors in these nerve fibers produces pain in the chest wall that feels superficial, sharp, and lancinating and is aggravated by laughing, coughing, and deep inspiration. The presence of a pleural friction rub establishes that the cause of a pleuritic-type pain involves the pleura and is not some other chest wall pain syndrome with respiratory variation in the intensity of the pain.

The causes of pleural disease are discussed in Chapter 64.

Chest Wall Pain. All structures in the thoracic wall, including the skin and subcutaneous tissues, are potential sources for chest pain. The muscles, ligaments, cartilage, and bone, which are the most common sources of chest wall pain, can be involved with trauma, strain, inflammation, malposition, or disease processes. The pain is most often a dull, aching soreness that varies in response to movement or local touch.

The *chest wall syndrome* is a catch-all term occasionally applied to anterior chest pain that arises from multiple causes, including cer-

vicothoracic nerve root irritation, inflamed tissues in the chest wall, or rib fracture. In this syndrome, chest tenderness can be evoked when firm, steady pressure is applied to the region of the chest where the spontaneous episodes of pain originate. Treatment is directed to the underlying abnormality.

Tumors of the ribs and soft tissues of the chest wall are not very common but are usually obvious when present. Traumatic intercostal neuritis, one of the more common painful afflictions of the intercostal nerves, can be produced by hypermobile costal cartilages (slipping rib syndrome) that pinch the intercostal nerve between the costal cartilages. Rib fractures are frequently unrecognized as the cause of chest pain. Strenuous coughing can be the culprit. Fractures may not be detected on roentgenograms until sufficient callus has formed. The deep, aching discomfort of herpes zoster (shingles) may precede the skin eruption. Myogenic chest pain (myodynia or fibromyositis) is represented by local areas of hyperirritability and tenderness located deep in various muscles, particularly the pectoralis muscles. Mondor's disease, superficial thrombophlebitis of the chest wall and breast, is a relatively uncommon cause of chest pain. The chief complaint is sudden pain in or near the breast, followed by the appearance of the thrombosed, tender, cordlike vein and its branches. The hypersensitive xiphoid syndrome (xiphoidalgia) may cause chest pain and local tenderness.

Tietze's syndrome (Tietze's disease, costal chondritis) is an unusual cause of chest pain in young adults and older children. On examination, a firm, fusiform or spindle-shaped swelling is confined to one or more of the upper four costal cartilages, usually the second. Tenderness is usually present, but heat and erythema are absent. The rare biopsies that have been done showed normal costal cartilage and no inflammation. The chief complaint is pain that is generally localized to the involved cartilage and is of mild to severe intensity. The pain is variously described as aching, gripping, sharp, dull, or neuralgic and may mimic that of angina pectoris, pleurisy, and intercostal neuritis. The pain tends to subside after several weeks or months, but the palpable swellings may persist. Treatment is essentially supportive with rest, reassurance, local heat, and analgesics.

Hemoptysis

Hemoptysis is the coughing or expectoration of gross blood or blood-tinged sputum. This symptom is always alarming to patients and almost inevitably brings them to seek medical attention quickly. Unlike dyspnea, cough, and sputum production, which are often insidious in onset, hemoptysis has an immediate psychologic impact, producing fear and anxiety. If sputum is usually swallowed, hemoptysis is often not detected. The source of blood in true hemoptysis may be the pulmonary parenchyma, larynx, or tracheobronchial tree. Bleeding from the mouth, throat, or nasopharynx must be carefully excluded. Blood from the gastrointestinal tract can create diagnostic confusion. Except when blood loss is extremely rapid, vomited blood is dark red, not frothy, and the pH is acidic. In contrast, hemoptysis is associated with coughing (not vomiting); a portion is often frothy because it is mixed with air and sputum. The color is usually (but not always) bright red. Hemoptysis may be followed by several days of blood-streaked sputum. The presence of blood in gastric secretions or even in the stool does not prove its origin in the gastrointestinal tract; it may represent blood from the respiratory tract that was swallowed.

Clinical Evaluation. Hemoptysis is a frightening occurrence and has to be investigated thoroughly to pinpoint its cause (Box 45-6). A careful history to ascertain the frequency and volume of blood expectorated and a physical examination to localize the source are required. Frothy sputum suggests pulmonary edema. Blood-tinged frothy sputum from a patient with mitral stenosis and heart failure must be distinguished from bright red blood coughed up by a patient with bronchiectasis or with an *Aspergillus* fungus ball in a residual lung cavity. An endobronchial neoplasm in the cigarette-smoking patient with hemoptysis is always a worrisome possibility, and fiberoptic bronchoscopy may be needed to inspect the airways and obtain histologic tissue for diagnosis. Bleeding can originate in the posterior nasopharynx and actually drip into the back of the throat, or it can be aspirated into the airways without the patient being aware. A careful examination of the nose and throat is thus very important for

---

BOX 45-6
Selected important causes of hemoptysis

Aspiration of blood
    Upper airway, esophageal, or gastric source
Bronchiectasis
Cardiac disease
    Left ventricular failure
    Mitral stenosis
Chronic bronchitis
Coagulation disorder
Diffuse alveolar hemorrhage
    Associated with glomerulonephritis
    Drug or chemical induced (D-penicillamine, trimellitic anhydride)
    Goodpasture's syndrome
    Idiopathic pulmonary hemosiderosis
    Pulmonary capillaritis
    Pulmonary vasculitis
Iatrogenic
    Bronchoscopy
    Needle biopsy
    Thoracic surgery
Infections
    Lung abscess
    Mycetomas
    Mycoses
    Parasitic diseases
    Pneumonia
    Tuberculosis
Miscellaneous
    Broncholithiasis
    Cystic fibrosis
    Endometriosis
    Intralobar sequestration
    Pulmonary arteriovenous malformation
    Sarcoidosis
    Tracheobronchial-arterial fistula
Neoplasms
    Bronchial carcinoid
    Bronchogenic carcinoma
    Secondary lung cancer
Pulmonary infarction
Trauma

---

rious disease and should rarely be the final study; half of patients with hemoptysis have a normal chest radiograph. Caution should also be exercised in attributing the site of bleeding to an obvious abnormality on a chest radiograph, as bronchoscopy may reveal that the bleeding site is different from this area seen on the radiograph. A blood cell count, clotting evaluation, and urinalysis are necessary. Sputum should be examined for malignant cells, tuberculosis organisms, and fungi. A tuberculosis skin test plus anergy controls should be applied.

Fiberoptic bronchoscopy is essential in the evaluation of a patient with hemoptysis, even if the chest radiograph is normal. There are a few exceptions, for example, a young, nonsmoking person with acute bronchitis, a few days of blood-streaked sputum associated with paroxysmal coughing, and complete clearing of the sputum when the bronchitis subsides. Fiberoptic bronchoscopy is diagnostic for the cause of hemoptysis in about 80% of lung cancer patients and in 60% of patients with a nonmalignant cause of hemoptysis. Early bronchoscopy (during hemoptysis or during the 48 hours after hemoptysis has ceased) is more likely to demonstrate active bleeding or localize the bleeding.

Thoracic CT can be valuable and should be part of the evaluation of hemoptysis if a chest radiograph is negative and fiberoptic bronchoscopy is not revealing. Thoracic CT may demonstrate an area of bronchiectasis, inapparent lung cavity, or broncholithiasis causing hemoptysis when these were not detected on the conventional chest radiograph. Ultrathin-section "slices" of 1.5 mm, instead of 1.0 cm, may be required to see bronchiectatic areas (high-resolution scan [HRCT]). This technique has rendered contrast bronchography, once the mainstay in the radiographic diagnosis of bronchiectasis, obsolete.

Other studies that are used in the appropriate situation include ventilation-perfusion lung scans, pulmonary angiograms, and selective bronchial artery angiography.

Treatment. The objectives of therapy for significant and ongoing hemoptysis are to stop bleeding, prevent airway obstruction, and support the patient's vital functions. Adequate suctioning capability and equipment for endotracheal intubation should be immediately available (a double-lumen tube should be included). If the bleeding site is known, it is best to place that side in a dependent position to reduce blood spilling over into the uninvolved lung. Drugs that significantly depress cough or respiration should be avoided because failure to clear the bronchi of blood may lead to airway plugging by blood clots. Antibiotics may be necessary to treat an underlying infection that may be causing hemoptysis. Oxygen may be indicated if hypoxemia is present, and transfusions should be considered to maintain the hematocrit above 30%. Mechanical ventilation should be initiated whenever respiratory failure is life threatening. Disorders of coagulation should be corrected quickly.

Bronchoscopy should be done as soon as possible to localize the site of bleeding. Patients with "massive" hemoptysis usually demonstrate a steady decrease of bleeding, with cessation of hemoptysis after 4 days. Many patients with serious hemoptysis can be successfully treated conservatively. In some situations, however, a pulmonary resection may be indicated. Selective embolization of bronchial arteries has also been found beneficial for treating life-threatening hemoptysis.

excluding this possible site of bleeding that can be mistaken as the source for hemoptysis. Telangiectasis on the lips or buccal mucosa may indicate Rendu-Osler-Weber disease.

Chronic bronchitis is the most common cause of hemoptysis in the United States. Intermittent, minimal blood streaking of the sputum regularly produced by the patient is typical, but larger amounts of blood may be noticed during exacerbations of COPD. Frank, bloody sputum is unusual with pulmonary embolus or infarction and with most forms of bacterial pneumonia. Rusty-colored sputum may signal bacterial pneumonia. Recurrent hemoptysis strongly suggests a lung tumor if chronic bronchitis, tuberculosis, sarcoidosis, and bronchiectasis are not the cause. Massive hemoptysis, arbitrarily defined as the coughing up of more than 200 to 600 ml of blood within 24 hours, is usually caused by bleeding from fungal cavities (mycetomas), tuberculous or sarcoidosis cavities, bronchiectasis, penetrating trauma, bronchogenic carcinoma, bronchial carcinoid tumors, or arteriovenous malformations. Hemoptysis may be fatal as a result of exsanguination or respiratory failure from filling the airway with blood and clots. Radiation-induced pneumonitis can cause brisk and recurrent hemoptysis that can be difficult to control and can be a distressing complication for the patient; in this case the cause is known, and in time the bleeding subsides. Rarely, hemoptysis concurrent with menstrual flow may suggest a focus of endometrial tissue in the bronchial wall. Bloody sputum mixed with white gritty material suggests broncholithiasis.

Diagnostic Studies. A careful history, physical examination, and chest radiographs (posteroanterior and lateral) are done first in nonemergent situations. A normal chest radiograph does not exclude se-

BIBLIOGRAPHY

Aisenberg J, Castell DO: Approach to the patient with unexplained chest pain, *Mt Sinai J Med* 61:476, 1994.
Bramen SS, Corrao WM: Cough: differential diagnosis and treatment, *Clin Chest Med* 8:177, 1987.
Butler DJ, Turkat NW: Great expectorations. A case of psychogenic throat clearing and expectoration, *Arch Family Med* 4:647, 1995.
Cahill BC, Ingbar DH: Massive hemoptysis. Assessment and management, *Clin Chest Med* 15:147, 1994.
Donat WE: Chest pain: cardiac and noncardiac causes, *Clin Chest Med* 8:241, 1987.
Hollingsworth HM: Wheezing and stridor, *Clin Chest Med* 8:231, 1987.
Irwin RS, Curley FJ: The treatment of cough. A comprehensive review, *Chest* 99:1477, 1991.
Irwin RS, Curley FJ, French CL: Chronic cough. The spectrum and frequency of causes, key components of the diagnostic evaluation, and outcome of specific therapy, *Am Rev Respir Dis* 141:640, 1990.
Irwin RS, French CL, Curley FJ et al: Chronic cough due to gastroesophageal reflux. Clinical, diagnostic, and pathogenetic aspects, *Chest* 104:1511, 1993.
Israel RH, Poe RH: Hemoptysis, *Clin Chest Med* 8:197, 1987.

Killian KJ, Jones NL: Mechanisms of exertional dyspnea, *Clin Chest Med* 15:247, 1994.

Loudon RG: The lung exam, *Clin Chest Med* 8:265, 1987.

Lundgren JD, Baraniuk JN: Mucus secretion and inflammation, *Pulmon Pharmacol* 5:81, 1992.

Mahler DA: Dyspnea: diagnosis and management, *Clin Chest Med* 8:215, 1987.

Mahler DA, Horowitz MB: Clinical evaluation of exertional dyspnea, *Clin Chest Med* 15:259, 1994.

Manning HL, Schwartzstein RM: Pathophysiology of dyspnea, *N Engl J Med* 333:1547, 1995.

Mulrow CD, Lucey CR, Farnett LE: Discriminating causes of dyspnea through clinical examination, *J General Intern Med* 8:383, 1993.

Murata GH: Evaluating chest pain in the emergency department, *West J Med* 159:61, 1993.

O'Donnell DE: Breathlessness in patients with chronic airflow limitation. Mechanisms and management, *Chest* 106:904, 1994.

Patel U, Pattison CW, Raphael M: Management of massive hemoptysis, *Br J Hosp Med* 52:74, 76-8, 1994.

Patrick H, Patrick F: Chronic cough, *Med Clin North Am* 79:361, 1995.

Pratter MR, Bartter T, Akers S et al: An algorithmic approach to chronic cough, *Ann Intern Med* 119:977, 1993.

Seamens CM, Wrenn K: Breathlessness. Strategies aimed at identifying and treating the cause of dyspnea, *Postgrad Med* 98:215, 1995.

Sharma OP: Symptoms and signs in pulmonary medicine: old observations and new interpretations, *Dis Mon* 41:577, 1995.

Stack LB, Morgan JA, Hedges JR et al: Advances in the use of ancillary diagnostic testing in the emergency department evaluation of chest pain, *Emerg Med Clin North Am* 13:713, 1995.

Widdicombe JG: Neurophysiology of the cough reflex, *Eur Respir J* 8:1193, 1995.

Zervanos NJ, Shute KM: Acute, disruptive cough. Symptomatic therapy for a nagging problem, *Postgrad Med* 95:153, 157, 163, 1994.

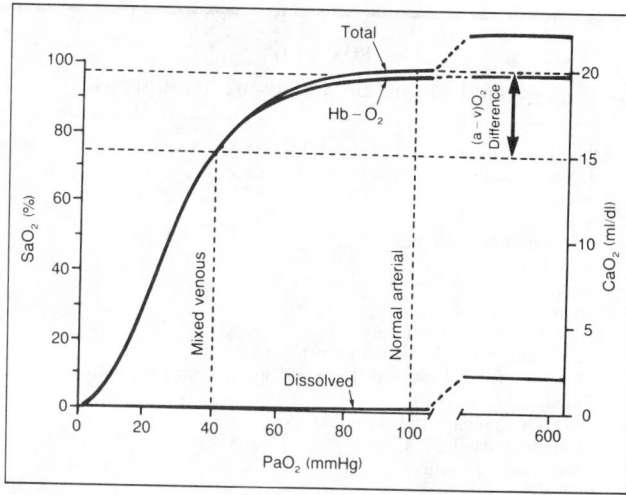

FIG. 46-1.   The oxygen-hemoglobin (O_2-Hb) dissociation curve, relating the partial pressure of oxygen in arterial blood (Pao_2) to arterial O_2 saturation (Sao_2) and to the O_2 content of arterial blood (Cao_2). A normal Hb concentration in milliliters per deciliter is assumed. The curve descends steeply below Pao_2 values of 50 mm Hg, indicating severely reduced O_2-carrying capacity by Hb below this Pao_2. The lower line represents O_2 in solution in the blood; the middle line depicts O_2 bound to the Hb at that Pao_2; the upper line shows O_2 bound to Hb plus O_2 dissolved. Note that dissolved O_2 contributes little to Cao_2 at a Pao_2 in the normal range.

(From Luce JM, Tyler ML, Pierson DJ: *Intensive respiratory care*, Philadelphia, 1984, WB Saunders.)

CHAPTER

46   Acute Respiratory Failure

Leonard D. Hudson

Acute respiratory failure (ARF) can be defined as the relatively sudden onset of failure of the respiratory system to carry out its major functions (i.e., the adequate delivery of oxygen into and adequate removal of carbon dioxide from the arterial blood) to a degree that causes a threat to life. Thus ARF is not a disease but rather a syndrome marked by abnormal physiologic functions that can be caused by a variety of disease processes. The process causing failure of function is not necessarily limited to the lungs themselves but may involve any part of the respiratory system: the ventilatory control system, the lungs (including the airways and the lung parenchyma), the lung vasculature, and the chest wall and muscles of respiration.

Acute respiratory failure can be more specifically defined by abnormalities of arterial blood gas values. The values used in any given definition are somewhat arbitrary. ARF is commonly defined by an arterial oxygen pressure (Pao_2) less than 55 mm Hg and/or an arterial carbon dioxide pressure ($Paco_2$) greater than 50 mm Hg with an accompanying acidemia. The defined limit of Pao_2 for ARF ranges from less than 50 to less than 60 mm Hg. This range is chosen because of its position on the oxygen-hemoglobin dissociation curve (Fig. 46-1). If the Pao_2 falls below 50 to 55 mm Hg, the oxygen saturation (and thus the oxygen content of the arterial blood) falls sharply. Therefore a Pao_2 below this level may be life threatening. With a Pao_2 above 60 mm Hg, saturation of the hemoglobin by oxygen is nearly complete. Raising the Pao_2 to higher values results in relatively little increase in arterial oxygen content.

A $Paco_2$ greater than 50 mm Hg is used as a limit because a sudden change from baseline normal $Paco_2$ (40 mm Hg) with a normal serum bicarbonate level (24 mEq/L) causes significant respiratory acidosis. Traditionally hypercapnia has been considered life threatening because of the associated acidosis. Acute onset of severe respiratory acidosis has been associated with higher mortality in some series of patients with chronic obstructive pulmonary disease (COPD) and ARF, compared with those with less severe acidosis. Chronic hypercapnia in which the pH is compensated by increased serum bicar-

bonate is not necessarily dangerous in itself. Recently the clinical importance of the respiratory acidosis per se has been questioned. Carbon dioxide pressure (Pco_2) has been allowed to rise in selected patients (to avoid potential complications associated with excessive minute ventilations delivered by mechanical ventilation), and the associated acidosis has apparently been well tolerated. The level of respiratory acidosis that is "safe" is not known. Since some patients with COPD may constantly have Pao_2 and $Paco_2$ values that fit these arbitrary definitions, the clinician must determine whether the observed abnormal blood gas values are chronic and stable or are associated with an acute clinical worsening.

The syndrome of ARF is analogous to acute functional failure in any other organ system, for example, cardiac, renal, or hepatic. The syndrome represents a severe functional abnormality that is potentially life threatening and requires immediate attention. Identification of the syndrome allows the clinician to consider a particular approach to diagnosis and management. Indeed, the principles of management are similar once a diagnosis of ARF has been established, despite the variety of diseases that may lead to this functional abnormality. Certain therapeutic measures can be initiated once ARF has been diagnosed. On the other hand, optimal management depends on establishing a more specific diagnosis of the disease or diseases that cause or precipitate the organ failure.

PATHOPHYSIOLOGIC CAUSES OF ACUTE RESPIRATORY FAILURE

Four pathophysiologic mechanisms can lead to ARF: hypoventilation, ventilation-perfusion ratio mismatch, shunt, and diffusion limitation. Only the first three mechanisms are important in clinical practice, since diffusion limitation is uncommon as a sole cause of significant hypoxemia. Thinking of ARF in terms of these mechanisms is useful in establishing the differential diagnosis of the cause of failure and facilitating management.

Hypoventilation

Alveolar hypoventilation is characterized by an elevation in $Paco_2$. Thus hypoventilation is present when alveolar ventilation is inadequate to meet the body's requirements for removal of carbon dioxide, and the $Paco_2$ level begins to rise. Hypoventilation may exist even when the absolute level of alveolar ventilation is increased above normal, if this increase is not adequate to compensate for an increase in carbon dioxide production. The resultant hypercapnia not only causes respiratory acidosis but is also associated with hypoxemia. Hypoxemia related to hypoventilation is a result of a decreased alveolar partial pressure of oxygen (Pao_2). The level of alveolar ventilation is not adequate to remove the carbon dioxide produced, and the amount of atmospheric air containing oxygen brought in to the alveolus is also reduced. Since Pao_2 is reduced, the Pao_2 in turn decreases. *If arterial hypoxemia is caused by hypoventilation alone,* the difference between the alveolar oxygen and the arterial oxygen, $P(A - a)o_2$, is normal. All other mechanisms resulting in hypoxemia are associated with an increased $P(A - a)o_2$ (Chapter 35).

The hypoxemia associated with hypoventilation can be corrected by administering supplemental oxygen. However, this oxygen has no direct effect on respiratory acidosis. The more physiologic way to correct both respiratory acidosis and hypoxemia is to improve alveolar ventilation. How this is best accomplished depends on the cause of the alveolar hypoventilation. When airflow obstruction is the cause of hypoventilation, bronchodilators and secretion removal are appropriate. When an overdose of sedatives has caused respiratory center depression, temporary mechanical ventilation may be warranted until drug metabolism or removal can be achieved.

Ventilation-Perfusion Mismatching

Ventilation-perfusion ratio ($\dot{V}/\dot{Q}$) mismatch is the most common explanation for hypoxemia. For hypoxemia to result, the mismatch must include lung regions where ventilation is decreased out of proportion to perfusion; this results in areas of increased $Paco_2$ and reduced Pao_2. Blood passing by these alveoli reflects the reduced oxygen tension. Also, less carbon dioxide is removed in these regions, and endcapillary blood has an increased Pco_2. However, an increase in ventilation to the areas of lung where ventilation and perfusion remain relatively normally matched provides enough carbon dioxide removal to compensate for the elevated Pco_2 from areas of mismatch. This effect is a consequence of the relatively linear shape of the carbon dioxide dissociation curve; an increase in ventilation in any local lung area strikingly lowers the carbon dioxide content of local pulmonary venous blood. However, increased ventilation of the relatively normally matched regions does not result in a significant increase in oxygen saturation or content because of the sigmoid shape of the oxygen-hemoglobin dissociation curve (Fig. 46-1). Thus increased ventilation does not compensate for the low $\dot{V}/\dot{Q}$ areas that result in hypoxemia.

Hypoxemia caused by $\dot{V}/\dot{Q}$ mismatching can be corrected by a relatively small increase in the fraction of inspired oxygen (FIo_2). This correction occurs because airways to poorly ventilated alveoli remain open, and if the gas mixture is administered for a long enough period, the increased pressure of inspired oxygen is eventually reflected by an increased Pao_2. Definitive therapy depends on reversal of the specific cause of the regional reductions in ventilation (e.g., bronchospasm).

Shunt

Intrapulmonary shunt can be thought of as one extreme of $\dot{V}/\dot{Q}$ mismatch. With shunt, however, there is *no* ventilation but perfusion continues, which, as with $\dot{V}/\dot{Q}$ mismatching, results in an increased $P(A - a)o_2$. Again, adequate carbon dioxide removal can usually be accomplished by increasing ventilation to areas of more normal $\dot{V}/\dot{Q}$ matching. The resulting normal $Paco_2$ does not mean that carbon dioxide removal is entirely normal, since a very high minute ventilation is often required to achieve a normal or low $Paco_2$. Shunt is distinguished from $\dot{V}/\dot{Q}$ mismatch by the magnitude of the increase in FIo_2 required to provide adequate arterial oxygenation. In an area of shunt, added oxygen cannot reach the alveoli, since there is no ventilation. Thus blood flowing past these areas of filled or collapsed alveoli have oxygen tensions that are equal to those of mixed venous blood. Administration of a high FIo_2 is still associated with hypoxemia and a greatly increased $P(A - a)o_2$.

Since processes that cause shunt must result in either alveolar fill-ing or collapse, these areas are usually recognizable on chest x-ray because they are airless.

Diffusion Limitation

Diffusion limitation is an uncommon cause of clinically significant hypoxemia. In normal circumstances blood flowing through the pulmonary capillary bed reaches nearly complete oxygen saturation of the hemoglobin in approximately one third of the total time available for exposure to the alveolar surface. Even when a limitation in diffusion of the oxygen is present, there is usually ample time for the hemoglobin to be saturated with oxygen. Exceptions can occur with exercise, with markedly increased cardiac output and associated markedly reduced capillary transit time, or at high altitudes. Diffusion limitation of oxygenation should not be confused with the pulmonary function test of diffusing capacity. The diffusing capacity is measured by using trace amounts of carbon monoxide and is chiefly influenced by the matching of alveolar blood and gas surfaces. Thus even a markedly abnormal diffusing capacity for carbon monoxide may not significantly affect oxygen transfer. Associated hypoxemia is more probably caused by $\dot{V}/\dot{Q}$ mismatch. For practical purposes, diffusion limitation is not a primary cause of ARF, although it could be a contributing factor in the critically ill patient with high cardiac output. When diffusion limitation of oxygenation does exist, hypoxemia can be corrected by administering an enriched oxygen mixture (increased FIo_2).

CLASSIFICATION OF ACUTE RESPIRATORY FAILURE

There are several possible classifications for ARF. None of these is entirely satisfactory for clinical purposes because none encompasses all the possible causes or types of ARF. Two of the commonly used classifications, taken together, can assist the clinician in planning a management approach to the patient with ARF. These classifications are based on (1) whether there is previous respiratory disease and (2) whether hypoxemia is associated with normocapnia or hypocapnia or with hypercapnia (Table 46-1). Appropriate classification of a patient with ARF aids in diagnosis and also helps in application of treatment principles. It is very important to determine a specific origin or cause so that treatment can be optimally designed.

DIAGNOSIS

The diagnosis of ARF can be considered in the following stages: (1) clinical suspicion that ARF might be present, (2) confirmation that ARF is present, and (3) identification of a specific cause.

Clinical suspicion that ARF might be present should develop from the clinical situation. Two particular settings are important to recognize. The first involves the patient with preexisting lung disease in whom there has been some relatively sudden clinical deterioration, for example, a patient with COPD with clinical worsening and a patient with neuromuscular disease with a superimposed respiratory or metabolic complication and overall clinical worsening. The second setting involves patients who may not have preexisting lung disease but have an acute injury or illness known to be associated with a high incidence of ARF, for example, the patient with septic shock, a circumstance known to be associated with a high incidence of acute diffuse lung injury (acute respiratory distress syndrome [ARDS]).

Compatible symptoms and signs may also suggest ARF and fall into two categories: those reflecting the acute disease process and those reflecting hypoxemia and/or acidosis. Symptoms and signs reflecting the precipitating disease usually suggest some acute lung disease or disorder. These symptoms include increased cough and sputum production and increased shortness of breath. Since these symptoms usually are related to the respiratory system, the possibility of ARF is usually considered and the diagnosis sought. Perhaps more important are the symptoms and signs reflecting hypoxemia and acidosis. These symptoms may be more subtle and difficult to relate to ARF, since they usually involve the central nervous system (CNS) or the cardiovascular system, or both. Central nervous system symptoms reflecting these physiologic abnormalities range from restlessness and irritability to confusion and coma. They may be as subtle as personality change in a patient with COPD, a change recognized by the fam-

Table 46-1   Classification of acute respiratory failure

CATEGORY	EXAMPLE	MECHANISM OF HYPOXEMIA	CHEST X-RAY
↓ Pao_2 with normal or ↓ $Paco_2$			
Preexisting lung disease	Restrictive lung disease (pulmonary fibrosis)	V̇/Q̇ mismatch with or without shunt	Diffuse interstitial infiltrate
	Asthma (until very severe)	V̇/Q̇ mismatch	Clear
No preexisting lung disease required (but could be superimposed on chronic disease)	Acute respiratory distress syndrome	Shunt	Diffuse alveolar-filling infiltrate
	Cardiogenic pulmonary edema	Shunt	Diffuse alveolar-filling infiltrate
	Pulmonary emboli	V̇/Q̇ mismatch and shunt	Clear (or localized infiltrate)
	Pneumonia	Shunt	Localized or diffuse alveolar-filling infiltrate
↓ Pao_2 with ↑ $Paco_2$			
Previous lung disease	COPD	Hypoventilation and V̇/Q̇ mismatch	Clear
	Asthma (very severe)	Hypoventilation and V̇/Q̇ mismatch	Clear
Normal lungs	Sedative drug overdose	Hypoventilation	Clear
	Neuromuscular disease (e.g., myasthenia gravis, Guillain-Barré syndrome)	Hypoventilation	Clear

ily but not necessarily by a stranger. Both hypoxemia and acidosis can cause CNS dysfunction. The CNS effects of respiratory acidosis are in part related to the vasodilatory effects of carbon dioxide, with accompanying central acidosis evident in the cerebrospinal fluid. Physical findings include papilledema and asterixis. Cardiovascular signs or symptoms can reflect either compensatory mechanisms to increase cardiac output and delivery of oxygen to the tissues or complications of hypoxemia and acidosis such as cardiac arrhythmia.

The clinical situation and symptoms and signs that provoke suspicion of ARF are obtained from appropriate history and physical examination. Diagnosis of this clinical syndrome is confirmed by arterial blood gas analysis. Measurement of arterial blood gases not only confirms the diagnosis but also provides information regarding the type of physiologic abnormality that causes the hypoxemia. Repeated arterial blood gas measurements following oxygen administration help separate V̇/Q̇ mismatch from shunt as possible mechanisms.

After the diagnosis has been established by arterial blood gas measurement, additional information can be obtained from a chest roentgenogram. The findings on the chest x-ray can help both with understanding the probable cause of hypoxemia and with diagnosis of the particular disease that is present. The chest roentgenogram can help determine the appropriate level of initial oxygen therapy by suggesting whether shunt or V̇/Q̇ mismatching is likely to be predominant. If shunt is present, usually there is evidence of alveolar filling or collapse; a density or infiltrate is caused by airless or edematous lung or lung filled with purulent secretions. If the chest x-ray is relatively normal, hypoventilation and V̇/Q̇ mismatching are more likely causes. Then the diagnoses to be considered include COPD with bronchitis, drug overdose, and neuromuscular diseases. If a diffuse alveolar-filling process involves most lung fields, ARDS or cardiogenic pulmonary edema must be considered and shunt is likely to be an important mechanism contributing to hypoxemia. If a localized airspace-filling abnormality is present, shunt is still the probable mechanism, but pneumonia must be considered. These examples are simplistic but are meant to illustrate only a few of the possible ways in which the chest roentgenogram is helpful in diagnosis (see Table 46-1).

PRINCIPLES OF MANAGEMENT

Establishing the diagnosis of ARF allows the application of general principles of management. These management principles apply to any type of ARF, although their specific application is greatly influenced by the type and specific cause of ARF. These principles are as follows.

Correction of Inadequate Oxygenation

The most life-threatening physiologic abnormalities should be corrected first. Hypoxemia does not have to be totally corrected to normal; the goal is improvement such that the acute threat to life is removed or greatly diminished. Since hypoxemia usually is the most

life-threatening abnormality, correction should be started immediately with supplemental oxygen administration.

Correction of Respiratory Acidosis

The importance of the level of carbon dioxide is related primarily to its effect on pH; thus treatment should be directed toward increasing pH above dangerously low levels, not correcting Pco_2 to normal values. If possible, treatment should be aimed at correction of the process that resulted in hypercapnia. The decision to use mechanical ventilation is based on clinical findings and is discussed later.

Maintenance of Cardiac Output and Tissue Oxygen Transport

Although ARF is defined by abnormal arterial blood oxygen tension, a goal of therapy is to maintain "adequate" oxygen delivery to the tissue and cellular level. The other important determinant of tissue oxygen transport (in addition to the arterial content of oxygen) is cardiac output. Some therapies used in ARF can decrease cardiac output. Thus even if there is an improvement in arterial oxygen content, the total amount of oxygen transported to the tissues might be adversely affected. Since hemoglobin concentration is an important determinant of arterial oxygen content, correction of anemia should be considered when planning therapy.

Treatment of the Underlying Disease

The first three principles of management are only supportive and temporizing. Definitive management depends on treatment of the processes that resulted in the initial physiologic abnormality. Table 46-2 outlines conditions that may precipitate ARF.

Avoidance of Preventable Complications

It is unusual for a patient with ARF to die of acute hypoxemia or respiratory acidosis with current methods of respiratory support. Death often occurs from other complicating factors such as infection or thromboembolism. For each clinical situation the common complications should be known and measures taken to avoid them. Some complications of management are outlined in Box 46-1.

Since ARF is by definition a life-threatening process and since therapy can be complicated and carries potential risk, any patient with ARF is best managed initially in an intensive care unit. The typical COPD patient with ARF may require only overnight management in such a unit, if there is a relatively rapid response to therapy, or may be managed on an acute care ward if personnel are experienced in the care of these patients and the patient's condition is relatively stable. In other situations (e.g., ARDS), critical care facilities may be required until the lung lesion has resolved.

Table 46-2 Factors that may precipitate acute respiratory failure

CATEGORY	PRECIPITATING FACTOR
I. Normal lungs	Central
	Head injury
	Stroke
	Drug overdose
	Bellows
	Guillain-Barré
	Rib fractures (flail chest)
	Airway
	Tracheal obstruction
II. Acute pulmonary disease (lungs previously normal)	Sepsis
	Shock
	Aspiration
	Pneumonia
	Edema
	Asthma
III. Acute pulmonary disease (lungs previously abnormal)	Pneumothorax
	Pneumonia
	Pulmonary embolism
	Factors in group II

BOX 46-1

Complications of management of acute respiratory failure

Infection (hospital-acquired)
Pneumothorax
Respiratory alkalosis
Cardiac arrhythmia
Thromboembolism
Tracheal injury
Sinusitis
Pulmonary oxygen toxicity
Decreased cardiac output

MEASURES TO IMPROVE OXYGENATION

The goal of measures to improve oxygenation is to increase the arterial oxygen saturation and thus arterial oxygen content. If possible, this increase should be accomplished while avoiding the risk of oxygen toxicity. Certainly it should be accomplished without producing clinically important decreases in cardiac output. A PaO_2 in the range of 60 mm Hg or above usually provides adequate oxygen saturation. However, if this level is achieved by administration of a high FIO_2, oxygen toxicity may damage the lung. The exact level of FIO_2 that represents a toxic threat is not known. It is known that oxygen toxicity is a time-dose relationship; that is, the higher the FIO_2 and the longer the time administered, the greater the risk. Data suggest that levels above 0.7 or 0.8 can be associated with parenchymal lung injury (similar to that seen with other causes of ARDS) after only a few days. Therefore the use of FIO_2 of 0.8 or higher for more than 1 day should be avoided *if possible*. It must be kept in mind, however, that the primary goal of therapy is to oxygenate the arterial blood adequately, and a dangerously high FIO_2 may be necessary. Evidence exists for other types of less severe oxygen toxicity at lower FIO_2. Ciliary action may be reduced, and bacterial killing by alveolar macrophages may be impaired. The clinical importance of these possible toxic effects has not been established.

Measures to improve oxygenation include administration of supplemental oxygen, use of positive end-expiratory pressure (PEEP) or continuous positive airway pressure (CPAP), improved ventilation or use of enhanced tidal volumes, and definitive therapy of the underlying pulmonary abnormality.

Supplemental Oxygen

The clinician must decide initially whether a high or low amount of supplemental oxygen is likely to be required. This estimate is based on knowledge of the clinical abnormality and the likely pathophysiologic mechanism involved, that is, whether the major mechanism of hypoxemia is shunt (requiring a high FIO_2) or hypoventilation and/or $\dot{V}/\dot{Q}$ mismatch (requiring only a small increment in FIO_2).

A low level of supplemental oxygen can be administered through nasal prongs. Nasal prongs are well tolerated by patients, since the prongs are relatively comfortable and allow the patient to cough out secretions and to eat or drink while receiving supplemental oxygen. If the nasal passages are open, nasal administration is effective even when a patient breathes through his or her mouth, since oxygen is entrained from the posterior nasopharynx during inspiration. The flow rate can be adjusted upward from 0.5 L/min to achieve the desired increase in PaO_2. Once a flow greater than 6 L/min is used, there is slight further augmentation of the actual FIO_2. High flows of nasal oxygen have a drying, irritating effect on the upper respiratory tract. Oxygen masks using the Venturi principle allow regulation of the FIO_2 at a given level and are particularly useful in transport or emergency situations in which it is important to maintain a known, relatively stable FIO_2 with a small amount of oxygen supplementation.

A higher FIO_2 can be provided with an appropriate oxygen mask, particularly one that has an oxygen reservoir so that all the oxygen inspired does not have to be provided by the flow rate delivered from the oxygen source. With such a mask the reservoir fills from the oxygen source during expiration and is available to provide an additional volume of oxygen during inhalation. It is difficult to ensure that masks stay in place; if a patient's condition is unstable and a high FIO_2 is required for more than several hours, it may be safer to place an endotracheal tube and administer oxygen through a closed system.

Positive End-Expiratory Pressure and Continuous Positive Airway Pressure

Positive end-expiratory pressure (PEEP) and CPAP are ventilatory maneuvers that are used to improve arterial oxygenation when specific indications are present. *PEEP* refers to the maintenance of positive pressure throughout the expiratory cycle when applied together with mechanical ventilation. *CPAP* refers to the maintenance of positive pressure throughout respiration during spontaneous breathing. The mechanism of improvement in oxygenation is the same with both PEEP and CPAP; they both increase the functional residual capacity (FRC, the amount of air in the lungs at the end of a resting exhalation). This increase in FRC improves oxygenation when lung volumes are low as a result of widespread lung injury associated with intrapulmonary shunt. PEEP either opens areas of microatelectasis, previously not ventilated but still perfused, or holds an edematous lung at a higher volume so that the fluid that previously totally filled alveolar sacs now occupies only a portion of the alveolus, allowing some ventilation. With both of these possible mechanisms, areas of shunt are converted to low or normal $\dot{V}/\dot{Q}$ regions and oxygenation is improved.

PEEP may not improve oxygenation if the abnormality is limited to one area of the lung. In this circumstance PEEP preferentially increases lung volume in the normal, more compliant areas of lung and may have little effect on focal abnormalities. A detrimental effect on oxygenation may even result, since high alveolar pressure in areas of normal lung (with an associated increase in lung volume and resistance to blood flow) can divert blood from the normal areas of lung to the diseased portions and actually increase the shunt effect. Thus a major indication for the use of PEEP/CPAP is ARDS, in which there is diffuse, acute lung injury resulting in widespread areas of microatelectasis and pulmonary edema. In this clinical situation the goals of the use of PEEP are to increase the PaO_2 to provide adequate oxygen saturation of hemoglobin and to allow a reduction in the FIO_2 below the potentially toxic range. There is little evidence that PEEP has other therapeutic effects on the lung or otherwise modifies the course of the disease.

Potential problems with PEEP include reduction in cardiac output, primarily through a decrease in venous return. This effect occurs as alveolar pressure is transmitted in part to the pleural space and mediastinum, impeding venous return. There is also a potential risk of barotrauma with resultant pneumothorax; this risk is increased by the concomitant use of mechanical ventilation with high tidal volumes. In general, airway pressure should be the least required to achieve the oxygenation required.

Increased Tidal Volume

The primary beneficial effects of mechanical ventilation are improvement of respiratory acidosis and reduced work of breathing, but *judicious use* can also improve oxygenation in selected patients. Although PEEP and CPAP are the primary methods to open areas of microatelectasis, the same effect can be achieved at times by use of mechanical ventilation with larger tidal volumes than the patient can generate spontaneously. To improve oxygenation in some animal models of lung injury (e.g., near-drowning in fresh water), it is necessary to apply both mechanical ventilation and PEEP. The potential role of large tidal volumes causing or enhancing lung injury is discussed later (see Acute Respiratory Failure Occurring With Adult Respiratory Distress Syndrome and Decisions in Ventilatory Support).

Definitive Therapy

Efforts directed at improving oxygenation are only supportive and temporizing. A permanent improvement in oxygenation requires definitive therapy for the underlying disease. If no definitive therapy is available, the normal healing or repair process must be given time to occur. In either case it is important to recognize which forms of treatment are merely supportive and which represent specific therapy directed at the cause of the oxygenation abnormality.

MEASURES TO CORRECT RESPIRATORY ACIDOSIS

The urgency for correction of respiratory acidosis and the type of therapy required depend on several factors, including the degree of acidosis, the time over which the acidosis has developed, and the specific cause of the respiratory acidosis. Each of these factors affects the risk-benefit relationship of the various types of treatment. Acidosis does not have to be totally corrected. Often partial correction suffices to remove the life-threatening aspects of respiratory acidosis, including impaired tissue functioning, impairment of enzyme systems, and presence or threat of severe cardiac arrhythmias.

Pharmacologic Compensation

Administration of bicarbonate partially corrects respiratory acidosis. If acidosis is severe and an acute threat to life, bicarbonate administration can provide rapid improvement and has the additional benefit of allowing other medications (such as bronchodilators) to act in a more optimal pH range. The major drawback of bicarbonate administration is the alkalosis and sodium overload that may follow correction of the underlying cause of the respiratory acidosis. Therefore bicarbonate administration is generally reserved for severe abnormalities, and in such cases relatively small amounts are given as a temporizing measure.

Attempts at pharmacologic stimulation of respiration generally are not useful.

Mechanical Ventilation

Mechanical ventilation usually corrects respiratory acidosis rapidly. Again the risk-benefit relationship must be carefully considered (see later discussion).

Treatment of the Underlying Disease

Treatment of the process that led to respiratory acidosis is obviously the most physiologic way to correct this abnormality. Once again, as with correction of oxygenation, administration of bicarbonate and mechanical ventilation are only temporizing supportive measures. Therapy aimed at correction of the underlying disease process may be the only treatment required to adequately improve respiratory acidosis. This is particularly true in COPD and asthma patients in whom aggressive administration of bronchodilators and help with secretion removal can result in sufficient improvement in both airflow and re-

spiratory acidosis within a few hours. In a patient with a sedative overdose, metabolism of the medication (or removal with dialysis when appropriate) requires more time, and correction of the acidosis with mechanical ventilation may be a more prudent approach.

DECISION TO USE MECHANICAL VENTILATION

Whether mechanical ventilation is indicated is a major management decision in patients with ARF. Although there are some guidelines to follow, generally the decision is based on the specific clinical situation. The general indications for mechanical ventilation are (1) to improve respiratory acidosis, (2) to reduce excessive work of breathing, and (3) to improve hypoxemia.

One primary goal is improvement of respiratory acidosis, but not all patients with respiratory acidosis require mechanical ventilation. There is no particular Pco_2 or pH value that warrants ventilation in all cases of respiratory acidosis. The decision to ventilate is based on an evaluation of anticipated benefits and possible risks. This evaluation, in turn, depends on the underlying disease causing the respiratory acidosis and the associated dangers of mechanical ventilation in the particular patient. For example, mechanical ventilation should be used readily for a patient with CNS depression caused by sedative overdose, since the benefits are substantial, the ventilation time is relatively short (until the sedative can be metabolized), and there are relatively few complications of intubation and mechanical ventilation in such a patient. On the other hand, mechanical ventilation should be reserved for the minority of COPD patients with ARF, since endotracheal intubation and mechanical ventilation are associated with higher risks in patients with COPD.

Even in the absence of respiratory acidosis, mechanical ventilation may be useful in the patient with very high work of breathing and high minute ventilation, particularly if a patient has not responded to other therapy and may continue breathing with a high minute ventilation for some time. There is no easy clinical way to measure work of breathing other than subjective clinical assessment.

In the patient with rapid, shallow breathing, hypoxemia may respond to increasing the tidal volume with mechanical ventilation. This improvement in hypoxemia is presumably caused by reopening atelectatic areas of lung and either reducing shunt or improving lung lesions with low $\dot{V}/\dot{Q}$.

ESTABLISHMENT OF AN ARTIFICIAL AIRWAY

One of the important decisions in the management of ARF is to determine whether an artificial airway is necessary. The indications for placing an artificial airway include (1) to protect the airway (especially from massive aspiration of gastric contents), (2) to close the system for delivery of an increased FIO_2, (3) to facilitate mechanical ventilation, and (4) to aid in control of secretions. It is rare that a patient requires establishment of an airway for secretion control alone. When suctioning is carried out through an artificial airway, only the trachea or one mainstem bronchus is usually accessible. Therefore the patient must be able to bring secretions up into the central airways, but intubation impairs cough and makes it difficult to clear secretions from the lower airways. Often, clearance can be facilitated by stimulation of cough during suctioning.

When an indication for an artificial airway exists, an endotracheal tube is placed. Placement of the tube should be done under the most controlled circumstances and by the most experienced person available. Whether an oral or a nasal tube is placed is largely a matter of individual preference, although one of the disadvantages of the nasotracheal tube is the increased risk of blocking drainage from paranasal sinuses and precipitating sinusitis. In fact, sinusitis should be considered as a possible source of infection in any patient with an endotracheal tube and fever; higher rates of sinusitis are associated with nasotracheal as compared with orotracheal tubes. Once the tube has been placed, physical examination should be performed to check for possible esophageal placement or placement in the right mainstem bronchus. Measurement of the level of exhaled carbon dioxide can help differentiate tracheal from esophageal intubation. Proper tube placement should be confirmed by a chest roentgenogram.

Currently available endotracheal tubes have low-pressure, high-volume cuffs, which have reduced the rate of complication at the cuff site. However, these cuffs do not prevent aspiration of small amounts of secretions or fluid. On the other hand, they should allow protection against massive aspiration of gastric contents, at least until the patient can be appropriately positioned so that aspiration of a large amount of material does not occur.

Whether a tracheostomy should be performed rather than continuing use of the endotracheal tube is decided by weighing the risks and benefits of each type of airway in the specific clinical situation. The cuff complications of both endotracheal and tracheotomy tubes are similar. The use of endotracheal tubes is associated with laryngeal and upper airway complications, including sinusitis. Tracheostomy has a low but definite mortality and is associated with late development of tracheal stenosis at the tracheostomy stoma site. Use of modern materials and improved respiratory therapy techniques to reduce the movement of the endotracheal tube in the larynx have reduced laryngeal complications. Currently it is common practice to leave an endotracheal tube in place for several weeks. The exact period of intubation associated with a rising incidence of laryngeal complications is not known. However, as a general guide, if a tracheal tube is to be in place for much longer than a month, tracheostomy is preferable. If this decision can be made early in the course of illness, tracheostomy should be performed as soon as possible. If it is believed that a patient can have extubation within 1 month, the endotracheal tube can be left in place and this decision reassessed on a weekly basis or as indicated.

MANAGEMENT OF SPECIFIC ACUTE RESPIRATORY FAILURE SYNDROMES

The principles of management remain the same for any ARF patient, regardless of the underlying cause. However, the specific application of these principles differs considerably depending on the cause.

Chronic Obstructive Pulmonary Disease With Acute Respiratory Failure

Most patients with COPD and ARF require only a small increase in supplemental oxygen to correct the oxygenation abnormality. This increase can be achieved by initially administering 1 to 2 L/min of oxygen by nasal prongs and then adjusting the flow rate according to the resulting arterial blood gas values. An alternative method of administration is a Venturi mask at 24% to 28%. In some patients with COPD, oxygen administration can be associated with worsening hypoventilation and respiratory acidosis. Previously this association was thought to result from removal of the hypoxic drive to breathe in patients with already diminished carbon dioxide ventilatory drive. Recent studies suggest that increased $PaCO_2$ related to the administration of oxygen results from changes in $\dot{V}/\dot{Q}$ with increased dead space ventilation.

Whatever the mechanism, an increased PaO_2 (usually greater than that necessary to achieve adequate oxygen saturation) can be associated with worsening respiratory acidosis. Three aspects of this phenomenon must be emphasized. (1) It occurs only in a minority of COPD patients with ARF. (2) The primary objective in any ARF patient is still to oxygenate the arterial blood adequately; the potential of increasing $PaCO_2$ does not justify allowing a patient to remain significantly hypoxemic. (3) A significant improvement in oxygenation (since the PaO_2 is usually in the steep portion of the oxygen-hemoglobin dissociation curve) can be achieved without a clinically important reduction in pH in nearly all patients by careful administration of oxygen and close monitoring, together with other forms of therapy aimed at the precipitating causes of ARF.

Some patients with COPD require a greater increase in FIO_2 than can be achieved with 2 L/min of nasal oxygen. In these patients there is usually an element of increased shunt, a result, for example, of pneumonia or congestive heart failure as the precipitating cause of respiratory failure.

Many COPD patients with ARF have significant respiratory acidosis. Experience with management of these patients has shown improved results if unnecessary application of mechanical ventilation is avoided and other means of improvement in acidosis are used. Coughing is extremely important for secretion removal in COPD patients with ARF. Effective mechanical ventilation requires placement of an endotracheal tube, which results in impairment of cough by preventing glottic closure. Also, mechanical ventilation often impairs mobi-

lization of the patient. Although this impairment can be avoided with a great deal of effort, it is often an undesired side effect.

Other risks of endotracheal intubation and mechanical ventilation are higher in the patient with COPD than in other patients with ARF. The COPD patient has increased lung compliance, which results in an increased risk of reduced cardiac output and barotrauma. In addition, the risk of infection in these patients is high. Therefore, unnecessary mechanical ventilation should be avoided.

When does mechanical ventilation become necessary in the COPD patient with ARF? This question can be answered in the negative sense as follows. If a patient is awake, can cough, and can cooperate with therapy (by taking inhaled bronchodilators and cooperating with measures to remove secretions), it is rarely necessary to use mechanical ventilation. Patients who meet these criteria should be given a trial of aggressive therapy before proceeding to mechanical ventilation. In these patients mechanical ventilation should be employed only if a patient is not improving or is clearly tiring. On the other hand, if a patient initially is obtunded and difficult to arouse, intubation and mechanical ventilation should be carried out even before knowing the degree of acidosis. Thus the decision to ventilate the lungs in a COPD patient is primarily based on clinical findings. Mental status is of prime importance. In most medical centers, less than 10% of COPD patients with ARF require mechanical ventilation.

Use of noninvasive methods of mechanical ventilation, which are applied via nasal or full-face mask, recently has been reported to be feasible in COPD patients with ARF and to reduce the need for endotracheal intubation. Patients receiving ventilatory support by mask should be awake, alert, and able to cooperate with treatment and should be managed in an intensive care unit or intermediate care unit allowing close observation. Noninvasive ventilation should be considered when a relatively short period of mechanical ventilation is anticipated. Patients with severe hypoxemia are not good candidates for noninvasive ventilation.

How should respiratory acidosis be treated in COPD patients? Therapy of respiratory acidosis is essentially the same as treatment of the underlying chronic disease. Worsening hypoventilation is usually associated with worsening airflow; potentially reversible elements of airflow obstruction are bronchospasm and increased secretions. Therefore treatment should be aimed at improving airflow with bronchodilators and aiding secretion removal. Aggressive bronchodilator therapy is indicated for potential improvement in airflow obstruction, even when a patient has not been previously shown to respond to bronchodilators in an outpatient setting. In most patients simultaneous treatment with inhaled β-adrenergic and/or anticholinergic agents and intravenous or oral corticosteroids is warranted. β-adrenergic agents should be given by inhalation, using metered dose inhalers (MDIs) or a nebulized solution. The bronchodilator effect of ipratropium bromide, an anticholinergic agent available by MDI or nebulized solution, is equivalent to and may even exceed that of β-adrenergic agents in patients with COPD. Although most studies in stable outpatients have failed to show added benefit if either agent is administered after a maximal dose of the other, a trial of administering both agents may be warranted in ARF.

In a study of patients receiving β-adrenergic agents and intravenous corticosteroids, addition of intravenous aminophylline had no beneficial effect on pulmonary function when compared with placebo. However, theophylline may have other beneficial effects including enhancement of recovery from respiratory muscle fatigue and stimulation of ventilatory drive; the clinical importance of these effects has not been established; therefore the current role of theophylline administration in patients with COPD and an acute exacerbation is unclear. If theophylline is given, it is usually first administered in the form of intravenous aminophylline with an intravenous loading dose, depending on whether the patient has been receiving long-term theophylline therapy. If the history indicates compliance with a reasonable outpatient theophylline regimen, the maintenance dose should be continued until therapy can be guided by measurement of the serum theophylline level. Since theophylline is well absorbed from the gastrointestinal tract, a change to an oral form can be carried out relatively early in the hospital course, after initial clinical improvement has occurred.

A well-controlled study of COPD patients with ARF caused by exacerbation attributable to acute bronchitis demonstrated significant improvement in airflow when corticosteroids were administered during the first 3 days of therapy. Corticosteroids were administered as methylprednisolone sodium succinate, 0.5 mg/kg body weight every 6 hours.

Promotion of secretion removal should be encouraged. Patients should be stimulated to cough, especially after inhalation of a bronchodilator. A trial of chest percussion and postural drainage may be warranted, with evaluation of results compared with those with cough alone. Hypoxemia may worsen in the lateral postural drainage positions, and a temporary further increase in FIO$_2$ may be required to counteract this change.

A randomized, controlled trial of antibiotic administration during an acute exacerbation in patients with COPD resulted in a slight but statistically significant improvement in the rate of successful outcomes in patients who received treatment with antibiotics. Antibiotic use was not associated with increased side effects when compared with placebo. Although the clinical importance of these results could be debated, it seems prudent to err on the side of using antibiotics in a patient whose exacerbation is severe enough to precipitate ARF. In the absence of evidence for a specific bacterial origin, any antibiotic that is effective against *Streptococcus pneumoniae* and *Haemophilus influenzae* is appropriate (Chapter 317).

Proper treatment of the underlying disease requires another diagnosis in addition to COPD—that of the cause precipitating ARF. Although the treatment described remains the same for the other aspects of COPD, specific therapy varies according to whether the acute illness is viral bronchitis, bacterial pneumonia, pulmonary embolism, congestive heart failure, or another condition.

Respiratory muscle fatigue may contribute significantly to the development of ARF. Clinical findings suggesting respiratory muscle fatigue include rapid, shallow respirations; paradoxical abdominal breathing; and respiratory alternans. The latter two are relatively specific for respiratory muscle fatigue. Paradoxical abdominal breathing is diagnosed by observing the abdomen move inward as the chest moves outward. Usually the abdomen and chest wall move out together during inspiration. Respiratory alternans is a more unusual finding. It consists of periods during which inspiratory muscle activity consists entirely of use of the chest wall muscles, alternating with periods of diaphragmatic breathing. At present, treatment of inspiratory muscle fatigue remains unclear; there is evidence that theophylline facilitates recovery, but the clinical importance of this observation is not yet known. It appears that rest is important in allowing recovery of the fatigued respiratory muscles; therefore mechanical ventilation allowing respiratory muscle rest may assume increasing importance in selected patients with evidence of recent onset of respiratory muscle fatigue as a major component of ARF.

Acute Respiratory Failure Occurring With Acute Respiratory Distress Syndrome

ARDS usually occurs in clinical situations involving severe underlying illness or injury and is associated with a variety of causes. The exact mechanism is not known but is generally believed to represent acute lung injury, either as a direct insult (e.g., from aspiration of gastric contents) or, more commonly, indirectly through activation of humoral or cellular mediators (such as with sepsis and severe multiple trauma). Treatment other than specific therapy aimed at the underlying causes is supportive.

Correction of the oxygenation abnormality in the ARDS patient requires a high FIO$_2$. The initial FIO$_2$ should be high to ensure adequate oxygenation and then should be adjusted downward as tolerated, with monitoring of blood gas values. PEEP and CPAP are employed either to provide an adequate PaO$_2$, if this has not already been achieved, or to lower the FIO$_2$ to reduce the risk of oxygen toxicity. Depending on the initial blood gas values and the initial FIO$_2$, the clinician must decide on a reasonable goal, but, at least, reducing the FIO$_2$ to 0.7 and preferably to 0.5 seems prudent, especially if this can be achieved with moderate (5 to 15 cm H$_2$O) levels of PEEP. The FIO$_2$ is reduced further as the PaO$_2$ improves, until the FIO$_2$ is down to 0.4 or 0.5. Then the PEEP can be progressively decreased by decrements of 5 cm H$_2$O.

Acute respiratory distress syndrome is rarely associated with respiratory acidosis. However, this does not mean that carbon dioxide removal is normal in these patients. Minute ventilation ($\dot{V}_E$) usually

is very high, producing a normal or often somewhat reduced PaCO$_2$. Mechanical ventilation may be indicated to reduce the work of breathing and to help improve oxygenation. Excessive tidal volumes and minute ventilations may be associated with auto-PEEP or intrinsic PEEP (and accompanying reductions in cardiac output) and the possible risk of creating or enhancing lung injury. Barotrauma with lung rupture and pneumothorax can also occur. To minimize these risks, limiting the size of the mechanically delivered tidal volume and the associated plateau (inflation hold) pressure has been recommended, even when this results in respiratory acidosis (so-called permissive hypercapnia). Whether this ventilatory support approach is superior to "conventional" or traditional approaches has not yet been proven. Several controlled trials comparing these two approaches are currently under way in North America, Europe, and South America.

Treatment of the underlying disease is mainly supportive. The one major exception is the treatment of sepsis. If sepsis is a likely possibility, appropriate cultures should be obtained and a thorough search for the source of possible infection should be made. Broad-spectrum antibiotics should be given until culture results are available. It is especially important to search for infections that may require surgical drainage, such as intraabdominal abscesses.

Infection represents the most important complication in the ARDS patient because it frequently leads to a clinical sepsis syndrome with hypotension and multiple organ failure and is associated with a very high mortality. In managing these patients, careful infection control measures, including compulsive hand washing between patient contacts, are mandatory.

Acute Respiratory Failure Without Lung Disease

Two categories of patients with ARF but no pulmonary abnormalities are those with suppressed central drive (most common are patients who have taken an overdose of sedative or tranquilizing drugs) and those with neuromuscular abnormalities leading to respiratory failure. Initial management of an overdose patient includes gastric lavage to remove any drug still in the stomach. If a patient is not awake, the airway should be protected during gastric lavage by endotracheal intubation. The decision to institute mechanical ventilation is based on both the patient's mental status and the presence of respiratory acidosis. If a patient is obtunded and respiratory acidosis is present, mechanical ventilation should be used until he or she is consistently awake. Aspiration of oropharyngeal or gastric contents is relatively common in the obtunded overdose patient. Antibiotic treatment of aspiration pneumonia is indicated only if evidence of a bacterial pneumonia develops, including purulent sputum with pathogenic organisms seen on Gram's stain. Prophylactic corticosteroids or prophylactic antibiotics are not warranted.

Patients with progressive neuromuscular disease should be followed up with serial measurements of vital capacity. As a general rule, ventilatory support should be considered when the vital capacity falls below 15 ml/kg body weight. Mechanical ventilatory support should be continued until muscle strength and spontaneous vital capacity improve and are adequate to sustain spontaneous ventilation without muscle fatigue.

DECISIONS IN VENTILATORY SUPPORT

Once it has been decided that mechanical ventilation is warranted, several other decisions must be made: the type of ventilator, the FIO$_2$, the mode of ventilation, the tidal volume and respiratory frequency, whether to use PEEP or CPAP, and what kind of monitoring should be performed. The FIO$_2$ should be the lowest necessary to achieve adequate arterial oxygenation; this level must be decided for each patient. It is best initially to use a high FIO$_2$ and then rapidly decrease it to the lowest level necessary as judged by arterial blood gas studies.

The modes of ventilation include controlled mechanical ventilation (CMV), assisted mechanical ventilation (AMV, also called *assist/control mode*), intermittent mandatory ventilation (IMV), pressure support ventilation (PSV), and pressure-controlled ventilation (PCV) with or without inverse ratio ventilation (IRV). With CMV the respiratory rate is set and the patient cannot adjust it by breathing spontaneously or by triggering additional breaths from the ventilator. Consequently the patient receiving controlled ventilation usually has to be sedated, given a muscle-paralyzing agent, or have ventilation with a frequency sufficiently high that respiratory alkalosis is produced. Both muscle paralysis and respiratory alkalosis have significant drawbacks; therefore CMV should be limited to specific clinical indications.

Most patients can be ventilated with either AMV or IMV. With AMV the ventilator rate is set slightly below the patient's intrinsic respiratory rate, and the patient is able to trigger some or all of the ventilator breaths. With IMV some breaths are given by the ventilator at a predetermined rate, and the patient is allowed to breathe spontaneously from a pressurized high-airflow circuit to meet the rest of the ventilatory requirements.

There is considerable debate regarding the relative advantages and disadvantages of AMV versus IMV. It is clear that the majority of patients requiring mechanical ventilation can be given effective ventilation by either ventilatory mode. Perhaps it is more important to be aware of specific clinical situations in which one of these modes may have particular advantages over the other. Intermittent mandatory ventilation can be useful in a patient who is "fighting the ventilator" while receiving CMV or AMV and in whom other causes for this so-called fighting (e.g., inadequate oxygenation, acidosis, or pain) have been ruled out. A change to IMV sometimes allows the patient to adjust to mechanical ventilation in a more comfortable fashion; each patient should be evaluated individually. In a patient with severe airflow obstruction progressive air trapping and auto-PEEP (positive alveolar pressure throughout exhalation) can develop during AMV. This phenomenon can be associated with significant reductions in cardiac output as positive alveolar pressure is transmitted to the pleural space and to the great veins, thus impeding venous return. Changing to IMV might allow dissipation of the positive alveolar pressure and air trapping during the periods of spontaneous breathing. Intermittent mandatory ventilation has a theoretical advantage in patients with marginal cardiac output because mean alveolar pressure tends to be lower, since some of the breaths are spontaneous; this lower pressure reduces the risk of impaired cardiac output. With the AMV mode, on the other hand, in the unstable critically ill patient with an already high minute ventilation requirement, further increased ventilatory demand could be met relatively easily by triggering the machine at a more rapid rate. With IMV in this situation the patient may not be able to meet this increased ventilatory demand by increasing spontaneous ventilation. In patients with high ventilatory demands the potential advantages of IMV may no longer exist if a high mandatory rate on IMV is used. Assisted mechanical ventilation is associated with a lower work of breathing than IMV (because of the component of spontaneous breathing with IMV). Some patients receiving AMV continue to actively inspire after they initiate the ventilator breath and continue to perform inspiratory muscle work. Thus the advantage of reducing work of breathing is not as great as it might seem. This phenomenon is particularly likely to occur if the inspiratory flow is relatively slow and unable to meet the patient's desired demands for inspiratory flow. There are no data to confirm that one mode has a clear advantage over the other in enhancing the process of weaning from mechanical ventilation.

Pressure support ventilation augments the patient's spontaneous breathing effort. As the patient triggers each breath, the airway pressure increases rapidly to the desired pressure setting and remains there until the flow rate decreases to a predetermined minimal flow or percentage of the peak flow, at which time the inspiratory flow of gas from the ventilator ceases. Thus part of the work of each breath is carried out by the patient and part by the ventilator. The amount of work contributed by the ventilator is determined by the set pressure and resulting tidal volume. Pressure support ventilation mainly has been recommended for weaning but can also be employed as a primary ventilatory mode. The patient has some control over the inspiratory pressure waveform, which appears to be associated with an improvement in patient comfort over other ventilatory modes in some patients. Use of PSV requires that a patient's ventilatory drive be intact.

Pressure-controlled ventilation involves setting a constant peak delivered pressure rather than a constant tidal volume, as in volume-controlled ventilation. The fundamental difference between these two approaches is demonstrable when the patient's compliance changes. An increase in compliance while receiving volume-controlled venti-

lation results in increased peak airway pressures, whereas a reduction in tidal volume would occur in the patient receiving PCV. The exact role for PCV is not yet clear. It is currently being used in patients with diffuse acute lung injury (ARDS), especially when compliance is especially abnormal. One advantage of PCV may be higher initial flow rates in delivery of a breath; this may result in lessening of the sensation of dyspnea in some patients.

Inverse ratio ventilation consists of lengthening the inspiratory time (with a resultant shorter expiratory time if respiratory rate is constant). It is usually applied in connection with the PCV mode. Anecdotal reports of improved oxygenation with lengthening inspiratory time have been reported. Several studies have suggested that reports of improved oxygenation with IRV may largely (although not entirely) be due to creation of auto-PEEP. Auto-PEEP in this regard has no advantage over set PEEP and may have some disadvantages, including more unequal distribution in the lungs. No controlled trials in patients have demonstrated any definite advantage of PCV with IRV over "conventional" ventilation. A current recommended approach in patients with ARDS is to first try ventilating with relatively low tidal volumes and modest levels of PEEP. If oxygenation is still inadequate (or the required F_IO_2 is considered to be excessive), a trial of lengthening the inspiratory time can be carried out, stopping when auto-PEEP (greater than set PEEP) develops. Inverse ratio ventilation carries the dangers of hemodynamic compromise and barotrauma (presumably associated with auto-PEEP and hyperinflation), and its application must be carefully monitored.

The tidal volume in a volume-controlled ventilatory mode and respiratory rate should be set so that the minute ventilation (their product) results in a normal pH (unless there are specific reasons for a different pH, for example, a temporary respiratory alkalosis in management of cerebral edema or if the technique of permissive hypercapnia is being employed). The tidal volume should be large enough to prevent progressive microatelectasis; however, this usually occurs only at low tidal volumes, less than 5 ml/kg body weight.

A tidal volume in the range of 6 to 10 ml/kg body weight is recommended initially. High tidal volumes have been associated with increased risk of pneumothorax and, extrapolating from animal model studies, may be associated with increased lung injury. As discussed earlier (see Acute Respiratory Failure Occurring With Adult Respiratory Distress Syndrome), the efficacy of limiting tidal volume and/or plateau pressure is under current investigation.

Rapid inspiratory flow rates shorten the inspiratory time and allow a longer exhalation time for any given respiratory rate in patients with chronic airflow obstruction. This reduces air trapping and is associated with improved oxygenation and a decrease in the dead space–to–tidal volume ratio (V_D/V_T). Therefore it is recommended that high inspiratory flow rates be used in COPD patients and that the inspiratory flow rate be adjusted on the basis of comfort for patients without COPD.

Positive end-expiratory pressure (with AMV or CMV) or CPAP (with IMV) should be applied if specific needs to improve oxygenation are present in patients with acute diffuse alveolar disease. Some investigators feel that a certain amount of PEEP or CPAP is "physiologic" in that lung volume and arterial blood gas measurements made on a low level of PEEP are similar to those made after extubation and slightly greater than measurements made while a patient is breathing without PEEP or CPAP with the endotracheal tube still in place. However, these differences are small and of doubtful clinical importance in most patients. It is not recommended that PEEP or CPAP be routinely applied to all patients. For example, PEEP or CPAP should not be applied in patients with possible increased intracranial pressure or in patients with increased risk for lung rupture, unless specific indications outweigh these risks.

It should be determined what monitoring is necessary for the patient receiving ventilatory support (see Chapters 44 and 49). In addition to general monitoring considerations, the patient receiving mechanical ventilation should have regular monitoring of the exhaled tidal volume, minute ventilation, peak and plateau (inflation hold) pressures, and the volume and pressure in the tracheal tube cuff required to occlude the airway. Occasional measurements of carbon dioxide production and dead space (V_D/V_T) can be useful, particularly in patients requiring prolonged ventilation with high minute ventilation requirements.

REMOVAL FROM MECHANICAL VENTILATION AND WEANING

In removing ventilatory support, cessation of mechanical ventilation should be considered as a separate step from removal of the endotracheal tube. Some patients are able to breathe spontaneously with adequate maintenance of arterial blood gas levels but continue to require endotracheal intubation for airway protection.

In most patients the term *weaning from mechanical ventilation* is applied incorrectly. Weaning implies gradual removal from mechanical ventilation. Most patients receiving ventilatory support can be readily removed from mechanical ventilation once their underlying problem has been corrected. In these patients a gradual process is not necessary. In determining which patients can be removed from mechanical ventilation, two separate questions should be asked. First, can the patient maintain adequate arterial oxygenation on the FIO_2 that can be achieved by nasal prongs or face-mask oxygen delivery? Second, can the patient maintain adequate ventilation spontaneously? A decision regarding the first question is made by interpretation of the PaO_2 in relation to the FIO_2. If the PaO_2 is adequate on an FIO_2 of 0.4, adequate oxygenation should be accomplished with an FIO_2 readily achievable after removal of the endotracheal tube. The second question is approached by measuring so-called ventilatory parameters during spontaneous breathing. These parameters should be used only as a guide to determining removal from mechanical ventilation because some patients, when breathing spontaneously in their chronic outpatient state, never meet the recommended criteria for removal from mechanical ventilation. However, if the criteria of ventilatory parameters *are* met and the patient's condition is otherwise stable, successful removal from mechanical ventilation can be virtually ensured.

Usual variables measured and guidelines for successful discontinuation of mechanical support include tidal volume (VT) greater than 5 ml/kg body weight, vital capacity (VC) greater than 10 ml/kg body weight, inspiratory force less than (more negative than) -30 cm H_2O, and minute ventilation ($\dot{V}E$) less than 10 L/min. Other measurements, including VD/VT, have been suggested but are used less frequently and are generally not necessary. Most of these criteria have not been subjected to critical study in a controlled trial. Respiratory rate (tachypnea) is a sensitive indicator of respiratory dysfunction. Recently an index of rapid shallow breathing, the frequency/tidal volume ratio (f/VT) was studied as a predictor of successful weaning in patients receiving mechanical ventilation. Using an f/VT threshold of 105 breaths/min per liter resulted in positive and negative predictive values for successful weaning of 0.78 and 0.95, respectively. Established criteria include $\dot{V}E$ less than 10 L/min per minute and the ability to double this minute ventilation value with a maximum voluntary ventilation (MVV) maneuver. All patients who met these criteria were able to be successfully removed from mechanical ventilation and have subsequent extubation. Of patients who did not meet these criteria, some had successful removal from mechanical ventilation, and others had to be returned to ventilatory support. Of those who did not meet the criteria but could have successful removal, several observations were helpful. Most of these patients had borderline values for the previously mentioned criteria. However, they had a greater mean inspiratory force than the patients who had to be returned to mechanical ventilation, with an absolute cut-off between the two groups of -24 cm H_2O. Once the endotracheal tube was removed, many of these patients who previously could not double their $\dot{V}E$ value with an MVV maneuver could now double or even triple this value. Thus it is apparent that in some of these measurements the endotracheal tube can add to airflow resistance, and these values might be improved once the tube has been removed. Tube sizes with an internal diameter less than 7.5 mm are particularly associated with increased resistance to airflow.

The resting minute ventilation must be interpreted in view of the patient's body size, muscle mass, and physical state before the onset of ARF. For example, attempts at stopping mechanical ventilation might not be warranted in a small elderly woman with COPD and possible muscle fatigue until the minute ventilation is less than 10 L/min, but a young, relatively large man in good health before the onset of ARDS might be removed from mechanical ventilation when the minute ventilation drops to 15 L/min. Once a patient is considered to be a candidate for removal from a ventilator, a trial of spontaneous breathing through a T piece usually is warranted. This trial should be relatively short (approximately 30 minutes), since ventilation will most likely be easier once the tube is removed. At the end of 30 minutes, arterial blood gas measurements are obtained. If these values are judged to be adequate, mechanical ventilation can be discontinued and a decision made regarding removal of the endotracheal tube.

In a patient who cannot be readily removed from the ventilator, a program of weaning must be started. The major methods of gradual withdrawal are (1) IMV with a progressively lowered mandatory rate until the patient is breathing entirely spontaneously, (2) PSV with a progressively lowered pressure until only the pressure required to overcome airway resistance of the endotracheal tube is reached, or (3) short T-piece trials that are progressively lengthened until the patient essentially is breathing spontaneously. Data regarding the superiority of any given method over another are conflicting.

Medical stability, appropriate nutritional status, and appropriate psychological preparation are extremely important when removing patients from mechanical ventilation. These aspects are probably more important than the specific method of weaning.

OTHER ASPECTS OF MANAGEMENT

If it is anticipated that the period of ARF might be prolonged, early attention should be directed at the nutritional state of the patient. Critical studies have not yet demonstrated whether early feeding favorably changes outcome or at what point in the course of ARF feeding should be started to produce the best outcome. However, most clinicians suspect that early administration of adequate nutritional support is important, especially in a catabolic patient.

The patient with ARF should not be limited to a supine position in bed, if at all possible. Moving from the supine to the sitting position improves lung volume. Moving to various positions is important in maintaining expansion of all areas of the lung and in enhancing secretion removal. In addition, sitting in a chair or walking helps maintain musculoskeletal function.

Attention to the psychological aspects of the patient with ARF is also important. These patients are often depressed. A patient with chronic underlying lung disease may be exhausted at hospital admission and irritable because of impaired sleep, in addition to any hypoxemia that might be present. Psychosocial support can be critical in influencing outcome.

All these aspects of care are even more important if a patient requires mechanical ventilation. Institution of mechanical ventilation often results in a patient being kept in bed rather than getting up to walk or sit in a chair, prevents feeding by mouth, and impairs communication. Thus these patients require more effort from the health care team.

BIBLIOGRAPHY

Bernard GR, Artigas A, Brigham KL, et al: The American-European Consensus Conference on ARDS: definitions, mechanisms, relevant outcomes, and clinical trial coordination, *Am J Respir Crit Care Med* 149:818, 1994.

Curtis JR, Hudson LD: Emergent assessment and management of acute respiratory failure on COPD, *Clin Chest Med* 15:481, 1994.

Fulkerson WJ, MacIntyre N, Stamler J, Crapo JD: Pathogenesis and treatment of the adult respiratory distress syndrome, *Arch Intern Med* 156:29, 1996.

Green KE, Peters JI: Pathophysiology of acute respiratory failure, *Clin Chest Med* 15:1, 1994.

Kollef MH, Schuster DP: Medical progress: the acute respiratory distress syndrome, *N Engl J Med* 332:27, 1995.

Marinelli WA, Ingbar DH: Diagnosis and management of acute lung injury, *Clin Chest Med* 15:517, 1994.

Marini JJ: Evolving concepts in the ventilatory management of adult respiratory distress syndrome, *Clin Chest Med* 17:555, 1996.

Meyer TJ, Hill NS: Noninvasive positive pressure ventilation to treat respiratory failure, *Ann Intern Med* 120:760, 1994.

Parsons PE: Respiratory failure as a result of drugs, overdoses, and poisonings, *Clin Chest Med* 15:93, 1994.

Schmidt GA, Hall JB: Acute on chronic respiratory failure: assessment and management of patients with COPD in the emergent setting, *JAMA* 261:3444, 1989.

Tobin MJ: Mechanical ventilation, *N Engl J Med* 330:1056, 1994.

47 Multiple Organ Dysfunction in the Context of ARDS

Jean E. Rinaldo and Melissa Clark

RELEVANT PHYSIOLOGY AND PATHOPHYSIOLOGY

The adult respiratory distress syndrome (ARDS) is now believed to be a multisystem disorder. Manifestations in the lung include abnormal microvascular and epithelial permeability, resulting in lung edema, and abnormal regulation of ventilation-perfusion matching, resulting in hypoxemia. Concurrent extrapulmonary abnormalities that accompanied pulmonary dysfunction during ARDS are now well recognized. Extrapulmonary components of ARDS include but are not limited to hepatic dysfunction, renal dysfunction, altered mental status, coagulopathies, gastrointestinal bleeding and dysmotility, and a propensity to superinfection. Infection and evidence of extrapulmonary multisystem organ failure (MSOF) have emerged as the most important predictors of mortality in ARDS patients. Nomenclature has changed accordingly. Sepsis syndrome, sepsis, multiple organ dysfunction syndrome (MODS), systemic inflammatory response syndrome (SIRS), and multisystem organ failure (MSOF) have become common terms to denote the multisystem response. *ARDS* or *ALI* (acute lung injury) are the terms most commonly used to refer specifically to the pulmonary components.

The "mechanisms" of MODS are enormously complex and poorly understood. One mechanism—that MODS is a pansystemic response linked to the activation of cytokine cascades—underlies most current clinical investigation. Cytokines are signaling peptides, which act as "hormones" of inflammation. The cytokines are generally protein molecules that are not stored in cells but rather are rapidly upregulated at the level of gene transcription in response to infection. These peptides are synthesized and released by many cells but especially by cells that are differentiated as specialists in orchestrating inflammation (i.e., macrophages and lymphocytes). The peptides bind with high specificity to cell surface receptors on many effector target cells. Binding to receptors induces a functional change in the target cells through a signal response coupling mechanism involving an array of second messenger systems such as intracellular calcium, cyclic nucleotides, and phospholipases. Examples of the myriad number of functional changes include leukocyte priming and activation; activation of transcription factors such as nuclear factor kappa B, which stimulate transcription of other cytokines (hence cytokine cascades or networks); production of prostaglandins that alter regional blood flow; synthesis of chemotactic factors that call in other inflammatory cells; and induction of cell division or of programmed cell death (apoptosis). *Cascade* means that there is sequential elaboration of cytokines: Some are "immediate" and evanescent, such as tumor necrosis factor (TNF), whereas others appear later and last longer, such as interleukin 6 (IL-6). The functional changes signaled by cytokines can be autocrine (the cell responds to its own cytokine product), paracrine (the cytokine acts locally to signal-modulated local inflammatory response in neighboring cells), or endocrine, meaning the cytokines are turned loose into the bloodstream and induce signaled changes in distant target cells that possess the requisite surface receptors.

How might activation of cytokine cascades cause multisystem end organ injury? There are likely to be three broad categories of mechanisms: (1) effects on blood vessels, which alter regional blood flow, leading to widespread regional hypoperfusion; (2) direct cytotoxicity to parenchymal cells; or (3) disruption of extracellular matrix by proteases, leading to permeability changes or cellular detachment. Vasoocclusive effects arise as a result of perturbations in vasomotor responsiveness or luminal plugging by leukocyte and platelet aggregates. Important vasoocclusive mediators that have been implicated include thromboxane, a cyclooxygenase metabolite of arachidonic acid released by platelets, and endothelin, a peptide released by endothelial cells. Synthesis of vasodilating mediator substances such as prostacyclin or PGE_2 may be inhibited, producing a net vasoconstrictor effect. Vasoocclusive mechanisms commonly involved cytokine-signaled changes in lipid mediator synthesis. This mechanism appears to result in sepsis-induced acute renal failure. Cell injury may result from signaled apoptosis or from accidental assault on bystander targets by proteases and free radicals from activated neutrophils; the second mechanism can also cleave cell surface proteins and degrade extracellular matrix components.

Cytokines serve important homeostatic host defense roles when lipopolysaccharide (LPS) is present in a local inflammatory milieu, but circulating bacterial LPS signals a cascade of unopposed physiologic reactions that threaten the host. In experimental studies, LPS causes the release of cytokines into the circulation and causes a constellation of symptoms that mimic the sepsis syndrome: fever or hypothermia, leukocytosis or leukopenia, hyperventilation and hypoxemia, and hypotension. The most widely investigated cytokines implicated are TNF, interleukin-1 (IL-1), interleukin-6 (IL-6), interleukin-8 (IL-8), and interferon γ. These cytokines appear in the blood of patients with sepsis; the levels are higher in patients with septic shock. Antibodies, inhibitors, or receptor blockade for these cytokines blunts these physiologic effects in experimental models, leading to attempts to develop effective therapeutic anticytokine agents for human use.

LABORATORY AND OTHER DIAGNOSTIC TESTS

There is no specific diagnostic test for either ARDS or MODS. ARDS is a physiologic syndrome characterized by lung edema that cannot be explained by clinical evidence of heart failure, along with concurrent hypoxemia. Recently, an international consensus conference has proposed standard physiologic criteria for milder ALI; ARDS is reserved for more severe cases. Similarly, MODS is a syndrome of multisystem organ dysfunction the observer cannot otherwise explain. MODS is suggested by demonstration of concurrent onset of otherwise unexplained pulmonary, central nervous system (CNS), renal, hepatic, and hematologic functional abnormalities in an appropriate clinical setting, usually one involving either infection or noninfectious inflammation or tissue injury. Respiratory abnormalities are often recognized first, prompting a clinical diagnosis of ARDS. Evidence of extrapulmonary involvement may be much more subtle. Injury to the lung microvasculature has immediate life-threatening clinical manifestations arising from pulmonary edema. In contrast, other organs may maintain functional integrity despite activation of inflammatory cascades. Some of the early signs of extrapulmonary dysfunction are confusion, glucose intolerance, unexplained volume requirement, diminished urine output, mild thrombocytopenia, slight prolongation of the prothrombin time, and mild elevation of creatinine and bilirubin. Clinical laboratory measurements are relatively insensitive indicators of renal and hepatic failure. Urine output and serum creatinine continue to be the most readily available and useful variables to detect alterations in renal function; serum bilirubin, prothrombin time, and serum albumen are used to monitor changes in hepatic functional activity. If the underlying predisposition is self-limited or effectively treated, the extrapulmonary organ dysfunctions may never be detected by these crude measurements. Inability to reverse the inciting event permits MODS to progress until elevations in creatinine, abnormal liver function studies, gastrointestinal hemorrhage, or other overt extrapulmonary manifestations occur. This sequence seems more common in immunosuppressed patients in whom infections are harder to eradicate.

Monitoring arterial oxygen saturation by pulse oximetry has become standard care in ALI. The ubiquity of the pulse oximeter has greatly diminished the need for frequent arterial blood gas samples. Frequent chest roentgenographs are necessary to ensure proper positioning of life support devices, to detect pneumothorax in patients receiving ventilation, and to gauge the accumulation of lung edema and appearance of new focal infiltrates. Hemodynamic monitoring by Swan-Ganz catheter continues to be common and is occasionally very useful to assess intravascular volume status and cardiac output; but no improvement in clinical outcome has been ascribable to this technique. Improvements in other technologies such as echocardiography and in clinical acumen by a generation of seasoned intensivists seem to have made it more frequently dispensable.

DIFFERENTIAL DIAGNOSIS

Many other clinical scenarios involve multiorgan dysfunctions. These often masquerade as MODS. Primary disorders such as thrombotic thrombocytopenic purpura (TTP) (characterized by fever, thrombocytopenia, renal failure, altered mental status) or myeloma (characterized by fever, renal failure, anemia, infection) may mimic MODS. Some infections, such as rickettsial disease, cause multisystem abnormalities. More commonly in the intensive care unit setting, a concurrent combination of primary organ system dysfunctions may mimic a multisystem process. Unrecognized prerenal azotemia; volume overload contributing to pulmonary edema; and/or drug toxicity, such as aminoglycoside-induced renal failure, toxicity for cholestatic drugs, and coagulation abnormalities induced by some cephalosporins, may coincide, mimicking MODS. Or there may be a combination of dysfunctional organ systems that are loosely causally linked. For example, concurrent liver disease predisposes patients to sepsis by impairing host defenses, to pulmonary edema by reducing colloid oncotic pressure, and to renal failure because of intravascular volume depletion. This is not MODS. Similarly, renal failure presents formidable logistical problems in volume management that may result in pulmonary edema and prolong the need for invasive respiratory support and for invasive central vascular access for dialysis, leading to nosocomial infections. This tangle of multisystem problems carries a high mortality, but it is not MODS.

Because so many of the causes of concurrent organ failure are iatrogenic or treatable, it is perhaps best to not even think of MODS as a *diagnosis* but rather as a *concept* that helps explain multisystem organ failure in some patients. Causes for each organ dysfunction should be sought independently, as if MODS did not exist. When the physician is faced with evidence of MODS, the diagnostic strategy is to uncover and treat the underlying etiology of each organ dysfunction as a separate entity and to prevent, identify, and treat primary or secondary infection. Medications should be reviewed to uncover nephrotoxic, hepatotoxic, or marrow-suppressing drugs administered singly or in combination. In the case of renal dysfunction, diagnostic workup should be undertaken to exclude prerenal and postrenal abnormalities such as intravascular hypovolemia, low cardiac output, and urinary obstruction. If the cause is still unexplained, MODS might be entertained as a diagnosis of exclusion. In that circumstance, infection should be suspected as the inciting event. Evaluation for occult sources of infection usually includes cultures of blood, sputum, urine, pleural fluid and ascites fluid if present; computerized tomography (CT) of the sinuses; abdominal ultrasound and/or CT; lumbar puncture; and evaluation of all invasive lines as a potential nidus of infection.

MANAGEMENT

As noted previously, the first key to management is to diagnose and treat all underlying conditions that predispose to MODS and to investigate independently each organ system that appears dysfunctional; concurrent factors may be involved. The second key to management is to provide assiduous supportive care, including maintenance of tissue perfusion and oxygen delivery; provision of nutritional support; avoidance and recognition of iatrogenic complications of ventilatory support such as oxygen toxicity and barotrauma; prevention, diagnosis, and appropriate antibiotic and/or surgical therapy of predisposing and secondary infections; support of critically impaired organ functions as needed, such as with mechanical ventilation or dialysis; and hemodynamic monitoring with volume or pressor therapy as indicated.

The first goal is identification of the underlying etiologic factors. MODS is most commonly associated with systemic infections. Noninfectious events may also cause MODS, including pancreatitis, extensive cutaneous burns, ischemia-reperfusion events, skeletal fractures and crush injuries, and hypovolemic or cardiogenic shock, but these should be considered diagnoses of exclusion and the patient evaluated for occult infection. In the case of burns and crush injuries, devitalized tissue should be aggressively débrided as early as possible. There is a growing population of immunosuppressed patients with profound impairments of host defense that predispose them to recurrent and/or ineradicable infections. This group includes patients with human immunodeficiency virus, patients with end-stage organ failure awaiting transplantation, organ transplantation recipients, pa-

tients who have received marrow ablative chemotherapeutic agents for hematologic malignancies, and debilitated, alcoholic, and/or malnourished patients. In these patients MODS may appear to result from occult infection even though the source of infection is difficult to identify, and empiric antibiotic therapy is usually used.

A second goal is the maintenance of tissue perfusion and oxygen delivery. It is important that *flow* rather than *blood pressure* be emphasized. Normalization of the blood pressure by vasoconstriction may promote MODS by enhancing tissue ischemia, especially in the kidney. Reduced cardiac output measured by thermodilution, mixed venous oxygen denaturation, and/or arterial blood lactate levels may provide evidence that tissue oxygen delivery is inadequate. Restoration of intravascular volume should be the initial therapeutic approach. After fluid resuscitation is complete, careful titration of peripheral vasoconstrictors may increase cerebral, renal, and coronary perfusion if there is a significant reduction in systemic vascular resistance that results in refractory hypotension despite euvolemia. Although it is important to normalize oxygen delivery, recent studies have shown that attempts to elevate oxygen delivery to supranormal levels using inotropic agents such as dobutamine, in order to "force" perfusion of regionally underperfused areas, does not improve outcome. As an adjunct measure to support renal perfusion specifically, low-dose dopamine (2 to 5 μg/kg/min) may provide renal vascular dilation, preserving renal blood flow. Although infusions may be needed initially to restore intravascular volume, exuberant overhydration or persistent positive fluid balance for days is a poor prognostic factor. After stabilization from septic shock, diuresis must be induced to permit weaning from mechanical ventilation.

After initial stabilization, nutrition should be instituted. A major advance in supportive care of critically ill patients in recent years has been the emphasis on provision of early adequate nutritional support. The three major goals of such therapy are the provision of adequate caloric support, the provision of adequate protein to maintain positive nitrogen balance whenever possible or to minimize proteolysis even when positive nitrogen balance cannot be achieved, and to maintain integrity of the gastrointestinal mucosa through enteral feeding. Total enteral nutrition has been shown to reduce the incidence of septic complications in trauma patients. Some but not all studies show superiority of enteral over parenteral nutrition. It has been proposed that enteral nutrition provides substrate that contributes to maintenance of gastrointestinal mucosal villous morphology and prevents mucosal breakdown. It is further argued that mucosal breakdown plays a part in translocation of intestinal flora and endotoxins into the systemic circulation, which sustains sepsis syndrome, leading to MODS. Although this hypothesis remains controversial, it seems prudent to provide some enteral nutrition if it can be tolerated, supplementing this with parenteral nutrition to fulfill caloric and protein requirements. Currently it is recommended to provide 25 to 35 kcal/kg/day (3 to 5 g/kg/day of glucose and 0.5 to 1 g/kg/day of fat, and 1.5 to 2.0 g/kg/day of protein. Some recommend assessment of caloric needs by indirect calorimetry and monitoring urinary nitrogen excretion to assess nitrogen balance.

Common iatrogenic complications include oxygen toxicity, barotrauma, catheter-related sepsis, and nosocomial pneumonia. Oxygen toxicity may be more common than usually appreciated. Animal models indicate that use for 72 hours of an FiO_2 of 0.5 may cause the injured lung to develop fibrosis during the repair phase of injury even though this dose of oxygen does not cause detectable injury to the normal lung. Thus an important aspect of care is to expeditiously and assiduously decrease the FiO_2 to the lowest level that provides hemoglobin oxygen saturation of 87% to 90%. The routine use of bedside pulse oximetry has greatly simplified this task. Positive endexpiratory pressure (PEEP) is routinely used to permit the FiO_2 to be lowered to <50%. When this is done, it is important to verify that cardiac output has not been inadvertently decreased by the preloadreducing effect of positive intrathoracic pressure such that oxygen delivery is actually lower although the Po_2 is higher.

Barotrauma is another complication. It may be overt, as in the case of tension pneumothorax, or covert, as in the case of high distention injury to the lung. Because PEEP significantly raises mean airway pressure, most believe that PEEP should be used at the lowest level needed to minimize the exposure to toxic oxygen concentrations. Balancing the complications of hyperoxia and PEEP requires careful titration to achieve a moderate level of both. Recently, modes of ventilatory support have been developed that achieve adequate alveolar ventilation without alveolar overdistention through pressure or volume limitation. *Permissive hypercapnia* is one such approach in which reduction in the delivered tidal volume is used to minimize alveolar overdistention. The $PaCO_2$ is allowed to rise above 40 mm Hg and no attempts are made to correct the pH. *Pressure controlled ventilation* limits airway pressure to a preset value. Inspiratory and cycle times are also set. Recent studies have demonstrated that patients with severe ARDS can improve PaO_2 and ventilation/perfusion matching with pressure-limited rather than volume-controlled ventilation. *Inverse ratio ventilation* is a strategy whereby the inspiratory time is prolonged so that the I:E ratio is greater than 1. This modality is thought to improve the distribution of ventilation, minimizing ventilation-perfusion ratio (V/Q) mismatch while minimizing inspiratory pressure. Outcome improvements using these measures have not been demonstrated.

Catheter-related sepsis arises as a frequent complication because of the need for continuous vascular access for delivery of drugs and for monitoring. Strict aseptic technique should always be used. Lines placed during emergency conditions should be replaced promptly. Lines should be changed every 72 hours, during febrile episodes, or if signs of inflammation are visible at the entry site. Every effort should be made to discontinue use of indwelling vascular catheters as soon as they are no longer needed.

Nosocomial pneumonia is a fourth iatrogenic problem and a major cause of mortality in ARDS; it is the factor usually associated with the development of MODS. Endotracheal intubation predisposes patients to such infections because mucociliary clearance is impaired. Weaning and extubation should be accomplished as expeditiously as possible to minimize the risk of nosocomial pneumonia as a sustaining factor for MODS.

Specific Pharmacologic Therapies for ARDS and MODS

Because cytokine cascades have been emphasized as the keystones of pathogenesis, one might suppose that therapy aimed at their interruption might be the key to a specific pharmacologic therapy. Several recent clinical trials have tested this hypothesis, with negative results. It is worthwhile to review a few of them to convey the direction these studies have taken in the past and will likely continue to take. Clinical trials have been reported that test the efficacy of monoclonal antibodies against LPS, but to date the results are inconsistent and the studies have been halted. Anticytokine trials have tested four classes of agents directed toward cytokines: cytokine-specific antibodies, soluble inhibitors of the cytokines, receptor antagonists, and receptor-specific antibodies. The *inhibitors* are usually soluble molecules that resemble the cell surface receptors; they bind the cytokine so that it cannot interact with receptors on cells. The *receptor antagonists* are usually analogs of the cytokine; they bind to the specific cytokine cell surface receptors of target cells but do not signal the functional response. Several clinical trials focusing on antagonism of the effects of TNFα have been completed in patients with sepsis syndrome. A phase II multicenter trial with a murine monoclonal anti-TNF antibody in patients with severe sepsis failed to show a survival advantage. However, TNFα antibody was efficacious in a small subgroup of patients with increased TNF levels at study entry on retrospective analysis of the data. A recent phase II study with soluble recombinant human dimeric TNF receptor demonstrated a dose-related increase in mortality, raising concern about potential deleterious effects of anticytokine therapies. Studies of IL-1 antagonists have involved primarily IL-1ra. A phase III multicenter trial of human IL-1ra has recently been completed and failed to demonstrate a statistically significant difference in mortality rate between placebo and IL-1ra treated patients. Based on animal studies, IL-1 receptor antibodies (IL-1R) have also been proposed, but no human trials utilizing IL-1R have been completed to date.

Despite the multisystem concept, attempts continue to develop therapies directed specifically at respiratory failure, because ARDS often poses the most difficult clinical problem. As an example, clinical studies are in progress to determine the efficacy of exogenous surfactant replacement therapy in the lung. Abnormalities have been identified in alveolar surfactant in these patients; bronchoalveolar lavage (BAL) fluid has diminished surface tension–reducing properties,

✔ WHEN TO REFER

ARDS in either the presence or absence of MODS should be treated in an intensive care unit by physicians who have expertise in mechanical ventilation and hemodynamic monitoring, as well as broad experience in the diagnosis and therapy of a spectrum of diseases and complications that befall the critically ill. Careful observation, usually in an intensive care environment, is indicated early in the clinical course of ALI, when dyspnea and tachypnea are present but gas exchange is preserved. Respiratory failure commonly progresses rapidly. It is important to perceive the need for endotracheal intubation early enough so that the procedure can be instituted expeditiously in a controlled setting. MODS is one clinical setting in which it may be quite appropriate to obtain multiple specialty consultations because multiple interacting organ systems are involved, the differential diagnosis for each is wide, and the penalty for mistakes is high with respect to both resources consumption and mortality.

in part because of abnormalities in surfactant composition and metabolism. The surfactants that are currently used in clinical studies are of two types: mammalian preparations (low-molecular-weight surfactant proteins) and synthetic protein-free preparations (Exosurf, Infasurf, Survanta). Clinical trials of these surfactants indicate no sustained improvement in gas exchange or mortality in adults with ARDS.

Although no specific therapies for MODS have been found to date, the mortality rate for severe ARDS has declined from >70% to <50%. This reassuring trend likely reflects the cumulative effect of many small details in clinical care: improvements in imaging techniques such as CT scans and echocardiography, better antibiotics with less renal toxicity, aggressive nutritional support, and better computer-driven mechanical ventilators that minimize work of breathing and airway pressures. Perhaps it also reflects more expertise in management of the critically ill than was present a decade ago because of the maturation of the specialty of critical care medicine.

BIBLIOGRAPHY

Bernard GH, Artigas A, Brigham, KL et al: The American-European Consensus Conference on ARDS, *Am J Respir Crit Care Med* 149:818-824, 1994.

Christman JW et al: Strategies for blocking the systemic effects of cytokines in the sepsis syndrome, *Crit Care Med* 23:955-963, 1995.

Deitch EA: Multiple organ failure, pathophysiology and potential future therapy, *Ann Surg* 216(2):117-1134, 1992.

Gattinoni L, Brazzi L, Pelosi et al: A trial of goal-oriented hemodynamic therapy in critically ill patients, *N Engl J Med* 333:1025-1031, 1995.

Hickling KG et al: Low mortality rate in adult respiratory distress syndrome using low-volume, pressure limited ventilation with permissive hypercapnia: a prospective study, *Crit Care Med* 22:1568-1578, 1994.

Hudson LD, Molberg JA, Anardi D, Maunder J: Clinical risks for development of acute respiratory distress syndrome, *Am J Respir Crit Care Med* 151:293-301, 1995.

Jobe AH: Pulmonary surfactant therapy, *N Engl J Med* 328:861-868, 1993.

Milberg JA, Steinberg KP, Hudson LD: Improved survival of patients with acute respiratory distress syndrome: 1983-1993, *JAMA* 2273:306-309, 1995.

CHAPTER

48 Pulmonary Edema

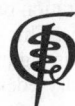

Arthur P. Wheeler, Gordon R. Bernard, and Kenneth L. Brigham

Heart failure and volume overload are prime examples of hydrostatic (increased pressure) pulmonary edema, and overall heart failure remains the most common cause of pulmonary edema. Edema secondary to lung microvascular injury (noncardiogenic pulmonary edema) has become a more prominent problem because of heightened sensitivity to the diagnosis and improved emergency care of patients at risk for the condition. In its most severe form, noncardiogenic pulmonary edema is referred to as the *acute respiratory distress syndrome* (ARDS).

The functional consequences of pulmonary edema are caused in part by the physical presence of excess fluid in the lungs, but, especially in ARDS, other abnormalities of airway and vascular function contribute to the failure of gas exchange. Bronchoconstriction and vasoconstriction are important functional abnormalities that may not be the direct result of edema. In fact, in some forms of pulmonary edema, the amount of water in the lungs is not the critical issue.

Pulmonary edema caused by heart failure is pathogenically different from that caused by lung injury, but there are many similarities in diagnosis and treatment. Comprehending the clinical problem requires understanding the pathophysiology so that an otherwise bewildering list of etiologic factors can be managed similarly.

Strictly defined, *pulmonary edema* is excess fluid in the lungs outside of the circulation. Increased intravascular volume (congestion) is commonly present, especially when edema is caused by heart failure, but vascular congestion and edema are distinct phases of the process.

RELEVANT PATHOPHYSIOLOGY

In the lungs, extravascular fluid may accumulate in two major compartments. The interstitial compartment includes the thin interstitium of the alveoli but also the potential spaces around larger airways and blood vessels. The interstitial compartment is the initial site of fluid accumulation, resulting in "cuffing" of fluid around vessels and airways, which causes increased prominence of the bronchovascular shadows on chest radiographs (interstitial edema). Edema fluid may accumulate in the interstitium without flooding alveoli or producing significant alterations in gas exchange at rest, but it increases the lung volume at which small airways collapse and may alter the distribution of blood flow in the lungs. The second compartment, the air spaces, represents an enormous potential space for fluid accumulation; the air spaces flood only after the interstitial compartment is filled and the recruitable mechanism for lung water clearance (lymphatic drainage) is overwhelmed. When air space flooding occurs, significant deterioration of ventilation and oxygenation rapidly follows. In some forms of edema, the epithelial barrier lining the alveoli is injured. Normally, this epithelial layer is very tight and prevents movement of fluid into air spaces. When this barrier is breached, filling of alveoli can occur without filling of the interstitial compartment because fluid filtered from capillaries could enter directly into alveoli.

Box 48-1 attempts to place many of the causes of pulmonary edema into pathophysiologically similar groups. As a practical matter, understanding the etiologies responsible for the edema is not terribly useful in that treatment is dictated more by the pathophysiology than by etiology.

The physical forces determining the rate of fluid filtration across capillaries are usually called *Starling forces*. The four Starling forces are hydrostatic pressure inside and outside exchange vessels (capillary pressure and interstitial pressure, respectively) and the oncotic (protein osmotic) pressure inside and outside exchange vessels. The sum of these forces adjusted by the filtration coefficient ("leakiness" of the capillary membranes) determines the rate of fluid filtration into the pulmonary interstitium.

Any abnormality that interferes with blood flow distal to the lung capillaries can result in increased capillary pressure. The most common such abnormality is failure of the left ventricle, which results in elevated left ventricular diastolic pressures, elevated left atrial pressures, and thus elevated pressure in pulmonary veins and capillaries. Fixed obstructions to flow proximal to the left ventricle, such as mitral stenosis and pulmonary vein occlusion, also elevate filtration pressures, as may variable constriction of the pulmonary veins. This latter mechanism may be operative in pulmonary edema occurring after injury to the central nervous system (neurogenic pulmonary edema) or in sepsis.

Decreases in plasma oncotic pressure resulting from hypoproteinemia can predispose to pulmonary edema. Whether it is possible for edema to result from hypoproteinemia in the absence of elevated capillary pressure in human disease is not clear because elevated pulmonary vascular pressures are commonly present in these same situations.

When capillary endothelium is injured, permeability is increased and excess fluid filters into the interstitium, resulting in edema without any derangement in the Starling forces. As indicated in Box 48-1, increased permeability pulmonary edema occurs in a large and diverse group of clinical disorders. The mechanism of microvascular injury is unclear, but some evidence shows that a common pathogenic sequence is shared by many of these disorders. In practice, the diagnosis usually depends on demonstration of edema by chest radiograph with a normal pulmonary arterial wedge pressure (PAWP). Increased permeability also results in edema fluid with higher protein concentration than in cardiogenic edema. Measurements of protein concentration in suctioned edema fluid have been used experimentally to distinguish between high- pressure and high-permeability edema but are not practical for routine care.

Sepsis and aspiration are the most common causes of increased permeability edema (ARDS), accounting for more than half of the cases. Experimental work has clearly implicated cytokines and prostanoids as mediators of some of the abnormalities in lung function. Marked alterations in lung mechanics and pulmonary hypertension after endotoxemia appear to be mediated by increased production of cyclooxygenase products of arachidonic acid, and, at least experimentally, these changes are inhibited by cytokine antagonists and nonsteroidal antiinflammatory agents.

Although the diagnosis of noncardiogenic pulmonary edema usually requires demonstration of normal left heart pressures, there is no a priori reason why increased permeability cannot occur in the presence of heart failure. In the absence of some specific measurement of pulmonary vascular permeability, diagnosis of ARDS in the presence of increased left heart pressures is difficult. Investigational techniques for measuring capillary endothelial or airway epithelial permeability exist, but none of these is available for routine clinical use. Until such methods are available, the diagnosis of mixed forms of edema must depend on the history and clinical course.

BOX 48-1

A pathophysiologic classification of pulmonary edema by etiology

I. Alterations in Starling forces
   A. Increased hydrostatic pressure (heart failure, mitral stenosis, neurogenic pulmonary edema, volume overload, lymphatic disruption)
   B. Decreased plasma oncotic pressure (malnutrition, hepatic failure, massive crystalloid infusion)
II. Altered pulmonary microvascular membrane permeability
   A. Shock (septic, hemorrhagic, neurogenic, cardiogenic)
   B. Infections (viral, fungal, tuberculosis, rickettsial)
   C. Multiple trauma (fat embolism, head trauma)
   D. Inhalation injury
      1. Gastric aspiration
      2. Near-drowning
      3. Hydrocarbons
      4. Irritant and poisonous gases (nitrogen dioxide, ammonia, phosgene, chlorine, cadmium, ozone), smoke
      5. Oxygen toxicity
      6. Hypersensitivity pneumonitis
   E. Drug-related (heroin, aspirin, paraquat)
   F. Hematologic disorders (disseminated intravascular coagulation, transfusion, cardiopulmonary bypass, pulmonary embolism)
   G. Metabolic disorder (pancreatitis, ketoacidosis)
   H. Immunologic disorders (systemic lupus erythematosus, Wegener's granulomatosis, Goodpasture's syndrome)
III. Miscellaneous and poorly understood conditions
   A. Uremia
   B. Eclampsia
   C. Radiation pneumonitis
   D. High-altitude pulmonary edema
   E. Reexpansion of unilateral collapsed lung

DIAGNOSTIC LABORATORY TESTS

In most cases, the arterial blood gas, plain chest radiograph, and electrocardiogram are sufficient to confirm a clinical diagnosis of pulmonary edema and pinpoint its cause. The electrocardiogram is most useful when it demonstrates an acute pattern of ischemia or infarction, suggesting left ventricular failure of dysfunction.

In severe pulmonary edema blood gases universally show hypoxemia and usually demonstrate hypocapnia. Abnormal oxygenation is the hallmark of ARDS. A PaO_2/FIO_2 ratio less than 200 is a widely accepted diagnostic criterion, but again there is no universally accepted level of hypoxemia. The $PaCO_2$ can, however, be elevated when severe alveolar flooding increases dead space or when respiratory failure has developed as the result of respiratory muscle fatigue. In situations in which cardiac output is compromised, systemic metabolic acidosis may be seen.

In well-established edema, the chest radiograph usually shows diffuse bilateral interstitial and alveolar infiltrates. The radiographic diagnosis can be subtle, however, especially in the early stages of ARDS. Attempts to reliably distinguish noncardiogenic from cardiogenic pulmonary edema by radiograph have met with little success. Early reports indicating that these two entities could be segregated by chest radiograph alone have not been widely reproducible. Even though it is of limited diagnostic value, a pattern of cardiomegaly, with pleural effusions, Kerley B lines, and a gravitional distribution of edema, suggests cardiac pulmonary edema. Usually the pattern seen in ARDS is more patchy and asymmetric. Kerley lines are rare, as are signs of central vascular congestion (cardiomegaly and a widened vascular pedicle).

DIFFERENTIAL DIAGNOSIS

The presence of pulmonary edema is suggested when a patient acutely develops dyspnea, anxiety, pallor, and cyanosis. The physical examination and clinical setting are important in differentiating the many possible etiologies. Cardiac edema is usually associated with valvular or ischemic myocardial disease and may be heralded by drenching sweats, nausea, distended neck veins, hepatojugular reflux, tachycardia, a third heart sound (S_3) gallop, and often the murmur of mitral regurgitation. The pulmonary examination reveals diffuse crackles that are usually more pronounced in the dependent portions of the lung. Occasionally wheezing is heard. The extremities may be cold, clammy, and sometimes cyanotic (low-cardiac-output state).

The patient with ARDS, on the other hand, does not typically display signs of heart failure and may have a normal chest examination or only very fine crackles and no orthopnea. The patient, however, is anxious, dyspneic, and cyanotic, and usually has evidence of an underlying entity associated with ARDS. Clinical history is crucial because more than 80% of ARDS victims will have a clear predisposing event (Box 48-2) noted within 24 hours of the onset of the disease. At least initially, cardiac output is usually normal or increased. Computed tomography of the chest is not superior to plain radiograph in diagnosing or characterizing the etiology of pulmonary edema.

Given a typical clinical setting and a preponderance of differentiating clinical signs, distinguishing cardiac from noncardiac pulmonary edema can be relatively simple. However, the two entities often overlap sufficiently to make diagnosis difficult, and the two processes can occur simultaneously in the same patient. Because the diagnosis is not clear in most cases, additional data are required for optimal patient management.

BOX 48-2

Common causes of acute respiratory distress syndrome

Sepsis
Aspiration
Pulmonary contusion
Multiple transfusions

Similarly, in most cases it is not difficult to distinguish other potentially catastrophic cardiopulmonary illnesses from pulmonary edema. Pneumonia usually has a more prominent cough and fever and commonly a predominantly unilateral radiographic appearance. Pulmonary embolism, although abrupt and profound in onset like pulmonary edema, is often associated with chest pain and rarely has a chest radiograph that could be confused with pulmonary edema. Pneumothorax, again symptomatically similar to pulmonary edema, is readily distinguished by the physical findings of deceased breath sounds, absence of rales, and its classic hypodense radiographic appearance.

Data supporting a diagnosis of cardiac edema include electrodiographic evidence of myocardial ischemia or infarction, elevated cardiac enzymes, relatively small calculated pulmonary shunt, and a bronchial fluid protein concentration less than 50% of plasma protein concentration. Data supporting a diagnosis of ARDS include a very large pulmonary shunt and edema fluid protein concentration greater than 70% of plasma protein concentration. Finally, a critical measurement for differentiating cardiac from noncardiac edema is the PAWP. A high PAWP (>18 mm Hg) indicates heart failure or volume overload as the etiology of the edema until proved otherwise. A PAWP <18 mm Hg in the face of progressive pulmonary edema suggests ARDS. There are pitfalls in this logic because during left ventricular failure, the PAWP can be reduced rapidly with nitrates, diuretics, digoxin, and oxygen such that by the time the PAWP can be measured, it may have returned to the normal range. Usually if this is the case, the pulmonary edema and hypoxemia rapidly subside. As stated earlier, there is no prohibition to heart failure superimposed on ARDS.

Thus any evidence of pulmonary edema (usually by chest radiograph) accompanied by an elevated PAWP is consistent with cardiogenic pulmonary edema. With ARDS, several other criteria must be met. There must be evidence of pulmonary edema by chest radiograph, and typically the pattern is of diffuse interstitial and alveolar infiltrates. However, the characteristics of the radiographic pattern may be diverse, as in the case of viral or *Pneumocystis* pneumonia (diffuse pattern), lung contusion (localized or patchy), and unilateral pulmonary edema. Unfortunately, only a rough consensus exists as to what the chest radiograph should look like in ARDS: "bilateral infiltrates consistent with pulmonary edema."

Although widely used in the past as a diagnostic criterion, reductions in lung compliance in ARDS are of little diagnostic value and probably more accurately reflect a reduced lung volume rather than a reduced compliance. Static lung compliance is measured by dividing tidal volume (ml) by plateau airway pressure (obtained by occluding the exhalation port of the ventilator after delivery of a tidal breath) minus whatever level of positive and expiratory pressure may be present at the time.

MANAGEMENT

The management of cardiac pulmonary edema is essentially the management of heart failure, a subject discussed in Chapter 19. When cardiac pulmonary edema causes severe respiratory embarrassment requiring mechanical ventilation, its management is similar to that for noncardiac pulmonary edema. Therefore, this discussion concentrates on the therapy of noncardiac edema.

Oxygen Therapy

Supplemental oxygen is first-line therapy for the patient with pulmonary edema and in the critically ill should be initiated in the highest practical concentration (e.g., a nonrebreathing 100% oxygen mask). Pulse oximetry can rapidly assess the adequacy of oxygenation but reveals little about ventilation. Hence, in most cases direct blood gas measurements are necessary, at least during the initial period of instability. Blood gases guide oxygen administration and provide useful information regarding acid-base status and the effectiveness of ventilation, thereby influencing the decision to institute mechanical assistance. Inspired oxygen fractions (FIO_2) of 1.0 are generally considered safe if used for less than 24 hours, and it is safer to err on the side of too much oxygen rather than to risk hypoxemia. If supplemental oxygen is essential for survival, endotracheal intubation should be considered. An endotracheal tube permits precise, consistent oxygen delivery and easy suctioning of airway secretions and maintains a reliable route for the institution of mechanical ventilation, if, and more likely, when, the need arises. Figure 48-1 depicts the rate of reversal of arterial blood gas criteria in a large group of patients with noncardiogenic pulmonary edema randomized to receive corticosteroids early in their illness.

Mechanical Ventilation and Positive End-Expiratory Pressure

Mechanical ventilation is usually required in the management of severe pulmonary edema. The ventilator controls oxygen delivery and maintains positive end-expiratory pressure (PEEP), but these functions can be performed by other means. The most important function of the ventilator is to provide adequate ventilation without requiring large energy expenditure by the patient. Work of breathing in patients with severe edema may rise tenfold above resting requirements and is increased for at least three reasons. First, early in the disease course the lungs are stiff (decreased compliance) because of accumulated edema fluid; later fibrosis may develop (Fig. 48-2). Second, the airways may be obstructed by edema fluid, mucus, or bronchospasm. Third, severe ventilation-perfusion mismatch increases physiologic dead space, which may require very large increases in minute ventilation to maintain alveolar ventilation. Mechanical ventilation is generally indicated when respiratory rates exceed 35 to 40 breaths per minute because this level of respiration exhausts ventilatory reserve and even slight complications (such as a mucus plug or aspiration) may result in respiratory arrest. Furthermore, the overall work required to sustain such a respiratory rate can rarely be maintained for more than a few hours.

Once intubated and ventilated, a patient with noncardiac edema may survive with severely abnormal gas exchange for weeks, although either death or significant improvement usually occurs in 7 to 14 days. Methods of assessing the course of such patients include chest radiographs, arterial blood gases, and hemodynamic measurements. To follow the efficiency of gas exchange, measurement of a derived variable that takes into account both alveolar oxygen tension (PAO_2) calculated from the alveolar gas equation and arterial oxygen tension (PaO_2) is useful. One widely used index of the efficiency of oxygenation is the calculation of pulmonary shunt. The shunt calculation requires knowledge of the FIO_2, PaO_2, mixed venous oxygen tension (PvO_2) and saturation (SvO_2), arterial PaO_2 and saturation (SaO_2), and $PaCO_2$. Because these values are not always readily obtainable, alternative indices have been derived, including PaO_2/PAO_2 ratio, PaO_2/FIO_2 ratio, A-aDO_2 (alveolar to arterial oxygen difference). Each has its limitations, but for ease of calculation, the PaO_2/FIO_2 ratio is simplest. Figure 48-2 shows the trends in oxygenation, chest radiograph score, and static lung compliance in a large group of patients with ARDS.

Although brief periods of exposure (<24 hours) to high oxygen concentrations are considered safe, longer periods may not be. Therefore, when inspired oxygen concentrations exceed 50% (a level gen-

erally accepted as safe for long periods), other manipulations should be made in an attempt to reduce FIO_2. PEEP is often used for this purpose. PEEP redistributes extravascular lung water, recruits atelectatic lung units, and discourages repetitive opening and closing of poorly compliant alveoli. Through these mechanisms, venous admixture or shunt can be reduced in most patients with pulmonary edema. Adverse effects of PEEP include hypotension, decreased cardiac output, and barotrauma. Whether PEEP is of benefit depends on its relative effects on hemoglobin saturation and cardiac output. For example, if PEEP increases hemoglobin saturation from 90% to 92% (roughly a change in PaO_2 of 60 to 70 mm Hg) but reduces cardiac output by 30%, oxygen delivery has been severely reduced despite the increase in saturation. In patients with pulmonary artery pressure catheters in place, arterial saturation and cardiac output should be obtained before and after each PEEP change to determine if a beneficial effect on oxygen delivery has occurred. As a general rule, PEEP should be increased in a stepwise fashion in increments of 3 to 5 cm H_2O until saturation is acceptable, the FIO_2 is below 0.5 to 0.6, and cardiac output is adequate. There are few data to suggest that PEEP levels higher than the 20 to 25 cm H_2O range are more effective than lesser levels, and typically a PEEP of 10 to 15 cm H_2O permits a reduction in FIO_2 to ≤50%.

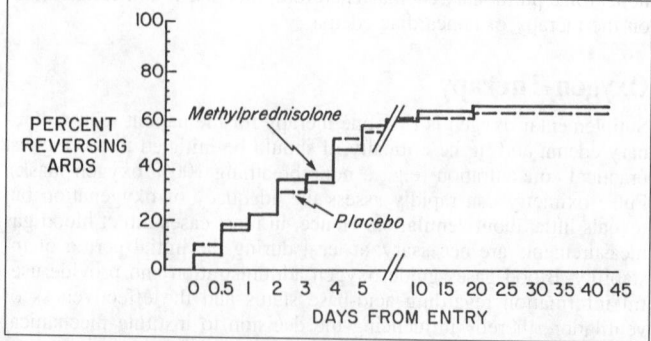

FIGURE 48-1 Trends in arterial blood gas reversal in ARDS patients randomized to receive either methylprednisolone (30 mg/kg × four doses 6 hours apart) (N = 50) *(solid line)* or placebo (N = 49) *(dashed line)*. No difference occurred in the mortality rate by treatment group; $p > 0.05$.

(From Bernard GR et al: *N Engl J Med* 317:1565, 1987.)

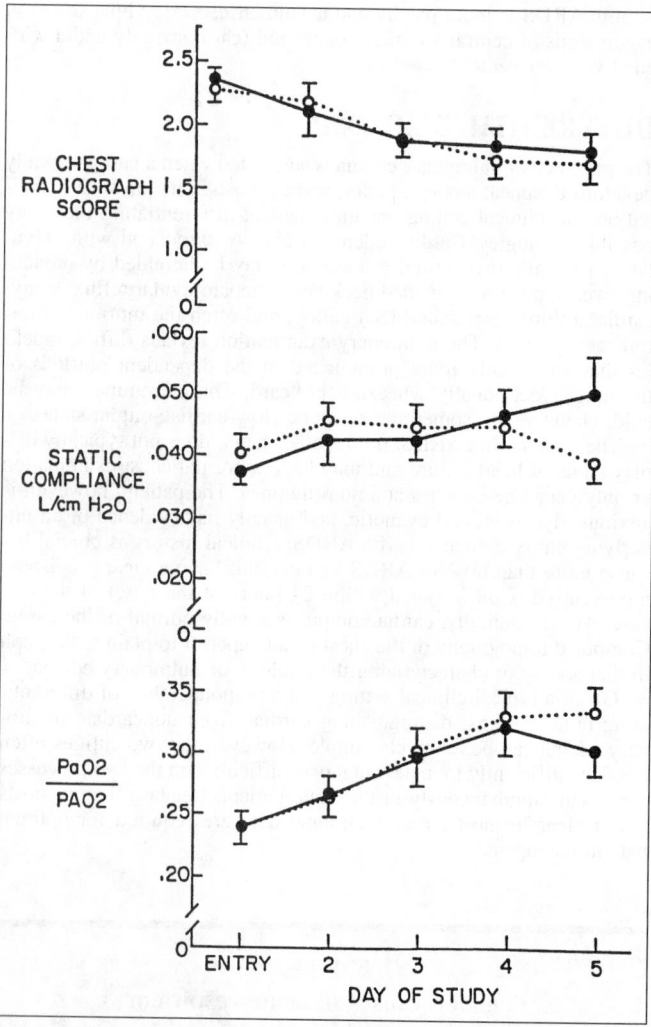

FIGURE 48-2 Chest radiograph score (0, normal; 1, mild; 2, moderate; 3, severe pulmonary edema), total thoracic static compliance, and arterial to alveolar PaO_2 ratio (PaO_2/PAO_2) in 99 patients randomized to receive either methylprednisolone 30 mg/kg every 6 hours for 24 hours *(solid line)* (N = 50) or placebo (N = 49) *(dashed line)*. There were no significant differences based on treatment group either at time of entry or at any point in the 5 days of close follow-up; $p > 0.05$.

(From Bernard GR et al: *N Engl J Med* 317:1565, 1987.)

Although it provides many benefits, the mechanical ventilator can exact a severe price. The cost of mechanical ventilation is often the creation of pressure-stretch–induced lung damage, barotrauma. Although macroscopic injury can occur in many forms (e.g., pneumothorax, air embolism, interstitial emphysema), subtle, microscopic injury can also result from overstretching the lung. Animal studies suggest this damage regularly occurs when transpulmonary pressure, best characterized as peak static inflation or plateau pressure, exceeds that necessary for inflation of a normal lung to total lung capacity. In humans this pressure has a value of 30 to 35 cm H_2O. Hence a third important variable—plateau pressure—must be balanced against an adequate saturation and cardiac output. Recent uncontrolled studies in ARDS suggest that a strategy that limits inflation pressure while providing adequate oxygen delivery results in the highest likelihood of survival. The potential downside of limiting airway pressures in patients with pulmonary edema is that some degree of carbon dioxide retention ensues.

Balancing Oxygen Delivery and Consumption

Even in the normal state, stress or activity reduces mixed venous hemoglobin saturation (SvO_2). Because normal individuals have little shunt, however, the lower SvO_2 has very little effect on arterial oxygen levels (i.e., even severely desaturated blood can be fully reoxygenated during a brief pass through a well-functioning alveolar-capillary unit). In patients with severe pulmonary edema, shunt can increase to extremely high levels (25% to 35% is common). This degree of shunt allows a significant volume of desaturated mixed venous blood to enter the arterial circulation, lowering the oxygen content of arterial blood. Treatable causes of increased oxygen consumption (Vo_2) include thyrotoxicosis, fever, pain, and agitation; the latter three are very common in patients with pulmonary edema. Fever is most effectively treated with antipyretics; cooling blankets are rather ineffective in reducing temperature in this setting, and the shivering they induce may actually increase Vo_2. Pain and agitation should be treated with some combination of narcotics, benzodiazepines, and neuroleptics, adding a paralyzing agent such as pancuronium only if absolutely necessary. If the latter is used, sedation must be used in an attempt to render the patient unaware.

With Vo_2 minimized, consideration should be given to increasing oxygen delivery (Do_2). Based on observational and limited interventional studies, the practice of boosting oxygen delivery (Do_2) to an empirically derived supranormal level has been tried in a variety of critically ill patients. Although it is clear that a Do_2 that is less than the Vo_2 will lead to an anaerobic state, it is far from certain that a greater than normal oxygen delivery prevents or reverses anaerobic metabolism or improves patient outcome. To the contrary, recent randomized controlled trials suggest the opposite. Possibly the most reasonable conclusion to draw from studies of augmented Do_2 are that patients with the cardiovascular reserve capable of generating an increased Do_2 represent an overall healthier subgroup of patients. Box 48-3 lists medically attainable means of increasing oxygen transport.

Fluid Management

In both cardiac and noncardiac pulmonary edema, a balance must be sought between the beneficial effect of relatively high PAWP on car-

diac output and its negative effect on lung fluid balance. Left ventricular filling pressure cannot be reliably estimated on physical examination or on measurement of central venous pressure. For these reasons, the flow-directed pulmonary artery catheter, which generally provides reliable estimates of left ventricular filling pressure, has become commonplace in the management of pulmonary edema. It is generally accepted that PAWP should be in the range of 15 to 18 mm Hg in patients with normal pulmonary vascular permeability and a failing left ventricle to maximize cardiac performance. Although it is reasonable to maintain patients with noncardiogenic pulmonary edema at the lowest left ventricular filling pressure producing an adequate cardiac output, substantial controversy continues with regard to the value of volume restriction/diuresis in ARDS. Several observational studies indicate a better outcome for ARDS patients who receive less fluid or experience less weight gain. Unfortunately, such studies leave unanswered the critically important question of whether it is the practice of providing less fluid that is beneficial, or if the patients who "require" less fluid for hemodynamic support simply have a better outcome. The correct balance between risk of increasing lung water and decreasing oxygen delivery has not been defined and probably varies on an individual basis. A proper clinical trial examining this important clinical question is needed.

Controversy remains over the relative merits of crystalloid versus colloid solutions in patients with pulmonary edema. In cardiac edema, infusions of albumin (especially if the serum albumin is low) can mobilize interstitial fluid. When pulmonary vascular permeability is increased, however, albumin readily crosses the microvascular barrier and therefore fails to increase the oncotic gradient, promoting interstitial fluid resorption. Clearly in hydrostatic pulmonary edema, all fluids should be minimized, and in noncardiogenic pulmonary edema, both colloid and crystalloid, will leak into the interstitium.

When intravascular volume must be reduced, the primary therapy should be volume restriction, diuretics, and, when necessary, hemodialysis/hemofiltration. Vasodilators such as nitroglycerin and nitroprusside may rapidly decrease pulmonary vascular pressures but can increase pulmonary shunt by paralyzing hypoxic vasoconstriction, the autoregulatory process that maintains ventilation-perfusion matching.

Corticosteroids

Based on animal studies and the inflammatory infiltration seen in lung biopsy specimens of ARDS victims, there has been a long-held belief that corticosteroids might be a useful treatment. However, studies have shown that early use of corticosteroids neither prevents septic patients from developing ARDS nor affects the course of gas exchange, chest radiograph, and lung compliance abnormalities in patients with established disease (see Figs. 48-1 and 48-2), and corticosteroids do not reduce overall mortality in patients with established ARDS even when treated early (Fig. 48-3). Several small un-

---

BOX 48-3
Methods for optimizing oxygen transport

Improve cardiac output
Maintain normal hemoglobin
Rightward shift of oxygen-hemoglobin curve
    Prevent hypothermia
    Increased 2,3-diphosphoglycerate
    Avoid alkalosis
    Avoid low Pco_2
Reduce oxygen consumption

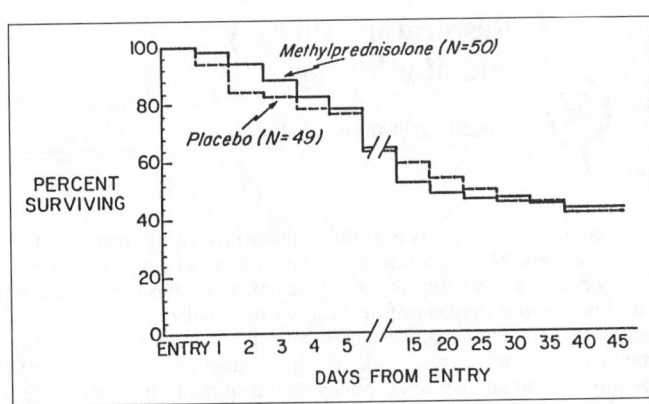

FIGURE 48-3 Cumulative survival of patients with ARDS randomized to receive either methylprednisolone (30 mg/kg $\times$ four doses 6 hours apart) or placebo. No difference occurred in the rate of reversal by treatment group; $p > 0.05$.

(From Bernard GR et al: *N Engl J Med* 317:1565, 1987.)

✔ *WHEN TO REFER*

The care of profoundly hypoxemic pulmonary edema victims is a complicated process of managing sophisticated technology, complex treatment strategies, and often the simultaneous failure of multiple organ systems. For most patients, the key clinical event that should trigger involvement of a pulmonary critical care specialist is institution of mechanical ventilation. The subtleties of mechanical ventilation (especially when using newer complex ventilators) and the interaction of the ventilator with the cardiovascular and renal systems are difficult to master. Because of the complexity and amount of time the physician must spend at the bedside, the assistance of an experienced critical care practioner should be enlisted in the care of most patients receiving mechanical ventilation.

controlled series report improvements in gas exchange and compliance of ARDS patients treated with corticosteroids in the so-called fibroproliferative phase (7 to 21 days after onset), but confirmation by studies using rigorous methodology is needed.

BIBLIOGRAPHY

Bernard GR et al: High-dose corticosteroids in patients with the adult respiratory distress syndrome, *N Engl J Med* 317:1565, 1987.

Bone RC et al: A controlled clinical trial of high-dose methylprednisolone in the treatment of severe sepsis and septic shock, *N Engl J Med* 317:653, 1987.

Brigham K, editor: Pulmonary edema, *Semin Respir Med* 4:267, 1983.

Britto M et al: Beneficial effects of the "open lung approach with low distending pressures in acute respiratory distress syndrome, *Am J Respir Crit Care Med* 152:1835,1995.

Hayes MA et al: Elevation of systemic oxygen delivery in the treatment of critically ill patients, *N Engl J Med* 330:1717, 1994.

Hickling KG et al: Low mortality using low volume pressure limited ventilation with permissive hypercapnia in ARDS: a prospective study, *Crit Care Med* 22:1568, 1994.

Meduri GU et al: Corticosteroid rescue treatment of progressive fibroproliferation in late ARDS: patterns of response and predictors of outcome, *Chest* 105:1516, 1994.

Mitchell JP et al: Improved outcome based on fluid management in critically ill patients requiring pulmonary artery catheterization, *Am Rev Respir Dis* 145:990, 1992.

Pepe P et al: Clinical predictors of the adult respiratory distress syndrome, *Am J Surg* 144:124, 1982.

Sznajder JI, Wood LDH: Beneficial effects of reducing pulmonary edema in patients with acute hypoxic respiratory failure, *Chest* 100:890, 1991.

Wheeler AP, Bernard GR: Minimal positive end expiratory pressure (PEEP): a safe, effective, defensible practice, *Clin Intensive Care* 3:175, 1990.

CHAPTER

49 Respiratory Therapy and Monitoring

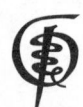

David H. Ingbar and Linda Nici

Respiratory therapy is a useful adjunct in treating many pulmonary disorders. The spectrum of respiratory care is broad, encompassing normobaric and hyperbaric oxygen therapy, postural drainage, chest percussion, delivery of medications by nebulization or aerosols, ventilator care, pulmonary rehabilitation, and noninvasive respiratory monitoring. However, respiratory therapy is labor intensive and costly. In only a small number of situations have respiratory treatments been scientifically proven to be of benefit, although few have been rigorously tested. The practitioner must be aware of the indications and contraindications for each modality of treatment and should work closely with the respiratory therapist to continually reevaluate the patient's response to therapy.

RESPIRATORY CARE TREATMENT MODALITIES
Oxygen Therapy

Many hospitalized patients are administered supplemental oxygen either as treatment for documented hypoxemia (measured arterial oxygen pressure (PaO_2) <60 mm Hg or oxygen saturation SaO_2 <92%), or prophylactically to prevent hypoxemia in patients who have symptoms of myocardial ischemia or who are undergoing certain procedures (e.g., bronchoscopy). Before initiating oxygen therapy, an arterial blood gas (ABG) sample should be obtained to determine the baseline values of $PaCO_2$ and PaO_2 unless the patient is in severe respiratory distress. Hypoxemia is regarded as life-threatening when the PaO_2 is below 55 mm Hg or the SaO_2 is below 85%, because in this range the steep hemoglobin-oxygen dissociation curve results in a large decrease in hemoglobin saturation with any further small decrement of PaO_2.

Oxygen Delivery Devices. The choice of an oxygen delivery device for a specific patient largely depends on how high and how constant an inspired fraction of oxygen (FIO_2) is necessary. In the hospital, the maximal FIO_2 that can be delivered to the trachea is limited by the maximal flow rate from the wall outlet (usually 15 to 20 L/min). As the patient's inspiratory flow rate increases above that from the oxygen delivery device, a larger fraction of the inspired gas consists of entrained room air. During respiratory distress or tachypnea, the inspiratory flow rate often increases markedly from the normal resting value of 20 L/min, and decreases the delivered FIO_2.

Nasal Prongs. Nasal prongs are used to deliver 0.5 to 6 liters of oxygen per minute. Higher flow rates dry the nasal mucosa and may lead to epistaxis. Even the patient who appears to be breathing through the mouth entrains oxygen through the nasopharynx. The FIO_2 varies with the patient's inspiratory flow rate but usually is between 0.22 and 0.40. This delivery method is useful for patients with hypoxemia resulting from ventilation-perfusion mismatching, such as those with chronic obstructive pulmonary disease (COPD) and asthma, because their hypoxemia is responsive to small increases in FIO_2. In COPD patients with carbon dioxide retention, supplemental oxygen may worsen respiratory acidosis because it either suppresses hypoxic respiratory drive or alters the dead space/tidal volume ratio. In these patients it is important to limit the increase in FIO_2 to the minimum that achieves an adequate SaO_2. Some authorities strongly advocate that nasal prongs should not be used in patients with CO_2 retention because the FIO_2 achieved varies with the patient's inspiratory flow rate. Other authorities are skeptical that these fluctuations of FIO_2 are clinically important and believe that this relative disadvantage may be outweighed by many patients' reluctance to wear face masks continuously.

Nasal prongs usually are the delivery device of choice for long-term oxygen therapy. Several oxygen-conserving devices are available that provide either a reservoir of oxygen or inflow only during inspiration. An alternative method of long-term oxygen delivery is via a transtracheal oxygen catheter. This Silastic catheter is placed through the cricothyroid membrane directly into the trachea. It can be used to deliver higher FIO_2 levels and greater flow rates. Thus it may be beneficial for selected patients with hypoxemia that is resistant to therapy with 2 to 3 L/min of oxygen by nasal cannulae, such as patients with pulmonary fibrosis. In addition, some patients prefer this method since it avoids the stigma of wearing easily visible nasal prongs.

Aerosol Face Masks. Masks that cover the nose and mouth deliver a humidified mixture of oxygen and room air with a wide range of possible FIO_2 values. Because the mask has side air holes and is not tightly fitted, a variable amount of room air is inhaled around or through the mask. As the set FIO_2 is increased, the flow rate provided from the mixing jet nebulizer falls because the mixed gas is more rich in oxygen. The patient may then need to entrain more room air to meet the inspiratory flow demand. Consequently, a setting of "100% oxygen" usually achieves a tracheal FIO_2 of only 50% to 70% oxygen.

A very high FIO_2 sometimes is required for patients with hypoxemia from shunt physiology, as in multilobar pneumonia, pulmonary edema, or severe atelectasis. Three strategies have been used to increase the maximum FIO_2 delivered without intubating the patient. First, the mask's side holes can be covered with flaps that close the holes during inspiration but permit exhalation. Second, a bag can be attached to the mask to provide a reservoir of oxygen-rich gas. A one-way valve makes this bag fill with pure oxygen while the patient exhales. When the patient inhales at a rate greater than the rate at which gas is delivered into the mask, this valve opens and the oxygen from the reservoir bag is inhaled instead of room air. This mask is called a nonrebreather reservoir mask because the patient's exhaled gas does not enter the reservoir bag. The combination of these two methods achieves FIO_2 values in the range of 70% to 90%, depending on how well the mask fits the patient. Partial rebreather masks fill the reservoir bag with the exhaled dead space gas that is oxygen-rich, but they are less reliable. Third, the oxygen from two wall outlets can be yoked together into one mask to provide a total flow of 30 L/min of pure oxygen. This system provides an FIO_2 in the trachea of up to 80% to 90%.

Air-entrainment or Venturi face masks direct a jet of oxygen through orifices engineered to entrain a fixed proportion of room air. By changing the orifice size, this mask can deliver a high flow of gas with a precise FIO_2 of 24%, 28%, 32%, 36%, or 40%, depending on the orifice selected. This mask is used for COPD patients with CO_2 retention to provide a controlled amount of FIO_2 rather than using nasal prongs. Its disadvantages are that the inspired gas is not completely humidified, and it must fit the face snugly.

Prescription of Oxygen. Oxygen may be prescribed for continuous use, for use during exertion, or for nocturnal use, depending on when the patient is hypoxemic. It should never be given to patients for prophylactic or as-needed use at home. Some patients recuperating from an acute illness may be given short-term home oxygen to treat hypoxemia while their underlying disease improves. The need for long-term oxygen should be determined after the patient is at baseline and on maximal medical therapy.

Third-party payers, including Medicare, have very stringent guidelines for reimbursement of long-term oxygen therapy because of its high cost. Medicare requirements for long-term oxygen are that patients breathing ambient air either (1) have a $PaO_2 < 55$ mm Hg *or* $SaO_2 < 88\%$ or (2) have a PaO_2 56 to 59 mm Hg *and* either cor pulmonale on electrocardiogram or a hematocrit $> 55\%$. In patients with COPD and hypoxemia at rest despite optimal therapy, continuous oxygen (24 hr/day) is more effective than shorter daily durations of treatment at improving survival and neuropsychologic function. The prescribing physician must document the need for oxygen, determine the appropriate flow rate and frequency, and specify the oxygen delivery system. Documentation of continued need for home oxygen in spite of maximal medical therapy is required at frequent intervals.

For patients with hypoxemia only while asleep or with exercise, oxygen should be prescribed for use during sleep or with exertion, respectively, but not at rest. Nocturnal hypoxemia commonly occurs in patients with many lung diseases, even in the absence of sleep apnea. Exertional oxygen also is indicated in patients who are able to be more active when using oxygen, but this improvement should be documented by a 6-minute walk test or exercise oximetry.

Home oxygen can be supplied from liquid oxygen tanks, compressed gas tanks, or oxygen concentrators. Home care companies are reimbursed a fixed amount based on the oxygen flow rate and therefore have a disincentive to provide more expensive oxygen systems that may be of maximal benefit to the patient. The physician must clearly specify and insist on the delivery system that is best for the patient. Tanks are more expensive and require frequent replacement, but small portable "walking tanks" can be filled from the main stationary tank, allowing the patient to leave home and be active. Despite the added cost, liquid oxygen systems are preferred for ambulatory patients, but the prescription must specify the therapeutic purpose and document some benefit. Concentrators are electrically driven devices that concentrate oxygen from the air and provide low-flow oxygen (<2 to 3 L/min) only. For patients who are primarily home bound or bed bound, an oxygen concentrator with extension tubing is adequate and is generally less expensive than tanks. However, the nonreimbursable, added cost of electricity to power these units is sig-

nificant and sometimes must be considered. Small oxygen cylinders that can be used for short excursions out of the home or in case of a mechanical or electrical failure of the concentrator usually should be provided along with a concentrator.

Secretion Clearance and Lung Expansion

Atelectasis—the loss of lung volume—impairs gas exchange, increases the work of breathing, and probably leads to a higher incidence of pneumonia. A variety of therapies attempt to reverse atelectasis by enhancing secretion clearance and by increasing and sustaining inspiratory lung volume. Simple treatments include coughing, deep breathing, mobilizing the patient, incentive spirometry, humidification, and tracheal suctioning. Increasing the tidal volume of breaths by sighs, intentional deep breathing, or incentive spirometry recruits atelectatic alveoli. Dependent regions of the lung are especially prone to atelectasis because they are partially compressed, less well ventilated, and do not spontaneously drain their secretions with gravity. Frequent changes of position distribute the tidal breaths to these previously dependent portions of the lung and assist in clearing secretions. Having the patient sit upright in a chair significantly increases both tidal volume and vital capacity relative to the supine position.

Cough. Cough is probably the most effective way to clear excess secretions from the airway. Aggressive encouragement of coughing by nursing, medical, and respiratory therapy staff is more important than most of the treatment techniques discussed later. Special cough techniques such as quadriplegic coughing or "huff coughing" may be helpful to teach some patients to improve their cough efficacy.

In the past, ultrasonic nebulization of small particles of water or saline commonly was used to induce cough because the particles stimulate tracheal irritant receptors. Many hospitals have discontinued offering this treatment because it is not very effective, it is expensive, and it has the significant side effect of triggering bronchospasm. However, ultrasonic nebulization of hypertonic saline increases the diagnostic yield of sputum induction for *Pneumocytis carinii* and *Mycobacterium tuberculosis*. It also may be worth an empiric trial of ultrasonic saline nebulization to induce cough in comatose patients.

Tracheal Suction. Suctioning of the trachea through the nose or mouth may help patients who cannot cough effectively by both stimulating cough and removing excess secretions that are within reach of the catheter. Harmful side effects include (1) tracheal damage that may result in bleeding or predispose to infection, (2) hypoxemia, (3) arrhythmias resulting from autonomic reflexes, (4) apnea, and (5) contamination of the lower respiratory tract. The right mainstem bronchus is more frequently entered than the left, but by turning the head to the right and/or using a special angled suction catheter, the left mainstem bronchus can be entered more easily.

Humidification. The upper airway provides very efficient humidification of gases reaching the lower airway, preventing mucosal drying and inspissation of mucus. For patients who are intubated or have a tracheotomy, inspired gas must be fully saturated with molecular (nonparticulate) water. For nonintubated patients, systemic hydration is probably the best way to avoid dessication of secretions. Patients with bronchospasm may benefit from using heated jet nebulizers to humidify their supplemental oxygen because of the higher water vapor pressure and content in the warm gas. Inadequately humidified air may trigger airway hyperreactivity. Nebulized saline, a suspended particulate, does not thin secretions or aid in their clearance. Nebulized water, hypotonic saline, or hypertonic saline do not thin secretions, and all can precipitate bronchospasm.

Incentive Spirometry. Incentive spirometers permit the patient to visually judge inspiratory effort. The patient is encouraged to inhale rapidly for as long as possible, thereby achieving a maximal inspiratory volume. This is one of the best ways to reverse or prevent atelectasis. Once taught properly, the motivated patient can use it with little supervision. In the motivated patient, it is as effective at preventing postoperative pulmonary complications as other more complicated and time-consuming measures. A recent adaptation is to place a one-way valve on the device that blocks expiration. This allows the patient to make several "stacked" inspiratory efforts, leading to a higher cumulative lung volume, a strategy that may be particularly useful in patients with respiratory muscle weakness.

Positive Airway Pressure (PAP) and Intermittent Positive Pressure Breathing (IPPB). These modalities expand the lung and augment the functional residual capacity either by continuous PAP (CPAP) or by augmenting the inspiratory effort with IPPB. CPAP uses a tight-fitting facial or nasal mask to continuously apply PAP and decrease lung collapse during expiration. Nasal CPAP also is used to treat sleep apnea.

With IPPB a pressure-limited ventilator delivers a rapid inflow of gas into the mouth until the preset pressure limit is reached, but the volume of gas administered is not regulated. IPPB once was widely used for patients with COPD or atelectasis, especially to nebulize aerosol medications; little or no objective benefit either of IPPB alone or as a method of medication delivery was shown in controlled studies. Consequently, it should be used only for the cooperative patient who is too weak to inspire effectively and who has a documented increase of tidal volume during and/or after treatment. With an increased tidal volume, IPPB can help reverse atelectasis, rest the respiratory muscles, or transiently prevent the need for intubation. Contraindications to IPPB include pneumothorax, bullous lung disease, asthma, recent esophageal or gastric surgery, cardiac dysfunction, and an uncooperative patient.

Recently, nasal or face masks have been used to deliver several new types of IPPB. Tight-fitting CPAP masks have been connected to mechanical ventilators and have provided positive pressure ventilation for 24 to 48 hours to treat nonintubated patients with rapidly reversible respiratory failure or congestive heart failure. Newer compact pressure ventilators provide different levels of inspiratory and expiratory pressure (bilevel PAP or Bi-PAP) to either nasal or face masks. Bi-PAP machines can provide nocturnal ventilation for patients with respiratory muscle fatigue or chronic respiratory failure, thereby avoiding tracheotomy. They also may obviate the need for intubation of some patients with acute respiratory failure by resting the respiratory muscles.

Postural Drainage. Postural drainage (PD) involves having the patient lie down in positions that encourage passive gravity drainage of secretions from either the segmental or lobar bronchi. It is frequently combined with chest percussion or vibration, but this is not required. Sometimes PD is applied selectively to drain secretions from a region that has pneumonia, atelectasis, or a lung abscess. At other times it is applied to all of the lung segments in sequence.

Postural drainage is reasonable to use for patients with the following:

1. COPD, who produce more than 30 ml/day of sputum
2. Bronchiectasis
3. Cystic fibrosis
4. Pneumonia, who cannot cough or spontaneously clear their secretions, especially with neuromuscular disorders or a depressed level of consciousness
5. Atelectasis not reversed by incentive spirometry and other simple measures
6. Lung abscess

If these conditions are chronic, these patients and their families should be taught these techniques for regular outpatient use. Prophylactic treatment of intubated patients with PD to compensate for their diminished ability to cough is sometimes done, but this has not been rigorously demonstrated to be helpful. For hospitalized patients with one or more of the preceding indications, PD should be given as an empiric trial and discontinued if there is no beneficial response. There is no clear benefit of PD beyond incentive spirometry, deep breathing, and coughing for most patients with COPD, pneumonia, or routine postoperative care.

Some patients do not tolerate the positions required to achieve effective PD and may become very dyspneic or hypoxemic, especially with addition of percussion or vibration. Increased intracranial pressure is another contraindication to PD.

Chest Percussion and Vibration. These techniques frequently are used in conjunction with PD. They can increase the velocity of tracheal mucus movement up the tracheobronchial tree. However, they also may worsen hypoxemia, especially in patients with hemodynamic instability, low cardiac output, or arrhythmias. Their clinical benefit beyond that from PD has not been established. Rib fractures or recent hemoptysis are additional contraindications. In rare cases, patients with a bacterial lung abscess suddenly drain abscess fluid or blood during PD. If this material spills throughout the tracheobronchial tree, respiratory failure may result.

Mucolytic Agents. Several agents, such as N-acetyl cysteine, disperse mucus plugs in vitro. Direct instillation of this agent through a bronchoscope onto a visible plug may disrupt it. However, N-acetyl cysteine may injure epithelial tissue, especially the cilia, and often stimulates tracheal irritant receptors, causing bronchospasm. Nebulization of mucolytic agents has not been effective in several randomized studies of patients with COPD. Consequently, N-acetyl cysteine should be used cautiously, if at all, in patients with asthma or COPD. If used, treatment should be limited to only a few doses and should be accompanied by bronchodilators. It often is used chronically for patients with cystic fibrosis, but the evidence supporting this practice is not strong.

Extracellular DNA contributes to the viscosity of mucus in chronic lung diseases. Recently, the FDA approved use of aerosolized recombinant human DNAse for treatment of patients with cystic fibrosis because it improves secretion clearance and pulmonary function tests and decreases the frequency of exacerbations requiring hospitalization. Although it also may be useful for some COPD patients, the high cost of regular therapy necessitates careful demonstration of significant benefit.

Iodinated glycerol is an oral agent that increases expectoration of respiratory tract secretions and may aid liquification of mucus in patients with chronic bronchitis. It improved cough frequency and severity and eased clearing of secretions in a randomized, double-blind controlled study, although there were no improvements in objective measures of pulmonary function. The lack of improvement in pulmonary function may be related to concomitant stimulation of mucus secretion by this drug. Other expectorants, such as guaifenesin and supersaturated solutions of potassium iodide (SSKI), stimulate sputum clearance but also increase bronchial gland mucus production and secretion. Their overall clinical efficacy, however, has not yet been defined with careful clinical studies.

Nebulized and Aerosolized Medications

Aerosolized β-adrenergic, anticholinergic, and steroid medications are mainstays of therapy of asthma and other forms of obstructive airways disease. They also are indicated for some parenchymal lung diseases. Nebulized ribavirin is used for treatment of respiratory syncytial virus, pentamidine is used as prophylaxis against *Pneumocystis* pneumonia in HIV-infected patients, and aerosolized surfactant compounds are used for neonatal respiratory distress syndrome. Use of specific drugs is discussed in chapters focusing on the diseases treated.

Three different delivery systems are available: nebulizers (jets and ultrasonics), metered dose inhalers (MDIs), and dry-powder inhalers (DPIs). Each method has advantages and disadvantages, the delivery system must be individualized for the specific patient and medication.

The deposition of aerosolized medications in the lung is affected by the characteristics of the particle generated, the ventilatory pattern, and the airway geometry. Particles with a mass median aerodynamic diameter (MMAD) between 2 and 5 μm are optimal to deliver drugs to the airways, whereas particles with an MMAD of between 0.8 and 3 μm are optimal for drug delivery to the alveoli. Particles larger than 5 μm are filtered by the upper airway. Inspiratory flow rates of approximately 0.5 liters appear to be best for aerosols generated by MDIs and nebulizers, whereas higher flow rates are required for DPIs. Aerosol deposition is adversely affected by the decreased airway diameter present in patients with airflow obstruction. Endotracheal tubes significantly decrease the delivery of aerosolized medications to the lower respiratory tract.

MDIs are the delivery system of choice for most outpatients because of their convenience, relatively high lung deposition (10% to

15%), and low cost. Holding chambers or spacers reduce oropharyngeal deposition of drug and make timing easier to coordinate. Spacers limit the systemic absorption of inhaled corticosteroids and decrease the incidence of steroid-induced oral candidiasis and dysphonia. Spacers with MDIs may be as effective as nebulizers in cooperative hospitalized patients with acute airflow obstruction. The major disadvantage of MDIs is that most devices require the patient to coordinate actuation with the initiation of inspiration and then to perform a 4- to 10-second breath-hold. Other limitations include the limited number of available medications, the inconvenience associated with higher dosage regimens, and the dependence on chlorofluorocarbons as propellants. Their ease of use may promote overusage and side effects, particularly from β-adrenergic agonists.

DPIs, such as "spinhalers," are actuated as the patient initiates inspiration, improving the ease of administration, but they require an inspiratory flow rate higher than what some patients are able to generate. Deposition appears to be equivalent to a properly used MDI. The disadvantages of DPIs are (1) limited numbers of medications are available for use with this system, (2) heavy oropharyngeal deposition may occur, and (3) high-humidity environments may cause clumping of the particles, preventing the use of DPIs in humidified ventilator circuits.

Nebulizers can deliver larger volumes and higher doses of medication than MDIs or DPIs and can be used in patients who are too ill or who otherwise are unable to effectively use an MDI. A larger number of medications are available for nebulization, and medications intended for parenchymal deposition (pentamidine and ribavirin) must be delivered by a nebulizer. However, the fractional lung deposition is low (2% to 10%), requiring longer administration time, more medication, and therefore increased cost. There is also the risk of microbial contamination of the aerosol or aerosol generator.

Both MDIs and nebulizers can be used in intubated patients, but dose adjustments are probably necessary to compensate for the deposition of drug in the circuit and on the endotracheal tube.

Pulmonary Rehabilitation

Pulmonary rehabilitation incorporates a multispecialty, interdisciplinary approach to treating patients with respiratory disease and their families, with the goals of achieving maximal independence and function in the community. Components include exercise conditioning, breathing retraining, education, smoking cessation, oxygen therapy, optimizing medication therapy, and psychosocial support. Evidence indicates that pulmonary rehabilitation improves quality of life and function in patients with COPD, but its benefit for other pulmonary diseases and its impact on health care utilization require further study. Unfortunately, many insurers do not cover the cost of pulmonary rehabilitation.

RESPIRATORY MONITORING

Noninvasive respiratory monitoring has increased markedly in the last 10 years. New methods monitor the pattern of breathing, including respiratory rate, tidal volume, and activity and synchrony of chest wall and abdominal muscles. Most useful are noninvasive determinations of the arterial blood percentage saturation with oxygen (SaO_2 and the end-tidal CO_2 level).

Oximetry

This technique uses the different absorption spectra of oxyhemoglobin and deoxyhemoglobin to determine the percentage of heme sites occupied with oxygen. Light of several wavelengths is passed through thin tissues of the earlobe, finger, toe, or nasal bridge to obtain this ratio. Pulse oximetry uses plethysmographic techniques to eliminate the absorption contributed by nonpulsatile blood in the tissue. This direct measurement of hemoglobin SaO_2 avoids the problems encountered in using calculated saturations from ABG results. However, special situations may result in erroneous oximetric SaO_2 measurements. Poor tissue perfusion, strenuous exertion, the presence of other pigments in the skin or blood, and pulsatile venous blood flow all may cause inaccurate readings. Abnormal hemoglobin levels also may affect the accuracy of the saturation measurement.

Measurements may be made continuously or at a single point in time as a substitute for ABG studies. Because oximetry does not accurately distinguish PaO_2 levels above 60 torr, its utility is restricted to ensuring that a patient does not have life-threatening hypoxemia or titrating the FIO_2 in a patient with a low SaO_2. It is useful for monitoring patients during anesthesia or procedures and for detecting nocturnal hypoxemia during sleep. It is not appropriate, however, as a replacement for an ABG in the initial assessment of dyspneic patients with lung or heart disease or of patients with significant metabolic derangements because it does not provide information about the pH or $PaCO_2$. Large changes in PaO_2 above 70 torr are not detected because hemoglobin is fully saturated in this range. Finally, in monitoring the patient who is difficult to wean from a ventilator or who has recently been extubated, oximetry alone is not sufficient because it will not detect CO_2 retention. Nonetheless, oximetry is extremely useful and decreases the need for ABG measurements, as long as it is used appropriately.

Capnography or End Tidal CO₂ Measurement

Methods to continuously measure the exhaled CO_2 pressure using either mass spectrometry or absorption of infrared light are becoming widespread, especially for intubated patients. The end-tidal PCO_2 ($P_{et}CO_2$) closely approximates the arterial PCO_2 if (1) there is complete equilibration of CO_2 across the alveolar capillary unit, (2) there is little physiologic right-to-left shunt, (3) there is uniform mixing of the exhaled gas, and (4) alveolar dead space is not significantly increased. A tracing of the exhaled wave form of PCO_2 over time should have a late expiratory plateau, indicating complete mixing. In the presence of severe lung disease or sepsis, there may be incomplete equilibration, resulting in an arterial to end-tidal CO_2 gradient. The CO_2 wave form may be altered in characteristic ways in different types of lung disease that suggest, for example, the presence of physiologic dead space resulting from pulmonary embolism. Capnography is a useful adjunct to oximetry in monitoring intubated patients during ventilator changes, weaning, procedures, or anesthesia. Better methods for obtaining reliable measurements of $P_{et}CO_2$ in nonintubated patients will be useful in caring for patients with COPD or neuromuscular disorders.

Other Monitoring Techniques

The evaluation of respiratory muscle strength and endurance is important in assessing the risk of respiratory failure in patients with neuromuscular disease such as Guillain-Barré syndrome, polymyositis, and muscular dystrophy. Maximal inspiratory airway pressure (MIP) and vital capacity (VC) are global measures of respiratory muscle strength that can be repeatedly measured at the bedside of these patients. Significant reductions in VC (<600 ml) and MIP (<20 cm H_2O) indicate severe impairment of respiratory muscle function and may be more sensitive indicators of the need for intubation than ABG studies in these patients. However, these measurements require standardized techniques and full patient cooperation.

Abnormal respiratory patterns may also predict impending respiratory failure. Respiratory inductive plethysmography provides a noninvasive method of continuously monitoring the respiratory pattern in spontaneously breathing patients. The simultaneous recording of movements of both the rib cage and abdominal compartments can detect abnormal patterns such as paradoxical motion (abdomen and rib cage moving in opposite directions) or asynchrony (time lag between motion of the rib cage and the abdomen). Indices that quantitate the degree of abnormal breathing may be useful in monitoring patients with respiratory impairment, but the equipment is expensive, and the bands placed around the rib cage and abdomen are easily dislodged.

BIBLIOGRAPHY

Aerosol Consensus Statement, *Chest* 100(4):1106-1109, 1991.
ATS Statement: Standards for the diagnosis and care of patients with chronic obstructive pulmonary disease, *Am J Respir Crit Care Med* 152:S78-S121, 1995.
Bach JR: Update and perspective on use of respiratory muscle aids. Part 1: The inspiratory aids and Part 2: The expiratory aids, *Chest* 105:1230-1240, 1538-1544, 1994.
Brochard L et al: Noninvasive ventilation for acute exacerbations of chronic obstructive pulmonary disease, *N Engl J Med* 333:817-822, 1995.

Celli BR: Pulmonary rehabilitation in patients with COPD, *Am J Respir Crit Care Med* 152:861-864, 1995.

Eid N et al: Chest physiotherapy in review, *Respir Care* 36:270-282, 1991.

Marini JJ, Pierson DJ, and Hudson LD: Acute lobar atelectasis: a prospective comparison of fiberoptic bronchoscopy and respiratory therapy, *Amer Rev Respir Dis* 119:971-978, 1979.

Nelson HS: Beta-adrenergic bronchodilators, *N Engl J Med* 333:499-506, 1995.

O'Donohue WT: Prescribing home oxygen therapy, *Arch Intern Med* 152:746-748, 1992.

Pierson DJ, Kacmarek RM, editors: *Foundations of respiratory care,* New York, 1992, Churchill Livingstone.

Tarpy SP, Celli BR: Long term oxygen therapy, *N Engl J Med* 333:710-714, 1995.

Tobin MJ: Respiratory monitoring in the intensive care unit, *Am Rev Respir Dis* 138:1625-1642, 1988.

50 Pulmonary Rehabilitation

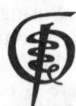

Barry J. Make

Many of the patients with lung disease encountered by internal medicine physicians during the course of daily office practices have chronic and incurable illnesses. Chronic obstructive pulmonary disease (COPD) and asthma are two such pulmonary disorders. Although asthma is potentially reversible with appropriate medications, the symptoms of dyspnea, cough, and sputum production seen in patients with COPD are often substantially unchanged with standard bronchodilator therapy. Pulmonary rehabilitation employs ancillary health care professionals, such as respiratory therapists, physical therapists, occupational therapists, and nurses, to apply scientific therapeutic principles to decrease the impact of the disease on these patients. Pulmonary rehabilitation has recently been defined by a National Institutes of Health Workshop as a "multidimensional continuum of services directed to persons with pulmonary disease and their families, usually by an interdisciplinary team of specialists, with the goal of achieving and maintaining the individual's maximum level of independence and functioning in the community." There are several important concepts embodied in this definition. First, pulmonary rehabilitation should not be considered as only a single limited intervention but rather as incorporating a lifelong set of therapies based on the patient's needs. Second, implicit in this definition is the recognition that the treatment of each patient is unique, the rehabilitation program being tailored to each individual. The practice of pulmonary rehabilitation requires that success be defined for each individual. Goals desirable for one person may be unattainable or undesirable for another. A third corollary is that the whole patient is treated, and as a result, improvement may occur in several spheres simultaneously, making it difficult to attribute increased functional capacity to any single rehabilitation component.

Broad goals for pulmonary rehabilitation may be defined. In general, attention is directed toward achieving maximum reversibility of airflow limitation, preventing and treating complications of the patient's underlying disease, and improving quality of life. An argument can be made that these are in fact the goals of any internist treating lung disease, and that formal rehabilitation programs are therefore unnecessary. Indeed, the principles of pulmonary rehabilitation should be considered in the management of all patients with respiratory disease. Although many of the medical and educational aspects of pulmonary rehabilitation may be applied by any well-trained internist, a formal program may involve input from a large number of highly specialized personnel who devote a significant portion of their time and effort to pulmonary rehabilitation. For a single practitioner to duplicate that input is enormously time-consuming on a per patient basis and may not represent optimal use of his or her time. Moreover, formal programs usually have concentrated patient educational resources and have developed efficient teaching techniques based on their experiences. Such programs are most often under the direction of a pulmonary specialist whose major interest lies in this area and who devotes significant amounts of time to patients undergoing rehabilita-

tion. Clearly, decisions regarding when and whether to refer are colored by multiple factors. Among these factors are availability of such programs in the area, patient financial resources, patient willingness to participate in a program, and desire of the individual practitioner to take advantage of a formal program instead of providing similar services himself or herself.

BENEFITS OF PULMONARY REHABILITATION

The distressing and fear-provoking symptom of shortness of breath likely leads to depression. Moreover, anxiety and emotions can precipitate shortness of breath. In addition, patients seek to reduce dyspnea by limiting their activity, which leads to deconditioning and actually increases dyspnea associated with activity. This sequence of events has been termed the *vicious cycle of dyspnea* (Fig. 50-1). Well-designed trials have demonstrated improvement as a result of both outpatient and inpatient pulmonary rehabilitation programs in the areas shown in Box 50-1. For example, a study reported from southern California demonstrated that pulmonary rehabilitation improves exercise capacity and reduces dyspnea in patients with COPD compared with patients who received education without exercise training (Fig. 50-2). The improved maximum exercise capacity and exercise endurance demonstrated by objective exercise testing leads to an improvement in more functional physical activities such as walking. Pulmonary rehabilitation is also associated with improved perception of quality of life in patients with COPD.

BOX 50-1
Benefits of pulmonary rehabilitation

Decreased respiratory symptoms
Decreased shortness of breath with activity and exercise

Improved exercise capacity
Increased peak oxygen consumption
Increased exercise duration
Decreased lactate production during exercise
Reduced ventilatory demand during exercise
Improved functional capacity (e.g. for walking)

Improved health-related quality of life
Increased perception of physical function
Improved sense of control over illness
Decreased anxiety
Decreased depressive symptoms

Decreased hospitalizations

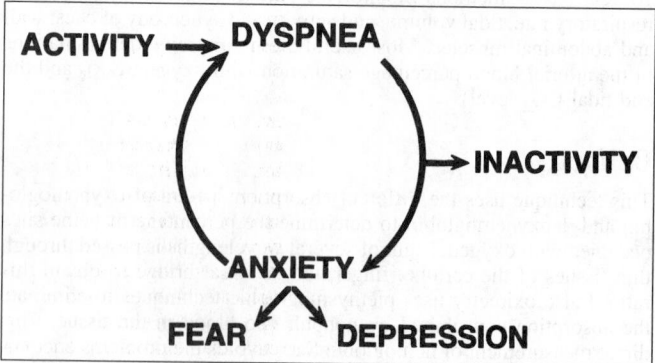

FIGURE 50-1   The vicious cycle of dyspnea. In patients with COPD, activity results in dyspnea; avoidance of dyspnea leads to inactivity, with subsequent deconditioning. Emotions result in dyspnea; dyspnea leads to anxiety, fear, and depression.

(From Make B: *Am Fam Physician* 43:1315, 1991.)

Although it has been clearly shown that chronic use of supplemental oxygen therapy in COPD patients with severe hypoxemia improves survival, there is no convincing evidence that comprehensive pulmonary rehabilitation has any impact on mortality. However, some reports have shown a decrease in hospitalizations following pulmonary rehabilitation. The decreased costs of medical care associated with reduction in hospital days may be substantial.

REFERRAL FOR PULMONARY REHABILITATION

When should patients be referred for pulmonary rehabilitation? The American Thoracic Society's published standards for the management of COPD has adopted a management algorithm that incorporates pulmonary rehabilitation (Fig. 50-3). Based on the benefits of pulmonary rehabilitation outlined previously, pulmonary rehabilitation should be considered in patients with COPD who remain symptomatic after optimal medical therapy including bronchodilators, smoking cessation, and oxygen therapy when appropriate. Because no objective measures of quality of life and dyspnea are universally used as criteria for pulmonary rehabilitation, the patient's perception of these factors is appropriate to determine the need for pulmonary rehabilitation. Although not firmly established, it is reasonable to expect better outcomes over a longer period for those with COPD who receive intervention earlier in the course of their illness. However, it has been clearly shown that rehabilitation benefits even those with very severe disease (forced expiratory volume in 1 second [FEV_1] < 0.5 liters), and these patients have a greater degree of improvement (i.e., a greater percentage change from baseline) than patients with less severe disease. Patients with other respiratory diseases such as cystic fibrosis and asthma have also been shown to benefit from pulmonary rehabilitation.

PROGRAM STRUCTURE

Pulmonary rehabilitation may be conducted on either an inpatient or outpatient basis. The latter is less expensive, yields results similar to those of inpatient programs, and is more cost effective in most circumstances. Inpatient programs allow multiple resources to be applied in a way that is convenient to both the patient and the multiple specialists participating and may be most beneficial for those with severely decreased functional ability. Pulmonary rehabilitation programs should not be thought to be the exclusive province of tertiary care referral hospitals; community-based and even home programs have clearly demonstrated and reported their success.

A typical pulmonary rehabilitation team in a formal program includes a variety of health care professionals. The director is most often a physician respiratory specialist with a particular interest in pulmonary rehabilitation. The day-to-day management of the program may appropriately reside in the hands of a clinical nurse specialist with expertise in respiratory care. A physical therapist may be in charge of a general conditioning program, breathing retraining, chest physical therapy, and an exercise program that may emphasize upper extremity and accessory respiratory musculature as well as standard walking or cycling. Occupational therapists bring special expertise to vocational counseling, and techniques and devices for energy conservation in daily activities. A respiratory therapist with particular interest in the area may be very effective in teaching the use and management of oxygen, inhaled medications, and ancillary equipment. Nutritional expertise may be appropriate not only for patients who are malnourished, but also for those who are affected by postprandial dyspnea. The complexities of medical reimbursement, home assistance, and available community resources may best be managed by a medical social worker. Last, the problems of anxiety, depression, and appropriate use of psychoactive medication may be greatly expedited by consultation with a psychiatrist and an ongoing support group with other patients.

When physician, hospital, and/or community resources are insufficient to support such a personnel-intensive approach, yet a need for pulmonary rehabilitation exists without conveniently available refer-

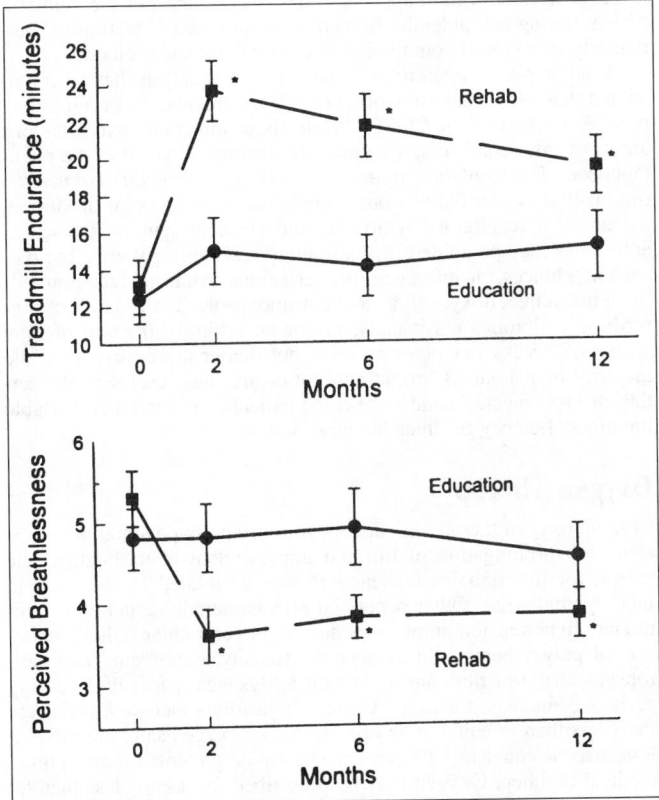

FIGURE 50-2 Improved endurance for walking on a treadmill *(upper panel)* and reduced perception of breathlessness at the end of exercise *(lower panel)* in patients following pulmonary rehabilitation compared with patients receiving an education-only intervention. *, *p* <0.05 for within-group change from preintervention baseline.

(From Ries AL, Kaplan RM, Limberg TM, Prewitt LM: *Ann Intern Med* 122:823, 1995.)

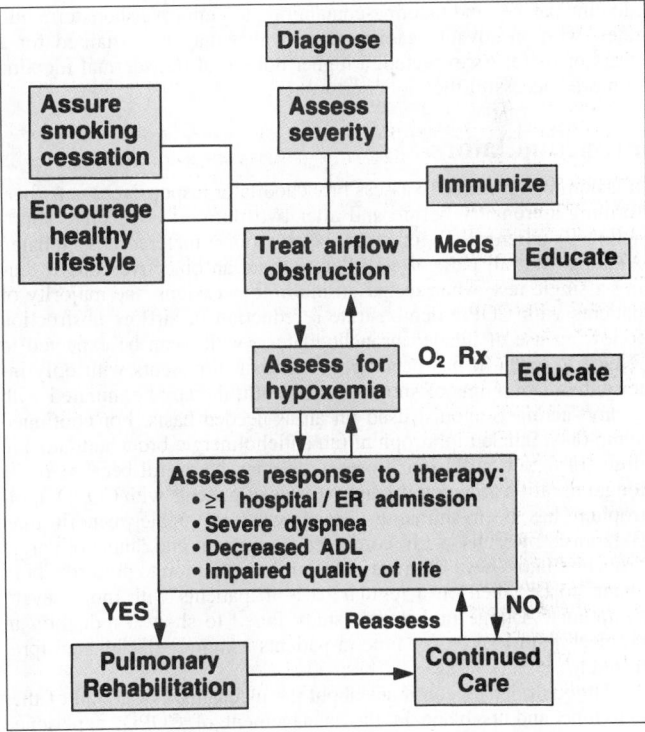

FIGURE 50-3 General management algorithm for patients with COPD.

(Courtesy Barry Make, MD, and National Jewish Medical Center, 1994.)

ral, it may be possible for a smaller number of health care professionals to assume the multiple roles described previously. There is no a priori reason that this cannot be successful; however, the advantages of scale will be lost, the nonspecialist will necessarily have a smaller proportion of time to devote to such a program, and these personnel will likely have less experience and expertise in this area.

MEDICAL INTERVENTION
Baseline Evaluation

Each patient should undergo a thorough baseline evaluation on entry. A careful history and physical examination, chest radiograph, laboratory tests indicated by the history and physical, pulmonary function tests before and after bronchodilator administration, and an exercise test that will provide guidance on the initial exercise intensity, exclude coronary artery disease, and assess hypoxemia constitute an acceptable minimum.

Smoking Cessation

Smoking cessation is of paramount importance. Beneficial effects include a diminished rate of decline of pulmonary function over time and occasional outright improvement; diminished respiratory symptoms, particularly cough; diminished risk of influenza and other viral respiratory infections; and reduced carboxyhemoglobin concentration with subsequent improved oxygen saturation and reduced oxygen requirements in the hypoxemic. Many programs exclude from participation and refer for smoking cessation therapy those who continue to smoke. The ability to end nicotine addiction may be a barometer of motivation and implies greater motivation and compliance with the rehabilitation process. Attempts at smoking cessation may be tailored to the individual's desires and personality. At one extreme, unsupervised efforts may be augmented by written self-help materials such as those available from the American Lung Association. Supervised programs may be medical, with physician advice and monitoring and prescription of medication to reduce symptoms leading to relapse, or primarily psychotherapeutic with group or individual emphasis and adjunctive use of biofeedback, hypnosis, aversive conditioning, and group support. All approaches have reasonable short-term success in motivated individuals, but the recidivism rate is high, and no clear advantage of one approach over another has emerged. Transdermal nicotine patches and nicotine-containing gum improve short-term quit rates, with an advantage over placebo that may be sustained for 2 years or more. As expected, a higher dosage of transdermal nicotine is more successful than a lower dosage.

Bronchodilators

It is common practice to assess bronchodilator responsiveness by performing spirometry before and after two puffs of a selective short-acting β_2-adrenergic agonist delivered from a metered-dose inhaler. Although not all patients will demonstrate an objective benefit during a single test, when tested on multiple occasions, the majority of patients with COPD demonstrate a reduction in airflow obstruction following use of inhaled bronchodilators, which can be expected to reduce dyspnea. It has been suggested that in patients with only intermittent symptoms of shortness of breath, therapy be initiated with a short-acting β-agonist used on an as-needed basis. For continued symptoms, inhaled ipratropium (an anticholinergic bronchodilator) at doses of 4 to 6 puffs four times a day may be useful because of its longer duration of action. In most studies of patients with COPD, ipratropium has been shown to be of equal or greater benefit than β-agonists. Results with combined β-agonist and anticholinergic bronchodilators have been variable, but it is common to prescribe both agents to be taken on a regular basis in patients with more severe symptoms. A large multicenter study failed to show a reduction in the decline in FEV_1 over time in patients using regular inhaled ipratropium.

Although debate continues about the mechanism of action of theophylline and its place in the management of COPD, experience shows that it clearly benefits many patients. Several controlled trials show benefits that include decreased airflow obstruction, increased respiratory muscle strength, and a variable improvement in dyspnea.

Multiple preparations are available; in general, compliance is improved with less frequent administration and minimization of side effects. The former can best be achieved with the use of long-acting preparations and the latter by cautious dosing, aiming for levels somewhat lower (10 to 15 mg/dl) than those traditionally recommended.

Corticosteroids

Although inhaled corticosteroids have clear benefits in patients with asthma by improving airflow and reducing exacerbations, their use in patients with COPD is more controversial. Inhaled antiinflammatory steroids may improve FEV_1 and decrease the number of exacerbations in patients with COPD. Although they may reduce inflammation in the airways, there is no reduction in the decline in FEV_1 over time with the use of inhaled steroids. Several large-scale studies are being conducted to more precisely define the role of these agents.

Patients for whom chronic oral corticosteroids are prescribed indiscriminately may experience adverse effects—Cushing's syndrome, myopathy, hyperglycemia, cataracts, and osteoporosis—without significant benefit. However, 10% to 20% of patients with stable nonasthmatic COPD show objective benefit from corticosteroids. Because it is difficult to predict which individuals will respond, a clinical trial remains the most useful way to select those who should receive steroids. The patient should receive 0.5 mg/kg/day of prednisone for a predetermined length of time, usually 2 to 4 weeks. If no objective pulmonary function benefit occurs, the prednisone should be tapered and discontinued. If, however, clear improvement results, the dose should be gradually reduced to the lowest effective level.

Infectious Complications

Prevention of infection may help to reduce exacerbation of disease. Influenza vaccination given each fall is indicated for this high-risk group of patients; concern regarding elevation of serum theophylline levels postimmunization appears to be unnecessary. For the high-risk patient during an epidemic, flumadine prophylaxis is warranted, particularly in a closed community of the predominately elderly.

A large placebo-controlled trial and metaanalysis have demonstrated that antibiotics are worthwhile in the treatment of acute infectious exacerbations of COPD. While these infectious exacerbations are most often viral, empiric antibiotic therapy directed at the pneumococci, *Haemophilus influenza,* and *Branhamella catarrhalis* (moraxella) is justifiable from a cost-effectiveness point-of-view at the onset of respiratory symptoms and purulent sputum. Choice of antibiotics may be guided by community resistance patterns, but reasonable choices for infrequent exacerbations would include ampicillin, tetracycline, doxycycline, and cotrimoxazole. The practice of prescribing antibiotics chronically, or for an arbitrary fraction of time such as 2 weeks out of every 4, is not demonstrably useful in the majority of patients. Chronic antibiotics are most useful in the setting of bronchiectasis and in selected patients with common variable immunodeficiency or other humoral deficiencies.

Oxygen Therapy

Chronic oxygen therapy in patients with severe hypoxemia is associated with prolongation of life and improvement of its quality. The reason for this remains unclear but may be related to reduction in fatal dysrhythmias. Other beneficial effects include reduction of pulmonary hypertension, improvement in right ventricular failure, reduction of polycythemia and associated viscosity, improvement of neuropsychiatric function, and reduction in dyspnea, particularly during periods of increased activity. Current indications include a persistent PaO_2 less than or equal to 55 mm Hg (or an oxygen saturation [SaO_2] less than or equal to 88%) in chronic stable patients on an optimal medical regimen. Oxygen may be prescribed for a PaO_2 less than 60 mm Hg or an SaO_2 of 89% in those with edema or other physical findings consistent with cor pulmonale, P pulmonale on electrocardiogram (ECG) (P wave greater than 3 mm in leads II, III, and AVF), mental dysfunction, or polycythemia (hematocrit greater than or equal to 56%). Patients with exercise-related desaturation to a PaO_2 $\leq$55 mm Hg or an SaO_2 $\leq$88% are also eligible for chronic oxygen therapy during activity. Individuals who have desaturation to a similar level during sleep and have the end-organ dysfunction listed previously may be candidates for nocturnal oxygen supplementation. A typical oxygen prescription is written for oxygen by nasal cannula at a flow rate sufficient to produce a PaO_2 greater than or equal to 65 mm Hg. Because nocturnal desaturation is common, the flow rate is arbitrarily increased by 1 L/min at night unless recording sleep oximetry demonstrates a different requirement. Because oxygen desaturation is usually worsened by exercise, it is prudent to assess oxygen requirements during activity as well as at rest. Pulse oximetry is a simple and noninvasive method of titrating oxygen flow during activity to ensure a saturation of 90%. In patients with severe hypoxemia, oxygen therapy should be used continuously throughout the day and night and at rest and with activity. As noted in Fig. 50-4, use of continuous oxygen therapy is associated with a reduction in mortality compared to oxygen therapy only used at night.

Home oxygen use is widespread and expensive. As many as 800,000 individuals in the United States may be recipients. Medicare supports approximately 60% of home oxygen use, and as a result, increasing government regulation has been the rule. Reimbursement for chronic oxygen therapy is fixed by Medicare at approximately $300 a month, regardless of the method of delivery. The rate of reimbursement is increased in patients who require higher flows, and a small additional supplement is provided when patients require portable oxygen. Health maintenance organizations are increasingly providing home oxygen through capitated contracts with home care companies.

Because of these considerations, many durable medical equipment vendors prefer to provide the lowest cost system possible. An oxygen concentrator is least costly for the homebound patient requiring low flow rates, and home oxygen delivery is never required. However, because the concentrator is dependent on electricity, a back-up system or home generator may be required in rural areas, and a separate portable system is required to enhance mobility. Compressed gas is widely available and is moderately expensive at low flow rates. Small portable cylinders are available that can provide up to 11 hours of oxygen when low flow rates are used. It is the most expensive method at higher flow rates and requires frequent home deliveries (a large H cylinder lasts about 4½ days at 1 L/min, and correspondingly less at higher flow rates). Liquid oxygen has the advantage of providing a longer-lasting supply (a reservoir may last 2 weeks at 1 L/min). The associated portable system is the lightest, longest-lasting, and thus most compatible with the goals of pulmonary rehabilitation. Although the small "stroller" compressed gas tanks are "portable," they are much less compatible with ambulation than the over-the-shoulder liquid oxygen containers. However, liquid oxygen is expensive, and as a result, in many rural areas liquid oxygen is not available. An additional problem with the liquid oxygen system is that re-filling the portable supply from the main reservoir may be difficult for the relatively infirm.

Patient compliance with continuous oxygen therapy is often limited, in part because of the high cost and symptoms related to mucous membrane drying. For these reasons methods to conserve oxygen have been developed. The most common are nasal cannulae with oxygen reservoirs, which collect the continuously flowing oxygen during patient exhalation and make it available during inhalation, allowing lower flow rates as well as less drying of the nose. Devices that pulse oxygen delivery only during inspiration also reduce oxygen needs, thereby allowing greater patient mobility. Patient compliance may be related to self-consciousness about visibility of oxygen tubing; in such cases systems that conceal or camouflage the reservoir and delivery system are best accepted. According to some investigators, transtracheal catheter oxygen delivery has very high acceptance because of enhanced appearance as well as reduction in oxygen needs and lack of mucous membrane drying. Minute ventilation and work of breathing are clearly reduced by transtracheal administration of oxygen. This method has the disadvantage of requiring a minor surgical procedure, and long-term follow-up from multiple centers is lacking.

EDUCATION

This goal is most effectively achieved when optimal health-related behaviors are enhanced by an education program that incorporates information about the appropriate use of medications including specific information about their dose and timing and instruction in the methods of medication administration. To achieve optimal outcomes, patients should assume responsibility for their health and actively participate in their health care in a cooperative effort with their physician, a process referred to as *collaborative self-management*. Although education alone is ineffective in improving outcomes in patients with COPD, most pulmonary specialists believe education is a necessary component of a comprehensive pulmonary rehabilitation program. In patients with asthma, education has been shown to reduce hospitalizations and use of emergency health care resources.

EXERCISE CONDITIONING

An exercise program is important in rehabilitation as it can clearly increase exercise capacity and reduce dyspnea at a given activity level in COPD (Fig. 50-5). The mechanism(s) for this improvement is

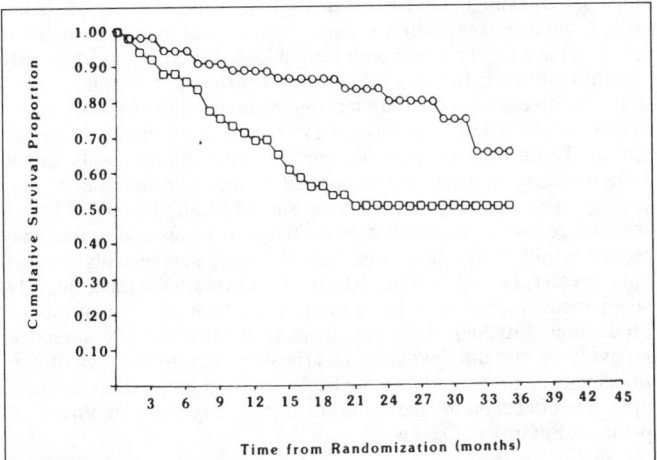

FIGURE 50-4 Cumulative survival of patients with COPD and severe hypoxemia. Use of continuous oxygen therapy *(open circles)* is associated with improved survival compared to use of nocturnal oxygen therapy *(squares)*. (From Nocturnal Oxygen Therapy Trial Group: *Ann Intern Med* 93:391, 1980.)

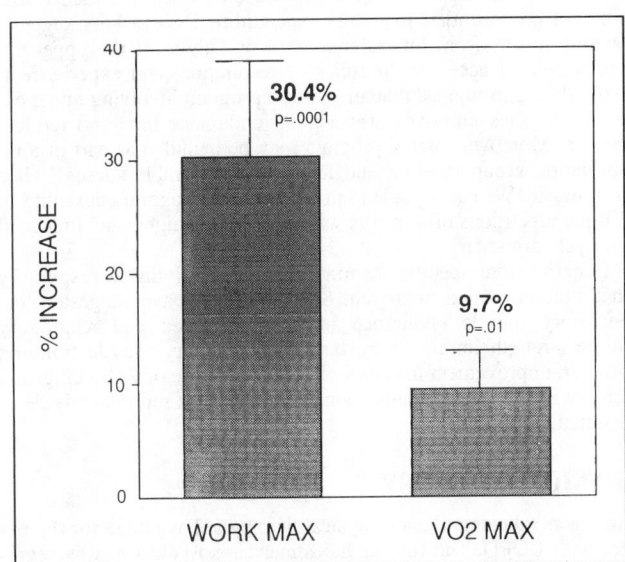

FIGURE 50-5 Improvement in exercise capacity following pulmonary rehabilitation. There was a 30.4% increase in maximum work and 9.7% increase in maximum oxygen consumption on bicycle ergometry testing in 26 COPD patients completing a 3-week rehabilitation program at the National Jewish Medical and Research Center.

Table 50-1   Advantages and disadvantages of exercise training methods

METHOD	ADVANTAGES	DISADVANTAGES
Treadmill	Effective	Expensive
	Easy to learn	Labor intensive
	Direct supervision required	Equipment is physically large
Bicycle	Effective	Moderately expensive
	Cheaper than treadmill	Moderately labor intensive
	May be used at home	
12-minute walk	Effective	Less supervision required
	Simple	Requires more patient self-motivation
	Inexpensive	
	No equipment required	
	Home or hospital based	

From Make BJ, O'Brien R: Pulmonary rehabilitation: an adjunct to the management of patients with chronic obstructive pulmonary disease. In Brody JS, Snider GL, editors: *Current topics in the management of respiratory diseases,* New York, 1985, Churchill Livingstone.

somewhat unclear, as improvement occurs at levels of exercise not ordinarily associated with a training effect in individuals without lung disease. Traditional programs concentrate on lower extremity exercise, in various combinations of free walking, treadmill walking, and stationary cycling. Each has advantages and disadvantages (Table 50-1). Improvement in one form of exercise may transfer poorly to other forms, and thus the advantage of free walking is that it is a useful activity in daily life, with improved capacity resulting in concrete benefits. Walking also requires no special equipment, and improvement is easy to measure as the distance achieved in either 6 or 12 minutes of continuous walking. An exercise prescription should be formulated after a baseline exercise study that includes at least heart rate, electrocardiographic monitoring, and oximetry for detection of exercise oxygen desaturation. A typical training schedule should involve performance of the selected exercise repetitively to the level of dyspnea, for at least 20 minutes four times weekly. Three weeks or more should be allowed for improvement and a maintenance exercise regimen followed thereafter. Figure 50-5 depicts the results of the National Jewish rehabilitation program.

Increasing interest has focused on the benefits of upper extremity exercise. It has long been noted that activities of daily life involving elevation of the upper extremities produce dyspnea in patients with COPD disproportionate to energy expenditure. Recent work suggests that this results from interference with or fatigue of the upper extremity–related accessory muscles of respiration, and experience is accumulating to suggest that an exercise program involving upper extremity muscles improves arm activity endurance time and reduces dyspnea. Moreover, such a program may be included as part of a rehabilitation group meeting and has had considerable success when set to music. We use a graded upper extremity program consisting of multiple repetitions of arm lifts with very light weights and unloaded arm cycle ergometry.

Benefits from specific inspiratory muscle training in respiratory rehabilitation remain unproven. Several studies have suggested that ventilatory muscle endurance may be enhanced and respiratory muscle strength improved by targeted inspiratory muscle training; however, improvement in exercise capability, sense of well-being, and increase in activities of daily living have not been reproducibly demonstrated.

PHYSICAL THERAPY

Three general categories of physical therapy are available for the patient with COPD. The first includes measures to clear airway secretions. Removing excess poorly cleared sputum is theoretically attractive, as it may reduce airway resistance, decrease ventilation-perfusion mismatch, improve oxygenation, and perhaps prevent infection. The most frequent methods are postural drainage alone or with chest percussion and/or vibration. Available evidence does not demonstrate fewer hospitalizations, diminished morbidity, or lesser

mortality in those receiving chest physical therapy and is supportive of its use only in those producing more than 30 ml of sputum daily, a situation uncommon in COPD. These techniques may be aided by reduction of viscosity with adequate hydration and perhaps mucolytics, reduction of airway irritation by elimination of tobacco and other inhalant exposure, and improving mucociliary clearance with theophylline and inhaled β_2 agonists.

A second category of physical therapy is breathing retraining. Although exercises aimed at emphasizing "diaphragmatic" breathing have been used for more than 40 years, little objective evidence is available to show improved function. A variety of postures and exercises have been described but appear to be useful chiefly in giving the patient a sense of control over dyspnea. Pursed-lip breathing is likewise standard. It diminishes minute ventilation with a larger tidal volume but lower respiratory rate and may be useful in allowing exhalation to a lower functional residual capacity by diminishing airway collapse, with the result being more advantageous respiratory muscle position and reduced work of breathing. Its most useful role is to reduce dyspnea.

Last, relaxation techniques such as internal visualization of a pleasant setting may be useful in giving patients another tool to control episodic nonexertional dyspnea.

OCCUPATIONAL THERAPY

Energy conservation techniques allow the COPD patient to accomplish more with less energy expenditure. Occupational therapists are experts in teaching patients how to plan tasks to eliminate unnecessary or duplicative effort, to work in the most efficient posture, and to proceed at a realistic pace. Evaluation of the patient's activities at work or at home may allow the use of work-reducing assistive devices. For example, kitchen work may be performed using a high chair with the opportunity to support the upper extremities on either the counter or the chair arms, rather than standing. Power kitchen appliances such as an electric can opener may reduce dyspnea-producing upper extremity work. The shelf storage may be rearranged to reduce walking and reaching, and long-handled gripping devices may be substituted for climbing. Similar principles may be applied to many other forms of work and activities of daily living.

NUTRITIONAL EVALUATION AND THERAPY

More than 30% of patients with severe COPD have evidence of significant protein-calorie malnutrition. The causes for this malnutrition are poorly understood and probably multiple. Patients with severe hyperinflation commonly have increased dyspnea after a meal, and the resultant decrease in intake may contribute to poor nutrition. Although no data show that nutritional repletion reduces mortality in COPD, it is clear that malnutrition has multiple negative effects on pulmonary function. Diaphragmatic and other respiratory muscle function is impaired, immune competence is compromised, and overall mortality is increased in COPD patients with weight loss. Actual versus ideal body weight (assuming freedom from edema) provides a simple, reasonably sensitive screen for long-term nutritional status. Patients whose actual weight is less than 90% of ideal need more thorough investigation. Those patients who become dyspneic during meals should have oximetry to detect the occasional patient who becomes hypoxemic with eating. Nutritional therapy should ideally be guided by nutritional consultation. Smaller, more frequent meals and snacks may reduce mealtime dyspnea. High-calorie dietary supplements may enable greater calorie intake. Relatively low-carbohydrate, high-fat supplements may reduce the respiratory quotient and carbon dioxide production. Although these supplements are theoretically attractive, no evidence currently available clearly shows long-term benefit. Optimization of the underlying medical condition and minimization of drug side effects on the gastrointestinal tract may allow improved appetite and nutritional status.

PSYCHOSOCIAL MANAGEMENT

The vicious cycle of dyspnea evoking anxiety, which provokes further dyspnea, is familiar to most clinicians. Decreased physical activity leads to an increasingly reclusive life-style, and the patient's social circle becomes progressively restricted. Diminished self-esteem is frequent and is made worse if employment is no longer possible. Reactive depression is thus very common (42% in the Nocturnal Oxygen Therapy Trial). Life-threatening depression is uncommon and is best approached by formal psychiatric evaluation and therapy. The much more common anxiety and reactive depression are more usefully managed by specific rehabilitation measures and support. However, an experienced psychiatric consultant often provides great help in separating the two groups, guiding psychopharmacotherapy, and identifying psychosocial obstacles to rehabilitation. Rehabilitation, as described previously, and breathing retraining may help the patient regain a sense of control, reducing anxiety. Both education and exercise training may result in desensitization to symptoms. Meditation as an approach to relaxation training may be useful. Group meetings provide for the sympathetic support of the rehabilitation staff as well as the opportunity to share experiences, problems, solutions, and often friendship with similarly afflicted peers.

SPECIALIZED PULMONARY REHABILITATION

Patients with problems other than COPD may benefit from the services of specialized pulmonary rehabilitation units. Those with early respiratory failure from skeletal and chest wall deformities (e.g., kyphoscoliosis and thoracoplasty) and neuromuscular disease (e.g., postpolio syndrome, muscular dystrophy, and high spinal cord injury) may be helped to remain at home with partial ventilatory support. Although negative pressure ventilation retains a role in this regard, its use is complicated by difficulties of application, particularly in the neuromuscularly impaired, and by its proclivity for inducing upper airway obstruction during sleep. A growing body of literature demonstrates that noninvasive positive-pressure ventilation, most often delivered via nasal mask, may be a reasonable nocturnal substitute for a significant number of these patients. Nocturnal hypoventilation is prevented, and respiratory muscles are rested. Patients may become demonstrably stronger during the daytime, and gas exchange often returns toward normal during waking hours. Moreover, quality of life may be significantly improved. A smaller proportion of these patients may benefit from nocturnal ventilation via tracheostomy. Last, as respiratory failure progresses, these patients may have very productive lives with complete, tracheostomy-delivered positive-pressure ventilation. Portable ventilators and motorized wheelchairs allow considerable mobility, and many patients may have normal speech during mechanical ventilation through the use of a variety of techniques.

A real but more limited role exists for home management of partially or completely ventilator-dependent patients with COPD. Medical intensive care has resulted in an increasing number of these chronically ventilator-dependent patients; as they become otherwise medically stable, options for continued care include an acute care hospital, a chronic care hospital, a skilled nursing facility, or their own home. It is estimated that there are more than 11,400 ventilator-dependent patients in U.S. hospitals. The care and maintenance of such individuals in the home is a labor-intensive effort that requires the coordinated skills of many of the individuals mentioned earlier in this chapter, with overall care directed by a skilled and motivated pulmonary subspecialist.

FOLLOW-UP CARE

Patients who have completed the formal rehabilitation program need continued follow-up. Those with relatively stable COPD may be seen regularly in the outpatient setting by a physician and/or nurse clinician. In addition to standard management of the lung disease, each visit should be used to reinforce the teachings of the formal program. Retention of knowledge and skills should be gently tested and emphasis given where needed. Those requiring home oxygen and home respiratory devices require periodic visits and assessment by the responsible home care company, whose reports should be examined by the physician. Patients who need physical therapy, or whose status is more tenuous, benefit from regular assessment and care from the personnel of the local visiting nurse association. Their services may allow the patient to remain in the home, and thoughtful attention to their reports and calls facilitates this.

BIBLIOGRAPHY

Anthonisen NR et al: Antibiotic therapy in exacerbations of chronic obstructive pulmonary disease, *Ann Intern Med* 106:196, 1987.

Anthonisen NR, Connett JE, Kiley JP et al: Effects of smoking intervention and the use of an inhaled anticholinergic bronchodilator on the rate of decline of FEV₁: the lung health study, *JAMA* 272:1497, 1994.

Callahan C, Dittus RS, Katz BP: Oral corticosteroid therapy for patients with stable chronic obstructive pulmonary disease: a meta-analysis, *Ann Intern Med* 114:216, 1991.

Celli BR, Snider GL, Heffner J et al: Standards for the diagnosis and care of patients with chronic obstructive pulmonary disease, *Am J Respir Crit Care Med* 152:S77, 1995.

Fishman AP: NIH workshop summary: pulmonary rehabilitation research, *Am J Respir Crit Care Med* 149:825, 1994.

Foster S, Thompson HM: Pulmonary rehabilitation in lung disease other than chronic obstructive pulmonary disease, *Am Rev Respir Dis* 141:601, 1990.

Goldstein RS, Gort EH, Stubbing D et al: Randomised controlled trial of respiratory rehabilitation, *Lancet* 344:1394, 1994.

Koltke TE, Battista RN, DeFriese GH: Attributes of successful smoking cessation interventions in medical practice: a meta-analysis of 39 controlled trials, *JAMA* 259:2882, 1988.

Make B: Collaborative self-management strategies for patients with respiratory disease, *Respir Care* 39:566, 1994.

Niederman MS et al: Benefits of a multidisciplinary pulmonary rehabilitation program. Improvements are independent of lung function, *Chest* 99:798, 1991.

Nocturnal Oxygen Therapy Trial Group: Continuous or nocturnal oxygen therapy in hypoxemic chronic obstructive lung disease, *Ann Intern Med* 93:391, 1980.

Ries AL: Scientific basis of pulmonary rehabilitation, *J Cardiopulmonary Rehabil* 10:418, 1990.

Ries AL, Kaplan RM, Limberg TM, Prewitt LM: Effects of pulmonary rehabilitation on physiologic and psychosocial outcomes in patients with chronic obstructive pulmonary disease, *Ann Intern Med* 122:823, 1995.

Saint S, Bent S, Vittinghoff E, Grady D: Antibiotics in chronic obstructive pulmonary disease exacerbations: a meta-analysis, *JAMA* 273:957, 1995.

Smith K, Cook D, Guyatt GH et al: Respiratory muscle training in chronic airflow limitation: a meta-analysis, *Am Rev Respir Dis* 145:533, 1992.

Wedzicha JA: Inhaled corticosteroids in COPD: awaiting controlled trials (editorial), *Thorax* 48:305, 1993.

Weill D, Make B: Oxygen-conserving devices. In O'Donohue WJ, editor: *Long-term oxygen therapy: scientific basis and clinical application*, New York, 1995, Marcel Dekker.

IV SPECIFIC DISEASE ENTITIES

CHAPTER

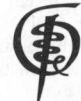

51 Chronic Obstructive Pulmonary Disease

Gordon L. Snider

DEFINITION

The term *chronic obstructive pulmonary disease* (COPD) has recently been defined by the American Thoracic Society as a disease state characterized by the presence of airflow obstruction due to chronic bronchitis or emphysema; the airflow obstruction is generally progressive, may be accompanied by airways hyperreactivity (Chapter 188), and may be partially reversible.

Chronic Bronchitis

Chronic bronchitis is defined as the presence of chronic productive cough that does not result from a medically discernible cause (e.g., tuberculosis, lung cancer) and that has been present for an extended period. For clinical purposes, "extended period" may be defined as the presence of symptoms in the patient half of the time for 2 years. This definition is based on symptoms. No known specific basis should exist for the sputum production that is the defining characteristic of chronic bronchitis.

Emphysema

Emphysema is defined as abnormal permanent enlargement of the air spaces distal to the terminal bronchioles accompanied by destruction of their walls and without obvious fibrosis. *Destruction* is defined as nonuniformity in the pattern of respiratory air space enlargement; the orderly appearance of the acinus is disturbed and may be lost.

AIRFLOW OBSTRUCTION

Chronic bronchitis and emphysema may occur with or without airflow obstruction. However, it is airflow obstruction that causes disability and death, and the diagnosis of COPD is made only if airflow obstruction is present. Asthma, by definition (Chapter 188), is always

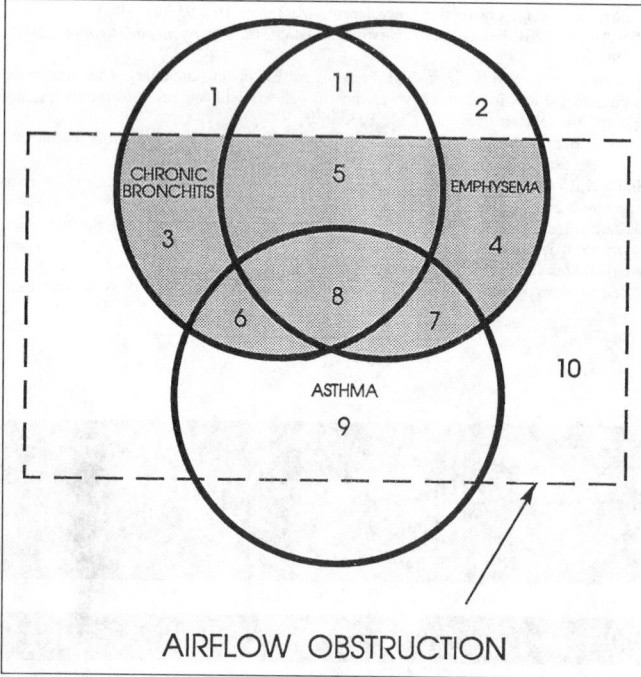

AIRFLOW OBSTRUCTION

FIGURE 51-1 Schema of chronic obstructive pulmonary disease (COPD). This nonproportional Venn diagram shows subsets of patients with chronic bronchitis, emphysema, and asthma. The subsets comprising COPD are shaded. Subset areas are not proportional to actual relative subset sizes. Asthma is by definition associated with reversible airflow obstruction, although in variant asthma special maneuvers may be necessary to make the obstruction evident. Patients with asthma whose airflow obstruction is completely reversible *(subset 9)* are not considered to have COPD. Because in many cases it is virtually impossible to differentiate patients with asthma whose airflow obstruction does not remit completely from persons with chronic bronchitis and emphysema who have partially reversible airflow obstruction with airway hyperreactivity, patients with unremitting asthma are classified as having COPD *(subsets 6, 7,* and *8).* Chronic bronchitis and emphysema with airflow obstruction usually occur together *(subset 5),* and some patients may have asthma associated with these two disorders *(subset 8).* Individuals with asthma exposed to chronic irritation, as from cigarette smoke, may develop chronic productive cough, a feature of chronic bronchitis *(subset 6).* Such patients are often referred to in the United States as having asthmatic bronchitis or the asthmatic form of COPD. Persons with chronic bronchitis, emphysema, or both conditions without airflow obstruction *(subsets 1, 2,* and *11)* are not classified as having COPD. Patients with airflow obstruction resulting from diseases with known etiology or specific pathology, such as cystic fibrosis or obliterative bronchiolitis *(subset 10),* are not included in this definition.

(From American Thoracic Society Statement, Standards for the diagnosis and care of patients with chronic obstructive lung disease, *Am J Respir Crit Care Med* 152:S77-S120:1995.)

associated with airflow obstruction. Remission of the airflow obstruction, either spontaneously or in response to treatment, is the hallmark of asthma. Patients with asthma whose airflow obstruction is completely reversible are diagnosed as having asthma and are not included in COPD. On the contrary, the airflow obstruction of COPD tends to be nonremitting. Patients whose asthma has become nonremitting cannot be differentiated from patients with COPD who have airways hyperreactivity, and such asthmatics are included within COPD. Patients whose airflow obstruction results from a specific cause (e.g., bronchiectasis, cystic fibrosis, obliterative bronchiolitis) are not included under the rubric COPD. These complex interrelations are shown in Fig. 51-1.

EPIDEMIOLOGY
Prevalence and Mortality

In 1994 an estimated 16 million persons in the United States suffered from COPD, representing an increase of 60% since 1982. In 1993, 95,910 deaths were attributed to COPD in the United States, representing the fourth most frequent cause of death and an increase of 103% over the 47,335 deaths from this cause in 1979. Prevalence, incidence, and mortality rates for COPD increase with age. Overall the age-adjusted death rate increased from 14.0 in 1979 to 20.0 in 1993, an increase of 43%; during this time the death rate for cardiovascular disease declined. These data reflect that, in contrast to cardiovascular mortality rates, COPD mortality rates are relatively insensitive to smoking cessation.

Risk Factors

Tobacco Smoking. Tobacco smoking and age account for more than 85% of the risk of developing COPD in the United States. Only homozygous α_1-protease inhibitor (API) deficiency presents a comparable risk, but this factor accounts for less than 1% of patients with COPD in the United States. Data from longitudinal, cross-sectional, and case control studies show that compared with nonsmokers, cigarette smokers have higher COPD mortality. They also have higher prevalence and incidence of productive cough, other respiratory symptoms, and spirometrically shown airways obstruction. A dose-response relationship exists for tobacco smoking; differences between smokers and nonsmokers increase as daily cigarette consumption and number of years smoked increase. Pipe and cigar smokers have higher COPD mortality and morbidity than nonsmokers, although their rates are lower than those of cigarette smokers. For reasons not known, only about 15% of cigarette smokers develop clinically significant COPD.

Passive Smoking. Passive, or involuntary, smoking, also known as environmental smoking and "second-hand smoking" is the exposure of nonsmokers to cigarette smoke indoors. Cigarette smoke in indoor air can produce eye irritation and may incite wheezing in asthmatic persons. An increased prevalence of respiratory symptoms and disease and small but measurable decreases in lung function have been shown in the children of smokers as compared with nonsmoking parents. However, the significance of these findings for the future development of COPD is unknown. Despite these uncertainties, children should be protected from environmental tobacco smoke.

Air Pollution. It is established that high levels of environmental air pollution are harmful to persons with chronic heart or lung disease. Although the exact role of air pollution in producing COPD is unclear, its role is small compared with that of cigarette smoking. The use of solid fuels for cooking and heating without adequate ventilation may result in high levels of indoor air pollution and lead to the development of COPD.

Sex, Race, and Socioeconomic Status. Prevalence and mortality rates are higher in males than females and are higher in whites than nonwhites. Incidence and mortality are generally higher in blue-collar workers than white-collar workers and in those with fewer years of formal education. Increasing evidence indicates that COPD aggregates in families independently of the occurrence of α_1-antiprotease deficiency.

Occupation. Working in an occupation in which the air is polluted with chemical fumes or a biologically inactive dust leads to increased prevalence of chronic airflow obstruction, increased rates of decline in forced expiratory volume for 1 second (FEV_1, a measure of ventilatory capacity) (Chapter 41), and increased mortality from COPD. Interaction between cigarette smoking and exposure to hazardous dust such as silica or cotton dust results in increased rates of COPD. In all studies, however, smoking effects are much greater than occupational effects.

Hyperresponsive Airways. It has been proposed but not proved that the atopic state or nonspecific airways hyperresponsiveness (usually measured as responsiveness to methacholine inhalation) predisposes smokers to the development of airways obstruction. In the absence of asthma, studies of what has come to be known as the "Dutch hypothesis" have failed to show a relation of manifestations of COPD in smokers to standardized levels of IgE, eosinophilia, or skin test reactivity to allergens. Airway hyperreactivity in COPD is inversely related to FEV_1 and is predictive of an increasing rate of decline of FEV_1 in smokers. However, it is not clear whether airway hyperreactivity is a cause of development of airflow obstruction or results from the airway inflammation that occurs in smoking-related airflow obstruction. Nonspecific airway hyperreactivity occurs in a significantly higher proportion of women than men.

PATHOLOGY
Chronic Bronchitis

Various structural changes, none of which is specific to chronic bronchitis, have been described in the airways of long-time cigarette smokers. The submucosal glands are enlarged and their ducts dilated. Focal areas of squamous metaplasia replace the pseudostratified columnar epithelium. Neutrophils and lymphocytes infiltrate the mucous membranes but are sparse and not a prominent feature. Airway smooth muscle may be hypertrophied. The terminal and respiratory bronchioles show varying degrees of secretory obstruction, goblet cell metaplasia, inflammation with a predominance of macrophages, increased smooth muscle, and distortion from loss of alveolar attachments and fibrosis.

Emphysema

Emphysema is classified according to the portion of the acinus involved by mild disease (Box 51-1). The acinus comprises the respiratory tissues arising from a single terminal bronchiole. Centriacinar emphysema begins as enlargement of the respiratory bronchioles and adjacent air spaces with breakdown of air space walls. Focal emphysema is a form of centriacinar emphysema that occurs in individuals who have had heavy exposure to a biologically inactive dust such as coal dust. The lesions are widespread through the lungs and are infiltrated by pigment-laden macrophages. Panacinar emphysema (PAE), which in diffuse form is the type of emphysema occurring in homozygous API deficiency, involves all the acinus.

Centrilobular emphysema (CLE), a form of centriacinar emphysema, is the most common form of emphysema in smokers. The lesions involve the upper and posterior portions of the lungs more than the lung bases. Focal PAE, which often accompanies CLE in smokers, occurs at the lung bases. About 25% of smokers have pure CLE, 25% have pure PAE, and about 50% have both types. Mild CLE shows an increase in collagen concentration, which is accompanied in severe disease by a loss of elastin concentration. In PAE, elastin concentration is consistently decreased. The air spaces of mild CLE tend to have decreased compliance; those of PLE have increased compliance.

Distal acinar emphysema, also known as paraseptal or subpleural emphysema, occurs subpleurally or along fibrous interlobular septa. The remainder of the lung is often spared, so pulmonary function may be well preserved despite the presence of many foci of locally severe disease. This is the type of apical emphysema that causes spontaneous pneumothorax in young people and may give rise to giant bullae. Air space enlargement with fibrosis, formerly called paracicatricial emphysema, may be an inconsequential lesion adjacent to a scar or it may be severe and clinically important, complicating fibrosing diseases such as tuberculosis, silicosis, or sarcoidosis.

Bullae. Bullae are defined as air spaces that are 1 cm or more in diameter; but they may reach huge proportions, filling an entire hemithorax. They may be entirely empty air spaces, or they may be areas of locally severe emphysema with strands of lung tissue traversing them. The latter may be recognizable radiographically but not pathologically as bullae. Bullae that are not a part of generalized emphysema may rarely become large enough to severely impair lung function; resection of such lesions may result in marked improvement.

Implications of Types of Emphysema. The anatomic classification of emphysema has little importance for clinical medicine. However, the variable predilection of the various types of emphysema for different regions of the lungs and the differences in their connective tissue concentrations and volume pressure relations suggest that there are differences in their etiology and pathogenesis. The lung consists of 300 million air cells circumscribed by a complexly organized vascular tissue; emphysema appears to represent one of its stereotyped responses to injury.

Structure-Function Correlations. Bronchial gland enlargement encroaches minimally on the airway lumen and correlates poorly with airflow obstruction. Mild respiratory bronchiolitis, which is the earliest lesion described in smokers, does not cause airflow obstruction. However, as the lesion increases in severity and is accompanied by terminal bronchiolitis, airflow obstruction supervenes.

Emphysema becomes evident at about the same time as the terminal bronchiolitis and increases steadily in severity as COPD progresses. It is the predominant lesion in most patients with end-stage COPD. Bronchiolitis also increases in severity as COPD runs its course. Bronchiolar inflammation contributes to the reversible elements of airflow obstruction, both by mechanical means and by generating mediators that cause bronchial muscle contraction.

ALPHA$_1$-PROTEASE INHIBITOR DEFICIENCY

Alpha$_1$-protease inhibitor, also known as α_1-antitrypsin, is a serum protein (molecular weight, 52 kD) and is normally found in the lungs. It inhibits several serine proteases, but its main role in the body is inhibition of neutrophil elastase; the deficient state is associated with the premature development of emphysema. API is a glycoprotein composed of 394 amino acids, which is coded for by a single gene on chromosome 14. The serum protease inhibitor phenotype (Pi type) is determined by the independent expression of the two parental alleles. The API gene is highly pleomorphic. About 75 alleles are known, and they have been classified into *normal* (associated with normal serum levels of normally functioning API), *deficient* (associated with serum API levels lower than normal), *null* (associated with undetectable API in the serum), and *dysfunctional* (API present in normal amount but not functioning normally).

BOX 51-1
Respiratory air space enlargement*

I. Simple air space enlargement
 A. Congenital (Down syndrome)
 B. Acquired (contralateral lung after pneumonectomy; aging lung)
II. Emphysema
 A. Centriacinar emphysema
 1. Focal emphysema (coal workers' pneumoconiosis)
 2. Centrilobular emphysema (main lesion of smokers)
 B. Panacinar emphysema (main lesion in α_1-protease inhibitor [API] deficiency)
 C. Distal acinar emphysema
III. Air space enlargement with fibrosis (sarcoidosis)

*Examples of each type are given in parentheses.

The variants of API occur because of point mutations that result in a single amino acid substitution. For example, the Z variant results from the substitution of a lysine for a glutamic acid in the M protein. The substitution changes the charge of the molecule and therefore its electrophoretic mobility. The normal M alleles occur in about 90% of persons of European descent with normal serum API levels; their phenotype is designated PiMM. Normal values of serum API are 150 to 350 mg/dl (commercial standard) or 20 to 48 μM (true laboratory standard).

More than 95% of persons in the severely deficient category are homozygous for the Z allele, designated PiZZ, and have serum API levels of 2.5 to 7 μM (mean, 16% normal). Most of these persons are Caucasian of northern European descent because the Z allele is rare in Asians and blacks. Rarely observed phenotypes associated with low levels of serum API include PiSZ and persons with nonexpressing alleles, Pi null. The latter occur in homozygous form, Pi null-null, or in heterozygous form with a deficient allele, PiZ null. Persons with phenotype PiSS have API values ranging from 15 to 33 μM (mean, 52% of normal). The threshold protective level of 11 μM, or 80 mg/dl (35% of normal), is based on the knowledge that PiSZ heterozygotes, with serum API values of 8 to 19 μM (mean, 37% of normal), rarely develop emphysema. PiMZ heterozygotes have serum API levels that are intermediate between levels for normal PiMM and homozygous PiZZ (12 to 35 μM; mean, 57% of normal) and are not at increased risk for emphysema.

Homozygous (PiZZ) API Deficiency and Lung Disease

Homozygous API deficiency is accompanied by the premature development of severe emphysema, with chronic bronchitis occurring in about half of patients. The onset of pulmonary disease is greatly accelerated by smoking; dyspnea begins at a median age of 40 years in smokers compared with a median age of 53 years in nonsmokers. Radiographically, panacinar emphysema, which predominates in PiZZ patients, usually begins at the lung bases (Fig. 51-2).

The natural history of API deficiency is incompletely known. PiZZ smokers have an earlier onset of dyspnea and a lower life expectancy than PiZZ nonsmokers; the latter have a lower life expectancy than PiMM persons. Severity of lung disease varies greatly; lung function is well preserved in some PiZZ smokers and severely impaired in some PiZZ nonsmokers. Nonindex persons (those discovered in population surveys) tend to have better lung function, whether or not they smoke, than index persons (those discovered because they have lung disease). Nonindex persons may live into their eighth or ninth decade. Airflow obstruction occurs more frequently in men than in women; asthma, recurrent respiratory infections, and familial factors are also risk factors for airflow obstruction. The most common cause of death is emphysema; cirrhosis, often with hepatic carcinoma, is the second mosy common.

Diagnosis

The diagnosis of API deficiency is made by measuring serum API level, followed by Pi typing for confirmation. The tests should be ordered in patients with premature onset of COPD and in nonsmokers with COPD. A predominance of basilar emphysema should suggest the genetic defect, as should the development of nonremitting asthma in a person under age 50 years and cirrhosis without apparent risk factors.

Augmentation Therapy

Augmentation therapy with purified human API for patients with severe API deficiency is based on the concept that a deficient protein is being restored to protective levels. It is presumed, but not proved, that augmentation therapy will halt the progression of emphysema. Because emphysema produces a permanent structural change, augmentation therapy cannot improve lung structure or function. The cost of the drug for 1 year of augmentation therapy in a 70 kg patient is about $25,000. Augmentation therapy should be reserved for patients with lung disease whose serum concentration of API is less than 11 μM; it is not indicated for patients with cigarette smoking–related

emphysema who have normal or heterozygous phenotypes. PiZZ persons with normal lung function should be followed but not treated; augmentation therapy should be considered when lung function is abnormal and especially if serial studies show deterioration.

For severely impaired persons under age 50, lung transplantation should be considered. The prospect of gene therapy for patients with API deficiency is under investigation.

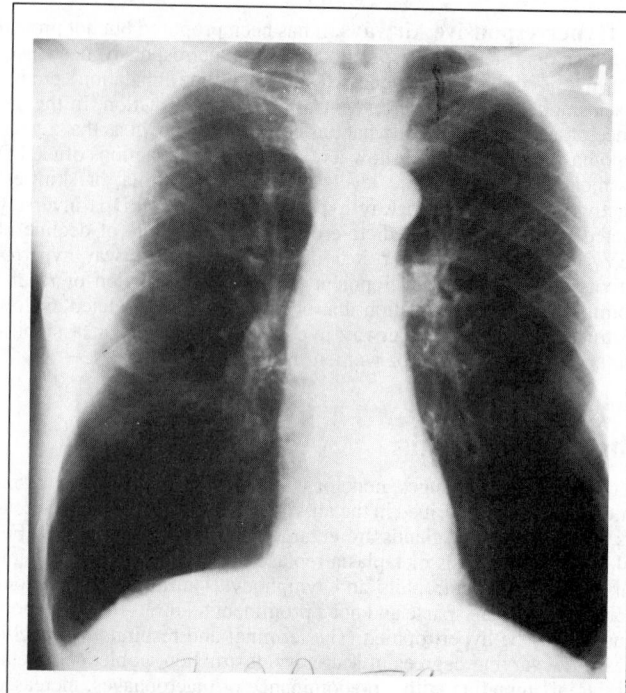

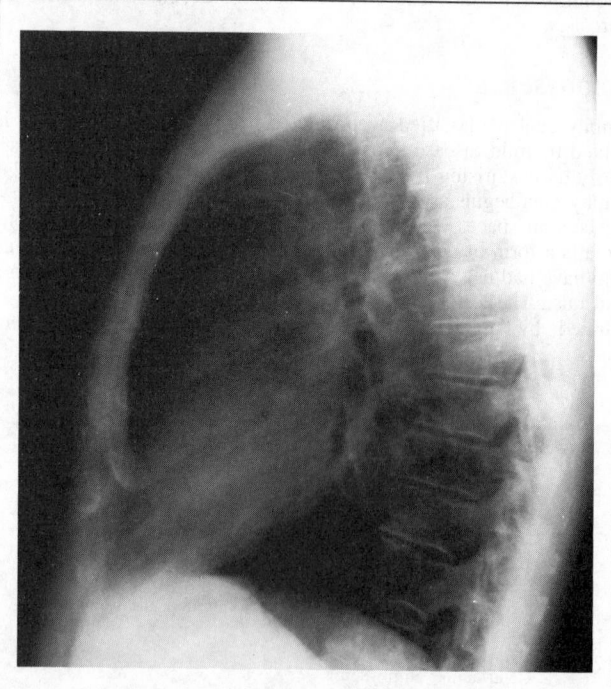

FIGURE 51-2 Chest radiograph of a 66-year-old man with homozygous α_1-protease inhibitor (API) deficiency. **A,** Frontal view shows a depression and flattening of the diaphragmatic shadow. Areas of hypertransradiancy with poorly defined upper borders occupy the lower lung zones and are patchy in the midlung zones. The cardiac silhouette is narrow. **B,** Lateral view shows marked flattening of the diaphragm and an increase in the retrosternal air space.

PATHOGENESIS
Emphysema

It has been known since the turn of this century that lung parenchymal elastic fibers are ruptured and frayed in emphysema. The discovery of the association of premature onset of emphysema with homozygous API deficiency in 1963 soon spawned the hypothesis that the emphysema was induced by the digestion of lung parenchymal elastic fibers by the individual's own neutrophil elastase because the API deficiency in the lungs failed to provide a sufficient antielastase shield. The observation that free elastase is found in the bronchoalveolar lavage fluid of PiZZ persons who smoke supports this hypothesis.

Extensive experimental evidence indicates that elastic fiber destruction leads to emphysema: Only enzymes with elastolytic properties, including human neutrophil elastase, induce emphysema when instilled into the lungs of animals. Emphysema-like changes occur in animals whose elastic fibers do not cross-link normally, either because of a genetic or an induced defect in the cross-linking mechanism. Emphysema has also been induced in animals by repeated induction of pulmonary neutrophilia, especially if at the same time the amount of API is diminished or its functional integrity impaired.

Much work relates the elastase-antielastase hypothesis (Fig. 51-3) to cigarette smoking. The number of cells that can be lavaged from the lungs is about fivefold higher in smokers than in nonsmokers. The proportion of neutrophils remains at 1% to 3%, but their absolute numbers increase fourfold to fivefold. In vitro studies have shown that API can be oxidatively inactivated by oxygen radicals derived either from cigarette smoke or from the neutrophils' myeloperoxidase system. Immunoultrastructural studies are purported to show elastase bound to elastin in the lungs of smokers. Biologic markers of elastin degradation (urinary desmosine or plasma or urinary elastin peptides) are higher in smokers than in people who never smoked and highest in persons with COPD. Thus, compelling although indirect evidence supports the concept that elastase-antielastase imbalance is responsible for emphysema in smokers with adequate protective levels of API.

There are also animal models of emphysema in which elastin degradation is not believed to occur. Emphysema has been produced experimentally by hyperoxia and cadmium chloride. In both of these models there is excess collagen without degradation of elastin. Emphysema in these two models is due to the combined effects of inflammation and fibrosis (Fig. 51-4).

As noted earlier, mild CLE demonstrates excess collagen, and only in severe disease is there evidence of loss of elastin. In PAE, elastin loss is noted in even mild disease. Thus it seems reasonable to suggest that CLE is due to a combination of inflammation and fibrosis and elastase-antielastase imbalance; PAE is due to only elastase-antielastase imbalance (Fig. 51-5).

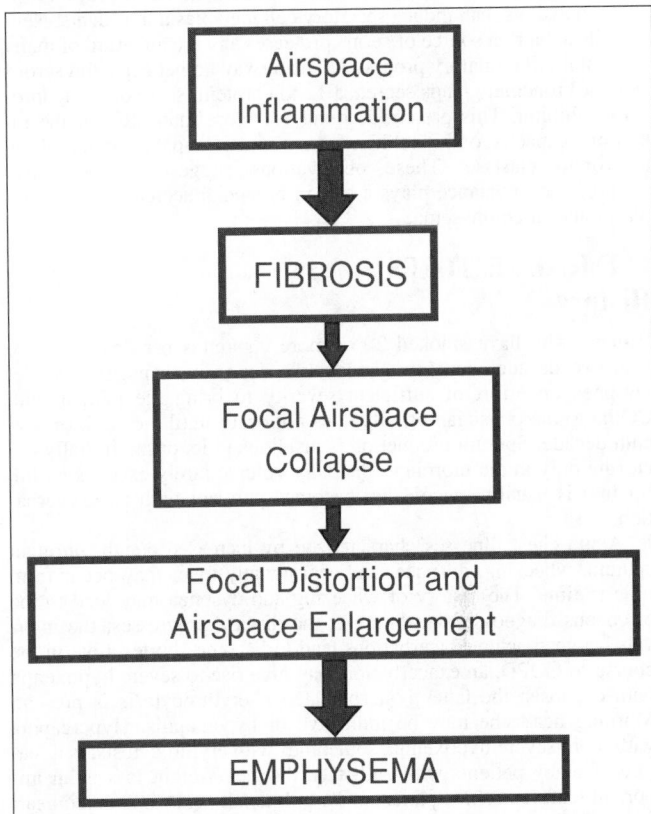

FIGURE 51-4 Schema of the inflammation-fibrosis hypothesis of pathogenesis of emphysema. Inflammation in which there is damage to alveolar epithelium or capillary endothelium gives rise to fibrosis and alveolar collapse. The redistribution of forces within the parenchyma causes focal distortion and enlargement of air spaces with destruction of tissue, or emphysema. Elastin degradation need not occur with this form of emphysema.

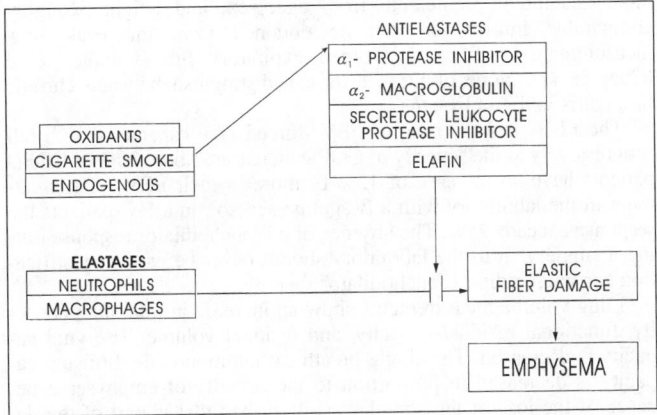

FIGURE 51-3 Schema of the elastase-antielastase hypothesis of pathogenesis of emphysema. Elastases, capable of damaging elastin, derive from neutrophils and macrophages in the lungs. The number of these cells is increased fourfold to fivefold in smokers. Elastic fiber damage results in emphysema. Antielastases prevent elastic fiber damage by elastases. α_1-protease inhibitor is the main antineutrophil elastase but, as shown, there are other antielastases in the lungs. Oxidants present in cigarette smoke or deriving from neutrophils may inactivate α_1-protease inhibitor, thus damaging the antielastase shield of the lungs.

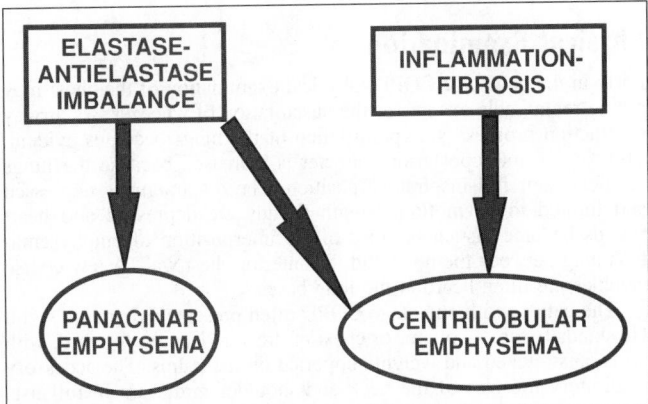

FIGURE 51-5 Schema of types of emphysema in smokers and their probable pathogenesis. In about 25% of smokers, emphysema is exclusively centrilobular or panacinar; in about 50% both types of emphysema are present. Current evidence indicates that panacinar emphysema is caused by elastase-antielastase imbalance; centrilobular emphysema is caused by both inflammation-fibrosis and elastase-antielastase imbalance.

Chronic Bronchitis

Experimental chronic bronchial injury has been produced with a variety of irritant gases. Sulfur dioxide produces a predominantly central lesion, with submucosal gland and goblet cell metaplasia. Cigarette smoke produces secretory cell metaplasia in both central and peripheral airways. Chronic exposure to low-dose ozone induces injury of the terminal bronchiole and the adjacent respiratory airway.

Serine proteases, which need not be elastolytic but must be enzymatically active, can induce secretory cell metaplasia in rodents. Neutrophils are a rich source of serine proteases and are a feature of many bronchial inflammatory processes. The airway goblet cells and serous cells of bronchial glands secrete a 12 kD protein, secretory leucoprotease inhibitor. This protein accounts for more than 80% of the inhibitory capacity of bronchitic sputum and is capable of inhibiting neutrophil elastase. These observations suggest that protease-antiprotease imbalance plays a role in bronchial secretory cell metaplasia and in emphysema.

CLINICAL FEATURES
History

Patients who have smoked 20 or more cigarettes per day for more than two decades develop a productive cough in their fifth decade. Dyspnea on effort of sufficient severity to bring the patient with COPD to the physician usually does not occur until the sixth or seventh decade. Sputum production is insidious in its onset, initially occurring only in the morning. The daily volume rarely exceeds 60 ml. Sputum is usually mucoid but becomes purulent with an exacerbation.

Acute chest illnesses characterized by increased cough, purulent sputum, wheezing, dyspnea, and occasionally fever may occur from time to time. The history of wheezing and dyspnea may lead to the erroneous diagnosis of asthma. As the disease progresses, the intervals between acute exacerbations tend to become shorter. Late in the course of COPD, an exacerbation may give rise to severe hypoxemia with cyanosis; the latter is accentuated if erythrocytosis is present. Morning headache may be indicative of hypercapnia. Hypercapnia with more severe hypoxemia, sometimes with erythrocytosis, is a feature of many patients with end-stage disease. Weight loss is an important feature in some patients. Cor pulmonale with right-sided heart failure and edema may complicate the course of patients with hypoxemia and hypercapnia.

Because bronchogenic carcinoma occurs with increased frequency in smokers with COPD, an episode of hemoptysis raises the possibility that carcinoma has developed. However, most episodes of hemoptysis complicating chronic bronchitis are caused by mucosal erosion and not by carcinoma. Indeed, mucosal erosion in chronic bronchitis is currently the most common cause of hemoptysis in the United States. The need for bronchoscopy and other studies to exclude carcinoma when hemoptysis occurs is evident.

Physical Examination

Early in the course of COPD, physical examination of the chest may not be remarkable except for the auscultation of wheezes. As airway obstruction progresses, hyperinflation of the lungs becomes evident. The chest's anteroposterior diameter is increased because the lungs are near their full inspiratory position. The diaphragm is depressed and limited in its motion. Breath sounds are depressed and heart sounds become distant because of the interposition of emphysematous lung between the heart and the anterior chest wall. A few coarse crackles are often heard at the lung bases.

The patient with end-stage COPD often presents a dramatic sight. He stands before a counter or chest of drawers leaning forward, with arms outstretched and weight supported on the palms. The accessory respiratory muscles of the neck and shoulder girdle are in full use. Expiration often occurs through pursed lips. The chest appears overinflated both because of the large total lung capacity of emphysema and because the chest is held near full inspiration. Paradoxical indrawing of the lower interspaces is often clearly evident. Cyanosis may be present.

The signs of pulmonary hypertension and right ventricular hypertrophy are usually not detectable on physical examination in patients with COPD because of the interposition of emphysematous lung between heart and chest wall. An enlarged tender liver indicates heart failure; neck vein distention, especially during expiration, may be observed in the absence of heart failure because of increased intrathoracic pressure. Asterixis may be seen with severe hypercapnia.

LABORATORY FINDINGS
Chest Radiography

Because emphysema is defined in anatomic terms, the chest radiograph provides the clearest evidence of its presence (see Fig. 51-2). Emphysema is consistently diagnosed radiographically when the disease is severe, is not diagnosed when the disease is mild, and is diagnosed in about half the instances when the disease is moderately severe. Persistent, marked overdistention of the lungs, indicated by a low, flat diaphragm in the frontal view and widening of the retrosternal air space and increase in the angle formed by the sternum and the diaphragm from acute to 90 degrees or greater in the lateral view, is strongly suggestive of emphysema. The heart shadow tends to be long and narrow. Excessively rapid tapering of the vascular shadows is a sign of emphysema, but it may be difficult to identify unless it is accompanied by obvious hypertransradiancy of the lungs. Bullae, appearing as radiolucent areas larger than 1 cm in diameter and surrounded by arcuate hairline shadows, are proof of the presence of emphysema. However, bullae reflect only locally severe disease, and their presence does not necessarily indicate widespread emphysema. Computed tomography (CT) especially high resolution CT (1 to 3 mm thick sections) clearly shows the hypovascular areas and bullae of emphysema. Because the accurate diagnosis of emphysema does not change management, CT has no place in routine management.

The complication of COPD by right ventricular hypertrophy does not result in an increased transverse diameter of the heart. Comparison with previous chest radiographs may show that the transverse cardiac shadow, although still within normal limits, is wider than previously. The heart shadow may be seen to encroach on the retrosternal space as it enlarges anteriorly. The hilar vascular shadows are prominent.

Pulmonary Function Tests

Pulmonary function measurements are helpful in diagnosing, assessing the severity of, and following the progress of COPD. Airflow obstruction is an important indicator of impairment of the whole person and of the likelihood of blood gas abnormalities. The FEV_1 is an easily measurable index of airflow obstruction that has less variability than other measurements of airways dynamics and that is more accurately predictable from age, sex, and height. Roughly comparable information can be obtained from the peak flow measurement or from the forced expiratory flow–volume curve (Chapter 41). None of these tests can distinguish between chronic bronchitis and emphysema.

The FEV_1 and the ratio of FEV_1/forced vital capacity (FVC) fall progressively as the severity of COPD increases. About 30% of COPD patients have an increase of 15% or more in their FEV_1 after treatment in the laboratory with a β-agonist aerosol; in a few patients the response exceeds 25%. The absence of a bronchodilator response during a single visit to the laboratory should never be used as justification for withholding bronchodilator therapy.

Lung volume measurements show an increase in total lung capacity, functional residual capacity, and residual volume. The vital capacity is decreased. The single-breath carbon monoxide diffusing capacity is decreased in proportion to the severity of emphysema because of the loss of the alveolar capillary bed that is part of the destructive process of emphysema. The test is not specific and cannot detect mild emphysema.

Arterial blood gas measurement reveals mild or moderate hypoxemia without hypercapnia in the early stages of COPD. As the disease progresses, hypoxemia becomes more severe and hypercapnia supervenes. Hypercapnia is observed with increasing frequency as the FEV_1 falls below 1 L. Blood gas abnormalities worsen during acute exacerbations and may worsen during exercise and sleep.

Troublesome erythrocytosis is infrequently observed in patients living at sea level who have arterial oxygen tension (PaO_2) levels greater than 55 mm Hg; the frequency of erythrocytosis increases as PaO_2 levels fall below 55 mm Hg. The reasons for failure of the bone marrow to respond to mild or moderate levels of hypoxemia are complex. Matched hypoxemic patients with and without erythrocytosis have no differences in blood erythropoietin levels or in the sensitivity of bone marrow red cell precursors to erythropoietin. Single measures of blood oxygenation are not representative of a patient's mean daily saturation. Intermittent hypoxemia, as during sleep, is a potent stimulus for erythropoietin production. Elevated levels of carboxyhemoglobin contribute to polycythemia in smokers. Given the many factors that influence oxygen delivery to the tissues (hemoglobin concentration, red cell 2,3-diphosphoglycerate concentration, blood carboxyhemoglobin concentration, cardiac output, blood pH and carbon dioxide tension, local tissue blood flow), a variable relation between blood oxygen level and red cell mass in COPD is not surprising.

Sputum Examination

In patients with stable chronic bronchitis, sputum is mucoid and the predominant cell is the macrophage. With an exacerbation, sputum usually becomes purulent, and microscopic examination shows an influx of neutrophils. The Gram stain usually shows a mixture of organisms, often gram-positive diplococci, characteristic of *Streptococcus pneumoniae,* and pleomorphic fine gram-negative rods, characteristic of *Haemophilus influenzae.* These are the most frequent pathogens cultured from the sputum. Other oropharyngeal commensal flora such as *Moraxella catarrhalis,* which have been recently shown occasionally to cause exacerbations, can be recovered. However, cultures and even Gram stains are rarely necessary before instituting antimicrobial therapy in outpatients. In hospitalized patients, Gram stains and cultures may reveal infection with a gram-negative rod or, rarely, a staphylococcus.

DIAGNOSIS

The history and physical examination suggest the possibility of COPD. A chest radiograph excludes other diagnoses (e.g., tuberculosis, lung cancer) that can give rise to the same symptoms and may reveal the findings of emphysema or of a complicating pneumonia. Forced expiratory spirometry and arterial blood gas measurements provide the basic physiologic assessment needed to quantify airflow obstruction and the presence and severity of hypoxemia and hypercapnia. A postbronchodilator improvement of the FEV_1 by more than 25% suggests that a trial of corticosteroids may be helpful. Measurements of lung volumes, diffusing capacity, or physiologic responses to exercise usually add little unless the diagnosis is in doubt or surgical risk is being assessed.

TREATMENT

The ambulatory management of patients with COPD is considered here under three headings: specific, symptomatic, and secondary therapy. The management of acute respiratory failure complicating COPD is briefly discussed under that heading; the reader should also refer to a detailed discussion of acute respiratory failure (Chapter 46).

Specific Therapy

Specific therapy may deal with the root causes of COPD. Support during smoking cessation and evaluation and counseling regarding environmental irritants in the workplace or elsewhere fall into this category. Influenza vaccine should be given annually because of the greater risk of serious complications of influenza in these patients. Although some question surrounds its efficacy in COPD, pneumococcal vaccine should be given and may be repeated after 6 years.

Smoking Cessation. Every effort should be made to help the patient with COPD stop smoking, especially if airways obstruction is mild or moderate. Many strategies have been tried to accomplish this aim; hypnotism, behavior modification techniques, group sessions, and nicotine given transdermally or as gum are all in use. No single "best" technique exists. However, it is important to stress the importance of the physician as the initiator of a smoking cessation effort. About 5% of patients stop smoking simply in response to 1 or 2 minutes of such advice. The cessation rate is higher if this advice is supplemented by a self-help manual, such as the one distributed by the American Lung Association, *Freedom From Smoking.* Physicians should consider referring patients to services in their community that offer smoking cessation programs. Of patients seeking help in smoking cessation programs, only 25% to 39% are not smoking 1 year later.

After smoking cessation, cough and expectoration diminish over a period of a few months; sputum may become more viscid. Understanding what happens to lung function is more complex. Longitudinal studies show that ventilatory function, as measured by the FEV_1 in nonsmokers, declines by 25 to 30 ml/year, along a curvilinear path, beginning at about age 30 (Fig. 51-6). The rate of decline for smokers is steeper than for nonsmokers, averaging up to 60 ml/year. Ventilatory function of middle-aged smokers whose FEV_1 is diminished on entry into the study declines at a more rapid rate than that of the general population of smokers. These persons reach an FEV_1 of 0.8 L, the level at which dyspnea during activities of daily living supervenes, in their seventh decade, whereas most smokers and normal persons do not reach this level even in their tenth decade. After smokers give up the habit, the rate of decline of FEV_1 first increases and then follows a path that is similar to that of nonsmokers. Lost lung function is not regained, but smoking cessation delays the time of onset of dyspnea on effort and the risk of dying of COPD.

Symptomatic Therapy

Symptomatic therapy is directed against the reversible elements of airflow obstruction. These result from bronchiolar inflammation, luminal secretions, and smooth muscle spasm.

Bronchodilator Drugs

Sympathomimetics. Although most of the airways obstruction in patients with COPD is fixed and irreversible, there is a high prevalence of partial reversibility with 250 µg of inhaled isoproterenol. The amount of reversibility of the FEV_1 averages 15% of the baseline

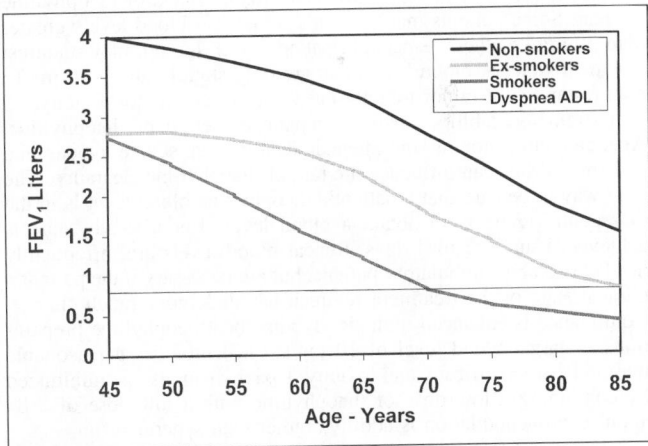

FIGURE 51-6 Relation among smoking status, FEV_1, and age. Three matched cohorts, followed from age 45 to 85 years are depicted. The nonsmokers show decline of FEV_1 along a curvilinear path but at age 85 years have not reached an FEV_1 of 0.8 L *(horizontal line),* the level at which dyspnea generally occurs during activities of daily living. The ex-smokers, who smoked at least 20 cigarettes a day for 25 years or more and who stopped smoking at age 45 years, show no decline of FEV_1 for 5 years and then decline at a rate parallel to normal subjects. They do not reach FEV_1 0.8 L until age 85 years. The group who continue to smoke decline at a rate much steeper than the normal subjects or ex-smokers and reach FEV_1 0.8 L by age 70. In their seventh and eighth decades, the smokers become dyspneic on mild effort and begin to populate chest clinics and intensive care units and to die of COPD. Smoking cessation at age 45 years delays this process by about 15 years.

value, with about one third of patients showing responses of 20% or greater. COPD patients with the greatest bronchodilator responses have the lowest annual decline in FEV_1 and the greatest 5-year survival. There is no evidence that regular bronchodilator therapy slows deterioration of lung function.

The β₂-*adrenergic agonists* have less cardioaccelerator effect for a given amount of bronchodilation than the less selective β-agonists; some examples are metaproterenol, albuterol, terbutalene, and pirbuterol. Administration of the β₂ agonists by inhalation produces a more rapid onset of action and greater bronchodilator effect than oral administration and does so with fewer side effects, such as skeletal muscle tremor. The preferred mode of administration is the metered-dose inhaler (MDI). Patients should be taught to inhale the aerosol slowly, starting at the resting end-expiratory position, with a brief breath-hold at the end of a full inhalation. For patients with poor coordination, the aerosol should be inhaled after delivery into a small chamber or spacer.

Anticholinergics. Anticholinergic agents are time-honored in the treatment of asthma. Their mode of action is not clearly understood; they may act by inhibiting normal, cholinergically mediated bronchomotor tone. The quaternary ammonium compound *ipratropium bromide* is poorly absorbed, does not impair mucociliary clearance, and has few side effects. In comparative studies, ipratropium has generally had a statistically greater bronchodilating effect than β₂ agonists in COPD, but this may be due to the doses selected for study. Because of delayed onset of action of ipratropium, a β₂ agonist must be prescribed for as-needed use. It seems preferable to start by prescribing a β₂ agonist for COPD unless side effects occur or bronchodilator response is not satisfactory.

Theophylline. The mode of action of theophylline is poorly understood but appears to be different from that of either the sympathomimetics or the anticholinergics. Theophylline decreases smooth muscle spasm, enhances mucociliary clearance, improves right ventricular function, and decreases pulmonary vascular resistance and arterial pressure. Its role in improving diaphragmatic function and dyspnea on exercise is controversial.

The toxicity of theophylline is weakly related to its blood levels. Sleeplessness and gastrointestinal upset occur often at blood levels less than 20 mg/L and tend to subside with time. More serious toxicity, such as supraventricular and ventricular arrhythmias and seizures, tends to occur at blood levels greater than 20 mg/L. However, individual variation in susceptibility to toxic effects of theophylline is great. Some patients manifest little toxicity at blood levels greater than 30 mg/L; others, especially patients over age 60, may manifest serious toxicity at blood levels that are only slightly above 20 mg/L; manifestations of minor toxicity need not precede major toxicity.

Extreme variability exists in hepatic excretion of theophylline. Age, cigarette smoking, diet, hepatic dysfunction, severe hypoxemia, and some drugs can influence the rate of theophylline clearance. The only way to be sure that a patient's theophylline blood level is in the therapeutic range is to obtain a blood level after a steady state is achieved, usually 2 to 4 days. Repeat blood levels are infrequently needed in stable, ambulatory patients but are necessary if the patient's clinical state or the treatment regimen has undergone much change. Compliance is enhanced with slowly absorbed theophylline preparations. A target blood level of 10 mg/L (± 3) provides a reasonable margin between efficacy and toxicity. Toxicity can also be minimized by combining a low dose of theophylline with a low dose of a β₂ agonist; bronchodilation is additive rather than synergistic.

Corticosteroids. Most patients with COPD do not respond to corticosteroids when they are in the chronic stable state. However, 15% to 20% of patients show sizable objective responses in ventilatory function after corticosteroid administration. The responders are generally those with improvement of the FEV_1 of 25% or more after use of a bronchodilator aerosol. A trial of oral corticosteroid therapy should be initiated only after patients have been on an optimal treatment regimen. A 2- to 4-week trial of prednisone in a dose of 0.5 mg/kg body weight (or equivalent) should be instituted. The drug should be continued only if objective evidence of improvement exists. The dose should then be reduced to the lowest level that maintains improvement. The use of aerosolized corticosteroids in patients with COPD remains experimental.

Antibiotics. It is unclear in many exacerbations of COPD whether the bronchial inflammation manifested by the development of purulent sputum is caused by infection or has some other basis, such as exposure for several days to heavily polluted air. Furthermore, it is not usually clear whether the infection is bacterial or viral, and about 25% of exacerbations are believed to be viral. Nevertheless, most clinicians prescribe antibiotics for these exacerbations. Controlled trials in general show that antibiotic-treated exacerbations are briefer and less likely to have serious consequences than are placebo-treated exacerbations. Routine cultures are not indicated before instituting treatment. Patients should be taught to recognize the change in sputum character from mucoid to purulent and to institute a 10- to 14-day course of antibiotic therapy on their own. Long-term antibiotic prophylaxis should be considered only in patients who have repeated exacerbations on an intermittent regimen.

Frequently used oral antibiotics to manage a COPD exacerbation include ampicillin (250 to 500 mg four times a day), tetracycline (250 mg four times a day), doxycycline (100 to 200 mg a day), and trimethoprim (160 mg) plus sulfamethoxazole (800 mg) twice a day. Because of the high prevalence of tetracycline-resistant *S. pneumoniae* and a low but increasing frequency of *H. influenzae* resistant to ampicillin (both β-lactamase and non–β-lactamase related), it is logical to use trimethoprim-sulfamethoxazole for most exacerbations. Amoxicillin-clavulanate (Augmentin), ofloxacin (Floxin), and cefuroxime axetil (Ceftin) are also effective against β-lactamase–producing strains of *H. influenzae* and *M. catarrhalis,* but these agents are much more expensive than trimethoprim-sulfamethoxazole and should be reserved for the most seriously ill patients.

Thinning and Mobilization of Secretions. Viscid secretion in peripheral airways is an important mechanism of airways obstruction in COPD. Unfortunately, no drugs, whether administered orally or by inhalation, are effective in thinning secretions. Dehydration causes secretions to become thick, but aggressive hydration does not favorably affect sputum characteristics. It is reasonable to advise patients to drink enough fluid to keep the urine pale except for the first morning voiding. Inhaling steam from hot water in the bathroom sink may help patients expectorate secretions. Controlled coughing, consisting of two or three coughs in succession after a deep inhalation, assists in sputum mobilization. Chest wall percussion with cupped hands or an electromechanical percussor may provide additional assistance in sputum mobilization in the most difficult cases.

Secondary Therapy

Secondary therapy is treatment designed to improve the function of the whole person while having little effect on the underlying pulmonary disease. A carefully integrated rehabilitation program, which helps the patient accommodate to physiologic limitations while at the same time providing realistic expectations for improvement, is important in managing patients with severe COPD. The patient's acceptance of responsibility for the treatment regimen is important.

Long-Term Oxygen Therapy. It is now firmly established that long-term oxygen therapy (LTOT) prolongs life in hypoxemic COPD patients. A 24-hour regimen is better than a 12-hour nocturnal regimen. In addition, LTOT results in a decrease in hematocrit toward normal levels, moderate neuropsychologic improvement, and amelioration of pulmonary hemodynamic abnormalities. Pulmonary O_2 toxicity is not a problem, and increases in arterial carbon dioxide tension ($PaCO_2$) in patients with hypercapnia are minimal.

Indications. The criteria for LTOT are summarized in Box 51-2. LTOT should be prescribed for hospitalized patients who meet the criteria as soon as they are ready for discharge from the hospital. Their room air PaO_2 should be reassessed after 30 days to determine whether they still meet the criteria for LTOT.

Decreases in PaO_2 during brief exercise are probably not harmful. The diffusing capacity for carbon monoxide may be used to predict desaturation with exercise in patients with COPD; desaturation occurs only when the single-breath diffusing capacity is less than 55% of predicted values. It seems reasonable to limit exercise testing to COPD patients with limited exercise tolerance who have a diffusing capacity less than 55% of predicted values, whose room air PaO_2 is

---

BOX 51-2

Indications for long-term oxygen therapy

Obligatory

In a patient who has been stable on an optimal medical regimen for
at least 30 days: PaO_2 ≤55 mm Hg or SaO_2 ≤88%*

In the presence of cor pulmonale or erythrocytosis (hematocrit
>55%): PaO_2 55 to 59 mm Hg or SaO_2 ≤89%*

Optional

Exercise or sleeping room air PaO_2 ≤55 mm Hg or SaO_2 ≤88%;
severe dyspnea relieved by low-flow oxygen: PaO_2 ≥60 mm Hg
or SaO_2 ≥90%*

---

*Arterial oxygen levels measured at rest during air breathing.

≥60 mm Hg (SaO_2 ≥90%) and who are highly motivated to work or
exercise. O_2 may be prescribed for patients in these categories who
desaturate on low-level exercise to a PaO_2 ≤55 mm Hg (SaO_2 ≤88%).

The consequences of nocturnal desaturations include erythrocytosis, transient periods of pulmonary hypertension, and an increase in
ventricular ectopy, along with electrocardiographic (ECG) changes of
prolonged QT interval, ST-T depression, and bundle branch block. A
sleep study should be considered only for patients with advanced
COPD who do not meet the criteria for LTOT but whose clinical assessment suggests the ill effects of hypoxemia. Nocturnal O_2 may be
prescribed if a sleep study reveals episodic desaturation to 80% or
less for more than 5 minutes, because it would be imprudent to assume that such episodes are harmless.

Modes of oxygen administration. O_2 is administered by nasal
cannula at a flow rate sufficient to achieve a PaO_2 greater than 60
mm Hg or saturation more than 90%; this usually requires a flow of
3 L/min or less with the patient at rest. O_2 is supplied by electrically
driven O_2 concentrators, as liquid O_2 systems, or in cylinders of compressed gas. Concentrators are the method of choice for patients who
spend most of their time at home, as this system is the least expensive of the three. Such patients require small O_2 tanks as backup in
the event of an electrical failure and for portable use while walking.

A liquid system is preferable if patients spend much time out of
their homes. The portable canisters that are part of liquid systems are
easier to carry and have more O_2 capacity than portable cylinders of
compressed gas. Large cylinders are the most expensive way of providing O_2 for LTOT and should be used only if no other source is
available. All patients must be taught the dangers of smoking during
O_2 use.

A variety of devices have been developed that conserve the amount
of O_2 used by the patient. These O_2-conserving devices operate either by use of a reservoir system or by permitting O_2 flow only during inspiration. They have been shown to be equivalent to continuous-
flow systems.

Exercise Programs. Patients who are sedentary because they
are dyspneic on exercise or who have undergone a prolonged period
of inactivity because they have been hospitalized for respiratory failure develop severe skeletal muscle deconditioning. As a result, they
have increased ventilatory and cardiovascular requirements during exercise. These effects can be ameliorated by a program of graded exercise. In seriously deconditioned patients with end-stage COPD,
supplemental O_2 therapy must generally be used. Training of the respiratory muscles seems to have little advantage over exercise training of the whole person. Based on the observation that unsupported
arm exercise results in dyspnea and fatigue at a much lower O_2 uptake than exercise performed by the lower extremities, upper extremity exercises appear to be helpful in relieving dyspnea.

COPD patients should be taught methods of energy conservation
during activities of daily living. Difficulties in sexual function should
be explored and advice given on the use of energy-conserving positions for sexual intercourse or noncoital alternatives for sexual gratification.

Nutrition. Many patients with advanced COPD experience major but slowly progressive weight loss, and some of them become
frankly cachectic. In others the weight loss occurs stepwise, seemingly precipitated by a superimposed acute illness or hospitalization.
These patients show no evidence of protein malnutrition; lean body
mass is preserved, and serum albumin is normal. The cause of this
excessive weight loss is mainly a 15% to 25% increase in resting energy expenditure, perhaps the result of a greatly elevated work of
breathing. Increased diet-induced thermogenesis, a higher energy cost
of daily activities, and a reduced caloric intake relative to need may
be other important factors. One consequence of this excessive weight
loss is reduced respiratory muscle strength.

Improved nutrition can restore respiratory and general muscle
strength and endurance, but such improvement occurs only after clear-
cut weight gain. Unfortunately, this has been consistently accomplished only within a controlled hospital environment, with little success in patients living at home.

Pulmonary Rehabilitation. Pulmonary rehabilitation may be
defined as a program designed to improve the functioning of the
whole person once everything possible has been done to improve the
function of the lungs. Many elements of a rehabilitation program for
COPD patients have already been discussed. It is important to educate the patient and the family about the nature of the illness and
how to care for it. The patient should take as much responsibility for
personal care as possible. The benefits of rehabilitation are improved
independence and quality of life, decreased number of hospital days,
and improved exercise capacity. Lung function is not improved.

Every physician who treats end-stage COPD will organize a rehabilitation program for the patient. Many hospitals and health care organizations have developed formal, multidisciplinary rehabilitation
programs with an intensive, focused approach. These programs are
especially important for persons who remain ventilator-bound after
an episode of acute respiratory failure. Many such patients can attain
a few hours per day off the ventilator and can be taught to participate
in their own care; some can even be sent home on a ventilator.

STAGING OF THERAPY AND WHEN TO REFER

As noted later, the best correlation with mortality and morbidity in
COPD is with the FEV_1, which is the basis of a staging scheme recently presented by the American Thoracic Society. The staging
scheme is defined and its use in planning the work-up and therapy
and providing guidance in the caregiver's expertise in managing patients with COPD is given in Table 51-1.

LUNG TRANSPLANTATION FOR EMPHYSEMA

With the advent of heart-lung or double-lung transplantation, considerable progress has been made over the last 10 years in lung transplantation for obstructive airways disease. Most of the patients who
have received transplants had API deficiency. Since 1989, single-lung
transplantation has largely replaced double-lung transplantation in
these patients. Single-lung transplantation is a much easier procedure
to perform than double-lung transplantation. Cardiac bypass is usually not necessary. The surgical, early, and late morbidity and the mortality are lower in single-lung than in double-lung transplantation.
However, the FVC and FEV_1 are lower after single-lung than after
double-lung transplantation. Arterial blood gases are similarly improved in the two procedures. Single-lung transplantation is more applicable to an older population than double-lung transplantation.

COMPLICATIONS
Sleep and COPD

A slight decrease in alveolar ventilation is normal during sleep. This
is manifest as a 5 to 6 mm Hg increase in $PaCO_2$ and a slightly greater
decrease in PaO_2. Patients with COPD have a greater decrease in alveolar ventilation with sleep than normal persons; the increase in
$PaCO_2$ and decrease in PaO_2 are also greater than in normal individuals. Since awake PaO_2 is on the shoulder of the oxyhemoglobin dissociation curve in many COPD patients, the decrease in saturation
will be much greater in the COPD patient than in the normal person.

Table 51-1 Staging of therapy for COPD and when to refer

STAGE	STAGE I	STAGE II	STAGE III
Defined	$FEV_1 \geq 50\%$ predicted	FEV_1 35% to 49% predicted	$FEV_1 \leq 39\%$ predicted
Additional pulmonary function studies	Hypoxemia is mild and ABG are not needed. Postbronchodilator spirometry is optional.	ABG studies are essential to determine severity of hypoxemia and the presence and severity of hypercapnia. Postbronchodilator spirometry is useful in deciding corticosteroid use. Lung volumes and diffusing capacity are optional.	
PA, lateral chest film	Required at all stages to exclude other diseases such as lung cancer and pneumonia.		
Smoking cessation	Undertaking a smoking cessation program is worthwhile at every stage of COPD.		
Infection prevention	Influenza vaccine should be given annually and pneumococcal vaccine approximately every 6 years at every stage of COPD.		
Pharmacotherapy	β_2-agonist MDI or slowly absorbed oral theophylline preparation.	In addition to the β_2-agonist MDI and oral theophylline, ipratropium MDI may be tried. Prescribe oral corticosteroids if there is a >25% bronchodilator response of FEV_1. Start antibiotics at home with exacerbation.	
Long-term oxygen therapy	Unnecessary.	Infrequently necessary.	Commonly necessary.
Rehabilitation program	Unnecessary.	Education and prescription of regular exercise and other elements of rehabilitation by the physician usually suffice.	A multidisciplinary rehabilitation program, coupled with chest physical therapy to help mobilize secretions, is indicated.
Expertise of physician	Patients are readily cared for by a generalist.	After evaluation by a respiratory specialist, can be cared for by a generalist with as-needed consultation.	Generally best cared for by a respiratory specialist.
When to refer	At any stage, hemoptysis, spontaneous pneumothorax, severe pneumonia, or acute respiratory failure requires consultation by a respiratory specialist.		

ABG, arterial blood gases during air breathing; *MDI*, metered dose inhaler.

The decrease in blood O_2 level is greatest during rapid eye movement (REM) sleep and also tends to become greater as the night progresses, perhaps as a result of retention of secretions and worsening ventilation-perfusion relations. Patients with COPD may have hypopnea, but episodes of apnea are distinctly uncommon. The quality of sleep is impaired. Severe nocturnal hypoxemia is associated with increased frequency of cardiac arrhythmias and development of pulmonary hypertension. Nocturnal oxygen should be used in COPD patients who have meaningful periods of $Sao_2 \leq 88\%$ during sleep.

Acute Respiratory Failure

Acute respiratory failure in patients with COPD may be defined as an exacerbation that is accompanied by a Pao_2 less than 50 mm Hg or a $Paco_2$ greater than 50 mm Hg. Respiratory depressant drugs, abdominal or thoracic surgery, or complications such as pneumothorax are additional precipitating factors. It is unusual for the $Paco_2$ to rise above 80 mm Hg unless the patient has received O_2 therapy. The patient's clinical state during an episode of acute respiratory failure is highly variable. Mental state ranges from alert, anxious, agitated, and distressed to somnolent, stuporous, or comatose. Cyanosis is usually present unless the patient is receiving O_2 therapy. Diaphoresis and a hyperdynamic circulation typically occur. Breathing is labored, and the accessory muscles are in full use.

The first goal in treatment is to improve hypoxemia and prevent tissue hypoxia. This goal may be quickly reached by administering low, controlled concentrations of O_2 sufficient to raise the Pao_2 to 55 to 60 mm Hg (arterial O_2 saturation, 88% to 90%), which will prevent tissue hypoxia but not completely abolish hypoxic ventilatory drive. The small increase in Pao_2 occurs on the steep part of the oxyhemoglobin dissociation curve, resulting in a large increase in saturation. A Venturi mask that delivers 24% to 28% O_2 or a nasal cannula with an O_2 flow of 1 to 2 L/min may be used. A slight increase in $Paco_2$ may occur, but because blood bicarbonate levels usually have risen in response to chronic hypercapnia, worsening of acidemia will be slight. Increases in $Paco_2$ that do not cause decreases in pH below 7.25 are tolerable.

The next step in management is to institute therapy to overcome reversible airway obstruction. Hydration should be started, along with intravenous aminophylline and corticosteroids. Appropriate antibiotic therapy should be given after a Gram stain and culture of sputum have been done. Inhalation therapy with a β_2 agonist should be instituted. Reevaluation of the patient should be carried out clinically and by blood gas measurement at least every 4 hours. The pH and $Paco_2$ are the important indices to follow.

A high proportion of patients can be managed by a conservative regimen. Slightly worsening hypoxemia and acidemia are not themselves an indication for instituting mechanical ventilation, as long as they are associated with a stable or improving clinical state. The role of noninvasive methods of mechanical ventilation using intermittent positive pressure by face mask is under investigation. Deterioration in blood gases associated with clinical deterioration, especially the development of progressive fatigue and difficulty in cooperation, indicates the need for instituting endotracheal intubation and mechanical ventilation.

Once the patient is on a ventilator, it is important not to ventilate so vigorously that the $Paco_2$ decreases rapidly. Because blood bicarbonate levels are usually high, a steep decrease in $Paco_2$ may result in severe alkalemia, with convulsions, coma, and death. Careful attention should be paid to nutrition. Weaning from mechanical ventilation should be carried out as soon as possible, often within a few days. With a good rehabilitation program, many patients can be restored to their former level of function. Patients can be managed with endotracheal tubes for 3 to 4 weeks before a tracheostomy is done.

In managing ambulatory patients who have COPD with severe obstruction, it is important to determine in advance whether, in the event of acute respiratory failure, the patient wishes to be mechanically ventilated and take the risk of having a tracheotomy and becoming dependent on a ventilator.

Chronic Cor Pulmonale

Chronic cor pulmonale may be defined as right ventricular hypertrophy caused by pulmonary hypertension. Pulmonary arterial pressures may rise to a mean of 30 to 40 mm Hg at rest and higher on exercise, as opposed to the normal value of 10 to 20 mm Hg. Although loss of capillary bed resulting from emphysema may play some part, the major cause of the pulmonary hypertension in COPD patients is hypoxic vasoconstriction. Acidemia augments hypoxemia and may be important during sleep and exacerbations. Transmission of increased intrathoracic pressure is reflected in pulmonary arterial pressure measurement. Increased viscosity of blood from erythrocytosis is of minor importance, but hypervolemia may play some role. Left ventricular dysfunction is a minor contributor.

Short of right-sided heart catheterization, the diagnosis of pulmonary hypertension and cor pulmonale in COPD is difficult. An R or R' wave greater than or equal to the S wave in lead V_1, an R wave less than the amplitude of the S wave in lead V_6, and right-axis deviation greater than 110 degrees without right bundle branch block all support the diagnosis of cor pulmonale. Two-dimensional echocardiography, especially with an esophageal transducer, and pulsed Doppler techniques to estimate mean pulmonary arterial pressure are recently developed modalities to assess pulmonary hypertension and right ventricular function. Left ventricular size and performance are generally normal in patients with COPD in the absence of other associated cardiac abnormalities. The right ventricular ejection fraction is frequently abnormal, especially on exercise. The radiographic diagnosis of cor pulmonale is discussed earlier in this chapter.

The treatment of cor pulmonale is the treatment of the underlying lung disease. Correction of hypoxemia by long-term O_2 therapy is essential. Diuretics are useful for the control of edema. Digitalis should be reserved for the management of a supraventricular tachyrhythmia.

Pneumothorax

Unlike the benign nature of simple spontaneous pneumothorax occurring in a young person with localized bullae, pneumothorax complicating COPD often precipitates severe dyspnea and acute respiratory failure. This condition should be suspected in any patient with sudden worsening of pulmonary status. Physical examination is of limited help because diminished breath sounds, the cardinal sign of a small pneumothorax, also occur with emphysema. The diagnosis is readily made from the chest radiograph. Even a small pneumothorax can cause severe respiratory insufficiency in COPD patients with marginal pulmonary reserve.

Because it is often accompanied by a persistent bronchopleural fistula, pneumothorax complicating COPD is difficult to treat. Most bronchopleural fistulas close after several days of tube thoracostomy, although negative pressures of 30 cm H_2O or more may be required to expand the lung. If this fails to occur, surgical closure of the fistula, along with bullectomy, pleurodesis, or a parietal pleurectomy, is often necessary. When pulmonary function is severely impaired, surgery may be judged too hazardous to undertake. An attempt to obliterate the pleural space with the instillation of doxycycline is a useful alternative approach.

Giant Bullae

Impairment of Function. Large bullae that involve a third or more of one or both hemithoraces may severely disrupt lung function in the involved hemithorax and may even encroach on the opposite lung. Resectional surgery under these circumstances may produce a marked improvement in symptoms and lung function. The functional results of surgery are related to the amount of normal or minimally diseased lung tissue that was compressed by the resected bullae. In general, patients do best when they have large bullae and an FEV_1 of about half the predicted normal value. Serial chest radiographs and CT are most useful in making a decision as to whether compression of viable lung by bullae is responsible for a patient's current functional state or whether the process is part of generalized emphysema. Since 1994, the use of volume reduction surgery has been explored in severely emphysematous patients without giant bullae. Patients have been highly selected. Although some have had impressive improvements in lung function and quality of life, the duration of improvement is unknown.

Infection. Infection with pyogenic organisms or with a fungus such as *Aspergillus* species, causing a mycetoma, may rarely occur within bullae. Treatment with appropriate antibiotics is indicated for pyogenic infection. Mycetomas rarely require therapy unless they are associated with life-threatening hemoptysis. In that event, resectional surgery or bronchial arterial embolization should be considered. Antifungal therapy is not indicated for mycetomas unless clear evidence exists of tissue invasion by the fungus.

COPD and Commercial Air Travel

Because commercial airliners pressurize their flight cabins to an altitude of 5000 to 10,000 feet, COPD patients who fly in the stratosphere are subjected to the added stress of a significantly reduced inspired O_2 partial pressure. At an altitude of 5000 feet, the equivalent inspired fractional concentration of O_2 (FIO_2) is 17.1% and at 10,000 feet, 13.9%. This may substantially worsen hypoxemia, because COPD patients have limited ability to increase their resting ventilation. Eucapnic COPD patients with a sea level PaO_2 greater than 68 mm Hg will generally have a flight PaO_2 greater than 50 mm Hg and will not require supplemental O_2. All COPD patients with hypercapnia, as well as those with significant anemia (hematocrit <30) or co-existing cardiac or cerebrovascular disease, should use supplemental O_2 during long flights.

When making their reservation, patients should notify the airline concerning their diagnosis and the need for in-flight O_2. Patients are not permitted to use their own O_2. The airlines will provide a chemically generated O_2 system. Patients should bring their own nasal cannulas because airlines usually provide only face masks.

PROGNOSIS AND COURSE

Not surprisingly, in view of what has already been said about the importance of airways obstruction in causing death and disability, the severity of airways obstruction is related to survival in patients with COPD. Mortality slightly increases at 10 years in persons with moderate airway obstruction but with an FEV_1 greater than 1.0 L. In persons with FEV_1 values less than 0.75 L, the approximate mortality rate at 1 year is 30% and at 10 years, 95%. Hypercapnia is an adverse prognostic factor. Recent data suggest that marked reversibility of airways obstruction is a favorable prognostic factor.

Longitudinal studies from several centers have shown that some patients with severe airways obstruction may survive for many years beyond the average, some for as long as 15 years. The reason for this appears to be that death in patients with COPD generally occurs because of some medical complication, such as acute respiratory failure, severe pneumonia, pneumothorax, cardiac arrhythmia, or pulmonary embolism. It is important for these patients to be able to enter the medical care system easily when they are acutely ill. Careful management of COPD patients can be rewarding not only because the physician's involvement in medical care relieves suffering, but also because it prolongs life.

BIBLIOGRAPHY

American Thoracic Society: Standards for the diagnosis and care of patients with chronic obstructive pulmonary disease, *Am J Respir Crit Care Med* 152:S77-S120, 1995.

Anthonisen NR: Prognosis in chronic obstructive pulmonary disease: results from multicenter clinical trials, *Am Rev Respir Dis* 133:S95, 1989.

Buist AS et al: Guidelines for the approach to the individual with severe hereditary alpha-1-antitrypsin deficiency: an official statement of the American Thoracic Society, *Am Rev Respir Dis* 140:1494, 1989.

Clausen JL: The diagnosis of emphysema, chronic bronchitis and asthma, *Clin Chest Med* 11:405, 1990.

Curtis JR, Hudson LD: Emergent assessment and management of acute respiratory failure in COPD, *Clin Chest Med* 15:481, 1994.

Donahoe M, Rogers RM: Nutritional assessment in chronic obstructive pulmonary disease, *Clin Chest Med* 11:487, 1990.

Douglas NJ, Flenley DC: Breathing during sleep in patients with obstructive lung disease, *Am Rev Respir Dis* 141:1055, 1990.

Celli BR: Pulmonary rehabilitation in patients with COPD, *Am J Respir Crit Care Med* 152:861, 1995.

Hodgkin JE: Prognosis in chronic obstructive pulmonary disease, *Clin Chest Med* 11:555, 1990.

Jenkinson SG, Levine SM: Lung transplantation, *Dis Mon* 40:1, 1994.

Kanford SL et al: Predicting smoking cessation: who will quit with and without the nicotine patch, *JAMA* 271:589, 1994.

Knoell DL, Wewers MD: Clinical implications of gene therapy for alpha 1-antitrypsin deficiency, *Chest* 107:535, 1995.

Lee EW, D'Alonzo GE: Cigarette smoking, nicotine addiction and its pharmacologic treatment, *Arch Intern Med* 153:34, 1993.

Lucey EC, Stone PJ, Snider GL: Consequences of proteolytic injury. In Crystal RG et al, editors: *The lung: scientific foundations*, ed 2, New York, 1996, Raven.

MacNee W: Pathophysiology of cor pulmonale in chronic obstructive pulmonary disease, *Am J Respir Crit Care Med* 150:833, 1158, 1994.

Schwartz JL: Methods of smoking cessation, *Med Clin North Am* 76:451, 1992.

Sherrill DL, Lebowitz M, Burrows B: Epidemiology of chronic obstructive pulmonary disease, *Clin Chest Med* 11:375, 1990.

Snider GL: Pulmonary disease in alpha-1-antitrypsin deficiency, *Ann Intern Med* 111:957, 1989.

Snider GL: Emphysema—the first two centuries—and beyond, *Am Rev Respir Dis* 146:1334, 1615, 1992.

Snider GL, Faling LJ, Rennard SI: Chronic bronchitis and emphysema. In Murray JF, Nadel JA, editors: *Textbook of respiratory medicine*, ed 2, Philadelphia, 1993, WB Saunders.

Tarpy SO, Celli BR: Long-term oxygen therapy, *N Engl J Med* 333:710, 1995.

52 Interstitial Lung Disease

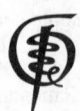

Jack D. Fulmer* and K. Randall Young, Jr.

The interstitial lung diseases are diverse disorders grouped together because of common clinical, roentgenographic, and pathologic features. Most patients come to medical attention with exertional dyspnea, and if the underlying pathologic process is unchecked, destruction of gas exchange units leads to end-stage lung disease.

The nomenclature for these diseases has varied. This chapter uses the term *interstitial* because most of these diseases result in the development of scar tissue in the alveolar interstitium. This term is only partly correct, however, since airways disease, alveolar filling disease, vascular disease, and pleural disease all can coexist with the interstitial disease. The term *infiltrative lung disease* also seems appropriate in some of these diseases, since it implies an abnormal accumulation of cells and noncellular elements in lung tissue. This is particularly applicable in the neoplastic diseases and in some metabolic or inherited interstitial lung diseases.

The objectives of this chapter are to present an overview of the pathologic, pathogenetic, pathophysiologic, and clinical features of these diseases. A rational approach to the decision making in the diagnosis and management of these diseases is presented. Specific diseases are briefly discussed. This chapter's overall emphasis, however, is on the interstitial pneumonias.

LUNG PATHOLOGY

An understanding of the pathologic features of the interstitial lung diseases, particularly the acute injury patterns and the chronic interstitial pneumonias, is critical to diagnosis and management. The histologic features of these diseases are remarkably similar and at times difficult for pathologists to classify. In almost all, there is an accumulation of cells within alveolar septae and air spaces, as well as alveolar septal fibrosis with destruction and revision of gas exchange units. Depending on the origin or cause, chronicity, and several poorly understood modulating factors, the severity of the alveolitis, degree of fibrosis, and actual tissue destruction vary. In general, early-stage disease is characterized by an active alveolitis with minimal alveolar septal fibrosis and destruction. In contrast, advanced disease is associated with minimal alveolitis but widespread alveolar destruction and fibrosis. If the disease is progressive, end-stage or "honeycomb" lung disease results. The use of the term *alveolitis* may be unfortunate in some cases, because inflammation may actually begin in the interstitial compartment of the lung. Nonetheless, the term has gained currency in discussions of early pathogenetic events in this group of disorders.

Various pathologic classifications have been used and, when possible, the pathologist makes an etiologic or specific histologic diagnosis. Examples include many of the inorganic dust diseases, the infectious and neoplastic infiltrative diseases, the pulmonary vasculitides, and the pulmonary hemorrhage syndromes. Further, although special techniques may be required, information can be provided on both the natural and the treated history of many interstitial diseases. Some interstitial diseases have a specific histologic pattern, but only through careful clinical and radiographic correlation can a correct diagnosis be made.

The pathologic classification of the interstitial pneumonias has been controversial. One useful classification (Box 52-1), which is a modification by Liebow, is now widely used and can be applied to the idiopathic interstitial pneumonias or the interstitial pneumonias of known origin. This classification, however, incorrectly includes bronchiolitis obliterans–organizing pneumonia (BOOP). This is pri-

*The authors gratefully acknowledge the contributions of the late Jack D. Fulmer.

> ### BOX 52-1
> ### Pathologic classification of interstitial pneumonias
>
> **Acute**
> Acute interstitial pneumonia (AIP)
> Bronchiolitis obliterans–organizing pneumonia (BOOP)
>
> **Chronic**
> Usual interstitial pneumonia (UIP)
> Desquamative interstitial pneumonia (DIP) (respiratory bronchiolitis)
> Chronic interstitial pneumonia–NOS (CIP)
> Lymphoid interstitial pneumonia (LIP)
> Giant cell interstitial pneumonia (GIP)

NOS, Not otherwise specified.

marily an airways disease, not an interstitial disease; BOOP is included because some view it as part of the spectrum of the interstitial diseases, and often an interstitial pattern is evident on the chest roentgenogram. This classification also includes giant cell interstitial pneumonia (GIP), a rare, poorly understood entity. Giant cell interstitial pneumonia probably is a form of organic dust disease caused by inhalation of heavy metals; this chapter does not discuss this disease further. A description of the interstitial pneumonias is presented in the following sections.

Acute Interstitial Pneumonia

Acute interstitial pneumonia (AIP) is a rare form of interstitial pneumonia corresponding to the lesion described by Hamman and Rich in 1944. The pathologic appearance of AIP is identical to that observed in diffuse alveolar damage (DAD), the pathologic appearance of the adult respiratory distress syndrome (ARDS). A single injury seems to occur at one point, after which an orderly sequence of events takes place. Initially there is an exudative phase, which involves capillary congestion, interstitial edema, and alveolar exudation with the formation of hyaline membranes. After approximately 1 week type II epithelial cells proliferate, and by the second week fibroblasts proliferate, resulting in an organizing phase. Interstitial fibrosis with the formation of end-stage lung disease can occur after 3 to 4 weeks. Thrombi are common in small arteries. The appearance of AIP, depending on the stage when biopsy is performed, usually corresponds to the organizing stage of DAD. Examples of AIP were previously lumped with cases of usual interstitial pneumonia (UIP). However, AIP can be distinguished on histologic examination by the uniformity of the lesions, reflecting an acute injury occurring at a single time.

Bronchiolitis Obliterans–Organizing Pneumonia

Previously classified with the chronic interstitial pneumonias, BOOP is primarily a disease in which the fibrosing process involves air spaces, not alveolar interstitium. However, some alveolar septal thickening with an inflammatory cellular infiltrate, as well as type II epithelial hyperplasia, may occur. Ultrastructural studies have demonstrated alveolar epithelial necrosis and collapse, indicating that BOOP is an acute form of lung injury.

The fibrosing process in BOOP is characterized by polypoid plugs of loose connective tissue containing spindle-shaped fibroblasts and a chronic inflammatory cellular infiltrate with a loose, myxoid matrix. These plugs are present in distal bronchioles, alveolar ducts, and peribronchiolar air spaces. These polyps may be covered by a lining of bronchiolar or alveolar epithelial cells. These polypoid lesions may be a minor feature of some other interstitial pneumonia (e.g., UIP), the eosinophilic pneumonias, and Langerhans' cell granulomatosis (eosinophilic granuloma); the presence of these lesions, however, should not mislead the pathologist to make the diagnosis of BOOP. BOOP is usually a steroid-sensitive disease, and it is likely that many cases of steroid-responsive UIP in the past literature represent examples of BOOP.

Usual Interstitial Pneumonia

Usual interstitial pneumonia is the most common pathologic type of chronic interstitial pneumonia. The characteristic features are microscopic areas of normal lung alternating with areas of active alveolitis and varying degrees of fibrosis. The cellular infiltrate consists of macrophages, lymphocytes, and plasma cells. Although neutrophils are frequently seen on lung lavage cellular analysis, neutrophils are rarely present in tissue. Usual interstitial pneumonia does not represent a specific clinical diagnosis, and the natural history of UIP varies depending on the clinical syndrome. Usual interstitial pneumonia is a common histologic diagnosis in many of the collagen vascular diseases, radiation lung disease, and the late stages of sarcoidosis and some dust diseases. Patients with UIP who have a progressive bibasilar interstitial pattern on chest roentgenogram and no evidence of a systemic illness usually have idiopathic pulmonary fibrosis (IPF).

Desquamative Interstitial Pneumonia

Desquamative interstitial pneumonia (DIP) is characterized by a homogeneous filling of the alveolar air spaces with macrophages and a few type II epithelial cells. There is minimum alveolar septal infiltration with cells and connective tissue. This lesion was initially thought to represent an early stage of UIP but more likely represents a rare response to some type of parenchymal injury. Most cases are idiopathic, but DIP has been described in drug-induced interstitial disease and in some collagen vascular disorders. Rarely, DIP may progress to end-stage lung disease. Some other interstitial diseases may have an accumulation of macrophages in scattered areas with a "DIP-like reaction," but these differ from DIP by the coexistence of significant interstitial fibrosis and destruction of gas exchange units, a feature not present in DIP.

Although primarily a disease of the airways and more correctly grouped with the inhalation disorders, respiratory bronchiolitis may produce an interstitial pattern on the chest roentgenogram. A disease of smokers, respiratory bronchiolitis is characterized by numerous pigmented macrophages in respiratory bronchioles and neighboring alveolar ducts. Alveolar septae may show some fibrous thickening, and some type II epithelial cell hyperplasia may be present. Although most patients do not have progression, it has been suggested that DIP may represent a late stage of a progressive form of respiratory bronchiolitis. It has been reported, however, that some patients with respiratory bronchiolitis may show clinical and roentgenographic improvement with cessation of smoking.

Chronic Interstitial Pneumonia–Not Otherwise Specified

A small but significant number of interstitial pneumonias cannot be classified using the previous criteria (not otherwise specified [NOS]). Now called chronic interstitial pneumonia (CIP), this lesion was previously classified along with cases of UIP. On histologic study CIP is characterized by a temporally uniform interstitial pattern without the skip areas of normal lung tissue that are seen in UIP. The interstitial infiltrate consists of chronic inflammatory cells, fibroblasts, and variable degrees of fibrosis. This pattern can be associated with the collagen vascular disorders, drug reactions, organic and inorganic dust diseases, bone marrow transplantation, or acquired immunodeficiency syndrome (AIDS). Chronic interstitial pneumonia can also be idiopathic.

Lymphoid Interstitial Pneumonia

Lymphoid interstitial pneumonia (LIP) was first described as an interstitial disease with a cellular infiltrate consisting of lymphocytes, plasma cells, and an occasional immunoblast. It is now known that LIP usually is a lymphoproliferative disorder, probably a low-grade lymphoma. Some cases of LIP do represent a response to a viral infection; others are associated with an autoimmune disorder. This pattern has also been associated with AIDS, particularly in children. Infrequently, LIP is idiopathic, and progression to end-stage lung disease has been reported.

BOX 52-2
Clinicopathologic classification of interstitial lung diseases

Known origins for interstitial diseases

Occupational and environmental inhalants
  Inorganic dusts
  Organic dusts
  Gases, fumes, vapors, aerosols
Drugs
Poisons
Infectious agents
Radiation
Allergy
Trauma
Neoplastic diseases
Hemodynamic/cardiac diseases
Metabolic disorders
Miscellaneous disorders

Interstitial diseases of unknown origin

Acute interstitial pneumonia (Hamman-Rich syndrome)
Idiopathic pulmonary fibrosis
Collagen vascular diseases
Sarcoidosis
Pulmonary vasculitis
Hemorrhage syndromes
Langerhans' cell granulomatosis (eosinophilic granuloma)
Lymphoid infiltrative disorders
Bronchiolar diseases
Eosinophilic pneumonias
Inherited diseases
Non–collagen vascular immune diseases
Pulmonary venoocclusive disease
Alveolar proteinosis
Lymphangioleiomyomatosis
Unclassified interstitial diseases

CLINICOPATHOLOGIC CLASSIFICATION

To approach the interstitial diseases in an orderly manner, some type of clinical or clinicopathologic classification is needed. Ideally a classification should be based on causes or origins, but only about half of these diseases have a defined origin; the remainder must be classified by careful clinical, laboratory, and pathologic correlation (Box 52-2). This classification is flawed because several of these diseases share overlapping clinicopathologic features. For example, many of the collagen vascular disorders, Wegener's granulomatosis, and several occupational lung diseases can become evident with diffuse alveolar hemorrhage. In addition, several alveolar filling diseases can ultimately progress to chronic interstitial fibrosis; these include the eosinophilic pneumonias, pulmonary alveolar proteinosis, and idiopathic pulmonary hemosiderosis.

PATHOGENESIS

Regardless of whether the origin of the interstitial disease is known or unknown, current concepts suggest that a common pathogenetic scheme is involved (Fig. 52-1). Initially some type of stimulus causes injury to epithelial or endothelial cells, resulting in edema or cellular death. As a result of the injury, there is activation of resident lung cells and exudation of serum and cellular debris into alveolar air spaces. Release of cytokines, with serum and cellular breakdown products, recruits inflammatory and immune effector cells into the alveolar interstitium and air spaces (e.g., an alveolitis). The eventual degree of lung injury is a consequence of the initial events triggering the cascade, as well as damage mediated by proteases, toxic oxygen species, cationic proteins, and other substances released by inflammatory cells recruited to the site of injury. Repair processes are also activated shortly after the injury and serve to limit the damage to the gas exchange unit by repairing damage to the basement membrane

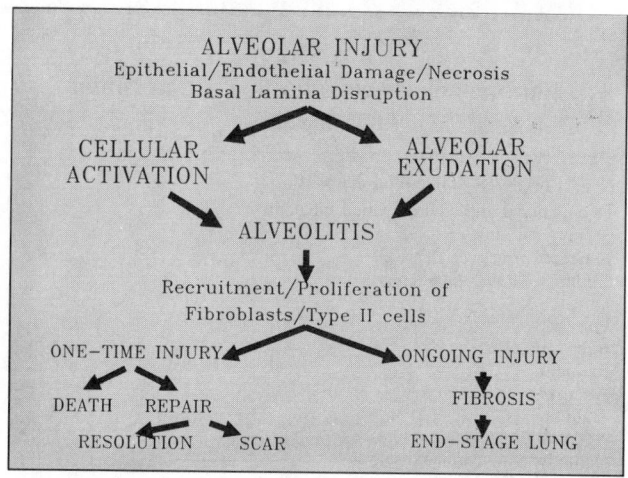

FIGURE 52-1   Pathogenesis of interstitial lung disease.

and stimulating proliferation of new alveolar lining cells. With a one-time injury lung repair can be complete, or some residual scarring may occur. In the chronic interstitial pneumonias there are continuous foci of alveolar injury, inflammation, destruction, and repair.

The injurious agents in these diseases are complex and poorly understood. In some of the interstitial lung diseases, parenchymal injury is initiated by deposition of immune complexes or tissue-specific or cytotoxic antibodies. In the majority of these disorders, however, little is known about the identity of specific inciting events. Substantial research has focused on cellular and molecular interactions triggered by known and unknown stimuli. Early damage to resident cells including alveolar macrophages and alveolar epithelial cells leads to the release of cytokines such as interleukin-1 and tumor necrosis factor, which seem important to the initiation of the alveolitis in several types of experimental disease. In some acute and chronic interstitial diseases the alveolar macrophage appears to be central in both the exudative phase and the reparative phase. Previously viewed as only phagocytic cells, macrophages can secrete a variety of polypeptides, complement components, enzymes, lipids, and extracellular matrix proteins. Many of these products appear important in the pathogenesis of the interstitial diseases. Alveolar macrophages harvested from patients with chronic interstitial pneumonias secrete a variety of chemoattractants, including interleukin-8, fibronectin, and members of the chemokine family. These chemoattractants are responsible for inducing the migration of fibroblasts into injured lung and for attracting inflammatory cells such as neutrophils and monocytes from the circulation into tissue. Additional cytokines such as transforming growth factor beta and platelet-derived growth factor, a potent mitogenic polypeptide for fibroblasts, recruit, activate, and induce proliferation of fibroblasts, type II epithelial cells, and endothelial cells (Fig. 52-1).

Lung architectural revision and the development of fibrosis have been intensively studied. Whether alveoli can be repaired depends on the intactness of the basement membrane; without it, no scaffolding exists for replacement of denuded cells. Also, proteinases appear to be important in destroying critical connective tissue macromolecules. Mechanisms of fibrosis are multiple, and the fibroblast is the key cell producing the connective tissue macromolecules. Recruitment of fibroblasts can occur into the alveolar exudate with subsequent synthesis of collagen and other connective tissue macromolecules. As an alternative, fibroblasts may increase in the alveolar interstitium, with increased connective tissue biosynthesis. With loss of epithelial cells lining alveoli, alveolar collapse or atelectatic induration and development of fibrosis and volume loss may occur. The result in all these situations is a disorderly deposition of collagen with the formation of epithelial-lined cystic spaces, often called "the honeycomb lung."

Ongoing investigation in several laboratories suggests that the appearance of fibrin in the alveolar space may be an important feature of the development of pulmonary fibrosis. Transudation of fibrinogen from serum into alveoli fosters the deposition of a fibrin "scaffolding" into which fibroblasts can migrate and elaborate fibrous tissue. This process depends on the balance of factors that either promote or inhibit fibrogenic responses, including plasminogen activators and inhibitors of plasminogen activation, and therapeutic strategies designed to alter this balance in favor of fibrin breakdown may have a beneficial effect by decreasing the extent of fibrotic reaction.

PATHOPHYSIOLOGY

The classic physiologic features of the interstitial diseases are a reduction in lung volumes and compliance, decreased carbon monoxide diffusing capacity (D_{LCO}), and exercise-induced hypoxemia. Airflow obstruction may be present in some patients but is not a common feature.

The earliest physiologic alteration in many patients is a reduction in D_{LCO} and exercise-induced hypoxemia with widening of the alveolar-arterial oxygen gradient. Some patients have a normal roentgenogram and normal lung volumes. Because of thickened alveolar septae, it was initially thought that the major cause of hypoxemia was a diffusion barrier to oxygen. Subsequent research indicated that ventilation-perfusion imbalance was a major cause. Recent reexamination of the origins of hypoxemia in these diseases, however, suggests that impaired oxygen diffusion may be a significant component of both resting and exercise-induced hypoxemia. As the disease process progresses, loss of gas exchange units from destruction or atelectasis results in increased elastic recoil, causing reduced lung volumes and increased work of breathing.

Vital capacity (VC) and total lung capacity (TLC) are reduced at midcourse in these diseases. Among the alveolar filling diseases and the acute diseases, increased elastic recoil and reduced lung volumes may occur quite early. In the chronic interstitial diseases, residual volume (RV) may be reduced to a greater or lesser extent than VC, the RV/TLC ratio may be increased, decreased, or unchanged. Lung compliance is also reduced midcourse in these diseases, and the volume-pressure relationship is shifted downward and to the right.

Some of the interstitial diseases show morphologic and functional evidence of airways disease. Small airways disease (airways <2 mm in diameter) may be present in patients with IPF, sarcoidosis, and some collagen vascular diseases. Intraluminal bronchial obstruction caused by granulomatous lesions may be seen in sarcoidosis and in Wegener's granulomatosis. Reversible airflow obstruction may occur in patients with the Churg-Strauss syndrome, in some with eosinophilic pneumonia, and occasionally in those with other interstitial diseases (e.g., sarcoidosis). A few of these diseases may show a major obstructive defect on routine spirometry. These include cystic sarcoidosis, Langerhans' cell granulomatosis, chronic organic dust disease, and lymphangioleiomyomatosis. Exercise-induced hypoxemia is characteristic of early interstitial disease, but resting hypoxemia is typical of advanced disease. In general, most patients with interstitial disease have elevated minute ventilation with hypocapnia. As the disease advances, hypercapnia may result, and large right-to-left intrapulmonary shunts may develop so that oxygenation may be impossible. Pulmonary hypertension with cor pulmonale often occurs in advanced interstitial lung disease.

CLINICAL FEATURES

Most patients come to medical attention with exertional breathlessness. Depending on the type of interstitial disease, other symptoms may be seen. Some patients may have fever, including some with AIP or BOOP or diseases caused by infectious disorders. Fever may also occur with acute organic dust disease, drug-induced disease, some collagen vascular disorders, and some pulmonary vasculitides, and infrequently in IPF. Cough is common at midcourse and in advanced interstitial disease. Wheezes can be auscultated in patients with Churg-Strauss syndrome and eosinophilic pneumonias. Digital clubbing often occurs in the advanced stages.

The physical examination of patients with early interstitial disease may be totally normal. As the disease advances, auscultation may reveal diffuse bronchovesicular breath sounds with bibasilar, coarse crackles. These are often described as "Velcro" crackles by analogy to the sound made by pulling Velcro apart. Interestingly, patients with sarcoidosis can have extensive interstitial disease on the chest roentgenogram but show few physical signs on auscultation. Exertional cyanosis may be present at midcourse in these diseases, but resting cyanosis with tachypnea and the use of accessory muscles usually signifies advanced disease. Accentuation of the pulmonic closure sound may initially be present only during exercise, but as the disease advances, pulmonary hypertension and findings of cor pulmonale develop. Right ventricular failure is a late manifestation of these diseases.

IMAGING TECHNIQUES

Some patients with interstitial disease have a normal chest roentgenogram. More often, however, the chest roentgenogram is abnormal and there are minimal symptoms. Four basic roentgenographic patterns have been described: "ground glass," nodular, reticulonodular, and reticular. In most of these diseases the infiltrate is predominantly in the lower lobes. A few diseases, such as silicosis sarcoidosis, and some connective tissue disorders, may have a predominantly upper lobe predilection. The roentgenographic pattern in patients with Langerhans' cell granulomatosis typically shows sparing of the costophrenic angles. The ground-glass pattern is characterized by a homogeneous haze of the lung, usually at the bases. This is thought to be produced by confluence of tiny nodular opacities and may represent an early stage of these diseases. A purely nodular pattern is rare but is best described by the pattern of miliary tuberculosis. Nodules can range from a few millimeters to greater than 10 cm in diameter, as seen in some pulmonary vasculitides. The reticular pattern consists of a network of linear shadows, a series of curvilinear opacities that form rings. This pattern can be further described according to the size of the opacities, using the terms fine, medium, and coarse. A coarse reticular pattern with intervening air spaces 2 to 10 mm in diameter is typical of honeycomb lung. This pattern corresponds to the presence of thick-walled, epithelial-lined cystic spaces and is mainly seen in advanced IPF, scleroderma, and Langerhans' cell granulomatosis.

The routine chest roentgenogram remains a valuable way to define the lung anatomy, but it is imprecise. In recent years computer application to lung imaging has enormously improved the precision of diagnostic imaging. High-resolution computed tomography (CT) is currently being investigated as both a diagnostic tool and a staging tool in the interstitial diseases. It is both sensitive and highly specific in demonstrating interstitial and pleural disease. Several diagnostic patterns appear to be emerging, including those associated with lymphangioleiomyomatosis, lymphangitic carcinomatosis, and asbestos-associated pleural disease. Some authorities suggest that high-resolution CT may provide diagnostic information of sufficient specificity to obviate the need for open or thoracoscopic lung biopsy in cases of suspected IPF, but this remains controversial. Pending further studies, we believe that the majority of patients with undiagnosed interstitial lung disease require lung biopsy.

Thoracic magnetic resonance imaging (MRI) and nuclear medicine imaging are being investigated but should currently be viewed as research tools. Extensive experience with gallium-67 scanning of the lung in disorders such as sarcoidosis and IPF has suggested that this technique is not sufficiently sensitive or specific to be helpful in diagnosis or staging.

DIAGNOSIS AND MANAGEMENT

Accurate diagnosis of specific interstitial diseases requires careful clinical, roentgenographic, and laboratory correlation; many cases require lung biopsy. Advances in imaging and other laboratory tests have greatly improved diagnostic accuracy and in some cases reduced the need for lung biopsy. Most of the interstitial diseases of known origin can be diagnosed by a very careful history and physical examination along with correlation with imaging techniques. The need for an exhaustive search for an etiologic agent cannot be overemphasized. If a specific cause can be identified and removed, the disease may regress. High-resolution CT appears to be useful in the diagnosis of some of these diseases. New techniques for detecting antibodies in the collagen vascular disorders have proved to be useful adjunctive measures, and the presence of antineutrophilic cytoplasmic antibody (ANCA) can be helpful in decision making in patients with the pulmonary vasculitides.

Considerable interest continues in the use of bronchoalveolar lavage (BAL) cell and fluid analysis in both the diagnosis and the management of interstitial diseases. The procedure has a very low morbidity and has proved to be valuable in the diagnosis of pulmonary infections, particularly in the immunosuppressed patient. BAL cell analysis has been useful in diagnosing some interstitial diseases when ultrastructural studies have been performed or when specific monoclonal antibodies to certain cells have been used. In the majority of cases, however, BAL should be reserved for research purposes and the diagnosis of infectious disorders.

If an accurate diagnosis cannot be established by noninvasive means, lung biopsy is indicated. Lung biopsy provides a histologic and at times an etiologic diagnosis and allows for assessment of disease activity and prediction of the natural or treated history of the disease. The latter is of great importance to both patients and families. The initial procedure of choice is fiberoptic bronchoscopy with transbronchial lung biopsy. In patients with suspected IPF or diffuse disease associated with the collagen vascular disorders, some clinicians proceed directly to open lung biopsy because UIP is the most common pathologic pattern and transbronchial biopsy is not reliable in making that diagnosis. Further, almost all pulmonologists would proceed to open lung biopsy in patients with pulmonary hemorrhage or pulmonary vasculitis. This is done to prevent delay in diagnosis and to provide the pathologist with adequate tissue. However, anecdotal reports reveal that these diseases are being diagnosed by transbronchial lung biopsy. If an open lung biopsy is required, areas of severely fibrotic lung should be avoided. Because this is an expensive, invasive procedure, our services use intraoperative frozen sections to ensure that diagnostic tissue has been obtained. It is important for the clinician to provide all clinical and roentgenographic data to the pathologists to make maximal use of the pathologist's diagnostic skills.

The increasingly widespread practice of *video-assisted thoracoscopic lung biopsy* has had an impact on the diagnostic approach to patients with suspected interstitial lung disease. Some surgeons believe that this technique offers a means for decreasing the morbidity and length of hospital stay for patients requiring lung biopsy.

The general principles of management of the interstitial diseases are to suppress inflammation to prevent further destruction and fibrosis of lung parenchyma and to palliate the complications of the disease. In some of the acute interstitial diseases avoidance of injurious agents and supportive measures may be sufficient. In other interstitial diseases the use of corticosteroids and/or cytotoxic agents may be required to suppress the inflammatory response. Interstitial diseases associated with circulating antibodies may require plasmapheresis.

In the acute and chronic interstitial pneumonias, once the decision is made to treat the patient, corticosteroids continue to be the mainstay of therapy. The initial treatment of choice is prednisone, 1 mg/kg ideal body weight per day (up to 80 mg) given as a single morning dose. Treatment is continued for 6 to 8 weeks at that dosage and then tapered by 5 mg weekly to a maintenance dose of 15 to 20 mg daily. Pulmonary function studies and chest imaging should be obtained serially at intervals of 6 to 8 weeks and are the only objective way to follow patients. Treatment is continued until pulmonary function studies have been stable for 1 year; then the prednisone is slowly tapered off. For patients whose disease progresses while receiving prednisone therapy or patients who cannot tolerate corticosteroids, cytotoxic or immunosuppressive agents have been advocated as alternative therapy. Oral cyclophosphamide at dosages of 1 to 2 mg/kg ideal body weight per day has been suggested as being useful. Although statistical data supporting the use of cyclophosphamide are lacking, there are anecdotal reports on its usefulness. Azathioprine has also been recommended as an alternative, as have a variety of other agents such as antimalarials; all are of unproven value. In some patients treatment with colchicine may prove beneficial in limiting disease progression, although this remains controversial.

Given that prednisone therapy alone is infrequently associated with significant clinical response in patients with chronic interstitial pneumonia, some authorities advocate beginning both prednisone and cyclophosphamide therapy initially, followed by gradual withdrawal of prednisone over the first few months. Data from controlled clinical trials are not available to permit direct comparison of one therapeutic regimen against another.

Preventive and palliative measures are also important in reducing the morbidity and mortality of these diseases. The structural changes constitute a host defense problem, and bacterial pneumonia may be a cause of death. Influenza and pneumococcal vaccines are recommended, and acute bronchitis should be treated. Some patients can have a component of reversible airways obstruction that should be treated with bronchodilators. Supplemental oxygen is recommended for patients who have an arterial oxygen tension of less than 55 mm Hg at rest or exercise, if this therapy has been found to improve oxygenation. Patients with cor pulmonale and right ventricular failure or those with significant hypoxic organ dysfunction (e.g., erythrocytosis) should also be treated. Recurrent pneumothoraces can complicate advanced interstitial disease, and at times, chemical pleurodesis is necessary.

Lung transplantation is now an accepted therapy for selected individuals who are unresponsive to medical therapy. In most patients, single-lung transplantation is used; however, double-lung transplantation has been used in patients with AIP. The timing of transplantation in patients with progressive disease may be difficult to decide, but the development or worsening of pulmonary hypertension and right ventricular dysfunction as evidenced by clinical or echocardiograhic findings suggests that end-stage is approaching.

KNOWN ETIOLOGIC FACTORS FOR INTERSTITIAL DISEASES
Occupational and Environmental Inhalants

Inhalation of a variety of organic and inorganic dusts, vapors, fumes, and aerosols can cause acute or chronic interstitial lung disease. Development of disease depends on the agent's physical properties allowing it to bypass upper airway host defenses and be deposited in gas exchange units. These properties include size, shape, and solubility. In the acute occupational and environmental lung diseases a short, predictable timetable exists between each exposure and development of lung disease. This predictability, correlated with environmental exposures, may be helpful in diagnosing organic dust disease. In the chronic lung diseases a lag time of 15 to 20 years often occurs between exposure and development of disease. Chapter 54 discusses the organic dust diseases, and Chapter 57 presents the other occupational and environmental lung diseases.

Drugs

See Chapter 58 for discussion of drug-induced lung diseases.

Poisons

The major poison of clinical significance is the herbicide paraquat. Accidental or deliberate ingestion of this agent causes diffuse alveolar damage and adult respiratory distress syndrome (ARDS). The pathogenesis of the injury is unclear, but it may be caused by the generation of reactive oxygen species. The mortality associated with paraquat-induced lung disease approaches 50%, and treatment is supportive.

Infectious Agents

Infections are a common cause of acute interstitial diseases. These are usually self-limited, and patients do not require hospitalization. Diagnosis of viral infections has become important as more effective therapy has become available. In the immunosuppressed host, cytomegalovirus is a common pathogen. Acute diffuse interstitial disease is common in AIDS patients. Chapter 334 discusses opportunistic infections in AIDS. Cases of both viral and mycoplasma pneumonias progressing to chronic interstitial disease have been reported.

Radiation

Long recognized as a cause of pneumonitis and fibrosis, most cases of radiation-induced interstitial disease are localized infiltrates from therapeutic radiation for lymphomas or carcinomas. The incidence of radiation-induced lung disease is unknown, but with current refined techniques clinically significant disease has greatly diminished in frequency. Since diffuse lung disease can result from medical or nuclear-related accidents, it is important to recognize the features of this disease. In addition, current data indicate that injury can be amplified by the administration of oxygen or certain cytotoxic drugs. The histologic appearance of radiation-induced lung disease does not differ significantly from that of AIP or, if the disease is chronic, from that of UIP. Clinical features of pulmonary radiation injury consist of an acute phase occurring 6 to 12 weeks after exposure, which is characterized by cough, fever, and breathlessness; remission follows. Chronic interstitial disease develops 6 to 12 months later. Acute radiation-induced pneumonitis can be improved by corticosteroid therapy. However, corticosteroids do not prevent progression to chronic interstitial fibrosis.

Neoplastic Diseases

Several neoplasms that invade lymphatics, alveolar air spaces, or pulmonary vasculature can become evident with a roentgenographic pattern of interstitial disease. Most have a reticular pattern; some have a nodular pattern. Lymphangitic adenocarcinoma generally demonstrates a reticular pattern. A nodular or reticulonodular pattern is more frequently seen in bronchoalveolar carcinomas and lymphomas. Lymphomas are particularly common in treated Hodgkin's disease. Kaposi's sarcoma can become evident with a diffuse reticular or nodular pattern. Infrequently, mycosis fungoides and some leukemias may demonstrate a diffuse interstitial pattern.

Hemodynamic and Cardiac Diseases

Chronic pulmonary venous hypertension from mitral stenosis, cor triatriatum, or chronic left ventricular failure can result in a progressive restrictive defect with roentgenographic evidence of interstitial disease. Unless associated with other causes of interstitial disease, primary pulmonary hypertension does not produce detectable pulmonary infiltrates on chest roentgenograms.

Metabolic and Miscellaneous Disorders

Chronic uremia can result in alveolar inflammation and fibrosis. Typically the roentgenogram shows bilateral perihilar infiltrates. Hypercalcemia can result in deposits of calcium in the alveoli and may rarely be evident on the chest roentgenogram as a ground-glass pattern. Metastatic calcification is seen in some patients undergoing dialysis and can result in diffuse alveolar calcification. Alveolar amyloidosis is a rare cause for a diffuse reticular pattern; more often, pulmonary amyloidosis is a nodular or airway disease process. Acute allergic reactions and trauma rarely cause diffuse interstitial disease.

INTERSTITIAL DISEASES OF UNKNOWN ORIGIN
Acute Interstitial Pneumonia

Acute interstitial pneumonia occurs infrequently and corresponds to what is usually referred to as the Hamman-Rich syndrome (or disease). The mean age of onset varies, ranging from 13 to more than 70 years of age. In one series, mean age was less than 30 years, and in another, 50 years. No sex predilection has been found. Most patients have a prodromal illness for 1 to 3 weeks. The prodrome consists of a flulike illness that progresses to cough and ultimately to progressive dyspnea. Fever, myalgias, and arthralgias often occur. On initial examination most patients are tachypneic and cyanotic. The chest roentgenogram shows progressive alveolar filling. Corticosteroids and antibiotics are almost always prescribed, and anecdotal reports are positive concerning their use. The prognosis is variable but generally is considered to be poor, with less than 50% of patients surviving. Many who survive can ultimately have normal or nearly normal pulmonary function.

Bronchiolitis Obliterans–Organizing Pneumonia

Previously confused with UIP or cases of obliterative bronchiolitis, BOOP is a distinct clinical and pathologic entity. Although BOOP is a disease of airways, it is often grouped with interstitial pneumonias (see previous section on pathology); thus a brief discussion is presented here. BOOP is a specific histologic diagnosis and has been associated with a variety of infections, toxic inhalants, drugs, and other disorders. It is often confused with obliterative bronchiolitis, which is characterized by progressive narrowing and scarring of small airways but without the typical fibrous plugs that are seen in BOOP. This discussion addresses idiopathic BOOP or BOOP associated with the collagen vascular disorders.

Most patients with BOOP are 40 to 60 years of age and have a flulike illness with fever, sore throat, myalgias, and progressive dyspnea. The duration of symptoms is usually 2 to 10 weeks but in some patients has exceeded 3 months. The chest roentgenogram typically shows bilateral, patchy, air space opacities. Lesions are variable on the roentgenogram, however, and can be focal and progressive or nonspecific. The diagnosis often requires open lung biopsy and very careful clinicopathologic correlation. Treatment is with corticosteroids, and the prognosis is usually good, with a high response rate to therapy. Exacerbations of the disease after discontinuation of corticosteroids have been reported; these patients may require corticosteroid therapy for an indefinite period.

Idiopathic Pulmonary Fibrosis

A common chronic interstitial disease, IPF mainly affects patients in the sixth or seventh decade of life but can occur at any age. No sex predilection exists, and most patients have insidious exertional breathlessness. At times, patients have a constant, nonproductive cough. Although there are reports of a prodromal period with a flulike illness followed by fever and other constitutional symptoms, many of these reports preceded our current understanding of interstitial pneumonias. Therefore many cases may represent AIP, BOOP, or possibly an undeclared connective tissue disease. Most patients with IPF, however, probably do have fever and constitutional symptoms. Survival can range from 1 to 2 years to longer than 20 years. The mean survival, however, is 4 to 5 years after presentation. Idiopathic pulmonary fibrosis represents the prototype of the chronic interstitial pneumonias (see previous section on clinical features for physical findings). Digital clubbing is a late feature of IPF but rarely may antedate the onset of the lung disease.

Initially the chest roentgenogram may be normal or show a bibasilar reticular or reticulonodular pattern. As IPF advances, infiltrates progressively involve more lung parenchyma, and in the absence of cigarette abuse with coexisting chronic obstructive pulmonary disease (COPD) progressive loss of lung volumes and development of end-stage honeycomb lung occur. Pleural effusions and lymphadenopathy are not features of IPF and, if present, suggest a complication or an alternative diagnosis. The pathologic appearance of IPF is UIP. Decision making in IPF is outlined in the previous section on diagnosis and management. Open lung biopsy is generally recommended, but recent use of high-resolution CT holds promise as a useful tool in the diagnosis and staging of IPF. Young patients with minimal fibrosis and active alveolitis appear most responsive to corticosteroid therapy; up to 90% survive 5 years. By contrast, among patients with severe pulmonary fibrosis with minimum cellularity, less than 25% survive 5 years.

Sarcoidosis

See Chapter 53.

Collagen Vascular Disorders

The collagen vascular disorders are a diverse collection of diseases in which the major disease or disorder is inflammation of blood vessels and connective tissue. Thoracic involvement varies and ranges from chest wall disease to parenchymal disease to diaphragmatic disease. Almost every collagen vascular disease can be associated with diffuse interstitial involvement. The pathologic appearance in most is that of UIP. The pathogenesis of these diseases is poorly understood but appears to be autoimmune. Although it has been stated that the prognosis in most of these patients is similar, adequate data are not available to support this. Some of the diseases have a course similar to that of IPF and are progressive, whereas others are not progressive and lung disease rarely limits survival. In general, management of progressive disease is as for patients with IPF. Initial treatment is with

corticosteroids, and if this is not tolerated or the disease is progressive, cyclophosphamide is added.

Rheumatoid Arthritis (see Chapter 192). Several thoracic manifestations of rheumatoid arthritis exist; pleuropulmonary manifestations are the most common. Approximately 20% of patients have roentgenographic evidence of diffuse interstitial disease. These patients are predominantly men in the sixth decade of life and usually have high titers of rheumatoid factor. The lung disease rarely may antedate the joint disease but usually occurs 5 or more years after the development of rheumatoid arthritis. Prognosis in patients with diffuse interstitial disease varies, but reports indicate that it parallels that of IPF.

Systemic Lupus Erythematosus (see Chapter 194). Becoming evident with fever, tachypnea, and hypoxemia with diffuse or patchy infiltrates, acute lupus pneumonitis is a well-described entity. In up to 50% of patients lupus pneumonitis may be the initial presentation of systemic lupus erythematosus (SLE). The incidence of pulmonary infection in SLE far exceeds that of lupus pneumonitis, so it is critical to exclude a treatable microbe. Lung biopsy may be necessary for an accurate diagnosis. Once the diagnosis of acute lupus pneumonitis is made, the disease is generally treated with high-dose intravenous corticosteroids. The addition of cyclophosphamide and/or azathioprine in progressive disease has been reported. Chronic interstitial disease is rare in SLE and is thought to develop from recurrent episodes of acute pneumonitis. When present, it is sometimes responsive to corticosteroids. The pathologic appearance is that of UIP. Death from end-stage chronic interstitial disease appears to be exceedingly rare.

Progressive Systemic Sclerosis (see Chapter 197). Interstitial lung disease is common in progressive systemic sclerosis (PSS); it is clinically evident in up to 50% of patients and is seen at autopsy in almost 100%. Generally a poor correlation exists between the cutaneous manifestations of this disease and the development of interstitial disease. The pathologic appearance is that of UIP, and data on treatment are scarce. Currently the disease is thought to be generally acellular, and corticosteroids are not useful. Some data suggest that penicillamine or cyclophosphamide may be efficacious. Lung and renal disease are the primary conditions that limit survival.

Dermatomyositis-Polymyositis (see Chapter 199). Diffuse interstitial disease can be seen in up to 5% of patients with dermatomyositis-polymyositis. Among patients who develop progressive interstitial disease, no correlation exists between the pulmonary disease and the severity or duration of the muscle disease. In general, patients with extremely cellular disease respond quite well to steroids and management should be similar to that for IPF.

Sjögren's Syndrome (see Chapter 193). Often coexisting with other connective tissue disorders, Sjögren's syndrome can be associated with several types of interstitial diseases, including UIP and LIP. Lymphoid interstitial pneumonia is considered to be a low-grade lymphoma. Few data are available on the natural history of cases with pathologic findings conforming to the UIP pattern, but management in patients with progressive interstitial disease should be similar to that for IPF.

Mixed Connective Tissue Disease (see Chapter 195). Becoming evident with signs and symptoms of several connective tissue disorders, diffuse interstitial disease is frequent in mixed connective tissue disease. There appears to be a female predilection and a trend toward developing many features of SLE. The diagnosis is generally made with clinical correlation and the presence of serum antibodies to extractable nuclear antigens composed of soluble ribonuclear protein and a glycoprotein called SM antigen. Antinative DNA antibodies are rarely present. The clinical course of the interstitial disease in this disorder is variable, and if it is progressive, management should be similar to that for IPF.

Ankylosing Spondylitis (see Chapter 200). Ankylosing spondylitis is characterized by inflammation and sclerosis of the sacroiliac joints, spine, and costovertebral joints. In patients with ankylosing spondylitis progressive upper lobe fibrocystic disease can develop. The cysts are susceptible to the development of aspergillomas or other mycetomas, but invasive aspergillosis may also develop. Amphotericin B and more recently itraconazole have been used to treat aspergillomas, but without clear benefit. If invasive disease develops, intravenous amphotericin is indicated. Resection or embolization may be necessary to control massive hemorrhage, a major complication of mycetomas. An identical pattern of upper lobe fibrocystic disease has been described in psoriatic arthritis and seropositive rheumatoid arthritis.

Pulmonary Vasculitis

The pulmonary vasculitic syndromes are a diverse group of diseases with overlapping clinical and pathologic features. Most are part of a disseminated vasculitic process, but in a few the lung is the major organ involved. The prototype of these diseases is Wegener's granulomatosis. Only a few of the pulmonary vasculitides become evident with progressive interstitial disease, but in most, significant pulmonary fibrosis can ultimately develop. Vasculitides in which the lung is the major organ involved include Wegener's granulomatosis, the Churg-Strauss syndrome (allergic angiitis and granulomatosis), and necrotizing sarcoid granulomatosis. Previously, lymphomatoid granulomatosis has been classified with this group; however, it is now known that it is a T-cell lymphoma. Pulmonary vasculitis may exist also as part of a diffuse vasculitic process (e.g., Henoch-Schönlein syndrome). Pulmonary vasculitis may be only part of a diffuse spectrum of lung disorders or diseases, such as with the collagen vascular disorders.

The pathogenesis of the pulmonary vasculitides is not known, but by analogy with other vasculitic syndromes one cause is believed to be immune-complex vascular injury with resulting vasculitis and tissue destruction. Circulating immune complexes have been identified in many of the pulmonary vasculitides, including Wegener's granulomatosis, Behçet's disease, rheumatoid arthritis, and others. In most cases the antigens are unknown, but in several the antigen appears to be molecules derived from microbes. Several factors determine whether immune-complex disease develops. These include the type and size of the immune-complex, the immune complex load, and the ability to handle immune complexes. Recent data suggest that when complement deficiencies are present or when defects in complement receptors or immunoglobulin G–Fc (IgG-Fc) receptors exist, the body is unable to handle immune complexes, so disease is more likely to develop. Mechanisms for localization of immune complexes are also poorly understood. Experimental data indicate that agents which alter vascular permeability (e.g., histamine) promote deposition of immune complexes. Once immune complexes are deposited, complement is activated, producing cleavage products that recruit polymorphonuclear leukocytes and cause degranulation of basophils, releasing other soluble mediators, proteolytic enzymes, and toxic radicals. Ultimately the vessel is infiltrated with polymorphonuclear leukocytes, producing vasculitis and vascular necrosis with tissue damage.

The hallmark of the initial stages of the vasculitides is endothelial cell activation and subsequent endothelial cell damage and sloughing. A prominent feature in some of these diseases is activation of the coagulation cascade with thrombogenesis. Less is known about the chronic granulomatous vasculitides. Evolution from an acute vasculitis is possible, but the development of cell-mediated immunity seems more likely.

Wegener's Granulomatosis. See Chapter 56.

Churg-Strauss Syndrome. See Chapter 56.

Pulmonary Hemorrhage Syndromes

The diffuse alveolar hemorrhage syndromes are characterized by hemoptysis, alveolar filling opacities on chest roentgenograms, dyspnea, hypoxia, and often nephritis with progressive renal failure. The following major disease groups are associated with alveolar hemorrhage:
1. Anti–glomerular basement membrane (anti-GBM) antibody disease
2. Alveolar hemorrhage associated with vasculitis
3. Alveolar hemorrhage associated with collagen vascular diseases
4. Idiopathic pulmonary hemosiderosis (IPH)
5. Alveolar hemorrhage associated with exogenous agents
6. Alveolar hemorrhage associated with idiopathic, rapidly progressive glomerulonephritis

Principles of diagnosis of these diseases are as follows: (1) document the presence of alveolar hemorrhage, (2) evaluate renal status, (3) search for the presence of serologic abnormalities (anti-GBM antibody, antinuclear antibody [ANA], ANCA, immune complexes), (4) perform biopsy of kidney if vasculitis is not suspected, and (5) perform lung biopsy if no diagnosis is made. All biopsy material should be studied by light and electron microscopy and by immunofluorescence techniques.

Anti–Glomerular Basement Membrane Antibody Disease. Previously termed Goodpasture's syndrome, anti-GBM antibody disease is a disorder in which antibodies bind to collagen in pulmonary and renal basement membranes, causing diffuse alveolar hemorrhage and progressive glomerulonephritis in the most common presentation of the disease. The disease can affect both sexes and all ages, but it typically occurs in white men in the third decade of life. Hemoptysis is the most common initial sign, and most patients have cough and dyspnea. Some patients have subclinical or mild pulmonary hemorrhage and iron-deficiency anemia. Most patients have evidence of nephritis initially, and in virtually all patients progressive renal failure develops. Serologic assays for anti-GBM antibody are positive in more than 95% of patients, but in many the diagnosis must be confirmed by immunofluorescence studies of renal tissue. Lung biopsy is usually not necessary.

The origin of anti-GBM antibody disease is unknown, but an association appears to exist between development of this disease and infection with influenza and also with inhalation of hydrocarbons. Renal disease appears to be the most commonly life-threatening facet of the disorder. The treatment of choice is suppression of pathogenic antibody formation and pulmonary and renal inflammation with corticosteroids and cytotoxic therapy, coupled with plasmapheresis for removal of circulating antibody. The latter is performed daily or three times weekly until the serum levels of anti-GBM antibodies are not detectable. High-dose intravenous corticosteroids for 2 to 3 days are generally recommended for life-threatening alveolar hemorrhage. There are reports of successful renal transplantation in patients with undetectable anti-GBM antibodies.

Alveolar Hemorrhage Associated With Vasculitis. Diffuse alveolar hemorrhage as a presentation of Wegener's granulomatosis occurs infrequently. Reported cases usually involve patients with extensive parenchymal hemorrhage and rapid renal failure. Skin disease, arthritis, and upper airways disease can coexist. The diagnosis is established from lung biopsy and shows a capillaritis; a granulomatous vasculitis may sometimes coexist. Renal biopsy is usually nonspecific. High-dose corticosteroids and cyclophosphamide are recommended for this presentation. The prognosis, however, is poor.

Diffuse alveolar hemorrhage may occur in the Henoch-Schönlein syndrome. In reported cases the extrapulmonary features of this disease were present with palpable purpura and at times nephritis. Limited studies have shown immunoglobulin A (IgA) granular deposits along the lung's basement membrane. Recommended therapy in life-threatening alveolar hemorrhage is intravenous high-dose corticosteroids. Pulmonary vasculitis with alveolar hemorrhage is also well described in Behçet's disease. Small vessel vasculitis and necrotizing vasculitis of muscular arteries with aneurysm formation and rupture have been described.

Infrequently becoming evident as a pure disease, polyarteritis nodosa is usually associated with a diffuse immune-complex vasculitis. Pulmonary artery involvement is rare but has been reported and can result in alveolar hemorrhage. Alveolar hemorrhage with nephritis has been reported in essential mixed cryoglobulinemia.

De Remee and others have recently reported on the association of alveolar hemorrhage and nephritis in patients with the perinuclear form of ANCA (p-ANCA). These patients do not have classic Wegener's granulomatosis, which is more commonly characterized by circulating cytoplasmic ANCA (c-ANCA).

Alveolar Hemorrhage Associated With Collagen Vascular Diseases. Diffuse alveolar hemorrhage has been well described in most of the collagen vascular syndromes. The prototype is SLE and, unlike in other alveolar hemorrhage syndromes, hemoptysis is rarely the presenting feature. Most patients with SLE have active disease with fever, arthritis, nephritis, and hypocomplementemia. Infections may complicate the hemorrhage. Alveolar hemorrhage associated with SLE is thought to be caused by immune complexes; however, immune complexes along alveolar septae have only rarely been described. Treatment with high-dose intravenous corticosteroids is usually recommended, but mortality is high.

Idiopathic Pulmonary Hemosiderosis. Characterized by recurrent bouts of subclinical or clinical alveolar hemorrhage, IPH has no extrapulmonary manifestations. Mainly a disease of children and young adults, IPH can affect all ages. Patients may come to medical attention with a single episode of life-threatening alveolar hemorrhage but more often have multiple episodes leading to progressive interstitial fibrosis. Most have iron-deficiency anemia and during bleeds have fever, hyperbilirubinemia, and reticulocytosis. The diagnosis must be established by excluding other causes of alveolar hemorrhage. The pathogenesis of IPH is unknown. The natural history varies, and remissions have been described. Corticosteroids are recommended in high doses during active bleeding and in low maintenance doses until the disease becomes quiescent.

Alveolar Hemorrhage Associated With Exogenous Agents and Idiopathic, Rapidly Progressive Glomerulonephritis. Inhalation of trimellitic anhydride fumes or dust can produce pulmonary hemorrhage. This agent is widely used in the manufacture of plastics, epoxy resins, and paints. Most patients have anemia and pneumonitis, whereas others have recurrent fever, hemoptysis, and hypoxemia. The origin is unclear but is thought to be immune-related, with the anhydride functioning as a hapten. Corticosteroid therapy appears useful, but avoidance of the anhydride is recommended. Alveolar hemorrhage has also been described after lymphangiography, as a toxic manifestation of penicillamine therapy, and with the use of cocaine.

Alveolar hemorrhage has been reported in association with idiopathic, rapidly progressive glomerulonephritis. Cases with and without immune complexes have been described. The cause is unknown but may represent part of a spectrum of vasculitis or of the collagen vascular disorders. In general, management of the condition is similar to that for lupus nephritis and alveolar hemorrhage.

Langerhans' Cell Granulomatosis

See Chapter 55.

Lymphoid Infiltrative Disorders

This infrequently occurring group of diseases was formerly thought to be benign, with some rarely progressing to lymphoma; current data suggest that many are low-grade lymphomas. These include lymphomatoid granulomatosis, a T-cell lymphoma; immunoblastic lymphadenopathy; lymphocytic angiitis and granulomatosis; and LIP associated with Sjögren's syndrome or other collagen vascular diseases, or as an idiopathic disorder. Treatment varies according to the disease. Patients with lymphomatoid granulomatosis generally receive aggressive treatment as for T-cell lymphoma, whereas those with lymphocytic angiitis and granulomatosis generally receive treatment with chlorambucil. Idiopathic LIP, if progressive, is usually treated with corticosteroids.

Bronchiolar Diseases

Several chronic bronchiolar diseases can become evident with roentgenographic evidence of interstitial disease, usually in the form of a reticular or reticulonodular pattern. BOOP and respiratory bronchiolitis have previously been discussed, but several other bronchiolar diseases can also have similar roentgenographic patterns. A disease described mainly in Japan, diffuse panbronchiolitis, is characterized by chronic inflammation of respiratory bronchioles. Usually the chest roentgenogram shows hyperinflation, and pulmonary function studies show an obstructive pattern with gas trapping. Some cases, however, show roentgenographic evidence of a bibasilar nodular infiltrate, whereas others show a linear reticular pattern, often with "tram" lines that are consistent with bronchiectasis/bronchiolectasis. Gram-negative bronchial infections develop in most patients, and the prognosis is poor.

Follicular bronchitis/bronchiolitis is a poorly described disease that occurs primarily in patients with collagen vascular disorders or in immunosuppressed patients. Familial cases also have been reported, and in some patients there appears to be an association with an allergic phenomenon. Most patients have a reticular or reticulonodular infiltrative pattern. Pulmonary function studies may show an obstructive or restrictive pattern or a combined restrictive-obstructive defect. Lung pathologic studies show reactive lymphoid germinal centers along bronchi and bronchioles, and prominent peribronchial and peribronchiolar fibrosis may be seen. There is no evidence of chronic bronchitis. Therapy is uncertain, with a variable response to corticosteroids.

Lymphangioleiomyomatosis

Lymphangioleiomyomatosis is a rare disease of young women in the third or fourth decade of life and is characterized by proliferation of smooth muscle in a lymphatic distribution without evidence of cancer. The abnormal smooth muscle is seen around the airways, blood vessels, and lymphatic vessels. Lymphatic involvement mainly involves lung, thorax, abdomen, and occasionally lymph nodes. Although lymphangioleiomyomatosis is mainly a disease of women of childbearing age with a survival of less than 10 years, disease in postmenopausal women has been reported. These latter patients may have a prolonged survival. The clinical features of this disease are progressive dyspnea, hemoptysis, cough, and repeated spontaneous pneumothoraces and chylous effusions. The chest roentgenogram typically shows a diffuse fibrocystic pattern with normal or increased lung volumes. Pulmonary function studies reveal a typical emphysematous presentation. The origin of lymphangioleiomyomatosis is unknown, but the occurrence of the disease during childbearing years has focused research on sex hormones. Disease remission has been reported after treatment with progesterone, oophorectomy, and synthetic hypothalamic analogs, which produce a medical castration. Successful single-lung transplantation in patients with this disease has been performed. Recurrent pneumothoraces and chylous effusions may require chemical pleurodesis.

Eosinophilic Pneumonias

Acute eosinophilic pneumonia can occur in association with a variety of drugs and parasites. Diffuse or patchy infiltrates are related to the migration of parasitic larvae through lungs. The term Löffler's syndrome is typically applied to patients with transient pulmonary infiltrates and with peripheral eosinophilia in which no clear cause is evident. Some of these patients may have clinically occult parasitic infestations. Asthma may be an associated symptom. Chronic eosinophilic pneumonia is a discrete disease characterized by fever, night sweats, exertional breathlessness, and occasional wheezing and peripheral eosinophilia. The chest roentgenogram typically shows peripheral, nonsegmental, fixed infiltrates; however, nodules with cavities and a chronic interstitial infiltrate also have been described. Exquisitely sensitive to corticosteroids, peripheral infiltrates tend to recur in the same location if the disease exacerbates.

Pulmonary Alveolar Proteinosis

Pulmonary alveolar proteinosis (PAP) is characterized by the deposition of a granular eosinophilic material within alveoli that is positive on and periodic acid–Schiff stain. Pulmonary alveolar proteinosis is mainly a disease of the fourth and fifth decades of life. There is a male predominance, and PAP is often associated with dust exposure or respiratory infections. Clinical features are progressive breathlessness, cough, fatigue, and malaise. The chest roentgenogram typically shows bilaterally symmetric, alveolar-filling opacities that spare the costophrenic angles and the apices. Laboratory data are nonspecific, but an elevated lactate dehydrogenase concentration is often present and appears to arise from the lung.

A pathologic reaction resembling PAP has been described in a variety of dust exposures, malignancies, and infections. Acute silicoproteinosis is a well-described entity. In animal models a PAP-like reaction can be produced by inhalation of silica, aluminum, and various other dusts. Pulmonary alveolar proteinosis associated with dust exposure is often termed secondary PAP. Pulmonary alveolar proteinosis is idiopathic, but pathogenetic theories speculate that abnormal production or metabolism of surfactant occurs. Some type of derangement seems to exist in either the production or the clearance of the surfactant material produced.

The diagnosis of PAP is established by clinical and pathologic data, often requiring lung biopsy. Treatment is with whole-lung lavage using 40 to 60 L of fluid. Corticosteroids have no value and may increase the incidence of lung infections. Spontaneous remissions have been frequently reported, but progression to advanced fibrotic disease has also been reported.

Other Interstitial Diseases

Diffuse interstitial disease can occur in a variety of inherited disorders, and a familial form of IPF exists. von Recklinghausen's disease is associated with progressive interstitial lung infiltrates, with lung biopsy showing UIP. Interstitial disease has been described in Gaucher's disease, Neimann-Pick disease, tuberous sclerosis, and the Hermansky-Pudlak syndrome. Various rare and unusual types of interstitial diseases have been described in relatively common illnesses, including ulcerative colitis, Crohn's disease, primary biliary cirrhosis, chronic active hepatitis, and renal tubular acidosis. The pathologic features of these diseases have not been well characterized, but in some cases a vasculitis appears to exist, whereas in others a nonspecific inflammation-fibrotic reaction occurs. Several unclassified interstitial pneumonias exist, and often in the course of patient evaluation diffuse nonprogressive interstitial pneumonia can be identified. These diseases may represent previous infections or cases of respiratory bronchiolitis. Lung biopsy is not indicated unless the disorder is progressive. Chronic interstitial pneumonia is a frequent feature of patients after transplantation and has been increasingly recognized in those with AIDS.

BIBLIOGRAPHY

Burkhardt A: Alveolitis and collapse in the pathogenesis of pulmonary fibrosis, *Am Rev Respir Dis* 140:513, 1989.

Crouch E: Pathobiology of pulmonary fibrosis, *Am J Physiol* 259:L159, 1990.

Daniele R et al: Clinical role of bronchoalveolar lavage in adults with pulmonary disease, *Am Rev Respir Dis* 142:481, 1990.

DeRemee RA, Homburger HA, and Specks U: Lesions of the respiratory tract associated with the finding of anti-neutrophil cytoplasmic autoantibodies with a perinuclear staining pattern, *Mayo Clin Proc* 69:819, 1994.

Fulmer JD, Katzenstein AA: The interstitial lung diseases. In Bone RC, editor: *Comprehensive textbook of pulmonary disease,* vol 2, St Louis, 1993, Mosby.

Gauldie J, Jordana M, Cox G: Cytokines and pulmonary fibrosis, *Thorax* 48:931, 1993.

Helmers RA, Humminghake GW: Bronchoalveolar lavage in the nonimmunocompromised patient, *Chest* 96:1184, 1989.

Katzenstein AA, Askin F: Surgical pathology of nonneoplastic lung disease, *Major Probl Pathol* 13:9, 1990.

Katzenstein AA et al: Bronchiolitis obliterans and usual interstitial pneumonia, *Am J Surg Pathol* 10:373, 1986.

Kennedy JI, Fulmer JD: Collagen vascular diseases. In Kassirer JP, editor: *Current therapy in internal medicine,* Philadelphia, 1991, BC Decker.

Kennedy JI, Fulmer JD: Pulmonary vasculitis and interstitial lung disease. In Schwartz MJ, King TE, editors: *Interstitial lung disease,* Philadelphia, 1993, BC Decker.

King TE Jr, Mortensen RL: Cryptogenic organizing pneumonitis: the North American experience, *Chest* 102:8S-13S, 1992.

Kuhn C III et al: An immunohistochemical study of architectural remodeling and connective tissue synthesis in pulmonary fibrosis, *Am Rev Respir Dis* 14:1693, 1989.

Kumar RK, Lykke AW: Messages and handshakes: cellular interactions in pulmonary fibrosis, *Pathology* 27:18, 1995.

Leatherman JW: Immune alveolar hemorrhage, *Chest* 91:891, 1989.

Muller NL, Ostrow DN: High-resolution computed tomography of chronic interstitial lung diseases, *Clin Chest Med* 12:97, 1991.

Olson J, Colby T, Elliott C: Hamman-Rich syndrome revisited, *Mayo Clin Proc* 65:1538, 1990.

Taylor JR et al: Lymphangioleiomyomatosis: clinical course in 32 patients, *N Engl J Med* 323:1254, 1990.

Wagner PD, Rodrigues-Roisin R: Clinical advances in pulmonary gas exchange, *Am Rev Respir Dis* 143:883, 1991.

Weissler JC: Southwestern Internal Medicine Conference: idiopathic pulmonary fibrosis—cellular and molecular pathogenesis, *Am J Med Sci* 297:91, 1989.

53 Sarcoidosis

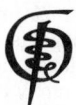

Geoffrey McLennan and Gary W. Hunninghake

DEFINITION

Sarcoidosis is a multisystem disorder of unknown etiology characterized pathologically by the presence of epithelioid granulomas. The diagnosis remains one of exclusion, resting entirely on the demonstration of multiple organ involvement and the absence of other conditions associated with granulomatous disease (Box 53-1). For these reasons, a careful history is essential. Special stains and culture of the biopsied tissue are frequently necessary to exclude granulomatous diseases of known cause.

PATHOPHYSIOLOGY

The epithelioid granuloma is the pathologic hallmark of sarcoidosis. The epithelioid granuloma contains two zones: a central compact zone consisting of mature mononuclear phagocytes, epithelioid cells, and giant cells admixed with lymphocytes of the CD4+ type; and a peripheral loose zone consisting of macrophages, monocytes, fibroblasts, and lymphocytes, which, in addition to the CD4+ type, are also of the CD8+ type. Morphologically, both the mononuclear phagocytes and the lymphocytes appear activated. The granulomas of sarcoidosis are sometimes associated with inclusion bodies, such as Schaumman's bodies and asteroid bodies, and/or small amounts

---

BOX 53-1
Differential diagnosis of granulomatous lung disease

Infections
Bacteria
  Brucella
  Francisella tularensis
  Yersinia enterocolitica
Mycobacteria
  Tuberculosis
  Atypical tuberculosis
Fungi
  Histoplasma capsulatum
  Blastomyces dermatitidis
  Coccidioides immitis
Spirochetes: *Treponema*

Nonfectious compounds
Organic: hypersensitivity pneumonitis
Inorganic
  Beryllium
  Talc
Drugs
  Methotrexate
  Dilantin
Neoplasms
  Lymphoma
  Germ cell cancer

Idiopathic
Sarcoidosis
Wegener's granulomatosis
Primary biliary cirrhosis
Crohn's disease
Ulcerative colitis

of necrosis, none of which is specific for this disease. Once formed, the granulomas can persist, resolve without residua, or undergo fibrotic change.

In the lung, granulomas are primarily localized to areas that parallel lymphatic drainage, including the peribronchial and mediastinal lymph nodes, pleural tissue septa, and along blood vessels. Although compression of the vasculature can occur, frank vasculitis is unusual.

Sarcoidosis is associated with the immunologic persistence of activated monocytes and activated CD4+ lymphocytes at sites of disease. The activated mononuclear cells can affect the host by regulating the initiation, maintenance, and resolution of local granuloma formation and by releasing a variety of mediators that potentially have systemic effects on the host.

The precursor to granuloma formation in sarcoidosis is alveolitis. In the lung this inflammatory process is localized to the interstitium and is reflected in the cells recovered by bronchoalveolar lavage. In normal people, alveolar macrophages make up greater than 85% of the cells, whereas lymphocytes constitute less than 15% of the cells, and both lymphocytes and macrophages are not activated. In contrast, patients with sarcoidosis have greater numbers of both macrophages and lymphocytes in bronchoalveolar lavage, with lymphocytes constituting a much larger percentage of the cells. The lymphocytes recovered are predominantly T-helper cells. Furthermore, both sarcoid alveolar macrophages and lymphocytes are activated and possess the ability to initiate and maintain granuloma formation. The activated sarcoid alveolar macrophages have an increased ability to release spontaneously a variety of mediators that attract and activate helper T lymphocytes (interleukin 1 [IL-1], tumor necrosis factor [TNF], interleukin 8 [IL-8]). Likewise, activated sarcoid lymphocytes spontaneously proliferate and also release monocyte chemoattractants, monocyte activators (gamma interferon, granulocyte-monocyte colony-stimulating factor), and interleukin 2 (IL-2). The activated mononuclear cells subsequently organize and differentiate under the control of these mediators into the sarcoid granuloma. The formed granuloma may alter the lung by local destruction and impingement on nearby structures. The resolution of the granuloma can also affect organ function if fibrosis predominates. Activated sarcoid macrophages and lymphocytes may participate in the fibrotic process by releasing mediators that can up-regulate fibroblast proliferation and collagen release.

Activated macrophages and activated lymphocytes can also affect the host by releasing a variety of potent systemically active mediators. The macrophages from patients with sarcoidosis spontaneously release IL-1 and TNF, which can act as pyrogens and stimulate weight loss and acute-phase reactant synthesis. In addition, they can release large quantities of 1,25-dihydroxycholecalciferol. Likewise, activated CD4+ lymphocytes can nonspecifically activate B lymphocytes to differentiate into immunoglobulin-secreting cells in a polyclonal manner. The resultant hypergammaglobulinemia is a common manifestation of sarcoidosis.

In sarcoidosis, granuloma formation is often compartmentalized to specific sites of disease activity. For example, although both macrophages and T-helper lymphocytes are increased in number and activated in the lungs of patients with sarcoidosis, these same patients often have a reduction in the circulating number of T-helper cells. Furthermore, these patients often exhibit anergy on skin testing despite an exaggerated immune response in the lung. Even within the lung, high-resolution computed tomographic (CT) scanning often reveals disease localized around the central bronchovascular bundles without peripheral parenchymal disease (Fig. 53-1).

ETIOLOGY

Despite advances in our understanding of the immunology of sarcoidosis, the etiology of this disease remains unknown. It is also not known if sarcoidosis is caused by a single agent or by multiple agents that trigger a similar type of granulomatous disease. Various studies examining T-cell receptor expression on lymphocytes isolated from the lungs of patients with sarcoidosis support an immunologic reaction to a single agent. These studies have shown that the T lymphocytes from patients with sarcoidosis have a bias toward expression of a specific receptor type on their surface in a subgroup of patients. This suggests that T-cell proliferation in sarcoidosis may be directed to a single specific antigen. Potential antigens that have been implicated in stimulating this disease include both exogenous antigens, such as infectious agents (mycobacteria, cell wall deficient cornyebacteria, the agent of Whipple's disease, *Yersinia enterocolitica,* herpes viruses, fungi) and respirable particles (inhaled organic or inorganic antigens), as well as endogenous antigens, such as latent viral or tumor antigens (e.g., germ cell neoplasms). No evidence, however, indicates that any of these agents is the cause of sarcoidosis. Epidemiologic studies also suggest a likely infectious cause, with a latent period of 2 years. Sarcoidosis has also been shown to occur in some families and in some identical twins, suggesting that genetic factors also play a role in expression of this disease.

CLINICAL PRESENTATION

Sarcoidosis is heterogeneous in distribution, presentation, and course. Although worldwide in distribution, sarcoidosis has a predilection for temperate environments. The prevalence in New York has been estimated at 40 per 100,000 population. Likewise, sarcoidosis can occur in any age, race, or sexual group. Classically, however, sarcoidosis appears to be found more frequently in younger people (>70% <40 years of age), blacks, and within the black race, females. These figures, however, represent rough estimates of the true prevalence of sarcoidosis within each group and region, the result of the high prevalence of clinically silent and unrecognized disease.

Sarcoidosis can affect any organ of the body. The disease can present acutely, subacutely, or chronically and can affect a single organ, an organ compartment, or multiple organs (Table 53-1).

The patient's ethnic background has been demonstrated to influence the mode of presentation, organ involvement, and clinical course in sarcoidosis. Women of Swedish, Puerto Rican, and Irish backgrounds often have Löeffler's syndrome, an acute disorder characterized by erythema nodosum, polyarthritis, iritis, and/or fever that has a good prognosis. In contrast, people of West Indian background in London have a later onset of disease and more generalized organ involvement, including the respiratory, ocular, and reticuloendothelial systems, than do Caucasians. Sarcoidosis also has a more chronic presentation with a poorer prognosis in blacks compared with whites in the United States.

Likewise, an individual's genotype may influence disease expression. Human leukocyte antigen B8 (HLA-B8), for example, has been

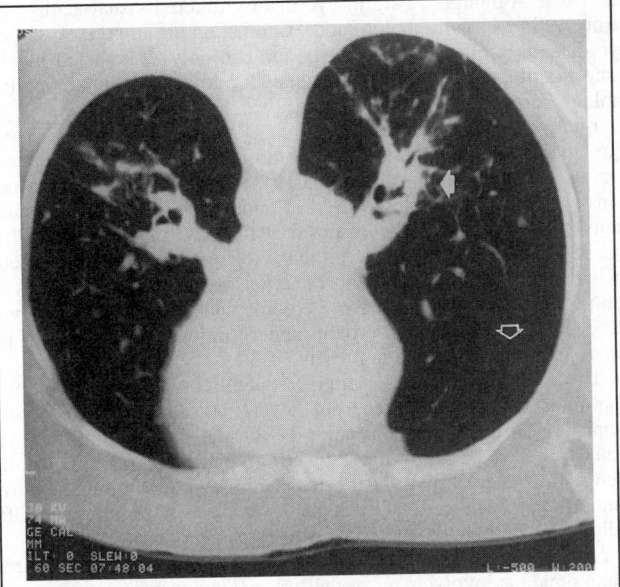

FIGURE 53-1   High-resolution computed tomographic (CT) scan of the lung from a patient with sarcoidosis. Disease is localized around the central bronchovascular bundles *(solid arrow),* with sparing of the peripheral parenchyma *(open arrow).*

Table 53-1   Organ system involvement in sarcoidosis

ORGAN SYSTEM	CLINICAL INCIDENCE (% PATIENTS)
Thoracic	
Pulmonary	90-95
Hilar nodes	75
Parenchyma	50
Cardiac	5-10
Extrathoracic	
Dermatologic	20-50
Erythema nodosum	15-20
Endocrine	10-50
Hypercalcemia	2-5
Hypercalciuria	20-50
Gastrointestinal	1-2
Genitourinary	1-2
Musculoskeletal	10-20
Nervous system	3-5
Ophthalmologic	20-50
Reticuloendothelial	20-30
Liver	20
Lymph nodes	20
Spleen	20
Upper respiratory	5-15
Number of involved organ systems	
Three or more	35
One or two	65

Data from Mayock RL et al: *Am J Med* 35:67, 1963; and Siltzbach LE et al: *Am J Med* 57:847, 1974.

Table 53-2   Radiographic stage of sarcoidosis and prognosis

STAGE	RESOLUTION (%)	PROGRESSION (%)
I	54	7
II	31	13
III	4	10

Modified from Siltzbach LE et al: *Am J Med* 57:847, 1974.

associated with erythema nodosum, arthritis, and early resolution, whereas HLA-B27 is found in a greater percentage of patients with uveitis.

Generalized fatigue, weakness, malaise, weight loss, anorexia, fevers, and sweats are some of the constitutional symptoms that represent the most common presentation of symptomatic sarcoidosis. Generally regarded as benign, sarcoidosis can also involve a number of vital structures, including those in the respiratory, cardiac, endocrine, ophthalmologic, and central nervous systems, with potential life-threatening implications.

The respiratory system is the most frequently involved organ system. Up to 90% of patients with sarcoidosis have pulmonary involvement at some time during the course of their disease. Of these, 60% may develop symptoms of cough, wheezing, or dyspnea. By international convention, chest radiographs are grouped into the following stages: stage 0, normal; stage I, bilateral hilar adenopathy; stage II, bilateral hilar adenopathy with diffuse parenchymal infiltrates; and stage III, diffuse parenchymal infiltrates without bilateral hilar adenopathy. Although useful for communication, the different radiographic stages have not been useful in determining the degree of a patient's symptoms, the progression of the underlying disease, or the histology of the biopsy specimen. The discrepancy between radiographic stage and disease progression partly results from the nonspecific information obtained by the plain chest radiograph. The plain chest radiograph is unable to distinguish fibrosis from alveolitis (see section on prognosis) and also is a two-dimensional representation of a three-dimensional object, the lung. With respect to sarcoidosis, although they may appear as diffuse parenchymal nodules on the plain chest film, with high-resolution CT scanning and autopsy data (see Fig. 53-1) these nodules are localized most frequently to the peribronchovascular bundles, which may be a more accurate representation of disease. The stages demonstrated on chest radiographs do predict resolution of infiltrates in large population studies (Table 53-2).

Progressive pulmonary sarcoidosis occurs in up to 20% of patients. The resultant physiologic abnormalities are those seen in most restrictive lung diseases. Some patients may also have an added obstructive component resulting from endobronchial disease. Often, however, static pulmonary function tests do not correlate with the degree of dyspnea. Exercise testing may be useful in delineating the cause of dyspnea in patients with sarcoidosis. Extrapulmonary factors may cause dyspnea in these patients (e.g., cardiac disease, anemia, myopathy). Finally, although pulmonary function tests do not appear to

correlate with the radiographic stage, symptoms, or histology in sarcoidosis (see section on prognosis), they appear to be a sensitive way to follow the course of disease.

The upper airway can also be involved with sarcoidosis, including the nasopharynx, larynx, vocal cords, paranasal sinuses, and nasal bones. Critical narrowing may result in upper airway obstruction, dyspnea, and cough.

Cardiac sarcoidosis, although infrequent, is important because it can be potentially lethal and a major source of symptoms, including dyspnea and cough, without clinical evidence of disease elsewhere. Similar to that of the lung, granulomatous involvement of the heart is patchy. The degree of cardiac compromise depends not only on the extent but also on the location of the disease. Granulomas localized to the conduction system potentially can result in heart block or arrhythmias. Likewise, extensive myocardial involvement may cause a restrictive and dilated cardiomyopathy. The mortality from cardiac sarcoidosis approaches 20% to 30%. Attempts to identify patients with early cardiac involvement, such as by thallium scanning with dipyridamole infusion, exercise testing with β-blockers, and magnetic resonance imaging (MRI), have resulted in detection of cardiac abnormalities in patients with sarcoidosis at a rate similar to that observed with postmortem examination (25% to 50%). Whether these detected abnormalities contribute to clinical disease remains to be determined.

In addition to direct cardiac involvement, the heart's electrical system also may be altered by hypercalcemia. The mechanism for both the hypercalcemia and the hypercalciuria in sarcoidosis is an increase in 1,25-dihydroxycholecalciferol concentration (see section on pathogenesis), which results in an increase in intestinal calcium absorption. In addition, chronic renal insufficiency from nephrolithiasis and nephrocalcinosis may be the result of a persistent hypercalcemia.

Ocular sarcoidosis, often clinically asymptomatic, can result in blindness. The most common structure involved is the anterior uveal tract. Involvement of any of the ocular structures, however, has been described. Although a careful eye history (altered visual acuity, watering, redness, photophobia) and examination are important, sarcoid eye disease is often asymptomatic and can only be detected by slit-lamp examination. Therefore annual eye examinations by an ophthalmologist are recommended.

Likewise, sarcoidosis can involve any portion of the nervous system, including the cranial nerves (most often VII), the peripheral nerves, the skeletal muscle, the basal meninges, and the central nervous system (CNS) in the form of inflammation or mass lesions. Lesions are more frequently localized at the base of the brain and, if localized to the hypothalamic/pituitary region, may result in diabetes insipidus or galactorrhea/amenorrhea. Seizures are a marker of severe central nervous system disease. Cerebrospinal fluid is typically lymphocytic with an elevated protein concentration, and in 20% of patients, hypoglycorrhachia is present.

The reticulendothelial system is frequently involved in sarcoidosis. The liver may be enlarged, but severe hepatic dysfunction with esophagogastric variceal formation is unusual. In addition, these patients may have an unexplained fever or a presentation similar to that seen with primary biliary cirrhosis. The lack of an antimitochondrial antibody has been used to distinguish sarcoidosis from cirrhosis. Finally, splenic enlargement may result in pancytopenia.

Skin manifestations from sarcoidosis can be the result of direct granulomatous involvement of the tissue (lupus pernio, skin plaques, cutaneous nodules) or the result of a vasculitic response. The latter is the mechanism responsible for erythema nodosum in these patients. Lupus pernio is a chronic violaceous lesion of the face that, in contrast to erythema nodosum, has been associated with multiple organ involvement, laryngeal sarcoidosis, and a poor prognosis.

✔ *WHEN TO REFER*

Patients may need to be referred for transbronchial or other biopsies to confirm the diagnosis of sarcoidosis. If the diagnosis is already established, it is important to have the following baseline investigations, some of which may require referral: blood for liver function; cell counts and calcium levels; full ophthalmic assessment; lung function tests, specifically spirometry with bronchodilator response; diffusing capacity for carbon monoxide; and arterial blood gas measurements. During the course of the sarcoidosis, any symptomatic ophthalmic, cardiac, CNS, renal, skin, or pulmonary involvement should be referred for an appropriate opinion and management.

Sarcoidosis can also affect the skeletal, gastrointestinal, and urinary systems. Involvement of the parotid or lacrimal glands in combination with uveitis and fever has been termed *uveoparotid fever* or *Heerfordt's syndrome.*

DIAGNOSIS

The diagnosis of sarcoidosis is made on the basis of the history and radiographic and pathologic findings, with careful exclusion of identifiable causes (see Box 53-1). Fiberoptic bronchoscopy with transbronchial biopsy is the procedure of choice to obtain tissue in patients with suspected pulmonary involvement. This is usually positive even in the presence of stage I disease. In the patient with asymptomatic bilateral hilar adenopathy, uveitis, and erythema nodosum, the diagnosis presents few uncertainties and usually does not require tissue confirmation.

Patients with suspected myocardial or central nervous system sarcoidosis present a unique dilemma. These patients have a potentially life-threatening disease that requires specific therapy, and biopsy of symptomatically uninvolved tissue may yield the diagnosis. The Kveim test has been used to confirm the diagnosis of sarcoidosis in some patients. However, the 4- to 6-week delay before test interpretation, the 20% false-negative rate, the number of false-positive results, and the lack of a commercially available reagent in the United States make this test impractical for routine use.

COURSE AND PROGNOSIS

The course of sarcoidosis is unpredictable and often organ dependent. Pulmonary sarcoidosis is usually a self-limited condition, with about 50% of patients showing some improvement and 25% remaining unchanged. However, sarcoidosis can progress in 20% of patients and result in pulmonary scarring and fibrosis. Up to 10% of patients may die from their disease. In general, patients with multiple organ involvement, a slower onset of disease, and a more advanced stage on chest radiography (see Table 53-2) do poorly.

In the individual patient, however, conventional clinical, radiographic, and pulmonary function parameters at diagnosis are unreliable in predicting the course of pulmonary sarcoidosis. The failure of chest radiographs and pulmonary function studies to predict the course of sarcoidosis is easily understood in the context of the disease's pathogenesis. The reversible lesion in the lung is the alveolitis, whereas the fibrosis is irreversible. Chest radiographs and pulmonary function tests are nonspecific studies that measure the combined effects of all processes affecting the lungs and do not distinguish alveolitis from fibrosis.

To quantify the degree of alveolitis, investigators have measured markers of alveolar macrophage activation (angiotensin-converting enzyme [ACE] levels, ^{67}Ga scanning) and directly quantified the alveolitis (bronchoalveolar lavage) present in a patient. In general, these studies cannot be recommended for general use to predict the course of disease.

ACE is elevated in up to 80% of patients with sarcoidosis because of the ongoing production of the enzyme by epithelioid cells in the granulomas. ACE levels are not specific for sarcoidosis and are elevated in a variety of other disorders. As such, ACE levels in sarcoidosis may reflect the total granuloma load present in a patient. The latter often differs from disease progression that depends on granuloma location. Progressive sarcoidosis can occur in the absence of elevated ACE levels.

Finally, in an effort to measure local disease activity directly, bronchoalveolar lavage has been used to assess the degree of lymphocytic alveolitis in these patients. In general, the presence of a lymphocytic alveolitis has reflected disease of shorter duration and does not indicate which patients have functional deterioration. Whether serially performed bronchoalveolar lavages will identify the patient with ongoing pulmonary inflammation and who is more likely to develop progressive disease is unknown.

TREATMENT

Individualizing therapeutic regimens is particularly important in patients with sarcoidosis because the disease has such a heterogeneous presentation and course. Most patients, because of the disease's self-limited nature, do not require therapy but rather simple observation. Occasionally, nonsteroidal antiinflammatory agents may be symptomatically useful in this group of patients, especially for arthralgia.

Antiinflammatory therapy is indicated for individuals who have either severe or progressive disease. To determine if progressive disease is present, individuals should be followed at least at 3-month intervals for the first year, to observe for evidence of progressive disease. From that point they can be followed every 6 months if they are clinically and physiologically stable. Pulmonary function testing is particularly useful in this regard. Some patients must be treated immediately. These patients usually have critical organ involvement (cardiac disease, central nervous system disease, ocular disease, persistent hypercalcemia) or disfiguring skin lesions. Many patients with pulmonary disease need to be treated immediately if progressive pulmonary functional impairment is already evident.

Glucocorticoids are currently the principal antiinflammatory agents used. Unfortunately, glucocorticoids have several side effects that limit both dosage and duration of therapy. In an attempt to overcome this, glucocorticoid analogs with less toxicity (inhaled steroids) or alternative antiinflammatory agents (e.g., methotrexate, cyclophosphamide) have been used.

Whom, when, and how long to treat are all unknown. Presently, we observe patients with noncritical organ involvement, including stage I pulmonary sarcoidosis without pulmonary function impairment, at 6-month intervals with serial pulmonary function studies. Patients with critical organ involvement or with evidence of disease progression receive prednisone (1 mg/kg/day) for 4 to 6 weeks, with a rapid tapering (0.25 mg/kg/day) for 3 months more. The prednisone is then tapered to an alternate-day regimen to reduce systemic side effects or to as low a dosage as the patient tolerates. If disease progresses despite prednisone therapy, disease recurs after tapering the prednisone, or severe glucocorticoid-related side effects occur, we institute alternative antiinflammatory therapy with the agents previously noted.

BIBLIOGRAPHY

Crystal RG et al: Pulmonary sarcoidosis: a disease characterized and perpetuated by activated lung T-lymphocytes, *Ann Intern Med* 94:73, 1981.
Gilbert SR, Hunninghake GW: Bronchoalveolar lavage in sarcoidosis. In Baughman RP, editor: *Bronchoalveolar lavage,* Cincinnati, 1992 Year Book.
Hunninghake GW: Staging of pulmonary sarcoidosis, *Chest* 89:178S, 1986.
Hunninghake GW et al: Outcome of the treatment of sarcoidosis, *Am J Respir Crit Care Med* 149:893, 1994.
Mayock RL et al: Manifestations of sarcoidosis, *Am J Med* 35:67, 1963.
Moller DR et al: Bias toward use of a specific T-cell receptor B-chain variable region in a subgroup of individuals with sarcoidosis, *J Clin Invest* 82:1183, 1989.
Muller NI, Miller RR: Computed tomography of chronic diffuse infiltrative disease, *Am Rev Respir Dis* 142:1440, 1990.
Newman LS et al: Sarcoidosis: medical progress, *N Engl J Med* 336:1224-1234, 1997.
Siltzbach LE: Sarcoidosis: clinical features and management, *Med Clin North Am* 51:483, 1967.
Siltzbach LE et al: Course and prognosis of sarcoidosis around the world. *Am J Med* 57:847, 1974.
Thomas PD, Hunninghake GW: Current concepts of the pathogenesis of sarcoidosis, *Am Rev Respir Dis* 135:747, 1987.
Winterbauer RH, Hutchinson JF: The use of pulmonary function tests in the management of sarcoidosis, *Chest* 78:640, 1980.

CHAPTER

54 Hypersensitivity Pneumonitis

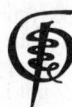

Herbert Y. Reynolds and Timothy J. Craig

Repeated inhalation of a variety of small organic particles (as powder or dust or as aerosolized droplets) can cause hypersensitivity pneumonitis (HP), also known as *extrinsic allergic alveolitis*. These dusts can be bacteria or spores from saprophytic fungi that contaminate vegetables, wood bark, water reservoir vaporizers, or dairy and grain products. They can be derived from animal excreta or can be dander. Although the antigen is usually organic, it may be inorganic, such as diphenylmethane di-isocyanate, which acts as a hapten and conjugates with self-proteins, causing a hypersensitivity reaction. Colorful, descriptive names for the diseases underscore the frequent occupational or home environmental nature of exposure (Table 54-1). Two phenomena are implied in these diseases: (1) the affected subject has acquired heightened immunologic reactivity to the inciting agent, and (2) the inflammatory response that occurs is located primarily in the alveolar air exchange portion of the lung and not in the larger conducting airways, which are usually involved in asthmatic diseases. This distinction is important, for extrinsic immunoglobulin E (IgE) antibody–mediated allergic asthma is also a form of hypersensitivity lung disease, which is often associated with airborne organic antigens, not infrequently to the same antigen(s) implicated in the hypersensitivity pneumonitis group of diseases.

CLINICAL PRESENTATION

Hypersensitivity pneumonitis is a syndrome with a spectrum that varies from acute to chronic, depending on the frequency of antigen exposure. It may vary from mild to severe and even fatal disease depending on the intensity of the immunologic response, the concentration of inhaled antigen, the patient's age, and the duration of exposure. Although many persons can be exposed to these common antigens and many develop specific serum antibodies to them (precipitins are present in 5% of exposed office workers and 30% to 50% of grain handlers, dairy workers, and pigeon or bird handlers), relatively few subjects manifest respiratory disease. Sensitization to an organic dust is often insidious. Repeated exposure can produce lung changes of a lymphocytic alveolitis, but the subject may remain

---

Table 54-1   Hypersensitivity pneumonitis diseases with major antigens and exposure or source

DISEASE	MAJOR ANTIGENS	EXPOSURE OR SOURCE
Thermophilic bacteria		
Farmer's lung	*Faenia rectivirgula (Micropolyspora faeni)*	Moldy hay
Grain handler's lung	*Thermoactinomyces faeni*	Moldy grain
Mushroom worker's lung	*M. faeni, Thermoactinomyces vulgaris*	Mushroom compost
Bagassosis	*Thermoactinomyces sacchari*	Moldy sugar cane (bagasse)
Humidifier or air conditioner lung	*T. vulgaris, M. faeni*	Heated water reservoirs
	Aureobasidium pullulans	
Other bacteria		
Detergent worker's lung	*Bacillus subtilis*	Water
Humidifier lung	*Bacillus cereus*	Water reservoir
Machine operator's lung	*Pseudomonas fluorescens*	Aerosolized metalworking fluid
True fungi		
Maple bark stripper's lung	*Cryptostroma corticale*	Moldy bark
Malt worker's lung	*Aspergillus clavatus*	Moldy malt, barley
Sequoiosis	*A. pullulans* and *Graphium* species	Moldy redwood dust
Paprika splitter's lung	*Mucor stolonifer*	Moldy paprika pods
Cheese worker's lung	*Penicillium caseii*	Cheese mold
Suberosis	*Penicillium frequentans*	Moldy cork dust
Aspergillosis	*Aspergillus* spores	Water reservoir
Summer-type hypersensitivity	*Trichosporon cutaneum*	House dust, bird droppings
Animal proteins		
Bird breeder's lung	Avian proteins (serum, excreta)	Pigeons, parakeets
Chicken plucker's lung	Chicken feathers (serum)	Chickens
Turkey handler's lung	Turkey feathers (serum)	Turkeys
Duck fever	Duck feathers	Ducks
Rodent handler's disease	Rat urine (serum)	Rats
Pituitary snuff-taker's lung	Porcine and bovine pituitary protein	Pituitary snuff
Ameba		
Humidifier lung	*Acanthamoebea castellani*	Water
	Naegleria gruberi	
Bacterial products		
Byssinosis	Lipopolysaccharide	Cotton bract
Bleomycin hypersensitivity (in contrast to fibrosis)	*Streptomyces verticillus* glycopeptides	Bleomycin
Insect products		
Miller's lung (wheat weevil disease)	*Sitophilus granarius*	Contaminated grain
Chemicals		
Chemical worker's lung	Trimellitic anhydride	Plastics
	Toluene di-isocyanate	Polyurethane foam or rubber manufacture
	Methylene di-isocyanate	
Epoxy resin lung	Phthalic anhydride	Heated epoxy resin

Modified from Reynolds HY: *Lung,* 169:S109, 1991.

asymptomatic. Unique host susceptibility or resistance may influence the individual response, especially in younger patients. Chronic exposure, however, can result in an interstitial, granulomatous, and fibrotic lung disease that is debilitating.

Clinically, three syndromes can occur. First, an acute reaction, occurring 4 to 8 hours after heavy exposure, develops, with dyspnea, cough, chills, fever (up to 40° C), and myalgias (Fig. 54-1). In the absence of a repeat exposure, spontaneous recovery occurs in 12 to 24 hours. On physical examination during an acute episode, the patient is dyspneic and has bibasilar crepitant crackles. Leukocytosis, with a left shift in the polymorphonuclear (PMN) differential count, and bibasilar alveolar infiltrates on chest radiographs are common. Pulmonary function tests during an acute attack demonstrate decreases in total lung capacity, vital capacity, and diffusing capacity. Between antigenic exposures, patients are usually asymptomatic and all clinical tests are normal.

Second, an asymptomatic or subclinical phase of illness may ensue. It is uncertain whether all subjects exposed to an appropriate aerosol antigen manifest the acute symptoms just described or can become sensitized without noticeable respiratory and systemic effects. Because many people will develop serum precipitins to the environmental antigens encountered in dairy and farming operations or after contact with, for example, domesticated birds, a primary host immunologic response may occur without prominent illness. However, when asymptomatic, nonsmoking dairy farmers with serum-precipitating antibodies to *Micropolyspora faeni* antigen were investigated with bronchoalveolar lavage to sample alveolar cells, they had an increased recovery of lung cells and a higher-than-normal percentage of lymphocytes. Thus these ostensibly sensitized but asymptomatic subjects had subclinical evidence of lymphocytic alveolitis. The long-term effects of this low-grade immunologic response in the lung were apparently well tolerated for up to 2 and 3 years despite continued antigenic exposure. When a group of such farmers was followed with repeat bronchoalveolar lavage analysis, the lymphocytic alveolitis was usually still present. Therefore an unsuspected, asymptomatic phase of illness could be more widespread than clinically evident and represents a reservoir from which some of the chronic-phase patients emerge with much more evidence of lung involvement, with fibrosis and a granulomatous reaction.

Third, if antigen exposure is protracted, a chronic form of disease develops that may no longer feature the acute exacerbation of respiratory symptoms, fever, and so on with reexposure. Instead, patients can develop breathlessness, dyspnea with exertion, and cough; these symptoms are indistinguishable from those found in many other forms of interstitial pulmonary diseases. Fatigue, poor appetite, and loss of weight can be significant in this stage of disease. Symptoms and evidence of constitutional effects of disease can be evident for months and occasionally for years before the subject comes for evaluation. The chest radiograph is abnormal and has telltale reticulolinear markings attributed to interstitial fibrosis. Pulmonary function tests are characterized by a restrictive ventilatory pattern and a decreased diffusing capacity for carbon monoxide. As bronchiolitis obliterans develops, a mixed obstructive restrictive pattern may be evident on pulmonary function tests. Such patients with this chronic form of inhalational hypersensitivity disease can be difficult to separate diagnostically from patients with other forms of interstitial lung disease of unknown etiology, unless the exposure history is obvious. A serum antibody precipitin screen for hypersensitivity antigens will not establish a diagnosis but, if positive, might direct the clinician to consider a possible environmental exposure. An environmental survey of the home or workplace may be needed to establish exposure.

IMMUNOPATHOLOGIC FINDINGS

Most of the pathologic lung samples and bronchoalveolar lavage samples made of cells and immunoglobulins that have been studied have been obtained from patients with chronic disease. Often an open lung biopsy is needed to provide an adequate specimen for histologic diagnosis, so these tissue changes are reviewed first.

If biopsy tissue is obtained from patients with established disease, chronic changes are present in lung tissue. The pathologic findings cited by Reyes and colleagues included 60 biopsies secured from patients with farmer's lung (caused by a variety of thermophilic actinomycetes). All biopsies contained interstitial pneumonitis, described as a patchy infiltrate of the alveolar walls consisting primarily of lymphocytes and plasma cells and occasionally other inflammatory cells. When the infiltrate was extensive, similar cells were seen within the alveolar spaces. The pathologic pattern was patchy, not uniform, and intervening pulmonary parenchyma did not appear to be involved. In 27 of the 60 biopsies, the degree of interstitial pneumonitis was graded as extensive (3+), and all biopsy samples contained some evidence of it. Unresolved pneumonia, featuring a fibrinous exudate and PMN leukocytes, was observed in two thirds of the specimens. Large histiocytes with foamy cytoplasm were observed in more than half of the biopsies. Granulomas were usually present; however, none was seen in 18 of 60 biopsies. Other prominent findings in the farmer's lung specimens included interstitial fibrosis (in 65%); bronchiolitis obliterans (in 50%); granulomas that contained giant cells that in turn contained foreign body material, as determined by polarized light examination (70%); and pleural fibrosis (about 50%). Unfortunately, the biopsies were not separated on the basis of clinical stage of disease as to recent versus chronic.

Bronchoalveolar Fluid

Although it is generally accepted that HP is an immunologic disorder, the exact immunopathogenic mechanisms are unknown. The most characteristic immunologic feature of hypersensitivity pneumonitis is the presence in serum of precipitating antibody against the causative antigen. These precipitins are usually IgG, but IgA and IgM have also been reported. It is important to note that the presence of precipitins is not diagnostic. An occasional patient with hypersensitivity pneumonitis will not have precipitating antibody; however, in these patients, use of concentrated serum or more sensitive assays such as radioimmunoassays usually will detect antibody. A significant percentage of exposed asymptomatic individuals will have serum precipitins, usually of lower titer than in symptomatic patients.

Bronchoalveolar lavage fluid has been studied in symptomatic pigeon breeders and those with farmer's lung in subacute or chronic stages of disease without recent exposure to antigen. Principal changes in blood and lung secretions are given in Box 54-1. Peripheral blood values are generally normal, in contrast to cellular and protein changes in alveolar lavage fluid. The recovery of respiratory cells is increased, which reflects a substantially higher percentage of T lymphocytes than is found in normal persons. Whereas the subtypes of T cells in normal persons are in a ratio of about 1.5:1.0 for CD_4^+ (T-helper) lymphocytes to CD_8^+ (T suppressor) lymphocytes (Chapter 39), a slight excess of T-suppressor cells in hypersensitivity pneumonitis can decrease the ratio to less than 1. This decrease has been documented in several studies. In contrast, T-helper cells are often found in greatly increased numbers in patients with active alveolitis of sar-

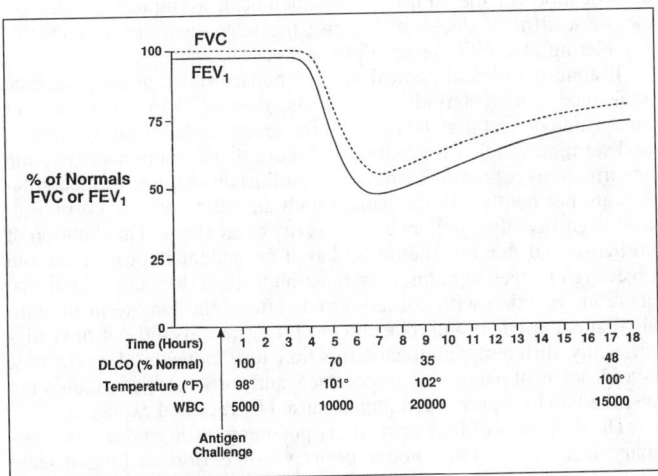

FIGURE 54-1 Changes that occur to the pulmonary function studies (forced vital capacity *[FVC]* and forced expiratory volume in 1 second *[FEV₁]*), the *diffusing capacity (DLCO),* temperature and white blood cell count *(WBC)* during the hours following an antigen challenge in a patient with hypersensitivity pneumonitis.

BOX 54-1

Immunologic features of blood and bronchoalveolar lavage fluid in chronic stage of hypersensitivity pneumonitis

Blood

Normal blood cell counts
Normal immunoglobulin levels, usually
Positive serum precipitins (IgG)

Bronchoalveolar lavage fluid

Lung cell recovery increased
High lymphocyte percentages (50% to 70% of bronchoalveolar lavage cells)
   T lymphocytes predominate
   May have increased number of cytotoxic T-suppressor cells (slight reversal of T-helper/T-suppressor cell ratio)
   T-cell division high (10% to 15% in replicating phase)
   Natural killer lymphocytes increased; enhanced cytotoxicity evident; gamma/delta receptors
Large and foamy macrophages, minimum eosinophils, and increased number (up to 1% of all lavage cells) of basophils
Total protein increased
   Elevated IgG and IgM levels
   IgG and IgA antibodies present
   Abnormal surfactant composition

coidosis such that the ratio may be in the 4 to 8 range. Cytotoxic lymphocytes can be activated in this stage of hypersensitivity disease as well. About 10% of the alveolar macrophages are large and have a peculiar appearance of vacuolated cytoplasm, which have been termed *foamy* macrophages.

Although the classic findings in HP from bronchoalveolar lavage analysis is a predominance of T-suppressor (CD_8^+) lymphocytes, there is considerable variation, depending on the duration between bronchoalveolar lavage (BAL) and last exposure. Early after exposure, a predominance of neutrophils occurs. Within 1 to 2 days CD_8^+ cells become the dominant cell type. With avoidance for approximately a week, a transition occurs and T-helper lymphocytes (CD_4^+) become the dominant cell recovered in BAL fluid. Because of the cellular kinetics in this transition, it is often difficult to distinguish this disease from other interstitial lung diseases by BAL alone.

Total protein content in lavage fluid is increased but without a disproportionate increase in albumin, which would indicate a significant leak of protein across the endothelial-alveolar barrier. Elevated immunoglobulin content accounts for a portion of the protein with IgG and IgM levels being increased; special elevation of IgG_4 was noted in pigeon breeders. Specific antibody activity in IgG and IgA classes can be identified. Apparently, surfactant has an unusual composition in hypersensitivity pneumonitis. Lavage shows increased levels of phosphatidylinositol compared with phosphatidylcholine, but levels of phosphatidylethanolamine and glycerol are decreased.

DIAGNOSIS

The diagnosis of a typical presentation of acute hypersensitivity pneumonitis can usually be made by history of exposure, subsequent signs and symptoms, chest radiographs, confirmatory serologic studies, and a trial of avoidance. Often the physician may never see someone in an early phase, because an alert person might recognize the precipitating cause and voluntarily remove it from the environment. Because of the fever that may occur with acute exposure, patients may be inappropriately diagnosed as having an infection such a psittacosis.

The chronic, insidious forms of hypersensitivity pneumonitis are often more difficult to diagnose. The differential diagnosis includes usual interstitial pneumonitis, chronic eosinophilic pneumonia, idiopathic hemosiderosis, sarcoidosis, pulmonary alveolar proteinosis, and interstitial pulmonary disorders caused by infectious agents, mineral dust, chemical fumes, neoplasia, drugs, and collagen vascular disease (Chapter 56). Hypersensitivity pneumonitis involves the lung

only; therefore extrapulmonary signs such as hepatosplenomegaly are not compatible with a diagnosis of hypersensitivity pneumonitis. If a specific diagnosis cannot be made by noninvasive tests, a lung biopsy may be required to differentiate hypersensitivity pneumonitis from other forms of interstitial pulmonary disease. Establishing the diagnosis may require considerable detective work, even going into the subject's working or home environment for clues, and may necessitate assessing fellow workers for illness.

High-resolution lung CT (HRCT) scan may be helpful in the differential diagnosis in difficult cases. Findings that favor hypersensitivity pneumonitis include poorly defined micronodules, widespread ground-glass attenuation, and predominance of disease in the upper and middle lung zones. The latter two findings were not specific for HP. Poorly defined micronodules had the strongest correlation with chronic hypersensitivity pneumonitis and can often allow this disease to be distinguished from idiopathic pulmonary fibrosis. Acute and subacute HP could not be reliably separated from idiopathic pulmonary fibrosis (IPF) by CT scan findings alone. Because there is a lack of certainty of the HRCT to diagnose hypersensitivity pneumonitis, other criteria, such as lung biopsy, are indicated in questionable cases.

Occasionally a challenge with the antigen is indicated for diagnosis. This challenge should be done only if history, physical examination, pulmonary function, chest radiograph, avoidance trial, and antibody tests have failed to establish a diagnosis. Moreover, challenges should be performed only on patients who have recovered lung function and only under the careful supervision of a physician experienced in these procedures. Because patients may become very ill as a result of deliberate challenges, physicians should initiate them with caution and with appropriate plans for observation and therapy in the event that severe immediate or late reaction occurs (see Fig. 54-1). Care must be taken in preparing the extract used in the challenge; if it contains endotoxins, a nonspecific reaction may occur, leading to an inappropriate diagnosis.

TREATMENT AND PROGNOSIS

Once the offending antigen has been identified, avoidance should be the primary modality of treatment. In a patient with a contaminated ventilation system, for example, cleaning to remove the thermophilic organisms is essential. With HP secondary to bird exposure, the bird should be removed from the home and cleaning performed. Even with cleaning, the antigen may persist for prolonged periods after the bird is removed. Because many exposures that cause hypersensitivity pneumonitis are occupational, such measures as improved ventilation, masks, or change in job duties or work site may suffice. Often, however, a change of occupation is necessary to prevent progression to irreversible lung damage. However, some workers can have an unsuspected lymphocytic alveolitis but remain asymptomatic despite continued antigen exposure. Whether to recommend a change in job or avocation for the subject with subclinical, asymptomatic disease can be a difficult decision, because the lung seems to tolerate this smoldering alveolitis for several years at least.

If abnormalities in clinical and pulmonary function occur despite avoidance, corticosteroids in moderate doses (30 to 40 mg/day of prednisone orally) may be required for several weeks or even months to determine whether reversibility of clinical and pulmonary function abnormalities is possible. Cromolyn, antihistamines, and bronchodilators are not helpful. In the patient with an acute episode, corticosteroids significantly ameliorate the severity of an attack. The duration of corticosteroid therapy should be based on patient improvement and objective changes in pulmonary function tests. It does not appear that acute intervention with corticosteroids affects the long-term prognosis. Patients treated with placebo or corticosteroids did not have significantly different pulmonary function tests 5 years after therapy. Avoidance is of paramount importance, and corticosteroids should not be relied on to suppress symptoms caused by repeated exposure.

The prognosis of hypersensitivity pneumonitis depends on two primary factors: (1) the amount of irreversible fibrotic lung disease present at the time of diagnosis and (2) the patient's capability to avoid further antigen exposure. In patients with the acute form of the disease, all clinical abnormalities will reverse and no further attacks will occur if avoidance is practiced. In patients with more chronic forms of the disease, avoidance and corticosteroids produce variable degrees of improvement. Those with permanent, irreversible pulmonary damage from fibrosis or bronchiolitis obliterans unfortunately will have little improvement. This problem underscores the importance of both early detection of clinical disease and identification and avoidance of the causative antigen.

BIBLIOGRAPHY

Bernstein DF et al: Machine operator's lung: a hypersensitivity pneumonitis disorder associated with exposure to metalworking fluid aerosols, *Chest* 108:636, 1995.

Campbell JM: Acute symptoms following work with hay, *Br Med J* 2:1143, 1932.

Cormier Y et al: Abnormal bronchoalveolar lavage in asymptomatic dairy farmers: study of lymphocytes, *Am Rev Respir Dis* 130:1046, 1984.

Cormier Y et al: Persistent bronchoalveolar lymphocytosis in asymptomatic farmers, *Am Rev Respir Dis* 133:843, 1986.

Costabel U et al: Ia-like antigens on T-cells and their subpopulations in pulmonary sarcoidosis and in hypersensitivity pneumonitis: analysis of bronchoalveolar and blood lymphocytes, *Am Rev Respir Dis* 131:337, 1985.

Fournier E et al: Early neutrophil alveolitis after inhalation challenge in hypersensitivity pneumonitis, *Chest* 88:563, 1985.

Kokkarinen JI et al: Effect of corticosteroid treatment on the recovery of pulmonary function in farmer's lung, *Am Rev Respir Dis* 145:3, 1992.

Leatherman JW et al: Lung T cells in hypersensitivity pneumonitis, *Ann Intern Med* 100:390, 1984.

Lynch et al: Can CT distinguish hypersensitivity pneumonitis from idiopathic pulmonary fibrosis, *AJR* 165:807, 1995.

Patterson R et al: IgA and IgG antibody activities of serum and bronchoalveolar fluid from symptomatic pigeon breeders, *Am Rev Respir Dis* 120:113, 1979.

Reed CE et al: Pigeon breeder's lung, *JAMA* 193:261, 1965.

Reyes CN et al: The pulmonary pathology of farmer's lung disease, *Chest* 81:142, 1982.

Reynolds HY: Concepts of pathogenesis and lung reactivity in hypersensitivity pneumonitis, *Ann NY Acad Sci* 465:287, 1986.

Reynolds H: Hypersensitivity pneumonitis: correlation of cellular and immunologic changes with clinical phases of disease, *Lung* 169:S109, 1991.

Reynolds HY et al: Analysis of cellular and protein components of bronchoalveolar lavage fluid from patients with idiopathic pulmonary fibrosis and hypersensitivity pneumonitis, *J Clin Invest* 59:165, 1977.

Schuyler M et al: Experimental hypersensitivity pneumonitis: effect of Thy 1.2^+ and $CD8^+$ cell depletion, *Am J Resp Crit Care Med* 151:1834, 1995.

Semenzato G et al: Lung T cells in hypersensitivity pneumonitis: phenotypic and functional analyses, *J Immunol* 137:1164, 1986.

Trentin L et al: Mechanisms accounting for lymphocytic alveolitis in hypersensitivity pneumonitis, *J Immunol* 145:2147, 1990.

CHAPTER

55 Langerhans' Cell Granulomatosis (Histiocytosis X, Eosinophilic Granuloma)

Allan J. Hance, Abdellatif Tazi, and Françoise Basset

DEFINITION AND NOMENCLATURE

Langerhans' cell granulomatosis (LCG) is defined pathologically by the presence of characteristic destructive granulomatous lesions containing Langerhans' cells. A wide spectrum of clinical manifestations can be encountered, depending on the number of tissues involved and the specific sites of involvement. Involvement of multiple tissues, ranging from diffuse involvement of visceral organs to multifocal involvement of two or more tissues, is more frequently observed in infants and young children. LCG localized to a single tissue (usually bone or lung) is the most common form of LCG observed in older children and adults.

Various names are used for this disease, which may cause confusion. The name *Langerhans' cell granulomatosis* has the virtue of emphasizing the essential role of Langerhans' cells in initiating the process and the granulomatous nature of the lesions. *Histiocytosis X* (HX) and *Langerhans' cell histiocytosis* are also frequently used terms. *Letterer-Siwe disease, Hand-Schüller-Christian syndrome,* and *eosinophilic granuloma* are often used, respectively, to describe patients with diffuse visceral and systemic manifestations, multifocal involvement of two or more tissues, or LCG localized to a single organ.

This discussion is limited to the adult pulmonary form of LCG.

Although pulmonary LCG usually is classified among the interstitial lung diseases, the granulomas are centered on small bronchioles, and it may be preferable to consider the process as a bronchiolitis.

EPIDEMIOLOGY

No precise data are available concerning the prevalence of localized pulmonary LCG. Since its description as a discrete nosologic entity in 1951, the disease is being recognized with increasing frequency and probably represents about 1% of all cases of interstitial lung disease. The disease appears to be less common among blacks. All age-groups can be affected, although most patients are 20 to 40 years old. The relative frequency of pulmonary HX in men and women has been quite variable in different series. There is a strong association between pulmonary LCG and cigarette smoking. More than 90% of patients are smokers, and patients with LCG tend to smoke more heavily than persons in the general smoking population. Daily cigarette consumption is a more important risk factor than total pack-years, since many patients have smoked for only a limited time.

PATHOGENESIS
Dendritic Cells and Langerhans' Cells

The initiation of immune responses depends on the participation of "accessory cells," which are required to present antigens to T-helper lymphocytes. Two different populations of accessory cells are present in the normal lung: those of monocyte/macrophage lineage (alveolar macrophages) and those of dendritic cell/Langerhans' cell lineage. As with the alveolar macrophages, cells of dendritic cell/Langerhans' cell lineage are derived from bone marrow precursors and probably arrive in the lung through the peripheral circulation. Dendritic cells, present within the alveolar parenchyma and peribronchiolar tissues, have a folded nucleus and multiple long dendritic processes; they contain few phagocytic inclusions. Langerhans' cells, found almost exclusively *within* the bronchiolar epithelium of normal nonsmokers, are morphologically similar to dendritic cells but contain characteristic pentalaminar platelike cytoplasmic organelles called *Birbeck granules,* which can be seen only by electron microscopy. Langerhans' cells also express surface antigens that react with anti-CD1a (T6) monoclonal antibodies. Most pulmonary dendritic cells are CD1a negative but do express CD1c surface antigens. Langerhans' cells are thought to be derived from dendritic cells, and this transformation in lung and other tissues is associated with close contact between the Langerhans' cells and epithelial cells. The differences between the functional capacities of dendritic cells and Langerhans' cells are still under investigation.

Langerhans' Cell Granulomatosis

Langerhans' cells are known to accumulate at sites of pulmonary epithelial hyperplasia and infiltrate some lung carcinomas because of the release of cytokines such as GM-CSF by the epithelial cells. Thus bronchiolar epithelial abnormalities may predispose to the development of LCG by modifying the number and/or activity of Langerhans' cells present, and could account for heavy cigarette smoking (a common cause of epithelial hyperplasia) being a strong risk factor for this disease.

Because very few smokers develop LCG, additional factors must be involved. Recent studies have demonstrated that Langerhans' cells present in other forms of LCG are of clonal origin, suggesting that somatic mutations of Langerhans' cell precursors contribute to the pathogenesis. The bronchocentric distribution, the rarity of cells in mitosis within the lesions, and the virtual absence of Langerhans' cells in late lesions refute the idea that the disorder is a malignancy or results from the "uncontrolled proliferation" of Langerhans' cells. Thus if clonal Langerhans' cells are also present in pulmonary LCG, abnormalities producing increased lymphostimulatory activity may be more likely in these cells than in those resulting in increased proliferative potential.

The evolution of the pathologic lesions of pulmonary LCG (see following discussion) is highly reminiscent of a granulomatous process and is the most compelling argument that the disease results from an uncontrolled immune response initiated by Langerhans' cells. The nature of the antigen(s), if any, involved in LCG remains unknown.

No associations between LCG and environmental exposures or infectious agents have been reported.

PATHOLOGY

Pulmonary involvement by LCG is typically generalized throughout both lungs. However, the process is not diffuse in the sense that the lesions occur almost exclusively adjacent to terminal and respiratory bronchioles and are separated from each other by apparently normal lung tissue. The pathologic appearance of LCG lesions changes considerably as the process evolves. Although the pulmonary lesions in a single biopsy frequently show a spectrum of evolutionary changes, the pathologic appearance of lung tissue is useful in assessing the activity of the process. The center of early lesions is composed primarily of clusters of Langerhans' cells, which are surrounded by variable numbers of lymphocytes, eosinophils, and neutrophils. These foci form adjacent to terminal or respiratory bronchioles and destroy the preexisting bronchiolar epithelium and wall, from the earliest respiratory bronchiole to the last alveolar duct, in the involved acini.

As the lesions progress, the number of Langerhans' cells usually decreases and other cell types predominate, especially macrophages, eosinophils, and neutrophils. Fibrotic changes begin to appear at this stage. Most often, scarring results in fibrotic walls, limiting cystic lesions. At other sites, fibrosis develops in the center and results in stellate scars often surrounded by traction emphysema. Scarring predominates in end-stage lesions, and few infiltrating cells are present, although lymphoid aggregates and lipid-laden macrophages may remain; Langerhans' cells are present in very small numbers or may be entirely absent. Although granulomatous lesions of all stages frequently appear cavitary, this does not usually result from necrosis of the center of the granulomatous lesions. Rather, destruction of the wall of bronchioles adjacent to the granulomas typically occurs, such that the distorted lumen of the now unrecognizable bronchiole appears as a cavity. The erosion of such peripheral cavities into the pleural space accounts for the high incidence of pneumothorax seen in patients with pulmonary LCG.

CLINICAL MANIFESTATIONS

Pulmonary LCG may manifest in a variety of ways. The most common presentations include (1) the insidious onset of cough, fatigue, and progressive dyspnea, with or without constitutional symptoms; (2) the discovery of diffuse pulmonary abnormalities on a routine chest roentgenogram; and (3) the occurrence of one or several episodes of spontaneous pneumothorax. More rarely, patients can present with systemic symptoms only (e.g., weight loss, malaise, fever) or are identified during evaluation of a patient with extrapulmonary LCG. Only a few adult patients with pulmonary LCG have involvement of other tissues. The most frequent forms of extrapulmonary involvement include isolated bone lesions, skin lesions, and diabetes insipidus resulting from involvement of the hypothalamic/pituitary axis.

In most patients the physical examination of the chest is normal. Crackles are present in a minority of patients (approximately 10%), but wheezing is rare. Clubbing is also uncommon but may occur in patients with advanced disease.

Characteristic radiographic findings in the early stages of pulmonary LCG are the presence of bilateral micronodular, reticular, or reticulonodular infiltrates that are most marked in the upper and middle zones and usually spare the costophrenic angles. In later stages, cystic lesions or small cavitary nodules can be seen. Multiple cystic lesions are often observed in advanced cases, frequently associated with the presence of larger bullous changes. Pleural abnormalities are rare, except in patients with a prior history of pneumothorax or thoracotomy. Enlargement of hilar lymph nodes is extremely rare. Recent studies have shown that high-resolution computed tomography (HRCT) is particularly useful in identifying patients with LCG. HCRT permits the detection of characteristic cystic lesions in essentially all patients, even when chest radiographs are interpreted as normal or showing a reticular pattern. Nodular lesions (usually <5 mm diameter) are also identified by HCRT in most patients. Most patients have both nodular and cystic lesions, and their simultaneous presence is highly suggestive of pulmonary HX. ^{67}Ga scans of the thorax are usually normal.

The results of the routine blood tests are often normal, although mild anemia and leukocytosis may be present. Eosinophilia is absent. Increased immunoglobulins and low titers of antinuclear antibodies, rheumatoid factor, and circulating immune complexes have been described in some patients, but these are of no diagnostic use.

Pulmonary function tests are quite variable and can show an obstructive, restrictive, or mixed pattern. Vital capacity is usually reduced; the residual volume/total lung capacity ratio is frequently increased, especially in patients with cystic changes on chest radiographs. The diffusing capacity is reduced in most patients. Evidence of overt airflow limitation is more common in LCG than in most other interstitial lung diseases. Hypoxemia can occur at rest and is seen more commonly with exercise.

Cells recovered by bronchoalveolar lavage from patients with pulmonary LCG typically include clearly increased numbers of eosinophils and neutrophils and a moderate increase in the number of T lymphocytes. Large numbers of alveolar macrophages are also often present but probably reflect that most patients are cigarette smokers; increased numbers of alveolar macrophages need not be present in lavage fluid from nonsmokers with pulmonary LCG. The identification of Langerhans' cells in lavage fluid by immunohistochemical techniques has been suggested to be useful in diagnosis. Although Langerhans' cells are rarely recovered by lavage from normal individuals, moderate numbers of Langerhans' cells can be recovered from cigarette smokers and patients with other interstitial lung diseases. Furthermore, the percentage of Langerhans' cells recovered by lavage from patients with pulmonary LCG can vary considerably and may depend on the activity of the process. Thus the test's sensitivity and specificity depend on the threshold used to define a positive result, and this question has not been systematically evaluated. In an appropriate clinical context, however, the presence of more than 5% Langerhans' cells is highly suggestive of LCG. This threshold will be attained in few patients; therefore a negative result does not eliminate the diagnosis.

DIAGNOSIS

The presenting signs and symptoms of pulmonary LCG are usually nonspecific, and it is often difficult to differentiate pulmonary LCG from other, more common forms of interstitial lung disease. Useful differential points in the history include the presence of interstitial lung disease in young patients, especially cigarette smokers; the occurrence of one or more pneumothoraces; or the presence of extrapulmonary involvement. Characteristic findings on chest radiographs or HCRT may raise suspicion of the process. Finally, the presence of obstructive abnormalities on pulmonary function testing also suggests involvement by pulmonary LCG.

Nevertheless, none of these clinical findings is specific. Histologic examination of lung tissue is required to firmly establish the diagnosis and is best obtained by thoracotomy or videothoracoscopy. HRCT should be used to identify sites containing "active" (i.e., nodular) lesions and to avoid tissue with extensive cystic or fibrotic changes. Samples of any biopsy should be processed to permit evaluation using electron microscopy and immunofluorescent techniques, which may be helpful in difficult cases. Transbronchial biopsy has a low diagnostic yield and carries a risk of pneumothorax because cystic lesions are frequently present beneath the visceral pleura.

The decision to perform open lung biopsy must be made on a case-by-case basis. In patients with atypical presentations or for whom treatment is anticipated, biopsy is generally appropriate. Conversely, patients with extensive cystic lesions, who are at higher risk for complications and unlikely to respond to treatment, and asymptomatic individuals with typical clinical and HRCT features may not require biopsy. Extrapulmonary lesions (e.g., skin and bone) can also be biopsied to support the diagnosis if the pulmonary manifestations are otherwise highly suggestive of pulmonary LCG.

EVOLUTION

The natural history of pulmonary LCG varies considerably. Approximately 25% to 50% of patients remain asymptomatic or become symptom free with accompanying regression of the radiologic abnormalities. The remaining patients experience a more progressive course, which may be punctuated by periods of remission or relative stability. Although the disease may arrest at any stage, patients with progressive disease are likely to experience persistent respiratory symptoms and have permanent loss of pulmonary function resulting from fibrosis, extensive remodeling of the lung parenchyma, and/or formation of bullous defects. As a general rule, bullous formation with evidence of air trapping and/or airflow obstruction appears to be more common than a purely restrictive defect in patients with significant sequelae. The clinical course is complicated by pneumothorax in 10% to 20% of patients. Unrelenting progression culminating in death from respiratory failure and/or cor pulmonale occurs in few patients.

A variety of factors appear to influence the evolution of pulmonary LCG. Very young or advanced age is often associated with a poor prognosis. The extent of clinical symptoms, radiologic abnormalities, and physiologic impairment at presentation also correlate to some extent with eventual outcome. In particular, repeated episodes of pneumothorax are by themselves a poor prognostic sign, at least partly because they lead to repeated surgical procedures and sometimes to superinfection. The association of pulmonary involvement with evidence of LCG in other tissues, especially cutaneous lesions or diabetes insipidus, can be a particularly ominous sign. However, the association of pulmonary LCG with bone lesions is of less significance, especially when such bone lesions are not widespread.

MANAGEMENT

Because of the strong association between cigarette smoking and LCG, cessation of tobacco use is imperative, although the effect of discontinuing smoking on the evolution of established LCG has not been studied. In view of the favorable prognosis in most patients, asymptomatic individuals or patients with little functional impairment should be managed conservatively. Similarly, patients whose lung pathology shows only inactive "late" lesions are unlikely to respond to treatment. Systemic corticosteroids (e.g., prednisone 1 mg/kg/day for several months followed by gradually tapering doses) are the usual treatment for patients with progressive symptoms and active pathologic lesions. Although anecdotal reports of favorable responses have been published, corticosteroids have never been proved to improve the course of pulmonary LCG. Respiratory superinfections, a common cause of decompensation, should be treated aggressively. Recurrent pneumothoraces are adequately treated by pleurodesis. Lung transplantation has been performed on a small number of patients who developed respiratory insufficiency.

BIBLIOGRAPHY

Friedman PJ, Liebow AA, Sokoloff J: Eosinophilic granuloma of lung: clinical aspects of primary pulmonary histiocytosis in the adult, *Medicine* 60:385, 1981.
Grenier P et al: Chronic diffuse interstitial lung disease: diagnostic value of chest radiography and high resolution CT, *Radiology* 179:123, 1991.
Hance AJ et al: Pulmonary and extrapulmonary manifestations of Langerhans' cell granulomatosis (histiocytosis X), *Semin Respir Med* 9:349, 1988.
Tazi A, Hance AJ: Pulmonary histiocytosis X. In Walters EH, duBois RM, editors: *Immunology and management of interstitial lung diseases*, (pp. 305-318), London, 1995, Chapman & Hall.
Travis WD et al: Pulmonary Langerhans cell granulomatosis (Histiocytosis X). A clinicopathologic study of 48 cases, *Am J Surg Pathol* 17:971, 1993.

CHAPTER

56   Primary Granulomatous Pulmonary Vasculitis

Stephen B. Sulavik and Nav T. Singh

Granulomatous vasculitis is the most common clinically apparent form of *primary* blood vessel inflammation affecting the lung. *Vasculitis* represents the initial and dominant inflammatory tissue reaction and may be defined as "a cellular infiltration with inflammation of the blood vessel walls involving at least the vascular media." Primary blood vessel involvement, which is mainly associated with vascular endothelial proliferation (e.g., scleroderma), vascular wall replacement (e.g., amyloidosis), or sustained pulmonary hypertension, therefore is not included.

A granulomatous tissue response is characterized by the presence of at least two of the following cell types: histiocytes (tissue macrophages), lymphocytes, plasma cells, giant cells, eosinophils, or lymphoreticular cells. The predominent cell type or types identify the specific disorder in most cases. This tissue response may take the spatial configuration of a three-dimensional, compact, organized collection of cells (granuloma/granulomata) or that of a loosely arranged, amorphous proliferation of cells (granulomatous response). Necrosis, usually fibrinoid, of the vessel wall may or may not result; therefore the qualifying terms *necrotizing* or *non-necrotizing* may be used and thus be contrasted to a primary vascular inflammatory response that is predominantly rich in neutrophils (e.g., hypersensitivity angiitis [of Zeek] or periarteritis nodosa [PAN]), as originally described by Kussmaul and Maier.

It may reasonably be postulated that the immunopathogenesis and etiology of these varied histologic responses differ. Unfortunately, the cause of most granulomatous vasculitides is not known, and pathogenetic mechanisms are at best poorly understood and therefore are not available for the purpose of accurate classification. Although histopathologic interpretation alone at times may be nondiagnostic, when interpreted in conjunction with the chest radiographic appearance and certain distinctive clinical and laboratory manifestations, rather clear clinical diagnoses generally emerge. Because considerable information is known regarding prognosis and treatment of many of these often life-threatening disorders, clinical suspicion of their presence and accurate diagnosis are essential. For these reasons, we have used a combined histologic, chest radiographic, and clinical-laboratory approach to classify and diagnose these disorders while continuing to retain important historic eponyms (Table 56-1).

In attempting to understand the pulmonary vasculitides, considerable confusion exists concerning PAN and its relationship to the lung. After careful, extensive review of patients reported to have PAN with "pulmonary" involvement, it is strikingly evident that virtually all would fit the histologic, radiographic, and clinical criteria for either Churg-Strauss syndrome (CSS) or Wegener's granulomatosis (WG), bearing no resemblance to the original gross and histopathologic description of PAN by Kussmaul and Maier.

EOSINOPHILIC GRANULOMATOUS VASCULITIS
Churg-Strauss Syndrome

Clinical and Laboratory Findings. CSS *(allergic granulomatosis, allergic vasculitis , Harkavy syndrome)*, is a multisystem disorder, the precise mechanism(s) and etiologic factors of which are unknown. Men and women are affected equally, with a mean age of onset of approximately 35 years. Clinically, CSS is characterized by the following:

1. The presence and/or history of bronchial asthma (rarely "cough equivalent" asthma)
2. Peripheral blood eosinophilia (PBE), usually in excess of 15%
3. Extrapulmonary signs and/or symptoms resulting from small and medium-sized blood vessel vasculitis with infarction
4. Characteristic "lateralizing" lung densities.

The erythrocyte sedimentation rate (ESR) and serum immunoglobulin E (IgE) levels are usually elevated, particularly during the "vasculitic" phase of the illness; at this time, anemia, weight loss, temperature elevation, sweats, weakness, and malaise are typically present.

The organ systems most involved clinically in CSS include the respiratory tract (100%), nervous system (65%), skin (60%), gastrointestinal tract (60%), and cardiovascular system (25%). *Respiratory tract* symptoms are dominated by bronchial asthma, with manifestations of other organ involvement usually occurring within the first 2 to 5 years after its onset, although much longer durations have been noted. Because asthma may not be clinically present at the onset of other systemic manifestations, a history of prior asthma assumes diagnostic importance. Sinorhinitis, often accompanied by nasal polyps, typically occurs. Chest pain caused by eosinophilic pleuritis may

Table 56-1   Primary granulomatous pulmonary vasculitis

DOMINANT HISTOPATHOLOGY	CHEST RADIOGRAPH	UNIQUE CLINICAL FEATURES
Eosinophilic GPV		
Churg-Strauss syndrome	"Lateral" densities*	Asthma
		Peripheral blood eosinophilia
Mononuclear (plasma cell)–giant cell GPV		
Wegener's granulomatosis		
Complete form (CWG)	Nodule(s),* mass lesion(s)*	Lung; kidney; upper respiratory tract, eye or ear, positive C-ANCA
Limited forms (LWG)	Nodule(s),* mass lesion(s)*	Variations of complete form, positive C-ANCA
Secondary to *Dirofilaria immitis*	"Solitary" nodule	Limited to lung
Lymphocytic GPV		
"Benign" lymphocytic angiitis	Nodules, infiltrates	Limited to lung
Behçet's disease/Hughes-Stovin syndrome	Pulmonary artery aneurysms	Eye involvement, phlebitis, orogenital ulcers, systemic phlebitis
	Pulmonary artery thrombosis	
Atypical lymphoreticular GPV		
Lymphomatoid granulomatosis	Nodule(s),* mass lesion(s)*	Central nervous system and skin involvement
Histiocytic (epitheloid) granuloma GPV		
Necrotizing sarcoid	Nodules, hilar adenopathy	Symmetric nodules are diagnostic
Schistosoma mansoni	Increased size of pulmonary arteries and heart	Pulmonary hypertension
Secondary to talc or starch	Same as above	Same as above
Giant cell GPV		
Takayasu's arteritis	Pulmonary artery narrowing and occlusion	"Aortic branch" syndromes, pulmonary hypertension

*May have transient-successive radiographic densities.
C-ANCA, diffuse, granulated cytoplasmic staining pattern.

also occur. Paresthesias, pain, and weakness, mainly resulting from mononeuritis multiplex, are the most common clinical expressions of *nervous system* involvement. Cerebral infarction and hemorrhage, although fortunately rare, are among the more common causes of death. *Skin* manifestations often occur in crops and include purpura (usually palpable), urticaria and angioneurotic edema, and cutaneous or subcutaneous nodules. Biopsy, particularly of the nodular type of lesion (necrotizing CSS granuloma), is often diagnostic. *Gastrointestinal* involvement should be suspected if signs and/or symptoms of ischemia and infarction occur. Angiographic studies of the abdominal arterial system may confirm the diagnosis of vasculitis if aneurysmal dilation of vessels is found. *Cardiac* manifestations include eosinophilic pericarditis, endomyocardiopathy, and coronary vasculitis, with congestive heart failure being the most frequent cause of death. *Renal* failure, quite responsive to corticosteroid therapy, occurs in less than 5% of patients. However, proteinuria and microscopic hematuria, suggesting mild nephritis, typically occur. Arthritis, arthralgia, lymphadenopathy, myositis, and prostatitis may also be observed.

Although tissue biopsy may provide definitive histologic evidence for CSS, in most patients the diagnosis can be made on clinical grounds alone.

Radiographic Appearance. Because bronchial asthma is an integral part of CSS, radiographic abnormalities frequently associated with asthma may occur. In addition, in those individuals who develop pericardial, myocardial, or endomyocardial involvement, radiographic changes consistent with such cardiac complications may also be observed.

As the result of massive eosinophil infiltration of the lung parenchyma, distinctive radiographic patterns emerge and serve to differentiate CSS from the other vasculitides. All these patterns have cloudy, shadow-like infiltrations that reside almost exclusively in the *lateral* aspects of the posteroanterior (PA) chest radiograph (Figs. 56-1 and 56-2). These infiltrations are observed in approximately 40% to 60% of patients at some time during the course of the disease and may assume any of the following patterns:

1. Transient-successive (i.e., on successive radiographs); some densities regress or disappear, whereas others increase in size or new lesions appear

2. Bilateral, symmetric, lateralizing densities extending from the lung apex to base
3. Symmetric variations of pattern 2, involving only the upper, middle, or lower lung fields
4. Unilateral lateralizing densities extending from the apex to the base
5. Multiple lateralizing densities in various lobes and segments (this pattern may also be observed in an idiopathic *intraluminal* organizing pneumonia referred to as *cryptogenic organizing pneumonia*)

Although over time all these patterns tend to wax and wane, this aspect may not be appreciated on initial presentation because they can remain unchanged for considerable periods. These patterns are also characteristic of chronic eosinophilic pneumonia (CEP), and the transient-successive pattern is the hallmark of Löffler's syndrome (LS). Although bronchial asthma and peripheral blood eosinophilia may also be present in CEP and LS, they differ in that no extrapulmonary manifestations exist, and significant vasculitis and necrotizing eosinophilic granulomas are absent. These radiographic features, in addition to peripheral blood and lung eosinophilia, provide a common thread, suggesting a relationship among the clinically benign Löffler's syndrome, the more severe CEP, and the potentially life-threatening CSS. The physician must have a high degree of clinical awareness of the possible presence of CSS in patients with peripheral blood eosinophilia (PBE) and bronchial asthma alone or in those patients with CEP who develop extrapulmonary manifestations consistent with CSS.

Pathology and Immunology. Aneurysmal dilation of medium-sized arteries may be observed on gross inspection. Other than the usual findings in bronchial asthma, characteristic histopathology includes:

1. *Infiltration* (predominantly by eosinophils) *of blood vessel walls* (venules, arterioles, medium-sized arteries). These lesions are segmental, and different stages, ranging from early eosinophil infiltration with fibrinoid necrosis to more nonspecific scarring, may be observed. The importance of elastic tissue staining to assess the presence and degree of vasculitis in this disease, as well as in all the pulmonary vasculitides, cannot be overemphasized.
2. *Necrotizing eosinophilic granulomas.* These are composed of an

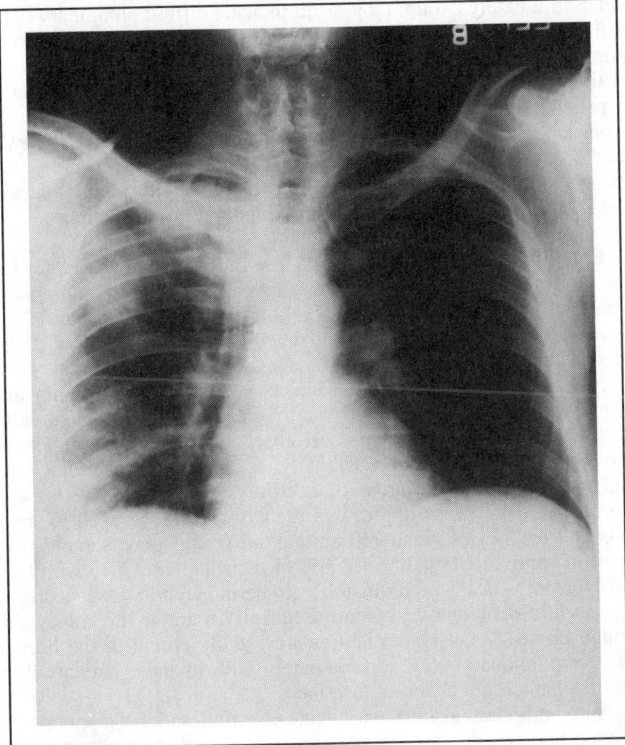

FIGURE 56-1   Churg-Strauss syndrome: "Cloudy," lateralizing, homogeneous densities occupying the right upper and lower lung fields.

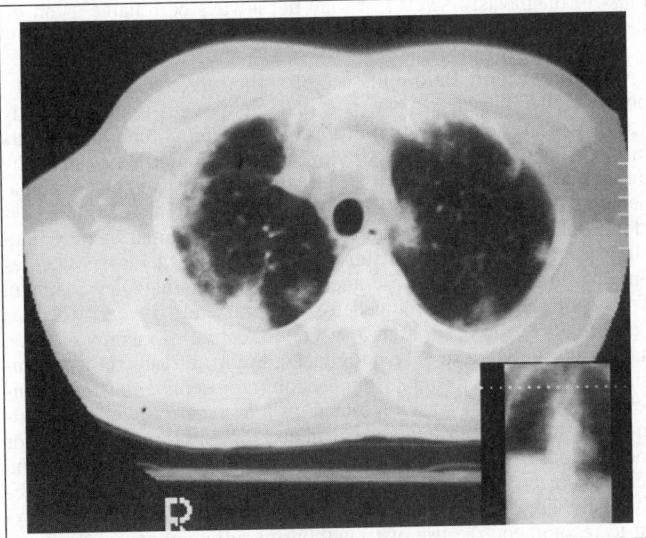

FIGURE 56-2   Churg-Strauss syndrome: thoracic CT with lateralizing densities.

eosinophilic fibrinoid necrotic core surrounded by radially arranged histiocytes and occasional giant cells. The cellular infiltrate surrounding the granuloma consists largely of eosinophils. They are most often found extravascularly, but occasionally are seen within walls of the larger blood vessels.

3. *Nonvascular tissue infiltration* (predominantly by eosinophils).
It is important to emphasize that these histopathologic lesions are randomly distributed throughout the various organs involved, so biopsy of a single organ rarely demonstrates all three histopathologic

changes. The intense tissue eosinophilia readily distinguishes CSS from the other pulmonary vasculitides.

Management. The ultimate mortality rate from CSS in untreated patients probably exceeds 80% to 90%. The use of corticosteroids and immunosuppressive therapy has reduced this mortality rate to less than 10% when the disease is diagnosed and treated early. This further emphasizes the importance of accurate, early diagnosis. Most patients respond well to prednisone (60 to 80 mg a day), particularly if heart failure has not supervened. Residual neurologic defects often remain despite therapy. Monitoring of the ESR, eosinophil count, and serum IgE, if initially detected, provides useful laboratory guidelines for management. Relapses can occur, requiring reinstitution of therapy or an increase in the administered dose. Prolonged therapy of 9 months to 1 year is recommended after an appropriate maintenance dose has been established. For those patients not responding to corticosteroid therapy, cyclophosphamide (2 mg/kg) has proved effective.

MONONUCLEAR (PLASMA CELL)–GIANT CELL GRANULOMATOUS VASCULITIS
Wegener's Granulomatosis

Wegener's granulomatosis is a multisystem disorder that, as classically described, consists of necrotizing vasculitis and aseptic necrosis of (1) the lung and (2) the upper respiratory tract with (3) focal glomerulonephritis of the kidney (complete form [CWG], Wegener triad). Since Wegener's original description, however, patients with identical histopathology, natural history, and response to therapy have been reported with limited clinical manifestations (LWG): (1) lung alone or with associated skin involvement; (2) upper respiratory tract, eye, or ear (URTE); (3) lung and URTE; (4) lung and kidney; and (5) kidney and URTE. Because focal glomerulonephritis occurs in many other disorders, a diagnosis of CSS based on kidney involvement alone cannot be made. Any of these formes frustes may evolve into another limited form or the classic triad. Because the mortality rate from these limited forms in untreated patients is exceedingly high, prompt recognition and appropriate therapy are essential.

Clinical and Laboratory Findings. Men are affected more frequently than women, with a mean age at onset of approximately 40 years. A significant number of patients (20%) are younger than age 25, and important clinical differences exist in this younger age-group. Typically in CWG, chronic sinusitis or rhinitis, refractory to usual therapy, heralds the onset of the disease. Lung involvement may already be present at this time or may follow the upper respiratory tract manifestations. Signs of kidney damage, often culminating in fulminant renal failure, may be present at initial diagnosis but usually occur later in the course of the disease to complete the triad. The ESR is significantly increased, and the C-ANCA is usually positive. Mild anemia and thrombocytosis may be found; however, significant peripheral blood eosinophilia is absent.

The following organ systems are the most frequently involved in CWG and LWG. In the *upper respiratory tract,* granulomatous invasion of large bronchi can lead to varying degrees of bronchial, tracheal, or laryngeal stenosis. Chronic ulcerative lesions of the oral mucosa (buccal, palatal, gingival) are particularly frequent in younger patients. Rhinitis (frequently with epistaxis) refractory to usual therapy, with or without ulceration or perforation of the nasal septum, typically occurs. Occasionally, a "saddle" nose deformity resulting from cartilage destruction is observed. Chronic sinusitis, also refractory to usual therapy, frequently occurs. Although ulcerations of these areas may be extensive, unlike other granulomatous diseases affecting the midline of the face, WG rarely extends to destroy the overlying skin. Biopsy of bronchial, tracheal, or laryngeal lesions often provides a specific diagnosis. Nasal or sinus biopsy is usually nondiagnostic because of the high prevalence of secondary bacterial infection, which may result in a contiguous secondary vasculitis. Other organs of the head may also be involved in WG, mainly the eyes and ears. Because sinorhinitis is so often observed in the general population, recognition of eye or ear involvement may distinguish WG from the other pulmonary vasculitides in which involvement of these or-

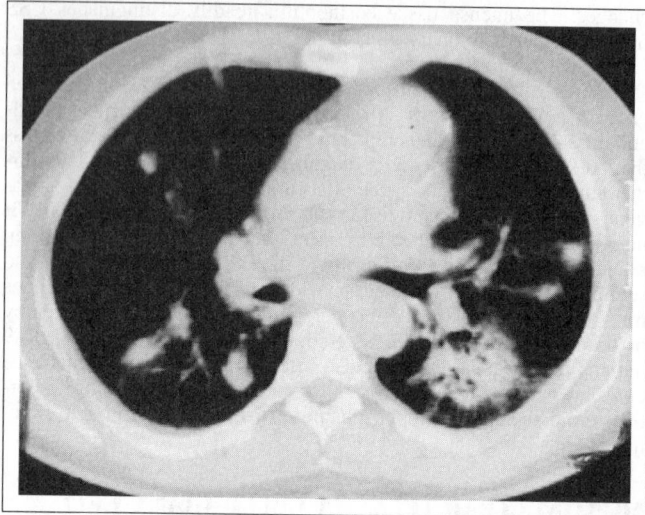

FIGURE 56-3   Wegener's granulomatosis: CT showing multiple nodules and one cavitating mass lesion.

gans is exceedingly rare. *Eye* manifestations occur in approximately 40% of patients but rarely signal the onset of disease. Proptosis, unilateral or bilateral, caused by orbital granulomatous inflammation (orbital pseudotumor) is the finding most suggestive of WG. Visual loss from corneal scarring, complications of uveitis, or retinal and optic nerve damage can lead to total blindness. *Otologic* manifestations are not only frequent but may herald the disease onset (20% to 40%). Chronic serous or purulent otitis media not responding to therapy is the most common ear manifestation. Mastoiditis, often with destructive bone lesions and associated cranial nerve abnormalities, external otitis, or rarely, ear lobe perforation have also been observed. Such involvement usually results in varying degrees of ear pain and sensorineural deafness.

Symptoms of *lung* involvement include cough, dyspnea, chest pain, or hemoptysis (occasionally massive). In many patients, however, symptoms are absent even in the presence of multiple pulmonary lesions. When present, *renal* abnormalities always appear to follow or occur with lung and/or upper respiratory tract disease. Renal disease may pursue an incredibly fulminant course within even days of onset and is the leading cause of death in patients with this disorder. *Skin* lesions are observed in approximately 40% of patients and include subcutaneous nodules (often resembling erythema nodosa), purpura (usually palpable), and chronic ulcerations. *Nervous system* involvement occurs in fewer than one fourth of patients. Peripheral nerve (mononeuritis multiplex) and cranial nerves are affected equally. Younger patients appear to have a much higher prevalence of central nervous system manifestations. *Cardiac* involvement, relatively infrequent and occurring in less than 10% of patients, manifests as acute pericarditis or, more rarely, coronary arteritis. Congestive heart failure is rare. Nondeforming *arthritis* and *arthralgia,* usually of large joints, occur in two thirds of patients.

Radiographic Appearance. Wegener's granulomatosis, lymphomatoid granulomatosis, "benign" lymphocytic granulomatous vasculitis, and necrotizing sarcoid granulomatosis generally have similar radiographic patterns (i.e., nodule[s] or mass lesion[s]) and therefore cannot be distinguished radiographically from one another. These patterns may mimic primary or metastatic cancer and certain noninfectious and infectious diseases, particularly those associated with a granulomatous reaction. The most common pattern in WG is *bilateral multiple nodules,* (oval or round densities ≤4 cm in diameter of varying size and often cavitated) either alone or associated with multiple or single mass lesions (diameter >4 cm), which also frequently cavitate (Fig. 56-3). Although radiographic presentation as a solitary pulmonary nodule occurs, a thoracic computed tomography (CT) scan almost always reveals more than one lesion. In addition, a diffuse "pneumonic" type of infiltration caused by small vessel vasculitis,

which fortunately is rare, may result in acute diffuse pulmonary hemorrhage. When this presentation is associated with nephritis, it may mimic Goodpasture's syndrome or "acute lupus lung." The most suggestive radiographic change, however, occurring in about one fourth of patients, is the spontaneous regression of a nodule or mass lesion in one area while in another area a lesion is increasing in size or newly develops (i.e., transient-successive) (Fig. 56-4). This peculiar sequence of events may also occur in lymphomatoid granulomatosis. Pleural effusion is observed in approximately 20% of patients.

Pathology and Immunology. The most reliable source for tissue diagnosis is the lung. The gross appearance suggests pulmonary infarction, however, lesions of a yellow or white-yellow color and should call attention to the possible diagnosis of WG at surgery. These three lesions are often pleural based and show multiple or single cavities. Microscopically, numerous plasma cells are found within and around both medium-sized and small veins and arteries; giant cells, mainly of the foreign body type, are characteristically present. Eosinophils are observed only occasionally, as are neutrophils, which are usually seen within the areas of necrotic debris. The granuloma is characterized by dense aggregates of plasma cells, as well as giant cells and histiocytes. Scattered epithelioid granulomas (sarcoid-like) occur in approximately 20% to 30% of patients with LWG with lung involvement. Focal granulomatous glomerulonephritis and necrotizing vasculitis of larger vessels are frequently found in the kidney. Although clinical renal abnormalities are usually absent in the limited form of pulmonary WG, approximately 40% of these patients have the histopathologic changes described.

Autoantibodies against extranuclear cytoplasmic components of polymorphonuclear leukocytes have been detected in patients with WG. These autoantibodies are directed against proteinase-3 of the neutrophil cytoplasmic azurophil granules, resulting in a diffuse, granulated *cytoplasmic* staining pattern (C-ANCA). C-ANCA has been found to be both sensitive and relatively specific (although not diagnostic) for WG, particularly when the disease is in an "active" phase. Therefore C-ANCA appears to be a quite useful clinical *adjunct* to diagnosis; however, it may not always be reliable as an indicator of "activity."

Management. Before the use of corticosteroids and cyclophosphamide, the 1-year survival rate of patients with CWG was only 15%. With the administration of these drugs, initial remission occurs in more than 90% of patients, with an ultimate mortality caused by the disease of approximately 20%. Although rare, complete spontaneous remissions may occur. Prednisone (60 to 80 mg a day) and cyclophosphamide (2 mg/kg) are recommended as initial therapy until clinical manifestations have subsided. Prednisone therapy is then reduced to a maintenance dose and then to an alternate-day regimen. Treatment should be continued for approximately 1 year. Relapses (25% to 30%) can occur after a successful course of therapy or when the corticosteroid dose is being reduced. Medical treatment is recommended even when a solitary lung lesion (representing the *only* manifestation of LWG) has been resected, as lung recurrence or renal failure may supervene in untreated patients. Proteinuria may persist for long periods in patients who are otherwise in complete remission. The serum C-reactive protein and ESR are useful monitors of disease activity in these patients. At present, sufficient information does not exist to recommend the use of trimethoprim sulfamethoxazole.

Dirofilaria immitis Granulomatous Vasculitis

Pulmonary dirofilariasis is essentially a benign condition that may have histologic features resembling more serious entities. The geographic distribution of *Dirofilaria immitis* (dog heartworm) in the United States is considerable. It not only extends along the seaboard from Maine to Texas but also includes the western coastal states; it penetrates inland to the Mississippi River valley, southern Great Lakes states, and the eastern midwestern states.

Circulating dog microfilaria (infective larval stage) are transported by and injected in the skin of the human by a mosquito vector. The nematode then penetrates the subcutaneous tissue and muscle sheaths. After 3 to 4 months, the infective larvae migrate to and reside in the right ventricle. Because the human environment is an unsuitable host

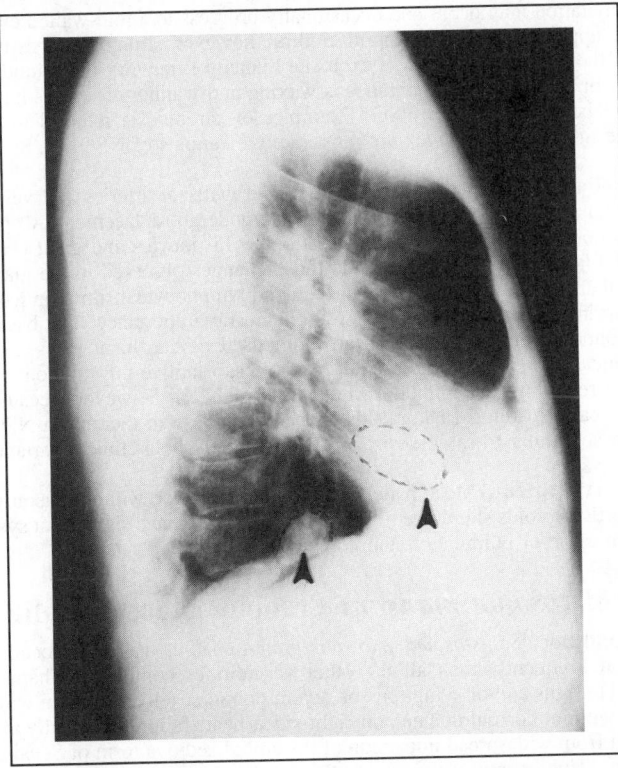

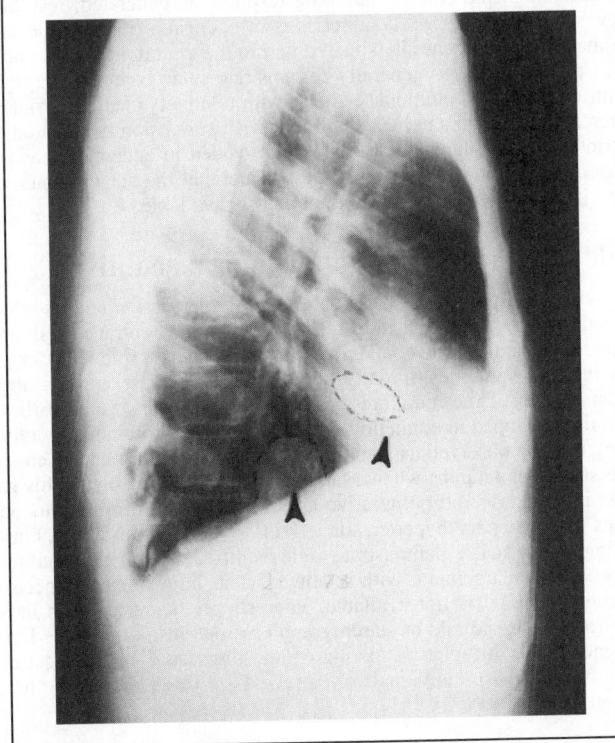

FIGURE 56-4   Wegener's granulomatosis. **A,** Nodular densities in lower and middle lung lobes. **B,** Six weeks later, lower lobe density has increased in size, whereas the middle lobe density has decreased in size. No treatment had been administered.

for larvae to develop to adulthood, the larvae die, embolize, and lodge in a branch of the pulmonary artery. Most patients remain asymptomatic; however, some may develop symptoms of pulmonary embolism with infarction (e.g., chest pain, hemoptysis).

The most common radiographic finding is a solitary pulmonary nodule. Pathologically, a granulomatous vasculitis develops at the impaction site and may closely resemble the vascular histologic changes of WG or the granulomatous reaction observed in tuberculosis, histoplasmosis, or coccidioidomycosis, all of which may present as an asymptomatic solitary pulmonary nodule. The differentiating feature of dilofilariasis is detection of the larvae on *thorough* histologic examination of the excised nodule.

LYMPHOCYTIC GRANULOMATOUS VASCULITIS
"Benign" Lymphocytic Angiitis and Granulomatosis

This disorder shares clinical, radiologic, and therapeutic similarity to LWG (characterized by lung involvement alone). Pathologically, however, lymphocytic angiitis appears to represent a more benign expression of a spectrum observed in angiocentric immunolymphoproliferative lesions (AIL) of T cell type. Necrosis within the lesions is unusual, and although arteries and veins may be heavily infiltrated by lymphocytes, the lumen usually remains patent. Giant cells and atypical lymphoreticular cells are exceedingly rare or absent. Although the prognosis generally appears to be quite good with current therapy, particularly chlorambucil, the process may rarely progress to malignant lymphoma.

Behçet's Disease and Hughes-Stovin Syndrome

Although Behçet's disease (BD), occurs worldwide, it has been reported mainly in young men in the Middle East, Eastern Mediterranean basin, and Japan. BD is characterized by relapsing ocular lesions, mainly iridocyclitis with hypopyon, often progressing to blindness, and ulcerations of the mouth and genitalia (Behçet's triad). Many other organ systems, however, including skin, gastrointestinal tract, joints, the blood vessels of the lung, and the systemic veins, may be involved (Chapter 244). Pulmonary involvement is characterized by a necrotizing, predominantly lymphocytic vasculitis of capillaries and all sizes of pulmonary arteries and veins and fortunately is observed in only 5% of patients. Patients who have lung involvement appear to develop fewer eye complications; however, a higher prevalence of relapsing systemic phlebitis is observed in this group of patients.

Clinical manifestations of BD include pulmonary arterial aneurysms; thromboses of pulmonary arteries and veins; obstruction of systemic veins, including those within the mediastinum (e.g., superior and inferior vena cava); and pulmonary infarction. Recurrent hemoptysis or death caused by massive hemoptysis as a result of pulmonary artery aneurysm and bronchial erosion is the frequent outcome, making pulmonary vascular involvement one of the most serious prognostic manifestations of BD. The finding of pulmonary aneurysms by angiography in the appropriate extrapulmonary clinical setting is diagnostic. Perfusion lung scans reveal multiple perfusion defects in most patients, and pulmonary hypertension is noted in approximately 50% of patients at diagnosis. Chest radiographs reveal pleural effusion, unilateral or bilateral infiltrates, or round densities representing pulmonary artery aneurysms. If these densities are parahilar, they may mimic hilar lymphadenopathy. Although BD exhibits clinical and immunologic (T and B lymphocyte abnormalities) features of autoimmune disease, the precise etiology and mechanism are unknown.

Immunomodulation (corticosteroids, immunosuppressives) therapy or surgical excision if the disease is localized to one area of the lung are recommended forms of treatment. Anticoagulants have not proved useful and may be harmful in patients with BD, as well as in those with Hughes-Stovin syndrome.

Hughes-Stovin syndrome (HSS) is characterized by pulmonary artery aneurysms and pulmonary vessel thromboses associated with systemic venous thrombosis, often involving the large mediastinal and neck veins and cerebral venous sinuses. Because the clinical, angiographic, and histopathologic (vasculitic) aspects of the vascular manifestations and the clinical course are so similar in BD and HSS, HSS probably represents an incomplete expression or variant of BD. Systemic phlebitis represents an important clinical finding, differentiating BD and HSS from the other pulmonary vasculitides.

ATYPICAL LYMPHORETICULAR GRANULOMATOUS VASCULITIS
Lymphomatoid Granulomatosis

The most enigmatic of the atypical lymphoreticular granulomatous vasculitides is lymphomatoid granulomatosis (LYG), which clinically and radiologically may resemble LWG but histologically has affinities with lymphoma. It appears to manifest as a spectrum of responses from spontaneous remission to evolution into true lymphoma. However, a propensity to cellular invasion and necrosis of veins and arteries in the lung is a striking feature, allowing for inclusion in the pulmonary vasculitides. Clinical features of LYG important in differentiating LYG from WG and typical lymphoma are the frequency of central nervous system involvement and the rarity of lymphadenopathy, upper respiratory tract involvement, and clinical glomerulonephritis.

Clinical and Laboratory Findings. Men are affected more than women at a ratio of 2 or 3 to 1, with a mean age at onset of 45 years. All patients with LYG have *lung* involvement, and symptoms of cough, chest pain, and dyspnea are usually the presenting manifestations. The *skin* is often involved in the form of rash or nodules. The nodules are typically tender, truncal in location, and often resemble erythema nodosum. *Central nervous system* signs and/or symptoms are particularly prevalent (20%) and, with cranial and peripheral neuropathy, make up the neurologic features. *Lymphadenopathy* only is rarely the first manifestation, and glomerulonephritis is rarely observed. Laboratory values are variable and of limited use in diagnosis.

Radiographic Appearance. The chest radiograph is abnormal in all patients with LYG. The most frequent finding is that of multiple bilateral nodules. Unilateral nodules, mass lesions, or a single nodule or mass lesion may also be seen, and cavitation may be noted in any of these patterns. These lesions tend to be more vague and irregular than in WG. A thoracic CT scan often reveals the nodular character better than the chest radiograph. The radiodensities in LYG may also wax and wane and thus may be indistinguishable from the radiographic patterns observed in WG. Occasionally, a diffuse reticulonodular pattern is seen. Pleural effusion is noted in approximately 20% of patients.

Pathology and Immunology. *Vasculonecrosis,* pleomorphic proliferations of atypical cellular elements of the lymphoreticular system (often plasmacytoid) around and within the walls of muscular arteries and/or veins and within the lung parenchyma, characterizes the histology of LYG. Epithelioid granulomas and giant cells are absent. The pathologic process in some patients may arrest or remit; in others it may progress to fulminant lung and/or central nervous system involvement, leading to death, or evolve into a true lymphoma involving lymph nodes. At present the immunopathogenesis of this lymphoproliferative disorder is unknown.

Treatment. Prolonged spontaneous remissions occur in approximately 10% to 15% of patients with LYG. Therapy with corticosteroids and immunosuppressants, although often inducing initial remission, ultimately fails in most patients; the mortality rate even in treated patients is as high as 60%. Further experience with various antilymphoma regimens appears warranted.

HISTIOCYTIC (EPITHELIOID) GRANULOMA GRANULOMATOUS VASCULITIS
Necrotizing Sarcoid Granulomatosis

Necrotizing sarcoid granulomatosis (NSG) is a comparatively benign disorder, mainly confined to the lung, more frequently seen in women, and with a mean age at onset of approximately 48 years. Approximately half of all patients are asymptomatic.

Radiographic Appearance. Multiple bilateral nodules of varying size represent the most common pattern. Unilateral nodules, a solitary nodule, or solitary or multiple mass lesions may also be observed.

Cavitation may occur and occasionally progress to a thin-walled cystic appearance. A radiographic finding, however, strongly suggestive of the diagnosis of NSG is exquisite bilateral symmetry of the nodular or mass lesions. Spontaneous waxing and waning of lesions have not been observed in NSG. Examples of sarcoidosis referred to in the literature as *nodular* are most likely examples of NSG.

Pathology and Immunology. The walls of arteries and veins of small and medium-sized vessels may undergo replacement by epithelioid granulomas and/or infiltration by histiocytes and giant cells (the latter may closely resemble those changes observed in the giant cell arteritides) or diffuse plasma cell and lymphocyte infiltration with varying degrees of necrosis. Of diagnostic importance, the background parenchymal lesions are composed of confluent masses of noncaseating epithelioid granulomas. No substantive information exists regarding the immunopathogenesis of NSG. However, because the basic histology, natural history, and response to therapy in NSG are so similar to sarcoidosis, NSG may merely be a clinical variant.

Treatment. Most patients with NSG recover without therapy. Corticosteroids should be reserved for those who have significant systemic and/or pulmonary symptoms.

Schistosoma mansoni Granulomatous Vasculitis

Worldwide, *Schistosoma mansoni* granulomatous vasculitis occurs more frequently than all the other vasculitides combined (Chapter 281). Signs and/or symptoms of severe pulmonary hypertension with or without cor pulmonale and right-sided heart failure eventually result from widespread impaction of the embolized ova form of *S. mansoni.* This occurs in the precapillary arterioles of the lung, where a noncaseating epithelioid granuloma response is generated, resulting in vascular damage and complete vessel occlusion. Finding the egg remnants, usually centrally situated within the granuloma, is diagnostic. Chest radiographs generally demonstrate enlargement of the right ventricle and main pulmonary artery, with relatively clear lung fields. Therefore those patients with pulmonary hypertension not related to intrinsic heart or lung disease who had resided in endemic areas for *S. mansoni* should be suspect. Unfortunately, at the stage of pulmonary hypertension, no specific treatment is available.

Talc and Starch Granulomatous Vasculitis

Signs and symptoms of severe pulmonary hypertension and its complications may also occur in drug abusers who have intravenously injected oral medications containing talc or starch as a filler. Talc crystals or starch granules, initially intraluminal in the precapillary arteriolar system of the lung, are ultimately found in the walls of these vessels, entrapped in epithelioid granulomas of the foreign body type. They may be observed as spindlelike crystals (talc) or maltese crosslike structures (starch) when examined with polarized light. This results in a widespread obliterative arteriolitis resulting in various degrees of pulmonary hypertension. As in *S. mansoni* vasculitis, chest radiographs usually demonstrate right ventricular and main pulmonary artery enlargement, with relatively clear lung fields. A specific effective therapy is not available. Interestingly, some patients have only a widespread talc or starch granulomatous response in the lung parenchyma, with relative sparing of the lung vasculature. Chest radiographs in these individuals often reveal a diffuse, infiltrating lung lesion.

GIANT CELL GRANULOMATOUS VASCULITIS
Takayasu's Arteritis

Takayasu's arteritis (pulmonary Takayasu's disease, pulmonary pulseless disease) is mainly observed in young Asian women and is associated with narrowing and/or occlusion of the pulmonary artery or its branches in approximately 50% of patients. Varying degrees of pulmonary hypertension are present in most patients with pulmonary vessel involvement. Symptoms of dyspnea and hemoptysis are occasionally observed. The diagnosis of Takayasu's arteritis is initially suggested by the presence of aortic branch occlusion syndromes. Pulmonary vessel involvement is suggested by loss of lung vasculature on

✔ *WHEN TO REFER*

Because of (1) the potentially life-threatening nature of the pulmonary granulomatous vasculitidies (with the exception of dirofilaria and NSG), (2) their relative rarity, and (3) the need to provide biopsy evidence for accurate diagnosis in many instances, when any of these entities are suspected it is most prudent to obtain consultation from one who has had extensive clinical experience in the diagnosis and management of these disorders.

chest radiographs and may be documented by pulmonary angiography.

BIBLIOGRAPHY

Carrington CB, Liebow AA: Limited forms of angiitis and granulomatosis of Wegener's type, *Am J Med* 41:497, 1967.
Cordier JF et al: Pulmonary Wegener's granulomatosis, *Chest* 97:906-912, 1990.
Cortes FM, Winters WL: Schistosomiasis cor pulmonale, *Am J Med* 31:808, 1961.
Erkan F, Cavdar T: Pulmonary vasculitis in Behçet's disease, *Am Rev Respir Dis* 146:232-239, 1992.
Hoffman GS: Advances in Wegener's granulomatosis, *Hosp Pract* April 15, 1995.
Hughes JP, Stovin PGI: Segmental pulmonary artery aneurysms with peripheral venous thrombosis, *Br J Dis Chest* 53:19, 1959.
Kerr GS et al: Takayasu arteritis, *Ann Intern Med* 120:919-929, 1994.
Lanham JG et al: Systemic vasculitis with asthma and eosinophilia: a clinical approach to the Churg-Strauss syndrome, *Medicine* 63:65, 1984.
Liebow AA: The J. Burns Amberson Lecture: pulmonary angiitis and granulomatosis, *Am Rev Respir Dis* 108:1, 1973.
Maskell GF, Lockwood CM, Flower CDR: Computed tomography of the lung in Wegener's granulomatosis, *Clin Radiol* 48:377-380, 1993.
Risher WH et al: Pulmonary dirofilariasis, *J Thorac Cardiovasc Surg* 97:303, 1989.
Saldana MJ, Israel HL: Necrotizing sarcoid granulomatosis, benign lymphocytic angiitis, and granulomatosis: do they exist? *Semin Respir Med* 10:182, 1989.
Savige JA, Davies JD, Gatenby PA: Anti-neutrophil cytoplasmic antibodies (ANCA): their detection and significance: report from workshops, *Pathology* 26:186-193, 1994.
Sneller MC: Wegener's granulomatosis, *JAMA* 273:1288-1291, 1995.
Wendt VE et al: Angiothrombotic pulmonary hypertension in addicts, *JAMA* 188:755, 1964.

CHAPTER

57 Occupational Lung Diseases

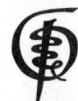

Akshay Sood, J. Bernard Gee, and William S. Beckett

Most major categories of respiratory disease may be produced by occupational exposures. Substances in the workplace may produce airway disease; alveolitis; infectious pneumonia, hypersensitivity pneumonitis, or alveolar proteinosis; and primary cancer of the lung or the pleura. The one major category of pulmonary diseases not associated with occupational exposures is the primary disease of the pulmonary arteries.

Occupational lung diseases result from the direct consequences of the exposure to a causative agent and the host defense responses. Because the normal respiratory system has substantial reserve, considerable injury or loss of function may occur before an individual becomes aware of the symptoms and seeks medical attention. Particularly for cancer and the pneumoconioses, a long latency period may elapse between the beginning of exposure and the manifestation of disease. This latency is sometimes measured in decades, and for some diseases, the process typically progresses even after all exposure has ceased. Because there is no effective therapy for most of these diseases, prevention is essential. The alert clinician must recognize that for each case diagnosed, many other cases may be about to occur in the same workplace and can be prevented by prompt identification of the cause and the population at risk.

A careful work history is critical to the diagnosis, management, and prevention of these diseases. Information on industrial materials can, by law, be obtained from Material Safety Data Sheets by employees and their physicians in the United States and Canada. Upon diagnosis of an occupational disease, notification (with the patient's prior permission) should be made to co-workers, physicians, and relevant health authorities. If the workplace standards are not being met, the physician may report the workplace to the local office of the federal Occupational Safety and Health Administration (OSHA), while maintaining the patient's confidentiality.

Workers' compensation is a separate health insurance system covering illness and loss of earning power caused by a work-related illness. It depends on the physician accurately identifying the workplace determinants of illness, informing the patient when the illness is work related, and sometimes acting as his or her advocate.

AIRWAY DISEASES

Airway diseases include rhinitis, occupational asthma, chronic bronchitis, and chronic obstructive pulmonary disease (COPD).

Occupational Asthma

Occupational asthma has become the most common occupational lung disease. The two categories of asthma in the workplace are occupational asthma arising de novo and preexisting or concurrent asthma aggravated in the workplace. Occupational asthma is characterized by variable airflow limitation, bronchial hyperresponsiveness, or both, due to conditions in a particular work environment. About 250 agents can cause occupational asthma. Table 57-1 lists some of the more frequently encountered causative agents by major categories. Isocyanates are responsible for the most common form of this disease. They are used in the production of flexible and rigid foam, body parts, and finish coatings used in the manufacture of automobiles, airplanes, and trains.

Two types of occupational asthma can be distinguished by the presence of a latency period. Occupational asthma *with* latency is the most common type. This develops after a period of exposure that may vary from a few weeks to several years. Occupational asthma with latency can be further subdivided into those that are immunoglobulin E (IgE) dependent and those that are IgE independent. Occupational asthma *without* latency follows exposure to high concentrations of irritant gases, fumes, or chemicals on one or several occasions. Most allergens are classic allergic sensitizers, having a molecular weight greater than 1000 Daltons and producing a specific IgE antibody response. On repeat challenge, this antibody binds to the antigen and leads to the release of mediators from inflammatory cells resulting in bronchoconstriction and mucus production. However, a sizable number of agents of low molecular weight (less than 1000 Daltons) produce a similar clinical picture without a specific IgE antibody, presumably since the agent acts through a separate mechanism or forms a new antigenic complex with a serum protein.

As with nonoccupational asthma, the patient's history alone most frequently leads to the correct diagnosis of occupational asthma. When asthma is caused by a workplace sensitization, the patient will give a history of asymptomatic exposure for months or even years before the gradual onset of symptoms. Once sensitization has occurred, reexposure may produce an immediate response (within minutes of exposure), a delayed response (several hours after exposure), a dual response combining the immediate and delayed responses, or a recurrent nocturnal response for several nights after a single exposure. With the delayed response, the presenting symptoms may be only a recurrent nocturnal cough and minor wheezing, which, if unrecognized as manifestations of asthma, may progress to daytime wheezing and breathlessness. Improvement on weekends or vacations may be the most helpful clue to a workplace etiology of asthma but is not invariably present. For certain occupational allergens, cigarette smoking appears to be a risk factor that increases the probability of becoming sensitized.

Although the demonstration of an IgE antibody specific to the workplace agent by intradermal skin tests may be confirmatory, skin testing is not typically required. Correlating airflow obstruction (as measured by a self-administered peak airflow meter) with workplace

Table 57-1   Listing of selected substances causing occupational asthma

AGENTS	INDUSTRIES/OCCUPATIONS	AGENTS	INDUSTRIES/OCCUPATIONS
High-molecular-weight compounds		Wood dust	
Laboratory animals		Western red cedar *(Thuja plicata)*	Carpentry, construction, cabinet-
Rat	Laboratory workers	California redwood *(Sequoia*	making, sawmill
Mouse	Veterinarians	*sempervirens)*	
Rabbit	Animal handlers	Cedar of Lebanon *(Cedra libani)*	
Guinea pig		Cocabolla *(Dalbergia retusa)*	
Birds		Iroko *(Chlorophora excelsa)*	
Pigeon	Pigeon breeders	Oak *(Quercus robur)*	
Chicken	Poultry workers	Mahogany *(Shoreal* species)	
Budgerigar (parakeet)	Bird fanciers	Abiruana *(Pouteria)*	
Insects		African maple *(Triplochiton*	
Grain mite	Grain workers	*scleroxylon)*	
Locust	Research laboratory	Tanganyika aningre	
River fly	Power plants along rivers	Central American walnut	
Screw worm fly	Flight crews	*(Juglans olanchana)*	
Cockroach	Laboratory workers	Kejaat *(Pterocarpus angolenisis)*	
Cricket	Field contact	African zebra wood *(Microber-*	
Bee moth	Fish bait breeders	*linia)*	
Moth and butterfly	Entomologists	Metals	
Plants		Platinum	Platinum refinery
Grain dust	Grain handlers	Nickel	Metal plating
Wheat/rye flour	Bakers, millers	Chromium	Tanning
Buckwheat	Bakers	Cobalt	Hard metal industry
Coffee bean	Food processors	Vanadium	
Castor bean	Oil industry	Fluxes	
Tea	Tea workers	Aminoethyl ethanolamine	Aluminum soldering
Tobacco leaf	Tobacco manufacturing	Colophony	Electronic
Hops *(Humulus lupulus)*	Brewery chemists	Drugs	
Biologic enzymes		Penicillins	Pharmaceutical
Bacillus subtilis	Detergent industry	Cephalosporins	Pharmaceutical
Trypsin	Pharmaceutical	Phenylglycine acid chloride	Pharmaceutical
Pancreatin	Pharmaceutical	Piperazine hydrochloride	Chemist
Papain	Laboratory	Psyllium	Laxative manufacturers
	Packaging	Methyldopa	Pharmaceutical
Pepsin	Pharmaceutical	Spiramycin	Pharmaceutical
Flaviastase	Pharmaceutical	Salbutamol intermediate	Pharmaceutical
Bromelin	Pharmaceutical	Amprolium hydrochloride	Poultry feed mixers
Fungal amylase	Manufacturing, bakers	Tetracycline	Pharmaceutical
Vegetables		Sulphone chloramides	Manufacturers, brewery
Gum acacia	Printers	Other chemicals	
Gum tragacanth	Gum manufacturing	Dimethyl ethanolamine	Spray painting
Other		Persulfate salts and henna	Hairdressing
Crab	Crab processing	Ethylene diamine	Photography
Prawn	Prawn processing	Azodiacarbonamide	Plastics and rubber
Hoya	Oyster farm	Dioazonium salt	Photocopying and dye
Silkworm larva	Sericulture	Hexachlorophene (sterilizing	Hospital staff
		agent)	
Low-molecular-weight compounds		Formalin	Hospital staff
Di-isocyanates		Urea formaldehyde	Insulation, resin
Toluene di-isocyanate	Polyurethane, plastics, varnish	Freon	Refrigeration
Diphenylmethane di-isocyanate	Foundries	Paraphenylene diamine	Fur dying
Hexamethylene di-isocyanate	Automobile spray painting	Furfuryl alcohol	Foundry mold making
Anhydrides			
Phthalic anhydride	Epoxy resins, plastics		
Trimellitic anhydride	Epoxy resins, plastics		
Tetrachlorophthalic anhydride	Epoxy resins, plastics		

Reprinted with permission of the authors and publisher from Chan-Yeung M, Lam S: *Am Rev Respir Dis* 133:686-782, 1986.

exposures may be extremely helpful when the history alone is not sufficient. The demonstration of airway hyperresponsiveness on methacholine challenge testing may help distinguish asthma from other forms of airway disease. Inhalation challenge with the substance in question carries the risk of inducing severe bronchospasm or even hypersensitivity pneumonitis and is best performed in specialized centers where exposures can be carefully controlled. The algorithm for the investigation of a suspected case of occupational asthma is outlined in Fig. 57-1. The differential diagnosis for occupational asthma includes nonoccupational asthma, industrial bronchitis, and hypersensitivity pneumonitis.

Some patients with sensitizer-induced asthma who continue in their workplace despite symptoms will have persistent asthma even after exposure has ceased completely. The likelihood of cure may be

greater if the exposure is ended sooner. Therefore it is essential that the physician recognize occupational causes of asthma early and work on the patient's behalf to end exposure, while at the same time protecting the patient's livelihood.

Chronic Bronchitis (Industrial Bronchitis)

The clinical definition of chronic bronchitis involves daily cough with mucus production for 3 or more months of the year for 2 or more years. It may be produced by cigarette smoking, as well as the occupational inhalation of dust by miners, steel foundry workers, cement workers, cotton and other textile workers, and welders. In cigarette smokers, an interaction may occur between the effects of smoke and dust. Chronic bronchitis may occur without any airway obstruction and is not life

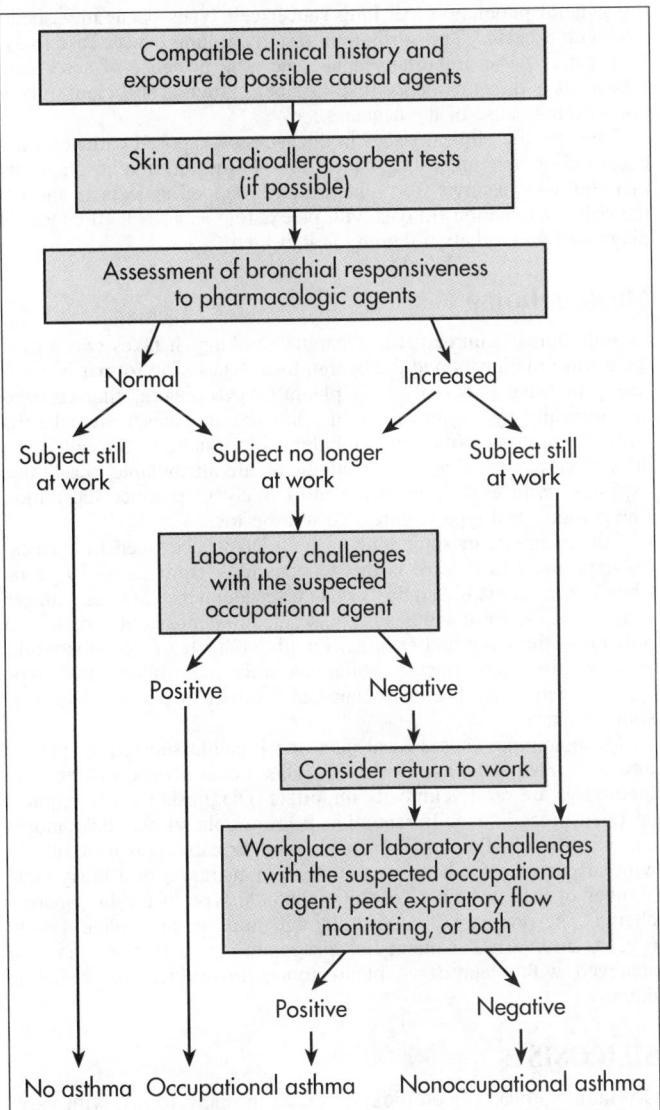

FIGURE 57-1 Algorithm for the clinical investigation of occupational asthma.
(From Chan-Yeung M, Malo J: *N Engl J Med* 333:107,1995.)

threatening. Therapy includes management of acute bacterial superinfections with a short course of a broad-spectrum oral antibiotic and the prevention of further exposure to the offending agent.

Chronic Obstructive Pulmonary Disease

Chronic obstructive pulmonary disease may occur alone or simultaneously with industrial bronchitis. The earliest finding on spirometry may be a decreased maximum mid-expiratory flow (MMEF). In large epidemiologic studies of certain working groups, small excesses over the normal age-related declines in airflow have been reported in relation to some dust exposures (independent of the effects of cigarette smoking). In the absence of complicating pneumoconiosis, this effect is generally small and clinically unimportant unless other lung diseases coexist. An exception is cadmium oxide dust, which some studies have associated with marked emphysema after prolonged exposure.

PARENCHYMAL DISEASE
Acute Toxic Exposures

In acute toxic exposures, both the small airways and the alveoli may be affected together as a bronchoalveolar unit. A single overwhelm-

ing exposure may cause either acute or chronic airway inflammation, pulmonary edema, and sometimes irreversible pulmonary fibrosis.

The acute disorders result from the inhalation of gases (chemically or thermally active), mists (liquid droplets), or fumes (solid-phase constituents). The depth of penetration, which determines whether alveolar leaks and thus pulmonary edema will occur, depends on the gas solubility in aqueous media or the size of the droplets or fume, with less than 10 μm being critical. Most such materials affect the conjunctival, oronasal, laryngeal, and major bronchial mucosae first; thus their effects are readily apparent by visual examination of the upper airways. Some fume materials (e.g., magnesium, cadmium, chromium) cause few upper respiratory effects but can have major pulmonary and systemic effects. On the other hand, some gases may cause neither external nor intrapulmonary effects but produce systemic disorders. Examples are organic solvents (which may cause central nervous system manifestations), hydrogen sulfide, carbon monoxide, and oxygen deprivation, which are major hazards for firefighters.

Patients with acute toxic pulmonary edema exhibit the usual manifestations of dyspnea, cough, expectoration, often blood-tinged sputum, profound oxygen desaturation, and patchy radiologic opacification. Cough and sputum from irritation of the upper respiratory tract are more obvious with the more soluble gases (e.g., sulfur dioxide, ammonia) and pulmonary edema with the less soluble ones (e.g., nitrogen dioxide). Many agents produce delayed effects that require observation for up to 24 to 48 hours. Both airway inflammation and obstructive effects are produced by the overtly irritant gases: ammonia, chlorine, nitrogen oxides (from fires, silo filling, shot firing, welding in confined spaces, chemical industries), ozone, formaldehyde, sulfur dioxide, fluoride, sulfuric acid, hydrochloric acid mists, metal fumes (including zinc, copper, magnesium, cadmium, manganese, and occasionally tin and lead), and paraquat. One particular form of hemorrhagic edema results from trimetallic anhydride, a compound used in plastic manufacturing. Finally, some of the isocyanates can occasionally cause a hypersensitivity pneumonitis.

Pathologically, acute toxic exposures, especially with ammonia, may be associated with inflammation and mucosal denudation, most prominent in the larynx and the major airways. The alveoli may rapidly develop a profound protein leak, fluid transudation, and the mobilization of neutrophils, which themselves contribute to oxidant endothelial and probably alveolar type 1 cell damage and may cause further pulmonary edema.

Management consists of supportive therapy, bronchodilators, oxygen, and immediate removal from the noxious agent. The role of corticosteroids is unclear. Fortunately, most patients recover completely with no demonstrable long-term lung function defects. However, long-term complications that do occur include persistent nonobstructive bronchitis, more rarely bronchiolitis obliterans (notably with nitrogen dioxide, as in silo filler's disease), and occasionally bronchiectasis.

Metal fume fever is an acute febrile illness caused by inhalation of freshly formed metal fume (metal that has been evaporated by very high temperature and then condensed in air into fine particles). The fever, rigors, diaphoresis, metallic taste in the mouth, and respiratory symptoms that accompany this illness often occur 4 to 6 hours after exposure and usually resolve 24 hours later. Zinc oxide fume is usually the causative agent. The diagnosis is clinical. Most workers are able to recognize it, partly because it is relatively frequent and partly because they have seen their co-workers with repeated attacks, and the condition is well known to them.

ASBESTOS-RELATED DISEASES

Asbestos was of immense social and economic value, but because its use has recently been restricted in most industrialized countries (but less so in some developing countries), asbestos-related diseases now largely reflect the legacy of its past poorly regulated use. These fibrous silicates exist in two general forms: the serpentine (chrysotile) and the amphiboles (i.e., crocidolite, amosite, tremolite, anthophyllite). Asbestosis, or pulmonary fibrosis, results from all these types of asbestos. However, considerable variation exists in their ability to produce mesothelioma. The major risks of asbestos-related disorders occur in workers in insulation industries, shipyards, construction, asbestos textiles, mining, and some chemical industries. The risk from asbestos to the general population is minimal, even though in some circumstances, judicious, careful asbestos abatement may be appropriate. The disorders associated with asbestos affect the pleura, lung, and peritoneum. Evidence that asbestos causes laryngeal cancer or gastrointestinal cancer is weak or lacking.

Benign Pleural Disease

All forms of asbestos probably cause pleural reactions. The fibrohyaline plaques found on the parietal pleura are the most common. These frequently involve the midportion of the thoracic wall, the diaphragm, and occasionally the pericardium. The lesions rarely coalesce but typically calcify. Although these radiologic manifestations usually progress, their generally discrete nodular nature by itself does not cause a restrictive loss of lung function. Plaques are most evident on the lateral aspects of the chest radiograph, but, when seen *en face*, may occasionally need to be distinguished from parenchymal disease by oblique films or computed tomographic (CT) scanning. Plaques are markers of asbestos exposure but, per se, have little prognostic import. Occasionally they can invade the subjacent lung and cause a nodular mass lesion from lung entrapment known as *rounded atelectasis;* this may require a differentiation from pleural-based lung tumors. Diffuse pleural thickening without asbestosis occurs less often than plaques and may rarely lead to a cuirass effect, producing restriction of lung function.

Benign pleural effusions also occur, usually 5 to 15 or more years after exposure. These effusions do not generally cause symptoms, but pleuritic pain does sometimes occur. The fluid is usually an exudate, occasionally bloody and often eosinophilic. The diagnosis is made by the exposure history and the exclusion of other causes of effusions. These effusions usually resolve spontaneously but can recur and are rarely associated with pleural fibrosis.

Asbestosis

The term *asbestosis* should be reserved for fibrosing alveolitis caused by asbestos deposition in the lung. The clinicophysiologic features are those of other forms of fibrosing alveolitis, even though pathologically the earliest fibrotic lesions occur at the level of the respiratory bronchioles. The process preferentially involves the bases of the lungs. Clubbing occurs uncommonly and suggests a poor prognosis. Asbestosis is characterized radiologically by the development of irregular small opacities. Although a detailed radiologic classification of stages of asbestosis exists, the radiologic features are similar to the other forms of interstitial fibrosis. In the absence of other causes of such fibrosis, an appropriate exposure history is sufficient for a presumptive diagnosis of asbestosis. Lung biopsies are rarely required to rule out other differential diagnoses. Histologically, asbestosis is characterized by the presence of numerous iron-staining asbestos bodies in association with fibrosis of the lung.

Although some cases progress slowly, those with a low radiologic category of disease frequently remain stable for more than 10 years. Among heavily exposed populations, a small subgroup may develop rapidly progressive fibrosis. Currently there is no effective treatment. Smoking cessation should be encouraged.

Lung Cancer

The risk of lung cancer in workers at various types of asbestos industries over the general population varies widely. In a comparison of the US industries using asbestos, it is highest among the South Carolina asbestos textile and insulation workers and only minimally increased in miners and millers, and not increased in friction product manufacturing. Relatively few lung cancers have been reported among nonsmoking workers in epidemiologic studies. A common view is that asbestos interacts with tobacco smoke carcinogens such as the polycyclic hydrocarbons. Epidemiologic studies of asbestos workers show an increase in lung cancer risk that varies from one-fold to threefold over smoking control populations. By contrast, a lifelong smoker of more than two packs per day with asbestos exposure carries up to a 70-fold risk as compared with the unexposed nonsmok-

ing general population. All lung cancer cell types occur in association with asbestos. The attribution of a given lung cancer case to asbestos may be an important legal issue. The presence of associated asbestosis is direct evidence that the fiber burden is sufficient to be a contributing cause of the cancer.

The specific clinical issues in the asbestos-exposed patient with a chest radiograph suggesting cancer are (1) the differential diagnosis of radiologic shadows from plaques and rounded atelectasis and (2) the risks of radiation fibrosis with preexisting asbestosis, if cancer is diagnosed and radiation therapy is indicated.

Mesothelioma

Mesothelioma is unrelated to cigarette smoking. It takes two forms: the diffuse malignant and the benign focal types. The former is a diffusely invasive tumor of either pleura or peritoneum, characterized histologically by combinations of epithelial and mesenchymal cells with fibrous tissue, often with tubulopapillary pattern. Overall, up to 70% of cases of malignant mesothelioma are attributable to asbestos exposure, with crocidolite being most likely to produce the tumor. The benign focal type is unrelated to asbestos.

For malignant mesothelioma, a long latency between first asbestos exposure and disease is the general rule—from 20 to 30 years. The disease occurs in certain Turkish Cappadocian and Greek villages in an epidemic form and has been ascribed to deposits of asbestiform minerals—tremolite and erionite. Family contacts of asbestos workers have also been affected. Mutations in the neurofibromatosis type 2 (NF2) gene have been associated in a subset of patients with mesotheliomata.

Mesothelioma causes local pain and breathlessness from the tumor mass and/or the associated effusions. Local invasion is the rule; metastases are rarely clinically important. Diagnosis usually requires an open procedure. Differentiation from peripheral adenocarcinoma can be difficult. Perhaps the most useful investigation in a subject with suspected mesotheliomata is the demonstration of a fairly large number of asbestos fibers of the amphibole type in the lung parenchyma. The prognosis is poor, although some patients have a 4- to 6-year survival. Treatment is disappointing; palliation may be achieved with pleurodesis, pleurectomy, doxorubicin, or radiation therapy.

SILICOSIS

Crystalline silica (silicon dioxide) exists in many forms, with varying toxicity. Exposures occur in mining (gold, coal, flint, bentonite production) and in sandblasting. Thus quarry workers, granite workers, road builders, stone polishers, foundry workers, and those employed in metal casting, ceramics, refractory insulating brick construction, glass making, and slate use are frequently exposed. Silicosis exists in three general forms: acute silicosis, chronic simple silicosis, and progressive massive fibrosis.

Acute Silicosis

Acute silicosis is relatively rare, occurs in subjects with heavy but relatively short exposure to silica, and has a fatal course in several months to a few years. It is seen in ceramic workers, silica flour or silica soap workers, and those in poorly regulated tunneling operations. A ground-glass appearance is seen on radiograph, and an irregular nodular fibrosis can ensue. There is no treatment, but lung transplantation should be considered.

Chronic Simple Silicosis

Chronic simple silicosis, the most usual form of silicosis, occurs after many years of exposure to relatively low levels of dust. Patients with chronic simple silicosis have few if any symptoms. Lung function shows little or no impairment; the best recent studies of Vermont granite workers show minimal or little acceleration of the normal age-related decline in forced expiratory volume in 1 second (FEV_1). This contrasts sharply with the striking chest radiograph that shows dense pinpoint nodulation in the upper lobes initially. The nodulation increases both in size and in profusion with increasing dust exposure, sometimes even after the cessation of exposure. Pleural abnormalities are not as impressive radiologically as are those in asbestos exposure. On radiograph, "eggshell" calcification frequently appears in the central lymph nodes, in contrast to its rarity in sarcoidosis. Silicosis is characterized pathologically by the silicotic nodule, which comprises of whorls of fibrous tissue, yielding an onionskin-like pattern. Rarely, and for inapparent reasons, the disorder can have an accelerated course. It has also been suggested that silicosis produces an increased risk for bronchogenic carcinoma.

Progressive Massive Fibrosis

Progressive massive fibrosis (PMF, complicated silicosis), although less common than in coal worker's pneumoconiosis, is disabling and life threatening. It arises on a background of chronic, simple silicosis and is radiographically characterized by the development of bilateral, usually symmetric, progressive mass opacifications greater than 1 cm in diameter in the upper third of the lungs. These may extend and are associated with severe architectural distortion of the unaffected lung with compensatory emphysema. Lung function becomes progressively deranged, with restrictive and obstructive components. Arterial desaturation and ultimately cor pulmonale supervene. The fibrotic material is subject to ischemic necrobiosis with expectoration—*melanoptysis* (black sputum)—in silicotic coal workers. The mechanism involved is unknown. The material contains not only collagen but also large amounts of glycosaminoglycans and fibronectin. Therapy, other than general measures, is ineffective.

Tuberculosis

The major complication of silicosis is tuberculosis. Because silica is cytotoxic for alveolar macrophages, and macrophages are the lung's main defense against *Mycobacterium tuberculosis,* the connection between the two diseases is not surprising. Necrobiotic cavitation can release entrapped tubercle bacilli, causing serious bronchogenic spread of tuberculosis. The diagnosis of tuberculosis in a setting of silicosis is difficult. There may be no symptoms, but loss of weight, increased cough, hemoptysis, and rapid radiologic change should alert the physician. Many authorities recommend isoniazid prophylaxis for patients with silicosis who have a positive tuberculin reaction, regardless of their age. In areas where the incidence of tuberculosis in patients with silicosis is high, as in Hong Kong, empiric antituberculous prophylaxis is recommended, regardless of skin test results. Some authorities recommend a prolonged course of antituberculous therapy during active disease from *M. tuberculosis* in silicotic patients because of a higher relapse rate when treated with standard regimens.

Immune Phenomena

More studies of immune reactions in patients with silicosis are needed, but several associated disorders are recognized. Scleroderma frequently occurs. Caplan has described the appearance of somewhat larger, occasionally cavitating nodules preceding or coinciding with the development of rheumatoid arthritis (Caplan's syndrome).

Because no effective therapy for silicosis exists, prevention is the key. When exposure is heavy, a positive-pressure external air supply respirator is essential. Careful observation of the health-protecting air standards can be successfully achieved in mining, although there is less effective monitoring in sandblasting.

COAL WORKER'S PNEUMOCONIOSIS

Coal mining has recently become much more mechanized, reducing the overall risks to workers. Nonetheless, those at the coal face (hard-headers) remain at risk.

Pathologically, the hallmark of coal workers' pneumoconiosis (CWP) is the coal macule, usually less than 4 mm in diameter. These macules include focal macrophage accumulation, with surrounding reticulin and collagen fibrosis. This leads to bronchiole dilation and patchy focal emphysema. In those miners exposed to hard-rock coal mining, silicosis may also develop.

On radiograph, simple CWP appears as fine pinpoint nodulations, usually involving the upper zones, which at later stages may become more profuse. In the simple form of CWP, symptoms are similar to those of industrial bronchitis, and lung function changes are few and subtle. In studies of nonsmoking miners, up to 20% increases in residual volume, variable losses of diffusing capacity, little change in the alveolar to arterial oxygen tension gradient or in static compliance, and minor reductions in dynamic compliance were observed. The effect of coal dust exposure on FEV_1 in simple CWP, if present, varies from a small acceleration in the age-related FEV_1 loss to an effect (in those most heavily exposed) comparable to that of chronic cigarette smoking; this loss is ascribed to the centrilobular emphysema. Patients with simple CWP have no major changes in exercise capacity. Unfortunately, PMF, as in silicosis, is a common problem. This generally occurs in patients with more rapidly progressive CWP. PMF is characterized radiologically by lesions 1 cm or more in diameter. By the time PMF occurs, airway obstruction, increase in residual volume, loss of diffusing capacity, and uneven gas/blood distribution are all evident. Pulmonary hypertension and cor pulmonale may ultimately supervene. No specific therapy exists.

As in patients with silicosis, immunologic abnormalities may occur, notably Caplan's syndrome.

BERYLLIUM DISEASE

Beryllium is used in the nuclear, aerospace, and missile industries. Inhalation of the metal beryllium or its compounds may lead to either acute or chronic beryllium disease. Acute beryllium disease is an immediate toxic response to high beryllium exposures, characterized by nasopharyngitis, tracheobronchitis, or pneumonitis. Chronic beryllium disease, quite different from the acute form, may occur as a result of lower levels of prolonged exposure after a latency period of 10 to 15 years. It is a systemic, granulomatous disease involving the lung predominantly and has many features of a T-cell–mediated chronic hypersensitivity lung disease. HLA-DPB1 glutamate at residue 69 has been recently suggested to have a role in conferring susceptibility to this disease and may have the potential to be used as a genetic marker in preemployment screening. Pathologically, it is an inflammatory disorder with non-necrotizing epithelioid granulomas involving one or more organs. On physical examination the patient may have no abnormal findings or may have clubbing of the fingers, granulomatous skin lesions, crackles, pleural friction rubs, or an enlarged liver. In cases involving the kidney, hypercalciuria and hypercalcemia may be found. The chest radiograph most frequently shows bilateral, diffuse, small opacities in either a miliary or fibrotic pattern with bilateral hilar adenopathy. Pulmonary function testing may show a restrictive ventilatory defect with impairment of gas exchange (as seen in a decreased diffusing capacity or lowered arterial oxygen tension). It may be extremely difficult to distinguish chronic beryllium disease from sarcoidosis. Patients with chronic beryllium disease have not been found to have uveitis and the cystic bone abnormalities sometimes seen in sarcoidosis.

A marked lymphocyte proliferation response of the patient's peripheral blood or lavaged lung lymphocytes when cultured in vitro with beryllium salts are usually considered diagnostic of beryllium disease in patients whose exposure history and clinical presentation are consistent.

Specific therapy for patients with acute and chronic beryllium disease consists of prolonged high-dose oral corticosteroids. The degree of response to this therapy depends in part on how far the inflammatory and fibrotic lung processes have advanced at the time treatment is started. Chronic beryllium disease may have a worse prognosis than sarcoidosis.

HARD METAL DISEASE

"Hard metal" is an alloy of tungsten carbide and cobalt. It has great importance in tool grinding, diamond polishing, and manufacture of ferromagnets and alloys ("high-speed steels"). Three respiratory effects are produced by hard metal: (1) reversible airways obstruction, (2) hypersensitivity pneumonitis, and (3) pulmonary fibrosis. All three are relatively uncommon. The currently available evidence suggests that cobalt rather than tungsten is responsible for hard metal disease. The interstitial fibrosis described with hard metal is characterized by multinuclear giant cells pneumonitis. Some improvement results from ending exposure, but progression to severe disability typically occurs.

OTHER PNEUMOCONIOSIS

Many other mineral dusts also may cause pneumoconiosis. Some radiopaque dusts (barium, antimony, tin, iron oxides) produce a strikingly abnormal chest radiograph but have little or no measurable effect on pulmonary function. Others (e.g., cement dust) may produce pulmonary fibrosis. Phylosilicate dusts (talc, kaolin, and others) are composed of crystalline silica bound to mineral cations. Kaolin appears to be less fibrogenic than either silica or asbestos, but all of these may produce pneumoconiosis with sufficient doses.

Siderosis is the pneumoconiosis resulting from the inhalation of ferric oxide dust. By itself it appears to have little effect on lung function. Siderosis may occur in electric arc welders and oxyacetylene cutters. Metal fume fever, chronic bronchitis, asthma, and hypersensitivity pneumonitis have also been described in welders.

LUNG CANCER

Bronchogenic carcinoma attributable to occupational exposures may currently be the most important cause of occupational lung disease mortality in the United States and Canada; an estimated 4% to 5% of the total lung cancer deaths annually in the United States may be occupationally derived (Chapter 60). Asbestosis, silicosis, and heavy exposure to polycyclic aromatic hydrocarbons, chloroethers, mustard gas, arsenic, and radon daughters (decay products) have all been variably associated with small to sizable lung cancer risk. Hexavalent chromium has been associated with nasal and bronchogenic carcinomas. All these cancers are characterized by a long latent period between first exposure to the carcinogen and the eventual clinical appearance of the disease. Thus the tumor may be recognized years or even decades after exposure to the causative agent(s) has ceased. It is suspected that many occupational agents interact with cigarette smoke, producing an increased risk for developing lung cancers. Efforts to reduce lung cancer mortality by regular chest radiographs and sputum cytology in middle-aged cigarette-smoking men have not been successful.

In general the lung cancers produced by occupational exposures are indistinguishable histologically from other cancers. An association with occupation is established only by a careful review of the patient's exposure history. The role for workplace causes of these generally fatal cancers may easily be overlooked if the treating physician limits the exposure history to questions about cigarette smoking.

Because these substances continue to be used worldwide without appropriate regard to their dangers, the potential for preventing deaths from these causes by reducing the amount of exposure at the workplace is currently unrealized. The identification of radon daughters as a cause of lung cancer in miners of both uranium and nonuranium minerals has raised the likelihood that domestic exposure to radon daughters (entering homes through basement walls) may also cause some increase in lung cancer, but the magnitude of this effect is not known.

BIBLIOGRAPHY

Chan-Yeung M, Lam S: Occupational asthma: state of the art, *Am Rev Respir Dis* 133:686, 1986.

Chan-Yeung M, Malo J: Current concepts: occupational asthma, *N Engl J Med* 333: 107, 1995.

Cugell D, Morgan W: The respiratory effects of cobalt, *Arch Intern Med* 150:177, 1990.

Harber P, Schenker MB, Balmes JR, editors: *Occupational and Environmental Respiratory Disease*, ed 1, St Louis, 1996, Mosby.

International Agency for Research on Cancer: Silica, *IARC Monogr Eval Carcinog Risk Chem Hum* 42:39-143, 1987.

Morgan WKC, Seaton A, editors: *Occupational lung diseases*, ed 3, Philadelphia, 1994, WB Saunders.

Mossman BT, Gee JBL: Asbestos-related diseases (medical progress), *N Engl J Med* 320:1721, 1989.

Parkes WR: *Occupational lung disease*, ed 2, London, 1982, Butterworth.

Richeldi L, Sorrentino R, Saltini C: HLA-DPB1 glutamate 69: a genetic marker of beryllium disease, *Science* 262:242-244, 1993.

Ziskind M, Jones RN, Weill H: Silicosis, *Am Rev Respir Dis* 113:643, 1976.

CHAPTER

58 Adverse Pulmonary Reactions to Drugs and Other Therapeutic Modalities

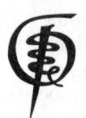

J. Allen Cooper, Jr.

Administration of various therapeutic modalities has been associated with respiratory alterations (Boxes 58-1 and 58-2) ranging from severe parenchymal destruction to reversible chronic cough. Drugs, irradiation, or oxygen therapy can adversely affect the lung. This chapter discusses clinical manifestations of these reactions.

PNEUMONITIS WITH FIBROSIS

Pneumonitis with fibrosis occurs after administration of several drugs and in association with thoracic irradiation. Patients most often have insidious progression of dyspnea and nonproductive cough occurring over weeks or months. Similar symptoms may rarely progress more rapidly. The most common physical finding is bilateral, late inspira-

---

BOX 58-1

Drugs or drug groups that cause pulmonary parenchymal reactions*

Cytotoxic antibiotics
  Bleomycin
  Mitomycin
Alkylating agents
  Cyclophosphamide
  Busulfan
  Chlorambucil
  Melphalan
Nitrosoureas
  Carmustine (BCNU)
  Lomustine (CCNU)
  Methyl-CCNU
  Chlorozotocin
Anticonvulsants
  Diphenylhydantoin
  Carbamazepine
Antimicrobials
  Nitrofurantoin
  Numerous antibiotics

Antiarrhythmics
  Amiodarone
  Tocainide
  Lidocaine
Antiinflammatory drugs
  Aspirin
  Other NSAIDs
  Gold salts
  Penicillamine
Opiates
  Heroin
  Propoxyphene
  Methadone
Miscellaneous
  Vinca alkaloids
  Hydrochlorothiazide
  Procarbazine
  Colchicine
  Oxygen
  Radiation
  Cytokines
  All-trans retinoic acid

*Numerous drugs not listed can sporadically cause hypersensitivity pneumonitis.
NSAIDs, Nonsteroidal antiinflammatory drugs.

BOX 58-2

Drug groups that induce bronchospasm or cough

β-adrenergic antagonists
Aspirin
Other NSAIDs
Cholinergic agents
Angiotensin-converting enzyme inhibitors

NSAIDs, Nonsteroidal antiinflammatory drugs.

tory crackles. Chest radiographs usually demonstrate bibasilar reticular infiltrates; diffuse alveolar infiltrates occur less frequently. Pulmonary function tests show reduced lung volumes consistent with a restrictive ventilatory defect and a decreased diffusing capacity. Because similar findings can occur from other processes that may affect this patient population, however, abnormal pulmonary function tests are not sufficient for the definitive diagnosis of pulmonary drug reactions. Pathologically, endothelial damage is an early manifestation of drug-induced pneumonitis. This is followed by type I pneumocyte destruction and type II pneumocyte proliferation with dysplastic changes. Finally, parenchymal inflammation and significant interstitial fibrosis with thickening of the interstitial space occur; the degree of fibrosis probably correlates with irreversibility of the syndrome.

HYPERSENSITIVITY (EOSINOPHILIC) PNEUMONITIS

Patients with drug-induced hypersensitivity pneumonitis have symptoms of cough, fever, and dyspnea that develop over several days. Systemic manifestations, including eosinophilia, hepatitis, dermatitis, or nephritis, may also be present. However, some patients may have isolated pulmonary hypersensitivity reactions. Chest radiographs show bilateral alveolar infiltrates that may be peripheral and rarely migratory. Pleural effusions may also be present. Lung tissue shows infiltration of acute inflammatory cells, including eosinophils and neutrophils, into parenchyma with minimum fibrosis. A similar syndrome induced by methotrexate may be associated with pulmonary granulomatous inflammation. The prognosis for patients with drug-induced hypersensitivity pneumonitis is favorable, especially for those with reactions caused by drugs other than methotrexate. Virtually all patients recover with no residual pulmonary abnormalities if the agent is withdrawn and corticosteroids are instituted. The mortality rate for patients who develop hypersensitivity pneumonitis from methotrexate may approach 10%.

NONCARDIOGENIC PULMONARY EDEMA

Noncardiogenic pulmonary edema can be induced by several drugs and is also a manifestation of pulmonary oxygen toxicity. When associated with drug ingestion, the syndrome usually occurs after overdose. Prognosis is variable but generally better than in patients with other causes of noncardiogenic pulmonary edema, presumably because the offending agent can be removed. Histopathologic specimens from patients with the syndrome show protein and inflammatory cellular exudation into the alveolar space.

COUGH

Recently it has been documented that angiotensin-converting enzyme (ACE) inhibitors can induce cough in as many as 10% of treated patients. Cough in these patients is generally nonproductive and may be slow in clearing after discontinuation of the drug.

BRONCHOSPASM

Certain drugs also precipitate bronchospasm (see Box 58-2) by varied mechanisms. Nonsteroidal antiinflammatory drugs (NSAIDs) that inhibit the cyclooxygenase enzyme or arachidonic acid metabolism induce bronchospasm in approximately 15% of adult asthmatic patients. One report indicated an increased incidence of HLA-DQw2 antigen in aspirin-sensitive asthmatic patients. Intolerance to these agents increases with age, may be associated with peripheral eosinophilia, is frequently associated with nasal polyposis and rhinitis, and develops more frequently in women. The associated triad of asthma, nasal polyposis, and aspirin sensitivity was initially described by Samter and Beers. Onset of bronchospasm occurs 30 to 90 minutes after ingestion of the drug. Treatment is similar to that for other forms of bronchospasm. Progressive desensitization with aspirin may be attempted, but this can induce severe bronchospasm if done incorrectly.

Cholinergic agents, typically used in the treatment of urologic and ocular disorders, may also occasionally induce bronchospasm in asthmatic patients when these drugs are administered locally to the eye or systemically. Treatment of bronchospasm in these patients consists of drug withdrawal and administration of atropine, parenterally or by inhalation, in addition to other bronchodilators.

β-adrenergic antagonists may also induce bronchospasm, primarily in patients with preexisting obstructive airways disease, although apparently normal persons may also rarely be susceptible. The association of timolol with this syndrome is particularly important because patients react to this drug after local ocular treatment, a situation that can be easily overlooked. Symptoms of wheezing and dyspnea occur 1 hour after use of the β-blocker and may be severe. Treatment includes supportive measures, withdrawal of the drug, and administration of bronchodilators. In these patients, anticholinergic bronchodilators such as atropine or ipratropium are the agents of choice since β-adrenergic agents may be ineffective because of blocked adrenergic receptors.

RESPIRATORY MUSCLE DYSFUNCTION

Antibiotics, including aminoglycosides, penicillin, polymixin, and occasionally other drugs, can cause acute respiratory failure secondary to respiratory muscle dysfunction. Signs and symptoms include severe dyspnea, orthopnea, hypoxemia, and reduced motion of the diaphragm. The chest radiograph may show an elevated hemidiaphragm and reduced lung volumes. Treatment involves supportive measures, including artificial ventilation. Occasionally, some improvement may occur with calcium or neostigmine therapy.

OTHER SYNDROMES

Pulmonary arterial hypertension can occur after administration of certain agents. Aminorex, an anorectic agent no longer in use, caused a high incidence of such reactions. Granulomatous lung disease with pulmonary hypertension may occur with intravenous injection of talc-containing preparations intended for oral use. The incidence of pulmonary venoocclusive disease also increases after administration of certain cytotoxic agents. Bronchiolitis obliterans occurs rarely after penicillamine therapy and is manifested primarily by airway obstruction, as documented by pulmonary function testing, although a restrictive component may also be apparent. Finally, a pulmonary-renal syndrome similar to Goodpasture's syndrome has been reported to occur infrequently after penicillamine therapy.

SPECIFIC DRUGS
Bleomycin

The polypeptide antibiotic bleomycin causes pneumonitis with fibrosis in approximately 4% of patients receiving the drug. The incidence of pulmonary reactions to this drug increases with certain well-defined risk factors, including age, oxygen administration, radiotherapy, use of multidrug regimens, and cumulative doses exceeding 450 total units. However, patients developing pulmonary reactions to bleomycin after only one dose have been reported. Although bleomycin most often causes a syndrome of pneumonitis with fibrosis, the drug also rarely induces a hypersensitivity (eosinophilic) pneumonitis. The chest radiograph of patients with pneumonitis/fibrosis caused by bleomycin commonly shows bibasilar subpleural reticular infiltrates. Chest computed tomography (CT) scans may show abnormalities before they are noted on plain radiograph.

The diagnosis of bleomycin-induced pulmonary disease usually requires lung biopsy to rule out other causes of lung disease, such as infection or underlying neoplasm. No pathognomonic histologic pattern exists for bleomycin-induced pulmonary damage. Screening for early diagnosis of bleomycin-induced pneumonitis/fibrosis is difficult. Currently, no tests can accurately identify patients at an early stage before onset of irreversible changes. Pulmonary functions tests are either too sensitive or are nonspecific, as in the case of carbon dioxide diffusing capacity (DLCO). A percentage of patients who show a decrease in DLCO will never develop clinical bleomycin-induced pneumonitis. In contrast, although relatively more specific, lung volumes are insensitive. Patients with clinical bleomycin-induced pneumonitis generally have reduced total lung capacity, but this occurs late in the process and may indicate irreversibility. Mortality from bleomycin-induced pulmonary disease approaches 50% overall, although the prognosis for patients who develop bleomycin-induced hypersensitivity lung disease is good. Corticosteroids appear to be useful in the treatment of both syndromes of pulmonary toxicity associated with bleomycin.

Methotrexate

This folate antagonist induces pulmonary disease in approximately 7% of patients who receive the drug. High doses used in the treatment of malignancy and lower doses used as part of an antiinflammatory regimen have been associated with pulmonary toxicity, the latter probably at a lower incidence than when used to treat malignancy. Pulmonary reactions have occurred after intravenous (IV) or intrathecal administration of methotrexate. Multidrug regimens, increased frequency of administration, and tapering of corticosteroids or previous adrenelectomy increase the risk of developing pulmonary disease from methotrexate. As noted, the most common clinical syndrome associated with methotrexate is hypersensitivity pneumonitis. However, noncardiogenic pulmonary edema, pneumonitis with fibrosis, and acute pleurisy have also been associated with methotrexate therapy.

Mitomycin

Pulmonary toxicity of the cytotoxic antibiotic mitomycin is manifested by several clinical syndromes. First, the combination of mitomycin with *Vinca* alkaloid treatment can result in acute bronchospasm in the presence or absence of pulmonary infiltrates. The incidence of pulmonary reactions to regimens containing this combination may be as high as 39%. Second, mitomycin can cause a syndrome of microangiopathic hemolytic anemia, pulmonary infiltrates, and uremia that is precipitated by blood transfusions. Finally, mitomycin may induce a pneumonitis with fibrosis that is histopathologically indistinguishable from that caused by other cytotoxic drugs, except for an increased degree of interstitial mononuclear cell infiltrates. The presence of these cells may correlate with the relative responsiveness of patients with this form of mitomycin toxicity to corticosteroid therapy.

Nitrosoureas

Carmustine and other nitrosoureas frequently cause pneumonitis with fibrosis. Symptoms usually progress insidiously, but a few reports have documented a rapid progression. Recently, emphasis has been on the late sequelae of therapy with these agents; reports of pulmonary fibrosis several years after discontinuation of treatment with these agents are relatively frequent. Risk factors for development of nitrosourea-induced pulmonary disease probably include cumulative dose, preexisting lung disease, younger age, and use of the nitrosourea in multidrug chemotherapy regimens.

Other Chemotherapeutic Agents

Several alkylating agents have been reported to cause pulmonary injury. In fact, busulfan was the first chemotherapeutic drug to be associated with pulmonary toxicity. Cyclophosphamide causes pneumonitis with fibrosis when used as a single agent and is also an important component of pulmonary-toxic multidrug regimens. Melphalan and chlorambucil rarely cause pulmonary toxicity.

Cytosine arabinoside induces noncardiogenic pulmonary edema in a cumulative dose-dependent manner. Azathioprine and mercaptopurine rarely cause hypersensitivity pneumonitis. Procarbazine has been reported to cause a pulmonary hypersensitivity reaction, with peripheral and pulmonary eosinophilia and skin rash in some patients.

Recent reports have documented pulmonary effects of newer anticancer therapy. Cytokine therapy, particularly with interleukin-2 (IL-2) can result in massive fluid accumulation that can involve the lungs. Rarely, patients require intubation and mechanical ventilation because of respiratory failure after IL-2 therapy. All-trans retinoic acid, a new therapy for acute myelogenous leukemia, can also result in noncardiogenic pulmonary edema in conjunction with total body fluid accumulation.

Amiodarone

The antiarrhythmic agent amiodarone causes a syndrome of pneumonitis with fibrosis in 5% to 10% of exposed patients. Elimination half-life of amiodarone from the body may be 30 days. Thus pulmonary toxicity from amiodarone must be recognized promptly and the drug discontinued early in the course of the illness. Risk factors that increase the incidence of pulmonary toxicity to amiodarone are the maintenance dose and previous pulmonary disease. Recent evidence also suggests that the combination of amiodarone and general anesthesia or cardiopulmonary bypass is synergistic for development of acute lung injury. As with bleomycin, pulmonary function tests are relatively poor predictors of early pulmonary disease caused by amiodarone. However, the D_{LCO} is useful in distinguishing between amiodarone pulmonary toxicity and congestive heart failure, a common malady in this patient population. If the D_{LCO} is normal, it is unlikely that pneumonitis resulting from amiodarone is present.

Chest radiographs of patients with amiodarone-induced pulmonary disease typically show both bilateral reticular infiltrates and patchy acinar infiltrates. Infrequent radiographic presentations are focal consolidation, nodular lesions, and isolated pleural effusions. The chest radiograph may be particularly useless in this patient population because of the common occurrence of cardiogenic edema. Positive gallium scans have been reported in several patients with amiodarone-induced pneumonitis, but gallium scans may also be negative. Chest CT may show high-attenuation abnormalities, but it is uncertain whether this is pathognomonic for lung injury associated with the drug.

Histologic findings in patients with amiodarone-induced pulmonary disease are relatively nonspecific, except for the presence of "foamy," phospholipid-laden macrophages. However, the presence of these cells is not pathognomonic for amiodarone-induced lung disease. Moreover, similar abnormal cells may be recovered from patients receiving the drug who have no apparent pulmonary disease. Other pulmonary histopathologic findings associated with amiodarone are pneumocyte atypia, interstitial thickening, and mononuclear cell infiltration.

Mortality in patients who develop amiodarone-induced pneumonitis is high. However, this is caused by the severity of their cardiac disease as much as by the pulmonary reaction to the drug. Many patients who develop amiodarone-induced pneumonitis cannot have the drug discontinued because it is life-saving for them. In these patients a reduction in dosage of amiodarone and institution of corticosteroid therapy may reverse the pulmonary sequelae.

Nitrofurantoin

The urinary antiseptic nitrofurantoin causes two distinct clinical syndromes: (1) a hypersensitivity (eosinophilic) pneumonitis or (2) chronic pneumonitis with fibrosis. The acute syndrome occurs within 1 month of drug initiation and does not predispose to the more chronic syndrome, which occurs after 2 months to 5 years of nitrofurantoin therapy. Both syndromes have been associated with pulmonary tissue eosinophilia and interstitial inflammation, although fibrosis is a more common finding in the chronic form of the disease. Acute pulmonary toxicity from nitrofurantoin carries a lower mortality rate, and residual pulmonary abnormalities occur infrequently compared with the chronic syndrome.

Gold Salts

Chrysotherapy for patients with rheumatoid arthritis may cause hypersensitivity pneumonitis. A more chronic process consistent with pneumonitis/fibrosis or bronchiolitis obliterans has also been described. Approximately 40% of patients with rheumatoid arthritis who develop gold salt–induced pulmonary disease are rheumatoid factor negative. In addition, a recent study has demonstrated a strong association between HLA and complement phenotype and occurrence of pulmonary reactions to gold salts. Lung tissue from patients with gold-induced pulmonary reactions demonstrates interstitial and alveolar infiltration by inflammatory cells, including histiocytes, lymphocytes, and plasma cells. Patients with gold-induced pneumonitis are often responsive to corticosteroid treatment, in addition to discontinuation of the drug.

Sulfasalazine

Sulfasalazine, used in the treatment of inflammatory bowel disorders, has been associated rarely with pulmonary hypersensitivity reactions. The drug also rarely causes chronic pneumonitis with fibrosis, bronchiolitis obliterans, or isolated bronchospasm.

Antiepileptics

Dilantin and carbamazepine have been implicated as causes of pulmonary hypersensitivity reactions. All patients had a similar presentation with cough, myalgia, fever, and peripheral eosinophilia, and most had a maculopapular rash. Some patients developed severe lymphadenopathy and hepatitis. In fact, liver biopsy has been used to diagnose the syndrome.

Opiates

An overdose of heroin, methadone, codeine, or propoxyphene causes noncardiogenic pulmonary edema. Pulmonary abnormalities develop acutely over several hours after exposure to the opiate. Signs and symptoms include lethargy, cyanosis, pulmonary crackles, and occasional fever.

Terbutaline and Ritrodine

These two tocolytic agents cause noncardiogenic pulmonary edema in less than 1% of patients receiving the drugs for premature labor. Risk factors for developing the syndrome are unclear, although concurrent corticosteroid use, aggressive fluid replacement, and abrupt withdrawal of terbutaline or ritrodine may be important.

Nonsteroidal Antiinflammatory Agents

Supratherapeutic serum concentrations of aspirin cause noncardiogenic pulmonary edema. Besides overdose, risk factors include age, a history of smoking, and chronic ingestion of salicylates. Aspirin and other NSAIDs also induce bronchospasm in approximately 0.3% of the normal population, as well as 4% to 20% of asthmatic patients (see previous section on bronchospasm). NSAIDs other than aspirin have also been associated with pulmonary hypersensitivity reactions.

Other Agents Used for Benign Conditions

Hydrochlorothiazide rarely causes a syndrome of noncardiogenic pulmonary edema. Several patients had previously noted milder symptoms after ingesting the drug, and in all patients, pulmonary symptoms developed within 1 hour of drug ingestion. Penicillamine therapy is associated with pneumonitis/fibrosis, bronchiolitis obliterans, bronchitis, hypersensitivity lung disease, and a pulmonary renal syndrome in less than 1% of the patients at risk, although the role of the underlying disease, usually rheumatoid arthritis, remains to be resolved. Tocainide, an antiarrhythmic agent, has produced three well-documented cases of pneumonitis with fibrosis. Captopril and other angiotensin-converting enzyme inhibitors induce cough in approximately 10% of treated patients. β-adrenergic antagonists can induce bronchospasm in asthmatic patients as well as in apparently normal individuals.

OXYGEN THERAPY

Delivery of partial pressures of oxygen (O_2) greater than ambient air is associated with lung injury, usually manifested by a syndrome of noncardiogenic pulmonary edema. However, chronic manifestations may occur if the patient survives. It is unclear what O_2 partial pressure is nontoxic to the human lung, although early studies in normal individuals suggest less than 0.50 fraction of O_2 is safe. Concurrent or previous therapy with bleomycin or possibly other cytotoxic agents may lower the tolerance of the lung to O_2 therapy; the lowest possible fraction of O_2 that can be used should be used at all times. Pathologically, the lungs of patients with O_2 toxicity demonstrate an early exudative phase, with loss of normal alveolar lining cells and exudation of protein, and a later proliferative phase, with proliferation of type II pneumocytes and interstitial thickening caused by a fibrotic

✔ WHEN TO REFER

Patients developing respiratory symptoms during treatment with any of the drugs mentioned should be referred to a pulmonary specialist for further evaluation. Early recognition of these diseases and discontinuation of the offending drug are important to prevent chronic pulmonary insufficiency. Although pulmonary function tests may be useful to screen patients prone to pulmonary drug reactions, no single test can identify these patients at an early stage. If pulmonary function test abnormalities are noted, a pulmonary specialist should be consulted.

reaction. To date, no effective therapy exists for pulmonary O_2 toxicity; prevention by use of the lowest possible fraction of O_2 is the best method to avoid the syndrome.

RADIOTHERAPY

Irradiation of the lung causes pulmonary alterations in approximately 10% of patients at risk. Factors that increase the risk of radiation lung injury are dose of radiation and previous or concurrent chemotherapy. The most common clinical manifestation of radiation-induced pulmonary disease is pneumonitis, occurring 1 to 3 months after initiation of radiation therapy. In most patients the pulmonary abnormalities resolve with or without steroid therapy. A few patients progress to chronic irreversible pulmonary alterations. A helpful radiographic manifestation of radiation pneumonitis is the presence of infiltrates only in the location of the irradiation port.

BIBLIOGRAPHY

Cooper JAD Jr, White DA, Matthay RA: State of the art: drug-induced pulmonary disease, *Am Rev Respir Dis* 133:321, 488, 1986.
Heffner JE, Sahn SA: Salicylate-induced pulmonary edema: clinical features and prognosis, *Ann Intern Med* 95:405, 1981.
Jackson RM: Molecular, pharmacologic, and clinical aspects of oxygen-induced lung injury, *Clin Chest Med* 11:73, 1990.
Kennedy JI Jr: Clinical aspects of amiodarone pulmonary toxicity, *Clin Chest Med* 11:119, 1990.
Rosenow EC: The spectrum of drug-induced pulmonary disease, *Ann Intern Med* 77:977, 1972.
Rosiello RA, Merrill WW: Radiation-induced lung injury, *Clin Chest Med* 11:65, 1990.
Slepian IK, Mathews KP, McLean JA: Aspirin-sensitive asthma, *Chest* 87:386, 1985.
Vahdat L, Maslak P, Miller WH Jr, et al: Early mortality and the retinoic acid syndrome in acute promyelocytic leukemia: impact of leukocytosis, low-dose chemotherapy, PMN/RAR-alpha isoform, and CD13 expression in patients treated with all-trans retinoic acid, *Blood* 84:3843-3849, 1994.
White RL, Schwartzentruber KJ, Guleria A, et al: Cardiopulmonary toxicity of treatment with high dose interleukin-2 in 199 consecutive patients with metastatic melanoma or renal cell carcinoma, *Cancer* 74:3212-3222, 1994.

CHAPTER

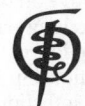

59 Cystic Fibrosis and Bronchiectasis

Pamela B. Davis and Michael D. Infeld

CYSTIC FIBROSIS
Pathophysiology

From 1970 to 1990, the proportion of patients over 18 years of age with cystic fibrosis (CF) has increased fourfold. The changing epidemiology of CF requires increased participation from internists in CF care. Although CF is a multisystem disease, most of the morbidity and mortality are due to its pulmonary manifestations.

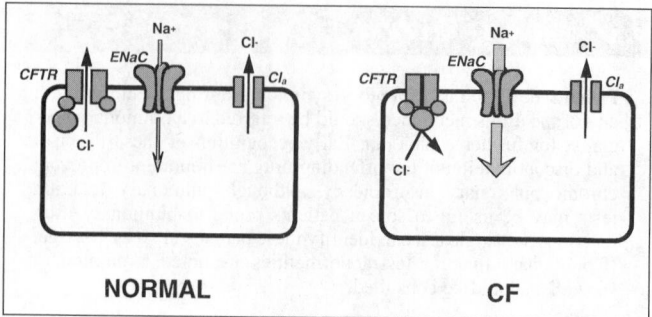

FIGURE 59-1 Schematic representation of some apical membrane ion transporters in airway epithelial cells. In normal cells, increases in intracellular cAMP activate protein kinase A (PKA) to phosphorylate the regulatory domain of cystic fibrosis transmembrane conductance regulator (CFTR). That, coupled with binding of ATP to nucleotide binding domains, opens the channel, permitting chloride to cross the plasma membrane. In cystic fibrosis, CFTR fails to secrete chloride in response to cAMP. At the same time, the solution reabsorption activity of the epithelial sodium channel *(ENaC)* is greatly increased. An "alternative" chloride conductance *(Cl$_a$)*, regulated by Ca^{++}, exists in the apical membrane and is a possible therapeutic target.

CF is an autosomal recessive disease resulting from the inheritance of two mutant alleles at the locus on chromosome 7 encoding the cystic fibrosis transmembrane conductance regulator (CFTR). It is the most common lethal inherited disease in the American Caucasian population, with an incidence of 1:2000 live births and a heterozygote frequency of 1 in 20. In the African-American population, the incidence is 1:17,000 live births, and CF is even more rare in Asian-Americans and native Americans.

CFTR is a 1480 amino acid integral membrane glycoprotein that functions as a cyclic adenosine monophosphate (cAMP)-regulated chloride channel. Its 12 transmembrane domains form an anion channel regulated by the binding and hydrolysis of adenosine triphosphate (ATP) by two cytoplasmic nucleotide binding domains and the phosphorylation of serine and threonine residues in a cytoplasmic regulatory (R) domain. Increased intracellular cAMP promotes protein kinase A–mediated phosphorylation of CFTR, which increases the open probability of the channel. As the chloride ions are transported across the plasma membrane, water follows. Interactions between CFTR and an epithelial sodium transporter may regulate transcellular sodium flux (Fig. 59-1). CFTR has been implicated in the secretion of fluid in the respiratory and gastrointestinal tracts, hydration and appropriate glycosylation of mucous glycoproteins, reabsorption of electrolytes in the sweat ducts, and maintaining the patency of the developing vasa deferentia.

Over 400 mutations in the 250 kilobase CFTR gene are associated with manifestations of CF. The most common mutation, present on 70% of CF chromosomes in the United States, is a three base pair deletion eliminating a phenylalanine residue at position 508 in CFTR (ΔF508). Different CF mutations are associated with different phenotypes. For example, patients homozygous for the ΔF508 mutation are more likely to be pancreatic insufficient than those hemizygous for ΔF508 and a less severe mutation such as A455E, and patients homozygous for an arginine to histidine substitution at amino-acid 117 (R117H) may present with only congenital bilateral absence of the vas deferens. Severity seems to be correlated with the relative amount of CFTR function at the plasma membrane. However, the lung damage in CF seems to be related to chronic bacterial infection of the airways and its attendant inflammation. The precise relationship between abnormal chloride transport and persistent airway infection is not completely clear.

The airways of most patients become colonized with bacterial pathogens early in life. Although *Staphylococcus aureus* and *Haemophilus influenzae* are common during childhood, *Pseudomonas* species are the most important pathogens in adults. As the disease advances, the *Pseudomonas* evolves a mucoid colony morphology by secreting an alginate-containing polysaccharide coating that protects the organism from host defense mechanisms in vivo. Acquisition of rarer pathogens such as *Xanthomonas maltophilia* and *Burkholderia*

BOX 59-1

Clinical scenarios suggestive of cystic fibrosis in adolescents and adults

Persistent cough, chronic bronchitis
Asthma with persistent radiographic abnormalities
Recurrent pneumonia with interval radiographic abnormalities
Unexplained lobar collapse
Bronchiectasis
Hemoptysis
Sputum culture positive for mucoid *Pseudomonas aeruginosa*
Allergic bronchopulmonary aspergillosis
Nasal polyposis
Pancreatitis
Unexplained cholelithiasis
Unexplained intestinal obstruction
Rectal prolapse
Cirrhosis
Infertility (azoospermia in males)
Unexplained delayed menarche
Heat prostration
Family history of cystic fibrosis

cepacia may be an ominous prognostic sign. The inflammatory response to these endobronchial pathogens is a crucial determinant of disease progression. Inflammation is dominated by neutrophils and creates a local protease/antiprotease imbalance. Proteolytic digestion of opsonins such as C3bi and immunoglobulins as well as opsonic receptors such as CR1 produces an opsonin-receptor mismatch, preventing phagocytosis and promoting persistent infection. Elastases also stimulate goblet cell hyperplasia and mucus secretion, which fosters airway obstruction. The vicious cycle of proteolytic damage causing bronchiectasis, which further impairs pulmonary defenses, is the final common pathway for lung destruction in CF.

Histologically, goblet cell and submucosal gland hyperplasia, airway obstruction by thick secretions, and subepithelial matrix thickening with hypertrophy of the bronchial vasculature and smooth muscle progress to cystic bronchiectasis. The airway infection can spread distally, resulting in purulent bronchiolitis and chronic pneumonia, but emphysematous lung destruction is rare. Impaired clearance in abnormal airways makes the CF patient vulnerable to opportunistic pathogens such as nontuberculous mycobacteria and fungi. Profound airway damage also leads to the common pulmonary complications of CF: pneumothorax, massive hemoptysis, atelectasis, and respiratory insufficiency.

The pathology in other organ systems is also characterized by ductal plugging. Early pancreatic lesions include ductular obstruction by eosinophilic concretions with relative sparing of the acini, but later normal parenchyma is entirely replaced by fibrosis and fat. Hepatic steatosis and focal biliary cirrhosis due to plugged biliary ductules are common autopsy findings in the CF population, but less than 5% of CF patients progress to diffuse multilobular cirrhosis. Although the mechanism is not completely clear, the patency of the vasa deferentia during development depends on normal functioning of CFTR. The majority of male CF patients have obstructive azoospermia resulting from an absent or atretic epididymal body and vasa deferentia.

Laboratory and Other Diagnostic Tests

Although 95% of CF patients are diagnosed in their preteen years, occasional patients, usually with milder disease, will remain undiagnosed into adulthood. These patients commonly have a history of recurrent pneumonias, sinusitis or "asthma." Patients with minimal pulmonary symptoms may come to medical attention with gastrointestinal manifestations or infertility. Asymptomatic patients may present because of a family history of CF (Box 59-1). Routine laboratory tests do not generally help in diagnosing CF. Hypochloremic metabolic alkalosis may be seen in children. Coagulation abnormalities and hemolytic anemia associated with fat-soluble vitamin deficiencies are

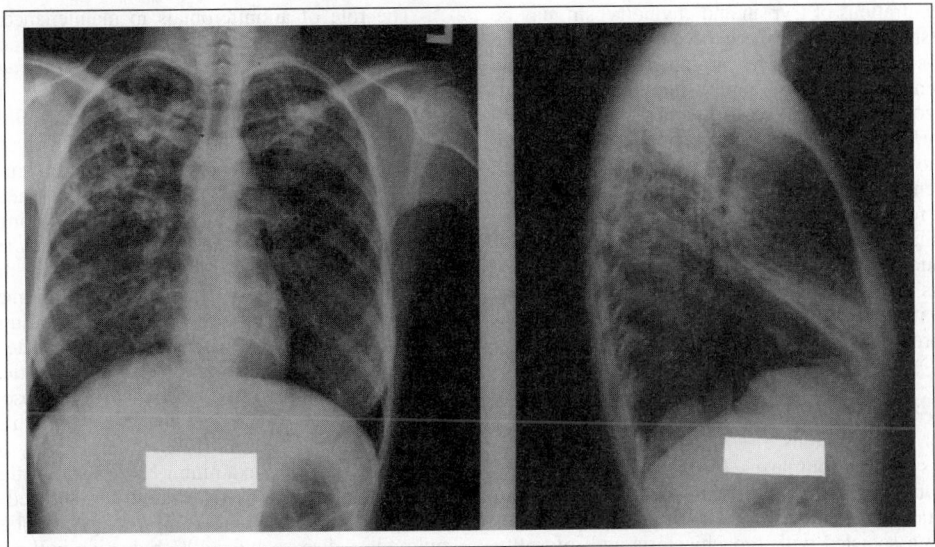

FIGURE 59-2 Posteroanterior and lateral chest radiographs of a 20-year-old female patient with cystic fibrosis. Increased interstitial markings, hyperinflation, and bronchiectasis are noted, with an upper lobe predominance.

unusual. Despite chronic pulmonary infection, leukocytosis is rare. The chest radiograph is usually abnormal. Increased interstitial markings, cystic bronchiectatic changes, hyperinflation, and mucus plugging are common. Upper lobe predominance of these findings is typical (Fig. 59-2).

The sheer number of different CFTR mutations makes definitive genotyping in large numbers of patients impractical. Therefore CF remains a clinical diagnosis. Most diagnostic criteria require the presence of characteristic abnormalities in at least two organ systems including abnormal sweat chloride concentration, obstructive ventilatory defect associated with chronic infection, exocrine pancreatic insufficiency, and azoospermia or a family history of classic cystic fibrosis.

The sweat chloride concentration is the most specific test for CF apart from a completely informative genotype. For this test, the secretogogue pilocarpine is administered by iontophoresis and sweat is collected on filter paper, weighed, and titrated electrically to measure chloride concentration. Two chloride concentrations of >60 mEq/L in children and >80 mEq/L in adults measured on separate days on at least 100 mg sweat constitute an abnormal test. Sweat chloride concentrations exceed 80 mEq/L in less than 5% of non-CF adults and less than 1% of CF patients fall below 60 mEq/L (Fig. 59-3). Conditions such as hypoadrenalism, hypothyroidism, diabetes insipidus, dehydration, ectodermal dysplasia, and glycogen storage diseases may cause elevated sweat chloride concentrations. CF patients with a cytidine to thymidine substitution in intron 19 of CFTR (3849 + 10kb C to T) have sweat chloride concentration <60 mEq/L, so a normal sweat chloride test does not necessarily rule out the diagnosis.

Abnormal pulmonary function is common in adults with CF. Decreased maximal mid-expiratory flow ($FEF_{25\%-75\%}$) and increased residual volume to total lung capacity ratio (RV/TLC) occur early. The forced expiratory volume in 1 second (FEV_1) is reduced out of proportion to the forced vital capacity (FVC), and eventually evidence of hyperinflation and air-trapping are noted. As many as 25% of CF patients have a component of reactive airway disease with a significant response to the acute inhalation of bronchodilators. The combination of an obstructive ventilatory defect and *Pseudomonas aeruginosa* isolated from the sputum makes a CF diagnosis more likely.

Several tests have been used to establish pancreatic insufficiency. The "gold standard" is measurement of enzyme and bicarbonate concentrations in the duodenal aspirate after hormonal stimulation of pancreatic secretion. A simpler approach is to document fat malabsorption with a Sudan black B fat stain for stool fat or quantitation of fat in a 72-hour stool collection. When stool fat is related to fat intake, a coefficient of fat absorption (normally >93%) can be calculated. Fe-

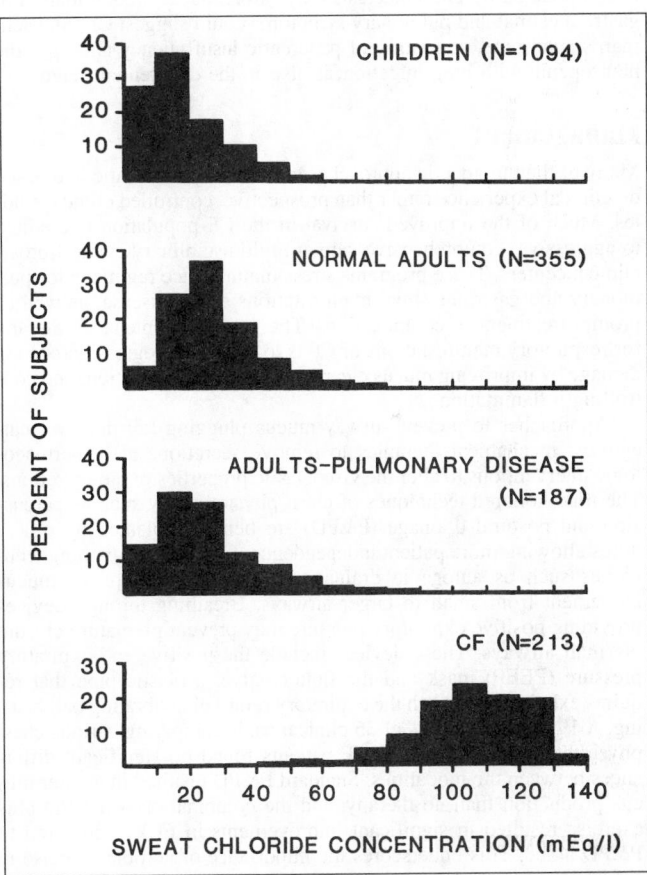

FIGURE 59-3 Distribution of values for sweat chloride in both normal and ill children who do not have cystic fibrosis *(CF)*, normal adults who do not have CF, adults with non-CF pulmonary disease, and patients with CF. (From Davis P, di Sant'Agnese P: *Chest* 85:802-809, 1984.

cal and/or serum concentrations of trypsin and chymotrypsin may be helpful. Indirect assessment of pancreatic exocrine function may be made by levels of fat-soluble vitamins or carotene. Estimates of the chymotrypsin-dependent breakdown of orally administered benzyl-tyrosyl-paraaminobenzoic acid (b-t-PABA) to its absorbable metabolite PABA as recovered in a timed urine collection have also been used. Azoospermia can be detected by routine semen analysis with documentation of absent vasa deferentia by physical examination. A careful family history for CF is mandatory.

Commercially available genotyping establishes the diagnosis if both alleles demonstrate one of the 70 most common mutants tested for in the screen. This test identifies about 85% of clinically diagnosed CF patients, but its lack of sensitivity makes population screening using genotypes problematic.

Differential Diagnosis

The broad spectrum of manifestations of CF place it in the differential diagnosis of many symptom complexes. In contrast, relatively few disease entities mimic the combined pulmonary, gastrointestinal, and genitourinary manifestations of classic CF. The dyskinetic cilia syndromes are commonly associated with bronchiectasis and infertility but not digestive problems. Patients with Young's syndrome, a disease of unknown etiology, also share these manifestations. Patients with α-1-proteinase inhibitor (α-1-Pi) deficiency, especially those with ZZ genotypes, may have cirrhosis and pulmonary disease, but emphysema is the primary lung lesion. Inflammatory bowel disease is complicated by bronchiectasis only rarely, but this combination of gastrointestinal and pulmonary symptoms could suggest CF. Schwachman's syndrome, consisting of pancreatic insufficiency and episodic neutropenia with lung infection, is also in the differential diagnosis.

Management

Many of the therapeutic approaches to CF are symptomatic and based on clinical experience rather than prospective, controlled clinical studies. Much of the improved survival in the CF population is credited to aggressive, comprehensive care at multidisciplinary cystic fibrosis clinical centers. These programs stress maintenance regimens for pulmonary and gastrointestinal manifestations of the disease, as well as prompt treatment of complications. The goal of maintenance therapy for respiratory manifestations of CF is to slow the progression of lung damage by improving mucus clearance, restraining infection, and controlling inflammation.

Approaches to prevent airway mucus plugging fall into two categories: mechanical therapies to remove secretions and pharmacologic interventions to alter the viscoelastic properties of the secretions. The time-honored techniques of chest physiotherapy such as percussion and postural drainage (P&PD) are being supplanted by procedures allowing more patient independence. Controlled breathing techniques such as autogenic drainage and "huffing" improve mucus movement from small to larger airways. Breathing through devices providing positive expiratory pressure may prevent premature closure of small airways. These devices include the positive end-expiratory pressure (PEEP) mask and the flutter valve, a plastic pipe that requires exhalation through the expiratory retard of a vibrating ball bearing. A 1995 metaanalysis of 35 clinical trials comparing various chest physiotherapy techniques in CF patients found no significant differences between the modalities. Standard P&PD resulted in greater mucus production than no therapy, and the combination of P&PD plus exercise resulted in significant improvements in FEV_1 compared to P&PD alone. This underscores the importance of aerobic exercise in enhancing mucus clearance, as well as exercise tolerance.

Attempts to thin CF airway secretions have included aerosolized N-acetylcysteine and bovine deoxyribonuclease (DNase), but side effects prevented wide acceptance of these therapies. Aerosolization of recombinant human DNase (rhDNase) showed reduced side effects compared to the bovine product and has gained popularity. Because much of the viscosity in CF sputum arises from sticky DNA released by necrotic cells, its degradation by 2.5 mg of aerosolized rhDNase per day resulted in better pulmonary function than placebo aerosols in a large multicenter study. However, with only small differences in clinical outcomes such as days hospitalized, the cost-effectiveness of this therapy has yet to be determined.

The role of antimicrobials in maintenance regimens is not well established. Because viral infections are associated with pulmonary deterioration, yearly influenza vaccination is clearly indicated. Short-term administration of 600 mg of tobramycin by aerosol three times a day resulted in significant increases in pulmonary function compared to placebo in a multicenter trial. However, the bacterial flora in nearly 15% of patients acquired tobramycin resistance during the study. The appropriate role of oral, aerosol, and intravenous antibiotics in maintenance therapy has not been definitively determined.

Medications to attenuate the inflammatory response to chronic airway infection have the potential to interrupt the vicious cycle of inflammation and lung destruction in CF. Convincing evidence supporting a role for inhaled corticosteroids or sodium cromoglycate in CF is lacking. A multicenter study of alternate day oral prednisone showed that the rate of spirometric deterioration is slowed; however, side effects such as growth retardation, glucose intolerance, and cataracts caused termination of the study for a high-dose group (2 mg/kg) and will likely limit the long-term utility of systemic corticosteroids in CF. A trial examining the effects of the non-steroidal antiinflammatory drug (NSAID) ibuprofen showed an 88% reduction in FEV_1 decline over 4 years in young, compliant patients with mild pulmonary disease and a 40% reduction in the overall group. Because high serum levels of ibuprofen appear to be important, each patient should have pharmacokinetic studies performed before beginning therapy with careful dosage adjustment and monitoring for side effects.

The role of bronchodilators in CF is controversial. Inhaled β-adrenergic agonists improve peak expiratory flow rates in the subset of CF patients with reactive airways disease. However, they may increase dead space, impair gas exchange during exercise, and promote collapse of compliant airways. Inhaled anticholinergic agents are probably as effective as sympathomimetics, and combination results in greater bronchodilation than either agent alone. The side effects of methylxanthines probably outweigh their therapeutic advantages for most CF patients.

Exacerbations in pulmonary disease will occur during the course of maintenance therapy. Symptoms defining exacerbation in research protocols usually include increased cough, sputum production, dyspnea, exercise intolerance, reduced appetite, or weight loss. Objective correlates of these symptoms include alterations in vital signs, gas exchange, and sputum flora and unexpected findings on lung examination, pulmonary function tests, and chest radiograph. Exacerbation is treated with intensification of the mucus clearance regimen and antimicrobial therapy guided by the in vitro sensitivities of the patient's respiratory flora on recent sputum cultures (Box 59-2). If initial oral and/or aerosolized antibiotics do not restore baseline status, intravenous antibiotics are indicated. Because most adult patients harbor *Pseudomonas* species, double antibiotic coverage with an antipseudomonal β-lactam-like agent (including aztreonam or imipenem-cilastin) and an aminoglycoside is routine. In the setting of aminoglycoside resistance, ciprofloxacin or colistimethate (a polypeptide antipseudomonal antibiotic) may be substituted. CF patients have increased volume of distribution and clearance of numerous medications. Their peculiar pharmacokinetics mandate antibiotic dosing as much as 100% higher than non-CF patients and careful monitoring of drug levels. These special circumstances normally require at least initial hospitalization, although some patients can complete their intravenous antibiotic therapy at home. The goal of therapy is not eradication of the respiratory flora but the restoration of the baseline respiratory condition. Nearly three fourths of patients achieve these goals after 2 weeks of therapy.

Sinusitis and nasal polyps commonly complicate CF. They are treated with antibiotics, vasoconstrictors, and topical antiinflammatory drugs, with surgery reserved for failure of conservative treatment. Pneumothorax occurs in up to 16% of adults. Although up to 25% resolve without thoracostomy tube drainage, high recurrence rates led to recommendations for early pleurodesis in the pre–lung transplant era. Because previous pleurodesis is a contraindication to transplantation in some centers, more conservative management is often tried initially. Lobar atelectasis, which occurs in up to 5% of adults with CF, can usually be managed by intensification of the mucus clearance regimen. Massive hemoptysis, defined as >240 ml blood expectorated over 24 hours, has a 1% annual incidence in the CF population. Most episodes resolve with conservative management, includ-

---

BOX 59-2
Guidelines for treatment of respiratory exacerbations in cystic fibrosis

Defining Respiratory Exacerbations
Increase in cough and/or sputum production
Dyspnea and/or decreased exercise tolerance
Weight loss and/or loss of appetite

Oral antibiotics
For *Staphylococcus:* Dicloxacillin 25 mg/kg q6h
For *Pseudomonas:* Ciprofloxacin 10 mg/kg q8-12h
(If patient fails to respond, aerosolized antibiotics may be added or substituted)
Aerosolized antibiotics
Tobramycin 40-600 mg q8-12h
Colistimethate 37.5-75 mg q12h
(If patient fails to respond, intravenous antibiotic therapy is indicated)

Intravenous antibiotics
For *Staphylococcus:* Nafcillin 50-75 mg/kg q4h (maximum 5 g/dose)
For *Pseudomonas:* Ceftazidime 30-75 mg/kg q6-8h
Piperacillin 65-100 mg/kg q4-6h (maximum 6 g/dose)
Tobramycin 3.3 mg/kg q8h
Colistimethate 1.5-2.3 mg/kg q8h (maximum 100 mg/dose)

Antibiotic therapy should be guided by in vitro sensitivities of the individual patient's flora when available. Doses may require alteration in event of renal insufficiency.

---

ing rest, antitussives, antibiotics, and vitamin K. Ongoing bleeding may require bronchial artery embolization or surgical resection of the affected lobe. The diagnosis of allergic bronchopulmonary aspergillosis (ABPA) is difficult in CF patients who already have bronchiectasis and are commonly colonized with aspergillus. A fourfold elevation of serum IgE and increased aspergillus-specific IgG and IgA coupled with clinical deterioration not responsive to antibiotics help establish the diagnosis. Most patients respond to treatment with corticosteroids. Nontuberculous mycobacteria colonization (usually *Mycobacterium avium* complex) is common in CF adults, but few colonized patients have clinical deterioration attributable to mycobacterial infection and require treatment with antimycobacterial drugs.

Most CF patients will eventually develop respiratory insufficiency. Although one study found little benefit to supplemental oxygen in CF patients with mild hypoxemia, the study was severely limited by a small sample size. Mechanical ventilation support for end-stage CF was rarely used in the pretransplantation era but is gaining favor because some programs offer high-priority transplantation to these patients. These issues must be discussed with the patient and family when a decision is made to pursue the option of a lung transplantation. Double lung transplantation is the definitive treatment for end-stage CF lung disease but is limited by donor availability and problems with chronic rejection. Transplantation is usually considered when the FEV_1 is <30% of predicted, significant hypoxemia or hypercarbia develops, or hospitalizations become frequent or prolonged. Some transplantation centers exclude patients with multiply resistant organisms, steroid dependence, previous pleurodesis, or severe malnutrition. Posttransplantation survival in CF patients is similar to that of recipients from other disease categories, although the abnormal pharmacokinetics of cyclosporine complicate its administration in the CF population.

Pancreatic insufficiency, present in 95% of adults with CF, is treated by exogenous pancreatic enzyme supplements with pH-sensitive microencapsulated preparations of porcine proteases, amylase, and lipase, which are released in the small intestine. The goal of enzyme supplementation is to prevent symptoms of steatorrhea, abdominal pain, flatulence, and frequent stools and to maintain normal weight for height. Initial dosage is 1000 to 2000 units of lipase/kg/meal. If symptoms persist at doses above 2000 lipase units/kg/

✔ WHEN TO REFER

The median survival in CF patients has improved to nearly 30 years of age. Much of the improved prognosis has been attributed to aggressive management in the multidisciplinary CF care centers. The Cystic Fibrosis Foundation recommends that all patients be registered and receive care in Foundation-accredited centers. Patients remote from centers are often cared for by primary care practitioners in close cooperation with center physicians.

---

meal, addition of cimetidine, ranitidine, or omeprazole one half hour before meals may help by increasing the duodenal pH and improving enzyme activity. Vitamin supplementation is recommended with special emphasis on fat-soluble vitamins that are malabsorbed in CF: 5000 to 20,000 IU vitamin A daily, 200 IU water-miscible vitamin E daily, 400 to 800 IU vitamin D daily, and 5 mg of oral vitamin K per week. Vitamin K is especially important in patients with liver disease or previous bowel resections, or those receiving long-term antibiotic therapy.

Frequent nutritional assessments are part of the multidisciplinary approach to the management of CF. Inadequate caloric intake is usually associated with deteriorating pulmonary status and improves with recovery of pulmonary function. Nutritional supplementation may be helpful in the later stages of the disease when either nocturnal tube feeding or hyperalimentation has been used to augment oral intake. CF patients may suffer abdominal pain because of partial or complete obstruction of the distal ileum and ascending colon with abnormal intestinal contents called either distal intestinal obstruction syndrome (DIOS) or meconium ileus equivalent (MIE). Persistent obstruction may require oral administration of 10% N-acetylcysteine solution or polyethylene glycol solutions, meglumine diatrizoate (gastrograffin) enema, or surgical intervention. Although DIOS is the most common cause of abdominal pain, volvulus, intussusception, and periappendiceal abscess, which occurs at increased frequency in CF, must be considered. In addition, colonic strictures associated with high doses of pancreatic enzymes have been reported.

CF patients are often troubled by hemorrhoids and rectal prolapse, which usually improve with symptomatic treatment. Acute pancreatitis has been reported in pancreatic-sufficient CF patients. The incidence of cholelithiasis is several-fold higher in CF patients than in the general population, but its management is similar. Ursodeoxycholic acid was ineffective in preventing and dissolving stones in this patient population. Although uncommon, cirrhosis is a major source of morbidity and mortality when present and is treatable only by liver transplantation. An abnormal response to oral glucose tolerance testing is present in up to 40% of CF patients, but insulin requiring diabetes develops in only about 5%.

There are numerous approaches to the reproductive problems of CF patients. In males, retrieval of epididymal sperm with subsequent artificial insemination has been tried. Because pregnancy may be deleterious to the mother's health unless her pulmonary status is very stable, contraception is generally recommended in the sexually active female. Reports of in vitro fertilization coupled with selection of fertilized ovum without CF alleles have been published.

BRONCHIECTASIS
Pathophysiology

Bronchiectasis is an abnormal dilation of the large conducting airways. It results from stromal remodelling of the airways as a consequence of either congenital structural anomalies or inflammatory or mechanical stresses. Although the incidence of this problem has declined with the advent of antibiotics and vaccinations to prevent severe respiratory infections in early life, for those afflicted it remains a serious chronic problem.

Reid described three classes of bronchiectasis, representing a spectrum of severity or evolution of the bronchial abnormality. Cylindrical bronchiectasis is a potentially reversible, uniform bronchial dilation, whereas varicose bronchiectasis indicates increased bronchial caliber with distortion of the bronchial contour. Cystic bronchiectasis denotes a balloonlike dilation with peripheral increases in bronchial caliber.

On histologic examination, ectatic bronchi show thickening of the bronchial wall with submucosal inflammation and fibrosis that can extend to the neighboring parenchyma. Bronchial lumens may be occluded with mucus and downstream bronchioles obliterated. The bronchial vessels can be massively hypertrophied. Cartilage may be completely absent in aneurysmal areas.

With progressive impairment of mucociliary clearance resulting from aberrant bronchial anatomy, cough becomes the primary clearance mechanism for these areas and hence is the cardinal symptom of bronchiectasis. Long-standing, daily, productive cough is common, sputum is typically purulent, and the quantity of sputum can exceed 500 ml/day. With hypertrophied bronchial vessels near the airway surface and the development of pulmonary-bronchial arterial anastomoses, hemoptysis accompanying the chronic cough may become massive. Recurrent pneumonias may also occur. The progressive ventilatory defects result in gas exchange abnormalities, exercise intolerance, and dyspnea. Physical findings include coarse crackles localized over involved areas, possibly accompanied by wheezing. Evidence of situs inversus and/or sinusitis may be noted in patients with congenital bronchiectasis. Digital clubbing may occur in more severe cases.

Laboratory and Other Diagnostic Tests

Routine blood work is not likely to yield specific clues to the diagnosis. Leukocytosis may signal acute exacerbations. On the chest radiograph, thickening of bronchial walls may be evident as a "signet ring" sign in airways projecting on end and as "tram tracking" in airways perpendicular to the x-ray beam. Multiple ectatic airways extending from the hila to the periphery give a "finger in glove" appearance typical of central bronchiectasis. Discrete cysts may have air-fluid levels and be confused with lung abscesses. Peribronchial fibrosis may produce vascular crowding and eventually a "honeycomb" appearance in the adjacent lung. Sputum cultures often reveal chronic infection with organisms such as *Staphylococcus aureus, Haemophilus influenzae,* anaerobes, or pseudomonads. Opportunists such as mycobacteria and fungi are not uncommon. Pulmonary function testing may initially be normal despite severe localized bronchiectasis. As the disease progresses, obstructive, restrictive, or combined restrictive and obstructive ventilatory defects can be seen depending on the extent of the peribronchial fibrotic reaction. Blood gases show hypoxemia and hypercarbia late in the process.

High resolution computed tomography (CT) has largely replaced bronchography as the standard for establishing the diagnosis of bronchiectasis. With autopsy as the criterion standard, this technique demonstrated a sensitivity of 87%. No universally accepted criteria for the CT diagnosis of bronchiectasis exist, but the failure of bronchi to taper along their longitudinal aspect and increased wall thickness, rendering airways detectable in the lung periphery, are two commonly used signs. Airway luminal diameter greater than that of adjacent vessels is also used. A beaded "string of pearls" appearance connotes varicose bronchiectasis. Cystic bronchiectasis can appear as grape-like clusters of hyperlucency, which may be differentiated from emphysematous blebs by their thicker walls, more linear arrangement, and accompanying blood vessels. Different classes of bronchiectatic changes can coexist in the same patient (Fig. 59-4). Once the diagnosis has been established, the next task is to determine the cause of the bronchiectasis. .

Differential Diagnosis

Etiologies of bronchiectasis fall into two broad categories, congenital disorders and acquired processes. Inherited diseases associated with bronchiectasis include CF, dyskinetic cilia disorders such as Kartagener's syndrome (including the triad of *situs inversus,* sinusitis, and bronchiectasis), α-1-Pi deficiency and defects of the humoral immune system like immunoglobulin deficiency or Job's syndrome (hyperimmunoglobulin E with recurrent staphylococcal infections). Developmental anomalies of the airway like tracheal bronchus, bronchial webs, sequestrations, and Swyer-James syndrome (unilateral hyperlucent lung) can be associated with bronchiectasis. Less frequent heritable causes include Young's syndrome, Williams-Campbell syn-

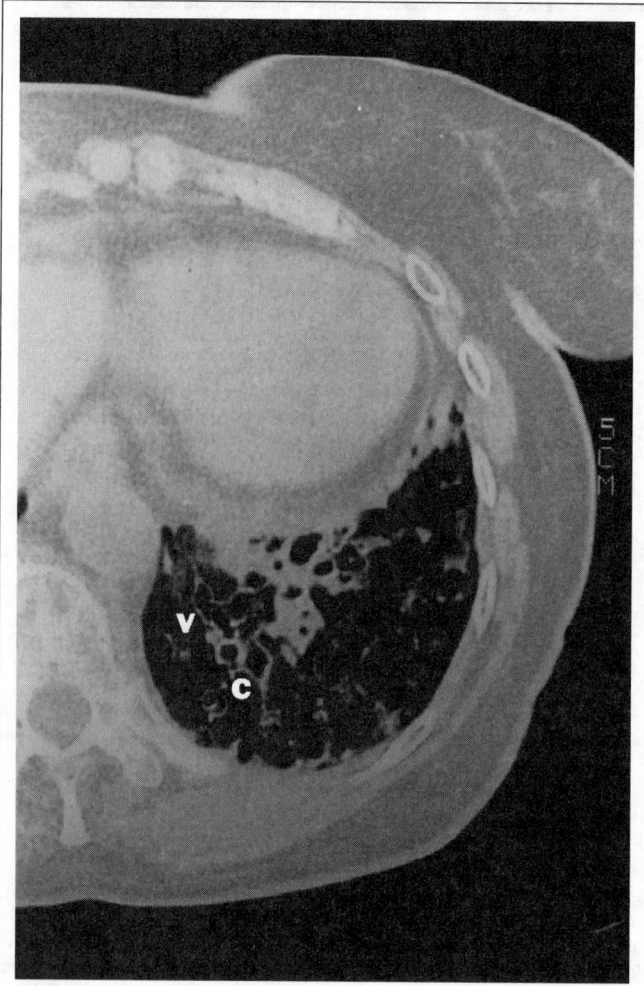

FIGURE 59-4 High resolution CT scan of the chest of a patient with bronchiectasis. Varicose bronchiectasis with lack of airway tapering and abnormal airway contour is evident *(V).* Areas of cystic dilation are also seen *(C).*

drome caused by a generalized bronchial cartilage deficiency, the tracheobronchomegaly of Mournier-Kuhn syndrome, and yellow nail syndrome when bronchiectasis is associated with discolored nails, lymphedema, and pleural effusions.

Bronchiectasis may be acquired after severe infection or chronic endobronchial obstruction. Common infectious culprits include adenovirus, measles, mumps, pertussis, and mycobacteria. Bronchiectasis has been described following influenza, mycoplasma, and other community-acquired pneumonias, as well as complicating human immunodeficiency virus infection and chronic aspiration pneumonitis. The allergic reaction to airway colonization with *Aspergillus* (ABPA) and other fungi can cause a diffuse central bronchiectasis. Localized postobstructive bronchiectasis can result from foreign bodies, tumors, broncholiths, or granulomas occluding the airway. Inhalational injury from smoke, ammonia, and paraquat can cause bronchiectasis. Some chronic inflammatory conditions such as inflammatory bowel disease, rheumatoid arthritis, relapsing polychondritis, and Sjögren's syndrome can result in bronchiectatic airway changes, although the causal relationship remains a mystery.

Unless the patient's history or physical examination defines the etiology, a thorough laboratory evaluation is mandated. The extent of lung involvement evident on CT may help limit the differential diagnosis. Most inherited anomalies will have a diffuse distribution whereas postobstructive acquired disorders will show focal involvement (Fig. 59-5). Measurement of immunoglobulins and IgG subclasses and assessment of neutrophil number and function are important. Sputum cultures may reveal tuberculosis, *Aspergillus,* or mucoid

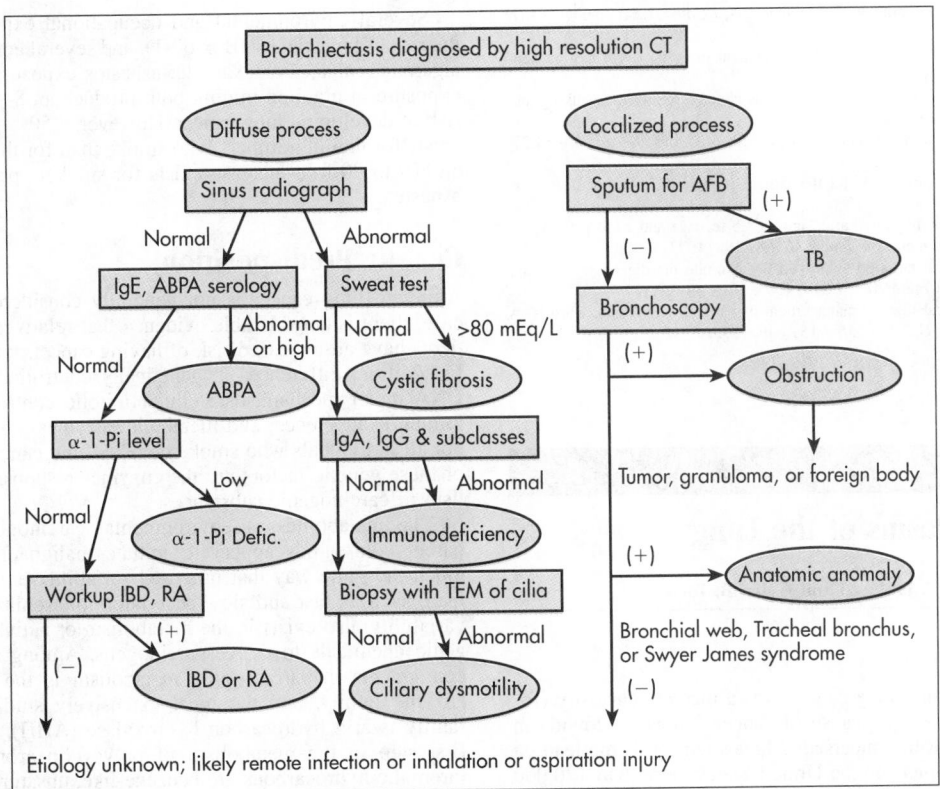

FIGURE 59-5   Algorithm for the workup of a patient with bronchiectasis when the etiology is not apparent after thorough history and physical examination. *ABPA,* Allergic bronchopulmonary aspergillosis; α-*1-Pi,* alpha-1-proteinase inhibitor; *IBD,* inflammatory bowel disease; *RA,* rheumatoid arthritis and other rheumatologic conditions, including Sjögren's syndrome and relapsing polychondritis; *TEM,* transmission electron microscopy, *AFB,* acid-fast bacilli.

✔ WHEN TO REFER

Surgical resection is indicated only if a localized process is associated with moderate to severe symptoms refractory to medical therapy in a patient with sufficient pulmonary reserve to ensure reasonable postoperative functional status. Massive hemoptysis not amenable to arteriographic embolization constitutes an emergent surgical indication. In most series, removal of ectatic segments required lobectomy more often than either segmentectomy or pneumonectomy. Operative mortality ranges from 1% to 8%, and postoperative morbidity, including empyema and bronchopleural fistula, occurs in up to 38% of cases. Although patients with a successful surgical outcome reported greater symptomatic improvement than medically managed control subjects in one study, there was no survival advantage. Bilateral lung transplantation is a surgical option for patients with severe diffuse disease. However, the prognosis has improved such that only about 5% of patients with non-CF bronchiectasis succumb to their pulmonary disease.

cally to remove the obstruction. Inflammatory conditions such as ABPA, sarcoid, rheumatologic, and inflammatory bowel disease may be amenable to antiinflammatory therapies. α-1-Pi deficiency can be treated with intravenous administration of the protein.

Permanently damaged airway segments can be managed medically or surgically. The mainstays of medical regimens are mucus clearance techniques, infection prophylaxis with vaccination (pneumococcal vaccine and yearly influenza vaccination), and aggressive antibiotic treatment of respiratory exacerbation guided by in vitro sensitivities of the individual patient's respiratory flora. Bronchodilators and inhaled or parenteral antiinflammatory drugs are usually limited to situations in which reactive airways are demonstrated. In the later stages, meticulous attention to nutritional status and supplemental oxygen therapy may be of benefit.

BIBLIOGRAPHY

Andersen MP et al: Demonstration that CFTR is a chloride channel by alteration of its anion selectivity, *Science* 253:202, 1991.

Annest LS et al: Current results of treatment of bronchiectasis, *J Thorac Cardiovasc Surg* 83:546, 1982.

Collins FS: Cystic fibrosis: molecular biology and therapeutic implications, *Science* 256:774, 1992.

de Groot R, Smith AL: Antibiotic pharmacokinetics in cystic fibrosis. Differences and clinical significance, *Clin Pharmacokinet* 13:228, 1987.

di Sant'Agnese PA, Davis PB: Cystic fibrosis in adults: 75 cases and a review of 232 cases in the literature, *Am J Med* 66:121, 1979.

FitzSimmons S: The changing epidemiology of cystic fibrosis, *J Pediatr* 122:1, 1993.

Fuchs HJ et al: Effect of aerosolized recombinant human DNase on exacerbations of respiratory symptoms and pulmonary function in patients with cystic fibrosis, *N Engl J Med* 331:637, 1994.

Knowles MR et al: A controlled trial of adenoviral-vector-mediated gene transfer in the nasal epithelium of patients with cystic fibrosis, *N Engl J Med* 333:823, 1995.

Koch C, Hoiby N: Pathogenesis of cystic fibrosis, *Lancet* 341:1065, 1993.

Konstan MW et al: Effect of high dose ibuprofen in patients with cystic fibrosis, *N Engl J Med* 332:848, 1995.

Pseudomonas characteristic of CF. Ultrastructural evaluation of cilia can be performed on nasal or tracheobronchial cells but may be confounded by changes acquired because of inflammation. The diagnostic approach should focus on etiologies that are amenable to therapy.

Management

Treatment of the underlying etiology is important to prevent disease progression. Postobstructive bronchiectasis can be approached surgi-

Naidich DP et al: Computed tomography of bronchiectasis, *J Comp Assist Tomogr* 6:437, 1982.

Ramsey BW et al: Nutritional assessment and management in cystic fibrosis: a consensus report, *Am J Clin Nutr* 55:108, 1992.

Rommens JM et al: Identification of the cystic fibrosis gene: chromosome walking and jumping, *Science* 245:1059, 1989.

Shennib H et al: Double lung transplantation for cystic fibrosis, *Ann Thorac Surg* 54:27, 1992.

Stern RC: The primary care physician and the patient with cystic fibrosis, *J Pediatr* 114:31, 1989.

Stern RC et al: Cystic fibrosis diagnosed after age 13: 25 teenage and adult patients including three asymptomatic men, *Ann Intern Med* 87:188, 1977.

Stewart B et al: Normal sweat chloride values do not exclude the diagnosis of cystic fibrosis, *Am J Respir Crit Care Med* 151:899, 1995.

Thomas J et al: Chest physical therapy management of patients with cystic fibrosis. A meta-analysis, *Am J Respir Crit Care Med* 151:846, 1995.

CHAPTER

60 Neoplasms of the Lung

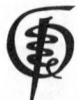

Michael C. Iannuzzi and Galen B. Toews

At the turn of this century, lung cancer was a medical curiosity. Today it has become the leading cause of cancer deaths worldwide in both men and women; it has superseded breast cancer as the leading cancer killer among women. In the United States more than 170,000 new cases of lung cancer are detected each year, with lung cancer accounting for more than 150,000 deaths at an annual health care cost of more than $12 billion.

The causal relationship between smoking and lung cancer was clearly established in case-control and cohort studies reported in the 1950s and 1960s. Tobacco smoking accounts for about 90% of all lung cancers. More recent studies show that differences in smoking behavior affect lung cancer risk and that passive smoking increases risk. It is also becoming increasingly evident that genetic susceptibility plays a role in lung cancer risk.

The diagnosis of lung cancer is generally not difficult. Management focuses on two questions: Is the tumor resectable? and What therapy is suitable to the patient's cardiopulmonary status? Treatment may then be directed at either potential cure or palliation, although cure is largely limited to patients with non–small cell carcinoma that is resected at an early stage. Despite the progress made in understanding and treating lung cancer, the overall 5-year survival for patients with lung cancer ranges from 10% to 13%. This dismal fact is particularly disturbing when one recognizes that lung cancer is a preventable disease.

ETIOLOGY AND PATHOGENESIS

The most important etiologic factor in lung cancer is cigarette smoke. The dramatic increase in cigarette smoking that is responsible for the current lung cancer epidemic began during the first two decades of this century and was due to the invention of machines that allowed mass manufacturing of cigarettes and the development of techniques that allowed mass marketing. Cigarette smoke contains more than 4000 chemical constituents and produces disease through diverse mechanisms. Some of the more important classes of carcinogens in cigarette smoke include polycyclic aromatic hydrocarbons, nitrosamines, aromatic amines, and adelyhydes. It should be noted that tar, which varies with the pattern of inhalation, is not a good measure of the dose of toxic or carcinogenic agents received by the individual smoker.

Epidemiologic studies have examined the effect of passive smoking on lung cancer risk. The most common approach in these studies has been to evaluate risk in nonsmokers who are married to smokers. There appears to be a statistically significant increase in the lung cancer risk of about 20% to 30% in the nonsmoking spouse with risk even greater to those who are married to heavy smokers.

Several environmental and occupational exposures also increase the risk of lung cancer (Box 60-1), and several act synergistically with cigarette smoke. For example, asbestos exposure and radon particle exposure in uranium mining both produce an 8- to 10-fold increased risk of developing lung cancer. However, a 50- to 60-fold greater risk exists for uranium miners who smoke than for those who do not, and an 80- to 90-fold increase exists for smokers previously exposed to asbestos.

Genetic Predisposition

Although lung cancer is not generally considered an inherited disease, there is considerable evidence that relatives of lung cancer patients have an increased risk of having cancer, including lung cancer. In addition, differences in genetically controlled processes, such as DNA repair mechanisms, cellular mitotic control, protease activity, immunocompetence, and metabolic enzymes are likely reasons why not all individuals who smoke develop lung cancer. The best defined of these genetic factors are the enzymes responsible for the metabolism of carcinogenic substances.

The metabolites of environmental carcinogens rather than the parent compounds appear to initiate malignant transformation. In much the same way that inherited variability exists in drug metabolism, such as fast and slow acetylators of isoniazid (INH), inherited variability also exists in the metabolism or activation of procarcinogenic chemicals to active carcinogens. Among the most important components in carcinogenic metabolism is the cytochrome P-450 enzyme family, and the most extensively studied enzyme in this family is aryl hydrocarbon hydroxylase (AHH). AHH catalyzes the first step in the metabolism of polycyclic aromatic hydrocarbons (aromatic hydrocarbons are benzene-like, unsaturated, six-membered carbon rings), the metabolites of which cause DNA mutations. Several studies have compared the metabolism of the antihypertensive drug debrisoquine in lung cancer cases and controls and found an eightfold higher risk of lung cancer in extensive metabolizers. Debrisoquine has only one metabolite, 4-hyroxy-debrisoquine, and debrisoquine metabolism correlates with the metabolism of many other chemicals, some of which are thought to be carcinogens that are present in tobacco smoke.

Besides enzymes involved in carcinogen metabolism, certain inherited cancer genes appear to predispose patients to lung cancer. For example, abnormalities in the tumor suppressor gene, the retinoblastoma susceptibility gene (rb), have been found in small cell lung cancer (SCLC). Studies of more than 4000 relatives of patients with retinoblastoma revealed a 15-fold increased risk of lung cancer.

BOX 60-1
Risk factors for lung cancer

Cigarette smoke
Carcinogens
Radon particles: uranium mining

Cocarcinogens
Arsenic: smelters, glass workers, manufacture of pesticides
Asbestos: insulation workers, textile workers, asbestos users
Coal dust: road workers, coke oven workers, roofers
Chromium: leather, ceramic, and metal workers, tanners
Chloromethyl methyl ether: chemical plant workers
Vinyl chloride: plastic workers

Pulmonary fibrosis
Scleroderma
Interstitial pulmonary fibrosis
Pneumoconiosis
Bronchiectasis
Scars attributable to infarcts
Mycobacterial disease
Lung abscess

PATHOLOGY

The histologic classification of primary lung cancer recommended by the World Health Organization is listed in Box 60-2. Four histologic types of lung cancer make up 95% of all primary lung neoplasia, and the frequency of the various histologic types has been changing. Adenocarcinoma has become the most frequent histologic type, accounting for 40% to 50% of all lung cancer. Squamous cell carcinoma accounts for about 30%; small cell, 20%; and anaplastic large cell, less than 10%. It is important to distinguish the cell types because of differences in their natural history and response to treatment. The following is a brief review of the characteristic histologic and pathologic features of each of the lung cancer cell types.

Squamous cell or epidermoid carcinoma, once the most prevalent lung carcinoma, has been surpassed by adenocarcinoma. Squamous cell carcinoma arises from the central bronchi in about 80% of cases. Because these cells tend to exfoliate, this tumor can be detected at an earlier stage by sputum cytologic examination. These tumors tend to be slow growing and it is estimated that up to 4 years are required from the development of in situ carcinoma to clinically apparent tumor. On light microscopy the neoplastic cells appear flattened to polygonal, tend to stratify, and form intercellular bridges. The presence of keratin "pearls" indicates well-differentiated to moderately differentiated growth. Squamous cell lung cancer makes up more than half of the superior sulcus tumors (Pancoast's tumors) and is the most common tumor to cavitate. Cavities are generally thick walled, usually without air fluid levels, and portend a poor prognosis. Squamous carcinoma tends to metastasize late. Lymph nodes, adrenal gland, and liver are the favored sites of metastases; bone metastases are lytic and infrequent.

Small cell carcinoma is distinguished by a proliferation of cells with dark, round to oval nuclei that are more than twice the size of a lymphocyte. These cells have meager cytoplasm in relation to their nuclei, so molding (indentation of one nucleus pressed by another) of adjacent cells occurs, with arrangement of the cells in ribbons, nests, and sheets. The meager cytoplasm is also thought to be responsible for frequently finding "crushing" on biopsy. Like squamous cell carcinoma, small cell carcinoma tends to be a central lesion. Small cell lung cancer is characterized by rapid development, frequent metastases, and low resectability. At presentation more than 80% of patients have had symptoms for less than 3 months. This is in contrast to patients with squamous cell lung carcinoma, in whom average symptom duration is as long as 8 months, and to those with adenocarcinoma, nearly 25% of whom are asymptomatic at presentation. At diagnosis more than 70% of patients with SCLC have widely metastatic disease.

Adenocarcinoma forms acinar and glandular structures with or without mucin formation. In addition to cigarette smoking, adenocarcinoma is the cell type most closely linked to pulmonary fibrosis and may arise in areas of previous scars in the lung. Unlike squamous cell and small cell carcinoma, most adenocarcinomas occur in the periphery of the lung. The metastatic pattern of adenocarcinoma is not much different from that of small cell carcinoma. Distant metastases occur early and frequently. Bone metastases are frequently blastic.

Bronchioloalveolar carcinoma (BAC) is a variant of adenocarcinoma that constitutes about 5% of all lung carcinomas. It is the only histologic type of lung cancer that is not closely linked to smoking. BAC is a peripheral, well-differentiated neoplasm that tends to spread locally throughout the air spaces. Because it may be difficult to distinguish BAC from metastatic adenocarcinoma, other supporting criteria that aid diagnosis include the absence of a primary endobronchial carcinoma and the absence of other organ involvement. The cell of origin for this tumor has been controversial. Potential cells of origin are the mucin-secreting bronchial epithelial cells, nonciliated secretory bronchiolar cells, and type II alveolar epithelial cells. Other unusual features of this neoplasm include a more common occurrence in women, who account for 30% to 50% of all cases, and a chest x-ray that may demonstrate multinodular lesions which indicate multicentric origin or diffuse, fluffy infiltrates.

Large cell carcinoma is a category used for lung cancer cells that lack light microscopic evidence of glandular or squamous differentiation that allows them to be typed as either squamous or adenocarcinoma. As molecular techniques for identifying the different lung cancer cells types have been improved, fewer lung cancers are placed in this category. The cells are large, bizarre, pleomorphic, multinucleated, and round or spindle shaped. Large cell carcinoma generally arises in the lung periphery and is often necrotic and quite large. Large cell carcinoma may invade locally or metastasize widely.

Any combination of the four main cell types may occur. Adenosquamous carcinoma, which is the most common (1% to 2%) tends to occur more peripherally than does squamous cell carcinoma.

MOLECULAR BIOLOGY OF LUNG CANCER

The importance of cytogenetic abnormalities and the role of oncogenes in lung cancer are presently being defined. A consistent chromosomal abnormality has been described SCLC, namely a deletion in the short arm of chromosome 3. Chromosome 3 deletions have also been identified in renal tumors, ovarian carcinoma, Wilm's tumor and rhabdomyosarcoma. What role the loss of the chromosome 3 segment plays in the malignant process in SCLC is not yet known. One hypothesis is that a gene or gene family in the deleted DNA segment codes for some factor which suppresses a growth-regulating gene or group of genes elsewhere in the genome. This is analogous to mechanisms proposed in the childhood cancer retinoblastoma. Multiple chromosomal abnormalities have been seen in non–SCLC; however, a specific, recurring chromosome defect has not been noted.

Various growth factors secreted by malignant cells in culture have been identified. Some of these growth factors and their receptors are encoded by oncogenes. The endogenous production of growth factors, called autocrine secretion, appears to free the cell from external physiologic controls that normally inhibit growth and thus serves as a constant stimulus for cell division. Other mechanisms for uncontrolled growth include production of defective growth factor receptors that are constitutively activated, increased number of receptors occurring as a consequence of gene amplification, and defective intracellular signal transducers transmitting growth-promoting signals without any external stimulus. Bombesin, a tetradecapeptide initially isolated from amphibian skin, is one example of an autocrine growth factor for SCLC cells, and monoclonal antibodies to bombesin, as well as to other growth factors and their receptors, may offer potential therapy in lung cancer.

Members of two families of oncogenes, myc and ras, appear to be important in the development of lung cancer. The myc family of oncogenes codes for nuclear proteins, and the ras gene family codes for proteins, that bind guanine nucleotides (G proteins) involved in growth-signal transduction. Members of the myc family of protooncogenes (c-myc, L-myc, and N-myc) are frequently amplified and overexpressed in SCLC and have been associated with more aggressive and drug-resistant tumors. The ras oncogene has been found to be activated in some adenocarcinoma specimens; however, the significance of this is not yet defined. The importance of oncogenes in cancer is discussed further in Chapters 70 and 99.

CLINICAL PRESENTATION

More than 75% of lung cancer patients are affected in the fifth to sixth decade of life. Lung cancer rarely occurs in persons under 35

BOX 60-2

World Health Organization (WHO) classification of malignant neoplasms

  I. Squamous (epidermoid) carcinoma
 II. Small cell carcinoma
III. Adenocarcinoma
 IV. Large cell carcinoma
  V. Combined cell types
 VI. Carcinoid tumors
VII. Bronchial gland tumors
      A. Cylindromas
      B. Mucoepidermoid
VIII. Papillary tumors

years of age. The initial signs and symptoms (Box 60-3) are variable and depend on the location of the tumor, the cell type, rapidity of growth, whether metastasis has occurred, the ectopic production of peptides and hormones, and the presence of underlying pulmonary disease. Systemic symptoms are common and include weight loss and malaise. In a small percentage of patients (5% to 15%) lung cancer is detected before the onset of symptoms, usually by routine chest radiography. Following are the common signs and symptoms of lung cancer.

Cough is the most frequent initial symptom of lung cancer, but since it is a common symptom in many chronic respiratory disorders, it is often overlooked. Cough may be produced by an endobronchial mass acting as a foreign body or by invasion and ulceration of the bronchial mucosa. Patients who have a persistent cough, particularly if they are 40 years of age or older, should have a chest radiograph. The production of sputum along with cough is of diagnostic value because it provides material for cytologic examination.

Hemoptysis occurs in about 35% to 45% of patients with bronchogenic carcinoma and may vary from blood-streaked sputum to more significant amounts. Massive hemoptysis in lung cancer is rare. Of all patients who come to medical attention with hemoptysis, lung cancer is responsible in about 20%. The absence of roentgenologic abnormalities should not discourage the clinician from ruling out an underlying malignancy, since the cancer may erode the bronchial wall and vessels early, before becoming apparent on radiographic examination.

Chest pain, most commonly ipsilateral to the tumor, is usually described as a dull, intermittent ache lasting minutes to hours, but may be severe, constant, penetrating and pleuritic, indicating metastatic involvement of the pleura. Shoulder and arm pain that is constant may be caused either by a superior sulcus (Pancoast's tumor) or by tumor invading the diaphragm. Other signs of superior sulcus tumors include weakness of the hand and Horner's syndrome. Horner's syndrome,

the result of involvement of the sixth cervical segments, consists of a drooping upper eyelid, constricted pupil, and narrowed palpebral fissure.

Hoarseness because of left-side vocal cord paralysis attributable to carcinoma or nodal metastases involving the left hilum or aortic arch is common. The long, tortuous intrathoracic course of the left recurrent laryngeal nerve makes it more susceptible than its counterpart on the right to tumor involvement.

Wheezing, when it is unilateral and present in certain body positions, suggests partial bronchial obstruction. A localized wheeze may be heard in the absence of chest roentgenologic abnormalities.

Superior vena cava syndrome is most frequently caused by lung cancer (75% to 80%). The clinical manifestations vary with how quickly obstruction develops. Patients may complain of headache, a feeling of fullness in the head, visual difficulties, dyspnea, cough, dysphagia, or syncope. Physical findings include dilated neck veins, conjunctival edema, plethora and edema of the face and neck, swelling of the arms, and distended veins over the chest. Diagnosis may be confirmed by ultrasonography or contrast-enhanced computed tomography (CT) of the chest. Venography is generally unnecessary and potentially hazardous. Recent studies have emphasized the relative safety in pursuing a definitive diagnosis rather than initiating emergent empiric treatment. If signs and symptoms are mild and chronic and no evidence of increased intracranial pressure exists, histologic diagnosis may be obtained safely by sputum cytologic examination, fiberoptic bronchoscopy, or mediastinoscopy before treatment.

Pleural involvement with effusion may result in dyspnea (60%) and cough (40%). Lung cancer is the most common cause of malignant pleural effusion, followed by breast cancer and lymphoma. The effusion in lung cancer is most often ipsilateral to the tumor mass, exudative (a ratio of pleural fluid protein to serum greater than 0.5 and a ratio of lactate dehydrogenase (LDH) in pleural fluid to serum greater than 0.6), and frequently hemorrhagic. A low pleural fluid pH (<7.3) correlates with a greater diagnostic yield on cytologic examination, a worse prognosis, and a poorer response to pleurodesis. Since direct pleural involvement is a contraindication to curative surgery, other mechanisms that may cause pleural effusion in patients with lung cancer should be kept in mind. These other mechanisms include mediastinal lymph node involvement with impaired lymphatic drainage, disruption of the thoracic duct with chylothorax formation, bronchial obstruction with atelectasis or postobstructive pneumonia, and pulmonary embolism.

Cardiac and pericardial involvement is frequent, underdiagnosed, and noted at autopsy in up to 20% to 25% of patients with SCLC and less frequently in patients with non-SCLC. Patients may complain of dyspnea, which is often mistakenly attributed to coexistent pleural effusion.

Electrocardiograms usually show only sinus tachycardia with changes in voltage that are often subtle and recognized only after comparison with previous tracings. Enlargement of the cardiac silhouette on chest x-ray is also often subtle and appreciated only after comparison with previous x-rays. Other signs of cardiac involvement include atrial arrhythmias, hypotension, pericardial friction rub, pulsus paradoxus, and, if cardiac tamponade develops, Kussmaul's sign (increase in jugular venous pressure on inspiration).

THE PARANEOPLASTIC SYNDROMES

Paraneoplastic syndromes are metabolic and neuromuscular disturbances unrelated to the primary tumor, metastasis, or effects of therapy. They are diverse and occur with all the lung cancer cell types, although they are seen most frequently with SCLC. The most common syndromes are the syndrome of inappropriate antidiuretic hormone secretion (SIADH), Cushing's syndrome from ectopic adrenocorticotropic hormone (ACTH) production, hypercalcemia, hypertrophic osteoarthropathy, neuromyopathies, and the Eaton-Lambert syndrome.

SIADH is caused by neoplasms in more than 50% of patients, and SCLC accounts for the vast majority of these neoplasms. SIADH results from the persistent, excess release of antidiuretic hormone (ADH, arginine vasopressin) and is characterized by hyponatremia, volume expansion without edema, renal sodium loss, hypouricemia, and inappropriately high urine osmolarity. SIADH is diagnosed by

---

BOX 60-3
Clinical presentation and signs and symptoms of lung cancer

Local tumor growth
Cough
Dyspnea
Hemoptysis
Wheezing
Pneumonia
Fever

Local extension
Chest pain
Hoarseness
Dysphagia
Superior vena cava obstruction
Pancoast's syndrome
Horner's syndrome

Metastasis
Bone pain
Headache
Abdominal pain
Pericardial effusion
Lymphadenopathy
Hepatomegaly
Pleural effusion

Paraneoplastic syndromes
Cushing's syndrome
Hypercalcemia
Hypertrophic osteoarthropathy and clubbing
Syndrome of inappropriate antidiuretic hormone secretion (SIADH)
Neuromyopathies
Eaton-Lambert syndrome
Trousseau's syndrome (venous thrombosis)

first excluding hypovolemia and by determining that thyroid and adrenal function is normal. Normal to decreased serum blood urea nitrogen (BUN) and creatinine levels, a urinary sodium concentration that exceeds 30 mEq/L, and a fractional excretion of sodium (FENa) greater than 1% indicate that the patient is euvolemic or has slight volume expansion. The inappropriate secretion of ADH in this clinical setting is then recognized by a urine osmolality greater than 120 to 150 mOsm/kg of water in association with reduced serum osmolality. Treatment of SIADH, as is the case for all the paraneoplastic syndromes, is best managed by effective therapy for the underlying disease. For the patient who has symptoms of hyponatremia (somnolence or confusion) or a serum sodium concentration less than 125 mEq/L, it is prudent to restrict water intake to 600 to 800 ml/day or to administer demeclocycline (300 mg three times daily). Demeclocycline, a tetracycline derivative, produces a reversible partial nephrogenic diabetes insipidus by antagonizing the renal tubular effect of ADH. Since compliance with fluid restriction is often difficult, demeclocycline is the usual treatment of choice.

In ectopic ACTH syndrome, hypokalemic metabolic alkalosis and muscle weakness are usually the predominant manifestations, although clinical and laboratory features may be subtle, such as glucose intolerance, mild hypertension, hyperpigmentation, and hirsutism. Physical changes such as moon facies, "buffalo hump," and striae are uncommon, perhaps because of the relatively short survival of these patients. SCLC is the cell type most frequently associated with ectopic ACTH syndrome. ACTH levels are very high and, unlike in classic Cushing's syndrome associated with pituitary adenoma, ACTH levels are not suppressible by high doses of dexamethasone. Like SIADH, the ectopic ACTH syndrome is best managed by effective therapy for the underlying disease; however, severe hypokalemia or hypertension may occur and requires immediate treatment.

Gynecomastia occurs in about 2% of patients with SCLC and has been reported in a few patients with non-SCLC. Gynecomastia may be caused by decreased testosterone or excessive gonadotropins.

Hypercalcemia is a common finding in patients with lung cancer (overall frequency is 12.5%) and varies with the histologic type (25% with squamous, 13% with large cell, and 3% with adenocarcinoma). Hypercalcemia is not associated with SCLC, and if found, another etiologic factor should be sought, such as hyperparathyroidism. Hypercalcemia was thought to occur because of direct bone destruction by cancer cells, but it is now evident that hypercalcemia, even in patients with extensive osteolysis, is mediated by factors either released or induced by malignant cells. Hypercalcemia is not due to bone metastasis. In fact, while bone metastases are frequent in SCLC (66%) and adenocarcinoma (50%), hypercalcemia is infrequent. Hypercalcemia in the majority of solid tumors appears to be caused by a parathyroid-like hormone (PLP) or PTH-related hormone that shares an N-terminal sequence similar to PTH in its first 13 amino acids. The clinical features of hypercalcemia include lethargy, psychiatric disturbances, anorexia, nausea, vomiting, abdominal discomfort, constipation polyuria, thirst, and renal insufficiency. Treatment of malignant hypercalcemia depends on its degree of severity and is discussed further in Chapter 312.

Hypertrophic osteoarthropathy (HOA) is most commonly seen in lung cancer patients and is characterized by the presence of periosteal new bone formation, arthritis, and clubbing of the digits. Hypertrophic osteoarthropathy occurs in up to 30% of patients with lung cancer, although it is rare in SCLC. HOA may precede the diagnosis of lung cancer in up to one third of patients. The symptoms are nonspecific and include joint pain, soft tissue swelling, and limitation of motion. Radionuclide bone scans typically demonstrate increased uptake at the distal ends of the affected long bones with sparing of the spine. Various mechanisms for HOA have been suggested, but none has been proven. Symptoms may respond to nonsteroidal antiinflammatory agents and are usually relieved by removal of the primary tumor.

Neuromyopathies may occur in association with lung cancer and includes encephalopathy, myelopathy, sensory and mixed sensorimotor neuropathies and polymyositis. Autoimmune, infectious, nutritional, and toxic causes have all been suggested.

Eaton-Lambert syndrome, or myasthenic syndrome, is closely associated with SCLC and may precede the appearance of the tumor by more than a year. Patients generally have easy fatigability and proximal muscle weakness, predominately in the pelvic girdle and lower extremities. Patients show weakness on first attempts at muscle contraction, but unlike in myasthenia gravis, repeated efforts increase their muscle strength. Other associated symptoms include dry mouth, muscle discomfort, impotence, and paresthesias. Electromyograms show a pathognomonic increase in amplitude on repetitive stimulation. Successful treatment of the tumor is often associated with relief from the Eaton-Lambert syndrome. Guanididine hydrochloride and plasmapheresis may be beneficial.

NERVOUS SYSTEM METASTASIS

Nervous system metastases are a major cause of morbidity and mortality in patients with lung cancer and may be the sole metastatic site. The incidence of brain metastasis by histologic type of lung cancer is listed in Table 60-1. For SCLC the risk increases as survival is prolonged; brain metastasis occurs in 80% of patients living for more than 2 years after diagnosis. The signs and symptoms are not different from those in patients with other metastatic tumors. Symptoms may have an abrupt onset and include headache, change in mental status, ataxia, focal weakness, and aphasia. Leptomenigeal metastases most frequently occur in SCLC and become evident with involvement of multiple areas of the neuraxis. Symptoms include headache, cranial nerve palsies, and altered mental status. Lung cancer is also the most common tumor to metastasize to the spine and accounts for up to 30% of these patients. Pain occurs in more than 90% of patients with spinal cord compression, and the onset of pain usually precedes the development of weakness, sensory changes, and autonomic dysfunction by days or weeks. However, once these later symptoms and signs develop, the course is rapid and the chances for reversing the neurologic changes with treatment greatly diminish.

DIAGNOSIS AND STAGING

The goal of diagnosis and staging is to answer the following questions: What is the histologic type? Is the tumor resectable? and Is the patient physically able to withstand treatment? This process begins with a thorough history, physical examination, and chest radiograph. The signs and symptoms of lung cancer are discussed earlier. The following is a discussion of the radiographic signs of lung cancer and the techniques used for diagnosis and staging.

The earliest radiographic signs of lung cancer are often overlooked. As many as 90% of peripheral cancers and 75% of central tumors have been reported to be visible in retrospect on prior radiographs. These early signs include enlargement of one hilum, a small homogenous density with sharp or poorly defined borders, a streaked infiltrate, and signs of volume loss (e.g., atelectasis, displacement of a fissure). Other radiographic findings of lung cancer include solitary pulmonary nodule, rounded peripheral mass, cavitary lesion, and pneumonia. A recurrent, persistent, or incompletely resolved infiltrate also suggests malignancy. Lack of air bronchograms in an opacified segment of lung should direct attention to the central bronchi in search of an endobronchial lesion. Volume loss in a consolidated lobe or a large pleural effusion with ipsilateral volume loss suggests bronchial obstruction and should raise suspicion of malignancy.

Computed tomography has added to the diagnosis and staging of lung cancer. Computed tomography can confirm the presence of a lung mass that was suspected from chest x-ray, define its extent, determine the presence of additional lung lesions, and demonstrate the location of enlarged mediastinal and hilar lymph nodes.

Sputum cytologic examination, bronchoscopy and percutaneous needle biopsy are the most common tests used to obtain histologic

Table 60-1 Incidence of brain metastases in lung cancer

TUMOR	INCIDENCE (%)
Squamous cell	15
Adenocarcinoma	25
Large cell	28
Small cell	30

diagnosis. Sputum cytologic study is a useful, relatively inexpensive, noninvasive test that is effective when at least three consecutive specimens are obtained and read by an experienced cytopathologist. Respiratory therapists or physiotherapists can frequently help to obtain satisfactory material for sputum examination by using techniques to induce sputum production, such as percussion and inhalation of aerosolized saline solutions. The yield is 30% in the absence of symptoms, 50% when cough is present, and 70% when hemoptysis is present; however, the yield drops to 15% to 20% for peripheral lesions. The yield of sputum cytologic study is also influenced by the histologic type and is most commonly positive with squamous cell carcinoma and least likely with small cell carcinoma. This occurs because squamous cell grows as a fungating endobronchial mass, whereas small cell carcinoma grows as a submucosal plaque. An important factor affecting the yield of sputum cytologic study is the training and experience of the cytopathologist who reads the results.

Fiberoptic bronchoscopy has proved very useful in the diagnosis of lung cancer. Combining bronchial washings, brushings, and forceps biopsy at the time of bronchoscope gives a yield of 85% to 95% for bronchoscopically visible lesions. About two thirds of lung cancer are seen through the fiberoptic scope. For peripheral masses not visible through bronchoscopy, transbronchial biopsy under fluoroscopic guidance is used. The yield with this procedure is a function of tumor size: about 30% for masses less than 2 cm and 65% to 70% for those larger than 2 cm. Thin-needle aspiration via a transtracheal or transbronchial approach has extended the role of bronchoscopy. This method is useful for identifying subcarinal, paratracheal, and parabronchial nodal disease and for aspirating peripheral nodules. The complications of fiberoptic bronchoscopy are minimal with a reported mortality of 0.02% and significant morbidity (arrhythmias, bronchospasm, drug reactions, hemorrhage, hypotension, and pneumothoraces) in less than 0.5% of patients.

Percutaneous fine-needle aspiration (FNA), performed under fluoroscopic or CT guidance, may be used to obtain material for cytologic examination, particularly for lesions that are not readily accessible by flexible fiberoptic bronchoscopy, such as small peripheral nodules. The yield is 90% to 95% but the incidence of pneumothorax requiring chest tube placement is higher with percutaneous FNA than with bronchoscopic biopsy.

When pleural effusion is detected on radiographic examination, thorocentesis may allow diagnosis if the pleural effusions arose because of direct pleural invasion or metastatic involvement. It should be noted that pleural effusions may also arise as a result of postobstruction pneumonitis, central lymphatic obstruction, or pulmonary embolism. A positive cytologic diagnosis can be made from pleural fluid in 40% to 75% of cases. If cytologic examination of the pleural effusion is normal, the diagnostic yield of thorocentesis may be increased by repeating thorocentesis. The pleural fluid obtained on repeat thorocentesis often contains freshly denuded cells, which aids cytologic diagnosis. Pleural biopsy increases the diagnostic yield only slightly, by about 5%. Pleural biopsy has a low diagnostic yield because metastasis generally involves only small areas of the pleural surface, making it highly unlikely that the involved area will be hit by blind pleural biopsy, and in about 50% of patients the costal parietal pleura is not involved.

Routine biopsy of nonpalpable scalene or supraclavicular nodes produces a very low diagnostic yield and is not recommended. However, with palpable supraclavicular nodes the yield for detection of metastasis is about 90%. The information gained can be valuable for both diagnosis and staging.

A variety of enzyme and hormone tumor products have been investigated as tumor markers. If sensitive, specific tumor markers could be found, they would be useful in screening high-risk populations, diagnosis, staging, prognostication, and monitoring of therapy. At present tumor markers that would be helpful in the diagnosis of lung cancer do not exist.

Staging guides the physician in assessing prognosis, designing treatment, and comparing treatment protocols between studies and study groups. The approach to staging lung cancer depends on the cell type. In patients with non-SCLC the tumor, node, and metastasis (TNM) system, which emphasizes the extent of tumor involvement of surrounding structures, is applied. Stages I and II disease is considered operable and stage III disease, in general, inoperable, although

some patients with stage III disease, because of their young age and cardiopulmonary status and the anatomic location of tumor, may be considered for resection. A reciprocal correlation exists between the anatomic extent of the primary tumor and survivability. In non-SCLC (for $T_1N_0M_0$) patients with all three cell types (squamous, adenocarcinoma, and large cell) have a 60% to 80% 5-year survival. For $T_2N_0M_0$, 50% of patients with squamous carcinoma and 40% with adenocarcinoma or large cell type survive 5 years. Survival dramatically decreases with nodal involvement and with metastasis: 20% to 40% for stage IIA disease and less than 20% for stage IIIB.

The TNM system is not useful in SCLC, primarily because more than 85% of patients have stage III disease at presentation. For SCLC a simple two-stage classification is used. Patients are classified as having either limited or extensive disease. Limited disease is defined as disease confined to one hemithorax and the mediastinum with or without supraclavicular lymph node involvement. The limited-stage group also includes patients with pleural effusions and contralateral hilar and contralateral supraclavicular lymph node involvement. The presence of any one or all of these findings does not appear to alter prognosis. Extensive disease is defined as any disease more advanced than limited. Staging and therapy of lung cancer are discussed in detail in Chapter 99.

SCREENING

Once the diagnosis of lung cancer has been made, a staging evaluation eliminates 85% to 90% of patients from curative resection. Because early detection is necessary for cures, several studies have evaluated the role of screening populations at high risk for lung cancer. These studies have examined the role of chest radiographs every 6 months and chest radiographs combined with sputum cytologic study and have demonstrated that aggressive use of these screening tests can lead to the early detection of limited-stage cancer in a high-risk population, but screening does not decrease overall mortality compared with unscreened groups. These studies have been criticized because they were performed in the 1970s, before the increase of lung cancer in women became apparent, and so were limited to male cigarette smokers; the groups compared may not have been balanced with regard to lung cancer risk; and the studies were insufficiently powered to detect a benefit below a 50% improvement in overall survival. Therefore at this time, although insufficient proved benefit exists to recommend intensive mass screening of all high-risk individuals, the decision to screen patients is left to the individual physician and patient. Innovative early detection tools using sputum immunocytochemisty techniques and in situ polymerase chain reaction are now being developed that may improve the use of sputum cytologic examination to detect early-stage lung cancer.

TREATMENT

Treatment is based on the cell type, the stage of disease, and the patient's general condition. The individual roles of chemotherapy, surgery, radiation therapy, and immunotherapy are discussed in Chapter 99. Surgical removal of the tumor is the preferred therapy for patients with non-SCLC. The overall operative mortality is less than 4%. The operative mortality for pneumonectomy is presently about 6% and for lobectomy, 3%. Staging evaluation eliminates 85% to 90% of patients from curative resection. All potentially operable patients should have thorough evaluation to determine their ability to undergo lung resection. Despite numerous studies, no firm guidelines are available for criteria that prohibit resectional surgery.

Prior history of cardiac disease doubles the risk of major operative morbidity (20% vs. 10%) and pulmonary function may be further compromised by removal of pulmonary tissue. Therefore the preoperative evaluation for any patient in whom surgery is contemplated includes a thorough evaluation of the cardiac and respiratory systems. Box 60-4 lists a general approach for determining surgical risk based on clinical assessment, lung spirometry, and arterial blood gas determinations. Traditionally patients are suitable candidates for pneumonectomy if forced expiratory volume in 1 second (FEV_1) is greater than 1.2 L. For patients with marginal lung function, further studies may be necessary. Exercise physiology studies help further define the significance of mildly abnormal arterial blood gas values. Ventilation-

---

BOX 60-4
Candidates for surgery

Should probably not undergo resection
Elevated partial pressure of carbon dioxide (Pco_2)
Dyspnea at rest
Predicted postoperative forced expiratory volume in 1 second (FEV_1)
  <0.8 L
Pulmonary hypertension
Cor pulmonale

Should undergo further pulmonary evaluation
Hypoxia
Moderate dyspnea on exertion
Predicted postoperative FEV_1 of 0.8 to 1.2 L
Heart disease

Eligible for resection
Normal arterial blood gas values
Good exercise tolerance
FEV_1 >50% predicted

BOX 60-5
Uncommon "benign" neoplasia in the lung

Bronchial adenoma
Hamartoma
Papilloma
Fibroma
Lipoma
Hemangioma
Teratoma
Leiomyoma
Chondroma
Endometriosis
Pseudolymphoma

---

perfusion scanning may aid in determining the effect of surgical resection on lung function and can be used to help predict the postoperative lung function.

For patients with unresectable primary lung carcinoma or who are unable to withstand surgery, radiation therapy can achieve complete local control of primary tumor in up to 75% of patients, resulting in prolonged survival. Radiation therapy may also be useful as adjuvant therapy together with chemotherapy for SCLC and before and after surgery for non-SCLC. Radiation therapy palliates regional symptoms and distant metastasis and is used for superior vena cava obstruction and superior sulcus tumors, pain control, neurologic complications such as brain metastases and spinal cord compression, pericardial effusion, and hemoptysis.

A common problem during the course of lung cancer is *endobronchial obstruction* with postobstructive pneumonitis. Radiation therapy is often helpful in relieving obstruction and is generally used for the first occurrence of obstruction. Frequently, endobronchial obstruction is due to recurrence of neoplasia in an area that had been previously irradiated. Surgical resection is usually contraindicated in these cases because of extent of tumor or poor pulmonary function, and further radiation therapy may not be possible. The development of laser treatment via the bronchoscope has allowed for a new approach to this problem. Endobronchial tumors respond quickly to laser therapy, and patients can have relief from obstruction. The potential complications, however, are serious and include bleeding, perforation, and fistula formation. This procedure is also limited by the rapid recurrence of the tumor. Despite these complications and limitations, it is possible to palliate disease in patients who have failed other therapies and have significant difficulties, particularly dyspnea, because of obstructing tumors.

PREVENTION

The greatest impact on the prevention of lung cancer can be made by helping patients who smoke to quit; after cessation of smoking for 10 to 15 years the risk for lung cancer decreases to near that of nonsmokers. Tobacco dependence is best conceptualized as a chronic disease, which requires that the patient be informed of the medical risks of continued smoking, as well as the medical benefits that can be expected from stopping. A treatment plan should be designed according to the individual's needs and may include medication, use of a self-help manual, behavior modification, and support groups. Several studies have recently shown that nicotine substitution, such as by transdermal nicotine patches, can facilitate tobacco withdrawal by alleviating or even preventing abstinence symptoms.

Chemoprevention, the use of nutrients or pharmacologic compounds to inhibit or reverse carcinogenesis, is actively being investigated in patients at risk for lung cancer. The impetus for the search of chemopreventive agents comes primarily from epidemiologic studies in which individuals who consumed large amounts of food rich in vitamin A and beta-carotene, such as carrots and vegetables, are at significantly reduced risk for lung cancer. Potential agents that are being evaluated include vitamins such as A, C, E and folate; minerals such as calcium, molybdenum, and selenium; natural products such as carotenoids; and synthetics such as N-acetyl-cysteine. Further research aimed at identifying molecular and cytogenetic markers to detect early precancerous changes may provide effective techniques to identify high-risk individuals, making chemoprevention practical.

UNCOMMON "BENIGN" NEOPLASIA IN THE LUNG

There are a several uncommon and rare neoplasms that may arise in the lung (Box 60-5). These tumors arise from the epithelium or mesenchyme of lung tissue. Although many of these tumors appear benign on histologic examination, many are potentially malignant. The radiologic and clinical manifestations depend on the relationship of the neoplasm to the airway. Thus there may be obstructive or nonobstructive findings and symptoms.

Bronchial Adenoma

The bronchial adenomas, which make up about 1% of all primary lung neoplasms, represent a heterogeneous group of lesions with differences in pathogenesis, morphologic features, and malignant potential. The term "bronchial adenoma" is a misnomer, since these tumors can metastasize to regional lymph nodes and more distal sites. Three histologic categories exist: carcinoid adenoma, mucoepidermoid bronchial tumor, and cylindroma or adenoid cystic carcinoma. Carcinoid adenoma or bronchial carcinoid occurs most frequently and makes up over 80% of the adenomas.

Bronchial carcinoids arise from Kulchitsky's or K cells, which are located between columnar epithelial cells in the basal part of the bronchial epithelium. K cells are also thought to be the cell of origin for SCLC and have amine precursor uptake and decarboxylation (APUD) properties. Adenoid cystic carcinomas arise from the bronchial glands, which predominate in the proximal airways. Bronchial carcinoids are classified as typical or atypical. The atypical carcinoids differ from the typical carcinoids by the their greater nuclear atypia and mitotic activity. Atypia is associated with an increased incidence of lymph node and distal metastasis.

Most bronchial adenomas occur in the mainstem bronchi or in the proximal portion of lobar bronchi, although they may arise more peripherally in the terminal bronchioles. Patients have intermittent cough, hemoptysis, and postobstructive pneumonia. The most frequent physical finding is localized dullness with decreased or absent breaths sounds and decreased fremitus caused by bronchial obstruction. A chest radiograph confirms the physical findings, demonstrating volume loss and consolidated lung parenchyma. This is similar to obstructing bronchogenic carcinoma. Diagnosis is made either at bronchoscopy or thoracotomy. Endobronchial biopsy may be accompanied by moderate to severe hemorrhage in up to one fourth of patients. However, this complication is generally not associated with the need for transfusion or thoracotomy and does not preclude diagnosis by bronchoscopy.

Bronchial carcinoid infrequently causes the carcinoid syndrome, but when it does, these symptoms are similar to those of intestinal carcinoid. Unlike intestinal carcinoid tumors, which rarely metastasize to bone and skin and which produce the carcinoid syndrome when liver metastases are present, bronchial carcinoid more often involves the bone and skin and produces the syndrome in the absence of metastases. Substances elaborated by carcinoid tumors may produce sclerosis of cardiac valves downstream from the site of their origin or metastases, that is, right-side heart valves with abdominal tumors, and left-side heart valves with lung tumors. Symptoms and signs that constitute the clinical carcinoid syndrome include episodic flushing, anxiety, tremulousness, diarrhea, lacrimation, salivation, wheezing, tachycardia, facial edema, and hyperthermia.

Bronchial adenomas are treated by surgical resection, preserving as much normal lung tissue as possible. The 10-year survival for patients with carcinoid without metastasis is 98% compared with 22% for patients with metastasis.

Hamartomas

Hamartomas, the most common benign tumors of the lung, result from developmental malformations and are composed of tissues normally found in the lung: cartilage, bronchial epithelia, bronchial glands, smooth muscle, fibrous tissue, and fat. Pulmonary hamartomas are usually diagnosed in patients between the fourth and seventh decades of life, but may occur in much younger persons. A 2:1 to 3:1 male preponderance has been reported in most studies. Most patients are asymptomatic with the tumor detected incidentally on chest x-ray. Almost all hamartomas lie in the peripheral parenchyma, and less than 10% are found endobronchially. The chest radiograph usually shows a well-circumscribed solitary nodule, usually less than 4 cm in diameter. Calcification is uncommon (5% to 25% of patients), but a "popcorn" pattern strongly suggests the diagnosis. Hamartomas may enlarge slowly, but more rapid growth can occur, causing a new nodule to appear in adult life. Because the tumor is infrequently found endobronchially, diagnosis is made either by transthoracic needle aspiration or thoracotomy.

Papillomas

Papillomas, caused by human papillomavirus (HPV) types 6 and 11, most often become evident as laryngeal tumors in children but may become evident in adulthood. A benign neoplasm on histologic examination, papilloma can be either solitary or, in its most troublesome form, multiple. The sites involved are in the larynx and include the true vocal folds, epiglottis, and false vocal folds. Tracheobronchial papillomatosis rarely develops without a prior history of tracheotomy or laryngeal lesions. Papillomas contain vascular connective tissue covered by stratified squamous epithelium and occasionally, ciliated respiratory epithelia. These tumors characteristically obstruct airways, resulting in peripheral atelectasis and obstructive pneumonia.

PULMONARY METASTASIS

The lung, with its rich vascular and lymphatic networks, is a frequent site of metastasis for a variety of tumors. Lung metastasis usually occurs by way of hematogenous dissemination of tumor emboli arising from invasion of thin-walled capillaries with delivery into the lung through the pulmonary artery. Other pathways include lymphatic spread, endobronchial metastases by way of bronchial invasion from a parenchymal or mediastinal mass, and bronchial arterial spread. About 30% of all cases of neoplastic disease metastasize to the lung. The estimated occurrence of pulmonary metastases by primary malignancy is given in Table 60-2. Metastasis may become evident as a solitary nodular lesion, but in 75% of cases the lesions are multiple. Certain primary tumors are more likely than others to become evident as solitary metastasis: sarcomas; melanoma; and kidney, colon, testicular, and breast carcinomas. Endobronchial metastasis is less common than parenchymal metastasis and occurs with breast, kidney, colon, and rectal carcinomas; melanoma; and cancers of the thyroid, female genital tract, testes, prostate, and pancreas. Lymphangitic pulmonary metastasis is most frequently seen with cancers of the breast, stomach, thyroid, and pancreas.

Because of the peripheral or subpleural locations of metastases, 85% to 95% of patients are asymptomatic. Cough and hemoptysis are very uncommon, since metastatic lesions rarely erode the bronchial wall. The most common respiratory symptom is dyspnea, which may occur from airway obstruction, pleural effusion, or lymphangitic spread. The treatment of pulmonary metastases includes surgical excision, radiotherapy, and chemotherapy, or a combination of these. Surgical excision results in improved survival when the tumor has a long doubling time (>40 days).

SUMMARY

Lung cancer is the predominant fatal neoplasm in the United States and is almost totally preventable, since it is largely due to smoking. Other risk factors may act alone or synergistically with tobacco smoke to produce lung cancer and can be identified by eliciting a thorough occupational and past medical history. Although a greater understanding of genetic influences on lung cancer susceptibility may also help to identify patients who are particularly at risk for the carcinogenic effect of tobacco smoke, the physician can have a major impact on this disease by helping all patients who smoke to quit.

The presentation and means of diagnosis have been reviewed. Knowledge of the pathologic classification and natural history of the different histologic types of lung cancer is important for deciding which treatment course is best for individual patients. Determining the extent or stage of disease and assessing the cardiac and respiratory status are necessary to decide on either an aggressive or a supportive course. A small percentage of patients may be cured of their disease, but the vast majority will have intractable, recurrent disease. Certain complications, such as the paraneoplastic syndromes, the superior vena cava syndrome, and endobronchial obstruction with obstructive pneumonia, require specific measures for palliation. Methods for early detection and more effective therapy are desperately needed.

BIBLIOGRAPHY

American Cancer Society (1993) Cancer Facts and Figures, Atlanta, 1993, American Cancer Society.

Carbone DP, Minna JD: The molecular genetics of lung cancer, *Adv Intern Med* 37:153-171, 1992.

Greenwald P, Kelloff, G, Burch-Whitman C, Kramer BS: Chemoprevention, *CA Cancer J Clin* 45:31-49, 1995.

Ihde DC: Small cell lung cancer, *Chest* 107:243S-248S, 1995.

Lin AY, Ihde DC: Recent developments in the treatment of lung cancer, *JAMA* 267:1661-1664, 1992.

Mountain CF: The new international staging system for lung cancer, *Surg Clin North Am* 67:925-935, 1987.

Mulshine JL, Treston AM, Scott FM et al: Lung cancer: rational strategies for early detection and intervention, *Oncology* 5:25-32, 1991.

Pass HI: Bronchial adenoma, *Ann Thorac Surg* 52:1201-1203, 1991.

Rusch VW: Pulmonary metastasectomy, *Chest* 107:322S-331S, 1995.

U.S. Centers for Disease Control and Prevention: Tobacco or health, *MMWR* 42:12, 1993.

Table 60-2 Estimated occurrence of pulmonary metastases by primary malignancy

PRIMARY MALIGNANCY	OCCURRENCE (%)
Choriocarcinoma	80
Osteosarcoma	75
Kidney carcinoma	70
Thyroid carcinoma	65
Malignant melanoma	60
Breast carcinoma	55
Prostatic carcinoma	45
Nasopharyngeal carcinoma	20
Gastrointestinal tract	20
Gynecologic carcinoma	20

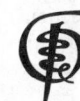

61 Solitary Pulmonary Tumor

Thomas Y. Sullivan

DEFINITION AND ETIOLOGY

A *solitary pulmonary nodule* is a small (no more than 5 cm in diameter), rounded, intrapulmonic density with more or less smooth margins. The original term used to describe a solitary nodule, *coin lesion,* has generally been abandoned because the mass is spheric rather than flat. A solitary pulmonary nodule is found in 1 in every 2000 chest radiographs, making this lesion a frequent diagnostic and therapeutic problem. The nodule itself seldom produces symptoms and is often discovered as an incidental finding on a routine chest radiograph.

Many different processes can produce a solitary pulmonary nodule (Table 61-1), and the frequency of each differs among reported series. If the series includes only persons participating in a community chest radiograph screening program, the incidence of lung cancer is very low. If the series includes only patients suspected of having cancer and referred for surgical resection, the incidence of lung cancer is understandably much higher. Benign lesions are usually granulomas associated with tuberculosis, other mycobacteria, or fungi.

The likelihood that a solitary nodule is lung cancer is directly related to the patient's age. Only 1% of solitary nodules are malignant in patients less than 35 years old, but 50% to 60% are malignant in patients age 50 or older. The likelihood that a nodule is lung cancer is also directly related to the amount of previous cigarette smoking. All cell types of lung cancer can present as a solitary nodule, but most malignant nodules are adenocarcinoma or squamous cell carcinoma.

The average 5-year survival of patients who have resection of a malignant solitary nodule is 30% to 50%. This is clearly better than the 10% survival rate of patients who have surgical resection of more advanced lung cancer. Therefore each solitary nodule represents a potentially resectable and curable lung cancer. In the evaluation it is essential to determine whether the lesion is suspicious for a malignancy and should be removed promptly, or whether it has features that strongly favor a nonmalignant process that can be managed without resection.

Table 61-1 Causes of solitary pulmonary nodules

CAUSE	RANGE OF REPORTED INCIDENCE (%)
Malignant tumors	
Bronchogenic carcinoma	16-52
Bronchial adenoma (certain cell types seem benign and have benign courses)	1-2
Metastatic carcinoma	1-10
Benign tumors	5-12
Hamartoma	1-2
Fibroma	0-1
Granulomas	
Histoplasmosis	5-38
Tuberculosis	10-15
Coccidioidomycosis	2-14
Cryptococcosis	0-1
Miscellaneous	
Bronchogenic cyst	1-3
Arteriovenous malformation	0-1
Bronchopulmonary sequestration	0-1
Sclerosing hemangioma	0-1
Intrapulmonary lymph node	0-1

DIAGNOSTIC EVALUATION

Separation of benign from probably malignant lesions relies heavily on the chest radiograph. If serial chest radiographs show the development of a nodule during resolution of pneumonia, pulmonary contusion, or pulmonary infarction, the lesion is clearly benign. If vessels are seen entering a nodule, an arteriovenous fistula should be suspected. Other radiographic findings suggesting benignity include small size, increased density, smooth borders, calcification, and absence of growth during a reasonable period of observation.

Reliable radiographic indicators of benign disease are certain calcification patterns noted within the nodule and absence of growth demonstrated by no change on chest radiographs taken 2 or more years apart. The patterns of calcification that indicate benignity include diffuse speckled or "popcorn" pattern (Fig. 61-1), large central nidus (Fig. 61-2), and concentric calcification (Fig. 61-3). A large central nidus or concentric calcification is found in granulomas; popcorn calcification occurs in hamartoma. A small fleck of calcium in the center or periphery of a nodule is a common finding in a granuloma; therefore this type of calcification suggests a benign disease. However, rarely lung cancer may develop a fleck of calcification or engulf a nearby calcified granuloma. Also, metastatic osteogenic sarcoma may calcify. Because of these unusual examples, a small fleck of calcium within a nodule is not a completely reliable sign of benignity.

Growth rate of a solitary nodule can be estimated from change in size on serial chest radiographs. A small increase in diameter indicates a greater increase in volume. A mass doubling in diameter has increased in volume eightfold, and a mass has doubled in volume when its diameter has increased by about one-fourth. Fig. 61-4 shows how the serial diameter of a nodule can be plotted on semilogarithmic paper against the number of days of observation to determine the doubling time. Doubling time of lung cancer ranges from 15 to

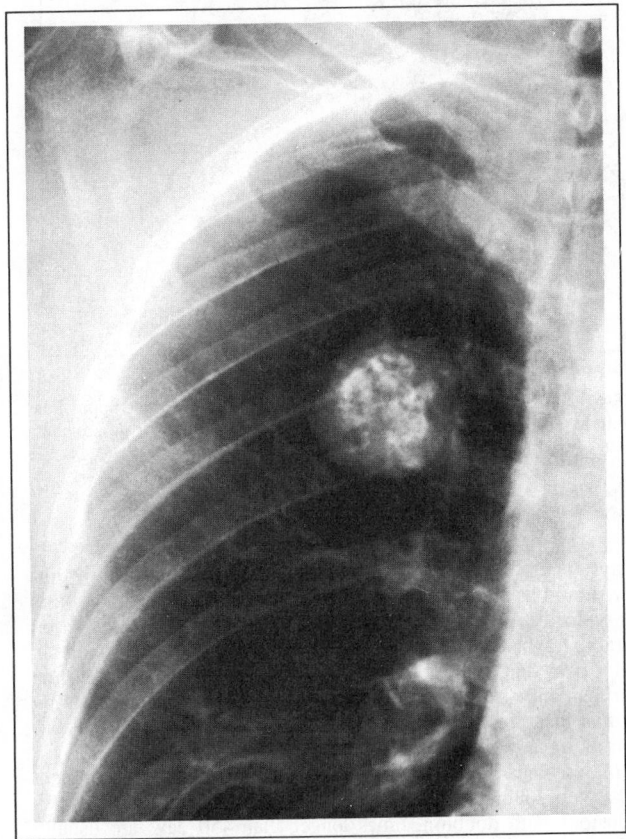

FIGURE 61-1 Standard chest radiograph demonstrating a right upper lobe nodule in an asymptomatic patient with diffuse "popcorn" calcification characteristic of a benign hamartoma.

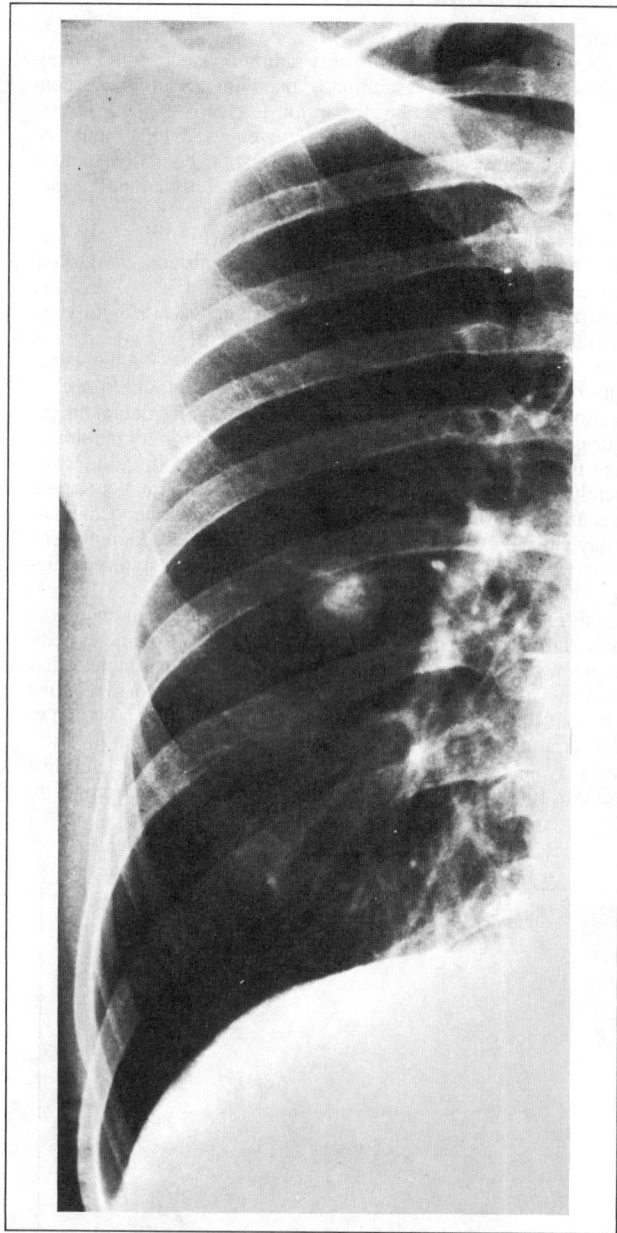

FIGURE 61-2   Standard chest radiograph demonstrating a right upper lobe nodule in an asymptomatic patient with a large central nidus of calcium characteristic of a granuloma.

450 days. Thus, if a lesion is malignant, a detectable increase in diameter should be expected within 2 years. Doubling time is the basis of the typically used practice of comparing the size of the lesion on chest radiographs taken 2 or more years apart. Lack of any change in diameter over that time indicates that the lesion has a doubling time greater than 450 days and therefore should be considered benign. Any lesion that increases in diameter during a 2-year period must be considered malignant until proved otherwise.

Benign lesions have their own natural histories and development periods, with doubling times that overlap those of lung cancer. However, lesions with doubling times longer than 450 days are usually granulomas. Lesions with very rapid doubling times (less than 15 days) are almost always inflammatory processes such as pneumonia or vasculitis, if primary or metastatic sarcoma can be excluded.

Several other clinical tests have been used to help decide whether a solitary nodule is benign or malignant. Skin tests for tuberculous and fungal serologies are often done but may reflect concomitant disease or previous exposures and are not reliable indicators of the etiology of a nodule. Sputum examinations for tuberculosis and fungi may give more specific and reliable information but are seldom positive because small numbers of organisms exist within infectious granulomas. Sputum smears are obtained for cytologic examination but also do not have a high diagnostic yield even in proved cases of malignant solitary nodule.

Two additional diagnostic procedures have become useful in the evaluation of a solitary nodule: fiberoptic bronchoscopy with transbronchial brushing, needle biopsy, or forceps biopsy; and transthoracic needle biopsy. Fiberoptic bronchoscopy with transbronchial biopsy has a diagnostic yield of 20% to 40% in patients with malignant nodules. Success decreases with decreasing size of the lesion, more peripheral location, and upper lobe lesions. Risk of hemorrhage or pneumothorax with transbronchial brushing is 5% and increases to 10% to 15% with a forceps biopsy. Transthoracic needle biopsy has an 80% to 95% diagnostic yield in patients with malignant nodules. Risk of pneumothorax is slightly greater than with bronchoscopic biopsy and is much greater if the patient has underlying bullous emphysema. To ensure a high diagnostic yield with needle biopsy, it is helpful for a cytopathologist to be present during the aspiration, immediately examine the specimen, and advise the physician performing the aspiration if repeat sampling is indicated.

Characteristics of the borders of the lesion and calcification may be defined with tomograms or computed tomography (CT) (see Fig. 61-3). With CT, density is expressed as relative CT units. Density of the nodule can also be compared with density of a "phantom" nodule with known calcification placed in the scanner. Lesions with calcification density are likely granulomas; less dense lesions can be either benign or malignant. Chest CT may also show other small nodules that were not apparent on the routine chest radiograph, suggesting metastatic malignancy or a variety of other diseases, including Wegener's granulomatosis, fungal infections, and occasionally sarcoidosis.

In nonmalignant conditions, the diagnostic yield of bronchoscopic or needle biopsies varies with the interest and skill of physicians performing the procedures and examining the specimens. The false-negative rate of a cytologic diagnosis of "benign disease" is unclear but of major concern. If acid-fast or fungal organisms are found, one can be secure in a diagnosis of nonmalignant disease; however, a finding of "inflammatory cells" is nonspecific and might be misleading because these types of cells can be found at the edge of a malignancy. Perhaps the major usefulness of biopsy procedures, especially transthoracic needle biopsy because of its higher yield, is in speeding the diagnosis of lung cancer. A rapid diagnosis will decrease the time and cost of hospitalization and prevent delaying necessary surgical resection.

CLINICAL MANAGEMENT

When dealing with a solitary nodule, a logical and sequential management scheme is essential (Fig. 61-5). The first step is examination of previous chest radiographs. It may be possible to show that the lesion has not changed in more than 2 years and therefore can be considered benign. If there are no previous films for comparison, or if a lesion has increased in size within 2 years and does not show any of the patterns of benign calcification, the lesion must be presumed to be cancer. Age and smoking history are important determinants of management. Older patients who smoke should be presumed to have malignant nodules.

The next consideration is that a solitary nodule may represent metastasis from a primary cancer elsewhere in the body. The primary cancer may not be apparent, and the clinician must be suspicious of any symptom or abnormality detected on physical examination. Abnormal laboratory tests or bleeding into the stool or urine prompt evaluation for an occult malignancy. However, an extensive search for a nonlung cancer that may have metastasized to the lung should be done only when there is a symptom, abnormal physical finding, or other simple clue. Extensive evaluation for occult malignancy in all patients with a solitary nodule is otherwise too often unrewarding and quite expensive.

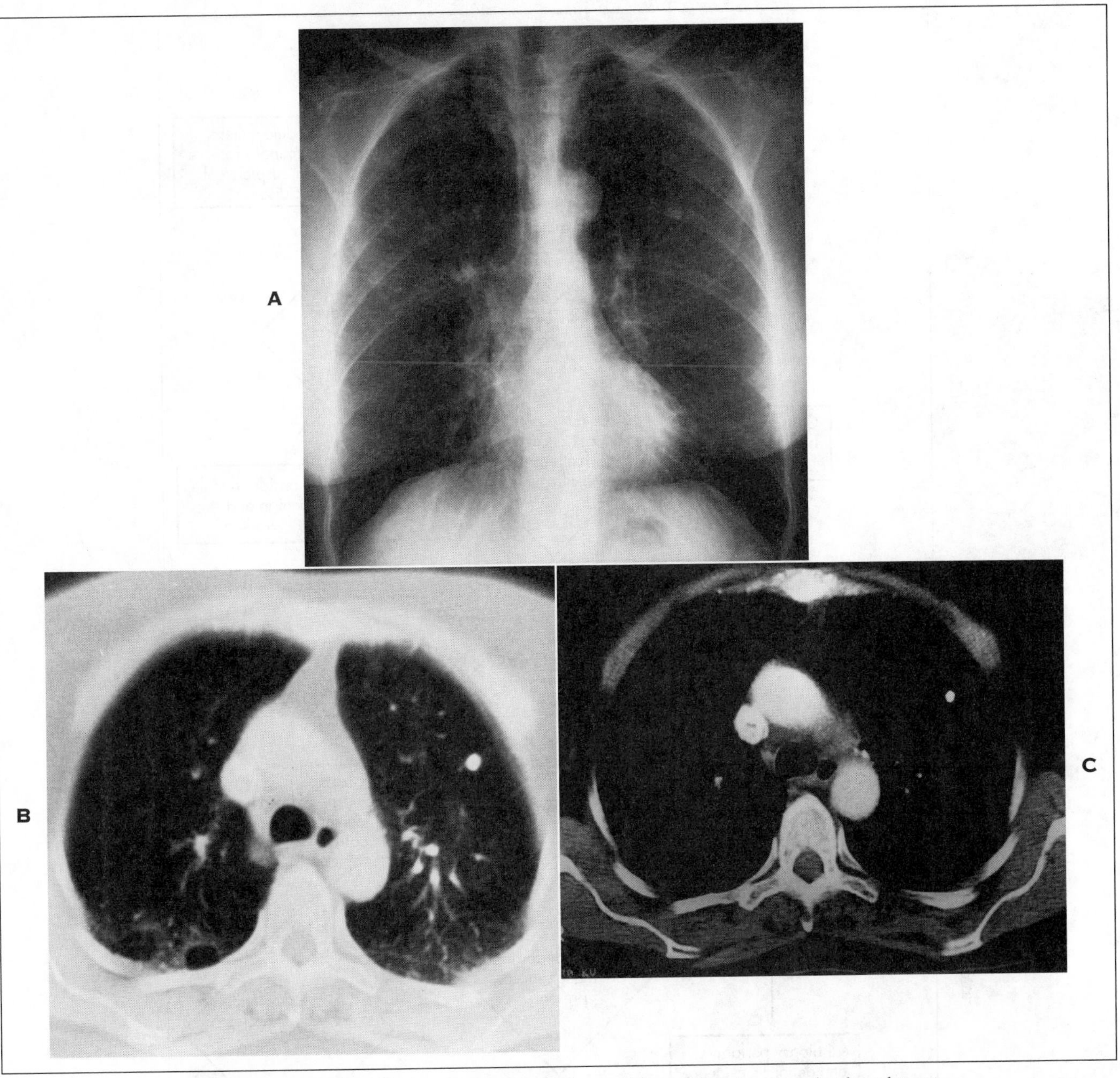

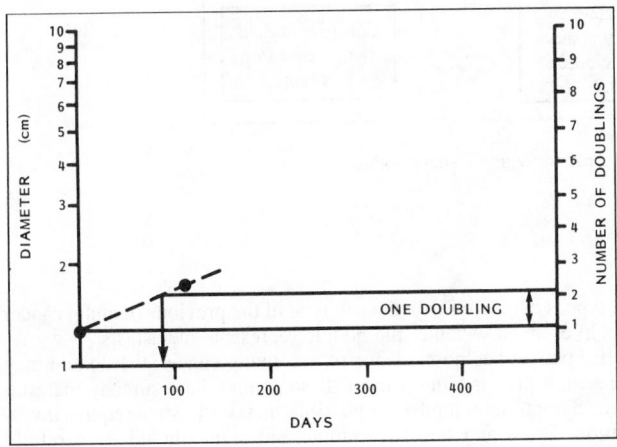

FIGURE 61-3   **A,** Chest radiograph showing a small left upper lobe nodule that is somewhat dense but not obviously calcified. **B,** Chest CT scan showing calcification on lung windows. **C,** Chest CT scan with mediastinal windows again showing dense calcification of the nodule.

FIGURE 61-4   Plot of diameter of a nodule in centimeters and number of doublings on chest radiographs taken 110 days apart. The nodule has increased in diameter from 1.3 to 1.6 cm, indicating that it has a doubling time of approximately 90 days. This lesion should be considered malignant until proved otherwise.

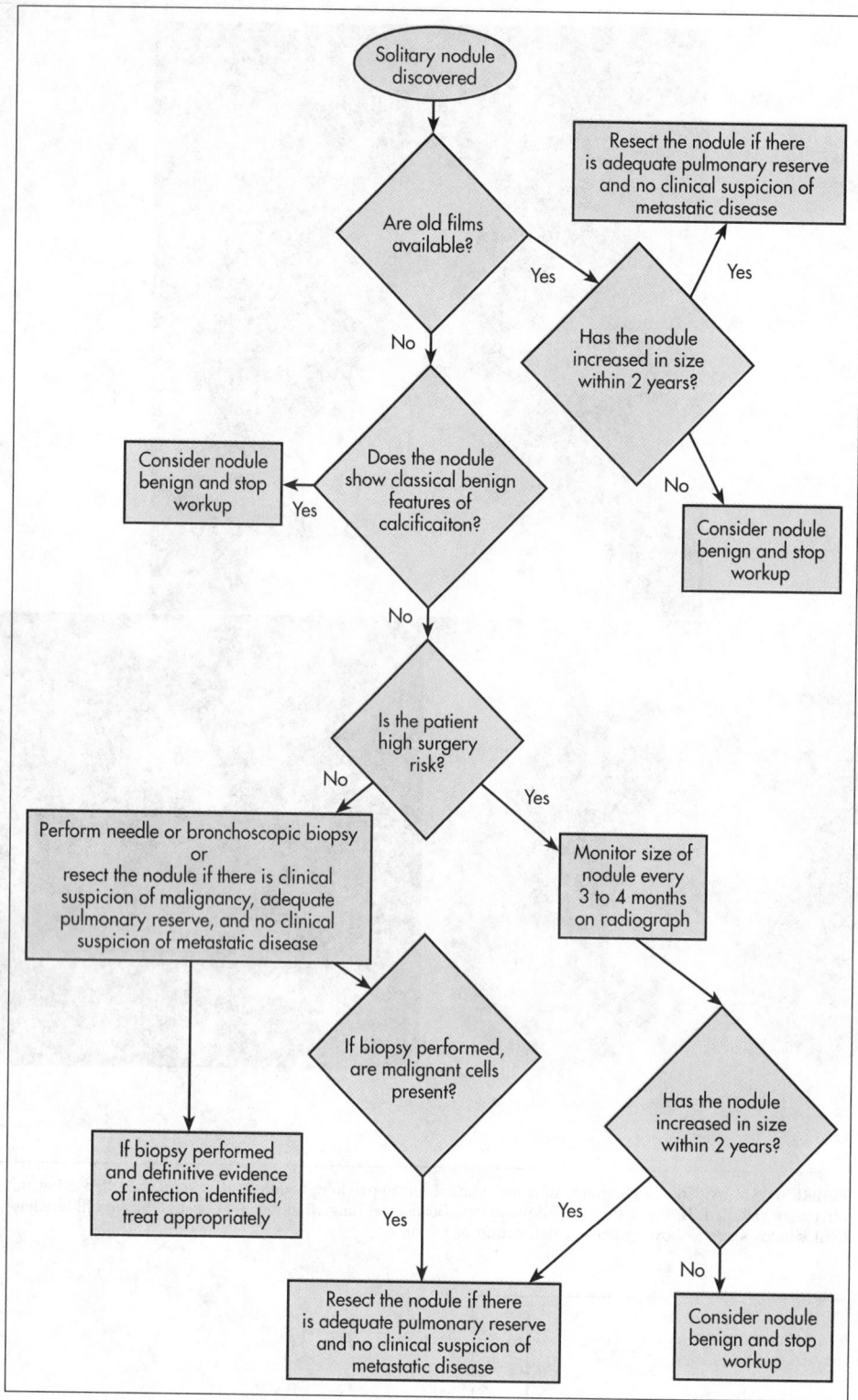

FIGURE 61-5   Algorithm for approach to the patient with a solitary nodule.

A solitary nodule occurring in a patient with known nonlung cancer may represent a metastasis but is a second cancer—a primary lung cancer—in slightly more than half the cases. In patients with a solitary nodule and history of previously treated nonlung cancer, it is appropriate to proceed with bronchoscopic or transthoracic needle biopsy without delay. If the cytology from the biopsy shows malignancy, the cell type is compared with the cell type of the previous nonlung cancer to help establish whether the nodule represents metastasis.

If a patient has no evidence of a nonlung cancer, the nodule may represent a primary lung cancer. If so, it may have already metastasized. Symptoms referable to possible metastatic sites require investigation. Brain and bone symptoms and signs should be carefully sought. Liver chemistries and blood calcium are checked. If no symptoms and no abnormal physical findings or blood tests exist, an extensive search for metastasis is generally unrewarding and not recommended. At that point in the evaluation, it is often apparent that the solitary nodule may represent a primary lung cancer without obvious metastasis.

Because the treatment of primary lung cancer is surgical resection, it is imperative to determine the patient's ability to withstand surgery. The patient's general medical health must be evaluated, and many have other medical problems, especially chronic obstructive pulmonary disease. Pulmonary function tests should be measured, and a forced expiratory volume at 1 second (FEV_1) greater than 2000 ml and absence of elevated arterial carbon dioxide tension ($Paco_2$) indicate that the patient can probably tolerate a lobectomy or pneumonectomy. Patients who have lower values of FEV_1 should be evaluated with nuclear lung scan techniques that determine regional lung function. It is important to be certain that lung function is not distributed so that the part with good function may be resected and the poorly functioning part left in the patient. Using these techniques, it is possible to predict postresection pulmonary function, and a predicted postoperative FEV_1 greater than 800 ml is likely adequate to proceed with surgery. If a patient has evidence of significant obstructive lung disease, it is prudent to treat aggressively with bronchodilators and then repeat pulmonary function tests before making a decision about surgery.

If the patient's pulmonary function is adequate to withstand surgical resection of the nodule, it must be decided (1) if the patient should go to surgery promptly, (2) if an attempt should be made to obtain tissue from the lesion to establish a diagnosis, or (3) if the lesion could be watched with serial chest radiographs (i.e., "watchful waiting"). The first approach, prompt resection of the nodule, is often advocated. A factor always important to consider is the morality and morbidity associated with thoracotomy. Mortality is unusual in young healthy patients but may approach 10% in patients with significant underlying cardiopulmonary disease, and all patients experience significant chest pain and the risk of developing postoperative pneumonia. Selective use of surgery for only malignant lesions is the ideal approach but may or may not be possible. It is often helpful to proceed with either bronchoscopic or needle biopsy. If no specific benign diagnosis is obtained, lung cancer is sufficiently likely that diagnostic/therapeutic surgical resection of the nodule is then appropriate.

Occasionally a patient with a nodule may be at high risk for surgery. Examples might be a patient with a recent myocardial infarction or a patient with multiple medical problems and only marginal pulmonary function to tolerate lung resection. In these extreme cases surgery may be delayed and the nodule followed with repeat chest radiographs. For example, the film could be repeated in 2 weeks. If no change occurs in the size of the nodule, the film is repeated in 4 weeks. The interval between radiographs is progressively increased until a total of 2 years of follow-up has accumulated. If the nodule does not increase in size during that time, it is assumed to be benign. If the nodule increases in size, it likely is malignant, and a decision about surgery must be made. The risk of cancer spreading during such "watchful waiting" is unknown.

FUTURE CONSIDERATIONS

The solitary pulmonary nodule will continue to be a difficult problem for the patient and physician. The smoking habit of the population ensures that concern about lung cancer will be present for many years, and success with treatment for most lung cancers has advanced little over the past 50 years. Since the best results in treatment occur if lung cancer is resected while it is localized as a solitary nodule, there will continue to be keen interest in removing a nodule whenever the clinical picture is not diagnostic of a benign process.

The most promising clinical developments will probably include further standardization and acceptance of CT evaluation of solitary nodules. These may include improvements in CT densitometry techniques, especially nodule simulators or so-called phantom nodules that allow density calibration on each CT scanner. Such developments may allow confident separation of nodules that are very unlikely to be malignant from those that may or may not be malignant. Another

development that may prove useful is combining information from the CT with that from bronchoscopic or needle biopsy. A CT-directed biopsy has the advantage of proving that the specimen came directly from the nodule. This might increase the diagnostic yield, especially in nonmalignant nodules, and increase the level of confidence in a cytopathologic diagnosis of "chronic inflammation." Immunologic staining techniques that identify the etiology of previous fungal or other infectious granulomas could also be helpful.

BIBLIOGRAPHY

Harvey JC, Beattie EJ: Surgical treatment of solitary and multiple metastatic tumors to the lung, *Compr Therapy* 19(5):238, 1993.
Higgins GA: The solitary pulmonary nodule: ten-year follow-up of Veterans Administration—Armed Forces Cooperative Study, *Arch Surg* 110:570, 1975.
Lillington GA: Management of solitary pulmonary nodules, *DM*, May 1991.
Pugatch RD: Radiologic evaluation in chest malignancies. A review of imaging modalities, *Chest* 107(6 Suppl):294S, 1995.
Steele JD, Buell P: Asymptomatic solitary pulmonary nodules: host survival, tumor size, and growth rate, *J Thorac Cardiovasc Surg* 65:140, 1978.

CHAPTER

62 Pulmonary Hypertension: Primary and Secondary Causes

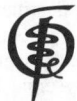

Lewis J. Rubin and Barbara J. Kircher

The pulmonary circulation is normally a low-resistance, high-flow circuit that has a remarkable capacity for vasoregulation to optimize intrapulmonary gas exchange. Conditions that produce elevations in the pulmonary artery pressure can be classified as either precapillary or postcapillary, based on the primary site of the circulation that is affected (Box 62-1). Disorders that raise pulmonary venous pressure *(postcapillary)* secondarily raise pulmonary artery pressure. In contrast, *precapillary* pulmonary hypertension is caused by diseases that affect the pulmonary arterial network, either as the primary site of injury or as a consequence of a more widespread process involving the lung parenchyma.

Pulmonary hypertension is not a disease per se, but rather a hemodynamic abnormality that is common to a variety of diseases. Although the severity of hemodynamic dysfunction may vary among

---

BOX 62-1

Classification of pulmonary diseases based on site of primary injury

Precapillary

Parenchymal lung diseases
Restrictive chest wall disease
Thromboembolic disease
Primary pulmonary hypertension
Persistent fetal circulation
Congenital heart disease
Pulmonary vasculitis
High-altitude disease
Peripheral pulmonic stenosis
Pulmonary arteriovenous fistula

Postcapillary

Left ventricular failure
Mitral valve disease
Left atrial myxoma or thrombus
Venoocclusive disease

these different conditions, the persistent pressure overload that confronts the right ventricle often leads to right ventricular failure and death. The term *cor pulmonale,* which is often used to describe overt right ventricular failure, is actually better defined as pulmonary hypertension in the absence of valvular, ischemic, or congenital heart disease. Right-sided heart failure is a late manifestation of cor pulmonale and need not be present for the diagnosis of cor pulmonale to be considered.

PRIMARY PULMONARY HYPERTENSION

Primary pulmonary hypertension (PPH) is an uncommon disease characterized by extreme elevations in pulmonary artery pressure in the absence of a demonstrable cause. The diagnosis of PPH requires the confirmation of precapillary pulmonary hypertension by cardiac catheterization and the exclusion of congenital heart disease, valvular or ischemic heart disease, significant parenchymal lung disease, other conditions that interfere with gas exchange (e.g., sleep apnea), and thromboembolic disease. Although PPH is more frequently found in young or middle-aged women, it can be seen in individuals of either sex and at any age.

PULMONARY HYPERTENSION SECONDARY TO CHRONIC LUNG DISEASE

Pulmonary hypertension can complicate a variety of chronic respiratory diseases, either by reducing the total cross-sectional surface area of the pulmonary circulation as a result of a generalized destructive process or as a result of pulmonary vasoconstriction and subsequent vascular remodeling. The former condition is most frequently seen in diffuse interstitial lung disease, extensive bullous emphysema, and other destructive processes. The latter is characteristic of chronic obstructive lung diseases, sleep-disordered breathing syndromes, or chronic high-altitude exposure. Clearly, overlap between these two mechanisms occurs, particularly as progressive lung destruction leads to greater contribution of hypoxic pulmonary vasoconstriction. This is frequently the sequence of events in patients with cystic fibrosis who survive into adulthood.

It has been known for many years that alveolar hypoxia produces precapillary pulmonary vasoconstriction and that acidosis or hypercarbia potentiates this phenomenon. Although vasoconstriction to a small region of alveolar hypoxia would optimize ventilation-perfusion ratios by diverting blood to well-ventilated lung units, diffuse alveolar hypoxia produces widespread pulmonary hypertension. Although the mechanism responsible for hypoxic vasoconstriction remains un-

known, enhanced calcium entry into the pulmonary vascular smooth muscle cells is an integral feature of the vasoconstrictor response to hypoxia that can be ameliorated with calcium channel blocking agents.

Patients may complain of increasing dyspnea, particularly with exertion, fatigue, and swelling. Physical examination may show cyanosis, jugular venous distention, hepatomegaly, ascites, and edema, particularly in the late stages. A prominent right ventricular impulse may be palpated in the subxiphoid region in individuals with severe obstructive airways disease and hyperinflation.

The presence and severity of pulmonary hypertension in chronic lung disease correlate with the severity of abnormalities in pulmonary function. Pulmonary hypertension is likely to present, at least during exercise, in patients with restrictive lung disease when the vital capacity falls below 50% of predicted values. In patients with obstructive airways disease, pulmonary hypertension is almost invariably present when the forced expiratory volume at 1 second (FEV_1) falls below 1 L. Pulmonary hypertension is also likely to be present when the arterial oxygen tension (PaO_2) falls below 55 mm Hg; the more severe the hypoxemia, the more severe the pulmonary hypertension.

Several other noninvasive tests may be used to suggest the presence of cor pulmonale. The electrocardiogram (ECG) may show an extreme right-axis deviation $\geq$ 110 to 120 degrees or right ventricular hypertrophy; the chest radiograph may show right-sided heart enlargement and enlarged main pulmonary arteries; and the right ventricular ejection fraction, measured by radionuclide angiocardiography, is depressed. Echocardiography is always indicated to exclude a structural abnormality responsible for pulmonary hypertension, such as a congenital lesion, valvular disorder, or left ventricular dysfunction. It is also valuable as a tool for following the hemodynamic and anatomic consequences of the disease process. The right atrium and right ventricle are usually enlarged, and increased thickness of the right ventricular wall is seen particularly well in subcostal views. Pulmonary artery dilation can be seen in the short-axis view.

Normally the interventricular septum is displaced toward the right ventricle in late diastole and early systole. With right ventricular pressure overload, the septum flattens or even bows toward the right ventricle (Fig. 62-1). A measurement of the degree of curvature of the septum in the short-axis view is an index of severity of right ventricular pressure elevation.

An estimation of the right ventricular systolic pressure can be obtained by applying the modified Bernoulli equation to the maximum velocity of the tricuspid regurgitation flow. By adding this pressure gradient to the right atrial pressure obtained from examination of the jugular venous pulse or degree of inspiratory collapse of the inferior

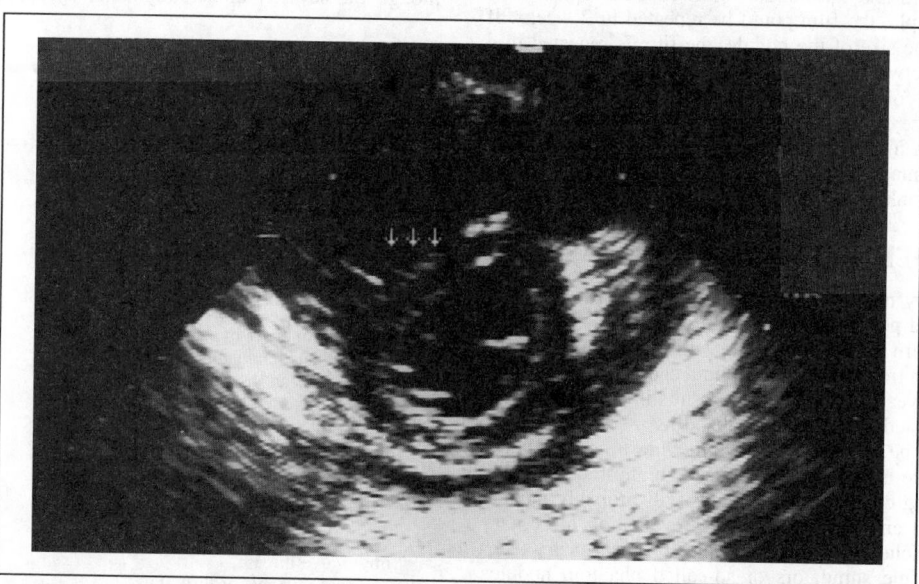

FIGURE 62-1   Two-dimensional short-axis echocardiogram demonstrating abnormal septal flattening *(arrows)* at end-diastole in the presence of right ventricular systolic hypertension.

vena cava on subcostal views, the right ventricular systolic pressure is determined. The tricuspid regurgitation signal can be augmented by intravenous injection of agitated saline during imaging, a technique that is especially helpful in measuring the pulmonary pressure response to exercise.

A fairly specific but not sensitive sign of pulmonary hypertension is a midsystolic drop or notch in the pulmonary systolic flow velocity curve caused by resistance to right ventricular ejection. The pulmonary artery pressure also correlates with a rapid acceleration time from the onset of pulmonic flow to peak velocity. Since Doppler measurements depend on loading conditions, heart rate, contractility, and compliance, they cannot be substituted for invasive hemodynamic measurements of pulmonary artery pressure when following acute or chronic responses to therapy.

Therapy should be aimed at improving gas exchange with bronchodilators, chest physiotherapy, corticosteroids, respiratory stimulants, and mucolytics, as appropriate. Low-flow supplemental oxygen in hypoxemic patients prolongs survival, although its hemodynamic effects are variable. Oxygen should be titrated to achieve a PaO_2 of 60 mm Hg or greater and should be used for at least 18 hours a day to minimize hypoxic vasoconstriction. Vasodilators, particularly the calcium channel blockers, have been shown to reduce pulmonary hypertension in some patients, but their role remains uncertain. Vasodilators can worsen gas exchange by increasing blood flow to poorly ventilated lung units, as well as producing systemic hypotension and salt and water retention.

Diuretics should be used cautiously in patients with cor pulmonale. Although they are useful in controlling excess volume retention, their use can decrease intravascular volume and compromise right ventricular function. In addition, the hypokalemia and alkalosis induced by excessive diuretic use are poorly tolerated by these patients.

Patients with severe pulmonary hypertension caused by primary pulmonary hypertension, congenital heart disease, or severe obstructive or restrictive lung disease may be candidates for lung transplantation. Patients with pulmonary hypertension and nonreparable, complex congenital heart disease will likely require combined heart-lung transplantation.

MISCELLANEOUS CAUSES

Pulmonary hypertension can be seen in patients with a variety of connective tissue disorders, including scleroderma, systemic lupus erythematosus, and rheumatoid arthritis. Rarely, vasculitis can involve the pulmonary vasculature either solely or in combination with a systemic vasculitis. Parasites, such as *Schistosoma mansoni,* can also produce pulmonary hypertension.

PULMONARY ARTERIOVENOUS FISTULA

Pulmonary arteriovenous (AV) fistula can occur singly, multiply, with hereditary telangiectasia (Osler-Weber-Rendu disease), or as an independent entity. AV fistula should be suspected when cyanosis and hypoxemia occur without evidence of cardiopulmonary disease. The hypoxemia is not corrected by breathing 100% oxygen. Usually no associated pulmonary hypertension or cardiac enlargement occurs unless the patient also has anemia, substantial systemic AV fistulas, or profound hypoxemia.

Particularly when associated with hereditary telangiectasia, AV fistulas may be multiple when discovered, or additional lesions may develop over time. Hemoptysis, pulmonary hemorrhage, and brain abscess may occur as associated complications.

Physical examination may disclose cyanosis and, if the fistula is sufficiently large, a venous hum, which increases with Müller's maneuver and decreases with Valsalva's maneuver. Chest radiography may demonstrate nodular or diffuse vascular lesions with or without connections to the hilum. The lesions generally enhance when visualized by contrast-enhanced computed tomographic (CT) scanning. Diagnosis depends on pulmonary angiography.

Selective embolization of thrombotic material, wire springs designed to induce local thrombosis, or catheter-introduced balloons have been used to close fistulas. Conventional therapy depends on surgical removal either by lobectomy or by wedge resection. In pa-

tients with hereditary telangiectasia, surgical therapy should be conservative because of the propensity for development of additional fistulas over time.

BIBLIOGRAPHY

Dawkins KD: Long-term results, hemodynamics, and complications after combined heart and lung transplantation, *Circulation* 71:919, 1985.
Fuster V et al: Primary pulmonary hypertension: natural history and the importance of thrombosis, *Circulation* 70:580, 1984.
Hughes JD, Rubin LJ: Primary pulmonary hypertension: an analysis of 28 cases and a review of the literature, *Medicine* 65:56, 1986.
Matthay RA, Berger HJ: Cardiovascular function in cor pulmonale, *Clin Chest Med* 4:269, 1983.
Pasque MK et al: Single-lung transplantation for pulmonary hypertension, *Circulation* 84:2275, 1991.
Rich S, Brundage BH: High-dose calcium blocking therapy for primary pulmonary hypertension: evidence for long-term reduction in pulmonary arterial pressure and regression of right ventricular hypertrophy, *Circulation* 76:135, 1987.
Schiller NB: Pulmonary artery pressure estimation by two-dimensional and Doppler echocardiography, *Cardiol Clin* 8:277, 1990.
Terry PB et al: Pulmonary arteriovenous malformations: physiologic observations and results of therapeutic balloon embolizations, *N Engl J Med* 308:1197, 1983.

CHAPTER

63 Pulmonary Thromboembolism

Charles K. Chan and Richard A. Matthay

Pulmonary thromboembolic disease is a common finding at autopsy. Mortality statistics indicate that pulmonary thromboembolism is the principal cause of death for more than 100,000 patients annually in the United States, and only 10% have any form of treatment for thromboembolism before death. Because not all pulmonary thromboembolic events result in death, the true incidence of pulmonary thromboembolism is probably greater than 500,000 per year in the United States. The difficulty in making a firm and correct diagnosis of pulmonary thromboembolism is predominantly because of the lack of specific signs and symptoms. Available data suggest that 25% to 30% of untreated patients die from pulmonary embolism, contrasted with a mortality rate of 5% to 8% in treated patients. Accordingly, improvement of our ability to accurately diagnose acute pulmonary embolism would have a much greater impact on reducing the associated mortality than would improvements in drug therapy.

This chapter provides an overview of current concepts of the pathogenesis, pathology, and pathophysiology of pulmonary thromboembolism. It also includes a discussion of the clinical manifestations, currently available diagnostic techniques to be utilized in a diagnostic algorithm, and appropriate therapy for pulmonary thromboembolism. Finally, prevention of this entity is emphasized.

PATHOGENESIS

Epidemiologic and autopsy data indicate that most pulmonary thromboemboli arise as detached portions of venous thrombi from the deep veins of the lower extremities. Less common sources are the right-sided heart chambers, pelvic veins, and central venous catheters. Several factors have been associated with an increased risk of venous thrombosis: (1) hemostasis, (2) hypercoagulable state, and (3) blood vessel wall abnormalities. Rarely a patient has a hypercoagulable state associated with an inborn error of metabolism, such as antithrombin III deficiency or protein C or S deficiency. More common hematologic conditions associated with thromboembolic disease include polycythemia, thrombocytosis, and sickle cell crisis. Less common systemic illnesses associated with hypercoagulable state are systemic lupus erythematosus (SLE) and infection with the human immunodeficiency virus (HIV), which have both been associated with antiphospholipid antibodies.

PATHOLOGY

Autopsy studies reveal that pulmonary thromboemboli are usually multiple and bilateral, and are found mainly in the lower lobes. Fewer than 10% of pulmonary thromboemboli cause pulmonary infarction or pulmonary hemorrhage, which occurs when a distal branch of the pulmonary vasculature is totally occluded. Infection and left ventricular failure increase the likelihood of pulmonary infarction.

On histologic examination, a pulmonary infarction appears as an area of coagulative necrosis of alveolar walls with erythrocyte extravasation into alveolar spaces and a mild acute inflammatory response. This type of infarction correlates with an infiltrate on chest radiograph that lasts longer than a week and frequently leaves a linear scar. An incomplete infarction manifests as a transient infiltrate on the chest radiograph and usually clears within a week, leaving no residual scar.

PATHOPHYSIOLOGY

Regardless of the source of the embolic material, the acute pathophysiologic results of sudden pulmonary arterial branch obstruction caused by pulmonary thromboembolism are similar and have been well defined. A total cessation of blood flow to the distal lung zone is the initial effect of embolic obstruction, and this invariably leads to respiratory and hemodynamic consequences.

Respiratory Consequences

Embolic obstruction is followed by three primary respiratory events: (1) establishment of an area of lung that is ventilated but not perfused (i.e., alveolar dead space); (2) pneumoconstriction, which is a result of the alveolar hypocapnia after cessation of pulmonary capillary flow; and (3) loss of alveolar surfactant that leads to alveolar collapse and segmental atelectasis in 24 to 48 hours after cessation of pulmonary capillary flow.

In addition to the three primary respiratory abnormalities induced by pulmonary thromboembolism, a secondary consequence is arterial hypoxemia. Arterial hypoxemia is not present in all patients with pulmonary thromboembolism, and accordingly, its absence does not exclude the diagnosis. However, a wide alveolar-arterial oxygen tension difference ($PA-aO_2$) and reduced arterial oxygen tension (PaO_2) are common findings, particularly after massive embolism. The principal mechanism responsible for hypoxemia in the early stage of pulmonary thromboembolism is ventilation-perfusion mismatching (i.e., alveolar dead space and pneumoconstriction in the embolized areas of lung). With massive embolic occlusion, arterial hypoxemia may result partly from a reduction of cardiac output and a subsequent drop in mixed venous oxygen content. Later, when emboli begin to resolve, some hypoxemia may persist because of reperfusion of poorly ventilated or nonventilated lung (i.e., intrapulmonary shunt).

Hemodynamic Consequences

The principal hemodynamic consequence of pulmonary thromboembolism is a decrease in the functional cross-sectional area of the pulmonary arterial bed, causing increased resistance to blood flow through the lungs. A significant increase in pulmonary vascular resistance requires high pulmonary arterial pressures to maintain pulmonary blood flow at the previous level. To maintain the same flow at higher pulmonary artery pressures, the right ventricle must work harder to compensate for the increased afterload. Thus pulmonary thromboembolism causes an increase in pulmonary vascular resistance, pulmonary arterial pressures, and right ventricular stroke work. Acute right ventricular strain often leads to a decline in cardiac output and a compensatory increase in heart rate.

The severity of these hemodynamic consequences depends on (1) the extent of embolic occlusion of capillary beds, (2) the operation of reflex vasoactive and/or bronchospastic mediators, and (3) the cardiopulmonary status of the patient before the episode of thromboembolism. Because of the large reserve capacity of a normal pulmonary capillary bed, the mean pulmonary artery pressure rarely exceeds 40 mm Hg (normal, ≤ 18 mm Hg) in acute pulmonary embolism. Thus pulmonary artery pressures greater than 40 mm Hg usually indicate the presence of concomitant or preexisting pulmonary vascular disease or suggest chronic pulmonary thromboembolism.

Infarction

Pulmonary infarction, ischemic necrosis of the parenchyma of the lung, occurs in less than 10% of all patients with pulmonary emboli. The infrequency of infarction is not surprising because the lung has three sources of oxygen: the pulmonary arterial system, the bronchial arterial system, and the airways. Prior studies indicate that the development of a pulmonary infarction is related to the extent of occlusion of the embolized artery and the adequacy of systemic bronchial collateral blood flow in the first few days after the embolic event. Total occlusion of a distal branch of the pulmonary arteries by an embolus occurs infrequently, and usually some blood flows around the embolus to the distal lung zones. Because this flow is often substantial, the continued perfusion inhibits infarction and moderates the cardiopulmonary events described earlier. Infarction is most common in patients with preexisting left ventricular failure with underlying pulmonary disease, since bronchial collateral arterial flow and ventilation are most likely to be compromised simultaneously in these individuals. Occasionally and for unclear reasons, infarction does appear in patients without overt cardiopulmonary disease.

Most chest radiographic densities that appear after pulmonary thromboembolism are caused by areas of congestive atelectasis rather than pulmonary infarction. The atelectatic changes usually occur within 72 hours after embolic occlusion, and tissue necrosis does not occur because of the bronchial collateral arterial supply. Histologic studies have revealed restoration of normal parenchyma to such lung zones after several weeks as the embolus resolves.

Resolution of Pulmonary Thromboembolism

As with venous thrombi, pulmonary thromboemboli resolve rapidly. As in deep vein thrombosis, fibrinolysis and organization control the removal of embolic material from the vascular bed. Whatever the mechanisms involved in the removal of embolic material, vascular patency is generally restored to normal. Studies in dogs have demonstrated substantial resolution within hours and have established that administration of heparin can accelerate the rate of resolution. Radionuclide perfusion lung scans and angiographic studies in humans have confirmed that resolution of pulmonary thromboemboli begins within a few days and is well advanced within 2 to 4 weeks. Permanent embolic residuals do occur, although the actual incidence is not known. Fewer than 10% of patients appear to retain perfusion defects on radionuclide perfusion lung scan after 6 weeks. The rate and degree of resolution observed in humans are probably related to thrombus composition and volume and individual difference in fibrinolytic activities. It is noteworthy that even massive emboli are likely to be resolved within days or weeks, particularly in otherwise young and healthy persons without coexisting cardiopulmonary disease. Two groups of patients may develop late pulmonary hypertension: (1) those with major "central" obstruction of main or lobar arteries and (2) those with obstruction of multiple distal vessels that supply a large capillary bed. These embolic events are not always recognized clinically, and incorrect diagnoses ranging from chronic lung disease to primary pulmonary hypertension are made. Early detection of this precapillary form of pulmonary hypertension is often difficult, and the disorder may be recognized only when dyspnea on exertion, effort-related syncope, or overt right ventricular failure develop.

CLINICAL FEATURES

To make a diagnosis of pulmonary thromboembolism, a high index of suspicion is necessary, especially in patients with the associated risk factors (Chapter 86). Acute onset of unexplained dyspnea is by far the most common and perhaps the most prominent symptom of pulmonary thromboembolism, followed by pleuritic chest pain, apprehension, cough, hemoptysis, syncope, and substernal chest pain.

Characteristic findings on physical examination associated with pulmonary embolism are few. Tachypnea and tachycardia are generally present, but, as in dyspnea, both may be transient. Other less common physical signs are a reduction in breath sounds and audible

BOX 63-1

Clinical features of pulmonary thromboembolism

Symptoms
Dyspnea
Pleuritic pain
Apprehension
Cough
Hemoptysis
Syncope
Substernal chest pain
Sweats

Signs
Tachypnea
Tachycardia
Reduced breath sounds
Wheezes
Crackles
Pleural rub
Elevated jugular venous pressure
Right ventricular gallop
Right ventricular lift
Loud pulmonic second sound
Pulmonary outflow tract murmur

wheezing. Atelectasis in the embolic areas may be associated with localized crackles, but in most patients, the lungs are clear to auscultation. If atelectasis or infarction occurs, additional confirmatory findings may include pleural friction rub, presence of a pleural effusion, and fever.

In the event of massive embolism, cardiac findings suggestive of pulmonary outflow tract obstruction may be present. These include a right ventricular diastolic gallop (S_3), a right ventricular "lift," prominent A waves in the jugular venous pulse, a scratchy systolic murmur in the pulmonary outflow area, and an accentuated pulmonic second sound. It is prudent to emphasize that none of these physical findings is specific for pulmonary thromboembolic disease because the same clinical syndrome can be present in other cardiopulmonary diseases and other pulmonary embolic disease, such as tumor, septic, and amniotic fluid embolism. Therefore to establish the diagnosis of pulmonary thromboembolism, clinical features alone cannot be confidently relied on (Box 63-1). It is necessary to obtain additional but crucial paraclinical data.

DIAGNOSIS
Laboratory Investigations

Arterial Blood Gases. Most patients with acute pulmonary embolism have an acute respiratory alkalosis. As stated, $PA - aO_2$ is typically widened because of an increase in alveolar dead space. Even though 85% of patients with angiographically proved pulmonary thromboembolism have a PaO_2 on room air of less than 80 mm Hg, a PaO_2 within the normal range is not sufficient to exclude this diagnosis. On the other hand, a reduced PaO_2 is by no means specific for this entity.

Electrocardiogram. More than 80% of patients with pulmonary thromboembolic disease have an abnormal electrocardiogram (ECG); however, the abnormalities are usually minor and nonspecific. In patients with massive pulmonary embolism, a classic $S_1Q_3T_3$ pattern, with or without a right bundle branch block pattern, may be present. These changes may be transient and disappear within a few hours.

Chest Radiography. Although the chest radiograph is usually abnormal, about 10% of patients with pulmonary thromboembolism have a normal film. A parenchymal infiltrate or pleural reaction and/or effusion may be seen. Parenchymal densities, which vary from patchy infiltrates to platelike atelectasis to round nodular lesions, are present in up to 75% of patients. Comparing vessels in both lungs may re-

veal discrepancy in size, and a "rat-tail" appearance of a major pulmonary artery may be indicative of an organizing thrombus within it. Oligemia of a lung zone, particularly in association with increased flow to other lung zones, may also suggest embolic obstruction. A unilateral pleural effusion is found in about 45% of the patients, but bilateral effusions are rare.

Thoracentesis. No specific diagnostic pleural fluid finding has been observed for pulmonary thromboembolism. The effusions can range from transudative to exudative to grossly bloody. However, the size of the effusion is usually small. The major role of thoracentesis is to exclude an empyema or a malignant effusion.

Other Tests. Increased fibrin degradation products are usually found in patients with angiographically proved pulmonary thromboemboli; however, the positive predictive value of this finding is low. Clinical studies evaluating the diagnostic usefulness of circulating cross-linked fibrin degradation products (D-dimers) and plasma thrombin-antithrombin III (TAT) complexes have shown that these two noninvasive diagnostic tests cannot distinguish between patients regarding the likelihood of pulmonary embolism after radionuclide lung scanning. Nonspecific elevations in serum lactic dehydrogenase, glutamic oxaloacetic transaminase, and/or bilirubin have also been described. However, these paraclinical tests have limited diagnostic value in most individuals suspected of having sustained pulmonary thromboemboli.

Diagnostic Imaging Strategies for Pulmonary Thromboembolism

Clinical features and routine diagnostic tests excluding radionuclide lung scan have clearly been shown to be of little assistance in the diagnosis of pulmonary embolism. The combination of a suggestive history in an individual with a known risk factor(s), together with consistent changes on arterial blood gases, ECG, and chest radiograph may be persuasive for a highly probable diagnosis, but the diagnosis is only correct in 68% to 78% of the patients.

To establish the diagnosis confidently, more specific diagnostic information is needed. Usually the next diagnostic step after clinical assessment and routine diagnostic tests is to perform a radionuclide ventilation-perfusion (V/Q) lung scan, which provides a reasonably high degree of sensitivity and reliability in the diagnosis of pulmonary thromboembolism.

Radionuclide Lung Scans. Perfusion lung scans are obtained by γ-camera imaging of the distribution of intravenously injected technetium 99m–labeled macroaggregates of albumin. The γ-emitting radioactive particles are trapped in the pulmonary capillary bed. At least six views from different projections are obtained to help confirm suspected perfusion defects. Normal perfusion scans show homogeneous distribution of radioactivity throughout both lungs, smooth margins, and configurations that correspond to the normal anatomy of the lungs.

The perfusion lung scan is a sensitive detector of changes in regional blood flow. However, any process that destroys or constricts pulmonary arterial vessels can cause perfusion defects, such as pneumonia, emphysema, or regional hypoventilation. Therefore a good-quality, normal perfusion lung scan virtually excludes the diagnosis of pulmonary thromboembolism, but deviations from normal simply represent an abnormality in blood flow distribution and are not diagnostic for pulmonary thromboembolic obstruction.

An abnormal perfusion lung scan must be interpreted cautiously. The extent of perfusion abnormalities can range from one small subsegmental defect to multiple segmental or even lobar defects, and in these circumstances, a ventilation lung scan is usually performed to determine if ventilation abnormalities exist in the same locations. A ventilation lung scan is performed by having patients breathe a radioactive gas such as xenon-133. The radioactive gas is expected to distribute evenly throughout both lungs. Unfortunately, in patients with obstructive airways disease, the xenon-133 is usually trapped in the proximal airways and poorly distributed to the peripheral lung zones, making the interpretation very difficult in those patients. A good-quality ventilation lung scan is expected to be normal or mismatched in the regions of perfusion defects because of pulmonary thromboemboli and to be abnormal or matched in the regions of perfusion defects caused by obstructive airways disease.

Data from the Prospective Investigation of Pulmonary Embolism Diagnosis (PIOPED) study help to define the diagnostic usefulness of V/Q lung scans. The positive predictive value of the V/Q lung scan for pulmonary embolism, using angiography as the gold standard, was 88% for high-probability scans, 33% for intermediate-probability scans, 16% for low-probability scans, and a surprisingly high 9% for normal or near-normal scans. Thus the PIOPED data indicate that lung scans cannot replace the conventional gold standard, pulmonary angiography. However, the PIOPED results also demonstrate that if clinical features and routine diagnostic test results are factored into the interpretation of the lung scans, the diagnostic usefulness of lung scans is enhanced substantially. Specifically, a high level of clinical suspicion coupled with a high-probability lung scan brings the likelihood of pulmonary embolism to 96%. Conversely, a low index of clinical suspicion with a low-probability lung scan yields a 4% likelihood of pulmonary embolism. Except for these extreme settings, all other patients should go onto B-mode ultrasonic imaging of the lower extremities or straight to pulmonary angiography (see Diagnostic Strategy for Pulmonary Thromboembolism). Also, patients with chronic thromboembolic disease need pulmonary angiography to clarify the development of new embolic episodes.

Pulmonary Angiography. Although it is widely accepted that the traditional pulmonary angiogram is the best available method of visualizing the pulmonary vasculature and thus the diagnostic "touchstones" for pulmonary thromboembolism, angiography is subject to interpretive and technical limitations. Current techniques cannot show obstruction in small subsegmental arterial branches, and thus many small peripheral emboli may be missed. The abrupt cutoff of a major vessel because of an impacted clot is easy to detect. However, by far the more common finding is a filling defect caused by flow of contrast medium around a partially occluded thrombus or an area of segmental hypoperfusion in the lung. Other angiographic signs include "pruning" or "tapering" or absence of small branches, delayed venous emptying, and dilation of the right ventricle and great vessels. None of these findings is as specific as cutoff and filling defects, particularly in the presence of coexisting cardiopulmonary disease. A well-performed pulmonary angiogram with augmentation techniques, such as subselective injections, magnification radiography, and balloon occlusion angiography, can visualize emboli down to 1 mm in diameter. However, standard angiographic technique without augmentation may completely miss occlusive emboli 2.5 mm in diameter. It is widely accepted that a negative good-quality angiogram confidently excludes pulmonary thromboembolism. The false-negative rate is less than 2%.

The only investigative procedure for pulmonary embolism that is associated with morbidity or mortality is pulmonary angiography. In high-risk patients (i.e., those with an allergy to contrast material, right ventricular end-diastolic pressure >20 mm Hg, or amiodarone-induced pulmonary toxicity), the use of low-osmolality contrast material may enhance patient safety and comfort. Low-osmolality contrast virtually abolishes the heat sensation and urge to cough, which in turn maximizes the quality of the images. Use of a "pigtail" catheter can also reduce the risk of inadvertent perforation of the right ventricle. In tertiary referral centers, the associated morbidity is only 3% to 4%, and the mortality should not exceed 0.3%. These data attest to the clinical usefulness and safety of this procedure in patients with suspected pulmonary emboli.

Diagnostic Tests for Peripheral Deep Venous Thrombosis

An alternative diagnostic route in patients with suspected pulmonary thromboembolism who have a nondiagnostic V/Q lung scan is to search for peripheral deep venous thrombosis (Chapter 31). Because the initial treatment for both conditions is identical (i.e., anticoagulation), if the presence of proximal venous thrombosis in the lower extremities is documented by a less invasive technique, therapy can be started without performing a pulmonary angiogram. This noninvasive

diagnostic step is rapidly becoming the preferred test following an inconclusive V/Q lung scan, not only for cost-effectiveness reasons, but also because of the lack of ready access to pulmonary angiography at some centers.

The diagnosis of proximal venous thrombosis has been made historically by means of contrast venography. However, this procedure is invasive, may cause considerable discomfort, and has been implicated in the generation of venous thrombosis. Critical evaluations of two noninvasive techniques for the detection of proximal venous thrombosis in the legs have been performed. The results of these evaluations suggest that the combination of iodine-125–fibrinogen leg scanning and impedance plethysmography (IPG) can be used as an alternative to venography, with respectable sensitivity and specificity in patients with clinically suspected venous thrombosis. In more recent years, high-resolution B-mode ultrasound in combination with color Doppler imaging has been widely applied for the assessment of deep leg veins. At most centers, B-mode ultrasound has become the diagnostic test of choice for assessing proximal venous thrombosis in the legs.

If the noninvasive venous imaging technique reveals proximal venous thrombosis, there is no need for pulmonary angiography because there is sufficient indication to initiate anticoagulation therapy. On the other hand, if the thrombus is localized below the calf or if no thrombus is revealed, pulmonary thromboembolism cannot be excluded with confidence because more than 20% of patients with pulmonary thromboembolism have no evidence of proximal venous thrombosis at diagnosis. Pulmonary angiography is necessary to exclude pulmonary embolism in these patients.

Diagnostic Strategy for Pulmonary Thromboembolism

A stepwise diagnostic strategy is outlined in Fig. 63-1. Results from the PIOPED study indicate that careful clinical evaluations together with routine diagnostic tests are quite helpful in excluding pulmonary thromboembolism. Specifically, based on clinical data, blood gas results, chest radiograph, and ECG findings, if the assessing physicians are confident that pulmonary embolism is unlikely, they are correct more than 90% of the time. But in all other scenarios, the risk of pulmonary embolism warrants further sequential workups as recommended.

DIFFERENTIAL DIAGNOSIS

The differential diagnosis for clinical syndromes suggestive of pulmonary thromboembolism can be subdivided into two parts: infarction and embolism without infarction.

Infarction

The differential diagnosis for pulmonary infarction includes bacterial pneumonia and pleurisy caused by either an infective process (e.g., viral) or an immunologic abnormality (e.g., postmyocardial infarction Dressler's syndrome).

Embolism Without Infarction

Pulmonary embolism may result from nonthrombotic material, presenting with the same clinical syndrome as thromboembolism. The differential diagnosis includes septic, tumor, air, fat, bone marrow, and amniotic fluid embolism.

A catastrophic clinical presentation of pulmonary embolism may include circulatory collapse, which usually occurs when a large cross section of the pulmonary vascular tree is obstructed acutely. The differential diagnosis for this condition includes other forms of circulatory collapse, such as acute myocardial infarction, the hyperventilation syndrome, and tension pneumothorax.

Recurrent pulmonary embolism may simulate primary pulmonary hypertension or vasculitis affecting the pulmonary vasculature. Also, patients with acute pulmonary thromboembolism without a clear-cut underlying medical condition or risk factor may have an occult malignancy. Finally, younger patients with acute pulmonary thromboembolism may have an unrecognized specific deficiency of antithrom-

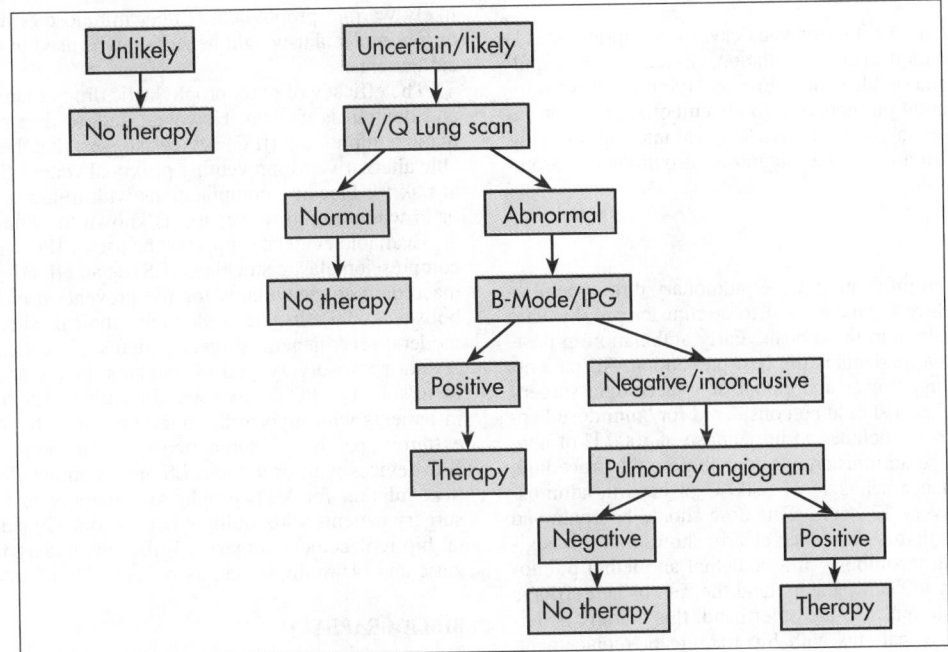

FIGURE 63-1   Algorithm for diagnosis and treatment of pulmonary embolism. *V/Q,* Ventilation/perfusion; *B-mode,* B-mode ultrasonic imaging; *IPG,* impedance plethysmography.

botic proteins, such as protein S, protein C, or antithrombin III, abnormal forms of fibrinogen, collagen vascular disease, or HIV infection.

TREATMENT
Anticoagulation With Heparin

Current strategies in anticoagulation therapy for venous thromboembolic disease is covered in detail on p. 85. In addition to heparin or low-molecular-weight heparin, additional supportive measures may be necessary in the acute period (Chapter 86). If the patient has arterial hypoxemia, oxygen should be administered. Mild sedation or analgesia may be required to alleviate anxiety or pain, and in the event of circulatory collapse, inotropic agents should be administered; dopamine and isoproterenol are most often used.

Thrombolytic Therapy

It has been demonstrated that streptokinase and urokinase, both widely available, are capable of rapidly lysing pulmonary thromboemboli. It is not clear, however, whether these agents should be used in patients with proved pulmonary thromboembolism, even if the pulmonary vascular occlusion is severe enough to cause persistent vascular collapse and profound hypotension. Although long-term studies have shown that stimulation of the plasmin system with enzymes such as streptokinase and urokinase accelerates reversal of physiologic derangements caused by massive embolism, no impact on mortality has been demonstrated. Clinical studies on recombinant tissue plasminogen activator (rt-PA) indicate that rt-PA is safer and has more favorable adverse reaction profile than the conventional thrombolytic agents.

Patients in whom thrombolytic therapy may be appropriate are those with massive proximal pulmonary thromboembolism associated with persistent systemic hypotension and those with very little cardiopulmonary reserve. The rationale for thrombolytic therapy is to speed up the lysis of thrombi to restore normal cardiac output and to minimize obliteration of limited pulmonary capillary bed. If streptokinase is used, the dosage is usually 250,000 units (U) given intravenously over 30 minutes, followed by 100,000 U/hr for 24 hours. The dosage for urokinase is 4400 U/kg as a loading dose over 10 minutes, followed by 2200 U/kg/hr for 12 hours. The recommended protocol for rt-PA is 100 mg as a continuous intravenous infusion administered over 2 hours. No dosage adjustment is necessary, and heparin is not given concomitantly. After termination of the thrombolytic agent, heparin can be started when the activated partial thromboplastin time or thrombin time has fallen below twice the control value.

Pulmonary Embolectomy

Surgical embolectomy is rarely indicated in acute pulmonary embolism but may be considered in patients with massive proximal thromboembolic loads. Usually, patients for whom it would be useful die before the surgical team can be mobilized, and those who survive long enough for the procedure to be done usually achieve a stable state before actual embolectomy. Pulmonary embolectomy by a catheter device in selected patients may be a viable alternative at tertiary referral centers, but its widespread use remains to be critically assessed.

Long-Term Therapy

After the initiation of anticoagulation with heparin, the patient should be changed to maintenance therapy, which should consist of either oral warfarin or adjusted-dose subcutaneous heparin. Traditionally, warfarin is begun on day 3 to 5 after the initiation of heparin therapy. However, convincing clinical data clearly show that warfarin can be initiated concurrently with heparin, substantially reducing the length of stay in the hospital without any significant increase in coagulation complications.

An alternative to oral anticoagulation is to maintain patients on adjusted dose subcutaneous heparin, usually at about 10,000 U every 12 hours, with the dose tailored to maintain the activated partial thromboplastin time about 1.5 to 2.0 times the control value. This mode of maintenance anticoagulation therapy is perhaps ideal for patients who are pregnant because the heparin molecule does not cross the placenta.

Although no precise data define the necessary duration of anticoagulation, it is prudent to continue this therapy indefinitely in patients who have an ongoing predisposing condition or who have sustained more than one episode of thromboembolism separated by more than a few weeks. On the other hand, it usually seems appropriate to stop anticoagulants after 6 to 8 weeks in patients who are otherwise healthy and have self-limiting predisposing medical problems.

Vena Caval Interruption

Well-accepted indications for inferior vena caval interruption are (1) an absolute contraindication to anticoagulation, (2) recurrence of pulmonary embolism or major bleeding while receiving effective anticoagulation, and (3) septic pulmonary thromboembolism from an infected pelvic focus. It is unwise to undertake caval interruption without angiographic confirmation of the diagnosis of pulmonary thromboembolism.

PREVENTION

The principal strategy in preventing acute pulmonary thromboembolism is to identify high-risk patients and to administer prophylactic measures to prevent deep vein thrombosis. Early ambulation in postpartum and postoperative patients is the best prevention. All patients over age 40 who undergo lower abdominal or gynecologic surgery requiring general anesthesia should be considered for "minidose heparin" therapy. The protocol includes an initial dose of 5000 U of heparin subcutaneously to be administered 2 hours before the procedure, followed by a maintenance schedule of 5000 U of heparin administered subcutaneously every 12 hours. This dose should be continued until the patient is ambulatory. Evidence clearly shows that this regimen prevents deep vein thrombosis and nonlethal and lethal pulmonary thromboembolism in such patients, and the risk of hemorrhage with this protocol is minimal. On the other hand, this therapy is neither effective nor safe in patients with hip fracture or replacement, in major trauma patients, or in those undergoing prostatic surgery. Data on low-molecular-weight heparin administered once daily seem to be comparable to data on conventional minidose or adjusted-dose heparin for the established clinical indications. The principal agent used for the prevention of deep vein thrombosis in patients undergoing total hip replacement is warfarin. Warfarin is started preoperatively and the daily dosage is adjusted to maintain the prothrombin time at about 14 to 16 seconds or International Normalized Ratio (INR) of 2 to 3. This "low-dose warfarin" protocol is as effective as higher dosage protocol but is associated with fewer bleeding complications. More recently, low-molecular-weight heparin has been proven to have similar effectiveness in the prevention of deep vein thrombosis in total hip replacement surgery, and thus can be used as an alternative.

Current data are not definitive regarding the prevention of nonlethal and lethal pulmonary thromboembolism in other groups of patients known to be at high risk of venous thrombosis. These groups include patients with congestive heart failure, myocardial infarction, varicose veins, and marked obesity, as well as those in the postpartum state and individuals immobilized because of severe illness. Accordingly, the application of heparin prophylaxis should be individualized for such patients. Obese patients with myocardial infarction and congestive heart failure would probably be good candidates, and a postpartum patient with a history of deep vein thrombosis would

likely warrant prophylaxis. Either minidose or adjusted-dose heparin or low-molecular-weight heparin can be used in these high-risk medical patients.

The efficacy of other prophylactic drugs such as antiplatelet agents and dextran is unclear. However, data to date on intermittent pneumatic compression (IPC) devices suggest that they can serve as a suitable alternative for preventing proximal venous thrombosis in patients at risk for bleeding complications with minidose heparin or warfarin or in whom minidose heparin is known to be ineffective.

Available evidence supports the use of IPC with or without graded compression elastic stockings (ES) as an effective alternative to pharmacologic anticoagulants for the prevention of venous thromboembolism (VTE) in the following clinical situations: (1) low- to moderate-risk general surgery patients, (2) patients undergoing intracranial neurosurgery, and (3) patients undergoing total knee replacement surgery. IPC devices with or without ES are probably effective in patients with myocardial infarction or ischemic stroke with lower extremity paralysis when anticoagulation cannot be used (Box 63-2). IPC devices with or without ES are recommended as adjuvant to anticoagulation for VTE prophylaxis therapy in (1) high-risk general surgery patients with multiple risk factors, (2) patients undergoing total hip replacement surgery, (3) patients undergoing hip fracture surgery, and (4) multiple trauma patients.

BIBLIOGRAPHY

Alpert JS et al: Mortality in patients treated for pulmonary embolism, *JAMA* 236:1477, 1976.

Chan CK et al: Pulmonary tumor embolism: a critical review of clinical, imaging and hemodynamic features, *J Thorac Imaging* 2:4, 1987.

Clagett GP et al: Prevention of venous thromboembolism, *Chest* 108:312S, 1995.

Dalen JE: Clinical diagnosis of acute pulmonary embolism. When should a V̇/Q̇ scan be ordered? *Chest* 100:1185, 1991.

Dalen JE, Alpert JS: Natural history of pulmonary embolism, *Prog Cardiovasc Dis* 17:259, 1975.

European Fraxiparin Study (EFS) Group: Comparison of a low molecular weight heparin and unfractionated heparin for the prevention of deep vein thrombosis in patients undergoing abdominal surgery, *Br J Surg* 75:1058, 1988.

Francis CW et al: Comparison of warfarin and IPC in prevention of venous thrombosis after total hip replacement, *JAMA* 267:2911, 1992.

Fulkerson WJ et al: Diagnosis of pulmonary embolism, *Arch Intern Med* 146:961, 1986.

Gallus A et al: Safety and efficacy of warfarin started early after submassive venous thrombosis or pulmonary embolism, *Lancet* 2:1293, 1986.

Geerts WH et al: A prospective study of venous thromboembolism after major trauma, *N Engl J Med* 331:1601, 1994.

Gillum RF: Pulmonary embolism and thrombophlebitis in the United States 1970-1985, *Am Heart J* 114:1262, 1987.

Goldhaber SZ: Recent advances in the diagnosis and lytic therapy of pulmonary embolism, *Chest* 99:173S, 1991.

Grant BJB: Noninvasive tests for acute venous thromboembolism, *Am J Respir Crit Care Med* 149:1044, 1994.

Henschke CI, Mateescu I, Yankelevitz DF: Changing practice patterns in the workup of pulmonary embolism, *Chest* 107:940, 1995.

Hull R et al: A comparison of subcutaneous low-molecular-weight heparin with warfarin sodium for prophylaxis against deep-vein thrombosis after hip or knee implantation, *N Engl J Med* 329:1370, 1993.

Imperiale TF, Speroff T: A meta-analysis of methods to prevent venous thromboembolism following total hip replacement, *JAMA* 271:1780, 1994.

Kearon C, Hirsh J: Starting prophylaxis for venous thromboembolism postoperatively, *Arch Intern Med* 155:366, 1995.

Killewich LA, Nunnelee JD, Auer AI: Value of lower extremity venous duplex examination in the diagnosis of pulmonary embolism, *J Vasc Surg* 17:934, 1993.

Leitha T et al: Pulmonary embolism: efficacy of d-dimer and thrombin-antithrombin III complex determinations as screening tests before lung scanning, *Chest* 100:1536, 1991.

Lund O et al: Pulmonary embolism: long-term follow-up after treatment with full-dose heparin, streptokinase or embolectomy, *Acta Med Scand* 221:61, 1987.

Nyman U: Diagnostic strategies in acute pulmonary embolism, *Hemostasis* 23(suppl 1):220, 1993.

Ondkerk M et al: Cost-effectiveness analysis of various strategies in the diagnostic management of pulmonary embolism, *Arch Intern Med* 153:947, 1993.

Petti DB, Strom PL, Melon KL: Duration of warfarin anticoagulant therapy and the probability of recurrent embolism and hemorrhage, *Am J Med* 81:255, 1986.

PIOPED investigators: Value of the ventilation/perfusion scan in acute pulmonary embolism, *JAMA* 263:2753, 1990.

Stein PD et al: Strategy for diagnosis of patients with suspected acute pulmonary embolism, *Chest* 103:1553, 1993.

Steiner RA et al: A prospective randomized trial of low molecular weight heparin-DHE and conventional heparin-DHE (with acenocoumarol) in patients undergoing gynecological surgery, *Arch Gynecol Obstet* 244:141, 1989.

Timsit JF et al: Pulmonary embolectomy by catheter device in massive pulmonary embolism, *Chest* 100:655, 1991.

BOX 63-2

Risk factors for venous thromboembolism (VTE)

- Advanced age (≥40 years)
- Prolonged immobility/paralysis
- Prior VTE
- Cancer
- Major surgery (abdomen, pelvis, lower extremities)
- Obesity
- Varicose veins
- Congestive heart failure
- Myocardial infarction
- Stroke
- Fractures of the pelvis, hip, leg
- Hypercoagulable status
- High-dose estrogen use.

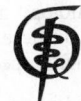

64 Pleural Diseases

Ian R.G. Dowdeswell

ANATOMY AND PHYSIOLOGY

The pleura is a thin membrane lining the interior surface of the chest wall, the superior surface of the diaphragm, and the lateral aspect of the mediastinum (*parietal* pleura), and enveloping the lungs (*visceral* pleura); the interlobar fissures are also lined by visceral pleura. The visceral and parietal pleurae become continuous at the hila, creating two anatomically distinct potential spaces in each side of the thorax. Each of these pleural spaces contains a small quantity of lubricant fluid, which allows the pleural surfaces to glide smoothly over each other during the movement of respiration. In healthy individuals, this fluid is probably less than 10 ml in each pleural space; the fluid contains 1.5 to 2 g of protein/dl and about 4500 cells/ml (predominantly mesothelial cells, monocytes, lymphocytes, and a few granulocytes).

The pleura consists histologically of single-cell-thickness mesothelial cells supported by layers of connective tissue, in which networks of lymphatics and capillaries are present. The parietal pleura is supplied by the systemic arterial circulation by way of the intercostal, internal mammary, and phrenic arteries; the visceral pleural capillaries are derived from the pulmonary and bronchial arterial systems. The parietal pleural vessels drain into the intercostal veins, and vessels from the visceral pleura drain into the pulmonary veins. Both parietal and visceral pleurae are liberally supplied with lymphatics, which drain toward the lower mediastinal lymph nodes and hilar nodes, respectively. The parietal pleura derives a rich supply of sensory nerve fibers from intercostal nerves, whereas the visceral pleura is virtually devoid of sensory innervation.

Fluid is formed continuously. Its transport in and out of the pleural space depends on the balance of hydrostatic and oncotic pressures in the capillary networks in the parietal and visceral pleurae. In healthy individuals, the oncotic pressures are equal, but the higher hydrostatic pressure in the parietal pleura results in fluid's being transferred to the pleural space, where it is reabsorbed by the lower-pressure visceral pleural system. The lymphatics play an important part in removing protein from the pleural space. Even though 600 to 800 ml is formed in healthy individuals each day, the pleural space is kept relatively free of fluid. Excess fluid accumulates if the balance of formation and absorption is upset to favor fluid formation. Excess fluid, or pleural effusion, is formed in the following situations: (1) when excessive hydrostatic pressure in the visceral pleura exists (e.g., cardiac failure), (2) when reduced osmotic pressure decreases reabsorption of fluid (e.g., nephrotic syndrome), (3) when the lymphatics draining the visceral pleura are obstructed (e.g., central carcinoma), and (4) when the permeability of the visceral or parietal pleura is disrupted (e.g., inflammation, carcinomatous involvement). The first two situations characteristically produce a transudate, but the latter two produce an exudate.

The pleura is normally kept free of gas because the combined partial pressures of oxygen, nitrogen, and carbon dioxide in venous blood lining the pleura are about 54 mm Hg less than atmospheric pressure.

Hydrostatic pleural pressure at functional residual capacity is about 2 mm Hg less than atmospheric pressure. Thus when air is introduced into the intact pleural space, causing a pneumothorax, it will be reabsorbed steadily by the pleural venous system.

The function of the pleural space is obscure because the parietal pleura can be removed surgically without impairing pulmonary function. However, lining this potential space with stretchable mesothelial cells provides the lungs and other intrathoracic organs with great flexibility to expand, retract, and deform. In addition, the presence of this space allows the development of pleural effusions or pneumothorax in a variety of situations, sometimes with serious or cata-strophic results. Large quantities of air or fluid may need to be drained as an emergency, and failure to remove pus or blood from the pleural space may lead to the formation of a fibrothorax with "trapped lung" and subsequent impairment of pulmonary function.

PLEURISY AND PLEURAL EFFUSION

The most common manifestation of pleural disease is pleural effusion, but inflammation of the pleura (pleurisy, or *pleuritis*) can occur in the absence of effusion.

Clinical Description

The predominant clinical manifestation of pleural disease is *pleuritic pain,* which is characteristically "sharp" or "cutting" and associated with respiration. Pleuritic pain is often abrupt in onset and is sufficiently severe to induce the patient to seek medical attention. The pain increases on inspiration and decreases on expiration, and respiration may be associated with an expiratory grunt in an attempt to "splint" the chest. Deep breathing, coughing, and sneezing are particularly painful and are often suppressed, but pain may also be exacerbated by body movement. The pain is generally well localized to the adjacent area of disease, but because the lower intercostal nerves supply the abdominal wall as well as the chest, pleuritic pain may be referred to the abdomen. The central portion of the diaphragm has afferent nerve fibers from the phrenic nerve; therefore pain originating in this area may be referred to the shoulder. The combination of low chest pain and ipsilateral shoulder pain is highly suggestive of diaphragmatic pleural disease.

It is important to differentiate pleuritic pain from other causes of chest pain that appear to be related to respiration. Musculoskeletal disorders produce pain exacerbated by breathing, but this type of pain is usually less well localized and less severe than pleuritic pain unless it is caused by a fractured rib; in the absence of a history of trauma, a rib fracture may result from forceful coughing.

Pain from irritation of inflamed bronchi is dull and more prolonged and is usually associated with coughing rather than with normal respiration. Mediastinal pain tends to be midline and less severe and radiates to the back. Pericardial pain may be associated with respiratory movements but is usually substernal and may be relieved by leaning forward. Myocardial pain may generally be differentiated by its well-known characteristics. When pleuritic pain presents with its classic characteristics, it is generally not difficult to determine its origin, but it may be mistaken for an extrathoracic, particularly subdiaphragmatic, pathologic condition.

Other symptoms frequently associated with pleural disease are dyspnea, cough, and fever. *Dyspnea* may be the presenting symptom, since pleuritic pain may have been transient or not present at all in patients with chronic effusions. Dyspnea is often more severe if the effusion has collected rapidly or if a large effusion exists, such as when compression of the lung results in a restrictive ventilatory defect. Dyspnea and cough are often manifestations of "mediastinal shift," when the mediastinal contents are shifted to the unaffected side. *Cough,* when present, produces little or no sputum unless concomitant parenchymal disease is present. *Fever* often accompanies infection but may also be a manifestation of pulmonary infarction or neoplastic or collagen vascular disease.

DIAGNOSTIC TESTS
Physical Examination

Examination of the chest should be accompanied by a thorough general examination, including the recording of lymphadenopathy, finger clubbing, skin lesions, signs of cardiac failure, or abdominal features that would help determine the cause of pleural involvement. Examination of the chest may be unrevealing if a small pleural effusion exists, but once the accumulated fluid is more than 500 to 600 ml, there are usually detectable clinical signs: decreased excursion of the chest on the affected side, "dullness" or "flatness" to percussion over the fluid (at the base of the lung when the patient is sitting or upright), diminished breath sounds on the affected side, and decreased vocal fremitus and resonance. Sometimes a creaky *pleural friction rub* is audible during the respiratory cycle, present in both inspiration and expiration; and egobronchophony may be heard over the level of the pleural fluid.

Radiologic Manifestations

Conventional radiology is the first approach in evaluating pleural disease but can be aided by ultrasound or computed tomographic (CT) scans in confusing situations. The pleura is generally too thin to be recognized on radiographs unless its layers are doubled or abnormally thickened. The horizontal fissure on the right may be seen in as many as 50% of normal posteroanterior (PA) chest films, and the major (oblique) fissures are often visible on lateral views. If pleural disease develops, pleural effusion is the most common radiologic manifestation. On PA films, at least 300 ml of fluid must be present before the costophrenic angle becomes blunted, although a lateral film may reveal a haziness in the posterior costophrenic angle before any abnormality is seen on the PA chest radiograph.

By the time the typical appearance of a small effusion develops in the erect adult, at least 1 L of fluid is present. On radiograph, this appearance includes the loss of the contour of the diaphragm, which is now replaced by a concave opacity located where the upper border of the diaphragm is hazy. In the presence of a large effusion, half the hemithorax or more may be opacified, and the consequent increased pressure may result in displacement of the mediastinum to the contralateral side. A subpulmonic or infrapulmonary effusion is sometimes seen when the hemidiaphragm appears to be elevated; on the left, the distance between the diaphragm's upper border and the stomach bubble is increased.

Fluid may be confirmed by a lateral decubitus film with the patient lying on the affected side. In this position, effusions of 100 ml or less may be detected. Atypical appearances of effusions occur when there are pleural adhesions, when the fluid loculates, or when air and fluid are within the pleural cavity (a hydropneumothorax). Occasionally, fluid is present in the interlobar fissures and may form a pseudotumor, which disappears when the fluid is reabsorbed.

Pleural Ultrasound

Pleural ultrasound is most often used to elucidate better an abnormality seen on chest radiograph. It is a particularly useful technique for determining the location of fluid in the presence of loculated effusions to help in draining either pus or blood from the pleural space. Also, ultrasound is a sensitive means of detecting fluid in ill patients in whom use of conventional radiography is limited.

Computed Tomography

CT is now widely available and is particularly valuable in evaluating pleural disease in areas not well visualized on conventional radiographs, such as the paraspinous regions, the anterior mediastinum, and apical areas. The extent of pleural effusions can be well defined, and mass lesions frequently can be distinguished from fluid to guide needle biopsy or drainage of fluid.

Although conventional radiology remains the main diagnostic procedure in pleural disease, the judicious use of both ultrasound and CT helps in delineating the extent of disease, guiding therapeutic maneuvers, and performing diagnostic procedures such as needle biopsy.

Thoracentesis, Pleural Biopsy, and Thoracoscopy

Thoracentesis should be performed when the cause of the pleural effusion is not apparent, if empyema (accumulation of pus in the pleural space) is suspected, or if the effusion is producing dyspnea. The gross appearance of the fluid is important, particularly in determining if the fluid is uniformly blood stained; a traumatic tap has probably occurred if the fluid clears as more fluid is withdrawn. Empyema or chylous effusions may be recognized at the time of the procedure. The importance of the initial thoracentesis is to differentiate between a *transudate*, which does not require further investigation, and an *exudate*, which indicates inflammation or malignancy. If the

cause of an exudate is not determined by initial examination of the fluid, pleural needle biopsy should be undertaken to provide more material for histologic examination and culture. Thoracoscopy, a procedure that provides direct visualization of the visceral and parietal pleura, both on the lateral and the diaphragmatic areas, is being increasingly used to evaluate effusions of undetermined etiology and thus increase the diagnostic yield. If these measures are unsuccessful, a limited thoracotomy is sometimes needed to acquire large specimens for analysis.

Despite thorough investigation, 5% to 15% of pleural effusions remain undiagnosed or nonspecific in nature.

SPECIFIC DISEASES

The predominant causes of pleural effusions are congestive heart failure, neoplastic disease, and infections. Box 64-1 gives a comprehensive list of the causes. Classification into transudate or exudate and specific diagnosis are important to allow appropriate therapy.

BOX 64-1
Classification of pleural effusions

I. Transudates
   A. Increased hydrostatic pressure
      1. Congestive heart failure
      2. Constrictive pericarditis
      3. Superior vena caval obstruction
   B. Decreased oncotic pressure
      1. Hypoalbuminemia
         a. Nephrotic syndrome
         b. Cirrhosis
      2. Intraabdominal disease
         a. Cirrhosis with ascites
         b. Peritoneal dialysis
II. Exudates
   A. Infections
      1. Parapneumonic empyema or effusion
      2. Tuberculosis
      3. Fungi
      4. Parasites
      5. Viral
      6. *Mycoplasma*
   B. Neoplasms
      1. Bronchogenic carcinoma
      2. Metastatic carcinoma
      3. Lymphoma and leukemia
      4. Mesothelioma
   C. Pulmonary emboli and infarction
   D. Intraabdominal disease
      1. Subdiaphragmatic abscess
      2. Pancreatitis
      3. Meigs' syndrome
   E. Connective tissue and hypersensitivity disease
      1. Rheumatoid arthritis
      2. Lupus erythematosus
      3. Dressler's syndrome
      4. Drug reaction
   F. Miscellaneous
      1. Esophageal rupture
      2. Familial Mediterranean fever
      3. Lymphedema
      4. Myxedema
      5. Atelectasis
      6. Uremia
      7. Benign asbestos related
   G. Idiopathic
III. Hemothorax
IV. Lipidic
   A. Chylous
   B. Cholesterol or pseudochylous

Transudates

Congestive heart failure is the leading cause of transudative pleural effusions. Effusions resulting from congestive heart failure are frequently bilateral, but if unilateral, the right side is more frequently affected. If the effusion has been present for some time or if sampled after diuresis, the fluid protein content may be greater than 3 g/dl. However, if the signs of cardiac failure are florid, thoracentesis is not necessary unless another cause is suspected. Effusions secondary to cardiac failure usually decrease with successful treatment of the underlying disease.

Constrictive pericarditis and *superior vena caval obstruction* may be associated with either transudate or exudate.

Transudates caused by a reduced oncotic pressure *(hypoalbuminemia)* are seen in nephrotic syndrome or cirrhosis. Ascites is usually present. Patients with *nephrotic syndrome* usually have bilateral effusions that reaccumulate after thoracentesis unless the underlying cause is treated. The effusion associated with ascites resulting from *cirrhosis* is right sided in two thirds of patients, left sided in one sixth, and bilateral in another sixth. Occasionally, thoracentesis is necessary, but the effusions usually respond to diuretic therapy or to improvement in the liver disease. The fluid is transported through the diaphragm, so paracentesis may be helpful in relieving the pleural effusion.

Small pleural effusions may develop in patients undergoing peritoneal dialysis. The fluid is similar to the dialysate and is reabsorbed when dialysis is terminated.

Exudates

Infections. Parapneumonic effusions frequently occur with bacterial pneumonias and may also accompany lung abscess or bronchiectasis. These effusions may be sterile or may contain infectious organisms. By definition, an *empyema* is pus in the pleural cavity and frequently contains organisms that may be cultured before therapy is instituted. It is important to examine a parapneumonic effusion early to determine whether it is likely to resolve with appropriate antibiotic therapy or whether tube drainage is required; sterile effusions can usually be managed with thoracentesis alone. A white blood cell count greater than 15,000/dl or a pH less than 7.3 suggests that tube drainage will decrease the morbidity produced by the effusion. Early antibiotic therapy may obviate the need for pleural drainage. Once empyema has developed, drainage of the pleural space is almost always necessary to effect a bacteriologic cure and preserve pulmonary function; however, fibrinous adhesions in the pleural space may complicate adequate drainage. The use of thrombolytics and videoassisted thoracoscopy has helped in effecting satisfactory resolution and reducing the need for operative thoracostomy.

The common organisms responsible for empyema reported in recent series are anaerobes (often more than one organism), *Staphylococcus aureus, Pseudomonas* species, and *Escherichia coli. Streptococcus pneumoniae* is less often identified as a causative organism since the advent of effective antibiotics, although parapneumonic effusions are seen in 40% to 60% of patients with pneumococcal pneumonia.

Empyema may also be a complication of thoracic surgery, trauma, or ruptured esophagus. Recognition of the underlying condition and drainage of the pleural space are important in the successful management of these patients.

Tuberculosis may produce either a serous exudative effusion or a frank tuberculous empyema. The former is associated with a small inoculation of tubercle bacilli into the pleural space when a subpleural, caseous focus ruptures; usually the pulmonary parenchyma appears normal on chest radiograph. Serous exudative effusion occurs within 3 to 6 months of the primary infection, and most patients are reactive to intermediate-strength tuberculin (purified protein derivative [PPD]), although a negative skin test does not exclude the diagnosis. Clinically the presentation may be acute, with fever and chest pain of a few days' duration, or subacute, with symptoms of up to a month's duration; more frequently the symptoms may have persisted for longer. In the vast majority of patients the effusion is small to moderate in size and unilateral.

Although tuberculous pleurisy is becoming less common in the United States, it is still a frequent finding in the developing world. It is also an important diagnosis to make because, although the natural history of tuberculous pleurisy results in resolution in the early phase, 45% to 65% of patients will proceed to active pulmonary tuberculosis if untreated. The diagnosis is confirmed by culturing sputum, pleural fluid, or pleural biopsy material for mycobacteria. The yield of sputum and pleural fluid cultures is usually about 10% and 25%, respectively. Analysis of the fluid usually shows a very high protein content (more than 5 g/dl) and a lymphocyte predominance in the white cells. Occasionally, a polymorphonuclear predominance is seen early in the disease; an eosinophilia of more than 10% is suggestive of another diagnosis. Glucose and lactate dehydrogenase (LDH) levels are not helpful in distinguishing tuberculous from malignant effusions. Needle biopsy of the pleura is particularly helpful and is positive in about 60% of patients; repeat biopsies may increase the yield to as high as 80%.

In contrast, tuberculous empyema occurs in patients with overt pulmonary tuberculosis and is the result of a bronchopleural fistula. The fluid is occasionally green in color and is less viscid than frank pus, or it may appear to be indistinguishable from empyema caused by other organisms. The bacteria are usually seen on direct acid-fast smear; cultures are positive. Tube drainage is necessary and may need to be prolonged. (Specific chemotherapy of tuberculosis is discussed in Chapter 273.)

Fungal diseases are an infrequent cause of small pleural effusions. About 5% of patients with coccidioidomycosis are reported to have pleural effusion. Effusion is not frequently reported in blastomycosis, cryptococcosis, and aspergillosis but may be more common in histoplasmosis than previously recognized.

Pulmonary infections caused by *Actinomyces israelii* and *Nocardia asteroides* are frequently associated with an empyema that may penetrate through the chest wall to present as a subcutaneous swelling or a draining sinus. Both are subacute or chronic diseases; *N. asteroides* is more common in immunosuppressed patients. The diagnosis of *A. israelii* is suggested by the presence of sulfur granules in the pleural fluid or draining sinuses, and confirmation is obtained by culture. Nocardiosis may be associated with hematogenous dissemination and a less favorable outcome. Patients with actinomycosis are best treated with high-dose penicillin but also respond to prolonged tetracyline or lincomycin therapy. Those with nocardiosis are treated with sulfonamides.

Viral diseases and *Mycoplasma* pneumonias may be infrequently accompanied by effusions that are usually small and resolve without specific therapy. Rarely, *Mycoplasma* pneumonia is associated with a larger effusion, and thoracentesis is required to exclude the development of empyema. Coxsackievirus B infection producing pleurodynia may be associated with a small pleural effusion for which no specific therapy is required.

Parasitic infections that may produce pleural exudates include amebiasis when the right-sided effusion is the result of either sympathetic effusion or rupture of a liver abscess through the diaphragm to produce an empyema. The diagnosis may be suspected in endemic areas and confirmed by demonstrating a liver abscess in the presence of indirect hemagglutination tests. Treatment is usually satisfactory with antiamebic drugs, but occasionally surgical drainage is required. Hydatid disease of the lungs or liver, caused by *Echinococcus granulosus,* may sometimes be complicated by pleural involvement, as may paragonimiasis, which is caused by the lung fluke *Paragonimus westermani.*

Malignant Pleural Effusion. Malignant pleural effusion is the most common cause of exudative effusion, particularly in older patients and when the effusion is moderate to massive in extent. The leading cause of malignant effusion is lung cancer, followed by breast carcinoma and then lymphoma; ovarian and other carcinomas, sarcomas, and pleural tumors are less frequent causes. If bilateral effusions are present, the cause is more likely metastatic carcinoma than bronchogenic carcinoma. The mechanisms responsible for malignant effusion are increased permeability, caused by pleural metastases involving visceral or parietal pleura, and lymphatic obstruction, resulting in impaired pleural lymphatic drainage. Atelectasis may also contribute to pleural fluid collection, as may pericardial involvement and postobstructive pneumonia. Most malignant effusions are symptomatic, the most common symptoms being cough, chest pain, and dyspnea; other nonspecific symptoms include anorexia, weight loss, and general malaise.

The diagnosis of malignant pleural involvement may be confirmed by cytologic examination of the fluid or by pleural biopsy. Repeat aspiration and biopsy result in a diagnostic yield of up to 80%. Diagnostic thoracoscopy has increased the yield to more than 90% in some centers. It is important to establish whether malignant cells are present in the effusion because this indicates that curative surgery is not feasible. However, if cytologic findings of the fluid and pleural biopsy are negative in the presence of a proximal tumor, the tumor may be resectable in a small number of cases.

Management of patients with malignant effusion caused by lung cancer depends on the identification of the primary tumor; if the primary tumor is likely to be responsive to chemotherapy, this treatment may provide cure or long-term palliation. If the primary tumor is not chemosensitive and the effusion is causing symptoms, drainage of the pleural space may be helpful. Determining the rate of reaccumulation of fluid helps determine whether pleurodesis should be attempted. Surgical removal of the pleura is seldom indicated but is usually successful in patients who are found to have malignant pleural involvement at thoracotomy. If the lung reexpands well with thoracentesis, chemical pleurodesis is worth attempting in selected patients. Various chemical irritants have been tried, including tetracycline, bleomycin, and doxycycline, with similar results. More recently, insufflation of talc at thoracoscopy has been reported to be very effective in producing pleurodesis. Occasionally, radiation therapy to the mediastinum is useful when lymphatic obstruction plays a significant role in the pathogenesis of the effusion.

The management of patients with metastatic carcinomas and lymphomas producing pleural effusion depends on the treatment of the primary tumor. Chemical pleurodesis or radiation therapy may be useful in controlling symptoms. Small effusions that do not produce significant symptoms do not need specific therapy.

Pulmonary Infarction. Pulmonary infarction, which occurs in 30% to 50% of patients with pulmonary embolism, is often accompanied by a pleural effusion. Pleuritic chest pain, usually of abrupt onset and associated with dyspnea, is present in about 80% of these patients. On radiograph, the effusion may be associated with a parenchymal infiltrate, and bilateral effusions may be seen. The fluid usually has the characteristics of an exudate and is blood stained in 50% of patients. (Further details of diagnosis and management are discussed in Chapter 63.)

Intraabdominal Diseases. Diseases of the gastrointestinal tract sometimes produce exudative pleural effusion. *Pancreatic disease* is frequently complicated by effusion; acute pancreatitis is associated with pleural effusion in nearly 20% of patients. The effusion is most often on the left but may be right sided or bilateral. The mechanism may be either transdiaphragmatic transfer of fluid arising from the pancreatic inflammation or a sinus tract formation between the pancreatic bed and the pleura. The fluid, which is often serosanguineous, frequently has amylase levels that are elevated for longer than the serum amylase levels and may be very high. Persistence of the effusion after the pancreatitis has resolved suggests the possibility of pancreatic abscess or pseudocyst. In these patients the effusion may be resolved only by a surgical approach to the pancreatic disease; if a sinus tract is found, it should be ligated or excised.

Subphrenic abscess is a complication of gastrointestinal surgery, splenectomy, and exploratory laparotomy for trauma. Approximately 50% of subphrenic abscesses are associated with a pleural effusion, which usually has a high white blood cell count and is sterile. CT scan or ultrasound may be helpful in demonstrating the subphrenic fluid collection. If a right-sided effusion is present, the possibility of intrahepatic abscess, either pyogenic or amebic, should be considered.

Meigs' syndrome is the association of a pelvic neoplasm with ascites and pleural effusion. It was originally described with benign fibromas of the ovary but has been associated with other benign pelvic tumors as well. The exudative effusion is characteristically right sided but may be bilateral. The ascites is not always detected clinically unless the pelvic tumor is large. The syndrome resolves after removal of the tumor.

Connective Tissue Disease. Connective tissue diseases may be associated with pleural effusion during the course of the disease. About 1% of patients with *rheumatoid arthritis* develop pleural effusions annually; this finding is more common in males and in older patients with a long history of arthritis and subcutaneous nodules. The effusion characteristically produces symptoms of pleuritic pain and usually is small to moderate in size and unilateral. One third of patients have associated intrapulmonary manifestations of rheumatoid arthritis. The fluid generally is yellow and may be turbid; lymphocytes predominate. Characteristically, the fluid glucose level is very low (usually <20 mg/dl), the pH is low (<7.20), and LDH and rheumatoid factor titers are high. Another interesting feature is that the fluid tends to contain cholesterol crystals or high levels of cholesterol. Closed pleural biopsy is of limited value in diagnosing rheumatoid disease because of the infrequency of finding rheumatoid nodules but may be useful in excluding other etiologies for effusion. Rheumatoid effusions tend to resolve slowly and respond poorly to therapy; occasionally, decortication is required.

Both systemic lupus erythematosus (SLE) and *drug-induced LE* may affect the pleura, producing an effusion in 16% to 40% of patients, although almost 60% report episodes of pleuritic chest pain during the course of their disease. The effusions tend to be small, evanescent, and recurrent; they are frequently bilateral. The fluid is a yellow exudate in which either polymorphs or lymphocytes may predominate; complement levels are usually low. Unlike rheumatoid pleuritis, glucose level and pH tend to be near serum levels, and antinuclear antibody (ANA) may be demonstrated. Also, in contrast to those with rheumatoid effusion, patients with pleural disease of SLE respond to corticosteroid therapy.

Drug hypersensitivity reactions account for only a small percentage of all pleural effusions, but it is an important cause to consider in the differential diagnosis of an exudate because there is usually rapid resolution after withdrawal of the drug. In addition to drugs that induce a lupus syndrome (i.e., hydralazine, procainamide, phenytoin, isoniazid), nitrofurantoin, methysergide, procarbazine, and methotrexate have been reported to produce pleural reactions.

Dressler's syndrome is characterized by pericarditis, pleuritis, and pneumonitis occurring after pericardial injury caused by trauma, surgery, or myocardial infarction. Pleural effusion may develop; the fluid is yellow or sanguineous. The diagnosis is suggested in the appropriate clinical setting and is confirmed by excluding pulmonary infarction or pneumonia. The patient's symptoms usually respond to nonsteroidal antiinflammatory drugs.

Miscellaneous Disorders. *Asbestos* exposure has been associated with benign exudative pleural effusions that are sometimes persistent or recurrent and may lead to pleural fibrosis; occasionally, these effusions are followed by the development of mesothelioma. The diagnosis is one of exclusion.

Esophageal rupture, although infrequent, should always be considered in the differential diagnosis of pleural effusion because the mortality is very high if the condition is not treated rapidly. The diagnosis should be suggested if the fluid examination reveals a high amylase (salivary) level, a low pH, squamous epithelial cells, and occasionally, food particles.

Other, less common causes of pleural effusion are listed in Box 64-1. Even after intensive diagnostic efforts, the etiology in some patients remains obscure, and it may be necessary to follow the clinical course of these patients. If the only positive finding has been a positive tuberculin skin test in the absence of other confirmatory evidence for tuberculosis, it is appropriate to give a course of antituberculous therapy followed by serial radiographs.

Hemothorax

Hemothorax occurs when a significant amount of blood is present in the pleural space, as opposed to a serosanguineous effusion. The hematocrit is usually more than 50% of the blood level. The most common cause of hemothorax is trauma, either penetrating or nonpenetrating, and is often associated with a pneumothorax. Occasionally, spontaneous pneumothorax is complicated by a small hemothorax. Iatrogenic hemothorax is being reported more frequently with placement of central venous catheters; thoracentesis or pleural biopsy is

✔ *WHEN TO REFER*

Patients with transudative pleural effusions or exudative effusions, which are characteristic of the the course of the disease, can be managed by the general internist. When the etiology of an exudative effusion is unclear or complicated, requiring invasive diagnostic procedures or surgical drainage, however, referral to a pulmonologist or thoracic surgeon is indicated.

BOX 64-2
Classification of pneumothorax

Spontaneous pneumothorax
  Primary (no previous lung disease)
  Secondary
    Preexisting lung disease
    Catamenial
Traumatic pneumothorax
  Chest trauma
    Penetrating
    Nonpenetrating
  Iatrogenic

---

occasionally complicated by hemothorax. Nontraumatic hemothorax occurs infrequently but is seen in metastatic pleural disease and as a complication of anticoagulant therapy. Rupture of an aortic aneurysm rarely presents as hemothorax. Treatment is directed to the underlying condition and to evacuating the blood from the pleural space, usually via intercostal tube drainage, so that blood loss can be monitored and development of a secondary *empyema* or subsequent fibrothorax can be prevented. Occasionally, bleeding persists and a thoracotomy is necessary.

Lipid Effusions

When high levels of lipid accumulate in the pleural space, the fluid appears milky or turbid. Lipid effusions occur in two situations: (1) a *chylothorax* forms when the thoracic duct is disrupted and chyle enters the pleural space, and (2) in long-standing effusions, large amounts of cholesterol or lecithin-globulin complexes accumulate to produce a chyliform effusion, and the patient is said to have a *pseudochylothorax*. It is important to distinguish between these two conditions because the etiology and management are completely different.

The most common cause of chylothorax is tumor, predominantly lymphoma. The second most frequent cause is trauma, generally in a postoperative situation following cardiovascular surgery. In about 15% of patients, the cause is said to be idiopathic, including congenital. Chyle is bacteriostatic, so infection occurs infrequently. Symptoms of chylothorax are related to the presence of space-occupying fluid, and patients develop dyspnea. The fluid is milky white and odorless, and the constituents can be confirmed by staining with Sudan III and analyzing the triglyceride content, which is usually greater than 150 mg/dl. The demonstration of chylomicrons in the fluid establishes the diagnosis. The pleural surfaces are normal. Treatment is directed to the cause because the fluid tends to recur after aspiration. Repeated aspiration is not advisable because the patient may become nutritionally depleted. Treatment of patients with progressive chylous effusions includes dietary modification and thoracic duct ligation if conservative measures fail.

The pathogenesis of pseudochylothorax is not known, but most patients with chyliform effusion have long-standing effusion with thickened, occasionally calcified pleura. The fluid is negative when stained with Sudan III dye and has a high cholesterol content, sometimes greater than 1000 mg/dl. These effusions may result from rheumatoid arthritis or tuberculosis but are often idiopathic. Treatment is directed toward the underlying condition; occasionally, decortication is indicated.

Pneumothorax

Pneumothorax is defined as the presence of air in the pleural space, occurring either spontaneously or as a result of trauma. A classification of pneumothorax is shown in Box 64-2.

Pathogenesis. *Spontaneous* pneumothorax, which occurs without antecedent trauma, may be classified as primary pneumothorax or secondary pneumothorax; the latter occurs with associated underlying lung disease. *Primary* spontaneous pneumothorax results from rupture of subpleural blebs, which are usually located at the apices. The cause of these blebs and the reason for their rupture are unclear, but patients with this disorder have been reported to be taller and thinner than age-matched control subjects. It is reported that primary

spontaneous pneumothorax is more common in smokers. *Secondary* spontaneous pneumothorax occurs most often in patients with chronic obstructive lung disease, including asthma, and less frequently in patients with granulomatous disease such as tuberculosis or sarcoidosis. Bronchogenic carcinoma, suppurative lung disease, and pulmonary fibrosis may also be associated with pneumothorax. Rarely, pneumothorax is associated with menstruation (*catamenial* pneumothorax).

Traumatic pneumothorax may be iatrogenic in origin or may result from penetrating or nonpenetrating injuries. Iatrogenic pneumothorax is becoming increasingly common with the widespread use of invasive procedures such as transbronchial biopsy, percutaneous fine-needle aspiration of the lung, mechanical ventilation with positive end-expiratory pressure, and subclavian vein catheterization. Nonpenetrating trauma causing pneumothorax may be associated with fractured ribs and thus laceration of the lung. Sudden compression of the chest is thought to cause raised intraalveolar pressure and rupture. Occasionally, the trachea or major bronchi are ruptured, and it is important to recognize this complication because surgical repair is often necessary. This complication is usually associated with severe trauma involving fracture of one or more of the first three ribs.

Clinical Manifestations. The symptoms and physical findings depend largely on the volume of gas in the pleural space and the extent of any underlying lung disease. The onset of dyspnea and pleuritic chest pain is usually sudden, with chest pain usually localized to the affected side. Primary spontaneous pneumothorax occurs most often in thin, asthenic men 30 to 40 years of age and, interestingly, occurs infrequently during vigorous exercise. Many of these patients do not seek medical attention immediately. Dyspnea is more prominent if the pneumothorax is large, and the clinical signs of decreased excursion of the affected hemithorax, with diminished breath sounds in the presence of normal or hyperresonant percussion, are characteristic. Arterial hypoxemia may be present early, but a subsequent decrease of both perfusion and ventilation to the affected lung may result in almost-normal arterial blood gases in subjects with otherwise healthy lungs.

Patients with secondary spontaneous pneumothorax, however, more frequently seek assistance early because symptoms are more severe. The severity of the symptoms appears out of proportion to the size of the pneumothorax, particularly in those with obstructive pulmonary disease, and the clinical signs are more difficult to elicit. In patients being supported by positive-pressure ventilation, the development of a pneumothorax is frequently associated with positive end-expiratory pressure and is manifested by the development of high peak inspiratory pressure with decreased lung compliance. Chest radiographs are essential to confirm the diagnosis and to quantitate the volume of the pneumothorax.

Treatment. For patients with primary spontaneous pneumothorax, treatment depends on the severity of symptoms and the size of the pneumothorax. Air leaks usually seal spontaneously, and the air is gradually reabsorbed. However, recurrence develops in about 50% of patients after the first pneumothorax; after the second the recurrence rates increase. If the pneumothorax is more than 40%, tube thoracostomy is required to allow the lung to reexpand and to seal the air leak. In recurrent pneumothorax or if an air leak persists, thora-cotomy, with oversewing of the blebs and pleural scarification, is effective in preventing further episodes. The role of chemical pleurode-sis remains controversial, but this approach should be considered in managing patients with secondary pneumothorax who are poor surgical candidates. More recently the use of the thoracoscope for chemical pleurodesis or pleural scarification provides the opportunity to avoid a thoracotomy; subpleural blebs may also be resected or oversewn using this technique. Iatrogenic pneumothorax can be managed conservatively unless the pneumothorax is large or the patient is on a positive-pressure ventilator, in which case tube thoracostomy is mandatory. Also, it may be necessary to reduce positive end-expiratory pressure to allow the air leak to seal.

Complications

Tension pneumothorax. A tension pneumothorax is present when air in the pleural space exceeds atmospheric pressure during expiration and often during inspiration. This abnormality produces major collapse of the lung and displacement of the mediastinum to the unaffected side, progressing to shock, which is probably on the basis of hypoxemia rather than decreased venous return. The progression of tension pneumothorax is thought to be caused by a one-way valve effect, resulting in air entering the pleural space during inspiration and being trapped during expiration. Although tension pneumothorax occasionally develops after spontaneous pneumothorax, it occurs more often after traumatic pneumothorax or when a patient is attached to a positive-pressure ventilator. The clinical manifestations include tachypnea, central cyanosis, and a larger hemithorax on the affected side, with a shift of the trachea to the contralateral side. Tension pneumothorax is a medical emergency and requires prompt decompression with a needle, catheter, or tube thoracostomy.

Pulmonary edema. Pulmonary edema can occur after rapid reexpansion of a lung following drainage of either a pneumothorax or a pleural effusion. The mechanism remains obscure, but controlled removal of air or fluid from the pleural space is likely to reduce the incidence of pulmonary edema.

Pyopneumothorax is seen as a complication of suppurative lung disease, tuberculosis, or ruptured esophagus. Large-tube thoracostomy drainage is required to prevent the development of fibrothorax. *Hemopneumothorax* may occur after trauma to the chest, and chest tube drainage is required, as for hemothorax.

Malignant Mesothelioma

Malignant mesothelioma is a rare tumor being recognized more frequently because of its association with asbestos exposure and the widespread use of asbestos until 1970. It occurs most frequently in asbestos workers, particularly in the manufacturing industries (Chapter 57). The interval between first exposure and presentation with the tumor is usually 25 to 45 years, but periods varying from 10 to 60 years have been reported. Pathologically, marked variation within a single tumor is characteristic, and differentiation from the much more common adenocarcinoma may be difficult, particularly early in the disease. Histologically, these tumors have been classified as epithelial, mesenchymal (sarcomatoid), or mixed. Initially, discrete plaques and nodules of firm, grayish tumor occur in the pleura; these progress to produce adherent parietal and visceral pleura, which encases and constricts the lung. Invasion of the chest wall or pericardium may occur. Lymphatic or hematogeneous spread is a late feature, but at autopsy, peritoneal involvement is not unusual. The diagnosis may be confirmed only by extensive sampling or at open biopsy. Special stains and electron microscopy may be necessary to differentiate the tumor from adenocarcinoma.

Clinical presentation usually occurs in patients older than age 40, with insidious onset of dyspnea, chest pain, or both. Weight loss and a dry, hacking cough develop with progression of the disease. Clinically and radiologically, a pleural effusion usually is found. After drainage, irregular pleural thickening may be seen in association with loss of volume of the underlying lung. This may be better visualized on a chest CT scan, when pericardial or mediastinal involvement can also be appreciated. The pleural fluid is yellow or serosanguineous and contains a mixture of normal mesothelial cells

with other cells of varying differentiation. It is seldom possible to confirm the diagnosis on cytologic examination alone. Direct video-assisted biopsy at thoracoscopy has improved the diagnostic yield. The outlook is generally poor because these tumors are relatively unresponsive to chemotherapy or irradiation. On occasion, excision of the pleura is successful in prolonging survival, and this modality should be considered if an open biopsy is undertaken. Although these tumors may metastasize, death usually results from intrathoracic complications.

Benign mesotheliomas remain localized and produce large, well-circumscribed globular masses, and only 10% are associated with pleural effusions. About 50% of these tumors are asymptomatic, but 20% are associated with hypertrophic osteoarthropathy. Diagnosis is made at thoracotomy, when the treatment is surgical excision; the lung parenchyma sometimes must be resected as well. Recurrence has been reported.

Pleural Calcification

Unilateral pleural calcification may develop after hemothorax, empyema, and tuberculous effusions. Calcified plaques, often on the diaphragmatic surface, may be seen in subjects exposed to asbestos and talc or in association with asbestosis.

BIBLIOGRAPHY

American College of Physicians, Health and Public Policy Committee: Diagnostic thoracentesis and pleural biopsy in pleural effusions, *Ann Intern Med* 102:799, 1985.
Chretien J et al, editors: *The pleura in health and disease,* New York, 1985, Marcel Dekker.
Light RW: *Pleural diseases,* ed 3, Baltimore, 1995, Williams & Wilkins.
Mathur PN, Loddenkemper R: Medical thoracoscopy: role in pleural and lung diseases, *Clin Chest Med* 16(3):487, 1995.
Sahn SA: The pleura—state of the art, *Am Rev Respir Dis* 138:184, 1988.

CHAPTER

65 Diseases of the Mediastinum

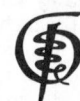

Ian R.G. Dowdeswell

ANATOMY AND PHYSIOLOGY

The mediastinum comprises the part of the thorax that lies between the lungs. Its contents can become involved in various diseases. The mediastinum is bounded superiorly by the thoracic inlet, anteriorly by the sternum, laterally by the parietal pleura, inferiorly by the diaphragm, and posteriorly by the spine and ribs. Within the mediastinum lie the heart and central vessels, the major airways, the esophagus, phrenic nerves, vagus nerves, sympathetic trunks, lymph nodes, and the main channel of the lymphatic system. All these structures can be affected primarily or secondarily by diseases involving the mediastinum.

Classically the mediastinum is divided into three compartments. The anterior, or anterosuperior, mediastinum extends from the thoracic inlet superiorly, along the anterior spinal ligament of the first four vertebrae posteriorly, and forward to the anterior aspect of the pericardium and small portion of the anterior diaphragm inferiorly; it is bounded by the sternum anteriorly. The middle mediastinum extends from the level of the fourth thoracic vertebra superiorly and is bounded by the posterior pericardium, diaphragm, and anterior pericardium. The posterior mediastinum lies behind the middle mediastinum, extending up to the anterior mediastinum, and is bounded by the posterior chest wall. The contents of each compartment are listed in Box 65-1.

The mediastinum is not a rigid compartment and may be displaced from its central position if the pressures in the pleural spaces are dis-

---

BOX 65-1
Contents of the mediastinum

Anterior or anterosuperior
Thymus gland
Aortic arch and major branches
Innominate veins
Lymphatic and areolar tissue
Thyroid gland (occasionally)
Upper trachea and upper esophagus

Middle
Heart
Pericardium
Trachea
Hilum of each lung
Tracheobronchial lymph nodes
Phrenic nerves

Posterior
Esophagus
Vagus nerves
Sympathetic nerve chains
Thoracic duct
Descending aorta
Azygos and hemiazygos venous systems
Paravertebral lymph nodes

BOX 65-2
Manifestations of compression and invasion by mediastinal masses

Cough
Hemoptysis
Stridor
Dyspnea, especially with phrenic nerve palsy
Hoarseness (vocal cord paralysis)
Superior vena caval obstruction
Pain (usually retrosternal)
Dysphagia
Pleural effusion, including chylothorax
Spinal cord compression
Pericarditis and pericardial tamponade
Horner's syndrome

Table 65-1 Systemic syndromes associated with mediastinal tumors

TUMOR	SYNDROME
Thymoma	Myasthenia gravis, red cell aplasia, hypogammaglobulinemia, Cushing's syndrome
Germ cell tumor	Gynecomastia
Substernal goiter	Thyrotoxicosis
Lymphoma (e.g., Hodgkin's disease)	Fever of undetermined origin, hypercalcemia
Neurofibroma, neurilemmoma	Osteoarthropathy
Pheochromocytoma	Hypertension
Ganglioneuroma	Hypertension, diarrhea
Parathyroid adenoma	Hypercalcemia

---

rupted, such as by tension pneumothorax, pleural effusion, or pneumonectomy. Abrupt displacement of the mediastinum can impair cardiorespiratory function, but insidious growth of a mediastinal mass can also compress vital structures, producing symptoms indicative of cardiorespiratory impairment. The elasticity and compliance of the mediastinum decrease with age or disease (e.g., neoplasm, chronic inflammation).

CLINICAL MANIFESTATIONS

Symptoms of central chest pain, cough, hoarseness, stridor, or dyspnea may indicate mediastinal abnormality. In adults, almost 50% of mediastinal masses are asymptomatic; inflammatory disease is more likely to be symptomatic. In children, however, mediastinal lesions are more likely to cause symptoms and findings. About 50% of symptomatic mediastinal masses prove to be malignant, whereas about 90% of asymptomatic masses are benign.

The most frequent symptoms are chest pain, cough, dyspnea, recurrent respiratory infection, and dysphagia, all usually resulting from compression by a mediastinal lesion or invasion of adjacent structures. Less frequent local symptoms include superior vena caval obstruction, vocal cord paralysis, Horner's syndrome, and spinal cord compression. A few patients have tumors or cysts that impinge on the heart or great vessels and produce symptoms simulating cardiac disease (e.g., pericardial involvement, pericardial tamponade). The presence of cough, hemoptysis, or stridor with a mediastinal mass suggests malignancy; hemoptysis is particularly suggestive of a bronchogenic carcinoma. Inspiratory stridor may occur with narrowing of the extrathoracic trachea or bilateral vocal cord paralysis and is an ominous finding. Usually, tumors grow to a large size before pain develops, but retrosternal pain suggests malignancy or inflammatory disease. Dyspnea may be caused by compression of the major airways, involvement of the phrenic nerve paralyzing diaphragmatic function, or a concomitant pleural effusion. Box 65-2 lists manifestations of local compression or invasion.

Some patients have systemic symptoms. These symptoms may result from endocrine secretion by the tumor, such as manifestations of hyperthyroidism caused by intrathoracic thyroid adenoma, hypercalcemia secondary to parathyroid adenoma, and systemic hypertension in association with neurogenic tumor. Myasthenia gravis occurs with thymoma, and fever occurs with Hodgkin's disease (Table 65-1).

Superior Vena Caval Obstruction

Obstruction of the superior vena cava produces a characteristic syndrome that often appears abruptly with headache, swelling, and venous engorgement of the face, chest, and arms. Patients with superior vena caval obstruction have distended, nonpulsatile jugular veins and often prominent upper thoracic collateral venous circulation. Obstruction below the junction of the azygos vein usually produces greater obstructive symptoms and results in more extensive collateral routes through the abdominal wall to enter the drainage system of the inferior vena cava. Obstruction above the azygos veins results only in the development of collateral drainage into the azygos system and thus the right atrium. Conjunctival edema and even chemosis can occur when obstruction has been rapid in onset.

Caval obstruction is usually readily apparent clinically, but identification of the cause of the obstruction may be more difficult. In patients with a history of cigarette smoking, especially middle-aged men, the diagnosis is almost always bronchogenic carcinoma. Attempts to confirm the diagnosis histologically must be undertaken with care because of the risks of bleeding from the engorged and extensive venous bed. Sputum cytologic examination may be helpful. If cytologic findings are negative, bronchoscopy may be undertaken with reasonable safety. Evidence of disease elsewhere, such as in lymph nodes, should be sought because scalene lymph node biopsy or mediastinoscopy may be accompanied by bleeding. However, fine-needle aspiration of supraclavicular nodes or of a mediastinal mass has been shown to be safe in these patients. Venography is seldom indicated unless the signs are equivocal, since it may be complicated by chemical phlebitis resulting from sluggish flow in the obstructed venous system.

In younger patients, in patients with bilateral hilar masses, or in those with findings compatible with lymphoma elsewhere, it is particularly important to establish a histologic diagnosis because therapy depends on a specific diagnosis. In such patients, more material for histologic examination is necessary than can be obtained by fine-needle aspiration, and tissue from extrathoracic sites should be sought. In young patients without an identifiable mass, fibrosing mediastinitis is possible. This condition may be associated with pulmonary artery or venous involvement, which may be demonstrated by angiography or perfusion lung scans. Fibrosing mediastinitis has been attributed to histoplasmosis, and therefore serologic evidence should be sought.

Once the diagnosis of caval obstruction has been established, treatment is determined by the nature of the primary disease. Adjunctive therapy includes elevation of the head of the bed, diuretic therapy, and corticosteroids. Emergency treatment with chemotherapy or radiotherapy is often advocated for this condition, but satisfactorily controlled trials to substantiate benefit are lacking. As with other thoracic malignancies, therapy should be dictated by cell type and stage rather than site, although caval obstruction does indicate an inoperable condition. Whatever form of therapy is used, relief of obstructive symptoms is usually satisfactory because collateral vessels develop, even in the absence of resolution of the caval obstruction.

Surgical relief of caval obstruction in patients with nonmalignant disease is tempting and has been tried with occasional success. In general, however, surgical procedures offer little therapeutic help. It is best to allow collateral routes to provide relief of symptoms. Sometimes surgical exploration is indicated to confirm the diagnosis of fibrosing mediastinitis or to exclude other etiologies.

Hoarseness

Hoarseness associated with a mediastinal mass usually results from paralysis of the left recurrent laryngeal nerve. This paralysis is most often associated with malignancy but is occasionally caused by an aortic aneurysm and, rarely, by an enlarged pulmonary artery from pulmonary hypertension.

Horner's Syndrome

Tumors of the anterior mediastinum may produce Horner's syndrome: unilateral pseudoptosis, enophthalmos, constricted pupil, and warmth and dryness of the face on the affected side. In the mediastinum, Horner's syndrome results from involvement of the inferior cervical or superior thoracic sympathetic ganglia. The most common cause of Horner's syndrome is bronchogenic carcinoma.

DIAGNOSTIC TESTS

Diagnostic studies are aimed at localizing the lesion, determining its site of origin, and obtaining a tissue diagnosis. With the expanding number of diagnostic modalities, the investigation of mediastinal lesions should follow a logical sequence from simpler, less expensive techniques to more complex, more expensive, and sometimes less comfortable techniques.

Because localization is of major importance, radiographic techniques play a crucial role in the evaluation of mediastinal lesions. A good chest film, particularly the lateral view, is the initial diagnostic test, providing information on the size and anatomic location of the mass; calcification may also be identified. Although oblique views and fluoroscopy can be helpful in equivocal chest radiographs, computed tomography (CT) is most valuable because masses of different density can be identified, and fatty tissue and cysts can be delineated. With the use of contrast agents, vascular lesions can be distinguished from nonvascular structures. CT is widely used to assess mediastinal lymphadenopathy and is particularly valuable in the posterior mediastinum. A barium contrast study of the esophagus may distinguish intrinsic pathology from extrinsic compression or may demonstrate a fistula. Magnetic resonance imaging (MRI) may be useful in providing information when the vertebral bodies or major vessels are involved in the disease process. Additional tests include angiography for suspected vascular lesions and radiolabeled iodine scans for thyroid tumors.

Nonvascular mediastinal masses usually require a histologic diagnosis; several techniques are available for obtaining tissue. In the ap-

propriate setting, not only may bronchoscopy and esophagoscopy reveal compression, but a biopsy may also be obtained if invasion of these structures has occurred. Transthoracic fine-needle aspiration for cytology is a useful technique because it is accompanied by relatively minor morbidity, and it may obviate the need for more invasive procedures. However, the small amount of material obtained is less useful for diagnosing lymphoma or benign lesions.

Mediastinoscopy is performed through an incision just above the sternal notch and is a valuable procedure for obtaining adequate amounts of tissue for specific diagnosis. Only lesions in the upper anterior mediastinum can be explored by this technique, and it is less useful on the left side because the great vessels interfere with the procedure. Lesions beyond the reach of the mediastinoscope can be approached by anterior mediastinotomy. This approach does not preclude a thoracotomy for resection of a cyst or tumor, if indicated, or if the diagnosis is not yet established. A period of observation for a patient with an undiagnosed mediastinal lesion is seldom indicated, and chemotherapy or irradiation should not be prescribed without a tissue diagnosis. In general all patients with mediastinal masses should be referred to a pulmonologist or thoracic surgeon.

SPECIFIC DISEASES
Tumors

The location of mediastinal tumors is important in diagnosis because of the predilection of certain mediastinal lesions to arise in specific compartments of the mediastinum. Box 65-3 summarizes the common tumors found in the three divisions of the mediastinum.

Anterior mediastinal tumors. *Thymoma* is the most common tumor originating in the anterior mediastinum. Benign and malignant thymomas are distinguished by their invasive features rather than by their microscopic appearance. About 30% of thymic tumors are malignant and tend to invade locally rather than by hematogeneous spread. Approximately 70% of thymomas are associated with systemic symptoms, of which the most common is myasthenia gravis, associated with up to 50% of thymomas; conversely, 10% to 15% of patients with myasthenia have a thymoma. The treatment of choice for a thymoma is surgical removal. A patient with myasthenia has a significant chance of improvement. Malignant thymomas may re-

---

BOX 65-3
Classification of mediastinal masses

Anterior or anterosuperior

Thymoma
Germ cell tumor
Lymphoma
Substernal goiter
Enlarged fat pad or lipoma
Aneurysm of ascending aorta
Parathyroid adenoma

Middle

Bronchogenic carcinoma
Bronchogenic cyst
Lymphoma
Metastatic tumor
Systemic granuloma (sarcoid, histoplasmosis, tuberculosis)
Pericardial cyst

Posterior

Neurogenic tumor
Bronchogenic cyst
Enteric cyst
Aneurysm of descending aorta
Diaphragmatic hernia
Paravertebral abscess
Meningocele
Achalasia

spond to radiation therapy, occasionally used in conjunction with surgery.

Germ cell tumors of the mediastinum occur primarily in adolescents or young adults and may be classified into benign teratomas, malignant teratomas (e.g., embryonal carcinomas, teratocarcinomas, choriocarcinomas), and seminomas. About 20% of these tumors are malignant and occur more frequently in males. The cystic teratomas, or *dermoids,* are usually benign, whereas almost one third of solid tumors are malignant. Benign teratomas may be identified because calcification, hair, or teeth are found within the cyst. Occasionally, the cysts rupture into a bronchus or the pericardium, causing severe symptoms. Ninety percent of patients with malignant teratomas have elevated levels of β-human chorionic gonadotropin or α-fetoprotein; these tumor markers should be measured in young male patients with masses in the anterior mediastinum. Benign teratomas are usually easily resected, but complete removal of malignant teratomas may be impossible. Treatment for malignant teratomas is primarily with chemotherapeutic agents. Seminoma is the most common form of malignant germ cell tumor to affect the mediastinum primarily and the anterior compartment exclusively. Treatment of patients with seminoma should include surgical extirpation and radiation therapy; chemotherapy is usually reserved for those patients with advanced disease or recurrence.

Substernal goiters are an important cause of anterior mediastinal masses. The routine chest film is occasionally diagnostic, with evidence of displacement and/or compression of the trachea, a smooth outline, and some calcification within the mass. Radioisotope scanning is often helpful, but some substernal goiters are nonfunctional. CT is often most helpful, demonstrating continuity of the mass with the cervical thyroid and confirming calcification. Calcification does not exclude malignancy, which is present in about 2% of patients with substernal goiters; hyperthyroidism also occurs infrequently. Surgical excision is the treatment of choice unless surgical risks are unacceptable.

Aneurysms of the ascending aorta, now usually arteriosclerotic in origin, usually present as anterior mediastinal masses; occasionally, aneurysms of the subclavian or innominate arteries also appear in this compartment. They are characterized by a smooth border, and continuity with other vascular structures may be recognized on the plain chest film. Angiography is often required to define the full extent of the aneurysm and assess the feasibility of surgery.

Patients with spontaneous or iatrogenic Cushing's syndrome often have radiographic evidence of fullness of the anterior mediastinum, best visualized on the lateral chest film. This fullness is usually caused by an enlarged mediastinal fat pad, and no therapy is indicated. CT is particularly useful in identifying fatty tissue in these patients or when a lipoma is present.

Lymphomas may present as anterior mediastinal masses because of forward growth of the mediastinal node group. Diagnosis must be confirmed histologically. Fibromas, hemangiomas, and lymphangiomas are rare, usually benign masses that require surgical excision to confirm the diagnosis.

Middle Mediastinal Tumors. *Lymph node enlargement* is a common cause of a mass in the middle mediastinum and is seen in many conditions. Many patients with mediastinal lymph node involvement have malignancies, either lymphoma or metastatic carcinoma. Small cell carcinoma of the lung may also present as a middle mediastinal mass, with a central bronchial tumor and mediastinal lymph node involvement. Benign disorders involving mediastinal nodes include sarcoidosis, histoplasmosis, coccidioidomycosis, and primary tuberculosis. These conditions should always be considered when investigating patients with mediastinal disease; evidence for disease elsewhere should be sought and appropriate serologic studies undertaken. When the diagnosis cannot be made by noninvasive means, mediastinoscopy is often successful in obtaining adequate tissue for histology.

Congenital Cysts. Cysts, including those of pericardial, bronchogenic, enteric, thymic, and thoracic duct origin, account for about 20% of mediastinal masses. Most are discovered incidentally on routine chest radiographs in asymptomatic individuals and are confirmed on CT scan to be cystic.

Pericardial cysts are the most common congenital cysts of the mediastinum. They seldom produce symptoms even though they occasionally contain several liters of fluid. They are usually solitary and characteristically are seen in the right cardiophrenic angle. Pericardial cysts may appear teardrop shaped on lateral projection; their contour may alter with respiration or positional change. The clear fluid they contain accounts for the term *springwater cysts.* CT and ultrasonography assist in the diagnosis. Surgical excision is usually undertaken.

Bronchogenic cysts occur in the lung or mediastinum. In the adult they are usually asymptomatic, whereas in children they may cause tracheobronchial compression with cough, stridor, wheezing, dyspnea, and occasionally atelectasis. Cysts sometimes become secondarily infected and produce a mediastinal abscess. Surgical removal of the cyst is indicated to exclude malignancy and to relieve compression of adjacent structures.

Enteric cysts are located adjacent to the esophagus in the posterior mediastinum. They are lined with esophageal, gastric, intestinal, or respiratory epithelium but rarely communicate with the esophageal lumen. Enteric cysts lined with gastric epithelium may develop peptic ulceration and bleed or perforate. More than 50% of enteric cysts are found in infants and produce symptoms by compressing adjacent structures. They have a solid appearance with a smooth contour radiographically. Barium swallow may be helpful because a localized defect in the lumen is common. Surgical extirpation is indicated in symptomatic patients and to establish a diagnosis.

Thymic cysts and those of thoracic duct origin are rare; they occur in the anterior and posterior mediastinal compartments, respectively. The diagnosis is established at surgery.

Posterior Mediastinal Tumors. *Neurogenic tumors* are the most common posterior mediastinal tumors, accounting for about one fifth of all mediastinal tumors. Less frequently seen are enteric cysts, esophageal tumors, achalasia, and lesions of the thoracic spine. Neurogenic tumors include all benign and malignant neoplasms arising from the intercostal nerves, sympathetic ganglia, and chemoreceptor cells. These tumors can occur at any age; however, in adults, most are asymptomatic and benign, whereas in children, 50% are symptomatic and malignant. Symptoms are occasionally caused by hormonal activity of the tumor (e.g., pheochromocytoma). The neural tumors are differentiated by the cells of their origin, (e.g., neurilemmoma, neurofibroma, ganglioneuroma, neuroblastoma [predominantly in children], pheochromocytoma). On radiographic examination, neurogenic tumors are smooth, rounded, homogeneous, and well circumscribed and are seen in the paravertebral sulcus; occasionally, calcification is seen. Erosion of the vertebral bodies or ribs can occur, and enlargement of the spinal neural foramen is a useful diagnostic sign. About one third of these neural tumors become malignant; therefore all should be excised.

Pneumomediastinum

Pneumomediastinum, or mediastinal emphysema, is the presence of gas in the interstices of the mediastinum. It can occur spontaneously, from trauma, or from dissection of air from the neck or retroperitoneal space. Infections with gas-forming organisms are very rare and are usually related to trauma.

Spontaneous Pneumomediastinum. In the absence of an obvious cause, pneumomediastinum is said to be spontaneous. Air is thought to leak from alveoli under high pressures into the interstitium of the lung and then into the perivascular sheaths, the hilar regions, and subsequently the mediastinum. The condition may be precipitated by a sudden rise in intrathoracic pressure during vigorous coughing or after a Valsalva maneuver.

Spontaneous pneumomediastinum is relatively common in the newborn and is associated with mucus or meconium plugging, respiratory infections, and use of positive-pressure ventilators. In adults, this condition can occur in young, otherwise healthy individuals, or it may be associated with asthma, pneumonia, bronchitis, emphysema, or pulmonary fibrosis. Pneumomediastinum can also occur during obstetric labor or as a result of rapid decompression while diving, and it may be a complication of positive-pressure ventilator therapy.

The air may spread from the mediastinum to the subcutaneous tissues of the neck or axilla, producing subcutaneous emphysema; and it may leak into the pleural space, producing pneumothorax.

Patients with spontaneous pneumomediastinum may be asymptomatic or have retrosternal chest pain and dyspnea; occasionally, sore throat is present because of dissection of air to the retropharyngeal space. Physical examination may demonstrate distant heart sounds and a crunching sound synchronous with the heart (Hamman's sign). Both these signs may accompany pneumothorax without evident mediastinal emphysema. Evidence for subcutaneous emphysema in the neck and axilla should be sought.

The diagnosis is usually made by radiography. A thin line of air is seen along the border of the mediastinum; sometimes this line of air is more clearly seen on the lateral chest film. Occasionally, large amounts of air produce mediastinal widening. The presence of a concomitant pneumothorax should be sought.

Most patients with spontaneous pneumomediastinum do not require specific therapy; occasionally, however, severe symptoms develop, with signs of cardiac decompensation and tamponade. Decompression is then indicated and may be accomplished by either needle aspiration or mediastinotomy.

Traumatic Pneumomediastinum. The most common cause of traumatic pneumomediastinum is rupture of the esophagus, which can occur during an episode of severe vomiting or, less frequently, after esophagoscopy. Traumatic pneumomediastinum can also occur after penetrating wounds of the chest or after fracture of the trachea or main bronchus after blunt trauma to the chest.

Rupture of the esophagus is usually associated with severe, boring chest pain and may be complicated by acute mediastinitis. Traumatic pneumomediastinum requires thoracotomy, with repair of the esophagus or tracheobronchial tree. Esophageal rupture is associated with high morbidity and mortality, which may be reduced if surgery is undertaken promptly.

Mediastinitis

Acute Mediastinitis. Acute infections of the mediastinum are usually the result of introduction of organisms into the mediastinum after perforation of the esophagus during vomiting or examination with an instrument. The diagnosis should be suspected when substernal pain, fever, and radiographic evidence of mediastinal air develop after a bout of vomiting or instrument examination. This setting represents an emergency that requires antibiotic therapy directed at gram-positive, gram-negative, and anaerobic organisms, as well as early surgical drainage and repair. On occasion, mediastinal lymph nodes perforate, with drainage into the mediastinum and consequent acute suppurative mediastinitis. This situation is rare, however, and most often is discovered only at autopsy. Perforation of mediastinal lymph nodes should be suspected if a patient with mediastinal lymphadenopathy develops substernal chest pain, fever, and hypotension. Therapy should include antibiotics to cover both gram-positive and gram-negative organisms and surgical exploration. An important consideration in the differential diagnosis is bleeding from or further dissection of an aneurysm.

Chronic Mediastinitis. Chronic mediastinitis is a condition, usually of unknown cause, that produces fibrosis in the mediastinum, with compression and restriction of vascular structures entering and leaving the mediastinum. Occasionally, bronchial obstruction occurs. It was previously thought that tuberculosis was the chief cause of chronic fibrosing mediastinitis, but other granulomatous diseases, particularly histoplasmosis, may also cause this syndrome. Precise etiologic diagnosis is seldom possible because the initial infection may precede the chronic condition by months or years. Symptoms are nonspecific and include chest pain. Superior vena caval obstruction may develop, and bronchial obstruction with distal infection and cough may be troublesome. Pulmonary hypertension from constriction of the pulmonary arteries can occur, and regional venous hypertension from focal venous obstruction is sometimes a feature.

Full evaluation of the patient includes bronchoscopy and ventilation-perfusion lung scans, in addition to skin testing for tuberculosis and complement-fixation tests for histoplasmosis. Treatment

is very limited once vascular obstruction has developed, although surgical decompression has been attempted. Often, however, fibrosis is too advanced to be amenable to surgical repair.

Mediastinal fibrosis is sometimes a complication of methysergide therapy.

BIBLIOGRAPHY

Adkins RB, Maples MD, Hainsworth JD: Primary malignant mediastinal tumors, *Ann Thorac Surg* 38:648, 1984.

Brown K et al: Current use of imaging in the evaluation of mediastinal masses, *Chest* 98:466, 1990.

Cohen AJ et al: Primary cysts and tumors of the mediastinum, *Ann Thorac Surg* 51:378, 1991.

Davis RD Jr, Odham HN Jr, Sabiston DC Jr: Primary cysts and neoplasms of the mediastinum: recent changes in clinical presentation, methods of diagnosis, management and results, *Ann Thorac Surg* 44:229, 1987.

Lloyd JE et al: Mediastinal fibrosis complicating histoplasmosis, *Medicine* (Baltimore) 67:295, 1988.

Newell JD: Evaluation of pulmonary and mediastinal masses, *Med Clin North Am* 68:1463, 1984.

CHAPTER

66 Pulmonary Transplantation

**James H. Dauber, Penny A. Williams,
and David R. Nunley**

DEFINITION OF PULMONARY TRANSPLANTATION

The term *pulmonary transplantation* is used to cover three major operations: single lung, double lung, and heart-lung allografting. The indications and operative techniques for each have become better defined in the last 10 years but are still evolving. The impetus to emphasize single lung transplantation emanates from the ever-increasing disparity between the numbers of candidates and donors. This has forced a reconsideration of earlier dictums about the utilization of scarce resources. Whereas heart-lung allografting was the principal form of pulmonary transplantation in the early to mid 1980s, it is a much less commonly performed procedure in the 1990s. Were it not for cystic fibrosis, for which a double lung allograft is mandatory, the great majority of pulmonary transplantation procedures today would use just one lung.

INDICATIONS

Indications for the three forms of pulmonary transplantation continue to evolve, and some differences of opinion amongst principal transplantation centers still remain. Table 66-1 matches diseases to forms of pulmonary transplantation based on the current consensus. Clinical judgment is still required in many instances.

Single Lung Allograft

Single lung allografting is suitable for advanced parenchymal lung diseases that are not complicated by chronic infection or irreversible cardiac dysfunction. Restrictive diseases from a wide array of causes and obstructive disease from emphysema or lymphangioliomyomatosis fall into this category. Primary pulmonary hypertension (PPH) and many types of secondary pulmonary hypertension are also amenable. The foremost considerations in patients with pulmonary hypertension are adequacy of cardiac reserve, ability to correct the associated cardiac anomaly, and the function of other vital organs. If these factors are favorable, single lung transplantation for vascular disease produces the same short-term survival rate as seen in uncomplicated end-stage parenchymal lung disease. In older recipients with compromised function of other organs, and the heart in particular, a double lung allograft is advisable.

Table 66-1   Matching diseases to forms
of pulmonary transplantation

PROCEDURE	ESTABLISHED INDICATIONS	CLINICAL JUDGMENT REQUIRED

Single lung	Pulmonary fibrosis
	  Idiopathic
	    Collagen vascular diseases
	    Pneumoconioses
	    Sarcoidosis
	    Histiocytoses
	  Emphysema
	  Lymphangioliomyomatosis
		Pulmonary hypertension
		  Primary with good LV function
		
		Secondary with correctable cardiac defect

Double lung	Septic lung disease
	  Cystic fibrosis
	  Bronchiectasis
		Pulmonary hypertension
		  with systemic pressures
		Emphysema from α-1-antitrypsin deficiency

Heart-lung	Eisenmenger's syndrome
	  with uncorrectable
	  cardiac defect
	End-stage lung or pulmonary vascular disease
	  with irreversible cardiomyopathy	

LV, left ventricle.

Double Lung Allograft

Double lung allografting is reserved principally for end-stage septic lung disease. The principal disease requiring this procedure is cystic fibrosis. Living related lobar donations are being used in a few centers for this disease as well. In this instance single lobes from two large donors are transplanted into a small recipient in place of two whole lungs. Bronchiectasis, which is not a result of cystic fibrosis, also requires double lung allografting. Whether transplantation will be successful in patients with bronchiectasis secondary to an immunologic deficiency requires further clinical testing. Some programs use a double lung allograft in patients with pulmonary vascular disease who are older and have pulmonary artery pressures that reach systemic levels. In this group there is concern that injury to the single lung from high pressures and flow rates in the early postoperative period prolongs recovery in the early postoperative course.

Heart-Lung Allograft

Heart-lung allografting is indispensable for patients with intractable heart and lung disease. The cardinal indication is Eisenmenger's syndrome with an uncorrectable cardiac defect. Other lung diseases complicated by inadequate left ventricular function require this approach as well.

SELECTION OF DONOR AND RECIPIENT
Donor

There are relatively few requirements for suitable donors, but they are stringent enough so that the number of donors does not exceed 1000 per year in the United States. Only one in five donors of other solid organs such as kidney, liver, and heart will provide a suitable lung. Lung function in the donor must must meet the criteria shown in Box 66-1 and the donor must be free of overt lung injury, severe airflow obstruction, neoplastic disease, and infection with HIV and hepatitis B and C viruses. Preferably there should be no history of heavy smoking, but many donors have smoked. The age cutoff is typically 40 years, but lungs from older donors occasionally are used.

Recipient

Although many more requirements seem to exist for a suitable recipient than for the ideal donor (Box 66-2), the number of candidates

---

BOX 66-1
Indicators of adequate function in donor lung

1. Normal chest radiograph
2. PaO_2 >300 torr with FiO_2 of 100%
3. No significant chest wall contusion
4. No evidence of recent aspiration by bronchoscopy
   a. Blood
   b. Cerebrospinal fluid
   c. Food
   d. Foreign bodies

BOX 66-2
Criteria for recipient selection

1. Age
   a. Less than 65 for single lung allograft*
   b. Less than 60 for double lung allograft*
   c. Less then 50 for heart-lung allograft*
2. Adequate function of left ventricle for lung allograft
3. Between 80% and 120% of ideal body weight
4. Never smoker or ex-smoker (stopped smoking at least 3 month before listing)
5. No substance abuse
6. Receiving <20 mg/day of prednisone
7. No severe osteoporosis
8. No evidence of active tuberculosis, hepatitis B, or HIV infection
9. No hepatic or renal insufficiency
10. No evidence of active neoplastic disease (long-term remission from previous neoplastic disease is acceptable)
11. No severe psychiatric disease
12. Adequate support group at home
13. Available within 4 hours of being called†

*See text for recommendations regarding acceptability of previous thoracotomy for each type of allograft.
†Some centers require that the candidate live in the local area.

---

far exceeds the number of donors. Consequently, criteria for selection of recipients must be stringent and consistently applied to ensure the most favorable outcome. The criteria listed here are widely followed, but the degree to which they are adhered to varies from center to center. A previous thoracotomy or pleurodesis is an absolute contraindication for heart-lung transplantation because of the risk of severe perioperative hemorrhage from anticoagulation. Cardiopulmonary bypass is not required for most single lung transplantations and may be avoided in double lung transplantation when bilateral "sequential" single lung transplantations are done. Diabetes mellitus per se is not an absolute contraindication, but secondary end-organ damage, particularly to the kidney, may disqualify the candidate. Potential candidates must be evaluated systematically and criteria applied consistently to ensure proper selection. Once selected, candidates must be monitored closely for developments that might complicate transplantation or disqualify them altogether. In addition, rehabilitation during the waiting period should be practiced whenever feasible. The entire selection process is best handled by a qualified team of health care providers with relevant expertise.

Operative Considerations

Heart-lung transplantation requires cardiopulmonary bypass, which subjects the recipient to risks of hemorrhage and air embolism. Phrenic and vagal nerve injury occasionally leads to diaphragmatic paralysis and gastric atony. These complications cause difficulty in weaning and erratic absorption of oral drugs in the early postoperative period.

Single lung transplantation rarely requires cardiopulmonary bypass but demands a wide thoracotomy. The large incision causes considerable pain, which interferes with pulmonary toilet and early mobilization of the recipient. Epidural anesthesia is useful for pain control, but parenteral narcotics and local nerve block may also be required. Vigorous pulmonary toilet is essential for prevention of atelectasis and infection of the graft. Extensive injury to the graft results in severe respiratory insufficiency, which may require differential mechanical ventilation through a double-lumen tube to prevent overinflation of the highly compliant native lung.

Double lung transplantation is performed as bilateral sequential single lung transplantations whenever possible to avoid cardiopulmonary bypass. This can be achieved if one native lung and the first allograft sufficiently oxygenate the recipient's blood during surgery. This approach requires continuous bilateral thoracotomies (referred to as a "clam shell" procedure). Incisional pain is substantial, and without proper fixation, the sternum may be unstable. These complications interfere with pulmonary toilet. Injury to the phrenic and vagal nerves is less frequent than with heart-lung transplantation.

Bronchoscopic examination in the early postoperative period serves three important functions. First, it detects significant injury to the donor airway and bronchial anastomoses, which might lead to dehiscence and infection with fungi. Second, it aids in clearance of retained secretions in the lower airways and relief of atelectasis. Third, it provides excellent specimens for culture if infection is suspected; this can be performed easily just before extubation and should be done within the first week in recipients with a history of septic lung disease complicated by colonization with *Aspergillus.*

IMMUNOSUPPRESSION
Induction

Most regimens begin with a combination of agents given intravenously: cyclosporin A or tacrolimus (formerly FK-506) to achieve whole blood levels of 500 to 1000 ng/ml or 10 to 20 ng/ml, respectively (by radioimmunoassay), azathioprine 1 to 2 mg/kg/day and methylprednisolone 125 mg IV every 8 hours for two to three doses. Use of antilymphocyte globulins at this time is more controversial, but a minority of centers continue to use them for induction. A variety of antisera have been used that appear to be effective. As they may cause lung injury, serum sickness, and enhanced susceptibility to infection, however, their use is generally confined to recipients in whom adequate levels of cyclosporin A or tacrolimus cannot be achieved safely in the immediate postoperative period. Prednisone, 0.3 mg/kg, and azathioprine are generally given enterally as soon as the recipient can tolerate oral intake. Before that time, equivalent doses of both agents are given intravenously. Controlled trials that compare the efficacy and toxicity of various induction regimens are needed.

Maintenance

Most centers use a combination of oral cyclosporin A, azathioprine, and prednisone. Cyclosporin A is administered every 12 hours to achieve a trough level between 500 and 750 ng/ml (measured by radioimmunoassay) in whole blood. A new formulation of cyclosporin A (Sandimmune Neoral) appears to provide more uniform absorption from the gut and consequently more stable blood levels than its predecessor. Tacrolimus may be used in place of cyclosporin A with equivalent and possibly superior control of rejection and an equivalent profile of adverse reactions. Therapeutic levels range from 10 to 20 ng/ml. A single daily dose of azathioprine is given, which maintains the total white blood cell count (WBC) above 5000/dl. The dose of prednisone varies from 5 to 15 mg/day. Lower doses are preferable for recipients with corticosteroid-induced complications. A new agent for the prevention of rejection that holds considerable promise is mycophenolate mofetil, a relatively selective inhibitor of T- and B-cell proliferation. It is effective when used in place of azathioprine in both renal and cardiac transplantation but has not been tested in pulmonary transplantation.

Maintenance immune suppression based on cyclosporin A and tacrolimus is associated with a number of side effects. The two most important are increased susceptibility to infection and impairment of re-

---

> **BOX 66-3**
> ## Drugs that increase or decrease the blood level of cyclosporin A and tacrolimus
>
> **Increased levels**
> Diltiazem
> Verapamil
> Ketoconazole
> Fluconazole
> Itraconzaole
> Macrolide antibiotics
>   Erythromycin
>   Clarithromycin
>   Azithromycin*
>
> **Decreased levels**
> Rifampin
> Phenobarbitol
> Phenytoin

*Azithromycin usually has a much lesser effect than the other macrolides and can be used safely in the majority of recipients without causing striking increases in blood levels.

---

nal function. Because there currently are no markers for an adequacy of immune suppression other than toxicity and rejection, it is important to follow the blood levels of cyclosporin A or tacrolimus on a regular basis and monitor the recipient closely for signs of toxicity and rejection, particularly in the first postoperative year. The frequency of monitoring of blood levels depends on the clinical status of the recipient. In stable recipients who have been followed for several years, the interval ranges from 1 to 3 months. In less stable recipients during the early postoperative period, it will be much shorter. A number of other drugs used to treat complications in recipients have important interactions with cyclosporin A and tacrolimus (Box 66-3). The physician treating recipients should be familiar with these interactions and monitor blood levels of tacrolimus or cyclosporin A closely whenever a new drug is begun. The treating physician should also work closely with the recipient's transplantation center to prevent such interactions, which may lead to severe toxicity or acute rejection.

OUTCOME

Recipient survival is essentially equivalent to graft survival, for if the allograft fails, the outcome is usually death, given the scarcity of donor lungs for retransplantation. Survival at 1, 2, and 3 years is 75%, 65%, and 55%, respectively, according to recent registry data from the International Society for Heart and Lung Transplantation. Long-term survival rates are less reliable given the relatively small number of recipients who are still alive more than 3 years after surgery. Present trends, however, point to continuing loss of life from infection and rejection in the late postoperative period, leading to a 5-year survival rate of about 50%.

COMPLICATIONS
Introduction

The next section focuses on problems that internists and medical subspecialists are most likely to encounter: preservation injury, infection, and rejection. The lung allograft appears to have a greater susceptibility to infection than do other solid organ allografts due in large part to its direct exposure to the environment. These three complications may occur contemporaneously in the early postoperative period, and later infection and rejection are often intertwined. Distinguishing between them is essential for proper therapy.

Preservation Injury

Sometimes referred to as the *reimplantation response,* this complication occurs very early in the postoperative course. Characteristically, diffuse interstitial and alveolar radiographic infiltrates develop in the first 12 to 72 hours, particularly after cessation of positive pressure ventilation. They are often associated with a decline in lung function. The pathogenesis remains incompletely defined but is believed to involve several mechanisms. The inciting event probably is an ischemia-reperfusion injury that is aggravated by disruption of pulmonary lymphatics and potentially by pulmonary venous hypertension from volume overload. Stenosis of pulmonary venous anastomoses, although uncommon, should always be considered and excluded with a transesophageal echocardiogram. Histologic abnormalities include hyaline membrane formation, intraalveolar edema, and hyperplasia of type II pneumocytes (collectively referred to as *diffuse alveolar damage*). These acute changes eventually give way to organization, which is followed by resolution if infection does not supervene.

The differential diagnosis includes acute rejection and infection. Careful monitoring for infection and rejection, institution of broad-spectrum antibacterial prophylaxis, and early specific therapy for infection or rejection are essential. Bronchoalveolar lavage is useful to evaluate for infection, but a lung biopsy is required to exclude acute rejection. Reducing the level of immunosuppression by maintaining cyclosporin A and tacrolimus blood levels in the range of 500 to 750 and 10 to 15 ng/ml, respectively, helps to prevent and control infection but necessitates vigilance for rejection. Fortunately, the allograft afflicted with mild to moderate injury does not seem more prone to acute rejection than an uninjured allograft. This syndrome is usually self-limited. Even in the face of severe injury, the allograft usually achieves normal function. Rarely, overwhelming injury of this type leads to graft and multisystem organ failure. If new lungs are not implanted, the recipient will eventually succumb.

Bacterial Pneumonia

Time Course. Bacterial pneumonia is the most common infection in the early postoperative period, but intensive prophylaxis and pulmonary toilet have reduced the rate to below 5%. Most cases are associated with severe preservation injury and preexisting septic lung disease. Bacteria are also the most common cause of pneumonia after the first postoperative year. In this setting bacterial pneumonia often is associated with chronic rejection, which is described later.

Agents. Most bacterial pneumonias are due to gram-negative rods. In the early postoperative period a number of species have been implicated, whereas in the late postoperative period, *Pseudomonas* predominates. In recipients with cystic fibrosis, the allograft may become infected with *Pseudomonas* species, which continue to colonize the upper airways after transplantation. This is particularly threatening if the organism is resistant to antibiotics. In fact, colonization with resistant bacteria in the pretransplantation period is a relative if not absolute contraindication to transplantation because of the possibility of these organisms causing pneumonia in the early postoperative period. A smaller but still substantial proportion of pneumonias are due to *Staphylococcus aureus*. This pathogen must be respected because it produces a highly destructive pneumonia. Finally, *Streptococcus pneumoniae* is a common cause of community-acquired pneumonia in healthy lung recipients.

Diagnosis. Culturing the trachea of the donor lung at harvest may provide useful information about subsequent infectious complications in the recipient. Isolation of mouth flora indicates an aspiration event before harvest and is often associated with subsequent preservation injury. Isolation of *S. aureus* from the donor airway is a harbinger of infection with this agent in the allograft in the early postoperative period. Isolation of *Candida* species deserves attention and is discussed later in this section.

Sputum and blood should be obtained for culture whenever a pneumonia is suspected. The sputum must also be examined for bacteria by conventional stains and the direct fluorescent antibody technique for *Legionella* species. Not infrequently, this information is sufficient for an accurate bacteriologic diagnosis. When the pneumonia occurs in the setting of preservation injury or diffuse radiographic infiltrates from other causes, more invasive techniques for obtaining secretions from the lower airways are required. If properly standardized, bron-

choalveolar lavage (BAL) can yield valuable information about not only bacterial but also viral and protozoal pathogens. Quantitative bacterial cultures of specimens obtained by protected brush catheter may also be utilized.

Prophylaxis. Some form of prophylaxis should be used in all recipients in the early postoperative period. Initially a combination of ceftazadine and clindamycin is sufficient (Table 66-2). This regimen should be used until results of cultures from the donor trachea become available. At this point, prophylaxis should be modified to cover potential pathogens recovered from the donor trachea or stopped if donor cultures reveal no potential pathogens. The presence of gram-negative rods in donor cultures warrants addition of a second antipseudomonal agent until the sensitivities of the isolates are established. Prophylaxis should be continued for longer than 3 days if there are positive donor trachea cultures, severe ischemic injury to the allograft, or clinically significant infection. In the latter two instances, the regimen should be tailored to the sensitivities of bacteria isolated from the lung allograft. If *S. aureus* is recovered from the donor trachea, antistaphylococcal agents should be given for 7 days. Because most of these isolates are sensitive to methicillin, vancomycin should be reserved for resistant strains and not given routinely. If the recipient underwent transplantation for septic lung disease associated with *Pseudomonas* species, prophylaxis with two antipseudomonal drugs for 1 to 2 weeks is indicated (see Table 66-2). Three agents may be used if there is more than one type of gram-negative rod, and one of these species is partially resistant to antibiotics. Culturing secretions from the *recipient's* native lungs at explant also provides information about potential pathogens in the postoperative period and should be done routinely for septic lung disease. Prophylaxis for recipients with a history of multiply resistant organisms in their native lungs is controversial, but giving specific antipseudomonal prophylaxis to prevent infection with sensitive organisms is justifiable.

Therapy of Established Infection. Specific antibiotics are the backbone of treatment for bacterial pneumonia. For infections due to *Pseudomonas*, two drugs to which the organisms are sensitive are indicated, with one being either an aminoglycoside or ciprofloxacin. Antibacterial agents alone are insufficient therapy in the early postoperative period. The contribution of airway injury and denervation to pathogenesis of infection cannot be underestimated. Postural drainage and chest percussion should be used routinely. Repeated therapeutic fiberoptic bronchoscopy appears to be helpful in recipients with poor cough and large volumes of sputum. When bacterial pneumonia is extensive or occurs with moderate to severe preservation lung injury, maintenance immunosuppression should be reduced and the allograft monitored closely for rejection.

Bacterial pneumonia in the late postoperative period frequently occurs in concert with chronic rejection (also called bronchiolitis obliterans syndrome [BOS] as described later). Colonization of the airways with bacteria is common once BOS has become established. Most often the organisms are gram-negative rods, with *Pseudomonas* species dominating. *S. aureus* may also colonize the airway and cause infection in this setting. Treatment is similar to that for infection in the early postoperative period. In addition, antibacterial "suppression" in the form of regularly scheduled courses of oral or inhaled agents in recipients who experience repeated infections seems to lessen the tendency to new infection. Such regimens usually consist of oral antibiotics to which previous pathogens were sensitive or inhaled aminoglycosides such as tobramycin and colistin. They may be given for the first 10 to 14 days of each month or at other intervals that prove to be effective in reducing the rate of relapse. Chronic postural drainage is also helpful. Regulation of maintenance immunosuppression in these individuals is complex. Transient reductions may be possible to hasten recovery from infection, but intermittent augmentation is often necessary to control exacerbations of BOS.

Outcome. In the early postoperative period, the mortality rate from bacterial pneumonia is about 25%, making it one of the leading causes of death in this time frame. It is also a leading cause of death in the late postoperative period; recipients with far advanced chronic rejection are its principal victims. Because the number of long-term

Table 66-2 Prophylaxis for infection

ORGANISM	PEAK PREVALENCE IN POSTOPERATIVE PERIOD	STARTING POINT	ANTIMICROBIAL AGENTS	DOSAGE	DURATION
Bacteria	Day 1-14	Postoperative day 0	Ceftazidime Clindamycin	1 gm IV q8h 600 mg IV q 8h	3-14 Days (see text)
Herpes simplex virus	Day 1-7	Postoperative day 1	Acyclovir*	400 mg PO tid	3 Months unless gancyclovir given for CMV
Candida sp.	Day 7-30	As soon as organisms identified in donor trachea or isolated from lower airway of allograft	Amphotericin B* 5-Flucytosine*† Fluconazole	25 mg IV daily 1 gm PO bid 400 mg IV/PO qd	21 Days With amphotericin 4-6 Weeks
Toxoplasma (heart-lung transplant only)	Day 7-60	When mismatch identified (positive donor to negative recipient)	Pyrimethamine Folinic Acid	25 mg PO qd 15 mg PO qd	Initial 6 weeks
CMV‡	Day 30-40	Postoperative day 5 Postoperative day 20	Gancyclovir*†	5 mg/kg IV bid 5 mg/kg IV daily	14 Days Day 15-90 for negative recipients of a CMV positive donor§
			Acyclovir*	800 mg PO qid	3 Months for CMV-positive recipients
P. carinii	Month 3	Postoperative day 30	TMP/SMX 160 mg/800 mg Dapsone‖	1 tab qod or bid 7 day/mo or bid for 2 wk/3 mo 100 mg PO 3 days/week	Indefinite Indefinite
M. tuberculosis	?	Before transplant or immediately after surgery	INH	300 mg PO qd	1 Year

*Dosage adjustment required for renal insufficiency.
†Dosage adjustment required for leukopenia.
‡Role of CMV immune globulin in prophylaxis is still under investigation.
§Some centers recommend gancyclovir 5 mg/kg IV 3 times/week for 3 months for recipients who are R$^+$ and/or D$^+$ for CMV.
‖Not the first-line drug for prophylaxis of *P. carinii*.

survivors who develop chronic rejection is increasing, this complication will continue to have a major impact on recipient well-being and survival in the near future.

Cytomegalovirus Infection

Prevalence. Infection with cytomegalovirus (CMV) may be detected as early as 3 weeks after transplantation in recipients who do not receive prophylaxis. Before the advent of effective prophylaxis, the onset was most often around the fortieth postoperative day. Prophylaxis delays the onset of infection with the degree of delay proportional to the duration and intensity of prophylaxis and the amount of treatment for allograft rejection. *Primary* CMV infection occurs in recipients who were seronegative at transplantation and receive an organ or blood products from seropositive donors. CMV infection in recipients who were seropositive before transplantation usually represents reactivation of latent virus and is called *secondary* infection. Infection in a seropositive recipient may also be due to a new strain of virus acquired from the donor but is still considered a secondary infection. The prevalence of infection depends on the serologic status of both the recipient and donor pools and the extent to which primary infection is prevented by using allografts and blood products from CMV negative donors in CMV negative recipients. In the past the bulk of primary infections arose through the use of CMV-positive blood products in seronegative recipients. Restricting exposure of seronegative recipients to CMV positive blood products has greatly reduced the overall rate of primary infections. Because no effort is presently made to match the CMV status of the donor organ and recipient at most transplantation centers, primary infection will continue to arise through this mechanism in virtually all recipients at risk for primary infection. In the absence of prophylaxis, about 80% of seropositive recipients will contract a secondary infection. Thus without effective prophylaxis, the vast majority of lung recipients will develop infection with this agent. For this reason prophylaxis for this infection is of paramount importance.

Clinical Manifestations. About 25% of infections are totally asymptomatic, with virus being isolated from either the buffy coat, urine, or bronchoalveolar lavage fluid. Most asymptomatic infections

are due to a secondary infection from reactivation of latent virus. Whenever infection is associated with symptoms, the diagnosis is usually referred to as CMV disease. About two thirds of cases of CMV disease are due to infection of the lung allograft. The majority of lung recipients with CMV pneumonia have a primary infection. The remainder of cases of CMV disease are associated with a viral syndrome, esophagitis, gastritis, colitis or disseminated disease involving more than one organ. Overall, the severity of symptoms and organ dysfunction tends to be greater in primary infection than in secondary infection. The rate of CMV pneumonia in the lung allograft greatly surpasses the rate of CMV pneumonia in other solid organ recipients.

Diagnosis. Diagnosis of CMV infection is confirmed by isolating virus from blood, urine, or bronchoalveolar lavage (BAL) fluid. Diagnosis of disease requires demonstration of specific inclusion bodies in cytologic or histologic preparations from affected organs. In patients with a primary infection, the diagnosis of CMV disease may be made with less stringent criteria, requiring only a compatible clinical syndrome and evidence of viral replication in an organ or peripheral blood based on a positive culture. For the lung allograft, fiberoptic bronchoscopy with transbronchial lung biopsy is the preferred approach to diagnose pneumonia. It should be used when infection is suspected on clinical grounds. In complex situations in which several processes may coexist in the allograft, an open lung biopsy may be required to demonstrate the presence of CMV. Sometimes a surveillance transbronchial biopsy will reveal CMV pneumonitis in an asymptomatic recipient. This result and the striking predilection of the lung allograft to infection with CMV rationalize the performance of surveillance bronchoscopy during periods when the recipient is at risk for CMV infection, that is, within the 3 months after CMV prophylaxis was stopped and following treatment of rejection with augmented immune suppression during the first 2 postoperative years.

Treatment. Prophylaxis with intravenous gancyclovir is highly effective in preventing CMV infection in the early postoperative period when this infection has the greatest potential to cause morbidity and mortality. Although there is uncertainty about the optimal duration of treatment and the frequency at which it is administered, there is universal agreement that it delays the onset of infection. Whether it truly prevents infection, particularly in a seronegative recipient who receives an organ from a seropositive donor, has not been established. Doses and duration of prophylaxis are outlined in Table 66-2. It should be noted that "breakthrough" infection with gancyclovir prophylaxis rarely occurs if the recipient has been compliant. The oral form of gancyclovir that has recently been released offers advantages in cost and convenience compared to the IV preparation, but its efficacy as a prophylactic agent for CMV infection in the lung transplantation recipient remains to be established. The roles of acyclovir and immune globulin for prophylaxis in this setting are also still under investigation.

Symptomatic infection is treated with the same regimen of gancyclovir as that outlined in Table 66-2, except for the addition of CMV immune globulin 150 mg/kg IV every other day for 7 doses. For life-threatening CMV disease or severe retinitis, foscarnet may be combined with gancyclovir. The level of immunosuppression is reduced unless there is evidence of clinically significant acute rejection. As subclinical infection may linger in the allograft for weeks, follow-up bronchoscopy 2 to 4 weeks after therapy has been completed is indicated to asses the response to treatment. Persistence of inclusion bodies on cytology or histology or continuation of viral shedding in a patient with primary infection early after transplantation requires another course of gancyclovir because CMV disease may relapse without it. Foscarnet is the drug of choice when resistance to gancyclovir is documented or strongly suspected.

Outcome. Before the availability of gancyclovir, prevention and treatment were relatively ineffective and the mortality rate from pneumonia in primary infection exceeded 50%. Prophylaxis with gancyclovir has dramatically reduced the prevalence of CMV disease, and specific therapy with this drug for pneumonia is highly effective in inducing a remission. Consequently, the overall mortality rate has declined from 22% before the availability of gancyclovir to less than 5%. Nonetheless, CMV disease and CMV pneumonia in particular continue to be an important cause of morbidity. CMV pneumonitis may also be a risk factor for chronic rejection. For these reasons, efforts to eliminate CMV infection in lung allograft recipients must continue.

Pneumocystis carinii Pneumonia

Before aggressive prophylaxis with trimethoprim (TMP) and sulfamethoxazole (SMX) (co-trimoxazole), clinically significant pneumonia due to *P. carinii* was not uncommon. Infection is first encountered around the third to fourth postoperative month. It can occur at any time later if adequate prophylaxis is not being delivered, but with effective prophylaxis, it is a rarity. Most of the recipients who contract it today have not been compliant with prophylaxis. Properly prepared specimens from bronchoalveolar lavage fluid reliably detect the presence of these organisms. Transbronchial or open lung biopsy is rarely necessary to confirm a suspected infection. Subclinical infection responds to oral cotrimoxazole, one double strength (DS) tablet of 160 mg TMP and 800 mg of SMX twice a day. Clinically significant infection requires intravenous therapy with sulfa drugs or pentamidine. A variety of prophylactic regimens have proven successful (Table 66-2). To date, inhaled pentamidine has not been widely used for prophylaxis.

Herpes Simplex

For the most part, infection with herpes simplex is clinically insignificant. Herpetic lesions of mild severity commonly develop on the lips and buccal mucosa during the first postoperative week and should be treated with acyclovir. In the occasional recipient with no previous exposure, a primary infection can produce a devastating pneumonia in the allograft. To prevent such a disaster, the recipient's serologic status for this virus should be routinely established before transplantation and the serologic status of the donor established when the potential recipient is seronegative. Seronegative recipients who receive an organ from a seropositive donor and do not require gancyclovir for CMV prophylaxis should be given acyclovir for the first 3 months beginning on the second postoperative day (see Table 66-2).

Epstein-Barr Virus and Posttransplant Lymphoproliferative Disease

The principal rationale for discussing Epstein-Barr virus (EBV) is the striking association between primary infection and posttransplant lymphoproliferative disease (PTLD). The frequency of primary infection depends primarily on the proportion of recipients who are seronegative at the time of transplantation. Virtually all such recipients will seroconvert in the early postoperative period. Primary infection manifests as a self-limited mononucleosis syndrome of variable severity in the second to fourth month but usually goes unrecognized. As many as 75% of recipients with primary infection will subsequently develop PTLD, which, in up to two thirds of cases, presents in the allograft. The next most common site is the small bowel, followed by the liver, then by abdominal and peripheral lymph node groups. Confirmation of the diagnosis by biopsy is essential. It reveals B cell proliferation, which is polyclonal or monoclonal in origin. EBV is usually detected in pleomorphic cells residing in areas of focal necrosis. Histologic distinction between a benign proliferative process and PTLD in this setting is often difficult, but usually the clinical presentation of recipients with PTLD helps to establish the diagnosis.

PTLD usually involutes quickly after the level of immunosuppression is drastically reduced. Unfortunately this manipulation usually causes acute rejection, the treatment of which demands augmentation of immunosuppression. In such instances PTLD may recur. If PTLD fails to respond to reduction of immunosuppression or if there is relapse after the treatment of rejection, more aggressive therapies may be considered. These include infusion of recipient-derived, lymphokine-activated killer (LAK) cells generated in vitro, radiation therapy, and/or chemotherapy. The response to LAK cells in the few instances tried has been encouraging, but the response to radiation and chemotherapy has been disappointing. Given the magnitude of the problem with PTLD, efforts to avoid and treat primary infection with EBV are clearly warranted, but to date no highly effective measures have been reported. Some transplantation centers will no longer perform transplantations in patients who are EBV seronegative because of the unacceptable risk of PTLD and its consequences.

PTLD may also develop much later in the postoperative course. In this setting latent EBV infection may be present, but association with clinical infection usually is less obvious and reduction of immunosuppression less effective in producing a remission. Radiation and chemotherapy may be used, but usually they, too, fail to induce a meaningful remission.

Fungal Infections

***Candida* Species.** Isolation of *Candida* organisms from the donor airways at the time of harvest and colonization of the recipient's native airways are risk factors for infection in the recipient during the early postoperative period. Colonization of the native airway is more common than expected when the recipient has been treated in the immediate preoperative period with corticosteroids and broad-spectrum antibiotics. Other factors permissive to infection in the early postoperative period include ischemic injury to the airway mucosa and lung, prolonged use of broad-spectrum antibiotics, generalized debility of the recipient, prolonged central venous catheterization, and oral thrush. Most infections are relatively superficial and clinically insignificant, but these organisms can invade the aortic anastomoses of the heart-lung allograft, creating a mycotic pseudoaneurysm that is usually fatal. They also have caused mediastinal abscesses around dehisced bronchial anastomoses, but this type of infection usually responds to therapy. Multiple parenchymal abscesses are rare and develop in the lung allograft only with disseminated infection.

Prophylaxis with fluconazole for the risk factors described earlier is usually adequate for *Candida albicans*. When there is heavy growth of yeast in cultures from one or more sites and visible involvement of the airways, however, inhaled amphotericin B should be added. Intravenous amphotericin B should be given prophylactically in a dose of 25 mg daily for up to 3 weeks when *Torulopsis glabrata* is the colonizing agent (see Box 66-3). Prophylaxis for thrush and esophagitis with antimonilial troches or mouth washes is advisable during the initial hospital stay, particularly in recipients who were treated with broad-spectrum antibiotics before transplantation. Prospective bronchoscopic examination of all recipients, and particularly those with risk factors for *Candida* infection, is advisable within the first 10 postoperative days to detect unsuspected infection of the donor airways and bronchial anastomosis. Deep-seated but isolated infection and disseminated infection demand treatment with intravenous amphotericin B in concert with 5-flucytosine. The latter can be given only by the oral route. Doses of 5-flucytosine lower than recommended usually achieve adequate serum levels in the recipient. This combination is continued until the infection appears to be under control both clinically and by cultures. At this time therapy may be continued with fluconazole alone if the strains causing the infection are sensitive to this agent.

***Aspergillus* Species.** Infection with *Aspergillus* organisms at any site, including the allograft, is rare in the early postoperative period. One notable exception is an ischemic airway anastomosis in recipients who were colonized preoperatively. Patients with cystic fibrosis are particularly prone to colonization with this organism and should be closely monitored for this before undergoing transplantation. Patients who are colonized at the time of transplantation should be carefully monitored for infection of the anastomoses in the first 3 postoperative weeks, with frequent bronchoscopic examinations. After the third postoperative month, however, organisms are detected in the lavage fluid of about 15% to 20% of all recipients who typically have no signs or symptoms of infection. Some of these recipients will develop clinical infection in the allograft at a later time, but there presently are no reliable markers to predict such an event. One source of organisms that leads to colonization of the allograft that may be overlooked is the native lung in the recipient of a single lung. If the native lung contains cystic spaces or cavities, *Aspergillus* may initially colonize these poorly defended regions and eventually disseminate endobronchially into the allograft. Some centers elect to treat colonized recipients with itraconazole or inhaled amphotericin, which appears to reduce the rate of disseminated infection without totally eradicating the organism. Optimal therapy for recipients with colonization of the allograft airways, however, remains to be defined.

Recovery of *Aspergillus* in lavage fluid from recipients with pulmonary infiltrates and symptoms of infection is ominous, and confirming that the infiltrates are due to infection with this agent may prove difficult. Transbronchial lung biopsy usually does not document invasive disease, and even an open lung biopsy may fail to do so. Invasive pulmonary aspergillosis in lung recipients is usually not the fulminant process it is in patients with profound leukopenia from chemotherapy, but it is still a life-threatening infection. When the diagnosis is suspected, intravenous amphotericin B should be given until infection is excluded. An established infection requires high doses of amphotericin B (at least 1 mg/kg/day) until there is strong evidence of a clinical response. In addition, the level of immune suppression should be lowered to permit native immune defense mechanisms to be more effective. During this time the allograft should be monitored for evidence of rejection. Once an adequate clinical response has been achieved, itraconazole may replace the amphotericin B, but recipients should be monitored to ensure therapeutic serum levels of itraconazole. Long-term maintenance of itraconazole seems warranted in *all* survivors of deep-seated *Aspergillus* infection, since it is likely that acute therapy does not completely eradicate this opportunistic organism.

Other Infections. Opportunistic organisms that occasionally cause clinically significant infection include *Cryptococcus neoformans*, *Rhizopus* spp, *Pseudoallscheria boydii*, *Nocardia* spp, *Dactylaria gallopava*, and *Mycobacterium abscessus* (which causes deep skin infection that may disseminate along surgical wounds). If unusual opportunistic agents are isolated from the allograft or *the remaining native lung*, they should never be considered contaminants. Infections with these organisms respond to early, aggressive, and specific treatment, but the duration of therapy may need to be prolonged. Toxoplasmosis infrequently causes illness in lung recipients, but it may be transmitted from the donor heart into recipients of a heart-lung allograft. For this reason the serologic status of the donor and recipient of a heart-lung allograft should be established and prophylaxis provided when such a mismatch occurs (see Table 66-2). The frequency of pulmonary tuberculosis has been low, with only a handful of cases reported to date. Careful screening of potential recipients and appropriate prophylaxis in the preoperative period appear to be the reason. Treatment of active disease is similar to that for nonimmunocompromised hosts, but the duration of therapy may need to be longer. Acute sinusitis is a recurrent problem in some recipients, particularly those receiving transplants because of cystic fibrosis. Strong consideration should be given to culturing material obtained by direct puncture and to early surgical drainage in any lung recipient with this type of infection.

ALLOGRAFT REJECTION
Introduction

The human lung allograft is a highly immunogenic organ that will reject rapidly in the absence of either an identical match or immune suppression. Because living related donor programs for pulmonary transplantation in adults will likely never become a major source of organs and the supply of adult organs is too limited to attempt close matching for human lymphocyte antigen (HLA) loci, immunosuppression will be essential to prevent rejection of mismatched organs in most recipients for the foreseeable future. Even with intense immunosuppression, the rate of rejection in the first postoperative month exceeds 75%. The pathogenesis of acute rejection involves the infiltration of the graft by lymphocytes that recognize antigens of the donor. The principal donor antigens that initiate acute rejection are the HLA DR subsets of the class II major histocompatibility complex (MHC). Antigens of the class I MHC type (HLA-A, B, and C) and other yet to be defined "minor transplant antigens" probably play a role as well, particularly in the pathogenesis of graft dysfunction in the late postoperative period, which is often called chronic rejection.

The histologic and clinical manifestations of rejection appear to take two forms. In acute rejection the endothelium and surrounding vessels seem to be the main target. As the intensity of this response escalates, it spills out into the interstitium. In the early postoperative period these changes are associated with a decline in pulmonary compliance, diffuse radiographic infiltrates, and symptoms of graft dysfunction, but later they may occur with few or no changes in lung function and the chest radiograph. The response to augmentation of immunosuppression is typically brisk and substantial. Relapse is not uncommon, but additional therapy nearly always brings this form of rejection under control, restoring allograft function.

As early as 3 months posttransplantation but typically after the first year, a different form of inflammation, often referred to as chronic rejection and more recently as bronchiolitis obliterans syndrome, or BOS, supervenes and eventually afflicts up to half of all long-term survivors. The target in this response is principally the airways, and the bronchioles in particular. Histologically, the defining abnormality is bronchiolitis obliterans. Physiologically, the prominent finding is obstruction to airflow. The chest radiograph reveals no new abnormalities until late in the course. Response to augmented immunosuppression is variable, with only a minority of treated recipients regaining the majority of lost lung function. Relapse is the rule and the response to additional therapy is often unsatisfying. A progressive decline in graft function despite therapy occurs in about 25% of afflicted recipients who will eventually die from respiratory failure and/or infection unless they receive a second transplant.

Acute Rejection

Time Course and Frequency. Acute rejection is encountered as early as the third postoperative day but most commonly presents in the second to third week. It can also be seen much later if there is a dramatic decrease in the level of immunosuppression. The prevalence depends on a number of factors. The most important appears to be the intensity of the induction and maintenance phases of immunosuppression. The degree of mismatch at HLA loci, the method for detecting rejection, and the philosophy about treatment also influence frequency of reported acute rejection. Despite minor differences from center to center, acute rejection is universally a common event, occurring in more than 90% of recipients who survive more than 3 months. After this time histologic changes consistent with acute cel-

BOX 66-4
Histologic grading of acute cellular rejection*

Grade I: minimal acute rejection
Infrequent lymphocytic infiltrates surrounding blood vessels, but principally venules. Lymphocytes have variable appearance, with some undergoing transformation.

Grade II: mild acute rejection
Frequent perivascular infiltrates of activated lymphocytes, macrophages, and eosinophils, which invade vessel walls and alter appearance of endothelial cells ("endothelialitis").

Grade III: moderate acute rejection
Perivascular infiltrates extend into alveolar septi and airspaces adjacent to bronchioles and vessels. Eosinophils are more prominent and neutrophils may be seen.

Grade IV: severe acute rejection
Diffuse infiltration of interstium and airspaces with alveolar pneumocyte injury, alveolar hemorrhage, and hyaline membrane formation (acute alveolar damage). A necrotizing vasculitis may cause infarction.

*All grades may be associated with inflammation and injury of cartilaginous bronchi, and bronchioles.

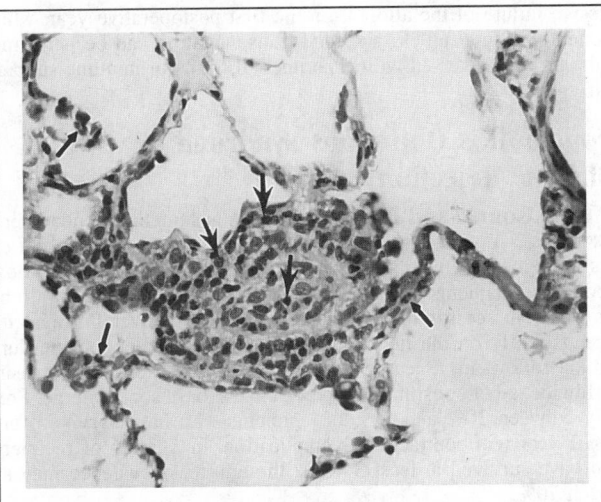

FIGURE 66-1 Histologic grade III acute rejection. A small vein is infiltrated by inflammatory cells that extend into the alveolar interstitium. Most of the infiltrating cells are lymphocytes *(broad arrows)*, which have a pleomorphic appearance characteristic of cellular activation. Occasional polymorphonuclear leukocytes are also seen *(thin arrows)*.

lular rejection may still be detected but at a much lower frequency. They usually are not associated with systemic symptoms or new radiographic infiltrates but often cause a decline in spirometric values. In such recipients there should be great concern for underlying BOS, which has not yet been confirmed histologically or by the usual clinical criteria described later.

Clinical Manifestations and Diagnosis. Recipients with acute rejection in the early postoperative period may be asymptomatic, but the majority experience one or more of the following: cough, dyspnea, chest tightness, fever, fatigue, and malaise. Fulminant acute rejection even mimics bacterial sepsis. The most sensitive laboratory abnormality is a decline in the arterial oxygen tension. Leukocytosis with a left shift is common, as are new interstitial radiographic infiltrates and pleural effusions. Pulmonary function tests demonstrate a decline in lung volumes with preservation of the forced expiratory volume at 1 second/forced vital capacity (FEV_1/FVC) ratio. None of these routine evaluations possesses sufficient specificity, however, to permit a clear-cut diagnosis in all instances. For this reason, a lung biopsy is usually obtained. The transbronchial route is sufficient if the specimens are adequate in quantity and quality. Six to eight generous pieces should be obtained from upper and lower lobes. The availability of a pathologist who is experienced with interpretation of these specimens favorably influences the diagnostic yield. If the recipient is too ill to undergo a transbronchial biopsy or there are other extenuating circumstances, and open lung biopsy may be required. Results from BAL are helpful in establishing the presence of infection, but presently there are no markers in lavage fluid that are specific for acute rejection. In selected instances, however, the clinical picture is sufficiently compelling that a clinical diagnosis is made in the absence of a confirmatory tissue specimen.

The histologic changes encountered in the rejecting lung allograft have been classified and graded in severity. This scheme, which has been widely adopted (Box 66-4), is useful for following a single recipient longitudinally and for facilitating comparisons of recipients within a single center and between different centers. The histologic abnormalities in moderate acute cellular rejection are shown in Fig. 66-1. Mononuclear inflammatory cell infiltrates are found mainly around and in the wall of the blood vessel but also occur in large and small airways. Granulation tissue and more mature scar tissue in the latter sites are rare, however. Generally there is a good correlation between the histologic score of rejection and the clinical manifestations it causes.

Treatment. Clinically evident acute rejection associated with grade III or IV changes on biopsy requires treatment with acute augmentation of immunosuppression. Most centers give methylprednisolone, 15 mg/kg, or up to a maximum of 1 g IV daily for 3 days. Symptoms may begin to lessen within hours of the first dose. Radiographic and laboratory abnormalities revert more slowly but usually resolve by several days after completion of therapy. A repeat biopsy 14 to 21 days after completion of therapy is indicated to assess the histologic response. This interval should be shorter if the clinical response has not been satisfying. An adequate clinical response is usually associated with almost complete clearing of the perivascular infiltrates on repeat biopsy. A less favorable clinical response that is associated with persistent histologic infiltrates of grade II or higher on biopsy requires a second course of corticosteroids. In many recipients, two and even three courses of corticosteroids are required to control acute rejection adequately within the first postoperative year. If the rejection does not resolve with repeated pulses of corticosteroids, the next step at most centers is treatment with antilymphocyte globulins. This sequential approach to therapy quells acute rejection in more than 90% of recipients. The remainder have what is called refractory acute rejection and often suffer irreversible injury to the allograft from this disorder or go on to contract an aggressive form of BOS.

Treatment of subclinical acute rejection associated with grade II histologic changes found after the first year is somewhat controversial. Many centers elect to withhold therapy and repeat the biopsy at a later time, particularly if symptoms or a decline in spirometry supervene. In the recipient who recently received pulsed doses of corticosteroids for histologic grade III acute rejection, the finding of persistent grade II rejection on follow-up biopsy is usually considered a treatment failure, which warrants additional therapy.

Outcome. Acute rejection produces morbidity in the early postoperative period but rarely is fatal. Consequently, care must be exercised not to immunosuppress the recipient too greatly to avoid opportunistic infection and the emergence of PTLD in susceptible hosts. If serious infection is not encountered and only one or two courses of treatment brings the episode under control, the outcome is uniformly good, with most recipients showing excellent long-term tolerance to the allograft. Recipients with recurrent episodes of acute rejection that requires multiple courses of treatment seem to be at greater risk for developing chronic rejection or BOS, as discussed later. Recipients with refractory acute rejection that never truly responds to augmented immune suppression usually experience progressive failure of the allograft in the first postoperative year, which frequently is fatal unless a second transplantation can be performed or the process reversed with experimental forms of immune suppression.

Bronchiolitis Obliterans Syndrome (Chronic Rejection)

Time Course and Prevalence. BOS is sometimes encountered as soon as 3 months after transplantation, but more commonly it occurs after the first year. The time of onset is highly variable, however. Some recipients with excellent early and intermediate graft function will contract it in the fourth to sixth year. The overall prevalence depends partly on the number of long-term survivors and the duration of follow-up. Because these numbers are steadily increasing worldwide, a better estimate of prevalence should soon emerge. Presently between 30% and 50% of recipients who have survived for a least 1 year will contract this complication. In a group of recipients who have survived at least 3 years, though, the prevalence may approach 70%.

Clinical Findings and Diagnosis. The onset of BOS is usually insidious. Not uncommonly the afflicted recipient will first notice only a decline in flow rates that they usually monitor with handheld spirometers in the home. The earliest symptoms are cough and dyspnea. The cough initially is productive of mucoid sputum, but as the disorder progresses, the sputum may become purulent. Dyspnea is usually encountered only with exertion. Physical examination in early disease is normal. In more advanced disease, rhonchi and expiratory wheezes may be heard. The chest radiograph remains unchanged from baseline until late in the course when both nodular and reticular interstitial markings appear. Segmental infiltrates usually indicate superimposed bacterial or fungal infection. Pulmonary function testing reveals a combined obstructive and restrictive impairment with a variable decline in diffusing capacity and increase in the alveolar-arterial oxygen gradient. Most often the decline in FEV_1 exceeds that of the FVC, resulting in reduced FEV_1/FVC ratio. Despite relatively large declines in the FVC, lung volumes on chest radiograph typically are well preserved, suggesting air trapping.

Although these findings are indicative of BOS, they lack diagnostic specificity. Infection with bacteria and CMV produce similar clinical and physiologic abnormalities and obviously require different therapy. Ideally, the diagnosis is confirmed with a lung biopsy. The transbronchial route is usually adequate, but since the histologic abnormalities have a patchy distribution, this approach will not always yield the diagnosis. In some circumstances it may be advisable to perform a thoracoscopic or open lung biopsy. There is growing sentiment, though, that such an invasive approach is not always necessary. If results from bronchoscopy exclude infection but the transbronchial biopsy specimens do not exhibit the typical histopathology, a clinical diagnosis may be made by exclusion. The constellation of findings required by most pathologists to make a diagnosis includes lymphocytic bronchiolitis, denudation of bronchiolar epithelium, plugs of granulation tissue in the lumen of the bronchioles, and collections of foamy macrophages in the alveoli of affected lobules (Fig. 66-2, *A*). The presence of perivascular lymphocytic infiltrates of the type seen in acute rejection is variable. However, lymphocytic infiltrates around arteries may be prominent along with sclerosis of veins. In addition, large airways may show lymphocytic infiltrates subepithelial fibrosis, and injury to cartilage. The number of neutrophils in the inflammatory infiltrates is typically small. Prominence of these cells suggests infection, in which case special stains for bacteria and fungi should be performed. Even in the absence of infection, the proportion of neutrophils in lavage fluid is usually greater than expected. The presence of bacteria in these cells (Gram stain) and isolation of bacterial pathogens from lavage fluid indicate superimposed infection, which may occur simultaneously with BOS or may be the actual cause of these histologic changes.

Clinical Staging. To assess the clinical severity of BOS and its response to treatment, an expert panel recently proposed a system based on decline in lung function and the presence or absence of his-

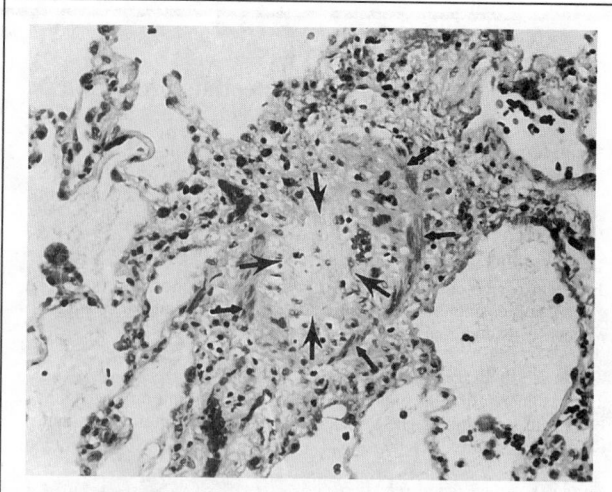

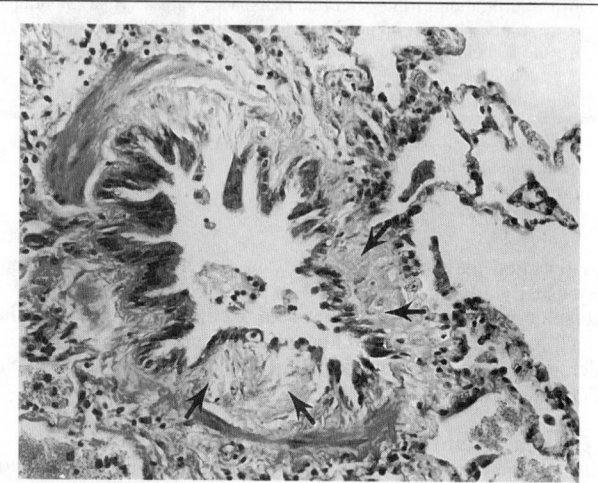

FIGURE 66-2   A, Posttransplant bronchiolitis obliterans. The lumen of this small bronchiole, which is surrounded by a mononuclear inflammatory infiltrate, is totally occluded by granulation tissue *(broad arrow).* The epithelium is virtually absent in this section. The smooth muscle cells *(thin arrows)* indicate that this destructive process involves a small airway. **B,** Inactive bronchiolitis obliterans. The lumen of this airway no longer contains granulation tissue, and the epithelium is basically intact. Nonetheless, eccentric collections of mature fibrous tissue *(broad arrows)* narrow the lumen. This histologic abnormality is usually associated with an obstructive impairment of lung function.

tologic bronchiolitis obliterans. Severity is scored on the degree to which the FEV_1 has declined compared to the best postoperative baseline value. The latter is determined by taking the average of two previous best measurements separated by 3 to 6 weeks. The new baseline is established by averaging the two most recent lower readings taken at least 1 month apart. The degree of decline is expressed as a percentage of the best baseline (Box 66-5). Four stages have been proposed (Stage 0 through Stage 3). Within each stage there are two subcategories. Subcategory "a" indicates that there is no confirmation of histologic bronchiolitis obliterans, whereas subcategory "b" indicates documentation of this abnormality. Once bronchiolitis obliterans has been confirmed histologically, the recipient will always retain the subcategory "b," even in the absence of a significant decline in the FEV_1 (Stage 0-b) or lack of this finding on subsequent biopsies. The panel has also recommended that the system be applied to recipients of a single lung allograft even though the nature of the disease in the native lung could influence the staging of BOS. Their preliminary analysis suggested that BOS was the principal process that led to clinically significant and persistent dysfunction of the lung

BOX 66-5
Clinical staging of bronchiolitis obliterans syndrome (chronic rejection)

Stage 0: no significant abnormality
FEV$_1$ is 80% of the best baseline value or greater.
 a. Without pathologic obliterative bronchiolitis
 b. With pathologic obliterative bronchiolitis

Stage 1 mild BOS
FEV$_1$ is 66% to 80% of best baseline value.
 a. Without pathologic obliterative bronchiolitis
 b. With pathologic obliterative bronchiolitis

Stage 2 moderate BOS
FEV$_1$ is 51% to 65% of best baseline value.
 a. Without pathologic obliterative bronchiolitis
 b. With pathologic obliterative bronchiolitis

Stage 3 severe BOS
FEV$_1$ is 50% of best baseline or lower.
 a. Without pathologic obliterative bronchiolitis
 b. With pathologic obliterative bronchiolitis

allograft in the late postoperative period. This system is becoming more widely adopted but will require reassessment as experience with the diagnosis and treatment of BOS matures.

Pathogenesis. Whether BOS has a unique immunologic pathogenesis is still unknown. Recipients of a lung allograft are susceptible to recurrent infection and repeated aspiration, both of which are causes of bronchiolitis obliterans. In addition, the bronchial circulation is disrupted during harvest but is not reestablished during engraftment. Loss of this blood supply likely plays a role. This factor is not the principal cause, though, because not all recipients contract BOS, and yet their bronchial circulation is nearly always compromised. Despite the potential importance of nonimmunologic factors, there is a growing consensus that BOS results from a chronic immunologic reaction to donor antigens for the following reasons:

1. Allogeneic bone marrow transplantation recipients with graft-versus-host disease develop bronchiolitis obliterans
2. Lymphocytes that recognize donor-derived antigens and exhibit proliferation and cytotoxicity in vitro can often be detected in BAL fluid and grown from transbronchial lung biopsy specimens of recipients with BOS.
3. Lymphocytes that show a high response to donor antigens are more frequently found in the blood of recipients with BOS than in recipients without this complication who demonstrate hyporesponsiveness to donor antigens
4. Recipients with recurrent acute rejection, which is difficult to control, are more prone to BOS than recipients with good graft tolerance
5. Augmentation of immunosuppression frequently stems the decline of lung function associated with BOS.

Taken together, these findings strongly support a role for alloreactivity in the pathogenesis of this disorder, but the mechanism(s) leading to BOS may differ fundamentally from that causing acute cellular rejection. Recipients with ischemic airway injury in the early postoperative period, pneumonitis with CMV, and bacterial pneumonia in the late postoperative period also seem to have a greater than expected risk for contracting BOS. It is possible these complications contribute to late dysfunction of the allograft either directly or by influencing the underlying immunopathogenesis. That they are merely associated with other factors that are the true cause of BOS is an alternative explanation that remains to be proved or disproved.

Treatment and Outcome. There is general agreement that stages 1 to 3 of BOS, i.e., those associated with a significant decline

in lung function, require treatment with augmented immunosuppression. Untreated BOS of this severity nearly always results in a progressive deterioration in graft function, which may be fatal. Preferred therapies at present include corticosteroids (100 mg orally of prednisone initially then tapered by 10 mg per day until maintenance dose is reached, or 1 g methylprednisolone IV daily for 3 days) and cytolytic agents (horse antihuman thymocyte globulin, ATGAM, or mouse monoclonal antihuman T lymphocyte antibody, OKT-3). Often corticosteroids are used initially, particularly in milder cases, with cytolytic therapy reserved for more advanced cases. Maintenance immune suppression is usually raised to tolerance.

There is growing evidence that corticosteroids are relatively ineffective because the response is either short-lived or not apparent at all. Consequently, reliance on cytolytic therapy seems to be growing, but this form of treatment does not consistently effect significant improvement in lung function. More often it stabilizes lung function for only a variable period, with relapse being common. A small but still meaningful proportion of recipients fail to show any response.

The rate of improvement in graft function differs for the two major treatments. The physiologic response to corticosteroids, when seen, usually becomes apparent within 2 weeks, whereas there is a lag of up to 6 weeks with polyclonal antilymphocyte globulins. On follow-up biopsy there may be resolution of inflammation and fibrosis, but this is not the rule. More often inflammation resolves, but fibrosis persists, causing narrowing or total occlusion of the lumens of small airways (Fig. 66-2, B). In the later case, flow rates, although higher than their lowest values, usually do not return to premorbid levels. If the follow-up biopsy reveals residual inflammation, another course of augmented immunosuppression should be given. The duration of remission is variable, but the majority of recipients will require additional therapy for relapse. When this approach fails to stem bronchiolar inflammation and fibrosis, other forms of therapy may be tried. These include mycophenolate mofetil, a recently released inhibitor of lymphocyte proliferation, total nodal irradiation, colchicine, and other cytotoxic drugs such as methotrexate. To date none have shown much promise. Preliminary trials with inhaled cyclosporin A have been encouraging. The vast majority of recipients who failed to respond to conventional therapy demonstrate stabilization of lung function and improvement in rejection histology after several months of this treatment. Controlled, randomized trials in which deposition of inhaled immunosuppressants is measured are needed to clarify the feasibility and efficacy of this form of treatment. The overall mortality rate from BOS seems to be in the range of 30% of afflicted recipients. As the number of long-term survivors increases, the prevalence of BOS will likely continue to increase and extract an even heavier toll until more effective measures are developed to control and eventually prevent this complication.

Retransplantation is the ultimate treatment for end-stage BOS. Because the number of recipients who have undergone retransplantation for BOS is presently very small, the feasibility and overall efficacy of this approach with its many medical and ethical implications remain to be defined. Preliminary results suggest that morbidity and mortality after retransplantation for BOS is higher than with the initial transplantation. This is not surprising in light of the poor medical condition of most recipients with advanced BOS. In addition, there is substantial risk for recurrence of severe BOS in recipients who underwent retransplantation for late graft dysfunction from this complication.

Augmentation of immunosuppression in recipients with BOS is not without risk. The airways of most of these individuals, and particularly those with cystic fibrosis, become colonized with bacteria, principally *P. aeruginosa* and *S. aureus,* which frequently cause clinically significant pneumonia. A staphylococcal pneumonia in this setting is nearly always life threatening and often irreversibly injures the allograft. Accordingly, efforts to limit the burden of bacteria in these recipients are indicated. Such measures include suppressive antibacterial therapy consisting of oral or inhaled antibiotics delivered for the first 10 days of each month and repeated surgical drainage of the paranasal sinuses when recurrent acute exacerbations of chronic sinusitis are documented. Reactivation of CMV following augmentation of immune suppression typically is clinically insignificant, but it may accelerate or promote the rejection process and has caused fatal disease in a small proportion of recipients afflicted with BOS. Recipients with PTLD, which has previously gone into remission, may experience a relapse with devastating consequences. Finally, invasive fungal infection occasionally supervenes. The high risk of superinfection in recipients with far advanced BOS is often a deterrent to additional immunosuppressive therapy. It also raises a question about the need to treat stage 0 BOS as aggressively as more advanced stages. Whether the option of withholding treatment in recipients with asymptomatic chronic rejection is viable remains to be proved.

FUTURE TRENDS IN LUNG TRANSPLANTATION

The achievement of an acceptable 3-year survival rate for pulmonary transplantation has ensured its future as a treatment for end-stage cardiopulmonary disease. The extent to which pulmonary transplantation eventually is adopted depends principally on the supply of organs. Demand continues to outstrip supply. Consequently, many suitable candidates in the near term will die before they can receive transplants. Efforts to improve the rate of donation are clearly warranted. A more efficient exploitation of the existing donor supply must also be achieved. Improved preservation would permit longer ischemic times and better distribution of organs. Implantation of a single lung must be performed whenever possible to maximize the number of recipients from a single donor. Strategies for the prevention of infection and rejection and organ damage from immune suppression (particuarly the kidney) must improve. The role of retransplantation for graft failure from BOS must be better defined. Finally, the impact of transplantation on the quality of life of recipients and the cost of medical care must be better defined. Despite the daunting challenges posed by these problems, their achievement in the future is realistic. Although it is fashionable these days to emphasize the prevention of chronic lung diseases and downplay the importance of expensive forms of therapy for them, control of such diseases may prove more difficult than anticipated. For this reason, pulmonary transplantation will likely continue to be the preeminent treatment for end-stage pulmonary and cardiopulmonary disease for many years to come, especially if it improves the quality of life and proves to be cost effective.

BIBLIOGRAPHY

Armitage JM, Kormos RL, Stuart RS et al: Posttransplant lymphoproliferative disease in thoracic organ transplant patients: ten years of cycolosporine-based immunosuppression, *J Heart Lung Transplant* 10:877-887, 1991.

Bando K, Paradis IL, Konishi H et al: The impact of pulmonary hypertension on outcome after single lung transplantation, *Ann Thorac Surg* 58:1336-1342, 1994.

Bando K, Paradis IL, Konishi H et al: Obliterative bronchiolitis after lung and heart-lung transplantation: an analysis of risk factors and management, *J Thorac Cardiovasc Surg* 110:4, 1995.

Cooper JD, Billingham M, Egan T et al: A working formulation for the standardization of nomenclature and for clinical staging of chronic dysfunction in lung allografts, *J Heart Lung Transplant* 12:713-716, 1993.

Dauber JH, Paradis IL, Dummer JS: Infectious complications in pulmonary allograft recipients, *Clin Chest Med* 11:291-308, 1990.

Guilinger RA, Paradis IL, Dauber JH et al: The importance of bronchoscopy with transbronchial biopsy in the management of lung transplant recipients, *Am J Respir Crit Care Med* 152:2037-2043, 1995.

Hosenpud JD, Novick RJ, Breen TJ et al: The registry of the International Society for Heart and Lung Transplantation: twelfth official report—1995, *J Heart Lung Transplant* 14:805-815, 1995.

Iacono AT, Keenan RJ, Duncan SR et al: Brief communication: aerosolized cyclosporine in lung recipients with refractory chronic rejection, *Am J Respir Crit Care Med* 153:1451-1455, 1996.

Keenan RJ, Konishi H, Kawai A et al: Clinical trial of tacrolimus versus cyclosporine in lung transplantation, *Ann Thorac Surg* 60:580-585, 1995.

Paradis IL, Yousem SA, Griffith BP: Airway obstruction and bronchiolitis obliterans after lung transplantation, *Clin Chest Med* 14:751-763, 1993.

Rabinowich H, Zeevi A, Yousem SA et al: Alloreactivity of lung biopsy and bronchoalveolar lavage-derived lymphocytes from pulmonary transplant patients: correlation with acute rejection and bronchiolitis obliterans, *Clin Transplant* 4:376-384, 1990.

Reinsmoen NL, Bolman M, Savik K et al: Improved long-term graft outcome in lung transplant recipients who have donor antigen-specific hyporeactivity, *J Heart Lung Transplant* 13:30-37, 1994.

Snell GI, Esmore DS, Williams TJ: Cytolytic therapy for the bronchiolitis obliterans syndrome complicating lung transplantation, *Chest* 109:874-878, 1996.

Sundaresan S, Trulock EP, Mohanankumar T et al: Prevalence and outcome of bronchiolitis obliterans syndrome after lung transplantation, *Ann Thorac Surg* 60:1341-1347, 1995.

Yousem SA, Berry GJ, Brunt EM et al: A working formulation for the standardization of nomenclature in the diagnosis of heart and lung rejection: lung rejection study group, *J Heart Lung Transplant* 9:593-601, 1990.

CHAPTER

67 Sleep-Related Respiratory Disorders

Laurel Wiegand

Periodic breathing events during sleep such as *apneas* and *hypopneas* contribute to a variety of clinical disorders, including the obstructive sleep apnea, central sleep apnea, and central alveolar hypoventilation syndromes. In addition, patients with pulmonary or cardiac dysfunction can experience sustained hypoventilation or periodic respiration during sleep. Sleep-related *apneas, hypopneas,* and *sustained hypoventilation* produce asphyxia and sleep disruption, the severity of which determines the systemic effects and clinical sequelae of the respiratory events.

This chapter focuses on obstructive sleep apnea (OSA), a disorder with serious medical, social, and economic consequences. Although described for centuries, OSA has only recently received widespread recognition, since symptoms develop slowly over years and the breathing abnormality is evident only during sleep in most patients. In the past, we have also neglected the importance of routinely taking a good sleep history to identify these patients in general clinical practice. Well-designed epidemiologic studies are beginning to define just how common the problem is. For example, the Wisconsin Sleep Cohort Study recently demonstrated that 4% of men and 2% of women in a middle-aged working population have OSA.

DEFINITIONS: APNEA AND HYPOPNEA

Apnea is commonly defined as airflow cessation for at least 10 seconds. Apneas may be central, mixed, or obstructive (Fig. 67-1). During central apneas, no effort is made to breathe, the diaphragm is inactive, and ventilation ceases. Mixed apneas begin with a pause in respiratory activity followed by efforts to breathe against an obstructed airway. During obstructive apneas, airflow is impeded by an obstructed upper airway despite continued efforts to breathe.

The term *hypopnea* is applied when airflow decreases enough to lower oxygen saturation. Hypopneas may be obstructive, mixed, or central. During obstructive hypopneas, the upper airway partially collapses. The patient does not fully compensate for the added breathing resistance, and hypoventilation results in oxyhemoglobin desaturation.

Apneas and hypopneas are referred to as *sleep-disordered breathing events.* They cause asphyxia and provoke arousal from sleep. The severity of asphyxia depends on baseline gas exchange and the duration of the apnea or hypopnea. Apneas and hypopneas are terminated by arousal, which serves a protective function but also disrupts sleep. Duration of the apnea or hypopnea depends on the patient's arousal threshold, which can vary. Apneas, hypopneas, and sustained periods

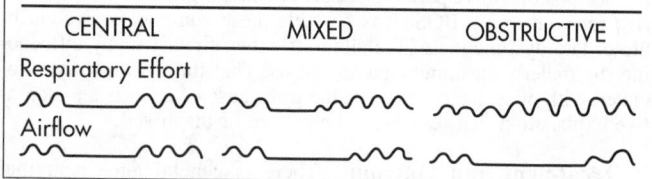

FIGURE 67-1 Three types of apnea.

of hypoventilation may occur in any sleep stage. They tend to be most severe during rapid eye movement (REM) sleep, when ventilation is most irregular.

NORMAL SLEEP AND RESPIRATION

Many neurophysiologic changes occur during sleep. Normal sleep has complex architecture, with several stages of non-REM sleep alternating with periods of REM sleep. Each sleep stage is defined by characteristic electrophysiologic patterns. Normal sleep begins with a progression from *light* (stage 1) through *deep* (stages 3 and 4) non-REM sleep, which is also called slow wave sleep due to the slow (low frequency), highly synchronized electrical activity recorded over the brain cortex by surface electroencephalography (EEG). REM sleep follows the non-REM sleep period, and this cycle is repeated several times a night. Except for the diaphragm, there is generalized skeletal muscle atonia in REM sleep. However, the REM sleep EEG resembles the EEG of wakefulness. Rapid eye movements on the electrooculogram (EOG) and skeletal muscle atonia on chin electromyography (EMG) recordings help identify REM sleep. REM sleep is also known as dream or paradoxical sleep because the brain cortex is active but the somatic musculature is inactive.

Important changes in respiration occur during sleep. Ventilation declines and arterial carbon dioxide increases, despite a lower metabolic rate during sleep. Although respiratory drive may decline during sleep, the sleep-related fall in alveolar ventilation may be better explained by sleep-related changes in upper airway mechanics. For instance, with sleep onset, partial pharyngeal collapse causes an increase in inspiratory resistance. Hypoventilation results if this added resistive "load" is not compensated for by increased respiratory effort.

It is not fully understood why the human pharynx partially collapses during normal sleep. In humans, the pharynx is unsupported by rigid structures and depends on muscle forces to maintain patency. Muscle groups that influence pharyngeal patency include the geniohyoid, genioglossus, and tensor veli palatini muscles, controlling the hyoid, tongue, and palate regions, respectively. These muscles are activated slightly before and in synchrony with the diaphragm, presumably to prepare the collapsible pharynx for the inspiratory fall in intraluminal pressure generated by diaphragm contraction. In contrast to the diaphragm, however, most upper airway muscles are less active during sleep, which may render the pharynx more collapsible. Sleep-associated changes in the relative timing and force of upper airway versus thoracic muscle activation could account for the increase in upper airway resistance.

Ventilation during sleep is also more dependent on autonomic carotid and brain stem chemoreceptor control systems because of the loss of awake behavioral input. Because cortical influences are diminished, compensatory responses to perturbations such as partial pharyngeal collapse are slower during sleep than during wakefulness.

PATHOPHYSIOLOGY OF OBSTRUCTIVE SLEEP APNEA

In OSA patients, upper airway obstruction during sleep occurs in the pharynx behind the soft palate or tongue base. We do not fully understand why OSA patients experience frequent pharyngeal occlusion during sleep, whereas nonapneic individuals do not. OSA patients may have abnormalities in upper airway structure, nonstructural factors, or respiratory control mechanisms. For example, obstructive apneas and hypopneas may result from normal sleep-induced changes in the muscular control of pharyngeal patency in individuals with a small or excessively collapsible pharynx.

Small pharyngeal lumens have been demonstrated in OSA patients by several imaging techniques, although few well-controlled studies are available. Some OSA patients do have abnormal upper airway structure on physical examination. Nasal obstruction, large tonsils and adenoids, an elongated soft palate, micrognathia, and macroglossia have all been associated with OSA. These anatomic abnormalities result in airway narrowing, requiring greater effort to achieve adequate airflow. Collapse occurs when the fall in intraluminal pressure exceeds the dilating muscle forces. Surgical correction of these structural problems can improve OSA. However, visual inspection does

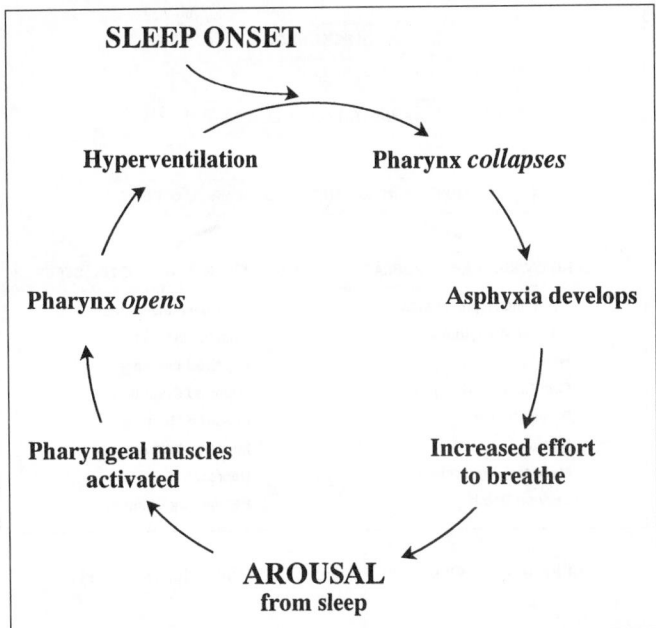

FIGURE 67-2   Obstructive sleep apnea (OSA) syndrome.

not reveal specific upper airway abnormalities in many OSA patients.

Obesity may predispose to apnea via many mechanisms, which could include altered tissue compliance and muscle function from fatty infiltration, elastic loading by fatty tissue around the upper airway, and metabolic and endocrine changes that might affect upper airway mechanics during sleep.

The OSA syndrome involves the events illustrated in Fig. 67-2. With the initial onset of sleep, the pharynx collapses and airflow decreases despite continued efforts to breathe. Hypoventilation causes progressive asphyxia, which stimulates breathing efforts. However, the airway often remains occluded until arousal occurs. With arousal, there is a surge in upper airway muscle activity, the upper airway opens, and airflow is restored. Hyperventilation in response to the accumulated hypercapnia and hypoxia initially follows restoration of airway patency. The subsequent hyperventilation-induced hypocapnia, along with sleep onset, is followed by a decrease in upper airway muscle activity and recurrent pharyngeal collapse. This sequence can occur hundreds of times a night in patients with severe OSA.

CONSEQUENCES OF SLEEP-DISORDERED BREATHING

Although occasional apneas and hypopneas during sleep may be normal, prolonged exposure to frequent apneas and hypopneas results in clinical problems that define the OSA *syndrome*. The clinical sequelae in OSA (Fig. 67-3) are related to periodic nocturnal asphyxia and sleep disruption.

Excessive daytime sleepiness and related sequelae stem from chronically disrupted sleep patterns and possibly nocturnal asphyxia. Apneas and hypopneas are frequently terminated by brief arousals less than 15 seconds in duration. Patients are usually unaware of these events, despite markedly disrupted sleep architecture. In severe cases, patients never achieve sustained or deep sleep and experience the symptoms of chronic sleep disruption, which include depression, personality changes, cognitive impairment, decreased vigilance, and irresistible sleepiness (see Fig. 67-3). These problems can compromise the individual's quality of life, family relations, job performance, and safety. Public safety is also of concern. For example, OSA patients have a higher rate of motor vehicle accidents.

Cardiovascular abnormalities (see Fig. 67-3) are related to repeated episodes of asphyxia and to fluctuations in intrathoracic pressure and autonomic activity during obstructed breaths. Sustained pulmonary and systemic hypertension and biventricular dysfunction may

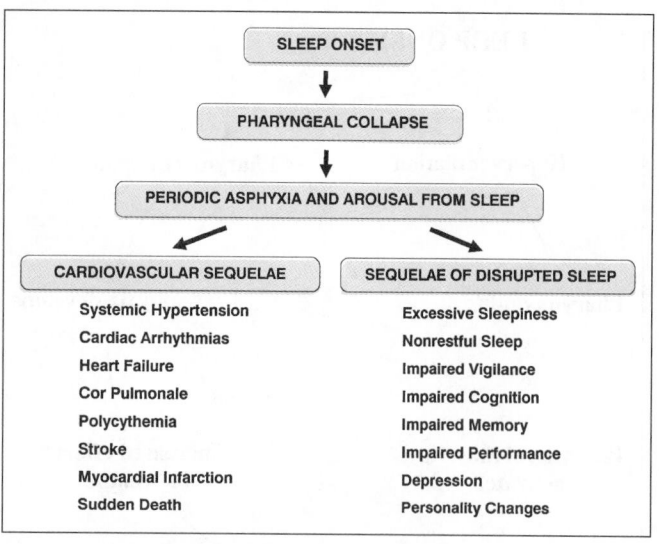

FIGURE 67-3   Obstructive sleep apnea (OSA) clinical sequelae.

eventually develop. Several recent studies suggest that a strong causal relationship exists between OSA and systemic hypertension. OSA patients may be at increased risk for malignant cardiac arrhythmias. Sinus and atrial arrhythmias, atrioventricular blocks, and ventricular arrhythmias occur primarily during apneic spells. It is not known how often apnea-related cardiac arrhythmias are life threatening. The incidence of cerebrovascular accidents and myocardial infarction are reportedly increased in OSA patients. One retrospective study reported a higher mortality in OSA patients with more severe sleep-disordered breathing. In that study, effective treatment appeared to have a positive influence on cumulative survival rates. Large population studies of OSA morbidity and mortality, however, are not available.

RISK FACTORS FOR OBSTRUCTIVE SLEEP APNEA

Important risk factors for OSA include obesity, male gender, and upper airway structural abnormalities (Fig. 67-4). The majority of OSA patients are overweight, with more than 75% reported to be at least 20% over ideal body weight. A thick neck (circumference of more than 17 inches) has been correlated with sleep apnea risk in men. The male predominance of OSA suggests that there may be important gender differences in upper airway anatomy and mechanics. Several studies have reported that many women with OSA are postmenopausal, suggesting that hormonal influences may be important. Premenopausal women with OSA are often morbidly obese. OSA can affect any age-group but appears to be most common in the middle-age years (30 to 70). In the Wisconsin Sleep Cohort Study, 4% of the men and 2% of the women in a middle-aged working population had symptomatic sleep apnea. Families with a high incidence of OSA have been reported, which may reflect genetic influences on body weight, upper airway structure, or respiratory drive. There is also a higher incidence of OSA in patients with hypothyroidism, acromegaly, and various congenital disorders (Down and Pierre Robin syndromes).

CLINICAL EVALUATION OF POTENTIAL SLEEP APNEA PATIENTS

It is important to take a good sleep history in any patient with risk factors or clinical features suggesting the possibility of OSA (see Fig. 67-4). Patients may notice several symptoms during wakefulness. Excessive daytime sleepiness is the most common complaint. Initially, daytime sleepiness may be mild and develops during relaxing activities such as reading or watching TV. As the disorder progresses, daytime sleepiness becomes more irresistible. Unwanted sleep may eventually interrupt activities such as driving a motor vehicle. By-products of excessive daytime sleepiness such as inability to concentrate,

memory and judgment impairment, irritability, depression, and personality changes also become more common as the disorder progresses. Decreased libido and impotence are common complaints, although the etiology is unknown. Early morning headache is occasionally reported and may be related to the nocturnal episodes of hypercapnia causing increased cerebral blood flow and edema.

Patients do not always realize that their sleep quality is poor and disrupted by frequent, brief arousals. However, they may complain of restless sleep or being awakened by their own snoring or a choking sensation. The sleeping partner usually describes loud snoring, although not all snorers have sleep apnea. It is more helpful if the sleeping partner has observed frequent apneas associated with snoring cessation and terminated by snorting, gasping, or restless movement.

On physical examination, patients are often overweight. The neck may be short and thick. The upper airway should be examined for nasal obstruction, large tonsils, an elongated palate, macroglossia, micrognathia, or pharyngeal tumor. Systemic hypertension may be present. Signs of left ventricular dysfunction, pulmonary hypertension, right heart failure, polycythemia, and chronic alveolar hypoventilation may develop in severe OSA. Neurologic examination may reveal excessive sleepiness and impaired memory and cognition in severe cases.

Routine laboratory tests are of limited value in the diagnosis of OSA. Screening tests for hypothyroidism and acromegaly should be performed if these disorders are suspected based on clinical findings. A minority of patients with very severe OSA have polycythemia or an elevated arterial carbon dioxide tension on awake arterial blood gas testing.

DIAGNOSIS OF OBSTRUCTIVE SLEEP APNEA

When OSA is suspected, polysomnography is indicated to establish the diagnosis. Standardized overnight polysomnography performed in a sleep laboratory by a trained technician is recommended as the best diagnostic approach. Polysomnography involves recording electrophysiologic variables such as the brain activity EEG, eye movements (EOG), and chin muscle tone (EMG). This information allows sleep quantity and quality to be characterized. The electrocardiogram is also recorded. Standard measurements of respiration include recordings of chest displacement, nasal and oral airflow, and arterial oxyhemoglobin saturation. The number of apneas and hypopneas, their type and duration, and their sequelae, such as the amount of hypoxia and associated sleep fragmentation, can then be quantified. Periods of sustained hypoventilation may also be identified. By defining the type and severity of sleep-disordered breathing and associated sleep fragmentation, polysomnographic data help the clinician to develop a therapeutic plan. Polysomnography should also be used to assess the response to therapy in OSA patients.

There has been interest in developing simplified diagnostic techniques. Proposed approaches include home monitoring with oximetry or abbreviated polysomnographic montages. However, the sensitivity, specificity, and cost-effectiveness of such approaches require further study before recommendations can be made regarding their routine use.

WHO REQUIRES TREATMENT?

The spectrum of clinical disorders related to sleep-induced upper airway obstruction is illustrated in Fig. 67-5. Unfortunately, we lack good prospective studies characterizing the long-term clinical consequences of simple heavy snoring or mild sleep-disordered breathing in untreated individuals. Accordingly, we do not know exactly what indices of apnea frequency, oxyhemoglobin desaturation, and sleep fragmentation require treatment. Most symptomatic patients with more than 20 apneas and hypopneas per hour of sleep or severe oxyhemoglobin desaturation should be treated. However, symptomatic patients with fewer sleep-disordered breathing events may also benefit from treatment. These patients may have debilitating sleepiness because of frequent arousals from sleep provoked by breathing efforts against a partially collapsed pharynx but few actual apneas or hypopneas. This is the so-called *upper airways resistance syndrome* (see Fig. 67-5). On the other hand, levels of sleep-disordered breath-

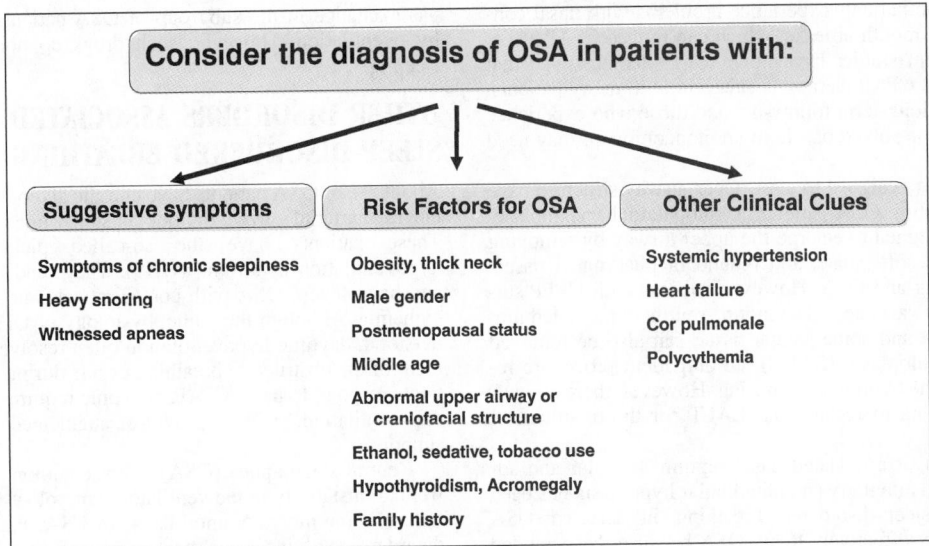

FIGURE 67-4 Risk factors for obstructive sleep apnea (OSA).

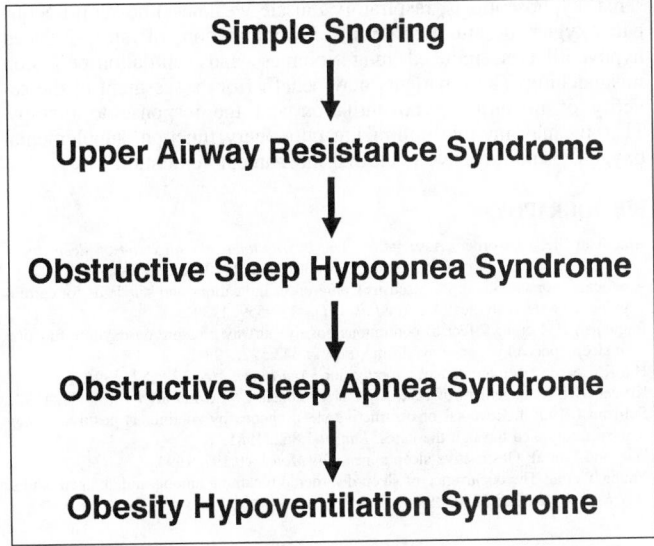

FIGURE 67-5 Clinical spectrum of sleep-induced upper airway obstruction.

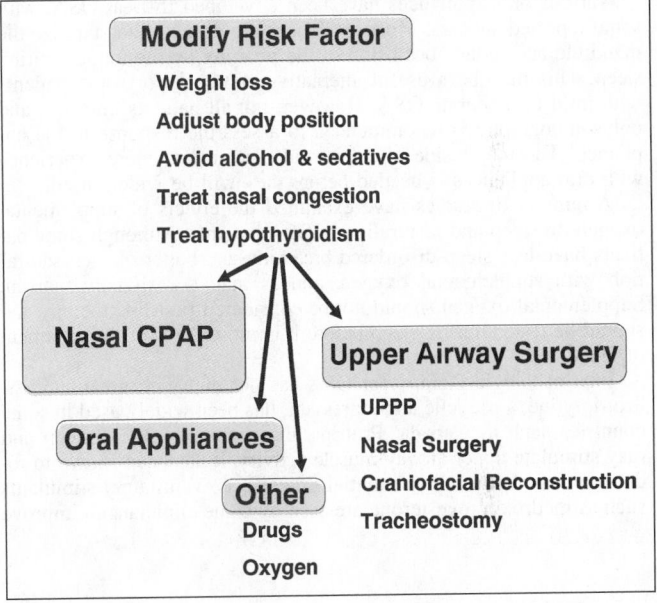

FIGURE 67-6 Obstructive sleep apnea (OSA) treatment.

ing formerly considered pathologic (>5 apneas/hour of sleep) have been reported in healthy, asymptomatic persons, especially with aging. Therefore the decision to treat must be based on an overall assessment of the severity of sleepiness and related symptoms, cardiac sequelae, *and* the severity of sleep-disordered breathing and sleep fragmentation documented on polysomnography.

THERAPY FOR OBSTRUCTIVE SLEEP APNEA

The first step in OSA therapy involves a search for reversible factors that worsen sleep-disordered breathing (Fig. 67-6). For example, OSA patients should avoid ethanol and sedative hypnotics, since these agents increase apneas in most patients. Weight loss is recommended for obese patients and may reduce apneas and improve oxygen saturation, particularly if the obesity is moderate. However, dietary weight reduction is difficult to achieve and maintain. Surgical procedures such as gastric stapling may help morbidly obese patients. Some patients benefit from adjustment of sleeping body position; many patients have fewer apneas when sleeping on their side than when supine. Reversible causes of nasal obstruction such as chronic rhinitis should be treated. Thyroid replacement may improve sleep-disordered

breathing in hypothyroid patients with sleep apnea. Most patients, however, require additional therapy beyond these steps.

Nasal continuous positive airway pressure (CPAP) has become the major treatment modality for OSA (see Fig. 67-6). Introduced by Sullivan and co-workers in 1981, nasal CPAP is produced by a high-flow blower that delivers a continuous stream of room air into a sealed nasal mask, which the patient wears during sleep. The positive pressure created in the circuit pneumatically splints the pharynx open. Nasal CPAP can abolish apneas and hypopneas, oxygen desaturation, and apnea-related sleep fragmentation in most patients. Patients should be studied in the sleep laboratory to determine the optimal CPAP level, which will vary with individual upper airway characteristics. CPAP pressures ranging from 5 to 15 cm H_2O are most commonly required. After the initiation of effective nasal CPAP therapy, patients experience a marked rebound of deep non-REM sleep and REM sleep. Sleep patterns gradually normalize over the first few weeks of therapy in association with symptomatic improvement, particularly daytime sleepiness and function. Side effects are generally minor but may affect compliance. Some patients experience problems with nasal congestion and mask and mouth airleaks, which can reduce CPAP effectiveness. Several recent studies have now clearly demonstrated that compliance with nasal CPAP therapy is suboptimal in many patients. OSA patients require long-term follow-up, and those who experience problems that cannot be solved or whom are noncompliant may need additional therapy.

Surgical procedures designed to alter upper airway structure have proved helpful in treating OSA patients. Uvulopalatopharyngoplasty (UPPP) surgery is designed to enlarge the upper airway by removing the uvula, part of the soft palate, and redundant pharyngeal tissue. UPPP can cure snoring and OSA. However, success with UPPP surgery for sleep apnea is variable and cannot be routinely predicted preoperatively. The uvula and some palatal tissue can also be removed with laser-assisted uvuloplasty (LAUP), an outpatient procedure recently developed for the treatment of snoring. However, there are currently no published data to recommend LAUP for the treatment of sleep apnea.

Surgical correction of a deviated nasal septum, tonsillar and adenoid hypertrophy, and maxillary and mandibular hypoplasia has been shown to improve sleep-disordered breathing in selected OSA patients. Tracheostomy effectively treats OSA because the occluded pharynx is by-passed. Patients can plug the tracheostomy tube while awake and sleep with it open. However, tracheostomy is now reserved for morbidly ill patients or those who do not respond to less invasive options.

Various oral appliances have been developed to treat OSA, with some reported success. Most appliances are designed to stabilize the mandible and reduce occlusion of the pharynx by the tongue during sleep. This may be a useful alternative approach for some patients with mild to moderate OSA. However, not all patients improve, and polysomnography is recommended to assess the response to the appliance. The major side effect is oral discomfort. More experience with oral appliances is needed before they will be widely used.

A number of studies have examined the effects of supplemental oxygen on sleep and respiration in OSA patients. Although some patients have less sleep-disordered breathing and better oxygen saturation with supplemental oxygen, apneas may occasionally worsen. Supplemental oxygen should not be considered first-line therapy and should be tested during sleep before it is prescribed for the treatment of OSA.

Pharmacologic therapy for OSA has not met with great success. Protriptyline, a tricyclic antidepressant, has been widely used in some countries such as Canada. Protriptyline suppresses REM sleep and may stimulate upper airway muscle activity. It has been shown to reduce apneas, but it has substantial side effects. Ventilatory stimulants such as medroxyprogesterone are used by some clinicians to improve gas exchange in the subgroup of OSA patients with awake alveolar hypoventilation. However, such drugs do not predictably improve sleep apnea.

OTHER DISORDERS ASSOCIATED WITH SLEEP-DISORDERED BREATHING

About 5% of OSA patients have chronic alveolar hypoventilation with elevated arterial carbon dioxide tension while awake (see Fig. 67-4). These patients have the so-called pickwickian or obesity-hypoventilation syndrome (OHS). They tend to be morbidly obese and have severe OSA with cor pulmonale and, in some cases, polycythemia. Although the pathophysiology of OHS remains poorly understood, daytime hypoventilation often resolves after effective treatment of the obstructive breathing events during sleep. Some OHS patients respond to nasal CPAP, but some require noninvasive mechanical ventilation, which provides augmented inspiratory pressure support.

Central sleep apnea (CSA) is not common. Central apneas result from an instability in the ventilatory control system. Congestive heart failure is the most common cause of CSA. Patients with neurologic disorders involving brain stem respiratory control centers may have CSA. The clinical sequelae of CSA are similar to those described for OSA. Supplemental oxygen, acetazolamide, or noninvasive nocturnal mechanical ventilation may help some patients.

Many patients with compromised pulmonary function (emphysema, kyphoscoliosis, respiratory muscle weakness) develop nocturnal oxygen desaturation from a combination of sleep-induced hypoventilation, reduced lung volumes, and ventilation-perfusion mismatching. These patients may benefit from assessment of the severity of nocturnal hypoventilation and the response to therapy. Therapy may involve optimizing pulmonary function, supplemental oxygen, or noninvasive nocturnal mechanical ventilation.

BIBLIOGRAPHY

American Sleep Disorders Association: *The international classification of sleep disorders: diagnostic and coding manual,* Lawrence, KS, 1990, Allen Press.
American Thoracic Society Consensus Conference: Indications and standards for cardiopulmonary sleep studies, *Am Rev Respir Dis* 139:559, 1989.
Engleman HM et al: Effect of continuous positive airway pressure on daytime function in sleep apnoea/hypopnea syndrome, *Lancet* 343:572, 1994.
Hla KM et al: Sleep apnea and hypertension, *Ann Intern Med* 120:382, 1994.
Kryger MH: Management of obstructive sleep apnea, *Clin Chest Med* 13(3):481, 1992.
Sullivan CE et al: Reversal of obstructive sleep apnoea by continuous positive airway pressure applied through the nares, *Lancet* 1:862, 1981.
Wiegand L et al: Obstructive sleep apnea, *Dis Month* 40:197, 1994.
Young T et al: The occurrence of sleep-disordered breathing among middle-aged adults, *N Engl J Med* 328:1230, 1993.

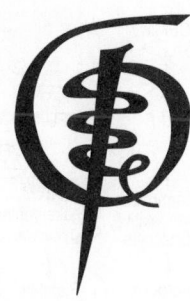

PART FOUR

Hematology
and
Oncology

68 Molecular and Cellular Biology of Hematopoiesis

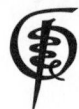

David A. Williams

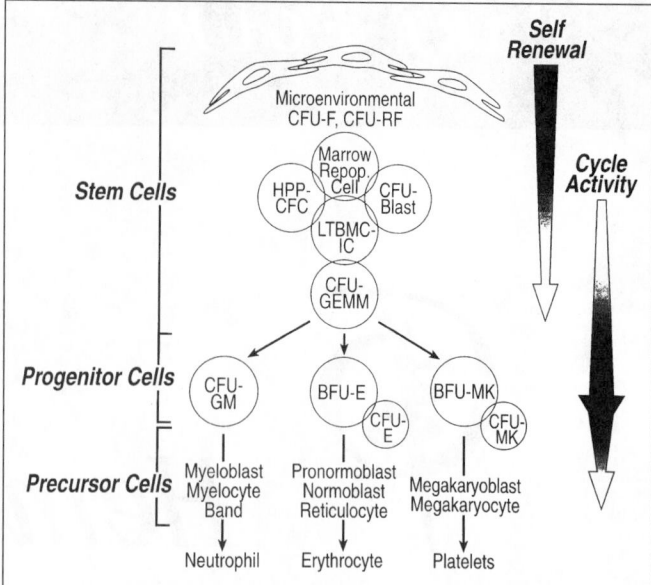

FIGURE 68-1 Schematic presentation of cellular events that occur during normal human hematopoiesis. *CFU*, Colony-forming unit; *CFU-B1, CFU-Blast* unit; *CFU-F*, CFU–fibroblast; *CFU-RF*, CFU–reticular fibroblast; *LTBMC-IC*, long-term bone marrow culture–initiating cell; *HPP-CFC*, high-proliferative-potential colony-forming cell; *CFU-GEMM*, CFU–granulocyte, erythrocyte, macrophage, megakaryocyte; *CFU-GM*, CFU–granulocyte, macrophage; *BFU-E*, BFU–erythrocyte; *CFU-E*, CFU–erythrocyte, *BFU-MK*, BFU–megakaryocyte; *CFU-MK*, CFU–megakaryocyte.

HEMATOPOIESIS

Human blood contains a variety of cells, each providing a vital function needed to sustain normal life. Red cells transport oxygen throughout the body, whereas platelets are required to promote clotting. White cells (granulocytes, monocytes, lymphocytes) combat attack by viruses, bacteria, fungi, and likely tumor cells. Quantitative or qualitative abnormalities of any of these blood cell types lead in a predictable manner to human disease. The life span of most blood cells is extremely short, ranging from hours to days, although some exceptions exist in the lymphoid compartment. The need for continued blood cell production requires the constant regeneration of the blood cell pool throughout life. In addition, various conditions such as bleeding or infection require that the bone marrow be able to respond quickly to produce additional cells. The term *hematopoiesis* refers to the system by which the body continuously produces blood cells. Blood cells ultimately arise from the bone marrow as the result of the proliferation and differentiation of primitive cells capable of maturation into all blood cell types. These primitive cells are termed *pluripotent hematopoietic stem cells*. Blood cell production is believed to be regulated in part by a series of glycoprotein hormones.

The vast majority of cells present in a healthy individual's bone marrow are bone marrow precursor cells (Color Plate IV-1). From 60% to 70% of these cells are myeloid precursors, 20% to 30% are erythroid precursors, and the remaining 10% include lymphocytes, plasma cells, and macrophages. In addition, four to five megakaryocytes are normally found per 1000 nucleated bone marrow cells. The normal ratio of myeloid to erythroid precursors is 3 to 3.5:1. Alterations in these numbers are difficult to determine with bone marrow aspirates because of variations in dilution with peripheral blood. Bone marrow biopsy is the preferred method of quantitation of marrow cellularity and precursor frequency.

Hematopoietic Stem Cells

Hematopoiesis can be viewed as being composed of a continuum of cell populations with differing self-renewal, proliferative, and differentiation capacities (Fig. 68-1). The most primitive cell in this hierarchy is the pluripotent hematopoietic stem cell, which is characterized by its extensive self-renewal capacity and its capability of giving rise to all hematopoietic cell lineages. The stem cell is a quiescent cell with extensive proliferative capacity. Self-renewal of the stem cell ensures the existence of an adequate pool of sustaining stem cells. Stem cells must undergo a *commitment process* to differentiate to different classes of progenitor cells, which are characterized by a progressive loss of self-renewal capacity and multipotentiality, leading to the production of multipotent, bipotent, and eventually unipotent progenitor cells. Unlike stem cells, a much greater proportion of progenitor cells are mitotically active. The decision to remain quiescent, undergo self-renewal, or proceed with commitment is a critical step in the determination of a stem cell's fate. Once the commitment decision is made, an irreversible movement toward production of blood cells occurs, which inevitably results in the loss of stem cell self-renewal capacity and ultimately the stem cell phenotype. It re-

mains unknown whether this decision is a random process (*stochastic hypothesis*) or whether it can be influenced by cytokines, matrix proteins, or marrow accessory cells present within the marrow microenvironment (*instructional hypothesis*).

Several models have also been constructed that give insight into the clonal organization of hematopoietic cells. If stem cell self-renewal capacity is unlimited and stem cells are truly immortal, they could likely function for an individual's entire lifetime. Stem cell immortality would confer stability on the clonal composition of an animal's hematopoietic system. On the other hand, stem cell self-renewal capacity could also be much more limited. Under these circumstances, only a portion of the total stem cell population would be active at any given time, and new stem cells would be required to contribute to active blood cell production to replace dying cells. This constant turnover in the active stem cell population would likely lead to changes in the clonal makeup of the different hematopoietic lineages over time. Hematopoiesis then would be maintained by a succession of short-lived clones (*clonal succession model*). The concept of short-lived stem cells is supported by the finding that the hematopoietic systems of irradiated, reconstituted animals undergo clonal changes with time. Equally convincing evidence, however, indicates that at least a subpopulation of stem cells are long lived, able to function for prolonged periods, and able to expand clonally during the regeneration of a new hematopoietic system.

Resolution of these theories that deal with stem cell fate and life span is extremely important to further our understanding of the basic biologic properties of stem cells. Such accomplishments would allow further insight into the pathobiology of bone marrow failure and the origins of hematologic malignancies. Greater knowledge of the stem cell is likely necessary if the full therapeutic potential of bone marrow transplantation and somatic gene therapy is ever to be achieved. New insight into the biology of stem cells and progenitor cells will surely occur with the recent ability of several research groups to obtain highly enriched populations of not only murine but also human stem cells.

Advances in our understanding of hematopoiesis have occurred following the development of several assays to measure stem cell and progenitor cell number and function. Stem cells and the numerous classes of marrow progenitor cells can be assayed using a variety of in vitro clonal assays performed in semisolid media (colony assays) or by using long-term marrow cultures. The time required for hematopoietic colonies to develop in vitro depends on the stage of differentiation of the cell from which they are derived. The most mature human progenitor cells produce small colonies after less than 7 days of incubation, whereas the more immature progenitor cells give rise to larger colonies after 14 to 28 days.

The overwhelming majority of morphologically identifiable cells within the marrow are precursor cells that have no self-renewal capacity, are unipotent, and are capable of limited mitosis. These cells exhibit well-described nuclear and cytoplasmic characteristics that allow the clinical hematologist to identify them as belonging to a particular cell lineage. Because of the quantity of precursor cells, in spite of their limited proliferative capacity considerable amplification of cell number occurs at this stage of development, resulting in a steady supply of functional blood cells that egress from the marrow.

Hematopoietic Microenvironment

Hematopoiesis occurs in a complex environment within the marrow cavity, termed the *hematopoietic microenvironment*. The marrow cavity is extremely vascular. Branches of a central longitudinal artery traverse the interior of the bone and cortex, either joining directly to venous sinuses or communicating indirectly through the *haversian* canals into bone cortex. These vascular connections define groups of developing hematopoietic cells termed *hematopoietic cords,* where stem cell self-renewal and commitment occur. Blood cells leaving the marrow cavity traverse the hematopoietic cords, pass through endothelial cells, eventually enter venous sinuses, and are rapidly transported into central longitudinal veins and arrive in the general circulation.

Various accessory cells contribute important functions to the hematopoietic microenvironment. Adventitial reticular cells cover most *abluminal* vascular surfaces and provide a reticular network that supports developing hematopoietic cells. Adventitial cells and preadipocytes probably also affect hematopoiesis by direct cell contact or local secretion of cytokines or other growth-regulatory proteins. Such marrow accessory cells normally contain fat and extend into the hematopoietic cord space. During periods of hematopoietic stress, these cells become flattened and devoid of fat globules, providing additional space for active hematopoiesis.

The hematopoietic microenvironment provides more than passive support for hematopoietic cells. Preferential localization of blood cell production to specific microenvironments is thought to affect stem cell differentiation, leading to the hypothesis that specific locations or "niches" within the marrow provide an inductive microenvironment for stem cell self-renewal and differentiation. The cellular and biochemical basis of such niches has yet to be defined, but the development of in vitro long-term marrow culture systems that mimic the marrow microenvironment has provided further insight into this process. Such cultures are composed of a complex adherent cell layer, termed the *stromal cell layer,* which contains endothelial cells, fibroblasts, macrophages, and preadipocytes. Hematopoiesis occurs within the adherent cell layer, and hematopoietic cells are continuously shed into the overlying media. Using this system, hematopoietic niches have been shown possibly to involve direct communication of stromal cells with stem cells through cell-to-cell contact, localization of growth factors and stem cells at the point of cell-to-cell contact, prevention of growth factor degradation by binding cytokines to extracellular matrix proteins, or secretion of growth factors that both stimulate and downregulate hematopoiesis. These interactions define a *local area network* (LAN) for hematopoiesis.

Stem Cell Assays

Attempts to assay stem cells began in the early 1960s, when Till and McCulloch injected lethally irradiated mice with marrow cells. These marrow cells contained CFU-S (colony-forming unit–spleen), which lodged in the spleens of injected animals and formed macroscopic nodules within 7 to 12 days. The splenic nodules were derived from a single cell and consisted of differentiating cells belonging to several hematopoietic lineages. In addition, such splenic nodules contained cells capable of generating additional splenic colonies when

transferred into secondarily irradiated hosts. Cells (CFU-S$_{12}$) that give rise to splenic nodules arising after 12 to 14 days contain larger numbers of CFU-S than splenic colonies that appear in 8 to 10 days (CFU-S$_8$). The biologic properties of the CFU-S led to speculations that this cell represented a hematopoietic stem cell. However, both CFU-S$_8$ and CFU-S$_{12}$ have recently been shown to be a more differentiated class of stem cells. Stem cells are currently being defined by their marrow-repopulating ability.

Stem cell function is now thought to be best quantitated by such cells' ability to reconstitute hematopoiesis in lethally irradiated recipients. Marrow-reconstituting ability of stem cells is optimally measured by the use of long-term in vivo assays. The use of retroviral-mediated gene insertion has enhanced investigators' ability to track the progeny of individual stem cells in vivo. This approach has been useful in quantitating murine stem cells, but obviously the human system does not lend itself to this form of experimental freedom. In vivo xenograft systems, however, have been recently developed that may allow assay of the marrow-populating capacity of human stem cells by transferring these cells into immune-deficient mice or immune-tolerant fetal sheep. In vitro assays for various primitive hematopoietic progenitor cells that resemble stem cells have also been developed: the colony-forming unit—blast (CFU-Bl), the high-proliferative-potential colony-forming cell (HPP-CFC), and the long-term bone marrow culture–initiating cell (LTBMC-IC). These assays detect cells with extensive proliferative and multilineage differentiation capacity. Using such in vitro and in vivo assays, human stem cells have now begun to be phenotypically characterized. However, the relationship of these primitive cells identified by in vitro assays to marrow-repopulating cells in vivo remains unknown.

Erythropoiesis

The immediate progeny of differentiated stem cells are several classes of progenitor cells, including the colony-forming unit–granulocyte, erythrocyte, macrophage, megakaryocyte (CFU-GEMM) (Color Plate IV-2); the burst-forming unit–erythroid (BFU-E); and the colony-forming unit–erythroid (CFU-E). This hierarchy of progenitor cells is characterized by a progressive loss of proliferative capacity and further restriction in differentiation potential (CFU-GEMM→BFU-E→CFU-E). These progenitor cells each can be detected by their ability in semisolid media to form erythroid colonies in the presence of appropriate growth factors. Each of these assays requires the presence of erythropoietin. The most differentiated erythroid progenitor cells, CFU-E, produce a variety of erythroid precursor cells.

The first identifiable and also largest erythroid precursor is the *pronormoblast* (Color Plate IV-3, *A*), which has a diameter of 14 to 19 μm and a large, homogeneously staining (violet) oval nucleus with indistinct nucleoli. The cytoplasm is deeply basophilic, with lighter-staining areas usually near the nucleus, reflecting the position of the Golgi and lipid-containing mitochondria. Maturation to the basophilic normoblast is accompanied by reduction in cell size and pronounced changes in the nuclear chromatin structure. The *basophilic normoblast* (Color Plate IV-3, *B*) is 12 to 17 μm in diameter, with basophilic cytoplasm and nuclear chromatin characterized by coarsening and prominent clumping, referred to as a "spoked wheel" or "cartwheel" appearance. Nucleoli are generally not visualized. The *polychromatic normoblast* (Color Plate IV-3, *C*) is nearly the same size as the basophilic normoblast. The accumulation of hemoglobin is accompanied by progressively less basophilia and increasing muddy gray coloration of the cytoplasm on Wright-Giemsa staining. The nucleus is almost black because of further condensation. The most differentiated nucleated red cell precursor is the *orthochromatic normoblast* (Color Plate IV-3, *C*). This cell's diameter approaches that of a reticulocyte (8 to 12 μm) and has an eosinophilic staining cytoplasm containing almost a complete complement of hemoglobin. The nucleus is fully condensed and pyknotic. Extrusion of the nucleus results in formation of a *reticulocyte,* a cell slightly larger than a fully mature erythrocyte. The reticulocyte is characterized by the presence of a fine granular or reticular network of ribosomal ribonucleic acid (RNA) (Color Plate IV-4, *J*). Such cells are rarely present in peripheral blood but are increased in response to hemolysis or blood loss. The final stage of erythroid maturation is the *erythrocyte*. The cell is a biconcave, relatively flat, nonnucleated disk with a diameter of 7 to 8 μm.

Myelopoiesis

Neutrophils and monocytes are closely related cells that arise from a common committed progenitor cell, the colony-forming unit–granulocyte macrophage (CFU-GM), which may give rise to a CFU–granulocyte (CFU-G) or CFU–macrophage (CFU-M); these progenitors have a unipotential differentiation capacity. Progenitor cells of basophil-mast cells and eosinophils have also been identified.

The earliest identifiable precursor cell of the myeloid lineage is the *myeloblast.* The cell is approximately 12 to 14 μm in diameter, with a round or oval nucleus and a cytoplasm that lacks granules. Nuclear chromatin is fine, and nucleoli are easily visible and number one to five per cell. The nucleus often stains reddish. *Promyelocytes* are the most frequent and largest of the primitive myeloid precursors (Color Plate IV-1). Promyelocytes are variable in nuclear shape, with less prominent nucleoli and coarse chromatin. The cytoplasm is deeply basophilic and contains variable numbers of peroxidase-positive granules. These granules distinguish the promyelocyte from the myeloblast. *Myelocytes* are characterized by round-to-oval nuclei with characteristic nuclear indentations, indistinct nucleoli, and unevenly stained, coarse chromatin structure. The cytoplasm stains pale gray-brown or pink-brown with numerous specific granules covering the nucleus and throughout the cytoplasm. The myelocyte is also characterized by the appearance of specific granules and is the final stage of myelopoiesis in which the cells are capable of cell division. The metamyelocyte, band neutrophil, and segmented neutrophil show progressive condensation and restriction of the nucleus. The *metamyelocyte* exhibits a characteristic bean-shaped nucleus, the *band neutrophil* a horseshoe-shaped or S-shaped nuclear structure without recognizable constrictions, and the *segmented neutrophil* the characteristic nuclear segmentations for which it is named that divide the nucleus into two to five lobes. These myeloid forms exhibit similar cytoplasmic characteristics to the myelocyte, with progressive reduction in overall cell size.

The marrow contains a large reserve of band and segmented neutrophils. In the peripheral blood, neutrophils are equally divided between circulating and marginal pools. A large reserve of neutrophils is therefore available in the marrow and the marginal pool to respond quickly to infection or inflammation. The mature neutrophil remains in the circulation for approximately 10 to 14 hours before entering tissues and performing its phagocytic function. This limited survival of granulocytes dictates that myelopoiesis be a highly dynamic biologic process.

Megakaryocytopoiesis

Progenitor cells for megakaryocytes can be cultured at low frequency from the bone marrow. These colony-forming cells are termed burstforming unit–megakaryocyte (BFU-MK) and colony-forming unit—megakaryocyte (CFU-MK). Development of platelets follows maturational steps that are unique in the hematopoietic system. In this process, called *polyploidization,* successive nuclear divisions occur without cytoplasmic divisions. The resulting megakaryocytes contain 1 to 32 nuclei (2N-64N nuclear content). The megakaryoblast is a distinctly large cell with a high nuclear/cytoplasmic ratio containing a nucleus that may possess nucleoli. The nucleus frequently shows convolutions. The cytoplasm is deep blue. The promegakaryocyte contains a lobulated nucleus without nucleoli, the cytoplasm contains some granules, and platelets may be seen forming at the surface of the cell. Mature megakaryocytes are the largest hematopoietic cells in the bone marrow and can easily be distinguished on low magnification. The nucleus is distinctly lobulated and contains coarse chromatin. The number of nuclei varies from four to eight. Megakaryocyte cytoplasm is basophilic with azurophilic granules, and platelets are frequently seen on the surface of the cell. Megakaryocytes are present at low (0.1%-0.5%) frequency in the bone marrow of normal individuals.

HEMATOPOIETIC REGULATORY MOLECULES

Hematopoiesis is sustained by a family of glycoproteins, the hematopoietic growth factors. The term *cytokine* refers to a bioactive cell secretion, whereas the term *growth factor* refers to a growth-regulatory molecule and is a more specific term encompassing eryth-

ropoietin, the colony-stimulating factors, and the interleukins. Many cytokines serve as hematopoietic growth factors. The nomenclature of these growth factors was first defined operationally. The initial factors described were identified by their ability to stimulate progenitor cells to form in vitro colonies composed of particular types of cells and were therefore referred to as granulocyte colony-stimulating factor (G-CSF) or granulocyte-macrophage colony-stimulating factor (GM-CSF). The interleukins derived their names initially from their cellular sources as well as their actions on leukocytes. The biologic activity of erythropoietin was first detected using a variety of rodent animal models. Erythropoietin was subsequently shown to stimulate in vitro erythropoiesis. The genes for many of the hematopoietic growth factors have now been cloned and their respective recombinant proteins produced and purified. The availability of these purified recombinant biomolecules has permitted determination of their actions, cellular origins, and actual therapeutic use (Table 68-1).

Each of the hematopoietic growth factors exhibits multiple biologic activities, most affecting several hematopoietic lineages. GM-CSF, for example, promotes CFU-GM proliferation but also influences the development of CFU-GEMM, HPP-CFC, CFU-B1, LTMBC-IC, and CFU megakaryocyte (CFU-MK). This cytokine stimulates the functional activation of such differentiated cells as eosinophils, macrophages, monocytes, and neutrophils. Many activities of the hematopoietic growth factors are either additive or synergistic. For example, both GM-CSF and interleukin-3 (IL-3) are capable of stimulating HPP-CFC–derived colonies, and their actions are additive. The c-kit ligand, on the other hand, has no colony-stimulating activity by itself but synergistically interacts with the combination of GM-CSF and IL-3 to optimize cloning efficiency of HPP-CFC in vitro, in addition to enhancing the cloning efficiency of many other classes of progenitor cells.

Some growth factors act directly on hematopoietic progenitors, whereas others induce the expression of a wide variety of other interleukins and growth factor genes by marrow accessory cells. Specific membrane receptors for various hematopoietic growth factors

Table 68-1 Potentially clinically useful hematopoietic growth factors

GROWTH FACTOR	POTENTIAL CLINICAL USES
Interleukin-6 (IL-6)	Stimulates platelet production; lessens degree of granulocytopenia/thrombocytopenia after bone marrow transplantation or chemotherapy
Interleukin-11 (IL-11)	Stimulates platelet production; lessens degree of granulocytopenia/thrombocytopenia after bone marrow transplantation or chemotherapy; stimulates recovery of small intestine after chemotherapy
Granulocyte-macrophage colony-stimulating factor (GM-CSF)	Lessens degree of granulocytopenia after bone marrow transplantation or chemotherapy; mobilization of peripheral blood stem cells
Granulocyte colony-stimulating factor (G-CSF)	Lessens degree of granulocytopenia after bone marrow transplantation or chemotherapy; treatment of chronic neutropenic disorders; mobilization of peripheral blood stem cells
Macrophage colony-stimulating factor (M-CSF)	Adjunctive therapy for fungal infections after bone marrow transplantation or chemotherapy; antitumor therapy when administered with monoclonal antibodies
Erythropoietin	Treatment of anemias of chronic renal disease, chronic inflammation, cancer, and human immunodeficiency virus 1 (HIV-1) infection; treatment of anemia of prematurity
c-kit ligand (stem cell factor [SCF])	Mobilization of peripheral blood stem cells
c-Mpl ligand (ML)	Stimulates platelet production
IL-3/GM-CSF fusion (Pixie)	Lessens degree of granulocytopenia after bone marrow transplantation or chemotherapy, stimulates platelet production

(IL-3, GM-CSF, G-CSF, erythropoietin, M-CSF, IL-11, c-kit ligand) are restricted to undifferentiated and maturing cells of the appropriate target cell lineages. By contrast, other growth factors have no colony-stimulating activity but affect hematopoiesis indirectly. For instance, IL-1 has no known colony-stimulating activity itself but induces G-CSF and GM-CSF expression by a variety of cells, including fibroblasts, endothelial cells, thymic epithelial cells, and T-lymphocytes. Such indirect-acting growth factors can have profound effects on in vivo and in vitro hematopoiesis.

Understanding growth factor physiology is an important step in optimizing their therapeutic use and furthering our knowledge of the biogenesis of many hematologic disorders. This information is available only for a few growth factors. Erythropoietin physiology is the best understood. Under steady-state conditions, erythropoietin is elaborated by either proximal tubules or peritubular cells of the kidney's inner cortex in response to a hypoxic stimulus or anemia. The oxygen sensor that monitors blood oxygen content is now thought to be a heme protein that controls the expression of erythropoietin messenger-RNA (mRNA) in an unknown way and results in the elaboration of erythropoietin. With the correction of the hypoxia or anemia, erythropoietin production ceases, except in cells that constitutively produce this hormone. Inadequate elaboration of this growth factor results in anemia, whereas excessive erythropoietin production leads to polycythemia.

Cytokines act in an indirect way and play a role in the development of the hematologic consequences of several systemic diseases. IL-1 and tumor necrosis factor (TNF) have been shown to play important roles in producing the clinical features associated with acute and chronic inflammatory states and other serious illnesses, including septic shock and cachexia. For example, TNF and IL-1 produced by resident macrophages during an inflammatory response promote IL-6, G-CSF, and GM-CSF production by marrow accessory cells. These secondarily elaborated cytokines account for many hematologic consequences of bacterial infections. IL-6, G-CSF, and GM-CSF promote myelopoiesis, leading to granulocytosis and likely monocytosis. Increased IL-6 levels promote megakaryocyte maturation and contribute to the development of secondary thrombocytosis. Overexpression of IL-6 also plays a role in the biogenesis of Castleman's disease. TNF has been shown to be an important factor in the biogenesis of the anemia of chronic inflammation. TNF directly suppresses erythroid development, leading to progressive anemia.

CONTROL OF CELL EXIT FROM MARROW

The movement of erythroid marrow cells from the marrow into the bloodstream has been studied using radiolabeled iron (Fe). After initial uptake of ^{59}Fe by the marrow, newly synthesized erythrocytes are released into the blood in 4 to 6 days. The generation time of proliferating erythroid precursors (pronormoblasts, basophilic and polychromatic normoblasts) averages about 24 hours at each stage of maturation. Nonmitotic erythroid precursor cells (orthochromatic normoblasts, reticulocytes) reside in the marrow cavity for approximately 48 hours each. The maturation process includes an average of four divisions and the generation of 8 to 16 cells from each pronormoblast. During periods of stress, red cells can exit the marrow prematurely after skipping several divisions. These cells maintain characteristics of more primitive red cells, such as macrocytosis, elevated fetal hemoglobin, and persistence of i (versus I) antigen on the cell surface. Red cell maturation time may also be shortened by decreasing the duration of each mitosis or by decreasing the maturation time of nondividing erythrocyte precursors. The red blood cell mass may be further elevated by increasing the number of erythrocytes actually entering the bloodstream. The last mechanism could result either from less destruction of red cell precursors (termed *ineffective erythropoiesis*) in the marrow cavity (normally about 10%) or from an expanded number of primitive cells entering the erythroid maturational sequence. The latter appears to be the usual mechanism of expansion of the erythroid compartment during times of increased requirement for red cells as a result of chronic hemolysis or blood loss.

Insight has recently been gained into the molecular basis of erythroid cells' movement out of marrow. Erythroleukemic cells have been shown to bind specifically to the extracellular matrix protein *fibronectin*. These cells' ability to adhere to fibronectin diminishes dur-

ing their differentiation. Subsequent studies have demonstrated that binding to fibronectin involves a specific sequence in the fibronectin molecule, Arg-Gly-Asp-Ser (RGDS). This interaction is mediated by a receptor on the surface of erythrocytes, VLA-5, a member of the integrin supergene family of receptors. Loss of adhesion of differentiating erythrocytes is associated with the functional absence of this receptor at the reticulocyte stage. Similar interactions of maturing normal erythroid precursors are thought to play a role in red cell release.

The mechanisms responsible for the release of myeloid cells from the marrow have not yet been elucidated. However, it is clear that the marrow compartment consists of both a mitotic pool (consisting of myeloblasts, promyelocytes, and myelocytes) and a storage pool of granulocyte precursors (metamyelocytes and band forms) and granulocytes. Stress and steroid administration produce a mobilization of granulocytes into the blood. The storage pool in the marrow is significantly larger than the peripheral blood pool of granulocytes. The maturation time for cells of the neutrophil series is approximately 8 days. The peripheral blood pool of granulocytes is made up of both circulating and marginating compartments of cells, with a distribution of approximately 50% in each compartment. Administration of epinephrine and stress-related endogenous release of cortisol induce rapid demargination of neutrophils, with subsequent doubling of the peripheral leukocyte counts within 30 minutes.

In order for hematopoietic cells to egress from the marrow and gain entry into the venous system, hematopoietic cells must pass through or between the endothelial cells lining the marrow venous sinuses. The point at which hematopoietic cells move through the endothelial cells is frequently near endothelial cell junctions. Pores can be observed in the endothelial lining of the venous sinus, but it is unclear whether these are permanent features of the surface or are present in response to specific signals from departing cells. In addition, areas of marked attenuation of the endothelial cell thickness have also been observed in scanning electron micrographs. Cells departing the hematopoietic cord must deform to a considerable degree to gain entry into the venous sinus. These observations, along with physical measurements of cell deformability, have led to the theory that increasing deformability associated with differentiation in both the erythroid and the myeloid lineages is an important component of the normal physiology of hematopoietic cell egress from the marrow.

Recent observations have led to the clinical use of growth factors to mobilize hematopoietic stem and progenitor cells from the bone marrow to the peripheral blood. In normal individuals, few primitive hematopoietic cells are present in the circulating blood. However, large numbers of hematopoietic stem and progenitor cells are present in the peripheral blood during the recovery phase postchemotherapy after the use of agents such as cyclophosphamide. The number of such cells can be further increased by administration of growth factors, such as G-CSF, SCF, and GM-CSF. These factors, used alone, also mobilize hematopoietic stem and progenitor cells to a degree. Peripheral blood hematopoietic stem and progenitor cells can be harvested from the blood using apheresis methods, and such cells are being increasingly used as alternative sources of hematopoietic stem cells for autologous hematopoietic rescue after high-dose chemotherapy and even primary sources of stem cells in transplantation protocols. Hematopoietic stem cell transplantation is discussed in Chapter 77.

Effects of Marrow Disruption

Abnormalities in blood cell production can occur if significant qualitative or quantitative alterations take place in hematopoietic growth factor production, in the hematopoietic stem cell and progenitor cell pools, and in the marrow microenvironment. Aplastic anemia, a clinical disorder characterized by pancytopenia and an acellular or hypocellular bone marrow, results from the total failure of hematopoiesis caused by disruption in any of these processes. The etiology of this disorder is likely multifactorial and is discussed in more detail in Chapter 90. Single cell deficiencies, such as pure red cell aplasia, pure white cell aplasia, and selective amegakaryocytic thrombocytopenia, are associated with a normocellular marrow and a selective deficiency of a single lineage of marrow precursors and the resultant cytopenia. These disorders can result from a variety of insults to the marrow progenitor cell and precursor pool, such as cytotoxic antibodies, viruses, suppressor T-cells, or natural killer cells. By contrast, the anemia of chronic renal failure is caused by defective growth factor production. This inevitable consequence of chronic renal failure largely results from a deficiency in the production of erythropoietin.

The hematopoietic microenvironment may also be important in pathologic conditions affecting hematopoiesis. Murine mutants exhibiting bone marrow failure, such as the *steel* mouse, exhibit characteristics attributable to defective microenvironments, including the hematopoietic microenvironment. Phenotypically the *steel* mouse is a black-eyed, white animal with reduced fertility and macrocytic anemia. Careful study has revealed defects in all hematopoietic lineages. The hematopoietic abnormalities of the *steel* animal are not cured by transplantation of congenic normal marrow. However, the anemia can be partially corrected by transplantation of intact spleens into the peritoneal cavity, which indicates that the hematologic abnormality resides in the hematopoietic microenvironment. In support of this view, long-term marrow cultures from *steel* mice do not support hematopoietic cells from normal congenic mice in vitro. The *steel* gene has recently been mapped to chromosome 10, the gene sequences cloned, and the molecular basis of the *steel* mutation characterized.

Although no congenital human bone marrow failure syndrome has been shown to result from a microenvironmental defect, the failure of engraftment of transplanted marrow in some patients with aplastic anemia suggests that such abnormalities may exist. The use of newer molecular methods, probes for growth-regulatory proteins, and more powerful genetic approaches to study affected kindreds may define abnormalities in the hematopoietic microenvironment associated with some congenital bone marrow failure syndromes.

CLINICAL IMPLICATIONS OF STEM CELL BIOLOGY

Knowledge of basic stem cell biology has influenced our understanding of the pathobiology of most hematologic malignancies, including the myeloproliferative disorders, the acute leukemias, and the lymphomas. The concept that a hematopoietic stem cell is capable of ultimately giving rise to each formed element of the blood has permitted further insight into the origins of each of these disorders. Using several techniques, such as analyses of blood cell isoenzymes, marker chromosomal abnormalities, and restriction fragment polymorphisms, normal hematopoietic cells have been shown to be replaced by a single neoplastic cell population that produces granulocytes, red blood cells, platelets, monocytes/macrophages, eosinophils, basophils, some B-lymphocytes, and perhaps T-lymphocytes, but not bone marrow fibroblasts, in some myeloproliferative disorders. The neoplastic cell population is clonally derived because it presumably arises following a series of oncogenic events affecting a single neoplastic hematopoietic stem cell. These events, leading to a neoplastic transformation, are thought to occur at the level of the stem cell, since only this primitive hematopoietic cell is capable of differentiating into multiple hematopoietic lineages.

Using similar investigative methods, acute myelogenous leukemia (AML) has been shown to also be a clonal disorder characterized by aberrant hematopoietic cellular proliferation and maturation. AML may involve each of the hematopoietic cell lineages, but it frequently has a more restricted pattern of involvement, presumably because of the distinct level of maturation along the hierarchy of hematopoietic development at which the initial oncogenic event occurs. In some elderly patients, peripheral blood granulocytes, red cells, and platelets possess the clonal features characteristic of the leukemia, indicating that the malignancy probably originated in a single hematopoietic stem cell. In other patients, predominantly children and young adults, red cells and platelets are frequently generated by normal residual stem cells. This situation likely comes about because the oncogenic event(s) occurred in a more differentiated progenitor cell that does not have the multipotentiality of a stem cell. Alternatively, such limited lineage involvement in AML could result from the effect of the neoplastic process on the stem cell, resulting in its inability to commit to erythroid and megakaryocytic pathways. In support of the former hypothesis, data obtained by immunologically phenotyping AML progenitor cells have shown that some leukemic progenitors express a stem cell phenotype, whereas others resemble that of committed myeloid progenitor cells.

Both allogeneic and autologous marrow transplantation can be

thought of as "stem cell rescue" of a patient who has received lethal doses of chemoradiotherapy (Chapter 77). The successful long-term engraftment of donor cells requires the transfer to the recipient of cells that possess marrow-repopulating ability. At present, at least two phases of engraftment are thought to occur after bone marrow transplantation. Early engraftment results from the differentiation of a subset of early progenitor or stem cells in the graft. A second delayed but sustained engraftment then occurs, which is likely the result of more primitive stem cells within the graft. These two phases of engraftment usually overlap and are not clinically distinguishable. The phenomenon of late graft failure after either allogeneic or autologous marrow transplantation in the presence of large numbers of assayable progenitors within the graft probably is caused by an absence from the graft of stem cells responsible for establishing long-term hematopoiesis.

GROWTH FACTORS AS THERAPEUTIC AGENTS

The synergistic relationship during the last decade between protein chemistry, molecular biology, and hematopoiesis research has resulted in growing numbers of hematopoietic growth factors becoming available for clinical use (see Table 68-1). Erythropoietin, the physiologic regulator of erythropoiesis, is now used regularly to treat the anemia of chronic renal disease, anemia of chronic infection and inflammation, anemia of cancer, and anemia associated with HIV-1 infection. G-CSF, on the other hand, has had a major impact on accelerating granulocyte recovery after chemotherapy for neoplastic diseases and is used to treat several congenital neutropenic syndromes. This cytokine has resulted in some cases in a decrease in the number of life-threatening bacterial infections in patients with these diverse clinical conditions. GM-CSF is currently used for accelerating marrow recovery after autologous marrow transplantation. The use of GM-CSF in these patients has resulted in a decreased incidence of bacterial infections after marrow transplantation. Unfortunately, neither G-CSF nor GM-CSF accelerates platelet recovery after cytotoxic therapy. Currently a growing number of growth factors, such as IL-6, GM-CSF/IL-3 fusion protein, c-Mpl ligand, IL-11, and c-kit ligand are undergoing evaluation in order to define their clinical uses. At present, combination therapy with several of these cytokines administered either simultaneously or in sequence is thought to be required pharmacologically to promote hematopoiesis optimally. Growth factors have recently proved useful in the mobilization of hematopoietic stem and progenitor cells for use in stem cell transplantation (Chapter 77). The clinical uses of these remarkably powerful agents will likely result in important advances in therapy.

BIBLIOGRAPHY

Bartelez SH, Andrews RG, Bernstein ID: Uncovering the heterogeneity of hematopoietic repopulating cells, *Exp Hematol* 19:861, 1991.
Grush WW, Quesenberry PJ: Recombinant human hematopoietic growth factors in the treatment of cytopenias, *Clin Immunol Immunopathol* 62:525, 1992.
Long M: Blood cell adhesion molecules, *Exp Hematol* 20:286, 1992.
Spangrude GL et al: Murine hematopoietic stem cells, *Blood* 78:1395, 1991.
Witte ON: Steel locus defines new multipotent growth factor, *Cell* 63:5, 1990.

CHAPTER

69 Hemostasis and Fibrinolysis

James N. George

Normal hemostatic mechanisms can be divided into two basic reactions. Primary hemostasis involves the immediate response of platelet adhesion to exposed subendothelial fibers at the site of vessel injury. This is followed by aggregation of platelets and vessel contraction that can effectively seal a small lesion. Secondary hemostasis involves the formation of fibrin that reinforces the initial platelet aggregate, thereby preventing bleeding from larger lesions. Although this distinction is helpful as a framework for understanding the symptoms and signs of bleeding disorders, these reactions are intimately related. Platelets provide a critical surface on which the reactions occur to generate thrombin, which catalyzes the formation of fibrin from fibrinogen. Thrombin is also the most potent agonist for platelet secretion, and platelet secretion of fibrinogen and calcium provides the substrate and a cofactor for fibrin formation. Also, several platelet-secreted products cause blood vessel contraction, further promoting hemostasis.

Each of these reactions is regulated by effective control mechanisms. The integrity of the normal vascular endothelium prevents the interaction between circulating platelets and subendothelial fibers that initiates further aggregation and secretion. Plasma proteins, such as protein C and antithrombin III, can develop activity to inhibit fibrin formation. The formation of the enzyme plasmin by the fibrinolytic system exerts the final control mechanism, with the proteolysis of fibrin restricting the clot to its essential location and beginning the process of restructuring the vessel lumen.

PRIMARY HEMOSTASIS: PLATELETS AND BLOOD VESSELS

Blood platelets are continually involved in microscopic hemostasis, sealing the gaps that occur normally in capillary and venule endothelium. Because they are the least dense blood cells, platelets are displaced laterally by the flowing red cells and circulate adjacent to the endothelium. Their role in maintaining endothelial integrity is shown by the result of their absence: with sudden, severe thrombocytope-

nia, innumerable petechial hemorrhages quickly appear, concentrated in dependent regions where hydrostatic pressure within the superficial capillaries is greatest. Microscopic analysis of capillaries and venules in thrombocytopenic animals demonstrates diminished thickness of the endothelial cell layer and an increased frequency of gaps and fenestrations.

Disruption of vascular integrity results in a standard sequence of platelet reactions. First, platelets adhere to subendothelial fibers. This contact interaction causes platelets to change from their circulating shape as compact disks to a more spherical form with long, extended pseudopodia that facilitate further contact with the subendothelium and adjacent platelets (Fig. 69-1). As the platelets change shape, their secretory granules move to the cell's center, fuse with the deeply invaginated surface membrane of the open canalicular system, and discharge their contents.

Platelet Development From Megakaryocytes

Platelets are derived from marrow megakaryocytes, which in turn are derived from pluripotent hematopoietic stem cells. Therefore platelets share a common ancestry with red cells, granulocytes, and lymphocytes.

Although megakaryocyte development can be influenced by multiple cytokines, thrombopoietin is the primary regulator of platelet production (Chapter 68). Pluripotent progenitor cells mature to cells committed to megakaryocyte development, or colony-forming unit–megakaryocyte (CFU-MK), and the number of megakaryocyte progenitor cells expands in response to interleukin-3 (IL-3) and stem cell factor. As megakaryocyte proliferation diminishes and differentiation

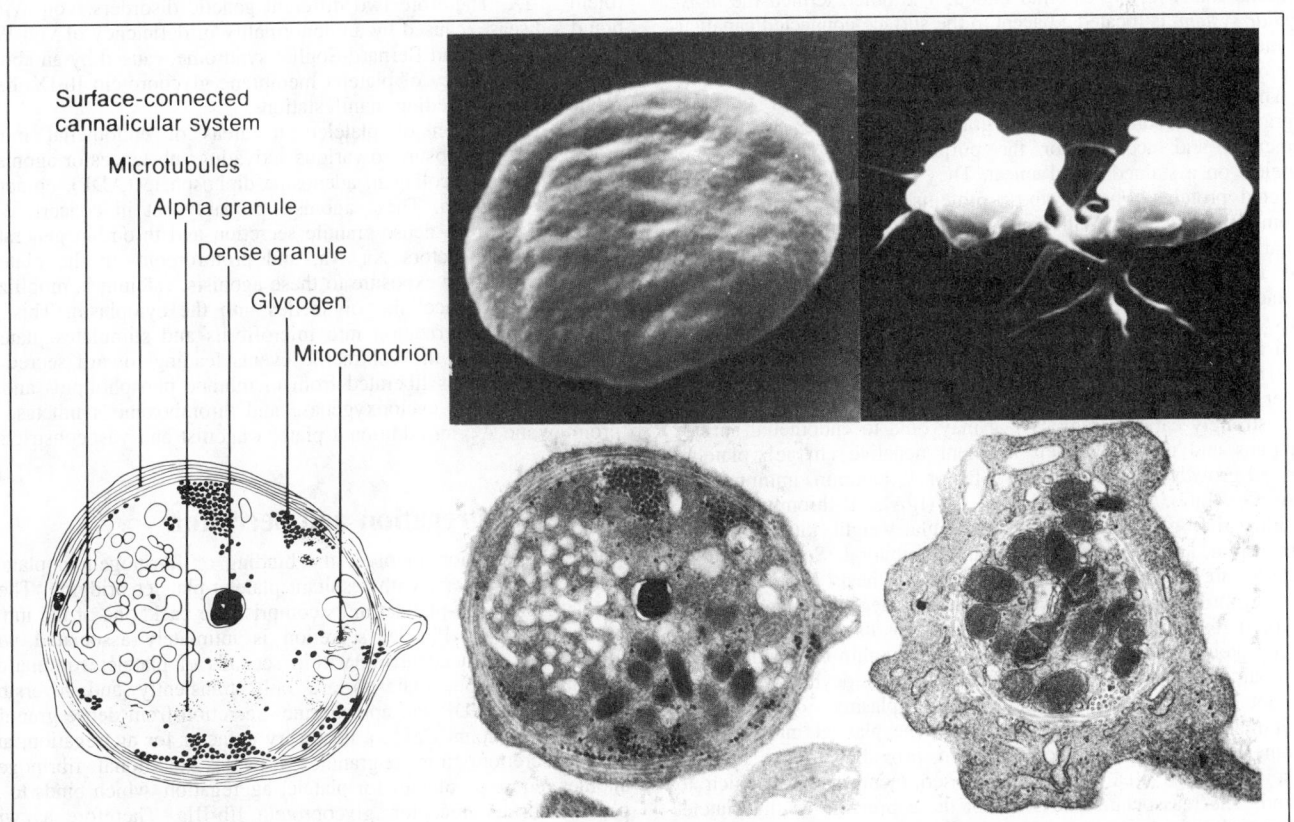

Surface-connected cannalicular system
Microtubules
Alpha granule
Dense granule
Glycogen
Mitochondrion

FIGURE 69-1   Electron micrographs of resting and activated platelets. The top figures are scanning electron micrographs demonstrating the disk shape of normal circulating platelets (*left,* ×20,000) and the more spherical form of activated platelets with many long pseudopodia (*right,* ×10,000). The bottom left photograph is a transmission electron micrograph of the cross section of a resting platelet (×21,000) with a matched drawing (*far left*) labeling the normal subcellular structures. In the bottom right photograph (×30,000) of an activated platelet, the constriction of the microtubular ring around the centralized granules and the formation of pseudopodia can be seen.

Electron micrographs courtesy James G White, MD, and Marcy Krumwiede.

begins, manifested by nuclear endoreduplication, enlargement of cell size, and acquisition of complex membrane systems demarcating zones of nascent platelets, thrombopoietin becomes the dominant hormone driving platelet production. As megakaryocytes mature in the marrow, the vast amount of cytoplasm develops into several thousand distinct sections that correspond to individual platelets, each containing all the organelles present in mature platelets. In the marrow, megakaryocytes occupy positions adjacent to vascular sinus walls, and some observations suggest that large portions of cytoplasm or even intact megakaryocytes move into the sinus and then to the pulmonary capillaries, where they are trapped and fragment into individual platelets. However, the mechanism and site of platelet release from megakaryocytes are unknown.

Once delivered to the circulation, platelets survive about 10 days. Within the normal circulatory system, about one third of platelets are transiently sequestered in the spleen. Repeated vessel wall encounters with loss of pseudopods and alteration of surface structures may contribute to the decreased functional capability of older platelets and eventual senescence.

Platelet Structure and Contents

Figure 69-1 demonstrates platelet ultrastructure and the shape change that accompanies activation. Circulating platelets have a disk shape that is maintained by a coiled ring of microtubules, composed of polymerized tubulin. Microfilaments, composed primarily of polymerized fibrous actin, are seen in activated platelets, causing the shape change and pseudopod formation. Two distinct membrane systems are present within the cytoplasm of platelets. One, termed the *surface-connected canalicular system,* is merely an extension of the surface plasma membrane and results from deep, tortuous invaginations that communicate with the external milieu. The other, termed the *dense tubular system,* is located adjacent to the surface-connected canalicular membranes and contains specialized membranes that are the site of prostaglandin and thromboxane synthesis.

Three types of secretory granules are present in platelets: α-granules, lysosomes, and dense granules. α-Granules are the most numerous and account for the purple granular appearance of platelets on a stained blood smear. They contain a large variety of secreted proteins. Four of these proteins (fibrinogen, fibronectin, thrombospondin, von Willebrand factor) share physical and functional properties and are termed *adhesive proteins.* They are large and filamentous; they are glycosylated, which facilitates their contact with other molecules; they are synthesized by a variety of cells, including megakaryocytes, endothelial cells, and vessel adventitial cells, and also are present in the plasma and vessel wall; and they are involved in platelet adhesion and aggregation reactions. Other secreted α-granule proteins include platelet factor 4 (a protein with strongly cationic regions that may bind to endothelial surface heparans and neutralize their repellent negative charge), platelet-derived growth factor, coagulation factor V, albumin, immunoglobulin G (IgG), immunoglobulin A (IgA), β-thromboglobulin, histidine-rich glycoprotein, high-molecular-weight kininogen, α$_2$-antiplasmin, and plasminogen activator inhibitor-1. Some α-granule proteins are the product of endogenous synthesis by megakaryocytes. Fibrinogen is not synthesized by megakaryocytes but is acquired by endocytosis after binding to its surface receptor, glycoprotein IIb-IIIa. Other plasma proteins within α-granules, such as albumin, IgG, and IgA, are acquired by pinocytosis, and their platelet concentration parallels their plasma concentration. α-Granule secretion occurs deep within the platelet into the long channels of the open canalicular system, providing for the secreted proteins a large area of surface-exposed membrane on which to rebind. The reassociation of some of these proteins on the platelet surface allows their concentration and organization to facilitate hemostatic reactions. Lysosomes, containing acid-hydrolase enzymes, are morphologically indistinguishable from α-granules except by specific histochemical reactions. The function of these enzymes is unknown, but they are probably involved in the clearance of cellular debris after hemostasis. Dense granules are the least frequent cellular organelle. They contain a high concentration of calcium and pyrophosphate ions (which cause the intrinsic electron density of these granules), as well as serotonin and adenine

nucleotides. As with α-granules, dense granules fuse with the plasma membrane after platelet activation. The exocytosed granule contents, particularly adenine nucleotides, in turn stimulate adjacent platelets, leading to amplification of the platelet response.

Platelet membrane glycoproteins, in addition to the structural proteins that control platelet shape and the secretory granules, are a third important element necessary for normal platelet function. Although a number of such proteins have been identified, the best characterized are the surface receptors for the adhesive molecules von Willebrand factor and fibrinogen, glycoprotein Ib-IX and glycoprotein IIb-IIIa, respectively. These molecules are abundant components of the platelet membrane and serve the principal functions of platelets, adhesion and aggregation. Congenital absence of either glycoprotein Ib-IX (Bernard-Soulier syndrome) or glycoprotein IIb-IIIa (Glanzmann's thrombasthenia) is associated with a significant bleeding diathesis. These molecules are also interesting because of their close structural resemblance to other adhesive protein receptors on other cells, making platelets the prototypical adhesive cell.

Platelet Adhesion to Subendothelium

The initial reaction of hemostasis is the adherence of circulating platelets to subendothelial fibers exposed by endothelial damage. Collagen is the principal fiber involved, and von Willebrand's factor is also required for platelet attachment. Von Willebrand's factor is synthesized by both megakaryocytes, for storage within platelet α-granules, and endothelial cells, from which it is secreted into the plasma and also back into the subendothelium. Through a structural alteration, von Willebrand's factor adsorbed onto a fibrillar surface can interact with circulating platelets. The platelet receptor that binds von Willebrand's factor to promote adhesion is the surface membrane glycoprotein Ib-IX. Therefore two different genetic disorders, von Willebrand's disease, caused by an abnormality or deficiency of von Willebrand's factor, and Bernard-Soulier syndrome, caused by an abnormality or deficiency of platelet membrane glycoprotein Ib-IX, have similar clinical bleeding manifestations.

The localization of platelets to areas of endothelial injury promotes their exposure to various activating substances or agonists. Among these are collagen, adenosine diphosphate (ADP), epinephrine, and thrombin. These agonists probably act in concert, with ADP derived from dense-granule secretion and thrombin generated by coagulation factors Xa, Va, and prothrombin on the platelet surface. Early after exposure to these agonists, calcium is mobilized from platelet intracellular organelles into the cytoplasm. This allows actin polymerization into microfibrils and stimulates platelet shape change and the contractile events leading toward secretion. Arachidonic acid is liberated from membrane phospholipids and is then converted by cyclooxygenase and thromboxane synthetase to thromboxane A$_2$, an additional platelet agonist and vasoconstricting agent.

Platelet Aggregation and Secretion

Platelet aggregation involves the binding of fibrinogen to platelet membrane receptors, with resultant platelet-platelet bridging. These platelet-fibrinogen-platelet units comprise the backbone of the initial hemostatic plug. Platelet secretion is intimately associated with aggregation, both occurring within seconds of platelet stimulation. Without secretion, platelets are only transiently and reversibly aggregated by ADP and epinephrine. Secretion from dense granules provides additional Ca^{2+}, a necessary cofactor for aggregation, and ADP. Secretion from α-granules provides additional fibrinogen, another required cofactor for platelet aggregation, which binds to its platelet surface receptor, glycoprotein IIb-IIIa. Therefore as with platelet adhesion, platelet aggregation is defective in two different genetic disorders. Congenital afibrinogenemia, absence of the specific plasma protein, and Glanzmann's thrombasthenia, an abnormality or deficiency of platelet membrane glycoprotein IIb-IIIa, both cause a lifelong bleeding disorder. With activation by ADP or thrombin, the surface membrane glycoprotein IIb-IIIa can also bind other platelet-secreted adhesive proteins—fibronectin and von Willebrand's factor. These large proteins may also have a role in stabilizing the platelet aggregate.

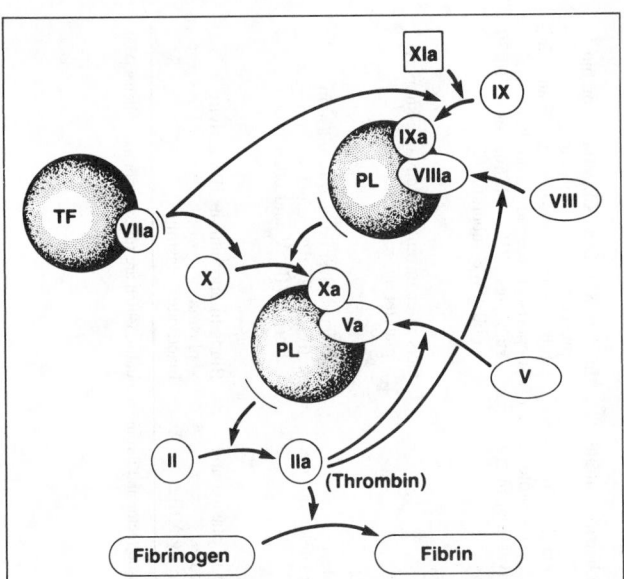

FIGURE 69-2   Plasma coagulation reactions in normal hemostasis. In this diagram, factor XII, prekallikrein, and high-molecular-weight kininogen are omitted because they are not required for normal in vivo hemostasis. The role of factor XI is uncertain because some patients with absent plasma factor XI activity can have apparently normal hemostasis. The vitamin K–dependent factors are all similar in structure and are indicated by the small circles. Factors V and VIII, large molecules that are similar to each other in structure and function, are indicated by the ellipses. Three distinct reactions occur on lipoprotein surfaces that are shown as large spheres: the binding of factor VII to tissue factor *(TF)* on the surface of perivascular cells and the activation of factor X and prothrombin (factor II) on the surface of platelets *(PL)* or platelet membrane microparticles.

Platelet Involvement in Thrombin Generation

Platelets have long been recognized to play a role in coagulation by accelerating the generation of thrombin and the consequent formation of fibrin. This property resides in the phospholipid structure of the platelet membrane, providing a specific surface favoring the reactions leading to thrombin formation. Platelets, particularly platelet membrane microparticles shed during activation, can bind and organize the enzyme-cofactor-substrate complexes in two key coagulation reactions: (1) the activation of factor X by factor IXa (enzyme) plus factor VIIIa (cofactor), and (2) the activation of prothrombin by factor Xa (enzyme) plus factor Va (cofactor) (Fig. 69-2). The effectiveness of these platelet surface–dependent reactions is hundreds-fold greater than a soluble reaction. The occurrence of thrombin formation on the platelet surface within the developing aggregate serves to protect the activated coagulation factors from their plasma inhibitors and to localize the fibrin formation to the immediate area of vessel damage. Platelets also have a specific surface receptor for thrombin, which is not only the key enzyme in coagulation reactions but also the most potent agonist for platelet activation and secretion.

SECONDARY HEMOSTASIS: COAGULATION

The reactions that lead to the formation of a fibrin clot, termed *coagulation,* are a cascade of sequential enzymatic reactions that are progressively amplified to generate the final key enzyme, thrombin. Within this sequence of reactions are many control loops; some accelerate thrombin formation, and others inhibit coagulation. The integration of these reactions and their controls effectively generates fibrin that is strictly localized to the site of hemostasis.

Traditionally, coagulation reactions have been divided into two pathways: one termed *intrinsic* because the major reactants are within the plasma, and the other termed *extrinsic* because the initiation requires tissue factor, a component not normally present within circulating blood. This distinction helps to define the laboratory assess-

ment of hemostasis because the two basic clinical assays, the partial thromboplastin time and the prothrombin time, measure the components of the intrinsic and extrinsic systems, respectively (Chapter 75). A normal partial thromboplastin time also requires the presence of several proteins that are not necessary for in vivo coagulation: factor XII (Hageman's factor), prekallikrein, and high-molecular-weight kininogen. For this reason, the coagulation scheme shown in Fig. 69-2, the sequence of in vivo coagulation, differs from that in Fig. 75-2, in vitro coagulation reactions measured by the standard laboratory assays. The proteins required for the development and control of normal plasma coagulation are described in Table 69-1.

Sequence of Reactions Leading to Thrombin Formation

Coagulation reactions are sequential activations of the plasma procoagulant proteins from their precursor (zymogen) form to active proteolytic enzymes, which are designated by a lowercase *a.* For example, factor X is the inactive zymogen found in normal plasma, and factor Xa is the active enzyme, a two-chain molecule resulting from the proteolytic cleavage by either factor VIIa–tissue factor or factors IXa-VIIIa (see Fig. 69-2). The triggering reaction that initiates blood coagulation in vivo is the exposure of tissue factor to plasma. Tissue factor, a cofactor for both factor VII activation and factor VIIa activity, is a specific cell surface protein that is constitutively expressed on perivascular fibroblasts, creating a hemostatic envelope poised to activate coagulation. At the site of vessel injury, exposed tissue factor selectively binds factor VII, causing it to become exquisitely sensitive for proteolytic activation by the normal trace plasma concentrations of factors VIIa or Xa. The tissue factor–factor VIIa complex then becomes the explosive force that activates factors IX to IXa and X to Xa. The coagulation system has many amplification steps: the appearance of factor Xa increases factor VII activation, and the first traces of thrombin convert cofactors V and VIII to more active forms (see Fig. 69-2). The need for both pathways of factor X activation is demonstrated by the occurrence of bleeding disorders with deficiencies of factors VII, VIII, or IX. The sequence of coagulation is also consistent with the absence of clinical bleeding in patients deficient in factor XII, prekallikrein, or high-molecular-weight kininogen, even though they have very abnormal partial thromboplastin times. The role of factor XI is less clear because not all patients with severe plasma factor XI deficiency have clinically important bleeding problems. In vivo, factor XI may also be activated by thrombin, allowing an additional pathway of factor IX activation after tissue factor–factor VIIa is inhibited by tissue factor pathway inhibitor.

Important similarities exist in the structural and complex-forming properties of the different coagulation factors. Four of these procoagulant proteins are vitamin K–dependent for normal structure and function: factors VII, X, IX, and prothrombin (also termed *factor II*). They are similar in size, and all become serine active-site proteases when activated from their zymogen form. Factor XIa is a larger molecule and is also a serine protease. Factors VIII and V are both very large molecules with extensive sequence homology. They do not have intrinsic enzymatic activity but function as cofactors for serine proteases (for factors IXa and Xa, respectively) in the form of a complex with phospholipid and Ca^{2+}.

Once formed, thrombin becomes the key coagulation enzyme in amplifying and promoting and also in inhibiting coagulation. Thrombin catalyzes the final steps in coagulation: the conversion of fibrinogen to fibrin and the activation of factor XIII to XIIIa, a transglutamase enzyme that converts the initial fibrin polymer to a covalently linked structure. It amplifies its own formation by directly activating cofactors VIII and V and also factor XI, and it stimulates platelet secretion and aggregation. In addition, thrombin, in combination with factor Va and an endothelial cell surface protein named *thrombomodulin,* activates plasma protein C, the zymogen of a coagulation inhibitor, to activated protein C, designated as *APC* or *protein Ca* (Fig. 69-3).

Fibrin Formation

Fibrinogen is a large molecule present in high concentrations in plasma and platelet α-granules. Its rod shape, made up of three pairs

Table 69-1   The major proteins of hemostasis and fibrinolysis*

PROTEINS	PRIMARY TISSUE SYNTHESIS	MOLECULAR WEIGHT (DALTONS)	PLASMA CONCENTRATION (MG/DL)	PLASMA HALF-LIFE (HOURS)	STRUCTURAL PROPERTIES	FUNCTION
Proenzymes of coagulation						
Factor XI	Liver	143,000	0.5	70	Unique	Activated by thrombin; activates IX
Factor IX	Liver	57,000	1.0	24	Vitamin K dependent	Activated by TF-VIIa and XIa; activates X
Factor VII	Liver	50,000	0.1	2-5	Vitamin K dependent	Activated by Xa and VIIa; activates IX and X
Factor X	Liver	59,000	1.0	36	Vitamin K dependent	Activated by TF-VIIa, and VIIIa-IXa; activates prothrombin
Prothrombin	Liver	72,000	2.0	72	Vitamin K dependent	Activated by Va-Xa; cleaves fibrinogen
Factor XIII	Liver	320,000	3.0	240	Proenzyme of transglutamase	Covalently cross-links fibrin gel
Cofactors of coagulation						
Tissue factor (TF)	Perivascular cells	30,000	—	—	Transmembrane protein	Required for VII activation and VIIa activity
Factor VIII	Liver	330,000	0.1	12	Homologous to V; bound to VWF in plasma	Activated by thrombin; cofactor for IXa
Factor V	Liver	330,000	2.0	12	Homologous to VIII	Activated by thrombin; cofactor for Xa
Regulatory proteins of coagulation						
Thrombomodulin	Endothelium	75,000	—	—	Transmembrane protein	Required for protein C activation
Protein C	Liver	62,000	0.4	8	Vitamin K dependent	Activated by thrombin; digests VIII and V
Protein S	Liver	80,000	3.0	17	Vitamin K dependent; inhibited by C4b-bp†	Cofactor for protein C
Antithrombin III	Liver	54,000	20.0	24	Binds to endothelial heparin sulfate	Inhibits XIa, IXa, Xa, VIIa, thrombin in presence of proteoglycan
Tissue factor pathway inhibitor	Liver	36,000	0.009	1	Associated with plasma lipoproteins	Inhibits VIIa in presence of TF and Xa
Von Willebrand's factor (vWF)	Endothelium, megakaryocytes	Subunit: 260,000 Molecule: 500,000-15,000,000	2.0	12	Giant filamentous adhesive protein; also component of perivascular matrix	Supports platelet adhesion; binds and stabilizes VIII in plasma: one VIII/30 to 60 VWF subunits
Structural protein of coagulation						
Fibrinogen	Liver	340,000	300.0	96	Adhesive protein	Gels after thrombin cleavage; supports platelet aggregation
Enzyme/proenzyme of fibrinolysis						
Tissue plasminogen activator (tPA)	Endothelium	68,000	0.0006	0.1	Bound to PAI-1 in plasma	Activates plasminogen to plasmin
Plasminogen	Liver	86,000	20.0	50	Binds to fibrin and platelet surface	Activated by tPA; digests fibrinogen, fibrin, VIII, V, and other proteins
Regulatory proteins of fibrinolysis						
Plasminogen activator inhibitor-1 (PAI-1)	Endothelium	52,000	0.0005	0.1	Bound to vitronectin in plasma and platelet alpha granules	Binds to and inhibits tPA activity in plasma
α_2 antiplasmin	Liver	60,000	5.0	60	Cross-linked to fibrin by XIIIa	Inactivates plasmin

*The principle structural and functional properties of selected proteins involved in hemostasis and fibrinolysis are presented. All are soluble plasma proteins except tissue factor and thrombomodulin, which are transmembrane proteins. Von Willebrand factor is both a soluble plasma protein and a component of the subendothelial matrix.
†C4b-bp, Plasma binding protein for the complement component 4b.

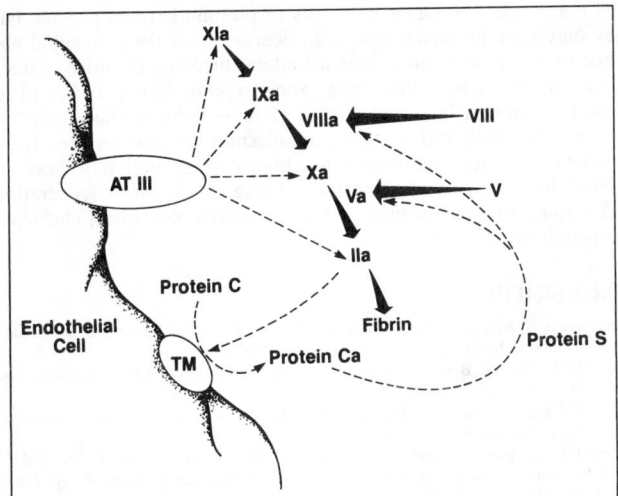

FIGURE 69-3 Natural coagulation inhibitors: antithrombin III *(AT III)* and protein C. The solid arrows represent the procoagulant reactions; the broken arrows represent the anticoagulant reactions. AT III inhibits the active serine protease enzymes, factors XIa, IXa, Xa, and IIa (thrombin). The inhibitory activity of AT III is greatly enhanced by heparin-like molecules on the endothelial cell surface. Factor VIIa is also inhibited by AT III, but it is more effectively neutralized by another plasma protein, tissue factor pathway inhibitor. Protein C is activated to a proteolytic enzyme, protein Ca, by thrombin with an endothelial cell protein, thrombomodulin *(TM)*, serving as a cofactor. Protein Ca then specifically inactivates factors Va and VIIIa, with protein S as a required cofactor.

of polypeptide chains (designated α, β, and γ), allows it to polymerize spontaneously by both end-to-end and side-to-side hydrogen bonds after thrombin cleaves off four small peptides. These peptides are derived from the amino termini of the α- and β-chains, at the center of the molecule, and are designated *fibrinopeptides A and B*. This initial fibrin polymer is neither properly oriented nor strong enough to provide permanent hemostasis or to allow clot retraction until the fibrin molecules are covalently linked by the transglutamase enzyme, factor XIIIa. Factor XIII zymogen is a molecule of a size similar to fibrinogen, consisting of a tetramer of two a chains and two b chains. In plasma, factor XIII circulates bound to fibrinogen, which allows it to be simultaneously activated by thrombin and directly incorporated into the fibrin clot. Platelets contain the factor XIII a chains, and it is the a-chain dimer that forms the enzyme, factor XIIIa. The active enzyme, factor XIIIa, but not the zymogen, binds specifically to thrombin-stimulated platelets, and this is an additional indication of the interactions between the fibrin clot and the platelet aggregate during hemostasis. Once the fibrin polymer is converted to a stable structure by the formation of covalent bonds between γ-chains and then α-chains on adjacent molecules, the coagulation sequence is completed.

Controls of Coagulation

Some activation of plasma coagulation factors occurs continuously, possibly by slight endothelial breaks or by circulation of plasma coagulation factors through extravascular tissues. This is normally controlled primarily by dilution in flowing blood and hepatic clearance of the activated enzymes. However, an enzymatic system that is as potentially explosive as these coagulation reactions must be regulated by a series of tight controls at each step. These control mechanisms are outlined in Box 69-1 and Fig. 69-3. The increased risk for thrombosis associated with defects in these control mechanisms is shown in Box 82-4 in Chapter 82.

An important control mechanism is the clearance and inactivation of the activated coagulation factors. Swiftly flowing blood is probably the most effective means of dispersing any activated factors not incorporated into the platelet aggregate and evolving clot. The protective effect of flowing blood is most clearly demonstrated by the

---

BOX 69-1

Control mechanisms for blood coagulation

I. Clearance of activated coagulation factors
  A. Dispersal by flowing blood
  B. Liver catabolism
II. Inactivation of activated coagulation factors
  A. Antithrombin III, a plasma protein, inactivates factors XIa, IXa, Xa, and VIIa, and thrombin. This reaction is accelerated by complex formation with endothelial cell surface heparin-like molecules.
  B. Protein C, a plasma protein, is activated to a serine protease (protein Ca) by thrombin plus thrombomodulin. Thrombomodulin is a protein present on the luminal surface of endothelial cells. Protein Ca proteolytically inactivates both factors VIIIa and Va, with protein S as a cofactor.
  C. Heparin cofactor II, a plasma protein, inactivates thrombin in the presence of heparin or dermatan sulfate. In contrast to antithrombin III, it does not inactivate factors XIa, IXa, and Xa.
  D. Tissue factor pathway inhibitor (TFPI), a plasma protein synthesized by endothelium and liver, binds to and inhibits the function of the factor VIIa–tissue factor complex in the presence of factor Xa.
  E. Thrombin bound to thrombomodulin is inactive regarding its procoagulant and platelet activation effects.
  F. Fibrin binds thrombin and inhibits its proteolytic activity.
III. Fibrinolysis by plasmin degrades and clears the fibrin clot.

---

increased risk for thrombosis associated with blood stasis. Circulation through the liver specifically removes activated coagulation factors from the plasma.

Antithrombin III and protein C are plasma proteins that are important for the inactivation of the activated coagulation factors generated during the coagulation reactions. Antithrombin III binds irreversibly to some serine protease enzymes (factors XIa, IXa, Xa, VIIa; and thrombin) and blocks their activity. Inhibition by antithrombin III alone is relatively slow, but its inhibitory activity is dramatically accelerated by heparin and heparin-like proteoglycan molecules. This acceleration is the basis for the therapeutic effect of heparin, and in normal hemostasis a similar role is performed by the proteoglycan heparan sulfate on the luminal surface of vascular endothelium.

Protein C is a vitamin K–dependent protein that is cleaved to form a serine protease, protein Ca, by thrombin when the thrombin is bound to an endothelial surface protein, thrombomodulin. Activated protein C inhibits factors VIIIa and Va by proteolytic degradation. The activity of protein Ca requires the presence of another vitamin K–dependent plasma protein, protein S, as a cofactor.

In addition to neutralization by antithrombin III, thrombin is also inactivated in its effect on factor V, fibrinogen, and platelets when it becomes bound to thrombomodulin on the endothelial surface or to the surface of polymerized fibrin. Another plasma protein termed *heparin cofactor II* can also inactivate thrombin in the presence of heparin.

Tissue factor pathway inhibitor (TFPI) is synthesized and secreted constitutively by endothelial cells and binds firmly to the complex of factor VIIa and tissue factor in the presence of factor Xa and calcium. TFPI does not bind to factor VIIa or tissue factor individually, and binding requires the intact activated factor Xa molecule. This allows the newly formed factor Xa to feed back and control further activity of the factor VIIa–tissue factor complex. Sustained factor X activation may then require factor XIa and the intrinsic pathway.

FIBRINOLYSIS

Digestion of the fibrin clot by the enzyme plasmin in the process of fibrinolysis is the ultimate coagulation control mechanism. This process helps to restrict the clot to the site of hemostasis and to clear away the fibrin as the process of wound healing begins. If the sequence of coagulation reactions is pictured as a cascade of enzyme activation resulting in the formation of thrombin, fibrinolysis can be pictured as a mirror-image cascade resulting in the formation of the proteolytic enzyme plasmin (Fig. 69-4). Plasmin is formed from a circulating zymogen, plasminogen, by an enzyme released from endothelial cells termed *tissue plasminogen activator* (tPA). Once formed, plasmin has a broad spectrum of protein substrates. Other enzymes are capable of activating plasminogen to plasmin: urokinase (often designated uPA), which is present in most tissues; and streptokinase, a therapeutic material derived from streptococci. tPA appears to be the physiologic intravascular activator of plasminogen in the process of fibrinolysis. In contrast, the primary activity of urokinase appears to be the activation of plasminogen to plasmin in extravascular tissues, where proteolysis by plasmin is involved in such widely diverse functions as cell migration during inflammation and tumor cell metastasis, ovulation, and embryonic organogenesis and organ involution.

As in coagulation, surface binding of the reactants serves to localize the reaction to the specific site where the activated enzyme is required. In this case, fibrin itself serves as a potent cofactor for the action of tPA on plasminogen. tPA associates only weakly with soluble plasminogen and fibrinogen but binds strongly to fibrin. The complex of tPA with fibrin forms a site that in turn binds plasminogen with high affinity. Therefore plasmin is formed almost exclusively within the fibrin clot. As with coagulation, significant control mechanisms exist for the fibrinolytic reactions. These control mechanisms include the restriction of tPA activity to the fibrin surface and the presence of plasma inhibitors of tPA and plasmin. *Plasminogen activator inhibitor-1* (PAI-1) is synthesized and secreted by endothelial cells, and most tPA circulates in an inactive complex with PAI-1. Both tPA and PAI-1 appear to be released from endothelial cells constitutively as well as after a variety of stimuli. Among the several other plasminogen activator inhibitors that have been characterized, PAI-2, a selective inhibitor of uPA produced primarily by placental tissue, is notable because of its high concentrations in plasma during late pregnancy.

Any plasmin that escapes the fibrin clot is immediately neutralized by α_2-*antiplasmin,* a protein present in normal plasma. Plasmin bound to fibrin is 100-fold less sensitive to α_2-antiplasmin than when it is free in plasma. Other inhibitors of plasmin exist in plasma, but they may have no physiologic significance, since the congenital absence of α_2-antiplasmin causes a lifelong bleeding disorder characterized by excessive fibrinolysis. Some α_2-antiplasmin is bound to fibrin by factor XIIIa, where it acts as a more intimate check on plasmin activity. Both PAI-1 and α_2-antiplasmin are also secreted from platelet α-granules, contributing to a higher concentration of these inhibitors in the milieu of hemostasis. These checks on the generation and activity of plasmin may protect the developing fibrin clot from premature dissolution.

BIBLIOGRAPHY

Bauer KA et al: Aging-associated changes in indices of thrombin generation and protein C activation in humans, *J Clin Invest* 80:1527, 1987.

Collen D, Lijnen HR: Basic and clinical aspects of fibrinolysis and thrombolysis, *Blood* 78:3114, 1991.

Davie EW, Fujikawa K, Kisiel W: The coagulation cascade: initiation, maintenance and regulation, *Biochemistry* 30:10363, 1991.

Esmon CT: The protein C anticoagulant pathway, *Arterioscler Thromb* 12:135, 1992.

Furie B, Furie BC: Molecular and cellular biology of blood coagulation, *N Engl J Med* 326:800, 1992.

Gailani D: Advances and dilemmas in factor XI, *Curr Opinion Hematol* 1:347, 1994.

Gilbert GE et al: Platelet-derived microparticles express high affinity receptors for factor VIII, *J Biol Chem* 266:17261, 1991.

Hajjar KA: Changing concepts in fibrinolysis, *Curr Opinion Hematol* 2:345, 1995.

Kaushansky K: Thrombopoietin: the primary regulator of platelet production, *Blood* 86:419, 1995.

Krishnamurti C, Alving BM: Plasminogen activator inhibitor type 1: biochemistry and evidence for modulation of fibrinolysis in vivo, *Semin Thromb Hemost* 18:67, 1992.

Kroll MH, Schafer AI: Biochemical mechanisms of platelet activation, *Blood* 74:1181, 1989.

Mann KG et al: Surface-dependent reactions of the vitamin K–dependent enzyme complexes, *Blood* 76:1, 1990.

Rapaport SI, Rao VM: Initiation and regulation of tissue factor–dependent blood coagulation, *Arterioscler Thromb* 12:1111, 1992.

Sadler JE: von Willebrand factor, *J Biol Chem* 266:22777, 1991.

Wendling F, Vainchenker W: Thrombopoietin and its receptor, the protooncogene c-mpl, *Curr Opinion Hematol* 2:331, 1995.

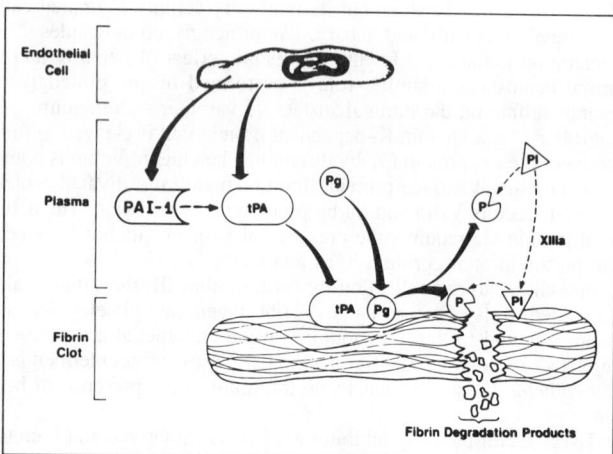

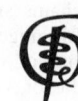

FIGURE 69-4 Mechanism and control of endogenous fibrinolysis. Once the fibrin clot is formed, it becomes the active cofactor for its own dissolution by providing the specific surface on which fibrinolytic reactions occur. Tissue plasminogen activator *(tPA)* is secreted from endothelial cells. In plasma, tPA circulates in an inactive complex with another endothelial cell–secreted protein, plasminogen activator inhibitor-1 *(PAI-1)*. tPA binds avidly to fibrin, where it becomes a binding site for plasminogen *(Pg)* from the plasma. Thus plasminogen is converted to the active fibrinolytic enzyme plasmin *(P)* directly on the fibrin surface. Plasmin digests fibrin into multiple soluble fragments, termed *fibrin degradation products.* Any plasmin escaping into the plasma is immediately neutralized by α_2-plasmin inhibitor *(PI;* α_2-antiplasmin). α_2-Antiplasmin is also covalently linked to fibrin by factor XIIIa. Thus the complete sequence of plasmin production and control is organized within the developing fibrin clot. The solid arrows indicate the profibrinolytic reactions. The broken arrows indicate the reactions inhibiting fibrinolysis.

CHAPTER

70 The Genetics of Cancer

Joanna Groden

Understanding the ways in which normal somatic cells become neoplastic will aid in the prevention and treatment of cancers by providing therapeutic targets for intervention and the means to identify individuals who may be at risk for particular tumor types. Therefore much of the recent research in cancer biology has been directed toward the identification of the genes, and therefore the proteins, that are crucial in signal transduction, cell growth, and differentiation. The study of families with predisposition to site-specific tumors and to cancer in general has been instrumental in this gene identification process. Genetic analyses of tumors also have led to the delineation of some of the molecular alterations that are present in malignant cells and that disrupt normal processes of cell growth and differentiated function.

All somatic cells, whether dividing or not, are subject to the acquisition of random or directed mutation. Some mutations arise spontaneously; some occur in response to radiation, chemicals, viruses, or other environmental agents. Some occur in response to particular environmental influences that induce a directed mutagenesis. These then result in heritable changes in the genome that in turn, if the cell is still viable and capable of undergoing mitosis, are passed on to the descendants of that cell. When present in the correct number, combination, or type, these accumulated mutations alter a cell and its descendants and allow a tumor to form. Therefore the identification of environmental agents that increase the incidence of cancer is an important focus of recent research.

The accumulation of mutations in cells, whether these errors are sporadic or occur in response to particular environmental agents, can be due to deficiencies in the components of systems required for DNA maintenance or repair. This is seen clinically by an increase in tumor incidence in individuals with such a deficiency. The identification of the genes that are altered in such individuals has resulted in the simultaneous identification of the components of human DNA repair systems. These new discoveries highlight the importance of maintaining the integrity of genetic information in the cell and have refocused research efforts to improve our understanding of basic cellular processes of DNA recombination, replication, and repair.

Although much remains to be learned, we now have insight into the genetic events that accompany malignant transformation. With this knowledge comes the potential for understanding how environmental agents might interact with cellular systems in the neoplastic process and therefore how we might interrupt or restore the aberrant processes in malignant cells.

THE GENETIC TARGETS OF TUMOR FORMATION

The statement that cancer is a genetic disease has entertained scientists and clinicians for more than a century. This statement has two implications: first, that a tumor is a clone of somatic cells that is genetically distinct from other cells of the same individual by the acquisition of mutations that are advantageous in some way; and secondly, that the factors allowing some cells to evolve into a tumor may be determined by the genotype of the individual. This implies that some individuals are prone to the development of cancer (site-specific or all types) because they carry a familial (germline) trait that determines cancer predisposition. Such a trait can be one of the specific and necessary gene mutations required for a pathway of tumorigenesis. The inheritance of this altered genotype would then push every cell one genetic step closer to the final genotype required for the formation of a tumor. Or the trait can affect the overall mutation frequency in the DNA of cells and thereby increase the likelihood that somatic cells acquire mutations in general as well as the necessary subset of mutations required for loss of growth control in a particular cell.

Cell growth is subject to both positive and negative regulatory influences. Genes that encode proteins that play positive, active, or dominant roles in the process of growth control are known as *oncogenes*. Genes that encode proteins that function primarily in the inhibition or down-regulation of growth are known as *tumor suppressor genes*. The interaction of these two types of regulatory gene products in normal cells determines appropriate cell growth and differentiation in response to particular signals. The disruption of one or both of these gene classes is associated with tumorigenesis.

Oncogenes and Their Normal Function

The existence of specific cellular genes that when disrupted are capable of directing malignant transformation was first established by the study of retrovirus-induced tumors. Retroviruses infect cells from many vertebrate species and can rapidly produce a variety of leukemias, lymphomas, sarcomas, or carcinomas. Numerous distinct viral genes have been identified in different retroviral isolates that are directly responsible for the tumor-producing capability of each retrovirus. Many tumorigenic retroviruses first acquired their "oncogene" by capturing and altering a normal cellular gene, or protooncogene, from the host cell in which the virus grew. Therefore a cellular oncogene, or protooncogene, in its new association with the virus, is corrupted in some way to become a viral oncogene. Other viruses induce deleterious changes in the expression of protooncogenes by integrating into the DNA adjacent to that protooncogene. Other protooncogenes were identified when their normal function in cells was disrupted by specific chromosome abnormalities present in some tumors. See Box 70-1 for a partial list of known oncogenes.

Protooncogenes have been highly conserved throughout evolution. For example, *ras* protooncogenes homologous to those in the human genome are found not only in other vertebrates but also in fruit flies and yeast. Therefore protooncogenes must represent important components of cell regulatory systems since their sequences have been carefully maintained. Experimental evidence suggests that these gene products normally play a role in the regulation of cell proliferation by serving as elements of a multicomponent signal transduction apparatus.

Growth-promoting signals from the microenvironment are communicated to cells through receptor structures associated with the plasma membrane. The most thoroughly studied of these are receptors with an external ligand-binding domain, a transmembrane domain, and a cytoplasmic domain possessing tyrosine kinase activity. In addition to such tyrosine kinase receptors, other distinct classes of molecules are thought to participate in signaling. These include receptors coupled to G proteins (guanosine triphosphate- or GTP-binding proteins with intrinsic GTPase activity) that can modulate the activity of such entities as adenylate cyclase and ion channels; ion channels themselves that can be activated by a variety of endocrine factors; receptors with intrinsic guanylate cyclase activity; as yet uncharacterized receptors for numerous lymphokines, cytokines, and growth factors for which no mechanism has been determined; receptors with phosphotyrosine phosphatase activity that may represent systems antagonistic to the tyrosine kinase receptor class; and the nuclear receptors of the steroid hormone receptor supergene family that bind such ligands as estrogens, glucocorticoids, and thyroid hormone as the first step in the direct control of gene transcription. Finally, growing evidence suggests that adhesion molecules expressed on the surface of cells, such as the products of the integrin gene family, communicate with the microenvironment in ways that have important consequences for cell growth and differentiation.

Signal transduction through a typical tyrosine kinase receptor is depicted in Fig. 70-1. Binding of a growth factor ligand results in activation of the cytoplasmic tyrosine kinase and autophosphorylation of that same cytoplasmic domain. For some receptors, such as the platelet-derived growth factor or PDGF receptor, ligand binding leads to receptor dimerization and intermolecular phosphorylation on key tyrosine residues. One of the consequences of tyrosine phosphorylation is the docking of kinase substrates, the downstream elements of the signal apparatus. These substrates recognize and bind to the cytoplasmic domain of the receptor through the newly phosphorylated tyrosine residue and are subsequently phosphorylated. In this set of interactions, the signal is thus transmitted from the extracellular to the cytoplasmic side of the plasma membrane.

Further stages of signal transduction require the participation of many protooncogenes with distinct functions. For example, some transmembrane receptors activate G proteins, which then propagate signals by the binding of GTP. Current evidence suggests the participation of still other protooncogenes, called *nucleotide exchange factors*, in the loading of G proteins with GTP. Signal transmission then occurs until G proteins hydrolyze the bound GTP to guanosine diphosphate (GDP). Inhibitory regulation of G proteins is accomplished by interaction with a cognate GTPase activating protein or GAP. In up-regulating the intrinsic GTP hydrolytic activity of G proteins, GAPs remove them from the activated state. Therefore signal transmission depends on the balance between activation of a G protein by its binding of GTP (facilitated by nucleotide exchange factors) and inactivation of the protein by GAP-induced GTP hydrolysis. Chief among these G proteins for growth factor receptors are members of the *ras* protooncogene family.

The *ras* protooncogenes (*H-ras, K-ras,* and *N-ras*) encode low molecular weight GTP-binding proteins that have been implicated in numerous signal transduction pathways for cellular growth and differentiation. Signals from activated RAS propagate through the cytoplasm to nuclear effectors by a cascade of serine/threonine kinases, culminating in activation of the mitogen-activated protein kinase MAPK. MAPK can further regulate cellular functions by controlling the transcription of a large number of genes by modifying the activity of transcription factors such as FOS. Under normal circumstances, the active GTP-bound form of RAS contains a weak GTPase activity that converts GTP to GDP and consequentially deactivates RAS. This GTP hydrolysis activity is enhanced 10^5-fold by interactions with GTPase-activating proteins or GAPs. This signal transduction cascade is an important regulator in the cell because many of the components of this cascade are protooncogenes (encoded by *raf-1, fos, jun*). Mutations leading to constitutive activation of this pathway yield an inappropriate growth signal that can contribute to the loss of cell growth control characteristic of tumor cells.

BOX 70-1

Oncogene compendium

Oncogenes are classified according to the functional properties of their corresponding protein product. Oncogenes listed in uppercase letters were discovered after their incorporation into retroviruses. Several oncogenes were discovered after their activation by the adjacent insertion of retroviruses (e.g., *pim*, several *wnt* genes, *mdm*).

Growth factors
  egf
  fgf (5)
  gro
  igf (2)
  SIS
  tgf-α
  tgf-β (many)
  wnt (many)
Hematopoietic factors (many)
Tyrosine kinases serving as transmembrane receptors
  ERBB1
  erbB2 (her2/neu)
  FMS
  KIT
  RET
  ROS
  sea
  trk
Tyrosine kinases associated with inner plasma membrane and cytoskeleton
  ABL
  FGR
  FPS
  lck
  SRC
  YES
Serine-threonine kinases
  MOS
  pkc
  pim-1
  RAF

G proteins (guanosine triphosphate binding and hydrolysis)
  gip
  gsp
  H-RAS
  K-RAS
  N-ras
  rho
Transcriptional regulatory factors
  ERBA
  ETS-1
  ETS-2
  FOS
  fosB
  gli-1
  hox
  JUN
  junC
  junD
  lyl-1
  max
  mdm
  MYB
  myl (pmi)
  MYC
  L-myc
  N-myc
  pbx
  rar-α
  REL
  relB
  scl
  SKI
  spi
  tal
  vav
Others
  bcr
  bcl-2
  bcl-3
  CRK
  dbl
  mas

More distal events after RAS protein activation include the hydrolysis of phosphatidyl inositol to yield diacylglycerol (DAG) and inositol diphosphates and triphosphates (PIP and PIP_2). These products continue signal propagation through DAG activation of protein kinase C (PK_C) and PIP_2 mobilization of intracellular calcium. As described next, PK_C may interact directly with transcription factors; changes in intracellular calcium lead to signal propagation through calmodulin kinases.

Propagation of a signal from this point requires activation of many transcriptional regulatory proteins. Several distinct mechanisms are activated for this purpose. First, signals proceeding from growth factor receptors (e.g., that of PDGF) often result in the expression of high levels of mRNA production for transcription factors such as FOS and JUN. The duration of this response is limited by the short half-lives of mRNA encoding these factors. In addition, mitogenic and differentiation signals often result in the posttranslational modification of already existing transcriptional regulatory proteins. For example, phosphorylation and dephosphorylation of various functional domains of both the FOS and JUN proteins are required for full activation of these factors. In other cases, transcription factors sequestered in the cytoplasm by inhibitory binding proteins are released for translocation into the nucleus as the result of signaling. The *rel*-related gene product, NFκB, is bound to an inhibitor IκB, until signals mediated by PK_C result in phosphorylation and release of the inhibitor. NFκB then migrates to the nucleus, where it binds specific DNA sequences near the promoters of genes that require this factor for transcription.

These few examples demonstrate the wide range of regulatory consequences that can be triggered by a signaling cascade.

The positive control of cell growth involves two other regulatory processes with relationships to signal transduction that are not completely understood. The first, cell cycle regulation, refers to control points at several critical boundaries between phases of the cell cycle. The most important of these are entrance into G_1 from the resting state, G_0; the passage from G_1 into DNA synthesis, S; and the transition from G_2 into mitosis. Several protooncogene products, such as SRC and MOS, have been implicated in the control of these critical transition points, particularly G_2/M. The products of several other genes (e.g., $p34^{cdc2}$ and the cyclins) are also important in this regulatory process, as are several tumor suppressor gene products (see later discussion).

Protooncogene products also are thought to play a role in another process of growth regulation known as *programmed cell death* or *apoptosis*. In many tissues, cells generated by the stem cell compartment proceed to terminal differentiation and ultimately to cell death. This process is particularly important in tissue with high cell turnover rates, such as hematopoietic and lymphopoietic organs, as well as the gastrointestinal tract. Apoptosis eventually results in the cessation of cell division and the orderly degradation of the cell's genetic material. The 25 kD product of the *bcl-2* protooncogene is located in the mitochondrial membrane and forestalls apoptosis, particularly in lymphoid cells. The continued expression of this oncogene (see later discussion) is the key consequence of a chromosome translocation

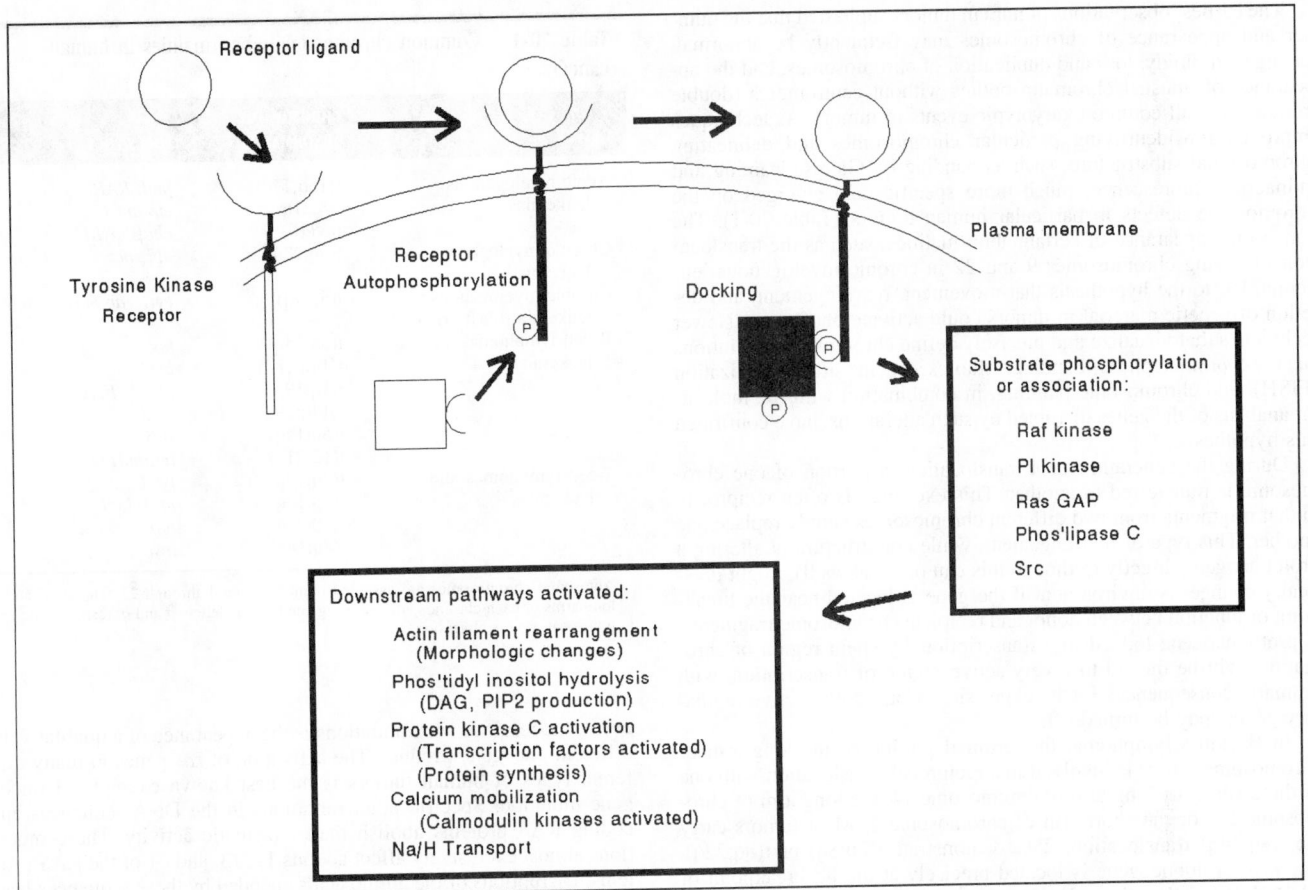

FIGURE 70-1   Oncogenes in signal transduction. Binding of a growth factor to its cognate transmembrane receptor results in activation of the cytoplasmic domain of the receptor *(thin black rectangle)*. This activation is accompanied by autophosphorylation of several tyrosine residues. One of these phosphorylation events activates the "docking" process, whereby cytoplasmic substrates of the receptor's kinase domain are themselves phosphorylated on tyrosine residues. Transmission of the signal continues by the resulting activation of the substrate *(solid black square)*. Recently identified substrates of tyrosine kinase receptors are listed in the right-hand box. Subsequent events in the signal cascade are listed in the center box. *Phos'lipase C,* Phospholipase C; *Phos'tidyl inositol,* phosphatidyl inositol.

present in human follicular lymphomas. The tyrosine kinase product of the *abl* protooncogene also may function in the control of apoptosis.

In the examples just described, each protooncogene product is considered to bear a single functional activity. Recently, protooncogene proteins with the potential to perform multiple functions have been defined. One of these, derived from the *bcr* protooncogene, possesses an amino terminus characteristic of a serine kinase, a carboxy terminus with GAP homology, and an intervening domain with strong homology to the DBL nucleotide exchange factor. Although the precise roles of multifunctional protooncogenes have not yet been elucidated, it seems possible that they function as bridges between distinct components of the mitogenic regulatory apparatus.

Disruption of Oncogenes During Tumor Formation

If protooncogenes function in normal cells to regulate growth and differentiation, what changes take place to activate these genes in cancer cells? As discussed earlier, retroviruses carrying altered forms of protooncogenes or retroviruses that integrate into DNA adjacent to protooncogenes can produce tumors in animals. However, retroviral infection or activation of cellular protooncogenes is thought to occur very rarely, if at all, in humans. Activation of protooncogenes by other types of viruses (hepatitis B virus, Epstein-Barr virus) has not been demonstrated directly but remains a possibility in some kinds of tumors (see later discussion). The alteration of the function of protoon-

cogenes, or oncogene activation, does occur in human tumors by a number of other mechanisms.

Inappropriate expression of a normal oncoprotein can be found in some tumorigenic cells. Some tumorigenic cells can synthesize too much of an oncoprotein or synthesize it at the wrong stage of the cell cycle. Alternatively, the protein may appear improperly at a given stage of differentiation. Finally, an otherwise normal oncogene product may appear in a cell type that does not usually express the gene. All these events lead to the same result: a stimulus for cell proliferation under inappropriate circumstances.

Cancer cells utilize several mechanisms for achieving the alterations just described. Overexpression of an oncogene product may result from amplification of the gene. By increasing the number of copies of an oncogene, sometimes by more than 100-fold, protein production can be greatly augmented. This mechanism often leads to cytogenetic abnormalities (see later discussion), such as double minutes and homogeneously staining regions that are prominent features of many tumor cell karyotypes. Amplification of the *myc* gene has been detected in many leukemias, small cell lung carcinomas, neuroblastomas, and neuroendocrine tumors of colonic origin. Glioblastoma tumors demonstrate amplification of *erbB1*, which encodes the epidermal growth factor (EGF) receptor. An increased number of EGF receptors are detected on the cell surface in some of these tumors and also in some epidermoid carcinomas. Expression of altered forms of EGF receptors also is observed in some glioblastomas. The amplification of *erbB2* occurs in breast cancers and is associated with a poor prognosis.

The earliest observations of human tumors suggested that the number and appearance of chromosomes may frequently be abnormal. Changes in ploidy, loss and duplication of chromosomes, and the appearance of unusual chromatin bodies without centromeres (double minutes) are all common karyotypic events in tumors. As techniques improved for identifying particular chromosomes and delineating chromosomal substructure, such as banding by Giemsa staining and quinacrine fluorescence, much more specific data emerged on the chromosome defects in particular human tumors (Table 70-1). The consistent appearance of certain abnormalities, such as the translocation involving chromosomes 9 and 22 in chronic myelogenous leukemia, led to the hypothesis that movement, rearrangement, and deletion of genetic material in tumors could activate oncogenes. Newer techniques that visualize and precisely define chromosome alterations such as prometaphase banding, fluorescent in situ hybridization (FISH), and chromosome painting, in combination with the molecular analysis of the genes disrupted by such alterations, have confirmed this hypothesis.

During the generation of a translocation, a portion of one chromosome is transferred to another. This exchange is often reciprocal, in that fragments from two different chromosomes simply replace one another. This type of rearrangement, while not structurally altering a protooncogene directly (although this can occur as well), might drastically change its environment if the gene is located near the breakpoint or junction between donor and recipient chromosome fragments. A protooncogene lodged in a transcriptionally silent region of chromatin might be moved to a very active region of transcription, with dramatic consequences for its expression. Conversely, active regulatory genes may be turned off.

In Burkitt's lymphoma, the terminal portion of the long arm of chromosome 8 (8q) is involved in a reciprocal translocation with one of three sites: the long arm of chromosome 14, the long arm of chromosome 22, or the short arm of chromosome 2. Most tumors carry the t(8q;14q) translocation; 25% demonstrate t(2p;8q) or t(8q;22q). The *myc* protooncogene is located precisely at the 8q breakpoint of all Burkitt translocations. Furthermore, the breakpoints on the other chromosomes represent the map locations of the κ-immunoglobulin light chain gene (2p), the immunoglobulin heavy chain locus (14q), and the λ-light chain gene (22q). Therefore, in a B-lymphocyte tumor, a protooncogene is moved to a position of active transcription, that is, one of the three immunoglobulin gene loci. The result of the translocation is not only the transcriptional activation of *myc* but also the uncoupling of its transcriptional regulation from events of the cell cycle; signals then go unheeded that might ordinarily result in downregulation of *myc* expression. As a consequence, this continuous *myc* expression drives cell proliferation as the cells no longer respond to signals for the cessation of cell division.

Several other B-lymphocyte lymphomas are characterized by translocations in which different oncogenes are brought into proximity of the heavy chain locus (see Table 70-1). Once again, the result is transcriptional activation of previously silent genes. One prominent example, the t(14q;18q) of follicular lymphoma, leads to the continued expression of the *bcl-2* gene product, which, as described earlier, prevents the onset of programmed cell death. Translocations also occur that are T-lymphocyte–specific (see Table 70-1).

As discussed, an important mechanism resulting in the inappropriate expression of protooncogenes is the rearrangement of these genes that occurs when chromosome translocations or inversions are generated. Other instances of overproduction or inappropriate production of oncogene proteins are known, although the means by which such aberrant expression occurs are not yet understood. For example, certain sarcomas elaborate PDGF, which in turn stimulates cell division within these tumors. Hematopoietic malignancies often produce many growth factors that provide mitogenic stimulation to tumor cells. The process whereby tumor cells synthesize and secrete growth factors to which they respond is called *autocrine stimulation,* a mechanism that may play an important role in tumor cell proliferation.

Somatic mutation of protooncogenes also can occur in cells and lead directly to malignant transformation. These more subtle mutations permanently alter that gene in a cell and in all its progeny. Physical and chemical carcinogens are known mutagens; perhaps several viruses associated with human cancer also act as mutagens. In any

Table 70-1   Common chromosomal abnormalities in human cancers.

CANCER	CHROMOSOME ABNORMALITY	LOCUS/LOCI
Acute myelogenous leukemias	t(15q;17q)	*pml, RAR*
	t(8;21q)	*eto/aml1*
	inv(16)	*chpβ/myh11*
Chronic myelogenous leukemia	t(9q;22q)	*abl; bcr*
Chronic myelogenous leukemia (blast crisis)	t(3;21q)	*evi1/eap/mds1; aml1*
B-cell lymphomas and leukemias	t(8q;14q)	*myc*
	t(14q;18q)	*bcl2*
	t(1q;19p)	*pbx-1, E2A*
	t(14q;19q)	*bcl3*
	t(5q;14q)	*II-3*
	t(12;21q)	*tel;aml1*
T-cell lymphomas and leukemias	t(7q;19p)	*lyl-1*
	t(1p;14q)	*tal,scl,tcl*
	t(10p;14q)	*hox*
	t(8q;14q)	*myc*

Autosomal chromosomes are assigned numbers from 1 through 22. The short and long arms of each chromosome are designated by the letters *p* and *q*, respectively; *t*, translocation; *inv*, inversion.

event, the result of such mutations is the appearance of a qualitatively different oncogene product. The activation of *ras* genes in many different types of human tumors is the best known example of oncogene mutation. Specific point mutations in the DNA sequences encoding RAS proteins abolish their enzymatic activity. These mutations almost exclusively affect codons 12, 13, and 61 of the RAS proteins. Disruptions of the amino acids encoded by these sequences lead to a constitutively active form of the RAS protein that ultimately affects signal transduction. Mutations in *ras* have been identified in roughly 50% of colorectal carcinomas; the majority of these occur in K-*ras*. Fifty percent of adenomas larger than 1 cm also contain *ras* mutations. However, *ras* mutations were found in only 9% of adenomas smaller than 1 cm. This implies that *ras* mutations have an early role in this tumorigenic pathway, but are not initiating events. Several animal models of radiation and chemical carcinogenesis have demonstrated that *ras* mutation is the probable event by which these agents initiate malignant transformation.

Another mechanism for the activation of protooncogenes is a combination of others: namely, rearrangement of genetic material that, rather than increasing the expression of a normal gene product, produces an entirely different one. Therefore in addition to activating the expression of a protooncogene, chromosome translocations in tumors can result in the creation of entirely novel genes. The Philadelphia chromosome of chronic myelogenous leukemia (CML) is the product of a reciprocal translocation of 9q and 22q. As a result, part of the *bcr* gene on chromosome 22 is fused with part of the *abl* protooncogene from chromosome 9. When this chimeric gene is expressed, the gene product is a novel fusion protein composed of the amino-terminal domain of BCR and the carboxy-terminal domain of ABL; this novel fusion protein is characterized by elevated tyrosine kinase activity. When translocation occurs further upstream in *bcr*, acute lymphocytic leukemia results (Fig. 70-2). The fusion product of this latter translocation retains the tyrosine kinase of the ABL parent at its C-terminus and the serine kinase domain of the BCR parent at its N-terminus. However, it lacks the nucleotide exchange (DBL-like) domain present in BCR and in the CML-specific translocation gene product. Evidently, the omission of these internal amino acid residues represents the difference between an oncogene product with specificity for a myeloid cell that retains the ability to differentiate (giving rise to a chronic leukemia) and a shorter product with specificity for a lymphoid precursor that has lost its capacity to differentiate (giving rise to an acute leukemia).

Several other spectacular examples show the power of translocation for creating new genes by fusing together fragments of preexisting ones. In the t(15q;17q) translocation of acute promyelocytic leu-

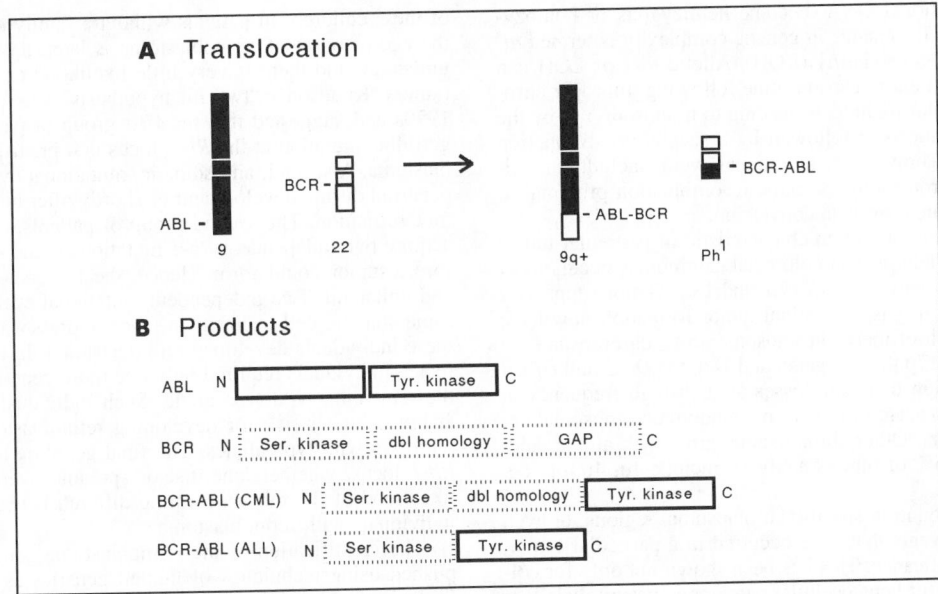

FIGURE 70-2   The Philadelphia chromosome translocation. **A,** Chromosomes 9 and 22 undergo a reciprocal exchange of genetic material through nonhomologous recombination. The Philadelphia chromosome, Ph[1] or 22q(−), bears a head-to-tail fusion *(bcr-abl)* of the *bcr* and *abl* oncogenes. The reciprocal chromosome, 9q(+), also contains a gene fusion *(abl-bcr)*, but the significance of this hybrid product is unknown. **B,** The protein products of the protooncogenes, *bcr* and *abl,* are depicted schematically, as well as the chronic myelogenous leukemia (CML) and acute lymphocytic leukemia (ALL) fusion proteins. *N* stands for the amino terminus of the protein; *C* for the carboxy terminus of the protein. Distinct functional domains are indicated by the rectangles. Because the ALL translocation occurs slightly more upstream in chromosome 22, the DBL-like domain of BCR is absent in the resulting fusion protein. The N-terminal domain of ABL may specify subcellular localization and/or substrate specificity.

kemia, a retinoic acid receptor gene *(RARκa)* is truncated and fused to the *PML* locus. The result is a chimeric gene product (PML-RARκa) that is apparently capable of dominant negative interference with the function of both the parental or wild-type products. In the t(1q;19p) translocation of acute pre–B cell leukemia, the *E2A* gene, which encodes a B cell–specific transcriptional regulatory factor, is fused to the homeobox gene *PBX1*. Homeobox genes, encoding proteins with homeodomains, specify DNA-binding proteins important in development and differentiation. The PBX1-E2A fusion product therefore has the transcriptional activating potential of the B-cell factor E2A, fused to the DNA-binding domain of the homeobox gene. This redirects the transcriptional regulation of one gene product (E2A) to the site of action, or gene targets, of the other (PBX1).

The analysis of leukemia-associated translocations has resulted in the identification of a number of transcription factors implicated in the normal regulation of hematopoiesis. An example of this is the acute myeloid leukemia 1 (AML-1)-core binding factor β (CBFβ) heterodimeric transcription factor complex. AML-1 was identified by analysis of the acute myeloid leukemia (AML)-associated t(8;21) translocation, found in about 15% of AML cases. AML1 is a transcription factor that binds DNA through a core region with homology to the *Drosophila* developmental gene *runt;* the DNA-binding activity of AML1 is enhanced by dimerization with CBFβ. The target genes of the complex are believed to be hematopoietic-specific genes, including those encoding the T-cell antigen receptor, granulocyte-macrophage colony-stimulating factor, and a variety of other cytokines. Via the t(8;21) translocation, AML1 is fused with a zinc finger-containing transcription factor ETO. The chimeric AML1-ETO is thought to alter the transcriptional regulation of AML1 target genes. In another 15% to 18% of AML cases, chromosome 16 is inverted (inv[16]); this alteration fuses CBFβ with a smooth muscle myosin heavy chain gene and produces a chimeric protein that retains its ability to interact with AML1 but alters the transcriptional activation ability of the AML1-CBFβ complex. The t(3;21) that occurs in rare cases of myelodysplasia and the blast crisis of chronic myelogenous leukemia (CML) results in at least three alternative AML1-fusion proteins, depending on the exact position of the trans-

location. Analysis of the t(12;21)-positive B-cell progenitor in childhood acute lymphoblastic leukemias (ALL) showed that a portion of AML1 becomes fused to the amino terminal helix-loop-helix domain of Tel, a member of the Ets-like family of transcription factors. In at least 25% of pediatric ALL cases, this chimeric transcript has been identified, whether or not the translocation is cytogenetically visible. In summary, perturbation of the transcriptional role of AML1 may be one of the most common mechanisms of transformation in human leukemias.

The general implications of these types of genetic rearrangements are two-fold. First, regulatory and structural domains of oncoproteins may be mixed to produce new products with entirely distinct specificities, producing functional activity in entirely inappropriate cell lineages. The net result is often abnormal proliferation, accompanied by improperly timed or absent differentiation. The second implication is that fusion genes, being specific to the tumors in which they arise, potentially serve as targets for tumor-specific therapeutic strategies.

Tumor Suppressor Genes

The second type of genetic target in tumorigenesis includes the genes that normally repress cell proliferation. Such genes are called *tumor suppressors* because the loss of such genes results in a tumorigenic phenotype. Both copies or alleles of a tumor suppressor gene must be inactivated by mutation before changes in growth control are apparent. Therefore unlike the dominant mutations that lead to the activation of protooncogenes by a gain of function in one allele, two mutations must occur at one locus (one in each allele) in order to eliminate the normal function of tumor suppressors. These mutations then are considered to be recessive.

Tumor suppressor genes can be mapped to particular chromosomal regions by genotyping tumors. Loss of genetic information in these candidate regions is a marker for the loss of tumor suppressor genes located in these same regions. These changes are detected using polymorphic DNA sequences in the genome that are heterozygous (each of the sequences on each chromosome is unique from the other) in normal cells from the same individual with the tumor. These loci, heterozygous in constitutional DNA, become hemizygous or homozygous in tumor DNA. This change in genetic complexity is termed *allelic loss* or *loss of heterozygosity* (LOH). Allelic loss or LOH can occur by the loss of an entire chromosome following improper chromosomal segregation during mitosis, leading to monosomy; or by the loss of an entire chromosome followed by a second nondisjunction event, leading to isodisomy. Other mutational events include interstitial deletion of the chromosome, somatic recombination proximal to the locus being evaluated, or gene conversion.

Patterns of allelic loss are often characteristic of particular tumor types. For example, allelic loss in colorectal carcinomas occurs most frequently on chromosome arms 5q, 17p, and 18q. Tumor suppressor genes that play a role in gastrointestinal tumor formation now have been identified on each of these chromosome arms: chromosome 5q carries the *APC* gene, 17p the *p53* gene, and 18q, the *DCC* and *DPC4* genes. The identification of allelic losses at such high frequency at these regions sparked a search for other nonrandom chromosomal deletions in colon cancers. Other chromosomal arms with allelic deletion in greater than 25% of tumors analyzed include 1q, 4p, 6p, 6q, 8p, 9q, 18p, and 22q.

In addition, LOH found in specific chromosomal regions, or even the number of LOH events that have occurred in a particular tumor, are of prognostic significance. This has been shown not only for colorectal carcinoma, but for hepatocellular carcinoma, where allele loss on chromosome 1q occurs early in tumor formation and on 13q, 16q, and 17p in advanced stages; allelic losses on 8q and 16q are associated with tumor progression. In general, the higher the frequency of LOH events in a tumor, the poorer the prognosis.

Fragile sites are chromosomal regions that form breaks or gaps when cells are exposed to specific reagents or tissue culture conditions. It has been proposed that these fragile sites also are the regions of the genome that undergo chromosomal rearrangement during tumor formation. One of the most common constitutive aphidicolin-inducible fragile sites is found in the region of chromosome 3p14.2. Allelic loss of this region is found in a variety of tumors; in addition, a t(3;8) breakpoint in this same region was found in an unusual family with hereditary renal cell carcinoma. Positional cloning identified the *FHIT* gene and demonstrated homozygous deletions of *FHIT* in multiple tumor-derived cell lines and in more than 50% of uncultured esophageal, stomach, and colon cancers. Evidence suggests that the *FHIT* gene is a tumor suppressor whose normal mode of action is unknown.

Tumor suppressor genes have been identified by analyzing tumors for common regions of genetic alteration. A second approach to gene identification has been to utilize inherited syndromes that predispose affected individuals to site-specific cancers. In its rarest forms then, the occurrence of cancer in an individual is due to familial or genetic factors. Such affected individuals are characterized by tumors that are usually site-specific, have an early age of onset, are bilateral or multifocal, and most importantly, although often difficult to distinguish from a background of common environmental or other risk factors, also have occurred in other family members. One of the earliest known examples of inherited, site-specific cancer is that which affected the family of Napoleon Bonaparte, where Napoleon, one of his sisters, and his father were each known to have died of gastric carcinoma. In addition, gastric carcinoma was suspected as the cause of death for two other sisters, a brother, and a grandfather. Such anecdotal reports suggested that the inheritance of particular genes could influence the likelihood of developing some tumors. In addition, the discovery of particular mouse strains that were susceptible to tumor formation further supported the idea that predisposition to cancer could be inherited. Affected individuals carry germline mutations of one gene that directly influence the likelihood that a particular tumor will form. It is from these inherited mutations that we can learn, even more precisely than via mutational analysis of tumors, which genes are commonly involved in sporadic tumor formation. In addition, the study of these affected families using the techniques of linkage analysis and positional cloning has resulted in the discovery of numerous tumor suppressor genes.

Retinoblastoma is a childhood tumor of the eye that occurs in infants from families with a history of the disease or in slightly older children without a family history. In familial cases, these tumors are almost always bilateral; often more than one tumor arises in the eyes

of these children. In patients without a family history of the disease, the age of onset of retinoblastoma is later, the tumors are primarily unilateral, and there is very little likelihood of independent multiple tumors. Knudson's "two hit hypothesis" was proposed in the early 1970s and suggested that the first group of patients had inherited a germline mutation at the *Rb-1* locus that predisposed them to retinoblastoma. A second, and somatic, mutational event at the *Rb-1* locus occurred during development or shortly after birth and resulted in tumor formation. The second group of patients, meanwhile, needed to acquire two independent *Rb-1* mutations in the same somatic cell before a tumor could form. Hence, the tumors were usually unifocal and unilateral. Two independent mutational events must occur in the same somatic cell to inactivate the suppressor effect of *Rb-1* before these individuals developed retinoblastoma. In the familial cases, affected individuals required only one more genetic lesion to inactivate the remaining wild-type allele. Such individuals were consequently at much higher risk for developing retinoblastoma than individuals with two wild-type alleles. The final genotypes of the tumors at the *Rb-1* locus, whether inherited or sporadic, were identical; only the likelihood of the tumors forming differed between the two types of individuals with retinoblastoma.

The identification of the retinoblastoma gene, *Rb-1*, was accomplished using techniques of human genetics as well by the genetic analysis of tumors. Clues to the location of the gene came from cytogenetic analyses of tumors that showed the deletion of a particular region of chromosome 13q. This same region also displayed allelic loss when polymorphic DNA markers were examined. Rare individuals with retinoblastoma and mental retardation were studied and shown to carry constitutional deletions of the same region of 13q. Positional cloning then identified a candidate gene from this region that was shown to carry more subtle alterations in constitutional DNA from individuals with familial retinoblastoma (one *Rb-1* mutation) as well as in tumor DNA from sporadic retinoblastomas (two *Rb-1* mutations). The presence of these subtle inactivating mutations proved that this gene was *Rb-1*, the retinoblastoma gene. Other tumors also have been shown to carry *Rb-1* mutations. Some of these tumors are found at an increased incidence in individuals with germline mutations of *Rb-1* (such as osteosarcomas); others are not (such as breast cancers).

The *Rb-1* gene encodes a nuclear protein (RB-1) with DNA-binding capability that is phosphorylated at the restriction point of the G_1 phase of the cell cycle. Unphosphorylated retinoblastoma protein interacts with a member of the E2F family of transcription factors through its pocket domain and then releases this factor upon phosphorylation. It is believed that the release of E2F promotes entry of the cell into S-phase by activating the transcription of E2F target genes. RB-1 remains hyperphosphorylated through the remainder of the cell cycle until the cell reenters G_1. Retinoblast differentiation, rather than proliferation, is the outcome of *Rb-1* expression. When this gene is deleted, the absence of its inhibitory function favors cell proliferation and eventually tumorigenic transformation. Interestingly, the oncoproteins produced by adenoviruses (E1A), SV40 (large T), and human papilloma viruses (E6, E7) all possess the capability of interacting directly with the pocket domain of RB-1, thereby promoting entry of the infected cell into S-phase by freeing the E2Fs. The product of the *abl* protooncogene also has the ability to interact with the RB-1 protein.

The retinoblastoma model of how tumor suppressors function and can be disrupted genetically is the paradigm for understanding other syndromes of cancer predisposition, the tumor suppressor genes that are mutated in each, and therefore the mutational targets in sporadic tumors of the same type. Germline alterations of specific tumor suppressor genes are now known to be responsible for a variety of site-specific cancer predispositions (Box 70-2). These syndromes include Wilms' tumor, adenomatous polyposis coli, familial breast and ovarian cancer, multiple endocrine neoplasia (many types), neurofibromatosis (type 1 and 2), Li-Fraumeni syndrome, von Hippel-Lindau syndrome, and others. Each of these disorders is an autosomal dominant predisposition to a particular tumor type; tumors form when the normal copy of the tumor suppressor is lost in somatic cells. The functions of the tumor suppressors vary for each of the genes and proteins already identified.

The *Nf-1* gene, mutations in which are responsible for the dominant cancer-predisposing disorder neurofibromatosis type I, also has

BOX 70-2

Tumor suppressor gene compendium

Tumor suppressor genes are classified according to the functional
properties of their corresponding protein product.
  Cell cycle regulatory proteins
    E2F-1 (perhaps other E2Fs)
    p53* (also listed under transcription factors)
    p107 (RB family)
    p130 (RB family)
    Rb-1* (also listed under transcription factors)
  Cyclin-dependent kinase inhibitors
    p15*
    p16*
    p21
    p27
  GTPase activating proteins
    Nf-1*
  Transcription factors
    p53*
    Rb-1*
    Wt-1*
  Others
    APC*
    Brca-1*
    Brca-2*
    FHIT
    Nf-2*
    ret*
    vhl*

*Tumor suppressors that are associated with an inherited syndrome of cancer
predisposition.

cyclin-dependent kinase inhibitor that negatively affects cell cycle progression by inhibiting the phosphorylation of proteins necessary to promote DNA replication. *p53* is upregulated in the G_1 phase of the cell cycle in response to radiation-induced DNA damage. Cells containing wild-type *p53* arrest in G_1 following γ-irradiation, or undergo apoptosis; cells lacking *p53* function fail to arrest in response to DNA damage or hypoxia. p53 is therefore described as the guardian of the genome.

As discussed previously, common chromosomal abnormalities in tumors are interstitial deletions and translocations that, in addition to activating protooncogenes, can inactivate tumor suppressor genes. Such deletions may be inherited in a variety of familial tumor syndromes, such as Wilms' tumor (11p-) or retinoblastoma (13q-). Additionally, characteristic tumor-specific deletions arise somatically in a wide range of human solid tumors, such as small cell carcinoma of the lung (3p-). In addition to interstitial deletions, inactivation of tumor suppressors can occur by point mutation in critical domains of the proteins. These mutations can also be dominant negative mutations as in the case of p53, which normally functions as a homodimer. Here, mutant protein produced from the mutated allele may bind to and inactivate normal protein produced from the normal allele. Thus mutation of only one *p53* allele may be sufficient to remove the function of the gene product from the normal homologue of the gene. This is in contrast to deletion of one homologue, where the remaining normal allele must still be damaged to eliminate functional activity of the tumor suppressor locus.

A Multistep Genetic Pathway to Tumor Formation

The development of cancer is considered to be a multistep process. Histopathologic observations, for example, have documented the sequence of changes from hyperplasia or dysplasia through carcinoma in situ to invasive metastatic cancer for a number of different tumors. In addition, genetic and epidemiologic analyses have suggested that multiple events are required for expression of the malignant phenotype. Recent experimental research, using both tissue culture and the breeding of laboratory mice with mutations in tumor suppressor genes, also supports the multistep hypothesis and provides a framework for further investigation into the genes that are responsible for normal growth control and differentiation.

The transfer of activated oncogenes to cells in culture with normal growth properties has determined some combinations of oncogenes that are required to generate a cancer cell. Several independent studies have shown that a cell that harbors a mutated *ras* gene may assume the abnormal morphologic features of a cancer cell but is not fully tumorigenic when inoculated into animals. The further addition of an activated *myc* gene is required for tumor formation to occur in vivo.

Interestingly, even two oncogenes are not sufficient for generating the full-blown cancer phenotype. The tumors resulting from transfer of activated *myc* and *ras* into normal cells do not invade and metastasize. Clearly, further steps and, presumably, other genetic alterations are required. The frequent appearance of deletions and mutations inactivating tumor suppressor genes strongly suggests that these changes must also accompany oncogene activation.

Mouse strains have been constructed that carry mutations in tumor suppressor genes known to predispose humans to particular tumors. The retinoblastoma mouse, although it carries a germline alteration of the *Rb-1* gene, does not develop retinoblastomas. However, if the animal is bred to strains of mice that lack one or both copies of the *p53* gene, as well as other genes that encode other RB family members (p130 or p107), retinal dysplasias develop.

Some of the most compelling evidence for the multistep model of tumor formation comes from the correlation of genetic alterations with distinct histologic stages in the progression of colorectal cancer. Colorectal tumors usually progress from benign adenomas to malignant carcinomas to metastases, and thus provide an excellent model in which to study the genetics of tumorigenesis. In addition, the study of age-dependent cancer incidence suggests that colorectal tumor development requires four to six independent genetic events.

As noted earlier, colorectal carcinomas demonstrate a high frequency of allelic loss of 5q, 17p, and 18q. These allelic alterations suggest the mutation of both copies of *APC, p53,* and an as yet un-

been cloned and characterized. Unlike the products of the *Wt-1* and *Rb-1* loci, which encode DNA-binding proteins, the *Nf-1* gene product, neurofibromin, contains a GAP-related domain that has been shown to catalyze RAS-GTP to RAS-GDP. Neurofibromin presumably functions by downregulating the activated state of its corresponding G protein(s). Germline mutations in *Nf-1* include premature stop codons, frameshifts, missense mutations, deletions, and chromosomal translocations that disrupt the gene. Specific point mutations also have been identified in a variety of tumors that alter a lysine residue within the GAP-related domain of the protein; these mutant neurofibromins have a much reduced GAP activity. The reduction of neurofibromin's GAP activity may result in upregulated RAS signaling, thus providing a similar effect as activating or dominant mutations in *ras* genes. Such results demonstrate that tumor suppressors can play a role in the inhibition of the cytoplasmic portion of the signal transduction apparatus.

The *APC* tumor suppressor encodes a cytoplasmic protein that interacts directly with β-catenin. Therefore it is thought that the protein may control β-catenin levels in the cell and consequently affect a β-catenin-specific signal transduction pathway; the ability of cells to interact by cadherin/catenin complexes also may be regulated in part by APC. Germline mutations in *APC* lead to the development of hundreds to thousands of adenomatous polyps of the colon and rectum, which then progress to carcinomas. Somatic *APC* mutation is an early event in colorectal tumor formation.

The tumor suppressor gene that is most frequently mutated in human cancers is *p53,* located on the short arm of chromosome 17. The product of this locus, a 53 kD nuclear protein, was originally identified by its ability to bind to the SV40 large T antigen; this binding results in the inactivation of p53 protein and direct tumorigenic consequences for the cell infected by this DNA tumor virus. Inherited mutations of the *p53* gene have been described in the Li-Fraumeni syndrome. Patients with this familial syndrome are at risk for malignant tumors in a variety of organs.

The C-terminal region of p53 contains a highly charged basic domain capable of binding DNA. p53 regulates the transcription of other genes critical to the control of the cell cycle, such as *p21*. p21 is a

confirmed gene (or genes) on 18q, such as *DCC* or *DPC4*. Mutations of *Ki-ras* also often occur. In the smallest of tumor lesions (adenomas less than 1 cm) very few *ras* mutations can be detected, although *APC* mutations are present. Furthermore, early adenomas infrequently demonstrate alterations of 17p/*p53* and 18q. Only advanced adenomas and carcinomas possess frequent changes of a gene or genes on 18q. From these correlations, we conclude that oncogene activation must be accompanied by genetic changes that inactivate other growth regulatory genes. The order of these events seems to follow a pattern in that *APC* and *ras* mutations appear early while *p53* and 18q alterations occur later. Exceptions have been identified, suggesting that although a preferred order exists, it is the accumulation of genetic events that is most important in colorectal tumor development.

The acquisition of somatic mutations leading to cancer development would predict that neoplasms have a monoclonal composition. A study of 20 different colorectal carcinomas and 30 adenomas from females displayed a monoclonal composition based on their X-inactivation patterns. Normal tissue, meanwhile, displayed polyclonal patterns. This suggests that a single colonic cell acquires a growth advantage over its neighbors and develops into a benign neoplasm.

Another characteristic of colorectal carcinomas is DNA hypomethylation. In normal human cells, CG repeats are methylated at about 70% of cytosines. However, a substantial hypomethylation of DNA was observed in both colon adenomas and carcinomas through the evaluation of methyl-sensitive endonuclease restriction sites. These restriction sites can be cleaved only in nonmethylated DNA, thus the levels of methylation can be analyzed by determining the amount of DNA digestion that occurs when treated with a specific endonuclease. Although the implications for this observation in tumorigenesis are unknown, the pattern is interesting. Some genes are upregulated when surrounding CG islands are demethylated by treatment with 5-azacytidine. This upregulation might lead to the overexpression of genes that affect cell growth and proliferation. More recently, breeding of a mouse strain with a germline mutation of the mouse *APC (mApc)* gene with a mouse strain lacking the ability to methylate DNA resulted in the reduction of expected intestinal tumors. This result, although unexplained, is intriguing because it suggests that other genes, in this case one encoding a methylase, may have the ability to modify the expressivity of other deleterious genes.

ENVIRONMENTAL AGENTS AND TUMOR FORMATION

Cancer is a disease that occurs via the accumulation of mutations in specific target genes in the same somatic cell. These mutations accumulate over time, often in response to environmental exposures. Therefore cancer is considered to be an environmental disease. Identification of the environmental agents that increase the likelihood that cancer will form has resulted in the delineation of some of the following agents and processes. These are shown in Table 70-2.

Ionizing radiation, in the form of x-rays or particle beams, causes cancer in direct proportion to the dose applied. Although the sensitivity of tissues varies, all forms of cancer can result from exposure to radiation. The mechanism by which neoplastic transformation is accomplished is via the generation of lesions or alterations in the structure of DNA, eventually leading to sequence alterations or mutations when the lesions are repaired improperly by cellular enzymes or not repaired at all. Large-scale damage to chromosomes, with subsequent rearrangements and deletions of genetic material, may also be important, although extreme damage may prevent a cell from replicating or surviving at all.

Other physical agents that are associated with increased tumor formation are listed in Table 70-2. Ultraviolet (UV) radiation induces skin cancer, including melanoma, again in direct proportion to the duration and intensity of the exposure. DNA damage with the subsequent introduction of mutation is the probable mechanism. In individuals with disorders characterized by deficient DNA repair, such as xeroderma pigmentosum, UV-induced skin cancer is more prevalent. This will be discussed more fully in the next section.

Foreign bodies are also carcinogenic in some circumstances. Asbestos fibers are the most prominent example of this group, with an

Table 70-2 Environmental agents implicated in carcinogenesis

AGENTS	SITE(S)
Biological agents	
Epstein-Barr virus	Burkitt's lymphoma (Africa); nasopharyngeal carcinoma (China)
Helicobacter pylori	Gastric carcinoma
Hepatitis B	Hepatocellular carcinoma
Papillomavirus	Cervical carcinoma
Schistosoma haematobium	Squamous cell carcinomas of the bladder
T-cell leukemia viruses (HTLV; HIV)	Leukemia; lymphoma; Kaposi's sarcoma
Chemical agents	
Alcohol	Esophageal; head and neck; liver
Aflatoxin	Liver
Alkylating agents	Hematopoietic system
Aniline dyes	Bladder
Benzols	Hematopoietic system
Diethylstilbestrol	Uterus; vagina
Lye (strictures)	Esophagus
Metal compounds	
Arsenic	Lung; skin
Asbestos	Lung; pleura
Cadmium	Kidney; prostate
Chromium	Lung
Nickel	Lung
Phenytoin	Lymphoreticular system
Tobacco (tars and metabolites)	Bladder; upper gastrointestinal tract; head and neck; lung
Vinyl chloride	Blood vessels; liver; lung
Physical agents	
Foreign bodies	
Asbestos (glass fibers)	Lung, pleura
Ionizing radiation	Skin
Ultraviolet radiation	Skin

increase of lung and pleural malignancies following exposure. Implantation of prostheses has very rarely been associated with sarcoma. The mechanisms underlying foreign body carcinogenesis are not understood.

An increased risk of cancer also exists for individuals with several chronic gastrointestinal inflammatory diseases, such as Barrett's esophagus, *Helicobacter pylori* infection of the gastric mucosa, and inflammatory bowel disease. In particular, individuals with long-standing ulcerative colitis have an increased risk for the development of colorectal carcinoma. This increased risk for ulcerative colitis begins approximately 7 years following disease onset and increases with the extent and duration of the inflammatory process. Squamous cell carcinoma of the bladder is strongly associated with the chronic inflammatory state induced by bladder infestation with *Schistosoma haematobium*.

A partial list of chemical carcinogens is provided in Table 70-2. Alcohol-related and tobacco-related cancers (head and neck, respiratory and upper gastrointestinal tracts, bladder) are among the most prevalent forms of malignant disease in the developed countries of the West. Such cancers are now increasing in the developing countries of Africa and Asia and in women. Cancer risk from other chemicals was formerly associated only with industrial exposure (aniline dyes, benzols, vinyl chloride). However, environmental contamination from both sanctioned and illegal toxic waste sites may yield in the future a significant number of chemically induced cancers. It should be noted, however, that current epidemiologic data do not support the hypothesis that cancer incidence is now increasing because of these environmental sources of carcinogens. In developing countries, aflatoxin-induced hepatocellular carcinoma, resulting from fungal contamination of grain stores, remains a significant public health problem.

With the exception of the response to chronic inflammation, the known biologic agents of cancer in human beings are viruses (see

Table 70-2). In the Western world, virus-induced cancer (with the possible exception of papillomavirus and cervical carcinoma) is rare. In other parts of the world, however, viruses have been strongly implicated in the major forms of cancer. Hepatocellular carcinoma following hepatitis B virus infection and nasopharyngeal carcinoma and its association with Epstein-Barr virus are the prominent examples.

Human retroviruses (human T-cell leukemia viruses), have been described that induce T-lymphocyte malignancies. Although many animal models of retrovirus-induced tumors are well characterized, the means by which human T-cell leukemia viruses cause leukemia have not yet been determined. Papillomavirus, a DNA virus associated with cutaneous warts, is now strongly suspected as the etiologic agent of human cervical carcinoma. Lastly, following infection by the human immunodeficiency virus (HIV), a number of cancers increase in frequency, including lymphomas and Kaposi's sarcoma. The balance between the tumorigenic contributions made by suppressed immune surveillance and mutation by viral factors remains unclear.

GENETIC STABILITY AND TUMOR FORMATION

Recent discoveries have highlighted the importance of DNA repair mechanisms in inherited predisposition to cancer. However, the discovery by cytogeneticists and clinicians of human disorders characterized by chromosome instability and cancer predisposition suggested, for many years before these recent discoveries, that the ability to maintain the genetic information of a cell was vital in preventing mutation and tumor formation. That responses to specific DNA-damaging agents or enzymatic deficiencies affecting DNA replication or recombination, proposed for xeroderma pigmentosum and Bloom's syndrome, respectively, could affect mutation rates and tumor formation, was predicted by study of chromosomes. The identification of the genes associated with the hereditary nonpolyposis colon cancer syndromes, the Li-Fraumeni syndrome, and many of the chromosome breakage syndromes has proven that the proteins responsible for normal DNA manipulations in the cell are required for adequate protection against tumor formation. Their discovery has reemphasized the importance of the ideas written years ago by Boveri: that disruption of the integrity of the genetic material can lead to developmental anomalies and can be characteristic of malignant clones of cells.

The chromosome breakage disorders include ataxia telangiectasia (AT), Bloom's syndrome (BS), Fanconi's anemia (FA), Werner's syndrome (WS), and xeroderma pigmentosum (XP). Each is an autosomal recessive disorder with a unique clinical presentation. Somatic cells from each type of patient are characterized by an increase in chromosome breakage as well as by other unique types of chromosome abnormalities. Lymphocytes from persons with AT are characterized by chromosome-specific translocations and inversions of the 7s and 14s; cells from persons with BS are characterized by an increase in sister chromatid exchange and the presence of quadriradial chromosome configurations; cells from persons with FA (any of the complementation groups) are characterized by triradial chromosome configurations; cells from persons with WS are characterized by variegated translocation mosaicism. Lastly, cells from persons with XP (any of the complementation groups) are sensitive to radiation. Therefore the tumors that develop in persons with XP affect the areas of the body that are exposed to sunlight, such as the skin and the tip of the tongue. Persons with AT have a high incidence of lymphoid malignancies; the tumors that form in persons with BS include those of all types and sites; FA tumors are often myeloid leukemias as well as those of the lymphoid system; tumors in persons with WS include a high frequency of sarcomas. The disease genes for the chromosome breakage syndromes are now being identified. Most of the gene products are those that seem to have important roles in the normal processes of repair, replication, recombination, or transcription of DNA, such as the recQ-like helicases of BS and WS. The loss of function of these genes leads to an increase in genomic instability and cancer predisposition.

Another type of site-specific heritable cancer first described by Henry Lynch is called *hereditary nonpolyposis colon cancer* (HNPCC) and is characterized by flat, broad tumors primarily of the proximal colon that, as the name indicates, do not seem to be preceded by adenomatous polyps. Other tumors can sometimes occur in association with these colon cancers: these include urothelial tumors, gastric tumors, and endometrial cancers. An interesting characteristic of HNPCC tumors, as well as a percentage of sporadic tumors from the same sites, is the presence of instability at short repeat sequences called *microsatellites*. The basis of this instability is a biochemical defect in DNA mismatch repair.

The DNA mismatch repair system was first examined in *Escherichia coli;* if a DNA sequence mismatch is created during DNA replication, it is identified and corrected by a series of enzymes that include the products of the *mutH, mutL,* and *mutS* genes. A number of homologues of the *mutL* and *mutS* genes have been identified in both yeast and humans. The human homologues were identified as the genes responsible for HNPCC through linkage analysis and mutation screening in affected family members. Mutations in at least four genes are associated with HNPCC: *PMS1, PMS2, hMLH1,* and *hMSH2.*

Alterations of these genes are inherited in families in an autosomal dominant manner; however, similar to tumor suppressors, the second allele at an HNPCC locus must be mutated somatically before DNA mismatch repair is impaired, before microsatellite instability appears, before mutations occur at a high frequency, and before tumors appear. The loss of the ability of a somatic cell to repair errors that accumulate, most likely under normal circumstances, leads to the formation of tumors.

The idea that mutations in repair genes and genes that encode proteins required for the appropriate manipulation of DNA increase the chances of a cell accumulating more mutations is compatible with the mutator phenotype theory of tumor formation. The accumulation of multiple mutations in a cancer cell should be a rare event, considering the low frequency of mutation in human cells, estimated at 1.4×10^{-10} per generation. The concept of a somatic mutator phenotype suggests that each genetic alteration in a cancer cell leaves that cell more susceptible to the acquisition of further mutation. One alteration may not only increase proliferation, increasing the number of cell divisions, but also increase the frequency of mutations per cell division. Gene amplification occurs at a much higher frequency in cells that lose both normal *p53* alleles. NIH-3T3 cells that have been stably transfected with activated *Ha-ras* have an increased frequency of chromosome breaks and rearrangements. Such studies have supported the idea that once some tumor-associated mutations are acquired, other mutational events in these cells occur more rapidly.

CONCLUSIONS

The idea that cancer is a genetic disease is well accepted. The cells that compose a cancer are derived from a clone of somatic cells that have acquired the mutations (some can be inherited) that are necessary to release that cell from the strict controls that govern its ability to divide or differentiate appropriately. The identification of the target genes that are mutated (both the positive and negative regulators of growth), the agents that increase mutation frequency, and the processes that decrease mutation frequency are important elements in understanding how tumors form. Genetic factors inherited in families influence the likelihood that somatic mutations important for transformation will occur (or are already present) and that a cell will evolve into what we see clinically as a cancer. Therefore, updating our ideas about how cells regulate their growth, differentiation, and the maintenance of their genetic material is important for all who are interested in understanding, preventing, and treating cancer.

BIBLIOGRAPHY

Fearon ER, Vogelstein B: A genetic model of colorectal tumorigenesis, *Cell* 61:759, 1990.

Hunter T, Pines J: Cyclins and cancer II: cyclin D and CDK inhibitors come of age, *Cell* 79:573, 1994.

Ko LJ, Prives C: p53: puzzle and paradigm, *Genes Dev* 10:1054, 1996.

Peter M, Herskowitz I: Joining the complex: cyclin-dependent kinase inhibitory proteins and the cell cycle, *Cell* 79:181, 1994.

Rabbitts TH: Chromosomal translocations in human cancer, *Nature* 372:143, 1994.

Sherr C: G1 phase progression: cycling on cue, *Cell* 79:551, 1994.

Weinberg R: The retinoblastoma protein and cell cycle control, *Cell* 81:323, 1995.

71 Principles of Cancer Treatment

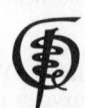

Beverly S. Mitchell

EPIDEMIOLOGY

According to American Cancer Society estimates, approximately 1.4 million new cancer cases exclusive of basal and squamous cell skin cancers will be diagnosed in 1996, accompanied by an estimated number of cancer deaths of 554,000. The distribution of cancers by site is shown in Table 71-1. As an overall cause of mortality, cancer is second only to heart diseases and accounted for 24% of total deaths in the United States in 1991. Trends in cancer death rates from 1930 through 1991, the last year for which valid data are available, have demonstrated a marked increase in the age-adjusted death rate for lung cancer in both males and females, while deaths from gastric and endometrial cancers have significantly declined. The incidences of other malignancies have remained rather stable when adjusted for age, but the advancing median age of the population clearly predicts a future increase in the total number of malignancies diagnosed.

It has been estimated that as many as 80% of cancers in the United States may result from environmental factors based on studies of the relative distribution of malignancies among different world populations, the variable incidences of cancer over time, and the effects of

Table 71-1   Estimated cancer incidence and death rates in the United States by site for 1996*

	NEW CANCER CASES	CANCER DEATHS
All Sites	1,359,150	554,740
Lung	177,000	158,700
Breast	185,700	44,560
Prostate	317,000	41,400
Colorectal	133,500	54,900
Pancreas	26,300	27,800
Kidney and bladder	83,500	23,700
Leukemias	27,600	21,000
Lymphoma/myeloma	74,600	35,210

*Data from the American Cancer Society's thirtieth annual compilation of cancer incidence, survival, and mortality data. Data exclude basal and squamous cell cancers and in situ carcinomas except bladder.

Table 71-2   Environmental causes of malignancy

AGENT	MALIGNANCIES
Aflatoxin	Liver
Alcohol	Head and neck, esophagus, liver
Aromatic amines	Bladder
Asbestos	Lung, pleura, peritoneum
Benzene	Leukemia
Drugs	
Alkylating agents, VP16	Secondary leukemias
Diethylstilbestrol	Vagina, cervix
Immunosuppressive	Non-Hodgkin's lymphoma
Tobacco smoke	Lung, larynx, mouth, esophagus, bladder, pancreas, leukemia
UV radiation	Skin
Viruses	
Epstein-Barr virus	Lymphomas, nasopharyngeal
Hepatitis B and C	Hepatocellular
HIV	Non-Hodgkin's lymphomas, Kaposi's sarcoma
Papillomaviruses	Cervix, anogenital
HTLV I	T-cell leukemia/lymphoma
Vinyl chloride	Liver angiosarcoma

migration on cancer incidence. Since carcinogenesis is a multistep process at the genetic level and since many of the genetic factors predisposing to and protecting from malignancy have not yet been determined, however, it is frequently difficult to pinpoint many of the environmental factors of importance. Exposure to carcinogens may occur many years prior to the diagnosis of malignancy and the dose and/or nature of exposure is difficult to determine in retrospect. Despite this caveat, a number of environmental causes have been defined, as outlined in Table 71-2. Tobacco smoking is felt to account for 40% of all cancer deaths in men and 20% in women and has been shown to increase the incidences of oral, esophageal, kidney, cervical, and stomach cancers and acute leukemias, as well as of lung cancer. Dietary risk factors are receiving increasing attention. The relationship between high dietary fat intake and colon cancer is the best established, with one study of a large cohort of nurses demonstrating a 1.9-fold relative increase in risk in individuals consuming diets high (>65 g/day) as compared to low (<39 g/day) in animal fat. Although high dietary fat intake has also been linked to an increased incidence of breast and prostate cancers, strong epidemiologic data to support causal relationships is lacking. Chronic alcohol intake is strongly associated with cancers of the oropharynx, larynx, and esophagus and appears to act synergistically with tobacco smoking in the pathogenesis of these diseases. Alcohol is also a risk factor for liver cancer and may play a role in cancers of the stomach, pancreas, colon, and breast. A number of associations between unusual carcinogens and rare malignancies have been identified, allowing a direct causal relationship to be directly established. Examples include the link between diethylstilbestrol administration during pregnancy and vaginal cancer in female offspring and the relationship between vinyl chloride exposure and hepatic angiosarcomas. Although a clinical history cannot encompass all possible carcinogenic exposures, a thorough history of occupational and drug exposures is an important component of the initial evaluation of patients with cancer.

PREVENTION

Once an environmental cause of cancer has been determined, the major approach to cancer prevention is avoidance of the precipitating agent. At the cellular level, however, it is possible to define sequential steps in the carcinogenic process and the long interval between the initiating carcinogenic insult and the appearance of malignancy provides an opportunity for the development of pharmacologic interventions to prevent this progression. The term *chemoprevention* has been coined to define the use of nutrients or compounds to decrease the incidence of malignancy resulting from either an initial carcinogenic insult or the progression of events that would subsequently result in a cancer. A striking example of effective chemoprevention is the use of *cis*-retinoic acid in patients with oral leukoplakia, lesions that have a high propensity for neoplastic progression, to reduce dramatically the incidence of head and neck cancers in a population of smokers. Similarly, *cis*-retinoic acid administration significantly decreases the incidence of second primary tumors in treated patients with head and neck cancer, although it has little effect on the recurrence or extension rates of the primary disease. Clinical trials are now in place to determine whether tamoxifen, an estrogen receptor agonist, will decrease the incidence of breast cancer in individuals at high risk for this disease and whether aspirin or other nonsteroidal antiinflammatory agents will decrease the incidence of colon cancer in individuals at high genetic risk. Cancer prevention represents an area of intense investigative interest that will assume even greater importance as the genetic risk factors for specific types of neoplasia continue to be identified. The development of animal models for neoplasia and a basic understanding of the molecular events in neoplastic progression are pivotal for the future development of this field.

DIAGNOSIS AND STAGING

The optimal treatment of any cancer is dependent on the accuracy of the pathologic diagnosis and a precise determination of the extent of disease. Although the presence of specific physical findings and/or diagnostic tests may point to the diagnosis, the pathologic determination of the cell of origin of the tumor and the degree of differentiation are critical determinants of the prognosis and appropriate treatment. Of additional major import is the extent of disease at diagnosis. Approximately two thirds of tumors will be localized at diagnosis and amenable to surgery and/or radiation therapy. Of individuals with these tumors, two thirds will be cured and the remainder will develop recurrent disease. Individuals with disseminated or extensive disease are candidates for systemic chemotherapy treatment, as are those with localized disease who are highly likely to have a recurrence. In order to determine sites of disease at presentation and to follow reponse to therapy, patients undergo clinical staging procedures in which a series of noninvasive radiographic or other tests are performed to identify sites of tumor involvement. In addition, a precise determination of the extent of tumor invasion of tissues within or around the primary site at the time of surgery allows assignment of a pathologic stage. The overall stage of the tumor is then indicated by a classification system that is either idiosyncratic for a given type of tumor or is defined by the parameters of tumor size or extent (T), lymph node status (N), and presence or absence of metastatic disease (M). The TNM assignment, which is becoming used with increasing frequency, will correlate with the stage of a tumor, but will vary with the type of tumor. Such classifications have considerable therapeutic and prognostic import for the patient. Accurate pathologic diagnosis and comprehensive staging are both critically important parameters for the optimal management of patients with cancer and for assessing the relative efficacy of different treatment regimens in clinical trials.

BIOLOGY AND GENETICS: RELEVANCE TO CANCER TREATMENT

There has been a recent explosion of knowledge of the genesis and cellular biology of cancer which, while not currently altering the standard approaches to cancer therapy, will have a major impact on our classification and treatment of cancer in the future. Molecular and biologic origins of cancer are discussed in Chapter 70. Since the major goal of cancer treatment is to rid the body of malignant cells with minimal toxicity to normal tissues, a greater understanding of the differences between normal and malignant cells will allow more selective and effective approaches to diagnosis and treatment.

The molecular alterations that give rise to malignancy originate as mutations in DNA that affect the nature or quantity of gene products that are important in regulating cellular proliferation. In order for a cell to proliferate autonomously, in general, a series of alterations in gene expression must take place over time in a single cell. This requirement for "multiple hits" for malignant transformation explains in part the long interval between exposure to carcinogens such as cigarette smoke or irradiation and the development of cancer.

The diversity of gene products that are important in regulating cell growth is great, although specific gene alterations are commonly associated with specific tumors. Aberrant cellular proliferation may result from the overexpression or altered structure of a category of growth-promoting genes or oncogenes. These gene products include a variety of transcription factors, growth factor receptors, GTP-binding proteins, and other signaling molecules. In addition, loss of expression of certain tumor suppressor gene products, such as the p53 and Rb proteins, leads to increased cell growth and frequently occurs as a late step in tumorigenesis. As an example, loss of p53 function through deletion and/or point mutations in both alleles is found in approximately 75% of colorectal cancers.

Of increasing importance to cancer therapeutics is an understanding of the molecular events controlling progression of cells through the cell cycle. Normal cell division depends on the progression of cells from a stationary phase (G_0) through G_1 into DNA synthesis (S phase). Once DNA has been replicated, cells undergo a second interval (G_2) prior to the onset of mitosis and reentry into G_1. Three major checkpoints have been defined that are critical for the regulation of normal cell division and are under the control of the cyclin family of proteins and their associated protein kinases. The G_1 checkpoint is directly regulated by the Rb gene product, which, in its phosphorylated state, releases the transcription factors necessary for cells to progress into S phase. Thus hypophosphorylation of Rb protein prevents cell cycle progression, whereas absence of Rb leads to loss of this checkpoint. A series of inhibitory proteins belonging to the p21 family also act to invoke cell cycle arrest in G_1. Of particular impor-

tance to cancer pathogenesis and treatment is the regulation of p21 by the tumor suppressor gene p53. Damage to DNA induced by drugs or radiation leads to increased expression of the p53 protein, induction of p21, and cell cycle arrest in G_1 (Fig. 71-1). This cascade is of importance in preventing cells from replicating damaged DNA, and loss of the G_1 checkpoint due to loss of p53, p21, Rb, and other factors has been associated with "genomic instability," an increased propensity for gene amplification, and the eventual development of chromosomal aberrations and aneuploidy. At the present time, factors controlling checkpoints in G_2 and M are not as well defined as those involved in the G_1 to S phase transition.

The molecular bases for hereditary predisposition to cancers have now been defined for an increasing number of disorders and include the BRCA1 and BRCA2 genes in breast cancer, the APC (adenomatous polyposis coli), DCC (deleted in colon cancer), and HNPCC (hereditary nonpolyposis colorectal cancer) tumor suppressor genes, and a chromosome 16 mutation associated with melanoma and pancreatic cancer. As the mechanisms of oncogenesis and tumor specificity of these mutations are further delineated, the opportunity to develop more specific diagnostic and therapeutic approaches to malignancy comes closer. Of concern, however, is the question of who should be screened for specific genetic defects that predispose to malignancy and what should be done with the information obtained. It is currently recommended that genetic screening be carried out in centers where trained cancer geneticists are available for counseling and where the genetic and molecular data obtained can be used to answer questions about natural history and the effects of medical and/or surgical interventions.

CURABILITY

The ability to cure a patient of a malignant disease is in general a function of tumor size and location and tumor cell biology. The early diagnosis of small localized tumors that are amenable to surgical resection confers the best prognosis. Malignancies that are disseminated at presentation and thus not optimally treated with surgery or radiation therapy may also be cured with chemotherapy alone or with combinations of surgery, radiation therapy, and chemotherapy, but the de-

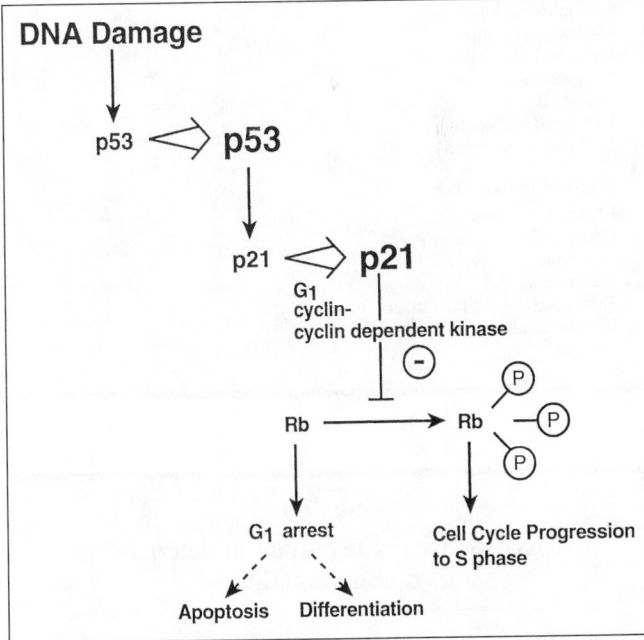

FIGURE 71-1 Induction of arrest in cell cycle progression by primary DNA damage. Increased expression of the p53 tumor suppressor gene leads to the inhibition of the G_1 cyclin-dependent kinase required for cell cycle progression into S phase. Loss of the p53 or Rb tumor suppressor genes by mutation and/or deletion is associated with loss of the G_1 "checkpoint" and may be associated with resistance to cancer treatment.

gree of curability depends in large part on tumor type and its intrinsic susceptibility to chemotherapeutic drugs and ionizing radiation. A listing of selected tumors according to their curability is shown in Box 71-1.

Prognostic factors that are important in determining the overall response of a tumor to cancer treatment are shown in Box 71-2 and result from information on the physiology of tumor cell growth, as well as on mechanisms of both chemosensitivity and drug resistance. Increased tumor size has several ramifications: first, according to the Goldie-Coldman hypothesis, tumor cells will develop a drug-resistant phenotype with a probability determined by the intrinsic mutation rate and the number of tumor cells. Thus larger tumors will contain more drug-resistant cells. In addition, larger tumors require several logs more cell kill to achieve a complete clinical response, generally defined as clinically undetectable disease with tumor cell mass less than 10^9 cells. Finally, larger tumors containing areas of central necrosis and hypoxia are more resistant to both drugs and radiation and will be more difficult to cytoreduce. An increased growth fraction or per-

centage of cells undergoing DNA synthesis has long been known to correlate with a better response to chemotherapeutic agents. Tumors such as small cell carcinoma of the lung and high grade lymphomas such as Burkitt's lymphoma respond rapidly to drugs that interfere with DNA synthesis, whereas tumors with low DNA synthetic fractions tend to have less dramatic responses.

Resistance to chemotherapeutic drugs is the most important parameter dictating overall tumor response to drug treatment. A number of cellular mechanisms have been defined as mediating drug resistance including drug transport, activation, and degradation. The widespread use of combination chemotherapy was initiated to circumvent the development of resistance to single agents and remains a major precept of drug therapy for cancer. The identification of a family of membrane transport proteins (multidrug resistance or mdr proteins) capable of pumping a large number of unrelated drugs out of the cell in an energy-dependent fashion has explained the phenomenon of multidrug resistance whereby cells rendered resistant to a single drug are cross-resistant to completely different classes of drugs that share no common structural characteristics. The increased expression of the P-glycoproteins responsible for this activity has been clearly demonstrated to be a negative prognostic variable for acute leukemia, multiple myeloma, and a number of solid tumors. Finally, mutations in the p53 tumor suppressor gene have been shown to decrease the apoptotic response to DNA damage induced in tumor cells by both chemotherapeutic drugs and radiation. Since p53 mutations are the most common genetic defect in malignancies, this mechanism may explain a number of therapeutic failures in cancer treatment. The availability of growth factors to alleviate myelosuppression and autologous marrow transplantation with stem cell reconstitution have made possible the use of chemotherapeutic agents at higher doses than were tolerated with conventional drug treatment. The use of dose-intensive treatments with standard chemotherapeutic agents such as alkylating agents has increased the response rate in a number of refractory and thus presumably drug-resistant neoplasms and the overall effects of this approach in improving the curability of relapsed or refractory lymphomas, breast, and testicular cancers are being assessed.

SCREENING AS AN APPROACH TO EARLY DIAGNOSIS

Since early diagnosis and smaller tumor burdens are the best predictors of cure for many tumors, the issue of when and how to screen asymptomatic individuals for malignancy is an important one. Any evaluation of screening efficacy will have to include an assessment of the cost and relative risks of the procedures used in relation to the benefit of early diagnosis to the population at large. Benefit is best defined as a reduction in mortality from the cancer, since earlier diagnosis will introduce several biases into an evaluation of length of survival after tumor diagnosis. Among these are the increased observation time that will result from earlier diagnosis and the propensity of screening procedures to identify more slowly growing tumors not associated with systemic symptoms, as well as "borderline" malignancies with different natural histories. Finally, the sensitivity and specificity of each screening procedure need to be carefully documented to provide the optimal interpretation of positive or negative results to the individual undergoing the test. Because of these stringent requirements to demonstrate efficacy, universal agreement on the utility of many screening procedures has been difficult to obtain.

Screening procedures have been demonstrated to be useful in the early diagnosis of breast and colon cancer, while data on prostate cancer remain more controversial. Routine mammography for the early detection of breast cancer is strongly recommended for women in the 50- to 69-year-old age-group where a 30% reduction in mortality has been demonstrated. There is ongoing debate about the role of mammography in reducing overall mortality in the 40 to 49 age-group and in women over 70 years of age. Screening for colorectal cancer in individuals over the age of 50 appears to reduce mortality through both the early identification of tumors and the identification and removal of premalignant polyps. The use of either flexible sigmoidoscopic or colonoscopic examination of the entire colon provides the most specific diagnostic approach. Evidence also supports the utility of fecal occult blood testing using hydrated stool specimens, but 1% to 5% of unselected persons tested in this manner will have positive

---

BOX 71-1

Curability of selected tumors with chemotherapy

Potentially curable with chemotherapy
Choriocarcinoma
Childhood acute lymphoblastic leukemia
Hodgkin's disease
Certain non-Hodgkin's lymphomas
Testicular cancer
Acute myelogenous leukemias
Wilm's tumor
Ovarian cancer

Potentially curable with adjuvant chemotherapy
Breast cancer
Osteogenic sarcoma
Colorectal cancer
Small cell lung cancer

Responsive to chemotherapy but not curable
Multiple myeloma
Gastric carcinoma
Head and neck cancers
Prostate cancer
Breast cancer
Carcinoid tumors
Soft tissue sarcomas

Resistant to treatment
Pancreatic cancer
Renal cell carcinomas
Colorectal cancer
Melanoma
Non–small cell lung cancer
Hepatocellular carcinoma
Glioma

BOX 71-2

Prognostic factors important in determining cancer curability

Tumor size
Tumor growth fraction
Intrinsic resistance to chemotherapy
    Multidrug resistance
    p53 Deficiency
Intrinsic resistance to radiation therapy

results. Of these, approximately 10% will have cancer and 20% to 30% benign adenomas, demonstrating the low specificity of the test. Data obtained on prostate cancer screening to date have not demonstrated a decrease in cancer-related mortality as a result of earlier diagnosis using digital rectal examinations alone or in conjunction with a serum prostate-specific antigen (PSA) and rectal ultrasound. Additional data are needed that incorporate the biologic features of this disease as important predictors of subsequent clinical outcome, since a large number of patients with prostate cancer will have a relatively benign course in the absence of medical intervention. Data supporting a reduction in mortality from screening for lung cancer by chest x-ray and for ovarian cancer by ultrasound, pelvic exam, or serum markers such as the Ca-125 antigen are currently lacking.

MODALITIES OF CANCER TREATMENT
Principles of Surgical Oncology

Surgery is the most commonly used diagnostic and therapeutic modality in cancer treatment and, as an isolated therapeutic approach, accounts for the majority of cancer cures. Increasingly, however, the optimal treatment of malignancies requires an interdisciplinary approach involving the participation of surgeons, medical oncologists, and radiation oncologists in an effort to prevent recurrences and to spare patients from radical and potentially deforming or debilitating surgical procedures. The diagnosis of solid tumors requires tissue, which can be obtained by aspiration, needle biopsy, incisional biopsy, or excisional biopsy depending on the tumor location, size, and possible tumor type. In general, the malignancy of the lesion is determined by frozen section before proceeding with resection. The surgical procedure commonly involves resecting nearby lymph nodes and tissues for pathologic evaluation and as part of the overall staging procedure and treatment. The extent of the surgery may also be influenced by prior clinical staging procedures such as CAT scans, x-rays, bone scans, routine blood chemistries, and serum tumor markers. The pathologic diagnosis and final pathologic stage of the tumor are the major determinants of what, if any, subsequent treatment is required.

Postoperative radiation therapy and adjuvant chemotherapy may each play a role in the treatment of tumors that may have spread beyond the local area, but that are not detectable by clinical evaluation. The application of these modalities has reduced the need for more radical surgery in breast cancer, for example, where local excision followed by radiation and/or adjuvant chemotherapy has obviated the need for radical mastectomies. Conversely, surgery may be used for metastatic disease that is localized to relatively few sites. Removal of isolated liver metastases in colorectal cancer with no other evidence of metastases may be curative in approximately 25% of patients. Finally, surgical approaches are of value for palliation of disease when tumor bulk results in mechanical problems or intractable pain and when debulking may facilitate a response to subsequent chemotherapy or radiation therapy.

Principles of Radiation Therapy

Radiation is used as a single therapeutic modality or combined with surgery for the cure or palliation of localized disease and in combination with chemotherapy with or without surgery for the treatment of tumors with high risk of systemic disease. Since the curative potential of radiation, as with surgery, depends on the effective treatment of areas of tumor involvement, meticulous staging and knowledge of the natural history of the disease are of critical importance to the success of treatment.

Ionizing radiation used in cancer therapy either is derived from the decay of radioactive isotopes (γ-radiation) or is electrically generated (x-rays). The ability of radiation to ionize air is measured in roentgens (R). The unit of measurement that indicates the amount of energy absorbed per unit mass is the *rad* (radiation absorbed dose) and the unit of measurement in current clinical use is the gray (Gy), where 1 gray = 100 rads. Ionizing radiation produces biologically active free radical intermediates within the cell that damage deoxyribonucleic acid (DNA) and interfere with its replication. This DNA damage is the primary mechanism of radiation-induced cell killing and recent work has demonstrated that a DNA damage–monitoring system exists within normal cells that leads to cell cycle arrest and/or apoptosis and ultimately cell death through a unique signaling pathway. Thus irradiation results in increased levels of expression of the p53 gene and several members of the *gadd* (growth *a*rrest and *D*NA *d*amage) gene families. Activation of these pathways and subsequent decisions about growth arrest versus apoptosis ultimately determine which cells will die as a result of radiation and are important in the relative killing of cells in tumors as opposed to normal tissues. Of potential major clinical relevance is the demonstration that mutations in the p53 tumor suppressor gene result in relative resistance to radiation treatment.

The type of equipment used in therapy has a significant impact on the therapeutic and toxic effects. Orthovoltage machines (rarely used at present) deliver the maximum radiation dose superficially with a rapid decrease in dose as the radiation beam penetrates into tissue, and skin burns are the dose-limiting acute toxicity. In contrast, the higher energy supervoltage equipment delivers maximum radiation at greater depths and the rate of decrease of dose delivery with depth in tissue is much slower than for orthovoltage. The most frequently used means for delivering radiation to tissues is by external beam, wherein the desired area to be treated is mapped out with appropriate shielding of vital organs. This composite of treated and shielded areas is called the *port* or *treatment field*. The total dose of radiation to be given over time is divided into a series of small doses that cumulatively equal the desired total dose (dose fractionation). The biologic effect of divided radiation doses is less than the same dose given in a single fraction (i.e., 400 cGy in one dose is biologically more effective than 200 cGy given twice), so doses cannot be simply added to obtain biologic equivalence. New computer-modeling techniques based on CAT scan images of tumors have allowed a more sophisticated approach to their three-dimensional imaging and treatment. This approach may allow more accurate dosing of radiation and better sparing of surrounding normal tissues.

Radiation administered to a tumor with curative intent requires that the radiation dose sterilize the tumor while producing reversible and tolerable toxicity to surrounding normal tissues. An understanding of the intrinsic radiation sensitivity of a tumor is an important part of this equation, again relating to aspects of tumor cell biology that are still incompletely understood. Radiation sensitivity is enhanced by increased oxygen tension and high proliferative rate. Tumors that have poor vascularization and are relatively hypoxic will produce fewer free oxygen radicals that act as intermediates in inducing DNA damage and are less sensitive to radiation. The tumor cell content of endogenous thiols, which act as free radical scavengers and reduce radiation sensitivity, can also influence tumor response. Efforts are underway to selectively increase the radiation sensitivity of tumors using radiosensitizing drugs such as 5-fluorouracil. In addition, drugs that accept electrons and form free radicals can enhance radiation damage to hypoxic cells. Conversely, sulfhydryl compounds could protect normal tissues from radiation damage and drugs of this class are currently under development.

Radiation therapy is used alone or in combination with surgery as primary therapy for a number of cancers including those of the oral cavity, pharynx, larynx, breast, certain non–small cell cancers of the lung, basal and squamous cancers of the skin, early stage Hodgkin's lymphoma, cancer of the cervix, soft tissue sarcomas, and brain tumors. It is combined with chemotherapy in the primary management of many breast tumors, anorectal cancers, small cell lung cancer, and esophageal cancer. Radiation therapy also has a major role in the palliation of painful bone metastases, brain metastases, and obstructing tumor masses. The major acute toxicity from radiation is generally due to damage to the rapidly turning over cell populations and is predominantly due to damage to epithelial cells. Thus damage to the mucosa of the oral cavity, pharynx, and larynx can result in painful mucositis, damage to gastric mucosa can cause nausea or vomiting, damage to colonic epithelium can result in diarrhea or tenesmus, and damage to bladder epithelium produces cystitis. These effects are usually transient with symptoms improving with epithelial repopulation. An additional major toxicity is bone marrow suppression. Dose-limiting neutropenia or thrombocytopenia is more likely to occur following systemic chemotherapy or as a result of large radiation fields that encompass bone marrow. Concomitant administration of growth factors with radiation therapy enhances the cytotoxicity to hematopoietic progenitors and may exacerbate neutropenia. Late radiation damage to organs results from killing of the functional cells and subsequent replacement with fibrosis and loss of function in organs such as kidney, liver, and lung. If a relatively small percentage of the organ has been irradiated, no clinical long-term result may be apparent. Damage to larger volumes can result in decreased functional capacity of these organs.

Principles of Chemotherapy

Principles of Cytotoxic Chemotherapy. The systemic administration of drugs to kill tumor cells has clearly improved duration of survival in many forms of cancer and resulted in the cure of others. Drugs effective in the treatment of cancer have generally been identified by screening compounds against tumor cell lines that have rapid doubling times. Consequently many of the chemotherapeutic agents in clinical use have generalized antiproliferative effects that render them most effective against rapidly growing tumors and lead to the side effects of toxicity to the bone marrow, gastrointestinal tract, and skin. A major advance in the use of chemotherapeutic drugs resulted from the practice of combining drugs with different mechanisms of action and with different toxicities for normal tissues. The rationale for combination chemotherapy lies in the observation that chemotherapeutic failures frequently result from the development of drug resistance. Drug combinations are designed both to circumvent the resistance of tumors to single agents and to prevent the use of drugs that have overlapping toxicities.

A second approach to preventing the development of drug resistance is the administration of the full and optimal dose of chemotherapeutic agents with relatively short time intervals between treatments. Dose reductions may be required for many serious toxicities such as renal insufficiency and gastrointestinal damage, but the use of hematopoietic growth factors following the administration of chemotherapy has allowed the administration of doses of chemotherapeutic agents that might previously have been limited by neutropenia or thrombocytopenia. Hematopoietic growth factors have also allowed the escalation of doses of drugs used in conventional chemotherapy and facilitated the use of dose-intensive regimens requiring the harvesting of peripheral blood or marrow stem cells prior to the administration of chemotherapy and restitution of cells following the treatment (autologous bone marrow transplantation).

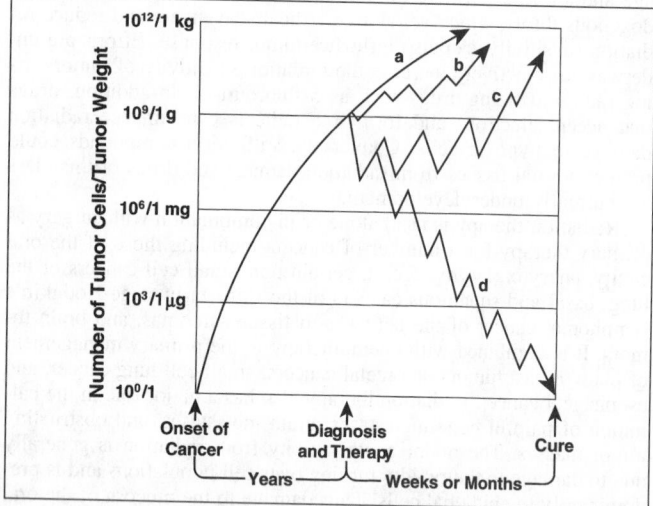

FIGURE 71-2   The relationship of tumor cell burden to diagnosis and treatment strategies. The growth of tumor cells slows with increased tumor size (*a*). Tumors that are sensitive to drugs or radiation will have a progressive reduction in tumor mass with each subsequent treatment and are curable (*d*). Tumors that are initially sensitive to treatment may develop drug or radiation resistance while clinically undetectable (<10⁹ cells) and subsequently emerge as recurrent disease (*c*). Tumors that are initially drug or radiation resistant will not enter clinical remission (*b*).

Modified from Stockdale FE: Cancer growth and chemotherapy. In *Scientific American Medicine*, New York, 1996, Scientific American.

Tumor cell kill by chemotherapy, as well as radiation therapy, follows first-order kinetics such that a given fraction of tumor cells is killed with each treatment (Fig. 71-2). The frequent administration of drugs will sequentially decrease the tumor burden and must be continued after the tumor is no longer clinically evident to achieve a cure. As a corollary, the lower the initial tumor burden and the greater the log kill with each treatment, the greater the probability of cure. Occasionally, large tumors or locally invasive cancers may be treated initially with systemic chemotherapy for cytoreduction in order to make them amenable to local treatment such as surgical excision or radiation. This approach has been termed *neoadjuvant* chemotherapy and has been found to be useful in some esophageal cancers and locally advanced breast cancer. In contrast, *adjuvant* chemotherapy involves the systemic administration of drugs following the local removal of a tumor that has a reasonably high probability of recurrence but where no residual disease can be measured.

Development of New Chemotherapeutic Drugs. Many promising chemotherapeutic agents have been identified by screening for cytotoxic activity against a panel of tumor cell lines. The National Cancer Institute has characterized a large number of such cell lines for potentially important markers for tumor response including such parameters as tumor suppressor gene expression, loss of cell cycle checkpoints, and expression of cytoskeletal proteins. In some instances, there is a correlation between the cytotoxic effects of specific classes of drugs and tumor cell biologic characteristics. These studies may make it possible in the future to predict, based on a biologic profile of a tumor, which drugs or classes of drugs might be particularly effective. At present, the clinical development of any drug with promising in vitro characteristics is dependent on first determining the maximal tolerated dose of the drug in Phase I clinical trials in which the dose is gradually escalated and any associated toxicities are documented in individuals with refractory malignancies. The pharmacokinetic data obtained from such studies, along with any suggestive therapeutic responses, allow further development in Phase II clinical trials where the type and degree of response of specific tumors are documented. Finally, Phase III clinical trials compare the reponses to new drugs and/or therapeutic regimens with those to standard treatments or to placebo where no treatment is effective. Since there are many tumors for which effective treatment is not available, it is very important that eligible patients be informed of the availability of clinical trials and be involved in the decision as to whether to participate in them.

Chemotherapy Administration. The majority of chemotherapy is administered intravenously, and the need to administer drugs recurrently that may damage veins or cause severe inflammation if extravasation occurs has led to the frequent use of indwelling catheters inserted directly into the subclavian vein that can be left in place for the entire course of chemotherapy. The majority of chemotherapeutic drugs do not penetrate the blood-brain barrier, and the central nervous system (CNS) constitutes a sanctuary site where certain tumors may recur or persist despite systemic treatment. It is therefore necessary to administer a select number of chemotherapeutic drugs directly into the CNS, either by lumbar puncture or through a reservoir inserted into the lateral ventricle, to treat tumors that have demonstrated meningeal involvement or disorders such as acute lymphoblastic leukemia that have a high potential for relapsing in the CNS. Regional administration of drugs to tumors through direct intraarterial administration has been used for the treatment of head and neck cancers, hepatic metastases, brain tumors, and bone sarcomas. Finally, chemotherapeutic agents may be directly administered into the pleural and peritoneal cavities.

Hormonal Treatments. Hormonal manipulation of tumors has been useful for malignancies in which the cell of origin is regulated in its growth by an endocrine mechanism, such as breast and prostate cancer. The use of hormones is predicated on the existence of appropriate receptors on the tumor cells and generally results in a cytostatic, rather than cytotoxic, response. Thus hormonal agents that bind as partial agonists or as antagonists to specific receptors are generally administered over a long period. An antiestrogen, tamoxifen, has been of major use in the treatment of postmenopausal women with estrogen and/or progesterone receptor–positive breast cancer. Similarly, prostate cancer may be responsive to antiestrogens and antiandrogens in combination with gonadotropin-releasing hormone agonists. Glucocorticoids such as prednisone and dexamethasone are of major use in the treatment of several types of lymphoproliferative disease and are used in high doses to reduce the swelling that is associated with tumors of the central nervous system or spinal cord.

Biologic Therapies. A number of biologic agents that are useful in the normal host immune response or have been engineered to mimic aspects of naturally occuring host defense mechanisms have been tried in the treatment of cancer. This class of agents, also termed *biologic response modifiers,* includes monoclonal antibodies that have been developed against cell type–specific or tumor antigens, cytokines that stimulate normal effector cells of the immune system, tumor cell vaccines developed against tumor cell–specific molecules, and inducers of cellular differentiation. Monoclonal antibodies may be administered alone to cause tumor cell lysis through complement fixation or as conjugates linked to drugs, radionuclides, or toxins that are themselves cytotoxic. Although the clinical use of monoclonal antibodies remains largely investigational, efficacy has been demonstrated in certain refractory B-cell lymphomas using antibodies to B cell–specific surface antigen either alone or conjugated to ^{131}I, and this approach may be of use in an adjuvant setting. The interferons constitute a family of related, naturally occuring antiviral proteins (α, β, and γ) with differing cells of origin. Interferon-α has been demonstrated to be effective in the treatment of certain hematologic malignancies and may be of use in renal cell carcinoma. Although the mechanism of action of this agent is not well defined, it has demonstrated efficacy in prolonging the survival of chronic myelogenous leukemia patients and has activity against certain lymphomas, multiple myeloma, and Kaposi's sarcoma. Use of the cytokine interleukin-2 to activate the immune system, either by systemic administration or through in vitro incubation with harvested peripheral blood leukocytes, has resulted in partial responses of certain tumors including renal cell carcinoma and melanomas. The recently acquired ability to delineate and purify specific tumor peptides or epitopes that are instrumental in initiating a cytolytic T-lymphocyte response to the tumor could well lead to major advances in the immunotherapy of malignancy. Phase I clinical trials using defined peptides as immunogens are underway for several tumors including melanoma. Finally, the demonstrated ability of the Vitamin A isomer, all-*trans* retinoic acid, to induce the differentiation of acute promyelocytic leukemic cells has led to the recognition that retinoids, by interacting with receptor molecules, may regulate the expression of certain genes that are important in overcoming a specific block to cellular maturation. A search for additional biologic and chemical agents that can induce cellular differentiation in the face of malignant transformation is underway.

Novel Therapies for Cancer. The ability to deliver potentially cytotoxic gene products to tumor cells by gene transfer techniques has led to a number of clinical trials in the area of gene therapy for malignancy. The most commonly used approach has been to transfer the cDNA encoding a nonmammalian enzyme that will selectively activate a prodrug to a cytotoxic compound within the tumor cells expressing the enzyme. Thus herpes virus thymidine kinase has been expressed in tumor cells and shown to render the prodrug gancyclovir, an antiviral compound activated by the enzyme, toxic to tumor cells. Additionally, tumor cells have been engineered to produce cytokines such as interleukin-2 that may induce a local immune response to the tumor. Finally, efforts are under way to supply wild-type tumor suppressor genes such as p53 to tumor cells in which this gene has been mutated. Although the therapeutic potential of this approach will be heavily dependent on the future development of improved delivery systems for the genes of interest that will efficiently and selectively target the tumor cell population, and the means for directing tumor-specific gene expression, cancer does represent an important target for the gene therapy approach.

The elucidation of mechanisms regulating cell cycle progression and facets of the pathways leading to cellular apoptosis (see Fig. 71-1) has created an entirely new series of targets for chemotherapy drug development. It is inevitable that the knowledge of specific molecular defects underlying carcinogenesis and tumor cell progression, in combination with knowledge of the mechanisms that induce cell differentiation and cell death, will lead to the development of novel interventions that will exploit these mechanisms and lead to enhanced selectivity of chemotherapy for tumor cells.

BIBLIOGRAPHY

Boone CW, Wattenberg LW: Current strategies of cancer chemoprevention, *Cancer Res* 54:3315, 1994.
Chabner BA, Collins JM: *Cancer chemotherapy: principles and practice,* Philadelphia, 1990, Lippincott.
Fisher DE, Fung CY: p53: from molecular mechanisms to prognosis in cancer, *J Clin Oncol* 13:808, 1995.
La Thangue NB, editor: Cell cycle regulation and cancer. In *Seminars in cancer biology,* vol 6(2), 1995.

II LABORATORY TESTS

CHAPTER

72 Evaluation of Peripheral Blood and Bone Marrow Cells

John C. Winkelmann

One of the most common problems facing clinicians is the evaluation of blood cell abnormalities, both quantitative and qualitative. Valuable information can be gleaned from automated blood counts. Additional, complementary data are obtained through microscopic examination of the peripheral blood smear. In certain situations, bone marrow aspirate and biopsy are required to establish a diagnosis. Newer methods based on flow cytometry and immunocytochemistry have become clinically useful tools. This chapter reviews the assessment of blood and bone marrow cells, emphasizing practical clinical application of the various laboratory techniques.

AUTOMATED BLOOD CELL ANALYSIS

Erythrocytes (RBCs), leukocytes, and platelets are all counted by automated laboratory counters with a high degree of accuracy, whether electrical impedance or optical methods are used. Furthermore the size of RBCs and platelets can be directly measured and the cell population displayed as a histogram. Newer equipment can perform automated leukocyte differential counts that are reliable and accurate.

Erythrocytes

The key erythrocyte measurements obtained by automated laboratory equipment are the red blood cell (RBC) count, the RBC size or mean cell volume (MCV), and the hemoglobin (Hgb) concentration. The hematocrit is calculated from the RBC count and the MCV. Since the hematocrit is a calculated value, clinicians should learn to "think" of patient values in terms of the hemoglobin level. The mean cell hemoglobin concentration (MCHC) and mean cell hemoglobin (MCH) are calculated from the hemoglobin and hematocrit, and the hemoglobin and the RBC count, respectively (Box 72-1). The RBC distribution width (RDW) is a measure of the variation of RBC size. The higher the RDW, the greater the RBC size variation.

The hemoglobin and MCV (and occasionally the RBC count) are the most clinically useful RBC parameters. Automated equipment gives a much more accurate and reliable measurement of the MCV than does morphologic analysis of the peripheral blood smear. Most

---

BOX 72-1
Red blood cell indices

Hematocrit (%) (calculated by automated counters):	MCV (femtoliters) $\times$ RBC count ($\times 10^6/\mu$l) $\times 10$
MCH:	[Hgb (g/dl)/RBC count ($\times 10^6/\mu$l)] $\times 10$
MCHC:	[Hgb (g/dl)/hematocrit (%)] $\times 100$

---

microcytic, macrocytic, and normocytic anemias can be easily recognized by examining only the hemoglobin and the MCV. The MCHC is occasionally useful in assessment of iron deficiency (decreased), thalassemia (decreased), and spherocytosis (increased). The RDW occasionally provides a hint that a patient's RBCs are abnormal in the presence of other measurements that are unremarkable. For example, the RDW is a sensitive indicator of iron deficiency and is useful in distinguishing iron deficiency (increased) from thalassemia trait (normal).

When there is a significantly abnormal RBC count or hemoglobin concentration on automated blood cell analysis, most hematologists recommend microscopic examination of the peripheral blood smear and measurement of reticulocytes to assist in the diagnosis (see later discussion). Together with the MCV, these data allow the clinician to quickly narrow down the possible explanations for an abnormal hemoglobin level.

Clinicians must appreciate that automated laboratory equipment gives erroneous or misleading information in certain circumstances. For example, cold agglutinins can cause RBC clumping in the test tube. Agglutinated RBCs may not be recognized individually and measurements of the MCV may be falsely increased. Reticulocytosis in response to bleeding or hemolysis increases the MCV because immature RBCs are considerably larger than typical RBCs. Automated equipment does not distinguish reticulocytes from mature RBCs, so the uncritical observer may falsely suspect a macrocytic anemia. In addition, severe hyperglycemia may falsely increase the MCV.

Leukocytes

In recent years, the automated assessment of peripheral blood leukocytes has become very sophisticated. As a result, it is possible to obtain accurate, limited leukocyte differential counts in addition to total leukocyte counts. Regardless of the method or equipment used, the data obtained are less prone to the field selection error of the traditional 100 cell manual leukocyte differential count. When abnormal leukocyte differential counts are obtained by automated equipment, many laboratories routinely examine a manual differential to confirm the data or detect aberrant cells that are not appreciated by machines. Such cells include nucleated erythrocytes, immature granulocytes, or nonneutrophilic granulocytes such as eosinophils and basophils. When the clinical laboratory does not routinely perform this examination, it is up to the physician to request it.

Patients with abnormal leukocyte differential counts that have aberrant cells of any kind should have a microscopic examination of peripheral blood leukocyte morphology by a physician (see later discussion). Automated leukocyte analysis is blind to several specific morphologic alterations of diagnostic significance such as nuclear hypersegmentation, toxic granulations, Döhle bodies, Pelger-Huët anomaly, Sézary cells, and presence of leukemic cells and immature cell populations (Color Plates IV-5 and IV-6).

Platelets

The total platelet count is the most clinically valuable platelet measurement obtained by automated laboratory equipment. This is generally much more accurate than manual platelet counts, regardless of the method used. The mean platelet volume (MPV) is determined by several automated devices and is clinically useful is some situations. Increased MPV values suggest the presence of destructive or congenital thrombocytopenias. Normal or decreased MPV levels are seen in hypoproductive thrombocytopenias. MPV alterations may also be seen in patients with regenerating bone marrow or myeloproliferative disorders. MPV measurements should never be taken, in isolation, as diagnostic of a clinical condition.

Physicians should be aware that platelet counts are less reliable in the thrombocytopenic range and lose linearity between 5,000 and 20,000 platelets/μl. Consequently, manual platelet counts should be performed to correlate with significantly thrombocytopenic measurements. If the clinical laboratory does not perform such confirmations automatically, the clinician must order them.

The most common reason for an erroneous platelet count is inadequate anticoagulation of the patient's blood specimen leading to partial clotting and aggregation of platelets producing a falsely low count. Another cause for a falsely low platelet count is platelet clumping resulting from EDTA anticoagulation that exposes platelet epitopes recognized by patient antibodies in some individuals. Platelet counts in heparinized blood or fingerstick specimens are normal in these patients.

Finally, most hematologists recommend microscopic examination of the peripheral blood platelet morphology (see later discussion) in patients with abnormally high or low platelet counts. This approach can help distinguish, for example, benign reactive thrombocytosis from thrombocytosis secondary to a myeloproliferative disorder.

EXAMINATION OF THE PERIPHERAL BLOOD SMEAR

The skillful microscopic examination of the peripheral blood smear is not the exclusive domain of the hematologist. Primary care physicians can become proficient in the clinical evaluation of peripheral blood cell morphology. In the contemporary practice of medicine, increased use of centralized laboratory facilities is making it more difficult for the office physician to examine peripheral blood smears. For this reason, it is essential for primary care physicians to become proficient at extracting the maximum information from automated blood count reports (see earlier discussion). Fortunately, it is usually convenient to obtain and examine peripheral blood smears in the hospital setting, while doing so in the outpatient clinic may be problematic. Nevertheless, it is important for clinicians to identify procedures to allow them to examine peripheral blood cell morphology in outpatients with abnormal blood cell counts without an obvious explanation (like iron deficiency). A hematologist should be consulted to assist when (1) the clinician is unsure of the morphology he or she is examining, (2) for logistic reasons the clinician is unable to evaluate the smear of a patient with an unexplained blood cell abnormality, or (3) the clinician identifies morphologic abnormalities that require the specialized diagnostic or therapeutic assistance of a subspecialist.

Erythrocytes

While the MCV and RDW may provide diagnostic hints in some patients, automated laboratory equipment cannot recognize morphologic abnormalities such as spherocytes, elliptocytes, target cells, schistocytes, teardrop cells, acanthocytes, macroovalocytes, sickle cells, polychromasia, malaria parasites, and erythrocyte inclusions (Color Plate IV-4). Clinicians can and should learn to recognize gross abnormalities of erythrocytes to aid in the diagnosis of anemia. Erythrocyte morphology is best appreciated between the feather edge of the blood smear on the microscope slide and the thick portion of the smear where red cells overlap.

Young erythrocytes, reticulocytes, retain RNA that is lost as these cells mature into normal discocytes. Stains such as new methylene blue reveal the cellular RNA and are useful in manually enumerating the percentage of erythrocytes that are reticulocytes. The application of flow cytometry to the measurement of reticulocytes (see later discussion) produces a more accurate count. The most useful clinical values are the reticulocyte index, which normalizes the reticulocyte percentage to the hemoglobin, and the absolute reticulocyte count. These values most reliably represent the erythroid activity of the bone marrow. Reticulocytosis is observed in recovery from bone marrow suppression due to toxic, therapeutic, nutritional, infectious, or idiopathic etiology. Reticulocytosis is also characteristic of physiologic compensation for blood loss or hemolysis. Hypoproductive anemias are generally associated with a low absolute reticulocyte count.

Heinz bodies are formed by denatured hemoglobin that is most often produced in oxidant-mediated hemolysis or in patients with unstable hemoglobins. Heinz bodies are detected microscopically in erythrocytes stained with crystal violet (Color Plate IV-4, P). They cannot be visualized on standard blood smears, so the clinician must order the Heinz body preparation in patients suspected to have oxidant hemolysis. Heinz bodies can be transient in patients with intermittent hemolysis, so their absence does not rule out oxidant hemolysis.

Special preparation of the peripheral blood smear is also helpful in the detection of intracellular erythrocyte parasites such as malaria species and *Babesia microti*. The thick film blood smear is more sensitive than standard techniques. The clinician should enlist the aid of an experienced observer to distinguish among the various different malaria parasites.

Leukocytes

There are numerous clinical conditions with characteristic peripheral blood leukocyte morphology (Color Plate IV-5 and IV-6). Many of these are benign conditions, such as leukemoid reactions and megaloblastic anemias. Many clinical disorders with abnormal leukocytes are neoplastic, such as acute and chronic leukemias, myelodysplastic syndromes, myeloproliferative disorders, and lymphomas with circulating cells. Some, such as large granular lymphocytosis and hypereosinophilic syndrome, may tread on either side of the line between reactive and neoplastic processes. An example of one common clinical scenario in which examination of the peripheral smear by a primary care physician frequently plays an important role: in assessing a patient with neutrophilia or neutropenia, increased band forms, metamyelocytes, toxic granulations, Döhle bodies, and/or neutrophil vacuolization suggest an infectious or septic etiology that may even be clinically occult.

Primary care physicians must learn to recognize abnormal cells and enlist the assistance of a hematologist to evaluate patients in whom they are identified. The application of cytochemistry, enzyme histochemistry, and immunohistochemistry using an ever-expanding repertoire of antibody reagents to peripheral blood leukocytes allows the hematologist and hematopathologist to characterize abnormal cell populations with great precision.

Platelets

Examination of platelet morphology is often helpful in differentiating reactive thrombocytosis from myeloproliferative disorders such as essential thrombocythemia (ET). In ET, platelets may be hypogranular and may vary considerably in size and shape. Circulating megakaryocyte fragments may also be seen in ET. In reactive thrombocytosis, platelets are typically bland in appearance. Platelet morphology is not usually helpful in the evaluation of patients with thrombocytopenia, except to exclude artifactual causes such as platelet clumping.

EXAMINATION OF THE BONE MARROW
Clinical Indications

Several clinical situations necessitate the evaluation of bone marrow cellular morphology, iron stores, or cytogenetics. Flow cytometry or microbiologic culture may also be helpful (Box 72-2). Culture of hematopoietic progenitor cells is a research tool and is not available in most clinical laboratories. In adults, bone marrow specimens are usually obtained under local anesthesia from the the posterior superior iliac spine of the pelvis. Physicians should be aware of factors, such as prior pelvic irradiation, that require selection of another site for biopsy. In most centers, both bone marrow aspirate and core biopsy specimens are taken in all cases where both are obtainable. Each provides complementary information (Box 72-3). Both aspirate and biopsy may be procured using a Jamshidi needle, preferably from separate sites in the bone.

In advance of performing bone marrow aspirate and biopsy procedures, careful consideration must be given to the specimens to be

---

> **BOX 72-2**
> ### Clinical indications for bone marrow aspirate and biopsy
>
> Evaluation of unexplained peripheral blood cytopenias
> Evaluation of excessive peripheral blood cell counts
> Evaluation of suspicious cells in the peripheral blood
> Evaluation of paraproteinemia
> Staging of patients with lymphoma or certain cancers
> Evaluation of patient iron stores when other tests are ambiguous
> To obtain cells for cytogenetic, flow cytometry, or immunocyto-
>   chemistry studies in patients with lymphoid or myeloid neoplasms
> Evaluation of patients with fever of unknown origin
> Microbiologic culture

> **BOX 72-3**
> ### Diagnostically useful information from bone marrow aspirate and biopsy
>
> **Aspirate**
> Hematopoietic precursor cell morphology and relative abundance
> Hematopoietic neoplasm morphology
> Cytochemistry, immunocytochemistry, flow cytometry, and cytoge-
>   netic analysis of bone marrow cells
> Iron stores
> Some metastatic carcinomas
> Microbiologic culture and stains
>
> **Biopsy**
> Bone marrow cellularity or aplasia
> Granulomatous disease
> Leukemic infiltration, especially with dry marrow aspirate (including
>   touch preparation of biopsy specimen)
> Lymphoma infiltration, especially when patchy or paratrabecular
> Cytochemistry and immunocytochemistry, correlated with bone mar-
>   row architecture
> Metastatic carcinoma
> Myelofibrosis
> Vasculitis
> Amyloidosis
> Platelet microthrombi
> Metabolic bone disease

---

collected. This is because the handling of flow cytometry, cytogenetics, microbiologic culture, bone marrow aspirate, core biopsy, and touch preparation specimens is different and may require extra steps in the procedure and extra equipment at the bedside.

It is often unnecessary to examine a bone marrow specimen when an explanation for a peripheral blood abnormality is obtained using noninvasive tests. Examples of such situations include clear-cut iron deficiency anemia, folate deficiency, pernicious anemia, Gaucher's disease, hairy cell leukemia, chronic myelogenous leukemia, chronic lymphocytic leukemia, and most forms of hemolytic anemia.

Analysis of Bone Marrow Cells

Bone Marrow Aspirate Smears. Bone marrow cell morphology is best appreciated on stained smears of bone marrow aspirate specimens. Regardless of the technique used to prepare bone marrow aspirate smears (squash preparations of bone marrow particles, direct smears made from anticoagulated aspirates, or smears of cellular concentrates from bone marrow aspirates), the information obtained is largely the same. The observer systematically examines the cells in all three hematopoietic lineages: erythroid, myeloid, and megakaryocytic (Color Plates IV-1 and IV-3). The relative abundance of hematopoietic precursor cells in each lineage is determined. Tools to quantify these relationships are the bone marrow cell differential count and the myeloid:erythroid ratio. Within each hematopoietic lineage, the relative abundance of immature and mature precursors is analyzed. Abnormal cellular forms of hematopoietic precursor cells are noted, for example, megaloblastic precursors (Color Plate IV-7), myeloblasts containing Auer rods (Color Plate IV-6), or dysplastic erythroblasts. Infiltration of the bone marrow by lympho plasmacytic elements can signify a reactive, inflammatory process or a neoplastic disorder such as lymphoma or multiple myeloma (Color Plate IV-8). Occasionally, metastatic carcinoma cells are visualized on bone marrow aspirate specimens.

When leukemic cells are identified on bone marrow aspirate smears, special stains are used to explore the cytochemistry and enzyme histochemistry of the abnormal cell population. These are often used to distinguish acute myelogenous from acute lymphoblastic leukemias or to subtype myelogenous leukemias. The application of immunocytochemistry and flow cytometry to bone marrow aspirate specimens is very useful in the analysis of lymphoid neoplasms and myeloid leukemias (see later discussion). Cytogenetic analysis of bone marrow aspirate cells has proven to be clinically relevant in myeloid and lymphoid leukemias, lymphomas, myelodysplastic, syndromes, and, occasionally, myeloproliferative disorders. In the future, the application of new cytogenetic methods such as fluorescent in situ hybridization is likely to become routine.

Iron stains are routinely performed on bone marrow aspirate specimens using, for example, Prussian blue dye (Color Plate IV-9). This technique can aid the physician in assessing total body iron stores. This is especially useful in patients with conflicting laboratory data concerning iron status and in whom definitive knowledge of iron stores would affect treatment decisions. In addition, cellular iron accumulation can assume characteristic patterns of diagnostic importance. For example, the presence of ringed sideroblasts among a patient's erythroid precursors can suggest the diagnosis of primary or secondary sideroblastic anemia (Color Plate IV-9).

Some sense of the bone marrow cellularity is gleaned from analysis of aspirates, but the observer must always reserve judgment with respect to cellularity until the biopsy is examined. For example, a patient with a fibrotic myeloproliferative syndrome or hairy cell leukemia may have a scant number of aspirable cells but significant cellularity on bone marrow biopsy sections.

Bone Marrow Biopsy Sections. Examination of stained bone marrow biopsy sections is possible after specimens undergo a decalcification step in the laboratory. The time required for decalcification means that biopsy sections are not usually available until 2 days after the aspirate has been examined. In spite of this fact, optimal diagnosis requires that both specimens be examined coordinately. This is because unique information concerning bone marrow architecture and cellularity are gleaned from the biopsy specimen. There are circumstances, however, in which treatment decisions must be made based on the aspirate alone. In autoimmune thrombocytopenic purpura and acute leukemia, for example, this is frequently the case and adverse consequences are rare. However, in some situations such as non-Hodgkin's lymphoma and aplastic anemia, the information obtained from the aspirate may be misleading or wrong. This is because patchy pathologic processes such as metastatic cancer, lymphoma, or infections may elude sampling by aspiration and are, therefore, best appreciated on biopsy. For this reason, bone marrow biopsies performed to stage lymphomas are typically bilateral, to further increase the chance of sampling diseased areas. Finally, non-Hodgkin's lymphoma may exhibit a paratrabecular distribution that is only visible upon examination of bone marrow biopsy sections.

Special stains for iron, reticulin, myeloperoxidase, lysozyme, chymotrypsin, and terminal deoxynucleotidyl transferase (TdT) may also be performed on bone marrow biopsy sections. Immunohistochemistry studies can delineate immunoglobulin heavy chain class, B-lymphocyte markers, T-lymphocyte markers, and monocyte markers. Due to the handling of core biopsy specimens, including decalcification, the repertoire of special stains and immunohistochemistry studies that can be reliably performed is considerably less than for aspirated cells or sections of bone marrow clots. As reagents improve, the list of available tests is likely to lengthen.

ANALYSIS OF PERIPHERAL BLOOD AND BONE MARROW CELLS BY FLOW CYTOMETRY AND IMMUNOHISTOCHEMISTRY

In recent years, analysis of blood and bone marrow cells using the complementary techniques of flow cytometry and immunohistochemistry has become an essential clinical tool. There is an extremely wide range of applications for these methods, from detection of reticulocytes to platelet-associated antibodies to cell surface phenotyping in leukemia. As immunologic reagents evolve and technology improves, the utility of these approaches will continue to expand for several years. While the interpretation of complex immunophenotyping data is outside the scope of primary care practice, a familiarity with the most common applications of these techniques is essential for the generalist.

Flow Cytometry

Methodology. At the simplest level, a flow cytometer is an instrument that delivers single cells in a fluid medium into a reading system that measures their light scatter and/or fluorescence properties. This is accomplished by passing individual cells through a focused excitation beam that is used to probe the properties of interest. If the cell is labeled with a fluorescent dye, which may or may not be attached to a specific monoclonal antibody, the cell will emit fluorescent light. If the cell is unlabeled, the light is scattered by the cell in a forward direction or perpendicular to the beam (side scatter). Fluorescent and/or nonfluorescent light of various wave lengths is measured for each cell.

Applications
Analysis of erythrocytes. Flow cytometry has been applied to the clinical analysis of erythrocytes in various ways. For example, the measurement of maternal-fetal hemorrhage, direct Coombs' autoantibodies, glucose-6-phosphate dehydrogenase, and certain hemoglobinopathies are readily accomplished using this approach. One of the most widely applied techniques is the measurement of reticulocytes using fluorescent dyes that associate with erythrocyte RNA. This method is superior to manual reticulocyte counting and is standard in many laboratories. Further information that may be valuable in the clinical assessment of anemia includes the reticulocyte maturity index. This index measures the proportion of reticulocytes that are younger and therefore have more RNA than more mature reticulocytes. True hypoproductive anemias have both a low absolute reticulocyte count and a low maturity index.

Antiplatelet antibodies. The most widely applied use of flow cytometry in the clinical evaluation of peripheral blood platelets is the measurement of platelet-associated immunoglobulin by labeling them with fluorescent antibodies. A variety of laboratory techniques have been developed that measure platelet-associated antibodies. There are disparate opinions about the clinical usefulness of the test, but the flow cytometry–based technique is at least as good as the others and may be superior in some ways. Some investigators have reported excellent sensitivity and specificity data in the differentiation of immune and nonimmune thrombocytopenia by this method.

Lymphoid clonality. Perhaps the most important clinical question asked when a lymphocytic infiltration is detected in peripheral blood or bone marrow concerns whether the cells stem from a polyclonal or monoclonal proliferation. A common application of clinical flow cytometry and immunocytochemistry (see later discussion) is to determine whether populations of B-lymphocytes are monoclonal. This procedure takes advantage of the fact that polyclonal surface immunoglobulins normally have a mixture of κ and λ immunoglobulin light chains. In contrast, monoclonal B-cell populations express a single light chain. These can be readily differentiated using fluorescent dye–labeled antibodies specific for light chain class.

Immunophenotyping of lymphoid neoplasms. One of the major achievements of modern immunobiology and hematopathology is the use of immunophenotyping to dissect the complex lymphocyte subpopulations that comprise the immune system. This has been made possible by an expanding wealth of antibody reagents that recognize cell surface antigens that define developmental stages and pathways of lymphoid cell development. The application of these methods to lymphoid neoplasms gives the clinician unprecedented detail in understanding the cellular origin of lymphoid leukemias and lymphomas.

Clinical reagents are available that distinguish B- from T-lymphocytes and mark different stages of development in each lineage. Certain neoplasms have characteristic surface markers. For example, in chronic lymphocytic leukemia the monoclonal B-cells express the CD5 antigen, otherwise unusual in B-cells. Similarly, non-Hodgkin's lymphomas, acute and chronic lymphoid leukemias, diverse T-cell neoplasms, plasmacytoid neoplasms, and natural killer cell proliferations can all be rigorously differentiated and subdivided based on immunophenotype.

Myeloid leukemias. The clinical application of flow cytometry to myeloid leukemias is rapidly expanding. Markers are available that mark, for example, early hematopoietic progenitors, monocytoid lineage cells, or erythroid lineage cells. Flow studies, together with immunocytochemistry, cytochemistry, and enzyme histochemistry, often help to differentiate acute lymphoblastic from acute myelocyte leukemias in which morphology is unhelpful. Specific subtypes of myeloid leukemia can also be differentiated by this technique.

Ploidy analysis. The DNA content of neoplastic cells can be measured by flow cytometry using fluorescent dyes that are avid for DNA. Genetic aneuploidy is readily assessed by this method. In addition, information concerning the cell cycle is also obtained, such as the fraction of cells in S phase. The percent of cells in S phase correlates, for example, with lymphoma grade by histology. Aneuploidy is often associated with certain types of leukemia and lymphoma and may affect disease prognosis.

Immunocytochemistry

The large and expanding repertoire of antibody reagents that is used to immunophenotype cells by flow cytometry is also available for immunocytochemical staining of peripheral blood and bone marrow cells. Immunofluorescence methods or immunoenzyme techniques are used to visualize bound antibodies by microscopy. The information obtained using this approach is complementary to flow cytometry data. One difference is that counterstaining techniques allow the observer to determine the morphology of the cell reacting with antibody. Small immunoreactive cell populations can be detected that might otherwise be missed in analysis of the entire bone marrow or blood specimen. These methods are most applicable to peripheral blood and bone marrow aspirate specimens. An increasing number of reagents are becoming useful in the study of bone marrow biopsy sections (see earlier discussion).

BIBLIOGRAPHY

Bauer KD, Duque RE, Shankey TV, editors: *Clinical flow cytometry,* Baltimore, 1993, Williams & Wilkins.

Hayhoe FGJ, Quaglino D: *Haematological cytochemistry,* ed 3, Edinburgh, 1994, Churchill Livingstone.

Hoffbrand VA, Pettit JE: *Color atlas of clinical hematology,* ed 2, London, 1994, Mosby-Wolfe.

CHAPTER

73 Molecular Diagnostics

Harold R. Schumacher

Advances in molecular biology hold promise to reveal the molecular basis of many human diseases. The tools of recombinant DNA technology are now being utilized in virtually every subspecialty of diagnostic medicine and pathology, including:

1. Sequencing of genes involved in human diseases, for example, cystic fibrosis, Duchenne's muscular dystrophy, and chronic myelogenous leukemia.

2. Antenatal and prenatal diagnosis of inherited disease.
3. Diagnosis and categorization of neoplastic disease with prognostic and therapeutic monitoring of the cancer patient.
4. Evaluation for minimal residual disease in leukemia.
5. Ascertainment of genetic susceptibility and predisposition to diseases such as atherosclerosis and diabetes.
6. Diagnosis of infectious diseases.
7. Evaluation of drug sensitivity and drug resistance in neoplastic and infectious disease.
8. Determination of concordance and identity in transplantation, paternity testing, and forensic medicine.

Undoubtedly, molecular diagnostics are likely to be involved in every aspect of patient management, from initial diagnosis, to prognosis, to monitoring therapeutic responses. Broad application of these techniques will result from their relatively inexpensive cost coupled with high speed, specificity, and sensitivity. Even though the economics and ethics of some molecular tests will spark intensive discussion, recombinant DNA technologies will play an ever-increasing role in disease diagnosis and will be an essential tool for the internist and hematologist to utilize effectively in diagnosis and treatment and for the pathologist to assimilate into the clinical laboratory. Pertinent to an understanding of molecular diagnostics in oncology is an understanding of the mechanisms of oncogenesis that are depicted in Fig. 73-1. Note that three general mechanisms are involved in oncogenesis: (1) fusion of protooncogenes to form oncogenes, (2) mutation of protooncogenes, and (3) loss of tumor-suppressing ability. Molecular diagnostics exploits these defects to enable clinicians to make diagnostic, prognostic, and therapeutic decisions.

CLONALITY AND MALIGNANCY

It is essential to understand the concept of clonality in order to comprehend the tests performed to analyze aberrant DNA that is expressed by malignant cells. A clone is a large number of identical cells or molecules derived from a single ancestor. Clonal cells have phenotypic and growth characteristics identical to those of the original precursor cell. Molecules derived from such clonal cells demonstrate identical structure. Normal T-lymphocytes are polyclonal proliferations that have their own unique structural and functional characteristics. Since such cells produce myriads of different molecules, as discussed in Chapter 174, none are in high enough concentration to be detected by molecular techniques. However, clonal proliferation of T-cells does give rise to large numbers of structurally identical cells, which can be detected by molecular techniques.

Clonality as a concept has been utilized for a long time. Monoclonal Ig expression has been used for years as the definitive marker for B-cell proliferations such as multiple myeloma, Waldenstrom's macroglobulinemia, chronic lymphocytic leukemia, hairy cell leukemia, and non-Hodgkin's lymphoma. Also cytogenetics has been employed for many years to analyze karyotypes and demonstrate clonality.

It is most important to realize that many clinically benign disorders may show clonality. These include a wide variety of benign lymphoproliferations, for example, Castleman's disease, AIDS, angioimmunoblastic lymphadenopathy with dysproteinemia, Sjögren's disease, and a large group of dermatologic disorders associated with lymphocytic infiltrates. For example, Staib and Sterry using the polymerase chain reaction (PCR) demonstrated a monoclonal lymphoid population in 59 out of 66 (89%) cases of pleomorphic cutaneous lymphoma; in 60 out of 78 (77%) patients with mycosis fungoides, in 11 out of 22 (50%) cases of parapsoriasis en plaques, in 5 out of 35 (14%) cases of pseudolymphoma, in 6 out of 15 (40%) patients with lymphomatoid papulosis, and in none of 64 patients with inflammatory skin diseases. Although higher percentages of patients with malignant disease showed clonality, a significant number of patients with clinically benign disorders also had clonal populations of cells.

MOLECULAR DIAGNOSIS: ANALYSIS OF DNA

Currently, molecular tools such as Southern blot hybridization, polymerase chain reaction (PCR), fluorescence in situ hybridization (FISH), and restriction fragment length polymorphisms (RFLP) are

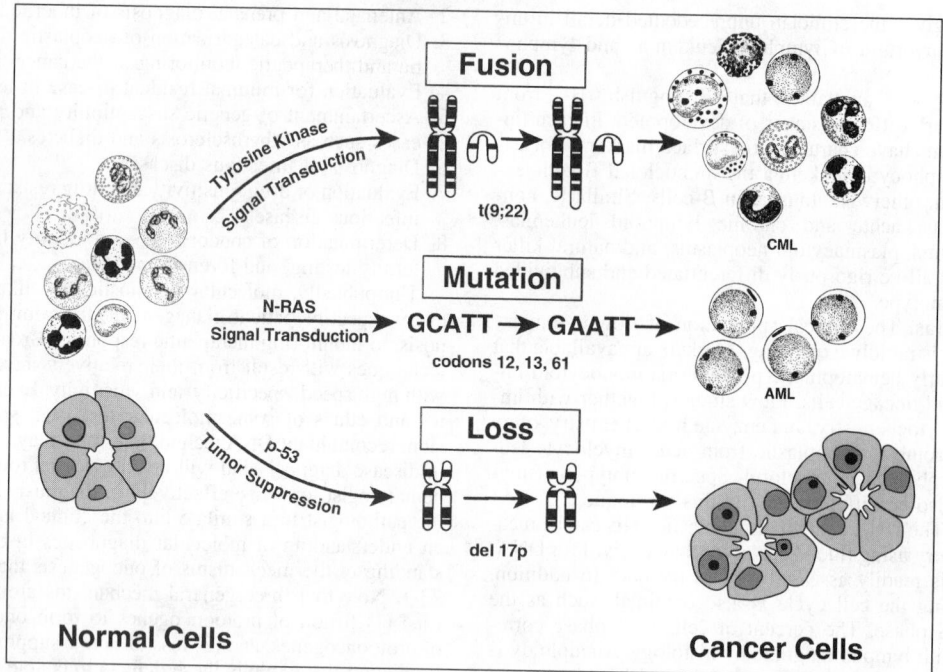

FIGURE 73-1   Mechanisms of oncogenesis showing normal protooncogenes that are altered by fusion, mutation, and loss. *Top,* t(9;22) translocation (C-ABL to BCR) in chronic myelogenous leukemia (CML). *Center,* Mutation in the N-RAS gene in acute myelogenous leukemia. *Bottom,* Loss of the p-53 tumor supressor gene in colon cancer. Tumor supressor genes may also be disrupted by rearrangements and mutations. Usually more than one event is necessary to produce cancer. Left arrows indicate type of gene involved *(above)* and function of the gene product *(below).*

used to detect clonality in malignant hematopoietic cells. RFLP represents a type of variation of DNA sequence between individuals; usually a point mutation in the DNA sequence that creates or abolishes a restriction enzyme recognition site, which results in a unique identifying DNA fragment (see later discussion).

Southern Blot Analysis

In Southern blot analysis, DNA from cells is purified and cut with various restriction enzymes (e.g., Eco RI, Hind III Bam HI, Bg1 II) that cleave DNA at very precise sites. The fragments, whose lengths are measured in kilobase (kb) pairs, are separated by agarose gel electrophoresis. Following electrophoresis, the separated fragments are transferred to nitrocellulose paper, where they are identified by hybridization to radio-labeled DNA probes (Fig. 73-2). The test is based on the principle that as a gene undergoes rearrangement, the relative position of restriction sites within the region of the rearrangement is affected. Consequently, a probe to the rearranged portion of the gene will detect a restriction fragment in a nongermline position if a sufficient number of cells (1% to 5% of the total) share the same rearrangement. Such a high percentage of genetically identical cells implies clonality. If lymphoid malignancies are being studied, the pattern of gene rearrangements may indicate either T- or B-cell lineage. Usually two sets of Southern blots are performed, one for immunoglobulin (Ig) gene rearrangement and the other for T-cell receptor (TCR) rearrangement. Details about rearrangements of normal Ig and TCR genes are presented in Chapters 173 and 174.

Although gene rearrangement analysis was thought initially to be the court of final appeal to identify clonal populations and the specific lineages of lymphoid cells, unfortunately this has not been the case. B-cells have demonstrated TCR rearrangements typical of T-cells; T-cells have shown IgH and IgL gene rearrangements typical of B-cells, and myeloid leukemias can occasionally have IgH and IgL gene rearrangements typical of lymphoid cells. In addition, RFLPs may be responsible for bands that appear to migrate like clonally rearranged DNA. Additional problems include false positives if the gene has only a few variable regions (TCR gamma gene) and false nega-

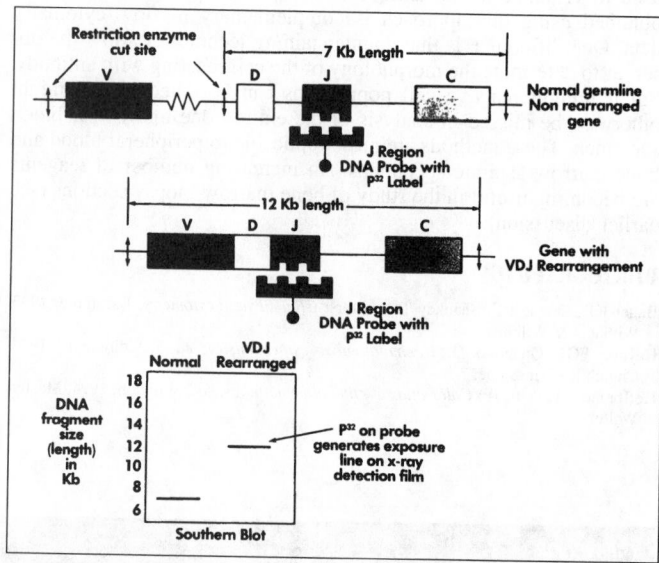

FIGURE 73-2   Southern blot analysis for gene rearrangement in T- and B-cells. Cellular DNA from blood specimens is cut with the appropriate restriction enzymes, and the size (length) of the fragments is analyzed by using a Southern blot format. Any deviation of fragment length, either larger or smaller from the germline, indicates that the genes are rearranged. The vertical arrows (↕) indicate restriction enzyme cut sites.

From Love JD et al: DNA probes to characterize leukemia and lymphoma cells, *Am Clin Prod Rev* 4:16, 1985.

tives because of lack of sensitivity, comigration, technical errors, deletion of both alleles, and antigen receptor rearrangements occurring over a long distance (TCR alpha gene). A practical approach to the interpretation of Southern blots to detect gene rearrangements in lymphoid cells is outlined in Box 73-1.

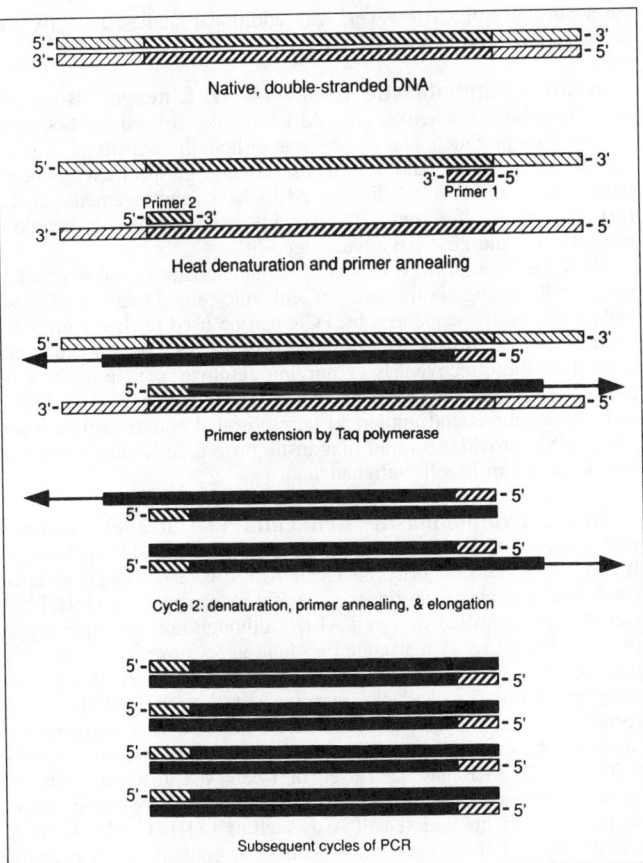

FIGURE 73-3 PCR demonstrating amplification of DNA sequence.
From Bunn FH: Molecular genetics: clinical and research use of polymerase chain reaction. In: *Hematology*, Education Program, Boston, 1990, American Society of Hematology.

BOX 73-1

Guidelines for the interpretation of Southern blots to detect gene rearrangements in lymphoid cells

DNA in germline configuration and no novel bands present
  Nonlymphoid tissue including nonlymphoid neoplasms
  Polyclonal lymphoid tissue
  Monoclonal cells in a quantity below limits of detection (1% to 5%)
DNA in germline and nongermline configuration
  Monoclonal lymphoid tissue mixed with nonlymphoid or reactive lymphoid tissue
  Homogeneous monoclonal tissue present with one germline and one rearranged allele
  Combinations of above two situations
Only novel bands present: No germline
  Homogeneous population of monoclonal lymphoid cells

Polymerase Chain Reaction (PCR)

The amount of genomic DNA required for the detection of single copy genes by typical Southern blot analysis is approximately 0.1 to 0.5 μg; therefore, when 10 μg of DNA is analyzed by such a technique, its sensitivity is limited to detecting a clone of cells representing approximately 1% to 5% of the cells in a heterogeneous population. PCR circumvents the problem of detecting small numbers of malignant cells by enzymatically amplifying target DNA sequences prior to electrophoretic analysis. PCR amplification has been utilized to:

(1) detect rare, malignant cells (1 in 100,000) with a particular molecular aberration, such as a mutation or chromosomal aberration, (2) identify infectious organisms, (3) amplify target DNA sequences from human hairs and blood for forensic identification, and (4) amplify target sequences for allele specific oligonucleotide probes, thereby improving Southern blot analysis.

The great paradox of PCR is that the major limitation comes from excess sensitivity. A common universal problem in laboratories performing PCR is the amplification of contaminants, most commonly the products of previous PCR experiments or the residual of plasmids that have been in high abundance in the laboratory and have spread indiscriminately to glassware, pipettors, common reagents, etc. Several measures can be taken to overcome these problems. They include: (1) distribution of all PCR reagents into small aliquots, (2) use of positive displacement pipettes, (3) performing PCR at a site distant from areas of contamination, and (4) meticulous inclusion of controls. The important point is that reliable molecular diagnostics require outstanding laboratory expertise of the highest quality.

PCR has been utilized to great advantage in diagnosing the hemoglobinopathies and hematologic malignancies. Since PCR of DNA does not accurately reflect the number of copies of the segment of interest, some investigators have gone to "nested" retrotranscriptase/polymerase chain reaction (RT-PCR). Such techniques more precisely detect minimal residual disease in hematologic malignancies, especially leukemia. A schematic of the PCR is depicted in Fig. 73-3.

FLUORESCENCE IN SITU HYBRIDIZATION (FISH)
Alpha Satellite DNA

The technologic advance that initially made interphase cytogenetic analysis possible was the development of chromosome-specific probes that could be used to generate strong hybridization signals, often being hybridized to interphase cells affixed to glass slides. These probes were specific to a type of DNA called α-satellite DNA. α-Satellite DNA is unique in three respects: (1) it is present at the (peri) centromeric region of each chromosome, (2) it is specific for each chromosome, and (3) it is present in high copy number. Since high copy numbers are present, fluorescinated avidin or avidin conjugated with a detector enzyme such as alkaline phosphatase can be utilized microscopically to detect a hybridized biotinylated probe.

In a metaphase spread, an α-satellite probe generates a signal that appears at the (peri) centromeric region of each copy of the targeted chromosome (Fig. 73-4). In an interphase cell, the signal, still associated with the targeted chromosome, appears as a distinct signal or spot within the chromatin of the nucleus. FISH has the advantage of: (1) enabling the investigator to evaluate large numbers of cells very rapidly, (2) not requiring special training, and (3) allowing some correlation of cytogenetic findings with morphology.

The cornerstone for application of FISH is that it allows the hematologist/hematopathologist to detect abnormalities in chromosomal number in terminally differentiated cells that are incapable of mitosis, and permits analysis of peripheral blood rather than bone marrow. The technique can be used in flow cytometry, evaluation of archival pathology specimens, and evaluation of previously stained slides.

Whole Chromosome Paint

Besides having probes specifically directed to α-satellite DNA of a specific chromosome, each chromosome has unique repetitive sequences that permit the labeling of the entire chromosome. Whole chromosome paint allows the hematologist/hematopathologist to identify translocations as well as numerical abnormalities in chromosomes. An example utilizing whole chromosome paint is shown in Fig. 73-5.

PRACTICAL APPLICATION TO HEMATOLOGIC DISEASE

Analysis of the DNA and mRNA from patients with hematologic disease has three important functions: (1) to establish clonality of a population of cells, (2) to determine cell lineage, and (3) to detect minimal residual disease.

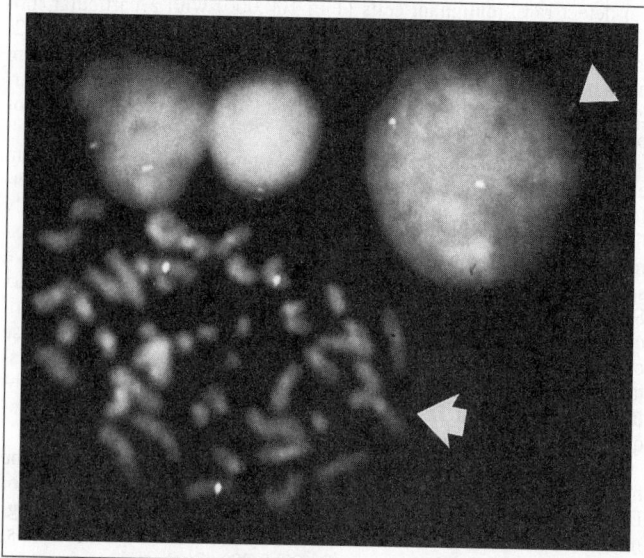

FIGURE 73-4 In situ hybridization of a biotinylated DNA probe to the α-satellite centromeric repeat sequences of chromosome 8. The hybridized probe was detected with fluorescinated avidin. Three signals are noted in some of the interphase cells *(arrow head)* and in the metaphase spread *(arrow)*. Patient has acute myelogenous leukemia FAB M2 (×1000).

Courtesy of Dr Jan C Liang, Department of Laboratory Medicine, Cytogenetics Research, University of Texas, MD Anderson Cancer Center, Houston, Texas.

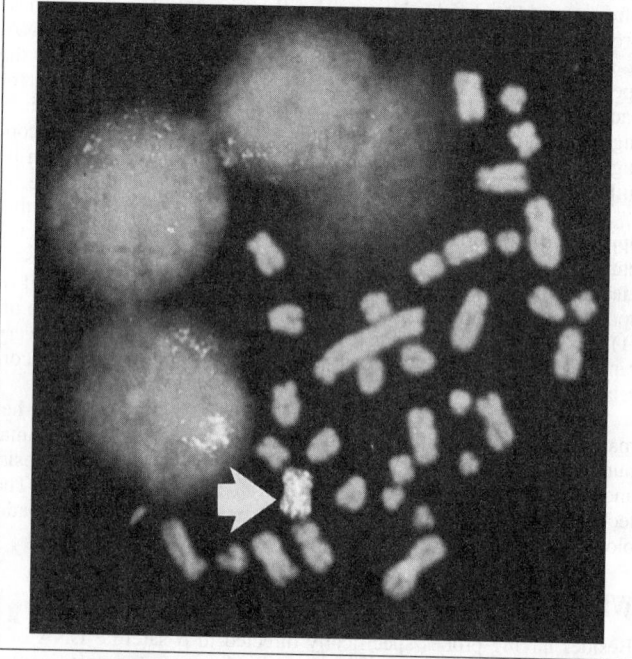

FIGURE 73-5 In situ hybridization using whole chromosome paint to chromosome 7. The patient has monosomy 7, which appears as a single chromosome marker in the metaphase *(arrow)*. The patient has acute myelogenous leukemia FAB M1 (×1000).

Courtesy of Dr Jan C Liang, Department of Laboratory Medicine, Cytogenetics Research, University of Texas, MD Anderson Cancer Center, Houston, Texas.

Acute Leukemia

The analysis of the Ig and TCR genes in acute leukemia has provided a large amount of data concerning the development of both leukemia and lymphoid precursor cells. Initially, such studies were thought to clearly and precisely define clonality and lineage within

the acute leukemias. However, with additional studies the early enthusiasm has been tempered.

Acute Lymphoblastic Leukemia (B-Lineage). B-lineage acute lymphoblastic leukemias (ALLs) as determined by Southern blot analysis provide a classic example of both the sensitivity of gene rearrangement studies and lack of absolute lineage specificity. Ninety-eight percent of all B-cell lineage ALLs have rearrangements of the IgH chain gene; 28% and 17% have Igk rearrangement or deletion, respectively; and 20% have rearranged Igλ.

PCR has been utilized to identify characteristic clonal rearrangements in immunoglobulin genes of leukemic cells. Detection of these leukemia-specific sequences by PCR can be used to detect minimal residual disease in patients who have been treated for leukemia, and to analyze the effectiveness of purging autologous bone marrow of clonal malignant cells. FISH has been used in B-lineage ALL to detect translocations and numerical chromosomal abnormalities. Interphase FISH provides a rapid diagnostic procedure to detect specific translocations in B-cell malignancies.

Acute Lymphoblastic Leukemia (T-Lineage). Southern blot analysis of T-cell ALLs has demonstrated similar findings to B-cell ALLs. The majority of T-cell ALLs have rearrangements of the δ, and β genes. Non–lineage-specific rearrangements (IgH 14%) can also be identified in T-cell ALLs, although not as frequently as in B-lineage ALLs. A rearranged L chain gene, however, is virtually diagnostic of a B-cell rather than a T-cell process. A small subset of early prethymic T-cells lacks rearrangements of any of the T-cell receptor genes. They characteristically express a very early immunophenotype comprising CD7, cytoplasmic CD3, and occasionally CD5 or CD2. PCR has been used in T-cell ALL to detect minimal residual disease. FISH has been used to detect cytogenetic abnormalities in patients with T-cell ALL such as t (1;14) and trisomy 8. Morphology of the bone marrow cells that contain the cytogenetic alterations can be studied by concomitant staining with May-Grunwald-Giemsa.

Acute Myelogenous Leukemia. The reported frequency of gene rearrangements in acute myelogenous leukemia (AML) varies widely. Approximately 2% of patients with AML have rearrangement of Igk, supposedly a specific B-cell lineage marker. PCR has been used to advantage in a number of acute myelogenous leukemias to detect minimal residual disease and to predict outcome. The t(8;21)(q22;q22) translocation is a recurring chromosomal abnormality observed in 20% to 40% of AML-FAB M2 patients. The translocation produces a new hybrid gene, AML1-ETO, which produces a fusion transcript. This transcript can be detected by RT-PCR. Interestingly, even patients in long-term remission may have residual cells (presumably malignant) expressing the AML1-ETO transcripts with polyclonal bone marrow reconstitution.

Acute promyelocytic leukemia, FAB M3, has a t(15;17) (q22;q12) translocation in most if not all patients. RT-PCR can be used to detect the fusion PML-RARA transcript and the reciprocal RARA-PML transcript. Contrary to FAB M2 above, remission is marked by undetectable fusion transcripts. However, in hyperleukocytic patients, PCR negativity does not seem to predict long-term remission. Hematologic relapse was preceded by PCR positivity in the bone marrow by 3 months.

FISH has been used in AML to circumvent the need for metaphase preparations and can detect numeric chromosomal abnormalities, which occur with some frequency in AML. Residual leukemic cells with chromosomal abnormalities can be detected by FISH more sensitively than residual blasts can be detected by routine stains of marrow. Whether treatment should be modified when such cells are detected by FISH is not clear.

Chronic Leukemia

Chronic Myelogenous Leukemia. Chronic myelogenous leukemia (CML) is associated with a specific chromosomal abnormality t(9;22) (q34;q11), which results in a shortened chromosome 22, termed the Philadelphia chromosome Ph[1]. The Ph[1] abnormality is the result of the translocation of the c-ABL protooncogene from chromosome 9 onto chromosome 22. The chromosomal break usually oc-

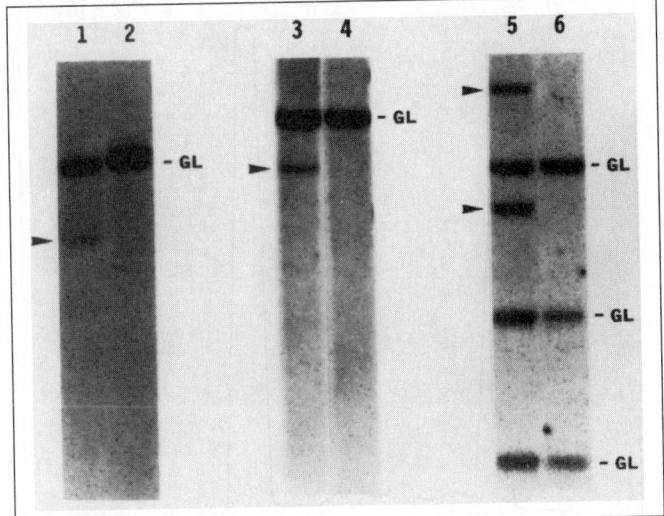

FIGURE 73-6 Southern blot analysis of clonal Ig gene rearrangements and BCR-ABL translocation in a case of CML in lymphoid blast crisis. Patient DNA is present in lanes 1, 3, and 5; control DNA is present in lanes 2, 4, and 6. Lanes 1 and 3 show clonal rearrangements of the IgH and κ-IgL genes, respectively. Lane 5 demonstrates a reciprocal translocation of the bcr of the BCR gene and the abl fragment of the ABL gene. Germline positions of the genes are designated *GL*, and clonal rearrangements are indicated by arrows.

From Schumacher HR, Cotelingam JD: Gene rearrangement and polymerase chain reaction. In: *Chronic leukemia: approach to diagnosis*, New York, 1993, Igaku-Shoin.

curs within a limited 5.8-kb region of the break point cluster region (BCR) gene, designated the break point cluster region (bcr). The well-defined area of the bcr locus permits detection of this translocation by Southern blot analysis. The translocation can be detected in most cases by screening digests of DNA from hematopoietic cells with the universal bcr probe. Since karyotypic analysis will not detect a Ph[1] chromosome in 5% of patients with clinical CML, Southern blot analysis to detect a BCR-ABL rearrangement can be utilized to advantage. About half of these Ph[1]-negative patients will demonstrate a BCR-ABL rearrangement in the DNA from leukemic cells. Such an abnormal fusion of the c-ABL and BCR genes results in the production of a fusion p210 protein with tyrosine kinase activity believed to be responsible for this disease at the molecular level. Even though the turnaround time for bcr analysis by Southern blot or PCR may be slightly longer than karyotypic analysis, the molecular techniques can detect bcr-positive, Ph[1]-negative patients with CML and determine the breakpoint site that may have prognostic significance. A Southern blot analysis showing a BCR-ABL rearrangement in a CML patient is depicted in Fig. 73-6.

PCR has been utilized primarily to detect minimal residual disease in CML patients following bone marrow transplant. However, the data have been difficult to interpret. The persistence of positive results of PCR in CML in a high number of patients in remission for over 6 months after bone marrow transplant has not been predictive of imminent relapse. Complete eradication of the leukemic clone may not be a necessary prerequisite for long-term remission or cure. However, an increase in the number of cells containing the translocation over time, as determined by serial quantitative PCR, may prove useful in predicting relapse.

Chronic Lymphocytic Leukemia. Chronic lymphocytic leukemia (CLL) is the most frequent leukemia in Western countries and is usually easy to recognize morphologically and clinically. With Southern blot analysis, CLL will almost uniformly have rearrangements of IgH and IgL chain genes, which would be expected for a mature B-cell malignancy. Occasionally (<10%) TCR β-chain rearrangements have been found in B-CLL. PCR amplification of IgH gene V-D-J junctional variability (IgH PCR) is increasingly replacing genomic Southern blot analysis for the detection of clonal lymphoid populations. PCR is more sensitive than dual marker flow cytometry for detection of minimal residual disease, but the significance

of minimal residual disease is not known and does not at present affect choice of therapy.

FISH has been helpful in detecting minimal residual disease in CLL patients since 50% have cytogenetic abnormalities. Specifically, these include trisomy 12, abnormalities of chromosome 13 at band q14, 14q+, and deletions of chromosomes 6 or 11. These karyotypic abnormalities are better detected by FISH than by conventional cytogenetic analysis. Karyotypic evolution, usually associated with disease progression, occurs in 15% to 40% of patients with CLL.

Hairy Cell Leukemia. The cell of origin of hairy cell leukemia (HCL) has remained an enigma for many years. Studies of cell surface markers using monoclonal antibodies and of molecular gene rearrangements using DNA probes have confirmed its B-cell origin. Hairy cells show 100% Ig H, 95% Igk, and 30% Igλ chain gene rearrangements. Only rare cases (5%) have had simultaneous rearrangement of the TCR β gene.

Malignant Lymphoma

Molecular analysis of gene rearrangements has had significant diagnostic impact in the non-Hodgkin's lymphomas. Molecular studies have been utilized to identify clonal proliferations (especially peripheral T-cell lymphoma); analyze organs and tissue for residual disease, postchemotherapy or posttransplantation; confirm lineage of a lymphoproliferation, and evaluate atypical hyperplasias for the presence or absence of a clonal population when routine morphologic or immunologic methods are equivocal.

B-Cell Non-Hodgkin's Lymphoma. Studies of gene rearrangements in B-cell non-Hodgkin's lymphoma have demonstrated 90% to 100% of the cases have Ig H and Ig L chain rearrangements. Although Ig H chain gene rearrangement has not been considered specific for B-cell processes, Ig L chain gene rearrangements have been considered highly specific. Nonetheless, rare cases of T-cell malignancies with kL chain gene rearrangements have been reported. Despite these rare reports, detection of an Ig L chain gene rearrangement is very strong evidence for a monoclonal B-cell process.

PCR has been extensively used to detect the t(14;18) translocation of follicular B-cell lymphoma as a test for minimal residual disease. Application of PCR for detection of these translocations makes use of oligonucleotide primers complimentary to nucleotide sequences lying on either side of the breakpoint at which the two chromosomal fragments are joined. PCR has permitted the detection of residual disease in patients who have been treated for follicular B-cell lymphoma. Interestingly, the t(14;18) translocation may be observed in peripheral blood B-cells of normal individuals. It is possible that B-cells with the t(14;18) translocation are regularly generated in normal individuals, but that only very few cells with the translocation will acquire the additional oncogenic hits necessary to establish the malignant phenotype.

FISH has been used to detect translocation of the BCL-2 gene in B-cell malignancies in both metaphase spreads and in interphase nuclei. It has also been used to detect unique chromosomal abnormalities in a variety of other non-Hodgkin's lymphomas.

T-Cell Non-Hodgkin's Lymphoma. Analysis of gene rearrangements has been useful in studying the T-cell lymphoma subgroup of non-Hodgkin's lymphoma. T-cell lymphoma cannot always be diagnosed on morphologic data alone and is often dependent on additional immunologic and genotypic data. The evaluation of T-cell lymphomas has been made more difficult by lack of a specific clonal marker. Nevertheless, some investigators demonstrated immunophenotypic aberrancy in T-cell lymphomas as indirect evidence of a T-cell malignancy. The ability to demonstrate clonal T-cell receptor rearrangements provides direct laboratory evidence of monoclonality, and useful diagnostic information. Most peripheral T-cell lymphomas exhibit rearrangements of the δ, and β chain genes. The detection of minimal disease in T-cell malignancies is limited by poor sensitivity, and/or complexity.

Hodgkin's Disease. The diagnostic Reed-Sternberg cells and their variants (RS/HV cells), are presumed to be the neoplastic cells of Hodgkin's disease. Immunophenotypic analysis provides strong evidence that the RS/HV cells in nodular lymphocytic predominance HD belong to the B-cell lineage, but controversy continues for the other subtypes.

Southern blot analysis of DNA from lymphoid cells in Hodgkin's disease has been done, but interpretation has been limited by its low sensitivity and inability to determine which cell population gives rise to a clonal band. A limited number of cases with large numbers of RS/HV cells, as well as enriched RS/HV populations, have been studied and the incidence of clonal Ig H rearrangements is high. However, the signal strength is often not proportional to the number of RS/HV cells, suggesting variability of genotype in the cell population.

Individual Reed-Sternberg cells have been isolated from classic Hodgkin's disease of B-cell immunophenotype and characterized with regard to rearranged immunoglobulin variable-region heavy-chain genes. Three patterns emerged when comparing cells from the same patient: identical rearrangements; unrelated and unique rearrangements; and both identical and unrelated rearrangements. Interestingly, half the patients who have been studied have RS cells that are polyclonal cells, whereas the other half are monoclonal or of mixed clonality. Polyclonal HD can present as widespread lymphoma. These kinds of discoveries expand our understanding of the already apparent morphologic and clinical heterogeneity of Hodgkin's disease.

BIBLIOGRAPHY

Biondi A, Rambaldi A: Polymerase chain reaction (PCR) approach for the evaluation of minimal residual disease in acute leukemia, *Stem Cells* 12(4): 394-401, 1994.

Gulley ML, Dent GA, Ross DW: Classification and staging of lymphoma by molecular genetics, *Cancer* 69(6): 1600-1606, 1992.

Hanson CA: Clinical applications of molecular biology in diagnostic hematopathology, *Lab Med* 24: 562, 1993.

Head DR, Downing JR: Pathology and immunology of leukemia, *Curr Opin Oncol* 4(1): 14-23, 1992.

Hollan S: Molecular genetics—new horizons in haematology, *Haematologia* 24(3): 167-188, 1991.

Hughes TP et al: Clinical value of PCR in diagnosis and follow-up of leukemia and lymphoma: report of the third Workshop of the Molecular Biology/BMT study group, *Leukemia* 5(6): 448-451, 1991.

Hummel M et al: Hodgkin's disease with monoclonal and polyclonal populations of Reed-Sternberg cells, *N Engl J Med* 333:901, 1995.

Potter MN et al: Molecular evidence of minimal residual disease after treatment for leukaemia and lymphoma: an updated meeting report and review, *Leukemia* 7(8): 1302-1314, 1993.

Seriu T et al: Improved detection of minimal residual leukemia through modifications of the polymerase chain reaction analyses based on clonospecific T cell receptor junctions, *Leukemia* 9:316, 1995.

Staib G, Sterry W: Use of polymerase chain reaction in the detection of clones in lymphoproliferative diseases of the skin, *Rec Adv Cancer Res* 139:239, 1995.

Westbrook CA: The role of molecular techniques in the clinical management of leukemia: lessons from the Philadelphia chromosome, *Cancer* 70(6): 1695-1700, 1992.

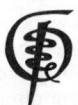

CHAPTER

74 Evaluation of Monoclonal Proteins in Serum and Urine

Robert A. Kyle

Each monoclonal protein (M protein, paraprotein) consists of two heavy-chain polypeptides of the same class and subclass and two light-chain polypeptides of the same type (Chapter 173). The different monoclonal proteins are designated by capital letters that correspond to the class of their heavy chains, which are designated by Greek letters: γ in immunoglobulin G (IgG), α in IgA, μ in IgM, δ in IgD, and ϵ in IgE. Their subclasses are IgG1, IgG2, IgG3, and IgG4, or IgA1 and IgA2, and their light-chain types are κ and λ.

A monoclonal protein is characterized by a narrow peak (resembling a church spire) (Fig. 74-1, *A*) or a localized band on electrophoresis; by a thickened, bowed arc on immunoelectrophoresis; and by a localized band on immunofixation. Many different entities are

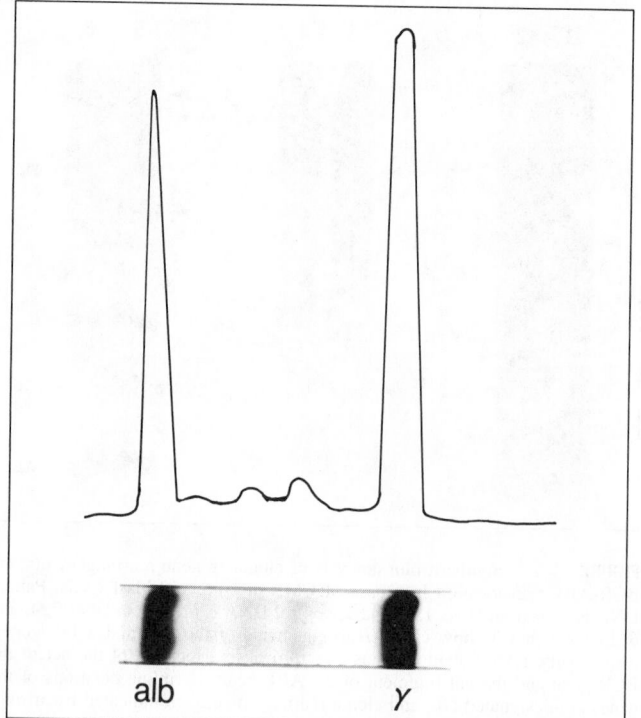

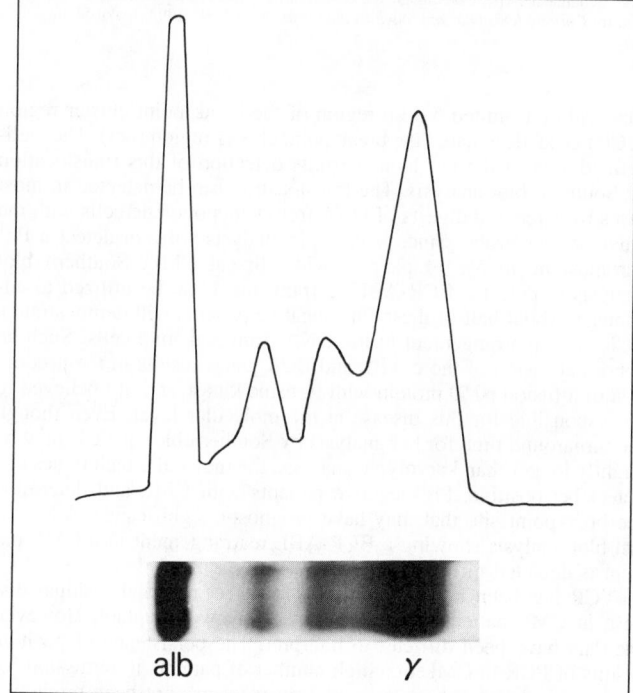

FIGURE 74-1 **A,** *Top,* Monoclonal pattern of serum protein from densitometer tracing after electrophoresis on cellulose acetate (anode on *left*): tall, narrow-based peak of γ mobility; *bottom,* monoclonal pattern from electrophoresis of serum on cellulose acetate (anode on *left*): dense, localized band representing monoclonal protein in γ area. **B,** *Top,* Polyclonal pattern of serum protein from densitometer tracing after electrophoresis on cellulose acetate (anode on *left*): broad-based peak of γ mobility; *bottom,* polyclonal pattern from electrophoresis of serum on cellulose acetate (anode on *left*): γ band is broad.

From Kyle RA, Garton JP: *Semin Oncol* 13:310, 1986.

associated with monoclonal proteins (monoclonal gammopathies) (Box 74-1).

In contrast to a monoclonal protein, a polyclonal protein consists of one or more heavy-chain classes and *both* light-chain types. A polyclonal protein is characterized by a broad peak or band, usually of γ

BOX 74-1
Differential diagnosis of monoclonal gammopathies

I. Malignant monoclonal gammopathies
  A. Multiple myeloma (IgG, IgA, IgD, IgE, and free light chains)
    1. Overt multiple myeloma
    2. Smoldering multiple myeloma
    3. Plasma cell leukemia
    4. Nonsecretory myeloma
    5. Osteosclerotic (POEMS) myeloma
  B. Plasmacytoma
    1. Solitary plasmacytoma of bone
    2. Extramedullary plasmacytoma
  C. Malignant lymphoproliferative diseases
    1. Waldenström's (primary) macroglobulinemia
    2. Malignant lymphoma
  D. Heavy-chain diseases
    1. γ heavy-chain disease
    2. α heavy-chain disease
    3. μ heavy-chain disease
  E. Amyloidosis
    1. Primary
    2. With myeloma
    (Secondary, localized, and familial amyloidoses have no monoclonal protein.)
II. Monoclonal gammopathies of undetermined significance (MGUS)
  A. Benign (IgG, IgA, IgD, IgM, and, rarely, free light chains)
  B. Associated with neoplasms of cell types not known to produce monoclonal proteins
  C. Biclonal gammopathies of undetermined significance (BGUS)

From Kyle RA: In Rose NR, Friedman H, Fahey JL, editors: *Manual of clinical laboratory immunology,* ed 3, Washington, 1986, American Society for Microbiology.

BOX 74-2
Differential diagnosis of polyclonal gammopathies

Connective tissue (autoimmune) diseases
Chronic liver disease, especially chronic active hepatitis
Chronic infections
Lymphoproliferative diseases
Normal

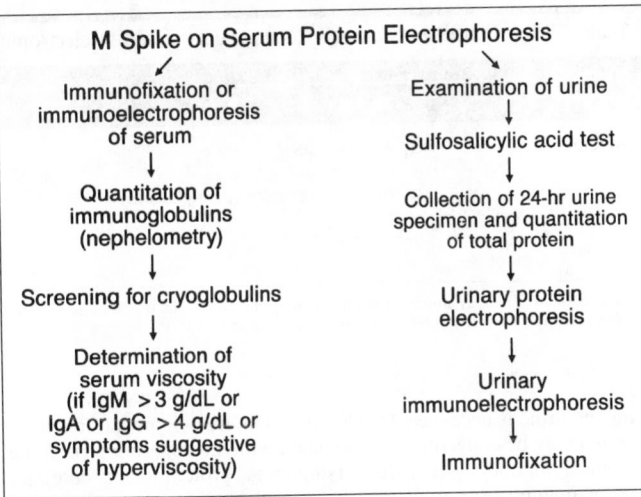

FIGURE 74-2 Sequence of immunologic testing for monoclonal proteins.

confirm the presence of a monoclonal protein and distinguish its immunoglobulin class and light-chain type (Fig. 74-2).

ANALYSIS OF SERUM FOR MONOCLONAL PROTEIN
Electrophoresis

In electrophoresis the basic principle is that particles in solution migrate according to their charge, albumin toward the anode (positive pole) and globulin toward the cathode (negative pole). Serum protein electrophoresis should be done on all patients in whom multiple myeloma, macroglobulinemia, or amyloidosis is known or suspected. The test is also indicated for any patient with unexplained weakness or fatigue, anemia, elevation of the erythrocyte sedimentation rate, back pain, osteoporosis or osteolytic lesions or fractures, immunoglobulin deficiency, hypercalcemia, Bence Jones proteinuria, renal insufficiency, or recurrent infections. Serum protein electrophoresis also should be performed on adults with peripheral neuropathy, carpal tunnel syndrome, refractory congestive heart failure, nephrotic syndrome, orthostatic hypotension, or malabsorption, because a localized band or spike is strongly suggestive of primary amyloidosis.

Several proteins are found in each of the peaks on electrophoresis (Table 74-1). Although immunoglobulins (IgG, IgA, IgM, IgD, IgE) make up the γ component, they are also found in the β-γ and β regions, and IgG extends to the α_2-globulin area. Thus an IgG monoclonal protein may range from the slow γ region to the α_2-globulin region.

Decrease in the α_1-globulin component is usually because of a deficiency of α_1-antitrypsin. The decrease may be associated with recurrent pulmonary infections and chronic obstructive pulmonary disease. A large peak in the α_2-globulin area may represent free hemoglobin–haptoglobin complexes resulting from hemolysis. In this situation the serum is often pink. Large amounts of transferrin in patients with iron deficiency anemia may produce a peak in the β region.

Fibrinogen appears as a discrete band between the β and γ peaks. It may be present because the sample has not clotted completely or the patient has received heparin. Therefore the specimen should be examined for a clot; if there is no clot, either thrombin should be added to the sample or fibrinogen may be detected by immunodiffusion using fibrinogen antisera. If no evidence of fibrinogen is found, immunoelectrophoresis should be done because the β-γ band might represent a small monoclonal protein.

Hypogammaglobulinemia (gamma globulin <0.6 g/dl) is characterized by a definite decrease in the γ component and should be confirmed by quantitative determination of the immunoglobulin levels. Hypogammaglobulinemia is seen in about 10% of patients with multiple myeloma and in approximately 20% of patients with primary systemic amyloidosis. In both diseases, Bence Jones proteinuria is often present, and immunofixation or immunoelectrophoresis of the se-

---

mobility, on electrophoresis (Fig. 74-1, *B*); by thickening and elongation of all heavy- and light-chain arcs on immunoelectrophoresis; and by the absence of a localized band on immunofixation. A list of the conditions in the differential diagnosis of polyclonal gammopathies is given in Box 74-2.

Although monoclonal proteins have long been considered abnormal, studies during the past several years have strongly suggested that they are only excessive quantities of normal immunoglobulins. Each heavy-chain subclass and light-chain type in a monoclonal protein has its counterpart among normal immunoglobulins and among antibodies. Monoclonal proteins are individual antibodies and are products of a single clone of plasma cells. Although some monoclonal proteins represent known antibodies, most do not; however, it is almost certain that more monoclonal proteins will be found to have antibody activity. The generation of antibody diversity is complex (Chapter 173). The one-cell one-immunoglobulin concept is supported by the finding that almost all individual plasma cells contain either κ or λ light chains, but not both.

Analysis of the serum and urine for monoclonal proteins requires a sensitive, rapid, dependable, inexpensive screening method to detect the monoclonal protein and a specific assay to identify its heavy-chain class and light-chain type. Electrophoresis on agarose gel is preferable for detecting monoclonal proteins. After screening, immunofixation or immunoelectrophoresis, or both, should be used to

Table 74-1 Constituents of major components of serum electrophoretic pattern*

(ANODE) ← ALBUMIN	α_1-GLOBULIN	α_2-GLOBULIN	β-GLOBULIN	→ (CATHODE) γ-GLOBULIN
Albumin	α_1-ANTITRYPSIN	α_2-Macroglobulin	β-Lipoprotein	IgG
	α_1-Lipoprotein	α_2-Lipoprotein	Transferrin	IgA
	α_1-Acid glycoprotein (orosomucoid)	Haptoglobin	Plasminogen	IgM
		Ceruloplasmin	Complement	IgD
	α-Fetoprotein	Erythropoietin	Hemopexin	IgE
		Lactate dehydrogenase		

*Immunoglobulins may migrate from the slow γ-globulin to the α_2-globulin region.
Modified from Kyle RA and Griepp PR: *Mayo Clin Proc* 53:719, 1978.

rum and urine is necessary for identification. Also, hypogammaglobulinemia may be congenital or associated with the nephrotic syndrome, chronic lymphocytic leukemia, lymphoma, protein-losing enteropathy, or malnutrition; or it may be caused by corticosteroid therapy. The point of application of the specimen in the cathodal area may be confused with a monoclonal protein. In 4% of sera, an additional monoclonal protein of a different immunoglobulin class is seen; this condition is designated *biclonal gammopathy* (Chapter 94).

A monoclonal protein may be present when the total serum protein concentration, β and γ globulin levels, and quantitative immunoglobulin levels are normal. The agarose gel must be examined visually because the densitometer tracing may not detect a small monoclonal protein. A small monoclonal protein also may be concealed among the β or γ components and be missed. A monoclonal light chain (Bence Jones proteinemia) is rarely seen on the tracing. In IgD myeloma the serum peak sometimes is small or not evident. Occasionally a sharp peak is seen in μ heavy-chain disease but is never seen in α heavy-chain disease. In γ heavy-chain disease, a broad band is often seen on electrophoresis. A monoclonal protein may appear as a rather broad band on the agarose gel or as a broad peak in the densitometer tracing and can be mistaken for a polyclonal increase in immunoglobulins. Presumably the broad band is caused by aggregates or polymers. Therefore immunofixation or immunoelectrophoresis is necessary to identify a monoclonal protein.

For follow-up after the diagnosis of a monoclonal protein in the serum, a densitometer tracing of the agar gel electrophoresis or quantitation of the immunoglobulins should be used. The quantitative immunoglobulin level may be 2000 mg/dl or more higher than that in the densitometer tracing. It is essential to follow the size of the monoclonal protein with densitometry or quantitation of the immunoglobulins, but methods should not be changed from one to another.

Immunofixation

This test should be performed when a sharp peak is found on the agarose gel tracing or when myeloma, macroglobulinemia, amyloidosis, or a related disorder is suspected (see Fig. 74-2). An appropriately diluted serum sample is placed in a small trough in 1% agarose. Electrophoresis is performed, and immediately afterward, monospecific antiserum is placed over the electrophoresed proteins. The excess protein is removed by washing, and bands corresponding to an antigen-antibody complex remain. The preparation is stained and read. A sharp, well-defined band with a single heavy-chain class and light-chain type is indicative of a monoclonal protein (Fig. 74-3). A polyclonal increase in immunoglobulins appears as a broad, diffuse, heavily stained band with all heavy-chain antisera and both κ and λ antisera. Care is necessary because overdilution of the sample results in loss of a monoclonal band, whereas an inadequate dilution may obscure the presence of a small monoclonal heavy or light chain in serum with normal background immunoglobulins. A prominent polyclonal band may be misinterpreted as a monoclonal protein.

Immunofixation is helpful when a monoclonal protein is suspected and only bowing of a single heavy-chain class or a single light-chain type is found on immunoelectrophoresis. A bowed light-chain arc may be absent when a monoclonal IgG, IgA, or IgM arc is present. Immunofixation is most helpful in the recognition of a biclonal gammopathy (Fig. 74-4) and for the detection of a small monoclonal protein in the presence of normal or polyclonal immunoglobulins. It is

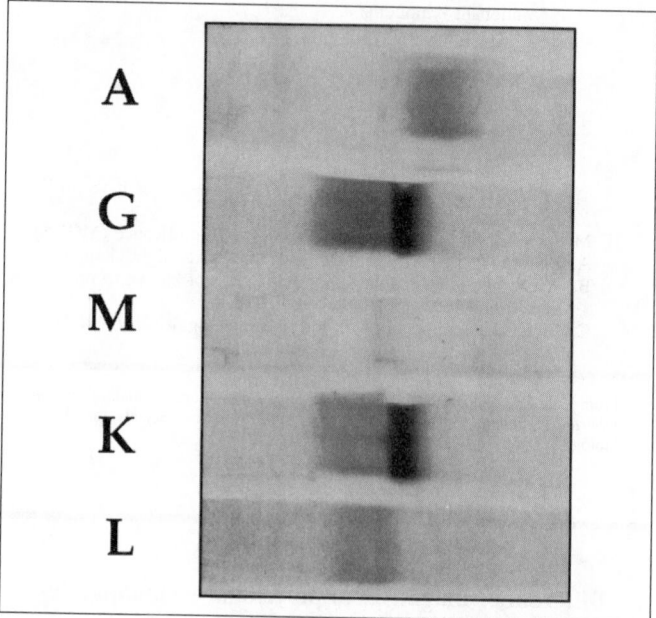

FIGURE 74-3 Immunofixation obtained in macroglobulinemia. Monospecific antisera to IgA, IgG, IgM, κ, and λ show a dense, localized band with IgG and κ indicating an IgG κ monoclonal protein. *K, κ; L, λ.*

particularly useful in successfully treated myeloma or macroglobulinemia when no spike occurs on electrophoresis, in suspected amyloidosis, or in an apparently solitary plasmacytoma after radiation.

Immunofixation is more sensitive than immunoelectrophoresis and therefore helpful in recognizing small monoclonal proteins. Despite the obvious advantages of immunofixation, immunoelectrophoresis is useful as the initial procedure because it is technically easier and less expensive.

Immunoelectrophoresis

The serum sample is placed in wells on microscope slides covered with 1% agar or agarose. Electrophoresis separates the various proteins, and a trough is cut parallel to the line of migration and filled with monospecific antisera. Proteins from the electrophoresed sample (antigen) and from the antisera (antibody) are then allowed to diffuse toward each other and form precipitin lines or arcs where they meet. In multiple myeloma, monospecific antisera to IgG, IgA, IgD, IgE, κ, or λ produce a localized thickening or bowing of both the heavy-chain arc and the light-chain arc.

In Waldenström's macroglobulinemia, IgM antisera produce a bowed, thickened arc, and a similar arc is seen with monospecific κ or λ antisera. Occasionally, no diagnostic light-chain arcs are seen, and a mistaken diagnosis of μ heavy-chain disease may be considered. Immunofixation is usually diagnostic in this situation. Another approach is to use a reducing agent such as dithiothreitol (DTT), which often makes an IgM κ or an IgM λ monoclonal protein iden-

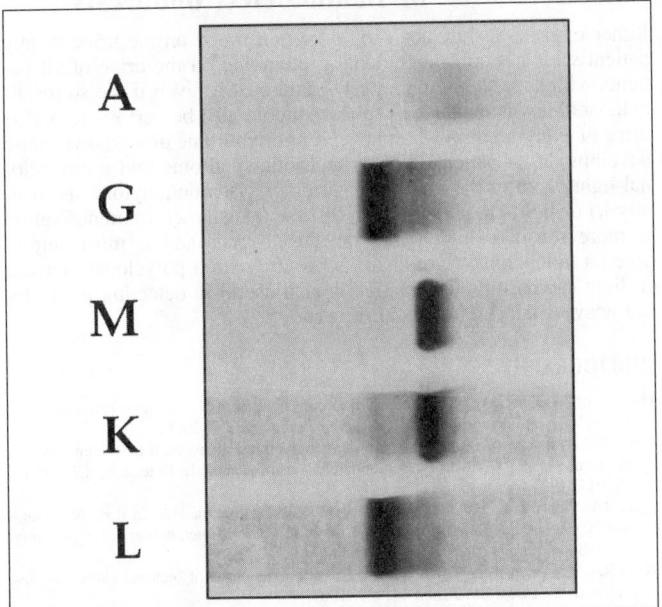

FIGURE 74-4   Immunofixation of serum with antisera to IgG, IgA, IgM, κ, and λ shows a dense, localized IgG band and a similar λ band as well as a dense, localized IgM band and a similar κ band. This is indicative of a biclonal gammopathy (IgG λ plus IgM κ). *K, κ; L, λ.*

tifiable with immunoelectrophoresis. Occasionally a monoclonal IgM protein may precipitate (euglobulin) near the application well without producing diagnostic arcs. The problem may be solved by immunofixation, by adding a reducing agent (e.g., DTT), or by repeating immunoelectrophoresis with a buffer of lower ionic strength.

If a bowed κ or λ arc is seen without an accompanying abnormality of the IgG, IgA, or IgM arcs, the possibility of a free monoclonal light chain or an IgD or IgE monoclonal protein must be considered. Bence Jones proteinemia is more common than an IgD or an IgE monoclonal protein. Ouchterlony immunodiffusion with IgD and IgE antisera should be performed when only a monoclonal light chain is found. All sera that form a precipitin band should then be studied by immunoelectrophoresis with monospecific antisera to IgD and IgE as well as to κ and λ. The presence of an additional light-chain arc (double bowing) without a similar change in the heavy-chain arc indicates a free monoclonal light chain (Bence Jones proteinemia) or a component of a biclonal gammopathy in which the associated heavy-chain arc has not been detected. Immunofixation is often helpful in this setting.

Identification of Monoclonal Proteins With a Rate Nephelometer

Monoclonal proteins can be identified without immunoelectrophoresis or immunofixation. The rate nephelometer, with use of monospecific anti-κ and anti-λ and the appropriate heavy-chain antisera, has been used successfully to detect the light-chain type of large monoclonal gammopathies. However, small monoclonal proteins will have a normal κ:λ ratio and will not be recognized. Thus small monoclonal proteins, particularly IgG κ, may be overlooked in a determination of κ:λ ratios with a rate nephelometer. Furthermore, in patients with biclonal gammopathy, the diagnosis frequently will be incorrect.

Immunoblotting

In combination with high-resolution electrophoresis on agarose, immunoblotting may detect monoclonal proteins in concentrations as low as 0.5 mg/L. In one series, immunoblotting detected a monoclonal protein in three fourths of patients older than 95 years in whom electrophoresis and immunofixation failed to find a monoclonal protein.

Quantitation of Immunoglobulins

For the diagnosis of hypogammaglobulinemia, the quantitation of immunoglobulins is more useful than either immunoelectrophoresis or immunofixation. The use of a rate nephelometer is practical for quantitation of immunoglobulins. In this system the degree of turbidity produced by antigen-antibody interaction is measured by nephelometry in the near-ultraviolet region. Because the method is not affected by molecular size of the antigen (as is radial immunodiffusion), the nephelometric technique accurately measures 7S IgM, polymers of IgA, and aggregates of IgG.

Radial immunodiffusion is tedious and subject to spurious abnormalities and is not recommended. For example, low-molecular-weight (7S) IgM will produce a spuriously elevated value because its rate of diffusion is greater than that of the 19S IgM used as a standard. Alternatively, spuriously low levels for IgA may occur because of polymeric IgA, which produces less diffusion than the 7S IgA used as a standard.

Serum Viscometry

Serum viscometry should be measured in every patient with more than 3 g/dl of IgM monoclonal protein or more than 4 g/dl of IgA or IgG protein and in any patient with oronasal bleeding, blurred vision, or neurologic symptoms suggestive of a hyperviscosity syndrome. The Ostwald-100 viscometer is a satisfactory instrument for this purpose. Distilled water and serum are made to flow separately through a capillary tube; the quotient of the flow duration (serum divided by water) is the viscosity value (normal, <1.6). The Wells-Brookfield viscometer is preferred because it is more accurate and requires less serum (about 1.0 ml) and because the procedure can be done quickly and performed at different shear rates and different temperatures. Symptoms of hyperviscosity are rare unless the value is more than 4 centipoises (normal, <1.8). Some patients with a value of 10 centipoises or more do not have symptoms of hyperviscosity.

ANALYSIS OF URINE FOR MONOCLONAL PROTEINS
Screening Tests

When patients with serum gammopathies are studied, the urine should also be analyzed (Chapter 102). The use of sulfosalicylic acid, or Exton's test, is best for the detection of protein. Sulfosalicylic acid detects albumin and globulin, Bence Jones protein, polypeptides, and proteases. False-positive reactions may be induced by penicillin or its derivatives, tolbutamide metabolites, sulfisoxazole metabolites, and organic roentgenographic contrast media.

Dipstick tests are used in many laboratories to screen for protein. The dipstick is impregnated with a buffered indicator dye that binds to protein in the urine and produces a color change proportional to the amount of protein bound to it. However, dipsticks are often insensitive to Bence Jones protein and should not be used when a possibility of Bence Jones proteinuria exists. Almost from the time of the discovery of the unique thermal properties of urinary light chains (Bence Jones protein), screening tests have been used for their detection. All such tests have serious shortcomings, and the heat test is not recommended. Both false-positive and false-negative results occur. The diagnosis of Bence Jones proteinuria depends on the demonstration of a monoclonal light chain by electrophoresis and either immunoelectrophoresis or immunofixation of an adequately concentrated aliquot from a 24-hour urine specimen (Fig. 74-5; see Fig. 74-2).

Electrophoresis

Electrophoresis of urine should be performed on all patients with a large monoclonal serum protein or the diagnosis of suspected multiple myeloma, macroglobulinemia, amyloidosis, or related diseases.

Before electrophoresis, a 24-hour urine collection is needed to determine the total amount of protein excreted per day. This collection is important when following the course of a patient because the amount of urinary monoclonal protein (size of spike on densitometer tracing × g protein/24 hr) correlates directly with the size of the plasma cell burden.

A urinary monoclonal protein appears as a dense, localized band on the cellulose strip and as a tall, narrow peak on the densitometer tracing

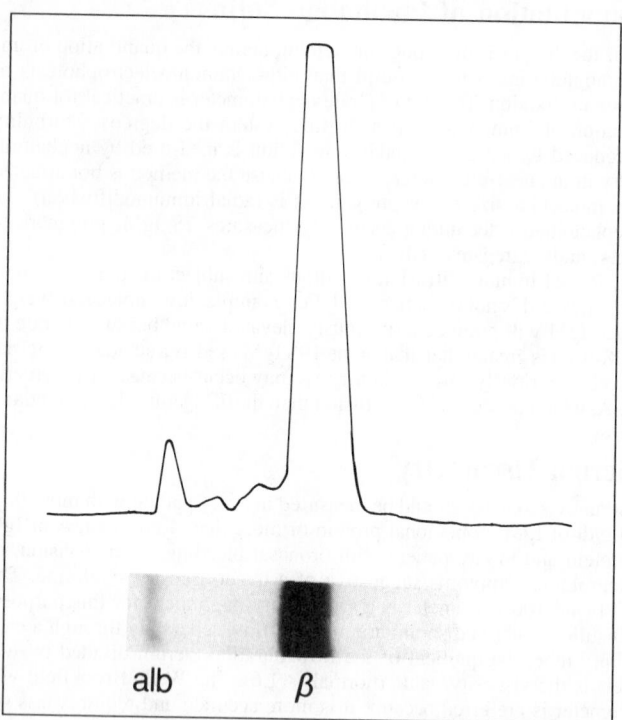

FIGURE 74-5   Monoclonal urine protein. *Top,* Densitometer tracing showing a tall, narrow-based peak of β mobility; *bottom,* cellulose acetate electrophoretic pattern showing a dense band of β mobility. This is consistent with a monoclonal urine protein (Bence Jones protein).

From Kyle RA, Garton JP: *Semin Oncol* 13:310, 1986.

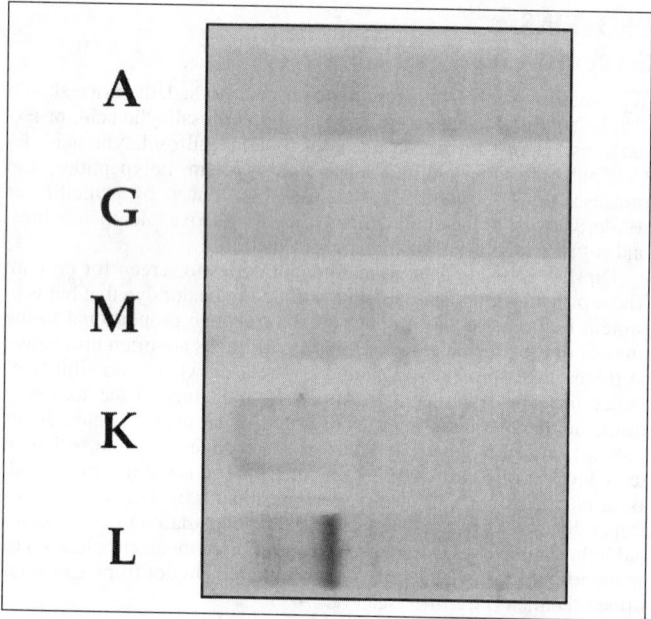

FIGURE 74-6   Immunofixation of urine with monospecific antisera to IgG, IgA, IgM, κ, and λ shows a small, discrete λ band indicating the presence of a monoclonal light chain (λ). *K,* κ; *L,* λ.

From Kyle RA, Garton JP: *Semin Oncol* 13:310, 1986.

(see Fig. 74-5). Immunofixation shows a discrete band with light-chain antisera (Fig. 74-6). Occasionally, two discrete globulin bands are seen, and these may represent either monomers and dimers of the monoclonal light chain or a monoclonal light chain plus a monoclonal immunoglobulin fragment from the serum. Rarely, two monoclonal light chains (κ and λ, biclonal) have been found in the urine.

Immunofixation or Immunoelectrophoresis

Either of these techniques should be performed on the urine of any patient with a serum monoclonal protein and on the urine of all patients with suspected monoclonal gammopathy, even if the sulfosalicylic acid test is negative. The tests should also be performed on the urine of every adult in whom a nephrotic syndrome of unknown cause develops. Most patients with a nephrotic syndrome and a monoclonal light chain in the urine have primary systemic amyloidosis (usually λ) or light-chain deposition disease (usually κ). Immunofixation is more sensitive than immunoelectrophoresis and is most helpful when a monoclonal light chain is present with a polyclonal increase in light chains. Immunofixation is also useful in detecting monoclonal heavy-chain fragments in the urine.

BIBLIOGRAPHY

Howerton DA, Check IJ, Hunter RL: Densitometric quantitation of high resolution agarose gel protein electrophoresis, *Am J Clin Pathol* 85:213, 1986.

Jones RG et al: Use of immunoglobulin heavy-chain and light-chain measurements in a multicenter trial to investigate monoclonal components. I. Detection, *Clin Chem* 37:1917, 1991.

Kyle RA: Classification and diagnosis of monoclonal gammopathies. In Rose NR, Friedman H, Fahey JL, editors: *Manual of clinical laboratory immunology,* ed 3, Washington, 1986, American Society for Microbiology.

Kyle RA, Robinson RA, Katzmann JA: The clinical aspects of biclonal gammopathies: review of 57 cases, *Am J Med* 71:999, 1981.

Kyle RA et al: Primary systemic amyloidosis: clinical and laboratory features in 474 cases, *Semin Hematol* 32:45, 1995.

Radl J, Wels J, Hoogeveen CM: Immunoblotting with (sub)class-specific antibodies reveals a high frequency of monoclonal gammopathies in persons thought to be immunodeficient, *Clin Chem* 34:1839, 1988.

Roberts RT: Usefulness of immunofixation electrophoresis in the clinical laboratory, *Clin Lab Med* 6:601, 1986.

Whicher JT, Wallage M, Fifield R: Use of immunoglobulin heavy- and light-chain measurements compared with existing techniques as a means of typing monoclonal immunoglobulins, *Clin Chem* 33:1771, 1987.

Whicher JT et al: The laboratory investigation of paraproteinaemia, *Ann Clin Biochem* 24:119, 1987.

Wolf PL: Interpretation of electrophoretic patterns of serum proteins, *Clin Lab Med* 6:441, 1986.

CHAPTER

75 Evaluation of Hemostasis and Thrombosis

James N. George

The laboratory methods used to confirm the clinical diagnosis of a bleeding disorder are well established, and a specific etiology should be detected in every patient with severe bleeding. Patients with mild bleeding symptoms may be difficult to define by laboratory studies. Many of these patients may simply have variations of normal bleeding. In contrast, laboratory evaluation of patients with excessive thrombosis is less likely to yield an explanation for the abnormality, even when the history clearly indicates a recurrent, severe disease. Recent investigations have more clearly defined the natural control mechanisms of coagulation, and congenital abnormalities of this control system that cause an increased risk for thrombosis are now being diagnosed with increased frequency.

PLATELETS AND PLATELET FUNCTION
Platelet Number

The normal platelet count is typically 150 to 350 × 10⁹/L. With the use of automated particle counters for all blood cell counts, including platelets, many more patients are being detected with mild asymptomatic thrombocytopenia. However, the automated particle counters may report falsely abnormal platelet counts. Falsely low platelet counts can occur with in vitro clumping caused by innocent antibodies that agglutinate platelets in the presence of the standard EDTA anticoagulant or at temperatures less than 37° C. Also, the particle counter may not detect very large platelets in patients with hereditary giant platelet syndromes. Falsely high platelet counts may occur if other cellular fragments, such as leukocyte fragments in leukemia, are not distinguished from platelets by the particle counter. Therefore examination of a routine stained blood smear is essential to confirm an abnormal platelet count. On the proper area of the smear, where the red cells just begin to overlap and their morphology is best, there should be about 7 to 20 platelets per oil immersion (×1000) field. This figure is derived from the fact that in this area there should be about 200 red cells per oil immersion field and that the normal red cell/platelet ratio in whole blood is about 10 to 30:1.

Evaluation of Thrombocytopenia

The first step must be to distinguish decreased marrow production from increased peripheral destruction or splenic sequestration as the cause of thrombocytopenia. In some disorders of increased platelet destruction the appearance of large platelets on the peripheral blood smear has been reported, but this observation is not consistent. An examination of the bone marrow may be helpful in some patients, but in many patients other clinical and laboratory data are sufficient. Megakaryocytes, the large precursor cells of platelets, are easily identified on marrow smears, but they cannot be quantified without special techniques. However, estimates of megakaryocyte frequency are sufficient. If megakaryocytes are difficult to locate in an adequately cellular marrow smear, thrombocytopenia is most likely caused by decreased production. If megakaryocytes are plentiful, it is assumed that they are functioning normally and that thrombocytopenia is caused by peripheral platelet destruction or splenic sequestration, but this may not always be true. In some diseases, such as HIV infection, megakaryocytes appear normal yet the thrombocytopenia is predominantly due to decreased platelet production.

Bleeding Time

The template bleeding time is performed with devices that make a reproducible skin incision 1 mm deep and several millimeters long. With these small wounds, the primary hemostatic mechanisms involving platelets and blood vessels can stop the bleeding almost independently of coagulation reactions. For standardization, a blood pressure cuff is inflated to 40 mm Hg to cause capillary filling and to ensure bleeding. Normal values are about 3 to 8 minutes. A platelet count of more than 75×10^9/L is sufficient to allow a normal bleeding time. A bleeding time test is rarely indicated when the platelet count is less than this because bleeding time is often prolonged and rarely yields clinically useful information. A normal bleeding time provides confidence that platelet function is normal.

Prolonged bleeding times are difficult to interpret. Elderly or malnourished patients may have a long bleeding time because of poor cutaneous elasticity. Some normal people may have a prolonged bleeding time because of aspirin or certain antibiotics and yet have a normal hemostatic response to surgical trauma. Although the bleeding time is clearly an important *diagnostic* aid for disorders affecting platelet function, such as von Willebrand's disease, its value in *predicting* the risk of bleeding in normal subjects is unknown. In some typical situations, such as uremia and the use of high doses of penicillin and related β-lactam antibiotics, a prolonged bleeding time does *not* predict an increased risk for hemorrhage.

Evaluation of von Willebrand's Factor Concentration, Structure, and Function

Abnormal platelet function may result from an intrinsic platelet defect or a deficiency or abnormality of plasma von Willebrand's factor, which is required for normal platelet adhesion to subendothelium. Therefore investigation of a disorder of primary hemostasis must include an evaluation of plasma von Willebrand's factor. Von Willebrand's factor is a very large multimeric protein, reaching the enormous molecular size of 12 million daltons and potential length, 1.5 μm. The concentration of von Willebrand's factor in plasma can be measured by immunoassays. In some genetic variants of von Wille-

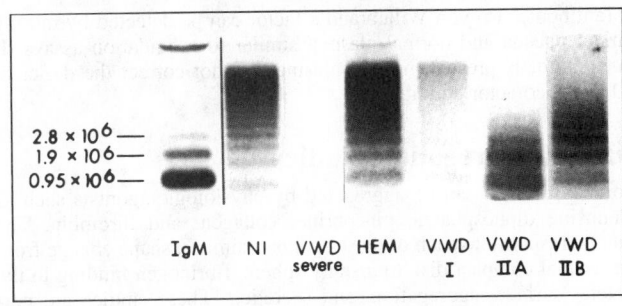

FIGURE 75-1 The polymer pattern of human plasma von Willebrand's factor analyzed by sodium dodecyl sulfate (SDS)–agarose electrophoresis. The migration of proteins proceeds from the top to the bottom of these gels, with smaller molecules moving farther toward the bottom. Immunoglobulin M (IgM) and IgM polymers are shown in the left gel, and their molecular weights are noted. After electrophoresis of plasma samples, the gels were incubated with ^{125}I-labeled rabbit anti–human von Willebrand's factor, and the plasma von Willebrand's factor was identified by autoradiography. From the left, these plasma samples are from (1) a normal individual *(NI)*, with a predominance of high molecular weight polymers; (2) a patient with severe von Willebrand's disease *(VWD)* and no demonstrable plasma von Willebrand's factor; (3) a patient with severe hemophilia A *(HEM)*, factor VIII deficiency, and normal plasma von Willebrand's factor; (4) a patient with type I VWD and a diminished concentration of plasma von Willebrand's factor that has the normal polymer size distribution; (5) a patient with type IIA VWD with a selective deficiency of the large and intermediate-size polymers of plasma von Willebrand's factor; and (6) a patient with type IIB VWD with a selective deficiency of the largest polymers of plasma von Willebrand's factor.

From Hoyer LW: *Blood* 58:1, 1981.

brand's disease, the highest molecular-weight multimers—the most hemostatically effective molecules—are missing, even though the plasma concentration is in the normal range. This can be assessed by sodium dodecyl sulfate agarose gel electrophoresis of the plasma sample and identification of the von Willebrand's factor multimers by autoradiography after incubating the gel with ^{125}I-labeled anti–von Willebrand's factor. Figure 75-1 demonstrates this technique and illustrates the abnormalities of von Willebrand's factor in different variants of von Willebrand's disease.

The function of von Willebrand's factor is assessed indirectly by the use of ristocetin-induced platelet agglutination. Ristocetin is an antibiotic that was withdrawn from clinical use more than 30 years ago because of its association with thrombocytopenia. Later it was recognized that ristocetin in vitro agglutinated all platelets except those from subjects with a severe deficiency of von Willebrand's factor and subjects with Bernard-Soulier syndrome, who lack platelet membrane glycoprotein Ib-IX-V, a receptor for von Willebrand's factor. Ristocetin-induced platelet agglutination using the patient's platelet-rich plasma can be used as a screening test. The standard ristocetin concentration of 1.5 mg/ml should cause rapid agglutination of normal platelets. Paradoxically, in some variant forms of von Willebrand's disease, such as type IIB, increased reactivity with ristocetin is clearly abnormal; platelet agglutination is strong at ristocetin concentrations of 0.3 to 0.5 mg/ml, well below the concentrations necessary to induce the agglutination of normal platelets.

Von Willebrand's factor function is more accurately evaluated by measurements with the patient's plasma, referred to as *ristocetin-cofactor assays*. Normal platelets fixed with formalin provide a stable reagent. (The term *agglutination* is used because ristocetin causes clumping of formalin-fixed platelets, in contrast to *aggregation*, which requires active metabolic participation of the platelets.) In this assay the washed normal formalin-fixed platelets are mixed with a dilution of patient plasma and ristocetin, and platelet clumping is evaluated by aggregometer tracings or simply by determining the time required for the formation of visible clumps. The principle is the same as that used for assays of coagulation factors except that the end-point is platelet clumping rather than fibrin clot formation. By comparing different dilutions of patient plasma with normal plasma, a result can be expressed as a percentage of normal ristocetin cofactor (von Willebrand's factor) activity. The rare patients with acquired inhibitors of (antibodies to) von Willebrand's factor can be detected by mixing patient plasma and normal plasma, similar to coagulation assays. If an inhibitor is present, normal plasma will not correct the deficient ristocetin cofactor activity.

Platelet Aggregation Studies

Normal platelets can be aggregated by physiologic agonists such as adenosine diphosphate, epinephrine, collagen, and thrombin. The platelet response to each of these agents is similar: shape change from the normal compact disk to a spiny sphere, fibrinogen binding to the platelet surface, aggregation, and secretion. These studies are performed in platelet-rich plasma prepared from citrate-anticoagulated whole blood, which is placed in a cuvette and mechanically stirred at 37° C. The response is detected by an increase in light transmission through the cuvette as the platelet clumping causes clearing of the plasma. Platelet aggregation studies are performed in patients who are suspected of having abnormal platelet function, for example, those who have a prolonged bleeding time and a normal or near-normal platelet count.

Aspirin and other inhibitors of platelet thromboxane synthesis prevent normal platelet secretion and aggregation by low concentrations of agonists. Since aspirin has an irreversible effect on platelets, patients must be studied after they have refrained from taking aspirin or related drugs for 10 days, the survival time of normal platelets. This is a difficult requirement because aspirin is ingested so frequently. The most striking abnormality of platelet aggregation occurs in the rare hereditary membrane glycoprotein IIb-IIIa (the fibrinogen receptor) defect, Glanzmann's thrombasthenia, in which no macroscopic aggregation occurs in response to any of these four agonists.

Although they are popular in many laboratories, the usefulness of platelet aggregation studies is difficult to assess. The ubiquitous use of aspirin must be emphasized, platelets from some normal people may not respond well to epinephrine or collagen, and the response to each agonist depends on its concentration. No standardized method of quantitation exists. Finally, it is not known if abnormal aggregation predicts an increased risk for clinically important bleeding.

Platelet Coagulant Activity

Although the role of platelets in accelerating in vivo coagulation is clear, demonstration of this property in vitro is difficult. With certain in vitro conditions in which platelets are disrupted or activated by contact with a foreign surface, platelet-rich plasma clots more rapidly than platelet-free plasma. Part of this platelet property seems attributable to membrane phospholipid and is possibly related to the specific interaction between platelets and coagulation factors VIIIa and IXa in the activation of factor X and factors Va and Xa in the activation of prothrombin. Tests of platelet coagulant activity can be interpreted only qualitatively.

The simplest test to perform in a clinical laboratory, and therefore the best screening assay, is the serum prothrombin time (PT), which seems to reflect primarily the platelet contribution to coagulation. The PT is measured in serum after whole blood is allowed to clot in a glass tube for 1 hour at 37° C. In normal subjects the serum PT is more than twice as long as the PT time in plasma (i.e., >25 seconds), whereas in disorders of platelet coagulant activity the serum PT may be similar to the PT time with plasma. In another common test, referred to as *platelet factor 3 availability,* citrate-anticoagulated platelet-rich plasma is activated by kaolin, and the clotting time is measured after recalcification.

PLASMA COAGULATION

Laboratory evaluation of plasma coagulation is based on a series of tests that activate the coagulation sequence at different sites. The activating substances have been developed empirically and their use established by clinical experience. However, it should never be forgotten that these in vitro assessments of plasma coagulation are useful artifacts and that they may be very different from the in vivo events. The coagulation scheme as tested by typical coagulation assays is shown in Fig. 75-2. Note the differences from the coagulation scheme

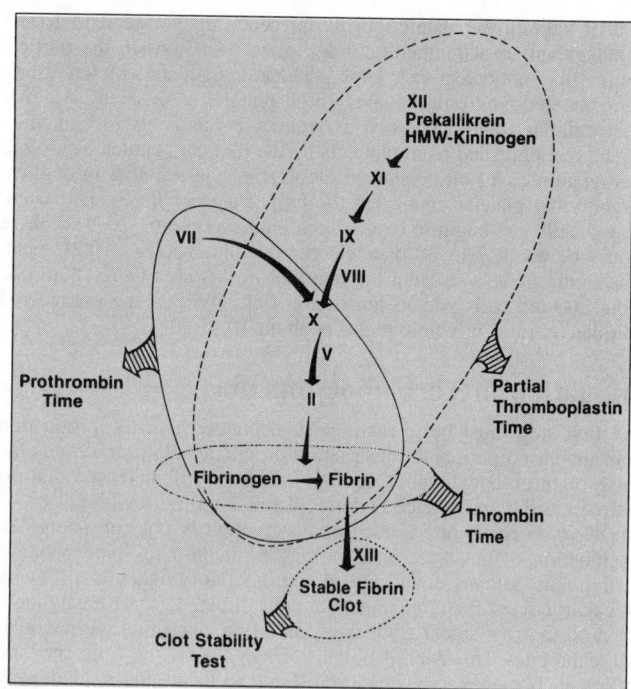

FIGURE 75-2 Plasma coagulation reactions in in vitro laboratory assays. Note the differences between this diagram and Fig. 69-2. Factor XII, prekallikrein, and high molecular weight kininogen are required for a normal partial thromboplastin time but not for normal in vivo hemostasis. Also, plasma factor XI may not always be required for normal in vivo hemostasis. Platelets and tissue factor are required for normal in vivo hemostasis but are supplied by exogenous reagents in the laboratory assays. This diagram outlines the coagulation factors required for each of four basic tests.

presented for normal in vivo hemostasis in Fig. 69-2. The activators used for the partial thromboplastin time (PTT) initiate the reaction at factor XII, and a normal PTT requires three factors that are unnecessary for hemostasis in vivo: factor XII, prekallikrein, and high-molecular-weight kininogen. Moreover, platelets are not required in these reactions because exogenous phospholipid is supplied. The PTT and the PT have different sensitivities to the same defect in their common pathway. For example, the PTT is more sensitive to the inhibitory effect of heparin (which inactivates thrombin and factor Xa, as well as factors IXa, XIa, and VIIa) and the inhibitor that occurs in systemic lupus erythematosus (which inhibits phospholipid-dependent reactions), whereas the PT is often more sensitive to the abnormalities in liver disease (which can reduce the concentration of all coagulation factors). In addition, the sensitivities of the PTT and PT to coagulation factor deficiencies also vary, depending on the commercial source of the reagents. Despite these problems, both tests are valuable contributors to the evaluation of hemostasis because they usually become abnormal at levels of coagulation factor deficiencies that are associated with clinical bleeding.

For all coagulation assays, blood collection is critical. Citrate anticoagulant is used to provide mild calcium chelation. EDTA is a stronger calcium chelator used as the routine anticoagulant for blood counts; it reduces the calcium concentration to a level that irreversibly inactivates factors V and VIII and thereby prevents subsequent assessment of plasma coagulation. Since some coagulation factors are labile, the assays must be performed on fresh or fresh-frozen plasma.

Partial Thromboplastin Time

The name of this test was derived from studies of various "thromboplastins" 50 years ago, when it was thought that these tissue extracts represented in vivo coagulation factors. Therefore when certain extracts were shown to correct the coagulation defect of hemophilic plasma, it was thought that missing factors were replaced, and these materials were termed *complete thromboplastins* (e.g., the current prothrombin time). Extracts that did not correct the hemophilic defect were termed *partial thromboplastins*. Subsequently these different tissue extracts were shown to activate the coagulation sequence at different points, factors VII and XII, respectively.

The PTT is a good screening test for coagulation abnormalities except for factors VII and XIII. Its level of sensitivity is best known for factor VIII because it is usually prolonged when factor VIII levels are below 20%. Since this is also the factor VIII concentration associated with a risk of bleeding after trauma, the PTT is a good screening test for detecting mild hemophilia and is presumably also an effective screening test for other coagulation disorders. However, patients with mild hemophilia, who may have significant bleeding after trauma, may sometimes have a normal PTT. The normal values for the PTT depend on the specific reagent used and the incubation conditions, and the normal range is relatively broad, usually about 20 to 40 seconds. The PTT is used for the control of heparin anticoagulation as it is much more sensitive than the PT.

Prothrombin Time

The PT was originally described by Quick in 1935, when the other factors involved in this test (factors VII, X, and V) were unknown. This is a highly reproducible assay with a normal value of about 9 to 13 seconds using the conventional American tissue factor reagent, an acetone extract of rabbit brain that is very rich in tissue factor. Based on Fig. 75-2, a combination of an abnormal PT with a normal PTT appears to be diagnostic of a factor VII abnormality. This is not necessarily true, however, as this observation is common in patients with liver disease or vitamin K deficiency in whom multiple coagulation factors are deficient. The only explanation is the difference in inherent sensitivities of these two assays.

The PT is used for the control of warfarin anticoagulation because the results are very reproducible. However, commercial PT thromboplastin reagents vary widely in their sensitivity to warfarin-induced deficiencies of factors II, VII, IX, and X activity. Therefore all reagents are now standardized by an International Sensitivity Index (ISI), and an accurate description of the intensity of warfarin anticoagulation must express the PT as a derivative of the ISI, termed the *International Normalized Ratio* (INR) (Chapter 85).

Thrombin Time

The thrombin time is simply the measurement of the fibrin clotting time after the addition of bovine thrombin. In theory this test may seem to be unnecessary, since both the PTT and the PT involve fibrin formation. In fact, the thrombin time is much more sensitive than either of the other two assays to abnormalities of the thrombin-fibrinogen interaction and subsequent fibrin polymerization. For example, the thrombin time is very sensitive to heparin anticoagulation (too sensitive to be clinically useful), deficiencies of fibrinogen, and abnormalities of fibrin polymerization such as those caused by fibrin degradation products, myeloma paraproteins, or congenital dysfibrinogenemias.

Fibrinogen Concentration

The plasma concentration of fibrinogen is measured by comparing the thrombin time of various dilutions of patient plasma with a standard reference plasma sample of known fibrinogen concentration, similar in principal to the assay of specific coagulation factors described below. When heparin is present or abnormalities of fibrinogen are suspected, immunoassays can be done.

Clot Stability Test

All the standard coagulation tests measure the time needed to form an initial fibrin clot. The subsequent conversion of this fibrin polymer into a permanent, covalently bonded structure is essential to form a firm clot in vivo but is not required for a normal PTT, PT, or thrombin time. The clot stability test evaluates the function of factor XIII, the enzyme that catalyzes the formation of covalent bonds within the fibrin polymer. Citrate plasma is clotted and the clot is then incubated with urea or monochloroacetic acid, agents that can dissolve the hydrogen bonds of the initial fibrin polymer but cannot break co-

valent bonds. This test may also be abnormal in the presence of inhibitors of factor XIII or with abnormal fibrin polymerization.

Specific Coagulation Factor Assays

These assays are based on the PTT (for prekallikrein, high molecular weight kininogen, factors XII, XI, IX, and VIII) or the PT (for factors VII, X, V, and II). In each case the assay requires a plasma sample that is deficient in the single coagulation factor to be measured. Then various dilutions of the patient plasma or a standard reference plasma are added, and the clotting time is measured. Curves are constructed, and the activity of the patient plasma is compared to the reference plasma. Data are expressed as a percent of normal, with the normal range being typically 50% to 150%, or as units (normal, 0.5 to 1.5 U/ml). For example, to assay factor VIII, a series of PTTs is performed. Each assay tube contains plasma from a patient with severe hemophilia (less than 1% of normal factor VIII activity) and dilutions of normal or patient plasma, usually between 1:10 and 1:500. If the patient has a 50% level of factor VIII (0.5 U/ml), the clotting time with a 1:10 dilution of plasma will be the same as the clotting time of a 1:20 dilution of normal plasma. If the patient has a 5% level of factor VIII (0.05 U/ml), the clotting time of his or her 1:10 diluted plasma will be the same as the clotting time of normal plasma diluted 1:200.

Screening Test for Coagulation Inhibitors

An abnormality of any coagulation factor can be caused by a deficiency of activity of the factor or by an inhibitor of the activated factor. The inhibitors may be antibodies to a coagulation factor, heparin-like molecules, or proteins that interfere with fibrin polymerization, such as fibrin degradation products or myeloma paraproteins. In some patients, both a deficiency and an inhibitor are present, as in the 10% of patients with severe hemophilia who develop antibodies to normal factor VIII after repeated transfusions. The detection of an inhibitor is critical because replacement therapy is difficult or impossible when an inhibitor is present. For example, a patient with a very prolonged PTT may have a deficiency of factor VIII and/or an acquired inhibitor of factor VIII. When the PTT is repeated using a 1:1 mixture of patient and normal plasma, the abnormality is corrected if only a deficiency exists and the clotting time is similar to that of a 1:1 mixture of normal plasma and saline (see Box 82-2 in Chapter 82). An inhibitor will inactivate some or all of the factor VIII activity in the normal plasma, just as it will the factor VIII in the patient's plasma, and therefore the clotting time of the mixture will be prolonged.

Screening Test for Fibrinolysis: Measurement of Fibrin Degradation Products

Plasmin activation is most easily assessed by measuring the products of plasmin digestion of fibrin. The simplest assays are based on most fibrin degradation products not being incorporated into a fibrin clot and remaining soluble in serum. Therefore the blood samples are collected in special tubes that have excess thrombin to ensure complete clotting, plus an inhibitor of in vitro fibrinolysis. Serum is collected, and fibrinogen-related antigens are measured by an immunoassay. This is not an entirely satisfactory assay, however, and the artifacts that may occur during serum preparation can be avoided by performing the immunoassays on whole plasma, using antibodies that recognize new antigens that are formed or exposed during plasmin digestion of fibrin and are specific for fibrin degradation products, such as the dimer of fibrin fragment D.

SCREENING TESTS FOR THROMBOTIC DISORDERS

Risk factors for thrombotic disease are primarily abnormalities of blood flow or blood vessels; abnormalities of blood coagulation are less frequent. In most persons with thrombosis, specific laboratory variations indicating blood coagulation abnormalities cannot be identified. However, in some patients, screening tests for abnormal regulation of coagulation may be indicated: patients with recurrent thrombotic disease without clinically apparent risk factors, with thrombosis in an unusual site, with thrombosis at an early age, or with a familial tendency for recurrent thromboembolism. Even in these carefully defined populations, however, abnormalities of the blood coagulation system that may contribute to an increased risk for thrombosis are identified in less than 10% of patients.

Among the coagulation factors recognized as important for the regulation of hemostasis, commercially available assays are available for antithrombin III, protein C, and protein S. These assays can measure the plasma concentration of these proteins and their functional activity. Assay for the "lupus anticoagulant" is also performed in the evaluation of persons with recurrent thrombotic disease. Unfortunately, interpretation of these assays' results can be equivocal, and indiscriminate use must be discouraged. For example, levels of antithrombin III fall after administration of therapeutic heparin, and levels of protein C and protein S fall after therapeutic administration of warfarin. Analysis of these proteins' levels after therapeutic anticoagulation therefore is difficult, if not impossible. A second major problem is that abnormalities of these proteins are well documented in normal asymptomatic subjects. The need for therapy must be determined on the basis of clinical, not laboratory, data.

BIBLIOGRAPHY

Bauer KA, Rosenberg RD: The pathophysiology of the prethrombotic state in humans: insights gained from studies using markers of hemostatic system activation, *Blood* 70:343, 1987.

Burns ER, Goldbert SN, Wenz B: Paradoxic effect of multiple coagulation factor deficiencies on the prothrombin time and activated partial thromboplastin time, *Am J Clin Path* 100:94, 1993.

Garcia-Suarez J et al: EDTA-dependent pseudothrombocytopenia in ambulatory patients: clinical characteristics and role of new automated cell-counting in its detection, *Am J Hematol* 39:146, 1992.

George JN, Shattil SJ: The clinical importance of acquired abnormalities of platelet function, *N Engl J Med* 324:27, 1991.

Lind SE: The bleeding time does not predict surgical bleeding, *Blood* 77:2547, 1991.

Mielke CH: Aspirin prolongation of the template bleeding time: influence of venostasis and direction of incision, *Blood* 60:1139, 1982.

Rodgers RPC, Levin J: A critical reappraisal of the bleeding time, *Semin Thromb Hemost* 16:1, 1990.

Suchman AL, Griner PF: Diagnostic uses of the activated partial thromboplastin time and prothrombin time, *Ann Intern Med* 104:810, 1986.

III SPECIAL TOPICS

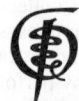

76 Blood Transfusion

Jay E. Menitove

WHOLE BLOOD AND RED CELL TRANSFUSION
Whole Blood

Whole blood units contain approximately 450 to 500 ml of phlebotomized blood and 63 ml of anticoagulant preservative solution. The hematocrit is 35% to 40%.

Whole blood repletes oxygen-carrying capacity and intravascular volume in patients who are deficient in these factors despite crystalloid or colloid solution administration. Whole blood may be stored for up to 35 days at refrigerated temperatures.

Packed Red Blood Cells

Red blood cells (RBCs) refers to plasma-depleted whole blood. That is, whole blood subjected to centrifugation to separate red cells and

plasma, followed by plasma removal. Frequently a 100-ml solution containing saline and nutrients is added to the red cells, resulting in an approximately 325-ml volume with a hematocrit of 55% to 65%. Red blood cells are stored at refrigerated temperatures for up to 42 days. In nonbleeding adults, the posttransfusion hematocrit or hemoglobin increases 3% or 1 g/dl, respectively, per unit infused.

RBC transfusions compensate for deficiencies in oxygen-carrying capacity and alleviate signs and symptoms of anemia: syncope, cerebral hypoxia, dyspnea, postural hypotension, tachycardia, or angina.

Current guidelines emphasize transfusion avoidance in the absence of signs or symptoms attributable to anemia, rather than a preset hematocrit level or "transfusion trigger." Treatment with iron, cyanocobalamin, folate, or recombinant erythropoietin in selected patients, should precede transfusion unless anemia renders the patient unstable. Patients with cardiovascular disorders, advanced age, significant pulmonary disease, or cerebrovascular insufficiency may show symptoms at higher hematocrit/hemoglobin levels, but most patients tolerate hemoglobin concentrations of 7 to 9 g/dl.

Leukocyte-Reduced Red Blood Cells

Adhesion filters decrease the leukocyte content of whole blood or red blood cells to less than 5×10^6 white blood cells per unit. Reducing the leukocyte content to less than 5×10^8 cells per unit prevents a recurrence of most febrile, nonhemolytic transfusion reactions caused by interaction of recipient leukoagglutination antibodies and donor leukocytes. Leukocytes produce variable amounts of tumor necrosis factor α, interleukin (IL)1-β, IL-6, and IL-8 during storage. Chills, fever, and general discomfort follow infusion of blood components containing elevated levels of these cytokines. In general, filters are attached to the blood bag at the bedside or in the laboratory immediately before transfusion. However, leukocyte reduction shortly after blood collection, that is, prior to storage, might prevent these reactions by reducing cytokine accumulation, but data for making definite conclusions are inconclusive at this time.

Leukocyte reduction to less than 5×10^6 cells per unit precludes or delays development of HLA (human leukocyte antigens) alloimmunization in multitransfused patients, for example, those with acute leukemia or aplastic anemia. The filters reduce the risk of cytomegalovirus (CMV) transmission to levels similar to that observed following transfusion of CMV seronegative blood.

Washed Red Blood Cells

RBCs washed with normal saline retain only small amounts of plasma. The leukocyte content is approximately 5×10^8 per unit. Saline-washed RBCs are used to prevent recurrence of severe allergic reactions or urticaria. Leukocyte reduction filters remove more white blood cells than occurs with washing.

Frozen Deglycerolized Red Blood Cells

Freezing red cells at $-65°$ C with a cryoprotective agent, glycerol, maintains viability for up to 10 years. Frozen red cells are used for creating repositories of units lacking high frequency red cells antigens for patients with antibodies against such phenotypes. Occasionally, autologous units are frozen to extend their availability beyond the normal dating period, for example, when a scheduled surgical procedure is postponed.

Autologous Transfusion

Autologous transfusion involves collection and subsequent reinfusion of a patient's own blood by one or a combination of techniques: preoperative blood donation, perioperative blood salvage, or acute normovolemic hemodilution. Preoperative collections begin, optimally, at least 2 weeks before a scheduled surgical procedure and are repeated as often as every 3 days provided the patient's hemoglobin level is greater than 11 g/dl. Procedures for which autologous predonation programs are likely to reduce allogeneic blood exposure include orthopedic, coronary artery bypass graft, and major vascular surgery; selected neurologic procedures; hepatic resections; and radical prostatectomy. Obstetric patients with placenta previa may also benefit. Overall, only 50% of predeposited autologous units are transfused to the patient/donor. Since unused autologous units are not made available for allogeneic transfusion, presurgical autologous blood donation should be restricted to patients likely to require a transfusion.

Perioperative blood salvage involves the collection and reinfusion of blood lost during and immediately after surgery. Instruments are available for washing blood for reinfusion. Intraoperative blood salvage is not used if the operative field is grossly contaminated with malignant cells or if bacteria are present, for example, from spillage of intestinal contents, bacterial peritonitis, abscesses, or osteomyelitis.

Acute normovolemic hemodilution involves removal of blood immediately before surgery with simultaneous infusion of crystalloid or colloid solutions to maintain vascular volume. After surgery the removed blood is reinfused. This option is not offered to patients with anemia, renal dysfunction, or limited ability to increase cardiac output.

Directed Donation

A directed or designated donation refers to blood provided by persons selected by the patient, usually family members or friends. Many patients believe such donations are less likely to transmit bloodborne infections than those from routine donors. However, available data do not support this hypothesis.

Compatibility Testing

Compatibility testing includes donor and recipient ABO and Rh determination; investigating patient samples for RBC alloantibodies; and, documentation and discrepancy resolution procedures. If no "unexpected" alloantibodies, for example, anti-Kell, anti-Kidd, anti-Duffy, are detected, donor blood with the same or compatible ABO and Rh type as the recipient and patient serum are centrifuged and then examined for agglutination or hemolysis. In the absence of these laboratory findings, ABO compatibility is assumed and the blood is released for transfusion. If "unexpected" antibodies are present, donor blood lacking the corresponding antigens is selected.

"Computerized" crossmatching provides an alternative approach to traditional compatibility testing. Rather than mix patient and donor samples, patient and donor test results are entered into a computer and electronic algorithms are used to ensure compatibility.

PLATELET TRANSFUSION

Platelet transfusions are prepared by separating platelets from whole blood (platelet concentrates) or by apheresis techniques using semiautomated blood cell separators (single donor platelets). Therapeutic doses are prepared by pooling 1 unit of platelet concentrates for each 12 kg of the recipient's body weight or by providing single donor platelets that are equivalent to approximately 6 units of pooled platelet concentrates. The ABO blood group of the platelet donor and recipient should be compatible, although this is not required. Compatibility testing is not performed routinely. The expected posttransfusion platelet count increment is approximately 50×10^9/L per transfusion.

Prophylactic platelet transfusions are used to prevent bleeding in patients with severe thrombocytopenia secondary to aplastic anemia, acute leukemia, or other disorders associated with megakaryocyte hypoproliferation. Several cancer chemotherapy protocols consider a platelet count less than 20×10^9/L as an indication for platelet transfusion. This may be appropriate in patients with severe mucositis, emesis, and other acute toxic effects of chemotherapy. However, stable patients tolerate platelet counts as low as 5 to 10×10^9/L without significant hemorrhage.

Patients undergoing surgical or invasive procedures are not considered at risk for significant microvascular bleeding if the platelet count is $>50 \times 10^9$/L and thrombocytopenia is the sole abnormality.

Platelet transfusion efficacy relates directly to the etiology of thrombocytopenia. Patients with bone marrow hypoplasia are most likely to benefit from platelet transfusions, whereas those with immune-mediated thrombocytopenia or processes that consume platelets, such as disseminated intravascular coagulation (DIC), are less likely to achieve significant posttransfusion platelet count increments.

Normally the spleen sequesters approximately one third of the circulating platelets. Achieving significant posttransfusion platelet count increments in patients with splenomegaly is difficult because an increased percentage of platelets pool in the enlarged spleen.

The posttransfusion platelet count obtained 10 to 60 minutes after transfusion provides information about platelet recovery. It is diminished in alloimmunized patients and those with splenomegaly and severe DIC. The 18- to 24-hour posttransfusion platelet count provides information about platelet survival and is decreased in patients with consumptive processes such as mild DIC, sepsis, fever, and other inflammatory states.

Alloimmunization and Refractoriness to Platelet Transfusion

Approximately one quarter of patients requiring long-term platelet support develop antibodies against HLA and/or platelet-specific antigens and become refractory to platelet transfusions. Fifty percent to sixty-five percent of platelet transfusions collected from donors who are HLA-matched to the patient or are found to be crossmatch compatible provide adequate posttransfusion platelet count increments.

Reducing the leukocyte content of platelets and red cells to less than 5×10^6 per transfusion significantly decreases the incidence of alloimmunization in patients not previously sensitized by transfusion or pregnancy. In addition, leukocyte reduction immediately after platelet concentrate collection reduces cytokine accumulation during storage that causes some "chill-fever" reactions. Antibodies against platelet and leukocyte alloantigens also cause febrile reactions and chills. As noted previously, the optimal timing of leukocyte reduction is under investigation.

PLASMA TRANSFUSION

Plasma separated from whole blood and frozen within 8 hours of collection contains all coagulation factors. Fresh frozen plasma (FFP) increases clotting factor levels in patients with demonstrated deficiencies and is used to correct such deficiencies when the prothrombin time is greater than 1.5 times the midpoint of the normal range or a partial thromboplastin time is greater than 1.5 times the upper limit of the normal range. FFP rapidly reverses the anticoagulant effect of warfarin but should be reserved for patients who are bleeding actively or require emergency surgery and cannot wait approximately 12 hours for the therapeutic effect of vitamin K. FFP is indicated for patients receiving massive blood transfusion replacement provided laboratory evidence supports a coagulation factor deficiency. FFP is the preferred replacement fluid for patients undergoing therapeutic plasma exchange therapy for thrombotic thrombocytopenic purpura. FFP is used also to treat deficiencies of factors II, V, VII, X, XI, or XIII. Clotting factor concentrates treated to inactivate viruses are available for replacing factors VIII and IX.

Dose calculations for FFP aim for 30% coagulation factor levels; usually 10 to 20 ml/kg body weight. If platelet transfusions are given concomitantly, the FFP dose should be revised to reflect the approximate 1 unit of plasma contained in 6 unit platelet pools. Some locations maintain liquid plasma inventories in addition to FFP. Liquid plasma, stored at 1 to 6° C, rather than -18° C, is relatively deficient in the labile coagulation factors, V and VIII.

Fibrinogen replacement for patients with hypofibrinogenemia is accomplished by giving 1 unit of cryoprecipitate/5 kg of body weight.

The FDA is currently evaluating viral inactivation of FFP by the solvent/detergent (S/D) method. Plasma subjected to S/D maintains coagulation factor activity and effectiveness in treating TTP. S/D inactivates enveloped viruses such as HIV and hepatitis B and C. However, economic considerations require pooling plasma from 2500 donors before addition of S/D. The increased number of donor exposures theoretically increases the risk of contamination with infectious agents.

GRANULOCYTE TRANSFUSION

Granulocyte transfusions are used infrequently because antibiotic therapy is effective, the length of neutropenia following chemotherapy has been decreased by hematopoietic growth factor administration, and the transfusion dose is relatively small compared with normal daily neutrophil production. However, some experimental programs address the latter issue by administering G-CSF to blood donors to

Table 76-1 Acute transfusion reactions

ADVERSE EFFECT	SIGNS/SYMPTOMS	APPROXIMATE FREQUENCY PER COMPONENT
Hemolytic reaction	Fever, fever and chills, nausea, vomiting, chest pain, facial flushing	1 : 12,000-33,000
Febrile, nonhemolytic reaction	Fever and chills, headache, chilliness, rigors 15 to 60 minutes after transfusion	RBCs 1 : 200 Platelets 1 : 3-20 transfusions
Transfusion-related lung injury	Dyspnea, cyanosis, cough, blood-tinged sputum, fever, pulmonary edema, hypoxemia within 4 hours of transfusion	1 : 5000
Allergic reactions	Hives, pruritus	1 : 30-100
Anaphylactic reactions	Apprehension, chest pain, facial flushing, urticaria, laryngeal edema, wheezing, dyspnea, hypotension	1 : 20,000-150,000

Bacterial sepsis	Severe chills, rigors, nausea vomiting, lethargy, fever, hypotention	RBCs 1 : 1,000,000
		Platelets
		  contamination 1 : 900-2000
		  clinical symptoms 1 : 2000-12,000

augment granulocyte counts and subsequent granulocyte yield. Neutropenic patients (absolute granulocyte count $<0.5 \times 10^9$/L) with documented sepsis not responsive to initial antibiotic therapy, who are likely to have a prolonged period of neutropenia, comprise the majority of patients receiving granulocyte transfusion. Transfusions are given daily for at least 4 days, until the infection is controlled, or there is evidence of granulocyte recovery.

THERAPEUTIC APHERESIS

Therapeutic apheresis involves the removal of plasma or blood cells for treatment of a disease process.

Plasma Exchange

Plasmapheresis combined with infusion of normal saline, plasma protein fraction, albumin, FFP, or a combination of these solutions is referred to as a plasma exchange procedure. A one–plasma volume exchange removes two thirds of the initial plasma in 2 to 3 hours. Procedures are repeated at 1 to 2 day intervals. Therapeutic plasma exchange is considered acceptable as a treatment modality for chronic inflammatory demyelinating polyneuropathy, cryoglobulinemia, Goodpasture's syndrome, Guillain-Barré syndrome, homozygous familial hypercholesterolemia, hyperviscosity syndrome, posttransfusion purpura, Refsum's disease, and thrombotic thrombocytopenic purpura.

Conditions for which plasma exchange therapy is reported to be beneficial as a second-line therapy include cold agglutinin disease, drug overdose and poisoning with protein-bound toxins, Eaton-Lambert syndrome, hemolytic uremic syndrome, pemphigus vulgaris, quinine/quinidine thrombocytopenia, rapidly progressive glomerulonephritis, and systemic vasculitis related to rheumatoid arthritis or systemic lupus erythematosus. Efficacy is not demonstrated conclusively for treatment of patients with many other conditions, including those where plasma exchange may be appropriate after other interventions have failed.

Cytapheresis

Cytapheresis involves the reduction of cellular blood components and is considered appropriate therapy for leukemia with hyperleukocytosis syndrome, peripheral blood progenitor cell collections for hematopoietic reconstitution, sickle cell syndromes (with the possible exception of prophylactic use in pregnancy), and systemic thrombocytosis. Cytapheresis is probably effective in the treatment of a cutaneous T-cell lymphoma and hyperparasitemia (e.g., fulminant malaria). Its efficacy is less certain when used for treating other disorders.

ADVERSE EFFECTS OF TRANSFUSION THERAPY
Acute Reactions

Acute reactions occur within minutes to hours after infusion of blood or components (Table 76-1). Significant overlap in presenting signs and symptoms necessitates the use of appropriate laboratory testing for making an accurate assessment.

Hemolytic Reactions. Fever (elevation of at least 2° F [1° C]) or fever and chills are seen in almost all patients with a hemolytic transfusion reaction. Severe reactions are manifest by shock, dyspnea, chest pain, back pain, headache, and/or coagulopathy. Anti-A, anti-B, anti-K, anti-Jk^a, anti-Jk^b, and anti-Fy^a, cause most severe hemolytic reactions. The pathophysiology involves generation of TNF, IL-1, and IL-8; and complement and Hageman factor activation. ABO-incompatible transfusions occur at an estimated frequency of 1 per 33,000 units. The mortality rate is 1 per 600,000 units. Most occur as a result of errors in clinical rather than laboratory areas.

If a hemolytic reaction is suspected, the infusion must be stopped immediately and the transfusion service notified to conduct a clerical check for determining whether the patient was given the intended unit. The laboratory investigation includes a direct antiglobulin test and examination of a postreaction serum or plasma sample for a pink or red tinge. The color change occurs because destruction of only 5 to 10 ml of RBCs renders a hemolytic hue to plasma. In addition, a urine specimen should be examined for the presence of free hemoglobin.

Acute interventions are directed at correction of hypotension with fluid administration, control of bleeding, and prevention of acute tubular necrosis. If vasopressors are needed, dopamine is preferred.

Febrile Nonhemolytic Reactions. These reactions are characterized by fever and chills without hemolysis. Some of the reactions are caused by antibodies against transfused lymphocytes, granulocytes, or platelets. The "threshold" leukocyte content for evoking a chill/fever reaction in susceptible patients is approximately 5×10^8 white cells per component. Passive infusion of cytokines produced during blood or platelet concentrate storage appears to be another etiologic factor. Since the initial manifestation of a hemolytic transfusion is similar to a chill/fever reaction, the transfusion should be discontinued and a laboratory evaluation for hemolysis initiated.

A diagnosis of a febrile nonhemolytic reaction is made on the basis of the clinical findings, the absence of hemoglobinemia, and a negative direct antiglobulin test in the postreaction specimen. Treatment consists of supportive measures, including orally administered antipyretics. Since only 15% of patients with a febrile reaction have a recurrence, components with reduced numbers of leukocytes are not provided until a second reaction occurs. Reactions attributed to cytokine infusion are prevented by prestorage leukocyte reduction or by washing to remove plasma containing cytokines.

Lung Injury. Passive infusion of antibodies against recipient leukocytes occasionally causes a noncardiogenic pulmonary edema–like syndrome. The patients require respiratory support, but recovery occurs usually within 48 hours.

Allergic Reactions. Hives and pruritus, and occasionally fever, occur after plasma-containing blood component infusions. Treatment with an antihistamine is usually sufficient to alleviate symptoms. Removal of plasma from RBCs and/or platelet transfusions by washing with saline is recommended for preventing recurrences in severely affected patients.

Anaphylactic reactions, mediated by anti-IgA antibody, require im-

Table 76-2   Delayed transfusion reactions

ADVERSE EFFECT	SIGNS/SYMPTOMS	APPROXIMATE FREQUENCY PER COMPONENT
Delayed hemolytic reaction	Anemia, fever, hemoglobinuria and/or jaundice 3 to 21 days after transfusion	Serologic: 1:1600-3000 Hemolytic: 1:5400-9000
Graft-versus-host disease	Fever, erythema, diarrhea, liver function abnormalities, pancyto-penia 4 to 30 days after transfusion	1:17,700-39,000
Iron overload	Endocrine, cardiac, and liver dysfunction	Chronically transfused patients (~120 units of blood)
Immunosuppression	Increased postoperative infection rate Increased recurrence rate after tumor resection	Unknown

mediate treatment with sympathomimetic drugs. If subsequent transfusions are required, cellular components should be washed to remove plasma.

Bacterial Sepsis. *Yersinia enterocolitica* and *Staphylococcus* are the primary pathogens contaminating red cells and platelets, respectively. Septic transfusions cause approximately nine deaths per year in the United States. When transfusion-associated sepsis is suspected, the transfusion should be discontinued immediately and not restarted. An aliquot should be examined for bacteria by appropriate staining and culture techniques; broad-spectrum antibiotics and supportive measures should be administered promptly.

Delayed Transfusion Reactions (Table 76-2)

Hemolytic Reactions. Delayed hemolytic transfusion reactions are the result of alloantibody-mediated RBC destruction by an antibody that was not detected by pretransfusion testing. Alloantibodies, usually a secondary or amnestic response, are produced 6 to 8 days (range: 3 to 21 days) after transfusion. Fortunately, the consequences of the reaction are not life-threatening, and only supportive therapy is required.

Graft-Versus-Host Disease. Graft-versus-host disease (GvHD) occurs when viable, infused T-lymphocytes recognize and react against recipient (host) tissues. The syndrome usually occurs in immunosuppressive clinical situations such as severe combined immunodeficiency and Wiscott-Aldrich syndrome; bone marrow transplantation; premature newborns and neonates undergoing exchange transfusion who previously received intrauterine transfusions; and patients undergoing chemotherapy for Hodgkin's disease, non-Hodgkin's lymphoma, acute leukemia, and neuroblastoma. Immunocompetent patients receiving transfusions from donors with closely matched HLA types (e.g., blood relatives) are at increased risk for transfusion-associated GvHD. The mortality rate is approximately 90%. Prevention is accomplished by exposing blood and components to 2500 cGy γ irradiation.

Iron Overload. Adult patients infused with 60 to 210 (mean, 120) units of blood may develop endocrine, cardiac, and liver dysfunction as a result of iron overload. Iron chelation therapy has been used successfully to decrease iron stores in some patients.

Immunosuppressive Effects. An increased frequency of cancer recurrence, a shorter disease-free interval after surgical resection of malignant tumor, and an increased incidence of postoperative infection have been reported in transfused patients. Investigations are ongoing to determine whether these postulated effects are related causally to transfusion, whether these effects can be prevented by removing leukocytes from infused blood components, and which patients are at highest risk for these events.

Transfusion-Transmitted Diseases (Table 76-3)

Hepatitis. Despite extensive testing, transfusion-associated hepatitis B occurs because hepatitis B surface (HbsAg) antigenemia is transient, some patients are infectious without antigenemia, and some viral variants are not recognized by current tests.

Testing for hepatitis B core antibody (anti-HBc) detects some do-

Table 76-3   Transfusion-transmitted infections/diseases

INFECTION/DISEASE	INFECTION RISK PER UNIT
Hepatitis A	Infrequent
Hepatitis B (56, 24-128 days)*	1:66,500
Hepatitis C (82, 54-192 days)	1:103,000
Hepatitis non-A,B,C	?
HIV - 1/2 (16, ?-32 days)	1:676,000
HTLV (51, 36-72 days)	1:641,000
Cytomegalovirus	Variable
Syphilis	Rare
Lyme disease	No transfusion-associated cases reported
Babesiosis	Infrequent
Malaria	1:4,000,000
Chagas' disease	Rare in North America
Creutzfeldt-Jacob disease (CJD)	No transfusion-associated cases reported

*Estimated length of seronegative window period and range in days is presented in parentheses.

nors infected chronically with hepatitis B who are hepatitis B surface antigen (HbsAg) negative or donors with acute hepatitis B who are in the "window period" between HbsAg disappearance and detectable hepatitis B surface antibody (anti-HBs).

In 1995, alanine aminotransferase (ALT) testing, a surrogate for detecting donors with non-A, non-B hepatitis, became optional as a result of the effectiveness of hepatitis C assays.

Infectious cases of transfusion-associated non-A,B,C hepatitis are emerging. Some may be related to a flavivirus, hepatitis G (HGV). Other cases may be caused by flaviviruses GBV-A/B or by hepatitis B detected only by HBV DNA.

Occasionally, patients with posttransfusion hepatitis A are reported. A carrier state does not occur; posttransfusion hepatitis A cases result from donations made during the acute, asymptomatic phase.

Retroviruses. The risk of transfusion-associated HIV infection decreased significantly after the introduction of HIV antibody testing in 1985 and subsequent improvements in donor screening and blood testing. Before introduction of HIV p24 antigen testing in January 1996, the HIV 1/2 antibody test "window period," that is, the time between HIV infection and HIV serodetection, was 22 to 25 days. HIV p24 antigen testing in combination with HIV 1/2 antibody testing reduced the "window" by approximately 6 days. The predicted result was a 25% decrease in HIV transmission (5 to 10 fewer infections) per year in the United States.

Human T-cell leukemia/lymphoma viruses I and II (HTLV-I, HTLV-II) are transforming retroviruses that cross-react serologically. Testing for these agents was introduced in December 1988. Approximately 40% to 60% of HTLV seropositive blood donors are infected with HTLV-II. Transmission of HTLV-I and HTLV-II by transfusion is restricted to cellular components. Current tests are more sensitive for HTLV-I detection than HTLV-II.

Cytomegalovirus. Immunocompetent patients rarely develop significant illness as a result of CMV infection through transfusion. However, CMV poses a risk for CMV-seronegative pregnant women because a primary CMV infection places the fetus at risk. Immuno-compromised patients at risk for a significant CMV infection include premature infants weighing less than 1200 g born to CMV-seronegative mothers, CMV-seronegative recipients of allogeneic bone marrow transplants from CMV-seronegative donors, and CMV-seronegative patients receiving renal, heart, liver, or lung transplants from CMV-seronegative donors.

Approximately 28% to 57% of CMV-seronegative marrow transplant recipients receiving standard blood components develop CMV infection. Approximately 30% become symptomatic with pneumonia, gastroenteritis, and other manifestations. CMV-seronegative screened blood reduces the incidence of infection to 1% to 4% in at risk patients. Third generation leukocyte reduction filters remove latently infected white cells. In one large, prospective, nonblinded, randomized trial, seronegative transplant patients receiving CMV seronegative marrow were given either CMV-seronegative or bedside-filtered blood components. There was no difference in CMV infection (1.3% versus 2.4%, respectively). Of note, CMV disease occurred in none of the seronegative blood recipients compared to 1.2% of those receiving filtered blood (p = 0.25). Seronegative blood appears to be the option of choice, but filtered blood is an acceptable substitute if seronegative components are not available. CMV transmission has not been reported after plasma or cryoprecipitate infusion.

Spirochete Infections. Syphilis is an extremely infrequent complication of blood transfusion as a result of donor screening, blood testing, and possibly the organism's lack of viability for more than 96 hours at 4° C. Transfusion-transmitted Lyme borreliosis has not been reported.

Parasitic Infections. The transfusion-transmitted malaria risk is 0.25 cases per million units of blood. Donations are not accepted from persons who travelled to malarious areas during the preceding 12 months; from residents of malaria endemic areas, or from those with a history of malaria until 3 years after leaving the endemic area and remaining asymptomatic. Transfusion-associated babesiosis is a potentially fatal complication in immunocompromised, asplenic, or elderly patients. Blood is not accepted from potential donors with a history of babesiosis.

Acute Chagas' disease (*Trypanosoma cruzi*) cases attributed to transfusion have been reported in North America. Transfusion-associated Chagas' disease is a longstanding problem in South America. Epidemiologic studies indicate blood donors from Chagas' disease endemic areas currently reside in the United States and may be parasitemic. These data may lead to changes in donor screening or blood testing procedures in the future.

Other Infections. Reports that a few blood donors later developed Creutzfeldt-Jakob disease (CJD) raised speculation about possible transmission of the etiologic prion by transfusion. Although there are no known transfusion-associated CJD cases, CJD has been transmitted by transplanted dura mater and corneas, and infected pituitary-derived growth hormone. Approximately 10% of CJD cases are familial. No laboratory tests are available for blood donor testing. In 1995, the Food and Drug Administration recommended that blood donors be questioned about a family history of CJD and whether they received dura mater transplants or pituitary-derived growth hormone. If affirmative answers are obtained, the donors are deferred and previous recipients are notified.

BIBLIOGRAPHY

Bowden RA et al: A comparison of filtered leukocyte-reduced and cytomegalovirus (CMV) seronegative blood products for the prevention of transfusion-associated CMV infection after marrow transplant, *Blood* 86:3598-3603, 1995.

Capon SM, Goldfinger D: Acute hemolytic transfusion reaction, a paradigm of the systemic inflammatory response: new insights into pathophysiology and treatment, *Transfusion* 35:513-520, 1995.

College of American Pathologists Taskforce: Practice parameter for the use of fresh-frozen plasma, cryoprecipitate, and platelets, *JAMA* 271:777-781, 1994.

Heddle NM et al: The role of the plasma from platelet concentrates in transfusion reactions, *N Engl J Med* 331:625-628, 1994.

Herbert PC et al: Transfusion requirements in critical care, *JAMA* 273:1439-1444, 1995.

Schreiber GB et al: Current risk of transfusion-transmitted viral infections and impact of new donor screening tests, *N Engl J Med* 334:1685-1690, 1996.

CHAPTER

77 Hematopoietic Stem Cell Transplantation

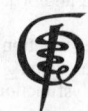

Frederick R. Appelbaum

Until recently, the term *bone marrow transplantation* was used to describe the process of transferring hematopoietic stem cells from one individual to another. With the recent demonstration that peripheral blood and umbilical cord blood can also be used as sources of stem cells, *hematopoietic stem cell transplantation* can be substituted as a more inclusive term.

The first suggestion that hematopoietic stem cell transplantation might be possible was made in 1949, when Leon Jacobson demonstrated that if a mouse spleen was shielded during total body irradiation, the otherwise lethal myelosuppressive effects of the radiation could be averted. Shortly thereafter, a similar radioprotective effect was demonstrated when bone marrow from one mouse was given intravenously to a radiated recipient of the same strain. By the mid-1950s, several laboratories, using cytogenetic markers, had shown that the radioprotective effect of spleen or marrow cells was accompanied by replacement of the original hematopoietic system of the host with cells of donor origin. The extent of replacement was shown to include all myeloid, lymphoid, and macrophage elements. The potential clinical implications of hematopoietic stem cell transplantation were immediately obvious, but the application of this technique had to await a better understanding of the major histocompatibility complex in humans and the development of improved methods of intensive supportive care. Advances in both these areas have been accompanied by a steady increase in the number of long-term healthy recipients of stem cell transplants and the application of this approach to an increased number of diseases.

INDICATIONS

Hematopoietic stem cell transplantation has been used to treat a variety of nonmalignant and malignant diseases.

Immunodeficiency States

Transplantation can successfully establish a normal immune system in infants with all forms of severe combined immunodeficiency. Similarly, the lymphoid and platelet abnormalities of the lethal sex-linked disorder, the Wiskott-Aldrich syndrome, can be corrected with transplantation.

Nonmalignant Disorders of Hematopoiesis

Patients with acquired severe aplastic anemia can achieve long-term survival in 70% of cases if previously transfused or 80% if not transfused. Similarly, transplantation can cure more than 70% of children with β-thalassemia and has been successfully used as treatment for sickle cell anemia, other hereditary hemoglobinopathies, and various congenital aregenerative anemias.

Enzymatic Disorders

Hematopoietic stem cell transplantation has been used to provide patients with normal enzyme systems in such disorders as the mucopolysaccharidoses and Gaucher's disease.

Malignant Diseases

Patients with acute myelogenous leukemia or acute lymphoblastic leukemia in relapse after failure of combination chemotherapy or in blastic crisis of chronic myelogenous leukemia can still be cured in 10%

to 30% of cases with transplantation. If transplantation is carried out earlier in the course of these diseases, the results are better. For patients with acute myelogenous leukemia or acute lymphoblastic leukemia in first remission or chronic myelogenous leukemia in the chronic phase, 5-year disease-free survival is seen in at least 55% of cases. Transplantation has been successfully applied to patients with myelodysplastic syndromes, non-Hodgkin's lymphoma, Hodgkin's disease, chronic lymphocytic leukemia, hairy cell leukemia, myelofibrosis, multiple myeloma, and neuroblastoma. Experimental studies are being conducted in patients with other chemosensitive tumors such as breast cancer.

Source of Hematopoietic Stem Cells

Hematopoietic stem cells used for transplantation can be categorized according to the relationship between the donor and the recipient, or according to their anatomic source.

Donor Selection

Hematopoietic stem cells used for transplantation can be categorized as autologous, syngeneic, or allogeneic. With *autologous* transplantation, a portion of the patient's own stem cells are removed, the patient is treated with intensive chemotherapy and/or radiotherapy, and the patient's stem cells are reinfused. Autologous transplantation has generally been used as a means of treating patients for malignancies with higher doses of chemoradiotherapy than would normally be tolerated. *Syngeneic* transplantation refers to transplantation of stem cells from a normal genetically identical twin. *Allogeneic* transplantation is transplantation of hematopoietic stem cells from a normal genetically different donor.

Most allogeneic transplants have been performed between siblings with identical human leukocyte antigens (HLA). HLA identity implies identity for HLA-A and HLA-B, as determined by serotyping, and identity for HLA-D, as demonstrated by either cellular techniques such as mixed leukocyte culture (MLC), or, what is now currently used, molecular techniques such as sequence-specific oligonucleotide probe (SSOP) hybridization (Chapter 172). The HLA genes are located on chromosome 6. Because their products are codominantly expressed, the chance that any two siblings will be HLA identical is one in four. Because patients have an average of slightly more than one sibling, the chances that a matched sibling can be identified for any one patient are 30% to 40%. Efforts to expand the donor pool include using donors who are genotypically identical for one HLA haplotype but only partially matched for the other. In general, survival following allogeneic transplantation from a family member donor mismatched with the patient for a single A, B, or D locus results in survival similar to that seen with a fully matched sibling, but survival following transplantation using family member donors mismatched for two or three antigens has been significantly worse.

Donors who are totally unrelated to the patient but are matched for HLA-A, HLA-B, and HLA-D have been used with promising results. The formation of a National Bone Marrow Donor Registry has led to an increase in the use of matched unrelated donors. Currently, more than 1,700,000 normal individuals have volunteered to serve as marrow donors in the United States alone. The odds of finding an A, B, and D matched unrelated donor are now approximately 50%. Major ABO incompatibility is not a barrier to successful transplantation. However, to avoid hemolysis, incompatible red blood cells must be removed from the stem cell inoculum by centrifugation or sedimentation, or alternatively, isoagglutinins must be removed from the patient's blood by immunoadsorption or plasma exchange.

Anatomic Sources of Hematopoietic Cells

Because bone marrow is rich in hematopoietic stem cells, it has in the past been the usual site from which stem cells have been harvested for transplantation. Marrow is usually obtained from the donor's anterior and posterior iliac crests using standard aspiration needles with the donor under general or spinal anesthesia. To obtain as many marrow cells with as little peripheral blood contamination as possible, each aspirate site is limited to 3 to 5 ml. Approximately 10 to 15 ml of marrow per kilogram body weight is obtained, so for

a normal adult male donor this means 700 to 900 ml of marrow and 100 to 200 aspirations. The marrow is placed in heparinized tissue culture media and then filtered through screens of 0.30- and 0.20-mm diameter to remove bony spicules and fat globules. The marrow is then either cryopreserved for later autologous transplantation or, in the case of allogeneic transplantation, taken to the patient's room and infused intravenously. In certain experimental studies the marrow may be treated before infusion, for example, to test whether removal of T-cells from the marrow can prevent graft-versus-host disease (GvHD) or whether tumor cells can be removed from marrow before autologous transplantation. The risk associated with marrow donation is small; among 1220 marrow donations in Seattle, no fatal complications were seen, but six serious complications occurred (three cardiopulmonary, two infectious, one cerebrovascular accident). Although small, this risk must be weighed carefully when considering the use of matched unrelated donors.

Hematopoietic stem cells circulate in the peripheral blood, although in very small numbers. During recovery from chemotherapy-induced cytopenias or after exposure to hematopoietic growth factors such as granulocyte-macrophage or granulocyte colony-stimulating factor (GM or G-CSF), the number of hematopoietic stem cells in the peripheral blood increases dramatically. With the use of these mobilizing techniques followed by leukapheresis, it is possible to collect sufficient numbers of stem cells from the peripheral blood for transplantation. Because peripheral blood has a higher proportion of T-cells than marrow, the first trials of peripheral blood stem cell (PBSC) transplantation took place in the setting of autologous transplantation where graft-versus-host disease was not a concern. These studies demonstrated that PBSC transplantation not only was possible, but resulted in much faster engraftment than seen using marrow. Recent pilot studies of the use of G-CSF mobilized PBSC for allogeneic transplantation between matched siblings suggest that this may be possible without a marked increase in the incidence of acute GvHD despite transfusing at least 1 log more T-cells.

Umbilical cord blood has been shown to be rich in hematopoietic stem cells and has been used successfully as a source of stem cells for transplantation. Cord blood has relatively few mature T-cells and, as a consequence, the risk of GvHD with cord blood appears somewhat less than with marrow, while the risk of graft rejection may be somewhat greater.

PREPARATIVE REGIMEN

The form of treatment administered to the patient directly before transplantation depends on the disease being treated. Patients with severe combined immunodeficiency often require no pretransplant therapy because there is no malignant cell population to eradicate and the patients are, by the nature of their disease, so immunoincompetent that they rarely reject the infused marrow. In other patients who are relatively immunocompetent, the preparative regimen must be immunosuppressive enough to prevent the patient from rejecting the marrow. In treating a patient for aplastic anemia where there is no malignancy to eradicate, high-dose cyclophosphamide is often used as the preparative regimen. When transplantation is applied to the treatment of leukemia or other malignancy, the regimen must be both immunosuppressive and capable of eradicating the malignancy. In these patients, other forms of therapy (e.g., high-dose total body irradiation) or chemotherapeutic agents (e.g., busulfan) are added to cyclophosphamide for their cytotoxic effects. Hematopoietic stem cells are generally transplanted 24 to 48 hours after the completion of the preparative regimen.

ENGRAFTMENT

After the preparative regimen and stem cell transplantation, a period of profound myelosuppression ensues. Within 1 to 2 weeks of transplant, however, the peripheral leukocyte count begins to increase, signifying engraftment (Fig. 77-1). If bone marrow is the source of stem cells, the granulocyte count reaches 0.1×10^9/L in about 16 days and 1.0×10^9/L by about day 26. The platelet count recovers simultaneously with or shortly after recovery of granulocytes. Administration of GM-CSF can accelerate the recovery of peripheral granulocyte counts by as much as 1 week. If growth factor mobilized PB-

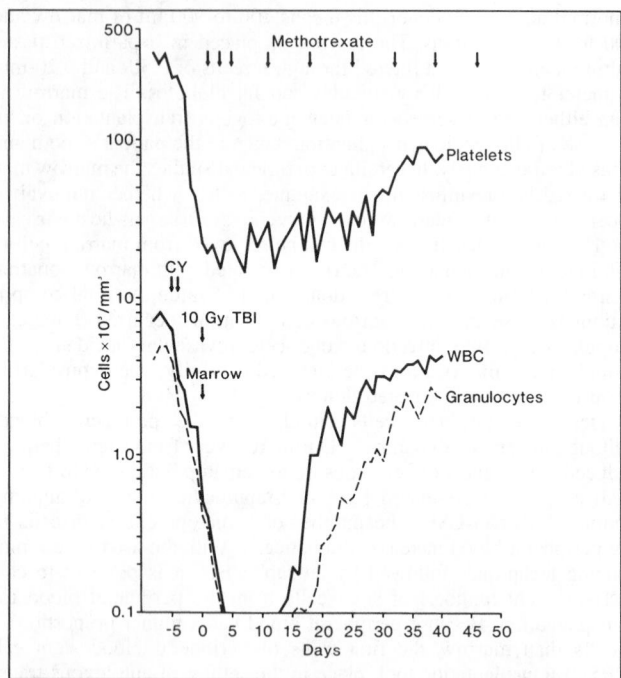

FIGURE 77-1   Peripheral blood cell counts of a patient treated for acute leukemia with cyclophosphamide, total body irradiation, and marrow transplantation from an HLA-identical sibling. Platelet transfusions were administered from day 3 through day 24; methotrexate was given in an effort to reduce or prevent graft-versus-host disease.

SCs are used instead of marrow, granulocyte and platelet recovery can be expected by day 12 to 14. Engraftment of allogeneic marrow can be documented using cytogenetic techniques or red cell antigens and isoenzymes. Cytogenetics is most easily done when donor and recipient are of different sexes. When they are of the same sex, unique chromosomal polymorphisms can be identified by banding techniques, thus allowing for the identification of chromosomes as being of host or donor origin in approximately half of same-sex donor-recipient pairs. With the use of deoxyribonucleic acid (DNA) restriction fragment length polymorphisms (RFLP) or using an analysis of variable nucleotide tandem repeats (VNTR), the origin of a population of cells can now be determined in virtually all cases. Molecular markers are discussed in Chapter 73. Polymorphic red cell enzymes can be used to monitor engraftment provided the patient has not received recent red cell transfusions.

COMPLICATIONS
Graft Rejection

In some patients the transplanted stem cell graft functions briefly, but after a period of days or weeks, marrow function is lost, and myeloid elements are absent on marrow biopsy. In most patients, graft rejection is thought to be the result of residual host immunity to the donor. Graft rejection occurring in recipients of HLA-identical marrow is thought to be the result of the patient having been sensitized to unshared non-HLA antigens of the donor by prior transfusions. Among recipients of HLA- identical marrow, graft rejection is seen most often when the patient has received prior transfusions and when the preparative regimen is less immunosuppressive, such as with the use of cyclophosphamide alone before transplantation for aplastic anemia. If patients are not transfused or if total body irradiation is used, graft rejection occurs less frequently.

Graft-Versus-Host Disease

GvHD is thought to be the result of allogeneic T-cells that were transfused with the graft or developed from it and reacted against targets of the genetically different host. Acute GvHD develops within the first 3 months of transplantation and presents with characteristic lesions of the skin, liver, and gastrointestinal tract. An erythematous maculopapular skin rash that favors the palms and soles is usually the first sign of GvHD (Color Plate IV-3). This is followed by diarrhea, often with abdominal pain and ileus, and liver disease characterized by rises in bilirubin, transaminases, and alkaline phosphatase. Pathologic features include lymphocytic and monocytic infiltration into perivascular spaces in the dermis and the dermoepidermal junction of the skin, into the epithelium of the oropharynx, tongue, and esophagus, into the base of the intestinal crypts of the small and large bowel, and into the periportal areas of the liver with secondary necrosis of cells in infiltrated tissues. In animal models, immunosuppressive therapy given immediately after transplantation can diminish or prevent GvHD, and based on these studies, in the past most patients were treated after transplantation with methotrexate. Despite methotrexate prophylaxis, 20% to 50% of patients receiving HLA-identical marrow from family member donors developed acute GvHD, and 20% to 40% of those died of GvHD and/or associated infections.

Other immunosuppressive agents such as steroids, antithymocyte globulin, or cyclosporine have also been used in attempts to prevent GvHD. Randomized trials have shown that cyclosporine is as effective as methotrexate and that the use of both agents in combination is more effective than the use of either agent alone. With the combination of methotrexate and cyclosporine, significant acute GvHD develops in only about 30% of HLA-identical transplants and lethal acute GvHD is the exception, occurring in fewer than 10% of patients. The incidence of acute GvHD is higher in older individuals and in recipients of partially matched or unrelated transplants. Another approach to prevention of acute GvHD, based on animal studies, is removal of T-cells from donor marrow. While this approach is effective in reducing the incidence of GvHD, it has also been associated with an increased incidence of graft rejection and recurrence of malignant disease.

Methods of treating established acute GvHD have included prednisone, antithymocyte globulin, cyclosporine, cyclophosphamide, and monoclonal antibodies against T-cells. Responses have been seen with each, but no one approach has yet been shown to be superior.

Chronic GvHD affects 20% to 40% of patients surviving more than 6 months after transplantation and resembles a collagen vascular disease, with skin changes that include malar erythema, sclerodermatous changes, and cutaneous ulcers, alopecia, sicca syndrome, polyserositis, and liver dysfunction characterized by bile duct degeneration and cholestasis. Two factors that are closely associated with the development of chronic GvHD are increasing age and a preceding episode of acute GvHD. Prednisone alone or in combination with either azathioprine or cyclophosphamide is effective in controlling chronic GvHD in 50% to 70% of patients. Thalidomide results in a complete response in 30% of patients not responsive to conventional therapy. Patients with chronic GvHD are susceptible to bacterial infections and should receive antibiotic prophylaxis (see later discussion).

Infectious Complications

The first 2 or 3 weeks after transplantation are complicated by severe granulocytopenia, fever, and in about 50% of patients, at least one episode of bacteremia. Therefore at virtually all transplant centers, febrile granulocytopenic patients are treated empirically with broad-spectrum antibiotics, and in many centers, antibiotics are begun once patients become granulocytopenic, even if afebrile. Fungal infections also occur often among this group of patients. The use of fluconazole prophylaxis reduces the incidence of both superficial and invasive fungal infections. Patients who become or remain febrile despite broad-spectrum antibiotics and have no obvious source of infection are usually treated with amphotericin. Both prophylactic granulocyte transfusions and laminar airflow isolation have been demonstrated to be effective in preventing early infections, but neither has been shown to affect survival. With current methods of supportive care, the risk of death from infection during the early granulocytopenic posttransplant period is about 5%.

Herpes simplex (HSV) infection can contribute to the severity of early oral mucositis and in some patients can result in esophagitis, bronchopneumonia, and rarely, encephalitis. Systemic acyclovir, 250

✔ *WHEN TO REFER*

On encountering a patient who may be a candidate for a stem cell transplant, the physician should contact a transplant center as soon as possible. The center can provide the physician with valuable information about the relative risks and benefits of transplantation, the process by which a donor can be identified, and the mechanism of transferring the patient for transplantation. For patients with nonmalignant disorders, stem cell grafting should be considered early in the course of disease before multiple transfusions have been given. Transfusions from family members should especially be avoided because of the increased risk of graft rejection. For patients with leukemia, the best results have also been obtained if transplantation is carried out early in the course of disease.

The ultimate choice of whether and when to undergo transplantation rests with the patient. Therefore the physician is obligated to provide the patient and family with up-to-date, reliable information to help in making the decision.

mg/m² every 8 hours intravenously, is highly effective in the treatment of established HSV infection after marrow transplantation. If used as prophylaxis starting 1 week before transplant and continuing for 4 weeks after transplant, acyclovir can prevent HSV reactivation in more than 90% of seropositive patients.

If patients have detectable antibody to cytomegalovirus (CMV) before transplantation, in 50% to 75% of cases the virus can be recovered from the throat, urine, or stool during the first 100 days after transplant. In approximately 50% of these patients, CMV reactivation is asymptomatic, but in the other 50%, reactivation of CMV is followed by the development of CMV pneumonia or CMV gastrointestinal disease. In the past, CMV pneumonia occurred in about 15% of patients receiving an allogeneic marrow transplant and had a case fatality rate of 80%. Primary CMV infection in patients with no detectable antibody to CMV before transplant can be prevented by the sole use of CMV-seronegative blood products or by the use of blood products that have been filtered to remove all leukocytes. In patients with antibody to CMV before transplant, the use of prophylactic ganciclovir, starting either at the time of initial engraftment or at the time of CMV reactivation, can substantially reduce the risk of CMV disease. Recently it has been shown that transfusing the patient posttransplant with CMV-specific cytotoxic T-cells isolated from the donor and expanded in vitro can restore CMV immunity in the patient and protect against CMV-mediated disease.

Pneumonia caused by *Pneumocystis carinii,* although previously a problem seen in 5% to 10% of transplant recipients, can be prevented by treating patients with oral trimethoprim-sulfamethoxazole for 1 week before transplant and resuming treatment 2 days per week once the granulocyte count exceeds 0.5×10^9/L.

Late infections (more than 3 months after the transplant) are usually caused by varicella-zoster virus (VZV) or, in patients with chronic GvHD, recurrent bacterial or fungal infections. The use of prophylactic trimethoprim-sulfamethoxazole and/or penicillin can reduce the incidence of late bacterial infections.

Chemoradiotherapy Toxicities

After the standard cyclophosphamide–total body irradiation preparative regimen, the immediate toxicities include nausea, vomiting, fever, parotitis, and mild skin erythema. Unusual toxicities associated with high-dose cyclophosphamide include hemorrhagic cystitis and, rarely, acute hemorrhagic carditis. Five to 7 days after total body irradiation most patients develop oral mucositis, and by 2 weeks most patients have developed complete but reversible alopecia. Also by this time, all patients are profoundly pancytopenic, with the resultant risks of bleeding and infection.

Venoocclusive disease (VOD) of the liver can be seen within 1 to 4 weeks of transplantation and presents with ascites, tender hepatomegaly, and jaundice. VOD is seen in approximately 10% of transplant recipients and is fatal in one third of these. Patients with abnormal liver function before transplant have a higher incidence of VOD.

Idiopathic interstitial pneumonia, which is thought to be a direct chemoradiotoxicity, is seen in 5% to 10% of patients between 30 and 90 days after transplant. The disease has an approximately 50% case fatality rate; no clearly effective therapy exists. Increasing age, preexisting lung disease, and prior exposure to chest radiotherapy increase the incidence of this complication, whereas the use of fractionated instead of single-dose irradiation decreases its incidence.

Late complications attributable to the cyclophosphamide–total body irradiation preparative regimen include decreased growth velocity in children and delayed development of secondary sex characteristics. Most postpubertal women develop ovarian failure, and few men regain spermatogenesis. Approximately 40% of patients develop cataracts within 2 years of transplantation, although this incidence may be less if fractionated irradiation is used. Thyroid dysfunction, usually well compensated, has been reported as well.

BIBLIOGRAPHY

Barrett AJ, Horowitz MM, Pollock BH et al: Bone marrow transplants from HLA-identical siblings as compared with chemotherapy for children with acute lymphoblastic leukemia in a second remission, *N Eng J Med.* 19:1253-1258, 1994.

Bearman SI: The syndrome of hepatic veno-occlusive disease after marrow transplantation, *Blood* 85:3005-3020, 1995.

Bensinger WI, Weaver CH, Appelbaum FR et al: Transplantation of allogeneic peripheral blood stem cells mobilized by recombinant human granulocyte colony-stimulating factor, *Blood* 85:1655-1658, 1995.

Biggs JC, Horowitz MM, Gale RP et al: Bone marrow transplants may cure patients with acute leukemia never achieving remission with chemotherapy, *Blood* 80(4):1090, 1992.

Buckner CD, Clift RA, Appelbaum FR et al: Treatment of chronic myeloid leukemia by marrow transplantation, *Blood* 82:1954, 1993 (editorial).

Crawford SW, Hackman RC: Clinical course of idiopathic pneumonia after marrow transplantation, *Am Rev Respir Dis* 147:1393-1400, 1993.

Ferrara JLM, Deeg HJ: Graft-versus-host disease, *N Engl J Med* 324:667-674, 1991.

Gahrton G, Tura S, Ljungman P et al: Allogeneic bone marrow transplantation in multiple myeloma, *N Engl J Med* 325:1267-1273, 1991.

Goodman JL, Winston DJ, Greenfield RA et al: A controlled trial of fluconazole to prevent fungal infections in patients undergoing bone marrow transplantation, *N Engl J Med* 326:845-851, 1992.

Goodrich JM, Bowden RA, Fisher L et al: Ganciclovir prophylaxis to prevent cytomegalovirus disease after allogeneic marrow transplant, *Ann Intern Med* 118:173-178, 1993.

Kernan NA, Bartsch G, Ash RC et al: Analysis of 462 transplantations from unrelated donors facilitated by The National Marrow Donor Program, *N Engl J Med* 328:593-602, 1993.

Lucarelli G, Galimberti M, Polchi P et al: Marrow transplantation in patients with Thalassemia responsive to iron chelation therapy, *N Engl J Med* 329:840-844, 1993.

Philip T, Guglielmi C, Hagenbeek A et al: Autologous bone marrow transplantation as compared with salvage chemotherapy in relapses of chemotherapy-sensitive non-Hodgkin's lymphoma, *N Eng J Med* 333(23):1540, 1995.

Wagner JE, Kernan NA, Steinbuch M et al: Allogeneic sibling umbilical-cord-blood transplantation in children with malignant and non-malignant disease, *Lancet* 346:214-219, 1995.

Zittoun R, Mandelli F, Willemze R et al: Prospective phase III study of autologous bone marrow transplantation (ABMT) v. short intensive chemotherapy (IC) v. allogeneic bone marrow transplantation (ALLO-BMT) during first complete remission (CR) of acute myelogenous leukemia (AML): results of the EORTC-GIMEMA AML 8A trial, *N Engl J Med* 332:217-223, 1995.

CHAPTER

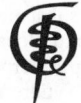

78   Complications of Cancer and Cancer Therapy

Sara L. Zaknoen

Cancer is the clinical consequence of unregulated cell proliferation. Because nearly every cell in the body retains some proliferative potential, from those with high proliferative potential such as bone marrow and the gastrointestinal (GI) tract to those of low proliferative potential such as neuronal tissue, every organ system is at risk for the development of cancer. The clinical manifestations of cancer are legion. Complications resulting from cancer and cancer therapy can be as inconsequential as the surgical removal of a small basal cell carcinoma to the life-threatening complications and management challenges of acute leukemia. For detailed information about specific cancers, the reader is referred to the appropriate chapters in this text. This chapter deals with the complications of cancer and its therapy in two parts. The first is a symptom-oriented approach to the problems faced by patients, and the second, a more specific discussion of toxicities from paraneoplastic syndromes and cancer treatments with chemotherapeutic agents and radiation.

PAIN

Pain is perhaps the most feared symptom when a diagnosis of cancer is made. The advances made in understanding the pathophysiology of pain have not translated into optimal control of pain, especially in cancer patients. Patients, patients' families, and physicians bring to the situation a host of personal, cultural, and emotional factors that must be taken into consideration when assessing and planning treatment to alleviate pain in the cancer patient. The diagnosis of breast cancer in a woman may call to mind memories of her grandmother dying with painful bony metastases. She may fear that this is the fate in store for her. Fear of addiction to narcotic analgesics may keep a patient from adequately controlling his or her pain by not taking the medications as prescribed.

Other barriers to the optimal management of cancer pain may relate to inadequate knowledge of pain management and poor assessment of pain on the part of health care professionals. The physician may have concerns about prescribing controlled substances, including fear of patient addiction and tolerance and concern about side effects of narcotic analgesics. Overcoming these barriers by involving the patient and family in the development of the treatment plan and education about pain and its management is the greatest reassurance that the physician can give that the patient's pain will be well controlled with minimal side effects.

Cancer pain may be due to a number of causes, including tumor progression and related pathology, operations and other diagnostic and therapeutic procedures, toxicities of chemotherapy and radiation, infection, and pain unrelated to the malignancy or its treatment. The clinician treating cancer patients requires a thorough understanding of the pathophysiology of pain. Frequent reevaluation of the patient's pain status is necessary to separate cancer-related pain from unrelated pain and detect new, potentially morbid occurrences such as pulmonary embolism or pathologic fractures.

The sensation of pain is relayed through the peripheral and central nervous system to higher centers, where the individual perceives that a painful event has occurred. Peripheral mediators of pain include substances released as part of the inflammatory response and form the rationale for the clinical use of nonsteroidal antiinflammatory drugs (NSAIDs). These substances include prostaglandins, bradykinin, histamine, serotonin, and substance P. NSAIDs such as aspirin and ibuprofen block the enzyme cyclooxyogenase. This inhibits the conversion of the arachidonic acid found in the phospholipid bilayer of cell membranes into prostaglandins, thereby decreasing the inflammatory response and the release of mediators of pain, especially when inflammation is present. Steroids such as prednisone and dexamethasone have also been found to decrease local inflammation and can often be used in low doses as adjuncts to other analgesics in the relief of pain from inflammatory lesions and bony metastases. Treatment with the topical agent capsaicin is based on the local release of substance P from sensory nerve terminals. Capsaicin initially produces a burning pain as a result of enhanced release of substance P but ultimately relieves pain through depletion of this peptide locally. Capsaicin has been shown to be effective in the relief of postherpetic neuralgia and postmastectomy and postthoracotomy pain syndromes.

Local painful stimuli are conducted through the afferent limb of the system into the spinal cord, where they synapse with cells in the dorsal root ganglion. In the dorsal horn, neurotransmitters that are produced locally activate nociceptive spinal neurons. Ascending fibers originating from these nociceptive neurons terminate in numerous areas of the brain stem and thalamus. A number of peptides and excitatory amino acids have been postulated to function as probable neurotransmitters, including adenosine triphosphate, aspartate, calcitonin gene-related peptide, cholecystokinin, glutamate, neuropeptide Y, substance P, and vasoactive intestinal polypeptide. Other substances

within the dorsal horn serve as inhibitory mediators. Endogenous opioids such as enkephalin, as well as exogenously administered opioids such as morphine, block the release of these excitatory neurotransmitters and suppress the transmission of pain within the region of the dorsal horn. Opioid analgesics perform the lion's share of work in relieving moderate to severe cancer pain. Other drugs that act outside the pain-conducting system but are effective in treating cancer pain syndromes include the tricyclic antidepressants, which are effective for chronic neuropathic pain. Antidepressives and anxiolytics help relieve the heightened anxiety in patients that can increase the perception of pain.

The previously mentioned classes of drugs, including NSAIDs, steroids, opioids, tricyclics, and neuroleptics, as well as topical capsaicin, have been organized by the World Health Organization (WHO) into a three-step analgesic ladder in which opioids are added to nonopioid analgesics with or without other adjuvant drugs such as neuroleptics or steroids in a stepwise manner until the patient is free of pain and the side effects are at a minimum.

For mild to moderate pain, the initial drugs used are members of the NSAID group, including acetaminophen, ibuprofen, indomethacin, and aspirin. The drugs are available primarily in oral form; however, rectal suppositories of indomethacin are now available. Ketorolac (Toradol), an NSAID available as an intramuscular injection and recently approved for intravenous use, is also available for acute pain with an inflammatory component. All of the nonsteroidal drugs share gastritis and GI tract toxicity as their major side effects, and patients should be watched closely for side effects including gastritis, duodenitis, and the development of gastric ulcers. When adequate doses of NSAIDs—with or without adjuvant analgesics—no longer control pain, the next step is the addition of an opioid analgesic. Morphine serves as the prototype drug of this class. When given subcutaneously, intravenously, or intramuscularly at a 10-mg dose, it reaches its peak effect at approximately 30 minutes to 1 hour and has a duration of effect of 3 to 6 hours. All other opioid drugs are dosed in quantities sufficient to give the same analgesia as 10 mg of morphine and exhibit a similar duration of effect (Table 78-1). Regimens of weaker opioids including codeine, oxycodone, and hydrocodone are often begun initially, and in conjunction with an NSAID can control moderate pain quite well. It is important to accurately calculate doses when switching from oral to intramuscular or intravenous forms of these drugs and when switching from weaker to stronger opioids.

Special attention should be given to methadone, which has a much longer half-life (from 15 to more than 150 hours) than other drugs of its class. The duration of analgesia is not prolonged. However, in the face of repeated dosing or in patients with renal dysfunction, accumulation of the drug may cause toxic effects such as excessive sedation and respiratory depression. The use of meperidine (Demerol) is not recommended for the management of cancer pain. Accumulation of its active metabolite (normeperidine) causes central nervous system (CNS) irritability and may lead to seizures. This problem is exacerbated in patients with renal dysfunction.

The major drugs in the weak and strong opiate classes are available in oral, intravenous, intramuscular, and now transdermal preparations. When possible, the oral route is preferred. Sustained-release preparations of morphine now available with durations of action of 8 to 12 hours allow for decreased frequency of dosing and free the patient from cyclic episodes of increasing pain resulting from the short duration of action. A common strategy is a dose of sustained-release morphine given every 12 hours, which is adequate to control pain but leaves the patient able to go about his or her daily activities. Doses of immediate-release morphine are given on an as-needed basis if the patient has exacerbations of pain in association with activities or procedures. If patients are unable to tolerate oral formulations of drugs, fentanyl is available in a transdermal formulation lasting 72 hours.

As patients become unable to take oral medication or in patients who are unable to swallow, intramuscular and intravenous doses of drugs given on a schedule that provides sustained analgesia should be instituted. Continuous infusions of morphine and hydromorphone and patient-controlled analgesia with pump devices are helpful. Other formulations available to patients unable to swallow pills include sublingual, elixir, and suppository forms of morphine. It is important to educate patients and family members on the side effects of the narcotic

Table 78-1   Opioid analgesics used in cancer pain

DRUG	ROUTE	EQUIANALGESIC DOSE TO 10 MORPHINE (MG)	FREQUENCY (HOURS)	COMMENT
Morphine	PO	30-60	q 3-4	
Morphine, sustained release (MS Contin, Oramorph)	PO	60-120	q 12	
Morphine	SQ/IM/IV	10	q 2-4	
Hydromorphone (Dilaudid)	PO/PR	7.5	q 3-4	
	SQ/IM/IV	1.5	q 2-4	
Levorphanol (Levo-Dromoran)	PO	4	q 6-8	Drug accumulation may occur
	IV/IM	2	q 6-8	
Methadone (Dolophine)	PO	20	q 6-8	Drug accumulation may occur
	IV/IM	10	q 6-8	
Meperidine (Demerol)	PO	300	q 2-3	Not recommended due to central nervous system toxicity
	IV/IM	100	q 3	
Fentanyl	TD	0.1	q 72	
	IV/IM	0.1	q 2-3	
Codeine	PO	200	q 3-4	
	IV/IM	130	q 3-4	
Oxycodone	PO	30	q 3-4	Parenteral formulation not available
Hydrocodone	PO	30	q 3-4	Available in fixed combinations with aspirin or acetominephen

IM, Intramuscular; *IV*, intravenous; *PO*, oral; *PR*, per rectum; *q*, every; *SQ*, subcutaneous; *TD*, transdermal.

analgesics. These include sedation, respiratory depression, nausea, vomiting, and constipation. Patients receiving long-term narcotic analgesic therapy should also be placed on an effective bowel regimen to prevent constipation that may lead to bowel obstruction and unnecessary hospitalization. Tolerance to narcotic analgesics develops and can be countered by slowly increasing the doses of the same drug or by changing to equally potent doses of different analgesic drugs. The addition of other drugs, including low doses of steroids, neuroleptics, or anxiolytics, may also control pain without increasing doses of narcotics. What is important for the physician to remember is that the size of the dose should not be the primary concern as long as the therapeutic/toxic ratio remains high and the patient's pain is well controlled.

In addition to pain management with nonnarcotic and narcotic analgesics and other adjuvant drugs, various ablative and invasive therapies have been used with success. These include nerve blocks, such as a celiac plexus block that is used to relieve the pain in pancreatic cancer, epidural blocks, dorsal rhizotomy, and cordotomy. These neurosurgical methods may be effective in patients with well-defined, localized pain but in general have limited application.

The use of drug therapy must go hand in hand with the psychologic support of patients and family during an often very stressful period of illness. Education is often the most potent analgesic when patients realize that their pain will be relieved. Referrals to appropriate counseling centers, including group therapy, support groups, and individual counseling, help many patients and families. Nonpharmacologic modalities such as hypnosis, biofeedback, and meditation have been reported to be helpful in controlling cancer pain. Appropriate diagnosis of depression and anxiety with treatment is also important. The patient with cancer pain provides the opportunity for the physician to combine the science of medicine with the art of medicine. Skillful diagnosis of acute and chronic pain with appropriate treatment, along with a team approach to the education and management of patients and their families, should be at the core of pain management care in cancer patients. Physicians should follow a stepwise process of drug treatment beginning with NSAIDs and adding weak and then strong opiates with the adjuvant use of such drugs as low-dose steroids, tricyclic antidepressants, and neuroleptic drugs. Physicians should remember that the simple act of sitting, listening, and holding a patient's hand in reassurance can go a long way toward relieving the pain of cancer.

NAUSEA AND VOMITING

Nausea and vomiting is second only to pain as a symptom that is dreaded by patients with cancer and those undergoing chemotherapy. The origin of nausea and vomiting in cancer patients is multifactorial

and should not be ascribed solely to side effects from chemotherapy. Nausea and vomiting may occur as a result of many factors: (1) obstruction of a viscus, (2) gastritis or duodenitis, (3) increased intracranial pressure caused by central nervous system disease, (4) metabolic abnormalities such as hypercalcemia, and (5) side effects from nonchemotherapy drugs such as narcotic analgesics. A careful assessment of the patient is necessary for the treatment of nausea and vomiting, whether chemotherapy-induced or not.

The emetogenic response is the result of a complex interaction of receptors throughout the peripheral and central nervous systems and is coordinated by the emetic center located in the lateral reticular formation of the brain. The emetic center receives afferent impulses from several sites, including the visceral afferents lining the GI tract, receptors in the midbrain that detect intracranial pressure, the limbic system, the vestibular system, and the chemoreceptor trigger zone located in the floor of the fourth ventricle. The neural network that constitutes the emetic center sends efferent signals to the salivary, vasomotor, and respiratory centers, as well as the nerves that control the abdominal musculature, diaphragm, esophagus, and stomach and participate in the physical act of vomiting. Neurotransmitters believed to be involved with the emetic response include dopamine, histamine, acetylcholine, the opioids, and more recently serotonin. Serotonin now appears to be the principal mediator of the emetogenic response. Of the three groups of serotonin receptors to be identified, the type III receptor appears to play a pivotal role in emesis. These receptors are abundant on the visceral afferent neurons and other neurons in the GI tract. They have also been identified in the area postrema and the nucleus tractus solarus which define the emesis center. Blockade of the type III serotonin receptors with serotonin antagonists ameliorates cisplatin-induced nausea and vomiting. This pathway is the basis for development of two potent antiemetic drugs, ondansetron (Zofran) and granisetron (Kytril). The severity of chemotherapy-induced vomiting depends on a number of factors. The first is the intrinsic emetogenicity of the chemotherapy agents themselves. They range from potent emetogenic agents such as cisplatin to those with a very low emetogenic potential such as bleomycin (Box 78-1). The dose of the drug and the mode of administration also play a role. Higher doses of drugs are more emetogenic than lower doses. Also, continuous infusion of certain drugs appears to be less emetogenic than bolus administration. Characteristics of the patients themselves must also be taken into account. Younger people tend to have more trouble with chemotherapy-induced nausea and vomiting, as do women.

Chemotherapy-induced nausea and vomiting can occur as an acute toxicity, usually within 1 to 2 hours of administration of the drug, or as a delayed toxicity occurring, particularly with cisplatin, 5 to 7 days after administration of the drug. Anticipatory nausea and vomiting,

---

BOX 78-1

Emetogenic potential of common chemotherapeutic drugs

High
Cisplatin
Dacarbazine
Mechlorethamine

Moderate
5-Fluorouracil
Doxorubicin
Daunorubicin
Cylophosphamide
Ifosfamide
Actinomycin D
Melphalan
Mitoxantrone

Low
Bleomycin
Hydroxyurea
Etoposide
Vinblastin
Vincristine
Chlorambucil

---

which is a learned response conditioned by the severity and duration of previous nausea and vomiting, must be treated in a different manner.

Classes of drugs used in treating chemotherapy-induced nausea and vomiting include phenothiazines, corticosteroids, anticholinergic drugs, butyrophenones, canabinoids, benzodiazipines, substituted benzamides, antihistamines, and serotonin antagonists. Currently, however, the most commonly used and effective drugs include drugs from the phenothiazine class, such as prochlorperazine (Compazine), promethazine (Phenergan), thiethylperazine (Torecan), corticosteroids including dexamethasone (Decadron), butyrophenones including haloperidol (Haldol), canabinoids including dronabinol (Marinol), benzodiapines including lorazepam (Ativan), substituted benzamides including metoclopramide (Reglan), cisapride (Propulsid), and the serotonin antagonists ondansetron (Zofran) and granisetron (Kytril). For mild to moderate nausea and vomiting the phenothiazines and butyrophenones are the most effective. The butyrophenones have fewer of the extrapyramidal side effects that are seen with the phenothiazines. These side effects can be adequately treated with low doses of antihistamines such as diphenhydramine (Benadryl). For more severe nausea and vomiting, combinations including a substituted benzamide such as metoclopramide with an antihistamine and a corticosteroid have been replaced by combinations including a serotonin antagonist in combination with dexamethasone.

Corticosteroids on their own have weak antiemetogenic potential and are usually used in combination with other drugs. For drugs with moderate to high potential for severe nausea, such as cisplatin, high-dose cytarabine, and dacarbazine, a combination such as granisetron 1 mg and dexamethasone 10 mg given intravenously before the chemotherapy or ondansetron 30 mg and dexamethasone 10 mg given in the same manner are equally effective in preventing acute nausea and vomiting in more than 90% of patients. In the delayed nausea and vomiting seen with cisplatin, the mechanism of action may be direct bowel inflammation due to the drug itself. In a randomized trial combinations of antiemetic drugs effective in preventing acute nausea and vomiting decreased the frequency of delayed vomiting as compared with placebo. Anticipatory vomiting is much more difficult to treat and can be avoided by the addition of a mild benzodiazepine with its anxiolytic, sedative, and amnesic properties. Primary prevention of acute nausea and vomiting is the best treatment for anticipatory nausea and vomiting.

Regardless of the regimen chosen to prevent chemotherapy-induced nausea and vomiting, the drug should be given appropriately approximately 30 minutes before the administration of chemotherapy. Patients receiving chemotherapy with highly emetigenic drugs should be sent home with scheduled antiemetics to be taken for several days to prevent the occurrence of nausea and vomiting in the 1 to 2 days following administration of the drug after the primary antiemetic effect of the preventive drugs has ended. The regimen of choice must be individualized for each patient and should be assessed with each session of chemotherapy to ensure that adequate antiemesis is maintained.

NEUTROPENIA AND FEVER

Infections and fever are a common occurrence in patients with cancer and those undergoing treatment for cancer and are not solely the consequence of chemotherapy-induced neutropenia. Factors involving the cancer itself, the pathogenic organism, and the host all play a role in infections in cancer patients. Postobstructive pneumonia caused by a bronchogenic carcinoma is very different from the pneumonia of an immunocompromised acquired immunodeficiency syndrome (AIDS) patient with lymphoma who is undergoing chemotherapy. A meticulous assessment with careful history and physical examination, as well as culture of appropriate material, must occur in every cancer patient with infection and fever.

Let us first consider factors related to the cancer itself. These factors may be local, as in obstruction of a bronchus or viscus, or systemic, as with cachexia and weakness or paraneoplastic neurologic syndromes that prevent patients from adequately resisting infection. Local tumor growth may lead to obstruction and postobstructive infections including pneumonia or pyelonephritis. Erosion of tumors into pleural or retroperitoneal spaces or involvement of these spaces with extending infections may lead to empyema and retroperitoneal abscess formation. Obstruction or perforation of abdominal visera may lead to peritonitis. In all of these instances emergent treatment with surgical drainage and antibiotics is necessary. Other examples of localized complications include tumors of the skin, head, neck, and genitourinary tract, which cause local erosion, and polymicrobial infection, which may require debridement and antibiotics.

Mechanisms that decrease the patient's resistance to infection include (1) general debilitation resulting from weight loss or cachexia; (2) muscle weakness due to paraneoplastic syndromes or atrophy, which decreases mobility and may impair the cough and gag reflexes; (3) altered mental status resulting from central nervous system involvement with tumor or metabolic complications; and (4) immune suppression as a result of involvement of the bone marrow or immune suppression intrinsic to the cancer. Patients with infections who are not neutropenic and in whom other immune suppression is not evident should be treated with surgical drainage when necessary and appropriate antibiotics before chemotherapy or local radiotherapy is instituted. Patients with fever who *are* neutropenic constitute a true medical emergency. Management of these patients is described in Chapters 229 and 243.

PARANEOPLASTIC SYNDROMES

In general, the signs and symptoms of cancer are those of the local effects of tumor and tumor progression, as well as metastases and metastatic progression leading to invasion of structures, obstruction, hemorrhage, or organ destruction. Paraneoplastic syndromes are signs and symptoms that occur at a distance from the tumor or its metastatic sites. In some patients this "action at a distance" caused by the tumors may be responsible for significant morbidity and a decrease in quality of life. Therefore it is important to recognize paraneoplastic syndromes because they may be the first sign or symptom of a malignancy, they may cause significant morbidity, and they may serve as markers for response to therapy and/or progression of disease.

The pathogenesis of the paraneoplastic syndromes may occur by several mechanisms. The tumors may produce biologically active proteins such as hormones or their precursors, growth factors, cytokines, prostaglandins, or immunoglobulins. Immunoglobulins may cause autoimmunity or immune complex formation and may mediate immune suppression, as may growth factor, interleukin, and cytokine production. By far the most common paraneoplastic syndromes are those caused by ectopic production of hormones. These hormones may be

Table 78-2   Endocrine paraneoplastic syndromes

SYNDROME	MEDIATOR	ASSOCIATED MALIGNANCY
Hypercalcemia	Parathyroid hormone (parathormone, PTH) or PTH-like substance Osteoclast-activating factors Prostaglandins Tumor growth factor (TGF), alpha Interleukin-1 (IL-1) Tumor necrosis factor Lymphotoxin	Breast cancer Squamous cell carcinoma of lung, head and neck, esophagus Multiple myeloma Renal cell carcinoma
Syndrome of inappropriate secretion of antidiuretic hormone (SIADH)	Antidiuretic hormone (ADH)	Small cell carcinoma of lung Head and neck carcinomas Hodgkin's disease Non-Hodgkin's lymphoma
Hypoglycemia	Insulin Insulin-like peptides	Insulinoma Mesenchymal tumors, including mesothelioma, fibrosarcoma, neurofibrosarcoma, rhabdomyosarcoma
Zollinger-Ellison syndrome	Gastrin	Gastrinoma
Ectopic secretion of human chorionic gonadotropin	Human chorionic gonadotropin (HCG)	Germ cell tumors containing trophoblastic elements
Cushing's syndrome	Adrenocorticotropic hormone (ACTH)	Lung carcinoma

---

BOX 78-2
Nonendocrine paraneoplastic syndromes

Cutaneous
Dermatomyositis
Acanthosis nigricans
Sweet's syndrome
Erythema gyratum repens
Systemic nodular panniculitis (Weber-Christian disease)

Renal
Nephrotic syndrome
Nephrogenic diabetes insipidus

Neurologic
Subacute cerebellar degeneration
Progressive multifocal leukoencephalopathy
Subacute motor neuropathy
Sensory neuropathy
Ascending acute polyneuropathy (Guillain-Barré)
Myasthenic syndrome (Eaton-Lambert)

Hematologic
Microangiopathic hemolytic anemia
Migratory thrombophlebitis (Trousseau's syndrome)
Anemia of chronic disease

Rheumatologic
Polymyalgia rheumatica
Hypertrophic pulmonary osteoarthropathy

---

normally produced by the tissue but may be produced in abnormally large amounts such as the excessive corticosteroid production in adrenalcorticocarcinoma. The production of hormones may be ectopic, resulting from the malignant transformation of a cell not normally producing the hormone. Secretion of polypeptide hormones by tumors has been recognized for the last several decades as a cause of paraneoplastic syndromes. However, in the past decade, many previously unknown hormones have been discovered. The function of many of these hormones remains unknown. Table 78-2 lists the most commonly occurring endocrine paraneoplastic syndromes.

Hormone levels are easily detected and followed with routine laboratory evaluation, usually radioimmunoassay. These include adrenocorticotropin hormone (ACTH), antidiuretic hormone (ADH), parathormone (PTH), erythropoietin, gastrin, and vasoactive intestinal peptide (VIP). These products mediate such syndromes as Cush-

ing's syndrome, the syndrome of inappropriate antidiuretic hormone (SIADH), hypercalcemia, and the polycythemia associated with malignancy. The secreted hormones may not be identical to natural hormone but may contain areas of amino acid identity sufficient to be biologically active. Parathyroid hormone–related protein (PTHRP), the most frequent cause of paraneoplastic hypercalcemia, is an example of this. The gene for PTHRP is expressed in many normal tissues and does not appear to be related to systemic calcium homeostasis. Eight of the first 13 amino acids are identical with parathormone, making PTHRP an agonist for the biologic activity of parathormone. Immunologic identification of ectopic hormone production, even when the products formed are biologically inactive precursors or fragments, may still be useful as tumor markers. Levels decrease as the tumor resolves, and increasing levels may herald a relapse before it is clinically detectable. Non-hormone–mediated paraneoplastic syndromes cover a spectrum of diseases, including skin, rheumatologic, and neurologic manifestations and renal and hematologic manifestations in which the pathophysiology is not as clearly understood as the endocrine neoplastic syndromes. Box 78-2 presents an abbreviated list of some of the more commonly recognized nonendocrine paraneoplastic syndromes.

COMPLICATIONS OF THERAPY

Most cytotoxic chemotherapeutic agents kill rapidly proliferating cells. They are toxic drugs with a narrow therapeutic index, and the benefits of their use must be carefully balanced against acceptable toxicity to normal tissues. Normal tissues with high proliferative rates are almost universally affected by chemotherapy drugs. These include bone marrow, skin, GI tract, and the genitourinary (GU) tract. Bone marrow toxicity has proved to be the dose-limiting toxicity in the vast majority of chemotherapeutic drugs. However, with the use of colony-stimulating factors (CSFs) and bone marrow rescue, chemotherapy drugs are now used in higher doses and in combination with each other so that toxicity to other organ systems has become dose limiting. The severity of toxicity depends on factors related to the drug and to the patient. Drug-related factors include dose, route of administration, and mode of administration. For example, the anthracycline doxorubicin has less cardiac toxicity when given as a continuous infusion rather than a bolus injection. Patient factors include underlying renal and hepatic dysfunction, nutritional status, and level of debilitation. The side effects of chemotherapy drugs can be classified as occurring early or late. Early toxicities include nausea and vomiting and those occurring early in the course such as leukopenia and alopecia. Delayed toxicities include those which occur months to years after exposure to the drug and include, for example, doxorubicin-induced cardiomyopathy, the peripheral neuropathy associated with *Vinca* alkaloids, decreased fertility, and the development of second malignancies.

CARDIOTOXICITY

The anthracyclines are the class of drugs most commonly associated with cardiotoxicity. However, cardiotoxicity has also been reported with 5-fluorouracil, cyclophosphamide, ifosfamide, and paclitaxel. Doxorubicin is the drug most commonly associated with anthracycline-induced cardiotoxicity. All currently available anthracyclines produce some degree of cardiac toxicity. Anthracycline-induced cardiotoxicity may be acute, subacute, or chonic. Acute effects occur during administration or shortly thereafter and include predominantly electrocardiographic (ECG) changes and ventricular and atrial ectopy. These changes do not appear to be dose dependent and usually do not result in discontinuation of the drug. Subacute toxicity, including myocarditis and pericarditis, occur rarely. Chronic toxicity from anthracyclines is manifested by congestive heart failure. Congestive heart failure usually does not develop if the total dose is less than 450 mg/m^2. In patients with preexisting heart disease and treatment with other cardiotoxic chemotherapy agents or mediastinal radiation, congestive heart failure may develop at cumulative doses less than 450 mg/m^2. The radionuclide cardiac scan or multiple gated acquisition (blood pool scan; MUGA) has allowed close monitoring of systolic function in the form of a left ventricular ejection fraction. All patients receiving anthracyclines should be followed with MUGA scans, especially those with preexisting heart disease. Newer members of the anthracycline class, including epirubicin and idarubicin, appear to be just as cardiotoxic as doxorubicin. The anthracenedione mitoxantrone may be less cardiotoxic. Several agents have been developed as cardioprotectants for patients receiving treatment with doxorubicin. ICRF-187 is an iron-chelating agent; others are of the class of free radical scavengers. Cyclophosphamide and ifosfamide are toxic at the high doses used in bone marrow transplantation conditioning regimens. Both have been reported to cause ECG changes, as well as congestive heart failure. Death within 2 weeks as a result of acute myocardial necrosis has been reported with cyclophosphamide. Paclitaxel, a new antineoplastic agent that affects microtubular organization, is reported to induce arrhythmias including ventricular tachycardia and atrioventricular conduction abnormalities such as sinus bradycardia and heart block. Therapy need not be discontinued unless these arrhythmias are associated with clinically significant hemodynamic changes.

PULMONARY TOXICITY

Pulmonary toxicity has been associated with several classes of antineoplastic agents, including antitumor antibiotics and the nitrosoureas. Although initial damage may include interstitial and alveolar infiltrates, edema, and eosinophilia, the final common expression appears to be pulmonary fibrosis. Pulmonary fibrosis remains a serious complication of treatment with nitrosoureas. The drug most frequently associated with pulmonary toxicity is the antitumor antibiotic bleomycin. Signs and symptoms may include fever, dry cough, and fine bibasilar crackles. Chest x-ray findings generally show fine interstitial infiltrates, and patients are generally hypoxemic. Pulmonary function testing reveals a decrease in the diffusing capacity as measured by carbon monoxide diffusion in the lung (DLCO). Toxicity of bleomycin appears to be dose dependent, occurring infrequently at doses below 400 to 500 U/m^2. However, in patients undergoing treatment with other chemotherapy agents, those receiving radiation to the lung, and those with underlying lung disease, pulmonary toxicity from bleomycin can occur at much lower doses. Serial measurement of the diffusing capacity is necessary in patients treated with bleomycin, because significant toxicity can occur before patients become clinically symptomatic. Unlike the rare hypersensitivity reaction to bleomycin, which becomes evident with fever, shortness of breath, diffuse infiltrates, and eosinophilia, the interstitial fibrosis related to bleomycin has not been successfully treated with steroids. The nitrosourea bischlorethylinitrosourea (BCNU), used almost exclusively with central nervous system tumors but now more frequently used in conditioning regimens before bone marrow transplantation in Hodgkin's disease, carries an incidence of pulmonary toxicity of approximately 30% in patients receiving more than 1000 mg/m^2 total dose. Clinical presentation is similar to that of bleomycin-induced pulmonary toxicity, and there is no effective therapy. A recent report described pulmonary fibrosis developing in patients as many as 17 years after exposure to BCNU. Busulfan was the first chemotherapeutic agent to be associated with pulmonary toxicity. It occurs much less frequently than that seen with BCNU, and rare dystrophic calcifications and pulmonary ossification have been reported. The signs and symptoms are similar to those of bleomycin toxicity. Other chemotherapeutic agents, including cyclophosphamide, methotrexate, mitomycin-C, and chlorambucil, have all been associated with pulmonary toxicity.

RENAL AND METABOLIC TOXICITY

Renal and metabolic toxicities include toxicities specific to the kidney, as well as the abnormalities seen in the tumor lysis syndrome. Tumor lysis syndrome is seen in a variety of tumors that are so sensitive to chemotherapy that treatment causes a large amount of cellular necrosis with release of cellular contents. Tumor lysis syndrome can cause a constellation of metabolic abnormalities including hyperkalemia, hyperphosphatemia, hyperuricemia, and hypocalcemia that can be life threatening. Tumor lysis syndrome can be avoided by the institution of allopurinol and vigorous intravenous hydration of the patient 12 to 24 hours before the beginning of chemotherapy.

Antineoplastic agents that have direct toxic effects on the kidneys include methotrexate, streptozotocin, cisplatin, and cyclophosphamide. Methotrexate is primarily excreted through the kidney, with more than 90% of the delivered dose recoverable from the urine unchanged. The nephrotoxicity of methotrexate appears to be related to the precipitation of the drug in the renal tubules and collecting ducts. Infusions of high-dose methotrexate exceed the solubility at pH 5 and promote drug precipitation. The 7-OH metabolite of methotrexate, which is two to three times less soluble than the parent compound, may also mediate some of this toxicity. Much of the renal toxicity caused by high-dose infusions of methotrexate can be avoided by alkalinization of the urine and a brisk diuresis during administration of the drug. Renal toxicity resulting from methotrexate is usually transient and recovers within several weeks after withdrawal of the drug. Cisplatin, an inorganic platinum complex used with remarkable success over the past decade in the treatment of testicular cancer, ovarian cancer, and non–small cell lung cancer, is dose limited by its nephrotoxicity. Azotemia occurs in nearly 30% of patients treated with a single 50 mg/m^2 dose but is usually mild and reversible. Higher doses and multiple courses of cisplatin, however, are more toxic to the kidney and may lead to chronic renal dysfunction. Pathologic damage to the kidney includes extensive renal tubular necrosis with extensive glomerular damage. Renal damage by cisplatin can be ameliorated by induction of a brisk diuresis during administration of the drug.

Intravenous saline and mannitol sufficient to maintain a urine output of at least 100 ml/hour have been shown to decrease nephrotoxicity. Cisplatinum also appears to produce a defect in magnesium reabsorption, and urinary magnesium wasting results. Life-threatening hypomagnesemia and hypokalemia can occur and should be monitored closely in patients receiving cisplatin. Streptozotocin, a nitrosourea used in the treatment of pancreatic islet cell tumors, may cause hypocalcemia, proximal renal tubular acidosis, and Fanconi's syndrome, as well as proteinuria of up to 10 g in a 24-hour period. Reversible proteinuria is the earliest manifestation of renal toxicity in patients treated with streptozotocin. Cyclophosphamide and vincristine may both cause transient azotemia and SIADH. Cyclophosphamide may also cause hemorrhagic cystitis as a result of accumulation of toxic metabolites in the urine. Patients treated with very high doses of cyclophosphamide require continuous bladder irrigation with an indwelling Foley catheter.

GASTROINTESTINAL TRACT TOXICITY

The GI tract is lined with rapidly proliferating cells and is especially sensitive to most chemotherapeutic agents. These agents produce stomatitis, glossitis, esophagitis, and oral ulceration that may decrease oral intake and have severe impact on quality of life. Methotrexate, 5-fluorouracil, and the antitumor antibiotics, particularly actinomycin D and doxorubicin, are most frequently associated with stomatitis. The severity of stomatitis associated with methotrexate depends on dose and schedule. Lower doses given on a weekly schedule rarely produce mucositis, whereas high doses and methotrexate given as a continuous infusion may produce severe mucositis. In patients receiving methotrexate, toxicity to the GI tract may be diminished if leucovorin is given within 24 hours of administration. Monitoring methotrexate plasma levels may identify patients at risk because of decreased clearance mechanisms. Prolonged elevated levels may be seen in patients with pleural effusions or ascites. GI toxicity with 5-fluorouracil is also dose and schedule dependent. Bolus injections given on a weekly schedule produce much less toxicity than prolonged continuous infusions or doses given on the 5-day regimens. Stomatitis resulting from chemotherapy may be worsened by the presence of oral candidiasis. Treatment of stomatitis remains symptomatic and includes mouth rinses and topical anesthetics such as viscous xylocaine. Measures such as continuous morphine sulfate drip to control pain may be needed. Although stomatitis may be severe with methotrexate, diarrhea is not as much of a problem. 5-Fluorouracil, especially when used in conjunction with high doses of leucovorin and given as a continuous infusion or on a daily basis for 5 days, may cause diarrhea in approximately 30% of patients. It is rarely bloody diarrhea but may become clinically significant in elderly patients, and hospitalization may be required for treatment of dehydration and electrolyte imbalances. Patients may be treated with loperamide (Imodium), diphenoxylate hydrochloride with atropine sulfate (Lomotil), and bismuth subsalicylate/bismuth subgallate (Pepto-Bismol). Autonomic nerve dysfunction may cause crampy abdominal pain and constipation, especially in elderly patients receiving vincristine. Adynamic ileus is a serious complication. Constipation should be treated prophylactically with mild laxatives and stool softeners.

HEPATOTOXICITY

Liver functions may be abnormal in cancer patients for a number of reasons, including liver involvement with the tumor; toxicity from medication other than chemotherapeutic agents; radiation therapy; infection, especially with hepatitis viruses; and underlying liver disease, including alcoholic liver disease. A number of chemotherapeutic agents are metabolized by the liver; however, no clear-cut guidelines exist for dose reduction in the face of abnormal liver functions. Hepatic venoocclusive disease, which results in the obliteration of small intrahepatic veins and becomes evident with a triad of jaundice, hepatomegaly, and weight gain, is increasing in frequency as higher doses of chemotherapy drugs are used in combination with radiation therapy in patients undergoing bone marrow transplantation. Venoocclusive disease is seen more commonly in patients who have received previous hepatotoxic chemotherapy agents and radiation therapy and have abnormal liver function. The clinical severity of hepatic venoocclusive disease can range from mild elevations in bilirubin levels to life-threatening hepatic failure. Treatment is supportive.

Agents such as busulfan and cyclophosphamide, when given in standard doses, are rare causes of hepatic toxicity. However, given in the high doses such as for bone marrow transplantation, both have been reported to cause venoocclusive disease in as many as 20% of patients. The antimetabolite 5-fluorouracil is largely metabolized by the liver when administered intravenously; however, reports of hepatic toxicity when 5-fluorouracil is used as a single agent are rare. Fluorodeoxyuridine, a derivative of 5-fluorouracil administered intraarterially for hepatic metastasis from colorectal cancer and hepatoma, causes a chemical hepatitis and a sclerosing cholangitis. 5-Fluorouracil given with its modulators leucovorin and N-phosphonoacetyl-L-aspartate (PALA) has also been reported to cause liver dysfunction. Methotrexate is probably the most frequently implicated chemotherapeutic agent in the development of hepatic toxicity. Fatty change, focal hepatitis, and portal fibrosis have all been reported in patients receiving low doses of methotrexate for rheumatologic diseases. High-dose methotrexate therapy results in an acute rise in hepatic transaminases that is transient and reversible. Of the antitumor antibiotics, dactinomycin and doxorubicin have both been implicated in hepatic toxicity, and both agents should be dose reduced in the face of hepatic insufficiency.

OTHER TOXICITY

Other organ systems affected by chemotherapy include the neurologic system. Toxicities include peripheral neuropathy, most commonly

with the *vinca* alkaloids and cisplatinum; ototoxicity, with cisplatinum; cerebellar toxicity with ataxia, with high dose cytarabine; and encephalopathy, with intrathecal methotrexate. A number of chemotherapy drugs are known to cause hypersensitivity reactions, and patients are often premedicated before administration of the drug. These include asparaginase, paclitaxel, teniposide, etoposide, and procarbazine. Vascular toxicity includes pulmonary venoocclusive disease leading to pulmonary hypertension that is seen rarely in patients treated with bleomycin. Hepatic venoocclusive disease occurs predominantly in patients receiving bone marrow transplantation who have been heavily pretreated with other chemotherapy drugs. Skin toxicity includes Raynaud's phenomenon resulting from bleomycin, thrombotic thrombocytopenic purpura as a result of mitomycin-C, and acral erythema that is seen with high-dose cytosine arabinoside.

Special mention should be made of fertility issues and gonadal function. In men with Hodgkin's disease and testicular cancer up to 75% may have oligospermia or azoospermia at the time of diagnosis. Recovery of spermatogenesis after treatment with combination chemotherapy in testicular cancer is generally good. In Hodgkin's disease, however, sterility remains a problem. Sperm banking should be offered to all men before chemotherapy or radiation therapy treatments for their cancers. New techniques such as in vitro fertilization may allow successful pregnancy even with stored sperm samples with low sperm count and decreased motility. Unlike in men with Hodgkin's disease, pretreatment gonadal dysfunction in young women is rare. The risk for developing ovarian failure after treatment for Hodgkin's disease is related to the age of the patient and the concomitant use of radiotherapy. Less than 30% of women younger than age 30 who receive treatment for Hodgkin's disease developed ovarian failure, whereas 70% to 80% of women over 30 years of age had menopausal symptoms and menstrual irregularity. Attempts to suppress spermatogenesis or follicular development with hormonal manipulation have not been successful. In women at high risk for ovarian failure, oocyte and embryo cryopreservation are feasible options.

COMPLICATIONS FROM RADIATION THERAPY

Radiation therapy was used to treat almost 500,000 cancer patients in 1990. As has been mentioned in previous sections, combinations of chemotherapy and radiation therapy can exacerbate the toxicity of both modalities. There are, however, toxicities specific to radiation therapy. The mechanism for radiation-induced cell death appears to be damage to the DNA resulting in double-stranded breaks in the DNA molecule. Radiation toxicity can be classified as early or late. In early toxicity rapidly growing tissue such as the GI tract, skin, and bone marrow, as well as reproductive tissue, is so affected that bone marrow suppression, mucositis, diarrhea, skin changes, and alopecia can be seen during therapy and in the few weeks after therapy. These effects are usually self-limited and resolve without complication after radiation therapy has been completed. Late complications result from accumulated injury to tissues with less repair and proliferative potential and include radiation fibrosis to the lung and pericarditis with a restrictive cardiomyopathy, as well as accelerated development of atherosclerotic coronary artery disease, myelitis with neurologic changes resulting from transverse myelopathy, and global encephalopathy. As radiation therapy techniques improve, less toxicity to normal tissues has been seen. However, physicians caring for patients who have received radiation therapy alone and in combination with chemotherapy should keep in mind that late complications can occur years after the therapy was given.

SECOND MALIGNANCIES

Great strides have been made in the cure of such malignancies as acute leukemia, Hodgkin's disease, non-Hodgkin's lymphoma, testicular cancer, and breast cancer. Survival has been prolonged and quality of life improved by the use of adjuvant chemotherapy and chemotherapy that is used in a palliative setting, and more children are living into adulthood having survived pediatric cancers. The price to be paid in these survivors is an increased risk of the development of secondary malignancies years after primary tumors have been cured. Survivors of curative therapy for Hodgkin's disease are at risk for the development of a number of malignancies years after their therapy. Patients treated with radiation therapy alone or treated with nitrosourea-containing compounds in low doses have a very low risk for the development of secondary malignancies. However, combinations of chemotherapy, especially nitrosoureas and alkalating agents at higher doses, and chemotherapy in combination with radiation therapy, greatly increase the risk of the development of a second malignancy. The most common second malignancy is acute myeloid leukemia that is often preceded by a prodromal myeolodysplastic syndrome. The incidence of the development of acute leukemia can be as high as 10%, and the development usually occurs within 3 to 10 years with a decrease in incidence after 10 years. These leukemias tend to be less sensitive to standard leukemia treatments. Non-Hodgkin's lymphoma, usually of B-cell type, occurs at a low but steady rate. The mean latency period is about 7 years, but there appears to be no plateau. Bone and soft tissue sarcomas that occur in radiated areas usually develop 6 to 10 years after treatment. Other cancers in Hodgkin's disease survivors include melanoma; lung cancer, even in patients who are nonsmokers; thyroid cancers; head and neck cancers; and breast cancer. There are now increased reports of the development of acute leukemia in women treated with cyclophosphamide- and adriamycin-based regimens for breast cancer. There is an increased risk of lung cancer in women receiving radiation therapy for breast cancer. Cancer survivors require lifelong screening for the development of second malignancies. Reports of successful treatment of second malignancies include bone marrow transplantation for treatment-related leukemia and surgical and chemotherapy cures for non-Hodgkin's lymphoma and secondary lung cancers.

BIBLIOGRAPHY

Cross SA: Pathophysiology of pain, *Mayo Clin Proc* 69:375-383, 1994.

Doria R, Holford T, Farber LR et al: Second solid malignancies after combined modality therapy for Hodgkin's disease, *J Clin Oncol* 13(8):2016-2022, 1995.

Grunberg SM, Hesketh PJ: Control of chemotherapy-induced emesis, *N Engl J Med* 329(24):1790-1791, 1993.

Hammack JE, Loprinzi CL: Use of orally administered opioids for cancer-related pain, *Mayo Clin Proc* 69:384-390, 1994.

Jacox A, Carr DB, Payne R: Management of cancer pain: clinical practice guideline no 9, AHCPR Pub No 94-0592, Rockville, MD, March 1994, Agency for Health Care Policy and Research, U.S. Department of Health and Human Services, Public Health Service.

Mitchell E: Gastrointestinal toxicity of chemotherapeutic agents, *Semin Oncol* 19(5):566-579, 1992.

Perry MC, editor: Toxicity of chemotherapy, *Semin Oncol* 19(5):452-610, 1992.

Portenoy RK, Coyle N: Controversies in the long-term management of analgesic therapy in patients with advanced cancer, *J Palliative Care* 7(2):13-24, 1991.

Rummans TA: Nonopioid agents for treatment of acute and subacute pain, *Mayo Clin Proc* 69:481-490, 1994.

Vieson KJ, Corcoran MB, Bradbur R: Cardiotoxicity secondary to cancer treatment, *Cancer Control* 1(4):390-395, 1994.

IV CLINICAL SYNDROMES

CHAPTER

79 Abnormal Hematocrit

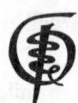

Emmanuel N. Dessypris

Under normal conditions the production of red blood cells (RBCs) is closely regulated so that the hematocrit remains in the range of 38% to 48% in women and 40% to 52% in men. The production of RBCs is controlled by *erythropoietin,* a glycoprotein hormone produced by

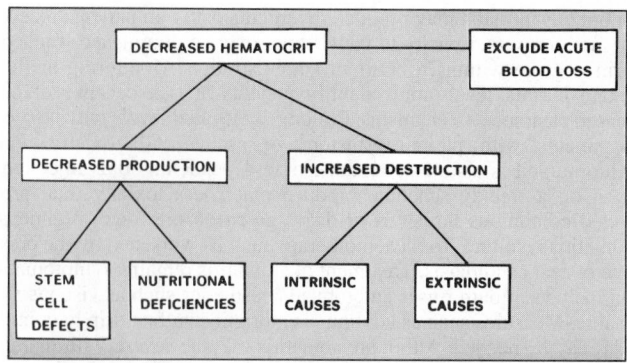

FIGURE 79-1   Simplified classification of anemias.

the interstitial cells in the kidneys. The concentration of erythropoietin in the blood is inversely related to the degree of oxygen delivery to the tissues by the blood. Hypoxia resulting from a decreased RBC mass leads to increased synthesis and release of erythropoietin by the kidney, which in turn stimulates RBC production by the bone marrow, thus restoring the RBC mass and tissue oxygenation back to normal levels. Under normal conditions the serum level of erythropoietin is low, but it is adequate to maintain a stable hematocrit.

The RBC *mass* is defined as the volume of RBCs per kilogram of body weight and can be accurately measured by the dilution technique using intravenously injected, autologous radiolabeled RBCs. By this technique the RBC mass is found to be 26 ml in women and 30 ml in men of RBCs per kilogram body weight, with a 10% variation among normal individuals. *Anemia* is a pathologic condition in which an absolute decrease occurs in the RBC mass. *Polycythemia* is an absolute increase of the RBC mass.

In clinical practice the RBC mass is assessed by the concentration of the hemoglobin in the blood or by the hematocrit, which measures the ratio of the RBC volume to the plasma volume. In general a close agreement exists between the RBC mass and the hematocrit or the hemoglobin concentration, except when a significant change occurs in the plasma volume. Thus dehydration of a patient with a normal RBC mass may lead to an elevation of hematocrit that may falsely be interpreted as a sign of polycythemia, whereas dehydration of an anemic patient may result in a normal hematocrit that drops precipitously on rehydration. In contrast, expansion of the plasma volume, as typically occurs during pregnancy, may result in an inappropriately low hematocrit in the presence of a normal RBC mass. In this chapter the terms *low* and *high* hematocrit refer to those circumstances in which the patient's hydration status and plasma volume are normal, so they can be considered synonymous with anemia and polycythemia, respectively.

LOW HEMATOCRIT

Anemia is one of the most common manifestations of disease. It should always be considered as a sign of an underlying disease and not a diagnosis in itself. Anemia can result from a reduction in the rate of RBC production, from an increase in the rate of RBC destruction in the peripheral blood, or from acute blood loss (Fig. 79-1). Blood loss can be easily ruled out by the history and clinical examination. Differentiation between decreased production and increased destruction of RBCs relies on the reticulocyte count. *Reticulocytes* are young RBCs that have recently been released from the bone marrow (Plate IV-4), and their number is expressed as a percentage of RBCs. Under normal conditions, only 1% to 2.5% of the RBCs are reticulocytes. In the presence of anemia, high levels of erythropoietin stimulate the marrow, and the release of reticulocytes increases manyfold. A reticulocyte count should be corrected for the degree of anemia. This correction is performed by multiplying the reticulocyte count by the patient's hematocrit and dividing by 45, which represents the average normal hematocrit. Using automated technology, the absolute number of reticulocytes in blood can be determined with great accuracy and is less labor intensive than manual methods (Chap-

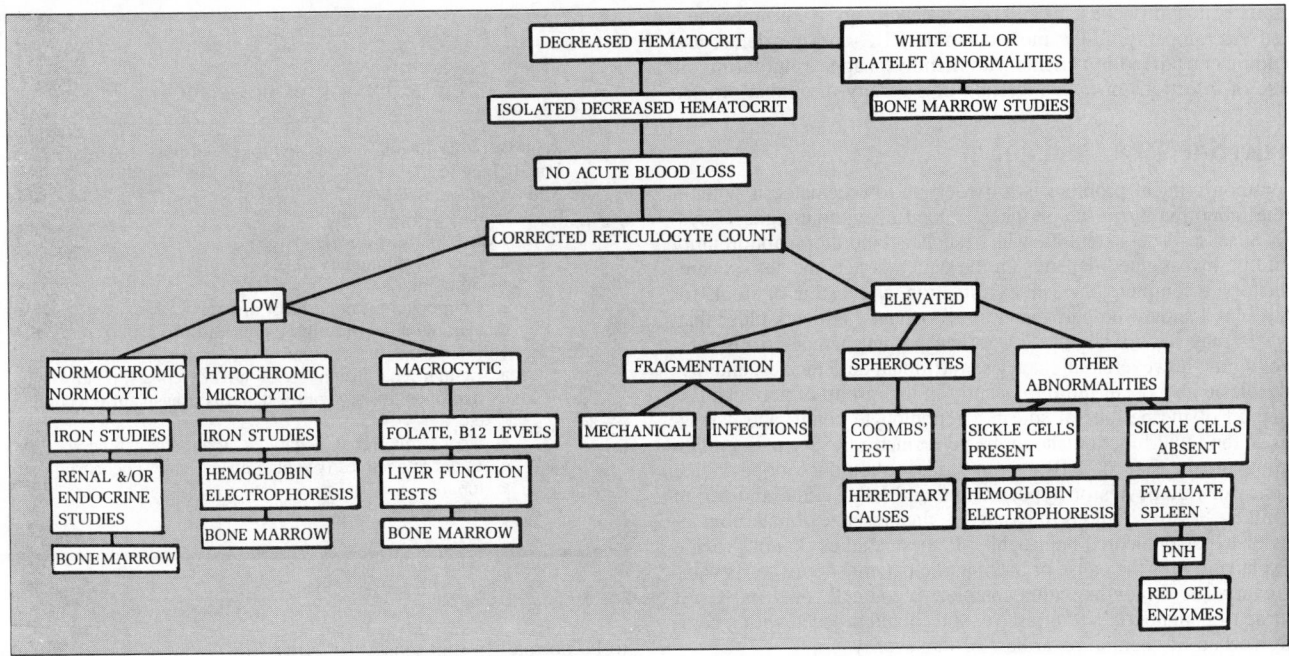

FIGURE 79-2   Evaluation of a patient with a low hematocrit.

ter 72). Figure 79-2 shows a diagnostic approach to the patient with a low hematocrit.

Decreased Reticulocyte Count

A corrected reticulocyte count of less than 1% or a low absolute number of reticulocytes is strong evidence that the anemia is caused by underproduction of RBCs by the bone marrow. This may result from erythropoietin deficiency secondary to renal failure, subnormal marrow response in the presence of an endocrinopathy, chronic inflammation or neoplasia, nutritional deficiencies (e.g., iron, folate, vitamin B_{12}), or a primary hematologic disease (e.g., marrow aplasia, dysplasia, myeloproliferation, leukemia). In the absence of abnormal white blood cell (WBC) or platelet counts, which usually indicate a primary hematologic disease and the need for bone marrow examination, further differentiation between nutritional deficiencies and other causes of underproduction anemia can be based on RBC size. Evaluation of RBC size requires both examination of the peripheral blood smear and direct measurement of mean corpuscular volume (MCV) by an electronic cell counter (Chapter 72). In iron deficiency the RBCs are microcytic and hypochromic, whereas in folate or vitamin B_{12} deficiency they are macrocytic and elongated (macroovalocytes). In general, other causes of reduced RBC production are associated with RBCs with a normal or near-normal MCV (*normocytic* RBCs) (Box 79-1).

Increased Reticulocyte Count

An elevated corrected reticulocyte count (>3%) or elevated absolute reticulocyte count in excess of 100,000 cells per μl indicates that the marrow has responded appropriately to anemia with an increase in RBC production and that the basic mechanism of anemia is accelerated destruction of the RBCs in the peripheral blood. Under normal conditions the RBCs survive in the blood for about 120 days. If their life span decreases to as low as 20 days, the bone marrow can produce RBCs in an accelerated manner so that the hematocrit can be maintained within the normal limits *(compensated hemolytic anemia)*. A further decrease in the RBC life span is associated with the development of anemia. An increase of the serum bilirubin, disappearance of serum haptoglobin, and an elevation of serum lactate dehydrogenase (LDH) add further confirmatory evidence to the existence of an underlying hemolytic process. In the patient with hemolytic anemia, examination of the peripheral blood smear (Plate IV-4) provides very

---

BOX 79-1

Disorders associated with decreased production or increased destruction of red blood cells (RBCs)

Decreased production
Renal failure
Chronic diseases (infectious, inflammatory, neoplastic)
Nutritional deficiencies (iron, folate, vitamin B_{12})
Myelodysplasia
Pure RBC aplasia
Endocrine hypofunction (thyroid, pituitary)
Hemoglobin with low oxygen affinity

Increased destruction
Hemolytic transfusion reaction
Infections
Immune hemolysis
RBC fragmentation
Hereditary spherocytosis
Hemoglobinopathies
Hypersplenism
RBC enzyme defects (glucose-6-phosphate dehydrogenase [G6PD], pyruvate kinase deficiency)
Paroxysmal nocturnal hemoglobinuria
Miscellaneous (severe burns, fresh water drowning)

---

important information that helps in the identification of the cause of hemolysis. Fragmented RBCs (schistocytes) are frequently seen in microangiopathic hemolytic anemia caused by the presence of a prosthetic heart valve or by disseminated intravascular coagulation. Spherocytes are seen in congenital spherocytosis and in acquired immune hemolytic anemia. The antiglobulin test (Coombs' test) result is negative in congenital spherocytosis and positive in autoimmune hemolytic anemia. The presence of sickle cells or severe anisocytosis with microcytosis or target cells suggests the presence of hemoglobinopathy, and a hemoglobin electrophoresis should be performed. In the absence of any prominent RBC morphologic abnormalities, one should consider the possibility of an RBC enzyme defect, hypersplenism, or of paroxysmal nocturnal hemoglobinuria. Glucose-6-

phosphate dehydrogenase (G6PD) deficiency, an X-chromosome–linked enzymopathy, is the most common RBC enzyme defect and should be considered in patients with hemolysis appearing during the course of infections or after ingestion of a variety of oxidant drugs.

Borderline Low Hematocrit

A common clinical problem is a borderline low hematocrit without another abnormality in the peripheral blood or without signs of systemic disease. The extent to which such a laboratory abnormality should be investigated depends on the patient's age and sex. A careful history, a complete physical examination, and testing of stools for occult blood should be performed in all patients. Patients older than 70 years may have a slightly lower-than-normal hematocrit as a result of aging; however, malignancies, nutritional deficiencies, and myelodysplasia also occur quite frequently in this group of patients. Examination of the peripheral smear, a reticulocyte count, and assessment of the renal function should be performed in every patient. Depending on the size of RBCs, iron studies should be done in the presence of microcytes or hypochromia, and RBC folate and serum vitamin B_{12} levels should be measured in the presence of macroovalocytes or hypersegmented neutrophils. If these studies do not provide an explanation for the cause of anemia, the patient should be reevaluated every 3 to 6 months with a complete blood cell count (CBC). If the drop of hematocrit is progressive, one should proceed with a complete workup of anemia, regardless of its severity.

Men of younger age should always have a complete investigation of a borderline low hematocrit. During their reproductive period, women frequently develop iron deficiency, which may present initially as a borderline low hematocrit. In the absence of any other abnormality, a therapeutic trial with oral iron is justified. If the hematocrit does not normalize within 4 to 8 weeks, a full investigation of anemia should be initiated.

Abnormal Red Blood Cell Indices in Nonanemic Patient

Occasionally in a patient with a normal hematocrit the RBC size is found to be abnormal. Such a finding must be confirmed by examination of the peripheral blood smear. Microcytosis without iron deficiency is a common manifestation of heterozygous thalassemia. In β-thalassemia, this can be confirmed by quantification of hemoglobin F and A_2. In α-thalassemia trait, hematologic studies of the patient's family members may confirm the familial nature of this finding. Isolated macrocytosis may be an early manifestation of folate or vitamin B_{12} deficiency, alcoholic liver disease, hypothyroidism, or myelodysplasia. Pseudomacrocytosis may occasionally be seen in patients with severe reticulocytosis resulting from compensated immune hemolytic anemia due to cold agglutinins with clinically insignificant thermoamplitude, and with cryoglobulinemia. Examination of the peripheral blood smear and measurement of folate and vitamin B_{12} levels are usually necessary for the patient's initial evaluation. In the absence of any abnormal finding indicating further investigation, the patient should be re-evaluated with a CBC at 3- to 6-month intervals.

HIGH HEMATOCRIT

A high hematocrit can result from hemoconcentration or an increased rate of RBC production by the bone marrow, which may be either autonomous or secondary to high serum erythropoietin levels. With hemoconcentration the RBC mass is normal, and the increased hematocrit is caused by decreased plasma volume. *Polycythemia* is defined as an absolute increase in the RBC mass that is appreciated clinically by a high hematocrit. In the absence of dehydration, a hematocrit greater than 60% is always associated with an increase of RBC mass and is diagnostic of polycythemia. For hematocrit values of 50% to 60%, the diagnosis of polycythemia requires direct measurement of the RBC mass. An RBC mass greater than 32 ml/kg in women and 35 ml/kg body weight in men confirms the diagnosis of polycythemia. A classification of polycythemia is shown in Box 79-2. Figure 79-3 illustrates a diagnostic approach to the patient with a high hematocrit.

In *relative* or *stress polycythemia* the patient has a high hematocrit because of decreased plasma volume, but the RBC mass is found

---

BOX 79-2
Classification of polycythemia

I. Relative polycythemia (stress, spurious, Gaisböck's syndrome)
II. True polycythemia
  A. Polycythemia vera
  B. Secondary polycythemia
    1. Decreased tissue oxygenation
      a. Chronic pulmonary disease
      b. Smoking
      c. Congenital cyanotic heart disease
      d. Hemoglobin with high oxygen affinity
    2. Normal tissue oxygenation
      a. Benign renal lesions (renal artery stenosis, renal cysts, hydronephrosis, nephrocalcinosis, transplant rejection, etc.)
      b. Neoplasms (renal, hepatic, ovarian, adrenal, cerebellar)
      c. Endocrinopathies (Cushing's syndrome, pheochromocytoma)
      d. Idiopathic

---

to be normal. In this sense the "stress" or "relative" polycythemia is a misnomer. This condition most often appears in anxious men, older than 50 years, who frequently are hypertensive and smokers with a high incidence of thrombotic episodes. Smoking and high blood pressure have been considered to be the cause of plasma volume contraction. Cessation of smoking, correction of hypertension, or switching from a diuretic to another antihypertensive medication may lead to normalization of the hematocrit. If these measures are not successful, and in the presence of any symptoms or signs of vascular insufficiency, treatment with phlebotomies to reduce the hematocrit to less than 45% is warranted.

Once the diagnosis of true polycythemia is established, the major differential diagnosis centers between polycythemia vera and secondary polycythemia (Table 79-1). *Polycythemia vera* is a myeloproliferative disorder in which the production of RBCs is not controlled by and is independent of erythropoietin (Chapter 92). Besides an elevated hematocrit, patients with this disease also have leukocytosis, thrombocytosis, splenomegaly, and a hypercellular bone marrow with trilinear hyperplasia. In early stages, however, a high hematocrit may be the only manifestation.

In *secondary polycythemia* the high hematocrit is always secondary to elevated levels of circulating erythropoietin, and the bone marrow remains normocellular. Neither leukocytosis nor thrombocytosis occurs, and the spleen size remains normal. Measurement of serum erythropoietin levels may help occasionally in the differential diagnosis. With a high hematocrit, a significantly elevated serum erythropoietin level favors the diagnosis of secondary polycythemia; however, a normal or mildly elevated value by itself cannot exclude the diagnosis of secondary polycythemia. Without an underlying disease or condition that can possibly cause hypoxia and elevated serum erythropoietin levels, and if the WBC and platelet counts are normal and the spleen size is not increased (as documented by spleen scan or abdominal computed tomography [CT]), examination of bone marrow is the only diagnostic procedure that can differentiate polycythemia vera from secondary polycythemia.

In secondary polycythemia the increase in the RBC mass is caused by an elevated serum erythropoietin level. This may represent a normal response to tissue hypoxia or may result from autonomous production of erythropoietin. Therefore the investigation of secondary polycythemia should focus on the identification of the cause of increased erythropoietin production. Chronic pulmonary disease resulting in a decrease of arterial oxygen tension (PaO_2) to less than 67 mm Hg is a frequent cause of secondary polycythemia. In patients with chronic obstructive lung disease and polycythemia in whom the PaO_2 is higher than 67 mm Hg while awake, oximetry during sleep may be necessary to detect periods of severe hypoxia during sleep. Severe cardiovascular disease may also lead to the development of hypoxia and polycythemia, particularly after years of chronic pulmonary congestion. Congenital cyanotic cardiac dis-

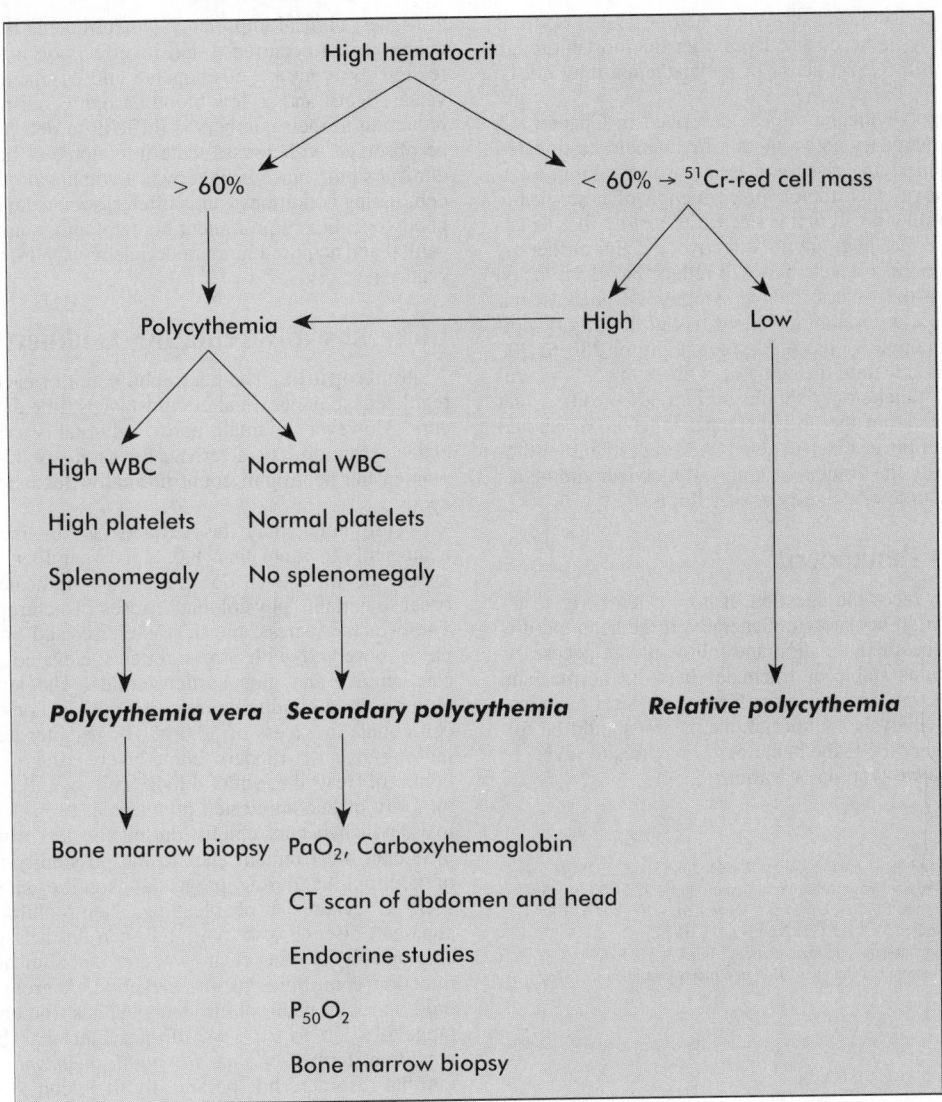

FIGURE 79-3   Evaluation of a patient with a high hematocrit.

Table 79-1   Differentiation among relative polycythemia, polycythemia vera, and secondary polycythemia

	RELATIVE POLYCYTHEMIA	POLYCYTHEMIA VERA	SECONDARY POLYCYTHEMIA
Hematocrit	H	H	H
Red blood cell mass	N	H	H
White blood cell count	N	H	N
Platelet count	N	H	N
Spleen size	N	H	N
Marrow cellularity	N	H	N

H, High; *N*, normal.

ease is a frequent cause of secondary polycythemia in children but is rare in adults.

In the absence of chronic lung disease, smoking by itself can cause polycythemia. Smoking not only causes an elevated level of carboxyhemoglobin (greater than 1%) but also shifts the oxyhemoglobin dissociation curve to the left, which results in an increased affinity of hemoglobin for oxygen (O_2). The latter is probably much more important in the pathogenesis of smokers' polycythemia than the conversion of a small percentage of hemoglobin to carboxyhemoglobin. The magnitude of the effect of smoking on O_2 delivery from hemo-

globin to tissues can be more accurately assessed by measuring the $P_{50}O_2$, which is usually less than 25 mm Hg. Rarely, secondary polycythemia is caused by an abnormal hemoglobin with high affinity for O_2. The presence of a positive family history for polycythemia appearing at an early age should lead to the measurement of $P_{50}O_2$. If abnormal, the type of abnormal hemoglobin can be identified by hemoglobin electrophoresis.

In some patients with secondary polycythemia, the elevation of serum erythropoietin levels is not the result of tissue hypoxia and thus is considered to be physiologically inappropriate. Such an elevation of erythropoietin leading to polycythemia has been described as a paraneoplastic manifestation of a variety of malignant or benign tumors, including tumors of the kidneys, liver, adrenal glands, ovaries, and cerebellum. More frequently, such an inappropriate elevation of serum erythropoietin is caused by benign focal lesions in the kidney that result in focal hypoxia stimulating erythropoietin production. Renal cysts, renal artery stenosis, hydronephrosis, nephrocalcinosis, transplant rejection, and a variety of other renal lesions may cause secondary polycythemia through this mechanism. Endocrinologic disorders characterized by high levels of androgenic steroids or catecholamines, such as Cushing's syndrome and pheochromocytoma, respectively, may directly or indirectly stimulate erythropoietin production by the kidney, resulting in polycythemia. In the absence of any clinically obvious cause of hypoxia, a CT scan of the abdomen is necessary for detection of pathologic conditions in the kidneys, liver, adrenal glands, or ovaries. If clinically indicated, a CT scan of the head and measurement of serum or urine 17-ketosteroids and catecholamines may be necessary. Even after the most thorough investigation, however, the exact cause of polycythemia may not be found.

The treatment of polycythemia vera is described in Chapter 92. The management of secondary polycythemia first should be directed toward the primary underlying disease. Cessation of smoking, long-term O_2 therapy, removal of a tumor, or correction of a surgically amenable renal lesion may be all that is needed to restore the hematocrit to normal. If these measures are not effective, the aim of therapy is to reduce the hematocrit to levels that will reduce blood viscosity, improve blood flow to the tissues, reduce symptoms from vascular insufficiency, and reduce a possibly increased risk of thrombotic episodes. This can be obtained by repeated phlebotomy of 250 to 400 ml of blood every other day until the hematocrit drops to 45%. Thereafter the frequency of phlebotomy should be individualized so that the hematocrit is kept within the normal range. Phlebotomy should be performed with caution in older patients with underlying cardiovascular disease. Usually the volume of removed blood should be replaced by an equal volume of colloids or oral fluids.

Borderline High Hematocrit

At times the physician faces the question of how extensively to investigate a borderline high hematocrit. Generally, if the hematocrit is 48% to 54%, only a repeat examination and follow-up are necessary. If the hematocrit remains stable or fluctuates between normal and slightly elevated levels, and if the clinical history, physical examination, and routine urine analysis are normal, the patient should be followed up at regular intervals. If the hematocrit increases to levels of 55% or higher, a complete workup is warranted.

BIBLIOGRAPHY

Beck WS: Diagnosis of megaloblastic anemia, *Annu Rev Med* 42:311-322, 1991.
Bilgrami S, Greenberg BR: Polycythemia rubra vera, *Semin Oncol* 22:307-326, 1995.
Cook JD: Iron deficiency anemia, *Baillière's clinical haematology* 7:787-804, 1994.
Finch CA, Cook JD: Iron deficiency, *Am J Clin Nutr* 39:471, 1984.
Golde DW: Polycythemia: mechanisms and management, *Ann Intern Med* 95:71, 1981.
Kellermeyer RW: General principles of the evaluation and therapy of anemias, *Med Clin North Am* 68:533, 1984.

80 Abnormal Nucleated Blood Cell Counts

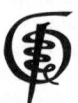

David H. Boldt

Patients frequently have alterations in numbers of leukocytes or abnormal nucleated blood cells in the peripheral circulation. Sometimes these changes may be discovered unexpectedly in an individual being seen for a routine examination. At other times the finding may be sought as part of the evaluation of a patient with debilitating systemic illness. In either case, blood is uniquely accessible and easily examined for the presence of underlying hematopathology. This chapter considers causes, clinical features, and approaches to diagnosis in patients who have abnormal peripheral nucleated blood cell counts. Specific disease entities are the subjects of other chapters.

QUANTITATIVE ALTERATIONS IN NORMAL NUCLEATED CELLS

Quantitative alterations—increases or decreases—in circulating leukocyte counts are encountered most often in clinical practice. Clinically important types of leukocytoses include neutrophilia, eosinophilia, basophilia, lymphocytosis, and monocytosis. The leukopenia

of highest clinical importance is neutropenia because of both the frequency of its occurrence and its effects on host susceptibility to infection. By contrast, eosinopenia and basopenia have no known adverse effects, and so few blood basophils normally are present that a reduction in their numbers is difficult to detect. Monocytopenia may be observed with stress, acute infections, or hairy cell leukemia. Its clinical significance is unknown. Lymphocytopenia occurs in chronic debilitating conditions and is often associated with malnutrition. Lymphocytopenia is a prominent hematologic manifestation of both congenital and acquired immunodeficiency syndrome (AIDS) and related syndromes.

Increases in Circulating Leukocytes

Neutrophilia. The neutrophil count of each individual is tightly regulated, so under usual circumstances little day-to-day variation occurs. However, a small normal diurnal variation and age-related changes that are characteristic for each sex have been described. In women the neutrophil count normally fluctuates with the menstrual cycle.

Neutrophilia may be defined as an increase in circulating neutrophils to more than 8.0×10^9 per liter. Neutrophil counts in excess of this level do not always indicate underlying disease because certain "physiologic" causes of neutrophilia are recognized. These include stress, physical exercise, and pregnancy. The neutrophilia observed with stress reflects elevated blood levels of catecholamines and glucocorticosteroids. The leukocytosis associated with all these conditions may be striking. For example, white blood cell counts in excess of 50.0×10^9 per liter have been documented in long-distance runners immediately after exercise. After several hours of rest the white blood cell count returns to normal. A minority of uncomplicated pregnancies are associated with leukocytosis, which occurs chiefly during the last trimester. However, the physician must remain alert to the possibility that the development of neutrophilia during pregnancy signifies a serious complication such as eclampsia or bleeding. Neutrophilia in the absence of apparent disease also may be seen in heavy cigarette smokers, although it is not clear whether subclinical bronchopulmonary infection contributes to this elevation. A group of individuals with mild chronic neutrophilic leukocytosis (neutrophil counts in the range of 12.0 to 20.0×10^9 per liter) has been described. This condition, termed *chronic idiopathic neutrophilia*, occurs both as a familial disorder and sporadically. It is considered benign and may represent the extremes of the normal range, but chromosomal abnormalities and organomegaly have been reported in some of these individuals. Some have also developed diseases such as vasculitis, rheumatoid arthritis, and Hodgkin's disease after prolonged follow-up. In other patients, however, long-term follow-up has failed to reveal evidence of any systemic illness.

Although neutrophilia may be a common host response to a variety of physiologic stimuli, it is more frequently encountered as a reaction to an underlying disease process (Box 80-1). The three major classes of disorders associated with neutrophilia are (1) infections and inflammatory diseases; (2) tissue destruction, as in myocardial or pulmonary infarction, major surgery, or shock; and (3) malignant disease. Other miscellaneous causes include hemorrhage, hemolysis, diabetic ketoacidosis, thyroid storm, eclampsia, or the administration of pharmaceutical agents such as lithium, glucocorticosteroids, or hematopoietic growth factors (granulocyte colony-stimulating factor [G-CSF] or granulocyte-macrophage colony-stimulating factor [GM-CSF]). Usually the underlying condition is obvious and the neutrophilia properly recognized as reactive.

Occasionally, however, neutrophilia may be the presenting sign of an occult process, and the physician must search for its cause. A diagrammatic approach to assessment of a patient with neutrophilia is given in Fig. 80-1. Bacterial infection is the most common cause of a neutrophilic leukocytosis, but neutrophilia may also be seen in fungal, viral, and parasitic infections. Presence of toxic granulations, Döhle's bodies, and/or cytoplasmic vacuolization in circulating neutrophils favors an infectious process, although none of these changes is specific. Occult sources of infections should be considered when diagnosis is difficult. These include bacterial endocarditis; deep-seated abscesses, especially in the abdomen; chronic fungal or myco-

---

BOX 80-1
Abnormal white blood cell counts:
diagnostic considerations

I. Quantitative abnormalities
  A. Increases in circulating leukocytes
    1. Neutrophilia
      a. Reactive: infections, inflammatory disorders, tissue destruction, malignancies, drug induced, hemorrhage, hemolysis, diabetic ketoacidosis
      b. Primary myeloproliferative disorders
      c. Physiologic
      d. Idiopathic
    2. Eosinophilia
      a. Reactive: allergies and hypersensitivity reactions, parasitic infections, immunologic disorders, malignancies
      b. Primary: hypereosinophilic syndromes
      c. Adrenal insufficiency
    3. Basophilia: myeloproliferative disorders
    4. Monocytosis
      a. Reactive: malignancies, immunologic disorders, infections
      b. Primary: monocytic leukemia
    5. Lymphocytosis
      a. Reactive: infection, especially viral, pertussis, acute infectious lymphocytosis, immunologic disorders
      b. Primary: lymphoproliferative diseases
  B. Decreases in circulating leukocytes
    1. Neutropenia
      a. Decreased production: bone marrow injury caused by ionizing radiation or drugs, marrow replacement, nutritional deficiencies, congenital stem cell defects
      b. Increased destruction/utilization/sequestration: hypersplenism, immune mechanisms, overwhelming infection
    2. Lymphocytopenia
      a. Decreased production: primary immunodeficiency diseases
      b. Increased destruction/utilization/loss: collagen vascular disease, acute infections or stress, ionizing radiation, cytotoxic drugs, antilymphocyte globulin, loss of lymph, human immunodeficiency virus (HIV) infection
      c. Unknown mechanism: malignancies, chronic infection
II. Qualitative abnormalities
  A. Immature granulocytes: leukemoid reactions, leukemia, myeloproliferative syndromes
  B. Morphologic alterations in granulocytes: toxic granulations, Döhle's bodies, vacuoles, Chédiak-Higashi syndrome, Pelger-Huët anomaly
  C. Abnormal lymphocytes
    1. Atypical lymphocytes: viral infections, immunologic reactions, toxoplasmosis
    2. Plasmacytoid lymphocytes: viral infections, immunologic reactions, Waldenström's macroglobulinemia
    3. Lymphoblasts: acute lymphoblastic leukemia
    4. Lymphosarcoma cells: lymphoma
    5. Sézary cells: cutaneous lymphomas
    6. Hairy cells: hairy cell leukemia
    7. Prolymphocytes: prolymphocytic leukemia

---

bacterial infections; and ascending cholangitis. In hospitalized patients, indwelling tubes and catheters are potential sites of infection.

Usually infection is accompanied by a *left shift* on the peripheral blood smear. This term refers to the presence in the circulation of increased numbers of neutrophil precursors. Two patterns of left shift may be encountered. In one form there are increased numbers of band forms (more than 0.45×10^9 per liter); in the other form, neutrophilic metamyelocytes, myelocytes, or promyelocytes are present. Cells less mature than band forms are not normally present on the peripheral smear. A granulocytic "leukemoid" reaction may be considered an extreme form of a reactive, left-shifted neutrophilia in which a very high neutrophil count and/or abundant neutrophil precursors may simulate the appearance of true leukemia in the peripheral blood. Features that aid in differentiation of such a leukemoid reaction from chronic myelogenous leukemia are listed in Table 92-3. Cytogenetic testing, leukocyte alkaline phosphatase (LAP) score, and presence of basophilia are the most helpful discriminating points. Granulocytic leukemoid reactions are seen most often in association with infections and malignancies.

When reactive neutrophilia has been excluded, consideration should be given to a primary myeloproliferative process. A neutrophilic leukocytosis consisting predominantly of mature segmented and band forms is a common feature of polycythemia vera and reflects that this disorder is a panmyelosis. In chronic myelogenous leukemia the neutrophilia is characteristically left-shifted, manifesting all stages of myeloid development from myeloblast to mature polymorphonuclear leukocyte in the peripheral blood. The neutrophilia in this disorder is frequently associated with basophilia. In myelofibrosis with myeloid metaplasia a neutrophilia is present in approximately 80% of patients. The neutrophilia, usually left-shifted as in chronic myelogenous leukemia, is often associated with circulating nucleated erythrocytes, a combination termed *leukoerythroblastosis*. There is usually concomitant anisocytosis and poikilocytosis. Teardrop-shaped red blood cells are usually prominent. In addition to careful examination of a peripheral blood smear, certain other clinical and laboratory features are helpful in the evaluation of a patient for a primary myeloproliferative syndrome. These include erythrocyte and platelet counts, LAP score, presence or absence of splenomegaly, and examination of bone marrow for presence of the Philadelphia chromosome or excessive fibrosis. Myeloproliferative diseases are discussed in Chapter 92.

Eosinophilia. Eosinophilia is diagnosed when the absolute blood eosinophil count is in excess of 0.5×10^9 per liter. The function of eosinophils is not well understood, but they are known to play a role in host defense against certain parasitic infestations and also to interact with immune complexes. Clinical conditions manifesting eosinophilia reflect these associations. Major diagnostic considerations are listed in Box 80-1. The most common cause for mild eosinophilia in hospitalized patients is drug allergy. Hypereosinophilic syndromes (Chapter 91) are associated with the most marked elevations of eosinophil counts.

Basophilia. Basophilia is rarely encountered. Its presence may be helpful in diagnosing a primary myeloproliferative disorder such as chronic myelogenous leukemia, polycythemia vera, or myelofibrosis.

Monocytosis. Peripheral blood monocytes are precursors of the tissue macrophages. The monocyte-macrophage system serves an important role in the body economy that may be summarized as (1) antigen uptake and presentation for generation of immune responses; (2) immune regulation; (3) phagocytosis and killing of microorganisms, macrophages being the first line of defense against various intracellular parasites such as *Mycobacterium tuberculosis, Listeria,* and *Brucella;* and (4) secretion of biologically active molecules, including complement, interferon and various cytokines, and hematopoietic growth factors. The presence of monocytosis (monocyte count in excess of 0.70×10^9 per liter) generally indicates an underlying neoplastic process, immunologic disease, or chronic inflammatory process (see Box 80-1). Monocytosis also may be associated with several primary hematologic disorders. These include drug-induced and other forms of neutropenia, hemolytic anemias, and dysmyelopoietic syndromes (preleukemia). In addition, monocytosis may be a feature of the early phase of bone marrow recovery from myelosuppression. Certain primary and secondary myelodysplastic syndromes as well as certain types of acute nonlymphoid leukemias may be characterized by the presence of abundant, well-differentiated monocytic cells in the circulation. When less well differentiated, these leukemic monocytes may be identified cytochemically by the presence of nonspecific esterase or expression of surface antigens characteristic of the monocyte-macrophage lineage. Their presence is also associated with increased levels of lysozyme in the serum and urine. The diagnosis of acute monocytic leukemia may be suggested clinically by the associated anemia, thrombocytopenia, and granulocytopenia. Gingival hypertrophy secondary to infiltration of the gums by leukemic cells is associated more frequently with acute monocytic leukemia than with other types of acute leukemia. (Acute leukemias are discussed in Chapter 92.)

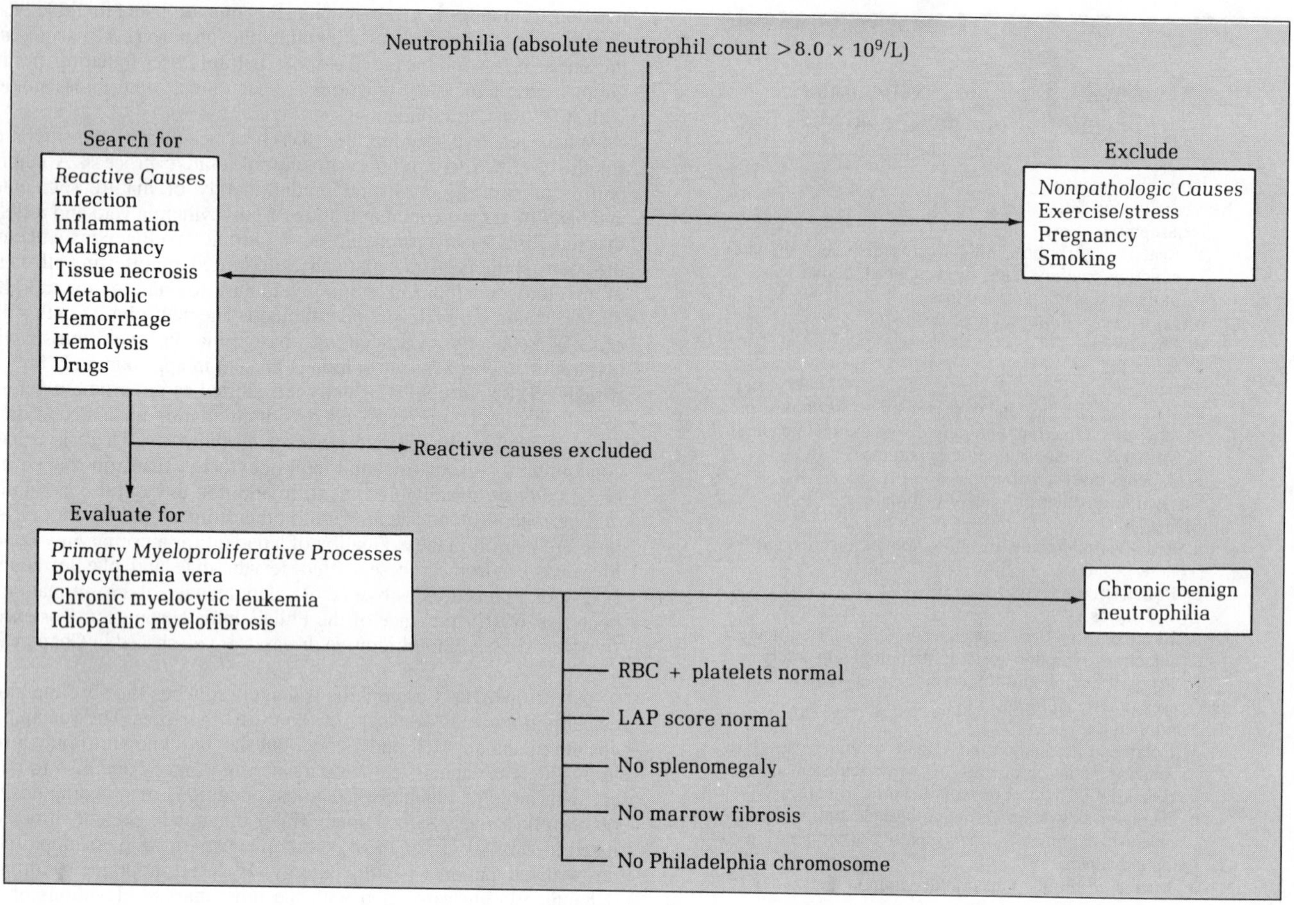

FIGURE 80-1   General approach to neutrophilia. *RBC,* Red blood cells; *LAP,* leukocyte alkaline phosphatase.

Lymphocytosis. It is necessary to distinguish between absolute and relative lymphocytosis. Absolute lymphocytosis may be defined as an increase in blood lymphocytes above 4.0×10^9 per liter. Relative lymphocytosis occurs when there is an increased percentage of circulating lymphocytes, but the absolute number does not exceed 4.0×10^9 per liter. An example of relative lymphocytosis occurs in patients with neutropenia, when the decreased granulocyte count produces leukopenia and most remaining cells are lymphocytes. The absolute number of lymphocytes, however, remains normal. Conditions that may be associated with elevated peripheral lymphocyte counts are listed in Box 80-1.

When assessing lymphocytosis, morphologic considerations are important. The normal lymphocyte and its morphologic variants are illustrated in Plate IV-5. A variety of morphologically distinct types of lymphocytes can be seen in normal peripheral blood. Approximately 80% of normal lymphoid cells are small lymphocytes 6 to 9 μm in diameter. These cells are characterized by nuclei containing compact clumps of chromatin surrounded by thin rims of clear blue cytoplasm. Most of the remaining lymphoid cells are of intermediate size, 10 to 15 μm in diameter, with more abundant cytoplasm and less compact nuclear chromatin. Some of these cells, referred to as *large granular lymphocytes* (LGLs), contain prominent intracytoplasmic azurophilic granules. LGL is the predominant cell type that mediates natural killer (NK) activity (Chapter 174). From 0.5% to 1% of lymphocytes are large, blastlike cells, up to 25 μm in diameter, whose nuclei may contain several nucleoli and finely dispersed chromatin. Frequently the cytoplasm of these cells may appear deeply basophilic and may contain vacuoles. Intermediate- and large-sized lymphoid variants including classic atypical lymphocytes are often referred to as *reactive lymphocytes.* Moderate increases in reactive lymphocytes are seen as a characteristic response to viruses and other infections, especially in children. Increases also occur in a wide va-

riety of other situations, including primary and secondary immune responses, hypersensitivity reactions, and autoimmune disorders.

The differential diagnosis of marked lymphocytosis composed solely of normal small lymphocytes is limited in scope. In the adult the major consideration is chronic lymphocytic leukemia. This diagnosis may best be confirmed by demonstrating the monoclonal B-cell nature of the proliferation and coexpression of the CD5 antigen by appropriate lymphocyte surface marker studies. In childhood and adolescence the chief considerations are pertussis and acute infectious lymphocytosis. In pertussis the lymphocyte count regularly reaches levels of 10.0 to 50.0×10^9 per liter during the early phase of the disease. Acute infectious lymphocytosis is a mild, asymptomatic, self-limited disease of childhood and adolescence. When symptoms do occur, they are transitory and may include fever, rash, coryza, cough, pharyngitis, or gastrointestinal complaints. Lymphocytosis may reach 100 to 150×10^9 per liter and generally persists for 3 to 5 weeks. Red blood cell and platelet counts are normal, and lymphadenopathy or hepatosplenomegaly does not occur. These features, as well as the mature morphology of the circulating lymphocytes, aid in differentiating acute infectious lymphocytosis from acute lymphoblastic leukemia. The absence of reactive or atypical lymphocytes and the extreme elevation of the lymphocyte count in acute infectious lymphocytosis allow its ready differentiation from infectious mononucleosis and other infectious conditions. The age distribution contrasts greatly with that of chronic lymphocytic leukemia, which is a disease of elderly persons. No treatment is indicated because the disease is uniformly self-limiting.

Lymphocytosis has been described in association with certain endocrine disorders, especially thyrotoxicosis and adrenal insufficiency. A small percentage of patients with thyrotoxicosis may display a relative lymphocytosis, sometimes associated with lymphoid hyperplasia, including splenomegaly. Lymphocytosis, usually relative, is seen

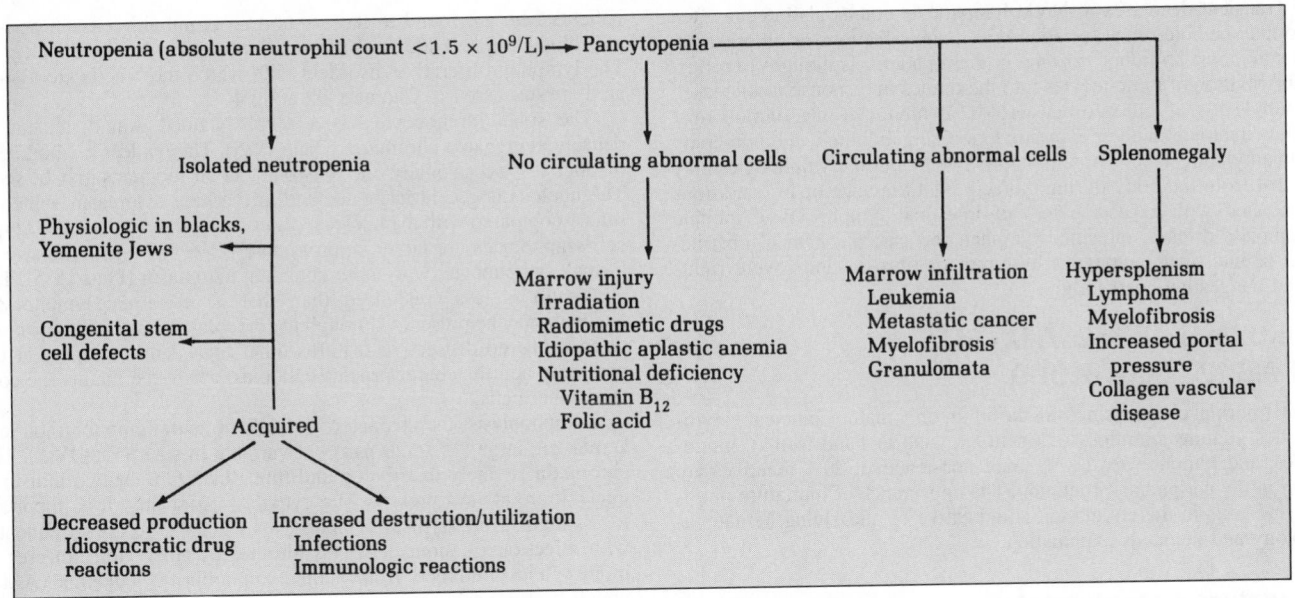

FIGURE 80-2 General approach to neutropenia.

in approximately half of patients with untreated Addison's disease. Lymphocytosis rarely may be impressive enough to simulate a lymphoid malignancy. Lymphoproliferative disorders associated with peripheral lymphocytosis are discussed later in this chapter.

Decreases in Circulating Leukocytes

Neutropenia. Neutropenia exists when numbers of circulating neutrophils are reduced below the normal range. Although neutrophil counts less than 2.0×10^9 per liter occur infrequently in normal individuals, some healthy, resting adults, particularly blacks and Yemenite Jews, may have counts as low as 1.0×10^9 per liter without evidence of disease.

Neutropenia may occur as an isolated condition or in association with decrease in other circulating elements, as in pancytopenia (Fig. 80-2). In either case the neutropenia is caused by one of the following major pathologic mechanisms: decreased production (i.e., a bone marrow problem) or increased destruction or removal from the circulation.

Decreased production may be secondary to ionizing irradiation, cytotoxic drugs such as nitrogen mustard or other alkylating agents, or idiopathic causes, as in aplastic anemia or myelodysplasia. Bone marrow replacement by leukemia, metastatic tumor, fibrosis, or granulomata is an additional consideration. Decreased production may result from nutritional deficiencies, particularly of vitamin B_{12} or folic acid. Hypersplenism is a cause of pancytopenia related to peripheral destruction or sequestration. This concept is discussed in Chapter 81.

The occurrence of isolated neutropenia secondary to failure of myelopoiesis implies a defect in the myeloid stem cell or in a committed progenitor such as the colony-forming unit (CFU)-GEMM (granulocyte, erythrocyte, megakaryocyte, monocyte) or CFU-GM (granulocyte, monocyte). Such a defect may be acquired, as in patients with certain idiosyncratic drug reactions, or it may be congenital, as in those with cyclic neutropenia. There are a variety of other poorly understood congenital disorders of myelopoiesis. Some of these disorders are associated with other abnormalities and constitute well-recognized clinical syndromes. In these congenital diseases, neutropenia is generally recognized during infancy, and fatal infections may supervene. A thorough drug and medication history should be obtained from all patients with acquired neutropenia. Idiosyncratic drug-induced neutropenia is discussed in Chapter 91.

Isolated neutropenia may be a sign of overwhelming infection, in which case it is caused by both rapid egress of neutrophils from blood to tissue sites and suppression of myelopoiesis. In certain instances,

isolated neutropenia may be caused by immunologically mediated granulocyte destruction. Recently, complement-induced granulocyte aggregation has been suggested as a cause of leukopenia in Felty's syndrome (neutropenia and splenomegaly in association with rheumatoid arthritis) and systemic lupus erythematosus. It might also be a mechanism for tissue damage caused by leukostasis in such diverse clinical settings as pulmonary dysfunction in hemodialyzed patients, myocardial infarction, or adult respiratory distress syndrome. Neutropenia is recognized increasingly as an accompaniment of infection by HIV. Although the precise mechanism remains unknown, most evidence does not support a direct role for HIV infection of granulocyte precursors. More likely, neutropenia in this setting is multifactorial, reflecting both the myelosuppressive effects of drugs (such as zidovudine) and HIV-induced alterations in the bone marrow microenvironment.

Diagnostic considerations in the evaluation of a neutropenic patient are charted in Fig. 80-2. Careful history, especially with respect to medications or other potential myelotoxins (e.g., alcohol), physical examination with attention to hepatosplenomegaly, evidence of portal hypertension, or manifestations of rheumatic disease, and routine hemogram including platelet count, red blood cell indices, and examination of a peripheral blood smear should point the way to appropriate additional studies. A bone marrow examination is essential to look for a marrow infiltrative process or destruction and to assess whether the differentiation of hematopoietic cells is normal. Other measurements usually necessary to identify the cause of neutropenia include serum levels of vitamin B_{12} and folic acid, rheumatoid factor, and serological tests for lupus. If an idiosyncratic drug reaction is suspected, it is advisable to discontinue the likely offending agent to avoid the development of severe neutropenia and subsequent serious infection. Radionuclide spleen scanning may demonstrate unsuspected splenic enlargement or help to resolve questions of equivocal splenomegaly or hypersplenism. These relatively straightforward tests resolve 90% of clinically encountered cases of neutropenia. Further evaluation requires expertise and research procedures generally available only at specialized centers.

Lymphocytopenia. An absolute lymphocytopenia occurs when the peripheral lymphocyte count is less than 1.5×10^9 per liter in adults, or less than 3.0×10^9 per liter in children. Major causes include immunodeficiency disorders, malignancy, collagen vascular diseases, and chronic infections (see Box 80-1). The most common cause of sustained lymphocytopenia is malignancy, followed by collagen vascular disease. Currently, infection with HIV has emerged as an important cause.

Transient decreases in blood lymphocyte counts also occur often and may be noted in association with acute infections or other stressful situations. Lymphocytopenia in these patients is thought to reflect redistribution of lymphocytes into the tissues in response to increased serum levels of glucocorticosteroids. Lymphocyte destruction may follow treatment with or exposure to ionizing radiation, chemotherapy with alkylating agents, or antilymphocyte globulin. Lymphocytes may be lost from the body during thoracic duct drainage or in conditions associated with excessive loss of intestinal lymph. These include Whipple's disease, intestinal lymphangiectasis, mechanical obstruction of intestinal lymphatics by tumor or fibrosis, and severe right-sided congestive heart failure.

ABNORMAL NUCLEATED CELLS IN PERIPHERAL BLOOD

Under normal circumstances in the adult, only mature anucleate erythrocytes, mature granulocytes (including stab or band forms), monocytes, and lymphocytes (80% small non-reactive, 20% reactive) are seen in the peripheral circulation. The appearance of immature or abnormal cells in the circulation is indicative of underlying hematopathology and demands explanation.

Immature Granulocytes

When immature granulocytes (blasts, promyelocytes, myelocytes, and/or metamyelocytes) appear in peripheral blood, the differential diagnosis is essentially between a leukemoid reaction and a primary myeloproliferative syndrome. Normal and pathologic granulocytes are illustrated in Plate IV-6. Presence of toxic granulations, Döhle's bodies, or cytoplasmic vacuoles suggests infection. Decreased or absent granulation may be seen in myelodysplastic syndromes. When blasts and promyelocytes make up more than a few percentages of the immature cells, a myeloproliferative syndrome or leukemia is likely. The presence of only one or two myeloblasts on routine peripheral blood smears is also highly suspicious for primary hematologic malignancy and should be evaluated by careful bone marrow examination. The presence of Auer rods in the blasts is virtually diagnostic of acute nonlymphocytic leukemia (Plate IV-6, *E*). Characteristics of morphology and cytochemistry of blast cells in acute leukemias are discussed in Chapters 73 and 92. It should be remembered that in acute leukemias the total leukocyte count may be elevated, normal, or low. It has been said that leukopenia is as suggestive of leukemia as leukocytosis. The peripheral blood smear in chronic myelogenous leukemia resembles a smear of bone marrow because all stages of myeloid maturation from blast through mature polymorphonuclear neutrophil leukocyte (PMN) can be found (Plate IV-6, *D*). A basophilia may also be present. Leukocyte alkaline phosphatase and cytogenetic analysis can confirm the diagnosis of chronic myelogenous leukemia.

In idiopathic myelofibrosis, immature myeloid cells are usually present in the setting of a leukoerythroblastic blood smear. A leukoerythroblastic blood picture may also be seen in other marrow infiltrative processes, such as tumor, granulomata, or myelofibrosis secondary to certain drugs.

The Pelger-Huët anomaly (Plate IV-6, *C*) is a hereditary condition in which mature granulocytes have two nuclear segments only. This condition has no pathologic significance because the granulocytes are normal in number and function. An acquired Pelger-Huët anomaly sometimes develops in myeloproliferative disorders, dysmyelopoietic syndromes, and severe infections.

Abnormal Lymphoid Cells

The variety of morphologic types of lymphoid cells that may be seen in normal blood has been discussed. The proportion and absolute number of reactive lymphocytes in the circulation may increase with certain conditions, such as infections and allergic reactions. It is important to distinguish such normal reactive variants from the variety of lymphoid cells that may enter the blood in malignant lymphoproliferative disorders (Table 80-1). Some of the malignant lymphocytes are illustrated in the photomicrographs in Plate IV-5, which allows for their comparison with normal and reactive lymphocytes. Table 80-1 lists helpful laboratory and clinical considerations in assessing

patients who are found to have abnormal lymphoid cells on peripheral blood films. Additional information is provided in Chapter 73. The lymphoproliferative disorders with which these cells are associated are discussed in Chapters 92 and 94.

The small lymphocyte has a deeply stained, round nucleus of densely aggregated chromatin (Plate IV-5). The nuclear membrane is distinct, and occasionally one or two nucleolar remnants may be seen. The nucleus is eccentrically located in the blue cytoplasm, which is scanty compared with the nucleus; often only a thin rim is seen. Atypical lymphocytes are larger, approximately 1½ to 3 times the size of a small lymphocyte, with more abundant cytoplasm (Plate IV-5). The chromatin is less condensed than that of a normal lymphocyte. Nucleoli may be present. Although the cytoplasm may be foamy, more often it has no distinctive features other than denser staining at the periphery and the characteristic scalloping where the membrane contacts other cells.

Lymphoblasts, the characteristic cells of acute lymphoblastic leukemia, are large (15 to 20 μm) but variable in size (Plate IV-5). The chromatin is finely distributed and threadlike. One or two indistinct nucleoli are always present. The cytoplasm is scanty. It is important to distinguish an atypical lymphocytosis such as occurs frequently with infectious mononucleosis syndromes or other viral illnesses in infancy and childhood from acute lymphoblastic leukemia (ALL), which has its peak occurrence in these same age-groups. Additional similarities are that both infectious mononucleosis and ALL may be acute in onset and may be associated with lymphadenopathy and splenomegaly. In addition to careful evaluation of a peripheral blood film for the morphologic features just discussed and shown in Plate IV-5, useful discriminatory points are the frequent presence in leukemia of anemia, granulocytopenia, and thrombocytopenia, as well as hyperuricemia and bone pain caused by accelerated cell turnover. Serologic features of the infectious mononucleosis syndromes are diagnostic. Diagnostic features of infectious mononucleosis are summarized Box 80-2. Cytochemical and immunologic features of lymphoblasts include presence of the enzyme terminal deoxynucleotidyl transferase (TdT), detection of the common ALL antigen, and an immunophenotype characteristic of B- or T-cell precursors.

Circulating lymphoma cells are sometimes seen in the peripheral blood of patients with non-Hodgkin's lymphoma. When these cells are so abundant as to cause a leukemic peripheral blood picture, the term *lymphosarcoma cell leukemia* has been applied. Various forms of lymphosarcoma cells have been described. These range from lymphoid forms, slightly larger and less mature looking than the usual forms, to blastlike cells that may be difficult to distinguish from the blasts of ALL. A characteristic morphologic feature of lymphosarcoma cells is a cleaved folded nucleus, which has led to the descriptive term *buttock cell* (Plate IV-5, *E*). Often there is a single, large, prominent nucleolus demarcated by a dense periphery of condensed chromatin. Lymphosarcoma cell leukemia frequently develops in middle-aged or older individuals as a late manifestation of lymphoma. In such patients its recognition and proper diagnosis are not difficult. At other times, lymphosarcoma cell leukemia may be an initial manifestation of lymphoma. In this setting it must be differentiated from chronic lymphocytic leukemia (CLL) (Plate IV-5, *D*) and prolymphocytic leukemia (Plate IV-5, *H*) on the one hand and ALL (approximately 20% of adult acute leukemias) on the other (Plate IV-5, *F*). The differentiation from CLL is best done by lymph node biopsy, whereas lymphocyte surface marker analysis, cytochemistry (TdT), and bone marrow examination in addition to lymph node biopsy will aid in the differentiation from ALL (Table 80-1). In ALL, bone marrow is diffusely infiltrated by the abnormal cells, whereas in lymphosarcoma cell leukemia, marrow involvement is patchy and has a characteristic distribution in association with bony trabeculae. In prolymphocytic leukemia the abnormal cells superficially may resemble lymphosarcoma cells but on close inspection appear intermediate in development between the cells of CLL and those of lymphosarcoma cell leukemia (Plate IV-5, *H*). Prolymphocytes lack the characteristic cleaved nucleus of lymphosarcoma cells. Patients with prolymphocytic leukemia typically are elderly and manifest marked splenomegaly without adenopathy and very high lymphocyte counts ($>100 \times 10^9$ per liter). Prolymphocytic leukemia may present de novo or as "prolymphocytoid" transformation in a patient with CLL.

In mycosis fungoides and other cutaneous lymphomas, character-

Table 80-1   Differential diagnosis of abnormal lymphocytes in peripheral blood

LYMPHOCYTE TYPE	USUAL DISEASE ASSOCIATION	CYTOLOGIC FEATURES	LABORATORY FEATURES	CLINICAL FEATURES
Small lymphocyte	Chronic lymphocytic leukemia	B-cell surface markers with low concentration of monoclonal surface immunoglobulin, CD5 antigen	Hypogammaglobulinemia in 50%; positive direct Coombs' test in 15%; on node biopsy, diffuse, well-differentiated lymphocytic infiltrate	Elderly adults; presentation runs gamut from asymptomatic with lymphocytosis only to bulky disease with adenopathy, splenomegaly, and "packed" bone marrow
Atypical lympho-cyte	Infectious mononucle-osis, other viral illnesses	Suppressor T-cell markers	Heterophil agglutinin; positive serology for Epstein-Barr virus, cytomegalovirus, toxoplasma, HBsAg	Pharyngitis, fever, adenopathy, rash, splenomegaly, palatal pe-techiae, jaundice
Plasmacytoid lymphocyte	Waldenström's macro-globulinemia	Cytoplasmic IgM, periodic acid–Schiff (PAS) positivity	IgM paraprotein, rouleaux, cryo-globulins	Adenopathy, splenomegaly, ab-sence of bone lesions, hypervis-cosity syndrome, cryopathic phenomena
Lymphoblast	Acute lymphoblastic leukemia (ALL)	Terminal transferase positivity, common ALL antigen, B- or T-precursor markers	Anemia, granulocytopenia, throm-bocytopenia, hyperuricemia, diffuse bone marrow infiltration	Peak incidence in childhood, acute onset, bone pain frequent
Lymphosarcoma cell	Lymphocytic lymph-oma	B-cell surface markers with high concentration of monoclonal surface immunoglobulin	Nodular, or diffuse, poorly differ-entiated lymphocytic lymphoma on node biopsy, patchy, peritra-becular bone marrow involve-ment	Middle-aged to older adults, gen-eralized adenopathy, constitu-tional symptoms
Sézary cell	Cutaneous lymph-omas	T-lymphocyte surface markers	Skin biopsy is diagnostic	Exfoliative erythroderma, cutane-ous plaques or tumors
Hairy cell	Hairy cell leu-kemia	B-lymphocyte markers, cytoplas-mic projections, tartrate-resistant acid phosphatase, interleukin-2 receptors, CD11 antigen	Pancytopenia	Middle-aged males, moderate to marked splenomegaly without adenopathy
Prolymphocyte	Prolymphocytic leukemia	B-cell surface markers with high concentration of monoclonal surface immunoglobulin, CD5 negative	Marked lymphocytosis (frequently $>100 \times 10^9$/L)	Elderly adults, massive spleno-megaly, minimum adenopathy, poor response to therapy

HBsAg, Hepatitis B surface antigen; *IgM,* immunoglobulin M.

istic *Sézary cells* may appear in the circulation (Plate IV-5, *I*). These cells may represent only a small percentage of circulating cells in these patients (1% to 20%) or, more rarely, may be the predominant peripheral cell present, leading to a leukemic peripheral blood pic-ture. The Sézary cell is large and contains a prominent, characteristic nucleus that occupies three fourths or more of the cell. The nucleus is lobulated and convoluted with numerous folds and clefts. The cy-toplasm is deep blue and may contain multiple small, round vacuoles sometimes rimming the nucleus. Electron microscopy is useful in demonstrating the convoluted pattern of the nucleus. Sézary cells are derived from T lymphocytes and express mature T-cell markers. The recognition of circulating Sézary cells in patients with advanced my-cosis fungoides is not difficult. Conversely, the appearance of classic Sézary cells in the peripheral blood of patients with nonspecific der-matologic lesions should suggest the possibility of cutaneous T-cell lymphoma. Definitive diagnosis should be pursued by biopsy of the appropriate lesions for histopathologic study.

The characteristic cell of hairy cell leukemia may also be con-fused with other lymphoid variants. The hairy cell is a large cell with an eccentrically located nucleus containing lacy-appearing chromatin (Plate IV-5, *G*). Nucleoli may be easily seen. The cytoplasm appears pale grayish blue and usually contains no granules. Characteristic fine filamentous projections are observed at the cytoplasmic border and may give the cell margins a serrated or fragmented appearance. These cells are prone to smearing artifacts with spreading and fusing of the cytoplasmic projections and loss of the hairy appearance. Further-more, they may make up only a small percentage of peripheral mono-nuclear cells in any given patient and thus may escape detection. Con-versely, artifactual hairy cells may be created on normal blood smears when blood is drawn and allowed to stand before smears are made. This is especially true if the blood is kept refrigerated. The diagnosis of hairy cell leukemia thus requires a high index of suspicion and careful examination of a peripheral blood smear. The typical patient is a middle-aged man with pancytopenia and splenomegaly. Hairy

cells are best demonstrated in wet mounts with supravital stains. Cy-tochemical staining for the tartrate-resistant isoenzyme of acid phos-phatase can provide important confirmatory information. In about 50% of patients the cells contain peculiar cylindric cytoplasmic in-clusions termed *ribosome lamella complexes*. As with the small lym-phocyte of CLL, the lymphosarcoma cell, and the prolymphocyte, the hairy cell usually is of B-lymphocyte origin. The characteristic hairy cell may be distinguished from other neoplastic B cells by the pres-ence of receptors for the lymphokine interleukin-2 (T-cell growth fac-tor) and expression of the CD11 antigen on surfaces of hairy cells.

Plasmacytoid lymphocytes may appear during infections (Plate IV-5, *C*) and are also the characteristic malignant cell seen in Wal-denström's macroglobulinemia. The diagnosis of Waldenström's mac-roglobulinemia is confirmed by demonstration of an immunoglobu-lin M paraprotein by serum protein electrophoresis and immunoelec-trophoresis. Patients with this disease frequently complain of cryo-pathic phenomena or give evidence of hyperviscosity syndrome (Chapter 94). Erythrocyte rouleaux are present on blood films (Plate IV-4, *F*), and a cryoglobulin may be detected in plasma and serum during routine blood processing. Mature plasma cells are not normally present in the circulation. A small number may be seen in association with multiple myeloma, and their presence in large number is diag-nostic of plasma cell leukemia, a rare complication of multiple my-eloma.

Nucleated Red Blood Cells

Nucleated red blood cells are not normally present in peripheral blood but may appear when the bone marrow is subjected to intense stimu-lation, as in response to acute hemorrhage, hypoxemia, or hemolytic anemia (Box 80-3). They may also be seen in asplenic individuals who lack the normal "pitting" function of the spleen. When present in substantial numbers, nucleated erythrocytes may produce spurious elevation of the leukocyte count because automated cell counters do

BOX 80-2
Diagnostic features of infectious mononucleosis syndromes

I. Clinical
   A. Fever, exudative tonsilitis, lymphadenopathy (98% to 100%)
   B. Splenomegaly (50% to 75%)
   C. Palatal petechiae (30% to 50%)
   D. Periorbital edema (30%)
   E. Hepatomegaly (10% to 20%)
II. Hematologic
   A. Relative and absolute lymphocytosis
   B. Atypical lymphocytes 20% or greater
III. Etiologic agents
   A. Epstein-Barr virus (EBV) (90%) (Chapter 255)
   B. Cytomegalovirus (CMV) (5%) (Chapter 255)
   C. *Toxoplasma gondii* (Chapter 279)
   D. Other viruses (e.g., adenovirus, hepatitis viruses, rubella)
IV. Serologic diagnosis
   A. For EBV syndrome, presence of one or more of the following:
      1. Heterophil antibodies (Monospot test)
      2. Immunoglobulin M antibodies to viral capsid antigen (VCA) that decline during convalescence
      3. Fourfold or greater rise in immunoglobulin G antibodies to VCA
      4. Transient antibody response to the diffuse component of the virus early antigen (anti-D)
   B. For CMV syndrome, negative heterophil plus one or more of the following:
      1. Seroconversion from anti-CMV negative to positive
      2. Fourfold or greater rise in anti-CMV antibodies
      3. Positive CMV buffy coat culture
   C. For other heterophil-negative syndromes, specific serologic tests for the following:
      1. *Toxoplasma gondii* (Chapter 279)
      2. Hepatitis viruses (Chapter 355)
      3. Adenovirus (Chapter 251)
      4. Rubella (Chapter 251)

BOX 80-3
Circulating nucleated erythrocytes: diagnostic considerations

I. Reactive secondary to intense erythropoietic stimulus
   A. Acute hemorrhage
   B. Hypoxemia
   C. Hemolytic anemia
   D. Megaloblastic anemia
II. Infiltrative processes in the bone marrow
   A. Metastatic malignancies
   B. Primary hematologic malignancies
   C. Myelofibrosis, either primary, secondary, or drug related
   D. Granuloma
III. Asplenic individuals

not distinguish between nucleated red and white blood cells. Examination of a peripheral blood smear will readily resolve such a discrepancy. Nucleated red blood cells also enter the blood in marrow infiltrative processes, which may result in a leukoerythroblastic blood picture. In the absence of a clear cause for nucleated red cells in the blood, bone marrow biopsy is indicated.

BIBLIOGRAPHY

Bessis M: *Blood smear reinterpreted,* New York, 1977, Springer Verlag.
Coates TD, Baehner R: Leukocytosis and leukopenia. In Hoffman R et al, editors: *Hematology: basic principles and practice,* ed 2, New York, 1995, Churchill-Livingstone.

Gurwith MJ et al: Granulocytopenia in hospitalized patients. I. Prognostic factors and etiology of fever, *Am J Med* 64:121, 1978.
Maldonado JE, Hanlon DG: Monocytosis: a current appraisal, *Mayo Clin Proc* 40:248, 1965.
Mintzer DM, Hauptman SP: Lymphosarcoma cell leukemia and other non-Hodgkin's lymphomas in leukemic phase, *Am J Med* 75:110, 1983.
Tomkinson BE, Sullivan JL: Epstein-Barr virus infection and infectious mononucleosis. In Gorbach SL, Bartlett JG, Blacklow NR, editors: *Infectious diseases,* Philadelphia, 1992, WB Saunders.
Ward PC: The lymphoid leukocytoses, *Postgrad Med* 67(2):217, 1980.
Ward PC: The myeloid leukocytoses, *Postgrad Med* 67(1):219, 1980.

CHAPTER

81   Lymphadenopathy and Splenomegaly

David H. Boldt

The immune system consists of various highly specialized cell types involved in carrying out the reactions of cell-mediated and humoral immunity (Chapter 171). These cells include the lymphocytes (T cells, B cells, and non-T, non-B cells), plasma cells, and mononuclear phagocytes. Most are produced in the bone marrow, but the lymphocytes may undergo programming in central lymphoid organs such as the thymus during fetal and neonatal life. After their differentiation has been completed, these cells populate peripheral lymphoid organs such as the lymph nodes and spleen. Anatomic localization in organs provides an organization to the immune system and serves to promote the generation of an immune response after antigenic challenge. Lymph nodes and spleen have blood and lymphatic supplies as well as internal architectures that facilitate antigen processing and cellular interactions, two prerequisites for normal immunologic function.

Because the immune system plays a central role in host defense against microbial and antigenic challenge, abnormalities of lymphoid organs are encountered frequently in clinical practice. Lymphadenopathy and splenomegaly are prominent features of a wide variety of diseases and in many instances serve as a focal point for subsequent clinical investigation. This chapter discusses the structure and function of lymph nodes and spleen as a basis for understanding clinical abnormalities, then focuses on etiologic considerations and guidelines for evaluation of patients with lymphadenopathy and/or splenomegaly.

LYMPHADENOPATHY
Lymph Node Structure and Function

Lymph nodes are distributed in clusters along the courses of lymphatic vessels throughout the body. They are ovoid and normally range in size from a few millimeters to more than a centimeter. Their architecture facilitates efficient filtration of lymph and promotes internal migration of cells, primarily lymphocytes and mononuclear phagocytes (Fig. 81-1). A lymph node consists of three anatomic zones. In the cortex of the node adjacent to the subcapsular sinus are aggregates of B lymphocytes termed *lymphoid follicles.* Some of the follicles contain germinal centers, areas of plasma cells, macrophages, and rapidly dividing lymphocytes actively engaged in protein synthesis. Among and adjacent to the follicles is the paracortical zone, consisting of sheets of T lymphocytes. Beneath the paracortex and occupying the central portion of the node is the medulla. Here the lymphocytes are arranged in cordlike arrays, termed *medullary cords,* that converge on the hilus.

Antigen is carried into the node by the afferent lymphatics and is engulfed and processed by cortical macrophages. A specialized type of cell, termed *dendritic cell,* is believed to play a major role in antigen presentation to lymphocytes. The lymph node serves to bring together all the elements necessary for initiating an immune response.

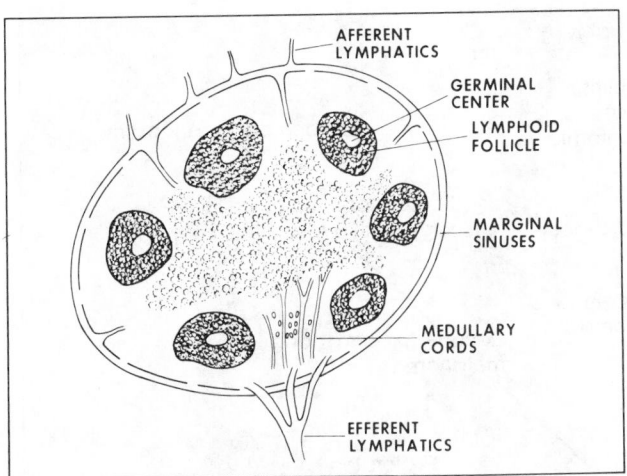

FIGURE 81-1   A lymph node. At the surface of the node the reticular fibers form a dense fibrous capsule. Afferent lymphatic vessels enter the node by piercing the capsular surface and empty into a subcapsular sinus. From there lymph flows inward along the channels formed by the reticular network and exits the node at the hilus via a single efferent lymphatic vessel. The lymphoid follicle consists of aggregates of B lymphocytes. Germinal centers are areas of plasma cells, macrophages, and rapidly dividing lymphocytes. Among and adjacent to the follicles is the paracortical zone of T lymphocytes.

T lymphocytes become activated by antigen in the paracortex. Activated B lymphocytes develop into antibody-secreting plasma cells in the germinal centers of lymphoid follicles. An intense immunologic reaction, as in a secondary immune response, will lead to proliferation of lymphoid follicles and formation of germinal centers. An increase in the number and size of lymphoid follicles secondary to such an immune response frequently results in clinically apparent lymphadenopathy.

The Patient With Lymphadenopathy: General Considerations

When one encounters a patient with lymphadenopathy, several considerations are important. One is the patient's age. The possibility that peripheral lymphadenopathy is caused by a benign process decreases with age. Reactive hyperplasia of lymphoid tissue in response to infectious or inflammatory processes is characteristic of infants and children. In a study of 925 adult patients undergoing diagnostic lymph node biopsies, approximately 80% of the lesions were benign in patients younger than 30, but only 40% were benign in patients older than 50. Conversely, 20% of lesions were malignant in patients under 30, and 60% were malignant in patients over 50.

Two questions are of primary importance in assessing lymphadenopathy. Is lymphadenopathy localized or generalized? What is the time course of its appearance? Lymphadenopathy in certain regions takes on special clinical significance. For example, palpable supraclavicular nodes are frequently associated with intrathoracic or intraabdominal malignancies and therefore demand careful evaluation. By contrast, isolated occipital lymphadenopathy seldom represents a malignant condition and usually reflects an infectious process of the scalp, such as ringworm or insect bites. Progressive enlargement of nodes over several weeks, especially if associated with complaints of fever, chills, night sweats, or weight loss, is suggestive of serious systemic illness such as chronic mycobacterial or fungal infection or a malignant lymphoproliferative disease.

Nodal tenderness is suggestive of an infectious process but does not adequately distinguish malignant from nonmalignant causes. For example, rapid lymph node enlargement in acute lymphoblastic leukemia may be associated with considerable discomfort. A peculiar symptom occasionally reported in association with Hodgkin's disease is the development of pain in enlarged lymph nodes after alcohol ingestion.

The consistency of enlarged nodes to palpation can provide clues

---

BOX 81-1
Causes of lymphadenopathy

   I. Infections: Bacterial, mycobacterial, fungal, viral, or parasitic
  II. Immunologic disorders
    A. Rheumatic disorders
    B. Serum sickness
    C. Sarcoidosis
    D. Drug reactions: Hydantoins
 III. Malignancies
    A. Hematologic
    B. Nonhematologic
  IV. Miscellaneous or of unknown origin
    A. Atypical lymphoproliferations of unknown cause: Angioimmunoblastic lymphadenopathy, angiofollicular lymph node hyperplasia (Castleman's disease), sinus histiocytosis with massive lymphadenopathy
    B. Dermatopathic lymphadenopathy
    C. Endocrinopathies: Thyrotoxicosis, adrenal insufficiency
    D. Lipidoses

to etiology. Tender, warm, erythematous nodes associated with fluctuance or lymphangitic streaking of adjacent skin are associated with local infectious processes. Stony, hard nodes fixed to the adjacent tissues are highly suggestive of malignancy, especially metastatic carcinoma or sarcoma, whereas rubbery, mobile nodes are suggestive of lymphomas. Conditions that may be associated with lymphadenopathy are listed in Box 81-1.

The Patient With Regional Lymphadenopathy

Figure 81-2 presents a clinical approach to patients with regional lymphadenopathy. Evaluation of a patient with localized adenopathy depends on knowledge of both the lymphatic drainage patterns of various portions of the body and the pathologic processes most likely to affect these areas. Lymphadenopathy in certain regions takes on special clinical significance that may allow for efficient direction of diagnostic investigation.

Cervical Lymph Nodes. Enlarged nodes confined to the neck may result from occult infection or malignancy. Because the cervical lymph nodes receive lymphatic drainage from the head, neck, and oropharyngeal cavities, infections that must be considered include soft tissue infections of the face, dental abscesses, otitis externa, and bacterial pharyngitis. Careful ears, nose, and throat examination and bacterial throat cultures, including use of special media and plating conditions for gonococci if recent orogenital contact is suspected, will aid in diagnosis. Infectious mononucleosis may also present with localized cervical lymphadenopathy and may be diagnosed by appropriate serologic tests and examination of a peripheral blood film for atypical lymphocytes (Chapter 80). The disorder is most common in young adults and is very rare after the age of 30. The occurrence of typical clinical and hematologic findings of infectious mononucleosis in the face of a negative heterophil reaction should suggest the possibility of infection by cytomegalovirus; another virus such as hepatitis, adenovirus, or rubella; or *Toxoplasma*. Diagnostic features of infectious mononucleosis syndromes are given in Box 80-2. Malignancies frequently presenting as localized cervical lymphadenopathy include Hodgkin's disease, non-Hodgkin's lymphomas, and squamous cell carcinomas arising from nasopharyngeal or laryngeal structures.

Axillary Nodes. Localization of lymphadenopathy to the axilla suggests a different spectrum of diagnostic possibilities. Axillary nodes drain the lymphatics of the upper extremities and the breasts. Axillary adenopathy should suggest infectious processes such as cat scratch fever, sporotrichosis, tularemia, and staphylococcal or streptococcal infections. Examination of the upper extremities for scratches, bites, suppurative lesions, or lymphangitis may provide im-

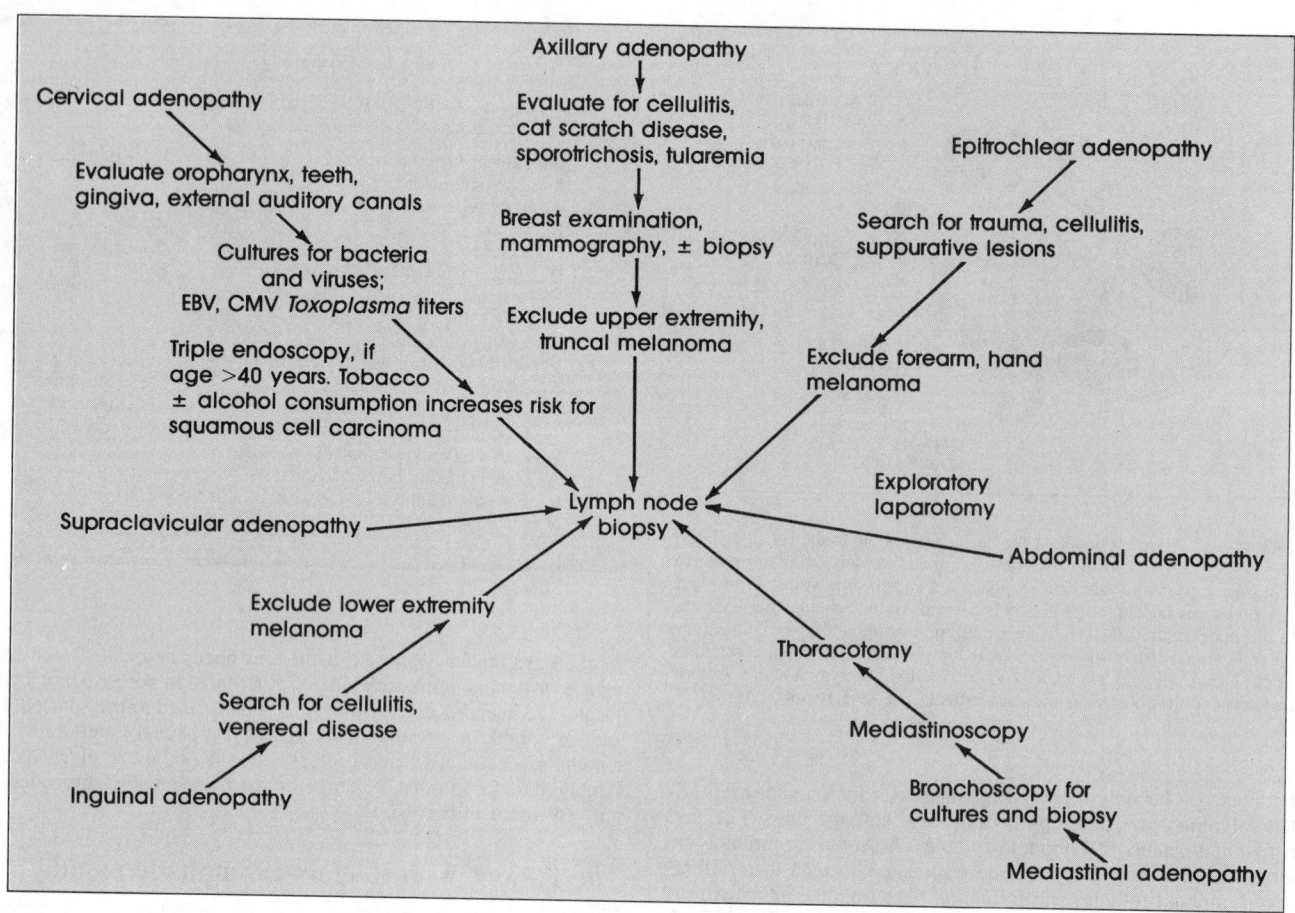

FIGURE 81-2   Clinical approach to the patient with localized lymphadenopathy.

portant diagnostic clues. Malignancies that may present with localized axillary adenopathy include lymphoma, melanoma, and carcinoma of the breast.

Epitrochlear Nodes. Bilateral, painless, epitrochlear lymphadenopathy may occur as a result of repeated minor trauma and/or infections in manual laborers. Its occurrence in other settings is suggestive of lymphoma.

Supraclavicular Nodes. Palpable supraclavicular lymph nodes are of ominous significance because of their frequent association with intrathoracic and intraabdominal malignancies and with breast cancer in women. Lymphatic drainage of the chest and mediastinum is to the supraclavicular nodes bilaterally. The thoracic duct carrying abdominal lymphatic drainage empties into the left innominate vein in the left supraclavicular region. This anatomic feature accounts for the well-known phenomenon of a left-sided supraclavicular sentinel node (Virchow's node) that heralds the presence of an occult abdominal neoplasm. Intrathoracic infections, usually chronic mycobacterial or fungal infections, may also present with localized supraclavicular lymphadenopathy, as may sarcoidosis. However, bacterial pneumonias or bronchial infections do not present in this manner. Early biopsy of localized enlarged supraclavicular nodes to establish a definitive diagnosis is usually indicated.

Inguinal Nodes. Localized inguinal lymphadenopathy may be most difficult to evaluate because virtually all adults manifest some degree of inguinal node enlargement as a consequence of repeated trauma and minor infections involving the genitalia and lower extremities. The inguinal nodes provide lymphatic drainage for the lower extremities and the skin of the lower abdomen, genitals, and perineum. An important point is that the internal pelvic organs and testes drain via the iliac nodes into the paraaortic chain, so deep pel-

vic infections or malignancies do not usually present as inguinal lymphadenopathy. Infectious considerations in a patient with inguinal lymphadenopathy include cellulitis of the lower extremities and venereal infections such as syphilis, chancroid, genital herpes, or lymphogranuloma venereum. Malignant conditions include lymphomas, metastatic melanomas arising in the lower extremities, and squamous cell carcinomas from primary sites in the penis or vulva.

Internal Nodes. Internal lymphadenopathy may come to the physician's attention on radiologic examination, for example, hilar or mediastinal adenopathy on chest radiographs. These nodes may be the principal manifestation of bronchogenic carcinoma or lymphoma. Hodgkin's disease is more often associated with hilar or mediastinal lymphadenopathy than are non-Hodgkin's lymphomas. Sarcoidosis, tuberculosis, or fungal infections are important non-malignant conditions that must be considered in the differential diagnosis. Bacterial infections in the lung are not usually associated with lymphadenopathy. Because there are so many different causes of intrathoracic adenopathy, aggressive workup, including bronchoscopy and/or mediastinoscopy for biopsy and establishment of a histopathologic diagnosis, is indicated.

Intraabdominal lymphadenopathy may be detected as a palpable mass on physical examination or it may come to attention indirectly, through obstruction or pressure effects on some adjacent organ such as a ureter. Various radiographic techniques must usually be employed to delineate fully the extent of intraabdominal or retroperitoneal lymphadenopathy. These include computed tomography, ultrasonography, magnetic resonance imaging, and/or lymphangiography. If lymphadenopathy is confined to the abdomen and peripheral tissue is not accessible, x-ray–guided needle aspiration may aid in establishing a diagnosis. As an alternative, exploratory laparotomy with excisional lymph node biopsy may be required for definitive diagnosis. Intraabdominal lymphadenopathy frequently signifies a malignant process such as Hodgkin's disease or non-Hodgkin's lymphoma. Hodgkin's disease typically involves pelvic and retroperitoneal nodes, while sparing mesenteric nodes. By contrast, non-Hodgkin's lymphomas frequently involve mesenteric nodes as well. Tuberculous mesenteric lymphadenitis may produce large, suppurative, abdominal lymph nodes that may calcify or rupture.

Superficial Nodes. Patients with a variety of dermatologic disorders, especially exfoliative dermatitis, may develop regional superficial lymphadenopathy. This condition, termed *dermatopathic lymphadenopathy,* is self-limited and regresses with improvement of the skin disease. On biopsy the involved nodes are characterized by the presence of large numbers of atypical reticulum cells and foamy cells containing lipoid material or melanin.

The Patient With Generalized Lymphadenopathy

Figure 81-3 presents a clinical approach to patients with generalized lymphadenopathy. In the adult, generalized lymphadenopathy usually signifies the presence of serious systemic illness, either infectious, immunologic, or malignant. Prompt biopsy of an involved lymph node is usually indicated. Nonetheless, it is important to exclude the possibility that the lymphadenopathy is related to drug ingestion. This relationship is best recognized in association with the phenytoin group of anticonvulsant drugs, hydralazine, and allopurinol. Clinical findings may include fever, rash, lymphadenopathy, hepatosplenomegaly, arthritis, and jaundice, all of which generally disappear rapidly once the offending agent has been discontinued. The clinical picture strongly resembles an immunologically mediated hypersensitivity reaction. Lymph nodes obtained at biopsy have architectural features that may be difficult to differentiate from malignant lymphoma. These atypical histologic findings have led to the use of the term *pseudolymphoma* for these lesions. Although true malignant lymphomas have developed in some of these patients, an etiologic relationship between the malignant transformation and either anticonvulsant therapy or the hypersensitivity reaction is not established.

Generalized adenopathy may be caused by systemic infections. The most common of these are probably the infectious mononucleosis syndromes, including those caused by Epstein-Barr (EB) virus, cytomegalovirus, other viruses, and *Toxoplasma.* Otherwise, generalized lymphadenopathy occurs infrequently in adults with infections except those infected with the human immunodeficiency virus (HIV), tuberculosis, or fungal infections such as histoplasmosis or coccidioidomycosis. Brucellosis, bacterial endocarditis, infectious hepatitis, or secondary syphilis also may cause generalized lymphadenopathy. Immunologic disorders to be considered in patients with generalized lymphadenopathy include sarcoidosis, rheumatoid arthritis, and systemic lupus erythematosus.

Generalized or localized lymphadenopathy may occur during the course of infection with HIV, the causative agent of acquired immunodeficiency syndrome (AIDS). HIV infections are discussed in Chapter 256. After infection, an initial asymptomatic period during which subjects exhibit serologic evidence of HIV may evolve into a symptomatic state that may be associated with a syndrome of generalized lymphadenopathy characterized by reactive lymph node hyperplasia on microscopic examination. In some of these patients a histopathologic syndrome of *progressive generalized lymphadenopathy* (PGL) may develop. PGL refers to a temporal histologic progression from benign hyperplasia through a stage of mixed follicular hyperplasia and involution and ultimately to complete follicular involution with lymphocyte depletion. Approximately one fourth of HIV-infected patients who develop non-Hodgkin's lymphomas have preexisting PGL, but this histologic finding does not appear to be predictive of lymphoma. It may, however, correlate with clinical symptoms, opportunistic infections, and overall survival. The diagnosis of full-blown AIDS is made clinically on the development of opportunistic infections, secondary malignancies, encephalopathy, or the HIV-associated wasting syndrome. Laboratory criteria for the diagnosis of AIDS in an HIV-infected individual are a CD4 T-cell count less than 200 cells/μL or a CD4 T-cell percentage less than 14%. At this stage of HIV infection, localized or generalized lymphadenopathy may represent viral, bacterial, mycobacterial, fungal, or parasitic infection or a lymphoma or a nonlymphomatous malignancy. Therefore lymph

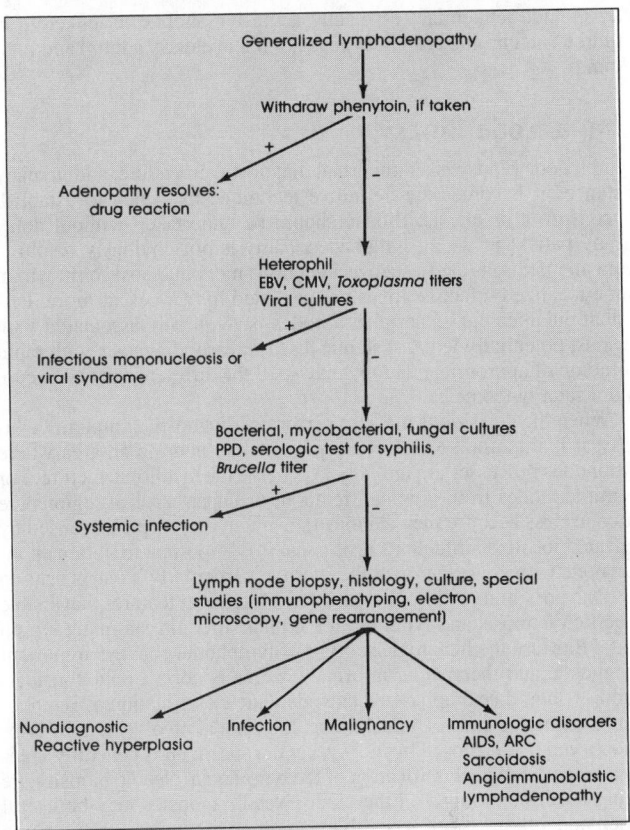

FIGURE 81-3 Clinical approach to the patient with generalized lymphadenopathy. *AIDS,* Acquired immunodeficiency syndrome; *ARC,* AIDS-related complex.

node biopsy should be strongly considered in any patient with suspected or documented HIV infection.

Several atypical lymphoproliferative disorders of unknown cause are increasingly recognized. A disorder termed *angioimmunoblastic lymphadenopathy* (AILD) seems to straddle a poorly defined border between immunologic hypersensitivity reactions and frankly malignant lymphoproliferative disorders. This condition frequently affects elderly individuals and is characterized by generalized adenopathy, hepatosplenomegaly, skin rash, and constitutional symptoms. Frequently, there is a history of recent drug exposure, insect bite, immunization, or other potential immunologic stimuli. Laboratory evaluation may reveal Coombs'-test–positive hemolytic anemia and polyclonal hypergammaglobulinemia. Histologic examination of the lymph nodes demonstrates a mixed cellular infiltration with immunoblasts, lymphocytes, plasma cells, and eosinophils. A characteristic feature is proliferation and arborization of small capillary blood vessels. Recent studies have identified clonal populations of T cells in AILD specimens, raising the concern that many cases actually may represent T-cell lymphomas. Patients with AILD usually follow a progressive downhill course, with a median survival of approximately 3 years. No effective treatment exists. In some patients the disease evolves into a true malignant lymphoma that is generally refractory to therapy.

Angiofollicular lymph node hyperplasia (Castleman's disease) usually presents with mediastinal lymphadenopathy. Two variants are recognized: hyaline vascular type (90%) and plasma cell type (10%). Often the disease is asymptomatic and discovered only by routine chest x-ray examination. Most cases are self-limited. Other cases may be associated with systemic symptoms of fever, sweats, fatigue, or weight loss and with anemia and hypergammaglobulinemia. The plasma cell variant tends to be more aggressive and may be associated with multicentric lymph node involvement and a progressive clinical course. Some cases may evolve into overt lymphoma. No effective therapy exists.

Malignant conditions associated with generalized lymphadenopathy include leukemias (especially acute lymphoblastic leukemia in children and chronic lymphocytic leukemia in elderly adults) and lymphomas.

Lymph Node Biopsy

Lymph node biopsy is an important diagnostic procedure, and in many instances it becomes the definitive technique by which to establish or confirm a diagnosis. Biopsy should be undertaken without delay in any patient in whom lymphadenopathy is not obviously resulting from an infectious cause such as infectious mononucleosis or in whom some localized infective focus has persisted for a week or more. Persistent enlargement of peripheral nodes is frequently associated with serious, potentially lethal systemic disease; early diagnosis with rapid initiation of appropriate therapy may spell the difference between cure and a fatal outcome.

When the decision is made to perform a diagnostic lymph node biopsy, it is important to select a representative node in an area where extraneous processes are unlikely to confuse the histologic picture. For example, nodes from inguinal, femoral, or upper cervical regions are often useless because they demonstrate reactive hyperplasia caused by repeated localized infectious processes. It is important to obtain an intact node with preservation of the capsule, particularly if one is dealing with the possibility of lymphoma. The architectural features that enable specific diagnosis and typing of a lymphoma require an intact lymph node. Because the histologic subtype of lymphoma conveys important prognostic and therapeutic information, this is not a trivial consideration. It should be emphasized that adequate classification of lymphomas can only be done on nodal tissue. Extranodal involvement by lymphoma can be diagnosed by biopsy, but the specimen is generally inadequate for detailed classification of the lymphoma. Needle biopsies are being used increasingly in the clinic. Needle biopsies may be useful when nodal tissue is not accessible, but otherwise are not preferable to excisional biopsy specimens for diagnosis.

At the time of node biopsy, a portion of the specimen is preserved in formalin for routine pathologic examination. Adequate material must be obtained for bacterial, fungal, and mycobacterial cultures, for special stains for these organisms, and under certain circumstances for special cytochemical stains and analysis of lymphocyte surface markers. In some instances, as in undifferentiated malignancies, electron microscopy may be helpful and a specimen may be preserved in special fixatives for this procedure. Several studies have demonstrated that lymph node biopsy will lead to a specific diagnosis in approximately two thirds of patients in whom it is undertaken.

Problem of Nondiagnostic Lymph Node Biopsy

In one third of lymph node biopsies, no specific diagnosis is established. Lymph nodes with atypical features suggestive but not diagnostic of malignancy are a continuing problem for the surgical pathologist. Traditionally this type of difficult biopsy has been called *atypical hyperplasia*. It is instructive to consider the fate of patients who have this diagnosis. In a 1957 study by Moore and others, 158 of 379 lymph node biopsies were nondiagnostic at the first attempt. Among these undiagnosed patients, 63 individuals developed either a malignancy or a rheumatic disorder over the ensuing decade. At the end of a decade, 47 of the 158 were alive and well, 56 were alive with serious disease, and 55 were dead. In a more recent study published in 1979 by Schroer and Franssila, 21 of 70 patients whose initial lymph node biopsy specimen demonstrated atypical hyperplasia developed a malignant lymphoproliferative disorder during a follow-up period of 2 to 13 years. Clearly, persistent lymph node enlargement is frequently associated with serious, often fatal, systemic illness and careful follow-up of patients with nondiagnostic lymph node biopsies is essential.

SPLENOMEGALY
Spleen Structure and Function

The spleen is the largest lymphoid organ in the body. It is well designed for accomplishing its major functions as a filter of the blood and generator of immune responses. When a fresh spleen is cut, it appears to consist of the relatively avascular white pulp and the vas-

cular red pulp. The white pulp, where immunologic function resides, consists of lymphoid aggregates associated with a central arteriole. This lymphoid tissue is organized into periarteriolar sheaths that are collections of T lymphocytes analogous to the paracortical regions of lymph nodes and lymphoid follicles that are collections of B lymphocytes. The marginal zone, a loosely organized collection of lymphocytes and reticuloendothelial cells, surrounds periarteriolar sheaths and follicles and is thought to play a major role in antigen uptake and processing. Antigenic challenge results in changes in the white pulp of the spleen analogous to those that occur in lymph nodes. There is hyperplasia of lymphoid follicles and formation of germinal centers, reflecting generation of immunologically competent T and B lymphocytes. These phenomena cause splenic hyperplasia and may result in palpable splenomegaly.

The red pulp occupies the largest portion of the spleen. It is within the unique vasculature of this region that the spleen's filtration function is accomplished. Here terminal arterial vessels empty into a reticular meshwork containing large numbers of macrophages. Blood cells must traverse this region to reach the venous sinuses, which they enter by passing between sinusoidal endothelial cells. In order to negotiate its passage through the red pulp, a cell must be sufficiently deformable to squeeze through the cords and sinuses and return to the systemic circulation. Inability to accomplish this passage results in sequestration of the cell in an environment of low oxygen tension and its ultimate phagocytosis and destruction by splenic macrophages. This is the normal mechanism for removal *(culling)* of effete erythrocytes or other cells that have been damaged by physical or immunologic mechanisms, or those that contain nuclear remnants, siderotic granules, denatured hemoglobin (Heinz bodies; Plate IV-4, *P*), or parasites such as malarial organisms. In certain instances, inclusions such as these may be removed from the red cell without its destruction, a process termed *pitting*. Absence of these normal pitting and culling functions of the spleen accounts for the characteristic peripheral blood picture of splenectomized patients. Nucleated red blood cells and Howell-Jolly bodies are frequently seen (Plate IV-4, *K*). In fact, absence of nucleated red blood cells and Howell-Jolly bodies from the peripheral blood of a patient who has had a splenectomy is evidence of a functional accessory spleen. The spleen normally contains large amounts of storage iron because of its role in red blood cell destruction. The spleen also plays a role in phagocytosis and disposal of foreign particles and microorganisms. It is normally the site of blood formation in utero, but after birth the presence of extramedullary hematopoiesis in the spleen always signifies a pathologic condition.

Patient With Splenomegaly

A list of conditions associated with splenomegaly is given in Box 81-2. The normal spleen weighs 150 g and is located in the left upper abdominal quadrant against the diaphragm and close to the

---

BOX 81-2
Differential diagnosis of splenomegaly

I. Associated with generalized lymphadenopathy
   A. Infections
   B. Inflammatory and immunologic diseases
   C. Hematologic malignancies
II. Not associated with lymphadenopathy
   A. Any condition listed above
   B. Hematologic disorders: chronic hemolytic anemias, megaloblastic anemias
   C. Congestive splenomegaly: portal hypertension or severe congestive heart failure
   D. Infiltrative processes: amyloidosis, storage diseases
   E. Other causes: splenic cysts, arteriovenous malformations, splenic artery aneurysms, splenic abscess
   F. Normal variation in young adults

abdominal wall. As enlargement occurs, the spleen retains its superficial location just beneath the abdominal wall, so deep palpation is usually not necessary to detect splenomegaly. However, substantial splenomegaly can occur in the absence of a palpable spleen by physical examination. Radionuclide scanning may be useful in resolving presence or absence of splenomegaly when the question is in doubt.

In evaluating causes of splenomegaly, it is convenient to divide them into two categories, depending on whether lymphadenopathy is present. Figure 81-4 presents a clinical approach to patients with splenomegaly. In general, any condition that can cause generalized lymphadenopathy can cause splenomegaly. These conditions include the chronic infections and the inflammatory and immunologic disorders discussed previously. In any of these conditions, splenomegaly may occur as an isolated finding without accompanying lymphadenopathy. Diagnostic considerations and approach to management of patients with both splenomegaly and lymphadenopathy are the same as approaches to lymphadenopathy discussed earlier in this chapter. Diagnosis is based on blood cell counts, morphology of cells in the peripheral blood, serologies, appropriate cultures, and in many instances, examination of a lymph node obtained at biopsy. In certain parasitic infections such as malaria or schistosomiasis, splenomegaly is frequently seen in the absence of significant lymphadenopathy. In kala-azar (leishmaniasis), massive splenomegaly may accompany modest lymphadenopathy. The occurrence of splenomegaly and leukopenia in association with rheumatoid arthritis is known as Felty's syndrome.

Malignancies associated with splenomegaly are predominantly the myeloproliferative or lymphoproliferative disorders. Hairy cell leukemia and prolymphocytic leukemia are examples of disseminated lymphoproliferative diseases marked by prominent splenomegaly without lymphadenopathy. Careful examination of the peripheral blood should allow recognition of these disorders. Although metastases to the spleen have been found in up to 50% of patients who died of carcinoma, these usually occur as a late event in the course of the disease and seldom cause clinically detectable splenomegaly. Splenomegaly in a setting of metastatic carcinoma is usually caused by portal hypertension secondary to obstruction by tumor deposits in the liver or elsewhere.

Splenomegaly in the absence of lymphadenopathy may be caused by nonmalignant hematologic disorders. These conditions are primarily hemolytic anemias such as congenital erythrocyte enzyme defects, hereditary spherocytosis, immune hemolytic anemia, or hemoglobinopathies. This has led to the concept of *work hypertrophy* of the spleen, which has been supported by experimental evidence. According to this hypothesis, the increased workload in terms of phagocy-

tosis and destruction of erythrocytes imposed on the spleen by a chronic hemolytic state leads to reticuloendothelial hyperplasia, a subsequent further increase in hemolysis, which may be followed by more hyperplasia and so on. For this reason, splenectomy may confer substantial benefit in many chronic hemolytic disorders. Other nonmalignant hematologic diseases that may be accompanied by splenomegaly are the megaloblastic anemias caused by nutritional deficiencies of folic acid or vitamin B_{12} (Chapter 87). Iron deficiency is associated with splenomegaly in the older literature, but this association is rarely, if ever, observed today. Besides these nonmalignant hematologic disorders, the other major cause of splenomegaly without lymphadenopathy is congestive splenomegaly. This type of splenomegaly is caused by portal hypertension, caused in turn by hepatic cirrhosis or, rarely, by severe congestive heart failure.

Evaluation of patients with isolated splenomegaly in the absence of lymphadenopathy is straightforward. Approximately 3% of adolescents and young adults have a palpable spleen as a normal finding on careful physical examination. Presence of chronic hemolysis, portal hypertension, or congestive heart failure usually is determined from the history and physical examination. Laboratory evaluation for hemolysis is discussed in Chapter 89. Rarely, isolated splenomegaly will be an incidental finding in an otherwise healthy adult. Such an individual may be screened for serious underlying disease by careful examination of a peripheral blood film (to rule out asymptomatic chronic lymphocytic or chronic myelocytic leukemias), spleen scan to look for splenic cyst or extrasplenic mass causing displacement of the spleen, and a noninvasive procedure such as sonography or abdominal computed tomography to search for occult abdominal masses, as in lymphoma.

Concept of Hypersplenism

The term *hypersplenism* refers to the occurrence of splenomegaly and peripheral cytopenias (anemia, leukopenia, or thrombocytopenia alone or in any combination) in the presence of normal or increased bone marrow activity, and the correction of the hematologic abnormalities by splenectomy. Any condition known to cause splenomegaly may be associated with hypersplenism, but conversely, splenomegaly is not always associated with the syndrome of hypersplenism.

The causes of the peripheral cytopenias in hypersplenism are multifactorial. Anemia is caused both by the dilutional effect of an increased splanchnic blood volume and also by a shortened survival of erythrocytes damaged during splenic pooling. Thrombocytopenia results mainly from splenic pooling, whereas granulocytopenia appears to reflect increased margination of granulocytes in the blood vessels of the spleen.

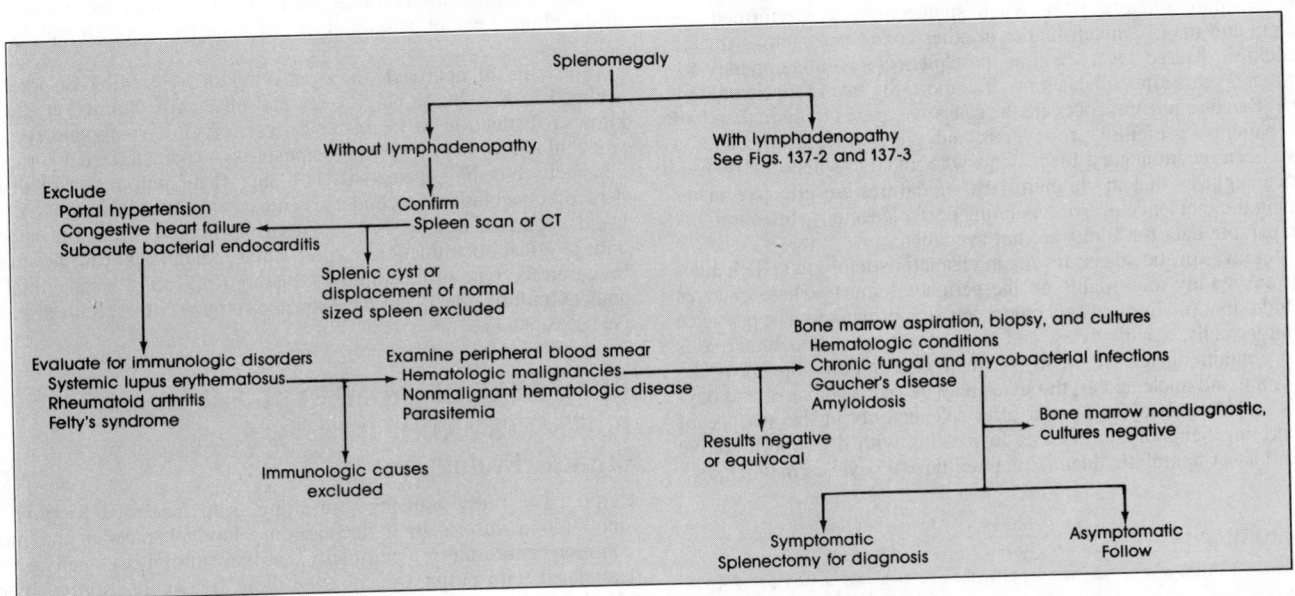

FIGURE 81-4   Clinical approach to the patient with splenomegaly.

Splenectomy for Treatment or Diagnosis

The physician managing a patient with splenomegaly must decide whether splenectomy is indicated and if so, when the procedure should be performed. It is important to recognize that most patients with splenomegaly will not require splenectomy but may benefit from specific therapy directed toward an underlying disease, for example, appropriate chemotherapy for lymphoma. Four indications for splenectomy can be identified. First, splenectomy is an important treatment option for patients with life-threatening cytopenias in whom the spleen may be responsible for persistence of the cytopenia. These conditions include hemolytic anemias, immune thrombocytopenia, myeloproliferative and lymphoproliferative diseases, and miscellaneous disorders such as Felty's syndrome. Indications for splenectomy in specific disease entities are discussed in the appropriate chapters. Splenectomy for hematologic diseases is not curative but may provide significant amelioration of symptoms by reducing or eliminating transfusion requirements and may improve prognosis by reducing the risk for complications such as sepsis or bleeding. In general, past experience provides the best guide to the utility of splenectomy in specific disease settings. Radionuclide studies to assess splenic sequestration or destruction of blood cells are not sufficiently reliable to provide useful information on which to base the decision for or against splenectomy. A second indication for splenectomy is the occurrence of a vascular or traumatic accident involving the spleen. Splenectomy may be life-saving in the setting of traumatic rupture of the spleen, and with splenic infarction it may provide symptomatic relief as well as prophylaxis against spontaneous splenic rupture. A third indication for splenectomy is mechanical encroachment by the enlarged spleen on other intraabdominal organs. Most often affected is the stomach with resultant symptoms of early satiety and sometimes prominent weight loss. Less frequently, obstruction to the left-side renal collecting system may occur. A fourth indication for splenectomy is for diagnosis. Evaluation of the patient with isolated splenomegaly or with splenomegaly and lymphadenopathy is discussed earlier (see Fig. 81-4). In some patients with isolated splenomegaly, careful evaluation by noninvasive means may fail to provide a diagnosis. In these patients, exploratory laparotomy for splenectomy and diagnostic lymph node and liver biopsies may be indicated. Three fourths of such patients will prove to have significant pathologic conditions approximately equally divided among lymphoproliferative diseases, inflammatory diseases, and congestive splenomegaly.

Asplenic Patient

Susceptibility to overwhelming infection is a well-recognized complication of splenectomy. Although this risk is magnified for splenectomy performed in infancy or early childhood, it remains significant in the adult. The incidence of overwhelming postsplenectomy infection is approximately 1.5% when splenectomy is performed for trauma and may be much higher in other conditions such as treated Hodgkin's disease. Overwhelming postsplenectomy infection may occur many years after splenectomy. The mortality rate is approximately 50%. Because pneumococci are the causative agents in more than half the patients, penicillin prophylaxis and pneumococcal vaccination have been recommended for patients who undergo splenectomy. Evidence suggests that in children these modalities are effective in reducing the incidence of overwhelming postsplenectomy infection, but comparable data for adults are not available.

Removal of the spleen results in characteristic blood cell changes that are readily identifiable on the peripheral smear. These changes include abnormalities in red blood cell shape, including appearance of target cells, acanthocytes, and fragmented cells. Red blood cells may contain nuclear remnants, termed *Howell-Jolly bodies* (Plate IV-4, *K*), and nucleated erythrocytes may be seen. Transient leukocytosis and thrombocytosis occur after splenectomy in the absence of underlying hematologic disease. In patients with myeloproliferative disorders or hemolytic anemia, marked thrombocytosis may persist.

BIBLIOGRAPHY

Abrahms DI: AIDS-related lymphadenopathy: the role of biopsy, *J Clin Oncol* 4:126, 1986.

Bowdler AJ: Splenomegaly and hypersplenism, *Clin Haematol* 12:467, 1983.

Eichner ER, Whitfield CL: Splenomegaly: an algorithmic approach to diagnosis, *JAMA* 246:2858, 1981.

Fijten GH, Blijham GH: Unexplained lymphadenopathy in family practice, *J Fam Pract* 27:373, 1988.

Greenfield S, Jordan MC: The clinical investigation of lymphadenopathy in primary care practice, *JAMA* 240:1388, 1978.

Moore RD, Weissberger AS, Bowerfind ES: An evaluation of lymphadenopathy in systemic disease, *Arch Intern Med* 99:751, 1957.

Schroer K, Franssila KO: Atypical hyperplasia of lymph nodes: a follow-up study, *Cancer* 44:1155, 1979.

CHAPTER

82   Excessive Bleeding and Clotting

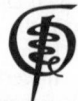

James N. George

Although the evaluation of patients who have excessive bleeding or thrombosis (or both simultaneously) is usually considered from the perspective of laboratory assessment, this chapter emphasizes that (1) the history and physical examination are the most important diagnostic aids, (2) laboratory studies are confirmatory and must be used selectively, and (3) laboratory analyses are necessarily artificial and may be misleading.

The initial discussion of bleeding disorders is organized in relation to the physiologic sequence of hemostasis. First, disorders of primary hemostasis, involving platelets and small vessels, are discussed, followed by disorders of secondary hemostasis involving plasma coagulation factors. The nature of the bleeding in these two categories of abnormalities can be clearly distinguished by the history and physical examination. In contrast to patients with bleeding disorders, evaluation of patients whose primary problem is an increased risk for thrombosis is often less clear. However, better understanding of the natural control mechanisms of hemostasis is improving the ability to diagnose specific abnormalities in thrombotic diseases. The assessment of patients anticipating surgery and the interpretation of laboratory assays of coagulation related to a potential risk of bleeding represent a special problem for hemostasis: not merely the diagnosis of an abnormality but the ensurance of normality. Here the sophistication of the laboratory evaluation is guided by the suspicion of a bleeding abnormality from the history. This chapter discusses the problem of patients who have a laboratory abnormality of hemostasis but no clinical bleeding, observations that further emphasize the importance of the clinical examination and the artificial nature of laboratory assays.

The clinical approach to a patient with a bleeding disorder is outlined in Box 82-1. The history and physical examination should allow a distinction to be made between disorders of platelets and small blood vessels (primary hemostasis)—characterized by mucocutaneous bleeding, petechiae, and superficial purpura—and disorders of coagulation (secondary hemostasis)—characterized by delayed, recurrent oozing and hematoma formation. From the history and physical examination a preliminary diagnosis can be made based on the type of bleeding, the history (indicating a congenital or an acquired disorder), and the expected frequency of certain diseases (see Box 82-1).

DISORDERS OF PRIMARY HEMOSTASIS: PLATELETS AND BLOOD VESSELS
Clinical Evaluation

Purpura (or "easy bruising") resulting from increased fragility of small blood vessels or a decrease in blood platelets is the most common hemostatic abnormality; milder thrombocytopenias not associated with purpura occur even more frequently. Normal blood platelets may function continuously to seal the small gaps in vascular endothelium that normally occur. Evidence for this is the

BOX 82-1
Clinical evaluation of a bleeding patient

I. History
  A. Type of bleeding
    1. Mucocutaneous, petechiae: suggests platelet disorder or vasculitis
    2. Delayed, recurrent oozing; hematoma: suggests plasma coagulation disorder
    3. Menorrhagia or gastrointestinal tract bleeding possible in either type of disorder
  B. Duration of bleeding
    1. Lifelong: indicates congenital defect of a single factor; confirm with family history of bleeding or presence of consanguinity for suspected recessive traits
    2. Recent onset: indicates an acquired disorder, usually defects of multiple factors; confirm by history of no bleeding with past trauma, surgery, teeth extractions, menses
  C. Systemic illnesses associated with bleeding: liver disease, malignant disease
II. Physical examination
  A. Petechiae and superficial mucocutaneous bleeding
    1. Dependent distribution, asymptomatic: indicates thrombocytopenia
    2. Clusters of palpable, pruritic petechiae: indicate vasculitis
  B. Deep hematomas or hemarthroses, which may be associated with extensive superficial purpura: indicate a coagulation disorder
III. Preliminary diagnostic categories
  A. Mucocutaneous bleeding, platelet-vessel defect
    1. Congenital
      a. von Willebrand's disease most likely
      b. Well-defined platelet function defects rare
      c. Thrombocytopenia rare
      d. Afibrinogenemia rare
    2. Acquired
      a. Severe thrombocytopenia most likely caused by idiopathic (autoimmune) thrombocytopenic purpura (ITP)
      b. Mild or moderate thrombocytopenia caused by splenic pooling in liver disease common
      c. Other thrombocytopenias caused by peripheral destruction (thrombotic thrombocytopenic purpura [TTP], disseminated intravascular coagulation [DIC], sepsis) or marrow failure less common
      d. Mild congenital von Willebrand's disease possible in an adult
  B. Hematomas and delayed bleeding, coagulation defect
    1. Congenital
      a. Hemophilia A most likely, hemophilia B one tenth as frequent
      b. Other coagulation defects rare
      c. Homozygous von Willebrand's disease with severe factor VIII deficiency rare
    2. Acquired
      a. Liver disease common
      b. DIC, vitamin K deficiency, coagulation factor VIII inhibitor, anticoagulant therapy
      c. Mild congenital hemophilia possible in an adult
IV. Proceed to laboratory evaluation

gingival bleeding, and bleeding that may seem excessive after trauma are both the hallmarks of abnormal primary hemostasis and part of the spectrum of normal bleeding.

The characteristic lesion of thrombocytopenia or vasculitis is the petechia. This dot hemorrhage does not blanch with pressure and evolves over days from bright red to yellow to brown with the catabolism of extravasated heme. These characteristics, although obvious, are critical in distinguishing petechiae from the vascular telangiectasias that are common in normal people. Petechiae are tiny because the endothelial lesion is contained by supporting perivascular tissue (Plate IV-10, *A*). However, if the same endothelial lesion occurs in an area of very loose tissue (buccal mucosa, conjunctiva), the small hemorrhage can readily dissect into a larger hemorrhagic bulla measuring a centimeter or more in diameter (Plate IV-10, *B*). In contrast, regions with stronger connective tissue support of small vessels have fewer petechiae, such as the sole of the foot in Plate IV-10, *A*. The distinction between thrombocytopenic and primary vasculitic petechiae is best made by the history and physical examination. With thrombocytopenia the appearance of petechiae is totally asymptomatic, whereas in vasculitis there are often prodromal symptoms of burning or stinging in the skin before the appearance of petechial hemorrhages. In addition, the petechiae of vasculitis may be palpable and may occur in clusters that are not necessarily distributed in dependent regions. Acute thrombocytopenia is usually unassociated with other systemic symptoms or diseases, whereas acute vasculitis usually occurs with symptoms in other organ systems or with a drug reaction. Whereas vasculitis usually causes only superficial petechiae, severe thrombocytopenia can cause severe and fatal internal hemorrhage. Thrombocytopenic bleeding may occur without trauma in the more vascular organs, resulting in nosebleed, gingival bleeding, menometrorrhagia, hematuria, and cerebral and gastrointestinal tract hemorrhage. Large, slowly developing hematomas in less vascular regions (such as the retroperitoneum) and hemarthroses, which are so characteristic of coagulation disorders, do not occur.

Purpura may refer to the appearance of many petechiae and is also frequently used to describe larger superficial hemorrhages. Purpura is distinct from the term *hematoma,* which implies a substantial mass of extravasated blood. The most common cause of purpura is the vascular fragility caused by atrophy of subcutaneous supporting tissue. *Senile purpura* is not a disease associated with other bleeding problems but an inevitable accompaniment of aging. The appearance of large, superficial, nonpalpable purple blotches on the back of the hands and forearms is predictable with thin, shiny, inelastic skin and the vulnerability of these areas to minor trauma. The same lesions accompany the cachexia of chronic illness and the peripheral subcutaneous atrophy of cortisol excess.

Laboratory Evaluation

The laboratory evaluation of congenital and acquired disorders of primary hemostasis is outlined in Figs. 82-1 and 82-2. The initial step in both evaluations is an estimation of platelet number; the absolute number is obtained by a platelet count with confirmation by examination of a peripheral blood smear. A platelet count of less than 150×10^9 per liter is abnormal; however, bleeding does not occur from thrombocytopenia alone until the platelet count is less than 50 to 100×10^9 per liter, and spontaneous bleeding with many petechiae does not occur until the platelet count is less than 10×10^9 per liter. A bone marrow aspiration to determine the presence or absence of megakaryocytes and thereby estimate the quality of platelet production is indicated only when the origin or cause of thrombocytopenia is not apparent from the clinical examination.

Congenital thrombocytopenias are rare; some are associated with specific disorders of platelet function (Bernard-Soulier syndrome) or abnormalities such as nephritis and deafness (Epstein syndrome), granulocyte inclusions (May-Hegglin anomaly), or immunodeficiency (Wiskott-Aldrich syndrome), whereas others manifest only a low platelet count. Since the most common acquired thrombocytopenia, idiopathic (autoimmune) thrombocytopenic purpura (ITP), is diagnosed only by excluding other causes, and since mild to moderate thrombocytopenia may cause minimal bleeding symptoms, congeni-

sudden, asymptomatic appearance of innumerable petechiae around the feet, ankles, and lower legs when severe thrombocytopenia develops (Plate IV-10, *A*). This distribution of petechiae in dependent regions parallels intravascular hydrostatic pressure and the greater vulnerability of these small vessels to endothelial breaks. This occurrence also emphasizes that disorders of platelets and blood vessels must be considered together and may initially be indistinguishable. The evaluation of patients with a suspected disorder of primary hemostasis may initially present an important but difficult differential diagnosis between normal and abnormal bleeding. Control groups in clinical studies have consistently documented that about 20% of subjects with normal hemostasis report mild to moderate bleeding symptoms. Easy bruising, epistaxis,

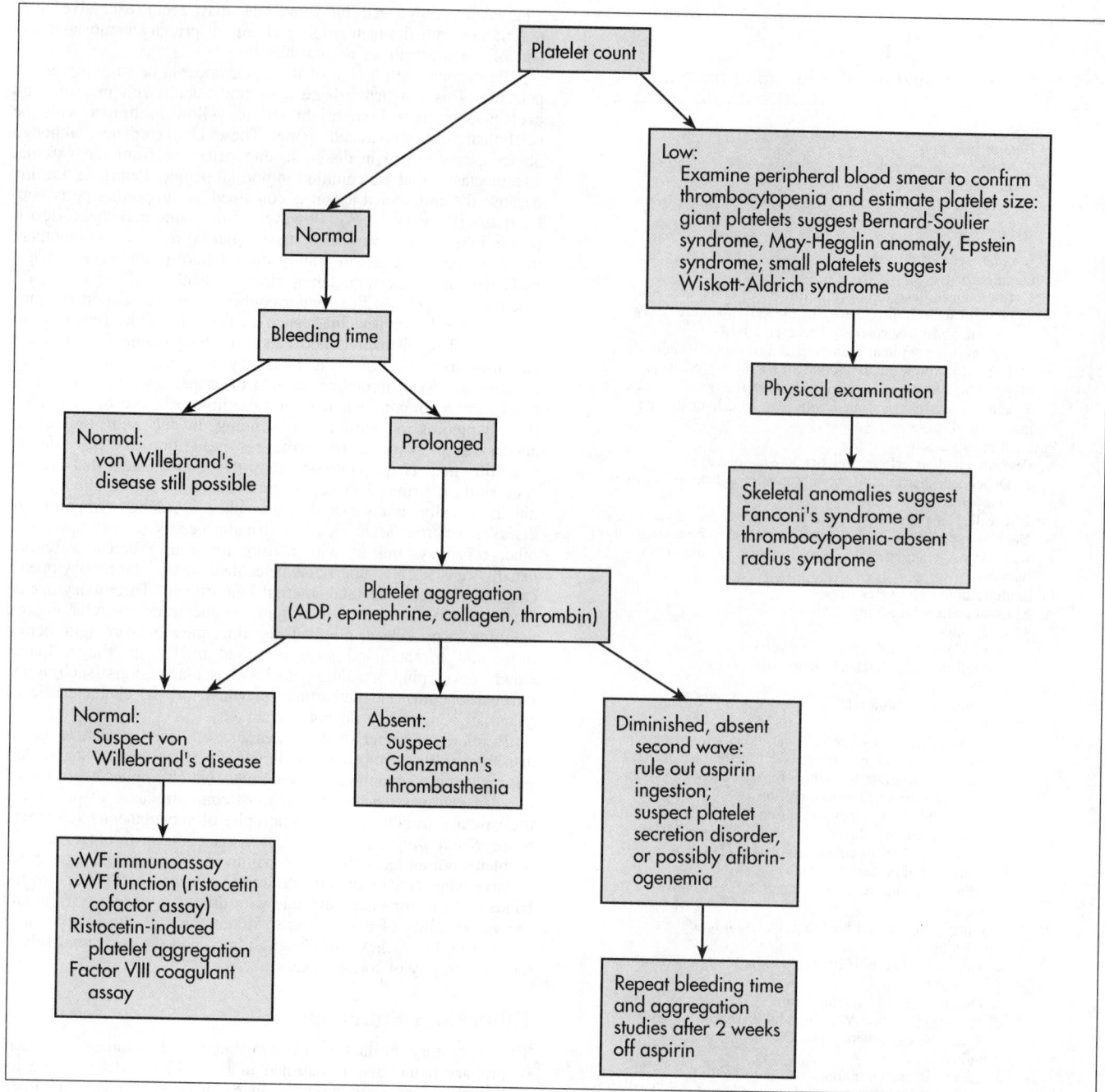

FIGURE 82-1 Algorithm for the laboratory evaluation of a patient with a bleeding disorder in whom the history and physical examination suggest a congenital disorder of platelets or small vessels. *ADP*, Adenosine diphosphate; *vWF*, von Willebrand's factor.

tal thrombocytopenia must be considered in the differential diagnosis of ITP. This is particularly important in the unusual cases of children who are thought to have chronic ITP.

The most common abnormality among congenital disorders of primary hemostasis is von Willebrand's disease. The incidence of von Willebrand's's disease is hard to define because in mildly affected patients laboratory test results may be variably abnormal, and even all test results may be normal at some times in some patients. Also, the pattern of laboratory abnormalities is not always consistent among family members, an unusual occurrence in a hereditary disease. In typical type I (heterozygous) von Willebrand's disease (defined and discussed in Chapter 84), the platelet count is normal but the bleeding time is prolonged because of a deficiency of von Willebrand's factor required for platelet adhesion to the damaged vessel wall. von Willebrand's factor deficiency can be measured by both immunoas-

says and functional assays (see Chapters 75 and 84 for a full description). In plasma, von Willebrand's factor functions as a carrier molecule for factor VIII; therefore the plasma factor VIII concentration may also be decreased. Patients with type III (homozygous or doubly heterozygous) von Willebrand's disease have severe abnormalities of all these values. Because of their very low factor VIII concentration, these patients may also have clinical bleeding problems characteristic of a coagulation defect. Other well-defined diseases among the group of congenital primary hemostasis disorders are rare (Fig. 82-1). The laboratory report of "mean platelet volume" cannot substitute for examination of the blood smear because giant platelets may not even be counted as platelets.

With rare exceptions, acquired disorders of primary hemostasis are caused by thrombocytopenia. The suspected cause depends on the associated medical problems. In an otherwise healthy person, ITP is the

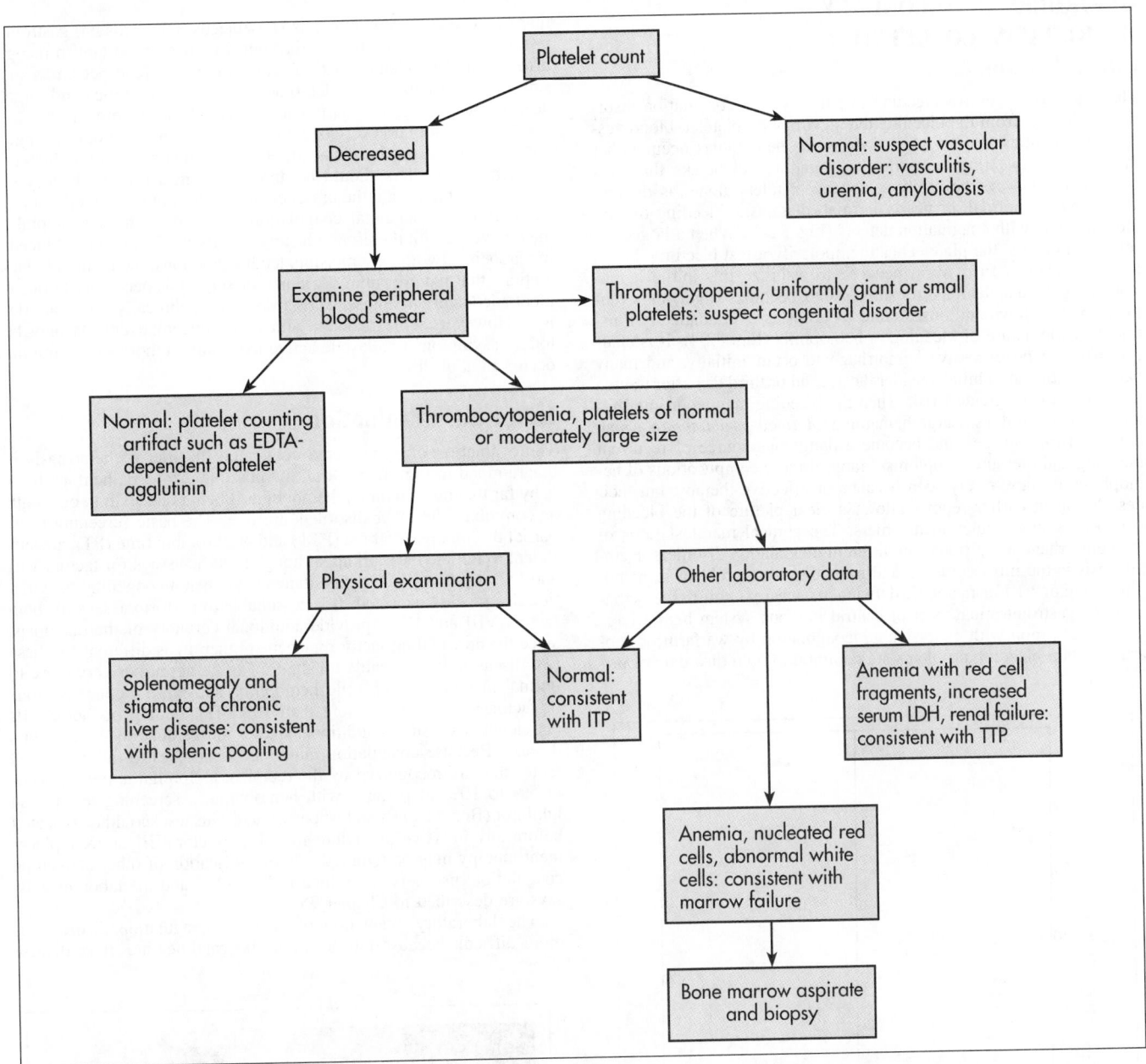

FIGURE 82-2 Algorithm for the laboratory evaluation of a patient with a bleeding disorder in whom the history and physical examination suggest an acquired disorder of platelets or small vessels. *DIC*, Disseminated intravascular coagulation; *ITP*, idiopathic (autoimmune) thrombocytopenic purpura; *LDH*, lactate dehydrogenase; *TTP*, thrombotic thrombocytopenic purpura.

most likely diagnosis for symptomatic thrombocytopenia and for asymptomatic, incidentally discovered thrombocytopenia. Thrombocytopenia resulting from marrow failure, with rare exceptions, is associated with other evidence of marrow disease. In patients with chronic liver disease the spleen becomes congested because of portal hypertension and thrombocytopenia occurs because of splenic pooling. In these patients the platelet count is rarely less than 30×10^9 per liter. Patients with marrow involvement by a malignant disease or folic acid or vitamin B_{12} deficiency or those who are receiving marrow-suppressive chemotherapy have expected thrombocytopenia, and these may be the most common causes of thrombocytopenia among hospitalized patients. Thrombocytopenia associated with human immunodeficiency virus (HIV) infection of long duration is an increasingly common observation.

Mild thrombocytopenia with no bleeding manifestations must be very common. Viral infections and acute alcoholism both can cause thrombocytopenia because of marrow suppression with decreased

megakaryocytes. It has been documented that in most children receiving live attenuated viral vaccines mild thrombocytopenia develops, although petechiae do not occur. These mild thrombocytopenias may be clinically important when they occur concurrently with another hemostatic abnormality.

An enormous number of drugs, foods, and spices can cause abnormal platelet function, but of these, only aspirin has been documented to cause a significantly increased frequency of bleeding. Even with aspirin, abnormal clinical bleeding is difficult to document, and most studies of major surgery in patients taking aspirin demonstrate no or minimally increased bleeding compared with control groups. Chronic renal failure also causes abnormal platelet function, but whether this causes clinically important bleeding is unknown. In a patient who has a history and clinical signs of a disorder of primary hemostasis but a normal platelet count and normal platelet function, vasculitis should be suspected and a cause of associated illness should be apparent.

DISORDERS OF SECONDARY HEMOSTASIS: COAGULATION
Clinical Evaluation

The nature of excessive bleeding in patients with coagulation disorders is distinct from the bleeding that occurs with platelet–blood vessel abnormalities. A few large, deep tissue hematomas occur rather than innumerable tiny hemorrhages. Small vessel breaks that may cause petechiae can be easily sealed by platelets alone, as demonstrated by the normal, or nearly normal, diagnostic bleeding time in most patients with coagulation defects (Fig. 82-3). When a large vessel lesion occurs, the platelets can temporarily arrest bleeding, but in the absence of a firm fibrin network to stabilize this initial hemostatic plug the platelet mass remains friable, becomes larger, and eventually breaks down and oozes more blood. This is dramatically illustrated by the nature of bleeding in hemophilia (Fig. 82-4). It is characteristic for no excessive hemorrhage to occur initially, and many patients with hemophilia consider the second or third day after trauma to be the time of greatest risk. Then the bleeding may recur intermittently for many days. Large hematomas, termed *pseudotumors,* may develop firm capsules and become a dangerous source of recurrent bleeding and pressure symptoms. Many of these complications of hemophilia are now rarely seen because of effective therapy, but their description in earlier reports allows a clear picture of the bleeding that occurs in coagulation disorders. The clinical manifestations of the hemorrhage are different in different coagulation disorders. Hemarthrosis is the most common and most disabling problem in hemophilia (factor VIII or factor IX deficiency), whereas soft tissue hematoma or gastrointestinal tract or central nervous system hemorrhage is more common with excessive anticoagulation by warfarin or heparin. Certain bleeding problems are common to both disorders of primary and secondary hemostasis (nosebleeds, menorrhagia, gastrointestinal tract bleeding, hematuria), but it is most important to recognize the distinct, characteristic features of each defect: petechiae and superficial purpura in platelet–blood vessel abnormalities and large, deep hematomas and hemarthroses in coagulation disorders.

It is most common for congenital defects to involve only a single coagulation factor, whereas acquired defects involve multiple factors. Congenital disorders should be apparent from a lifelong history of bleeding problems and the presence of similar problems in other family members. Congenital coagulation disorders such as hemophilia may be very mild; therefore a history specifying the amount of bleeding associated with circumcision, teeth extractions, menstruation, lacerations that require sutures, trauma, or surgery is necessary to document adequately the presence or absence of a clinically important defect. However, some patients with mild congenital defects may be totally asymptomatic, despite active lives, until a more severe trauma occurs in adult life.

Laboratory Evaluation

The evaluation of a suspected congenital disorder of hemostasis is diagrammed in Fig. 82-5. Of all the possible disorders, hemophilia A is by far the most common, hemophilia B being one sixth to one tenth as common. The other disorders are rare. The basic screening tests, partial thromboplastin time (PTT) and prothrombin time (PT), are sufficient to initiate the workup, although specific assays for factors VIII and IX are often ordered simultaneously when a congenital coagulation disorder is suspected. It is reasonable to perform assays for both factors VIII and IX to provide additional certainty of the diagnosis, since the coagulation factor replacement therapy is different for these two diseases. It is possible for the PTT to be normal or very close to normal in patients with mild hemophilia and plasma concentrations of factor VIII or IX of more than 10%. The finding of factor VIII deficiency necessitates additional studies to rule out von Willebrand's disease. Because coagulation inhibitors, antibodies to the transfused factor that are recognized by the recipient as foreign antigens, occur in 5% to 10% of patients with hemophilia, a screening test for an inhibitor (Box 82-2) should be performed. This test should be repeated before any invasive procedure for which factor VIII or IX replacement therapy may be required. The identification of other congenital coagulation disorders is outlined in Fig. 82-5, and the laboratory assays are described in Chapter 75.

The laboratory evaluation of acquired coagulation disorders is more difficult because the potential abnormalities are more diverse

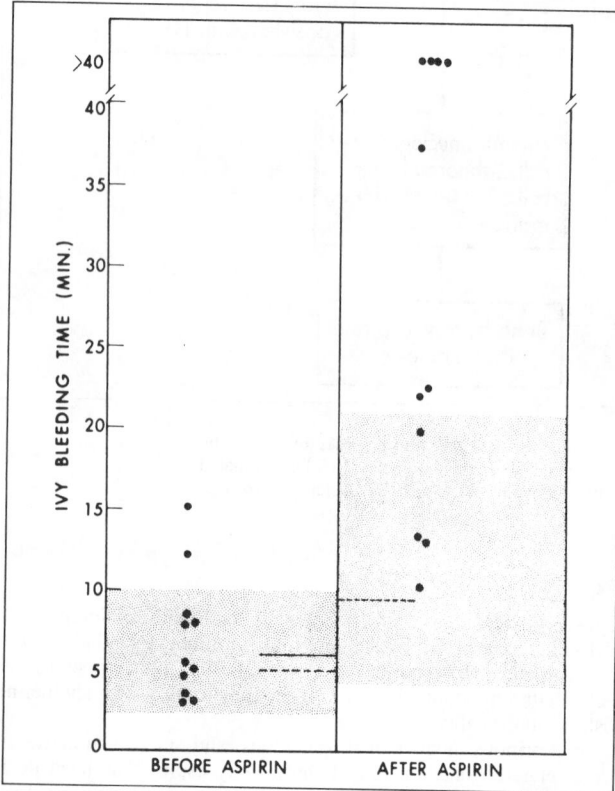

FIGURE 82-3 Ivy method bleeding time in 11 patients with severe classic hemophilia (factor VIII deficiency) before and 2 hours after ingestion of 1 g aspirin. The shaded areas represent the range of normal subjects. The dotted straight line is the normal mean, and the solid straight line is the mean for the patients. After aspirin ingestion, bleeding continued in four of the patients when the test was stopped at 40 minutes. In five patients, control of continued bleeding or rebleeding from the incisions eventually required the administration of either plasma or factor VIII concentrate.

(From Kaneshiro MM et al: *N Engl J Med* 281:1039, 1969.)

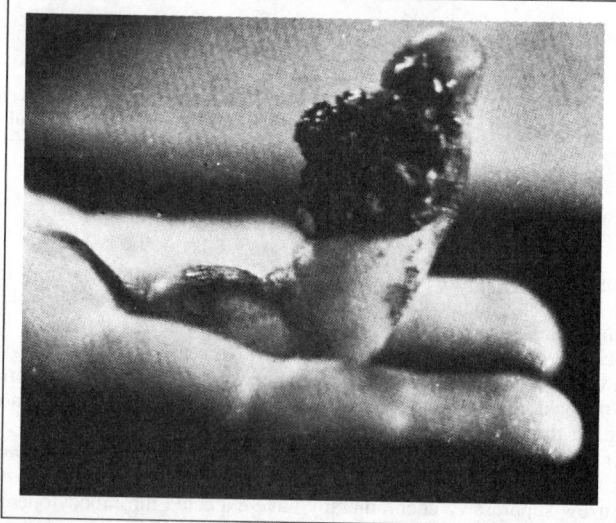

FIGURE 82-4 Ineffective clot with continual oozing after minor trauma in an untreated patient with severe hemophilia. The original figure legend stated that "the finger was cut on a blade of grass. The patient was put to bed and the hand elevated. A large clot formed, and blood continued to ooze from beneath the crust for 12 days."

(From Birch CL: *University of Illinois Bull,* vol 34, March 9, 1937.)

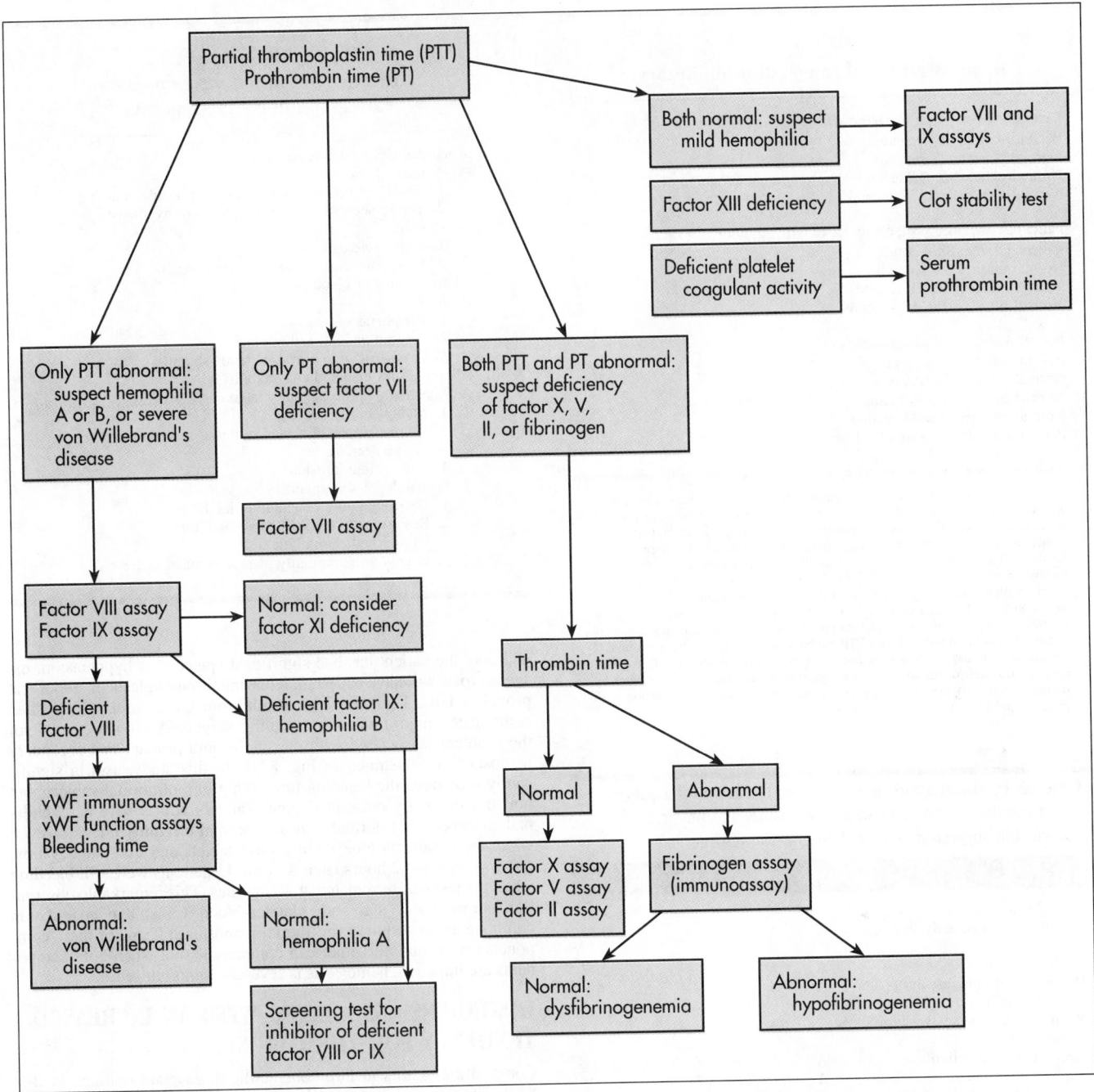

FIGURE 82-5   Algorithm for the laboratory evaluation of a patient with a bleeding disorder in whom the history and physical examination suggest a congenital coagulation disorder. *vWF*, von Willebrand's factor.

and a diagrammatic outline of the laboratory evaluation is much less clear. Table 82-1 shows the results of the most common laboratory assays for the major clinical disorders. In a patient with serious bleeding and no immediately apparent cause it is reasonable to order the entire group of these assays. Usually, however, a cause is clearly suspected from the history and physical examination. Liver disease occurs often; since all coagulation factors are synthesized by the liver, this is the most common cause of acquired coagulation disorders. In acute liver disease, such as infectious hepatitis, a coagulation abnormality may be evident only by a prolonged PT. No explanation exists for a simultaneously normal PTT other than the artifactual sensitivity of these tests and their reagents. As liver disease progresses to severe chronic cirrhosis, all studies may become abnormal. The synthesis of all plasma coagulation factors is diminished. Thrombocytopenia is the result of excessive pooling in an enlarged, congested spleen. Chronic disseminated intravascular coagulation (DIC) and fi-

brinolysis may occur in chronic liver disease because of the liver's failure to clear activated coagulation factors and because of a deficiency of plasmin inhibitors. DIC from other causes is discussed later. The coagulation inhibition that may be present in DIC is most likely caused by fibrin degradation products that interfere with normal fibrin polymerization and is most clearly demonstrated with the thrombin time. Vitamin K deficiency can occur in patients whose food intake is negligible. Unrecognized vitamin K deficiency may be a common cause of significant bleeding in severely ill, hospitalized patients. Fat malabsorption is also associated with vitamin K deficiency. Surreptitious or accidental administration of anticoagulant agents can present a difficult diagnostic problem. An acquired coagulation disorder caused by an autoantibody (inhibitor) against factor VIII is a rare but well-recognized condition (see Box 82-2). Inhibitors of other coagulation factors are extremely rare. The clinician must be aware that mild hemophilia can occur initially in an adult with severe bleed-

---

BOX 82-2

Demonstration of coagulation inhibitors

Patient 1: Hemophilia A (factor VIII deficiency), no inhibitor
Patient plasma, 72 seconds
Normal plasma, 28 seconds
Normal plus saline 38 seconds
Normal plus patient, 32 seconds

Patient 2: Acquired postpartum factor VIII inhibitor
Patient plasma, 88 seconds
Normal plasma, 28 seconds
Normal plus saline, 38 seconds
Normal plus patient, 62 seconds

Patient 3: Lupus anticoagulant
Patient plasma, 52 seconds
Normal plasma, 28 seconds
Normal plus saline, 38 seconds
Normal plus patient, 44 seconds
Patient plus platelet extract, 31 seconds

These assays, using a partial thromboplastin time (PTT) with patient or normal plasma or a mixture of equal volumes of patient and normal plasma, distinguish between an abnormality caused by a coagulation factor deficiency and an abnormality caused by an inhibitor of coagulation. In these examples the normal range for the PTT is assumed to be 21 to 34 sec. To identify inhibitors of factor VIII, incubation of the samples at 37° C for 2 hours is required. Addition of patient plasma with a severe coagulation factor deficiency may slightly prolong the coagulation time of normal plasma, even in the absence of an inhibitor. A control for this is a mixture of normal plasma plus saline. The lupus anticoagulant may initially be confused with a factor VIII inhibitor because the prothrombin time is usually normal and the lupus anticoagulant may interfere with the factor VIII assay at low plasma dilutions. It is distinguished from a factor VIII inhibitor by normal factor VIII activity at higher plasma dilutions and by correction with platelet lipid extracts.

Table 82-1 Diagram for the laboratory evaluation of a patient with a bleeding disorder in whom the history and physical examination suggest an acquired coagulation disorder

	PTT	PT	TT	INH	FDP	PLT
Liver disease						
Acute hepatitis, early liver disease		A				
Chronic liver disease	A	A	A		A	A
Disseminated intravascular coagulation (DIC)	A	A	A	A	A	A
Vitamin K deficiency, warfarin ingestion	A	A				
Heparin administration	A	A	A	A		
Lupus anticoagulant	A	*		A		
Acquired factor VIII inhibitor	A			A		

PTT, Partial thromboplastin time; *PT*, prothrombin time; *TT*, thrombin time; *Inh*, coagulation inhibitor screening test (see Box 82-2); *FDP*, fibrin degradation products; *Plt*, platelet count; *A*, abnormal result; ∗, the PT typically is normal.

---

ing after trauma, even when the past history indicates a normal experience with activities such as athletics and military service. However, when bleeding begins in a patient with mild hemophilia, it can be very difficult to control.

BLEEDING DISORDERS WITH MULTIPLE HEMOSTATIC DEFECTS

Bleeding problems resulting from multiple causes are seen frequently in hospital practice. An example is postoperative bleeding, in which it is often difficult to distinguish normal from excessive amounts and whether excessive bleeding is caused by a hemostatic abnormality or a structural defect such as an unligated vessel or a broken suture. If the patient has received many units of transfused blood, platelets and the labile coagulation factors (factors V and VIII) may be deficient. If, in

---

BOX 82-3

Increased risk for thrombosis: Pathophysiologic mechanisms

  I. Abnormalities of the vessel wall
    A. Acute
      1. Vasculitis caused by inflammation or infection
      2. Tissue necrosis caused by trauma or hypotension
    B. Chronic
      1. Atherosclerosis
      2. Prosthetic heart valve or vascular graft
  II. Abnormalities of blood flow
    A. Stasis
      1. Peripheral venous stasis
      2. Arterial or intracardiac stasis
    B. Liver disease with portal-systemic shunting
  III. Abnormalities of blood coagulability
    A. Injection of procoagulant material
      1. Malignant disease
      2. Uterine-placental abnormalities
      3. Tissue necrosis
      4. Therapeutic infusions
    B. Hematologic abnormalities
      1. Deficiency of a coagulation inhibitor
      2. Resistance to a coagulation inhibitor
      3. Diminished fibrinolytic activity
      4. Excess or abnormality of procoagulant factor

---

addition, the patient has had significant episodes of hypotension, tissue necrosis will have occurred, releasing thromboplastic material that provokes DIC. DIC may also result from bacteremia, which often complicates major trauma that requires surgery. A simpler example of the problems associated with defects in both primary and secondary hemostasis is illustrated in Fig. 82-3. In this study, aspirin significantly prolonged the bleeding time in a group of normal subjects but not to a clinically relevant degree. Patients with severe hemophilia had, as expected, a normal or nearly normal bleeding time. However, when these patients took three aspirin tablets and the bleeding time test was repeated 2 hours later, 4 of the 11 patients were still bleeding when the test was terminated at 40 minutes. This remarkable observation demonstrates that both platelet–blood vessel and coagulation components are required for normal hemostasis; if one of these components is normal, the other can compensate, but when both components are impaired, hemostasis is severely compromised.

DISORDERS ASSOCIATED WITH AN INCREASED TENDENCY FOR THROMBOSIS

Contributing factors to thromboembolic disease are outlined in Box 82-3. The three major categories are often termed Virchow's triad, in reference to the proposal by Rudolph Virchow in 1845 that these abnormalities were the principal mechanisms of thrombotic disease. Vessel wall damage can expose subendothelial matrix cells that constitutively display tissue factor on their membrane surfaces, and this, plus a trace amount of factor VIIa, can effectively trigger coagulation. Vessel surface abnormalities such as atherosclerosis and prostheses may initiate thrombosis by activating coagulation and/or causing formation of platelet aggregates, which then dislodge to obstruct distal circulation. Venous stasis contributes to thrombosis by less effective dilution and clearing of activated coagulation factors. Cardiac abnormalities may cause sufficient stasis to allow formation of atrial or ventricular wall thrombi. Turbulent arterial circulation may increase the risk for thrombosis because the high shear forces can damage endothelium and activate platelets. The portal-systemic shunting of chronic liver disease causes less effective catabolism of activated coagulation factors. This can be a critical problem when procoagulant material enters the circulation, as during malignant disease or obstetric complications, or with infusion of concentrates of the coagulation factors II, VII, IX, and X, which may contain activated coagulation factors or other procoagulant material. Patients with malignancies may be predisposed to severe recurrent thromboembolic dis-

BOX 82-4
Increased risk for thrombosis: Clinical conditions

I. Congenital disorders
  A. Deficient coagulation inhibitor activity
    1. Antithrombin III
    2. Protein C
    3. Protein S
  B. Resistance to coagulation inhibitor activity (factor V mutation)
  C. Deficient fibrinolytic activity
    1. Deficiency or abnormality of plasminogen
    2. Abnormality of plasminogen activator/plasminogen activator inhibitor balance
    3. Dysfibrinogenemia
  D. Blood or vessel wall disease
    1. Sickle cell anemia
    2. Homocysteinuria
II. Acquired disorders
  A. Primary hematologic disorders
    1. Proliferative diseases
      a. Myeloproliferative diseases with erythrocytosis and thrombocytosis
      b. Acute promyelocytic leukemia
      c. Paroxysmal nocturnal hemoglobinuria
      d. Macroglobulinemia, cold agglutinin disease
    2. Adverse reactions to therapy
      a. Factors II, VII, IX, and X concentrates
      b. Fibrinolysis inhibitors (e.g., epsilon-aminocaproic acid [EACA])
      c. Heparin-induced thrombocytopenia/thrombosis
      d. Warfarin-induced protein C and S deficiency
    3. Diverse causes
      a. Lupus anticoagulant
      b. Thrombotic thrombocytopenic purpura
      c. Disseminated intravascular coagulation
  B. Nonhematologic conditions
    1. Malignant disease
    2. Cardiac abnormalities (e.g., prosthetic valve, atrial fibrillation, dilated cardiomyopathy, ventricular aneurysm, congestive heart failure)
    3. Pregnancy, oral contraceptives
    4. Nephrotic syndrome
    5. Extremes of age
    6. Immobility

ease, a condition known as *Trousseau's syndrome.* Women with abnormal placental separation from the uterine wall at the time of delivery may have thromboses that are related to the presence of thromboplastic material from the placenta in the circulation.

The recognized clinical conditions that can predispose to thrombosis are outlined in Box 82-4. Defects of three proteins involved in the control of coagulation reactions—antithrombin III, protein C, and protein S—appear to allow increased thrombosis because of failure to inhibit activated coagulation factors (see Box 82-4). Some heterozygous-deficient subjects develop recurrent venous thromboembolism. In the rare patients with homozygous protein C or protein S deficiency, fulminant and potentially fatal thromboses develop in infancy. Abnormalities of other coagulation inhibitors, heparin cofactor II and tissue factor pathway inhibitor, have been less well or not yet described. Congenital abnormalities of fibrinogen and the fibrinolytic system have also been associated with an increased frequency of thrombosis because of the absence of effective fibrinolysis to control a developing clot.

Sickle cell anemia can predispose to thrombosis by the vascular obstruction caused by irreversibly sickled cells. Homocystinuria is associated with vessel wall damage that can result in venous or arterial thrombosis and accelerated atherosclerosis.

The acquired disorders that can increase the risk for thrombosis are much more frequent. Several of these factors often may coincide to result in a thromboembolic complication. For example, an elderly patient with congestive heart failure who is confined to bed has a significantly increased risk for thrombosis. Thrombocytosis may be

associated with thrombosis, but also many patients have extreme thrombocytosis (platelet counts of over 1000×10^9 per liter) for years with no evidence of thromboembolic complications. The lupus anticoagulant is an antibody to phospholipid that was originally described in patients with systemic lupus erythematosus but also occurs in other subjects with or without accompanying illnesses (see Box 82-2). These patients do not have excessive bleeding unless there is concomitant thrombocytopenia or a coagulation abnormality, but they may have an increased risk for thrombosis.

The number of specific abnormalities that may be associated with an increased risk for thrombosis is large and growing. As in the assessment of bleeding disorders, clinical evaluation must be the primary basis of diagnosis. For example, a discrete arterial embolism suggests a cardiac origin, and histologic study of the embolus may reveal a diagnosis of endocarditis or tumor. An isolated occurrence of deep venous thrombosis in the lower leg may have no apparent predisposing cause and not warrant a thorough investigation for a hemostatic defect. However, a recent onset of recurrent severe thromboembolic complications may suggest the possibility of an underlying malignancy, and a thorough workup is indicated. Patients with congenital hemostatic disorders that predispose to thrombosis often do not have a history of lifelong symptoms; many patients have a thrombotic episode only after a traumatic event. Affected relatives may then be identified who have had no apparent problems. For example, a recent survey of a normal population suggested a prevalence of protein C deficiency of 1 in 250 persons, although none of the identified subjects had a history of thrombotic disease. The most common congenital abnormality causing an increased risk for thrombosis is a mutation of factor V that limits its susceptibility to proteolysis by activated protein C. This mutant factor V is present in 3% to 5% of normal individuals and 50% of patients with venous thrombosis who also have a family history of thrombosis. A thorough laboratory evaluation should be reserved for patients who have recurrent thromboembolic disease with no obvious cause. With these selected patients, 60% may have an identifiable laboratory abnormality.

Disseminated Intravascular Coagulation

A clinical syndrome with both hemorrhage and thrombosis is DIC. The clinical spectrum of DIC extends from clinically insignificant laboratory abnormalities to uncontrollable hemorrhage and thrombosis. DIC has innumerable specific causes, but all are related to vascular damage with activation of plasma coagulation factors or entry of tissue thromboplastic material into the blood. Occasional patients have infarction of fingertips and toes, or renal failure may occur with thrombosis of cortical vessels. Bleeding is the most prominent clinical problem, and cerebral hemorrhage is the most common cause of death. In severe DIC, two mechanisms contribute to the bleeding. In severe DIC, thrombocytopenia and fibrinogen deficiency may be extreme. The coagulation abnormalities are comparable to the changes found in normal serum after in vitro clotting of whole blood: platelets, fibrinogen, prothrombin, and factors V and VIII are decreased; other coagulation factors may be decreased or may be present with even greater activity than in plasma. In the second mechanism, as a consequence of DIC, systemic fibrinolysis is activated, clot lysis is accelerated, and the soluble products of plasmin proteolysis of fibrin and fibrinogen are present in plasma. During severe DIC, alpha$_2$ antiplasmin can be consumed and allow fibrinolysis to be unchecked.

Laboratory evaluation of coagulation in DIC demonstrates abnormalities in the PTT, PT, and thrombin time (TT). Among these, the TT is the most sensitive test and is most prolonged because of interference with fibrin polymerization by the fibrin degradation products. A TT test performed on a mixture of patient and normal plasma yields results consistent with a coagulation inhibitor (see Box 82-2) produced by the fibrin fragments.

PREOPERATIVE ASSESSMENT TO ENSURE A PATIENT'S NORMAL HEMOSTASIS

A special problem in hemostasis is determining the clinical approach to the patient whose primary illness requires surgery and in whom evaluation must be effective to ensure normal hemostasis. Although this problem is often considered primarily from the laboratory perspective of screening assays, a careful history and physical examination are much more important. It is necessary to be sure that the patient has no current disease typically associated with acquired hemostatic defects, such as chronic liver disease. Previous bleeding episodes must be carefully documented, and specific questions are essential: menses (number of days and number of pads); teeth extractions (number of hours or days of bleeding, requirement for sutures or repacking); previous surgery (wound hematoma, reexploration, any requirement for transfusion). The history of any extraordinary bleeding in the family is important. The physical examination should focus on physical signs of a hemostatic defect or a systemic disease that could be associated with a hemostatic defect. If the history and physical examination are normal, only three basic laboratory tests are necessary to provide adequate reassurance of normal surgical hemostasis: platelet count, PTT, and PT. Several studies have documented that preoperative laboratory screening is not helpful in predicting postoperative hemorrhage in asymptomatic adults with a normal history. The obvious flaw in extrapolating these studies to everyday practice is that careful histories frequently are not performed. If the history suggests the existence of a significant bleeding problem, surgery must be postponed, even if the primary laboratory evaluation is normal. A more thorough laboratory evaluation must then be performed. However, it must be noted again that rare patients with mild congenital bleeding abnormalities may appear normal based on this evaluation but have serious bleeding complications after surgery.

LABORATORY ABNORMALITIES OF HEMOSTASIS NOT ASSOCIATED WITH CLINICAL BLEEDING PROBLEMS

Since laboratory studies of hemostasis are often ordered as part of an evaluation for another problem, unexpected abnormalities are occasionally found in patients who have no indication of any problem with excessive bleeding (Box 82-5). These observations further emphasize the artificial nature of these coagulation assays.

Pseudothrombocytopenia occurs in about 0.1% of patients having routine blood cell counts as a result of an EDTA-activated, or cold-activated, platelet-agglutinating antibody. Since EDTA is the conventional anticoagulant for laboratory platelet counts, the platelets agglutinate in the blood sample and the count is falsely low. Platelets are normal in number and morphologic appearance on the peripheral blood smear made from finger-stick blood. This is one example of the importance of examining the peripheral blood smear to confirm the presence of thrombocytopenia. These agglutinins have no clinical importance.

The initial coagulation reactions required for a normal PTT involve three proteins that are unnecessary for normal hemostasis in vivo: factor XII, prekallikrein, and high-molecular-weight kininogen. The association of each of these proteins with in vitro coagulation was originally recognized by the observation of a prolonged PTT in a subject with entirely normal hemostasis. A similar observation has been made in some patients with plasma factor XI deficiency, although other patients may have excessive bleeding. The lupus anticoagulant also causes a significant in vitro coagulation abnormality

(see Box 82-2) but no clinical bleeding, although it is associated with an increased risk for thrombosis (described earlier).

A simpler in vitro artifact is the abnormality of coagulation tests reported in patients with extreme erythrocytosis. A common example is the finding of abnormal PTT and PT as screening tests before cardiac catheterization in a patient with cyanotic congenital heart disease and a hematocrit greater than 65%. In these samples the ratio of the liquid sodium citrate anticoagulant to plasma is too great, and the standard amount of calcium added for the coagulation assay is inadequate. This problem can be corrected by removing an appropriate amount of the anticoagulant from the commercially prepared tube.

BIBLIOGRAPHY

Abilgaard CF et al: Serial studies in von Willebrand's's disease: variability versus "variants," *Blood* 56:712, 1980.
Alperin JB: Coagulopathy caused by vitamin K deficiency in critically ill, hospitalized patients, *JAMA* 258:1916, 1987.
Aster RH: Pooling of platelets in the spleen: role in the pathogenesis of "hypersplenic" thrombocytopenia, *J Clin Invest* 45:645, 1966.
Bell WR et al: Trousseau's syndrome: devastating coagulopathy in the absence of heparin, *Am J Med* 79:423, 1985.
Close HL et al: Hemostatic assessment of patients before tonsillectomy: a prospective study, *Otolaryngol Head Neck Surg* 111:733, 1994.
Dahlback B: Inherited thrombophilia: resistance to activated protein C as a pathogenic factor of venous thromboembolism, *Blood* 85:607, 1995.
Furie B, Limentani SA, Rosenfeld CF: A practical guide to the evaluation and treatment of hemophilia, *Blood* 84:3, 1994.
Gastineau DA et al: Lupus anticoagulant: an analysis of the clinical and laboratory features of 219 cases, *Am J Hematol* 19:265, 1985.
George JN, Caen JP, Nurden AT: Glanzmann's thrombasthenia: the spectrum of clinical disease, *Blood* 75:1383, 1990.
George JN, El-Harake MA, Raskob GE: Chronic idiopathic thrombocytopenic purpura, *N Engl J Med* 331:1207, 1994.
George JN, Shattil SJ: The clinical importance of acquired abnormalities of platelet function, *N Engl J Med* 324:27, 1991.
Hoyer LW: Hemophilia A, *N Engl J Med* 330:38, 1994.
Kitchens CS: Occult hemophilia, *Johns Hopkins Med J* 146:255, 1980.
Kitchens CS: Prolonged activated partial thromboplastin time of unknown etiology: a prospective study of 100 consecutive cases referred for consultation, *Am J Hematol* 27:38, 1988.
Miletich JP et al: Inherited predisposition to thrombosis, *Cell* 72:477, 1993.
Oski FA, Naiman JL: Effect of live measles vaccine on the platelet count, *N Engl J Med* 275:352, 1966.
Rodeghiero F, Castaman G, Dini E: Epidemiological investigation of the prevalence of von Willebrand's's disease, *Blood* 69:454, 1987.
Sramek A et al: Usefulness of patient interview in bleeding disorders, *Arch Intern Med* 155:1409, 1995.
Visentin GP, Aster RH. Heparin-induced thrombocytopenia and thrombosis, *Curr Opin Hematol* 2:351, 1995.

V SPECIFIC DISEASES

CHAPTER

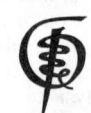

83 Thrombocytopenia and Disorders of Platelet Function

Andrew I. Schafer

DISORDERS OF PLATELET FUNCTION
Etiology

The formation of a hemostatic platelet plug at a site of vascular injury is initiated by disruption of the monolayer of endothelial cells that normally covers the intimal surfaces of blood vessels. This exposes circulating platelets to subendothelial structures such as colla-

---

BOX 82-5

Laboratory abnormalities of hemostasis not associated with clinical bleeding problems

I. Spurious thrombocytopenia caused by EDTA-activated platelet agglutinins
II. Coagulation abnormalities
   A. Prolonged partial thromboplastin time (PTT) caused by deficiencies of factor XII, prekallikrein, or high-molecular-weight kininogen; some patients with factor XI deficiency have normal hemostasis
   B. Prolonged PTT (and rarely prothrombin time [PT]) caused by the lupus anticoagulant, an antibody against phospholipid
   C. Prolonged PTT and PT caused by extreme erythrocytosis resulting in an increased ratio of citrate anticoagulant to plasma

gen and leads to the process of platelet *adhesion* (platelet-vascular interaction), in which platelets seal the site of vascular damage. Platelet adhesion is mediated by von Willebrand's factor, which binds to platelet surface receptors localized on membrane glycoprotein Ib (GpIb) to attach platelets to the subendothelium. After adhesion, platelets undergo the *release* reaction, during which they degranulate (secreting constituents of specific storage granules such as fibrinogen and adenosine diphosphate [ADP]) and also rapidly synthesize thromboxane A_2, a potent vasoconstrictor and platelet-activating derivative of arachidonic acid. Released granule constituents and thromboxane A_2 act in concert to mediate the process of platelet *aggregation* (platelet-platelet interaction), in which platelets stick to each other to form a platelet plug that occludes the damaged vessel lumen. Fibrinogen and von Willebrand's factor mediate aggregation, binding to platelet surface receptors localized on the membrane glycoprotein IIb-IIIa (GpIIb-IIIa) complex. Several disorders of platelet function are caused by specific defects in each of these steps in platelet plug formation, as shown in Fig. 83-1.

The most common disorder of platelet adhesion is *von Willebrand's disease,* an inherited (or rarely, acquired) quantitative deficiency or qualitative defect in plasma von Willebrand's factor (Chapter 84). The platelet counterpart of von Willebrand's disease is the *Bernard-Soulier syndrome,* a rare autosomal recessive disorder of platelets in which adhesion is defective because of a structural or functional loss of receptors for von Willebrand's factor on platelet membrane GpIb. This intrinsic platelet abnormality, the clinical manifestations of which mimic those of von Willebrand's disease, is associated with mild thrombocytopenia and circulating giant platelets. Using in vitro models of perfused vessels, platelet adhesion to subendothelium is greatly impaired in both von Willebrand's disease and Bernard-Soulier syndrome; however, the release reaction and the platelets' capability to aggregate remain preserved in these disorders.

Defects in the platelet release reaction can be caused either by the structural loss of platelet storage granules (i.e., *storage pool disease*) or by a *functional release defect* that is most often caused by impaired thromboxane A_2 formation. Both types of release defects can be either congenital or acquired. Some patients with congenital storage pool disease have associated abnormalities, such as oculocutaneous albinism in the Hermansky-Pudlak syndrome and immunodeficiency in the Wiskott-Aldrich syndrome. Acquired storage pool disease may develop in the course of various disorders, including the

myeloproliferative disorders and transiently in patients undergoing cardiopulmonary bypass. Functional platelet release defects caused by impaired production of thromboxane A_2 most frequently result from drugs that inhibit platelet cyclooxygenase. This enzyme oxygenates arachidonic acid to cyclic endoperoxides, which are then converted in platelets by thromboxane synthase to thromboxane A_2. *Aspirin* acetylates cyclooxygenase and irreversibly blocks its activity. Therefore, since platelets are incapable of resynthesizing new uninhibited enzyme, the aspirin-induced platelet release defect persists for the lifetime of the affected platelet (i.e., 7 to 10 days). A single, low dose of aspirin (one children's aspirin) thus produces a defect in platelet function for several days. *Nonsteroidal antiinflammatory agents* inhibit platelet cyclooxygenase reversibly, and their effects on platelet function are therefore lost with the clearance of the drugs from the circulation (i.e., within hours). Diets rich in omega-3 fatty acids or dietary supplementation with fish oils can produce a similar platelet release defect. They exert this action in part by causing the release of eicosapentaenoic acid (EPA) to compete with arachidonic acid (AA) for cyclooxygenase, producing EPA-derived functionally inactive thromboxane A_3 rather than AA-derived active thromboxane A_2. Rare cases of congenital cyclooxygenase deficiency, thromboxane synthase deficiency, and deficiency of platelet receptors for thromboxane/endoperoxides have also been described. The platelets of patients with storage pool disease and functional release defects are able to adhere normally to damaged vessels and can also aggregate normally in response to certain potent stimuli that bypass the requirement for the release reaction.

Functional platelet abnormalities that are specifically caused by defective aggregation are rare. Quantitative or qualitative disorders of fibrinogen, including afibrinogenemia and dysfibrinogenemia, are sometimes associated with abnormal platelet aggregation. *Glanzmann's thrombasthenia* is an unusual autosomal recessive disease involving an intrinsic platelet abnormality that is characterized by a structural or functional loss of receptors for fibrinogen and von Willebrand's factor on the platelet membrane GpIIb-IIIa complex. The platelet count and morphologic appearance are normal in this disorder.

Some acquired clinical conditions are associated with qualitative defects of primary hemostasis and platelet function, in which the pathophysiology of bleeding is more complex and poorly understood. The hemorrhagic disorder of *uremia* is characterized by a prolonged bleeding time, but no specific, reproducible functional platelet abnormalities can be demonstrated in vitro. Easy bruising is the most frequently encountered symptom, but more severe bleeding can occur. The hemostatic defect appears to be caused, at least in part, by dialyzable uremic toxins, since dialysis transiently improves or even completely corrects the prolonged bleeding time and the clinical bleeding tendency. For unclear reasons, amelioration of the anemia of renal failure, either by red blood cell transfusion or by administration of recombinant erythropoietin, also leads to improved hemostasis. Cryoprecipitate, deamino-8-D-arginine vasopressin (DDAVP), and conjugated estrogens have also been shown to have beneficial effects in uremic bleeding, although their mechanisms of action are largely unknown.

Bleeding and thrombosis are major causes of morbidity and mortality in the *myeloproliferative disorders* (Chapter 92). The thrombocytosis that occurs in many of these patients is generally not causally linked to the hemostatic complications. A variety of metabolic and biochemical platelet abnormalities have been identified in patients with myeloproliferative disorders, and these qualitative platelet defects that occur independent of platelet count are more likely to be responsible for the bleeding and thrombotic problems. Lowering of the platelet count in asymptomatic younger patients with thrombocytosis is generally not indicated. However, cytoreduction with hydroxyurea or interferon may reduce the risk of thrombosis in high-risk patients with thrombocytosis who are prone to thrombosis because of advanced age or previous thrombotic complications. Aspirin can promptly improve microvascular thrombotic manifestations in the cerebrovascular or peripheral circulation. Qualitative platelet abnormalities also occur in patients with acute leukemia and myelodysplasia and may exacerbate a bleeding tendency when they coexist with thrombocytopenia.

Platelet dysfunction occurs in patients with *dysproteinemias*

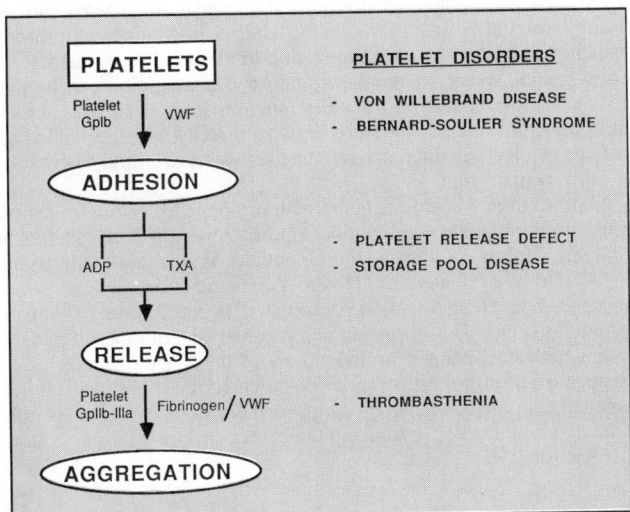

FIGURE 83-1   Biochemical basis of disorders of platelet function. Platelet adhesion is mediated by von Willebrand's factor *(vWf)* binding to platelet GpIb: defective adhesion is found in von Willebrand's disease (a plasma defect) and Bernard-Soulier syndrome (a platelet defect). The release reaction is mediated by adenosine diphosphate *(ADP)* and thromboxane A_2 *(TXA);* abnormal release is found in platelet-release defects (aspirin-like defects) and storage pool disease. Platelet aggregation is mediated by fibrinogen and vWf binding to platelet GpIIb-IIIa; defective aggregation is found in Glanzmann's thrombasthenia.

(Chapter 94), including multiple myeloma and Waldenström's macroglobulinemia, in whom the hemostatic problems tend to be related to the level of paraprotein and are improved by plasmapheresis. The bleeding problems in these patients may be complicated by other associated coagulopathies, including defective fibrin polymerization, thrombocytopenia, and hyperviscosity. The bleeding diathesis of chronic *liver failure* is highly complex and multifactorial, including components of thrombocytopenia secondary to hypersplenism, multiple coagulation factor deficiencies, dysfibrinogenemia, impaired clearance of activated coagulation factors causing intravascular coagulation, and increased fibrinolytic activity. Poorly defined defects in platelet function related to extracorpuscular plasma factors may contribute to these patients' hemorrhagic tendency. In addition to aspirin and nonsteroidal antiinflammatory agents, a variety of other drugs interfere with platelet function in vitro; however, only a few of these drugs have demonstrable clinical effects on hemostasis. High doses of penicillins, cephalosporins, and related antibiotics, including penicillin G, carbenicillin, ticarcillin, ampicillin, and moxalactam, cause prolongation of the bleeding time and interfere with platelet function by binding to platelets and blocking recognition of platelet membrane agonist receptors. Platelet dysfunction caused by antibiotics can contribute to serious bleeding complications when administered in the clinical setting of coexisting illnesses (e.g., renal and hepatic failure, malignancy, concomitant use of anticoagulants), which themselves may independently cause a bleeding diathesis. Alcohol, which itself does not affect the bleeding time, enhances the effect of aspirin on prolongation of the bleeding time. Newer antiplatelet agents exert more specific inhibitory actions on platelets. Ticlopidine inhibits platelet function by blocking platelet ADP receptors. Monoclonal antibody and peptide or peptidomimetic inhibitors of platelet GpIIb-IIIa produce a thrombasthenia-like defect.

Clinical Features

Patients with disorders of platelet function generally develop bleeding complications that are clinically distinguishable from those seen in patients with coagulation factor deficiencies. In contrast to the bleeding patterns associated with coagulopathies, which usually involve deep tissue and visceral hemorrhage and which often occur in a delayed manner after trauma, patients with platelet disorders characteristically exhibit superficial hemorrhage that develops either spontaneously or immediately after injury. Superficial bleeding may involve mucosal hemorrhage (e.g., epistaxis, gastrointestinal or genitourinary tract bleeding) or cutaneous hemorrhage in the form of ecchymoses (common bruises) and purpura. Petechiae are more typically seen in severe thrombocytopenic states. Patients with platelet adhesion or aggregation abnormalities generally have more severe bleeding tendencies than do those with platelet release defects.

Laboratory Features

The most valuable laboratory screening test of primary hemostasis is the *bleeding time*. This is determined by measuring the time to cessation of bleeding from a standardized incision on the volar aspect of the forearm. The bleeding time is prolonged in patients with (1) thrombocytopenia (platelets <100,000/μl), (2) disorders of platelet function, and (3) primary vascular defects. Generally, it is unnecessary to perform this test in patients with thrombocytopenia unless an associated qualitative platelet abnormality is suspected, in which case the bleeding time would be expected to be disproportionately prolonged for the degree of thrombocytopenia (Fig. 83-2). The bleeding time is usually unaffected by coagulation factor deficiencies or pharmacologic anticoagulation. Although it is a valuable diagnostic test, the bleeding time is prone to both falsely abnormal or falsely normal results when performed by improper technique. Furthermore, in patients without a known clinical history of bleeding problems, the bleeding time has been found to be unreliable as a routine screening test to predict the risk of excessive surgical hemorrhage.

In patients who exhibit a prolonged bleeding time associated with a normal platelet count, the presence of an intrinsic qualitative platelet defect can be evaluated by platelet aggregation studies. In vitro platelet aggregation induced by the addition of specific agonists to

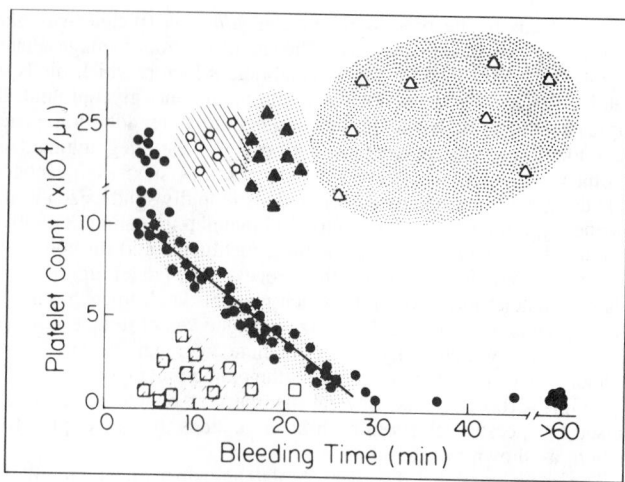

FIGURE 83-2   Relationship of bleeding time to platelet count. The bleeding time is inversely related to circulating platelet count in patients with thrombocytopenia because of decreased production (*closed circles,* which also include eight normal subjects) when the count is between 100,000 and 10,000 cells/μl. Platelet function defects (without thrombocytopenia) are represented by subjects taking aspirin (*open circles*) and patients with uremia (*closed triangles*) and inherited severe von Willebrand's disease (*open triangles*). Patients with idiopathic thrombocytopenic purpura may have platelets with increased hemostatic competence (*open squares*).

(From Thompson AR, Harker LA: *Manual of hemostasis and thrombosis,* Philadelphia, 1983, FA Davis.)

platelet-rich plasma is monitored by a turbidometric method in an aggregometer. The normal platelet response to epinephrine and certain concentrations of ADP demonstrates a biphasic pattern of aggregation, the second wave of which results from the release reaction; a single wave of aggregation is generally noted in response to collagen, arachidonate, and ristocetin (Fig. 83-3). In patients with adhesion defects (von Willebrand's disease or the Bernard-Soulier syndrome), only ristocetin-stimulated platelet aggregation may be affected. In patients with release defects caused by storage pool deficiency or a functional release abnormality (e.g., after aspirin ingestion), second-wave aggregation in response to epinephrine or ADP is lost, and arachidonate-induced aggregation may be entirely absent, particularly in subjects taking aspirin. In patients with thrombasthenia, complete loss of aggregation to all agonists is characteristically found. Specific patterns of abnormal aggregation can be pursued with more specialized platelet function studies, such as serotonin uptake and release, measurements of platelet adenine nucleotide content, or electron microscopy, but these tests are rarely necessary for clinical management.

Nonthrombocytopenic patients with prolonged bleeding times but with normal platelet aggregation studies pose difficult diagnostic problems. Unless they are using potentially implicated medications, they should be evaluated for (1) von Willebrand's disease, even when ristocetin-induced aggregation is normal, (2) renal failure, (3) hepatic dysfunction, and (4) dysproteinemia. A substantial number of patients remain with unexplained prolongations of the bleeding time, possibly because of a primary vascular disorder. In these patients, clinical management must depend on empiric therapeutic trials of platelet transfusions, DDAVP, cryoprecipitate, or occasionally, brief courses of corticosteroids.

Treatment

Most patients with disorders of platelet function do not require chronic treatment, and avoidance of the use of aspirin or other platelet inhibitory drugs may be the only intervention recommended. The prophylaxis or management of surgical or traumatic bleeding depends on the clinical severity and the specific type of qualitative platelet abnormality. Patients undergoing elective surgery should be advised to avoid aspirin- containing medications for at least 1 week before surgery. The definitive treatment for severe bleeding from an intrin-

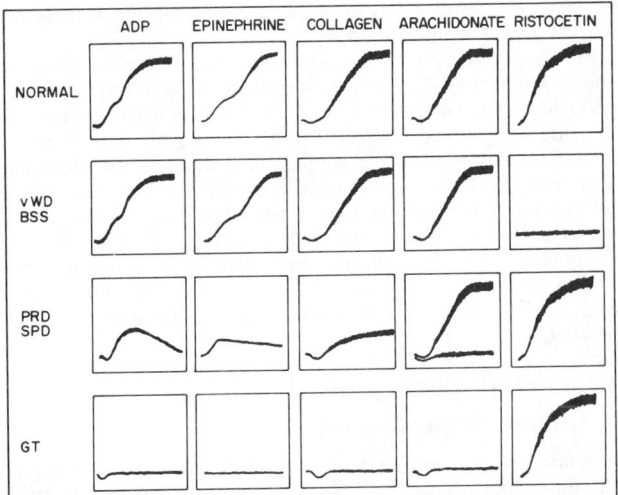

FIGURE 83-3   Normal and abnormal patterns of platelet aggregation in response to adenosine diphosphate (ADP), epinephrine, collagen, arachidonate, and ristocetin. In classic (type I) von Willebrand's disease *(vWD)* and Bernard-Soulier syndrome *(BSS),* platelet aggregation is normal with all agents except ristocetin. In platelet-release defects *(PRD)* and storage pool disease *(SPD),* only first-wave aggregation occurs in response to ADP and epinephrine, and collagen-induced aggregation is greatly blunted; arachidonate-induced aggregation may be abnormal but is always lost after aspirin ingestion. In Glanzmann's thrombasthenia *(GT),* the initial shape-change remains normal but aggregation is completely inhibited in response to all agents except ristocetin.

BOX 83-1
Major causes of thrombocytopenia

I. Decreased platelet production
   A. Megakaryocyte hypoplasia
      1. Aplastic anemia
      2. Myelofibrosis
      3. Leukemia
      4. Marrow invasion by metastatic tumor, granulomas
      5. Viral infection
      6. Radiation myelosuppression
      7. Toxic agents, drugs, antineoplastic chemotherapy
   B. Ineffective thrombopoiesis
      1. Vitamin B_{12} deficiency
      2. Folate deficiency
II. Splenic sequestration, hypersplenism
III. Increased platelet destruction
   A. Non–immune-mediated platelet destruction
      1. Disseminated intravascular coagulation (DIC)
      2. Prosthetic intravascular devices
      3. Extracorporeal circulation
      4. Thrombotic thrombocytopenic purpura (TTP)
   B. Immune-mediated platelet destruction
      1. Drug-induced immune thrombocytopenia
      2. Alloimmune thrombocytopenia
         a. Neonatal
         b. Posttransfusion purpura
      3. Autoimmune thrombocytopenia (ITP)
         a. Idiopathic thrombocytopenic purpura
         b. Secondary to rheumatic diseases, infections, lymphoproliferative disorders

---

sic platelet disorder is the transfusion of normal platelets. Cryoprecipitate may ameliorate bleeding and shorten the prolonged bleeding time not only in von Willebrand's disease, but also in uremia. The arginine vasopressin analog, DDAVP, infused intravenously at a dose of 0.3 μg/kg body weight over 15 to 30 minutes immediately before surgery, has been shown to shorten the bleeding time and improve hemostasis in patients with type I and, to a lesser extent, type IIA von Willebrand's disease. This drug has also demonstrated efficacy in shortening the bleeding time of some patients with uremia, as well as those with a variety of functional platelet disorders. The mechanism of clinical action of DDAVP is not clear, but it stimulates the release of von Willebrand's factor from vascular endothelial cells and may also exert nonspecific vasoactive effects to improve hemostasis. Rapid tachyphylaxis tends to occur, and second infusions of DDAVP 12 hours after the initial treatment generally result in suboptimal responses. Therefore, although DDAVP can obviate the need for blood products in many of these patients, its hemostatic actions tend to be short-lived. More sustained improvement in the prolonged bleeding time of uremic patients may be achieved with the use of conjugated estrogens. Partial correction of the anemia of renal failure (to a hematocrit of about 27% to 31%) with either red blood cell transfusions or erythropoietin is sufficient to normalize the bleeding time of most such uremic patients.

THROMBOCYTOPENIA

Thrombocytopenia is defined as a platelet count less than 150×10^9 per liter. The major causes of thrombocytopenia are outlined in Box 83-1. These can be broadly divided into three categories on the basis of platelet kinetics. Thrombocytopenia may be caused by (1) impaired production of platelets by the bone marrow, (2) platelet sequestration from splenomegaly, or (3) increased destruction of platelets in the peripheral circulation that exceeds the approximately eightfold capacity of the bone marrow to compensate by accelerated production. In patients receiving large volumes of rapidly administered platelet-poor blood products, thrombocytopenia may also develop on a dilutional basis. The destructive thrombocytopenias can be further subdivided into nonimmune and immune-mediated disorders; immune thrombocytopenias, in turn, may be caused by drug-induced antibodies, alloantibodies, or autoantibodies.

The clinical bleeding manifestations of thrombocytopenia depend on the severity of thrombocytopenia, its cause, and possible associated coagulation defects. In general, abnormal bleeding is unusual even after surgery or trauma, when the platelet count is greater than 100×10^9 per liter, unless complicating coexisting conditions are present. Patients with platelet counts of 20 to 100×10^9 per liter are at risk of excessive posttraumatic bleeding, whereas those with platelet counts less than 20×10^9 per liter may bleed spontaneously. For any given degree of thrombocytopenia, bleeding tends to be more severe when the cause is decreased production rather than increased destruction of platelets; in the latter situation, accelerated platelet turnover results in the circulation of younger, larger, and hemostatically more effective platelets. The types of clinical bleeding manifestations of thrombocytopenia are similar to those described previously for functional platelet abnormalities. In addition, severe thrombocytopenia is typically associated with the appearance of mucous membrane and cutaneous petechiae (Plate IV-10), particularly over dependent parts of the body (e.g., lower legs).

The laboratory evaluation of thrombocytopenia must begin with a careful examination of the peripheral blood smear. "Pseudothrombocytopenia" occurs when platelets clump in the test tube, leading to an artifactually low platelet count reading by automated machines that exclude large platelet aggregates. This phenomenon in some patients may be caused by the EDTA anticoagulant in tubes used for blood cell counts or a clinically insignificant platelet cold agglutinin that functions only at room temperature. Pseudothrombocytopenia should be suspected in patients who have unexpected reports of very low platelet counts in the absence of bleeding problems; it is confirmed by the finding of platelet clumps on the peripheral smear. In these patients, platelet counts obtained by finger-stick, from blood drawn into tubes containing alternative anticoagulants, or in promptly processed samples will reveal a normal concentration of platelets. Examination of the peripheral smear may also provide critical clues to the cause of the thrombocytopenia (e.g., fragmented red blood cells in thrombotic thrombocytopenic purpura).

Certain laboratory tests may provide guidance to the broad kinetic category of thrombocytopenia. In general the occurrence of a severe, selective thrombocytopenia (in the absence of anemia or leukopenia) strongly suggests that the origin involves increased peripheral platelet destruction by either a non–immune-mediated or immune-mediated mechanism. The finding of large platelets on the blood smear may likewise be an indication of increased platelet turnover. In patients with low platelet counts because of peripheral platelet destruction, an increased number of megakaryocytes is typically seen in the bone marrow, and bone marrow examination can often directly reveal the cause of thrombocytopenias caused by decreased platelet production (e.g., aplastic anemia, myelofibrosis, leukemia, tumor infiltration). Platelet survival studies, tracing the fate of autologous chromium-51-labeled platelets infused intravenously (Fig. 83-4), can be instructive but are rarely necessary clinically. A cruder but more practical clinical approach to this kinetic diagnosis of thrombocytopenia is the serial testing of platelet counts after a platelet transfusion. An expected level and duration of rise in the platelet count suggests that the thrombocytopenia results from decreased platelet production, whereas failure of an expected response suggests a mechanism involving increased platelet clearance.

Thrombocytopenia Caused by Decreased Platelet Production

Patients with congenital thrombocytopenia caused by decreased platelet production are rarely seen; they include those with constitutional aplastic anemia (Fanconi's syndrome) and congenital amegakaryocytic thrombocytopenia, which may be associated with skeletal malformations. Acquired disorders of platelet production are caused by either (1) hypoplasia of megakaryocytes or (2) ineffective thrombopoiesis. Megakaryocytic hypoplasia can result from a variety of conditions, including *marrow aplasia* (including idiopathic forms or myelosuppression by chemotherapeutic agents, toxins, or radiation therapy), *myelofibrosis, leukemia,* and invasion of the bone marrow by *metastatic tumor* or *granulomas.* In most of these patients, red blood cell and leukocyte production are also affected, and the diagnosis can be made on bone marrow biopsy. In some situations, *toxins, infectious agents,* or *drugs* may interfere with thrombopoiesis relatively selectively. Examples include transient thrombocytopenias caused by alcohol and certain viral infections and mild thrombocytopenia associated with the administration of thiazide diuretics. Ineffective thrombopoiesis secondary to megaloblastic processes (*folate*

or *vitamin B₁₂ deficiency*) can cause thrombocytopenia, usually with coexisting anemia and leukopenia.

Effective treatment of thrombocytopenias caused by decreased platelet production depends on identification and reversal of the underlying cause of the bone marrow failure. Platelet transfusions are generally reserved for patients with serious bleeding complications or for coverage during surgical procedures, since isoimmunization may lead to refractoriness to further platelet transfusions. Mucosal bleeding resulting from severe thrombocytopenia may be ameliorated by the oral or intravenous administration of an antifibrinolytic agent such as epsilon aminocaproic or tranexamic acid. Thrombotic complications may develop, however, if antifibrinolytic agents are used in patients with disseminated intravascular coagulation (DIC).

Thrombocytopenia Caused by Splenic Sequestration

Splenomegaly from any cause may be associated with mild to moderate thrombocytopenia. This phenomenon of *hypersplenism* results from expansion of the splenic platelet pool. This is a largely passive process of splenic platelet sequestration, in contrast to the active destruction of platelets by the spleen in patients with immune-mediated thrombocytopenia (discussed later). Although the most common cause of hypersplenism is congestive splenomegaly from portal hypertension caused by alcoholic cirrhosis, other forms of congestive, infiltrative, or lymphoproliferative splenomegaly are also associated with thrombocytopenia. Platelet counts generally do not fall below 50 × 10⁹ per liter as a result of hypersplenism alone, and coexisting anemia and leukopenia frequently occur. The size of the spleen does not clearly correlate with the degree of thrombocytopenia. Splenectomy, which is rarely indicated solely because of the thrombocytopenia, leads to an unpredictable rise in the platelet count.

Thrombocytopenia Caused by Non–Immune-Mediated Platelet Destruction

Thrombocytopenia can result from the accelerated destruction of platelets by various nonimmunologic processes. Disorders of this type include DIC, prosthetic intravascular devices, extracorporeal circulation of blood, and thrombotic microangiopathies such as thrombotic thrombocytopenic purpura (discussed in the next section). In all these situations, circulating platelets that are exposed to either artificial surfaces or abnormal vascular intima are either consumed at these sites or are damaged so that they are then prematurely cleared by the reticuloendothelial system. DIC is discussed in Chapter 84. A localized consumptive coagulopathy occurs in patients with *giant cavernous hemangiomas,* termed the *Kasabach-Merritt syndrome,* in which thrombocytopenia is usually associated with laboratory evidence of intravascular coagulation. *Intravascular prosthetic devices,* including cardiac valves and intraaortic balloons, can cause a mild to moderate destructive thrombocytopenia. Transient thrombocytopenia in patients undergoing *cardiopulmonary bypass* or *hemodialysis* may result from consumption or damage of platelets in the extracorporeal circuit. Successful treatment of these types of thrombocytopenia depends on the correction or removal of the underlying cause.

Thrombotic Thrombocytopenic Purpura

Thrombotic thrombocytopenic purpura (TTP) is a rare form of consumptive thrombocytopenia caused by widespread platelet thrombi that form in the microcirculation. This is a syndrome of largely unknown and probably multiple diverse causes that occurs predominantly in adults without evidence of antecedent illness. An association has been noted with HIV infection. Although infectious, genetic, or immunologic origins have been suspected in some patients, the cause of TTP usually is unknown. The underlying pathophysiology appears to involve abnormal interaction between platelets and vascular endothelium. Some laboratory observations have indicated that TTP may be caused by a primary endothelial cell disorder in which the thromboresistant properties of normal vascular intima are defective; this has been suggested by the finding of decreased endothelium-derived prostacyclin (PGI₂), impaired protein C activation, and de-

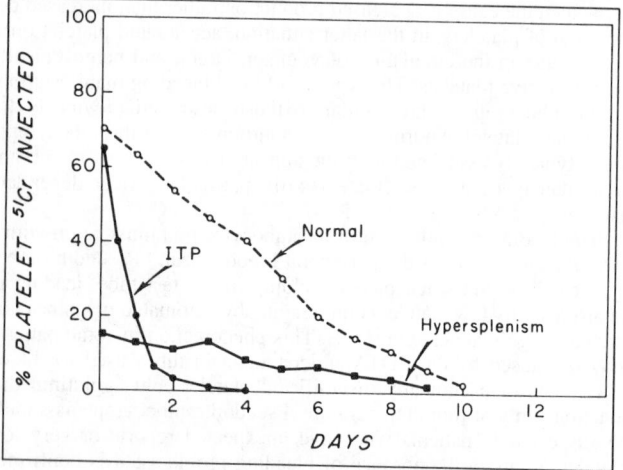

FIGURE 83-4   Platelet survival measured by chromium-51-labeled autologous platelets. Normal platelet survival is 10 days. The recovery of labeled platelets in the general circulation 2 hours after infusion is approximately only 70%. The remainder are reversibly sequestered in the spleen. In patients with immune thrombocytopenia the initial recovery may not be changed, but platelet survival is greatly shortened. In patients with hypersplenism the initial platelet recovery is decreased because of platelet pooling within the spleen, but platelet survival is normal.

(From Aster RH. In Williams WJ et al, editors: *Hematology,* New York, 1972, McGraw-Hill.)

fective fibrinolysis. A plasma defect has been implicated by the finding of a circulating platelet agglutinating factor in the plasma of some patients with TTP and the appearance in plasma of unusually large multimers of von Willebrand's factor during remission in patients with chronic relapsing TTP.

The major clinical manifestations of TTP are attributable to the disseminated occlusive microvascular platelet thrombi: (1) thrombocytopenia, which may be very severe and associated with bleeding; (2) microangiopathic hemolytic anemia, caused by red blood cell fragmentation during passage of blood through the disrupted microcirculation; (3) neurologic symptoms and signs, including nonspecific headache, mental changes, seizures, coma, and focal neurologic signs; (4) renal abnormalities, ranging in severity from proteinuria and microscopic hematuria to frank renal failure; and (5) fever. Not all these major manifestations of TTP may be present simultaneously. Other clinical features may include abdominal pain, nausea, vomiting, malaise, and weakness. The onset of symptoms is frequently abrupt, and the disease course may be fulminant and self-limited or fatal. Other patients may be characterized by an insidious onset or a chronic, relapsing course.

In patients with typical, acute disease the diagnosis of TTP should not pose difficulty. The constellation of laboratory findings include thrombocytopenia, red blood cell fragmentation on peripheral smear, evidence of intravascular hemolysis (including reticulocytosis, elevated serum levels of indirect bilirubin and lactate dehydrogenase, decreased level of haptoglobin), proteinuria, abnormal urinary sediment, or uremia. No activation of the coagulation system occurs in TTP; therefore laboratory manifestations of DIC (e.g. prolonged prothrombin time, partial thromboplastin time, elevated fibrin degradation products) should not be found. Diagnostic problems may arise in patients with more subtle disease, particularly when other conditions coexist to which some of the clinical and laboratory features could be attributed. Associated DIC, malignant hypertension, eclampsia or preeclampsia, or vasculitis may mimic some of the features of TTP. A tissue diagnosis, most conveniently obtained by gingival biopsy, is rarely necessary and should not delay therapy in fulminant cases. The characteristic pathologic features of TTP, consisting of microvascular hyaline thrombi, should be clearly distinguishable from the changes of vasculitis whenever the differential diagnosis is in doubt.

The design of rational therapy has been hindered by the lack of understanding of cause, the unpredictable natural history, and the rarity of patients with TTP. Nevertheless, prompt treatment of TTP has dramatically reduced mortality from rates of more than 90% in historically untreated patients to approximately 10% to 30%. In acute, fulminant TTP, two major therapeutic interventions are generally used simultaneously. First, prednisone at a dose of 1 to 2 mg/kg/day is started. Second, plasma exchange is begun without delay. Plasmapheresis is usually performed with a 2- to 3-L exchange daily for at least 7 days, using fresh-frozen plasma as replacement. In some patients who fail to respond to this treatment, the substitution of cryosupernatant for fresh-frozen plasma in the plasma exchange procedure has been found to be effective. Plasma exchange has been demonstrated to be more effective than simple plasma infusion in the treatment of TTP. Other, second-line treatments of largely unproven efficacy may include heparin, antiplatelet agents (aspirin, dipyridamole, prostacyclin), vincristine, and splenectomy. Platelet transfusions are contraindicated, even in the presence of severe thrombocytopenia, because transfused platelets may "fuel the fire" to exacerbate the thrombotic microangiopathy.

Most survivors of an acute episode of TTP recover completely. However, it has been projected that more than one third of patients who survive an acute episode of TTP will have at least one relapse during the following 10 years, which may occur several years following the original event. In some patients, chronic, relapsing TTP develops in which recurrent episodes are separated by months or years of health. Therefore, since relapses are common, close follow-up is recommended for survivors of TTP.

Several syndromes that are clinically and pathologically similar to TTP have been described. The *hemolytic-uremic syndrome* (HUS) is typically encountered in children and frequently follows viral infections. Gastroenteritis caused by a verotoxin-producing serotype of *Escherichia coli* or by *Shigella* may also cause a similar syndrome.

Thrombocytopenia and microangiopathic hemolytic anemia are prominent manifestations of HUS, but neurologic symptoms are unusual and renal complications, including frank renal failure, are more predominant features of HUS than TTP. Treatment of patients with HUS also centers around the use of plasma exchange. During the late stages of pregnancy, a preeclamptic TTP-like syndrome of microangiopathic hemolysis, elevated liver enzyme levels, and low platelet counts has been give the acronym "HELLP." An either fulminant or slowly progressive thrombotic microangiopathy that resembles TTP/HUS has been observed in some patients receiving chemotherapy with certain agents, including mitomycin, cyclosporine, and cisplatin.

Drug-Induced Immune Thrombocytopenia

More than 100 drugs have been implicated in immunologically mediated thrombocytopenia. However, only a small number of these, notably quinidine, quinine, gold, sulfonamides, cephalothin, and heparin, have been well characterized. Use of illicit drugs, including cocaine and heroin, also may be associated with immune thrombocytopenia. The mechanism of drug-induced immune platelet destruction depends in part on the offending agent. It may be mediated either through the binding of the drug (hapten)-antibody complex to platelets with subsequent complement fixation and platelet damage or, alternatively, the drug's binding to platelets to induce new and unstable immunogenic platelet surface antigens that are expressed only in the drug's presence and are stabilized on reaction with antibody. The mechanism of heparin-associated immune thrombocytopenia is unusual. Antibodies are formed against complexes between heparin and platelet factor 4 (PF4), a heparin-binding protein released by platelets. Immune complexes of heparin-PF4-antibody then cause platelet activation and aggregation by binding to platelet Fc receptors.

Drug-induced thrombocytopenia is frequently severe and typically occurs precipitously within days while patients are taking the sensitizing medication. These idiosyncratic reactions are generally not drug-dose dependent. For example, severe quinine-induced thrombocytopenia may be precipitated by drinking tonic water. Although clinical manifestations of drug-induced thrombocytopenias are common to the bleeding complications encountered in other forms of thrombocytopenia, heparin-associated thrombocytopenia has unusual features. As many as 10% of patients receiving heparin may develop thrombocytopenia, but this is usually dose related, not immune mediated, and mild, stable, and asymptomatic. The idiosyncratic form of heparin- associated thrombocytopenia, in contrast, tends to be more severe and precipitous and may be triggered by even the small doses included in intravenous flushes. These latter patients may develop serious venous or arterial thrombosis, presumably on the basis of in vivo platelet aggregation mediated by heparin-induced antibody. The thrombotic complications of heparin may also be related to heparin-dependent antibodies targeted to vascular endothelial cells. In most patients with any drug-induced thrombocytopenia, rapid recovery of the platelet count occurs within 7 to 10 days of removal of the offending agent. With some drugs that are metabolized and eliminated slowly, particularly gold, recovery may take weeks or even months. In the latter patients, the possible coexistence of autoimmune thrombocytopenia caused by the underlying rheumatic disease may complicate and confuse the clinical picture.

Specific laboratory tests may confirm the diagnosis with certain types of drugs; in vitro platelet immunoinjury or, in the case of heparin, platelet aggregation may be found when target platelets, patient serum (or plasma), and the suspected drug are mixed. However, the definitive demonstration is prompt recovery after withdrawal of the immunizing agent.

Treatment of drug-induced thrombocytopenia depends on immediate discontinuation of any suspected medication. In patients with severe bleeding complications, a short course of prednisone (1 to 2 mg/kg/day) may be of benefit. Platelet transfusions are indicated only for critical or life-threatening hemorrhage, since the transfused platelets are likely to be destroyed as rapidly as the recipient's own platelets. The management of patients with heparin-associated thrombocytopenia poses special problems if alternative antithrombotic treatment is required after discontinuation of the heparin or in choosing anticoagulation for the thrombotic complication caused by the heparin itself. Institution of an oral anticoagulant and interim antithrombotic therapy with a fibrinolytic agent has been suggested as one approach. Heparin-associated thrombocytopenia and thrombosis are more common in patients receiving treatment with unfractionated heparin than in those receiving treatment with low-molecular-weight heparin. Nevertheless, low-molecular-weight heparin should not be substituted for unfractionated heparin when this complication occurs because there is extensive cross-reactivity of these two forms of heparin. The appropriate management of heparin-induced thrombocytopenia and thrombosis is not clearly established.

Alloimmune Thrombocytopenic Purpura

Neonatal alloimmune thrombocytopenia and posttransfusion purpura are disorders of alloimmune platelet destruction that most commonly involve patients who are homozygous for the platelet antigen HPA-1b (Pl^{A2}). These individuals lack the platelet antigen HPA-1a (Pl^{A1}) and are therefore "Pl^{A1}-negative." About 2% of the white population is Pl^{A1}-negative (i.e., homozygous for HPA-1b).

In most cases of *neonatal alloimmune thrombocytopenia* the mother is homozygous for the HPA-1b antigen (Pl^{A1}-negative) and the fetus is a HPA-1a/HPA-1b heterozygote. The mother develops anti-HPA-1a antibodies, and transplacental transmission of the antibodies against this antigen, which is shared by the father and fetus, causes immune platelet destruction and thrombocytopenia in the neonate. This syndrome is a platelet counterpart of hemolytic disease of the newborn. Serologic diagnosis is made by maternal platelet typing and antibody detection. Until the maternal anti-HPA-1a antibodies are cleared from the neonatal circulation and thrombocytopenia recovers, the newborn is at risk for intracranial hemorrhage and other bleeding complications. During this period neonates frequently require support with transfusions of platelets from a donor who is homozygous for HPA-1b (Pl^{A1}-negative), most conveniently the unaffected mother herself. Treatment of the neonate with intravenous gamma globulin may shorten the duration of thrombocytopenia.

Posttransfusion purpura is a rare disorder that most commonly involves HPA-1b homozygous (Pl^{A1}-negative) adult recipients of blood products containing platelet material bearing the HPA-1a (Pl^{A1}-positive) antigen. Rare cases are associated with alloimmunization to other platelet antigens. The precipitating transfusion may be platelet concentrates, fresh or stored whole blood, packed red blood cells, or plasma. Affected patients are typically multiparous women who have been previously sensitized to the platelet antigen by prior pregnancy or blood transfusion. The mechanism of thrombocytopenia is unclear in this disorder, particularly since the recipient's platelets are destroyed by alloantibodies (anti-HPA-1a) to an antigen their platelets do not express. It has been considered that soluble HPA-1a or platelet fragments bearing HPA-1a released from lysed platelets in the donor blood bind to the surfaces of the HPA-1a-negative (Pl^{A1}-negative) platelets of the transfusion recipient, effectively converting them to HPA-1a positivity and permitting immune complexes to form. The clinical consequence is the development of acute, profound thrombocytopenia in some of these patients 7 to 10 days after the transfusion. Platelet counts of survivors generally return to normal within 10 to 14 days. Intracranial hemorrhage occurs in about 10% of cases. Currently used serologic tests of platelet alloantibody are likely to be replaced by DNA-based assays of HPA-1b homozygosity for individuals at risk for posttransfusion purpura (and mothers at risk for bearing children with neonatal alloimmune thrombocytopenia). Prompt administration of high-dose intravenous gamma globulin (1 g/kg/day for 2 days) is the treatment of choice in this life-threatening disease. It has largely replaced plasmapheresis and exchange transfusion as initial therapy. Prednisone may have an adjunctive role in improving the bleeding tendency of posttransfusion purpura. Platelet transfusions are ineffective and may cause severe transfusion reactions.

Immune (Autoimmune) Thrombocytopenic Purpura

Immune thrombocytopenic purpura (ITP) in adults is a chronic disease characterized by autoimmune platelet destruction. Adult ITP occurs predominantly in young women. The antiplatelet autoantibody is usually immunoglobulin G (IgG) that may or may not fix comple-

ment, although other immunoglobulins have also been reported. Although the autoantibody of ITP has been found to be associated with platelet membrane GpIIb-IIIa, the platelet antigen specificity has not been identified in most patients. Extravascular destruction of sensitized platelets occurs in the reticuloendothelial system of the spleen and liver. Although more than half of all cases of ITP are idiopathic, many patients have underlying rheumatic or autoimmune diseases (e.g., systemic lupus erythematosus) or lymphoproliferative disorders (e.g., chronic lymphocytic leukemia). ITP is also a frequent and often very early complication of human immunodeficiency virus (HIV) infection. However, thrombocytopenia in HIV-infected patients may be caused by factors other than immune destruction of platelets, including the suppressive effects of the viral infection on hematopoiesis, bone marrow infiltration with opportunistic microorganisms (e.g. tuberculosis, *Mycobacterium avium-intracellulare*) or tumor (e.g. lymphoma), and TTP.

Childhood ITP appears to be a distinctly different clinical entity. This is an acute, self-limited disorder, usually resolving spontaneously within a few weeks. It frequently follows minor viral infections, and the deposition of resultant immune complexes on platelets is considered to be the major mechanism of immune platelet destruction in these patients. There is no absolute separation of the two clinical forms of ITP by age; occasionally, adults may develop acute "childhood" ITP, and children may have chronic ITP.

The onset of bleeding problems in patients with chronic ITP may be either insidious or abrupt and fulminant. The hemorrhagic complications of ITP are indistinguishable from those associated with other types of thrombocytopenia described earlier. Besides signs of bleeding, the physical examination is generally unremarkable. The finding of splenomegaly is distinctly unusual in idiopathic forms of ITP and strongly suggests the presence of an underlying rheumatic or lymphoproliferative disease.

Laboratory studies usually reveal a selective thrombocytopenia. In rare patients, autoimmune hemolytic anemia may coexist with ITP (an association known as *Evans's syndrome*). Bone marrow examination, which is not indicated in all patients, is typically normal except for the presence of an increased number of megakaryocytes that is characteristic of other types of destructive thrombocytopenias. Several laboratory tests for the detection of antiplatelet antibodies have been developed. However, interpretation of the results of many of these assays is complicated by both false-positive test results (e.g., from platelet adsorption of immunoglobulin in patients with hypergammaglobulinemia) and false-negative test results. Antiplatelet antibody assays are not essential for diagnosis or treatment. In making the diagnosis of ITP, other types of destructive thrombocytopenias must be rigorously excluded. DIC can be ruled out in most patients by the presence of a normal prothrombin time, partial thromboplastin time, and fibrin degradation products. TTP can be ruled out by the absence of red blood cell fragmentation on the peripheral smear and the lack of renal or neurologic involvement. Drug-induced thrombocytopenia must be ruled out by the discontinuation of any suspected medications.

The therapeutic approach to patients with ITP is dictated by the severity and urgency of the clinical situation. Some adult patients with only mild to moderate chronic thrombocytopenia and no bleeding problems may require no treatment. However, such patients may have transient precipitous decreases in platelet counts at times of even trivial viral infections. The standard approach in patients requiring treatment is to begin prednisone at a dose of 1 to 2 mg/kg/day as initial therapy. Even before a demonstrable platelet response to prednisone is noted, clinical bleeding manifestations are often promptly ameliorated, presumably by the beneficial effects of corticosteroids on microvascular fragility. Although some patients obtain a prolonged complete remission after a short course of prednisone, in most patients either the response is incomplete or relapse occurs when the prednisone dose is decreased. Splenectomy should be performed in patients who fail to respond after 2 to 3 weeks of prednisone or do not achieve sustained responses after discontinuation of prednisone. Patients who have even a transient response to prednisone tend to have better results with splenectomy. Splenectomy removes the major site of platelet destruction and a major source of autoantibody production in most patients. This procedure results in prolonged, treatment-free remissions in about two thirds of patients. The use of intravenous gamma globulin (IV IgG) has now been established as highly effective treatment and is particularly useful when rapid correction of the thrombocytopenia is required (e.g., with the threat of serious bleeding or for surgical coverage). The usual dose of IV IgG is 0.4 g/kg/day infused on 3 to 5 consecutive days. Platelet counts frequently begin to rise after only 2 to 3 days of this treatment. The emergency regimen of IV IgG is 1 g/kg, which can be repeated with a second dose on the following day. IV IgG has been found to be effective in patients with ITP refractory to prednisone or splenectomy and may be used as maintenance therapy in such patients. In RhD-positive patients, anti-RhD immune globulin may be as effective as IV IgG, with the advantages of lower cost and easier administration. Splenectomized patients do not respond to anti-RhD as well as those who have not undergone splenectomy. In patients who fail to respond to these therapies, second-line treatment modalities include other immunosuppressive drugs (azathioprine, vincristine, cyclophosphamide) and the synthetic androgen danazol (600 to 800 mg/day). More recently, patients with refractory ITP have been found to respond to cycles of chemotherapy agents that are used for the treatment of malignant lymphoproliferative disorders. These include combination chemotherapy with cyclophosphamide, prednisone and vincristine, procarbazine and/or etoposide, and pulsed high-dose dexamethasone.

The response to treatment of ITP in HIV-infected patients is not significantly different from that in uninfected patients. However, long-term corticosteroid therapy may cause further immunologic suppression in such patients. Many patients with HIV-associated thrombocytopenia have been found to respond to zidovudine (azidothymidine, [AZT]) with a significant increase in platelet count.

The management of pregnancy and delivery in patients with chronic ITP, which is not rare because ITP most frequently affects women of childbearing age, poses special problems. The unexpected discovery of mild thrombocytopenia in an asymptomatic, previously healthy, pregnant woman with no prior diagnosis of ITP should not be considered to be equivalent to the new diagnosis of ITP. Thrombocytopenia is detected incidentally in about 8% of normal pregnant women at term, and this is not associated with any adverse effects on either the mothers or their infants. In women who do have a history of ITP, maternal antiplatelet autoantibodies cross the placenta and can cause fetal platelet destruction. No reliable correlation exists between the maternal and neonatal platelet counts. Even mothers in apparent remission from ITP (e.g., after splenectomy) may give birth to thrombocytopenic infants. It has been previously recommended that, unless a prenatal fetal platelet count can be obtained, delivery should be performed by cesarean section to prevent the possibility of intracranial hemorrhage caused by head trauma during vaginal delivery. However, fetal platelet counts obtained from scalp-vein blood at the time of impending vaginal delivery may be artifactually low, and umbilical blood sampling percutaneously by cordocentesis before labor may be associated with serious fetal or neonatal complications. Furthermore, it has not been shown that vaginal delivery causes hemorrhage in thrombocytopenic fetuses or that cesarean delivery prevents it. In view of the very low risk of fetal thrombocytopenia and intracranial hemorrhage associated with maternal ITP, it has been recommended that routine fetal scalp sampling, cordocentesis, and cesarean section are not indicated in women with ITP.

BIBLIOGRAPHY

Aster RH: Heparin-induced thrombocytopenia and thrombosis, *N Engl J Med* 332:1374, 1995.
Berkman N et al: EDTA-dependent pseudothrombocytopenia: a clinical study of 18 patients and a review of the literature, *Am J Hematol* 36:195, 1991.
Burrows RF, Kelton JG: Incidentally detected thrombocytopenia in healthy mothers and their infants, *N Engl J Med* 319:142, 1988.
Burrows RF, Kelton JG: Fetal thrombocytopenia and its relation to maternal thrombocytopenia, *N Engl J Med* 329:1463, 1993.
Cortelazzo S et al: Hydroxyurea for patients with essential thrombocythemia and high risk of thrombosis, *N Engl J Med* 332:1132, 1995.
George JN, El-Harake MA, Raskob GE: Chronic idiopathic thrombocytopenic purpura, *N Engl J Med* 331:1207, 1994.
George JN, Shattil SJ: The clinical importance of acquired abnormalities of platelet function, *N Engl J Med* 324:27, 1991.
Leung L, Nachman R: Molecular mechanisms of platelet aggregation, *Annu Rev Med* 37:179, 1986.
Lind SE: The bleeding time does not predict surgical bleeding, *Blood* 77:2547, 1991.
Mannucci PM: Desmopressin: a nontransfusional hemostatic agent, *Annu Rev Med* 41:55, 1990.
Najean Y, Rain J-D: The mechanism of thrombocytopenia in patients with HIV infection, *J Lab Clin Med* 123:415, 1994.
Rao AK: Congenital disorders of platelet function, *Hematol Oncol Clin North Am* 4:65, 1990.
Rodgers RP, Levin J: A critical reappraisal of the bleeding time, *Semin Thromb Hemost* 16:1, 1990.
Rose M, Rowe JM, Eldor A: The changing course of thrombotic thrombocytopenic purpura and modern therapy, *Blood Rev* 7:94, 1993.
Samuels P et al: Estimation of the risk of thrombocytopenia in the offspring of pregnant women with presumed immune thrombocytopenic purpura, *N Engl J Med* 323:229, 1990.
Schafer AI: Bleeding disorders: finding the cause, *Hosp Pract* 19:88K, 1984.
Shumak KH et al: Late relapses in patients successfully treated for thrombotic thrombocytopenic purpura, *Ann Intern Med* 122:569, 1995.
Silver RM, Branch DW, Scott JR: Maternal thrombocytopenia in pregnancy: time for a reassessment, *Am J Obstet Gynecol* 173:479, 1995.

✔ WHEN TO REFER

General practitioners can initiate the screening evaluation of patients with suspected coagulopathies; surgeons can do likewise in preparation of patients for surgical procedures. The most important aspect of such evaluations is a careful and complete history, including specific questions about previous bleeding episodes, family history of bleeding, current medications, and prior responses to hemostatic challenges (e.g., surgery, dental extractions, injections, menstrual periods, trauma). The patient who has recently had surgery without excessive bleeding has undergone a much better assessment of hemostasis than any laboratory test can provide. Based on the history, screening laboratory tests may include a platelet count, bleeding time, prothrombin time, and partial thromboplastin time.

Patients with a bleeding tendency who have an unexplained prolongation of the bleeding time with a normal platelet count most likely have a qualitative platelet disorder or a disorder of platelet-vessel wall interactions. They should be referred to a hematologist for more specialized testing. In patients reported to have low platelet counts, particularly in those without clinical bleeding manifestations, the general practitioner should rule out "pseudothrombocytopenia." Patients with severe thrombocytopenia should be referred to a hematologist for specialized testing to determine cause, including consideration of bone marrow aspirate and biopsy, as well as guidance in management.

CHAPTER

84 Disorders of Blood Coagulation

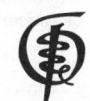

Gilbert C. White II

CONGENITAL DISORDERS

The most common inherited disorders of blood coagulation are the two sex-linked disorders, hemophilia A (factor VIII deficiency, classic hemophilia) and hemophilia B (factor IX deficiency, Christmas disease), and the autosomal disorder von Willebrand's disease (vWD). These disorders account for more than 95% of congenital disorders of blood coagulation. Deficiencies of other clotting factors are inherited in an autosomal recessive manner and are quite rare. These disorders are summarized in Table 84-1. The clinical and laboratory approach to the bleeding patient is discussed in Chapters 75 and 82.

Hemophilia A

Hemophilia A (classic hemophilia) is caused by a deficiency or abnormality of factor VIII procoagulant activity (VIII; Table 84-2 pro-

Table 84-1 Congenital disorders of blood coagulation

COAGULATION FACTOR	INHERITANCE	INCIDENCE (PER MILLION)	BLEEDING SYMPTOMS	ABNORMAL SCREENING TESTS	BIOLOGIC HALF-LIFE OF PROTEIN (HOURS)	TREATMENT
I (fibrinogen)	Autosomal recessive	1	Umbilical bleeding at birth, posttrauma hemorrhage	PT, PTT, TT	100	Cryoprecipitate
II (prothrombin)	Autosomal recessive	1	Similar to hemophilia	PT, PTT	72	FFP, rarely prothrombin complex concentrates
V	Autosomal recessive	1	Similar to hemophilia	PT, PTT	24	FFP, possibly platelet concentrates
VII	Autosomal recessive	1	Similar to hemophilia	PT	4-6	VII Concentrates
VIII (hemophilia)	Sex-linked recessive	100 (milder disease is much more common)	Hemarthrosis, hematoma, bruising, severe postoperative bleeding	PTT	12	VIII Concentrates
vWF (von Willebrand's factor)	Autosomal dominant or recessive	Probably as frequent as hemophilia A	Epistaxis, gingival bleeding, bruising, menorrhagia, severe postoperative bleeding	PTT	4-6, for correction of bleeding time	DDAVP, vWF-rich VIII concentrates
IX (hemophilia B)	Sex-linked recessive	20	Identical to hemophilia	PT, PTT	24	IX Concentrates
X	Autosomal recessive	1	Similar to hemophilia	PT, PTT	50	FFP, rarely prothrombin complex concentrates
XI	Autosomal recessive	1	Mild; however, severe postoperative hemorrhage can occur	PTT	60	FFP, level of 25% adequate for hemostasis
XII	Autosomal recessive	1	None	PTT	60	None
XIII	Autosomal recessive	1	Umbilical bleeding at birth, posttrauma hemorrhage, poor wound healing	—	120	FFP monthly, since level of 2% is adequate for hemostasis
Alpha$_2$ antiplasmin	Autosomal recessive	Unknown	Similar to hemophilia	—	Unknown	FFP
Plasminogen activator inhibitor (PAI-I)	Unknown	Unknown	Severe postoperative and posttrauma bleeding	—	Unknown	EACA
Passovoy	Autosomal dominant	Unknown	Similar to factor XI	PTT	Unknown	FFP

FFP, Fresh-frozen plasma; *PT*, prothrombin time; *PTT*, partial thromboplastin time; *TT*, thrombin (clotting) time; *DDAVP*, 1-deamino-8-D-arginine vasopressin; *EACA*, epsilon aminocaproic acid.

Table 84-2 Factor VIII and von Willebrand's factor (vWF) activities

FACTOR/ANTIGEN	ACTIVITY
VIII	Factor VIII procoagulant activity. Clot-promoting activity of factor VIII as determined by a coagulation assay. Circulates in plasma complexed with vWF.
VIII:Ag	Factor VIII procoagulant antigen. Antigenic expression of factor VIII as detected by monoclonal or patient antibodies.
vWF	Von Willebrand's factor activity. Supports platelet–vessel wall and platelet-platelet interactions. Most often measured by platelet agglutination in the presence of the antibiotic ristocetin, but also reflected in tests such as the bleeding time and platelet adhesion to glass bead columns. Previously called *factor VIII–von Willebrand's factor activity* (VIIIR:vWF) and *ristocetin cofactor activity* (VIIIR:RCoF). Circulates in plasma complexed with VIII.
vWF:Ag	Von Willebrand's factor antigen. Antigenic expression of vWF as detected by heterologous antibodies. Previously called *factor VIII–related antigen* (VIIIR:Ag).

vides a definition of factor VIII activities). Factor VIII, as measured by clotting activity, is diminished. In most patients, factor VIII procoagulant antigen (VIII:Ag) is diminished and is proportional to VIII activity, although some patients have levels of VIII:Ag in excess of VIII clotting activity and are said to have cross-reacting material

(CRM$^+$). von Willebrand's factor (vWF) and vWF:Ag activities are normal in hemophilia A. The bleeding time is usually normal or only minimally prolonged.

Diagnosis. The diagnosis of hemophilia A is suggested by a prolonged partial thromboplastin time (PTT) in association with a normal prothrombin time (PT) and thrombin (clotting) time (TT). Factor VIII activity assay is required for a specific diagnosis. One unit of VIII activity is defined as the activity present in 1 ml of a standard normal plasma pool. Levels in normal individuals range from 0.6 to 1.5 U/ml. In patients with hemophilia A, VIII levels are decreased (i.e., less than 0.5 U/ml). Because VIII can also be diminished in vWD (Table 84-3), vWF:Ag and vWF levels and a bleeding time should be determined in patients with no clear history of sex-linked hemophilia. In patients with mild VIII deficiency, a factor V level should also be measured to exclude combined factor V and VIII deficiency.

Molecular Defects. Factor VIII is synthesized as a linear polypeptide of 330,000 molecular weight. It circulates as a two-chain, calcium-linked molecule that consists of a variable heavy chain of 90,000 to 200,000 molecular weight and a light chain of 80,000 molecular weight (Fig. 84-1). Three structural domains have been identified. The A domain consists of three triplicated segments, each 350 amino acids in length, that are homologous with similar domains in the copper-binding protein ceruloplasmin and that may play a role in calcium binding. The C domain consists of two duplicated segments, each 150 amino acids in length, that may be important in phospholipid binding. The B domain is proteolytically removed from VIII during activation by thrombin.

Nearly half of individuals with severe hemophilia have a unique

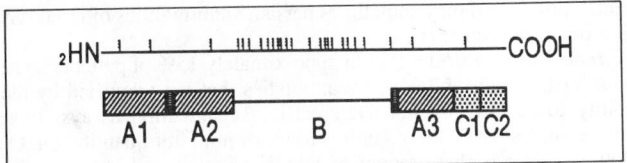

FIGURE 84-1 Factor VIII molecule. Linear representation of the factor VIII molecule. Carbohydrate chains are indicated by the curved lines. The hatched boxes indicate the segments of the A domain *(A1, A2, A3)*. The stippled boxes indicate the segments of the C domain *(C1, C2)*. The B domain separates the A2 and A3 segments of the A domain.

Table 84-3 Characteristics of hemophilia and von Willebrand's disease (vWD)

	HEMOPHILIA	vWD
Clinical bleeding	Joint, soft tissue	Mucous membranes
VIII	↓	↓
vWF	nl	↓
vWF:Ag	nl	↓
Bleeding time	nl	↑
Inheritance	X-linked	Autosomal
De novo synthesis	No	Yes

↓, Reduced factor levels in plasma; ↑, prolongation of bleeding time; *vWF*, von Willebrand's factor; *nl*, normal. This table is a comparison of clinical and laboratory findings in patients with hemophilia A and vWD. Clinical bleeding refers to the characteristic location of hemorrhages in each disorder. De novo synthesis refers to the delayed rise in factor VIII activity after administration of cryoprecipitate that is characteristic of vWD but does not occur in hemophilia. Although this has been termed *synthesis*, little evidence indicates whether the delayed rise results from synthesis, activation, or some other mechanism.

molecular defect in which there is a partial inversion of the factor VIII gene that disrupts normal transcription. This "flip-tip inversion" is due to homologous recombination between a small intronless "gene within a gene" in intron 22 of the factor VIII gene and one of two similar intronless genes at the tip of the X chromosome more than 400 kb distant. As a result of this inversion, the factor VIII that is produced is truncated and nonfunctional. The remainder of individuals with severe hemophilia and those with milder forms of hemophilia have a variety of molecular abnormalities, including deletions, insertions, and point mutations resulting in nonsense, missense, or splicing defects. A database of known mutations in hemophilia has been compiled by Tuddenham and others.

Genetics and Carrier State. Because hemophilia A is an X-linked disorder, almost all symptomatic individuals are males (X^hY). All daughters of affected males are obligate carriers (X^hX), whereas sons, who receive their father's Y chromosome, are unaffected. Daughters of carriers have a 50:50 chance of being carriers, and sons of carriers have a 50:50 chance of having hemophilia.

Initial methods for carrier detection, which are still valid, were based on two observations: (1) the abnormality in hemophilia is a deficiency of VIII, whereas vWF:Ag is normal; and (2) only one X chromosome in a given cell is expressed. Thus, in a carrier who possesses a hemophilia gene (X^h) from her father and a normal gene (X) from her mother, some of the VIII-producing cells (X) make normal amounts of VIII, whereas the rest of these cells (X^h) make no VIII. Thus, if there are equal numbers of X and X^h cells, the ratio of VIII to another unrelated protein such as vWF:Ag will be 0.5 in a carrier, whereas the ratio in a normal woman will be 1.0. However, according to the Lyon hypothesis, inactivation of the X chromosome in each cell is a random process, so, frequently, an unequal number of X-active and X^h-active cells results. Furthermore, the assays have an inherent variability. For these reasons, the ratio of VIII to vWF:Ag in carriers may vary from 0.1 to more than 1.0, whereas the ratio in normal persons may vary from 0.5 to 1.5 or more. Because of the overlap between carriers and normal persons, the laboratory data determine the likelihood that a subject is a carrier; then that likelihood ratio is combined with pedigree information to arrive at a final sta-

tistical probability that she is a carrier. These carrier detection tests are 90% to 95% accurate, but they are more accurate against normal than against carrier women.

Modern molecular biology techniques offer more precise carrier detection but are not universally applicable. If the molecular defect in a family is known, a probe specific for the defective portion of the genomic sequence for VIII is used to study an individual's DNA. This technique depends on recognition by the probe of the specific genomic defect, whether a deletion or a nucleotide change, and has the advantage of not requiring samples from family members if the precise defect has been established in the family in question. If the molecular defect in a family is not known, one takes advantage of restriction polymorphisms linked to the hemophilia gene. The DNA probes in this case identify independently segregating restriction polymorphisms close to a hemophilia A gene. The disadvantages of this technique are that key family members have to be available and the mother must be heterozygous for the restriction polymorphism. A weakness of the method is that only 50% of mothers are heterozygous for a specific polymorphism.

The object of carrier detection is to assist family planning and to allow the putative or obligate carrier the option of prenatal diagnosis. Two procedures are now available to help with prenatal diagnosis. First, *amniocentesis* and karyotyping can be performed to determine fetal sex. This can be done from weeks 13 to 16 of pregnancy. If the fetus is female, no further testing is required, although the female infant may prove to be a carrier, a fact that might possibly be specifically determined by one of the DNA methods just described. If the fetus is male, amnionic cells can be used for DNA analysis. DNA can be obtained earlier in pregnancy (between 9 and 12 gestational weeks) by *chorionic villus sampling*. If amniocentesis indicates the fetus is male but the DNA studies fail to establish a diagnosis of hemophilia, *fetal blood sampling* may be undertaken by either ultrasound-guided needle aspiration or fetoscopy. Fetal blood is tested by measuring VIII (usually VIII:Ag) and vWF:Ag ratios in fetal blood. The affected family members must first be tested to ensure that they have the type of hemophilia A in which VIII:Ag is reduced. Fetal morbidity with these procedures is 0.5% to 1.0%.

In cases of extreme inactivation of the normal (X) gene (termed *extreme lyonization*), VIII levels in carriers may be as low as 0.1 U/ml and may result in hemorrhage after major surgery, trauma, or tooth extractions. Factor VIII levels should therefore be obtained on all potential carriers so that treatment may be instituted as necessary.

Clinical Features. Hemophilia A is classified clinically as severe, moderate, or mild, depending on the frequency of hemorrhage, the severity of the hemorrhage, and the degree of trauma producing the hemorrhage. Clinical severity is usually related to the plasma level of VIII. Severely affected individuals may have two or three bleeding episodes per month, may frequently bleed spontaneously without noticeable trauma, may bleed profusely unless treated, and may have VIII levels of less than 0.01 U/ml (less than 1% of normal). Moderately affected individuals bleed perhaps five or six times per year but may have prolonged periods free of bleeding, usually bleed only with trauma, and have VIII levels of 0.01 to 0.05 U/ml (1% to 5% of normal). Mildly affected individuals bleed rarely (if at all) and then only with significant trauma or surgical stress. The disease in many of these individuals is so mild that it is undetected throughout their lives. Factor VIII levels are usually greater than 0.05 U/ml (5% of normal).

Although clinical symptoms closely parallel plasma levels of VIII, an occasional patient has clinically moderate or mild disease, yet has VIII levels of less than 0.01 U/ml. Conversely, patients with VIII levels of 0.05 to 0.10 U/ml occasionally, if trauma occurs, develop a joint bleed that recurs and becomes a "target joint" mimicking joint bleeds seen in severe hemophiliacs.

Hemarthroses are the most characteristic and among the most disabling of the hemorrhages that occur in hemophilia A. Any joint can be involved, but those most frequently affected in adults are the knees, elbows, and ankles. According to most hemophiliac patients, the initial manifestation of a joint hemorrhage is a "tingling" or "bubbling" sensation in the joint. This then progresses over a matter of hours to swelling and pain. Joint range of motion becomes limited. Since the joint is a closed space, bleeding is confined to the joint. Vessel and nerve compression do not occur, and the acute consequences of the joint bleeding are primarily pain and limitation of motion. When proper treatment is started, the hemorrhage abates promptly, and resolution of the joint hematoma is related to the quantity of the blood that accumulates in the joint.

The chronic consequences of joint hematomas are caused by the biochemical responses to blood in the joint space and are very similar pathophysiologically to joint changes in rheumatoid arthritis. Clinically, recurrent hemorrhages in the joint lead to proliferation of synovial tissue, which results in a swollen, boggy joint. The vascular synovial tissue has an increased tendency to hemorrhage, and the joint bleeding becomes cyclic. Eventually, collagenolytic enzymes begin to attack the joint, resulting in progressive loss of joint space. The final result is a collapsed joint with marked limitation or complete loss of motion (Fig. 84-2).

Muscle hematomas occur less often than joint hemorrhages but have more acute effects. Muscles of the arms and legs tend to be common sites. The initial manifestation is pain and swelling of the involved muscle. If the bleeding continues, a compartment syndrome may occur with compression of nerves and/or vessels.

Bleeding into the iliopsoas and iliacus muscles, called *retroperitoneal hematomas,* deserves special comment because these particular hemorrhages tend to cause nerve compression. The anatomic relation of the iliopsoas and iliacus muscles to the ischium means that hemorrhages in this muscle are prone to compartmentalization, which results in femoral nerve or lateral cutaneous nerve palsy.

Intracranial bleeds are among the most common causes of death in hemophiliac patients, and prompt treatment of possible intracranial hemorrhage is one of the main goals of home therapy. Any unusual or persistent headache in a person with severe hemophilia should arouse the strong suspicion of an intracranial bleed.

Hematuria occurs frequently, and whereas abnormalities of the collecting system by intravenous pyelogram may be seen during the acute episode and may sometimes persist, abnormalities of renal function occur infrequently.

Inhibitors to VIII develop in approximately 15% of patients treated with VIII. These inhibitors are antibodies that are identified by their ability to specifically inactivate VIII in coagulation assays. In the United States the Bethesda unit is used for inhibitor quantitation. One Bethesda unit is that amount of inhibitor which will inactivate half the VIII in 1 ml of normal plasma in 2 hours at 37° C. Several clinically distinct types of inhibitors may be observed. In a small number of patients with inhibitors the level of inhibitor is low (less than 10 Bethesda units) and remains low despite challenge with VIII. Other patients have *high-response inhibitors.* These are inhibitors that remain at low levels until stimulated by exposure to VIII. This exposure then leads to an anamnestic increase in antibody level, frequently to very high levels (up to 1000 to 2000 Bethesda units). The antibody level then starts to fall and continues to fall until the next exposure to VIII. In some individuals the inhibitor may become undetectable before the next treatment. A final group of patients has antibody levels that are high (greater than 20 Bethesda units) and remain high even in the absence of VIII administration.

Antibodies should be described according to their anamnestic response to VIII (high or low response) and by their level (high or low titer). Thus an inhibitor that is currently 5 Bethesda units but has previously been shown to increase to 200 Bethesda units after administration of VIII is a *high-response, low-titer inhibitor.* After treatment with VIII, the inhibitor in this patient might rise to 125 Bethesda units and, accordingly, be termed a *high-response, high-titer inhibitor.*

Although it was initially postulated that inhibitors would be found in patients with deletions of the VIII gene, who would therefore "see" VIII as a foreign protein, present data indicate that inhibitors can oc-

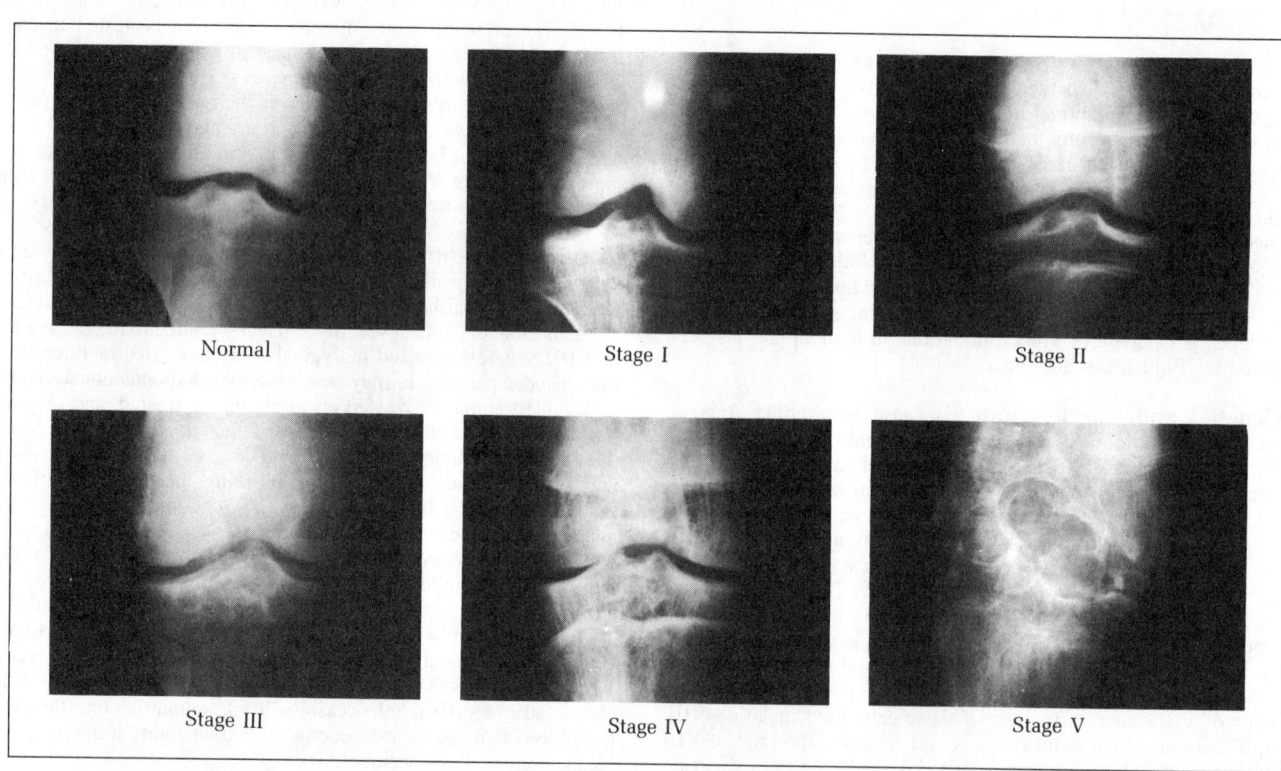

FIGURE 84-2   Radiologic joint changes in hemophilia A. Knee joints illustrating the various stages of hemophilic arthropathy.

   Stage I: No skeletal abnormalities, soft tissue swelling caused by bleeding in and around joint
   Stage II: Osteoporosis and epiphyseal overgrowth; joint space intact; no bone cysts
   Stage III: Subchondral cysts; minor irregularities of the joint surface; joint space is preserved
   Stage IV: Cysts and joint surface irregularities more prominent; joint space is narrowed as a result of cartilage damage
   Stage V: Loss of joint space; marked epiphyseal overgrowth

Radiographs courtesy of Bonner Guilford, MD.

cur in patients who have partial deletions of the VIII gene as well as in patients with point mutations.

Patients with inhibitors are subject to the same type and frequency of hemorrhage as are patients without inhibitors, but they differ in that when the antibody level is greater than 10 Bethesda units, they respond poorly, if at all, to treatment with VIII. Patients should be tested for inhibitors when a surgical procedure is contemplated or response to therapy is diminished.

Treatment. Treatment consists of replacement VIII. In the United States, this is accomplished with fresh-frozen plasma, a blood bank–prepared cryoprecipitate fraction of fresh plasma, or commercial concentrates of VIII. Several different types of commercial concentrates have now been developed (Table 84-4) including synthetic factor VIII produced by recombinant DNA technology. In contrast to plasma and cryoprecipitate, which must be frozen, commercial concentrates are lyophilized and are stable at ambient temperatures. More than 90% of the VIII given in the United States is in the form of commercial concentrate because of its high potency and ease of administration.

Calculation of the dose of VIII is performed as follows:

$$VIII_i = (VIII_f - VIII_s) \times PV$$

where VIII_i is the amount of VIII to be infused in units; VIII_f is the desired peak VIII level in units per milliliter; VIII_s is the initial VIII level in units per milliliter; and PV is the plasma volume in milliliters, which is calculated as 5% of body weight. The half-life of VIII in plasma is approximately 12 hours. To maintain a specific level of VIII usually requires that half the loading dose be administered every 12 hours. Factor VIII may be administered by either intermittent boluses or continuous infusion.

The following are intended as general guidelines for replacement therapy for patients with severe disease. Relatively minor bleeding episodes such as hemarthroses are treated with sufficient concentrate to bring the VIII level to 0.30 U/ml (30% of normal). If bleeding continues, the dose is repeated in 12 to 24 hours. Minor muscle bleeds may be treated the same way, but muscle bleeds with incipient neurovascular compromise and retroperitoneal bleeds should be treated with higher doses to bring the VIII level to 0.5 to 1.0 U/ml (50% to 100% of normal) for up to 5 to 7 days. Intracranial hemorrhage and hemorrhage in the neck or throat with potential airway compromise are major medical emergencies and are treated with sufficient concentrate to raise the VIII level to 1.0 U/ml (100% of normal) for 10 to 14 days.

Patients with severe hemophilia can best treat minor bleeding episodes at home. The advantage of home therapy is that treatment can be instituted as soon as the patient suspects bleeding. It is not yet certain if the development of joint deformities can be avoided by this approach. However, it reduces time away from work or school and has clear advantages in potentially life-threatening bleeds such as in-

tracranial and neck bleeds. Because of the great cost of the commercial concentrates, the cost of treatment for a patient with severe hemophilia can easily exceed $50,000 per year.

Patients with mild forms of hemophilia A may occasionally need treatment for surgery or traumatic injuries. Although concentrates or cryoprecipitate may be used, there is still a small risk of hepatitis and/or acquired immunodeficiency syndrome (AIDS). Intravenous infusion of a vasopressin analog, 1-deamino-8-D-arginine vasopressin (DDAVP), increases VIII levels twofold or threefold and provides an alternative to plasma products and their risks. DDAVP is the treatment of choice in patients with mild hemophilia who require treatment.

The type of treatment of bleeding episodes in patients with inhibitors is determined by the titer of the antibody at the time treatment is required, the antibody response to administration of VIII, and the severity of the bleed. Patients with low-response inhibitors can be treated with VIII for all bleeding episodes, although doses of up to 4000 U or more may be required to achieve VIII levels of 30%. In patients with high-response, high-titer inhibitors, it becomes impossible to infuse sufficient VIII to achieve hemostasis. For these individuals, several alternative treatment modalities are available, including porcine VIII, activated or nonactivated prothrombin complex concentrates, plasmapheresis, and immunosuppressive agents, although none works as well as VIII in patients without inhibitors. Patients with high-response, low-titer inhibitors can be treated with human VIII, but this treatment is likely to result in an anamnestic increase in inhibitor titer. For this reason, use of VIII in these patients is often reserved for life-threatening bleeding episodes. For other hemorrhages, such as joint bleeds or hematuria, treatment with prothrombin complex concentrates is sometimes effective but is less likely to produce an anamnestic increase in inhibitor titer. Patients with inhibitors should generally be referred to specialized centers for care.

Complications of Treatment. Before introduction of viral inactivation methods, transfusion-associated *hepatitis* occurred in a large percentage of hemophiliac patients receiving replacement therapy. Almost 80% of hemophiliac patients treated prior to 1990 demonstrate at least intermittent abnormalities of liver function tests, although only about 10% offer a history of symptoms. The chronic consequences of transfusion-associated hepatitis—cirrhosis, hepatosplenomegaly, portal hypertension, esophageal varices, hypersplenism, and hepatocellular carcinoma—occur in a small number of those at risk. Both hepatitis B and C viruses have been implicated in the liver disease in hemophilia.

Treatment of hepatitis in hemophiliac patients should conform to the guidelines outlined in Chapter 355. Patients should continue to take VIII as needed. In chronic hepatitis, thrombocytopenia from hypersplenism may be especially troublesome because of the underlying bleeding defect. Hepatitis B virus vaccine should be given to patients who have never been treated before or who demonstrate nega-

Table 84-4   Comparison of various sources of factors VIII and IX

	VOLUME TO 100%*	EASE OF USE	RISK OF HEPATITIS B OR C	RISK OF AIDS	RISK OF HEMOLYSIS	RISK OF THROMBOSIS
Factor VIII						
Plasma	3000	—	+	+	±	—
Cryoprecipitate	750	+	+	+	±	—
VIII Concentrate						
Intermediate purity	50	4+	—	—	4+	—
Monoclonal	20	4+	—	—	—	—
Recombinant	20	4+	—	—	—	—
Factor IX						
Plasma	6000	—	+	+	±	—
PCC	50	4+	—	—	—	4+
IX Concentrate	50	4+	—	—	—	—

*Calculated for a 60-kg individual.
± to 4+, Degree of increasing risk or ease of use; —, no risk.
This table is a general assessment of the relative risks of treatment sources available for treating hemophilia A and B. Plasma and cryoprecipitate are usually obtained from the American Red Cross or blood banks, whereas VIII and IX concentrates are usually obtained commercially. Intermediate-purity factor VIII concentrates, prothrombin complex concentrates (PCCs), and monoclonal factor VIII and factor IX concentrates are prepared from donors screened for human immunodeficiency virus-1 (HIV-1) and either heat treated or extracted with solvent-detergent mixtures to inactivate viruses, including HIV-1 and hepatitis B and C viruses. Monoclonal factor VIII and IX concentrates are ultrapure products prepared using affinity chromatography. Recombinant factor VIII is a synthetic product prepared in hamster cells.

tive hepatitis B serology. Current VIII concentrates, including solvent-detergent-extracted VIII, monoclonal VIII, and synthetic preparations, appear to be free of hepatitis B and C.

Before the development of heat treatment and donor screening, factor VIII concentrate use was associated with infection with human immunodeficiency virus (HIV). Thus many patients with hemophilia are HIV antibody positive, and many have developed AIDS. Current VIII concentrates are free of HIV.

With intermediate-purity VIII concentrates, antibodies to red cell blood group substances are isolated with VIII and can cause red blood cell *hemolysis* in intensively treated patients. Blood typing should be performed before intensive treatment, and concentrates containing low isoagglutinin titers should be used in susceptible individuals.

Hemophilia B

Hemophilia B (Christmas disease), as is true with hemophilia A, is an X-linked recessive disease. However, hemophilia B is caused by an abnormality in factor IX, one of the vitamin K–dependent factors. Factor IX protein (as detected by immunologic tests) may be absent (CRM$^-$), present in reduced amounts (CRM^r), or present in normal amounts but with greatly decreased clot-promoting activity (CRM$^+$). The molecular defect responsible for hemophilia B has been determined in more than 500 patients.

Diagnosis. As in hemophilia A, the PTT is prolonged, and the PT and TT are normal. The diagnosis of hemophilia B is made by specific factor IX assay. As in hemophilia A, the factor IX levels are predictive of the severity of the bleeding tendency. The normal level of factor IX is 1.0 U/ml. Levels less than 0.01 U/ml indicate severe disease, levels of 0.01 to 0.05 indicate moderate disease, and levels greater than 0.05 indicate mild disease.

Carrier State. Hemophilia B is an X-linked disorder, and all affected males are X^{h}Y and carriers are X^{h}X. All daughters of affected males are carriers, and daughters of carriers have a 50:50 chance of being carriers. Because of random inactivation of the X chromosome, carriers have a spectrum of factor IX activity levels that ranges from levels as low as those in patients with mild hemophilia (0.10 U/ml) to normal levels. Diagnosis of the carrier state can sometimes be made on the basis of factor IX activity levels alone. Detection of carriers may be improved by measuring factor IX antigen levels in families that have a CRM$^+$ defect, but measuring the antigen adds no useful information to measuring the activity alone in CRM$^-$ kindred. Carriers of hemophilia B are more likely to be symptomatic from low IX levels than are carriers of hemophilia A from low VIII levels.

Carrier detection by gene detection or gene tracking is also applicable to hemophilia B and with appropriate probes should permit carrier assignment in CRM$^-$, CRM^r, and CRM$^+$ variants.

Clinical Features. The types and complications of hemorrhages in hemophilia B are similar to those in hemophilia A.

Inhibitors to factor IX occur infrequently, in approximately 3% of severely affected individuals. Preliminary studies suggest that those most likely to develop inhibitors are CRM$^-$ individuals who demonstrate partial or complete deletion of the factor IX gene.

Treatment. Factor IX concentrates, prothrombin complex concentrates (PCCs) which are rich in factor IX, and fresh-frozen plasma are available for treatment of hemophilia B (Table 84-4). Although more expensive, IX concentrates appear to be safer than PCCs, with less risk of thrombosis. Because factor IX distribution is approximately twice the plasma volume, it takes twice as much factor IX as VIII to achieve a given level. The half-life of factor IX is approximately 18 hours.

Commercial PCCs are associated with a high risk of thrombosis and diffuse (disseminated) intravascular coagulation (DIC) because of activated clotting factors in the concentrates. Factor IX concentrates appear to have little risk of thrombosis. As a result, factor IX concentrates are the current treatment of choice in hemophilia B. Hemolytic reactions do not occur with PCCs.

von Willebrand's Disease

This is probably the most frequently diagnosed inherited bleeding disorder in adults. The exact prevalence of vWD is unknown because precise criteria for its diagnosis and classification are only now being evolved.

Inheritance. In contrast to hemophilia A and B, vWD is inherited in an autosomal manner (Table 84-3). The vWF gene is located on chromosome 12. The more common varieties (types 1 and 2) are autosomal dominant. However, the most severe form of this disorder is recessive and is expressed only in homozygous or doubly heterozygous subjects.

von Willebrand Factor. vWF is currently thought to circulate in plasma as a complex with VIII. Its role in hemostasis is to act as a carrier for VIII and to promote adhesion of platelets to the subendothelium and to one another. Thus vWF plays an important role in primary hemostasis. Abnormalities of vWF are expressed as an abnormality of platelet function, as reflected in a prolonged bleeding time. vWF is present in endothelial cells, megakaryocytes, platelets, and plasma. The subunit protein has a molecular weight of 220,000, but it is found in cells and in plasma as multimers ranging in molecular weight from approximately 800,000 to between 10 and 14 million or more, in increments of 800,000 to 1 million (Chapter 75). Factor VIII appears to be able to complex with any size of multimer. However, the large-molecular-weight multimers are the most effective in supporting the interaction between platelets and the vessel wall and are necessary for a normal bleeding time.

Diagnosis. The diagnosis of vWD should be suspected in patients who demonstrate an abnormality of one or more of the following: bleeding time, VIII, vWF, and vWF:Ag (Table 84-3). Because these tests may be somewhat variable in vWD and because an isolated bleeding time prolongation and isolated reduction in VIII may be confused with a platelet defect and hemophilia, respectively, testing of patients should be performed on more than one occasion in cases that are unclear. Different forms of vWD can be distinguished using vWF multimer analysis and other special tests (Fig. 84-3).

Type 1. Type 1 vWD results from decreased production of a structurally normal vWF molecule. The most common form of vWD, it is inherited in an autosomal dominant pattern. Plasma levels of vWF, vWF:Ag, and VIII are variably reduced, usually concordantly. All sizes of vWF multimers are present but are reduced in concentration.

Type 2. Type 2 vWD results from functionally abnormal vWF molecules. The defect may be in the interaction with the platelet glycoprotein Ib receptor, in the assembly of vWF into high-molecular-weight multimers, or in the stabilization of factor VIII. The following are the major forms of type 2 vWD.

Type 2A. This variant form of vWD is inherited as an autosomal dominant trait and is characterized by an absence of the large and medium-sized multimers from plasma and platelets. vWF activity is greatly reduced and is lower than vWF:Ag and VIII, which may be decreased or normal. Ristocetin-induced platelet aggregation is reduced.

Type 2B. In this variant, only the high-molecular-weight multimers are absent from plasma. All multimers are present in platelets, and the plasma levels of vWF, vWF:Ag, and VIII may be normal or decreased. The distinguishing characteristic of type 2B vWD is the finding that ristocetin-induced aggregation is increased rather than decreased. This observation and the finding that type 2B vWF demonstrates increased ristocetin-induced binding to normal platelets has suggested that the defect in type 2B disease is a qualitative abnormality of vWF causing increased affinity of the large-molecular-weight multimers for cellular binding sites on platelets. Therefore deficiency of the large multimers results from increased utilization, not reduced production. Inheritance of type 2B disease is autosomal dominant.

Type 2M. Variant vWD characterized by reduced platelet-dependent function and normal vWF multimers. In the small number of cases reported, VIII and vWF:Ag levels are normal but vWF activity is reduced. Ristocetin-induced platelet aggregation is reduced but aggregation with botrocetin, a snake venom derived coagglutinin, is normal. The bleeding time is prolonged.

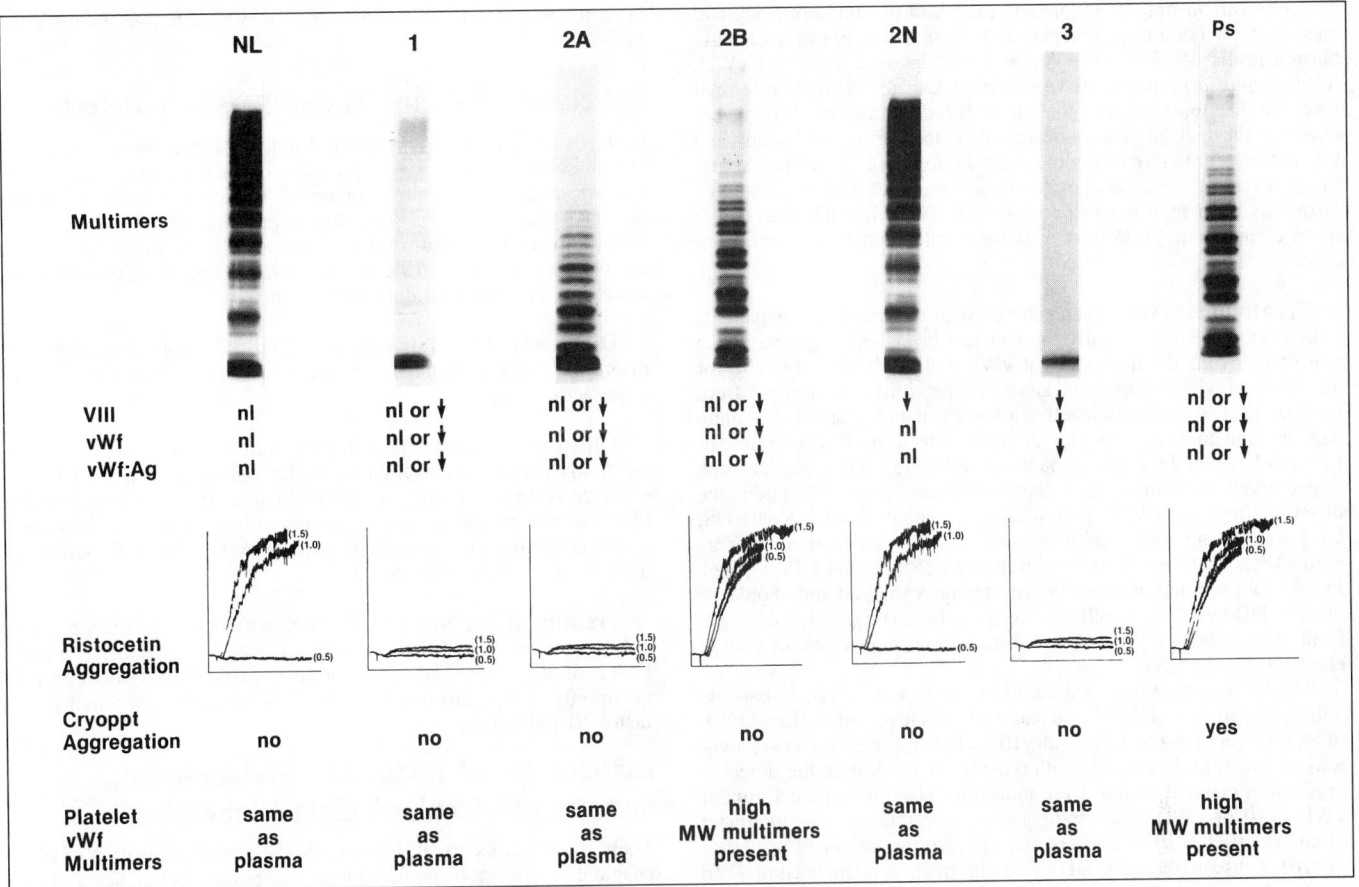

FIGURE 84-3   Classification of von Willebrand's disease (vWD). Multimeric von Willebrand's factor (vWf) patterns; levels of VIII, vWf, and vWf:Ag; patterns of ristocetin aggregation; response of patient platelets to normal cryoprecipitate in vitro; and the multimeric pattern of vWf in patient platelets are shown for normal, type 1 vWD, variant vWD (types 2A, 2B), type 3 or homozygous vWD, and pseudo-vWD or platelet-type vWD, individuals.

In type 1 individuals the characteristic laboratory findings are variably reduced vWf, vWf:Ag, and VIII. The multimeric pattern and ristocetin aggregation abnormalities are proportional to the reduction in vWf, vWf:Ag, and VIII.

In type 2A individuals the characteristic finding is the absence of high- and middle-molecular-weight multimers. Factor VIII, vWf, vWf:Ag, and ristocetin aggregation abnormalities may be indistinguishable from those in type 1 individuals.

In type 2B individuals the characteristic finding is absence of the high-molecular-weight multimers and increased ristocetin aggregation.

Type 3 individuals show a profound reduction in VIII, vWf, and vWf:Ag, and this profound reduction is reflected in the pattern of vWf multimers and ristocetin aggregation.

In pseudo-vWD the distinguishing feature is aggregation of patient platelets by normal cryoprecipitate. Otherwise, this variant is similar to type 2B vWD.

The vWf multimer patterns courtesy of Z.M. Ruggeri, MD, and T.S. Zimmerman, MD.

Type 2N. Type 2N vWD masquerades as an autosomal form of mild to moderate hemophilia A. VIII levels are reduced, typically in the range of 5% to 15%, with normal levels of vWF and vWF:Ag. The molecular defect in type 2N vWD is in the region of vWF involved in binding factor VIII and results in impaired formation of the vWF/VIII complex. As a result, the half-life of VIII in the circulation is markedly shortened.

Type 3. This is severe homozygous or doubly heterozygous, autosomal recessive vWD. Plasma levels of vWF and vWF:Ag are undetectable, and VIII levels are less than 10%. The bleeding time is invariably prolonged. Ristocetin-induced platelet aggregation is absent. Bleeding in this form may be severe and may involve joints and soft tissues.

Pseudo–von Willebrand's disease. This condition is similar in many respects to type 2B vWD. There is a deficiency of the high-molecular-weight multimers in plasma but not in platelets. Plasma levels of vWF, vWF:Ag, and VIII are decreased or normal. Ristocetin-induced aggregation is increased. However, vWF from these patients does not demonstrate increased binding to normal platelets. Instead, platelets from these patients show increased ristocetin-induced binding of normal vWF. The presumed defect is a platelet abnormality, and the absence of large vWF multimers results from increased utilization, as in type 2B vWD. Two additional features which help to distinguish this condition from type 2B vWD are that (1) many pseudo-vWD patients have chronic or intermittent thrombocytopenia and (2) cryoprecipitate causes aggregation of pseudo-vWD platelets in vitro but not of platelets from type 2B.

Clinical Features. The bleeding in vWD is usually much less severe than that in hemophilia. Massive bleeding into joints and tissues occurs only in patients with type 3 forms of the disease, but bleeding from mucous membranes (nasal, intestinal, uterine mucosa) and easy bruising are common and are characteristic of patients with other forms of the disease. Bleeding typically follows minor injury or surgery. Major surgical procedures or trauma may result in serious bleeding. The tendency to bleed appears to decrease later in life.

Menorrhagia may be severe and may lead to iron deficiency and anemia. Oral contraceptives may reduce menorrhagia and increase plasma levels of vWF, vWF:Ag, and VIII in some forms of vWD. *Angiodysplasia* of intestinal vessels may lead to recurrent intestinal bleeding. Demonstration of the site of bleeding is often difficult because of the lack of radiologically detectable structural lesions and the intermittent nature of the bleeding. Endoscopic procedures sometimes reveal telangiectasia of the bowel mucosa. *Mitral valve prolapse* has been reported in patients with vWD, but whether this is more common in vWD than in the general population is questionable.

Treatment. Several agents are used in the treatment of patients with vWD. The traditional treatment has been with cryoprecipitate that contains all the multimers of vWF and is effective therapy for all forms of vWD. However, since cryoprecipitate is derived from plasma but has no virus inactivation step, it has a small but finite risk of transmitting hepatitis or HIV infection. Concentrates of factor VIII contain large amounts of vWF:Ag, but most lack the larger vWF multimers and therefore have little effect on the bleeding time in vWD. Two products, Humate-P and Koate-HS, have some large vWF multimers and can be used to treat patients with vWD. Both are treated to inactivate hepatitis and HIV viruses. In addition, concentrates of vWF are being developed and should be useful. DDAVP, the synthetic vasopressin analog, releases vWF from storage sites in endothelial cells and thus provides an endogenous source of vWF.

The form of treatment is dictated by the type of vWD. In patients with type 1 disease, DDAVP increases plasma levels of VIII and vWF of all multimeric sizes. Levels of VIII and vWF can be increased twofold to threefold. In patients with type 2A or 2B disease the defect is production of an abnormal vWF molecule. Thus, in variant forms of vWD, VIII or vWF concentrates (when available) are the treatment of choice. VIII or vWF concentrates are also the treatment of choice in type 3 disease because DDAVP is ineffective in increasing vWF release. In pseudo-vWD the platelet is defective, and treatment should be with platelets. Administration of VIII concentrate, vWF concentrates, or DDAVP to these patients may trigger sudden aggregation of platelets and cause severe thrombocytopenia.

Treatment of vWD, when required, is aimed at correction of both the bleeding time and the VIII level. If major surgery is undertaken, VIII level and bleeding time should be monitored. Treatment should be aimed at keeping both within normal limits in the perioperative period.

Complications of Treatment. DDAVP may cause water retention and lead to symptomatic hyponatremia. Plasma sodium levels should be monitored. Inhibitors (antibodies) to vWF develop only in the most severely affected individuals.

Congenital Deficiencies of Factors II, V, VII, and X

Deficiencies of these clotting factors are inherited as autosomal recessive traits and are quite rare. Deficiencies may reflect either absence of the clotting factor or its presence in a dysfunctional form.

Diagnosis. A deficiency of any one of these clotting factors results in a prolonged PT. With factors II, X, and V, the PTT is also prolonged. However, in factor VII deficiency the PTT is normal. Diagnosis is made by specific factor assays.

Clinical Features. The severity of symptoms varies considerably among individuals, and severity does not uniformly correlate with factor levels.

Treatment. Milder episodes are best treated with fresh-frozen plasma, even though plasma levels can only be brought to 20% because of the limitation of the volume of plasma that can be infused. The PCCs used to treat factor IX deficiency also contain variable quantities of factors VII, X, and II, and higher plasma levels can be obtained with them. However, the risk of hepatitis and thrombosis is significant. These concentrates do not contain significant quantities

of factor V. Platelet transfusions have been used to treat factor V deficiency.

Deficiency of Factor XI and Passovoy Defect

Factor XI deficiency is the result of a decreased quantity of this protein in some individuals; the presence of an inactive clotting factor appears to be responsible in others. It is inherited in an autosomal recessive manner. The abnormality in patients with Passovoy defect is not known at this time, but it is presumed to be a deficiency of an as-yet unidentified plasma protein. Passovoy defect appears to be inherited in an autosomal dominant manner.

Diagnosis. The PT is normal and the PTT is prolonged in both disorders. Precise diagnosis of factor XI deficiency requires a specific factor assay.

Clinical Features. The clinical picture in both disorders is similar. Many patients are asymptomatic throughout their lives, and others have relatively mild bleeding problems. However, postoperative bleeding may be severe even in patients without previous hemorrhagic symptoms. Inhibitors to factor XI in patients with factor XI deficiency have been described but are rare.

Treatment. Treatment for factor XI deficiency is usually required only for surgery. Fresh-frozen plasma is the only modality available. Levels of 30% appear adequate for hemostasis. Repeat doses need be given only every third day because of the unusually long half-life of factor XI (64 hours).

Deficiencies of Factor XII, Prekallikrein, and High-Molecular-Weight Kininogen

These three factors are all involved in the contact activation of blood coagulation, fibrinolysis, and kinin generation. Deficiencies are inherited in an autosomal recessive fashion.

Diagnosis. The PTT is prolonged in the absence of any of these factors. Specific factor assays are required for precise diagnosis.

Clinical Features. No clinical abnormalities have been associated with deficiency of any of these proteins. However, correct diagnosis is necessary to exclude other causes of a prolonged PTT.

Factor XIII Deficiency

The function of factor XIII is to cross-link fibrin monomers to one another by transamidation, thus stabilizing the fibrin clot. Factor XIII also cross-links fibronectin (cold-insoluble globulin, LETS protein) to fibrin and to collagen. The latter process is important for migration of macrophages into sites of injury, and absence of this function may be responsible for the poor wound healing sometimes seen in factor XIII deficiency.

Inheritance of factor XIII deficiency is clearly autosomal recessive in some families. In others the only affected individuals have been males, suggesting a sex-linked pattern.

Diagnosis. The PTT, PT, and TT are normal in factor XIII deficiency. The diagnosis is suggested by demonstrating solubility of the fibrin clot in either 5 M urea or 1% monochloroacetic acid.

Clinical Features. Clinical features differ from those of hemophilia A and B in that hemarthroses are rare. Bleeding after separation of the umbilical cord is characteristic of this disorder. Intracranial hemorrhage, often fatal, has been reported in several patients. Spontaneous abortions have been a serious problem in adult women. Bleeding is common after trauma but is often delayed. Wound healing may be poor, with resultant gaping scars.

Treatment. Treatment is relatively simple because the half-life of factor XIII is relatively long (4.7 days), and levels of only 2% of normal provide satisfactory hemostasis. Monthly plasma transfusions are therefore sufficient to prevent spontaneous bleeding.

Fibrinogen Abnormalities

Congenital disorders of circulating fibrinogen include both quantitative (afibrinogenemia or hypofibriniogenemia) and qualitative (dysfibriniogenemia) defects. Qualitative disorders may also be acquired and are discussed elsewhere in this chapter.

Diagnosis. Patients with severe fibrinogen abnormalities may have prolonged PTT, PT, and TT, since all three depend on formation of a fibrin clot as an end point, but these screening tests are only sensitive to fibrinogen levels less than approximately 100 mg/dl (normal fibrinogen levels in most laboratories are 150 to 250 mg/dl). The diagnosis of a quantitative abnormality is confirmed by direct measurement of fibrinogen by clotting, chemical, or immunologic techniques. In patients with congenital dysfibrinogenemias, the clotting screening tests may be normal or abnormal, or the abnormality may be limited to the TT, which is the most sensitive screening test of fibrinogen defects. The diagnosis depends on either the demonstration of reduced functional levels of fibrinogen with normal levels by physiochemical or immunologic techniques, or, in patients with normal clotting times on screening tests, the demonstration of a functional or electrophorectic defect.

Genetics. Congenital afibrinogenemia is an autosomal recessive disorder. Affected individuals are homozygous or doubly heterozygous; heterozygous individuals are clinically asymptomatic, although some may have mild or moderately reduced plasma fibrinogen levels. Congenital dysfibrinogenemias, on the other hand, are inherited in an autosomal dominant manner in most patients, although in a few cases a recessive pattern of inheritance has been suggested.

Clinical Features. Clinical symptoms in patients with abnormal fibrinogens are highly variable. Patients with congenital afibrinogenemia have a moderately severe bleeding diathesis. Spontaneous hemorrhage in soft tissues and from mucous membranes occurs, and bleeding caused by trauma or surgery may be severe. Clinical symptoms in dysfibrinogenemias range from those described in patients with afibrinogenemia to none at all. Defects in wound healing with wound dehiscence and subsequent keloid formation are prominent in some dysfibrinogenemias. A small number of patients with dysfibrinogenemia have been reported to have a thrombotic tendency. Fibrinogen inhibitors are rare. Platelet function tests may be abnormal in afibrinogenemia. In approximately 25% of reported cases, mild thrombocytopenia has been described.

Treatment. Bleeding problems in the afibrinogenemic patient are treated with transfusions of cryoprecipitate. In most patients the fibrinogen circulates with a normal half-life. Normal hemostasis in congenital afibrinogenemia is achieved with fibrinogen levels of 100 mg/dl or higher.

Hemorrhagic Disorders Associated With Inherited Deficiencies of Protease Inhibitors

Recently, deficiencies of alpha$_2$ plasmin inhibitor and plasminogen activator inhibitor (PAI) have been reported in association with a severe bleeding disorder. Presumably, bleeding is the result of dissolution of fibrin clots by plasmin. The diagnosis is suggested by rapid lysis of whole blood clotted in a glass tube. Specific diagnosis may be made by immunologic measurement of alpha$_2$ plasmin inhibitor or PAI concentration. At present, infusions of fresh-frozen plasma are the only therapy.

ACQUIRED DISORDERS
Vitamin K Deficiency

Vitamin K is a fat-soluble vitamin that catalyzes the postribosomal modification of glutamic acid residues in certain proteins to γ-carboxyl glutamic acid (Gla). Proteins known to contain Gla residues include clotting factors II, VII, IX, and X (called vitamin K–dependent clotting factors); protein C and protein S (involved in the control of coagulation); protein Z; protein M; and the skeletal proteins, bone Gla aprotein (osteocalcin) and bone matrix Gla protein. Vitamin K–dependent clotting factors that contain Gla residues bind ionic calcium and, as a result, are able to efficiently assemble procoagulant complexes on the surface of platelets (Chapter 69). How the vitamin K–dependent proteins are targeted for postribosomal modification by vitamin K is not completely understood; protein sequences in both the pre-pro portion of the protein and in the Gla-rich domain of the mature protein may be involved. For example, hemophilia B$_{Cambridge}$ is a CRM$^+$ factor IX variant characterized by mutation of Arg to Ser at position −1 in the propeptide and by defective γ-carboxylation of glutamic acid. Similarly, hemophilia B$_{San Dimas}$ and hemophilia B$_{Oxford}$ are CRM$^+$ variants characterized by mutation of Arg to Gln at position −4 in the propeptide and by defective γ-carboxylation of glutamic acid.

Several forms of vitamin K exist. Vitamin K$_1$, or phytonadione (2-methyl-3-phytyl-1,4-naphthoquinone), is a naturally occurring compound that has a 20-carbon side chain attached to the naphthoquinone nucleus. It is found primarily in green leafy plants and vegetables. Vitamin K$_2$, or menaquinone, has a 20-60-carbon side chain and is produced by bacteria as a metabolic product. Vitamin K$_3$, or menadione, has no side chains. Vitamin K is absorbed in the small intestine and transported to the liver, where the vitamin is obligatorily oxidized by a microsomal enzyme, vitamin K epoxidase, to vitamin K-2,3-epoxide (Fig. 84-4). The vitamin is stored in the liver as the epoxide. To become catalytically competent, vitamin K must be reduced by other microsomal enzymes, vitamin K-2,3-epoxide reductase and quinone reductase, to vitamin K$_1$, which is the active form of the enzyme. Vitamin K$_1$ catalyzes the γ-carboxylation of glutamic acid by a hepatic carboxylase.

Etiology. The causes of vitamin K deficiency are listed in Box 84-1. Most cases are acquired and result from either reduced absorption of the vitamin or a block in the metabolism of vitamin K.

Hemorrhagic disease of newborn. In the newborn, levels of vitamin K–dependent clotting factors are lower than in adults, perhaps in part because of poor transplacental transfer of maternal vitamin K, the absence of vitamin K–synthesizing intestinal flora, and immature hepatic protein synthesis. In a small number of infants, especially premature infants and those who are breast-fed, severe reduction of one or more of the vitamin K–dependent clotting factors to levels of less than 10% may occur with the development of severe hemorrhagic symptoms. Onset of bleeding occurs typically within 2 or 3 days of birth and may be severe, with a significant risk of intra-

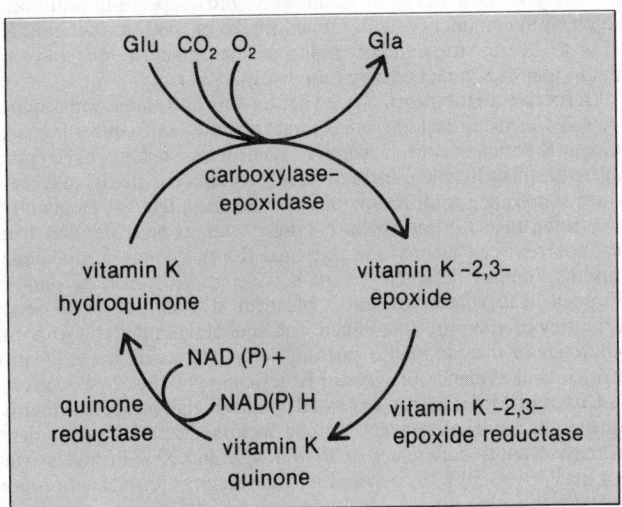

FIGURE 84-4 The vitamin K cycle. γ-carboxylation of glutamic acid (*Glu*) residues to γ-carboxylation acid (*Gla*) residues is catalyzed by a hepatic microsomal carboxylase in a reaction that is coupled to the conversion of vitamin K hydroquinone to vitamin K-2,3-epoxide by vitamin K epoxidase. Vitamin K-2,3-epoxide is reduced by a series of reactions involving vitamin K-2,3-epoxidase, vitamin K quinone reductase, and NAD(P). Both vitamin K-2,3-epoxide reductase and vitamin K quinone reductase appear to be inhibited by coumarin drugs.

BOX 84-1
Causes of deficiency of vitamin K-dependent clotting factors

Abnormal or inadequate absorption
Hemorrhagic disease of newborn
Dietary deficiency
Parenteral nutrition
Malabsorption
Biliary tract obstruction
Liver disease
Drugs (broad-spectrum antibiotics)

Abnormal metabolism
Congenital
Drugs (coumarins, hydantoin)

---

cranial hemorrhage. Before institution of routine prophylactic administration of vitamin K to newborns, hemorrhagic disease occurred in up to 1% of births, with a mortality of up to 30%. Today, however, hemorrhagic disease of the newborn occurs rarely and almost exclusively in infants who have not received vitamin K prophylaxis.

Drug induced. The therapeutic administration of coumarin drugs in patients with venous or arterial thrombosis is the most common cause of vitamin K deficiency. Coumarin and its various congeners act as anticoagulants by interfering with the regeneration of vitamin K_1 from vitamin K-2,3-epoxide. As a result, II, VII, IX, and X cannot be γ-carboxylated, and inactive, decarboxy forms of the vitamin K–dependent clotting factors circulate in plasma. Surreptitious use of coumarin drugs, especially in health care workers and poisoning by administration of rat poison are other causes of coumarin-associated coagulopathy and should be considered in the differential diagnosis of vitamin K deficiency. Newer superwarfarins are especially potent and may have prolonged effects on metabolism of vitamin K. Hydantoin anticonvulsants and salicylates are also vitamin K antagonists.

Broad-spectrum antibiotics suppress vitamin K–synthesizing intestinal flora and may cause vitamin K deficiency. However, in most patients taking antibiotics, dietary sources of vitamin K are sufficient to maintain body levels and prevent vitamin K deficiency. Vitamin K deficiency is most likely to result when broad-spectrum antibiotics are given in conjunction with limited intake of food or a vitamin K–deficient diet. In vitro evidence indicates that cephalosporins may also affect vitamin K metabolism in the liver.

Defective absorption. Since vitamin K is fat soluble and requires bile salts for its absorption, biliary tract obstruction frequently causes vitamin K deficiency. Malabsorptive syndromes, such as celiac sprue, pancreatic insufficiency, ulcerative colitis, regional ileitis, and short bowel syndrome, produce vitamin K deficiency, but less frequently.

Inadequate dietary intake. Since vitamin K is derived from dual sources (i.e., dietary and intestinal flora), vitamin K deficiency caused by dietary deficiency alone is unusual. Vitamin K is found in all green leafy vegetables and is plentiful in a normal diet. Dietary deficiency of vitamin K combined with concomitant therapy with oral antibiotics or disease of the gastrointestinal tract will generally produce clinical evidence of vitamin K deficiency within 1 to 3 weeks.

Congenital defects. Congenital γ-carboxylation defects involving the vitamin K–dependent clotting factors are rare. Patients demonstrate variable deficiency of II, VII, IX, and X with levels from less than 1% to 50%. In general, all four factors are reduced proportionately. Levels respond poorly or not at all to large doses of vitamin K_1. The defect is presumed to be in the vitamin K cycle, either in the epoxidase/carboxylase or the reductase step. Inheritance appears to be autosomal recessive.

Diagnosis. The hallmark of vitamin K deficiency is a prolonged PT and PTT with a normal TT. Since factor VII has a half-life of approximately 4 hours and the other vitamin K–dependent clotting factors have longer half-lives, patients with early or mild vitamin K deficiency may demonstrate only minimum prolongation of PT (14 to 17 seconds with control of 12 seconds). With more advanced deficiency, both the PT and PTT are prolonged. In severe cases, prolongation of the PT and PTT may be marked. Measurement of clotting factor levels will reveal variably reduced levels of II, VII, IX, and X, depending on the degree of vitamin K deficiency.

The differential diagnosis of prolonged PT and PTT includes liver disease, the lupus inhibitor, and deficiency of clotting factors of the final common pathway such as V and X. Liver disease can be identified by tests of liver function (Chapter 53), but liver disease and vitamin K deficiency may coexist, especially in alcoholics and in patients with metastatic disease to the liver. In such patients the only way to demonstrate vitamin K deficiency may be to administer a trial of vitamin K.

Clinical Features. With mild vitamin K deficiency, bleeding is minimal, and oozing after venipuncture or easy bruising may be the only manifestation. With more severe deficiency, spontaneous hemorrhage may be evident. Hematomas, hematuria, gingival bleeding, and gastrointestinal tract bleeding may occur.

Treatment. Deficiency of vitamin K is treated with vitamin K_1, either orally or parenterally. For patients with mild prolongation of the PT and no hemorrhagic tendency, 5 mg oral vitamin K_1 daily for 3 days is usually sufficient to restore vitamin K levels to normal. The dose can be repeated at weekly intervals if it is anticipated that deficiency will persist. For mild hemorrhage, administration of larger doses of vitamin K_1 (15 to 20 mg) usually results in cessation of hemorrhage within 24 to 36 hours. For intracranial and other serious hemorrhages, 25 mg of parenteral vitamin K_1 should be administered immediately by the subcutaneous or intramuscular route. Vitamin K may be administered intravenously but should not be given in doses greater than 1 mg and only when other routes are not feasible. In addition, since vitamin K_1 may take 6 to 24 hours to have an effect, 2 units of fresh-frozen plasma should be given to provide an immediate source of II, VII, IX, and X. Fresh-frozen plasma should be given every 4 to 6 hours until the PT and PTT demonstrate response to vitamin K. Prothrombin complex concentrates, which contain II, VII, IX, and X, should be avoided because of a high frequency of hepatitis and because they have been reported to cause thrombosis and diffuse intravascular coagulation. In patients with coumarin drug overdose, the same general rules just described apply, except that it may be advantageous to avoid administration of vitamin K_1 if coumarin anticoagulation is to be continued.

Hemorrhagic disease of the newborn is prevented by parenteral administration of 1 mg of vitamin K_1 to the child on the day of birth. Patients in whom prolongation of PT is caused by liver disease will not respond to administration of vitamin K_1.

Complications of Treatment. In rare instances, intravenous vitamin K may cause anaphylaxis, and it should always be given with epinephrine at the bedside.

Liver Disease

Liver disease may cause hemostatic abnormalities through several mechanisms. First, the liver is the site of production of fibrinogen, II, VII, VIII, IX, X, XI, XII, and XIII, as well as antithrombin III, protein C, and protein S. Liver disease may result in variably impaired synthesis of any or all of these factors. Although in general, defective synthesis correlates with the severity of the liver disease, the vitamin K–dependent factors, II, VII, IX, and X, are most sensitive to hepatocellular disease and may be the only abnormalities in mild forms of liver disease. In contrast, V and VIII are most resistant to hepatocellular disease and are only decreased in fulminant hepatitis and severe liver failure. Synthesis of both procoagulant and anticoagulant proteins may be affected, resulting in hemorrhagic or thrombotic tendencies. Second, deficiency of plasminogen or alpha$_2$ plasmin inhibitor may cause alterations in plasma fibrinolytic activity and increased levels of fibrin(ogen) degradation products (FDP). Third, vitamin K deficiency may occur in liver disease, especially in binge alcoholics with limited nutritional intake. In addition, in severe hepatic parenchymal disease with severe jaundice, intrahepatic biliary obstruction may be present and cause vitamin K deficiency. Fourth, synthesis of functionally abnormal molecules of fibrinogen characterized by increased sialic acid content occurs in some forms of liver disease, especially hepatocellular carcinoma, chronic active hepatitis, and some types of cirrhosis. Functionally, these abnormal molecules, called dysfibrinogens, demonstrate delayed fibrin monomer polymerization, resulting in marked prolongation of TT. Fifth, small amounts of activated clotting factors generated during normal homeostasis are cleared through the activity of the hepatic reticuloendothelial system. In liver disease, clearance of these activated factors may be impaired, and circulation of these factors may predispose to diffuse (disseminated) intravascular coagulation (DIC) or thrombosis. Sixth, in patients with cirrhosis and increased portal pressure, splenomegaly occurs and may cause sequestrational thrombocytopenia. In addition, alcohol itself may have a suppressive effect on thrombopoiesis and cause thrombocytopenia, as may nutritional defects, especially folate deficiency. Qualitative platelet defects may occur in liver disease with bleeding times that are mildly or moderately prolonged in the absence of or out of proportion to the degree of thrombocytopenia.

Diagnosis. The diagnosis of hemostatic abnormalities in liver disease is based on routine screening tests of coagulation: the PT, PTT, TT, and tests of platelet function. In *acute liver failure,* which may occur in toxic or fulminant viral hepatitis, the PT, PTT, and TT are all extremely prolonged. The PTT mix is normal, but the TT mix may be prolonged by FDP. Assays for specific coagulation factors show severely reduced levels of those factors synthesized in the liver, including V and VIII. Levels of FDP are initially very high but may decrease as levels of fibrinogen decrease from synthetic failure and fibrinolysis. The platelet count is moderately decreased. In *chronic liver disease* a spectrum of coagulation abnormalities may occur. The PT, PTT, and TT may be variably prolonged or may be normal. Since the vitamin K–dependent factors are more sensitive to hepatocellular disease, PT is often more prolonged than PTT. Measurement of clotting factor levels in patients with chronic liver disease will often reveal reduced levels even when the screens are normal. In contrast, VIII may be increased in patients with less severe liver disease. In *acute hepatitis,* the coagulation screening tests are usually normal. Prolongation of the PT in patients with acute hepatitis is a bad prognostic sign.

Although hemostatic abnormalities can be simply diagnosed with routine screening tests, the nature of the abnormality can be difficult to determine. For example, since II, VII, IX, and X are sensitive to hepatocellular disease, it may be difficult to diagnose vitamin K deficiency in patients with liver disease. In many patients a trial of vitamin K may be needed to make the diagnosis. It is also difficult to diagnose DIC in patients with liver disease. Since V and VIII are resistant to hepatocellular disease and are rapidly consumed in DIC, reduced levels of these factors may suggest the presence of DIC. Another way to diagnose DIC in liver disease is to measure serial platelet counts and levels of fibrinogen, V, and VIII. Progressive decline in these parameters is consistent with DIC. Patients with the lupus inhibitor have a prolonged PT and PTT, but such patients can be distinguished from those with coagulopathy of liver disease because the TT is normal and the PTT mix is prolonged.

Clinical Features. Bleeding in patients with acute liver failure may be catastrophic. Spontaneous hemorrhage from mucous membranes, skin, and other sites can be prominent, and bleeding from varices, gastritis, Mallory-Weiss tears, and other structural sites may be greatly aggravated by the hemostatic abnormalities in liver disease. Bleeding is typically from multiple sites. Petechiae may be present in patients who are thrombocytopenic or have a qualitative platelet defect. In patients with chronic liver disease, bleeding signs are less prominent.

Treatment. Treatment of hemostatic defects in liver disease is complicated by the defect's global nature and the short half-life of some clotting factors, especially VII. To maintain correction of the hemostatic defect may require administration of 2 to 4 units of fresh-frozen plasma every 3 to 4 hours. This and the administration of other products, such as platelet concentrates, cryoprecipitate, and red blood cells, can quickly lead to severe volume overload in patients who already have difficulty with fluid balance. For this reason, a major question in the treatment of hemostatic defects in liver disease is often not how to treat but whether to treat.

For patients who are not actively bleeding, vitamin K should be administered orally; treatment with fresh-frozen plasma and other products should be reserved for bleeding episodes. In such patients, minor procedures, such as liver biopsy, should be covered with 2 units of fresh-frozen plasma immediately before the procedure. Platelets may also be given for minor procedures if the platelet count is less than 50,000/μl, and cryoprecipitate if the fibrinogen is less than 75 mg/dl. A single bag of cryoprecipitate contains approximately 150 mg of fibrinogen and will raise the plasma concentration of fibrinogen by about 5 mg/dl.

For patients with significantly abnormal coagulation screening test results who have generalized or severe localized bleeding, therapy should be considered. Vitamin K and folate should be administered initially. Two units of fresh-frozen plasma are given and the coagulation screens repeated after the second bag. This therapy is then repeated until the bleeding stops or the screens are normal. For patients with severe fluid retention, plasma exchange should be considered. Red blood cells and platelets are given as needed, and cryoprecipitate is given if the fibrinogen level is decreased. Prothrombin complex concentrates have been associated with a high incidence of DIC or thrombosis in liver disease and should not be used.

Disseminated Intravascular Coagulation

Disseminated intravascular coagulation (also called diffuse intravascular coagulation or DIC) is a catastrophic bleeding disorder caused by the generation of excessive thrombin in the circulation. DIC has innumerable specific causes (Box 84-2), but all are related either to (1) vascular damage with activation of plasma coagulation factors, leading to thrombin generation by the intrinsic coagulation pathway or (2) entry of tissue thromboplastic material into the blood and generation of thrombin by the extrinsic coagulation pathway.

The consequences of thrombin generation in blood on the coagulation system are shown in Fig. 84-5. Thrombin causes platelets to aggregate, converts fibrinogen to fibrin, activates coagulation factors V and VIII, activates protein C, converts plasminogen to plasmin, activates factor XIII, and combines with and is inactivated by antithrombin III. Thus thrombin simultaneously promotes thrombosis by activating platelets, fibrinogen, V, VIII, and XIII; promotes the dissolution of any thrombi that form by generating plasmin; and inhibits hemostasis by producing thrombocytopenia and by consuming fibrinogen, V, and VIII. The net effect is a hemorrhagic tendency from deficiency of the consumed coagulation factors. For this reason, DIC is also called *consumptive coagulopathy.*

Diagnosis. Laboratory evaluation of coagulation in DIC demonstrates abnormalities in PTT, PT, and TT. Among these, TT is the most sensitive test and is most prolonged because of interference with fibrin polymerization by FDP. A TT performed on a mixture of patient and normal plasma yields results consistent with a coagulation inhibitor produced by the fibrin fragments. Platelets are also decreased, sometimes to very low levels; this is often an early indicator of DIC. The blood smear may show fragmented red blood cells, called *schistocytes,* in about half of patients. The diagnosis is confirmed by factor assays showing decreased fibrinogen, V, and VIII and elevated FDP, although the latter may be increased with surgery and trauma and in other patients and are therefore not specific for a diagnosis of DIC.

Clinical Features. The clinical spectrum of DIC ranges from clinically insignificant laboratory abnormalities in mild cases to uncontrollable hemorrhage in patients with severe disease. The bleeding manifestations of DIC are very characteristic. In contrast to structural bleeding, hemorrhage in DIC is typically from multiple sites. Bleeding from small wounds, such as venipuncture sites, continues without stopping for hours or days. In contrast to patients with thrombocytopenia alone, the bleeding in patients with DIC is not arrested with local pressure that would normally allow fibrin formation. Even in patients with severe thrombocytopenia, bleeding from a deep

BOX 84-2
Causes of disseminated (diffuse) intravascular coagulation (DIC)

Obstetric complications
Amniotic fluid embolism
Abruptio placentae
Retained dead fetus
Eclampsia
Septic abortion
Induced abortion
Hydatidiform mole

Shock
Hemorrhagic
Traumatic
Septic
Anaphylactic

Carcinoma
Prostate
Lung
Pancreas
Stomach
Ovary
Colon
Sarcoma

Infections
Bacterial (gram positive and negative)
Viral (herpes)
Rickettsial (Rocky Mountain spotted fever)
Fungal (aspergillosis)
Parasitic (malaria)
Granulomatous (tuberculosis)

Vascular and pulmonary
Pulmonary embolism
Hyaline membrane disease
Crush syndrome
Malignant hypertension
Cardiopulmonary bypass pump
Thoracic surgery
Giant hemangioma
Fat embolism

Hematologic
Promyelocytic leukemia
Acute leukemia
Tranfusion reaction
Acquired hemolytic anemia
Sickle cell crisis

Renal
Transplant rejection
Glomerulonephritis
Acute renal failure

Miscellaneous
Hepatic cirrhosis
Acute pancreatitis
Allergic drug reaction
Snakebite
Decompression sickness
Amyloidosis
Heatstroke

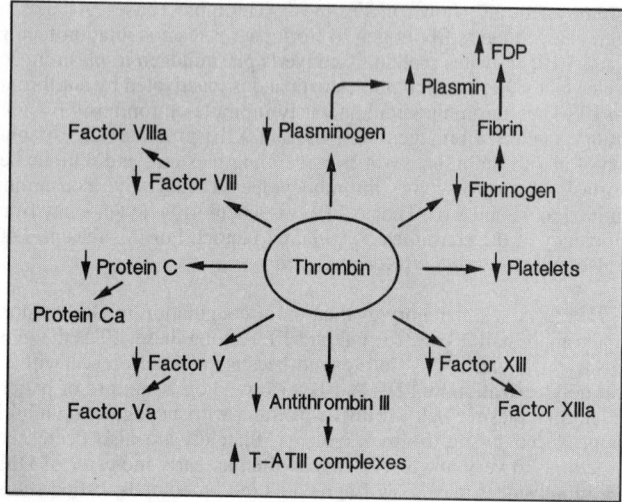

FIGURE 84-5 Consequences of thrombin generation in diffuse (disseminated) intravascular coagulation (DIC). Thrombin has multiple effects on the coagulation system, activating cellular, humoral, and fibrinolytic components. Down arrows indicate reduced plasma concentrations of factors. Up arrows indicate increased plasma concentrations of factors. *FDP,* Fibrin(ogen) degradation products.

nent appears to be either deficient or insufficient, and microthrombi develop. These unusual patients demonstrate the importance of the fibrinolytic component in DIC and provide a strong argument against the use of antifibrinolytic agents in the treatment of DIC.

Treatment. When DIC occurs, it is important to remove the provoking cause: correct the hypotension, control the sepsis, or deliver the placenta or dead fetus. The treatment of DIC itself consists of replacement of consumed coagulation factors and alpha$_2$ antiplasmin with fresh-frozen plasma, replacement of fibrinogen with cryoprecipitate, and platelet transfusions. Because of the short half-life of some of the clotting factors, fresh-frozen plasma must be given as often as every 30 minutes or so to patients with severe DIC. Antithrombin III concentrates are now available and may be used in the treatment of DIC. Intravenous heparin is also used to increase neutralization of thrombin, but it should be used in very low doses and may increase the bleeding in patients with DIC.

Acquired Inhibitors of Blood Coagulation

Acquired inhibitors are endogenous substances, usually polyclonal antibodies, that interfere with normal blood coagulation. Most are immunoglobulin G (IgG) immunoglobulins, but some are IgM or mixtures of IgG and IgM. In most patients the antibody is directed against a site at or near the active site of a single coagulation factor and either inhibits the participation of that factor in coagulation or interferes with normal circulation of the protein. Most acquired inhibitors are directed against VIII, but antibodies to fibrinogen, II, V, IX, X, XI, XIII, and vWF have been reported.

Factor VIII Inhibitors. Spontaneous inhibitors of factor VIII have been reported in a variety of clinical settings (Box 84-3). More than half of spontaneous inhibitors occur in individuals over the age of 40 without any associated underlying disorder. Autoimmune disorders, including rheumatoid arthritis, systemic lupus erythematosus, temporal arteritis, dermatomyositis, polymyositis, myasthenia gravis,

wound such as that caused by marrow aspiration is easily controlled with local pressure. In contrast to patients with only a defect in coagulation, the bleeding in DIC is not initially delayed and is not arrested intermittently by platelet aggregates.

Rarely, patients with DIC have peripheral, symmetric infarction of fingertips and toes, or renal failure may occur with thrombosis of small renal cortical vessels. In these patients the fibrinolytic compo-

and Sjögren's syndrome, may be found in 10% to 15% of patients with VIII inhibitors. Inhibitors occur infrequently in patients with neoplasms, particularly lymphoproliferative disorders and cancer of the prostate and lung, and may be the initial manifestation of a malignancy. It is therefore important to search for occult malignancies in otherwise asymptomatic patients with inhibitors. Postpartum factor VIII inhibitors typically appear after the birth of a normal child, usually the first. The inhibitor becomes manifest weeks to months after delivery, but intervals of up to 1 year have been reported. In about half of such patients the anticoagulant disappears within 12 to 18 months and does not recur during subsequent pregnancies. Other conditions associated with VIII inhibitors include ulcerative colitis; dermatologic disorders such as psoriasis, pemphigus, and exfoliative dermatitis; asthma, especially when treated with corticosteroids; and drugs, including penicillin, sulfa, diphenylhydantoin, and phenylbutazone.

The course of VIII inhibitors is variable. Low-titer inhibitors and those in postpartum women may disappear spontaneously or after a course of corticosteroid therapy. It has been estimated that approximately one third may disappear spontaneously within 2 years. High-titer inhibitors and inhibitors in patients with autoimmune disorders are more persistent and are unlikely to spontaneously resolve. Some will improve or disappear after treatment with corticosteroids in combination with alkylating agents.

Lupus Inhibitor. The "lupus anticoagulant" is an antibody with affinity for negatively charged phospholipids, perhaps in a complex with beta$_2$ glycoprotein I, that inhibits phospholipid-dependent coagulation reactions by preventing the normal interaction of clotting factors with the phospholipid surface. Thus the phospholipid-dependent conversion of prothrombin to thrombin and factor X to Xa is inhibited. Recent studies indicate that although the lupus inhibitor inhibits the catalytic action of the negatively charged phospholipids used in the PTT and PT, it may have little effect on the catalytic action of the platelet surface in these reactions. This may explain why the lupus inhibitor is an in vitro inhibitor but does not have anticoagulant effects in vivo.

Clinically, patients with the lupus inhibitor have a thrombotic tendency. Up to 50% of patients with the lupus inhibitor have clinically detectable thrombosis. In addition, in women of childbearing age the lupus inhibitor is associated with a syndrome of recurrent spontaneous abortions. A strong correlation exists between the presence of the lupus inhibitor, the tendency to thrombosis, and the presence of antibodies to cardiolipin, the lipid used in most serologic tests for syphilis. Based on retrospective studies, cardiolipin antibodies have been shown to predict thrombosis correctly in nearly 90% of patients, but the specificity of the test is lower (approximately 70%). In women with the lupus inhibitor and the syndrome of recurrent spontaneous abortions, the risk of abortion is related to the level of anticardiolipin antibody.

A corollary of the presence of anticardiolipin antibodies is that many patients with the lupus inhibitor have a false-positive test result for syphilis. Tests based on detection of treponemal antigens (i.e., fluorescent treponemal antigen, or FTA) should be used to distinguish a false-positive from a true-positive serologic finding.

Although the lupus inhibitor may be seen in the absence of any underlying disorder, several associated diseases have been described (Box 84-3). Nearly half of patients with the lupus inhibitor have systemic lupus erythematosus (but only 10% of patients with systemic lupus erythematosus have the lupus inhibitor). The lupus inhibitor has also been reported in patients with drug-induced lupus, rheumatoid arthritis, rheumatic fever, Raynaud's phenomenon, hypothyroidism, AIDS, neoplasms, prostatic hypertrophy, and atherosclerotic cardiovascular or peripheral vascular disease.

Other Inhibitors. The prevalence of inhibitors directed against coagulation factors other than factor VIII is much lower. With a single exception, all reported examples of inhibitors of factor V have appeared in patients who were previously normal. The persistence of the inhibitor is usually short. The occurrence of inhibitors to factor V seems to be associated with surgical procedures or the administration of streptomycin or penicillin. Inhibitors to either factor XIII activation or factor XIII transamidase activity have been

---

BOX 84-3
Conditions associated with coagulation inhibitors*

Factor VIII inhibitors
Autoimmune disorders (SLE, RA, TA)
Neoplasms (lymphoma, prostate, lung)
Postpartum
Inflammatory bowel disease
Skin diseases (psoriasis, pemphigus, exfoliative dermatitis)
Drugs (penicillin, sulfa, phenylbutazone)
Asthma
Idiopathic

Acquired von Willebrand's disease
Lymphoma
Autoimmune disorders (SLE)
Idiopathic

Factor XI inhibitor
Autoimmune disorders (SLE)
Drugs (prednisone)
Idiopathic

Factor V
Drugs (streptomycin)
Surgery

Fibrinogen
Ulcerative colitis?
Sarcoidosis?

Factor XIII
Drugs (isoniazid, diphenylhydantoin)

Lupus inhibitor
Autoimmune disorders (SLE, RA, Raynaud's disease)
Acquired immunodeficiency syndrome
Drugs (phenothiazines)
Hypothyroidism
Neoplasms
Atherosclerotic cardiovascular disease
Idiopathic

*Excluding inhibitors occurring in inherited coagulopathies.
SLE, Systemic lupus erythematosus; *RA,* rheumatoid arthritis; *TA,* temporal arteritis.

---

described, especially in association with antituberculous drugs. Inhibitors against vWF also have been described. The blood of some patients with dysproteinemias also demonstrates inhibition of various tests of blood coagulation (and platelet function). This apparently results from an interaction between an abnormal protein and certain plasma proteins involved in blood coagulation. In contrast to the previously described examples of circulating anticoagulants, in this instance inhibition results from a presumed physicochemical rather than an immunologic interaction. Hemorrhagic symptoms are seen only rarely and are more likely caused by increased blood viscosity secondary to high levels of abnormal proteins or decreased platelet function.

Clinical Features. Patients with spontaneous VIII inhibitors typically experience the sudden appearance of a severe hemorrhagic defect when they were previously free of a bleeding tendency. Bleeding is usually spontaneous and profuse. Bleeding is primarily from mucous membranes, the gastrointestinal tract, and the genitourinary tract. Joint bleeds occur less frequently than in patients with hemophilia A.

The lupus inhibitor may become manifest in several ways. In many patients the presence of the inhibitor is an incidental finding in a patient admitted for other reasons. There may be a history of remote thrombosis. Patients with the lupus inhibitor may also have thrombosis. Both deep venous thrombosis, primarily in the lower extremities, and superficial venous thrombosis may occur. Arterial thrombosis, especially cerebral thrombosis, is less often encountered but may also occur. Women with the lupus inhibitor may have spontaneous abortion or a history of recurrent spontaneous abortion. Patients with the lupus inhibitor and systemic lupus erythematosus may bleed when thrombocytopenia or a coexisting specific inhibitor to VIII, XI, or other clotting factors is present.

Diagnosis. Diagnosis of an inhibitor to a specific coagulation factor is suggested by a history of a coagulopathy of recent onset and the presence of an abnormal screening test result. In such patients, it is important to try to obtain the results of past clotting tests to ascertain that the abnormality is new. The pattern of abnormal screening tests depends on the clotting factor to which the antibody is directed and will be similar to the pattern seen in deficiency of that factor (Table 84-1). For example, an inhibitor to VIII is characterized by a prolonged PTT and normal PT and TT, whereas an inhibitor to XIII is characterized by a normal PTT, PT, and TT. The presence of an inhibitor is confirmed by demonstration of an abnormal mixing test result. When plasma from a patient with an inherited clotting factor deficiency is mixed with normal plasma, the normal plasma supplies sufficient amounts of that clotting factor to correct the clotting time in the deficient plasma. In contrast, when plasma from a patient with an inhibitor is mixed with normal plasma, the inhibitor neutralizes the target clotting factor in the normal plasma, and the clotting time of the mixture remains prolonged. With most inhibitors, this neutralization is rapid, and abnormal mixing studies are immediately apparent. With VIII inhibitors, however, the neutralization of VIII in the normal plasma is enhanced by incubation of the mixed plasmas at 37° for 2 hours. The specificity of the inhibitor is determined by demonstrating reduced levels of the target clotting factor by specific assay.

Diagnosis of the lupus inhibitor is based on the presence of a prolonged PTT with an abnormal mix, a variably prolonged PT, and normal TT. The PTT is typically two or three times the control value but may be minimally prolonged. Individual clotting factor assays may be normal or slightly reduced and show an inhibitory pattern. Numerous clotting tests have been proposed for the specific diagnosis of the lupus inhibitor. The platelet neutralization procedure is based on the ability of platelet phospholipids to correct the PTT. Other tests include the kaolin clotting time, the dilute Russell's viper venom time, and the tissue thromboplastin inhibition index, but the number of tests that have been used attests to the uncertainty of each.

Treatment. Bleeding in patients with spontaneous inhibitors to VIII can be treated according to the guidelines outlined for treatment of hemophilic inhibitors in the previous section on hemophilia A. The same principles apply except that the patient usually has not been previously exposed to plasma products, and immunization with hepatitis B vaccine should be started before administration of plasma products. Treatment of the inhibitor itself should be considered. Although some inhibitors may disappear without therapy, a course of corticosteroids may hasten disappearance of the inhibitor. Intravenous gamma globulin has also been reported to be effective in some patients with acquired VIII inhibitors. For patients who do not respond to corticosteroids or intravenous gamma globulin, a trial of alkylating agents may be considered. When an underlying disease or drug is associated with a circulating anticoagulant, therapy should be directed at the basic disease or discontinuation of the potentially causative drug.

Patients with inhibitors to V or XIII have been successfully treated with either plasma or transfusion of platelet concentrates. Those with inhibitors to II, IX, and X may respond to prothrombin complex concentrates. Patients with inhibitors to vWF may respond at least transiently to intravenous gamma globulin. Treatment of the associated disease may result in permanent disappearance of the inhibitor.

Thrombosis associated with the lupus anticoagulant can be successfully controlled with anticoagulants. In women with recurrent spontaneous abortions, corticosteroids and antiplatelet agents have been reported to improve fetal mortality. Coumarins appear to be less effective and can produce fetal malformations, especially if administered during the first trimester.

BIBLIOGRAPHY

Aledort LM: Inhibitors in hemophilia patients: current status and management, *Am J Hematol* 47:208, 1994.

Berntorp E: Methods of haemophilia care delivery: regular prophylaxis versus episodic treatment, *Haemophilia* 1(suppl 1):3, 1995.

Bloom AL: Management of factor VIII inhibitors: evolution and current status, *Haemostatsis* 22:268, 1992.

Brettler DB: Recombinant coagulation factor products, *Haemophilia* 1:155, 1995.

Francis RB Jr: Clinical disorders of fibrinolysis: a critical review, *Blut* 59:1, 1989.

Furie B, Limentani S, Rosenfield CG: A practical guide to the evaluation and treatment of hemophilia, *Blood* 84:3, 1994.

Hoyer LW: Hemophilia A, *N Engl J Med* 330:38, 1994.

Kazazian HH: The molecular basis of hemophilia A and the present status of carrier and antenatal diagnosis of the disease, *Thromb Haemost* 70:60, 1993.

Khamashta MA et al: The management of thrombosis in the antiphospholipid antibody syndrome, *N Engl J Med* 332:993, 1995.

Kunkel LA: Acquired circulating anticoagulants, *Hematol Oncol Clin North Am* 6:1341, 1992.

Lakich et al: Inversions disrupting the factor VIII gene are a common cause of severe haemophilia A, *Nature Genet* 5:236, 1993.

Lusher JM: Considerations for current and future management of haemophilia and its complications, *Haemophilia* 1:2, 1995.

Makris M, Preston FE: Chronic hepatitis in haemophilia, *Blood Rev* 7:243, 1993.

Mammen EF: Congenital coagulation disorders, *Semin Thromb Hemost* 9:1, 1981.

Mannucci PM: Viral safety of plasma-derived and recombinant products used in the management of haemophilia A and B, *Haemophilia* 1(suppl 1):14, 1995.

Morrison AE, Ludlam CA: Acquired haemophilia and its management, *Br J Haematol* 89:231, 1995.

Naylor JA et al: Characteristic mRNA abnormality found in half the patients with severe haemophilia A is due to large DNA inversions, *Hum Mol Genet* 2:1773, 1993.

Rickard KA: Guidelines for therapy and optimal dosages of coagulation factors for treatment of bleeding and surgery in haemophilia, *Haemophilia* 1(suppl 1):8, 1995.

Roberts HR: Molecular biology of hemophilia B, *Thromb Haemost* 70:1, 1993.

Roberts HR, Cederbaum AI: The liver and blood coagulation: physiology and pathology, *Gastroenterology* 63:297, 1972.

Roubey RA: Autoantibodies to phospholipid-binding plasma proteins: a new view of lupus anticoagulants and other "antiphospholipid" antibodies, *Blood* 84:2854, 1994.

Sadler JE et al: Molecular mechanism and classification of von Willebrand disease, *Thromb Haemost* 74:161, 1995.

Sutor AH: Vitamin K deficiency bleeding in infants and children, *Semin Thromb Hemost* 21:317, 1995.

Suttie JW: Synthesis of vitamin K–dependent proteins, *FASEB J* 7:445, 1993.

Thompson AR: Progress towards gene therapy for the hemophilias, *Thromb Haemost* 74:45, 1995.

Triplett DA: Protean clinical presentations of antiphospholipid protein antibodies, *Thromb Haemost* 74:329, 1995.

Triplett DA, Harris EN: Antiphospholipid antibodies and reproduction, *Am J Reproduct Immunol* 21:123, 1989.

Tuddenham EGD et al: Haemophilia A: database of nucleotide substitutions, deletions, insertions and rearrangement of the factor VIII gene, *Nucl Acids Res* 19:4821, 1991.

CHAPTER

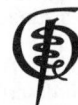

85 Thrombosis and Anticoagulation

Russell D. Hull, Graham F. Pineo, and Gary E. Raskob

This chapter provides an overview of the management of patients with arterial and venous thromboembolic disease and reviews the role of heparin, oral anticoagulant therapy, thrombolytic therapy, and venous interruption procedures in the treatment of patients with established thromboembolism.

VENOUS THROMBOEMBOLISM
Etiology and Pathogenesis

Venous thromboembolism (venous thrombosis and/or pulmonary embolism) usually complicates the course of sick, hospitalized patients but may also affect ambulatory and otherwise apparently healthy individuals. Pulmonary embolism remains the most common preventable cause of hospital death and is responsible for approximately

150,000 to 200,000 deaths per year in the United States. Most patients who die of pulmonary embolism succumb suddenly or within 2 hours after the acute event, before therapy can be initiated or can take effect. Effective prophylaxis against venous thromboembolism is now available for most high-risk patients. The use of prophylaxis is more effective for preventing death and morbidity from venous thromboembolism than is treatment of the established disease. Furthermore, numerous studies have shown that it is more cost effective to prevent postoperative venous thrombosis than it is to treat the complications when they occur.

Venous thrombi are composed predominantly of fibrin and red blood cells with a variable platelet and leukocyte component. The formation, growth, and dissolution of venous thromboemboli represent a balance between various thrombogenic stimuli and several protective mechanisms. The factors that predispose to the development of venous thromboemboli are venous stasis, activation of blood coagulation, and vascular damage. The protective mechanisms that counteract these thrombogenic stimuli include (1) the inactivation of activated coagulation factors by circulating inhibitors (e.g., antithrombin III, protein C including activated protein C resistance, protein S), (2) clearance of activated coagulation factors and soluble fibrin polymer complexes by the reticuloendothelial system and by the liver, and (3) dissolution of fibrin by fibrinolytic enzymes derived from plasma, endothelial cells, and circulating leukocytes. Activated protein C resistance has been identified as the most common hereditary abnormality predisposing to venous thrombosis. The defect is due to a replacement of arginine for glutamine at residue 506 on the factor V gene, rendering activated factor V resistant to inhibition by activated protein C. Up to 20% of patients with activated protein C resistance that is evident by the coagulation abnormality do not have the factor V mutation (Leiden mutation), suggesting that other mutations may be detected in the future.

Various risk factors predispose to the development of venous thromboembolism (Box 85-1). Other conditions that have been reported to be associated with a high risk of venous thromboembolism include hereditary or acquired defects in the metabolism of homocystine, polycythemia vera, paroxysmal nocturnal hemoglobinuria, and the antiphospholipid antibody syndrome.

Pulmonary embolism originates from thrombi in the deep veins of the leg in 90% or more of patients. Other less common sources of pulmonary embolism include the deep pelvic veins, renal veins, inferior vena cava, right side of the heart, or axillary veins. Most clinically important pulmonary emboli arise from thrombi in the popliteal or more proximal deep veins of the leg (proximal-vein thrombosis).

Pulmonary embolism occurs in 50% of patients with objectively documented proximal-vein thrombosis; many of these emboli are asymptomatic. Usually only part of the thrombus embolizes, and 50% to 70% of patients with angiographically documented pulmonary embolism have detectable deep vein thrombosis of the legs at presentation. Therefore strategies for the detection of venous thromboembolism (pulmonary embolism or deep vein thrombosis) can include tests for the detection of pulmonary embolism in the lung (ventilation/perfusion lung scanning or pulmonary angiography) or deep venous thrombosis in the legs (single or serial noninvasive testing with compression ultrasound or impedance plethysmography, or venography). The clinical significance of pulmonary embolism depends on the size of the embolus and the patient's cardiorespiratory reserve.

Clinical Features

The clinical features of venous thrombosis include leg pain, tenderness and swelling, a palpable cord (i.e., a thrombosed vessel that is palpable as a cord), discoloration, venous distention and prominence of the superficial veins, and cyanosis. The clinical diagnosis of venous thrombosis is highly nonspecific because none of the symptoms or signs is unique, and each may be caused by nonthrombotic disorders (Table 85-1). The rare exception may be the patient with phlegmasia cerulea dolens, in whom the diagnosis of massive iliofemoral thrombosis usually is obvious on clinical examination; this syndrome occurs in less than 1% of patients with symptomatic venous thrombosis. In most patients who have clinically suspected venous thrombosis the symptoms and signs are nonspecific, and in more than 50% of these patients the clinical suspicion of venous thrombosis is not confirmed by objective testing. Further, patients with relatively minor symptoms and signs may have extensive deep venous thrombi, whereas in patients with florid leg pain and swelling, suggesting extensive deep vein thrombosis, objective testing may produce negative results. In prospective studies patients who came to medical attention with the clinical diagnosis of deep vein thrombosis were assessed for clinical probabilities of the diagnosis before they underwent objective testing. With the use of predefined criteria, patients with high and moderately high pretest probability were more likely to have proven deep vein thrombosis than those in the low pretest probability group. The authors recommended venography for patients with discordant pretest probability and noninvasive leg test results. At present, an investigative algorithm that uses serial leg testing must still be used to establish the diagnosis and management of a large proportion of patients with suspected deep vein thrombosis.

Pulmonary embolism may become evident on clinical examination in a variety of ways, depending on the size, location, and number of emboli and on the patient's underlying cardiorespiratory reserve. The clinical manifestations of acute pulmonary embolism generally can be divided into the following syndromes that overlap considerably: (1) transient dyspnea and tachypnea in the absence of other associated clinical manifestations; (2) the syndrome of pulmonary in-

---

BOX 85-1
Risk factors predisposing to development of venous thromboembolism

Clinical risk factors
Surgical and nonsurgical trauma
Age (>40 years)
Previous venous thromboembolism
Immobilization
Malignant disease
Heart failure
Myocardial infarction
Leg paralysis
Obesity
Varicose veins
Estrogens
Parturition

Inherited abnormalities
Antithrombin III deficiency
Protein C deficiency
Protein S deficiency
Dysfibrinogenemia

Table 85-1 The alternative diagnosis in 87 consecutive patients with clinically suspected venous thrombosis and negative venograms*

DIAGNOSIS	PATIENTS (%)
Muscle strain	24
Direct twisting injury to leg	10
Leg swelling in paralysed limb	9
Lymphangitis, lymphatic obstruction	7
Venous reflux	7
Muscle tear	6
Baker's cyst	5
Cellulitis	3
Internal abnormality of knee	2
Unknown	26

*The diagnosis was made once venous thrombosis had been excluded by the finding of a negative venogram.

farction or congestive atelectasis (also known as *ischemic pneumonitis* or *incomplete infarction*), including pleuritic chest pain, cough, hemoptysis, pleural effusion, and pulmonary infiltrates on chest radiographs; (3) right-sided heart failure associated with severe dyspnea and tachypnea; (4) cardiovascular collapse with hypotension, syncope, and coma (usually associated with massive pulmonary embolism); and (5) a variety of less common and highly nonspecific clinical features, including confusion and coma, pyrexia, wheezing, resistant cardiac failure, and unexplained arrhythmia. For a detailed discussion of the clinical features and diagnosis of suspected acute pulmonary embolism see Chapter 63.

It is now widely accepted that the clinical diagnosis of pulmonary embolism is highly nonspecific. Multiple studies indicate that in more than half of all patients with clinically suspected pulmonary embolism this diagnosis is not confirmed by objective testing. Attempts to determine the clinical probability of pulmonary embolism using certain pretest criteria have been more useful in excluding pulmonary embolism than in establishing the diagnosis. Therefore objective testing is mandatory to confirm or exclude the presence of pulmonary embolism.

Laboratory Features

Various laboratory abnormalities have been associated with venous thromboembolism, including a decrease in the activated partial thromboplastin time (APTT) and a group of nonspecific laboratory changes that make up the acute-phase response to injury. Tissue injury is associated with a systemic response, including elevated levels of fibrinogen, factor VIII, and alpha$_1$ antitrypsin and increases in both the leukocyte and the platelet counts. Tissue injury is also associated with systemic activation of blood coagulation and fibrin formation: increase in the plasma concentration of prothrombin fragments 1 and 2 (F1.2), fibrinopeptide A (FpA), and complexes of thrombin-antithrombin 3 (TAT) and increased levels of plasma D-Dimer. All the preceding changes are highly nonspecific and may occur as a result of surgical or nonsurgical trauma, infection, inflammation, or infarction. Patients with venous thromboembolism frequently have other comorbid conditions, and it is not surprising that the laboratory changes reported to be associated with venous thromboembolism are highly nonspecific. Currently no evidence exists to indicate that any of the reported laboratory changes associated with venous thromboembolism can be used to predict the development of venous thromboembolism.

The D-Dimer assay has been evaluated in several studies of patients with clinically suspected venous thromboembolism, which was later confirmed by objective testing. The D-Dimer can be measured by the enzyme-linked immunosorbent assay (ELISA) or by a latex agglutination assay. Using the appropriate cut-off value, the negative predictive value of these tests is very high in patients with suspected venous thromboembolism. Several of these assays have a rapid turnaround time and some of them are quantitative, so these assays can now be studied in a prospective fashion in patients with suspected venous thromboembolism.

Differential Diagnosis

The differential diagnosis in patients with clinically suspected venous thrombosis includes muscle strain (usually associated with unaccustomed exercise), muscle tear, direct twisting injury to the leg, vasomotor changes in a paralyzed leg, venous reflux, lymphangitis, lymphatic obstruction, Baker's cyst, cellulitis, internal derangement of the knee, hematoma, and venous insufficiency. An alternate diagnosis is frequently not evident at presentation, and without objective testing (Table 85-2), it is impossible to exclude venous thrombosis. The cause of symptoms can often be determined by careful follow-up once a diagnosis of venous thrombosis has been excluded by objective testing. In some patients, however, the cause of pain, tenderness, and swelling remains uncertain even after careful follow-up.

Treatment

General Considerations. The objectives of treatment in patients with venous thromboembolism are (1) to prevent death from pulmonary embolism, (2) to prevent recurrent venous thromboembolism, and (3) to prevent the postphlebitic syndrome.

Initial therapy with intravenous (IV) heparin is the treatment of choice for most patients with pulmonary embolism or proximal-vein thrombosis. IV heparin given in doses that maintain the APTT greater than 1.5 times the control value is highly effective and associated with a low frequency (2%) of recurrent venous thromboembolism. Failure to follow the initial course of heparin with adequate long-term anticoagulant therapy exposes patients with proximal-vein thrombosis to a 40% to 50% risk of recurrent venous thromboembolism. This risk is reduced to 2% with adequate long-term anticoagulant therapy with warfarin sodium. Adjusted subcutaneous heparin is an effective alternative to warfarin sodium for long-term treatment, with a low risk (2%) of bleeding, and is preferred in selected patients (see section on long-term subcutaneous heparin therapy).

Thrombolytic therapy is indicated in patients with life-threatening massive pulmonary embolism and in selected patients with acute massive proximal-vein thrombosis (e.g., phlegmasia cerulea dolens with impending venous gangrene). Besides these indications, the role of thrombolytic therapy remains uncertain.

The relative and absolute contraindications to anticoagulant therapy are listed in Box 85-2. Inferior vena caval interruption using a transvenously inserted filter (Greenfield filter) is the management of choice for preventing pulmonary embolism in patients with proximal-vein thrombosis in whom anticoagulant therapy is absolutely contraindicated, as well as in the very rare patient in whom anticoagulant therapy is ineffective. In patients with proximal-vein thrombosis who have relative contraindications to anticoagulant therapy the preferred treatment is carefully controlled continuous IV heparin, maintaining the anticoagulant effect near the lower limit of

Table 85-2 Frequency of recurrent venous thromboembolism according to whether activated partial thromboplastin time (APTT) response was above or below 1.5 times the value control

TREATMENT GROUP	FREQUENCY OF RECURRENT VENOUS THROMBOEMBOLISM (NO. OF PATIENTS [%])		
	APTT RESPONSE <1.5	APTT RESPONSE ≥1.5	*P* VALUE
Subcutaneous	10/36 (27.8)	1/21 (4.8)	0.041
Intravenous	3/17 (17.6)	0/41	0.022
All patients*	13/53 (24.5)	1/61 (1.6)	<0.001

From Hull R et al: *N Engl J Med* 315:1109, 1986.
*The relative risk of recurrent venous thromboembolism was 15 times higher in patients with an APTT response below the lower limit (1.5 times the control value) of the prescribed range for 24 hours or more from the start of therapy than in patients with an APTT response at or above the lower limit.

BOX 85-2
Contraindications to anticoagulant therapy

Absolute contraindications
Subarachnoid or cerebral hemorrhage
Serious active bleeding (postoperative, spontaneous or associated trauma)
Recent brain, eye, or spinal cord injury
Malignant hypertension

Relative contraindications
Recent major surgery
Recent cerebrovascular accident (stroke)
Active gastrointestinal tract hemorrhage
Severe hypertension
Hemorrhagic diathesis
Bacterial endocarditis
Severe renal failure
Severe hepatic failure

the therapeutic range (see later discussion), or interruption of the inferior vena cava.

The optimal management of patients with calf vein thrombosis has not been completely resolved. Two approaches are currently available: (1) initial heparin therapy followed by long-term anticoagulant therapy and (2) surveillance with serial objective testing for proximal-vein thrombosis (e.g., using impedance plethysmography or duplex ultrasound) to detect and treat proximal extension. If untreated, approximately 20% of calf vein thrombi extend into the proximal venous segment. Pulmonary embolism is unlikely in the absence of proximal-vein thrombosis. Recent prospective clinical trials in patients with suspected venous thrombosis indicate that anticoagulant therapy can be safely withheld if the results of the impedance plethysmography (which is insensitive for calf vein thrombosis but highly sensitive for proximal-vein thrombosis), remain negative on repeated testing over 10 to 14 days. Negative findings by serial impedance plethysmography are associated with a low risk of clinically important pulmonary embolism (less than 1%) or recurrent venous thrombosis (2%). Thus surveillance with serial impedance plethysmography can be used to separate the 20% of patients with calf vein thrombosis who develop proximal extension (and require treatment) from the 80% who do not have extension, in whom the risks and costs of anticoagulant therapy may outweigh the benefits. Patients with calf vein thrombosis who cannot be monitored for extension by the use of noninvasive tests should be given treatment initially with heparin and then with adequate long-term anticoagulant therapy.

Anticoagulant Therapy for Venous Thromboembolism.

Heparin. Heparin continues to be the initial treatment of choice for most patients with venous thrombosis or pulmonary embolism because it is both effective and relatively safe. Heparin can be administered intravenously or subcutaneously. Continuous IV infusion is the preferred approach. Intermittent IV injection is associated with a greater risk of bleeding and should be reserved for patients in whom continuous infusion and anticoagulant monitoring is not possible.

Recent clinical trials have improved our knowledge of the relations among heparin dose, anticoagulant response, and effectiveness of heparin therapy for preventing recurrent venous thromboembolism. Low doses of subcutaneous (SC) heparin (5000 U every 12 hours) provide effective prophylaxis against venous thromboembolism in moderate- to high-risk general surgical patients but are not effective for preventing recurrent venous thromboembolism in patients with established proximal-vein thrombosis. This difference in the dose of heparin required for the prevention and treatment of proximal-vein thrombosis is probably caused by the biochemical amplification that occurs with each successive step in the blood coagulation pathway. Consequently, much lower doses of heparin are required to prevent thrombin generation and the formation of venous thrombi than are required to inhibit thrombin activity and to prevent extension or recurrence of established thrombosis.

The laboratory test most commonly used to monitor heparin dosage is the APTT. This test is widely available, it is inexpensive, and the relationship between APTT and heparin levels is approximately linear over the therapeutic heparin range. Heparin levels can be measured using either protamine sulphate titration assays or chromogenic anti–factor X^a assays. Therapeutic levels of heparin by the protamine sulphate titration assay are 0.2 to 0.4 U/ml, and 0.35 to 0.70 U/ml for the anti–factor X^a heparin levels. The recommended therapeutic range for heparin is an APTT ratio of 1.5 to 2.5 times the mean of the APTT control. There is a wide variability in the APTT values with different thromboplastin reagents, and in a recent study of several reagents an APTT of 1.5 times the control corresponded to subtherapeutic heparin levels. Therefore, rather than using a fixed ratio of APTT, an APTT equivalent to a plasma heparin level of 0.2 to 0.4 U/ml by the protamine sulphate titration assay should be used for the therapeutic range.

It has been established from experimental studies in clinical trials that the efficacy of heparin therapy depends on achieving a critical therapeutic level of heparin within the first 24 to 48 hours of treatment. Patients receiving heparin either by continuous IV infusion or intermittent SC injection who do not achieve therapeutic APTT values during initial therapy have an increased risk of recurrent venous

thromboembolism during follow-up over the subsequent 3 to 12 weeks.

Whereas there is a strong correlation between subtherapeutic APTT values and recurrent thromboembolism, the relationship between supratherapeutic APTT and bleeding (APTT ratio of 2.5 or more) is less definite. Indeed, bleeding during heparin therapy is more closely related to underlying clinical risk factors than to APTT elevation above the therapeutic range. Recent studies confirm that age greater than 65 years and female gender increase the risk of bleeding when receiving heparin.

Numerous audits of heparin therapy indicate that administration of IV heparin is fraught with difficulty and that the clinical practice of using an ad hoc approach to heparin dose titration frequently results in inadequate treatment. These problems can be overcome with the use of a prescriptive heparin nomogram, and to date three of these have been reported; two of these reports have included clinical outcome data.

In one clinical trial patients were given either IV heparin alone followed subsequently by warfarin sodium or IV heparin and simultaneous warfarin sodium in the treatment of proximal venous thrombosis. This heparin nomogram is summarized in Table 85-3 and Box 85-3. Less than 2% of patients were subtherapeutic for more than 24 hours, and recurrent venous thromboembolism occurred infrequently in both groups. These findings demonstrate that subtherapy was avoided in most patients and that the heparin protocol resulted in effective delivery of heparin therapy. In the other clinical trial a weight-based heparin dosing nomogram was compared with a standard care nomogram (Table 85-4). In the weight-adjusted group, 89% of patients achieved the therapeutic range within 24 hours, compared with 75% in the standard care group. The risk of recurrent thromboembolism was greater in the standard care group. This study included patients with unstable angina and arterial thromboembolism, in addition to venous thromboembolism, indicating that the principles applied to a heparin nomogram for the treatment of venous thromboembolism may be generalizable to other clinical conditions.

It has become standard clinical practice to start IV and heparin simultaneously for all patients with venous thromboembolism who are medically stable. Exceptions include patients who require immediate medical or surgical intervention, or patients at very high risk of bleeding. The length of the initial intravenous heparin therapy has been reduced to 5 days, thus shortening the hospital stay and leading to significant cost savings.

Heparin currently in use clinically is polydispersed unmodified heparin, with a mean molecular weight ranging from 10,000 to 16,000 daltons. In recent years, low-molecular-weight derivatives of commer-

Table 85-3 Intravenous heparin dose-titration nomogram for activated partial thromboplastin time (APTT)

APTT (SECONDS)	INTRAVENOUS INFUSION		ADDITIONAL ACTION
	RATE CHANGE, ML/HOUR	DOSE CHANGE, U/24 HOURS*	
≤45	+6	+5760	Repeated APTT† in 4-6 hours
46-54	+3	+2880	Repeated APTT in 4-6 hours
55-85	0	0	None‡
86-110	−3	−2880	Stop heparin sodium treatment for 1 hour; repeated APTT 4-6 hours after restarting heparin treatment
>110	−6	−5760	Stop heparin treatment for 1 hour; repeated APTT 4-6 hours after restarting heparin treatment

From Hull RD, Raskob GE, Rosenbloom D et al: *Arch Intern Med* 152:1589, 1992.
*Heparin sodium concentration, 20,000 U in 500 ml = 40 U/ml.
†With the use of Actin-FS thromboplastin reagent (Dade, Mississauga, Ontario, Canada).
‡During the first 24 hours, repeated APTT in 4 to 6 hours. Thereafter the APTT will be determined once daily, unless response is subtherapeutic.

BOX 85-3

Heparin protocol

1. Initial intravenous heparin bolus: 5000 U
2. Continuous intravenous heparin infusion: commence at 42 ml/ hour of 20,000 U (1680 U/hour) in 500 ml of two-thirds dextrose and one-third saline (a 24-hour heparin dose of 40,320 U), except in the following patients, in whom heparin infusion will be commenced at a rate of 31 ml/hour (1240 U/hour) (i.e., a 24-hour dose of 29,760 U):
   a. Patients who have undergone surgery within the previous 2 weeks
   b. Patients with a previous history of peptic ulcer disease, gastrointestinal tract or genitourinary tract bleeding
   c. Patients with recent stroke (i.e., thrombotic stroke within 2 weeks previously)
   d. Patients with a platelet count $<150 \times 10^9$ cells per liter
   e. Patients with miscellaneous reasons for a high risk of bleeding (e.g., hepatic failure, renal failure, or vitamin K deficiency)
3. Heparin dose adjusted using the activated partial thromboplastin time (APTT). The APTT test is performed in all patients as follows:
   a. Four to 6 hours after commencing heparin; the heparin dose is then adjusted according to the nomogram (Table 85-3)
   b. Four to 6 hours after implementing the first dosage adjustment
   c. The APTT is then performed as indicated by the nomogram for the first 24 hours of therapy
   d. Thereafter the APTT will be performed once daily, unless the response is subtherapeutic, in which case the APTT will be repeated 4 to 6 hours after increasing the heparin dose

From Hull RD, Raskob GE, Rosenbloom D et al: *Arch Intern Med* 152:1589, 1992.

Table 85-4   Comparison of standard care and weight-based heparin dosing nomograms

STANDARD CARE	WEIGHT-BASED
Initial dose	80 U/kg bolus, then 18 U/kg per hour
APTT, <35 seconds (<1.2 × control)	80 U/kg bolus, then 4 U/kg per hour
APTT, 35-45 seconds (1.2-1.5 × control)	40 U/kg bolus, then 2 U/kg per hour
APTT, 46-70 seconds (1.5-2.3 × control)	No change
APTT, 71-90 seconds (2.3-3.0 × control)	Decrease infusion rate by 2 U/kg per hour
PTT >90 seconds (>3.0 × control)	Hold infusion 1 hour, then decrease infusion rate by 3 U/kg per hour

From Raschke RA, Reilly BM, Guidry JR et al: *Ann Intern Med* 119:874-881, 1993.
PTT, Partial thromboplastin time; *APTT,* activated PTT.

---

cial heparin have been prepared that have a mean molecular weight of 4000 to 5000 daltons. Low-molecular-weight heparins have a number of advantages over unfractionated heparin: they have greater bioavailability when given by subcutaneous injection; the duration of anticoagulant effect is greater, permitting once- or twice-daily administration; the anticoagulant response (anti-X^a activity) to low-molecular-weight heparin is highly correlated with body weight, permitting administration without laboratory monitoring; and there is less bleeding with equivalent antithrombotic effect.

Several different low-molecular-weight heparins and one heparinoid are available for the prevention and treatment of venous thromboembolism in various countries. In North America, three low-molecular-weight heparins have been approved for clinical use; two in the United States and three in Canada. A large number of clinical trials of deep vein thrombosis prophylaxis have been carried out in general and orthopedic surgery in both Europe and North America.

Metaanalyses indicate that low-molecular-weight heparins are at least as effective as unfractionated heparin or warfarin in the prevention of postoperative deep vein thrombosis with the added convenience of once-daily administration. However, the incidence of postoperative bleeding may be somewhat higher than with low-dose, unfractionated heparin or warfarin. Low-molecular-weight heparin has become the prophylaxis of choice for patients undergoing high-risk surgery, such as total hip or total knee replacement.

Subcutaneous, unmonitored, low-molecular-weight heparin has been compared with continuous IV heparin in a number of clinical trials for the treatment of proximal venous thrombosis. In one clinical trial conducted in North America there was a significant decrease in major bleeding and in mortality rate in patients treated with low-molecular-weight heparin as compared with unfractionated heparin. There was also a trend to decreased recurrent thromboembolism. Four other clinical trials, which also used long-term follow-up as an outcome measure rather than repeat venography, showed that low-molecular-weight heparin was at least as effective and safe as unfractionated heparin, although the differences were not significant. When all five studies were combined, there was a significant advantage with low-molecular-weight heparin with respect to recurrent venous thromboembolism, major bleeding, and mortality. Data from ongoing studies indicate that low-molecular-weight heparin is equally effective in the treatment of patients who come to medical attention with pulmonary embolism. Two recently completed randomized clinical trials show that selected patients with venous thromboembolism can safely be given treatment as outpatients with low-molecular-weight heparin. Cost analyses indicate that low-molecular-weight heparin is cost-effective in both the prevention and treatment of venous thromboembolism, when compared with standard treatment. When these agents become more available for treatment, they will undoubtedly replace IV unfractionated heparin in the initial management of patients with venous thromboembolism, as well as in the management of other patients in whom IV heparin is currently used.

Long-term subcutaneous heparin therapy. Adjusted-dose SC heparin is the long-term anticoagulant regimen of choice in pregnant patients, patients at high risk of bleeding, and patients who return to geographically remote areas in which long-term anticoagulant monitoring is unavailable or impractical (in whom the heparin dose is adjusted during the first few days of long-term therapy and then fixed). The starting dose of long-term SC heparin is determined from the patient's initial IV heparin dose requirement. A starting SC dose equivalent to one third of the patient's 24-hour IV heparin dose is administered every 12 hours. For example, if the patient required 30,000 U/24 hours of continuous IV heparin to maintain the APTT greater than 1.5 times the control value, the starting dose of long-term SC heparin would be 10,000 U every 12 hours. The SC dose is adjusted during the first few days of long-term therapy to maintain the midinterval APTT (determined 6 hours after injection) at 1.5 times the control value. This level of anticoagulant response is usually achieved with a dose of 8000 to 12,000 U every 12 hours (mean dose, 10,000 U every 12 hours). In pregnant patients larger doses may be required, and continued monitoring is desired because of changes in heparin requirements throughout the course of pregnancy.

Adverse effects of heparin therapy. The side effects of heparin therapy include bleeding, thrombocytopenia with arterial or venous thromboembolism, osteoporosis, hypersensitivity, hypoaldosteronism, and elevated liver enzyme levels.

Bleeding, the most common side effect of heparin, occurs in 5% to 10% of patients during initial continuous IV heparin therapy. At particular risk are those patients who have been exposed to recent surgery or trauma and those with an underlying hemostatic defect or predisposing clinical risk factor (e.g., unsuspected peptic ulcer or occult carcinoma). The risk of bleeding complications is greater in patients who receive IV heparin by intermittent injection than in those who receive continuous infusion.

Immune heparin-induced thrombocytopenia is a well-recognized complication of heparin therapy that usually occurs 5 to 10 days after heparin prophylaxis or treatment has commenced, but it may occur earlier in patients who have been previously exposed to heparin. This complication has been seen with the low-molecular-weight heparins, but the incidence and severity may be less than with unfractionated heparin. Approximately 1% to 2% of patients receiving unfractionated heparin have a fall in the platelet count to less than the normal range. In the majority of cases this appears to be a direct effect of heparin and is of no consequence. However, approximately 0.1% to 0.2% of patients receiving heparin develop an immune thrombocytopenia, which is mediated by an immunoglobulin G (IgG) antibody directed against a complex of platelet factor IV (PF$_4$) and heparin. The syndrome may be accompanied by the extension of preexisting venous thromboembolism or the development of new arterial thrombosis, and these complications may precede or coincide with a fall in the platelet count. Heparin-induced thrombocytopenia has been associated with a high incidence of limb amputation and a high mortality rate. Therefore it is mandatory that heparin in all forms be discontinued when the diagnosis of heparin-induced thrombocytopenia is made on clinical grounds. The laboratory diagnosis of heparin-induced thrombocytopenia is often not achievable because the definitive platelet activation assays are not widely available and are limited by a slow turnaround time. The more readily available PF$_4$ immunoassay does not appear to have the same sensitivity and specificity as the serotonin release assay, and the heparin platelet aggregation (HEPA) test lacks sensitivity and specificity.

For patients with heparin-induced thrombocytopenia who have an ongoing need for anticoagulation, alternative approaches are available. However, the use of these alternatives is not supported by randomized clinical trials. These include commencement of warfarin therapy, insertion of an inferior vena cava filter, and the use of alternative anticoagulants such as Ancrod (Arvin), a defibrinogenating extract of snake venom, the heparinoid Danaparoid sodium (Orgaran), or specific antithrombin agents such as hirudin or Argatroban. In case series Arvin and Danaparoid sodium have been shown to be useful. Randomized clinical trials are currently underway, comparing specific antithrombin agents with the currently available agents.

Osteoporosis occurs rarely in patients receiving long-term SC heparin therapy (>20,000 U/day for longer than 6 months). The earliest clinical manifestation of heparin-associated osteoporosis is usually the onset of nonspecific low-back pain primarily involving the vertebrae or ribs; patients may also have spontaneous fracture in these areas. There is some evidence that the development of osteoporosis may occur less frequently with the use of low-molecular-weight heparin as compared with unfractionated heparin.

Hypersensitivity to heparin occurs infrequently and may take the form of a skin rash or, less often, anaphylaxis. Alopecia has been reported as a rare complication of heparin therapy. Serum transaminase levels may be moderately raised. Rarely, a bluish discoloration of the toes associated with a burning sensation has been reported. Hyperkalemia develops in some patients as a result of heparin-induced hypoaldosteronism.

Antidote to heparin. The anticoagulant effect of heparin can be immediately neutralized by the IV injection of protamine sulfate. The appropriate neutralizing dose depends on the dose of heparin, its route of administration, and the time it is given. If protamine sulfate is used within minutes of an IV heparin injection, a full neutralizing dose (1 mg protamine sulfate/100 U heparin) should be given. Because the plasma half-life of IV heparin is approximately 60 minutes, an injection of protamine sulfate in a bolus of more than 50 mg is seldom required. An occasional hypotensive response to protamine sulfate has been reported; therefore it should be injected slowly over 10 to 30 minutes. Treatment with protamine sulfate may need to be repeated because protamine is cleared from the blood more quickly than heparin. After an SC injection of heparin, repeated small doses of protamine may be required because of prolonged heparin absorption from the SC depot.

Patients who bleed while receiving low-molecular-weight heparin should receive protamine sulphate in a similar fashion. Protamine sulphate decreases anti-X^a activity and has been noted to decrease clinical bleeding, presumably by neutralizing the high-molecular-weight components of these agents.

Oral Anticoagulant Therapy. There are two distinct chemical groups of oral anticoagulants: the 4-hydroxy coumarin derivatives (e.g., warfarin sodium) and the indane-1, 3-dione derivatives (e.g., phenindione). The coumarin derivatives are the oral anticoagulants

of choice because they are associated with fewer nonhemorrhagic side effects than are the indanedione derivatives.

The anticoagulant effect of warfarin is mediated by the inhibition of the vitamin K–dependent γ-carboxylation of coagulation factors II, VII, IX and X. This results in the synthesis of immunologically detectable but biologically inactive forms of these coagulation proteins. Warfarin also inhibits the vitamin K–dependent γ-carboxylation of proteins C and S. Protein C circulates as a proenzyme that is activated on endothelial cells by the thrombin/thrombomodulin complex to form activated protein C. Activated protein C inhibits activated factor VIII activity directly, and in the presence of protein S it also inhibits activated factor V. Therefore vitamin K antagonists such as warfarin create a biochemical paradox by producing an anticoagulant effect due to the inhibition of procoagulants (factors II, VII, IX, and X) and a potentially thrombogenic effect by impairing the synthesis of naturally occurring inhibitors of coagulation (proteins C and S). Heparin and warfarin treatment should be overlapped by 4 to 5 days when initiating warfarin treatment in patients with thrombotic disease.

The anticoagulant effect of the warfarin is delayed until the normal clotting factors are cleared from the circulation, and the peak effect does not occur until 36 to 72 hours after drug administration. During the first few days of warfarin therapy the prothrombin time (PT) reflects mainly the depression of factor VII, which has a half life of 5 to 7 hours. Equilibrium levels of factors II, IX, and X are not reached until about 1 week after the initiation of therapy. The use of small initial daily doses (e.g., 7.5 to 10 mg) is the preferred approach for initiating warfarin treatment. The dose-response relationship to warfarin therapy varies widely between individuals and therefore the dose must be carefully monitored to prevent overdosing or underdosing.

Laboratory monitoring and therapeutic range. The laboratory test most commonly used to measure the effects of warfarin is the one-stage PT test. Prothrombin time is sensitive to reduced activity of factors II, VII, and X but is insensitive to reduced activity of factor IX. Confusion about the appropriate therapeutic range has occurred because the different tissue thromboplastins used for measuring the PT vary considerably in sensitivity to the vitamin K–dependent clotting factors and in response to warfarin. Rabbit brain thromboplastin, which is widely used in North America, is less sensitive than is standardized human brain thromboplastin, which has been widely used in the United Kingdom and other parts of Europe. A PT ratio of 1.5 to 2.0 using rabbit brain thromboplastin (i.e., the traditional therapeutic range in North America) is equivalent to a ratio of 4.0 to 6.0 using human brain thromboplastin. Conversely, a two- to three-fold increase in the PT using standardized human brain thromboplastin is equivalent to a 1.25- to 1.5-fold increase in the PT using rabbit brain thromboplastin such as Simplastin or Dade-C.

To promote standardization of the PT for monitoring oral anticoagulant therapy, the World Health Organization (WHO) has developed an international reference thromboplastin from human brain tissue and has recommended that the PT ratio be expressed as the International Normalized Ratio (INR). The INR is the PT ratio obtained by testing a given sample using the WHO reference thromboplastin. For practical clinical purposes, the INR for a given plasma sample is equivalent to the PT ratio obtained using a standardized human brain thromboplastin known as the Manchester Comparative Reagent, which has been widely used in the United Kingdom.

Oral anticoagulants (warfarin sodium) protocol. Warfarin is administered in an initial dose of 7.5 to 10 mg per day for the first 2 days, and the daily dose is then adjusted according to the INR. Heparin therapy is discontinued on the fourth or fifth day following initiation of warfarin therapy, provided the INR is prolonged into the recommended therapeutic range (INR 2.0 to 3.0). The selection of the correct dosage of warfarin must be individualized, since some individuals are either fast or slow metabolizers of the drug. Therefore, frequent INR determinations are required initially to establish therapeutic anticoagulation.

Once the anticoagulant effect and patient's warfarin dose requirements are stable, the INR should be monitored every 1 to 2 weeks throughout the course of warfarin therapy for venous thromboembolism. However, if there are factors that may produce an unpredictable response to warfarin (e.g., concomitant drug therapy), the INR should be monitored more frequently to minimize the risk of complications due to poor anticoagulant control.

Long-Term Treatment of Venous Thromboembolism.
Patients with established venous thrombosis or pulmonary embolism require long-term anticoagulant therapy to prevent recurrent disease. Warfarin therapy is highly effective and is preferred in most patients. In patients with proximal-vein thrombosis (popliteal, femoral, or iliac vein thrombosis), long-term therapy with warfarin reduces the frequency of objectively documented recurrent venous thromboembolism from 47% to 2%. The less intense warfarin regimen (INR 2.0 to 3.0) markedly reduces the risk of bleeding (from 20% to 4%) without loss of effectiveness when compared with more intense warfarin. It is recommended that all patients with the first episode of venous thromboembolism receive warfarin therapy for 12 weeks. Attempts to decrease the treatment to 4 or 6 weeks resulted in higher rates of recurrent thromboembolism than seen with either 12 or 26 weeks of treatment.

Warfarin treatment for more than 3 months is indicated for patients with recurrent venous thromboembolism or in patients in whom there is a continuing risk factor for venous thromboembolism. The optimal duration of therapy in patients with recurrent venous thromboembolism is the subject of clinical trials currently underway. Until those trials are completed the current recommendation is to continue oral anticoagulant therapy for 12 months in patients with a first recurrence and indefinitely for those who have more than one recurrence.

In patients with a continuing risk factor that is potentially reversible (e.g., prolonged bed rest), long-term therapy should be continued until the risk factor is reversed. Anticoagulant therapy should probably be continued indefinitely in patients with an irreversible risk factor, such as a deficiency of antithrombin III or protein C. It is unknown at present whether patients who have activated protein C resistance and venous thromboembolism require anticoagulant treatment for more than 3 months. This is an active area of research, and the evidence should become available within the next few years.

Adverse Effects of Oral Anticoagulants.
The major side effect of oral anticoagulant therapy is bleeding. Bleeding during well-controlled oral anticoagulant therapy is usually caused by surgery or other forms of trauma or by local lesions such as peptic ulcer or carcinoma. Spontaneous bleeding may occur if warfarin sodium is given in an excessive dose, resulting in marked elevation of the INR; this bleeding may be severe, even life threatening. The risk of bleeding can be substantially reduced by adjusting the warfarin dose to achieve a less intense anticoagulant effect than has traditionally been used in North America (INR 2.0 to 3.0).

Nonhemorrhagic side effects of oral anticoagulants differ according to whether the coumarin derivatives (e.g., warfarin sodium) or indanediones are administered. Nonhemorrhagic side effects of coumarin anticoagulants occur infrequently, and the coumarins are the oral anticoagulants of choice. Nonhemorrhagic side effects occur more frequently with the indanedione derivatives and include skin necrosis, dermatitis, and a syndrome of painful blue toes. Hypersensitivity reactions have been reported to occur in 1% to 3% of patients receiving indanedione derivatives and include rash, fever, hepatitis, leukopenia, renal failure, and diarrhea; these side effects are sometimes fatal. The indanedione derivatives also produce red discoloration of the urine in many patients, which may be confused with hematuria.

Coumarin-induced skin necrosis is a rare but serious complication that requires immediate cessation of oral anticoagulant therapy. It usually occurs 3 to 10 days after therapy has commenced, is more common in women, and most often involves areas of abundant subcutaneous tissues such as the abdomen, buttocks, thighs, and breast. The mechanism of coumarin-induced skin necrosis, which is associated with microvascular thrombosis, is uncertain but appears to be related, at least in some patients, to the depression of protein C. Patients with congenital deficiencies of protein C or S may be particularly prone to the development of coumarin skin necrosis. To avoid the development of skin necrosis in patients with protein C or S deficiency who require anticoagulant therapy, IV heparin should be commenced and then warfarin should be initiated without a loading dose. The heparin should be continued until the INR is therapeutic for at least 2 consecutive days.

Oral anticoagulants cross the placenta and may cause fetal malformations when used during pregnancy. Two specific fetopathic syndromes are associated with oral anticoagulant administration during pregnancy. Treatment with oral anticoagulants during the sixth to twelfth weeks of gestation may induce the syndrome of *warfarin embryopathy* in the fetus. This syndrome consists of skeletal abnormalities ranging from stippled epiphyses to frank skeletal hypoplasia. Although most reported cases have occurred in infants of mothers receiving warfarin, it has also been reported as a result of phenindandione or acenocoumarin administration. Oral anticoagulant administration during the second or third trimester of pregnancy may result in central nervous system abnormalities in the fetus, including abnormalities of the ventricular system (Dandy-Walker malformation), dorsal midline dysplasia, and optic atrophy. Therefore the use of oral anticoagulants is contraindicated at any time during pregnancy, and they should not be used in women planning a pregnancy. Adjusted-dose SC heparin is the treatment of choice for venous thromboembolism during pregnancy.

Factors That Interact With Oral Anticoagulant Therapy.
Many drugs interact with oral anticoagulants and may produce either a prolongation or a reduction in the anticoagulant effect. In a recent critical review of the literature, foods and drugs interacting with warfarin were classified as highly probable, probable, possible, or doubtful. In Table 85-5, the foods and drugs with a probable interaction with warfarin are shown. Special care should be taken to adjust the dose of oral anticoagulant during the time that other drugs are being taken, to minimize the risk of inadequate anticoagulant control.

Table 85-5   Drug and food interactions with warfarin by level of supporting evidence and type of interaction

LEVEL OF EVIDENCE	POTENTIATION	INHIBITION	NO EFFECT
Highly probable	Alcohol (if concomitant liver disease), amiodarone, cimetidine, clofibrate, co-trimoxazole, erythromycin, fluconazole, isoniazid (600 mg daily), metronidazole, miconazole, omeprazole, phenylbutazone, piroxicam, propafenone, propranolol, sulfinpyrazone	Barbiturates, carbamazepine, chlordiazepoxide, cholestyramine, griseofulvin, nafcillin, rifampin, sucralfate, high vitamin K–content foods and enteral feeds, large amounts of avocado	Alcohol, antacids, atenolol, bumetanide, diflunisal, enoxacin, famotidine, felodipine, fluoxetine, ketorolac, metoprolol, moricizine, naproxen, nitrazepam, nizatidine, psyllium, ranitidine
Probable	Acetaminophen, anabolic steroids, aspirin, chloral hydrate, ciprofloxacin, dextropropoxyphene, disulfiram, itraconazole, quinidine, phenytoin, simvastatin, tamoxifen, tetracycline, influenza vaccine	Dicloxacillin	Ibuprofen, ketoconazole, ketoprofen

Modified from Wells PS, Holbrook AM, Crowther NR, Hirsh J: *Ann Intern Med* 121(9):676-683, 1994.

Increased sensitivity to oral anticoagulants occurs in vitamin K deficiency, impaired liver function, and thyrotoxicosis because of the more rapid metabolism of the vitamin K–dependent clotting factors.

Antidote to Oral Anticoagulants. The antidote to the vitamin K antagonists is vitamin K_1. If the INR is excessively increased, treatment depends on the level of the INR and whether the patient is bleeding. If the increase is mild (INR < 6.0) and the patient is not bleeding, no specific treatment is necessary other than reduction of the warfarin dose. The INR can be expected to decrease during the next 24 hours with this approach. With more marked increase of the INR in patients who are not bleeding, treatment with small doses of vitamin K_1 given either orally or by SC injection (2.5 to 5.0 mg) could be considered. With very marked increase of the INR (>10.0), particularly in a patient who is either actively bleeding or at risk of bleeding, vitamin K_1 should be given.

Second-generation rodenticides known as "super warfarins" have an extremely long half-life. Accidental or intentional consumption of these agents requires repeated injection of vitamin K and fresh-frozen plasma for up to 1 to 2 years to overcome their effects completely.

Reported side effects of vitamin K include flushing, dizziness, tachycardia, hypotension, dyspnea, and sweating. Intravenous administration of vitamin K_1 should be performed with caution to avoid inducing an anaphylactoid reaction. The risk of anaphylactoid reaction can be reduced by giving vitamin K_1 slowly, at a rate no faster than 1 mg/minute IV. In most patients IV administration of vitamin K_1 produces a demonstrable effect on the INR within 3 to 4 hours and corrects the prolonged INR within 6 to 8 hours. Because the half-life of vitamin K_1 is less than that of warfarin sodium, a repeat course of vitamin K_1 may be necessary. If bleeding is very severe and life threatening, vitamin K therapy can be supplemented by using concentrates of factors II, VII, IX, and X.

Thrombolytic Therapy for Venous Thromboembolism.
The frequency of clinically evident recurrent venous thromboembolism is very low during anticoagulant therapy, and this remains the treatment of choice in most patients. Theoretically, however, anticoagulant therapy is not ideal because it does not induce thrombolysis. Thus, although anticoagulant therapy is highly effective in reducing the important immediate complications of venous thromboembolism, it may be relatively ineffective at preventing the late sequelae (e.g., postphlebitic syndrome). For these reasons, thrombolytic therapy is recommended in selected patients with acute massive venous thrombosis or massive pulmonary embolism.

Advocates of thrombolytic therapy point out that it may achieve the following objectives of ideal management: (1) lysis of the thrombi and emboli with circulation restored to normal, (2) rapid reduction of hemodynamic disturbances, and (3) prevention or minimizing of damage to the pulmonary vascular bed, reducing the likelihood of persistent pulmonary hypertension. In patients with venous thrombosis the use of thrombolytic therapy is based on the premise that thrombolysis can minimize or prevent venous valvular damage and prevent the postphlebitic syndrome.

Thrombolytic agents currently available for clinical use (U.S. Food and Drug Administration [FDA] approved) in patients with venous thromboembolism include streptokinase, urokinase, and tissue plasminogen activator (tPA). Streptokinase, a product of hemolytic streptococci, combines with plasminogen, producing a conformational change that exposes an active site, which in turn converts noncomplexed plasminogen to plasmin by proteolytic cleavage. Streptokinase is antigenic in humans and stimulates the production of neutralizing antibodies. Urokinase, which is isolated from human urine or from cultures of human embryonic kidney cells, is nonantigenic. Recombinant tissue plasminogen activator (rtPA), 100 mg by IV infusion over 2 hours, has been approved by the FDA for the treatment of pulmonary embolism, but clinical trials using shorter-duration therapy have also been reported.

Thrombolytic therapy with streptokinase, urokinase, or tPA is more effective than heparin for inducing rapid resolution of recent venous thrombi and pulmonary emboli. The use of thrombolytic agents followed by conventional anticoagulant therapy is indicated in patients with massive pulmonary embolism. In patients with massive pulmonary embolism, the degree of lysis can be striking. The use of strep-

tokinase or urokinase for 12 to 24 hours followed by conventional anticoagulant therapy is indicated in patients with massive pulmonary embolism. Thrombolytic therapy should also be considered in patients with pulmonary embolism and underlying severe cardiac or pulmonary disease in whom even a small or moderate embolus may be life threatening.

Thrombolytic therapy may benefit selected patients with acute massive venous thrombosis, such as those with phlegmasia cerulea dolens. In most patients with acute deep vein thrombosis, however, the indication for thrombolytic therapy remains controversial. Currently, randomized clinical trials have yielded no definitive evidence that thrombolytic therapy is associated with improved benefit by prevention of the postphlebitic syndrome.

The following guidelines are recommended for patient selection for thrombolytic therapy:
1. The presence of an appropriate clinical indication, including an objectively documented diagnosis and evidence that the venous thromboembolic event is of recent origin (less than 7 days)
2. Careful evaluation of contraindications (Box 85-4)

Before thrombolytic therapy is begun, the diagnosis of venous thromboembolism should be established by objective means. If pulmonary angiography is performed to confirm a diagnosis of pulmonary embolism, the angiography catheter should be inserted into an arm vein, where hemostasis is easier to achieve than in the femoral vein. Acute massive pulmonary embolism can be diagnosed with the use of B-mode echocardiography, which significantly decreases the bleeding risk with thrombolytic therapy.

Complications of thrombolytic therapy. The major complication of thrombolytic therapy is hemorrhage. Thrombolytic therapy produces lysis of fibrin in hemostatic plugs in wounds; therefore bleeding occurs more frequently than with heparin. Intracranial bleeding is of most concern. In patients who receive treatment with thrombolytic agents for venous thromboembolism the risk of intracranial hemorrhage is 0.5% to 1%. Serious retroperitoneal hemorrhage may occur, particularly if the femoral artery is inadvertently punctured during pulmonary angiography. Retroperitoneal hemorrhage is serious because the bleeding is often massive and difficult to diagnose. Bleeding may also occur in the genitourinary or gastrointestinal tract. Bleeding complications can be reduced by careful selection of patients and avoidance of treatment of those with contraindications.

Fever occurs in approximately 25% of patients receiving streptokinase. Allergic reactions occur in 10% of patients treated with streptokinase, usually in the form of pruritus or urticaria, but ana-

---

BOX 85-4
Contraindications to thrombolytic therapy

Absolute contraindications
Active internal bleeding
Recent (within 2 months) cerebrovascular accident or other active intracranial processes

Relative major contraindications
Recent (<10 days) major surgery
Recent obstetric delivery
Recent organ biopsy
Recent previous puncture of noncompressible vessels
Recent serious gastrointestinal bleeding
Recent serious trauma
Severe hypertension (systolic blood pressure >200 mm Hg, diastolic blood pressure >110 mm Hg)

Relative minor contraindications
Recent minor trauma, including cardiopulmonary resuscitation
High likelihood of left-sided thrombus (e.g. mitral stenosis with atrial fibrillation)
Bacterial endocarditis
Diabetic hemorrhagic retinopathy
Pregnancy
Age >75 years

phylactic reactions may develop in approximately 1% to 2% of patients. The allergic reactions to streptokinase can be promptly reversed by standard therapy, including epinephrine, IV corticosteroids, and antihistamines. Allergic and febrile reactions are not problems with the use of urokinase or tPA.

Antidote to thrombolytic therapy. If bleeding is life threatening, the fibrinolytic process can be rapidly reversed by the infusion of 5 g of epsilon-aminocaproic acid (EACA, Amicar) given over a half-hour period and followed by 1 g/hour until hemostasis has been achieved. Antifibrinolytic therapy with EACA frequently must be supplemented with transfusions of fresh plasma or cryoprecipitate.

Management of massive pulmonary embolism. Most patients who die of pulmonary embolism do so within 2 hours. In patients who survive for more than 2 hours the prognosis with standard anticoagulant therapy is usually excellent. Thrombolytic therapy produces rapid lysis of pulmonary emboli and helps patients with cardiorespiratory decompensation by promoting more rapid resolution of the pulmonary emboli during the first few days than does standard anticoagulant therapy. Thrombectomy or catheter-directed clot disruption may be required in selected patients with acute massive pulmonary embolism who have contraindications to thrombolytic therapy.

Inferior vena caval filter. Indications for the insertion of an inferior vena caval filter include the following:

1. In the patient with acute venous thromboembolism and an absolute contraindication to anticoagulant therapy (Box 85-2)
2. In the rare patient with massive pulmonary embolism who survives but in whom recurrent embolism may be fatal
3. In the very rare patient who has objectively documented recurrent venous thromboembolism during adequate anticoagulant therapy

The inferior vena caval filters in current use are associated with few complications and can be readily inserted through the femoral or jugular venous route.

MANAGEMENT OF SUPERFICIAL THROMBOPHLEBITIS

Superficial thrombophlebitis may occur with or without associated deep venous thrombosis. In the absence of associated deep vein thrombosis the treatment of superficial thrombophlebitis is usually confined to symptomatic relief with analgesia and rest of the affected limb. The exception is the patient with superficial thrombophlebitis involving a large segment of the long saphenous vein, particularly when it occurs above the knee; these patients should be treated with either heparin therapy or superficial venous ligation.

Patients in whom superficial thrombophlebitis occurs in association with deep vein thrombosis should be treated with full-dose heparin therapy followed by long-term oral anticoagulant therapy (see previous sections on heparin protocol and oral anticoagulant protocol).

ARTERIAL THROMBOEMBOLISM
Etiology and Pathogenesis

Arterial thrombi (white thrombi) are composed predominantly of platelets and fibrin, in contrast to venous thrombi (red thrombi), which consist primarily of red blood cells and fibrin. Arterial thromboemboli usually occur when platelets come into contact with exposed subendothelium at the site of vascular injury or with a prosthetic surface. The platelets adhere, undergo the release reaction, and aggregate; if these aggregates are sufficiently large or if the atherosclerotic stenosis is severe, an occlusive thrombus may form. Frequently, however, the platelet aggregates embolize to obstruct the arterial circulation distally. Thus the clinical manifestations of arterial thromboembolism may be the result of occlusive thrombus formation (e.g., acute coronary thrombosis), which usually occurs on a background of ruptured or ulcerated atherosclerotic plaque, or the result of peripheral embolization of platelet-fibrin aggregates (e.g., transient cerebral ischemic attacks).

Systemic embolism is an important clinical sequela of arterial thrombosis. Prosthetic cardiac valves, prosthetic vascular grafts, and implanted catheters are sites for arterial thrombus formation and are

important sources of systemic emboli. The introduction of a prosthetic material into the circulation exposes blood to a foreign surface that may induce platelet adhesion, aggregation, and embolization of the aggregated platelets. Furthermore, foreign surfaces may induce the activation of blood coagulation. Systemic embolism also occurs from left ventricular thrombi that form as a result of transmural myocardial infarction. Atrial fibrillation and valvular heart disease (e.g., rheumatic mitral stenosis) may also lead to systemic embolism (Chapter 25). Thrombi originating in the right side of the heart or on the surface of central venous catheters may lead to pulmonary embolism.

The various risk factors for atherosclerosis and arterial thromboembolism that have been identified include age, sex, hypertension, diabetes mellitus, smoking, obesity, hypercholesterolemia, and the inherited hyperlipidemic disorders.

A tendency to arterial thrombosis, which may be massive, may be seen in patients with the anticardiolipin syndrome or in those in whom heparin-induced thrombocytopenia and thrombosis develop.

Clinical Features

The clinical manifestations of arterial thromboembolism are organ specific and depend on the particular area of the circulation affected.

Atherosclerotic narrowing of the coronary arteries with ruptured or ulcerated plaque may lead to thrombus formation; if a sufficient area of the lumen is occluded, myocardial infarction may result (Chapter 23). Left ventricular mural thrombosis frequently complicates the course of patients with transmural anterior myocardial infarction and poses the risk of systemic embolism.

Severe atherosclerosis of the carotid artery may progress to thrombotic occlusion and subsequent cerebrovascular accident (CVA, stroke); the junction of the vertebral and basilar arteries and the main bifurcation of the middle cerebral artery are also common sites for thrombosis (Chapter 144). Atherosclerotic narrowing of the carotid arteries may serve as a nidus for repeated formation and embolization of platelet aggregates to the cerebral circulation or to the eye. Repeated "showers" of platelet-fibrin emboli result in transient, reversible episodes of cerebral ischemia or episodes of amaurosis fugax (Chapter 144). These emboli usually lyse and disperse spontaneously, with resolution of the neurologic deficit during a period of hours.

Atherosclerosis frequently affects the large- to medium-sized arteries of the lower limbs (e.g., distal aorta; iliac, femoral, and popliteal arteries); these lesions may serve as foci for the development of occlusive thrombi or as a source of distal embolization. Acute thrombotic occlusion of the large- or medium-sized arteries of the leg results in limb-threatening ischemia; untreated, it may progress to ischemic necrosis. Distal embolization of platelet-fibrin thrombi from the proximal arteries of the leg may result in multiple discrete areas of localized tissue necrosis.

For a detailed discussion of the clinical features associated with atherosclerosis and thromboembolism in the coronary arteries, cerebral vasculature, and peripheral vessels, see Chapters 22, 144, and 31, respectively.

Laboratory Features

A variety of laboratory abnormalities have been reported in patients with arterial thromboembolism, including elevated plasma levels of beta thromboglobulin and platelet factor 4 (indicating that platelets have undergone the release reaction) and elevated plasma levels of thromboxane B_2 (indicating that the platelet prostaglandin pathway has been activated). The continuous process of platelet adhesion, aggregation, and embolization may result in an increased platelet turnover (decreased survival), which can be detected by measuring the survival of isotopically labeled platelets injected intravenously. Although these laboratory tests have been useful research techniques that have provided important information about the pathophysiology of arterial thromboembolic disease, they currently have no role in patient management. Furthermore, these laboratory changes are nonspecific because many nonthrombogenic stimuli (e.g., trauma, infection, inflammation, infarction) may interact with platelets, inducing platelet release and prostaglandin formation and producing decreased platelet survival.

Treatment

Role of Anticoagulant Therapy. The objective of treating patients with arterial thromboembolism with anticoagulants is to prevent the clinical sequelae that occur as a consequence of thrombosis and systemic embolism. Historically the role of anticoagulants in the treatment of patients with arterial thromboembolism has been less certain than in the setting of venous thromboembolic disease. More recently, however, clinical trials have confirmed that anticoagulants also have a major role in patients with arterial thromboembolism, such as patients with unstable angina and myocardial infarction, and for preventing systemic embolism in patients with atrial fibrillation or prosthetic cardiac valves.

Antiplatelet agents, primarily acetylsalicylic acid (ASA), have been used in patients with cardiovascular diseases as an adjunct to thrombolytic therapy, in the prevention of myocardial infarction in patients with unstable angina, as secondary prophylaxis after an initial myocardial infarction, and as primary prophylaxis. When compared with placebo or no treatment, ASA has been shown to be superior in all these situations. A metaanalysis performed by the Antiplatelet Trialists Collaboration Group reviewed 25 randomized trials of antiplatelet treatment in patients with a history of transient ischemic attacks, occlusive CVA, unstable angina, or myocardial infarction. Vascular mortality and occurrence of a nonfatal vascular event (CVA or myocardial infarction) were reduced. The addition of dipyridamole to aspirin had no benefit.

Recent data indicate that both anticoagulants and antiplatelet agents will have an important place in the management of patients with arterial thromboembolism. Further, both pathophysiologic evidence and clinical trial data exist, supporting the concept that combined anticoagulant and antiplatelet therapy may be preferred in certain clinical settings of arterial thromboembolism. The relative roles of anticoagulants, antiplatelet agents, and combined treatment in the different clinical syndromes of arterial thrombosis is currently undergoing extensive evaluation by clinical trials. The role of anticoagulant therapy in the management of individual clinical disorders of arterial thromboembolism is discussed in the next sections.

Traditionally patients with arterial thromboembolism have received treatment using a more intense oral anticoagulant regimen (PT 2.0 to 2.5 using rabbit brain thromboplastin, INR 4.0 to 10.0) than that used with patients with venous thromboembolism. Randomized clinical trials support the use of a less intense therapeutic range (INR 2.0 to 3.0) for the prevention of systemic embolism in patients with myocardial infarction, atrial fibrillation, and bioprosthetic cardiac valves.

Myocardial Infarction. Anticoagulant therapy was recommended as part of the routine management of patients with myocardial infarction in the 1950s but later fell into disrepute because of the fear of bleeding complications and doubt about its effectiveness. The objectives of anticoagulant treatment in patients with myocardial infarction are (1) to improve survival; (2) to prevent recurrent infarction, mural thrombosis, and systemic embolism; and (3) to prevent the complication of venous thromboembolism (Chapter 23). Although there is consensus that anticoagulant therapy should be used for preventing systemic embolism, the use of long-term anticoagulant therapy for improving survival and preventing recurrent infarction has been controversial. The findings of recurrent randomized clinical trials have reopened this long-standing debate and have rekindled interest in the role of long-term anticoagulant therapy after myocardial infarction. The Sixty-Plus Reinfarction Study Research Group reported a 50% reduction in fatal and nonfatal reinfarction in elderly patients (over 60 years of age) who received treatment with long-term oral anticoagulant therapy after myocardial infarction. In a more recent trial warfarin treatment was associated with a 24% reduction in total mortality over 3 years (from 20% to 15.5%). The beneficial effect of warfarin persisted in patients who were also taking beta blockers on a long-term basis. Both trials evaluating long-term warfarin therapy after myocardial infarction used relatively intense warfarin therapy (INR 2.7 to 4.8), and trials are currently under way using less intense warfarin or very-low-intensity warfarin plus low-dose ASA (aspirin) in this setting.

Anticoagulant therapy is effective for preventing systemic embolism in patients with myocardial infarction. Cerebral embolism occurs in 2% to 4% of nonanticoagulated patients after myocardial in-farction. Patients with transmural anterior myocardial infarction are at particularly high risk of mural thrombosis (30%) and systemic embolism (2% to 6%) and should be treated with anticoagulant therapy for the period of risk. Full-dose continuous IV heparin followed by warfarin sodium for 3 months to up to 1 year is a current practical regimen. Further studies are required to establish definitively the most appropriate duration of anticoagulant therapy. Heparin is administered in full therapeutic doses to maintain the APTT at 1.5 to 2.0 times the control value; the protocol for heparin administration and the adverse effects of heparin are the same as those outlined previously for the treatment of venous thromboembolism. Therapeutic doses of heparin are used because the effectiveness of low-dose SC heparin for preventing systemic embolism is currently uncertain. Warfarin sodium is overlapped with IV heparin for 4 or 5 days and then continued long-term. Warfarin is administered according to the protocol outlined previously for venous thromboembolism to maintain the INR between 2.0 and 3.0.

The application of thrombolytic therapy in the management of patients with acute myocardial infarction has been the subject of intensive investigation in recent years. Intravenous thrombolysis is effective for inducing coronary thrombolysis and reperfusion and reducing mortality in patients with acute myocardial infarction. Recent clinical trials have also clarified the relative roles of streptokinase, tPA, and the anisoylated-plasminogen-streptokinase activator complex (APSAC) in patients with myocardial infarction. Anticoagulant therapy with IV heparin has an important role as adjunctive treatment to thrombolysis with tPA. Clinical trials are currently evaluating the relative roles of IV heparin and the direct thrombin inhibitor, recombinant hirudin, as adjunctive treatment to thrombolysis in patients with acute myocardial infarction. For further details on thrombolytic therapy of acute myocardial infarction see Chapter 23.

Unstable angina. Both antiplatelet therapy with aspirin and anticoagulant therapy with IV heparin are effective for preventing myocardial infarction in patients with acute unstable angina. Intravenous heparin is more effective than aspirin for reducing the incidence of refractory angina in patients who have received optimal antianginal therapy. Recent clinical trial data in patients with unstable angina and non–Q-wave myocardial infarction indicate that combined treatment with IV heparin and aspirin is more effective than aspirin alone for reducing the composite outcome of new myocardial infarction, death, or recurrent ischemia. A recent metaanalysis suggests a 56% risk reduction in the incidence of myocardial infarction for patients treated with combined IV heparin and aspirin compared with those who receive aspirin alone. Thus treatment with both aspirin and IV heparin is indicated for patients with unstable angina. In patients who receive heparin alone, there is a 13% incidence of myocardial infarction or recurrent unstable angina between 2 and 18 hours after stopping heparin; these events are prevented when aspirin is given concurrently with heparin and continued after heparin is stopped. Thus patients with unstable angina should receive aspirin (160 to 325 mg/day) as soon as possible, and also IV heparin adjusted to maintain the APTT between 1.5 to 2.0 times the control. Heparin should be continued for 3 to 4 days or longer if needed, until the unstable pain pattern resolves. Low-molecular-weight heparin is currently being evaluated by clinical trials in patients with unstable angina. Low-molecular-weight heparin may be potentially more effective and safer and is more practical than IV heparin, with the potential for continued treatment for weeks to months on an outpatient basis. The role of long-term treatment with warfarin is currently uncertain.

Atrial fibrillation. Atrial fibrillation is an important independent risk factor for systemic (cerebral) embolism. The prevalence of atrial fibrillation increases with age and rises sharply after the age of 65 years. About 50% of all patients with atrial fibrillation are over the age of 75. In the past, atrial fibrillation was most commonly found in patients with rheumatic valvular heart disease, and it was erroneously believed that antithrombotic therapy was not required among patients with nonvalvular atrial fibrillation. This belief has now been shown to be incorrect. The effectiveness of warfarin treatment for reducing the incidence of stroke among patients with nonvalvular atrial fibrillation has been unequivocally established by the findings of randomized clinical trials performed over the past 10 years. It is estimated that atrial fibrillation is the cause of about 10% of all strokes in the United States. Anticoagulant therapy with warfarin reduces the risk of stroke by two thirds among patients with atrial fibrillation. The appropriate application of this anticoagulant therapy to patients with atrial fibrillation could have a marked impact on the disease burden from stroke in the community and could prevent 30,000 to 40,000 strokes each year in the United States.

The relative benefits and risks of treatment with warfarin or aspirin, particularly in elderly individuals, have been clarified by a recent analysis of the data from clinical trials. The Atrial Fibrillation Investigators analyzed the pooled data from five randomized trials evaluating the effectiveness and safety of warfarin or aspirin. Warfarin consistently decreased the risk of stroke (a 68% risk reduction) with a low risk (1.3% annually) of major bleeding. The evidence for the effectiveness of aspirin was less consistent than for warfarin.

The European atrial fibrillation trial compared the effectiveness and safety of warfarin, aspirin, and placebo for stroke prevention in patients with atrial fibrillation who had had a recent stroke or transient ischemic attack. The warfarin dose was adjusted to achieve an INR of 2.5 and the aspirin dose was 300 mg/day. Warfarin was more effective than aspirin and resulted in a 60% risk reduction in annual stroke rate (from 10% to 4% annually).

The Stroke Prevention and Atrial Fibrillation (SPAF) II trial provided new information regarding the risks of intracranial hemorrhage in very elderly patients (greater than 75 years of age) with atrial fibrillation. These patients are at increased risk of intracranial bleeding with warfarin but are also at substantially higher risk of embolic stroke than younger patients. The SPAF II trial evaluated the target therapeutic range for warfarin approximately equivalent to an INR of 2.0 to 4.5. The mean INR value for the 13 patients who had intracranial hemorrhage with warfarin in this trial was 3.5. It is possible that a tighter, less intense range (INR of 2.0 to 3.0) would have been associated with a lower rate of intracranial bleeding in these elderly patients. The earlier trials evaluated treatment within a narrower, less intense INR range (INR 1.4 to 3.0). Among the patients greater than 75 years of age in these clinical trials the annual rate of intracranial bleeding was only 0.3%.

Antithrombotic therapy is indicated for most patients with atrial fibrillation. Antithrombotic therapy is indicated for all patients older than 65 years, and for patients younger than 65 who have any of the following risk factors: a previous transient ischemic attack (TIA) or stroke, hypertension, heart failure, diabetes, clinical coronary disease, mitral stenosis, or thyrotoxicosis. The exception to the need for antithrombotic therapy may be patients less than 65 years of age without any of the preceding risk factors, but this group makes up less than 5% of all patients with atrial fibrillation.

Warfarin is the antithrombotic regimen of choice for most patients. The recommended therapeutic range is an INR of 2.0 to 3.0. Aspirin (325 mg/day) is indicated for patients in whom warfarin is contraindicated. Age alone should not be a contraindication to warfarin. Warfarin treatment should be monitored closely and the INR kept below 3.0, particularly in the very elderly. Ongoing clinical trials should further clarify the role of aspirin and combined therapy with very-low-dose warfarin and aspirin, as well as the optimal intensity of warfarin treatment. Ambulatory patients with atrial fibrillation can be started on warfarin therapy without the need for concurrent heparin treatment, and clinical trials support the safety of this approach in patients who have no ongoing thrombotic process (e.g., left atrial or mural thrombus).

Prosthetic Cardiac Valves. The goal of anticoagulant therapy in patients with artificial cardiac valves is to prevent thrombus formation on the valve surface and subsequent systemic embolism (Chapters 25 and 144). In the absence of anticoagulant treatment patients with prosthetic cardiac valves have a yearly risk of systemic embolism of approximately 5% to 30% or more, depending on the type of valve and its position. Mechanical valves are associated with a higher frequency of systemic embolism than are tissue (bioprosthetic) valves. Mitral prosthetic valves are associated with a greater risk of systemic embolism than are aortic valves. The risk of systemic embolism is increased by the presence of coexistent atrial fibrillation. The frequency of systemic embolism in anticoagulated patients with mechanical valves is approximately 4% per year for valves in the mitral position and 2% per year for aortic placement.

The clinical practice of treatment of patients with prosthetic heart valves with long-term oral anticoagulant therapy is now well established. The use of warfarin sodium to maintain an INR of 2.0 to 3.0 is the standard approach for patients with bioprosthetic (tissue) valves. In the past an INR of 3.0 to 4.5 has been recommended for patients with mechanical valves. Clinical trials indicate that less intense regimens of warfarin alone (INR 1.9 to 3.6) or warfarin (INR 2.0 to 3.0) plus ASA and dipyridamole are associated with fewer bleeding complications and may be as effective as the traditional, more intense therapy. The addition of aspirin, 100 mg/day, to warfarin (INR 3.0 to 4.5), when compared with warfarin alone, resulted in a marked reduction in mortality and systemic embolism without an increase in major bleeding or cerebral hemorrhage. The optimal intensity of warfarin treatment, either alone or in combination with aspirin, in patients with mechanical valves is currently uncertain. Ongoing clinical trials will determine whether combined warfarin and aspirin treatment at less intense INR ranges (INR 2.0 to 2.5) will retain efficacy, with a reduced incidence of bleeding complications. At present the approach that maximizes efficacy for preventing systemic embolism and for survival is warfarin maintained at an INR of 3.0 to 4.5, combined with aspirin in a dose of 100 mg/day.

The risk of bleeding complications associated with long-term anticoagulant therapy in patients with prosthetic heart valves has been reported to range from 1% to 40%. Major bleeding ranged from 0% to 7%, and fatal bleeding from 0% to 4.1%. The addition of aspirin to warfarin increases the risk of bleeding. However, when low doses of aspirin are used (100 mg/day), this increase is due mainly to minor bleeding episodes, without an increase in major bleeding. The combined approach of warfarin at an INR of 3.0 to 4.5 plus aspirin 100 mg/day is associated with major bleeding at a rate of 4% per year, but this is offset by clinically important risk reductions in the rate of systemic embolism and mortality from all causes.

In pregnant patients with prosthetic heart valves, SC heparin in therapeutic doses (e.g., 15,000 U every 12 hours) that maintain the APTT to 1.5 to 2.0 times the control value is a practical anticoagulant regimen that avoids the risk of fetopathic effects associated with warfarin therapy during pregnancy. To date, however, the effectiveness of this regimen for preventing systemic embolism in patients with prosthetic valves has not been formally evaluated by randomized clinical trials. A recent study indicates that lower doses of SC heparin (5000 U every 12 hours) are ineffective in preventing valve thrombosis and systemic embolism in pregnant women with prosthetic cardiac valves. The use of long-term SC heparin exposes the patient to the potential risk of osteoporosis (see previous section on adverse effects of heparin).

Cerebrovascular Disease. For practical purposes, patients with thromboembolic cerebrovascular disease can be divided into the following categories: (1) those with attacks of transient cerebral ischemia, (2) those with CVA-in-evolution (progressing thrombotic CVA), and (3) those who have had a completed CVA (thrombotic infarction).

The aim of treating patients who have had TIAs with anticoagulants is to prevent further episodes of transient cerebral ischemia, prevent CVA, and to improve survival (Chapter 144). The use of anticoagulant therapy in patients with TIAs is highly controversial because of doubt about its effectiveness and the fear of bleeding complications. Further clinical trials are required to establish definitively the role of anticoagulant treatment in patients with TIAs. Antiplatelet therapy with aspirin is partially effective for preventing CVA and death in patients with TIAs. Ticlopidine is more effective than aspirin but has more nonhemorrhagic side effects and causes severe neutropenia in 1% of patients.

In patients with CVA-in-evolution the objectives of treatment with anticoagulants are to arrest the thrombotic process, prevent its progression to completed infarction, and improve survival. The effectiveness of IV heparin for these purposes is currently uncertain. Recent data indicate that thrombolysis with rtPA and anticoagulant therapy with low-molecular-weight heparin are effective approaches for reducing the proportion of patients with CVA-in-evolution who end up with permanent major disability. In patients with completed CVA, anticoagulant therapy is without benefit and is potentially dangerous.

Review of the published literature indicates that the risk of bleeding complications associated with long-term anticoagulant therapy in patients with established cerebrovascular disease ranges from 12% to 40% (mean, 29%). It is important that the risk of fatal bleeding ranges from 2% to 7% (mean, 5%); most fatal bleeding episodes are caused by intracranial hemorrhage. The risk of cerebral bleeding is increased approximately 2.5-fold in patients with documented hypertension.

Because of the lack of effectiveness and the documented high risk of both fatal bleeding and serious major hemorrhage, long-term anticoagulant therapy should be reserved for patients who have systemic embolism and should not be used routinely for preventing further episodes of arterial thrombosis and CVA in patients with established cerebrovascular disease.

Peripheral Vascular Disease. The role of anticoagulant therapy in the management of patients with arterial occlusive disease of the legs is limited. Anticoagulant therapy is effective in preventing recurrent distal embolism in patients with acute arterial occlusion. Continuous IV heparin (see previous heparin protocol) should be commenced immediately in patients with acute arterial occlusion of the limb and continued postembolectomy until full therapeutic oral anticoagulation with warfarin is accomplished (see next section). The role of long-term anticoagulant therapy in the management of patients with intermittent claudication or ischemic rest pain is uncertain. Anticoagulant therapy may be effective in improving the long-term patency of peripheral arterial bypass procedures (e.g., femoropopliteal bypass), particularly procedures involving prosthetic graft materials, but further studies are required to adequately assess its role in this context. A recent randomized trial suggests that long-term oral anticoagulant therapy improves survival after femoropopliteal bypass surgery by reducing mortality from associated cardiovascular disease (e.g., coronary artery disease).

Recurrent Systemic Embolism. Anticoagulant therapy is effective in preventing recurrent embolism in patients who have had an episode of systemic embolism. Recurrent embolism occurs early in the clinical course of patients with systemic embolism. In the absence of anticoagulant therapy, approximately 10% to 15% of patients with cerebral embolism from a defined source have a second embolic event within 2 weeks. For this reason, anticoagulant therapy should be commenced immediately once a diagnosis of systemic embolism is established. In patients with cerebral embolism, computed tomographic scanning should be performed immediately and before commencing anticoagulant therapy to exclude the presence of hemorrhagic infarction.

Full-dose continuous IV heparin is the preferred approach to achieve an immediate and sustained anticoagulant effect; the heparin dose is adjusted to maintain the APTT at 1.5 to 2.0 times the control. The protocol for administering heparin is the same as that outlined previously for the treatment of venous thromboembolism. Heparin therapy is continued for 5 to 6 days and is followed by long-term oral anticoagulant therapy, with warfarin sodium adjusted to maintain the INR between 2.0 and 3.0.

BIBLIOGRAPHY

Anderson FA, Wheeler HB, Goldberg RJ et al: A population-based perspective of the hospital incidence and case-fatality rates of deep vein thrombosis and pulmonary embolism, *Arch Intern Med* 151:933, 1991.

Boston Area Anticoagulation Trial for Atrial Fibrillation Investigators: The effect of low-dose warfarin on the risk of stroke in patients with nonrheumatic atrial fibrillation, *N Engl J Med* 323:1505, 1990.

Brill-Edwards P, Ginsberg JS, Johnston M, Hirsh J: Establishing a therapeutic range for heparin, *Ann Intern Med* 119:104, 1993.

Cruickshank MK, Levine MN, Hirsh J et al: A standard nomogram for the management of heparin therapy, *Arch Intern Med* 151:333, 1991.

Dahlback B: New molecular insights into the genetics of thrombophilia: Resistance to activated protein C caused by Arg (506) to Gln mutation in factor V as a pathogenic risk factor for venous thrombosis, *Thromb Hemost* 74:138, 1995.

Gallus AS, Jackaman J, Tillett J et al: Safety and efficacy of warfarin started early after submassive venous thrombosis or pulmonary embolism, *Lancet* 2:1293, 1986.

Goldhaber SZ, Agnelli G, Levine MN: Bolus Alteplase pulmonary embolism group: Reduced-dose bolus Alteplase vs. conventional alteplase infusion for pulmonary embolism thrombolysis—an international multicentre randomized trial, *Chest* 106:718, 1994.

Hirsh J, Dalen JE, Daken D et al: Oral anticoagulants: mechanism of action, clinical effectiveness and optimal therapeutic range, *Chest* 108(4):231S, 1995.

Huisman MV, Buller HE, ten Cate JW et al: Serial impedance plethysmography for suspected deep-vein thrombosis in outpatients, *N Engl J Med* 314:823, 1986.

Hull RD, Delmore T, Carter C et al: Adjusted subcutaneous heparin versus warfarin sodium in the long-term treatment of venous thrombosis, *N Engl J Med* 306:189, 1982.

Hull RD, Raskob GE, Pineo GF et al: Subcutaneous low-molecular-weight heparin compared with continuous intravenous heparin in the treatment of proximal-vein thrombosis, *N Engl J Med* 326:975, 1992.

Hull RD, Hirsh J, Jay R et al: Different intensities of oral anticoagulant therapy in the treatment of proximal vein thrombosis, *N Engl J Med* 307:1676, 1982.

Hull RD, Raskob GE, Hirsh J et al: Continuous intravenous heparin compared with intermittent subcutaneous heparin in the initial treatment of proximal-vein thrombosis, *N Engl J Med* 315:1109, 1986.

Hull R, Raskob G, Rosenbloom D: Heparin for 5 days as compared with 10 days in the initial treatment of proximal venous thrombosis, *N Engl J Med* 322:1260, 1990.

Hull RD, Raskob GE, Rosenbloom DR et al: Optimal therapeutic levels of heparin therapy for patients with venous thrombosis, *Arch Intern Med* 152:1589, 1992.

Iturbe-Alessio I, del Carmen Fonseca M, Mutchinik O et al: Risks of anticoagulant therapy in pregnant women with artificial heart valves, *N Engl J Med* 315:1390, 1986.

Kakkar VV, Cohen AT, Edmonson RA et al: Low-molecular-weight versus standard heparin for prevention of venous thromboembolism after major abdominal surgery, *Lancet* 341:259, 1993.

Lansing AWA, Prins MH, Davidson BL, Hirsh J: Treatment of deep venous thrombosis with low-molecular-weight heparins, *Arch Intern Med* 155:601, 1995.

Pineo GF, Hull RD: Adverse effects of coumarin anticoagulants, *Drug Safety* 9(4):263, 1993.

Raschke RA, Reilly BM, Guidry JR et al: The weight-based heparin dosing nomogram compared with a "standard care" nomogram, *Ann Intern Med* 119:874, 1993.

Saour JN, Sieck JO, Mamo LAR et al: Trial of different intensities of anticoagulation in patients with prosthetic heart valves, *N Engl J Med* 322:428, 1990.

Schulman S, Rhedin AS, Lindmarker P et al: A comparison of 6 weeks with 6 months of oral anticoagulant therapy after a first episode of venous thromboembolism, *N Engl J Med* 332:1661, 1995.

Smith P, Arneson H, Holme I et al: The effect of warfarin on mortality and reinfarction after myocardial infarction, *N Engl J Med* 323:147, 1990.

Turpie AGG, Gunstensen J, Hirsh J et al: Randomized comparison of two intensities of oral anticoagulant therapy after tissue heart valve replacement, *Lancet* 1:242, 1988.

Warkentin TE, Levine MN, Hirsh J et al: Heparin-induced thrombocytopenia in patients treated with low-molecular-weight heparin or unfractionated heparin, *N Engl J Med* 332:1330, 1995.

Wells P, Hirsh J, Anderson D et al: Accuracy of clinical assessment of deep vein thrombosis, *Lancet* 345:1326, 1995.

Wells P, Holbrook AM, Crowther R, Hirsh J: Warfarin and its drug/food interactions: a critical appraisal of the literature, *Ann Intern Med* 121:676, 1994.

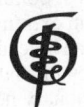

86 Iron Deficiency Anemia, Anemia of Chronic Disease, Sideroblastic Anemia, and Iron Overload

Robert T. Means, Jr.

NORMAL PHYSIOLOGY OF IRON REGULATION
Iron Absorption

For normal individuals the total iron content of the body is fairly constant, being approximately 50 mg/kg in men and 37 mg/kg in women. This homeostasis is maintained by regulation of iron absorption from the gastrointestinal tract. The average amount of iron absorbed from the diet reflects daily iron losses: 0.6 mg daily for men and 1.2 mg daily for women (the difference reflects the need to replace iron lost in menses). A number of dietary factors and local conditions in the gastrointestinal tract influence iron absorption. Iron in the form of myoglobin or other heme compounds is readily absorbed into the intestinal mucosa and bound to transferrin at the serosal surface. Non-heme iron must be taken up by the intestinal brush border epithelium and borne through the cell by specific intracellular carrier proteins before delivery to transferrin at the serosal surface. Gastric acidity enhances iron absorption, as does administration of ferrous as opposed to ferric iron salts. Obviously, surgical resection of the duodenum or proximal jejunum (the sites of iron absorption) or local inflammation will reduce iron absorption. The status of iron stores influences the rate of iron absorption. Iron-deficient individuals absorb a greater proportion of dietary iron than do iron-replete persons.

Iron Stores and Iron Mobilization

Absorbed iron not taken up by transferrin remains in the mucosal cell and is lost when the mucosal cell sloughs off into the intestinal lumen. Transferrin is the primary iron transport protein in the blood and delivers iron from the mucosal cell either to the marrow for incorporation into erythroid precursors or to storage. Storage iron mobilized for erythropoiesis is also carried by transferrin.

In the human body the vast majority of iron is in the form of hemoglobin in red blood cells (31 mg iron/kg in men and 27 mg iron/kg in women). Five to six milligrams of iron per kg is stored in structural proteins such as myoglobin or enzymes of intermediary metabolism such as the cytochromes. The remainder (13 mg/kg in men and 4 mg/kg in women) is stored as either hemosiderin or ferritin in the reticuloendothelial cells of the bone marrow, liver, and spleen and in the liver parenchyma. These molecules provide the basis for two of the most useful tests for evaluating iron stores: Prussian blue staining of tissue reveals hemosiderin iron, and the serum ferritin level is generally indicative of reticuloendothelial iron status. Iron may be readily mobilized from either hemosiderin or ferritin for erythropoiesis.

Iron for erythropoiesis is delivered to the erythroid precursors by transferrin. A fully saturated transferrin molecule carries two iron atoms. The iron-transferrin complex binds to a specific receptor and undergoes endocytosis. Efficiency of this process is enhanced by regulation of transferrin receptor affinity: fully saturated transferrin is bound with high affinity, monoferric transferrin with lower affinity, and iron-free transferrin (apotransferrin) with least affinity. In addition, the number of transferrin receptors per erythroid precursor is significantly increased in iron deficiency.

The life span of a red blood cell under normal conditions is 120 days. At the end of this period, the senescent cell is phagocytosed by the reticuloendothelial system, and the hemoglobin iron extracted and recycled for either storage or erythropoiesis. This process is not perfectly efficient, so a small amount of iron is lost in the recycling process and must be absorbed from the diet. This recycling loss, as well as the minute quantities of iron lost when dead skin or mucosal cells are sloughed, makes up the daily iron requirement.

ANEMIAS ASSOCIATED WITH DECREASED SERUM IRON LEVELS
Etiology and Pathophysiology

Iron Deficiency Anemia. Iron deficiency is the most common cause of anemia encountered in clinical medicine and is an extremely significant epidemiologic problem in developing nations. The causes of iron deficiency anemia are listed in Box 86-1. Although malabsorptive syndromes and more exotic entities such as pulmonary hemorrhage (such as is seen in Goodpasture's syndrome) and hemosiderinuria from intravascular hemolysis may result in iron deficiency, it cannot be too strongly emphasized that the overwhelming majority of cases of iron deficiency in Western adults result from blood loss. This blood loss may result from a physiologic process as in menses or pregnancy, from a pathologic state such as gastrointestinal malignancy or angiodysplasia, or from iatrogenic causes such as blood loss associated with surgery or hemodialysis.

The degree of iron depletion can be estimated from the volume of blood lost. One milliliter of red blood cells represents approximately 1 mg of iron. For example, a women with a hematocrit of 40% who loses 50 ml of blood during the menstrual cycle loses 20 mg iron (50 ml blood × 0.40 ml red blood cells/ml blood × 1 mg iron/ml red blood cells). Divided over the 28 days of the menstrual cycle, the additional iron required as a result of this blood loss (0.7 mg/day) accounts for the difference between the iron requirements of men and women. The same calculation can be made using the hemoglobin concentration (hemoglobin is 0.35% iron by weight), but the numbers are less easy to remember.

Gestational iron deficiency deserves special mention. An uncomplicated, full-term vaginal delivery is associated with a loss of approximately 850 mg iron, and 85% of women who do not receive iron supplements during pregnancy have no detectable marrow iron stores. For these reasons, iron supplementation should be administered during pregnancy.

BOX 86-1
Causes of iron deficiency anemia

I. Blood loss
  A. Menstrual
  B. Gastrointestinal
    1. Stomach
      a. Hiatal hernia
      b. Esophageal varices
      c. Peptic ulcer disease
      d. Acute gastritis
      e. Drugs
      f. Carcinoma of the stomach
    2. Large bowel
      a. Carcinoma of the colon/rectum
      b. Benign polyps
      c. Angiodysplasia
      d. Diverticular disease
      e. Ulcerative colitis
    3. Small bowel
      a. Hookworm
      b. Crohn's disease
      c. Milk allergy
  C. Iatrogenic
    1. Blood donation
    2. Phlebotomy (diagnostic or therapeutic)
    3. Surgery/procedures
    4. Hemodialysis
  D. Other
    1. Epistaxis
    2. Hematuria
    3. Coagulopathy
    4. Decubitus ulcers
II. Malabsorption
  A. Achlorhydria
  B. Total gastrectomy
  C. Gastrojejunostomy
  D. Celiac disease and spruelike syndromes
  E. Pica
III. Inadequate intake or increased requirements
  A. Dietary (rare)
  B. Pregnancy and lactation
  C. Growth and development
IV. Miscellaneous
  A. Pulmonary hemorrhage
  B. Hemosiderinuria (usually secondary to intravascular hemolysis)

Most individuals with iron deficiency anemia are asymptomatic, and symptoms that do occur are related to the degree of anemia. In rats, iron deficiency results in depletion of iron-containing enzymes and in reduced exercise capacity independent of the degree of anemia; however, it is not clear that these findings apply in humans. In a recent study the exercise tolerance and maximal oxygen consumption did not differ between nonanemic iron-deficient college students and iron-replete students.

Anemia of Chronic Disease. The anemia of chronic disease is traditionally defined as the anemia associated with chronic infectious diseases such as tuberculosis or infective endocarditis, chronic inflammatory diseases such as rheumatoid arthritis, or neoplasms. However, new insights into its pathophysiology have suggested that it may be observed in any disorder associated with cytokine activation (Box 86-2). The anemia of chronic disease is second in frequency only to iron deficiency as a cause of anemia. After gastrointestinal bleeding, hemolysis, and hematologic malignancies were excluded, 52% of anemic patients admitted to the medical wards of a county hospital met laboratory criteria for this syndrome. It is also observed in approximately 25% of outpatients in rheumatology clinics.

The disorders associated with the anemia of chronic disease share the common feature of cytokine activation, either as a primary result of the disease (as with cytokine secretion by myeloma cells) or as

BOX 86-2

Diseases associated with the anemia of chronic disease

Acute infections
Bacterial, fungal, or viral

Chronic infections
Tuberculosis
Infective endocarditis
Osteomyelitis
Human immunodeficiency virus
Chronic urinary tract infection
Chronic fungal diseases (histoplasmosis and others)

Chronic noninfectious inflammatory disorders
Rheumatoid arthritis
Collagen vascular diseases
Polymyalgia rheumatica
Decubitus ulcer
Sarcoidosis
Other inflammatory arthropathies

Malignancy
Disseminated nonhematologic malignancies
Lymphoproliferative malignancies

BOX 86-3

Pathophysiologic processes in anemia of chronic disease

Shortened red blood cell survival
Impaired marrow response to shortened red blood cell survival
Impaired erythropoietic activity
    Blunted erythropoietin response to anemia
    Inhibition of erythroid progenitor proliferation and differentiation
Impaired iron mobilization and utilization
    Shift of iron from transferrin to ferritin
    Impaired mobilization of reticuloendothelial iron stores
    Downregulation of transferrin receptors on erythroid precursors

part of the body's defensive response to the disease, such as in infections. The anemia of chronic disease results from the interplay of a number of pathophysiologic processes (Box 86-3). First, there is a modest shortening of red blood cell survival. Anemia develops because the marrow is unable to increase red blood cell production, because of direct inhibitory effects on erythropoiesis and erythropoietin production, and also because of impairment of iron mobilization from the reticuloendothelial system and of iron utilization by erythroid precursors. All of these processes are induced by the activation of cytokines such as tumor necrosis factor, interleukin-1, and γ-interferon.

In 75% of cases the anemia of chronic disease is a mild anemia with a hemoglobin level of 9 g/dl or greater or a hematocrit greater than 30%. In these cases the patients' symptoms are those of the associated disease rather than of the anemia. For the patients with more severe anemia, symptoms related to the reduced hematocrit may complicate those of the underlying chronic disease.

Laboratory Tests in the Evaluation of Anemias With Low Serum Iron Levels

Serum Iron, Total Iron Binding Capacity, and Total Iron Binding Capacity Saturation. A low serum iron level is characteristic of either iron deficiency or the anemia of chronic disease and, taken by itself, cannot distinguish the two syndromes. The serum iron level is most useful in association with the serum total iron binding capacity (TIBC), particularly when used to determine the TIBC saturation. (In some laboratories, the TIBC is expressed as serum transferrin concentration. For practical purposes the values are interchangeable.) Serum TIBC is typically elevated in iron deficiency and decreased in the anemia of chronic disease. Reduced TIBC saturation is characteristic of iron deficiency. TIBC saturation greater than 15% is not consistent with iron deficiency, while TIBC saturation less than 10% is strongly suggestive of iron deficiency. Certain caveats must be noted. Ingestion of iron tablets, transfusion, or hemolysis results in acute transient elevation of serum iron level and hence of TIBC saturation. Also, if the serum TIBC is less than the lower limit of normal (usually 200 ng/ml), a low TIBC saturation value is not dependable as a marker for iron deficiency.

Serum Ferritin. The serum ferritin level is the most useful chemical test for the evaluation of iron status. The serum ferritin level, in the absence of inflammation or cytokine activation, reflects the quantity of iron stored in the reticuloendothelial system. A low serum ferritin value (usually <20 ng/ml) is diagnostic of iron deficiency. However, the serum ferritin level may be elevated out of proportion to iron stores when cytokine activation is present. For this reason, iron deficiency cannot be ruled out by a normal serum ferritin level in patients with significant concurrent illness. An elevated serum ferritin level (>200 ng/ml) confirms that the patient has iron present. A review of the experience at the University of Cincinnati Medical Center evaluated patients who had had both serum ferritin determinations and histologic evaluation of bone marrow iron status. Using a low serum ferritin level as the indication of iron deficiency and serum ferritin level greater than 200 ng/ml as the indication for adequate iron stores resulted in a correct diagnosis in 73% of cases.

Mean Corpuscular Volume. Microcytosis, or a decreased mean corpuscular volume (MCV), is a characteristic feature of iron deficiency anemia. The decrease in MCV begins after iron stores are completely depleted and the hemoglobin concentration or hematocrit has begun to decline. Although red blood cells in the anemia of chronic disease are typically of normal size, 20% of patients with this syndrome exhibit microcytosis. The electronically determined MCV may be falsely elevated by processes resulting in red blood cell agglutination or aggregation, and patients with concurrent megaloblastic anemia and iron deficiency may exhibit a normal MCV.

Red Blood Cell Morphology. In the evaluation of anemia it is always useful to examine a Wright-stained peripheral blood smear. The peripheral blood smear in iron deficiency shows microcytic, hypochromic red blood cells with striking variation in size and shape (anisocytosis and poikilocytosis; see Plate IV-4B). This is in contrast to the relatively normal findings on blood smear observed in the anemia of chronic disease.

Erythrocyte Protoporphyrin. In the absence of adequate iron for erythropoiesis, protoporphyrin IX accumulates in erythrocytes. The free erythrocyte protoporphyrin level is elevated in iron deficiency, but also in the anemia of chronic disease.

Bone Marrow Examination. The gold standard for the identification of iron stores available for erythropoiesis is the examination of a bone marrow aspirate stained with Prussian blue. Iron appears as small blue granules in reticuloendothelial cells. Iron stains performed on a marrow core biopsy specimen may be less satisfactory, since a certain amount of iron may be chelated and removed during decalcification and processing of the biopsy specimen; however, there is generally a good correlation between aspirate and biopsy specimen.

Bone marrow examination yields other useful information as well. Iron-deficient marrow typically shows erythroid hyperplasia, while the marrow of patients with the anemia of chronic disease is either unremarkable or exhibits a slight, nonspecific increase in plasma cells and lymphocytes.

Other Tests. The reticulocyte response to anemia is increased in anemia caused by acute blood loss, but is decreased in the anemia of chronic disease and iron deficiency. The coefficient of variation of the red blood cell distribution width (RDW) is typically elevated in both iron deficiency and the anemia of chronic disease. An elevated platelet count is often observed in iron deficiency, particularly when it is the result of gastrointestinal blood loss.

As noted earlier, iron is taken up by erythroid precursors through the interaction of iron-bearing transferrin with specific cell surface receptors. The number of these receptors per cell increases in iron deficiency. The serum transferrin receptor concentration is directly related to the total mass of cellular transferrin receptors, and it has been observed that this value is significantly elevated in iron deficiency. This is the opposite of what is observed in the anemia of chronic disease. It has been proposed that the serum transferrin receptor concentration is a useful, sensitive, and specific test for iron deficiency; however, since serum transferrin receptor concentration is also elevated in conditions associated with reticulocytosis (such as hemolysis) or with marrow erythroid hyperplasia (such as vitamin B$_{12}$ or folate deficiency), its diagnostic utility remains to be demonstrated.

Changes in Laboratory Test Results in the Development of Iron Deficiency Anemia

Iron deficiency anemia evolves through three stages: iron depletion, iron-deficient erythropoiesis, and frank iron deficiency anemia. The stage of iron depletion is a period in which iron stores are depleted through blood loss. During this time (unless the blood loss is very brisk), the hematocrit and hemoglobin concentration remain normal, although with an elevated reticulocyte count, and the MCV remains normal. The serum iron and ferritin levels decrease, and the TIBC begins to rise, resulting in a decrease in TIBC saturation.

In the next stage, iron-deficient erythropoiesis, iron stores are depleted, but the quantity of iron contained in red blood cells as hemoglobin and the MCV are still normal. At the beginning of this phase, serum iron and ferritin values are below the lower limit of the normal range, and the TIBC saturation is 15% or less. The iron contained in red blood cells as hemoglobin is recycled by the reticuloendothelial system for use in erythropoiesis, but this process is not perfectly efficient, resulting in a steady decline in red blood cell hemoglobin production and in hematocrit and hemoglobin concentration. As the patient becomes anemic, the stage of frank iron deficiency anemia begins. The MCV is initially normal until the hemoglobin concentration falls below 13 g/dl in men or 11 g/dl in women, at which point microcytosis develops.

Differential Diagnosis

The differential here is between iron deficiency and the anemia of chronic disease. In simplest terms, iron deficiency is defined by the absence of reticuloendothelial iron stores, and the anemia of chronic disease by a low serum iron level with adequate or elevated iron stores. In most cases the two syndromes are easily distinguished

Table 86-1   Iron deficiency anemia versus anemia of chronic disease: typical features

	IRON DEFICIENCY	ANEMIA OF CHRONIC DISEASE
Serum iron level	Low	Low
Serum total iron binding capacity (TIBC)	Typically increased	Decreased
TIBC saturation	<10%	>16%
Serum ferritin level	Low	Normal or elevated
Mean corpuscular volume	Decreased	Normal (80% of cases)
Red blood cell distribution width	Elevated	Elevated
Free erythrocyte protoporphyrin	Elevated	Elevated
Serum transferrin receptor concentration	Increased	Normal
Marrow iron stores	Absent	Present

(Table 86-1). For example, anemia with microcytosis in a young woman of childbearing years is almost certainly iron deficiency. In the presence of significant concurrent illness, there may be confusion between these syndromes. In these cases the serum ferritin level may be elevated in the absence of iron stores, suppression of the TIBC may make the TIBC saturation useless for the diagnosis of iron deficiency, and microcytosis may be observed in the anemia of chronic disease. In these cases bone marrow examination for the definitive determination of iron status is required.

Management

Iron Deficiency Anemia. The management of iron deficiency anemia consists of two components: iron repletion and identification of the causes of iron deficiency. The diagnosis of iron deficiency should be clearly established prior to initiating iron therapy. A "therapeutic trial" of iron replacement should be used only in a setting where the probability of iron deficiency is extremely high: the menstruating or postpartum woman. Iron is most effectively replaced orally. The most inexpensive, safest, readily available source of iron replacement is the nonenteric-coated ferrous sulfate tablet. A 325-mg tablet contains 65 mg of elemental iron and should be administered three times daily, preferably on an empty stomach. On this regimen, reticulocytosis should be noted after 2 weeks (in the absence of ongoing blood loss), and increments in the hemoglobin concentration or hematocrit should be noted approximately 2 weeks after that.

Failure to respond to oral iron replacement typically reflects either poor compliance or a mistaken diagnosis. Ferrous sulfate therapy is associated with some upper abdominal discomfort and with constipation. The darkening of stools noted after 2 to 3 days of therapy provides a useful index of compliance. The abdominal discomfort associated with oral iron therapy can often be reduced by using an enteric-coated preparation or administering iron preparations with food; however, these maneuvers interfere with iron absorption and result in a slower response to therapy. Alternative iron salts, such as ferrous gluconate or ferrous fumarate, are available and may be better tolerated, but contain less iron per tablet and result in slower responses. Some patients who do not tolerate ferrous sulfate tablets respond well to ferrous sulfate elixir.

In the setting of iron deficiency, iron absorbed from the gastrointestinal tract is promptly utilized for erythropoiesis. Oral iron therapy should be continued for 3 to 6 months after correction of anemia to replete iron stores.

Intravenous iron dextran replacement may be indicated for the rare patient who fails to respond to oral iron therapy or who is truly unable to tolerate it. There is a small but real risk of anaphylaxis associated with this therapy, and virtually all patients experience a flushing sensation with or without an urticaria-like reaction, so its use must be undertaken carefully. The total iron deficit (the depleted stores plus the deficit in red blood cell hemoglobin iron) should be calculated prior to initiating therapy, to determine the total dose requirements. Replacement of the total iron deficit by a single dose or in a few large doses has been used safely for many years, but the manufacturers of this product currently recommend administration of much smaller quantities at short intervals. Premedication with diphenhydramine and acetaminophen is often useful. Administration of intravenous iron dextran does not result in a more rapid correction of anemia but does replete iron stores more rapidly. Intramuscular iron dextran should not be used, as only small quantities of iron can be administered, the injections are painful, and prolonged discoloration of the skin overlying the gluteal muscles results.

It should be emphasized that iron deficiency anemia is a syndrome, not a disease: the diagnosis of iron deficiency implies an obligation to identify a source of blood loss. In the menstruating or postpartum woman, iron deficiency can be attributed to menstrual or gestational blood loss, but a careful history and examination should still be carried out. In all men and in postmenopausal women, an origin or cause of blood loss must be sought, particularly in the gastrointestinal tract. More than 60% of iron-deficient patients have identifiable lesions in the upper (37%) or lower (26%) gastrointestinal tracts. Overall, an origin or cause of blood loss can be identified in more than 75% of carefully evaluated patients.

Anemia of Chronic Disease. For the most part, therapy of the anemia of chronic disease should be directed at the associated chronic disease. Iron therapy is not useful. For specific patients, particularly those who are sufficiently anemic to require transfusion or who wish to donate autologous blood for transfusion at elective surgery, recombinant human erythropoietin may be useful and has been shown to be effective.

SIDEROBLASTIC ANEMIAS

Sideroblastic anemia refers to a state of ineffective erythropoiesis characterized by the presence of significant numbers of erythroid precursors containing mitochondria with stainable iron granules, called ringed sideroblasts (Plate IV-11). These cells result from a disruption of mitochondrial heme synthesis, typically at point at which iron is incorporated into protoporphyrin IX. This results in iron accumulation in mitochondria and the characteristic morphologic finding on Prussian blue stain. In a number of circumstances, the cellular defect resulting in ringed sideroblast formation can be corrected by administration of pyridoxine, since pyridoxal-5-phosphate is a necessary cofactor for δ-aminolevulenic acid synthase, a key enzyme in the porphyrin pathway.

The sideroblastic anemias are classified in Box 86-4. It should be noted that very small numbers of ringed sideroblasts can be observed in a variety of states associated with bone marrow dysfunction; however, these sideroblasts appear to be a consequence of hematopoietic suppression and not a cause thereof, so they are not considered in this chapter.

Sideroblastic anemia may be suspected in patients who have anemia with microcytic red blood cells, elevated serum iron level, and elevated erythrocyte protoporphyrin value; however, the diagnosis requires the demonstration of ringed sideroblasts in a Prussian blue–stained marrow specimen, usually with significant erythroid hyperplasia.

✔ *WHEN TO REFER*

As discussed earlier, the diagnosis of iron deficiency anemia or the anemia of chronic disease can be made by any careful physician in most cases. Referrals may be required for patients requiring bone marrow examination for definitive diagnosis, for patients who do not respond to oral iron replacement, or for patients in whom erythropoietin therapy is being considered. Iron-deficient patients typically require referral to a gastroenterologist for endoscopy.

BOX 86-4
Classification of the sideroblastic anemias

Hereditary
X-linked (recessive)
  Pyridoxine responsive
  Pyridoxine refractory
Autosomal recessive

Acquired
Idiopathic (myelodysplastic)
  Pyridoxine responsive
  Pyridoxine refractory
Secondary (toxic)
  Heavy metal poisoning (lead, arsenic)
  Zinc toxicity
  Alcohol
  Copper deficiency
  Antibiotics (chloramphenicol, isoniazid, cycloserine, pyrazinamide)

Hereditary Sideroblastic Anemias

The hereditary sideroblastic anemias are most commonly X-linked, although autosomal recessive forms have been identified. Patients typically come to medical attention as young adults, although presentations in infancy, childhood, or midlife are reported. The clinical syndrome observed is a microcytic hypochromic anemia often associated with iron overload. The iron overload state, as discussed subsequently, may be associated with hepatomegaly or splenomegaly. In a number of families with X-linked sideroblastic anemia, a defect has been noted in the erythroid-specific δ-aminolevulenic acid synthase gene; the anemia in many of these patients responds to pyridoxine therapy.

Idiopathic (Myelodysplastic) Sideroblastic Anemia

Sideroblastic anemia can also be one of the myelodysplastic or preleukemic syndromes. These syndromes typically occur after the fifth decade of life. The myelodysplastic sideroblastic anemias are characterized by a dimorphic red blood cell population consisting of both normocytic red blood cells and microcytic red blood cells. These latter cells arise from the abnormal clone. Refractory anemia with ringed sideroblasts, in addition to meeting the diagnostic criteria described earlier, also exhibits varying degrees of dysplasia in the myeloid and megakaryocytic cell lineages. There is a small risk that in these patients the condition will evolve to acute myelogenous leukemia. There is also an entity, sometimes called "pure sideroblastic anemia," in which myeloid and megakaryocytic changes are not observed, and which carries a good prognosis. Patients with this syndrome often exhibit thrombocytosis.

Toxic Sideroblastic Anemias

A variety of drugs and chemical agents induce sideroblastic anemia. Ringed sideroblasts are observed in 30% to 50% of bone marrow specimens from chronic alcohol abusers; this phenomenon is attributed to impaired conversion of pyridoxine to pyridoxal phosphate by erythroid cells in the presence of alcohol. The marrow changes resolve in a few days following cessation of alcohol intake. Heavy metals such as lead or arsenic are also associated with sideroblastic anemia; lead inhibits a variety of enzymes involved in porphyrin synthesis, such as pyrimidine nucleotidase, porphyrobilinogen synthase, ferrochelatase, and coproporphyrin oxidase. Copper is required for incorporation of iron into heme, so copper deficiency results in ringed sideroblast formation; zinc causes sideroblastic anemia by inducing a copper deficiency. (Copper becomes bound to the zinc-induced protein metallothionein). Chloramphenicol induces sideroblastic anemia by inhibiting ferrochelatase. The antimycobacterial agents isoniazid, cycloserine, and pyrazinamide induce sideroblastic anemia by interfering with pyridoxine metabolism; this can be avoided by prophylactic administration of pyridoxine.

Differential Diagnosis

The differential diagnosis is that of microcytic anemia: sideroblastic anemia versus iron deficiency, the anemia of chronic disease, or hemoglobinopathies/thalassemias. Sideroblastic anemias are typically associated with an elevated serum iron level, which allows separation from anemia of chronic disease and iron deficiency. The hemoglobinopathies and thalassemias are identifiable by abnormal hemoglobin electrophoresis and (in most cases) characteristic red blood cell morphologic findings. The diagnosis of sideroblastic anemia is confirmed by the demonstration of ringed sideroblasts on bone marrow examination. Hereditary sideroblastic anemias are identified by family studies. Toxic sideroblastic anemias may be identified by a medication history or by identification of abnormal levels of lead, arsenic, zinc, or copper.

Management

Patients with hereditary or idiopathic sideroblastic anemia should receive a 4- to 6-week trial of oral pyridoxine at doses of 50 to 200 mg/day. A response typically consists of partial (but rarely complete) correction of anemia. Responding patients should be maintained on pyridoxine at the lowest dose that sustains the response; patients who fail to respond should not continue on pyridoxine therapy. Patients with hereditary or idiopathic sideroblastic anemia who do not respond to pyridoxine typically require supportive care, often including transfusions. Attention should be paid to the potential for iron overload (discussed later). A number of individuals with idiopathic sideroblastic anemia may respond to therapy with recombinant human erythropoietin.

Sideroblastic anemia due to chloramphenicol or to alcohol spontaneously resolves with cessation of the inciting agent. Patients with sideroblastic anemia resulting from lead, arsenic, or zinc toxicity should receive the standard therapy for those disorders. Sideroblastic anemia due to isoniazid, cycloserine, and pyrazinamide should be treated with pyridoxine.

IRON OVERLOAD

As discussed in the beginning of this chapter, body iron status is regulated at the level of absorption. Should an excessive quantity of iron accumulate in the body as a result of abnormal iron absorption or parenteral administration of iron or of red blood cells, there is no physiologic mechanism for its removal. Hemochromatosis refers to a state of systemic iron overload associated with deposition of iron in parenchymal cells with resultant organ damage. The most common sites of this damage are the liver, heart, and endocrine organs.

Hereditary Hemochromatosis

Hereditary hemochromatosis is condition in which iron is absorbed in excess of body requirements. It is discussed in detail in Chapter 359.

Secondary Hemochromatosis

The tragedy of secondary hemochromatosis is that it is largely a preventable iatrogenic disorder. Although patients with anemia and marrow erythroid hyperplasia, such as individuals with chronic hemolytic anemias or myelodysplastic syndromes, exhibit an increased plasma iron turnover and a slightly increased proportional dietary iron absorption, the major cause of secondary hemochromatosis is iron administered as transfused red blood cells. Patients with ineffective erythropoiesis or hemolysis, in contrast to individuals with blood loss, recycle the hemoglobin iron from damaged red blood cells, and, when transfused, progressively accumulate iron. In these patients iron accumulates in much the same pattern as in hereditary hemochromatosis, and a very similar clinical picture is presented (see Chapter 359). In contrast, patients with aplastic marrow typically accumulate excess iron only in the reticuloendothelial system.

Diagnosis

A TIBC saturation of less than 50% is strongly against the diagnosis of iron overload from any cause. In contrast, a TIBC saturation equal to or greater than 70% is virtually diagnostic of iron overload in the case of a chronically transfused patient. Serum ferritin levels are invariably greater than 500 ng/ml; the degree of ferritin elevation, reflecting predominantly reticuloendothelial iron stores, may lead to an underestimation of actual iron overload. Liver biopsy with quantitation of tissue iron concentration may also be helpful. Hepatic or myocardial dysfunction, hypogonadism, arthritis, and/or diabetes may be observed in patients with severe iron overload. Urinary iron excretion following deferoxamine is also elevated in these patients.

✔ WHEN TO REFER

Referral to a hematologist may be necessary for the diagnosis of sideroblastic anemia and, in the cases of hereditary or idiopathic syndromes, for the development of a therapeutic plan. However, the therapeutic plan can be carried out by a primary care physician in association with the hematologist.

Management

The most effective management of secondary iron overload is prevention. Prophylactic administration of deferoxamine to patients beginning a chronic transfusion program (children with severe thalassemia, adults with myelodysplastic syndromes) should be strongly considered, since chelation therapy is more effective in preventing iron accumulation than in dispersing iron stores. If organ damage from iron is already present (see Chapter 359), chelation therapy should be administered with the goal of preventing further organ damage. Patients in whom iron overload already exists but in whom organ damage has not yet occurred should also be treated aggressively with deferoxamine.

Deferoxamine is most effective when administered in daily 12-hour infusions by subcutaneous pump but can also be administered as a rapid intravenous infusion immediately following transfusion.

BIBLIOGRAPHY

Borgna-Pignatti C, Castriota-Scandberg A: Methods for evaluating iron stores and efficacy of chelation in transfusional hemosiderosis, *Haematologia* 76:409, 1991.

Cazzola M et al: Natural history of idiopathic refractory sideroblastic anemia, *Blood* 71:305, 1988.

Cohen A: Treatment of transfusional iron overload, *Am J Pediatr Hematol Oncol* 27:86, 1990.

Cotter PD et al: Late-onset X-linked sideroblastic anemia, *J Clin Invest* 96:2090, 1995.

Lee MH, Means RT: Extremely elevated serum ferritin levels in a university hospital: associated diseases and clinical significance, *Am J Med* 98:566, 1995.

Massey AC: Microcytic anemia: differential diagnosis and management of iron deficiency anemia, *Med Clin North Am* 76:549, 1992.

Means RT: Clinical application of recombinant erythropoietin in the anemia of chronic disease, *Hematol Oncol Clin North Am* 8:933, 1994.

Means RT, Krantz SB: Progress in understanding the pathogenesis of the anemia of chronic disease, *Blood* 80:1639, 1992.

Mittelman M, Lessin LS: Clinical application of recombinant erythropoietin in myelodysplasia, *Hematol Oncol Clin North Am* 8:993, 1994.

Rockey DC, Cello JP: Evaluation of the gastrointestinal tract in patients with iron-deficiency anemia, *N Engl J Med* 329:1691, 1993.

Saxena S et al: Iron deficiency anemia: a medically treatable chronic anemia as a model for transfusion overuse, *Am J Med* 94:120, 1993.

CHAPTER

87　Megaloblastic Anemia

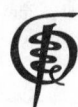

Robert T. Means, Jr.

The term "megaloblastic anemia" describes a state in which anemia results from impaired maturation of erythroid precursors in the bone marrow (ineffective erythropoiesis). This abnormal erythropoiesis results from impaired synthesis of deoxyribonucleic acid (DNA), which appears morphologically as asynchrony between nuclear and cytoplasmic maturation (nuclear/cytoplasmic dissociation). These large erythroid precursors with immature nuclei and mature cytoplasm are called megaloblasts. Although the syndromes resulting in this phenomenon are typically called megaloblastic anemias, in fact these are systemic processes; abnormalities of the white blood cell count and platelet count are commonly observed, and cells scraped from the buccal mucosa of patients with megaloblastic anemia also exhibit megaloblastic changes. Deficiencies of vitamin B_{12} (cobalamin) or folate (pteroylmonoglutamate) are responsible for most cases of megaloblastic anemia.

PHYSIOLOGY OF VITAMIN B_{12} AND FOLATE ABSORPTION

Vitamin B_{12} is produced by microorganisms that contaminate plant surfaces. It accumulates in animal proteins, and this is the major source of vitamin B_{12} in the Western diet. Daily requirements for vitamin B_{12} are low (1 to 2 μg/day) and stores of vitamin B_{12} (2 to 5 mg in adults) are large relative to these requirements, so that interruption of vitamin B_{12} intake may not result in deficiency for years.

Vitamin B_{12} in animal proteins is found as a cofactor bound to enzymes, and acidic proteolysis is required for its release. The released vitamin B_{12} becomes bound to salivary R protein in preference to intrinsic factor (IF), which is released from parietal cells. In the duodenum, however, pancreatic proteolytic enzymes digest R proteins, and vitamin B_{12} becomes bound to IF. IF-B_{12} becomes bound to specific receptors on the microvilli of distal ileal mucosal cells and is internalized. This freshly absorbed vitamin B_{12} subsequently appears in the portal circulation bound to the transport protein transcobalamin II. Previously absorbed vitamin B_{12} is predominantly bound to a circulating storage molecule, transcobalamin I.

Folate, in contrast, is synthesized by plants as well as by microorganisms, and the primary dietary sources are leafy green vegetables. The daily folate requirements range from 400 µg/day for pregnant or lactating women to 50 µg/day for other adults or children. The quantity of folate in storage is sufficient for fewer than 4 months. Folates in food occur as polyglutamates. These are broken down to pteroylmonoglutamate and rapidly absorbed in the jejunum. In the jejunal mucosa folate is reduced to tetrahydrofolate (H_4-folate), and methylated to 5-methyl (5-CH_3)-H_4-folate, in which form it is released into serum.

CELLULAR METABOLISM OF VITAMIN B_{12} AND FOLATE

After uptake into cells, vitamin B_{12} is converted to methyl (CH_3-)-B_{12} and to deoxyadenosyl-B_{12}. In the mitochondria, methylmalonyl CoA mutase converts methylmalonyl coenzyme A (CoA) to succinyl CoA in the presence of deoxyadenosyl-B_{12}. In the cytoplasm, CH_3-B_{12} is a coenzyme for methionine synthase, donating a methyl group to convert homocysteine to methionine; the reduced CH_3-B_{12} then becomes Cob(I)alamin. In the same reaction, 5-CH_3-H_4-folate donates a methyl group to Cob(I)alamin, regenerating CH_3-B_{12} and also H_4-folate.

As previously noted, 5-CH_3-H_4-folate is converted to H_4-folate by methionine synthase. This H_4-folate then undergoes polyglutamation (which is required for retention in the cell) and is converted to 5,10-methylene-H_4-folate. This compound in turn may participate in the thymidylate synthase reaction, generating deoxythymidine monophosphate for thymidine and DNA synthesis, and dihydro (H_2)-folate, which is in turn converted to H_4-folate; or it may be converted to 5-CH_3-H_4-folate, which will be utilized in the methionine synthase reaction as described earlier. These three major enzymatic reactions are summarized in Fig. 87-1.

As Fig. 87-1 indicates, vitamin B_{12} and folate interact in the reactions of cellular metabolism. In the absence of vitamin B_{12} the methionine synthase reaction does not occur. Conversion of 5-CH_3-H_4-folate to H_4-folate does not occur, with failure of folate polyglutamation and loss of folate from the cell. In addition, 5,10-methylene-H_4-folate is not generated, interrupting conversion of deoxyuridine monophosphate to deoxythymidine monophosphate and leading to an arrest of the cell cycle.

This phenomenon is represented on morphologic study in the bone marrow by erythroid hyperplasia with arrested nuclear maturation (Plate IV-7). The erythroid precursors in megaloblastic anemia are large and show immature nuclei and karyorrhexis. These cells then undergo programmed cell death (apoptosis). In in vitro models of folate deficiency, addition of thymidine (bypassing the blocked thymidylate synthase reaction) prevents apoptosis in folate-deficient erythroblasts.

CAUSES OF MEGALOBLASTIC ANEMIAS

A variety of causes of megaloblastic anemia are described in Box 87-1. Vitamin B_{12} deficiency may result from insufficient intake or insufficient mobilization from the gastrointestinal tract. Insufficient mobilization may result from impaired acid proteolysis (as in achlorhydria or hypochlorhydria), impaired separation of vitamin B_{12} from R proteins (as in pancreatic insufficiency), or insufficient IF production. Insufficient IF production due to parietal cell atrophy is the basis for pernicious anemia, the most common cause of vitamin B_{12} deficiency, but similar findings are observed following surgical removal of parietal cells at gastrectomy. Abnormalities of IF receptor number (ileal surgery, ileal infiltration or inflammation) or function (Immerslund-Gräsbeck syndrome) also result in cellular vitamin B_{12} deficiency. Human immunodeficiency virus (HIV) infection may be associated with transcobalamin II deficiency and impaired vitamin B_{12} delivery to cells. Intraluminal contents, such as bacteria in the blind loop or stasis syndrome, the parasite *Diphyllobothrium latum,* or medications such as cholestyramine may compete with IF receptors for vitamin B_{12} uptake. Prolonged exposure to the inhalational anesthetic nitrous oxide inhibits methionine synthase and produces a megaloblastic anemia often reversible by high doses of vitamin B_{12}.

Since the daily folate requirement is relatively high and folate stores are sufficient for only a few months, poor dietary intake is the major cause of folate deficiency. In lactating or pregnant women the daily folate requirement increases eightfold, greatly increasing the likelihood of folate deficiency in the patient not receiving dietary supplementation. The major risk in pregnancy is not, however, anemia, but rather is development of neural tube defects in utero. Patients who have chronic, long-standing elevations of reticulocyte counts, as in chronic hemolysis, are at significant risk of folate deficiency because of increased demand. Malabsorption is a less common cause of folate deficiency than of vitamin B_{12} deficiency.

A number of drugs interfere with folate metabolism. The best known of these agents, methotrexate, is an inhibitor of dihydrofolate reductase. The sulfonamides also interfere with dihydrofolate reductase activity. Hematologic syndromes caused by these drugs can be reversed by treatment with folinic acid (leucovorin, citrovorum factor) without loss of their antibacterial or antineoplastic effects. The anticonvulsant diphenylhydantoin interferes with folate absorption. Alcohol abuse is associated with impaired folate utilization by hematopoietic cells; the generally poor dietary habits associated with alcohol abuse probably contribute to this effect.

A variety of other processes producing abnormal DNA synthesis results in morphologic changes similar to those seen in vitamin B_{12} or folate deficiency. The erythroid changes observed in the myelodysplastic syndromes (see Chapter 90) or during treatment with or recovery from myelosuppressive drugs resemble the erythroid changes seen in vitamin B_{12} or folate deficiency but do not exhibit the characteristic myeloid changes (discussed later). Therefore some hematologists and pathologists categorize these changes as "megaloblastoid" rather than "megaloblastic."

CLINICAL PRESENTATION OF VITAMIN B_{12} OR FOLATE DEFICIENCY

The clinical presentation of vitamin B_{12} or folate deficiency can vary considerably. Patients with full-blown megaloblastic anemia may have severe anemia and pancytopenia. The very gradual onset

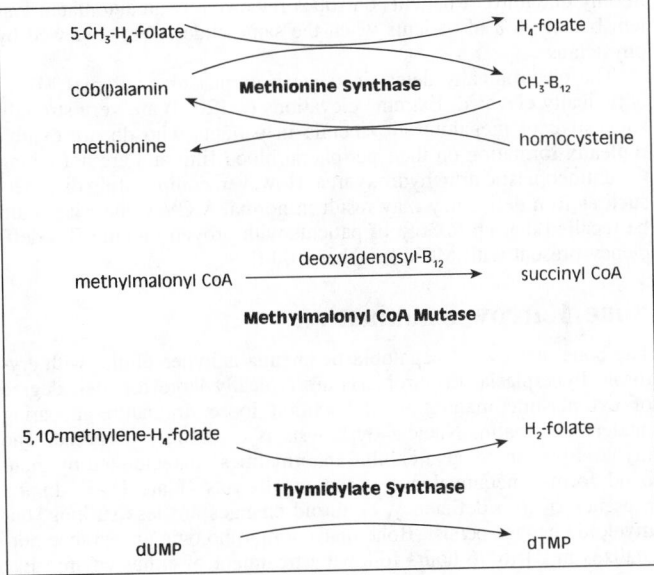

FIGURE 87-1 Major metabolic reactions involving vitamin B_{12} or folate.

BOX 87-1
Causes of megaloblastic anemias

I. Vitamin B_{12} deficiency
  A. Insufficient vitamin B_{12} intake: Vegetarians, vegans, breast-fed infants of mothers with pernicious anemia
  B. Inadequate proteolysis of food vitamin B_{12}: Atrophic gastritis, partial gastrectomy with hypochlorhydria, suppression of acid secretion (ranitidine, cimetidine, omeprazole)
  C. Deficient intrinsic factor (IF) production: Total or partial gastrectomy, pernicious anemia, gastric scarring
  D. Pancreatic protease insufficiency: Pancreatic insufficiency, Zollinger-Ellison syndrome
  E. Competition of microorganisms for vitamin B_{12}
    1. Bacterial overgrowth syndromes: Blind loops, pouches of diverticulosis, strictures, fistulas, anastomoses, scleroderma, pseudoobstruction, hypogammaglobulinemia
    2. *Diphyllobothrium latum*
  F. Disorders of ileal mucosa/IF receptors
    1. Diminished or absent IF receptors: Ileal bypass, resection, or fistula
    2. Abnormal mucosal architecture or function: Tropical or nontropical sprue, Crohn's disease, tuberculosis ileitis, infiltration by lymphomas, amyloidosis
    3. IF-receptor or post–IF-receptor defects: Immerslund-Gräsbeck syndrome, transcobalamin II deficiency (primary or in human immunodeficiency virus [HIV] infection)
    4. Drug-induced effects: Slow-release potassium, biguanides, cholestyramine, colchicine, neomycin, valproic acid
  G. Disorders of plasma vitamin B_{12} transport:
    1. Congenital transcobalamin II deficiency, defective binding of transcobalamin II-B_{12} to transcobalamin II receptors (rare)
  H. Metabolic disorders
    1. Inborn enzyme errors (rare)
    2. Acquired disorders: Nitrous oxide toxicity

II. Folate deficiency
  A. Nutritional causes
    1. Decreased dietary folate intake: Kwashiorkor, marasmus; institutionalized individuals (psychiatric hospitals, nursing homes); chronic debilitating disease; special diets or dietary habits (weight reduction, cultural or ethnic cooking techniques, ingestion of goat's milk)
    2. Increased folate requirements, with or without decreased intake
      a. Physiologic: Pregnancy and lactation, prematurity, infancy
      b. Pathologic: Chronic hemolytic anemias (autoimmune hemolytic disease, hemoglobinopathies/thalassemia, hereditary spherocytosis, paroxysmal nocturnal hemoglobinuria)
  B. Folate malabsorption
    1. With normal intestinal mucosa
      a. Some drugs (controversial)
      b. Congenital folate malabsorption (rare)
    2. With mucosal abnormalities: Tropical and nontropical sprue, regional enteritis
  C. Defective cellular folate uptake: Familial aplastic anemia (rare)
  D. Inadequate cellular utilization
    1. Folate antagonists (methotrexate, sulfonamides, triametrexate)
    2. Hereditary enzyme deficiencies involving folate
  E. Drugs: Alcohol, diphenylhydantoin, barbiturates, cigarette smoking

III. Miscellaneous megaloblastic anemias (not caused by vitamin B_{12} or folate deficiency)
  A. Congenital disorders of DNA synthesis (rare): Orotic aciduria, Lesch-Nyhan syndrome, congenital dyserythropoietic anemia
  B. Acquired disorders of DNA synthesis: Thiamine-responsive megaloblastosis (rare)
  C. Myelodysplastic syndromes or myelosuppressive drugs ("megaloblastoid")

---

of the anemia means that these patients often remain asymptomatic until their hemoglobin concentration is extremely low. Leukopenia and/or thrombocytopenia is found in approximately one third of patients and may be severe also. Intramedullary hemolysis of erythroid progenitors may result in a modest elevation of the bilirubin concentration with jaundice, and an elevated lactate dehydrogenase concentration. Megaloblastic mucosal changes are observed in the mouth, producing the classic "beefy red tongue," and may also be noted in the gastrointestinal and urogenital tracts. Megaloblastic changes of the intestinal mucosa may produce malabsorption. Modest splenic enlargement may also be noted. A variety of neuropsychiatric manifestations are also present in approximately one third of patients (discussed later). The presentation of vitamin B_{12} and folate deficiency is very individual; any combination of these manifestations may be present.

The neuropsychiatric manifestations of vitamin B_{12} or folate deficiency are numerous. Cerebral syndromes may range from irritability, forgetfulness, dementia/delirium ("megaloblastic madness"), or visual problems to (rarely) coma. Demyelination observed predominantly in vitamin B_{12} deficiency begins with distal loss of vibration sense and proprioception and may progress to subacute combined degeneration of the spinal cord. Ataxia, paresthesias, orthostatic hypotension, bowel/bladder dysfunction, and abnormal reflexes may be observed. Neuropsychiatric manifestations may accompany hematologic abnormalities or may occur alone, although the more severe deficits tend to be observed in patients with significant anemia.

Patients with vitamin B_{12} deficiency may also remain asymptomatic for prolonged periods. A study in which asymptomatic elderly individuals were screened with urinary methylmalonic acid levels suggested a 3% to 5% frequency of vitamin B_{12} deficiency in this population.

LABORATORY STUDIES
Peripheral Blood Morphology

The red blood cells in megaloblastic anemia are large and typically oval ("macroovalocytes"). The frequency of hypersegmented (≥ 5 lobes) neutrophils varies depending on how the blood films are reviewed. In one large series hypersegmented neutrophils were reported in only one third of patients on slides reviewed by an automated system but in 94% of patients when the same slides were reviewed by physicians.

The electronically determined mean corpuscular volume (MCV) is typically elevated. Extreme elevations (>120 fl) are very strongly suggestive of megaloblastic anemia in patients who do not exhibit rouleaux formation on their peripheral blood film and are not taking the antineoplastic drug hydroxyurea. However, complicating disorders such as iron deficiency may result in normal MCV values; it should be recalled that up to 36% of patients with proven vitamin B_{12} deficiency present with MCV less than 100 fl.

Bone Marrow Examination

The bone marrow in megaloblastic anemia is hypercellular with erythroid hyperplasia. Erythroblasts are typically large for their degree of cytoplasmic maturation and exhibit loose, immature-appearing nuclear chromatin. Nuclear dyskinesis is commonly observed. The myeloid precursors also exhibit abnormalities characterized by giant band forms, metamyelocytes, and myelocytes (Plate IV-7). In the presence of iron deficiency, erythroid changes are less striking, but myeloid changes persist. Bone marrow morphologic appearance normalizes in 24 to 96 hours following treatment of either vitamin B_{12} or folate deficiency.

Serum Vitamin B$_{12}$ Levels

The use of serum vitamin B$_{12}$ levels as the initial test for vitamin B$_{12}$ deficiency has been questioned by a number of investigators. In a review of patients followed at a Veterans Affairs Medical Center, 16 of 84 patients with serum vitamin B$_{12}$ levels less than or equal to 180 pg/ml proved to be vitamin B$_{12}$ deficient, whereas none of 168 patients with normal levels proved to be deficient. However, an advantage of the serum vitamin B$_{12}$ assay is that it is readily available in most clinical settings, whereas other tests may require the use of a reference laboratory. In patients in whom a clinical picture consistent with vitamin B$_{12}$ deficiency is present, a low serum vitamin B$_{12}$ level is probably an adequate indication for therapy. In other patients consideration should be given to the use of more definitive tests, such as methylmalonic acid determination. The serum vitamin B$_{12}$ level may be falsely low in folate deficiency and in hypergammaglobulinemia (as with multiple myeloma) and may be elevated out of proportion to tissue status in liver disease and myeloproliferative or lymphoproliferative diseases. Red blood cell transfusion does not alter the serum vitamin B$_{12}$ level.

Serum and Red Blood Cell Folate Values

The serum folate level is influenced by recent dietary intake but should be the first test used for folate deficiency, since it is readily available and inexpensive. A low serum folate level reliably indicates folate deficiency; a normal serum folate level may does not necessarily rule out deficiency. In patients in whom the serum folate level is normal but clinical suspicion is high, a red blood cell folate test should be ordered. The red blood cell folate value indicates the average folate status during the red blood cell life span. Since vitamin B$_{12}$ deficiency causes folate leakage from the red blood cell, a serum vitamin B$_{12}$ level should be ordered simultaneously. An advantage of the red blood cell folate value is that it will not be altered by short-term therapy. If the serum folate result is equivocal, a red blood cell folate test can be ordered at that time. The obvious exception would be if red blood cell transfusion is required by the patient. Red blood cell folate testing after transfusion would reflect the donor's folate status; serum folate levels would not be changed.

Methylmalonic Acid and Homocysteine

As discussed earlier, deficiency of either vitamin B$_{12}$ or folate impairs conversion of homocysteine to methionine, with consequent accumulation of homocysteine; vitamin B$_{12}$ deficiency impairs conversion of methylmalonyl CoA to succinyl CoA, with accumulation of methylmalonic acid. Methylmalonic acid and homocysteine levels may be measured in either serum or urine and indicate true tissue deficiency of vitamin B$_{12}$ and/or folate. These values are probably the most definitive chemical indicators of deficiency. They are readily available through commercial reference laboratories. However, they should probably be used as confirmatory tests or in unclear clinical situations. Homocysteine is elevated in either vitamin B$_{12}$ or folate deficiency; the red blood cell folate value probably provides a better indication of folate deficiency. Methylmalonic acid elevation is unique to vitamin B$_{12}$ deficiency and can be used when the clinical picture strongly suggests vitamin B$_{12}$ deficiency but the serum vitamin B$_{12}$ value is normal.

Schilling Test

The dictum which prevailed several years ago, that no one should be treated for vitamin B$_{12}$ deficiency without an abnormal Schilling test result, reflected an assumption that nearly all cases of vitamin B$_{12}$ deficiency resulted from malabsorption. The Schilling test is not a test for vitamin B$_{12}$ deficiency but rather a means of identifying the way a patient became vitamin B$_{12}$ deficient. The Schilling test identifies inability to absorb crystalline vitamin B$_{12}$ (used in the standard test) from the gastrointestinal tract; the phase II Schilling test identifies cases of malabsorption that are due to IF deficiency. In fact, a number of elderly individuals with achlorhydria or hypochlorhydria or patients who have had surgery impairing either acid secretion or gastric motility have failure to absorb vitamin B$_{12}$ from food but have normal Schilling test results. This is because these patients can absorb crystalline vitamin B$_{12}$ but cannot extract it from food, as shown by performing a Schilling test in which the radiolabeled vitamin B$_{12}$ is bound to egg albumen and administered as either scrambled eggs or eggnog. It should also be noted that megaloblastic changes in the intestinal mucosa may result in a falsely abnormal test result in patients with other causes of vitamin B$_{12}$ or folate deficiency.

The role of the Schilling test in the routine evaluation of vitamin B$_{12}$ deficiency is unclear. It may be very helpful in evaluating patients who are receiving long-term vitamin B$_{12}$ replacement whose original diagnosis was unclear; since it is a test of absorption and not tissue deficiency, an abnormal Schilling test result persists even in the vitamin B$_{12}$–replete individual.

Other Studies

A number of other tests (serum gastrin levels, antiparietal cell antibody tests, thyroid function tests) are often ordered in vitamin B$_{12}$–deficient patients, usually to identify conditions associated with pernicious anemia. The routine use of these tests cannot be recommended, although they may be helpful in individual, selected patients.

DIFFERENTIAL DIAGNOSIS

Vitamin B$_{12}$ and/or folate deficiency should be suspected in patients with macrocytic anemias (particularly when the MCV is $\geq$120) but, since the manifestations of these syndromes are so diverse, may also be a possibility in a wide variety of syndromes. The approach to patients is predicated on a small number of assumptions. First, the clinical syndromes of vitamin B$_{12}$ and folate deficiency are generally indistinguishable, so both deficiencies should be evaluated. Second, in significantly anemic patients with vitamin B$_{12}$ deficiency, treatment with folate rather than vitamin B$_{12}$ may result in progressive neurologic deficits; therefore vitamin B$_{12}$ deficiency should be ruled out definitively. Third, in a setting where clinical suspicion of vitamin B$_{12}$ or folate deficiency is high, normal levels should not necessarily be taken as the end of the workup. An approach to the diagnosis of vitamin B$_{12}$ and folate deficiency is outlined in Table 87-1.

MANAGEMENT

Pending a definitive diagnosis, empiric vitamin B$_{12}$ *and* folate therapy can be initiated without harm after diagnostic tests are ordered. Vitamin B$_{12}$–deficient patients may show a partial hematologic improvement when receiving folate therapy alone, but folate therapy alone may lead to progression of neurologic disease in these patients. This is primarily a problem with severely anemic patients.

There are a variety of different ways to initiate treatment in vitamin B$_{12}$–deficient patients: none of them are wrong. Vitamin B$_{12}$ may be administered daily for 5 to 7 days, weekly for 3 to 6 weeks, or every other day for five to seven doses. The usual dose is either 100 or 1000 μg subcutaneously or intramuscularly, although responses have been reported with daily or weekly doses less than or equal to 30 μg. Correction of marrow abnormalities is noted within 24 to 72 hours; reticulocytosis is noted within 5 days, and increases in hemoglobin or hematocrit follow. The rapid maturation and differentiation induced by vitamin B$_{12}$ causes a rapid cellular uptake of potassium and may result in severe hypokalemia in patients with severe deficiency. Serum potassium should be followed in the first few days following initiation of treatment.

The maintenance regimen is typically vitamin B$_{12}$ 100 to 1000 μg subcutaneously each month for the duration of the patient's life, but alternatives are available in individual cases. Patients in whom vitamin B$_{12}$ deficiency developed as a result of a limited process (i.e., medications no longer taken, local mucosal problems no longer active, anatomic defects that have been corrected) can probably stop maintenance therapy after several months but should be monitored quarterly or biannually for early evidence of deficiency. Methylmalonic acid determinations are ideal for this purpose. Patients can be taught to administer their injections at home. Some patients who will require lifelong maintenance can be successfully maintained on a regimen of oral vitamin B$_{12}$ (cyanocobalamin) 500 to 1000 μg/day after several months of parenteral maintenance; however, this should be reserved for highly motivated, compliant patients with less severe de-

Table 87-1 Diagnostic approach to vitamin B$_{12}$ and folate deficiency

1. Serum vitamin B$_{12}$, serum folate determinations
2. If transfusion indicated, order RBC folate test

HIGH SUSPICION FOR VITAMIN B$_{12}$/FOLATE DEFICIENCY (ANEMIA, MEAN CORPUSCULAR VOLUME >110 FL, HYPERSEGMENTED POLYMORPHONUCLEAR NEUTROPHILS)	LOW SUSPICION FOR VITAMIN B$_{12}$/FOLATE DEFICIENCY

Initiate vitamin B$_{12}$ and folate therapy

1. B$_{12}$ low, folate normal: Continue B$_{12}$, stop folate

2. B$_{12}$ normal, folate low: Continue folate; stop B$_{12}$ and order MMA; if MMA elevated, resume B$_{12}$

3. B$_{12}$ low, folate low: B$_{12}$ and folate therapy

4. B$_{12}$ normal, folate normal

1. B$_{12}$ low, folate normal: B$_{12}$ therapy; order MMA; if normal, stop B$_{12}$

2. B$_{12}$ normal, folate low: Folate therapy

3. B$_{12}$ low, folate low: B$_{12}$ and folate therapy; order MMA; if normal, stop B$_{12}$

4. B$_{12}$ normal, folate normal: Consider other diagnoses

No response to therapy
Consider other diagnoses

Responding to therapy
Continue both, order MMA, RBC folate
Discontinue B$_{12}$ if MMA normal
Discontinue folate if RBC folate normal

Reevaluate patients receiving vitamin B$_{12}$ or folate therapy if no response in 1 month

MMA, Methylmalonic acid determination (serum or urine); *RBC folate,* red blood cell folate determination.

ficiency. In the author's experience, patients find it easier to remember a monthly injection than a daily pill.

Folate deficiency should be treated with oral folic acid 1 mg daily. The time course of hematologic response is similar to that of vitamin B$_{12}$ deficiency. Much like the situation in vitamin B$_{12}$ deficiency, the duration of therapy depends on the cause of the deficiency. Some persons may require indefinite maintenance on folate therapy. Patients who became deficient during a limited period of malnutrition, during a pregnancy, or due to a medication they no longer take can stop therapy after several months but should be periodically monitored for a time. Because folate stores are only sufficient for a few months, the monitoring interval should be no longer than 3 months. However, patients who show no evidence of recurrent folate deficiency after a year off therapy probably do not require further follow-up.

Patients with neurologic manifestations may exhibit a variable response. In general, abnormalities of short duration (particularly those not likely to result from demyelination) tend to respond readily; others may respond slowly or not at all. The response in an individual patient cannot be predicted, but defects persisting after 6 to 12 months of therapy are likely to be permanent.

Three special topics require mention. Concurrent iron deficiency may be unmasked by correction of vitamin B$_{12}$ or folate deficiency. This is reflected by a failure of the hemoglobin and hematocrit to correct and is readily identifiable because of a steady decline in MCV and disappearance of hypersegmented neutrophils. Many physicians routinely treat patients who have chronic hemolytic disorders (hereditary spherocytosis, sickle cell disease, prosthetic valve hemolysis, etc.) with prophylactic folate because of the increased folate requirements of these patients. It has recently been suggested that this practice may do some patients a disservice by masking unsuspected vitamin B$_{12}$ deficiency and allowing treatable neurologic abnormalities to develop and progress. While this is a legitimate concern, it remains to be seen whether it is a real problem. It has been suggested that

✔ *WHEN TO REFER*

As outlined in this chapter, megaloblastic anemia can generally be diagnosed and treated by the primary care physician. Referral would be indicated for confirmation of the diagnosis in patients who fail to respond to appropriate therapy or when the diagnosis cannot be clearly established. Bone marrow examination is generally not necessary in the diagnosis of megaloblastic anemia but may be helpful in ruling out concurrent iron deficiency or myelodysplastic syndromes that may resemble the megaloblastic anemias.

patients with vitamin B$_{12}$ deficiency due to pernicious anemia have an increased risk for gastric carcinoma and should be screened for this disease. Large population-based studies suggest that there is no firm indication for screening; the risk of gastric carcinoma appears to be the same as that of age-matched controls.

BIBLIOGRAPHY

Carmel R et al: Food cobalamin malabsorption occurs frequently in patients with unexplained low serum cobalamin levels, *Arch Intern Med* 148:1715, 1988.

Healton EB et al: Neurologic aspects of cobalamin deficiency, *Medicine* 70:229, 1991.

Lindenbaum J et al: Frequency of neuropsychiatric disorders caused by cobalamin deficiency in the absence of anemia or macrocytosis, *N Engl J Med* 318:1720, 1988.

Matchar DB et al: Performance of the serum cobalamin assay for the diagnosis of cobalamin deficiency, *Am J Med Sci* 308:276, 1994.

Norman EJ, Morrison JA: Screening elderly populations for cobalamin (vitamin B$_{12}$) deficiency using the urinary methylmalonic acid asssay by gas chromatography/mass sprectrometry, *Am J Med* 94:589, 1993.

Savage DG et al: Sensitivity of serum methylmalonic acid and total homocysteine determinations for diagnosing cobalamin and folate deficiencies, *Am J Med* 96:239, 1994.

Schafer LW et al: Risk of development of gastric carcinoma in patients with pernicious anemia: a population-based study in Rochester, Minnesota, *Mayo Clin Proc* 60:444, 1985.

Schilling RF, Williams WJ: Vitamin B$_{12}$ deficiency: underdiagnosed, overtreated? *Hosp Pract* 30:47, 1995.

Stabler SP et al: Clinical spectrum and diagnosis of cobalamin deficiency, *Blood* 76:871, 1990.

Werler MM, Shapiro S, Mitchell AA: Periconceptual folic acid exposure and the risk of occurent neural tube defects, *JAMA* 269:1257, 1993.

CHAPTER

88 Hemoglobinopathies and Thalassemias

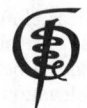

Martin H. Steinberg

Hemoglobinopathies and thalassemias result from mutations in the globin genes of the hemoglobin (Hb) molecules or in regulatory areas near these genes. In hemoglobinopathies (e.g., sickle cell anemia) a mutation in the protein-coding part of the gene leads to the synthesis of sickle hemoglobin, a structurally abnormal globin. Thalassemia, in contrast, results from mutations that reduce the amounts of globin produced.

The molecular abnormalities and genetics of Hb disorders are well understood. Genes for the gamma chains of fetal hemoglobin (HbF), the delta chain of adult hemoglobin A$_2$ (HbA$_2$), and the beta chain of adult hemoglobin (HbA) are closely linked in a cluster on the short arm of chromosome 11 (Fig. 88-1, *A*). Duplicated alpha-globin genes (Fig. 88-1, *B*) that have identical coding sequences are at the telomere of the short arm of chromosome 16. Interspersed among active globin genes are pseudogenes representing inactive remnants of ancient gene duplications (Fig. 88-1). Beta- and alpha-gene cluster haplotypes define the chromosomal milieu inherited with these genes. Haplotypes are delineated by polymorphic restriction endonuclease cleavage sites

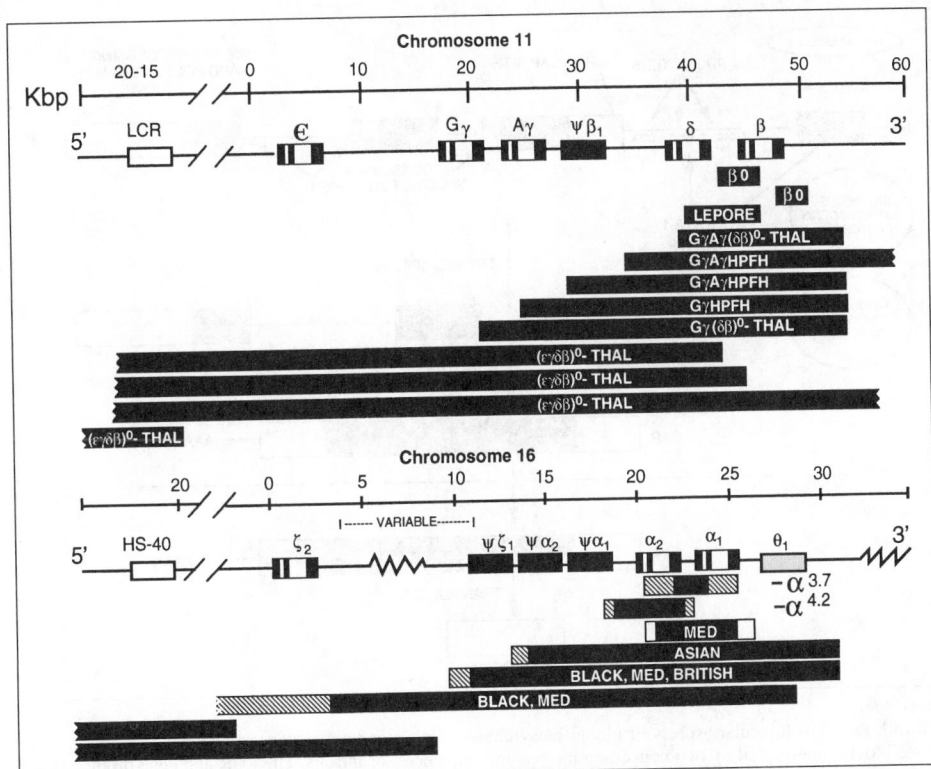

FIGURE 88-1 Globin-gene arrangement and some deletion types of thalassemia. **A,** The betalike genes (epsilon, ^Ggamma, ^Agamma, delta, and beta) are found in a 50-kb cluster on the short arm of chromosome 11. About 20 kbp 5′ to the epsilon gene lies the locus control region (LCR), which interacts with the betalike gene promoters to allow high-level gene expression. The pseudobeta gene is not expressed, the epsilon gene is expressed in the embryo, and the paired gamma genes are active mainly in fetal life. The gamma-globin gene products differ by a single amino acid at residue 136: glycine (^Ggamma) or alanine (^Agamma). Deletions described in some forms of hereditary persistence of fetal hemoglobin (HPFH), hemoglobin (Hb) Lepore, delta-beta thalassemia, a type of beta⁰ thalassemia found in Asian Indians, and small deletions in the 5′ portion of the beta gene associated with very high adult hemogloin A_2 (HbA_2) levels, are shown. A rare mutation spares the betalike genes but removes the LCR, so these gene cannot be expressed. **B,** The alpha-gene cluster including the zeta gene, pseudogenes, the paired alpha-globin genes, and the theta gene are on the short arm of chromosome 16. The alpha HS-40 region serves as an alpha-gene–specific enhancer. Extensive homology between alpha-globin genes makes crossing over and gene deletion the most common causes of alpha thalassemia. The zeta gene is normally expressed only in embryonic and fetal life. A theta-gene product has not been detected. The extent of some deletions causing alpha thalassemias is shown below. The two common uppermost deletions remove only one gene (alpha thalassemia-2, α^+); the remainder deletes both genes or the HS-40 enhancer that is required for gene expression (alpha thalassemia-1, α^0). *Med,* Mediterranean population; *Asian,* Southeast Asian population.

within and about these genes. Globin genes are compact, and each contains three exons and two introns (Fig. 88-2). *Cis*-acting elements and *trans*-acting transcription factors that control globin gene expression have been identified. Gene transcription depends on phylogenetically conserved nucleotides 5′ to the coding portion, called promoters. These ensure the fidelity and influence the rate of gene transcription (Fig. 88-2). Remote from the epsilon gene lies the beta–locus control region (LCR), a group of deoxyribonuclease (DNase) hypersensitive sites containing binding sites for generic and erythroid-specific transcription factors (Figs. 88-1 and 88-2). The LCR interacts with the promoters of the betalike genes, permitting access to transcription factors and allowing high levels of tissue-specific and developmentally regulated gene expression. Another upstream regulatory element (HS-40) regulates alpha-globin gene expression. Several erythroid-specific transcription factors have been found. The most active is called GATA-1, after the nucleotides that form the core of its recognition sequence. GATA-1 plays an important role in erythroid development and the transcription of other nonglobin erythroid-specific proteins. Other important erythroid transcription factors are NF-E2 and beta-globin gene-specific EKLF.

Globin polypeptide synthesis is outlined in Fig. 88-2. Gene transcription results in a large intranuclear pre–messenger ribonucleic acid (pre-mRNA) (Fig. 88-2). This is processed to a smaller mRNA by excision of introns, splicing together the translated sequences, or ex-

ons, and adding special nucleotides 5′ and 3′ to the coding sequence (Fig. 88-2). The latter enhance the translatability and stability of the mRNA. Processed mRNA is exported to the cytoplasm where, on polyribosomes, it is enzymatically translated into protein. Alpha and beta chains are produced on separate ribosomes in nearly equal quantities. Globin chains acquire heme groups and form alpha/nonalpha heterodimers, which rapidly self-associate into a tetrameric hemoglobin molecule.

Both globin gene clusters undergo developmental switches in utero (Fig. 88-3). Embryonic epsilon and zeta globins are normally made only in the earliest stages of gestation. The epsilon-globin chain is soon replaced by gamma- and beta-globin, constituents of the predominant hemoglobin of the fetus (HbF) and adult (HbA), respectively. The alpha-globin chain, common to all adult and fetal hemoglobins, begins accumulating during the first trimester and persists at high levels throughout life (Fig. 88-3). In normal adults, hemoglobin A, composed of two alpha- and two beta-globin chains, makes up about 97% of the total hemoglobin. Therefore in adults, only abnormalities affecting the alpha- or beta-globin chain have clinical significance. Although the general features of all globin genes are similar, amino acid sequence differences exist. The similarities among the betalike genes are greater than those between the betalike and alpha genes. Hemoglobin switching during development may be governed by competitive interactions of the LCR with different globin gene pro-

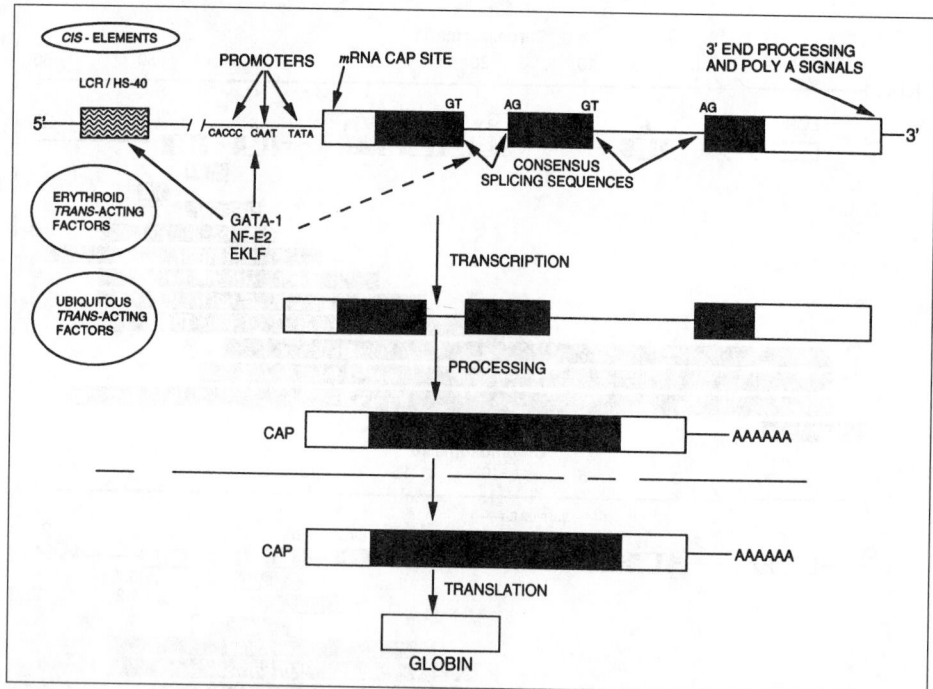

FIGURE 88-2   Molecular aspects of globin biosynthesis. Globin coding sequences, or exons, are arranged in three blocks, interrupted by two noncoding intervening sequences, or introns. The LCR and gene promoters are rich in binding sites for erythroid-specific and generic transcription factors, and all these elements interact to permit developmental and tissue-specific regulation of globin gene expression. A series of nucleotides located 5' to the messenger RNA (mRNA) capping site are the *cis*-acting promoters of gene expression. At the 3' end are signals for chain termination and mRNA polyadenylation. Removal of introns depends in part on conserved GT and AG dinucleotides at their 5' (donor) and 3' (acceptor) extremities. The entire gene is enzymatically transcribed into a pre-mRNA containing untranslated sequences and introns. mRNA is processed by excision of introns and ligation of exons, capping of the 5' end by a special nucleotide, and polyadenylation. The latter two processes enhance the translatability and stability of mRNA; mRNA is then exported to the cytoplasm for translation. mRNA is translated to a globin polypeptide on ribosomes via the interplay of groups of initiation and elongation factors and transfer RNAs that convey amino acids to the growing polypeptide. Completed alpha and beta chains acquire heme groups and form dimers that associate to make a completed hemoglobin tetramer. *EKLF*, erythroid Kruppel-like factor.

moters, as well as the interplay of positive and negative *trans*-acting regulatory factors.

Hemoglobin is a globular protein with a molecular weight of about 64,000 (Fig. 88-4). Oxygen transport is mediated by the heme groups, which are cradled within a protected niche of each globin chain. Heme groups bind and release their oxygen sequentially, and loading or unloading of each oxygen molecule depends on the number of oxygen molecules already bound. This property of hemoglobin is termed *cooperativity*, or *heme-heme interaction*. It is a result of specific interactions among the four globin chains of the tetramer. Cooperativity is responsible for the familiar sigmoid shape of the hemoglobin-oxygen dissociation curve. It allows blood to be oxygenated in the lungs and then to release oxygen to the tissues. The point on this curve where hemoglobin is half saturated with oxygen is called the P50. Neither a dimeric globin molecule, such as myoglobin, nor a tetramer of a single type of globin chain, such as hemoglobin H (HbH) (beta-4) or Bart's Hb (gamma-4) have the property of cooperativity. Some hemoglobin mutants have an abnormal P50, and this alters oxygen transport and erythropoiesis. Temperature, pH, erythrocyte metabolism, 2,3-bisphosphoglycerate (2,3-BPG) levels, and blood phosphate concentration may all influence the P50 of normal hemoglobin.

The expression of globin disorders is usually not clinically significant unless the affected person is a homozygote or compound heterozygote. However, in cases of unstable hemoglobins, or variants with altered oxygen affinity, heterozygotes are affected clinically. Clinical expression thus depends on the globin-gene product, which in turn is usually readily detectable by widely available tests. Hemoglobin disorders are transmitted autosomally, and their inheritance obeys mendelian laws.

THALASSEMIA

Thalassemias—the most common single gene-inherited disorder of humankind—are widely distributed throughout the world population and result from a reduction in or absence of normal globin synthesis. In some locales, over half the population carry a thalassemia gene. The thalassemic phenotype encompasses microcytosis, hypochromia, reticulocytosis, anemia, ineffective erythropoiesis, and splenomegaly. Depending on the thalassemia-causing mutation, these features may be insignificant or flagrant. Clinically important thalassemias are due to failures in beta- or alpha-globin chain biosynthesis.

BETA THALASSEMIA

In some regions of Italy, Greece, and Southeast Asia the frequency of beta thalassemia carriers is nearly 20%, but beta thalassemia may appear sporadically in any ethnic group. In the United States beta thalassemia is found mainly in descendants of immigrants from areas of high disease prevalence. About 0.5% to 1% of black Americans are beta thalassemia heterozygotes.

Etiology

In beta thalassemia, reduced beta-globin synthesis leads to redundant alpha-globin chains and reduced cellular hemoglobin. Alpha-globin chains are insoluble, precipitate intracellularly as Heinz bodies, and damage the developing cell, leading to intramedullary hemolysis and ineffective erythropoiesis. Unbalanced hemoglobin synthesis and membrane injury, caused in part by oxygen radical generation and Heinz bodies, curtail the erythrocytes' life span. These cells are de-

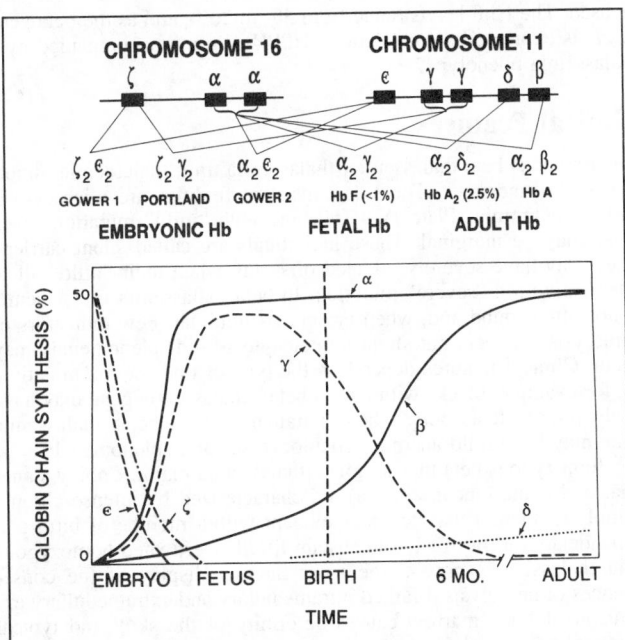

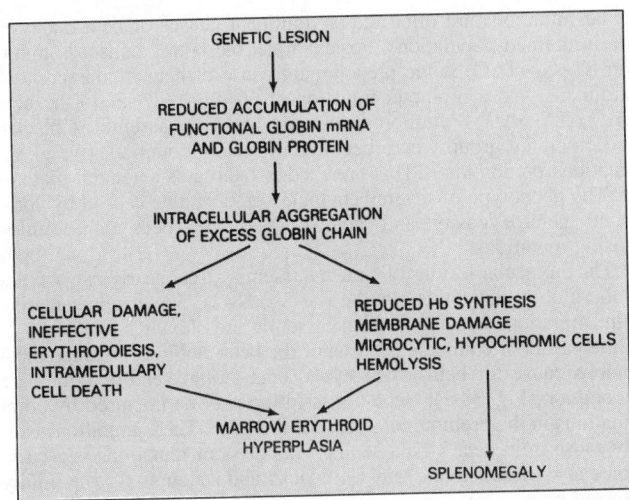

FIGURE 88-3   Developmental switching of globin synthesis and the globin chain composition of human hemoglobins. Switching of gene expression within the betalike and alphalike gene clusters leads to the synthesis of different hemoglobins in the embryo, fetus, infant, and adult. *Top,* The globin-gene–containing chromosomes and their contributions to the hemoglobin molecules of the embryo, fetus, and adult. *Bottom,* Embryonic epsilon and zeta chains rapidly disappear and are replaced by fetal gamma and adult alpha chains. Gamma-chain synthesis peaks in midgestation and reaches its adult level at 6 months of age. There is a progressive rise in beta-chain synthesis from the first trimester to its peak at 6 to 12 months of age. The small amounts of delta chain synthesized peak at about 12 months.

FIGURE 88-5   Pathophysiology of thalassemia. The genetic lesion of thalassemia results in absent or insufficient accumulation of globin messenger RNA (mRNA) and absent or reduced globin synthesis. Redundant globin chains, a product of the nonthalassemic genes, cause injury to the developing and mature cells by virtue of their aggregation into insoluble Heinz bodies and promotion of oxidant-induced damage to the cell membrane and contents. The damaged cells either undergo intramedullary cell death or are removed from the circulation by the spleen.

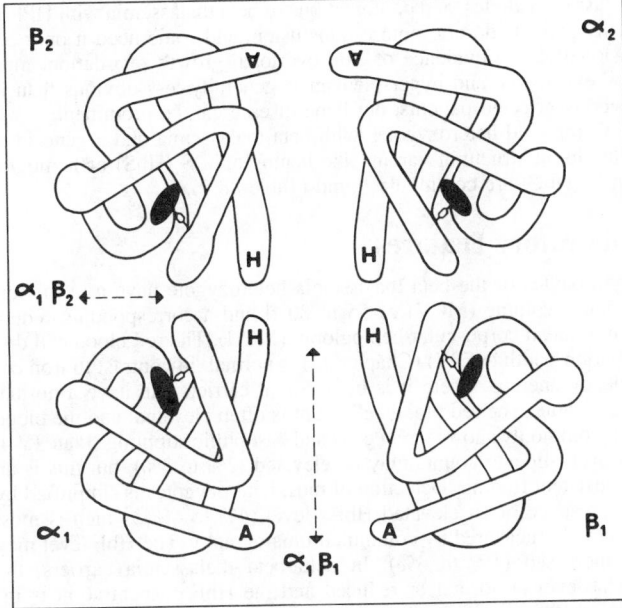

FIGURE 88-4   A schematic diagram illustrating the relationships of the four globin chains and heme groups to form the hemoglobin tetramer. Each chain consists of eight helical segments (A to H) joined by short nonhelical regions. The important areas of contact, alpha$_1$, beta$_1$, and alpha$_1$, beta$_2$, are indicated by the arrows. Blackened ovals within each chain represent heme groups.

From White JM, Dacie JV: *Prog Hematol* 7:69, 1971.

BOX 88-1
Thalassemias

I. Beta thalassemia
   A. Beta$^+$ thalassemia (suboptimal beta-globin synthesis)
   B. Beta^0 thalassemia (total absence of beta-globin synthesis)
   C. Delta-beta thalassemia (total absence of both delta- and beta-globin synthesis)
   D. Lepore hemoglobin (total absence of normal delta- and beta-globin synthesis with synthesis of small amounts of a fused delta-beta-globin chain)
   E. Gene deletion hereditary persistence of fetal hemoglobin (HbF) (reduction or absence of delta- and beta-globin synthesis and increased HbF synthesis)
II. Alpha thalassemia
   A. Silent carrier, heterozygous alpha thalassemia-2 (three alpha-globin genes present; $-\alpha/\alpha\alpha$)
   B. Alpha thalassemia trait, heterozygous-alpha thalassemia-1, homozygous alpha thalassemia-2 (two alpha-globin genes present; $-\alpha/-\alpha$ or $--/\alpha\alpha$)
   C. HbH disease (usually one alpha-globin gene present; $-\alpha/--$)
   D. Hydrops fetalis (usually no alpha-globin genes present; $--/--$)
   E. Hb Constant Spring (elongated alpha-globin chain; α^{CS})
III. Thalassemic hemoglobinopathies
   A. Hb Terre Haute, Hb Quong Sze (reduced synthesis produced by extreme instability)
   B. HbE, Hb Knossos (reduced hemoglobin synthesis produced by abnormal mRNA splicing)

---

stroyed in the spleen, which in turn hypertrophies to meet the demand for removing abnormal cells from the circulation (Fig. 88-5). Within each broad category of beta thalassemia (Box 88-1) there is considerable clinical and hematologic heterogeneity. This heterogeneity can be accounted for by the multitude of thalassemia-causing mutations. Patients may be heterozygotes, homozygotes, or compound heterozygotes for these mutations.

Beta thalassemia mutations either prevent (beta^0) or inhibit (beta$^+$) the production of normal beta globin. So far, more than 125 molecular lesions have been associated with beta thalassemia. Particular mutations are often the predominant causes of beta thalassemia in defined populations. For example, the beta[39] nonsense mutation (CAG→TAG) is the predominant cause of beta[0] thalassemia in Sardinians, and a promoter mutation at position −29 5′ to the beta gene (ATA→ATG) often produces mild beta[+] thalassemia in blacks. In each ethnic group where beta thalassemia is common, five or six mutations predominate. This knowledge facilitates antenatal diagnosis. The phenotype of severe beta thalassemia can be caused by compound heterozygosity and homozygosity for beta thalassemia–causing mutations.

The molecular lesions of beta thalassemia affect nearly every point of the globin biosynthetic pathway (Fig. 88-2). Some representative point mutations causing beta thalassemia are shown in Table 88-1. While partial or complete deletion of the beta-globin gene is the most obvious cause for beta[0] thalassemia, beta globin gene deletions are uncommon (Fig. 88-1). Gene transcription may be impaired by point mutations in the promoter elements of the gene. These mutations usually cause mild beta[+] thalassemia. This class of mutations is a common cause of beta thalassemia in blacks and accounts for the mildly affected homozygotes who have the phenotype of thalassemia intermedia (discussed later). To assemble a functional mRNA, the introns must be excised from the initial transcript and the exons ligated to produce a contiguous coding sequence. Mutations that involve the splicing sites at the intron-exon borders can thwart this process—totally or partially—and cause beta[0] or beta[+] thalassemia. Other mutations introduce a base change that causes a "cryptic" splicing site to be activated and an abnormal mRNA to be transcribed. Mutations that introduce a premature termination codon (nonsense mutation) into the coding region lead to a truncated and useless globin. The discovery of mutations that simultaneously produce a structurally abnormal hemoglobin and a thalassemia phenotype has blurred the distinction between thalassemias and hemoglobinopathies. These "dominantly" inherited disorders have been called thalassemic hemoglobinopathies. They are often caused by mutations that occur in the third exon of the globin gene and create a globin with such marked instability that no detectable protein accumulates. Their severe phenotype—in distinction to the minimal consequences of heterozygosity for most common mutations—is due to the deleterious effects of both the abnormal, unstable globin and the redundant alpha-globin chain. Lepore hemoglobins, resulting from nonhomologous crossing over between the delta-and beta-globin genes, are characterized by a delta-beta fusion chain and deletion of the normal beta-globin gene from the affected chromosome. This hybrid gene is under the regulation of the weak delta-gene promoter and is poorly expressed. About 5% of carefully studied thalassemias lack identifiable mutations in *cis*. Mutations remote from the gene, or in *trans*-acting elements that regulate gene expression, might explain these special cases.

High HbF levels in adults are also due to mutations in the beta-globin gene complex. Most delta-beta thalassemias and pancellular hereditary persistence of fetal hemoglobin (HPFH) syndromes result from large deletions that remove both the beta- and delta-globin genes (see Fig. 88-1). Homozygotes have 100% and heterozygotes, 10% to 30% HbF. A class of HPFH is produced by a variety of mutations in the promoters of the gamma genes. These mutations lead to increased transcription of either [G]gamma or [A]gamma genes, in contrast to the deletion forms of HPFH, where, usually, both gamma chains are increased. The HbF levels range from 3% to 20%, and as the beta gene in *cis* is expressed, "nondeletion" HPFHs are not accompanied by a thalassemia phenotype.

Clinical Features

Heterozygous beta thalassemia (thalassemia trait; thalassemia minor) is usually innocuous. The sole consistent findings are microcytosis and hypochromia (Plate IV-4, *M*), and with "mild" mutations even these may be marginal. These individuals are called silent carriers. They may have severely affected offspring when their "mild" allele interacts with a "severe" mutation. In beta thalassemia trait, anemia is not often found and, when present, is minimal. Few indicators of hemolysis are seen, but slight reticulocytosis and splenomegaly may occur. Clinical features depend on the type of thalassemia mutation, so, for example, blacks with a mild beta[+] thalassemia gene may have slight microcytosis only, whereas Italians with a beta[0] thalassemia gene may have mild anemia, reticulocytosis, and splenomegaly.

Homozygous beta thalassemias (thalassemia major, Cooley's anemia, or Mediterranean anemia) are characterized by intense chronic hemolytic anemia that becomes evident within months of birth and dependency on transfusion to sustain life. Undertreated homozygous beta thalassemias present the most flagrant display of the consequences of hemolysis. Marked intramedullary and extramedullary expansion of bone marrow causes deformity of the skull and typical "mongoloid" facial characteristics, bowing and rarefaction of long bones, and extension of marrow into paraspinal or intraabdominal tumors. Massive enlargement of the liver and spleen can occur. Iron overload, produced by excessive intestinal absorption and transfusion, leads to cardiac failure and endocrinopathies that include diabetes mellitus and hypogonadism. Growth is retarded, sexual maturation delayed or absent, infections common, and gallstones prevalent. When untreated, patients with homozygous beta thalassemia die within the first two decades of life. With modern management this tragic spiral to dissolution need not transpire.

Thalassemia intermedia, a phenotype between that of thalassemia major and thalassemia minor, is caused most often by combinations of beta and alpha thalassemia, compound heterozygosity for beta thalassemia and delta-beta thalassemia, homozygosity for mild beta[+] thalassemia alleles, and combinations of beta thalassemia with HPFH. Many patients do not require transfusion, and some need it only occasionally. The evidence of iron overload, growth retardation, marrow expansion, and hypersplenism is generally less obvious than in severely affected patients, but bone disease can be prominent.

Compound heterozygotes with beta thalassemia and a gene for a beta-globin structural variant like hemoglobin S (HbS) or hemoglobin C (HbC) are commonly found (Table 88-2).

Laboratory Features

Erythrocytes of the beta thalassemia heterozygote have a mean corpuscular volume (MCV) of 55 to 80 fl and a corresponding reduction in mean corpuscular hemoglobin (MCH). The red blood cell distribution width (RDW) (Chapter 72) is normal, in contrast to iron deficiency anemia, where it is high. Silent carriers can have a normal MCV value. The red blood cell count is often elevated, and the blood film commonly shows target cells and basophilic stippling (Plate IV-4, *M*). Reticulocyte counts may be elevated (2% to 3%), but this is an inconsistent finding. Detection of most heterozygotes is simplified by the presence of an elevated HbA_2 level (4% to 6%), which is most accurately measured by column chromatography. The HbF level may be increased (1% to 3%). In delta-beta thalassemia carriers, the HbA_2 level is normal or reduced and the HbF concentration is increased (5% to 20%).

Homozygotes are severely anemic with hemoglobin levels of less than 5 g/dl without transfusion. Values for MCV and MCH are reduced, and the reticulocyte count strikingly elevated. The blood film findings are characterized by nucleated red blood cells, Pappenheimer and Howell-Jolly bodies, marked anisocytosis, poikilocytosis, and polychromatophilia (Plate IV-4, *L*). The bone marrow is hypercellular with marked erythroid hyperplasia and increased iron stores. Heinz bodies can be demonstrated by special staining methods (Plate IV-4, *P*). Fetal hemoglobin is the major hemoglobin component, with

---

Table 88-1   Molecular causes of beta thalassemia

MUTATION CLASS	LOCATION	PHENOTYPE
Nonsense mutations	Codon 39 C→T	beta[0]
	Codon 121 G→T	beta[0]
Frameshift mutations	Codon 6, A deleted	beta[0]
mRNA processing mutants	IVS-1, G→A	beta[0]
	IVS-2, A→G	beta[0]
	IVS-1 pos 5, G→C	beta[+]
	IVS-1 pos 110, G→A	beta[+]
Transcriptional mutants	−88 C→T	beta[+]
mRNA Cleavage site mutants	AATAAA→AACAAA	beta[+]
Hyperunstable globins	Codon 106 T→G (leu→arg)	beta[0]

absent or very reduced levels of HbA. The HbA_2 level shows considerable variation. Other indicators of chronic hemolysis are present, such as unconjugated hyperbilirubinemia, elevated lactate dehydrogenase (LDH) level, and decreased haptoglobin. Radiography of the skull may show the "hair on end" appearance of an enlarged diploic space, and other bones may appear osteoporotic.

Differential Diagnosis

The heterozygous beta thalassemias may be confused with iron deficiency and other microcytic anemias (Fig. 88-6; see Chapter 86). There are few disorders that may be confused with the severe homozygous beta thalassemias. Improperly managed patients with serious growth retardation, impaired nutrition, and marked hepatosplenomegaly superficially resemble individuals with advanced cirrhosis of the liver or malignancy.

Treatment

Heterozygous beta thalassemias require only recognition so that iron is not injudiciously administered, and carriers can be offered counseling. Screening programs based on the detection of microcytosis and presence of elevated HbA_2 levels are practical in groups with high disease prevalence. When a family is at risk for having homozygous

offspring, prenatal diagnosis is possible (discussed later). In parts of Greece, Italy, and Cyprus, screening, counseling, and prenatal diagnosis have led to a nearly 100% reduction in the numbers of homozygotes born.

Intensive transfusion therapy and chelation of excessive iron have improved the management of severe disease. When transfusion is started very early in life and the hemoglobin levels are kept at 9 to 10 g/dl, erythropoiesis is suppressed, marrow expansion does not occur, severe hemolysis is not present, and growth and development are near normal. Besides the usual complications of transfusion, such as alloimmunization and transmission of retroviral infection, the iron burden (deposited in tissues because of the destruction of transfused blood) must be removed by chelation to prevent the development of transfusion-induced hemochromatosis. Desferrioxamine (Desferal), a chelating agent, is given by prolonged subcutaneous or intravenous infusion, 8 to 12 hours nightly, 5 to 6 days weekly, at doses of 2 to 6 g/day using a portable infusion pump. The regimen must be tailored to each individual, since the amount of iron excreted varies. Optimum chelation therapy can induce negative iron balance. Keeping the iron burden low (serum ferritin level <1000 μg/L) is associated with the best prognosis. Even established cardiac disease is benefited by intense chelation. Ideally, chelation should be started in young children before the acquisition of excessive iron stores. Serum ferritin levels may not reflect accurately the iron content of liver biopsy speci-

Table 88-2   Sickle hemoglobinopathies

	HEMATOCRIT	MCV (Fl)	HBA (%)	HBS (%)	HBA$_2$ (%)	HBF (%)	VASOOCCLUSIVE SEVERITY
Sickle trait	Normal	Normal	60	40	2.5	<1	0
Sickle trait alpha thalassemia	Normal	70-80	65-75	25-35	2.5	<1	0
Sickle–beta$^+$ thalassemia	25-40	60-75	10-30	70	>3.5	<3	++
Sickle cell anemia	15-30	80-100	0	>85	2.5	5-15	++++
Sickle–beta^0 thalassemia	20-35	60-80	0	>85	>3.5	5-15	++++
Sickle cell anemia alpha thalassemia	20-35	70-90	0	>85	>3.5	5-15	++++
Sickle–delta-beta thalassemia	25-35	60-80	0	>80	2.5	10-20	++
Sickle–hereditary persistence of HbF	Normal	80-90	0	>70	2.5	20-30	0
HbSC disease	25-45	70-90	0	50	2.5	1-5	+++
Normal	38-55	80-95	97	0	2.5	<1	0

Hb, Hemoglobin; *HbSC disease*, compound heterozygosity for HbS and HbC.

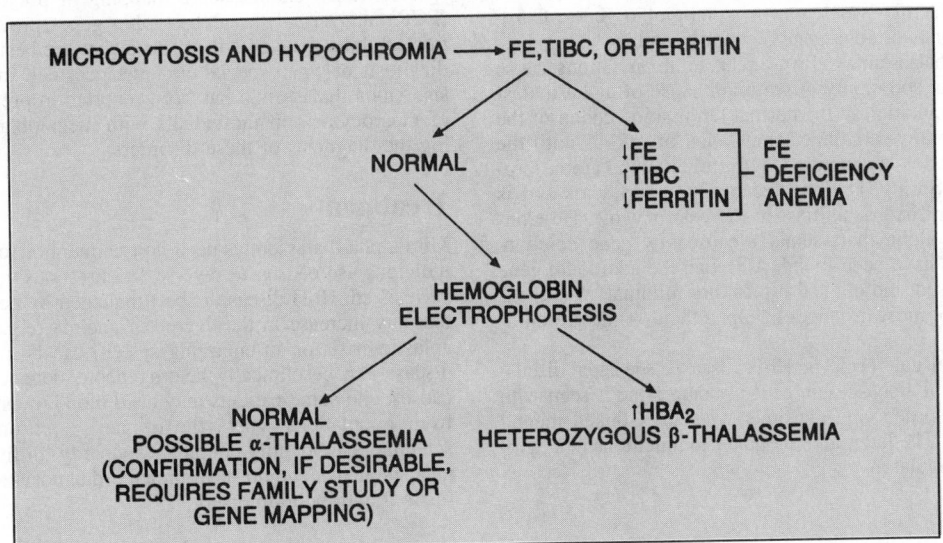

FIGURE 88-6   The evaluation of microcytosis and mild thalassemias. Microcytosis, best detected by electronic cell counters, may result from many causes. Iron deficiency is excluded by measuring serum iron level and iron binding capacity or ferritin level. If these values are normal, hemoglobin electrophoresis should be performed, with measurement of the level of adult hemoglobin A_2 (HbA_2) and fetal hemoglobin (HbF). An elevated HbA_2 level is consistent with heterozygous beta thalassemia. If HbA_2 and HbF levels are normal, microcytosis with minimal or no anemia suggests alpha thalassemia. This diagnosis is more likely in populations where the prevalence of this disorder is high.

mens, and some experts recommend measuring the latter. Low doses of vitamin C may increase the excretion of iron by desferrioxamine and can be used in vitamin C–depleted individuals while they are receiving chelation treatment. An oral chelating agent that provides relief from the arduous regimen of subcutaneous infusion is under investigation. Although effective, it has worrisome toxicities and may not remove iron as efficiently as desferrioxamine.

Splenectomy may be performed when the red blood cell survival shortens. This reduces the excessive red blood cell destruction and cytopenias of hypersplenism and lengthens the interval between transfusions. Severe postsplenectomy infection is a risk that must be weighed and argues for delaying surgery as long as possible. Polyvalent pneumococcal, *Haemophilus influenzae* and *Neisseria meningitidis* vaccine should be given before surgery, and prophylactic penicillin afterward.

Bone marrow transplantation has been employed in severe beta thalassemia, and considerable experience has been gained in Italian centers. It is the sole way to eradicate the disease. However, the best candidates are the youngest children, as older, more heavily transfused patients are less likely to become engrafted and have higher morbidity and mortality. Because transfusion and effective chelation can allow normal development and a decent quality of life for many years, and since bone marrow transplantation still has appreciable short-term mortality, the decision to recommend this therapy has been difficult. However, in children who have little or no liver disease as a result of efficient chelation, transplantation using haploidentical donors results in a disease-free survival rate of 90%. If these results are replicable, early transplantation may be the most efficacious and cost-effective method of treatment and free the patient who has a suitable donor from the lifelong burden of transfusions and chelation.

Hydroxyurea and 5-azacytidine—perhaps with the addition of erythropoietin—may increase HbF and raise the hemoglobin level in some individuals with beta thalassemia. Few patients have been treated, and the results are unpredictable. Further over the horizon are means of compensating for the genetic defect of thalassemia by gene therapy.

ALPHA THALASSEMIA
Etiology

Alpha thalassemia results from a reduction in the synthesis of alpha chains so that insufficient amounts are available for combining with nonalpha globins and assembling a hemoglobin tetramer. The usual cause of alpha thalassemia is deletion of alpha-globin genes. Chromosomes with one or two alpha-gene deletions combine to produce the different alpha thalassemias (Box 88-1). Point mutations cause alpha thalassemia less commonly. A common cause of alpha thalassemia in Asians is a mutation in the normal termination codon of the 5′-alpha gene. This allows continued translation of mRNA until the next termination codon is encountered. The variant alpha globin produced, Hb Constant Spring, is elongated by 31 amino acids and is made in greatly diminished quantities. In the heterozygote, Hb Constant Spring mimics alpha thalassemia-1 caused by gene deletion. Triplicated alpha loci have been found. Although the additional gene appears to be expressed, the clinical effects are minimal. While extraordinarily common, most instances of alpha thalassemia are clinically trivial.

There are two unusual forms of HbH disease (see later discussion), both with normal alpha-globin gene structure; one is seen with myeloproliferative disorders and the other with an X-linked mental retardation syndrome. The latter are secondary to mutations in a "global" transcriptional regulator.

Clinical Features

The prevalence of a single deleted alpha-globin gene ($-\alpha/\alpha\alpha$) may be near 90% in some southwest Pacific Islanders and is 30% in black Americans. In this population clinically significant disease is seldom seen because the chromosome lacking two alpha genes (α^0 or $--/$) is rare. Southeast Asians have a high prevalence of both the $-\alpha/$ and $--/$ chromosomes. Therefore the clinically important alpha thalassemias, HbH disease and hydrops fetalis, are most often seen in this

✔ *WHEN TO REFER*

On diagnosis, patients with thalassemia major, thalassemia intermedia, and HbH disease should have a plan of care established in a center experienced in the treatment options for and complications of these disorders. Here the needed genetic, diagnostic, and counseling services can be arranged, hypertransfusion and chelation regimens initiated and monitored, and psychosocial support provided.

region. However, HbH disease is found in Mediterranean populations and occurs rarely in blacks.

Lack of a standard nomenclature for alpha thalassemia is reflected in the clinical and genetic terminology (Box 88-1).

Loss of one or two alpha-globin genes is clinically inconsequential. Single gene deletions are virtually undetectable, and loss of two genes results in microcytosis only. HbH disease, in which only a single alpha gene is active, is a mild to moderately severe hemolytic anemia with microcytic erythrocytes and splenomegaly. Total loss of four functional alpha genes is incompatible with life and causes stillbirth of hydropic fetuses. Pregnancies carrying hydropic fetuses are complicated by a high incidence of toxemia.

Laboratory Features

Diagnosis of mild forms of alpha thalassemia is hindered by lack of a simple test. In populations where the prevalence of this disorder is high, suspicion of its presence can be raised by finding microcytosis and a normal RDW (Chapter 72) with minimal or no anemia, in the absence of iron deficiency or beta thalassemia (Fig. 88-6). Bart's Hb and HbH are produced by tetramerization of excessive gamma and beta chains, respectively. Both have very high oxygen affinity and are of no value in oxygen transport. The levels of Bart's Hb in cord blood of individuals with alpha thalassemia are proportionate to the reduction of functional alpha genes, but considerable overlap in levels precludes this from being a facile method of diagnosing alpha thalassemia in neonates. In HbH disease, HbH can be detected by electrophoresis and by special staining of erythrocytes. Bart's Hb and HbH predominate in hydropic fetuses.

Restriction endonuclease mapping or polymerase chain reaction (PCR) analysis of the alpha-globin genes provides definitive detection of alpha-gene deletion. These tests are best reserved for prenatal diagnosis or when special circumstances call for a definitive diagnosis. Alpha thalassemia has been reported to prevent the development of macrocytosis in individuals with megaloblastic anemias, impairing the diagnosis of these disorders.

Treatment

Mild alpha thalassemias need no treatment or follow-up care. The injudicious use of iron to reverse a nonresponsive microcytosis should be resisted. HbH disease is best managed by periodic observation so that any increase in the degree of anemia (e.g., from a supervening aplastic crisis or an enlarging spleen) can be properly treated. HbH disease can be clinically heterogeneous depending on its molecular causes, and some patients may need blood transfusion. In individuals from populations where the α^0 or $--/$chromosome is common, screening can identify couples at jeopardy for hydropic fetuses. Pregnancies at risk should have prenatal diagnosis and, if a hydropic fetus is found, be terminated.

SICKLE CELL DISEASE

Sickle hemoglobin (HbS; beta^6 glu→val) results from a GAG→GUG mutation in the codon for the sixth amino acid of beta globin. This mutation had four distinct origins in Africa 2000 to 3000 years ago. Its high prevalence in blacks and selected other ethnic groups results from the survival advantage of the heterozygote under the selective pressure of *Falciparum malaria* infestation that blossomed about that time. Natural selection has also led to the high prevalence of alpha and beta thalassemia, HbC and hemoglobin E (HbE), ovalocytosis, and glucose-6-phosphate dehydrogenase deficiency where malaria was endemic.

Etiology

Sickle hemoglobin polymerizes when deoxygenated. Accumulation of HbS polymer within the erythrocyte distorts the cell and injures its membrane. Potassium and water leak from the cell, and it becomes dense and inflexible. Travel through the microcirculation, where capillary diameter is often only 2 to 3 μm, is slowed because considerable cellular deformability is a requisite for successful passage. Lodging of cells retards flow, reducing oxygen tension and causing further hemoglobin polymerization and tissue ischemia or infarction. These events may be initiated by subpopulations of dense cells within the community of sickle erythrocytes. In contrast to the uniformity of normal erythrocytes, the erythrocytes in sickle cell anemia (hemoglobin SS [HbSS]) are very heterogeneous, with a spectrum of density, deformability, membrane injury, hemoglobin content, and life span.

Adherence of some cells to endothelium may allow vasoocclusion to occur before their escape into large vessels. Deoxygenation-induced polymerization of HbS is reversible with reoxygenation. But, after a number of sickle-unsickle cycles, permanent damage to the cell membrane occurs, leaving the cell distorted, whatever the quantity of intracellular polymer. These irreversibly sickled cells (ISCs) are seen on the blood film (Plate IV-4, *H*) and are diagnostic of sickle cell disease. Their numbers vary widely among patients, but in an individual they remain relatively constant. However, early during a painful episode, ISC levels and dense cell fractions fall, only to rebound to higher levels as the crisis resolves.

Hemoglobin F concentration is the major prognostic factor in HbSS. Its high postnatal level is responsible for the benignity of this period. X-chromosome–linked genes and genetic elements marked by the haplotype of the beta-globin gene cluster regulate, in part, HbF levels. A higher HbF level is associated with fewer episodes of pain and longer survival.

Clinical Features

Sickle cell trait (HbAS; heterozygotes for the beta^S gene)—present in about 8% of African-Americans—is asymptomatic. Carriers have none of the hemolytic or vasoocclusive events typical of patients with HbSS or other severe sickling disorders (Table 88-2). Their sole clinical complication is hematuria, which is usually mild and self-limiting and needs no treatment. Hyposthenuria—nearly always present—is clinically unimportant. Both renal abnormalities result from sickling in the hypertonic, hypoxic, acidotic environment that typifies the normal renal medulla. There is no valid reason to restrict the activities or occupation of individuals with HbAS.

Hemoglobin SS is present in about 1 in 600 African-American newborns, and hemoglobin SC (HbSC) disease is found in 1 in 800. All of the complications of HbSS can be present in HbSC disease, albeit with a reduced incidence. The beta^S gene is often present in compound heterozygotes with genes for beta thalassemia or other beta-globin mutants, such as HbC, HbD, HbE, and HbO. Alpha thalassemia is commonly found with HbAS and HbSS (Table 88-2). Examples of the inheritance of HbSS and HbS–beta^0 thalassemia are shown in Fig. 88-7 and illustrate the mendelian transmission of all globin-gene abnormalities. Pathophysiologic and clinical features of sickling disorders can be separated into those that result from hemolysis of sickle cells and those that result from vasoocclusive episodes due to sickle cells. The former are common to all chronic hemolytic anemias, are amenable to management, and are generally benign. The latter typify the sickling disorders, are difficult to manage, and are the major cause of morbidity and mortality.

Hemolysis in sickle cell disease occurs largely extravascularly and even in HbSS is usually only moderate. The symptoms of anemia per se are not the hallmark of this disease. Some severely anemic patients have an element of renal failure, or anemia can develop acutely because of acquired marrow failure. Plasma volume in HbSS may be expanded 20% to 40%, making it difficult to predict the red blood cell mass from the hemoglobin level. Most patients tolerate chronic

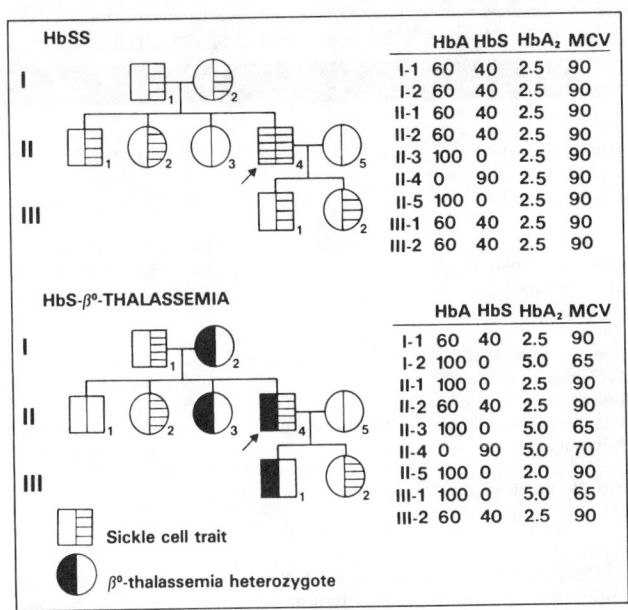

FIGURE 88-7   Genetics of sickle cell disease. Pedigrees and hematologic data in two typical families with a proband who has the "sickle hemoglobin (HbS) only" pattern on hemoglobin electrophoresis. In the first family the proband (↗) is homozygous for the beta^S gene and has sickle cell anemia. Both his parents have the sickle trait. In the idealized family of four offspring, two have the sickle trait, one is normal, and one has sickle cell anemia (HbSS). If the mother is normal, all offspring of the proband will have the sickle trait. In the second family the proband (↗) is a compound heterozygote for the beta^S gene and a beta^0 thalassemia gene (HbS-beta^0 thalassemia). One parent has sickle trait and the other has heterozygous-beta^0 thalassemia. The idealized family of four offspring contains one normal, one sickle trait, one beta^0 thalassemia trait, and one HbS-beta^0 thalassemia individual. The offspring of the proband, given a normal mother, have either sickle trait or beta^0 thalassemia trait.

hemoglobin levels of 5 to 7 g/dl exceptionally well. Persistent hyperbilirubinemia, a consequence of hemolysis, is associated with a high prevalence of gallstones. Stones may appear in patients at remarkably young ages and are present in nearly half of all adults.

Vasoocclusive events of the sickling disorders can occur acutely, producing dramatic clinical findings, or be chronic but, nevertheless, disabling (Table 88-3). The recurrence and duration of painful episodes vary markedly among patients. A minority have monthly episodes that last for 3 to 10 days and require hospitalization for management. Others never describe a serious pain crisis. The frequency of painful episodes is directly related to the total hemoglobin concentration and inversely related to the HbF level. Numerous painful crises are a poor prognostic sign.

The heart is usually enlarged, and systolic murmurs are common. Contractility is normal, and overt congestive heart failure is uncommon. Children with sickle cell disease may develop "hand-foot" syndrome—a sickling-induced periostitis of metacarpal and metatarsal bones that mimics acute rheumatoid arthritis.

Hemoglobin level remains quite constant over time unless erythropoiesis is depressed. Bacterial infection may transiently reduce erythropoiesis. Dramatic but transient falls in hemoglobin level can occur in association with infection by the human B19 parvovirus. This agent preferentially attacks erythroid precursors and is the major cause of aplastic crisis. In aplastic crisis, the bone marrow has few primitive red blood cells and reticulocytes may be absent. Recovery occurs in 1 to 2 weeks. Children with HbSS and splenomegaly and, less often, adults with HbSC disease or HbS–beta thalassemia may have splenic sequestration crisis—the sudden pooling of red blood cells in a damaged spleen. The spleen rapidly enlarges as the hemoglobin level plummets, and transfusion may be lifesaving. Rarely, when severe anemia develops, megaloblastic arrest of erythropoiesis is found. This is usually due to marginal nutrition that causes folic acid deficiency.

Table 88-3 Vasoocclusive consequences of sickle cell disease

EVENT	INCIDENCE	FEATURES
Acute		
Painful episodes	More than 50% of patients with HbSS and HbS–beta thalassemia	Mild to severe pain, one or several areas
Chest syndrome	10%-20% of adults	Difficult to distinguish from pneumonia; may involve entire lung
Priapism	10%-40% of males	Can have a more chronic form; causes impotence
Cerebrovascular accidents	1%-10% of children	Usually subarachnoid bleeds in adults
Hepatopathy	<2% of adults	Bilirubin may reach level >80 mg/dl
Chronic		
Aseptic bone necrosis	10%-25% of adults	Hips and shoulders: also seen in HbSC
Proliferative retinopathy	50% of adults with HbSC, <5% HbSS	Can lead to retinal detachment
Leg ulcers	10%	Can be severe and disabling
Functional asplenia and autosplenectomy	Starts in infancy >90% of adults with HbSS	Predisposes to sepsis
Nephropathy	Renal failure in older patients	Nephrotic syndrome, renal failure

HbS, Hemoglobin S (sickle hemoglobin); *HbSC,* hemoglobin SC disease; *HbSS,* hemoglobin SS (sickle cell anemia).

Infection is the major cause of death in children in the first years of life, and the most common offending agent is *Streptococcus pneumoniae.* Sepsis produced by this bacterium claims a quarter of its victims. Osteomyelitis caused by *Salmonella* organisms is typical of sickle cell disease. During the course of HbSS, and to a lesser extent in HbSC and HbS–beta thalassemia, splenic function decreases and is ultimately lost because of repetitive infarction. Early in life the spleen may be large but hypofunctional. It then atrophies and disappears. The rate of splenic regression is related to the natural reduction in HbF levels that occurs during postnatal development and can be readily detected by the appearance of intraerythrocytic inclusions such as Howell-Jolly bodies (Plate IV-4, *K*). Hyposplenic patients are susceptible to infection with encapsulated bacteria such as *S. pneumoniae* and *Haemophilus influenzae.* Sepsis, pneumonia, meningitis, and otitis are most frequent, and infection can progress with devastating rapidity. Sepsis in adults is often due to *Escherichia coli* and associated with urinary tract infection. Defects of the alternative complement pathway, other opsonins, and the antibody response to capsular polysaccharides may also increase the susceptibility to infection.

Causes of death in adults are more varied. About 20% of deaths are related to organ failure, but often death is unexpected and occurs in the midst of an acute event like a pain crisis. In the United States the median age at death is about 45 years in HbSS and about 65 years in HbSC disease. Survival past childhood is still unusual in underdeveloped lands.

A general feature of sickle cell disease is its clinical heterogeneity. Some patients have very mild disease and others have many complications. It is this latter group—actually the minority of patients—that frequents the emergency department and clinic and gives most physicians their portrait of this disease. We still do not fully understand the reasons for this phenotypic diversity, but genetic and environmental modulators are the most likely cause.

Laboratory Features

Typical hematologic findings in sickle cell diseases are listed in Table 88-2. The cornerstone of diagnosis is the detection and quantification of the level of HbS. Hemoglobin solubility tests can only confirm the presence of HbS and should not be used for primary diagnosis. The blood film (Plate IV-4, *H*) shows ISCs, Howell-Jolly bodies, and Pappenheimer bodies in most patients with HbSS. In HbSC disease, only target cells may be seen (Plate IV-4, *D* and *N*), and in HbS–beta thalassemia, hypochromia, microcytosis, and target cells are present (Plate IV-4, *M*). For the evaluation of compound heterozygous conditions (Table 88-2; Fig. 88-7), family studies are vital.

Differential Diagnosis

Diagnosis of a sickle hemoglobinopathy is not difficult, but in some cases differentiating among these disorders can be confusing. Useful points of distinction are shown in Table 88-2. The spectrum of clinical events that occur in these patients makes sickling-induced complications a great mimic of many other diseases.

Treatment

Sickle cell disease is a chronic disorder, and attention should be given to good nutrition, immunizations, and avoidance of extremes of temperature and activity. Nonexertional work should be encouraged. Increased rates of red blood cell production and inadequate nutrition have led to the routine use of supplemental folic acid, 1 mg daily. Although polyvalent pneumococcal vaccine provides only limited protection in children, it should be used. Its value in adults is not proved. *H. influenzae* vaccine should also be employed in infancy. Prophylactic penicillin should be started at 3 to 4 months of age. Children less than age 3 years should receive 125 mg of oral penicillin twice a day, and older children, 250 mg orally twice a day. This treatment has reduced the incidence of pneumococcal sepsis and death. If severe pneumococcal disease has not occurred, and if the patient is enrolled in a comprehensive care program, prophylactic penicillin can be safely discontinued at age 5 years. An alarming increase in the resistance of *S. pneumoniae* to penicillin should prompt continuing surveillance of the efficacy of this life saving treatment.

Painful episodes are the most common acute clinical events; an approach to management is outlined in Box 88-2. Infrequently given, inadequate doses of analgesics are the most common deficiency in their treatment.

Acute chest syndrome—characterized by fever, chest pain, cough, and lung infiltrates—affects a third of all HbSS patients. The cause varies. Chest syndrome is most common but least severe in young children, in whom it often results from infection. In adults, pain often precedes this event and mortality is higher than in children. Fat embolism is a common cause of the most severe events during which hemoglobin and platelet levels fall and the leukocyte count increases.

When treating infection, antimicrobial agent selection need not deviate from the general practice in non–immune-suppressed-individuals. However, it should be recalled that pneumococcal infection is the scourge of childhood, salmonella osteomyelitis has a high incidence in HbSS, and gram-negative infections are most common in adults.

Replacement of sickle blood with normal blood is conceptually the most specific form of treatment. Used routinely, however this approach is impractical because of the problems of transfusional hemosiderosis, alloimmunization, venous access, viral infection, and expense. However, transfusion of red blood cells at times can be lifesaving and at other times may be useful. For chronic situations such as severe symptomatic anemia or stroke prophylaxis simple transfusions are preferred. Acute events like stroke or acute chest syndrome are better handled with exchange transfusion. Transfusions increase partial pressure of oxygen in arterial blood and oxygen saturation in acute chest syndrome. Anemia is rarely an indication for transfusion.

BOX 88-2
Management of pain in sickle cell disease

Identify a cause if possible.
  If infection is present, treat with antibiotics.
  Treat dehydration with fluids.
Ensure optimal hydration, 3 to 4 L of fluids per day.
  If possible, replace fluids orally.
  When necessary, give fluids intravenously.
Treat acute, severe vasoocclusive pain.
  Give morphine, meperidine, or hydromorphone parenterally in full
    therapeutic doses at 2-4-hour intervals.
  Avoid as-needed analgesics.
  Consider patient-controlled analgesia and adjunctive drugs like
    hydroxyzine and promethazine.
Treat mild to moderate acute and chronic pain.
  Consider fentanyl patches for prolonged, moderate to severe pain.
  Give reliable patients acetaminophen-codeine for mild to moderate
    pain that can be managed at home.
  Use nonsteroidal antiinflamatory drugs for chronic pains of osteo-
    necrosis or backache.

✔ *WHEN TO REFER*

Since for many primary care physicians these are rare disorders, on diagnosis a referral to a hematologist or sickle cell center may help establish the needed level of continuing care. Because of the implications for genetic counseling, individuals in whom the genotypic diagnosis is unclear should be examined by a laboratory expert in the complexities of hemoglobin disorders. Management of stroke and the acute chest syndrome is best handled by experienced hematologists. The choice of whether to begin treatment with hydroxyurea and how to adjust the dose requires knowledge of this drug and its effects in HbSS, a clear notion of the desired end points, and the laboratory capacity for reliable HbF measurements. Transfusion programs require laboratory support to fractionate HbS and HbA levels and the means to follow the effectiveness of iron chelation therapy. Difficult pain problems are helped by consultation with individuals with special expertise in pain management and mental health professionals.

With aging and incipient renal failure, severe anemia may become symptomatic. Transfusion may then become necessary. Judicious use of very high doses of erythropoietin aimed at restoring the hemoglobin level to values customarily seen in HbSS may substitute for transfusion in the expanding group of patients with renal insufficiency.

Packed red blood cells are often needed during the acute and very severe anemia of aplastic and splenic sequestration crisis. In splenic sequestration normal erythrocytes appear to reverse the hypoxic injury to the splenic vasculature. Sequestration crises do recur, and splenectomy is indicated after the first recurrence. Repeated thrombotic cerebrovascular accidents can be prevented by prophylactic transfusion. Here the aim is to rapidly—by exchange transfusion—reduce the proportion of HbS to 20% to 30% and maintain a hemoglobin level of about 10 g/dl. It is not clear how long prophylactic transfusion should be continued or what is the lowest effective HbA concentration. After keeping the HbS level at 20% to 30% for several years, some authorities believe that the frequency of transfusion may be readjusted to maintain about 50% HbS. Iron chelation may be needed in patients receiving chronic transfusion. Transcranial Doppler measurement of cerebral blood flow can identify patients at greatest risk for stroke, raising the issue (now under study) of whether they could be candidates for primary prevention by transfusion. That "silent" infarction associated with cognitive defects is twice as prevalent as overt stroke emphasizes the potential utility of this approach. Hemorrhagic stroke is the most prevalent cerebrovascular accident in adults. In this case the value of prophylactic transfusion is unknown. Intensive transfusion to reduce HbS levels should be performed before angiographic studies of the cerebral vasculature.

Transfusions are often used without the benefit of critical studies that confirm their merit. Refractory severe leg ulcers may respond to intensive transfusion but often recur when the HbS level rises. Severe sickle hepatopathy and episodes of acute chest syndrome with hypoxia have also been managed by transfusion. In these cases reduction of the HbS level is most rapidly achieved by red blood cell exchange using a cell separator to prevent hypervolemia. The goal of 20% to 30% HbS concentration can then often be maintained by transfusion of 1 or 2 units of packed red blood cells every 2 to 4 weeks. Alloimmunization occurs in about a fourth of frequently transfused patients. In the presence of multiple alloantibodies it may be difficult to find compatible blood. This high incidence of alloimmunization is a result of underrepresentation of blacks in the blood donor pool and antigenic differences that exist between erythrocytes of white donors and black recipients. To reduce the risk of sensitization, the recipient's red blood cell antigen phenotype should be determined and the most compatible blood provided. An alternative is to transfuse racially identified blood, as this will reduce the chance of exposure to units containing new antigens. Surgery can be safely performed in sickle cell disease. Simple transfusion to a hemoglobin level of about 10 g/dl before surgery under general anesthesia is as effective in preventing complications as an aggressive regimen that reduces HbS levels to 30% or less and exposes patients to half as much blood. Despite the regimen used, complications—often minor—happen in about a third of surgeries; acute chest syndrome, a major problem, occurs in 10%. Still unclear is the complication rate of surgery without routine transfusion. Random transfusions for painful episodes and most other acute or chronic events are not helpful and expose the patient to the previously discussed risks.

Pregnancy in sickle cell disease is associated with a high rate of obstetric complications. Spontaneous abortion has a 1% to 20% incidence, even with the best management. This is presumably a result of placental insufficiency. In controlled studies, patients managed with intrapartum transfusion or meticulous obstetric care without prophylactic transfusion had similar outcomes. There is no general indication for sterilization or interruption of pregnancy in women with HbSS. Folic acid should be given, iron supplements employed if there is evidence of reduced iron stores, and transfusions given only when the clinical and hematologic status indicates their necessity. The usual methods of birth control can be used, although contraceptive pills might be avoided by older women.

The management of gallstones is problematic. Many events can provoke right upper quadrant pain in HbSS, often making a firm diagnosis of cholecystitis difficult. When stones are asymptomatic or symptoms and laboratory findings are equivocal, it is probably best not to perform cholecystectomy. Laparoscopic cholecystectomy could, because of its minor morbidity, change the approach to stones.

The pain of osteonecrosis is sometimes relieved by nonsteroidal antiinflamatory agents. As destruction progresses, however, pain becomes severe, and function is lost, the affected joint—most often the hip—needs replacement. Leg ulcers usually heal spontaneously with rest and careful local hygiene. At times they become huge, exceedingly painful, and disabling and defy all simple therapeutic measures. Intensive transfusion, hydroxyurea (see later discussion), local oxygen application, and skin grafting all have been used with some success.

By inhibiting HbS polymerization, HbF diminishes the severity of HbSS. Both clinical and laboratory features of HbSS are influenced by HbF concentration. Patients with higher HbF levels have fewer pain episodes and longer survival. Hydroxyurea can increase the level of HbF in some patients with HbSS. In a group of severely affected individuals who had at least several crises yearly, hydroxyurea reduced by nearly half the incidence of pain crisis and acute chest syndrome, frequency of hospitalization, and use of blood transfusion. Sickled red blood cells became less dense, hemolysis was reduced, and the hemoglobin level increased. When this treatment is carefully monitored, toxicity, mainly granulocytopenia, is minor. At present this treatment should be reserved for patients whose complications are sufficiently severe to warrant the bother of this potentially hazardous treatment and who are capable of complying with the treatment regimen. Therapy should be started with 500 mg of hydroxyurea daily.

Table 88-4   Clinical syndromes produced by hemoglobinopathies

SYNDROME	EXAMPLES	CLINICAL AND HEMATOLOGIC FINDINGS	DIAGNOSIS
Unstable hemoglobin (Hb)	Hb Zürich Hb Köln	Hemolytic anemia May be drug induced Heinz bodies	Hb electrophoresis Heat instability Isopropanol test Often a new mutation
High O_2 affinity	Hb Chesapeake Hb Yakima	Polycythemia Normal mean corpuscular volume Normal white blood cell count	Hb electrophoresis Hb-O_2 dissociation curve (P50)
Methemoglobinemia	Hb M-Boston Hb M-Iwate	Cyanosis Mild hemolysis	Hb electrophoresis Hb absorption spectra

After 6 to 8 weeks, if blood cell counts are stable, the dose may be increased to 1000 mg per day. Most patients who respond to hydroxyurea with an increase in HbF maintain tolerable blood cell counts at doses of 1000 to 2000 mg daily. The therapeutic end point should strike a balance between a nontoxic dose of hydroxyurea and increases of HbF. The MCV increases along with HbF and may be used as a surrogate measure. Until a stable dosage is achieved, counts should be monitored biweekly. Even when a final dose is reached, monthly counts should be obtained to forestall complications from the occasional capricious fall in blood cell counts. A poor response to hydroxyurea in patients who take the drug as directed may be associated with a lack of bone marrow "reserve" and the inability to safely suppress the marrow—a necessity for hydroxyurea to have an effect on HbF. Patients should be explicitly counseled that it may take months to reach the best dose of drug, that medication must be taken exactly as directed with frequent blood tests, that response differs among patients, and that the very long-term toxicities and effects of treatment are unknown. Studies of hydroxyurea in young children or even adolescents, where its therapeutic effects are likely to reap the greatest benefits, are just beginning. Efforts to minimalize the effective dose of hydroxyurea seem justified because of the possible long-term hazards of a drug that may have carcinogenic potential.

Bone marrow transplantation has been used in HbSS, but results in less than 100 patients have been reported. Early results are encouraging, but parental acceptance of this procedure may be low. Current trials focus on young patients with the poorest prognosis—individuals with strokes, repeated acute chest syndrome, and intractable pain. Central nervous system events were a troublesome complication in patients receiving transplants because of an earlier cerebrovascular accident.

PRENATAL DIAGNOSIS AND SCREENING

Prenatal diagnosis of thalassemia and hemoglobinopathies is a feasible option. This should be carried out in the context of selected heterozygote screening and education of high-risk groups. The major goal of these programs is family counseling about the risks, options, and potential outcomes of pregnancy. Cord blood screening programs for sickle cell disease, in contrast, are directed at the detection of neonates with clinically severe sickle hemoglobinopathies. These programs are cost effective in high-risk populations. Early detection allows the institution of continuing care and prophylactic penicillin. More than 40 states screen neonates for sickle hemoglobinopathies.

DNA technology has revolutionized prenatal diagnosis and is likely to be the method of the future for sickle cell screening programs. Prenatal diagnosis can now be made from chorionic villi that can be obtained at 10 weeks of gestation or on fetal DNA from amniotic fluid cells at 16 weeks of gestation. Both procedures increase fetal loss by less than 1%. The HbS gene can be detected by use of restriction endonucleases that cut at the site of this mutation or by direct examination of the mutation using allele-specific oligonucleotide probes. Alpha thalassemia hydrops fetalis is diagnosed by finding a complete absence of alpha genes. Because beta thalassemia–causing mutations cluster in different racial and ethnic groups, direct detection of the mutations in fetal DNA, using gene amplification and groups of oligonucleotide probes specific for the mutations common in the patients' ethnic group, has become the standard means of rec-

ognition. Unusual or new mutations can be ascertained by direct DNA sequencing. Quantum leaps in technology have characterized the past decades' work in molecular biology. It is well within our current expectations that most common genetic diseases will be rapidly and inexpensively discovered before or at birth.

OTHER HEMOGLOBINOPATHIES

Other hemoglobinopathies can produce clinical disorders. These are summarized in Table 88-4. Several hundred hemoglobinopathies have been characterized, but those causing clinically recognizable disorders are a minority. Amino acid substitutions involving heme-binding residues may lead to irreversible iron oxidation, methemoglobinemia, and cyanosis. Substitutions at contacts between globin subunits may alter the affinity of hemoglobin for oxygen. When hemoglobin-oxygen affinity is increased, less oxygen is available in tissues, erythropoietin production is enhanced, and erythrocytosis results. If hemoglobin-oxygen affinity is reduced, anemia or cyanosis may result. Hemoglobin instability produced by several molecular mechanisms including introduction of proline residues into the alpha helix, substitutions near the heme ring, and deletion or addition of amino acids often causes hemolysis.

HbC (beta[6] glu→lys) and HbE (beta[26] glu→lys) are common beta-globin variants. The former is present in about 2% of blacks, and the latter is seen in Asians; its prevalence in Southeast Asians may reach 60%. Heterozygotes with either mutation are asymptomatic. Even homozygotes for these variants have virtually no clinical disease, only mild hematologic abnormalities like microcytosis, target cells, and in HbC, mild anemia. When HbE and beta thalassemia interact, a syndrome similar to homozygous beta thalassemia is produced as a consequence of the intrinsically "thalassemic" nature of the HbE gene. HbE heterozygotes have the phenotype of mild beta thalassemia trait. In certain Southeast Asian groups where HbE, alpha, and beta thalassemia are prevalent, heterozygote screening can identify couples who are likely to have severely affected offspring.

BIBLIOGRAPHY

Brittenham GM et al: Efficacy of deferoxamine in preventing complications of iron overload in patients with thalassemia major, *N Engl J Med* 331:567, 1994.

Cao A, Galanello R, Rosatelli MC: Genotype-phenotype correlations in β-thalassemias, *Blood Rev* 8:1, 1994.

Charache S et al: Hydroxyurea and sickle cell anemia: clinical utility of a myelosuppressive "switching" agent, *Medicine* 75:300, 1996.

Embury SH, Hebbel RP, Mohandas N, Steinberg MH: *Sickle cell disease: basic principles and clinical practice*, New York, 1994, Raven.

Hebbel RP: Beyond hemoglobin polymerization: the red blood cell membrane and sickle disease pathophysiology, *Blood* 77:214, 1991.

Platt OS et al: Pain in sickle cell disease: rates and risk factors, *N Engl J Med* 325:11, 1991.

Platt OS et al: Mortality in sickle cell disease: life expectancy and risk factors for early death, *N Engl J Med* 330:1639-1644, 1994.

Steinberg MH: Genetic modulation of sickle cell anemia, *Proc Soc Exp Biol Med* 209:1, 1995.

Vichinsky EP et al: A comparison of conservative and aggressive transfusion regimens in the perioperative management of sickle cell disease, *N Engl J Med* 333:206, 1995.

Wayne AS, Kevy SV, Nathan DG: Transfusion management of sickle cell disease, *Blood* 81:1109, 1993.

Weatherall DJ: The thalassemias. In Stamatoyannopoulos G, Nienhuis AW, Majerus PW, Varmus H, editors: *The molecular basis of blood diseases*, Philadelphia, 1994, WB Saunders.

CHAPTER

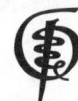

89 Hemolytic Anemia

John C. Winkelmann

Hemolytic anemias are pathologic conditions that sufficiently shorten the survival of red blood cells (RBCs) in the circulation to decrease their steady state concentration. Because the bone marrow can be stimulated physiologically to produce erythrocytes 8 to 10 times faster than the normal rate, hemolytic processes must reduce RBC survival considerably below the normal life span of 115 days to generate a significant clinical problem.

Regardless of their cause, hemolytic disorders exhibit several common features that facilitate diagnosis. The most helpful of these is an increased reticulocyte index stemming from enhanced RBC production to compensate for the accelerated rate of destruction. Because reticulocytes are larger than mature RBCs, significant reticulocytosis is usually accompanied by a high RBC mean cell volume (MCV) that may be mistaken by the clinician for evidence of macrocytic anemia. Furthermore, reticulocytosis is not specific for hemolysis. Increased reticulocytes are seen in patients who are bleeding or recovering from bone marrow suppression. Conversely, the absence of increased reticulocytes does not rule out hemolysis. Acute hemolysis may become evident prior to the time required to produce new reticulocytes (3 to 5 days). Also, patients with suppressed bone marrow function or impaired erythropoiesis due to nutrient deficiencies, B19 parvovirus infection, or inflammation may have a blunted reticulocyte response to hemolysis.

Several biochemical changes occur in hemolytic states. Clinically significant hemolysis usually produces increased serum levels of indirect (unconjugated) bilirubin that result from the degradation of heme in destroyed RBCs. In hemolysis, lactate dehydrogenase (LDH) is released from RBCs and is detectable in the serum. Haptoglobin is a serum glycoprotein that binds to hemoglobin and facilitates its uptake by the liver. Haptoglobin levels are usually decreased in hemolysis. None of these chemical alterations is specific for hemolysis. Indirect hyperbilirubinemia is characteristic of Gilbert's disease and megaloblastic anemia. LDH may be increased due to damaged hepatocytes (or other cell types), lymphoma, or ineffective erythropoiesis. Haptoglobin may be decreased due to hepatocyte dysfunction or a congenital absence of this molecule.

Several diagnostic test results are characteristic of hemolysis occurring within the circulation (intravascular hemolysis). Plasma free hemoglobin, hemoglobinuria, and urine hemosiderin are produced by intravascular hemolysis. Plasma free hemoglobin may be very transient and is easily missed. Also, shearing of RBCs during phlebotomy can give falsely positive measurements. Hemoglobinuria only occurs after serum haptoglobin and renal tubular absorption are saturated and may also be transient. In contrast, urine hemosiderin may be detectable for several days after a hemolytic episode. Therefore analysis of urine hemosiderin is of diagnostic value in cases of intermittent or low-grade intravascular hemolysis.

EVALUATION OF THE PATIENT WITH HEMOLYTIC ANEMIA

When should a clinician consider hemolysis as a possible diagnosis in a patient with anemia? Box 89-1 lists circumstances in which a patient should be evaluated for hemolysis. The clinical presentation of patients with acute hemolysis may differ substantially from patients with chronic hemolysis. Causes, however, often overlap. For example, conditions that produce chronic hemolysis may become evident initially as an acute hemolytic process. Regardless of the cause, an acute hemolytic event may become evident as a precipitous drop in hemoglobin with marked symptoms of anemia and new jaundice. Hemoglobinuria is indicative of an intravascular process. Chronic hemolytic anemias are often well tolerated symptomatically and may even be incidental discoveries. Erythropoietic compensation is usually re-

---

BOX 89-1
When to consider the diagnosis of hemolytic anemia

Acute hemolysis
Unexplained drop in hemoglobin level
Acute jaundice due to indirect hyperbilirubinemia
Hemoglobinuria (if intravascular hemolysis)
Clinical situation associated with acute hemolysis
  Recent transfusion (hemolytic transfusion reaction)
  Oxidant stress (acute hemolysis in glucose-6-phosphate dehydrogenase deficiency)
  Mycoplasma pneumoniae infection (cold agglutinin hemolysis)
  Recent cardiac valve surgery (red blood cell [RBC] shearing hemolysis due to perivalvular leakage)
  Wilson's disease (copper-mediated oxidant hemolysis)
  Clostridia sepsis (toxin-mediated hemolysis)
  Drug abuse with volatile nitrites (oxidant hemolysis)
  Infection with verocytotoxin-producing *Escherichia coli* (hemolytic uremic syndrome [HUS])
  Freshwater drowning (osmotic hemolysis)
  Burn (thermal damage to RBCs)
  Marching, jogging (mechanical trauma to RBCs)

Chronic hemolysis
Chronically low hemoglobin level with high reticulocyte index (may increase RBC mean cell volume)
Persistent indirect hyperbilirubinemia
Splenomegaly (helpful if present)
Family history of hemolysis, anemia, or splenectomy
Clinical condition associated with chronic hemolysis
  Systemic lupus erythematosis (autoimmune hemolytic anemia [AIHA], thrombotic thrombocytopenic purpura [TTP])
  Lymphoproliferative disorders (AIHA, cold agglutinin hemolysis)
  Alcoholic liver disease (spur cell hemolytic anemia)
  Antiphospholipid antibody syndrome (AIHA)
Medication associated with chronic hemolysis
  Penicillin (hapten-mediated, drug-induced immune hemolysis)
  Quinidine (immune complex–mediated, drug-induced immune hemolysis)
  Alphamethyldopa (AIHA)
  Cephalosporins (hemolysis via nonimmune protein adsorption)
  Cyclosporin A (TTP)
  Interferon (AIHA)
  Intravenous immunoglobulin (AIHA)

---

flected by reticulocytosis. Splenomegaly is associated with many causes of chronic hemolysis. The absence of splenic enlargement, however, does not rule out hemolysis. Family history, past medical history and clinical circumstances may provide important hints to implicate a hemolytic process. Furthermore, a detailed history concerning alcohol use, illicit drug use, human immunodeficiency virus (HIV) risk, therapeutic medications, transfusions, travel, occupational exposure, and diet is required.

As in all patients with anemia, the clinician must first obtain a complete blood cell count (CBC) and reticulocyte count and examine the peripheral blood smear. Structural alterations in RBC morphologic appearance are common in hemolytic states and often provide critical clues regarding the condition's origin. Table 89-1 describes the appearance of RBCs in hemolytic anemias of diverse cause. Further evaluation of an individual patient must be guided by morphologic information. Even bland or nondescript RBC morphologic appearance has potential diagnostic value in this setting.

It is useful to classify hemolytic disorders mechanistically into hemolysis resulting from either intrinsic RBC defects or extrinsic defects. In general, the former constitute inherited conditions and the latter are acquired. Because there are so many different inherited hemolytic anemias, a family and ethnic history is important to the evaluation of hemolysis. Many conditions (e.g., glucose-6-phosphate dehydrogenase [G6PD] deficiency, sickle cell anemia, hemoglobin C, hemoglobin E, thalassemia, hereditary elliptocytosis, and Southeast

Table 89-1 Peripheral blood morphology (Wright's stained smears)* as a guide to evaluation of patients with suspected hemolytic disease

| | DIFFERENTIAL DIAGNOSIS | | |
BLOOD SMEAR FINDINGS	CONGENITAL	ACQUIRED	FURTHER TESTS (IN ORDER OF PRIORITY)
Spherocytes	HS, Hb CC	Immune, burns	Direct Coombs, osm. fragil., Hb electrophoresis
Elliptocytes, poikilocytes	HE, HPP	Myelodysplasia	Osm. fragil., specialized membrane studies
Hypochromic microcytes, "leptocytes"	Thalassemia, Hb Lepore, sideroblast	Iron defic., lead poisoning sideroblast	Fe/TIBC, Hb A$_2$ and F, Hb electrophoresis, marrow, DNA probes
Sickle cells	SS, SC	—	Hb electrophoresis
Target cells (normocytic)	AC, SC, CC	Obstructive jaundice, post splenectomy	Hb electrophoresis
Acanthocytes	PK defic., abetalipoproteinemia	Liver disease, spur cell anemia	PK screen, LFTs, lipid panel
Stomatocytes	Hydro-cytosis or xerocytosis, Rh null, hereditary stomatocytosis	Liver disease, alcohol	Red cell Na/K and water content, specialized membrane studies
Erythrophagocytosis, clumped red blood cells	—	Immune	Direct Coombs, D-L test, cold agglutinins
Schistocytes	Kasabach-Merritt syndrome	TTP, HUS, DIC, heart valve defects, myelodysplasia, carcinoma	Cardiac asucultation, coagulation tests
Blister cells, eccentrocytes, "bite" cells	G6PD defic., unstable Hb	Oxidant poisoning	G6PD screen, test for unstable Hb
Heavy basophilic stippling	pyr-5'-nucleot. defic.	Lead poisoning	Lead screen, specialized enzyme assay
Nondescript or no changes	G6PD defic., most glycolytic defects	PNH, internal bleeding†, recovering marrow†	Sucrose lysis test, acid lysis test, G6PD screen, PK screen, specialized enzyme assays, test for unstable Hb, specialized membrane studies

*Many of these abnormalities are illustrated in Plate IV-4.
†These conditions may simulate hemolytic disease because both feature the combination of anemia and a high reticulocyte count.
HS, hereditary spherocytosis; *HE,* hereditary elliptocytosis; *HPP,* hereditary pyropoikilocytosis; *HUS,* hemolytic uremic syndrome; *osm. fragil.,* osmotic fragility; *sideroblast.,* sideroblastic anemia; *Hb,* hemoglobin; *SS, SA, SC, CC, A$_2$, F,* hemoglobin variants; *Fe/TIBC,* iron and iron-binding capacity; *PK,* pyruvate kinase; *defic.,* deficiency; *LFTs,* liver function tests, *D-L test,* Donath-Landsteiner test; *TTP,* thrombotic thrombocytopenic purpura; *DIC,* disseminated intravascular coagulation; *G6PD,* glucose-6-phosphate dehydrogenase; *pyr-5'-nucleot,* pyrimidine-5'-nucleotidase; *PNH,* paroxysmal nocturnal hemoglobinuria; *Rh null,* congenital absence of Rh antigens.

BOX 89-2

Situations in which the diagnosis of hemolysis may be difficult

Acute hemolysis prior to reticulocyte response
Impaired compensation blunting the reticulocyte response to chronic hemolysis, such as B19 parvovirus infection, folate deficiency, bone marrow suppression, and renal insufficiency
Nonhemolytic reasons for indirect hyperbilirubinemia, increased lactase dehydrogenase level, low haptoglobin level, altered red blood cell morphology, or reticulocytosis
Hemolytic conditions with bland peripheral blood red blood cell morphology such as hereditary nonspherocytic hemolytic anemia and paroxysmal nocturnal hemoglobinuria
Imperfect sensitivity of the direct antiglobulin (Coombs') test and other diagnostic tests
Conditions such as hemophagocytic syndromes and ineffective erythropoiesis, which may exhibit clinical or laboratory features of hemolysis
Coexistence of hemolysis with other conditions such as multisystem organ failure, bleeding, myelodysplasia, iron deficiency, thalassemia, Gilbert's disease, and liver failure
Low-grade hemolysis

Asian ovalocytosis) are more common among members of particular ethnic groups. Further subclassification of hemolytic conditions into acute and chronic processes or intravascular and extravascular hemolysis is useful in certain instances.

Clinicians must consider many factors to accurately diagnose hemolysis in difficult cases. Box 89-2 lists problems that may be encountered in evaluating patients with suspected hemolytic anemia. For example, it is important, but difficult, to recognize chronic hemolysis that becomes evident initially as profound reticulocytopenic anemia caused by B19 parvovirus infection that destroys erythroid progenitors in the bone marrow. In rare instances conflicting diagnostic test data may raise sufficient doubts about whether hemolysis contributes to a patient's anemia that a chromium 51 RBC survival test is helpful. When considering this approach, it is important to note that occult bleeding also shortens RBC survival measured using this method.

HEREDITARY HEMOLYTIC ANEMIAS

Inherited, intrinsic abnormalities of erythrocytes that lead to their premature destruction can be subdivided into hemoglobin defects, enzyme defects, and membrane defects. Genetic disorders of hemoglobin are discussed elsewhere and are considered here only in relationship to other hemolytic processes.

Enzyme Defects

Deficient metabolic enzymes in the erythrocyte may lead to episodic hemolysis resulting from increased RBC sensitivity to oxidant stress, chronic hemolysis of varying severity, and chronic hemolysis punctuated by acute exacerbations (Table 89-2). Chronic hemolytic anemias secondary to hereditary enzymopathies often exhibit bland or nondescript RBC morphologic features. Consequently these conditions are sometimes called hereditary nonspherocytic hemolytic anemias to distinguish them from the common RBC membrane defect, hereditary spherocytosis. Some cases that seem to fit into the hereditary nonspherocytic hemolytic anemia category are actually caused by unusual membrane defects or unstable hemoglobins.

The mechanism by which erythrocytes with deficient metabolic enzymes are prematurely destroyed has been extensively studied. In the course of normal oxygen transport, RBCs generate reactive oxidant molecules including superoxide anions and hydroxyl radicals. These agents can damage proteins through thiol oxidation and lipids through peroxidation. One major function of RBC glucose metabolism is to develop a biochemical buffer against damage by these endogenous oxidants and exogenous oxidant stress. The hexose monophosphate (HMP) shunt is a critical component of this buffer system. Together with superoxide dismutase, catalase, and vitamin E, the HMP shunt protects RBCs from oxidant damage. The HMP shunt is an alternative pathway of glucose-6-phosphate metabolism that can replace the first steps of anaerobic glycolysis. In contrast to glycoly-

Table 89-2   Some inherited red blood cell enzymopathies that lead to hemolytic anemia

ENZYME AFFECTED	MODE OF INHERITANCE	COMMENTS
Glucose-6-phosphate dehydrogenase	SL	Most common; see text discussion
Pyruvate kinase	AR	Next most common; echinocytes may be seen on blood smear; possible benefit from splenectomy
Hexokinase	AR	
Glucose phosphate isomerase	AR	
Triose phosphate isomerase	AR	Associated severe neuromuscular disease
Phosphoglycerate kinase	SL	Associated neurologic disease
Pyrimidine-5' nucleotidase	AR	Heavy basophilic stippling of red blood cells.

SL, Sex-linked; *AR,* autosomal recessive.

BOX 89-3
Drugs known to cause hemolysis in patients with G6PD deficiency

Acetanilid	Sulfacetamide
Nalidixic acid	Sulfapyridine
Nitrofurantoin	Trinitrotoluene
Phenylhydrazine	Primaquine
Sulfanilamide	Niridazole
Toluidine blue	Pentaquine
Methylene blue	Sulfamethoxazole
Naphthalene	Thiazolesulfone
Pamaquine	

G6PD, Glucose-6-phosphate dehydrogenase.

sis, the HMP shunt does not generate adenosine triphosphate (ATP). Its primary function is the reduction of the oxidized form of nicotinamide adenine dinucleotide phosphate (NADP$^+$) to reduced NADP (NADPH). NADPH functions primarily to facilitate the reduction of oxidized glutathione via glutathione reductase. Reduced glutathione is used to detoxify hydrogen peroxide that forms spontaneously or by the action of superoxide dismutase on superoxide radicals. Therefore defects in HMP shunt enzymes lead to RBC destruction by endogenous and/or exogenous oxidants. Hemolytic anemia due to HMP shunt enzyme deficiencies may be intermittent or chronic with intermittent acute exacerbations associated with oxidant stress.

Having no mitochondria, RBCs are totally dependent on anaerobic glycolysis for energy production. Therefore deficient glycolytic pathway enzymes lead to decreased RBC ATP concentrations. Without adequate ATP, vital cellular functions are disrupted, such as ion transport via the sodium/potassium adenosine triphosphatase (ATPase). Clinically significant defects in glycolytic pathway enzymes usually produce chronic hemolytic anemia.

Hemolysis may also accompany abnormalities of RBC nucleotide metabolism. Interestingly, not every example is the result of an enzyme deficiency. Hyperactivity of erythrocyte adenosine deaminase is associated with hemolysis. Like glycolytic pathway defects, clinically significant abnormalities of nucleotide metabolism produce chronic hemolysis.

Glucose-6-Phosphate Dehydrogenase Deficiency

Pathophysiology. The most common enzyme deficiency that results in oxidative damage to RBCs affects the HMP shunt enzyme G6PD. G6PD deficiency is the most common known human enzymopathy and affects approximately one tenth of the world's population. The reason for the prevalence of G6PD deficiency is likely due to selection of affected individuals by resistance to *Plasmodium falciparum.* The frequent occurrence of G6PD deficiency in regions with endemic malaria supports this hypothesis, as does other evidence.

Approximately 300 electrophoretically separable variants of G6PD have been reported. The normal "wild type" enzyme is termed G6PD-B. Two common variants of G6PD occur in patients of African descent, G6PD-A and G6PD-A$^-$. G6PD-A is characterized by normal levels of catalytic activity, but G6PD-A$^-$ has reduced activity and becomes increasingly unstable with increased RBC age. Individuals with the G6PD-A$^-$ variant are susceptible to episodic hemolysis. The gene frequencies for G6PD-A and A$^-$ among black Americans are 20% to 25% and 10% to 13%, respectively. Because the G6PD gene is located on the X chromosome, G6PD deficiency is inherited in an X-linked recessive manner. Therefore males who are hemizygous for G6PD deficiency make up the large majority of affected patients. Females who are homozygous for G6PD deficiency are rare. Most female heterozygotes are clinically normal. Due to ran-

dom X chromosome inactivation, about 50% of a heterozygote's RBCs have an enzyme deficiency. Sometimes, by chance, X chromosome inactivation happens in such a way that most of a heterzygous female's RBCs are affected. This can lead to a clinically significant G6PD deficiency state.

The normal African isozyme (G6PD-A) results from a single amino acid substitution and has normal catalytic activity and other biochemical properties of G6PD-B. The G6PD-A$^-$ variant differs by an additional amino acid substitution that markedly decreases the catalytic activity and alters its biochemical properties. The Mediterranean isozyme is the most common G6PD variant in white populations, and this variant is associated with favism. The Mediterranean variant has markedly decreased catalytic activity, but hemolysis is seen only in patients who are exposed to certain drugs, infections, surgery, or fava beans.

Numerous other mutations causing G6PD deficiency have been described in various ethnic groups. These produce a range of phenotypes from chronic hereditary nonspherocytic hemolytic anemia to intermittent oxidant-stimulated hemolysis.

Clinical features. Black patients with G6PD-A$^-$ usually have normal RBC survival. Hemolysis occurs only when these patients experience an oxidant stress. Several drugs are known to produce such a stress. Offending agents are listed in Box 89-3. Other oxidative stressors are acute infection or sepsis, diabetic ketoacidosis, and hepatitis. In patients with G6PD-A$^-$ the enzyme activity rapidly declines in mature RBCs, whereas in reticulocytes the enzyme activity is normal. Thus when patients with G6PD-A$^-$ have a hemolytic episode and large numbers of reticulocytes subsequently appear in their circulation, measurement of G6PD may reveal normal activity because the older, more susceptible RBCs have been rapidly destroyed during the hemolytic episode. In contrast, patients who have the Mediterranean variant of G6PD deficiency are hematologically normal in the absence of oxidative stress. However, because the mutant enzyme is catalytically defective, G6PD levels are deficient in both young and old RBCs in patients with the Mediterranean variant. Therefore the intensity and duration of their hemolytic episodes are both greater than in the G6PD-A$^-$ variant. A severe chronic hemolytic anemia can be seen in a subgroup of patients with unusual G6PD variants with extremely low enzyme activity. Interestingly, fava beans, which cause intense hemolytic anemia in patients with the Mediterranean variant of G6PD deficiency, have little or no effect on patients with the G6PD-A$^-$ variant.

Patients with G6PD deficiency have widely variable signs and symptoms. These range from an intermittent mild anemia to life-threatening episodes of hemoglobinuria, shock, profound anemia, and acute renal failure. Some individuals have chronic nonspherocytic hemolytic anemia that may be punctuated by occasional hemolytic exacerbations. Hemizygotes for G6PD deficiency are believed to be particularly vulnerable to the lethal consequences of infections with *Rickettsia rickettsiae,* the cause of Rocky Mountain spotted fever.

Laboratory features. Most clinical laboratories can rapidly screen for G6PD deficiency by measuring enzyme activity in hemolysates. As noted, patients with G6PD-A$^-$ deficiency may have near-

BOX 89-4
Drugs that can be safely given to patients with G6PD deficiency of the A⁻ type

Acetaminophen	Probenecid
Acetophenetidin	Procainamide
Ascorbic acid	Pyrimethamine
Aspirin	Quinidine
Chloramphenicol	Quinine
Chloroguanidine	Streptomycin
Chloroquine	Sulfacytine
Colchicine	Sulfadiazine
Diphenhydramine	Sulfaguanidine
Isoniazid	Sulfamerazine
Levodopa	Sulfamethoxypyridazine
Menadione	Sulfisoxazole
Menaphthone	Trimethoprim
p-Aminobenzoate	Tripelennamine
Phenylbutazone	Vitamin K
Phenytoin	

G6PD, Glucose-6-phosphate dehydrogenase.

normal levels of G6PD activity after a recent hemolytic episode because the susceptible older RBCs, which have low levels of G6PD and were sensitive to oxidative stress, were lysed during that episode. Reticulocytes, which have near-normal levels of G6PD activity, are proportionally increased. The blood smear of patients who are undergoing hemolysis may have "blister cells" with a lopsided distribution of hemoglobin (Plate III-4, *O*), spherocytes, poikilocytes, and reticulocytes. If hemolysis has been severe, nucleated RBCs may be seen. Heinz bodies, which represent precipitated hemoglobin adhering to the RBC membrane, are usually not seen in Wright's stained blood smears but can be seen with supravitally stained peripheral blood using methylene blue or brilliant cresyl violet (Plate III-4, *P*). In patients with intact spleens, Heinz bodies may not be seen but "bite cells" may be present that appear to have had a bite taken out of them. G6PD variants that become evident as hereditary nonspherocytic hemolytic anemia may have a nondescript RBC morphologic appearance and laboratory evidence of chronic hemolysis.

Management. The primary treatment of patients with G6PD deficiency is prevention of exposure to agents that trigger hemolysis. Box 89-4 lists agents that may safely be given to patients. Once hemolysis has begun, patients should be kept well hydrated and the inciting agent removed. Splenectomy is of little value in most patients with common types of G6PD deficiency because they have periodic acute hemolytic episodes that are usually self-limited. Splenectomy has been helpful in some patients with chronic hemolytic anemia caused by severe G6PD deficiency but cannot be viewed as a reliable treatment. In patients with chronic hemolysis, folate supplementation is indicated.

Pyruvate Kinase Deficiency. Pyruvate kinase (PK) catalyzes the conversion of phosphoenolpyruvate to pyruvate with the generation of two molecules of ATP. Decreased PK activity results in loss of ATP, elevated concentrations of 2,3 diphosphoglycerate, and decreased NAD⁺/NADH concentrations. Decreases in erythrocyte PK are the second most common RBC enzymopathy, after G6PD deficiency. The severity of the PK deficiency and the corresponding anemia may vary from mild to very severe with transfusion dependence. Severe PK deficiency usually becomes evident as a chronic hemolytic anemia early in childhood and may cause hydrops fetalis. Clinical manifestations include splenomegaly, icterus, indirect hyperbilirubinemia, decreased haptoglobin level, and reticulocytosis with marrow erythroid hyperplasia. Infections, pregnancy, and surgery can exacerbate the chronic hemolysis. B19 parvovirus infections may result in an aplastic crisis in these patients. Splenectomy has been used to treat PK-deficient patients and may result in a decreased transfusion requirement.

Other Enzyme Defects. In addition to PK deficiency there are many other enzyme deficiencies that produce hemolytic anemia. These conditions can be categorized as glycolytic enzyme defects, HMP shunt defects, and nucleotide metabolism defects. Examples are hexokinase deficiency, glucose phosphate isomerase deficiency, triose phosphate isomerase deficiency, phosphoglycerate deficiency, and pyrimidine 5′ nucleotidase deficiency (Table 89-2). These patients usually have chronic hemolysis that varies in severity from mild to severe. Except for phosphoglycerate kinase deficiency, these defects have an autosomal recessive pattern of inheritance. Severely affected patients may require transfusional support.

Red Blood Cell Membrane Defects

An important characteristic of the RBC is its capacity to repeatedly and reversibly deform in the microcirculation. The strength, resilience, elasticity, and durability required for the erythrocyte to survive its full life span are provided by the membrane skeleton. The RBC membrane skeleton is a specialized assembly of structural proteins arranged into a lattice attached to the inner face of the RBC membrane's lipid bilayer. The main protein constituents are α spectrin, β spectrin, ankyrin, protein 4.1, protein 4.2, and short actin filaments (Fig. 89-1). Several spectrin αβ heterodimers attach to each short actin filament to form a junctional complex. This interaction is facilitated by the binding of protein 4.1 to spectrin. Spectrin heterodimers self-associate into tetramers. Both ends of each tetramer are linked to short actin filaments. Spectrin is tethered to the lipid bilayer by interacting with ankyrin which, together with protein 4.2, binds to an integral membrane protein called band 3, the anion channel. Protein 4.1 joins the junctional complex to the lipid bilayer by binding to glycophorin C, an integral membrane glycoprotein. Quantitative and qualitative defects in membrane skeleton proteins and their interactions lead to hereditary hemolytic anemias (Table 89-3). In fact, known defects in each of the constituents just described lead to hemolysis. These conditions vary in severity from subclinical to lethal.

Hereditary Spherocytosis.

Pathophysiology. Hereditary spherocytosis (HS) is the most common inherited hemolytic anemia affecting individuals of northern European descent (>1/5000), although it occurs frequently in all ethnic groups. HS is caused by a diverse array of mutations affecting several different RBC membrane and membrane skeleton proteins. These mutations are typically inherited in an autosomal dominant fashion (~75%), although recessive (~20%) and sporadic (~5%) forms of HS occur. The unifying abnormality that leads to the phenotype of spherocytosis is spectrin deficiency. While various mutations of ankyrin (most common), band 3, spectrin, and protein 4.2 can produce HS, each results in spectrin deficiency. The degree of spectrin deficiency correlates with clinical severity, regardless of the molecular cause. Rare cases of recessive HS have profound spectrin deficiency and exhibit lethal or nearly lethal hemolysis.

Spectrin deficiency leads to loss of erythrocyte surface area, which produces spherical RBCs. Spherocytic RBCs are culled rapidly from the circulation by the spleen. Consequently patients with HS develop splenomegaly. Hemolysis is primarily confined to the spleen and therefore is extravascular. This fact has diagnostic and therapeutic implications.

Clinical features. Patients with HS may come to medical attention early in life with severe anemia or may go through adulthood with undiagnosed, compensated hemolysis. The most common forms of HS produce mild hemolytic anemia that may become evident as an incidental finding of anemia, splenomegaly, or mild jaundice during an acute illness, or as an aplastic crisis due to B19 parvovirus infection of folate deficiency. In an aplastic crisis, compensation is impaired and profound, life-threatening anemia can develop. Bilirubin gallstones may develop at an early age, and, rarely, chronic leg ulcers may develop. A past history of neonatal jaundice and a family history of anemia and/or splenectomy may provide clues to the diagnosis of HS. Occasionally, patients with HS carry the erroneous diagnosis of Gilbert's disease.

Laboratory features. Anemia, reticulocytosis (except in aplastic crisis), and spherocytosis on peripheral blood smear examination provide strong hints to suggest the diagnosis of HS. Spherocytes are

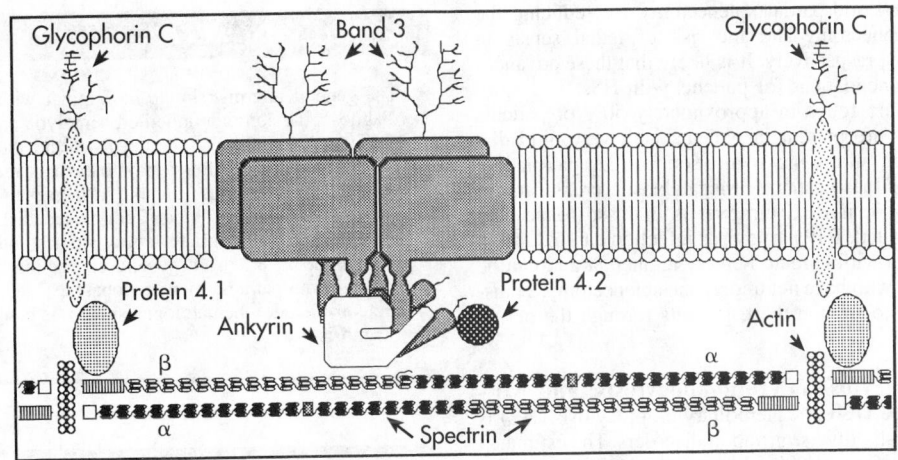

FIGURE 89-1   Molecular organization of the erythrocyte membrane skeleton. The main protein constituents of the red blood cell membrane skeleton (labeled) are depicted in relation to the lipid bilayer. Mutations affecting each of the proteins shown, except actin, are known to cause hereditary hemolytic anemia. Other important constituents, for which disease-causing mutations have not been identified, are omitted.

Table 89-3   Hereditary hemolytic anemias due to red blood cell membrane defects

CONDITION	FREQUENCY	MOLECULAR DEFECTS	INHERITANCE	DIAGNOSTIC TESTS	CLINICAL EXAMINATION	TREATMENT
Hereditary spherocytosis	1/5000	Ankyrin Band 3 Spectrin Protein 4.2	Autosomal dominant (25% nondominant)	Blood smear, osmotic fragility, (−) Coombs' test	Variable severity, usually mild-moderate splenomegaly	Splenectomy if moderate to severe
Hereditary elliptocytosis	1/2000-1/4000 (some forms regionally common)	Spectrin Protein 4.1 Glycophorins C and D Band 3	Autosomal dominant	Blood smear	Variable severity, usually very mild	None, occasionally splenectomy if severe
Hereditary pyropoikilocytosis	Rare	Spectrin (hereditary elliptocytosis mutations, low-production allele)	Autosomal recessive	Blood smear	Severe	Splenectomy occasionally, transfusions
Hereditary stomatocytosis	Rare	Unknown ?Protein 7.2b	Autosomal dominant	Blood smear	Variable severity	Splenectomy if severe

characterized by a lack of central pallor, decreased mean corpuscular diameter, and increased density (Plate III-4, *G*). Other biochemical changes of hemolysis are also present, including increased LDH, increased unconjugated bilirubin, and decreased serum haptoglobin. Red blood cell indices show an increase in mean corpuscular hemoglobin concentration (MCHC). Spherocytic RBCs are not specific to HS. For example, autoimmune hemolytic anemia (AIHA) may also produce spherocytosis (see later discussion). Usually, however, the spherocytosis of HS is more bland, uniform, and monotonous than in AIHA. In AIHA one usually sees microspherocytes side by side with normal-appearing RBCs. A negative direct antiglobulin (Coombs') test usually rules out AIHA. RBC morphologic appearance in more severe HS, such as in recessive cases, shows more poikilocytosis, microspherocytosis, polychromasia (reflecting more reticulocytosis), and RBC fragmentation than is seen in typical HS patients.

Tests for RBC osmotic fragility, performed by placing patient RBCs in hypotonic solutions, demonstrate increased RBC lysis upon swelling compared with normal RBCs. The increased osmotic fragility results from the decreased amounts of membrane per RBC. Thus these RBCs cannot compensate for the increase in intracellular volume that occurs in hypotonic solutions. Increased osmotic fragility is a characteristic of all spherocytic anemias and is not unique to HS. The increased osmotic fragility persists in patients who have undergone splenectomy because splenectomy does not change the basic membrane defect. In patients who have very mild HS, overnight incubation of the cells at 37° C may be required to demonstrate the

increased osmotic fragility. Bone marrow examination is not required to make the diagnosis of HS. Interestingly, results of specialized tests of RBC membrane mechanical fragility are normal in patients with HS.

Management. Splenectomy is the treatment of choice for patients with HS and is curative in most patients with the disease. However, the indications for splenectomy are not always clear. There is little doubt that patients with more severe anemia and symptoms and complications of HS should undergo splenectomy. Similarly, splenectomy can be safely deferred in patients with mild, uncomplicated HS (hemoglobin level >11). There are no good studies upon which to base clinical judgments in patients with moderate, asymptomatic HS (hemoglobin level, 8 to 11). Therefore recommendations must be individualized. When splenectomy is performed, a simultaneous cholecystectomy in patients with bilirubin stones may eliminate future complications and the need for a second operative procedure. After splenectomy, RBC survival improves dramatically, enabling most HS patients to maintain a normal hemoglobin level. Ideally splenectomy should not be performed until after the age of 3 or 4 years because of the increased incidence of postsplenectomy infections with encapsulated organisms such as *Streptococcus pneumoniae* and *Haemophilus influenzae* in young children. Patients should be immunized against *S. pneumoniae, H. influenzae,* and *Neisseria meningitidis* at least 1 month before splenectomy. Patients at increased risk for these types of infections should be considered candidates for lifelong treatment with prophylactic penicillin. Newer surgical techniques such as laparoscopic splenectomy and partial splenectomy are reducing the acute morbidity of splenectomy and the risk of lethal sepsis in postsplenectomy patients, respectively. It is likely that these advances will affect future recommendations for patients with HS.

Bilirubin gallstones are found in approximately 50% of patients with HS and frequently are present in patients with very mild disease. Therefore periodic ultrasonic evaluation of the gallbladder should be performed for these patients. Megaloblastic crisis can develop during pregnancy or if RBC turnover is high, so folate acid supplementation is indicated. B19 parvovirus infection can induce an aplastic crisis in patients with chronic hemolytic anemia and can be seen in patients with HS who have not undergone splenectomy. Transfusion is often required to support these patients through the period of erythroid aplasia.

Hereditary Elliptocytosis, Pyropoikilocytosis, and Miscellaneous Membrane Defects.

Hereditary elliptocytosis (HE) is a clinically and etiologically diverse group of disorders. The estimated frequency of HE is 1/2000 to 1/4000, although the incidence in certain ethnic groups is much higher. In some parts of Africa, HE occurs in 1% of individuals. An asymptomatic variant of HE, Southeast Asian ovalocytosis, is present in up to 30% in some locales. Resistence to malaria is thought to account for this high prevalence. Mutations that lead to HE affect the genes encoding spectrin, protein 4.1, glycophorins C and D, and band 3 (Southeast Asian ovalocytois) and are inherited in an autosomal dominant fashion. The cellular pathophysiologic features of HE are increased RBC membrane fragility and decreased deformability (not osmotic fragility!). After defective erythrocytes traverse the microcirculation, they fail to reassume their normal shape. As a result, the peripheral blood smear reveals the characteristic elliptocytic RBC morphology (Plate III-4, *R*). The clinical severity of HE may vary from a mild, asymptomatic condition to a moderately severe chronic hemolytic anemia with splenomegaly. Similarly to HS, the most severe cases benefit from splenectomy, cholecystectomy, and folate supplementation.

Hereditary pyropoikilocytosis (HPP) is an unusual condition that typically becomes evident as a severe anemia in childhood, although diagnosis in adults is seen occasionally. Spectrin mutations affecting dimer self-association into tetramers are almost universally identified in HPP. Interestingly, these same mutations are seen in patients with HE. Therefore HPP is sometimes a recessive form of HE, either homozygous or compound heterozygous for HE-causing spectrin mutations. Other cases of HPP have one HE-causing mutation coinherited with a "low-expression" spectrin allele. RBC morphology in HPP is remarkable for impressive RBC fragmentation, extreme poikilocytosis, spherocytes, and other misshapen cells. Hemolysis is ameliorated by splenectomy but not eliminated.

Other hereditary RBC membrane defects include hereditary stomatocytosis that manifests an increased RBC passive sodium leak and decreased protein 7.2b, hereditary xerocytosis in which RBCs are markedly dehydrated, Rh null disease that shows spherostomatocytic characteristics, various serum lipid abnormalities that affect RBCs secondarily (abetalipoproteinemia and Tangier disease), and McLeod's syndrome in which RBCs lack Kell blood group antigens. Some membrane defects, including some mutations of protein 4.2, become evident with a syndrome that resembles hereditary nonspherocytic hemolytic anemia.

ACQUIRED HEMOLYTIC ANEMIAS
Erythrocyte Fragmentation Syndromes

Microangiopathic and Macroangiopathic Hemolytic Anemia

Pathophysiology. Erythrocyte fragmentation occurs when RBCs pass through abnormal microvasculature (microangiopathy) or abnormal vascular structures such as prosthetic heart valves, cardiac anomalies, aneurysms, large vessel grafts, or arteriovenous malformations (macroangiopathy). In the former case erythrocytes are damaged on fibrin strands within small vessels. In the latter, RBCs are subjected to excessive mechanical shearing forces that cause them to break. Several causes are listed in Box 89-5. In both microangiopathy and macroangiopathy damaged RBCs are usually recognizable on the peripheral blood smear (Plate III-4, *E*). These may be schistocytes (small, irregular RBC fragments that have one to three sharp projections),

✔ *WHEN TO REFER*

The general internist should be familiar with, and readily able to diagnose, the common inherited hemolytic anemias such as G6PD deficiency, hereditary spherocytosis, and the more prevalent hemoglobinopathies. After a new patient is identified, consultation with a hematologist is valuable to help plan therapy and identify any unusual features. Input from a specialist may also be helpful in performing appropriate family studies and identifying patients that might benefit from genetic counseling. When the less common enzymopathies, membranopathies, and hemoglobinopathies are considered, a hematologist should be consulted to assist in the diagnosis.

BOX 89-5
Erythrocyte fragmentation syndromes

Disseminated intravascular coagulation (DIC)
Hemolytic uremic syndrome (HUS)
Thrombotic thrombocytopenic purpura (TTP)
Malignant hypertension
Eclampsia
Vasculitis
Glomerulonephritis
Solid organ transplant rejection
Post–bone marrow transplantation thrombotic microangiopathy
Disseminated carcinoma, especially adenocarcinoma
Cavernous hemangioma
Hepatic hemangioendothelioma
Drugs
   Mitomycin C
   Cyclosporin A
   Quinidine
Aortic stenosis
Ruptured chordae tendinae
Aortic aneurysm
After surgical repair of heart and large vessel defects
Perivalvular leak
March hemoglobinuria

---

helmet cells, or microspherocytes. In both microvascular and macrovascular categories, intravascular hemolysis is demonstrable and damaged cells are prematurely cleared by the reticuloendothelial system.

Clinical features. The clinical spectrum of this group of disorders is extremely broad (Box 89-5). As a result, the clinical features often stem from the underlying disorder. For example, disseminated intravascular coagulation (DIC; see Chapter 84) may become evident with acute sepsis, abruptio placentae, acute promyelocytic leukemia, or any of its other many causes. The coagulopathy may be more clinically threatening than the anemia, but RBC transfusion may be required to treat these patients. Thrombotic thrombocytopenic purpura (TTP; see Chapter 84) may become evident with fever, central nervous system impairment, anuria/hematuria, bleeding due to thrombocytopenia, and symptomatic anemia. Hemolytic uremic syndrome (HUS; see Chapter 83) becomes evident with renal failure, thrombocytopenia, and anemia. Other causes such as adenocarcinoma (especially stomach, breast, and lung), vasculitis, and eclampsia have similarly diverse clinical characteristics and varying degrees of anemia. Recently the entity of post–bone marrow transplantation thrombotic microanigiopathy has been recognized.

The macroangiopathic hemolytic anemias may have an acute onset in patients who develop a postoperative anatomic lesion such as a perivalvular leak. Patients may develop acute hemoglobinuria and marked, sudden anemia. These entities may also become evident as chronic anemia with reticulocytosis and variable levels of compensation. March hemoglobinuria is caused by mechanical RBC damage incurred while running or marching long distances. Patients with this disorder typically presents with a mild, compensated anemia, as iron deficiency from hemoglobinuria, or as acute hemoglobinuria after strenuous activity.

Laboratory features. The severity of the clinical findings in patients with microangiopathic hemolytic anemia is proportional to the severity of the underlying disease. The peripheral blood smear consistently shows fragmented RBCs and occasional microspherocytes (Plate III-4, *E*). The reticulocyte count is usually elevated, and occasional nucleated RBCs may be seen. In patients with sepsis, the leukocyte count may be elevated. The platelet count is reduced if consumption of platelets is an associated feature (e.g., DIC, HUS, TTP). If the hemolytic process is severe, there is evidence of intravascular hemolysis with elevated plasma hemoglobin levels, decreased or absent haptoglobin, hemoglobinuria, and hemosiderinuria. A characteristic finding in patients with march hemoglobinuria is hemosiderin in the urine. These patients are usually not severely anemic and have a mildly elevated reticulocyte count. They may have iron deficiency anemia caused by iron loss in their urine. In DIC there is evidence of a consumptive coagulopathy with elevation of the prothrombin and activated thromboplastin times, decreased fibrinogen levels, and increased fibrin degradation products.

Differential diagnosis. The erythrocyte fragmentation syndromes must be distinguished, first, from other anemias and, second, from other hemolytic anemias. After the diagnosis of hemolysis is established (as discussed earlier), the peripheral blood smear is typically adequate to implicate a fragmentation syndrome. A thorough history, physical examination, and basic laboratory evaluation are usually sufficient to narrow the focus on one of the known causes of erythrocyte fragmentation (Box 89-5). Occasionally the cause remains obscure. Such cases may be due to occult arteriovenous fistulae, unsuspected cardiac anomalies, medications not commonly associated with RBC fragmentation, or occult carcinoma.

Management. Treatment of erythrocyte fragmentation syndromes should be directed primarily at the underlying disease process (Table 89-5). For example, TTP and HUS respond to plasma exchange. Eclampsia responds to emergent delivery of the infant. DIC improves with the treatment of sepsis, leukemia, and so forth. Effective chemotherapy for disseminated breast cancer may ameliorate the attendant hemolysis. Removal of the offending drug, treatment of rejection, replacement of the vascular valve, and repair of the vascular anomaly may all be effective treatments. Introduction of padded footwear can improve march hemoglobinuria. In patients whose underlying disease cannot be treated, transfusions and replacement of iron and folate may be required.

Hemolytic Anemia Caused by Infectious Agents

As noted, hemolysis can occur in the course of a variety of infectious diseases in which disseminated intravascular coagulation is present with deposition of fibrin strands in the microvasculature. Some of these infections are also associated with splenomegaly, which may be responsible for the increased destruction of RBCs. Several infectious agents, however, directly invade the RBC and damage the RBC membrane. Malaria, caused by the parasites *Plasmodium malariae, Plasmodium vivax,* and *Plasmodium falciparum,* is the most common cause of hemolytic anemia in the world (Chapter 279). These parasites are transmitted by the *Anopheles* mosquito. The merozoites enter the erythrocytes and grow intracellularly. The osmotic fragility of the RBC is increased in uninfected as well as infected cells. The infected RBCs are removed by the spleen, so splenomegaly is a common finding in chronic malarial infections (tropical splenomegaly). Infection with the *P. falciparum* form of malaria is associated with severe hemolysis and may occasionally result in the syndrome of blackwater fever, in which patients pass dark urine. The diagnosis of malaria requires the demonstration of the parasites on a blood film. Treatment of malaria includes quinine, chloroquine, sulfones, and pyrimethamine. Care should be take in administering these drugs, because they may induce a hemolytic episode in G6PD-deficient patients.

Babesiosis is caused by an intracellular parasite *(Babesia microtia)* that causes symptoms similar to malaria. This organism is endemic to coastal New England and is transmitted by ticks. In patients with splenectomy, life-threatening hemolysis with renal failure may occur.

Other infections that can cause hemolysis include *Bartonella ba-cilliformis,* which is a bacterium transmitted by the sandfly. This organism infects the RBC by adhering to the cell membrane rather than growing within the cell. The infected RBCs are rapidly removed from the circulation by the spleen and liver. Fever, chills, and hemolysis occur within 2 to 3 weeks of transmission. Bartonellosis (Oroya fever) responds to antibiotics but may be lethal without treatment. *Clostridium perfringens* infection can induce massive hemolysis as a result of the production of a bacterial α-toxin, a lecithinase that reacts with RBC membranes to release lysolecithin, a potent hemolysin (Chapter 271). The resulting hemolysis can be dramatic and is frequently fatal.

Hemolysis Associated With Liver Disease

Patients with severe liver disease may have anemia from any of several causes, including folate deficiency, blood loss, hypersplenism, iron deficiency, and bone marrow suppression. Hemolysis may also occur. Typically, erythrocytes of patients with liver disease include many target cells (Plate III-4, *D*). Target cells are not usually associated with hemolysis. One recognizable hemolytic syndrome, referred to as "spur cell anemia," is characterized by brisk hemolysis and acanthocytic erythrocytes. Acanthocytes have an increased cholesterol/phospholipid ratio. These cells are cleared by the spleen. Splenectomy is beneficial to some patients with severe hemolysis and favorable surgical risk. Zieve and others have described a syndrome characterized by alcoholic fatty liver, hypertriglyceridemia, jaundice, and spherocytic hemolytic anemia. Hemolysis most probably results from acute congestive splenomegaly, which is observed frequently in patients with fatty livers, rather than from changes in the composition of the RBC membrane. Hypophosphatemia (<0.2 mg/dl) may develop in acute alcoholics, cirrhotics, diabetics, and patients on total parenteral nutrition or phosphate binding antacids. Hypophosphatemia leads to depletion of RBC ATP, producing increased cellular rigidity, loss of surface area, and premature clearance by the spleen.

The diagnosis of hemolytic anemia associated with liver disease can be made on the basis of the clinical setting, examination of the blood smear, abnormal liver function, and clinical and laboratory evidence of hemolysis. In patients with end-stage liver disease, treatment of the hemolytic anemia is frequently difficult and repeated transfusion of RBCs may be necessary.

Hemolytic Anemia Caused by Drugs, Chemicals, and Toxins

Drugs and chemicals induce hemolysis by several mechanisms that can be broadly divided into immune (see later discussion) and nonimmune. Agents producing nonimmune hemolysis can be categorized as oxidative and nonoxidative.

Drugs and Chemicals That Cause Oxidative Hemolysis.
Numerous agents are capable of inducing oxidative hemolytic anemia. Dapsone and other sulfones, sulfasalazine, phenazopyridine (Pyridium), nitrofurantoin, and para-aminosalacylic acid are therapeutic agents responsible for cases of hemolysis. Abuse drugs such as volatile nitrites can produce oxidant hemolysis. Naphthalene mothballs, paraquat, hydrogen peroxide, and many other agents induce oxidant hemolysis.

The pathophysiology of oxidant hemolysis involves the formation of methemoglobin (by the conversion of Fe^{+2} to Fe^{+3}) and oxidation of RBC membrane components. Damaged cells are cleared from the circulation by the reticuloendothelial system or may lyse in the bloodstream. Severe methemoglobinemia becomes evident as cyanosis. The peripheral blood morphologic appearance is nonspecific but may resemble G6PD deficiency. Denatured hemoglobin may form Heinz bodies that assist in diagnosis. Measurement of methemoglobin is essential in suspected cases. Methemoglobinemia in excess of 20% to 30% may be treated with intravenous methylene blue.

Drugs and Chemicals That Cause Nonoxidative Hemolysis.
Lead poisoning causes a modest shortening of the RBC life span and interferes with normal production of erythrocytes. Lead blocks several enzymes of the heme synthetic pathway, especially aminolevulinic acid (ALA) dehydrase and heme synthetase. Lack of

heme probably causes abnormal synthesis of alpha and beta globin chains. Blockade of heme synthetase probably is responsible for elevation of free erythrocyte protoporphyrin levels in these patients. Examination of the peripheral smear reveals coarse basophilic stippling, which represents abnormally aggregated ribosomes in the RBCs. The diagnosis of lead poisoning can be inferred by finding basophilic stippling on the peripheral blood smear coupled with the presence of lead lines on the teeth at the gumline. Twenty-four-hour urine collection for heavy metal analysis should be performed to confirm lead intoxication.

Inhalation of arsine gas (arsenic hydride) produces hemolysis in exposed individuals. The setting of exposure is typically industrial. Patients may come to medical attention with severe jaundice, anemia, and hemoglobinuria. The mechanism of hemolysis is not well understood.

Hemolysis From Stings, Bites, and Venoms. Hemolysis can occur after bee and wasp stings and snake and spider bites. Bites from black widow and brown recluse spiders can produce hemolysis, although most of the associated reaction is local. Numerous bee and wasp stings can result in hemolysis. The venom of the cobra contains phospholipases that destroy RBCs; other snake venoms, including rattlesnakes and other pit vipers, induce DIC (Chapter 84) with an associated microangiopathic hemolytic anemia.

Hypersplenism

In pathologically enlarged spleens, cell transit time is increased; the increase can cause the reduction of one or more of the circulating blood elements. Splenomegaly can result from a large number of disease processes and may decrease RBC mass. Hypersplenism is discussed in Chapter 81.

Paroxysmal Nocturnal Hemoglobinuria

Paroxysmal nocturnal hemoglobinuria (PNH) is an acquired disorder affecting the hematopoietic stem cell that results in the clonal expansion of cells with an inability to form glycosyl-phosphatidylinositol (GPI) linkages that anchor certain membrane proteins to glycolipids. Acquired mutations in the gene encoding PIG-A, a protein involved in the formation of GPI linkages, are responsible for PNH. One clinically important consequence of this defect is that RBCs become sensitive to lysis by complement. Therefore patients with PNH come to medical attention with intravascular hemolytic anemia that may be episodic or chronic. Other clinical features of the syndrome include a venous thrombotic diathesis and deficient hematopoiesis that may evolve into bone marrow failure resembling idiopathic aplastic anemia. The erythrocyte morphology in PNH is nondescript. Diagnostic evaluation should include the sucrose lysis test, which, if the result is positive, should be followed by the more specific Ham's test. Both of these tests evaluate the susceptibility of PNH RBCs to complement-mediated hemolysis. Treatment of PNH includes glucocorticoids, iron (when deficient through urinary hemosiderin), and folate. Erythropoietin and transfusion have been used with success. Thrombosis is treated with anticoagulants. Bone marrow hypoplasia may be treated by bone marrow transplantation or antithymocyte globulin.

Miscellaneous Causes

Thermal Injury. In patients with severe, third-degree burns, involving greater than 15% to 20% of the skin, intravascular hemolysis develops that may destroy 30% of the RBC mass. This hemolysis is usually complete by the third day after the burn. No specific treatment is available, although transfusion may be required to support these patients.

Freshwater Drowning. Freshwater drowning has been associated with hemolysis. This is caused by severe decrease in the osmolality in the lung blood vessels resulting in osmotic lysis of the RBCs. Similarly, osmotic swelling and lysis of RBCs can occur during transurethral resection of the prostate, when the prostatic bed is washed with large amounts of distilled water.

Cardiopulmonary Bypass. Occasional patients have the postperfusion syndrome following cardiopulmonary bypass. These patients have a febrile illness associated with leukopenia and acute intravascular hemolysis. Acute lung injury may develop. The mechanism of hemolysis is thought to involve complement activation during cardiopulmonary bypass followed by complement-mediated RBC lysis. This condition is treated supportively.

Immune Hemolytic Anemias

Immune hemolytic anemias include several distinct clinical entities that share the common characteristic that damage to RBCs is mediated by immune effectors such as antibodies and complement. These disorders can be subclassified as autoimmune (AIHA), either primary (25%) or secondary (60% to 65%), or drug-induced. Secondary AIHA results from neoplasms, infections, or systemic immunologic disorders. Drug-induced immune hemolysis stems either from the elaboration of drug-dependent antibodies or the stimulation of autoimmunity by the drugs (10% to 15% of AIHA). Alloimmune hemolysis may occur in transfused patients, but is beyond the scope of this discussion.

AIHA, whether primary, secondary, or drug induced, results from the binding of autoantibodies to antigens on the RBC membrane, which causes premature removal of the RBCs from the circulation. Three major types of antierythrocyte antibodies cause these diseases: (1) warm antibodies that bind to the RBC membrane at 37° C, (2) cold agglutinins that are usually immunoglobulin M (IgM) antibodies and clump RBCs at temperatures below 37° C, and (3) Donath-Landsteiner antibodies that are immunoglobulin G (IgG), fix to RBC membranes in the cold, and then activate the complement cascade when the cells are warmed to 37° C. About 75% of anti-RBC antibodies are warm-reacting antibodies of the IgG class, and about 25% are cold-reacting antibodies.

Warm-Reacting Antibody Hemolytic Anemia
Pathophysiology. The elaboration of warm-reacting IgG autoantibodies directed against erythrocyte surface antigens initiates a chain of events that can lead to AIHA. Typically these are not very active complement-fixing antibodies. Rather, they coat the RBC surface, most often bound to epitopes that are part of the Rh blood group antigen. The fragment crystallizable (Fc) portions of the bound antibodies interact with macrophage Fc receptors, leading to ingestion of RBCs and their destruction in the reticuloendothelial system. This process produces extravascular hemolysis that occurs primarily in the spleen, where coated erythrocytes are trapped in the hemoconcentrated microcirculation and interact with splenic macrophages. Most commonly the macrophages only remove small bits of the erythrocyte membrane, producing a microspherocyte. These microspherocytes have a more rigid cell membrane, are more prone to osmotic lysis, and are destroyed more easily during repassage through the spleen. The amount of antibody bound to the RBC surface, which depends on the avidity of antibody for the erythrocyte autoantigen and the capacity of the antibody to fix complement, contributes to the rapidity and efficiency of RBC clearance by the splenic macrophages. It is important to recognize that antibody-coated erythrocytes are not always opsonized and ingested. The presence of autoantibodies is not synonymous with AIHA.

Clinical features. Symptoms in these patients are directly related to the severity of the hemolytic process and the underlying diseases that are often associated. Primary warm-reacting antibody AIHA is more common in women than in men and occurs most frequently in midlife, but can occur at all ages. The incidence of warm-reacting antibody–induced autoimmune hemolytic anemia is approximately 10 cases per 1 million population per year. On presentation the patient may complain of increasing shortness of breath, decreased exercise tolerance, or other symptoms of anemia. Physical examination may rarely reveal signs of congestive heart failure, but this is usually in patients in whom autoimmune hemolytic anemia has developed rapidly. Splenomegaly is found in approximately one third of patients.

Underlying diseases that produce secondary AIHA include neoplasms, especially lymphoproliferative disorders such as chronic lymphocytic leukemia and non-Hodgkins lymphoma. Patients with systemic autoimmune diseases such as systemic lupus erythematosis, antiphospholipid antibody syndrome, inflammatory bowel disease, rheumatoid arthritis, and vasculitis can also develop warm-reacting antibody AIHA. Viral infections and sarcoidosis are associated with warm-reacting antibody AIHA. Acquired immunodeficiency syndrome (AIDS) patients may come to medical attention with autoimmune thrombocytopenia or AIHA. Following bone marrow transplantation or solid organ transplantation, AIHA may develop as a result of transferred immunity from the graft. The clinical characteristics of these disorders are diverse, but the symptoms of AIHA are similar.

Laboratory features. Microspherocytes are a hallmark of this process and can be seen on examination of the peripheral blood smear (Plate III-4, *G*). The reticulocyte index is increased. In severe cases the peripheral blood smear may reveal polychromatophilia, microspherocytes, occasional RBC fragments, and nucleated RBCs (Plate III-4, *E*). Examination of the bone marrow is not usually indicated but shows erythroid hyperplasia. As in other causes of hemolysis, the indirect serum bilirubin level is elevated. Hemolysis is usually extravascular, meaning that plasma free hemoglobin, hemoglobinuria, and hemosiderinuria are not typically detectable. This disorder is diagnosed by the direct antiglobulin (Coombs') test, which detects the presence of IgG and/or complement on the patient's RBC surface (Table 89-4). The IgG autoantibodies that are present on the RBCs in warm-reacting antibody hemolytic anemia are usually subclass IgG_1 or IgG_3. In addition, the proteolytic fragment of C3 of the complement cascade may also be bound to the RBCs. If the direct Coombs' test result is positive, it should be repeated with more specific reagents against IgG or complement. In a small minority of patients who have warm-reacting antibody autoimmune hemolytic anemia, the standard Coombs' test result is negative, because (1) antibodies are of low affinity, leading to a decreased amount of bound antibody on RBCs, (2) antibodies are not IgG, and (3) antibodies are directed against antigens that are not affixed to the erythrocyte surface. In patients who have both IgG and C3 bound to the RBC membrane the diagnosis of systemic lupus erythematosus should be considered. In about 80% of patients with autoimmune hemolytic anemia autoantibodies are present in the serum as well as on the RBC membrane. These antibodies, detected by the indirect antiglobulin test, may be used to determine the antibody specificity. As an alternative, antibodies eluted from the patient's erythrocytes can by analyzed for specificity.

In rare patients autoantibodies may be directed against RBC precursors as well as mature RBCs and produce pure RBC aplasia. Despite ongoing hemolysis, the reticulocyte count is low. Pure RBC aplasia is difficult to treat and carries a serious prognosis.

Table 89-4 The direct antiglobulin test in immune hemolytic anemia

CONDITION	ANTIBODY	ANTIBODY SPECIFICITY	DIRECT ANTIGLOBULIN TEST
Warm-reacting antibody AIHA	IgG	Rh	IgG IgG + C′ C′
Cold agglutinin	IgM	Ii	C′
Paroxysmal cold hemoglobinuria	IgG	Pp	C′
Alloimmune	IgG IgM	Blood group	IgG IgG + C′ C′
Drug-induced			
Hapten type	IgG	Drug	IgG
Immune complex	IgG IgM	Drug	C′
AIHA type	IgG	Rh	IgG IgG + C′ C′

AIHA, Autoimmune hemolytic anemia; *IgG,* immunoglobulin G; *IgM,* immunoglobin M.

Management. Therapy of warm-reacting antibody AIHA is directed toward eradication of the autoantibody and/or the reduction of the rate of RBC destruction. Glucocorticoids are the usual initial therapy for patients with warm-reacting antibody AIHA. Oral prednisone is usually given at doses of 1 to 2 mg/kg per day, with the higher doses given at the outset in more severe cases. Patients with milder hemolysis may be started on 1 mg/kg and increased to 2 mg/kg if there is no improvement in 1 to 2 weeks. Responses are detected by an increase in the hematocrit and a fall in the reticulocyte count. Prednisone decreases both the expression and the function of macrophage Fc receptors, and this accounts for the early effects of prednisone. Prednisone also decreases autoantibody production, but the half-life of IgG in the circulation is approximately 3 weeks. Once a response is noted, prednisone dosage is slowly tapered over the next 2 to 3 months, and the patient is closely monitored by measuring hemoglobin level, reticulocytes, and peripheral smear microspherocytes. Approximately 75% of patients who have the primary form of autoimmune hemolytic anemia respond to prednisone. Approximately 25% of these responsive patients maintain a sustained remission after glucocorticoids have been tapered and discontinued. Fifty percent require continued maintenance therapy with 5 to 20 mg of prednisone per day. The remainder of corticosteroid-responsive patients require unacceptably high doses of prednisone to maintain a satisfactory hemoglobin. These patients, as well as corticosteroid-unresponsive patients, should undergo splenectomy. Splenectomy removes the major site of RBC destruction in warm-reacting antibody AIHA and also eliminates a source of autoantibody production. Sixty-five percent to 80% of patients have a beneficial response to splenectomy. Splenectomy may be curative in up to 50%. Many patients who respond to splenectomy, however, still require low doses of glucocorticoids to maintain control of the AIHA. If the necessary corticosteroid doses are acceptably low, no further treatment is necessary. Folate administration is required in AIHA patients with chronic hemolysis.

Approximately 10% of patients are unresponsive to glucocorticoids or splenectomy and require immunosuppressive drugs such as azathioprine, cyclophosphamide, or vinca alkaloids to impair macrophage function and decrease antibody production. However, immunosuppressive agents that are cytotoxic can induce numerous side effects, including marrow suppression. Therefore danazol, a synthetic androgen that has been found to be beneficial in some patients, may be tried in doses of 400 to 600 mg/day. Danazol has benefited a limited number of patients with refractory hemolytic anemia, with remissions lasting for up to 1 year. In case reports, intravenous gamma globulin has been used in a way similar to its use in immune thrombocytopenia. Intravenous IgG therapy appears to be effective in some patients with autoimmune hemolytic anemia associated with lymphoproliferative diseases.

In patients with life-threatening hemolytic anemia, transfusion of RBCs may be necessary. Cross-matching is made difficult by the presence of autoantibodies and may take a longer time to perform. If urgent transfusion is required before cross-matching can be completed, patients should receive type-specific blood or type O, Rh-negative blood under close clinical supervision. Relatively small quantities of RBCs may alleviate the signs and symptoms of anemia (½ to 1 unit of packed RBCs) so that large amounts of blood need not be transfused in these patients. The major goal of transfusion therapy is to support the patient until other forms of treatment can control the hemolytic process.

Cold Agglutinin Disease

Pathophysiology. Cold agglutinins are complement-fixing IgM antibodies that react with the Ii antigen system on RBCs. Normal individuals have low titers of cold agglutinins (<1:16 at 4° C) that have low thermal amplitude and do not bind to RBCs at 20° to 37° C. In cold agglutinin disease, the antibody titers measured at 4° C are greatly increased (up to $1:1 \times 10^6$) and the thermal amplitude of the antibody is increased, so the antibody binds to the surface of RBCs at temperatures as high as 28° to 32° C. Monoclonal cold agglutinins may occur in lymphoproliferative diseases; polyclonal cold agglutinins may be produced in patients with *Mycoplasma pneumoniae* infection, Epstein-Barr virus infection, or lupus erythematosus.

Clinical features. Patients with primary, chronic cold agglutinin disease usually have moderate anemia and attacks of acrocyanosis that are precipitated by exposure to the cold. This acrocyanosis usually results from intraarterial agglutination of RBCs in the tips of the fingers, toes, ear lobes, and nose. Most patients with chronic cold agglutinin disease are elderly (70 to 80 years of age) and many have lymphomas, Waldenström's macroglobulinemia, or chronic lymphocytic leukemia. Cold agglutinin–mediated AIHA secondary to lymphoproliferative disease may become evident as hemolytic anemia or from other manifestations of the underlying condition. Uncommonly, patients with cold agglutinin disease may exhibit Raynaud's-like reactions or hemoglobinuria. Because the site of erythrocyte destruction is often the liver, splenomegaly is less common than in warm-reacting antibody autoimmune hemolytic anemia. Hemolysis is usually extravascular, with varying degrees of intravascular hemolysis mediated by complement fixation.

A subset of patients have cold agglutinin disease of acute onset associated with *M. pneumoniae* or infectious mononucleosis. These patients tend to be younger than those who have the chronic form of the disease and usually have an abrupt onset of hemolysis as the infection wanes. The cold agglutinin produced in patients with *M. pneumoniae* has anti-I specificity, whereas the antibody in infectious mononucleosis has anti-i specificity. These cases of cold agglutinin disease improve as the patient recovers from the infection.

Laboratory features. The peripheral blood smear shows RBC agglutination, reticulocytosis, polychromatophilia, and spherocytosis. Automated blood cell counts may be inaccurate because of erythrocyte agglutination that increases the MCV and thereby distorts the calculated hematocrit. Typical of hemolysis, the serum indirect bilirubin and LDH levels are elevated. The severity of the anemia in these patients is directly correlated with the thermal amplitude of the autoantibody. The higher the temperature at which the cold agglutinin can react with the RBC, the more rapid the destruction of the cell. The direct Coombs' test result is positive because the RBCs are coated with C3b. Results of tests with the anti-IgG reagents are usually negative, as is the result of the indirect Coombs' test. Extravascular hemolysis occurs because membrane receptors for C3b on hepatic macrophages allow binding and ingestion of C3b-coated RBCs. Hepatic clearance of these cells predominates because there is no plasma C3b to inhibit macrophage binding competitively.

Management. Prednisone is usually not useful in treatment of cold agglutinin disease because corticosteroids do not impair macrophage binding of C3b-coated RBCs. Splenectomy usually is not beneficial because hepatic clearance of RBCs predominates. No treatment is usually required for the self-limited episodes associated with this disease except avoidance of cold. If the patient requires transfusion of RBCs, the cross-match must be done at 37° C to find compatible units of blood. The blood must be warmed to body temperature before transfusion. Rapid infusion of blood at room temperature results in dramatic hemolysis because the autoantibody reacts well at low temperatures. Cytotoxic agents and plasmapheresis are sometimes used to reduce cold agglutinin titers. Treatment of the undelying disorder may be beneficial in patients with seconday cold-reacting antibody AIHA.

Paroxysmal Cold Hemoglobinuria

Paroxysmal cold hemoglobinuria (PCH) has been reported in patients with tertiary congenital syphilis and in children who have viral infections. It is an extremely rare disease and accounts for less than 2% of cases of acquired hemolytic anemia. Currently it is most often associated with chickenpox and mumps. The Donath-Landsteiner antibody responsible for paroxysmal cold hemoglobinuria is of the IgG subclass. It binds to RBCs at 4° C and fixes complement at 37° C. It has an anti-P specificity and does not agglutinate RBCs in the cold. Patients with PCH have a positive Coombs' test result. The antibody is hemolytic in vivo and in vitro and can bind to RBCs at temperatures as high as 32° C. Symptoms of patients with paroxysmal cold hemoglobinuria include fever, malaise, anorexia, and flank pain. The urine contains hemoglobin, and paroxysms of hemolysis are followed by jaundice. Treatment consists of bed rest, avoidance of the cold, and treatment of the primary disease process. Prednisone therapy and cytotoxic drugs may be helpful, but splenectomy and intravenous gammaglobulin are not. Transfusion is made difficult by the presence of an antibody to a nearly universal antigen.

Drug-Induced Immune Hemolytic Anemia

Drug-induced immune hemolytic anemia is produced by three different mechanisms (Table 89-4). In the first, the drug acts as a hapten and binds the RBC membrane. Circulating antibodies that are directed against the drug then develop, and the drug-antibody interaction occurs on the RBC surface (e.g., penicillin) and causes RBC destruction. The patient's antidrug antibodies may fix complement and cause severe anemia and hemoglobinuria. These episodes of hemolysis usually occur during the first 3 weeks of therapy with the drug but may occur after longer intervals. In the case of penicillin, hemolytic anemia occurs only with administration of large doses of the drug. With lower doses of penicillin, a positive direct Coombs' test result without hemolytic anemia is not unusual. Discontinuation of the drug stops the hemolytic process. In this type of hemolytic anemia, antibodies eluted from the patient's RBCs do not react with a panel of RBCs from normal donors, showing that the antibodies are not directed against normal RBC antigens. The diagnosis is often made by showing that the antibody eluted from the patient's RBCs and the patient's serum itself reacts with penicillin-coated RBCs.

The second mechanism responsible for drug-induced hemolytic anemia is immune complex deposition on the RBC surface. The offending drug often binds to plasma Ig, forming an immune complex. This complex then binds to the RBC membrane, and the antidrug antibody that is present may bind complement. The clinical picture may include intravascular hemolysis with hemoglobinemia, hemoglobinuria, and rarely renal failure. This is the most common type of drug-induced immune hemolytic anemia. In this type of drug-induced hemolytic anemia, the direct Coombs' test result reveals complement bound to the RBC surface. The patient's serum reacts with RBCs in the presence of the offending drug. The patient's RBC eluate usually does not react with normal RBCs. Therapy is discontinuation of the offending drug.

The third mechanism involved in drug-induced hemolysis is induction of authentic autoantibodies against RBC antigens by a drug. Methyldopa is the classic example, in which patients develop an RBC autoantibody with specificity against the Rh system. AIHA has also been described in patients taking newer drugs such as interferon, fludarabine, pentostatin, ciprofloxacin, and ranitidine. The serologic findings in these patients are indistinguishable from those of primary autoimmune hemolytic anemia. Patients have positive direct and indirect Coombs' test results, and their serum reacts with normal erythrocytes. In 15% to 20% of patients who take alpha methyldopa a positive direct Coombs' test result develops, but hemolytic anemia develops only in a few individuals. The Coombs' test demonstrates IgG alone on the RBC surface. Patients who have this disorder usually have been taking alpha methyldopa for several months. The antibody that binds to the RBCs does not fix complement. Once the drug is stopped, the hemolysis often improves over 1 to 2 weeks. However, the titer of the autoantibody declines slowly and it requires 3 to 6 months before the Coombs' test result becomes negative. Therapy for these drug-induced autoantibodies to RBCs is to discontinue the drug. Patients may require transfusions if the anemia is severe. It may take several months for the Coombs' test result to return to normal.

✔ WHEN TO REFER

General internists should be able to diagnose fragmentation hemolysis and immune hemolysis. In a community setting patients with life-threatening thrombotic microangiopathy or severe autoimmune hemolysis must often be emergently evaluated without the input of a hematologist. Coupled with the usual clinical and laboratory findings of hemolysis, the peripheral blood smear and direct antiglobulin (Coombs') test allow accurate diagnosis in most circumstances. Nevertheless, for all patients with clinically severe acquired hemolysis such that transfusion is considered, a hematologist should be consulted to assist in diagnosis and treatment. Even the most seemingly straightforward case can exhibit unusual features that may be apparent only to the subspecialist.

BIBLIOGRAPHY

Beutler E, Westwood B, Prchal JT et al: New glucose-6-phosphate dehydrogenase mutations from various ethnic groups, *Blood* 80:255, 1992.

Brown KE, Young NS: Parvovirus B19 infection and hematopoiesis, *Blood Rev* 9:176, 1995.

Delaunay J: Genetic disorders of the red cell membranes, *FEBS Lett* 369:34, 1995.

Hillmen P, Lewis SM, Bessler M et al: Natural history of paroxysmal nocturnal hemoglobinuria, *N Engl J Med* 333:1253, 1995.

Izui S: Autoimmune hemolytic anemia, *Curr Opin Immunol* 6:926, 1994.

Jeffries LC: Transfusion therapy in autoimmune hemolytic anemia, *Hematol Oncol Clin North Am* 8:1087, 1994.

Melnyk AM, Solez K, Kjellstrand CM: Adult hemolytic-uremic syndrome, *Arch Intern Med* 155:2077, 1995.

Miwa S: Molecular basis of red cell enzymopathies associated with hereditary nonspherocytic anemia, *Hematologia* 22:215, 1989.

Palek J, Jarolim P: Clinical expression and laboratory detection of red blood cell membrane protein mutations, *Semin Hematol* 30:249, 1993.

Petz LD: Drug-induced autoimmune hemolytic anemia, *Transfusion Med Rev* 7:242, 1993.

Rosse WF, Ware RE: The molecular basis of paroxysmal nocturnal hemoglobinuria, *Blood* 86:3277, 1995.

Tarr PI: *Escherichia coli* 0157:H7: clinical, diagnostic and epidemiological aspects of infection, *Clin Infect Dis* 20:1, 1995.

Winkelmann JC, Forget BG: Erythroid and nonerythroid spectrins, *Blood* 81:3173, 1993.

CHAPTER

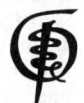

90 Bone Marrow Failure and Myelodysplasia

Frederick R. Appelbaum

The term *bone marrow failure* describes the clinical situation in which peripheral blood cytopenias develop because of the failure of bone marrow stem cells to produce mature progeny. A wide range of diseases can result in bone marrow failure (Box 90-1). This chapter discusses three relatively specific categories of bone marrow failure: bone marrow failure associated with aplastic anemia, with the myelodysplastic syndromes, and with myelofibrosis.

APLASTIC ANEMIA
Definition

Aplastic anemia is defined by the presence of pancytopenia in the peripheral blood and a bone marrow that is markedly hypocellular and largely replaced by fat. Although a similar condition regularly occurs in patients receiving chemotherapy or radiotherapy for malignant disease, such patients quickly recover and are not considered to have aplastic anemia. Aplastic anemia may be categorized as mild or severe. *Severe aplastic anemia* has been defined by the International Aplastic Anemia Study Group as follows: (1) a marrow of less than 25% marrow cellularity and (2) at least two of the following three peripheral blood values: granulocytes less than 0.5×10^9 per liter, platelets less than 20×10^9 per liter, and anemia with reticulocytes less than 1% (corrected for the hematocrit). Within this group, those with extreme neutropenia ($<0.2 \times 10^9$ per liter) have the worst outlook. *Mild aplastic anemia* is defined as marrow hypoplasia with cytopenias in two or more cell lines, but not severe enough to meet the preceding criteria.

Etiology

In the majority of cases the cause of aplastic anemia is unknown. In others a possible cause can be identified on the basis of a statistical or temporal relationship. However, the existence of such a relationship is not equivalent to proving cause and does not explain the mechanisms involved. An etiologic classification of aplastic anemia is presented in Box 90-2.

Drugs. Two types of marrow suppression produced by drugs can be distinguished. Many drugs have the potential to suppress prolif-

---

✔ WHEN TO REFER

Patients with bone marrow failure should always be referred to a hematologist to provide a definitive diagnosis and plan of therapy. Management of these patients is complex, and initial decisions such as whether to transfuse can seriously affect prognosis. Once a firm plan is developed by the subspecialist in collaboration with the patient and the referring physician, the appropriate roles of the primary internist and the subspecialist can be defined to be convenient and cost effective for the patient while providing the best possible care.

BOX 90-1
Causes of pancytopenia

Pancytopenia with hypocellular bone marrow
  Acquired aplastic anemia (see Box 90-2)
  Constitutional aplastic anemia (see Box 90-2)
  Exposure to chemical or physical agents, including ionizing irradiation and chemotherapeutic agents
  Some hematologic malignancies, including myelodysplasia and aleukemic leukemia
Pancytopenia with normal or increased cellularity of hematopoietic origin
  Some hematologic malignancies, including myelodysplasia, and some leukemias, lymphomas, and myelomas
  Paroxysmal nocturnal hemoglobinuria
  Hypersplenism
  Vitamin B_{12}, folate deficiencies
  Overwhelming infection
Pancytopenia with bone marrow replacement
  Tumor metastatic to marrow
  Metabolic storage diseases
  Osteopetrosis
  Myelofibrosis

BOX 90-2
Classification of aplastic anemia by cause

Idiopathic
Drugs
  Chloramphenicol
  Phenylbutazone and related antiinflammatory drugs
  Quinacrine and related antiprotozoals
  Sulfonamides
  Cimetidine
  Gold salts
  Hydantoins
Chemicals
  Benzene and benzene-containing solvents
  Insecticides including dichlorodiphenyltrichloroethane (DDT)
Viral
  Hepatitis
  Epstein-Barr virus
  Human immunodeficiency virus
Immunologic
  Graft-versus-host disease
  Systemic lupus erythematosus
  Eosinophilic fasciitis
  Thymoma
Pregnancy
Congenital
  Fanconi's anemia
  Dyskeratosis congenita
  Shwachman-Diamond syndrome
  Reticular dysgenesis

eration of one or more cell lines in all individuals in a dose-related fashion, a form of suppression that is not considered aplastic anemia. Rather, drug-induced aplastic anemia is an idiosyncratic reaction that occurs relatively independent of dose and affects only a very small population of patients receiving the drug. The true incidence of drug-induced aplastic anemia is unknown. But in about 20% of cases of severe aplastic anemia a suspected agent can be identified. Historically the broad-spectrum antibiotic chloramphenicol was the most commonly identified drug. Other drugs with the strongest association to aplastic anemia include phenylbutazone, quinacrine, sulfonamides, phenytoin (Dilantin), and gold salts. Gold salts deserve special mention because when they are given, a falling neutrophil count may presage the development of aplasia and careful monitoring of blood cell counts may prevent the disease.

Chemicals. Benzene and benzene-containing compounds such as kerosene and carbon tetrachloride cause marrow damage that may take the form of aplastic anemia, myelodysplasia, or acute leukemia. The frequency of marrow damage is related to the extent of benzene exposure. Benzene is widely used in industry, particularly in organic synthesis and as a solvent, and makes up 1% of unleaded gasoline. Exposure to a number of other chemicals has been temporally associated with the development of severe aplastic anemia, particularly the insecticides dichlorodiphenyltrichloroethane (DDT) and lindane and derivatives of toluene.

Viral Causes. Approximately 5% of cases of aplastic anemia occur in the wake of a preceding viral infection. Severe aplasia is a rare complication of otherwise typical non-A, non-B, non-C hepatitis, but is seen more commonly in recipients of liver transplants for fulminant seronegative hepatitis. Aplastic anemia also has been associated with hepatitis A and, rarely, hepatitis B. Other viral infections, including Epstein-Barr virus and human immunodeficiency virus (HIV), have been implicated in aplastic anemia. Parvovirus B19 can cause temporary cessation of red blood cell production but is not generally considered a cause of aplastic anemia.

Immunologic Causes. In immunodeficient children and other immunosuppressed individuals who receive unirradiated blood products and have graft-versus-host disease caused by the inadvertent engraftment of donor T cells, aplasia may develop. Aplastic anemia also rarely develops in association with other immunologically based diseases such as systemic lupus erythematosus, myasthenia gravis, and eosinophilic fasciitis.

Congenital Causes. Fanconi's anemia is the most common inherited form of aplastic anemia and is caused by one of several autosomal recessive genes. The disorder is associated with a broad spectrum of congenital abnormalities, the most consistent of which are small stature; skeletal defects, especially hypoplastic thumbs or radii; and renal abnormalities. Patients frequently have pancytopenia during the first or second decade of life and also have a high incidence of myelodysplasia and leukemia. Patients with Fanconi's anemia have a defect in deoxyribonucleic acid (DNA) repair and are particularly sensitive to the toxic effects of chemotherapy. Because the physical anomalies of Fanconi's anemia may be subtle or absent, some investigators believe the incidence of the disorder may be higher than generally appreciated and recommend that all young patients with aplastic anemia be screened for Fanconi's anemia before undergoing marrow transplantation. If evidence of Fanconi's anemia is found, the doses of chemotherapy in the transplant preparation regimen should be reduced. Rare cases of aplastic anemia are associated with dyskeratosis congenita, Shwachman-Diamond syndrome, or reticular dysgenesis.

Pathogenesis

A consistent feature of all cases of aplastic anemia is the marked reduction in marrow hematopoietic progenitor cells. The mechanisms causing this are not understood. In perhaps 50% of cases it seems likely that an ongoing immunologic mechanism is responsible. Evidence for this view includes the observation that about 50% of patients respond to therapy with immunosuppressants such

as antithymocyte globulin (ATG) or cyclosporine, and that only about 50% of patients with aplastic anemia who receive infusions of bone marrow cells from their normal genotypically identical twin without intensive preconditioning recover. In the other 50% of cases the mechanisms leading to aplastic anemia are less well understood, but could be a previous, no longer active immune attack or some other direct toxic insult to marrow stem cells. In cases of immune-mediated aplastic anemia, hematopoietic failure is likely mediated by cytotoxic T lymphocytes, which can be detected in the blood and marrow of some patients. These cells produce α-interferon and tumor necrosis factor B, which inhibit marrow function. These cells also are cytotoxic to marrow progenitors, perhaps by inducing Fas-mediated apoptosis. In occasional cases of otherwise typical aplastic anemia, clonal hematopoiesis has been demonstrated, suggesting that in those cases the disease might be due to the replacement of normal stem cells by a clone of cells incapable of normal proliferation and differentiation.

Clinical Features

The clinical features of aplastic anemia are the consequences of the anemia, neutropenia, and thrombocytopenia that result from bone marrow failure. Anemia leads to weakness, easy fatigability, and pallor. Neutropenia may result in recurrent infections, most frequently of the gingiva, throat, and perirectal area. Petechiae, easy bruising, bleeding from the nose and gums, and heavy menses in women are results of thrombocytopenia. Findings other than those attributable to marrow failure are rare. Thus bone pain, lymphadenopathy, or hepatic or splenic enlargement suggests a disease other than aplastic anemia. The clinical history should carefully document all exposures to drugs, solvents, or other causative agents and any symptoms related to previous viral illnesses. A family history of anemia or congenital abnormalities may disclose unsuspected cases of Fanconi's anemia.

Laboratory Findings

Patients with severe aplastic anemia have less than 0.5×10^9 neutrophils per liter, less than 20×10^9 platelets per liter, a corrected reticulocyte count of less than 1%, and a hypoplastic or aplastic bone marrow biopsy result (Fig. 90-1). The anemia is usually normocytic and normochromic with normal-appearing red blood cells. Likewise, the neutrophils and platelets, although severely diminished in number, are normal in their individual structure. The bone marrow biopsy result shows less than 25% of normal cellularity. There is, on occasion, an increase in plasma cells, but marrow fibrosis or replacement by malignant cells is not seen. Occasionally foci of active hematopoiesis persist and by chance may undergo biopsy. In such cases repeat biopsy procedures may be required to establish the diagnosis. Although not usually required, magnetic resonance imaging can provide an accurate method of determining the extent of fatty replacement of the marrow. Cytogenetic studies of bone marrow are useful to distinguish aplastic anemia, which has normal cytogenetic findings, from hypoplastic myelodysplasia, in which clonal abnormalities such as trisomy 8 or monosomy 7 may be seen.

Differential Diagnosis

As listed in Box 90-1, mild to moderate pancytopenia occurs in many situations, but severe pancytopenia is markedly less common. The diagnosis of aplastic anemia generally rests on the marrow biopsy specimen's demonstration of the characteristic findings previously mentioned. The most difficult distinction is between severe aplastic anemia and hypoplastic myelodysplasia. Cytogenetic study may be helpful in making the distinction.

Therapy

An important first step in therapy is determining whether patients have mild or severe aplastic anemia because the prognosis differs so greatly. If aplasia is judged to be mild, the appropriate course is to remove any possible offending agents and provide supportive care as necessary. Most patients spontaneously recover; in others mild aplasia remains for years. However, in some patients mild aplasia may

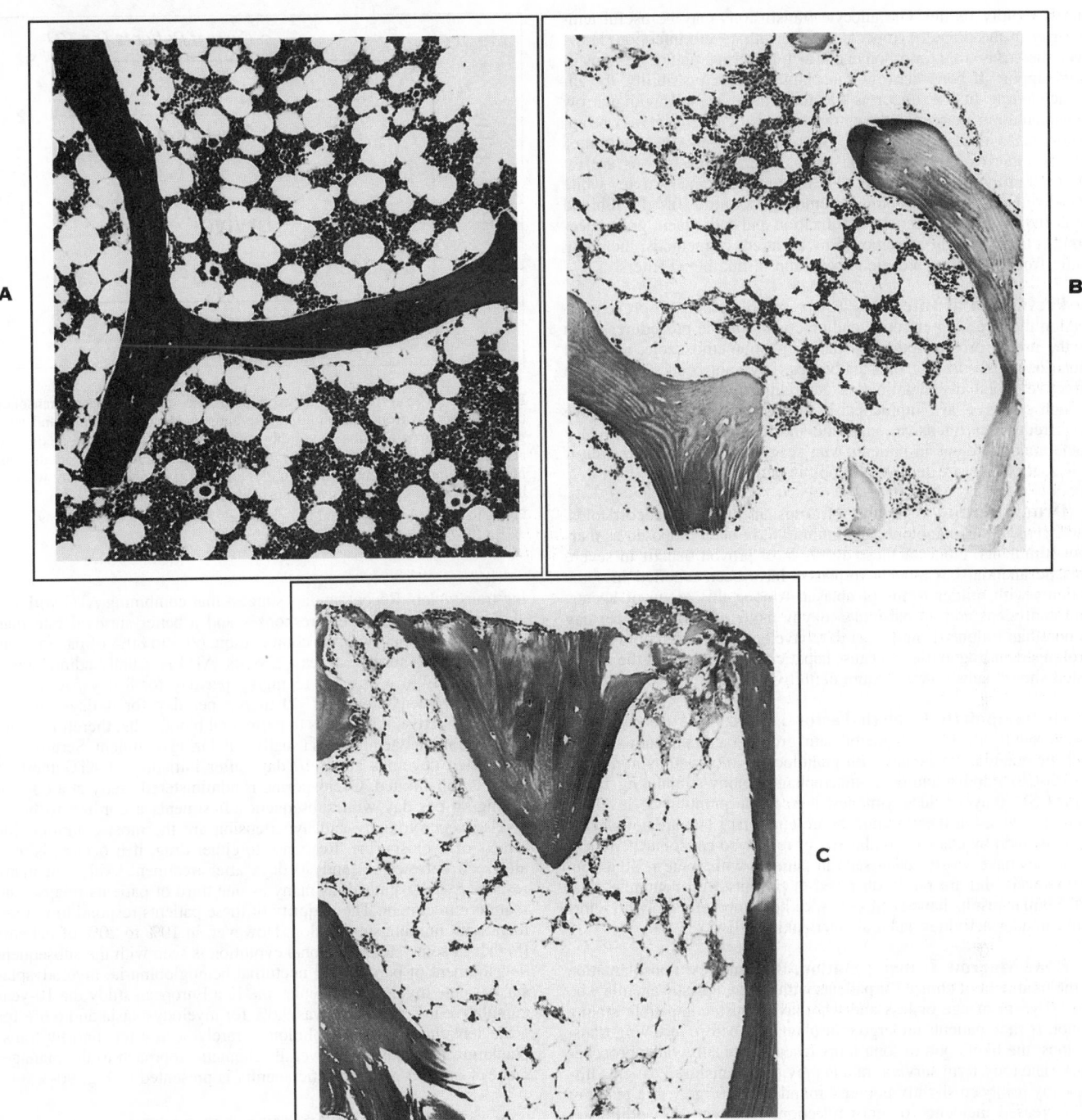

FIGURE 90-1   Bone marrow biopsy specimens. **A,** From a normal person. **B,** From a person with mild aplastic anemia. **C,** From a person with severe aplastic anemia. In the normal individual the marrow cavity between bony trabeculae contains approximately 50% nucleated cells and 50% fat. Megakaryocytes are large and easily seen. Hematopoietic cells are absent in the aplastic marrow.

progress to severe aplastic anemia. Patients who are judged to have severe aplasia, on the other hand, have a poor prognosis if no specific therapy is given. Fifty percent of patients die within 3 months of diagnosis, and the overall mortality rate is estimated to be approximately 80%. As for mild aplastic anemia, a first step in therapy is removal of offending agents. The next steps are providing supportive care and then administering specific therapy designed to restore normal hematopoiesis.

Supportive Care. Anemia is easily reversed with packed red blood cell transfusions. Thrombocytopenia can likewise be reversed,

at least temporarily, with platelet transfusions. However, with repeated transfusions of random donor platelets most patients become sensitized to human leukocyte antigen (HLA) and other antigens on the platelet surface, leading to rapid destruction of the transfused platelets. In most cases, with the use of carefully selected HLA-matched platelet donors, good platelet increments can be produced even in sensitized patients. Platelet transfusions are obviously warranted for any patient with thrombocytopenia and signs of bleeding. Whether platelets should be given prophylactically is less settled, but such transfusions can generally be recommended for patients with a demonstrated bleeding tendency and in those with less than 20×10^9 platelets per liter and a count that is rapidly falling. Granulocyte transfusions may be useful temporarily in the granulocytopenic patient with severe infection. However, there is no role for prophylactic or long-term granulocyte transfusion support. If bone marrow transplantation is a possibility, the approach to transfusion support is affected. The best results with marrow transplantation are seen in the untransfused patient. Thus it may be appropriate to defer transfusions, if possible, until it is determined whether marrow transplantation is possible. If transfusions are required, family member donors should be avoided and as many white blood cells as possible should be removed from transfused red blood cells and platelets to prevent sensitization and subsequent graft rejection. Leukocytes can be removed by a variety of methods, including using frozen, washed red blood cells and in-line blood filters.

Prevention of Infection. There are no methods to prevent infection that are both effective and practical. Simple procedures, such as the use of prophylactic trimethoprim-sulfamethoxazole, modified diets, or nonabsorbable oral antibiotics, have not been shown to be effective. Total decontamination and laminar airflow isolation, although effective, are impractical in the long run. Patients who have fever require an intensive diagnostic and therapeutic approach. Once bacteremia develops in patients with severe aplastic anemia, even if it is successfully treated, the outlook is particularly grave.

Drug Therapy. A number of drugs, including glucocorticoids, androgens, etiocholanolone, and lithium, have been proposed as marrow stimulants. None of these agents is of proven benefit in severe aplastic anemia, but modest responses have been reported in some patients with milder forms of aplasia. Among this group of agents, oral androgens and, in particular, oxymetholone at 3 mg/kg per day or norethandrolone, 1 mg/kg per day, have been most commonly used. Prolonged androgen use can cause hepatic toxicity. None of the agents listed should substitute for more definitive therapy.

Hematopoietic Growth Factors. There is no clearly established role for the use of hematopoietic growth factors in patients with aplastic anemia. Treatment with granulocyte colony-stimulating factor (G-CSF) and granulocyte-macrophage colony-stimulating factor (GM-CSF) may produce a modest increase in granulocyte levels in some patients, but these responses are temporary and are not usually accompanied by changes in platelets or red blood cells. Further, these responses have mostly been seen in patients with some residual hematopoiesis and are rarely observed in patients with complete aplasia. Similar results have been seen with hematopoietic growth factors with broader activities, such as interleukin-3 (IL-3).

Bone Marrow Transplantation. Bone marrow transplantation is the treatment of choice for patients with severe aplastic anemia who are 50 years of age or less and who have a histocompatible sibling donor. If such patients undergo transplantation before receiving transfusions, the likelihood of long-term, disease-free survival approaches 90%. The long-term survival rate in previously tansfused patients historically has been slightly poorer (around 70%), largely as a result of an increased incidence of graft rejection. However, the addition of antithymocyte globulin (ATG) to the usual cyclophosphamide conditioning regimen appears able to improve survival in transfused patients to close to 90% as well (Fig. 90-2). Patients less than age 50 years who lack an HLA-identical sibling can still be cured with transplantation using either a partially matched family member or a matched, unrelated donor. However, the likelihood of a successful outcome is considerably less with these alternative donors, and such transplantations should be restricted to patients in whom immunosuppressive therapy with ATG and/or cyclosporine has failed. The principles of marrow transplantation are presented in Chapter 77.

Immunosuppressive Therapy. For patients who are not candidates for immediate transplantation, because they either are above age 50 years or lack an HLA-identical sibling donor, immunosuppression has emerged as the treatment of choice. Approximately 50% of patients treated with either antithymocyte globulin (ATG) or cyclosporine respond with an increase in granulocytes to a safe level and an increase in platelets and red blood cells to levels no longer requir-

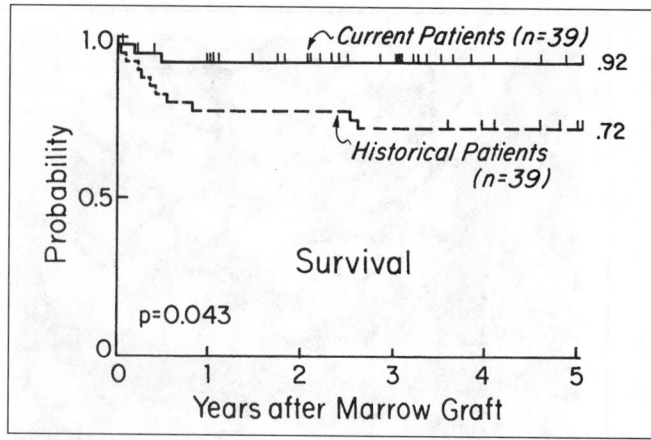

FIGURE 90-2 Survival of patients with aplastic anemia who had transplantation in Seattle from human leukocyte antigen–identical siblings and were given graft-versus-host disease prophylaxis with cyclosporine and methotrexate after transplantation. *Current patients* were prepared for transplantation using a combination of antithymocyte globulin and cyclophosphamide, whereas historical patients received cyclophosphamide alone.

From Storb R, Etzioni R, Anasetti C, Appelbaum FR et al: *Blood* 84(3):941-949, 1994.

ing transfusion. Recent studies suggest that combining ATG with cyclosporine produces more responses and a better survival rate than either agent alone. With the combination, 60% to 80% of patients can be expected to survive at least 3 years. ATG is usually administered intravenously at a dose of 15 mg/kg per day for 8 days. A shorter, more convenient course of 40 mg/kg per day for 4 days appears equally effective. ATG binds to peripheral blood cells; therefore platelet and granulocyte numbers usually fall during treatment. Serum sickness often develops about 10 days after initiation of ATG therapy, but it is self-limited. Cyclosporine is administered orally at a dose of 12 mg/kg per day with subsequent adjustments according to blood levels. Nephrotoxicity and hypertension are the most common side effects of cyclosporine. Response to either drug, if it occurs, is usually seen between 30 and 90 days after treatment. Although many responses are sustained, as many as one third of patients relapse and require retreatment. The majority of these patients respond to retreatment with immunosuppression. However, in 10% to 20% of patients (higher in some studies), clonal evolution is seen with the subsequent development of paroxysmal nocturnal hemoglobinuria, myelodysplasia, or acute myelogenous leukemia. In a European study the 10-year cumulative incidence rate was 9.6% for myelodysplasia and 6.6% for acute leukemia. Clonal evolution is rarely seen after marrow transplantation for aplasia. An overall schematic approach to the management of patients with aplastic anemia is presented in Fig. 90-3.

APLASIAS OF SINGLE CELL LINEAGES

In contrast to aplastic anemia, in which all three cell lines are affected, patients sometimes have aplasia restricted to a single cell lineage. Such patients lack both the marrow precursors and the mature circulating cells of the affected lineage, a situation different from those syndromes such as hemolytic anemia or immune-mediate thrombocytopenia in which the problem is one of destruction of the mature blood element rather than its production.

Pure Red Blood Cell Aplasia

Pure red blood cell aplasia (PRCA) occurs as a congenital or an acquired syndrome. The congenital form, Diamond-Blackfan syndrome, usually becomes evident as an isolated anemia during the first 2 years of life. The disease is thought to be transmitted as an autosomal recessive trait and in 25% of cases is associated with other minor congenital anomalies. The disorder responds to glucocorticoids in 50% to 75% of cases, and occasionally patients who fail glucocorticoid

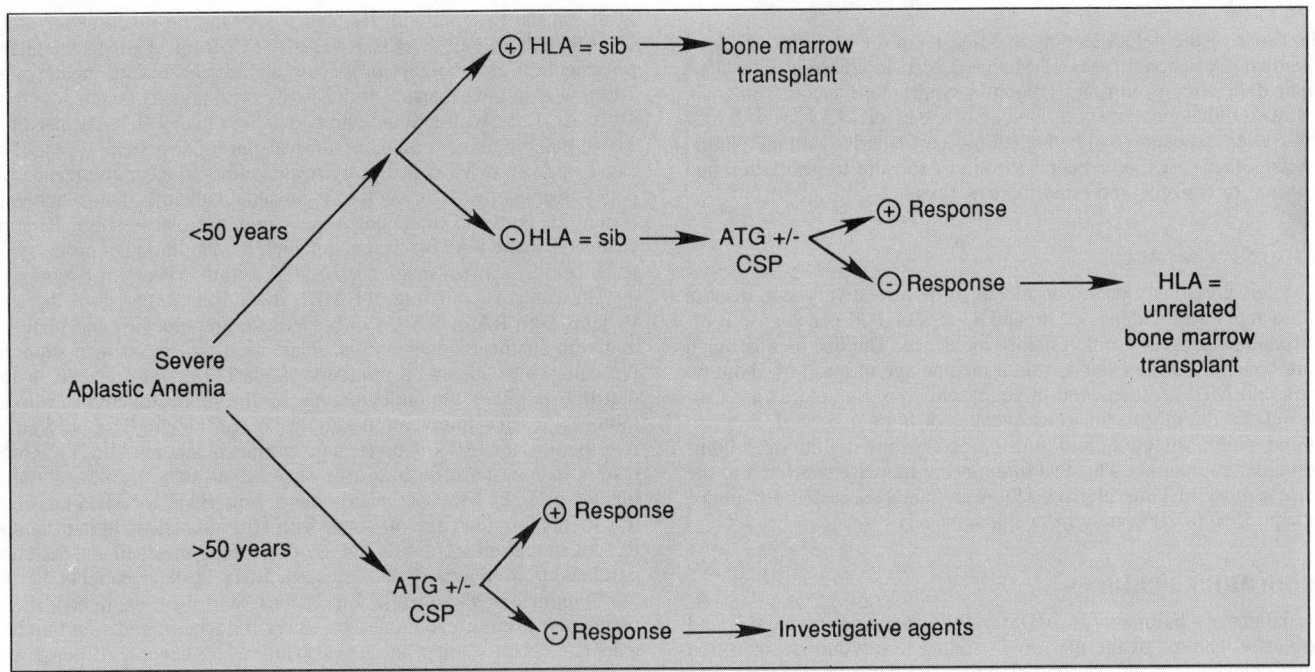

FIGURE 90-3   Management of patients with severe aplastic anemia. Appropriate therapy depends on patient age, availability of a human leukocyte antigen–identical sibling (HLA = sib), and response to antithymocyte globulin (ATG) therapy. ATG is combined with cyclosporin (CSP) in some treatment regimens.

therapy respond to other immunosuppressants. Marrow transplantation has been used in corticosteroid-resistant patients and can cure the disease.

Primary acquired PRCA has both acute and chronic forms. The acute form of PRCA is most often seen in young patients with underlying hemoglobinopathy or hemolytic anemia. The disease often follows a relatively mild viral infection, most often with parvovirus. The disease is usually self-limited; therefore the appropriate management involves maintaining an adequate hemoglobin level with red blood cell transfusions during the period of severe anemia and administration of folic acid 1 mg/day during the regenerative phase to prevent folate deficiency. The chronic form of PRCA is usually seen in patients aged 20 to 50 years, becoming evident as a slowly progressive anemia. Thymomas are sometimes found in cases of PRCA. While the exact incidence of thymoma in PRCA is unknown, most studies put the incidence at 15% to 20%. Most often these tumors are of the spindle cell type and behave as benign tumors. PRCA is sometimes associated with other diseases such as chronic lymphocytic leukemia or systemic lupus erythematosus and rarely occurs with the same groups of drugs associated with aplastic anemia. In many patients complement-fixing immunoglobulin G (IgG) selectively cytotoxic to marrow erythroblasts can be detected and is thought to be causative. Management of patients with PRCA begins with discontinuation of any suspected offending agent followed by a search for a thymoma. Thymectomy induces remission in 50% of patients with an enlarged thymus but is not effective in those with normal-sized thymuses. For patients without thymoma or for whom thymectomy fails, a trial of immunosuppressive therapy is warranted. Glucocorticoid or cyclosporine is usually the first agent of choice; ATG and cytotoxic immunosuppressants such as cyclophosphamide and azathioprine are reserved for treatment failures.

Pure White Blood Cell Aplasia

Pure white blood cell aplasia is a very rare condition with parallels to PRCA in that it appears to have an immune basis and is sometimes associated with thymoma, whereas in other cases it appears to be drug-related. Management, like that of PRCA, involves removal of any identified offending agent, thymectomy if an enlarged thymus

is found, and immunosuppressive therapy with glucocorticoids or cyclosporine for patients in whom the first two maneuvers are inappropriate or unsuccessful.

Pure Amegakaryocytic Thrombocytopenic Purpura

Pure amegakaryocytic thrombocytopenic purpura (PATP) is a rare syndrome characterized by severe thrombocytopenia associated with a total absence or a marked reduction of bone marrow megakaryocytes. Changes in other cell lines are minimal or absent. PATP has been attributed to viral infections, toxin or drug exposure, or immune-mediated suppression of megakaryocytopoiesis. Patients generally have symptoms caused by cutaneous or mucous membrane hemorrhage. Physical examination findings are otherwise normal. Laboratory evaluation findings reveal severe thrombocytopenia with normal or small platelets, as opposed to the large platelets of idiopathic thrombocytopenic purpura (ITP), and bone marrow that is normal except for the virtual absence of identifiable megakaryocytes. Therapy is directed at removal of all possible offending agents and administration of platelet transfusion support. Responses to other therapies, such as those using corticosteroids, gamma-globulin infusions, cyclosporine, and cyclophosphamide, are largely anecdotal.

MYELODYSPLASIA

The myelodysplastic syndrome (MDS) includes a group of clonal hematopoietic diseases characterized by impaired maturation of hematopoietic precursors with the development of progressive peripheral cytopenias. MDS is now understood to be the result of the neoplastic transformation of a cell at a level of differentiation close to that of the hematopoietic stem cell. Unlike in acute leukemia, the abnormal clone expands only gradually and retains the ability to differentiate, albeit not entirely normally. With time, the abnormal clone completely suppresses normal hematopoiesis and becomes increasingly abnormal, a process referred to as clonal evolution, which reflects the inherent genetic instability of the abnormal clone. The final result is development of either progressively severe and ultimately fatal pancytopenia or progression to an acute leukemia-like state.

Etiology

The cause of the defect leading to MDS is, in the majority of cases, unknown. Occasional cases of MDS are seen in children with DNA repair deficiency syndromes (Bloom's syndrome, Fanconi's anemia, and ataxia-telangiectasia). A number of cases of MDS arise 3 to 7 years after exposure to chemotherapy, particularly with alkylating agents. Other cases have been seen after exposure to irradiation and exposure to benzene and other marrow toxins.

Clinical Features

MDS has previously been considered to be a relatively rare disease with a reported incidence of around 1 per 100,000 per year, but recent studies suggest a much higher incidence. The disorder is much more common in the elderly, with a median age of onset of about 60 years, but MDS is seen even in young children. Symptoms are usually related directly to the consequences of bone marrow failure, so fatigue, pallor, infection, and bruising or bleeding are the most common chief complaints. Physical findings are likewise restricted to the consequences of bone marrow failure, although occasional patients, perhaps 15% to 20%, may have splenomegaly.

Laboratory Features

The laboratory hallmarks of MDS are peripheral pancytopenias and dysplastic features of the marrow including dyserythropoiesis, often with ringed sideroblasts, dysgranulopoiesis with hypogranulation, and dysmegakaryocytopoiesis with micromegakaryocytes. The French/American/British Cooperative Group (FAB) recognizes five distinct forms of MDS, which are based predominantly on pathologic findings (Table 90-1). In refractory anemia (RA), anemia is invariably seen and the reticulocyte count is usually low. Peripheral blood granulocytes and platelets may be normal or diminished. Leukemic blasts are rarely seen in the periphery and make up less than 5% of marrow cells. Refractory anemia with ringed sideroblasts (RARS) has features essentially like those of RA except that ringed sideroblasts make up 15% or more of the marrow cellularity. In refractory anemia with excess blasts (RAEB), blasts make up from 5% to 20% of the marrow cells and can make up as much as 5% of the peripheral white blood cells. Thrombocytopenia is common. RAEB in transformation (RAEB-t) is similar to RAEB, but the blast count is greater than 5% in the peripheral blood or greater than 20% but less than 30% in the marrow. If more than 30% marrow blasts are seen, the diagnosis of acute leukemia is made. Chronic myelomonocytic leukemia (CM-MoL) shows features similar to those of RAEB, but circulating monocytes are greater than 1.0×10^9 per liter.

Clonal chromosomal abnormalities are found in 50% to 75% of patients (see Chapter 73 for a discussion of methods of studying these abnormalities). The most common abnormalities are loss of part or all of chromosome 7, trisomy 8, isochrome 17, 5q−, and 20q−. These abnormalities are also seen in some cases of acute myelogenous leukemia (AML) and in that setting are associated with a poor prognosis. Mutations in the RAS protooncogene family, particularly N-RAS, are found in 20% to 50% of cases and appear to be more common in the more aggressive forms of MDS (Chapter 70).

Course and Treatment

The prognosis of patients with MDS is extremely variable: some patients survive beyond a decade, whereas others die within the first year of diagnosis. Patients with RA and RARS have a much better prognosis than those with RAEB, RAEB-t, or CMMoL. Patients who have a particularly unfavorable prognosis include those with greater than 10% blasts in their marrow at diagnosis, with platelet counts less than 40×10^9/L, or with granulocyte counts less than 1.0×10^9 per liter. These patients have a median survival rate of less than 1 year. The cause of death in MDS is usually related either to the consequences of pancytopenia or to the evolution to an acute leukemia. Once leukemia occurs, response to treatment is poor and survival is short. Patients with RAEB and RAEB-t have a much higher likelihood of progression to leukemia, with an incidence of 50% within 2 years of diagnosis.

The category and stage of MDS dictate the appropriate therapy. Patients with RA or RARS with adequate granulocytes and platelets and with anemia as their only problem are best treated with supportive care. Once increased numbers of blasts (>5%) are seen in the marrow or either granulocytopenia or thrombocytopenia develops, more aggressive intervention should be considered. The only curative therapy for MDS is bone marrow transplantation (BMT), which results in long-term, disease-free survival in 40% to 50% of transplanted patients. Most of the experience with BMT for MDS has been in patients less than age 50 years with HLA-matched sibling donors. Recent studies are exploring the use of partially matched and matched unrelated donors as well as the use of BMT in older patients.

A number of therapeutic approaches have been explored for patients who are not candidates for BMT. Glucocorticoids and androgens have been studied but are probably of no benefit. Although occasional responses have been reported after treatment with differentiating agents such as 13-*cis* retinoic acid, controlled randomized studies have failed to show any advantage with their use. Low-dose subcutaneous cytosine arabinoside (20 mg/m² per day) has been studied extensively. A survey of numerous reports and the results of one randomized study indicate a complete response rate to low-dose cytosine arabinoside of about 15%, but these studies have failed to find any effect on overall survival. Patients with RAEB or RAEB-t have a slightly higher response rate to this therapy. Intensive combination chemotherapy, similar to that used in acute myelogenous leukemia, results in complete responses in 30% to 60%. The highest complete response (CR) rates occur in younger patients with primary MDS. The average duration of complete response is less than 12 months, and few patients are cured. These results are inferior to what is seen with the use of similar chemotherapeutic approaches in patients with de novo acute myelogenous leukemia.

More recently the use of hematopoietic growth factors has been studied in patients with the hope that these factors might increase normal cell counts in pancytopenic patients both by stimulating normal cell production and by inducing abnormal progenitors to differentiate more normally. Recombinant human erythropoietin has been used to treat patients with anemia resulting from RA or RARS, and a 20% to 30% response rate has been seen. Both G-CSF and GM-CSF increase the granulocyte counts in the majority of neutropenic MDS patients. Occasionally patients given treatment with hematopoietic growth factors have a sudden increase in the number of circulating blasts, a change that is usually but not always reversed when administration of the growth factor is discontinued. There are no data to indicate whether the use of growth factors affects survival in patients with MDS.

MYELOFIBROSIS

Myelofibrosis is characterized by fibrosis of the bone marrow space with development of extramedullary hematopoiesis. These changes

Table 90-1 Classification of myelodysplasia MDS by the French/American/British Cooperative Group

CLASSIFICATION	MARROW BLASTS (%)	PERIPHERAL BLOOD BLASTS (%)	RINGED SIDEROBLASTS >15% OF BONE MARROW	MONOCYTES >1000/μL
Refractory anemia	<5	≤1	−	−
Refractory anemia with ringed sideroblasts	<5	≤1	+	−
Refractory anemia with excess blasts	5-20	<5	−/+	−
Refractory anemia with excess blasts in transition	20-30	>5	−/+	−/+
Chronic myelomonocytic anemia	≤20	<5	−/+	+

can occur as a response to other disorders or as a primary hematologic disease. Cancer metastatic to the bone marrow; infectious agents such as fungi, mycobacterium, or leishmaniasis; granulomatous disorders such as sarcoidosis; and metabolic disorders such as Gaucher's disease have all been reported to cause myelofibrosis. The following section deals predominantly with primary myelofibrosis, also termed *idiopathic myelofibrosis* (IMF) or *agnogenic myeloid metaplasia* (AMM) with myelofibrosis. This disorder is now understood to be the result of a clonal proliferation of an abnormal hematopoietic progenitor and as such is usually categorized as one of the myeloproliferative disorders.

Etiology

The cause of IMF is unknown, but as in the other myeloproliferative syndromes, an increased incidence is seen after exposure to irradiation, benzene, and other marrow toxins. Although marrow fibrosis is the hallmark of the disease, recent studies have demonstrated that the disorder is a result of a clonal proliferation of cells of hematopoietic origin and that the fibroblasts that are seen, although increased in numbers, are not clonal. Rather, the marrow fibrosis is a reactive process of nonclonal fibroblasts, possibly mediated by platelet-derived growth factor and transforming growth factor–B released by, or as a response to, the malignant clone.

Clinical Features

The majority of patients with IMF are in their mid-fifties, but occasionally children are affected. The disease evolves slowly; as many as 25% of patients are asymptomatic and diagnosis is made because an abnormality is found during a routine physical examination or blood cell count. In most patients the chief symptoms are produced by anemia with weakness and/or pallor; others have abdominal fullness caused by an enlarged spleen. Fever, night sweats, anorexia, and weight loss are other common complaints. The most common physical findings are pallor and splenomegaly: splenomegaly is present in 90% of cases, and in 50% the spleen extends at least 6 cm below the rib cage. In an occasional patient, the spleen may be remarkably large, filling most of the abdomen. Hepatomegaly is present in 50% to 70% of cases. Purpura caused by thrombocytopenia occurs in 10% to 20% of cases. Often patients have mild jaundice produced by low-grade hemolysis.

Laboratory Features

Most patients have mild to moderate anemia that becomes more severe as the disease progresses. The anemia is due to a combination of ineffective erythropoiesis and low-grade hemolysis. The peripheral leukocyte count is increased in approximately half of patients, is normal in about one fourth, and is low in the remainder. Immature myeloid precursors including blasts are usually present in the blood smear, platelets are increased in one third of patients, and the same fraction are normal or thrombocytopenic. As the disease progresses, thrombocytopenia becomes more severe. The peripheral smear invariably demonstrates a leukoerythroblastic pattern with "teardrop" poikilocytosis, nucleated red blood cells, and immature myeloid elements all present. Bone marrows are usually not aspirable, and on bone marrow biopsy bone marrow fibrosis and osteosclerosis are the rule. Large numbers of blast cells are usually not seen in the marrow and, if present, suggest that the diagnosis might instead be M7 acute myelogenous leukemia (AML), a disease that in the past has sometimes been called acute myelofibrosis or acute myelosclerosis. Although no single cytogenetic abnormality is associated with IMF, approximately 40% of patients have a clonal chromosomal abnormality, frequently of chromosomes 1, 5, 7, 9, 11, or 13. A new, second chromosomal abnormality often heralds the conversion to an acute leukemia-like condition.

Differential Diagnosis

The clinical findings of pallor and splenomegaly, along with a complete blood cell count and smear showing a leukoerythroblastic pattern, usually suggest a diagnosis of IMF, and a biopsy specimen of the marrow disclosing diffuse fibrosis helps confirm that impression. Fibrosis resulting from other diseases must be excluded. Hairy cell leukemia (Chapter 92) may be characterized by splenomegaly, neutropenia or pancytopenia, and a dry tap when the marrow is aspirated. Hairy cell leukemia can be excluded by examination of the blood and staining of the blood and marrow lymphocytes for tartrate-resistant acid phosphatase. Chronic myelogenous leukemia (CML) with fibrosis can look very much like IMF, but a decreased leukocyte alkaline phosphatase score and the presence of the Ph chromosome distinguish CML from IMF. Large numbers of myeloblasts in the marrow help distinguish M7 AML from IMF. More rapid disease onset and lack of splenomegaly also favor a diagnosis of M7 AML.

Course and Treatment

Survival after the diagnosis of IMF is quite varied, ranging from 1 to 30 years and averaging approximately 5 years. Not surprisingly, a poor prognosis is associated with the presence of increasingly severe anemia, thrombocytopenia, hepatomegaly, and B symptoms at diagnosis. Many investigators view the disease as comprising two groups, one with a fulminant course and a median survival of less than 2 years and a separate group accounting for about half the patients, with a median survival of approximately 10 years. The asymptomatic patient with IMF requires no treatment. Therapy of the disease is aimed at treating the anemia, the thrombocytopenia, and the problems associated with an enlarged spleen, including pain, portal hypertension, and hypersplenism. Anemia is usually treated with transfusion therapy, and in one third of patients androgens appear to decrease transfusion requirements. Corticosteroids are used in patients with a hemolytic component of the disease. Patients with IMF may have difficulty with either thrombocytosis or, later in the course of the disease, thrombocytopenia. If thrombocytosis is severe and thrombosis occurs, platelet count can be lowered by platelet pheresis, by the administration of oral hydroxyurea at 500 to 1500 mg/day, or by the use of anagrelide (Chapter 92). Patients with thrombocytopenia receive treatment with platelet transfusions, but long-term, effective replacement is usually not possible because of poor transfusion increments, in part as a result of hypersplenism, as well as development of alloimmunization. Treatment of splenic enlargement in IMF is controversial, and splenectomy, splenic irradiation, and administration of busulfan and α-interferon have all been used. Splenectomy is effective in alleviating splenic pain and portal hypertension in most patients, but only about 50% of patients have improvement in either red blood cell requirements or platelet counts. Irradiating the spleen may result in a transient decrease in spleen size and alleviation of splenic pain but only rarely has a beneficial effect on anemia and thrombocytopenia. Busulfan, likewise, can control splenic pain but leads to a decrease in peripheral cell counts. Marrow transplantation has been used in a handful of patients, and long-term survival has been reported in several of them. In most patients with IMF, refractory thrombocytopenia and neutropenia eventually develop, leading to death as a result of bleeding or infection. Approximately 15% to 20% of patients die after evolution to an acute leukemia-like state.

BIBLIOGRAPHY

Anderson JE et al: Allogeneic bone marrow transplantation for 93 patients with myelodysplastic syndrome, *Blood* 82:677-681, 1993.

Frickhofen N: Treatment of aplastic anemia with antithymocyte globulin and methylprednisolone with or without cyclosporine, *N Eng J Med* 324:1297-1304, 1991.

Socie G et al: Malignant tumors ocurring after treatment of aplastic anemia, *N Engl J Med* 329:1152-1157, 1993.

Storb R et al: Cyclophosphamide combined with antithymocyte globulin in preparation for allogeneic marrow transplants in patients with aplastic anemia, *Blood* 84:941-949, 1994.

Visani G et al: Myelofibrosis with myeloid metaplasia: clinical and haematological parameters predicting survival in a series of 133 patients, *Br J Haematol* 75:4, 1990.

Young NS: Aplastic anaemia, *Lancet* 346:228-232, 1995.

Young NS et al: The treatment of severe acquired aplastic anemia, *Blood* 85:3367-3377, 1995.

CHAPTER

91 Abnormalities of Phagocytes, Eosinophils, and Basophils

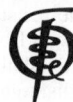

David H. Boldt

Granulocytes-neutrophils, eosinophils, basophils, and monocytes together account for the majority of leukocytes circulating in the blood of normal individuals. These cells pass through the blood during their migration from the bone marrow to the tissues, where they carry out their specific roles in host defense. Neutrophils and monocyte-macrophages constitute the two major phagocytic systems in the body. Although the functions of eosinophils and basophils are not so well understood, many important clinical disorders are associated with abnormalities of these cell types.

ABNORMALITIES OF NEUTROPHILS

Abnormalities of neutrophils are listed in Box 91-1. They are divided conveniently into three groups: (1) quantitative abnormalities—neutropenia or neutrophilia, the most frequently encountered group of neutrophil disorders; (2) qualitative abnormalities—inherited or acquired functional defects in spite of normal neutrophil numbers; (3) neoplastic abnormalities—as in the myelocytic leukemias. Diagnostic considerations and approaches to patients with neutropenia or neutrophilia are addressed in Chapter 80.

Neutropenia

Neutropenia refers to a reduction below the normal range of absolute numbers of circulating neutrophils. In the adult this is generally below 2.0×10^9 per liter.

Clinical Features. The clinical manifestations of neutropenia result from an increased susceptibility to infection. Generally, no increase in infection occurs until the neutrophil count falls below 1.0×10^9 per liter; the risk of infection is moderately increased when the count is 0.5 to 1.0×10^9 per liter and greatly increased when the count is below 0.5×10^9 per liter. Infections in neutropenic patients are most often caused by encapsulated gram-negative or gram-positive bacteria, which normally are controlled by opsonization and phagocytosis. When the course of neutropenia is prolonged beyond a few weeks, opportunistic infections caused by fungi such as *Candida* or *Aspergillus* become increasingly prevalent.

Because neutrophils are responsible for most clinical findings during acute infection, the classic signs of infections may be diminished or absent in a severely neutropenic patient. Evaluation for infections should include extensive cultures for both bacteria and fungi. During examination of the neutropenic patient, particular attention should be given to the sinuses, skin, and perirectal region, in addition to the usual sites of lung, nasopharynx and oropharynx, urinary tract, and central nervous system. Because of the potential for rapid and fatal progression of any infection, broad-spectrum antibiotic coverage should be provided the febrile, neutropenic patient pending the outcome of cultures, at which point a more specific therapeutic regimen may be devised. In addition, treatment with the hematopoietic growth factors, granulocyte colony-stimulating factor (G-CSF), or granulocyte-macrophage colony-stimulating factor (GM-CSF) may shorten the period of severe neutropenia in some patients with transient marrow suppression (as in drug-induced cases) or ameliorate the clinical

---

BOX 91-1
Abnormalities of neutrophils

I. Quantitative abnormalities
  A. Neutropenia (Chapter 80)
    1. Decreased production
      a. Predictable drug-induced marrow suppression
      b. Irradiation injury
      c. Idiosyncratic drug-induced marrow suppression
      d. Bone marrow replacement by tumor, hematologic neoplasm, granulomatous reaction, or myelofibrosis
      e. Nutritional deficiencies: Malnutrition, starvation, vitamin B_{12} or folic acid deficiencies
      f. Immunologically mediated marrow suppression caused by antibodies or T lymphocytes
      g. Stem cell defects (hereditary): Cyclic neutropenia, Kostman's hereditary neutropenia, reticular dysgenesis, Schwachman-Diamond syndrome, dyskeratosis congenita, lazy leukocyte syndrome, cartilage-hair hypoplasia, Chediak-Higashi syndrome
    2. Excessive destruction, utilization, or sequestration
      a. Idiosyncratic drug-induced granulocyte destruction (usually immunologically mediated)
      b. Immunologically mediated granulocyte destruction: Isoimmune neonatal neutropenia, autoimmune neutropenia (primary or secondary)
      c. Overwhelming infection (utilization)
      d. Hypersplenism
      e. Sequestration in lungs or spleen caused by complement activation during hemodialysis, sepsis, adult respiratory distress syndrome
    3. Unknown or multiple causes: Chronic idiopathic neutropenia, Felty's syndrome

  B. Neutrophilia (Chapter 80)
    1. Infections
    2. Malignancies
    3. Inflammatory disorders: Rheumatoid arthritis, vasculitis, inflammatory bowel disease, gout
    4. Hematologic disorders: Acute hemolysis, transfusion reactions, rebound from myelosuppression, postsplenectomy state
    5. Drugs: Corticosteroids, epinephrine, etiocholanolone, lithium
    6. Metabolic conditions: Diabetic ketoacidosis, thyroid storm
    7. Tissue destruction: Myocardial infarction, pulmonary infarction, bowel infarction
    8. Pregnancy
    9. Physiologic: Exercise, stress
    10. Chronic idiopathic neutrophilia
II. Qualitative abnormalities (Chapter 230)
  A. Intrinsic
    1. Chronic granulomatous disease
    2. Job's syndrome
    3. Myeloperoxidase deficiency
    4. Chediak-Higashi syndrome
    5. Lazy leukocyte syndrome
  B. Extrinsic
    1. Complement and immunoglobulin abnormalities
    2. Hypophosphatemia
    3. Sickle cell anemia
    4. Diabetes mellitus
    5. Alcoholism
    6. Corticosteroid administration
III. Neoplastic abnormalities (Chapter 92)
  A. Acute nonlymphocytic leukemia
  B. Chronic myeloproliferative disorders: Chronic myelogenous leukemia, polycythemia vera, idiopathic myelofibrosis

severity in patients with chronic neutropenia. The CSFs also have the potential benefit of enhancing the phagocytic and cytotoxic activities of neutrophils. At this time blanket recommendations about the use of CSFs in neutropenic patients cannot be made, but their application should be individualized on a case-by-case basis. The management of the neutropenic patient is discussed in detail in Chapter 236.

Etiology. Pathophysiologically, the causes of neutropenia (Box 91-1) can be broadly divided into two groups: decreased production and excessive destruction, utilization, or sequestration.

Drug-induced neutropenia. There are two types of drug-induced neutropenia. First, predictable neutropenias, usually occurring in association with anemia and thrombocytopenia, are regularly caused by many agents used for cancer chemotherapy or immunosuppression. These drugs inhibit cellular proliferation and include alkylating agents, antimetabolites, nitrosoureas, antibiotics, and certain vinca alkaloids (Chapter 71). Irradiation of the bone marrow and exposure to benzene also have predictable myelotoxicity. Examination of the bone marrow of affected individuals reveals hypoplasia with decreased or absent neutrophil precursors.

The second type of drug-induced neutropenia is an idiosyncratic reaction to drug administration. A hallmark of this disorder is its unpredictable occurrence. As a general rule, any drug should be considered capable of causing neutropenia in a susceptible individual, but certain agents have been especially prominent. These are the phenothiazines, phenylbutazone, antithyroid drugs, sulfonamides, and chloramphenicol.

Two basic mechanisms are believed to account for drug-induced neutropenia. These are direct marrow suppression and immune-mediated granulocyte destruction. In drug-induced marrow suppression the onset is insidious and occurs in subjects who have been receiving the drug over an extended period, usually many weeks. The classic example is the neutropenia associated with phenothiazine administration. Typically, the neutropenia occurs 2 to 10 weeks after initiation of the drug and after a total dose of 10 to 20 g. By contrast, immune-mediated granulocyte destruction often begins abruptly after 1 to 2 weeks. Symptoms including fever, chills, arthralgias, and prostration may be due to neutrophil lysis.

Bone marrow examination in the patient with idiosyncratic drug-induced neutropenia may reveal either hypoplasia or a hypercellular marrow. Myeloid precursors may be absent, normal, or increased. Because of their rapid release from the marrow, mature neutrophils are often markedly reduced, giving a false picture of maturation arrest. A hypercellular marrow containing an abundance of myeloid precursors suggests that neutropenia is due to peripheral destruction, utilization, or sequestration.

Management of patients with suspected drug-induced neutropenia consists in withdrawal of all drugs that are not absolutely essential, particularly those known to be associated with neutropenia. The condition then usually resolves within 2 to 3 weeks. Some patients may benefit from treatment with hematopoietic growth factors to shorten the period of severe neutropenia.

Felty's syndrome. In Felty's syndrome (Chapter 192) neutropenia is associated with rheumatoid arthritis and splenomegaly. Hypersplenism, circulating antineutrophil antibodies, complement-mediated granulocyte aggregation, inhibitory T lymphocytes, and bone marrow failure may all be involved in causing the neutropenia. The degree of neutropenia in Felty's syndrome is variable but may be profound, and infectious complications may be frequent and severe. Splenectomy leads to improvement of the neutrophil count in about half the patients. Such improvement is most likely to occur in patients with normal or hypercellular bone marrows and is less likely to occur in patients with hypocellular marrows or marrows infiltrated with lymphocytes. Responses to corticosteroids or lithium therapy have also been reported.

Human cyclic neutropenia. Human cyclic neutropenia is a unique disorder characterized by regular oscillations of the blood neutrophil count with periodic disappearance of neutrophils from the circulation. The oscillations are based on cyclic changes in bone marrow production and release of neutrophils. The diagnosis of cyclic neutropenia rests on the demonstration of regular, recurrent episodes of profound neutropenia. The periodicity is usually about 21 days but may be as short as 14 days or as long as 30 days. It is not unusual for neutrophil counts to fall to zero and to remain below 0.2×10^9

per liter for 3 to 5 days. The disease is often familial, and clinical manifestations usually occur before the age of 10 but can occur later in life. An association has been noted between adult-onset cyclic neutropenia and increased numbers of large granular lymphocytes. Symptoms attributable to infection typically occur during the period of neutropenia and last from 3 to 10 days. Treatment of infections with antibiotics decreases their severity and reduces the likelihood of dissemination and death. Recent data from a multicenter, randomized, controlled trial indicate that long-term treatment with G-CSF can be effective in cyclic neutropenia and should be considered for patients with recurrent severe infection. Previous reports indicted that androgens, lithium, or splenectomy may be successful in selected cases. In addition, corticosteroid therapy may correct neutrophil cycling in some patients with the adult-onset form of the disease.

Chronic idiopathic neutropenia. The term *chronic idiopathic neutropenia* has been used to refer to patients in whom blood neutrophil counts of less than 2.0×10^9 per liter persist for months or years and in whom other known causes of neutropenia are excluded. Some patients follow a benign clinical course and no specific therapy is required. In this condition, referred to as chronic benign neutropenia, patients can mobilize neutrophils from the bone marrow reserve pool in response to corticosteroid administration, an occurrence that may account for their ability to deal appropriately with infections. Other patients have a more aggressive clinical course marked by frequent, severe infections. These patients do not respond to corticosteroid administration with an increased neutrophil count, and they may benefit from treatment with hematopoietic growth factors.

Immunologically mediated neutropenia. In certain instances, neutropenia may be due to immunologic mechanisms that cause granulocyte destruction or that interfere with neutrophil production by interacting with precursor cells in the bone marrow. Antibody-mediated neutrophil destruction analogous to immune thrombocytopenia or immune hemolytic anemia has been described. It may occur as a primary condition, as a complication of an underlying lymphoproliferative disorder or collagen-vascular disease, or in response to to administration of certain drugs. Secondary immune neutropenia may respond to appropriate therapy of the underlying condition or to discontinuation of the offending medication. Primary immune neutropenia has been managed by administration of short, intensive courses of corticosteroids and/or splenectomy. However, such therapy is risky, and the indications are not well established.

Inhibitory T lymphocytes have been shown to be responsible for granulopoietic failure in 20% of a large group of patients with neutropenia and hypocellular bone marrows. Affected patients had a variety of underlying conditions, including rheumatic diseases, preleukemic syndromes, acquired or congenital immunodeficiency diseases, and idiopathic acquired neutropenia. A high percentage of subjects with T-cell–mediated neutropenia responded to corticosteroids.

The association of lymphocytosis of large granular lymphocytes (LGLs) with neutropenia has been described. Anemia is also common in affected patients with red blood cell precursors decreased or absent from the bone marrow. In vitro tests often demonstrate suppression of erythroid progenitor growth by the LGL in this condition, but similar suppression of myeloid progenitors has been difficult to demonstrate. Affected patients generally follow a chronic course marked by hyperlymphocytosis, neutropenia, and frequent, mild infections. The syndrome often occurs in association with rheumatoid arthritis, and patients may have positive rheumatoid factor and antinuclear antibody test findings as well as polyclonal hypergammaglobulinemia. Lymphocytes in this disorder express the CD8 surface antigen characteristic of the cytotoxic suppressor T-lymphocyte subset, and the cells may display antibody-dependent cellular cytotoxicity and variable natural killer activity. In some cases the lymphocyte proliferation is monoclonal and the disease may manifest some features of a malignancy, such as organ infiltration; but in other cases the disease is polyclonal and organ infiltration does not occur. Treatment of this syndrome with corticosteroids or cytotoxic agents has been largely ineffective.

Neutrophilia

Causes of neutrophilia are listed in Box 91-1. Evaluation of patients with neutrophilia is discussed in Chapter 80.

Qualitative Neutrophil Abnormalities

Functional defects of neutrophils may be hereditary or acquired, extrinsic or intrinsic to the cell. Some of these abnormalities are discussed in Chapter 230.

Neoplastic Abnormalities of Neutrophils

Myeloid leukemias and myeloproliferative diseases are discussed in Chapter 92.

ABNORMALITIES OF MONOCYTES AND MACROPHAGES

Abnormalities of monocytes and macrophages are listed in Box 91-2. Similar to neutrophil disorders, quantitative, qualitative, and proliferative abnormalities are recognized. In addition, storage disorders resulting from inability of the monocyte-macrophage properly to dispose of organic materials may lead to accumulation of tissue macrophages containing an overabundance of various ingested substances. These storage disorders, caused by hereditary deficiencies of certain lysosomal enzymes, are discussed in Chapter 309. Monocytosis and reactive hyperplasia of macrophages are the abnormalities most commonly encountered. In general, diseases that cause a peripheral blood monocytosis are also associated with macrophage proliferation in tissues. Causes of monocytosis and reactive macrophage hyperplasia are given in Box 91-2.

Proliferative abnormalities of monocytes and macrophages may be benign or malignant. The latter category includes monocytic and myelomonocytic variants of acute myelogenous leukemia (Chapter 92), true histiocytic lymphoma (Chapter 93), and malignant histiocytosis. The clinical behavior of malignant histiocytosis resembles that of the malignant lymphomas. Common features are fever, weight loss, lymphadenopathy, hepatosplenomegaly, and progressive pancytopenia. Diagnosis is based on demonstration of malignant macrophages in involved tissues. In many patients abnormal histiocytes may be seen by examination of the peripheral blood. Untreated, the disorder is rapidly fatal but recent studies report successful treatment with combination chemotherapy. In such patients the 5-year actuarial survival rate is approximately 40%.

Langerhans' cell histiocytosis is the currently preferred terminology for the group of histiocytic syndromes formerly known as eosinophilic granuloma, Hand-Schüller-Christian disease, Letterer-Siwe disease, and histiocytosis X. These disorders most commonly affect infants and young children but may be seen in adults. The signs and symptoms vary, depending on which organs are infiltrated by histiocytes. In addition to the usual visceral sites, involvement of bones and skin may be especially troublesome. For example, involvement of the skull may lead to dental impairment, chronic otitis media, loss of vision, or diabetes insipidus. Extent of involvement ranges from solitary bone lesions to massive systemic involvement with multiorgan failure. Prognosis is related to age, extent of disease, and presence of organ dysfunction. Treatment must be tailored to the needs of individual patients and may require no or only supportive care, irradiation therapy of solitary lesions, systemic corticosteroids, or single-agent or multiagent chemotherapy. Young age (less than 2 years), involvement of four or more organ systems, and dysfunction of three organ systems—lungs, liver, and bone marrow—are poor prognostic features. Approximately 25% of all patients die of disease progression or complications of treatment such as infections. Most of the remaining patients respond to therapy and eventually stabilize without need for further treatment. Long-term follow-up observation is required for these patients to manage disabilities resulting from the histiocytic syndrome itself and to observe for secondary malignancies that may be associated with chemotherapy and/or radiotherapy.

Sinus histiocytosis with massive lymphadenopathy is a benign condition characterized by painless and massive lymphadenopathy usually involving cervical lymph nodes. Other node groups and extranodal sites also may be involved. The cause is unknown. Lymph node biopsies show sinusoidal dilation and follicular hyperplasia with abundant foamy histiocytes and multinucleated giant cells within the sinuses. A characteristic finding is "emperipolesis," the presence of intracellular lymphocytes apparently engulfed by histiocytic cells. As

---

BOX 91-2
Abnormalities of monocytes and macrophages

I. Monocytosis and reactive macrophage hyperplasia
   A. Infectious diseases: especially tuberculosis, syphilis, brucellosis, malaria, leprosy, listeriosis, schistosomiasis, leishmaniasis, histoplasmosis, cryptococcosis, toxoplasmosis, bacterial endocarditis
   B. Neoplastic diseases: myelomonocytic leukemia, lymphoproliferative and myeloproliferative disorders, preleukemia, other malignancies
   C. Hematologic diseases or conditions: hemolytic anemia, recovery from neutropenia, postsplenectomy state
   D. Rheumatic disorders: rheumatoid arthritis, systemic lupus erythematosus, others
   E. Gastrointestinal disorders: inflammatory bowel disease, cirrhosis
   F. Miscellaneous disorders: sarcoidosis, drug reactions, reactive macrophage hyperplasia to chemicals such as beryllium, silica, or organic substances
II. Proliferative disorders
   A. Neoplastic: monocytic and myelomonocytic leukemia, histiocytic lymphoma, malignant histiocytosis
   B. Reactive or of uncertain cause: Langerhans' cell histiocytosis, sinus histiocytosis with massive lymphadenopathy, virus-associated hemophagocytic syndrome
III. Storage diseases (Chapter 309), Gaucher's disease, Niemann-Pick disease, Tay-Sachs disease, Fabry's disease, sea-blue histiocyte disorders
IV. Monocyte-macrophage dysfunction syndromes
   A. Congenital: chronic granulomatous disease, myeloperoxidase deficiency, Chediak-Higashi syndrome
   B. Acquired: alveolar macrophages in smokers, macrophages in lepromatous leprosy, miliary tuberculosis, disseminated fungal infections

---

disease manifestations commonly resolve spontaneously, no treatment is usually necessary. However, massive adenopathy in strategic locations may cause serious or fatal complications, such as tracheal or epidural compression, and treatment may become necessary under special circumstances. In these instances, local excision, irradiation, corticosteroids, or chemotherapy may be used but results have been inconsistent.

A virus-associated hemophagocytic syndrome has recently been described in immunosuppressed subjects with herpesvirus infections. It may also occur in some previously healthy subjects. Clinically the disorder may mimic malignant histiocytosis with hepatosplenomegaly, lymphadenopathy, skin rash, and pancytopenia. Involved tissue shows macrophage infiltration with prominent erythrophagocytosis. Differentiation from malignant histiocytosis is based on the morphologic appearance of the macrophages. They are neoplastic and poorly differentiated in malignant histiocytosis but well differentiated and reactive in the hemophagocytic syndrome. The hemophagocytic syndrome is a self-limited disorder and usually resolves within several weeks or months when patients are given appropriate supportive care.

ABNORMALITIES OF EOSINOPHILS AND BASOPHILS

Eosinophils and basophils are the least numerous of the circulating leukocytes. Clinically important disorders of these cell types are eosinophilia and basophilia (Box 91-3). In most of these conditions the eosinophilia or basophilia is a reactive phenomenon and may result from secretion by activated lymphocytes or other cells of hematopoietic growth factors that stimulate production of eosinophils (interleukin-3 [IL-3], IL-5, GM-CSF) or basophils (IL-3).

A small subset (approximately 5%) of patients with acute myelogenous leukemia (AML) have a variant termed acute myelomonocytic leukemia with abnormal eosinophils (M4Eo). In addition to myelo-

---

BOX 91-3
Causes of eosinophilia and basophilia

I. Eosinophilia
  A. Metazoan infestation, especially amebiasis, ascariasis, schisto-somiasis, strongyloidiasis, trichinosis, visceral larva migrans
  B. Allergic conditions: bronchial asthma, allergic rhinitis, eczema, acute allergic reactions to drugs or food, insect bites
  C. Skin diseases: especially atopic dermatitis, acute urticaria, pemphigus, pemphigoid, eczema
  D. Pulmonary eosinophilias: tropical eosinophilia, visceral larva migrans, ascariasis, fungal infections, inhalation of allergens, Churg-Strauss allergic granulomatosis
  E. Neoplastic diseases: acute myelogenous leukemia, Hodgkin's and non-Hodgkin's lymphomas, solid tumors, especially carcinoma of the lung
  F. Immunologic disorders: polyarteritis nodosa, rheumatoid arthritis, angioimmunoblastic lymphadenopathy
  G. Idiopathic hypereosinophilic syndrome
II. Basophilia
  A. Allergic conditions: drugs, foods, inhalants
  B. Myeloproliferative disorders
  C. Miscellaneous conditions: myxedema, ulcerative colitis, systemic mast cell disease
  D. Basophilic leukemia

✔ WHEN TO REFER

Alterations in numbers of neutrophils are commonly encountered in clinical practice. Neutrophilia is most common and the cause is usually apparent. Consultation will most frequently be sought to aid in the differentiation of a leukemoid reaction from myeloproliferative disease. In this instance, presence of splenomegaly, immature myeloid cells with or without nucleated erythrocytes or basophils in the circulation, and a decreased or absent level of leukocyte alkaline phosphatase would point strongly to the diagnosis of myeloproliferative disease. Bone marrow aspiration and biopsy with cytogenetic studies would be definitive. Because treatment options for patients with myeloproliferative diseases, especially chronic myelogenous leukemia, are complex, a specialist should be involved early in the course of management.

Severe neutropenia (absolute neutrophil count <1000 cells/μl) is a life-threatening condition. The goals in managing this problem should include prompt diagnosis of cause and, where appropriate, initiation of effective therapy as well as intensive supportive care. Involvement of appropriate specialists in the management of these patients is critical to achieving a successful outcome.

Proliferative disorders of monocytes and macrophages (such as Langerhans' cell histiocytosis), the idiopathic hypereosinophilic syndrome, and mastocytosis are very uncommon disorders and are all most appropriately cared for by physicians experienced in their management. By contrast, patients with reactive monocytosis or eosinophilia constitute the majority of individuals with these abnormalities and may frequently receive diagnosis and treatment from the general internist.

---

blasts with characteristic features of French/American/British (FAB) class M4 (Chapter 92), bone marrows of these patients are infiltrated by up to 30% atypical eosinophils. The abnormal morphologic and cytochemical features of these eosinophils suggest that they may be derived from the leukemic clone, but this has not yet been rigorously proved. M4Eo typically is associated with cytogenetic abnormalities of the long arm of chromosome 16. Patients with the M4Eo variant of AML have a favorable prognosis for response and survival with current therapies.

The idiopathic hypereosinophilic syndrome appears to represent a primary disorder of eosinophils. It may be defined according to the following criteria: (1) persistent eosinophilia of at least 1.5×10^9 per liter for longer than 6 months or fatal termination within 6 months; (2) lack of evidence of parasitic, allergic, or other known causes of eosinophilia (Box 91-3); and (3) signs and symptoms of organ involvement or dysfunction either directly related to eosinophilia or unexplained in the given clinical setting.

The onset of disease typically occurs between the ages of 20 and 50 years, and there is a strong male predominance. Involvement of the heart and nervous system is responsible for the most important clinical findings. Cardiac involvement produces congestive heart failure, valvular dysfunction, conduction defects, and myocarditis. Congestive heart failure secondary to endocardial fibrosis is a frequent cause of death. Central neurologic findings may include altered behavior and cognitive function, spasticity, and ataxia.

Prognosis in the idiopathic hypereosinophilic syndrome historically has been poor, with median survival of approximately 1 year. However, chemotherapy has recently been reported to produce 70% survival at 10 years.

A recently described disorder, eosinophilia-myalgia syndrome, is a chronic multisystem disease with a spectrum of clinical manifestations ranging from self-limited myalgias and fatigue to a progressive, occasionally fatal illness characterized by scleroderma-like skin changes, peripheral and central nervous system abnormalities, and pulmonary hypertension. Peripheral eosinophilia is a universal feature. The illness has been related to ingestion of L-tryptophan. Corticosteroids may ameliorate acute symptoms, but they have not been consistently effective, and their role in the long-term management of patients with progressive disease is undefined.

Basophilia refers to an increase in the absolute peripheral basophil count above 0.15×10^9 per liter. Basophilia can accompany myxedema, ulcerative colitis, Hodgkin's disease, and hemolytic anemias. Significant basophilia is also seen with the myeloproliferative disor-

ders—chronic myelogenous leukemia, polycythemia vera, and myeloid metaplasia. Basophilic leukemia is a very rare disorder.

Mastocytosis

The mast cell is a connective tissue cell widely distributed throughout the body. Mast cells are involved in allergic reactions and immunoglobulin E (IgE)-mediated immune phenomena. Although the basophil and mast cell share many histologic, biochemical, and physiologic properties, they probably represent two distinct cell lines. Abnormalities of mast cells include urticaria pigmentosa and systemic mastocytosis. Urticaria pigmentosa is a benign, self-limiting disorder characterized by focal cutaneous infiltrates of mast cells. Bone lesions may also occur. In systemic mastocytosis infiltration of mast cells occurs in many organ systems. Signs and symptoms reflect this multisystem involvement and may include weight loss, fever, flushing, bronchospasm, hypotension, diarrhea, gastrointestinal bleeding, rhinorrhea, palpitations, and dyspnea. When large numbers of mast cells appear in bone marrow and peripheral blood, the condition is designated mast cell leukemia. Treatment of systemic mast cell disorders is usually symptomatic with the aim of alleviating symptoms. Antihistamines, H_2 receptor blockers, and cromolyn sodium may be effective for this purpose. Prognosis is quite variable. Some patients follow a prolonged stable course. However, mast cell leukemia and clinically aggressive mast cell disorders do not respond to conventional chemotherapeutic regimens. The prognosis in this setting is poor with rapid progression of disease and death.

BIBLIOGRAPHY

Bagby GC Jr, Lawrence HJ, Neerhout RC: T-lymphocyte–mediated granulopoietic failure, *N Engl J Med* 309:1073, 1983.
Coates TD, Baehner R: Leukocytosis and leukopenia. In Hoffman R et al, editors: *Hematology: basic principles and practice,* ed 2, New York, 1995, Churchill Livingsone.
Fauci AS et al: The idiopathic hypereosinophilic syndrome: clinical, pathophysiologic, and therapeutic considerations, *Ann Intern Med* 97:78, 1982.
Loughran TP Jr: Clonal diseases of large granular lymphocytes, *Blood* 82:1, 1993.
Osband ME, Pochedly C: Histiocytosis-X, *Hematol Oncol Clin North Am* 1:1, 1987.
Parker RI, Metcalfe DD: Systemic mastocytosis. In Hoffman R et al, editors: *Hematology: basic principles and practice,* ed 2, New York, 1995, Churchill Livingstone.
Spry CJ, Kay AB, Gleich GJ: Eosinophils: 1992, *Immunol Today* 13:384, 1992.

CHAPTER

92 The Leukemias and Polycythemia Vera

John J. Hutton

LYMPHOID LEUKEMIAS

Lymphoproliferative disorders may originate either in the bone marrow or in extramedullary sites such as lymph nodes and thymus. Those primarily involving bone marrow are classified as lymphoid leukemias and are discussed in this chapter. The remainder are classified as lymphomas and are discussed in Chapter 93. Three of the most common lymphoid leukemias are presented here. Of these, acute lymphoblastic leukemia (ALL), if untreated, is rapidly fatal, whereas chronic lymphocytic leukemia (CLL) and hairy cell leukemia run a more indolent clinical course.

Acute Lymphoblastic Leukemia

Etiology. The clonal origin of ALL has been demonstrated by studies of cytogenetic abnormalities, immunoglobulin and T-cell receptor gene rearrangements, and glucose-6-phosphate dehydrogenase isoenzymes in leukemic cells. The concept of clonality is discussed in Chapters 70 and 73.

The cause of malignant transformation of a normal lymphoid cell to a leukemic cell is not known. Retroviruses have long been implicated in the induction of leukemia and lymphoma in animals. There is no evidence that typical human ALL is caused by a retrovirus, although a member of the family of human T-cell lymphotropic viruses, HTLV-I, is consistently associated with an aggressive T-cell lymphoma (Chapter 93) that can have a leukemic phase. The malignant T cell in this disease is more differentiated than is typical of blasts in ALL. The clinical presentation of the acute adult T-cell leukemia-lymphoma syndrome resembles that of mycosis fungoides-Sézary syndrome (Chapter 228). Lytic bone lesions and hypercalcemia are common. Patients with subclinical infection are almost entirely asymptomatic and are frequently from the Caribbean, Japan, or sub-Saharan Africa where the virus is endemic. In the United States HTLV-I is found mainly in black Americans. Human T-cell leukemia-lymphoma is not considered further in this chapter.

Chromosomal translocations are seen in approximately half of patients with adult ALL (Table 92-1). Genes located near the breakpoint of a translocation are in a new environment. This may affect the regulation of gene expression so that its products are made inappropriately, thereby affecting cellular proliferation and differentiation. There is a concordance between the breakpoint of translocations or deletions, for example, and the chromosomal locations of genes that encode growth factors, receptors that convey signals from the cell membrane to the nucleus, or proteins that are involved in programmed cell death (apoptosis). The exact relationship between the rearrangements of genes and leukemogenesis is not always clear, but it is likely that the rearrangements are the cause of the leukemia rather than a result of the abnormal cellular proliferation in the disease. For example, blasts from certain patients with ALL have been found to have a reciprocal translocation between chromosomes 9 and 22. The breakpoint on chromosome 22 occurs within the breakpoint cluster region (bcr), and the breakpoint on chromosome 9 occurs within the c-abl protooncogene. This creates a fusion gene with juxtaposition of bcr and c-abl deoxyribonucleic acid (DNA) sequences. The abnormal c-abl protooncogene messenger ribonucleic acid (RNA) that is produced encodes a chimeric tyrosine kinase with abnormally high enzymatic activity. The increased tyrosine kinase activity increases cell proliferation by unknown mechanisms. A similar translocation occurs in chronic myelogenous leukemia (CML), but the exact sites of the breakpoints differ between ALL and CML, presumably accounting for the differences in biologic behavior. Causes of cancer are further discussed in Chapter 70.

Clinical Features. Signs and symptoms of acute leukemia are caused by infiltration of normal tissues by leukemic cells. Marrow infiltration is most prominent and results in the failure of normal hematopoiesis. Fatigue, weakness, pallor, and weight loss are common. Easy bruising and bleeding develop in patients with thrombocytopenia. Pneumonia, urinary tract infection, and perirectal abscess occur in those with granulocytopenia. Enlargement of the spleen, thymus, liver, and lymph nodes is common. Meningeal leukemia with headache and cranial nerve dysfunction is seen in 5% to 10% of patients.

The differential diagnosis of ALL includes infections and other malignancies. Infections that produce lymphocytosis and lymphadenopathy include toxoplasmosis and viral infections such as cytomegalovirus and infectious mononucleosis (Chapter 255). These infections do not seriously distort bone marrow structure. Analysis of viral antibody titers and the results of the heterophil and monospot tests should establish the correct diagnosis. Malignant diseases that may mimic ALL include acute myelogenous leukemia (AML), neuroblastoma, small cell or oat cell carcinoma of the lung, Ewing's sarcoma, CLL, non-Hodgkin's lymphoma in leukemic phase, and lymphoid transformation of CML.

Laboratory Features. Leukemia is diagnosed on the basis of laboratory tests rather than clinical findings. The hallmark of acute leukemia is the presence of an increased percentage (generally a minimum of 30%) of blasts in the bone marrow. In most patients with ALL, the peripheral white blood cell count exceeds 10×10^9 cells per liter, but it ranges from 1 to 1000. An occasional patient is leukopenic. Unlike the situation in AML, the blasts in lymphoblastic leukemia do not tend to aggregate, so high leukocyte counts are rarely associated with signs of leukostasis in the patient. Anemia, granulocytopenia, and thrombocytopenia are common.

Lymphoblastic and myelogenous leukemias are distinguished on the basis of the cytochemical and immunologic features of the leukemic blasts. The presence or absence of specific cytogenetic abnormalities or gene rearrangements can provide definitive diagnoses (Table 92-1; see Chapter 73). The distinction is critically important because of differences in therapy. Lymphoblasts do not contain myeloperoxidase or Auer rods. This means that they do not stain for peroxidase and do not contain granules that stain with the lipophilic dye, Sudan black. Lymphoblasts, but not myeloblasts, typically contain clumps of material that stain with the periodic acid–Schiff (PAS) re-

Table 92-1   Biology of acute lymphoblastic leukemia

SUBTYPE	TYPICAL MARKERS	APPROXIMATE PERCENTAGE OF PATIENTS	GENE REARRANGEMENTS	TYPICAL CYTOGENETIC ABNORMALITY, IF PRESENT	PROGNOSIS
Early Pre-B	CD19, SIg$^-$, CIg$^-$	50	Ig	t(4;11), t(9;22)	Favorable
Pre-B	CD19, SIg$^-$, CIg$^+$	20	Ig	t(1;19), t(4;11), t(9;22)	Moderately unfavorable
B	CD19, SIg$^+$, CIg$^-$	4	Ig	t(8;14), t(8;22), t(2;8)	Unfavorable
Pre-T	CD7, cCD3	6	TCR	Involves TCR genes on chr 7 or 14	Unfavorable
T	CD7, sCD3, CD4	20	TCR	Involves TCR genes on chr 7 or 14	Favorable

Modified from Copelan EA, McGuire EA: *Blood* 85:1151, 1995.
C or *c*, Cytoplasmic; *CD*, differentiation antigens detected with commercial monoclonal antibodies; *chr*, chromosome; *S* or *s*, surface; *Ig*, immunoglobulin; *TCR*, T-cell receptor.

agent (PAS reaction). Examples of the cytochemical properties of blasts are shown in Plates III-5 and III-6.

Acute lymphoblastic leukemia can be further classified according to immunologic reactivity, presence or absence of terminal transferase, and arrangement of immunoglobulin genes (Chapter 73). The subgroups appear to represent clonal expansions of lymphocytes that are partially blocked in their capacity to differentiate. They differ in prognosis and may require different types of treatment (Table 92-1). The prognostic relevance of the immunologic subtypes varies with type of therapy and is continuously changing as therapy evolves. Markers are most commonly defined by commercially available monoclonal antibodies directed against antigens such as those characteristic of T and B cells (Table 92-1). They are usually detected by flow cytometry. Classifications by immunologic subtype have changed over time. For example, cases previously classified as "null" are now known to be pre-B in phenotype. The enzyme terminal deoxynucleotidyl transferase helps to distinguish myelogenous from lymphoblastic leukemias. It is present in most lymphoblasts, but not in myeloblasts. Immunoglobulin genes are rearranged from germ line configuration in blasts corresponding to stages of B-cell differentiation, but not T-cell differentiation. Conversely, T-cell receptor genes rearrange during T-cell differentiation in a way that is analogous to the changes in immunoglobulin genes during B-cell differentiation. It is through studies of gene rearrangements that most non-T–, non-B–marked ALLs have been proved to represent clonal proliferation of committed precursors of B lymphocytes. The leukemic blasts always possess rearranged immunoglobulin heavy (H) chain genes, and approximately half also have light (L) chain rearrangements. The recombination of individual segments from multiple alternative variable (V), diversity (D), and joining (J) gene segments generates a specific rearrangement pattern unique to each patient's disease.

Treatment. Prolonged survival in patients with acute leukemia is correlated with the ability to eradicate detectable leukemic cells. This is termed a complete remission. Initial attempts to achieve a remission, termed the induction phase, involve the administration of multiple drugs over weeks to months. Most induction regimens include vincristine, prednisone, and an anthracycline. If a remission is achieved, the next step is to attempt to prolong its duration by the cyclic administration of additional drugs. This is referred to as the consolidation phase. Subsequently, lower doses of drugs may be given over months to years during the maintenance phase. Other phases of treatment may include late intensification and central nervous system prophylaxis. The entire treatment regimen is extraordinarily toxic and must be carried out in specialized centers.

As the intensity of therapy has increased, the proportion of patients achieving a complete remission and the median duration of complete remission have increased. The continuation of therapy in remission of ALL appears to be essential, although the optimal intensity and duration of such therapy are not known. Current regimens require intensive therapy for 2 to 3 years after achievement of complete remission and include central nervous system prophylaxis.

Approximately 80% of adults with ALL achieve complete remission when intensively treated. Approximately 40% of good-risk adults remain free of disease at 5 years, when optimally managed, but patients can relapse many years after initial remission. Disease-free survival for 5 years does not necessarily indicate cure. It is estimated that fewer than 20% of adults can actually be cured by chemotherapy. Relapse of disease is a grim prognostic indicator, and essentially all adults who have relapse die of their disease, unless receiving stem cell transplantation. Survival is worse in patients over the age of 35 years and is particularly poor in those over 50 years. Other indicators of a poor prognosis include mature B-cell phenotype and presence of chromosomal translocations t(9;22) or t(4;11). Extramedullary masses, a high initial blast count, and T-marked blasts were associated with a poor prognosis in regimens developed several years ago but are not always detrimental with more recent intensive treatment regimens.

Chemotherapy reduces spermatogenic activity in men and secondary follicles in women. Patients who have been treated for leukemia usually recover gonadal function and may have a normal child, particularly if they do not have chemotherapy for several years.

Allogeneic bone marrow transplantation has not proved superior to chemotherapy alone in primary treatment of adults with ALL and favorable prognostic indicators (Table 92-1). Broader use of allogeneic bone marrow transplantation has been hindered by the morbidity and mortality of graft-versus-host disease, the poor ability of patients over the age of 55 years to tolerate the procedure, and the high frequency of relapse in patients prepared for grafting by total body irradiation (Chapter 77). Patients who relapse while receiving primary chemotherapy have a very poor prognosis with secondary chemotherapy. If they are under the age of 55 years and have a histocompatible donor, they should be considered candidates for allogeneic transplantation.

Hairy Cell Leukemia

Etiology. Hairy cell leukemia is a rare neoplasm but is important because it responds well to appropriate treatment. It was formerly called *leukemic reticuloendotheliosis*. The cause of the leukemia is not known. There is no association with exposure to chemicals or radiation, and it is not hereditary. In most patients the disease appears to represent the clonal expansion of a cell committed to the B-lymphocyte lineage. The best evidence for this is the rearrangement of immunoglobulin genes in hairy cells in a way thought to be pathognomonic of B-cell differentiation. These cells circulate in the blood, where they have prominent cytoplasmic projections. They also infiltrate the bone marrow and spleen in a characteristic fashion.

Clinical Features. The typical patient with hairy cell leukemia is a middle-aged man with a palpable spleen. The median age of occurrence is the mid-50s, although the disease occurs in patients from 20 to 80 years of age. There is a 4:1 male predominance. In half of patients the presenting complaints are vague weakness, lethargy, and fatigue. In one fourth of patients the presenting complaints are severe infection or bruising. These symptoms are related to the neutropenia and thrombocytopenia that are so characteristic of the disease. In the remainder of patients the diagnosis of hairy cell leukemia is made incidentally, usually as a result of a routine blood cell count.

The characteristic physical finding is palpable splenomegaly, which is found in 90% of patients. Mild hepatomegaly may be present. Peripheral lymphadenopathy and infiltration of skin are not characteristic.

Laboratory Features. At least 80% of patients have cytopenia of one or more elements of blood. The differential diagnosis of peripheral cytopenias is discussed in Chapter 80. A pancytopenia involving erythrocytes, neutrophils, and platelets is most common, although isolated cytopenias of one element may occasionally occur. The cytopenias are secondary to both increased destruction by hypersplenism and decreased production because of marrow infiltration by hairy cells. Hairy cells account for 2% to 80% of cells in the peripheral blood, but they are easily missed. Hairy cells are large cells with irregular, fine, filamentous cytoplasmic projections that can be seen by both light and electron microscopy (Plate IV-5, *G*). The projections are redundant plasma membranes. Hairy cells are best demonstrated in wet mounts with supravital stains. Cytochemical staining for the tartrate-resistant isoenzyme of acid phosphatase can provide confirmatory information, although it is not diagnostic. The enzyme is present in hairy cells from 95% of patients. It can sometimes be seen in other lymphoproliferative disorders such as Sézary syndrome and chronic lymphocytic leukemia. In about 50% of cases the hairy

---

✔ **WHEN TO REFER**

A patient with ALL should be referred to a specialist for confirmation of the diagnosis and plan of therapy. For most adults this is a fatal illness, but if properly managed there is a small but real chance of long-term survival or cure. Under most circumstances treatment should be in specialized clinical research centers that are studying the biology of the disease and the efficacy of new treatment strategies.

cells contain peculiar cylindric cytoplasmic inclusions termed ribosome-lamella complexes that are best seen by electron microscopy. The differential diagnosis of abnormal lymphocytes in peripheral blood is listed in Chapter 80.

Bone marrow biopsy is recommended as a diagnostic procedure in all patients. Bone marrow aspiration usually results in a nondiagnostic "dry tap." The biopsy specimen shows the presence of hairy cells and other specific morphologic changes. The histopathologic examination of spleen is also diagnostic. Because of splenomegaly, the spleen is frequently removed before the underlying diagnosis of hairy cell leukemia has been made. The correct diagnosis is usually made by an experienced pathologist, even if the diagnosis has not been suspected clinically.

Treatment. Hairy cell leukemia is a chronic disorder. The clinical course of the disease is extremely variable, and treatment must be individualized. Approximately 10% of patients have minimal splenomegaly and mild cytopenias. They may remain asymptomatic for many years with minimal progression and no need for therapy. The remaining 90% require therapy at some time during the course of their disease. Median survival of patients who do not receive chemotherapy is 53 months. In the past, the accepted indications for therapy have included an absolute neutrophil count below 0.5×10^9 cells per liter, a platelet count below 50×10^9 cells per liter, symptomatic anemia requiring red blood cell transfusions, life-threatening infection, symptomatic splenomegaly, or splenic infarction. Splenectomy was the treatment of choice in the past and produced a return of all blood cell counts to the normal range in 40% of patients.

Two purine nucleoside analogs, 2-deoxycoformycin (2-dCF) (Nipent, Parke-Davis, Morris Plains, N.J.) and 2-chlorodeoxyadenosine, (2-CdA) (Leustatin, Ortho Biotech) are highly effective in treatment of hairy cell leukemia. They have changed the approach to therapy in two ways. First, therapy is initiated early in the symptomatic phase of the disease to eliminate the need for repeated transfusions of blood products and to reduce the risk of fatal infection. Second, splenectomy is no longer primary therapy. 2-chlorodeoxyadenosine is administered at a dose of 0.1 mg 2-CdA/kg per day as a continuous intravenous infusion for 7 consecutive days. Using this protocol, 50% to 75% of patients show a complete hematologic response with normal peripheral blood cell counts and no hairy cells in their bone marrows. Approximately 90% of patients who are treated have a complete or partial response. The most common adverse effects are nausea, granulocytopenia, and infection. The average duration of complete responses is not well defined, although most patients achieve very long remissions of their disease. Patients who have symptomatic relapse generally respond to retreatment with 2-CdA. A European clinical trial reported that subcutaneous injections of 2-CdA at a dose of 3.4 mg/m^2 body surface area administered for 7 consecutive days were as effective as intravenous therapy, but were more convenient.

2-Deoxycoformycin is also approved for the treatment of hairy cell leukemia. At doses of 4 mg/m^2 of body surface area given intravenously as a bolus every other week for 3 to 6 months it has induced, with minimal toxicity, long-lasting complete hematologic remissions in 60% of patients. It appears to be equally effective in previously untreated patients and in those who have progressive disease after splenectomy or administration of interferon. Clinical trials have established that 2-CdA and 2-dCF are more effective than interferon alfa-2a in treatment of hairy cell leukemia, although interferon does produce hematologic responses in most patients. A comparison of the efficacy of 2-CdA with 2-dCF as therapy of hairy cell leukemia has not been made. Of particular importance is the duration of hematologic responses that are achieved with each agent and a test of their effectiveness when administered in combination with other drugs.

A cautionary note must be sounded about the use of 2-CdA and 2-dCF in the treatment of hairy cell leukemia, and particularly about the danger of simultaneously administering a corticosteroid. Results of therapy with purine nucleosides are excellent in terms of the percentage of patients who achieve long-term clinical improvement. However, these drugs can cause prolonged immunosuppression to levels similar to those observed in acquired immunodeficiency syndrome (AIDS), as well as short-term granulocytopenia. Opportunistic infection with a wide variety of organisms is common, especially if an

✔ *WHEN TO REFER*

Hairy cell leukemia is a chronic, ultimately fatal illness. Frequently the diagnosis is difficult to make. Patients should be referred to a specialist for confirmation of the diagnosis and plan of therapy. Most medical management can be carried out by a primary care physician in consultation with a specialist. If patients are profoundly immunosuppressed or granulocytopenic, life-threatening opportunistic infections can occur. These require specialized laboratory and medical expertise for successful management.

immunosuppressive corticosteroid has been administered with the purine nucleoside. Patients should remain in regular long-term contact with a knowledgeable physician after treatment. The physician must remain alert to the possibility of serious infection and must not delay appropriate evaluation and therapy.

Chronic Lymphocytic Leukemia

Etiology. Chronic lymphocytic leukemia is a disease of the elderly and is the most common type of leukemia in the population aged 50 years and over. In more than 95% of patients the disorder represents the accumulation of slowly proliferating, long-lived B lymphocytes derived from a single clone. The remainder of patients have an aggressive T-cell leukemia that is refractory to therapy and rapidly fatal. The T-cell disorder is not discussed here further.

The cause of B-cell CLL is unknown. It is not associated with prior exposure to radiation or chemicals. A trisomy of chromosome 12 is present in malignant cells from 40% of patients and may play some role in causing the disordered cellular kinetics that characterize the disease.

Humoral immunodeficiency occurs in all patients with CLL and becomes worse as the disease progresses. Neoplastic CD5+ B lymphocytes accumulate in CLL, possibly because of a failure of programmed cell death (apoptosis). Normal CD5+ B cells are increased in autoimmune diseases. Immunologic abnormalities in CLL may reflect the presence of the neoplastic CD5+ cells. Autoimmune disorders are frequently observed in CLL. For example, 10% to 25% of patients have autoimmune hemolytic anemia at some time during the course of their disease.

Malignant lymphocytes can invade the blood of patients with poorly differentiated lymphocytic lymphoma and other types of non-Hodgkin's lymphomas. The resulting leukemia is usually called lymphosarcoma cell leukemia and may be confused with, but is not, CLL (Plate IV-5, *D* and *E*).

Clinical Features. Ninety percent of patients with CLL are above the age of 50 years. Twice as many men as women are affected. The presenting symptoms and signs of CLL are extremely variable. In one fourth of patients the diagnosis is made incidentally at the time of a routine physical examination or blood cell count. Common presenting complaints are fatigue, weight loss, repeated infections, and enlarged lymph nodes. On physical examination the most common abnormality is lymphadenopathy, usually generalized with small, discrete, movable, nontender nodes. Localized masses of matted nodes may also be seen. Bone marrow failure is common in the advanced stages of the disease, so signs of anemia and thrombocytopenia occur. Signs of infection, mostly pyogenic, are also common because of humoral immunodeficiency that becomes worse as the disease progresses. Relationships between clinical and laboratory features of the disease and survival are outlined in Table 92-2.

Laboratory Features. Chronic lymphocytic leukemia is a laboratory diagnosis. The minimal requirement is a sustained absolute increase of well-differentiated lymphocytes in the peripheral blood and bone marrow not attributable to other causes (Plate IV-5, *D*; see Chapter 80). Disorders most commonly confused with CLL include non-Hodgkin's lymphoma, hairy cell leukemia, Waldenström's macroglobulinemia, and viral infections. There is controversy about the degree of sustained lymphocytosis necessary to make the diagnosis. A minimum of 5×10^9 cells per liter lymphocytes in peripheral blood is accepted in some schemes; 15×10^9 cells per liter is required in others. If a sustained peripheral lymphocyte count of 10×10^9 cells per liter is present, documentation of either bone marrow involvement or a B-cell phenotype typical of chronic lymphocytic leukemia serves to make the diagnosis. If the peripheral blood cell count is less than 10×10^9 cells per liter, both bone marrow involvement and a typical B-cell phenotype should be documented. For bone marrow, 30% or more of the nucleated cells must be well-differentiated lymphocytes. The abnormal lymphocytes in the marrow and peripheral blood are fragile and easily traumatized, resulting in the presence of ruptured "smudge" cells on the peripheral blood smear. Surface immunoglobulin (SIg) is present on the surface of the leukemic lymphocyte and is decreased in amount compared with normal B lymphocytes. The SIg is usually immunoglobulin M (IgM), frequently with coexpression of immunoglobulin D (IgD), and is rarely immunoglobulin G (IgG). Because the population is clonal, the light chain is either lambda or kappa, not both. There is clonal rearrangement of heavy- and light-chain immunoglobulin genes (Chapter 73). The concentration of immunoglobulins in the serum is markedly decreased. The Coombs' antiglobulin test result is positive in 15% of patients. The majority of these patients do not have signs of hemolysis, although autoimmune hemolytic anemia is a well-known complication of CLL.

Treatment. Chronic lymphocytic leukemia cannot be cured by current therapy, so palliation is the goal. The course of the disease varies from patient to patient. Because the patients cannot be cured, it is critically important to observe each patient over a period of time to ascertain the pace of the disease. This information is necessary if therapeutic interventions are to be made at appropriate times without increasing the patient's morbidity.

Criteria for assessing the stage of disease at diagnosis are listed in Table 92-2. The stage is related to prognosis, but it does not predict the rate of progression of the disease in the individual patient. Stages 0, I, and II should not be treated if the patient is asymptomatic. Randomized clinical trials have shown that treatment of such good-prognosis patients with daily chlorambucil slows the progression of the disease to more advanced stages, but ultimate survival is shorter. Early treatment is harmful because treated patients have short survival after disease progression and an increased incidence of fatal epithelial cancers, when compared with untreated patients. Indications for treatment include progressive marrow failure, debilitating symptoms such as weakness, symptomatic bulky disease, autoimmune phenomena such as hemolytic anemia, and progressive lymphocytosis with a peripheral lymphocyte count above 100×10^9 cells per liter. Stages III and IV generally do require treatment. Some patients may initially exhibit stage III or IV disease, whereas others may progress to these stages from earlier stages. Initial therapy is usually an alky-

✔ WHEN TO REFER

Chronic lymphocytic leukemia is a common disease. The diagnosis is generally easy to make. The challenge is to avoid inappropriately aggressive management while the disease is indolent (Rai stages O, I, and II). The patient should be referred to a specialist for consultation if chemotherapy is contemplated or if complications such as autoimmune hemolytic anemia occur. In patients with Rai stages III and IV disease management is generally difficult, so consultation with a specialist is advised.

lating agent such as chlorambucil, 6 to 10 mg/day orally for 1 to 2 weeks, followed by maintenance at lower doses, such as 2 to 6 mg/day. Usually treatment is stopped when the patient has achieved a good, stable response and then restarted when there is significant progression.

Approximately 75% of patients respond to therapy, but in only 10% to 20% is there complete remission. Response is usually slow and is monitored both in the peripheral blood and by the size of the lymph nodes. The peripheral lymphocytosis should decrease; the platelet count and hematocrit should increase. Because bone marrow function is compromised, the possibility of dangerous marrow suppression by chemotherapy must be borne in mind. The most serious toxic effect is usually progressive thrombocytopenia, which is a relative contraindication to further therapy with alkylating agents. Some clinical trials have produced evidence that chlorambucil given as a pulse of 0.4 to 0.6 mg/kg of body weight once every 2 to 4 weeks induces remissions with less toxicity than daily dosage produces. If chlorambucil therapy is inadequate or if autoimmune phenomena occur, a glucocorticoid (typically prednisone 60 mg/day initially, tapering to 10 to 20 mg every other day) is added to the alkylating agent. Local radiotherapy may be used to treat isolated symptomatic masses of nodes. Progressive advanced disease may respond to combination chemotherapy, but the long-term prognosis is grim, with a median life expectancy of 1 to 2 years.

Fludarabine is a newly approved drug that is useful in the treatment of CLL. When used alone at doses of 25 mg/m² body surface area intravenously for 5 days every 4 weeks, fludarabine induces a partial or complete hematologic remission in 80% of previously untreated and 40% to 90% of previously treated (alkylating agents) patients. Remissions are generally 2 to 3 years in duration. Fludarabine clearly has a role in the treatment of CLL, but its place as compared with chlorambucil is not yet defined. Similarly, 2-CdA, as described for hairy cell leukemia, is active in CLL but probably is not as effective as fludarabine. The major toxic effects of the purine nucleoside analogs are myelosuppression and immunosuppression. The effect of the agents on long-term survival is not known. Tumor lysis syndrome with hyperuricemia and renal failure has occasionally been reported when purine nucleoside analogs are administered to patients with bulky lymphoid disease.

Most patients with CLL eventually die of infection, usually bacterial, but sometimes mycobacterial or fungal. In patients with IgG levels below 50% of the lower limit of normal or with a history of serious bacterial infection, intravenous IgG (250 mg/kg of body weight) every 3 or 4 weeks reduces the frequency of infection. However, treatment is extremely expensive and inconvenient and results in very little, if any, increase in life expectancy. Transformation of chronic lymphocytic leukemia to an immunoblastic sarcoma (Richter's syndrome) or to an acute leukemia is rare but can occur. Each is resistant to therapy.

MYELOPROLIFERATIVE DISORDERS

The myeloproliferative disorders are clonal neoplasms arising in a pluripotent hematopoietic stem cell and characterized either by excessive production of phenotypically normal mature cells (chronic myeloproliferative disorders) or by impaired or aberrant maturation of hematopoietic precursor cells (acute myeloproliferative and myelodysplastic disorders) (Box 92-1).

Table 92-2   Clinical staging and prognosis of chronic lymphocytic leukemia

RAI STAGE	FEATURES	MEDIAN SURVIVAL FROM DIAGNOSIS (YEARS)
0	Lymphocytosis of peripheral blood (lymphocytes $>5 \times 10^9$/L) and bone marrow only	>15
I	Lymphocytosis plus enlarged nodes	8
II	Lymphocytosis plus enlarged spleen and/or liver; nodes may or may not be enlarged	6
III	Lymphocytosis plus anemia (hemoglobin <11 g/dl); nodes, spleen, and liver may be enlarged	3
IV	Lymphocytosis plus thrombocytopenia (platelets $<100 \times 10^9$/L); nodes, spleen, and liver may be enlarged; anemia may be present	2

These criteria for clinical staging of chronic lymphocytic leukemia are a modification of those first proposed by Rai KR et al: *Blood* 46:219, 1975.

BOX 92-1

Classification of the myeloproliferative disorders

I. Chronic myeloproliferative disorders (excessive production of mature cells)
   A. Chronic myelogenous leukemia (chronic granulocytic leukemia)
   B. Idiopathic myelofibrosis (agnogenic myeloid metaplasia)
   C. Essential thrombocythemia (essential thrombocytosis)
   D. Polycythemia vera
II. Acute myeloproliferative and myelodysplastic disorders (impaired maturation or dysplasia of hematopoietic cells)
   A. Acute myelogenous leukemia (acute nonlymphocytic leukemia)
   B. Myelodysplastic syndromes
      1. Refractory anemia
      2. Refractory sideroblastic anemia
      3. Chronic myelomonocytic leukemia
      4. Refractory anemia with excess blasts
      5. Refractory anemia with excess blasts in transformation

---

Table 92-3   Distinguishing features of chronic myeloproliferative disorders

	CML	IMF	PV	ET
Leukocytes	↑↑↑	↑/N/↓	↑	N/↑
Hematocrit	↓	↓	↑↑↑	N
Platelets	↑↑	↑/N/↓	↑↑	↑↑↑
LAP score	↓	↑/N/↓	↑↑↑	N/↑
"Teardrop" red blood cell	–	↑↑↑	–	–
Marrow fibrosis	±	↑↑↑	–	–
Ph¹ chromosome	+	–	–	–

CML, chronic myelogenous leukemia; *IMF,* idiopathic myelofibrosis; *PV,* polycythemia vera; *ET,* essential thrombocythemia; *LAP,* leukocyte alkaline phosphatase; *Ph¹,* Philadelphia.
↑↑↑, Marked increase; ↑↑, moderate increase; ↑, slight increase; ±, variable; +, present; –, absent; N, normal; ↓, decrease.

The evidence for the clonal nature of these disorders is derived from studies on the expression of isoenzymes of glucose-6-phosphate dehydrogenase (G6PD) and from chromosomal analyses. Women who are heterozygous for isoenzymes of G6PD have two populations of cells, one containing type A isoenzyme and the other, type B. When a neoplastic disease develops, cells containing only one enzyme (A or B) are present, indicating that the neoplasm is derived from a single cell. In the myeloproliferative disorders single isoenzymes are present in granulocytes, erythrocytes, monocytes, and megakaryocytes, indicating that the neoplasms arise in a stem cell common to the different cell lineages. In some, the single enzyme is also present in lymphocytes, indicating that the disease arises in a more primitive pluripotent stem cell common to both the myeloid and lymphoid cell lines. Similarly, identical marker chromosomes are present in erythroid, myeloid, and megakaryocytic precursor cells, but not in marrow stromal fibroblasts.

The exact nature of the defects is unknown but differs in the two groups of disorders. In the chronic disorders there appears to be a loss of regulatory signals that control the production of mature cells, whereas in the acute disorders the major defect is in cell maturation. The differential diagnosis of an elevated blood neutrophil count is discussed in Chapter 80.

Chronic Myeloproliferative Disorders

The chronic myeloproliferative disorders include chronic myelogenous leukemia (CML), essential thrombocythemia (ET), polycythemia vera (PV), and idiopathic myelofibrosis. Distinguishing features are listed in Table 92-3. This chapter focuses on CML, ET, and PV; myelofibrosis is discussed in Chapter 90. These are clonal neoplasms of a pluripotent stem cell with an overproduction of one or more formed elements of the blood. The variation in patterns of cellular proliferation and differentiation can be explained by a clonal mutation of pluripotent stem cells with different lineage potentials. PV arises from a stem cell with a high erythroid potential, and CML may arise in a stem cell with a high neutrophil potential. Stem cells with equal potential for neutrophils and megakaryocytes may be involved in CML and ET. The diseases are interrelated, and one may evolve into another during its course. PV and ET may evolve into myelofibrosis, and all may evolve into acute leukemia.

Chronic Myelogenous Leukemia

Chronic myelogenous leukemia is a clonal neoplasm arising in a pluripotent stem cell that is characterized by extreme leukocytosis with an increase in immature and mature granulocytes and by splenomegaly. It occurs most frequently in young and middle-aged adults, with a slightly higher incidence in men. A distinctive chromosome abnormality, the Philadelphia (Ph¹ or Ph) chromosome, a shortened G-22

chromosome resulting from the reciprocal translocation of genetic material between chromosomes 9 and 22, appears in 95% of patients with CML. This abnormality is present in granulocytes, erythrocytes, and megakaryocytes, indicating that CML arises from a pluripotent stem cell. The disease follows two distinct courses: a mild chronic phase lasting approximately 3½ years and an acute phase (blast crisis) that results in death in 90% of patients within several months.

Etiology. The cause of CML is unknown, but its incidence is increased in atom bomb survivors and in patients who have received irradiation for ankylosing spondylitis. Of significance is that the breakpoint of the translocation between chromosomes 9 and 22 occurs in the region of the cellular oncogene, c-abl on chromosome 9. c-abl is the cellular homolog of the transforming gene of the Abelson murine leukemia virus, which causes pre–B-cell leukemia in mice. c-abl is translocated to a specific region of chromosome 22, the breakpoint cluster region (bcr). This translocation results in a hybrid bcr/abl gene that is unique to CML. Its product is a 210-kD fusion protein with greater tyrosine phosphokinase activity than normal. The abnormal kinase may be responsible for the development of the disease. The causes of cancer are discussed further in Chapter 70. Translocations are discussed in Chapters 70 and 73.

In 5% of patients with features resembling CML, the Ph¹ chromosome is not detected. In some of these patients there is a translocation between chromosomes 9 and 22, even though there is no microscopically detectable chromosomal abnormality, and in most there is rearrangement of the bcr gene. A number of patients considered to have Ph¹-negative CML were found on reevaluation to have features more consistent with a myelodysplastic disorder (chronic myelomonocytic leukemia) than with CML.

The Ph¹ chromosome is found in a number of adults and children with acute lymphoblastic leukemia (ALL). Some of these may represent CML presenting in the acute phase.

Clinical Features. The chronic phase of CML is characterized by a stable overproduction of leukocytes. The acute phase (blast crisis) is an aggressive form of the disease similar to acute myelogenous leukemia, and 90% of patients with CML die as a consequence of transformation to the acute phase. Transformation occurs at a rate of 25% per year after the first year after diagnosis but can occur at any time during the disease. Survival from diagnosis of the chronic phase is approximately 3½ years.

Chronic Phase. The onset of CML is insidious, and 20% of patients are asymptomatic at the time of diagnosis. Most symptoms are related to anemia (fatigue, weakness) or to splenomegaly (discomfort or a mass in the left upper quadrant of the abdomen). Less common are bleeding or thrombotic episodes, arthralgias, and bone pain. Some patients have fever, sweating, and weight loss produced by hypermetabolism. Splenomegaly and pallor are the major findings on examination. The spleen is palpable in more than 90% of patients and ranges in size from those that are barely palpable to those that fill the entire left side of the abdomen. Spleen size is directly correlated with the height of the peripheral leukocyte count. In 50% of patients the liver

BOX 92-2
Findings associated with onset of the acute phase of chronic myelogenous leukemia

Clinical observations

Rapidly increasing spleen size
Resistance to previously effective doses of chemotherapy
New and unexplained fever
Lymph node enlargement
Skin infiltration
Lytic bone lesions

Laboratory data

Progressive basophilia
Progressive thrombocytosis
Thrombocytopenia
Progressive anemia
Normalization of the leukocyte alkaline phosphatase (LAP) score
Progressive myelofibrosis
Increasing percentage of blast forms in peripheral blood and bone marrow
Cytogenetic clonal evolution
Hypercalcemia

is enlarged at diagnosis; 20% have purpura; and a few have lymphadenopathy or infiltration in the skin.

Acute Phase. Onset of the acute phase (blast crisis) occurs randomly but most often at about 3½ years after diagnosis. Transformation to the acute phase may be insidious, occurring over several months, or abrupt. Any change in symptoms or signs or in blood findings during the chronic phase that are unrelated to chemotherapy usually indicates that transformation to the acute phase has occurred (Box 92-2). Symptoms usually include fever, weight loss, increasing size of the spleen, worsening anemia and thrombocytopenia, bone pain, and purpura. Additional cytogenetic abnormalities are commonly seen, such as a second Ph[1] chromosome, monosomy 7, trisomy 8, and trisomy 19. Transformation in most patients is to acute myelogenous leukemia or to one of its variants. In 20% transformation is to an acute lymphoblastic leukemia.

Laboratory Features. Leukocytosis is the most prominent feature; the peripheral leukocyte count ranges between 50×10^9 cells per liter and 200×10^9 cells per liter at the time of diagnosis but can exceed 1000×10^9 cells per liter. The entire spectrum of neutrophils from myeloblasts (<5%) to mature polymorphonuclear leukocytes is present (Plate IV-6, *D*). Numbers of eosinophils and basophils are increased. Most patients have a normochromic, normocytic anemia resulting from decreased erythropoiesis. Platelet numbers are increased in 50% of patients; they function normally, and thrombotic events are uncommon. The marrow is hypercellular, with a marked increase in the ratio of myeloid to erythroid cells caused by the marked increase in granulocytes and their precursors. The marrow contains more immature granulocytes than the blood, but the concentration of blasts is less than 5% in the chronic phase. In some patients mild fibrosis of the marrow is present and may increase during the course of the disease.

Leukocyte alkaline phosphatase (LAP) score is decreased in neutrophils in more than 90% of patients. It may return to normal after treatment or increase with acute transformation. The serum vitamin B_{12} level and vitamin B_{12} binding proteins are increased and correlate with the degree of leukocytosis. Hyperuricemia may result from increased cell turnover.

The acute phase is accompanied by a variety of changes in the blood and marrow (Box 92-2), including an increase in blasts and promyelocytes in the blood and marrow; worsening of the anemia and increasing leukocytosis, thrombocytosis, or thrombocytopenia; increase in basophils; and increase in fibrosis of the marrow. The Ph chromosome persists, and additional chromosomal abnormalities may be detected.

✔ WHEN TO REFER

For patients under the age of 55 years with chronic myelogenous leukemia the critical decisions at diagnosis are whether and when to perform stem cell transplantation. This requires consultation with a specialist. Choice of interferon versus chemotherapy also requires the advice of a specialist. Treatment with interferon is extremely expensive and inconvenient in comparison with hydroxyurea, although it appears to prolong survival. Because the disease is rapidly fatal for most patients, referral to a clinical research center where the patient has the opportunity to participate in the evaluation of new therapies is encouraged.

Treatment. Chronic myelogenous leukemia cannot be cured by chemotherapy. Chronic-phase CML progresses inexorably to blastic phase or myelofibrosis and death. At diagnosis all patients with CML should be offered allogeneic bone marrow transplantation (BMT) (Chapter 77) if they are eligible (age under 55 years, availability of a suitably compatible donor). BMT in early chronic phase offers a 55% chance of cure. BMT in accelerated phase/blast crisis offers a 10% to 30% chance of cure.

Interferon-alfa is the drug of choice for initial therapy of CML. It is extremely expensive, and treatment is usually accompanied by significant malaise and sometimes by changes in memory. Approximately 80% of patients in early chronic phase have a hematologic remission when given 5 MU/m² per day of interferon-alfa. At best, approximately 20% of these patients also achieve a complete cytogenetic remission with disappearance of the Ph chromosome for periods of 2 to 8 years. A cytogenetic remission is a favorable prognostic indicator.

Hydroxyurea and busulfan are the drugs most widely used to treat CML. Clinical trials have proved that interferon-alfa and hydroxyurea are both superior to busulfan in prolonging survival of patients with CML. Hydroxyurea is sometimes combined with interferon-alfa. Although there is no evidence that the combination is more effective in promoting long-term survival than either drug alone, hydroxyurea can be helpful in reducing the leukocyte count and other signs of bulk disease while interferon-alfa takes effect. Hydroxyurea is an active agent affecting cells in DNA synthesis; continuous oral administration of 1 to 3 g/day is required to control the disease. Higher doses can be administered when a very high leukocyte count must be quickly reduced. Leukocyte counts increase and decrease rapidly as doses of hydroxyurea are modified, so frequent peripheral blood cell counts are necessary during therapy. A remission in symptoms and blood cell counts can occur, but the Ph chromosome persists in cells in the marrow. Treatment with aggressive combination chemotherapy in an attempt to eradicate the leukemic clone has not resulted in an increase in survival. Busulfan is an alkylating agent that is less effective than interferon-alfa or hydroxyurea. It can be given intermittently or continuously. It is given in a dose of 4 to 6 mg/day orally until the peripheral leukocyte count decreases to 10 to 15×10^9 cells per liter, at which time it is discontinued. The disease may be controlled for months after a single course of therapy, and patients may receive repeated courses of treatment. Side effects of busulfan include myelosuppression, increased skin pigmentation, pulmonary fibrosis, and, rarely, adrenal insufficiency.

Patients who do not receive BMT eventually progress to myelofibrosis with bone marrow failure (Chapter 90) or to blast crisis, a form of acute leukemia; 80% have myeloid blasts and 20% have lymphoid blasts. Treatment of the acute phase (blast crisis) of CML is unsatisfactory, and the disease is less responsive to therapy than the de novo acute myelogenous or acute lymphoblastic leukemias. The overall median survival from onset of blast crisis is approximately 18 weeks unless BMT can be performed.

Essential Thrombocythemia

Essential thrombocythemia (essential thrombocytosis [ET]) is the least common of the myeloproliferative disorders and is characterized by a marked increase in circulating platelets, usually in excess of 1000×10^9 cells per liter. It occurs most frequently in the sixth and seventh decades and affects men and women equally. With the advent of automated platelet counts, the disorder is seen with increasing frequency as an incidental diagnosis in young adults. The major criteria for a diagnosis of ET are (1) persistent elevation of platelet count, usually more than 1000×10^9 cells per liter; (2) marked increase in megakaryocytes in the marrow; (3) absence of other chronic myeloproliferative disorders; and (4) absence of an underlying condition responsible for reactive thrombocytosis, such as infection, chronic inflammatory disease, iron deficiency, malignancy, or prior splenectomy.

Clinical Features. Symptoms are related to thromboembolic phenomena in 50% of patients and to bleeding in 10%. Nearly half remain asymptomatic. Bleeding results from abnormal platelet function and may take the form of easy bruising, nosebleed, or gastrointestinal bleeding. Thrombotic events often include vascular ischemia of the central nervous system manifested by transient ischemic attacks, dizziness, visual problems, and headaches; or peripheral vascular ischemia, including deep vein thrombosis, pulmonary emboli, and emboli of digital vessels leading to painful ischemia of the toes. In approximately 40% of patients the spleen is palpably enlarged, although not to the extent seen in other myeloproliferative disorders.

Laboratory Features. Platelet counts are increased to more than 600×10^9 cells per liter, usually exceed 1000×10^9 cells per liter, and can be as high as 5000×10^9 cells per liter. Platelet function is abnormal. The leukocyte count is elevated in 50% of patients but seldom exceeds 40×10^9 cells per liter. Leukocyte alkaline phosphatase level is normal or increased, but not to the extent seen in PV. Megakaryocytes are markedly increased in the marrow. Serum vitamin B_{12} and uric acid levels are usually increased. Pseudohyperkalemia may result from the increase in circulating platelets that release potassium during the preparation of serum.

Treatment. Treatment is directed at controlling the platelet level and relieving symptoms. In asymptomatic patients with mild thrombocythemia (less than 600×10^9 cells per liter), treatment is not indicated. However, treatment should be given if platelets exceed 1000×10^9 cells per liter or if patients are symptomatic at lower levels. The disorder is not benign, even in young people. Nearly half of patients have bleeding or thrombosis, or both, although complications are rarely life threatening. Previously, treatment included administration of alkylating agents and radioactive phosphorus (phosphorus 32). Although these are effective forms of therapy, they are associated with an increased risk of leukemia or other neoplasm. Therefore it seems more appropriate to treat patients with hydroxyurea, anagrelide, or interferon-alfa. Hydroxyurea at an oral dose of 1 to 3 g/day generally maintains the platelet count at near-normal levels. The dose of hydroxyurea must be adjusted to prevent inducing severe neutropenia and anemia. The peripheral blood cell count should generally be checked every week or two for patients receiving hydroxyurea because the drug can rapidly change the blood cell count. If hydroxyurea is ineffective, anagrelide can be used. Anagrelide is an orphan drug that can be obtained through the Office of Orphan Products Development of the U.S. Food and Drug Administration. Induction doses of 1 mg every 6 hours orally usually reduce the platelet count to near-normal levels within 1 to 2 weeks. Maintenance doses generally range from 1 to 4 mg/day. Anagrelide is not cytotoxic to bone marrow. Side effects are generally mild but can include headache, nausea, palpitations, fluid retention, and diarrhea.

The course of the disease in most patients is rather benign and resembles that of PV. ET may evolve into other myeloproliferative disorders and in some cases into acute leukemia, which may be secondary to treatment with phosphorus 32 or alkylating agents.

Polycythemia Vera

Polycythemia vera in most cases can be easily distinguished from secondary polycythemia by the presence of leukocytosis, thrombocytosis, basophilia, splenomegaly, and trilinear hyperplasia of the marrow with clustering of megakaryocytes. The polycythemias are discussed in Chapter 79. Polycythemia vera is a clonal disease in which the primary production of increased red blood cells by the bone mar-

row depresses erythropoietin levels to normal or below normal values (<30 mU/ml). The clonal cells overgrow the normal population of red blood cell precursors that may still be present as a minority of cells. The incidence of PV is highest in patients who are 60 to 70 years old, but it may occur in individuals ranging in age from adolescence to 90 years. The male-to-female ratio is 1.2:1.0, and all races are affected. Some reports indicate a higher than expected incidence in Jews. In addition to the signs and symptoms common to all cases of polycythemia, there is severe pruritus that may be related to elevated blood levels of histamine and/or increased numbers of skin mast cells. Thrombotic and hemorrhagic complications are frequent as a result of the high blood viscosity. The overall incidence of thrombotic events in untreated patients is 3.4 per 100 patients per year, ranging from 1.8 in patients under 40 years of age to 5.1 in patients over 70 years. The most common thrombotic events are myocardial infarction, transient ischemic attack, and venous thrombosis. Some patients with virulent disease have marked symptoms of hypermetabolism. Clinical gout can result from hyperuricemia accompanying increased hematopoietic cell turnover.

Treatment. With optimum therapy, mortality resulting from the hyperviscosity can be greatly reduced, allowing patients with PV to have prolonged median survival times of 10 to 15 years. In 15% of patients acute leukemia eventually evolves. This is most often myelogenous but may occasionally be monocytic or lymphocytic. The incidence of leukemia is 4 times higher in patients who have been treated with alkylating agents than in those who receive phlebotomy alone. Fifteen percent to 30% of cases evolve into myelofibrosis with myeloid metaplasia (Chapter 90). The evolution may take the form either of a primary marrow fibrosis with consequent pancytopenia or of a rampant myeloid metaplasia with extramedullary hematopoiesis throughout the body that produces marked splenomegaly and hepatomegaly with portal hypertension. In this case a marked leukocytosis may produce a blood state like that of chronic myelogenous leukemia. A variety of cytogenetic abnormalities have been reported, but none is characteristic.

Because patients with PV who have not been treated have an extremely poor prognosis (median survival, 1.5 years) as a result of massive thrombotic and hemorrhagic complications, it is extremely important to reduce the hematocrit. Because thromboembolic events increase precipitously in patients with PV when the hematocrit is greater than 44%, this level is the therapeutic end point for therapy. Patients undergoing surgery without such control have extremely high morbidity and mortality rates, whereas those whose hematocrits have been under good control for more than 3 months have a normal course.

Patients 40 years old or less without evidence of severe vascular disease whose primary manifestation is erythrocytosis and whose hematocrit can be controlled by phlebotomy should continue to have this form of therapy. The administration of aspirin or dipyridamole has been recommended to reduce thrombosis, but clinical trials show that these anti–platelet-aggregating agents do not reduce the incidence of thrombotic events associated with phlebotomy. They do increase morbidity from bleeding. Older individuals with poor blood vessels have a very high incidence of thrombotic complications and should be treated with chemotherapy or interferon-alfa, in addition to phlebotomy, to suppress the bone marrow activity. This therapy produces better long-term control of the disease than phlebotomy alone. Hydroxyurea is recommended as chemotherapy because it has not been

---

✔ *WHEN TO REFER*

Consultation with a specialist to confirm the initial diagnosis of polycythemia vera and to plan therapy is recommended. Phlebotomy is preferred as primary management. If clinically significant abnormalities in the leukocyte or platelet counts occur, consultation is recommended before choosing chemotherapy or administration of interferon. Interferon is expensive, inconvenient, and not fully evaluated as therapy. At this time it should be administered only as part of formal clinical trials.

reported to increase the frequency of acute leukemia, unlike phosphorus 32 and the alkylating agents. During the first week, 30 mg/kg per day of hydroxyurea is given orally in divided doses, followed by 15 mg/kg per day orally the second week; the dose is then individualized to maintain normal blood cell counts. Periodic phlebotomy is continued as necessary to keep the hematocrit in the normal range. Hydroxyurea can produce marrow aplasia in a short time, and patients taking it must be followed up very carefully. Marrow suppression is reversible. In uncontrolled clinical trials interferon-alfa has been reported to eliminate the need for phlebotomy and to control the symptoms and signs of PV. An indication for starting therapy in addition to phlebotomy, is severe pruritus not controlled by histamine (H_1-, H_2-)-receptor–blocking agents (either alone or in combination), symptomatic splenomegaly, severe hypermetabolism, or history of thrombotic or hemorrhagic events.

ACUTE MYELOPROLIFERATIVE AND MYELODYSPLASTIC DISORDERS

In contrast to the chronic myeloproliferative disorders, which are characterized by excessive production of mature functional cells, the acute myeloproliferative disorders are marked by a defect in maturation of hematopoietic precursors (see Box 92-1). Generally by the time the diagnosis of the disorder is made, the clone of abnormally maturing cells has suppressed the normal marrow cells. This results in symptoms of bone marrow failure and cytopenias. If failure of maturation occurs rapidly, immature precursor cells (blasts) may be dominant in the marrow with features of acute myelogenous leukemia (AML). As an alternative, defects in maturation may be minimal initially and progress slowly over many years, with the marrow showing only variable degrees of dysplasia. In some of these patients clonal evolution occurs with increasingly more malignant characteristics in the marrow until, eventually, a large number of blasts are present, as in classic AML.

Acute Myelogenous Leukemia

Acute myelogenous leukemia, also referred to as acute nonlymphocytic leukemia (ANLL) or acute myeloblastic leukemia, is a malignant disorder arising in a stem cell capable of differentiating along the granulocytic, erythrocytic, and megakaryocytic cell lines. In some patients the malignant clone is expressed in all three cell lines, whereas in others expression may be restricted to erythrocytes and granulocytes or to granulocytes and macrophages. Malignant transformation occurs at different stages of differentiation, leading to morphologically different subtypes. These are listed in Table 92-4, as classified by a French-American-British (FAB) group.

In all subtypes the malignant clones of immature myeloid cells (primarily blasts) proliferate but do not differentiate to mature functional end cells. Blasts eventually replace the marrow, circulate in the blood, and invade most tissues in the body. Suppression of normal hematopoiesis by leukemic cells or their products results in anemia, neutropenia, and thrombocytopenia. These cytopenias are responsible for the symptoms of the disease. All subtypes except acute promyelocytic leukemia are similar in regard to course and response to treatment. In untreated cases survival is less than 3 months. With therapy, prolonged survival and cure can be achieved. Although AML may occur at any age, the incidence increases with advancing years. The disease is more common in men.

Etiology. The exact cause of AML is unknown, but certain factors are associated with an increased incidence of the disease. These factors include exposure to ionizing radiation (atom bomb survivors), chemicals (benzene), or chemotherapy with alkylating agents and nitrosoureas. Genetic factors also predispose to AML. Identical twins have an increased incidence of disease that occurs before the age of 6 years. Diseases with chromosome instability, including Down syndrome, Bloom's syndrome, Fanconi's anemia, neurofibromatosis, and Wiskott-Aldrich syndrome, convey greater risk for developing leukemia. Chronic myeloproliferative diseases may evolve to AML, as may the myelodysplastic syndromes. Acute promyelocytic leukemia (APL) is associated with a specific chromosomal abnormality, the translocation of a portion of the long arm of chromosome 17 onto the long arm of chromosome 15. The chromosomal breakpoints from several patients have been clustered within the gene on chromosome 17 that encodes the nuclear retinoic acid receptor (RAR-alpha) and within the PML gene on chromosome 15. The translocation results in the production of a hybrid fusion messenger RNA that contains portions of both the RAR-alpha and the PML transcripts. This fusion transcript appears to represent an abnormal transcription factor that affects the expression of genes in myeloid cells. The results are abnormal growth and differentiation of myeloid precursors with consequent clinical APL. Remission of APL can be induced by treatment of patients with all-trans-retinoic acid, a ligand that binds to the receptor encoded by RAR-alpha. Presumably the retinoic acid binds to the abnormal transcription factor in APL cells and inhibits its ability to induce abnormal growth and differentiation of myeloid precursors.

Clinical Features. Signs and symptoms are similar in all subgroups of AML and result from suppression of normal hematopoiesis. Symptoms are usually present for less than 3 months and are related to anemia (fatigue, pallor, tachycardia, dyspnea), neutropenia (infection), or thrombocytopenia (bruising, bleeding, petechiae). Several of the subgroups are associated with distinctive features. Acute promyelocytic leukemia (M3) is associated with disseminated intravascular coagulation (DIC) and bleeding caused by procoagulants released from the cytoplasmic granules of promyelocytes. Myelomonocytic (M4) and monocytic (M5) subtypes are associated more frequently with skin infiltration and gum hypertrophy. The spleen is enlarged in approximately one third of patients, and rarely there is enlargement of the liver or nodes. Approximately 25% of patients with AML have a history of myelodysplasia or "preleukemia."

Laboratory Features. Anemia, neutropenia, and thrombocytopenia are present in most patients and may be severe. The peripheral nucleated blood cell count is increased in 50% of patients, and this increase is nearly always due to circulating blasts. The blasts may contain Auer rods (rod- or string-shaped abnormal aggregation of lysosomal granules in the cytoplasm) (Plate IV-6, *E;* Figs. 92-1 and 92-2), which are pathognomonic for AML. The marrow is usually hypercellular, with blasts being the predominant cell type. Differentiation of AML subtypes and acute lymphocytic leukemia (ALL) is based on morphologic appearance and uses specific cytochemical stains or monoclonal antibodies. Serum uric acid level may be increased, and serum and urine muramidase levels are increased in the monocytic and myelomonocytic subtypes.

Nonrandom chromosome abnormalities are found in more than 80% of patients with AML. Specific abnormalities are associated with certain morphologic subtypes and are correlated with prognosis. For example, chromosomal translocation t(15;17) is associated with M3 and inverted 16 with M4. Translocations are discussed in Chapter 70.

Table 92-4 Subtypes of acute myelogenous leukemia

SUBTYPE	PREDOMINANT CELL IN MARROW	FAB CLASSIFICATION	PREVALENCE (%)
Myeloblastic (AML)	Myeloblast	M1, M2	45
Promyelocytic (APL)	Promyelocyte	M3	10
Myelomonocytic (AMML)	Myeloblasts, monoblasts	M4	30
Monocytic (AMMOL)	Monoblasts, promonocytes	M5	10
Erythroleukemia (AEL)	Pronormoblasts, myeloblasts	M6	5
Megakaryocytic (AMgL)	Megakaryoblasts	M7	3

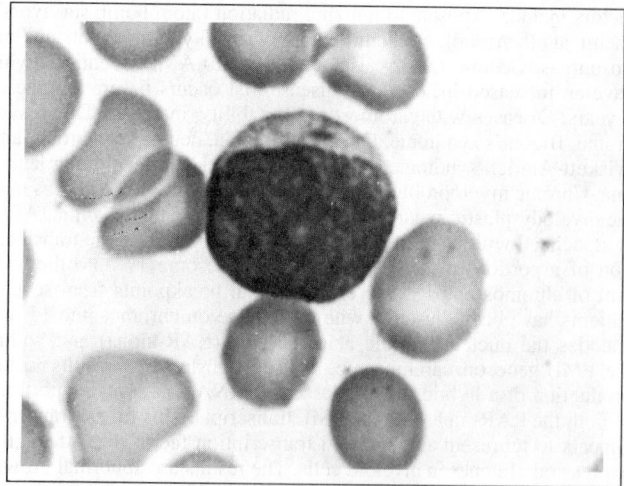

FIGURE 92-1   Stained smear of blood from a patient with acute myelogenous leukemia. The nucleated cell is a myeloblast that contains a dark-staining cytoplasmic body known as the Auer rod.

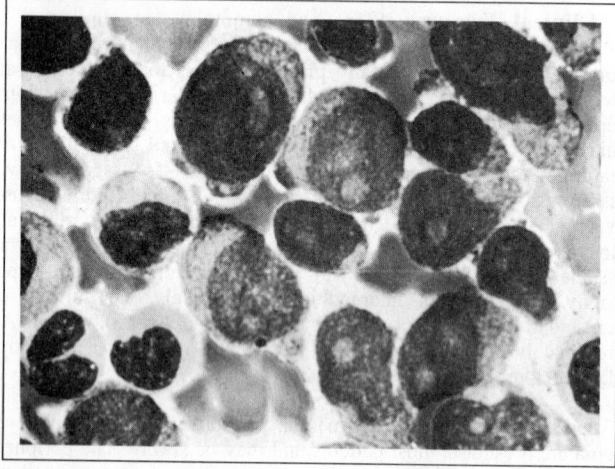

FIGURE 92-2   Stained bone marrow aspirate from a patient with acute myelogenous leukemia. The predominant cell type, the myeloblast, has a high nuclear/cytoplasmic ratio and has large nucleoli (compare with normal marrow, Color Plate IV-1).

Treatment. The goal of treatment is to induce a complete remission by eradication of the leukemic clone and restoration of normal hematopoiesis. A *complete remission* is defined as disappearance of signs and symptoms related to AML and a return to normal of blood cell counts and marrow, with less than 5% blasts in the marrow. The two most effective agents for inducing a remission are daunorubicin, an anthracycline antibiotic, and cytosine arabinoside, a pyrimidine antimetabolite (Chapter 71). In a typical treatment protocol induction therapy, given in a 7-day schedule as shown in Table 92-5, results in complete remission after one or two cycles of therapy in 60% to 80% of patients. Duration of survival depends on the length of the first remission, which usually lasts between 12 and 18 months. Cure is a possibility, but only 20% of patients survive 5 years or more. Attempts to prolong the duration of remission and survival are carried out through various programs of maintenance therapy or consolidation therapy for periods ranging from several months to 1 to 2 years. Repeated courses of multidrug consolidation over a period of 4 to 8 months have resulted in 30% to 40% disease-free survival rates at 3 to 5 years. These results are encouraging and suggest that all patients should receive postinduction consolidation therapy. There is little evidence to indicate that maintenance therapy has improved the duration of remission or survival.

Table 92-5   Drugs commonly used to induce a remission in acute myelogenous leukemia

DRUG	DOSE (MG/M²)	ROUTE	SCHEDULE*
Cytosine arabinoside	100-200	Intravenous	Continuous infusion days 1 to 7 of 7-day cycle
Daunorubicin	30-60	Intravenous	Single dose, days 1, 2, 3, of 7-day cycle

*May require two cycles to induce a complete remission.

In nearly all instances the marrow must be made aplastic to achieve a remission with induction therapy because the chemotherapeutic agents do not distinguish between leukemic and normal cells. The exception is APL, in which complete remission can be induced without marrow aplasia. During periods of marrow aplasia (2 to 3 weeks) aggressive support must be given to prevent fatal infections or bleeding. Infections with gram-negative bacilli or gram-positive cocci and fungi are common in patients with severe neutropenia. Neutropenic, febrile patients should receive broad-spectrum antibiotic coverage with an aminoglycoside and a semisynthetic penicillin (Chapter 236). If fever persists or recurs after 1 week of antibiotics, amphotericin B should be given, because *Aspergillus* and *Candida* infections are common in this setting. Platelet transfusions must be given to prevent bleeding, and platelet counts should be maintained above 20×10^9 cells per liter (Chapter 76). If patients become sensitized to random donor platelets, single-donor or human leukocyte antigen (HLA)–matched platelets must be given.

A different approach to therapy has proved effective in acute promyelocytic leukemia. All-trans-retinoic acid administered orally at a dose of 45 mg/m² of body surface area per day induces a complete remission in more than 80% of patients. Aplasia of the bone marrow does not occur, and abnormalities of coagulation (DIC) resolve promptly. Patients eventually relapse. Ongoing clinical trials are examining combinations of conventional chemotherapy, treatment with all-trans-retinoic acid, and allogeneic bone marrow transplantation (BMT). The aim is to cure a higher percentage of patients with APL, who generally have a more favorable prognosis than patients with other types of AML.

Bone marrow transplantation is an effective therapy for AML, with a 50% to 60% long-term survival rate and probable cure. This option is limited primarily to those patients less than age 55 years with an identical twin or an HLA-identical sibling, although use of HLA-matched unrelated donors is increasing (Chapter 77). The morbidity and mortality rates associated with BMT are significant because of graft-versus-host disease, interstitial pneumonitis, and other infections. This raises the question of when BMT should be performed. The best results are obtained in patients less than 30 years of age during first remission. Compared with chemotherapy, BMT in first remission appears to improve survival rate. Results are also encouraging for BMT in very early relapse. Therefore, because of the increasing survival and possible cure in some patients with chemotherapy, it may be appropriate to defer BMT until the first sign of relapse. A comparison of survival rate after chemotherapy or BMT in adults is shown in Fig. 92-3. As BMT procedures and techniques are further improved and complications are better controlled, BMT should become available to more patients. Results with autologous transplants after removal of the marrow and cleansing with monoclonal antibodies or cytotoxic agents in vitro have been associated with prolonged survival in several reports. However, the latter procedure requires further study and a longer follow-up period of observation.

Myelodysplastic Syndromes

The myelodysplastic syndromes (MDSs) are stem cell disorders characterized by a defect in maturation of hematopoietic precursors to functionally mature cells. The defect in maturation leads to ineffective hematopoiesis, which results in variable degrees of cytopenia or even pancytopenia, leading to infection and hemorrhage. There may

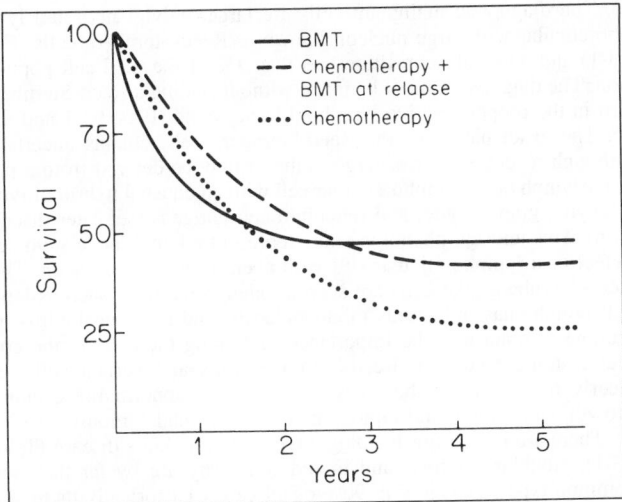

FIGURE 92-3   Survival of adults with acute myelogenous leukemia receiving either allogenic bone marrow transplants in first remission, postremission chemotherapy, or postremission chemotherapy with bone marrow transplants at relapse.

From Champlin RE, Gale RP: *Semin Hematol* 24:55, 1987.

✔ WHEN TO REFER

For patients under the age of 55 years the key initial decisions for patients with AML are whether and when to perform bone marrow transplantation. All aspects of therapy of AML are complex. If the patient is to be treated aggressively, this should be done in specialized centers, preferably as part of clinical research protocols aimed to evaluate new therapies.

---

be gradual expansion of the abnormal clone of cells over many years with concomitant suppression of normal hematopoiesis. In some cases the clonal evolution increases with progressive malignant characteristics in the marrow. Eventually there is a large number of blasts and, consequently, a classic picture of AML. The classification of MDS is complex and confusing. MDS encompasses disorders ranging from those with a low likelihood of evolution to leukemia (refractory anemia, refractory sideroblastic anemia) to those with a high propensity for developing into leukemia (refractory anemia with excess blasts in transformation). Myelodysplastic syndromes are seen in older adults, occur at a median age of 60 years, and are more frequent in men. Because chronic failure of hematopoiesis with anemia, leukopenia, and thrombocytopenia is prominent, these syndromes are discussed in Chapter 90.

BIBLIOGRAPHY

Anagrelide Study Group: Anagrelide: a therapy for thrombocythemic states—experience in 577 patients, *Am J Med* 92:69, 1992.
Cline MJ: The molecular basis of leukemia, *N Engl J Med* 330:328, 1994.
Copelan EA, McGuire EA: The biology and treatment of acute lymphoblastic leukemia in adults, *Blood* 85:1151, 1995.
Degos L et al: All-trans-retinoic acid as a differentiating agent in the treatment of acute promyelocytic leukemia, *Blood* 85:2643, 1995.
Devine SM, Larson RA: Acute leukemia in adults: recent developments in diagnosis and treatment, *CA Cancer J Clin* 44:326, 1994.
Grignani F et al: Acute promyelocytic leukemia: from genetics to treatment, *Blood* 83:10, 1994.
Gruppo Italiano Studio Policitemia: Polycythemia vera: the natural history of 1213 patients followed for 20 years, *Ann Intern Med* 123:656, 1995.
Kantarjian HM, Deisseroth A, Kurzrock R et al: Chronic myelogenous leukemia: a concise update, *Blood* 82:691, 1993.
Rozman C, Montserrat, E: Chronic lymphocytic leukemia, *N Engl J Med* 333:1052, 1995.
Silver RT: Interferon-α 2b: a new treatment for polycythemia vera, *Ann Intern Med* 119:1091, 1993.
Tallmann MS, Hakimian D: Purine nucleoside analogs: emerging roles in indolent lymphoproliferative disorders, *Blood* 86:2463, 1995.
Wetzler M, Kantarijian H, Kurzrock R, Talpaz M: Interferon-α therapy for chronic myelogenous leukemia, *Am J Med* 99:402, 1995.

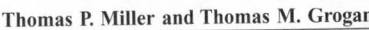

93 Hodgkin's Disease and Non-Hodgkin's Lymphoma

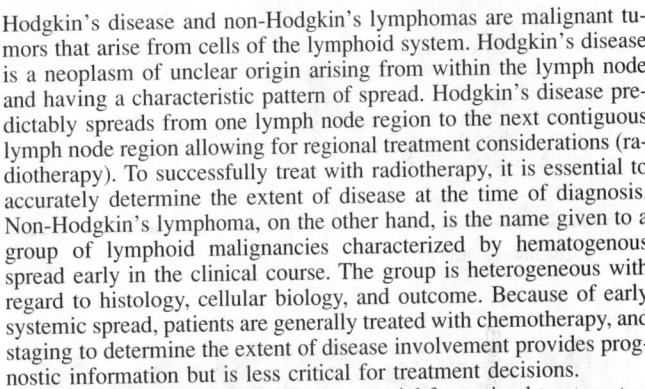

Thomas P. Miller and Thomas M. Grogan

Hodgkin's disease and non-Hodgkin's lymphomas are malignant tumors that arise from cells of the lymphoid system. Hodgkin's disease is a neoplasm of unclear origin arising from within the lymph node and having a characteristic pattern of spread. Hodgkin's disease predictably spreads from one lymph node region to the next contiguous lymph node region allowing for regional treatment considerations (radiotherapy). To successfully treat with radiotherapy, it is essential to accurately determine the extent of disease at the time of diagnosis. Non-Hodgkin's lymphoma, on the other hand, is the name given to a group of lymphoid malignancies characterized by hematogenous spread early in the clinical course. The group is heterogeneous with regard to histology, cellular biology, and outcome. Because of early systemic spread, patients are generally treated with chemotherapy, and staging to determine the extent of disease involvement provides prognostic information but is less critical for treatment decisions.

A correct histologic diagnosis is essential for optimal treatment of lymphoma and requires adequate tissue sampling. Although technical advances may allow clinicians to make a diagnosis based on needle biopsy specimens using endoscopic or computed tomographic (CT) guidance, small samples are frequently inadequate and even misleading. In general, the morphology of malignant lymphomas is not homogeneous at the cellular level and sampling errors can be significant. Further, small biopsy samples seldom provide adequate tissue for additional studies using immunohistochemistry or molecular analysis when the diagnosis is in doubt. Consequently, the initial approach to patients with suspected lymphoma should involve a surgeon to perform an excisional lymph node biopsy or obtain an adequate sampling of involved extranodal disease to clearly establish a diagnosis. A portion of all biopsy specimens should be kept fresh and snap-frozen in liquid nitrogen to allow subsequent immunohistochemical or molecular studies as indicated. On occasion, single cell suspensions and flow cytometry are used, but this technique is fraught with problems because lymphomas are composed of a mixture of malignant and reactive cells. Further, the malignant cells may be a minority component. Even a laparotomy may be justified to obtain adequate tissue rather than base months of toxic treatment and a lifetime prognosis on inadequate needle biopsy findings. Many of these diseases are curable, and mistaken diagnosis can compromise that expectation (Box 93-1).

HODGKIN'S DISEASE
Etiology

The cause of Hodgkin's disease is unknown. Historically, it was thought to be an infectious illness. Hodgkin's disease occasionally is seen in clusters, either geographic or familial, leading to speculation that there might be a causative virus. Recently the Epstein-Barr virus (EBV) has been implicated as an etiologic agent by finding elevated serologic features, EBV genomic material, and messenger RNA in the neoplastic Reed-Sternberg cells using in situ hybridization techniques. Whether EBV is playing a primary pathologic or secondary "passenger stand-by" role is not certain. There is evidence of a genetic susceptibility because an occasional relationship between Hodgkin's disease and certain human leukocyte antigens (HLAs) has been found.

However, the overall risk of Hodgkin's disease in members of affected families is only slightly higher than that in the general population.

Histology

The diagnosis of Hodgkin's disease is based on pathologic review of a tissue biopsy specimen, usually of a lymph node. Hodgkin's disease is unusual among neoplasms in that only a small proportion of cells are malignant. The great majority of cells are normal reactive cells (lymphocytes, plasma cells, fibroblasts, and eosinophils; Fig. 93-

---

BOX 93-1

Lymphomas that may be curable

Hodgkin's disease (all subtypes and stages)
Malignant lymphoma
   Childhood lymphomas
   Diffuse small noncleaved cell
   Lymphoblastic
   Diffuse large cell (including immunoblastic)
   Diffuse mixed
   Follicular large cell (?)*
   Follicular mixed (?)*

---

*(?), Controversial data exist.

---

1). The diagnostic malignant cells are large, polylobated, and lymphoreticular with large nucleoli known as Reed-Sternberg cells (Fig. 93-1) and generally constitute less than 1% of the total cell population. The diagnosis cannot be made without finding a Reed-Sternberg cell in the proper reactive lymphoid background (Figs. 93-1 and 93-2). The exact nature of the Reed-Sternberg cell remains uncertain, although recent evidence suggests that it may be derived from a primary lymph node lymphoreticular cell with an unusual hybrid of lymphocytic, granulocytic, and reticulum cell antigens (see later discussion). This unusual phenotype may represent a lymph node stem cell defect or a lymphoreticular cell with aberrant gene expression. That Reed-Sternberg–like cells are seen in other conditions, such as large cell lymphomas, infectious mononucleosis, and cytomegalovirus infections, emphasizes the importance of finding the cells in the correct histologic context. Reed-Sternberg cells and variant cells are clearly malignant on the basis of karyotypic abnormalities, clonal growth, and growth and tumorgenicity in the "nude" mouse.

There are four major histologic types of Hodgkin's disease (Table 93-1). Nodular sclerosis and mixed cellularity are by far the most common types, constituting 90% of all cases. Historically there was a difference in prognosis related to the histologic subtype of Hodgkin's disease, but with modern treatment this difference has been largely obliterated.

Immunohistochemical analysis is a major aid to diagnosis and provides a useful adjunct to light microscopy, thereby reducing errors in diagnosis. Using immunohistochemical techniques, the neoplastic Reed-Sternberg cells and variants have been shown to have a complex array of phenotypic properties including sometimes coexpression of lymphoid activation (CD30, Ki1), granulocyte (CD15, Leu M1), and reticulum cell antigens. The neoplastic cells in Hodgkin's disease are characteristically positive for Ki1 and Leu M1 and negative for leucocyte common antigen (CD45). This CD 30+15+45− phenotype occurs in 80% of Hodgkin's disease cases. A majority of

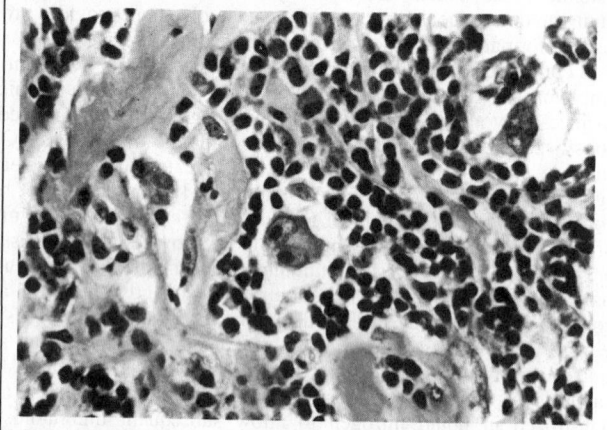

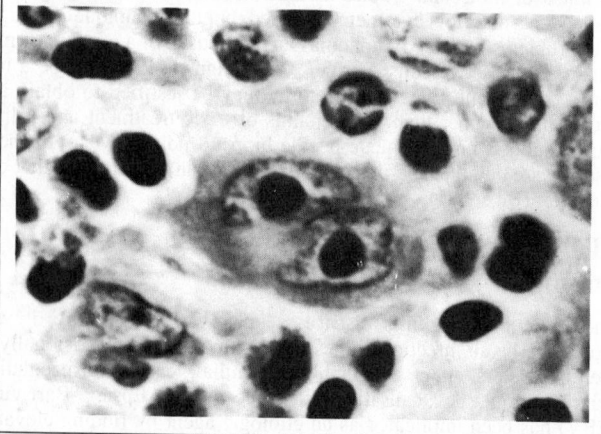

FIGURE 93-1 **A,** Reed-Sternberg cell in "proper" cellular background consisting of small round lymphoid cells and plasma cells (magnification ×400). **B,** High-power details of Reed-Sternberg cell. Prominent nucleoli, distinct nuclear envelopes, and polylobated nucleus are evident (magnification × 1000).

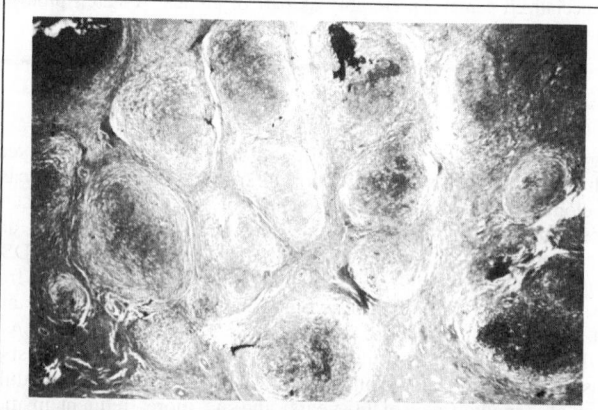

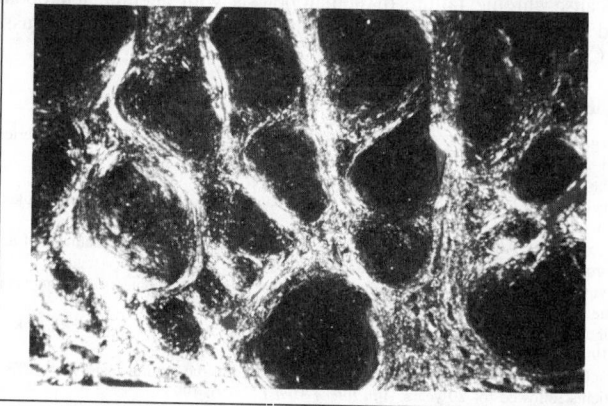

FIGURE 93-2 **A,** Low-power view of nodules in nodular sclerosing Hodgkin's disease (magnification × 100). **B,** Polarized light demonstrates birefringent collagen surrounding nodules (magnification × 100).

Table 93-1 Clinical and pathologic features of Hodgkin's disease subtypes (Lukes-Butler classification)*

HISTOLOGIC SUBTYPE	FREQUENCY (%)	USUAL CLINICAL FEATURES	RELATIVE PROGNOSIS
Lymphocytic predominance—lymphocytic infiltrate; rare Reed-Sternberg cells	5-10	Often quite localized in cervical regions; teenage males predominate	Excellent
Nodular sclerosis—broad bands of fibrosis (collagen); "lacunar" cells; rare Reed-Sternberg cells	40-70	Usually localized; 70% have mediastinal masses; young women predominate	Usually excellent
Mixed cellularity—abundant Reed-Sternberg cells, histiocytes; can be confused with diffuse large cell lymphoma	20-40	Tends to be widespread; occurs in older population; males predominate	Usually good
Lymphocytic depletion—fibrosis; abundant Reed-Sternberg cells; may be easily mistaken for diffuse large cell lymphoma; very rare	5	Frequent in older patients; often widespread at discovery	Good to poor

*The comments regarding prognosis associated with particular types of Hodgkin's disease illustrate only a general relationship and may not apply to individual patients. Effective treatment may be curative in patients with any stage or type of Hodgkin's disease.

Hodgkin's disease of the lymphocyte predominant subtype cases show Pan-B cell antigen (CD20) expression, indicating that some Hodgkin's disease subtypes may be specifically of B-cell origin.

Clinical Features

Hodgkin's disease primarily affects younger patients than does malignant lymphoma. The majority of patients are between the ages of 15 and 40, and a second, smaller peak occurs about age 50. Hodgkin's disease can occur in childhood. The presenting symptom is usually an enlarged lymph node, often in the cervical or supraclavicular regions. Only about 15% of patients have subdiaphragmatic disease. Lymph nodes characteristically are firm, mobile, and "rubbery." Lymph nodes 2 cm or larger suggest the diagnosis of lymphoma, particularly when they are located in the supraclavicular or axillary region. Hodgkin's disease rarely involves epitrochlear or popliteal lymph nodes. Tender lymph nodes more often have infectious or inflammatory causes than lymphomas, but occasionally rapidly enlarging lymph nodes can be tender. Rock-hard or fixed lymph nodes are more common with carcinoma than with lymphoma. The evaluation of patients with lymphadenopathy is fully discussed in Chapter 81.

Hodgkin's disease frequently involves mediastinal and/or hilar lymph nodes. Patients may have cough or shortness of breath. Hemoptysis and the superior vena cava syndrome are very rare. Pleural effusions are sometimes found in association with mediastinal involvement but rarely contain malignant cells.

Because Hodgkin's disease generally spreads to contiguous lymph node regions, abdominal lymph nodes may also be involved. Within the abdomen, the disease often first involves the spleen, although the spleen rarely is massively enlarged. With splenic involvement the splenic hilar lymph nodes commonly are involved; so too, eventually, are the paraaortic lymph nodes. The disease may spread farther down the lymph node chains to involve the iliac or inguinal lymph nodes or farther up the lymph node chains to involve celiac or porta hepatis nodes. Mesenteric lymph node involvement, even with widespread Hodgkin's disease, is rare. Eventually, Hodgkin's disease may involve the liver and bone marrow. The frequency of sites of involvement found during pretreatment staging is shown in Table 93-2.

Symptoms associated with Hodgkin's disease are non-specific. Three symptoms are considered "constitutional" or "B" symptoms: unexplained fever, drenching night sweats, and weight loss of more than 10% of body weight. Any of the "B" symptoms portend a worse prognosis. Occasionally, fever is periodic (Pel-Ebstein fever). These constitutional symptoms may mimic an infectious disease. In addition, generalized pruritus may be a presenting symptom of Hodgkin's disease, but it does not constitute one of the B symptoms and does not influence prognosis. Pruritus abates with satisfactory treatment of disease. Rarely, patients may experience a peculiar syndrome of alcohol-induced pain at sites involved by disease. This rare symptom is virtually pathognomonic for Hodgkin's disease.

A severe defect in cell-mediated (T-cell) immunity exists in patients with even the most limited forms of Hodgkin's disease. This T-cell defect leads to anergy and a propensity for infection with opportunistic organisms, particularly tuberculosis, fungi, and viruses.

Table 93-2 Approximate frequency of involvement by Hodgkin's disease of various sites

SITE	FREQUENCY (%)
Mediastinal lymph nodes	40-70
Hilar lymph nodes	25-50
Abdominal lymph nodes	
Paraaortic	40
Mesenteric	5
Portal	5
Splenic hilar	30-40
Liver	10
Spleen	35-40
Bone marrow	5

Herpes zoster is commonly seen during the course of Hodgkin's disease and can be a life-threatening illness. In addition, patients who have undergone splenectomy as part of staging are at increased risk of overwhelming bacterial septicemia (Chapter 81.) Despite successful treatment of Hodgkin's disease, the immune defect persists for life. Patients should be cautioned against receiving live virus vaccinations, such as smallpox or yellow fever, that might prove fatal.

Laboratory Features

No specific laboratory abnormalities are associated with Hodgkin's disease. Routine peripheral blood evaluation often indicates a mild neutrophilic leukocytosis, a slightly increased platelet count, and a mild normochromic normocytic anemia. Very rarely, Coombs' test–positive hemolytic anemia is found. A number of nonspecific serum protein abnormalities are present and account for an increased erythrocyte sedimentation rate and increased ceruloplasmin and copper levels. None of these abnormalities is diagnostic or particularly useful in following patients. Mild abnormalities of liver function are sometimes noted. With bulky disease, hyperuricemia may be present, but it is less common than with non-Hodgkin's lymphomas. Hypercalcemia is rarely a feature of Hodgkin's disease except occasionally as a terminal event. Rare patients may have nephrotic syndrome. Because bone marrow involvement is uncommon, pancytopenia caused by marrow replacement is unusual.

Differential Diagnosis

Hodgkin's disease may mimic many infectious diseases. In addition, other malignancies including leukemia and carcinoma can sometimes be characterized by lymphadenopathy, and the diagnosis can be established only through biopsy and histologic review. The most important differential diagnosis is between Hodgkin's disease and other malignant lymphomas. In particular, pleomorphic large cell lymphomas with scattered Reed-Sternberg–like cells may be histologically problematic. In such a circumstance, snap-frozen tissue section phenotyping can be useful.

Staging

The proper treatment for patients with Hodgkin's disease is predicated on knowledge of the exact extent of disease before treatment. The usual pretherapy evaluation includes a careful history and physical examination, paying particular attention to all of the lymph node areas and the abdomen. Routine chest radiographs may show the presence of mediastinal or hilar adenopathy. Whole lung and mediastinal tomography or a CT scan of the chest is indicated to rule out pulmonary nodules and adenopathy not apparent on plain chest radiographs. For patients with B symptoms or evidence of at least stage III disease (Table 93-3) a bone marrow core biopsy is useful for ruling out involvement of the bone marrow. An abdominal imaging procedure should be performed to rule out abdominal lymph node involvement. CT scanning of the abdomen is used to screen for enlarged paraaortic or iliac lymph nodes. Ultrasonography is somewhat less reliable for screening for enlarged abdominal lymph nodes. Neither ultrasonography nor CT scanning can reliably detect involvement of the liver or spleen. Bipedal lymphangiography remains an extremely useful procedure in defining paraaortic and iliac lymph node involvement in Hodgkin's disease. The results of this initial evaluation usually provide enough information to make a decision about the most appropriate form of initial therapy, although staging laparotomy and splenectomy are required in some patients. In general, radiotherapy with curative intent is utilized for patients with limited disease (stage I or II) without potentially adverse prognostic features (Box 93-2). Alternatively, chemotherapy with curative intent is employed for patients with more advanced stages of disease (stage III or IV). Certain special situations require the use of radiotherapy and chemotherapy together (combined modality treatment).

Therapy

With the development of modern radiotherapy (Fig. 93-3), localized Hodgkin's disease has been treated successfully, with cure rates of 60% to 90% depending on the experience of the radiotherapist and the presence or absence of several prognostic indicators (Box 93-2). Radiotherapy should be performed only in centers in which the radiation oncologists have extensive experience with Hodgkin's disease to minimize acute and long-term side effects and to optimize the chances for cure.

The prognostic factors listed in Box 93-2 are usually believed to have an adverse impact on the outcome when radiotherapy is employed as the only treatment modality. Thus the ideal patients for treatment with radiotherapy alone are those without the adverse factors listed, and cure is achieved in 70% to 90% of patients. If any of the adverse factors listed in Box 93-2 is present, the chance of cure with radiotherapy alone drops significantly, and consideration should be given to chemotherapy or chemotherapy plus radiotherapy (combined modality treatment). For patients with stage III_2, IIIB, or IV disease, chemotherapy is the mainstay of treatment. Some groups advocate the use of radiotherapy along with chemotherapy. Chemotherapy is curative in 50% to 70% of patients with advanced Hodgkin's disease.

In the 1960s, the major form of treatment for recurrent or advanced Hodgkin's disease was single-agent chemotherapy, but complete responses were rarely observed. A major breakthrough in the drug treatment of Hodgkin's disease occurred in the mid-1960s, when investigators at the National Cancer Institute combined four agents (nitrogen mustard, vincristine, procarbazine, and prednisone) in what is now known as the MOPP program. In patients without prior chemotherapy, complete remissions are regularly achieved in 70% to 80% of patients with 6 to 10 courses (months) of therapy. Among patients who achieve complete remission, approximately 70% remain in long-term remission and are cured. Since the first reports of treatment with the MOPP regimen appeared, considerable clinical research has been invested in attempts to define new or improved regimens to supersede MOPP. The first of these alternative regimens combined doxorubicin, bleomycin, vinblastine, and dacarbazine (ABVD). The ABVD regimen has been shown to be effective in patients relapsing after MOPP treatment and appears to be more active than MOPP in previously untreated patients. Further, the ABVD regimen causes less long-term toxicity, including a decreased frequency of treatment-related leukemia, ovarian failure, and sterility. Over the past decade investigators have combined MOPP and ABVD in attempts to exploit the advantages of each regimen, reduce the toxicities of each, and overcome multidrug resistance. The MOPP regimen has been alter-

Table 93-3   Ann Arbor staging* classification of Hodgkin's disease

STAGE	CLASSIFICATION
I	Involvement of a single lymph node region (I) or single extralymphatic site (I_E)
II	Involvement of two or more lymph node regions on the same side of the diaphragm (II), which may also include the spleen (II_S), localized extralymphatic involvement (II_E), or both (II_{SE}), if confined to the same side of the diaphragm
III	Involvement of lymph node regions on both sides of the diaphragm (III), which may also include the spleen (III_S), localized extralymphatic involvement (III_E), or both (III_{SE})
IV	Diffuse or disseminated involvement of extralymphatic sites (e.g., bone marrow, liver, or multiple pulmonary metastases), with or without lymph node involvement

*The presence of fever, night sweats, or unexplained weight loss of 10% or more of body weight over 6 months is designated by the letter *B*. The letter *A* indicates absence of these symptoms.

Clinical staging (CS) refers to the use of noninvasive tests; pathologic staging (PS) refers to staging based on invasive or surgical procedures (e.g., laparoscopy or laparotomy with splenectomy). Thus a patient with CSIIA Hodgkin's disease may prove to have $PSIV_{S+He+}$ on the basis of positive liver and splenic biopsies.

BOX 93-2

Potentially adverse prognostic features of Hodgkin's disease to be defined through careful staging

Constitutional or B symptoms (fever, night sweats, weight loss)
"Bulky" disease (usually defined as a mediastinal mass greater than one third of the chest diameter on a chest radiograph or an abdominal mass greater than 10 cm in diameter)
Hilar adenopathy
Extranodal (E) spread
Extensive splenic involvement (more than four nodules of Hodgkin's disease)
Substage III_2 (pelvic node involvement)

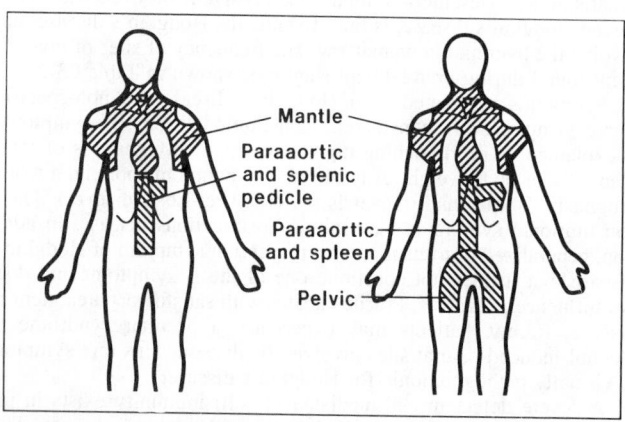

FIGURE 93-3   Standard radiotherapy ports used for treating Hodgkin's disease with curative intent (with *[left]* or without *[right]* splenectomy).

nated with the ABVD regimen, and the combination (MOPP/ABVD) has been shown to be better than MOPP alone. Two hybrids formed by combining elements of MOPP and ABVD (MOP-BAP and MOPP-ABV) have also been tested. The MOP-BAP regimen was shown to be better than MOPP in a randomized trial and the MOPP-ABV regimen was recently compared to MOPP followed by ABVD. Further follow-up evaluation of patients is required in this latter study. However, it appears that regimens containing doxorubicin and vinblastine are superior to and less toxic than classical MOPP. Drug doses and schedules for several of these regimens are shown in Table 93-4. This type of intensive multiagent chemotherapy is associated with considerable acute toxicity, such as nausea, vomiting, myelosuppression, hair loss, and predisposition to infection. The use of these multidrug regimens is complicated and should be overseen only by experienced physicians. In addition to acute toxicity, two important types of long-term toxicity are associated with combination chemotherapy—sterility and carcinogenesis. Sterility occurs in about 50% of women and in 80% to 90% of men. Secondary malignancies occur in about 1% of long-term survivors, although in certain high-risk groups, the projected actuarial risk of leukemia or undifferentiated lymphomas may be as high as 8%.

Hodgkin's disease has become a model of a curable neoplasm. Its cure depends on close cooperation among a team of experienced cancer specialists, including hematopathologists, diagnostic radiologists, surgeons, medical oncologists, and radiation therapists. Should Hodgkin's disease recur after initial therapy, often a second and perhaps even a third major treatment effort may result in cure. In younger patients with normal heart and lung function, second-line treatment usually includes high-dose chemotherapy with autologous stem cell or bone marrow rescue.

NON-HODGKIN'S LYMPHOMAS
Etiology

A specific cause of most non-Hodgkin's lymphomas cannot be identified. However, several distinct types of non-Hodgkin's lymphomas have been associated with a viral cause (Chapter 256). For example, the Burkitt's lymphoma of Africa is a unique clinical entity that is strongly associated with the EBV. More recently, a family of T lymphotropic retroviruses has been isolated from humans, and one member of this family, the human immunodeficiency–related retrovirus (HIV-III), is strongly associated with a distinct type of lymphoma called adult T-cell leukemia-lymphoma. HIV-III is endemic in southern Japan, the Caribbean islands, Africa, and the southeastern United States, and there is strong seroepidemiologic evidence linking HIV-III and the adult T-cell leukemia-lymphoma. A second member of this retrovirus family, HIV-I, has been linked to the pathogenesis of acquired immunodeficiency syndrome (AIDS), an immunodeficiency disease that frequently predisposes to life-threatening infections, Kaposi's sarcoma, and lymphoma (Chapters 227, 248, and 256). Malignant lymphomas can develop in association with a wide range of other immunologic disorders. In as many as 10% of patients with Sjögren's syndrome lymphoma eventually develops. Immunosuppressive therapy for heart, liver, or kidney transplant patients using azathioprine plus prednisone or cyclosporine is associated with development of malignant lymphoma in approximately 4% to 10% of patients.

The addition of anti–T-cell serum to these immunosuppressive drugs greatly increases the risk of development of lymphoma, and the risk is related to the dosage of the immunosuppressive agent(s) used. The EBV genome is associated with lymphomas that develop in both the posttransplant immunosuppressed patient and the human

Table 93-4 Chemotherapeutic regimens useful in the treatment of Hodgkin's disease

MOPP

REGIMEN*	DOSE	1	2	3	4	5	6	7	8	9	10	11	12	13	14
M = nitrogen mustard	6 mg/m² IV	x							x						
O = vincristine (Oncovin)	1.4 mg/m² IV (max. 2mg)	x							x						
P = procarbazine	100 mg/m² PO	x	x	x	x	x	x	x	x	x	x	x	x	x	x
P = prednisone	40 mg/m² PO	x	x	x	x	x	x	x	x	x	x	x	x	x	x

ABVD

REGIMEN*	DOSE	1	2	3	4	5	6	7	8	9	10	11	12	13	14	15
A = doxorubicin (Adriamycin)	25 mg/m² IV	x														x
B = bleomycin	10 mg/m² IV	x														x
V = vinblastine	6 mg/m² IV	x														x
D = dacarbazine (DTIC)	375 mg/m² IV	x														x
MOPP/ABVD	Monthly courses alternating two regimens															

MOP-BAP

REGIMEN*	DOSE	1	2	3	4	5	6	7	8	9	10	11	12
M = nitrogen mustard	6 mg/m² IV	x											
O = vincristine (Oncovin)	1.4 mg/m² iv (max. 2 mg)	x							x				
P = procarbazine	100 mg/m² PO			x	x	x	x	x	x	x	x	x	
B = bleomycin	2 mg/m² IV	x							x				
A = doxorubicin (Adriamycin)	30 mg/m² IV								x				
P = prednisone	40 mg/m² PO			x	x	x	x	x	x	x	x	x	

MOPP-ABV (repeat every 4 weeks)

REGIMEN*	DOSE	1	2	3	4	5	6	7	8	9	10	11	12	13	14
M = nitrogen mustard	6 mg/m² IV	x													
O = vincristine (Oncovin)	1.4 mg/m² IV (max. 2 mg)	x													
P = procarbazine	100 mg/m² PO	x	x	x	x	x	x	x							
P = prednisone	40 mg/m² PO	x	x	x	x	x	x	x	x	x	x	x	x	x	x
A = doxorubicin (Adriamycin)	35 mg/m² IV								x						
B = bleomycin	10 mg/m² IV								x						
V = vinblastine	6 mg/m² IV								x						

*MOPP is the standard regimen most often used, and ABVD is the regimen most often used for MOPP failures. MOPP/ABVD is a program that has produced superior results to MOPP alone in one trial. MOP-BAP was shown to be superior to MOPP-bleomycin in one trial. MOPP-ABV is commonly used, but a comparative trial with MOPP has not been completed. In general, each regimen is repeated on a 4-week basis. Most physicians administer a maximum of 2 mg of vincristine per dose in these regimens.

immunodeficiency viral syndrome patient. Whether the virus is causative or simply an associated finding in immunocompromised hosts is unclear. Malignant lymphomas are also rarely observed as a second malignancy after chemotherapy for Hodgkin's disease. There is indirect evidence that chronic "immunostimulation" such as occurs with inflammatory bowel disease, with drugs such as phenytoin, or with lymphoproliferative disorders such as angioimmunoblastic lymphadenopathy may predispose to the development of malignant lymphomas.

Histology

The diagnosis of malignant lymphoma is based on the morphologic appearance of an excised lymph node. The normal architecture of the lymphomatous lymph node is frequently replaced by a monomorphic infiltrate of neoplastic lymphoid cells. However, the pathologic diagnosis is often complicated by the finding of incomplete effacement of the lymph node and residual follicles with normal-appearing architecture. In addition, the infiltrate may be polymorphic, and the degree of cellular atypia may be subtle. In such cases it is often difficult to determine whether the lymph node represents neoplastic growth or benign reactivity. At other times a lymph node may be replaced with such an extreme degree of cellular atypia that the lymphoid nature of the neoplasm cannot be determined on the basis of morphologic characteristics alone. In such difficult cases the diagnosis often requires expert review by an experienced pathologist, or application of newer diagnostic processes such as immunohistochemical or molecular biologic techniques to demonstrate gene rearrangements.

In the majority of instances the diagnosis of a non-Hodgkin's lymphoma is made on morphologic criteria, and the histologic subtype is classified according to the Working Formulation. Until recently, many systems were used to classify non-Hodgkin's lymphomas. All of these systems are based on the morphologic appearance of the lymphoma, and all have some clinical utility for determining response to treatment and prognosis. The Working Formulation is an attempt to accommodate the terminology of these different systems. Before adoption of the Working Formulation, the Rappaport classification was most often used in the United States. Many textbooks and journal articles still use the terminology of the Rappaport classification. Table 93-5 summarizes these two systems and divides the histologic subtypes of each system into two clinically useful subgroups based on prognosis. The terms favorable and unfavorable have gained wide clinical acceptance and are useful for discussing general aspects of these complex diseases.

Morphologically, malignant lymphomas may appear as follicular (nodular) or diffuse (Fig. 93-4). This difference in architecture is both the most reproducible histologic feature and the most important variable affecting survival. Approximately 50% of patients have lymphomas with a follicular pattern, and these patients in general have a more favorable prognosis. In addition to the architectural pattern, malignant lymphocytes can be categorized on the basis of size as small (lymphocytic) or large (histiocytic) (Fig. 93-5). This distinction is helpful but does not suffice to subdivide patients into groups with different prognoses. Malignant lymphocytes can be characterized as to their degree of cellular atypia (poorly differentiated or well differentiated). These three morphologic determinations (architectural pattern, cell size, and cellular atypia) determine the histologic subtype of the lymphoma.

Immunophenotypic and genetic analysis has further subdivided lymphomas into biologically relevant subgroups. Immunohistochemical evaluation of snap-frozen biopsy tissues, in particular, has delineated specific clinicopathologic entities. As an example, high-grade lymphoblastic lymphomas were initially separated from the lower-grade, small cleaved-cell category on the basis of an immature T-cell phenotype that mimics the chemical characteristics of immature cortical thymocytes found in the thymus. Clinically, lymphoblastic lymphomas commonly occur in the mediastinum (thymic area) in teenage males consistent with their thymic lineage. As another example, the follicular lymphomas have immunoglobulin and pan–B-cell antigen expression consistent with their origin from germinal centers. Typically, there is a monoclonal immunoglobulin-bearing pattern with light and heavy chain restriction. Genotypic assay using Southern blotting reveals a comparable monoclonal rearrangement of the immunoglobulin genes. Beside B- and T-cell lineage, other markers are useful in lymphoma categorization, including markers of (1) proliferative status, (2) histocompatibility (HLA) status, (3) cell adhesion molecule and "homing" receptor status, and (4) immunosurveillance

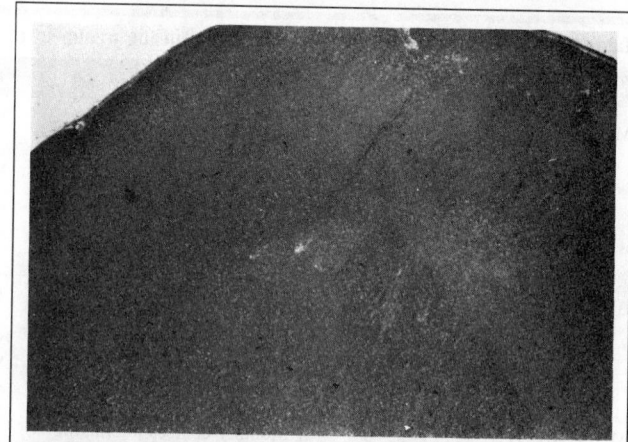

A

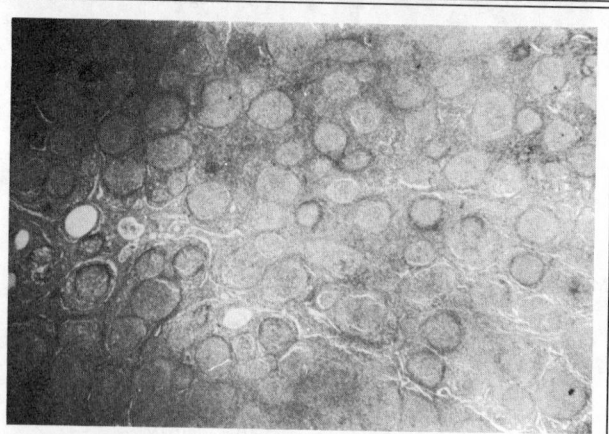

B

FIGURE 93-4 **A,** Diffuse effacement of node by lymphoma (magnification × 100). **B,** Follicular effacement of node by follicular (nodular) lymphoma (magnification × 100).

Table 93-5   Nomenclature of non-Hodgkin's lymphomas

NEW WORKING FORMULATION	OLD RAPPAPORT CLASSIFICATION
Low grade: Favorable types	
1. Small lymphocytic	1. Diffuse, lymphocytic, well-differentiated
2. Follicular, small cleaved cell	2. Nodular, poorly differentiated lymphocytic
3. Follicular, mixed small cleaved and large cell	3. Nodular, mixed, lymphocytic and histiocytic
Intermediate grade: unfavorable types	
4. Follicular, large cell	4. Nodular, histiocytic
5. Diffuse, small cleaved cell	5. Diffuse, poorly differentiated lymphocytic
6. Diffuse, mixed small and large cell	6. Diffuse mixed, lymphocytic and histiocytic
7. Diffuse, large cell	7. Diffuse, histiocytic
High grade: Unfavorable types	
8. Large cell immunoblastic	8. Diffuse, histiocytic
9. Lymphoblastic	9. Lymphoblastic
10. Small noncleaved cell	10. Burkitt's undifferentiated

status as measured by the quantity of infiltrating T cytotoxic/suppressor cells. For example, the proliferative status varies from 1% to 3% in low-grade categories to greater than 80% in high-grade categories. A proliferative rate of 20% to 25% identifies patients with low-grade lymphomas having a poor prognosis. Genotypic markers have also proved relevant to biologic subcategorization. In particular, the BCL-2 oncogene product, which in physiologic circumstances confers long-lived status on "memory B cells" by preventing normal B-cell death, may be overexpressed in some of the low-grade lymphomas. BCL-2 overexpression in these lymphomas immortalizes the neoplastic lymphoid cells in the resting state. The overexpression of BCL-2 in low-grade lymphomas has been specifically related to a distinct chromosomal translocation t(14, 18), which results in a fusion gene readily detected by immunoblotting and the polymerase chain reaction. At the other end of the proliferative spectrum are the high-grade lymphomas. In this instance, the greater than 80% proliferative rate may be associated with a translocation t(8, 14), and upregulated expression of the MYC oncogene. The upregulated MYC oncogene is a nuclear mitogenic factor accounting for the loss of proliferative control. Immunoblotting may also be used to detect MYC rearrangement or amplification.

New Lymphoma Entities

Recently several new non-Hodgkin's lymphoma entities have emerged using combinations of morphologic, immunologic, genotypic and clinical features (Box 93-3). Mantle cell lymphoma derives from B lymphocytes in the mantle zone surrounding the germinal center. The cells of this lymphoma have an alteration of the bcl-1 oncogene due to a characteristic chromosomal translocation (t 11; 14) which results in overexpression of a proliferative protein, cyclin D1.

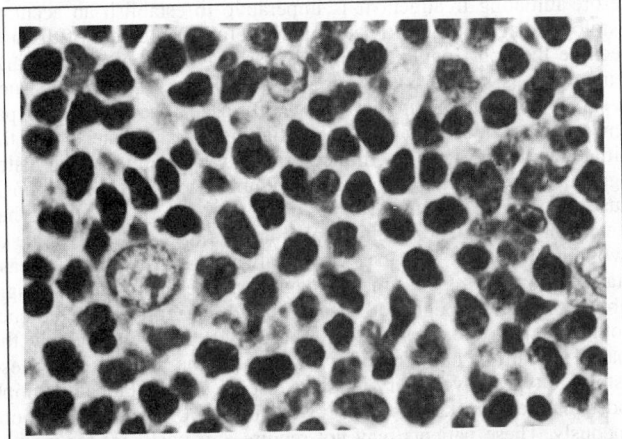

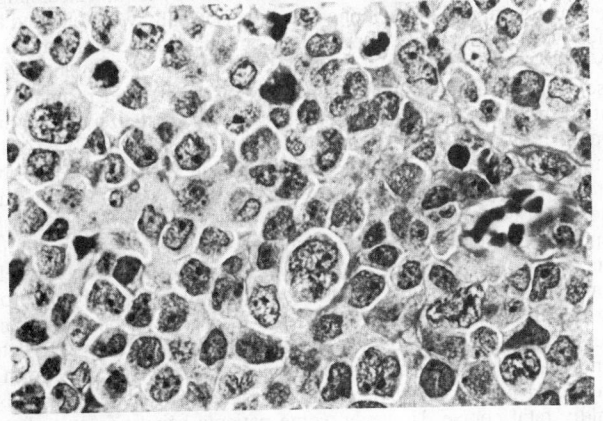

FIGURE 93-5   Small cleaved-cell lymphoma (magnification × 600). **B,** Large cell lymphoma. Mitoses are evident (magnification × 600).

These genetic changes result in a more proliferative lymphoma than its small lymphoid appearance would suggest. The clinical consequence is a lymphoma associated with shortened survival. Marginal zone lymphomas derive from the B cells in the marginal region outside the mantle zone and are divided into two types. Mucosa-associated lymphoid tissue (MALT)-omas are associated with mucosal surfaces and monocytoid B lymphomas are lymph-node based. MALTomas are diffuse, small lymphocytic proliferations occurring in such sites as the salivary glands, lacrimal glands, thyroid, respiratory epithelium, and gut mucosa. In the stomach and duodenum, in particular, a high association with *Helicobactor pylori* has been described. Most important, remission of some of these lymphomas is possible with triple antibiotic therapy. Monocytoid B lymphomas have the peculiar morphologic feature of having a nucleus of a small lymphocyte and the cytoplasm of a monocyte. The disease is remarkably indolent. Anaplastic large cell lymphoma is characterized by large, bizarre, blastic cells sometimes found in large cohesive groups and visually simulating carcinoma. The large neoplastic cells overexpress CD30 (Ki1 antigen) and are associated with a chromosomal translocation (t2; 5). Clinically the response rate and survival appear to be similar to other intermediate- and high-grade non-Hodgkin's lymphoma.

Clinical Features

Malignant lymphomas are a group of diseases having as a common feature the malignant transformation of a lymphocyte. The diseases are, however, relatively distinct with regard to clinical presentation and natural history.

The favorable histologic subtypes of malignant lymphomas are most often seen in older patients and are present in equal frequency in both sexes. The median age of onset is during the sixth decade, and the diseases are rare in patients less than 30 years of age. Patients usually seek medical attention because of unexplained or persistent adenopathy. These patients often feel well, but systemic symptoms may be present in 15% at the time of diagnosis. Frequently, patients recall having enlarged lymph nodes for months or even years before diagnosis. The adenopathy is frequently generalized and may involve any peripheral lymph node site including the epitrochlear, inguinal, and femoral lymph node. Less commonly, patients present with symptoms related to anemia that is usually caused by bone marrow involvement with lymphoma, which is present in 50% to 70% of patients at diagnosis. Involvement of other extranodal sites of disease at the time of diagnosis may occur in 15% to 30% of patients, frequently including the liver, spleen, or, less often, the gastrointestinal tract. Follicular small cleaved-cell lymphoma is the most common type of lymphoma with favorable histologic features. After diagnosis, the course of disease may be variable but is often indolent (i.e., does not require treatment for periods of time). In 20% to 30% of patients, these diseases are slowly progressive or occasionally undergo spontaneous regression (decrease in size of the involved lymph nodes). When treatment is required, these diseases are often quite responsive, sometimes for years. Eventually they become more aggressive and refractory to treatment. A repeat lymph node biopsy at such a time frequently reveals a change in morphology to a more aggressive histologic subtype. Documentation of this transition from a favorable to an unfavorable lymphoma portends a poor prognosis and requires a change in treatment strategy. The median survival of patients with favorable histologic subtypes of malignant lymphoma is

---

BOX 93-3
New lymphoma entities

Mantle cell
Marginal zone
    Mucosa-associated lymphoid tissue (MALT)
    Monocytoid B
Anaplastic large cell

approximately 6 years, and as many as 25% of patients are alive after 12 years.

The unfavorable histologic subtypes of malignant lymphomas can occur at any age, including childhood. However, the majority of patients are older, and the median age of onset is in the sixth decade. These diseases affect men more often than women. Patients frequently seek medical attention because of symptoms related to a rapidly enlarging tumor mass. The disease usually begins in a recognized lymph node area but may form an extranodal mass in 20% of patients. After a thorough evaluation, extranodal disease can be documented in 75% of patients. The most common sites of extranodal involvement, in decreasing order of frequency, include the gastrointestinal tract, bone marrow, liver, spleen, nasopharynx, lung, and skin. Any extranodal site can be involved with malignant lymphoma, and case reports abound describing patients who have lymphoma involving such organs as the thyroid gland, testicle, kidney, and ovary.

Patients may have diffuse adenopathy at presentation, but clinically localized disease is much more common in patients with unfavorable histologic types than in those with the more indolent histologic features. Approximately 30% to 40% of patients are found to have localized disease (stages I or II; see Table 93-3) after careful clinical staging. The malignant lymphomas of unfavorable histologic types are characterized by a rapid doubling time and a propensity for early hematogenous spread. Consequently, even patients with clinically localized disease at the time of diagnosis frequently have microscopic metastatic disease. The clinical course of these patients is rapidly progressive, and very few patients survive 2 years without treatment. However, combination chemotherapy has substantially affected the prognosis of these patients, and a discussion of the natural history is no longer relevant unless one includes an assessment of the impact of treatment. The major determinant of prognosis for patients treated with systemic chemotherapy is the extent of disease at the time of diagnosis. The most common unfavorable histologic subtype is diffuse large cell lymphoma (Fig. 93-5, *B*). The cure rates are 90% to 95% of patients with stage I diffuse large cell lymphoma, 75% to 85% of patients with stage II disease, and 30% to 50% of patients with stage III or IV disease. In general, patients who respond to treatment do so quickly, and detectable disease completely disappears within 2 or 3 months. Relapses after 5 years of follow-up observation can occur but are unusual. Patients who do not respond to initial therapy or who relapse after completion of therapy most often die of their disease. Second-line therapy using standard drug regimens is rarely successful. Consequently, these patients are often considered for experimental approaches, including high-dose chemotherapy with autologous marrow rescue, new cytotoxic drugs, or immunomodulators. Relapses after therapy may occur at any site but most frequently involve sites of initially bulky disease.

The unfavorable histologic subtypes of malignant lymphoma may involve the central nervous system. Rarely, diffuse large cell lymphomas may appear as a localized brain mass. More frequently, these lymphomas involve the central nervous system during the course of therapy with diffuse meningeal involvement, resulting in symptoms of headache and multiple cranial nerve palsies. The histologic subtypes most likely to have meningeal involvement are lymphoblastic lymphoma and diffuse large cell lymphoma.

Laboratory Features

No laboratory findings are specific or diagnostic of non-Hodgkin's lymphoma. However, several laboratory features are variably present and may be important in determining prognosis or helpful in managing complications of therapy. The peripheral blood cell counts are usually normal at the time of diagnosis, but anemia, leukopenia, or thrombocytopenia may occur. Abnormalities of the peripheral blood cell counts are usually the result of bone marrow infiltration with lymphoma. Occasionally lymphoma cells are found in the peripheral blood (leukemic phase) at diagnosis but more commonly as a terminal event. However, excessive destruction of any blood cell line may occur, most commonly through immune-mediated destruction or hypersplenism. Increases in serum enzyme levels usually reflect involvement of bone or liver with lymphoma but are not sensitive indicators of involvement of these organs. Elevation of the serum lactic dehydrogenase (LDH) level is nonspecific, but higher levels have been associated with a worse prognosis, particularly in large cell lymphoma. Hyperuricemia is common in patients with high tumor burdens or rapidly proliferating tumors. Rarely, bulky disease may cause jaundice or azotemia. Hypercalcemia is unusual at the time of diagnosis except in patients who have lymphoma associated with the HIV-III virus. Hypogammaglobulinemia or serum monoclonal protein spikes are occasionally observed.

Staging

The extent of disease before treatment is determined in patients with malignant lymphoma to assess prognosis, to establish a baseline for gauging response to treatment, and to make certain that tumor masses have not compromised organ function. Because malignant lymphomas have a propensity for early hematogenous spread and are usually systemic at the time of diagnosis, staging has less importance for determining proper treatment than in Hodgkin's disease. The stage of disease is usually assigned as in Hodgkin's disease (see Table 93-3). All patients should have a careful history and physical examination, a chest radiograph, a complete blood cell count, and measurements of serum enzyme levels. Bone marrow aspiration should be done and a biopsy obtained, because they frequently reveal lymphoma. A CT scan of the abdomen should be performed; it is preferred to a lymphangiogram because the mesenteric lymph nodes and visceral organs within the abdomen are involved relatively frequently. A lumbar puncture with a cytocentrifuge preparation for morphologic examination is recommended for patients with unfavorable histologic subtypes if central nervous system symptoms are present. More invasive procedures such as a liver biopsy or staging laparotomy are generally not required, and patients are usually assigned a stage on the basis of clinical findings.

Treatment

Before initiating treatment it is imperative to establish an accurate histologic diagnosis and to determine carefully the extent of disease. Because the non-Hodgkin's lymphomas have a propensity for early hematogenous spread, locally or regionally directed treatment such as surgery or radiotherapy is infrequently used. The majority of patients receive chemotherapy as the initial therapy. The intensity of the initial chemotherapy is determined primarily by the presenting histologic diagnosis. For this reason it is emphasized that the diagnosis must be established with certainty, usually by a pathologist who has considerable experience with lymphomas. Patients with low-grade or favorable histologic subtypes almost always have systemic disease (stages III or IV) at the time of diagnosis. The favorable histologic subtypes are not thought to be curable with currently available chemotherapy or radiotherapy (see Table 93-5), and consequently the goal of therapy is palliation of symptoms. Some patients with these histologic types have a very indolent disease course. Palpable lymph nodes may remain stable, wax and wane in size, or even regress spontaneously. These patients may not require any treatment for months or even years. Once it is established that therapy is indicated, single-agent chlorambucil or cyclophosphamide is usually well tolerated and effective in the majority of patients. Combination chemotherapy with CVP (cyclophosphamide, vincristine, and prednisone; Table 93-6) is also usually well tolerated and probably offers a higher response rate but no survival advantage over single-agent chemotherapy. Other drug combinations do not have any proven advantage over CVP. A systemic form of radiation (total body irradiation [TBI]) has been advocated by some, but its use is not widespread. At some point, usually after several years of observation and palliative therapy, in most patients with favorable histologic subtypes a more aggressive clinical course develops. Previously responsive areas of disease may develop clinical resistance to drugs, existing sites of tumor may begin growing rapidly, or new sites of disease may develop in spite of ongoing chemotherapy. These are all indications for a repeat biopsy to determine whether histologic transformation to a more aggressive form of lymphoma has occurred. Histologic progression usually portends a rapidly fatal course. However, some patients benefit from a change in chemotherapy to one of the more aggressive drug regimens that are used for treating the unfavorable histologic types of lymphoma.

Malignant lymphomas of favorable histologic type occur in localized forms (stage I or II) in only 10% of cases. Accordingly, the approach to localized disease is less well defined than the approach to disseminated disease. Observation without treatment, involved field radiotherapy, total nodal radiotherapy, and chemotherapy have all been advocated, but none is clearly the treatment of choice for localized disease. Involved field radiotherapy is probably the least harmful of these approaches.

Treatment of advanced stages of malignant lymphoma of unfavorable histologic subtype (stages III and IV; some experts would include patients with stage II disease in the "advanced" stage category) re-quires chemotherapy with drug regimens of proven curative potential. These drug regimens usually include doxorubicin and cyclophosphamide (Tables 93-6 and 93-7). The most commonly used regimen is the CHOP (cyclophosphamide, Adriamycin, Oncovin, prednisone) combination, which produces a complete response rate of 50% to 68%. For patients who achieve a complete response, treatment is normally discontinued after 6 months. After treatment with CHOP, approximately 30% to 50% of patients experience a relapse and eventually die of their disease. Most relapses occur within the first 2 years, and relapses after 5 years are uncommon. Maintenance chemotherapy has

Table 93-6 Chemotherapeutic regimens useful in the treatment of malignant lymphomas

REGIMEN*	DOSE	1	2	3	4	5	6	7	8	9	10	11	12	13	14	15
CVP (repeat every 21 days)																
C = cyclophosphamide	400 mg/m^2 po	x	x	x	x	x										
V = vincristine (Oncovin)	1.4 mg/m^2 IV (max. 2.0 mg)	x														
P = prednisone	100 mg po	x	x	x	x	x										
C-MOPP (repeat every 28 days)																
C = cyclophosphamide	650 mg/m^2 IV	x								x						
O = vincristine (Oncovin)	1.4 mg/m^2 IV	x								x						
P = procarbazine	100 mg/m^2 po	x	x	x	x	x	x	x	x	x	x	x	x	x	x	
P = prednisone	40 mg/m^2 po	x	x	x	x	x	x	x	x	x	x	x	x	x	x	
CHOP (repeat every 21 days)		1	2	3	4	5										
C = cyclophosphamide	750 mg/m^2 IV	x														
H = doxorubicin (Adriamycin)	50 mg/m^2 IV	x														
O = vincristine (Oncovin)	1.4 mg/m^2 IV	x														
P = prednisone	100 mg IV	x	x	x	x	x										

*CVP and single-agent chlorambucil are the standard regimens most often used for favorable histologic subtypes of malignant lymphoma. CHOP is the standard regimen most often used for intermediate grades of unfavorable histologic subtypes. C-MOPP is useful for patients with unfavorable histologic types who have preexisting heart disease, for whom doxorubicin may be contraindicated. Regimens for the high grades of unfavorable histologic subtypes have not been standardized.
IV, Intravenously; *po,* by mouth.

Table 93-7 Developmental chemotherapeutic regimens frequently used to treat malignant lymphomas of unfavorable histology

REGIMEN*	DOSE	SCHEDULE (DAYS)
m-BACOD (repeat every 21 days)		
m = methotrexate (followed by leukovorin rescue)	200 mg/m^2, IV	8,15
B = bleomycin	4 mg/m^2, IV	1
A = doxorubicin (Adriamycin)	45 mg/m^2, IV	1
C = cyclophosphamide	600 mg/m^2, IV	1
O = vincristine (Oncovin)	1.4 mg/m^2, IV	1
D = dexamethasone	6 mg/m^2, PO	1-5
ProMACE-CytaBOM (repeat every 21 days)		
Pro = prednisone	60 mg/m^2, PO	1-14
A = Adriamycin (doxorubicin)	25 mg/m^2, IV	1
C = cyclophosphamide	650 mg/m^2, IV	1
E = etoposide	120 mg/m^2, IV	8
Cyta = cytarabine	300 mg/m^2, IV	8
B = bleomycin	5 mg/m^2, IV	8
O = vincristine (Oncovin)	1.4 mg/m^2, IV	8
M = methotrexate (followed by leukovorin rescue)	120 mg/m^2, IV	8
MACOP-B (one 12-week course)		
M = methotrexate (followed by leukovorin rescue)	400 MACOP/m^2, IV	8,36,64
A = Adriamycin (doxorubicin)	50 mg/m^2, IV	1,15,29,43,57,71
C = cyclophosphamide	350 mg/m^2, IV	1,15,29,43,57,71
O = Oncovin (vincristine)	1.4 mg/m^2, IV (max. 2.0 mg)	8,22,36,50,64,78
P = prednisone	75 mg/m^2, PO	1-84
B = bleomycin	10 mg/m^2, IV	22,50,78

*These regimens are frequently used to treat non-Hodgkin's lymphomas with unfavorable histologic features. However, a study directly comparing these regimens to CHOP has recently been completed demonstrating similar response rates and overall survival, but with increased toxicity and costs. The schedules are complex, and morbidity rate can be significant. Thus expert consultation is required to adjust doses, prescribe prophylactic antibiotics, and administer the leukovorin rescue.

✔ WHEN TO REFER

Patients having adenopathy without an identifiable cause that persists longer than 2 weeks and patients with progressive adenopathy should be referred for an excisional biopsy. The referral for biopsy should include a request for a portion of the excised node to be snap-frozen in the event that immunophenotypic studies or molecular analysis is needed. Clinicians should also request that all lymphoid malignancies be reviewed by an experienced hematopathologist, as mistaken diagnoses are common. Once the diagnosis is secure and initial staging procedures obtained (peripheral blood cell counts, serum chemistries, chest radiograph, and abdominal CT scan), all patients should be evaluated for treatment by a medical oncologist.

not been shown to be helpful for prolonging the complete response. In recent years there have been a number of attempts to improve on the complete response rate and the duration of response achieved using the CHOP combination (Table 93-7). These more aggressive regimens are associated with increased morbidity and a treatment-related mortality as high as 6%. However, a recently completed national cooperative group study directly comparing CHOP to m-BACOD, ProMACE-CytaBOM, and MACOP-B demonstrated remarkable similarity among regimens. In this randomized study of 1138 patients, response rates, failure-free survival rate, and overall survival rate were similar. However, CHOP was associated with the fewest fatal toxicities (1%) and is the least expensive regimen to administer.

Malignant lymphomas of unfavorable histologic subtypes appear as apparently localized disease (stage I or II) in approximately 30% to 40% of patients. Traditionally these patients have been treated with radiotherapy alone, with a cure rate of approximately 40% to 50%. More recently, the strategy of using chemotherapy of proven curative potential in advanced disease, such as CHOP, as initial therapy for localized disease has increased the proportion of patients who are apparently cured of disease to approximately 80%. Patients with very localized disease (stage I) can be treated with initial chemotherapy after clinical staging or with involved field radiotherapy after pathologic staging with equal success. Approximately 90% to 95% of these patients are cured of disease.

There are many exceptions to the general guidelines for treatment as outlined. For example, patients with T-cell lymphoblastic lymphoma are seldom cured using conventional drug regimens such as CHOP. These patients frequently have bone marrow involvement. Standard regimens often fail because central nervous system disease develops. More successful approaches to these patients include intensive induction therapy and central nervous system prophylaxis similar to the treatment strategies used in acute lymphoblastic leukemia (Chapter 92). The intensive multiagent chemotherapy programs used to treat childhood malignant lymphomas have resulted in a marked improvement in prognosis for these adult patients.

BIBLIOGRAPHY

Croce CM, Nowell PC: Molecular basis of human B cell neoplasia, *Blood* 65:1, 1985.

Diel V et al: The cell of origin in Hodgkin's disease, *Semin Oncol* 17:660, 1990.

Fisher RI et al: A clinical analysis of two indolent lymphoma entities: mantle cell lymphoma and marginal zone lymphoma (including the mucosa-associated lymphoid tissue and monocytoid B-cell subcategories)—a Southwest Oncology Group study, *Blood* 85:1075, 1995.

Fisher RI et al: Phase III comparison of CHOP vs. m-BACOD vs. ProMACE-CytaBOM vs. MACOP.B in patients with intermediate or high-grade non-Hodgkin's lymphoma: results of SWOG 8516, the national high-priority lymphoma study, *N Engl J Med* 378:1002, 1993.

Grogan TM, Miller TP: New biologic markers in non-Hodgkin's lymphomas, *Hematol Oncol Clin North Am* 5:925, 1991.

Harris NL et al: A revised European-American classification of lymphoid neoplasms: a proposal from the International Lymphoma Study Group, *Blood* 84:1361, 1994.

Horning SJ, Rosenberg SA: The natural history of initially untreated low-grade non-Hodgkin's lymphomas, *N Engl J Med* 311:1471, 1984.

Miller TP et al: P-glycoprotein expression in malignant lymphoma and reversal of clinical drug resistance with chemotherapy plus high dose verapamil, *J Clin Oncol* 9:17, 1991.

Urba WJ, Longo DL, Hodgkin's disease, *N Engl J Med* 326:678, 1992.

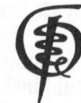

94 Multiple Myeloma and the Dysproteinemias

Robert A. Kyle

Multiple myeloma (plasma cell myeloma, myelomatosis, Kahler's disease) and related disorders are characterized by a neoplastic or potentially neoplastic proliferation of a single clone of plasma cells engaged in the production of a specific immunoglobulin. This immunoglobulin is monoclonal—one class of heavy chains (gamma, alpha, mu, delta, or epsilon) and one type of light chains (kappa or lambda)—and often is referred to as monoclonal protein (*M* protein or paraprotein). This group of disorders is classified in Box 94-1.

MULTIPLE MYELOMA
Etiology and Epidemiology

The cause of multiple myeloma is unknown. Radiation may be a factor in some cases. Exposure to asbestos, benzene, or industrial and agricultural toxins; a genetic element; and viruses have all been considered possible causes, but proof is meager.

Multiple myeloma accounts for about 1% of all types of malignant disease and slightly more than 10% of hematologic malignancies. The incidence of multiple myeloma is 4 per 100,000 per year. The apparent increase of rates in recent years is probably related to increased availability and utilization of medical facilities and improved diagnostic techniques.

Clinical Findings

The onset of multiple myeloma usually occurs in older persons with a median age of approximately 65 years. Only 3% of patients are younger than 40 years of age. It is slightly more common in men than in women. The incidence of multiple myeloma in blacks is almost twice that in whites. At diagnosis, bone pain, particularly in the back or chest, is present in more than two thirds of patients. Pain is usually induced by movement and does not occur at night, except with change of position. Weakness and fatigue are common and often are associated with anemia.

Some renal insufficiency occurs in about half of patients. This is often due to "myeloma kidney," in which the distal and collecting tubules become obstructed by large laminated casts consisting mainly of Bence Jones protein (Chapter 118). Hypercalcemia is also a common preventable cause of renal insufficiency. Hyperuricemia, amyloid deposition, acute or chronic pyelonephritis, infiltration of the kidney by plasma cells, and increased blood viscosity may all contribute to renal insufficiency. Acute renal failure has occurred after dehydration, infection, hypercalcemia, and intravenous urography.

Neurologic involvement is most often manifested by root pain from nerve compression. Compression of the spinal cord or cauda equina, usually produced by myeloma arising in the marrow cavity of a vertebra and extending to the extradural space, occurs in about 5% of patients with myeloma. This compression produces back pain with radicular features, weakness or paralysis of the lower extremities, and bowel or bladder incontinence. Peripheral neuropathy may occur but is usually associated with amyloidosis.

Patients with multiple myeloma have an increased susceptibility to bacterial infections, particularly pneumococcal pneumonia, although the incidence of gram-negative infections has recently increased. The greatest risk of infection occurs during the first 2 months after the initiation of chemotherapy. The incidence of herpes zoster is increased in myeloma. Bleeding may be a prominent feature. Qualitative platelet abnormalities, inhibition of coagulation factors from the monoclonal protein, and thrombocytopenia are major causes. Intravascular coagulation, amyloid deposition, and hepatic or renal insufficiency also may contribute to bleeding.

BOX 94-1

Multiple myeloma and related disorders

I. Multiple myeloma
II. Variant forms of myeloma
   A. Smoldering myeloma
   B. Plasma cell leukemia
   C. Nonsecretory myeloma
   D. Osteosclerotic myeloma (polyneuropathy, organomegaly, endocrinopathy, M protein, skin changes [POEMS] syndrome)
   E. Solitary plasmacytoma of bone
   F. Extramedullary plasmacytoma
III. Waldenström's macroglobulinemia
IV. Heavy-chain diseases
   A. Alpha heavy-chain disease
   B. Gamma heavy-chain disease
   C. Mu heavy-chain disease
V. Monoclonal gammopathy of undetermined significance (MGUS, benign monoclonal gammopathy)
VI. Biclonal gammopathies
VII. Cryoglobulinemia
VIII. Primary amyloidosis (Chapter 210)

BOX 94-2

Minimal criteria for the diagnosis of multiple myeloma

Bone marrow with ≥10% plasma cells OR
Plasmacytoma plus one of the following:
   Monoclonal protein in serum (usually >3 g/dl)
   Monoclonal protein in urine
   Lytic bone lesions
Usual clinical features of myeloma
Exclude connective tissue diseases, chronic infections, carcinoma, lymphoma, and leukemia

Pallor is the most common physical finding. The liver is palpable in about 20% of patients and the spleen in 5%. Extramedullary plasmacytomas are uncommon except in the late stages of the disease. Amyloidosis, which occurs in 10% of patients, may produce such diverse findings as defects of cardiac conduction, congestive heart failure, macroglossia, swelling of the joints, and peripheral neuropathy.

Laboratory Findings

At diagnosis, two thirds of patients have a hemoglobin value less than 12 g/dl. A normocytic, normochromic anemia eventually occurs in nearly every patient with multiple myeloma. The anemia is due mainly to inadequate production of red blood cells. Increased plasma volume from the osmotic effect of a large amount of monoclonal protein may produce a spurious decrease of hemoglobin and hematocrit values.

Serum electrophoresis reveals a peak or discrete band in 80% of cases, hypogammaglobulinemia in 10%, and no apparent abnormality in the remainder. A monoclonal protein is detected in the serum in about 90% of cases. The laboratory evaluation of monoclonal proteins is discussed in Chapter 74. Approximately 50% of the proteins are immunoglobulin G (IgG), 20% immunoglobulin A (IgA), 17% light chain only (Bence Jones proteinemia), 2% immunoglobulin D (IgD), and 1% biclonal. Electrophoresis of urine shows a globulin peak in 80% of cases, mainly albumin in 5%, and a normal pattern in 15%. Immunoelectrophoresis or immunofixation shows a monoclonal protein in 75% of cases. The kappa/lambda ratio is 2:1. Nearly all patients (98%) with multiple myeloma have a monoclonal protein in the serum or urine at diagnosis.

The serum creatinine level is elevated initially in about one half of patients and is greater than or equal to 2 mg/dl in one fifth. The serum calcium level is elevated in 25% of patients at diagnosis, and 15% have a calcium value of more than 11 mg/dl. Conventional radiographs show abnormalities consisting of punched-out lytic areas, osteoporosis, or fractures in 75% of patients at diagnosis. The vertebrae, skull, thoracic cage, pelvis, and proximal humeri and femurs are the most frequent sites of involvement. There is a positive correlation between the production of osteoclast-activating factors by bone marrow cells and the extent of skeletal destruction. Technetium-99m bone scans are inferior to conventional radiographs for detecting lesions in myeloma. Computed tomography (CT) or magnetic resonance imaging (MRI) is helpful in patients with myeloma who have skeletal pain but normal radiographic findings.

The peripheral blood of patients with myeloma shows a reduction of OKT4$^+$ cells (helper T lymphocytes) and an increased percentage of OKT8$^+$ cells (suppressor T lymphocytes). An aneuploid myeloma cell population is found in approximately three fourths of cases. Chromosome abnormalities are detected in about half of patients, but no specific abnormality has been demonstrated.

The demonstration of the monoclonal protein idiotype and the production of the patient's monoclonal protein by peripheral blood lymphocytes or plasma cells indicate that they are part of the malignant clone. This is supported by the demonstration of heavy- and light-chain immunoglobulin gene rearrangements in circulating blood cells.

Interleukin-6 (IL-6) is an important growth factor for myeloma cells. It induces a polyclonal proliferation of plasma cells. Elevated levels of IL-6 have been reported in patients with active multiple myeloma, in contrast to those with benign monoclonal gammopathy.

Differential Diagnosis

The differential diagnosis of monoclonal gammopathies is listed in Chapter 74. Bone pain, anemia, and renal insufficiency constitute a triad that is strongly suggestive of multiple myeloma. The diagnosis depends on the demonstration of increased numbers of plasma cells in the bone marrow (Plate IV-8). Identification of a monoclonal immunoglobulin in the plasma cells by immunofluorescence or immunoperoxidase is useful in differentiating multiple myeloma from reactive plasmacytosis and also in recognizing myeloma cells that have unusual morphologic features. Minimal criteria for the diagnosis of multiple myeloma are listed in Box 94-2. Because of differences in prognosis and therapy, variant forms of myeloma, such as smoldering multiple myeloma (SMM) and monoclonal gammopathy of undetermined significance (MGUS), must be distinguished from typical progressive multiple myeloma.

Prognosis

The plasma cell labeling index using a monoclonal antibody to 5-bromo-2-deoxyuridine is helpful in distinguishing patients with overt multiple myeloma from those with stable monoclonal gammopathies. The labeling index is low in MGUS, in SMM, and in successfully treated multiple myeloma (plateau phase) but is often elevated in overt multiple myeloma at the time of diagnosis and in patients with myeloma in relapse.

In 1975, Durie and Salmon devised a clinical staging system based on a combination of factors that correlated with the myeloma cell mass (Table 94-1). The median survival is approximately 5 years in patients with stage IA disease and approximately 3 years in those with stage IIIA disease. Renal insufficiency is associated with shorter survival. Patients with stage IIIB disease have a median survival of slightly more than 1 year.

Elevation of the plasma cell labeling index and the uncorrected beta-2-microglobulin level are two very important independent prognostic factors in multiple myeloma. In addition, elevations of thymidine kinase, lactic dehydrogenase, and C-reactive protein levels; advanced age; plasmablastic morphology; hypodiploidy; low RNA content of plasma cells; elevation of serum creatinine level; hypercalcemia; and stage IIIB disease are all associated with shortened survival.

Table 94-1   Clinical staging system for multiple myeloma

STAGE	CRITERIA
Stage I	Low cell mass ($<0.6 \times 10^{12}/m^2$)
	All of the following:
	Hb >10 g/dl; IgG <5 g/dl; IgA <3 g/dl; calcium normal
	Urinary monoclonal protein <4 g/24 hr
	No generalized lytic lesions
Stage II	Intermediate (neither stage I nor stage III)
Stage III	High cell mass ($>1.2 \times 10^{12}/m^2$)
	Any one of the following:
	Hb <8.5 g/dl; IgG >7 g/dl; IgA > 5 g/dl; calcium >12 mg/dl
	Urinary monoclonal protein >12 g/24 hr
	Advanced lytic bone lesions
Subclasses	A if creatinine level is <2 mg/dl and B if level is ≥2 mg/dl

From Durie BGM, Salmon SE: *Cancer* 36:842, 1975.

Chemotherapy

Chemotherapy is the preferred initial treatment for overt symptomatic multiple myeloma. Patients with SMM or MGUS (benign monoclonal gammopathy) should not be treated. The patient's symptoms, physical findings, and all laboratory data must be considered when determining whether to begin chemotherapy. If there is doubt in the physician's mind, it is usually better to withhold therapy and to reevaluate the patient in 2 or 3 months.

In most instances, analgesics, together with chemotherapy, can control the pain. This combination is preferred to local irradiation because the bone marrow reserve of many patients is limited and focal irradiation does not benefit systemic disease. The major controversy is whether a single alkylating agent or a combination of alkylating agents should be used.

The oral administration of melphalan (Alkeran) (0.15 mg/kg daily for 7 days) and prednisone (20 mg three times a day) for the same 7 days every 6 weeks is a satisfactory regimen that produces objective responses in 50% to 60% of patients. Leukocyte and platelet counts must be determined at 3-week intervals and the dose of melphalan altered to achieve modest cytopenias at midcycle because the absorption of melphalan is variable.

Because of the obvious shortcomings of melphalan and prednisone therapy, various combinations of therapeutic agents have been tried. A useful combination, VBMCP (M-2), consists of vincristine (1.2 mg/m^2 intravenously on day 1), 1,3-bis-(2-chloroethyl)-1-nitrosourea (BCNU) (20 mg/m^2 intravenously on day 1), melphalan (8 mg/m^2 orally on days 1 to 4), cyclophosphamide (400 mg/m^2 intravenously on day 1), and prednisone (40 mg/m^2 orally on days 1 to 7). In a recent Eastern Cooperative Oncology Group (ECOG) study, the addition of alpha$_2$-interferon to VBMCP produced a higher percentage of complete responses, but the overall survival was the same as for VBMCP. In a metaanalysis of 18 published trials, no difference in efficacy was shown between melphalan/prednisone and combination chemotherapy. However, there was an implication that melphalan and prednisone therapy was superior for patients with a good prognosis and inferior to combination chemotherapy for those with a poor prognosis.

Chemotherapy should be continued until the patient reaches a plateau phase, which is defined as a stable monoclonal protein level in the serum and urine and no evidence of progression of myeloma. The plateau state is prolonged and relapses are fewer with administration of alpha$_2$ interferon, but overall survival rate is probably not altered. Chemotherapy must be reinstituted when relapse occurs.

Treatment of Refractory Myeloma

The highest response rates reported for patients with multiple myeloma that are resistant to alkylating agents have been with the following VAD regimen: vincristine (0.4 mg/day) plus Adriamycin (doxorubicin) (9 mg/m^2 per day) by continuous infusion for 4 days, plus dexamethasone (40 mg each morning for 4 days beginning on days 1, 9, and 17 of each 28-day cycle). Most of the activity of VAD is from dexamethasone. If the patient has pancytopenia or does not

want to take VAD, methylprednisolone in a dosage of 2 g intravenously three times weekly for a minimum of 4 weeks produces a response in about one third of refractory patients. We find fewer side effects from methylprednisolone than from dexamethasone. If there is a response, administration of methylprednisolone is reduced to once or twice weekly. A regimen of vincristine, BCNU (carmustine), Adriamycin (doxorubicin), and prednisone (VBAP regimen) has produced some benefit in approximately 30% of patients.

Other Therapeutic Approaches

The reversal of resistance to chemotherapeutic agents is an important area of research. The use of verapamil or quinine to reverse the resistance to doxorubicin has been disappointing. An analog of cyclosporine, PSC 833, is being investigated in an effort to reduce multidrug resistance (MDR) to vinca alkaloids and anthracyclines. PSC 833 appears to be a much more effective inhibitor of MDR than cyclosporine A. Taxol has been disappointing in that it produces an objective response in about 25% of patients but is associated with considerable neutropenia. Topotecan has also produced some objective responses. The use of monoclonal antibodies to IL-6, a potent growth factor for plasma cells, has produced some response in patients with advanced multiple myeloma and plasma cell leukemia, but this is not a practical approach. New agents for the treatment of multiple myeloma are needed.

Peripheral Blood Stem Cell or Bone Marrow Transplantation

Bone marrow transplantation from an identical twin donor (syngeneic) has been associated with occasional prolonged survival, but most patients die of myeloma. Allogeneic bone marrow transplantation is advantageous in that the graft contains no tumor cells that can subsequently lead to a relapse. However, only modest numbers of patients with multiple myeloma are eligible for this procedure because a human lymphocyte antigen (HLA)–compatible donor is available in only one third of patients, 80% are greater than 50 years of age, and renal insufficiency (creatinine level >2 mg/dl) occurs in 20%. Consequently, only 5% to 10% of patients with multiple myeloma are eligible for an allogeneic bone marrow transplantation. In addition, the significant mortality of 25% within 6 months, the risk of graft-versus-host disease, and the eventual relapse in most patients make allogeneic bone marrow transplantation of limited use.

Autologous peripheral blood stem cell or bone marrow transplantation is applicable to more patients because the age limit is higher and a matched donor is unnecessary. Two major problems exist: (1) eradication of multiple myeloma from the patient usually does not occur even with large doses of chemotherapy and irradiation and (2) reinfusing autologous peripheral blood stem cells or bone marrow contaminated by myeloma cells or their precursors is a major concern. Selection of CD34+ LIN− THY+ stem cells may be a useful approach. Purging of the marrow in vitro with a combination of monoclonal antibodies or cytotoxic agents is not effective for routine clinical use. Prospective studies comparing transplantation and chemotherapy are under way in a number of centers.

Management of Complications

Hypercalcemia must be suspected if the patient has anorexia, nausea, vomiting, polyuria, increased constipation, weakness, confusion, stupor, or coma. Treatment is urgent because renal insufficiency commonly develops. Hydration, preferably with isotonic saline, is essential. In addition, oral prednisone in an initial dose of 25 mg four times daily should be given, but the dose must be reduced and discontinued as soon as possible. If these fail to control the hypercalcemia, pamidronate disodium (Aredia), etidronate disodium (Didronel), or gallium nitrate is useful. Maintenance of a high fluid intake (3 L/24 hours) is important in preventing renal failure. Allopurinol is necessary if hyperuricemia is present. Patients with acute renal failure should be treated promptly with fluid and electrolyte correction and then with hemodialysis if indicated. Peritoneal dialysis is preferable in some patients. Plasma exchange may be helpful for regaining renal function, but patients with severe myeloma cast formation or other irreversible renal changes are not likely to benefit from plasmapheresis. Renal transplantation for myeloma kidney has been followed by prolonged survival.

Prompt and appropriate treatment of bacterial infections is necessary. Pneumococcal and influenza vaccines should be given to all patients, despite their suboptimal antibody response. Intravenously administered gamma globulin may be helpful for patients with recurrent infections, but it is very expensive for long-term therapy. Prophylactic daily oral penicillin often benefits patients with recurrent pneumococcal pneumonia infections. Patients should be encouraged to be as active as possible because confinement to bed increases demineralization of the skeleton. Trauma must be avoided because even mild stress may result in multiple fractures. Fixation of long bone fractures or impending fractures with an intramedullary rod and methyl methacrylate has given excellent results. Bisphosphonates may be of benefit for demineralization of the skeleton. Erythropoietin is helpful for most patients with symptomatic anemia when the plateau state has been reached.

Symptoms of hyperviscosity include oronasal bleeding, blurred vision, neurologic symptoms, and congestive heart failure. Hyperviscosity is more common in IgA myeloma than in IgG myeloma. Vigorous plasmapheresis promptly relieves the symptoms of hyperviscosity. If spinal cord compression is suspected, MRI, CT, or myelography must be done immediately to determine whether an extradural mass is causing the symptoms. Radiation therapy to the lesion is usually beneficial.

VARIANT FORMS OF MYELOMA
Smoldering Multiple Myeloma

The diagnosis of SMM depends on the presence of a monoclonal protein concentration greater than 3 g/dl in the serum, more than 10% atypical plasma cells in the bone marrow, and the absence of anemia, renal insufficiency, and skeletal lesions. Often, a small amount of monoclonal protein is found in the urine, and the concentration of uninvolved immunoglobulins in the serum is decreased. Clusters or aggregates of plasma cells are often seen in the biopsy specimen of the bone marrow. The plasma cell labeling index is low. These patients should be observed without treatment because, in some, overt symptomatic multiple myeloma has not developed for years. Biologically, patients with SMM have a "benign" monoclonal gammopathy (MGUS), but it is difficult to accept that diagnosis initially when the monoclonal protein concentration is greater than 3 g/dl and the bone marrow contains more than 10% plasma cells.

Plasma Cell Leukemia

Plasma cell leukemia is characterized by more than 20% plasma cells in the peripheral blood and an absolute plasma cell count of at least 2000 cells/μl. It is classified as primary when it is diagnosed in the leukemic phase (60%) and as secondary when there is leukemic transformation of a previously recognized multiple myeloma (40%). Patients with primary plasma cell leukemia are younger and have a greater incidence of hepatosplenomegaly and lymphadenopathy, a higher platelet count, fewer lytic bone lesions, a smaller serum monoclonal protein component, and a slightly longer survival than those who have secondary plasma cell leukemia. Treatment is generally unsatisfactory, but administration of combinations of alkylating agents or melphalan and prednisone frequently produces a response; however, the median survival is only 7 to 9 months. High-dose therapy followed by peripheral blood stem cell rescue may be beneficial. Secondary plasma cell leukemia rarely responds to chemotherapy because the patients have already been treated for myeloma and are resistant.

Nonsecretory Myeloma

In approximately 1% of patients with multiple myeloma, a monoclonal protein cannot be detected in either the serum or the urine; this disorder has been designated nonsecretory myeloma. To confirm the diagnosis, a monoclonal protein should be identified in the plasma cells by the use of immunoperoxidase or immunofluorescence. More than a dozen patients with nonsecretory myeloma have been reported in whom a monoclonal protein cannot be found within the cells—a finding that suggests a lack of synthesis. Patients with nonsecretory myeloma have longer survival than do those with typical multiple myeloma.

Osteosclerotic Myeloma

Osteosclerotic myeloma (POEMS syndrome) is characterized by *p*olyneuropathy, *o*rganomegaly, *e*ndocrinopathy, *m*onoclonal protein, and *s*kin changes. The major clinical features are a chronic inflammatory-demyelinating polyneuropathy with predominantly motor disability and sclerotic skeletal lesions. The diagnosis is confirmed by the finding of a plasmacytoma on a biopsy specimen of a bony lesion. Hyperpigmentation and hypertrichosis may be striking. Gynecomastia, atrophic testes, and clubbing of the fingers and toes may occur. Papilledema is common. Hepatomegaly, splenomegaly, and lymphadenopathy may develop. In contrast to that in multiple myeloma, the hemoglobin level is usually normal or polycythemia is present. Thrombocytosis occurs in more than half of patients. A monoclonal protein is found in the serum in most patients, but it is usually small and is almost always of the lambda class. Immunoglobulin A is common. The presence of a monoclonal light chain in the urine is infrequent; when it is present, it is of modest amount. The bone marrow usually contains less than 5% plasma cells. Renal insufficiency and hypercalcemia are rare. Irradiation for single or multiple lesions in a limited area benefits more than half of patients. If the patient has widespread osteosclerotic lesions, chemotherapy with melphalan and prednisone may be helpful.

Solitary Plasmacytoma (Solitary Myeloma) of Bone

The diagnosis of solitary plasmacytoma of bone depends on histologic confirmation, absence of other lesions in the skeletal radiographs, no evidence of multiple myeloma in the bone marrow, and absence or small amounts of monoclonal protein in the serum or urine. More than half of patients have involvement of the vertebral column. Treatment consists of radiation to the local lesion in the range of 45 Gy (4500 rad). The patients must be closely followed because in approximately half, overt multiple myeloma develops and in approximately 10%, new solitary bone lesions or local recurrence develops. Progression usually occurs within 3 to 4 years. Approximately half of patients survive 10 years. There is no evidence that adjuvant chemotherapy affects the incidence of conversion to multiple myeloma.

Extramedullary Plasmacytoma

Extramedullary plasmacytoma is a plasma cell tumor that arises outside the bone marrow. The upper respiratory tract, including the nasal cavity and sinuses, nasopharynx, and larynx, is the most frequent site, but it may also occur in the gastrointestinal tract, central nervous system, urinary bladder, breast, testes, thyroid, parotid gland, and lymph nodes. Epistaxis, rhinorrhea, and nasal obstruction may occur. There is a predominance of IgA monoclonal protein in extramedullary plasmacytomas. The diagnosis is based on the finding of a plasma cell tumor in an extramedullary site and on the absence of multiple myeloma (determined from bone marrow examination, skeletal films, and examination of the blood and urine). Treatment consists of tumoricidal irradiation (40 to 50 Gy). The prognosis is favorable; regional recurrences develop in 25% of patients. Development of typical multiple myeloma is uncommon.

WALDENSTRÖM'S MACROGLOBULINEMIA

This malignant lymphoplasma cell proliferative disorder produces a high concentration of immunoglobulin M (IgM) monoclonal protein. The condition bears similarities to multiple myeloma, lymphoma, and chronic lymphocytic leukemia.

Etiology

Although the cause of Waldenström's macroglobulinemia is unknown, the disease may be more frequent in certain families. Studies of relatives of patients with macroglobulinemia reveal an increased frequency of IgM monoclonal proteins as well as quantitative immunoglobulin abnormalities.

Clinical Findings

Macroglobulinemia has a predilection for older men, and the onset is usually insidious. Weakness, fatigue, and bleeding (especially oozing from the oronasal region) are common presenting symptoms. Blurring or other impairment of vision affects some patients. In contrast to multiple myeloma, bone pain is rare. Dyspnea, weight loss, recurrent infections, or congestive heart failure may occur. Pallor, mild splenomegaly, hepatomegaly, and peripheral lymphadenopathy are the most frequent physical findings. Retinal abnormalities, including hemorrhages, exudates, and venous congestion with vascular segmentation ("sausage" formation), may be striking.

Pulmonary involvement is manifested by diffuse pulmonary infiltrates, isolated masses, or pleural effusion. These lesions consist of plasmacytoid lymphocytes. Peripheral neuropathy may be the initial symptom and usually involves both sensory and motor modalities. Sudden deafness, progressive spinal muscular atrophy, and multifocal leukoencephalopathy have all been noted. Renal failure rarely occurs. Systemic amyloidosis may be associated with Waldenström's macroglobulinemia.

Laboratory Findings

Almost all patients have a normocytic, normochromic anemia. Spuriously low hemoglobin and hematocrit levels may result from the increased plasma volume produced by a large amount of monoclonal protein. Occasionally, there is a Coombs'-test–positive hemolytic anemia. Rouleau formation is striking on the peripheral blood smear (Plate IV-4, *F*), and erythrocyte sedimentation is greatly increased. Mild lymphocytosis or monocytosis is not uncommon. The serum cholesterol value is frequently very low. The bone marrow aspirate is usually hypocellular, but fixed sections are hypercellular and extensively infiltrated with lymphoid and plasma cells. The number of mast cells is usually increased.

An IgM monoclonal protein, often at a concentration greater than 3 g/dl, is found in all cases. Approximately 75% of light chains are kappa. Both 7S and 19S IgM are present. About 10% of macroglobulins are cryoprecipitable. Most often, the bones are normal, but diffuse osteoporosis may be seen, and in rare instances lytic lesions develop. Almost 80% of the patients have a monoclonal light chain in the urine, but the amount is usually small. Elevation of serum viscosity is common, but most patients have no symptoms of hyperviscosity.

Differential Diagnosis

The combination of typical symptoms and physical findings, IgM monoclonal protein, and lymphoplasma cell infiltration of the bone marrow provides the diagnosis of Waldenström's macroglobulinemia. The major problem in the differential diagnosis centers around the distinction from multiple myeloma, chronic lymphocytic leukemia, lymphoma, undifferentiated lymphoproliferative disease, and monoclonal gammopathy of undetermined significance (MGUS) of the IgM type. To differentiate MGUS of the IgM class from early Waldenström's macroglobulinemia, the patient must be carefully observed for an indefinite period.

Treatment

Specific treatment should be directed against the abnormal proliferation of lymphocytes and plasma cells. Therapy should be withheld until the patient is symptomatic. Nucleoside analogs, fludarabine and 2-chlorodeoxyadenosine, produce response in more than 80% of patients previously untreated. Only one third of patients who are resistant to alkylating agents respond. Chlorambucil, in an initial daily oral dose of 6 to 8 mg, is a useful agent. The dosage of chlorambucil must be altered, depending on the results of leukocyte and platelet counts, which should be determined every 2 weeks.

Chlorambucil also may be given in a dosage of 0.3 mg/kg daily for 7 days plus prednisone in a dosage of 60 mg daily for the same 7-day period and repeated every 4 to 6 weeks. The dosage must be altered depending on the leukocyte and platelet levels. Cyclophosphamide or combinations of alkylating agents such as the M2 protocol (vincristine, BCNU, melphalan, cyclophosphamide, and prednisone) also have been beneficial. There have been no prospective studies comparing fludarabine or 2-CDA with chlorambucil. Chemotherapy should be discontinued when the patient's monoclonal protein level decreases and reaches a stable state and there is no other evidence of active disease. Transfusions of packed red blood cells should be given for symptomatic anemia. Erythropoietin may be of benefit for patients in the plateau state with symptomatic anemia. Patients must be followed up and treatment reinstituted in the event of relapse. The symptoms of hyperviscosity must be treated with vigorous plasmapheresis. The median survival is approximately 5 years after diagnosis.

HEAVY-CHAIN DISEASES
Gamma Heavy-Chain Disease

This lymphoplasma cell proliferative syndrome produces a monoclonal gamma heavy chain with extensive deletions of amino acids. The median age at diagnosis is approximately 60 years, although the condition has appeared before the age of 20 years. Patients with gamma heavy-chain disease usually have a lymphoma-like illness, although the clinical findings are diverse, ranging from an aggressive lymphoproliferative disease to an asymptomatic state. Hepatosplenomegaly and lymphadenopathy occur in about 60% of patients; anemia occurs in about 80%. Serum electrophoresis frequently shows no localized band or spike. Proteinuria consisting of gamma heavy chains is usually modest in amount. Increased numbers of plasma cells, lymphocytes, or plasmacytoid lymphocytes are seen in biopsy specimens of bone marrow and lymph node. Treatment is not indicated for the asymptomatic patient. The combination of cyclophosphamide, vincristine, and prednisone (CVP) that is useful in the treatment of lymphoma (Chapter 93) has been beneficial. If there is no response to this regimen, doxorubicin should be added (cyclophosphamide, doxorubicin, Oncovin, and prednisone [CHOP]).

Alpha Heavy-Chain Disease

The majority of patients with alpha heavy-chain disease are from the Mediterranean area and have involvement of the digestive tract with severe malabsorption, loss of weight, diarrhea, and steatorrhea. The duodenum and jejunum are almost always involved. The diagnosis is most often made in persons who are in the second and third decades of life, and approximately 60% of patients are men. The serum protein electrophoretic pattern is normal in half the cases; in the remainder, an unimpressive broad band may appear in the alpha₂ or beta region. Bence Jones proteinuria does not occur. The diagnosis depends on the recognition of a monoclonal alpha heavy chain. Immunoproliferative small intestinal disease or "Mediteranean" lymphoma is identical to alpha heavy-chain disease except for the absence of staining with alpha heavy-chain antisera. Most often, alpha heavy-chain disease is progressive and fatal, but responses occur with antibiotics or with chemotherapy, such as melphalan, cyclophosphamide, and prednisone.

Mu Heavy-Chain Disease

In mu heavy-chain disease, chronic lymphocytic leukemia or a lymphoma-like picture is most common. The presence of vacuolated plasma cells in the bone marrow may be a helpful finding. A stable, asymptomatic state also has been noted. The clinical spectrum of mu heavy-chain disease should broaden, as it has in gamma heavy-chain disease. Serum electrophoresis usually reveals hypogammaglobulinemia; a localized spike occurs in less than half of patients. Bence Jones proteinuria has been found in two thirds of patients. Treatment with alkylating agents and corticosteroids has produced some benefit. The course of mu heavy-chain disease is variable; median survival is approximately 2 years.

MONOCLONAL GAMMOPATHY OF UNDETERMINED SIGNIFICANCE (BENIGN MONOCLONAL GAMMOPATHY)

Serum monoclonal proteins have been found without evidence of myeloma, macroglobulinemia, amyloidosis, or related diseases in approximately 3% of persons more than 70 years of age in Sweden and the United States. Currently at the Mayo Clinic, of the patients with newly recognized monoclonal proteins, less than 20% have multiple myeloma, whereas more than one half have MGUS.

Of 241 patients with a monoclonal protein but no evidence of multiple myeloma, macroglobulinemia, amyloidosis, or lymphoma (benign monoclonal gammopathy) who were followed for more than 20 years, in 24.5% myeloma, macroglobulinemia, amyloidosis, or related diseases developed; 9.5% had an increased monoclonal protein concentration to more than 3 g/dl, but myeloma and macroglobulinemia did not develop; 47% died of unrelated causes; and only 19% had no increase in the monoclonal protein concentration and fulfilled the criteria for the diagnosis of benign monoclonal gammopathy.

The actuarial rate for the development of multiple myeloma, macroglobulinemia, amyloidosis, or a malignant lymphoplasma proliferative process at 10 years was 17% and was 33% at 20 years. There was no difference in the actuarial rate for development of serious disease with IgG, IgA, or IgM proteins.

The interval from the recognition of monoclonal gammopathy to the diagnosis of multiple myeloma ranged from 2 to 29 years (median, 10 years). After multiple myeloma was diagnosed, the median survival was 34 months. The median interval from the recognition of monoclonal gammopathy to the diagnosis of macroglobulinemia was 8 years, whereas the median interval from the recognition of monoclonal gammopathy to the diagnosis of systemic amyloidosis was 9 years.

Differential Diagnosis

Patients with MGUS have less than 3 g/dl of monoclonal protein in the serum and no or small amounts of Bence Jones proteinuria, less than 5% plasma cells in the bone marrow aspirate, and no anemia, hypercalcemia, renal insufficiency, or osteolytic lesions (unless caused by other diseases). The only basis for deciding that the patient has MGUS is the absence of an increase in the monoclonal protein concentration or the development of a lymphoplasma cell proliferative disease during long-term follow-up observation. The differentiation of benign monoclonal gammopathy from myeloma or macroglobulinemia may be difficult at the time when the monoclonal protein is found. The following may be helpful: the amount of the serum monoclonal protein, levels of normal polyclonal or background immunoglobulins, the presence and amount of Bence Jones proteinuria, the number of plasma cells in the bone marrow, the presence of osteolytic lesions, plasma cell labeling index, the serum beta$_2$ microglobulin level, the presence of J chains in plasma cells, and the presence of circulating plasma cells.

At the time of recognition of a monoclonal protein, patients in whom multiple myeloma and related disorders will develop cannot be differentiated from those with MGUS on the basis of age, sex, presence of organomegaly, the initial hemoglobin level, size of the serum monoclonal protein peak, IgG subclass type, levels of uninvolved immunoglobulins, serum albumin level, presence of small amounts of monoclonal light chain in the urine, and number of plasma cells in the bone marrow. The most reliable means of distinguishing a benign course from a malignant one is serial measurement of the monoclonal protein concentration. Periodic examinations must be performed to determine whether the disorder is benign or the initial manifestation of multiple myeloma, systemic amyloidosis, macroglobulinemia, or other malignant lymphoproliferative disorders.

Although MGUS frequently exists without any other abnormalities, certain diseases are associated with it, as would be expected in an older population. Therefore studies of such an association must include a control group to determine whether the association is merely a coincidence. Monoclonal proteins have been noted in lymphoma, leukemia, and a wide variety of hematologic conditions. Rheumatic diseases and neurologic disorders such as peripheral neuropathy have been seen. Lichen myxedematosus has frequently been noted with an IgG lambda monoclonal protein, whereas pyoderma gangrenosum is often associated with an IgA monoclonal protein.

The monoclonal protein may exhibit high specificities to dextran, antistreptolysin O, antinuclear activity, von Willebrand's factor, thyroglobulin, insulin, double-stranded DNA, apolipoprotein, thyroxin, various antibiotics, actin, calcium, and copper.

Biclonal Gammopathies

Two monoclonal proteins (biclonal) occur in approximately 4% of patients with a gammopathy. Electrophoresis often shows only a single localized band, and the second monoclonal protein is recognized only when immunofixation or immunoelectrophoresis is done. The most frequent combinations are IgG and IgA, followed in frequency by monoclonal IgG and IgM. The clinical findings are similar to those seen in monoclonal gammopathy, and most patients have biclonal gammopathy of undetermined significance. Approximately one third of patients have multiple myeloma, macroglobulinemia, or other malignant lymphoproliferative disease. Triclonal gammopathies have been found.

Cryoglobulins

Cryoglobulins are proteins that precipitate when cooled and dissolve when heated. To test for cryoglobulins, 5 ml of fresh centrifuged serum, kept at 37° C, is placed in a graduated centrifuge tube and incubated at 1° C (in an ice bath in a refrigerator or cold room) for 7 days. The precipitate is washed, and immunoelectrophoresis is performed.

Cryoglobulins may be classified as type I (monoclonal, consisting of IgG, IgM, IgA, or rarely, free light chains), type II (mixed, two or more immunoglobulins, of which one is monoclonal), or type III (polyclonal, no monoclonal protein found).

In most cases, monoclonal cryoglobulins are IgM or IgG, but IgA and Bence Jones cryoglobulins have been reported. Unexpectedly, many patients with large amounts of cryoglobulin are completely asymptomatic, whereas others with monoclonal cryoglobulin levels of 1 to 2 g/dl may, because of high thermal insolubility, have pain, purpura, Raynaud's phenomenon, cyanosis, and even ulceration and sloughing of skin and subcutaneous tissues on exposure to the cold.

✔ WHEN TO REFER

Patients with multiple myeloma or their variants, Waldenström's macroglobulinemia, or the heavy-chain diseases should be referred to a hematologist-oncologist or a tertiary medical center that has a special interest in these disorders. This is necessary for confirmation of the diagnosis and for outlining the course of therapy. Patients may fulfill the minimal diagnostic criteria for multiple myeloma or macroglobulinemia but have a smoldering or indolent process. These patients should be recognized and not treated because they may remain stable for many years. If it is not feasible to refer the patient, the physician should consult with a person or facility with expertise in the disease. Because multiple myeloma and the dysproteinemias are not curable diseases and since investigators are searching for better treatment, patients should be referred to a center where protocol studies are available. Prospective studies have led to more effective therapy over the years and will continue to do so.

Patients with MGUS (benign monoclonal gammopathy) are challenging because the presence of a monoclonal protein may indicate primary amyloidosis, early multiple myeloma, macroglobulinemia, lymphoproliferative disease, solitary or extramedullary plasmacytomas, or osteosclerotic myeloma syndrome (POEMS). If the patient has any features of these diseases, if other laboratory abnormalities are present, or if the monoclonal protein concentration is greater than 2.5 g/dL, the patient should be referred to a hematologist or an oncologist.

Cryoglobulinemia may produce a spurious elevation of the leukocyte count on the model S Coulter counter. Monoclonal cryoglobulins are associated with monoclonal MGUS (benign monoclonal gammopathy), macroglobulinemia, multiple myeloma, and lymphoproliferative disease.

Most commonly, mixed cryoglobulins (type II) consist of IgM-IgG, but IgG-IgG and IgA-IgG combinations have been reported. Usually, the quantity of mixed cryoglobulin is less than 0.2 g/dl and may not reach maximal amounts for 7 days. The serum protein electrophoretic pattern either is normal or shows diffuse hypergammaglobulinemia. Patients with mixed cryoglobulinemia frequently have vasculitis, glomerulonephritis, or lymphoproliferative or chronic infectious processes. Hepatic dysfunction and serologic evidence of previous infection with hepatitis C virus are common.

Type III (polyclonal) cryoglobulinemia is not associated with a monoclonal component. It is found in many patients with infections or inflammatory diseases and is of no clinical significance.

BIBLIOGRAPHY

Dimopoulos MA, Alexanian R: Waldenström's macroglobulinemia, *Blood* 83:1452, 1994.

Dimopoulos MA et al: Curability of solitary bone plasmacytoma, *J Clin Oncol* 10:587, 1992.

Durie BGM, Salmon SE: A clinical staging system for multiple myeloma: correlation of measured myeloma cell mass with presenting clinical features, response to treatment, and survival, *Cancer* 36:842, 1975.

Fermand JP, Brouet JC: Marrow transplantation for myeloma, *Annu Rev Med* 46:299, 1995.

Fermand JP et al: Gamma heavy chain "disease": heterogeneity of the clinicopathologic features—report of 16 cases and review of the literature, *Medicine* 68:321, 1989.

Gahrton G et al: Prognostic factors in allogeneic bone marrow transplantation for multiple myeloma, *J Clin Oncol* 13:1312, 1995.

Gregory WM, Richards MA, Malpas JS: Combination chemotherapy versus melphalan and prednisolone in the treatment of multiple myeloma: an overview of published trials, *J Clin Oncol* 10:334, 1992.

Kelly JJ Jr et al: Osteosclerotic myeloma and peripheral neuropathy, *Neurology (NY)* 33:202, 1983.

Kyle RA: Multiple myeloma: review of 869 cases, *Mayo Clin Proc* 50:29, 1975.

Kyle RA: 'Benign' monoclonal gammopathy: after 20 to 35 years of follow-up, *Mayo Clin Proc* 68:26, 1993.

Kyle RA, Garton JP: The spectrum of IgM monoclonal gammopathy in 430 cases, *Mayo Clin Proc* 62:719, 1987.

Kyle RA, Gertz MA: Second malignancies after chemotherapy. In Perry MC, editor: *The chemotherapy source book*, Baltimore, 1992, Williams & Wilkins.

Kyle RA, Greipp PR: Plasma cell dyscrasias: current status, *CRC Crit Rev Oncol Hematol* 8:93, 1988.

Kyle RA, Greipp PR: Smoldering multiple myeloma, *N Engl J Med* 302:1347, 1980.

MacLennan ICM et al: Combined chemotherapy with ABCM versus melphalan for treatment of myelomatosis, *Lancet* 339:200, 1992.

Noel P, Kyle RA: Plasma cell leukemia: an evaluation of response to therapy, *Am J Med* 83:1062, 1987.

Rambaud JC et al: Immunoproliferative small intestinal disease (IPSID): relationships with α-chain disease and "Mediterranean" lymphomas, *Springer Semin Immunopathol* 12:239, 1990.

Wahner-Roedler DL, Kyle RA: μ–Heavy-chain disease: presentation as a benign monoclonal gammopathy, *Am J Hematol* 40:56, 1992.

Westin J et al: Interferon alfa-2b versus no maintenance therapy during the plateau phase in multiple myeloma: a randomized study, *Br J Haematol* 89:561, 1995.

CHAPTER

95 Breast Cancer

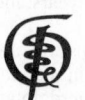

C. Kent Osborne

ETIOLOGY AND EPIDEMIOLOGY

Breast cancer is the leading cause of cancer death in women in the United States and Western Europe. In one of every nine women born in the United States breast cancer will develop during her lifetime. An estimated 182,000 new cases were detected in the United States in 1995, and an estimated 46,000 women die of the disease. Surpris-

ingly, breast cancer is the most common cause of death of disease in young women between the ages of 25 and 35, and the most common cause of death of all causes in women between the ages of 35 and 50. In older women breast cancer mortality rate is third only to death caused by cardiovascular disease and death from lung cancer. Recent trends suggest that, after increasing for decades, breast cancer mortality is now declining.

The cause of breast cancer is unknown, although various risk factors have been identified that provide clues to its genesis (Table 95-1). Hormonal regulation of the breast is clearly related to the development of breast cancer, but the mechanisms are poorly defined. Early menarche or late menopause prolongs exposure to estrogen and is associated with increased risk. Prolonged estrogen administration for menopausal symptoms is also associated with a slightly increased risk of breast cancer, although an increased risk has not yet been observed consistently with use of oral contraceptives. In contrast, early castration reduces the risk of breast cancer. Parity and age at the time of the first full-term pregnancy are also related to breast cancer risk. Early pregnancy reduces the incidence, whereas nulliparity and, especially, late pregnancy increase the risk. These data, together with studies in experimental model systems, suggest that sex steroid hormones may act as tumor promoters or cocarcinogens in concert with initiating agents to induce malignant change. For unclear reasons obese and/or tall women are at increased risk for breast cancer. This risk may relate to dietary or hormonal factors.

Living in Western societies also increases the risk of breast cancer. Specific factors have not been identified, although high dietary intake of fat and dairy products and/or high caloric intake has been implicated. Immigrants to the United States from areas of low breast cancer incidence have little change in incidence rates, but with succeeding generations the incidence rate approaches that of the U.S. female population.

Family history of breast cancer increases the risk to a variable extent. In first-degree relatives (mother, sister, or daughter) the risk is a function of whether the cancer was bilateral (5.4-fold increase) and whether it occurred during the premenopausal (3-fold increase) or postmenopausal (1.5-fold increase) period. The highest risk (8.8-fold increase) is observed in relatives of patients with bilateral breast cancer that develops in the premenopausal years. Obviously these women require careful monitoring because of the high risk of breast cancer development at a relatively young age.

Hereditary breast cancer, in which a germ-line mutation in a tumor-suppressor gene gives rise to increased susceptibility for breast

Table 95-1   Risk factors influencing the occurrence of breast cancer

RISK OF BREAST CANCER	FACTOR
Increased	Increasing age
	Early menarche
	Late menopause
	Nulliparity
	Late pregnancy (above age 30)
	Interrupted first pregnancy
	Western culture (? diet)
	Family history of breast cancer
	Benign breast disease with atypical epithelial hyperplasia
	Obesity
	Ionizing radiation
	Prolonged postmenopausal use of estrogens
	Prior diagnosis of breast cancer, colon cancer, endometrial cancer, major salivary gland cancer
	Alcohol intake
Decreased	Full-term pregnancy (before age 24)
	Early oophorectomy
No effect	Breast feeding (lactation)
	Oral contraceptive use
	Benign breast disease without epithelial hyperplasia

and other cancers, accounts for 10% of all breast cancers. Two genes, BRCA-1 and BRCA-2, have been identified, and genetic testing is now available. Patients who have these genes have an 85% lifetime risk of developing breast cancer.

BIOLOGY

The majority of breast carcinomas arise from large-, medium-, or small-sized duct epithelium. Tumors originating from duct epithelium but still confined to the duct lumen without invasion into adjacent stroma are called intraductal, or ductual carcinoma in situ (DCIS) tumors. These tumors rarely metastasize, and they have a high cure rate with local surgical therapy. Carcinomas invading adjacent stromal tissues are called infiltrating duct carcinomas. These tumors have a propensity for early metastasis and a worse prognosis.

The concept of how a primary breast carcinoma spreads to distant sites has changed during the past 20 years. In the late nineteenth century, when William Halsted developed the radical mastectomy, it was assumed that breast cancer spread through the lymphatics, under the skin, and along fascial planes to involve the regional lymph nodes first. The lymph nodes were thought to provide a temporary barrier to further dissemination. With these principles in mind, Halsted reasoned that "en bloc" dissection of the primary tumor, adjacent normal tissue, and the regional lymph nodes (radical mastectomy) would result in a high cure rate. It is now clear that the major contribution of this procedure was a reduction in the local-regional recurrence rate with little impact on overall survival rate. Recurrent disease in distant metastatic sites eventually develops in about half of all women with primary operable breast cancer and nearly 90% of those with significant numbers of axillary lymph nodes involved with cancer at the time of radical mastectomy, indicating early hematogenous dissemination of the tumor. Thus breast cancer is already a systemic disease in many women at the time of presentation. Ultimate survival of patients depends on the net interaction between tumor and host defense factors. This concept led to the development of two new alternative treatment strategies—conservative breast cancer surgery to improve the cosmetic result and adjuvant chemotherapy or hormonal treatment after local therapy to attempt to eradicate distant micrometastases.

The natural history of breast cancer varies considerably from patient to patient. The disease can be indolent and slowly progressive with about 5% of patients surviving 10 years even without treatment. In other patients the disease takes a fulminating, relentless course resistant to all therapy and resulting in death within a few months of diagnosis. Several variables have been recognized as important prognostic factors for individual patients. The most important prognostic marker is axillary lymph node status. The actual number of positive lymph nodes represents a continuum of rising risk for later recurrence of disease after mastectomy. Histopathologic evidence of the degree of tumor differentiation is another important prognostic factor. Tumors displaying morphologic features reminiscent of those of normal breast tissue (well differentiated) carry a lower risk of recurrence. Tumor size also correlates with risk of recurrence. Tumors less than or equal to 1 cm in diameter with no axillary node involvement have a 10-year recurrence rate of only 10% to 12%.

The presence of hormone receptors for estrogen and progesterone is biochemical evidence of tumor differentiation and indicates a relatively good prognosis. Abnormal deoxyribonucleic acid (DNA) content (aneuploidy) determined by flow cytometry reflects poor tumor differentiation and a higher risk for recurrence. An index of the proliferative potential of the tumor can be obtained by cell kinetic analysis to determine the fraction of cells in S phase of the cell cycle. Patients with high S-phase fraction tumors have a higher risk for recurrence and a shorter survival. Certain cellular oncogenes have also been identified in human breast cancer tissue. Amplification or overexpression of the c-erb B-1 oncogene, which codes for the membrane receptor for epidermal growth factor, or the related c-erb B-2 (HER-2/neu) oncogene is associated with a higher risk of recurrence after mastectomy. The latter may also predict for resistance to certain chemotherapy drugs. Knowledge of these prognostic factors is playing an increasing role in the design of appropriate therapy for the patient with breast cancer.

METHODS OF EARLY DETECTION AND SCREENING

Evidence suggests that the earlier a breast cancer is detected, the better the survival prospect of the patient. Preinvasive intraductal carcinomas are highly curable, and patients with small invasive cancers have a better survival rate than those with large tumors. Numerous methods have been developed to detect breast cancer at an early, potentially curable stage. However, the only screening method for asymptomatic women with documented survival benefit is mammography combined with regular physical examination of the breast by physician and patient. It is clear that this technique can detect cancers in the preinvasive and nonpalpable stage. Thermography, ultrasound, computed tomography (CT), magnetic resonance imaging (MRI), and diaphanography have not yet proved useful as screening tools and remain experimental. The widespread use of screening mammography has been controversial because of cost considerations and because of the potential for carcinogenesis with repeated exposure to radiation. However, with modern equipment and proper expertise the radiation dose to the breast is low, and the estimated carcinogenic risk is infinitesimally small relative to the natural risk of the disease. A prudent approach recommended by the American Cancer Society and the American College of Radiology is to obtain a baseline mammogram at age 35 and then to begin annual mammography in women after age 50. Women between the ages of 40 and 50 should be considered for periodic mammography every 1 or 2 years, depending on the presence of risk factors outlined in Table 95-1. Extremely high-risk women (multiple risk factors, previous breast cancer) may be considered for periodic mammography and close physician follow-up observation at an earlier age. In general, however, mammography is less useful in younger women because of increased breast density, and because the younger breast may be more susceptible to the carcinogenic effects of radiation. Furthermore, screening studies have not yet consistently demonstrated a significant reduction in mortality in women less than 50 years of age, although most of these studies were not specifically designed to evaluate benefit in this subset. Screening in this age-group remains a controversial issue. Decisions about routine screening should be made after a thorough discussion with the patient.

HISTOLOGIC FEATURES

Most breast cancers are infiltrating adenocarcinomas that arise from the ductal or lobular epithelium. Invasive duct or lobular carcinomas of no special type have similar prognoses, whereas medullary carcinoma, colloid carcinoma, tubular carcinoma, and papillary carcinoma have a much better prognosis. If the axillary nodes are not involved by tumor at diagnosis, these tumors have less than a 15% chance of recurrence at 10 years. These patients may not need adjuvant therapy. Paget's disease of the breast is characterized by eczematoid changes in the nipple caused by neoplastic involvement of the epidermis. Inflammatory carcinoma is an uncommon clinical entity characterized by extensive erythema, edema, and induration of the breast caused by invasion of the dermal lymphatics by tumor cells. Prognosis is so poor that it must be treated as a systemic disease even when it is apparently localized.

CLINICAL FEATURES

Breast cancer is frequently discovered by the patient as a painless mass in the breast. Although it may appear as a vague thickening in what is otherwise an area of physiologic nodularity, most carcinomas are hard and have an irregular border that can be relatively well defined. The term *dominant mass* is sometimes used to identify highly suspect lesions that have distinct character and margins. Breast pain, skin dimpling, nipple discharge, retraction, or erosions occasionally lead to diagnosis. Fixation of the cancer to the skin or pectoral fascia, skin edema or ulceration, satellite nodules, and presence of large axillary metastases are all signs of more advanced breast cancer and are uncommon at presentation. Rarely, patients show signs of metastatic disease without a palpable mass in either breast.

LABORATORY FEATURES

The diagnosis of breast cancer may be suggested by the presence of a hard, irregular dominant mass or by suspect mammographic findings. Confirmation of the diagnosis depends on histologic examination of tissue obtained by needle aspiration cytologic evaluation, needle biopsy, or incisional or excisional biopsy. With the advent of breast conservation surgery, the biopsy should be performed with the ultimate definitive therapeutic options in mind, so that appropriate tissue can be obtained without compromising the optimal cosmetic results and eliminating the need for repeated general anesthesia. Needle aspiration cytologic testing or core needle biopsy of palpable masses has become popular for patients desiring breast conservation. In experienced hands these techniques are accurate and rapid and can be done under local anesthesia on outpatients. Needle biopsy of nonpalpable lesions is often possible with ultrasound guidance or stereotactic mammography. Some lesions may require surgical excision after placement of a guide wire with mammography for localization.

Except when lesions are small (all such lesions should be sent for diagnostic pathologic examination), tumor tissue should always be sent for estrogen receptor (ER) and progesterone receptor (PgR) analyses. Knowledge of receptor status provides important prognostic information and serves as a guide to treatment strategy. Growing evidence also suggests that cell kinetic analysis by flow cytometry and oncogene expression by immunohistochemistry are helpful prognostic indicators. In the near future these techniques may be widely applied, although currently they should still be considered experimental.

Tumor markers measured in serum are not helpful in establishing the diagnosis of breast cancer. No markers specific for breast cancer have been discovered, and those currently available lack the sensitivity and specificity for early detection of disease. Carcinoembryonic antigen, the breast cancer–associated antigen CA 15-3, human chorionic gonadotropin, and ferritin levels are elevated in some patients with primary breast cancer and in the majority with metastatic disease and are sometimes helpful in monitoring response to therapy.

DIFFERENTIAL DIAGNOSES

Many benign lesions of the breast may mimic clinically the symptoms and signs of breast carcinoma (Box 95-1). Acute bacterial mastitis may easily be confused with inflammatory cancer. Fat necrosis may appear as a firm, irregular dominant mass. Mammary dysplasia usually presents diffuse changes (lumps) in the breast but may present a single suspect mass. Benign tumors can also be confused with carcinoma clinically. The majority of breast lumps prove to be benign, especially those in premenopausal women. Nevertheless, if there is any clinical question of the diagnosis, evaluation, including biopsy, should continue. Mammography and ultrasound are sometimes helpful in differentiating benign from malignant breast disease. It is important to emphasize, however, that suspect masses should receive biopsy evaluation even if the mammogram finding is unremarkable. Ten to twenty percent of cancers cannot be seen mammographically. Needle aspiration of suspected cysts is also helpful. If nonbloody fluid is obtained and the lump regresses with aspiration and does not re-

cur, the physician can be confident that the process is benign. The rare cystic carcinoma can sometimes be detected by cytologic evaluation of the cyst fluid. Solid dominant masses usually require definitive tissue diagnosis by aspiration cytologic examination, needle biopsy, or open excisional biopsy. These can be done as outpatient procedures. If the biopsy result is positive for carcinoma, a second definitive procedure can be planned after discussion with the patient. This two-step procedure is preferred to the older one-step operation in which women with suspect lumps went to the operating room for general anesthesia with biopsy, frozen section diagnosis, and definitive surgery. Many patients found this process psychologically debilitating. Patients with "lumpy" breasts who have associated breast cancer risk factors pose a difficult management problem. Regular breast self-examination coupled with frequent breast examination (two to three times per year), including detailed mapping of all lesions by an experienced physician, is required. Mammography may not be helpful in such patients because of the density of the breast tissue. Some patients require repeated biopsy procedures over a period of years to exclude malignant change.

STAGING AND PROGNOSIS

Once a histopathologic diagnosis of breast cancer has been established, the physician must determine the stage of the disease before planning therapy. Tables 95-2 and 95-3 summarize the relationship between the stage of disease and prognosis. The extent of staging before treatment of the primary tumor depends on the initial clinical stage of the patient. In a patient with clinical stage I and II disease without symptoms of metastases, mammography, complete blood cell count, and screening panel of blood chemical features (such as an

---

BOX 95-1
Differential diagnosis of breast mass

Inflammatory disease
   Acute bacterial mastitis
   Chronic mastitis
   Fat necrosis
Mammary dysplasia (benign breast disease)
   Adenosis
   Cystic disease
   Duct ectasia
Benign tumors
   Fibroadenoma
   Papilloma
Malignant tumors

Table 95-2 Survival of women with breast cancer relative to clinical stage

CLINICAL STAGING (AMERICAN JOINT COMMITTEE)	CRUDE 5-YEAR SURVIVAL (%)	RANGE OF SURVIVAL AT 5 YEARS (%)
Stage I	85	82-94
Tumor less than 2 cm in diameter		
Nodes, if present, not believed to contain metastases		
Without distant metastases		
Stage II	66	47-74
Tumors less than 5 cm in diameter		
Nodes, if palpable, not fixed		
Without distant metastases		
Stage III	41	7-80
Tumor more than 5 cm		
Tumor any size with invasion of skin or attached to chest wall		
Nodes in supraclavicular area		
Without distant metastases		
Stage IV	10	—
With distant metastases		

From Henderson I, Canellos GP: *N Engl J Med* 302:17, 1980.

Table 95-3 Survival of women with breast cancer relative to histologic stage (treatment with surgery only)

HISTOLOGIC STAGING (NATIONAL SURGICAL ADJUVANT BREAST PROJECT)	CRUDE SURVIVAL (%) 5-YEAR	CRUDE SURVIVAL (%) 10-YEAR	5-YEAR SURVIVAL (%)
All patients	63.5	45.9	60.3
Negative axillary lymph nodes	78.1	64.9	82.3
Positive axillary lymph nodes	46.5	24.9	34.9
1-3 positive axillary lymph nodes	62.2	37.5	50.0
More than 4 positive axillary lymph nodes	32.0	13.4	21.1

From Henderson I, Canellos GP: *N Engl J Med* 302:17, 78, 1980.

SMA-12) are sufficient. Chest x-ray, bone scan, and liver studies are not required unless symptoms or laboratory tests suggest metastases. For patients with clinical stage III or IV disease, bone scans are recommended, as well as any other tests required to assess symptoms or abnormal laboratory values. Bone marrow biopsy is generally unnecessary unless the patient has unexplained bone marrow dysfunction, such as the presence of anemia or nucleated red blood cells on the peripheral blood film.

TREATMENT OF LOCALIZED BREAST CANCER

Twenty-five years ago radical mastectomy was performed immediately after biopsy and frozen section diagnosis in the majority of women with primary localized breast cancer. With the change in our understanding of the mechanisms of breast cancer metastases and the recognition that survival is predetermined in most patients by distant micrometastases, clinical trials of more conservative, cosmetically appealing local therapies were initiated. Modified radical mastectomy has now become the most frequent operation performed in the United States in women with clinical stage I or II breast cancer. This procedure still involves en bloc removal of the breast and axillary contents, but the preservation of the pectoral muscles and the horizontal scar result in a more pleasant appearance of the upper chest wall. There is also convincing evidence now from retrospective studies as well as prospective randomized clinical trials that even less radical breast conservation procedures provide excellent local control without jeopardizing survival. Segmental mastectomy or lumpectomy involves excision of the breast mass, usually with a small rim of adjacent normal tissue. Axillary dissection must be done on all patients treated by breast conservation operations both for local control in the axilla and for pathologic staging purposes. Radiation therapy to the breast frequently with a "boost" dose to the area of excision is then given. With proper planning, patient selection, and technical expertise, these procedures can produce excellent cosmetic results. Patients with very large tumors, small breasts, or multicentric lesions identified by mammography are poor candidates for segmental mastectomy and are best treated by modified radical mastectomy followed by reconstructive surgery for optimum cosmetic results. Patients with active collagen vascular diseases are also poor candidates for breast irradiation because of increased risk of local complications. Despite extensive data indicating the safety of breast conservation, only 30% of patients in the United States have breast-sparing surgery compared to 50% to 65% in other industrialized countries. Most authorities now agree that postoperative chest wall and regional lymph node irradiation is not necessary for most patients undergoing modified radical mastectomy. Exceptions might be patients at very high risk for local recurrence such as those with tumor involvement at the margin of surgical resection, those with grossly involved axillary lymph nodes or many positive nodes, or those with large central or medial primary tumors with more than four positive axillary lymph nodes. Combined surgery plus irradiation is useful for local control in patients with more advanced stage III or IV primary tumors.

ADJUVANT CHEMOTHERAPY FOR PRIMARY BREAST CANCER

On the basis of the concept that breast cancer is frequently already a systemic disease at the time of diagnosis, which assumes that many patients with stage I and, especially, stage II disease have micrometastatic disease in occult sites, the practice of early administration of systemic therapy after surgery to eradicate micrometastases has evolved. This treatment, commonly called adjuvant chemotherapy, involves the administration of chemotherapy and/or endocrine manipulation in patients at high risk for early recurrence and poor survival. More than 100 clinical trials in both axillary node-positive, and node-negative patients have been completed in the past 25 years.

The first-generation studies now have a minimum of 20 years of patient follow-up observation, and several conclusions can be drawn. First, combination chemotherapy using two to five drugs together is superior to the use of single agents. Evidence suggests that aggressive therapy with high drug doses is required for optimal results. Second, the optimal duration of therapy has not yet been established for all regimens, although 6 months appears adequate for the popular

CMF regimen (cyclophosphamide, methotrexate, and 5-fluorouracil), and 3 to 4 months of doxorubicin regimens may suffice. Third, disease-free and overall survival rates are significantly improved by treatment, although many patients continue to relapse despite therapy. In the initial clinical trials, benefit of adjuvant chemotherapy was confined to premenopausal women. More recent trials, however, suggest that postmenopausal patients also benefit from adjuvant chemotherapy. In contrast, postmenopausal patients receive the most benefit from adjuvant endocrine therapy with the antiestrogen tamoxifen. Fourth, the ER and PgR status of the primary tumor may be useful in identifying high-risk patients requiring intensive therapy (receptor-negative) as well as patients who may benefit from the addition of endocrine therapy (receptor-positive). Clinical trials involving chemotherapy combined with endocrine therapy have shown no benefit for chemotherapy plus tamoxifen compared with either treatment alone in premenopausal patients. There is some evidence to suggest that the combined approach is superior in postmenopausal patients. Both node-negative and node-positive patients benefit from adjuvant treatment. An overview analysis of all randomized trials suggests that about one in five to one in four deaths at 10 years can be prevented by appropriate adjuvant therapy. The toxicity of adjuvant chemotherapy is acceptable: nausea, vomiting, alopecia, and myelosuppression are common but reversible, and death caused by drug toxicity is rare. Permanent ovarian dysfunction is an important long-term side-effect that occurs in many premenopausal patients. A very small increase in the risk of leukemia has been observed with some chemotherapy regimens, but the benefit in reducing breast cancer recurrence far outweighs this risk. The incidence of other solid tumors is not increased by chemotherapy. Commonly used adjuvant chemotherapy regimens are similar to those used for advanced disease and are shown in Table 95-4. Chemotherapy is now standard treatment for most premenopausal and certain postmenopausal patients with a sufficiently high risk of recurrence to warrant its use.

ADJUVANT ENDOCRINE THERAPY FOR PRIMARY BREAST CANCER

Many breast cancers, especially those containing the estrogen receptor protein, are stimulated by estrogen. Endocrine therapy designed to reduce estrogen levels in premenopausal patients (ovarian ablation)

Table 95-4   Commonly used chemotherapy regimens

REGIMEN	DOSE	SCHEDULE
CMF* (repeat every 28 days)		
C = cyclophosphamide	100 mg/m² PO	Days 1-14
M = methotrexate	40 mg/m² IV	Days 1 and 8
F = 5-fluorouracil	600 mg/m² IV	Days 1 and 8
CMFVP (continuous for 1 year)		
C = cyclophosphamide	60 mg/m² PO	Daily
M = methotrexate	15 mg/m² IV	Weekly
F = 5-fluorouracil	400 mg/m² IV	Weekly
V = vincristine	0.625 mg/m² IV	Weekly × 10 weeks only
P = prednisone	30 mg/m² PO	Days 1-14
	20 mg/m² PO	Days 15-28
	10 mg/m² PO	Days 29-42, then discontinue
AC (repeat every 21 days)		
A = Adriamycin	60 mg/m² IV	Day 1
C = cyclophosphamide	600 mg/m² IV	Day 1
FAC (repeat every 21 days)		
F = 5-fluorouracil	500 mg/m² IV	Days 1 and 8
A = Adriamycin	50 mg/m² IV	Day 1
C = cyclophosphamide	500 mg/m² IV	Day 1
A × 4 → CMF × 8 (started after the 4 cycles of A)		
A = Adriamycin	75 mg/m² IV	Day 1, every 21 days × 4
C = cyclophosphamide	600 mg/m²	Day 1, every 21 days × 8
M = methotrexate	40 mg/m²	Day 1, every 21 days × 8
F = 5-fluorouracil	600 mg/m²	Day 1, every 21 days × 8

*Prednisone is sometimes used at a dose of 40 mg/m² po days 1-14. The CAF regimen is identical except Adriamycin 30 mg/m² IV days 1 and 8 is substituted for methotrexate and F is reduced to 500 mg/m² IV days 1 and 8.

po, By mouth; *IV,* intravenously.

or to inhibit estrogen's effects by blocking ER (tamoxifen) has been studied in patients with primary breast cancer after surgery. Ovarian ablation reduces breast cancer mortality by 20% to 25%, similar to the benefit with chemotherapy in premenopausal patients. Current trials investigating medical castration are under way. Despite the favorable results, oophorectomy has not yet become a popular approach, perhaps because the database supporting its use is small compared with that for chemotherapy or tamoxifen. If the ongoing trials around the world confirm the positive results from the earlier studies, this ovarian ablation may become standard for certain subsets of patients.

The antiestrogen tamoxifen has been studied in more than 30,000 patients with primary breast cancer, and firm conclusions can be drawn. Tamoxifen reduces mortality by about 20% (1 in 5 deaths annually is avoided by treatment). The benefit is greater in patients with high ER-positive tumors. Patients with low ER-positive tumors may also receive a more modest mortality reduction (about 10%). Studies of treatment duration suggest that 5 years is optimal. Recently completed trials indicate that prolonging treatment beyond 5 years may not offer additional benefit. The incidence of contralateral breast cancer is reduced by 30% to 40% by tamoxifen adjuvant therapy. Other benefits include a reduction in cholesterol and maintenance of bone density. These surprising effects may be due to the estrogen-like qualities of tamoxifen in certain tissues. The most frequent side effects of tamoxifen are menopausal symptoms. Much like estrogen replacement therapy, the drug is also associated with a small risk of endometrial cancer requiring close monitoring by a gynecologist. Tamoxifen is now standard treatment for many postmenopausal and premenopausal patients with ER-positive tumors.

SYSTEMIC TREATMENT OF METASTATIC BREAST CANCER

The two major kinds of systemic therapy for the treatment of metastatic breast cancer are endocrine manipulation and cytotoxic chemotherapy. Other systemic therapies, such as immunotherapy or whole body hyperthermia, remain experimental. Similarly, the use of cytotoxic drugs combined with endocrine therapy has not yet proved superior to the sequential administration of each modality and thus should be avoided. Tables 95-4 to 95-6 list the endocrine therapies and cytotoxic regimens most commonly used in the treatment of advanced breast cancer. Choosing between endocrine therapy and cytotoxic chemotherapy requires an understanding of the natural history of the disease and careful evaluation of the individual patient. The hormone receptor status of the patient's tumor is of paramount importance in making this choice. Only about 30% of all breast cancers are hormone dependent and respond to endocrine therapy. Hormone

manipulation is unlikely (less than 10% response rate) to benefit a patient whose tumor lacks ER or PgR. If the tumor is ER-positive, the patient has a 50% chance of responding. If the tumor has a high concentration of ER and/or also contains PgR, the chance of response is increased to 70% to 80%. Patients with receptor-positive tumors also tend to have a more indolent course with prolonged survival, and they have a predominance of bone and soft tissue metastases compared to those with ER-negative tumors, who have frequent visceral metastases and shorter survival. Care must be taken in interpreting the receptor assay results. False-negative values may arise from assay of very small tissue biopsy specimens, or from hormone receptor occupancy in patients taking exogenous estrogens, or in premenopausal patients with high endogenous progesterone levels during the luteal phase of the menstrual cycle.

A variety of other factors, in addition to the hormone receptor status of a tumor, may affect the choice of therapy. These factors include the length of time between removal of the original primary tumor and its recurrence (disease-free interval), site of metastatic disease, age of patient, and response to previous therapy. For example, it is widely recognized that a short disease-free interval (less than 2 years) between primary treatment and subsequent metastatic disease is associated with a rapidly growing tumor. Such patients tend to respond poorly to hormonal manipulation and may be more appropriately treated with cytotoxic chemotherapy. Conversely, a very long disease-free interval is often associated with a better response to hormonal manipulation than to cytotoxic chemotherapy. The site of metastatic disease may influence the choice of systemic treatment. Metastatic disease in the soft tissues, skin, regional lymph nodes, pleural space, or bone may respond well to endocrine manipulation, whereas metastatic tumor involving abdominal visceral organs or the brain rarely responds to such treatment. Endocrine manipulation may be especially effective in elderly women, whereas cytotoxic chemotherapy tends to be poorly tolerated by this group of patients. A good response to oophorectomy or other hormonal manipulation is also useful in predicting a good response to other kinds of endocrine treatment. Indeed, patients may pass successively from one form of endocrine manipulation to another when the disease is relatively indolent and restricted to either soft tissues or bone.

Before specific programs of treatment are discussed, several general principles underlying the management of patients with disseminated breast cancer must be stressed. First, cure is not possible with current treatment modalities, so optimal palliation with the least toxicity is the primary therapeutic goal. Second, only one form of therapy at a time is employed. An exception to this rule is irradiation of a

Table 95-5   Cytotoxic regimens useful in the treatment of advanced breast cancer

	OBJECTIVE RESPONSE RATE (%)
Single agents	
Cyclophosphamide	34
Methotrexate	34
5-Fluorouracil	26
Phenylalanine mustard	22
Chlorambucil	20
Vincristine	21
Vinblastine	40
Doxorubicin	35
Mitomycin-C	21
Taxol	50
Taxotere	50
Combinations*	
CMF	34-62
CMFP	63
CMFVP	48-73
FAC	43-82

*C, cyclophosphamide; M, methotrexate; F, 5-fluorouracil; P, prednisone; A, Adriamycin (doxorubicin).

Table 95-6   Endocrine therapies useful in the treatment of advanced breast cancer

THERAPIES	DOSE
Additive therapy	
Estrogens	
Diethylstilbestrol	5 mg po, tid
Ethinyl estradiol	1 mg po, tid
Antiestrogens	
Tamoxifen	10 mg po, bid
Toremefene	60 mg po, qd
Progestins	
Megestrol acetate	40 mg po, qid
Androgens	
Fluoxymesterone	10 mg po, tid
Aromatase inhibitors	
Aminoglutethimide plus hydrocortisone	250 mg po, qid 20 mg pohs, 10 mg po AM and PM
Arimidex	1 mg po, qd
Ablative therapy	
Oophorectomy	
Zoladex	3 mg sc, q month
Lupron	7.5 mg IM, q month

*bid, Twice daily; IM, intramuscularly; po, by mouth; pohs, by mouth at bedtime; q, every; qid, four times a day; sc, subcutaneous; tid, three times daily.

destructive lesion in a weight-bearing bone in combination with other modalities of treatment. Third, therapy is changed only if the disease is advancing, not if it is static or regressing. This approach is especially important in patients with bone metastases only, because such lesions are notoriously difficult to evaluate. Fourth, endocrine therapy might even be considered in ER- or PgR-negative patients despite the small chance of benefit, especially in the elderly patient or the patient with indolent disease who cannot tolerate or who is no longer responsive to chemotherapy. Endocrine therapy should be considered for initial therapy in most receptor-positive or receptor-unknown patients, unless life-threatening visceral metastases are present. Fifth, after initiating endocrine therapy, patients should be observed for a minimum of 6 to 12 weeks. Tumor regression may be quite delayed in certain patients. Sixth, patients failing an initial course of endocrine therapy usually should be considered to have endocrine-unresponsive tumors that require chemotherapy. An exception to this rule is the patient with an indolent receptor-positive tumor that is not life-threatening. About 20% of such patients may respond to a second attempt at hormone manipulation. In contrast, patients responding to an initial course of hormone therapy should be considered for sequential second- or third-line therapies when the disease progresses. Such patients have an excellent chance for additional responses, although the duration of remissions tends to become shorter with each treatment. Initial responses generally last from 10 months to 2 years; occasional patients have remissions lasting many years. Seventh, newer forms of endocrine therapy such as antiestrogens or aromatase inhibitors have largely replaced the need for the more radical major ablative procedures of surgical adrenalectomy and hypophysectomy. Eighth, some patients demonstrate a transient "flare" in their disease with hypercalcemia or increased bone pain during the first 2 weeks of additive hormonal therapy. Therapy should not be stopped in such patients (unless the flare is life-threatening); patients should be observed and symptoms controlled, and many enjoy tumor regression with continued therapy.

ENDOCRINE MANIPULATION

Menopausal status determines the precise type of endocrine therapy for patients whose tumors are known to be ER-positive and those whose receptor status is unknown. The initial choice of endocrine manipulation is commonly called primary hormonal manipulation. Subsequent manipulation is called secondary or even tertiary therapy. Doses of drugs for these regimens are summarized in Table 95-6.

Premenopausal Patients

Patients who are menstruating or who have appropriate serum levels of estrogen and gonadotropins are considered premenopausal.

Primary Endocrine Manipulation. Bilateral oophorectomy is still an acceptable initial therapy in premenopausal patients with metastatic disease who are candidates for endocrine therapy. This treatment is presumed to work by the ablation of ovarian estrogen and estrogen precursors that may stimulate the growth of breast cancer. Oophorectomy causes objective regression in approximately one third of all premenopausal women. The response rate is approximately 50% in those who have ER-positive disease and less than 10% in those who have ER-negative disease. Castration can also be achieved medically with the use of superagonists or antagonists of luteinizing hormone-releasing hormone. These agents may supplant surgical castration in the future when comparative studies are completed.

Some clinicians consider the antiestrogen tamoxifen to be preferable to oophorectomy as initial treatment. The frequency of response to tamoxifen is similar to that of oophorectomy. Patients who fail to respond to tamoxifen are less likely to benefit from oophorectomy. Thus tamoxifen may represent an effective initial therapy that may be supplemented subsequently by oophorectomy in responding patients whose disease progresses later.

Secondary Endocrine Manipulation. Patients who do not respond to oophorectomy usually proceed to treatment with cytotoxic drugs. Those who respond to oophorectomy and then relapse may respond to tamoxifen. An alternative in this setting is an aromatase in-

hibitor such as aminoglutethimide or the newer, less toxic, Arimidex. This therapy further reduces serum estrogen levels in postmenopausal patients (surgical or natural) by inhibiting the enzyme aromatase, which converts androgens to estrogens in peripheral tissues. This regimen may also be used as tertiary therapy in patients responding to tamoxifen. Other effective secondary or tertiary therapies use megestrol acetate or fluoxymesterone. Patients who no longer respond to endocrine manipulations or in whom rapidly progressing visceral disease develops are candidates for chemotherapy.

Postmenopausal Patients

Patients whose last menstrual period occurred more than 1 year before the development of metastatic disease are considered postmenopausal. A subgroup of patients who are 1 to 5 years postmenopausal may also be identified as perimenopausal.

Primary Endocrine Manipulation. The initial treatment of choice for most postmenopausal women with metastatic breast cancer who are candidates for endocrine manipulation is tamoxifen or toremefene, a similar antiestrogen agent. A response rate of 16% to 52% has been reported, with an average of 32% for unselected women. In patients with ER-positive tumors the response rate is approximately 50%. Conversely, fewer than 10% of ER-negative tumors respond. In the past, diethylstilbestrol (DES) was used to treat these patients. However, tamoxifen is less toxic than DES and has largely supplanted the older agent.

Secondary Endocrine Manipulation. Patients who respond to tamoxifen and then experience a relapse are candidates for secondary endocrine manipulation. Aromatase inhibitors, megestrol acetate, DES, or androgens are effective secondary and/or tertiary therapies. The choice of treatment is partially dependent on the individual patient and the relative toxicities of the agents. Younger women may reject androgen therapy because of the virilizing effects. Elderly patients, especially those with cardiovascular disease, are not good candidates for DES because of fluid retention and other cardiovascular side effects.

CHEMOTHERAPY

Cytotoxic chemotherapy is the initial treatment of choice for most patients with ER-negative tumors or individuals who have aggressive, life-threatening disease, regardless of receptor status. In patients with receptor-positive or receptor-unknown tumors, chemotherapy is withheld until the patient is shown to be refractory to endocrine treatment. Although partial responses can be obtained frequently with cytotoxic chemotherapy in advanced breast cancer, complete responses are uncommon, and chemotherapy rarely induces a long-term disease-free state.

Single Agents

A variety of single agents with different mechanisms of action and different toxicities are effective in this disease (see Table 95-5). Among the most active and frequently used agents are doxorubicin (Adriamycin), cyclophosphamide, methotrexate, and 5-fluorouracil. Single agents usually induce remission durations of only a few months, and complete remissions are rare. Taxol and Taxotere are new agents with response rates approaching 50%.

Combination Chemotherapy

Combination chemotherapy was developed on the rationale that combining agents with different mechanisms of action and different toxicities might increase the response rate without increasing morbidity. It has had considerable success, particularly in the hematologic malignancies. Combination chemotherapy for advanced breast cancer has been studied extensively since 1969, when Cooper reported a high response rate to the five-drug combination of cyclophosphamide, methotrexate, 5-fluorouracil, vincristine, and prednisone (CMFVP). This report generated numerous clinical trials testing CMFVP or a modification of it against single agents. In general, the response rate, particularly the complete response rate, is higher for the combination regimens (Table 95-6). However, clear survival advantage has not been consistently demonstrated for the combination regimens compared to that for sequential use of the same agents except in patients with extensive visceral involvement. Nevertheless, combination chemotherapy has become standard for the initial treatment of advanced breast cancer in this country. Although there are numerous modifications of the original CMFVP regimen, no major differences in response rate or duration exist. Objective response rates range between 34% and 73%, and median response durations are consistently less than 1 year. Complete response rates average about 15%. Side-effects of these regimens include transient bone marrow suppression, occasional mucositis, alopecia, and nausea and vomiting. Doses of drug are modified according to individual patient characteristics and toxicity encountered. Cytotoxic drugs should be given only by physicians experienced in their administration. Commonly used regimens are described in detail in Table 95-4.

The introduction of doxorubicin (Adriamycin) is considered to be a major advance by some oncologists. However, the incorporation of this agent into combination regimens (such as FAC) has failed to achieve a significant improvement in response rate, response duration, or duration of survival, despite its high activity as a single drug (Table 95-6). Nausea, vomiting, and alopecia are more severe with the Adriamycin regimens, and cardiac toxicity is a potential dose-limiting problem. There are no convincing data demonstrating that one combination regimen is superior to another in advanced breast cancer.

Patients who fail initial combination chemotherapy or who are not candidates for this more aggressive approach may be treated with single agents used alone in sequence. The use of drug combinations as second-line treatment offers no proven advantage. In general, secondary chemotherapy for advanced breast cancer is of modest benefit: responses usually last no more than a few months. The use of high-dose chemotherapy with autologous bone marrow transplantation in the treatment of metastatic and high-risk primary breast cancer is now under investigation. Patients should not be treated with this approach outside a clinical trial.

INTEGRATION OF TREATMENT MODALITIES

The management of breast cancer is in a state of flux; recommendations must be made within the context of the results of current therapeutic research. The evolving nature of the situation makes for some disagreement among experienced physicians about the specific management of some patient groups. In addition, it should be remembered that each patient has a distinct socioeconomic and psychologic background, spectrum of associated organ dysfunctions, and stage of disease activity. The tumor may also be distinctive in terms of the rate of growth, areas of dominant disease, and presence or absence of estrogen and progesterone receptors. The experienced physician individualizes therapy when appropriate. Nevertheless, it is useful to have a generalized approach to treatment as a guide. Figure 95-1 presents one such scheme.

PSYCHOLOGIC FACTORS AND REHABILITATION

Through the Reach to Recovery Program, the American Cancer Society has pioneered efforts to help the woman who has undergone mastectomy adjust to an altered body image. Breast reconstruction should also be considered in some patients who are not candidates for breast conservation procedures to augment psychologic adaptation. Whatever approach to rehabilitation is chosen, it is critical to employ a sensible and attentive manner in dealing with a patient's emotional concerns. Most patients do adjust, but the speed of adjustment can be markedly influenced by an attentive and sensitive physician.

MALE BREAST CANCER

Breast cancer in men is rare, comprising less than 1% of all breast carcinomas. The fact that men have approximately 1% as much breast tissue as women suggests that the difference in incidence of breast cancer in men and women may relate to the volume of tissue susceptible to neoplastic change. There are multiple reports of familial male breast cancer, and altered estrogen metabolism has been proposed as a possible etiologic factor. However, with the exception of idiopathic

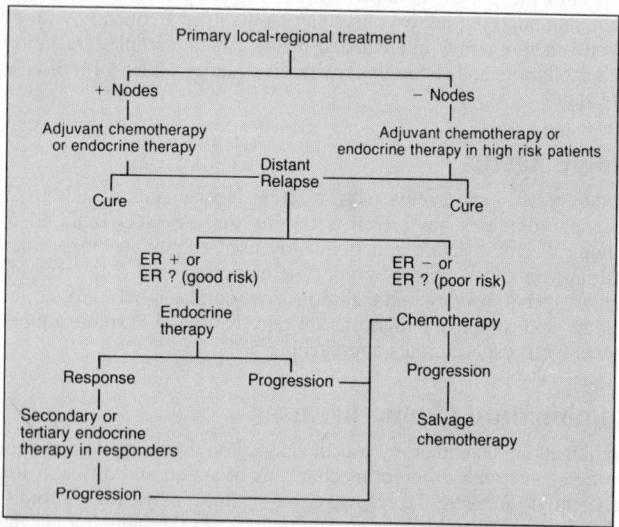

FIGURE 95-1   A sequential program of treatment for women with breast cancer. Key: + *Nodes,* regional lymph nodes contain metastatic carcinoma; − *Nodes,* regional nodes free of tumor; *ER +,* the tumor contains estrogen receptor in its cytoplasm; *ER −,* the tumor has either very low or no detectable estrogen receptor; *Er ?,* estrogen receptor status is unknown.

Modified from Haskell CM, Sparks FC, Thompson RW. In Haskell CM, editor: *Cancer treatment,* Philadelphia, 1980, WB Saunders.

> ✔ *WHEN TO REFER*
>
> Patients with a suspicion of breast cancer based on physical findings or on mammography should be sent to a surgeon with experience and expertise in diagnosing and treating breast disease. These specialists are best suited to plan the appropriate diagnostic and therapeutic approaches in the most efficient manner. This is preferable even in centers where mammographically directed sterotactic biopsies are available. A physician experienced in breast disease may conclude that a biopsy at that time is unnecessary or that a different type of biopsy procedure would be optimal in a particular case. At the time of breast cancer diagnosis, it is often helpful for the patient to also be seen by a medical oncologist and sometimes a radiation oncologist—especially if breast preservation surgery is being considered. The management of breast cancer is multidisciplinary, and it is useful to obtain opinions prior to definitive surgery. Adjuvant chemotherapy or tamoxifen should be administered only by experienced medical oncologists. It is optimal for the surgeon and medical oncologist to follow patients on a long-term basis often in concert with the internist in order to detect recurrent or new contralateral breast cancers at their earliest stage. The medical oncologist will by necessity usually become the patient's primary physician after she develops metastatic breast cancer. The sequential therapies required in such patients are complicated and require considerable experience and judgment.
>
> A history suggestive of familial or hereditary breast cancer should always be sought. Although hereditary breast cancer only accounts for 10% of all breast cancer, it is important to recognize potentially affected families so that relatives can be appropriately evaluated. Clues to hereditary breast cancer are the following: breast cancer occurring at a young age (<40 years of age), breast and/or ovarian cancer in multiple family members, or bilateral breast cancer. Such patients are candidates for genetic testing for BRCA-1 and BRCA-2 when the tests become widely available in conjunction with appropriate screening, genetic counseling, and prevention programs.

gynecomastia and Klinefelter's syndrome, predisposing conditions for the development of male breast cancer are poorly defined.

Numerous reports have confirmed a high frequency of estrogen receptors and progesterone receptors in male breast cancer tissue. Furthermore, the disease mimics female breast cancer in histologic features, clinical presentation, and tendency to metastasize to bone. Therapeutic considerations are also similar, although complete concordance does not exist. Specifically, it would appear that men with breast cancer should be treated with endocrine manipulation as the initial approach, even in fairly advanced disease. Primary endocrine manipulation in the male generally consists of orchiectomy or a luteinizing hormone–releasing hormone agonist to cause medical castration. As an alternative, one may consider tamoxifen and, less frequently, androgens or DES. Although few data exist, combination chemotherapy seems to provide the same benefit to men as to women.

BIBLIOGRAPHY

Bonadonna G, Valagussa P: Chemotherapy of breast cancer: current views and results, *Int J Radiat Oncol Biol Phys* 9:279, 1983.

Bonadonna G et al: Ten-year experience with CMF-based adjuvant chemotherapy in resectable breast cancer, *Breast Cancer Res Treat* 5:95, 1985.

Clark GM et al: Progesterone receptors as a prognostic factor in stage II breast cancer, *N Engl J Med* 309:1343, 1983.

Early Breast Cancer Trialists' Collaborative Group: Effects of radiotherapy and surgery in early breast cancer: an overview of the randomized trials, *N Engl J Med* 333:1444-1455, 1995.

Early Breast Cancer Trialists' Collaborative Group: Systemic treatment of early breast cancer by hormonal, cytotoxic, or immune therapy, *Lancet* 339:1, 71, 1992.

Fisher B et al: The pathology of invasive breast cancer: a syllabus derived from findings of the National Surgical Adjuvant Breast Project (protocol no. 4), *Cancer* 36:1, 1975.

Fisher B et al: Ten year results from the National Surgical Adjuvant Breast and Bowel Project (NSABP) clinical trial evaluating the use of L-phenylalanine mustard (L-Pam) in the management of primary breast cancer, *J Clin Oncol* 4:929, 1986.

Fisher B, Anderson S, Redmond CK et al: Reanalysis and results after 12 years of follow-up in a randomized clinical trial comparing total mastectomy with lumpectomy with or without irradiation in the treatment of breast cancer, *N Engl J Med* 333:1456-1461, 1995.

Fletcher SW, Black W, Harris R et al: Report of the International Workshop on Screening for Breast Cancer, *J Natl Cancer Inst* 85:1644-1656, 1993.

Harris JR, Lippman ME, Veronesi U, Willett W: Breast cancer. I. *N Engl J Med* 327:319-328, 1992.

Harris JR, Lippman ME, Veronesi U, Willett W: Breast cancer. II. *N Engl J Med* 327:390-398, 1992.

Harris JR, Lippman ME, Veronesi U, Willett W: Breast cancer. III. *N Engl J Med* 327:473-480, 1992.

Ingle JN et al: Randomized clinical trial of diethylstilbestrol versus tamoxifen in postmenopausal women with advanced breast cancer, *N Engl J Med* 304:16, 1981.

Kelsey JL, Gammon MD: The epidemiology of breast cancer. *CA Cancer J Clin* 41:146-165, 1991.

Kopans DB: Screening for breast cancer and mortality reduction among women 40-49 years of age, *Cancer* 74:311-322, 1994.

Miki Y, Swensen J, Shattuck-Eidens D et al: A strong candidate for the breast and ovarian cancer susceptibility gene BRCA1, *Science* 266:66-71, 1994.

Osborne CK et al: Modern approaches to the treatment of breast cancer, *Blood* 56:745, 1980.

Osborne CK et al: The value of estrogen and progesterone receptors in the treatment of breast cancer, *Cancer* 46:2884, 1980.

Osborne CK, Clark GM, Ravdin PM: Adjuvant systemic therapy of primary breast cancer. In Harris JR, Lippman ME, Morrow M, Hellman S, editors: *Diseases of the breast*, New York, 1996, Lippincott-Raven.

Santen RJ et al: Aminoglutethimide as treatment of post-menopausal women with advanced breast carcinoma, *Ann Intern Med* 96:94, 1982.

able to these diseases. Coordination of care by a gynecologic oncologist, an individual specifically trained to operate on, administer chemotherapy to, and manage the surgical and medical complications experienced by women with cancer of the reproductive tract, is an important component of the comprehensive care of these women.

ENDOMETRIAL CANCER
Relevant Physiology and Pathophysiology

Among cancers of the female genital tract, adenocarcinoma of the endometrium is the most common and is also associated with the best overall survival rate. It is primarily a disease of postmenopausal women, although one fourth of cases are diagnosed in premenopausal women.

This neoplasm has been associated with a number of different risk factors (Box 96-1), many of which are associated with excessive stimulation of the endometrium by estrogen. However, this cancer also occurs in women who do not exhibit any of these risk factors, suggesting that other variables are also operative in the pathogenesis of this disease.

Painless postmenopausal vaginal bleeding, regardless of the amount or duration, is the sentinel warning sign of endometrial cancer. Premenopausal and perimenopausal women may have menstrual irregularities and intermenstrual spotting. Advanced-stage disease is often associated with anemia secondary to vaginal bleeding, inguinal adenopathy, lymphedema, and deep venous thromboses of the lower extremities, urinary retention resulting from suburethral metastases, and weight loss.

Laboratory and Diagnostic Tests

The symptom of abnormal vaginal bleeding should always prompt further evaluation. A pelvic examination is performed in an effort to localize the site of bleeding. A Papanicolaou (Pap) smear should be obtained, although this test is not specific for endometrial cancer. Endometrial cancer cells are detected in only approximately 50% of cervical cytology specimens obtained from women with endometrial cancer. Endometrial biopsy, which is routinely performed as an office procedure, should always be part of the diagnostic evaluation of abnormal vaginal bleeding. This procedure compares favorably with formal uterine dilation and curettage performed in the operating room in terms of diagnostic accuracy, sensitivity, and specificity.

After the histologic diagnosis of endometrial cancer, chest radiography is performed to provide a baseline study and to exclude metastatic disease. Because the patient who has uterine cancer is at increased risk of breast cancer, mammograms should be obtained. In addition, patients with any change in bowel habits or those with stools positive for occult blood should undergo evaluation of the colon because the risk of colon cancer is also increased in patients with endometrial cancer.

Differential Diagnosis

The differential diagnosis for abnormal vaginal bleeding includes pregnancy-related complications, disorders of the cervix, irregular uterine bleeding secondary to hormonal disturbances, and bleeding

---

96 Gynecologic Cancers

Vicki V. Baker

Cancers of the endometrium, cervix, and ovary are diagnosed in approximately 68,000 women each year and result in 22,000 cancer-related deaths. Cancer screening, prompt recognition of symptoms, and advances in therapy have reduced the number of deaths attribut-

---

BOX 96-1

Risk factors for endometrial cancer

Obesity
Unopposed estrogen hormone replacement therapy
Diagnosis of colon cancer
Diagnosis of breast cancer
Chronic anovulation
Low parity
Late menopause
Complex atypical hyperplasia of the endometrium

Table 96-1   Staging and 5-year survival rate in endometrial cancer

STAGE	DESCRIPTION	5-YEAR SURVIVAL (%)
I	Tumor confinement to uterine corpus	75
II	Tumor extension to endocervix or cervical stroma	55
III	Tumor extension to uterine serosa, retroperitoneal node biopsies positive for metastatic disease, vaginal metastases, positive peritoneal cytologic findings	30
IV	Tumor invasion of the bladder or bowel or presence of distant metastases	10

BOX 96-2
Current recommendations concerning cervical cancer screening

Annual Papanicolaou smears after age 18 or the onset of sexual activity, whichever occurs first

After three consecutive normal smear results, subsequent screening is based on the presence of risk factors for cervical dysplasia/neoplasia

"At-risk" patients should be screened annually

Low-risk patients should be screened every 3 years

---

from the bladder, urethra, and anus that is mistaken for vaginal bleeding by the patient.

Management

The staging and primary treatment of endometrial cancer are surgical, consisting of abdominal hysterectomy, bilateral salpingo-oophorectomy, and selected biopsies of pelvic and paraaortic lymph nodes. Peritoneal washings should be obtained for cytologic study. Radiation therapy as primary treatment is reserved for patients who are not surgical candidates.

Prognosis is directly related to stage of disease (Table 96-1). Other prognostic indicators include steroid hormone receptor status, ploidy, S-phase fraction, and overexpression of the HER-2/neu protooncogene by the malignant cells. After surgery, recommendations for additional therapy are based on the presence of high-risk factors such as poorly differentiated or deeply invasive neoplasms, positive surgical margins, metastatic disease, and positive peritoneal cytologic results.

In an effort to control extrauterine pelvic disease, whole pelvic radiation therapy, consisting of 45 to 50 Gy, is administered over a 4- to 5-week period in an outpatient setting. Chemotherapy is reserved for patients with distant metastatic disease and for those who have recurrence after radiation therapy. Single-agent chemotherapy is associated with modest response rates of variable duration. Clinical responses in as many as 42% of patients treated with cisplatin (50 mg/m^2 intravenously (IV) once every 3 weeks) have been reported. Doxorubicin (Adriamycin) (50 mg/m^2 IV once every 3 weeks) is associated with an objective response rate of 37%. 5-Fluorouracil (1000 mg/m^2 IV once every 3 to 4 weeks) is associated with a response rate of 23%, and cyclophosphamide (Cytoxan) (1000 mg/m^2 IV once every 3 to 4 weeks) induces a response rate on the order of 21%. There is no evidence that combination chemotherapy is superior to single-agent therapy. Although complete response rates may be achieved with aggressive chemotherapy in a small number of patients who have advanced or recurrent disease, this rarely translates into curative therapy.

Hormonal therapy with high-dose progestational therapy, such as megestrol acetate (Megace) (80 mg by mouth twice daily) or antiestrogen therapy with tamoxifen (20 mg by mouth twice daily) may benefit patients with metastatic disease. Response rates of 13% to 42% are reported, although this therapy is not considered curative.

CERVICAL CANCER
Relevant Physiology and Pathophysiology

Invasive cervical cancer is preceded by a premalignant phase, cervical dysplasia. The transit time between the premalignant and malignant conditions is estimated to be 5 to 10 years in most cases. This interval, which gives ample opportunity for therapeutic intervention, in addition to accessibility of the cervix for inspection and testing, has contributed to the decline in the number of deaths resulting from invasive cervical cancer.

Risk factors for cervical cancer include young age at first sexual encounter, multiple male partners, or a male partner with multiple consorts. These observations provide circumstantial evidence that cervical cancer is a sexually transmitted disease. The identification of specific subtypes of human papillomavirus (HPV), which is a sexually transmitted disease, in a significant proportion of both dysplastic and neoplastic lesions of the cervix has strengthened this hypothesis. Although it has been postulated that HPV alone is the causative agent of cervical dysplasia and neoplasia, there is no conclusive evidence to support this contention. In addition, the dramatic increase in HPV infections of the cervix noted during the past decade has not been accompanied by a parallel increase in the number of premalignant and malignant lesions, suggesting that other causative factors contribute to the development of neoplastic cervical disease. Potential cofactors include the mutagens found in cigarette smoke that are selectively concentrated in cervical mucus, nutritional deficiencies, and the use of oral contraceptives. Alterations of the host immune system also appear to play an important role in predisposing patients to the development of cervix dysplasia and neoplasia. For example, renal transplant patients exhibit a 40-fold increased risk of cervical cancer, emphasizing the need for periodic gynecologic examinations and Papanicolaou smears in these patients. There are also recent reports suggesting that the incidence of cervical dysplasia and neoplasia may be increased in patients infected with human immunodeficiency virus (HIV).

Laboratory and Other Diagnostic Tests

Largely as a result of effective cervical cancer screening programs using the Papanicolaou smear, the goal of which is premalignant disease detection, the incidence of invasive cervical cancer and the number of deaths attributable to this disease have demonstrated a steady decline over the past two decades. Current recommendations by the American College of Obstetricians and Gynecologists concerning the frequency of Papanicolaou smear screening are provided in Box 96-2.

To obtain a Papanicolaou smear, an unlubricated speculum is inserted into the vagina to expose the cervix. An Ayre spatula is rotated 360 degrees around the cervix to sample ectocervical cells, which are then promptly smeared onto a clean glass slide. A cytobrush is inserted into the endocervical canal and rotated to collect endocervical cells, which are also transferred to a glass slide. Once the cells are placed on the slide, they must be promptly fixed to prevent drying artifact.

A Papanicolaou smear is considered adequate when sufficient numbers of endocervical cells and squamous cells are present. The diagnosis of cytologic abnormalities is based on alterations in cell morphologic character, size, and nuclear appearance. The nomenclature for cervical cytologic reports is detailed in Table 96-2. Although the Papanicolaou smear currently provides the best cancer screening test available, a variable percentage of cases of dysplasia and carcinoma is not detected. Improper preparation of the smear, inaccurate interpretation, and presence of inflammatory cells or red blood cells that obscure visualization of the cervical cells contribute to false-negative results. It is important that any suspicious-appearing lesion on the cervix receive biopsy evaluation, regardless of the cervical cytologic finding report.

Table 96-2   Nomenclature for cervical cytologic reports

BETHESDA SYSTEM	WORLD HEALTH ORGANIZATION SYSTEM
Normal	Normal
Reactive or reparative changes	Atypia
Squamous epithelial abnormality of undetermined significance	Dysplasia
Low-grade intraepithelial lesion (includes mild dysplasia and HPV)	Mild
	Moderate
	Severe
High-grade intraepithelial lesion (includes moderate and severe dysplasia and carcinoma in situ)	Carcinoma in situ
	Invasive squamous cell carcinoma
Squamous carcinoma	Adenocarcinoma
Glandular cell abnormalities	

HPV, Human papillomavirus.

Treatment of dysplasia is never based solely on the results of a Papanicolaou smear. Colposcopy with directed biopsies of the cervix must first be performed to obtain a histologic diagnosis. Colposcopy involves inspection of the cervix at fourfold to sixfold magnification after the application of 3% acetic acid solution to the cervix. Biopsy specimens should be obtained from areas demonstrating abnormal vascular patterns such as punctation and mosaicism, as well as areas of white epithelium, all of which are often associated with dysplastic epithelial changes. In addition, an endocervical curettage is performed to evaluate the endocervical canal for the presence of dysplasia. To formulate a treatment plan after the diagnosis of invasive cervical carcinoma, the extent of disease must first be determined. In addition to a careful pelvic examination to assess the palpable extent of disease, select radiographic tests are helpful. A radiograph of the chest is obtained to detect pulmonary metastases. An intravenous pyelogram is performed to detect hydronephrosis or a nonfunctioning kidney, either one of which indicates advanced-stage disease. Patients with large lesions that extend anteriorly beneath the bladder or posteriorly toward the rectosigmoid should be further evaluated by cystoscopy and sigmoidoscopy, respectively. Although computed tomography (CT) and magnetic resonance imaging (MRI) studies provide additional information about the extent of disease, this information is not incorporated into the clinical staging system currently used for cervical cancer (Table 96-3).

Both cervical dysplasia and early invasive carcinoma of the cervix are asymptomatic conditions. Patients with more advanced disease may have vaginal discharge, postcoital spotting, and intermenstrual spotting. Patients with disease beyond the cervix may have profuse vaginal bleeding, malodorous vaginal discharge, unilateral lower extremity edema or pain, and weight loss. Uremia secondary to bilateral ureteral obstruction caused by advanced disease extension into the paracervical tissue is not uncommon.

Management

After histologic confirmation of the diagnosis of dysplasia, the treatment options include cryotherapy, laser vaporization, excision of the transformation zone, and hysterectomy. The location and extent of the lesion seen at the time of colposcopy and the patient's wishes concerning future fertility determine which option(s) is appropriate.

In general, cervical cancer is treated with radiation therapy. Whole pelvic radiation, consisting of 50 to 60 Gy, is given in 1.8- to 2-Gy fractions per day, 5 days a week for 4 to 5 weeks. Intracavitary irradiation, in which radioactive sources are placed in close proximity to the cervix and parametriae, is also incorporated into the treatment plan.

Patients with small lesions confined to the cervix, who are surgical candidates, may be treated by radical hysterectomy and pelvic lymphadenectomy. These patients exhibit comparable 5-year survival rates to those who are treated with radiation therapy.

After completion of therapy, patients should be seen at 3- to 4-month intervals for the first 2 years, followed by visits at 6-month

Table 96-3   FIGO staging and 5-year survival in cervical cancer

STAGE		DESCRIPTION	5-YEAR SURVIVAL (%)
0		Carcinoma in situ	100
I		Carcinoma confined to uterus	90
	Ia	Preclinical invasive carcinoma, diagnosed by microscopy	
	Ia1	Minimal stromal invasion	
	Ia2	Invasion <5mm in depth and <7 mm horizontally	
	Ib	Any lesion >Ia2	
II		Carcinoma beyond uterus, but not to sidewall or to lower third of vagina	70
	IIa	No parametrial invasion	
	IIb	Parametrial invasion	
III		Carcinoma to sidewall or to lower third of vagina	44
	IIIa	Tumor extension to lower third of vagina, but not to pelvic sidewall	
	IIIb	Tumor extension to pelvic sidewall or hydronephrosis or nonfunctioning kidney	
IV		Distant disease or invasion into adjacent organs	<14
	IVa	Tumor invasion of bladder or rectum	
	IVb	Distant metastases	

FIGO, International Federation of Gynecology and Obstetrics.

intervals for the next 3 years. At each visit, a careful physical examination, including pelvic examination and Papanicolaou smear, should be performed. The value of periodic chest radiographs, intravenous pyelograms, and CT has not been established.

Recurrent disease is most commonly diagnosed in the first 2 years after completion of therapy. Treatment options are determined by the location and extent of the recurrence and the patient's general medical condition. Recurrent disease in the nonirradiated pelvis is treated with radiation therapy with salvage rates of 30% to 40%.

When radiation therapy is not an option, recurrent disease in the pelvis that is surgically resectable may be treated by pelvic exenteration, in which the uterus, cervix, vagina, bladder, and rectosigmoid are removed. Although the morbidity and mortality rates of this operation are appreciable, it represents the patient's only realistic chance for cure.

Treatment of metastatic and recurrent, surgically unresectable disease with cisplatin chemotherapy (50 to 100 mg/m^2 IV every 3 weeks) is associated with response rates that range from 10% to 30%, but cures are anecdotal. Most patients die within 1 year of the diagnosis of metastatic disease.

The 5-year survival of cervical cancer is directly related to stage of disease at the time of diagnosis (Table 96-3). Implementation of Papanicolaou smear testing has been the single greatest advance in the management of this disease, permitting disease diagnosis in premalignant stages when the cure rates approach 100%.

OVARIAN CANCER
Relevant Physiology and Pathophysiology

Ovarian cancer holds the distinction of being the most lethal gynecologic cancer. Approximately 17,000 new cases of ovarian cancer were diagnosed in 1993, and 12,000 women died of this disease. A woman's cumulative lifetime risk of development of ovarian cancer is 1 in 76. Epithelial ovarian cancer, which is the most common histologic type, is generally a disease of postmenopausal women, although this cancer is also diagnosed in women during the third and fourth decades of life. The use of oral contraceptives is associated with a decreased risk of ovarian cancer. Factors associated with increased risk of epithelial ovarian cancer include low parity, delayed childbearing, and diagnosis of breast cancer. Hereditary factors increase the risk of ovarian cancer in a small subset of women. Approximately

5% of women with ovarian cancer can be classified by a currently recognized inherited ovarian cancer syndrome.

Less common ovarian neoplasms include germ cell and stromal cell tumors of the ovary. Germ cell tumors usually occur in prepubescent and adolescent patients with the exception of dysgerminoma, which is more common in the third decade. Stromal cell tumors are diagnosed in reproductive age and postmenopausal women.

Survival in ovarian cancer is clearly a function of stage of disease (Table 96-4). The disparity between 5-year survival rate of women with stage I and II disease and that of those with stage III and IV disease provides the rationale for the development of effective methods of early disease detection. As a cancer screening method, pelvic examination is insensitive and nonspecific. Although transabdominal and transvaginal ultrasound are useful radiographic tests that aid in the differentiation of benign and malignant pelvic masses, the applicability of these tests to cancer screening in the general population has not been demonstrated. Similarly, ovarian cancer screening tests based on measurement of serum tumor antigens such as the CA125 antigen, which is produced by over 85% of nonmucinous epithelial neoplasms of the ovary, exhibit sensitivities and specificities that are unacceptably low, given the limited prevalence of ovarian cancer in the general population. At this time, no screening strategies for ovarian cancer have been endorsed as public health policy.

Differential Diagnosis

No pathognomonic signs are associated with early-stage neoplasms of the ovary. The detection of asymptomatic, early-stage ovarian cancer is usually serendipitous. Patients with advanced-stage ovarian cancer typically have a variety of nonspecific signs and symptoms, including abdominal distention, early satiety, nausea and vomiting, and weight loss.

The differential diagnosis of an ovarian mass is in part determined by the patient's age, although considerable overlap occurs (Table 96-5). In general, young girls are at risk for malignant germ cell tumors and postmenopausal women are at risk for epithelial neoplasms. However, ovarian cancer of virtually every cell type has been diagnosed in girls and women of all ages.

Laboratory and Other Diagnostic Tests

The radiographic characteristics of the mass also assist in the preoperative differentiation of benign versus malignant masses. In general,

malignant epithelial ovarian neoplasms are bilateral, exhibit cystic and solid components, and may be associated with ascites. The CA125 antigen value is typically elevated in most women with advanced-stage nonmucnous epithelial ovarian cancer. It is important to recognize that this test is not particularly useful in premenopausal women who have a pelvic mass, since elevated values may also occur in the presence of endometriosis and uterine leiomyomata.

Management

The cornerstone of therapy for women with ovarian cancer is surgery, consisting of abdominal hysterectomy, bilateral salpingo-oophorectomy, omentectomy, surgical staging, and resection of all obvious disease. Because of the low incidence of bilaterality, unilateral adnexectomy and surgical staging without hysterectomy may be appropriate for patients with germ cell tumors when future fertility is of concern.

Regimens for germ cell tumors include vincristine-actinomycin D-cyclophosphamide, vinblastine-bleomycin-cisplatin, and bleomycin-VP16-cisplatin.

With the exception of stage I, well-differentiated ovarian neoplasms in patients who have undergone a thorough and complete staging operation, malignant epitheial ovarian neoplasms require additional therapy after surgery. Taxol and platinum-based combination chemotherapy is the first-line regimen that is typically offered to women with advanced-stage epithelial ovarian cancer.

Response to chemotherapy is assessed by monitoring of serum tumor marker levels when applicable, in addition to pelvic examination before each cycle of therapy. The use of radiographic studies such as CT and MRI must be individualized. Second-look laparotomy to assess response to chemotherapy is generally reserved for patients participating in clinical research protocols.

Germ cell tumors were once considered uniformly lethal, but the administration of aggressive combination chemotherapy has resulted in striking improvements in prognosis. Although there is some reason for cautious optimism for the patient diagnosed with a germ cell tumor, that is not generally the case for the patient with epithelial ovarian cancer. Despite aggressive, multiagent chemotherapy, most women with advanced-stage ovarian cancer have persistent or recurrent disease. Although a variety of agents are used to treat these women, response rates are modest, ranging from 20% to 35%, and cures are rare. Death is usually the result of starvation secondary to a carcinomatous ileus.

Table 96-4   Staging and 5-year survival rate for epithelial ovarian cancer

STAGE	DESCRIPTION	5-YEAR SURVIVAL RATE (%)
I	Carcinoma limited to ovaries	55
II	Carcinoma with extension to pelvis	40
III	Carcinoma with implants outside the pelvis or positive retroperitoneal nodes	5
IV	Distant metastases (positive pleural effusion, lung metastases, hepatic parenchymal metastases)	<5

✔ WHEN TO REFER

Causes of abnormal vaginal bleeding must always be definitively diagnosed. Any patient with a known or suspected cancer of the female reproductive system should be referred to a gynecologic oncologist for evaluation and treatment planning. A gynecologic oncologist is the only specialist trained in both women's health care in general and the comprehensive management of gynecologic cancer.

Table 96-5   Differential diagnoses of ovarian masses with respect to age

NEONATE	PREPUBESCENT/ADOLESCENT	REPRODUCTIVE AGE	POSTMENOPAUSAL	MASSES ARE
Simple cyst	Mature teratoma (dermoid) Cystadenoma	Functional cyst Endometrioma Mature teratoma	Fibroma Thecoma Cystadenoma	Benign
Primary ovarian cancer very rare	Germ cell tumors	Epithelial ovarian neoplasm Germ cell tumors Sex cord/stromal tumors	Epithelial ovarian neoplasm	Malignant

BIBLIOGRAPHY

DiSaia PJ, Creasman WT, editors: *Clinical gynecologic oncology,* St Louis, 1993, Mosby.

Lindahl B: Endometrial carcinoma: current concepts and future perspectives, *Crit Rev Oncol Hematol* 10:315, 1990.

NIH Consensus Conference: Ovarian cancer: Screening, treatment, and follow-up—NIH Consensus Panel on Ovarian Cancer, *JAMA* 273:491-497, 1995.

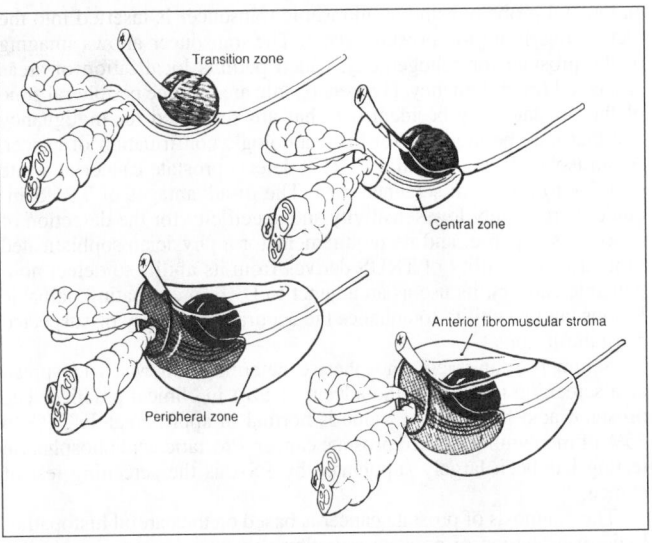

FIGURE 97-1   Zonal anatomy of the prostate from the work of McNeal. Benign prostatic hypertrophy occurs most often in the transition zone, while most prostate cancer arises in the peripheral zone.

From Greene DR et al: Urologic ultrasonography. In Walsh PC, Retik AB, Stamey TA, Vaughan ED, editors: *Campbell's urology,* ed 6, Philadelphia, 1992, WB Saunders.

97 Cancer of the Prostate and Testis

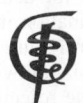

Geoffrey R. Weiss

PROSTATE CANCER

The primary care internist is likely to be confronted with an abnormal finding on digital rectal examination of the prostate gland or an elevated prostate-specific antigen value during the routine examination of patients. The frequency of prostate cancer in the general population and the sensitivity of prostate cancer to medical therapy warrant a review of its management for the internist. An estimated 334,500 cases of prostate cancer will be discovered in 1997, and 41,800 deaths are expected in the same year. As a consequence, prostate cancer represents the second most common cause of cancer (behind skin cancer) and the third most common cause of cancer death (behind lung cancer and colorectal cancer) in males in the United States.

Relevant Physiology and Pathophysiology

Male gender and age are the most important risk factors for prostate cancer. Although extraordinarily rare in men under the age of 40, prostate cancer reaches a prevalence of 10% in men during the sixth decade of life and nearly 40% by the ninth decade. However, most prostate cancer is occult; only 1% to 2% of men in the ninth decade of life annually manifest clinical evidence of new prostate cancer. Ambient plasma androgen concentrations appear to correlate with the incidence of prostate cancer. Castrated men, men with chronic liver disease who have elevated levels of plasma estrogen, and men with inborn defects of dihydrotestosterone production have lower or negligible risks of prostate cancer. Plasma testosterone concentrations appear to account in part for racial differences in prostate cancer incidence. Black men have the highest incidence of prostate cancer worldwide, American white men have intermediate risk, and Asian men the lowest risk; these trends in risk correlate with racial differences in inherent androgen concentrations.

The histopathologic precursor for prostate cancer is prostatic intraepithelial neoplasia (PIN) or carcinoma in situ. Benign prostatic hyperplasia (BPH) is not a risk factor for prostatic malignancy. Benign prostatic hyperplasia occurs most commonly within the prostate transition zone, a superficial and relatively small proportion of the gland near the prostatic urethra (Fig. 97-1). In contrast, PIN and prostate cancer most often arise within the peripheral zone of the gland, the largest component of the gland located near the base of the gland and extending to its apex. More than 95% of prostate cancers are adenocarcinomas originating from the glandular acinae and their proximal ducts; tumors arising from these structures are typically responsive to hormonal therapy. The less common histopathologic types of prostate cancer include small cell cancer, carcinoid tumors, adenoid-cystic cancer, mucinous cancer, and sarcomas, which are not typically sensitive to hormonal therapies.

The most useful clinical-pathologic system for classifying prostate cancer is the Gleason grading system (Fig. 97-2). The surgical pathologist examining the biopsied or resected prostatic adenocarcinoma evaluates the primary or dominant degree of differentiation of the tumor and the secondary or next most common degree of differentiation of the tumor. A score (1 to 5) is applied to each of these areas of tumor, and the scores are added. The sum of the scores provides the most consistent assessment of prognosis, with a higher score correlating with a greater frequency of mortality. More recent work has sought to associate other biologic characteristics of prostate carcinomas with clinical behavior and prognosis. Excess DNA content (ploidy); abnormalities of chromosomes 7, 8, 10, or 12; and expression of oncogenes or mutated tumor suppressor genes are beginning to yield important leads to the understanding of prostate cancer carcinogenesis, prognosis, and tumor biology.

Laboratory and Other Diagnostic Tests

Recent advances have been made in the clinical screening for prostate cancer. Because prostate cancer frequently occurs as an occult condition, may be curable when still localized to the gland, and remains resistant to cure when locally advanced (extending beyond the capsule of the gland) or metastatic to pelvic lymph nodes, distant organs, or bones, there is strong motivation to improve the early detection capability. Annual digital rectal examination (DRE) and serum prostate-specific antigen (PSA) determination remain the chief components of screening recommendations by the American Urological Association and the American Cancer Society. Onset of screening is recommended for all men over the age of 50 years. For black men and men with a family history of prostate cancer, onset of screening is recommended at age 40.

DRE is a simple procedure whose sensitivity for prostate cancer is 86% but whose specificity is only 44%. The rate of detection of prostate cancer by DRE alone in asymptomatic men ranges from 0.2% to 2.2%.

PSA is a serine protease found exclusively in benign and malignant prostate tissue. Elevation of serum PSA may occur in BPH, inflammation or infection of the prostate, or prostate cancer. PSA elevations above 10 ng/ml usually reflect malignant disease of the gland and are rarely observed in individuals with benign conditions. PSA determination with a value of 4 ng/ml as an upper limit of normal provides a 79% sensitivity and a 59% specificity for the detection of prostate cancer. The rate of detection of prostate cancer using PSA determination alone in asymptomatic men is 2.2% to 2.6%. Estimates of PSA concentration in prostatic tissue (PSA density), the rate of rise of PSA values over time (PSA velocity), or the creation of age-specific normal reference ranges for PSA may have greater discriminatory value for cancer detection, particularly for men with PSA values in the troublesome range of 4 to 10 ng/ml.

Transrectal ultrasound (TRUS) is a screening method whereby an endorectal probe housing an ultrasonic transducer is inserted into the rectum overlying the prostate gland. The transducer allows imaging of the prostate for echogenicity, which permits localization of areas suspected for malignancy. Hypoechogenic areas in the peripheral zone of the prostate may be identified that are suspected for malignancy and that may be biopsied for histopathologic confirmation of cancer. As an isolated screening tool, TRUS detects prostate cancer at a rate of 1.7% to 20.6% in screened men. The disadvantages of TRUS include its relatively low sensitivity and specificity for the detection of cancer, its expense, and its requirement for a physician sophisticated in its use. The utility of TRUS derives from its ability to detect non-palpable cancers, its use as an adjunct to DRE in evaluating palpable lesions, and its ability to enhance the accuracy of biopsy of suspected prostatic lesions.

Serum prostatic acid phosphatase determination was widespread as a screening test before the advent of PSA in clinical practice. The prostatic acid phosphatase value is normal in approximately 57% to 75% of men with localized prostate cancer. Prostatic acid phosphatase testing has been largely supplanted by PSA as the screening test of choice.

The diagnosis of prostate cancer is based on the careful histopathologic examination of prostate resection specimens or specimens collected from prostate biopsy. In the examination of tissue obtained from patients with suspected localized prostate cancer, Gleason scoring should be sought (Fig. 97-2). The probability of extension of cancer beyond the prostatic capsule and into pelvic lymph nodes increases with increasing Gleason score. Once the diagnosis of pros-

tate cancer is confirmed by histopathologic examination, noninvasive evaluation of the patient for metastatic disease should be conducted. The radionuclide bone scan is the most sensitive method for the detection of bone metastases, the most common site of extrapelvic advanced disease in the prostate cancer patient. Plain x-rays of bone in areas showing uptake of radionucliude should be obtained, particularly if in weight-bearing sites or if correlated with pain. Metastasis to visceral or solid organs is relatively uncommon in prostate cancer, whereas metastases to pelvic and abdominal lymph nodes is a frequent route of dissemination. In the 25% of men with metastatic prostate cancer who have pulmonary metastases, routine chest x-ray is a useful procedure. Chest x-ray may not only delineate pulmonary abnormalities but may also detect bone metastases. Computed tomography (CT) and magnetic resonance imaging (MRI) are relatively expensive, low-yield, and insensitive screening procedures for detecting advanced prostate cancer at these sites. PSA determination may be used in the therapeutic management of prostate cancer. Failure of an elevated preoperative PSA value to decline to normal following prostate resection is strong indirect evidence of incomplete resection or disseminated disease. Serial PSA determinations allow the clinician to assess the progress of the patient with disseminated disease receiving systemic therapy.

Differential Diagnosis

The principal diagnostic mandates for the practitioner who screens patients for prostate cancer are (1) differentiation of prostate cancer from benign prostatic disease and (2) detection of prostate cancer when it is still localized to the gland, a clinical circumstance most amenable to curative therapy. The greatest diagnostic dilemma is presented by the asymptomatic patient with elevated PSA values. Benign prostatic hyperplasia and acute or chronic prostatitis may elevate the PSA. Indeed, up to 20% of men with biopsy-proven BPH may have abnormal PSA levels. In addition, some experts believe that occult prostate cancer detected by elevated PSA values may be biologically unaggressive and represent little threat to survival. Nevertheless, the PSA determination remains at the heart of accepted screening practice for prostate cancer. In the event that PSA alone is elevated, TRUS is recommended. If TRUS examination is normal, random biopsies of the prostate are often performed if the PSA level is greater than 4 ng/ml. If TRUS examination reveals abnormal (hypoechoic) areas, directed biopsies of these areas are performed. If biopsies do not reveal cancer, follow-up with annual PSA determination and DRE is continued.

Annual PSA screening should be performed in conjuction with DRE. DRE may detect 16% to 20% of prostate cancers in men whose PSA level is normal. In any circumstance in which a suspected palpable prostatic abnormality is perceived, TRUS and biopsy should be sought. Such abnormalities may include a nodule in one or both lobes of the prostate, asymmetry of the prostate, or induration of a lobe of the prostate. It is a daunting realization that up to 50% of apparently localized palpable abnormalities of the prostate ultimately shown to be cancer will be upstaged and extend beyond the capsule of the gland.

The presence of prostatic symptoms offers little assistance in differentiating patients with BPH from those with prostate cancer. PSA and DRE have some value in making this distinction. Cancer is more probable in men with elevated PSA levels or a palpable abnormality of the prostate. The emergence of symptoms of bone pain, weight loss, renal dysfunction, or anemia has little diagnostic value for prostate cancer. If prostate cancer is demonstrated in the setting of these symptoms, advanced, incurable disease is the rule.

Management

There is no known preventive therapy of prostate cancer. A large national cooperative trial of the daily administration of finasteride, an inhibitor of 5α-reductase which converts testosterone to the multifold more potent dihydrotestosterone, is currently in progress. The study seeks to determine whether finasteride reduces the prevalence of biopsy-proven prostate cancer in men 55 years of age or older who have taken the drug for 7 years.

The election of specific therapy for prostate cancer requires the histopathologic diagnosis of the disease. Because the therapies of

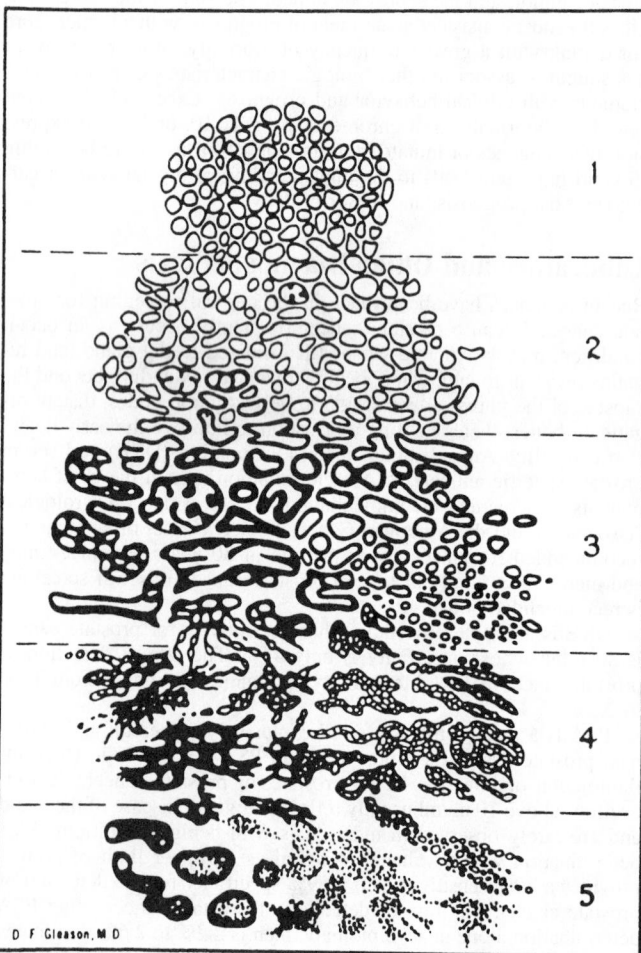

FIGURE 97-2   Drawing by Gleason of the grading system assigned to histologic patterns of prostatic carcinoma differentiation. Cytologic detail has been removed to highlight the histologic pattern of tumor and its relation to prostate stroma.

From Gleason DF: Histologic grading of prostatic adenocarcinoma. In Tannebaum M, editor: *Urologic pahology: the prostate,* Philadelphia, 1977, Lea & Febiger.

prostate cancer may induce important disabilities or toxicities, the ensurance of the presence of malignancy is paramount. In addition, the occasional identification of atypical forms of prostate cancer (e.g., sarcomas or small cell tumors) may warrant the avoidance of hormone ablation therapies in favor of other management approaches.

It is important that the management of prostate cancer is linked to the presenting stage of the disease (Tables 97-1 and 97-2). In general, surgery or radiation therapy is applied to disease that is still confined to the prostate gland. For cancer that has transgressed the capsule of the gland, spread to pelvic lymph nodes, or disseminated to bone or other organs, hormonal ablation or systemic chemotherapy is often used. For patients anticipating receipt of local therapy for prostate cancer, staging pelvic lymphadenectomy is recommended. This procedures has no intrinsic therapeutic value but provides important evidence of disease dissemination to pelvic (obturator and iliac) lymph nodes and ultimately to occult distant sites.

Patients commonly have clinically occult prostate cancer detected on pathologic examination of tissue obtained during transurethral resection of the prostate for BPH (T_{1a} or T_{1b}; stage A) or following needle biopsy of the prostate following elevated PSA level (T_{1c}; stage A).

For stage A1 (T_{1a}) prostate cancer, progression of disease is infrequent and removal of the prostate has not been shown to provide a survival benefit. Observation is a reasonable approach in such individuals unless the patient is young (<60 years of age). If the patient is otherwise expected to live many additional years, radiation may eradicate microscopic residual disease.

For stage A_2/B (T_{1b}, T_{1c}, T_2) prostate cancer, radical prostatectomy and irradiation (external beam with or without interstitial therapy) are essentially equivalent therapies. Adequate comparisons of radiotherapy versus surgery that provide convincing evidence of survival differences in balanced patient samples have not been performed. Both therapies can cause substantial morbidities: prostatectomy is accompanied by risks of anesthesia and surgical complication, urinary incontinence, and/or sexual impotence; radiation may induce prolonged proctitis, cystitis, urethral stricture, and/or sexual impotence. Procedures with potentially less morbidity and results equivalent to prostatectomy or external beam radiotherapy include transperineal brachytherapy or cryosurgery. Data about long-term overall and disease-free survivals for these latter techniques are pending. In addition, these techniques require comparison in clinical trials to the standard management of early-stage prostate cancer before they may be accepted as a standard of care.

Stage C (T_3) prostate cancer represents a substantial therapeutic predicament for the treating physician. Attempted radical prostatectomy often reveals evidence of extracapsular extension of cancer (pathologic stage C). Clinical examination of the prostate may also suggest extracapsular extension (clinical stage C). The best therapy for this stage is unknown, and local therapies are regarded as beneficial to a minority of such patients, since most are destined to relapse. Surgery appears to have limited effectiveness in this setting due to a high frequency of positive surgical margins following attempted resection.

Radiation is not uncommonly applied to patients with stage C cancer, either alone or as adjunct to surgical resection. Hormonal ablation is frequently employed, particularly in the elderly individual for whom surgical management or radiation therapy risks serious morbidity.

Stage D_1 (any T, N_{1-3}) is characterized by the presence of metastases to pelvic lymph nodes. The detection of pelvic lymph node metastases defines an expectation of disseminated prostate cancer within 5 years. Currently controversy exists about the need for early or delayed therapy in patients with stage D_1 disease. It has not been definitively shown that patients have any detrimental survival outcome with delay of hormonal ablation therapy until the appearance of disseminated disease. Consequently, expectant observation is a common approach following pelvic lymphadenectomy and detection of lymph node metastasis.

Stage D_2 prostate cancer encompasses metastatic disease to all extrapelvic sites. This stage of cancer is classically managed in its initial phases with androgen ablation. Bilateral orchiectomy remains the standard against which all alternative hormone ablation methods are compared. The advantages of orchiectomy include accomplishment of androgen ablation with a single procedure, immediate effect, and avoidance of continued therapy to sustain its effectiveness. No competing ablative therapy has been shown to exceed orchiectomy for long-term effectiveness. As an alternative, prostate cancer patients with metastatic disease may elect "total androgen blockade" (Table 97-3). Total androgen blockade utilizes a parenterally administered luteinizing hormone–releasing hormone (LHRH) agonist (goserelin acetate or leuprolide acetate) plus an orally administered antiandrogen (flutamide or bicalutamide). The LHRH agonist diminishes LH and follicle-stimulating hormone blood levels and ultimately yields castrate blood levels of androgens. The antiandrogens block androgen receptors and thereby block the modest androgenic contribution from adrenal hormone synthesis. Although the major hormone ablation therapies may accomplish dramatic tumor regression, symptom

---

Table 97-1   TNM staging system for prostate cancer of the American Joint Committee on Cancer (1992)

T_x Primary tumor cannot be assessed
T_0 No evidence of primary tumor
T_1 Clinically inapparent tumor not palpable or visible by imaging
   T_{1a} Tumor incidental histologic finding in 5% or less of tissue resected
   T_{1b} Tumor incidental histologic finding in more than 5% of tissue resected
   T_{1c} Tumor identified by needle biopsy
T_2 Tumor confined within the prostate
   T_{2a} Tumor involves half of a lobe or less
   T_{2b} Tumor involves more than half a lobe but not both lobes
   T_{2c} Tumor involves both lobes
T_3 Tumor extends through the prostatic capsule
   T_{3a} Unilateral extracapsular extension
   T_{3b} Bilateral extracapsular extension
   T_{3c} Tumor invades the seminal vesicles
T_4 Tumor is fixed or invades adjacent structures other than the seminal vesicles
   T_{4a} Tumor invades any of bladder neck, external sphincter, or rectum
   T_{4b} Tumor invades levator muscles and/or is fixed to the pelvic wall
N_x Regional lymph nodes cannot be assessed
N_0 No regional lymph node metastasis
N_1 Metastasis in a single lymph node, 2 cm or less in greatest dimension
N_2 Metastasis in a single lymph node, more than 2 cm but not more than 5 cm in greatest dimension; or multiple lymph node metastases, none more than 5 cm in greatest dimension
N_3 Metastasis in a lymph node more than 5 cm in greatest dimension
M_x Presence of distant metastasis cannot be assessed
M_0 No distant metastasis
M_1 Distant metastasis
   M_{1a} Nonregional lymph nodes
   M_{1b} Bone metastases
   M_{1c} Other metastatic sites

Table 97-2   Whitmore staging system

WHITMORE SYSTEM	AMERICAN JOINT COMMITTEE ON CANCER
A	T_1
B	T_2
C	T_3
D_1	Any T, N_{1-3}
D_2	Any T, any N, M_1

Table 97-3   Total androgen blockade

AGENT	REGIMEN
Leuprolide	7.5 mg intramuscularly, every 28 days
Flutamide	250 mg orally, twice a day

relief, and perhaps survival benefits, most patients are destined to develop resistance to such therapies. Resistance to hormone ablative therapy (i.e., hormone refractory) has ominous meaning insofar as restoration of antitumor response with alternative therapies occurs in a minority of patients, and survival expectation is materially truncated. Alternative hormone ablation therapies include diethylstilbestrol, aminoglutethimide with hydrocortisone, flutamide withdrawal, or ketoconazole.

Chemotherapy is reserved for those patients who are hormone refractory (defined as failure to manifest antitumor response following one or two hormone ablative therapies). Objective antitumor responses are infrequent with chemotherapy, and survival is rarely impacted. Agents that have shown some utility include estramustine, paclitaxel (Taxol), vinblastine, doxorubicin, cisplatin, and etoposide.

Important palliative approaches for patients with symptomatic bone metastases include radiopharmaceuticals such as strontium 89 (Metastron). Antitumor agents with some promise in the treatment of advanced prostate cancer include suramin, an antitrypanosomal agent that inhibits growth factor binding to receptors on prostate cancer cells.

TESTICULAR CANCER

Germ cell tumors of the testis are the most common cancer in young men between the ages of 15 and 35 years. Before 1970, the young man with recurrent testicular cancer following orchiectomy was destined to have rapid progression and death from disseminated disease. With the development of sophisticated high-voltage radiation therapy technology and the application of aggressive multiagent chemotherapy since the early 1970s, this cancer is routinely cured in young men entering the most productive phase of life. Consequently, the internist caring for the testicular cancer patient in whom durable remission and long-term survival are anticipated must recognize the impact of the disease and its therapy on fertility, employability, insurability, and delayed morbidity. In 1997, an estimated 7200 new cases of testis cancer will be diagnosed, yet only 350 deaths from the disease are expected. Testicular cancer is infrequent, occurring with an incidence of approximately 2 per 100,000 males. The incidence has been rising in white males while remaining stable in black males.

Relevant Physiology and Pathophysiology

The major risk factors for the development of testis cancer are male gender and cryptorchidism. However, maldescent of the testis does not seem to be causal in the development of testicular cancer but rather a marker for some genetic or dysgenic event in embryonic or fetal life. The opposite normally descended testis develops cancer in about one quarter of cryptorchid testis cancer patients. Orchiopexy fails to restore normal cancer risk to the patient with testicular mal-

descent, but it does allow adequate examination of the testis for development of cancer. Other risk factors include various genitourinary abnormalities such as inguinal hernia, ureteral duplication, abnormal lobulation or orientation of the kidney, and testicular hydroceles.

Germ cell tumors of the testis represent greater than 90% of all tumors of the testis. These tumors appear to arise from a pluripotent germ cell capable of differentiating into embryonic structures (teratoma and embryonal carcinoma), placental structures (yolk-sac tumor and choriocarcinoma) or seminoma (the most primitive germ cell tumor). Germ cell cancers may express features of only one of these histopathologies or mixtures of two or more. Other malignancies of the testis include lymphoma (the most common non–germ cell cause of testicular malignancy in elderly men), metastatic cancer or leukemia, tumors of the testicular stroma, and other rare tumors.

Laboratory and Other Diagnostic Tests

The diagnosis of germ cell tumor of the testis requires histopathologic examination of tissue obtained from an orchiectomy specimen. Inguinal orchiectomy, rather than transcrotal biopsy, is the preferred surgical approach for retrieval of diagnostic testicular tissue. The risk of contamination of the scrotal skin followed by local recurrence of cancer or risk of distribution of microscopic metastases to inguinal lymphatic drainage is circumvented. Because the tumor may contain histologic mixtures of several germ cell elements, it is essential that a total orchiectomy specimen plus a generous margin of spermatic cord be provided the pathologist. Occasionally extragonadal germ cell tumors may present within the mediastinum or retroperitoneum without an identifiable testicular tumor. A major proportion of patients with these unusual malignancies may expect cure with systemic chemotherapy. As a consequence, representative incisional biopsy rather than wholesale excision of these frequently bulky tumors is sufficient to guide therapeutic recommendations. Ultrasonography of the testes should be performed in the event that there is doubt about which testis may harbor the tumor, that bilateral tumors are suspected, or that there is an extragonadal presentation of a germ cell tumor.

The availability of sensitive serum assays for α fetoprotein (AFP) and for the β-subunit of human chorionic gonadotropin (β-HCG) has markedly enhanced the accurate and aggressive management of patients with germ cell tumors. AFP is produced by embryonal carcinoma, yolk sac, and occasionally teratomatous components of germ cell tumors. The half-life of this glycoprotein is 5 to 7 days. β-HCG is produced by syncytiotrophoblastic cells found in seminoma, choriocarcinoma, and embryonal carcinomas. The half-life of this glycoprotein is 18 to 24 hours. Elevation of either one or both markers before orchiectomy provides some insight into the possible representative germ cell elements in the tumor. If these markers are detectable before orchiectomy, they may be used to assess adequacy of resection. If AFP and β-HCG fail to normalize postoperatively consistent with their serum half-lives, one may be concerned about the presence of residual disease. During follow-up of patients who have undergone orchiectomy with curative intent, reappearance of the markers in serum suggests recurrent disease. Indeed, in the absence of objective evidence of recurrent cancer, marker elevation alone represents sufficient evidence of recurrent disease to warrant the intitiation of salvage treatment. Elevated tumor markers in the patient with disseminated germ cell cancer serve as an additional tool for the assessment of response to treatment. Several cautions must be kept in mind when using these markers for assistance in treatment decisions. β-HCG may be falsely elevated in patients who smoke marijuana. High levels of LH induced by hypogonadal states may produce cross-reactions with reagents used in the assay for β-HCG, producing spuriously high results. AFP can be elevated by non–germ cell malignancies (hepatocellular carcinoma and other gastrointestinal malignancies), by benign conditions (hepatitis, cirrhosis), and by mature teratoma following treatment of germ cell cancers.

Formal diagnostic evaluation for metastatic dissemination of germ cell tumors of the testis may await the confirmation of diagnosis by orchiectomy. Germ cell tumors of the testis spread in characteristic sequence to pelvic lymphatics, retroperitoneal lymphatics, and mediastinal lymphatics. Once the diagnosis is confirmed, chest x-ray and CT (or MRI) of the abdomen, pelvis, and chest should be performed. Until recently, bipedal lymphangiography has been a commonly used diagnostic study in patients with an established diagnosis of germ cell

---

✔ WHEN TO REFER

The internist engaged in general practice is likely to have ample opportunity to engage in screening procedures (PSA determination and DRE) leading to the detection of prostate cancer. Indeed, the detection of prostate cancer that is restricted to the gland is a clinical diagnostic challenge where the internist may have important impact on the survival of individual patients and ultimately on the public health. PSA determination and DRE remain the gold standards for screening. It behooves the clinician to become proficient in prostate examination by DRE. Abnormalities of the gland (asymmetry, localized induration, nodules) should be recognizable and, whether or not the PSA value is elevated, lead to prompt referral to a urologist for confirmation and further diagnostic evaluation. In addition, any PSA elevation greater than 4 ng/ml in a man over 40 years of age should prompt consultation with a urologist. Although prostate cancer is extremely uncommon in individuals younger than 50 years of age, elevation of PSA level in such men, particularly if a family history of prostate cancer in a first-degree relative is provided or if the individual is black, requires consultation with a urologist.

cancer. Both CT and lymphangiography provide only fair sensitivity in the detection of nodal metastases. Nevertheless, CT is the most commonly and conveniently used staging and follow-up method for the majority of patients. In patients with disseminated cancer, lung metastases are commonly observed. Metastases are less frequently observed in liver, brain, and other solid organs and viscera, usually representing late manifestations in patients with prolonged survival or delayed recurrence after systemic therapy. Consequently, other radiologic studies (e.g., bone scans, CT of the brain, gallium studies) should be reserved for patients with symptoms suggesting that disease is likely to be detected by these means.

Differential Diagnosis

The cardinal diagnostic finding in the patient with testis cancer is a mass in the substance of the testis. Unilateral enlargement of the testis with or without pain in the adolescent or young adult male should raise concern for testis cancer. The differential diagnosis includes hydrocoele, spermatocoele, epididymitis, testicular torsion, or infectious orchitis. Epididymitis, orchitis, and testicular torsion tend to be acutely painful conditions, unlike testis cancer, which produces sensations of heaviness or aching. The inflamed epididymis can usually be differentiated from testis cancer by physical examination. Transillumination or ultrasonography of the testis differentiates the solid mass of testis cancer from the fluid densities of spermatocoele and hydrocoele. Metastatic testis cancer is often associated with back, flank, or chest pain from massively enlarged lymph nodes. Extragonadal germ cell tumors are a common cause of superior vena cava syndrome. These tumors may also produce chest pain, dyspnea, or difficulty swallowing. Extragonadal germ cell cancers are often identified by elevated serum tumor markers in a patient with a mediastinal or abdominal mass and biopsy evidence of poorly differentiated cancer.

Management

The management of established testis cancer is closely allied with its clinical stage. The inguinal orchiectomy is a therapeutic operation, in addition to its importance as a diagnostic procedure. Whether additional interventions are required in the patient with newly diagnosed testis cancer depends on evidence of more advanced cancer yielded by ancillary diagnostic studies and the known risk of recurrence for each stage of cancer at presentation. A variety of staging systems of testis cancer are used in clinical practice. For the purpose of this discussion, the Memorial Sloan-Kettering staging system will be used (Table 97-4).

For patients with clinical stage A nonseminomatous germ cell tumor (confined to the testis), inguinal orchiectomy may be sufficient therapy for selected individuals. It must be realized that patients with clinical stage A disease with no evidence of metastatic disease by noninvasive evaluation (negative CT scans and normal serum markers) sustain a 30% risk of relapse. Since most first recurrences of testis cancer involve the retroperitoneal lymph nodes, retroperitoneal lymph node dissection (RPLND) lends substantial accuracy to the detection of microscopic lymph node disease at the time of cancer presentation. Some controversy remains regarding the necessity for RPLND in all patients, since (1) the procedure harbors some risk for surgical morbidity (retrograde ejaculation) and (2) salvage chemotherapy is sufficiently effective that cure may be anticipated in the vast majority of patients with recurrent cancer. A reasoned approach might involve the application of RPLND for patients with clinical stage A cancer for whom follow-up reliability is in question, for whom the prospect of a 30% recurrence rate is intolerable, or for whom histopathologic prognostic factors (presence of embryonal carcinoma or yolk sac elements, lymphatic or vascular invasion, or extension of tumor beyond the testis) suggest adverse outcome. Expectant follow-up after orchiectomy may be entirely warranted for individuals who are likely to adhere to intensive follow-up and for whom avoidance of the risk of surgical morbidity is desired.

For patients with stage B disease (involvement of retroperitoneal lymph nodes) discovered at RPLND (pathologic stage B_1 or B_2), the risk of later relapse is a nearly intolerable 50%. Such patients are usually offered two to four courses of cisplatin-based chemotherapy followed by an expectation for cure in the vast majority. Patients with radiologic evidence of retroperitoneal lymph node involvement (clinical stage B_2) are most often treated with chemotherapy. RPLND is not performed for clinical stage B_2 patients in whom resection of a residual mass will be required following chemotherapy. This approach achieves long-term survival in more than 90% of patients with stage B_{1-2} nonseminomatous testicular cancer. Patients with bulky (stage B_3) cancer are rarely candidates for primary surgery. Multiagent cisplatin-based chemotherapy is routinely used in this setting with the goal to achieve complete radiologic and serologic (tumor marker) remission. RPLND is then undertaken for any residual tumor mass. In the event that tumor markers remain elevated or that the tumor does not respond to systemic treatment, salvage chemotherapy may be implemented (see later discussion).

The treatment of patients with pure seminoma of the testis relies heavily on primary or adjunctive radiotherapy following diagnostic biopsy. For greater than 90% of patients with clinical stages A to B_2 seminoma, irradiation of the infradiaphragmatic lymph nodes at relatively low doses (2500 cGy) accomplishes remission and long-term survival. For patients with bulky abdominal disease (clinical stage B_3), chemotherapy is favored and produces remission and cure in approximately 90% of such individuals.

For the patient who comes to medical attention with advanced (clinical stage C) disease in supradiaphragmatic lymph nodes, viscera, solid organs, soft tissues, and/or bone (a rare event in patients with seminoma), chemotherapy remains the mainstay of treatment. The chemotherapeutic management of patients with testicular cancer represents one of the most important advances in cancer treatment, contributing to reliably curative multidisciplinary therapy for approximately 96% of testis cancer patients diagnosed annually. A chemotherapy regimen developed at Indiana University utilizing cisplatin, etoposide, and bleomycin (PEB) has received wide acceptance as a safely administered and highly effective means to treat advanced or recurrent cancer (Table 97-5). Three to four courses of this regimen are curative for greater than 90% of patients with "good-risk" disseminated nonseminomatous germ cell cancer or pure seminoma. For patients manifesting "poor-risk" characteristics such as large-volume, bulky cancer, nonlung visceral organ involvement, and high levels of lactate dehydrogenase (LDH), AFP, and β-HCG, initial management may include PEB chemotherapy or participation in ongoing clinical trials. Thirty-five to forty percent of patients with poor-risk disseminated cancer relapse after such therapy. Additional methods for improving the disease management and survival of relapsing patients include the liberal use of surgery to resect residual tumor masses, salvage chemotherapy, and, rarely, high-dose chemotherapy with or without autologous bone marrow or peripheral stem cell rescue.

Table 97-4 Memorial Sloan-Kettering staging system for non-seminomatous germ cell tumors

STAGE	DESCRIPTION
Stage A	Tumor confined to the testis
Stage B	Spread to regional nodes
	B_1 <5 cm
	B_2 >5 cm
	B_3 >10 cm (bulky)
Stage C	Spread beyond retroperitoneal nodes (mediastinal lymph nodes, bone, brain, or solid organs)

Table 97-5 Indiana University cisplatin, etoposide, and bleomycin (PEB) chemotherapy regimen

AGENT	REGIMEN
Cisplatin	20 mg/m² intravenously, days 1-5
Etoposide	100 mg/m² intravenously, days 1-5
Bleomycin	30 units intravenously, days 2, 9, and 16

Repeat cycles of treatment every 21 days.
A total of 3 to 4 cycles is given in good-risk patients.

✔ WHEN TO REFER

The primary care internist may only occasionally be confronted with a young patient with a scrotal mass. In general, most acute clinical conditions of the testis or its adnexae may be differentiated by physical examination and by the judicious application of noninvasive ultrasonography. However, the clinician must remain aware of the frequency of testicular cancer as a cause of testicular disease, of the effectiveness of therapy, and of the necessity for early recognition and management of this rapidly growing malignancy. Transscrotal biopsy of any testicular lesion should be avoided at all cost, and prompt referral to a urologist should be sought. The internist involved in the care of an individual recently treated for germ cell cancer of the testis must be prepared to pursue a rigorous follow-up schedule (monthly for the first year of follow-up, every 2 months for the second year, with a more liberal schedule only after 2 years of uneventful follow-up). The patient who has completed treatment for germ cell cancer may face delayed clinical problems, including (1) late recurrence (greater than 2 years after remission) of cancer, particularly to the central nervous system or the opposite testis, (2) diminished fertility due to RPLND or chemotherapy, and (3) prolonged toxicity of chemotherapy (e.g., bleomycin lung injury, etoposide-related acute leukemia). Early referral for evaluation of suspected recurrent cancer may be lifesaving, since aggressive salvage therapy may cure many patients.

BIBLIOGRAPHY

Anscher MS, Marks LB, Shipley WU: The role of radiotherapy in patients with advanced seminomatous germ cell tumors, *Oncology* 6:97-104, 1992.

Catalona WJ, Bigg SW: Nerve-sparing radical prostatectomy: evaluation of results after 250 patients, *J Urol* 143:538-544, 1990.

Crawford ED, Eisenberger MA, McLeod DG et al: A controlled trial of leuprolide with and without flutamide in prostatic carcinoma, *N Engl J Med* 321:419-429, 1989.

Donohue JP, Thornhill JA, Foster RS et al: The role of retroperitoneal lymphadenectomy in clinical stage B testis cancer: the Indiana University experience (1965 to 1989), *J Urol* 153:85-89, 1995.

Einhorn LH: Treatment of testicular cancer: a new and improved model, *J Clin Oncol* 8:1777-1781, 1990.

Forman D, Chilvers C, Oliver R et al: The aetiology of testicular cancer: association with congenital abnormalities, age at puberty, infertility and exercise, *Br Med J* 308:1393-1399, 1993.

Harlan L, Brawley O, Pommerenke F et al: Geographic, age, and racial variation in the treatment of local/regional carcinoma of the prostate, *J Clin Oncol* 13:93-100, 1995.

Slawin KM, Ohori M, Dilglugil O, Scardino PT: Screening for prostate cancer: an analysis of the early experience, *CA Cancer J Clin* 45:134-147, 1995.

Williams SD, Birch R, Einhorn LH et al: Treatment of disseminated germ-cell tumors with cisplatin, bleomycin, and either vinblastine or etoposide, *N Engl J Med* 316:1435-1440, 1987.

Williams S, Stablein D, Einhorn L et al: Immediate adjuvant chemotherapy versus observation with treatment at relapse in pathological stage II testicular cancer, *N Engl J Med* 317:1433-1438, 1987.

Woolf SH: Screening for prostate cancer with prostate-specific antigen: examination of the evidence, *N Engl J Med* 333:1401-1405, 1995.

CHAPTER

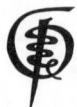

98 Head and Neck Cancer

Jack L. Gluckman and Michael Farrell

The term *head and neck cancer,* if strictly applied, encompasses all cancers involving the head and neck region, including those involving the skin, brain, eyes, upper aerodigestive system, salivary glands, thyroid, and so forth. In actuality, this term is used to describe cancers arising from the mucosa of the upper aerodigestive tract, and for the purposes of this chapter it is these tumors that will be highlighted.

The involved mucosa is that of the nose, paranasal sinuses, oral cavity, nasopharynx, oropharynx, hypopharynx, larynx, and cervical esophagus. While many histologic types of cancer may occur in these areas, by far the most common is squamous cell cancer.

SQUAMOUS CELL CARCINOMA OF THE UPPER AERODIGESTIVE TRACT
Incidence

Squamous cell cancers of the upper aerodigestive tract are a significant global problem with 380,000 new cases diagnosed worldwide in 1980. Almost three quarters of these cases occur in developing countries, and in some countries (e.g., India, Pakistan, Bangladesh) these cancers may account for almost 25% of all cancers. In parts of India, this figure may rise to almost 50%. In developed countries the incidence is less common, ranking this type as the eighth most common cancer; however, the incidence varies from country to country (e.g., in some areas of France it is extremely common). In the United States, the incidence of these cancers has stabilized, comprising 3% of all cancers in men and 2% in women, and results in 2% of all cancer deaths in males and 1% in females. In general, the incidence is greater in males than in females, and these cancers are more common in the elderly, although the disease is being seen more commonly in females and in younger patients.

Etiology

The exact origin or cause of squamous cell cancer is not well understood, but it appears to develop in a susceptible host, with the process being precipitated by environmental factors. These include tobacco, alcohol, radiation, drugs, diet, pollution, viral infections, and other unknown factors. Of these, tobacco (smoked or smokeless) is the most important, with the majority of cases occurring in those who use tobacco products. Tobacco and alcohol appear to have a synergistic effect in the development of these cancers. There is some suggestion that there exists a genetic predisposition to the carcinogenic effects of tobacco products. Other factors (e.g., radiation exposure, syphilis, viral infections, lichen planus, vitamin deficiencies) all may be implicated but appear to have a lesser role.

Pathology

As already stated, not all cancers of the upper aerodigestive tract are squamous cell cancers, and cancer may arise from minor salivary glands (e.g., adenocarcinoma, adenoid cystic carcinoma) or from the underlying submucosal tissue (various sarcomas and others). However, the vast majority are squamous cell carcinoma. Macroscopically, these cancers usually become evident late as an exophytic or fungating mass or as a superficial or deeply infiltrating ulcer with or without evidence of cervical lymphatic metastases.

Premalignant lesions are less easily identifiable but occasionally are noted. Of these, the most common is leukoplakia, which presents as a white patch (Plate IV-12). It should be appreciated, however, that the incidence of malignant transformation in these lesions is extremely rare (0.13% to 6%) and undue concern is inappropriate if these legions are identified, although they may require biopsy and careful follow-up. Of greater significance is the presence of erythroplakia, which presents as a red patch. These patches have an extremely high incidence of malignant transformation (almost 100%). The erythroplastic character is related to a submucosal vascular proliferation and round cell infiltrate secondary to the malignant squamous cells (Plate IV-13). These cancers have a propensity to multicentricity within the field of growth (i.e. the mucosa of the upper aerodigestive tract), and it is not unusual to identify further cancers presenting either simultaneously or later during follow-up. Histologically the degree of differentiation has been shown to have no real practical significance, although these tumors are usually described as well, moderately well, and poorly differentiated. Probably of greater value in determining tumor behavior is whether the tumor infiltrates in a broad base or in columns of cells and depth of infiltration into the underlying soft tissue. Many histologic variants of squamous cell carcinoma have

BOX 98-1

American Joint Committee on Cancer TNM classification for squamous cell cancer of the oral cavity (1993)

Definition of TNM

Primary tumor (T)

T_x Primary tumor cannot be assessed
T_0 No evidence of primary tumor
T_{is} Carcinoma in situ
T_1 Tumor 2 cm or less in greater dimension
T_2 Tumor more than 2 cm but not more than 4 cm in greater dimension
T_3 Tumor more than 4 cm in greatest dimension
T_4 (lip) Tumor invades adjacent structures (e.g., through cortical bone, tongue, skin of neck)

Regional lymph nodes (N)

N_x Regional lymph nodes cannot be assessed
N_0 No regional lymph node metastasis
N_1 Metastasis in a single ipsilateral lymph node, 3 cm or less in greatest dimension
N_2 Metastasis in a single ipsilateral lymph node, more than 3 cm but not more than 6 cm in greatest dimension; or in multiple ipsilateral lymph nodes, none more than 6 cm in greatest dimension; or in bilateral or contralateral lymph nodes, none more than 6 cm in greatest dimension
  N_{2a} Metastasis in single ipsilateral lymph node more than 3 cm but not more than 6 cm in greatest dimension
  N_{2b} Metastasis in multiple ipsilateral lymph nodes, none more than 6 cm in greatest dimension
  N_{2c} Metastasis in bilateral or contralateral lymph nodes, none more than 6 cm in greatest dimension
N_3 Metastasis in a lymph node more than 6 cm in greatest dimension

Distant metastasis (M)

M_x Presence of distant metastasis cannot be assessed
M_0 No distant metastasis
M_1 Distant metastasis

been described, including lymphoepithelioma, a tumor that arises in the lymphoid-bearing areas (i.e., the nasopharynx, faucial and lingual tonsils) and is exquisitely radiosensitive. Verrucous carcinoma is a cancer that is so well differentiated that it is difficult to establish the diagnosis histologically; it is preferably treated with surgery. These tumors tend to increase in size locally, infiltrating the surrounding structures, and metastasize to regional cervical nodes and then, in advanced stage, distantly to lung, liver, and bone.

The staging system used is that designed by the American Joint Committee on Cancer, which is updated every few years (Box 98-1). This tumor staging system takes into account the surface dimensions of the tumor and infiltration into the surrounding structures, the presence and extent of nodal metastases, and the presence of distant metastases. In general, tumors of the oral cavity and oropharynx are staged by their surface dimensions and tumors of the larynx, hypopharynx, and nasopharynx by their local extension. While quite useful as a means of standardization of description for reporting, the system does not take into account tumor behavior. For this reason, much effort has been directed to the identification of both histologic (e.g., tumor-host interface, tumor thickness, perineural and vascular invasion, angiogenesis) and molecular factors, to determine meaningful prognostic indicators.

Clinical Features

The clinical features of these cancers are determined by the site of origin, the local extent at presentation, and whether there are metastases. While the tumors are easily accessible in most instances to direct visualization and therefore should be amenable to early diagno-

sis, most of these cancers become evident at a late stage with not only advanced primary cancers, but also cervical nodal metastases.

Oral cavity cancers usually become evident with a mass or painful ulcer in the mouth (Plate IV-14). As the tumor advances, the tongue may become infiltrated causing dysarthria and dysphagia. Infiltration into the mandible causes severe pain, and, of course, there may be evidence of nodal metastases, usually to the submental, submandibular, and upper deep cervical nodes.

Oropharyngeal cancers become evident with odynophagia or foreign body sensation or evidence of cervical metastases, even at an early stage. Trismus and a persistent sore throat occur as the disease progresses.

Nasopharyngeal cancer is usually relatively asymptomatic at an early stage. However, nasal obstruction, unilateral serous otitis, cervical metastases, facial pain, and an ipsilateral sixth nerve palsy are findings as the tumor progresses. Cancer of the hypopharynx may achieve significant size before giving symptoms. Painful and obstructive dysphagia, referred otalgia, and hoarseness are all symptoms of advanced disease.

Laryngeal cancer, particularly if it arises from the vocal cords, presents with hoarseness as an early symptom; pain on swallowing and nodal metastases develop with advancing stage.

Cancer of the nose and paranasal sinuses may become evident with unilateral rhinorrhea, nasal obstruction, facial pain, and loose teeth, depending on the site of origin. A late finding is evidence of orbital dysfunction and includes diplopia and impaired visual activity. Because the cavities are air-filled, significant growth of the cancer may occur before causing symptoms. In addition, the early symptoms and signs are nonspecific and mimic common ailments (e.g., cold or allergy). This, together with the low index of suspicion because of the rarity of these cancers, contributes to the late presentation.

Diagnosis

It is indeed a tragedy that even today the vast majority of these cancers are diagnosed at a late stage, given their characteristic symptoms; the fact that well over 90% occur in a high-risk population (i.e., tobacco and alcohol abusers); and how easily accessible most of these lesions are to clinical evaluation. If possible, all patients who are at high risk (e.g., heavy smokers) should be examined on a regular basis to detect premalignant lesions or early malignancies.

Clinical examination of the head and neck should be carried out in a systematic manner. First, the neck should be examined for any evidence of cervical metastases, and the thyroid and salivary glands palpated. All nodal groups should be carefully examined. Involvement of certain nodal groups may indicate the site of the primary tumor (e.g., posterior triangle nodes are more likely to enlarge with nasopharyngeal cancer) and, conversely, primary cancers at certain sites are more likely to spread to certain groups (e.g., oral cancer to submental, submandibular, and upper deep cervical nodes), although this does not always hold true.

Examination of the oral cavity and oropharynx can easily be accomplished by direct inspection, but palpation, particularly of the base of the tongue, should always be performed, as a carcinoma may be almost entirely submucosal and not visible on examination. Evaluation of the nasopharynx, hypopharynx, and larynx can be accomplished by indirect mirror examination or more easily by using a fiberoptic endoscope. Likewise, examination of the nasal cavity can be accomplished using a nasal speculum for anterior rhinoscopy and rigid or fiberoptic scopes for posterior endoscopy.

Imaging may be used to augment the physical examination in evaluating areas not accessible to direct or indirect visualization. To this end, chest x-ray, an esophagram, and computed tomography (CT) scan of the sinuses are most useful. Other imaging studies are ordered at the discretion of the clinician and depend on the clinical problem. It is our belief that CT or magnetic resonance imaging (MRI) scans or other contrast studies should be ordered only to obtain information essential to the therapeutic decision-making process and not performed indiscriminately or routinely (e.g., CT scan can evaluate mandible and base of skull erosion; MRI can accurately determine the extent of tongue invasion). An extensive metastatic workup above and beyond x-ray chest and blood chemistry is usually not indicated unless the patient is symptomatic or the locoregional disease is extensive.

If at all possible, an examination under anesthesia should be performed before making the appropriate therapeutic decision for a particular cancer. The purpose of this is to more accurately delineate the extent of the tumor; take adequate and, if necessary, multiple biopsy specimens; and exclude the possibility of a simultaneously developing second cancer, which is present in 8% to 10% of cases. To this end, concomitant laryngoscopy, bronchoscopy, esophagoscopy, and even nasopharyngoscopy, if appropriate, are recommended. Biopsy is obviously necessary to establish diagnosis, and an adequate sample should always be taken. Fine-needle aspirate biopsy is useful for diagnosis of nodal, salivary gland, and thyroid masses.

Treatment

At the outset it should be stated that there exists no ideal treatment for these cancers. The primary aim is, of course, cure. However, a quality of life issue is always paramount in making the appropriate therapeutic decision. If at all possible, mutilation and profound impairment of function should be avoided unless deemed absolutely necessary. A classic example is a patient with carcinoma of the larynx, which might have been treated with a total laryngectomy in years gone by; today every effort is made to preserve function by using radiation therapy or performing a conservation laryngectomy. Because of the difficulty in making these decisions, it is essential that these patients be managed only by the most experienced oncologists, preferably in a multidisciplinary setting.

Primary prevention of these cancers is theoretically an achievable goal by eliminating or significantly limiting tobacco and alcohol consumption. However, this obvious solution continues to elude us, despite increased public awareness. Various attempts at chemoprevention continue to be investigated, using various antioxidants, particularly vitamin A derivatives, but definitive studies have not yet been conclusive as to their efficacy.

The ideal treatment for an individual patient depends on tumor, physician, and patient factors. Tumor factors include site, size, histologic variant, and tumor behavior. Patient factors include the general medical condition, emotional status (i.e., ability to tolerate radical therapy), and the support system available (i.e., home circumstances and family support). Physician factors include the philosophy and experience of the oncologist and the facilities available for treatment. The accepted modalities available include surgery, radiation therapy, and chemotherapy, either on their own or in various combinations. In general, early cancers are treated with surgery or radiation therapy with equal survival rates, with the therapy in any given patient depending on the previously mentioned factors. Exceptions include lymphoepithelioma, which is treated with radiation therapy, irrespective of size and site, with good results, and verrucous carcinoma, which conversely is treated with surgery, irrespective of size. Advanced cancers usually require combination therapy with surgery followed by postoperative radiotherapy being the standard approach.

In general, the basic surgical premise is to remove the cancer with an adequate margin of normal tissue, reconstructing the defect created by primary closure, skin graft, and regional or revascularized distant flaps. Frequently these resections and reconstructions permit the patient almost normal residual function and adequate quality of life. Sometimes these operations may be mutilating (e.g., total laryngectomy or total glossectomy). These situations have stimulated contemporary oncologists to attempt organ preservation approaches using a combination of chemotherapy and radiation therapy. However, it still remains unclear whether this trend ultimately will result in equal or better cure rates or whether the adjunct chemotherapy is in fact superfluous.

The treatment of the cervical lymph nodes is likewise mired in controversy with overt nodal metastases usually treated with a neck dissection—selective, modified radical, or radical removal of the involved nodes. If no palpable nodal metastases are noted, radiation therapy, observation, or neck dissection is employed, depending on the size, site, and type of primary tumor and the philosophy of the oncologist.

Adequate rehabilitation is the key to the management of these patients with emphasis on physical, functional, psychosocial, and occu-

✔ WHEN TO REFER

Prevention and early diagnosis by the primary care physician are key to improved outcome in head and neck cancer. High-risk patients (significant tobacco and alcohol consumption, history of previous aerodigestive tract cancer) with one of the following symptoms of undue duration (±3 weeks) and refractory to conservative therapy should be referred to a specialist capable of visualizing the whole upper aerodigestive tract:

Sore throat
Irritation (foreign body sensation) in throat
Nonhealing ulcer or mass in mouth
Chronic cough
Lump in neck
Unilateral nasal obstruction
Unilateral nasal discharge
Unilateral facial pain of unknown origin

pational rehabilitation. This requires a team approach of dedicated health care professionals including physical therapists, speech and swallowing therapists, psychologists, social workers, nurses, and prosthodontist.

All patients should be followed up for life with frequent visits, particularly in the first 2 years, when the risk of recurrence is greatest. There is always a risk for the development of a second cancer up to 20 years later, particularly if the patient continues to smoke.

Prognosis

The 5-year survival of these cancers is approximately 50% for all sites and stages. Early cancers have a 75% survival, whereas advanced cancers have a 35% survival. Some sites have a very poor prognosis (e.g., cervical esophagus), despite our best efforts, whereas others (e.g., cancer of the glottic larynx) have good survival rates, particularly if diagnosed early enough.

BIBLIOGRAPHY

Centers for Disease Control and Prevention: Reducing the health consequences of smoking: 25 years of progress—a report of the Surgeon General, U.S. Department of Health and Human Services publication no. 89-8411, Washington, DC, 1989, Public Health Service.

Gluckman JL, Crissman JD: Survival rates in 548 patients with multiple neoplasms of the upper aerodigestive tract, *Laryngoscope* 93:71-74, 1983.

Mashberg A, Roffetta P, Winkelman R, Garfinkel C: Tobacco smoking, alcohol drinking and cancer of the oral cavity and oropharynx among U.S. Veterans, *Cancer* 72:1369-1375, 1993.

Mashberg A, Samit A: Early diagnosis of asymptomatic oral and oropharyngeal squamous cancers, *CA Cancer J Clin* 45:328-351, 1995.

Shirinian MH, Weber RS, Lippman S: Laryngeal preservation by induction chemotherapy plus radiotherapy in locally advanced head and neck cancer: the MD Anderson Cancer Center experience, *Head Neck* 16:39-44, 1994.

Wingo PA, Tong T, Bolden S: Cancer statistics: 1995, *CA Cancer J Clin* 45:8-30, 1995.

CHAPTER

99 Lung Cancer

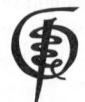

Manuel Valdivieso

The epidemiologic features and causes, general clinical picture, and diagnostic considerations in primary lung cancer are discussed in Chapter 60. The focus of this chapter is on staging, treatment, pathophysiology, and prognosis.

Lung cancer remains among the most common malignancies in men and women combined and is also among the most aggressive.

Table 99-1 Staging of carcinoma of the lung

TNM definitions

Primary tumor (T)

T_x Tumor proved by the presence of malignant cells in bronchopulmonary secretions but not visualized roentgenographically or bronchoscopically, or any tumor that cannot be assessed as in a retreatment staging

T_0 No evidence of primary tumor

T_{is} Carcinoma in situ

T_1 A tumor that is 3 cm or less in greatest dimension, surrounded by lung or visceral pleura, and without evidence of invasion proximal to a lobar bronchus at bronchoscopy

T_2 A tumor more than 3 cm in greatest dimension, or a tumor of any size that either invades the visceral pleura or has associated atelectasis or obstructive pneumonitis extending to the hilar region; at bronchoscopy, the proximal extent of demonstrable tumor must be within a lobar bronchus or at least 2 cm distal to the carina; any associated atelectasis or obstructive pneumonitis must involve less than an entire lung

T_3 A tumor of any size with direct extension into the chest wall (including superior sulcus tumors), diaphragm, or mediastinal pleura or pericardium without involving the heart, great vessels, trachea, esophagus, or vertebral body, or a tumor in the main bronchus within 2 cm of the carina without involving the carina

T_4 A tumor of any size with invasion of the mediastinum or involving heart, great vessels, trachea, esophagus, vertebral body or carina or presence of malignant pleural effusion

Nodal involvement (N)

N_0 No demonstrable metastasis to regional lymph nodes

N_1 Metastasis to lymph nodes in the peribronchial or the ipsilateral hilar region, or both, including direct extension

N_2 Metastasis to ipsilateral mediastinal lymph nodes and subcarinal lymph nodes

N_3 Metastasis to contralateral, mediastinal lymph nodes, contralateral hilar lymph nodes, ipsilateral or contralateral scalene or supraclavicular lymph nodes

Distant metastasis (M)

M_0 No (known) distant metastasis

M_1 Distant metastasis present—specify site(s)

Stage grouping of TNM subsets

Occult carcinoma	T_x	N_0	M_0
Stage 0	T_{is}	Carcinoma in situ	
Stage I	T_1	N_0	M_0
	T_2	N_0	M_0
Stage II	T_1	N_1	M_0
	T_2	N_1	M_0
Stage IIIa	T_3	N_0	M_0
	T_3	N_1	M_0
	T_{1-3}	N_2	M_0
Stage IIIb	Any T	N_3	M_0
	T_4	Any N	M_0
Stage IV	Any T	Any N	M_1

According to the American Cancer Society, there will be 178,100 new diagnoses of lung cancer and approximately 160,400 deaths from this cancer in the United States in 1997. Eighty percent of new cases (142,480) correspond to the so-called non–small cell lung cancer (NSCLC) varieties that include predominantly the epidermoid, adenocarcinoma, and large cell lung cancer histologies. Adenocarcinoma is the most common lung cancer cell type, accounting for approximately 40% of all lung tumors. Other histologies are less frequent: epidermoid, 30%; large cell, 10%; and small cell, 20%.

Lung cancer is epidemiologically associated with smoking and other industrial and environmental factors. Smoking is associated with 80% of all forms of lung carcinoma, although this association is less striking with the adenocarcinoma cell type. Other important epidemiologic factors include exposure to arsenic, asbestos, beryllium, chloromethyl ethers, chromium, hydrocarbons, mustard gas, nickel, and radiation. Mechanisms of carcinogenesis are discussed in Chapter 70.

STAGING

The fundamental purpose of staging in any disease is to determine the most appropriate therapy for a given patient and to assist in the determination of the patient's prognosis. Staging represents a quantitative assessment of disease burden. A secondary benefit is that accurate staging allows comparisons of outcome of therapy across many groups of patients and improves the interpretation of clinical trials. Accurate staging is of critical importance in patients with lung cancer.

Non–Small Cell Lung Cancer

The different forms of NSCLC are classed together for the purposes of staging and treatment because of similarities in clinical behavior.

Surgical resection remains the mainstay of treatment for NSCLC. The International Staging System, developed by the American Joint Commission on Cancer in conjunction with the International Union Against Cancer, is a reflection of that fact. Staging is based on assessment of the size, location, and extent of invasion of the primary tumor (T), the degree of lymph node invasion (N), and the presence or absence of distant metastatic disease (M). Each increase in T, N, or M correlates with a worsening prognosis, as does each increment in stage (Table 99-1).

Once a diagnosis of NSCLC has been made, the cost-effective staging process begins with an accurate history and physical examination. Only 20% of consecutive cases of NSCLC become evident with local disease amenable to surgical resection. The remaining patients have disease that is already advanced. Squamous cell tumors tend to arise more centrally than other forms of NSCLC. Adenocarcinomas and large cell tumors tend to arise more peripherally and can invade the pleura and chest wall. Adenocarcinomas may metastasize earlier in the course of disease than squamous cell tumors. Constitutional symptoms such as weight loss, poor appetite, and bone pain raise the likelihood of disseminated disease and in themselves worsen the prognosis. Palpable adenopathy and organomegaly may direct attention to sites of metastatic disease and spare the patient unnecessary invasive diagnostic procedures. Fine-needle aspiration of suspected metastatic disease is widely available and can be used to establish diagnosis or to confirm the presence of metastases.

Baseline laboratory investigations are desirable and may further guide the diagnostic evaluation. A posteroanterior and lateral chest roentgenogram, complete blood cell count, and serum electrolyte values are appropriate and complement the history and physical examination.

If disseminated disease is not suspected after initial evaluation of the patient, additional testing is indicated. The goal is to identify patients who may benefit from surgical resection, primarily those with stages I and II and some patients with stage IIIa disease. In approximately 60% of patients with NSCLC clinical staging can be determined by paying attention to history and physical examination, chest roentgenographs, and biochemical profile (SMA) determination. The remaining 40% of patients require additional testing. Computed axial tomography (CT scan) of the chest, abdomen, and brain is often necessary to better determine the extent of disease under these circumstances. The accuracy of CT scan is determined heavily by the experience of the interpreter of the examination and the clinical situation under consideration. In most instances CT scanning provides a reasonable assessment of the lesions and their relation to the adjacent anatomy. While the evaluation of the mediastinum by CT remains controversial, it is reliable when the involved lymph nodes are larger than 1 cm in diameter.

Some authors consider CT scanning to be of limited benefit in the staging of patients with NSCLC because of its low specificity (88%) and sensitivity (71%). CT scanning also is not always capable of distinguishing the presence of malignant chest wall involvement. Despite the limitations of CT scans, their use remains popular. An emerging consensus is to omit mediastinoscopy and proceed with definitive surgery in patients whose mediastinum is "uninvolved" by chest CT scan criteria, but to proceed with mediastinal node sampling in patients whose mediastinal nodes are "abnormal" on CT scan. Enlargement of mediastinal nodes is caused by benign processes approximately as often as by neoplastic processes. Patients should not be denied definitive surgical therapy without histologic confirmation of metastatic disease as the cause of enlarged mediastinal nodes. In many institutions the adrenal glands are often included in the chest CT scanning, which could be beneficial to rule out metastasis. Asymptomatic adrenal metastases may be present in 10% to 15% of patients with NSCLC, more commonly in patients with adenocarcinoma and poorly differentiated tumors than in those with squamous cell carcinomas. Solitary adrenal masses may be benign adenomas or metastases. Fine-needle aspiration may be required to establish the diagnosis. CT scanning of the abdomen is helpful in assessing liver and/or adrenal metastasis. Routine radionuclide scans of bone in asymptomatic patients have very low yield.

All patients without known stage IV disease should be offered bronchoscopy, if not already performed for diagnosis. Rigid bronchoscopy remains a valuable tool for certain situations, although the use of flexible fiberoptic bronchoscopes has become standard. Bronchoscopy permits an accurate assessment of the proximal extent of endobronchial involvement and thus assists in determination of the appropriate T designation. Tumors more than 2 cm from the carina are designated T_1 or T_2; those less than 2 cm from the carina, but not involving it, are T_3. Tumors that involve the carina are classified T_4, which establishes the patient's disease as at least stage IIIb and therefore not appropriate for surgical intervention.

For patients with tumors staged T_3 or less, biopsy of relevant nodes is generally indicated. The purpose of such biopsies is to identify patients who have N_3 disease (stage IIIb) and who therefore are not candidates for surgical resection. Mediastinoscopy and anterior mediastinotomy remain the most popular methods; many centers use cervical mediastinoscopy for direct evaluation of the paratracheal, tracheobronchial, and anterior subcarinal nodes. Lesions in the left upper lobe are better evaluated by left anterior mediastinotomy. In skilled hands these procedures have low morbidity rates. Patients with N_0 or N_1 and some patients with N_2 disease are candidates for surgical resection via thoracotomy. Sampling of multiple hilar and mediastinal nodes at the time of operation completes the staging process. The site of sampling of mediastinal nodes should be appropriately identified to ensure an accurate surgical staging. Meticulous mediastinal lymph node dissections for the purpose of cure remain of questionable value.

Small Cell Lung Cancer

Approximately 20% of primary lung cancers are so-called small cell lung cancer (SCLC) tumors. These tumors differ from the other histologic subtypes of primary lung cancers in that early, widespread hematogenous dissemination is the rule, not the exception. In addition, SCLC is not considered a surgically treatable disease, except in the

infrequent case when it is manifested as a solitary pulmonary nodule (Chapter 61). This fact was established more than 20 years ago by a Medical Research Council study that randomized patients to surgical excision or chest irradiation without surgery. Surgery did not improve the survival rate. Other studies, however, suggest that stage I patients have a high cure rate (30% to 60%) when initial surgical resection is followed by appropriate postoperative therapy. For disease stage II or IIIa, routine surgical exploration is not indicated. TNM staging has not been prognostically or therapeutically evaluated in cases of SCLC and generally is not applied. Rather, SCLC is "staged" on the basis of its extent vis-è-vis the thoracic cavity. "Limited-stage" SCLC consists of disease confined to the ipsilateral hemithorax and/or the regional lymph node drainage. All of the disease should fit within a single radiation port. The presence of malignant pleural effusion does not increase the patient's stage. "Extensive-stage" cancer encompasses all other patients who have SCLC that is not classified as "limited."

A careful history and physical examination are as important in cases of SCLC as in those of NSCLC. Careful consideration should be given to the appropriate staging of the disease by the addition of tests such as chest roentgenographs and CT scans of the chest and abdomen. The CT scan of the abdomen is helpful because it discloses disease in liver and adrenal glands, which is more common than in NSCLC. Particular attention should be paid to the central nervous system because of the high frequency of metastases to the brain. About 10% of patients have asymptomatic central nervous system metastases at the time of diagnosis. Brain metastasis occurs in up to 50% of patients during the duration of the illness. CT scan and magnetic resonance imaging (MRI) of the brain are excellent tests to evaluate for brain metastasis. However, MRI is more sensitive and more expensive. Fine-needle aspiration cytologic study of suspect findings can establish the presence of disease outside the chest. Bone marrow examination may be indicated, particularly in the presence of cytopenias in the routine complete blood cell count. Unilateral aspiration and core biopsy of bone marrow are adequate, although bilateral sampling increases the yield by about 20%. The presence or absence of anemia does not correlate with marrow involvement, but nucleated red blood cells may be present on the peripheral blood smear when tumor is in the marrow. Radionuclide bone scanning can be helpful in detecting metastatic lesions and should be obtained in most patients. Serum electrolyte determinations should be part of the evaluation of patients with SCLC. Hyponatremia and hypochloremia suggest an underlying syndrome of inappropriate secretion of antidiuretic hormone, a complication commonly associated with SCLC.

THERAPY
Non–Small Cell Lung Cancer

Patients with stages I and II NSCLC are candidates for surgical resection (Table 99-2; Fig. 99-1). Intraoperative histologic assessments are required to determine the appropriate scope of the surgery. Lobectomy is the procedure of choice for localized lesions within a pulmonary lobe. Wedge resections are often recommended for patients with limited pulmonary function and patients who could be disabled by loss of a lobe. Limited resections, however, are associated with a higher chance for local recurrence. More extensive resections to in-

Table 99-2 Surgical staging by tumor, node, and metastasis (TNM) and survival in non–small cell lung cancer at 5 years with surgery with or without radiation therapy

STAGE	TNM	SURVIVAL AT 5 YEARS (%)
I	$T_1N_0M_0$	60
	$T_2N_0M_0$	50
II	$T_1N_1M_0$	40
	$T_2N_1M_0$	30
IIIa	$T_3N_0M_0$	20-50
	$T_3N_1M_0$	15-20
	$T_{1-3}N_2M_0$	15-20

clude pneumonectomy are required sometimes to remove the tumor. Postoperative chemotherapy or radiotherapy has not proved of definite benefit for patients with stage I or II NSCLC and cannot be considered standard therapy at this time.

Management of Patients With Stages IIIa and IIIb Non–Small Cell Lung Cancer

This is a heterogenous group that includes patients with different disease manifestations and outcomes. An extreme of this spectrum is represented by patients who have malignant pleural effusions (T_4 lesions and therefore stage IIIb disease) and for whom systemic chemotherapy, chest tube drainage, and pleurodesis are appropriate treatment options. The other extreme is represented by patients who have chest wall tumors (T_3 lesions) and negative locoregional or distant metastases (N_0M_0) or stage IIIa disease and for whom en bloc chest wall resection alone is the treatment of choice. More often, however, the physician is confronted with the spectrum of patients in between, and for whom ipsilateral mediastinal (N_2) or contralateral mediastinal (N_3) adenopathy is the common denominator. Under these circumstances, single treatment modality is of questionable value and combined modality therapy is becoming increasingly important.

Surgical resection of cancer in patients with mediastinal disease has not been rewarding. Resection in patients with ipsilateral mediastinal disease (stage IIIa) has produced cure rates in up to 8% for adenocarcinoma and 12% for squamous cell histologies. More often than not, however, the cure rate for these patients falls in the range of 0% to 5%. Isolated series with cure rates in the 30% range have been reported in patients with limited, often microscopic, involvement of the mediastinum. In more favorable stage IIIa patients, such as those with chest wall involvement and no local or distant metastases ($T_3N_0M_0$), results of surgical resection are excellent with a favorable cure rate in up to 50% of patients.

The long-term results of radiation therapy in stage III patients are also discouraging. Fifty percent to 80% of patients are expected to respond favorably to chest irradiation alone. However, the response is usually partial, its duration is limited, the median survival of patients is usually in the range of 8 to 10 months, and the cure rate is between 5% and 10%. Best results have been observed in patients receiving higher total doses of chest irradiation. Although chest irradiation alone has limited value as definitive therapy for patients with stages IIIa and IIIb NSCLC, irradiation has considerable palliative benefit in patients with complications from disease such as lung collapse from endobrachial tumor, superior vena cava compression, brain metastasis, or painful bone metastasis.

Available systemic chemotherapy is also of limited value in NSCLC. Best combination chemotherapy programs contain cisplatin, etoposide, or vinblastine and produce responses in 30% to 50% of patients, with best responses in patients with less disease bulk. Responses, however, are transient and are associated with median survival duration of 12 to 15 months. Survival beyond 2 or 3 years is unusual.

Based on experimental and clinical evidence of synergism between radiation therapy and certain chemotherapeutic agents (e.g., cisplatin, 5-fluorouracil, anthracyclines, hydroxyurea), chemotherapy and radiation therapy are being considered in the treatment of patients with locally advanced lung cancer. In fact, randomized, comparative trials conducted by the Lung Tumor Study Group in the United States have demonstrated a survival advantage for cyclophosphamide, doxorubicin, and cisplatin when combined with radiation therapy to the chest in patients with microscopic and macroscopic residual adenocarcinoma and large cell forms of lung cancer. Other trials have expanded on these studies and have suggested that the administration of sequential or concomitant systemic chemotherapy and chest irradiation produces an objective tumor response in 50% to 75% of patients with NSCLC to the point of making two thirds of cancers in initially inoperable patients resectable and with an apparent survival advantage of 10% to 30% at 3 years. Most

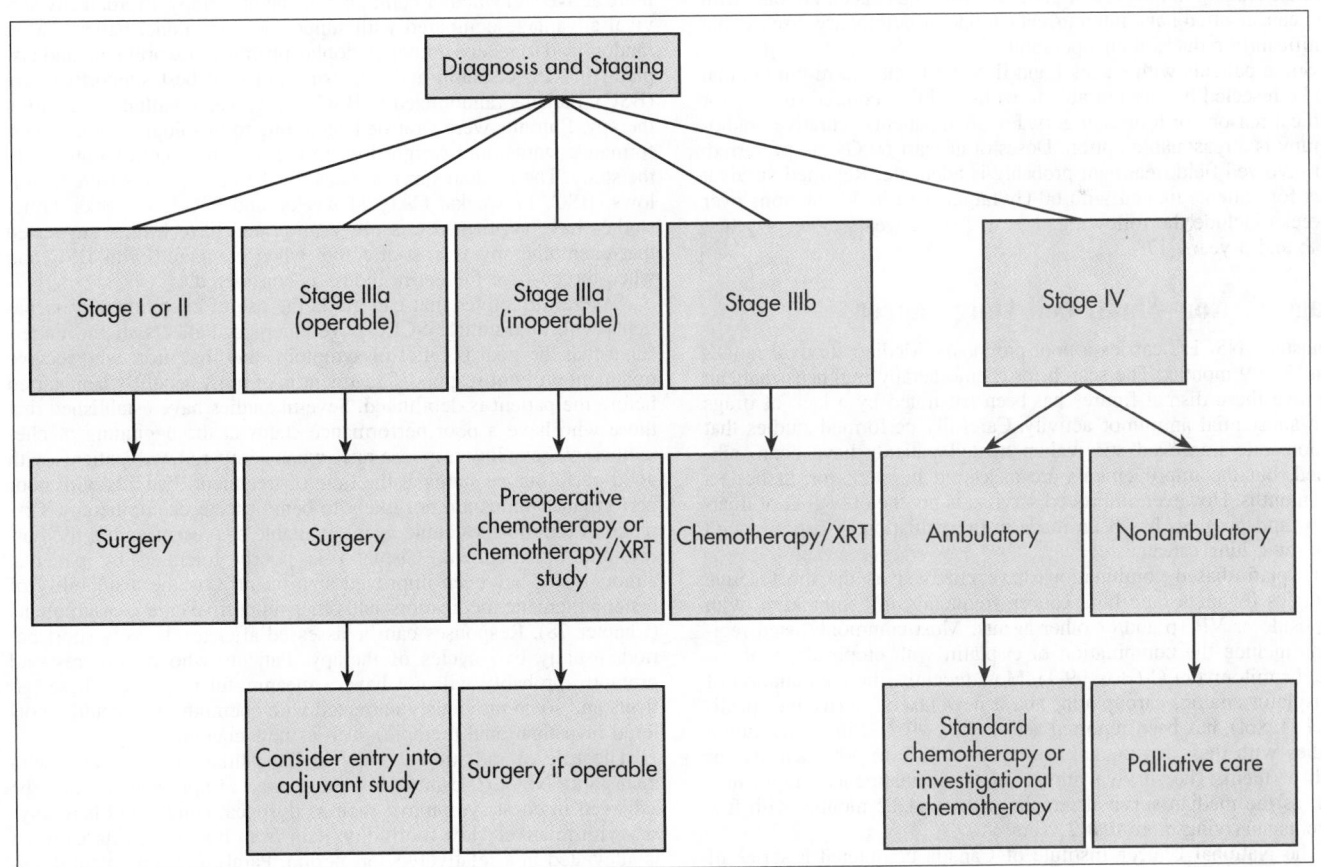

FIGURE 99-1 Algorithm for management of patients with non–small cell lung cancer. *XRT,* Radiation therapy.

patients selected for these trials have gross ipsilateral mediastinal disease prior to treatment and otherwise adequate cardiopulmonary status for potential lung cancer surgery. A close evaluation of these trials, however, raises questions concerning patient selection and the contribution of each treatment modality to the outcome of the study. Prospective randomized trials are in progress that are evaluating the importance of each of the components of this combined treatment in patients with stages IIIa and IIIb disease. Survival advantage for combined chemotherapy and chest irradiation over radiation therapy alone has been demonstrated in two randomized studies. Patients received chest irradiation (65 Gy) with or without vindesine, cyclophosphamide, cisplatin, and lomustine chemotherapy. The chemoradiation therapy group had a better median survival (12 vs. 10 months) and a higher percentage surviving 2 years (21% vs. 14%). In a second study, patients received chest irradiation (60 Gy) with or without cisplatin and vinblastine. The combined modality group achieved a better median survival (13.7 vs. 9.6 months) and percentage survival at 2 years (26% vs. 13%). Therefore the administration of combined modality therapy appears promising for patients with locally advanced, stages IIIa and IIIb NSCLC. High initial tumor response has been associated with a greater rate of resectability of residual disease and encouraging survival. Since the overall significance of this approach remains under study, eligible patients should be encouraged to participate in clinical trials designed to evaluate this mode of therapy.

Resectable Tumors in Inoperable Patients

Resectability refers to the anatomic extent of disease and the fact that a surgical cure can be accomplished; *operability,* on the other hand, is the patient's ability to withstand the procedure required to remove all of the cancer. A patient's tumor might be anatomically removable with a lobectomy, but because of poor pulmonary or cardiac reserve the patient may not be able to tolerate more than a wedge resection. Such a patient would be resectable but inoperable. Preoperative evaluation of pulmonary function and cardiac reserve is as important as accurate staging in the care of patients with lung cancer. Patients with lung cancer often have intercurrent cardiac or pulmonary disease that significantly reduces their operability.

Some patients with stages I and II NSCLC may have tumors that can be resected but are not able to withstand the required surgery for medical reasons or refuse surgery. For such patients "curative" radiotherapy is a reasonable option. Doses of at least 60 Gy are preferred, and involved field treatment probably is adequate. Reported survival rates for patients treated with 60-Gy target dose in 30 fractions over 6 weeks include the following: 1 year, 57%; 2 years, 36%; 4 years, 17%; and 5 years, 17%.

Stage IV Non–Small Cell Lung Cancer

Metastatic NSCLC carries a poor prognosis. Median survival ranges from 6 to 9 months. The search for chemotherapy regimens that can improve these dismal figures has been frustrated by a lack of drugs with substantial antitumor activity. Carefully performed studies that demonstrate improved survival in treated patients have been published, but the improvements are measured in weeks or, at best, a few months. However, improved survival is not the only goal of treatment, and progress has been made in the palliation of patients with metastatic lung cancer.

Cisplatin-based combinations have emerged as the most active therapies for metastatic lung cancer, frequently in combination with etoposide or VP-16 and/or other agents. Most commonly used regimens include the combination of cisplatin with etoposide, vinblastine, or mitomycin C (Box 99-1). Most recently, the combination of a cisplatin analog, carboplatin, and a new taxene derivative, paclitaxel (Taxol), has been reported active (Box 99-2). Single-institution studies with these regimens have reported 30% to 50% activity for each of them. The survival impact of these treatments remain limited, as the median survival remains at around 12 months with few patients surviving more that 2 years.

The National Cancer Institute of Canada completed a series of studies in patients with stage IV NSCLC. The purpose of these studies was to determine which of two commonly used regimens was

---

BOX 99-1

Most commonly used chemotherapeutic regimens in lung cancer

Non–small cell
- Cisplatin-etoposide
- Cisplatin-velban
- Cisplatin-velban-mitomycin C
- Carboplatin-paclitaxel

Small cell
- Cisplatin-etoposide (VP)
- Cyclophosphamide-doxorubicin-cisplatin (CAP)
- Alternating VP and CAP
- Weekly cisplatin, vincristine, doxorubicin, and etoposide (CODE)

BOX 99-2

Promising new chemotherapeutic agents against lung cancer

- Paclitaxel
- Taxotere
- CPT-11
- Topotecan
- Navelbine
- Gemcitabine

---

more active and whether combination chemotherapy afforded any survival advantage compared with supportive care alone. Patients were randomized to receive either cyclophosphamide, doxorubicin, and cisplatin (CAP); cisplatin and vindesine (VP); or best supportive care (BSC). Patients randomized to BSC could receive palliative radiation therapy. Entrants were stratified according to histologic features, performance status, and weight loss in the 3 months before entry onto the study. The median survival rates for the three groups were as follows: BSC, 17 weeks; CAP, 24 weeks; and VP, 32.6 weeks. Other studies have confirmed this observation and have further suggested that chemotherapy is cost-effective when compared with BSC and when the cost for the entire illness is considered.

Several principles that can guide the use of chemotherapy in patients with metastatic NSCLC have emerged. Patients should understand that the goal is relief of symptoms and that most who receive treatment will not respond. Treatment is of most benefit when started before the patient is debilitated. Several studies have established that those who have a poor performance status at the beginning of chemotherapy have low response rates when compared with patients with good performance status at the time of treatment. Patients with poor performance status are not likely to benefit from chemotherapy. Cisplatin is the most valuable agent available at present and is the cornerstone of treatment. Cisplatin is poorly tolerated by patients, although this has been improved significantly by the availability of better antiemetic medications and other supportive care measurements (Chapter 78). Responses can be assessed after a relatively short period, usually two cycles of therapy. Patients who do not respond promptly probably will not have a meaningful response. These patients and some previously untreated with chemotherapy could be offered investigational therapies such as new chemotherapy.

The role of radiation therapy in the palliation of patients with metastatic NSCLC cannot be overlooked. Improvement may be achieved in chest symptoms, such as dyspnea, cough, and hemoptysis, with relatively low morbidity. Pain from boney metastases often is alleviated in a relatively short period. Paralysis from epidural spinal cord compression and devastating neurologic deficits from cerebral metastases also may be prevented if treatment is promptly instituted. Because of the wide availability of radiotherapy equipment and the low morbidity rate associated with limited treatment ports, few patients are unable to be treated.

Small Cell Lung Cancer

Chemotherapy is the mainstay of treatment for SCLC, regardless of stage. There exist a number of chemotherapeutic agents which, alone or in combination, are capable of significant tumor responses in 30% to 80% of patients, respectively. Most significant responses, complete remissions, are inversely related to disease extent. As a result, long-term survival is most likely in limited-disease patients.

Limited-Disease Small Cell Lung Cancer

Limited disease SCLC is usually treated with systemic chemotherapy alone or frequently with the addition of chest irradiation. As stated earlier, most commonly used chemotherapeutic regimens are shown in Box 99-1. As in the case of NSCLC, cisplatin is a key element of these regimens, and it is usually administered with etoposide or with doxorubicin and cyclophosphamide. The strategy of administration of these varies between monthly and weekly administration of a single treatment regimen or the administration of alternating treatment regimens to minimize the possible emergence of drug resistance. Best single-institution studies with all of these approaches give similar results. The complete response rate is in the 40% to 50% range; partial responses are seen in an additional 30% for an overall response rate of 70% to 80%. The median duration of response is approximately 40 weeks with median survival of about 1 year.

The role of irradiation to the primary tumor and mediastinum in patients with limited-stage SCLC appears established. Greater tumor control and improved long-term survival rate have been established in several trials. The optimum technique to use is less clear. Some authors prefer the so-called sandwich technique, in which several cycles of chemotherapy are given initially, followed by a break for irradiation, and chemotherapy resumed at the end of irradiation. Others are inclined toward the simultaneous use of chemotherapy and radiation therapy with the irradiation given as a single daily dose or as a multiple daily fraction (hyperfractionated radiation). Most commonly used regimens use the simultaneous administration of chemotherapy and chest irradiation from the very beginning. Encouraging results with 30% survivorship at 3 years have been reported with these approaches. Most series, however, report half that many long-term survivors.

Prophylactic whole-brain irradiation in a dose of 30 Gy has been, on and off, standard treatment for patients with limited disease who have a complete response to therapy. The long-term morbidity because of secondary neurologic problems, most commonly dementia, can be considerable, and some authors have questioned the wisdom of routine use of this treatment. In fact, there is no consensus to date as to whether patients should be given prophylactic brain irradiation.

Other treatment approaches have included the administration of more intense doses of chemotherapy alone or in the setting of autologous bone marrow transplantation. The data to date, however, has not shown the superiority of these approaches over more conventional forms of therapy.

The success achieved in the treatment of SCLC, albeit limited, has opened a new set of challenges for these patients. In addition to the neurologic sequelae associated with therapy, there is increasing evidence that most patients die as a result of a second malignancy, usually an NSCLC, and that the mortality rate is greater among patients who continue to smoke.

Extensive-Disease Small Cell Lung Cancer

Chemotherapy is also the initial treatment for patients with extensive SCLC. Generally the same regimens and many of the same chemotherapy strategies are used as for limited disease. Responses are less common in extensive than in limited disease; however, 5% to 20% attain complete response and 40% to 60% partial response, for an overall response rate in the range of 50% to 80%. Median duration of response is shorter than for patients with limited disease, as is overall survival (8 to 10 months). Two-year survival is uncommon for patients who have extensive disease, although up to 5% long-term survival has been reported.

Irradiation to the primary tumor and mediastinum does not improve overall response or survival rate and is not indicated. Similarly, whole-brain irradiation is reserved for patients in whom symptomatic brain metastases develop.

BIBLIOGRAPHY

Bonomi P: Non–small cell lung cancer chemotherapy. In Pass HI, Mitchell JB, Johnson DH, Turrisi AT, editors: *Lung cancer: principles and practice*, Philadelphia, 1996, Lippincott-Raven.

Dillman R et al: A randomized trial of induction chemotherapy plus high-dose radiation versus radiation alone in stage III non–small cell lung cancer, *N Eng J Med* 323:940, 1990.

Grilli R, Oxman AD, Julian JA: Chemotherapy for advanced non–small cell lung cancer: how much benefit is enough, *J Clin Oncol* 11:866, 1993.

Liu RJ: Chemotherapy outcomes in advanced non–small cell lung carcinoma, *Semin Oncol* 20:296, 1993.

McCracken JD et al: Concurrent chemotherapy/radiotherapy for limited small cell lung carcinoma: a Southwest Oncology Group study, *J Clin Oncol* 8:892, 1990.

Perez CA et al: Impact of tumor control on survival in carcinoma of the lung treated with irradiation, *Int J Radiat Oncol Biol Phys* 12:539, 1986.

Rapp E et al: Chemotherapy can prolong survival in patients with advanced non–small cell lung cancer: report of a Canadian multicenter randomized trial, *J Clin Oncol* 6:633, 1988.

Rowinsky EK, Ettinger DS: Drug development and new drugs for lung cancer. In Pass HI, Mitchell JB, Johnson DH, Turrisi ST, editors: *Lung cancer: principles and practice*, Philadelphia, 1996, Lippincott-Raven.

Shields TW et al: Surgical resection in the management of small cell carcinoma of the lung, *J Thorac Cardiovasc Surg* 84:481, 1982.

Talton BM, Constable WC, Kersh CR: Curative radiotherapy in non–small cell carcinoma of the lung, *Int J Radiat Oncol Biol Phys* 19:15, 1990.

Turrisi AT, Glover DJ: Thoracic radiotherapy variables: influence on local control in small cell lung cancer limited disease, *Int J Radiat Oncol Biol Phys* 19:1473, 1990.

✔ *WHEN TO REFER*

At the time of initial diagnosis, patients with lung cancer should be referred to a cancer center where they can be evaluated by a multidisciplinary team of surgeons, medical onoclogists, and radiation oncologists. An appropriate plan of staging and therapy can be developed by experts. The primary care phsycian generally plays a collaborative role in long-term follow-up.

CHAPTER

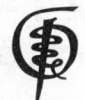

100 Cancer of Unknown Primary Site

Stephen C. Schwartz, Jared Klein, and William P. Peters

EPIDEMIOLOGY AND NATURAL HISTORY

Unknown primary cancers represent between 5% and 10% of all newly diagnosed malignancies. Clinically, patients are often debilitated and exhibit constitutional signs and symptoms including weight loss, cachexia, and fatigue. Initial presentations of patients with unknown primary cancers include parenchymal metastasis involving lung, liver, or lymph nodes, osseous metastasis, and malignant pleural effusions or ascites. Rarely, patients possess solitary sites of disease involving cutaneous structures or the central nervous system. More commonly, unknown primary cancers become evident with disseminated multiorgan involvement. The most frequently identified sites of origin include lung, breast, and colon.

The diagnostic evaluation for a cancer of unknown primary site serves as a paradigm for the assessment of all newly diagnosed malignancies. Two tasks are incumbent upon the clinician in this setting. First, a diagnosis of malignancy must be established on pathologic grounds. Second, an origin or primary site is sought to permit classification of the malignancy. This will allow for prognostication and suggest a therapeutic direction. Biopsy of the most accessible site should be performed early. Open biopsies have proven their superiority over fine-needle aspiration, as the former demonstrates improved maintenance of histologic features and provides abundant tissue for immunohistochemical, cytogenetic, and electron microscopic analysis.

PATHOLOGY

Pathologic assessment of a cancer of unknown primary site begins with light microscopy. The primary objective of this assessment is the identification of a treatable malignancy. This technique allows for the placement of the malignancy into one of five distinct categories, which include adenocarcinoma, squamous carcinoma, poorly differentiated malignant neoplasms, poorly differentiated carcinoma, and poorly differentiated adenocarcinoma. Approximately 60% of patients are placed into the category of adenocarcinoma of unknown primary site. Adenocarcinomas from various organs are not usually distinguishable by conventional light microscopy and require other means to be categorized specifically. Five percent of all cancers of unknown primary site are recognizable as squamous cell carcinomas.

Light microscopy does not provide information regarding tumor lineage in the remaining 35% of patients assessed. Pathologic analysis suggests poorly differentiated neoplasm, poorly differentiated carcinoma, or poorly differentiated adenocarcinoma. Malignancies carrying these diagnoses should undergo further pathologic assessment, as identification of specific tumor types may allow for curative therapy to be instituted in some cases. This caveat is especially important with regard to poorly differentiated neoplasms, as 30% to 70% of these cases ultimately are diagnosed as non-Hodgkin's lymphomas. Lymphomas are considered chemosensitive tumors and are potentially curable with present therapies (Chapter 93).

The tissue of origin for poorly differentiated carcinomas and poorly differentiated adenocarcinomas is not identified by further analysis in a majority of cases. However, because approximately 20% of these cases will also be diagnosed as non-Hodgkin's lymphomas, full analysis should be carried out. On occasion, patients demonstrate classic histologic features for specific tumors other than the five aforementioned distinct classifications. These cases should be staged appropriately and treated in accordance with the particular tumor type involved (i.e., sarcomas or melanoma).

IMMUNOHISTOCHEMISTRY

Patients whose pathologic examination suggests poorly differentiated malignancy, poorly differentiated carcinoma, or poorly differentiated adenocarcinoma should have specimens assessed by immunohistochemistry (immunoperoxidase staining). This method, which relies on the detection of cell components or products by immunologic methods (monoclonal and polyclonal antibodies), allows for the characterization and classification of cancers (Fig. 100-1).

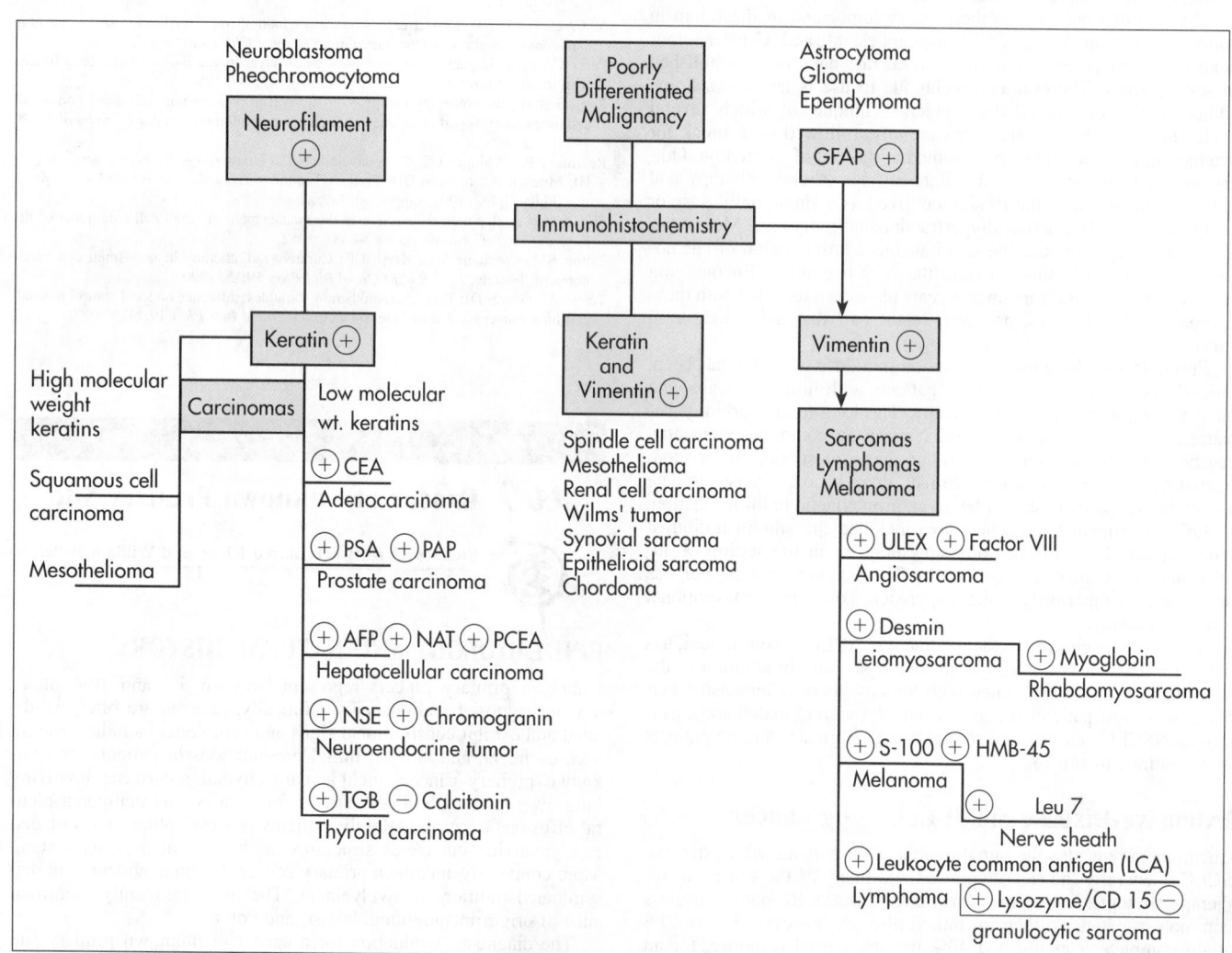

FIGURE 100-1   Algorithm for the characterization and classification of cancers based on immunohistochemistry.

Specimens staining positive for *cytokeratin* represent carcinomas or mesotheliomas. A distinction between mesothelioma, squamous cell carcinoma, and other carcinomas is made on the basis of molecular weight. Squamous cell carcinomas and mesotheliomas have high molecular weight keratins, while adenocarcinomas, hepatocellular carcinoma, neuroendocrine tumors, and thyroid and renal cell carcinomas have low molecular weight keratins. Epithelial membrane antigen (EMA) has found a role in serving to confirm the presence of an epithelial cell–derived malignancy. While it is often not feasible to determine the primary site for most carcinomas, several specific stains exist which may lead to their identification. These include stains for prostate-specific antigen in prostate carcinoma, thyroglobulin in follicular thyroid carcinoma, calcitonin in medullary thyroid carcinoma, neuron-specific enolase and chromogranin in neuroendocrine tumors, and human chorionic gonadotropin (HCG) and α-fetoprotein (AFP) in germ cell tumors. While these stains may be specific in the appropriate clinical setting, only prostate-specific antigen carries enough specificity to confirm the diagnosis based on the results of the stain alone.

Antibodies to the *leukocyte common antigen (LCA)* detect lymphocytes and other associated hematopoietic elements, thus making it an invaluable tool in the identification of malignant lymphomas. If the clinical setting warrants, patients whose specimens stain positive for LCA should be treated for lymphoma accordingly. Granulocytic sarcoma or chloromas are rare extramedullary myeloid malignancies that become evident as solid tumors. They also stain for LCA, lysozyme, and CD15. Histologically, large cell anaplastic lymphomas may be confused with metastatic carcinoma. The former often express CD30, which is detected by the Ki-1 antibody. The distinction between these two entities is critical, as effective therapy is available for this lymphoma variant.

Although some lymphomas stain positive for *vimentin,* this cellular component is most often associated with sarcomas. The particular variety of sarcoma may also be identified by immunoperoxidase staining. Rhabdomyosarcomas stain positive for desmin, myoglobin, and smooth muscle actin. Angiosarcomas often express factor VIII antigen and binding sites for the lectin ULEX. Melanomas invariably stain for S-100 and HMB-45. Melanomas frequently stain for vimentin, while spindle cell carcinomas, mesotheliomas, renal cell carcinomas, Wilms' tumor, synovial sarcoma, epithelioid sarcoma, and chordoma often stain for both keratin and vimentin.

Specimens initially identified as adenocarcinoma or squamous carcinoma may occasionally benefit from immunohistochemical analysis. However, the majority of these cancers are not placed in a specific subgroup and remain adenocarcinomas and squamous carcinomas of unknown primary site.

ELECTRON MICROSCOPY AND CYTOGENETICS

Electron microscopy (EM) may reveal specific ultrastructural features that may aid in the diagnosis of cancer of unknown primary site. Electron microscopy allows the pathologist to distinguish carcinoma from lymphoma. It may also identify neuroendocrine tumors by the presence of neurosecretory granules or suggest melanoma by the presence of premelanosomes. Adenocarcinoma is identified by the presence of intracellular lumina or microvilli, while squamous cell carcinoma demonstrates tonofilaments.

Cytogenetics may define the malignancy when chromosomal abnormalities exist which are specific for a particular tumor type. Multiple cytogenetic abnormalities exist in lymphomas. The (14,18) translocation is present in a high percentage of cases of follicular lymphoma, while (8,14), (8,2), and (8,22) translocations are common to high-grade lymphomas of the Burkitt's variety. Immunoglobulin and T-cell receptor gene rearrangements also provide evidence for the presence of lymphoma (Chapter 73).

The (11,22) translocation in Ewing's sarcoma and the isochromosome 12 in germ cell tumors are two distinct cytogenetic abnormalities specific for solid tumor malignancies. The latter is most important when being considered in the context of a poorly differentiated carcinoma arising in a midline structure of a male patient less than 50 years of age. As more specific cytogenetic abnormalities and tumor-associated oncogenes are identified, techniques such as the polymerase chain reaction (PCR) and fluorescent in situ hybrid-

ization (FISH) will be employed to identify various tumor types. When tumor type cannot be identified solely by immunohistochemistry, electron microscopy, cytogenetic, and molecular analysis may be useful adjuncts in establishing tumor type.

IDENTIFICATION OF THE PRIMARY SITE

After pathologic assessment of relevant biopsied tissue has been completed, the search for the primary site may be undertaken. The diagnostic strategy employed relies heavily on the patient's signs and symptoms, confirmed disease, and distribution of metastasis. The initial workup should commence with a detailed history and thorough physical examination. Pelvic and rectal examinations are mandatory. Routine laboratory analysis including complete blood cell count, electrolyte levels, and screening profile should be obtained, as should a chest x-ray and computed axial tomography (CAT) scan of the abdomen and pelvis. If a primary site cannot be established by these means, further pursuit of the primary site may be unnecessary and nonproductive. The use of further diagnostic imaging, invasive procedures, or random tumor marker determination is not prudent. However, in patients with relevant history or positive radiographic findings, further studies may be warranted. For example, patients whose chest x-rays exhibit positive findings (parenchymal or mediastinal lesions) should be considered for further imaging and/or bronchoscopy. Primary sites are identified in 10% to 30% of all cases of unknown primary cancers. The paramount goal that ultimately guides the diagnostic workup for an unknown primary site should be the detection of a treatable malignancy.

TREATMENT PARADIGMS

When the origin of a cancer of unknown primary site is subsequently identified, treatment is initiated based on best therapy available for the particular stage of the primary cancer. While the vast majority of patients with cancer of unknown primary site do not benefit from intervention save for supportive care, there is a small percentage of patients for whom potentially curative therapy is available. In the approach to therapy for a truly unknown primary, patients are separated into four representative histologic groups, including adenocarcinoma, squamous carcinoma, poorly differentiated carcinoma and poorly differentiated adenocarcinoma (Box 100-1). It is assumed that poorly differentiated malignancies will be

---

BOX 100-1

Treatable subgroups for cancers of unknown primary site based on histologic study

Adenocarcinoma

Axillary metastasis in female patients in the absence of a breast mass

Solitary peripheral lymph node sites without ostensible primary

Peritoneal carcinomatosis with papillary features without identifiable ovarian primary

Metastatic sites staining for prostate-specific antigen (PSA) or males with metastatic sites who possess elevations in level of serum PSA

Squamous cell carcinoma

Cervical lymph node sites in patients without identifiable head and neck primaries

Inguinal lymph node sites in patients without identifiable anal or perirectal primaries

Poorly differentiated carcinoma/poorly differentiated adenocarcinoma

Lesions arising in midline structures (extragonadal germ cell tumors)

Lesions ultimately confirmed or suspected to represent lymphoma, neuroendocrine tumors, or anaplastic carcinoids

Lymph node metastasis representing anaplastic melanoma with occult primary

assigned into one of these four histologies based on light microscopy and immunohistochemical analysis. Each of the aforementioned histologic groupings has a series of treatable subgroups based on the patient profile and the site of disease. Each subgroup in turn has a particular approach to therapy.

ADENOCARCINOMA

Patients with adenocarcinomas represent the largest of the unknown primary site groups. Initial presentations include metastatic disease to liver, lung, or bone. Bronchogenic and pancreatic primaries represent the majority of primary sites (40%). Other gastrointestinal malignancies such as colon and gastric adenocarcinomas are seen occasionally; adenocarcinomas of the breast, ovary, and prostate, only rarely. The following potentially treatable subgroups are recognized:

1. Women with axillary nodal metastases
2. Women with peritoneal carcinomatosis
3. Men with tumors staining for prostate-specific antigen (PSA) or who have elevations in serum PSA levels
4. Patients who possess a solitary peripheral nodal metastasis

Women who possess *axillary nodal metastases* or who have them in combination with other metastatic sites are likely to have breast cancer. Patients having only axillary nodal disease (stage II breast cancer) may be treated with intent to cure. Data support modified radical mastectomy and axillary nodal dissection in these patients, even in the setting of negative mammogram findings and physical examination. This approach stems from the 40% to 60% of patients who ultimately have an occult breast cancer identified. The use of adjuvant chemotherapy and/or hormonal therapy has been recommended in this subset. The prognosis for these patients is similar to that for patients who have routinely diagnosed stage II breast cancer. Patients who have axillary nodal metastasis in conjunction with other sites may benefit from treatment for metastatic breast cancer, which may include chemotherapy, hormonal therapy, or both, depending on the clinical setting (Chapter 95).

Women with *peritoneal carcinomatosis* whose disease is consistent with adenocarcinoma and in whom histologic findings reveal papillary features often have ovarian cancer. There remains a segment of this subgroup in whom an ovarian primary cannot be detected. These women have a pathologic finding identical to that of ovarian cancer. This denotes a syndrome referred to as peritoneal papillary serous carcinoma or multifocal extraovarian serous carcinoma. This presentation is based on the embryologic development of the ovarian epithelium, which is derived ultimately from elements of the peritoneum. Women who come to medical attention with peritoneal carcinomatosis identified as adenocarcinoma (with papillary features) with or without an identifiable ovarian source should undergo surgical cytoreduction. These same patients should be treated with chemotherapeutic regimens that are active against ovarian cancer. Response rates ranging from 30% to 40% have been described for patients treated in such fashion (Chapter 96). Patients who have adenocarcinomas not demonstrating papillary features on histologic examination or whose tumors stain for mucin may have other malignancies known to have a predilection for peritoneal carcinomatosis (i.e., gastric adenocarcinoma). This distinction remains critical in light of the added morbidity associated with an unnecessary attempt at surgical cytoreduction in patients with gastrointestinal malignancies misdiagnosed as ovarian carcinoma or peritoneal papillary serous carcinoma.

Men who have metastatic lesions in the setting of an elevated PSA or whose tumors are positive for PSA by immunohistochemical means may have metastatic prostate cancer. These patients should receive a trial of hormonal therapy appropriate for prostate cancer. In the elderly age cohort, patients who develop osteoblastic metastasis whose tumors do not stain for PSA, or whose serum levels of PSA remain normal, may also be considered for a trial of hormonal therapy directed at prostate cancer (Chapter 97).

Patients who have an isolated peripheral lymph node in the cervical, axillary, or inguinal region revealing adenocarcinoma by pathologic study may benefit from an excisional procedure, radiation therapy, or a combination of both. These measures have produced long-term survival in a small proportion of these patients.

Patients who come to medical attention with adenocarcinomas not falling into one of the four categories just mentioned may be consid-

ered for a trial of chemotherapy. It must be pointed out that response rates for these patients have been generally poor to date, with approximately 20% of patients achieving some type of response. Chemotherapy should be reserved for patients with an adequate performance status, which in the setting of unknown primary tumors may be a small population of patients. Chemotherapeutic agents including cis-platinum, 5-fluorouracil, adriamycin, etoposide, and mitomycin have been used alone or in various combinations. It has been suggested that two cycles of chemotherapy be administered and adequacy of response assessed. If response is poor, best supportive care may be instituted. Patients who are responders may continue therapy for up to 6 months if response is maintained. There remains no documented benefit in extending therapy for a longer duration in this patient cohort.

SQUAMOUS CELL CARCINOMA

The majority of patients who possess squamous cell carcinomas of unknown primary site have disease isolated to cervical or inguinal lymph nodes. It is important that these entities be recognized, as they represent treatable and potentially curable malignancies. Patients with cervical lymph nodes containing squamous cell carcinoma may have either head and neck or lung primaries. If a primary site cannot be established by panendoscopy; CAT examination of the head, neck, and chest; and a thorough otolaryngeal evaluation, treatment is based on the level of nodal involvement and should be directed toward the involved neck region. Patients with upper cervical or midcervical involvement should be treated by both radical neck dissection and radiation therapy. Each modality has proven to be the other's equal in terms of survival; however, higher recurrence rates (approximately 30%) are observed in patients not receiving postoperative irradiation. Therefore radiation therapy is administered in conjunction with radical neck dissection and should be given in the same field and dosage as that given to known primaries of head and neck cancer (Chapter 98). Low cervical and supraclavicular nodes containing squamous cell carcinoma are more likely to represent lung primaries. The limited disease-free and overall survival inherent to these patients is probably a reflection of their bronchogenic origin. These patients should be assessed for disease below the clavicle. If no site is found, treatment should follow guidelines established for patients with midcervical and high cervical disease.

Patients who have inguinal lymph nodes containing squamous cell carcinoma may have anal or perirectal tumors. If a thorough workup fails to disclose a primary, these patients should be treated by inguinal lymph node dissection and radiation therapy. Long-term survival has been reported in patients so treated.

POORLY DIFFERENTIATED CARCINOMA AND POORLY DIFFERENTIATED ADENOCARCINOMA

Patients whose initial pathologic examination by light microscopy reveals poorly differentiated carcinoma or poorly differentiated adenocarcinoma may be given new diagnoses after immunohistochemical analysis. The most often revealed new diagnosis is lymphoma; however, the vast majority of patients continue to carry diagnoses of poorly differentiated carcinoma and poorly differentiated adenocarcinoma. Patients with poorly differentiated carcinomas (anaplastic carcinomas) limited to lymph node metastasis may have melanoma from an occult skin primary or a primary that was excised in the past and not identified as malignant melanoma. An occasional patient under the age of 50 years has features of a germ cell tumor with disease arising in the mediastinum or retroperitoneum and concomitant elevations in serum B-HCG and/or AFP. The finding of an isochromosome 12 in germ cell tumors by cytogenetic analysis has helped to identify germ cell tumors initially diagnosed as poorly differentiated carcinomas and poorly differentiated adenocarcinoma of unknown primary origin. Patients who are isochromosome 12 positive respond well overall to platinum-based compounds. Neuroendocrine tumors can sometimes be identified by their neurosecretory granules on electron microscopy. The origin of these tumors is not well established. They are, however, chemoresponsive, especially to cis-platinum–based regimens.

Patients with lymphoma, melanoma, suspected germ cell tumors,

cycles may be given. Prognostic factors used to predict a positive response to platinum-based chemotherapy include localization of tumor to the retroperitoneum, peripheral lymph node involvement, less than two sites of metastasis, young age, and no past history of tobacco exposure.

✔ *WHEN TO REFER*

The paramount goal that guides the diagnostic evaluation of a patient with metastatic cancer from an unknown primary site is to determine whether the malignancy is treatable. This is not a trivial task because many disseminated cancers (e.g., lymphoma, seminoma, breast) can be highly responsive to appropriate therapy, whereas others such as adenocarcinoma of the stomach do not respond. Referral to a multidisciplinary team of cancer specialists ensures close cooperation among the surgeon, pathologist, and oncologist. This is necessary to be certain that diagnosis and therapy are customized to treat the treatable, but to ensure palliative therapy only to those who will not respond to aggressive management.

and other specifically identified malignancies initially diagnosed as poorly differentiated carcinomas or poorly differentiated adenocarcinoma should be treated for their appropriate tumor. Treatment for patients with poorly differentiated carcinomas and poorly differentiated adenocarcinomas has evolved significantly over the last 10 years. The introduction of platinum-based regimens to this group of patients has resulted in complete response rates in the 50% range. Approximately 20% of these patients had long-term disease-free survival. It is theorized that this group of responders represents a heterogeneous group of patients with malignancies that include atypical germ cell tumors, neuroendocrine carcinomas, and anaplastic carcinoids.

Patients who are not placed in a specific category and have poorly differentiated carcinomas and poorly differentiated adenocarcinomas should receive a trial of platinum-based therapy. Two cycles are given initially to assess response. If a response is achieved, two additional

BIBLIOGRAPHY

Allhoff EP, Proppe KH et al: Evaluation of prostate-specific acid phosphatase and prostate-specific antigen in identification of prostate cancer, *J Urol* 129:315-318, 1983.

Bosl GJ, Dmitrosky E, Reuter V et al: Isochromosome of chromosome 12: clinically useful marker for male germ cell cancer, *J Natl Cancer Inst* 81:1874-1878, 1989.

Dalrymple JC, Bannatyne P et al: Extraovarian peritoneal serous papillary carcinoma: a clinicopathologic study of 31 cases, *Cancer* 64:110-115, 1989.

Gatter KC, Alcock C, Heryet A, Mason DY: Clinical importance of analysing malignant tumors of uncertain origin with immunohistochemical techniques, *Lancet* 2:1302-1305, 1985.

Hainsworth JD, Greco FA: Treatment of patients with cancer of unknown primary site, *N Engl J Med* 329(4):257-263, 1993.

Hainsworth JD, Johnson DH et al: Poorly differentiated neuroendocrine tumor of unknown primary site: a newly recognized clinicopathologic entity, *Ann Intern Med* 109:364-371, 1988.

Hainsworth JD, Wright EP: Poorly differentiated carcinoma of unknown primary site: clinical usefulness of immunoperoxidase staining, *J Clin Oncol* 9:1931-1938, 1991.

Mohit-Tabatabai MA, Dasmahapatra KS et al: Management of squamous cell carcinoma of unknown origin in cervical lymph nodes, *Am Surg* 52:152-154, 1986.

Nystrom JS, Weiner JM et al: Metastatic and histologic presentations in unknown primary cancer, *Semin Oncol* 4:53-58, 1974.

Patel J, Nemoto T, Rosner D et al: Axillary lymph node metastases from an occult breast cancer, *Cancer* 47:2923-2927, 1981.

Shildt RA, Kennnedy PS et al: Management of patients with metastatic adenocarcinoma of unknown origin: a Southwest Oncology Group study, *Cancer Treat Rep* 67:77-79, 1983.

Spiro RH, DeRose G, Strong EW: Cervical node metastasis of occult origin, *Am J Surg* 146:441-446, 1983.

Strnad CM, Grosh WW et al: Peritoneal carcinomatosis of unknown primary site in women: a distinctive subset of adenocarcinoma, *Ann Intern Med* 111:213-217, 1989.

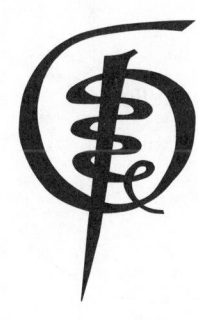

Renal
and Electrolyte
Disorders

CHAPTER

101 **Principles of Renal Physiology**

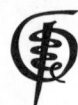

Jay H. Stein and George L. Bakris

RENAL PHYSIOLOGY

The kidney modulates sodium, water, hydrogen, and potassium balance. In a normal setting sodium intake can be varied from negligible amounts to 500 mEq per day without the formation of edema or substantial changes in systemic hemodynamics. Urinary osmolality may be varied from 40 to 1200 mOsm/kg of water (H_2O), whereas hydrogen ion excretion may be increased several-fold after the ingestion of an acid load. A large exogenous potassium load, which potentially could cause life-threatening hyperkalemia, can be excreted rapidly by the normally functioning kidney.

This section reviews the composition of body fluids and the factors that maintain their constancy, the determinants of glomerular filtration, and the renal functional events that are involved in the regulation of sodium, water, hydrogen, and potassium balance.

Composition of Body Fluids

Water and the major electrolytes are distributed among the various body fluid compartments on the basis of a complex series of transport and diffusional processes. Water accounts for 45% to 75% of total body weight, depending on the amount of adipose tissue, which is a function of the person's age and sex. Water is distributed between two basic compartments, extracellular and intracellular (Fig. 101-1), which are separated by the cellular membrane. Cell water accounts for approximately 60% of total body water. The extracellular compartment has been divided, somewhat artificially, into four subcompartments: plasma; interstitial fluid (including lymph); fluid within dense connective tissue, cartilage, and bone; and transcellular fluid (e.g., gastrointestinal tract secretions, urine, cerebrospinal fluid, sweat). Interstitial fluid makes up approximately half of the extracellular fluid (ECF).

Table 101-1 lists the electrolyte content of plasma, plasma water, interstitial fluid, and skeletal muscle intracellular water. As can be noted, sodium is the only major cation in ECF, whereas chloride and bicarbonate are the principal anions. In contrast, the intracellular concentration of sodium is one tenth that in ECF, whereas the cellular potassium concentration is approximately 150 mEq/L. Further, intracellular chloride and bicarbonate concentrations are low, with the anionic content of cells consisting primarily of inorganic and organic phosphates and proteins.

The differences between the composition of plasma and interstitial water are the consequence of the much higher concentration of proteins in plasma compared with that in interstitial fluid. When a concentration difference exists for a given impermeable charged particle across a membrane, the ionic particles to which the membrane is permeable (e.g., sodium and chloride) are distributed in a mathematically predictable manner. This is the so-called Gibbs-Donnan effect.

The mechanisms responsible for the compositional differences between extracellular and intracellular fluid are more complex. The values listed in Table 101-1 for intracellular electrolyte content are taken from skeletal muscle. In addition, the complex structure of the cellular matrix may markedly alter the activity of these various electrolytes. For example, it has been proposed that the chemical activity of

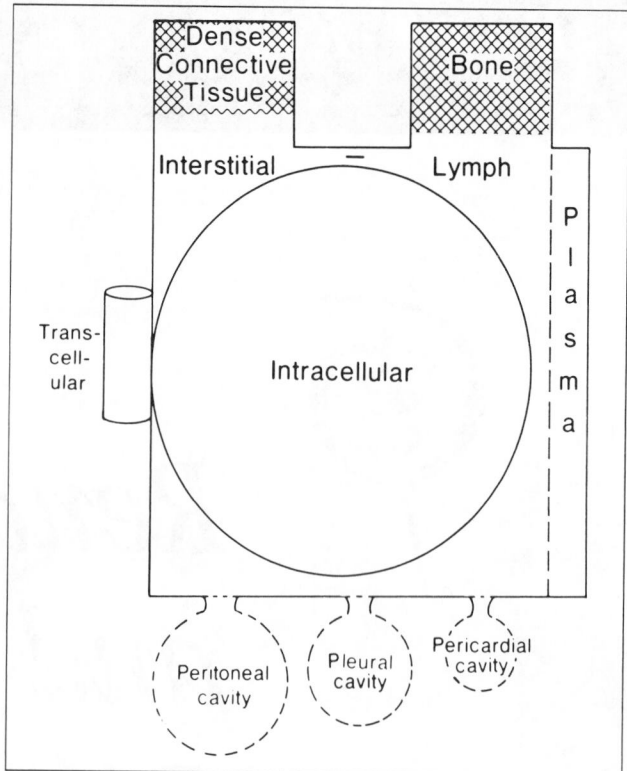

FIGURE 101-1 Compartmentalization of body water.

From Maffly RH. In Brenner BM, Rector FC Jr, editors: *The kidney,* ed 2, Philadelphia, 1981, WB Saunders.

Table 101-1 Ionic composition of the body water compartments

ION	PLASMA (mEq/L)	PLASMA WATER (mEq/L)	INTERSTITIAL FLUID (mEq/L)	SKELETAL MUSCLE CELL (mEq/L)
Cations				
Na^+	142.0	152.7	145.1	12.0
K^+	4.3	4.6	4.4	150.0
Ca^{2+}	2.5	2.7	2.4	4.0
Mg^{2+}	1.1	1.2	1.1	34.0
Total	149.9	161.2	153.0	200.0
Anions				
Cl^-	104.0	111.9	117.4	4.0
HCO_3^-	24.0	25.8	27.1	12.0
HPO_4^{2-}, $H_2PO_4^-$	2.0	2.2	2.3	40.0
Proteins	14.0	15.0	0.0	54.0
Other	5.9	6.3	6.2	90.0
Total	149.9	161.2	153.0	200.0

intracellular potassium is markedly reduced because of the attraction of the cation to cell protein anions.

The electrolyte content of the different transcellular fluids is also variable. The potassium concentration averages 4 mEq/L in biliary and pancreatic fluid but may reach 20 mEq/L in saliva and cecal fluid. Further, the bicarbonate concentration is essentially zero in gastric juice and as high as 90 mEq/L in pancreatic secretions. Although the pH of most transcellular fluid is close to 7.4, gastric juice may have a pH as low as 1.0.

Osmotic equilibrium exists between the plasma and the interstitial and intracellular compartments. Thus the size of each space is determined by the number of osmotically active particles present. Sodium and its attendant anions are the primary solutes in ECF, whereas potassium salts are the principal intracellular osmoles. A water load administered to a patient is rapidly distributed across all these major compartments until osmotic equilibrium is again reached. An isosmotic infusion of sodium chloride is distributed only in ECF and expands the extracellular volume without altering the tonicity. A solution of hypertonic sodium chloride also is distributed in ECF but also causes a rapid loss of intracellular water until the osmotic pressure is the same in all compartments. After these initial alterations in body fluid dynamics, the renal excretion of salt or water and changes in antidiuretic hormone release and in the thirst mechanism restore the previous steady-state condition.

The exchange of fluid between the plasma and interstitial compartments also is determined in great part by the Starling forces across the capillary wall. The net flow across the capillary is determined by the differences between the capillary and the interstitium in the oncotic and hydrostatic forces, or:

$$\text{Net flow} = K_f[(P_{cap} + \pi_{IF}) - (\pi_{cap} + P_{IF})]$$

where K_f refers to the ultrafiltration coefficient across the capillary; P_{cap} and P_{IF} are the hydrostatic pressures in the capillary and interstitium, respectively; and π_{cap} and π_{IF} are the oncotic processes in the capillary and interstitium. Because π_{IF} and P_{IF} are substantially less than π_{cap} and P_{IF} and approximately equal, net filtration is determined by the difference between P_{cap} and π_{cap}. At the arterial end of the capillary, P_{cap} exceeds π_{cap} by about 7 mm Hg, and net filtration occurs. On the venous end of the capillary, the reverse is true ($\pi_{cap} > P_{cap}$), and reabsorption of fluid back into the capillary occurs. The pathophysiologic significance of this phenomenon is discussed in other sections.

Glomerular Ultrafiltration

The production of an ultrafiltrate of plasma across the glomerulus occurs by a process entirely analogous to that discussed in the preceding section on transcapillary fluid movement. The net driving force affecting ultrafiltration of fluid across the glomerular capillary wall ($\overline{P}_{uf}$) is given by the difference between the transcapillary hydraulic pressure (ΔP) and the corresponding change in oncotic pressure ($\Delta\pi$). Thus the rate of ultrafiltration along a glomerulus (GFR) is given by

$$GFR = K_f\overline{P}_{uf} \text{ or}$$
$$GFR = K_f(\Delta P - \Delta\pi)$$

where K_f is the ultrafiltration coefficient (the product of the hydraulic permeability coefficient and the surface area); ΔP is equal to the difference between the hydraulic pressure within the glomerular capillary ($\overline{P}_{GC}$) and the pressure in Bowman's space (P_T); and $\Delta\pi$ is the difference between the mean oncotic pressure within the glomerular capillary ($\overline{\pi}_{GC}$) and that in the glomerular ultrafiltrate.

Direct measurements of these variables have been obtained in the rat. Several points are worthy of note. First, the pressure drop between the aorta and glomerulus is much greater than had been believed, with $\overline{P}_{GC}$ averaging approximately 45 mmHg. Since the plasma oncotic pressure is approximately 25 mmHg and P_T is 10 mm Hg, $\overline{P}_{uf}$ at the afferent end of the glomerulus is only 10 mm Hg. As ultrafiltration occurs, $\overline{\pi}_{GC}$ increases substantially and may, in fact, equal ΔP. When ΔP and $\Delta\pi$ become equal, filtration ceases and a state of filtration equilibrium is present. When filtration equilibrium is present, filtrate formation is markedly dependent on renal plasma flow. Thus the various factors that affect renal resistance (e.g., intrinsic tone, sympathetic activity, humoral release of various vasoactive substances, renin-angiotensin system, prostaglandin release, kinin release) are major determinants of GFR in a setting in which filtration equilibrium exists at the end of the glomerulus. Whether this phenomenon occurs in humans is, of course, not known.

It should be emphasized that K_f may have a major effect on GFR. Recent work has demonstrated that angiotensin II, antidiuretic hormone, cyclic adenosine monophosphate (AMP), and other agents may decrease the K_f. Further, K_f has been shown to be reduced in various experimental models of acute glomerulonephritis and acute renal failure.

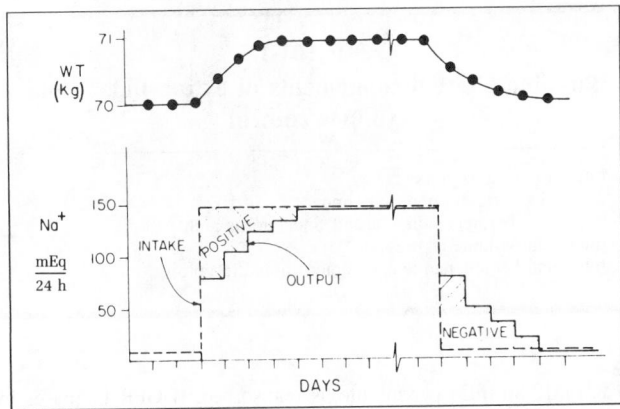

FIGURE 101-2   Normal sodium balance. An abrupt increase in dietary sodium intake results in a period of positive sodium balance and concomitant weight gain lasting 3 to 5 days. Thereafter, urinary sodium excretion equals sodium intake and weight stabilizes. When dietary sodium intake is reduced, negative sodium balance occurs and body weight decreases until, after 3 to 5 days, a steady state is again achieved.

(From Reineck HJ, Stein JH. In Maxwell M, Kleeman CR, editors: *Clinical disorders of fluid and electrolyte metabolism*, ed 3, New York, 1980, McGraw-Hill.)

Sodium Balance

Because sodium salts constitute more than 90% of the total solute content in the ECF, the net transport of these ions by the kidney is the primary determinant of the status of ECF volume. In the steady state, sodium intake and urinary excretion are approximately equal. If sodium intake is acutely increased, urinary sodium excretion increases, but it may take 3 to 5 days for a new steady state to be established (Fig. 101-2). In this interval there will be a concomitant weight gain and a period of positive sodium balance until intake and output are again equivalent. It is assumed that the increase in sodium intake expands ECF volume, which in some manner leads to an increase in sodium excretion and the eventual attainment of a new steady state at a higher level of ECF volume. Although this concept seems simple, the components of the afferent and efferent limbs responsible for this critical homeostatic mechanism are still far from being clearly understood.

Afferent Limb

The status of the ECF volume should be viewed in terms of the relationship between the volume of fluid contained in that compartment and the holding capacity of that compartment. The latter is determined by the capacity of the vascular tree and the compliance of the interstitial space. The vasodilation that accompanies normal pregnancy results in sodium retention, not because of an absolute deficit of ECF volume but because of the expanded ECF capacity. Cirrhosis, arteriovenous fistula, and assumption of the upright posture are other examples of conditions of relative volume depletion that result in sodium retention. Conversely, exposure to cold and immersion in water are instances in which relative increases in ECF volume occur, enhancing sodium excretion.

If the kidney is to respond appropriately to either absolute or relative changes in ECF volume, there must be some mechanism for sensing these changes. The possible components of the afferent limb are summarized in Box 101-1. It seems likely that there is more than a single afferent receptor and that the kidney itself may be intimately involved in sensing the "fullness" of the ECF space.

Efferent Limb

Glomerular Filtration Rate. The urinary excretion of sodium is determined by the difference between the rates of filtration and tubular reabsorption. In normal humans the filtered load of sodium equals approximately 14 mEq per minute. The urinary excretion rate is about 1% of this amount, or 0.14 mEq per minute, indicating that

---

BOX 101-1

Possible afferent components of extracellular fluid volume control

Intravascular receptors
   Cardiac atrial natriuretic hormone
   Arterial baroreceptors (carotid sinus, aortic arch)
Interstitial volume or pressure
Intrarenal hemodynamic and compositional receptors

BOX 101-2

Possible efferent components of extracellular fluid volume control other than glomerular filtration rate and aldosterone

Peritubular capillary forces: Hydrostatic and colloid osmotic pressures
Medullary blood flow
Redistribution of renal blood flow or glomerular filtrate
Humoral substances: "Atrial natriuretic peptide"
Sympathetic nerve activity

99%, or 13.86 mEq per minute, is reabsorbed. If GFR increases by as little as 1% and reabsorption remains unchanged, urinary sodium excretion doubles.

Conversely, small decreases in GFR would be associated with a relatively large decrease in sodium excretion if there were not some type of coupling between filtration and sodium reabsorption. Yet, there is abundant evidence of a relationship between filtration and reabsorption. In other words, an increase in GFR is associated with a comparable increase in tubular sodium reabsorption. Conversely, a decrease in GFR leads to a parallel reduction in absolute sodium reabsorption.

Thus under normal circumstances there is a direct relationship between filtration rate and tubular sodium reabsorption, which would tend to minimize changes in sodium excretion as the filtered load is varied.

Aldosterone. Aldosterone is necessary for the maintenance of normal sodium balance. This is illustrated by renal salt wasting in adrenal insufficiency. Because volume depletion stimulates aldosterone secretion and ECF expansion suppresses it, it has been attractive to credit this hormone with an important regulatory role in controlling urinary sodium excretion and ECF volume. Indeed, clearance, in vivo micropuncture, and in vitro microperfusion studies have demonstrated the importance of this hormone in the tubular reabsorption of sodium, especially along the distal nephron, where it affects potassium secretion as well. Several observations, however, indicate that aldosterone is not solely responsible for regulating sodium excretion. Most important, the chronic administration of mineralocorticoid causes only a transient period of salt retention, after which sodium balance is restored ("desoxycorticosterone [Doca] escape" phenomenon). Interestingly, atrial natriuretic peptide and transformation growth factor β impair the kidney's ability to "escape" from these sodium-retaining effects. The mechanism for this action by atrial natriuretic peptide is through guanylate cyclase–coupled natriuretic peptide receptor activation.

After mineralocorticoid is administered, a period of sodium and water retention ensues that lasts for 3 to 5 days. Then, despite continued mineralocorticoid administration, a natriuresis occurs, and balance is restored, albeit at a higher level of extracellular volume. This indicates that the sodium-retaining action of mineralocorticoid is overcome by a factor or factors that become operative as ECF volume is expanded.

Thus factors other than GFR and aldosterone play an important role in the regulation of sodium balance. In fact, it has been demonstrated that a natriuresis occurs after expansion of the ECF volume, despite a reduction in GFR and maintenance of high levels of exogenous aldosterone. Proposed mechanisms to explain this finding are summarized in Box 101-2.

Peritubular Capillary Forces. An increase in postglomerular capillary oncotic pressure or a decrease in hydrostatic pressure would increase the uptake of fluid from the interstitium into the capillary. Conversely, opposite changes in the Starling forces would lead to a net decrease in proximal tubular reabsorption. This mechanism has been suggested to be a regulator of sodium transport primarily in the proximal convoluted tubule and to be responsible, at least in part, for the alteration in sodium transport that occurs with expansion of ECF volume. Because these physical factors seem to operate only in the proximal tubule, it would appear that other mechanisms must affect sodium transport in more distal nephron segments.

Medullary Blood Flow. In addition to the alterations in net transport in the proximal tubule that may occur by purely passive means, hemodynamic alterations may change sodium transport in the distal nephron. An increase in medullary blood flow occurs during extracellular volume expansion, leading to a dissipation of the usual hypertonicity of the medullary interstitium. As a consequence of this change in the medullary environment, sodium excretion may increase in certain settings.

Redistribution of Blood Flow and/or Filtrate. The anatomy of the kidney is complex, and various differences have been noted between nephrons in the outer and inner cortex and their vascular supply. Primarily because of these anatomic differences, many studies have been done to determine whether blood flow or filtrate redistribution occurs in various pathophysiologic states. In addition, microperfusion techniques have been used to compare various functional aspects of transport in superficial and juxtamedullary nephrons. Although many interesting findings have been noted in these studies, their relevance to the regulation of sodium balance is still not clear.

Natriuretic Peptides. Atrial natriuretic peptide (ANP) is produced mainly in the heart and released into the circulation in response to atrial stretch. The circulating peptide is 28 amino acids long, with a 17-member cystine-cystine ring. Exogenous administration of synthetic analogs of atrial natriuretic peptide increases the GFR through an increase in the glomerular capillary hydrostatic pressure and possibly an increase in the glomerular capillary permeability coefficient, K_f. The capability of ANP to increase the GFR, together with its direct effects on the collecting tubule, results in profound natriuresis and diuresis.

In addition to its natriuretic-diuretic effect, atrial natriuretic peptide has been shown to inhibit almost all vasoconstrictors tested so far, including norepinephrine, angiotensin II, and vasopressin. It inhibits renin and aldosterone secretion both directly and indirectly. The action of aldosterone on the cortical collecting tubular cells is also inhibited by ANP. Circulating levels of this hormone are elevated in congestive heart failure, cirrhosis, and renal insufficiency and are normal or low in nephrotic syndrome, volume depletion, and possibly idiopathic edema.

Related natriuretic peptides such as brain natriurteic peptide (BNP) and the C type of natriuretic peptide have all been identified and characterized as contributing in some way to sodium homeostasis. However, their precise role is unclear.

Sympathetic Activity. Altered adrenergic nervous activity can modify urinary sodium excretion by influencing the Starling forces in the peripheral capillary bed, by affecting the central blood volume and thus the distribution of ECF, or by changing renal hemodynamics. A more direct effect of autonomic nervous activity on increasing renal tubular sodium reabsorption also has been demonstrated. It should be noted, however, that patients with a renal transplant (i.e., a denervated kidney) seem to handle a sodium load normally. An increase in sympathetic tone and arterial pressure may also result in a "pressure natriuresis." This results from a decrease in sodium reabsorption in the deep nephrons of the loop of Henle and questionably the proximal tubule. Thus further studies are needed for a better understanding of the role of the renal nerves in the physiologic control of urinary sodium excretion.

Water Metabolism

Normal persons possess a remarkable ability to maintain the tonicity of body fluids within very narrow limits, ranging from 285 to 295 mOsm/kg H_2O. This regulatory function requires the complex coordination of a variety of factors. When plasma osmolality begins to rise, mechanisms required to prevent further increases include stimulation and perception of thirst, release of antidiuretic hormone (ADH), and the renal expression of that hormone that permits maximum concentration of the urine. Conversely, small decreases in tonicity are corrected by suppression of thirst, inhibition of ADH release, and subsequent elaboration of a maximally dilute urine. The regulation of thirst and ADH release are discussed in Chapter 350. The following section describes the renal handling of water.

Renal Concentrating and Diluting Mechanisms. Even in the presence of intact thirst and ADH-releasing mechanisms, maintenance of normal water balance requires that the kidney be capable of maximum dilution or concentration of the urine. The ability to concentrate and dilute the urine is indicated by maximum and minimum urine osmolality (U_{osm}), respectively. During water deprivation and maximum ADH release, U_{osm} approaches 1200 mOsm/kg H_2O; during water diuresis with total suppression of ADH, normal persons can lower U_{osm} to nearly 50 mOsm/kg H_2O. Although clinically useful, U_{osm} is a purely quantitative term and does not necessarily indicate a normal ability to excrete a water load or retain water. The former is determined by measurement of free water clearance (C_{H_2O}), which indicates the amount of solute-free water that the kidney can excrete per unit time. C_{H_2O} is calculated by the following formula:

(EQ. 1)

$$C_{H_2O} = V - C_{osm}$$

where V = urine volume and C_{osm} = osmolar clearance, calculated as follows:

(EQ. 2)

$$C_{osm} = \frac{U_{osm}}{P_{osm}} \times V$$

where U_{osm} = urine osmolality, and P_{osm} = plasma osmolality. Combining (EQ. 1) and (EQ. 2),

(EQ. 3)

$$C_{H_2O} = V \left[\frac{U_{osm}}{P_{osm}} \times V \right]$$

Several important points regarding C_{H_2O} deserve comment. First, from close scrutiny of this equation, it is apparent that the maximum amount of free water that can be excreted depends on solute load as well as on ADH suppression and minimum urine osmolality. For instance, if a person with a plasma osmolality of 300 mOsm/kg H_2O ingests and excretes 1500 mOsm of solute per day $(U_{osm} V)$ and can reduce U_{osm} to 50 mOsm/kg H_2O, V is 30 L per day, and C_{osm} is 5 L per day. Therefore C_{H_2O} is, 25 L per day, meaning the person can ingest 30 L of water per day without dilutional hyponatremia developing. This quantity contrasts with the maximum fluid intake for a person ingesting and excreting 600 mOsm of solute per day. With the same dilute urine (50 mOsm/kg H_2O), V = 12 L per day and C_{osm} = 2 L per day; maximum C_{H_2O} is now only 10 L per day. Hyponatremia results with a fluid intake in excess of 12 L per day.

An important aspect of C_{H_2O} relates to the nephron site responsible for the generation of "free water." As is discussed in more detail later, urinary dilution involves removal of solute from the tubular fluid without extraction of water. In the mammalian kidney this process begins along the ascending limb of the loop of Henle at the point at which the osmolality of the tubular fluid becomes hypotonic relative to plasma. Distal to this point, further dilution of tubular fluid occurs and free water is generated. From this consideration it is obvious that maximum C_{H_2O} depends on quantitative delivery of filtrate to this nephron site, where free water formation begins.

The ability to conserve water maximally is quantitatively expressed by the term *free water reabsorption* $(T^C_{H_2O})$. This value is calculated by the following formula:

$$T^C_{H_2O} = C_{osm} - V \text{ or}$$
$$T^C_{H_2O} = \frac{U_{osm}V}{P_{osm}} - V$$

As can be seen, this expression is the opposite of free water clearance (C_{H_2O}) and is therefore sometimes termed *negative free water clearance*. The same principles that apply to maximum C_{H_2O} (i.e., dependence on maximum ADH release, solute excretion, and distal delivery) are also applicable to $T^C_{H_2O}$. Maximum $T^C_{H_2O}$ is physiologically important in preventing the development of water deficits. It should be stressed that once a water deficit is incurred (e.g., by profuse sweating or diarrhea), the thirst mechanism also must be activated to replace these losses.

As was noted earlier, the maintenance of normal water balance requires that the kidney be capable of responding to the extremes of ADH exposure. Maximum dilution of the urine is relatively straightforward and, as previously alluded to, requires removal of solute without water. In the absence of ADH the remainder of the nephron distal to this diluting segment is relatively impermeable to water and, as a result, a dilute urine is excreted.

The process of urinary concentration is more complex and is schematically represented in Fig. 101-3, A. Perhaps paradoxically, it, too, depends on the removal of solute without water from the ascending limb of the loop of Henle. This dependence is because this process is the driving force necessary for establishing a hypertonic medullary interstitium. As tubular fluid leaves the thick ascending limb, it enters the distal convoluted tubule and cortical collecting tubule, which, in the presence of ADH, are permeable to water but not to urea. Thus, as the initially dilute fluid traverses these segments, (in which interstitial tonicity is equal to that of plasma), water is removed and osmolality increases. The tubular fluid next enters the outer medullary collecting duct, which is also water permeable and urea impermeable. Because this segment lies in the hypertonic interstitium, as water is removed, the urea concentration and osmolality of the tubular fluid increase further. The fluid enters the inner medullary collecting duct, where further water extraction occurs. In addition, at the junction of the outer and inner medulla, the collecting duct epithelium becomes permeable to urea, which then diffuses passively down a concentration gradient, supplying solute to the inner medulla. The urea permeability of this segment is enhanced by ADH. As fluid enters the medulla from the proximal tubule, the characteristics of the thin descending limb allow for diffusion of water into the hypertonic interstitium without solute. As a result, the sodium chloride concentration at the bend of the loop of Henle is high.

In addition to the loop of Henle and the collecting duct, the vasa recta play an important role in maintaining urinary concentrating ability. As is shown in Fig. 101-3, B, these vascular capillary loops serve a dual function: they remove water that enters the medullary interstitium from the descending limb of the loop of Henle and the collecting duct and, by virtue of their permeability to sodium chloride and urea, they serve as countercurrent exchangers to maintain the hypertonicity of the medulla.

RENAL ACIDIFICATION

Under steady-state conditions the excretion of acid by the kidney precisely balances the acid that enters the ECF. As a consequence of the renal excretion of acid, the extracellular bicarbonate concentration is stabilized and the maintenance of systemic acid-base homeostasis is facilitated. The rate of nonvolatile acid production in the adult is estimated to be 1 mEq/kg body weight per day, or 70 mEq per 1.73 m^2. Because at the minimal urine pH only trivial amounts of hydrogen are present as the free ion, acid (hydrogen) excretion in the urine is buffered by ammonia or other buffers, particularly inorganic phos-

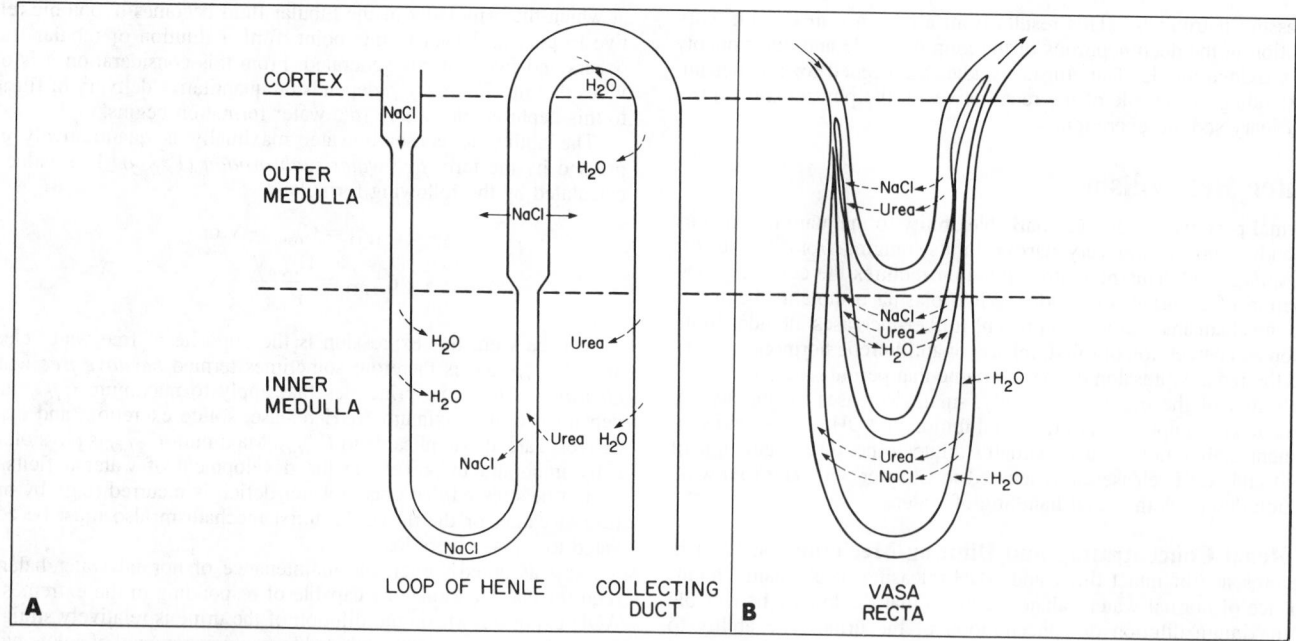

FIGURE 101-3   Urinary-concentrating mechanisms. **A,** The loop of Henle and collecting duct serve as a source of solute (NaCl and urea) to provide a hypertonic interstitium (see text for detailed explanation). **B,** The complex of vasa recta entering and leaving the medulla provides a mechanism for removing water from and trapping solute within the medullary interstitium.

phate, which is measured as titratable acid. The excretion of acid as ammonium accounts for about two thirds of the acid present in urine, whereas approximately one third of the acid is excreted as titratable acid. The magnitude of titratable acid excretion depends on the rate of excretion of the buffer involved, its pK, and the urinary pH. Net acid excretion by the kidney may be expressed as the sum of the ammonium and titratable acid excreted minus any bicarbonate that may be present in the urine.

The hydrogen ions that enter the ECF are primarily formed through catabolism of ingested food or tissue stores. Sulfuric acid produced as the neutral sulfur in sulfur-containing amino acids is oxidized. Similarly, the incomplete oxidation of carbon foodstuffs produces organic acids such as pyruvic, lactic, citric, and acetoacetic acid. The hydrolysis of organic orthophosphate and pyrophosphate gives rise to phosphoric acid, and the metabolism of nucleoproteins gives rise to uric acid. As these various nonvolatile acids dissociate, the hydrogen ions react with the body buffers (e.g., bicarbonate, dibasic phosphate, protein) to yield a neutral sodium salt and carbonic acid (H_2CO_3). The H_2CO_3 is excreted as carbon dioxide by the lungs.

As previously indicated, the renal contribution to systemic acid-base homeostasis is to regulate plasma bicarbonate concentration. This regulation is achieved by the appropriate reabsorption of filtered bicarbonate and the regeneration of the bicarbonate decomposed by reaction with nonvolatile acids, as has been discussed. As the neutral salts of the nonvolatile acids are presented to the kidney in the glomerular filtrate, the anion is excreted with hydrogen and the sodium, together with the newly formed bicarbonate, is returned to the ECF. The quantity of hydrogen excreted as titratable acid and ammonium is equivalent to the amount of bicarbonate regenerated.

As it is generally conceived, hydrogen ions are actively secreted at the luminal membrane into the tubular urine (Fig. 101-4). Associated with this secretion of hydrogen ions is the return of bicarbonate to the ECF. In the lumen the hydrogen ions react either with filtered bicarbonate to form H_2CO_3, which dehydrates to water and carbon dioxide, or, as discussed previously, with certain salts to form the acid salt (HA) and with ammonia to form ammonium (NH_4^+). The relative distribution of the reaction of hydrogen ions between filtered bicarbonate and nonbicarbonate buffers depends on the pH of the tubular urine. In more proximal nephron segments, where the luminal bicarbonate concentration is high, most of the hydrogen ion secreted

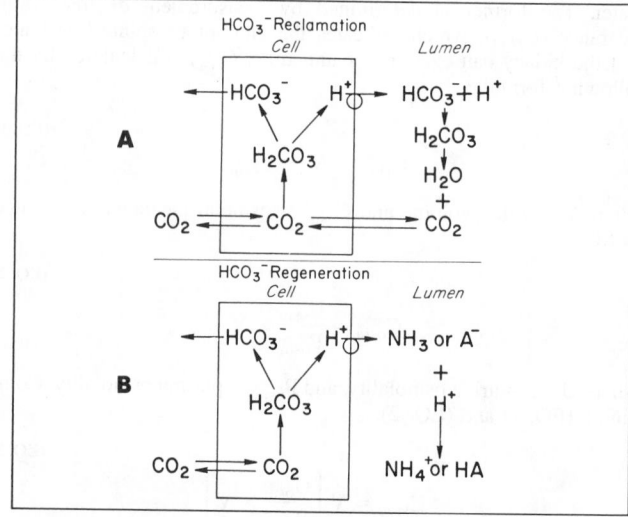

FIGURE 101-4   Tubular acidification. Hydrogen ions secreted at the luminal border effect **A,** bicarbonate reabsorption from the glomerular filtrate or, **B,** bicarbonate regeneration. The generation of hydrogen and bicarbonate ions may not occur precisely as shown, but the net effect is as illustrated.

results in bicarbonate reabsorption. As bicarbonate reabsorption nears completion, the luminal bicarbonate concentration decreases and an increasingly larger fraction of the secreted hydrogen reacts with the nonbicarbonate buffers. The enzyme carbonic anhydrase plays an important role in renal acid excretion in many portions of the nephron.

Renal acid excretion is influenced by a number of factors; some are capable of enhancing acidification, whereas others have the opposite effect. Angiotensin II is a factor known to stimulate proximal tubule acidification by activating both the sodium-hydrogen antiporter and the sodium bicarbonate cotransporter. This occurs through angiotensin receptor stimulation, mediated by activation of G proteins. In clinical practice the levels of ECF volume expansion, carbon dioxide tension, potassium, mineralocorticoids, and perhaps calcium, phosphorus, and parathyroid hormone have the greatest influence on renal acidification.

Clearance studies have suggested that potential renal bicarbonate reabsorption is inversely related to the degree of effective ECF volume expansion. Thus the addition of bicarbonate to the ECF in a patient with contraction of the effective volume results in a higher steady-state bicarbonate concentration than when it is given in the volume-replete state.

An acute increase in plasma partial pressure of carbon dioxide (PCO_2) stimulates renal hydrogen ion secretion. Because the quantity of bicarbonate in the glomerular filtrate is limited, however, bicarbonate reabsorption can only increase to the extent that tissue buffers are titrated, forming extra bicarbonate. More chronic (more than 24 hours) increments in the plasma PCO_2 result in increases in net acid excretion, adding new bicarbonate to the ECF. After a variable period, net acid excretion returns to normal as a new steady state is attained.

Mineralocorticoids and potassium have a complex and interrelated effect on renal hydrogen ion secretion. Current studies suggest that mineralocorticoid excess and potassium deficiency, when present as individual entities, have a very modest effect, if any, on net acid excretion and the extracellular bicarbonate concentration. Yet, the effect of combined potassium deficiency and mineralocorticoid excess in humans can lead to significant increases in net acid excretion and extracellular bicarbonate concentration. Mineralocorticoid deficiency results in a modest metabolic acidosis, as a consequence of a decrease in net acid excretion.

RENAL POTASSIUM TRANSPORT

In this section we present a brief description of the characteristics of potassium transport within individual nephrons and between different nephron populations.

Most of the filtered potassium is reabsorbed in the proximal nephron, that is, the proximal tubule and the loop of Henle. More distal portions of the nephron, namely, the distal tubule, the collecting tubule, and the collecting duct, are the sites where the final regulation of renal potassium transport occurs.

Proximal Nephron

Direct micropuncture study of the superficial proximal convoluted tubule of the mammalian kidney has shown that this segment reabsorbs filtered potassium in proportion to the amount of sodium and water reabsorbed. Under control circumstances this is 50% to 60% of the filtered load. The intraluminal concentration of potassium in the proximal tubule approximates the plasma level.

At the superficial early distal tubule, only about 10% to 15% of the filtered load of potassium remains. This indicates that reabsorption must take place in at least one distinct anatomic segment in the superficial loop of Henle. When potassium delivery to the bend of Henle's loop of juxtamedullary nephrons was measured in control circumstances, the amount of potassium present represented 113% of the filtered load, indicating that a net addition of potassium occurred between the glomerulus and the bend of Henle's loop. If the proximal convoluted tubule of juxtamedullary nephrons reabsorbs potassium, as does its superficial cortical counterpart, the addition of potassium must occur in the proximal straight tubule or the thin descending limb. Studies have suggested that the added potassium is derived, at least in part, from potassium reabsorbed in the collecting system.

Distal Nephron

Micropuncture studies of the superficial distal tubule have indicated that this nephron site is a major contributor to urinary potassium and the site where a number of factors that influence renal potassium excretion express their effect. The superficial distal tubule, like the loop of Henle, does not consist of a single anatomic or functional unit but is composed of a number of different segments. The initial superficial distal tubule contains, for the most part, the distal convoluted tubule, but later segments may have cells typical of the cortical collecting tubule. Between these two may be a segment where both histologic types are seen. The distal tubule can demonstrate either net reabsorption or secretion of potassium, with secretion being restricted to the distal half of this tubular segment. Therefore, although 10% to 15% of the filtered potassium may arrive at the early distal tubule, the amount present at its most distal portion, may be less than, equal to, or more than the amount that arrived at the early distal site.

The cellular mechanisms responsible for such divergent transport properties have been the subject of extensive study. The late distal tubular cell is assumed to be asymmetrically polarized, with the electrical potential difference across the peritubular membrane exceeding that across the luminal membrane. Potassium secretion is envisioned as comprising active and passive components. The active component takes place on the peritubular border, where potassium is moved into the cell by a process coupled with extrusion of sodium from the cell and associated with ($Na^+ + K^+$)–adenosine triphosphatase (ATPase). Potassium movement from cell to lumen is assumed to be passive, proceeding down a favorable electrochemical gradient. Viewed simply, the amount of potassium secreted depends on the rate of potassium uptake into the cell, the permeability of the luminal membrane, and the electrochemical gradient for potassium across the luminal membrane. Net potassium reabsorption also can be observed in the distal tubule when dietary potassium is restricted.

The collecting system comprises a number of different anatomic segments, including the cortical collecting tubule, the outer medullary collecting duct, and the papillary collecting duct. The cortical collecting tubule is capable of active potassium secretion but has not been observed to reabsorb potassium. The more terminal portions of the collecting duct have the potential to reabsorb or secrete potassium, depending on the experimental circumstance examined.

A number of factors—namely, potassium balance, mineralocorticoids, glucocorticoids, ADH, catecholamines, acid-base balance, and the delivery of sodium and water to distal nephron segments—appear to be capable of exerting profound effects on renal potassium transport.

Acute respiratory and metabolic alkalosis and potassium administration are known to increase the renal excretion of potassium. Conversely, both potassium deprivation and acute respiratory and metabolic acidosis may diminish the urinary excretion of potassium. The ability of mineralocorticoids to enhance potassium excretion may, at least in part, be mediated by their increasing the quantity of potassium incorporated into the cellular transport pool, thereby increasing the electrochemical gradient of potassium from cell to lumen. Mineralocorticoids also may increase the permeability of the luminal membrane to potassium. Glucocorticoids appear to affect potassium transport primarily by altering renal hemodynamics. Antidiuretic hormone directly stimulates distal potassium secretion. Epinephrine inhibits potassium secretion, an effect mediated by the beta$_1$-adrenergic receptor. The mechanism of this effect is still undergoing investigation. It has been known for some time that urinary potassium excretion may vary in parallel with the flow rate of urine and the delivery of sodium to the distal nephron. The potentiating effect of enhanced distal water and sodium delivery on potassium transport is also seemingly mediated through changes in the electrochemical gradient of potassium, although the precise nature of this relationship has yet to be clearly defined.

BIBLIOGRAPHY

Abraham WT, Schrier RW: Body fluid volume regulation in health and disease, *Adv Intern Med* 39:23-47, 1994

Bakris GL, Stein JH: Sodium metabolism and maintenance of extracellular fluid volume. In DeFronzo R, Arieff A, editors: *Fluids and electrolytes*, ed 2, New York, 1995, Churchill-Livingstone.

Ruiz OS, Qiu YY, Wang LJ, Arruda JAL: Regulation of the renal Na-HCO$_3$ cotransporter: mechanisms of the stimulatory effect of angiotensin II, *J Am Soc Nephrol* 6:1202-1208, 1995.

Rose BD: *Clinical physiology of acid-base and electrolyte disorders*, ed 4, New York, 1994, McGraw-Hill.

Tuunhorst RL, Lewis SJ, Johnson AK: Effects of sinoaortic baroreceptor denervation on depletion-induced salt appetite, *Am J Physiol* 267:121043-121049, 1994.

Yokota N, Bruneau BG, Kuroski deBold ML, deBold AJ: Atrial natriuretic factor significantly contributes to the mineralocorticoid escape phenomena, *J Clin Invest* 94:1938-1946, 1994.

II LABORATORY TESTS AND DIAGNOSTIC METHODS

102 Urinalysis and Renal Function Tests

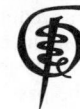

Charles R. Nolan, T. Dwight McKinney, and Marvin Forland

Table 102-1 Urine color alterations

COLOR	CAUSE
Black	Melanoma
Brown	Bilirubin (to olive green on standing), blood, cascara, hemoglobin, homogentisic acid (to black on standing), myoglobin, phenacetin, quinine
Greenish blue	Biliverdin, indigo blue, methylene blue, tetrahydronaphthalen (Cuprex)
Orange	Salicylazosulfapyridine (Azulfidine), phenazopyridine (Pyridium), rifampin
Purple	Porphyrin (on standing)
Red	Beets, free hemoglobin, fresh blood, phenolphthalein, phenytoin, vegetable dyes
Yellow	Quinacrine (Atabrine), riboflavin
White	Chyluria due to filariasis or thoracic duct obstruction

URINALYSIS

The urinalysis is one of the oldest, simplest, and most useful laboratory tests in clinical medicine. Traditionally it has been regarded as an extension of the physical examination, to be performed regularly as part of the periodic health evaluation and as an essential part of the evaluation of the sick patient. Despite its relatively low cost, it is a significant component of laboratory expenditure because of its widespread use. In many laboratories and hospitals routine urine microscopic examination is not performed unless an abnormality is detected on the screening reagent strip test (dipstick). Moreover, the cost-effectiveness of the urinalysis as a routine screening procedure or for preoperative evaluation has recently been questioned. Nonetheless, in the patient with a clinical picture suggesting renal disease, careful microscopic examination of the urine sediment by a well-trained clinician is imperative.

The *routine urinalysis* usually consists of a description of the urine, including its color and appearance, determination of specific gravity or osmolality, and the use of a multireagent test strip to semiquantitatively assess protein and glucose concentrations and to screen for the presence of blood or heme pigment. Semiquantitative measurement of ketones, bilirubin, and urobilinogen concentrations are often included. Reagent strip testing for leukocyturia is based on colorimetric detection of granulocyte leukocyte esterase. A complete urinalysis should also include microscopic examination for detection of formed elements such as red blood cells, white blood cells, and various casts.

Urine for examination must be freshly collected or refrigerated immediately if storage is required. If the examination is delayed, multiplication of bacteria results in pH alteration, leading to disintegration of cells and casts in alkaline urine. A specimen collected immediately after arising in the morning ("first morning specimen") is usually preferred for examination, since it has a lower pH and thus provides the best chance for observation of formed elements.

Color

The color of the urine may provide useful diagnostic clues. Many color alterations are due to drug ingestions. Table 102-1 summarizes the conditions or drugs that are responsible for some of the more common color alterations of the urine.

Specific Gravity and Osmolality

Plasma osmolality is maintained in a narrow range of approximately 285 ±5 mOsm/kg water (H_2O) because of the kidney's ability to reabsorb or excrete water as mediated by the tubular effect of antidiuretic hormone (ADH). Urinary osmolality (Uosm) and specific gravity reflect the activity of ADH and the sensitivity of the collecting ducts to its effects. The Uosm is the most accurate measure of urine concentration, whereas specific gravity provides only a rough estimate. Osmolality is a colligative property that reflects the total solute particle *number* per kilogram of water. It is a physiologically signifi-

cant measure of renal concentrating and diluting ability because it is unaffected by particle size and weight. Osmolality is usually determined by measuring freezing point depression with an osmometer based on the physical principle that a solute concentration of 1000 mOsm/kg depresses the freezing point of water by 1.86° C. The lack of one-to-one correlation between Uosm and urine specific gravity is due to the fact that the latter reflects not only the number of particles but also the *size* and *weight* (density) of urinary solutes. Specific gravity represents the weight of 1 ml of urine, a mixture of water and solute, compared to the weight of 1 ml of pure water. The possible range is 1.001 to 1.040 (the approximate specific gravity of serum is 1.010). The normal range is 1.003 to 1.025. High-molecular-weight particles present in abnormal amounts in the urine significantly elevate specific gravity with only a modest effect on Uosm. Intravenous contrast material is one of the most frequent causes of a marked dissociation between specific gravity and Uosm. Specific gravity is measured by a hydrometer or, as an alternative, a total solids meter, a simple instrument that measures refractive index and is calibrated to indicate specific gravity. A reagent strip is now available for determining urinary specific gravity based on a polyacid, the acidity of which is determined by the ionic strength of the urine. However, correlation of the reagent strip measurement with pyknometry or a total solids meter determination is altered by urinary pH greater than 6.5, albumin concentration over 100 mg/dl, and glucose concentration over 1000 mg/dl. The principal value of urine specific gravity measurement in routine urinalysis is to make certain the urine is not so markedly dilute as to permit false-negative values, particularly for proteinuria and formed elements. In a clinical setting suggesting renal or urinary tract disease, urinary abnormalities should not be ruled out unless the specific gravity of the specimen is over 1.015 or the Uosm is over 600 mOsm/kg.

Urinary pH

Because of the relative abundance of sulfur-containing protein in the human diet, the typical adult must excrete in the urine approximately 1 mEq of hydrogen ion/ kg of body weight each day to maintain acid-base balance. Because maximal urinary acidification can only lower the pH into the 4.5 to 5.0 range, net acid excretion is critically dependent on the presence of the urinary buffers, phosphate (titratable acidity) and ammonium. Normal urine is generally of acid pH except during the postprandial "alkaline tide," which may result in a transient rise in urine pH. Classic distal (type 1) renal tubular acidosis (RTA) is characterized by inability to reduce the urine pH below 5.3, despite the presence of systemic acidosis. Urine pH greater than 7 occurs with bicarbonaturia in the setting of systemic metabolic alkalosis caused by nasogastric suction or protracted (often surreptitious) vomiting. The upper physiologic limit of urine pH is approximately 8. Persistently alkaline urine may indicate an infection with a urea-splitting organism such as *Proteus mirabilis,* the usual cause for urine pH greater than or equal to 8.

Urine pH is most commonly measured using pH-sensitive color dye impregnated on multipurpose reagent strips. Nitrazine paper is frequently used by patients with uric acid nephrolithiasis whose urine pH is being regulated into the alkaline range as a therapeutic maneuver. The color changes permit estimation of pH in 0.5 unit increments. The more accurate result obtained with a pH meter is preferable for evaluation of patients with RTA. For the latter, the urine should be freshly voided, immediately aspirated into a syringe and, following evacuation of air, sealed tightly with a cork for transport to the laboratory to prevent diffusional loss of carbon dioxide resulting in erroneous elevation of the urine pH. The outdated practice of collection of the urine specimen under mineral oil is discouraged by most laboratories.

Proteinuria

Persistent proteinuria provides one of the best clues to the presence of primary renal disease or renal involvement in systemic illness. Proteinuria is often an initial manifestation of a renal abnormality during an early asymptomatic phase of disease and *always* requires further evaluation and clarification of its cause. Although approximately 180 L of plasma containing 12,000 g of plasma protein flow through the kidneys each day, the glomerular filtration barrier permits the passage of only a relatively small amount of protein into the ultrafiltrate. The 50 to 150 mg of protein found in the urine of normal individuals consists of a variety of components. Some of the proteins are identical to plasma proteins and presumably represent filtered plasma components that have escaped tubular reabsorption. Albumin is the major component in this fraction and represents 10% to 20% of the total excreted protein. The principal protein components in normal urine, representing one third of the total amount, are high-molecular-weight glycoproteins believed to be secreted by the more distal nephron segments. The Tamm-Horsfall glycoprotein is the major component and also a primary constituent of hyaline casts. The remaining urinary proteins are a heterogeneous mixture of as many as 30 components, which have the electrophoretic mobility of globulins. In pathologic states with proteinuria in excess of normal, albumin is the predominant component because of its high serum concentration and relatively low molecular weight as compared with other plasma proteins. Some individuals spill significant amounts of urine protein only while in the upright position but not while supine, a condition known as benign orthostatic proteinuria (see Chapter 105).

A number of methods are available to detect proteinuria on routine urinalysis. The reagent stick test is based on the reaction of tetrabromophenol blue plus citrate buffer, resulting in a color change when the stick is dipped into urine containing anionic proteins such as albumin. A trace reaction indicates approximately 20 mg/dl. The reagent strip does not react with tubular proteins or globulins, and the result may be negative in the face of massive proteinuria due to immunoglobulin light chains, as in multiple myeloma. Most nephrologists prefer the sulfosalicylic acid (SSA) method, which detects a broader range of proteins. Two to three drops of 20% SSA are added to 3 to 5 ml of clear urine, and the resulting degree of turbidity is estimated. Slight turbidity is reported as trace proteinuria and indicates approximately 4 to 10 mg protein/dl. The presence of a flocculent precipitate indicates 4+ proteinuria and generally reflects in excess of 500 mg of protein/dl. The intermediate ranges of turbidity are scaled from 1+ to 3+. False-positive readings may occur in urine that contains radiologic contrast material, tolbutamide, sulfisoxazole metabolites, or massive amounts of penicillin. Highly buffered alkaline urine may also give false-positive protein readings. The SSA method gives a positive result with Bence Jones proteinuria, since it detects the light-chain proteins that are missed with the reagent test strip. Significant proteinuria by SSA with negative or trace proteinuria by reagent strip provides a clinical clue to the diagnosis of multiple myeloma.

The recent availability of radioimmunoassays for detection of urinary albumin excretion rates at levels below the threshold for detection by the reagent strip or routine 24-hour urine protein assays has led to considerable interest in the clinical significance of "*microalbuminuria.*" In normal subjects urine albumin excretion rate rarely exceed 15 μg/minute, with a mean value of 5 μg/minute. Normal 24-hour excretion is up to 20 mg. Microalbuminuria is defined as an albumin excretion rate between 30 and 300 mg/day. Albumin excretion rates above this level can be detected by routine methods (macro-

scopic proteinuria). Microalbuminuria can also be defined by a single, untimed urine specimen with a microalbumin/creatinine ratio over 30 mg/g. A urine test strip providing semiquantitative immunoassay for microalbuminuria has also been introduced. A series of studies have demonstrated that the onset of microalbuminuria in individuals with insulin-dependent (type I) diabetes mellitus is highly predictive of the development of overt diabetic nephropathy with eventual progression to end-stage renal disease. Moreover, routine screening of type I diabetics for microalbuminuria is now recommended, since initiation of therapy with angiotensin-converting enzyme inhibitors has been shown to slow the progression of incipient as well as overt diabetic nephropathy.

Among individuals with non–insulin dependent (type II) diabetes mellitus, microalbuminuria is not as clearly predictive of the risk of developing overt diabetic nephropathy. However, in these patients as well as in nondiabetic hypertensive individuals the finding of microalbuminuria is associated with increased cardiovascular mortality and all-cause mortality. It is possible that microalbuminuria is a marker of renal vascular endothelial dysfunction or injury that is also present in other vascular beds, where it may predispose to atherosclerotic disease.

Glucose

Plasma glucose is freely filterable across the glomerulus and in normal individuals is almost completely reabsorbed in the proximal tubules. The transport maximum in men is approximately 375 mg/minute and is somewhat lower in women. The renal threshold at which glucose first appears in the urine is a plasma concentration of 160 to 180 mg/dl. Normal individuals excrete approximately 100 to 200 mg of reducing substances (principally glucose) in the urine in 24 hours. The presence of a positive test result for urinary glucose indicates either that the normal renal threshold has been exceeded by the plasma glucose level or that a reduction has occurred in the reabsorptive capacity of kidney as a result of proximal tubule dysfunction (renal tubular glycosuria).

Tablets for measuring sugar-reducing agents (Clinitest) have been largely replaced by enzyme-impregnated reagent strips that produce a color reaction when moistened with a glucose-containing solution. Because they contain glucose oxidase, the strips specifically test for glucose and not other reducing substances, and they detect glucose concentrations of 100 mg/dl or less. After rapid dipping, comparison is made with color standards on the container. Attention to timing is critical for accurate measurement.

Ketone Bodies

The ketone bodies, which include β-hydroxybutyric acid, acetoacetic acid, and acetone, are normal intermediary metabolites produced during fatty acid oxidation in the liver and other tissues. They are normally completely metabolized with negligible excretion in the urine. Normal blood levels are 1.5 to 2.0 mg/dl, and urine excretion is less than 1 mg/day. Ketosis occurs with the excessive formation and accumulation of ketone bodies in the blood. Diabetic ketoacidosis (DKA), alcoholic ketoacidosis (AKA) and rarely starvation ketosis lead to accumulation of all three ketone bodies with an accompanying anion gap metabolic acidosis. Isopropyl alcohol intoxication leads to ketosis without acidosis, since isopropanol is metabolized to acetone without formation of ketoacids. With ketosis, blood levels may reach 200 mg/dl with renal excretion of over 60 g/day.

Reagent strips for detection of ketones are impregnated with nitroprusside and react with urine or serum containing ketones to form a colored reaction product. These reagent test strips and Acetest tablets commonly used for ketone measurement react with acetoacetate and acetone but fail to detect β-hydroxybutyrate. In DKA with profound acidemia, DKA with superimposed lactic acidosis, or AKA almost all of the ketones are in the unmeasurable β-hydroxybutyrate form, and the diagnosis of ketoacidosis may be missed. Paradoxically, as the underlying condition is treated and the acidosis improves, the amount of serum and urine ketones may appear to increase as more ketones are converted to the measurable acetoacetate form.

Blood Pigments

A reagent stick test for heme pigment is included in most multire-agent urine dipsticks. The reaction is based on the principle that heme pigment catalyzes the oxidation of orthotolidine by peroxide, resulting in a blue product. This reaction may occur with red blood cells (hematuria), free urine hemoglobin, or urine myoglobin. The reagent strip test is most commonly used to screen for the presence of micro-hematuria. However, the test result may be negative if few red blood cells are present or if none are lysed, providing no free hemoglobin for the reaction.

The finding of a positive orthotolidine reaction in the absence of microhematuria by microscopic examination of the sediment occurs in the setting of intravascular hemolysis with hemoglobinuria or rhabdomyolysis with myoglobinuria. Acrylamide-gel electrophoresis or immunodiffusion can be used to definitively differentiate hemoglobin and myoglobin. However, examination of the color of the patient's serum usually allows for rapid clinical differentiation of intravascular hemolysis and rhabdomyolysis. Hemoglobin is a large molecule that binds to a serum protein (haptoglobin) and, when present in sufficient amounts in the serum to spill into the urine, results in a pink-tinged serum. Myoglobin is a much smaller molecule (not bound to haptoglobin), which is readily filtered and excreted in the urine, usually resulting in straw-colored serum with rhabdomyolysis.

Bilirubin and Urobilinogen

To be filtered at the glomerulus, bilirubin must be conjugated by the hepatic cell with glucuronic acid and excreted in the bile. Thus bilirubin appears in the urine only when plasma levels of conjugated (direct-acting) bilirubin are elevated. Urobilinogen is a colorless chromagen derived from conjugated bilirubin by bacterial metabolism in the bowel. Urobilinogen is partially reabsorbed in the small bowel and excreted in the urine in amounts up to 4 mg/day. Urinary urobilinogen excretion is elevated in states with increased bilirubin turnover such as hemolytic anemia. Urobilinogen may be decreased or absent from the urine with complete bile duct obstruction or with the use of broad-spectrum antibiotics that reduce intestinal bacteria capable of converting bilirubin to urobilinogen. Reagent strips are available for detection of both urinary bilirubin and urobilinogen.

MICROSCOPIC EXAMINATION OF THE URINE SEDIMENT

The urine sediment may be considered an "exfoliative biopsy specimen" of the genitourinary tract. It contains formed elements that may be derived from the renal parenchyma or elsewhere along the course of the urinary tract. Immediate examination of a concentrated, first-voided morning urine specimen yields the most reliable result.

A generally accepted method of preparation for examination of urine sediment is as follows: 15 ml of urine is placed in a clean conical tube and centrifuged at 2000 rpm for 3 to 5 minutes. The tube is inverted to allow the supernatant urine to run off, and the remaining urine is shaken gently to resuspend the sediment. A drop of this suspension is pipetted onto a slide, topped with a square cover glass, and examined while still wet. Using subdued light from a brightfield microscope, the slide is examined under low power (magnification ×10) initially and then under high power (magnification ×40). Quantitation of formed elements is accomplished by counting a minimum of 10 fields and averaging the number of casts per low power field and cells per high power field. Glitter cells and dysmorphic red blood cells are best seen with phase-contrast or interference-contrast microscopy. Oval fat bodies are most readily detected by the cross patté configuration under polarized light. Although motile rod-shaped microorganisms or budding yeast can be identified on the wet preparation, they are best identified by examination of a Gram's stain preparation.

White Blood Cells

Leukocytes in the urine must be differentiated from columnar epithelial cells originating from the tubules and squamous and transitional epithelial cells from the lower genitourinary tract (Fig 102-1). Normally two or fewer white blood cells are observed per high power field in cen-

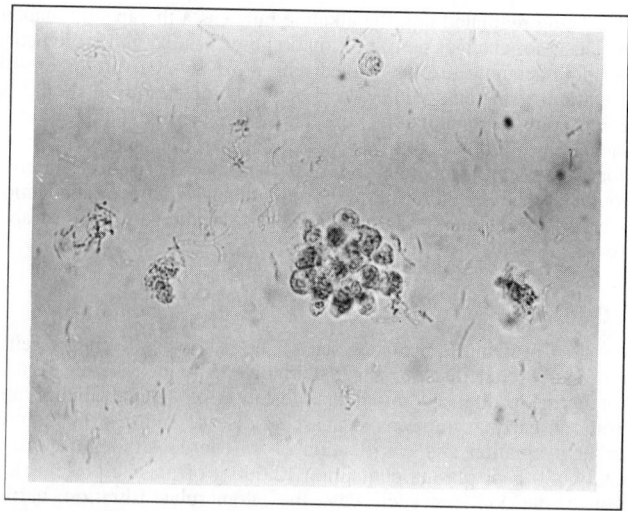

FIGURE 102-1   A cluster of white blood cells in a field containing numerous bacteria (magnification ×400).

trifuged urine sediment. In hypotonic urine white blood cells may take on the appearance of "glitter cells" with Brownian movement of their granules. Women are more likely to have urinary leukocytes than are men because of vestibular contamination. Significant pyuria is most often associated with bacterial infection of the urinary tract. The presence of leukocytes in the absence of bacteriuria by routine culture (sterile pyuria) may occur with Chlamydia infection, renal tuberculosis, acute glomerulonephritis, or systemic lupus erythematosus.

The presence of bilobed eosinophils with bright pink granules in a Hansel stain preparation of the urine sediment is a nonspecific finding that can occur in a number of primary renal parenchymal diseases. However, in the appropriate clinical setting the presence of eosinophiluria can help to support a diagnosis of drug-induced allergic acute interstitial nephritis, renal cholesterol embolization syndrome, or urinary schistosomiasis.

A number of epithelial cells may be seen in the urine as the result of normal urinary tract desquamation or vestibular contamination. These cells can usually be differentiated from leukocytes. Large, flat squamous epithelial cells with a single, small nucleus originate from the urethra or represent vaginal or vulvar contamination. Bladder or transitional epithelial cells are intermediate in size between white blood cells and squamous cells. They are often flat or cuboid and have a moderate-sized, round nucleus. Renal tubular epithelial cells are round, slightly larger than leukocytes, and have a large, single nucleus.

Red Blood Cells

Red blood cells normally appear as biconcave disks. Their form in urine partially depends on osmolality, and they may appear crenated, shrunken, or swollen. A few red blood cells may be found normally in the urine resulting from passage across the glomerular filtration barrier or renal tubules by diapedesis. Urine in adults often shows an occasional red blood cell per high-power field. More than two red blood cells per high power field is considered abnormal. Red blood cells must be differentiated from fat droplets, degenerated epithelial cells, yeast, and amorphous urates in an acid urine. The lysis of red blood cells by 2% acetic acid is often a useful differential feature.

The presence of red blood cells in the urine is usually indicative of renal parenchymal or genitourinary tract disease. Recent studies suggest that red blood cells of renal origin may exhibit a wide range of morphologic variation. These "dysmorphic" red blood cell forms contrast with the predominately uniform "isomorphic" cells characteristically seen with nonrenal sources of blood in the urine. Recognition of dysmorphic red blood cell forms in the urine is greatly facilitated by the use of phase-contrast or differential interference contrast microscopy.

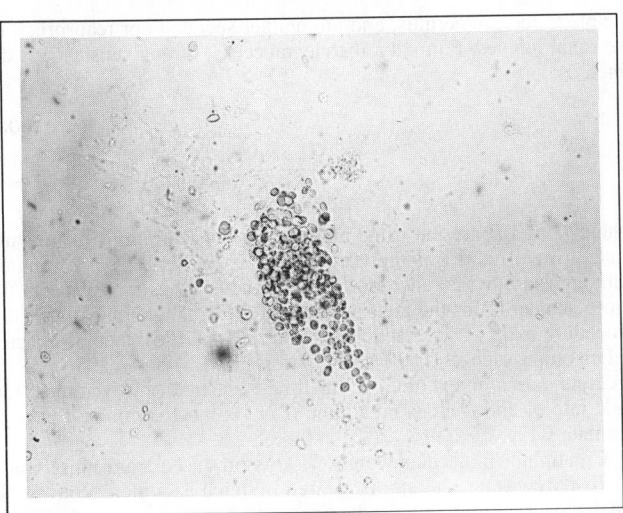

FIGURE 102-2   A red blood cell cast with clearly defined cells within a more extensively hyaline matrix (magnification ×400).

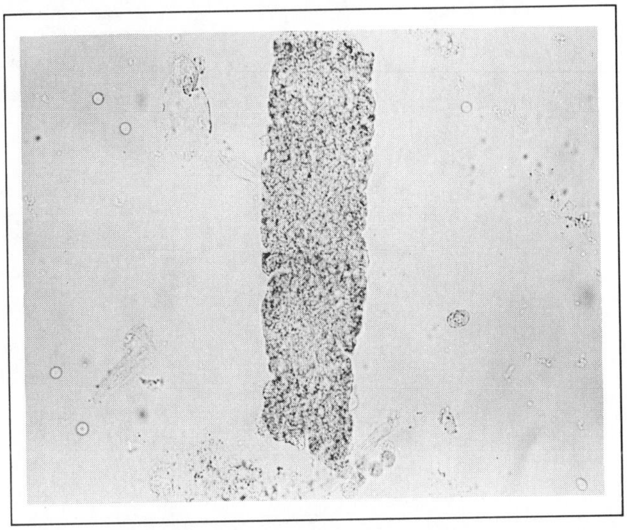

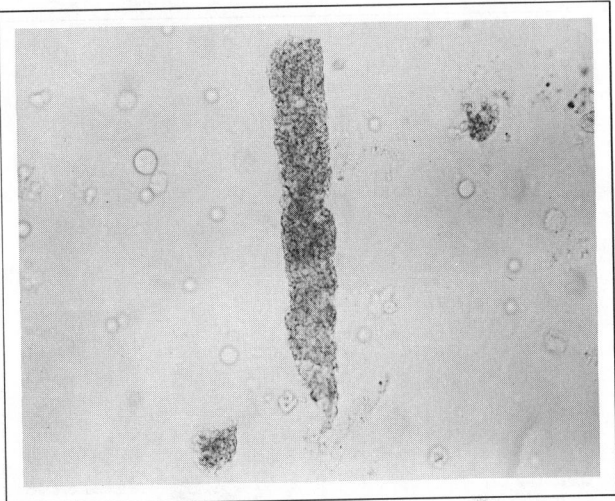

FIGURE 102-3   A broad, or renal failure cast with a finely granular matrix (magnification ×400).

Casts

Casts are cylindric masses of agglutinated material that represent a mold of a tubular lumen. They are usually formed in the distal convoluted tubule or collecting ducts. Addis found normal cast excretion rates to be in the range of 5000 to 10,000 casts/24 hours. The simplest type of cast is a *hyaline cast,* which is composed of Tamm-Horsfall mucoprotein. This is a low-molecular-weight protein whose tendency to precipitate is promoted by the presence of small quantities of urinary albumin and low urinary sodium concentration. Casts are best observed with subdued light and may be recognized by their parallel walls, squared ends, and faint pink staining with Sternheimer-Malbin stain. Casts may dissolve in alkaline solutions, hence the usefulness of attempting to collect an acid, first-voided morning urine specimen. The excretion of casts is increased with fever, exercise, and congestive heart failure.

Casts are often of critical diagnostic importance. *White blood cell casts* indicate the presence of a leukocytic response within the renal tubules. They are most commonly seen with renal parenchymal infection (pyelonephritis) or glomerulonephritis. Bacterial casts may occasionally be observed with upper tract infection. *Red blood cell casts* usually indicate the presence of glomerulonephritis, although they have occasionally been reported in acute interstitial nephritis (Fig 102-2). The red blood cells in casts may be distinct or may lyse and become incorporated in a homogeneous mass characterized by a rust or orange-red color. The latter are referred to as *blood casts.* In chronic renal disease, collecting ducts may become massively dilated. The so-called *renal failure casts* that form in these static collecting ducts are two to six times the normal diameter (broad casts), and they often have a homogenous, waxy appearance (Fig. 102-3). The presence of pigmenturia due to myoglobin, hemoglobin, or bilirubin may result in the staining of excreted casts (pigmented casts). Degeneration of cellular inclusions is thought to result in the commonly observed granular appearance of casts. Electron microscopy supports this sequence; however, some workers suggest that the granularity simply represents a modification of the basic fibrillar protein constituents (Figs. 102-4 and 102-5).

Urinary Fat

Free-floating fat droplets may be present in the urine as an external contaminant or from seminal vesicle or vaginal secretions. When fat droplets are observed within cells or casts, they are usually associated with massive proteinuria resulting in nephrotic syndrome. This type of lipiduria apparently is of dual origin: it may represent increased filtration of lipid in association with the hyperlipoproteinemia of nephrotic syndrome. A second mechanism appears to be the

FIGURE 102-4   A finely granular cast surrounded by red blood cells and white blood cells (magnification ×400).

increase in tubular reabsorption of protein associated with altered glomerular permeability, which results in tubular cell degeneration with the appearance of cholesterol esters in the tubules. These fatty droplets may be shed and make their way into casts (fatty casts).

Oval fat bodies are degenerated, swollen, fat-filled tubular cells that appear dark in subdued light but refractile in bright light (Fig 102-6). The presence of urinary fat may be suggested by the highly refractile appearance of the droplets. It is best confirmed with the use of polarized light. The doubly refractile element then appears as a brilliant white color that usually takes the characteristic shape of a Maltese cross or, more accurately, cross pattée (Fig. 102-6). Staining with Sudan III dye is also helpful for demonstrating fat particles.

Crystals

Crystals are often present in normal urine, particularly when pH is at the extremes of the normal range, and they may give the urine a cloudy appearance. The nature of urinary crystals becomes significant in evaluating the patient with demonstrated or suspected renal calculous disease.

With alkaline urine, phosphates are precipitated that can be readily

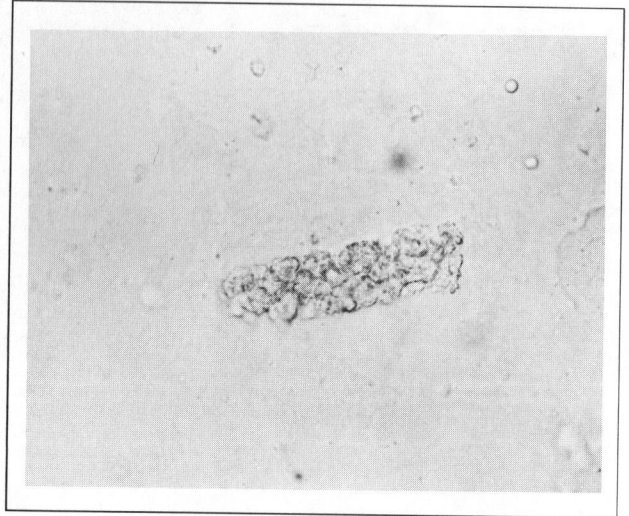

FIGURE 102-5 A coarsely granular cast with still recognizable cellular elements (magnification ×400).

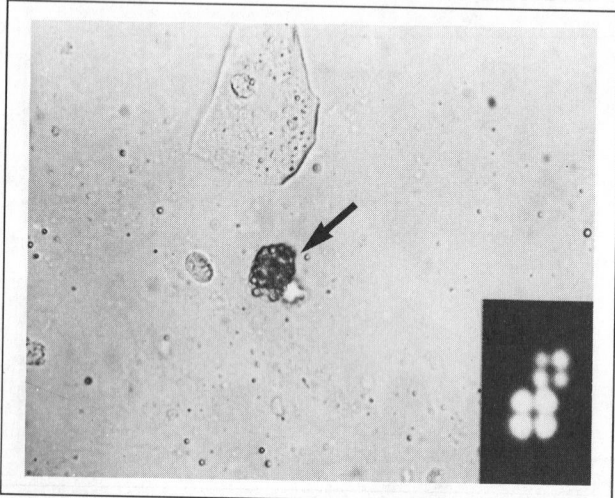

FIGURE 102-6 An oval fat body beneath a large squamous epithelial cell (magnification ×400). *Insert:* High-power view of lipid droplets under polarized light demonstrating the characteristic cross pattée pattern.

redissolved with the addition of dilute acetic acid. Triple phosphate crystals (ammonium, calcium, and magnesium phosphate) have a characteristic coffin-lid shape. Calcium carbonate and ammonium urate are also frequently present. With acid urine pH, uric acid crystals develop that appear as red, rhombic prisms or plates. Sodium urate appears as amorphous brown clumps, needles, or fan shapes. Calcium oxalate has the characteristic envelope shape. The finding of the hexagonal cystine crystals is highly significant, since it is usually indicative of cystinuria.

RENAL FUNCTION TESTS
Glomerular Filtration Rate

The most useful index of overall renal function is the glomerular filtration rate (GFR). In patients with renal disease serial measurements of GFR are used to assess progression of disease and response to therapy. The GFR is the amount of plasma ultrafiltered across glomerular capillaries per unit of time, expressed in milliliters per minute. GFR can be measured indirectly by determining the renal clearance of plasma-borne substances such as insulin, creatinine, or iothalamate, which are not bound to plasma proteins, are freely fil-

terable at the glomerulus, and are neither secreted nor reabsorbed by the renal tubules. Formally, the clearance (C) of any substance is defined as:

$$(EQ. 1)$$

$$C = \frac{U \times V}{P}$$

where U and P are the urine and plasma concentrations of the substance (mg/dl) and V is the urine flow rate (millimeters per minute). Although inulin clearance during continuous infusion represents the "gold standard" for the measurement of GFR, the complexity of this procedure makes it impractical for routine use. Clearance of injected radioisotope such as ^{125}I-iothalamate is used as a research tool for accurate measurement of GFR. In clinical practice, however, the clearance rate of endogenous creatinine (Ccr) is most commonly used to estimate GFR.

Creatinine (molecular weight 113) is produced from muscle at a relatively constant rate and is cleared by renal excretion. With stable renal function creatinine production and excretion are equal. Consequently, plasma creatinine concentration remains constant and Ccr is proportional to GFR. In an average-sized, normal man (70 kg, body surface area of 1.73m^2), serum creatinine concentrations range between 0.7 and 1.5 mg/dl, which corresponds to a GFR of approximately 125 mg/minute per 1.73m^2. The corresponding values in women are somewhat less—0.5 to 1.3 mg/dl and 115 ml/minute per 1.73m^2, respectively. However, the concept of a "normal range" for serum creatinine concentration is actually a misnomer, since the normal serum creatinine concentration depends on muscle mass as well as renal function. For any given level of GFR, muscular individuals have higher rates of creatinine production and excretion, as well as a higher serum creatinine concentration, than asthenic individuals. Thus a serum creatinine concentration of 1.8 mg/dl in a very muscular young man may not be associated with a reduced Ccr, whereas a serum creatinine concentration of 1.0 mg/dl in a frail, elderly woman may reflect significant impairment in renal function.

Creatinine clearance is determined by collecting all urine produced over a 24-hour period, obtaining a serum creatinine level once during this interval, and calculating clearance by the previously given equation (EQ. 1). Since incomplete collection of urine may lead to underestimation of Ccr, it is important to assess the adequacy of the collection. The total amount of creatinine excreted (creatinine index) should be in the range of 20 to 26 mg/kg per day for men and 15 to 20 mg/kg per day for women. The relationship between Ccr and serum creatinine concentration is shown in Fig. 102-7. Creatinine clearance normally declines with age beyond the fourth decade and with progressive renal disease. Once Ccr falls to 10 to 15 ml/minute, patients are usually in need of renal replacement therapy in the form of dialysis or renal transplantation (Chapter 110). As impairment of renal function progresses, the normally modest tubular secretion of creatinine comes to represent a much larger fraction of total creatinine excretion, so Ccr tends to overestimate GFR more in these patients than in normal individuals. Conversely, some drugs such as cimetidine, trimethoprim, and probenecid inhibit normal creatinine secretion, raise serum creatinine concentration, and decrease Ccr without changing GFR.

Because of the difficulties inherent in obtaining accurately timed urine collections, especially on a repeated basis, other methods have been devised to estimate Ccr. Once Ccr has been determined in the conventional manner outlined earlier, given the reciprocal relationship between the serum creatinine concentration and Ccr, subsequent changes in Ccr can be estimated from changes in serum creatinine concentration alone (assuming no major changes in muscle mass). For example, if a serum creatinine concentration of 1 mg/dl is associated with a Ccr of 100 ml/minute, increases of serum creatinine concentration to 2, 4, and 8 mg/dl will reflect Ccrs of 50, 25, and 12.5 ml/minute, respectively. It is also possible to estimate Ccr without the need for any urine collection, using the following formula:

$$(EQ. 2)$$

$$\text{Creatinine clearance} = \frac{(140 - \text{age}) \times \text{weight (kg)}}{72 \times \text{serum creatinine concentration (mg/dl)}}$$

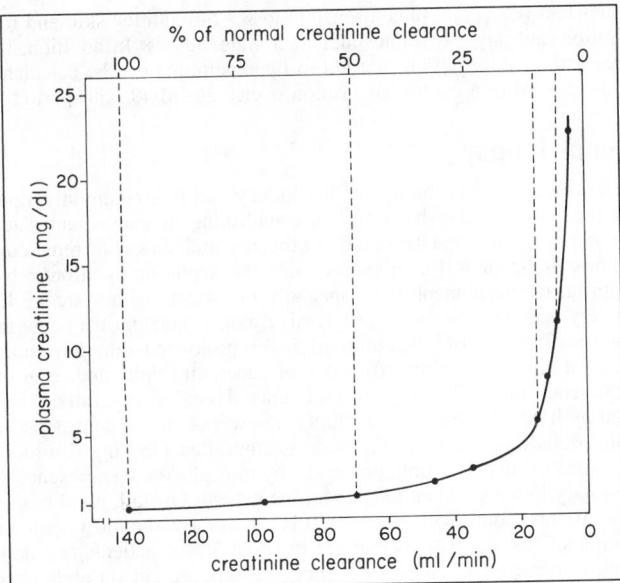

FIGURE 102-7   Relationship between creatinine clearance and plasma creatinine concentration. Note that at low concentrations of plasma creatinine, small changes in plasma creatinine concentration are associated with major changes in creatinine clearance. For example, as plasma creatinine rises from 0.7 to 1.4 mg/dl, creatinine clearance falls from 139 to 69 ml/minute (*dashed lines at 100% and 50%*). However, when levels are already elevated, large changes in plasma creatinine concentration are associated with only small changes in creatinine clearance. For example, as plasma creatinine rises from 5.6 to 11.2 mg/dl, creatinine clearance falls only from 17.4 to 8.7 ml/minute (*dashed lines at right*).

The result should be multiplied by 0.85 in women. Patients with marked obesity, ascites, or anasarca excrete less creatinine per kilogram of body weight, since their muscle mass represents a much smaller proportion of the weight than in normal individuals. Thus a correction of the weight used in the formula to lean or ideal body weight is advised for these patients. In normal or asthenic individuals actual body weight is used.

In the past the blood urea nitrogen concentration (BUN) and urea clearance rate were used to estimate GFR. Normally the ratio of BUN to serum creatinine concentration is 10. Although the BUN generally increases with a decline in GFR, numerous other factors may disproportionately elevate the BUN. These include tetracycline antibiotics, corticosteroids, gastrointestinal tract bleeding, urinary tract obstruction, high dietary protein intake, and prerenal azotemia. Conversely, liver disease and dietary protein restriction disproportionately lower the BUN. Consequently, the BUN per se is not a reliable index of renal function.

Fractional Excretion of Sodium

Under normal steady-state conditions urinary sodium excretion approximates intake. Determination of the fraction of sodium filtered by the glomeruli that is eventually excreted in the urine—the so-called factional excretion of sodium (FE_{Na})—is useful for evaluation of patients with an acute fall in urine output and/or a rise in serum creatinine concentration. Single blood and untimed urine samples can be used to calculate FE_{Na} as follows:

(EQ. 3)

$$FE_{Na} = \frac{\text{urine sodium concentration}}{\text{serum sodium concentration}}$$
$$\times \frac{\text{serum creatinine concentration}}{\text{urine creatinine concentration}} \times 100$$

To accurately interpret FE_{Na}, patients should not have recently received diuretics. FE_{Na} is greater than 1% and usually greater than 2% with acute tubular necrosis. It is generally less than 1% in pa-

tients with acute glomerulonephritis, hepatorenal syndrome, and states of prerenal azotemia such as congestive heart failure and volume depletion. The FE_{Na} in the setting of urinary tract obstruction is variable. It may be less than 1% with acute or partial obstruction or greater than 2% with severe or long-standing obstruction.

Determination of the fractional excretion of other substances relative to creatinine may also be useful for evaluating patient with disorders of calcium, phosphorus, bicarbonate, potassium, and uric acid metabolism.

Tests of Renal Acidification

The kidneys normally maintain blood pH and bicarbonate concentration within narrow ranges through tubular reabsorption of all bicarbonate from the glomerular filtrate and excretion of 1.0 to 1.5 mmol/kg per day of net acid in the form of titratable acid and ammonium chloride. The majority of bicarbonate reabsorption occurs in the proximal tubule. In contrast, net acid excretion requires the steep pH gradient from blood to tubular fluid that is present only in the distal nephron segments (distal convoluted tubules and, especially, collecting ducts). Forms of hyperchloremic metabolic acidosis referred to as *renal tubular acidosis* (RTA) may result from incomplete bicarbonate reabsorption with bicarbonaturia (*proximal* RTA) or from decreased net acid excretion (*distal* RTA) (Chapter 115). In addition to urinary bicarbonate wasting, some patients with proximal RTA excrete excessive amount of other solutes normally reabsorbed in the proximal tubule, including glucose, phosphate, amino acids, and uric acid. This condition of multiple proximal tubule abnormalities is referred to as *Fanconi's syndrome*.

The ability to maximally acidify the urine can be evaluated by an ammonium chloride (acid) loading test: 0.1 g ammonium chloride/kg body weight is ingested over 1 hour and urine samples are collected for the next 8 hours. Two hours following ammonium chloride ingestion, urine pH in normal individuals falls to 5.3 or less. Inability to lower the urine pH to this level, either spontaneously or after an acid load, suggests the possibility of classic distal (type 1) RTA, whereas an appropriate urinary acidification response excludes this diagnosis. In contrast, a normal urinary acidification response to ammonium chloride loading does not rule out proximal RTA. In proximal RTA, if significant metabolic acidosis occurs either spontaneously or with acid loading and the serum bicarbonate value falls below the abnormally low threshold for bicarbonate reabsorption in this disorder (serum bicarbonate concentrations below 15 to 18 mEq/L), reabsorption of filtered bicarbonate can be complete and normal distal acidification is possible. On the other hand, if the serum bicarbonate concentration is above the threshold, bicarbonaturia ensues and the urine pH exceeds 7.0. Proximal and distal forms of RTA can be differentiated by measuring the fractional excretion of bicarbonate (FE_{HCO_3}). Following exogenous alkali administration to normalize serum bicarbonate concentration, FE_{HCO_3}, calculated by the previous equation (EQ. 3), exceeds 10% in patients with proximal RTA, whereas values of less than 3% to 5% are observed in distal forms of RTA.

In certain forms of distal RTA other than classical type 1, such as type 4 or hyperkalemic distal RTA, urine can be acidified normally but urinary ammonium and therefore net acid excretion are diminished. (Chapter 115). Determination of urinary ammonium may be useful in differentiating these disorders from hyperchloremic acidosis that is due to gastrointestinal tract losses resulting from diarrhea or laxative abuse. Whether ammonium is present in the urine can be estimated by calculation of the urine anion gap (UAG) by the following formula:

(EQ. 4)

$$UAG = \text{Urine } (Na^+ \text{ conc.} + K^+ \text{ conc.} - Cl^- \text{ conc.})$$

Because ammonium (an unmeasured cation) in the urine is accompanied by an anion (predominantly Cl^-), when ammonium is present the UAG will be negative. A positive UAG indicates the absence of urinary ammonium, as is the case in hyperkalemic distal RTA. In contrast, with gastrointestinal tract disorders that are causing hyperchloremic acidosis the UAG is negative, implying appropriate excretion of acid in the form of ammonium.

Urinary Concentration and Dilution

Normal individuals are able to vary urine osmolality between approximately 50 and 1000 mOsm/kg H_2O under conditions of water loading and deprivation, respectively. This ability to either excrete or conserve water depends on proper renal and hypothalamic function and allows for maintenance of plasma osmolality in the narrow range of 280 to 298 mOsm/kg H_2O.

Disorders of urinary dilution lead to hyponatremia. Urinary diluting ability is tested by oral administration of water, 20 ml/kg over 30 minutes, with collection of urine samples every 30 minutes for the next 4 hours. Normal individuals excrete greater than 80% of the water load during this period and lower urine osmolality to less than 100 mOsm/kg H_2O. To avoid acute water intoxication, a water load should not be administered to individuals with serum sodium concentration less than 130 mEq/L.

Disorders of urinary concentration can become evident in two ways. In ambulatory adult patients mild defects in urinary concentration manifest as nocturia, whereas more profound defects lead to the development of polyuria and polydipsia. In these patients, as long as access to water is unimpaired, hypernatremia does not usually develop. In contrast, in children and hospitalized adults with impaired access to water, urinary concentrating defects manifest in the form of hypernatremia.

Polyuria, defined as a urine output greater than 3 L per day, can result from osmotic diuresis, water diuresis, or a combination of both. Determination of osmolar and free-water clearance in a timed urine collection is useful in the differential diagnosis of these disorders. The urine produced over a 24-hour period can be conceptualized as consisting of two components.

(EQ. 5)

$$V \text{ (urine flow rate, ml/minute)} = Cosm + C_{H_2O}$$

The first component, known as osmolar clearance *(Cosm)*, is the daily volume (ml/minute) of urine required to excrete the daily solute load at a urine osmolality equal to plasma osmolality. The second component, known as free-water clearance *(C_{H_2O})* is the daily volume of urine (ml/minute) excreted in excess of the Cosm. The formula for Cosm is analogous to that in the earlier equation (EQ. 1), where *U* and *P* are the urine and plasma osmolality and *V* is the urine flow rate (ml/minute). Since the typical daily solute load is roughly 600 mOsm, the normal Cosm is in the range of 1.4 ml/minute. By definition, if Cosm exceeds 3 ml/minute, an osmotic diuresis is present. Causes of osmotic diuresis include glucose, mannitol, increased urea excretion resulting from excessive protein intake, and increased sodium excretion resulting from excessive intake or diuretic administration. On the other hand, a large free-water clearance rate implies water diuresis, which may result from central or nephrogenic diabetes insipidus or primary polydipsia. The cause of water diuresis can be further evaluated by determining the maximal urinary concentration achieved in response to water deprivation and the magnitude of any additional increase in urine osmolality (Uosm) produced by exogenous administration of antidiuretic hormone.

The traditional formulas for osmolar and free-water clearance describe urinary water excretion in relation to total urinary solids and are primarily useful for differentiating osmotic and water diuresis as outlined earlier. However, in the evaluation of disturbances of plasma osmolality and plasma sodium concentration it is best to ignore non-electrolyte urinary solute and focus only on relative amounts of electrolyte and water excreted in the urine. In this regard, in patients with hospital acquired hypernatremia resulting from disorders of urinary concentration the magnitude of ongoing urinary losses of free water can be determined by calculation of electrolyte free-water clearance ($C_{H_2O\text{-}EF}$) in a timed urine collection using the following formula where V is the urine flow rate (ml/minute):

(EQ. 6)

$$C_{H_2O\text{-}EF} = V - \left[\frac{(\text{urine Na conc.} + \text{urine K conc.}) \times V}{(\text{serum sodium concentration})} \right]$$

The amount of daily water administration required to prevent further dehydration is the sum of the ongoing urinary electrolyte free-water loss ($C_{H_2O\text{-}EF}$), plus insensible losses through the skin and respiration and any gastrointestinal tract water losses. In addition, the preexisting water deficit that led to hypernatremia can be calculated and replaced in a controlled fashion over a 36- to 48-hour period.

Renal Biopsy

Percutaneous needle biopsy of the kidney and less commonly, open surgical biopsy, may be useful in establishing diagnosis and determining prognosis and as a guide to therapy in a variety of renal conditions. Indications for biopsy include the nephrotic syndrome; hematuria; glomerulonephritis, especially in patients with systemic lupus erythematosus; rapidly progressive glomerulonephritis; acute renal insufficiency of uncertain origin or prolonged duration; some cases of chronic renal insufficiency of uncertain origin; and renal insufficiency in renal transplant recipients. Tissue is generally examined by light, electron, and immunofluorescence microscopy. Contraindications to renal biopsy include uncontrolled bleeding disorders, uncontrolled hypertension, urosepsis, hydronephrosis, the presence of a solitary kidney, and an uncooperative patient. Overall, renal biopsy is a safe procedure with less than 0.1% mortality. The most common complications are gross hematuria in about 5% of patients and perinephric hematoma. The later complication is present on abdominal computerized tomography in up to 60% of patients but clinically apparent in only about 1%. Clinically significant arteriovenous fistulas and inadvertent laceration of adjacent organs are rare complications.

BIBLIOGRAPHY

Carlson JA, Harrington JT: Laboratory evaluation of renal function. In Schrier RW, Gottschalk CW, editors: *Diseases of the kidney*, ed 5, Boston, 1993, Little, Brown.
Perrone RD, Madias NE, Levey AS: Serum creatinine as an index of renal function: new insights into old concepts, *Clin Chem* 38:1933-1953, 1992.

CHAPTER

103   Imaging of Renal Disorders

Abraham A. Ghiatas

Diagnostic radiology makes a significant contribution to the evaluation of the urinary system. This chapter outlines the diagnostic methods available for evaluation of various urinary tract diseases and provides some diagnostic algorithms for the use of these imaging modalities.

METHODS OF EXAMINATION
Intravenous Pyelography

Intravenous pyelography (IVP) remains the most important imaging modality for evaluation of kidney and urinary tract disease. Intravenous contrast medium (iodinated products) is administered, which is then concentrated and excreted by the kidney. This process produces opacification of the renal parenchyma, collecting system, ureter, and bladder.

A scout view of the abdomen (kidneys, ureters, and bladder [KUB]) (Fig. 103-1) is an important part of the IVP. IVP should not be performed or interpreted without a scout view of the abdomen, which provides significant information regarding calcifications of the kidney and/or urinary tract (the presence of contrast media within the urinary tract may obscure calcifications). It also provides information regarding the bones (metastasis, fracture, etc.) and gas pattern. It is highly advisable to obtain a precontrast tomographic exposure of the kidneys for evaluation of the position, size, shape, and so forth.

After the intravenous administration of contrast medium several films of the abdomen and tomograms of the kidneys are obtained. Compression may be used to partially obstruct the ureters and achieve

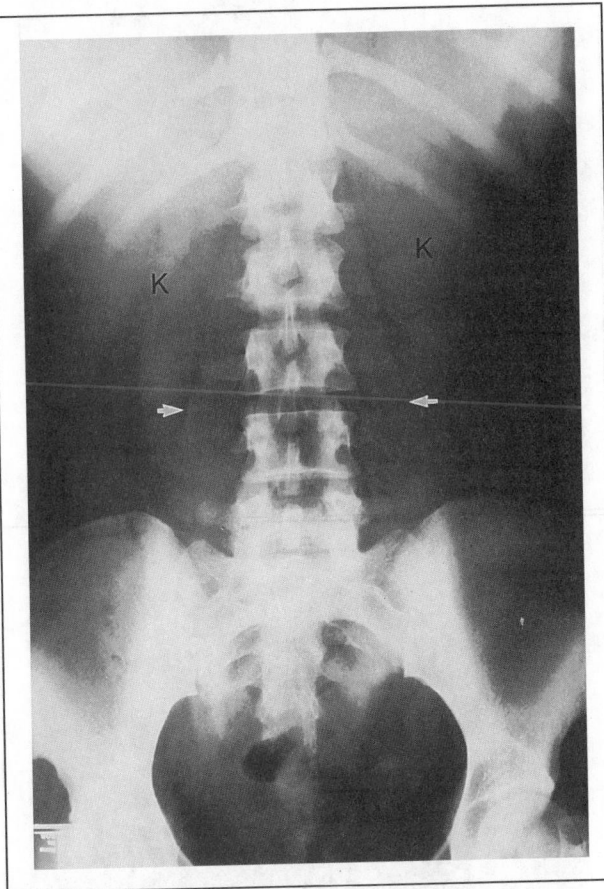

FIGURE 103-1   Normal view of kidneys, ureter, and bladder (KUB). *Arrows* indicate psoas muscles. *K,* kidneys.

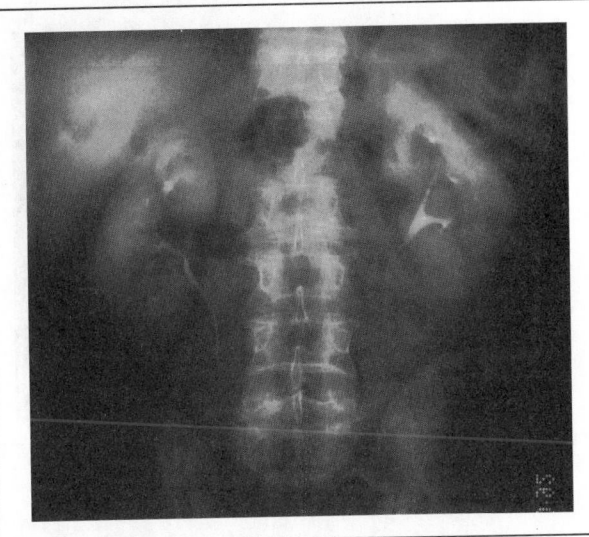

FIGURE 103-2   Normal intravenous pyelogram. Nephrogram and pyelogram phases are well demonstrated.

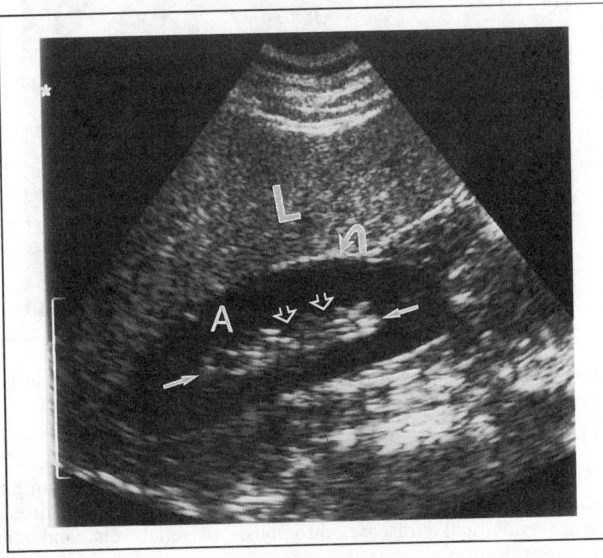

FIGURE 103-3   Normal ultrasonogram of kidney. Renal sinus *(arrows),* pyramids *(open arrows),* cortex *(A),* and retroperitoneal fat stripe *(curved arrow)* are evident. The renal cortex is of lower echogenicity when compared with the liver *(L).*

better visualization of the pyelocalyceal system (compression is contraindicated in urinary tract obstruction, abdominal aneurysms, and recent abdominal surgery).

The IVP has two phases. During the first phase, the nephrogram phase, the contrast medium is in the tubular space, which provides information about the renal parenchyma. During this phase the kidney appears homogeneously dense (white). During the second phase the pyelogram phase, the contrast media is in the pyelocalyceal system (Fig. 103-2). Approximately 3 minutes after the administration of contrast medium, the ureters are opacified and can be evaluated for defects indicating calculi, tumors, or blood clots. Their course and relationship to the psoas muscle and spine are also evaluated.

Abnormalities in the course of the ureters indicate the presence of extrinsic mass compressing on the ureters. In an IVP study dilation of the middle third of the ureter is a normal finding and is caused by compression of the ureter by the iliac vessels. In females there may be a vascular compression of the right ureter at the level L4-5 caused by the ovarian vein as it enters the inferior vena cava. The urinary bladder is evaluated (shape, position, contour, residual urine volume, filling defects) when filled with contrast medium, as well as when empty (on postvoid film). In females, compression of the dome of the bladder is usually caused by the uterus, whereas compression of the base of the bladder in males is caused by a hypertrophic prostatic gland.

Ultrasonography

Diagnostic ultrasonography (US) is an accurate, noninvasive, cost-efficient, and portable imaging modality that has become essential in the evaluation of the urinary system. Neither radiation nor contrast medium is needed for imaging. In cases where renal insufficiency or allergy to contrast media precludes the use of IVP or computed to-

mography (CT), sonography assumes a primary role in the evaluation of renal disease. US can accurately diagnose and grade hydronephrosis.

Renal masses are easily imaged by US, and differentiation of a cystic from a solid mass is mainly made by sonography. Cysts less than 1 cm in diameter and solid masses of approximately 2 cm in diameter can easily be evaluated by sonography.

In a normal renal sonogram the kidney appears as an ovoid (bean-shaped) solid structure with the following distinct sonographic zones:

1. Central zone: Renal sinus, fat, blood vessels, and pyelocalyceal system of high echogenicity
2. Peripheral zone: Sonolucent and consisting of the renal pyramids of the renal medulla
3. Outer zone: Represents the renal cortex (tubules, glomeruli, connective tissue) of medium-level echogenicity (Fig. 103-3).

In medical renal disease the echogenicity of the cortex is increased almost to the level of that of the liver (compare Fig. 103-4 with Fig. 103-3).

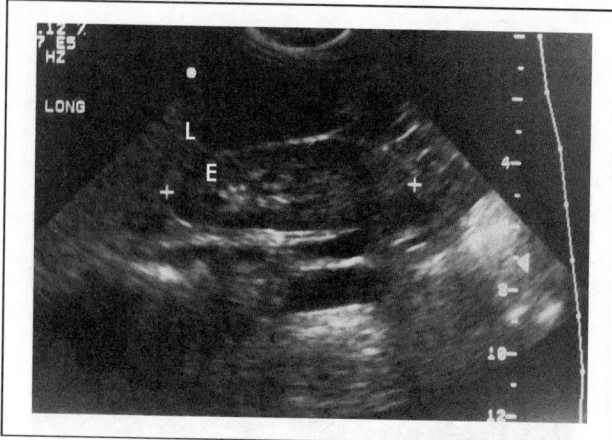

FIGURE 103-4　Medical renal disease. *E*, Cortex; *L*, liver.

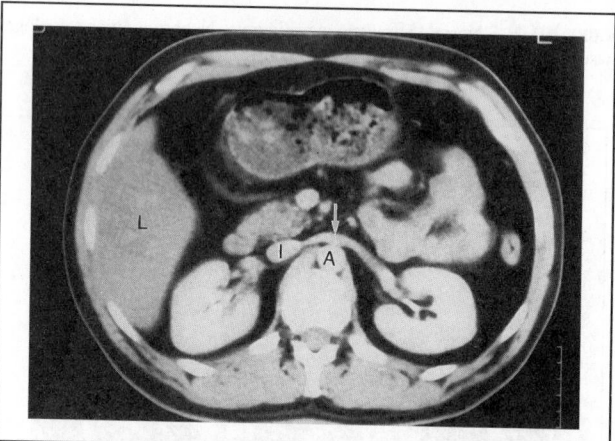

FIGURE 103-5　Normal enhanced computed tomography (CT) scan of kidneys. *I*, Inferior vena cava; *A*, aorta; *arrow*, renal vein; *L*, liver.

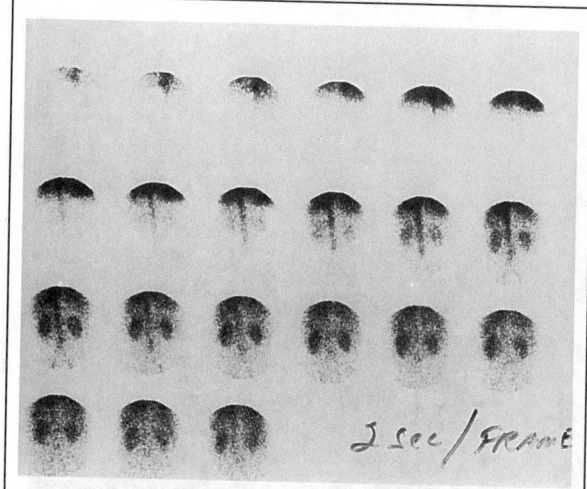

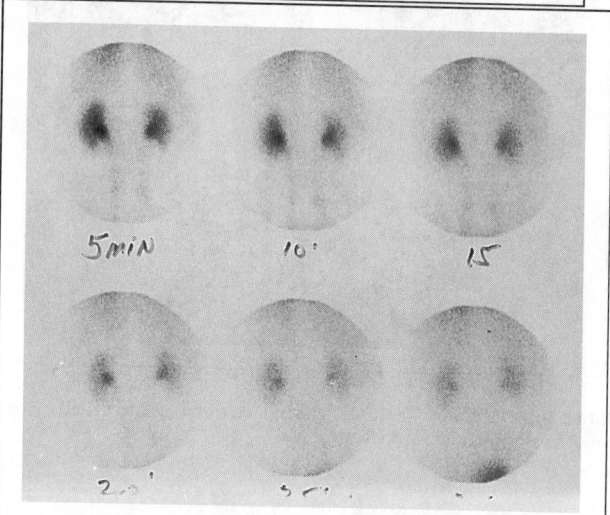

FIGURE 103-6　Normal radionuclide renal scan. **A**, Dynamic phase. **B**, Static phase.

The use of Doppler analysis of blood flow is rapidly becoming an important noninvasive modality in accessing renal vascular disease such as renovascular disease, thrombosis of renal vein, and renal transplant rejection.

Computed Tomography

The introduction of CT in the evaluation of the urinary system has been revolutionary. It is the examination of choice for detailed imaging of the kidneys, adrenals, perirenal spaces, and pararenal spaces (Fig. 103-5).

The kidneys are imaged before and during the intravenous administration of contrast medium, and 5- or 10-mm thick slices are obtained. Nonenhanced images provide information regarding calcifications involving the urinary system, which otherwise will be masked by contrast medium.

Renal masses/malignancies are primarily evaluated by CT, which significantly has replaced angiography as the primary imaging modality. The primary malignancy, possible vascular involvement, and proximal as well as distant metastasis are accurately evaluated by CT. CT adequately evaluates ureter and bladder disease.

Nuclear Medicine

Nuclear scintigraphy provides information about the function and anatomy of the kidney. It provides quantitative evaluation of the kidney, which cannot be provided by other radiographic techniques. The radiopharmaceutical agents used for renal evaluation/imaging are of low toxicity and low radiation. Technetium (Tc 99m)–DTPA is an agent used for imaging and evaluation of glomerular filtration (Fig. 103-6, *A* and *B*). For imaging only, especially in patients with renal failure, Tc 99m DMSA or Tc 99m glucoheptonate (GHA) can be used. Orthoiodohippurate (OIH) labeled with iodine 131 is used for tubular function evaluation. Visualization of the kidney by nuclear medicine requires minimal renal function.

Imaging by nuclear medicine is useful for evaluation of the function of each kidney separately to follow up the progress of obstruction, to evaluate the presence or absence of functioning renal parenchyma, to search for ectopic kidney, and to evaluate renal hypertension.

Magnetic Resonance Imaging

Magnetic resonance imaging (MRI), the newest imaging modality, uses electromagnetic forces to generate images. The patient is placed into a magnetic field (0.2 to 1.5 T), which magnetizes the patient's protons (mainly the hydrogen protons). A radiofrequency pulse stimulates the protons in the area of interest (of the body) by altering their orientation in relation to the main magnetic field. When the radiofrequency pulse ceases, the stimulated protons return to their baseline position by emitting a radiofrequency energy that generates the images.

MRI does not use ionizing radiation and has the capability of multiplanar imaging (coronal, axial, sagittal). At present the use of contrast medium is not necessary. Contraindications for performing MRI include cardiac pacemaker, certain prosthetic heart valves, cerebrovascular clips, and cochlear stimulators. MRI is a well-established imaging modality for the nervous and musculoskeletal systems, whereas in the chest and abdomen, cardiac, respiratory, and bowel motion create some deterioration of the images. Advanced MRI techniques such as respiratory and cardiac gating have improved the quality of the images.

In the genitourinary system, MRI provides adequate anatomic information. The corticomedullary differentiation is routinely seen on MRI. The renal artery, vein, and inferior vena cava (IVC) are easily assessed by MRI, which is one of the imaging modalities of choice for evaluation of the vascular pedicle of the kidney in renal malignancies. Although MRI is inferior to CT in spatial resolution, it is equal and in some instances superior to CT in the pelvis (bladder, prostate).

Angiography

The introduction of new imaging modalities such as CT and MRI has decreased the need for angiography in the evaluation of renal disease. This invasive imaging modality requires puncturing of the femoral artery and placing the tip of a catheter in the abdominal aorta above the orifices of renal arteries. Contrast medium is injected at this area, and information is gained for the aorta and renal arteries. Then the catheter is manipulated and placed into the orifice of each renal artery where contrast medium is injected selectively, providing detailed vascular information of each kidney.

Besides its diagnostic role, angiography is gaining importance as a therapeutic modality for preoperative embolization of renal tumors, angioplasty of renal artery stenosis, and stenting of renal arteries.

Retrograde Pyelography

Retrograde pyelography is an imaging modality in which the contrast medium is injected into the ureter in a retrograde fashion for visualization of the ureter and renal pelvis. This radiographic method is used for evaluation of the collecting systems and ureters in cases where IVP fails to optimally visualize these structures. It is also indicated for evaluation of filling defects in the ureter and/or pelvis.

Since the development of CT and US and improvement of IVP techniques, retrograde pyelography is performed less frequently.

PATHOLOGIC FINDINGS
Renal Mass

The work-up of a renal mass can include almost every imaging modality. Because IVP is the most frequently used imaging modality, most renal masses are first visualized by this modality. Renal masses have different presentations on IVP. They may be evident as a nephrogram defect, renal contour irregularity (bulge), calcifications, or abnormal position of the kidney. Involvement of the pelvicocalyceal system by a mass appears as distortion, amputation, invasion, clubbing, or displacement (Fig. 103-7). Renal carcinoma may narrow or obstruct the renal vein, resulting in hypofunctioning or nonfunctioning kidney.

A mass on IVP may be solid or cystic, and US is the study of choice for making the differentiation. A simple cyst needs no further evaluation because it is benign. A solid mass or a complex cyst requires further evaluation to determine whether it is benign or malignant. A simple cyst must meet *all* the following sonographic criteria (Fig. 103-8):

1. Echo free
2. Smooth wall with good through-transmission of the sound
3. Enhanced back wall

If any of these criteria are not met, the cyst cannot be classified as simple. A complex cyst on sonography demonstrates thick wall, calcifications, solid components, and/or mixed echogenicity (Fig. 103-9). Renal sonography for evaluation of a mass should always include the renal veins and IVC for the presence of thrombus.

Evaluation of a solid or complex cystic mass requires the use of CT. Renal cell carcinoma, the most common renal malignancy (83%), appears on CT as a mass of low density (as compared with the rest of renal parenchyma), which enhances after the intravenous adminis-

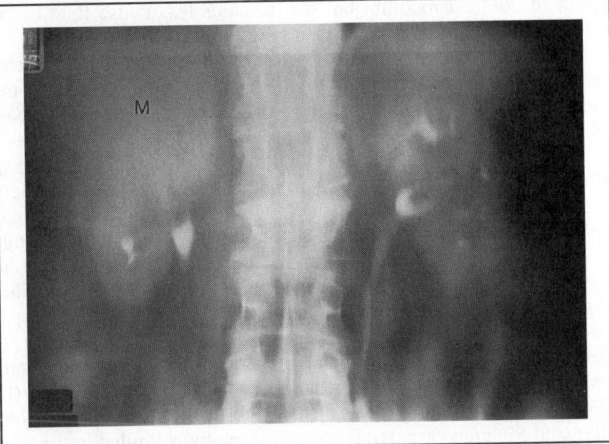

FIGURE 103-7 Nephrotomogram demonstrating a large mass *(M)* involving the upper aspect of the right kidney with amputation of the collecting system.

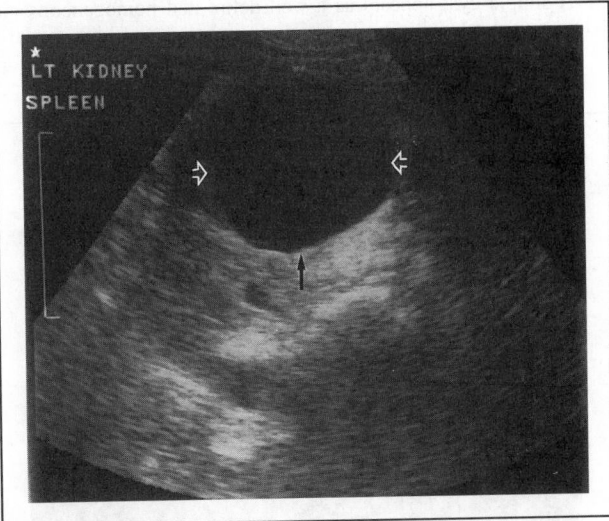

FIGURE 103-8 Simple cyst *(open white arrows)*. Smooth wall and enhanced back wall *(black arrow)* are evident.

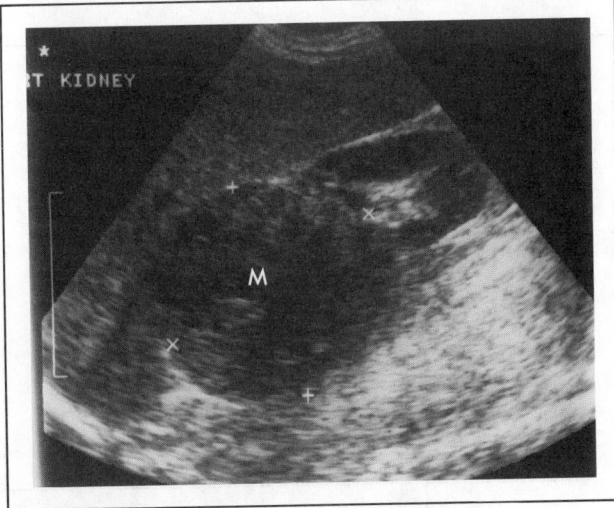

FIGURE 103-9 Large renal cell carcinoma. Inhomogeneous mass *(M)* arising from the upper pole of the right-side kidney.

tration of contrast medium but still remains less dense than the rest of the enhanced renal parenchyma (Fig. 103-10).

Staging of renal carcinoma is primarily performed by CT because this method has the ability to provide a global view of the abdomen. Local extension, lymphadenopathy, or distant metastases are easily delineated by CT.

The use of arteriography in evaluating renal masses and, more specifically, renal cell carcinoma, has decreased since the introduction of cross-sectional imaging (CT, US, MRI). The main role of angiography in diagnosis is to provide a preoperative vascular mapping of the mass (Fig. 103-11). Angiography may also be of significant help in embolizing the tumor to decrease its vascularity and to facilitate surgical removal. Renal cell carcinoma appears as a hypervascular mass (80%) demonstrating capillary blush, vascular encasement, tortuosity of vessels, early venous filling, and pooling of the contrast medium. Involvement of the renal vein is easily demonstrated (Fig. 103-12). Approximately 15% of renal cell carcinomas are hypovascular, and 5% are avascular. Renal scintigraphy is limited in the evaluation of renal mass because it demonstrates only the renal defect without differentiating between a benign and malignant lesion. The role of MRI has not yet been completely defined. A renal mass appears as an inhomogeneous mass of low signal intensity on T_1-weighted imaging and high signal intensity on T_2-weighted imaging (Fig. 103-13). A simple cyst appears as a well-delineated homogeneous mass of low signal intensity on T_1-weighted imaging and high signal in-

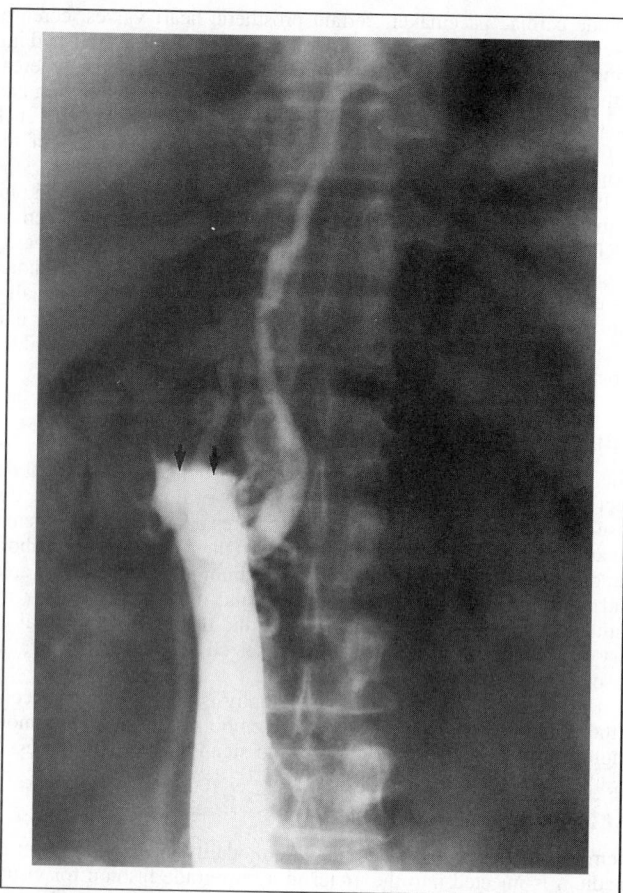

FIGURE 103-12 Renal cell carcinoma with involvement of the inferior vena cava *(arrows)*.

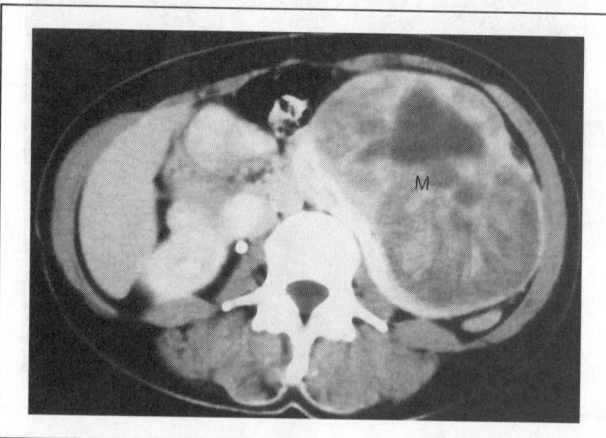

FIGURE 103-10 Large renal cell carcinoma. Large mass *(M)* containing areas of high enhancement, low enhancement, and necrosis.

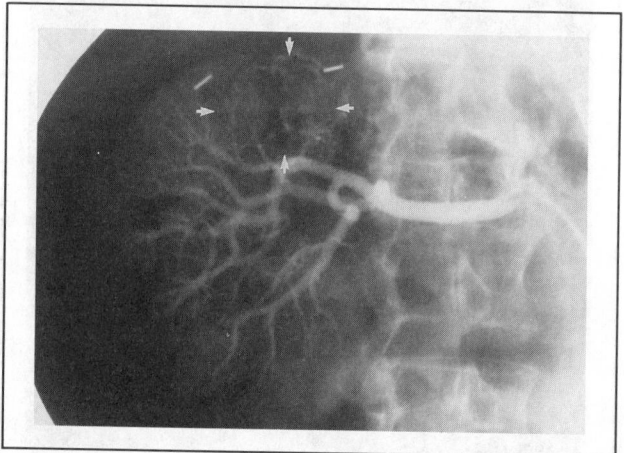

FIGURE 103-11 Renal cell carcinoma. Right-side renal angiography reveals a vascular mass *(arrows)* containing abnormal vessels and pooling of contrast medium.

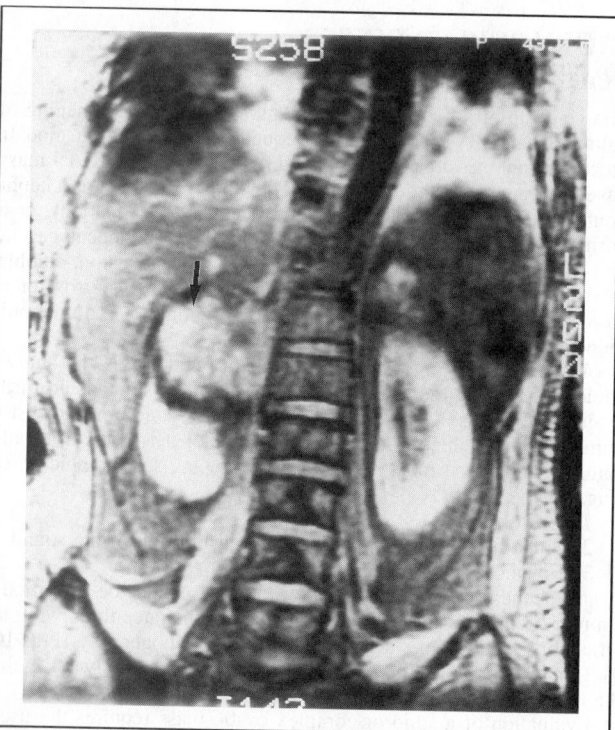

FIGURE 103-13 Coronal view of renal magnetic resonance imaging (MRI). Mass involves upper pole of right-side kidney *(arrow)*.

tensity on T$_2$-weighted imaging. The multiplanar imaging capabilities of MRI have increased the accuracy in staging renal malignancies. MRI is also helpful in assessing the patency of renal veins and IVC (Fig. 103-14).

Besides renal cell carcinomas, other tumors may involve the kidney. Benign neoplasms include the following:

1. Oncocytoma on cross-sectional imaging appears as a solid mass with a central scar. Angiography demonstrates a hypervascular mass with a "spoked wheel" pattern. Despite its characteristic appearance, malignancy cannot be totally excluded.
2. Adenomas are slow-growing solid tumors that may exhibit cystic areas and calcifications. Adenomas larger than 3 cm are considered potentially malignant.
3. Angiomyolipomas are solid tumors containing fat, muscle, and blood vessels. CT demonstrates fat as a low-density area (or mass); on ultrasound, fat appears echogenic (Fig. 103-15). The combination of CT and US findings of fat strongly suggests angiomyolipoma. (Fat on IVP appears radiolucent; on MRI fat appears as high signal intensity on T$_1$-weighted imaging and low signal intensity on T$_2$-weighted imaging.)

Other malignant tumors include metastases and lymphoma, which are difficult to differentiate from renal cell carcinoma. Transitional cell carcinoma is the most common malignancy involving the renal pelvis, ureters, and bladder. On IVP it appears as an irregular filling defect destroying the pelvicalyceal system. Hydronephrosis is frequently present. Similar findings are seen on the cross-sectional images. Fig. 103-16 provides a diagnostic algorithm for renal mass found on IVP.

Obstructive Uropathy (Hydronephrosis)

The radiologic evaluation of obstructive uropathy is clinically important because it provides significant information such as level and degree of obstruction and physiologic status of the involved kidney.

On IVP the KUB frequently demonstrates the level of obstruction by delineating a calcified calculus. In the acute phase of obstruction, the kidney may be of normal size or enlarged. A delayed, dense, and persistent nephrogram appears, which is followed by a moderate distention of the collecting system. On delayed views the level of obstruction may be demonstrated by a columnized and dilated ureter down to the level of obstruction (Fig. 103-17). Complete obstruction may cause forniceal rupture of the calyces (acting as a safety valve) and extravasation of the contrast medium. Chronic obstructive uropathy is manifested by a dilated collecting system filled by nonopacified urine, which appears lucent against the dense (by contrast media) renal parenchyma. This negative pyelogram sign later becomes positive when contrast medium enters the collecting system and displaces the nonopacified urine.

In long-standing and severe obstruction the renal parenchyma atrophies and appears during the parenchymal phase of the IVP as a thin, dense rim (the rim sign). US is a sensitive modality demonstrating various degrees of hydronephrosis (Fig. 103-18). Sonography's ability to visualize the kidney does not depend on the renal function, making this modality ideal for evaluating obstruction in patients with renal failure. It is an important imaging modality in the follow-up of the progression of hydronephrosis because it is sensitive in delineating

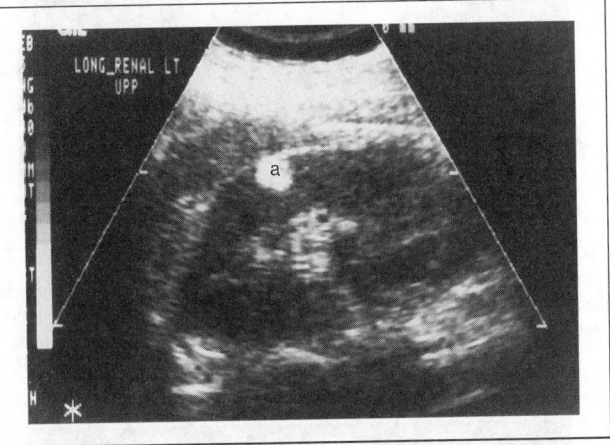

FIGURE 103-15   Renal sonogram demonstrating an angiomyolipoma *(a)*.

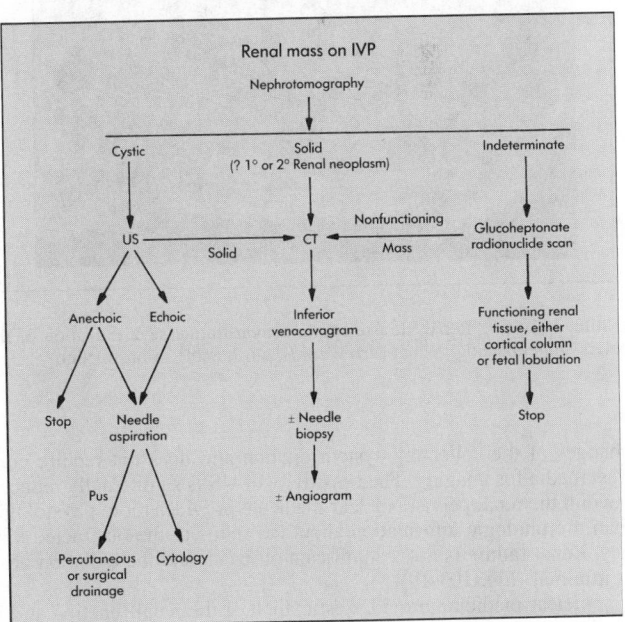

FIGURE 103-16   Diagnostic algorithm for renal mass on intravenous pyelography.

From Ferruci JT: *Radiology: diagnosis-imaging-intervention imaging algorithms for radiological diagnosis,* vol 1, Philadelphia, 1986, JB Lippincott.

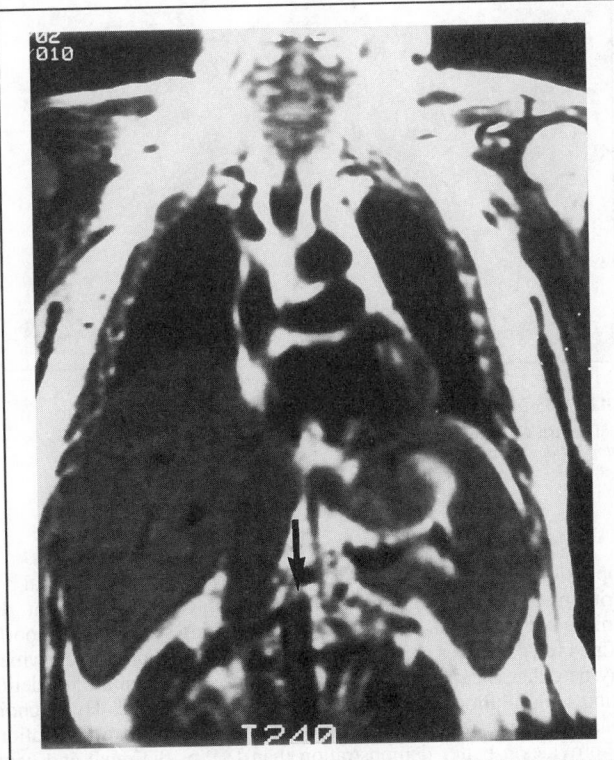

FIGURE 103-14   Same patient as in Fig. 103-12 on coronal view of renal MRI demonstrating involvement of inferior vena cava *(arrow)*.

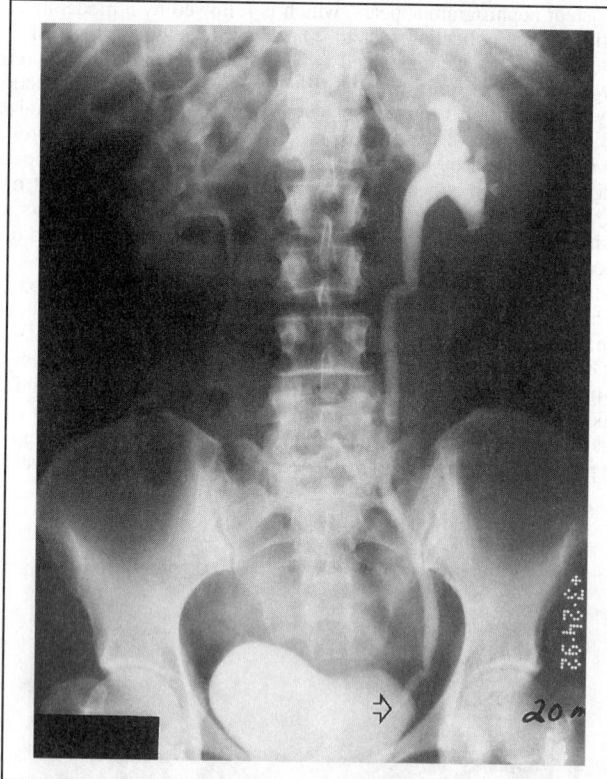

FIGURE 103-17   Left-side obstruction demonstrating dense nephrogram-dilated collecting system and ureter. Calculus of the ureterovesicle junction *(open arrow)*, is responsible for the obstruction.

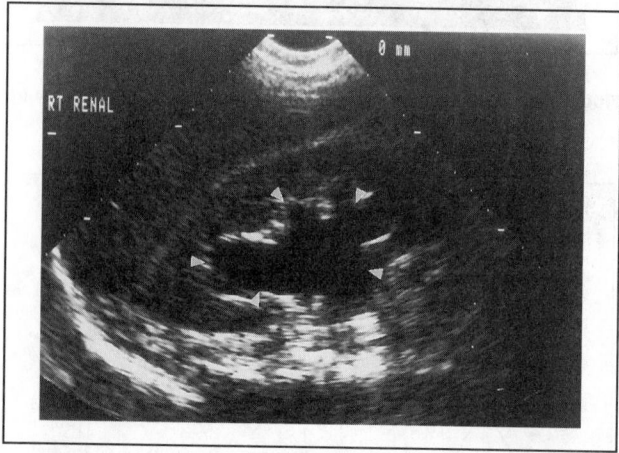

FIGURE 103-18   Renal ultrasonogram demonstrating severe dilation of the pelvis and collecting system *(arrowheads)* attributable to obstruction.

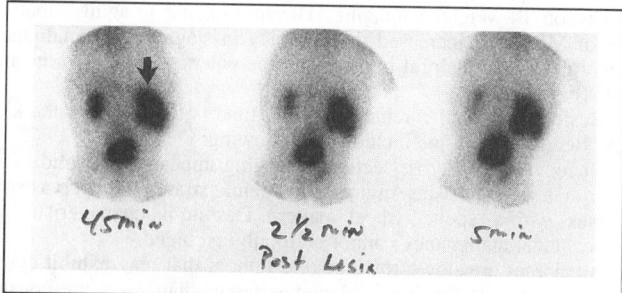

FIGURE 103-19   Renal radionuclide scan. Right-side hydronephrosis *(arrow).*

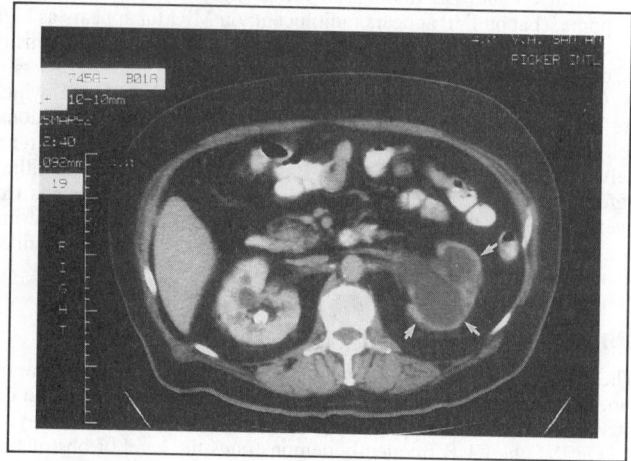

FIGURE 103-20   The rim sign is well demonstrated on CT *(arrows).*

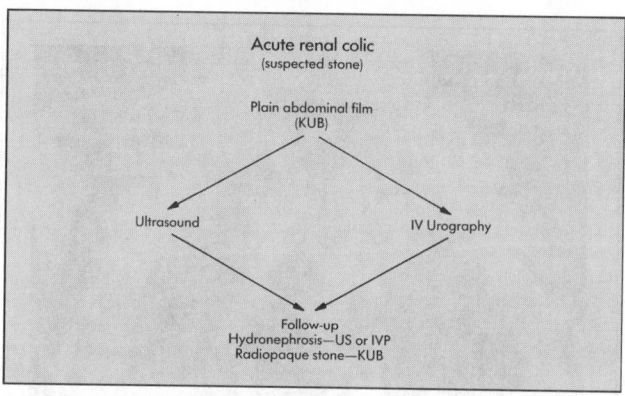

FIGURE 103-21   Diagnostic algorithm for acute renal colic.

From Ferruci JT: *Radiology: diagnosis-imaging-intervention imaging algorithms for radiological diagnosis,* vol 1, Philadelphia, 1986, JB Lippincott.

changes of the collecting system dilation and does not require contrast media for imaging. The sensitivity of US is significantly reduced beyond the renal pelvis. Nuclear medicine provides more physiologic than morphologic information about the status of the obstructed kidney. Renal failure is not a significant obstacle, and the radiation dose is minimal (Fig. 103-19).

Nuclear medicine provides estimation of the renal function and is used in the follow-up of the progression of hydronephrosis. CT demonstrates obstructed kidney and involved dilated ureter (Fig. 103-20). CT is not usually obtained for screening purposes but for determination of the cause of hydronephrosis and the extension of the process. Fig. 103-21 provides a diagnostic algorithm for acute renal colic.

Acute Inflammation

Approximately 25% of patients with acute pyelonephritis or focal nephritis manifest no urographic abnormalities. Renal enlargement, diminished nephrogram, alteration of the collecting systems, and poorly defined renal outlines are some of the urographic abnormalities, which may be either focal or diffuse. Sonography is not sensitive for delineating abnormalities and in many instances is normal. Hypoechoic areas within the renal parenchyma indicate edema or inflammation. CT provides a better demonstration than IVP of the renal and pararenal inflammatory changes.

Renal abscess appears as an area of diminished contrast enhancement on IVP and CT. If there is gas formation, it appears as small

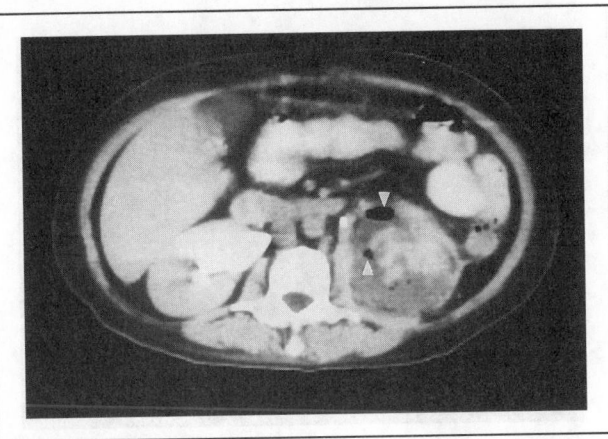

FIGURE 103-22 Enhanced renal CT scan. Left-side renal abscess with pockets of gas *(arrowheads)*.

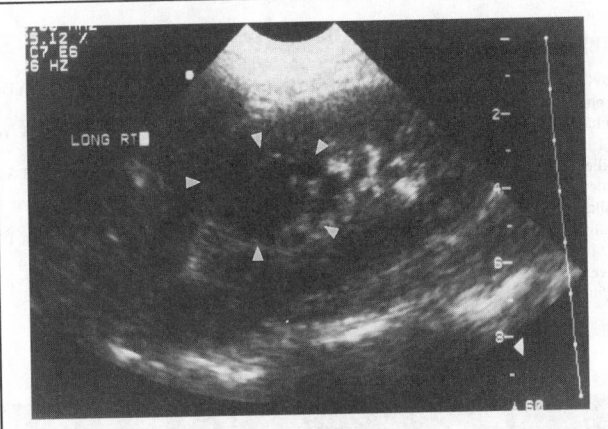

FIGURE 103-23 Renal sonogram demonstrating an inflammatory mass as an area of mixed echogenicity *(arrowheads)*.

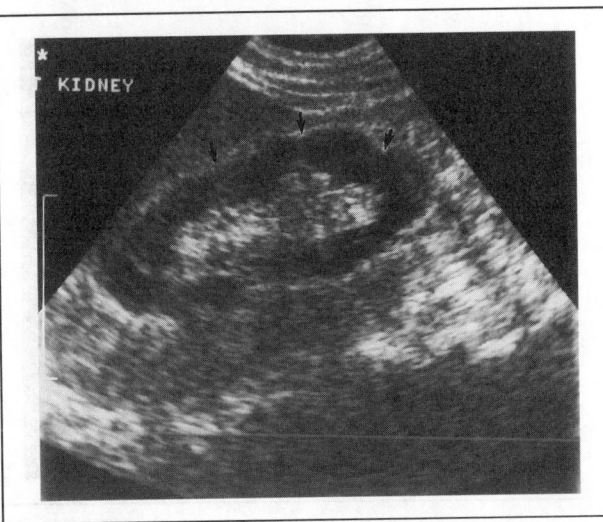

FIGURE 103-24 Scarring *(arrows)* involving the kidney as a result of pyelonephritis.

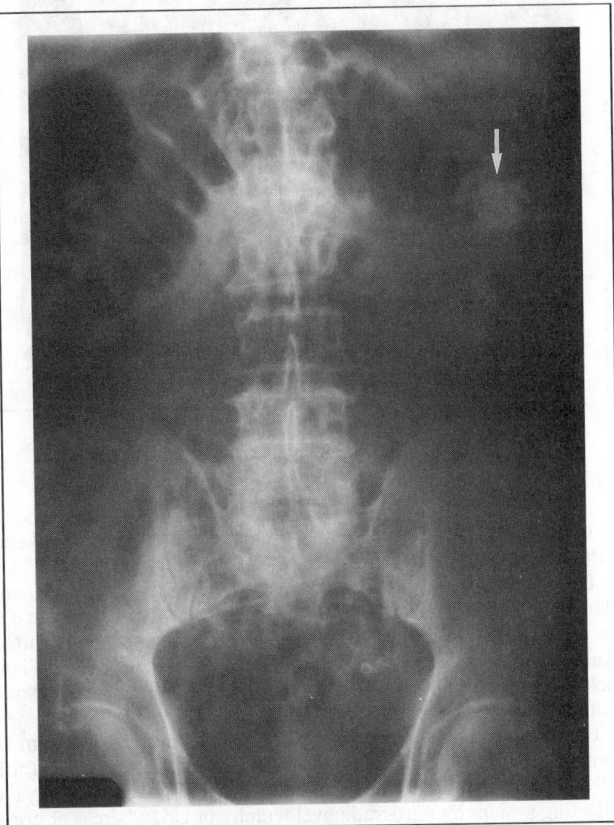

FIGURE 103-25 View of kidneys, ureter, and bladder (KUB). Slaghorn calculus *(arrow)*.

bubbles of air. CT has assumed a leading role because it can easily demonstrate the renal inflammatory process as well as its extension beyond the kidney (Fig. 103-22). US easily demonstrates an abscess as an area of mixed echogenicity, with gas appearing as echogenic focus with some shadowing (Fig. 103-23).

Chronic Inflammation

Chronic pyelonephritis is usually a focal disease manifested by alteration of the renal outlines resulting from the formation of scars. There is also dilation of the calyx at the proximity of the scar. The kidney is small. These findings are easily seen on IVP and CT. Sonography reveals the same findings, as well as echogenic kidney attributable to the stiffness of the parenchyma (Fig. 103-24).

Xanthogranulomatous pyelonephritis is a chronic inflammatory disease characterized by the presence of lipid-containing histiocytes. The diffuse form of the disease (85% to 90%) is characterized as an enlarged nonfunctioning kidney containing a staghorn calculus or a calculus in the renal pelvis (Fig. 103-25). The focal form is manifested by a focal mass involving a functioning kidney.

Renovascular Disease

Angiography is the main diagnostic modality for the evaluation of renovascular disease. Radionuclide renal scan offers a safe, easy, accurate screening method for evaluation of renovascular hypertension.

The most common vascular lesion is atherosclerosis, which involves the proximal aspect of the renal artery (usually 1 to 2 cm from its origin at the aorta). The lesions may be single or multiple (Fig. 103-26). Angiography accurately demonstrates the stenotic portion of the renal artery, collateral arteries in cases of severe stenosis, and poststenotic dilation.

Fibromuscular dysplasia, another cause of hypertension, occurs more frequently in women (80% of the cases). Bilateral lesions occur approximately 50% of the time; unilateral lesions more often oc-

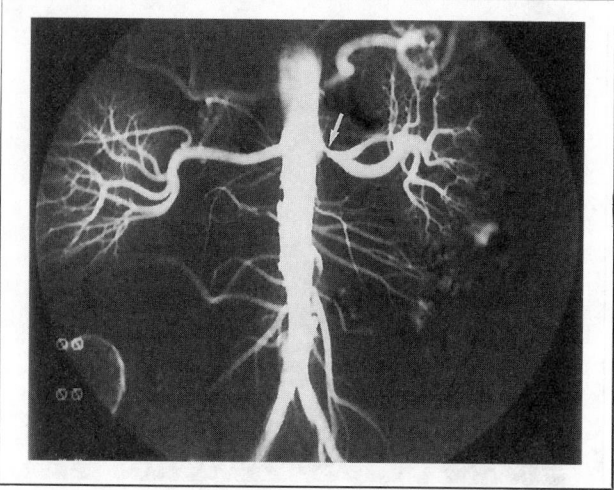

FIGURE 103-26   Left renal artery stenosis *(arrow)*.

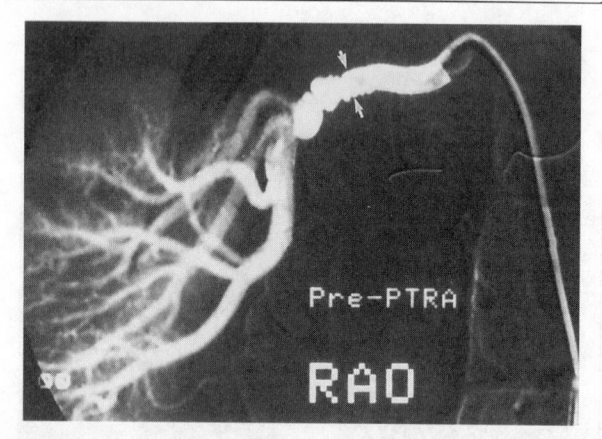

FIGURE 103-27   Right-side fibromuscular dysplasia *(arrows)*.

cur in the right artery. Typically the lesions appear as a string of beads in the middle and distal portions of the renal artery (Fig. 103-27).

Thrombosis of the renal artery may occur as a result of atherosclerosis, vasculitis, or trauma. In the acute form there is absence of excretion on IVP. In contrast, gradual occlusion of the renal artery results in diminished renal size and reduced excretion on IVP or nuclear medicine. Upon complete occlusion the kidney appears small without function.

Emboli to the renal arteries may originate from the left atrium (in the case of atrial fibrillation), cardiac vegetations, aorta, and so forth. IVP demonstrates absence of excretion with a normal-sized kidney and collecting system by retrograde pyelography or US, whereas arteriography demonstrates the obstruction of the renal artery or its branches.

Renal artery aneurysms may be diagnosed on plain radiography of the abdomen if they are calcified. (Approximately 30% of renal artery aneurysms are calcified.) Arteriography demonstrates the size, shape, and location of the aneurysm. Other renal vascular abnormalities include renal infarct and renal and perirenal hematoma.

Lower Urinary Tract

Bladder tumors can be visualized by IVP; however, CT and MRI are more sensitive because both imaging modalities evaluate the tumor from its extension within the wall of the bladder to the bowel and distant metastasis (Fig. 103-28). Diseases of the urethra are usually evaluated by cystourethrography or retrograde urethrography.

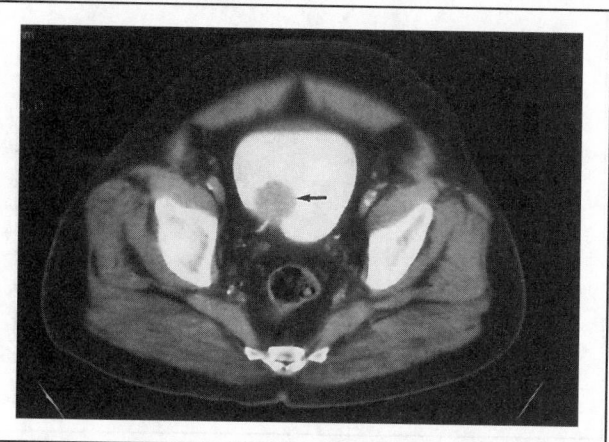

FIGURE 103-28   Enhanced CT scan of pelvis. Tumor involving the urinary system bladder *(arrow)*..

BIBLIOGRAPHY

Davidson AJ, Hartman DS: *Radiology of the kidney and urinary tract,* ed 2, Philadelphia, 1994, WB Saunders.

Kutcher R, Lautin EM: *Genitourinary radiology: a multimodality approach,* New York, 1990, Gower Medical.

Miller WT: *Seminars in roentgenology: renal neoplasms,* Philadelphia, 1995, WB Saunders.

Pollack HM: *Clinical urology,* vol 1, Philadelphia, 1990, WB Saunders.

Rumak CM, Wilson CM, Charboneau WJ: *Diagnostic ultrasound,* vol 1, St Louis, 1991, Mosby.

Taveras JM, Ferrucci JT: *Radiology: diagnosis-imaging-intervention, imaging algorithms for radiological diagnosis,* vol 1, Philadelphia, 1986, JB Lippincott.

III   BASIC CLINICAL SYNDROMES

CHAPTER

104   Hematuria

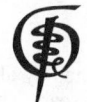

B.S. Kasinath

Hematuria is encountered frequently in general practice. Often it is recognized for the first time during routine health screening for employment or insurance purposes. It may occur in isolation or be associated with other abnormalities found on urinalysis such as proteinuria and cellular casts. It may be macroscopic or microscopic, intermittent or persistent.

DEFINITION

Since normally up to a million erythrocytes pass into the urine daily, it is not unusual to encounter some erythrocytes in the urine sediment. Most authorities agree that the presence of greater than three erythrocytes in a high-powered field in a centrifuged specimen of urine, confirmed on repeated urinalyses, qualifies as significant microscopic hematuria. Red urine does not always imply hematuria because several drugs, dyes, and coloring agents in food may discolor the urine.

Hematuria is detected on urinalysis by dipstick or microscopic examination. Dipsticks rely on chemical detection of hemoglobin that is present in the urine. A positive reaction on the dipstick should always be confirmed by microscopic examination of the urine sediment to ascertain the existence of intact erythrocytes because dipsticks can react with urinary myoglobin and hemoglobin in rhabdomyolysis and hemolysis, respectively. False-negative reactions may be seen in patients taking large amounts of vitamin C (ascorbic acid). Recently attention has been drawn to variations in size, shape, and hemoglobin content of urinary erythrocytes. These dysmorphic red blood cells favor glomerular origin of hematuria, whereas red blood cell morphologic appearance tends to be uniform in other causes of hematuria (e.g., malignancy). To gain maximum information, an early morning, freshly voided urine should be examined for hematuria and presence of red cell casts. It is important to avoid specimens obtained during menstruation or after recent instrumentation of the genitourinary tract.

ETIOLOGY

The causes of hematuria may be considered in two categories: nonrenal and renal parenchymal (Box 104-1). Although benign prostatic hypertrophy has been suggested to cause hematuria, because of its high prevalence another independent cause should be considered. Similarly, although anticoagulants or coagulation abnormalities can result in hematuria, underlying genitourinary tract disease should be excluded. Renal parenchymal causes could involve glomerular or nonglomerular structures. Box 104-1 lists some of the more common diseases. Recently, metabolic disorders such as hypercalciuria and hyperuricosuria have been implicated in hematuria. Strenuous exercise can lead to transient hematuria.

APPROACH TO DIAGNOSIS

The objective of investigating hematuria is to uncover potentially serious diseases such as malignancies or severe glomerulonephritides so that early therapeutic intervention can be instituted when possible. Proper evaluation of hematuria requires a detailed history, physical examination, and a thorough urinalysis including examination of a spun urine sediment by the physician, followed by appropriate investigations (Fig. 104-1). Urinalysis should exclude factitious hematuria (e.g., urine discoloration due to coloring agents in drugs and foods, myoglobinuria, porphyria).

The timing of hematuria during micturition may be helpful. Urethral diseases cause hematuria in the initial part of the stream, whereas terminal hematuria usually suggests bladder disease. Other origins usually cause hematuria throughout the stream.

Symptoms of dysuria, urgency, and increased frequency suggest infection of the urinary tract. Presence of symptoms of photosensitivity, rashes, arthritis, and Raynaud's phenomenon point to connective tissue disease as a possible cause (e.g., systemic lupus erythematosus). A thorough history should include inquiries of drugs, including over-the-counter formulations; family history of renal disease and stones, and foreign travel, especially to regions where infestation with *Schistosoma haematobium* is endemic. On physical examination one should search for hypertension, edema (suggests glomerular origin), and prostatic nodularity or enlargement; bimanual pelvic examination should be performed in women to search for invasive pelvic neoplasms. Signs of systemic diseases such as rashes, arthritis, and palpable purpura may point to connective tissue disease and/or vasculitis.

Strategies for laboratory evaluation depend on whether one has uncovered clues to the presence of renal parenchymal or extrarenal causes during a thorough initial evaluation consisting of history, physical examination, and urinalysis. For instance, presence of proteinuria (especially >3.5 g/day), dysmorphic erythrocytes, erythrocyte casts, hypertension, and renal insufficiency point to glomerular causes. Dysuria, fever, chills, leukocyturia, and bacteriuria suggest infection of the urinary tract. If these clues are not present, it is wise to exclude asymptomatic urinary tract infection by urine culture. Hematuria associated with "sterile" pyuria should prompt a search for genitourinary tract tuberculosis and interstitial nephritis. A negative urine culture should be followed by intravenous pyelography (IVP), which may delineate neoplasms, calculi, anatomic abnormalities, or cystic diseases of the urinary tract. In patients who are sensitive to contrast

---

BOX 104-1
Causes of hematuria

I. Nonrenal parenchymal causes
  A. Genitourinary tract diseases
    1. Calculi: Renal pelvis, ureter, bladder, urethra
    2. Neoplasms: Renal pelvis, ureter, bladder, prostate, urethra
    3. Infections: Bladder, prostate, urethra, epididymis
    4. Others: Congenital abnormalities, drugs (e.g., cyclophosphamide), foreign bodies, benign prostatic hypertrophy, endometriosis, trauma, strictures, vesicoureteral reflux
  B. Unrelated to genitourinary tract
    1. Coagulopathies
    2. Anticoagulation
II. Renal parenchymal causes
  A. Glomerular diseases
    1. Mesangial proliferative glomerulonephritis (e.g., immunoglobulin A nephritis)
    2. Acute proliferative glomerulonephritis (e.g., poststreptococcal nephritis)
    3. Glomerulonephritis due to systemic diseases (e.g., lupus erythematosus)
    4. Rapidly progressive glomerulonephritis (e.g., Goodpasture's syndrome)
    5. Membranoproliferative glomerulonephritis
    6. Vascular (e.g., malignant hypertension, vasculitides)
    7. Familial (e.g., Alport's syndrome, thin glomerular basement membrane disease)
    8. Miscellaneous (e.g., exercise, loin pain-hematuria syndrome)
  B. Tubulointerstital disease
    1. Infections (e.g., pyelonephritis, tuberculosis)
    2. Interstitial nephritis, acute (e.g., drugs) or chronic (e.g., analgesic abuse)
    3. Polycystic kidney disease, sickle cell nephropathy
    4. Vascular: Renal infarction, cortical necrosis, renal vein thrombosis, malformations
    5. Neoplasms: Renal cell carcinoma
    6. Others: Papillary necrosis, trauma, hypercalciuria, hyperuricosuria

---

media or in whom acute renal failure due to contrast media is considered a high probability, ultrasonography of the genitourinary tract may be performed in the place of IVP.

If ultrasound or IVP is equivocal or normal, cystoscopy is generally performed, especially in the elderly, to detect lower urinary tract disease, as well as to determine whether hematuria is originating from one or both kidneys. Retrograde pyelography may be needed to define ureteral lesions. A negative cystoscopic examination should lead to a search for hypercalciuria and hyperuricosuria and consideration of renal biopsy for renal parenchymal diseases or renal angiography to diagnose vascular malformations or neoplasms that are too small to be seen on IVP. Computerized tomography has been used to delineate the anatomic structure of mass lesions found on IVP or ultrasound or to visualize masses beyond the resolution of these imaging procedures. Urinary cytologic examination may help in the detection of malignant cells that suggests diagnosis of genitourinary tract malignancy.

Prognosis of hematuria necessarily depends on the underlying cause. A prospective study of patients with hematuria with or without mild proteinuria in whom urologic and systemic diseases were excluded has shown that immunoglobulin A nephropathy, thin glomerular basement membrane disease, and interstitial nephritis are commonly found; nearly 40% had no renal parenchymal disease. At a median follow-up of 11 years most of the patients retained normal renal function, but there was an increased prevalence of hypertension.

Some caveats should be kept in mind. Significant disease, particularly malignancies of the gentourinary tract, is more likely to be discovered in the elderly population, especially men. Although a thorough investigation may not reveal an identifiable cause in up to 12% of patients, urologic disease may still be present and periodic follow-up in such cases is recommended. Complications from reac-

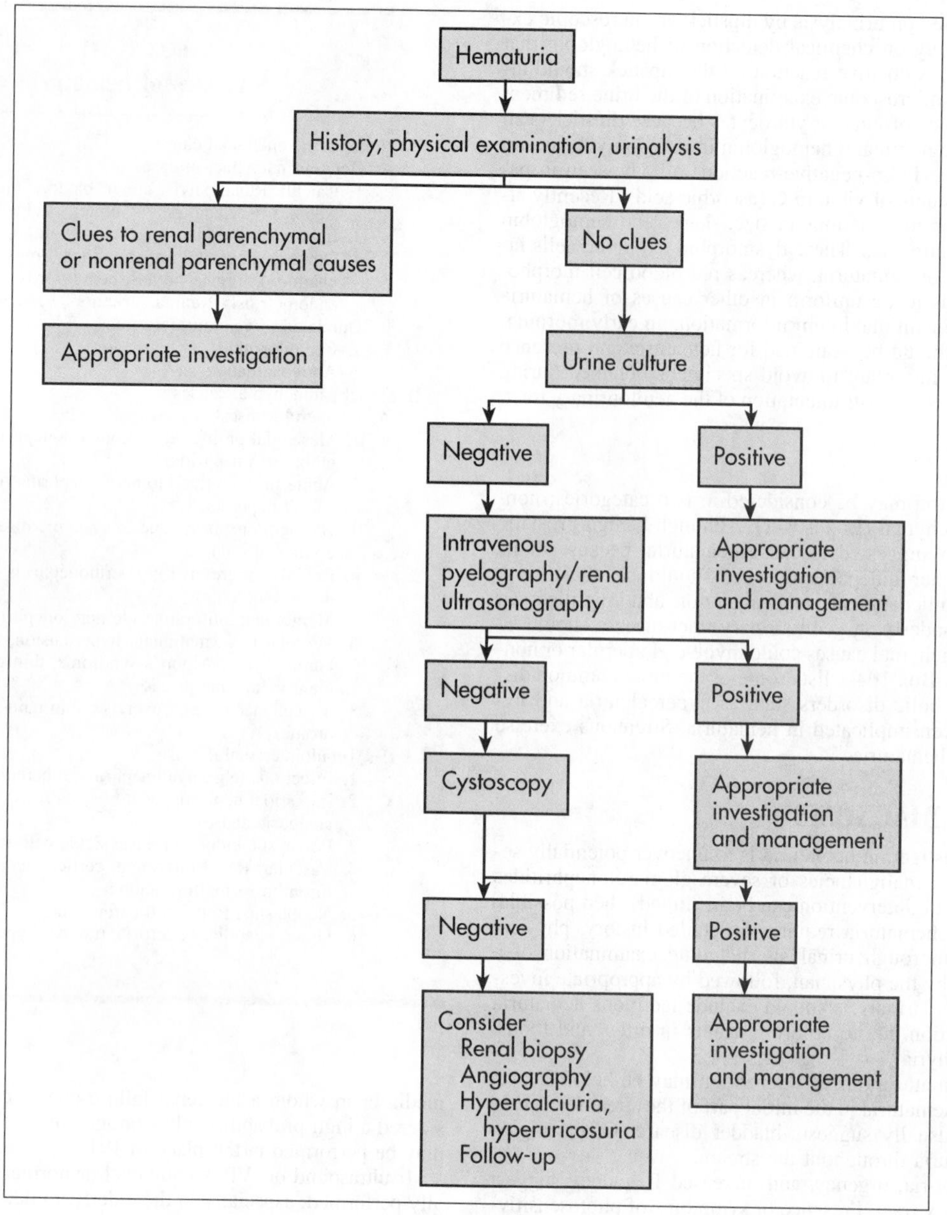

```
                        ┌──────────────┐
                        │  Hematuria   │
                        └──────┬───────┘
                               │
              ┌────────────────────────────────────┐
              │ History, physical examination, urinalysis │
              └────────────────┬───────────────────┘
                    ┌──────────┴──────────────────┐
        ┌───────────────────────┐          ┌────────────┐
        │ Clues to renal parenchymal │     │  No clues  │
        │ or nonrenal parenchymal causes │ └─────┬──────┘
        └───────────┬───────────┘                │
                    │                      ┌─────────────┐
        ┌───────────────────────┐          │ Urine culture │
        │ Appropriate investigation │       └──────┬──────┘
        └───────────────────────┘      ┌───────────┴─────────┐
                                  ┌──────────┐          ┌──────────┐
                                  │ Negative │          │ Positive │
                                  └────┬─────┘          └────┬─────┘
                             ┌──────────────┐        ┌──────────────┐
                             │ Intravenous  │        │ Appropriate  │
                             │ pyelography/renal │   │ investigation │
                             │ ultrasonography │     │ and management │
                             └──────┬───────┘        └──────────────┘
                               ┌──────────┐          ┌──────────┐
                               │ Negative │          │ Positive │
                               └────┬─────┘          └────┬─────┘
                             ┌──────────────┐        ┌──────────────┐
                             │  Cystoscopy  │        │ Appropriate  │
                             └──────┬───────┘        │ investigation │
                                                     │ and management │
                               ┌──────────┐          └──────────────┘
                               │ Negative │          ┌──────────┐
                               └────┬─────┘          │ Positive │
                             ┌──────────────┐        └────┬─────┘
                             │ Consider     │        ┌──────────────┐
                             │   Renal biopsy │      │ Appropriate  │
                             │   Angiography │       │ investigation │
                             │   Hypercalciuria, │   │ and management │
                             │     hyperuricosuria │ └──────────────┘
                             │   Follow-up  │
                             └──────────────┘
```

FIGURE 104-1   Strategy for investigation of hematuria.

✔ *WHEN TO REFER*

The primary care physician could easily perform the initial workup of hematuria including appropriate clinical evaluation, urinalysis, and renal sonography or IVP. If there is no evidence of renal parenchymal disease, referral to a urologist is appropriate, especially in the older patient. If the initial evaluation reveals evidence of renal parenchymal disease, consultation with a nephrologist is indicated.

tions to contrast media including acute renal failure in susceptible patients, untoward consequences of renal biopsy, the patient's underlying illness, and expenses of workup should be considered as factors that affect the investigation of individual cases of hematuria.

BIBLIOGRAPHY

Nieuwhof C, Doorenbos C, Grave W et al: A prospective study of the natural history of idiopathic nonproteinuric hematuria, *Kidney Int* 49:222-225, 1996.
Sutton JM: Evolution of hematuria in adults, *JAMA* 263:2479-2480, 1990.

---

105 Proteinuria

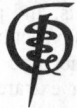

B.S. Kasinath and Manjeri A. Venkatachalam

An abnormal urinary excretion of protein, commonly termed proteinuria, is often a sign of primary intrinsic renal disease but can also be found in a multitude of other disorders.

Normally on average an adult excretes approximately 80 mg of protein daily and usually not more than 150 mg/day. The accepted normal value in adolescence and pregnancy is somewhat higher (up to 300 mg/day). In the healthy adult the protein excretion consists of approximately 40% albumin, 40% tissue protein, 15% immunoglobulins (5% to 10% immunoglobulin G or its fragments, 5% light chains, and 3% immunoglobulin A) and 5% other filtered plasma proteins. A portion of the tissue protein is Tamm-Horsfall protein (uromodulin), a glycoprotein produced by cells of the thick ascending limb of the

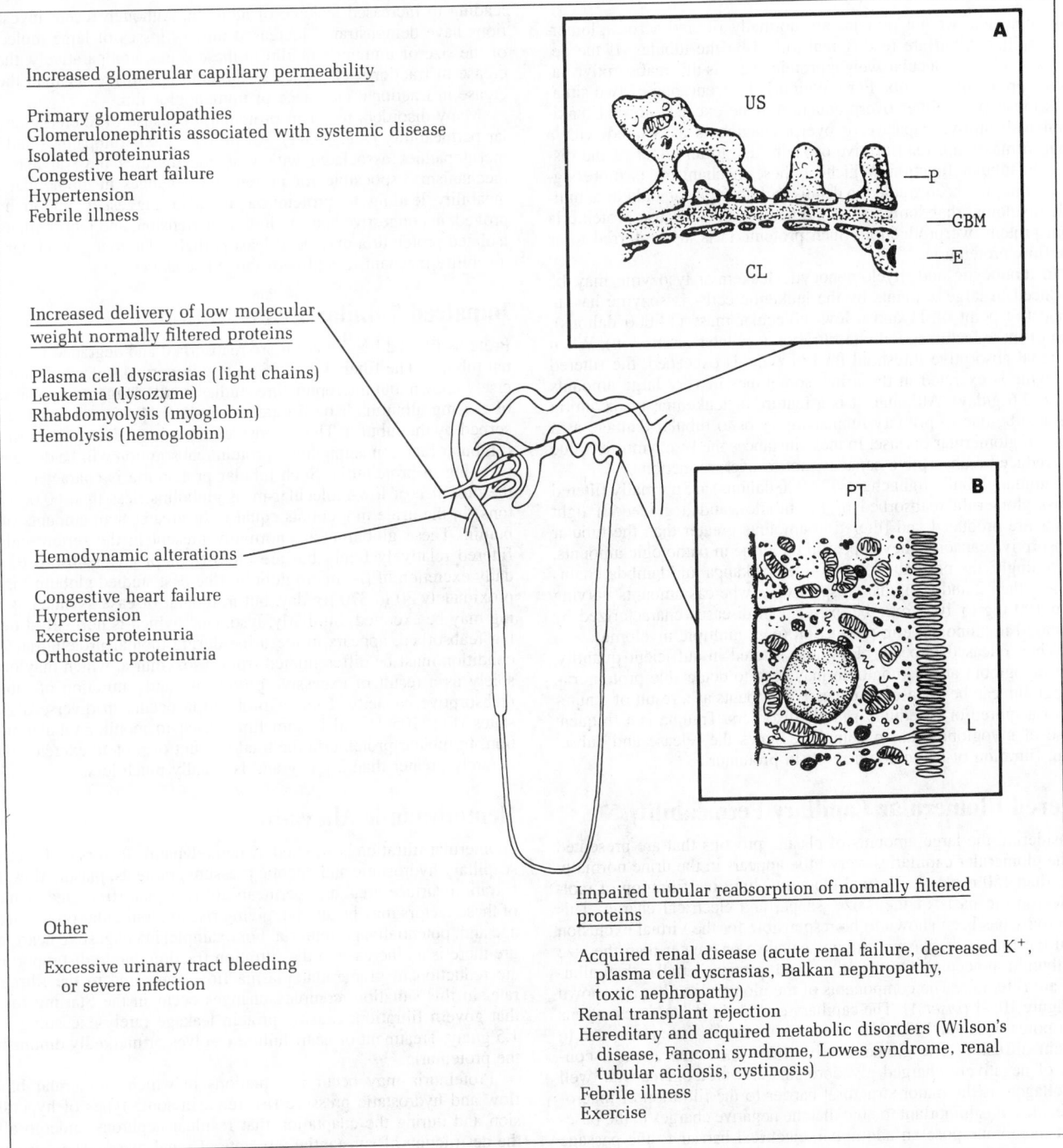

Increased glomerular capillary permeability

Primary glomerulopathies
Glomerulonephritis associated with systemic disease
Isolated proteinurias
Congestive heart failure
Hypertension
Febrile illness

Increased delivery of low molecular
weight normally filtered proteins

Plasma cell dyscrasias (light chains)
Leukemia (lysozyme)
Rhabdomyolysis (myoglobin)
Hemolysis (hemoglobin)

Hemodynamic alterations

Congestive heart failure
Hypertension
Exercise proteinuria
Orthostatic proteinuria

Other

Excessive urinary tract bleeding
or severe infection

Impaired tubular reabsorption of normally filtered
proteins

Acquired renal disease (acute renal failure, decreased K^+,
plasma cell dyscrasias, Balkan nephropathy,
toxic nephropathy)
Renal transplant rejection
Hereditary and acquired metabolic disorders (Wilson's
disease, Fanconi syndrome, Lowes syndrome, renal
tubular acidosis, cystinosis)
Febrile illness
Exercise

FIGURE 105-1   Mechanisms of proteinuria. The glomerular capillary wall and proximal tubular cell are depicted in expanded views. The glomerular capillary wall *(inset A)*, which separates the capillary lumen *(CL)* from the urinary space *(US)*, consists of endothelial cell *(E)*, glomerular basement membrane *(GBM)*, and foot process *(P)* of the glomerular visceral epithelial cell. In the proximal tubule *(inset B)* protein is reabsorbed from fluid in the tubular lumen *(L)* by the proximal tubular epithelial cell *(PT)*.

loop of Henle that may modulate activity of cytokines. It constitutes more than 80% of the mass of "casts" that are found in the urine in disease states (Chapter 102).

Urinary protein excretion in normal individuals varies under different circumstances and is markedly influenced by posture and exercise, proteinuria being greater in the erect posture and after exercise. Change in protein excretion with position has also been demonstrated in patients with pathologic protein loss in disorders such as pyelonephritis or glomerulonephritis. Renal hemodynamic changes induced by change of posture and exercise may underlie the concomitant alterations in protein excretion (see later discussion).

MECHANISMS OF PROTEINURIA

Enhanced urinary protein loss can occur by any of the following mechanisms (Fig. 105-1): (1) an increased delivery and filtration of low-molecular-weight proteins in the plasma, which overwhelms the reabsorptive capacity of the tubule to reclaim normally filtered proteins; (2) an increase in glomerular capillary permeability; (3) impaired capacity of the tubule to reabsorb normally filtered proteins; (4) hemodynamic alterations; and (5) extensive bleeding or severe infection in the urinary tract. Figure 105-1 illustrates the anatomic sites of these mechanisms and lists the most important conditions associated with each of them.

Increased Protein Delivery

Low-molecular-weight proteins are normally filtered across glomerular capillaries but are readily reabsorbed by the tubules. If the delivery of a low-molecular-weight protein exceeds this reabsorptive capacity, proteinuria results. For proteinuria to occur, one of two situations must exist: either overproduction alone exceeds normal maximum reabsorptive capacity or overproduction is associated with a reduced maximum reabsorptive capacity due to an effect of the disease on tubular function. Which of these mechanisms is more significant has not been studied in detail. Various types of leukemia, multiple myeloma, rhabdomyolysis, and hemolysis can cause proteinuria from protein overproduction. Such proteinuria is also referred to as overflow proteinuria.

In monocytic and myelomonocytic leukemia, lysozyme may be produced in large amounts by the leukemic cells. Lysozyme has an isoelectric point of 11 and a low molecular mass (14,000 daltons); both of these features facilitate filtration (see later discussion). When the renal absorptive threshold for lysozyme is exceeded, the filtered lysozyme is excreted in the urine, sometimes in very large amounts (up to 2.6 g/day). Although it is a feature of leukemia, lysozymuria can also be due to primary tubular injury or to tubular damage as a result of glomerular disease. In these instances the lysozymuria is due to a reduced reabsorptive capacity, not to overproduction.

Immunoglobulin light chains (22,000 daltons) are normally filtered across glomeruli, reabsorbed by the tubules, and degraded. If light chains are produced and filtered in amounts greater than the tubular reabsorptive capacity, they appear in the urine in pathologic amounts. Accordingly, the normal excretion rates of kappa and lambda chains are less than 2 and 1 mg/day, respectively, whereas amounts varying from 100 mg to 10 g may be excreted in diseases characterized by increased immunoglobulin production (e.g., multiple myeloma).

When released into the blood and filtered in sufficient quantity, both myoglobin and hemoglobin may lead to detectable proteinuria. Myoglobin can be released in excessive amounts as a result of a number of acquired or hereditary muscle disorders. Trauma is a frequent cause of myoglobinuria. In hemolytic states the release and subsequent filtration of hemoglobin result in proteinuria.

Altered Glomerular Capillary Permeability

Considering the large amounts of plasma proteins that are presented to the glomerular capillaries, very little appears in the urine normally (less than 150 mg/day). Normal glomeruli limit the filtration of molecules on the basis of their size, shape, and electrical charge. This selectivity has been shown to be responsible for the virtual exclusion from the filtrate of plasma proteins equal to or greater than the size of albumin molecules. On the other hand, proteins smaller than albumin are filterable. The components of the glomerular filter are shown in Figure 105-1 *(inset A)*. The capillary endothelium has fenestrations with pores of about 1000 Å in diameter that offer little resistance to protein diffusion. The glomerular basement membrane, which consists of negatively charged glycoproteins and proteoglycans as well as collagen, is the major structural barrier to the filtration of macromolecules. It is important to note that the negative charges in the basement membrane pose an additional, electrical barrier to the passage of negatively charged proteins. Further, structures called slit diaphragms, which bridge adjacent foot processes of the glomerular visceral epithelial cells, offer additional resistance to any proteins that may have penetrated the basement membrane.

Alterations in the selective permeability properties of glomeruli lead to glomerular proteinuria. Structural defects in the filtration pathway that increase the proportion of larger "pores" or molecular defects which give rise to abnormal electrical charge interactions, or both, may account for glomerular protein leakage. Defects in structure and alterations in proportion of large "pores," associated mostly with destructive and inflammatory processes, lead to loss of size discrimination. Therefore the filtrate and urine contain high-molecular-weight globulins and albumin in ratios that approach those of plasma. On the other hand, there are proteinuric glomerulopathies (such as lipoid nephrosis; see also Chapter 116) in which urinary protein is almost exclusively albumin. It would appear that the glomerular lesion in such cases is a decrease in the net negative charge of the filter and diminished repulsion of negatively charged albumin molecules

leading to increased leakage of albumin. Although recent investigations have demonstrated increased urinary losses of large molecules of the size of immunoglobulin in these states, comparatively, the increase in fractional clearance of albumin is still greater than the increase in fractional clearance of immunoglobulin.

Many disorders result in proteinuria because of altered glomerular permeability (Fig. 105-1). All primary glomerulopathies and glomerulopathies associated with systemic diseases have at least this mechanism responsible for proteinuria. Changes in glomerular permeability leading to proteinuria are also suggested, although not proved, in congestive heart failure, hypertension, and febrile illnesses. Isolated proteinuria may be at least partially due to a glomerular permeability mechanism and is discussed separately.

Impaired Tubular Reabsorption

Proteins filtered by glomeruli are reabsorbed and degraded by the renal tubules. The filtered load of protein in normal kidneys is not precisely known, but micropuncture studies in rats suggest an upper limit of 2.5 mg albumin/dl of filtrate. Almost all of this amount is reabsorbed by the tubules. These considerations immediately suggest that if tubular function is impaired, protein reabsorption will be decreased, resulting in proteinuria. Such tubular proteinuria is characterized by the presence of low-molecular-mass globulins (less than 60,000 daltons) in the urine in amounts equal to or greater than amounts of albumin. These globulins are normally present in the serum and are filtered relatively freely but are almost completely reabsorbed. The daily excretion of β_{-2} microglobulin (the best studied globulin) is approximately 30 to 370 μg/day, but in tubular disease as much as 100 mg may be excreted. Similarly, lysozyme, which is normally filtered but reabsorbed, appears in the urine during tubular proteinuria. This condition must be differentiated from lysozymuria, which may occur solely as a result of excessive production and saturation of tubular reabsorptive capacity. Tubular proteinuria occurs in diverse disease states (Fig. 105-1) and is sometimes used to monitor tubular function. In tubular proteinuria the total amount of protein excreted daily is rarely greater than 2 g/day and is usually much less.

Hemodynamic Alterations

Glomerular filtration is affected by hemodynamic factors such as transcapillary hydrostatic and oncotic pressure gradients, plasma flow, the filtration surface area, and permeability (Chapter 101). One or more of these factors may be altered, giving rise to glomerular protein leakage and, potentially, proteinuria. For example, in congestive heart failure there is an increase in the filtration fraction due to disproportionate reduction in glomerular plasma flow compared to the filtration rate. In this situation, complex changes occur in the Starling forces that govern filtration, causing protein leakage rarely exceeding 1 to 1.5 g/day. Treatment of heart failure resolves or markedly diminishes the proteinuria.

Proteinuria may occur in situations in which glomerular blood flow and hydrostatic pressure rise (e.g., in some types of hypertension and during the adaptation that residual nephrons undergo after the destruction of substantial amounts of renal mass). These intrarenal circulatory abnormalities may damage glomeruli and increase protein leakage. Proteinuria is usually moderate, reaching daily excretions of 2 to 3 g only in severe hypertension or unusual cases. Control of hypertension diminishes the proteinuria, in line with its postulated hemodynamic basis. In this regard, angiotensin-converting enzyme inhibitors are thought to be effective, not only as systemic antihypertensives but also as agents that specifically correct the altered glomerular hemodynamics that lead to proteinuria. Chronic, severe dietary restriction of protein intake is known to ameliorate proteinuria and retard the progression of nephron destruction in diverse experimental renal diseases. It is thought that correction of altered glomerular hemodynamics underlies this protection also. However, whether this type of nutritional intervention is beneficial in human disease is not proven.

The other forms of proteinuria that may be hemodynamically mediated include orthostatic proteinuria and exercise-induced proteinuria. Orthostatic proteinuria is abnormal protein excretion that occurs during erect posture and subsides on assumption of recumbent position (see Isolated Proteinuria). Totally reversible marked proteinuria may occur after severe exercise and, if not recognized as such, may cause undue concern.

Other Causes of Proteinuria

Extensive bleeding or severe infection of the urinary tract can be associated with excretion of abnormal amounts of plasma proteins and therefore must be taken into account in the evaluation of urinary protein excretion.

LABORATORY DETERMINATION OF PROTEINURIA

Initial determination of proteinuria is accomplished either by a protein precipitation method (i.e., sulfosalicylic acid test) or by a dipstick colorimetric method. The dipstick method has replaced precipitation methods in most clinical laboratories for initial screening because of its simplicity. Dipstick strips are sensitive to a protein concentration as low as 20 mg/dl. They react preferentially with albumin and are relatively insensitive to globulins and Bence Jones proteins. False-positive results on dipstick examination may be obtained when urine is highly concentrated or alkaline or in the presence of antiseptics (e.g., chlorhexidine). Protein precipitation methods flocculate all proteins and are useful in detecting nonalbumin proteins (e.g., in multiple myeloma).

Quantification of confirmed proteinuria is accomplished with a 24-hour urine collection. As mentioned, the upper limit in the adult, on average, is approximately 150 mg/day of protein. Several studies have shown that protein-creatinine or protein-osmolality ratios in urine samples voided randomly during waking hours correlate well with 24-hour protein values.

Further characterization of the proteinuria as to the selectivity of protein loss is possible by urine protein electrophoresis, but this differentiation has limited clinical application. Urine protein electrophoresis, along with immunodiffusion and immunoelectrophoresis (on concentrated urine), is required to characterize the immunoglobulins in proteinuria associated with plasma cell dyscrasias.

Microalbuminuria

Sensitive radioimmunoassays have determined that the rate of albumin excretion in normal individuals is less than 15 μg/minute. Albumin excretion rates greater than 30 μg/minute are pathologic but below the detection limit of conventional dipsticks used to detect protein in routine urinalysis. This degree of albumin excretion in urine has been termed microalbuminuria. Investigations in diabetic patients have identified microalbuminuria as an early marker of patients destined to develop progressive nephropathy and an index of increased cardiovascular mortality. Screening for early diabetic nephropathy by microalbuminuria is gaining popularity with the object of employing therapeutic interventions such as angiotension-converting enzyme inhibitors. Whether microalbuminuria can serve as an early marker of other progressive renal diseases is being investigated. Sensitive dipsticks and radioimmunoassays are employed in the detection of microalbuminuria.

EVALUATION OF PROTEINURIA

Proteinuria can occur in several different clinical settings: (1) renal disease occurring as a part of acquired or hereditary systemic disorders (e.g., in systemic lupus erythematosus and Alport's syndrome); (2) primary renal disease (e.g., glomerulonephritis); (3) protein overproduction due to plasma cell dyscrasias, leukemia, rhabdomyolysis, or hemolysis; (4) proteinuria resulting from renal hemodynamic alterations, as in congestive heart failure; and (5) patients having no evidence of disease by history, physical examination, or laboratory examination and having normal renal function except for proteinuria with a normal urinary sediment. The last-mentioned category is referred to as isolated proteinuria. The likelihood of an underlying disease is high if quantitative proteinuria exceeds 2 g/day. Proteinuria in excess of 3.5 g/day, consisting mostly of albumin, is considered to be in the range usually seen in the nephrotic syndrome (Chapter 108).

This amount of proteinuria (greater than 3.5 g/day) indicates glomerular disease at least as a component (assuming the proteinuria is not due to overproduction, as in multiple myeloma).

The first three categories of proteinuria are discussed in detail elsewhere (Chapters 108, 116, 117, and 118). Patients with proteinuria that is due to hemodynamic alterations usually have a profound reduction in protein excretion with appropriate treatment of the underlying disease. Otherwise healthy individuals with isolated proteinuria deserve special consideration.

ISOLATED PROTEINURIA

Isolated proteinuria is not a rare finding in practice, with the incidence reported between 0.55% and 5.8% of young servicemen or college freshmen. The range of protein loss can vary from less than 1 g/day to the values associated with the nephrotic syndrome. When the proteinuria is greater than 1 g/day, the likelihood of finding underlying glomerular disease increases and a renal biopsy may be indicated. Isolated proteinurias can be further divided into transient, intermittent, constant, and orthostatic. These patterns do not represent specific disease and may occur in the same patient at different times.

Transient proteinuria is defined as proteinuria present on initial examination of apparently healthy individuals and absent on subsequent urinalysis. It is a common type of proteinuria in children and young adults. Transient proteinuria can also be seen during exercise and fever. There is no evidence of renal disease in these patients.

Intermittent proteinuria does not define a specific group of patients. In one group of individuals with intermittent proteinuria studied by biopsy 30% demonstrated minimal or no change and 70% demonstrated either interstitial fibrosis or glomerular disease. Although a significant number of patients show some renal histologic changes, the prognosis for most patients in this group is good and proteinuria disappears in a few years in most patients. Persons under 30 years of age have mortality rates similar to comparable age-matched controls. In general, periodic follow-up is recommended, with evaluation of blood pressure, urine, and renal function.

The constant pattern of isolated proteinuria is associated with a higher mortality than the intermittent pattern and a greater risk of death resulting from renal disease. It should be distinguished from orthostatic proteinuria, which carries a very good prognosis. The constant pattern correlates with a variety of renal lesions on biopsy; thus a uniform prognosis cannot be predicted. Renal biopsy may show a normal pattern or mild mesangial proliferation (≈70%), definite glomerular lesions (20%), and/or interstitial nephritis (≈5%). In up to 50% of these patients hypertension may develop over a 5-year period, and renal insufficiency has occurred in up to 20% of patients during 10 years of follow-up.

Orthostatic proteinuria must be distinguished from the constant pattern. Urine samples are obtained in the morning on awakening, while the patient is still supine, and after 2 hours of continuous walking or standing. Orthostatic proteinuria is defined as proteinuria that is present only in the urine samples obtained in an upright position. Patients with orthostatic proteinuria have a low risk of development of renal insufficiency. In a 20-year follow-up study of young men, none had developed any evidence of renal functional impairment, and only a few continued to be proteinuric.

BIBLIOGRAPHY

Kasinath BS, Kanwar YS: Glomerular basement membrane: biology and physiology. In Rohrbach DH, Timpl R, editors: *Molecular and cellular aspects of basement membranes,* San Diego, 1993, Academic Press.

Kasiske BL, Keane WF: Laboratory assessment of renal disease: clearance, urinalysis and renal biopsy. In Brenner BM, editor: *The kidney,* ed 5, Philadelphia, 1996, WB Saunders.

Scandling JD et al: Glomerular permselectivity in healthy and nephrotic humans, *Adv Nephrol* 21:159-176, 1992.

106 Dysuria

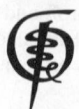

Marvin Forland

Dysuria literally means difficult urination, but in customary clinical usage it refers to the painful passage of urine, often accompanied by frequency, urgency, and a sense of incomplete bladder emptying. Although this symptom complex is characteristic of bacterial cystitis-urethritis, the differential diagnosis is broad (Box 106-1) but is usually readily narrowed by a careful history and physical examination, aided by a few easily obtainable laboratory data. Dysuria is a far more frequent complaint among women than among men, and we will consider the sexes separately.

DYSURIA IN WOMEN
Infectious Causes

Urinary Tract Infection. The presence of costovertebral or flank pain or tenderness and fever in association with dysuria strongly suggests upper urinary tract infection. In less acutely ill women, a distinction has been made between *internal dysuria*—perceived by the patient as inside the body and experienced with urethritis—and *external dysuria*—pain felt in the inflamed vaginal labia, induced by the stream of urine, and characteristic of vaginitis.

Urinary tract infection is confirmed by the culture findings of

---

BOX 106-1
Differential diagnosis of dysuria

I. Urinary tract infection
  A. Enterobacteriaceae
  B. Gram-positive organisms
  C. *Chlamydia trachomatis*
  D. *Mycobacterium tuberculosis*
II. Vaginitis
  A. Fungi *(Candida albicans)*
  B. Bacterial
    1. *Gardnerella vaginalis (Haemophilus vaginalis)*
    2. *Neisseria gonorrhoeae*
    3. *Treponema pallidum* (endourethral chancre)
    4. *Chlamydia trachomatis*
  C. Protozoa *(Trichomonas vaginalis)*
III. Genital infection
  A. Herpes simplex (genitalis)
  B. Condyloma accuminatum
  C. Paraurethral glands
IV. Estrogen deficiency
V. Interstitial cystitis (Hunner's ulcer)
VI. Reiter's syndrome
VII. Chemical irritants
  A. Douches
  B. Deodorant aerosols
  C. Contraceptive jellies
  D. Bubble bath
VIII. Impedance to flow
  A. Urethral caruncle or diverticula
  B. Meatal stenosis or stricture
  C. Transient urethral edema
  D. Chronic fibrosis after trauma
  E. Impaired synergy: bladder contraction and sphincter relaxation
IX. Regional disease
  A. Crohn's disease
  B. Diverticulitis
  C. Cervical radium implant
X. Bladder tumor

100,000 or more colonies per milliliter of urine obtained from a clean-voided midstream urine specimen. This widely used criterion was based largely on studies of women with acute pyelonephritis or asymptomatic bacteriuria. In a series of studies of symptomatic women, only one third to two thirds of the patients whose urine contained organisms on suprapubic aspiration or urethral catheterization met this standard. Finding 100 or more colonies per milliliter of urine was the diagnostic criterion providing the most useful sensitivity and specificity in this symptomatic population. The finding of pyuria is nonspecific, but in association with dysuria it strongly suggests an infectious origin. The presence of organisms on direct examination of the fresh, spun, preferably Gram-stained urine, is helpful, rapid confirmation.

The presence of pyuria in association with dysuria and in the absence of bacteriuria by standard techniques should alert the physician to the possibility of genitourinary tuberculosis. Tuberculin skin testing is appropriate, and, if the findings are positive, a series of first morning urine specimens should be cultured for *Mycobacterium tuberculosis*. Dysuria has been reported as a prominent symptom in 20% to 34% of patients with renal tuberculosis.

An additional consideration is *Chlamydia trachomatis* infection. This organism was implicated in more than half the women with dysuria and frequency, sterile bladder urine, and pyuria in a study using cell culture techniques for isolation of the organism. Sexual transmission appears likely. Diagnosis has been facilitated by the availability of rapid DNA probe testing.

Vaginitis. Vaginitis assumes a major role when dysuria is described as external and particularly when it is accompanied by an unusual or malodorous vaginal discharge, dyspareunia, or vulvar itching or discomfort. Dysuria is a less common symptom with vaginitis than with urinary tract infection but may be more often attributable to vaginitis in young women because vaginitis occurs far more frequently than urinary tract infection. *Candida albicans* is the most common cause of symptomatic vaginitis, and the fungal growth may be sustained by elevated estrogen levels. Consequently, it occurs more frequently in pregnancy or with the use of oral contraceptives, and the patient may experience premenstrual exacerbations. Candidal discharge is characteristically white, thick, curd forming, and adherent, and organisms are readily identifiable on wet mount.

Trichomonas vaginalis infection is associated with dysuria or frequency in about 25% of infected women. The discharge is classically described as profuse, yellowish green, frothy, and malodorous, but is highly variable. Identification of the organisms by wet mount is successful in 60% to 70% of infected women; culture provides a significantly higher yield.

Bacterial vaginosis is now the preferred term for the most prevalent vaginal infection in the reproductive years, previously called nonspecific vaginitis. The designation emphasizes its noninflammatory characteristics and its relationship to the interplay of several species of facultative anaerobic bacteria, genital mycoplasma, and suppression of the usually dominant *Lactobacillus*. A vaginal malodor, often described as fishy, is the major symptom. The discharge is small to moderate in amount, gray, malodorous, thin and adherent. While *Gardnerella vaginalis* may be a necessary pathogenic component, it is no longer considered the sole etiologic agent. However, its presence is an important diagnostic finding, evident on wet mount examination as tiny granules studding the vaginal epithelial cells, termed *clue cells*. Additional characteristic findings are a vaginal pH greater than 4.5 and a positive amine test result, established by elicitation of a fishy odor upon addition of 10% KOH to vaginal secretions. Bacterial vaginosis is associated with the preterm delivery of low-birth-weight infants independent of other recognized risk factors.

Gonorrhea continues to be a major consideration in the differential diagnosis of dysuria. This diagnosis was made in 8% to 29% of women with dysuria as an initial complaint and accounted for over 60% of those with "negative" urine cultures in one experience. The symptoms were similar to those in the group with urinary tract infection and sometimes included fever. Thus a preliminary diagnosis of acute pyelonephritis was not rare in those subsequently found to have gonorrheal infection. A complete pelvic examination and a Thayer-Martin culture or DNA probe test of an endocervical specimen play an important role in initial evaluation in populations at risk of gonorrhea.

Less common infectious causes include the presence of an endourethral chancre, herpes simplex (genitalis) usually located on the labia, or condyloma accuminatum. Infection localized to the small Skene's glands that empty into the urethra has been suggested as analogous to male prostatitis. Exudate may be expressed from the glands for smear and culture.

Noninfectious Causes

Atrophic Vaginitis. In the postmenopausal woman, dysuria may be a consequence of estrogen deprivation, resulting in senile or atrophic vaginitis with associated urethral irritation. Vaginal discharge, itching, and dyspareunia are frequent accompanying symptoms. The vaginal mucosa appears thin, often inflamed, and bleeds easily. Infections occur with increased frequency. A wet smear of vaginal cells shows a marked predominance of parabasal cells. Response to estrogen administration is usually rapid.

Interstitial Cystitis. Persistent dysuria with sterile cultures raises the possibility of interstitial cystitis, an uncommon bladder lesion of unknown etiology seen most often in women. The classic symptom complex includes continuous frequency and urgency and suprapubic pain relieved by voiding. Pyuria and hematuria are sometimes present but not uniformly, and the findings of exfoliative cytologic examination are negative. The diagnosis is made by cystoscopy, with the characteristic findings of reduced bladder capacity and the presence of superficial, often stellate Hunner's ulcers. In the earlier stages of the disease, however, only multiple petechiae-like hemorrhages (glomerulations) may be observed after second distention of the bladder on cystoscopy, and the capacity may be normal. Increased numbers of mast cells have been described on detrusor muscle biopsy of patients with presumed interstitial cystitis, but therapeutic results with mast cell stabilizing agents have been poor. Bladder surface alterations and autoimmune responses are among possible causes currently under investigation.

Urethral Syndrome. The urethral syndrome, or *frequency and dysuria syndrome,* is a term that has been used to describe the approximately 50% of women with these complaints who have either no growth or counts below 100,000 colonies per milliliter on repeated urine cultures. The majority of these symptomatic women with low colony counts on conventional cultures have been found to have pathogenic organisms present on cultures of suprapubic aspiration or urethral catheterization specimens. Response to antibacterial therapy is usually prompt.

A smaller subset of patients is defined by the presence of sterile urine and absence of correlation between symptoms and evidence of genitourinary tract inflammation. Measures effective for bacteriuric patients fail to relieve symptoms, among which frequency is often more prominent than dysuria. Diazepam (Valium) has been suggested as an effective agent for the symptomatic abacteriuric patient, the drug acting perhaps through a bladder mechanism rather than through its better-described psychopharmacologic effect.

The patient must be questioned concerning the possibility of a chemical irritant. These have included a variety of topical applicants such as douching agents, deodorant aerosols, and contraceptive jellies. Bathing preparations have also been implicated.

Impedance to urine flow may produce complaints of hesitancy, frequency, urinary straining, diminished caliber of the stream, and dribbling. The prominence of these symptoms, rather than burning pain, and the negative bacterial cultures suggest such an origin. Meatal stenosis or stricture, urethral caruncle, or diverticula may be responsible. Transient edema may be related to sexual activity or straddle-position injury. Functional lesions related to impaired synergy between bladder contraction and sphincter relaxation have also been described. Less common causes include infiltrating bladder tumors or inflammation secondary to regional disease such as Crohn's ileocolitis or diverticulitis.

DYSURIA IN MALES

Presentation with dysuria raises the possibilities of cystitis-urethritis or pyelonephritis, as in women, and the additional consideration of

prostatitis. Terminal dysuria, pyuria, or bacteriuria first evident or increased in expressed prostatic fluid or in a post–prostatic-massage voiding (third-glass collection) all suggest prostatic localization. This determination is of importance in deciding on the extent of diagnostic evaluation that is appropriate and in selecting antibacterial agents capable of concentrating within the prostatic parenchyma. Bacterial urinary tract infection is more likely to be associated with an underlying anatomic abnormality in the young male or with calculi or prostatic hypertrophy with obstruction in the older male; hence the need for thorough evaluation.

Dysuria, as well as a urethral discharge, is seen in approximately 80% of men with gonorrhea; 10% may be symptomatic without a discharge. The diagnosis is made on the basis of the characteristic intracellular diplococci found on urethral smear in 95% of patients. Thayer-Martin cultures or DNA probe testing confirm the diagnosis in the remaining few.

A number of organisms are suspected of playing a role in nonspecific urethritis. *C. trachomatis,* an obligate intracellular parasite, has been isolated in 30% to 50% of symptomatic males. It is found in only 3% of sexually active asymptomatic men. Its recovery from symptomatic women supports its pathogenicity. *Ureaplasma urealyticum* has been reported in up to 80% of men with nonspecific urethritis, but its presence in 60% of asymptomatic males has raised questions concerning its significance.

Trichomonas is seen in about 5% of men with nongonorrheal urethritis. It is best observed and cultured with a first morning urine specimen.

Dysuria may be related to balanitis-urethritis with Reiter's syndrome. The classic tetrad of this symptom complex also includes conjunctivitis, mucocutaneous lesions, and arthritis; however, more limited clinical expression is frequently observed.

BIBLIOGRAPHY

Hillier SL et al: Association between bacterial vaginosis and preterm delivery of a low-birth-weight infant, *N Engl J Med* 333:1737, 1995.

Krieger JN, Ross SO, Simonsen JM: Urinary tract infections in healthy university men, *J Urol* 149:1046, 1993.

Kunin CM, Van Arsdale White L, Hua Hua T: A reassessment of the importance of "low-count" bacteriuria in young women with acute urinary symptoms, *Ann Intern Med* 119:454, 1993.

Ratliff TL, Klutke CG, McDougall, EM: The etiology of interstitial cystitis, *Urol Clin North Am* 21:21, 1994.

Raz R, Stamm WE: A controlled trial of intravaginal estriol in postmenopausal women with recurrent urinary tract infections, *N Engl J Med* 329:753, 1993.

CHAPTER

107 Acute Nephritic Syndrome

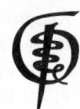

B.S. Kasinath

Glomerular diseases can become evident in the form of acute nephritis, nephrotic syndrome, or asymptomatic urinary abnormalities of hematuria and proteinuria. Acute nephritic syndrome is suggested by the sudden appearance of hematuria (gross or microscopic) often associated with erythrocyte casts with some or all of the following: variable degree of proteinuria (mild to nephrotic range), edema, hypertension, and renal insufficiency. A subset of these patients come to medical attention with rapidly progressive glomerulonephritis (RPGN), which is defined as 50% or greater loss of glomerular filtration rate within 3 months that is associated with extensive crescents usually involving 50% or more glomeruli as the principle finding on renal biopsy. The clinician should recognize acute nephritic syndrome, especially RPGN, without delay and assiduously pursue the underlying cause, as timely intervention can save renal function in many cases.

BOX 107-1
Common causes of acute glomerulonephritis

I. Hypocomplementemic glomerulonephritis
  A. Primary renal diseases
    1. Acute poststreptococcal glomerulonephritis
    2. Membranoproliferative glomerulonephritis
  B. Systemic diseases
    1. Systemic lupus erythematosus
    2. Infectious endocarditis
    3. Ventriculoatrial shunt infection–associated nephritis
    4. Cryoglobulinemia
    5. Hepatitis C–associated membranoproliferative glomerulo-
       nephritis
II. Normocomplementemic glomerulonephritis
  A. Primary renal diseases
    1. Immunoglobulin A nephritis
    2. Idiopathic, rapidly progressive glomerulonephritis
    3. Antiglomerular basement membrane disease
  B. Systemic diseases
    1. Vasculitis (e.g., Wegener's granulomatosis, polyarteritis
       nodosa, hypersensitivity vasculitis)
    2. Goodpasture's syndrome
    3. Henoch-Schönlein purpura
    4. Others (e.g., hemolytic-uremic syndrome, thrombotic
       thrombocytopenic purpura, visceral abscesses)

Modified from Madaio M, Harrington JT: *N Engl J Med* 309:1299-1302, 1983.

ETIOLOGY AND PATHOLOGY

A large variety of glomerular diseases can become evident as acute glomerulonephritis; the more common causes are shown in Box 107-1. In primary renal disease the original disease process first affects the kidney without involvement of other organ systems by the same process. Secondary renal diseases are characterized by multisystem organ involvement, including the kidneys, by a single disease process.

Renal pathology usually shows proliferation of glomerular mesangial or endothelial cells; "crescents" may be seen surrounding the glomeruli and are composed of proliferating glomerular epithelial cells and monocyte/macrophages. Evidence of focal or diffuse necrosis may be present. Vascular lesions may predominate in diseases such as hemolytic uremic syndrome. Immunofluorescence and electron microscopic examination may reveal evidence of immune reactants in mesangial, subendothelial, or subepithelial locations or in the glomerular basement membrane.

APPROACH TO DIAGNOSIS

A thorough history should include inquiry of infections. Recent infection of pharynx (postpharyngitic) or skin *preceding* acute nephritis is typically seen in poststreptococcal glomerulonephritis. In contrast, an ongoing pharyngeal (synpharyngitic) upper respiratory tract or gastrointestinal tract "infectious" process is commonly encountered in acute presentation of immunoglobulin A nephritis. Recurrent sinusitis and otitis resistant to therapy may be seen in Wegener's granulomatosis. Hemoptysis, dyspnea, and exposure to hydrocarbons may be relevant in pulmonary-renal syndromes (e.g., Goodpasture's syndrome). Symptoms suggestive of connective tissue disease such as rashes, photosensitivity, arthritis, and Raynaud's phenomenon should be sought. History of drug abuse is important, since infectious endocarditis can cause acute glomerulonephritis. Transfusion-related hepatitis C can be associated with membranoproliferative glomerulonephritis. Physical examination should focus on blood pressure, edema, evidence of congestive heart failure, and signs of connective tissue disease (e.g., arthritis, rashes). Roth spots, new cardiac murmurs, and splenomegaly suggest infectious endocarditis. Necrotizing lesions of the nasal mucosa, sinusitis, otitis, and palpable purpura may lead to considerations of vasculitis.

✔ *WHEN TO REFER*

Once the initial clinical evaluation including urinalysis reveals the presence of acute nephritic syndrome, an early consultation with a nephrologist is recommended while investigations are performed by the primary care physician as suggested. This strategy permits early recognition of serious glomerular diseases (e.g., crescentic glomerulonephritides) and allows institution of therapeutic intervention as soon as possible.

The next step is careful evaluation of a freshly voided urine sample, preferably obtained early in the morning. Urine sediment microscopy should reveal presence of erythrocytes in significant numbers; "dysmorphic" red blood cells with variations in size, shape, and hemoglobin content are suggestive of glomerular origin of hematuria (see Chapter 104). Erythrocyte casts are highly suggestive of acute glomerulonephritis. Proteinuria may be mild or nephrotic. Nephrotic proteinuria (nephritic-nephrotic presentation) as revealed by greater than 3.5 g protein excretion in urine over 24 hours can be seen (e.g., lupus erythematosus, membranoproliferative glomerulonephritis). Screening blood tests should include blood urea nitrogen (BUN) and serum creatinine values to assess the extent of renal functional impairment, serum electrolyte levels, and complete blood cell count including platelet count. The peripheral blood smear may reveal schistocytes, suggesting a microangiopathic process (e.g., thrombotic thrombocytopenic purpura). Microcytic, hypochromic anemia may be seen in pulmonary-renal syndromes due to hemoptysis (e.g., Goodpasture's syndrome). Measurement of serum complement components C3, C4, and CH50 has been found to be of great assistance. Presence of hypocomplementemia suggests a short list of causes of acute glomerulonephritis (Box 107-1). Serologic tests for antinuclear antibody, antibody against double-stranded DNA, cryoglobulins, antibodies against streptococcal antigens (antistreptolysin-O, antihyaluronidase, antideoxyribonuclease-B), blood cultures, and cultures of foci of infections (e.g., throat, skin) may be undertaken depending on the clues on clinical evaluation, although patients with lupus erythematosus may not always have characteristic constellation of symptoms. Detection of antibodies against glomerular basement membrane in the serum points to Goodpasture's syndrome as diagnosis.

Recently, presence of increased titers of antineutrophil cytoplasmic antibodies (ANCA) has been shown to correlate with the diagnosis of Wegener's granulomatosis and idiopathic (pauciimmune) RPGN. The precise histologic diagnosis can be established only by a renal biopsy. Close, daily monitoring of renal function is essential. It should be emphasized that in the face of a rapidly deteriorating renal function (e.g., RPGN) one should perform renal biopsy as soon as it is safely possible. In severe glomerulonephritis (e.g., crescentic nephritis), if therapy is not instituted at an early stage, renal function may be irrevocably lost. The histologic information and the assessment of reversibility of a particular lesion on renal biopsy help the clinician to decide whether to treat and, if a decision is made to treat, which therapeutic modality to choose.

BIBLIOGRAPHY

Cattell V: Macrophages in acute glomerular inflammation, *Kidney Int* 45:945-952, 1994.
Johnson RJ, Wilson R, Yamabe H et al: Renal manifestations of hepatitis C virus infection, *Kidney Int* 46:1255-1263, 1994.
Kallenberg CGM, Brouwer E, Weening JJ, Cohen Tervaert JW: Antineutrophil cytoplasmic antibodies: current diagnostic and pathophysiological potential, *Kidney Int* 46:1-15, 1994.

108 Nephrotic Syndrome

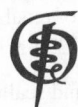

B.S. Kasinath

The nephrotic syndrome is characterized by urinary protein losses (consisting mostly of albumin) exceeding 3.5 g/1.73 m² of body surface area per day, accompanied by hypoalbuminemia, edema, hyperlipidemia, and lipiduria. Nephrotic syndrome occurs as a result of a severe defect in the glomerular selective permeability function (permselectivity). Therefore it is a useful clinical clue for the existence of glomerular disease. However, it must be emphasized that the quantitative definition of proteinuria of 3.5 g/day is arbitrary and that all causes of nephrotic syndrome can be associated with lesser degrees of proteinuria. Since many of the complications of nephrotic syndrome are due to hypoalbuminemia and decreased oncotic pressure, lesser degrees of proteinuria that are sufficient to cause hypoalbuminemia can result in the same consequences.

The diseases causing nephrotic syndrome may be considered in the broad categories of primary renal diseases in which kidneys are fundamentally involved in a disease process and secondary renal diseases, in which kidneys are involved in a systemic disease. Many systemic diseases can cause pathologic lesions that are usually associated with primary renal diseases causing nephrotic syndrome. For example, lupus nephritis can be evident as membranous nephropathy, which may be quite similar to primary membranous nephropathy on histologic examination. Box 108-1 lists common causes of nephrotic syndrome.

CLINICAL MANIFESTATIONS AND PATHOPHYSIOLOGY
Proteinuria

Although proteinuria can be due to a variety of glomerular and nonglomerular mechanisms, the massive degree of proteinuria encountered in nephrotic syndrome occurs primarily because of dysregulation of glomerular permselectivity. As reviewed in Chapter 105, the selective permeability function of the glomerulus regulates filtration of molecules based on their size, charge, and shape. Normal urine contains molecules spanning a wide range of molecular radii, including large molecules such as immunoglobulin G (IgG), suggesting that the glomerular capillary wall behaves like a heteroporous filter (i.e., having "pores" of different sizes). Pores that permit passage of large molecules such as IgG (molecular weight, 150,000) form a small fraction of the general population of pores. In addition, for molecules of identical size negatively charged species have less permeability across the glomerular capillary compared with neutral species. This charge barrier function is due to the presence of highly anionic molecules such as proteoglycans in the glomerular capillary wall. In nephrotic syndrome, changes in the size or charge-selective properties, or both, of the capillary wall may be seen. In minimal change disease, a common cause of nephrotic syndrome in children, the filtration of albumin greatly exceeds that of IgG. Plasma albumin at physiologic pH is anionic, and the selective loss of albumin in this disease suggests a selective impairment in the charge barrier function of the glomerulus. In other causes of the nephrotic syndrome an abnormal, nonselective leakage of small and large marker proteins is seen, implying an impairment in the size-selective barrier function of the glomerular basement membrane. In diabetic nephropathy, a common cause of nephrotic syndrome in adults, a relative increase in the proportion of large pores has been proposed as the mechanism of nonselective proteinuria.

Hypoalbuminemia

Normally albumin is synthesized by the liver (12 to 14 g/day). It is catabolized mainly by the endothelium and to a small extent by the

---

BOX 108-1
Classification of nephrotic syndrome

Primary renal diseases
Minimal change nephrtoic syndrome
Membranous nephropathy
Focal and segmental glomerulosclerosis
Membranoproliferative glomerulonephritis
Mesangial proliferative glomerulonephritis
Others

Secondary renal diseases
Genetic disorders: Alport's syndrome, congenital nephrotic syndrome, sickle cell disease
Metabolic diseases: Diabetes mellitus, amyloidosis
Autoimmune diseases: Systemic lupus erythematosus, Henoch-Schönlein purpura, vasculitides
Malignant diseases: Multiple myeloma; carcinomas of lung, colon, breast, stomach; leukemias, lymphomas
Infectious diseases
  Bacterial: Infectious endocarditis
  Viral: Human immunodeficiency virus, hepatitis B, hepatitis C
  Protozoal: Malaria
  Helminthic: Schistosomiasis
Others
  Drugs: Nonsteroidal antiinflammatory agents, gold, heroin, interferon-alfa, lithium, pencillamine, mercury, probenecid, captopril
  Pregnancy: Precclampsia
  Transplant rejection

---

proximal tubular epithelium of the kidney. Hypoalbuminemia, a characteristic feature of the nephrotic syndrome, results from a combination of several mechanisms including urinary losses. However, urinary losses alone do not account for reduction in plasma albumin levels, since hypoalbuminemia may be present even when albumin losses are modest—well below the nephrotic range. Catabolism of albumin in the kidney, which normally accounts for only 10% to 20% of overall albumin breakdown, is increased in nephrotic syndrome. However, as albumin catabolism in other organs is reduced, augmented renal breakdown of albumin is unlikely to be the main mechanism of hypoalbuminemia. The hepatic synthesis of albumin is increased in response to hypoalbuminemia, probably by regulating the amount of messenger RNA of albumin. The factors that are involved in transcriptional regulation of albumin are not well understood but may include decreased oncotic pressure and nutritional factors such as protein intake. The response of nephrotic patients to an increase in protein intake is complex. Although the rate of albumin synthesis increases, this is offset by augmentation of both urinary albumin losses and the catabolic rate of albumin. Serum albumin levels may actually fall when high-protein diets are administered to nephrotic patients. An adequate protein diet combined with intervention aimed at reducing protein excretion may be beneficial. In untreated cases, despite enhanced synthesis by the liver, the urinary losses of albumin are not fully compensated, perpetuating hypoalbuminemia.

In addition to hypoalbuminemia, alterations in plasma levels of a variety of proteins occur in the nephrotic syndrome. Levels of immunoglobulins G and A (IgG and IgA) are reduced, and these changes are only partly explained by urinary losses. IgM levels may be increased. Urinary losses of vitamin D–binding protein, thyroid-binding globulin, corticosteroid-binding globulin, and transferrin have been documented. However, nephrotic patients do not have thyroid hormone deficiency. Rarely, microcytic hypochromic anemia attributable to transferrin deficiency has been reported. Erythropoietin losses into urine have been reported in nephrotic patients and may contribute to anemia.

Edema

The cardinal manifestation of nephrotic syndrome is edema. Edema of the feet is commonly noted following ambulation; edema is seen around the eyes after recumbency. In severe nephrotic syndrome ana-sarca, with effusions in pleural, pericardial, or peritoneal spaces may be present. Two hypotheses have been proposed for pathogenesis of nephrotic edema. The "underfill theory" suggests that, because of hypoalbuminemia and decreased plasma oncotic pressure, there is a shift of water from the intravascular compartment to interstitial space (i.e., edema). This results in a state of intravascular volume depletion (underfill state) leading to activation of the renin-angiotension-aldosterone axis, stimulation of antidiuretic hormone (ADH) secretion, and augmentation of sympathetic neural activity. These factors enhance sodium and water retention by the kidneys, which further decreases the plasma albumin concentration and contributes to edema formation. The second mechanism, "the overfill theory," proposes a *primary* defect in sodium excretion by the nephron, resulting in increase in blood volume (overfill) and blood pressure. This leads to an elevation in the capillary hydrostatic pressure that is opposed even less than normally by the reduced oncotic pressure of the nephrotic state, resulting in edema formation. The nature of the primary renal defect is not clear, but resistance to atrial natriuretic peptide has been proposed.

Hyperlipidemia

Various lipid abnormalities have been described in patients with the nephrotic syndrome. During evaluation of hyperlipidemia in nephrotic patients the potential contributions of renal insufficiency, coincident diseases such as diabetes mellitus, familial hyperlipidemias, and the use of therapeutic agents that affect lipoproteins (such as corticosteroids) have to be taken into account. In patients with the nephrotic syndrome without the confounding factors mentioned earlier, elevation of low-density lipoprotein (LDL) and very-low-density lipoprotien (VLDL) concentrations has been reported as the most common abnormality in lipoproteins; elevated levels of serum LDL with normal VLDL levels may be present in one third of the patients; however, an elevated level of VLDL with normal LDL level is a rarity. The increment affects the cholesterol, triglyceride, and phospholipid constituents of LDL and VLDL. In addition, significant increases in serum levels of apoproteins B, C-II, C-III, and E are also seen. There are conflicting reports on the status of high-density lipoprotein (HDL) in the nephrotic syndrome. Although total plasma HDL levels remain normal, levels of HDL_2, which are thought to be protective against atherosclerosis, are decreased. Thus the LDL:HDL cholesterol ratio is increased. In addition, there is elevation of levels of another plasma lipoprotein—Lp(a)—associated with increased risk of cardiovascular disease independent of LDL. Lipiduria is commonly encountered in the nephrotic syndrome and is associated with lipid casts. Urinary lipids that may be ingested by the renal tubular epithelial cells are contained in casts and give a Maltese cross appearance under polarized light microscopy. Analysis of urinary lipids has shown abnormal excretion of apolipoprotein C-II, cholesterol, triglycerides, and phospholipids in the nephrotic syndrome. The pathogenetic mechanisms underlying hyperlipidemia are not well understood. There is evidence for increased synthesis of lipoproteins, including LDL and apolipoproteins, and decreased breakdown of VLDL. Reduced activity of lipoprotein lipase and diminished uptake of chylomicron remnant particles by the liver have been reported. The factors that trigger these changes probably differ for individual lipid abnormalities and include urinary protein losses, reduced oncotic pressure, and hypoalbuminemia.

Coagulation Abnormalities

Thrombosis is a well-known complication of the nephrotic syndrome and may occur in the venous vessels of the lower extremities, renal veins, or subclavian veins. Arterial thrombosis can also occur, especially in children. The frequency of renal vein thrombosis in several prospective studies ranges from 5% to 62%, with an average of 35%, whereas thrombosis in nonrenal circulation ranges from 8.5% to 44%, with an average of approximately 20%. Renal vein thrombosis was erroneously considered a cause of nephrotic syndrome in the past; now it is established as its complication. Renal vein thrombosis may be acute or chronic. *Acute renal vein thrombosis* usually becomes evident with flank pain and hematuria. It may be associated with fluctuation in the level of proteinuria and reduction in glomerular filtra-

tion rate, especially with bilateral involvement. *Chronic renal vein thrombosis* may be asymptomatic or may be associated with pulmonary emboli, backache, varicocele, and signs of inferior vena cava obstruction when the clot obstructs that vessel. Certain causes of the nephrotic syndrome are more commonly associated with renal vein thrombosis (e.g., membranous nephropathy). Other causes of renal venous obstruction such as malignancy should be considered in the differential diagnosis.

Intravenous pyelography may show enlarged kidneys and scalloping of the ureters. The latter finding is due to extensive collateral circulation that occurs in chronic renal vein thrombosis. Renal venography is the definitive test, although noninvasive techniques such as magnetic resonance imaging and Doppler-assisted sonographic studies have also been proposed. Occurrence of hemoptysis or dyspnea in a nephrotic patient should prompt a search for pulmonary embolism.

The pathogenesis of coagulation abnormalities in the nephrotic syndrome is multifactoral. Increased hepatic synthesis of high-molecular-weight procoagulant proteins such as fibrinogen and clotting factors V and VIII has been documented. In addition, excessive urinary losses of coagulation inhibitors such as antithrombin-III and proteins C and S also occur in the nephrotic syndrome. Other contributory factors include increased aggregation of platelets, increased plasma viscosity as a result of hyperfibrinogenemia, deficiency of fibrinolytic proteins, and steroid therapy. The pathogenetic relationship between these changes and clinical thromboembolism is not firmly established.

COMPLICATIONS

Many of the complications of nephrotic syndrome have been alluded to in our discussion of clinical manifestations and pathophysiology. The major untoward consequences of the nephrotic state are discussed here.

Accelerated Atherosclerosis

The lipid abnormalities of increased LDL and Lp(a) levels and LDL:HDL cholesterol ratio and decrease in HDL_2 levels, in association with hypercoagulability, would suggest that nephrotic patients are at an increased risk for atherosclerotic cardiovascular disease. However, the issue is controversial. Some studies have reported increased frequency of myocardial infarction and death from coronary artery disease compared with nonnephrotic controls after accounting for risk factors such as diabetes, smoking, and hypertension. Since the lipid abnormalities seen in nephrotic syndrome are associated with accelerated atherosclerosis in the general population, it is quite likely that they have the same implication in nephrotic patients. In addition, recent findings suggest that the previously mentioned lipid abnormalities may contribute to progression of renal disease.

Thromboembolism

As described earlier, thrombosis of lower-extremity veins, renal veins, subclavian vein, and arterial vessels can occur in nephrotic syndrome, particularly in association with membranous nephropathy. Pulmonary embolism should be considered in a nephrotic patient who comes to medical attention with dyspnoea or hemoptysis. The approach to diagnosis of thromboembolic complications has been discussed in the previous section of this chapter.

Increased Susceptibility to Infections

Deficiencies of IgG and the complement factor B contribute to increased susceptibility to bacterial infections and defective opsonization, respectively. Infectious complications are common, and encapsulated bacterial infections can be particularly virulent. Pneumonia, meningitis, peritonitis, and sepsis may be encountered. Although a variety of abnormalities in in vitro tests of humoral and cellular immunity have been described in the nephrotic syndrome, these patients do not seem to be at higher risk for malignancies or infections with unusual pathogens.

Bone Disease

Urinary losses of vitamin D–binding protein results in decreased plasma vitamin D levels. Hypocalcemia, including reduced ionized calcium levels, occurs in nephrotics. Rickets has been described in children. Elevation in parathyroid hormone secretion and secondary osteitis fibrosa have also been reported.

Other Complications

Malnutrition resulting from persistent urinary protein losses and a decrease in muscle mass are frequently present in nephrotic syndrome.

APPROACH TO DIAGNOSIS

A thorough history, physical examination, and analysis of a freshly voided urine specimen by an experienced examiner should enable the physician to develop a short list of diagnostic possibilities. A diagnostic approach to glomerular diseases (similar to that discussed in Chapters 342 and 345) may be adopted for nephrotic syndrome. The prevalence of diseases causing nephrotic syndrome varies with age, gender, and geographic location in the patient. In the Western hemisphere minimal change disease is most frequently encountered in children, whereas in adults idiopathic membranous nephropathy and diabetic nephropathy are the most common causes of primary and secondary nephrotic syndrome, respectively. Amyloidosis and multiple myeloma are seen with greater frequency in elderly individuals. Lupus nephritis is more commonly encountered in nephrotic women than men. Geographic location is also a determinant; for example, malaria is a common cause of nephrotic syndrome in African countries like Uganda.

Laboratory tests such as determinations of complement levels, antinuclear antibody, and antineutrophil cytoplasmic antibody, and tests for detection of monoclonal proteins and antibodies against hepatitis viruses or human immunodeficiency virus (HIV) should be guided by the data obtained by clinical evaluation. Renal biopsy is a powerful tool that can assist not only in the diagnosis of underlying disease but also in assessing its prognosis. It is usually not performed in diabetic patients when the clinical evaluation demonstrates retinal microangiopathy and the clinical features are consistent with the natural history of diabetic nephropathy. Renal biopsy is commonly performed in other patients. Renal biopsy is helpful in making a definitive histologic diagnosis, assessing the extent of irreversible injury, and deciding whether the disease is amenable to therapy. In nephrotic children, especially in the age-group of 3 to 7 years, renal biopsy is generally not performed because minimal change disease, an entity that readily responds to steroids, is the most common cause of the nephrotic syndrome. A therapeutic steroid trial is first attempted, and renal biopsy is considered if a salutary response is not obtained.

GENERAL MANAGEMENT

Whenever possible, the underlying disease should be treated, (e.g., lupus nephritis). Only general principles of management that apply to nephrotic patients, regardless of underlying causes, are discussed. Edema, the cardinal manifestation of nephrotic syndrome, is treated by restriction of dietary salt intake to 2 to 3 g/day and administration of diuretics. Mild edema should respond to dietary salt restriction and oral thiazide diuretics, provided the glomerular filtration rate is normal. More severe degrees of edema, especially when associated with impaired renal function, require loop diuretics. In resistant cases a combination of loop diuretics and metolazone may be helpful. It should be emphasized that large doses of loop diuretics or combinations of diuretics acting on different segments of nephron can elicit profound diuresis resulting in hypotension, acute renal failure, and serious hypokalemia. Patients with profound hypoalbuminemia may have diminished intravascular volume and are particularly prone to hypovolemia from aggressive diuresis. Serum potassium levels should be monitored when aggressive diuresis is undertaken. Potassium supplements or potassium-sparing diuretics may be used, but caution should be exercised in patients with impaired renal function. In patients who are resistant to the preceding approach and who have profound hypoalbuminemia and anasarca, infusions of concentrated salt-poor albumin combined with loop diuretics have been tried. This is

best performed in patients who are admitted to the hospital who can be monitored closely and have adequate urine flows. This is a temporary measure, since the infused albumin only transiently increases serum albumin and is promptly excreted in the urine.

Malnutrition can be addressed with a diet that provides protein of 1 g/kg, in addition to amounts equaling daily urinary protein losses. The protein in the diet should be of high biologic value and protected by adequate nonprotein calories (35 kcal/kg per day). Infusion of albumin to correct hypoalbuminemia or large protein intake may worsen proteinuria. To ensure that dietary protein is not lost in the urine, steps that reduce proteinuria may be added to the management plan. Nonsteroidal antiinflammatory agents and angiotensin-converting enzyme (ACE) inhibitors have been shown to reduce proteinuria in nephrotic syndrome of diverse causes. Although a complete remission of proteinuria is usually not obtained with these agents, a modest reduction in proteinuria, especially when levels of protein are below the nephrotic range, could be of significant benefit in managing edema, hyperlipidemia, and malnutrition. Side effects of these drugs, including hyperkalemia and worsening renal function, should be closely monitored. It may be necessary to modify protein intake if renal function deteriorates. Vitamin D administration is indicated in patients who have deficiency of that vitamin. Replenishment of iron, zinc, and copper may be necessary.

Hyperlipidemias are managed with diet and pharmacologic agents. Although a low-protein, vegetarian diet that contains soy protein, has a reduced fat content, and is enriched in monounsaturated and polyunsaturated fatty acids and fiber has been shown to reduce total and LDL cholesterol levels and reduce proteinuria in nephrotic patients, whether patients can comply with such a diet for long periods remains to be established. Omega-3 fatty acids have been shown to decrease plasma triglycerides and total cholesterol in uncontrolled trials. Of the many lipid-lowering agents that have been studied in nephrotic patients, 3-hydroxy-3-methylglutaryl coenzyme A (HMG CoA) reductase inhibitors have shown the most promise in prospective studies. Simvastatin and pravastatin decrease total cholesterol, LDL cholesterol, and triglycerides by nearly 30%, with variable effects on HDL cholesterol. These agents do not affect proteinuria. Fibric acid derivatives significantly reduce triglycerides in nephrotic patients with smaller effects on cholesterol levels. Side effects of lipid-lowering agents (e.g., hepatotoxicity and myositis) should be closely monitored, especially when these agents are used in combination and when renal function is impaired. Interestingly, in a double-blind study an ACE inhibitor fosinopril has been shown to reduce proteinuria, total and LDL cholesterol levels, and Lp(a) in patients with nephrotic syndrome. The effect of Lp(a) is of significance, since it does not respond to the usual lipid-lowering agents. Long-term studies are needed to identify the best strategies to manage nephrotic hyperlipidemias and to assess whether such interventions result in lowering the risk of atherosclerotic vascular disease.

Thromboembolic complications are managed by anticoagulation therapy, similar to management of major vein thrombosis in nonrenal patients. Whether diseases associated with an increased risk of thromboembolic complications (e.g., membranous nephropathy) should be managed with *prophylactic* anticoagulants is controversial. Infections should be promptly treated in nephrotic patients, and unnecessary instrumentation such as cystoscopy should be avoided. Alterations in drug kinetics should be kept in mind in nephrotic patients. As a result of urinary losses, the binding protein levels in plasma may fall, resulting in increased free drug levels (e.g., salicylates, phenytoin,

---

✔ WHEN TO REFER

The clinical evaluation of nephrotic syndrome can be initiated by the primary care physician. A renal consultation is recommended early in the course of the disease to make a definitive diagnosis of the underlying disease with renal biopsy, if indicated, and to put in place a comprehensive plan of management. Periodic follow-up by the nephrologist is prudent, particularly when renal function begins to deteriorate.

prednisone, and benzodiazepines). This could result in either increased drug activity (e.g., prednisone) or accelerated metabolism (e.g., phenytoin). The changes in metabolism of individual drugs should be considered.

BIBLIOGRAPHY

Anderson S, Kennefick TM, Brenner BM: Renal and systemic manifestations of glomerular disease. In Brenner BM, editor: *The kidney*, ed 5, Philadelphia, 1996, WB Saunders.

Glassock RJ, Cohen AH, Adler S: Primary glomerular diseases. In Brenner BM, editor: *The kidney*, ed 5, Philadelphia, 1996, WB Saunders.

Keilani T, Schlueter WA, Levin ML, Battle DC: Improvement of lipid abnormalities associated with proteinuria using fosinopril, an angiotensin-converting enzyme inhibitor, *Ann Intern Med* 118:246, 1993.

Perico N, Remuzzi G: Edema of the nephrotic syndrome: the role of atrial natriuretic peptide, *Am J Kidney Dis* 22:359, 1993.

Wanner C, Rader D, Bartens W et al: Elevated plasma lipoprotein (a) in patients with the nephrotic syndrome, *Ann Intern Med* 119:263, 1993.

Wheeler DC, Bernard DB: Lipid abnormalities in the nephrotic syndrome: causes, consequences and treatment, *Am J Kidney Dis* 23:331, 1994.

CHAPTER

109 Acute Renal Failure

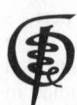

Satish Kumar and Jay H. Stein

Acute renal failure can be defined as a reduction in renal function of abrupt onset (less than 6 to 12 weeks). It is usually detected by elevation of urea or creatinine levels on blood chemistry. It is frequently but not always associated with oliguria (urine output less than 400 ml/day). Acute renal failure occurs in 2% to 5% of all hospitalized patients and in a third of patients admitted to the intensive care unit. Acute renal failure is associated with considerable morbidity and mortality.

ETIOLOGY

The etiology of acute renal failure can be divided into the following main categories: prerenal, postrenal, and intrinsic renal disease.

Prerenal Azotemia

Prerenal azotemia is the most common cause of a reversible increase in the creatinine and blood urea nitrogen (BUN) levels in hospitalized patients, accounting for 50% to 60% of all cases of acute renal failure. Common causes of prerenal azotemia are listed in Box 109-1. The common feature of all these conditions is a reduction in renal blood flow. If the decrement in renal blood flow is severe or prolonged, ischemic damage to the tubules may occur, leading to acute tubular necrosis.

Postrenal Azotemia

Postrenal azotemia accounts for 5% to 10% of all cases of acute renal failure and can be caused by obstruction to the flow of urine anywhere along the urinary tract. Common causes of urinary obstruction are listed in Box 109-2. Unilateral obstruction usually does not lead to detectable azotemia because of compensatory increase in glomerular filtration rate from the contralateral kidney and because a substantial change in plasma creatinine level may be accommodated within the normal range that extends from 0.6 to 1.4 mg/dl. Hence, obstructive lesions causing significant azotemia are often localized at or below the level of bladder. Neurogenic bladder and bladder neck obstruction are common causes of postrenal azotemia. In men prostatic enlargement is the most common cause of bladder outlet obstruction.

> ### BOX 109-1
> ### Prerenal causes of acute renal failure
>
> I. Decreased cardiac output
>   A. Congestive heart failure
>   B. Arrhythmias
>   C. Pericardial constriction or tamponade
>   D. Pulmonary embolism
> II. Hypovolemia
>   A. Gastrointestinal tract losses (vomiting, diarrhea, nasogastric suction)
>   B. Blood losses (trauma, gastrointestinal tract surgery)
>   C. Renal losses (diuretics, mineralocorticoid deficiency, postobstructive diuresis)
>   D. Skin losses (burns)
> III. Volume redistribution (decrease in effective blood volume)
>   A. Hypoalbuminemic states (cirrhosis, nephrosis)
>   B. Sequestration of fluid in "third" space (ischemic bowel, peritonitis, pancreatitis)
>   C. Peripheral vasodilation (sepsis, vasodilators, anaphylaxis)
> IV. Altered renal vascular resistance
>   A. Increase in afferent vascular resistance (nonsteroidal antiinflammatory agents, catecholamine infusion, liver disease, sepsis, hypercalcemia, cyclosporine)
>   B. Decrease in efferent arteriolar tone (angiotensin-converting enzyme inhibitors)

> ### BOX 109-2
> ### Postrenal causes of acute renal failure
>
> I. Ureter and renal pelvis
>   A. Intrinsic obstruction
>   1. Blood clots
>   2. Stones
>   3. Sloughed papillae: Diabetes, sickle cell disease, analgesic nephropathy
>   4. Inflammation: Fungus ball
>   B. Extrinsic obstruction
>   1. Malignancy
>   2. Retroperitoneal fibrosis
>   3. Iatrogenic: Inadvertent ligation of ureters
> II. Bladder
>   A. Prostatic hypertrophy or malignancy
>   B. Neuropathic bladder
>   C. Blood clots
>   D. Bladder cancer
>   E. Stones
> III. Urethral
>   A. Strictures
>   B. Congenital valves

Intrinsic or Parenchymal Renal Disease

Intrinsic renal diseases account for 40% to 50% of all patients with acute renal failure. A great variety of intrinsic renal lesions can be associated with the syndrome of acute renal failure (Box 109-3). They can involve any of the four major anatomic parts of the kidney: the vasculature, the glomeruli, the interstitium, or the tubules. Vascular lesions include systemic or renal-limited vasculitis. Glomerular lesions include the various types of glomerulonephritis—usually involving immune mechanisms. Interstitial lesions are generally categorized under the term tubulointerstitial nephritis. Drugs are the major cause of tubulointerstitial nephritis, especially penicillins and sulfonamides. Other antimicrobial agents, diuretics, anticonvulsants, nonsteroidal antiinflammatory agents, hypouricemic drugs, phenobarbitol, and cimetidine may also cause tubulointerstitial nephritis. Infectious pyelonephritis is a frequent manifestation of urinary tract infection and can sometimes be severe enough to cause acute renal failure. Renal failure can also result from interstitial infiltration by lymphoproliferative or granulomatous diseases. Major tubular causes of acute renal failure are tubular obstruction and acute tubular necrosis. Primary intratubular obstruction can occur with crystals of uric acid, oxalate, acyclovir, and methotrexate or with myeloma proteins. Acute uric acid nephropathy is seen most frequently in association with hematologic malignancies before or after chemotherapy. Intratubular deposition of calcium oxalate can occur following ethylene glycol ingestion or methoxyflurane anesthesia. Acute tubular necrosis (ATN) is the most common cause of intrinsic acute renal failure. The two major causes of ATN are ischemia and nephrotoxic agents. Ischemic ATN can result from any of the causes of prerenal azotemia if the stimulus is severe or prolonged enough. Common causes of ischemic ATN are hypotension and sepsis. Nephrotoxic causes of ATN are listed in Box 109-3. Aminoglycosides, amphotericin, and radiocontrast medium are common causes of nephrotoxic ATN. In hospitalized patients ATN is often multifactorial, combining ischemic and toxic causes.

PATHOPHYSIOLOGY
Prerenal Azotemia

In prerenal azotemia the kidneys are structurally normal, but their function is impaired as a result of a reduction in renal blood flow caused by decreased cardiac output or by altered renal arteriolar resistance. Reduced renal blood flow is accompanied by lower glomerular filtration pressure and a fall in glomerular filtration rate (GFR). The glomerular permeability may also be decreased as a direct effect of vasoconstrictive hormones such as catecholamines, angiotensin, and endothelin that are released in response to systemic hypotension. Autoregulatory mechanisms exist in the kidney that increase renal blood flow, maintain glomerular filtration, and prevent ATN by dilation of *afferent* arterioles in the glomerulus mediated by vasodilatory substances such as nitric oxide and prostaglandins. In addition, the *efferent* arteriolar resistance is increased by the vasoconstrictive effect of angiotensin. The net effect of dilation of the afferent arterioles and constriction of the efferent arterioles is to increase hydrostatic pressure in the glomerulus and to allow filtration of a higher fraction of the plasma flowing through the glomerulus (increased filtration fraction). Drugs that interfere with these autoregulatory mechanisms such as nonsteroidal antiinflammatory agents that decrease the synthesis of afferent vasodilatory prostaglandins or angiotensin-converting enzyme inhibitors that suppress the production of the efferent vasoconstrictor, angiotensin, can predispose to acute renal failure. This is especially common in conditions where renal blood flow and glomerular filtration might be particularly dependent on renal autoregulatory mechanisms, such as real or effective hypovolemia, bilateral renal artery stenosis, or unilateral stenosis in a solitary functioning kidney. The histologic appearance of the kidney remains normal in prerenal azotemia, but if the stimulus for prerenal failure is severe or prolonged, the decrease in renal blood flow can lead to ATN.

Postrenal Azotemia (see also Chapter 123)

In the early stages of obstruction, filtration continues and the ureteral and intratubular pressures rise progressively. Glomerular filtration is subsequently reduced by back pressure. The elevated tubular pressure also causes reflex vasoconstriction of the afferent arterioles leading to decrease in renal blood flow and in glomerular filtration. On pathologic study the kidneys show tubular dilation, varying degrees of interstitial edema, and fibrosis with time.

Intrinsic or Parenchymal Renal Disease

This group includes a variety of conditions and the pathophysiology depends on the specific cause. In diseases of renal arteries, blood flow to the kidney is reduced and renal function is impaired because of ischemia of the kidney. In renal vein thrombosis, a rare cause of acute renal failure, renal congestion is the presumed cause of poor function. In microscopic vasculitis and acute glomerulonephritis, glomerular filtration is impaired as a result of accumulation of inflamma-

---

BOX 109-3

Causes of acute renal failure due to intrinsic or parenchymal kidney disease

I. Abnormalities of the vasculature
   A. Renal arteries: Atherosclerosis, thromboembolism, large vessel arteritis
   B. Renal veins: Thrombosis
   C. Microvasculature: Microscopic vasculitis, thrombotic microangiopathy
II. Abnormalities of glomeruli (acute glomerulonephritis)
   A. Antiglomerular basement membrane disease (Goodpasture's disease)
   B. Immune complex glomerulonephritis: Lupus erythematosus, postinfectious, idiopathic, membranoproliferative
III. Abnormalities of interstitium (acute interstitial nephritis)
   A. Drugs
      1. Antibiotics: Penicillins, sulfonamides, cephalosporins, ciprofloxacin
      2. Nonsteroidal antiinflammatory agents
      3. Diuretics: Furosemide, thiazides
      4. Others: Allopurinol, cimetidine, anticonvulsants, clofibrate
   B. Infectious pyelonephritis
   C. Infiltrative: Lymphoma, leukemia, sarcoidosis
IV. Abnormalities of tubules
   A. Physical obstruction of tubules
      1. Crystals: Uric acid, oxalate, methotrexate
      2. Proteins: Light chains
   B. Acute tubular necrosis
      1. Ischemic (see causes of prerenal azotemia, Box 109-1)
      2. Toxic
         a. Antibiotics: Aminoglycosides, amphotericin, acyclovir, foscarnet
         b. Chemotherapy: Cisplatinum, ifosfamide
         c. Immunosuppressives: Cyclosporine
         d. Radiocontrast dyes
         e. Heavy metals: Mercury, lead, arsenic
         f. Endogenous: Myoglobin, hemolysed red blood cells

---

tory cells in the glomeruli and direct damage to the glomerular architecture. In interstitial nephritis the inflammatory reaction is localized predominantly in the interstitum. The tubules surrounded by the inflammatory exudate show various degrees of cellular damage, and the glomerular function is impaired as a result of the tubular damage.

In ATN renal function is impaired as a result of the following major mechanisms: (1) glomerular vasoconstriction, (2) transepithelial leakage of tubular fluid across damaged tubules, (3) tubular obstruction, and (4) reduced glomerular permeability (Fig. 109-1). Many cellular mediators of tubular injury have been described including adenosine triphosphate (ATP) depletion, loss of cell polarity, generation of oxygen free radicals, activation of phospholipases and proteases, increase in cytosolic calcium, and activation of leukocyte adhesion molecules. The tubular obstruction occurs because of plugging of tubules with cellular debris, exfoliated cells, and Tamm-Horsfall protein, which is a glycoprotein synthesized in the thick ascending limb of the loop of Henle. The mechanism of alteration in glomerular permeability is not clear. The tissue oxygen tension in the kidney normally decreases from cortex toward medulla because of countercurrent exchange of oxygen in the vasa recta. The balance of oxygen supply and demand is most tenuous in the outer medulla, which has a relatively high workload of tubular transport. Hence, the tubules in the outer medulla, especially pars recta of the proximal tubule and thick ascending limb of the loop of Henle, are most susceptible to ischemic injury. On histologic examination the kidney in ATN reveals patchy damage in the proximal tubules consisting of flattening of brush border, dilation of tubular lumen, and sloughing of epithelial cells. The distal nephron often shows tubular casts. The glomeruli appear normal. Findings in ischemic and toxic ATN are similar overall, but tubular cell damage is somewhat more prominent in toxic necrosis and cast formation more frequent in ischemic ATN.

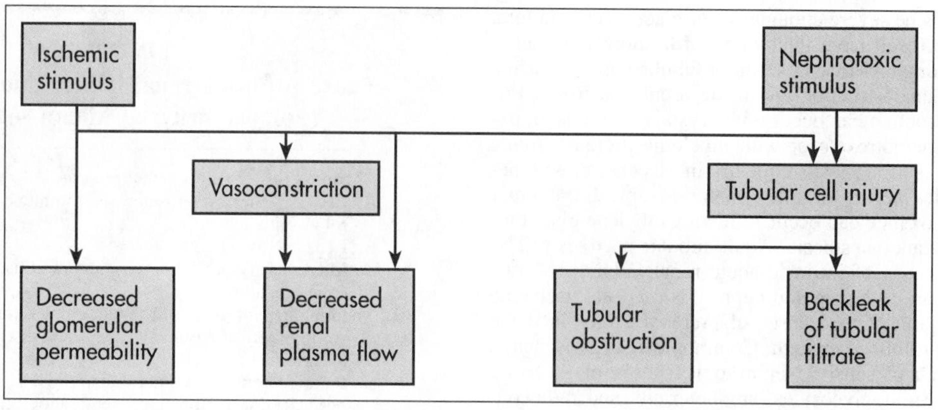

FIGURE 109-1   Pathogenetic mechanisms in acute tubular necrosis.

DIAGNOSIS

In patients with newly discovered azotemia the first step is to ascertain whether the renal failure is acute or chronic. Features that suggest chronic renal failure are the following: documented azotemia of more than 3 to 6 months, small kidneys, and renal osteodystrophy. Patients without these features should be considered to have acute renal failure. Patients with chronic renal failure who have an elevation of plasma creatinine levels above their stable baseline should also be evaluated for a cause of superimposed acute renal failure. Diagnostic evaluation of acute renal failure includes a careful history, physical examination, urinalysis, serum chemistry, measurement of postvoid bladder volume by Foley catheter, renal ultrasound, and under certain conditions a renal biopsy. Priority should be given to seeking possible causes of prerenal and postrenal azotemia because of their potential for reversibility.

Prerenal Azotemia

The cause of prerenal azotemia (Box 109-1) is, under most circumstances, obvious on history and physical examination. In some cases, however, more subtle clues must be sought, such as an increase in diuretic dosage in decompensated cirrhosis or congestive heart failure. The physical examination may suggest one of the etiologic categories listed in Box 109-1 or demonstrate evidence of hypovolemia. Weight loss, orthostasis, tachycardia, decreased skin turgor, and dry mucous membranes all suggest hypovolemia. Of these, acute weight loss and orthostasis (increase in pulse of more than 20 beats/minute or fall in systolic pressure of more than 10 mm Hg on moving from recumbent to upright posture) are the most useful signs. At times it may be necessary to measure central venous pressure or pulmonary capillary wedge pressure for an accurate assessment of the intravascular volume.

The kidney's response to a decrease in blood flow is to reabsorb salt and water avidly. Thus in prerenal failure in the absence of diuretics, urine sodium concentration is typically less than 10 to 20 mEq/L, the fractional excretion of sodium is less than 1%, the renal failure index (RFI) is less than 1 (see EQ. 2), and the urine osmolality is greater than 500 mOsm/L (Table 109-1). The fractional excretion (percentage) of sodium (FE_{Na}) is calculated as follows:

(EQ. 1)

$$FE_{Na} = \frac{\text{Sodium excreted}}{\text{Sodium filtered}} \times 100$$

$$FE_{Na} = \frac{U_{Na} \cdot V}{P_{Na} \cdot GFR} \times 100$$

$$GFR = \text{Creatinine clearance} = \frac{U_{Cr} \cdot V}{P_{Cr}}$$

Table 109-1   Urinary indices in acute renal failure

INDEX	PRERENAL AZOTEMIA	INTRINSIC ACUTE RENAL FAILURE
Urine osmolality (mOsm/L)	>500	<350
Urine sodium concentration (mEq/L)	<20	>40
Plasma urea nitrogen/creatinine ratio	>20	<10
Fractional excretion of sodium (%)	<1	>1
Renal failure index	<1	>1
Urine/blood urea nitrogen ratio	>8	<3
Urine/plasma creatinine ratio	>40	<20

$$FE_{Na} = \frac{U_{Na} \cdot V}{P_{Na} \cdot \dfrac{U_{Cr} \cdot V}{P_{Cr}}} \times 100$$

$$FE_{Na} = \frac{U_{Na} \cdot P_{Cr}}{P_{Na} \cdot U_{Cr}} \times 100$$

where U_{Na} and P_{Na} are urine and plasma sodium concentrations, respectively, in mEq/L, U_{Cr} and P_{Cr} are urine and plasma creatinine concentrations, respectively, in mg/dl, V is urine volume, and GFR is glomerular filtration rate.

The RFI is a simplification of FE_{Na} and does not include plasma sodium, which is usually normal in acute renal failure. RFI is expressed as a ratio and not as a percentage:

(EQ. 2)

$$RFI = \frac{\text{Sodium excreted}}{GFR}$$

$$= \frac{U_{Na} \cdot V}{\dfrac{U_{Cr} \cdot V}{P_{Cr}}}$$

$$= \frac{U_{Na} \cdot P_{Cr}}{U_{Cr}}$$

Since there is no parenchymal damage in prerenal azotemia, the urinalysis is typically normal; only fine granular casts and hyaline casts are present, and proteinuria is minimal. If significant numbers of red blood cells, white blood cells, or cellular casts are present, an alternate or additional abnormality must be considered. Creatinine is filtered at the glomerulus and is not reabsorbed. Therefore under conditions of avid water reabsorption, the urine creatinine concentration rises but its serum value remains relatively constant, resulting in a high urine/plasma creatinine ratio (Table 109-1). Urea, on the other hand, is both filtered and reabsorbed. Its reabsorption is flow depen-

Table 109-2   Urinalysis in acute renal failure

	PRERENAL	POSTRENAL	INTRINSIC ACUTE RENAL FAILURE		
			VASCULITIS AND ACUTE GLOMERULONEPHRITIS	ACUTE INTERSTITIAL NEPHRITIS	ACUTE TUBULAR NECROSIS
Dipstick					
Blood	−	−	+++	+	−
Protein	−	−	+++	+	−
Microscopy					
Red blood cells	−	−	+++	+	−
White blood cells	−	−	+	+++	−
Casts	Hyaline casts	−	Red and white blood cell casts	White blood cell casts	Brown casts
Other				Eosinophils	Tubular cells

dent; thus during low flow conditions more urea is reabsorbed, resulting in a high plasma urea/creatinine ratio. Water is, however, reabsorbed in excess of urea in this setting, and the urine/plasma urea ratio still rises.

Postrenal Azotemia

The history and physical examination may be helpful in delineating the duration of the symptoms and the location of the obstruction. Ureteral obstruction must either be bilateral or occur in a patient with previous renal dysfunction to result in detectable azotemia. The history may be suggestive when it includes an abrupt onset of ureteric colic or inability to void. Extrinsic compression of both ureters from retroperitoneal fibrosis or an intraabdominal mass can lead to a slower development of obstruction and a less symptomatic onset. Acute bladder outlet obstruction is usually symptomatic, but if it develops slowly, the diagnosis may be suspected only by palpation of an enlarged bladder or by the demonstration of a large prostate gland. The urinalysis may be normal. The urine flow rate may vary from anuria, as seen with complete obstruction, to polyuria, as may be seen in partial obstruction. Urine flow that fluctuates widely from day to day suggests the possibility of intermittent obstruction.

Laboratory findings depend on the time course and degree of obstruction. The renal response to acute obstruction is similar to that seen in prerenal azotemia, and similar laboratory indices are found, that is, high urine osmolality, low urine sodium concentration, and low fractional excretion of sodium (Table 109-1). After a few days of obstruction the indices change and the urine becomes isotonic with a high fractional excretion of sodium. A postvoid residual urine measurement by Foley catheter is a relatively simple and potentially revealing test that should be performed in any patient in whom obstruction is being considered. Renal ultrasonography has become the procedure of choice to screen for obstruction. Intravenous pyelography carries the risk of contrast nephrotoxicity and should be avoided. When ultrasonography shows obstruction and if retroperitoneal fibrosis or malignancy is suspected as the cause of obstruction, computed tomography can be helpful in clarifying the diagnosis.

Parenchymal Renal Disease

Following the exclusion of prerenal and postrenal causes of acute renal failure, intrinsic or parenchymal causes should be considered. Pertinent aspects of history may define the basis of the renal functional impairment. While the exact clinical presentation differs from patient to patient, several of the categories listed in Box 109-3 have characteristic constellations of symptoms and signs.

Patients with acute glomerulonephritis come to medical attention with a short history of dark-colored (smoky) urine, hypertension, and edema. Patients with vasculitis have a similar presentation but, in addition, often have symptoms and signs of vasculitis in other organs, particularly skin and lungs. Patients with interstitial nephritis have a recent history of having taken a drug—often an antibiotic or a nonsteroidal antiinflammatory agent—and come to medical attention with fever, rash, and, occasionally, arthralgia.

> ### BOX 109-4
> ### Intrinsic causes of acute renal failure with low fractional excretion of sodium
>
> - Acute tubular necrosis (ATN) in the setting of underlying prerenal azotemia (e.g., liver disease, heart failure)
> - ATN resulting from radiocontrast dye
> - Acute glomerulonephritis or vasculitis
> - First 48 hours of transition from prerenal azotemia to ATN
> - Nonoliguric ATN

Ischemic ATN occurs in the same settings as prerenal azotemia (Box 109-1), and the likely cause is often apparent by history and physical examination. Patients with nephrotoxic ATN usually have a history of being treated with one of the agents listed in Box 109-3. Oliguria is common in ischemic ATN but not in nephrotoxic ATN.

Urine electrolyte levels can be helpful in distinguishing between prerenal azotemia and intrinsic acute renal failure. Of the various indices listed in Table 109-1, urinary sodium and fractional excretion of sodium are most useful clinically, but these tests are not always definitive and fractional excretion of sodium can be low in certain causes of renal parenchymal disease (Box 109-4). Conversely, urine sodium concentration and fractional excretion of sodium can be high in prerenal azotemia if a diuretic has been administered recently.

Urinalysis on a freshly voided specimen can be very useful in distinguishing the major categories of intrinsic acute renal failure from each other (Table 109-2). In acute glomerulonephritis or vasculitis urine dipstick testing is positive for blood and protein, and microscopy shows red and white blood cells and cellular casts, especially red blood cell casts. In acute interstitial nephritis dipstick testing shows low levels of protein and blood and microscopy shows more white blood cells than red blood cells and often eosinophils. Hansel's stain is more sensitive than Wright's stain in the detection of eosinophils. In ATN urine dipstick testing is characteristically negative, and microscopy may show, somewhat inconsistently, brown casts, tubular cells, and tubular cell casts. Presence of envelope-shaped calcium oxalate crystals suggests ethylene glycol toxicity, and the presence of pleomorphic uric acid crystals is consistent with uric acid nephropathy.

Serologic tests are helpful in differentiation among the various causes of vasculitis and acute glomerulonephritis. These include antineutrophilic cytoplasmic antibodies (ANCA) for Wegener's granulomatosis, antiglomerular basement membrane antibodies for Goodpasture's disease, anti-DNAse and antistreptolysin (ASO) antibodies for poststreptococcal glomerulonephritis, antinuclear and anti-DNA antibodies for lupus erythematosus nephritis, cryoglobulins and hepatitis C antibodies for hepatitis C infection, and serum complement levels for systemic immune complex disease.

A renal biopsy is required to establish the diagnosis of vasculitis, acute glomerulonephritis, or acute interstitial nephritis with certainty and is indicated if these conditions are suggested by history, examination, urinalysis, and serologic test results.

CLINICAL COURSE, COMPLICATIONS, AND PROGNOSIS

The clinical course of acute renal failure depends in part on the underlying causes. Prerenal and postrenal azotemia, if diagnosed and treated promptly, are rapidly reversed with a return to normal or near-normal renal function. Intrinsic causes of acute renal failure are usually not reversed as quickly. The clinical course of ATN, the largest group in this category, may span a number of weeks and be associated with a variety of complications. The mortality in ATN has remained high at 50% to 60% for the past 50 years, largely as a result of the increasing complexity of clinical situations in which ATN now occurs. The cause of death is usually nonrenal; sepsis and cardiovascular causes predominate. The following discussion pertains primarily to patients with ATN.

About half the patients with ATN are oliguric (urine output <400 ml/day), and 5% to 10% are anuric (<50 ml/day). Anuria and oliguria are associated with a more prolonged course and more frequent complications than nonoliguric ATN. Volume overload may lead to hypertension and pulmonary edema. The course of oliguric ATN can be divided into the following phases: initiation, maintenance, and recovery. The initiation phase is often unrecognized. Maintenance phase is typically 7 to 14 days long but can be variable. During this phase plasma BUN level rises by 10 to 20 mg/dl daily and creatinine level by 0.5 to 1.0 mg/dl daily. The rise in BUN level may be more marked than that of creatinine in the presence of gastrointestinal tract bleeding, hypercatabolism, or volume depletion, and the rise in creatinine level may be disproportionately higher in cases of rhabdomyolysis or drugs that reduce tubular secretion of creatinine, such as cimetidine and trimethoprim-sulfamethoxazole. The recovery phase is characterized by increasing urine output and falling plasma BUN and creatinine levels.

Metabolic acidosis is almost universally present in acute renal failure unless the patient is receiving nasogastric suction. Only rarely, however, does the serum bicarbonate level fall to values less than 13 to 15 mEq/L. Normally, approximately 1 mEq of hydrogen ions per kilogram body weight is generated and excreted each day. This production is considerably higher in catabolic states, resulting in the liberation of large amounts of hydrogen ions, mostly in the form of sulfuric and phosphoric acids that are not excreted normally in acute renal failure. The retention of these compounds results in a decrease in serum bicarbonate concentration and high anion gap acidosis (see Chapter 115).

Hyperkalemia, hypocalcemia, hyperphosphatemia, and hyponatremia are the most common electrolyte disorders seen in acute renal failure. *Hyperkalemia* is a serious, life-threatening complication of acute renal failure. Because potassium excretion from the body occurs primarily in urine, potassium tends to be retained in acute renal failure, especially if oliguria is present. Hyperkalemia may be aggravated by an exogenous potassium load and by drugs that impair potassium handling, such as beta blockers, converting enzyme inhibitors, heparin, and potassium-sparing diuretics (see Chapter 110). Extensive tissue breakdown and metabolic acidosis may exacerbate hyperkalemia. The most serious complication of hyperkalemia is a cardiac arrhythmia. Figure 109-2 illustrates electrocardiographic al-

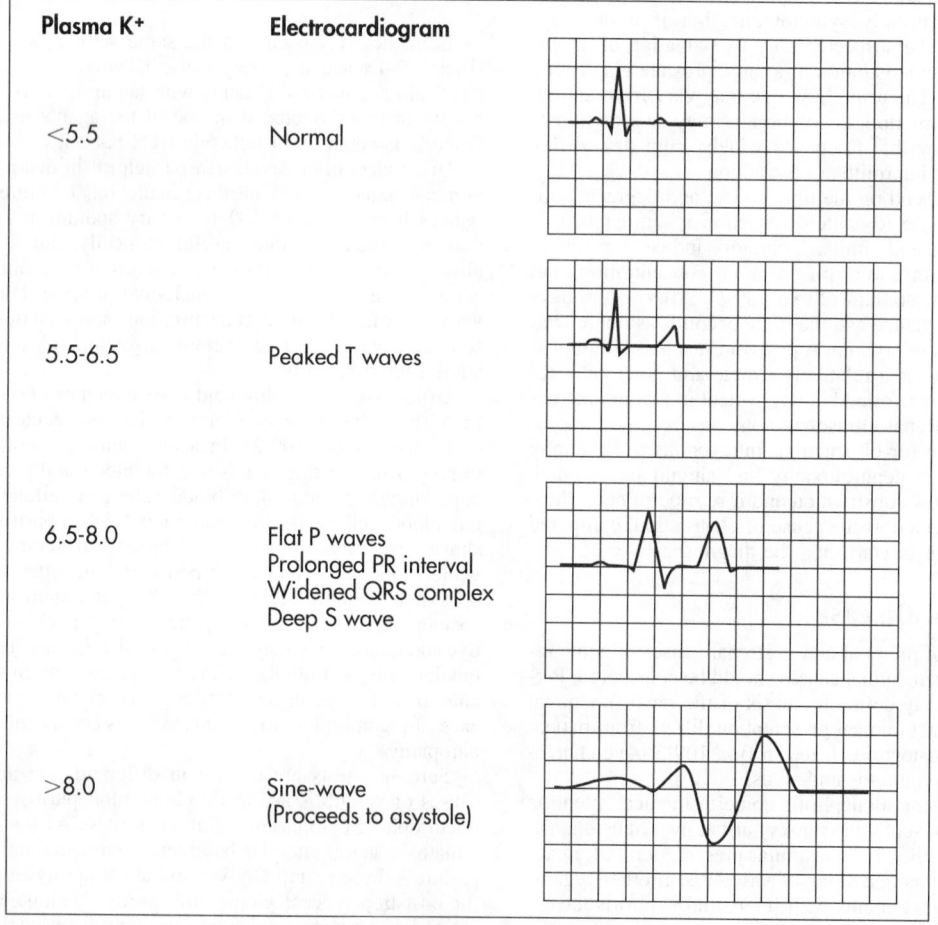

Plasma K+	Electrocardiogram	
<5.5	Normal	
5.5-6.5	Peaked T waves	
6.5-8.0	Flat P waves Prolonged PR interval Widened QRS complex Deep S wave	
>8.0	Sine-wave (Proceeds to asystole)	

FIGURE 109-2   Sequential electrocardiographic changes in hyperkalemia.

From Kumar S. Disorders of potassium homeostasis. In Kaufman CE, McKee PA, editors: *Essentials of pathophysiology,* Boston, 1996, Little, Brown.

terations that occur with hyperkalemia. The level at which a particular electrocardiographic change is seen depends on the rate of change in plasma potassium level, the acid-base status, and the level of other electrolytes. Very high potassium levels can cause neuromuscular effects such as paresthesia, weakness, and paralysis. *Hypocalcemia* is common in acute renal failure, although usually asymptomatic, partly because the coexistent acidosis of renal failure increases the ionized fraction of calcium. Reasons for hypocalcemia in acute renal failure include hypoalbuminemia, hyperphosphatemia, resistance to parathyroid hormone, and a reduction in the active component of vitamin D. If the serum calcium level falls below 6.5 mg/dl or if metabolic acidosis is rapidly corrected, hypocalcemia may produce symptoms of perioral paresthesia, muscle twitching, tetany, and seizures. Latent tetany can be elicited by Chvostek's (tapping of facial nerve over the mandible causes twitching of facial muscles) or Trousseau's maneuver (inflation of sphygmomanometer cuff on the arm to above systolic pressure for 3 minutes causes spasm of muscles in the hand). *Hyperphosphatemia* is common in acute renal failure and is predominantly due to decreased renal excretion of phosphate. It can be exacerbated by tissue breakdown and by continuing high dietary intake of phosphate. If the product of the plasma calcium value times the phosphate value (both in ml) exceeds 70, metastatic calcification may occur in tissues such as heart, vessels, skin, and cornea. Patients with rhabdomyolysis and acute pancreatitis are at particular risk of severe hypocalcemia because of extensive deposition of calcium salts in necrotic tissue. In patients with rhabdomyolysis, rebound *hypercalcemia* may also develop later in their course when blood returns to the severely damaged muscle and the calcium is reabsorbed back into the circulation. *Hyponatremia* is the result of decreased ability to excrete free water and is exacerbated by excessive water intake via oral or intravenous fluids. Other biochemical abnormalities include hypermagnesemia and hyperuricemia. *Hypermagnesemia* is frequent in patients with acute renal failure because the kidney is the main route of magnesium excretion from the body, but it is rarely significant clinically. *Hypomagnesemia* may occur in acute renal failure as a result of tubular toxins such as amphotericin, aminoglycosides, and cisplatinum, especially in the early stages. *Hyperuricemia* may accompany ATN, especially if extensive tissue breakdown is present.

In addition to the aforementioned electrolyte alterations, almost every organ system is frequently involved in ATN. Cardiovascular abnormalities occur mainly as the result of changes in electrolyte or volume balance. Hypertension, edema, and pulmonary congestion are the result of salt and water retention. Life-threatening arrhythmias can be caused or aggravated by electrolyte disorders. Pericarditis with pericardial effusion and tamponade can occur with severe azotemia.

A number of hematologic manifestations can complicate acute renal failure. These include anemia, bleeding diathesis, and abnormalities in the immune system. Anemia is frequent and results from a combination of factors that include decreased production of erythropoietin, hemolysis, shortened red blood cell survival, and blood loss. The bleeding diathesis appears primarily to be the result of alterations in platelet aggregation and adhesiveness. Immunologic abnormalities are diverse but somewhat poorly characterized. Defective chemotaxis, lymphopenia, and impaired cellular immunity have been described. Infection is a leading cause of death in patients with acute renal failure.

The gastrointestinal tract is commonly affected by acute renal failure. Hiccups, nausea, vomiting, or anorexia is frequent, and ileus or gastrointestinal tract bleeding may occur in up to one third of the patients. Gastrointestinal tract bleeding may be due to altered hemostasis or an increased incidence of gastrointestinal tract ulceration. Serum amylase levels may be up to twice normal in the absence of pancreatitis.

Neurologic complications of acute renal failure include disorientation, asterixis, seizures, coma, and peripheral neuropathy. Although subtle alterations are frequently seen, frank uremic encephalopathy is now uncommon because of early initiation of dialysis.

MANAGEMENT
Prerenal Azotemia

In prerenal azotemia renal function improves rapidly if renal blood flow can be improved. Drugs adversely affecting glomerular hemodynamics such as nonsteroidal antiinflammatory agents and angiotension-converting enzyme inhibitors should be stopped. Hypovolemia should be corrected by infusion of normal saline. Transfusion of red blood cells may be necessary with hemorrhagic losses. Measurement of serum electrolytes is usually necessary to guide selection of intravenous fluids. Fluid management is particularly challenging in patients who have total body volume overload and expanded plasma volume but reduced "effective" volume as a result of venous pooling, as may occur in congestive heart failure due to poor cardiac pump or in cirrhotic ascites due to splanchnic pooling of blood. In these patients renal failure may be precipitated by transient or minor reduction of the effective volume by excessive diuresis, vomiting, diarrhea, or bleeding. These events, if present, might necessitate careful saline infusion, but the risk of worsening pulmonary congestion or ascites is great. In severe congestive heart failure azotemia is often improved by effective diuresis.

Postrenal Azotemia

Once obstruction is diagnosed, referral to a urologist is usually necessary for definitive treatment. Since many causes of obstruction involve bladder neck obstruction, insertion of a bladder catheter usually relieves obstruction temporarily and allows amelioration of azotemia. Ureteric obstruction can be bypassed by a catheter placed percutaneously or cystoscopically in the ureter or renal pelvis above the obstruction. Following relief of obstruction some patients might have a transient postobstructive diuresis as a result of continued tubular dysfunction. If urinary losses are not replaced in these patients, volume depletion can develop.

Intrinsic Renal Failure

Management of vasculitis, glomerulonephritis, and interstitial nephritis is discussed in other chapters of this book. This section focuses on the management of ATN.

Prophylaxis of Acute Tubular Necrosis

Acute tubular necrosis can be prevented in a number of patients by careful attention to volume status, cardiac output, and the use of nephrotoxic agents. These measures are more important in patients in whom renal blood flow might already be compromised, such as the elderly or those with heart failure, liver disease, previous renal insufficiency, renal artery stenosis, and diabetes mellitus. In such patients, agents that impair autoregulation of renal blood flow, such as nonsteroidal antiinflammatory agents or angiotensin-converting enzyme inhibitors, should be used with caution. Nephrotoxic agents should be minimized and plasma levels measured to guide dosing of aminoglycosides and cyclosporine. Allopurinol decreases uric acid synthesis in patients with leukemia and lymphoma who are prone to uric acid nephropathy. Forced alkaline diuresis prevents blockage of renal tubules by uric acid or methotrexate in these malignancies, and by casts in rhabdomyolysis. Dimercaprol may prevent nephrotoxicity of heavy metals and ethanol of ethylene glycol.

Use of Diuretics and Dopamine in Acute Tubular Necrosis

The use of furosemide, mannitol, and low-dose dopamine in the prevention or reversal of ATN has been the subject of many experimental and clinical studies. The results of these studies have been somewhat inconsistent. Experience with the use of these agents to *prevent* renal failure has been studied in the setting of aortic surgery and the use of radiocontrast medium and has been disappointing. In *established ATN* in early stages, high doses of loop diuretics or mannitol increase the urine output in 25% to 30% of patients. Low-dose dopamine (1 to 3 µg/kg per minute, intravenous) is a renal vasodilator and in combination with furosemide (80 to 400 mg, one to three times a day, intravenous) has also been shown to initiate diuresis and possibly reduce the duration of azotemia in some uncontrolled human studies. The effect of these agents on reducing mortality, however, is not clear. The greatest benefit of these agents is to increase urine flow, which allows easier control of the patient's fluid and electrolyte status. Any benefit of low-dose dopamine or diuretics is usually apparent within 48 hours. If no effect is seen during that period, their continued use is not warranted. These compounds are not without risk. Both furosemide and ethacrynic acid can cause deafness, and mannitol can be associated with volume overload, hyperosmolality, and hyperkalemia.

Newer Therapies in Established Acute Tubular Necrosis

A number of novel therapeutic agents are being examined for potential use in experimental ATN. These include atrial natriuretic peptide, epidermal growth factor, antibodies to adhesion molecules, oxygen free radical scavengers, calcium channel blockers, amino acid infusions, and prostaglandins. None of these experimental therapies have yet been proven to be safe and effective for human use in acute renal failure. Current therapy of established ATN is aimed mainly at prevention and treatment of the associated complications.

Supportive Treatment of Acute Renal Failure

Hyperkalemia was a frequent cause of death in the past but has become less frequent with greater access to dialysis and with development of rapid, accurate laboratory procedures to identify and monitor the clinical course. The restriction of potassium in the diet and the avoidance of potassium-containing drugs are especially important. Patients who are oliguric, anuric or hypercatabolic may have a rapid increase in serum potassium level, and emergent treatment of hyperkalemia may become necessary. In these patients, diet should contain less than 40 mEq potassium per day. Therapy of hyperkalemia is dictated primarily by changes in the ECG. Emergency treatment of hyperkalemia (also see Chapter 114 and Table 114-2) includes the use of intravenous calcium in an attempt to antagonize the effect of the hyperkalemia at the cell membrane level. Furthermore, serum potassium level can be lowered by driving potassium into cells with sodium bicarbonate and/or an infusion of glucose and insulin. These emergency measures do not *remove* potassium from the body, and additional therapy is needed to remove potassium from the body. This can be accomplished with a sodium-potassium exchange resin such as sodium polystyrene sulfonate (Kayexalate) or by dialysis. Sodium polystyrene sulfonate resin given orally in the dose of 15 g in 50 ml of 20% sorbitol, one to four times a day, removes approximately 1 mEq potassium for each gram of the resin. The resin causes constipation, so sorbitol is added as an osmotic laxative. Sodium polystyrene sulfonate can also be given rectally, albeit with less effective results, in the dose of 30 to 50 g in 100 ml water as a retention enema. Dialysis provides a more rapid mode of removing potassium, and hemodialysis is more effective than peritoneal dialysis for the treatment of acute hyperkalemia. The serum potassium level should be maintained below 5 mEq/L in any patient with acute renal failure to ensure a safe margin for any unexpected alteration.

Abnormalities in water and sodium metabolism need careful management in acute renal failure. Daily weight, intake, and output should be measured. Insensible water loss approximates 400 to 800 ml/day. This is partially compensated by the 400 ml/day of water that is released from the metabolism of fat and protein. The oliguric patient's intake of fluid should be limited to 400 ml/day plus the previous day's urinary output unless physical signs of volume depletion or volume overload are present. Dietary sodium should be restricted to 2 g (87 mEq)/day. A patient with ATN, if not receiving hyperalimentation, is expected to lose 0.3 to 0.5 kg/day of weight. If this loss does not occur or if there is an actual weight gain, fluid therapy should be reevaluated. Hyponatremia may require stringent free-water restriction.

Acidosis occurs frequently in acute renal failure, although the serum bicarbonate level is usually above 12 to 15 mEq/L except in the hypercatabolic patient. Modest amounts of sodium bicarbonate may be administered if the serum bicarbonate level drops below 15 to 18 mEq/L, although the potential for volume overload should be recognized. Hyperphosphatemia should be treated with calcium carbonate (1 g with each meal or snack) or other phosphate binders. Hypermagnesemia may be exacerbated after an exogenous load of magnesium, and magnesium-containing antacids should be avoided. Severe hyperphosphatemia or severe hypermagnesemia can be treated with dialysis.

Nutritional support is an important aspect of the treatment of acute renal failure. It should be designed to give adequate calories without excessive volume. The caloric requirements in acute renal failure are relatively high, especially in patients who are hypercatabolic. Carbohydrate intake should be sufficient (more than 100 g per day) to avoid breakdown of endogenous protein for glucose. The protein requirements depend on the clinical status. With oral feedings one can start with a diet of 40 g/day of high-quality protein and increase it as deemed necessary. Meeting the nutritional needs of the patient may not be possible without dialysis, which allows larger quantities to be given. Enteral or parenteral alimentation may be necessary in the postoperative patient or in those with anorexia or vomiting. The use of essential amino acids or their keto analogs in the postoperative or trauma patient has been suggested but not proven to improve the outcome of acute renal failure. Doses of several drugs must be altered in patients with acute renal failure. These include drugs that are renally excreted or those whose pharmacokinetics are altered by azotemia or dialysis.

Dialysis: Indications and Options

Indications for dialysis are listed in Box 109-5. Dialysis is helpful in the treatment of complications and allows more extensive nutritional support. Early, intensive dialysis has been advocated but not proven to minimize the occurrence of complications. There are two main modes of dialysis, hemodialysis and peritoneal dialysis. Hemodialysis allows more rapid clearance of nitrogenous waste products but requires trained staff and specialized equipment. Hemodialysis using biocompatible membranes results in less activation of leukocytes and complement and leads to better outcome than that using older membranes made of cuprophane or cellulose. Peritoneal dialysis requires less specialized equipment but provides slower clearance and may be inadequate in the treatment of the severely catabolic patient. Slow continuous arteriovenous or venovenous hemofiltration is an alternative to conventional hemodialysis. Arteriovenous hemofiltration is driven by the patient's own blood pressure but requires an arterial catheter. Venovenous hemofiltration can be performed via a double lumen venous catheter but requires a pump in the circuit for ultrafiltration. These therapies are suitable when large volumes of fluid must be removed, but the clearance of nitrogenous waste products is modest. They cause less hypotension and are useful for patients with tenuous hemodynamic status.

ACUTE RENAL FAILURE IN SPECIFIC SITUATIONS
Acute Renal Failure in Liver Disease

In advanced liver disease, especially in presence of portal hypertension, effective blood volume is often low because of splanchnic vasodilation. Renal blood flow is diminished due to afferent vasoconstriction induced by cytokines and endotoxins that accumulate due to liver disease and by hormones such as catecholamines, angiotensin, and endothelin released in response to the effective hypovolemia. Hypovolemia can be exacerbated by vomiting, diarrhea, bleeding, aggressive diuresis, or large-volume paracentesis. Hence several factors exist in advanced liver disease that predispose to prerenal azotemia and ATN. Clinical esimation of intravascular volume may be difficult in patients with ascites, and measurement

---

BOX 109-5
Indications for dialysis in acute renal failure

1. Hyperkalemia
2. Fluid overload
3. Acidosis
4. Pericarditis
5. Uremic symptoms
6. Poisoning with certain toxins (ethylene glycol, methanol)
7. Blood urea nitrogen level >100 mg/dl, creatinine level >10 mg/dl (relative indication)

of central venous pressure may be required. Urine sediment can suggest the presence of ATN. Urine sodium often remains low, even in presence of ATN, and does not reliably distinguish prerenal azotemia from ATN. Management should consist of careful balance between fluid replacement and diuresis to optimize intravascular volume. Use of low-dose dopamine to increase renal blood flow remains controversial. Therapeutic paracentesis should be performed cautiously and with adequate replacement with intravenous albumin to prevent an abrupt shift of fluid from intravascular space into the peritoneal cavity. The term *hepatorenal syndrome* is reserved for cases in which an intense afferent renal vasoconstriction exists as a result of circulating endotoxins, cytokines, and hormones of liver disease in the absence of intravascular volume depletion or ATN. The kidneys have no intrinsic disease and have, indeed, been used for transplantation. Prognosis of true hepatorenal syndrome is poor, but clinical distinction among hepatorenal syndrome, prerenal failure, and ATN is usually difficult and management with an open differential diagnosis is often necessary.

Acute Renal Failure in Pregnancy

Acute renal failure is an uncommon but serious complication of pregnancy. Causes include severe preeclampsia, placental hemorrhage, septic absorption, and postpartum hemolytic uremic syndrome. It is important to recognize that in normal pregnancy, glomerular filtration is increased by about 50%. Therefore plasma creatinine (0.4 ± 0.13 mg/dl) and BUN (6.7 ± 1.5 mg/dl) levels are near the lower limit of the normal range. A BUN level above 20 mg/dl or plasma creatinine level above 1.0 mg/dl strongly suggests abnormal renal function in pregnancy. HELLP syndrome (hemolysis, elevated liver enzymes, and low platelet count) refers to a severe complication of preeclampsia that may be difficult to distinguish from hemolytic uremic syndrome and requires prompt termination of pregnancy. Patients with hemolytic uremic syndrome may benefit from plasma exchange. Acute renal failure in pregnancy places the fetus at considerable risk, and if the fetus is near maturity, serious consideration should be given to an early delivery.

Acute Renal Failure in Cancer

Patients with cancer are at increased risk for acute renal failure in each of the three (prerenal, renal, and postrenal) categories (Box 109-6). Prophylactic measures can prevent renal failure in several of these situations. Uric acid nephropathy refers to acute renal failure induced by physical obstruction of renal tubules by uric acid crystals in response to rapid tumor lysis before or after chemotherapy. It has been demonstrated most often in patients with rapidly growing tumors that are sensitive to chemotherapy, such as lymphoma or leukemia. The serum uric acid level is characteristically above 20 mg/dl, and urine to plasma uric acid ratio exceeds 1. Prophylactic and thera-peutic measures include allopurinol, vigorous volume repletion, forced alkaline diuresis, and hemodialysis.

Acute Renal Failure in Renal Allograft

With the increasing success with renal transplantation there are now numerous patients with functioning renal transplants (Chapter 110). Beyond the immediate postoperative phase, when acute renal failure may occur as a result of surgical causes such as arterial thrombosis or ureteric obstruction, acute renal failure in a previously functioning transplant is usually due either to drug nephrotoxicity or to rejection, and a renal biopsy may be necessary to clarify the diagnosis.

Rhabdomyolysis

Rhabdomyolysis is frequently associated with acute renal failure. Common causes of rhabdomyolysis include trauma, alcoholism, seizures, and exertional heatstroke. Less frequent causes include hypokalemia, hypophosphatemia, cocaine intoxication, hydroxymethylglutaryl coenzyme A (HMG-COA) reductase inhibitors such as lovastatin and human immunodeficiency virus infection. The pathogenesis is multifactorial and includes tubular obstruction by pigmented casts, direct tubular toxicity of heme, and glomerular ischemia. Acute renal failure in rhabdomyolysis has several characteristic features, including reddish urine, pigmented casts in urine, elevated plasma creatine kinase level and a disproportionate rise in creatinine level as compared with BUN level. Hyperkalemia, hyperphosphatemia, hyperuricemia, and hypocalcemia may be marked. Treatment consists of vigorous volume repletion to keep urine volume above 300 ml/hour and forced alkaline diuresis to keep urine pH above 6.5. Mannitol is often added to the bicarbonate infusion, but its benefit apart from its diuretic effect remains uncertain. One effective regimen that has been proposed is as follows: one half normal saline in 5% dextrose with 10 g mannitol and 50 mEq/L sodium bicarbonate at a rate of 500 ml per hour until the urine is free of myoglobin.

Radiocontrast Nephropathy

Acute renal failure resulting from radiocontrast dye occurs with increasing frequency in patients with preexisting renal insufficiency. Other risk factors that have been suggested but not proven are old age, diabetes mellitus, multiple myeloma, volume depletion, and dose of the contrast medium. The pathogenetic mechanisms are not well characterized. Urine sodium level is often low, suggesting a role for glomerular ischemia. Azotemia peaks in 3 days and is usually reversible by 7 to 14 days. Patients at risk for contrast nephrotoxicity should have volume repletion before the radiographic procedure, but the benefit of prophylactic mannitol or furosemide has been unconvincing. Use of low-osmolality, nonionic media does not substantially reduce the risk of nephrotoxicity.

Pulmonary-Renal Syndrome

Acute glomerulonephritis with hemoptysis is the classic presentation of Goodpasture's disease in which antiglomerular basement membrane antibodies attack the basement membranes both in the kidney and the lung. Other causes of vasculitis, particularly Wegener's granulomatosis, can also become evident with acute renal failure and pulmonary hemorrhage. Diagnostic evaluation includes serologic tests for antiglomerular basement membrane antibodies, antineutrophilic cytoplasmic antibodies (ANCA), complement levels, and a renal or lung biopsy.

Acute Renal Failure Following Bone Marrow Transplantation

Acute renal failure occurs in 40% of patients receiving bone marrow transplantation, and in half of these patients dialysis is required. A few patients can have acute renal failure the first 5 days after transplantation, either because of a tumor-lysis-like syndrome from cytoreduction resulting from high-dose radiochemotherapy or because of toxicity from infusion of marrow and the associated preservatives, especially dimethylsulfoxide. Most of the cases of acute renal failure following bone marrow transplantation occur 10 to 20 days after

---

BOX 109-6
Causes of acute renal failure in patients with cancer

I. Prerenal causes
  A. Anorexia
  B. Vomiting
  C. Diarrhea
  D. Bleeding
II. Intrinsic renal causes
  A. Glomerular: Hemolytic uremic syndrome
  B. Tubular
    1. Obstructive: Uric acid, light chains, methotrexate
    2. Toxic
      a. Chemotherapy: Cisplatinum, ifosfamide
      b. Antibiotics: Aminoglycosides, amphotericin
      c. Radiocontrast media
III. Postrenal causes: Pelvic or retroperitoneal masses

✔ *WHEN TO REFER*

When renal failure is first detected, the first step should be to look for causes of prerenal azotemia. In about half of the patients with new-onset renal failure a prerenal cause can be identified by history and physical examination, and its correction restores renal function. A Foley catheter should be inserted to exclude bladder neck obstruction, and a renal ultrasound performed to exclude hydronephrosis resulting from obstruction and atrophic kidneys from a cause of chronic renal failure. If these measures suggest obstruction, a referral to a urologist should be made for further diagnosis and management. All patients discovered to have chronic renal failure should be referred once to a nephrologist and then managed in consultation with the nephrologist until chronic dialysis becomes necessary, when the majority of their care is usually carried out by a nephrologist. Once prerenal and postrenal causes are excluded, a careful urinalysis and sediment analysis offer the best noninvasive tests for distinguishing among the various causes of intrinsic renal disease; a renal biopsy is indicated for definitive diagnosis. All patients suspected to have vasculitis, glomerulonephritis, or interstitial nephritis should be considered for renal biopsy and referred to a nephrologist. When the diagnosis of ATN is clear, a renal biopsy is not necessary.

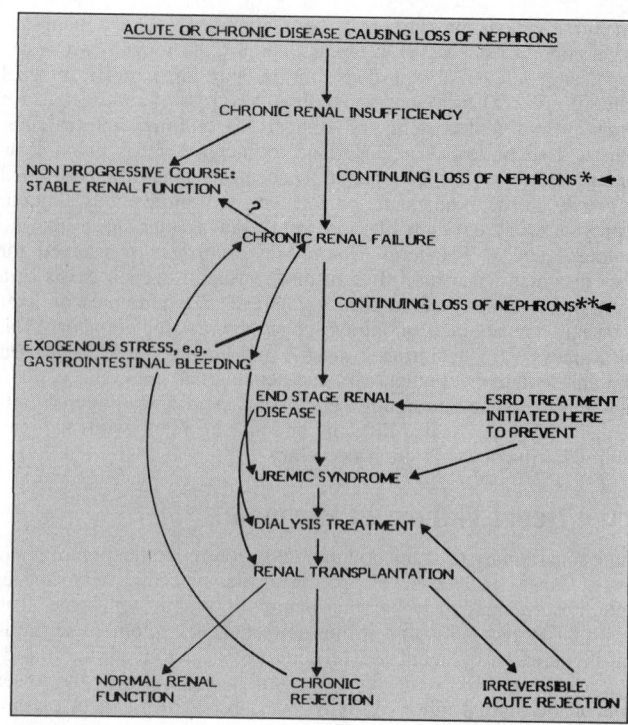

FIGURE 110-1 Course of chronic renal failure that is due to progressive nephron loss from chronic renal insufficiency to end-stage renal disease (ESRD), including therapy for ESRD. Treatment at *← may prevent progression and at **← may slow progression.

transplantation as a result of a hepatorenal-like syndrome associated with venoocclusive disease, sepsis, and the use of amphotericin. Therapy is largely supportive. Four to 12 months after bone marrow transplantation, hemolytic-uremic syndrome can occur, considered primarily to be a result of pretransplant total body irradiation. Plasma exchange is usually employed for hemolytic-uremic syndrome occurring after bone marrow transplantation, but its efficacy remains uncertain.

BIBLIOGRAPHY

Bellomo R, Boyce N: Acute continuous hemodiafiltration: a prospective study of 110 patients and a review of the literature, *Am J Kidney Dis* 21:508, 1993.
Conger JD: Interventions in clinical acute renal failure: what are the data? *Am J Kidney Dis* 26:565, 1995.
Denton MD, Chertow GM, Brady HR: "Renal-dose" dopamine for the treatment of acute renal failure: scientific rationale, experimental studies and clinical trials, *Kidney Int* 49:4, 1996.
Goligorsky M, Stein JH, editors: *Acute renal failure: new concepts and therapeutic strategies,* New York, 1995, Churchill Livingstone.
Hakim RM, Wingard RL, Parker RA: Effect of the dialysis membrane in the treatment of patients with acute renal failure, *N Engl J Med* 331:1338, 1994.
Lazarus JM, Brenner BM, editors: *Acute renal failure,* ed 3, New York, 1993, Churchill Livingstone.
Levy M: Hepatorenal syndrome, *Kidney Int* 43:737, 1993.
Thadani R, Pascual M, Bonventre JV: Acute renal failure, *N Engl J Med* 334:1448, 1996.
Zager RA: Rhabdomyolysis and myohemoglobinuric acute renal failure, *Kidney Int* 49:314, 1996.

CHAPTER

110 Chronic Renal Failure

Robert G. Luke, Charles E. Sanders, Jr., and John J. Curtis

Chronic renal failure can be defined as a permanent and significant reduction in glomerular filtration rate (GFR). In nearly all patients, once GFR is reduced to about one third of normal (GFR <30 to 40 ml/min, serum creatinine >3 mg/dl), progressive renal failure develops and leads eventually—but often slowly over as long as 20 to 30 years—to the *uremic syndrome* and *end-stage renal disease* (ESRD). *Chronic renal insufficiency* is present when the GFR is permanently and definitely reduced below normal, but progressive renal failure is not yet inevitable or established (serum creatinine in the range of 1.5 to 3 mg/dl). *Uremia* can be defined as the signs and symptoms associated with retention of the end products of nitrogen metabolism; in chronic renal failure it is eventually fatal unless *renal replacement therapy* (dialysis and/or renal transplantation) is introduced. The time of onset of the uremic syndrome is quite variable and unpredictable during the course of chronic renal failure, but its occurrence is unusual before the blood urea nitrogen (BUN) level reaches 60 mg/dl or the serum creatinine level 8 mg/dl (GFR <10 ml/min) and more commonly occurs at a BUN level of more than 100 mg/dl and a serum creatinine level of more than 12 mg/dl. It is good medical practice to initiate renal replacement therapy before the onset of uremic symptoms, usually when the GFR is 5 to 10 ml/minute. In making these assessments, it must be remembered that there is normally a reduction in GFR with aging; at age 85 to 90 years GFR is reduced to about 50% of normal. This reduction may not be associated with an elevation in serum creatinine because muscle mass and, consequently, creatinine production also fall with aging.

Because all patients in whom no contraindication exists now receive renal replacement therapy, at least in the United States and most Western countries, it is useful to consider dialysis treatment as an extension of the natural history of chronic renal failure (Fig. 110-1). Furthermore, in such patients early, aggressive treatment of risk factors for cardiovascular disease—especially hypertension—is essential if we are to reduce their high cardiovascular morbidity, which accounts for 50% of deaths in patients with ESRD. Dialysis treatment is equivalent to a GFR of only about 10 ml/minute. Hence some problems of patients with chronic renal failure are not completely resolved by chronic dialysis. Nevertheless, virtually all patients receiving chronic dialysis would otherwise not survive for long.

Discussed in detail later (see Pathophysiology) is the important concept that many patients with chronic renal failure progress along a final common path toward ESRD despite disappearance of the renal insult that initially led to the loss of some nephrons. If the pathogenetic mechanisms for the loss of remaining nephrons can be elucidated and then prevented or modified, a substantial proportion of cases of chronic renal failure might be converted to chronic renal insufficiency, or at least progression toward ESRD might be slowed. Because development of ESRD is most frequent in older patients, even the latter benefit might prevent the need for renal replacement therapy.

ETIOLOGY AND INCIDENCE

To see the relative importance of the various causes of chronic renal failure, let us look at ESRD, for which data are best established because the federal government assumes the heavy costs of such treatment. It should be noted, however, that because some diseases progress more slowly to ESRD than others, the data in Table 110-1 probably do not accurately reflect the relative prevalence in the community of chronic renal insufficiency or of chronic renal failure attributable to these diseases before ESRD. It is striking that 65% of cases of ESRD are now due to two systemic diseases—diabetes mellitus (diabetic glomerulosclerosis) and essential hypertension (hypertensive nephrosclerosis) (see Prevention). At present, the annual incidence of new ESRD patients continues to increase at a rate of 9% per year, with a predominance in patients older than 60 years of age.

There is an almost fourfold increase in ESRD (secondary to all causes except for congenital ones such as polycystic kidney disease) in blacks. The racial discrepancy is most marked for hypertensive nephrosclerosis in younger patients (e.g., a black:white ratio of ESRD of 20:1 in the age-group 25 to 45 years). Even after controlling for prevalence of primary and secondary causes before renal impairment, efficacy of treatment (e.g., glycemic or blood pressure control), and socioeconomic and demographic factors, the difference persists. It is possible that there is an increased renal susceptibility in blacks to primary or secondary hypertension. By the year 2000 it is estimated that 300,000 patients will be receiving renal replacement therapy. About 75% of these will be receiving some form of dialysis, and about 25% will have a functioning kidney transplant. In a city of 100,000 people one might anticipate that each year 24 patients would develop ESRD, 75 patients would be receiving some form of chronic dialysis, and a greater but unknown number would have chronic renal failure.

PATHOPHYSIOLOGY

The common clinical features of chronic renal failure and of the uremic syndrome relate to the diminishing number of nephrons that function relatively normally except for the increased excretion of solute per remaining nephron. This phenomenon is the *intact nephron hypothesis*. The process of chronic renal failure is essentially that of progressive loss of nephrons, irrespective of the primary site of attack (e.g., the glomerulus in glomerulonephritis and the medullary portions of the nephron in chronic pyelonephritis [reflux nephropathy]) on those nephrons. Ultimately, if damaged severely enough at any site, complete individual nephrons are destroyed. The site of primary damage, however, may be clinically evident and may help to indicate the type of disease process present: nephrotic syndrome indicates a primary or secondary glomerular disease (e.g., glomerulonephritis), whereas severe impairment of the renal concentrating mechanism out of proportion to the reduction of GFR may suggest a primary tubulointerstitial disease process (e.g., hypercalcemic nephropathy). Nevertheless, chronic renal failure manifests many of the same signs and symptoms, irrespective of the specific primary cause of nephron loss (the "final common path").

As nephrons are lost, the remaining undamaged or less severely damaged nephrons (both glomeruli and tubules) undergo "compensatory hypertrophy." In human kidneys there are normally 1 million nephrons in each kidney and GFR of 120 ml/minute. This would give a single nephron glomerular filtration rate (SNGFR) of 60 nl/minute if the SNGFR is homogeneous. Animal models of chronic renal failure suggest that as nephrons are lost, the SNGFR in remaining "intact" nephrons increases. Thus normal GFR could, at least theoretically, be maintained, despite the reduced number of nephrons, until the limits of increase of SNGFR are reached.

As nephrons are lost, if dietary intake remained the same, solutes such as sodium, chloride, potassium, and phosphate would accumu-

Table 110-1 Causes of annual incidence of new patients with end-stage renal disease ranked by percentage of total patients*

DISEASE	PATIENTS (%)
Diabetic glomerulopathy	36
Hypertensive nephrosclerosis	29
Glomerulonephritis	12
Tubulointerstitial†	5
Congenital‡	5
Collagen-vascular	2
Unknown	7
Total	100 (240)§

From the United States Renal Data System: *USRDS Annual Data Report,* Bethesda, Md, 1995, National Institutes of Health, National Institute of Diabetes and Digestive and Kidney Diseases.
*Data from 1993.
†Mainly obstructive and analgesic nephropathy.
‡Mainly polycystic kidney disease.
§Patients per million, U.S. population.

late in the body and cause symptoms if there were not *increased excretion of solute per remaining nephron.* Hyperkalemia, for example, is unusual until the GFR is reduced to less than 10 ml/minute. We have already seen that there is increased GFR per remaining nephron; this process is supplemented by diminished fractional reabsorption of those substances normally reabsorbed (e.g., sodium, chloride, phosphate) and increased secretion per nephron for those substances normally secreted after filtration (e.g., potassium; in late chronic renal failure, potassium clearance may exceed inulin clearance). This process prevents solutes from increasing in concentration in the blood (e.g., phosphate) until much later in the course of disease—either until GFR is reduced to about 25% of normal (often, for substances reabsorbed but not secreted) or until even greater reductions in GFR take place (for substances secreted [e.g., as noted, potassium]).

These *adaptations* in the function of remaining nephrons are aided by humoral, hormonal, and paracrine changes that either decrease absorption of a solute (e.g., parathyroid hormone for phosphate) or increase its secretion (e.g., aldosterone for potassium). There is also evidence for accumulation of a natriuretic factor, which impairs tubular reabsorption of sodium chloride, perhaps due to inhibition of $(Na^+ + K^+)$-ATPase (sodium potassium activated adenosine triphosphatase) in response to minor degrees of sodium chloride retention and expansion of extracellular fluid (ECF) volume.

Although these adaptations of remaining nephron function maintain the constancy of the internal environment, they severely limit the capacity of these same remaining nephrons to cope with an additional acute task such as a sudden increase in potassium, water, or acid load. In a sense each remaining nephron has already used its reserve capacity. Thus the patient with chronic renal failure loses the capacity or flexibility to deal with alterations in solute intake in response to dietary changes or in solute production in response to metabolic changes, for example, in response to infection or trauma. To avoid unnecessary or even iatrogenic illness (e.g., excess water intake causing hyponatremia) in these circumstances, the physician must anticipate the limited renal capacity to deal with such changes.

These beneficial compensatory adaptations in residual nephron function and in systemic hormonal secretion may ultimately "trade off" for harmful renal (the adapted nephron) and systemic (e.g., renal bone disease due to secondary hyperparathyroidism) effects (Fig. 110-2). Indeed "nephron trade-off" secondary to the adapted nephron (Fig. 110-3) is responsible for some of the clinical similarities of the "final common path" of chronic renal failure, irrespective of the primary cause of nephronal damage. Animal and some human studies suggest that important deleterious effects on the glomerulus relate to mechanical stress that is due to glomerular capillary hypertension and hyperperfusion with increased glomerular permeability to macromolecules into the mesangium; cytokine and growth-factor–induced proliferative effects (e.g., via transforming growth factor beta [TGF-β] and angiotensin II) on mesangial, epithelial, and endothelial cells with increased matrix protein and collagen formation; dyslipidemic endothelial and mesangial cell changes; and local coagulation abnormalities

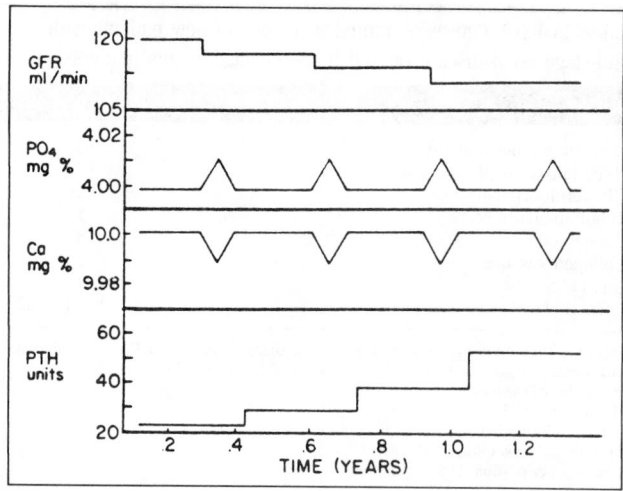

FIGURE 110-2   As glomerular filtration rate (GFR) falls, serum phosphate level rises, especially after eating; this leads to a fall in serum calcium level and thereby to an increase in parathyroid hormone (PTH) secretion, which reduces tubular reabsorption of phosphate and calcium to normal, but at the expense of an ever-increasing PTH level.

From Bricker NS, Slatopolsky E, Reiss E, Avioli LV: *Arch Intern Med* 123:543-553, 1969.

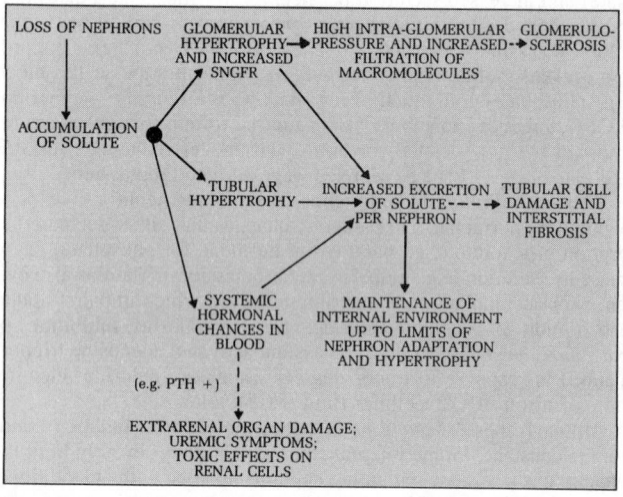

FIGURE 110-3   Response to loss of nephrons. Originally constituting a beneficial response to allow increased excretion per remaining intact nephron, these changes ultimately lead to continuing nephron loss independent of the initial injury or disease (nephron trade-off). *SNGFR,* Single nephron glomerular filtration rate; *PTH,* parathyroid hormone.

including platelet-endothelial interactions. Focal glomerulosclerosis is the prototypical glomerular lesion of nephron trade-off and is best seen in nephrons initially damaged by a primary tubulointerstitial process such as reflux nephropathy (chronic pyelonephritis). The similarity of glomerulosclerosis to atherosclerosis is noteworthy; hypertension, hyperlipidemia, and coagulation abnormalities are risk factors. Nephron trade-off also damages the tubules and interstitium by effects due to phosphate, urate, and ammonium excess per nephron and "hypermetabolic" effects in hyperperfused nephrons, especially when accompanied by ischemia due to primary and secondary renal arteriolonephrosclerosis. Therapeutic approaches in humans related to these pathogenetic mechanisms, such as reducing intraglomerular pressure via angiotensin-converting enzyme (ACE) inhibitors, have now been shown to be beneficial. Specific examples of the limitations imposed by progressive nephron loss and nephron adaptation on renal handling of water, sodium, potassium, and acid-base balance are considered next.

Water Excretion

With advancing renal disease there is progressive impairment in the urinary concentrating ability. Whereas in health the maximum urine osmolality may be about four times greater than that of plasma, in progressive renal disease the maximum urine osmolality approaches that of plasma. If the total solute requiring excretion remains at about 600 mOsm/day in uremia and the urine osmolality is fixed at slightly more than 300 mOsm/kg water, about 1 L of water will have to be excreted with every 300 mOsm of solute, and obligatory water excretion will approximate 2 L per day. This restricts the capacity of patients with chronic renal disease to lower water excretion during hydropenia to the levels seen in normal persons (500 ml/day at a urine osmolality of 1200 mOsm/kg water). With a decrease in the nephron population, there is also a restriction on the upper limit of water excretion that can be achieved. Although diluting ability is well preserved in chronic renal disease, the total amount of free water that can be excreted decreases as the nephron population and GFR fall. For example, if 10% of GFR can be excreted as free water, the capacity to excrete free water in response to water excess is 0.4 ml/minute (or 0.58 L/24 hours) in a patient with an insulin clearance of 4 ml/minute, compared with 12 ml/minute (or 17 L/24 hours) in a normal person.

The increased obligatory water excretion in chronic renal disease may lead to polyuria and nocturia. Occasionally, particularly when hypotonic fluids are administered, hyponatremia may result because of the diseased kidney's inability to increase water excretion appropriately. In conscious patients it is wiser to rely on the thirst mechanism, which is usually normal.

Sodium Excretion

As renal disease progresses, fractional sodium excretion increases appropriately and external balance is maintained until late in the course of renal disease; hence ECF volume is relatively well preserved. With changes in sodium intake, the fractional excretion of sodium has to change substantially to maintain sodium balance. For example, in a normal person increasing sodium chloride intake from 3.5 to 7.0 g/24 hours, the fractional excretion of sodium has to change from 0.25% to 0.5% to maintain balance. The same increment in salt intake may require a change in fractional sodium excretion from 8% to 16% to remain in balance in a patient with a GFR of 4 ml/minute. Hence, in renal failure, sodium excretion can be varied only over a restricted range, which progressively narrows as GFR declines.

With chronic renal disease, upper and lower limits of sodium excretion develop. At the lower limit, or "floor," the patient cannot conserve sodium maximally. Patients with renal disease fed a low-salt diet often cannot reduce sodium output over the usual time scale. A negative sodium balance ensues, and a corresponding volume of water is excreted. Plasma volume, ECF volume, and GFR fall. About 1% or 2% of patients with early chronic renal failure have a urine sodium leak, which causes sodium depletion even when salt intake is *normal.* Most of these patients have medullary cystic disease and analgesic nephropathy, but a few have obstructive uropathy, chronic interstitial nephritis, or polycystic kidney disease. They are typically normotensive and require a high sodium intake to maintain sodium balance.

Sodium retention is a more common problem than sodium depletion in chronic renal failure. It may occur as a result of associated nephrotic syndrome or cardiac failure or, in advanced chronic renal failure, because of lack of reduction of sodium chloride intake to match renal capacity to excrete those ions. The resulting positive balance in sodium chloride will expand ECF and plasma volume and may, in turn, lead to worsening hypertension and left ventricular or biventricular heart failure.

Potassium Excretion

Normally, about 90% to 95% of ingested potassium is excreted in the urine, with the remainder being excreted in the stool. In chronic renal failure a greater fraction of ingested potassium is excreted in the stool; 20% to 50% of the ingested amount may appear in the stool when the GFR falls below 5 ml/minute.

There is also a marked increase in potassium excretion per

nephron, and urinary potassium excretion approaches—and may even surpass—the filtered load of potassium. Therefore in chronic renal failure those adjustments in renal mechanisms that increase potassium excretion, together with the increased stool excretion of potassium, are enough to maintain a normal concentration of this cation in plasma, even on a normal intake of potassium (60 to 80 mEq/day), until the GFR falls below 10 ml/minute.

In contrast to sodium, potassium excretion depends on tubular secretion to maintain balance. In health, aldosterone and the distal tubular flow rate are major mediators of potassium secretion in the distal nephron. In chronic renal failure, increased basolateral sodium, potassium, (K)-ATPase in collecting duct principal cells, a rise in aldosterone levels, and increased flow of fluid through the distal tubule may be important factors increasing potassium excretion per nephron. Care with prescription of converting enzyme inhibitors for hypertension is needed because they may reduce aldosterone levels and precipitate hyperkalemia. Plasma potassium level may rise in chronic renal disease as a result of redistribution of potassium between intracellular and extracellular compartments, usually as a consequence of progressive acidosis, or the use of beta-blocking drugs.

The maintenance of normal excretion of potassium by the kidney when the number of functioning nephrons is decreased depends on a large increase in the distal tubular capacity to secrete potassium. At very low GFRs, the secretory rate of potassium may be near maximum to maintain the steady state. Thus very little functional reserve remains to respond to sudden changes in potassium intake. Situations such as oliguria, a sudden increase in potassium intake, sudden metabolic acidosis, or catabolic states may result in life-threatening hyperkalemia in patients with far-advanced renal insufficiency. A circulating inhibitor of $(Na^+ + K^+)$-ATPase (a natriuretic factor) and other effects of uremia may lead to increased cellular sodium content, decreased transcellular potential, and a decrease in intracellular potassium levels; hence total body potassium may actually be decreased, despite hyperkalemia.

Acid-Base Balance

The maintenance of acid-base balance in normal humans requires the renal reabsorption from the daily filtered load of approximately 4000 mEq of bicarbonate and the urinary excretion of 50 to 100 mEq of hydrogen ions in the form of ammonium and titratable acid (H^+ bound to phosphate and other buffer ions). Because of compensatory adaptations in acid excretion by the residual nephrons as renal function declines (except for a small group of patients with renal tubular acidosis associated with tubulointerstitial disease) most patients do not have significant acidemia attributable to renal disease until GFR falls below about 25% of normal.

Hydrogen ion excretion is impaired in chronic renal failure. Although ammonia excretion per residual nephron increases, total urinary ammonium excretion is lower than normal for the urinary pH. On the other hand, titratable acid excretion is normal or only slightly reduced, because the main buffers (phosphate and creatinine) are present in nearly normal amounts in the urine until very late in the course of renal disease. The result is decreased net acid excretion in the urine and a positive hydrogen ion balance; urinary pH, however, usually remains about 5.0.

A progressive fall in plasma bicarbonate level below 15 mEq/L usually does not occur in chronic renal failure until GFR values are quite low, presumably because buffers such as the carbonate of bone are then being utilized in buffering the hydrogen ion retention (positive H^+ balance) that occurs in such patients. In some patients there is also a urinary bicarbonate leak when the plasma levels are restored toward normal by the infusion of bicarbonate. When the infusion is stopped, the renal excretion of bicarbonate continues until plasma bicarbonate falls back to its previous level. This bicarbonate leak may have several causes, including an effect of high parathyroid hormone levels or of occult volume expansion on bicarbonate reabsorption in the proximal tubule.

Two types of acidosis have been observed in chronic renal disease: (1) hyperchloremic acidosis (normal anion gap acidosis), which occurs relatively early in the course of renal insufficiency and is mild, and (2) metabolic acidosis with an increased anion gap, which is due to the accumulation of phosphate, sulfate, and other anions usually not measured during routine laboratory determinations. If the anion gap is greater than about 20 mEq/L, other complicating events such as ketosis or lactic acidosis should be sought. In some patients with chronic renal disease and hyporeninemia, acidosis with hyperkalemia may occur (type IV renal tubular acidosis).

Magnesium

Most patients with chronic renal failure have normal or moderately elevated serum magnesium levels, which, however, seldom cause symptoms. The serum magnesium level rises further in response to acidosis, tissue trauma, and the administration of vitamin D and its analogs. Only in patients receiving occasional enemas or antacids containing magnesium are there marked increases in serum magnesium level. These elevations can lead to drowsiness, muscle weakness, and skin irritation. In patients with higher levels of magnesium, dramatic symptoms (muscle paralysis and respiratory failure) may occur.

Phosphate and Calcium

Urinary phosphate excretion remains unchanged as GFR falls, because of a progressive decrease in phosphate reabsorption, the consequences in part of increased levels of parathyroid hormone in serum (see Fig. 110-2). When the GFR falls below 30 ml/minute, however, even a marked decrease in phosphate reabsorption cannot compensate for the marked decrease in the filtered load of phosphate, and serum phosphate level rises. Hyperphosphatemia is therefore seen commonly in patients with a GFR of 25 ml/minute or less on an unrestricted diet. It is also at this level of GFR that decreases in serum calcium concentrations occur.

The fall in calcium concentration is due to several factors (Fig. 110-4). The increase in serum phosphate leads to a reciprocal decrease in serum calcium and decreased serum levels of 1,25(OH)$_2$-vitamin D$_3$ that are also due to nephron loss. These changes, in turn, decrease calcium absorption from the gastrointestinal tract. In addition, the ability of parathyroid hormone to mobilize calcium from bone is impaired, and this "skeletal resistance" to the action of the hormone also contributes to the development of hypocalcemia. The metabolic acidosis that is present tends to increase the fraction of ionized calcium and prevents some of the clinical consequences of hypocalcemia. Rapid correction of the acidosis in patients with chronic renal disease may lead to a fall in ionized calcium concentration and precipitate acute manifestations of hypocalcemia, including tetany and convulsions. A normal or elevated serum calcium concentration in patients not receiving vitamin D derivatives suggests severe secondary hyperparathyroidism or the syndrome of aluminum-induced bone disease.

Uremic Syndrome

The pathogenesis of the uremic syndrome is not precisely established but almost certainly has no single cause. Urea itself is relatively nontoxic, but measurement of blood urea (or BUN) offers the best single laboratory index of the likelihood of certain symptoms being "uremic" in origin; it represents an overall measure of the accumulation of products of protein metabolism. Restriction of dietary protein in association with maintenance of a caloric intake adequate to prevent gluconeogenesis frequently ameliorates uremic symptoms; likewise, a catabolic state often precipitates uremia at a GFR at which it would normally not occur (see Fig. 110-1). Hemodialysis, which most efficiently removes the many small-molecular-weight substances that are the end products of protein metabolism, also corrects the major manifestations of uremia, although there are some subtle persisting abnormalities, perhaps related to the less efficient clearance of "middle molecules" (molecular mass, 300 to 2000 daltons). Likely major contributing mechanisms to the uremic state are the following:

1. Accumulation of "toxins"
   a. Small-molecular-weight substances (e.g., urea, urate, sulfate, phosphate, which result from failure to excrete the end products of nitrogen metabolism)
   b. A whole series of substances such as phenols, guanidines, and low-molecular-weight polypeptides (however, evidence linking accumulation of any single substance to a specific uremic manifestation or organ dysfunction is weak)

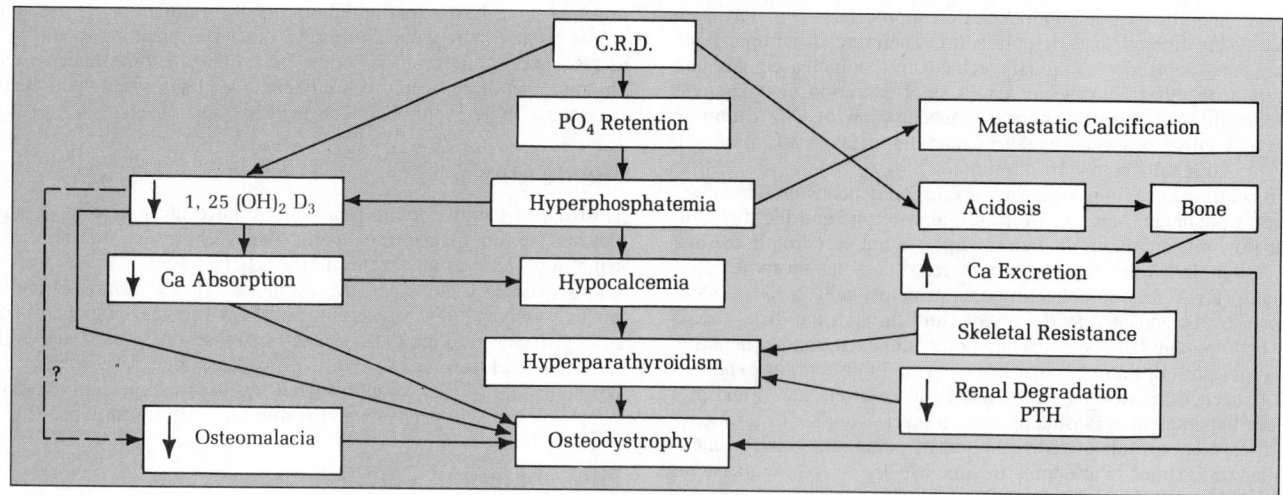

FIGURE 110-4 Pathogenesis of osteodystrophy in patients with chronic renal disease (CRD). The retention of phosphate leads to hyperphosphatemia and a decrease in serum calcium level (hypocalcemia). The hyperphosphatemia may also decrease the level of circulating 1,25 $(OH)_2$-vitamin D_3 by an effect on the renal 1-α-hydroxylase enzyme. The fall in the level of 1,25 $(OH)_2$-vitamin D_3 results in decreased gastrointestinal tract calcium absorption, which contributes to the hypocalcemia. The fall in serum calcium level leads to increased secretion of parathyroid hormone (PTH) hyperparathyroidism. The level of PTH also increases as a consequence of decreased degradation by the kidney (as renal mass decreases) and skeletal resistance. The acidosis of chronic renal disease promotes the removal of calcium carbonate from bone and contributes to the osteodystrophy. Increase in PTH results in bone changes (osteitis fibrosa cystica). A negative calcium balance and lowered levels of 1,25 $(OH)_2$-vitamin D_3 may result in osteomalacia.
From Slatopolsky E: *Kidney Int* 7:S253, 1975.

2. Extracellular and intracellular electrolyte and acid-base disturbances, including sodium, potassium, magnesium, and calcium. Inhibitors of Na, K, and ATPase are likely to impair cell function.
3. Accumulation of various hormones due to the following:
   a. Impaired renal degradation (growth hormone, glucagon)
   b. Responses to solute retention (natriuretic factor, parathyroid hormone)
   c. Impaired end-organ responses (follicle-stimulating hormone and luteinizing hormone)
4. Impaired production of renal hormones (e.g., erythropoietin, 1,25(OH)-vitamin D_3)

Specific organ dysfunctions in patients with chronic renal failure, uremia, and ESRD are considered in the next section. However, it is likely that these various mechanisms lead to diffuse defects of cellular function and metabolism in general, including energy production, cell membrane function, and ion pumps.

It is important for the physician to remember that there are many other causes of acute symptomatic deterioration in patients with chronic renal failure than uremia per se. Water excess (hyponatremia), drug intoxication that is due to accumulation of a drug in the presence of impaired renal excretion, congestive heart failure, and hypertensive encephalopathy are examples of complications that may need specific treatment to avoid premature acceptance that the patient has reached ESRD and uremia.

CLINICAL PRESENTATION AND DIAGNOSIS
Manifestations

Chronic renal failure may become evident in a myriad of ways and stages from chronic renal insufficiency to the uremic syndrome. Its secondary manifestations are often mistaken for primary problems in the affected organ system; common examples are mistaking essential hypertension for renal hypertension, peptic ulcer disease for gastrointestinal tract symptoms of uremia, and various anemias for renal anemia. Failure of the renal regulatory mechanisms to maintain the constancy of the internal environment ultimately produces symptoms and signs in every organ system, often in varying degrees in different patients.

Major modes of presentation of chronic renal failure are listed in Box 110-1. Only a small minority of patients come to medical attention with specific renal complaints; conversely, the vast majority of patients with specific complaints related to the urinary tract do not

---

BOX 110-1
Presentations of chronic renal failure

Renal symptoms
Nocturia, polyuria
Hematuria
Nephrotic syndrome

Routine urinalysis
Proteinuria with or without urinary casts, red blood cells, and white blood cells

Routine physical examination
Symptomatic or asymptomatic hypertension
Congestive heart failure
Cardiovascular disease

General symptoms
General malaise
Lassitude
Anemia
Anorexia
Pruritus, bruising
Halitosis

Specific extrarenal abnormalities
Impaired cognitive function
Peripheral neuropathy
Anemia
Renal bone disease
Gout or pseudogout
Pericarditis
Gastrointestinal tract bleeding

---

have chronic renal disease but, rather, have problems such as urinary tract infection. Similarly, most patients with proteinuria do not have progressive renal disease (Chapter 105). However, it is a rare patient with progressive renal disease who does not have proteinuric abnormalities, even though the proteinuria may be difficult to detect by

Table 110-2 Superimposed problems leading to acute deterioration of renal function in patients with chronic renal failure

PROBLEM	COMMENT
Volume depletion	Extrarenal losses or salt restriction: Excessive diuretic therapy, especially in nephrotic syndrome
Extracellular fluid (ECF) volume overexpansion with or without congestive heart failure	Salt loading, vasodilators, excess blood transfusion
Severe hypertension	Can also result from ECF volume expansion or renal artery stenosis
Obstruction	Renal stone, prostatic hypertrophy
Urinary tract infection	Most likely to cause fall in GFR in abnormal urinary tract
Drug toxicity	Aminoglycosides, cisplatin, prostaglandin inhibitors, contrast media, cyclosporine-converting enzyme inhibitors
Metabolic: Hypercalcemia, acute, severe hyperuricemia	Volume depletion, vitamin D analogs, tumor lysis
Endocrine deficiencies	Hypoadrenalism, hypothyroidism

BOX 110-2
Classification of causes of chronic renal failure

I. Hereditary
  A. Polycystic kidney disease
  B. Familial glomerulonephritis (Alport's syndrome)
  C. Medullary cystic disease
II. Systemic disease with potential for renal involvement
  A. Diabetes mellitus
  B. Connective tissue disorders
    1. Systemic lupus erythematosus
    2. Polyarteritis nodosa
    3. Scleroderma
    4. Wegener's granulomatosis
  C. Amyloidosis, myeloma kidney, gout
  D. Essential hypertension
  E. Chronic viral disease (e.g., HIV)
III. Primary glomerulonephritis (major progressive types)
  A. Membranous
  B. Membranoproliferative
  C. Focal glomerulosclerosis
IV. Primary tubulointerstitial renal disease
  A. Reflux nephropathy
  B. Analgesic abuse nephropathy
  C. Renal stone disease and nephrocalcinosis
V. Primary vascular renal disease
  A. Hypertensive nephrosclerosis
  B. Bilateral renal artery disease
VI. Obstructive uropathy
  A. Congenital
  B. Stone disease
  C. Prostatic disease

---

dipstick methods in patients with polyuria and tubulointerstitial disease rather than glomerular disease because the protein concentration in their urine is relatively low. An exception is medullary cystic disease, in which urinalysis may be completely normal.

By the time patients have general symptoms and specific extrarenal abnormalities (Table 110-2), usually at least 75% of renal function has been lost because of the efficacy of the compensatory mechanisms already discussed.

Hypertension may occur early in some patients with progressive renal disease, even before impaired renal function; this finding occurs in the more aggressive glomerulonephritides, in connective tissue disorders and vasculitides involving the kidney, in some patients with polycystic kidney disease, and in some with reflux nephropathy. Especially in white patients under the age of 35 years, the physician should remember to consider underlying renal parenchymal disease in patients presenting with even mild hypertension. Patients with evidence of hypertensive damage in brain, retina, or heart may also present with related symptoms and may have hypertension attributable to renal disease. At least two important risk factors for atherosclerosis are present in chronic renal failure—hypertension and hyperlipidemia; secondary hyperparathyroidism, with deposition of calcium in small blood vessels, may also contribute to the diffuse vascular disease that is not uncommonly found in patients who come to medical attention with chronic renal failure.

Common general presenting manifestations are listed in Box 110-1. Some, such as the alterations in cognitive function and lack of energy, develop so slowly that the patient often does not complain and, indeed, is not aware of them until improvement follows treatment. Sensory peripheral neuropathy is common and should be inquired for, as it may be the harbinger of motor neuropathy, which, unlike the sensory type, may not be reversible with therapy. Anorexia may be associated with vomiting and with negative nitrogen balance and malnutrition. A delayed presentation by the patient or a late diagnosis by the responsible physician prolongs treatment and inhibits rehabilitation, although almost all features of the uremic syndrome eventually respond.

Patients with a systemic illness causing chronic kidney disease most often come to attention because of the primary disease, such as diabetes mellitus, systemic lupus erythematosus, or scleroderma. Diabetic glomerulopathy (Chapter 117) is now the most common cause of ESRD. In insulin-dependent diabetes overt clinical renal disease with fixed proteinuria does not develop until 10 to 15 years after the onset of the disease. More patients (60%) have diabetic renal disease in association with type II diabetes because it is a much more common variety, but the true duration of disease before the development of renal disease is often difficult to quantitate.

Differential Diagnosis

When chronic renal failure is suspected, the physician should (1) rule out acute renal failure, especially that with a possibly reversible cause, (2) rule out reversible extrarenal or renal factors contributing to renal impairment independent of the underlying specific chronic renal disease (Table 110-2), and (3) seek a specific diagnosis. Late in the course of chronic renal failure, differentiation may not always be possible because specific diagnostic histologic features may have been obscured by the general changes of ESRD (the final common path of nephron adaptation).

Especially when presentation occurs with acute uremia, differentiation between acute and chronic disease can be difficult. *Acute* disease is more often associated with potential reversibility and always indicates a vigorous search for a specific diagnosis.

A history of nocturia or polyuria, or of previous nephrotic or nephritic syndrome, or of long-standing symptoms suggestive of late chronic renal failure (e.g., pruritus), together with findings of bilaterally small or scarred kidneys, severe anemia, hyperphosphatemia, or evidence for some of the chronic systemic complications of chronic renal failure such as renal osteodystrophy, all favor a *chronic* over an acute disease process.

Likely causes of acute deterioration in renal function in patients with chronic renal failure—which may well lead to the initial physician contact—are listed in Table 110-2; a search for these reversible influences is important. They are often caused by the restricted compensatory flexibility of the kidney with a substantially reduced number of nephrons, as discussed earlier. A very careful assessment of vascular and ECF volume and of the potential nephrotoxicity of any ingested drugs is especially necessary. Pathogenetic mechanisms of drug effects include hemodynamic (prostaglandin inhibitors, ACE inhibitors) superimposed acute tubular necrosis (aminoglycosides), or acute interstitial nephritis (methicillin), and protein catabolism (tetracyclines).

After treatment of any remediable factors and determination that stable renal failure persists, an orderly approach to specific diagnosis should follow (Boxes 110-2 and 110-3). While specific diseases are discussed in various chapters, some salient diagnostic points helpful in differential diagnosis are commented on here. History may reveal

BOX 110-3
An approach to diagnostic workup

History
Familial renal disease or systemic disease involving kidney
History of analgesic intake
Nephrotic or nephritic syndrome

Physical examination
Large "knobby" (polycystic) kidney
Evidence of systemic disease
Enlarged bladder with incomplete emptying
Rectal examination (prostate)
Renal artery bruit

Urinalysis, 24-hour urine protein, and endogenous creatinine (Cr) clearance
Proteinuria 3+ or 4+: glomerular disease
Proteinuria 1+: tubulointerstitial disease
Bence Jones proteinuria: myeloma kidney
Red blood cell casts: glomerular disease
White blood cell casts: tubulointerstitial disease
Impaired concentrating ability *early* in tubulointerstitial disease (e.g., hypercalcemia)
Proteinuria >5.0 g/dl: glomerular disease
Proteinuria <1.5 g/dl: tubulointerstitial disease
Urinary immunoelectrophoresis: myeloma kidney or light chain disease

Renal ultrasonography; excretory urogram (selected cases) for kidney size and symmetry
Obstruction, polycystic kidneys
Reflux nephropathy (chronic pyelonephritis)
Analgesic nephropathy (papillary necrosis)

Serology
Complement abnormalities: membranoproliferative glomerulonephritis, systemic lupus erythematosus
Antinuclear antibodies: systemic lupus erythematosus
Antineutrophil cytoplasmic antibodies: Wegener's granulomatosis or polyarteritis nodosa
Serum immunoelectrophoresis: myeloma
Serum chemistries: hypercalcemia; severe hyperuricemia
Viral studies
    Hepatitis B (membranous glomerulopathy, vasculitis)
    Hepatitis C (membranoproliferative glomerulonephritis, essential cryoglobulinemia)
    Human immunodeficiency virus (focal glomerulosclerosis)

Renal biopsy (selected cases)
Evidence for glomerular disease: relatively well-preserved kidney and symmetric kidney size are relative indications

Renal angiogram (highly selected cases)
Suspected bilateral renal arterial disease

a familial renal disease, including the need for renal replacement therapy in relatives, or of a systemic disease such as diabetes mellitus. Especially in the southeastern United States, a history of intake of illicit alcohol, gout, and long-standing hypertension is not infrequent, and lead nephropathy is often suspected, although definitive proof is difficult. Initial and persistent denial of analgesic abuse is common. Most patients with chronic glomerulonephritis do not have a history of acute nephritic syndrome preceding it. Renal disease as a presenting feature of diabetes is rare. Most patients with glomerular-level proteinuria continue to excrete large amounts of protein until late in the course of chronic renal failure, but this usually diminishes considerably at the end stage. In patients with progressive primary tubulointerstitial renal disease, especially reflux nephropathy and analgesic abuse nephropathy, a secondary focal glomerulosclerosis with associated glomerular-level proteinuria may develop as part of the adapted nephron syndrome (Fig. 110-3). Renal ultrasound is completely safe and should be the initial structural screening test. In some

patients pelvocaliceal details are needed for specific diagnosis, which requires an excretory urogram, and the potential risks of the nephrotoxicity of radiopaque contrast media must be considered. In reflux nephropathy a voiding cystourethrogram may permit diagnosis and thus avoid intravenous contrast medium injection. Renal stones, including staghorn calculi, and nephrocalcinosis are usually detectable on an abdominal film or on ultrasonography. Tophaceous gout may contribute to, but rarely is a sole cause of, chronic renal failure.

Renovascular renal failure is increasingly being recognized in elderly patients with hypertension, diffuse atherosclerosis and renal impairment, and recurrent "flash" pulmonary edema; in some patients acute renal deterioration occurs when they are receiving ACE inhibitors, even at acceptable blood pressure control levels. This ACE-induced, abrupt but reversible drop in GFR can also be seen in severe nephrosclerosis or cardiac failure when GFR has become dependent on angiotensin-II–maintained efferent arteriolar constriction. Renal arteriography should be reserved for carefully selected patients because of risk for atheroembolic renal disease and dye-induced acute tubular necrosis. Therefore the noninvasive screening test, magnetic resonance arteriography, is increasingly being used. Renal angioplasty or renovascular surgery may preserve function. Renal biopsy is occasionally indicated, especially if renal size is well maintained, to rule out parenchymal renal disease.

As should now be evident, the disease process is relatively slow and is silent unless the patient with chronic renal failure has an early-stage acute event such as edema or hematuria, or an incidental urinalysis or measurement of BUN or serum creatinine level. Renal symptoms are usually absent, except for nocturia, until uremic symptoms develop. After discussing prevention of ESRD, next, we will review the signs and symptoms relevant to each organ system in patients with late-stage renal failure both before and after dialysis treatment.

PREVENTION OR DELAY OF END-STAGE RENAL DISEASE

At present, if the diagnosis is made early enough, we have the ability to prevent progression in reflux nephropathy, analgesic nephropathy (if the patient discontinues intake), recurrent stone disease, and obstructive uropathy. We now know that tight euglycemic control of type I diabetes mellitus with insulin can reduce all microvascular complications by 30% to 50% (see Chapter 303). Treatment of any hypertension or early proteinuria (microalbuminuria) with ACE inhibitors can reduce the incidence and rate of progression of diabetic glomerulopathy. These measures eventually ought to reduce ESRD attributable to diabetes. Likewise, we are optimistic, but cannot yet prove, that control of blood pressure in essential hypertension to normal levels, especially in African Americans, will delay, prevent, or reduce the development of hypertensive nephrosclerosis. Control of hypertension does certainly reduce cardiovascular complications in chronic renal failure patients, who can be regarded as potential "vasculopaths."

An important question is whether the development of nephron trade-off in the adapted nephron syndrome can be modified or slowed, especially when the primary disease process is no longer active. In polycystic kidney disease, for example, cysts continue to enlarge and compress remaining nephrons, and in some glomerulonephritides there is continuing immunologic attack. Nevertheless, when the inciting pathologic condition is quiescent, it is a highly desirable goal to preserve the remaining nephrons; at any level of endogenous function above a GFR of 10 to 15 ml/minute, this is far preferable to dialysis.

The major documented beneficial intervention is careful control of blood pressure. ACE inhibitors and calcium channel blockers may offer additional advantages over other antihypertensives. It is likely that target blood pressure should be lower than 140/90 mm Hg—indeed, as close to normal levels as possible unless contraindicated—in patients with proteinuria greater than 3 g/24 hours, in diabetic glomerulosclerosis, and in African Americans. Falling proteinuria level in response to treatment, best documented with the use of ACE inhibitors, is associated with slowing of rate of progression. A high-protein diet should be avoided because of evidence that it increases intraglomerular flow and pressure. Control of serum phosphate, prevention of secondary hyperparathyroidism, and treatment of hyperlipidemia may all be indicated, but specific benefit in human disease is not yet documented. Expert nutritional support is essential to maintain an appropriate caloric, phosphate, and nitrogen intake and avoid negative nitrogen balance.

ORGAN SYSTEM COMPLICATIONS OF CHRONIC AND END-STAGE RENAL DISEASE
Hematologic Disorders

Anemia. A normochromic normocytic anemia is a consistent finding in chronic renal failure. As the GFR falls below 40 ml/minute, the hematocrit decreases in proportion to the degree of renal insufficiency until a value of approximately 20% is reached with ESRD. Decreased or absent erythropoietin is the primary event underlying the anemia. As renal mass decreases, erythropoietin level falls, leading to decreased red blood cell production by the bone marrow. Patients with polycystic kidney disease tend to have a higher hematocrit relative to the stage of renal failure, even while receiving dialysis. Recombinant human erythropoietin can now be used to treat renal anemia effectively and improve well-being in patients with chronic renal failure; however, it is expensive. Gastrointestinal tract bleeding is quite common and should be looked for, especially if the response to erythropoietin is less than anticipated. Erythropoietin is now used routinely (intravenously or subcutaneously) in dialysis patients if hematocrit does not reach 30% to 35%. Lack of response to erythropoietin should suggest a search for iron-deficiency, folic acid, aluminum-related, or hyperparathyroid bone disease; inflammatory or neoplastic disease; or malnutrition. The availability of erythropoietin constitutes one of the largest advances in treatment for dialysis patients.

Coagulation Abnormalities. A bleeding tendency manifested by epistaxis, menorrhagia, gastrointestinal tract bleeding, and prominent bruising after trauma is common in advanced renal failure. Patients with chronic renal failure have a qualitative defect in platelet function and abnormal factor VIII function. This condition is manifested as a prolonged bleeding time, although the partial thromboplastin time, prothrombin time, and clotting time are all within normal limits. The factors in uremic serum that induce the qualitative platelet defect are not well delineated, but dialysis does correct the defect; cryoprecipate, 1-deamino-8-D-arginine vasopression (DDAVP), and conjugated estrogens may also help to alleviate uremic bleeding. Anemia itself contributes to uremic bleeding, and erythropoietin has ameliorated this problem. The serum concentrations of the various proteins of the coagulation cascade are usually within normal limits unless the patient has the nephrotic syndrome in addition to chronic renal failure. However, plasma fibrinogen levels may be increased in renal failure, which may play a role in the increased erythrocyte sedimentation rate disproportionate to the anemia seen in uremia. Plasma fibrinolytic activity is decreased but improves after hemodialysis.

Hypertension

Hypertension may complicate chronic parenchymal renal disease even before azotemia develops, as in polycystic kidney disease or membranoproliferative glomerulonephritis. In most patients it develops later, and by end-stage it occurs in 80% of patients. As noted, essential hypertension may also cause nephrosclerosis and progressive renal disease, especially in blacks. Even in such patients in whom hypertension appears to be primary, however, there is evidence for participation of a functional or structural renal abnormality in the pathogenesis of essential hypertension (Chapter 32).

The treatment of hypertension in patients with chronic renal failure at all stages is important. Otherwise, it is very likely to become more severe and accelerate loss of nephrons via nephrosclerosis, and likely also contribute to the high intraglomerular pressures thought to cause glomerular loss (nephron trade-off). ACE inhibitors may offer some benefits by reducing intraglomerular pressure, especially in diabetic glomerulopathy.

Hypertension probably is due to elevated renin production in the kidneys and some sodium chloride retention, even though overt edema may not be present. Plasma renin levels are high for the degree of ECF volume expansion. Accordingly, treatment usually begins with modest salt restriction and then, if needed, a loop diuretic such as furosemide (thiazides lose their effectiveness as the GFR falls below 40 ml/minute). Other hypertensinogenic mechanisms include the failure of the diseased kidneys to produce physiologic vasodepressors (e.g., certain prostaglandins and a neutral lipid produced in the renal medulla), enhanced peripheral sympathetic activity attributable to afferent renal (? chemoreceptor) reflexes, and diminished nitric oxide formation resulting from inhibition of nitric oxide synthase by accumulated dimethyl arginine in renal failure.

At initiation of treatment, care must be taken not to superimpose prerenal azotemia, although a slight but usually reversible drop in GFR may occur early after blood pressure is restored to normal levels, especially in patients with more severe hypertension. In accelerated-phase or malignant hypertension, effective treatment of hypertension should be maintained, even though apparent ESRD develops and necessitates dialysis, because the risk of developing hypertension-induced cerebrovascular and cardiovascular problems is otherwise too great. In such patients recovery of renal function after a few months occasionally occurs and allows cessation of dialysis treatment, for at least some months or even years. This recovery is thought to be due to healing of fibrinoid necrotic lesions in small arterioles as blood pressure control is maintained.

Once dialysis therapy is initiated, blood pressure usually can be regulated again by control of plasma volume with dialysis, ultrafiltration, and modest dietary restriction of salt. Hypertension in anephric dialysis patients is almost always due to excess volume.

Renal hypertension can be very severe and resistant to hypotensive drugs; formerly, bilateral nephrectomy was sometimes required for control of blood pressure, even after successful renal transplantation. This is virtually never required now because of the efficacy of the ACE inhibitors, minoxidil, and the calcium channel blockers. If hypertension cannot be controlled by dialysis, hypotensive drugs can be used as in patients before dialysis. However, diuretic drugs have no place in patients receiving regular dialysis, and such patients may need to omit medications immediately before dialysis because of hypotension as ultrafiltration proceeds, especially in patients with autonomic nerve insufficiency that is due to either chronic renal failure per se or diabetes.

A well-functioning renal allograft can cure hypertension; nevertheless, hypertension recurs in about 50% of renal transplant recipients on follow-up as a result of cyclosporine (which leads to renal vasoconstriction), chronic rejection, allograft renal artery stenosis, and renin effects of the native kidneys on the allograft.

Cardiopulmonary Complications

Cardiovascular abnormalities are common in patients starting renal replacement therapy: left ventricular (LV) hypertrophy (40%), coronary artery disease, systolic left ventricular dysfunction, diastolic dysfunction (myocardial interstitial fibrosis is increased), and frank congestive heart failure (10%) are all much more common than in matched subjects without renal disease. Remarkable improvement in cardiac function sometimes follows successful renal transplantation. Coronary artery bypass surgery can be successfully performed in patients after they are adequately dialyzed and in stable condition, and in high-risk patients this should precede major surgery. Thus cardiovascular disease is the most important cause of death in patients on dialysis, and hypertension is the most important risk factor. Long-term survival (20 years) has now been demonstrated in chronic dialysis patients, and in all of these long-term survivors a normotensive state has been maintained. Other risk factors for atherosclerosis are hyperlipidemia, smoking, hyperparathyroidism with vascular calcification, carbohydrate intolerance, and hyperuricemia. It is unlikely that the dialysis procedure itself causes accelerated atherosclerosis. Other commonly seen cardiovascular abnormalities are uremic pericarditis and effusion, in some cases with cardiac tamponade, and arrhythmias, which are often associated with hyperkalemia.

The combination of hypertension, anemia, fluid overload, and acidosis all contribute to the uremic patient's increased tendency toward the development of congestive heart failure. Pulmonary edema may be the first manifestation of congestive heart failure in the patient with advanced renal disease, and this edema is often due to excess ECF volume. However, increased pulmonary capillary permeability, decreased oncotic pressure, and left ventricular dysfunction also may be present and contribute to the genesis of the disorder. Of course, cardiac disease of all types may coexist with renal failure and must be considered in patients with renal disease and congestive heart failure. The existence of a true uremic cardiomyopathy that is due to uremic toxins, independent of the previously mentioned causes of ventricular failure, is debated. Metastatic calcification of the lungs and heart can be seen in far-advanced renal failure and may relate to secondary hyperparathyroidism, hyperphosphatemia, or vitamin D administration.

Pericarditis occurs in approximately half of patients with chronic renal disease who do not receive dialysis in whom terminal uremia develops. Before dialytic and transplantation therapy became available, pericarditis in the several days before death from uremia was a common event; aggressive dialytic therapy is usually effective in reversing the clinical manifestations of pericarditis. *Uremic serositis* includes pericarditis, ascites, and pleural effusion; several or only one of these may become evident in a single patient. These effusions are characteristically exudates and are made worse by fluid overload; other causes must be considered, for example, infection or malignant disease, especially if the effusions are not controlled by dialysis and fluid removal as indicated. The pathogenesis of uremic serositis is unknown but may relate to an effect of uremic toxins on capillary permeability. Serositis with or without effusion also occurs in chronic dialysis patients and indeed is now more commonly seen in these circumstances, especially during periods of underdialysis and catabolic illness. The frequency of dialysis is often increased to daily, and the problem may then resolve. Because the pericardial effusion is most often hemorrhagic, heparin must be used with great caution. For increasing effusion and cardiac tamponade, the patient must be observed in the hospital. Tamponade requires pericardial stripping or pericardiocentesis and instillation of a nonreabsorbable steroid.

Neuromuscular Abnormalities

The central nervous system and peripheral nerves are affected, with diverse consequences. Nerve conduction time characteristically is prolonged; peripheral neuropathy may develop in advanced uremia; sleep patterns are disturbed; and asterixis, convulsions, and psychosis all may occur. The early changes of uremic encephalopathy are subtle. They consist of insomnia, inability to concentrate, lack of alertness, and slowing of cerebration. Ultimately, there may be loss of memory, confusion, hallucinations, and delirium or obtundation. Convulsions occur in about one third of the patients nearing terminal uremia. The electroencephalogram in uremia shows a "slow-wave pattern," which may be related to increased calcium in the brain, which in turn may be caused by high levels of circulating parathyroid hormone. Autonomic neuropathy occurs and can contribute to impotence in the male, absence of sweating, and dialysis hypotension. Cramps of various limb muscles, intermittent numbness and tingling of the hands and feet, and the "restless leg" syndrome (uncomfortable sensations in the legs occurring during rest and relieved by movement) are common in late chronic renal failure and during long-term hemodialysis. Shifts in water and electrolytes may in some way account for this syndrome and may also account for muscle cramps and distal limb paresthesias. With dialysis, overt clinical neuropathy is rare, and a subclinical form may be present in which only nerve conduction studies or special tests of cutaneous sensation are abnormal. Asymptomatic uremic neuropathy occurs in at least 50% of all patients who reach ESRD or who are receiving long-term hemodialysis.

Gastrointestinal Tract Disturbances

Gastrointestinal tract symptoms attributable to chronic renal failure usually do not appear until the GFR falls below 10 ml/minute. Early symptoms include anorexia, nausea, and vomiting; the latter two symptoms are most prominent in the early morning, when vomiting may be a daily event. Early morning vomiting usually alleviates fur-

ther nausea during the day, when appetite improves, allowing adequate oral intake.

Gastrointestinal tract bleeding is common in chronic renal failure. It may occur at any site, from the stomach to the rectum. The lesions found most commonly are shallow, small ulcers that bleed slowly. Mucosal ulcerations are a prominent feature of advanced uremia and occur along virtually the entire gastrointestinal tract. Superficial erosions of the buccal and gingival mucosa may occur; these lesions may also involve the tongue, lips, or larynx (uremic stomatitis). The stomach and the duodenum are also subject to superficial erosions and frequently are the site of chronic blood loss. More advanced peptic ulcerations are also observed in uremia, although gastric acid secretion is depressed in 40% of patients, while the other 60% have normal gastric acid secretion.

Immunoreactive plasma gastrin values increase progressively with renal failure. This increase may represent true gastrin or small peptides with gastrinlike antigen structure accumulating in plasma because of the inability of the diseased kidney to metabolize low-molecular-weight proteins.

Other gastrointestinal tract manifestations include colitis, ileus, parotitis, and, as already noted, ascites. Bloody diarrhea and abdominal cramps resulting from colonic ulcerations (uremic colitis) have been attributed to local irritation of the colonic mucosa by ammonia produced by the intestinal flora. Pancreatitis and parotitis occur with increased frequency in chronic uremia. The diagnosis is hampered by the frequent finding of elevated serum amylase in uremia as a result of decreased renal amylase clearance; however, a threefold increase is significant. Levels of gastrointestinal tract–related hormones, such as cholecystokinin, gastric inhibitory polypeptide, and glucagon, all are elevated in the serum of patients with chronic renal failure. These elevations may be due to increased secretion and/or to failure of the diseased kidney to metabolize these hormones or their constituents. Small bowel and colonic bleeding in chronic dialysis patients is sometimes recurrent and attributable to angiodysplastic lesions, which are difficult to diagnose and treat. Heparinization during hemodialysis may precipitate bleeding. Diverticular disease is increased in patients with polycystic kidneys.

After transplantation, two major life-threatening gastrointestinal tract complications occur. Upper gastrointestinal tract bleeding resulting from gastritis or peptic ulcer disease is seen in 5% to 10% of recipients, and bowel perforation attributable to ruptured diverticula is especially common in elderly patients. Symptoms may be masked by steroids.

Immunologic and Infectious Complications

Infection is a common cause of death in both acute renal failure and the terminal stages of chronic renal failure. Such patients are often malnourished or have other complications that predispose them to infection. Most infections in patients on dialysis are due to gram-positive organisms. Vascular and peritoneal accesses are common sites of infection. Pruritus may lead to skin infection by chronic scratching. The delayed wound healing seen in uremia probably plays a role in the increased incidence of postoperative and posttraumatic infections. However, additional factors that impair both cellular and humoral immunologic defenses are likely to underlie the increased incidence of infection in uremia.

Although granulocyte counts, total immunoglobulin level, and complement levels are usually normal, polymorphonuclear leukocyte, T-cell, and B-cell functions are impaired in ESRD. Hence, some antibody responses and cell-mediated, immune, chemotactic, and phagocytic abnormalities are present.

As a general rule, diminished immunity has been associated with the predisposition to viral and fungal diseases. Exposure to serum hepatitis virus in hemodialysis units has provided a unique setting for comparing the responses to viral infections in normal and uremic subjects. The course of the disease in staff members who contract hepatitis in these units is characterized by acute liver damage, elevations of enzyme and bilirubin levels, and liver tenderness and enlargement, and is followed by recovery within 1 to 2 months. On the other hand, subacute hepatitis with mild to moderate (or no) clinical evidence of liver damage often develops in patients with uremia, but the course is protracted, and viremia persists for years.

These observations suggest impairment of host immune defenses. Uremic patients as a group have mild but not grossly impaired antibody responses, opsonic activity, and in vitro phagocytic capacity. Immunization for hepatitis B and influenza viruses is less effective than in normal persons but should still be offered.

By far the most dreaded complication of transplantation is infection, the leading early cause of death among allograft recipients. During the first posttransplant month opportunistic infections are unusual, and the major infectious disease hazards are similar to those in other patients undergoing major urologic surgery (i.e., atelectasis with pulmonary wound, urinary tract, and intravenous line infections). The period between 1 and 6 months after transplantation, which coincides with attempts to reverse rejection episodes by high-dose immunosuppressive therapy, is when the most dangerous opportunistic viral, fungal, and protozoan infections occur. Often, infection with cytomegalovirus precedes infection with other, potentially more dangerous microbes such as *Pneumocystis carinii*. Cytomegalovirus infection is especially common in patients lacking circulating anticytomegalovirus antibodies who have received a graft from a donor previously infected with cytomegalovirus. If this situation cannot be avoided, hyperimmune globulin and acyclovir may be given prophylactically. Acyclovir and bactrim are often also given prophylactically after transplantation, especially for herpes simplex and *Pneumocystis* species. The dire consequences of imprecise or delayed treatment in these immunosuppressed hosts dictate early antibiotic therapy and an aggressive, exacting approach to identifying the organism, its susceptibility to antimicrobial agents, and the site or sites of infection. For example, lung infection usually indicates urgent bronchoscopy.

Chronic progressive liver disease, probably related to chronic hepatitis B or C viral infection, is an important and eventually usually lethal late (3 to 10 years) complication of transplantation.

Renal Osteodystrophy, Hyperphosphatemia, Hypocalcemia, and Bone and Joint Disease

For the reasons discussed earlier, progressive loss of renal mass ultimately leads to derangements in mineral and skeletal metabolism. Elevated levels of parathyroid hormone, a consequence of both increased secretion and decreased degradation, lead to increased bone reabsorption, especially subperiosteally, and reduced bone density may be found on x-ray examination. The serum levels of alkaline phosphatase are elevated. Decreased conversion of vitamin D to a more active form, $1,25(OH)_2$-vitamin D_3, results in decreased intestinal absorption of calcium and potentially in osteomalacia. Metabolic acidosis also contributes to bone disease by causing titration of the calcium carbonate salts of bone and leading to their dissolution. Calcium carbonate as a phosphate binder also provides alkali, but sodium bicarbonate may also be needed to maintain a normal serum bicarbonate level.

Renal osteodystrophy is a common complication of chronic renal disease both before and after dialysis (see Fig. 110-4) and is characterized histologically by several alterations in bone structure, including osteomalacia, secondary hyperparathyroidism, and, less commonly, osteosclerosis. Osteitis fibrosa cystica reflects the reabsorptive effect of increased osteoclastic activity resulting from secondary hyperparathyroidism, and osteomalacia, a defect in bone mineralization that is secondary, at least in part, to alterations in the metabolism of vitamin D and is characterized by a widening of the osteoid seam and an absent or abnormal mineralization front. Less commonly, osteoporosis is seen in uremic patients.

These abnormalities of bone, calcium and phosphorus, vitamin D metabolism, and parathyroid hormone secretion can have devastating effects on patients. In children there may be retardation of growth. In the adult, bone pain, fractures, collapse of vertebrae, necrosis of femoral heads, and skeletal deformities may occur. Along with osteitis fibrosa cystica, there may be metastatic calcification and medial calcification of arteries, with ischemic necrosis, calcification of soft tissues and skin, intractable pruritus, periarthritis from calcium hydroxyapatite precipitation, conjunctival calcification, and so on. This syndrome, calciphylaxis, may necessitate subtotal parathyroidectomy (removal of three and a half glands).

Attempts to prevent renal osteodystrophy optimally now start early in the course of chronic renal failure. Recommended measures include dietary phosphate restriction, often usefully combined with protein restriction, prescription of calcitriol with careful follow-up of serum calcium and phosphorus levels to avoid hypercalcemia, and use of intestinal phosphate binders as necessary. Parathyroid levels are monitored to assess success in avoiding or minimizing secondary hyperparathyroidism; because of skeletal resistance to parathormone, levels of three times normal may be best. Ensuring near-normal serum calcium and phosphorus levels also may help prevent progression of renal disease, as already discussed, as well as soft tissue and vascular calcification. The latter can be avoided by keeping the product of serum calcium and phosphorus levels (milligrams per deciliter) less than 65. Calcium carbonate or calcium acetate are preferred for phosphate binding because the use of aluminum-containing antacids as binders contributes to aluminum-related bone and muscle disease and microcytic hypochronic anemia.

Phosphate clearances on dialysis on an adequate protein and caloric intake are insufficient to control serum phosphate, and binders must be continued. Aluminum-containing antacids should only be used for short periods to aid in controlling severe hyperphosphatemia, which should then be controlled by calcium carbonate or acetate, with monitoring of serum calcium level to avoid hypercalcemia. If the latter remains a problem, dialysate calcium level can be lowered and/or judicious amounts of magnesium-containing antacids can be used. Persistent hypocalcemia should be treated with calcitriol to avoid secondary hyperparathyroidism. Intravenous calcitriol or oral "pulse" calcitriol can help when suppression of hyperparathyroidism is difficult. Recent work suggests relative resistance to suppression of parathyroid function in response to both vitamin D and ionized serum calcium. These preventive measures have much reduced symptomatic renal osteodystrophy and the need for subtotal parathyroidectomy. The latter is still occasionally required for hypercalcemia or in a noncompliant patient with severe bone disease or extraosseous calcification.

Before virtual cessation of the chronic use of aluminum-containing antacids and efficient removal of aluminum from dialysate water, dialysis dementia, myopathy, anemia, osteodystrophy (unresponsive to calcitriol or measures to reduce parathormone levels and sometimes associated with hypercalcemia and severe bone pain and fractures) were seen quite frequently. When they occur now, these consequences of aluminum intoxication can be treated with the chelating agent deferoxamine during hemodialysis. Calcium citrate must not be used as a phosphate-binding agent because it increases aluminum absorption from the gut.

In addition to hyperparathyroid bone disease, osteomalacia, and aluminum-related bone disease, a new form of renal osteodystrophy, aplastic (or adynamic) bone disease, is being seen. It requires bone biopsy for diagnosis, and to date we have no specific additional therapy other than maintaining higher than normal (three or four times normal) active parathormone levels.

After a successful renal transplantation, a phosphate diuresis promptly ensues. Usually the transplanted organ promptly converts vitamin D to $1,25(OH)_2$-vitamin D_3. In contrast, resolution of severe hyperparathyroidism is far more gradual. Posttransplantation osteodystrophy usually improves as normal vitamin D metabolism is restored, aluminum deposition secondary to intake of oral gels and hemodialysis reverses, and hyperparathyroidism resolves. In contrast, osteopenia resulting from steroid intake becomes manifest. A more feared complication, osteonecrosis, occurs in 5% of all patients; the head of the femur is the most common site.

Secondary gout may occur in chronic renal failure as a result of hyperuricemia, usually in those with a family history of gout. Allopurinol should not be used routinely for prophylaxis but only after gout has been firmly diagnosed (and it should be noted that the breakdown of azathioprine is much reduced in patients receiving allopurinol). Pseudogout mimics gout, but joint aspiration does not reveal uric acid but rather calcium pyrophosphate crystals; associated chondrocalcinosis is common, and, like gout, it responds well to prostaglandin inhibitors such as indomethacin.

Another new form of bone and joint disease recognized in patients receiving dialysis for 5 to 10 years or more is due to the accumulation of an amyloid-like substance formed from β_2 microglobulin (a normal protein of 11,800 daltons). The normal levels of the latter of 1 to 2 mg/L rise to 50 to 100 mg/L in late chronic dialysis patients because dialyzer clearance is inadequate. The clinical syndromes attributable to β-2 amyloidosis include carpal tunnel, destructive osteoarthropathy of large joints, bone cysts, and pathologic fractures. Visceral deposition appears to be less common, and the reason for the atypical distribution of deposits is not known. There is no specific treatment except for surgery (e.g., for carpal tunnel syndrome), but prevalence may be less in those receiving dialysis by more permeable membranes (e.g., polysulphone), which may also adsorb the protein. Transplantation halts progression but does not lead to regression of the bone lesions.

Nutritional and Metabolic Alterations

Disorders of Nitrogen Metabolism. Not only are the end products of protein metabolism the main culprits in the genesis of the uremic syndrome, but also protein metabolism is abnormal in both chronic renal failure and in dialysis patients. In individuals with stable BUN level and body weight and an adequate dietary intake, protein intake can be measured by urinary nitrogen excretion plus non–urea-nitrogen (which is constant at 0.031 g nitrogen/kg body weight per 24 hours). Patient estimates of protein intake are inaccurate; dietary protein intake in patients in stable condition is best measured as follows:

$$\text{(EQ. 1)}$$

(Urinary urea = nitrogen grams per 24 hours + body weight
$\times$ 0.031 g) $\times$ 6.25 + urinary protein (if >5 g/24 hours)

Positive nitrogen balance can be maintained in normal individuals and patients with chronic renal failure who are receiving dietary protein intakes as low as 0.6 g/kg per 24 hours if caloric intake is adequate (35 kcal/kg per 24 hours). To give some margin of error, minimum protein intake should be 0.8 g/kg per 24 hours, unless very careful nutritional expertise and supervision is available.

A high-protein diet is harmful and will accelerate the onset of the uremic syndrome. It should be avoided, even when nephrotic syndrome is present, because it increases urinary protein losses. There have been many controlled prospective studies to determine whether restriction of dietary protein, as in some experimental animal models, can retard loss of nephrons and progression of renal disease by modifying nephron adaptation, especially reduction of glomerular capillary hypertension. For the majority of patients with chronic renal failure any small decrease in rate of progression when dietary protein is reduced to 0.6 g/kg per 24 hours is balanced against the danger of negative nitrogen balance and malnutrition. The team supervising patients on such diets must include an experienced dietician.

Anorexia, an early, troubling symptom in patients with chronic renal failure, complicates such attempts to reduce protein intake but maintain adequate caloric intake, often combined with dietary salt restriction and other dietary modifications for hyperlipidemia, diabetes, and so forth. Most patients can avoid a high protein intake, and a goal of 0.8 g/kg per 24 hours is feasible and safe. There is now good evidence that patients spontaneously and progressively reduce their dietary protein intakes as GFR falls. Indeed, in one study unregulated intake fell to 0.5 g/kg per 24 hours when creatinine clearance was less than 20 ml/minute.

Malnutrition and negative nitrogen balance, demonstrated by weight loss, muscle atrophy and weakness, dryness and scaling of the skin, and falling serum albumin and transferrin levels, is a bad prognostic factor in patients with chronic renal failure, both before and after the initiation of renal replacement therapy. Morbidity and mortality are clearly increased. Good nutrition must be maintained, and dialysis is initiated if it cannot be. Rigid dietary protein restriction to levels less than 0.8 g/kg per 24 hours should be avoided unless dialysis is not available.

Once dialysis is initiated, protein intake is increased to 1.2 g/kg per 24 hours, in part because amino acids are lost during both hemodialysis (10 to 12 g per procedure) and peritoneal dialysis (12 g/24 hours, and more during peritonitis). Monitoring of adequacy of nutrition must continue; if the serum albumin level falls below normal, a considerable increase in mortality risk occurs.

Increased protein catabolism in renal failure is due in part to metabolic acidosis, and this should be treated with sodium bicarbonate or citrate, with care taken to avoid sodium overload. Metabolic acidosis

also contributes to renal bone disease because of buffering of protons in bone and loss of calcium hydroxyapatite. Secondary hyperparathyroidism also contributes to muscle protein catabolism; other hormonal disturbances, especially with action of insulin, probably also play a role. Plasma and intracellular amino acid levels are abnormal; levels of branched chain amino acids such as valine and leucine are low. Uremia also alters the distribution of amino acids and proteins between cells and extracellular fluids.

Disorders of Carbohydrate Metabolism. Fasting blood glucose level is normal or slightly elevated in uremia. However, after oral or intravenous administration of glucose loads, carbohydrate tolerance is impaired. Several factors may be responsible for this abnormality. Skeletal muscle shows resistance to the action of insulin on glucose uptake, and uremia reduces insulin release. Increased levels of growth hormone present in uremia may also contribute to the resistance of peripheral tissues to the action of insulin. Basal insulin levels in uremic patients are usually increased, presumably as a consequence of a decreased rate of renal removal of insulin. Although glucagon levels are elevated in uremia, their contribution to the glucose intolerance is not clear. In addition, increased gluconeogenesis and increased hepatic glucose release have also been proposed as mechanisms responsible for carbohydrate intolerance in uremic subjects. Other factors, such as acidosis, potassium depletion, hypermagnesemia, and increased levels of parathyroid hormone, may also play a role in the glucose intolerance of the uremic state.

It has been demonstrated that carbohydrate tolerance improves after hemodialysis and that the response of peripheral tissues to insulin is increased. Diabetic patients with progressive renal disease require diminishing doses of insulin as the disease progresses. Reduced caloric intake and weight loss, plus a reduced renal degradation of insulin, probably play a role in this decreased insulin requirement. Oral hypoglycemic agents must be employed with caution because both the reduced renal rate of excretion of the drug itself and the reduced rate of degradation of the insulin produced can, together, cause troublesome hypoglycemia. In patients with diabetes mellitus who are receiving dialysis, tight glucose control is difficult and postprandial levels greater than 250 to 300 mg/dl may have to be accepted.

Steroid-induced diabetes mellitus occurs in 5% to 10% of all graft recipients. Ketoacidosis is rarely noted, and the steroid-induced diabetes may remit with reductions of steroid dosage.

Disorders of Lipid Metabolism. Uremic patients have elevated serum levels of triglycerides and lipoproteins. Lp(a) level is elevated and may contribute to increased cardiovascular risk. There is a decreased rate of removal of triglycerides from the plasma, as well as decreased activity of lipoprotein lipase and increased hepatic synthesis of very-low-density lipoproteins (VLDLs). The plasma levels of high-density lipoprotein (HDL), alpha-lipoprotein, and low-density, cholesterol-rich lipoprotein (LDL) are decreased. Plasma cholesterol levels are usually normal in uremia but elevated after renal transplantation. In renal failure these abnormalities of carbohydrate and lipid metabolism presumably contribute to increased risk of atherogenesis, which may be troublesome in patients receiving long-term dialysis. No consensus on treatment exists. Disturbances of lipid metabolism also occur in nephrotic patients (Chapter 306) with and without chronic renal insufficiency. A majority of patients with uremia and hyperlipidemia, however, are not nephrotic; moreover, their lipid profile differs from that of nephrotic patients who have increased cholesterol levels.

Abnormalities in Endocrine Function

Uremia alters virtually all hormones in the body, either in amount or in their effect. The mechanisms of these disturbances are complex, involving decreased renal clearance, altered receptor activity, altered protein binding, and interference with feedback controls. Not only the hormones arising within the kidney are affected by renal failure, but also those being produced elsewhere. The levels of calcitonin in plasma, as determined by radioimmunoassay, are elevated, probably as a result of a decreased rate of metabolic clearance by the kidney.

Patients with renal failure can appear hypothyroid, and abnormalities in thyroid function tests are common; these abnormalities include normal free T4 but low free T3 levels (diminished T4-to-T3 conversion in periphery) and diminished binding of T4 to thyroid-binding globulin. A sensitive thyroid-stimulating hormone (TSH) assay is the most helpful test for true hypothyroidism.

Gonadal dysfunction is characteristic of ESRD. Menstrual irregularities are very frequent; menstruation often ceases completely in ESRD, and amenorrhea may persist on dialysis. Menorrhagia occasionally occurs as a result of the hemostatic defect if menses recur. When GFR values fall below 20 ml/minute, both conception and the ability to complete a pregnancy are severely impaired. Impotence and a diminished sperm count are common in men with chronic renal failure.

These abnormalities in both men and women are secondary to gonadal resistance to the effects of follicle-stimulating hormone and luteinizing hormone, to complex hypothalamic-pituitary disturbances, and to hyperprolactinemia. Men have diminished concentrations of testosterone in plasma, and both progesterone and estrogen are diminished in women. Gynecomastia is sometimes seen before, and despite, dialysis treatment. In men, administration of testosterone has been shown to suppress plasma luteinizing hormone, although with a slightly delayed response. Thus in the patient with chronic renal failure gonadal resistance to the effect of pituitary trophic hormones is a major factor in sexual inadequacy. Depression is not uncommon in dialysis patients, and it may contribute, along with insomnia and poor nutritional intake, to sexual dysfunction.

TREATMENT

Treatment for chronic renal failure can be divided into *conservative treatment* and, for ESRD, *renal replacement therapy.* After general and comparative discussion of treatment here, the sections Dialysis and Renal Transplantation take up these topics in more detail.

Conservative Treatment

Conservative treatment includes specific measures (e.g., an ACE inhibitor in diabetic nephropathy) for the disease causing chronic renal failure. Accurate measurement of rate of progression of renal disease, however, is difficult. Blood urea nitrogen levels reflect many variables other than GFR. Especially in the early stages of progressive renal diseases, changes in serum creatinine may be a poor early indicator of accelerating renal deterioration. Contrary to previous views, altering protein (meat) intake does alter serum levels. Creatinine clearance progressively overestimates GFR as serum creatinine level increases. Even measurement of true GFR may miss maintenance of the GFR by adaptation of remaining intact nephrons. Worsening proteinuria may indicate such an event. Increased activity of the urinary sediment may also indicate recurrent glomerular damage, as in lupus nephritis. In general, therapeutic measures that reduce proteinuria improve prognosis.

All patients receiving conservative therapy should have renal function, serum electrolytes, calcium and phosphorus, and hematocrit monitored regularly after serum creatinine exceeds 2.5 to 3.0 mg/dl. Individual patients with chronic renal failure tend to deteriorate at a constant rate; this may best be seen when the reciprocal of the serum creatinine level is plotted serially. An accelerated rate of deterioration should engender a search for remediable factors (see Table 110-2). Measures to prevent renal bone disease should be initiated. As discussed, even mild elevation of blood pressure must be treated: this is the single most valuable intervention to retard progression. In the absence of specific contraindications an ACE inhibitor and a loop diuretic are used initially, followed by a calcium channel blocker as needed. If serum bicarbonate level falls below normal, exogenous bicarbonate in small amounts is indicated (each 650-mg tablet of sodium bicarbonate contains 8 mEq each of sodium and of bicarbonate). Each gram of protein in the diet leads to production of approximately 1 mEq of hydrogen ions. Usually, in the absence of renal tubular acidosis and frank bicarbonate wasting, three or four sodium bicarbonate tablets per day are adequate.

Chronic metabolic acidosis should be treated for the reasons discussed, as well as to maintain plasma bicarbonate and prevent life-threatening acidemia if an acute problem develops that leads to catabolism and increased production of hydrogen ions.

Care must be taken with all potentially nephrotoxic drugs and in determining the dosage of all drugs that are excreted substantially by the renal route. Several useful drug dosage lists are maintained and should be consulted regularly by physicians seeing patients with chronic renal failure. If no alternative is available, potentially nephrotoxic drugs such as the aminoglycosides can be used with appropriate modification in dosage or dosing intervals; but, whenever feasible, monitoring of serum levels is indicated. Digoxin dosage always has to be reduced below normal maintenance levels. Glycoside-induced anorexia and vomiting can be confused with uremia.

Dietary salt restriction should be instituted only for management of edema, hypertension, or congestive heart failure. However, most patients with GFR approaching 10 to 15 ml/minute do require modest salt restriction (1 to 2 g sodium or 44 to 88 mEq Na$^+$ in the diet). Potassium restriction (40 to 50 mEq K$^+$) is usually not needed until GFR approaches 10 ml/minute unless specific tubular defects are present. As noted, however, increased potassium intake is tolerated poorly, and potassium supplements with diuretics and "potassium-sparing" diuretics such as spironolactone should generally be avoided. Beta blockers, nonsteroidal antiinflammatory drugs (NSAIDs), and ACE inhibitors also increase the risk of hyperkalemia.

Compliance with prescribed dietary protein restriction may be checked by observing the BUN:creatinine ratio, which should be less than the normal 10:1 in patients ingesting a low-protein diet with adequate caloric intake, and by measuring urinary urea excretion, as discussed earlier. A commonly used but never routinely prescribed diet in the later stages of conservative treatment is 0.8 g protein/kg body weight (plus an allowance for urinary protein losses if still high), 2 g Na$^+$ (88 mEq), and 40 mEq K$^+$. In some patients hyperkalemia also requires the oral administration of sodium-potassium exchange resins; 1 g of sodium polystyrene sulfonate (Kayexalate) binds approximately 1 mEq of potassium. However, the sodium-potassium exchange process results in a net gain of sodium, and dialysis must be instituted if hyperkalemia returns. Fluid restriction is not required unless there is significant hyponatremia, but fluid should not be pushed beyond what thirst dictates. Symptomatic anemia can be treated with subcutaneous erythropoietin.

Planning for renal replacement therapy should begin well before ESRD has been reached; ESRD begins usually at a GFR of 5 to 10 ml/minute (serum creatinine >7 to 8 mg/dl in women and >10 to 12 mg/dl in men). An arteriovenous fistula between radial artery and cephalic vein is constructed a few months before dialysis is required; if the vessels are unsuitable, a synthetic arteriovenous graft is used. These procedures are usually performed with the patient under local or regional anesthesia. Neither of these procedures offers immediately available access to the blood for dialysis and in emergency access is obtained via an internal jugular or femoral venous catheter. The former can be maintained for a few weeks or longer if a subcutaneous tunnel is used. A full explanation of the various treatment options available should be given to the patient. This procedure may require several visits to a renal treatment center. If live donor transplantation is feasible, arrangements are made for tissue typing of family members. Proper planning and preparation of the patient allows efficient initiation of renal replacement therapy and avoids complications and catastrophes. Patients who present late with uremic symptoms often require long hospitalizations and have delayed rehabilitation and even increased mortality rates.

Timing of initiation of renal replacement therapy requires careful, regular evaluation of patient well-being, nutrition, and cardiovascular status, as well as of serum chemistry studies, including serum albumin. The goal is to avoid, on the one hand, a uremic trough of illness, but, on the other hand, not to initiate expensive therapy prematurely. It is unusual for a patient not to need such treatment after the serum creatinine level is greater than 10 mg/dl in women and greater than 15 mg/dl in men. Congestive heart failure or fluid retention, severe anemia, severe hypertension, hyperkalemia, and sensory peripheral neuropathy all may indicate earlier initiation. Severe uremic complications (e.g., pericarditis and malnutrition) usually result from too long a delay in initiating renal replacement therapy. In patients with diabetic glomerulosclerosis, replacement therapy is initiated earlier (serum creatinine level, 5 to 8 mg/dl) than in primary renal disease because there is a compounding of many of the features of diabetic microangiopathy by uremia.

Renal Replacement Therapy

Although all patients with chronic renal failure nearing ESRD should be considered for renal replacement therapy, the obligation to the patient is not to provide such care uncritically but, rather, to determine if the patient will benefit from it. Patients with intractable, irremediable, severely disabling disease in other organ systems who would clearly not benefit from dialysis or transplantation should receive only conservative treatment. In cases of doubt as to benefit, and with the agreement of patient and family, a trial of dialysis can be initiated; later cessation of dialysis by mutual consent of physician, patient, and family is ethical. Chronic dialysis in patients with established acquired immunodeficiency syndrome (AIDS) and ESRD extends life in most patients by only a brief period and is, in general, not indicated; however, each patient should be evaluated individually. Chronic or acute dialysis, but not renal transplantation, is usually indicated for acute or chronic renal failure in asymptomatic human immunodeficiency virus (HIV) carriers.

The various options for renal replacement therapy are summarized in Fig. 110-5. To date the number of patients on chronic dialysis (currently approximately 200,000) has not reached a plateau because the annual mortality (23% if all age-groups are included) plus the annual successful transplantation rate (currently about 10,300 of the 12,000 performed) is less than the annual influx of about 60,000 new patients with ESRD. Median age at onset of ESRD is now 63 years, and 70% of the overall ESRD population is more than 45 years of age. The renal transplantation waiting list has 30,000 patients on it. Thus most patients will require some form of dialysis to survive. The various forms of renal replacement should be highly integrated (Fig. 110-5); many patients will receive various forms at different times. Some patients who receive live donor kidneys now do so without preliminary dialysis. Fifty percent of all ESRD patients ages 20 to 44 years have a functioning transplant as compared to 4% older than age 65 years. The growth of continuous ambulatory peritoneal dialysis (CAPD) has been dramatic and is substantially responsible for the 16% of patients receiving home dialysis. The patient should be fully informed about all appropriate options and involved in the choice of treatment. Important differences among the main treatment alternatives can be seen in Table 110-3.

Younger patients without major extrarenal disease fare well with all three modes of renal replacement treatment. Children are best managed by CAPD first, then renal transplantation when feasible (the incidence of children reaching ESRD is relatively small (12 million per year in the age-group 0 to 19 years). Live donor transplantation offers the best results in virtually all patients except the elderly, in the absence of contraindications to transplantation. However, there is no specific age limit for transplantation.

Patient education for CAPD takes about 1 week compared with 6 weeks for home hemodialysis. CAPD allows more mobility and does not require a partner, in contrast to home hemodialysis. These methods are cheaper than in-center hemodialysis and are encouraged by the Medicare program by financial incentives to the patient and the dialysis center. CAPD and transplantation offer specific advantages to patients with type I diabetes: intraperitoneal insulin offers good glucose control, and peritoneal dialysis avoids the need for vascular access in such patients, who often have peripheral vascular disease and may develop distal ischemia after a graft or fistula. In hemodialysis patients infection (most often, staphylococcal) and thrombosis of the vascular access are the most common causes of admission to the hospital, whereas in CAPD patients the most common cause is peritonitis. Thrombosis of a graft or fistula is often preceded by venous stenosis, which is detectable by venography and treatable by angioplasty. Problems associated with prednisone and other long-term immunosuppressive drugs after transplantation are discussed in the section Renal Transplantation.

Rehabilitation after renal replacement therapy is negatively influenced by increasing age, presence of systemic diseases such as diabetes mellitus, and a poor work record before ESRD and is best after successful renal transplantation at any age. This is counterbalanced, however, by some negative effects of failed renal transplants. In one survey of rehabilitation in dialysis patients, as many as 40% to 50% were poorly rehabilitated. The 1-year mortality rate for dialysis in all patients was 23% in 1992. It is markedly affected by age (e.g., 11% in the 20- to 44-year-old and 33% in the 65- to 74-year-old age-groups; for 5 years, the rates are 50% and 80%, respectively). Another major factor adversely affecting mortality is diabetes mellitus as a cause of ESRD. There is a lesser mortality rate in transplantation than in dialysis patients of the same age, but no strictly controlled prospective studies exist. The most important causes of death in dialysis patients are cardiovascular (myocardial infarction, congestive heart failure, and stroke); collectively, these causes are responsible for 55% of the deaths. Infection (15%) is also a significant cause of death. Withdrawal from dialysis by the patient or guardian, mainly because of dementia, cachexia, or malignancy, is not infrequent.

Overall, dialysis mortality (1996) is now improving as a result of increased attention to adequacy of dialysis clearance of small solutes (e.g., urea) and combined awareness of the importance of good nutrition and adequate control of hypertension.

An important new dialysis complication is *acquired renal cystic disease*. This occurs in as many as 90% of patients who receive dialysis for 5 to 10 years. It probably relates to growth factors responsible for the adaptation of nephrons in chronic renal failure and is important because malignancy and metastases can develop in a small but as yet uncertain percentage of cases. Histologic examination usually reveals a papillary type of tumor. Screening of all dialysis patients by renal ultrasonography is now recommended after 3 years of dialysis at 1- to 2-year intervals. Cysts often resolve after successful renal transplantation, but transplantation candidates must be screened for this disease.

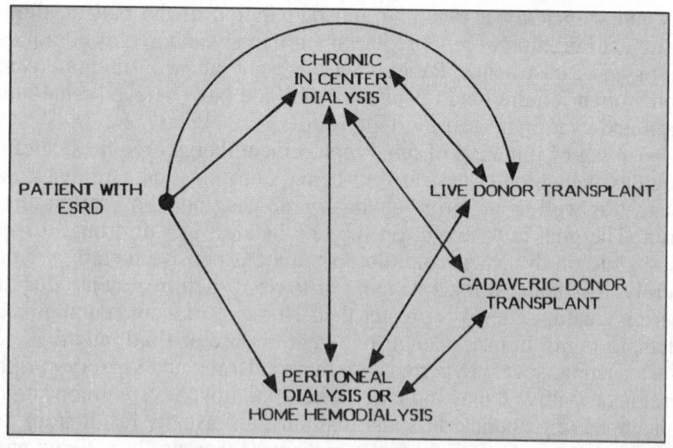

FIGURE 110-5 Interrelationships between types of renal replacement therapy. The success of transplantation is aided by the ready availability of dialysis if the allograft fails.

Table 110-3 Renal replacement therapy: Important clinical differences among major alternatives

	HEMODIALYSIS	CAPD*	TRANSPLANT
Dependence on machine	Yes	No	No
Excretory function	10% of normal	<10% of normal†	May be normal
Endocrine function	No‡	No	Yes
Major surgery	No	No	Yes
Immunosuppressive drugs	No	No	Yes
Vascular access problems	Yes	No	No
Peritoneal catheter problems and peritonitis	No	Yes	No
Regular exposure to heparin	Yes	No	No

*CAPD, continuous ambulatory peritoneal dialysis. Patients on continuous cycling (CCAD) do use an automatic cycler.
†Percentage is better for higher-molecular-weight substances, as compared with hemodialysis.
‡Erythropoietin and calcitriol can be replaced.

DIALYSIS
Principles of Dialysis Treatment

All forms of readily available dialysis depend on diffusion of small molecules across a semipermeable membrane, extracorporeal with a synthetic cellulose membrane in hemodialysis and intracorporeal with a biologic membrane in peritoneal dialysis. Dialysate must be sterile for peritoneal dialysis, but the semipermeable synthetic membranes exclude bacteria (though not endotoxin). Therefore the dialysate does not need to be sterile, although prescribed limits for bacterial counts exist.

The principles of dialysis are outlined in Fig. 110-6. Solute can be removed from the blood (or as appropriate to the chemical gradient, can enter the blood) by diffusion or by convection when fluid is removed from the blood either by an osmotic gradient (e.g., high glucose in the peritoneal dialysate fluid) or by a hydrostatic gradient (e.g., by negative pressure on the dialysate side). A typical dialysate composition would be Na^+ 140, K^+ 3 (variable), Cl^- 105, HCO_3^- 35, and Ca^{2+} 3.5 mEq/L; because only the ionized fraction exchanges, calcium diffuses into the blood in most patients; a lower-calcium dialysate can be used to treat hypercalcemia and is sometimes now necessary if a high intake of calcium-binding agents for phosphate is being used. In hemodialysis patients dialysate contains glucose at 100 mg/dl; in peritoneal dialysis patients dialysate contains large amounts of glucose (1.5 to 4.25 g/dl) as an osmotic agent; Na^+ is usually 132, and K^+ 0 mEq/L. Because the blood of dialysis patients is exposed to about 120 L of dialysate fluid per dialysis session, special preparation of the water is required to remove trace metals and other substances present in tap water. Reverse osmosis and deionization techniques are used to prepare dialysate water for chronic dialysis patients. Because this process has become routine, a syndrome of dialysis dementia attributable to aluminum intoxication has become very rare.

In all forms of dialysis water-soluble vitamins may be lost from the blood. Routinely, dialysis patients should receive vitamin supplements, including B vitamins, vitamin C, and folate. Oral iron is usually also required, especially in chronic hemodialysis patients, because small amounts of blood (5 to 10 ml) unavoidably remain in the dialyzer after the dialysis procedure.

Both hemodialysis and peritoneal dialysis can be used to remove certain poisons acutely and to treat acute renal failure (Chapter 109) or chronic renal failure with an acute superimposed problem (e.g., surgery) for periods of a few days to a few weeks. Temporary access can be obtained immediately by a femoral or subclavian catheter. The Scribner shunt permitted the introduction of long-term dialysis in the early 1960s, but is now replaced for long-term access by the arteriovenous fistula (often radiocephalic) or prosthetic graft. Short-term peritoneal dialysis can also be used for acute renal failure; a tempo-

rary catheter can be inserted at the bedside. Many nephrologists now prefer to use a Tenckhoff catheter from the beginning because of reduced risk of infection. Relative indications for peritoneal or hemodialysis in acute renal failure are discussed in Chapter 109.

Hemodialysis

A typical circuit for hemodialysis is shown in Fig. 110-7. An artificial kidney is made up of a dialysate delivery system, a blood pump to deliver blood at 150 to 450 ml/minute from the arterial needle inserted in the cannula or fistula, various safety monitoring devices, and a dialyzer, in which actual dialysis takes place. The major dialyzer now is the hollow fiber dialyzers; blood flow and dialysate flow (the latter usually at 500 ml/min) are countercurrent. Dialyzers are now commonly reused by the same patient for economic reasons. Patients require small amounts of heparin (3000 to 10,000 units) either intermittently or by infusion during the procedure. In some patients with severe coagulopathy or active bleeding it is possible with careful monitoring of activated clotting times to avoid the use of heparin. The usual duration of dialysis is 3 to 6 hours depending on patient size, level of persisting endogenous renal function, BUN level, creatinine level, and the like before dialysis, as well as on the amounts of ECF to be removed. The latter can be calculated from the ultrafiltration coefficient of the membrane and the net transmembrane hydraulic pressure; more than 3 L/hour can be removed. A physician's order for dialysis would normally indicate duration of dialysis, type of access, arterial flow rate, type of dialyzer (several are available with different dialysis characteristics and extracorporeal volumes), anticoagulant dose, type of dialysate, and "dry weight" of the patient. The dry weight is an important concept in the chronic dialysis patient: it is the postdialysis weight at which the patient has an acceptable blood pressure and a plasma volume adequate for avoiding diminished cardiac output and lung congestion. Most patients receiving long-term hemodialysis need dialysis three times weekly, and the predialysis BUN level in patients ingesting 1.2 g protein/kg should be less than 90 mg/dl for optimal management.

High-flux, high-efficiency dialysis uses synthetic (e.g., polyacrilonitrile [PAN]) membranes with increased solute clearance and hydraulic permeability and is best for selected patients with access blood flows of 300 ml/minute or more and interdialytic weight gains that are moderate (<4 L). Its principal advantages are diminished time requirements (as little as 2 hours for smaller patients) and fewer hypotensive complications, but it does require more expensive equipment and monitoring devices and higher rates of blood flow from the

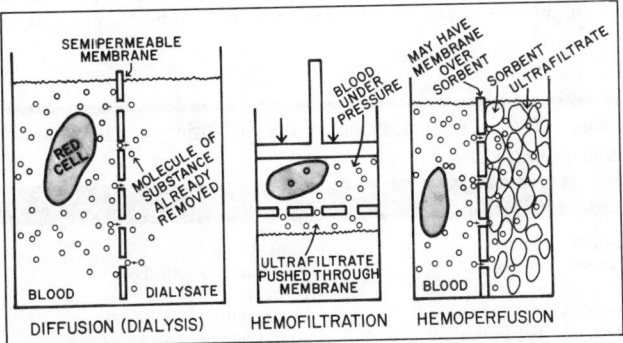

FIGURE 110-6   Mechanisms for removing substances from blood include diffusion of solute across a semipermeable membrane into a dialysis solution, or dialysate *(left)*, and convective movement of solute along with the bulk flow of water. The fluid movement (ultrafiltration) may be initiated by hydraulic or osmotic pressure *(middle)* or by absorption of solute to a sorbent *(right)*. The blood may be separated from the sorbent by a membrane coating; solute and water cross the membrane by diffusion and ultrafiltration.

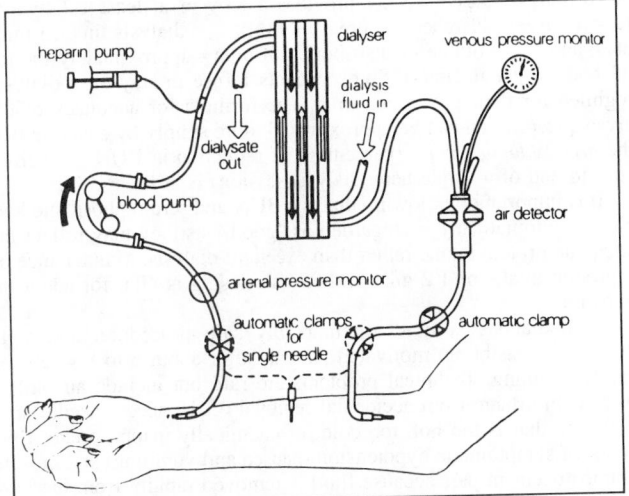

FIGURE 110-7   Essential components of an artificial kidney in use for hemodialysis. The apparatus for using a single needle for inflow and outflow of blood from the patient is shown by a dashed line.

From Drukker W, Parsons M, Maher JF, editors: *Replacement of renal function by dialysis,* ed 2, Boston, 1983, Martinus Nijhoff.

vascular access. The new membranes, in contrast to the older cellulose membranes, are not only more permeable but are more biocompatible. The latter relates to cell (lymphocytes, monocytes, polymorphonuclear leukocytes) membrane interactions during hemodialysis with resulting release of cytokines such as interleukin-1 (IL-1), tumor necrosis factor (TNF), and activation of complement with subsequent leukocyte sequestration in the lungs, associated in the first hour of dialysis with leukopenia. These may contribute to minor febrile effects during dialysis, to slight hypoxia, and even to a modest catabolic effect of dialysis itself. The new membranes substantially diminish or avoid these cell-activating effects, but their increased permeability may allow back-flux of small endotoxin molecules from dialysate.

Improved bioengineering now allows controlled rates of ultrafiltration of excess fluid so that fluid removal is much more predictable, and hypotension, nausea, and muscle cramps during the procedure are much reduced. As solutes are removed from plasma during hemodialysis, gradients are set up between, for example, muscle and brain cells and extracellular fluid, especially in too-rapid initial hemodialysis of a patient with chronic or acute renal failure with a high BUN level. When this happens, a dialysis disequilibrium syndrome can develop, with headache and even seizures and focal central nervous system signs. This problem is avoided by initial slow daily dialysis for shorter periods and with lower blood flow rates. In chronic dialysis patients symptoms are much less severe but can be minimized by controlling dialysate sodium concentration ("sodium modeling") so that it is initially high and combats the cell-plasma gradient. Too high a dialysate sodium level, however, can induce thirst, excess weight gain in the interdialytic period, and hypertension. Most dialyzers are now reused perhaps 4 to 20 times for cost reasons. Careful interdialytic storage and sterilization are critical. Reuse has diminished patient side effects such as "first use syndrome" (urticaria, back pain, and hypotension), which relates to plasma protein membrane interactions with high immunoglobulin E (IgE) levels in blood. This reaction is less likely because reuse is associated with "lining" of the membrane by the patient's own platelets and protein. Residual capacity of the dialyzer is tested before each use.

Together with erythropoietin, these upgrades in dialysis techniques have improved the dialysis patients' lives; there is less hypotension, nausea, and postdialysis "exhaustion," especially if the patient is compliant with minimizing interdialytic weight gain and maintains good nutrition.

With shorter dialysis times and an increased variety of dialyzers with different solute clearance and ultrafiltration capacities, more precise "prescription" of individualized dialysis for patients is necessary. It is now well established that *adequate dialysis* in patients who receive dialysis thrice weekly provides a Kt/v of at least 1.2 (where K = dialyzer clearance for urea [ml/min], t = dialysis time in minutes, and v = volume of distribution of urea—approximately the total body water in liters). Some patients refuse to stay on a dialysis regimen for their prescribed time. The formula for adequacy of dialysis prescription can be approximated more simply by ensuring that the *urea reduction ratio* (percentage of reduction in BUN level from start to end of a single hemodialysis session) is at least 60%.

It is important that low predialysis BUN and serum phosphate levels not automatically be regarded as "good," as they may reflect inadequate protein intake rather than excellent dialysis. Maintenance of a protein intake of 1.2 g/kg and 35 calories/kg is vital for adequate nutrition.

Hemodialysis is now a remarkably safe procedure, and self-dialysis is feasible in motivated patients after about 6 to 8 weeks of careful training. Technical problems are rare but include air embolism, hemorrhage from accidental removal of the access needle, and dialysate that is too hot, too cold, or chemically inappropriate. Episodes of symptomatic hypotension (nausea and vomiting) and muscle cramps occur in part because fluid is removed rapidly from the vascular compartment but then has to be mobilized from the extracellular space (analogous to overrapid diuresis with diuretics). Muscle cramps can usually be treated by slowing ultrafiltration and by infusion of small amounts of hypertonic mannitol, saline, or glucose. Atypical hypotension should raise the consideration of pericarditis or another cardiac event, sepsis, or bleeding.

During dialysis there is often an associated modest decrease in arterial oxygen levels. It has been shown that carbon dioxide is lost from the blood when acetate, not bicarbonate with bubbled carbon dioxide, is used in the dialysis solution; hypocapnia may result in slowing of respiration and a decrease in arterial oxygen level of 10 to 30 mm Hg. In a few patients with cardiac or respiratory tract disease, oxygen administration during dialysis is indicated. As noted, pulmonary sequestration of leukocytes may also contribute to hypoxia.

When dialysis is terminated, the artificial kidney is usually rinsed with saline and the blood is returned to the patient. However, a blood residue of up to 10 ml remains in the artificial kidney and so is lost to the patient. Over a prolonged period, total blood loss in the dialyzer may be substantial.

Viral hepatitis can be transmitted by blood. Thus carriers of the hepatitis virus expose dialysis personnel and other patients to an increased risk of viral hepatitis, particularly if any drops of blood are allowed to contaminate the surrounding area during the process of initiating hemodialysis or at the end of dialysis. Although hepatitis epidemics have occurred among patients and personnel in some dialysis programs, an epidemic can usually be avoided if proper precautions are taken. These universal precautions are also effective against blood transmission of HIV, which is much less infective than the hepatitis B virus. HIV carriers do not need to receive dialysis in separate facilities, but hepatitis B carriers should receive dialysis in that manner. Active immunization for hepatitis B should be given to all dialysis patients and staff who do not have immunity. It is likely that hepatitis C virus can also be transmitted by dialysis, and carrier rates are increased in dialysis patients.

Hemodialysis can pose some risk to patients who have cardiovascular instability. During hemodialysis, blood pressure may fall (primarily as a result of rapid removal of sodium and water from the vascular space), even though the patient has expanded extravascular ECF spaces and, often, obvious edema. As noted, removal of fluid and sodium from the vascular space may not be accompanied by rapid mobilization of edema fluid into the vascular bed. Rapid, severe blood pressure decreases may compromise blood flow through diseased coronary arteries or the cerebral circulation and result in myocardial infarction, seizure, or stroke. Such patients may be better managed by peritoneal dialysis.

Common complications of the hemodialysis procedure of potential interest to the generalist are listed (Table 110-4).

Peritoneal Dialysis

The Tenckhoff catheter for chronic intermittent or continuous peritoneal dialysis is about 25 cm long and consists of intraperitoneal (pelvic), subcutaneous, and extracorporeal sections. Patients receiving chronic intermittent peritoneal dialysis use this catheter for instillation of fluid into, and drainage from, the abdominal cavity. CAPD patients usually perform three to five exchanges per day of 1.5 to 3.0 L of dialysate. Solution is instilled from plastic bags. A connecting tube allows the empty bag to remain attached to the chronic catheter,

---

Table 110-4 "Complications" of dialysis during or a few hours after procedure*

CLINICAL	LABORATORY
Slight fever	Leukopenia
Muscle cramps	Respiratory alkalosis
Hypotension†	Hypoxia
Cardiac arrhythmia	Eosinophilia‡
Dialysis disequilibrium	Anion gap acidosis§
Rebound hypertension‖	Hypoglycemia#
Steal syndrome distal to access	Hypokalemia; "rebound" increase in blood urea nitrogen

*Transient unless otherwise indicated.
†Increased nitric oxide production possible.
‡May be chronic.
§Only with acetate as base in dialysate.
‖Only in renin-dependent hypertension.
#Only with glucose-free dialysate.

and the bag is used later for receiving drainage. The bag of drainage fluid is replaced with a fresh bag of solution and then is discarded. Y-shaped transfer sets have led to "bagless" CAPD. The bag is needed only for infusion and drainage. This technique provides continuous slow dialysis, which has the advantage that it maintains essentially steady-state body fluid levels and thus avoids rapid fluctuations in body fluid solute concentrations and too-rapid shifts in body fluid compartments. On average, patients on CAPD have one episode of peritonitis per each 9- to 12-month period of dialysis. Most of these episodes are mild, are due to gram-positive organisms from the skin, and respond to an increased rate of peritoneal exchange and to intraperitoneal or oral antibiotics. A modification of CAPD that uses an automatic cycling machine (cycler) at night during sleep with one CAPD exchange during the day (continuous cycling peritoneal dialysis or CCPD) is gaining in popularity, especially for those who wish to work or need help with their connections during exchanges.

CAPD, as compared with hemodialysis, has the additional advantages of avoiding the cardiovascular stress and eliminating the need for vascular access. Disadvantages include the high glucose load, which can cause obesity and aggravate hyperlipidemia, development of hernias, and the more likely eventual loss of peritoneal as compared with vascular access (one abdomen versus four limbs). Ostomies and marked obesity are strong relative contraindications.

An increasing number of patients are remaining on this treatment modality for 10 years or more. Ultrafiltration failure sometimes occurs after many episodes of peritonitis as a result of a sclerosing peritonitis. This complication usually necessitates transfer to hemodialysis. Peritoneal function can be tested by measuring dialysate/plasma ratios over time for urea and creatinine levels, rate of fall of peritoneal glucose concentration, and fluid ultrafiltration rates.

Peritonitis is most often due to gram-positive skin organisms. The peritoneal dialysate fluid becomes cloudy and has a cell count greater than 100 cells/mm^3 with more than 50% polymorphonuclear leukocytes. Multiple gram-negative or anaerobic organisms suggest a perforated viscus (but remember that subphrenic free air may occur in peritoneal dialysis patients "normally") or diverticulitis. An elevated peritoneal fluid amylase level suggests intraabdominal disease. Relapsing infections suggest a tunnel infection or catheter colonization. Fungal infection or relapsing infection usually requires catheter removal and a period of a few weeks of appropriate treatment while receiving hemodialysis. Protein losses increase considerably during episodes of peritonitis.

Adequacy of peritoneal dialysis is now measured as K_{pr} t/V, and 1.7 is the prescribed minimum (for a 70-kg man receiving CAPD at 2-L exchanges four times a day, dialysate collections of 10 L/day, and a dialysate–blood urea ratio of 1.0, $K_{pr}t$ = 70 L; V is the urea space [i.e., total body water, 42 kg]; and $K_{pr}t/V$ = 1.7). This value should be obtained on a dietary protein intake of 1.2 g/day and serum albumin level should be above 3.5 g/dl. Increases in dialysis clearance are obtained by increasing exchanges to five per day (or CCPD) and increasing exchange volume to 2.5 or 3 L.

A comparison of solute clearances by hemodialysis, intermittent peritoneal dialysis, CAPD, and the normal kidney is given in Table 110-5.

Other Forms of Dialysis

Other forms of dialysis include isolated ultrafiltration, in which no dialysate is used, for patients with a marked need for fluid removal. This approach is especially important if hypotension and diminished cardiac output are problems because hypotension is less when solute is not simultaneously removed by diffusion. Similarly, hemofiltration (see Fig. 110-6) occurs when fluid and solute are removed by ultrafiltration (not diffusion) across an unusually permeable synthetic membrane, similar to glomerular filtration in vivo. An arterial pump is not required, and this type of dialysis can be performed continuously at low rates in certain types of patients with acute renal failure, especially those with a very low cardiac output (continuous arteriovenous hemofiltration [CAVH]). In a more complex type of hemofiltration, which can be used for long-term therapy, immediately before or after this ultrafiltration process the cellular and protein components of the blood are diluted with a replacement solution that ideally contains the essential substances and none of the undesirable ones. This technique is used in Europe but rarely in the United States. To date, it appears to offer no distinct advantage over hemodialysis. Hemoperfusion (see Fig. 110-6) is used, especially, for the treatment of certain lipid-soluble poisons: membrane-coated activated carbon is commonly used in the blood path of a dialysis cartridge.

RENAL TRANSPLANTATION

During the last three decades improvements in immunosuppression, histocompatibility matching, and organ preservation have made transplantation the preferred mode of treatment for many patients with end-stage renal disease (ESRD). One-year allograft survival of 91% for living-related and 84% for cadaveric recipients is now possible, with less mortality than comparably matched patients remaining on a regimen of hemodialysis. This short-term success will allow more attention in the future to be focused on ways to improve long-term allograft survival, eliminate the need for chronic immunosuppression (i.e., tolerance), and obtain organs for those desiring transplantation.

Renal Donors

The major rate-limiting step toward transplantation for over 30,000 patients with ESRD in the United States is the supply of cadaveric kidneys. Cadaveric kidney donation rates have remained static since 1988, while an enlarging ESRD population and less stringent criteria for transplantation have magnified the demand.

The equitable distribution of cadaveric kidneys is overseen by the United Network for Organ Sharing (UNOS). Allocation is based on the desire to restore normal growth and development in pediatric ESRD patients, waiting time, and matching of major histocompatibility antigens (Chapter 172) between donors and recipients. Superior allograft survival for perfectly matched combinations is reflected by the UNOS policy requiring national sharing of these organs between transplantation programs. However, clinically significant survival advantages with lesser degrees of matching have been more difficult to demonstrate, and most of these organs are used locally.

The prolonged wait for a cadaveric organ can be avoided in patients with a suitable living donor. Living-related donor transplantation offers several advantages to the ESRD patient, including a lower risk of acute rejection, lower immunosuppression requirements, and superior long-term allograft survival. These beneficial effects are realized with minimal risk to the donor, provided that a careful screening evaluation is performed. Such an evaluation is provided by the transplantation center at no charge to the donor and designed to exclude underlying medical problems or unrecognized familial renal disease. The methods used to evaluate individual donors vary between institutions but generally include determinants of glomerular filtra-

Table 110-5 Clearances by different dialysis methods as compared with normal kidney

	WEEKLY DURATION	UREA CLEARANCE (ML/MIN)	INULIN CLEARANCE (ML/MIN)
Normal kidney	Continuous	60	120
Hemodialysis	3 × 4 = 12 hours	11 (160)	0.3 (4)
Continuous ambulatory peritoneal dialysis	Continuous	7 (70 L/week)	3

NOTE: Clearances are time-averaged and are exclusive of residual renal function. Figures in parentheses are actual clearances during the procedure. Note that urea (60 daltons) is cleared better during hemodialysis while inulin (5200 daltons) is cleared relatively better by peritoneal dialysis, because of increased permeability of the peritoneal membrane to higher molecular weight solutes. High-flux dialyzers also have increased clearance for larger solutes, such as β_2 microglobulin.

tion rate (GFR) and 24-hour urine protein excretion and an arteriogram to document normal renal anatomy and function. Individual donors are also counseled about the long-term sequelae of kidney donation, such as increases in systolic and diastolic blood pressure without an increase in the prevalence of hypertension, and an initial fall in GFR that increases with time.

The inability of cadaveric and living-related donor transplant donors to meet recipient demand and the recognition that excellent short- and long-term allograft survival is possible with ABO-compatible, living-unrelated transplant donors have led to increasing acceptance of these individuals as organ donors in the United States. Three-year allograft survival of 76% to 87% with living-unrelated donors is similar to that seen with parenteral living-donors and superior to the 70% survival in cadaveric transplant recipients. Despite growing acceptance, most transplantation programs require some degree of emotional attachment (usually spousal) between donor and recipient before serious consideration.

Renal Transplant Recipients

Referral of potential recipients for cadaveric transplantation should be made with the expectation of a 1- to 2-year waiting period for a suitable organ. Because of the uncertainty involved in the waiting process, plans for transplantation and dialysis should be made concomitantly. When potential living-related donors exist, there is greater opportunity to avert the need for dialysis. In such instances, referral should be considered 6 months in advance of the need for dialysis to allow evaluation of the recipient and donors and scheduling of the transplant operation.

Contraindications to renal transplantation are few and consist mainly of recently diagnosed malignancies and active infections that are exacerbated by immunosuppression (Box 110-4).

As a general rule, a 2-year disease-free interval from successful treatment to transplantation is required for any malignancy. In certain instances of breast cancer and malignant melanoma a longer delay may be advisable. No waiting period is necessary following treatment of basal cell carcinoma of the skin or carcinoma in situ.

Active bacterial infections such as peritonitis and catheter-related bacteremia require adequate treatment before transplantation. Patients who are seropositive for the human immunodeficiency virus (HIV) have no survival benefit with transplantation, and accelerated disease progression may develop with immunosuppression. Significant histologic damage from chronic hepatitis B and C infection is unaccompanied by abnormal liver function tests in many ESRD patients. Therefore a liver biopsy may be required in those with viremia before acceptance for transplantation. Patients with biopsy evidence of cirrhosis are excluded as candidates; those with chronic active hepatitis are counseled about the possibility of accelerated disease progression, future liver transplantation, or death. When indicated, alpha interferon (INF-α) should be administered before transplantation, since the immunomodulating effects of this drug may increase the risk of renal allograft loss.

Less common contraindications to transplantation include extensive peripheral vascular disease that precludes the technical success of the operation, coronary artery disease not amenable to bypass grafting, active systemic lupus erythematosus, and social factors that make close follow-up in the early posttransplantation period difficult. Examples of the latter are inadequate family support, psychiatric illness, and active alcohol or drug abuse.

Age is no longer considered an absolute contraindication to transplantation. Successful kidney transplantation in individuals older than age 65 years is possible, although allograft survival is lower than expected because of an increased incidence of death with a functioning graft.

Insulin-dependent diabetics referred for renal transplantation require special consideration, since up to one third have clinically silent coronary artery disease. This is especially true in patients older than age 45 years or in those with long-standing disease ($\geq$25 years), a smoking history, or an abnormal baseline electrocardiogram (ECG). Cardiac catheterization is often required in these individuals before acceptance for transplantation.

Immunosuppression

Many new immunosuppressive drugs with greater specificity of action are emerging and will change the management of future renal transplant recipients. Such an influx of drugs is unparalleled in the brief history of transplantation and makes it difficult to define the optimal regimen for today's recipient. The challenge for the future is to define those combinations with maximal efficacy and minimal toxicity.

Azathioprine has been a cornerstone of posttransplantation immunosuppression since the 1960s. Beneficial effect is derived from the inhibition of purine nucleotide synthesis, which is necessary for rapidly dividing cells such as lymphocytes mounting an immunologic attack. This beneficial action is also responsible for azathioprine's most common side effects, including leukopenia, thrombocytopenia, and anemia. Coadministration of allopurinol further accentuates these side effects and may lead to life-threatening bone marrow suppression. Newer immunosuppressive agents with greater specificity and less bone marrow toxicity are likely to dislodge azathioprine from its current position in immunosuppressive regimens of the future.

As previously mentioned, the combining of azathioprine and corticosteroids enabled successful renal transplantation between genetically disparate individuals. Today, prednisone remains an integral part of posttransplantation immunosuppression. Like azathioprine, prednisone is nonspecific in its actions, modulating the alloimmune response by impairing cytokine synthesis (interleukins 1 and 6 [IL-1 and IL-6], tumor necrosis factor alpha [TNF-α]), macrophage-killing capacity, and expression of major histocompatibility antigens on the surface of endothelial cells. These beneficial effects are accomplished at the expense of increased infections, glucose intolerance, poor wound healing, osteoporosis, growth retardation, and a cushingoid body habitus. Tapering the prednisone dose to a maintenance level of 5 to 10 mg/day in the first few months after transplantation is a primary goal of current immunosuppression protocols. Complete steroid withdrawal from most renal transplant recipients is associated with an unacceptable risk of acute rejection. As more potent immunosuppressive drugs are introduced, repeat attempts at prednisone reduction or withdrawal will undoubtedly be performed to avoid its toxic effects.

Polyclonal and monoclonal antilymphocyte antibodies are used in the immediate posttransplantation period and for the treatment of corticosteroid-resistant acute rejection. The only approved monoclonal preparation, and the most commonly used, is OKT3. OKT3 is a murine, antihuman antibody that binds to the CD3 receptor on the surface of T lymphocytes. Binding interferes with the process of foreign antigen recognition that is necessary for allograft rejection. OKT3 is administered intravenously for 7 to 14 days. Early doses are associated with significant side effects such as fever, chills, hypotension, dyspnea, tachycardia, and diarrhea. Development of anti-

---

BOX 110-4
Contraindications to transplantation

Malignancy
Active infections
Bacterial
Fungal
Mycobacterial
Human immunodeficiency virus
Cirrhosis (hepatitis B and C)

Atherosclerosis
Extensive peripheral vascular disease
Coronary artery disease not amenable to surgery

Active systemic lupus erythematosus
Social factors
Lack of family support
Psychiatric disease
Active alcohol or drug abuse

murine antibodies in recipients occasionally limits effectiveness or repeat administration.

Cyclosporine A (CsA) has gained widespread clinical use since its approval by the U.S. Food and Drug Administration in 1983. The result has been a 10% to 15% improvement in short-term renal allograft survival and the realization of successful heart, liver, and lung transplantation. CsA is now the forerunner of a growing armamentarium of immunosuppressive drugs with a specifically targeted mechanism of action. Therapeutic effect stems from its ability to inhibit IL-2 production, a critical cytokine necessary for proliferation of host lymphocytes directed at the donor organ. Efficacy is marred by erratic bioavailability and significant toxicity. Common side effects include nephrotoxicity, hypertension, hepatotoxicity, neurotoxicity, hyperglycemia, hyperkalemia, hypercholesterolemia, hirsutism, tremor, and gingival hypertrophy. Metabolism via the hepatic cytochrome P450 system provides the opportunity for a number of drug interactions that further complicate its use (Box 110-5). A new formulation of CsA (Neoral) with better bioavailability has recently been approved for use in transplant recipients. It is hoped that this preparation will allow more consistent dosing and alleviate the need for frequent drug-level monitoring, which hamper current administration.

Tacrolimus (FK506) use in renal transplantation remains experimental. Despite being structurally unrelated to CsA, its mechanism of action, metabolism, and propensity for drug interactions are similar. FK506 shares several side effects with CsA, such as nephrotoxicity, neurotoxicity, tremor, and hypertension. Hyperkalemia and hyperglycemia are more common; hypercholesterolemia, hirsutism, and gingival hypertrophy are not seen. FK506 is 10 to 100 times more potent than CsA in vitro, allowing for lower initial and maintenance dosing.

Mycophenolate mofetil (MM) was approved for use in renal transplantation in 1995. This drug inhibits purine nucleotide synthesis in a manner similar to azathioprine. Unlike azathioprine, inhibition can be bypassed in most cells using a salvage pathway that is lacking or insignificant in T and B lymphocytes. Therefore MM expressly targets those cells involved in allograft rejection, with a lower likelihood of bone marrow suppression. Uniform dosing, which does not require adjustment for body weight or surface area, simplifies administration in adults. Side effects are predominantly gastrointestinal tract related and responsive to dose reduction. Early clinical trials with substitution of MM for azathioprine, in combination with prednisone and CsA, report significant reductions in acute rejection and the need for antilymphocyte therapy within the first 6 months after renal transplantation. If continued clinical experience confirms these early findings, MM is likely to become an integral part of future immunosuppressive regimens.

Rapamycin has not yet been approved for use in transplantation. It shares some structural homology and binds to the same intracellular receptor as FK506. Unlike FK506 or CsA, rapamycin does not interfere with cytokine production but appears to impair cytokine-induced cellular responses. Early experience suggests that this drug has potent immunosuppressive properties which may make it a useful addition to future immunosuppressive regimens.

Many of the currently available immunosuppressive drugs are prohibitively expensive, forcing patients to rely on insurance coverage for continuous administration. Loss or cancellation of insurance and financially necessitated noncompliance on the part of the transplant recipient can have disastrous consequences. Some pharmaceutical companies have responded to this crisis by providing free drug to those in need. Such programs currently exist for azathioprine, CsA, and MM.

Allograft Dysfunction

Timely diagnosis and treatment of the transplant recipient with renal dysfunction are important steps in achieving the goal of long-term allograft survival. Arriving at the proper diagnosis can be facilitated by considering causes of renal dysfunction that are more common in the early (i.e., first 6 months) and late posttransplantation periods (Box 110-6).

Hyperacute rejection is characterized by rapid destruction of the allograft following revascularization. It is caused by preformed antibodies in the recipient's circulation to ABO blood group or major histocompatibility antigens—the latter acquired by previous transfusions, pregnancy, or transplantation. Today this complication is seldom seen because of pretransplantation ABO typing and crossmatching of recipient serum and donor lymphocytes. Lysis of donor lymphocytes, following addition of complement to recipient serum, heralds the presence of preexisting antibodies and aborts the transplantation operation. A more sensitive method of antibody detection using flow cytometry has been developed and is useful in recipients with high levels of preformed antibodies or those receiving repeat transplants.

Delayed allograft function is defined as the need for dialysis within the first week after transplantation. Incidence rates vary but are higher with prolonged preservation times (>24 hours) and repeat transplantations. Delayed function complicates the management of renal transplantation recipients and necessitates early administration of antilymphocyte antibodies to avoid the nephrotoxic effects of CsA or FK506. Recent evidence also suggests that delayed function detrimentally impacts allograft survival. This may be due to delays in recognizing acute rejection or the ability of ischemia to increase histocompatibil-

---

BOX 110-5
Cyclosporine drug interactions

Increase cyclosporine levels
Calcium channel blockers
 Verapamil
 Diltiazem
 Nicardipine
 Amlodipine
Antibiotics
 Erythromycin
 Ketoconazole, itraconazole, fluconazole
Bromocriptine
Danazol
Metoclopramide

Decrease cyclosporine levels
Antiepileptics
 Carbamazepine
 Phenobarbital
 Phenytoin
Rifampin
Trimethoprim/sulfamethoxazole

BOX 110-6
Causes of allograft dysfunction

Early
Hyperacute rejection
Delayed allograft function
Accelerated acute rejection
Obstruction
Acute cyclosporine or FK506 nephrotoxicity
Acute rejection
Vascular thrombosis
Recurrent glomerulonephritis

Late
Obstruction
Acute rejection
Chronic rejection
Chronic cyclosporine nephrotoxicity
Recurrent glomerulonephritis
Renal artery stenosis

ity antigen expression on donor cells, increasing their vulnerability to immunologic attack.

Accelerated acute rejection occurs in the first 1 to 2 weeks following transplantation. These episodes are often severe and probably are due to low levels of preformed antibodies in the recipient that were undetected by the cross-matching. Early, aggressive antirejection therapy may sometimes lead to reversal.

Sonographic evidence of mild to moderate pelvicalyceal dilation is often seen in renal transplant recipients in the absence of allograft dysfunction. However, marked dilation indicates functional obstruction, which in the early posttransplantation period is usually due to a collection of lymph or urine. Distinction between the two requires fluid sampling and analysis of creatinine content. Creatinine concentration in lymphatic fluid is similar to serum measurements, whereas urine creatinine level is significantly higher. If wound drainage is present, prompt discoloration following intravenous injection of indigo carmine green or methylene blue is also indicative of urinary leakage. Obstructing lymphoceles are drained by means of laparoscopy into the peritoneum. Urinomas are the result of distal ureteral necrosis and require surgical reimplantation into the bladder or reanastomosis to the native ureter. Rarely, retained blood clots in the bladder cause urethral obstruction necessitating resumption of catheter drainage and irrigation.

Acute CsA or FK506 nephrotoxicity occurs when vasoconstriction of afferent arterioles reduces glomerular blood flow. The rise in serum creatinine level that follows is inconsistently associated with drug levels and reversible when either agent is transiently withheld. In addition, both drugs have been implicated in rare examples of acute renal failure associated with the histologic characteristics of the hemolytic uremic syndrome. This disorder has been difficult to characterize in renal transplant recipients because of shared morphologic features with acute vascular rejection but serves to illustrate the importance of a renal biopsy in anyone with unexplained renal allograft dysfunction.

Acute rejection is seen in 30% to 50% of cadaveric renal transplant recipients. Most patients have a progressive rise in serum creatinine level 3 weeks to 3 months after transplantation. Associated symptoms of allograft tenderness and fever are less common with CsA use, emphasizing the need for vigilant monitoring of the serum creatinine level in the early posttransplantation period. Treatment consists of high-dose intravenous methylprednisolone for 3 to 5 days, followed by a tapering course of prednisone. Severe or corticosteroid-resistant episodes are treated with polyclonal or monoclonal antilymphocyte antibodies. With prompt recognition and treatment, 90% of acute rejection episodes are successfully reversed. However, acute rejection predisposes patients to future allograft loss from chronic rejection.

Vascular thrombosis accounts for 1% to 2% of early allograft loss and is ordinarily seen in the first 30 days after transplantation. This complication is generally the result of twisting or kinking of the renal artery or vein and is more common with disparate size between donor and recipient vessels, multiple vessels, or postoperative hypotension.

Ureteral obstruction in the late posttransplantation period is usually due to scarring from previous ischemia or rejection. Retrograde stenting is difficult because of poor visualization of the ureteral insertion into the bladder, and reoperation is usually required.

Although more common in the first 3 months, acute rejection can be seen at any time after transplantation. Such late episodes are frequently related to overzealous tapering of maintenance immunosuppression or patient noncompliance.

Chronic rejection is the most common cause of allograft loss after the first year of transplantation if death is excluded. Patients typically come to medical attention with slowly progressive renal dysfunction accompanied by proteinuria and worsening hypertension. Histologic hallmarks include vascular intimal hyperplasia, tubular atrophy, and interstitial fibrosis. Lack of effective therapy forecasts eventual renal failure and the resumption of dialysis. Azathioprine and CsA are discontinued following initiation of dialysis, and prednisone is tapered. Allograft nephrectomy can be avoided in most patients unless unexplained fever, allograft tenderness, or gross hematuria occurs.

Chronic CsA nephrotoxicity has been described in the native kidneys of heart and liver transplant recipients, patients with refractory rheumatoid arthritis, and diabetics receiving isolated pancreas transplants. However, histologic abnormalities similar to those encountered in chronic rejection make this disorder more difficult to characterize

in renal transplantation patients. Most transplantation programs continue to use long-term CsA but limit the dose to approximately 5 mg/kg per day after the first year. Delayed CsA withdrawal is associated with an increased risk of acute rejection; the effects on long-term allograft survival remain controversial.

Recurrent glomerulonephritis is seen in the early or late posttransplantation periods, accounting for less than 5% of overall allograft loss. Most instances can be categorized into those leading to graft loss or those that recur on histologic examination but seldom lead to loss. The former category includes focal segmental glomerulosclerosis (FSGS), mesangioproliferative glomerulonephritis (MPGN) type 1, hemolytic uremic syndrome, and possibly scleroderma, which recur in 20% to 30% of recipients. In addition, allograft loss to FSGS predicts its recurrence in 60% to 80% of subsequent transplantations. Diseases that recur on histologic examination but are often clinically insignificant include MPGN type 2, Henoch-Schönlein purpura, and immunoglobulin A (IgA) nephropathy.

Recurrent membranous glomerulonephritis infrequently recurs in 5% of patients. However, higher rates have been reported in recipients of living-related donor transplants. Histologic evidence of anti–glomerular basement membrane (anti-GBM) disease is seen in up to 50% of patients. Delaying transplantation for 12 months following the disappearance of circulating anti-GBM antibodies lessens the likelihood of a clinically significant recurrence.

Special consideration of Alport's syndrome and primary hyperoxaluria type 1 is required. Alport's patients have a defect in type IV collagen that is not present in the GBM of the donor organ. Rarely, antibody-mediated destruction of normal type IV collagen ensues with allograft loss from anti-GBM disease. Primary hyperoxaluria type 1 is no longer considered an absolute contraindication to renal transplantation. However, the disease is due to an inborn error of hepatic metabolism that can lead to widespread tissue oxalate deposition and multiorgan dysfunction. Patients losing an allograft to recurrent oxalosis or those with multiorgan involvement should be considered for combined liver and kidney transplantation to simultaneously correct the metabolic defect and renal failure.

Renal artery stenosis is an uncommon cause of late renal allograft dysfunction. This is particularly true in cadaveric transplant recipients, where the integrity of the renal artery is preserved by using a cuff of donor aorta for the vascular anastomosis. Doppler ultrasonography is the best noninvasive screening test for diagnosis. However, treatment is suboptimal with angioplasty and reoperation; each is associated with a significant risk of allograft loss.

Complications

Advances in immunosuppression have improved allograft survival without increasing infectious complications. Nevertheless, infection remains a common occurrence in many patients after renal transplantation. When considering the source of infection, it is important to note the time that has elapsed since transplantation and the cumulative amount of immunosuppression that the patient has received.

Bacterial infections dominate the very early (first 4 weeks) and late (after 6 months) posttransplantation periods—before and after the effects of the heaviest immunosuppression result. These infections usually originate from the urinary tract, lungs, or intravenous catheters and consist mainly of organisms encountered in the normal population. Urinary tract infections in the early period are more likely to be associated with pyelonephritis and require intravenous antibiotics. The prophylactic use of trimethoprim-sulfamethoxazole reduces this complication, with the added benefit of preventing most *Pneumocystis, Nocardia,* and *Listeria* species infections.

Viral, fungal, and other opportunistic infections are more common 1 to 6 months after transplantation. However, they may be encountered at any point while patients are receiving unusually heavy immunosuppression, such as in those with multiple acute rejections and suboptimally functioning allografts. Candidal species, mainly *Candida albicans* and *Candida tropicalis,* are the leading causes of fungal infection in renal transplant recipients. Prophylaxis against mucocutaneous infection with nystatin or clotrimazole is usually effective in the early posttransplant period. Rarely, fluconazole and amphotericin B are required for more serious manifestations such as esophagitis or disseminated infection.

Herpes viruses make up the majority of viral infections in renal transplant recipients. Herpes simplex types 1 and 2 are less common when prophylactic acyclovir is used for the first 3 to 4 months. Shingles resulting from varicella zoster is seen in 20% to 30% of recipients with a dermatomal distribution and response to high-dose acyclovir similar to the general population. In contrast, more serious sequelae often result from cytomegalovirus (CMV) and Epstein-Barr virus (EBV) infections.

Cytomegalovirus is the most important infection in transplant recipients. Modes of acquisition include primary infection (often from the transplanted kidney), reactivation of dormant infection, and superinfection with a previously unencountered strain. Patients typically present with generalized malaise, intermittent fever, and leukopenia. More severely affected persons have evidence of solid organ involvement including hepatitis, interstitial pneumonitis, encephalitis, chorioretinitis, and gastrointestinal tract ulceration. Diagnosis requires demonstration of viremia (by culture or polymerase chain reaction), antigenemia, or characteristic viral inclusions in histologic specimens from involved organs. Effective therapy is now available with intravenous gancyclovir for 14 to 21 days, accompanied by a modest reduction in immunosuppression. Because of the significant morbidity and cost of this complication, several strategies aimed at prevention are currently employed, including high-dose acyclovir, hyperimmune globulin, and preemptive gancyclovir during periods of increased immunosuppression.

Epstein-Barr viral infections are a consequence of today's more potent immunosuppressive regimens. Epstein-Barr virus (EBV) secondarily infects B lymphocytes, transforming them into immortal cells, which are ordinarily destroyed by specific, cytotoxic T lymphocytes. Excess immunosuppression impairs this destruction and can lead to uncontrolled proliferation of transformed B lymphocytes and the development of posttransplantation lymphoproliferative disease (PTLD). Posttransplantation lymphoproliferative disease encompasses a spectrum ranging from a benign, polyclonal collection of B cells to a highly malignant, monoclonal tumor. Presenting features include fever, leukopenia, and atypical lymphocytosis. Lymphadenopathy is less common than in the normal host with a predilection for primary gastrointestinal tract and central nervous system involvement. Diagnosis requires histologic confirmation and demonstration of EBV DNA within the abnormal B cells. Treatment in the early, polyclonal stages is curative and consists of reduction or withdrawal of immunosuppression with or without high-dose acyclovir. Once progression to a monoclonal tumor occurs, these measures are seldom effective and prognosis is poor, despite adjunctive chemotherapy or radiation therapy.

Yearly vaccination against influenza is recommended for all transplant recipients. In addition, pneumococcal antibody titers characteristically decline rapidly after transplantation, and revaccination after 6 years is required. When indicated, vaccination against hepatitis B before transplantation is preferable because of a greater likelihood of antibody response. In general, the use of live-viral vaccines should be avoided in all transplantation patients.

The association between malignancies and immunosuppression has been recognized since 1967. The most common neoplasms encountered in renal transplant recipients, in the order of their occurrence, are skin, lymphoma, renal, bladder, and bronchial cell carcinoma.

A unique feature of skin cancer is its tendency to increase over time. Similar to the general population, carcinoma of the skin is more common in fair-skinned individuals with above average sun exposure. Important differences in transplant recipients include a greater prevalence of squamous cell tumors and likelihood of metastases. Prevention comprises mainly avoiding excess sun exposure, liberal use of sunscreens, and periodic dermatologic evaluation. Metabolites of azathioprine have a photosensitizing effect on the skin, which necessitates a dose reduction or discontinuation in severely affected patients.

Most lymphomas in renal transplant patients are of the non-Hodgkin's variety. They are of B-cell lineage and related to EBV infection, as previously discussed.

Cardiovascular complications are the leading cause of death in renal transplantation patients. This is not unexpected in a population characterized by a high prevalence of hypertension, hyperlipidemia, and diabetes mellitus.

Hypertension is seen in 60% to 80% of renal transplant recipients and detrimentally affects patient and allograft survival. It can be pre-existing or due to several factors encountered in the posttransplantation period: immunosuppression (prednisone, CsA, FK506), allograft dysfunction, transplant renal artery stenosis, or excessive weight gain. Combination therapy is often required for adequate control; loop diuretics and calcium channel blockers are the most frequently prescribed agents.

Exacerbation of hypertension in association with posttransplantation erythrocytosis occurs in 10% to 15% of patients. This complication is most common in the first 2 years after renal transplantation and is invariably associated with excellent allograft function. Treatment with angiotensin-converting enzyme inhibitors is effective and should be given when the hematocrit exceeds 51% to 55% to prevent thromboembolic complications. Monitoring of serum creatinine and potassium levels is required in the early stages of therapy. In most instances a gradual decrease in hematocrit can be expected within 6 weeks of treatment onset.

Elevations in cholesterol and triglyceride levels are common after renal transplantation. Contributing factors include prednisone, CsA, obesity, and antihypertensive agents. Early-stage treatment strategies are limited to dietary restriction and weight control while immunosuppression is tapered to maintenance levels. Thereafter, low doses of 3-hydroxy-3-methyglutaryl coenzyme A (HMG CoA) reductase inhibitors are recommended as the drugs of first choice. Rare examples of rhabdomyolysis have been reported after combining higher doses of these agents with CsA.

Diabetes mellitus is the leading cause of ESRD in the United States. Corticosteroids, CsA, FK506, and increased metabolism of insulin in the functioning transplant all contribute to worsening glucose tolerance in the posttransplantation period. Oral hypoglycemic agents are seldom adequate for glucose control, and patients with non–insulin-dependent diabetes should be forewarned of the need for insulin administration. Greater morbidity and lower allograft survival rates in combined kidney-pancreas transplantation currently limit its use in many insulin-dependent diabetics.

Renal transplantation is associated with a number of musculoskeletal complications resulting from preexisting alterations in bone metabolism or the consequences of immunosuppression.

Secondary hyperparathyroidism is manifested by persistent hypercalcemia and usually corrects after successful renal transplantation. The rate of resolution is variable and correlates with the duration of dialysis and the size of the hyperplastic glands. Most studies recommend a conservative approach to management in the first year after transplantation in the absence of persistent hypercalcemia (≥ 12.5 mg/dl), deteriorating allograft function in conjunction with nephrocalcinosis, or severe osteitis fibrosa cystica.

In 15% of transplant recipients osteonecrosis develops within 3 years of renal transplantation. The femoral head is most often affected, although disease develops at two or more sites in many patients. Pathogenesis is poorly understood, with hyperparathyroidism and corticosteroids each suspected as playing a role. Presenting complaints are usually related to pain on weight bearing. Magnetic resonance imaging is presently the best noninvasive test for establishing the diagnosis. No specific therapy is available, and joint replacement is ultimately required for disabling pain. Tapering or discontinuing corticosteroids does not retard the process and risks precipitation of an acute rejection.

Hyperuricemia and gout are consequences of decreased urate excretion attributable to the combined effects of CsA, diuretics, and a reduction in GFR. Acute gout can be treated cautiously in most renal transplant recipients with a nonsteroidal antiinflammatory drug, whereas colchicine or a transient increase in prednisone is reserved for those with significant renal impairment. Long-term management of hyperuricemia is complicated by the ineffectiveness of uricosuric agents when the GFR is less than 50 ml/minute and the potentially life-threatening interaction between allopurinol and azathioprine.

Severe joint or bone pain similar to that encountered during a sickle cell crisis has recently been described in kidney, liver, lung, and pancreas transplant recipients. The pain usually involves the lower extremities and, in contrast to osteonecrosis, is worsened with recumbency. The pathophysiologic mechanisms of this new bone pain syndrome are not understood. However, significant relief of symptoms has been reported following treatment with calcium channel blockers.

✔ *WHEN TO REFER*

Whenever a diagnosis of chronic renal insufficiency or chronic renal failure is made, consultation with a nephrologist is indicated. An exception would be the patient with severe, progressive nonrenal disease that is likely to be fatal in the near future. The purpose of the referral is to determine cause of renal disease and its possible treatment, to rule out remediable factors, to institute a proper regimen and monitoring system for chronic renal failure, and to begin to plan for renal replacement therapy at the appropriate time. The primary care physician and nephrologist must determine a follow-up plan and partnership for provision of care. Live-donor transplantation and placement of appropriate vascular access for hemodialysis must be considered electively well before onset of the uremic syndrome. Initiating renal replacement therapy too late increases morbidity and cost. For most patients renal transplantation offers the best chance of rehabilitation, but the availability of kidneys is inadequate to meet the need.

Restoration of normal menstrual function after successful renal transplantation may be followed by a desire of women of childbearing age to conceive. Current guidelines to ensure the best possible outcomes for mother and child include a minimum waiting period of 2 years from transplantation to conception, stable allograft function with a serum creatinine level lower than 1.5 mg/dl, and absent or easily controlled hypertension. Cyclosporine levels often decrease during the initial stages of pregnancy because of accelerated metabolism and increases in volume of distribution. Careful attention to maintenance of stable CsA levels throughout pregnancy may limit the likelihood of acute rejection, currently estimated at 10%. Despite optimal management, pregnancy is associated with a 5% risk of allograft loss.

BIBLIOGRAPHY

Armenti VT et al: National transplantation pregnancy registry: outcomes of 154 pregnancies in cyclosporine-treated female kidney transplant recipients, *Transplantation* 57:502, 1994.

Bardin T et al: Dialysis arthropathy: outcome after renal transplantation, *Am J Med* 99:243, 1995.

Bergström J: Nutrition and mortality in hemodialysis, *J Am Soc Nephrol* 6:1329, 1995.

Brennan DC, Mohanakumar T, Flye MW: Donor-specific transfusion and donor bone marrow infusion in renal transplantation tolerance: a review of the efficacy and mechanisms, *Am J Kidney Dis* 26:701, 1995.

Burkart JM, Nolph KD: Peritoneal dialysis. In Brenner BM, editor: *The kidney,* ed 5, vol 2, Philadelphia, 1996, WB Saunders.

Diethelm AG et al: Progress in renal transplantation, *Ann Surg* 221:446, 1995.

First MR: Long-term complications after transplantation, *Am J Kidney Dis* 22:477, 1993.

Galla JH, Luke RG: Hypertension in renal parenchymal disease. In Brenner BM, editor: *The kidney,* ed 5, vol 2, Philadelphia, 1996, WB Saunders.

Gaston RS, Julian BA, Curtis JJ: Posttransplant erythrocytosis: an enigma revisited, *Am J Kidney Dis* 24:1, 1994.

Gauthier VJ, Barbosa LM: Bone pain in transplant recipients responsive to calcium channel blockers, *Ann Intern Med* 121:863, 1994.

Gaya SBM et al: Malignant disease in patients with long-term renal transplants, *Transplantation* 59:1705, 1995.

Hakim RM, Lazarus JM: Initiation of dialysis, *J Am Soc Nephrol* 6:1319, 1995.

Hruska KA, Teitelbaum SL: Renal osteodystrophy, *N Engl J Med* 333:166, 1995.

Ikizler TA: Spontaneous dietary protein intake during progression of chronic renal failure, *J Am Soc Nephrol* 6:1386, 1995.

Julian BA: Metabolic bone disease in renal transplant recipient, *Endocrinologist* 3:415, 1993.

Kasiske BL: Cyclosporine withdrawal after renal transplantation: does it affect graft loss? *J Nephrol* 8:65, 1995.

Kasiske BL, Bia MJ: The evaluation and selection of living kidney donors, *Am J Kidney Dis* 26:387, 1995.

Kasiske BL et al: The evaluation of renal transplant candidates: clinical practice guidelines, *J Am Soc Nephrol* 6:1, 1995.

Kasiske BL et al: Long-term effects of reduced renal mass in humans, *Kidney Int* 48:814, 1995.

Manske CL et al: Screening diabetic transplant candidates for coronary artery disease: identification of a low-risk subgroup, *Kidney Int* 44:617, 1993.

Markell MS et al: Hyperlipidemia and glucose intolerance in the post–renal transplant patient, *J Am Soc Nephrol* 4(suppl 1):S37, 1994.

Marple JT, MacDougall M, Chonko AM: Renal cancer complicating acquired cystic kidney disease, *J Am Soc Nephrol* 4:1951, 1994.

Meyer TW, Baboolal K, Brenner BM: Nephron adaptation to renal injury. In Brenner BM, editor: *The kidney,* ed 5, vol 2, Philadelphia, 1996, WB Saunders.

Mitch WE, Walser M: Nutritional therapy for the uremic patient. In Brenner BM, editor: *The kidney,* ed 5, vol 2, Philadelphia, 1996, WB Saunders.

Morbidity and mortality of renal dialysis: an NIH Consensus Conference statement, *Ann Intern Med* 121:62, 1994.

Muirhead N et al: Evidence-based recommendations for the clinical use of recombinant human erythropoietin, *Am J Kidney Dis* 26(2):S1-S24, 1995.

Owen WF et al: The urea reduction ratio and serum albumin concentration as predictors of mortality in patients undergoing hemodialysis, *N Engl J Med* 329:1001, 1993.

Peters DH et al: Tacrolimus: a review of its pharmacology and therapeutic potential in hepatic and renal transplantation, *Drugs* 46:746, 1993.

Peterson JC et al: Blood pressure control, proteinuria, and the progression of renal disease, *Ann Intern Med* 123:754, 1995.

Petitclerc T, Jacobs C: Dialysis sodium concentration: what is optimal and can it be individualized? *Nephrol Dial Transplant* 10:596, 1995 (editorial).

Pol S et al: Efficacy and tolerance of alpha-2b interferon therapy on HCV infection of hemodialyzed patients, *Kidney Int* 47:1412, 1995.

Ponticelli C et al: Hypertension after renal transplantation, *Am J Kidney Dis* 21(suppl 2):73, 1993.

Port FK et al: Comparison of survival probabilities for dialysis patients vs. cadaveric renal transplant recipients, *JAMA* 270:1339, 1993.

Ramos EL, Tisher CC: Recurrent diseases in the kidney transplant, *Am J Kidney Dis* 24:142, 1994.

Rostaing L et al: Treatment of chronic hepatitis C with recombinant interferon alpha in kidney transplant recipients, *Transplantation* 59:1426, 1995.

Rubin RH: Infectious disease complications of renal transplantation, *Kidney Int* 44:221, 1993.

Sollinger HW for the U.S. renal transplant mycophenolate mofetil study group: Mycophenolate mofetil for the prevention of acute rejection in primary cadaveric renal allograft recipients, *Transplantation* 60:225, 1995.

Starzl TE: The development of clinical renal transplantation, *Am J Kidney Dis* 16:548, 1990.

Terasaki PI et al: High survival rates of kidney transplants from spousal and living unrelated donors, *N Engl J Med* 333:333, 1995.

U.S. Renal Data System: *USRDS 1995 Annual Data Report,* Bethesda, Md, April 1995, National Institutes of Health, National Institute of Diabetes and Digestive and Kidney Diseases.

U.S. Renal Data System: *USRDS 1995 Annual Data Report,* Bethesda, Md, National Institutes of Health, National Institute of Diabetes and Digestive and Kidney Diseases, *Am J Kidney Dis* 22(suppl 2):S95, 1995.

Van Buren DH, Burke JF, Lewis RM: Renal function in patients receiving long-term cyclosporine therapy, *J Am Soc Nephrol* 4(suppl 1):S17, 1994.

CHAPTER

111 Nephrolithiasis

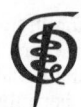

Stanley Goldfarb

By the age of 70, approximately 12% of men and 5% of women will have at least one symptomatic kidney stone and approximately one person per thousand in the United States will receive hospital care each year for kidney stones. Moreover, the incidence of renal calculi, principally stones composed of calcium oxalate, appears to be increasing in industrialized nations. Nephrolithiasis is frequently a recurrent malady among untreated patients. In a patient who has passed a first calcium stone, the likelihood of forming a second stone is approximately 15% at 1 year, 35% to 40% at 5 years, and 50% at 10 years, with a greater likelihood of recurrence in men.

A systematic approach to the treatment of nephrolithiasis requires a correct diagnosis, determination of the composition of the stone, and assessment of possible abnormalities in the composition of the urine that led to crystallization of the constituents of the stone within the urinary tract. Yet there is a great deal of uncertainty and controversy over the most cost-effective and clinically sound approach to the patient who has formed a kidney stone, particularly the first stone. Recent data that suggest that stones are very likely to recur have persuaded many clinicians to pursue an attempt at diagnosis and therapy, even in the patient who has formed a single stone. Even when an extensive evaluation is not performed, patients can benefit from careful analysis of risk factors for stone recurrence and some simple interventions aimed at reducing painful and costly repeated episodes.

PHYSIOLOGY AND PATHOPHYSIOLOGY OF NEPHROLITHIASIS
Crystal Nucleation and Stone Growth in the Urinary Tract

The formation of a kidney stone (Table 111-1) requires a number of physical steps in the transition from a single crystal of an insoluble compound within the urinary tract to the aggregation and further accumulation of crystals, growth of stones, attachment to the uroepithelium, and ultimate excretion in the final urine.

1. Abnormalities in the excretion of solutes may be a crucial factor in the initiation of crystal formation in the urine. Urine is supersaturated with a variety of solutes that precipitate and crystallize at typically normal pH, solute content, and rates of water excretion. Thus factors such as inhibitors of stone formation are important in preventing stones from occurring far more frequently than clinically observed. Most patients who form stones do not continually excrete excess amounts of these various stone-related solutes. Nonetheless, in a sizable minority of patients, increased amounts of calcium, oxalate, phosphate, uric acid, and cystine may contribute to the formation of stones, and specific therapies may be applied to this problem of excess excretion. Reduced excretion of water leading to increased urinary concentration of solute may be as important as increased total excretion of stone-forming solutes. A variety of clinical disorders (inflammatory bowel disease with diarrhea, eating disorders) or climatic conditions (tropical or desert environments) associated with chronically reduced urinary volume may lead to increased stone formation, particularly in susceptible individuals. Thus reduced urinary volume or increased solute excretion may raise the concentration of urinary solutes. These components and the deficiency of endogenous inhibitors may increase the frequency of crystal nucleation, the first stage in stone growth.

2. Alterations in normal diurnal variation in urinary pH (usually acid at night and in the early morning and relatively alkaline in the late morning and early afternoon) significantly affect the ionization of several sparingly soluble urinary constituents and thus their potential for crystallization. In only slightly acid urine of pH 6.8, about 50% of urinary phosphate is present as the HPO_4^{2-} ion ($H_2PO_4^- \rightleftharpoons HPO_4^{2-}$, $pK_2 = 6.8$), which readily reacts with calcium to form sparingly soluble brushite ($CaHPO_4, \cdot 2H_2O$; solubility in water about 1.8 mmol/L). However, when the urine pH is 5.5, only about 5% of urinary phosphate is present as the HPO_4^{2-} ion. Because the solubility of $Ca(H_2PO_4) \cdot 2H_2O$ (solubility in water about 7.1 mmol/L) is almost four times greater than that of brushite, the tendency for calcium phosphate precipitation is correspondingly reduced. On the other hand, the solubility of undissociated uric acid (pK_1 uric acid $\rightleftharpoons$ urate = 5.6) in maximally acid urine of pH 4.5 to 5.0 is about 100 mg/L, whereas the solubility of (sodium) urate at pH 7 is about 16 times greater (1700 mg/L). Thus crystallization of uric acid is more likely to occur if the urine is persistently very acid.

3. Normal urine contains inhibitors of crystal nucleation that form complexes with potentially insoluble urinary constituents. Citrate is the main urinary chelator of calcium. Hypocitraturia is a characteristic of all states of chronic acidosis and is the principle reason that kidney stones form in patients with renal tubular acidosis. Citrate is reabsorbed in the proximal tubule and is metabolized in the liver to bicarbonate via the Krebs cycle. Thus the reduction in urine citrate in acidosis serves to ameliorate the degree of acidosis but at the price of an increased risk of nephrolithiasis. Magnesium can form soluble complexes with oxalate. Hypocitraturia or hypomagnesuria may thus contribute to initial crystal nucleation.

4. Normal urine contains protein inhibitors of crystal growth. A number of such proteins have now been identified, including nephrocalcin—a glycoprotein containing γ-carboxyglutamic acid—and uropontin. Both are potent inhibitors of calcium oxalate crystal growth, but the recently described uropontin, similar to the bone protein osteopontin, is a more potent inhibitor of crystal growth. Urinary Tamm-Horsfall protein is another inhibitor of crystal aggregation. Abnormalities in the structure of these protein inhibi-

Table 111-1 Crystalline constituents of kidney stones

STONE TYPE	COMMENTS
Calcium Stones	75% of stones
Calcium oxalate	
Calcium oxalate monohydrate (whewellite) (predominant form)	
Calcium oxalate dihydrate (wedellite)	~50% of calcium stones
Calcium oxalate associated with apatite (hydroxyapatite) $[Ca_{10}(PO_4)_6(OH)_2]$ carbonate apatite$[Ca_{10}(PO_4)_6CO_3]$ (central nucleus apatite alone)	~50% of calcium-containing stones
Calcium monohydrogen phosphate dihydrate (brushite, $CaHPO_4 \cdot 2H_2O$)	<5% as principal constituent
Magnesium ammonium phosphate hexahydrate	
(struvite, $MgNH_4PO_4 \cdot 6H_2O$), always together with carbonate apatite	10% of stones
Uric acid	10% of stones
Cystine	2% of stones
Rare stones	
Xanthine stones (xanthine oxidase deficiency; allopurinol therapy, especially in patients with massive hyperuricosuria)	
2,6-dihydroxyadenine stones (adenine phosphoribosyltransferase deficiency)	
Stones composed of drugs	
triamterene (diuretic therapy)	

tors that reduce their capacity to inhibit crystal growth may contribute to the pathogenesis of stones. A few families have been described in whom this is the case.

5. Crystals must attach to the papillary collecting duct or pelvic surfaces to provide sufficient time for growth to the size of a clinically relevant stone because rates of renal tubular fluid flow are too rapid to permit time for such crystal growth. Recent studies have demonstrated specific and inhibitable binding of calcium oxalate, apatite, and uric acid to papillary collecting duct cells in tissue culture at specific sites. These observations suggest that alterations in uroepithelial surfaces may play a role in the formation of kidney stones. In addition, most kidney stones contain a protein matrix that may initiate crystal nucleation or, in addition, attach small crystals as they form and thus allow time for their growth.

6. Crystals of one substance may be the nucleus for precipitation of another. For example, seeding of otherwise stable saturated solutions of calcium oxalate with apatite crystals leads to the removal of calcium and oxalate ions from solution and growth of calcium oxalate crystals upon the seed crystal of apatite. This effect is termed *heterogeneous nucleation* or *secondary crystal growth* because the molecular structures of calcium oxalate and apatite differ significantly. Uric acid seed crystals are similarly able to induce calcium oxalate crystal growth. Because calcium oxalate dihydrate and uric acid crystal lattices and surfaces are of similar dimensions on an atomic level, this effect is termed *epitaxial nucleation*.

PATHOPHYSIOLOGY OF SPECIFIC CAUSES OF NEPHROLITHIASIS
Calcium-Containing Stones

Mechanisms of Hypercalciuria. Hypercalciuria occurs whenever the excretion of calcium is greater than 250 mg/24 hr in a female or 300 mg/24 hr in a male. While these levels are somewhat arbitrary, they do define patients at increased risk of stone formation. Hypercalciuria may result from one of several pathophysiologic mechanisms. Any hypercalcemic condition increases urine calcium excretion as the increased filtered load may not be entirely reabsorbed by tubular mechanisms. The most common cause of hypercalcemia that is associated with kidney stone formation is primary hyperparathyroidism. This is somewhat paradoxical in that parathyroid hormone (PTH) is a powerful stimulus to renal calcium reabsorption, in part through enhancing sodium-calcium exchange mechanisms in the distal nephron. However, the hypercalcemia induced by hyperparathyroidism typically results in a greater increment in filtered calcium load than in tubular reabsorption rates for calcium; hence renal calcium excretion rises. If hypercalcemia occurs in the absence of PTH, for example, during the ingestion of excess amounts of vitamin D or secondary to accelerated skeletal release of calcium in patients who are immobilized or paraplegic, the increment in urine calcium excretion is much greater for a given level of hypercalcemia than that seen for comparable degrees of hypercalcemia in hyperparathyroidism. Absence or suppression of PTH, provided that serum calcium is not greatly reduced, markedly enhances renal calcium excretion and increases the risk of kidney stone formation.

Tubular Factors in Secondary Hypercalciuria.

A reduction in tubular calcium reabsorption without an increase in filtered load can also produce hypercalciuria. As calcium is reabsorbed throughout the nephron in close association with sodium reabsorption, any maneuver or physiologic circumstance that exaggerates urine sodium excretion, including high dietary sodium, enhances calcium excretion. In a similar fashion, diuretics such as furosemide increase urinary calcium excretion. Primary, intrinsic reductions in tubular transport have also been postulated to cause hypercalciuria. However, hypercalciuria may be mistakenly attributed to a primary tubular disorder whenever PTH levels are depressed while serum calcium levels are in the normal range. Increased gastrointestinal (GI) calcium absorption or mildly increased bone resorption may also produce this effect. In fact, these latter two pathways may be the principal causes of the syndrome of idiopathic hypercalciuria.

Idiopathic Hypercalciuria.

Idiopathic hypercalciuria is defined as excess calcium excretion in the absence of hypercalcemia, any known cause of PTH suppression such as exogenous vitamin D use, or a condition known to directly inhibit renal calcium reabsorption such as use of loop-active diuretics. The pathophysiology of this disorder is probably complex and multifactorial. Animal models suggest that genetic factors that lead to enhanced sensitivity to vitamin D may underlie some forms of this condition. Other studies suggest that increased levels of vitamin D may occur in some proportion of hypercalciuric patients and lead to increased GI calcium absorption, secondary suppression of PTH, and increased urinary calcium excretion.

Recent clinical studies have shown that administration of small doses of 1,25-dihydroxy vitamin D_3 to normal volunteers produces a variety of patterns of hypercalciuria. Some subjects develop hypercalciuria while on a low-calcium diet; this suggests increased rates of bone resorption. Some subjects are hypercalciuric only when ingesting a high-calcium diet, suggesting enhanced GI calcium absorption as the source of hypercalciuria. This heterogeneous pattern of responses to exogenous vitamin D administration closely mimics that seen clinically in patients with hypercalciuria. Although the predominant form in hypercalciuric, stone-forming patients appears to be an enhanced GI calcium absorption, some patients do show hypercalciuria independent of dietary calcium intake, suggesting a primary role for increased skeletal calcium release. Therefore it is probably not useful to subdivide patients with idiopathic hypercalciuria into diet-dependent and diet-independent categories as they all may represent different forms of an abnormality in vitamin D sensitivity or synthesis of active forms of vitamin D.

Other factors that may induce hypercalciuria include the administration of vitamin D to prevent osteoporosis or to treat hypoparathyroidism. Hyperthyroidism either due to excess hormone replacement therapy or secondary to spontaneous disease is an important and easily overlooked cause of hypercalciuria.

Chronic acidosis has been associated with increased urinary calcium excretion. While the mechanisms have not been well defined, enhanced bone resorption with secondary suppression of PTH is probably an important contributing factor. In addition, direct tubular effects of acidosis may be present. As noted earlier, perhaps the most important cause of stone formation and chronic acidosis is not hypercalciuria per se but rather a reduction in urinary citrate excretion, the principal antagonist of calcium precipitation in the urine. Nonetheless, hypercalciuria is also an important feature of distal renal tubular acidosis.

Association of Diet, Hypercalciuria, and Stone Formation.

There has been a well-documented epidemic of calcium stone formation in affluent societies in the developed world. This highly prevalent disorder is closely correlated with household spending on food, which in turn is well correlated with intake of increased amounts of dietary animal protein.

Several aspects of diet may contribute to stone formation. Dietary protein rich in methionine residues has been shown to be associated with increased calcium excretion in long-term studies. There are several potential mechanisms for this phenomenon, including an enhanced glomerular filtration rate due to the vasodilatory actions of dietary protein (perhaps a result of increased nitric oxide synthesis) and an increased acid load resulting from protein metabolism. This effect leads to chronic bone resorption and enhanced renal calcium excretion. Through this latter effect, stone formation may be induced by hypocitraturia, a consequence of the acid load.

High dietary sodium intake is also associated with hypercalciuria and is found in a small subset of patients who are hypercalciuric and form kidney stones. In fact, hypercalciuria can be "cured" in some patients by lowering sodium intake from several hundred to less than 100 mEq/day.

Reduced fluid intake is a feature of certain environmental circumstances. Migration to tropical climates from northern Europe has been associated with increased stone formation rates and well documented in British soldiers during World War II. In addition, within small nations such as Israel, the local availability of water to maintain high fluid intake in the face of desert heat is closely associated with the risk of kidney stone formation. Clinical disorders such as chronic diarrhea produce a similar condition because extrarenal losses of fluid induce a low urine output unless fluid intake is augmented above the individual's usual pattern.

The deleterious effect of excess dietary calcium has been assumed by clinicians for many years. Early attempts at dietary advice on kidney stone formation invariably included suggestions to restrict dietary calcium intake. This recommendation is flawed; low dietary calcium has now been shown in both specific experimental trials and epidemiologic studies to be associated with an increased risk of kidney stones. The mechanism of this association has not been completely defined but likely is accounted for by the effect of low dietary calcium in allowing enhanced GI oxalate absorption, oxalate excretion, and formation of calcium oxalate stones, as will be discussed later.

An intriguing hypothesis states that patients who form kidney stones need not ingest excess amounts of dietary protein, calcium, or sodium but rather have an exaggerated hypercalciuric response to any level of protein or sodium intake. The underlying mechanism of this response has not been defined but could result from some intrinsic variability in renal tubular transport. Thus dietary factors including level of protein and sodium intake may be contributory to kidney stone formation even if excess intake cannot be documented.

Genetic Factors in Hypercalciuria.

Recent studies have suggested that a genetic component may underlie idiopathic hypercalciuria. There are multiple studies that show that hypercalciuria occurs in families, although the relative contributions of genetic factors and environmental influences such as adherence to a specific protein or sodium intake have not been well defined. Intestinal hyperabsorption of calcium due to enhanced sensitivity to vitamin D occurs in genetically defined strains of rats that demonstrate hypercalciuria. Recently studies have shown that a defect in a chloride channel may be the common genetic feature in families with high penetrance of idiopathic hypercalciuria. The mechanism whereby alterations in chloride transport may contribute to hypercalciuria and the localization of the genetic defect in bone, kidney, GI tract, or elsewhere have not been defined, but success in this endeavor holds the promise for major new insights into the mechanism of hypercalciuric syndromes.

Hyperoxaluria. Although emphasis has been placed on hypercalciuria as the most important metabolic disturbance leading to the formation of calcium oxalate–containing stones, evidence has suggested that increased oxalate excretion may be an even more important factor. Normal urinary oxalate in healthy adults, eating typical diets, ranges from 8 to 45 mg/day. There are several mechanisms whereby excess oxalate excretion may occur. First, some form of primary hyperoxaluria may be present. This condition is the result of a recessively inherited defect (type I: α-ketoglutarate:glyoxylate carboligase deficiency associated with increased urinary glyoxylate excretion; type II:D-glyceric dehydrogenase deficiency, associated with increased urinary L-glyceric acid excretion). The disorder usually begins in childhood in association with urinary oxalate excretion rates in the range of 90 to 270 mg/day and leads to renal failure because of nephrocalcinosis and repetitive episodes of ureteral obstruction that may be complicated by urinary infection. Less severe degrees of primary hyperoxaluria may result in only periodic passage of stones and prolonged survival. Acquired hyperoxaluria may be seen among gluttons for oxalate-rich foods (rhubarb, spinach, and other leafy vegetables; cashews; almonds; and strong tea). Also some patients produce excess amounts of oxalate when ingesting large doses of ascorbic acid.

Patients with intestinal disorders may develop secondary hyperoxaluria and recurrent nephrolithiasis. This condition arises in individuals with inflammatory bowel disease, typically with ileal involvement and with an intact colon. Several mechanisms have been proposed for this condition, including decreased intraluminal binding of oxalate by calcium as formation of calcium complexes with unabsorbed fat molecules reduces free calcium levels. Also, increased delivery of bile salts to the colon has been postulated to increase oxalate absorption across the colon.

Finally, patients with calcium hyperabsorption may also have hyperabsorption of oxalate. In a manner analogous to the mechanism of hyperoxaluria associated with intestinal disease, if GI calcium absorption is more complete, then the residual oxalate derived from dietary intake is more absorbable in the form of sodium oxalate salts. It is this enhanced solubility of oxalate that allows increased rates of absorption and further contributes to calcium stone formation. This latter point emphasizes the important role of prescribing adequate amounts of dietary calcium to patients with calcium nephrolithiasis to prevent this complication.

Hypocitraturia. Urinary citrate excretion ranges from approximately 350 to 1450 mg/day in health and, by complexing calcium, lowers urinary saturation with respect to calcium oxalate and apatite. Citrate excretion is higher in women than in men, and this may contribute to the lower incidence of nephrolithiasis in women. Citrate excretion is low among some patients with calcium stones, regardless of hypercalciuria and in the absence of systemic acidosis or even incomplete forms of renal tubular acidosis. The metabolic or transport abnormalities underlying this latter condition are unknown.

Hyperuricosuria. A subset of hypercalciuric patients has been described in whom the primary abnormality that could be identified has been an excessive urinary uric acid excretion rate. These patients typically have a rather severe form of stone disease with multiple recurrences and resistance to standard interventions. It is postulated that hyperuricosuria seen in these patients is a contributory factor to stone formation. This effect may occur through the mechanism of epitaxial crystal growth as outlined earlier or it may be the result of adsorption of other urinary small–molecular-weight inhibitors of crystal growth onto the surface of the uric acid crystals, thereby allowing calcium oxalate crystals to propagate. One convincing study has shown that reduction of urinary uric acid excretion with allopurinol therapy markedly reduces calcium oxalate stone formation in these hyperuricosuric calcium stone formers. Other studies support the idea that the etiology of hyperuricosuria in these individuals is the ingestion of a high purine intake.

Uric Acid Stones

Although uric acid stones occur relatively uncommonly, once present, the disorder recurs frequently; fortunately uric acid stone disease is particularly responsive to treatment. Although uric acid stones are typically radiolucent, they may be slightly radiopaque when there is a veneer of calcium crystals.

Most patients who form uric acid stones do not have hyperuricosuria. Typically serum uric acid levels and urinary acid levels are normal in patients with recurrent acid stones. Urine pH is actually a more important factor than the level of uric acid excretion. When urine pH decreases from 6.0 to 5.0, the concentration of undissociated uric acid (as opposed to the urate concentration) increases nearly six-fold, which leads to precipitation and uric acid stone formation. Undissociated uric acid becomes insoluble at a concentration >90 mg/L; because total excretion typically ranges between 500 and 600 mg/day, persistently acid urine will lead to uric acid stone formation.

Uric acid stones are common in patients with gout, increasing in frequency as urinary uric acid excretion increases, particularly among a subset of gouty patients who overproduce uric acid. Uric acid overproduction may occur as a result of rapid cell turnover and cytolysis, and uric acid stones may be an early symptom of underlying malignancy. Purine gluttony can result in hyperuricosuria and may occasionally be a cause of uric acid stones. A tendency towards uric acid crystal growth in this setting is probably a function of the high protein intake that increases fixed endogenous acid production and the ingestion of uric acid precursors.

It has been proposed that a persistently acid urine in patients with uric acid stones is secondary to an impairment in renal tubular ammonia synthesis. A reduction in urinary buffer excretion leads to the lower urinary pH level.

Struvite Stones

Struvite stones are composed of a combination of magnesium ammonium phosphate (struvite) and calcium carbonate-apatite. Struvite stone formation can be sustained only when ammonia production is increased and the urine pH is elevated to decrease the solubility of phosphate. Both of these requirements can occur only when urine is infected with a urease-producing organism, such as *Proteus* or *Klebsiella*. Urease metabolizes urea into ammonia plus carbon dioxide: Urea $\rightarrow 2NH_3 + CO_2$. The ammonia/ammonium buffer pair has a pK of 9.0, resulting in the combination of a highly alkaline urine, rich in ammonia.

Symptoms directly attributable to struvite stones are uncommon. More often a woman presents with a urinary tract infection, flank pain, or hematuria and is found to have a persistently alkaline urine pH (>7.0), often with multiple magnesium ammonium phosphate crystals in the urine sediment and a renal calculus that is radiodense, but less so than calcium oxalate. The stone may grow and develop into a staghorn or branched calculus involving the entire renal pelvis and calyces. Infection nearly always persists within the interstices of the stone. There is often focal parenchymal scarring with loss of cortex.

Cystine Stones

The formation of kidney stones composed of the amino acid cystine

$$^-OOC-CH-CH_2-S-S-CH_2-CH-COO^-$$
$$\quad\quad\;\; | \quad\quad\quad\quad\quad\quad\quad\quad\quad | $$
$$\quad\quad NH_3^+ \quad\quad\quad\quad\quad\quad NH_3^+$$

is the result of a genetic abnormality of amino acid transport. Cystinuria is an autosomal recessive trait resulting in defective renal tubular, as well as intestinal, transport of cystine, lysine, arginine, and ornithine. The genetic defect resides on chromosome 2, where a defective transport protein for a sodium-coupled cystine transporter is expressed. Urinary excretion rates of cystine, together with the other dibasic amino acids lysine, arginine, and ornithine, are increased. Because cystine is only sparingly soluble, the excessive excretion rate leads to cystine crystallization within the renal pelvis and the formation of stones.

Patients with cystinuria account for only about 1% to 3% of all patients with urolithiasis. Stone disease may begin at any age but appears most commonly in the second and third decades of life. The initial symptoms may be those of renal colic, with or without hematuria, but occasionally only vague backache is present, followed by the discovery of large pelvic staghorn calculi. The stones are radiopaque because of the sulfur contained in cystine, although they are not as radiodense as calcium-containing stones.

The diagnosis is suspected either when the typical hexagonal cystine crystals are observed in the urinary sediment (Fig. 111-1, *F*) or when the results of the urinary cyanide nitroprusside screening test, which detects cystine in a concentration exceeding 75 μg/mg creatinine (normal less than 70 μg cystine/mg creatinine), are positive. The diagnosis is confirmed by the analysis of a stone or by quantitation of 24-hour urinary cystine excretion in the range of 425 μg/mg creatinine among cystinuric patients compared with less than 70 μg cystine/mg creatinine in healthy subjects. The urinary excretion of lysine, arginine, and ornithine is also observed to be elevated.

LABORATORY AND DIAGNOSTIC TESTING STRATEGIES
Initial Stone Passage

The indications for metabolic evaluation of patients who have formed kidney stones remain to be completely defined. The risk of stone recurrence, as noted earlier, is substantial, and many patients will have symptoms of stone recurrence within 5 years. It has been estimated that approximately 50% of patients will form a second stone and the occurrence of kidney stones begets further stones, increasing the likelihood of more stone episodes in the future. This pattern suggests that patients would benefit from metabolic evaluation and careful follow-up even after the formation of a single stone. On the other hand, medical practice has generally been to withhold extensive clinical evaluation until stone activity is documented. Stone activity is defined as either the passage of a newly formed stone or the rapid growth of a stone already in situ. In fact, studies have suggested that a "stone clinic effect" is present in that patients who merely seek therapy at a center devoted to the evaluation and management of patients with recurrent kidney stones experience a dramatic reduction in the formation of new stones despite the fact that "specific" therapy was not applied. Rather these individuals were simply given dietary advice and suggestions for changes in fluid intake. This approach alone leads to a 75% reduction in stone formation rate over 5 years in hypercalciuric individuals.

These observations suggest that the patient who forms a first kidney stone should have a limited evaluation. Perhaps the most useful test that could be applied to a patient who passes a kidney stone is a crystallographic analysis of the kidney stone. The presence of particular crystal composition will strongly guide further analytic and therapeutic interventions. Assuming that the patient is found to have passed a calcium oxalate stone, testing should be focused on identifying abnormalities in calcium metabolism. This should include the measurement of plasma calcium on at least two occasions to assess the possibility of primary hyperparathyroidism and the careful evaluation of the patient's diet with recommendations to increase fluid intake to at least 2 L/day and to restrict dietary intake of sodium and protein while not limiting dietary intake of calcium. The rationale for this latter recommendation is based on the effects of adequate dietary calcium to limit intestinal oxalate absorption and to reduce the risk of stone formation on that basis. In addition, patients should be assessed for their intake of an unusual diet that contains large amounts of sodium or protein or the intake of large amounts of vitamin C or vitamin D, all of which can be associated with an increased risk of kidney stone formation. Urine should be examined for the signs of infection or for the presence of crystals (see Fig. 111-1). Thereafter the subjects should be monitored yearly, but no specific therapy should be instituted unless evidence of stone activity is present.

If the stone is not retrieved for analysis, uncommon forms of stone such as cystine or uric acid must be considered. A screening test for cystinuria should then be performed. Later sections deal with the pathophysiology that underlies the formation of various forms of kidney stone and the risk factors that lead to the production of nephrolithiasis of various crystalline composition. If uric acid, cystine, or struvite stones are found, then specific and detailed diagnostic studies are required, as will be discussed later.

Recurrent Stones

Once patients have formed multiple kidney stones, a detailed evaluation is necessary to identify the underlying cause and to institute appropriate therapy (Fig. 111-2). The initial evaluation should include crystallographic stone analysis as well as duplicate measurements taken at different times of the 24-hour urine levels of calcium, phosphate, uric acid, citrate, oxalate, cystine, creatinine, and urea nitrogen, as well as volume. These measurements should be carried out in patients maintaining their usual diet and fluid intake, although many patients will spontaneously modify that intake at the time that the measurements are made. At the same time, plasma should be assayed for calcium, phosphate, creatinine, uric acid, bicarbonate, and urea nitrogen. Urinary urea nitrogen will provide insight into the patient's dietary protein intake in grams if urea nitrogen excretion in grams is multiplied by a factor of six. Microscopic examination of the urine should be performed on fresh specimens to seek the presence of crystals (see Fig. 111-1). Radiologic studies should also be performed to localize the presence of stones, to document stone size, and to serve as a baseline for future therapy. Intravenous urography should be performed at some point and is the most sensitive and most specific approach to identifying stones. Once an intravenous urogram has established the presence or absence of kidney stones, patients may be followed with flat abdominal films, with or without tomography, to identify any changes in the size, number, and location of stones. The quality of the plain film is often improved if the patient undergoes a modest bowel prep the night before the study.

Fasting urinary pH should be measured in all patients with calcium-containing stones. If the fasting urinary pH is >6 in the absence of urinary tract infection, then an ammonium chloride acid-loading test (l00 mg/kg body weight using a 500 mg/5 ml oral solution) should be performed. If urinary pH does not fall to less than 5.4 when concurrently measured serum bicarbonate falls below 20 mEq/L, then classic distal renal tubular acidosis is likely.

DIFFERENTIAL DIAGNOSIS
Clinical Presentation of Kidney Stones

Patients with active passage of kidney stones generally present with the dyad of pain and hematuria. The pain is frequently colicky but may be unremitting. It typically begins as flank pain but may also originate in the midabdomen and be confused with acute GI disorders. The pain may then localize to the flank and radiate to the groin or into the urethra. While the site of pain may indicate the locus of the stone, this is not invariable. As stones pass into the terminal ureter, the symptoms may mimic urinary tract infections or cystitis. The pain associated with stone passage is not completely specific to that entity, and the possibility of a fungus ball in the immunocompromised patient, a clot originating from a neoplasm in the urinary tract, or a sloughed papilla associated with severe urinary tract infection or with use of large amounts of analgesic compounds over an extended time all must be considered. Hematuria, either gross or microscopic, is an almost invariant accompaniment of stone passage, and its absence should encourage the clinician to seek alternative diagnoses.

It must be stressed that stone passage complicated by urinary tract infection represents a medical emergency because the combination of infection and obstruction can lead to sepsis and to the rapid destruction of the affected kidney. Patients with urinary tract infection and active stone passage will generally require intravenous antibiotic therapy and rapid decompression of the obstructed portion of the urinary tract through percutaneous nephrostomy placement.

Radiologic studies play an important role in the diagnosis of active stone passage. A flat film of the abdomen may show the location of a radiopaque stone and may also provide evidence of an ileus, suggesting other diagnoses. Ultrasonography may detect radiolucent stones and can identify a urinary tract obstruction. However, ultrasonography may fail to identify very small stones and cannot precisely define the degree or site of obstruction. Intravenous urography remains the standard method for examining the urinary tract for obstruction in cases of stone passage. This study should be promptly performed in most patients with acute stone passage unless the patient has had multiple recent stone episodes and ultrasonography suffices to rule out obstruction, the patient is allergic to contrast media,

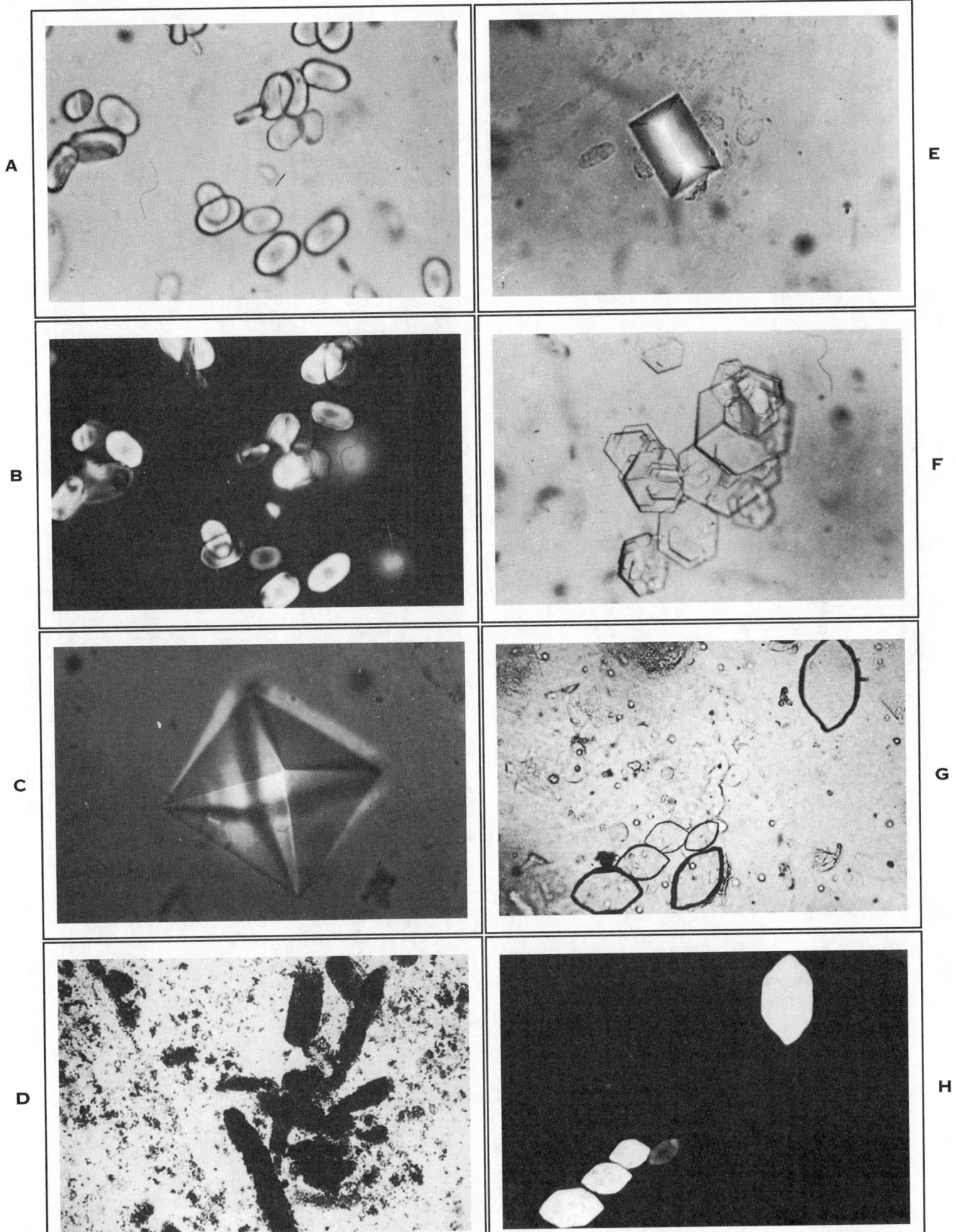

FIGURE 111-1   Crystals that may be seen in the centrifuged sediment from fresh, warm urine in patients with nephrolithiasis and that reflect the composition of the patient's stone. **A**, Calcium oxalate monohydrate (whewellite). **B**, Same as in **A** under polarized light. **C**, Calcium oxalate dihydrate (wedellite). **D**, Calcium phosphate (amorphous apatite), single crystals, in clusters, and in casts. **E**, Magnesium ammonium phosphate hexahydrate (struvite). **F**, Cystine. **G**, Uric acid. **H**, Same as in **G** under polarized light.

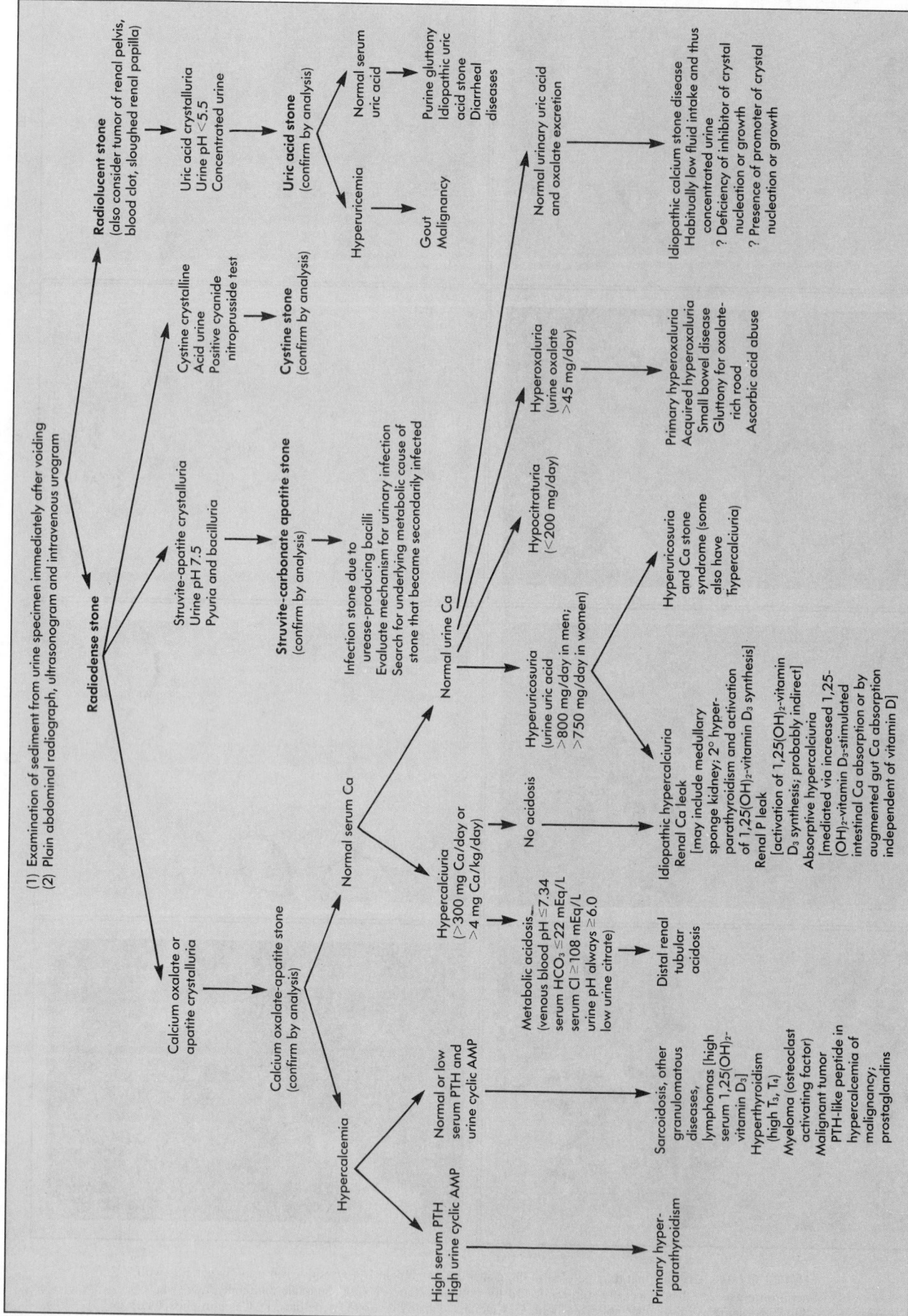

FIGURE 111-2   Evaluation of patients with suspected nephrolithiasis (flank pain, ureteral colic, hematuria, fever).

or the patient has a particular risk for contrast-associated nephropathy.

MANAGEMENT OF NEPHROLITHIASIS
Management of Acute Stone Event

The approach to the therapy of acute stone passage remains the subject of some controversy and variability in clinical pattern. The optimal treatment of a symptomatic stone depends upon both size and location. Spontaneous stone passage is unlikely with stones larger than 8 to 10 mm. Stone removal should be considered for stones causing significant urinary tract obstruction or for any stone associated with infection, particularly an infected struvite stone.

The most important first principle of management of acute stone passage is analgesia. While recent studies suggest that nonsteroidal antiinflammatory agents such as ketorolac may be effective, intravenous morphine remains the best initial analgesic. Intravenous fluids are often administered in large volumes, but there is no evidence that induction of a forced diuresis actually enhances acute stone passage. Patients can typically be managed in an outpatient setting provided that pain is controlled and complete urinary tract obstruction and/or infection is not present. The decision to intervene with invasive approaches to stone removal should be carried out in close consultation with radiologists and urologists.

Stones that become impacted in the distal ureter can be removed ureteroscopically with a stone basket or disrupted in situ with extracorporeal shock wave lithotripsy (ESWL). Stones impacted in the proximal ureter can be treated by in situ percutaneous methods such as ESWL or by ESWL after the stone is pushed up into the renal pelvis (via cystoscopic insertion of a ureteral catheter).

The most effective use of ESWL is in fragmenting small (<2 cm diameter) calcium stones, for which the success rate exceeds 80%. ESWL is now the treatment of choice for stones in the proximal ureter. Approximately one third of patients have transient mild fever, with obstruction by the stone fragments or urinary tract infection occurring in less than 10% of cases. There are few contraindications to ESWL. A bleeding diathesis, an obstructing lesion that might prevent passage of the stone fragments, and pregnancy are the major ones to consider. Unfortunately, after ESWL in patients with larger (>2.5 cm diameter) renal stones (including partial or complete staghorn struvite calculi), residual stone fragments are found about 40% of the time. Thus ESWL is best used in this instance to remove smaller fragments after the stone has been debulked by initial percutaneous nephrolithotomy.

Prevention of Chronic and Recurrent Calcium-Containing Stones

The initial strategy for treating patients with recurrent stone disease is to correct the underlying disturbance. In patients with specific disorders such as hyperparathyroidism, sarcoidosis, or vitamin D excess, therapies aimed at reducing the skeletal release of calcium or GI calcium hyperabsorption are specific to the underlying disturbance. In patients with distal renal tubular acidosis, alkali therapy is required. However, in the vast majority of patients with nephrolithiasis, either idiopathic hypercalciuria or no identifiable abnormality in calcium metabolism is found. In these conditions, various therapeutic options are available but few have been subjected to rigorous experimental validation.

Dietary Modification. There is evidence that a substantial benefit can be achieved with a nonpharmacologic, diet and fluid protocol as previously noted as the "stone clinic effect." Dietary modifications usually involve a reduction in dietary protein intake to no more than 1 g/kg/day, reduction in dietary sodium chloride intake to less than 120 mmole/day, and an increase in fluid intake to achieve 24-hour urine volume of 2 to 3 L. Recently a prospective study of 45,617 healthy men who did not have a history of kidney stones demonstrated that increased dietary calcium intake actually reduces the risk of symptomatic kidney stones, presumably through an action to reduce the availability and absorption of intestinal oxalate. Patients are thus encouraged to reduce their calcium intake only if it is excessive but to maintain it at a level of at least 1 g/day. Oxalate intake should be reduced as much as possible by avoiding foods with a high oxalate content.

Unfortunately the benefits of dietary therapy in patients with recurrent stone formation have not been rigorously tested in controlled studies. However, rigorous studies are also lacking for many pharmacologic therapies such as phosphates, cellulose phosphate, or citrate. Since there is no clear advantage of any specific pharmacologic agent in a majority of patients, it is prudent to utilize dietary modification before embarking on a long-term use of medications. In patients in whom such conservative therapy fails and in whom continued stone activity is demonstrated (radiologically documented new stone formation or stone growth), specific pharmacologic intervention may be required.

Hydrochlorothiazide. Fifty to 100 mg daily of hydrochlorothiazide effectively reduces urinary calcium excretion. The mechanism of this action is complex and involves both a mild reduction in extracellular fluid volume and a secondary enhancement of sodium and calcium reabsorption in the more proximal portions of the nephron to the site of action of thiazides. Because of the linkage of the hypocalciuric action of thiazides to sodium reabsorption pathways, augmentation of dietary sodium intake abrogates the hypocalciuric action of thiazides. Therefore dietary sodium restriction must be part of a thiazide treatment program. Since thiazides do *not* produce sustained reductions in extracellular fluid volume, the long-term benefits of thiazides to induce hypocalciuria must depend on other mechanisms in addition to stimulation of linked sodium-calcium transport. Direct stimulation of distal nephron calcium transport is likely and may secondarily result from the actions of thiazides to block sodium uptake in the distal nephron. This action may lead to an enhancement of sodium-calcium exchange in the basolateral membrane of the distal renal tubule and thereby enhance calcium uptake.

Although thiazides have been shown in at least three studies to be beneficial in reducing stone formation rates, it must be emphasized that the effect is only marginal since the benefits of fluid therapy and diet modification alone are substantial. In patients with an underlying disorder of calcium such as primary hyperparathyroidism or in those with excess vitamin D intake, thiazides may produce hypercalcemia. Serum calcium levels should thus be monitored for 2 months after initiating thiazide therapy.

Thiazide-associated potassium depletion leads to intracellular acidosis and causes hypocitraturia. Potassium levels should also be monitored following initiation of thiazides as persistent hypocitraturia may induce stone formation.

Amiloride. Amiloride acts to reduce urine calcium excretion through secondary stimulation of a sodium-calcium antiporter at the epithelial basolateral membrane which, in turn, leads to stimulation of calcium transport in the distal convoluted tubule. Amiloride reduces potassium excretion and prevents hypokalemia. It may be particularly useful as an adjunct to, or replacement for, thiazides in some patients. Thiazide therapy is contraindicated or ineffective in approximately 10% of patients; amiloride can be used in those cases.

Potassium Citrate. As noted earlier, some patients with calcium-containing stones have associated hypocitraturia. This abnormality may result from an underlying primary disorder or may be the result of one of the various forms of chronic metabolic acidosis. Some studies suggest that dietary supplements with citrate in the dose of 1 mEq/kg body weight raise the level of urinary citrate excretion. This occurs as the alkali load produced by citrate metabolism leads to a reduction in renal citrate reabsorption and secondarily enhances citraturia. Long-term studies suggest that citrate therapy effectively reduces the frequency of new stone formation. While therapy with an equivalent amount of bicarbonate could have the same effect, it is generally not as well tolerated by patients because of gastric bloating. Also the intake of sodium bicarbonate may have an adverse effect since the enhanced sodium intake stimulates calcium excretion.

Other Therapies. Neutral sodium or potassium phosphate has been suggested as an effective therapy for hypercalciuria. It acts by reducing bone resorption of calcium, promoting renal calcium reabsorption, and perhaps by reducing high 1,25-dihydroxy vitamin D_3

levels. Diarrhea is the most common short-term side effect and is a recurrent problem. Acid-containing phosphate salts should not be used because the effects of acidosis on bone and kidney to promote hypercalciuria may override the beneficial effects of phosphate salts. Cellulose phosphate has also been advocated as an effective treatment for hypercalciuria. Unfortunately, cellulose phosphate acts as a nonabsorbable cation-binding resin that complexes calcium in the GI tract and thereby increases the risk of oxalate hyperabsorption. Secondary hyperoxaluria has been documented to be a concomitant of cellulose phosphate therapy.

Therapy of Hyperoxaluria

In those patients with acquired hyperoxaluria from increased intake of oxalate-rich foods such as rhubarb, spinach and other leafy vegetables, cashews, almonds, and strong tea, management includes eliminating these foods from the diet. In addition, in those patients who have hyperoxaluria secondary to the abuse of ascorbic acid, a potential endogenous precursor for oxalate synthesis, this supplement should be discontinued. An important group of patients is those with inflammatory bowel disease and secondary hyperoxaluria. In this condition, additional intake of calcium as calcium carbonate, 500 mg of elemental calcium four times a day, may bind intestinal oxalate and reduce its absorption. Ion exchange resins such as cholestyramine can also be administered in a dosage of 4 g, two to four times daily. The resin binds bile acids, the free forms of which increase colonic absorption of oxalate by increasing its permeability across the intestinal wall. Cholestyramine may also bind oxalate in the intestinal lumen. A trial of pyridoxine 50 to 200 mg/day is also indicated in those cases in whom the dietary restriction of oxalate and increased calcium intake are not effective in reducing oxalate excretion. Adjunct therapy with magnesium oxide (400 mg once or twice daily taken with meals) may be useful because magnesium forms a soluble complex with oxalate.

Management of Uric Acid Stones

The therapy of uric acid nephrolithiasis is directed toward increasing the solubility of uric acid in urine and reducing the daily urine uric acid excretion, if elevated. Again, high fluid intake is a crucial component of therapy, and urine volume should be maintained at least 2 L/day. Water intake should be prescribed at a set rate during the day, and high urine flow at night is an important adjunct. Because maintenance of urinary pH in the vicinity of 6.5 markedly enhances uric acid solubility as urate, alkali therapy should be utilized. In general, approximately 70 mEq of sodium bicarbonate or Shohl's solution is sufficient when administered in divided doses four times per day. In addition, 250 mg of acetazolamide can be given at bedtime to maintain an alkaline urine pH at night. Patients should be taught to monitor urinary pH using pH paper at each voiding for several days after initiating alkali therapy to ensure that urine pH is maintained in the range of 6 to 6.5.

In patients whose urinary uric acid excretion exceeds 800 mg/day or in those in whom high uric acid excretion will be the result of cytolytic drug therapy as treatment for malignant disease, allopurinol should be used. Allopurinol is a competitive inhibitor of xanthine oxidase and blocks uric acid synthesis and inhibits purine biosynthesis. After allopurinol therapy, hypoxanthine and xanthine appear in the urine as predominate end products of purine metabolism. While these compounds are only sparingly soluble, since total purine biosynthesis falls after allopurinol use, risk of stone formation is markedly reduced. Usually 200 to 400 mg of allopurinol in a single daily dose suffices. On occasion, allopurinol causes skin rash, leukopenia, or cholestatic jaundice. Side effects, particularly rash, are common if allopurinol and ampicillin are taken concomitantly.

Management of Struvite Stones

Treatment of struvite stones with medical therapy alone is rarely if ever successful since bacteria live within the interstices of the stone, creating a persistently alkaline local environment and fostering continued deposition of struvite crystals despite apparent sterilization of the urine. Nevertheless, chronic administration of a culture-specific

antimicrobial can, in the occasional patient, prevent further stone growth. Acetohydroxamic acid, an inhibitor of the ectoenzyme urease, has been proposed as an experimental form of medical therapy. This agent can prevent further stone growth or even induce partial stone dissolution. However, it is associated with a number of side effects including thrombophlebitis, and its role, particularly in light of more definitive surgical and lithotriptic approaches, remains marginal.

Stone growth and declining renal function occur in almost all patients who do not undergo definitive invasive therapy. Extracorporeal shock wave lithotripsy and/or percutaneous nephrolithotomy or lithotripsy have become the most commonly used current therapies. These treatment modalities combined with hemiacidrin, a combination of relatively strong organic acids that serves to lyse the remaining stone fragments by lowering the in situ pH, have proven to be safe and effective. After stone removal, a 2- to 4-week course of organism-specific antibiotics should be administered to sterilize the urinary tract. This approach has produced a stone-free rate of approximately 80%.

The surgical removal of struvite stones has been a controversial form of therapy, but more recent surgical approaches have yielded impressive results. Struvite stone removal by anatrophic nephrolithotomy, chemolysis, and organism-specific antibiotics requires only one procedure and has a 90% to 100% success rate, even with large stones.

Following stone removal and after a suitable period of stabilization, patients should undergo a metabolic evaluation because they will frequently be found to have a disorder in the urine such as hypercalciuria to explain the initiation of the stone process before the onset of chronic infection.

Management of Cystine Stones

The frequency of stone recurrence and of complicating urinary obstruction tend to increase as urinary cystine excretion rates increase. As a consequence, ureteral obstruction and complicating urinary infection can lead to progressive renal failure as a result of hydronephrosis and pyelonephritis. Thus the initial phase of therapy involves the education of the patient and, in the case of a young child, the family, regarding the genetic basis for the cystinuria and the need for lifelong therapy. The immaturity of adolescent patients is a major obstacle to adherence to a rigorous pattern of fluid therapy and medications required to control this disorder.

Treatment of cystine stones is aimed at both increasing cystine solubility in urine and lowering cystine excretion. Animal protein intake, principally methionine-containing residues, should probably be limited to 1 g/kg body weight/day to reduce the source of dietary cystine intake. The solubility of cystine over the pH range 4.5 to 7.0 is limited to about 290 to 380 mg/L. Because cystinuric patients typically excrete more than 700 mg/day, urine volume of 3 L/day must be maintained with sufficient nocturnal water intake of at least 300 ml. Patients should monitor 24-hour urine volume regularly.

The solubility of cystine in urine rises sharply to about 790 mg/L as urinary pH rises from 7.0 to 8.0. Thus sustained alkalinization of the urine, in addition to a large urine volume, assists in maintaining cystine in solution. Approximately 2 mEq/kg body weight, or 150 mEq/day, of actual or potential bicarbonate, given in divided doses, is required to maintain the urine pH in the range of 7.5. This can generally be achieved by the administration of 35 to 50 mEq of sodium bicarbonate, or 40 to 60 ml of Shohl's solution, four times a day. Because dietary sodium chloride may enhance cystine excretion, it should be restricted, and some of the needed base should be administered as potassium citrate or potassium bicarbonate rather than sodium bicarbonate. In addition, 250 mg of acetazolamide may be given at bedtime to inhibit proximal tubular bicarbonate reabsorption and induce a nocturnal alkaline diuresis. When acetazolamide is administered, an additional dose of sodium bicarbonate or Shohl's solution should be given during the night when the patient arises to void, to check the tendency for serum bicarbonate levels to fall and the urine to become more acid as the action of acetazolamide develops and then wanes. Patients should check their urine pH at each voiding for several days, using phenaphthazine paper to ensure that the pH is 7.5 or higher.

Daily cystine excretion can be reduced by the administration of the SH-containing drugs, D-penicillamine, mercaptoproprionylglycine (MPG), or captopril. These drugs can undergo a disulfide exchange

✔ *WHEN TO REFER*

Patients with cystinuria and struvite stones should be referred for management by a consultant with experience utilizing the medications and techniques required for the proper treatment of these patients. Patients with recurrent nephrolithiasis and in the absence of a predisposing disorder such as sarcoidosis or hyperparathyroidism should be referred to a specialized center only if a conservative dietary program has failed and the patient, if hypercalciuric, has not responded adequately to thiazide therapy. Patients with uric acid nephrolithiasis do not typically require referral unless allopurinol therapy fails.

reaction with cystine to form the mixed disulfide of cysteine and the drug. These mixed disulfides are very much more soluble than cystine. D-penicillamine may result in significant toxic side effects that include fever, rash, leukopenia, thrombocytopenia, and the nephrotic syndrome. MPG appears to be less toxic. Captopril is effective, and although additional experience with its use is needed, recent reports have supported early claims for its efficacy in reducing stone growth and enhancing cystine solubility.

Collectively these therapeutic measures may sometimes result in the dissolution of nonobstructing cystine stones, but more often they appear to be most useful in preventing further growth of existing stones and the formation of new stones.

BIBLIOGRAPHY

Asplin JR, Favus MJ, Coe FL: Nephrolithiasis. In Brenner BM, editor: *Brenner and Rector's The Kidney,* ed 5, Philadelphia, 1996, WB Saunders.

Barcelo P, Wuhl O, Servitge E et al: Randomized double-blind study of potassium citrate in idiopathic hypocitraturic calcium nephrolithiasis, *J Urol* 150:1761, 1993.

Coe FL, Favus MJ, editors: *Disorders of bone and mineral metabolism,* New York, 1992, Raven Press.

Coe FL, Parks JH, Asplin JR: The pathogenesis and treatment of kidney stones, *N Engl J Med* 327:1141, 1992.

Drach GW: Urinary lithiasis. In Walsh PC et al, editors: *Campbell's urology,* ed 6, Philadelphia, 1992, WB Saunders.

Lemann J, Jr: Composition of the diet and calcium kidney stones, *N Engl J Med* 328:880, 1993 (editorial).

Robertson GL: Berl T: Pathophysiology of water metabolism. In Brenner BM, editor: *Brenner and Rector's The kidney,* ed 5, Philadelphia, 1996, WB Saunders.

Segura JW, Preminger GM, Assimos DG et al: Nephrolithiasis Clinical Guidelines Panel summary report with management of staghorn calculi, *J Urol* 151:1648, 1994.

Ziyadeh FN: Results of therapy of calcium renal calculi with the thiazides. In Puschett JB, editor: *Diuretics. IV. chemistry, pharmacology and clinical applications,* Amsterdam, 1993 Excerpta Medica.

IV DISORDERS OF ELECTROLYTE AND ACID-BASE BALANCE

CHAPTER

112 Disorders of Water Balance

Robert G. Narins, Mark D. Faber, and G. Gopal Krishna

Worsening weakness, lethargy, and nausea merge with progressive headache and obtundation to culminate in generalized seizures, coma, and, ultimately, death. This pernicious continuum of symptoms and signs describes equally well the deteriorating course of either hyponatremia or hypernatremia, the chemical hallmarks of disordered water balance. Disorders that spawn deranged water balance with its potentially lethal consequences are best understood in terms of the regulatory system that normally controls solute concentration *(osmoregulation)* with exquisite precision. Accordingly, after first outlining the chemical and physiologic principles that underlie the normal control of water balance, we develop a pathophysiologic approach to the classification, diagnosis, and therapy for the states of disordered osmoregulation. (See Chapter 101 for a more detailed discussion of solute and water balance.)

PRINCIPLES OF OSMOREGULATION
Definitions, Water Distribution, and Solute Concentration

Driven by osmotic forces, water moves freely across membranes from areas of low to high solute concentration, thereby dissipating concentration gradients. Because all cell membranes (except renal medullary structures) are freely permeable to water, the solute concentration, or osmolality, of intracellular fluid (ICF) always equals that of extracellular fluid (ECF).

Cell metabolism, membrane selectivity, and transport pumps create and sustain major qualitative differences in the solute composition of ICF and ECF (Fig. 112-1), whereas osmotic water movement ensures transcellular equality of concentration. In contrast to the low-molecular-weight, membrane-permeable anions in the ECF, intracellular anions are macromolecular and relatively nonpermeating. As defined by the *Gibbs-Donnan equilibrium* (Chapter 101), the compartment containing impermeable anions attracts more cations, which in turn leads to the osmotic attraction of more water. Cell swelling, dysfunction, and eventual rupture would occur if accrual of ions and water went unchecked. Membrane-associated cation pumps prevent cellular disruption by actively exporting sodium and importing potassium. Thus the $(Na^+ + K^+)$-ATPase (sodium-potassium activated adenosine triphosphatase) pump is responsible for potassium and sodium being the major cellular and extracellular solutes, respectively, and for negating passive cation and water entry into cells, thereby maintaining the stability of *cell volume.* The other prime determinant of cell volume is ECF osmolality. Dilution or concentration of ECF solute causes water to enter or leave cells, respectively, and thereby effects cell swelling or shrinkage (see later discussion). It follows therefore that osmoregulation is tantamount to control of cell volume. Indeed, most of hyponatremia's poisonous effect is secondary to brain cell swelling, whereas that of hypernatremia is due to brain cell shrinkage.

Addition of urea or ethanol, solutes that freely cross cell membranes, equally increases the solute concentration of the ECF and the ICF without provoking water movement. Urea and ethanol, therefore, are *ineffective osmols,* because their addition increases osmolality (solute concentration/kg water) without effecting water movement. Addition of sodium salts, which are largely restricted to the ECF, ini-

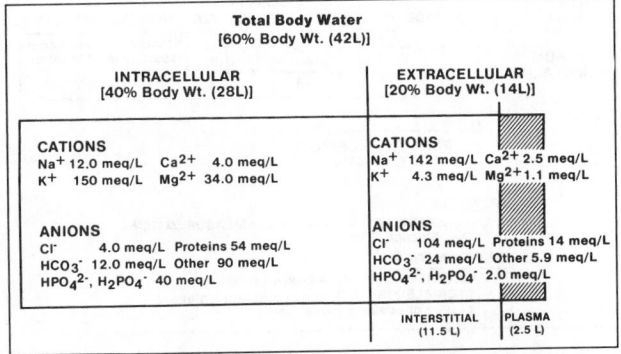

FIGURE 112-1 Body water and electrolyte distribution. Approximate distribution of body water and electrolytes in a 70-kg man. Extracellular fluid is divided into interstitial and plasma *(shaded)* components.

tially increases extracellular osmolality. This extracellular hypertonicity is minimized by solute-free water moving along osmotic gradients from the ICF to the ECF. Net water movement ceases when ECF and ICF osmolalities equalize at new, higher levels. Cell shrinkage resulting from this fluid redistribution can have disastrous effects (especially on the brain), but certain central receptor cells (see later discussion) respond by increasing thirst and the release of *arginine vasopressin* (AVP), the hormone that causes renal retention of acquired water. Retained exogenous water reexpands cells and normalizes the solute concentration of body fluid. Thus sodium salts are *effective osmols* because they increase osmolality and effect transfer of water. The term *tonicity* refers to the effective osmolality of serum. Hypertonic and hypotonic serums cause water to leave or enter cells, respectively. Addition of *ineffective* osmols (e.g., urea) to serum does not affect tonicity. Thus azotemic serum may be hyperosmolal without being hypertonic. Loss of sodium salts or the addition of water to the ECF transiently lowers ECF solute concentration, causing water to move into cells until ECF and ICF concentrations equalize at a new, lower value. Although resulting cellular expansion can be life-threatening, swelling of certain brain cells (see later discussion) diminishes thirst and water acquisition and suppresses AVP release, allowing the kidneys to excrete the excess water.

Measurements of *osmolality* define the concentration of all plasma solutes (per kilogram of water), that is, electrolyte and nonelectrolyte solute and effective and ineffective osmols. The electrolyte component is almost entirely accounted for by sodium and its accompanying anions, and may be estimated by doubling the serum sodium concentration (Fig. 112-2). Urea and glucose account for virtually all of the normally occurring nonelectrolyte solute. The concentration of either may be converted from mass units (mg/dl) to mmole/L (which is equivalent to mOsm/L), by dividing by its molecular weight. Because urea concentration is reported in terms of its nitrogen content (atomic weight 14) (i.e., blood urea nitrogen, or BUN), and because each mole of urea contains 2 mol of nitrogen, the osmolality of urea (mOsm/L) from the mass of urea (mg/L or /dl) is found by dividing as follows:

$$\text{(EQ. 1)}$$

$$\text{BUN (mOsm/L)} = \frac{\text{BUN (mg/L)}}{28} = \frac{\text{BUN (mg/dl)}}{2.8}$$

Because sodium, urea, and glucose are the principal contributors to plasma osmolality, it is logical to infer that calculated plasma osmolality should equal that measured in the laboratory. Indeed, under physiologic conditions the difference between measured and calculated osmolality, otherwise termed the *osmolal gap,* does not exceed 10 mOsm/L (see Fig. 112-2). Marked increases in plasma proteins and lipid levels cause underestimation of the plasma sodium concentration but do not interfere with the measured osmolality. Thus hyperlipidemia and hyperproteinemia spuriously increase the osmolal gap. A true increase in osmolal gap indicates the presence of an osmotically active solute not accounted for by sodium and its counterbalancing anions urea and glucose, but may be due to circulating etha-

nol, methanol, ethylene glycol, or other low molecular weight toxins. Modest increases in the osmolal gap occur in patients with chronic renal failure who are not receiving dialysis and in patients with lactic acidosis and/or ketoacidosis. Therapeutic administration of osmotically active compounds such as mannitol, sorbitol, or glycine increases the measured but decreases the calculated osmolality by lowering serum sodium levels and thus increases the osmolal gap.

Sodium accounts for more than 95% of the ECF solute and potassium exerts an equivalent effect in the ICF. Thus because total body solute is virtually equivalent to the body content of exchangeable sodium (Na_e) and potassium (K_e) salts, it follows that the *concentration* of solute (i.e., the osmolality) is equal to the sum of these two salts, with their respective anions, divided by the volume of total body water (TBW):

$$\text{(EQ. 2)}$$

$$\text{ECF osmolality} = \text{ICF osmolality} = \frac{2\,(Na_e + K_e)}{\text{TBW}}$$

As discussed later, loss of Na_e or K_e at constant TBW causes hypotonicity. Water retention while body solute content remains constant has a similar effect. Solute gain or water loss causes hypertonicity. Because sodium is the major ECF solute, with rare exception (see later discussion), hypotonicity is equivalent to hyponatremia. However, because such effective osmols as glucose or mannitol may accumulate in the ECF and cause hypertonicity with or without changing sodium concentration, hypertonicity is *not* equivalent to hypernatremia (but hypernatremia always means that hypertonicity is present).

Proportionate accumulation of solute and water causes *isotonic expansion* of body fluid. States of solute and water depletion may be isotonic (normal serum sodium concentration) if solute and water are lost in proportion, hypotonic (hyponatremia) if proportionately more solute than water is lost, or hypertonic (hypernatremia) if proportionately more water is lost. It follows therefore that the serum sodium concentration only defines the ratio of sodium to water and should imply nothing about the state of body sodium content or ECF volume.

As influenced by the aforementioned forces, body water is distributed into cellular and extracellular compartments, the latter being further subdivided into interstitial and intravascular spaces (see Fig. 112-2). Transcellular fluid encompasses such epithelial cell secretions as sweat, gastrointestinal secretions, saliva, bile, and cerebrospinal, ocular, and joint fluids. These fluids, at any instant, do not constitute a large space, but because their turnover is great, their continued loss can eventually lead to severe fluid depletion. Capillary permeability characteristics cause entrapment of albumin and other large molecules in the vascular space, ensuring that interstitial fluid has little protein and that approximately 25% of ECF is retained in the vascular space because of the osmotic (oncotic) effect of protein.

Forces controlling fluid distribution are further illustrated by tracking the distribution of various parenteral fluids (Table 112-1). Rapid catabolism of administered dextrose allows remaining water to distribute throughout all fluid spaces. Thus of the liter of dextrose and water (see Table 112-1), two thirds enters cells and only one fourth of the one third (i.e., $\frac{1}{12}$, or 83 ml) remaining extracellularly is kept in the vascular space. Because sodium is restricted to the ECF, the entire liter of isotonic saline remains in this space, and, according to Starling's forces, 25% (250 ml) remains in the vascular space. It follows that for volume expansion, saline is far superior to water but less effective than protein-containing solutions.

Osmoregulation: An Integrated Triarchy

Under control conditions normal humans can ingest and excrete up to 15 to 20 L of water daily with only a 1% to 3% reduction in serum osmolality. In this setting urine osmolality is reduced to 35 to 40 mOsm. Under conditions of severe water restriction with continued evaporative losses, a 2% to 3% increase in serum osmolality causes urine volume to decrease to 0.4 to 0.5 L/day, whereas urine osmolality increases to 1200 to 1400 mOsm. Thus, depending on the imposed demands for water conservation or excretion, urine volume can vary fifty-fold and urine osmolality thirty-five–fold (Fig. 112-3). Sev-

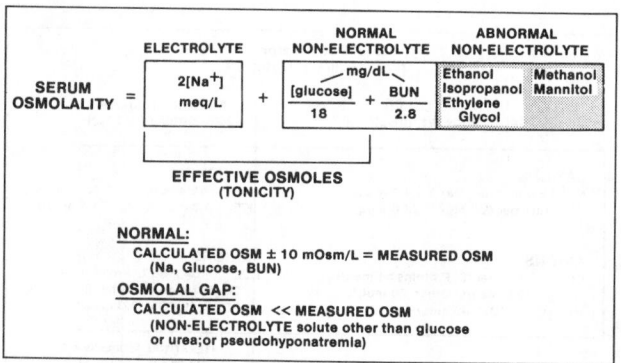

FIGURE 112-2　Calculated and measured serum osmolality. Total serum osmolality comprises electrolyte and nonelectrolyte solute. The effective osmoles are largely restricted to the extracellular fluid. The common contributors to the pathologic accumulation of solute are shown in the shaded box.

eral important clinical points follow from these observations. The renal capacity for water excretion is enormous, making it extremely difficult to imbibe enough fluid to overwhelm a normally operating osmoregulatory system. Exceptions are discussed later. With total abstinence from water, the kidney can strikingly lower urine volume, but it continues to excrete an obligatory 400 to 500 ml of urine, which, along with continuing evaporative losses, causes serum hypertonicity to progressively worsen. Failure of maximal renal water retention would, of course, accelerate the progression of hypertonicity in thirsting subjects. Figure 112-3 also emphasizes that the greatest water savings and reduction in urine volume occur when urine osmolality is increased from maximal dilution to isotonicity. The additional water conserved in maximizing urine concentration is much less (see Fig. 112-3).

The three key elements of the osmoregulatory system are *thirst, AVP*, and the *renal concentrating and diluting mechanism.* This system is exquisitely sensitive to small (1% to 2%) changes in effective ECF osmolality (tonicity) and is poised to maintain serum osmolality almost constant despite wide variations in water intake. Consequently, serum sodium concentration and cell volume are protected from disruptive and dangerously capricious changes in our daily water appetite. Contraction of intravascular volume requires that protective water retention occur to ensure vascular filling and continued perfusion of vital organs. Indeed the osmoregulatory system also responds to volume demands, but is less sensitive to hypovolemia than to hypertonicity. Whereas a 1% to 2% change in serum osmolality provokes appropriate and salutary changes in the system, an 8% to 10% reduction in blood volume is required to stimulate AVP release and water retention. Thus regulation of solute concentration takes precedence over volume regulation when ECF volume contraction or expansion is modest. With severe contraction, however, water is retained, giving volume requirements precedence over osmoregulation. Thus in hypovolemic states water may be retained and tissue perfusion protected despite worsening hypotonicity.

Integrated Overview of the Osmoregulatory System (Fig. 112-4). Changes in ECF tonicity are translated into appropriate increments or decrements in plasma AVP levels by hypothalamic osmoreceptors, which signal neighboring nuclei and the neurohypophysis to alter AVP synthesis and release. Water acquisition or rejection is also provoked by osmoreceptor signals to centrally located thirst-control centers. Thus *hypertonicity* elicits AVP release, which in turn stimulates renal retention of ingested water. Similarly, *hypotonicity* suppresses thirst and AVP release, enabling the kidney to excrete

Table 112-1   Distribution of 1 L of infused fluid

SOLUTION	SPACE OF DISTRIBUTION	CHANGE IN VOLUME*		
		ICW (ML)	ISF (ML)	PLASMA (ML)
1000 ml 5% dextrose in water	Total body water	665	250	85
1000 ml normal saline	Only in extracellular water	0	750	250
1000 ml half normal saline				
500 ml water	Total body water	335	125	40
500 ml normal saline	Only in extracellular water	0	375	125
1000 ml plasma	Restricted to plasma	0	0	1000

ICW, Intracellular water; *ISF*, interstitial fluid.
*Values rounded.

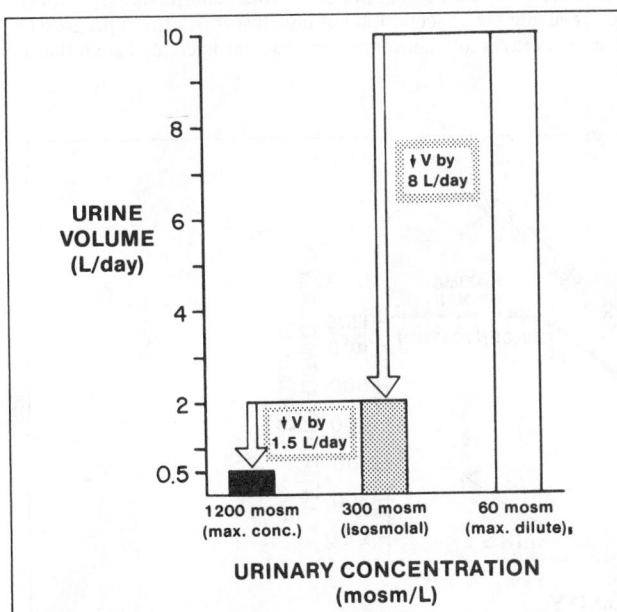

FIGURE 112-3   Urine volume *(V)* in relation to urine osmolality. The figure illustrates the changes in urine volume that are seen as a subject excreting 600 mOsm of solute daily concentrates his urine from maximum dilution to isosmolality to maximum concentration.

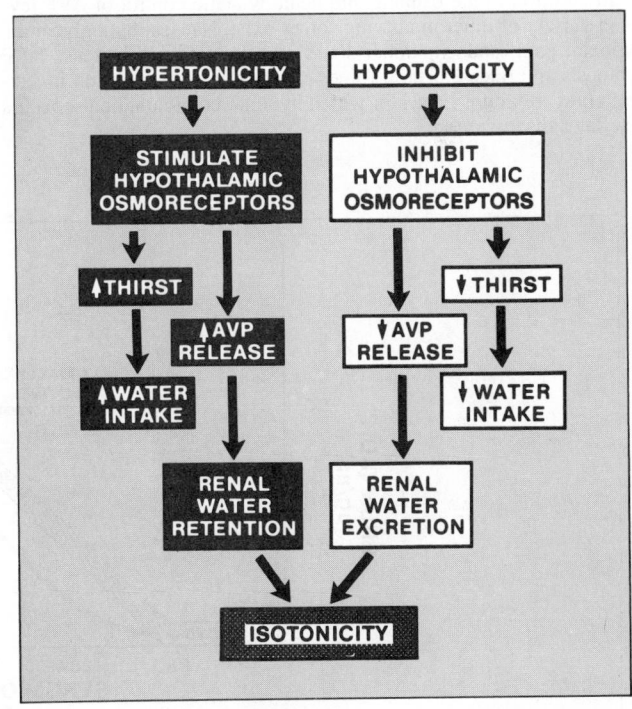

FIGURE 112-4   Osmoregulation. The diagram illustrates the interaction of serum tonicity with hypothalamic centers for thirst and arginine vasopressin *(AVP)* release. Resulting renal retention or excretion of water restores serum isotonicity.

solute-free water. Renal retention of water in the former setting or excretion of water in the latter, reestablishes ECF isotonicity.

Control of Arginine Vasopressin (Chapter 296)

Osmotic stimulation. Rapid intracarotid injections of hypertonic solutions caused water-loaded, diuresing, conscious dogs to abruptly reduce urine volume and increase urinary tonicity. Failure of ineffective osmols to elicit a similar antidiuretic response led Verney in the 1940s to hypothesize that osmoreceptor cells contract or expand in response to altered ECF tonicity, and signal release or suppression of an antidiuretic principle. Since then, Verney's conclusions and hypotheses have been refined and extended but rarely challenged. The supraoptic and paraventricular nuclei of the hypothalamus synthesize the hormone that is transported with its carrier portion, *neurophysin,* intraaxonally to its storage site in the neurohypophysis.

When the ECF osmolality is less than or equal to 280 mOsm, plasma AVP levels are undetectable, and the urinary osmolality is usually less than 150 mOsm (Fig. 112-5). In this setting, free-water excretion can be torrential, making 280 mOsm the lower limit of achievable ECF osmolality, given a system that is operating normally. Exceptions are discussed later. Plasma AVP levels increase linearly as serum osmolality rises. When serum osmolality reaches 290 to 294 mOsm, plasma AVP levels approximate 5 pg/ml and urinary osmolality approaches its upper limits of 1200 to 1400 mOsm (see Fig. 112-5). Further increments in plasma AVP concentration are not translated into greater degrees of renal water retention. Thus the entire range of maximal renal concentration and dilution is realized over a plasma AVP concentration that spans from undetectable to 5 pg/ml. Indeed, AVP levels of 2.0 to 2.5 pg/ml convert maximally dilute urine to isotonicity, thereby effecting the greatest conservation of water over the range of dilution and concentration (see Fig. 112-5.).

Nonosmotic stimulation. As noted earlier, *baroreceptors* located in the left atrium, aortic arch, and carotid sinus modify AVP release through signals carried by glossopharyngeal and vagal afferent nerves during periods of volume depletion and/or hypotension. In contrast to the linear relationship between osmolality and plasma AVP levels, the volume-AVP curve is exponential. Thus although relatively insensitive to changes in volume (see earlier discussion), the logarithmic increase in AVP levels allows for water retention and the establishment of the high concentrations required to achieve a pressor effect.

In addition to the osmotic and hemodynamic control of AVP levels, a variety of other modifying forces exist. Nausea, hypoglycemia, hypoxia, pain, and emotional stress can dramatically increase AVP synthesis and release. These forces can sustain AVP secretion in several clinical circumstances in which hyponatremia commonly occurs (see later discussion).

During pregnancy, plasma osmolality and the osmotic thresholds for the release of AVP and for thirst decrease by approximately 10 mOsm/L (i.e., AVP is released at lower levels of osmolality, and thirst is not extinguished until osmolality is below normal). These alterations in pregnancy appear to be independent of changes in effective plasma volume. Once hypotonicity reaches the new threshold level for thirst and AVP release, water intake and hormone secretion are extinguished, thereby establishing a new steady state. In addition to these changes in osmotic threshold, metabolic clearance of AVP is augmented from the tenth week of gestation to midterm. The latter phenomenon has been attributed to an increase in the plasma concentration of a cystine aminopeptidase enzyme termed *vasopressinase*. Vasopressinase is elaborated by the placental tissue and inactivates both oxytocin and AVP. Enhanced release of vasopressinase may explain the unmasking of central diabetes insipidus during pregnancy.

Renal Response to AVP. (See Chapter 101 for a more detailed discussion.) The volume of glomerular filtrate is reduced by approximately two thirds in the proximal convoluted tubule, but under all conditions remains isotonic through the last portion of this segment accessible to micropuncture analysis. The tonicity of fluid emerging from the thick ascending limb is always hypotonic, indicating that proportionately more solute than solvent is reabsorbed in Henle's loop. In the absence of AVP, the collecting tubules remain almost "waterproof," causing the final urine to be markedly hypotonic. Following the hormone's binding to its V2 receptor, AVP's primary action is to increase the number of selective water channels in the luminal membrane of cortical and medullary collecting ducts, thereby effecting osmotic communication between dilute luminal fluid and the hypertonic medullary interstitium. These water channels are termed *aquaporin-2* or *CHIP-28 pores*. Because medullary interstitial tonicity increases longitudinally from the isotonic corticomedullary junction (300 mOsm) to the hypertonic papillary tip (1200 mOsm), collecting duct filtrate, in the presence of AVP, loses water and becomes progressively more concentrated.

Medullary hypertonicity is created and maintained by the interaction of several forces. The reabsorption of sodium and potassium chloride without water from the thick ascending limb of Henle's loop at once renders luminal fluid dilute and medullary interstitium, in receipt of salt, hypertonic. The countercurrent exchange mechanism in medullary vasa recta (Chapter 101) prevents loss of medullary solute and allows for removal of reabsorbed water. In the presence of AVP, water is reabsorbed without urea in cortical and medullary collecting ducts, causing the concentration of unreabsorbed urea to progressively increase. A favorable concentration gradient is created such that urea

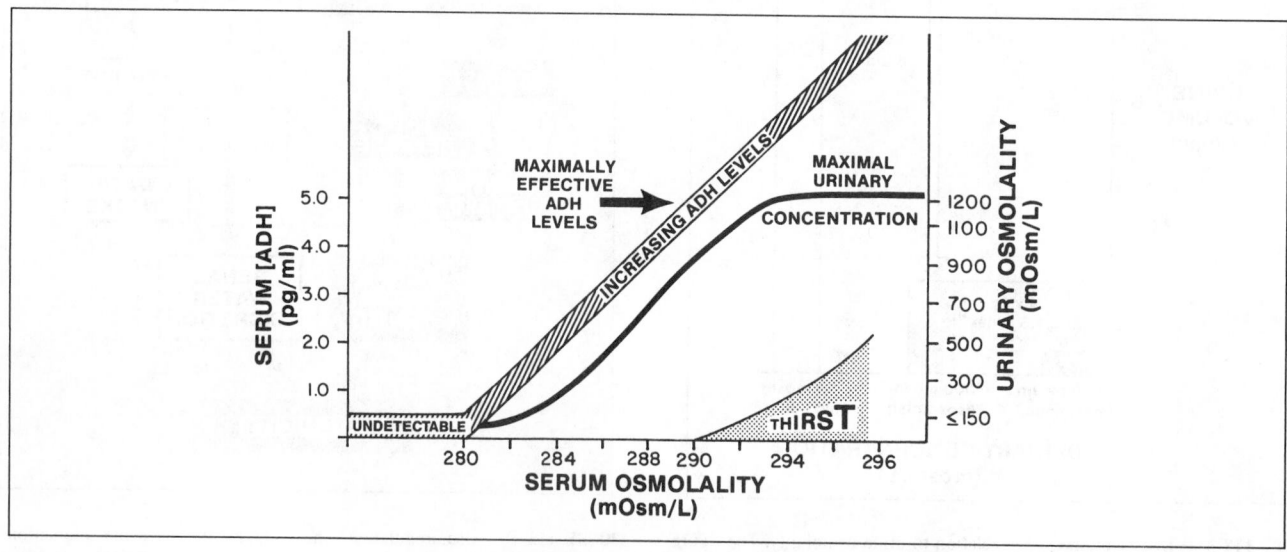

FIGURE 112-5 Integration of osmoregulatory forces. The diagram suggests an approximate correlation between serum antidiuretic hormone *(ADH)* levels, urine and serum osmolality, and thirst. See text for details.

diffuses from the inner medullary collecting duct fluid to the interstitium, further increasing medullary hypertonicity.

It follows that urinary dilution will be impaired and water retention favored when distal delivery of fluid and solute is reduced due to diminished glomerular filtration or to enhanced proximal reabsorption. Inhibition of salt reabsorption in the thick ascending limb and in more distal portions of the nephron, and failure to appropriately suppress AVP release will also limit maximal urinary dilution. These pathophysiologic forces find expression in the various forms of hyponatremia (see later discussion). Impaired maximal urinary concentration with consequent loss of body water may result from inhibited salt reabsorption in the thick ascending limb, from reduced medullary hypertonicity due to altered medullary blood flow or intrinsic renal disease, and from lack of AVP secretion or failure of the tubules to respond normally to the hormone. These pathophysiologic forces find expression in the various clinical forms of hypernatremia (see later discussion).

Thirst. Although there are many qualitative similarities between the control of AVP secretion and thirst, important quantitative differences exist. Both processes are stimulated by hypertonicity and by ECF volume contraction. Although the AVP response to these stimuli has been defined with relative precision, the quantification of thirst has proved more elusive. Social and cultural forces play importantly on the "ebb and flow of body fluid," rendering difficult the development of standard tests for thirst in humans.

Whereas changes in plasma osmolality of 1% to 2% elicit a large outpouring of AVP and excretion of hypertonic urine, most humans do not experience thirst until the serum osmolality exceeds 295 mOsm (see Fig. 112-5). Thus water ingestion is not stimulated until maximum renal water retention has developed. Speaking teleologically, thirst appears to function as a backup, or reserve, system for AVP-renal regulation of water balance. For a given increase in plasma osmolality, that caused by sodium stimulates thirst to a greater extent than does that caused by glucose.

It would also appear that thirst is less sensitive to hypovolemia than is AVP release, requiring a 20% reduction in blood volume for stimulation (compared with the 8% to 10% reduction needed for AVP release). Renal baroreceptors, located in the juxtaglomerular apparatus, seem to play a key role in stimulating thirst but do not significantly alter AVP secretion. Hypovolemia and reduced renal perfusion pressure activate the renin-angiotensin system, thereby generating angiotensin II, a central thirst stimulant. It is also true that angiotensin II is synthesized within the central nervous system and may play a more important role in controlling thirst than does peripheral angiotensin II.

In summary, the challenge of water excess is met primarily by suppression of AVP release with consequent renal excretion of solute-free water. Thirst is inhibited early in hypotonic states but seems to afford little protection above and beyond that contributed by the AVP-renal system. With progressive hypertonicity, thirst comes into play only late in the course. This stimulation of water ingestion in severe dehydration is clearly an important protective addition.

STATES OF ABNORMAL WATER METABOLISM
Hyponatremic States

Etiology and Pathogenesis. Because sodium accounts for more than 95% of ECF solute, hypotonic states are *always* associated with hyponatremia (see later discussion) (Fig. 112-6). The reverse, how-

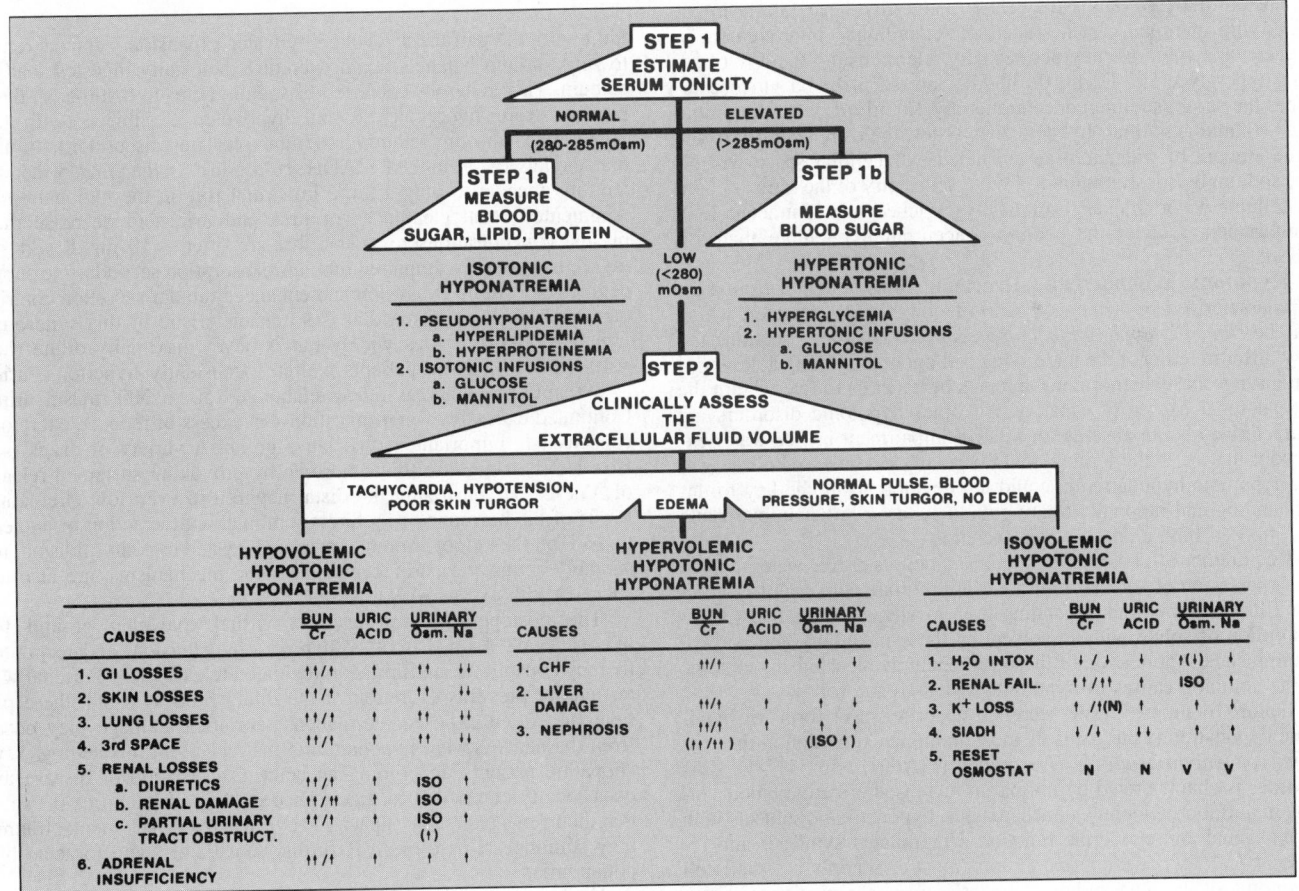

FIGURE 112-6 Differential diagnosis of hyponatremia. The figure integrates the classification of the hyponatremias with a clinical and laboratory approach to their diagnosis. See text for details. *CHF,* Congestive heart failure; *ISO,* isotonic; *N,* normal; *V,* variable.

Modified from Narins RG et al: Diagnostic strategies in disorders of fluid, electrolyte, and acid-base homeostasis, *Am J Med* 72:496, 1982.

ever, is not true (i.e., hyponatremia is not *always* associated with hypotonicity) (see later discussion). Thus the hyponatremias may be classified pathophysiologically into three variants: isotonic, hypertonic, and hypotonic. Tonicity is a calculated parameter; it is not directly measured (see Fig. 112-2). The serum concentrations of the common effective osmols, sodium and glucose, allow estimation of tonicity (see Fig. 112-2).

Isotonic hyponatremia. Isotonic hyponatremia occurs during the infusion of isotonic, sodium-free solutions or may be caused by a laboratory artifact. Administration of isotonic solutions of glucose (5%) or mannitol (5%) expands the ECF and dilutes serum sodium, and the hexose prevents water movement into cells. Eventual entry of glucose into cells and its subsequent metabolism allow two thirds of the infused water to enter cells. The hyponatremia is thus transformed from isotonic to hypotonic as the sugar is oxidized. Renal excretion of mannitol has the same effect. Hyperlipidemia or hyperproteinemia (e.g., in myeloma or macroglobulinemia) displaces water from each liter of plasma. Because sodium salts distribute only in the water phase, each unit volume of plasma will contain less water and therefore less sodium. The sodium concentration in remaining plasma water, and therefore its osmolality, remain unchanged, but clinical laboratories expressing sodium concentration per liter of whole plasma report spuriously low values. This set of chemical findings is termed *pseudohyponatremia*. Absorption of the mannitol or glycine solutions used as bladder irrigants during prostatic resections causes isotonic hyponatremia. If hypotonic solutions are used, an element of hypotonic hyponatremia adds to the fall in serum sodium concentration.

Hypertonic hyponatremia. Accumulation of effective osmols in the ECF dilutes serum sodium by causing the osmotic withdrawal of solute-free water from cells. Glucose and mannitol are the major clinically relevant osmols responsible for this effect. This solute-induced expansion of ECF volume may cause congestive heart failure in patients with marginal cardiac function. Accordingly, improvement in congestive symptoms may occasionally attend insulin therapy of severe hyperglycemia. Each 100 mg/dl increase in blood glucose reduces the serum sodium concentration by 1.6 mEq/L when the initial ECF volume is normal. In edematous states, the osmotic entry of the same amount of water into an expanded extracellular space will dilute sodium by a lesser amount. Conversely, entry of the same amount of cellular water into an osmotically enriched but contracted ECF compartment reduces the sodium concentration by more than 1.6 mEq/L.

Hypotonic hyponatremia. Hypotonic forms of hyponatremia are all characterized by a reduced ratio of body solute to water, which may be *clinically apparent or inapparent* (see Diagnosis section) and may differ in terms of the underlying pathogenesis. Rarely a deranged patient ingests such enormous amounts of water as to overwhelm the normal renal excretory capacity. All other hypotonic disorders are characterized by an absolute or relative impairment in free-water excretion; that is, if the kidney could normally excrete solute-free water, hypotonic hyponatremia could not develop. Thus the key to understanding and rationally treating these syndromes lies in clarifying the imposed limitation on water excretion.

Requirements for excreting maximal amounts of free water include (1) suppression of AVP secretion, (2) appropriate delivery of glomerular filtrate to the thick ascending limb of Henle's loop, and (3) reabsorption of solute without solvent by these medullary and cortical diluting sites. Application of these pathogenetic mechanisms to some of the common causes of hypotonic hyponatremia follows.

Failure to suppress AVP secretion underlies most forms of hypotonic hyponatremia but gains its most dramatic expression in the *syndrome of inappropriate ADH secretion* (SIADH) (Box 112-1). This disorder is characterized by normal to increased effective blood volume in normoproteinemic, nonedematous, hyponatremic subjects with normal renal and endocrine function. Unregulated synthesis and release of AVP by nonendocrine tumors (most commonly by small-cell carcinoma of the lung and/or its metastases) or the persistent stimulation of hypothalamic-hypophyseal release of AVP by a variety of pulmonary and cerebral disorders, accounts for the majority of reported cases of SIADH (see Box 112-1 and Fig. 112-6). Excessive AVP secretion causes retention of ingested water, two thirds of which expands the intracellular space while the remainder swells the ECF.

BOX 112-1

Differential diagnosis of the syndrome of inappropriate antidiuretic hormone (SIADH) secretion

Neoplasms

Lung (small cell in 80%), pancreas, duodenum, lymphoma, ureter, prostate, Ewing's sarcoma

Pulmonary

Infection (viral, bacterial, fungal), abscess, asthma, respirator therapy

Central nervous system

Trauma, neoplasms, infections, vascular, degenerative diseases (including aging), psychoses

Cardiac

Atrial tachycardias, post–mitral-commissurotomy syndrome

Metabolic

Myxedema, adrenal insufficiency, acute porphyria, anterior pituitary insufficiency, angiotensin II

Stress
Drugs

Hypoglycemic agents (chlorpropamide, tolbutamide), antineoplastic drugs (cyclophosphamide, vincristine), narcotics (morphine, barbiturates), psychotropics (phenothiazine derivatives)

Following the natriuresis evoked by water expansion, subjects return to zero sodium balance, again excreting their daily ingested load of sodium. This generous excretion of sodium helps to distinguish these patients from hypervolemic and hypovolemic subjects with hyponatremia who are retaining sodium (see later discussion). In animal models of prolonged SIADH, solute loss, rather than water retention, appears to play a more important role in the hyponatremia. Augmented renal clearances of urea and uric acid decrease their plasma concentrations to values that are often <10 mg/dl and <3 mg/dl, respectively. Impaired tubular reabsorption secondary to subtle degrees of volume expansion and enhanced tubular secretion contributes to the hypouricemia that is so characteristic of this syndrome. Urine osmolality varies widely but is never maximally dilute (i.e., <100 mOsm). Some patients excrete persistently hypertonic urine (>300 mOsm), whereas others elaborate 150 to 300 mOsm urine. Continued excessive water ingestion—in excess of reduced excretory capacity—is important in this latter group. A variety of drugs (see Box 112-1) can cause this syndrome by provoking sustained release of AVP or by sensitizing the distal nephron to even low circulating levels of the hormone or by directly mimicking the action of authentic AVP on the kidney. Adrenal insufficiency and hypothyroidism, presumably acting via baroreceptor-mediated mechanisms, are also associated with excess AVP release.

The postoperative setting is a virtual spawning ground for hyponatremia. Pain, narcotics, hypoxia, hypotension, and respirator therapy conspire to sustain the unregulated release of AVP. Renal water avidity prevents excretion of the dilute fluid to which these patients are often exposed. Permanent neurologic damage may occur from the acute, severe hyponatremia that occurs in this setting. Psychopathic patients undergoing an acute exacerbation of disease are occasionally compelled to ingest such enormous quantities of water that their renal excretory capacity is overwhelmed. The mental trauma may stimulate release of AVP, further sensitizing them to acute hyponatremia.

Hyponatremic disorders associated with reduced effective blood volume stimulate AVP release via the previously discussed baroreceptor mechanisms. Reduction of circulating volume by hemorrhage, gastrointestinal, or renal fluid loss, or redistribution of plasma into the interstitial space, triggers baroreceptor-mediated release of AVP. Hypoproteinemic states (cirrhosis, nephrosis) and congestive heart failure similarly stimulate release of the hormone. It follows that these disorders limit the excretion of free water and thus sensitize these patients to hyponatremia.

Delivery of filtrate to the distal diluting segments is dependent on adequate glomerular filtration, normal proximal nephron reabsorption, and ingestion of adequate amounts of solute. As renal failure progresses and the glomerular filtration rate declines, the absolute volume of filtrate reaching distal sites diminishes. With advanced disease, the maximum achievable volume of free water that can be generated and excreted is markedly reduced. Even modest increases in water intake may lead to hyponatremia in this setting. Disorders associated with diminished effective blood volume (see earlier discussion) (Fig. 112-6) often reduce the glomerular filtration rate and, through various hormonal and physical changes that alter renal transport, stimulate proximal sodium and water reabsorption. The reduced volume of filtered blood, coupled with increased proximal capture of filtrate, compromises distal delivery and free-water generation. As noted earlier, these disorders also may provoke excessive release of AVP, which further sensitizes subjects to hyponatremia.

Reduced solute ingestion will ultimately limit the volume of free water that can be excreted. For example, when a subject excreting 700 mosm of solute (ingested salts plus products of catabolism) in 24 hours undergoes a maximal water diuresis, urine osmolality may reach a nadir of 40 mOsm. Thus excretion of 40 mosm of solute in each liter requires 17.5 L of urine. Reduction of solute excretion to 200 mosm/day, as can occur when beer, a solute-poor fluid, constitutes the entire daily fare, allows for excretion of only 5 L of maximally dilute urine (40 mOsm/L). In this setting, ingestion of more than 5 L of solute-free water results in fluid retention and hyponatremia. "Beer-drinker's potomania" and hyponatremia are therefore due to limited water excretion coupled with excessive solute-free water intake. The virtue of pretzels, pizza, and potato chips in this setting should be apparent.

Even when filtration and distal delivery are well preserved, inhibition of sodium reabsorption in the thick ascending limb and cortical diluting site can strikingly limit free-water generation. The loop-active diuretics, furosemide, bumetanide, and ethacrynic acid, inhibit solute reabsorption in the thick ascending limb, thereby increasing salt and water losses but limiting solute–free water excretion. Some have argued that furosemide-stimulated synthesis of renal prostaglandins—peripheral antagonists of AVP—minimizes the incidence of hyponatremia in this setting. Thiazides and related diuretics inhibit solute reabsorption in the cortical diluting site and, like other diuretics, may provoke AVP secretion via baroreceptor mechanisms. Proximal reabsorption is eventually stimulated by diuretic-induced volume contraction, consequently limiting distal delivery and free-water generation. The greater incidence of hyponatremia from thiazides may relate to their inability to stimulate renal prostaglandin synthesis.

Symptoms. The clinical manifestations of the hyponatremic syndromes (Fig. 112-7) are largely determined by the rate and magnitude of decline in plasma tonicity and by the nature of any associated disorders. Symptoms and signs of the *isotonic hyponatremias* relate to the effects of the hyperlipidemia, hyperproteinemia, or reason for treating with large volumes of isotonic glucose or mannitol. Likewise, the *hypertonic hyponatremias* owe their chemical and clinical features to the effects of hyperglycemia or reasons for administering hypertonic mannitol. Neurologic signs and symptoms are the primary manifestations of the *hypotonic hyponatremias.*

Acute hyponatremia, developing over hours, causes brain cell swelling, which results in confusion, lethargy, anorexia, and nausea and may progress to headache, stupor, and coma. In time (hours to days) brain cells effect remedial changes in cell volume by exporting solute (sodium, potassium, various organic acids) and inactivating retained osmols. This loss of effective intracellular osmols allows the brain to achieve the required level of hypotonicity without the added danger of imbibing extracellular water. Slowly developing hyponatremia is less likely to be symptomatic, presumably because the aforementioned brain cell compensations keep pace with the falling serum sodium concentration. Associated hepatic, renal, and cardiac disorders with coexisting but variable changes in effective blood volume and cerebral perfusion further modify the emerging clinical picture.

SERUM Na+ (meq/liter)	SYMPTOMS	HYPOVOLEMIA	HYPERVOLEMIA
120-125	NAUSEA MALAISE	DIMINISHED BRAIN PERFUSION EXACERBATES SYMPTOMS	DIMINISHED EABV IN CHF, NEPHROSIS, CIRRHOSIS MAY REDUCE BRAIN PERFUSION AND EXACERBATE SYMPTOMS
115-120	HEADACHE LETHARGY OBTUNDATION		
<115	SEIZURES COMA		

FIGURE 112-7 Symptoms of hypovolemic and hypervolemic forms of hyponatremia. *CHF,* Congestive heart failure; *EABV,* effective arterial blood volume.

Focal neurologic signs are unusual unless the patient has an underlying cerebral disorder.

Diagnosis. The exact etiology of hyponatremia can be extracted from its myriad possible causes by application of the principles outlined earlier. The algorithm illustrated in Fig. 112-6 classifies the hyponatremias in terms of the prevailing serum tonicity and then subclassifies hypotonic hyponatremia on the basis of the clinically apparent state of ECF volume.

The serum osmolality usually need not be measured, because the isotonic and hypertonic hyponatremias are most often recognized from the history, physical examination, or blood glucose levels. Lactescent serum, lipemia retinalis, and fatty deposits in the skin suggest that hyponatremia may be secondary to hyperlipidemia, whereas hyperproteinemic states are characterized by a history typical for multiple myeloma or macroglobulinemia. The use of hypertonic mannitol in acute renal failure or cerebral edema, or for continuous washing of the bladder during prostatic surgery, should alert the physician to the possibility of hypertonic hyponatremia. Once the likely isotonic or hypertonic causes have been excluded, one of the forms of hypotonic hyponatremia must be present.

Blood pressure, pulse, and their changes with posture; the presence or absence of edema; and normalcy of skin turgor provide the basis for assessing the state of ECF volume. A history of drug ingestion or the presence of ongoing diseases known to predispose to hypotonic hyponatremia is of obvious importance. On this basis, these syndromes may be sorted into the hypovolemic, hypervolemic, or the clinically apparent isovolemic hypotonic hyponatremias.

Patients with *hypovolemic hyponatremia* have reduced their effective blood volume through external loss of salt and water (renal or gastrointestinal losses or hemorrhage) or redistribution of plasma volume into an inflamed organ (e.g., pancreatitis, burns, trauma). Hypotension, tachycardia with postural accentuation, and diminished skin turgor characterize this group. Urinary losses are usually hypotonic when caused by diuretic excess, glycosuria, ketonuria, partial urinary tract obstruction or other interstitial nephritides, or adrenal insufficiency. Hyponatremia develops only because resulting volume contraction provokes retention of subsequently ingested or administered water. *Hyponatremia never occurs unless the patient is exposed to excess free water.* Gastrointestinal, blood, and redistributional losses are either hypotonic or isotonic. Urinary tonicity is relatively low, and sodium concentration is high during renal fluid wasting and solute wasting (urinary sodium concentration is generally >20 mEq/L, fractional excretion >3%, and urine osmolality approximates that of serum), but with extrarenal losses tonicity is high and sodium excretion low (urine sodium concentration <20 mEq/L, fractional excretion <1%, and urine osmolality is greater than that of serum). Discontinuation of diuretics 12 or 24 hours before evaluation may cause the urine to assume the chemical characteristics of extrarenal sodium- and water-wasting syndromes. The history is key in the latter setting. Chemical screening of the urine for diuretics may be required in patients whose hyponatremia could be due to the surreptitious abuse of these drugs.

Edema is the hallmark of the *hypervolemic* syndromes. These hyponatremic disorders are characterized by reduced effective blood volume, which diminishes glomerular filtration rate, enhances proximal reabsorption, and stimulates the nonosmotic release of AVP. The synergy of these forces can markedly restrict free-water excretion. In general, however, a substantial degree of hyponatremia usually occurs late in the course of congestive heart failure and liver disease and suggests a poor prognosis. Hyponatremia is an unusual complication of untreated nephrotic syndrome; when present, it is usually associated with aggressive diuretic therapy. Urine in these sodium-avid states is characterized by increased osmolality and diminished volume and sodium concentration.

Typically the *isovolemic* hyponatremias are associated with retention of 3 to 5 L of water, of which two thirds remains in cells. Thus the degree of ECF expansion is usually inadequate to detect edema. SIADH and the pathologic ingestion of excessive amounts of water were described earlier. As discussed, patients with acute or chronic renal failure have limited ability to generate and excrete free water, predisposing them to isovolemic hyponatremia. Another syndrome in this category has been variously termed the *reset osmostat,* or *sick cell syndrome*. This functional disorder complicates a variety of chronic illnesses, including pulmonary tuberculosis and cirrhosis. It is characterized by a lowering or resetting of the level of ECF tonicity that evokes release of AVP. Apart from this resetting, the osmoregulatory system apparently operates normally. Thus instead of being poised to protect a serum osmolality of 285 mOsm (serum sodium concentration of 140 mEq/L), the system may now pathologically protect 250 mOsm (i.e., a serum sodium concentration of 125 mEq/L). When challenged with an exogenous water load, patients with a reset osmostat, in contrast to those with SIADH, appropriately dilute their urine, eliminate the administered water load, and sustain a low but unchanged serum sodium concentration. With water deprivation, a concentrated urine is elaborated in pathologic protection of a fixed degree of hyponatremia.

Loss of 200 to 500 mEq of body potassium stores is commonly seen in various hypokalemic disorders. Because the total ECF content of this cation is normally less than 70 mEq, intracellular potassium stores obviously must contribute the bulk of lost electrolyte. Because potassium is the prime intracellular solute, its loss should cause transient intracellular hypotonicity, which in turn should simultaneously cause cell water to enter the ECF and extracellular sodium to enter cells in partial replacement of lost cation. Hyponatremia results from this diluting translocation of water and cation. Why the kidney retains the requisite quantity of water to sustain this hyponatremia is unclear. Disorders causing potassium wasting (e.g., diuretics, vomiting) and perhaps reduced cell volume resulting from potassium loss provoke sustained release of AVP.

Severe potassium depletion also impairs vasopressin's action on the distal nephron, thus facilitating water loss. Enhanced prostaglandin synthesis induced by potassium depletion may partially explain this effect. The change in plasma sodium concentration during potassium depletion therefore reflects the net balance attained between transcellular water and sodium fluxes (which tend to lower the sodium levels) and renal water losses (which tend to increase these levels).

In summary, the history, physical examination, and blood glucose level are usually sufficient to identify or exclude the isotonic and hypertonic hyponatremias. The hypotonic syndromes are classified through clinical assessment of ECF volume and urinary sodium excretion. Thus rapid clinical evaluation coupled with a few simple blood and urine tests allows quick definition of the cause and development of a rational therapeutic approach to hypotonic hyponatremia.

Therapy. Fluid-electrolyte therapy is unnecessary in the *pseudohyponatremias* caused by hyperlipidemia and hyperproteinemia because serum tonicity remains normal in these disorders. Indeed, the inappropriate restriction of free water or administration of concentrated saline solutions could lead to dangerous degrees of hypertonicity. Therapy should be directed toward the abnormality of lipid or protein metabolism.

The *hypertonic hyponatremias* are best treated by eliminating the offending ECF osmol. Insulin therapy of hyperglycemia or the renal elimination of accumulated mannitol allows for the return to cells of water that had been osmotically displaced to the ECF. Resulting intravascular volume reduction should be buffered by administration of saline or colloid. Once intravascular volume has been stabilized, hypotonic solutions may be administered to replenish the loss of proportionately more water than sodium caused by glycosuria and mannitoluria (Chapter 303).

Glycine and sorbitol, used as irrigants for transurethral prostatic resection, may cause severe hyponatremia and neurologic symptoms (see earlier discussion). The component causes of the hyponatremia include the following. If a hypertonic irrigation solution is used, the induced hyperosmolality provokes movement of sodium-free cellular water into the ECF. If the irrigation fluid is hypotonic, electrolyte-free water is absorbed, and, of course, dilutes the serum sodium. Absorption of isotonic irrigation fluid does not immediately change serum osmolality but simply obligates the presence of absorbed water in the ECF. Glycine's eventual metabolism leaves free water behind. Acute hyperammonemia consequent to glycine metabolism may add to the neurologic deterioration in these patients.

Therapy of the *hypotonic hyponatremias* is dictated by the underlying pathophysiology. *Hypovolemic* disorders require reexpansion of ECF volume, which eliminates baroreceptor stimulation of AVP release and simultaneously restores glomerular filtration and the distal tubular delivery of filtrate. Normalization of renal free-water generation and excretion, coupled with sodium retention, reestablishes normonatremia. Attention to such precipitating causes as diuretic abuse, gastrointestinal fluid losses, and adrenal insufficiency (see Fig. 112-6) obviously must accompany fluid therapy.

Therapy of *hypervolemic* hypotonic hyponatremic syndromes usually entails water restriction and treatment of the precipitating heart, liver, or kidney disease (see Fig. 112-6 and earlier discussion). Addition of an angiotensin-converting enzyme inhibitor (ACEI) to diuretic therapy of heart failure reverses associated hyponatremia more rapidly. The ACEI increases renal plasma flow and glomerular filtration, which simultaneously enhance the distal delivery of solute and diuretic. Cardiac output improves after afterload reduction and suppresses AVP secretion, further enhancing solute-free water excretion. It is instructive to calculate the time required to restore the normal serum sodium concentration from 120 mEq/L in a 70-kg man with 10 L of edema secondary to cirrhosis of the liver. Assume daily evaporative losses of 500 ml and excretion of 1 L of urine containing 40 mEq of electrolyte (largely accounted for by sodium, potassium, and their accompanying anions). It is useful to divide the urine into its isotonic and free-water components. If the urinary electrolyte, 40 mEq/L, were suspended in only 0.33 L, its *concentration* would be 120 mEq/L (i.e., isotonic with existing plasma). The remaining 0.67 L of urine would then be electrolyte-free water. In this manner, 1170 ml of free water (500 ml from insensible loss plus 670 ml from urinary loss) and 330 ml of isotonic fluid are lost daily. If daily water intake were restricted to 500 ml and salt intake were limited to 40 mEq, isotonic electrolyte intake (330 ml) would equal its excretion, whereas subtraction of free-water intake (170 ml) from daily losses (1170 ml) defines a net water loss of 1000 ml daily. Since salt intake and excretion are identical, the body content remains unchanged. Apparent total body sodium is the product of total body water (60% body weight plus edema fluid or [70 kg × 0.6] + 10 L = 52 L) and serum sodium concentration (120 mEq/L). Thus the product of total body water (52 L) and serum sodium concentration (120 mEq/L) yields the apparent total body sodium content (6240 mEq). In what volume would these 6240 mEq have to be suspended to yield a concentration of 140 mEq/L (i.e., 6240 mEq/x L = 140 mEq/L)? These calculations indicate that with an unchanged body sodium content, the patient would have to reduce total body water by 7.4 L, from 52 L to 44.6 L (i.e., 6240 mEq of Na^+ in 44.6 L yields a concentration of 140 mEq/L). By losing 1 L of electrolyte-free water daily, slightly more than a week would be required to achieve normonatremia. Renal free-water excretion will improve as the associated heart, liver, or kidney disease is treated and thereby will reduce the time required for the shedding of retained water.

The *isovolemic* hypotonic hyponatremias are usually best treated by water restriction. An occasional patient with chronic hyponatremia may find water restriction too demanding, necessitating the addition of agents that enhance solute-free water excretion. This situation is seen most commonly in SIADH, and usually when the syndrome is associated with a malignancy. Increasing sodium intake combined with furosemide may allow for an increase in water intake without compromising serum sodium concentration. Demeclocycline, a peripheral inhibitor of AVP action, induces enough free-water excretion to allow such patients to comfortably liberalize their daily water intake. Administration of this drug in patients with cirrhosis may impair renal function. Lithium, another renal AVP-antagonist, is less often effective and is more likely to cause untoward reactions than is demeclocycline. These drugs take days to become effective and so are of no value in the emergency therapy of symptomatic hyponatremia.

Patients with symptomatic isovolemic hypotonic hyponatremia (see Fig. 112-6) occasionally require the emergency removal of body water to raise serum sodium to levels that reverse symptoms. Currently no drugs are available that can acutely and selectively increase renal free-water excretion. For now, the imperfect but effective loop-active diuretics may be used in this setting. These diuretics simultaneously cause both a water and a sodium diuresis. Returning shed sodium in small volumes of water (i.e., hypertonic solutions) to the patient allows for net water loss. For example, intravenous administration of 80 to 120 mg of furosemide every 1 to 2 hours causes loss of approximately 1000 ml of urine per hour with approximately 70 mEq of electrolyte. Return of these 70 mEq of NaCl in only 135 ml of water (i.e., as 3% saline) maintains body sodium content unchanged while allowing for net loss of 865 ml of water. In this manner, substantial volumes of solute-free water may be removed. Serum sodium concentration may be increased from 110 mEq/L to 120 mEq/L over 5 hours in a 70-kg man losing 865 ml of water hourly. This 5-hour correction is used only for purposes of illustration; see later discussion for the proper rate of repair. When normal, this 70-kg man has a total body water of 42 L (60% body weight) and a serum sodium concentration of 140 mEq/L. His apparent total body sodium content is 140 mEq/L × 42 L, or 5880 mEq. What volume of body water must be present to dilute this sodium content to 110 mEq/L (i.e., 5880 mEq/x L = 110 mEq/L)? Solving this equation gives a volume of 53.5 L. Thus retention of 11.5 L of water reduces his serum sodium concentration from 140 mEq/L to 110 mEq/L. How much of this retained water must be removed to raise the sodium level to 120 mEq/L? Again, the calculation is based on the estimated normal sodium content and the volume of body water required to create the desired concentration: 5880 mEq/x L = 120 mEq/L. The volume required is 49 L; thus 4.5 L (53.5 − 49 = 4.5) must be removed to increase the serum sodium concentration from 110 mEq/L to 120 mEq/L. With loss of 865 ml of water hourly, it will take 5.2 hours to shed these 4.5 L. Care must be taken to assay urinary sodium and potassium losses and restore them. Administration of excessive amounts of electrolyte risks volume overload and pulmonary edema, whereas underreplacement results in potassium depletion and hypovolemia. Addition of furosemide not only prevents volume overload due to infusions of hypertonic saline but also enhances solute-free water clearance.

Acute hyponatremia is a medical emergency that can cause obtundation seizures, permanent neurologic damage, or death. The treatment of chronic hyponatremia differs markedly, however, because as discussed, brain cells eventually adapt to hyponatremia by exporting solute and thereby avoid cerebral edema. Both the loss and eventual reconstitution of cell solute content takes 36 to 48 hours. If the rate of rise of serum sodium concentration exceeds the rate at which cell solute is replenished, cells will shrink, and this "osmotic shock" may cause permanent neurologic damage. Unduly rapid repair of chronic hyponatremia may cause central pontine myelinolysis (CPM). If chronic hyponatremia is corrected too rapidly, seizures, coma, and demyelinating lesions in the central nervous system may occur. The latter seems to occur much more commonly in the pons. Young women manifest these neurologic sequelae far more often than do men. Although the pathogenesis of this disorder has yet to be clarified, many believe it is caused by adaptation of the brain to chronic hyponatremia, which sensitizes it to dehydration if the serum osmolality is corrected too rapidly. Survival depends on reducing brain cell swelling. Active export of cellular potassium and various amino acids with obligate amounts of water accomplishes this life-saving effect. The resulting solute depletion then sensitizes cells to dehydration if the serum sodium level is raised too quickly.

Because the duration of hyponatremia is difficult to define in many patients, rapid correction, and certainly overcorrection, must be carefully avoided (Box 112-2). On balance, the literature would suggest that the initial correction rates in symptomatic hyponatremic patients should not exceed 0.5 mEq/L/hr. As improvement is noted or if the serum sodium level has been increased by 4 to 5 mEq/L, the rate of correction should be reduced so that the increment in sodium concentration does not exceed 10 to 12 mEq/L/24 hr. Patients suffering from alcoholism, malnutrition, and liver disease are predisposed to demyelinating syndromes and deserve special attention during therapy. In acute severe hyponatremia where adaptation has not yet occurred, more rapid correction may be used. Normonatremia may be achieved within 24 hours. In all patients, serum sodium concentration must be monitored frequently as repair progresses. Current concepts suggest that if these guidelines are followed, the neurologic sequelae from rapid correction of hyponatremia can be avoided.

Hypernatremic States

Because sodium is excluded from cells and is the major ECF solute, all hypernatremic states are at once *hyperosmolar* and *hypertonic* (see earlier discussion) (Fig. 112-8). Attraction of cellular water by ECF hypertonicity effects *ICF contraction* in all hypernatremic states regardless of whether ECF expansion or contraction coexists. Cerebral cells are unique exceptions to this rule by virtue of their ability to increase ICF osmolality by generating solute (idiogenic osmols) rather than losing water.

Indeed the brain content of a variety of organic compounds such as glutamine, taurine, urea, myoinositol, betaine, glycerophosphorylcholine, and phosphocreatinine increase within several days after the onset of hypernatremia. Intracellular generation of these osmotically active particles by brain cells minimizes cell shrinkage and the neurologic consequences of this metabolic disorder. Within 2 days of correcting hypernatremia, the concentration of these solutes decreases.

In contrast to the constancy of ICF volume contraction, the *ECF volume* in hypernatremic states is quite variable (see later discussion). Indeed, these changes in ECF volume serve to classify the syndromes of hypernatremia (see later discussion).

Etiology and Pathogenesis. The imbalance between body water and sodium content that characterizes all hypernatremic states may result from pure water loss or pure sodium retention. Since two thirds

---

BOX 112-2
Treatment of hyponatremia

I. **Hypertonic hyponatremia:** Replace salt losses from the osmotic diuresis and treat the underlying disorder (e.g., hyperglycemia, exposure to mannitol, glycine)

II. **Isotonic hyponatremia:** Recognize the potential roles of hyperproteinemia and hyperlipidemia, or exposure to isotonic, sodium-free solutions (e.g., 5% dextrose)

III. **Hypotonic hyponatremia:**
   A. **Hypovolemic states:** Restore ECF volume status with isotonic saline and treat underlying gastrointestinal, adrenal, renal conditions
   B. **Hypervolemic states:** Water restriction and treatment of the underlying disorders (e.g., congestive heart failure, liver disease, nephrosis)
   C. **Isovolemic states:**
      1. **Asymptomatic:**
         Water restriction, increased sodium intake with furosemide, (demeclocycline, lithium, if antagonism of ADH is deemed necessary)
      2. **Symptomatic:**
         a. Recognize predisposing causes for demyelination: women, elderly, alcoholism, liver disease, malnutrition.
         b. 3% saline with furosemide to achieve initial correction rates of 1.0 mEq/L/hr. Continue until symptoms abate or for 4 to 5 hours and then slow the rate of correction so as not to exceed increases of more than 10 to 15 mEq/L/24 hr.

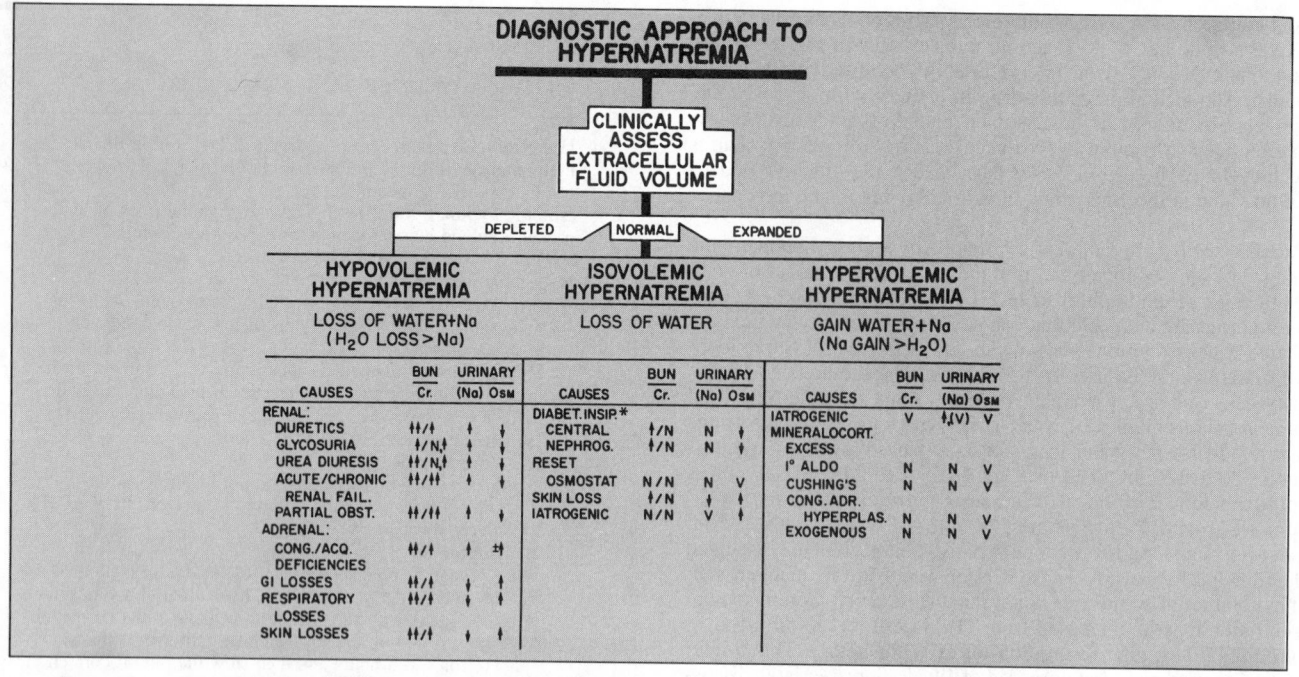

FIGURE 112-8   Differential diagnosis of hypernatremia: the clinical and laboratory approach to the classification and diagnosis of the hypernatremic disorders is illustrated. See text for details. *N*, Normal; *V*, variable; *INSIP*, insipidus.

From Narins RG et al: Diagnostic strategies in disorders of fluid, electrolyte, and acid-base homeostasis, *Am J Med* 72:496, 1982.

of body water resides intracellularly, pure water losses shrink both ICF and ECF, but reduction of the latter is usually clinically inapparent unless dehydration is severe (i.e., serum sodium concentrations in excess of 160 mEq/L). The hypernatremia caused by retention of salt without water simultaneously contracts the ICF and expands the ECF. The extracellular expansion is usually too modest to cause edema but may overload a previously compromised myocardium. The hypernatremia resulting from concomitant changes in sodium and water effects more striking changes in the ECF volume. Loss of hypotonic fluid (i.e., loss of proportionately more water than salt) reduces ECF volume in proportion to the loss of sodium, whereas a gain of hypertonic fluid (i.e., gain of proportionately more sodium than water) expands the ECF in proportion to the retained sodium.

As hypernatremia develops, thirst and AVP release are normally stimulated. The hormone AVP causes renal retention of ingested water, thereby reestablishing normal tonicity of body fluid. It follows that sustained hypernatremia could result from a defect in thirst, AVP synthesis or release, or failure of the kidneys to respond to normally elaborated hormone. Net loss of hypotonic fluid by kidneys, gastrointestinal tract, skin, or lungs or net retention of sodium from massive exposure could also cause hypernatremia. These different syndromes are conveniently classified on the basis of the associated changes in ECF volume (see Fig. 112-8) and are discussed here.

Hypervolemic hypernatremia. Pure sodium retention as a cause of hypernatremia is usually iatrogenic, being restricted to specific clinical circumstances. Use of hypertonic sodium bicarbonate solutions (each 50-ml ampule contains approximately 1000 mEq/L) in various forms of severe metabolic acidosis will cause hypernatremia unless enough water is added to ensure isotonicity. Intraamniotic injection of hypertonic saline (250 ml of a 25% solution), for a therapeutic abortion, is occasionally inadvertently misdirected into a vein, causing potentially catastrophic acute hypertonicity. Rarely, when infant feeding formula or dialysis solution is constituted with excess sodium, or when concentrated sodium salts are accidentally ingested in emetics or gargles, life-threatening hypernatremia results. Perhaps the most common iatrogenic form of hypernatremia occurs when patients dependent on parenteral fluids are given isotonic saline without free water to replace daily hypotonic insensible losses. In certain settings diuretics may cause hypernatremia. Hypotonic urine is gen-

erally excreted in response to vigorous diuretic therapy. Replacement of these losses with only free water commonly leads to hyponatremia, whereas replacement of sodium without free water results in hypernatremia. Indeed, most cases of edematous hypernatremia occur because incapacitated edematous patients receive diuretics while their access to water is restricted. The various syndromes of primary mineralocorticoid excess (Chapter 298) cause retention of sodium and water, and the resulting ECF volume expansion increases the threshold for AVP release. The latter provokes mild water loss, and a new steady state evolves that is characterized by mild hypernatremia. Potassium depletion and increased synthesis of prostaglandins may also contribute to the polyuria observed in these hypermineralocorticoid states. Prostaglandins, by antagonizing the effect of AVP on water reabsorption, impair the kidney's ability to elaborate a concentrated urine (see earlier discussion).

Hypovolemic hypernatremia. Loss of hypotonic solutions through the kidney, gastrointestinal and respiratory tracts, or the skin may result in hypernatremia (see Fig. 112-8). Such urinary losses are induced by pharmacologic and osmotic diuretics and by the obligatory relative polyuria that complicates acute or chronic renal failure. Glycosuria and the urea diuresis created by protein feeding in catabolic settings cause loss of sodium with large amounts of water. Failure to replace these losses results in hypovolemic hypernatremia. Partial urinary tract obstruction leads to distal tubular damage and a clinical syndrome characterized by polyuria, hyperkalemia, normal anion gap acidosis, and occasionally hypernatremia. Vomiting, diarrhea, lactulose therapy (for hepatic encephalopathy), and fistulous communications between the skin and gastrointestinal tract may cause hypotonic losses, which, when coupled with reduced free-water intake, provoke hypernatremia. Peritoneal dialysis removes hypotonic fluid and may increase the serum sodium concentration unless free water is returned in appropriate amounts.

Isovolemic hypernatremia. The free-water losses underlying most cases of isovolemic hypernatremia occur through the skin or the kidney (Fig. 112-8). Such renal losses are caused by either partial or complete failure to synthesize or release AVP (i.e., central diabetes insipidus) or from failure of the kidney to respond to normally elaborated AVP (i.e., nephrogenic diabetes insipidus) (Chapter 296).

Because the hypernatremia resulting from free-water loss stimulates thirst, most patients with diabetes insipidus have normal or only slightly increased serum sodium concentrations. It follows that hypothalamic lesions that concomitantly damage AVP synthesis and thirst provoke the worst degrees of hypernatremia.

Central diabetes insipidus (CDI) is discussed in Chapter 296.

Nephrogenic diabetes insipidus (NDI) occurs in two general forms. The first type is composed of acquired disorders causing structural renal damage that interferes with the generation of a properly functioning medullary countercurrent system. The second form is caused by familial and acquired disorders in the end-organ responsiveness to AVP. The forms of NDI caused by structural renal damage usually allow for excretion of isotonic urine and thus result in only mild polyuria (usually less than 8 L daily), whereas familial NDI often unleashes torrential volumes of urine.

The mild chronic polyuria and limited concentrating capacity attending most chronic renal diseases is well known. Rarely, *amyloidosis,* and occasionally, *partial urinary tract obstruction,* cause enough selective distal nephron damage to effect substantial degrees of polyuria. *Potassium depletion* and *hypercalcemia* interfere with AVP's action, causing usually mild polyuria. *Lithium carbonate* and *demeclocycline* also impair the cell's response to AVP. This interference is used to therapeutic advantage to treat SIADH with demeclocycline. Craniopharyngiomas, which often release an inhibitor of AVP's renal action, may cause NDI.

The rare *congenital forms of NDI* are inherited as X-linked recessive or dominant disorders with partial penetrance in females. Thus males are most severely afflicted. Hypotonic polyuria that is unresponsive to AVP characterizes this syndrome. The genetic defect in x-linked NDI includes a variety of V2-receptor gene mutations that can disrupt the binding, synthesis, or intracellular transport of the receptor. An autosomal disorder directly affecting the aquaporin-2 water channel has recently been described.

Disorders of thirst and of the sensitivity of osmoreceptors to hypertonic stimuli may also spawn hypernatremic syndromes. Aging impairs thirst, thereby sensitizing elderly patients, whose access to water may be limited, to developing dehydration and hypernatremia. Because high serum sodium concentrations in the elderly usually complicate serious underlying disorders, hypernatremia augurs a poor prognosis. *Primary hypodipsia* may reduce water intake so severely as to allow normal insensible and urinary losses to increase serum sodium concentration. Appropriate renal water retention accompanying more mild thirst defects may simply result in reduced urine volume and relatively normal serum sodium concentrations. Hypothalamico-hypophyseal or cerebrocortical lesions that impair thirst are also the same disorders that can independently cause CDI. The *reset osmostat syndrome* (i.e., essential hypernatremia) results from simultaneous "upward resetting" of the osmostat and proportional insensitivity of thirst. As a result of the former defect, a greater degree of serum hypertonicity is required to elicit a given level of AVP secretion. Resulting water loss causes hypernatremia, which is sustained by the associated thirst defect. In some settings, AVP release is not stimulated until enough water has been lost to cause hypovolemia. These patients behave as if their osmoreceptors are totally defective while volume-dependent hormone release is intact.

Symptoms and Signs. Irritability, lethargy, and weakness are early neurologic signs of acute hypernatremia. As serum sodium concentration climbs, cerebral dehydration worsens, soon provoking convulsive activity and eventuating in coma and death (Fig. 112-9). Contraction of brain cells stretches and distorts intracerebral and pericerebral veins, causing their rupture and eventually intracerebral and subarachnoid hemorrhage.

Within 24 to 36 hours of developing hypernatremia, idiogenic osmols form, causing water to return to and reexpand brain cells. Thus patients with chronic hypernatremia may be relatively asymptomatic. It also follows that excessively rapid therapy with water, before the involution of cerebral idiogenic osmols, may lead to symptomatic and potentially fatal brain edema.

The clinical picture will, of course, also be colored by the disorder precipitating the hypernatremia. Hypovolemic and hypervolemic disorders tend to be more symptomatic, which is perhaps related to associated alterations in cerebral perfusion.

SERUM Na+ (meq/liter)	SYMPTOMS	HYPOVOLEMIA	HYPERVOLEMIA
150-155	WORSENING WEAKNESS, LETHARGY,	DIMINISHED BRAIN PERFUSION EXACERBATES SYMPTOMS	DIMINISHED EABV IN CHF, CIRRHOSIS, NEPHROSIS MAY REDUCE BRAIN PERFUSION AND EXACERBATE SYMPTOMS; PULMONARY SYMPTOMS MAY DOMINATE IN CHF
>160	TWITCHING, SEIZURES, COMA DEATH		

FIGURE 112-9 Symptoms of hypovolemic and hypervolemic hypernatremia. *CHF,* Congestive heart failure; *EABV,* effective arterial blood volume.

Diagnosis. Clinical clues suggesting the presence of hypernatremia should stimulate the physician to measure serum electrolytes, which establishes the diagnosis. Clinical assessment of the ECF volume serves as a useful basis for the differential diagnosis of hypernatremia (see Fig. 112-8). Hypovolemic disorders are characterized by postural accentuation of tachycardia and hypotension from hypotonic fluid losses. Renal and gastrointestinal losses account for most cases of hypovolemic hypernatremia. The presence of edema is required to clinically diagnose hypervolemic forms of hypernatremia. Previously edematous patients suffering hypotonic fluid losses from diuretics, gastrointestinal disorders, or underreplaced evaporative losses account for most of these cases. Excessive retention of hypertonic fluids can also cause this syndrome. The euvolemic disorders of hypernatremia may present primarily as polyuric, polydipsic disorders with varying degrees of hypernatremia or with few clinical signs associated with the serendipitous finding of an increased serum sodium concentration. An extensive discussion of the differential diagnosis of polyuria is beyond the intended scope of this chapter. Briefly, however, polyuric disorders are best classified by the character of the excreted urine, and on this basis they fall into the following three major groups: those caused by increased solute excretion, those in which excessive free-water excretion underlies the increased urinary volume, and those caused by combined solute and water excretory excesses. Measurement of osmolality in plasma and in timed urine specimens allows for calculation of osmolal (C_{osm}) and free-water clearances (C_{H_2O}) (Chapter 101). Solute diureses are caused by excessive excretion of urea, NaCl, $NaHCO_3$, glucose, or mannitol, and are characterized by isotonic urine and a C_{osm} that is generally greater than 3 ml/min. Water diureses are typified by hypotonic urine and C_{H_2O} usually in excess of 1 to 2 ml/min. Combined disorders manifest hypotonic urine in the face of increased C_{osm}. This mixed diuresis is seen, for example, when a patient with CDI is inappropriately treated with large amounts of saline.

As noted earlier (and in Chapter 296), free-water diureses are caused by compulsive water drinking and by CDI and NDI. Serum sodium concentration in the diabetes insipidus syndromes is normal to increased, whereas in the primary polydipsic syndromes it is normal to reduced. Careful restriction of water intake until body weight is reduced by 2% to 3%, or until the serum osmolality has increased to 290 to 295 mosm/L, increases urine osmolality to values in excess of plasma in compulsive water drinkers who manifest no further increase when 5 units of aqueous pitressin are given subcutaneously at the end of the period of thirsting. Patients with NDI sustain a constant level of hypotonic polyuria that is unresponsive to exogenous AVP. Those with complete CDI also continue to excrete a relatively constant volume of hypotonic urine during thirsting, but AVP administration elicits a striking decrease in volume and increase in tonicity of urine. With partial CDI, urine volume declines with thirsting, and urinary tonicity increases but plateaus at levels inappropriately low as compared with that seen in thirsting normal persons. Because their tubules are exposed to less than maximum concentrations of endogenous AVP, administration of the hormone at the end of the period of thirsting significantly increases the urine osmolality.

In summary, clinical assessment of the state of ECF volume expansion allows for the rapid classification of the hypernatremias. The urinary response to thirsting and to the administration of AVP provides a simple means for further subclassifying the euvolemic polyuric syndromes.

Therapy. Because poor tissue perfusion is most threatening, treatment of patients with hypovolemic hypernatremia who manifest prerenal azotemia and hypotension is best initiated with isotonic saline. Once hemodynamic stability and adequate urine volume are achieved, hypotonic solutions may be administered and serum sodium concentration normalized. Therapy of associated gastrointestinal and renal disorders that precipitated the hypernatremia must of course proceed in parallel with the administration of salt and water.

Therapy of hypervolemic hypernatremic syndromes requires removal of sodium in excess of water and is best achieved by replacing diuretic-induced sodium and water losses with only water. Oral or parenteral fluids may be used to replenish losses. Obviously, attention must also be paid to treating the underlying cause of the edema. Dialysis will be required to remove excess sodium in hypervolemic patients with hypernatremia who also have severe acute or chronic renal failure.

Chapter 296 thoroughly discusses treatment of CDI and NDI. Replacement of water losses in clinically euvolemic hypernatremic patients requires the following assumptions: that serum sodium behaves as if it is distributed in total body water; that total body water is 60% of normal body weight; and that the patient's body sodium content remains normal. Thus the amount of water required in a 70-kg man with isovolemic hypernatremia and a serum sodium level of 155 mEq/L is calculated as follows: Normal total body water = 70 kg × 0.6 = 42 L. Normal total body sodium content = 42 L × 140 mEq/L = 5880 mEq. In what reduced volume must the 5880 mEq be distributed to increase the serum sodium concentration to 155 mEq/L (i.e., 5880 mEq/xL = 155 mEq/L)? Answer: 37.9 L. Thus loss of 4.1 L of water (42 − 37.9 = 4.1) accounts for the observed degree of hypernatremia. These 4.1 L should be replenished to restore normonatremia.

Some controversy exists as to how rapidly this fluid should be given. Most observers agree that the cerebral consequences from too rapid a rate of therapy can be avoided if the serum sodium concentration is reduced no faster than 1 to 2 mEq/L/hr. Ongoing water losses must be replenished along with deficits.

BIBLIOGRAPHY

Arief AI: Hyponatremia, convulsions, respiratory arrest, and permanent brain damage after elective surgery in healthy women, *N Engl J Med* 314:1529, 1986.
Ayus CL, Krothapalli RK, Arief AI: Treatment of symptomatic hyponatremia and its relation to brain damage, *N Engl J Med* 317:1190, 1987.
Berl T: Treating hyponatremia: damned if we do and damned if we don't, *Kidney Int* 37:1006-1018, 1990.
Bichet DG: Nephrogenic diabetes insipidus, *Semin Nephrol* 14:349, 1994.
Howard RL, Bichet DG, Schrier RW: Hypernatremic and polyuric states. In Seldin DW, Giebisch G, editors: *The kidney: physiology and pathophysiology*, ed 2, New York, 1992, Raven Press.
Morrison G, Singer I: Hyperosmolar states. In Narins RG, editor: *Clinical disorders of fluid and electrolyte metabolism*, New York, 1994, McGraw-Hill.
Verbalis JG: Hyponatremia: epidemiology, pathophysiology and therapy, *Curr Opin Nephrol Hyperten* 2:636, 1993.

CHAPTER

113 Disorders of Sodium Balance

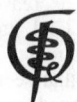

Murray Epstein

The sodium content of a healthy 70-kg man ranges from 4400 to 5600 mEq. Of this pool, approximately 2800 mEq is contained within the extracellular fluid (ECF). Much of the remaining sodium exists in a poorly exchangeable pool bound to the crystalline structure of the bone and is thus not an osmotically active solute. As a consequence of an active transport mechanism that results in the extrusion of so-

dium from the intracellular fluid to the ECF, most of the sodium resides in the ECF. Therefore sodium, with its accompanying anions, chloride and bicarbonate, constitutes more than 90% of the total solute contained in the ECF. It follows that sodium is the major determinant of ECF volume.

Under normal circumstances, ECF volume is maintained relatively constant. The kidney compensates for either a deficit or excess of salt and water with great precision, thereby ensuring that ECF volume is maintained within narrow limits. The ECF volume deviates from these normal constraints when excess sodium is retained (edematous states) or when significant quantities of sodium are lost as a result of the loss or sequestration of body fluids containing substantial quantities of sodium (sodium depletion states).

EDEMATOUS STATES

Edema is an excessive accumulation of fluid within the interstitial space. Irrespective of its cause, generalized edema requires two events for its development. First, an imbalance of Starling forces favors outward movement of fluid across the capillary wall into the interstitial space. Such a perturbation of the Starling forces must be accompanied by the renal retention of sodium as the kidney attempts to refill the diminished vascular space. In the absence of renal sodium retention, edema formation would be largely self-limited because the imbalance of Starling forces would tend to correct itself as fluid accumulation progressed. Thus the clinical consequences of generalized edema derive from the fact that renal sodium retention maintains the edematous state.

The major edematous states differ one from the other with regard to both anatomic and functional abnormalities, but they have in common a deranged regulatory mechanism for maintaining sodium homeostasis. Thus in cirrhosis of the liver the volume receptors appear to be intact and functioning normally, but circulating blood volume is maldistributed so that the kidney behaves as if it were underperfused. In another major edematous state, congestive heart failure, it has been proposed that sodium retention occurs because of damaged receptors that are incapable of adequately apprising the kidney that sodium excretion should be increased.

All the major edematous disease states are characterized by a continuing and unrelenting accumulation of salt and water. Even when the fluid retention has become massive, the kidney often continues to retain salt and water, behaving as though it were responding to a volume deficit. It has been proposed that the stimulus for sodium retention is a contraction of the "effective" blood volume, a feature common to all major edematous states. In this context, it is important to note that the term *effective plasma volume* refers to that part of the total circulating volume that is effective in stimulating volume receptors. The concept is somewhat elusive because the actual volume receptors remain incompletely defined. A diminished effective volume may reflect subtle alterations in systemic hemodynamic factors, such as decreased filling of the arterial tree, a diminished central blood volume, or both. In normal circumstances, effective blood volume correlates with total ECF volume; in contrast, in the major edematous states it does not. Despite massive retention of salt and water, effective blood volume remains functionally contracted because of a disturbance in the Starling forces that govern the distribution of fluid within the ECF compartment.

In the light of this formulation, it is possible to understand why the retained fluid in major edematous states fails to modify the stimulus for continuing sodium and water retention. Despite a progressive increase in total ECF volume, fluid is sequestered into one or more of the other fluid compartments without succeeding in normalizing effective blood volume. Only a normalization of the disturbance in the forces governing fluid distribution will permit a reexpansion of effective blood volume to normal.

In summary, it is apparent that in two of the major edematous disorders (congestive heart failure and cirrhosis), the kidney is not the culprit in this situation but rather is best visualized as an innocent victim: the kidney's response is appropriate to the information it receives. What is inappropriate in this setting are the signals being transmitted to the kidney.

Box 113-1 lists the conditions associated with generalized edema. This chapter does not cover the entire spectrum of edematous disor-

---

BOX 113-1
Causes of generalized edema

I. Common causes
   A. Congestive heart failure
   B. Cirrhosis of the liver
   C. Nephrotic syndrome
   D. Acute "nephritic" syndrome
   E. Pregnancy
      1. Normal pregnancy
      2. Toxemia of pregnancy
   F. Idiopathic edema
II. Unusual causes
   A. Arteriovenous fistulas
   B. Hypothyroidism
   C. Diabetes mellitus
      1. Associated with microangiopathy (rare)
      2. Associated with insulin treatment of ketoacidosis
   D. Drugs
      1. Nonsteroidal antiinflammatory drugs
      2. Estrogens
      3. Vasodilator antihypertensive drugs
      4. Hyperstimulation syndrome secondary to menotropins (Pergonal)

ders. Rather, consideration will be given only to three of the four major disorders encountered frequently in clinical practice.

CONGESTIVE HEART FAILURE

In congestive heart failure (CHF), impaired cardiac emptying results in a rise in ventricular end-diastolic pressure. As depicted in Fig. 113-1, the consequent high venous pressure promotes transudation of fluid out of the vascular channel through several mechanisms. First, the mean capillary hydraulic pressure is increased. Because the resulting rate of fluid transfer from peripheral capillaries to the interstitial space exceeds the rate of return of interstitial fluid to the intravascular compartment, edema formation ensues. Furthermore, an increased peripheral venous pressure may cause a neurogenic resetting of precapillary and postcapillary resistances, leading to increased capillary hydraulic pressure and transudation of fluid from the intravascular to the interstitial space. Third, an increase in systemic venous pressure often leads to hepatic congestion, which may depress both plasma renin clearance and the hepatic metabolism of aldosterone. Fourth, there is reason to believe that an increase in systemic venous pressure per se may contribute to sodium retention via afferent pathways. There is supportive evidence for the existence of volume receptors in the low-pressure central venous portion of the circulation (referred to as *low-pressure volume receptors*). It is thus possible that an increased venous pressure activates such receptors, leading to sodium retention by the kidneys. Furthermore, salt and water retention in CHF leads to a mild decrease in systemic plasma protein concentration, with a decrease in the oncotic pressure gradient, thereby favoring edema formation. Several lines of evidence suggest that the increase in central venous pressure in CHF retards lymph flow in the thoracic duct, with a resultant decrease in lymphatic drainage of peripheral interstitial spaces.

The decrease in cardiac output and sometimes in mean arterial pressure (MAP) characteristic of severe CHF may be associated with a reduction of the renal fraction of cardiac output and of both renal plasma flow (RPF) and glomerular filtration rate (GFR). Nevertheless, a close correlation between cardiac output and renal blood flow is not observed.

The adaptive activation of the renin-angiotensin aldosterone (RAA) system seen in CHF, with the resultant increases in circulating and intrarenal angiotensin II levels, results not only in better preservation of MAP but in a relative preservation of the GFR in the face of reduced renal perfusion, that is, an increase in the filtration fraction (FF), the ratio of GFR/RPF. The increase in FF, which augments GFR for any given level of RPF, is a consequence of the induction

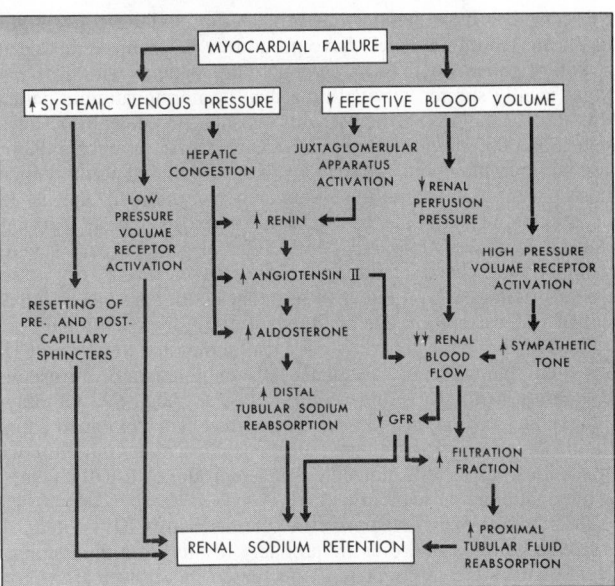

FIGURE 113-1 The major pathophysiologic mechanisms leading to renal sodium retention in congestive heart failure. The increased systemic venous pressure promotes transudation of fluid out of the vascular channel by several mechanisms. Concomitantly, a diminution in "effective" blood volume promotes renal sodium retention through a number of hormonal, hemodynamic, and neural mechanisms. *GFR*, Glomerular filtration rate.

Modified from Humes HD, Gottlieb MN, Brenner BM: The kidney in congestive heart failure. In Brenner BM, Stein JH, editors: *Sodium and water homeostasis,* New York, 1978, Churchill Livingstone.

of a greater increase of vascular resistance in the efferent than in the afferent arteriole by angiotensin II. This adaptive process minimizes the fall in glomerular capillary hydrostatic pressure that would otherwise occur. In very severe CHF, however, a marked increase in intrarenal angiotensin II may result in predominant constriction of the afferent arteriole, thereby contributing to a fall in GFR.

Patients with severe decompensated CHF typically have marked, complex activation of several neurohumoral systems. These neurohumoral changes include those that produce systemic and renal microvascular vasoconstriction, tending to cause renal sodium and water retention, for example, activation of the RAA system, and the sympathetic nervous system, and increased release of arginine vasopressin (AVP). Neurohumoral activation not only reflects the magnitude of CHF, but probably directly contributes to functional impairment and poor long-term prognosis.

Because of the contraction of effective blood volume, the kidneys respond by retaining salt by several different mechanisms. The reduced effective blood volume activates the RAA system, with enhanced sodium reabsorption in the distal segments of the nephron. Concomitantly, there is a decrease in renal blood flow that is attributable to several mechanisms (see Fig. 113-1). The decline in renal perfusion is usually associated with little or no concurrent decline in GFR, thereby resulting in a rise in the ratio of GFR/RPF (i.e., the FF), which in turn is thought to play a fundamental role in promoting the sodium retention encountered (Chapter 101).

Concomitantly, there is activation of the sympathetic nervous system as well as stimulation of vasopressin release. These systems maintain systemic blood pressure and promote renal sodium and water retention during acute cardiac decompensation. In the chronic "compensated" phase of cardiac failure, which is associated with expansion of ECF volume and restoration of blood pressure, the plasma levels of the previously mentioned hormones generally return to normal.

Many patients with chronic severe (class III or IV) cardiac failure exhibit hyponatremia. Serum sodium concentration has been shown to be a useful predictor of the state of the renin-angiotensin and sympathetic nervous systems in cardiac failure. An inverse correlation has been reported between serum sodium concentration and plasma renin activity.

Recent data have demonstrated that serum sodium concentration and plasma hormonal levels have prognostic value in predicting the survival of patients with CHF. Hyponatremic patients with CHF have a significantly shorter survival time than do normonatremic patients with cardiac failure. Patients with plasma norepinephrine levels greater than 800 pg/ml have a significantly worse prognosis than do those with plasma norepinephrine levels of 400 to 800 pg/ml. Patients whose plasma norepinephrine levels are nearly normal, that is, less than 400 pg/ml, have the best relative prognosis. These seemingly independent observations are clearly related: patients with severely decompensated heart failure have elevated levels of plasma vasoconstricting-sodium retentive hormones with consequent impairment of water excretion eventually resulting in hyponatremia.

Fluid restriction is generally not a useful measure to reverse CHF-associated hyponatremia. Similarly, discontinuation of furosemide alone rarely increases serum sodium level, although the withdrawal of thiazide-type diuretics may have this effect. The combined administration of an angiotensin-converting enzyme (ACE) inhibitor with furosemide (but usually not of either agent alone) usually reverses the hyponatremia, at least in part.

The reversal of hyponatremia in patients with CHF treated with both ACE inhibitor and diuretic probably results from the combined effects of the ACE inhibitor (e.g., decreased thirst, decreased proximal tubular resorption of sodium, interference with the hydroosmotic effect of AVP) and the loop diuretic (increased distal delivery of glomerular filtrate, reduction in urine osmolality) acting to offset the pathophysiologic factors causing impaired excretion of water.

As discussed earlier, enhanced sodium reabsorption mediated by these several different mechanisms expands the *total* blood volume to values usually far in excess of normal. Despite such increases in ECF, effective blood volume remains contracted because the cardiac output remains low, and the central venous pressure remains elevated. Consequently, the stimulus for salt retention persists.

Successful therapy of CHF consists of interrupting this vicious circle. Improvement of the pumping action of the heart increases effective blood volume and lowers systemic venous pressure. Consequently, the two major afferent mechanisms leading to salt and water retention in CHF are interrupted. Traditional therapy of CHF has consisted mainly in measures to strengthen the force of contraction and to reduce elevated ventricular filling pressures. Accordingly, patients have been treated with a combination of an inotropic drug (one of the digitalis compounds) to stimulate myocardial contractility and a diuretic to increase renal excretion of salt and water.

Although such an approach is often successful in restoring adequate ventricular function in a setting of mild CHF, the more severe CHF affecting patients with ischemic heart disease or cardiomyopathy is often refractory to such therapy. More than a decade ago a major change of approach in the management of heart failure began with the demonstration that vasodilator drugs, which have no direct cardiac action, could dramatically improve left ventricular performance. The underlying concept of vasodilator therapy is to unburden the failing heart. Because vasoconstriction and increased impedance to left ventricular (LV) ejection are hallmarks of CHF, the use of vasodilator drugs should be considered in all patients with CHF. In the past these drugs were used primarily to improve LV performance and relieve the symptoms of heart failure. Recent data indicate that they also can prolong survival in heart failure, probably by preventing progression of the ventricular dysfunction. The following regimens have proved to be effective in reducing mortality: (1) the combination of hydralazine and isosorbide dinitrate in mild to moderate heart failure in the Veterans Administration study (VHeFT); and (2) the converting enzyme inhibitor enalapril in severe heart failure in the Scandinavian CONSENSUS trial. Vasodilator therapy should be used in all patients unless there are major contraindications to its use such as hypotension accompanied by inadequate regional perfusion.

CIRRHOSIS

The clinical course in patients with decompensated Laenec's cirrhosis is often complicated by progressive impairment of renal sodium handling, leading to the formation of fluid in the peritoneal cavity (ascites) and peripheral edema (Chapter 354). It should be underscored that cirrhotic patients who are unable to excrete sodium will continue to gain weight and accumulate fluid as long as dietary sodium content exceeds maximum urinary sodium excretion. If access to sodium is not curtailed, the relentless retention of sodium may lead to the accumulation of vast amounts of ascitic fluid (on occasion, up to 20 L). Weight gain and ascites formation promptly cease when sodium intake is limited. It should further be noted that the impairment of renal sodium handling in such patients is not a static and unalterable condition. Rather, cirrhotic patients may undergo spontaneous diuresis followed by a return to avid salt retention.

Discussion of the pathogenetic events leading to the deranged sodium homeostasis of cirrhosis is simplified by considering the "afferent" and the "efferent" events that eventuate in this derangement.

Afferent Events

Traditionally it has been proposed that ascites formation in cirrhotic patients begins when a critical imbalance of Starling forces in the hepatic sinusoids and splanchnic capillaries causes an excessive amount of lymph formation, exceeding the ability of the thoracic duct to return this excessive lymph to the circulation. Consequently, excess lymph accumulates in the peritoneal space, with a subsequent contraction of circulating plasma volume. Thus as ascites develops, there is a progressive redistribution of plasma volume. Although total plasma volume may be increased in this setting, the physiologic circumstance may mimic a reduction in plasma volume (a reduced effective plasma volume). The diminished effective volume is thought to constitute an afferent signal to the renal tubule to augment salt and water reabsorption.

Although an imbalance of Starling forces in the hepatosplanchnic microcirculation is thought to contribute importantly to the relative decrease in effective blood volume, it should be emphasized that this is not the sole mechanism. An additional determinant is total peripheral resistance, which is diminished significantly in most patients with cirrhosis who are retaining sodium and water. This decrease in peripheral vascular resistance is no doubt partially related to anatomic arteriovenous shunts, but it has also been proposed that some undefined vasodilator (either produced by or not inactivated by the diseased liver) plays a role. Thus, despite an increase in *total* plasma volume, the relative "fullness" of the arteriovenous tree is diminished. Several hemodynamic events therefore act in concert to diminish the effective volume, thereby activating the mechanisms promoting sodium retention (Fig. 113-2). In summary, the traditional formulation suggests that the renal retention of sodium is a secondary rather than a primary event.

Recently an alternative hypothesis, termed the *peripheral arterial vasodilatation hypothesis,* has been proposed to account for the initiation of sodium and water retention in cirrhosis. One may regard

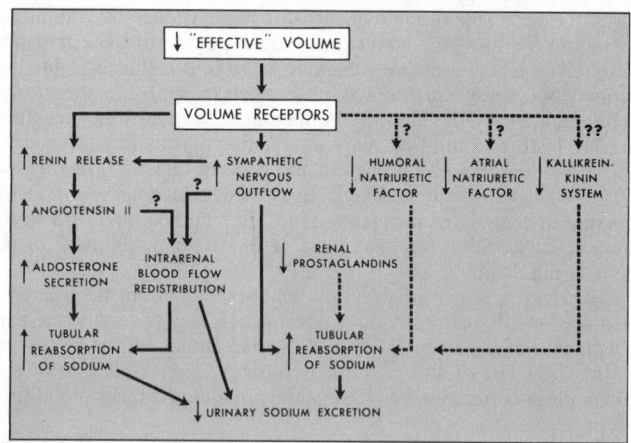

FIGURE 113-2 Possible mechanisms by which a diminished "effective" volume results in sodium retention in cirrhosis. The heavy arrows indicate pathways for which evidence is available. The dashed lines represent proposed pathways, whose existence remains to be established.

Modified from Epstein M: Renal sodium handling in liver disease. In Epstein M, editor: *The kidney in liver disease,* ed 4, Philadelphia, Hauley & Belfus, p. 12.

this theory as a revision of the underfill theory. The principal distinguishing feature of this newly proposed theory is that the decrease in effective blood volume is attributable primarily to an early increase in vascular capacitance. Thus peripheral vasodilation is the initial determinant of intravascular underfilling, and an imbalance between the expanded capacitance and the available volume constitutes a diminished effective volume. This formulation recognizes that total peripheral resistance is diminished significantly in most edematous cirrhotic patients.

Both underfill theories possibly explain why fluid retention may fail to attenuate the stimulus for continuing sodium and water retention. Despite a progressive increase in total ECF volume, fluid is sequestered into one or more of the other fluid compartments without normalizing effective blood volume (EBV). Only correction of the disturbance in the forces governing fluid distribution will permit a reexpansion of EBV.

Over two decades ago an alternative hypothesis was proposed. Lieberman and his associates postulated the "overflow" theory of ascites formation. In contrast to the traditional formulation, the overflow theory suggests that the primary event is the inappropriate retention of excessive sodium by the kidneys, with a resultant expansion of plasma volume. Studies in a canine model of cirrhosis have further supported this view. The mechanism(s) underlying a primary retention of sodium by the kidney has not been fully elucidated. In the setting of abnormal Starling forces (both portal venous hypertension and a reduction in plasma colloid osmotic pressure) in the portal venous bed and hepatic sinusoids, the expanded plasma volume is sequestered preferentially in the peritoneal space, with ascites formation. Thus according to this formulation, renal sodium retention and plasma volume expansion precede rather than follow the formation of ascites.

Although we believe that the presently available evidence favors a prominent role for diminished *effective* plasma volume in mediating the avid sodium retention of many cirrhotic patients with established cirrhosis, it should be emphasized that these two theories may not be mutually exclusive. As noted earlier, cirrhosis is not a *static* disease but rather a constantly evolving clinical disorder. Yet virtually all the available clinical studies of deranged sodium homeostasis were carried out on a single state of the disease, at a time when decompensation was well established, with little information about the incipient stage of sodium retention. In contrast, the studies with the canine cirrhosis model deal with the relatively early stage of sodium retention. Any theory suggesting that the same antinatriuretic forces are operative throughout the evolution of sodium retention in a cirrhotic patient is probably a marked oversimplification. Rather, one should adopt a more global view of the pathogenesis of abnormal sodium retention in cirrhosis in which differing forces participate in varying degrees as the derangement in sodium homeostasis evolves.

Efferent Events

Although initial attempts to explain the abnormalities of renal sodium handling focused on the decrement in GFR that occurs frequently in patients with advanced liver disease, it is clear that abnormalities of renal sodium handling occur despite preserved (and at times supranormal) GFR. These observations emphasize that the renal sodium retention accompanying cirrhosis is attributable primarily to enhanced tubular reabsorption rather than to alterations in the filtered load of sodium.

The mediators of the enhanced tubular reabsorption of sodium in cirrhosis and their relative participation in the avid sodium retention have not been elucidated completely. Many earlier formulations have attributed the deranged renal sodium handling primarily to abnormalities of aldosterone, but it is now clear that this is an oversimplification. Several lines of evidence have recently demonstrated that the enhanced tubular sodium reabsorption of cirrhosis occurs independently of elevated circulating aldosterone levels. The evidence currently available favors the postulate that the hyperaldosteronism of cirrhosis is a permissive factor only, and that the predominant component of the abnormal renal sodium handling is diminished distal delivery of filtrate. Only when distal filtrate delivery is enhanced by experimental or pharmacologic maneuvers does aldosterone play a major role in promoting sodium retention in cirrhosis.

The reappraisal of the role of aldosterone has prompted a search for additional effectors of sodium retention. Several hormonal, neural, and hemodynamic mechanisms have been implicated or suggested. The mechanisms, for which there is some evidence, and their interrelationships are summarized schematically in Fig. 113-2. The diminution of effective volume results in activation of the renin-angiotensin system. As a consequence, aldosterone secretion is augmented, with a resultant increase in sodium reabsorption in the distal segments of the nephron. It is also possible that activation of the renin-angiotensin system may contribute to sodium retention by producing a redistribution of intrarenal blood flow.

Simultaneously, an increase in sympathetic nervous system activity may contribute to the sodium retention. Activation of the sympathetic nervous system is commonly present in patients with cirrhosis. Many investigators have shown that patients with cirrhosis have elevated plasma concentrations of the sympathetic neurotransmitter norepinephrine and higher rates of norepinephrine spillover to plasma from the body as a whole and from individual organs and vascular territories such as the kidneys and the hepatomesenteric circulation. That sympathetic nerve firing rates are elevated in patients with cirrhosis has been confirmed by a study in which sympathetic nerve discharge rates were recorded directly using clinical microneurography. Recently, Esler and others reported that acute sympathetic inhibition, achieved by intravenously administered clonidine, was accompanied by potentially clinically beneficial effects: the lowering of renal vascular resistance, elevation of glomerular filtration rate, and reduction of portal venous pressure. Such observations suggest an important pathophysiologic role for increased sympathetic nervous activity in mediating the sodium retention of cirrhosis. It is now well established that alterations of the input of cardiopulmonary receptors induce changes in renal sympathetic activity. Thus a decrease in blood volume could alter the afferent input from the cardiopulmonary region, with a resultant increase in sympathetic nerve activity. Such an increase could contribute to the antinatriuresis of cirrhosis by (1) effecting a redistribution of blood flow into the kidney that favors increased net reabsorption of filtrate, and (2) a direct tubular effect of the renal sympathetic nerves on renal sodium handling.

Additional evidence has been marshaled to support the possibility that a diminution in endogenous prostaglandin production contributes to the sodium retention. A large body of evidence demonstrates that nonsteroidal antiinflammatory drugs (NSAIDs), which inhibit the endogenous production of prostaglandins, induce profound decrements of renal plasma flow, GFR, and sodium excretion in sodium-avid cirrhotic patients. Conversely, experimental manipulations that augment endogenous prostaglandins such as water immersion are associated with an increase in prostaglandin E and 6-keto prostaglandin $F_{1\alpha}$ excretion and a marked natriuresis and increase in creatinine clearance. In concert, these observations provide good evidence that renal prostanoid production contributes importantly to sodium retention. One can postulate that in the setting of cirrhosis, enhancement of prostaglandin synthesis is a compensatory or adaptive response to incipient renal ischemia. An important clinical corollary of this formulation is that the administration of agents inhibitory to prostaglandin synthesis may result in clinically important sodium retention and/or deterioration of renal function. Alterations in the kallikrein-kinin system, with diminished kinin formation, may contribute to the sodium retention encountered in liver disease.

Deficient production of endogenous natriuretic hormones has traditionally been suggested as another mechanism of sodium retention in cirrhosis. Two natriuretic hormones have been recognized: the atrial natriuretic peptide (ANP), mainly synthesized by atrial myocytes, and the so-called natriuretic hormone (NH), which is thought to be produced in the hypothalamus.

With the recent characterization of ANP and the demonstration that it participates in the regulation of volume homeostasis in both animals and humans, theoretic considerations suggest its possible role in the pathogenesis of sodium retention in cirrhosis. Nevertheless, recent evidence militates against an important role for atrial natriuretic factor (ANF) in mediating sodium retention. Experimental maneuvers such as water immersion have clearly demonstrated that cirrhotic patients augment plasma ANF to levels that either equal or exceed those of normal subjects studied under identical conditions, suggesting that sodium retention is not attributable to a diminished capacity to release ANF. Furthermore, recent studies during water immersion have demonstrated a striking dissociation between plasma ANF and the concomitant natriuretic response. In concert with data indicating that the natriuretic response to ANF infusion is markedly blunted or absent in approximately half of patients, these observations suggest that the sodium retention of cirrhosis may be related in part to a reduced renal responsiveness to ANF. It is conceivable that renal vasoconstriction mediated by diverse mechanisms, including the observed activation of the renin-angiotensin and probably the sympathetic nervous systems, impedes the ability of ANF to promote natriuresis.

The role of NH in mediating the sodium retention of cirrhosis is controversial, primarily because it is difficult to measure this hormone. The chemical nature of NH has not been established and can only be evaluated indirectly by assessing its biologic activities, namely the ability to inhibit sodium and potassium-activated (Na-K-) adenosine triphosphatase (ATPase) and ouabain binding in vitro, cross-react with antidigoxin antibodies, and induce a natriuresis when infused into experimental animals. Initial studies using bioassay techniques suggested a defect in the release of NH. In contrast, more recent studies, in which NH was specifically investigated in plasma and urine from cirrhotic patients with and without ascites by assessing digoxin-like immunoreactivity (DLIA) and the inhibition of ouabain binding, suggest that this hormone is not reduced but rather increased in these patients. These preliminary results have suggested that sodium retention in cirrhotic patients cannot be attributed to a deficiency in this hormone. As an alternative, the increased activity of natriuretic hormone in patients with cirrhosis and ascites may represent a compensatory response that is insufficient to antagonize the renal effects of sodium-retaining forces.

Recent investigative attention has focused on the role of nitric oxide as a mediator of both the hyperdynamic circulation and the sodium retention. Because patients with decompensated liver disease frequently have endotoxemia, the endotoxemia could induce nitric oxide synthase. The resultant increased nitric oxide synthesis and release could account for the associated hyperdynamic circulation. This formulation suggests that renal hypoperfusion and sodium retention are a result of a diversion of blood away from the kidney. Specific inhibitors of nitric oxide synthase theoretically should fac ilitate a more precise manipulation of nitric oxide synthesis and help to clarify the pathophysiologic importance of nitric oxide in endotoxemia and cirrhosis.

Management

The rational management of excessive salt and water retention in the cirrhotic patient should be grounded on the realization that ascites, unless massive, may not require intervention with diuretic agents. The initial goal of any treatment program should be an attempt to obtain spontaneous diuresis by consistent and scrupulous adherence to a well-balanced diet with rigid dietary sodium restriction (250 mg/day). It should be emphasized that the sodium intake prescribed for cardiac patients (1200 to 1500 mg/day) is not sufficiently restrictive for the cirrhotic patient, who continues to gain weight on such a program.

When the response to dietary management is inadequate, or when the imposition of rigid dietary sodium restriction is not feasible due to the cost or unpalatability of the diet, the use of diuretic agents may be considered. When diuretics are used, the therapeutic aim is a slow and gradual diuresis not exceeding the capacity for mobilization of ascitic fluid. Shear and others demonstrated that ascites absorption averages about 300 to 500 ml/day during spontaneous diuresis, with an upper limit of 700 to 900 ml/day. Thus any diuresis that exceeds 900 ml/day (in the ascitic patient without edema) must perforce be mobilized at the expense of the plasma compartment, with resultant volume contraction.

Because of the possible risk of hyponatremia, renal failure, and encephalopathy, therapeutic paracentesis has not enjoyed much popularity in the treatment of refractory ascites. Recently, several groups of investigators have evaluated the effects of large-volume paracentesis. They have suggested that therapeutic paracentesis, in the form of either repeated large-volume paracentesis or total paracentesis associated with an intravenous infusion of albumin (6 to 8 g/L of as-

citic fluid removed), is a rapid, effective, and safe therapy for refractory ascites in patients with cirrhosis.

NEPHROTIC SYNDROME

Normal adult humans excrete 100 to 150 mg of protein in the urine daily. In the setting of renal disease with involvement of the glomerulus, proteinuria (>150 mg/day) often supervenes. When the magnitude of proteinuria is great enough to exceed rates of albumin production by the liver, the concentration of albumin in plasma declines and the complex of symptoms recognized as the nephrotic syndrome develops (Chapter 108). The nephrotic syndrome may be defined as severe proteinuria (3.5 g or more), predominantly albuminuria, with concomitant hypoalbuminemia. Edema is the most prominent outward manifestation of the nephrotic syndrome and often provides the first evidence of disease noted by patients with some types of nephrotic syndrome.

Although the initiating event in these patients differs from that in patients with other edematous states, the overall pathogenetic cascade has many similarities. In contrast to patients with CHF and cirrhosis, patients with nephrotic syndrome frequently have a diminished total blood volume. The decrease in total blood volume (and thus in effective blood volume) is related to the hypoalbuminemia and diminished plasma oncotic pressure in the syndrome. Figure 113-3 summarizes the sequence of potential events that may contribute to the enhanced tubular reabsorption of sodium and edema formation. As a consequence of the diminished effective blood volume, the RAA system is activated, contributing to increased tubular reabsorption of sodium. As with cirrhotic patients, recent evidence suggests that the hyperal-

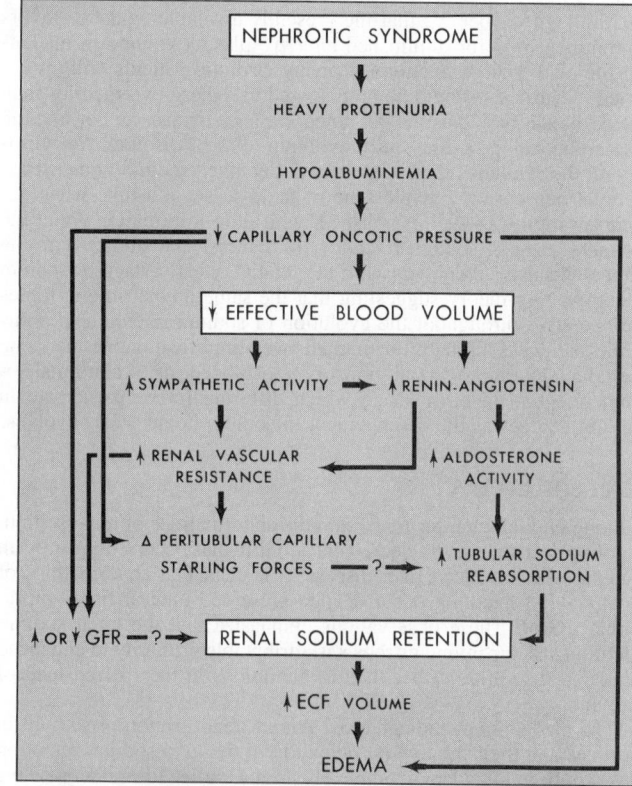

FIGURE 113-3   The major pathophysiologic mechanisms leading to renal sodium retention in the nephrotic syndrome. As a result of the massive proteinuria, hypoalbuminemia and decreased plasma oncotic pressure ensue, with resultant diminution in total blood volume and effective blood volume. Depicted here are the sequence of potential hormonal, hemodynamic, and neural events that may be activated as a consequence thereof and the manner in which they may interact to promote sodium retention. *ECF*, Extracellular fluid; *GFR*, glomerular filtration rate.

Modified from Schrier RW, Anderson RJ: Renal sodium In Schrier RW, editor: *Renal and electrolyte disorders*, ed 2, Boston, 1980, Little, Brown.

dosteronism of nephrotic syndrome is a permissive factor only and not the major determinant of the abnormal sodium retention. Concomitantly, several mechanisms act in concert to increase renal vascular resistance. Despite an increased renal vascular resistance, renal blood flow and GFR are not uniformly diminished, and in some instances GFR may actually be supranormal. The maintenance of the normal or increased GFR is thought to be related to the hypoalbuminemia, which decreases glomerular capillary oncotic pressure and therefore tends to increase net glomerular filtration pressure. In the presence of profound hypovolemia, however, the enhancement of GFR may be obscured by increased afferent arteriolar constriction, which diminishes glomerular capillary hydrostatic pressure.

The characteristics of the enhanced tubular reabsorption of sodium in patients with nephrotic syndrome may differ from those in CHF patients and patients with cirrhosis. It has been suggested that patients with nephrotic syndrome reabsorb less tubular sodium and water in the proximal tubule, perhaps due to the lowering of peritubular oncotic pressure with hypoalbuminemia. Accordingly, the main site for the enhanced sodium reabsorption in nephrotic syndrome might be localized to the distal nephron. Thus in the presence of blockade of distal reabsorption of sodium by large doses of ethacrynic acid and thiazide diuretics, nephrotic syndrome patients excrete a larger fraction of their filtered load of sodium than either cirrhotic patients or cardiac failure patients.

Aside from the administration of diuretics, several therapeutic considerations are unique to the nephrotic patient. Because the linchpin of the pathogenetic cascade responsible for sodium reabsorption is proteinuria, one may consider the administration of corticosteroids in an attempt to diminish or eliminate the proteinuria. Certain diseases causing the nephrotic syndrome, particularly lipoid nephrosis (nil disease), are amenable to such an approach (the diverse glomerulonephritides and their treatment are discussed in detail in Chapter 116). Although hypoalbuminemia is a salient feature of the nephrotic syndrome, the administration of albumin solutions is of little lasting value because the increase in plasma albumin concentration is only transient. In extremely severe hypoalbuminemia, however, an infusion of albumin may be a lifesaving maneuver in the management of a hypotensive episode.

ACUTE NEPHRITIC SYNDROME

The pathophysiology of sodium retention in the acute nephritic syndrome is discussed in detail in Chapter 107 and will not be considered further here.

IDIOPATHIC EDEMA

Idiopathic edema is a common disorder that occurs exclusively in women and is characterized by salt retention in the absence of cardiac, renal, or hepatic disease. Although the edema may be episodic and the disorder has been called cyclic edema, it can be persistent. In women afflicted with this disorder, edema of the face, hands, and feet develops rapidly, frequently accompanied by symptoms of headache, irritability, and depression. Some women can gain as much as 3 to 4 kg during a 24-hour period, with a concomitant decrease in urine output.

There is a significant postural component to the occurrence of edema. Although upright posture is associated with hyperaldosteronism and sodium retention in normal subjects, edema rarely occurs. In contrast, patients with idiopathic cyclical edema seem to have an exaggerated response to upright posture whereby the antinatriuresis of upright posture results in significant pitting edema of their lower extremities.

Another intriguing facet of the syndrome is its frequent association with *surreptitious* diuretic use. Many of the patients are obese women, and there frequently is great anxiety about appearance and weight. Such concern can lead some women with idiopathic edema to take diuretics constantly and surreptitiously. The clinical presentation then may not be edema but rather unexplained hypokalemia, urinary potassium wasting, and elevated plasma renin activity, which can lead to the mistaken diagnosis of Bartter's syndrome.

In a similar vein, administration of potent diuretics in patients with

idiopathic edema may have a deleterious effect by inducing ECF volume depletion, further exaggerating an already abnormal response to upright posture. The resultant hyperaldosteronism together with other mediators may induce sustained antinatriuresis for as long as 2 weeks after cessation of treatment. Furthermore, long-term diuretic therapy is associated with potassium depletion, which can potentiate the problem by producing symptoms of weakness, malaise, and irritability.

Despite much study, the mechanisms responsible for the sodium retention have not been established. Postulated mechanisms include a reduction in arterial blood pressure when standing, intermittent alteration in capillary permeability, increased aldosterone secretion, alteration in estrogen or progesterone secretion, and hypoproteinemia.

USE OF DIURETICS

When edema persists despite adequate treatment of the primary disease, diuretics may be required. It should be emphasized that the presence of edema alone is not a definite indication for diuretic treatment, and the physician must weigh any cosmetic value against the potential deleterious effect of the drug.

Once the decision is made to use diuretic agents to treat an edematous disorder, there are several guidelines for gauging the desired rate of diuresis. In general, it should approximate the rate of accumulation of the edema fluid. Thus acute pulmonary edema necessitates induction of a rapid diuresis, whereas less emergent edema formation is best treated with a more gradual diuresis. In either case, the rate of diuresis should be so limited that the potential rate of movement of interstitial fluid into the vascular compartment will not be exceeded to any large extent. If renal excretion does exceed the rate of mobilization of interstitial fluid, intravascular volume depletion and hypotension can result, even though ECF volume is still expanded. Intermittent diuretic therapy (e.g., alternate-day therapy) may be of value in avoiding intravascular volume depletion.

The rational basis of diuretic therapy lies in an understanding of the mechanism(s) and sites of action of the diuretic agent. Box 113-2 summarizes the primary sites of action of the available diuretic agents. The loop diuretics ethacrynic acid, furosemide, and bumetanide are the most potent diuretic agents available. The very steep dose-response relationship they manifest has led to the label *high-ceiling diuretics*. The inhibition of sodium and chloride reabsorption that these agents produce in the medullary ascending limb of the loop of Henle exceeds the rate-limited sodium reabsorption in the more distal nephron, and a maximal acute diuretic effect equivalent to 20% to

---

BOX 113-2
Classification of diuretics by site of action in the nephron

Osmotic diuretics
 Urea
 Mannitol
Proximal tubular diuretics
 Mannitol
 Acetazolamide
Loop of Henle diuretics
 Ethacrynic acid
 Furosemide
 Bumetanide
Distal tubular diuretics
 Potassium-losing diuretics
  Thiazides
  Chlorthalidone
  Metolazone
  Indapamide
 Potassium-sparing diuretics
  Triamterene
  Spironolactone
  Amiloride

25% of the filtered load of sodium may be achieved. These drugs are effective immediately after intravenous administration and exert an effect within 1 hour of oral administration. In patients with pulmonary edema the intravenous administration of furosemide not only induces a diuresis but also reduces the preload on the heart. The management of CHF is often complicated by an inability of orally administered furosemide to produce an effective diuresis, requiring intravenous furosemide to achieve the desired clinical response.

The distal tubular diuretics can be classified into two groups, namely, the potassium-losing and potassium-sparing diuretics. The thiazide-like diuretics chlorthalidone and metolazone, although chemically different, have diuretic effects similar to those of the thiazides. The diuretic effect of all of these compounds is attributable solely to the demonstrated inhibition of sodium and chloride reabsorption in the distal convoluted tubule. Consequently, these diuretics partially inhibit only urinary diluting capacity, not concentrating capacity. Thiazides are relatively safe and are the first-line drugs in patients with normal renal function. In contrast, they may exert little effect in patients with a GFR of less than 30 ml/minute. The use of these diuretics, which act proximally to the distal site of potassium secretion, is associated not only with a natriuresis but also with an increase in urinary potassium excretion.

The potassium-sparing diuretics act by blocking distal potassium-linked sodium reabsorption in the extreme distal tubule and collecting duct. Because these sites reabsorb relatively little sodium, these agents are weak diuretics, increasing fractional excretion of sodium to a lesser extent than the thiazide type of diuretics. Consequently, their primary usefulness is in the prevention or treatment of hypokalemia caused by other diuretics.

Because the specific attributes and usage of the various diuretics used to mobilize ascites and edema in patients with liver disease are reviewed elsewhere (Chapter 354), it might be helpful at this point to consider the appropriate role of diuretics in the management of one of the prototypical edematous states—chronic liver disease.

To produce its required pharmacologic effect, a loop diuretic has to be delivered into the renal tubule. Consequently, a major determinant of response to the agent is its access to the urine and to its site of action at the thick ascending limb of the loop of Henle. In some cirrhotic patients delivery of these agents into the urine is impaired, although to what degree and with what frequency have not been established. Consequently, it has been suggested that cirrhotic patients may require doses that are 2 to 2.5 times higher than normal to attain normal amounts at the site of action. I suggest the following algorithm for management of cirrhotic ascites (Fig. 113-4). Approximately 10% of cirrhotic patients with ascites can be managed with bed rest and sodium restriction. The next step is the use of spironolactone in doses of up to 200 to 300 mg/day. If this is insufficient, a cautiously used combination of diuretic therapy using spironolactone and loop diuretics (with or without addition of metolazone) may induce a response in some patients, although there is a growing awareness that the use of such combinations may be attended by a wide array of complications, including profound hypokalemia.

Occasionally a patient does not respond to conventional diuretic therapy, even when a loop diuretic is used. Several possible mechanisms may mediate such refractoriness and each can be treated in a specific way (Table 113-1).

Should the ascites be refractory to a combined diuretic regimen, a number of more intensive techniques are available. Probably the best known is the peritoneovenous shunt. Although peritoneovenous shunting alleviates ascites more rapidly than medical management does, overall experience with this technique has not been particularly favorable. Repeated large-volume paracentesis with concomitant infusion of expanders (e.g., human albumin, dextran 70) is a rapid, effective, and relatively safe therapy for mobilizing ascites in patients with cirrhosis. Because mobilization of ascites by paracentesis alone is associated with contraction of effective circulating blood volume with a consequent risk of inducing renal impairment, intravenous colloid administration must be an essential part of the treatment. Recently there have been increasing reports describing improvement in sodium excretion following insertion of a transjugular intrahepatic portosystemic shunt (TIPS). The rationale for this procedure is similar to that for the establishment of a side-to-side portacaval shunt, thereby creating a portal to systemic vascular pathway that serves to

Table 113-1 Treatment of refractory edema according to underlying mechanism

PROBLEM	TREATMENT
Excessive sodium intake	Measure urinary sodium excretion; if greater than 75 to 100 mEq/day, attempt more rigorous dietary restriction.
Decreased intestinal drug absorption	Switch to intravenous loop diuretic.
Increased distal reabsorption	Add thiazide type of diuretic and/or potassium-sparing diuretic.
Decreased loop delivery	Try to increase delivery out of proximal tubule with albumin.
Reduced delivery of furosemide to kidney because of severe hypoalbuminemia	Inject furosemide-albumin complex.
Decreased drug entry into tubule lumen	Administer massive doses of loop diuretic. If unresponsive, initiate extracorporeal techniques or the peritoneovenous shunt.

From Epstein, M: *The kidney in liver disease,* ed 4, Philadelphia, 1996, Hanley & Belfus, p. 455.

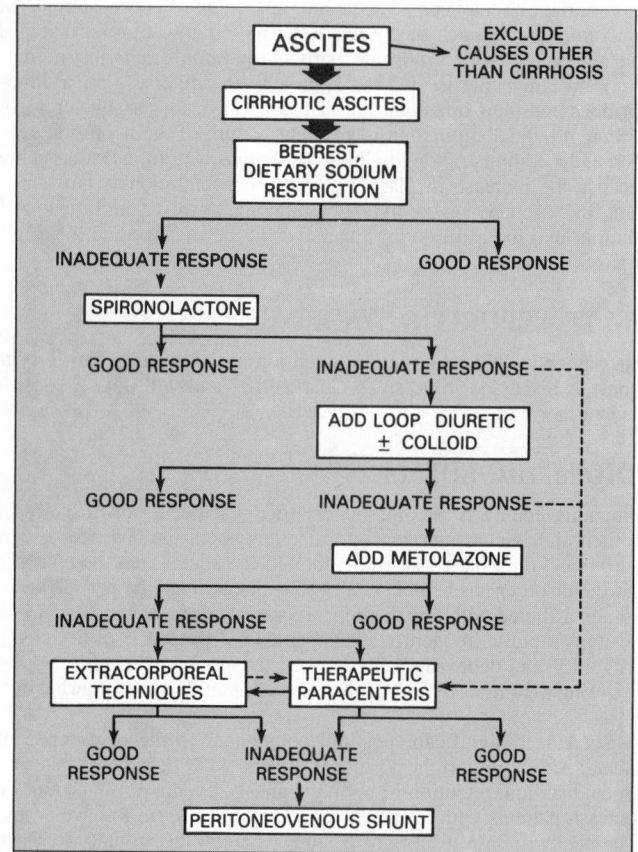

FIGURE 113-4 Algorithm for the comprehensive management of cirrhotic ascites and edema. The solid lines represent therapeutic options and sequences that I believe are well established. The interrupted lines indicate uncertainty regarding the appropriate positioning of paracentesis in the therapeutic sequence.

From Epstein M. In Epstein M, editor: *The kidney in liver disease,* ed 4, Philadelphia, 1996, Hanley & Belfus, p. 457.

BOX 113-3

Extrarenal causes of sodium depletion

I. Gastrointestinal tract sodium loss
  A. External loss of sodium
    1. Diarrhea
    2. Vomiting
    3. Small bowel suction
    4. Pancreatic, biliary, or intestinal fistula
  B. Sequestration of sodium
    1. Small bowel obstruction
    2. Pancreatitis
    3. Peritonitis
II. Skin sodium loss
  A. External loss of sodium
    1. Heat exposure
    2. Adrenal insufficiency
  B. Sequestration of sodium
    1. Burns
    2. Inflammatory disease
III. Miscellaneous sodium loss (external)
  A. Severe hemorrhage
  B. Central nervous system lesions (rare)
  C. Removal of large volumes of serous cavity fluid

Modified from Anderson RJ, Linas SL. In Brenner BM, Stein JH, editors: *Sodium and water homeostasis,* New York, 1978, Churchill Livingstone.

BOX 113-4

Renal causes of sodium depletion

I. Intrinsic renal processes
  A. Chronic renal failure
  B. Acute renal failure
    1. Nonoliguric acute renal failure
    2. Recovery from oliguric acute renal failure
  C. Salt-wasting nephropathy
    1. Relief of obstructive uropathy
    2. Nephrocalcinosis with interstitial nephritis
    3. Medullary cystic disease
    4. Polycystic kidney disease
    5. Proximal renal tubular acidosis
II. Extrinsic renal processes
  A. Solute diuresis/nonreabsorbable anion diuresis
    1. Endogenous (bicarbonate, urea, glucose)
    2. Exogenous (mannitol, dextran, urea, glycerol, radiocontrast media)
  B. Diuretic administration
  C. Mineralocorticoid deficiency
    1. Failure of steroidogenesis
    2. Failure of renin secretion
  D. Fasting
  E. Hypertensive hyponatremic syndrome
  F. Acute-phase vomiting

Modified from Anderson RJ, Linas SL: In Brenner BM, Stein JH, editors: *Sodium and water homeostasis,* New York, 1978, Churchill Livingstone.

---

decompress the portacaval system. Although TIPS obviates the need for performing major vascular surgery, the reported experience is preliminary. Randomized prospective studies are being conducted to delineate the future niche of TIPS in the therapeutic armamentarium.

In some patients, especially those with peripheral edema, therapeutic paracentesis may be a reasonable alternative. For the patient who is truly refractory to these maneuvers the therapeutic choices include extracorporeal techniques and the peritoneovenous shunt. The former include ascites reinfusion, dialytic ultrafiltration of ascites, or continuous arteriovenous hemofiltration (CAVH).

SALT-WASTING STATES

As noted at the beginning of the chapter, ECF sodium constitutes the major determinant of ECF volume. It follows that an inordinate loss of sodium would result in a decrease in ECF solute, with a resultant contraction of ECF volume. The relentless progression of this process can result in circulatory collapse. The ultimate hemodynamic consequences of sodium depletion depend on both the magnitude and the rapidity of the development of sodium loss. Acute, profound sodium depletion that results in a 20% to 40% decrement in ECF volume results in marked decrements in mean arterial pressure and cardiac output. In contrast, a more gradual rate of sodium depletion (i.e., as much as 500 mEq over 10 days) is associated with only slight alterations in arterial pressure and pulse rate, despite profound sodium deficits.

Sodium depletion results from the loss or sequestration of a variety of body fluids, ranging from gastrointestinal tract fluids to sweat, that contain substantial quantities of sodium. To afford a framework with which to approach this subject, it is worthwhile to classify these disorders of sodium depletion according to the source of the deficit (i.e., extrarenal and renal sources). Determining the urinary sodium concentration affords an easy means of classifying the source of sodium depletion. Urinary sodium concentrations of less than 10 mEq/L suggest an extrarenal source of sodium depletion (Box 113-3), whereas urinary sodium concentrations greater than 20 mEq/L (and usually exceeding 40 mEq/L) suggest a renal cause (Box 113-4).

EXTRARENAL SODIUM DEPLETION
Gastrointestinal Tract Origin of Sodium Loss

Because both the volume and sodium concentration of most gastrointestinal tract secretions are substantial, disturbances of the gastrointestinal tract have the potential for producing clinically significant sodium loss. In practice, gastrointestinal tract disturbances are responsible for extrarenal sodium depletion. As enumerated in Box 113-3, the mechanisms of gastrointestinal tract sodium loss are twofold: external loss of sodium and sequestration of sodium within the body.

Diarrhea is the most common gastrointestinal tract disturbance leading to sodium depletion through external losses. Any of the mechanisms that may result in diarrhea, including osmotic retardation of sodium and water reabsorption, abnormalities of sodium and water transport (as with *Vibrio cholerae* infection), and increased intestinal transport, can produce sodium depletion. Such losses can be marked, as exemplified by patients infected with *V. cholerae* who may manifest losses of up to 800 ml/hour of diarrhea fluid containing substantial concentrations of sodium. Sodium depletion can also occur from protracted vomiting and loss of gastrointestinal tract fluids through drainage of fistulas or ileostomies.

Another mechanism for gastrointestinal tract sodium loss is the sequestration of sodium-rich fluid within the gastrointestinal tract. Thus inflammatory diseases of the pancreas or peritoneum and mechanical small bowel obstruction can lead to sequestration of large volumes of sodium-containing fluid and resultant ECF volume depletion. Intraabdominal sequestration of ECF volume may be difficult to detect clinically.

Loss of Sodium Through Skin

It is not commonly appreciated that the skin may constitute an important source of sodium depletion. Physical labor at high ambient temperatures may be associated with as much as 5 L of sweat containing 60 to 70 mEq/L of sodium. Continuing loss of such a large quantity of sodium would be expected to result in volume depletion. In normal, acclimatized subjects the volume and sodium concentration of sweat is reduced, diminishing the risk of volume depletion. In contrast, in unacclimatized subjects and patients with adrenal insufficiency the volume and sodium concentration of sweat may fail to decrease, with resultant sodium depletion.

SODIUM DEPLETION OF RENAL ORIGIN

Because the kidney is the major organ that mediates sodium homeostasis, it is not altogether surprising that a failure of the kidney to conserve sodium will result in sodium depletion. Impaired renal sodium conservation is attributable to either intrinsic renal diseases or conditions extrinsic to the kidney (Box 113-4).

Intrinsic Renal Diseases

Patients with chronic renal failure of diverse causes fail to conserve sodium as efficiently as normal volunteers in response to dietary sodium restriction. Although in many patients with chronic renal failure urinary sodium excretion may eventually be lowered to equal intake, the interval required to attain sodium balance is markedly prolonged.

Aside from the mild sodium-wasting tendency of chronic renal failure, a relatively small number of patients with renal failure may manifest massive renal salt-wasting characterized by urinary sodium excretion of 100 to 300 mEq/day, despite negligible sodium intake. In general, the cause of the renal failure in these patients is either medullary cystic disease or interstitial renal diseases.

Several mechanisms have been postulated to explain the sodium wasting of intrinsic renal disease: anatomic damage to nephron segments involved in sodium reabsorption; an increased filtered load of solute per nephron, which could contribute to sodium wasting; and hyperperfusion of residual nephrons, which could result in the delivery of sodium in amounts that exceed the capacity of the distal nephron to reabsorb sodium. It has recently been proposed that an adaptive process as yet undefined (perhaps mediated through an NH) contributes to the progressive natriuresis per nephron.

Although the exact mechanism(s) responsible for the sodium-wasting tendency of renal failure remain undetermined, this salt-wasting tendency can have serious consequences for the patient. The withdrawal of sodium from the diet or the induction of extrarenal sodium losses can result in marked volume contraction, with a dramatic deterioration in renal function. Implicit in this formulation is the clinical aphorism that an unexplained decline in renal function in patients with previously stable renal failure and in whom clinical evidence of volume overload is absent should prompt a trial of volume repletion.

Renal Sodium Loss Due to Conditions Extrinsic to the Kidney

Osmotic Diuresis. An endogenous solute diuresis, such as that resulting from the glycosuria seen in patients with diabetic ketoacidosis or hyperosmolar, nonketotic coma, may result in significant renal sodium loss. Similarly, exogenous solutes such as mannitol, dextran, glycerol, or radiopaque dye may induce a solute diuresis, with the resultant loss of large volumes of urine containing as much as 70 mEq/L of sodium.

Mineralocorticoid Deficiency. The failure of the kidney to conserve sodium is a prominent, well-recognized feature of primary adrenal insufficiency. A variety of adrenal insufficiency syndromes can produce sodium depletion, including primary adrenal insufficiency, adrenogenital syndromes, and isolated deficiencies in aldosterone biosynthesis. Although these syndromes differ in their biochemical defects, they share in common mineralocorticoid deficiency and thus are capable of inducing salt wasting.

Among the several variants of the syndrome of isolated hypoaldosteronism are specific adrenal enzymatic defects that result in impaired aldosterone biosynthesis in the setting of an intact renin-angiotensin axis and diminished aldosterone production secondary to diminished renin secretion (syndrome of hyporeninemic hypoaldosteronism). Patients with hyporeninemic hypoaldosteronism present with mild to moderate degrees of renal insufficiency and with acidemia and hyperkalemia disproportionate to their modest decrement in renal function.

It should be noted, however, that a large proportion of patients with isolated hypoaldosteronism are not actually volume depleted or salt wasting. On the contrary, many have hypertension and mild volume overload, and the latter may in fact be one of the causes of the suppressed plasma renin and aldosterone levels.

Treatment. The mainstay of treatment of sodium depletion includes prompt restoration of ECF volume and correction of the cause of the sodium loss.

Table 113-2 Correlation of clinical signs with the magnitude of extracellular fluid volume contraction

SIGN	DEGREE OF DEHYDRATION		
	<5%	6%-10%	>10%
Skin			
Turgor	↓	↓↓	↓↓↓
Color	Pale	Dusky	Mottled
Mucosae	Dry	Very dry	Parchmentlike
Sympathetic overactivity			
Cremasteric contraction	+	++	++
Temperature of extremities	Cool	Cooler	Cold
Hemodynamics			
Pulse*	↑	↑↑	↑↑↑
Blood Pressure*	±↓	↓↓	↓↓↓

*Pulse and blood pressure changes augmented by posture.
Modified from Rudnick MR Narins RG. In Brenner BM Lazarus JM, editors: *Acute renal failure,* Philadelphia, 1983, WB Saunders.

The history and physical findings often provide significant clues in the assessment of patients with suspected volume depletion and prerenal azotemia. Table 113-2 summarizes the clinical signs of hypovolemia. As can be seen, ECF volume depletion will manifest itself by the following signs of increased sympathetic nerve activity: resting tachycardia worsened by sitting or standing, sustained cremasteric muscle contraction (testes held close to the perineum), and peripheral vasoconstriction with cool extremities. Sitting or standing blood pressure falls when intravascular volume is decreased by approximately 10%. Skin, axillae, and mucous membranes tend to be dry and skin turgor is diminished. Assessment of skin turgor is rather subjective and is influenced by loss of skin elasticity from aging and malnutrition. Nonetheless, with experience and by directing attention to the skin over the forehead and sternum (areas less influenced by age), one gains important insights into fluid status.

Because there is no reliable clinical method to determine the magnitude of sodium repletion necessary to achieve normovolemia, one may obtain a rough approximation of the underlying sodium deficit by computing the decrease in the patient's body weight (one may assume that each kilogram of body weight loss is equivalent to 1 L of 0.9% saline). If sodium depletion occurred in the absence of hemorrhage or hemolysis, one may calculate the sodium loss by utilizing the change in hematocrit.

Although alterations in the hematocrit and hemoglobin concentration may be helpful in approximating the degree of salt and water depletion, it should be emphasized that such computations constitute only a rough guide to management. A number of considerations should be borne in mind in the interpretation of such changes. First, it should be emphasized that red blood cell volume changes in accordance with changes in effective osmolality; hypoosmolality increases and hyperosmolality decreases red blood cell size. Thus only in isotonic volume depletion, in which red blood cell volume remains normal, will the hematocrit properly reflect reduction in plasma volume. In hypertonic dehydration, a decrease in plasma volume is accompanied by a decrease in red blood cell volume; therefore the hematocrit may remain close to normal. Conversely, in hypotonic dehydration, decrements in plasma volume are accompanied by increases in red blood cell volume, and the hematocrit tends to increase to a greater extent than one would anticipate from the degree of volume depletion. Because hemoglobin concentration does not change with alterations in osmolality, this variable should more accurately reflect alterations in intravascular volume. It is self-evident that hematocrit and hemoglobin levels are invalid indices of fluid loss when hemorrhage has occurred. From a practical standpoint, ECF volume repletion should be accomplished with careful and continuous clinical monitoring (preferably with central venous pressure determinations). A rapid or overly vigorous attempt at repletion may overcorrect, with resultant hypervolemia and cardiac failure. When hyponatremia coexists with volume depletion, consideration must be given to the rapidity with which serum sodium increases during therapy.

Although numerous reviews have suggested the use of a "fluid or diuretic challenge," their utility in the differentiation of prerenal and intrarenal azotemia is questionable. Not only does the use of diuretics provide minimal diagnostic insight, but their natriuretic effects worsen the condition of previously dehydrated patients.

BIBLIOGRAPHY

Buckalew VA Jr: Natriuretic hormone. In Epstein M, editor: *The kidney in liver disease,* ed 4, Philadelphia, 1996, Hanley & Belfus.

Cohn JN: Future directions in vasodilator therapy for heart failure, *Am Heart J* 121:969-973, 1991.

Epstein M: Atrial natriuretic factor in liver disease. In Epstein M, editor: *The kidney in liver disease,* ed 4, Philadelphia, 1996, Hanley & Belfus.

Epstein M: Diuretic therapy in liver disease. In Epstein M, editor: *The kidney in liver disease,* ed 4, Philadelphia, 1996, Hanley & Belfus.

Epstein M: Renal sodium handling in cirrhosis. In Epstein M, editor: *The kidney in liver disease,* ed 4, Philadelphia, 1996, Hanley & Belfus.

Epstein M: Role of the peritoneovenous shunt in the management of ascites and the hepatorenal syndrome. In Epstein M, editor: *The kidney in liver disease,* ed 4, Philadelphia, 1996, Hanley & Belfus.

Esler M et al: Increased sympathetic activity and the effects of its inhibition with clonidine in alcoholic cirrhosis, *Ann Intern Med* 116:446-455, 1992.

Gines P et al: Paracentesis with intravenous infusion of albumin as compared with peritonovenous shunting in cirrhosis with refractory ascites, *N Engl J Med* 325:829-835, 1991.

Glassock RJ: Pathophysiology of acute glomerulonephritis, *Hosp Pract* 23:163-178, 1988.

Kubo SH, Cohn JN: Approach to treatment of the patient with heart failure in 1994, *Adv Intern Med* 39:485-515, 1994.

MacGregor GA, DeWardner HE: Idiopathic edema. In Schrier W, Gottschalk CW, editors: *Diseases of the kidney,* ed 5, Boston, 1993, Little, Brown.

Oster JR, Materson BJ: Renal and electrolyte complications of congestive heart failure and effects of therapy with angiotensin-converting enzyme inhibitors, *Arch Intern Med* 152:704-710, 1992.

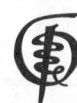

CHAPTER

114 Disorders of Potassium Balance

Richard H. Sterns and Robert G. Narins

Potassium, the most prevalent intracellular cation, resides primarily in skeletal muscle (60%) and bone (18%). Although tissues vary, the mean intracellular potassium concentration approximates 150 mEq/L. The distribution of potassium between cellular and extracellular fluid is largely determined by cell membrane–associated $(Na^+ + K^+)$-ATPase (sodium potassium–activated adenosine triphosphatase), which actively imports potassium in exchange for exported sodium. The extracellular fluid concentration of 4 to 5 mEq/L indicates that only 1% to 2% (70 mEq) of total body potassium resides outside cells. The cell's resting electrical potential difference is a function of the ratio of the concentrations of intracellular (K_i) to extracellular (K_e) potassium. Disturbances of potassium homeostasis alter this ratio because K_e changes proportionately more than K_i. Therefore hypokalemia tends to increase the ratio, thereby hyperpolarizing cell membranes, whereas hyperkalemia has the opposite effect (Fig. 114-1). These changes in membrane potential underlie many of the clinically important cardiac and neuromuscular manifestations of disordered potassium metabolism.

EXTERNAL POTASSIUM BALANCE

Approximately 10% of the 50 to 100 mEq of dietary potassium normally escapes intestinal absorption, whereas the remaining 45 to 90 mEq enters the extracellular fluid. In the steady state, in the absence of net anabolism or net catabolism, the absorbed potassium is excreted in the urine (Fig. 114-2).

The kidneys regulate external potassium balance by matching the cation's excretion to the host's metabolic needs. Thus closely regulated renal excretion limits the risk of potassium surplus or deficit from largely unregulated dietary intake and absorption. Even small increases of the plasma potassium concentration markedly stimulate urinary potassium excretion. This response is amplified by aldosterone, a kaliuretic hormone secreted in response to hyperkalemia. Thus

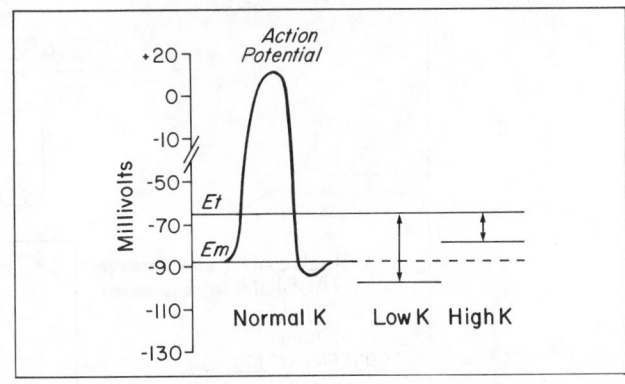

FIGURE 114-1 The influence of hypokalemia and hyperkalemia on membrane excitability. *Em,* Resting transmembrane electrical potential difference; Et, threshold potential.

Modified from Leaf A, Cotran R: Pathophysiology of potassium excess and deficiency. In *Renal pathophysiology,* ed 2, New York, 1980, Oxford University Press.

when renal function and aldosterone secretion are normal, accumulation of excess potassium is unlikely, even when intake of the cation is very large. Aldosterone secretion and renal potassium excretion are diminished by hypokalemia. However, renal potassium conservation during dietary restriction with hypokalemia is less efficient than the excretion of excess potassium during dietary loading and hyperkalemia. Because potassium cannot be totally eliminated from the urine, severe dietary restriction of the cation can eventually cause substantial deficits.

Abnormalities in the renal regulation of external potassium balance may cause potassium surfeits or deficits. Impairment of this regulatory function may be caused by diseases of the kidneys themselves, abnormalities in aldosterone secretion, acid-base disturbances, and pharmacologic agents.

INTERNAL POTASSIUM BALANCE

The distribution of potassium between extracellular and intracellular fluid compartments (internal balance) is a major determinant of the plasma potassium concentration. Extracellular leakage of only 70 mEq of the 4000 mEq of potassium contained in cells would result in lethal hyperkalemia (9 mEq/L), whereas intracellular translocation of only 45 mEq of the extracellular cation would cause severe hypokalemia (1.5 mEq/L). The membrane transport protein $(Na^+ + K^+)$-ATPase is ultimately responsible for potassium's normal asymmetric transcellular distribution. Both the number of transport molecules and their rate of transport are subject to regulation. Potassium itself plays a role in this regulation. For example, potassium depletion reduces the number of transporters, enabling cellular stores to replenish extracellular losses.

Insulin and *catecholamines* are the most important hormonal regulators of internal potassium balance. Both enhance cellular potassium uptake by stimulating the $(Na^+ + K^+)$-ATPase activity of skeletal muscle. Insulin's hypokalemic effect is dose-related, reaching a plateau at hormone levels many times greater than those required for maximum glucose utilization. Insulin deficiency impedes cellular uptake of excess potassium. The hypokalemic effect of catecholamines is mediated by cyclic-AMP and is promoted by β_2-adrenergic agonists. β-Adrenergic blockade can lead to hyperkalemia.

Acid-base disturbances may influence internal potassium balance. Acidemia provokes hyperkalemia by exchanging extracellular hydrogen ions for cellular potassium during tissue buffering. The reverse occurs in alkalemia or during correction of some types of acidemia. In general, metabolic acid-base disturbances exert greater effects on potassium distribution than do respiratory disorders. However, the hyperkalemic effect of metabolic acidosis depends on the anion accompanying the accumulated hydrogen ion. If the anion is chloride (which does not readily enter cells), a transmembrane electrochemical gradient favoring potassium egress is created when protons are buffered intracellularly. By contrast, organic anions such as lactate and ketones are able to penetrate cells in the buffering process so that potassium

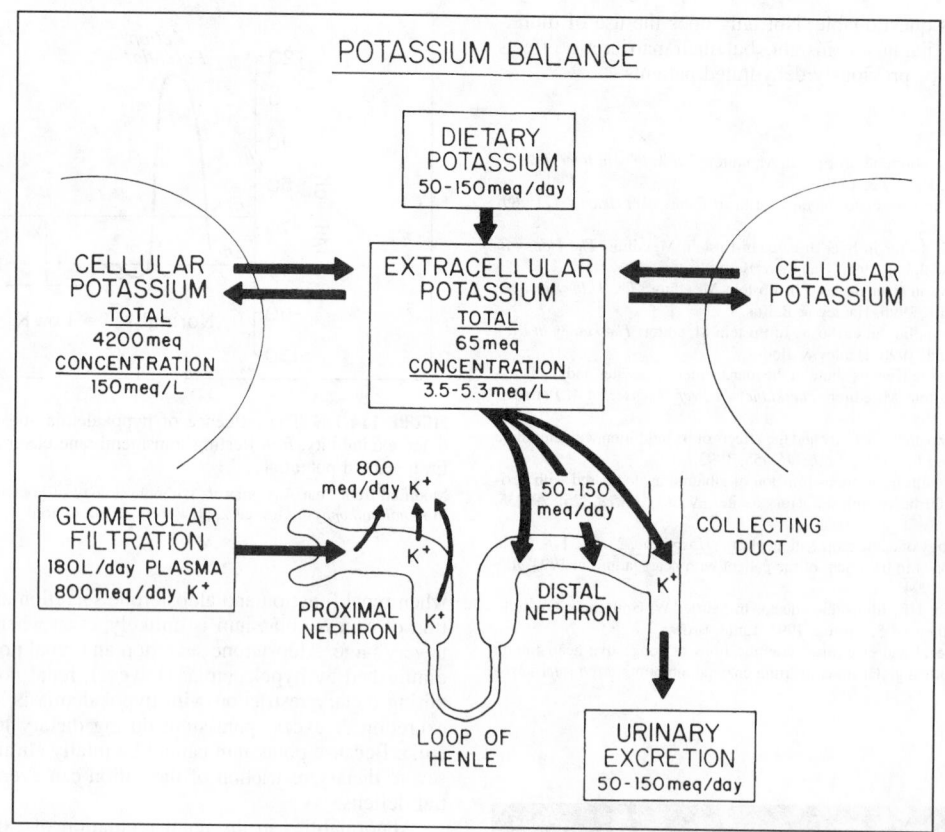

FIGURE 114-2   Overview of potassium balance. The figure ignores fecal potassium excretion, normally about 10% of dietary intake. See text for further details.
From Narins RG: *Am J Cardiol* 65:4E, 1990.

exchange is not promoted. Thus organic acidoses by themselves have only a minimal effect on internal potassium balance.

Hypertonicity provokes potassium diffusion out of cells, presumably by increasing the intracellular potassium concentration as cells become dehydrated. Hyperglycemia in diabetics with previously reduced renal potassium excretion is the most important example of this phenomenon. It also occurs when hypertonic mannitol or saline is infused into subjects with renal failure.

HYPOKALEMIA

Hypokalemia may result solely from disordered internal potassium balance, but more commonly it reflects potassium depletion from renal or extrarenal losses.

Spurious Hypokalemia

This rare in vitro phenomenon can occur in acute myelogenous leukemia if the blood sample remains at room temperature before separation, allowing metabolically active leukemia cells to absorb potassium.

True Hypokalemia Without Potassium Depletion

Transient hypokalemia may be caused by a shift of potassium into cells. This phenomenon should be suspected when hypokalemia resolves after little or no potassium replacement (Table 114-1).

Exogenous insulin can cause hypokalemia without potassium depletion (e.g., when excessive insulin is given with total parenteral nutrition). More commonly, however, insulin therapy unmasks or exacerbates hypokalemia in potassium-depleted patients with uncontrolled diabetes mellitus. Insulin-induced hypoglycemia reduces the plasma potassium concentration by virtue of the combined effects of insulin and the high levels of catecholamines released in response to the low blood sugar.

Table 114-1   Factors that alter internal potassium balance

INCREASED CELL K⁺ UPTAKE	INCREASED CELL K⁺ EFFLUX
Insulin	Insulin deficiency
Endogenous catecholamines	Beta₂-adrenergic blockers
Beta₂-adrenergic agonists	Hypertonicity
Hypokalemic periodic paralysis	Hyperkalemic periodic paralysis
Alkalosis (metabolic > respiratory)	Metabolic acidosis (mineral, not organic) and respiratory acidosis
Hypothermia	Vigorous exercise
Barium poisoning	Digitalis intoxication
Cell growth	Succinylcholine
	Arginine hydrochloride
	Cell lysis or catabolism

Endogenous catecholamines secreted in states of extreme stress (e.g., myocardial infarction, cerebral hemorrhage, and possibly delirium tremens) may cause transient hypokalemia. Exogenous catecholamines, particularly β₂-adrenergic agonists used in the treatment of asthma (terbutaline, albuterol, and salbutamol) or premature labor (ritodrine) may cause marked, transient hypokalemia by shifting potassium into cells. The effect peaks within 30 minutes, lasts 1 hour, and lowers serum potassium 0.3 to 1.5 mEq/L.

Hypokalemic periodic paralysis is a rare disorder characterized by intermittent episodes of muscle weakness associated with transient acute shifts of potassium into cells. Attacks, which may last from a few hours to a few days, are provoked by rest after exercise and carbohydrate-rich meals. Oral or intravenous potassium reverses acute attacks and acetazolamide is the most effective long-term prophylactic therapy. Mutations of the calcium channel α-1 subunit, also known as the dihydropyridine receptor, are responsible for the familial form of the disease, which is transmitted as an autosomal dominant trait. Sporadic acquired cases may complicate thyrotoxicosis, especially in

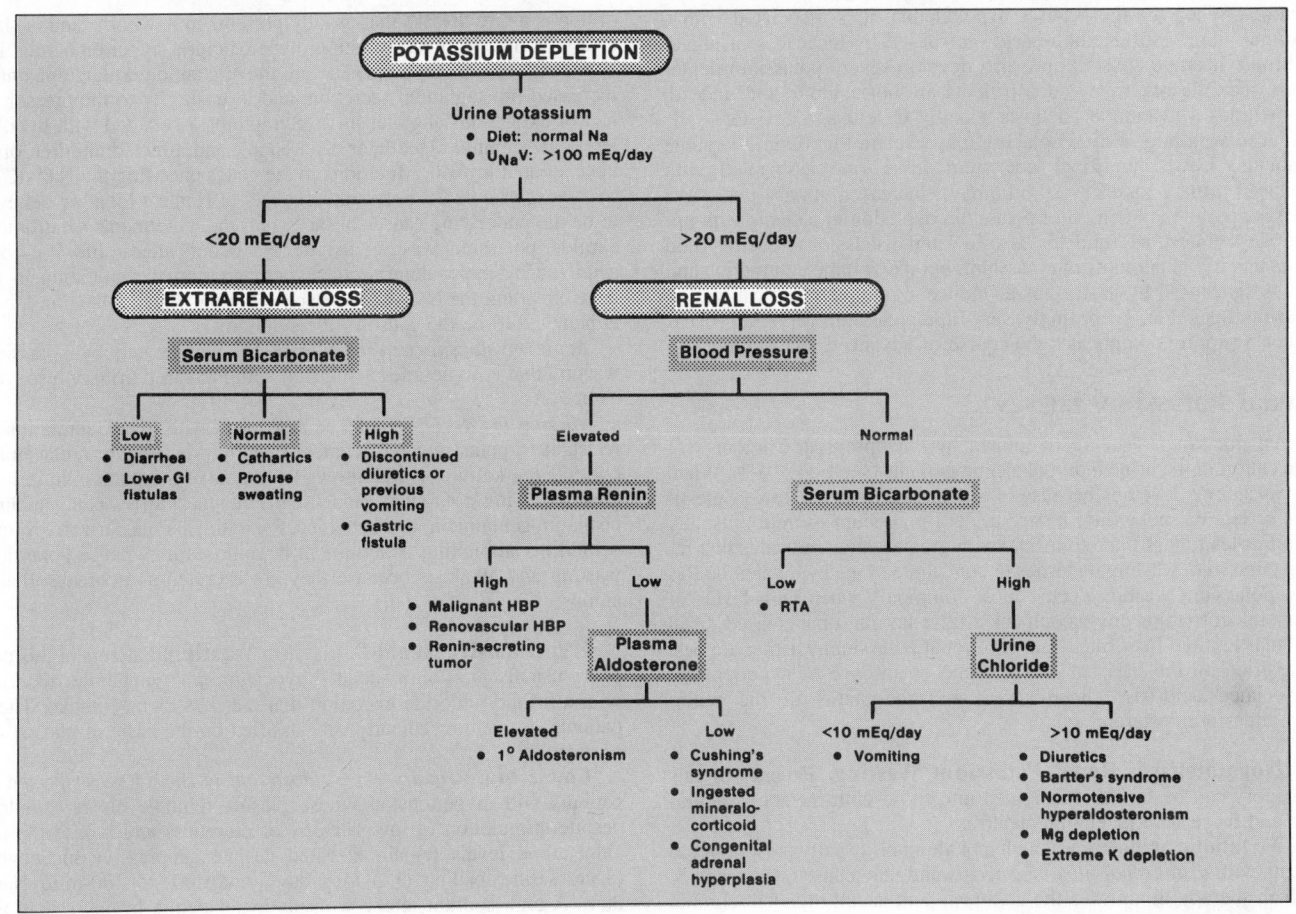

FIGURE 114-3 Diagnostic approach to hypokalemia. Because renal potassium wasting may improve during sodium restriction, diminished potassium excretion is indicative of extrarenal loss only when the diet (and therefore the urine) is rich in sodium.

Asian males. Clinical manifestations are similar to the familial disease and resolve when a euthyroid state is restored.

Alkalosis favors potassium entry into cells, but the effect is small. Only extreme degrees of respiratory alkalosis, caused by improper respirator settings, have caused substantial degrees of hypokalemia. The effect of metabolic alkalosis is greater and is usually associated with potassium depletion. The intracellular shift of potassium slightly exacerbates the hypokalemia in potassium-depleted, alkalotic patients.

Hypothermia may lower the plasma potassium to less than 3.0 mEq/L by potentiating potassium entry into cells. The effect is rapidly reversed during rewarming, and if potassium has been administered, "overshoot" hyperkalemia may result.

Barium poisoning caused by soluble barium salts (not those used in radiologic studies) is associated with a rapid and severe decrease in the plasma potassium concentration that appears to be caused by a shift of potassium into cells. Barium inhibits membrane potassium conductance channels, which traps the cation inside cells. Complicating vomiting and diarrhea also play a role.

Vitamin B$_{12}$ therapy of megaloblastic anemia rapidly increases net production of new blood cells, which incorporate extracellular potassium. Severe and potentially lethal hypokalemia may result. Thrombocytopenic patients with pernicious anemia seem especially prone to this form of hypokalemia. An analogous condition may occur during the *transfusion of frozen washed red blood cells*. Replenishment of the frozen cells' low intracellular potassium stores with the recipient's extracellular potassium causes the hypokalemia. Similarly, acute leukemias and rapidly growing lymphomas (especially Burkitt's lymphoma) may also divert extracellular stores into proliferating tumor cells.

Hypokalemia With Potassium Depletion

Once disordered internal potassium balance has been excluded (see Table 114-1), a cause of potassium depletion should be sought. Although diminished intake can occasionally be incriminated, most cases result from excessive extrarenal potassium losses or from defective renal potassium conservation; measurement of urinary potassium losses permits a distinction between these two major diagnostic possibilities (Fig. 114-3). Daily urinary potassium excretion can be estimated from the potassium and creatinine content of a "spot" urine sample. The potassium content per gram of creatinine approximates the daily excretion level.

Decreased Potassium Intake

Renal conservation of potassium is imperfect, allowing deficits to develop when dietary intake is low, particularly if protein and calorie intake continues. Patients treated with total parenteral nutrition may develop profound potassium depletion if supplements are inappropriately withheld. In some areas of the southern United States, clay ingestion *(geophagia)* is inexplicably common. White clay binds dietary potassium, preventing its absorption from the gut; because protein intake is preserved, profound hypokalemia may result. Interestingly, red clay is rich in potassium and may actually be a cause of hyperkalemia in patients with renal failure.

Extrarenal Potassium Losses

Diarrhea from any cause can result in large potassium losses (see Fig. 114-3). Hypokalemia is particularly profound in patients with diarrhea caused by villous adenomas or non–β-cell pancreatic islet cell tumors. When diarrhea causes hypokalemia, it is associated with a normal anion gap metabolic acidosis caused by fecal loss of alkali. Chronic laxative abusers may also develop severe potassium depletion. Inexplicably, many such patients are not acidotic and, indeed, sometimes a metabolic alkalosis actually develops. Coexistent self-induced vomiting or diuretic abuse may explain this finding in some patients. Lower intestinal potassium losses are associated with reduced urinary losses (<20 mEq/day). Increased urinary potassium losses are the major cause of potassium depletion in patients with upper gastrointestinal fluid losses (see later discussion). Gastric fluid contains trivial amounts of potassium, but the volume contraction and alkalosis caused by gastric losses induce a kaliuresis that causes potassium depletion. Accordingly, very little potassium depletion ensues when vomiting complicates the course of advanced renal failure.

Renal Potassium Losses

Renal potassium wasting is defined by "inappropriate" amounts of the cation in the urine in hypokalemic patients (see Fig. 114-3). When hypokalemia develops because of inadequate intake or lower intestinal or internal potassium losses, urinary potassium excretion usually diminishes to less than 20 mEq/day; a greater value indicates that renal potassium wasting underlies or contribute to the hypokalemia. Renal potassium wasting occurs most commonly when high levels of mineralocorticoids are accompanied by a normal or increased distal tubular luminal flow rate. Causes of renal potassium wasting are best classified on the basis of the presence or absence of hypertension, associated acid-base disturbances, and the status of the renin-angiotensin-aldosterone axis.

Normotensive Renal Potassium Wasting. Patients in this category can be further subdivided into those with metabolic acidosis and those with metabolic alkalosis.

Metabolic acidosis. Severe hypokalemia is usually present in patients with *distal renal tubular acidosis* and may cause quadriparesis. Alkali therapy diminishes the kaliuresis and usually renders chronic potassium replacement unnecessary as long as the acidosis is controlled. Hypokalemia is usually milder in patients with *proximal renal tubular acidosis,* and in this disorder renal potassium wasting is exacerbated by alkali therapy. The carbonic anhydrase inhibitor *acetazolamide* used in the treatment of glaucoma causes a similar proximal tubular phenomenon.

Metabolic alkalosis. *Active vomiting,* an important cause of hypokalemia and metabolic alkalosis, enhances renal excretion of potassium, sodium, and bicarbonate. Hypovolemic stimulation of NaCl reabsorption makes hypochloriduria a typical finding. With chronicity, $NaHCO_3$ reabsorption increases but the kaliuresis continues. Psychiatrically disturbed (bulimic) patients often deny self-induced vomiting. The finding of a urinary chloride concentration of less than 10 mEq/L in a persistently alkalotic patient is virtually diagnostic of gastric fluid loss, because it indicates that chloride (HCl) has been lost extrarenally.

Thiazide and loop diuretics (furosemide, bumetanide, and ethacrynic acid) are by far the most common causes of renal potassium wasting and alkalosis. Edematous conditions, although associated with high renin and aldosterone levels, do not by themselves cause potassium wasting. Increased proximal tubular reabsorption caused by the primary disorder reduces distal luminal flow, thereby limiting cation exchange. Diuretic therapy, however, by increasing distal sodium and fluid delivery, enables aldosterone to markedly increase urinary potassium losses. Surreptitious diuretic abuse must be excluded in all patients with normotensive renal potassium wasting of obscure etiology. Because diuretics may be taken intermittently, serial determinations of serum and urinary electrolytes may be helpful. While the diuretic is being taken, urinary chloride concentrations are high, but they decrease dramatically within hours after discontinuing the diuretic. Chromatography of the urine at the appropriate time will reveal the presence of the diuretic. Routine urinary screening tests will not identify bumetanide, a compound that requires a separate assay.

Hereditary transport disorders should be considered in normotensive alkalotic patients with renal potassium wasting in whom surreptitious vomiting and diuretic abuse have been excluded. Bartter's syn-

drome is a rare disease that usually presents in newborns and is characterized by severe salt wasting, hypercalciuria hyperreninemia, hyperaldosteronism, hyperplasia of the juxtaglomerular apparatus, increased prostaglandin secretion, and insensitivity to the pressor effect of exogenous angiotensin II. Symptoms associated with hypokalemia are common (see later discussion), and affected children often have stunted growth. Mutations in the genes encoding the Na^+-K^+-2 Cl^- transporter or the potassium channel in Henle's loop are believed to be the underlying causes of the syndrome. Gitelman's syndrome is a milder potassium wasting disorder that occurs later in life. It is characterized by hypocalciuria and hypomagnesemia; a mutation in the gene encoding the Na^+-Cl^- transporter in the distal collecting tubule is believed to be the cause of the syndrome.

Acute myelocytic leukemias may be complicated by potassium wasting that is sometimes associated with increased urinary lysozyme excretion.

Magnesium depletion may be associated with hypokalemia that is resistant to potassium replacement therapy. Magnesium replacement corrects the kaliuresis and allows for repair of the potassium deficit. *Drugs* causing potassium (and usually magnesium) wasting include cisplatin, gentamicin, and levodopa. Penicillin and its derivatives (carbenicillin, ampicillin, oxacillin) in large doses may cause potassium wasting and alkalosis because they are excreted as nonreabsorbable anions.

Hypertensive Renal Potassium Wasting. Patients in this category usually have an associated hypochloremic, metabolic alkalosis with a urinary chloride excretion that matches dietary intake. These patients can be conveniently subclassified on the basis of plasma renin activity.

Low renin. *Primary hyperaldosteronism* should be suspected in patients with hypertension whose plasma renin levels remain low despite stimulation (a low-salt diet or diuretics) and whose plasma aldosterone levels remain elevated despite suppressive maneuvers (acute saline loading or 5 to 7 days of a 200- to 300-mEq NaCl diet). A high sodium intake worsens hypokalemia by increasing the distal tubular luminal flow rate while hyperaldosteronemia persists. A single aldosterone-secreting adenoma (Conn's syndrome) is the most common cause of these findings, particularly in patients with clinically important hypokalemia. Patients with bilateral adrenal hyperplasia may also present with hypertension, but hypokalemia is usually milder. Elaboration of an aldosterone-stimulating factor may be the underlying cause of the hyperplasia. Urinary excretion of this factor may differentiate the surgically incurable hyperplasia from the curable adenoma. Because of the wide range of "normal" for blood pressure, occasional hypokalemic patients with Conn's syndrome may be normotensive, mimicking Bartter's syndrome and other causes of normotensive renal potassium wasting.

In familial *glucocorticoid remediable aldosteronism,* hormone synthesis and release is abnormally responsive to the diurnal secretion of ACTH, causing hyperaldosteronism. The "GRA" defect is in the 5′ regulatory region of the $P450_{11\beta}$ gene and is expressed in the zona fasciculata of the adrenal cortex. The gene product catalyzes a key step in the biosynthesis of aldosterone. Suppression of ACTH release with dexamethasone eliminates the mineralocorticoid excess.

Adrenogenital syndrome due to 11β-hydroxylase (masculinizing) or 17α-hydroxylase deficiency causes renal potassium wasting resulting from overproduction of deoxycorticosterone.

Liddle's syndrome is a rare familial disorder resembling Conn's syndrome except that plasma aldosterone levels are low. A mutation of the sodium channel results in continuously avid sodium reabsorption in the distal nephron, creating a negative electrical potential difference in the tubular lumen that promotes potassium secretion.

11 β-OH steroid dehydrogenase deficiency is another hereditary disorder that presents with low renin hypertension, hypokalemic renal potassium wasting, and low aldosterone levels. The enzyme, 11 β-OH steroid dehydrogenase, converts the glucocorticoid, cortisol (which can activate the minerals corticoid receptor), to its inactive 11-oxo form (cortisone). Deficiency of the enzyme allows physiologic levels of cortisol to flood mineralocorticoid receptors resulting in a syndrome of apparent mineralocorticoid excess. The disorder can be treated with dexamethasone, a pure glucocorticoid that suppresses cortisol production.

Sodium glycyrrhizinate found in chewing tobacco, European licorice, and certain liquors, inhibits 11 β-OH steroid dehydrogenase, thereby mimicking the hereditary enzyme deficiency. ACTH, at the extremely high concentrations seen only with ectopic production, inhibits 11 β-OH steroid dehydrogenase. This helps explain why hypokalemic renal potassium wasting uniformly complicates this form of Cushing's syndrome and not those associated with much lower or suppressed circulating ACTH levels.

High or normal renin. *Renovascular hypertension* is often complicated by mild degrees of hypokalemia, but this finding is not specific for the disorder because *malignant hypertension* and the *vasculitides* are also associated with high renin levels and may also cause hypokalemia. Rarely, *renin-secreting tumors,* including Wilms' tumor and small renal juxtaglomerular cell tumors, produce hypertension and hypokalemia. The hypertension of *Cushing's syndrome* is associated with a normal or high plasma renin level. Most cases with severe hypokalemia occur in adrenal carcinoma or ectopic ACTH secretion, most commonly caused by small-cell carcinoma of the lung (see earlier discussion).

Potassium Depletion Without Hypokalemia

The osmotic diuresis and kaliuresis associated with *diabetic ketoacidosis* or *nonketotic hyperglycemia* result in large potassium deficits. In ketoacidosis the potassium losses are particularly large because acetoacetate and β-hydroxybutyrate serve as nonreabsorbable anions, further enhancing renal potassium loss. Hypokalemia may be masked in these disorders because of abnormalities in internal potassium balance caused by insulin deficiency, hypertonicity, and catabolism. Ketoacidosis probably plays little role in masking the hypokalemia because organic acidoses do not appear to cause potassium exit from cells. Some patients may present with hyperkalemia despite potassium depletion. Because of changing internal balance, severe hypokalemia may emerge during insulin and fluid therapy.

CONSEQUENCES OF HYPOKALEMIA

The consequences of hypokalemia derive from potassium's role in regulating cellular metabolism and influencing the transmembrane electrical potential. In potassium depletion, the reduction in the cation's cellular concentration is proportionally less than the reduction in extracellular potassium levels causing the concentration ratio of intracellular to extracellular potassium to increase. Hypokalemia hyperpolarizes cell membranes, reducing membrane excitability and thereby provoking clinically important changes in the cardiac conducting system, skeletal and smooth muscle, and endocrine function.

Cardiac Effects

In hypokalemia, potassium losses are less marked in cardiac than in skeletal muscle, causing striking hyperpolarization of cardiac conduction tissue. Characteristic electrocardiographic changes result (Fig. 114-4) and include ST segment depression, decreased amplitude or inversion of the T wave, and increased height of the U wave (>1 mm). These changes usually reflect a plasma potassium concentration of less than 3.0 mEq/L and are seen in the vast majority of cases with values below 2.7 mEq/L. With more severe hypokalemia, increased amplitude of the P wave, prolongation of the PR interval, and widening of the QRS complex ensue. Severe hypokalemia may induce atrioventricular block and supraventricular and ventricular tachyarrhythmias, including ventricular fibrillation. The incidence of digitalis-induced arrhythmias is increased in hypokalemia. Indeed, hypokalemia reduces renal excretion of digoxin and increases its binding to the heart, further predisposing patients to digitalis toxicity. In the absence of digitalis, there is disagreement as to whether mild hypokalemia (plasma potassium 3 to 3.5 mEq/L) causes arrhythmias. When patients with myocardial infarction present with hypokalemia, they are more prone to ventricular arrhythmias. However, more severe infarctions may yield high levels of catecholamines, which may be the cause of both hypokalemia and arrhythmias. Based on the available data, it appears prudent to treat hypokalemia in patients with underlying ischemic heart disease. The use of potassium-sparing diuretics seems to reduce the incidence of sudden death in hypertensive patients.

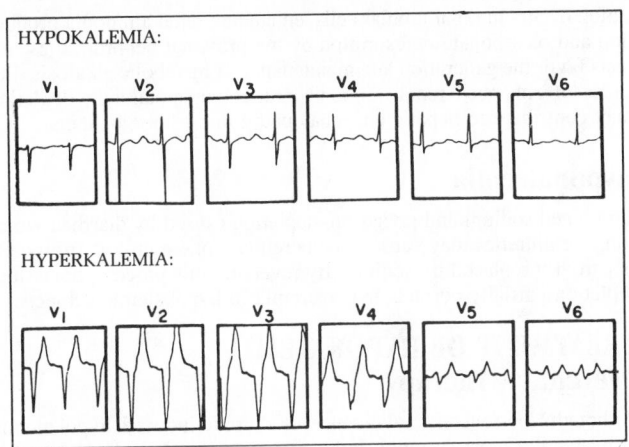

FIGURE 114-4 Electrocardiographic changes induced by hypokalemia and hyperkalemia. Hypokalemia changes include flattened T waves and the presence of U waves. Hyperkalemic changes include peaked T waves, decreased R wave amplitude, and widened QRS complexes.

From Gabow PA, Peterson LN: Disorders of potassium metabolism. In Schrier RW, editor: *Renal electrolyte disorders,* Boston, 1980, Little, Brown.

Muscle Dysfunction

Patients with mild hypokalemia commonly complain of muscle cramps and may suffer mild muscle weakness. Impaired smooth muscle function may cause intestinal ileus. Severe hypokalemia (less than 2.5 mEq/L) may cause marked weakness or frank paralysis of skeletal muscles. The proximal muscles of the lower extremities are typically affected first, whereas in more severe cases the trunk and respiratory muscles can become involved, leading to respiratory failure. Severe potassium depletion may also lead to disruption of skeletal muscle cells, particularly during exercise. The normal hyperemic response to exercise depends on the local release of potassium from muscle. In potassium-depleted muscle, the lack of potassium-induced vasodilation impairs muscle blood flow, leading to cramps, ischemic necrosis, and rhabdomyolysis.

Renal Dysfunction

Renal blood flow and glomerular filtration rate are moderately and reversibly reduced in hypokalemia. The ability to excrete a sodium load is impaired, and edema may occur in potassium-depleted subjects on a high-salt diet. Potassium depletion impairs the ability to maximally concentrate the urine and also directly stimulates thirst. Hence polyuria and polydipsia are common symptoms of hypokalemia. Chronic, severe hypokalemia causes vacuolar lesions in the epithelial cells of the proximal and distal tubule, which have been associated with chronic renal insufficiency in bulimic patients, and which may increase the sensitivity to acute tubular necrosis during exposure to nephrotoxic antibiotics. Rhabdomyolysis caused by severe hypokalemia may produce myoglobinuric acute renal failure.

Endocrine Dysfunction

Hypokalemia impairs the secretion of aldosterone, insulin, and possibly catecholamines. The impairment of insulin secretion may cause hyperglycemia even in patients without clinically apparent diabetes mellitus. Glucose intolerance is rapidly corrected by potassium replacement. Prostaglandin and renin synthesis are both increased in response to hypokalemia.

Metabolic Alkalosis

Many of the disorders that cause hypokalemia also increase acid losses from the body (e.g., vomiting, hyperaldosteronism, diuretics). In addition, hypokalemia itself affects acid-base balance. Hydrogen ions shift into potassium-depleted cells, causing intracellular acidosis and a slight degree of extracellular alkalosis. The same intracellular acidification occurs in renal tubular cells, enhancing renal ammonia production and bicarbonate reabsorption by the proximal nephron; these effects favor the generation and maintenance of metabolic alkalosis. Because of enhanced renal ammonia production, potassium depletion may contribute to hepatic encephalopathy in cirrhotic patients.

Hyponatremia

Combined sodium and potassium depletion caused by diarrhea, vomiting, or diuretics may cause hyponatremia. Potassium lost from cells is partially replaced by sodium. By reversing this process, potassium repletion partially corrects hyponatremia in hypokalemic subjects.

TREATMENT OF HYPOKALEMIA
Preventive Therapy

Although controversial, avoidance of diuretic-induced hypokalemia is by far the most common indication for potassium therapy in the United States. Routine administration of potassium or potassium-sparing diuretics should be discouraged in patients with renal disease, diabetes mellitus, or autonomic insufficiency, since the disordered external and internal potassium balances in these patients may predispose to life-threatening degrees of hyperkalemia. Only a small percentage of diuretic-treated patients develop severe hypokalemia (less than 3 mEq/L), and if the goal of potassium replacement were simply to avoid severe depletion, few patients would require therapy. A much larger percentage of diuretic-treated patients develop mild hypokalemia (3 to 3.5 mEq/L), which may indeed be arrhythmogenic. The incidence of hypokalemia can be reduced in hypertensive patients by using low doses of thiazide diuretics (the equivalent of 12.5 to 25 mg hydrochlorothiazide daily); higher doses cause greater kaliuresis with little additional antihypertensive effect. Hypokalemia can also be minimized by dietary sodium restriction (70 to 80 mEq/day), since high rates of sodium excretion promote urinary potassium losses. Encouraging intake of potassium-rich fruit is of dubious benefit. The calorie content is excessive, and since the potassium in fruit is associated not with chloride but with poorly reabsorbable anions, the cation is poorly retained. Effective therapy requires either high doses of KCl or a potassium-sparing diuretic (amiloride, triamterene, or spironolactone).

Correction of Potassium Depletion

When other variables affecting plasma potassium concentration have been avoided, metabolic balance studies show, deficits of 300 mEq/70 kg body weight (corrected for nitrogen) are required to lower the plasma potassium concentration by 1 mEq/L (Fig. 114-5). These estimates are valid only for chronic potassium depletion. When potassium is lost rapidly from the extracellular fluid (for example, by hemodialysis), loss of a mere 15 mEq can transiently lower the plasma concentration by 1 mEq/L. With time, cellular potassium partially replenishes extracellular fluid losses. The relationship between the potassium deficit and the plasma potassium concentration can be altered by factors that affect internal potassium balance. While it is difficult to quantify these effects, the presence of associated acid-base disorders, hormonal disturbances, and so forth, must be taken into account in planning therapy. Because the estimate of potassium deficits is crude, it is wise to remeasure the plasma potassium concentration frequently during the course of therapy. The administered dose should replace the patient's ongoing losses as well as correct the existing deficit. Once the deficit has been replaced, additional potassium may cause hyperkalemia, since the renal excretion and cellular uptake of excess potassium may not be efficient in chronically potassium-depleted subjects. As a consequence, potassium therapy should be slowed once normokalemia is approached, and then frequent measurements of plasma potassium levels are essential.

Route of Administration

Either oral or parenteral therapy is potentially dangerous, and treatment via either route requires careful attention. Oral potassium administration is more practical for repairing large deficits because intravenous therapy usually obligates the infusion of large amounts of

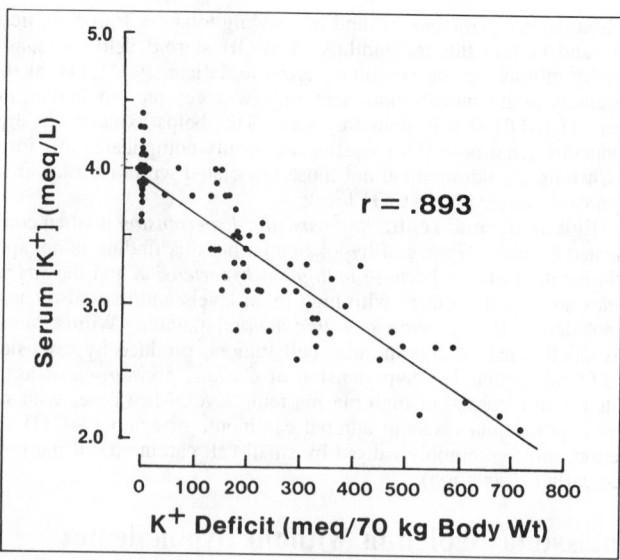

FIGURE 114-5   The effect of uncomplicated potassium depletion on serum potassium concentration, as defined by published potassium balance studies. The decrease in serum potassium concentration equals 0.27 mEq/L for every 100 mEq of potassium deficit (r = 0.893).

From Sterns RH et al: Internal potassium balance and the control of plasma potassium concentration, *Medicine* 60:339, 1981.

fluid. Attempts to limit the fluid load by increasing the concentration of potassium in intravenous solutions create two problems: (1) the infusion must be carefully monitored to avoid the inadvertent infusion of large volumes of concentrated potassium and (2) potassium concentrations greater than 60 mEq/L are painful if infused into a peripheral vein unless the rate of administration is slow (5 to 10 mEq/hr). On rare occasions when rapid intravenous infusion of concentrated potassium is required, it can be safely infused into a central vein, providing the patient is carefully monitored.

Rapid intravenous infusions of potassium are indicated only for the treatment of severe hypokalemia with such life-threatening complications as ventricular dysrhythmias or quadriparesis. When such rare emergencies occur, potassium can be infused for limited periods of time at a rate that exceeds the rate of ongoing external potassium losses by 20 to 60 mEq/hr. Infused potassium initially distributes in the extracellular fluid (20% of body weight), and with time most of the infused cation enters cells. Emergency therapy requires only that the plasma potassium concentration be raised to a safe level (usually an increase of approximately 1 mEq/L). This can be achieved by the infusion of only 15 mEq over a period of 15 minutes. Thereafter the deficit should be repaired more slowly. It is essential that the electrocardiogram be monitored for evidence of hyperkalemia and that the plasma potassium concentration be monitored at frequent intervals whenever it is administered aggressively.

HYPERKALEMIA

Hyperkalemic patients may be classified by the presence or absence of a potassium surfeit. It is important to note that patients with *chronic* hyperkalemia invariably suffer from a defect in renal potassium excretion. Extracellular translocation of potassium causes hyperkalemia only when it occurs suddenly or when there is an accompanying renal defect.

Spurious Hyperkalemia

Local Potassium Release. Local release of potassium from ischemic exercising muscle can increase the serum potassium concentration by 1 mEq/L or more when the patient's fist is repeatedly clenched with a tourniquet in place during blood drawing. Use of a tourniquet without fist clenching does not cause spurious hyperkalemia.

In Vitro Hemolysis. Hemolysis extensive enough to visibly discolor the plasma can give the spurious impression of severe hyperkalemia. When whole blood is used for emergency potassium determinations by electrode, hemolysis will not be apparent; therefore the sample must be centrifuged to allow examination of the plasma.

Pseudohyperkalemia. Marked thrombocytosis (usually $>1 \times 10^6/mm^3$) or leukocytosis (usually $>250 \times 10^3/mm^3$) may falsely increase the potassium level because of in vitro release of cellular potassium during blood clotting. A simultaneously drawn plasma potassium concentration or whole blood potassium concentration will be normal. In chronic lymphocytic leukemia, loss of potassium from "fragile" leukemic cells may raise both the plasma and serum potassium concentrations if the blood sample is allowed to stand before separation.

True Hyperkalemia Without a Potassium Surfeit

Increased Potassium Loss From Cells. Hyperkalemia may occur if potassium egress is rapid enough to overwhelm normal renal excretory function or if there is an associated defect in renal potassium excretion. *Tissue catabolism* after trauma, burns, ischemic muscle necrosis, or rapid lysis (particularly during chemotherapy of Burkitt's lymphoma) may rapidly release large amounts of potassium into the circulation. Hyperkalemia is more likely to be severe if acute renal failure develops.

Exercise causes release of potassium from skeletal muscle, and the plasma potassium concentration may increase transiently by more than 2 mEq/L after exhausting exercise. Nonselective β-adrenergic blocking agents (e.g., propranolol) cause leakage of potassium out of cells and may contribute to hyperkalemia in patients with compromised potassium homeostasis. This problem can be avoided by the substitution of $β_1$-antagonists (e.g., metoprolol) in such patients. Seizures, rhabdomyolysis, and renal failure caused by cocaine intoxication often result in hyperkalemia.

Diabetic hyperglycemia may cause hyperkalemia in patients with impaired renal function. In nondiabetic subjects, glucose infusion lowers the plasma potassium concentration by stimulating insulin release. In the patient with diabetes, insulin fails to respond normally to administered glucose and the hypertonicity dehydrates cells, raising intracellular potassium concentration, thereby promoting diffusion of the cation out of the cell. Infusion of hypertonic mannitol to subjects with renal failure may cause a similar phenomenon. In patients with defects in renal potassium excretion (such as hypoaldosteronism), serious hyperkalemia may result.

Uremic metabolic acidosis and *hyperkalemic renal tubular acidosis* also induce potassium loss from cells, exacerbating the hyperkalemia caused by potassium retention in these conditions. *Acute respiratory acidosis* causes potassium loss from cells, which becomes maximal in about 4 hours, and may elevate the plasma potassium concentration, particularly in patients with renal failure. *Arginine hydrochloride* can cause severe hyperkalemia when used to treat metabolic alkalosis in patients with renal failure. The hyperkalemia does not appear to be related to the correction of the acid-base disturbance but rather to displacement of cellular potassium by this cationic amino acid. Patients with advanced liver disease are especially sensitive to this effect.

Digitalis poisoning causes severe hyperkalemia, a finding to be expected from the known inhibitory effect of cardiac glycosides on $(Na^+ + K^+)$-ATPase. *Succinylcholine,* a depolarizing muscle relaxant used in anesthesia, causes potassium loss from cells by increasing the ionic permeability of muscle. Patients with burns, muscle trauma, spinal injury, tetanus, and certain neuromuscular diseases are most sensitive to this effect and may develop severe hyperkalemia when given this agent.

Hyperkalemic periodic paralysis is a rare familial disorder characterized by recurrent attacks of hyperkalemia and muscle weakness or paralysis. Attacks are precipitated by the ingestion of small amounts of potassium or by a variety of other apparently unrelated stimuli (relaxation after exercise, excitement, cold, fasting, infections, and general anesthesia). The disease has been linked to an inherited defect in the sodium channel.

BOX 114-1
Causes of sustained hyperkalemia

Combined aldosterone and glucocorticoid deficiency
  Addison's disease
  Other disorders destroying the adrenal cortex
  21 Hydroxylase deficiency
Selective aldosterone deficiency
  Addison's disease
  Hyporeninemic hypoaldosteronism
  Angiotensin-converting enzyme inhibitor therapy
  Prostaglandin synthetase inhibitors
  Corticosterone methyl oxidase deficiency
  Heparin therapy
Decreased response to aldosterone
  Renal failure
    Acute renal failure
    Advanced chronic renal failure
    Severe prerenal azotemia
  Renal tubular disorders
    Obstructive uropathy
    Sickle cell disease
    Renal transplantation
    Amyloidosis
    Systemic lupus erythematosus
    Tubulointerstitial nephropathies
  Potassium-sparing diuretics
  Pseudohypoaldosteronism
  Gordon's syndrome

True Hyperkalemia With a Potassium Surfeit

Body cells can function as a "sink" or as a source of potassium during periods of loading or depletion, respectively. Because cells are less able to take up potassium than to contribute it, hypokalemia is more effectively buffered than is hyperkalemia (Box 114-1). Consequently a much smaller change in external potassium balance is required to raise the plasma potassium concentration above normal levels than to lower it below normal levels. It has been estimated that in a 70-kg man, only 100 mEq of excess potassium increases plasma potassium concentration from 4 to 5 mEq/L and even less may be required to increase the plasma potassium concentration further. Fortunately, normal renal potassium clearance is profound. Even a slight increase in plasma potassium concentration causes a brisk kaliuresis. Rarely, this large renal excretory capacity can be briefly overwhelmed by a large rapid potassium intake. Chronic hyperkalemia is almost always associated with reduced renal clearance of potassium. Although a steady state may be achieved, allowing daily potassium intake to match urinary removal, potassium excretion remains far less than appropriate for the degree of hyperkalemia. These disorders can be divided into those characterized by aldosterone deficiency and those in which renal resistance to the hormone causes hyperkalemia.

Combined Aldosterone and Glucocorticoid Deficiency. Patients with combined mineralocorticoid and glucocorticoid deficiency present with the features of *Addison's disease.* Aldosterone deficiency causes renal sodium wasting and potassium retention, whereas glucocorticoid deficiency causes constitutional symptoms and water retention. These defects lead to hypotension, hyponatremia, and hyperkalemia. Plasma renin levels are elevated and plasma cortisol levels are low and unresponsive to ACTH stimulation. Addison's disease may result from destruction of the adrenals (by autoimmune disease, infection, or hemorrhage) or from bilateral adrenalectomy. Rarely, adrenal hormonal insufficiency results from congenital deficiency of 21-hydroxylase (congenital adrenal hyperplasia).

Selective Aldosterone Deficiency
Low renin. Hyporeninemic hypoaldosteronism is the most common cause of isolated aldosterone deficiency. Most patients have mild to moderate renal insufficiency secondary to tubular interstitial dis-

eases (in 50%) or diabetic nephropathy. In contrast to addisonian patients, these patients are usually fluid overloaded; hyponatremia is unusual because cortisol levels are normal. Low aldosterone levels are associated with low levels of renin, which fail to increase with stimulatory maneuvers. The cause of renin deficiency may be multifactorial: suppression of renin secretion by extracellular volume expansion, sclerosis of the renin-secreting cells of the juxtaglomerular apparatus, secretion of inactive prorenin, autonomic insufficiency, and decreased prostaglandin synthesis have all been proposed as factors in its pathogenesis. Moreover, renin secretion decreases with age, possibly accounting for the increased prevalence of the disorder in elderly patients. Low renin levels reduce angiotensin II formation and may explain the diminished responsiveness of the adrenal gland to hyperkalemia (normally a potent stimulus to aldosterone secretion). Alternatively, a defect in aldosterone biosynthesis may coexist with renin deficiency in some patients.

The hyperkalemia of hyporeninemic hypoaldosteronism is exacerbated by volume depletion, which, by reducing distal tubular luminal flow rate, worsens the potassium secretory defect. The majority of cases have an associated normal anion gap metabolic acidosis, termed *type IV renal tubular acidosis* (RTA) (Chapter 115). The acidosis and hyperkalemia respond to treatment with fludrocortisone, a potent synthetic mineralocorticoid. Assessment of the response to fludrocortisone may be helpful diagnostically. The dose required is usually several times that needed in Addison's disease, implying that patients with hyporeninemic hypoaldosteronism have some degree of renal resistance. Alternatively, liberal salt intake, combined with such diuretics as furosemide or metolazone, increases potassium excretion by increasing the luminal flow rate in the distal nephron and prevents the sodium retention and hypertension that commonly complicate fludrocortisone therapy. *Prostaglandin synthetase inhibitors* (indomethacin, ibuprofen, naproxen) inhibit renin release and may cause reversible hyperkalemia and type IV RTA, particularly in patients with renal insufficiency, in whom renin secretion may be marginal.

Converting enzyme inhibitors. The angiotensin-converting enzyme inhibitors captopril, enalapril, and lisinopril inhibit the conversion of angiotensin I to angiotensin II, thereby reducing aldosterone levels. Although these drugs have caused a few cases of reversible frank hyperkalemia, in most patients only a slight increase in serum potassium (0.3 mEq/L) develops, but in patients with renal disease severe hyperkalemia may result.

Abnormal aldosterone biosynthesis. Rare congenital deficiencies of the enzymes required for the final steps in aldosterone biosynthesis (corticosterone methyl oxidase) result in a syndrome of isolated mineralocorticoid deficiency characterized by salt wasting, hyperkalemia, and metabolic acidosis in infancy. Some cases of acquired isolated aldosterone deficiency in adult diabetics have also been reported to result from defects in aldosterone biosynthesis. *Heparin* therapy inhibits aldosterone secretion within a few days at doses as low as 5000 units twice daily; rare cases of marked hyperkalemia have been reported, primarily in the presence of additional factors that perturb potassium balance.

Decreased responsiveness to aldosterone

Renal failure. Patients with chronic renal failure are usually able to maintain potassium balance and normokalemia while on a normal diet until very late in their course. This adaptation appears to require increased aldosterone levels, implying that most patients with renal disease have some degree of "resistance" to mineralocorticoids. Relative hypoaldosteronism (i.e., when hyperkalemia fails to clearly increase plasma or urinary aldosterone levels) may respond to high doses of exogenous mineralocorticoids. Hyperkalemia is the rule in oliguric acute or chronic renal failure and may also be seen in oliguric patients with severe prerenal azotemia. In the latter circumstance, potassium excretion does not appreciably increase when exogenous mineralocorticoids are given.

Renal tubular disorders. A variety of disorders including lupus nephritis, allergic tubulointerstitial nephritis, and amyloidosis have been reported to cause mineralocorticoid-resistant potassium excretory defects with only mild azotemia. The plasma aldosterone level in these patients is usually high. Obstructive uropathy and sickle cell nephropathy may cause hyperkalemia and a normal anion gap metabolic acidosis. Although some patients with the aforementioned disorders have hyporeninemic hypoaldosteronism, others appear to have a mineralocorticoid resistant tubular defect analogous to that seen in

patients treated with amiloride and have normal or elevated aldosterone levels. Mineralocorticoid-resistant hyperkalemia has been reported in transplanted kidneys, and hyperkalemia may be particularly prevalent when cyclosporine is used for immunosuppression.

Potassium-sparing diuretics and trimethoprim. Spironolactone is a competitive inhibitor of aldosterone that impairs renal potassium excretion. Triamterene and amiloride also reduce potassium excretion but independently of aldosterone. Amiloride acts by blocking sodium channels in the distal luminal membrane; the transepithelial electrical potential is reduced, thereby impairing both potassium and hydrogen ion secretion. These agents are commonly combined with the thiazides or loop diuretics to avoid diuretic-induced hypokalemia. Administration of potassium supplements to patients receiving potassium-sparing diuretics is contraindicated. *Trimethoprim* in standard doses can cause severe hyperkalemia, especially in patients with renal insufficiency. The antibiotic acts as a potassium-sparing diuretic, reducing potassium secretion by blocking sodium channels in the renal cortical collecting duct.

Miscellaneous disorders. A number of rare disorders affecting renal potassium excretion have been reported. A syndrome known as *pseudohypoaldosteronism,* characterized by salt wasting, hyperkalemia, acidosis, and very high levels of renin and aldosterone, occurs in infants and improves with age. Another group of nonazotemic patients have been described in which hyperkalemia and acidosis are associated with hypertension and reduced renin and aldosterone levels. Renal potassium excretion in these patients does not respond to large doses of mineralocorticoids but does respond to thiazide diuretics (Gordon's syndrome). It has been proposed that the primary disturbance in these patients is an abnormally increased reabsorption of chloride in the distal nephron, which reduces the lumen's negative potential (thus decreasing potassium and hydrogen ion secretion) while augmenting distal sodium reabsorption, causing extracellular volume expansion, hypertension, and reduced levels of renin and aldosterone.

CONSEQUENCES OF HYPERKALEMIA

The most important effects of hyperkalemia derive from its action on cell membrane potentials. Because the intracellular potassium concentration increases minimally in hyperkalemia, the intracellular/extracellular potassium concentration ratio decreases, causing depolarization of the cell membrane; clinically important dysfunction of the heart and skeletal muscle results.

Cardiac Effects

A characteristic progression of electrocardiographic changes (see Fig. 114-4) is seen with progressively more severe hyperkalemia. The earliest manifestation of hyperkalemia is a peaking and narrowing of the T wave, which usually becomes prominent once the plasma potassium concentration exceeds 6 mEq/L. With more severe hyperkalemia, the QRS complex is prolonged, followed by a decreased amplitude, prolongation, and ultimately, disappearance of the P wave. With preterminal hyperkalemia, the markedly widened QRS complex merges with the T wave, giving the electrocardiogram a "sine wave" appearance. Soon thereafter, ventricular flutter, fibrillation, or standstill ensues.

Neuromuscular Dysfunction

With severe hyperkalemia (usually when the plasma potassium concentration exceeds 8 mEq/L), muscle weakness develops, beginning in the lower extremities and usually sparing the respiratory muscles. Skeletal muscle weakness is sometimes accompanied by symptoms of distal paresthesias; both symptoms (which may mimic hysteria and hyperventilation syndrome) are important clues to the presence of life-threatening hyperkalemia.

Metabolic Acidosis

Hyperkalemia is commonly associated with a normal anion gap metabolic acidosis. The uptake of excess potassium by cells displaces cellular hydrogen ions and causes a slight decrease in the plasma bicarbonate concentration. In addition, hyperkalemia impairs renal ammo-

Table 114-2   Emergency therapy for hyperkalemia

THERAPEUTIC AGENT AND MECHANISMS OF ACTION	DOSE AND ADMINISTRATION	ONSET	DURATION
Antagonize cardiac effects			
Calcium gluconate 10%	10-30 ml IV	1 minute	30-60 minutes
Redistribution			
Glucose and insulin	50 g glucose IV hourly	5-10 minutes	2 hours
	5 units regular insulin IV q15min		
Sodium bicarbonate	50-100 mEq IV	2 hours	3-6 hours
Albuterol	10-20 mg by inhaler	30 minutes	2 hours
Removal			
Sodium polystyrene sulfonate (Kayexalate)	15-60 g with sorbitol orally or 50-100 with retention enema (hold for 30-60 min)	1-2 hours	
Hemodialysis	Much more effective than peritoneal dialysis	Immediate	
Diuretics ("loop active")		At onset of diuresis	
Furosemide	40-240 mg IV over 30 min		
Ethacrynic acid	50-100 mg IV over 30 min		
Bumetanide	1-8 mg IV over 30 min		

nia production, thereby reducing net acid excretion. Aldosterone deficiency also contributes to metabolic acidosis by impairing renal hydrogen ion secretion.

Hypertension

Partly by causing sodium retention, potassium depletion increases blood pressure in normotensive and hypertensive subjects. An increased dietary potassium intake may reduce the need for antihypertensive medications.

TREATMENT OF HYPERKALEMIA

A 12-lead electrocardiogram should be obtained in all hyperkalemic patients to assess the urgency of therapy. Severe hyperkalemia unaccompanied by electrocardiographic changes should suggest one of the causes of spurious hyperkalemia. Peaked T waves are usually seen when the plasma potassium concentration exceeds 6.5 mEq/L. This finding demands a prompt effort either to remove potassium from the body or to reverse factors responsible for potassium loss from cells (insulin deficiency or acidosis) (Table 114-2). Prolongation of the QRS interval and more advanced electrocardiographic changes usually appear once the plasma potassium concentration exceeds 7 to 8 mEq/L. These findings demand emergency administration of calcium (see later discussion) as well as measures to lower the plasma potassium level.

Calcium

The administration of 10 ml of 10% calcium gluconate reverses the electrocardiographic findings of hyperkalemia rapidly (within seconds) and averts ventricular fibrillation or standstill. Calcium administration can also be helpful in determining whether the electrocardiographic abnormalities are caused by hyperkalemia. Calcium does not affect the plasma potassium concentration. An increased serum calcium concentration raises the threshold potential of neuromuscular tissue. By raising the threshold potential, calcium therapy reestablishes the difference between the resting and threshold potentials and restores cell excitability (see Fig. 114-1).

Insulin

Because the hypokalemic effect of insulin is dose-related, insulin should be administered as an intravenous bolus to achieve high plasma levels. Repeated injections of 5 units every 15 minutes accompanied by the infusion of 50 g of glucose per hour can achieve a maximal effect, usually without hypoglycemia.

Sodium Bicarbonate

Hyperkalemia is usually associated with a decreased plasma bicarbonate concentration. The administration of sodium bicarbonate promotes urinary potassium excretion and is also weakly effective in driving potassium into cells. Doses in excess of the usual 50 to 100 mEq may be used in severely acidotic patients. Isotonic solutions are preferred and can be prepared by adding three ampules (50 mEq/ampule) to a liter of 5% dextrose in water. In anuric subjects the full hypokalemic effect of bicarbonate may not be seen for 2 to 3 hours or more. Thus bicarbonate infusion alone is inadequate in hyperkalemic emergencies.

Beta-2 Adrenergic Agonists

Inhaled or parenteral β_2-agonists have been used successfully to treat attacks of familial hyperkalemic periodic paralysis. There is also a limited experience in hyperkalemic patients with renal failure. A substantial number of uremic patients do not respond, however, and given the potential risk for cardiac toxicity and the effectiveness of glucose and insulin, these agents may not be appropriate for first-line therapy.

Measures to Achieve Negative Potassium Balance

Because the uptake of excess potassium by tissues is relatively limited, small potassium surfeits can cause marked hyperkalemia. It follows that the treatment of hyperkalemia does not usually require removal of large amounts of potassium.

Reduced Intake. Potassium intake should be reduced, and "hidden" sources of potassium such as salt substitutes (10 to 13 mEq/g), potassium penicillin (1.7 mEq/million units), and stored blood should be sought.

Increased Renal Excretion. Potassium-sparing diuretics and (if the patient's cardiac condition permits) angiotensin-converting enzyme inhibitors should be discontinued. Negative potassium balance can be achieved by the repeated administration of a loop diuretic (e.g., furosemide), replacing urine losses with NaCl or $NaHCO_3$.

Kayexalate (Sodium Polystyrene Sulfonate). This cation exchange resin binds potassium secreted in the distal rectum. When given orally, it should be combined with sorbitol, an osmotic cathartic, to speed delivery to its site of action. As an alternative, it can be given by retention enema without sorbitol. Each gram of the resin binds approximately 1 mEq of potassium while yielding approximately 2 mEq of sodium. The potential side effect of sodium overload can be offset by sorbitol-induced diarrhea. In high doses, however, the cathartic can cause negative water balance and hypernatremia.

Dialysis. Hyperkalemia can be corrected within minutes by hemodialysis. Peritoneal dialysis removes potassium more slowly than Kayexalate.

BIBLIOGRAPHY

Agarwal R et al: Pathophysiology of potassium absorption and secretion by the human intestine, *Gastroenterol* 107:548, 1994.

Alappan R et al: Hyperkalemia in hospitalized patients treated with trimethoprim-sulfamethoxazole, *Ann Intern Med* 124:316, 1996.

Field MJ et al: Regulation of renal potassium metabolism. In Narins RG, editor: *Clinical disorders of fluid and electrolyte metabolism*, ed 5, New York, McGraw-Hill.

Fontaine B et al: Periodic paralysis and voltage-gated ion channels, *Kidney Int* 49:9, 1996.

Kamel KS et al: Disorders of potassium balance. In Brenner BM, editor: *The kidney*, Philadelphia, 1996, WB Saunders.

Kupin W, Narins RG: The hyperkalemia of renal failure: pathophysiology, diagnosis, and therapy, *Contrib Nephrol* 102:1, 1993.

Oster JR et al: Heparin-induced aldosterone suppression and hyperkalemia, *Am J Med* 98:575, 1995.

Simon DB, Lifon RP: The molecular basis of inherited hypokalemic alkalosis: Bartter's and Gitelman's syndromes, *Am J Physiol* 271:F961, 1996.

Steigerwalt SP: Unraveling the causes of hypertension and hypokalemia, *Hospital Pract* 30:67, 1995.

Walker BR et al: Mineralocorticoid excess and inhibition of 11β-hydroxysteroid dehydrogenase in patients with ectopic ACTH syndrome, *Clin Endocrinol* 37:483, 1992.

CHAPTER

115   Disorders of Acid-Base Balance

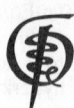

Susan R. DiGiovanni and George M. Feldman

Acid-base balance is assessed by measuring the hydrogen ion (H^+) concentration in blood or the pH of blood. Blood pH, which is equal to $-\log[H^+]$, is normally maintained within a narrow range from 7.35 to 7.45. Changes in blood pH can result from the addition or removal of H^+ ions or can result from the addition or removal of hydroxyl ions (OH^-). Disturbances in acid-base balance have numerous significant physiologic consequences. An acute decrease in blood pH (increase in H^+ concentration) or acidemia depresses myocardial function, decreases pulmonary blood flow, decreases the affinity of hemoglobin for oxygen, and can cause arrhythmias, central nervous system (CNS) depression, and hyperkalemia. In addition, chronic acidemia alters bone metabolism (resulting in osteopenia) and causes muscle wasting due to protein catabolism to sustain ammonia excretion (see later discussion). An increase in blood pH (decrease in H^+ concentration) or alkalemia can cause arrhythmias, decreases cerebral blood flow, decreases tissue delivery of oxygen by increasing the affinity of hemoglobin for oxygen, increases binding of calcium to proteins, and decreases the solubility of calcium salts, which may precipitate tetany or seizures. The term *acidosis* refers to the process that causes the body to accumulate H^+ ions or lose OH^- ions; the term *alkalosis* refers to the process that causes the body to lose H^+ ions or accumulate OH^- ions. This chapter reviews the physiologic processes, both respiratory and renal, that regulate blood pH. Then it discusses the primary disorders of acid-base balance and the compensatory processes that occur, finally considering the treatment of acid-base disturbances.

PHYSIOLOGY OF ACID-BASE HOMEOSTASIS
Production of Acids and Bases (Chapter 101)

Base, which is primarily present in the form of HCO_3^-, is generated metabolically by oxidation of dietary substances like citrate and acetate. If produced in excess, HCO_3^- is excreted by the kidneys. H^+ is also generated metabolically from dietary sources. Carbonic acid (H_2CO_3 or $CO_2 + H_2O$) is formed from the complete oxidation of carbon-containing compounds, whereas acids such as lactic acid, β-hydroxybutyric acid, and acetoacetic acid are produced from the incomplete oxidation of carbon-containing substances. Sulfuric acid (H_2SO_4) results from the oxidation of sulfur-containing amino acids such as methionine and cysteine. Because CO_2 is a gas, it is volatile and is excreted by the respiratory system. However, other acids such as sulfuric and lactic are nonvolatile or fixed acids that are excreted by the kidneys. The metabolic production of CO_2 is approximately 220 mmole/kg body weight per day. When a normal diet is eaten, the production of fixed acids predominates over base, yielding net H^+ production of approximately 1 mmole H^+/kg body weight per day.

Buffers

Buffers minimize pH changes that result from the addition or removal of H^+. There are several buffers, which are both intracellular and extracellular, that modify blood pH, and they include inorganic phosphates, plasma and intracellular proteins, and hemoglobin. The most important buffer, however, is the HCO_3^-/CO_2 buffer system. This is represented by the following equilibrium reaction:

(EQ. 1)

$$H_2O + CO_2 \leftrightarrow H_2CO_3 \leftrightarrow H^+ + HCO_3^-$$

The Henderson-Hasselbalch equation, derived from the law of mass action, demonstrates that it is the ratio of the HCO_3^- concentration to the CO_2 concentration, rather than their absolute values, which determines the H^+ concentration:

(EQ. 2)

$$pH = pK + \log\frac{[HCO_3^-]}{[CO_2]}$$

The equilibrium constant or pK for the HCO_3^-/CO_2 buffer system is 6.1. The concentration of CO_2 is determined by multiplying the partial pressure of CO_2 (P_{CO_2}) by the solubility coefficient (0.03). Using the normal values for $[HCO_3^-]$ (24 mEq/L) and P_{CO_2} (40 mm Hg), the ratio is normally 24/1.2 or 20, which, when substituted in the Henderson-Hasselbalch equation, yields a pH of 7.40.

Besides its abundance, what makes the HCO_3^-/CO_2 buffer pair such a powerful and biologically useful buffer system is that two separate organs independently control excretion of its components. HCO_3^- is regulated by the kidneys, whereas CO_2 is altered by the lungs. This allows one organ to regulate excretion in response to a disturbance by the other, thus allowing one organ system to compensate for the other and minimize the change in pH. Although other organ systems such as the gastrointestinal tract also handle large quantities of H^+ and HCO_3^-, only the respiratory and renal systems adjust excretion and thereby regulate systemic pH.

Regulation of P_{CO_2}

The respiratory rate and the tidal volume are the main determinants of P_{CO_2}. Although changes in P_{CO_2} are frequently associated with changes in respiratory rate, both rate and tidal volume are important for regulation of P_{CO_2}. Changes in blood pH are determined by sensors in the brain and periphery, and the respiratory rate and/or tidal volume is then increased or decreased appropriately. Primary disorders of the respiratory system are discussed in Chapters 51-67.

Compensation for metabolic disorders of acid-base homeostasis begins immediately but may take several hours to complete. Response to a metabolic acidosis (addition or decreased excretion of H^+) typically produces a pattern of hyperventilation whereby tidal volume increases and, to a lesser extent, so does the respiratory rate. This is called *Kussmaul's respiration*. The expected respiratory compensation to metabolic acidosis depends on the degree of acidosis and can be calculated by Winters's formula:

(EQ. 3)

$$\text{Expected } P_{CO_2} = 1.5 \times [HCO_3^-]_{current} + 8$$

A P_{CO_2} lower than expected indicates a concurrent respiratory alkalosis. Similarly the respiratory response to metabolic alkalosis (excess intake HCO_3^- or increased excretion H^+) can be calculated and depends on the degree of HCO_3^- excess:

(EQ. 4)

$$\text{Expected } P_{CO_2} = 0.9 \times [HCO_3^-]_{current} + 9$$

It should be noted, however, that compensation for a metabolic alkalosis is limited by the hypoxemia that develops with hypoventilation. Therefore the P_{CO_2} is often lower than expected. If, however, after sufficient time to allow full compensation has elapsed, the P_{CO_2} is higher than expected, a mixed disorder—respiratory acidosis and metabolic alkalosis—exists.

Renal Regulation of Acid-Base Homeostasis

Given a normal serum bicarbonate and glomerular filtration rate (24 mEq/L and 125 ml/min), about 4500 mEq of bicarbonate is filtered each day. This entire amount must be reabsorbed by the kidney tubules in order to maintain acid-base balance (Chapter 101). In addition, the 50 to 100 mEq of net H^+ produced each day must be excreted. Both processes, reclamation of filtered HCO_3^- and net excretion of H^+ (or regeneration of HCO_3^-), are accomplished by the secretion of H^+.

Renal Mechanisms to Reclaim Filtered HCO_3^-. Cells of the proximal tubule transport H^+ into the lumen via a Na^+/H^+ exchanger and possibly through an H^+-ATPase. In the lumen, the H^+ is titrated by HCO_3^-, forming H_2CO_3, which is then dehydrated to CO_2 and H_2O (Fig. 115-1). The rate of this reaction would be too slow in the absence of an enzyme, carbonic anhydrase, present in the brush border of the proximal tubule. The CO_2 thus formed diffuses across the apical cell membrane into the cell, where the opposite reaction occurs, forming more H^+ to be secreted and HCO_3^-, which exits the basolateral membrane via a Na^+/HCO_3^- transporter.

The kidney adapts to volume depletion, metabolic acidosis, respiratory acidosis, and hypokalemia by increasing the reabsorption of HCO_3^- in the proximal tubule. Angiotensin II increases the activity of both the Na^+/H^+ exchanger and the Na^+/HCO_3^- cotransporter. In volume depletion, this appears to be the mechanism of the increased reabsorption of HCO_3^- so characteristic of hypovolemia. Acetazolamide, an inhibitor of carbonic anhydrase, slows the dehydration of H_2CO_3, resulting in decreased reabsorption of HCO_3^-. Parathyroid hormone also decreases proximal tubule reabsorption of HCO_3^-.

Excretion of net H^+. The distal portion of the nephron can create a pH gradient from blood to lumen, with urinary pH going as low as 4.5. This is accomplished by H^+-ATPases present in the apical membrane of α-intercalated cells of the collecting duct (Fig. 115-2). The H^+ to be secreted is supplied by carbonic anhydrase forming H_2CO_3 from CO_2 and H_2O. The H_2CO_3 dissociates into H^+, which is secreted through the apical membrane, and HCO_3^-, which is exchanged for Cl^- across the basolateral membrane. Thus new HCO_3^- is formed to replace HCO_3^- that has been consumed by titrating acids in the blood.

Hydrogen ion secretion is stimulated by increasing Na^+ reabsorption, which increases luminal electronegative charge. Increasing delivery of Na^+ to the collecting tubule, such as is seen after administration of loop diuretics (e.g., furosemide), therefore is associated with increased H^+ secretion and HCO_3^- generation. Aldosterone stimulates H^+ secretion by stimulating the H^+-ATPase and by stimulating sodium reabsorption.

It is clear, however, that the amount of H^+ excreted in 1 to 2 L of urine daily, even at a pH of 4.5, is insufficient to accommodate the 50 to 100 mEq required to be excreted daily to maintain blood pH. Therefore the secreted H^+ must be buffered. There are two different types of buffers present in the urine, titratable acidity and ammonia (NH_3). The titratable buffers are predominantly phosphates. Because phosphate excretion depends on intake, excretion will vary little from day to day. Ammonia, on the other hand, is produced and excreted by the proximal tubule, and its production is regulated. Ammonia is formed by the deamination of glutamine. It is readily transported across membranes by nonionic diffusion. In the collecting tubule, NH_3 is titrated by secreted H^+ to form NH_4^+, which is nondiffusible and thus "trapped" in the tubule lumen. Ammoniagenesis is stimulated by metabolic acidosis, hypokalemia, and glucocorticoids. Metabolic alkalosis, hyperkalemia, and glucocorticoid deficiency have the opposite effect.

Renal Compensation for Primary Respiratory Disorders. The compensatory response for respiratory disorders occurs much more slowly than respiratory compensation for metabolic disorders. The renal response to a respiratory alkalosis (decreased Pco_2) is to decrease the serum HCO_3^- level over a period of 12 to 24 hours. The HCO_3^- decreases 2 to 4 mEq/L for each 10 mm Hg decrease in the Pco_2. The response to respiratory acidosis (retention of CO_2) may take 3 to 5 days to complete. The serum HCO_3^- can be expected to

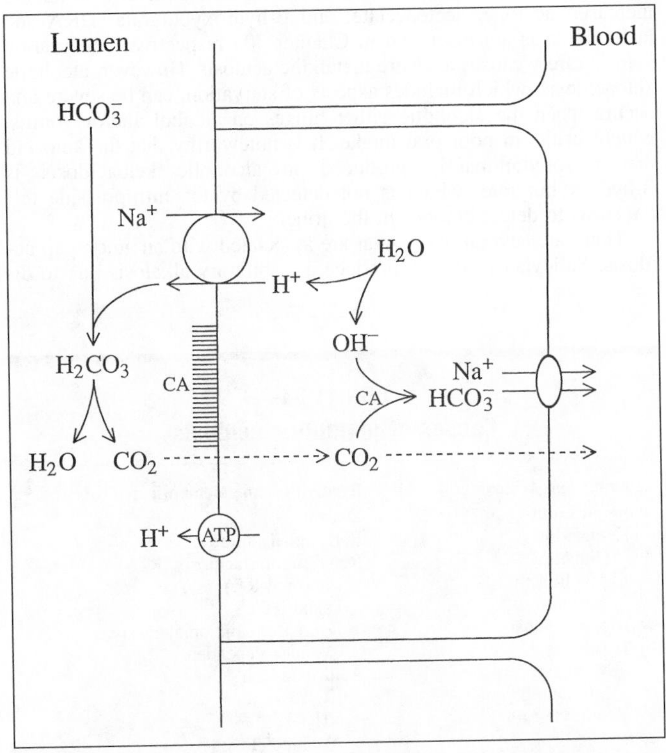

FIGURE 115-1 Bicarbonate reabsorption in the proximal tubule. Bicarbonate is reabsorbed by H^+ secretion via Na^+/H^+ exchange predominantly. An H^+-ATPase pump accounts for one third of the absorption. Carbonic anhydrase *(CA)* is located on the luminal brush border and intracellularly. A Na^+-coupled cotransporter mediates bicarbonate exit from the cell into blood.

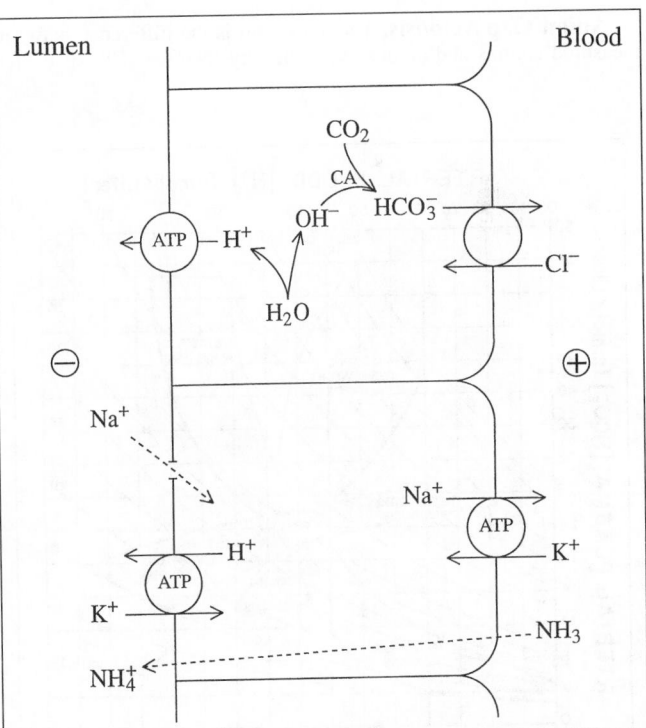

FIGURE 115-2 Acid secretion in the collecting tubule. Alpha-Intercalated cells *(top cell)* secrete H^+ pumped via an H^+-ATPase pump, and HCO_3^- exits the cell via Cl^-/HCO_3^- exchange. Principal cells *(bottom cell)*, which reabsorb Na^+, generate a lumen negative voltage, aiding H^+ secretion. In addition, H^+ secretion also occurs by a gastriclike H^+/K^+-ATPase pump. NH_3 diffuses into the lumen, where it is titrated to NH_4^+.

increase 1 to 3 mEq/L for every 10 mm Hg rise in Pco_2; this is accomplished by increasing H^+ secretion primarily by the collecting tubules. It should be noted that compensation is never complete, that is, the pH does not return to normal.

ACID-BASE DISORDERS

Both metabolic (altered HCO_3^- concentration) and respiratory (altered Pco_2) disorders can cause a disturbance in acid-base balance. Accumulation of H^+ or decreased excretion of H^+ causes an acidosis. Similarly, accumulation of or decreased excretion of base (HCO_3^-) causes an alkalosis. Respiratory compensation begins immediately and is maximal only a few hours after the metabolic disorder commences. Renal compensation for respiratory disorders, however, can take 12 to 24 hours to be complete in the case of the response to hyperventilation, or several days to fully compensate for a respiratory acidosis. Figure 115-3 is an acid-base nomogram demonstrating the primary acid-base disorders and the expected compensation for each disorder.

Mixed acid-base disorders are complex and occur when a primary metabolic disorder and a primary respiratory disorder develop at the same time or when two or more primary metabolic disturbances develop simultaneously. Two examples would be the tendency of a patient in diabetic ketoacidosis to also have vomiting and hypovolemia, which cause metabolic alkalosis; and patients with sepsis, who frequently have a concurrent lactic acidosis and a respiratory alkalosis. Mixed disorders can be diagnosed when there appears to be "overcompensation" or "undercompensation" to a primary disturbance.

Metabolic Acidosis

There are several mechanisms that produce metabolic acidosis; increased intake or production of fixed acids, decreased excretion of H^+, or loss of HCO_3^-. The common denominator of these disturbances is that the renal excretion of H^+ is insufficient to prevent acidosis. For convenience to aid in the diagnosis, metabolic acidosis may be classified into "anion gap" acidosis or hyperchloremic metabolic acidosis (HCMA) (Box 115-1).

Anion Gap Acidosis. The anion gap is the difference between measured cations and anions, calculated by ($Na^+ - (Cl^- + tCO_2)$).

The "missing" or unmeasured anions are predominantly negatively charged proteins such as albumin, or nonvolatile acids. The normal range is 8 to 14. The term tCO_2 represents the total CO_2 of the blood (i.e., the sum of HCO_3^- and dissolved CO_2). In addition, the tCO_2 is measured in venous blood. Thus the tCO_2 is 2 to 5 mmole/L higher than the arterial HCO_3^-. Although the anion gap formula uses the tCO_2, the formula for renal compensation of respiratory disorders uses the HCO_3^-. The anion gap is increased when there is accumulation of nonvolatile or fixed acids due to either increased production (e.g., lactate, acetoacetate, or β-hydroxybutyrate) or decreased renal excretion of fixed acid (e.g., phosphate and sulfate retention in renal failure).

There are several factors that alter the anion gap besides acid-base disturbances. Because the majority of unmeasured anions are proteins, change in the charge or quantity of protein greatly influences the anion gap. Hypoalbuminemia, which is commonly found in critically ill patients, decreases the "normal" anion gap. Because of this an anion gap acidosis can be overlooked. Paraproteinemias such as multiple myeloma also alter the anion gap. Other serum cations such as Ca^{2+} and Mg^{2+} or the presence of excessive lithium or bromide can result in a reduced anion gap. Respiratory alkalosis that alters the negative charge of albumin also increases the anion gap. Therefore, although helpful, the anion gap must be analyzed in conjunction with the patient's history and clinical condition as well as the components of the blood gas. When an abnormality is suspected, organic anions such as lactate or ketone bodies must be measured.

Renal disease can cause both an anion gap and a hyperchloremic metabolic acidosis. As renal function (creatinine clearance) declines, other aspects of renal function also decline, including the capacity to excrete H^+; hence metabolic acidosis occurs. In the earlier stages of renal failure the clearance of phosphate and sulfate is adequate and the metabolic acidosis is hyperchloremic. However, as renal function deteriorates further, phosphates and sulfates are retained and the anion gap widens. The renal tubular acidoses cause a hyperchloremic metabolic acidosis; this is discussed later.

Lactic acidosis and diabetic ketoacidosis are the most common causes of anion gap metabolic acidosis. In diabetic ketoacidosis (DKA), the inability of cells to use glucose for energy (due to lack of insulin) results in the metabolism of fatty acids, thereby producing increased acetone, acetoacetate, and β-hydroxybutyrate. DKA and lactic acidosis are discussed in Chapter 303 respectively. Starvation ketosis rarely causes a severe metabolic acidosis. However, alcoholic ketoacidosis, which includes aspects of starvation, can be severe and occurs when the alcoholic either binges on alcohol and/or vomits, which results in poor oral intake. It is noteworthy that the ketoacid that is predominantly produced in alcoholic ketoacidosis is β-hydroxybutyrate, which is not detected by the nitroprusside test (Acetest) to detect ketones in the urine.

There are several toxins that are associated with an anion gap acidosis. Salicylates initially produce a respiratory alkalosis due to di-

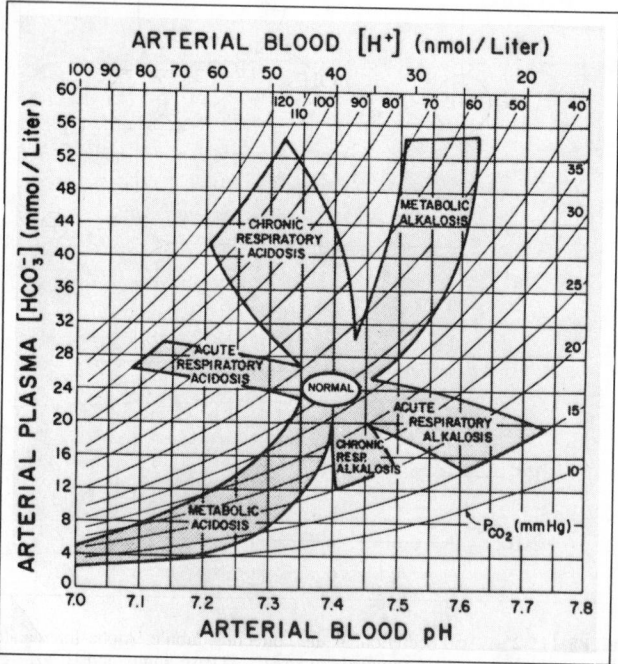

FIGURE 115-3   Acid-base nomogram. The labeled bands represent the 95% confidence limits for compensation for primary acid-base disturbances.

BOX 115-1
Causes of metabolic acidosis

Anion Gap Acidosis	Hyperchloremic Metabolic Acidosis
Renal failure	Diarrhea
Ketoacidosis	Early renal failure
Diabetes	Renal tubular acidosis (RTA)
Alcoholism	Proximal RTA
Starvation	Distal RTA
Lactic Acidosis	Decreased ammoniagenesis
Toxins	"Voltage dependent"
Methanol	Acid ingestion
Ethylene glycol	HCl
Salicylates	NH_4Cl
	ArginineCl
	LysineCl
	Anion exchange resins
	Ureteral diversions

rect stimulation of CNS respiratory centers. This is frequently complicated by a lactic acidosis. Administration of bicarbonate will "uncover" the underlying respiratory alkalosis and can result in alkalemia.

Ingestion of methanol or ethylene glycol can result in accumulation of organic acids when they are metabolized. Alcohol dehydrogenase, a liver enzyme that metabolizes alcohol, also metabolizes methanol to formaldehyde and formic acid. Likewise ethylene glycol is metabolized to glycolic, oxalic, and formic acids. In addition to the toxicity of formic acid, oxalate crystals can form in the kidneys, brain, heart, and lungs, resulting in multiple toxicities. The treatment of methanol and ethylene glycol ingestion is similar. Initial efforts are supportive and designed to decrease metabolism of the toxins. Ethanol is a competitive substrate for alcohol dehydrogenase, therefore the intravenous administration of alcohol slows metabolism of methanol and ethylene glycol. The second step is to remove the parent compound by hemodialysis.

Anion gap acidoses due to toxins, including ethanol, methanol, and ethylene glycol, are also associated with a widened osmolar gap because these toxins accumulate in the serum and contribute to the serum osmolality. Although the toxin-induced increment in osmolality is readily measured, it is not accounted for when the serum osmolality is estimated with the standard formula:

$$(\text{EQ. 5})$$

$$\text{Estimated osmolality} = 2 \times Na^+ + \frac{BUN}{2.8} + \frac{glucose}{18}$$

Therefore an osmolar gap (measured serum osmolality − estimated serum osmolality) of greater than 10 mOsm/kg is consistent with the presence of a toxin in the serum.

Hyperchloremic or "Non–Anion Gap" Metabolic Acidosis.

Unlike organic acids, which add unmeasured anions to the blood, in hyperchloremic metabolic acidosis (HCMA) the loss of bicarbonate is "matched" by the addition of chloride. An example would be the ingestion or administration of HCl or the chloride salts of ammonium, arginine, and lysine. These substances donate an H^+, which is buffered by HCO_3^-, and in the process Cl^- is released. Dilution of serum HCO_3^- by the rapid administration of saline can cause a *mild* acidosis acutely but never a severe or chronic acidosis. In the course of treatment of diabetic, alcoholic, or starvation ketosis HCMA can occur. Because saline administration improves renal perfusion, renal excretion of ketoacid anions is rapid and converts an anion gap acidosis to an HCMA.

Diarrhea is the most common cause of HCMA. Bicarbonate, which is secreted into the ileum and colon, is lost with the increased stool volume, and metabolic acidosis ensues. Laxative abuse must also be considered in these circumstances. Certain anion exchange resins (e.g., cholestyramine), if taken in excessive quantities, can also result in loss of HCO_3^- in the feces. It is not uncommon to see HCMA in patients who have undergone a ureteral diversion. Ureterosigmoidostomies and ileal conduits can result in significant HCO_3^- loss in the urine because the conduit secretes HCO_3^- in exchange for urinary chloride. These gut segments also absorb urinary ammonia, preventing the excretion of acid. Increased surface and increased duration of contact of the urine with the intestinal loop result in a more severe acidosis.

Acetazolamide and methazolamide, inhibitors of carbonic anhydrase, cause renal loss of bicarbonate. This effect is useful clinically in the case of metabolic alkalosis in a person with pulmonary disease. A patient with little pulmonary reserve or who already has retention of CO_2 can become hypoxic in the face of respiratory depression secondary to metabolic alkalosis. Especially in a patient who requires mechanical ventilation, treatment with acetazolamide can facilitate extubation.

The Renal Acidoses.

Renal tubular defects resulting in the failure to reclaim filtered bicarbonate or regenerate bicarbonate utilized in buffering body fluids cause a hyperchloremic metabolic acidosis. There are four categories of renal acidosis: proximal (Type II), distal (Type I), decreased ammoniagenesis, and "voltage-dependent" renal tubular acidoses.

Proximal renal tubular acidosis (pRTA). Defects in the ability of the proximal tubule to reabsorb filtered bicarbonate result in metabolic acidosis. Most commonly this is associated with other defects in proximal tubule function such as glycosuria and amino aciduria (Fanconi's syndrome). This can be inherited and present in childhood or can be acquired, such as is seen with heavy metal toxicity (Box 115-2). The proximal tubule defect results in a reduced tubular maximum (Tm) for the reabsorption of HCO_3^-. The function of the distal tubule to acidify the urine and secrete H^+, which is buffered by titratable acidity, and ammonia remains intact. Since the acidosis is sustained by urine HCO_3^- losses, the urine pH is often >5.5 in untreated patients. These patients develop a new equilibrium around a lower serum HCO_3^- level (14 to 18 mEq/L). Attempts to administer sodium bicarbonate to raise the serum HCO_3^- above this reabsorption threshold exaggerate bicarbonaturia. Diagnosis is made by calculation of the fractional excretion (FE) of HCO_3^-. To do this, the patient's serum bicarbonate must be within the normal range (or at least above the threshold). A random (spot) urine sample is sent for measurement of creatinine and HCO_3^-. The $FE_{HCO_3^-}$ is calculated from the following formula:

$$(\text{EQ. 6})$$

$$FE_{HCO_3^-} = \frac{(U_{HCO_3^-} \times P_{Cr})}{(P_{HCO_3^-} \times U_{Cr})}$$

where Cr is the creatinine, U is the concentration in the urine, and P is the concentration in plasma. A value less than 5% is normal and greater than 15% is indicative of decreased tubular reabsorption of HCO_3^-. Left untreated, children with pRTA develop rickets or osteomalacia due to the buffering action of bone over a long period of time. Treatment with bicarbonate is difficult because whenever the serum HCO_3^- is above the threshold level, bicarbonaturia occurs. Treatment with hydrochlorothiazide can be effective by creating a state of mild volume depletion that in turn increases proximal tubular reabsorption of HCO_3^-.

Type I or distal RTA. In distal RTA (dRTA), the reabsorption of filtered HCO_3^- is normal. The deficit is in the ability of the distal tubule to secrete sufficient quantities of H^+ to regenerate HCO_3^- consumed by buffering acids. The defect in patients with dRTA in theory could be gradient limited (either decreased secretion due to decreased luminal voltage or excessive back-leak of H^+) or rate limited (de-

---

BOX 115-2
Causes of proximal renal tubular acidosis

Primary
  Idiopathic
  Inherited
Secondary to inherited disease
  Cystinosis
  Hereditary fructose intolerance
  Lowe's syndrome
  Wilson's disease
  Carbonic anhydrase deficiency or dysfunction
  Pyruvate carboxylase deficiency
Drugs and toxic agents
  Heavy metals (lead, cadmium, copper, mercury)
  Carbonic anhydrase inhibitors
  Outdated tetracycline
  Arginine and lysine
Miscellaneous
  Hyperparathyroidism
  Multiple myeloma
  Sjögren's syndrome
  Amyloidosis
  Nephrotic syndrome
  Renal transplantation
  Hypervitaminosis D
  Deficiency of vitamin D
  Chronic active hepatitis

BOX 115-3
Causes of distal renal tubular acidosis

Primary
  Idiopathic
  Inherited
Secondary to inherited disease
  Osteoporosis
  Nerve deafness
  Carbonic anhydrase deficiency or dysfunction
  Hereditary fructose intolerance
Drugs and toxic agents
  Amphotericin B
  Lithium
  Toluene
  Amiloride
Disorders of calcium metabolism
  Nephrocalcinosis
  Idiopathic hypercalciuria
  Hypervitaminosis D
  Hyperparathyroidism
Systemic diseases
  Idiopathic hypergammaglobulinemia
  Multiple myeloma
  Systemic lupus erythematosus
  Sjögren's syndrome
  Hepatic cirrhosis
  Primary biliary cirrhosis
  Chronic active hepatitis
Interstitial renal disease
  Obstructive uropathy
  Rejection of renal transplant
  Sickle cell disease
  Medullary sponge kidney
  Analgesic nephropathy

BOX 115-4
Causes of impaired net acid excretion

Primary aldosterone deficiency
  Adrenal steroid deficiency
    Addison's disease
    Bilateral adrenalectomy
    Bilateral adrenal destruction (hemorrhage, carcinoma)
    Adrenal enzyme defects (21-hydroxylase deficiency, 3β-ol-
      dehydrogenase deficiency, desmolase deficiency, AIDS)
  Isolated aldosterone deficiency
    Familial hypoaldosteronism
    Primary zona glomerulosa defect
    Transient hypoaldosteronism of infancy
    Chronic hypoaldosteronism
    Heparin
    Persistent hypotension
  Inhibition of angiotensin I converting enzyme
    Primary
    Drugs (captopril, enalopril, etc.)
Hyporeninemic hypoaldosteronism
  Diabetic nephropathy
  Tubulointerstitial nephropathies
  Nephrosclerosis
  Nonsteroidal antiinflammatory drugs
  AIDS
Resistance to aldosterone
  With salt wasting
    In children
    In adults (methicillin, obstructive nephropathy, transplantation,
      cyclosporin A, sickle cell disease)
    Drugs (spironolactone, amiloride, triamterene)
  Without salt wasting
Chronic renal insufficiency

creased rate of H^+ secretion); most human studies indicate the latter mechanism. The acidosis in dRTA is often quite severe, with serum HCO_3^- often less than 10 mEq/L. When measured, the urine pH is always greater than 5.5. Diagnosis may require either a load of NH_4Cl as an acid challenge or treatment with bicarbonate, producing the opposite effects of pRTA. Another way of distinguishing pRTA from dRTA is in the measurement of the urine-to-blood P_{CO_2} gradient. When patients with pRTA are given sodium bicarbonate, H^+ secreted by the distal tubule forms carbonic acid (H_2CO_3), which in the distal tubule slowly dehydrates to CO_2. This results in a urine P_{CO_2} that is more than 40 mm Hg higher than arterial P_{CO_2}. In patients with dRTA, however, the decreased H^+ secretion results in a low urine-to-blood P_{CO_2} ratio.

Distal RTA can be inherited and develop in childhood or be acquired in adults due to renal manifestations of autoimmune disease or drug use (Box 115-3). The disorder is associated with hypercalciuria, nephrocalcinosis, and nephrolithiasis. Potassium wasting is also a significant problem. Children infrequently develop bone disease but are almost always growth-retarded. Patients with dRTA respond very readily to sodium bicarbonate therapy.

Decreased ammoniagenesis. As mentioned earlier, the synthesis of ammonia is essential to buffer H^+ secreted by the distal tubule. Decreased synthesis of ammonia results in decreased secretion of H^+, resulting in acidosis. Because the defect is in the buffering capacity of the urine and not the mechanism of H^+ secretion, urine pH will be below 5.5. Diagnosis can be made by measuring the urinary ammonia excretion. The urine "anion gap" can provide a quick, more readily available estimate of urinary ammonia excretion. The urine anion gap is calculated from spot urine Na^+, K^+, and Cl^-, and is calculated with the formula: urine anion gap = $(Na^+ + K^+)$ − Cl^-. In metabolic acidosis, the anion gap is usually negative due to the unmeasured NH_4^+ in the urine. In patients with decreased ammonia excretion, the anion gap is positive. It may also be positive when a large quantity of unmeasured anion appears in the urine: for

example, in patients with an anion gap acidosis due to DKA, ethylene glycol, etc.

Ammonia synthesis is inhibited by hyperkalemia and glucocorticoid deficiency. Aldosterone deficiency results in hyperkalemia and renal salt wasting. The hyperkalemia in turn decreases ammonia synthesis, thus causing an HCMA. A subgroup of patients with hyperkalemic metabolic acidosis have a syndrome of low renin hypoaldosteronism (also called type IV RTA). There are numerous proposed mechanisms as to why the secretion of renin is suppressed, which in turn suppresses aldosterone secretion. Hyperkalemia in these patients also fails to stimulate aldosterone secretion. In addition, these patients have reduced responsiveness to aldosterone. These patients respond to potassium restriction and treatment with anion exchange resins to reduce serum potassium.

Renal disease, resulting in reduced renal mass, decreases ammonia synthesis and excretion, which is one of the many reasons these patients are acidotic. As mentioned earlier, an anion gap metabolic acidosis due to retention of anions occurs when the renal disease is advanced. Sodium bicarbonate therapy readily corrects the acidosis.

Voltage-dependent RTA. Salt wasting associated with aldosterone resistance diminishes the lumen voltage in the distal tubule. The voltage in this segment due to sodium reabsorption is normally negative and thus facilitates H^+ secretion. A reduction in distal Na^+ reabsorption, as seen in salt wasting due to resistence to aldosterone, decreases the quantity of H^+ secreted. These patients therefore have a picture consistent with a dRTA. Treatment consists of salt and sodium bicarbonate supplementation.

These last two categories represent impaired net acid excretion, that is, a quantitative defect. Box 115-4 lists the disorders that can cause this type of problem.

Potassium and Metabolic Acidosis. Serum potassium is frequently elevated in patients with metabolic acidosis. Shift of intracellular potassium into the extracellular fluid can result in significant hyperkalemia in patients with acute HCMA. In some anion gap acidoses, such as lactic acidosis due to generalized seizures, the serum

K^+ is not altered. However, in other forms of anion gap acidoses, such as DKA and lactic acidosis due to shock or sepsis, the serum K^+ is influenced by numerous factors including volume status, insulin deficiency, oxygen delivery to tissues, aldosterone secretion, and renal potassium excretion, and hence the serum K^+ is difficult to predict. Chronic metabolic acidosis will not cause hyperkalemia unless there is a defect in renal potassium excretion.

Treatment of Metabolic Acidosis. The initial step is to determine the cause for the acidosis and eliminate it. In acute acidosis, treatment should be limited to those with a serum pH less than 7.2 and therapy should be aimed at increasing the pH above 7.2 and serum HCO_3^- above 10 mEq/L. The volume of distribution of HCO_3^- varies inversely with the plasma $[HCO_3^-]$, and the formula to calculate the dose of bicarbonate to administer takes into account this factor:

$$\text{Amount NaHCO}_3 = (0.4 + 2.4/[HCO_3^-]_{current}) \times wt \times (10 - [HCO_3^-]_{current}) \quad \text{(EQ. 6)}$$

The value of 10 is the $[HCO_3^-]$ that is desired after treatment. It is not the aim of therapy to normalize the serum bicarbonate, but to elevate the pH above the level that can cause manifestations of acidosis. It should be noted that this formula does not include a factor to correct for continued production of acid. Therapy, therefore, should be monitored with frequent blood gases and chemistries. Therapy may be limited by the large sodium load associated with sodium bicarbonate administration. In these circumstances and when there is renal insufficiency, dialysis may be beneficial. Due to the possibility of bone disease, patients with a chronic acidosis should be treated. The goal of therapy in patients with chronic acidosis should be to maintain the pH around 7.3 or an $[HCO_3^-]$ of 15 mEq/L.

Bicarbonate treatment is not without complications. As serum pH increases, symptoms of hypokalemia and hypocalcemia may ensue. In ketoacidosis and lactic acidosis, correction of the underlying problem results in metabolism of the respective anions, which may cause an alkalosis if a significant quantity of bicarbonate has been administered. In addition, lactic acid and ketoacid production may be stimulated by exogenous sodium bicarbonate and the resulting alkalinization. Changes in the affinity of oxygen to hemoglobin can cause tissue hypoxia. Finally, bicarbonate therapy can cause a paradoxic fall in CNS pH resulting in CNS depression. This is due to the fact that HCO_3^- penetrates the blood-brain barrier very poorly. CO_2, on the other hand, formed by the buffering of H^+ with the administered HCO_3^-, readily enters the CSF. As CO_2 enters the CSF, carbonic acid is formed, thus decreasing CSF pH.

Metabolic Alkalosis

There are two phases of any metabolic alkalosis; generation and maintenance. Either excess addition of alkali (e.g., bicarbonate, lactate, or citrate) or excess excretion of acid (either via the gastrointestinal tract or the kidneys) can cause a metabolic alkalosis (Box 115-5). In either case, if renal function was normal, excess bicarbonate would be rapidly excreted by the kidneys.

Renal bicarbonate excretion can be altered by several mechanisms. Decreased glomerular filtration rate (GFR) decreases the filtration of bicarbonate, and thus it can maintain the alkalosis. For the reasons outlined earlier, most renal failure patients have a predominant metabolic acidosis, but it is often a mixed disorder. In addition, when renal failure patients do develop frank alkalosis (through bicarbonate administration or other means), the alkalosis can be difficult to treat. If the alkalosis is severe, a special bicarbonate-poor dialysate must be used.

Volume depletion contributes to the maintenance of the alkalosis through several mechanisms. Activation of the renin-angiotensin-aldosterone system leads to a direct increase in proximal absorption of bicarbonate via angiotensin II effects. Aldosterone increases distal H^+ secretion, and aldosterone-induced hypokalemia stimulates ammoniagenesis and increases H^+ secretion.

Disorders Causing Maintenance and Generation of an Alkalosis. Vomiting or nasogastric suctioning of H^+-rich gastric se-

---

> **BOX 115-5**
> ## Causes of metabolic alkalosis
>
> Exogenous HCO_3^- load with renal failure (including milk-alkali syndrome)
> Reduced extracellular volume
>   Gastrointestinal
>   Vomiting and gastric aspiration
>   Chloride-rich diarrhea (congenital or acquired)
>   Villous adenoma
>   Renal
>   Diuretics
>   Potassium depletion
>   Posthypercapnic metabolic alkalosis
>   Recovery from organic acidosis
>   Refeeding following starvation
>   Bartter's syndrome
> Expansion of extracellular volume
>   High renin
>   Renal artery stenosis
>   Accelerated hypertension
>   Renin-secreting tumors
>   Estrogen treatment
>   Low renin
>   Primary aldosteronism (adenoma, hyperplasia, carcinoma, glucocorticoid-suppressible)
>   Adrenal enzyme defects (11 β-hydroxylase deficiency, 17 α-hydroxylase)
>   Cushing's syndrome (ectopic ACTH, adrenal carcinoma, adrenal adenoma, pituitary adenoma)
>   Other mineralocorticoids (licorice, carbenoxolone, chewing tobacco)

---

cretions generates an alkalosis due to loss of HCl and addition of HCO_3^- to the blood across the antiluminal side of the parietal cell. The volume depletion associated with this is what causes the maintenance of the alkalosis through the mechanisms outlined earlier. Initial attempts by the kidney to excrete the excess bicarbonate result in losses of Na^+ and K^+ in the urine, contributing to the volume depletion and enhancing aldosterone secretion. Between vomiting episodes, NaCl and HCO_3^- excretion is virtually nonexistent because of volume depletion, and urinary pH is low. Potassium wasting, however, continues because of aldosterone stimulation of K^+ excretion.

Chloride-rich diarrhea (chloridorrhea) is a less common cause of gastrointestinal-induced alkalosis. Diarrhea is usually HCO_3^- rich. Certain congenital disorders, infections, and villous adenomas can cause loss of large amounts of chloride in the stool and failure of the normal ileal and colonic mechanisms that secrete bicarbonate. Here too, activation of the renin-aldosterone-angiotensin system by volume depletion maintains the alkalosis.

Diuretics (thiazides and loop diuretics) are a very common cause of metabolic alkalosis due to volume and potassium depletion and activation of aldosterone. Loss of NaCl in the urine resulting in volume depletion is said to cause a "contraction" alkalosis because the same amount of HCO_3^- is now present in a smaller volume. In most clinical settings, however, the effect of contraction on the HCO_3^- concentration is trivial and without the effect of activation of the renin-angiotensin-aldosterone axis, the alkalosis would not be maintained.

An uncommon but much talked about cause of metabolic alkalosis is Bartter's syndrome. Patients with Bartter's present with metabolic alkalosis, potassium depletion, hypomagnesemia, hyperreninemia, and hyperaldosteronism. Patients are usually normotensive because vascular reactivity to angiotensin II is markedly reduced. However, the kidney biopsy is remarkable for hyperplasia of the juxtaglomerular apparatus. Some controversy exists as to the role of prostaglandins in this disorder, but there is general agreement that abnormal NaCl transport occurs in the thick ascending limb of the Henle's loop. Although the inheritance pattern is unknown, the disorder most commonly presents in childhood, but there are

Metabolic Alkalosis

Saline Responsive (Urine Cl⁻ < 20 mEq/L)	Saline Resistant (Urine Cl⁻ > 30 mEq/L)	
↓ ECFV	↔ or ↓ ECFV	↑ ECFV
Vomiting	Bartter's syndrome	Primary and secondary hyperaldosteronism
Gastric aspiration	K⁺ depletion (severe)	Licorice
Diuretics		
Posthypercapnia		
K⁺ depletion (mild to moderate)		
Refeeding alkalosis		
Recovery from organic acidosis		
Chloride diarrhea		

FIGURE 115-4   Diagnostic approach for metabolic alkalosis.

documented cases of acquired Bartter's syndrome in adults, with some cases being reported in association with gentamicin treatment. The differential diagnosis of Bartter's includes other causes of aldosterone activation: vomiting, diuretics, and laxative abuse. It can be distinguished from these disorders by the urinary chloride, which is elevated in Bartter's syndrome and normally very low in these other disorders (Fig. 115-4). Primary hyperaldosteronism is ruled out by the normal blood pressure and the mildly reduced plasma volume.

Mineralocorticoid excess states are associated with metabolic alkalosis because of the renal effects of increased H⁺ secretion, hypokalemia-induced ammoniagenesis, and in some instances angiotensin II effects. In these patients, however, there is volume expansion. Box 115-5 lists the various disorders that result in excess mineralocorticoid effect. Natural licorice flavoring, but not artificial licorice flavoring, is believed to interact with aldosterone receptors in the kidney, causing metabolic alkalosis. Chewing tobacco flavored with licorice has similar effects. Once the offending product is removed, the renal defects resolve.

Transient metabolic alkalosis can be seen after resolution of an organic acidosis (e.g., ketoacidosis or lactic acidosis). If bicarbonate therapy was administered, recovery associated with metabolism of the lactate or ketoacids results in a metabolic alkalosis, especially if renal failure, hypovolemia, or hypokalemia coexist. A mild acidosis is also seen after a period of starvation. During the period of deprivation, ketoacids are formed. When calories (in particular carbohydrates) are readministered, the ketoacids are metabolized to HCO_3^-. Again if volume depletion coexists this will cause an alkalosis. This "refeeding" phenomenon usually resolves by itself within a few days.

"Posthypercapnic" alkalosis can be a significant problem in the intensive care unit. In patients who have had respiratory depression or pulmonary disease resulting in retention of CO_2, renal compensation increases HCO_3^- reabsorption and regeneration to bring the pH back toward normal. When the hypercapnia is corrected, the kidneys should promptly excrete the excess HCO_3^-. If, however, hypokalemia or volume depletion (often due to diuretics) is not treated also, the kidneys will be unable to excrete the alkaline load. This will make weaning from a mechanical ventilator difficult, if not impossible. Treatment aimed at correcting the potassium deficit and the volume depletion can facilitate weaning. Acetazolamide, a carbonic anhydrase inhibitor, may be beneficial with the caveats that it might worsen hypokalemia and that its efficacy as a HCO_3^- losing diuretic is significantly blunted by volume depletion.

Finally, metabolic alkalosis is sometimes seen in hospitalized patients undergoing antibiotic therapy. This is due to certain antibiotics (e.g., carbenicillin) that have poorly resorbable anions. These "extra" negative charges in the urine increase the excretion of positive charges such as Na⁺, K⁺, H⁺, and NH₄⁺, generating and maintaining the alkalosis.

Treatment. Severe alkalosis can cause cardiac arrhythmias, tissue anoxia due to increased affinity of hemoglobin for oxygen, and decreased CNS blood flow; in addition, it may precipitate calcium salts, resulting in tetany and seizures. As in the treatment of all acid-base disorders, treatment should be aimed at correcting the primary disorder. In most cases the cause of alkalosis (e.g., vomiting, diuretics) will be obvious. Measurement of the urine chloride can be helpful (see Fig. 115-4). Finally, in cases of suspected diuretic or laxative abuse, drug screens can be helpful.

When extracellular volume depletion exists, treatment is centered on repletion of chloride and, when necessary, hypokalemia. Administration of normal saline and KCl will correct the alkalosis. In cases of volume expansion as seen in mineralocorticoid excess, diuretics, in particular aldosterone receptor blockers, such as spironolactone, and blockers of aldosterone-stimulated Na⁺ reabsorption, such as amiloride and triamterene, are useful.

In acutely symptomatic patients (i.e., those with seizures or tetany), rapid correction of the alkalosis can be achieved with the administration of HCl, arginine hydrochloride, and NH₄Cl. The latter two should be avoided in patients with liver disease. HCl may be ad-

---

BOX 115-6
Diagnostic approach to disorders of acid-base balance

Identify the medical problems
  History
    Symptoms (vomiting, diarrhea, polyuria, etc.)
    Diseases (diabetes mellitus, congestive heart failure, chronic obstructive pulmonary disease, etc.)
    Medications (diuretics, laxatives, sedatives, etc.)
    Treatment (ventilation, nasogastric suction, intravenous fluids, etc.)
  Physical examination
    Tetany, jaundice, cyanosis, respirations, blood pressure, fever, etc.
Consider influence of medical problems on acid-base balance
Laboratory evidence of acid-base disorders
  Routine laboratory data (liver disease, sepsis, renal disease, etc.)
  Electrolytes
    Serum total CO_2 (tCO_2)
      If abnormal, then at least a single disturbance
      If normal, there may be multiple disturbances
    Serum anion gap: $Na^+ - (Cl^- + tCO_2)$
      Widened anion gap suggests metabolic acidosis
      Normal anion gap suggests hyperchloremic acidosis or respiratory alkalosis
      Hypoalbuminemia may obscure widened anion gap
    Serum osmolar gap
      Measured serum osmolality $- 2\ Na^+ + BUN/2.8 + glucose/18$)
      Widened osmolar gap along with widened anion gap suggests toxin-induced metabolic acidosis
    Serum potassium
      Altered [K⁺] may predict pH: ↓K⁺ in alkalemia, ↑K⁺ in acidemia
    Urine anion gap ($U_{Na^+} + U_{K^+} - U_{Cl^-}$)
      Positive urine anion gap along with hyperchloremic metabolic acidosis suggests reduced urinary ammonium
      Positive urine anion gap along with widened serum anion gap is consistent with excess unmeasured urinary anion (same as in serum)
    Urine chloride (U_{Cl^-})
      Reduced U_{Cl^-} along with metabolic alkalosis indicates Cl⁻-sensitive alkalosis
      Normal U_{Cl^-} along with metabolic alkalosis indicates Cl⁻-insensitive alkalosis
  Arterial blood gas
    Evidence for respiratory disorder: primary versus compensatory
    Questions to ask
      Is the ABG consistent with the previous information?
      Is there a simple or mixed acid-base disturbance?
Integrate laboratory data with medical problem(s) and ask: Is the picture consistent?

✔ *WHEN TO REFER*

Most simple acid-base disorders are easily diagnosed and managed. However, if the patient has severe symptomatic alkalosis or acidosis, if the disorder is not corrected by therapy, or if there is difficulty in diagnosing the disorder, a nephrology consult can be useful. In particular, if volume overload is a concern about bicarbonate administration, dialysis can be initiated. This is especially important in the face of renal failure. Dialysis is also important in the treatment of drug toxicities and ingestion of ethylene glycol or methanol. Finally, diagnosis of renal acidoses should be made by a nephrologist.

---

ministered in a 0.1 to 0.2 M solution into a central vein and must be accompanied by frequent blood gas monitoring.

EVALUATION OF THE PATIENT WITH ACID-BASE DISORDERS

A systematic approach is necessary to diagnose a patient with disturbed acid-base balance. Such an approach is outlined in Box 115-6. It is likely to aid in the correct diagnosis of both simple and complex (mixed) acid-base disorders, that is, when more than one primary abnormality occurs simultaneously. Although there is no substitute for an arterial blood gas measurement in the patient with a suspected acid-base disorder, care must be taken in interpreting blood gas data with acid-base nomograms like that in Fig. 115-3. These nomograms describe only simple acid-base disorders and yield erroneous results when applied to a patient with a complex (mixed) acid-base disorder.

Following the approach outlined in Box 115-6 should be helpful, especially when dealing with a patient with a mixed acid-base disorder. On occasion, however, three or more acid-base disorders can occur simultaneously, and this level of complexity may be suspected when analyzing the patient's history and physical status. Laboratory evidence for such a diagnosis can be obtained by evaluating the relationship between the serum anion gap and the tCO_2. In the case of uncomplicated anion gap acidosis, the increment in the anion gap should equal the decrement in tCO_2, because the H^+ accompanying the unmeasured anion neutralizes bicarbonate in a stoichiometric fashion. Numerically, the change in the anion gap (Δ anion gap = observed anion gap − normal anion gap [i.e., 12]) approximates the change in the tCO_2 (Δ tCO_2 = normal tCO_2 [i.e., 28] − observed tCO_2), and the difference between these changes (Δ anion gap − Δ tCO_2) or Δ gap should approach 0 ± 6. Deviation of the Δ gap from the ideal value suggests the existence of an additional metabolic abnormality. For example, patients with alcoholic acidosis often have positive Δ gaps, because they also vomit, which induces a coexistent metabolic alkalosis, mitigating the severity of the acidosis.

BIBLIOGRAPHY

Alpern RJ, Rector FC Jr: Renal acidification mechanisms. In Brenner BM, editor: *The kidney,* ed 5, Philadelphia, 1996, WB Saunders.

DuBose TD Jr, Cogan MG, Rector JC Jr: Acid-base disorders. In Brenner BM, editor: *The kidney,* ed 5, Philadelphia, 1996, WB Saunders.

Fernandez PC, Cohen RM, Feldman GM: The concept of bicarbonate distribution space: the crucial role of body buffers, *Kidney Int* 36:747, 1989.

Kaehy WD, Anderson, RJ: Bicarbonate therapy of metabolic acidosis, *Crit Care Med* 22:1525, 1994.

116 Glomerular Diseases

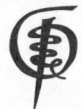

William G. Couser

Almost half of the 250,000 patients with end-stage renal disease in the United States suffer from some form of glomerular disease. Glomerular diseases may be primary or secondary due to glomerular involvement in a number of systemic illnesses.

The clinical manifestations of glomerular disease can be considered in two broad categories, with overlap between them. Some patients present with acute glomerulonephritis. Signs of glomerular inflammation include proteinuria (usually less than 3.5 g/day and not in the nephrotic range), red blood cells and red blood cell casts in the urinary sediment, and often a reduction in renal function that may be associated with sodium and water retention and hypertension. The clinical and pathophysiologic aspects of the acute nephritic syndrome are considered in Chapter 107. Currently recognized glomerular diseases that may cause this syndrome are discussed in detail in this chapter, and a summary of their distinguishing features is presented in Table 116-1. A second group of patients with glomerular disease present with nephrotic range proteinuria (greater than 3.5 g/day in adults) and usually other manifestations of nephrotic syndrome including hypoalbuminemia, edema, hyperlipidemia, and lipiduria. The pathophysiology of proteinuria and the nephrotic syndrome are discussed in Chapters 105 and 108. This chapter describes the clinical and pathologic features of the major glomerular diseases that cause the idiopathic nephrotic syndrome. The features of these diseases are summarized in Table 116-4.

In addition to distinguishing between acute glomerulonephritis and the nephrotic syndrome, it is also useful to separate patients with glomerular disease into those with a primary renal disease and those with some systemic disease associated with major extrarenal manifestations. Glomerular involvement in several systemic diseases is discussed at the end of this chapter.

MECHANISMS AND CONSEQUENCES OF IMMUNE GLOMERULAR INJURY

Most glomerular diseases are mediated by immune mechanisms involving deposition of antibody and/or immune complex formation in glomeruli. Diseases in which immune deposits are not seen, such as minimal change disease (MCD) or idiopathic crescentic glomerulonephritis, are also believed to be immunologically mediated, but the mechanisms are less well understood. Glomerular immune deposits may be continuous, or linear, as in anti-glomerular basement membrane (GBM) disease (see Fig. 116-5, *A*) or discontinuous and granular in various forms of immune complex nephritis (see Figs. 116-2, *B;* 116-3, *B;* 116-5, *B*). Linear deposits represent glomerular deposits of an autoantibody to a GBM antigen. Anti-GBM antibody disposition is relatively uncommon clinically and causes only Goodpasture's syndrome and anti-GBM nephritis without pulmonary hemorrhage.

Granular, or immune complex, deposits are much more common and may be seen at three different sites in the glomerulus: within the glomerular mesangium (immunoglobulin A [IgA] nephropathy, lupus nephritis; see Fig. 116-3, *B*); along with the inner, or subendothelial, surface of the capillary wall (lupus, type I membranoproliferative glomerulonephritis; see Fig. 116-10, *A*); and along the outer, or subepithelial, surface of the capillary wall as in membranous nephropathy (see Fig. 116-8, *C*). The locations of these different types of deposits are illustrated schematically in Fig. 116-1. Four factors determine the type of glomerular lesion that results from glomerular immune deposit formation: (1) site of the deposit formation (subepithelial deposits are noninflammatory; subendothelial and mesangial deposits incite inflammation), (2) mechanism of deposit formation (local immune complex formation is more nephritogenic than preformed complex trapping), (3) biologic properties of the antibodies deposited

Table 116-1 Summary of primary renal diseases that normally become evident as acute glomerulonephritis

DISEASES	POSTSTREPTOCOCCAL GLOMERULONEPHRITIS	IGA NEPHROPATHY	GOODPASTURE'S SYNDROME	IDIOPATHIC CRESCENTIC NEPHRITIS
Clinical manifestations				
Age (years) and sex	All ages, mean 7; 2:1 male	15-35; 2:1 male	15-30; 6:1 male	Mean 58; 2:1 male
Acute nephritic syndrome	90%	50%	90%	90%
Asymptomatic hematuria	Occasionally	50%	Rare	Rare
Nephrotic syndrome	10%-20%	Rare	Rare	Rare
Hypertension	70%	30%-50%	Rare	10-20%
Acute renal failure*	50% (transient)	Very rare	50%	25%
Other	1-3 week latent period	Follows viral syndromes	Pulmonary hemorrhage Iron-deficiency anemia	60% None
Recurs in transplants	No	Yes	Only if antibody present	No
Laboratory findings	ASO titers (70%) Positive streptozyme (95%) C3-C9, normal C1, C4	Increased IgA-fibronectin aggregates IgA in dermal capillaries	Positive anti-GBM antibody	Increased anti-neutrophil cytoplasmic antibody (ANCA)
Immunogenetics	HLA D "EN" (9)* ? DR4 (4)	DR4 (4), ? HLA Bw 35	HLA DR2 (16), B7 (5)	None established
Renal pathologic study				
Light microscopy	Diffuse proliferation	Focal proliferation	Focal diffuse proliferation with crescents	Crescentic glomerulonephritis
Immunofluorescence	Granular IgG, C3	Diffuse mesangial IgA, IgG	Linear IgG, C3	No immune deposits
Electron microscopy	Subepithelial humps	Mesangial deposits	No deposits	No deposits
Treatment	Supportive	Fish oil	Plasma exchange, steroids cyclophosphamide	Steroid pulse therapy, cyclophosphamide
Prognosis	95% resolve spontaneously 5% RPGN or slowly progressive	Slow progression in 25%-50%	75% stabilize or improve if treated early	75% stabilize or improve if treated early

*Relative risk.

ASO, Antitreptolysin O; *GBM,* glomerular basement membrane; *IgA, IgG,* immunoglobulins A and G; *HLA,* human leukocyte antigen; *RPGN,* rapidly progressive glomerulonephritis.

(complement-fixing antibodies produce more injury than non–complement-fixing), and (4) amount of antibody deposited.

The subepithelial immune complex deposits seen in membranous nephropathy are probably all formed locally, or in situ, by one of two mechanisms. An autoantibody response to an antigenic component of normal glomerular epithelial cells results in immune complex formation on the cell surface followed by capping and shedding of the immune complexes from the cell surface into the adjacent lamina rara externa to produce subepithelial deposits. Alternatively, exogenous, nonrenal antigens, particularly if they are positively charged or cationic, may first become localized in the glomerular capillary wall by binding electrically to heparin sulfate-proteoglycan anionic sites in the lamina rara externa (Fig. 116-1). Antibody binding to these antigens then results in subepithelial immune complex formation and proteinuria.

Regardless of whether subepithelial deposits contain renal or extrarenal antigens, they cause proteinuria by a mechanism that requires assembly of the complement C5b-9 membrane attack complex and does not involve inflammatory cell participation. The lack of inflammatory change is probably because the formation of deposits on the outer surface of the capillary wall renders them inaccessible to circulating neutrophils and macrophages.

Mesangial and subendothelial deposits usually contain exogenous antigens and occur together. Mesangial deposits are present in milder forms of diseases such as classes II and III lupus nephritis and IgA nephropathy. Subendothelial deposits appear, in addition to the mesangial deposits, when the disease is more severe (class IV lupus nephritis, severe IgA nephropathy). Deposits at both sites may be formed locally, or they can result from the passive trapping of performed immune complexes from the circulation.

Because subendothelial and mesangial deposits (and anti-GBM antibody deposits) are accessible to circulating inflammatory cells such as neutrophils and macrophages, these cells are attracted by chemotactic factors and chemokines and localize at the site of deposit formation by immune adherence mechanisms involving Fc or C3b receptors on the cell surfaces or by interaction with leukocyte adherence molecules expressed on the surface of endothelial cells in response to inflammatory cytokines. Activated inflammatory cells release proteolytic enzymes and reactive oxygen species believed to cause the capillary wall damage, which results in proteinuria, hematuria, and in some cases leakage of fibrin into Bowman's space to initiate glomerular crescent formation. Crescents represent proliferating parietal epithelial cells of Bowman's capsule and mononuclear cells in a bed of fibrin, which is deposited in part due to tissue factor released by macrophages that migrate through gaps in the capillary wall into Bowman's space. Thus crescents are markers of severe glomerular injury, but not causes of injury. These inflammatory changes are the histologic hallmarks of acute glomerulonephritis.

In addition to these morphologic changes, functional consequences of acute glomerular injury reduce the glomerular filtration rate (GFR). Immune reactions within the glomerulus result in glomerular vasoconstriction with a marked decrease in glomerular plasma flow. In addition to reduced plasma flow, a decrease in the filtering surface area (Kf, LpA) occurs due to the adherence of inflammatory cells to the capillary wall and endothelial cell damage. All of these processes in concert account for the decrease in GFR seen in acute glomerulonephritis.

Immune injury in one portion of the glomerulus may lead to increases in glomerular hydrostatic pressures and plasma flows in other capillary loops and in other glomeruli as a compensatory mechanism to preserve GFR. These increased intraglomerular pressures and flows (hyperfiltration) contribute to maintaining GFR in the short term but appear to induce glomerular damage and destruction over longer periods of time. The principal morphologic consequence of these adaptive changes is glomerulosclerosis, a lesion characteristic of the chronic stages of most progressive glomerular diseases.

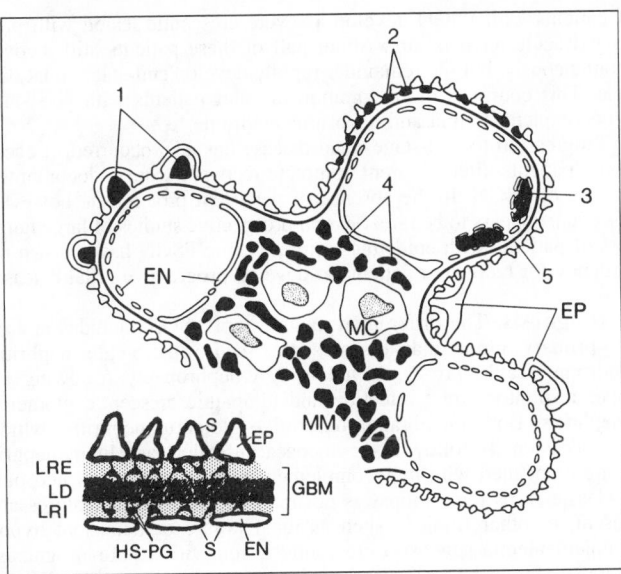

FIGURE 116-1 Schematic depiction of intraglomerular sites of immune complex formation. Subepithelial deposits such as those in postinfectious glomerulonephritis *(1)* or membranous nephropathy *(2)* apparently form by local, or in situ, mechanisms. Subendothelial *(3)* and mesangial *(4)* deposits are usually seen together and may form locally or result from the passive trapping of preformed immune complexes from the circulation. Anti-glomerular basement membrane (GBM) antibody deposits are in a linear pattern within the capillary wall itself *(5)*. The mechanisms of formation, composition, quantity, and relative accessibility of each of these deposits to circulating inflammatory cells are the major determinants of the type of lesion produced. The inset illustrates the three layers of the normal glomerular capillary wall, endothelial cells *(EN)*, GBM, and epithelial cells *(EP)*. The negative charge on the capillary wall results from the sialoproteins *(5)* coating the endothelial and epithelial cell surfaces and the heparin-sulfate proteoglycan (HS-PG) anionic sites in the lamina rare interna *(LRI)* and externa *(LRE)* of the GBM.

From Alder S, Couser WG: *Am J Med Sci* 289:55-60, 1985.

GLOMERULAR DISEASES THAT USUALLY PRESENT AS ACUTE GLOMERULONEPHRITIS
(Table 116-1)
Postinfectious Glomerulonephritis

Etiology and Incidence. The origin of postinfectious glomerulonephritis is a tissue-invading infection with a nephritogenic organism. Although poststreptococcal glomerulonephritis (PSGN) is the prototype of postinfectious glomerulonephritis, glomerulonephritis may occur after infection with a number of other agents including bacteria, viruses, fungi, protozoa, helminths, and spirochetes. Most of these organisms induce a proliferative glomerulonephritis associated with glomerular immune complex deposits. This section describes only PSGN in detail.

The incidence of PSGN varies considerably depending on the source and site of infection, but has diminished markedly in developed countries, due to improved hygiene and health care. PSGN may occur with streptococcal infection at any site, occurs primarily after exposure to a nephritogenic M type, and has a very variable attack rate. Nephritogenic streptococci are usually group A (beta-hemolytic) organisms. M type 12 is the most common source in the United States.

Pathogenesis and Pathophysiology. The glomerular injury observed is believed to be consequent to an inflammatory response generated by the formation of immune complex deposits that may contain streptococcal antigens in the mesangium and on the glomerular capillary walls. Several features of this disease including the latent period between the infection and the onset of nephritis, hypocomplementemia, and granular immune complex deposits in glomeruli suggest that the disease is similar to the acute bovine serum albumin (BSA)–serum sickness model in rabbits.

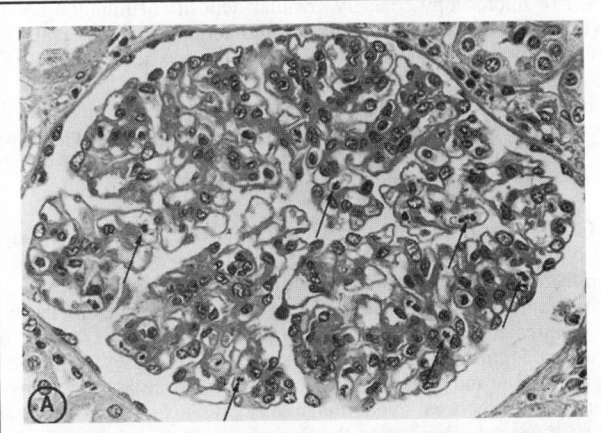

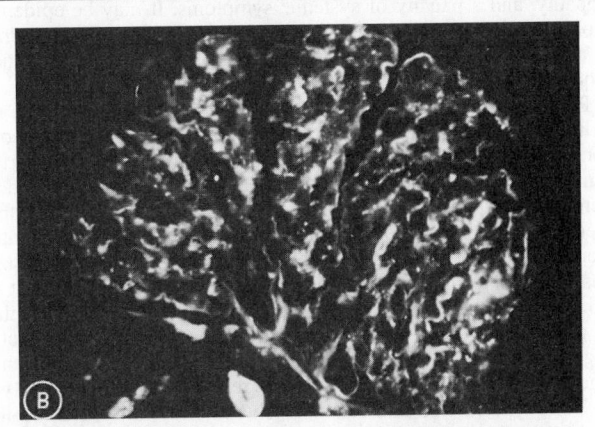

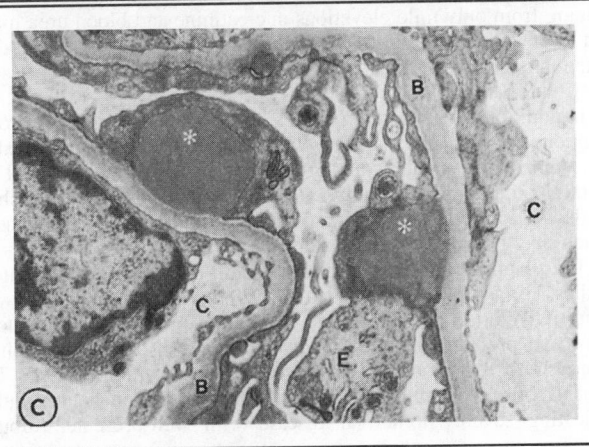

FIGURE 116-2 Renal biopsy findings from a patient with acute poststreptococcal glomerulonephritis. **A,** Light microscopy shows diffuse cellular proliferation with numerous neutrophils *(arrows)* in glomerular capillaries (hematoxylin-eosin stain; magnification ×375). **B,** Immunofluorescence shows diffuse coarsely granular deposits of immunoglobulin G on capillary walls and in the mesangium (magnification ×400). **C,** Electron microscopy demonstrates two large electron dense "humps" *(asterisks)* on the subepithelial surface of the capillary wall. *B,* basement membrane; *C,* capillary lumen, *E,* epithelial cell (uranyl and lead stain; magnification ×10,000).

Pathology. The characteristic features of PSGN by light microscopy, immunoflourescence microscopy (IF), and electron microscopy (EM) are illustrated in Fig. 116-2. By light microscopy the lesion is a diffuse proliferative glomerulonephritis (Fig. 116-2, *A*). All glomeruli exhibit a marked hypercellularity with narrowing or occlusion of capillary loops. In about 5% of patients, glomerular crescent formation similar to that in rapidly progressive glomerulonephritis (RPGN) (see later discussion) may be seen.

By IF microscopy coarsely granular deposits of immunoglobulin G (IgG) and C3 are seen along the glomerular capillary walls and less conspicuously in the mesangium in the acute phase (Fig. 116-2, *B*).

By EM the immune deposits are seen as discrete, subepithelial, electron-dense nodules, or "humps," (Fig. 116-2, *C*). Humps are usually present at the outset of the disease and persist for about 6 weeks before their gradual resolution makes identification difficult.

Clinical and Laboratory Features. The onset of clinical signs and symptoms of PSGN occurs after a 1- to 3-week latent period after infection with a nephritogenic strain of group A streptococcus. Nephritis due to a sporadic streptococcal pharyngitis develops in about 5% of infected patients after a latent period of about 10 days. It occurs most commonly in children between 3 and 12 years, usually during the winter and spring. Males are affected twice as commonly as females. Streptococcal pyoderma usually presents in the summer and fall with vesicular lesions on the skin of the extremities, regional adenopathy, and a paucity of systemic symptoms. It may be epidemic. Nephritis occurs in up to 50% of these patients after a latent period of about 3 weeks. Males and females are affected with equal frequency.

PSGN characteristically produces all the features of the acute nephritic syndrome, which is discussed in Chapter 107. The most common presenting features are the abrupt onset of gross hematuria and a smoky or coffee-colored appearance to the urine accompanied by edema and hypertension. The gross hematuria may last for 1 to 2 weeks, although microscopic hematuria can persist for months. Edema is often periorbital initially but may progress to generalized anasarca with ascites and pleural effusions. Proteinuria is almost invariably present, but daily urine protein excretion is usually less than 3.5 g. However, about 20% of patients will have transient nephrotic-range proteinuria at some time during their illness. Hypertension is largely volume-dependent due to renal retention of sodium and water. Both hypertension and edema resolve after the brisk diuresis that heralds recovery. Renal function is decreased to a variable degree ranging from only mild elevations in creatinine and blood urea nitrogen levels to acute oliguric renal failure requiring dialysis. Renal dysfunction is greater in older patients and patients with nephritis resulting from pharyngitis.

In addition to the classic features of the acute nephritic syndrome mentioned earlier, patients with PSGN may also exhibit other extrarenal signs and symptoms, including congestive heart failure and cerebral symptoms related to hypertension and cerebral edema such as headache, nausea and vomiting, and alterations in consciousness, which may progress to convulsions.

The diagnosis of acute PSGN is usually supported by laboratory studies. Urinalysis reveals evidence of glomerular inflammation with many red blood cells, red blood cell casts, occasional white blood cells, and protein. The need to examine a fresh urine specimen to demonstrate red blood cell casts cannot be overemphasized. The urine is often concentrated with a low urine sodium concentration indicating severe glomerular disease with well-presented tubular function.

Positive cultures for group A beta-hemolytic streptococci may be obtained from infected sites in about 25% of patients if treatment has not already been instituted. The most commonly measured serologic parameters are the antistreptolysin O (ASO) titer, which exceeds 200 Todd units within 1 to 3 weeks in about 70% of patients and persists for several months, and the streptozyme test, which is the most sensitive measure of antistreptococcal antibodies available.

Levels of C3 are low in over 95% of patients with PSGN during the first 2 weeks of the illness, whereas the classic pathway components C1, C4, and C2 are often normal, indicating activation predominantly of the alternate complement pathway. Neither the level of antistreptococcal antibody response nor the degree of hypocomplementemia correlates well with the severity or outcome of the renal disease.

With regard to prognosis, about 95% of patients recover normal renal function within 2 months of the onset of the disease, although abnormal proteinuria and hematuria may persist for 1 to 2 years. Spontaneous recovery is the rule even in patients with crescents and disease severe enough to require short periods of dialysis. About 5%

of patients with PSGN develop a severe crescentic lesion with prolonged acute renal failure. About half of these patients still recover spontaneously, but the remainder rapidly develop end-stage renal disease. This course is more common in older patients with persistent hypocomplementemia and nephrotic syndrome.

Progression to end-stage renal disease has also occurred in occasional patients after apparent complete recovery from a documented episode of PSGN. In the absence of persistent proteinuria, however, this event appears to be rare. Several prospective studies of large numbers of patients with epidemic forms of acute PSGN have shown no tendency for recovered patients to develop progressive renal disease.

Diagnosis. The differential diagnosis of PSGN includes any of the primary glomerular diseases that cause the acute nephritic syndrome (Table 116-1), including IgA nephropathy following an upper respiratory tract infection and idiopathic crescentic glomerulonephritis. Both membranoproliferative glomerulonephritis, which may occasionally follow a streptococcal infection, and lupus nephritis are associated with hypocomplementemia and must be ruled out. In classic cases renal biopsy is not required. If atypical features are present, or other findings such as renal failure or persistent hypocomplementemia suggest a crescentic lesion with a poor prognosis, a biopsy should be performed to determine if treatment for RPGN should be considered.

Treatment. The vast majority of patients recover spontaneously, regardless of the severity of the initial disease; therefore usually only supportive therapy is indicated. Antibiotic treatment is appropriate if evidence of persistent streptococcal infection is present. Early penicillin therapy may blunt rises in antistreptococcal antibody titers but does not reduce the incidence or severity of poststreptococcal nephritis. Sodium restriction and diuretics are critical in managing or preventing hypertension, edema, and congestive heart failure. Dialysis should be used if necessary. Spontaneous recovery has been reported following up to 31 days of oliguria.

Patients who have a severe, rapidly progressive course associated with extensive glomerular crescent formation have a form of rapidly progressive glomerulonephritis (RPGN) and may be considered for treatment as discussed later.

Other Postinfectious Glomerulonephritides

Subacute Bacterial Endocarditis (SBE). Some hematuria and proteinuria occur in about 70% of patients with SBE, but renal failure and nephrotic syndrome are uncommon. Renal involvement may be seen with infection of any heart valve and with a wide variety of organisms. Staphylococci and streptococci are most commonly involved. Renal lesions are most severe in patients with prolonged disease or right-sided cardiac involvement in which negative blood cultures may obscure the diagnosis. Associated laboratory abnormalities usually include reduced levels of both classic and alternate pathway complement components. The most common glomerular lesion is a focal proliferative glomerulonephritis often with necrosis and intracapillary thrombi associated with granular immune complex deposits of IgG, immunoglobulin M (IgM), and C3 by IF and mesangial and subendothelial deposits by EM. Both bacterial antigens and specific antibodies to them have been identified in the glomerular deposits of a few patients. Occasional patients with endocarditis develop a crescentic glomerulonephritis with rapid loss of renal function. The disease is usually not progressive, however, and resolves without specific therapy when the cardiac infection is eradicated.

Nephritis Associated With Visceral Abscesses. An association has been reported between bacterial abscesses at several sites, usually in the lung or abdominal cavity, with or without septicemia, and development of acute nephritis, often with oliguria, crescents, and acute renal failure. In contrast to the previously discussed diseases, patients with this condition commonly have normal serum complement levels, glomerular IF frequently is positive for C3 without immunoglobulins, and no bacterial antigens have been identified in the lesions. The pathogenesis of the glomerular lesion is not clear. The renal lesion is usually reversible if the septic site can be removed.

Immunoglobulin A Nephropathy

IgA nephropathy is usually a primary renal disease, but the same renal lesion can be associated with systemic manifestations (usually purpura, arthritis, and gastrointestinal tract involvement) in the Henoch-Schönlein syndrome, which is discussed later under glomerular involvement in systemic diseases. These two disorders probably present a spectrum of disease manifestations resulting from a common immunopathogenetic mechanism.

Etiology and Incidence. IgA nephropathy is the most common form of acute glomerulonephritis in the United States. It is even more common in Asian countries. The origin of IgA nephropathy is unknown.

Pathogenesis and Pathophysiology. The fact that IgA nephropathy frequently follows viral upper respiratory tract or gastrointestinal tract infections suggests a postinfectious process. The mechanisms leading to glomerular immune deposit formation are unclear but may involve a mucosal antibody response. IgA containing circulating immune complexes and IgA-fibronectin aggregates are often present, but it is not known if the mesangial deposits result from trapping of these macromolecules or from local immune complex formation in the mesangium. There is also evidence that an IgG autoantibody to a mesangial cell antigen may contribute to the disease. In some patients, extensive capillary wall deposits of IgA may occur and cause heavy proteinuria with a worse prognosis.

Pathology. Fig. 116-3 illustrates the typical light and IF findings in IgA nephropathy. The renal pathology in IgA nephropathy, Henoch-Schönlein purpura, and some cases of focal proliferative lupus nephritis are quite similar, but differentiation between these entities can usually be readily made by clinical criteria. The typical finding by light microscopy is a focal proliferative glomerulonephritis.

In contrast to the focal distribution of changes by light microscopy, IF reveals diffuse deposition of IgA, and often IgG and C3, in the mesangium of all glomeruli (Fig. 116-3, *B*). EM confirms mesangial deposits, and some extension to the subendothelial aspect of the capillary wall in paramesangial areas may be seen, usually in association with more severe glomerular histologic change and proteinuria.

Clinical and Laboratory Features. Half of all patients with IgA nephropathy come to medical attention with an acute nephritic syndrome usually characterized by gross hematuria that develops coincident with, or 24 to 48 hours after, an upper respiratory tract infection (50%), flulike illness (15%), or episode of gastroenteritis (10%). In contrast to PSGN, there is no significant latent period, and hypertension and edema during acute attacks are uncommon. The disease is one of younger patients, usually 15 to 35 years old, and affects males two to three times more often than females (see Table 116-1). The onset of gross hematuria may be accompanied by dull loin pain and occasionally vague constitutional symptoms. Although some decrease in renal function is common during attacks, acute renal failure is rare. Gross hematuria usually lasts 2 to 6 days. Proteinuria rarely exceeds 1 to 2 g/day; however, about 10% of patients can present with nephrotic syndrome. Some of these patients have extensive capillary wall immune deposits and a poor prognosis. Others have no capillary wall deposits, respond well to steroid therapy, and probably have nephrotic syndrome similar to MCD with superimposed incidental mesangial IgA deposits. Between episodes, persistent proteinuria and microscopic hematuria are common, and these abnormalities bring the remaining patients to medical attention. About half of the patients with gross hematuria have only a single recognized episode. The remainder have recurrent episodes that can continue for decades.

About 50% of patients with IgA nephropathy eventually have progressive loss of renal function. This course is more common in adults than children. Although no clinical or laboratory parameters can accurately predict prognosis, the presence of decreased renal function initially, hypertension early in the course, male sex, and proteinuria exceeding 3 g/day are all more common in patients with progressive disease. Occasional patients have extensive crescent formation and may follow a course similar to that described later for RPGN. Me-

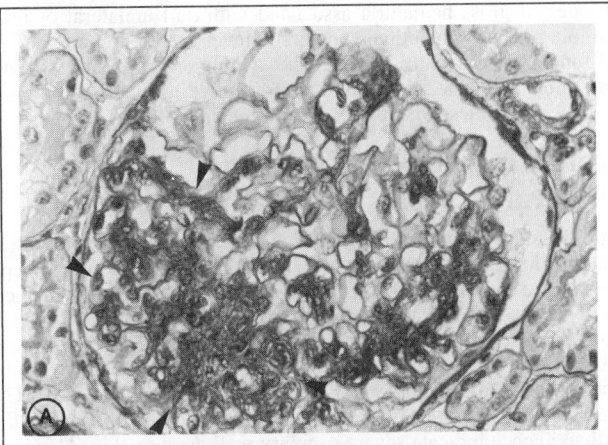

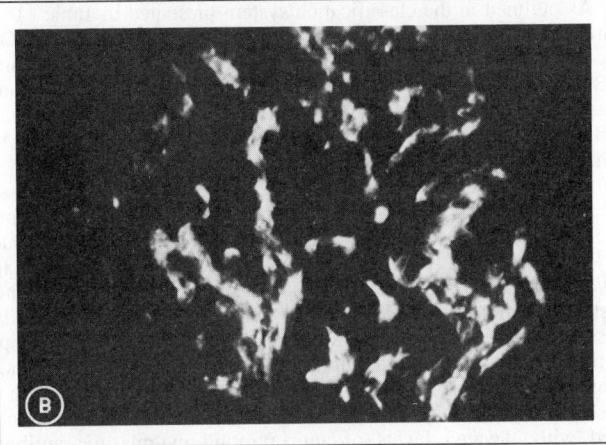

FIGURE 116-3   Renal biopsy findings from a patient with gross hematuria due to immunoglobulin A (IgA) nephropathy. **A,** Light microscopy shows a segmental area of cellular proliferation and mesangial matrix increase *(between arrowheads)* with sparing of adjacent capillary loops (periodic acid–Schiff stain; magnification ×465). **B,** Immunofluorescence shows nodular deposits of IgA confined to mesangial stalks (magnification ×400). Similar biopsy findings are present in the nephritis of Henoch-Schönlein purpura.

sangial IgA deposits have been shown to recur with high frequency in renal allografts, but they rarely cause acute nephritis or graft loss.

Most patients with IgA nephropathy or Henoch-Schönlein purpura have elevated levels of IgA-fibronectin aggregates. Serum complement levels are usually normal. About 50% of patients have elevations in serum levels of IgA.

Diagnosis. The diagnosis of IgA nephropathy is confirmed by the presence of focal nephritis associated with mesangial IgA deposits in a renal biopsy of a patient with nephritis without clinical or serologic evidence of systemic disease.

Treatment. The only therapy of established benefit in IgA nephropathy is oral fish oil, which may slow or halt slowly progressive disease. Hypertension may develop early in the course, before significant loss of renal function, and should be treated aggressively. In the rare patient who develops crescentic nephritis with a rapidly progressive course, treatment as discussed later for RPGN may be indicated. A subset of patients with nephrotic syndrome and mesangial IgA deposits may respond to oral steroid therapy, similar to patients with MCD (see later discussion).

Loin Pain–Hematuria Syndrome

A cause of recurrent gross hematuria that may be confused with IgA nephropathy is the loin pain–hematuria syndrome. This disorder, which generally affects young women, is characterized by recurrent episodes of gross hematuria associated with dull unilateral or bilateral loin pain and sometimes low-grade fever. Blood pressure and renal function are usually normal. The syndrome has been associated most often with the use of oral contraceptive agents and generally resolves when these agents are discontinued.

Rapidly Progressive (Crescentic) Glomerulonephritis

A third group of patients that may come to medical attention with an acute nephritic syndrome are those with RPGN. RPGN is not a separate disease entity but rather a clinicopathologic syndrome, which can occur with several systemic and primary renal diseases and may be initiated by several different pathogenetic mechanisms. Only diseases that produce rapid loss of renal function associated with extensive (usually over 50%) glomerular crescents are referred to as RPGN. Crescents develop after fibrin leakage across the glomerular capillary wall and hence indicate severe capillary wall damage (Fig. 116-4, *A*).

As outlined in the classification system presented in Table 116-2, patients with RPGN can be considered in three broad categories. One group (20%) has crescentic glomerulonephritis mediated by anti-GBM antibody deposition either with pulmonary involvement (Goodpasture's syndrome) or without pulmonary disease (idiopathic anti-GBM nephritis). These two groups of patients are discussed later. Another group (40%) has granular immune complex deposits in glomeruli. These patients may have a crescentic form of a primary renal disease such as PSGN, IgA nephropathy, or type I membranoproliferative glomerulonephritis (MPGN) or a systemic disease such as lupus nephritis, Henoch-Schönlein purpura, or essential mixed cryoglobulinemia. These diseases can usually be diagnosed by their distinctive clinical and pathologic or serologic features and are discussed in more detail elsewhere in this chapter. A third group of patients with crescentic glomerulonephritis (40%) have disease without glomerular immune deposits. Most of these patients have a form of vasculitis, which may be renal-limited or systemic, and are associated with elevated levels of antineutrophil cytoplasmic antibody (ANCA). Among ANCA-positive patients, those with primary renal disease are generally referred to as ANCA-positive glomerulor nephritis. Other terms sometimes applied to this group of patients include *pauciimmune glomerulonephritis, microscopic polyarteritis nodosa,* or, when the disease follows an initiating allergic event such as a drug reaction, *hypersensitivity vasculitis.* Systemic forms of ANCA-positive vasculitis that involve the kidney include classic polyarteritis nodosa and Wegener's granulomatosis, which are discussed later in the chapter (see Glomerular Involvement in Systemic Diseases). Occasional patients with a lesion similar to that in ANCA-positive glomerulonephritis do not have demonstrable ANCA antibodies (idiopathic RPGN). Although these patients may have a different disease process, they are clinically similar to ANCA-positive patients and are treated similarly.

RPGN Due to Antiglomerular Basement Membrane Antibody
Goodpasture's syndrome
Etiology and incidence. Goodpasture's syndrome is a rare disease characterized by a triad of pulmonary hemorrhage, iron deficiency anemia, and glomerulonephritis due to anti-GBM antibody deposition in the lungs and kidneys. It accounts for about 5% of all patients seen with RPGN and less than 1% of all cases of glomerulonephritis. The disease is due to the production and deposition of antibodies to antigens on the alpha-3 chain of type IV collagen. The events that initiate anti-GBM antibody production are not known. Several potential etiologic factors have been implicated, including influenza A viral infection and hydrocarbon solvent exposure. An increased incidence of human leukocyte antigen (HLA)-DRw2 and B7 antigens has been reported in Goodpasture's syndrome (relative risk 15 to 34 times normal) and is associated with a worse prognosis, suggesting that immunogenetic factors also play a role.

Pathogenesis and pathophysiology. The production of anti-GBM antibody results in the direct binding of IgG in a linear pattern by IF to GBM (Fig. 116-4, *A*). The immunologic and physiologic consequences of this process have been discussed earlier. In general, anti-GBM disease appears to be self-limited. Renal function can be pre-

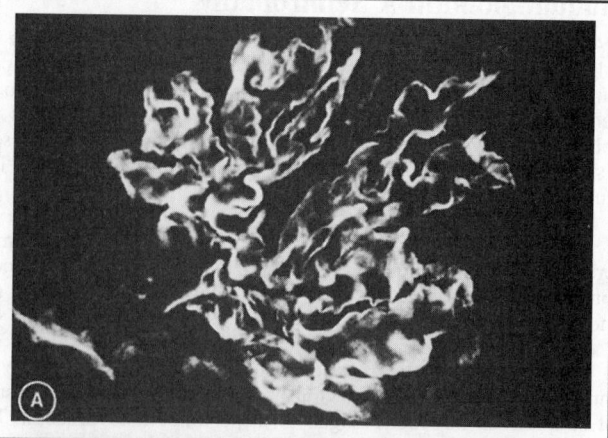
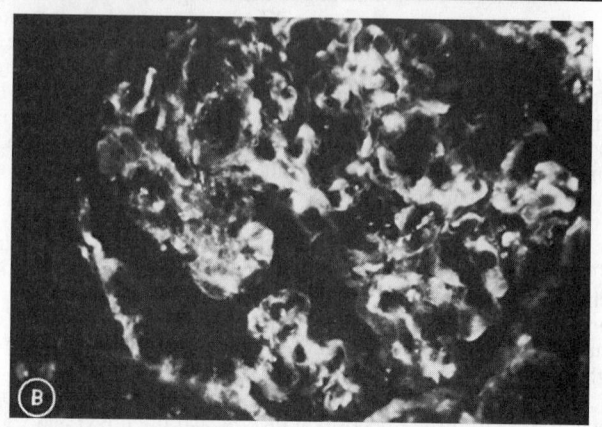
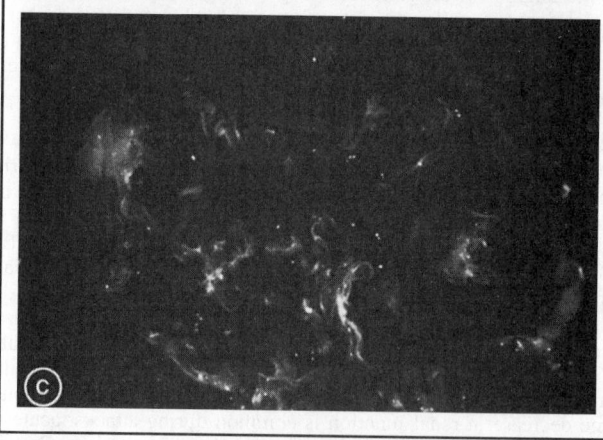

FIGURE 116-4   Immunofluorescent staining for immunoglobulin G in three patients with rapidly progressive glomerulonephritis illustrating the three immunopathogenetic mechanisms that may be present. **A,** Immunoglobulin G is deposited in the continuous, linear pattern along all capillary loops characteristic of anti-GBM antibody deposition. **B,** Coarsely granular immune complex deposits are present on capillary walls and in the mesangium in a patient with rapidly progressive glomerulonephritis resulting from systemic lupus erythematosus. **C,** There are no significant deposits of immunoglobulin G in a patient with crescentic glomerulonephritis and antineutrophil cytoplasm antibody (magnification ×325).

served if glomerular destruction can be minimized until production of pathogenic antibody ceases.

The pulmonary lesions in Goodpasture's syndrome also appear to be mediated by the same anti-GBM antibody that cross-reacts with alveolar basement membrane but gains access to alveolar basement membrane only if prior lung injury is present. For example, many patients with anti-GBM nephritis and pulmonary hemorrhage are

Table 116-2 Classification of crescentic glomerulonephritis

CATEGORY	PRIMARY RENAL	SYSTEMIC
I. Anti-GBM antibody mediated	Idiopathic Complicating membranous	Pulmonary-renal (Goodpasture's)
II. Immune complex mediated	Postinfectious GN IgA nephropathy MPGN type I	Lupus nephritis Henoch-Schönlein purpura Essential mixed cryoglobulinemia
III. No immune deposits		
a. ANCA-positive	ANCA-positive GN	Microscopic polyarteritis nodosa Wegener's granulomatosis
b. ANCA-negative	Idiopathic crescentic GN	

cigarette smokers or have a recent history of exposure to other respiratory toxins or of an influenza-like illness.

Pathology. The histology in Goodpasture's syndrome is that of an initial focal proliferative and necrotizing glomerular lesion that progresses rapidly to diffuse proliferation with crescents as described earlier. The IF findings are diffuse linear deposition of IgG (or rarely, IgA) in a continuous, uninterrupted pattern along the GBM (see Fig. 116-4, *A*) accompanied in most cases by C3 in a similar pattern. Many patients with Goodpasture's syndrome also show linear deposits of IgG along the tubular basement membranes. Anti-GBM antibody deposits cannot be identified by EM.

Clinical and laboratory features. Goodpasture's syndrome is primarily a disease of young white males (male/female ratio, 6:1 with a mean age of 21 years) who develop hemoptysis, iron-deficiency anemia, and RPGN associated with anti-GBM antibody deposits. In most cases the pulmonary manifestations appear first and range from mild hemoptysis with bilateral, fluffy alveolar infiltrates to severe, life-threatening pulmonary hemorrhage with hypoxemia and respiratory failure. About one third of patients with Goodpasture's syndrome die of pulmonary involvement. It must be emphasized that Goodpasture's syndrome is not the only glomerular disease in which both pulmonary and renal manifestations may occur. Other such diseases include systemic lupus erythematosus, Wegener's granulomatosis, Henoch-Schönlein syndrome, mixed cryoglobulinemia, and idiopathic crescentic glomerulonephritis. The term Goodpasture's syndrome is reserved only for those patients with the triad of iron-deficiency anemia, pulmonary hemorrhage, and glomerulonephritis mediated by anti-GBM antibody.

Anemia generally parallels the degree of pulmonary involvement and is secondary to blood loss and iron sequestration in the lungs. Although microscopic hematuria and proteinuria usually occur within 2 weeks of the onset of pulmonary disease, some patients may have several exacerbations and remissions of pulmonary disease before nephritis becomes apparent, and in occasional patients nephritis never develops.

Renal involvement in Goodpasture's syndrome is initially manifest as microscopic hematuria, which progresses to include proteinuria and decreased renal function. Although rare cases of mild renal disease with spontaneous recovery have been reported, the lesion is usually severe and progressive with rapid development of oliguria and renal failure. The mean time from diagnosis to renal failure is about 3 to 4 weeks. Nephrotic-range proteinuria and hypertension are usually not seen, and kidney size is normal.

In addition to the characteristic urinary abnormalities of the acute nephritic syndrome, laboratory abnormalities in Goodpasture's syndrome include circulating antibody to human GBM in the serum in most patients. Antibody levels roughly parallel activity of the renal disease and usually persist for several months. Serum levels of complement are normal. About 30% of patients with Goodpasture's syndrome also have elevated ANCA antibodies. These patients often have significant extra renal disease but respond well to treatment.

Diagnosis. The diagnosis of Goodpasture's syndrome is made in patients with pulmonary hemorrhage or alveolar infiltrates and glomerulonephritis associated with positive anti-GBM antibody assays or linear deposits of IgG by IF. The almost uniformly poor prognosis and potential benefit from early treatment in Goodpasture's syndrome make it imperative to establish an accurate diagnosis as quickly as possible. A presumptive diagnosis may be made by demonstrating anti-GBM antibody in the serum in the presence of clinically characteristic pulmonary and renal manifestations.

Treatment. Steroid pulse therapy as described later for idiopathic crescentic glomerulonephritis has been associated with a dramatic improvement in severe pulmonary hemorrhage but has less effect on the renal lesion. The current treatment of choice for renal involvement in Goodpasture's syndrome is plasma exchange therapy to remove circulating anti-GBM antibody combined with prednisone, 1 mg/kg/day, and cyclophosphamide, 2 to 3 mg/kg per day to inhibit further antibody production. Plasma exchanges of up to 4 L are performed on a daily or alternate-day basis until anti-GBM antibody is no longer detectable in the circulation and disease progression has halted. Therapy may require several weeks. Replacement is with albumin, or, when pulmonary hemorrhage is active, with fresh-frozen plasma. Overall survival in anti-GBM nephritis appears to be improved by plasma exchange therapy. However, the response rate in patients who are oliguric at the time of presentation or have serum creatinines exceeding 6 mg/dl is very low, again emphasizing the need for early diagnosis. In patients with end-stage renal disease due to anti-GBM nephritis, renal transplantation appears to be a safe and effective form of therapy if it is delayed until anti-GBM antibody is no longer detectable in the serum.

Anti-GBM glomerulonephritis without pulmonary involvement. Over 50% of patients with RPGN mediated by anti-GBM antibodies do not have the pulmonary hemorrhage characteristic of Goodpasture's syndrome and have no other extrarenal manifestations of their disease. In this group of patients the age and sex distribution and the clinical manifestations, course, and prognosis are essentially the same as those described for idiopathic crescentic glomerulonephritis, although patients in their 20s and 30s may be somewhat more commonly affected. Defining the anti-GBM antibody pathogenesis of this disease is essential to select the most appropriate therapy and to avoid recurrent anti-GBM nephritis in transplants. Diagnosis and treatment would be the same as that described for Goodpasture's syndrome.

ANCA-positive crescentic glomerulonephritis

Etiology and incidence. The most common cause of RPGN is a vasculitic process, which may be confined to the glomerular capillaries (ANCA-positive crescentic glomerulonephritis) or part of a systemic disease (microscopic polyarteritis nodosa). In both cases the disease is associated with elevated levels of antineutrophil cytoplasmic antibody (ANCA) and occurs in the absence of linear or granular immune deposits in the glomeruli. The origin of ANCA-positive glomerulonephritis is not known. In some cases the disease is preceded by a flulike illness with fever, weight loss, and malaise, reflecting a systemic vasculitis. The presence of elevated ANCA suggests that the disorder is autoimmune in nature.

Pathogenesis and pathophysiology. In the ANCA-positive glomerulonephritis, capillary wall injury results from some undefined mechanism, which is associated with increased levels of ANCA and does not produce glomerular immunoglobulin deposits. The mechanisms of tissue injury in ANCA-positive vasculitis are unclear. It seems likely that many severe cases of glomerulonephritis are also accompanied by some ischemic acute tubular necrosis. The degree of recovery of renal function depends on whether the underlying disease process resolves spontaneously or whether it can be modified by therapeutic intervention before irreversible glomerular alterations such as thrombosis, necrosis, sclerosis, and scar formation develop.

Pathology. The principal finding by light microscopy in crescentic glomerulonephritis of any cause is the presence of extensive glomerular crescent formation, often with compression of the glomerular tuft (Fig. 116-5, *A*). In most cases over 50% of glomeruli have crescents. Pathology in the glomerular tuft itself is variable. A common finding is a focal segmental necrotizing glomerular lesion. This lesion is generally regarded as indicative of a renal capillary vasculitis, particularly when it occurs in a setting of constitutional symp-

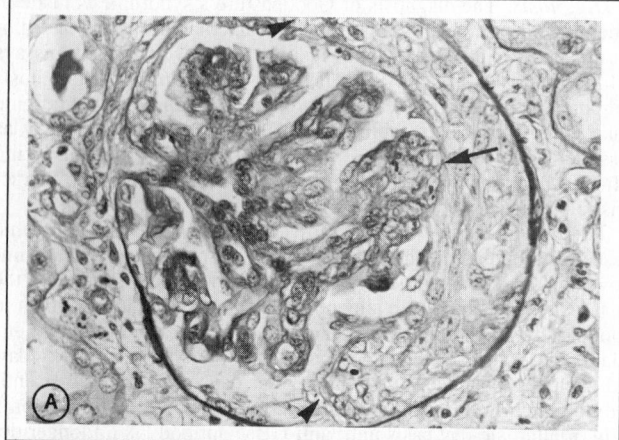

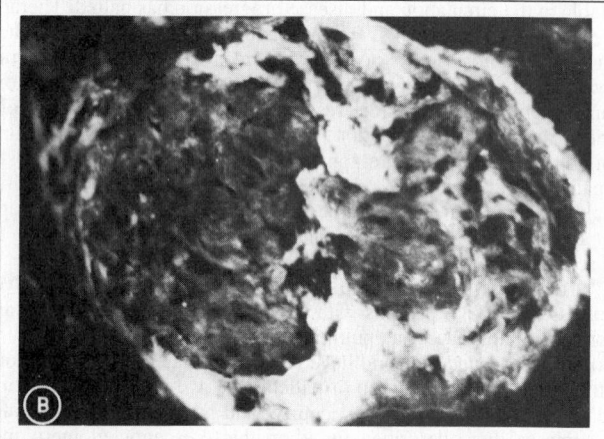

FIGURE 116-5 Renal biopsy findings from a patient with rapidly progressive glomerulonephritis. **A,** Light microscopy demonstrates a large crescent compressing the glomerular tuft, which shows an area of segmental necrosis *(arrow)* (periodic acid-Schiff stain; magnification ×325). **B,** Immunofluorescent staining shows fibrin deposition in the area of crescent formation (magnification ×350).

toms and no immune deposits. Studies have demonstrated that the clinical manifestations and response to therapy of patients with focal necrotizing glomerulonephritis and crescents are much the same, regardless of whether histologic evidence of extraglomerular small vessel vasculitis is present. Because many glomerular diseases (Table 116-2) may be accompanied by glomerular necrosis and crescent formation, these findings alone are not diagnostic of any specific disease entity. Other features in the biopsy, such as diffuse proliferative changes and humps in poststreptococcal glomerulonephritis or granulomata in Wegener's granulomatosis, may assist in the differential diagnosis.

In addition to the glomerular changes, an interstitial infiltrate of mononuclear cells is commonly present and occasionally may assume a periglomerular distribution. Both the severity of the interstitial changes and the percentage of glomeruli showing crescent formation correlate roughly with the clinical course and prognosis.

Most patients with ANCA-positive glomerulonephritis have no pathogenic glomerular immune deposits by IF (Fig. 116-5, *C*). In all patients, regardless of the underlying disease mechanism, fibrin-related antigens are easily demonstrable in glomerular crescents (Fig. 116-5, *B*).

Findings by EM confirm those by IF. No deposits are seen in anti-GBM disease or crescentic glomerulonephritis with negative IF.

Clinical and laboratory features. The onset of the disease is usually abrupt but can be insidious, and patients may come to medical attention either with an acute nephritic syndrome (50%) and rapidly deteriorating renal function or with oliguria, elevated serum creatinine levels, and the recent onset of signs and symptoms of uremia

(50%). The duration of disease from onset to severe renal failure varies from 1 to 2 weeks to a few months. Men are affected twice as often as women, and the median age is 58 years, although cases have been reported in children and in adults over 80.

Many patients give a history of a recent viral-like syndrome with fever, myalgias, and polyarthralgias. Transient pulmonary infiltrates by radiography or small amounts of hemoptysis are also common, but pulmonary manifestations are rarely of major clinical significance as they are in Goodpasture's syndrome (see earlier discussion). These clinical signs and symptoms are probably consequent to extrarenal vasculitis, which may be demonstrated in a renal biopsy. In the absence of volume overload, blood pressure is usually normal, edema is absent, and kidney size is normal. Renal failure is the only manifestation of the disease to cause significant morbidity, and the course and prognosis of the renal lesion is the same, regardless of whether other systemic manifestations of vasculitis are present.

All patients have proteinuria, hematuria, and usually red blood cell casts. Proteinuria in excess of 3 g/day is unusual, and nephrotic syndrome is rarely seen. A mild anemia is common, and the erythrocyte sedimentation rate is always elevated. Tests for complement anti-GBM antibody and circulating immune complexes are normal or negative. However, levels of ANCA are usually elevated in crescentic glomerulonephritis without immune deposits, and antibody levels may parallel disease activity.

Diagnosis. The differential diagnosis of crescentic glomerulonephritis includes all of the diseases listed in Table 116-2. When crescentic glomerulonephritis develops as a primary renal disease, patients can generally be divided into ANCA-positive and ANCA-negative groups. ANCA-negative causes of crescentic glomerulonephritis include diseases such as systemic lupus erythematosus, Henoch-Schönlein purpura, essential mixed cryoglobulinemia, and anti-GBM disease. These entities are discussed elsewhere in this chapter and can generally be readily diagnosed by available serologic tests and biopsy characteristics. ANCA-positive patients include those with Wegener's granulomatosis, polyarteritis nodosa, and the pauciimmune form of crescentic glomerulonephritis. Wegener's granulomatosis is characterized by upper respiratory tract and pulmonary disease, as well as nephritis and ANCA antibodies usually directed to proteinase 3 (C-ANCA).

Patients with polyarteritis nodosa demonstrate prominent multisystem dysfunction, usually with purpura and necrotizing vasculitis on biopsy. Patients with crescentic glomerulonephritis are usually ANCA positive with antibody usually specific for myeloperoxidase (P-ANCA), and have a variant of the syndrome with renal involvement invariably present, extrarenal disease less evident, and usually no extraglomerular vasculitic changes on renal biopsy.

Treatment. The natural history of RPGN is difficult to define because virtually all patients have received some form of therapy. Favorable prognostic factors include a young age at the time of onset, a history of a preceding infectious episode, absence of oliguria and hypertension, serum creatinine level below 6 mg/dl at presentation, and fewer than 50% crescents in the renal biopsy. Response rates approaching 75% have been reported in patients treated with either methylprednisolone pulse therapy or plasma exchange. In pulse therapy methylprednisolone, 30 mg/kg to a maximum of 3 g, is given intravenously over 20 minutes on a daily or alternate-day basis for three doses followed by oral prednisone, 2 mg/kg, which is tapered over several months. About 75% of patients, including some who were oliguric and on dialysis, have shown a dramatic response with a return of renal function to normal or near-normal levels. Responses have generally been evident within 5 to 10 days and continued over 4 to 6 weeks. Some patients, however, progress to renal failure later, despite an impressive initial response. Because of the vasculitic nature of crescentic glomerulonephritis, most patients are also treated with cytotoxic drugs, usually cyclophosphamide, 1 to 2 mg/kg per day, or pulse intravenous cyclophosphamide, 500 mg/M^2 per month. Any patient with signs or symptoms of a systemic vasculitic disease, positive ANCA, or vasculitis or focal necrotizing glomerulonephritis on renal biopsy should receive cytotoxic drug therapy. No data compare the efficacy of daily oral cyclophosphamide versus monthly pulse cyclophosphamide, but the latter appears to be efficacious and associated with fewer side effects in treating lupus nephritis.

The reported experience with renal transplantation in ANCA-positive crescentic glomerulonephritis is minimal, but the disease appears to recur rarely in allografted kidneys.

GLOMERULAR DISEASES THAT USUALLY PRESENT AS IDIOPATHIC NEPHROTIC SYNDROME

The pathophysiology of alterations in the glomerular capillary wall that result in proteinuria, various causes of proteinuria other than glomerular disease, and the clinical consequences of massive urinary protein loss have been discussed in detail in Chapters 105 and 108 and are not reviewed here. However, it is important to be aware that nephrotic syndrome may result from many different diseases. Although the diseases discussed earlier present most commonly as acute glomerulonephritis and those that follow are usually characterized initially by nephrotic syndrome, this separation is arbitrary. It is also arbitrary to designate a particular value for urine protein excretion, such as the traditional 3.5 g/day, as separating those diseases that usually cause nephrotic syndrome from other glomerular diseases. Thus nephrotic syndrome may be a manifestation of almost any glomerular disease. Moreover, all diseases that can cause nephrotic syndrome are sometimes seen in milder forms or earlier stages with proteinuria, which is not in the nephrotic range. Similarly, the development of the various clinical and biochemical derangements, such as hypoalbuminemia, edema, hyperlipidemia, and lipiduria, which are commonly seen in nephrotic syndrome, may be modified by a number of host factors such as GFR, nutritional intake, hepatic disease, and age.

In adults about one third of patients with nephrotic syndrome have a systemic disease such as diabetes, systemic lupus erythematosus, and amyloid. The remaining two thirds of patients have idiopathic nephrotic syndrome. Most patients with idiopathic nephrotic syndrome have one of three types of glomerular diseases: minimal change (focal sclerosis), membranous nephropathy, or membranoproliferative glomerulonephritis. The most common types are MCD or focal sclerosis in children and membranous nephropathy in adults. The approximate prevalence and clinical features of each of these lesions in large series of children and adults with idiopathic nephrotic syndrome is presented in Table 116-3.

Minimal Change Disease (Lipoid Nephrosis, Nil Disease)

Etiology and Incidence. Despite its relative frequency and association with several clinical events, the origin of MCD remains unclear. In occasional patients MCD develops with or without interstitial nephritis as an allergic reaction to various nonsteroidal antiinflammatory agents. The disease causes idiopathic nephrotic syndrome in about 75% of children and 15% of adults. The incidence varies somewhat in different parts of the world, but it is estimated to affect two to three patients per year per 100,000 population under age 16 years in the United States and Europe. Focal glomerular sclerosis (FGS), which is seen in about 10% of children and adults with idiopathic nephrotic syndrome, is treated here as a separate clinical entity (see later discussion). Many authors, however, now regard the histologic lesion of FGS as simply a marker of a more severe form of MCD, which results in structural glomerular damage and is often resistant to steroid therapy.

Pathogenesis and Pathophysiology. The pathogenesis of MCD is unknown. Recent evidence suggests that T cells from patients with active MCD produce a soluble factor that induces a similar lesion when infused into animals (see Chapter 108 for a discussion of the pathophysiology of the nephrotic syndrome that characterizes MCD).

Pathology. The biopsy changes in MCD are illustrated in Fig. 116-6. As suggested by the terms *minimal change,* or *nil* disease, glomeruli by light microscopy generally appear entirely normal (Fig. 116-6, *A*). By light microscopy alone the presence of normal glomeruli does not exclude the presence of FGS in unbiopsied glomeruli, nor does it distinguish this disease from early membranous

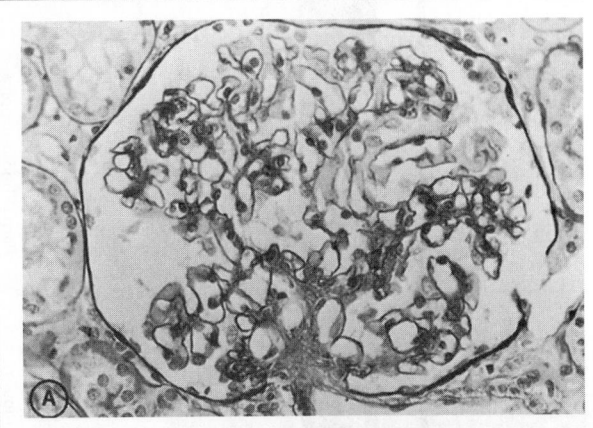
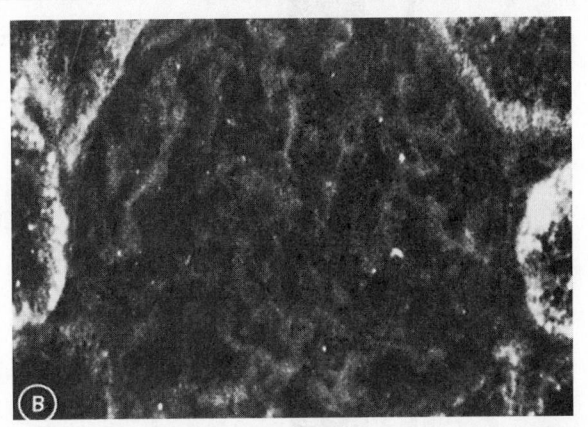
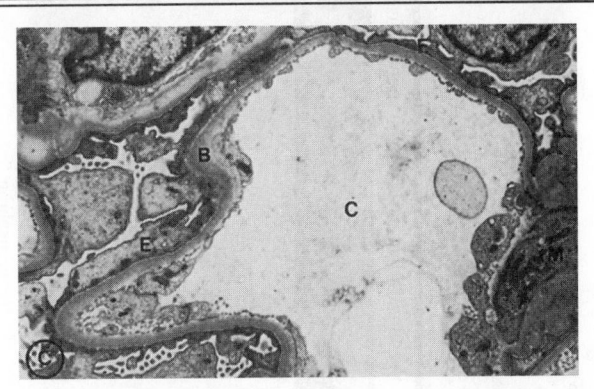

FIGURE 116-6   Renal biopsy findings in idiopathic nephrotic syndrome resulting from minimal change disease. **A,** By light microscopy the glomerulus is normal (periodic acid–Schiff stain; magnification ×600). **B,** Immunofluorescence shows no glomerular immune deposits (magnification ×500). **C,** Electron microscopy shows no deposits and diffuse effacement of epithelial cell *(E)* foot processes. B, Basement membrane; C, capillary lumen (uranyl and lead stain; magnification ×5600).

nephropathy. By IF there is no glomerular deposition of immunoglobulins or complement in typical MCD except for occasional traces of IgM or C3 in a nonspecific pattern in the mesangium of some glomeruli (Fig. 116-6, *B*). The only consistent abnormality is seen by EM, which reveals wide spread effacement, or "fusion," of epithelial cell foot processes (Fig. 116-6, *C*). Foot process fusion is characteristic of MCD but is not specific. It occurs in all glomerular diseases associated with significant proteinuria.

Clinical and Laboratory Features. MCD is primarily a disease of childhood with a peak incidence between 2 and 6 years of

Table 116-3 Summary of primary renal diseases that become evident as idiopathic nephrotic syndrome

DISEASES	MINIMAL CHANGE DISEASE	FOCAL GLOMERULAR SCLEROSIS	MEMBRANOUS NEPHROPATHY	MEMBRANOPROLIFERATIVE GLOMERULONEPHRITIS	
				TYPE I	TYPE II
Frequency*					
Children	75%	10%	<5%	10%	<5%
Adults	15%	35%	35%	10%	<5%
Clinical manifestations					
Age	2-6, some adults	2-6, some adults	40-50	5-40	5-20
Sex	2:1 male	1.3:1 male	2:1 male	2:1 female	2:1 female
Nephrotic syndrome	100%	90%	80%	60%	60%
Asymptomatic proteinuria	0	10%	20%	40%	40%
Hematuria	No	40%	20%	80%	80%
Hypertension	10%	20% early	Infrequent	35%	35%
Rate of progression	Does not progress	10 years	50% in 10-20 years	10-20 years	5-15 years
Associated conditions	Allergy to NSAIDs, Hodgkin's disease	Heroin nephropathy, AIDS	Renal vein thrombosis, cancer, SLE, hepatitis	Hepatitis C cryoglobulinemia	Partial lipodystrophy
Recurs in transplants	Yes	50%	Rarely	30%	90%
Laboratory findings	Manifestations of nephrotic syndrome	Manifestations of nephrotic syndrome	Manifestations of nephrotic syndrome	Low C1, C4, C3-C9; cryoglobulins; anti-HCV antibody	Normal C1, C4; low C3-C9; C3 nephritic factor
Immunogenetics	DR7 (6)†	DR4 (5-6)	DR3 (2-12)	None	DR7 (9)
Renal pathologic study					
Light microscopy	Normal	Focal sclerotic lesions	Thickened GBM, spikes	Thickened GBM, proliferation, lobulation	Same as type I
Immunofluorescence	Negative	IgM, C3 in sclerotic lesions	Fine granular IgG, C3	Granular IgG, C3	C3 only
Electron microscopy	Foot process fusion	Foot process fusion	Subepithelial deposits	Mesangial and subendothelial deposits	Dense deposits
Response to steroids	90%	20%-40%, may slow progression	Rare	Rare	None established
Other treatment	None	Cytotoxic drugs if steroid resistant	Steroids and cytotoxic drugs in high-risk patients	Alpha interferon if HCV positive	None

*Approximate frequency as a cause of idiopathic nephrotic syndrome. About 10% of adult nephrotic syndrome is due to various diseases that usually present with acute glomerulonephritis (Table 116-1).
†Relative risk.
GBM, glomerular basement membrane; IgG, IgM, immunoglobulins G and M; HCV, hepatitis C virus; NSAIDs, nonsteroidal antiinflammatory drugs; SLE, systemic lupus erythematosus.

age and is the cause of about 75% of childhood nephrotic syndrome (see Table 116-3). It may also occur in adults. Boys are affected twice as often as girls in childhood, but in adults the sex incidence is about equal. The disease virtually always presents as a severe nephrotic syndrome with heavy proteinuria, hypoalbuminemia, edema, hyperlipidemia, and lipiduria. Urine protein excretion exceeding 40 g/day and serum albumin levels of less than 1.0 g% are not unusual. In the absence of significant intravascular volume depletion, blood pressure and renal function are usually normal. However, severe volume contraction may occur and can produce hypotension, prerenal azotemia, and occasional acute oliguric renal failure, which is reversible with volume repletion. Acute renal failure, which may be due to intrarenal edema and may be reversible with diuretic therapy, has also been reported. Edema is common and often progresses to generalized anasarca.

Patients with MCD may have a variety of secondary complications of nephrotic syndrome including an increased susceptibility to infection, usually with gram-positive organisms, due to reduced serum levels of IgG; a tendency to form spontaneous thromboses in renal and peripheral veins and pulmonary arteries with thromboembolic phenomena; severe hyperlipidemia; and protein malnutrition due to negative nitrogen balance. In adult patients particular attention must be given to the possibility of an occult lymphoma, because MCD may be associated with Hodgkin's disease. In such patients the nephrotic syndrome often precedes clinical evidence of tumor.

There are no laboratory abnormalities specific for MCD, although most patients have unexpectedly low levels of antibodies to streptococcal antigens (ASO titers). Other abnormalities may occur with severe nephrotic syndrome of any cause. The urinalysis reveals nephrotic changes with proteinuria, free fat, oval fat bodies, and fatty casts. Microscopic hematuria is rare, and gross hematuria and red cell casts are not seen. Proteinuria is generally selective (greater than 90% albumin) in children, but may be nonselective in adults. Occasional patients exhibit proximal tubular dysfunction with wasting of phosphate, urate, bicarbonate, and amino acids, which results in lowered serum levels of these substances and occasionally leads to rickets or osteomalacia. Tubular dysfunction is presumably related to toxic effects of increased protein and lipid filtration and reabsorption. Levels of serum cholesterol, phospholipids, and triglycerides are elevated. Serum albumin and IgG levels are low. Alpha$_2$ macroglobulin, IgM, IgE, and clotting factors V, VII, VIII, X, and fibrinogen are often elevated. These elevations, along with the frequent thrombocytosis and hypovolemia, contribute to a hypercoaguable state. T3 resin uptake is often low because of urinary loss of thyroxin-binding globulin, but thyroid function is usually normal.

Diagnosis. In childhood the development of nephrotic syndrome with normal renal function, benign urine sediment, normal blood pressure, and normal complement levels makes the diagnosis of MCD so likely that steroid therapy may be initiated without performing a renal biopsy unless renal function deteriorates or there is no response to therapy. The diagnosis is confirmed if a typical complete remission occurs after steroid therapy. In adults the diagnosis is made by demonstrating the features of MCD in a renal biopsy.

Course and Treatment. The spontaneous remission rate has been variously estimated at 25% to 40%. Despite the relatively high spontaneous remission rate and the fact that MCD probably does not progress to renal failure, the mortality rate from this disease in children was over 50% at 5 years before the use of steroid therapy. Most deaths resulted from bacterial infections or thromboembolic events.

It has never been proved in a controlled study that steroid therapy improves survival in MCD. The response of MCD to steroids, however, is generally dramatic and has led to the widespread belief that such therapy is beneficial. Conventional doses of oral prednisone are 60 mg/M^2 per day for children and 1 mg/kg per day for adults, generally given on an alternate-day basis after remission is induced. At least four clinical courses can be identified in treated patients, which appear to be similar in both children and adults:

1. Nonresponders: Patients who do not become free of proteinuria after 8 to 12 weeks of therapy generally fail to respond thereafter. In most series this represents about 10% of all patients, and they usually have, or develop, evidence of structural glomerular damage in the form of focal glomerular sclerosis (FGS). The relationship of FGS to MCD is discussed later.
2. Primary responders (90%): Most patients (70%) enter remission and become protein-free within 4 weeks after starting steroid therapy, and more have remission within 12 weeks. Of these, about 15% remain protein free when steroids are tapered after several weeks of remission. The remaining 85% have one or more relapses. Two thirds have frequent relapses or remain dependent on steroids to maintain remission.
3. Frequent relapsers: Relapses occur more than twice a year when steroids are discontinued and persist for many years but are always steroid responsive. Eventually, spontaneous remission occurs in most of these patients.
4. Steroid-dependent: These patients always relapse when steroids are reduced below a certain level but respond when the dosage is increased.

In the latter two groups of patients (frequent relapsers and steroid dependent), steroid toxicity may force consideration of alternative approaches to therapy.

Patients who are frequent relapsers or steroid dependent may have long-term consequences of persistent nephrotic syndrome. Such patients can be treated with an alkylating agent, either cyclophosphamide, 2 to 3 mg/kg per day, or chlorambucil, 0.2 to 0.3 mg/kg per day, for 8 to 12 weeks. These agents clearly increase the frequency and duration of subsequent remissions and reduce the need for steroids. Over half of frequently relapsing and steroid-dependent patients treated with a second drug are reported to be in remission 4 years later. The use of such agents should be reserved for patients with severe nephrotic syndrome and steroid toxicity and must be undertaken with the full knowledge that susceptibility is increased to a host of complications, particularly gonadal failure and an increased incidence of leukemia and probably other malignancies in later life. The management of steroid-resistant nephrotic syndrome with MCD on biopsy is discussed with FGS later.

Mesangial Proliferative Disease

Some patients present with idiopathic nephrotic syndrome and varying degrees of mesangial cell proliferation by light microscopy in the absence of definite focal sclerotic changes. An additional subgroup develops diffuse mesangial deposits of IgM and C3 by IF. Some authors put such patients into separate diagnostic categories such as mesangioproliferative glomerulonephritis or IgM mesangial nephropathy. Mesangial changes tend to be accompanied by more hematuria, a tendency to hypertension, a relatively poor response to steroids, and progressive renal failure due to FGS. Although each of these entities may represent a different disease mechanism, I believe that pure MCD, the various degrees of mesangial disease seen in some cases of idiopathic nephrotic syndrome, and FGS probably represent a spectrum of increasingly severe glomerular injury and steroid unresponsiveness that are likely to be due to a common underlying mechanism. The approach to the therapy of patients with mesangial proliferation and/or IgM deposits is similar to that in MCD, although treatment is substantially less effective.

Focal Glomerular Sclerosis

Etiology and Incidence. FGS is a histopathologic term that refers to the presence on biopsy of unique sclerosing glomerular lesions in a focal and segmental distribution. Focal sclerotic lesions may be present in early biopsies of patients with idiopathic nephrotic syndrome who have changes in most glomeruli consistent with MCD. In this circumstance the lesions are associated with a progressive clinical course and poor response to therapy. A genetic association has been noted with HLA DR4. Patients with the clinical and histologic features of FGS account for about 10% to 15% of all patients with idiopathic nephrotic syndrome in both children and adults (Table 116-3).

Pathogenesis and Pathophysiology. The mechanism that causes the diffuse increase in glomerular permeability in FGS is unknown but may be similar to that in MCD discussed earlier. Studies of patients in whom recurrent FGS develops in renal allografts have

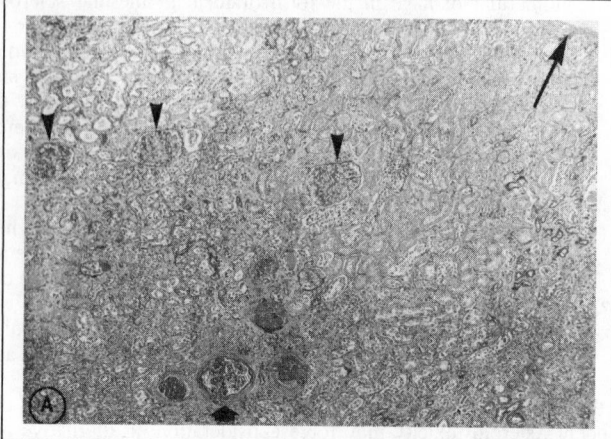

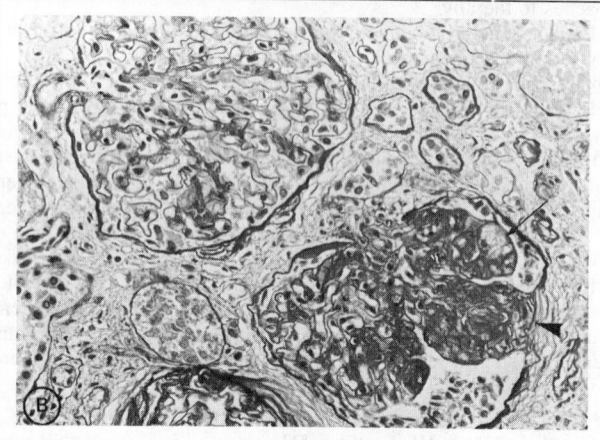

FIGURE 116-7   Renal biopsy findings in a patient with steroid-resistant idiopathic nephrotic syndrome and focal glomerular sclerosis. **A,** A low-power light micrograph illustrates the juxtamedullary distribution of sclerotic lesions. Several glomeruli in the deep cortex are totally sclerotic, and one *(short arrow)* has only segmental involvement. Superficial glomeruli *(arrowheads)* near the cortical surface, identified by the *long arrow,* are normal. There is also tubular atrophy and interstitial fibrosis (periodic acid-Schiff stain; magnification ×40). **B,** The glomerulus in the upper left is normal with adhesion to Bowman's capsule *(arrowhead)* and foamy cells *(small arrow)* (periodic acid-Schiff stain; magnification ×265).

demonstrated the presence of a circulating permeability factor that induces proteinuria in animals. The focal sclerotic lesions themselves, which ultimately result in glomerular destruction and loss of renal function, may result from injury to the glomerular epithelial cell by this process. These lesions may also occur as a consequence of hemodynamic changes, which produce local increases in glomerular hydrostatic pressure and plasma flow. The development of focal sclerotic glomerular lesions is characteristic of most forms of progressive glomerular disease. Deposits of IgM and C3 are usually seen in sclerotic lesions and probably represent trapping of serum proteins by nonimmune mechanisms in areas of tissue damage.

Pathology. The characteristic lesion of FGS is seen by light microscopy in only some glomeruli (focal). It appears first in juxtamedullary glomeruli and therefore may not be seen in biopsy specimens obtained from the superficial cortex (Fig. 116-7, *A*). Each individual lesion consists of intracapillary deposition of eosinophilic, periodic acid–Schiff (PAS)-positive hyaline material involving portions of one or two lobules in a glomerulus with the other lobules spared (segmental). As in MCD, variable amounts of diffuse mesangial proliferation may be seen and suggest a less favorable prognosis.

By IF, glomerular deposits of IgM and C3 are present only in the areas of glomerular sclerosis. EM reveals generalized effacement of foot processes in all glomeruli and may show areas of epithelial cell

detachment and thickening and folding of the GBM before sclerotic lesions are visible by light microscopy.

Clinical and Laboratory Features. The clinical features that distinguish FGS from MCD are the more frequent presence of hematuria and hypertension, relative resistance to steroid therapy, and progressive loss of renal function; however, there is a wide clinical spectrum in FGS. The mean age is about 20 years, and the ratio of men/women is about 1.3 : 1. Most patients present with idiopathic nephrotic syndrome, but persistent nonnephrotic proteinuria or hematuria may also be presenting features. Although some microscopic hematuria is seen in 80% of cases, red blood cell casts are rare. In patients with lesions of FGS on initial biopsies, hypertension and decreased renal function are present in 25% to 50% at the time of diagnosis, and steroid resistance is frequent. Progression to renal failure occurs in an average period of 10 years, although progression over 1 to 2 years ("malignant" focal sclerosis) is not uncommon. The rate of progression is related to the amount of proteinuria. Some patients with documented FGS, however, may retain renal function, despite persistent proteinuria, usually without nephrotic syndrome, for over 20 years. In general the prognosis is worse in adults than in children.

Approximately 30% of adult patients are initially steroid responsive, hypertension and hematuria are not prominent, and renal function is well preserved, although typical lesions of FGS are present on renal biopsies. Despite the presence of histologic lesions of FGS, the prognosis in patients with FGS who respond to steroids is good.

Diagnosis. The differential diagnosis of FGS is that of idiopathic nephrotic syndrome. The diagnosis is made by demonstrating the presence of typical focal sclerotic glomerular lesions on renal biopsy in the absence of other glomerular disease. In patients with biopsies characteristic of MCD who do not respond to steroid therapy, it is often assumed that lesions of FGS must be present in glomeruli not contained in the biopsy specimen. Several other diseases are associated with idiopathic nephrotic syndrome, progressive renal failure, and a glomerular lesion of FGS, including heroin nephropathy, acquired immunodeficiency syndrome (AIDS), and a nephropathy associated with idiosyncratic reactions to NSAIDs. These lesions are discussed briefly later.

Treatment. An initial trial of steroid therapy as described earlier for MCD is warranted in FGS because up to 30% of patients respond with a marked reduction in proteinuria as they do in MCD, and these patients have a good prognosis. At present the evidence that cytotoxic drugs are of benefit in inducing remission or preserving renal function in steroid-resistant patients with FGS is controversial. Occasional patients who do not respond to conventional oral steroids, however, have entered remission after short-term methylprednisolone pulse therapy or after a course of oral cyclophosphamide, chlorambucil, or cyclosporin. Final conclusions regarding the possible benefit of such therapy must await the outcome of prospective controlled studies. Nonsteroidal antiinflammatory agents, particularly meclofenamate, have also been reported to reduce protein excretion without lowering GFR in patients with steroid-resistant FGS. Angiotensin-converting enzyme inhibitors may also be useful in managing some patients with steroid resistant nephrotic syndrome, particularly if hypertension is present.

FGS may recur in the transplanted kidney. The likelihood of recurrence is influenced by the rapidity of progression of the original disease to renal failure, the presence of mesangial hypercellularity, and probably the receipt of a relatively well-matched, living, related donor kidney. Patients who progress to renal failure in less than 3 years are at particularly high risk for recurrent disease. In four antigen matches, the recurrence rate may approach 80%, although it is less than 50% for all patients transplanted with FGS. When the disease does recur, it may be manifest as severe proteinuria within hours of transplantation with biopsy evidence of MCD initially and lesions of FGS developing within days leading to graft failure. Such patients have elevated levels of a circulating permeability factor, and treatment with plasma exchange reduces proteinuria and may prevent graft loss.

Heroin Nephropathy

Renal disease in intravenous drug abusers may take several forms including immune complex nephritis related to bacterial endocarditis or visceral abscess, membranous nephropathy or MPGN related to antigen-positive hepatitis, glomerulonephritis as part of a generalized vasculitis, amyloid, AIDS nephropathy, and chronic interstitial nephritis. However, idiopathic nephrotic syndrome occurs with increased frequency in parenteral drug users, and the majority have a lesion similar to FGS. In some centers heroin nephropathy has accounted for over 25% of new cases of FGS seen in adults and over 10% of new cases of end-stage renal disease in young adults, but the entity is becoming less common. It is most commonly seen in African-American men between 18 and 45 years of age who have been heroin addicts for several years. Most patients have hypertension and impaired renal function, in addition to nephrotic syndrome, when first seen. The prognosis is poor, and progression to renal failure usually occurs within 4 years.

AIDS Nephropathy

Proteinuria has been reported in up to 50% of AIDS patients, and 10% may develop nephrotic syndrome. The disorder is more common in African-American patients and patients who have AIDS associated with intravenous drug abuse, but it has been observed in patients without a history of drug abuse and in children, suggesting that an AIDS-specific nephropathy exists. The glomerular lesion in AIDS nephropathy is FGS often accompanied by glomerular viral-like bodies, and the diagnosis of AIDS may be suggested by the renal biopsy. The course is one of progressive loss of renal function.

Adverse Reaction to NSAIDs

Occasional patients develop nephrotic syndrome as a consequence of an apparent allergic reaction to NSAIDs. In about half of cases, nephrotic syndrome is accompanied by acute renal failure with lesions of MCD accompanied by interstitial nephritis on biopsy. With persistent proteinuria, glomerular lesions of FGS and loss of renal function may occur.

Membranous Nephropathy

Etiology and Incidence. Although the inciting event is not known in most cases of membranous nephropathy, in a minority of patients the lesion occurs in association with a variety of identifiable conditions. The best established associations are with persistent hepatitis B and C antigenemia, autoimmune diseases including lupus, diabetes, thyroiditis, and mixed connective tissue disease, carcinoma, and treatment with several drugs, particularly gold, penicillamine, captopril, and rarely NSAIDs. Membranous nephropathy is rare in children but is the most common cause of idiopathic nephrotic syndrome in adults (Table 116-3).

Pathogenesis and Pathophysiology. Increased glomerular permeability in membranous nephropathy results from the formation of granular immune deposits containing IgG and complement along the subepithelial surface of the glomerular capillary wall and in filtration slit pores. The disease is most likely due to an autoimmune IgG antibody response to an antigen expressed on the surface of the glomerular epithelial cell. Proteinuria is induced by a complement-dependent mechanism that involves assembly of C5b-9 membrane attack complexes. There is also a strong association between idiopathic membranous nephropathy and HLA-DRw3 (relative risk 4), suggesting a genetic susceptibility to this disease, although familial cases are rare. Proteinuria is nonselective. Glomerular destruction occurs slowly due primarily to progressive thickening of the capillary wall, which results from accumulation of laminin and novel collagen chains along the subepithelial surface.

Pathology. The renal pathology in membranous nephropathy is illustrated in Fig. 116-8. By light microscopy glomeruli in early membranous nephropathy appear normal and cannot be distinguished from MCD (or FGS) unless IF and EM studies are performed. Biopsies

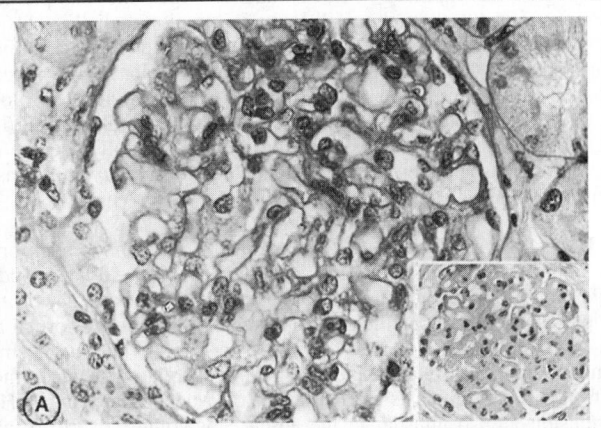

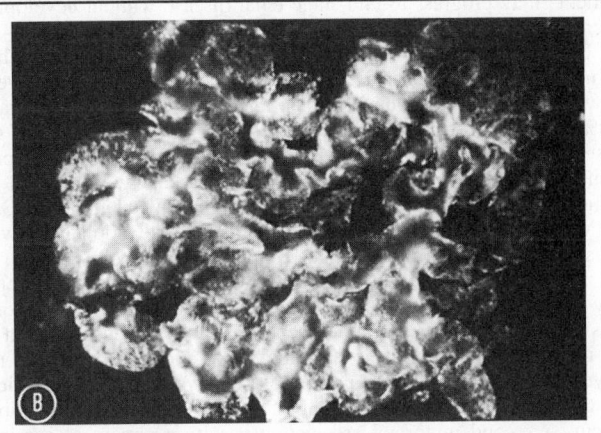

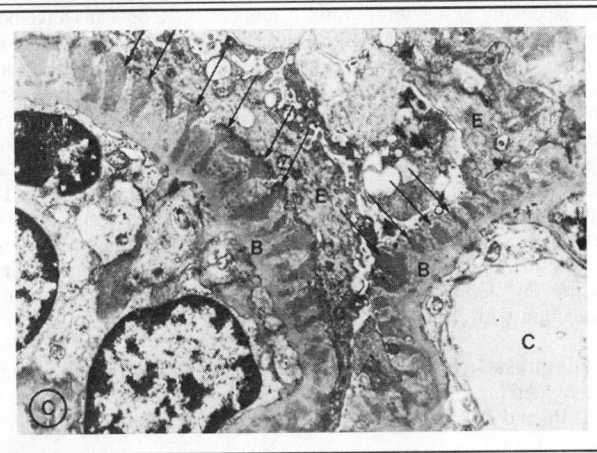

FIGURE 116-8   Renal biopsy findings from a patient with the idiopathic nephrotic syndrome resulting from membranous nephropathy. **A,** By light microscopy the glomerulus is essentially normal (periodic acid–Schiff stain; magnification ×500). As the disease progresses, there is diffuse thickening of the capillary walls without cellular proliferation (*inset;* hematoxylin-eosin stain; magnification ×125). **B,** By immunofluorescence finely granular deposits of immunoglobulin G IgG (and C3) are distributed evenly along all capillary loops (magnification ×450). **C,** Electron microscopy shows discontinuous electron dense deposits (*arrows*) along the subepithelial surface of the basement membrane *(B)* and in filtration slit pores with spikelike projections of basement membrane between the deposits. *C,* capillary lumen; *E,* epithelial cells (uranyl and lead stain; magnification ×500).

later in the course of the disease show an increase in capillary wall thickness but no inflammatory changes or cellular proliferation (Fig. 116-8, *A*). When stained with silver methenamine, a "spike and dome" pattern may be seen due to projections of excess basement membrane between the subepithelial deposits. By IF there is a characteristic, finely granular capillary wall staining for IgG and complement present uniformly throughout all loops in the glomeruli (Fig. 116-8, *B*). Mesangial deposits are usually not seen except in the membranous form of lupus nephritis (see later discussion). EM reveals electron-dense deposits in a discontinuous pattern exclusively along the subepithelial surface of the glomerular capillary wall (Fig. 116-8, *C*). As the disease progresses, the deposits may gradually become intramembranous and then resolve, leaving areas of lucency in the basement membrane.

Clinical and Laboratory Features. Membranous nephropathy is a disease of adults with a mean age of 40 to 50 years and a male predominance of 2 to 1. Most patients (80%) present with the insidious onset of idiopathic nephrotic syndrome and have normal renal function, although less severe or earlier cases with only asymptomatic proteinuria also occur. Hematuria is relatively uncommon (20%), and the urinalysis usually shows only nephrotic changes. Hypertension is also unusual in the absence of volume overload, and patients may progress to end-stage renal disease without developing increased blood pressure.

The natural history of membranous nephropathy is quite variable. Urine protein excretion may vary widely from day to day and week to week. The spontaneous remission rate is about 25% in adults and 50% in children, but spontaneous remission after the first year of the disease is uncommon. Another 25% of patients have persistent proteinuria but retain stable renal function for decades. About 50% of patients have a slow but progressive loss of renal function over 3 to 10 years. Rarely, previously stable patients may develop RPGN with crescents because of a superimposed anti-GBM antibody disease.

Three clinical conditions associated with membranous nephropathy warrant comment. The incidence of secondary renal vein thrombosis in idiopathic membranous nephropathy has been estimated to be up to 40%, but renal vein thrombosis does not appear to alter the severity or course of the renal disease. Renal venography and anticoagulant therapy are undertaken only if thromboembolic complications occur. A second important association is with a variety of carcinomas, especially of the lung, stomach, and colon. Neoplasms have been reported in up to 25% of patients over age 50 with membranous nephropathy. They are often occult when the nephrotic syndrome develops and should be searched for carefully in such patients. A lesion clinically and pathologically indistinguishable from idiopathic membranous nephropathy is seen in 15% of patients with lupus nephritis (see later discussion). These patients typically have low levels of antiDNA antibodies and may have negative antinuclear antibody test results and normal complement levels. This possibility must be kept in mind, particularly in young women presenting with apparently idiopathic membranous nephropathy. There are no laboratory findings specific for membranous nephropathy except as they may occur in association with the conditions listed earlier.

Diagnosis. The diagnosis of membranous nephropathy is made only by demonstrating the characteristic findings described above by light, IF, and EM studies of a renal biopsy specimen.

Treatment. Treatment of membranous nephropathy remains controversial. Patients with less than 8 g of proteinuria and normal renal function usually do well, especially if they are women, and may be treated symptomatically with angiotensin-converting enzyme (ACE) inhibitors and/or nonsteroidal antiinflammatory agents to decrease proteinuria. In patients with persistent nephrotic syndrome beyond 6 months and/or evidence of declining renal function, treatment with corticosteroids and a cytotoxic agent such as cyclophosphamide or chlorambucil is indicated. Some patients have also responded well to prolonged treatment with low-dose cyclosporine. In patients with membranous nephropathy resulting from hepatitis B or C, antiviral therapy with alpha-interferon may be useful.

Renal transplantation has been widely used in patients with end-stage renal disease caused by membranous nephropathy. Recurrent disease after transplantation has been rare and has occurred only in patients with unusually rapid courses who develop renal failure 3 years or less after diagnosis. Membranous nephropathy has also been reported to develop de novo in renal transplants and is a common cause of nephrotic syndrome in transplant recipients.

Membranoproliferative Glomerulonephritis

Two major subgroups of MPGN, type I and type II, are recognized. Although their clinical and light microscopic features are similar, differences in other features strongly suggest that different pathogenetic mechanisms are involved. These two subtypes are therefore discussed here as separate entities except in areas where no major distinction is apparent.

Type I

Etiology and incidence. Most cases of MPGN I are idiopathic, particularly in children. In adults a significant number of patients with MPGN I, especially when it is associated with hypocomplementemia and cryoglobulins, appear to have the disease as a consequence of hepatitis C infection. MPGN causes about 10% of all cases of nephrotic syndrome in both children and adults and may also become evident as acute glomerulonephritis in children.

Pathogenesis and pathophysiology. Characteristics of type I MPGN in adults include the presence of granular subendothelial and, sometimes, subepithelial immune complex deposits, often in a setting of hypocomplementemia.

In idiopathic type I MPGN the disease is likely to be one of chronic glomerular immune complex deposition similar to class IV lupus nephritis, but the relevant antigen antibody systems have not been identified. In cases associated with hepatitis C there is persistent hepatitis C virus antigenemia and evidence of hepatitis C virus antigen in glomerular deposits and circulating cryoglobulins, suggesting that the deposits are a consequence of circulating immune complex trapping, but other auto antibodies may also be involved. The lesion is probably complement-neutrophil–mediated with activated mesangial cells also playing a role.

Pathology. The pathologic findings in type I MPGN are illustrated in Fig. 116-9. Light microscopy reveals diffuse glomerular abnormalities with thickening of the capillary walls and enlargement of glomerular tufts, often in a lobular pattern (Fig. 116-9, *A*). Mesangial cells and matrix are increased, neutrophils are often present, and epithelial crescents may occasionally be seen. The thickened capillary wall is due to interposition of mesangial matrix between GBM and endothelial cells, which gives a characteristic splitting or double contour to the capillary wall ("tram-tracks") when stained with appropriate stains. IF reveals coarsely granular deposits of C3, and often C1q, C4, and properdin, in the mesangium and along the peripheral aspect of the capillary wall (see Fig. 116-9, *B*). These complement components are usually accompanied by IgG and IgM. By EM the typical findings are electron-dense deposits along the subendothelial surface of the peripheral capillary loops and in the mesangium, and the presence of mesangial interposition encircling the capillary loop to varying degrees and separating the lamina densa from endothelial cells with narrowing of the capillary lumen. In some patients the deposits by EM exhibit a fibrillar appearance consistent with deposited cryoglobulins. Occasionally, subepithelial deposits and humps such as those in poststreptococcal nephritis may be seen.

Clinical and laboratory features. The clinical manifestations of MPGN are much more variable than in other glomerular diseases causing the nephrotic syndrome, and there are no consistent differences between types I and II that permit differentiation on clinical grounds. MPGN is a disease of children and adolescents usually between the ages of 5 and 15 years, with only 10% of cases over age 30. MPGN is somewhat more common in females. Onset occurs after an upper respiratory tract infection in many patients. Some cases clearly follow streptococcal infections and may account for some of the reported cases of chronic poststreptococcal nephritis, but there is no evidence for a streptococcal origin in most cases. About 20% of all patients come to medical attention with an acute nephritic syndrome, and about 40% with nephrotic syndrome, with or without a nephritic component. Nephrotic syndrome develops in over 80% of patients sometime during the course of the disease, and persistent nephrotic syndrome is more common in type II disease. The remaining 40% of patients are detected by finding asymptomatic hematuria or proteinuria on routine examinations. Hypertension is a common early manifestation of MPGN and is present initially in 30% to 50% of patients. Renal function is impaired in about one third of patients at the time of diagnosis.

The course of MPGN, like the clinical presentation, is variable.

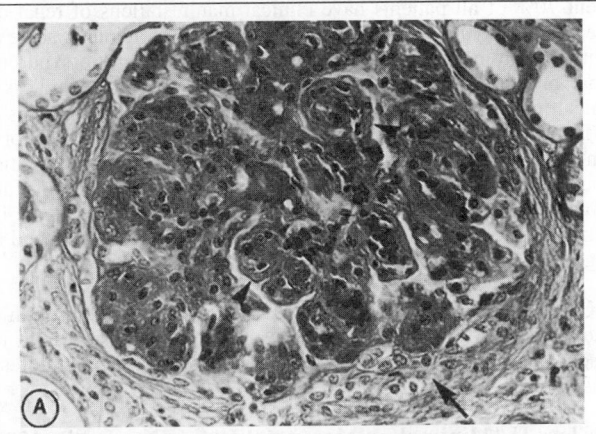

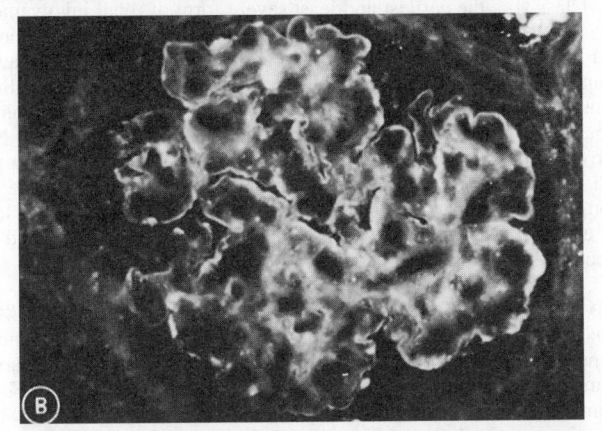

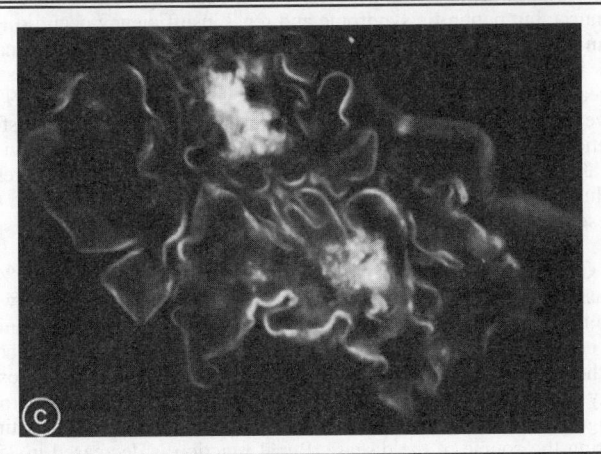

FIGURE 116-9 Histologic and immunofluorescence findings in membrano-proliferative glomerulonephritis. **A,** By light microscopy glomeruli show cellular proliferation, segmental basement membrane thickening, and accentuation of individual lobules. A capillary loop *(arrowhead)* shows the splitting, or double contour, of the basement membrane often seen in this disease. A small crescent is present *(arrow)* (periodic acid–Schiff stain; magnification ×325). **B,** In type I granular immune complex deposits of immunoglobulin G and C3 are present along peripheral capillary loops and in the mesangium (magnification ×350). **C,** In type II there is positive staining only for C3 along the capillary loops and in the mesangium (mesangial rings) (magnification ×550).

Within 6 to 10 years about one third of patients progress to chronic renal failure, one third have persistent nephrotic syndrome with relatively stable renal function, and one third have persistent nonnephrotic proteinuria or hematuria. Spontaneous remissions are rare. In the long term (10 to 20 years), at least 50% of patients will progress to end-stage renal disease.

The laboratory features of MPGN are not different from other diseases causing nephrotic syndrome except with respect to the complement abnormalities. In type I, serum levels of both classic and alternate-pathway complement are reduced at some point during the course of the disease in all patients, but levels tend to fluctuate. Hypocomplementemia is present on a single determination at the time of diagnosis in less than half of patients. There is no correlation between complement levels and disease severity, activity, or prognosis. In patients with type I MPGN associated with hepatitis C, 60% have type II mixed cryoglobulins containing an IgM rheumatoid factor that may occur in the absence of extrarenal manifestations of cryoglobulinemia. Seventy percent have laboratory evidence of liver disease, usually chronic active hepatitis or cirrhosis. Many patients come to medical attention with a primary glomerular disease without clinical evidence of either cryoglobulinemia or liver disease.

Diagnosis. The clinical manifestations of type I MPGN are indistinguishable from several other glomerular diseases, and the diagnosis can be made only by renal biopsy. The disease should be strongly suspected in adolescent patients with nephrotic syndrome, hematuria, and persistent hypocomplementemia or in patients with evidence of hepatitis C infection.

Treatment. There is no immediate response to oral steroid therapy in MPGN, although alternate-day steroid therapy for 2 years has been reported to be beneficial in preserving renal function in children. However, there is no consensus that any form of immunosuppressive therapy is beneficial in adults. In type I MPGN associated with hepatitis C infection, treatment with alpha-interferon, often for several months, is associated with reduction in proteinuria and improvement in renal function along with clearing of hepatitis C virus RNA from the serum, but relapse is common when interferon therapy is discontinued.

Both type I and type II MPGN have been reported to recur morphologically in transplanted kidneys (type I, 30%; type II, 90%). However, less than 25% of such patients develop nephrotic syndrome, and graft loss due to recurrent MPGN is rare.

Type II (Dense Deposit Disease). The clinical and light microscopic features of type II MPGN are very similar to those of type I, but the disease is not associated with cryoglobulins or hepatitis C and the origin is unknown. The incidence of type II MPGN in developing countries has declined significantly over the past decade, suggesting a potential infectious origin.

Immunofluorescence and electron microscopic studies reveal no glomerular immune complex deposits in type II MPGN, but rather a characteristic widened, electron-dense GBM that is due to replacement of lamina dense with a homogenous, osmiophilic material of uncertain composition, which may stain for C3 (Fig. 116-9, *C*). Hypocomplementemia is usually persistent and involves C3 and late-reacting complement components with normal levels of C1, C4, and C2. Most patients also have a circulating IgG antibody to the C3 convertase of the alternate-complement pathway called C3 nephritic factor, or C3 Nef. C3 Nef appears to stabilize the C3 convertase, resulting in persistent activation of C3. Type II MPGN is usually a more rapidly progressive disease than is type I and recurs in about 90% of transplanted kidneys, but graft loss due to recurrence is rare. There is no treatment of established benefit for this disease.

GLOMERULAR INVOLVEMENT IN SYSTEMIC DISEASES

The various forms of vasculitis are the most common systemic diseases resulting in glomerular involvement. Among the diseases referred to as systemic necrotizing vasculitis, a distinction is made between necrotizing vasculitis involving medium-sized and larger vessels (polyarteritis nodosa), and necrotizing vasculitis involving small vessels and capillaries (microscopic polyarteritis nodosa [PAN] plus several well-defined clinical syndromes including lupus nephritis, Henoch-Schönlein purpura, and mixed essential mixed cryoglobulinemia). The only other common vasculitic syndrome with renal involvement is Wegener's granulomatosis.

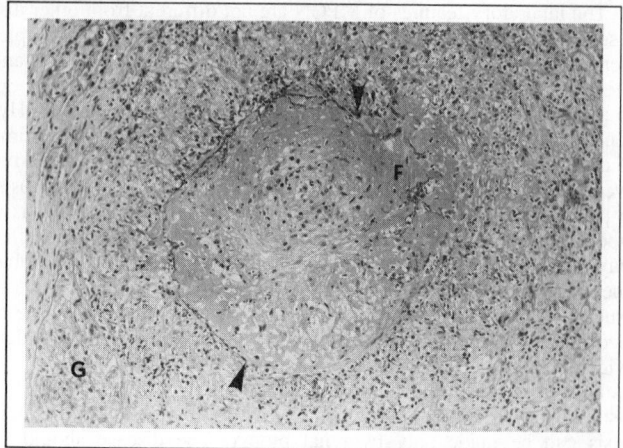

FIGURE 116-10   Renal biopsy finding from a patient with the classic form of polyarteritis nodosa. An arcuate artery shows extensive fibrinoid necrosis *(F)*, reduplication of the elastic lamina *(arrowheads)*, occlusion, and a perivascular inflammatory cell infiltrate. The glomerulus *(G)* is intact (periodic acid–Schiff stain; magnification ×375).

Systemic Necrotizing Vasculitis Involving Large Vessels

Polyarteritis Nodosa. Polyarteritis nodosa (PAN) is a disease of older patients, which may be associated with drug abuse (particularly amphetamines) and hepatitis B or C antigenemia. It is usually insidious in onset with arthralgias, weight loss, abdominal and testicular pain, fever, hypertension, and neurologic symptoms as prominent features. PAN is a disease of uncertain pathogenesis, which involves medium-sized blood vessels, and the kidney is affected in over 90% of cases. Pulmonary and skin lesions are rare. Histologically, there are acute inflammatory changes in medium-sized muscular arteries, particularly the arcuate and interlobular vessels with fibrinoid necrosis and subsequent aneurysms (Fig. 116-10). These lesions are generally not seen on renal biopsy and can best be demonstrated by abdominal angiography, which may demonstrate aneurysms in renal, hepatic, and mesenteric vessels.

Renal disease is usually evident first as hematuria with an active urine sediment and mild proteinuria. The glomerular lesion is primarily an ischemic one in 70% of cases resulting from vasculitic involvement of arcuate and interlobular arteries. In 30% of patients a focal necrotizing glomerulonephritis with crescents similar to the lesions in small vessel vasculitis may be seen, and most of these patients are ANCA-positive. Both types of glomerular involvement can occur in the same patient. Immune deposits are usually not found in the glomerulus, and the pathogenesis of the renal disease is uncertain.

Renal failure is a major cause of death. It may be slowly progressive or develop acutely, often associated with accelerated hypertension. In patients with PAN who develop hypertension and acute renal failure, renal cortical necrosis is common, and there is little reversibility. More commonly, the disease is slowly progressive. Vigorous control of hypertension, use of oral steroids, and the addition of cytotoxic agents such as cyclophosphamide have resulted in 5-year survival rates of over 80% in uncontrolled studies.

Systemic Necrotizing Vasculitis Involving Small Vessels

Microscopic Polyarteritis Nodosa. Microscopic PAN as a cause of ANCA-positive vasculitis with RPGN is discussed with idiopathic (pauciimmune) crescentic glomerulonephritis.

Systemic Lupus Erythematosus (SLE). The current diagnostic criteria and clinical manifestations of SLE are considered in more detail in Chapter 194. This section describes only the renal involvement in this common form of systemic necrotizing vasculitis.

About 70% of all patients have clinical manifestations of renal disease, which may include microscopic hematuria, proteinuria, acute nephritic syndrome with acute renal failure, and nephrotic syndrome. Renal biopsies reveal abnormalities in most patients regardless of clinical manifestations.

The most common classification system used for renal involvement in SLE is the World Health Organization (WHO) classification, which is based on histopathologic criteria (Table 116-4). In Table 116-4 the WHO classification is presented with the approximate frequency of each lesion, the associated clinical manifestations, and the prognosis.

Class I (Normal Kidneys, <5%). Only rare patients with diagnostic criteria for SLE have entirely normal kidneys by light microscopy, IF, and EM, as well as an absence of clinical manifestations of glomerular disease.

Class II (Minimal or Mesangial Lupus Nephritis, 15%). Class II is the earliest and least severe form of renal involvement in SLE. It is characterized by mesangial deposits of immunoglobulin and C3 with (class IIB) or without (class IIA) focal proliferative changes by light microscopy. These lesions are similar to those illustrated for IgA nephropathy in Fig. 116-3. Clinical manifestations of proteinuria and hematuria are present in two thirds of patients. Nephrotic syndrome and renal insufficiency, however, are uncommon and do not develop unless there is progression to a more severe lesion, which occurs in about 20% of such patients. Complement levels usually are normal. The 5-year survival rate exceeds 90%, and no specific therapy is indicated for the renal lesion.

Class III (Focal Proliferative Lupus Nephritis, 20%). This lesion is a stage in the continuum between mesangial lesions alone and diffuse proliferative lupus nephritis. Focal proliferative changes, as illustrated in Fig. 116-3, are present in less than 50% of glomeruli. Deposits are predominantly mesangial (Fig. 116-3, *B*), but occasional subendothelial deposits may be seen. All patients have proteinuria, but nephrotic syndrome and renal insufficiency occur in less than 20% and often remit after steroid therapy. Serologic abnormalities including hypocomplementemia are more severe than in class II disease. Long-term prognosis with this lesion is also good (90% 5-year survival), but there is a relatively high incidence of transformation to class IV disease resulting in a reduction in 5-year survival to about 70%, with almost half of the deaths occurring from renal failure. The most reliable predictor of progression is probably the presence of subendothelial deposits by EM.

Class IV (Diffuse Proliferative Lupus Nephritis, 50%). Class IV is the most severe form of glomerular disease in lupus, with proliferation seen in over 50% of glomeruli, frequently accompanied by crescent formation and necrosis. Extensive mesangial and subendothelial deposits can be seen by IF and EM. Subepithelial deposits may also be present. Proteinuria is seen in all patients, and nephrotic range proteinuria is present in 50% at onset and in 90% at some time during the course of the disease. Renal function is decreased in 75% of patients at the time of presentation, and serologic evidence of disease activity including hypocomplementemia, elevated levels of anti-DNA antibody, and circulating immune complexes are present in most patients. The long-term prognosis of this lesion has improved considerably. Survival rates of over 70% at 5 years are now common. Patients who exhibit a remission of nephrotic syndrome and normalization of serologic parameters within 1 year of starting therapy have the best prognosis.

Class V (Membranous Lupus Nephritis, 15%). About 15% of patients with SLE develop a glomerular lesion that can be indistinguishable from idiopathic membranous nephropathy. Unlike idiopathic membranous nephropathy, the subepithelial deposits usually contain all immunoglobulins ("full-house" IF) and C3, and some mesangial deposits are usually present. Nephrotic syndrome and slowly progressive renal disease are common. The level and avidity of anti-DNA antibody are often low in such patients, who may have undetectable levels of antinuclear antibody at the time of presentation. Some transformation can occur from class V to class

Table 116-4 Histologic class, clinical presentation, and prognosis in systemic lupus erythematosus (SLE)

HISTOLOGIC TYPE	WHO CLASS	FREQUENCY (%)*	PROTEINURIA (%)	NEPHROTIC SYNDROME (%)†	AZOTEMIA (%)‡	DEATH (%)	UREMIC DEATH (%)
Normal	I	<5	0	0	0	0	0
Mesangial	II	15	68	0	12	18	0
Focal proliferative	III	20	100	15	18	30	11
Diffuse proliferative	IV	50	100	87	75	58	36
Membranous	V	15	100	88	20	38	6

*% of patients biopsied with SLE who exhibit this lesion.
†Proteinuria exceeding 3.0 g/24 hours.
‡Level of serum creatinine >1.2 mg% or blood urea nitrogen >25 mg%.

IV, and vice versa, but the long-term prognosis for patients with this lesion does not differ significantly from those with class II disease. As in idiopathic membranous nephropathy, there appears to be an increased incidence of renal vein thrombosis. Therapy as discussed for idiopathic membranous nephropathy should probably be given to these patients.

Serologic Monitoring. Serologic tests that have been correlated with renal disease activity in SLE include measurements of antibody to double-stranded DNA, particularly if only complement-fixing antibodies are measured, and levels of C3, C4, and CH50, with C4 probably the most sensitive. Although reports of a general correlation between abnormalities in each of these laboratory parameters and disease activity in large numbers of patients have been published, the utility of such measurements in predicting renal disease activity and adjusting therapy in individual patients is minimal. The best parameters for following the activity of renal disease are the serum creatinine level, urine protein excretion, and careful examination of the urine sediment.

Treatment of Lupus Nephritis. There is general agreement that oral steroids are beneficial in treating lupus nephritis. Usually high-dose steroid therapy is given for a period of 4 to 6 weeks and subsequently tapered and adjusted according to response in renal function, serologic parameters, and extrarenal disease. In the two decades since the introduction of steroid therapy, survival rates have increased steadily to over 70% 5-year survival in class IV disease and 90% in other patients.

Benefits from immunosuppressive drug therapy are most apparent in patients with class IV disease. Use of cytotoxic agents should be considered in such patients, particularly when nephrotic syndrome persists, when azotemia does not improve after treatment with oral steroids, when steroid toxicity develops, or when renal function is rapidly deteriorating. Recent studies demonstrate that administration of cyclophosphamide as a monthly intravenous pulse is as efficacious as and less toxic than daily oral administration and improves renal survival significantly in patients with severe lupus nephritis. In the presence of crescents and rapidly deteriorating renal function, steroid pulse therapy as discussed for idiopathic crescentic glomerulonephritis may be more efficacious than high doses of oral steroids alone. Plasma exchange therapy does not appear useful in the routine management of lupus nephritis.

Henoch-Schönlein Purpura. This disease, also referred to as Henoch-Schönlein syndrome or anaphylactoid purpura, is another systemic necrotizing vasculitis of small vessels in which systemic manifestations include palpable purpura (100%) on the extensor surfaces of the legs, arms, and buttocks due to a leukocytoclastic vasculitis of dermal vessels; arthralgias of large joints, usually the knees and ankles (70%); gastrointestinal tract involvement with colic and bleeding (25%); and renal involvement. About 30% of patients have clinical evidence of renal disease in the form of hematuria or acute nephritic syndrome, and the disease is a common cause of glomerulonephritis before age 15. Except for the systemic manifestations, the disease is similar in its morphologic and clinical characteristics to IgA nephropathy, and the pathogenetic mechanisms are presumably similar. However, Henoch-Schönlein purpura is somewhat more severe, particularly in adults. The typical presentation is with an acute nephritic syndrome, usually without edema or hypertension, developing within 3 months of the onset of other systemic manifestations. In contrast to IgA nephropathy, up to 25% of adults may develop a severe crescentic lesion with RPGN. Nephrotic syndrome has been reported to develop in over 50% of patients and progressive renal failure occurs in at least 25% of patients. Predictors of progressive disease include presentation with an acute nephritic syndrome, nephrotic syndrome, and crescents. Most patients have self-limited episodes of renal involvement usually lasting 1 week or less; however, recurrences are common.

Laboratory features are not distinctive and do not differ from those described for IgA nephropathy. Elevated levels of IgA-fibronectin aggregates are often present. Renal biopsy may reveal a spectrum of lesions ranging from focal mesangial proliferation to diffuse crescentic glomerulonephritis, but the most characteristic lesion is a focal necrotizing glomerulonephritis in which necrosis and fibrin deposition are more common than in IgA nephropathy.

The pathogenesis of Henoch-Schönlein purpura is unknown. The various possible pathogenetic mechanisms are outlined in the discussion of IgA nephropathy. Reports of patients with typical IgA nephropathy who later develop systemic manifestations of this disease, IgA nephropathy and Henoch-Schönlein purpura in identical twins, and similar immunogenetic associations in the two diseases, as well as the clinical, histologic, and immunopathologic similarities, strongly implicate a common underlying disease.

No treatment has been shown to be of benefit in patients with recurrent episodes of acute nephritis or patients with slowly progressive loss of renal function. Short courses of steroids may be useful in controlling systemic manifestations but usually do not benefit the renal lesion. Patients who develop crescents and a clinical picture of RPGN should be treated as outlined for idiopathic crescentic glomerulonephritis. With focal necrotizing glomerular lesions and deteriorating renal function, the use of cytotoxic agents may be warranted.

Essential Mixed Cryoglobulinemia. Another systemic necrotizing vasculitis of small vessels that may affect the kidney is essential mixed cryoglobulinemia (EMC). Low concentrations of mixed cryoglobulins, usually type III with polyclonal IgG and IgM with rheumatoid factor activity, are seen in a variety of glomerular diseases, autoimmune disease, vasculitides, and neoplastic syndromes where they rarely produce symptoms. However, type II mixed cryoglobulins, which contain monoclonal rheumatoid factor and polyclonal IgG, are present in EMC associated with vascular purpura, Raynaud's phenomenon, arthralgias, weakness, and glomerulonephritis. The disease begins in middle age and affects women more than men. Most patients have evidence of hepatitis C infection with persistent antigenemia and hepatitis C virus RNA in serum and cryoprecipitates. Fifty percent of patients have renal involvement, which is usually preceded by purpura and arthralgias. The severity of renal disease ranges from microscopic hematuria and mild proteinuria to an acute nephritic syndrome with acute renal failure. Nephrotic syndrome may also be seen, and severe hypertension is common. Laboratory findings include a markedly elevated sedimentation rate, cryoglobulins, positive rheumatoid factor, hypocomplementemia, and often hepatitis B antigenemia or evidence of hepatitis C infection. The glomerular lesion resembles type I MPGN and is a diffuse proliferative and exudative glomerulonephritis, sometimes accompanied by vasculitis, with large PAS-positive proteinaceous subendothelial deposits present in many capillaries. The deposits are composed predominantly of IgG and IgM, presumably representing the cryoglobulins, with lesser amounts of C3 and fibrin, which exhibit a characteristic fibrillar or crystalloid appearance by EM. Patients with acute nephritic syndrome and renal failure have a poor prognosis. However, over 50% of patients with renal involvement recover with or without therapy, and the survival rate at 10 years is about 75%. No role for steroids or cytotoxic agents alone has been established in this disease, but recent reports suggest that plasma exchange therapy may improve the prognosis in patients with severe renal involvement.

Wegener's Granulomatosis. Wegener's granulomatosis is a granulomatous vasculitis, which usually involves the upper and lower respiratory tract and kidneys. The presenting signs are most often respiratory, but renal involvement eventually develops in over 50% of patients and is the cause of death in up to 30%. Hematuria, proteinuria, and mild renal impairment may be seen due to a focal necrotizing and proliferative glomerulonephritis, usually without immune deposits; however, severe necrotizing and crescentic glomerulonephritis may develop rapidly. Necrotizing granulomatous vasculitis may be seen in biopsy specimens of the respiratory tract but is often not evident in renal biopsy specimens. In Wegener's granulomatosis, ANCAs are usually positive with reactivity against proteinase 3 (C-ANCA), and titers parallel disease activity. Although the diagnosis can often be made on clinical grounds, a renal biopsy is generally performed early in the disease to identify potentially severe renal involvement, which may be clinically silent, as well as to distinguish Wegener's granulomatosis from other diseases with pulmonary and renal manifestations such as Goodpasture's syndrome, which would be treated differently.

In recent studies a remission rate of over 90% has been achieved in patients with Wegener's granulomatosis when steroids are used in combination with cyclophosphamide. Many patients have been able to maintain complete remissions and discontinue all drug therapy. Because therapy is more effective in preventing progression than it is in reversing the necrotizing glomerular lesion, early institution of treatment is particularly important with respect to the renal disease.

Thrombotic Microangiopathy (Hemolytic-Uremic Syndrome and Thrombotic Thrombocytopenic Purpura). Hemolytic uremic syndrome (HUS) and thrombotic thrombocytopenic purpura (TTP) can be referred to collectively as thrombotic microangiopathy, a term that emphasizes that the two diseases can be clinically indistinguishable, probably have a common pathogenesis, and respond to similar therapy.

Hemolytic-Uremic Syndrome. HUS is a syndrome of microangiopathic hemolytic anemia, thrombocytopenia, and renal impairment, which usually occurs abruptly in children 3 to 10 days after episodes of gastroenteritis often due to verotoxin-producing *Escherichia coli* 0157 or viral upper respiratory tract infections. A similar syndrome may occur in adults, often in association with complications of pregnancy or during the postpartum period (postpartum acute renal failure) or associated with oral contraceptives. Up to 60% of children develop acute renal failure, which usually resolves spontaneously with only supportive therapy. Chronic renal failure occurs in only 10% of patients. Laboratory features of the disease include microangiopathic hemolytic anemia, thrombocytopenia, increased reticulocytes, elevated bilirubin levels, reduced haptoglobin levels, and elevations in fibrin split products, usually with only minimal laboratory evidence of disseminated intravascular coagulation. The glomerular lesion is one of the intimal hyperplasia of arterioles and intracapillary fibrin thrombi, sometimes with areas of focal necrosis (Fig. 116-11). The anemia and thrombocytopenia presumably result from trapping of platelets and destruction of red blood cells in areas of capillary thrombosis. The pathogenesis of the syndrome is unknown but may result from glomerular endothelial cell injury due to an antiendothelial cell antibody with subsequent platelet aggregation, fibrin deposition, and thrombosis.

Children with typical HUS require only supportive therapy, including early dialysis, because the rate of spontaneous recovery is very high. In adults renal involvement is more severe and development of bilateral cortical necrosis more common. Severe disease is commonly seen in cases associated with pregnancy and oral contraceptives. No

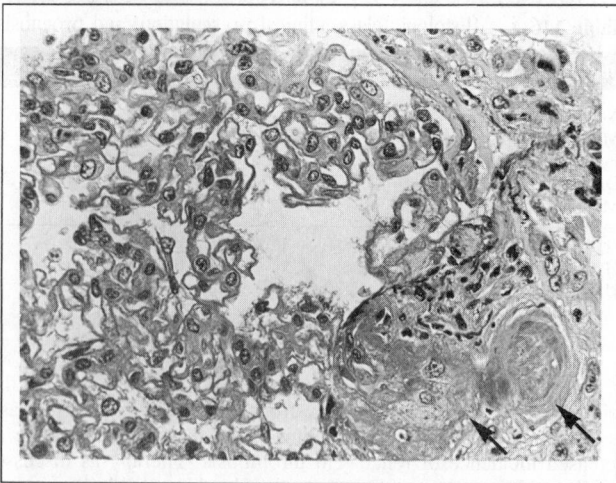

FIGURE 116-11   Renal biopsy finding from a patient with hemolytic-uremic syndrome showing fibrinoid necrosis and occlusion of an afferent arteriole by fibrinoid material *(arrows)*. The glomerulus is normal except for slight mesangial matrix increase (hematoxylin-eosin stain; magnification ×450).

✔ WHEN TO REFER

Patients with glomerular disease should be referred to the nephrologist under the following circumstances. If clinical evidence of acute glomerulonephritis is present and accompanied by a decrease in renal function or nephrotic-range proteinuria, rapid consultation is essential to determine whether a diagnostic renal biopsy is indicated. All adult patients with idiopathic nephrotic syndrome should be referred for diagnostic biopsy and treatment recommendations. Any patients with active glomerular disease undergoing therapy with steroids or cytotoxic agents should be managed primarily by a nephrologist. Similarly, patients with chronic glomerular disease and evidence of deteriorating renal function should be evaluated for possible renal-sparing therapies, as well as for management of the complications of chronic renal failure.

---

treatment has been established to be beneficial in HUS, although aspirin, antiplatelet agents, heparin, fresh-frozen plasma infusions, and plasma exchange have all been advocated by some authors. In adults with severe disease treatment with plasma exchange as described later for TTP, the addition of steroids, antiplatelet agents, and aspirin are probably indicated.

Thrombotic Thrombocytopenic Purpura. TTP is distinguished from HUS by its more common occurrence in young adults, frequent presence of fever, and neurologic abnormalities, which tend to predominate and cause death and a lesser degree of renal involvement. Acute renal failure occurs in only about 10% of cases. Hematuria is the most common manifestation of renal disease. Mild proteinuria and a serum creatinine level in excess of 2 mg/dl occur in only about 50% of cases. Histologically the renal lesion is the same as that in HUS. The prognosis in TTP is worse than in HUS, with about a 75% mortality rate within 3 months, and spontaneous recovery is rare.

A wide variety of therapeutic regimens have been used in TTP. The most promising results have been obtained with plasma exchange, often using fresh plasma, antiplatelet agents, and steroids. Dramatic clinical remissions have occurred in several patients with apparently severe disease. In refractory cases splenectomy may confer an additional benefit.

BIBLIOGRAPHY

Boumpas DT et al: Systemic lupus erythematosus: emerging concepts, *Ann Intern Med* 122:940-950, 1995.

Couser WG: Pathogenesis of glomerulonephritis, *Kidney Int* 44(suppl 42):S/19-S/26, 1993.

Donadio JV Jr et al: A controlled trial of fish oil in IgA nephropathy, *N Engl J Med* 331:1194-1199, 1994.

Glassock RJ: Treatment of immunology-mediated glomerular disease, *Kidney Int* 42(suppl 38):S/121-S/126, 1992.

Ibels LS et al: IgA nephropathy: analysis of the natural history, important factors in the progression of renal disease, and a review of the literature, *Medicine* 73:7910, 1994.

Johnson RJ et al: Membranoproliferative glomerulonephritis associated with hepatitis C virus infection, *N Engl J Med* 328:465-470, 1993.

Kallenberg CGM et al: Antineutrophil cytoplasmic antibodies: current diagnostic and pathophysiological potential, *Kidney Int* 46:1-15, 1994.

Kelly PT et al: Goodpasture syndrome: molecular and clinical advances, *Medicine* 73:171-185, 1994.

Pasquarielli A et al: Cryoglobulinemic membranoproliferative glomerulonephritis associated with hepatitis C virus, *Am J Nephrol* 13:300-304, 1993.

Ponticelli C et al: Treatment of the nephrotic syndrome associated with primary glomerulonephritis, *Kidney Int* 46:595-604, 1994.

Ponticelli C et al: A 10-year follow-up of a randomized study with methylprednisolone and chlorambucil in membranous nephropathy, *Kidney Int* 48:1600-1604, 1995.

Remuzzi G et al: Idiopathic membranous nephropathy, *Lancet* 342:1277-1280, 1993.

Ruggenenti P et al: Treatment of thrombotic microangiopathy, *J Nephrol* 8:255-272, 1995.

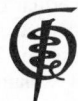

CHAPTER

117   Diabetic Nephropathy

Fuad N. Ziyadeh and Stanley Goldfarb

Diabetic nephropathy is currently the major cause of end-stage renal failure in the United States; approximately 33% of all patients entering dialysis programs have lost renal function as a result of diabetes. Although nephropathy is one of the most serious long-term complications of diabetes, only 25% of patients with insulin-dependent diabetes mellitus (IDDM) ever develop renal failure. Diabetic nephropathy develops in patients with IDDM and in those with non–insulin-dependent diabetes mellitus (NIDDM). The cumulative incidence of this diabetic microvascular complication is uncertain for NIDDM, but it, too, probably approaches 25% (with a lower incidence in whites and a higher incidence in blacks, Native Americans, Mexican Americans, and Asians). The frequency of diabetic nephropathy among patients with IDDM has declined from nearly 50% during the last several decades, perhaps because of improved glycemic and blood pressure control, but the total number of patients afflicted with IDDM and NIDDM appears to be increasing worldwide. The presence of even minor evidence of renal involvement, however, appears to convey a dramatically increased risk of other microvascular and macrovascular complications, so overall mortality is not reduced. The mechanism of the latter association has not been explained yet but probably reflects a generalized abnormality in small vessels or in organs such as kidney, nerve, or heart.

NATURAL HISTORY
Structural Lesions

Kidney structure is dramatically altered in diabetes in virtually all affected patients, even those not destined to develop full-blown diabetic nephropathy (as defined by proteinuria >500 mg/day and progressive decline in glomerular filtration rate [GFR]). These structural changes include kidney enlargement involving both the tubules and the glomeruli and occurring as early as the first few months after the onset of diabetes. This process involves predominantly hypertrophy (cell enlargement) and, to a much lesser extent, hyperplasia (cellular proliferation). The basement membrane of the tubules and the glomeruli also begin to thicken after 2 to 3 years of diabetes. After 3 to 5 years progressive expansion of the mesangial regions of the glomerulus and of the tubulointerstitial regions of the kidney begins. Renal hypertrophy and basement membrane thickening may play an important role in the pathogenesis of diabetic nephropathy but have been seen in all patients with long-standing diabetes and are not specific

signs of overt nephropathy or the potential for development of progressive nephropathy. Expansion of the mesangial region and tubulointerstitial fibrosis, however, do correlate well with progressive loss of renal function. These latter lesions are specific for the development of nephropathy as detected clinically by the appearance of hypertension, frank proteinuria, and reduced GFR.

The pathologically distinctive lesions of full-blown diabetic glomerulopathy require a longer time to appear. The most nearly pathognomonic lesion is nodular diabetic glomerular sclerosis, frequently termed the Kimmelstiel-Wilson lesion. This lesion consists of nodular enlargement of the mesangial compartment of the glomerulus. A roughly similar pattern may be seen in other renal diseases, notably light-chain nephropathy and amyloidosis; however, appropriate immunofluorescent staining, electron microscopy, and historical and laboratory information distinguish these conditions from the nodular glomerular sclerosis of diabetes. More prevalent, and perhaps of greater pathophysiologic significance, is the diffuse rather than nodular enlargement of the mesangium (diffuse glomerulosclerosis), which is a characteristic lesion of established diabetic nephropathy. The declining GFR most likely results from progressive expansion of the glomerular mesangium causing reduction in the glomerular filtering surface area. In addition, sclerotic glomeruli similar to those seen in kidneys with end-stage disease of any cause also develop in kidneys of patients with diabetic nephropathy. Another pathognomonic finding is the arteriosclerotic changes in the afferent and efferent arterioles. Although diabetic nephropathy is generally regarded as primarily a glomerular disease because of the presence of proteinuria and clear glomerular structural lesions, abnormalities of the vasculature and tubulointerstitium occur and correlate well with declining functional status. These lesions of the renal tubulointerstitium include chronic interstitial inflammation, fibrosis, and a predisposition to papillary necrosis. Global glomerulosclerosis associated with widespread vascular ischemic lesions and tubulointerstitial damage also contributes to a reduced GFR.

Clinical Course

Except for the renal functional abnormalities readily ascribable to the diabetic state, such as polyuria and ketoacidosis, renal function in the first years of IDDM is clinically unremarkable, although a substantial portion of these patients have abnormally high GFRs. When measured early in IDDM, the highest increments in GFR are often predictive of the later development of nephropathy. Clinically detectable glomerular injury does not develop until the diabetes has existed for approximately 10 years. Even then, diabetic nephropathy occurs in only a minority of patients. In patients with NIDDM, however, the onset of disease is difficult to date, hence the interval to renal disease is more uncertain. Recent studies of populations that are at high risk for developing NIDDM, such as the Pima Indians, have suggested that nephropathy occurs in 30% to 50% of patients and that increased GFR is also a common feature of the early stages of NIDDM.

Persistent microalbuminuria (i.e., urinary albumin excretion rates detectable by sensitive assays but below the level detectable by conventional clinical measurement, including dipstick) occurs in patients who later have clinical nephropathy and therefore has been advocated as a useful tool for identifying the patients with diabetes who are at risk for development of nephropathy. Such microalbuminuric patients have been designated as having *incipient* nephropathy. However, there is a great deal of variation in the rate of microalbuminuria in patients with incipient nephropathy; all patients with diabetes, even those who will not have later development of clinical nephropathy, have intermittent microalbuminuria at times of suboptimal glucose control or strenuous exercise. This variability has reduced the overall utility of the test. Disagreement also exists over the rate of microalbuminuria that represents incipient nephropathy, although in general the higher the amount of albuminuria within the microalbuminuric range, the greater the probability of later development of overt nephropathy. Normal, nondiabetic individuals excrete less than 15 μg/min of albumin. It is quite clear that in diabetic patients with excretion rates greater than 70 μg/min, gross proteinuria, a highly predictive marker for eventual renal failure, is very likely to develop within 5 years. Lesser rates of excretion, although above the normal range, are also predictive of a moderate to high likelihood of clinical nephropathy in the subsequent 5 to 10 years. Biopsy studies have shown that glomerular structural lesions are prominent in patients with microalbuminuria greater than 70 μg/min leading to the hypothesis that microalbuminuria is an *indicator* rather than a *predictor* of diabetic nephropathy. Therefore diabetes with microalbuminuria should lead physicians to carefully monitor such individuals for even minimal hypertension and to optimize diet and blood glucose control to improve long-term prognosis (see later discussion).

Frank proteinuria, which is detectable by the standard dipstick method, is the usual first indicator of *overt* diabetic glomerulopathy and occurs between 10 to 15 years after the diagnosis of IDDM. Over the next 7 to 10 years patients with proteinuria have a progressive decline in GFR leading to end-stage renal failure. The rapidity of this decline is quite variable, but on average, patients with overt diabetic glomerulopathy lose 1 ml/min of GFR per month. In most diabetic patients with declining GFRs obvious arterial hypertension simultaneously develops, although many may have had modest elevations in blood pressure before proteinuria and declining renal function developed. During the phase of declining GFR, proteinuria of nephrotic proportions with the common features of nephrotic syndrome develops in many patients.

The diagnosis of diabetic nephropathy is generally straightforward in patients with IDDM. The usual criteria are duration of diabetes greater than 10 years, proteinuria, arterial hypertension, and at least some degree of diabetic retinopathy. The urinalysis usually shows no cellular elements and consists merely of bland proteinuria. Rarely, patients with only diabetic nephropathy have hematuria and even red blood cell casts. Such an active sediment, however, is unusual enough that one should consider the possibility that the patient with hematuria has a renal disease other than diabetic nephropathy. Except in such unusual cases, renal biopsy is usually not required for diagnosis. In patients with NIDDM, however, the diagnosis is more complex. As many as 30% to 40% of patients with NIDDM and obvious renal dysfunction have other forms of renal disease, including membranous nephropathy and hypertensive nephrosclerosis, on renal biopsy.

In most respects the signs and symptoms of renal insufficiency in diabetic nephropathy are similar to those seen in other progressive, chronic renal diseases. However, several aspects of diabetes and its nonrenal chronic complications may adversely affect the diabetic patient with progressive renal insufficiency. For example, the propensity to extracellular volume overload that is often associated with renal disease, nephrotic syndrome, and hypertension may be poorly tolerated by a diabetic patient who has concomitant congestive heart failure. The kidney and retina in diabetes may be particularly susceptible to even slight elevations in blood pressure. The anorexia and nausea common to end-stage renal insufficiency are often exacerbated by intestinal autonomic neuropathy and gastroparesis in patients with diabetes. Visual impairment and peripheral vascular disease may further diminish the resiliency of these patients. Insulin therapy often must be altered owing to progressive renal disease because the kidney is a major site for catabolism of insulin. Thus in many patients with renal insufficiency, reductions in insulin dosage are required to maintain glucose control without hypoglycemia. Yet another metabolic complication in patients with diabetic nephropathy is the predisposition to hyperkalemia and normal anion gap acidosis out of proportion to the degree of renal insufficiency. Many of these people have low levels of renin and aldosterone secretion that account for these metabolic abnormalities (Chapter 114).

PATHOGENESIS

Hyperglycemia is the central biochemical abnormality of diabetes. The mechanism of tissue and organ dysfunction in diabetes is due to this central feature and is not the result of a discrete mechanism of injury inherited or acquired independently of the hyperglycemic milieu. However, since nephropathy does not develop in all diabetic patients, genetic and environmental factors, in addition to hyperglycemia, must be operative in patients at risk for development of diabetic nephropathy. Factors predicting a high risk, in addition to poor glycemic control, include duration of diabetes (typically more than 10 years), hemodynamic injury (systemic and intraglomerular hypertension), renal hypertrophy, smoking, familial or genetic factors, and racial predisposition.

Arterial hypertension is one of the most important risk factors for the progression and possibly the development of diabetic nephropathy. The combination of arterial hypertension and renal vasodilation would predictably lead to especially high intrarenal and glomerular capillary pressures, as described later. In IDDM, blood pressure increases parallel the rise in urine albumin excretion. Careful 24-hour blood pressure monitoring has demonstrated that increases in both systolic and diastolic pressure (even in the top range of traditionally accepted normal values) are associated with progression from normoalbuminuria to microalbuminuria. Diabetic patients with the complication of renal failure may have a coinherited predisposition to essential hypertension. The presence of a parent with hypertension triples the risk for development of diabetic nephropathy. Recent studies have suggested that this predisposition is marked by an increased activity of the sodium-lithium transporter in red blood cells, an abnormality also seen in subsets of nondiabetic essential hypertensives. This countertransport activity represents the physiologic sodium-hydrogen antiporter. Diabetic patients with proteinuria also have higher lymphocyte or skin fibroblast sodium-hydrogen antiporter activity than nonproteinuric diabetics or nondiabetic controls. However, a large overlap exists in transporter activities among subgroups of diabetic patients, and this severely limits the general utility of such tests as predictive markers of nephropathy.

Patients with early (during the first 10 years of the disease) IDDM tend to have GFRs greater than those of nondiabetics; indeed, many are above the range of normal subjects. This hyperfiltration of early diabetes is due to increases in plasma flow and, based on data obtained in diabetic animals, a concomitant increase in glomerular capillary hydraulic pressures. Thus the diabetic kidney initially sustains increased renal perfusion and glomerular capillary pressure. The mechanism of this change in tissue blood flow has not been explained, but a number of possible factors, including increased vasodilatory prostanoids; nitric oxide; and humoral vasodilators such as glucagon, atrial natriuretic peptide, and insulin-like growth factor 1 (IGF-1), have all been suggested. In addition, the glomerular capillary surface area available for filtration enlarges and contributes to the increase in filtration rate. The hemodynamic changes of diabetes may contribute to the ultimate occurrence of end-stage renal disease through the injurious effects of high capillary pressures.

The mechanistic link between high intraglomerular pressure and vascular injury has not been directly established but could be based on direct pressure injury to endothelium or on increased wall tension leading to altered capillary wall structure and function. The latter could be exacerbated by the increased glomerular size in diabetes. The kidneys of diabetic patients are increased in size, and this can be taken as an index of hyperfiltration. Mesangial expansion may be a specific example of how renal and, in particular, glomerular hypertrophy can be disadvantageous because disproportionate expansion of the mesangial areas appears to be an important contributor to ultimate filtration failure. Besides the crowding out of the filtering surface area by the expanded mesangial matrix, the increased diameter of the glomerular capillary early in the course of diabetes may confer a mechanical disadvantage through the LaPlace relationship (tension = transmural pressure × vessel radius). Through this relationship increased capillary diameter would increase wall tension, which may be another injurious component of diabetes-induced renal enlargement. It is also postulated that increased stretching of mesangial cells caused by increased intraglomerular pressure may increase the production of prosclerotic cytokines such as transforming growth factor–beta (TGF-β). A growing body of evidence from cell culture studies and experimental animals has provided support for the notion that high ambient glucose levels stimulate the production and activity of TGF-β by glomerular cells; this cytokine in turn promotes cellular hypertrophy and stimulates the production of extracellular matrix. Thus hyperglycemia and glomerular hemodynamic stress cooperate to stimulate TGF-β activity, a key mediator of renal hypertrophy and extracellular matrix production.

Studies of the alterations of extracellular matrix metabolism in diabetes all suggest that there is an increased production and reduced degradation; both processes may contribute to extracellular matrix accumulation. A number of observations in various tissues suggest that both animals with experimental diabetes and patients have an increased synthesis of a variety of extracellular matrix components including types I and IV collagens, as well as various noncollagenous proteins such as fibronectin and laminin. Glomerulosclerosis, vascular hyalinosis, and interstitial fibrosis could result from the actions of glucose to stimulate biosynthetic pathways for extracellular matrix synthesis. In general these effects of high glucose concentration may arise as a consequence of increased de novo synthesis of diacylglycerol and subsequent activation of protein kinase C, early or advanced nonenzymatic glycation reactions in target proteins, increased activity of the polyol pathway and disordered cellular myoinositol metabolism, or enhanced synthesis and/or response to hormones, cytokines, or growth factors such as TGF-β.

A series of recent studies has suggested an important role for the *nonenzymatic glycation* of various circulating and structural proteins in contributing to the altered function and structure of vascular and glomerular components when exposed to persistent elevation of extracellular glucose levels. Nonenzymatic glycation refers to the condensation reaction between a sugar aldehyde or ketone with the ε-amino group of lysine or hydroxylysine in proteins; the resultant aldimine (Schiff base) then undergoes a stable Amadori rearrangement to form an "early glycation product." The concentration of the Amadori product is increased in proportion to the glucose concentration. Glycation of circulating proteins such as albumin could lead to deposition in the glomerulus and increased trafficking across the mesangium. Studies in tissue culture and in experimental animals have shown that Amadori glycated albumin stimulates mesangial cell production of extracellular matrix and promotes proteinuria.

The Amadori product can undergo further, slow, and irreversible reactions in vivo to form an array of compounds known collectively as advanced Maillard products or "advanced glycation products." These products accumulate progressively in tissues of diabetic patients. Tissue levels are higher in diabetic patients with nephropathy than in those without renal disease, perhaps reflecting the homeostatic role of the normal kidney in clearing these compounds. It has been proposed that the increased fibrosis and exudative vascular hyalinoses that characterize long-standing diabetes in experimental animals, as well as in patients, could in part be a function of chronic exposure of extracellular matrix proteins to high ambient glucose levels and subsequent nonenzymatic glycation forming long-lived glycation products. In addition, binding of these products to putative cellular receptors may result in activation of a variety of cytokine systems, which may play a role in tissue responses of the diabetic state. Extracellular matrix proteins such as collagens are rich in lysine and hydroxylysine, have a long biologic half-life, and are continuously exposed to ambient levels of glucose in the extracellular fluid. These proteins are good candidates for undergoing substantial glycation in vivo. The advanced glycation end products so produced create extremely abnormal matrix proteins that are capable of trapping albumin within basement membranes, trapping immunoglobulin G in extracellular matrix, and decreasing the solubility and capacity for degradation of the now abnormally linked collagens. Aminoguanidine has effects to inhibit the formation and action of the advanced glycation end products, and clinical trials are in progress with this compound to attempt to reproduce the favorable results that have been observed in experimental animals.

One potential common mechanism for the early tissue dysfunction seen in diabetes is stimulation of activity of the *polyol pathway.* This series of biochemical reactions may be summarized as follows:

(EQ. 1)

$$\text{Glucose} \xrightarrow[\substack{\text{Aldose} \\ \text{Reductase}}]{} \text{Sorbitol} \xrightarrow[\substack{\text{Sorbitol} \\ \text{Dehydrogenase}}]{} \text{Fructose}$$

$$\underbrace{\qquad}_{\text{NADPH}+\text{H}^+ \quad \text{NADP}^+} \qquad \underbrace{\qquad}_{\text{NAD}^+ \quad \text{NADH}+\text{H}^+}$$

The intracellular accumulation of sorbitol was first thought to produce cellular injury because of osmotically induced cell swelling. This mechanism may be operative in the lens in diabetes and lead to cataract formation. The cellular content of sorbitol in most other tissues, however, does not exceed 200 to 300 μM, despite severe hyperglycemia, and therefore is a small osmotic burden. Rather, a large body of evidence suggests that increased sorbitol formation produces a fundamental disturbance in cellular *myo*inositol metabo-

lism and that this disturbance is the proximate cause of the cellular defect induced by polyol pathway activation, at least in the retina and nerve. Cellular dysfunction may also relate to the altered redox potential as a result of the enhanced rate of reduction of the oxidized form of nicotinamide adenine dinucleotide (NAD$^+$), and increased fructosylation of tissues, another form of the nonenzymatic glycation pathway described earlier. Treatment with inhibitors of aldose reductase, the rate-limiting enzyme, may ameliorate early features of retinopathy and neuropathy and may alter the hemodynamic abnormalities seen in the kidney in early experimental and clinical diabetes. However, there is no consistent evidence that aldose reductase inhibitors are effective in reducing late manifestations of nephropathy. Clinical trials of the long-term safety and efficacy of this class of drugs are in progress.

The pathogenesis of diabetic nephropathy probably results from several abnormalities of the diabetic milieu. Identified factors are increases in ambient glucose level, arterial hypertension, glomerular hyperfiltration and capillary hypertension, the production of early and late nonenzymatic glycation products, extracellular matrix synthesis and accumulation due to increased prosclerotic growth factor activity, and excessive renal growth.

PREVENTION AND THERAPY

Most clinical evidence suggests that the more closely glucose is maintained within the normal range, the less likely it is that diabetic nephropathy will occur. Increasing evidence supports a role for strict control to prevent the development of incipient nephropathy and its manifestations, including glomerular hyperfiltration, renal hypertrophy, and microalbuminuria. The Stockholm Diabetes Intervention Study and the much larger Diabetes Control and Complication Trial clearly demonstrated the beneficial effects of intensive insulin therapy on the development and progression of diabetic complications in IDDM patients. In the latter study mean adjusted risk of microalbuminuria (more than 28 μg/min) over a 9-year period was reduced by 34% in the primary prevention cohort (without baseline retinopathy) and by 43% in the secondary intervention cohort (with mild retinopathy). The mean hemoglobin A1c level in the intensively treated group was 7 mg/dl as compared with 9 mg/dl in the conventionally treated group. The risk of macroalbuminuria ("dipstick positive" or a value exceeding 200 μg/min) was reduced by 56% in the secondary intervention cohort. However, in the subset of patients in whom microalbuminuria was present at the onset of the study, intensive therapy did not significantly decrease the rate of progression to macroalbuminuria as compared with conventional therapy. Other clinical experience also indicates that once definite nephropathy with declining GFR occurs, strict glycemic control does not alter the rate of deterioration or the nature of the late structural lesions. Thus, in terms of prevention of diabetic nephropathy, intensive glycemic control is of paramount importance in the normoalbuminuric IDDM patient, but it is of less clear value in the IDDM patient with established microalbuminuria. Nevertheless, strict glycemic control is warranted to diminish the overall risk of long-term multisystem complications. The strict control of glucose by exogenous insulin is often difficult and may be attended by substantial risks, especially hypoglycemia. The effect of improved glycemic control has not yet been prospectively tested in large populations of NIDDM patients.

Control of arterial hypertension with antihypertensive drugs is the most important available measure for retarding the progression of established diabetic nephropathy and retinopathy. Relatively strict criteria for antihypertensive therapy should be applied. Thus careful, repeated follow-up of even minor elevations above average blood pressure levels for age should be standard care of all patients with diabetes. If elevation above average arterial pressure is confirmed, antihypertensive treatment should be promptly initiated. The specific antihypertensive regimen must be tailored to the patient's individual needs, but the overriding need to lower elevated arterial pressure with agents cannot be overemphasized. Several clinical trials have demonstrated that reductions of arterial pressure with standard antihypertensive agents can dramatically slow the progressive decline in GFR. Angiotensin-converting enzyme (ACE) inhibitors have recently emerged as the drugs of choice because they are relatively well tolerated and are effective not only in reducing systemic blood pressure but also in controlling proteinuria and slowing the progression of renal injury. In particular, they reduce early manifestations such as hyperfiltration and microalbuminuria and may be particularly effective in reducing intraglomerular pressure. A large, prospective, placebo-controlled multicenter trial conducted in IDDM patients with overt nephropathy, whose blood pressure was controlled by antihypertensive agents excluding ACE inhibitors and calcium channel blockers, has demonstrated that the addition of captopril reduced by 50% the risk of doubling of serum creatinine concentration, as well as the mortality or the need for dialysis. It is currently recommended that blood pressure be reduced to 130/85 mmHg or lower, preferably by relying on an ACE inhibitor. Diuretics in low dose can be added to achieve a sustained reduction of systemic blood pressure. Additional antihypertensive regimens may sometimes be necessary. The concomitant appearance of clinically significant autonomic neuropathy with diabetic nephropathy and hypertension can complicate the treatment because of symptomatic orthostatic hypotension. Beta-blocking agents may, in certain patients, mask the symptoms of hypoglycemia, but these agents can be used in many patients with careful instruction and frequent monitoring of glucose levels. Calcium channel blockers have been used effectively with minimal side effects, but their long-term efficacy in reducing the progression of diabetic nephropathy must be established by comparison with ACE inhibitors in prospective studies.

Proteinuria itself may be considered an independent "progression promoter" of kidney diseases including diabetic nephropathy. The mechanism of this action remains obscure. Nevertheless, use of ACE inhibitors in microalbuminuric but normotensive patients is currently recommended to decrease the rate of decline in GFR in both IDDM and NIDDM patients. ACE inhibition achieves a renoprotective response independent of (or in addition to) an antihypertensive effect. Additional benefits of ACE inhibitors include improved glucose tolerance and lipid profile. These agents, however, may cause hyperkalemia more frequently in diabetic patients with nephropathy. Diuretic therapy may ameliorate the hyperkalemia associated with ACE inhibitor therapy. In patients with associated renal artery stenosis (more commonly the non–insulin-dependent older patient) these agents may induce reversible acute renal failure. Hence, serum creatinine and potassium levels should be monitored during treatment with these drugs.

Dietary protein restriction appears to lessen the progression of a number of progressive renal diseases, including diabetic nephropathy. Available evidence suggests that restriction of dietary protein to the level of 0.8 g of high biologic value protein per kilogram body weight is safe. Careful education and follow-up, usually with the help of a dietitian, are required to effect such a dietary change successfully.

Delaying the onset of diabetes itself is the most logical maneuver in eliminating its long-term complications. This mostly pertains to NIDDM, whereby dietary prevention of obesity in genetically predisposed populations effectively delays or prevents the onset of overt hyperglycemia and insulin resistance.

BIBLIOGRPAHY

Bennett PH et al: Screening and management of microalbuminuria in patients with diabetes mellitus: recommendations to the Scientific Advisory Board of the National Kidney Foundation from an ad hoc committee of the Council on Diabetes Mellitus of the National Kidney Foundation, *Am J Kidney Dis* 25:107, 1995.

Brownlee M: Advanced protein glycosylation in diabetes and aging, *Annu Rev Med* 46:223, 1995.

Clark CM, Lee DA: Prevention and treatment of the complications of diabetes mellitus, *N Engl J Med* 332:1210, 1995.

Cohen MP, Ziyadeh FN: Role of Amadori-modified nonenzymatically glycated serum proteins in the pathogenesis of diabetic nephropathy, *J Am Soc Nephrol* 7:1-8, 1996.

Diabetes Control and Complications Trial Research Group: The effect of intensive treatment of diabetes on the development and progression of long-term complications in insulin-dependent diabetes mellitus, *N Engl J Med* 329:977, 1993.

Diabetes Control and Complications Trial Research Group: Effect of intensive therapy on the development and progression of diabetic nephropathy in the Diabetes Control and Complications Trial, *Kidney Int* 47:1703, 1995.

Gall MA, Borch-Johnsen K, Hougaard P et al: Albuminuria and poor glycemic control predict mortality in NIDDM, *Diabetes* 44:1303, 1995.

Leese GP, Vora JP: Clinical interventions in diabetic renal disease, *Curr Opin Nephrol Hypertension* 4:139, 1995.

✔ *WHEN TO REFER*

Referral to a nephrologist is indicated when the blood pressure becomes difficult to control and when there is evidence of the nephrotic syndrome or progressive decline in GFR. Discussion can also begin on the relative merits and advisability of various dialysis options or renal transplantation and to decide when to establish access to the circulation. Patients with end-stage renal disease have the same options for renal replacement therapy as do patients with other chronic renal diseases. In general, patients with diabetic nephropathy in general, do less well with both hemodialysis and peritoneal dialysis than do patients with nondiabetic uremia and have a generally poorer prognosis after renal transplantation. However, the survival rates for patients with diabetes with all these modes of therapy have improved. Renal transplantation for young IDDM patients not only offers a better quality of life and freedom from the encumbrances of regular dialytic therapy, it also achieves longer survival. A major difficulty for patients with diabetes is progressive vascular disease in other organs, notably the central nervous system and peripheral and coronary circulation; substantial mortality resulting from cardiovascular disease persists, even with successful dialysis or transplantation.

Lewis EJ, Hunsicker LG, Bain RP, Rohde RD: The effect of angiotensin-converting enzyme inhibition on diabetic nephropathy, *N Engl J Med* 329:1456, 1993.

Mogensen CE: Diabetic renal disease: the quest for normotension—and beyond, *Diabetic Med* 12:756, 1995.

Parving HH, Rossing P, Hommel E, Smidt UM: Angiotensin-converting enzyme inhibition in diabetic nephropathy: ten years' experience, *Am J Kidney Dis* 26:99, 1995.

Reichard P, Nilsson B, Rosenqvist U: The effect of long-term intensified insulin treatment on the development of microvascular complications of diabetes mellitus, *N Engl J Med* 329:304, 1993.

Sharma K, Ziyadeh FN: Hyperglycemia and diabetic kidney disease: the case for transforming growth factor–beta as a key mediator, *Diabetes* 44:1139, 1995.

Trevisan R, Viberti GC: Genetic factors in the development of diabetic nephropathy, *J Lab Clin Med* 126:342, 1995.

Ziyadeh FN: Mediators of hyperglycemia and the pathogenesis of matrix accumulation in diabetic renal disease, *Miner Electrolyte Metab* 21:292, 1995.

Ziyadeh FN, Goldfarb S: The diabetic renal tubulointerstitium. In Dodd S, editor: *Current topics in pathology,* Berlin, 1995, Springer-Verlag.

CHAPTER

118 Renal Manifestations of Dysproteinemias

Paul W. Sanders

MULTIPLE MYELOMA AND PLASMA CELL DYSCRASIAS (Chapter 94)
Physiology and Pathophysiology

In the century and a half following the initial description by Dr. Henry Bence Jones of an abnormal urinary protein excreted from a patient who had multiple myeloma, Bence Jones proteins have been identified as monoclonal immunoglobulin light chain proteins and demonstrated to possess the center stage in the pathogenesis of the renal lesions associated with plasma cell dyscrasias. Light chains are low-molecular-weight proteins of approximately 22 kD and are divided into two classes: kappa (κ) and lambda (λ). Each light chain protein possesses two globular domains: a constant region of 105 to 107 amino acids that is common to either κ or λ light chain and a variable domain, which comprises the remaining 110 to 120 amino acids. This variable segment makes each light chain molecule unique and forms part of the antigen-binding site of the immunoglobulin molecule. The constant region is a single gene product located on human chromosome 2 for κ light chain and on chromosome 22 for λ light chain. Multiple gene segments are used to produce the variable polypeptide region. Thus, despite similar chemical properties, no two light chains are identical. Plasma cells synthesize light chains independently of heavy chains and subsequently combine them in the endoplasmic reticulum to form the immunoglobulin molecule. However, excess light chains are often synthesized, as compared with heavy chains, allowing escape of free light chains into the circulation. Occasionally, if the heavy chain is unavailable, two light chains may combine by disulfide linkage to form a dimer before secretion. A plasma cell clone can release large amounts of homogeneous light chains. Because of their size, light chains are filtered readily through the glomerulus and are reabsorbed by the proximal tubule. As the reabsorptive process of the proximal tubule becomes saturated, light chain proteins appear in the distal nephron and finally in the urine as Bence Jones proteins. Causes of Bence Jones proteinuria are listed (Box 118-1).

Many light chains are nephrotoxic and during transit through the nephron damage nephrons by altering function of glomerular mesangial cells or proximal tubule epithelial cells, or by precipitating in the lumen of the distal nephron. The type of lesion produced depends on specific, yet poorly characterized, physicochemical properties of the light chain. The predominant renal lesions of plasma cell dyscrasias include cast nephropathy ("myeloma kidney"), light chain glomerulopathy (monoclonal light chain deposition disease) and the immunocyte-derived (AL) type of amyloidosis, although other renal lesions are associated with myeloma (Box 118-2).

The pathophysiology of the major renal lesions of light chains is now better understood. Light chain glomerulopathy (monoclonal light chain deposition disease) is characterized by deposition of light chains (approximately 10% have light and heavy chains) in granular deposits in the mesangium and subendothelial space. The mesangial space is increased by accumulation of these light chains and matrix proteins; sclerotic nodules are frequently seen in the glomeruli. The pathogenesis of this lesion is related to binding of certain light chains to mesangial cells to stimulate them to produce transforming growth factor-β. In turn, transforming growth factor-β serves as an autacoid to stimulate the mesangium to produce extracellular matrix proteins. Production of matrix proteins expands the mesangial space and compresses the filtering surfaces of the glomerulus. The result is progressive renal failure from nodular glomerulosclerosis.

The other glomerular lesion of light chains is the AL type of amyloidosis. *Amyloid* is a generic term applied to proteins that have unique tinctorial characteristics and a distinctive ultrastructural appearance (see also Chapter 210). Amyloid stains particularly with Congo red dye and thioflavin T. With electron microscopy amyloid appears as nonbranching fibrils 8 to 10 nm in diameter. Numerous different proteins, which are overproduced in heredofamilial or chronic inflammatory states and in plasma cell dyscrasias, can serve as precursors for amyloid. Certain immunoglobulin light chains, particularly the λ_{VI} type, are potentially amyloidogenic. The AL type of amyloidosis develops when mesangial cells are exposed to amyloidogenic light chains. These proteins are processed in the mesangial cell to form intracellular amyloid, which then is extruded into the extracellular space. Accumulation of amyloid in the mesangium results in loss of the filtering surface of the glomerulus; the result is progressive renal failure from formation of nodules of amyloid protein.

Intraluminal precipitation of light chain with subsequent obstruction of the tubule lumen is characteristic of cast nephropathy. The number of casts present correlates with reversibility of the renal failure. Cast nephropathy is initiated in the distal nephron, where cast-forming light chains bind to Tamm-Horsfall glycoprotein, a heavily glycosylated protein synthesized by cells of the thick ascending limb of the loop of Henle. Tamm-Horsfall glycoprotein forms the matrix of these intraluminal casts. Light chains bind noncovalently to a common site on Tamm-Horsfall glycoprotein, but with differing affinities, and form insoluble complexes that can obstruct the tubule lumen. Several factors can alter the clinical manifestation of this biochemical interaction (Box 118-3). Factors that enhance precipitation include a high concentration of light chain in the tubule lumen, a high

---

BOX 118-1

Causes of monoclonal light chain proteinuria

Multiple myeloma
Immunocyte-derived (AL) type of amyloidosis
Monoclonal light chain deposition disease
Waldenström's macroglobulinemia
Heavy chain (μ) disease
Monoclonal gammopathy of undetermined significance
Chronic lymphoproliferative disease
Rifampin therapy (rare)

BOX 118-2

Renal lesions associated with plasma cell dyscrasias

Glomerulopathies
    Immunocyte-derived (AL) type of amyloidosis*
    Monoclonal light chain deposition disease*
    Fibrillary glomerulonephritis
Tubulointerstitial lesions
    Fanconi's syndrome
    Proximal tubule necrosis
    Cast nephropathy ("myeloma kidney")*
    Inflammatory tubulointerstitial nephritis
Vascular (arterial) lesions
    AL type of amyloid
    Granular light chain deposition disease
Asymptomatic Bence Jones proteinuria
Plasma cell infiltration of the kidney
Urinary tract obstruction
Hypercalcemic nephropathy*
Hyperviscosity syndrome
Pyelonephritis

*Represents most common renal lesions.

BOX 118-3

Factors affecting cast formation

Amount and type of immunoglobulin light chain protein
Amount and carbohydrate composition of Tamm-Horsfall glycoprotein
Distal nephron milieu, including the following:
    Sodium chloride concentration
    Calcium concentration
    Tubule fluid flow rate
    Tubule fluid pH
    Presence of furosemide or radiocontrast agents

---

binding affinity with Tamm-Horsfall glycoprotein, high concentration and type of carbohydrate on Tamm-Horsfall glycoprotein, high concentrations of certain electrolytes (sodium and calcium), extracellular fluid volume depletion that decreases flow through the nephron, acidic pH, and presence of furosemide or radiocontrast agents.

Proximal tubule damage can also occur during the process of endocytosis and catabolism, when certain toxic light chains fill and distend lysosomes and often precipitate within these organelles; crystals can be identified in some cells. This process, if significant and widespread, can cause acute tubular necrosis. Renal tubule acidification defects and Fanconi's syndrome may also be seen.

Laboratory and Other Diagnostic Tests

The classic presenting features of multiple myeloma include skeletal pain, pathologic fractures, and diffuse osteoporosis (see also Chapter 94). Localized areas of osteolysis without osteoblastic reaction are characteristic. Normochromic, normocytic anemia, as well as other hematologic abnormalities including leukopenia, thrombocytopenia, and hemolysis, has been described. Hypogammaglobulinemia is not uncommon, and may be pronounced when only monoclonal light chains are produced ("light chain disease"). The capacity of B cells to secrete or produce normal immunoglobulins is frequently impaired. The combined effects of hypogammaglobulinemia, malnutrition, and renal failure make infections the most common cause of death in these patients.

The incidence of renal failure is related to the type of immunoglobulin produced and is highest in immunoglobulin D (IgD) type of myeloma. Acute or chronic renal failure is present in about 50% of all patients at presentation, and renal failure in the usual clinical setting of myeloma is almost a coincidental finding. Renal failure can also be triggered by use of nonsteroidal antiinflammatory agents. However, earlier clinical presentations of isolated renal involvement are occurring in part because of development of sensitive techniques that detect monotypical light chain deposition in kidney tissue. It is not uncommon to uncover a plasma cell dyscrasia after performing a renal biopsy to diagnose the nature of the renal disease. Progressive renal failure, nephrotic syndrome, nephrotic-range proteinuria, acute renal failure, and mild proteinuria with or without hematuria can be presenting manifestations of myeloma.

Electrolyte abnormalities may provide a clue to the diagnosis of multiple myeloma. Hypercalcemia is the most frequent and important electrolyte disturbance. Rarely, the myeloma protein can bind calcium and produce a syndrome of pseudohypercalcemia with normal ionized calcium concentration, despite elevated total serum calcium concentration. Similarly, some myeloma proteins bind phosphate and can produce spurious hyperphosphatemia when standard colorimetric assays are used. Multiple myeloma, particularly the immunoglobulin G (IgG) type, may also be associated with a low anion gap because large amounts of immunoglobulin that possess net positive electrostatic charges tend to reduce the normal "anion gap" by increasing the amount of neutralizing anions in the serum. Fanconi's syndrome, which is a severe proximal tubule injury that results in aminoaciduria, glycosuria, phosphaturia, and hyperchloremic metabolic acidosis, is found in a small number of patients and can be a presenting feature of myeloma.

Diagnosis and classification of multiple myeloma rest on the identification and quantification of the abnormal immunoglobulin molecule by immunoelectrophoretic analysis of serum and urine. Immunofixation electrophoresis, which is very sensitive, detects monoclonal proteins, including light chains, even in very low concentrations. However, the presence of a small amount of monoclonal light chain can be masked by coexistent tubulointerstitial disease that produces significant proximal tubule damage and therefore results in increased excretion of low-molecular-weight proteins that include polyclonal light chains. Despite problems with detection, a diagnostic hallmark of plasma cell dyscrasias has been Bence Jones proteinuria. In over two thirds of patients with myeloma a monoclonal gammopathy is detected in the serum. Quantitative assay of the abnormal immunoglobulin ("M" component) is one of the best indices to follow the progression of the disease and the response to treatment. Other important diagnostic tests include a bone survey to identify osteolytic lesions and examination of the bone marrow. Plasma cells that are more than 20% of nonerythroid cells, especially if they are vacuolated, bizarre, and multinucleated, support a diagnosis of multiple myeloma.

Differential Diagnosis

Virtually any compartment of the kidney can be damaged from monoclonal light chain overproduction (Box 118-2). However, the simultaneous occurrence of two or more of these lesions in the same patient is unusual (Fig. 118-1). The degree of proteinuria, which can be impressive and is related to excessive glomerular filtration of the light chain, cannot distinguish glomerular from tubular lesions. The presence of hypoalbuminemia, edema, and nephrotic-range albuminuria

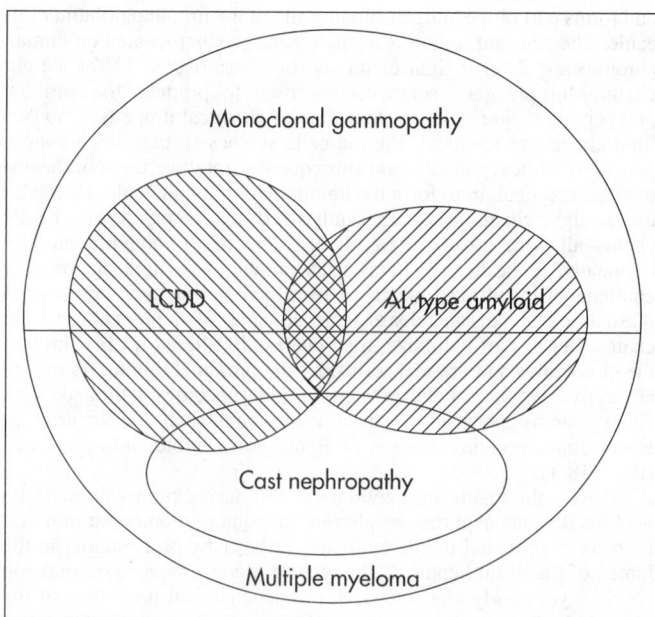

FIGURE 118-1   Diagram of the relationship of the three major renal lesions related to light chain deposition and association with plasma cell dyscrasias. Although most patients with cast nephropathy have multiple myeloma, significantly fewer patients with monoclonal light chain deposition disease *(LCDD)* and the immunocyte-derived (AL) type of amyloidosis have overt myeloma. Overlap among these three renal lesions occurs but is uncommon.

suggests a glomerular lesion such as monoclonal light chain deposition disease or the AL type of amyloidosis. Although exact identification of the nature of the renal failure requires percutaneous renal biopsy, there are several similarities and differences between monoclonal light chain deposition disease and the AL type of amyloidosis (Table 118-1).

Determining the nature of the plasma cell dyscrasia producing the renal lesion can be difficult. Although virtually all patients with cast nephropathy have multiple myeloma, the glomerular lesions can occur without other clinical manifestations of myeloma. An absent "M" component occurs in about one fifth of patients with monoclonal light chain deposition disease and the AL type of amyloidosis (Table 118-1). Metastatic bone surveys are also frequently normal in these patients. Bone marrow biopsy with immunophenotyping to document a monoclonal population of plasma cells may facilitate a diagnosis of multiple myeloma in these patients. A significant number of patients with monoclonal light chain deposition disease and AL type of amyloidosis do not have overt myeloma (Table 118-1). Thus a normal bone marrow biopsy and skeletal survey do not rule out the existence of a population of bone marrow cells producing abnormal light chains that are deposited in the kidney and cause renal failure. Overt multiple myeloma may develop in these patients over time. Patients with monoclonal gammopathy of undetermined significance and without evidence of clinical renal dysfunction should also be closely followed up because in as many as one fourth overt myeloma, amyloidosis, macroglobulinemia, or malignant lymphoproliferative disorder will eventually develop (see also Chapter 94).

Management

As a group the renal lesions responsible for renal failure are potentially reversible renal diseases. Virtually all lesions progress to end-stage renal failure if not treated. Because the common thread in these lesions is monoclonal light chain production, treatments designed to reduce circulating light chain levels should be the mainstay of therapy. The standard chemotherapeutic regimen that includes melphalan and prednisone ameliorates renal failure in over half of patients who have multiple myeloma and come to medical attention with renal failure.

Monoclonal light chain deposition disease is more resistant to che-

Table 118-1 Comparison of monoclonal light chain deposition disease (LCDD) and immunocyte-derived (AL) type of amyloidosis

RENAL PRESENTATION	LCDD RPGN, NEPHROTIC SYNDROME, PROTEINURIA, HEMATURIA	AL TYPE OF AMYLOIDOSIS NEPHROTIC SYNDROME, PROTEINURIA, HEMATURIA
Systemic deposition	Yes	Yes
Presentation with myeloma (%)	47	21
Absent "M" component in serum and urine (%)	20	18
Glomerular morphologic features	Nodular, "minimal change," membranoproliferative, mesangioproliferative, crescentic (rare)	Nodular, "minimal change"
Composition of nodules	Matrix + light chains (can contain heavy chains)	Light chains (heavy chain: one case)
Light chain component	κ > λ	λ > κ
Type of deposits	Granular, noncongophilic	Fibrillar, congophilic

*RPGN, Syndrome of rapidly progressing glomerulonephritis, characterized by worsening renal failure as the presenting manifestation.

motherapy but may remit when treatment is initiated before the serum creatinine concentration reaches 2 mg/dl (180 μmol/L). A 12- to 24-month course of alkylating agents and prednisone also decreases proteinuria, ameliorates nephrotic syndrome, and improves renal dysfunction in some patients with the AL type of amyloidosis. In addition, chemotherapy appears to prolong survival. The response rate to chemotherapy in amyloidosis approaches 20%. Generally, however, amyloid deposition continues and progressive renal failure is the rule.

Chemotherapy improves renal function in cast nephropathy but slowly reduces light chain levels. Plasmapheresis rapidly lowers the plasma concentration of light chains, improves outcome in acute renal failure, and has been recommended in the management of patients who come to medical attention with acute renal failure and have not received chemotherapy previously. Renal failure improves in perhaps half of patients during chemotherapy, but progressive loss of renal function subsequently occurs in many of these patients. For this reason, attention should be paid to correcting those factors known to aggravate nephrotoxicity of light chains by facilitating coprecipitation with Tamm-Horsfall glycoprotein (Box 118-3). Thus rapid correction of hypercalcemia, alkalinization of the urine, and increasing tubule fluid flow rates by recommending a daily intake of 2 to 3 L of dilute fluids (as tolerated) may prevent renal failure from light chains. In humans alkalinization of the urine by itself has not been shown to be readily beneficial but may be used in conjunction with other measures. Other prudent measures include avoidance of radiocontrast agents and other medications that enhance light chain toxicity. Because furosemide aggravates cast formation, this loop diuretic should be used with caution, especially when extracellular volume depletion is present. Nonsteroidal antiinflammatory agents are contraindicated, as they can precipitate acute renal failure in the setting of light chain proteinuria.

Allogeneic or autologous marrow transplantation is another potential therapy for overt myeloma but carries a high morbidity and mortality rate and should be performed at centers with expertise in bone marrow transplantation. Generally, allogeneic marrow transplantation is a potential therapy for patients who are less than 65 years of age and have not responded to standard therapy. Autologous marrow transplantation with intensive chemotherapy offers the hope of control of the disease. Controlled trials involving the use of bone marrow transplantation to manage monoclonal light chain deposition disease or the AL type of amyloidosis not associated with overt myeloma have not been reported.

Recovery of renal function sufficient to survive without dialysis occurs in as many as 5% of patients with multiple myeloma but requires months in some individuals. In addition, while multisystem involvement and advanced age at the time of diagnosis shorten life span, patients with disease generally limited to the kidney may achieve functional rehabilitation and survive more than 2 years. For these reasons renal replacement therapy (hemodialysis or peritoneal dialysis) may be recommended. The role of renal transplantation is less certain, but may be considered for the exceptional patient whose extrarenal manifestations of the disease are absent for more than 1 year. Suitable patients may then undergo successful transplantation and obtain prolonged survival. Renal transplantation in these individuals may be particularly beneficial if the clinical manifestation of the disease has remained limited to the kidney. In

> ✔ **WHEN TO REFER**
>
> Patients with plasma cell dyscrasias should be examined closely for renal involvement. Blood should be obtained for determination of serum albumin, calcium, urea nitrogen, creatinine, and electrolyte levels. A 24-hour creatinine clearance rate and a protein excretion rate should also be determined. Renal ultrasound estimates kidney size and excludes urinary tract obstruction. Periodic assessment of renal function, along with determination of progression of the plasma cell dyscrasia, is indicated in patients who do not have renal function abnormalities at presentation. Evidence of renal involvement dictates a thorough evaluation to determine the nature of the renal lesion and institution of appropriate therapy.

one large study of 62 patients, 15 of whom had the AL type of amyloidosis, 65% of patients were alive 5 years after renal allograft implantation. Although amyloid involved the graft in 10%, only 3% lost the graft as a direct result of this involvement. Transplant experience with monoclonal light chain deposition disease is even more limited, but the disease may also recur in the allograft and cause renal failure. Besides recurrent disease in the transplanted kidney, despite careful screening, myeloma may also recur after transplantation.

Despite treatment, the median survival of patients with renal failure and multiple myeloma is 20 months, versus 25 months for all patients with myeloma. Median survival is reduced to 4.3 months when the serum creatinine concentration exceeds 2 mg/dl (180 μmol/L). The course in monoclonal light chain deposition disease is variable. The 3-year survival approaches 76% but is reduced to 15 to 20 months when overt multiple myeloma is also present. The survival in the AL type of amyloidosis is 12 to 15 months but is similarly reduced with coexistent multiple myeloma.

WALDENSTRÖM'S MACROGLOBULINEMIA

Waldenström's macroglobulinemia (see also Chapter 94) is considered separately from the other plasma cell dyscrasias because the renal lesions are different from those described earlier. Macroglobulinemia is a B-cell neoplastic transformation that behaves more like lymphoma and, moreover, secretes monoclonal immunoglobulin M (IgM) (macroglobulin). The clinical manifestations are related to organ infiltration and hyperviscosity of blood. Osteolytic lesions are uncommon. Infiltration of the kidney can produce nephromegaly. Symptoms of increased blood viscosity are usually the presenting manifestation and include bleeding diathesis, neurologic disturbances, visual disturbances, renal failure, and congestive heart failure. Although Bence Jones proteinuria can be detected by immunologic methods in over 90% of patients, cast nephropathy is rarely seen and the AL type of amyloidosis is uncommon. A unique but infrequent renal feature of macroglobulinemia is intraglomerular capillary occlusion by IgM protein.

Hyperviscosity syndrome is an indication for plasmapheresis. Plasma viscosity can be followed to determine efficacy, and plasmapheresis may be required intermittently during the indolent, progressive course of the disease. Chemotherapy with alkylating agents may be beneficial, but whether this treatment prevents renal failure in this disease is unclear.

BIBLIOGRAPHY

Ganeval D et al: Treatment of multiple myeloma with renal involvement, *Adv Nephrol* 21:347-370, 1992.

Hartmann A et al: Fifteen years' experience with renal transplantation in systemic amyloidosis, *Transplant Int* 5:15-18, 1992.

Huang Z-Q et al: Bence Jones proteins bind to a common peptide segment on Tamm-Horsfall glycoprotein to promote heterotypic aggregation, *J Clin Invest* 92:2975-2983, 1993.

Huang Z-Q, Sanders PW: Biochemical interaction between Tamm-Horsfall glycoprotein and Ig light chains in the pathogenesis of cast nephropathy, *Lab Invest* 73:810-817, 1995.

Sanders PW, Booker BB: Pathobiology of cast nephropathy from human Bence Jones proteins, *J Clin Invest* 89:630-639, 1992.

Zhu L et al: Pathogenesis of glomerulosclerosis in light chain deposition disease: role for transforming growth factor-β, *Am J Pathol* 147:375-385, 1995.

CHAPTER

119 Drug- and Chemical-Induced Nephropathy

William M. Bennett and William F. Finn

Renal injury attributable to drugs and chemicals has become an important cause of a variety of nephrologic syndromes. Acute and chronic renal failure, fluid and electrolyte abnormalities, proteinuria, and aggravation of preexisting renal disease are frequently produced by the expanding list of drugs and chemicals in our environment. Any given nephrotoxin may produce a variety of clinical effects, depending on type of exposure and host factors. Thus it is prudent for the clinician to consider toxic renal diseases as a potential cause in any patient who comes to medical attention with an undifferentiated renal syndrome.

The susceptibility of the kidney to toxic agents is in large part a consequence of its intricate anatomic and functional relationships. For example, the blood flow to the kidney per gram of tissue weight is greater than that to any other organ, ensuring that exposure of the kidney to bloodborne toxins is great. Furthermore, the processes of glomerular filtration, tubular reabsorption, and secretion serve to concentrate toxic agents within the kidney itself. As a result of their sophisticated function, renal tubular epithelial cells are particularly vulnerable to the action of metabolic inhibitors. The kidney also possesses various mixed-function oxidases that are useful in the biotransformation of foreign compounds (xenobiotics) into nontoxic metabolites. At times these processes result in the production of more toxic metabolites.

The specific mechanisms for toxic renal injury are multiple, and more than one can coexist in a given patient. Direct toxic effects are determined by the specific chemical properties of the substances, the duration and extent of exposure, and the nature of the host response. They may be manifested as abnormalities in the renal vasculature, dysfunction of the glomerular capillary membranes, or changes in tubular epithelial cell function. Immunologic responses include cytotoxic reactions with complement activation, immune-complex reactions, and perhaps a delayed hypersensitivity response.

Host factors may alter renal toxicity by influencing the metabolism of xenobiotics, the renal concentration of toxic agents, the susceptibility to cell injury, or the capacity for repair. It is important to consider that exposure to several agents often produces a synergistic effect. Other important host factors are those related to growth and aging. Not only does renal susceptibility to toxic damage increase with age, but at the same time the ability to repair damaged tissue also fades.

Often disregarded is the role of the nutritional status of the individual in determining the susceptibility or tolerance to or the recovery from noxious agents. Certain disease states, particularly those independently involving the kidney, significantly enhance renal toxicity in response to various classes of agents.

The following discussion concentrates on the most important causes of environmental and occupational nephrotoxicity, along with the most common causes of nephrotoxicity caused by diagnostic and therapeutic agents.

EFFECT OF ENVIRONMENTAL AND OCCUPATIONAL AGENTS ON THE KIDNEY
Glycols

Glycols are used as industrial solvents in a variety of industries. *Ethylene glycol* is the main component in antifreeze and may be ingested by patients as a substitute for alcohol or in suicide attempts. Ethylene glycol is converted to glycoaldehyde with further metabolism to glycolic acid, glyoxylate, and eventual irreversible oxidation to oxalate. The initial reaction depends on alcohol dehydrogenase, so simultaneous ingestion of ethyl alcohol and ethylene glycol decreases the oxidation of the latter and modifies its toxicity. The initial manifestations of ethylene glycol poisoning involve the central nervous system and generally coincide with the greatest amount of aldehyde production. Later, pulmonary symptoms predominate and with the deposition of calcium oxalate crystals in the kidney, oxaluria and oliguric acute renal failure supervene. Severe hypocalcemia caused by chelation of calcium ions by oxalate and an overwhelming acidosis aggravated by the production of lactate are hallmarks of this condition. Pyridoxine deficiency markedly increases the amount of ethylene glycol metabolized to oxalate and thus adds to the toxicity. The lethal dose of ethylene glycol is 2 ml/kg, which represents 0.1 g/kg of oxalic acid. The diagnosis should be considered when alcohol-like intoxication without the odor of alcohol, coma with metabolic acidosis and a large anion gap, or massive calcium oxalate crystalluria is observed on examination of the urine. Crystalluria is demonstrated by needle-shaped crystals of calcium oxalate monohydrate or octahedral "envelopes" of calcium oxalate dihydrate. Treatment is designed to correct the acidosis, prevent the manifestations of hypocalcemia, supply adequate thiamine and pyridoxine, and remove ethylene glycol and its products by means of forced diuresis or dialysis, or both. With acute, massive exposure dialysis is indicated even in the absence of renal failure. In acute conditions intravenous treatment with ethyl alcohol, given in a loading dose of 0.6 to 1.0 g/kg over 1 hour, followed by a sustained infusion of 10 to 12 g/hr to maintain the blood level at 100 mg/dl, is effective by virtue of its competition with alcohol dehydrogenase. Other potentially toxic glycols include *ethylene glycol dinitrite, propylene glycol, ethylene dichloride,* and *diethylene glycol.* The latter has been used in the past as a medicinal vehicle in an elixir of sulfanilamide. It is a potent tubular toxin.

Organic Solvents

Carbon tetrachloride has been widely used as an industrial solvent and as a household cleaning agent. It is soluble in alcohol, and both hepatic and renal toxicity increase if ethyl alcohol is consumed during the period of exposure. Acute renal failure occurs as a consequence of ingestion or inhalation and exhibits several unusual characteristics. After exposure a reduction in urine volume may not be apparent for 7 to 10 days. During this time the individual may be symptom free but is more likely to complain of vomiting, abdominal pain, constipation, diarrhea, or fever. The oliguria lasts 1 to 2 weeks. Analysis of the urine reveals more red blood cells and protein than are present in other forms of nephrotoxic acute renal failure. Recovery is expected. *Chloroform* is used chiefly as a refrigerant and as an aerosol propellant and in the synthesis of fluorinated resins. It is also produced during the chlorination of water. Although its primary effect is on the central nervous system and liver, it can also be nephrotoxic. Chloroform is thought to be transformed into a toxic product by microsomal metabolism. On this basis the ingestion of diets high in polybrominated biphenyls, known to be inducers of microsomal enzyme activity, enhances chloroform nephrotoxicity. *Trichloroethylene* is chemically related to both carbon tetrachloride and chloroform and shares with them the propensity for liver and kidney damage. It has a number of industrial applications and has been used as an anesthetic agent for obstetric patients. Acute renal failure has followed inhalation by "solvent sniffers" and in those using cleaning solutions containing this agent. *Toluene* is an aromatic hydrocarbon that has widespread use as an organic solvent. Its potential for renal toxicity has been demonstrated by those who have sniffed toluene-containing substances such as model glues. The maximum allowable concentration of toluene is far exceeded when these compounds are inhaled from paper bags. Although renal damage is generally mild, severe metabolic renal tubular acidosis can be produced.

It has been suggested by epidemiologic studies that prolonged, excessive exposure to various *hydrocarbons,* interacting with as yet unidentified host factors, predisposes a patient to chronic glomerular disease. An apparent association with Goodpasture's syndrome with exposure to petroleum products has been reported. Some authors have found that previous exposure to hydrocarbon solvents is a common feature among some groups of patients with crescentic or proliferative glomerulonephritis. Remissions and exacerbations of the nephrotic syndrome are noted to follow removal from and reexposure to solvents. A temporal relationship between glomerulonephritis and exposure to gasoline vapors has also been described.

Heavy Metals

Arsenic is used in insecticides, ant poisons, weed killers, wallpaper, antifouling paint, ceramics, wood preservatives, and glass. The inorganic arsenicals such as arsenic trioxide are more toxic than the organic compounds. Absorption follows inhalation or ingestion. The soluble compounds are readily absorbed via skin and mucous membranes and excreted primarily in the urine. Repeated doses are cumulative. Toxicity results when arsenic combines with sulfhydral enzymes and interferes with cellular oxidative processes. When arsenic is ingested in large amounts, the initial symptoms include a dry, burning sensation in the mouth and throat. This is followed by crampy abdominal pain, severe vomiting, and diarrhea. Vertigo, delirium, and coma are quite obvious manifestations of central nervous system involvement. Death may be caused by circulatory collapse with liver and renal failure. Hemodialysis has been found to be effective treatment for renal failure in some studies. British antilewisite (BAL) (2, 3,-dimercapto-1-propanol or dimercaprol) is valuable in acute arsenic poisoning. *Arsine* is an extremely toxic gas produced by the action of acid on metal in the presence of arsenic. It is a hazard to workers in metallurgic industries who work with ore contaminated by arsenic. Acute renal failure may accompany arsenic poisoning, which is most likely caused by concomitant cardiovascular collapse and hemolysis. Oliguric acute renal failure is a common complication of arsine (AsH$_3$) inhalation.

Cadmium is a major by-product of industrial zinc production. It is used in nickel-cadmium batteries; in manufacture of alloys, paints, and glass; in electroplating and soldering; and as a stabilizer in plastics. Cadmium is found in cigarette smoke, seafood, and drinking water. As a result of widespread exposure and a half-life that may exceed 30 years, the body content of cadmium slowly accumulates and may eventually reach about 30 mg. Cadmium contamination of food is thought to be the major source of cadmium for the general population. After absorption, cadmium tends to accumulate in the liver and kidney. It is bound to metallothionein, a low-molecular-weight, cysteine-rich apoprotein. Accumulation in the kidney continues even as other tissue concentrations fall. It appears that a certain level of cadmium must accumulate within the kidney before overt damage is produced. Urinary excretion increases when defects occur in the tubular reabsorption of metallothionein. Later, as tubular injury progresses to the point of cell death, the renal cortical concentration of cadmium decreases. Thereafter renal cadmium levels may fall, despite the fact that liver concentrations continue to rise. Blood values greater than 0.7 μg/dl, urine values above 20 μg/L, and renal cortical concentrations exceeding 200 μg/g wet kidney weight are thought to be associated with nephrotoxicity.

Lead has been associated with at least two types of renal impairment. In the more acute form generalized defects in proximal tubular function result in Fanconi's syndrome with aminoaciduria, glycosuria, and phosphaturia. Serum uric acid levels are generally elevated because of a defect in the tubular secretion of uric acid. Occasionally

the urine contains cells with eosinophilic intranuclear inclusions composed of lead and protein. These abnormalities most often occur in children after several months of heavy lead ingestion with blood lead levels usually in excess of 150 mg/dl. Although this impairment is generally rapidly reversible, it is likely that some conditions progress to chronic lead nephropathy, a form of chronic interstitial nephritis. Various factors, such as a deficiency of calcium in the diet, iron deficiency, and exposure to sunlight and vitamin D, may increase the amount of lead absorbed and the severity of the disease.

Chronic lead nephropathy is qualitatively different from Fanconi's syndrome. It is an indolent disease that is difficult to separate from other forms of chronic, slowly progressive renal insufficiency. Evidence of excessive lead absorption is supplied by determining urinary lead excretion by the calcium disodium salt of ethylenediamine tetraacetic acid (EDTA) lead mobilization test. The test is performed by measuring the urinary lead excretion after the administration of EDTA. One gram of EDTA is given twice, 8 to 12 hours apart. During this time a 24-hour urine specimen is collected. An excessive body lead burden is indicated by excretion of more than 1000 μg of lead per day. As an alternative, 1 g EDTA in 250 ml of 5% glucose solution may be given intravenously over the course of 1 hour for 3 consecutive days. Excretion of more than 600 μg in 3 days is indicative of excess body lead. Long-term consequences of chronic lead exposure have been described in individuals with occupational exposure, gout, and primary hypertension. Treatment with chelation therapy is effective in cases of acute lead nephropathy and the early renal dysfunction associated with occupational lead exposure, but there is no evidence that such therapy can reverse the chronic interstitial disease. Therefore chelation therapy for chronic nephropathy should be instituted with specific guidelines in mind, such as normalization of the EDTA test result and restoration of organ function.

Mercury exists in the form of inorganic salts and gases and organic mercury compounds. In the organic form mercury is present either as the free metal or in an ionic form such as mercurous or mercuric salt. In the organic form mercury is bound covalently to at least one carbon atom. Chronic exposure to organic compounds primarily results in central nervous system manifestations, although several distinct renal lesions have been described. Poisoning with inorganic mercury was once a common cause of acute renal failure. Mercury tends to form highly undissociable linkages to sulfhydral groups. The toxic dose of mercuric chloride (HgCl$_2$) is 0.5 to 2.5 g (mean, approximately 1.5 g). After ingestion and before onset of acute renal failure patients should be treated with intravenous chelation therapy (BAL, dimercaprol) and induction of diuresis. Chronic exposure to mercury may also be associated with the development of an immune-complex nephropathy that is evident as mesangioproliferative glomerulonephritis or as membranous glomerulopathy.

Other heavy metals have been shown to produce clinical, acute renal failure; they include *antimony, bismuth, copper,* and *gold.* Bismuth compounds were once prepared as therapeutic agents. Copper ingestion may result from ingestion of fungicide-contaminated feed grains or use of corroded copper-containing hot water heaters. *Gold* has been implicated as a rare cause of acute renal failure, but proteinuria is much more common in association with therapy for rheumatoid arthritis.

Insecticides and Herbicides

Nephrotoxicity has been associated with the use of two major categories of insecticides: the organophosphorus compounds such as *parathion* and the chlorinated hydrocarbons such as *chlordane.* Bipyridinium compounds have been used as herbicides. *Paraquat* reacts with atmospheric oxygen to produce reactive oxygen species. The major toxic effect is on pulmonary tissue, although azotemia with evidence of renal tubular damage may be found.

Pigment Nephropathy

Myoglobinuria and hemoglobinuria can be produced by exposure to chemical agents. Illicit drug users may have this presentation, particularly in overdose situations. When hemoglobinuria and myoglobinuria accompany acute renal failure, it is difficult to define their role in the development of renal damage. Such coexistent factors as abnormalities in blood pressure and the adverse effects of the toxic agents tend to obscure the role of hemoglobinuria and myoglobinuria on renal function.

Radiation

The dose of radiation required to produce renal damage is thought to exceed 2300 R delivered to both kidneys within a 5-week period. A number of variables determine the renal response to radiation, including age, area, and technique of irradiation; extent of perirenal fat; and concomitant administration of chemotherapeutic agents. Radiation nephritis has been separated into five clinical categories: acute or chronic radiation nephritis, asymptomatic proteinuria, benign essential hypertension, and late malignant hypertension.

Carcinogenesis

Exposure to chemical agents has been implicated in the development of neoplasms of the renal parenchyma, renal pelvis and ureter, and urinary bladder. In the late nineteenth century it was first reported that men working in the aniline dye industry had an increased incidence of bladder cancer. Later it was appreciated that bladder cancer was linked to employment in the rubber and electric cable industries and that its development was related to exposure to a number of aromatic amines. Transitional cell carcinoma of the renal pelvis and ureter may be induced by the same exogenous carcinogens that produce bladder tumors. Workers in the aniline dye, rubber, textile, and plastic industries have a higher incidence of these tumors, which account for 7% to 8% of renal neoplasms. Smokers appear to have about twice the bladder cancer rate of nonsmokers. This may reflect increased exposure to such agents as polycyclic aromatic hydrocarbons, dialkylnitrosamines, and aromatic amines, all of which are present in cigarette smoke.

EFFECT OF DIAGNOSTIC AND THERAPEUTIC AGENTS ON THE KIDNEY
Antibacterial Agents

Aminoglycoside Antibiotics. The aminoglycoside antibiotics include streptomycin, neomycin, tobramycin, gentamicin, and the semisynthetic compounds netilmicin and amikacin. The aminoglycoside antibiotics are potent tubular toxins. A significant decline in renal function can be expected to occur in 10% to 15% of all patients who receive them, and they have been found to be responsible for 7% of all cases of hospital-acquired renal insufficiency. The nephrotoxicity of the aminoglycosides depends in large part on positively charged amino groups that promote binding to anionic, acidic phospholipids on the brush border membranes of proximal renal tubular epithelial cells. Once binding to the membranes of renal tubular epithelial cells occurs, the aminoglycosides undergo pinocytosis, are internalized, and are sequestered in lysosomes. Renal cortical concentrations may be 10 to 100 times that of plasma. Aminoglycoside toxicity is associated with an increase in the number and size of proximal tubular secondary lysosomes. These often contain myeloid bodies, which are lamellar structures consisting of concentrically arranged phospholipid material. Cytoplasmic vacuolization and dilation of the cisternae of the rough endoplasmic reticulum may occur with eventual mitochondrial swelling and tubular epithelial cell necrosis. An aminoglycoside-induced decline in renal tubular function precedes a decline in the glomerular filtration rate. Early tubular damage may be manifested by increased urinary excretion of tubular enzymes and increased excretion of low-molecular-weight proteins. This may be coupled by renal potassium and magnesium wasting and defects in urine concentrating ability, resulting in decreased urine osmolality and increased urine volume, as seen in nephrogenic diabetes insipidus. Consequently, the acute renal failure associated with aminoglycoside nephrotoxicity tends to be nonoliguric rather than oliguric. Frank tubular necrosis may occur 5 to 10 days after aminoglycoside therapy is begun but is often accelerated if other renal insults are present. The usual course of aminoglycoside nephrotoxicity is eventual resolution, which may be partial or complete. Several risk factors have been associated with aminoglycoside nephrotoxicity, including high doses and/or high serum drug levels (gentamicin or tobramycin peak levels >10 mg/ml and trough levels >2 mg/ml), long duration of therapy,

recent aminoglycoside therapy, advanced age, liver disease, preexisting renal insufficiency, and/or concurrent nephrotoxic insults. Extracellular fluid volume depletion is a potent risk factor for acute renal insufficiency resulting from aminoglycosides. Comparative studies suggest that gentamicin is relatively more toxic than tobramycin, followed by amikacin and netilmicin; however, these differences are minor in individual patients.

Beta-Lactam Antibiotics. The β-lactam antibiotics, which include the penicillins, cephalosporins, carbapenems, and monobactams, may produce a variety of hypersensitivity reactions, and it is by this mechanism that renal function is most likely to be impaired. Although the β-lactams are too small to be directly immunogenic, hypersensitivity occurs when their metabolites bind to larger molecules and act as haptens. In the kidney this may produce an immunologically mediated acute interstitial nephritis that is most commonly encountered with the penicillins. The most common clinical manifestations are fever, pyuria, eosinophiluria, eosinophilia, and azotemia. The detection of eosinophiluria may be increased by the use of Hansel's stain. On histopathologic examination penicillin-induced acute interstitial nephritis is characterized by a patchy interstitial infiltrate composed mainly of lymphocytes, plasma cells, and eosinophils. Complete recovery occurs in up to 90% of cases. Steroid therapy remains controversial. Acute interstitial nephritis has also been reported with first-generation (cephalothin, cephradine), second-generation (cephalexin), and third-generation (cefotaxime) cephalosporins, as well as with carbapenem and monobactams. Acute interstitial nephritis may recur at rechallenge with β-lactams other than the original offending agent.

Tetracyclines. Four types of renal dysfunction have been described with the tetracyclines: Fanconi's syndrome, demeclocycline-induced nephrogenic diabetes insipidus, demeclocycline-induced renal failure in cirrhotic patients, and acute interstitial nephritis. In addition, by inhibiting protein synthesis and producing a catabolic state, the tetracyclines may elevate the blood urea nitrogen concentration without changing the glomerular filtration rate, an effect that may worsen azotemia in patients with renal failure.

Macrolide Antibiotics. Although not directly nephrotoxic, erythromycin may produce cyclosporine nephrotoxicity by inhibiting hepatic mixed-function oxidases and increasing cyclosporine levels in cyclosporine-treated patients.

Rifampin. Many cases of acute interstitial nephritis have been attributed to rifampin. This complication may be more common in twice- or thrice-weekly therapy or when drug administration resumes after a medication-free interval than it is in continuous daily therapy. Eosinophilia and eosinophiluria may be less common in rifampin-induced acute interstitial nephritis than in methicillin-induced acute interstitial nephritis.

Quinolones. Nephrotoxicity is uncommon in ciprofloxacin and norfloxacin administration, although acute interstitial nephritis with nonoliguric acute renal failure has been reported to be associated with the former.

Sulfonamides. Many of the older sulfonamides were poorly soluble, especially at acid pH, and tended to crystallize in the renal tubules and collecting system, producing intrarenal and extrarenal obstruction with resulting renal colic, hematuria, and acute renal failure. Furthermore, their acetylated metabolites tended to be even less soluble and more likely to precipitate than the parent drug. Maintaining a high urine flow rate and alkalinizing the urine lessened this problem. The incidence of renal injury has declined greatly as more soluble sulfonamides have come into use. Sulfadiazine is poorly soluble, as is the acetylated metabolite of sulfamethoxazole. In patients who have preexisting renal insufficiency elevated serum drug levels develop if the dose is not reduced, increasing the risk of sulfonamide-induced nephrotoxicity.

Trimethoprim. Trimethoprim has been reported to block tubular creatinine excretion, increasing the serum creatinine concentration without changing the glomerular filtration rate. Acute interstitial nephritis has been reported to be associated with trimethoprim-sulfamethoxazole. With large doses that are used in patients with acquired immunodeficiency syndrome (AIDS) trimethoprim may produce hyperkalemia as a result of impaired tubular potassium excretion. This is particularly true in patients with preexisting renal dysfunction.

Antiviral Agents

Acyclovir. Acyclovir is active against herpes simplex viruses and against varicella zoster virus. Intracellular conversion to an active form by viral thymidine kinase results in inhibition of herpesvirus deoxyribonucleic acid (DNA) polymerase enzyme. A decline in renal function is more likely to occur in patients with increased serum creatinine concentrations or when acyclovir is given in conjunction with other nephrotoxic agents. Rapid intravenous infusion is a primary risk factor. Consequently, doses must be adjusted for renal function and given by slow infusion to prevent intrarenal precipitation and obstruction.

Foscarnet. Foscarnet is a pyrophosphate analog that inhibits DNA polymerase in herpes viruses and ribonucleic acid (RNA) polymerase in influenza viruses. Its use has been associated with a significant decline in renal function in up to 66% of patients. Examination of renal biopsy specimens has revealed extensive tubular epithelial cell necrosis. The protective effects of hydration with the infusion of 2.5 L saline solution per day during the night before the foscarnet therapy and throughout the course of treatment have been demonstrated.

Antifungal Agents

The polyene *amphotericin B* is nephrotoxic as a result of a direct toxic effect on renal tubular epithelial cells and renal vasoconstriction. The nephrotoxicity is characterized by potassium wasting, distal renal tubular acidosis, nephrogenic diabetes insipidus, and azotemia. Renal dysfunction occurs in almost all patients treated with this drug and is dose related. The tubular transport abnormalities tend to precede azotemia and are usually reversible. Sodium loading reduces amphotericin B nephrotoxicity by preventing the expected declines in renal blood flow and glomerular filtration rate. Patients receiving amphotericin B should be well hydrated, and the serum electrolyte, blood urea nitrogen (BUN), and creatinine levels should be closely monitored. Saline solution may reverse developing azotemia. In most regimens amphotericin B is withheld or given only on alternate days if the BUN concentration exceeds 50 mg/dl. The imidazoles such as *ketoconazole* and fluconazole are not directly nephrotoxic but may increase cyclosporine blood levels in cyclosporine-treated transplant patients, producing nephrotoxicity.

Antiprotozal Agents

A common side effect of parenteral *pentamidine isethionate* administration is reversible renal and/or hepatic toxicity in approximately 25% of patients. Hypovolemia and diarrheal states in patients with AIDS appear to be important risk factors for increased nephrotoxicity. Pentamidine has also been associated with myoglobinuria and acute renal failure. Renal dysfunction has also been noted with inhalation of this agent.

Antineoplastic Agents

Alkylating Agents

Cisplatin. *Cisplatin* is active against a broad range of solid tumors and is particularly useful in the treatment of testicular and ovarian tumors. It is freely filtered at the glomerulus and has great potential for tubular toxicity. Histologic lesions include dilated proximal and distal tubules lined by flattened epithelium and containing intraluminal cast material and sloughing of tubular cells. Necrosis of the epithelial cells lining the collecting ducts may also be seen. Cisplatin nephrotoxicity may result in hypomagnesemia, which stems from impaired tubular conservation of magnesium. It may be accompanied by hypocalcemia, hypokalemia, and sodium wasting. Proteinuria, albuminuria, aminoaciduria, and glucosuria may also occur, but they

tend to resolve after withdrawal of the drug. In contrast, the defects of tubular electrolyte handling may persist. The most serious side effect is an acute, dose-related decline in the glomerular filtration rate, which is not completely reversible after cessation of therapy. The toxicity is cumulative, so each cycle of treatment produces a progressive and often permanent decline in renal function. Proximal tubular cell injury and death may result from inhibition of DNA synthesis, adenosine triphosphate (ATP) synthesis, ATP utilization, or a combination of these. Mitochondrial damage may occur, and oxygen free radicals may play a role in the evolution of the injury. Volume expansion with intravenous sodium chloride solutions in association with mannitol- or furosemide-stimulated diuresis greatly reduces cisplatin-induced nephrotoxicity. For example, the administration of cisplatin in 250 ml of 3% saline solution over 30 minutes along with an intravenous infusion of normal saline solution with 20 mEq/L of potassium chloride at 250 ml/hr may be effective in reducing nephrotoxicity.

Nitrosoureas. *Streptozocin* is a glycosylated nitrosourea whose primary use is in the treatment of malignant pancreatic islet cell tumors. Unchanged streptozocin is excreted in the urine and concentrated within the kidney. Streptozocin produces renal dysfunction in 28% to 73% of treated patients. The most common abnormality is tubular dysfunction, producing some combination of proteinuria, hypophosphatemia, hypokalemia, renal tubular acidosis, renal glycosuria, and acetonuria. Nephrogenic diabetes insipidus occasionally occurs. In more severe cases acute tubular necrosis and azotemia develop. Streptozocin is uricosuric and frequently produces hypouricemia. Nephrotoxicity is poorly predictable but may be minimized by reducing the dose by 50% in patients in whom persistent proteinuria or mild elevations in the serum creatinine concentration develop. *Semustine* is a chloroethyl nitrosourea active against lymphomas, melanoma, and tumors of the brain and gastrointestinal tract. Semustine-induced renal failure is insidious and irreversible; the first indication of renal abnormalities appears at a median of 2 years after the start of therapy. Nephrotoxicity is manifested by a slowly rising serum creatinine concentration and by small kidney size as indicated by radiographic or ultrasonographic examination. Glomerular sclerosis, tubular atrophy, and interstitial fibrosis have been reported. *Cyclophosphamide* is a nitrogen mustard that at high doses may impair renal water excretion and produce a dilutional hyponatremia. This represents a self-limiting effect on renal tubular epithelial cells.

Antimetabolites. *Methotrexate* inhibits dihydrofolate reductase, blocking the conversion of dihydrofolate to tetrahydrofolate. Methotrexate is excreted by both glomerular filtration and tubular secretion, and as a result it has a renal clearance exceeding that of inulin. Precipitation of a poorly soluble drug metabolite, 7 hydroxymethotrexate, within the distal nephron produces intrarenal obstructive uropathy. This is a particular problem in high-dose therapy with leucovorin rescue protocols. The incidence of nephrotoxicity can be substantially reduced by hydration and urinary alkalinization, although most patients have a small, reversible decline in glomerular filtration rate. *Fluoracil* and *floxuridine* are not nephrotoxic but when used in combination with mitomycin C may be associated with the development of the hemolytic-uremic syndrome. *Thioguanine* may be associated with reversible renal failure in approximately 20% of patients receiving individual doses of 700 mg/m² or more.

Antitumor Antibiotics. *Mitomycin* is used in the palliative treatment of various solid tumors. Nephrotoxicity is a significant dose-related side effect. The renal failure is characteristic of the hemolytic-uremic syndrome with microangiopathic hemolytic anemia and thrombocytopenia. This occurs in approximately 9% of mitomycin-treated patients and is related to total cumulative dose and associated with concurrent fluorouracil treatment. The kidneys demonstrate arteriolar intimal hyperplasia with deposition of fibrin thrombi in the arterioles and glomerular capillaries. Mitomycin C–induced hemolytic-uremic syndrome (HUS) has a high fatality rate, and no treatment has proved effective. *Mithramycin* suppresses osteoclast activity and is most often used to treat tumor-associated hypercalcemia. When it is given on a daily basis, considerable nephrotoxicity occurs with necrosis of proximal and distal tubular cells. Glomeruli are not affected. *Bleomycin*-containing combination regimens may occasionally be associated with the HUS.

Other Agents. *Vincristine* is a vinca alkaloid that promotes antidiuretic hormone (ADH) release and hyponatremia resulting in the syndrome of inappropriate ADH. *Interleukin-2* is an immunotherapeutic agent whose use causes reversible azotemia accompanied by hypotension, sodium retention, and reduced urine volume in most patients. *Interferon* use is associated with reversible and usually mild proteinuria in 15% to 42% of patients. The enzyme *asparaginase* may produce prerenal azotemia.

Immunosuppressive Agents

Cyclosporine is a hydrophobic cyclic undecapeptide that has revolutionized solid organ transplantation by providing superior immunosuppression. The drug acts by inhibiting an intracellular enzyme, calcineurin phosphatase, which in turn inhibits interleukin-2 gene transcription.

The major side effect of cyclosporine is dose-related nephrotoxicity. This can have many clinical presentations, the most common of which is reversible acute renal dysfunction attributable to afferent arteriolar vasoconstriction. The precise mediator of the vasoactive effects of cyclosporine are unclear, but pharmacologic blockade of endothelin, thromboxane A2, and other potent mediators can enhance renal function. Acute cyclosporine nephrotoxicity is characterized by enhanced proximal tubular reabsorption of sodium, fluid retention, and systemic hypertension. Elevation of cyclosporine blood levels has a statistical relationship with acute cyclosporine nephrotoxicity; however, reversible renal dysfunction attributable to cyclosporine can be seen even in patients with "therapeutic" blood levels. Probably more important for the long-term use of cyclosporine is a chronic nephropathy consisting of afferent arteriolar myointimal damage associated with striped tubulointerstitial fibrosis. This form of chronic toxicity is only poorly correlated with cyclosporine dose and blood level. The lesion is most prominently observed in patients who receive treatment with cyclosporine for extrarenal organ transplants and autoimmune disease. In the kidney transplant patient the diagnosis of chronic nephropathy is difficult to make because of the confounding factor of chronic allograft rejection. The pathogenesis of chronic cyclosporine nephropathy is unclear. Recent data suggests that the intrarenal renin-angiotensin system and transforming growth factor–β may be important in the pathogenesis of this nephropathy. In approximately 5% to 10% of patients with chronic cyclosporine nephropathy end-stage renal disease develops, whether or not the cyclosporine is discontinued.

Cyclosporine is extremely hydrophobic; thus individual patient pharmacokinetic profiles are variable. The drug is extensively metabolized in the liver by cytochrome P450 3A4. As a result, there are many interacting drugs that block metabolism and raise blood levels, producing nephrotoxicity, or as an alternative, induce hepatic enzymes that diminishes the drug's immunosuppressive effects. The clinician caring for a patient with cyclosporine should ensure that any new medication prescribed for intercurrent conditions is appropriately dosed relative to cyclosporine.

Cyclosporine may be associated with arterial hypertension, either distinct from nephrotoxicity or associated with it. Plasma renin activities are low, similar to one-kidney, one-clip experimental hypertension. There is evidence that the intrarenal renin-angiotensin system is stimulated. Many antihypertensive drugs are used to treat cyclosporin A–associated hypertension; calcium channel blockers are the drugs of choice. This is largely on theoretic ground, since afferent arteriolar vasoconstriction mediated by endothelin, thromboxane, and angiotensin can be minimized by effective calcium channel blockade. Other cyclosporine-induced effects are hyperuricemia; hyperchloremic, hyperkalemic metabolic acidosis with impaired potassium secretion; and renal magnesium wasting.

A much more uncommon manifestation of cyclosporine nephrotoxicity is a syndrome that simulates the hemolytic uremic syndrome. This has been reported most often in bone marrow transplant recipients but can be seen when cyclosporine is used in other settings. There are fibrin thrombi throughout the glomeruli associated with thrombocytopenia and microangiopathic hemolytic anemia. Withdrawal of cyclosporine is necessary. Even if the drug is discontinued, renal dysfunction may progress. Several patients have been treated successfully with plasma exchange; however, there are no controlled studies regarding the management of this unusual complication of therapy.

Tacrolimus, another hydrophobic fungal product, has been introduced into many immunosuppressive regimens, particularly in the liver transplant setting. This drug, although chemically dissimilar to cyclosporine, has a mechanism of action that involves inhibition of calcineurin phosphatase. Like cyclosporine, this agent produces dose-related acute nephrotoxicity, as well as chronic nephropathic changes. Although it is difficult to compare these two agents, tacrolimus seems to produce less arterial hypertension than cyclosporine, although the clinical significance of this is unclear. *Rapamycin*, a chemically similar drug to tacrolimus, binds to the same intracellular binding protein but produces immunosuppression by different mechanisms. It is of interest that rapamycin and FK506 antagonize each other's immunosuppressive actions. Rapamycin is synergistic with cyclosporine for immunosuppression. Whether rapamycin will be synergistically nephrotoxic is unclear, since in animal species rapamycin produces less nephrotoxicity than cyclosporine or tacrolimus. Metabolic side effects of these immunosuppressive agents include neurotoxicity, hyperglycemia, and in the case of cyclosporine, hirsutism.

Nonsteroidal Antiinflammatory Drugs and Analgesics

The nonsteroidal antiinflammatory drugs (NSAIDs) are a group of carboxylic and enolic acid derivatives that are used by an estimated 40 million people in the United States for their antipyretic, antiinflammatory, and analgesic properties. As with other nonnarcotic analgesics, they are now available over the counter. Nonsteroidal antiinflammatory drugs exert their major effects through the inhibition of prostaglandin synthesis. In clinical situations involving increased activity of the renin-angiotensin system, acute renal failure may result from enhanced renal vasoconstriction unopposed by the vasodilatory effect of prostaglandins; this is the most common disorder associated with NSAIDs. Oliguria and a rise in serum creatinine concentration begin within 24 to 48 hours of drug exposure. The urinalysis finding is usually unremarkable, and the fractional excretion of sodium is less than 1%. Hyperkalemia disproportionate to the degree of renal failure may develop. Dialysis is rarely indicated, and renal function usually returns to baseline after discontinuation of the drug. Predisposing factors include congestive heart failure, cirrhosis, preexisting renal insufficiency, advanced age, volume depletion, hypertension, and previous diuretic use.

A less common complication of use of NSAIDs is the syndrome of nephrotic-range proteinuria or acute renal failure, or both, associated with acute interstitial nephritis. This syndrome appears to involve an older age-group and to have a time course to development of several months. The patients usually have cramps, edema, and oliguria. Recovery is slow and may take weeks to months. The efficacy of steroids is unclear. The renal biopsy result typically shows focal interstitial edema and fibrosis, diffuse or focal monocellular infiltrate, and eosinophils in 30% of specimens. The pathogenesis is still unknown, although current speculation implicates lymphokines or leukotrienes, or both. Nonsteroidal antiinflammatory drugs have been associated with sodium retention in as many as 25% of patients. This problem is usually transient and minor, except in patients with severe congestive heart failure or cirrhosis. Nonsteroidal antiinflammatory drugs may also cause diuretic resistance, impaired urinary diluting ability, and hyperkalemia. Hyperkalemia is more likely in patients with diabetes or renal insufficiency and in those receiving beta blockers. Chronic renal failure that is due to use of NSAIDs over a long period is characterized by papillary necrosis and chronic tubulointerstitial nephropathy.

Use of combination analgesics containing phenacetin, acetaminophen, and aspirin plus other ingredients such as caffeine and codeine can lead to progressive chronic renal insufficiency and renal papillary necrosis. The percentage of patients receiving maintenance hemodialysis who have this diagnosis varies throughout the world. In some European countries and Australia between 10% and 15% of all patients requiring renal replacement therapy have analgesic-associated nephropathy as their primary renal diagnosis. The pathogenesis of this disorder still remains unclear. Metabolism by prostaglandin synthase enzymes in the renal medulla and papilla to adducts, which cause cellular damage, combined with decreases in renal blood flow and possibly inhibition of glutathione synthesis by these combination products, leads to renal damage. These changes begin in the renal papilla and spread more proximally to involve the overlying renal cortex, resulting in kidneys with irregular contours and signs of papillary damage. Recently the use of objective criteria defined by computed tomography has permitted identification scanning with high specificity and sensitivity of those patients with chronic renal disease who have analgesic nephropathy as a primary diagnosis. There is weak epidemiologic evidence suggesting that acetaminophen alone causes renal disease or aggravates renal disease of other origins; however, the research in this area is flawed by various systematic biases. The major one results from the fact that physicians advise acetaminophen as the analgesic drug of choice in patients with preexisting renal disease. Avoidance of combination analgesic products and careful warning about the overuse of these agents on a regular basis should result in the disappearance of this entity in the future.

Anesthetic Agents

Methoxyflurane and other fluorinated anesthetics, which are metabolized in the liver to inorganic fluoride and oxalate, have been associated with nonoliguric acute renal failure and nephrogenic diabetes insipidus. The newer halogenated anesthetics in current use have dramatically reduced the incidence of this complication, although renal dysfunction may be produced with very high exposures.

Radiographic Contrast Media

Although many studies have identified radiocontrast dye as a cause of acute renal failure in hospitalized patients, the true incidence of this problem is still unknown. The incidence varies from 0.15% to 17%, depending on the type of radiographic procedure and the definition of acute renal failure, which ranges from a rise in serum creatinine concentration of 0.3 mg/dl to a rise of 2.0 mg/dl during the 24 to 48 hours after radiocontrast exposure. Although the list of predisposing risk factors is quite long, only preexisting renal insufficiency and diabetes mellitus are consistently recognized. Acute renal failure developed in approximately 50% of diabetic patients with a serum creatinine level greater than 1.5 mg/dl and in 76% with a level greater than 5 mg/dl.

Radiocontrast-induced acute renal failure may be oliguric or nonoliguric. Patients with preexisting renal insufficiency are more likely to have the oliguric form, which usually lasts for 2 to 5 days with recovery by the seventh day. The urinalysis result may be normal or may reveal multiple tubular epithelial cell and granular casts. The urinary sodium concentration (<10 mEq/L) and fractional excretion of sodium (<0.5%) may be extremely low. A persistent nephrogram for 24 to 48 hours is a characteristic feature. The pathophysiologic mechanisms responsible for the acute renal failure are still unclear. The best strategy to prevent this disorder is the maintenance of normal extracellular volume with saline loading if possible. In patients with preexisting renal insufficiency or diabetes mellitus, or both, consideration should be given to an alternative procedure (e.g., sonography, magnetic resonance imaging). Nonionic contrast agents, which are less nephrotoxic, should be used in these high-risk patients if contrast is necessary.

BIBLIOGRAPHY

Bennett WM: Drugs and the kidney. In Whitworth J, Lawrence J, editors: *Textbook of renal disease,* Edinburgh, 1994, Churchill Livingstone.

Bennett WM: The nephrotoxicity of immunosuppressive drugs, *Clin Nephrol* 43(suppl 1):53-57, 1995.

Berns JS et al: Renal aspects of antimicrobial therapy for HIV infection. In Kimmel PL, Berns JS, editors: *Renal and urologic aspects of HIV infection,* New York, 1995, Churchill Livingstone.

Elseviers MM et al: Evaluation of diagnostic criteria for analgesic nephropathy in patients with end-stage renal failure: results of the ANNE study, *Nephrol Dial Transplant* 10:808-814, 1995.

Finn WF: Disorders of the kidney and urinary tract. In Tarcher AB, editor: *Principles and practice of environmental medicine,* New York and London, Book Company, Plenum Medical, 1992.

Porter GA: Radiocontrast-induced nephropathy, *Nephrol Dial Transplant* 9(suppl 4):146-156, 1994.

Shuler C, Bennett WM: Antimicrobial nephrotoxicity. In Massry S, Glassock RJ, editors: *Textbook of nephrology,* Baltimore, 1995, Williams and Wilkins.

Swan SK, Bennett WM: Nephrotoxic acute renal failure. In Lazarus M, Brenner B, editors: *Acute renal failure,* New York, 1993, Churchill Livingstone.

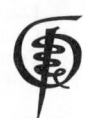

CHAPTER

120 Cystic Diseases of the Kidney

Jared J. Grantham

Cysts are the most common structural abnormalities encountered in adult kidneys. By definition, a *cyst* is an epithelium-lined cavity filled with fluid or semisolid material. Nearly all renal cysts are derived from nephrons or collecting duct elements. They begin as tiny hair-sized structures, enlarging in some instances to structures several centimeters in diameter that contain several hundred milliliters of fluid. Generalized cystic diseases are typified by cysts scattered throughout the cortex and the medulla of one or both kidneys. The term *polycystic* is reserved for kidney diseases in which the cysts are diffusely scattered throughout the renal cortex and medulla. In *medullary cystic diseases* the lesions occur principally in the medulla and papilla. The major types of renal cystic disease are outlined in Table 120-1.

SIMPLE OR SOLITARY CYSTS

About 25% to 50% of persons above the age of 50 years have one or more renal cysts. These cysts are usually found incidentally in the course of radiographic studies to evaluate hypertension, renal stone disease, hematuria, or urinary tract infection. They are rarely symptomatic. The presence of these cysts does not lead to chronic renal insufficiency. There is no known hereditary connection.

Pathologic Features

Simple cysts are usually seen on the outer portion of the kidney cortex, but they can be detected in the medullary and papillary regions. They usually contain a clear fluid that has a composition similar to that of an ultrafiltrate of plasma. Occasionally the cysts may contain blood or pus. They are lined by simple columnar or flat squamous epithelium. Microdissection studies show that the cysts originate from tubule segments. The mechanism of fluid accumulation in the cysts is unknown. Usually there are only a few simple cysts per kidney, but occasionally they may be so numerous as to be confused with autosomal dominant polycystic kidney disease or with acquired cystic disease. Cysts with diameters of 0.5 to 1.0 cm are common, but a diameter of 3 to 4 cm is not unusual.

Clinical and Diagnostic Features

Most simple cysts are found on routine urographic examinations. They are more common in adults than in children. Hypertension has been attributed to simple cysts in rare instances. The occasional infected cyst may cause flank pain, pleurisy, fever, and leukocytosis. In most cases, however, the simple cysts are asymptomatic, and the major problem is to differentiate them from malignant masses.

Simple cysts are only rarely associated with renal malignancy. When an asymptomatic renal cyst is discovered incidentally by urography or sonography, further evaluation by computed tomography (CT) may be indicated to rule out the possibility of an associated tumor mass. Sonography with cyst puncture has been used as the cornerstone of screening in the past, but further evaluation with CT has now become more accepted in some centers. Strict criteria for benign cysts by CT scanning are (1) a homogeneous attenuation value near that of water, (2) no enhancement with intravenous contrast material, (3) no measurable thickness of the cyst wall, and (4) smooth interface with renal parenchyma. If these criteria are met, the cystic

Table 120-1   Features of renal cystic diseases

| | CORTEX AND MEDULLA | | | | | MEDULLA |
| | | | POLYCYSTIC | | | |
	SIMPLE	ACQUIRED	DOMINANT	RECESSIVE	SPONGE KIDNEY	MEDULLARY CYSTIC
Prevalence	Common	>50% of dialysis patients	1:500-1:1000	Rare	1:5000-1:1000	Rare
Symptoms	Rare	Occasional	Common	Common	Occasional	Common
Inherited	No	No	Yes	Yes	Unknown	Dominant and recessive forms
Kidney size	Normal	Small to large	Large	Large	Normal	Small
Hypertension	Rare	Variable	Common	Common	Rare	Rare
Hematuria	Occasional	Occasional	Common	Occasional	Rare (except with stones)	Rare
Associated conditions						
Azotemia	No	Always	Common	Common	Rare	Common
Liver disease	No	No	40%-60%	100%	No	No
Arterial aneurysm	No	No	10%	No	No	No
Differential diagnosis	Tumor	ADPKD	ARPKD	ADPKD	Medullary cystic kidney	End-stage renal disease
	Diverticula of renal pelvis	Simple cysts	Tuberous sclerosis	Medullary sponge kidney	Renal tubular acidosis	Medullary sponge kidney
		Hippel-Lindau disease	Multiple simple cysts		Idiopathic nephrocalcinosis	

ADPKD, Autosomal dominant polycystic kidney disease; *ARPKD,* autosomal recessive polycystic kidney disease.

lesion can be followed by periodic sonographic evaluation. If the criteria are not met, the cyst falls into an indeterminant or solid category and surgical exploration is recommended. Calcification within cystic lesions should raise suspicion of malignancy.

Treatment

There is considerable diversity in the therapeutic approach to the simple cyst. With the use of modern diagnostic tests, most physicians do not advocate surgery if strict CT criteria are met and the mass is asymptomatic. The management of symptomatic renal cysts can take several forms. Most cysts are accessible to percutaneous aspiration for diagnosis. In some cases sclerosing agents can be injected to reduce the reaccumulation of cyst fluid. If the cyst is associated with hypertension and the renal vein renin levels are elevated above normal, drainage of the cysts may be associated with improvement of hypertension. Infected cysts have been drained by percutaneous approaches. Differentiation of infected cysts from renal abscess may be difficult. In this instance an operative approach is usually taken.

AUTOSOMAL DOMINANT POLYCYSTIC KIDNEY DISEASE

Autosomal dominant polycystic kidney disease (ADPKD) is usually recognized in adults between the third and fourth decades of life. The diagnosis is rarely made in infants. In most cases a family history of renal disease can be elicited on careful questioning. Approximately 85% of ADPKD cases are caused by a defective gene located on the short arm of chromosome 16p. A second mutated gene on chromosome 4q accounts for most of the remaining cases. The two genotypes of ADPKD are indistinguishable by conventional diagnostic methods. The disease exhibits autosomal dominant inheritance with nearly complete penetrance of the gene defect. It is found on all continents and in all races. The prevalence is estimated to be between 1 in 500 and 1 in 1000 individuals with an annual "attack" rate of about 6000 new cases per year in the United States. The disease causes renal insufficiency in 50% of individuals by the age of 70 years, accounts for 6% to 10% of dialysis patients in the United States, and is the third or fourth leading cause of renal failure in adults.

Pathologic Features

Polycystic kidneys are impressively enlarged. The cysts are scattered diffusely throughout the kidneys and may vary in size from a few millimeters to several centimeters in diameter. Most of the cysts are filled with straw-yellow fluid that resembles urine. Some cysts appear to be filled with blood or thick, putty-like material, which represents old blood. Both kidneys are involved by the process; unilateral polycystic kidney disease has been reported only rarely. Microdissection studies have shown that the cysts originate in all segments of the nephron, including Bowman's capsule, the proximal tubule, the loop of Henle, the distal tubule, the collecting tubule, and the papillary collecting duct. The cysts are lined by a single layer of epithelium that in some instances resembles that seen in the distal nephron. The cells are connected by junctional complexes resembling those seen in proximal and distal tubule segments. Marked hyperplasia of cells and polyp formation have been observed on the interior wall of cysts originating in all the portions of the nephron. Analysis of the cyst fluid reveals cyst fluid to plasma electrolyte concentration gradients for sodium, potassium, chloride, and hydrogen ions. Thus some of the cysts continue to function as nephron segments throughout the life of the patient.

The liver also contains cysts in about 40% to 60% of patients with ADPKD. Females seem to have a greater enlargement of the liver produced by cysts than do males. In some cases the liver cysts are so prominent as to cause portal hypertension or, in rare cases, obstruction of the common bile duct. Liver cysts rarely lead to parenchymal dysfunction.

Arterial aneurysms of the circle of Willis are found in about 10% of patients with polycystic kidney disease. These aneurysms may rupture, causing sudden death. Patients with ADPKD appear to have an increased incidence of aortic aneurysm, abnormalities of the mitral-valve, and inguinal hernia. Diverticulosis appears to be increased in patients with ADPKD.

Pathophysiology

Autosomal dominant polycystic kidney disease is clearly an inherited disorder. The responsible gene on chromosome 16p (PKD-1) encodes a large protein (polycystin) that is believed to regulate cell-to-cell and cell-to-matrix interactions in nephrons. The pathogenetic steps by which aberrant polycystin causes renal cysts to develop in renal tubules are unknown. Renal cysts can be found in utero and in neonates, but renal failure does not develop usually until the fifth or sixth decade of life. As one grows older there appears to be an increase in the size of cystic nephrons in both kidneys. There is associated atrophy and fibrosis of adjacent kidney tissue, which probably underlies the progression to renal insufficiency.

The mechanism by which the cysts enlarge is not known, but several hypotheses have been suggested, all of which incorporate abnormal growth as a central theme. One view holds that abnormal basement membrane material fails to retard the proliferation of the cells. Another suggests that the epithelial cells are more sensitive to normal levels of epithelial growth factors, such as epidermal growth factor; a third suggests that the cells making up the cyst walls are locked in a permanent state of immaturity. In all of these hypotheses, the fluid is thought to derive from glomerular filtrate and transepithelial fluid secretion. Thus the cysts enlarge progressively from the size of a human hair to that of oranges as a result of the proliferation of a thin layer of cells surrounding a large cavity filled with urine-like fluid.

Clinical and Diagnostic Features

Abdominal pain and hematuria are the most common initial symptoms in patients with ADPKD. Infected renal cysts, secondary to urinary tract infection, are also relatively common. Hypertension occurs in over 50% of patients with ADPKD and often antedates the diagnosis of the disease. Renal insufficiency occurs late in this disorder and is not a presenting feature. There are no distinguishing laboratory features. Patients at various stages of the disease have been found to have mild proteinuria and to excrete lipid bodies in the urine.

The diagnosis of ADPKD can be made by several radiographic tests in patients who are at risk. Sonography is the preferred screening test. When more than five cysts are found in each kidney in a patient with a family history of ADPKD, a secure diagnosis of autosomal dominant polycystic kidney disease can be made. If the sonogram result is equivocal, CT is recommended (Fig. 120-1). In advanced cases intravenous nephrotomography can be used to establish the diagnosis, but this is usually not definitive for patients in the early stages of the disease. Because it is important in many instances to exclude the diagnosis of polycystic kidney disease in a patient at risk, I recommend the use of CT when there is any doubt about the diagnosis of ADPKD. Angiography is seldom necessary except when tumor is suspected in a polycystic kidney. Carcinoma has been reported in patients with ADPKD, but this problem is rare. Retrograde pyelography is seldom indicated and should be avoided if at all possible because of the high risk of renal infection.

It is possible to diagnose ADPKD by means of genetic linkage markers on chromosome 4q and 16p. For this examination deoxyribonucleic acid (DNA) of at least two relatives (siblings, parent, grandparent, or children) with clinically apparent ADPKD is surveyed together with that of the subject at risk. Genetic markers that flank the ADPKD gene are examined by Southern blotting to determine the extent to which they are expressed in the individual without clinical ADPKD. In families in which the markers are informative, it is possible to determine an ADPKD genotype in the person at risk with an accuracy exceeding 95%. As a matter of practice, the linkage test has not been widely used because radiologic methods of diagnosis are highly sensitive in adults.

The clinical course of ADPKD is highly variable. Some patients experience minor symptoms throughout life and never progress to end-stage renal disease. More commonly, however, they have bouts of abdominal pain, hematuria, hypertension, or urinary tract infection, and in over half of patients, renal insufficiency develops between the fifth and the sixth decades of life. Gross hematuria in a patient with ADPKD is usually due to rupture of a cyst, but in some cases it may be secondary to infection in the kidney, renal stone, or, in rare cases, a renal tumor. In most patients bed rest, sedation, and hydration result in resolution of the hematuria in a few days. When hematuria persists, more extensive radiologic investigation is indicated.

Urinary tract infection should be treated promptly with bactericidal antibiotics. When a kidney cyst becomes infected, it is important to try to identify the offending organism. When identification is possible, bactericidal therapy should be administered parenterally for at least 2 weeks, followed by long-term oral therapy. Perinephric abscess has been reported in dialysis patients with ADPKD, and this complication requires surgical drainage. Occasionally nephrectomy may be indicated to control renal infection. Renal calculi are found with increased incidence in patients with polycystic kidney disease.

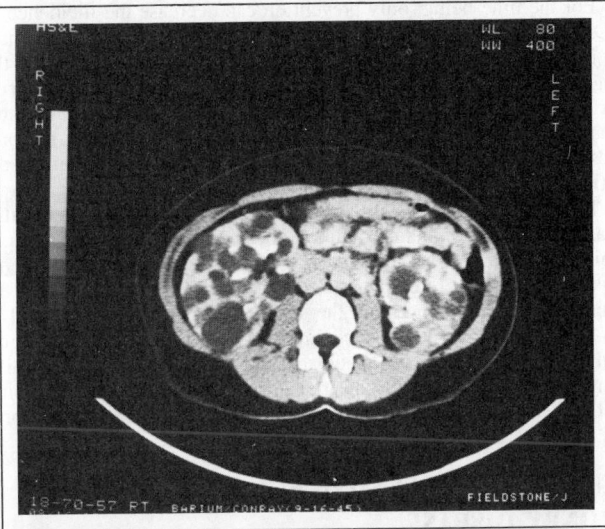

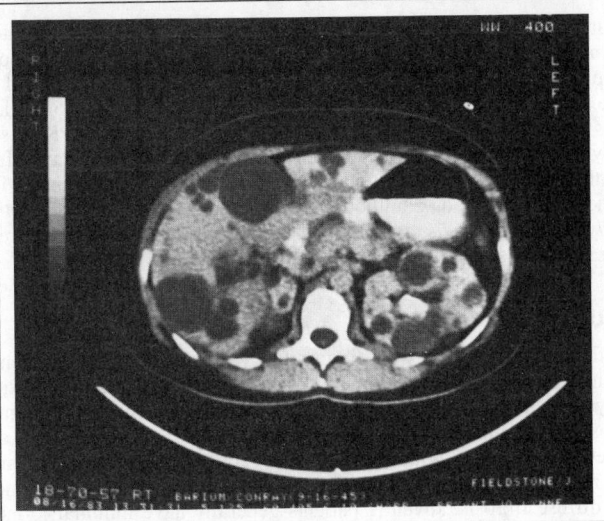

FIGURE 120-1   Tomogram of autosomal dominant polycystic kidney disease. **A,** Kidney cysts, **B,** Kidney and liver cysts.

Unique pathophysiologic characteristics have not been described for the formation of these calculi.

Most patients with ADPKD require no modification in physical activity or lifestyle unless they have unusual symptomatic disease. These patients should probably avoid contact sports in which direct blows to the abdomen may be incurred. Pain is managed by specific therapy for the underlying cause, such as stone or infection. Nonsteroidal antiinflammatory drugs should be avoided because of the risk of papillary injury. In difficult cases surgical unroofing of cysts has proved beneficial in managing renal pain.

Hypertension is usually of the volume-dependent variety. Sodium restriction is effective in the treatment of most patients, but in some it is necessary to add a vasodilator. Diuretics should be used cautiously because of the unknown effect of these drugs on the formation rate of renal cysts. Hemodialysis and peritoneal dialysis are effective means of treating end-stage ADPKD. These patients are also excellent candidates for renal transplantation. In most instances a cadaveric source is chosen because of the hereditary nature of the disease.

Treatment

There is no specific treatment for ADPKD. Control of blood pressure, urinary tract infection, and renal lithiasis is important to prolong kidney function. Pregnancy does not appear to have an adverse effect when kidney function is normal.

For the time being, only prevention can decrease the incidence of ADPKD. For prevention to be effective, patients with ADPKD must be identified in the early portion of their childbearing years. On the other hand, it is probably not advisable to evaluate all patients at risk for ADPKD to determine whether they have the disorder. One must bear in mind that nothing can be done presently to prevent the progression of the disease, and knowledge of the ailment may affect the patient's employment and insurability.

Patients who have established ADPKD should be advised that it is an autosomal dominant condition and that they can expect each of their children to have a 50-50 chance of inheriting the defective gene. It is also important to emphasize that if the child does not inherit the gene, there is no chance that the same disease will be expressed in his or her progeny. Patients should also be advised of the risk, signs, and symptoms of cerebral aneurysm. Once a patient shows a significant decrease in creatinine clearance, the prognosis for progression of the disease can be judged by the relationship between the reciprocal of the serum creatinine concentration and time.

AUTOSOMAL RECESSIVE POLYCYSTIC KIDNEY DISEASE

Autosomal recessive polycystic kidney disease (ARPKD) is inherited as an autosomal recessive trait attributable to a mutated gene on both copies of chromosome 6p. The disease is almost never recognized in the parents. Both parents carry the recessive gene, so each offspring has a one-in-four chance of having symptomatic disease. ARPKD usually causes the death of the patient within a few hours or days after birth. In milder forms the renal disease may not be detected until infancy, childhood, or adulthood. The commonly used term *infantile polycystic kidney disease* is technically incorrect; the more correct designation is *autosomal recessive polycystic kidney disease.*

Pathologic Features

Patients with ARPKD who die in infancy usually do not die of renal failure but of underdevelopment of the pulmonary system. The kidneys are enlarged symmetrically and have a spongy character. On microscopic examination the collecting ducts are seen to be widely dilated. In newborns with ARPKD the liver appears relatively normal on gross inspection but almost invariably shows microscopic evidence of diffuse fibrosis. Juvenile patients generally have minimal kidney involvement, with spherical cysts revealed by urography and CT scanning that are very difficult to differentiate from the cysts of ADPKD. However, these individuals have striking liver abnormalities produced by diffuse fibrosis. Portal hypertension is an important complication. Thus there appears to be a spectrum of renal hepatic involvement in ARPKD, with severe kidney disease and mild liver changes at the perinatal end and severe hepatic fibrosis with mild kidney changes in juveniles and young adults.

Clinical and Diagnostic Features

In children whose kidneys are found to be enlarged at birth, sonography and intravenous nephrotomography are important diagnostic tools. The typical sonogram shows enlarged kidneys with increased echogenicity in the cortex and medulla. In older patients microcystic changes can be observed by CT scanning in those patients who are able to cooperate with the test.

There is no known treatment for ARPKD. Patients who have renal insufficiency can be treated with hemodialysis and peritoneal dialysis. Renal transplantation has been used in selected cases. However, because of the associated fibrosing liver disorder, these patients must be classified as high-risk candidates for renal replacement therapy.

As with other cystic diseases, hypertension, edema, hepatic insufficiency, and urinary tract infection should be treated appropriately.

Parents who give birth to a child with ARPKD should be advised that each of their children will have a one-in-four chance of having the disease or a one-in-two chance of being a carrier of the abnormal gene.

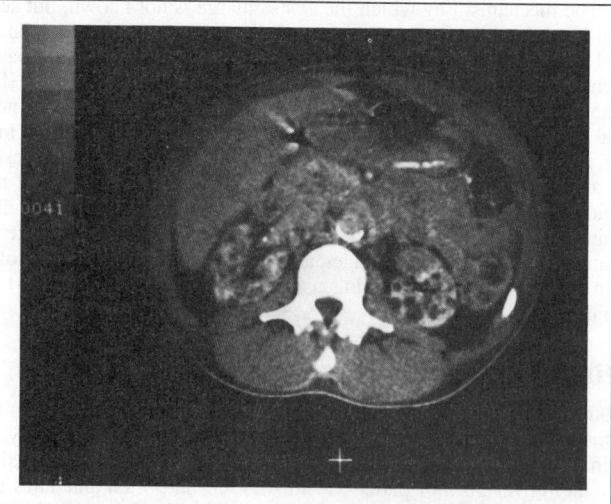

FIGURE 120-2   Acquired cystic disease.

ACQUIRED CYSTIC DISEASE

Patients who have been maintained on dialysis regimens, either hemodialysis or peritoneal dialysis, for several years have been observed to have a type of bilateral polycystic kidney disease. Patients with noncystic disorders, such as chronic glomerulonephritis, diabetes mellitus, and interstitial nephritis, who have end-stage renal disease and require dialysis treatment appear to have this peculiar diffuse polycystic kidney disease. In several studies, approximately 50% of patients who had been treated by dialysis longer than 3 years showed signs of acquired polycystic kidney disease. The cysts develop as a consequence of chronic renal insufficiency and may be clinically apparent long before dialysis is instituted.

Pathologic Features

Both kidneys are involved with diffuse cysts, which in some cases may be several centimeters in diameter. The cysts are usually filled with clear fluid, but in some instances they are hemorrhagic. Microscopic examination of the kidneys reveals hyperplasia of the cells lining the inside of many cysts. In some cases microadenomas are found in the cysts' walls, and adenocarcinomas may be found in about 5% of patients with acquired polycystic kidney disease. In several instances, the kidneys have contained adenocarcinoma with metastasis to regional lymph nodes and distant organs.

Clinical and Diagnostic Features

Recent studies indicate that in patients with long-standing chronic renal insufficiency acquired cystic disease may develop before they enter a dialysis program. In those who do not have acquired cystic disease at the time dialysis is started, the disease will almost certainly develop in a high proportion of patients who have dialysis for long periods. Major clinical manifestations of acquired cystic disease include flank pain and hematuria in association with rupture of hemorrhagic cysts into the urinary tract or into the perinephric region. There are no reported cases of infection in acquired polycystic kidney disease. These patients seem to be unusually susceptible to the development of oxalate stones in the pelvis of the kidney. Erythrocytosis has been associated with acquired cystic disease in a few cases.

The diagnosis is made by sonography in far advanced cases or by CT scan in instances in which the cysts are relatively small (Fig. 120-2). The cysts appear to regress in patients who have successful kidney transplantation and who become nonazotemic.

There is no specific treatment for acquired polycystic kidney disease. When the cystic lesions are associated with solid tumor formation, nephrectomy may be indicated. Kidneys that develop spontaneous bleeding may have to be removed to reduce the risks of severe hemorrhage in the course of hemodialysis and anticoagulation.

JUVENILE NEPHRONOPHTHISIS AND MEDULLARY CYSTIC DISEASE

There appear to be at least three diseases in humans that primarily involve the tubular structures of the renal medulla. Medullary cystic disease and juvenile nephronophthisis are familial disorders that appear to be separate and distinct disease entities. By contrast, medullary sponge kidney (discussed separately) occurs only occasionally in members of the same family.

Juvenile nephronophthisis is an autosomal recessive disorder that maps to chromosome 2p. By contrast, medullary cystic disease appears to be due to an autosomal dominant trait of unknown chromosomal location. Another condition, termed *renal-retinal dysplasia,* encompasses retinal degeneration, familial retinitis pigmentosa, and pigmentary optic atrophy with renal changes similar to those of juvenile nephronophthisis.

Pathologic Features

These various disorders cannot be separated by histologic techniques. In all cases the kidneys are moderately small, and on cut section thinning of the cortex and medulla is revealed. The cortical medullary junction is the site of a variable number of cysts, which range in size from barely perceptible to 2 cm in diameter. The cysts contain clear fluid that resembles normal urine. In some of these cases gross cysts are not visible. As in all cystic diseases, the cysts arise from renal tubules; however, in this instance they originate from medullary nephron structures and collecting ducts.

Clinical and Diagnostic Features

Within a family structure the disease appears to be inherited in a relatively uniform way. In juvenile nephronophthisis one usually obtains a history of polydipsia, polyuria, pallor, lethargy, and growth retardation. This disease usually progresses to the end-stage before the age of 20 years. In the medullary cystic form seen in adults, the clinical symptoms are similar except for growth retardation. Some cases have been discovered in the sixth and seventh decade of life. These patients may consume extraordinary amounts of water and sodium chloride to accommodate the renal salt and water losses.

The diagnosis is difficult to make by the usual radiographic techniques. Sonography and CT scanning have been useful in patients with clear-cut medullary cysts. But in the last analysis, open renal biopsy that includes medulla is probably the only certain way to make the diagnosis.

The uncertain genetic transmission of these conditions is a problem in genetic counseling. In these individual cases, it is extremely important to obtain a careful family history, so that the dominant or recessive character of the disorder can be ascertained within the family at risk.

MEDULLARY SPONGE KIDNEY

The diagnosis of medullary sponge kidney is usually not made until the fourth or fifth decade of life, when patients have secondary calcifications with passage of urinary stone or infective complications emerge. Progression to end-stage renal failure is uncommon. The incidence of this disease is approximately 1 in 5000 in the general population and perhaps as high as 1 in 1000 in patients studied in urology clinics. Males and females appear to be affected equally. Familial transmission of the disease has been reported on occasion, and there is an occasional association with other congenital problems.

Pathologic Features

The external surface of the kidney is normal in this condition, and only on cut section is the abnormality obvious. There is irregular enlargement of the medullary and interpapillary collecting ducts, giving a "Swiss cheese" appearance to the kidney in these regions. The

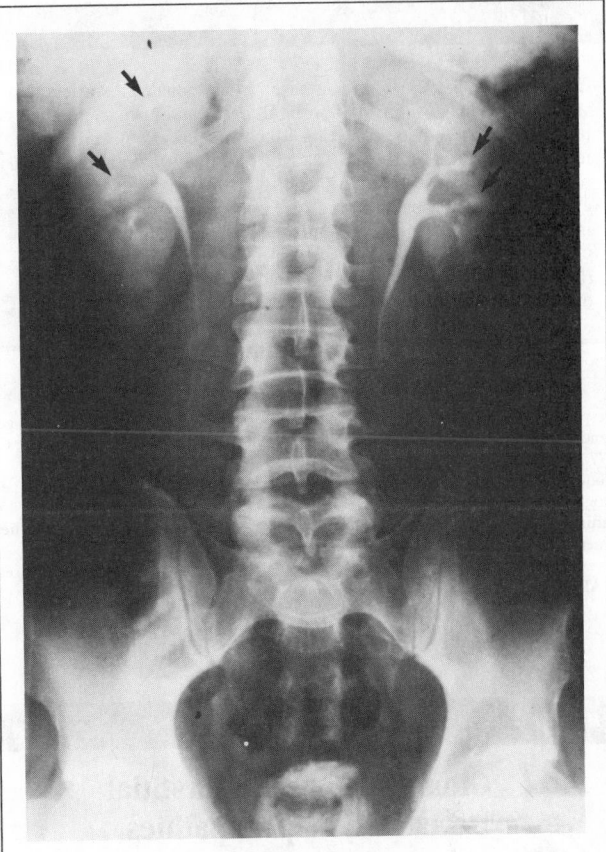

FIGURE 120-3   Typical striations in medullary sponge kidney. *Arrows,* Papillary tip calcifications.

papillary changes are bilateral in most cases. Within an individual kidney one or several papillae may be affected. In some cases the cavity of the cyst may be filled with calculi, but in other instances there is no evidence of calcification in the ectatic collecting ducts.

Clinical and Diagnostic Features

The disease is usually noticed in the fourth or fifth decade of life, when it may be associated with gross or microscopic hematuria. Nephrolithiasis with renal colic, loin pain, and secretion of small stones is also a prominent feature. The disease seldom progresses to end-stage renal failure; the most common abnormality is decreased urinary concentrating ability and in rare instances inability to acidify the urine maximally.

The diagnosis is made by intravenous urography, which shows the typical striations in the papillary portions of the kidney produced by the accumulation of contrast material in the dilated collecting ducts (Fig. 120-3). On plain films of the abdomen, calcium precipitates may also be observed in the papillary regions of the kidneys.

There is no known therapy. A causal association of parathyroid adenoma and medullary sponge kidney has been found in several reports. Among all calcium stone formers, women have a greater incidence of medullary sponge kidney than do men. Absorptive hypercalciuria is a common abnormality in sponge kidney that is associated with renal calcification. As a general rule patients should be advised to excrete over 2 L of urine a day to reduce the opportunity for calcium precipitation in the urine. If a patient has hypercalciuria, thiazide diuretics may decrease urinary calcium excretion.

BIBLIOGRAPHY

Antignac C et al: A gene for familial juvenile nephronophthisis (recessive medullary cystic kidney disease) maps to chromosome 2p, *Nature Genet* 3:342, 1993.

✔ *WHEN TO REFER*

On the whole, polycystic kidney diseases are unusual disorders that warrant referral for consultation in all cases and primary management by nephrologists, sometimes in conjunction with urologists, in many instances. In the early stages of polycystic kidney disease patients should be referred to nephrologists to establish a firm diagnosis that is the basis for genetic counseling and for determining prognosis. The management of intercurrent complications including hypertension, renal infection, renal stone, renal hemorrhage, renal pain, or progressive renal insufficiency should be under the direction of an experienced nephrologist.

European Polycystic Kidney Disease Consortium: The polycystic kidney disease 1 gene encodes a 14 kb transcript and lies within a duplicated region on chromosome 16, *Cell* 77:881, 1994.

Gabow PA, Grantham JJ: Polycystic kidney disease. In Schrier RW, Gottschalk CW, editors: *Diseases of the kidney*, ed 5, Boston, 1993, Little Brown.

Martinez JR, Grantham JJ: Polycystic kidney disease: Etiology, pathogenesis and treatment, *Disease a Month* 41:693, 1995.

Zerres K et al: Mapping of the gene for autosomal recessive polycystic kidney disease (ARPKD) to chromosome 6p, *Nature Genet* 7:429, 1994.

CHAPTER

121 Glomerular and Interstitial Hereditary Nephropathies

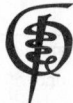

Gerald F. DiBona

Inherited renal disease is the cause of end-stage renal failure in approximately 10% of patients starting dialysis. Autosomal dominant polycystic kidney disease (Chapter 120) accounts for approximately 80% of these cases. This chapter deals with other hereditary nephropathies that have a documented or highly suggestive genetic pattern.

ALPORT'S SYNDROME

Alport's syndrome is a hereditary glomerulonephritis that is associated with sensorineural deafness and characteristic eye lesions affecting the lens and the macula. The gene frequency is approximately 1 in 5000 individuals.

Genetics and Pathogenesis

Pedigree analysis has identified three patterns of inheritance: X-linked dominant (most common), autosomal dominant, and autosomal recessive. The locus for the X-linked dominant form is on the long arm of the X chromosome (Xq22). Spear proposed that a genetic defect at a locus governing a structural protein common to the basement membrane of the glomerulus, the anterior lens capsule (Descemet's membrane), and the tectorial membrane of the organ of Corti in the cochlea could explain the association of renal, ocular, and auditory abnormalities. The responsible gene, COL4A5, is also located at Xq22 and encodes for the α5 chain of type IV collagen, which is abundant in glomerular basement membrane, Descemet's membrane, and tectorial membrane. Several mutations have been identified, including missense mutations, deletions, insertions and duplications; splice site mutations; and premature stop codons. These mutations can be considered to have serious effects on the assembly, folding, and cross-linking of the type IV collagen triple helix, increasing its susceptibility to proteolytic degradation. In some families with the X-linked dominant form the disorder is transmitted in association with leiomyomas in the esophagus or tracheobronchial tree. In these families there

is a deletion at the 5' ends of the paired COL4A5 and COL4A6 genes, suggesting that the COL4A6 mutation is responsible for the leiomyomatosis. The autosomal recessive form has been traced to mutations in the COL4A3 and COL4A4 genes that lie on chromosome 2. The autosomal dominant form has also been mapped to chromosome 2, in the region of the COL4A3 and COL4A4 genes.

Clinical and Laboratory Findings

The diagnosis can be made in any family in which at least three of the following criteria are fulfilled:
1. Positive family history of hematuria with or without chronic renal failure (i.e., more than one individual affected)
2. Electron microscopic evidence on renal biopsy of characteristic changes (i.e., thickening and splitting of the glomerular basement membrane with electron lucent areas containing small, dense granulations)
3. Characteristic eye findings on slit lamp ophthalmoscopy (i.e., anterior lenticonus, spherophakia, polar cataracts, perimacular pigmentation ["macular flecks"], and absence of macular reflex)
4. High-frequency sensorineural deafness that is usually progressive during childhood

Careful clinical examination of all at-risk relatives of the proband may be necessary before the requisite number of criteria is fulfilled.

In the X-linked dominant form males are more severely affected than females; severity of involvement is equal in males and females in the autosomal recessive form. Usual onset is in childhood or adolescence, being earlier in males. Initially there is intermittent or persistent microscopic hematuria. Gross hematuria may occur spontaneously, after exercise, or after a nonspecific upper respiratory tract infection. Associated with the hematuria are mild, intermittent proteinuria, which increases over time, and frequent occurrence of the nephrotic syndrome and hypertension. Renal insufficiency is progressive; in nearly all patients serum creatinine concentration is elevated by age 25 years and renal replacement therapy is required by age 30.

Some degree of hearing loss, produced by a bilateral symmetric sensory nerve defect, is an early symptom; deafness occurs in approximately two thirds of affected persons. Hearing loss can occur as an isolated manifestation or in association with ocular or renal abnormalities. Audiometric examinations are required to evaluate affected family members.

Kindreds with ocular abnormalities have a higher incidence of renal and auditory abnormalities, but any of the three major features (renal, auditory, and ocular abnormalities) may appear in a given patient.

Routine laboratory investigation for immunologic or urologic abnormalities yields consistently normal results. There is no specific biochemical marker of the syndrome in blood or urine.

Pathologic Features

By light microscopy the findings are nonspecific. In young children the renal biopsy result may be normal except for an increase in the number of immature glomeruli. Later, there is focal and segmental glomerular hypercellularity consisting of both mesangial and endothelial cells. The mesangial matrix is also increased. There is segmental and diffuse thickening with duplication of the glomerular capillary wall. Progressive glomerular disease is characterized by segmental and global glomerulosclerosis; crescent formation is unusual. The interstitium shows inflammatory cell infiltration, fibrosis, and tubular atrophy. Interstitial lipid-containing foam cells are seen, but their presence is not specific to Alport's syndrome. Immunofluorescence findings are usually normal.

Electron microscopy is the most reliable method of establishing a diagnosis. The earliest changes are focal thinning and thickening of the glomerular basement membrane. There is irregular thickening of the glomerular basement membrane, whose substructure is variously described as splitting, splintering, replication, reticulation, lamination, lamellation, or interweaving ("basket weave") of the lamina densa, and within which there are clear, electron-lucent zones containing small, round electron-dense granulations. Occasionally there are similar lesions of the basement membranes of Bowman's capsule and tu-

✔ *WHEN TO REFER*

With progressive deterioration of renal function that is usually associated with hypertension the patient should be referred to a medical center with capability for both dialysis (nephrologist) and renal transplantation (transplant surgeon).

bular cells. There is fusion of epithelial foot processes, but electron-dense deposits are absent. Diffuse, widespread splitting of the glomerular basement membrane is strongly indicative of Alport's syndrome.

Differential Diagnosis

In a patient with persistent hematuria, immunofluorescence and electron microscopic study of a renal biopsy specimen are clearly indicated. In a majority of cases a definitive diagnosis can be made with these techniques. The finding of characteristic glomerular basement membrane changes should lead the physician to perform further studies to confirm the diagnosis of Alport's syndrome in the patient and in family members. The X-linked dominant form may be diagnosed in males by immunohistochemical analysis of skin biopsy specimens that disclose an absence of staining of epidermal basement for COL4A5. Mosaicism in heterozygous females limits the utility of skin biopsy in making this diagnosis in women.

Berger's disease, or immunoglobulin A (IgA) nephropathy (Chapter 121), a common cause of hematuria in children, adolescents, and young adults, can be differentiated by renal biopsy. In IgA nephropathy the typical finding by light microscopy is an area of hypercellularity with increased mesangial cells and matrix, often involving only a single lobule in a given glomerulus and with sparing of some adjacent glomeruli. Immunofluorescence reveals diffuse deposition of immunoglobulins in the mesangium of all glomeruli. The principal constituent of these deposits is IgA, which must be demonstrated to establish the diagnosis. Deposition of lesser amounts of immunoglobulin G (IgG) is often seen as well. Electron microscopy confirms the immunofluorescence findings by demonstrating small, electron-dense deposits predominantly in the mesangium. In young patients the only abnormality may be glomerular basement membrane thinning, making it difficult to distinguish between Alport's syndrome and thin basement membrane nephropathy. This is an important distinction, since thin basement membrane nephropathy is not associated with apparent increase in morbidity or mortality.

Management

No form of therapy slows progression to end-stage renal failure. Prompt, aggressive treatment of urinary tract and ear infections is advisable. Dialysis and transplantation have been successfully used for patients with end-stage renal failure (Chapter 110). Stabilization of progressive hearing loss after successful transplantation and recurrence of the disease in the allograft have been reported. Corneal transplantation and lens extraction may be useful, but there is no treatment for the hearing loss.

THIN BASEMENT MEMBRANE NEPHROPATHY

Thin basement membrane nephropathy (familial benign essential hematuria) is characterized by persistent microhematuria with rare episodes of gross hematuria without proteinuria, impairment of renal function, or progression. Autosomal dominant transmission is speculated. Defining histologic findings consist of normal glomeruli or only minor glomerular abnormalities on light microscopy; normal immunofluorescence; and diffuse, widespread thinning of the glomerular basement membrane in which attenuation of the lamina densa is particularly prominent on electron microscopy. Berger's disease is excluded by normal immunofluorescence, and Alport's syndrome may be excluded by absence of diffuse, widespread splitting of the glomerular basement membrane and intramembranous deposits on elec-

tron microscopy. There is no apparent increase in morbidity or mortality.

NAIL-PATELLA SYNDROME

Nail-patella syndrome, or hereditary onychoosteodysplasia, is transmitted as an autosomal dominant trait. The responsible gene is located on the long arm of chromosome 9 in the region of 9q34.1, which is near the location (9q34.3) of the gene that encodes for the α1 chain of type V (fibrillar) collagen. The disorder is characterized by dysplasia of the nail beds, hypoplasia or absence of the patellae, accessory posterior iliac horns, and elbow deformities with increased carrying angle and limitation of supination and extension due to deformation or luxation of the head of the radius. About 50% of affected persons have proteinuria or abnormal urinary sediment, or both. Progression to end-stage renal failure occurs in approximately 25% of affected patients. The light microscopy findings are variable and resemble those of Alport's syndrome. The electron microscopy findings in all patients with skeletal abnormalities, regardless of urinalysis or renal function, consist of (1) an irregular nodular thickening of the glomerular basement membrane with intramembranous collagen-like fibrils and (2) localized translucent areas in the glomerular basement membrane and mesangium that have a moth-eaten appearance. The immunofluorescence findings are variable. There is no known specific therapy, but successful dialysis and transplantation have been reported. The disorder does not recur in the transplanted kidney.

FAMILIAL MEDITERRANEAN FEVER

Familial Mediterranean fever (FMF) is an autosomal recessive disease characterized by recurrent, brief but disabling, self-limited febrile attacks of peritonitis, synovitis, pleuritis, vasculitis, or an erysipelas-like erythema of the lower extremities. The responsible gene, MEF (the FMF gene), is located on the short arm of chromosome 16 in the region of 16p13.3. It is seen mainly in Sephardic Jews. Increases in serum monohydroxy and dihydroxy fatty acids known to cause neutrophil aggregation and serum amyloid A protein, as well as decreases in peritoneal fluid C5a-inhibitor, which antagonizes the chemotactic activity of the complement fragment C5a, may participate in the pathogenesis of the acute inflammatory attacks. Systemic amyloidosis (Chapter 210) with renal involvement is a common but insidious complication of FMF. Renal insufficiency is the major cause of mortality, and renal functional impairment can occasionally precede other features of the disease. Renal involvement, which peaks in the third decade, becomes manifest as proteinuria, at first intermittent, later constant and massive. Renal vein thrombosis is not unusual. The clinical course is progressive, with development of the nephrotic syndrome and eventually end-stage renal failure. Average survival is 7 years after onset of proteinuria and 3 years after the development of the nephrotic syndrome; survival beyond age 40 years is uncommon. Colchicine is effective in relieving the symptoms and frequency of acute extrarenal attacks. Colchicine therapy prevents amyloidosis (defined as proteinuria) and prevents additional deterioration of renal function in patients with amyloidosis who have proteinuria but not the nephrotic syndrome. Renal transplantation is an acceptable alternative to hemodialysis for the treatment of end-stage renal failure, although recurrence of amyloidosis in the renal transplant has been observed.

LIPODYSTROPHY

The syndrome of lipodystrophy is characterized by diminished subcutaneous fat, particularly of the face and upper arms; hirsutism; hyperpigmentation; splenomegaly; hypertension; and diabetes mellitus. Although there is familial aggregation of cases, the mode of transmission is unknown. The most common renal manifestation is asymptomatic proteinuria or the nephrotic syndrome. Renal biopsy reveals membranoproliferative glomerulonephritis, more frequently type II than type I, and there is decreased serum C3 concentration in association with circulating C3 nephritic factor (Chapter 116). The serum complement abnormalities may exist in the absence of clinical evidence of renal disease. The pathogenesis is unknown, and there is no known treatment. Renal transplantation has been successfully employed for patients who progress to end-stage renal failure.

ANDERSON-FABRY DISEASE

Angiokeratoma corporis diffusum, or Anderson-Fabry disease, is an inborn error of glycosphingolipid metabolism resulting from a deficiency of the enzyme α-galactosidase A. Inheritance is X-linked recessive, with carrier females displaying no or less marked features of clinical disease. The enzyme deficiency results in widespread tissue accumulation (including in the kidneys) of uncleaved glycososphingolipids, chiefly trihexosyl ceramide. Pain is often the first and usually the most characteristic symptom of the peripheral neuropathy. There are two forms: periodic "crises" of knifelike or burning pain in the limbs, particularly the hands and feet, and chronic acral paresthesias. In the first decade punctate dark blue, red, or black nonblanching macules, which evolve into blanching papules, appear in clusters on the skin of the lower trunk, thighs, and scrotum. Corneal opacities, posterior subcapsular cataracts, retinal abnormalities, premature cerebrovascular disease, cardiac involvement, and hypertension are frequently observed. Renal dysfunction is the rule and is evident by the third decade; end-stage renal failure occurs by the fifth decade. Early laboratory findings are hematuria and proteinuria. The urinary sediment may reveal lipid-containing foam cells that have a Maltese-cross appearance on polarizing light microscopy. Under electron microscopy the lipid is stored as concentric lamellar inclusions in the lysosomes of the podocytes. These structures have been termed myelin bodies because of the resemblance to the myelin that surrounds nerve fibers. These myelin bodies may be noted in several inborn errors of glycosphingolipid metabolism.

Light microscopy reveals lipid deposition in blood vessels, glomerular epithelial cells, Bowman's capsule, and the epithelium of Henle's loop and the distal convoluted tubule. Immunofluorescence findings are normal. Treatment with dialysis and transplantation produces excellent survival rates (83% surviving 33 months). Isolation and characterization of the gene for α-galactosidase A have permitted the identification of various molecular defects: partial deletion, duplication, and point mutations.

BIBLIOGRAPHY

Bodziak KA et al: Inherited diseases of the glomerular basement membrane, *Am J Kidney Dis* 23:605, 1994.

Kashtan CE, Michael AF: Alport syndrome, *Kid Int* 50:1445, 1996.

Matzner Y: Biologic and clinical advances in familial Mediterranean fever, *Crit Rev Oncol Hematol* 18:197, 1995.

Parfrey PS: Hereditary renal diseases, *Curr Opin Nephrol Hypertension* 2:192, 1993.

Sessa A et al: Alport syndrome: clinical, molecular and genetic aspects, *J Nephrol* 7:102, 1994.

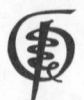

CHAPTER

122 Disorders of Renal Tubular Transport

Sidney Kobrin and Stanley Goldfarb

The production of an ultrafiltration of plasma across the glomerulus causes an enormous load of plasma components to reach the tubular lumen. The tubular cells reabsorb many of these filtered substances from the tubular lumen. Abnormal tubular handling of sodium (Chapter 113), potassium (Chapter 114), and components involved in acid-base homeostasis (Chapter 115) are discussed elsewhere. This chapter focuses on Fanconi's syndrome and selected isolated disorders of renal tubular function.

RENAL GLYCOSURIA
Pathogenesis

Renal glycosuria is defined as the presence of significant amounts of glucose in the urine in the absence of hyperglycemia. This abnormality may occur in a variety of settings. Primary renal glycosuria is an isolated heritable defect that occurs in the absence of other structural or functional abnormalities of the kidney. Congenital glucose-galactose malabsorption is a rare autosomal recessive inherited disorder. It is characterized by intestinal malabsorption of glucose and galactose and renal glycosuria and becomes evident with severe diarrhea at birth. Generalized proximal tubular dysfunction (Fanconi's syndrome) may include renal glycosuria. In addition, several more specific tubular defects, such as phosphate wasting and glycinuria, may also be associated with renal glycosuria. Renal glycosuria is commonly seen in pregnancy, the nephrotic syndrome, and, occasionally, advanced renal failure (glomerular filtration rate [GFR] less than 15 ml/min).

The exact mode of inheritance of the primary form remains to be determined. The early literature on glycosuria suggested that the defect was inherited as an autosomal dominant trait. However, these studies were confounded by investigators' use of different definitions and techniques of studying glucose handling, as well as the fact that the expression of the disease shows marked variability in severity even among members of the same family.

Pathophysiology

Glucose transport across epithelial cells of the kidney proximal tubule and the small intestine is mediated by brush border Na^+-coupled glucose transporters termed SGLT and basolateral facilitated glucose transporters (GLUT). In the mammalian kidney the major site for glucose reabsorption is the early S1 segment of the proximal convoluted tubule. In experimental studies in the rat, approximately 90% of the filtered glucose is reabsorbed by this tubule segment and only a small fraction of the filtered load reaches the straight tubule of the proximal nephron.

In human intestine and kidney the existence of a shared high-affinity Na^+/glucose cotransporter and of a second, kidney-specific, low-affinity Na^+/glucose cotransporter is supported by studies of patients with familial intestinal glucose-galactose malabsorption and renal glycosuria. Patients with renal glycosuria were found to have impaired renal but not intestinal glucose absorption, whereas patients with intestinal glucose-galactose malabsorption generally also have an associated mild glycosuria. Thus at least two gene loci must be present, to explain impaired glucose absorption in these diseases.

In normal persons, glucose is almost entirely reabsorbed in the proximal tubule, and less than 100 mg, well below the sensitivity of commonly used dipstick tests, appears in the urine. Glucose transport displays a transport maximum (T_mG); that is, below the saturating filtered load, or T_m, glucose is entirely reabsorbed, whereas the filtered load above T_m is passed into the urine. Theoretically one might expect glucose to appear in the urine only when filtered load exceeds T_m, but the minimal filtered load, or threshold at which glucose appears in the urine ($F_{min}G$), is usually 70% to 80% of T_m. T_m is normally about 325 mg/min/1.73 m^2, and threshold is about 220 mg/min/1.73 m^2 (equivalent to a blood glucose level of 180 mg/dl). This discrepancy accounts for the so-called splay in the glucose titration curve. Splay could be the consequence of nephronal heterogeneity for glucose reabsorption if filtered load exceeds the reabsorptive capacity of some nephrons before others. As an alternative, splay may be explained by Michaelis-Menten kinetics on the assumption that glucose and its carrier behave as substrate and enzyme, with a finite dissociation constant.

Recent studies have elucidated the molecular mechanisms underlying renal glucose transport in humans and have clarified the nature of the two glucose transport genes mentioned earlier. SGLT2 is the designation of the renal low-affinity, high-capacity Na^+/glucose cotransporter that is the major renal Na^+/glucose reabsorptive mechanism. SGLT1 is the high-affinity transporter in the kidney and intestine. A point mutation in the latter is responsible for the altered transport of glucose in patients with glucose-galactose malabsorption. It

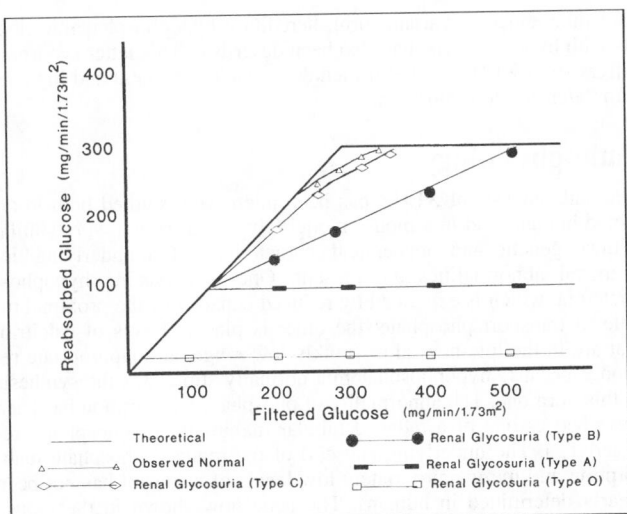

FIGURE 122-1 Patterns of glycosuria.

is likely that the more common form of hereditary renal glycosuria is due to a defect in the gene for SGLUT1.

In primary renal glycosuria, glucose titration studies have defined three pathogenetic mechanisms. In type A, T_m is reduced; in terms of the enzyme kinetic model, the number of glucose carriers is reduced but the affinity of each carrier for glucose is normal. In type B, T_m is normal but threshold is reduced, and the titration curve has an exaggerated splay. This variant is consistent with a normal number of carrier sites and reduced carrier affinity for glucose. In type O, there is virtual absence of renal tubular glucose reabsorption. On histologic examination the kidney is perfectly normal.

Three patterns of glycosuria have been described in patients with the nephrotic syndrome, including types A and B as described with the primary form, as well as a curve characterized by a low point of splay but an otherwise almost physiologic tracing (type C). The different patterns of glycosuria are displayed graphically in Fig. 122-1.

Diagnosis

The diagnosis of renal glycosuria depends on the following criteria: (1) true glycosuria in the absence of hyperglycemia, (2) a normal glucose tolerance test result, (3) excretion of at least 500 mg glucose/ 1.73 m² per day, and (4) exclusion of generalized tubular defects (Fanconi's syndrome).

Clinical Features

Primary renal glycosuria is generally a benign condition, with only occasional reports of development of hypoglycemia and ketosis during prolonged fasting. The major purpose of documenting the primary form of this condition is to exclude diabetes mellitus, the nephrotic syndrome, renal failure, and Fanconi's syndrome from the diagnosis. The early literature suggested that primary glycosuria was a harbinger of diabetes mellitus. However, recent studies suggest that this disorder does not evolve into diabetes mellitus.

AMINOACIDURIA

Amino acids are freely filtered at the glomerulus; more than 95% of these filtered amino acids are then reabsorbed by transport processes located in the proximal tubule. The finding of excessive amounts of amino acids in the urine does not specifically imply a renal disorder. Thus a primary increase in blood levels of amino acids can produce aminoaciduria either as a "spillover" phenomenon or as the result of competition for transport between two structurally similar amino acids. As an alternative, blood levels can be normal, and aminoaciduria can be due to a renal tubular transport defect that is either generalized or specific for a certain type of amino acid. Generalized amino-

Table 122-1   Aminoacidurias

AMINO ACID	CLINICAL DISORDERS	CLINICAL MANIFESTATIONS
Alpha-amino neutral tryptophan and others	Hartnup disease	Pellagra-like disorders
Dibasic Cystine Lysine Ornithine Arginine	Cystinuria	Recurrent nephrolithiasis
Dicarboxylic acid Glutamic acid Aspartic acid	Dicarboxylic aminoaciduria	Fasting hypoglycemia and ketoacidosis
Iminoglycines Hydroxyproline Glycine	Iminoglycinuria	No known disease

aciduria is usually part of Fanconi's syndrome. The substrate-specific amino acid transport systems in the kidney and the associated disorders are listed in Table 122- 1.

NEUTRAL AMINOACIDURIA: HARTNUP DISEASE
Etiology

Hartnup disease (named for the index family) is inherited as an autosomal recessive trait, and its incidence is 1 in 26,000 live births. The disease represents the apparent failure of synthesis of a transport protein that mediates the intestinal absorption and renal tubular reabsorption of monoaminomonocarboxylic amino acids with neutral or aromatic side chains. These include serine, alanine, threonine, valine, leucine, isoleucine, phenylalanine, tyrosine, glutamine, asparagine, histidine, and tryptophan.

Clinical and Laboratory Findings

The clinical features of Hartnup disease are similar to those characteristic of pellagra with the exception that the former is intermittent and usually less severe. Nicotinamide deficiency in Hartnup disease results from reduced availability of its precursor, tryptophan, because of both reduced gastrointestinal absorption and increased renal excretion. Patients have a red, scaly rash that is exacerbated by exposure to sunlight. Cerebellar ataxia, psychiatric disturbances, and diarrhea are common. Intermittent dystonia without ataxia has been reported. However, these clinical findings are highly variable, and patients in normal physical and mental health have been described. The clinical disorders are subject to exacerbations and remissions, and periods of poor nutrition and excessive sunlight may precipitate clinical attacks. It is also possible that some of the neuropsychiatric manifestations of the disease are due to the absorption of metabolites of the amino acids generated by bacterial action on malabsorbed amino acids within the gut.

Dietary history plus chromatographic analysis of the urine readily distinguishes Hartnup disease from classic pellagra resulting from dietary deficiency. The cornerstone of treatment is the administration of nicotinamide in dosages of 40 to 200 mg/day to prevent pellagra-like disturbances.

DIBASIC AMINOACIDURIA: CYSTINURIA

For a discussion of cystinuria see Chapter 111.

DICARBOXYLIC AMINOACIDURIAS

Increased renal excretion of glutamic and aspartic acids has been reported in only a few cases but has been detected by genetic screening programs and so may be more prevalent than has been believed. It is an autosomal recessive trait with two forms: type I is associated with reduced gastrointestinal and renal uptake. In type II gastrointestinal uptake is normal but renal uptake is impaired. Central nervous system deficiencies have been reported in affected children. Renal

BOX 122-1
Causes of renal phosphate wasting

Primary hyperparathyroidism
Secondary hyperparathyroidism
Vitamin D deficiency
Dietary
Malabsorption
Lack of 25-(OH)-vitamin D
Liver disease
Phenobarbital, phenytoin
Lack of 1,25-(OH)$_2$-vitamin D$_3$
Vitamin D–dependent rickets

Primary phosphate transport defect
X-linked hypophosphatemic rickets
Oncogenic hypophosphatemia
Idiopathic hypercalciuria

Fanconi's syndrome

clearance of glutamic and aspartic acids has been found to exceed that of inulin, so an alteration in the bidirectional transport of these compounds is present, with a definite secretory component. Recent studies have allowed the assignment of the gene coding for the human high-affinity glutamate transporter EAAC1 to chromosome 9.

One child described with this disorder was completely normal and the abnormality was detected by screening tests, whereas a second exhibited fasting hypoglycemia, ketoacidosis, and growth retardation. The symptomatic child had a type I defect, and it is postulated that reductions in gastrointestinal uptake combined with renal loss led to a more severe deficiency and consequent impairment of gluconeogenesis. The only available therapy is frequent feeding to prevent hypoglycemia and ketoacidosis.

IMINOGLYCINURIA

Iminoglycinuria is a rare, benign disorder characterized by the excretion in urine of excessive amounts of three amino acids, proline, hydroxyproline, and glycine. The underlying defect is believed to be reduced activity of a transport system in the proximal tubule that normally mediates the reabsorption of these amino acids. There are apparently no clinical consequences of this tubular defect.

RENAL PHOSPHATE WASTING SYNDROMES

Hypophosphatemia (Chapter 314) is most commonly seen in acutely ill patients and is usually a consequence of a combination of low dietary intake or malabsorption and a shift of phosphate into cells. Less commonly, hypophosphatemia is due to reduced renal reabsorption of phosphate (i.e., renal phosphate wasting). The causes of renal phosphate wasting are shown in Box 122-1. Primary or secondary hyperparathyroidism may be diagnosed fairly readily by the finding of elevated parathyroid hormone levels and by coexisting disturbances of serum calcium. Three uncommon causes of renal phosphate wasting—X-linked hypophosphatemic rickets, oncogenic hypophosphatemia, and Fanconi's syndrome, are discussed in the following sections in more detail.

X-LINKED HYPOPHOSPHATEMIC RICKETS
Definition and Etiology

Various forms of familial hypophosphatemic rickets have been described. The most common form is transmitted via a sex-linked dominant mode of inheritance and is referred to as X-linked hypophosphatemic rickets (XLHR). This syndrome is characterized by hypophosphatemia, inappropriately high urinary phosphate excretion, normocalcemia, normal to lower levels of calcitriol, and the occurrence of rickets in childhood, despite normal vitamin D intake. There are also sporadic forms of hypophosphatemic rickets that are probably new X-linked mutations, and rare instances of autosomal domi-

nant inheritance. A variant form, hereditary hypophosphatemic rickets with hypercalciuria, has also been described. This latter syndrome differs from XLHR in that it includes muscle weakness and high serum calcitriol concentrations.

Pathophysiology

The pathogenesis of XLHR has been intensively studied both in affected humans and in a mouse model (Hyp mouse) with very similar clinical, genetic, and biochemical characteristics. Two underlying biochemical abnormalities are present. One is persisting hypophosphatemia, which is explained by reduced capacity of the proximal tubule to transport phosphate; the other is plasma levels of calcitriol that are in the low-normal or frankly low range, an inappropriate response because hypophosphatemia normally stimulates the synthesis of this hormone. The abnormality of phosphate reabsorption has been described as one of a reduced tubular maximum for phosphate (reduced T_m). The underlying cause(s) of the reduced phosphate reabsorption and the inappropriately low levels of calcitriol has not been clearly determined in humans. The gene now shown in the mouse model to be responsible for the phenotypic expression of the syndrome does not encode the luminal sodium-phosphate cotransporter that is responsible for phosphate transport in the proximal tubule. Rather, the presence of this abnormal gene somehow secondarily leads to a lower rate of phosphate transport, in part through a lower rate of expression of the transport protein in the tubule. Thus a defect in the transport protein does not explain the genetic basis of this disorder. Moreover, despite this reduction in the expression of the phosphate transport protein, the clinical syndrome is not improved by transplanting a normal mouse kidney into an affected mouse. This finding suggests that an extrarenal factor is responsible for the defect. Several studies have indeed indicated the presence of a humoral phosphaturic factor derived from an extrarenal source in the mouse model. Some evidence has come from studies in patients with oncogenic osteomalacia. This sporadic acquired disease in adults caused by the secretion of a factor by mesenchymal vascular tumors almost completely mimics the inherited disorder. Extracts of the tumor can be shown to inhibit phosphate transport in renal epithelial cells and to produce both hypophosphatemia and reduced calcitriol production in experimental animals. This putative hormone differs from parathyroid hormone in that it has no effect on calcium metabolism, its action is not blocked by a parathormone (PTH) antagonist, and its effects do not appear to be mediated by the adenylate cyclase–cyclic adenosine monophosphate (AMP) system. In addition, recent studies of tumor cells in culture show the elaboration of a factor that impairs phosphate uptake in epithelial cells in culture.

The inappropriately low plasma calcitriol concentration in the presence of significant hypophosphatemia suggests that the X-linked mutation may also perturb the regulation of renal vitamin D metabolism. The Hyp mouse exhibits a blunted response to activators of calcitriol biosynthesis, as well as increased renal catabolism of this hormone. The increased catabolism is corrected by phosphate supplementation, suggesting that the abnormal vitamin D metabolism results from a disorder in cellular phosphate homeostasis. Interestingly, serum phosphate and calcitriol levels and the T_m for phosphate are very similar in affected males and females.

Bone changes, which include rickets or osteomalacia, stunted growth, and lower limb deformities, define the clinical expression of the disease in XLHR. These skeletal manifestations are caused by a dual abnormality: a renal defect combining phosphate wasting with altered calcitriol metabolism, as described previously, and a bone defect that decreases the ability of the bone-forming cells (osteoblasts and osteocytes) to control mineral deposition in the matrix. As is characteristic of a sex-linked dominant mutation, the bone lesions are fully expressed in male hemizygotes and variably expressed in female heterozygotes. There is no direct correlation between the severity of the bone disease and the degree of hypophosphatemia. Female subjects with hypophosphatemia and no evidence of skeletal involvement have been identified as "carriers" of the trait. These subjects provide evidence that the defect in renal phosphate transport alone cannot explain the abnormal bone phenotype. The reason for this sex-dependent difference in expression of the disease in bone and kidney is not clear, but it seems likely that two pathogenetic processes may be acting in parallel in kidney and bone.

Insufficient availability of calcium or phosphate similarly affects cartilage mineralization and induces rachitic changes. However, the effect on osteoid tissue calcification is somewhat different. Calcium deficiency provokes secondary hyperparathyroidism, which stimulates osteoclastic absorption, leading to a progressive decrease in bone mass and osteopenia. By contrast, the phosphate-deficient bone in XLHR is characterized by very little osteoclastic activity because these patients are normocalcemic and secondary hyperparathyroidism does not occur. Therefore, despite severe osteomalacia, trabecular bone mass is within the normal range in patients with XLHR. This finding may explain the rarity of fractures in these patients. The response to various forms of treatment provides another insight into the bone defect in XLHR. Patients who receive treatment with phosphate and vitamin D have correction of the rickets, but not osteomalacia. When calcitriol is substituted for vitamin D, there is a beneficial effect, including improved and even healed osteomalacia. Some form of osteoblast resistance to vitamin D that can respond only to supraphysiologic levels of calcitriol could explain these findings.

Clinical and Laboratory Features

The clinical consequence of the reduced serum phosphate level is rickets. Growth retardation to the point of dwarfism and rachitic deformities are primarily seen in the lower extremities. Rickets develops as the infant begins to place weight-bearing stress on the lower extremities. Myopathy, a typical feature of other forms of hypophosphatemia, is rarely seen in XLHR, but adults have a variety of rheumatic complaints, including arthralgias and bone pain. The teeth may also be affected by apical abscesses and early decay attributable to abnormal dentine and cementum formation. The dental lesions, analogously to the condition in bone, are more marked in males. Renal phosphate wasting is manifested by a low T_m phosphate/GFR ratio or inappropriately high clearance of phosphate for the reduced serum level. Other abnormalities of tubular or glomerular function are not usually seen, but glycosuria and glycinuria have occasionally been reported. The bone biopsy result shows rickets or osteomalacia, depending on the age of the patient. The features of rickets are fairly typical, but as discussed, the osteoclastic activity is less than in osteomalacia associated with hypocalemia and secondary hypoparathyroidism.

Treatment

Adequate treatment requires both oral phosphate and calcitriol administration. Treatment with calcitriol alone does not raise serum phosphate levels, whereas treatment with phosphate alone results in hypocalcemia and secondary hyperparathyroidism. Although the conclusions are still challenged by some authors, most studies have demonstrated that the combination of phosphate and calcitriol administration enhances intestinal absorption of phosphate, heals the lesions of rickets and osteomalacia, and, if given early enough in childhood, significantly improves the growth rate and dramatically decreases the need for corrective osteotomies. Successful phosphate supplementation requires the administration of several daily doses to maintain a normal serum phosphate concentration for most of the day and night. The major complication of this therapy is the induction of nephrocalcinosis, which may ultimately result in a decrease in renal function. Therefore frequent renal imaging and assessment of renal function are essential. This strategy may allow a timely decrease in the dosage or discontinuation of these agents. Whether the treatment should be continued after growth has ceased remains an open question.

FANCONI'S SYNDROME
Etiology and Pathogenesis

Fanconi's syndrome is a generalized disorder of proximal tubular transport characterized by excessive urinary excretion of amino acids, glucose, bicarbonate, uric acid, phosphate, potassium, and low-molecular-weight proteins. Incomplete expressions of the syndrome may lack one or more of these abnormalities. The syndrome is usually a secondary consequence of some toxic, immunologic, or metabolic insult. In children Fanconi's syndrome is usually due to an inborn error of metabolism, whereas in adults Fanconi's syndrome is usually acquired. Fanconi's syndrome may rarely arise in a primary

---

BOX 122-2
Causes of Fanconi's syndrome

Inborn
Cystinosis (cystine)
Wilson's disease (copper)
Galactosemia (galactose-1-phosphate)
Hereditary fructose intolerance (fructose-1-phosphate)
Tyrosinemia
Lowe's syndrome
Glycogenosis
Vitamin D–resistant rickets
Cytochrome *c* oxidase deficiency
Idiopathic

Acquired
Light chain deposition
  Multiple myeloma
  Monoclonal gammopathy
  Light chain nephropathy
Heavy metal poisoning
  Lead, mercury, cadmium, uranium
Vitamin D deficiency
Renal transplantation
Nephrotic syndrome
Amyloidosis
Sjögren's syndrome
Drugs
  Anydro-4-epitetracycline
  Methyl-5-chrome
  Maleic acid
  6-Mercaptopurine
  Glue sniffing
  Isofosfamide
  cis-Platinum

---

idiopathic form. The primary type may occur at any age. It is most commonly sporadic, but familial cases with variable patterns of inheritance also occur. Histologic examination may reveal no specific findings or tubulointerstitial atrophy and fibrosis. The prognosis is variable: some patients have shown only tubular dysfunction, whereas in others the condition has progressed to chronic renal failure over 10 to 30 years.

The various conditions that produce Fanconi's syndrome share the feature of deposition in the proximal tubule of a toxic substance, for example, a heavy metal, a normal metabolite that accumulates in excessive amounts, or an abnormal protein (Box 122-2). The precise mechanism by which transport is impaired is uncertain. A leading hypothesis at present is that increased membrane permeability allows enhanced back-leak of solutes from the proximal tubular cell or of peritubular fluid into the tubular lumen.

Cystinosis is the most common cause of Fanconi's syndrome in children (Chapter 308). It is characterized by deposition of cystine in the conjunctiva, lymph nodes, bone marrow, and kidney. The mechanism of the increased cystine deposition is uncertain but appears to be related to a combination of increased cellular uptake and impaired cystine egress from lysosomes. Inheritance is autosomal recessive. Three forms may be distinguished. The nephropathic form is manifested by tubular dysfunction in infancy and progresses to early renal insufficiency. The adult form is benign, not characterized by renal involvement, and may be detected only by slit lamp examination. An intermediate form appears in adolescence with mild nephropathy and slower progression than in the infantile type. The diagnosis of cystinosis is made by determination of cystine in leukocytes or fibroblasts; by detection of cystine crystals in the conjunctiva, bone marrow, lymph nodes, or rectal mucosa; or by the presence of retinal pigment degeneration. Specific treatment of cystinosis has been unavailing. Renal transplantation has been successful, however, and although cystine crystals have been detected in the transplanted kidney, Fanconi's syndrome has not recurred.

In other hereditary causes of Fanconi's syndrome the renal functional abnormality can be reversed by halting tissue accumulation of the toxic agent. Wilson's disease is due to copper toxicity, and Fanconi's syndrome, if not far advanced, can be ameliorated by penicillamine. Distal renal tubular acidosis (RTA) may also occur and may cause renal calculi, not otherwise a feature of Fanconi's syndrome. Hereditary fructose intolerance allows the accumulation of fructose-1-phosphate and is fully reversed by dietary fructose restriction. Similarly, galactosemia reflects the accumulation of galactose-1-phosphate, and Fanconi's syndrome is fully reversed by dietary galactose and sucrose restriction. A poorly characterized impaired glycogenolytic response has been associated with Fanconi's syndrome, but the specific enzymatic defect has not been defined. Unusually severe glucosuria and hypoglycemia are characteristic. Lowe's syndrome is an X-linked recessive disorder characterized by cataracts and glaucoma, mental retardation, Fanconi's syndrome, and ultimate renal failure. The biochemical basis is unclear.

In adults the most common cause of Fanconi's syndrome is injury to the proximal tubular cells by light chain deposition. In multiple myeloma or chronic overproduction of monoclonal light chains (Bence Jones protein), filtered light chain is reabsorbed by and accumulates in the proximal tubular cell; it can be identified in renal biopsy specimens by immunofluorescent staining using antisera against the appropriate light chain and on electron micrographs by the appearance of intracellular crystals, probably representing condensed light chains. Why proximal tubular injury and Fanconi's syndrome develop in only a small proportion of patients with paraproteins and Bence Jones proteinuria is not known. The diagnosis of Fanconi's syndrome may precede the recognition of myeloma, sometimes by many years.

Other dysproteinemic states, including amyloidosis and Sjögren's syndrome, are also associated with Fanconi's syndrome, and all these states frequently demonstrate distal tubular defects as well, such as distal RTA and nephrogenic diabetes insipidus (DI). Fanconi's syndrome in nephrotic syndrome may also be caused by tubular toxicity that is produced by filtered and reabsorbed protein, which in this case consists of massive quantities of albumin. However, Fanconi's syndrome is rare in nephrotic syndrome, and a majority of patients have normal amino acid excretion.

Heavy-metal intoxication is caused by lead, cadmium, mercury, and uranium. Acute lead poisoning has produced full-blown Fanconi's syndrome, but chronic lead nephropathy is typically associated with decreased uric acid clearance and hyperuricemia. Cadmium toxicity is typically associated with painful osteomalacia, nephrolithiasis, and characteristic hypouricemia in the presence of renal failure. Outdated tetracycline produced Fanconi's syndrome in the 1960s, but the pharmaceutical preparation has been modified so that the responsible degradation product (anhydro-4-epitetracycline) is not formed in currently available preparations. Thus this problem is no longer of clinical significance. Vitamin D deficiency states, including both nutritional deficiency and vitamin D–dependent rickets, have been associated with some features of Fanconi's syndrome, and the mechanism is presumed to be secondary hyperparathyroidism. Aminoaciduria, phosphaturia, and mild bicarbonate wasting (proximal RTA) may occur with both primary and secondary hyperparathyroidism.

Several drugs (Box 122-2) have been associated with Fanconi's syndrome. Recently the chemotherapeutic agent isofosfamide has been shown to induce Fanconi's syndrome in 4% of a population with underlying normal renal function. The incidence of Fanconi's syndrome may be even higher when preexistent renal function is impaired or other nephrotoxins such as *cis*-platinum have been administered simultaneously. Preliminary in vitro studies suggest that it is the metabolite chloracetaldehyde, rather than isofosfamide itself, that is the toxic agent. This could explain why cyclophosphamide itself has no nephrotoxicity. At equivalent doses the rate of chloracetaldehyde generation with isofosfamide is 40 times greater than with cyclophosphamide.

Clinical Features

Glycosuria in Fanconi's syndrome is similar to that seen in hereditary glycosuria and is of no clinical consequence, as long as it is recognized as being renal in origin and not indicative of diabetes mellitus. Neither uricosuria nor aminoaciduria has clinical consequences, but the former may cause hypouricemia, which can be readily detected biochemically.

The predominant clinical features of Fanconi's syndrome are acidosis produced by bicarbonate wasting, polyuria caused by osmotic diuresis and hypokalemia, sodium wasting resulting from bicarbonaturia, and rickets or osteomalacia generated by phosphate wasting and, probably, reduced production of calcitriol. Growth retardation in children is due to acidosis, potassium, and phosphate depletion and possibly to amino acid wasting. Depending on the underlying cause, distal tubular abnormalities, such as distal RTA and nephrogenic DI, and progression to renal insufficiency are frequently associated. Characteristically, tubular abnormalities such as hypokalemia, hypophosphatemia, and bicarbonate wasting dominate the early clinical course and are ameliorated or become relatively less important if and as GFR falls.

Proximal bicarbonate wasting produces proximal RTA, which is characterized by hyperchloremic acidosis and a tendency to hypokalemia; normal urinary acidification when serum bicarbonate is at or below its reduced threshold; normal citrate excretion; and high therapeutic alkali requirements. Distal acidification is usually intact but may be impaired by concomitant potassium depletion or a dysproteinemic state. Hypokalemia is of multifactorial origin and may reflect decreased proximal tubular reabsorption, increased distal delivery of sodium and bicarbonate (particularly after alkali therapy), chronic acidosis, and hyperaldosteronism attributable to volume contraction.

Metabolic bone disease also results from several factors, including phosphate depletion and chronic acidosis. In addition, the conversion of 25(OH)–vitamin D to 1,25(OH)$_2$–vitamin D$_3$ occurs in the proximal tubule and is inhibited in metabolic acidosis and in the maleic acid model of Fanconi's syndrome. Thus reduced 1,25(OH)$_2$–vitamin D$_3$ level may be a manifestation of intrinsic proximal tubular dysfunction or a consequence of acidosis and may contribute to metabolic bone disease. Muscle weakness caused by hypophosphatemia has been observed.

Diagnosis

The detection of any of the components of Fanconi's syndrome, including generalized aminoaciduria, proximal RTA, renal glycosuria, hypophosphatemia with renal phosphate wasting, and hypouricemia with increased fractional excretion of urate, should prompt a search for other components. In its full-blown form the diagnosis should be obvious, but when only two or three components are present, an incomplete Fanconi's syndrome must be distinguished from a more specific genetic defect, such as X-linked hypophosphatemia with glycosuria, and family studies may be helpful. Once Fanconi's syndrome is recognized, a specific cause must be sought among the possibilities listed in Box 122-2.

Treatment

Treatment of the underlying cause, when possible, may ameliorate the manifestations of Fanconi's syndrome. When the underlying disease fails to respond to therapy or primary Fanconi's syndrome is present, symptomatic therapy focuses on acidosis, hypokalemia, and hypophosphatemic bone disease. Full correction of acidosis, as judged by normalization of serum bicarbonate, is essential to prevent growth retardation in children. Because of bicarbonate wasting, proximal RTA requires alkali supplements far in excess of daily net acid production—up to or more than 2 to 10 mEq/kg per day as sodium bicarbonate or Shohl's solution. The ensuing bicarbonaturia markedly enhances urinary potassium losses, necessitating potassium supplementation, which is given as phosphate, citrate, or bicarbonate. In adults there is little evidence that proximal RTA requires treatment with oral alkali.

Similar to those who have X-linked hypophosphatemia (described previously), patients with Fanconi's syndrome and osteomalacia (or rickets) have both hypophosphatemia and reduced plasma levels of calcitriol. Treatment consists of both oral phosphate and calcitriol with the same precautions as when prescribed to patients with X-linked hypophosphatemia.

The renal dysfunction associated with isofosfamide can be minimized by the administration of mesna (sodium-2-mercaptothanesulfonate), a synthetic sulfhydryl-containing compound that can act in the urine to detoxify these metabolites. However, the protection may not be complete.

NEPHROGENIC DIABETES INSIPIDUS
Etiology (Chapter 296)

The causes of nephrogenic DI are listed in Box 122-3. This chapter focuses on familial nephrogenic diabetes insipidus (FNDI), an X-linked recessive disorder that is fully expressed in males. There is no male-to-male transmission, and mothers and half of the sisters of affected males are obligate heterozygotes, or carriers. However, as many as two thirds of female carriers manifest a more mild form of the disease and may have a concentrating defect; some have symptomatic polyuria and polydipsia. In addition, female carriers show a blunted response to infusions of desmopressin acetate (1-deamino-8-D-arginine vasopressin [DDAVP]) with smaller and briefer increases in plasma levels of factor VIIIc and von Willebrand's factor. This indicates that the genetic defect has variable penetrance in obligate heterozygotes. An interesting aspect of the disorder is that the ancestry of many apparently unrelated cases had been traced to the ship *Hopewell,* which landed in Nova Scotia in 1761. However, recent genetic studies have demonstrated that this apparently homogeneous disorder actually has many variants including multiple mutations in the Aquaporin-2 gene as well as the V2 receptor gene (see later discussion).

Pathophysiology

The pathogenesis of this syndrome is still not entirely clear. Normally vasopressin stimulates adenylate cyclase at the basolateral membrane, and the increased cyclic AMP production enhances water permeability by an incompletely understood mechanism. In patients with FNDI plasma vasopressin levels are appropriate to the serum sodium concentration and osmolality; that is, plasma vasopressin level rises linearly as plasma osmolality increases above a threshold level of approximately 280 mOsm/kg. However, urine osmolality remains low, despite high endogenous levels of vasopressin, and fails to increase in response to administration of either arginine vasopressin or DDAVP, a specific V_2 receptor agonist. (The V_2 receptor mediates the hydroosmotic effect of vasopressin on the renal tubule via generation of cyclic AMP, whereas the V_1 receptor mediates the vasoconstriction effect via phosphatidylinositol and intracellular calcium.) Although it is clear that the cause of the polyuria is tubular resistance to the action of vasopressin, the specific nature of the defect leading to resistance is not known. Urinary cyclic AMP levels have been reported to increase in response to vasopressin in some families, whereas in others they do not, so it is unclear at what step in the sequence of events that leads to increased water permeability the abnormality lies. In patients with familial nephrogenic DI, vascular responses to vasopressin, mediated by the V_1 receptor, are normal, but extrarenal responses to DDAVP, a selective V_2 agonist, are absent. For example, patients with this condition do not show the expected increase in plasma levels of factor VIIIc and von Willebrand's factor that normally follow infusion of DDAVP, suggesting that there is a generalized defect in the V_2 receptor in this condition.

Recently a second, autosomal recessive form of hereditary nephrogenic DI has been described. While the V_2 receptor and vasodilatory and coagulation factor responses to antidiuretic hormone (ADH) are intact, there is a defect in the function of the collecting duct water channels (called aquaporin-2). These channels are normally stored in the region of the cell immediately adjacent to the apical membrane. Under the influence of ADH, they fuse with the apical membrane, thereby allowing water to enter the cell and be reabsorbed down the favorable concentration gradient. Patients with nephrogenic DI appear to have impaired trafficking of the water channels, which do not fuse with the luminal membrane. In fact, urinary excretion of these channel proteins has been described in the normal response to ADH, and excretion of aquaporin-2 is deficient in nephrogenic DI. Measurement of urinary aquaporin-2 may become a standard test for nephrogenic DI.

Clinical and Laboratory Findings

Inability to produce concentrated urine leads to increased urine output, hyperosmolality, and thirst. The ability of the patient to avoid dehydration becomes dependent on his or her perception of thirst and access to water. Polyhydramnios may be present at birth, and marked polyuria and polydipsia may appear shortly afterward. In the infant, whose access to water is limited, severe dehydration with fever and circulatory collapse may ensue. Neurologic abnormalities range from lethargy to coma and reflect central nervous system cell shrinkage produced by the hypertonic state. An increased incidence of mental retardation in these patients presumably is due to repeated episodes of hypertonic dehydration in infancy. The main difficulty of those who survive infancy is the inconvenient urge for frequent drinking and voiding, but an intercurrent illness or event that limits access to water can be life threatening. Laboratory investigation reveals ADH-resistant hyposthenuria in the presence of plasma hypertonicity. The GFR is normal if the patient is not dehydrated, but hyperuricemia is typical even in well-hydrated adults and has been attributed to an increased filtration fraction and enhanced proximal tubular reabsorption. Hydronephrosis, hydroureter, and bladder enlargement may also result from the high urine flow.

Diagnosis

The approach to differentiating the various causes of polyuria is discussed in detail in Chapter 112. The diagnosis of familial nephrogenic DI is usually made in infancy in a child with polyuria and polydipsia who has a family history of the disorder and who fails to respond to exogenous vasopressin administration. This disorder can be differentiated from central DI by absence of response to exogenous vasopressin or by measurement of plasma vasopressin concentrations, which are inappropriately low or absent in central DI.

Other causes of a nephrogenic concentrating defect may be sought from determinations of levels of serum calcium, potassium, and glucose; results of renal function tests; examination of the urinary sediment; and a relevant drug history.

An unusual form of transient ADH resistance may occur during the second half of pregnancy. Pregnancy is associated with release of a vasopressinase from the placenta, leading to rapid degradation of endogenous or exogenous ADH, but not of DDAVP, since this agent is resistant to the vasopressinase.

Treatment

In infants with nephrogenic DI, control of solute intake with breast milk or low-solute formulas limits obligatory urine volume. For instance, if the maximum urinary concentration is 100 mOsm/L, an infant requires 3 L of urine to excrete a 300-mOsm diet but proportionately less if solute intake is reduced. It is also important that the infant's mother ensure a constant high-fluid intake to prevent potentially irreversible neurologic sequelae of dehydration.

BOX 122-3
Causes of nephrogenic diabetes insipidus

Familial (X-linked recessive)
Electrolyte disorders
Hypercalcemia
Hypokalemia

Tubulointerstitial disease
Obstructive nephropathy
Acute tubular necrosis
Sickle cell anemia
Amyloidosis
Fanconi's syndrome
Sjögren's syndrome

Drug-induced
Lithium
Demeclocycline
Amphotericin B
Methoxyflurane
Aminoglycosides
Cisplatin
Rifampin
Foscarnet

✔ WHEN TO REFER

In this heterogeneous group of disorders, a clear set of referral guidelines is difficult to define. Renal glycosuria is a benign disorder that rarely requires more than a diagnosis. The aminoacidurias are disorders that are either benign and represent no more than curiosities or are associated with significant impairments in growth and development. In either case, they are typically in the province of the pediatrician. In patients with vitamin D–resistant rickets or with oncogenic osteomalacia, referral to an endocrinologist is typically required because these patients are extraordinarily challenging in that one must be intimately familiar with the use of phosphate salts and with vitamin D metabolites in order to avoid the major complications of secondary hyperparathyroidism and nephrocalcinosis.

Agents that have been used to reduce the degree of polyuria in patients with nephrogenic DI include thiazide diuretics, amiloride, and prostaglandin synthetase inhibitors. Thiazide diuretics probably work by producing mild extracellular fluid volume contraction and thereby enhance proximal tubular fluid reabsorption. As distal delivery of filtrate is reduced, free-water excretion is limited. Recently the combination of a thiazide diuretic and amiloride has been found to have several advantages over a thiazide diuretic alone. The antidiuretic actions of thiazides and amiloride appear to be additive. The combination obviates the need for potassium supplementation, and long-term side effects are rare. The mechanism of the response to prostaglandin synthesis inhibitors such as indomethacin is unclear, but they probably also act by increasing reabsorption of filtrate at a site proximal to the collecting duct. Although polyuria may not be completely ameliorated by these agents, patient comfort is enhanced.

BIBLIOGRAPHY

Bichet DG, Arthus MF, Lonergan M et al: X-linked nephrogenic diabetes insipidus in North America and the *Hopewell* hypothesis, *J Clin Invest* 92:1262, 1993.

Cai Q, Hodgson SF, Kao PC et al: Brief report: inhibition of renal phosphate transport by a tumor product in a patient with oncogenic osteomalacia, *N Engl J Med* 330:1645, 1994.

Nesbitt T, Coffman TM, Griffiths R, Drezner MK: Cross-transplantation of kidneys in normal and Hyp mice: evidence that the Hyp mouse phenotype is unrelated to an intrinsic renal defect, *J Clin Invest* 89:1453, 1992.

Tenenhouse HS, Werner A, Biber J, Ma S et al: Renal Na(+)-phosphate cotransport in murine X-linked hypophosphatemic rickets: molecular characterization, *J Clin Invest* 93:671, 1994.

CHAPTER

123   Obstructive Uropathy

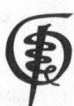

Saulo Klahr

Obstruction of the urinary tract (obstructive uropathy) affects renal function and structure. *Obstructive uropathy* refers to the structural or functional changes in the urinary tract that impair the flow of urine such that proximal pressure must be raised to transmit the usual flow through the point of anatomic or functional "narrowing." *Hydronephrosis* implies dilation of the urinary tract. The term *obstructive nephropathy* is used to describe the renal abnormalities that result from urinary tract obstruction. The degree, duration, and location of the obstruction (Box 123-1) condition the rapidity and extent of functional and pathologic changes in the kidney.

BOX 123-1

Factors that condition the rapidity and extent of renal abnormalities in obstructive uropathy

Degree of obstruction
Partial or incomplete ("low grade")
Total or complete ("high grade")

Duration of obstruction
Acute (hours or days)
Chronic (months or years)

Location of obstruction
Upper urinary tract
Ureteropelvic junction
Ureter
Ureterovesical junction
Lower urinary tract
Bladder
Urethra

INCIDENCE

Obstructive uropathy is a relatively common disorder that occurs at all ages. However, the postmortem incidence of hydronephrosis in children (about 2%), mostly due to congenital anomalies of the urinary tract, is less than that in adults. It was estimated that 166 patients per 100,000 population were hospitalized with a presumptive diagnosis of obstructive uropathy in 1985 in the United States. Obstructive uropathy was the fourth leading diagnosis at discharge (242 patients per 100,000 discharges) among male patients with renal and urologic disorders. In 1985, 387 patient visits per 100,000 population were ascribed to obstructive uropathy in the United States. Obstructive nephropathy accounted for 1.9% of new end-stage renal disease (ESRD) patients in the United States in 1992. The crude sex ratio was 3:1, reflecting the higher susceptibility of men to urinary tract obstruction. End-stage renal disease resulting from obstructive uropathy occurred at a stable, low rate until ages 55 to 59 years, when the incidence increased. The peak incidence occurred at ages 75 to 79 years.

PATHOGENESIS AND PATHOPHYSIOLOGY

Urine formation and flow depend on (1) hydrostatic pressure, which decreases progressively from the kidney to the bladder, and (2) ureteral peristalsis. Obstruction to urine flow anywhere in the urinary tract increases the pressure and volume of urine proximal to the obstruction. Significant obstruction impairs renal function, and if the obstruction is severe enough, the kidney may be destroyed. Renal injury is probably due to elevated ureteral pressure and decreased renal blood flow, causing ischemia, cellular atrophy, and necrosis. Ureteral peristalsis allows for the generation of the high intraluminal pressures that are necessary for the propulsion of a bolus of urine. Contraction of the circular muscular fibers of the ureter above the bolus of urine prevents the pressure from being transmitted to the kidney. With obstruction, this phenomenon, called *coaptation,* is lost, and high intraluminal pressures can be transmitted upward to the kidney. Hence, a rise in ureteral pressure leads to increased intratubular pressure. The rise in intratubular pressure in turn decreases the net hydrostatic filtration pressure. After 24 hours of obstruction intratubular pressures return to normal in animals with unilateral ureteral obstruction but remain elevated in animals with bilateral ureteral obstruction, although values are less than the peak levels observed at 3 to 6 hours after obstruction. Although there is an increase in renal blood flow initially (2 to 3 hours), this is followed by a progressive decrease such that renal blood flow in the obstructed kidney of dogs is only 20% of control values after 8 weeks of obstruction. The initial rise in renal blood flow is due to increased prostaglandin synthesis. The subsequent decrease in blood flow is mediated by increased release of the vasoconstrictors thromboxane A_2 and angiotensin II. After 24 hours of obstruction the decreases in renal blood flow and hydrostatic glomerular capillary pressure are the main mechanisms responsible for the fall in glomerular filtration rate (GFR). Inhibition of prostaglandin synthesis at this time results in further decreases in renal blood flow and GFR, suggesting that vasodilatory eicosanoids antagonize the vasoconstrictive effects of angiotensin II and thromboxane A_2. Partial obstruction of the urinary tract may lead to similar alterations in renal blood flow and GFR, but in addition tubular defects may be prominent. These include a concentrating defect and decreased excretion of potassium and hydrogen ions. The concentrating defect is due in part to the inability to generate a high osmolar gradient in the renal medulla as a consequence of decreased sodium reabsorption in the thick ascending limb of Henle. There is also a diminished osmotic water reabsorption in the collecting duct in response to vasopressin. The acidifying defect and the decreased potassium excretion are due to impaired proton and potassium secretion in the distal nephron, presumably as a consequence of decreased responsiveness of this segment to aldosterone.

CAUSES OF OBSTRUCTIVE UROPATHY

Obstructive lesions can occur throughout the urinary tract from the renal tubules (uric acid nephropathy) to the urethral meatus (phimosis) (Box 123-2). Obstruction may be due to intrinsic lesions of the urinary tract or to extrinsic causes. *Renal calculi* are the most common cause of *intraluminal obstruction* in the young adult male. Approximately 1 of every 1000 hospital admissions in the United States is related to renal stones, which are three times more frequent in males than in females and have a peak incidence in the second and third decades of life. Calcium oxalate stones are the most common and cause intermittent acute urinary obstruction, which is seldom associated with a significant decrease in renal function. Renal calculi most commonly cause obstruction at the calyx, the ureteropelvic or ureterovesical junction, or the pelvic brim, where the ureter is crossed anteriorly by the pelvic blood vessels and broad ligament. Most stones are passed spontaneously. If they are not, surgical removal or disintegration of the stones by mechanical means may be necessary. A less common cause of intraluminal obstruction is a sloughed papilla produced by papillary necrosis, which occurs in entities such as sickle cell trait or disease, analgesic abuse, renal amyloidosis, and acute pyelonephritis, particularly when associated with diabetes mellitus. *Intramural causes of obstruction* are either functional or anatomic. The *functional disorders* causing obstruction include ureterovesical reflux, adynamic ureteral segments (usually at the ureteropelvic or ureterovesical junction), and neurogenic dysfunction of the bladder and sphincters. Neurogenic vesical dysfunction (neurogenic bladder) can be caused by upper neuron damage, which may produce involuntary micturition (spastic bladder dysfunction), or by lower spinal tract injury, giving rise to a flaccid atonic bladder. In both settings a significant residual of urine may develop, resulting in ureterovesical reflux, ureteral dilation, and a significantly increased pressure in the upper urinary tract. Box 123-2 lists some of the entities that cause a neurogenic bladder. Certain drugs, such as tranquilizers (diazepam), anticholinergics, antihistaminics, or alpha-adrenergic stimulators, can cause bladder dysfunction and urinary retention. *Anatomic lesions* of the urinary tract resulting in obstruction are less common. *Ureteral strictures* are uncommon and may be due to retroperitoneal surgery or radiation therapy for cervical carcinoma. Rarely, strictures may develop with analgesic abuse or during treatment of genitourinary tuberculosis. *Urethral strictures* resulting from chronic instrumentation or gonococcal infections are an infrequent cause of obstructive uropathy. *Malignant* and *benign tumors* of the renal pelvis, ureter, and bladder are uncommon causes of obstructive uropathy.

The *extrinsic causes of urinary tract obstruction* are best classified in terms of the system from which the obstruction originates. Most of the extrinsic lesions that produce obstructive uropathy originate in the reproductive system. Ureteral dilation is common in pregnant females. The changes are reversible; ureteral dilation subsides 3 to 4 months after delivery. Pelvic malignancies, particularly carcinoma of the cervix, are a common cause of extrinsic obstruction. In males, prostatic hypertrophy is the most frequent cause of extrinsic obstruction. About 80% of men over 60 years of age have benign

---

BOX 123-2
Causes of obstructive uropathy

I. Intrinsic causes
  A. Intraluminal
    1. Intratubular deposition of crystals (uric acid, sulfas)
    2. Stones
    3. Papillary tissue
    4. Blood clots
  B. Intramural
    1. Functional
      a. Ureter (ureteropelvic or ureterovesical dysfunction)
      b. Bladder (neurogenic): Spinal cord defect or trauma, diabetes, multiple sclerosis, Parkinson's disease, cerebrovascular accidents
      c. Bladder neck dysfunction
    2. Anatomic
      a. Tumors
      b. Infection: granuloma
      c. Strictures
II. Extrinsic causes
  A. Originating in the reproductive system
    1. Prostate: Benign hypertrophy or cancer
    2. Uterus: Pregnancy, tumors, prolapse, endometriosis
    3. Ovary: Abscess, tumor, cysts
  B. Originating in the vascular system
    1. Aneurysms (aorta, iliac vessels)
    2. Aberrant arteries (ureteropelvic junction)
    3. Venous (ovarian veins, retrocaval ureter)
  C. Originating in the gastrointestinal tract: Crohn's disease, pancreatitis, appendicitis, tumors
  D. Originating in the retroperitoneal space
    1. Inflammations
    2. Fibrosis
    3. Tumor, hematomas

---

prostatic hyperplasia and some evidence of bladder dysfunction. Ten percent of these patients require surgery. In one large series 24% of the patients had the initial complaint of complete urinary retention. Carcinoma of the prostate is another important cause of obstructive uropathy. The combination of benign prostatic hypertrophy and carcinoma of the prostate accounts for the greater occurrence of obstructive uropathy in men than in women after the age of 60. Other lesions that may obstruct the ureter originate in the *vascular system,* the *gastrointestinal tract,* or the *retroperitoneal space* (Box 123-2). Diseases of the retroperitoneum may produce chronic obstruction with few clinical manifestations. Metastasis from tumors of the cervix, prostate, bladder, colon, ovary, and uterus account for 70% of the extrinsic causes of obstruction in the retroperitoneum. Retroperitoneal fibrosis is another cause of ureteral obstruction. A growing number of cases of so-called idiopathic retroperitoneal fibrosis, occurring with equal frequency in both sexes, have been described. The fibrosis usually involves the ureter in the middle third, pulling it toward the midline. In some cases administration of drugs such as methysergide or other ergot derivatives may account for the development of retroperitoneal fibrosis.

CLINICAL MANIFESTATIONS AND LABORATORY FINDINGS

Patients with obstructive uropathy may experience acute renal failure, with chronic and slowly progressive symptoms, or with virtually no symptoms or signs. The clinical presentation depends on the duration, severity, and location of the obstruction (Box 123-1) and on the presence of complications. Although the symptoms and signs of obstructive uropathy are often nonspecific, some clinical features are sufficiently distinctive, when present, to suggest the diagnosis of obstruction (Box 123-3).

Flank pain is a common complaint of patients with obstructive uropathy. It is secondary to stretching of the collecting system or renal capsule. Its severity correlates with the rate of distention rather

---

BOX 123-3
Findings that suggest the presence
of obstructive uropathy

Flank pain or an enlarged tender kidney
Changes in urine output (anuria, polyuria)
"Bladder symptoms" (decreased stream, hesitancy, incontinence)
Repeated urinary tract infections or infections refractory to "appropriate" treatment
Impaired renal function (elevated blood urea nitrogen or serum creatinine level)
Gross hematuria
Hypertension
Hyperchloremic metabolic acidosis with hyperkalemia

BOX 123-4
Procedures used to diagnose obstructive uropathy

Plain abdominal films (KUB)
Excretory or intravenous pyelography
Ultrasonography
Computed tomography
Antegrade or retrograde pyelography
Pressure flow studies (Whitaker test)

KUB, Kidneys, ureter, bladder.

than the degree of dilation. Pain is more common in acute than in chronic obstruction. Acute ureteral obstruction is characterized by a steady crescendo of flank pain radiating to the groin, testicles, or labia ("classic renal colic"). The acute attack may last less than half an hour or as long as 24 hours. Pain radiating into the flank during micturition is said to be pathognomonic of ureterovesical reflux. On physical examination an *enlarged tender kidney* may be noted. Long-standing obstructive uropathy may increase renal size with readily palpable kidneys. Such patients may have increased abdominal girth or a flank mass. Hydronephrosis is the most common cause of palpable *abdominal mass* in children. *Anuria* occurs with complete bilateral obstruction or with unilateral obstruction in a patient with a solitary kidney. However, with partial obstruction, urine output may be normal or increased (polyuria). A pattern of oligoanuria alternating with polyuria or the presence of anuria should strongly suggest obstructive uropathy. Obstructing lesions of the bladder neck may cause *difficulties in micturition* such as decrease in the force and/or caliber of the urinary stream, intermittency, postvoid dribbling, hesitancy, and nocturia. Urgency, frequency, and urinary incontinence (overflow incontinence) may result from an inability to empty the bladder completely. Infection is a frequent complication in lower urinary tract obstruction. Repeated infections without apparent cause should raise the suspicion of obstruction. Moreover, as long as the obstruction persists, eradication of the infection is exceedingly difficult. Therefore a history of repeated urinary tract infections or persistent infection refractory to antibiotic therapy requires a detailed investigation to exclude obstructive uropathy. A number of patients who have *renal insufficiency* (elevated blood urea nitrogen [BUN] and/or serum creatinine level) may have long-standing, unrecognized obstructive uropathy. Obstructive uropathy may occur in patients with underlying chronic renal disease of another cause and may become evident by a rapid change in the rate of progression of renal insufficiency. In other patients, however, obstructive uropathy is the sole cause of end-stage renal failure. Occasionally, in patients with retroperitoneal fibrosis, in whom the onset of obstruction is slow and progressive, far-advanced renal failure may be an initial presenting complaint. Urinary tract obstruction should be considered in uremic patients with no previous history of renal disease and a relatively benign urine sediment. *Gross hematuria* may be associated with obstructive uropathy, particularly when the obstruction is due to calculi. Acute or chronic hydronephrosis, either unilateral or bilateral, may be accompanied by a significant elevation in blood pressure. The hypertension could be coincidental or could be due to impaired sodium excretion with expansion of extracellular fluid volume or abnormal release of renin (renin-dependent hypertension). Obstruction may impair the ability of the kidney to excrete acid and potassium, resulting in the development of *hyperchloremic/hyperkalemic metabolic acidosis.* Obstructive uropathy should be considered in elderly individuals without diabetes who have hyperkalemic/hyperchloremic metabolic acidosis.

DIAGNOSIS

The diagnostic approach to a patient with obstructive uropathy depends on the clinical setting and presenting symptoms. The spectrum of the disease encompasses patients who have acute onset of pain to those with acute renal failure and anuria. Thus the approach and the urgency with which the diagnosis must be made are highly variable. When obstructive uropathy is suspected, it is important to inquire about a past history of similar symptoms, presence of urinary tract infection, symptoms of lower urinary tract obstruction, recent surgery, and ingestion of drugs. In hospitalized patients, it is important to characterize the pattern of urine output to determine whether it has changed abruptly, gradually declined, or fluctuates. Physical examination with emphasis on abdominal masses is important. Urinary outlet obstruction should be suspected in elderly patients with an enlarged prostate on palpation. Laboratory procedures provide little help in the diagnosis of urinary tract obstruction. The urine sediment may be normal. The presence of hematuria suggests that the obstructing lesion is a calculus, a sloughed papilla, or a tumor. The presence of bacteriuria, of course, heightens the suspicion of obstructive uropathy. The finding of uric acid crystals in the sediment suggests the diagnosis of acute uric acid nephropathy (Chapter 124). Once this information has been obtained, the diagnostic evaluation will vary depending on the symptom complex and the results obtained during the preliminary assessment of the patient.

In patients who have pain but no decrease in GFR, the next step is to determine the presence of a renal calculus. This determination can be made by obtaining plain films of the abdomen without injection of contrast media (the kidney, ureter, bladder [KUB] film (Box 123-4). If a calculus is found or if the clinical evidence suggests the passage of a stone, an intravenous pyelogram (IVP) should be performed next. This study helps to determine the degree of obstruction caused by the stone and ascertains whether there is a radiolucent stone. Once a diagnosis of an obstructing calculus has been made, radiologic techniques are essential in the follow-up care. A notable exception to the approach described applies to the pregnant patient with obstructive uropathy. In such a patient radiographic evaluation should be performed only when other diagnostic procedures such as ultrasound or renographic techniques have failed. When renal function is impaired and there is no apparent reason for the decline or when renal insufficiency exists for an apparent reason but abruptly declines, the diagnosis of ureteral obstruction should be considered. Diagnostic ultrasound is the preferred procedure to determine the presence of dilated calices or renal pelvis. Because this procedure is not invasive and is not affected by renal function, it is particularly useful to exclude hydronephrosis in patients with acute or chronic renal failure. Ultrasonography is extremely sensitive in the diagnosis of hydronephrosis, with a reported accuracy greater than 90%. Infrequently, ultrasonography may fail to recognize obstruction in certain conditions. Retroperitoneal fibrosis, for example, may cause significant obstruction with only minimal dilation. The major drawback of ultrasonography is its extreme sensitivity, resulting in a number of false-positive results. Computed tomography (CT) may be useful as a subsequent study to determine the cause of previously diagnosed obstructive uropathy. This procedure can provide detailed anatomic information but should not be used as an initial procedure because of its high cost, lack of widespread availability, and relatively large radiation dose. Other procedures useful in determining the site of the obstruction include antegrade or retrograde pyelography. Occasionally, pressure flow studies (Whitaker test) may be required to diagnose upper urinary tract obstruction. The test measures pressure differences between the pelvis and the bladder during the infusion at a known rate of fluid into the renal pelvis.

TREATMENT AND MANAGEMENT OF URINARY TRACT OBSTRUCTION

Once the diagnosis of urinary tract obstruction is established, a decision should be made as to whether to undertake surgical or instrumental procedures. High-grade or total bilateral obstruction requires intervention as soon as possible. In these patients, the site of obstruction frequently determines the approach. If clinical conditions permit, instrumentation or surgery should be carried out the same day. In some patients dialysis may be necessary before performing any procedure designed to overcome or bypass the obstruction. In some patients with partial unilateral obstruction, especially those with calculi, immediate intervention is not necessary, and attention should be given to the relief of pain, evaluation of renal function, follow-up of urine cultures to detect the presence of urinary infection, and treatment of such infections. Close follow-up observation using intravenous pyelograms may allow evaluation of the progression and location of stones. If infection is present together with obstruction, infections should be treated vigorously, and efforts to correct the obstruction should be made. Prompt relief of partial obstruction is indicated when (1) there are repeated episodes of urinary tract infection, (2) the patient has significant symptoms (flank pain, dysuria, voiding dysfunction), (3) there is urinary retention, and (4) there is evidence of recurrent or progressive renal damage. Patients with lower urinary tract obstruction (urethral and bladder neck obstruction) require surgery if they are ambulatory and have recurrent infections. Obstruction secondary to benign prostatic hyperplasia is not always progressive. Thus a patient with minimal symptoms, no infection, and a normal upper urinary tract may be observed periodically until he or she and the physician agree that surgery is desirable.

Proscar (Merck, Sharp & Dohme), an inhibitor of the 5-alpha-reductase (the enzyme responsible for the conversion of testosterone to dihydrotestosterone) is now available for the treatment of benign prostatic hyperplasia. In clinical trials this drug was shown to ameliorate the symptoms of "prostatism" in about 30% of patients with benign prostatic hyperplasia.

POSTOBSTRUCTIVE DIURESIS

A profound and sometimes prolonged diuresis may follow the relief of obstruction of both kidneys or of a solitary kidney. This diuresis is characterized by marked losses of water, sodium, and other solutes. The mechanisms underlying this syndrome, usually referred to as *postobstructive diuresis,* are not completely clear. Many factors may account for this phenomenon (Box 123-5). One is the volume status of the patient before the relief of obstruction. Individuals who have received large amounts of intravenous or oral fluids before the release of obstruction are often volume expanded. Thus the marked polyuria seen after relief of obstruction may represent a physiologic response to an expanded extracellular fluid volume. Another factor is the accumulation during the period of obstruction of substances such as urea, which are capable of causing an osmotic diuresis. Finally, the inappropriate natriuresis and diuresis observed after release of obstruction may be due in part to increased levels of circulating atrial peptide. This hormone may accumulate during the period of anuria and inhibit sodium and water reabsorption by the renal tubule after relief of the obstruction.

In summary, postobstructive diuresis may be due to the excretion of retained water and electrolytes, to the osmotic effect of retained urea, to the natriuretic effect of atrial peptide, or to a defect in the tubular reabsorption of sodium and water that occasionally results from obstructive uropathy and becomes apparent only after relief of the obstruction.

The management of postobstructive diuresis should include care-

---

BOX 123-5
Potential factors responsible for postobstructive diuresis

Physiologic

Excretion of excess salt and water retained during the period of obstruction

Excessive administration of salt and water after relief of obstruction

Osmotic diuresis resulting from urea retained during the period of obstruction

Pathologic

Excessive urine losses of salt and water unrelated to the volume status of the patient caused by:

  Intrinsic defect in the tubular reabsorption of sodium

  Increased circulating levels of atrial peptide

  Decreased hydrosmotic response of the distal nephron to antidiuretic hormone

---

✔ WHEN TO REFER

Calculi are the most common cause of ureteral obstruction. Renal pelvic or ureteral stones greater than 7 mm in diameter usually do not pass spontaneously. These stones should be surgically treated. Renal and upper ureteral stones are often treated by extracorporeal shock wave lithotripsy (ESWL). Patients with urinary tract stones greater than 7 mm in diameter should be referred to a urologist or a lithotripsy center. It should be remembered that renal stones greater than 2 to 5 cm in diameter require multiple treatments with ESWL. Patients who come to medical attention with anuria and acute renal failure as a consequence of bilateral ureteral obstruction or, in patients with a single kidney, obstruction of the ureter may need to be referred to a nephrologist for management of the acute renal failure. Such patients may require hemodialysis for severe azotemia and hyperkalemia before any surgical intervention. The use of nephrostomy for treatment of urinary tract obstruction may be considered. The technique involves the insertion of a tube into the kidney to provide drainage. Referral to a urologist or an interventional radiologist will then be required.

---

ful and adequate fluid replacement with frequent determination of body weight and plasma and urine electrolytes. These latter measurements provide a rational basis for the amount and composition of fluid to be administered. Urinary losses of fluid and electrolytes should be replaced only to the extent necessary to prevent hypovolemia, hypotension, hypokalemia, hypomagnesemia, and hyponatremia, or hypernatremia.

BIBLIOGRAPHY

Gillenwater JY: The pathophysiology of urinary tract obstruction. In Walsh PC, Retik AB, Stamey TA, Vaughan ED Jr, editors: *Campbell's urology,* ed 6, Philadelphia, 1992, WB Saunders.

Klahr S: Obstructive nephropathy. In Massry S, Glassock R, editors: *Textbook of nephrology,* ed 3, Orlando, 1995, Williams & Wilkins.

Klahr S: Pathophysiology of obstructive uropathy. In Coe F, Favus M, Parks J, Preminger G, editors: *Kidney stones: medical and surgical management,* New York, 1996, Lippincott-Raven.

Klahr S: Obstructive nephropathy: pathophysiology and management. In Schrier RW: *Renal and electrolyte disorders,* ed 5, Boston, Little, Brown (in press).

Klahr S, Ishidoya S, Morrissey J: Role of angiotensin II in the tubulointerstitial fibrosis of obstructive nephropathy, *Am J Kidney Dis* 26:141-146, 1995.

Resnick MI, Kursh ED: Extrinsic obstruction of the ureter. In Walsh PC, Retik AB, Stamey TA, Vaughan ED Jr, editors: *Campbell's urology,* ed 6, Philadelphia, 1992, WB Saunders.

124 Tubulointerstitial Renal Diseases

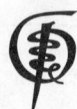

Shreeram Aradhye, Shelley Albert, and Eric G. Neilson

Tubulointerstitial damage is a prominent feature of all diseases leading to end-stage renal failure. Furthermore, it has been well documented that changes in glomerular filtration rate (GFR) correlate more strongly with the pathologic conditions of the tubulointerstitium than with glomerular morphologic features. This seeming curiosity is the combined result of interstitial fibrosis, destruction of peritubular capillaries, and reduced performance of the tubular nephron leading to decreased distal solute reabsorption and reduction of filtration via tubuloglomerular feedback. Although this chapter focuses on primary tubulointerstitial diseases, the aforementioned correlation should be borne in mind when assessing patients with other progressive glomerular or vascular diseases.

Primary tubulointerstitial diseases account for approximately 15% of lesions leading to acute renal failure and 25% of those leading to chronic renal failure. These disorders can be subdivided into acute and chronic forms, each with distinct origins, pathologic features, and clinical course. Acute interstitial nephritis is usually a reversible disease, but chronic tubulointerstitial nephritis often goes undetected and tends to lead to progressive renal failure.

In assessing a patient with suspected tubulointerstitial disease it is important to search for environmental and drug exposures and to uncover evidence of systemic infection or concurrent disease. Eosinophilia is seen in 80% and the classic triad of fever, rash, and eosinophilia in 30% of patients with drug-induced acute interstitial nephritis. However, the absence of these symptoms does not exclude a diagnosis of interstitial nephritis, particularly that caused by diuretics or nonsteroidal antiinflammatory drugs. The urinalysis of acute interstitial nephritis reveals mild to moderate proteinuria (usually less than 1 g/24 h), gross or microscopic hematuria, white blood cells, tubular cells and occasionally white blood cell casts. Eosinophiluria has been suggested as a marker of the hypersensitivity type of interstitial nephritis. A recent study confirmed the superiority of Hansel's stain over Wright's stain in examining the urine for eosinophils and noted that a finding of greater than 1% eosinophils in the urine yielded a sensitivity of 63% and specificity of 93% for acute interstitial nephritis. Renal ultrasound reveals normal-sized or enlarged kidneys with increased cortical echogenicity, and gallium scanning may show bilateral increased uptake, although this finding is nonspecific. In the absence of a clear-cut clinical picture, renal biopsy is often necessary to direct therapy.

In chronic tubulointerstitial nephritis the preceding findings are absent. The urinalysis is typically bland, with mild proteinuria, broad granular casts, and few cells. Chronic tubulointerstitial disease should be suspected when there is evidence of tubular dysfunction out of proportion to the decrement in GFR. This is often absent in the acute syndrome because of the rapid decline in renal function. Although much overlap exists, a specific cause of tubulointerstitial nephritis may be suggested by dysfunction of a specific segment of the tubule. The heavy metals and paraproteins often preferentially damage the proximal tubule. This becomes evident as a proximal renal tubular acidosis, which may be seen in association with one or more components of Fanconi's APOS syndrome (glycosuria in the absence of hyperglycemia, phosphaturia, amino aciduria, uricosuria, and ketonuria). Distal nephron defects include acidification disorders (due to impaired ammoniagenesis, hydrogen ion [H^+] adenosine triphosphatase [ATPase] impairment or H^+ back-leak), hyperkalemia related to aldosterone unresponsiveness, and concentrating defects and can be seen in virtually any of the causes of chronic tubulointerstitial nephritis. The nonanion gap metabolic acidosis from proximal renal tubular acidosis (RTA) can be distinguished from a distal acidification defect by the administration of a bicarbonate load that raises the urine pH above 7. In proximal RTA this will be accompanied by a low serum bicarbonate level and a high (>70 mm Hg) urine partial pressure of car-

bon dioxide (pCO_2) because of preservation of distal hydrogen ion secretion, which drives the reaction $H^+ + HCO_3^- \rightarrow CO_2 + H_2O$ in the distal lumen. In distal RTA the serum bicarbonate level normalizes and the alkaline urine pCO_2 depends on distal H^+ secretion. Volume depletion that is due to impaired distal sodium reabsorption (salt-wasting nephropathy) is unusual and is generally seen only in medullary cystic disease or obstructive nephropathy. Medullary lesions result in impaired concentrating ability, which is evident on clinical examination as polyuria and nocturia, and are commonly seen in the setting of analgesic nephropathy or sickle cell disease. Imaging studies that may be helpful in establishing a diagnosis include renal ultrasound, which may reveal hydronephrosis in obstruction, and intravenous pyelography, which can show abnormalities in the settings of reflux nephropathy, papillary necrosis, nephrocalcinosis, and renal tuberculosis. Serum and urine immunoelectrophoresis should be obtained in the older patient to rule out plasma cell dyscrasia.

PATHOLOGY

The hallmark of acute interstitial nephritis is the infiltration of inflammatory cells into the interstitial compartment with sparing of glomeruli. The infiltrating cells are mainly T cells and monocytes, but plasma cells and eosinophils may be seen. The tubules, rather than lying in close apposition, appear to be pushed away from each other as a result of the infiltrate and the accompanying interstitial edema. In severe cases the tubular basement membrane may be disrupted. Staining of the tubular basement membrane for immunoglobulin G or M (IgG or IgM) or complement may occasionally be seen by immunofluorescence; both linear and granular patterns have been reported.

In the chronic lesion the cellular infiltrate is largely replaced by interstitial fibrosis, which accounts for the irregular and contracted gross appearance of the kidney. The tubular epithelial cells are atrophied, and the tubular lumina are dilated. It should be noted that "chronic" is a relative term, since fibrotic changes can be seen within 7 to 10 days of initiation of an inflammatory process. Chronic vascular and glomerular changes, consisting of nephrosclerosis and glomerulosclerosis, are often present at later stages of the disease, so pathologic determination of the primary cause may be impossible.

Granulomatous interstitial nephritis constitutes a third pathologic category. In acute granulomatous interstitial nephritis, the granulomas are sparse and nonnecrotic, giant cells are rare, and an accompanying interstitial infiltrate is common. Chronic granulomatous lesions contain more giant cells, and if attributable to tuberculosis, may be necrotic. Drugs are a common cause of this lesion in the acute setting, and most of the drugs associated with acute interstitial nephritis have been reported to cause granuloma formation. Sarcoidosis or tuberculosis should be considered when granulomas are seen in chronic disease. When renal granulomas are seen in Wegener's granulomatosis, they are almost always accompanied by glomerular and vascular disease.

PATHOGENESIS

It is likely that the immune system plays a role in the pathogenesis of a variety of tubulointerstitial diseases, including some that are not traditionally thought of as being immunologic. Tubulointerstitial structures may become the target of immune attack by a number of possible mechanisms. Most of these mechanisms are recognized from work in experimental animals and assumed to hold true in human disease. Foreign proteins may bind to renal structures and act as a hapten initiating an antibody response against the "carrier," as noted in methicillin-induced acute interstitial nephritis with the development of anti–tubular basement membrane antibodies. Drugs or infectious agents that share immunoreactive epitopes with interstitial structures may induce production of cross-reactive antibodies or T cells, which can then attack those structures. Toxins may alter tubulointerstitial proteins or reveal new ones, leading to their recognition as foreign. Self proteins may become visible to the immune system through increased expression of class II major histocompatibility complex proteins on tubular cells, which are required for antigen recognition by CD4$^+$ T helper cells. Such increased expression has been seen in a variety of human tubulointerstitial nephritides, including some metabolic origins, and, indeed, tubular cells in vitro are capable of presenting antigen to T helper cells when class II expression is increased. The response against these renal antigens may be modulated by such systems as regulatory T-cell populations or idiotypic networks (antibodies and T cells directed against the antigen-binding site of autoantibodies), and only when these protective mechanisms are overcome or fooled does the autoimmune response ensue.

The effector limb of the nephritogenic immune response consists of several elements that may function individually or in combination in different human diseases. Humoral mediators, such as antibodies directed against continuous tubular basement membrane components or deposited in the tubulointerstitium as immune complexes, have been identified in isolated instances of human disease, including renal transplant rejection, lupus nephritis, and idiopathic tubulointerstitial nephritis. Cell-mediated immunity appears to predominate in most forms of tubulointerstitial nephritis. When eosinophils are attracted to the tubulointerstitium by chemotactic factors, their activation may lead to the release of various cytotoxic substances, including major basic protein, which has been detected in renal biopsy specimens in acute tubulointerstitial nephritis. T cells may damage tubules through direct cytotoxicity by release of cytolytic agents called perforins or through delayed hypersensitivity in which lymphokines are released to recruit monocytes and other inflammatory cells.

Numerous insults to the tubulointerstitium are capable of initiating the fibrogenic process. These include inflammatory events located primarily in either the tubulointerstitial or glomerular compartments, obstructing lesions, some drugs, and diabetes mellitus. The two most abundant resident cell types of the tubulointerstitium, the interstitial fibroblasts and, to a lesser extent, the tubular epithelial cells, are both capable of secreting types I and III collagen, the major components of the interstitial matrix. A complex array of mediators can modulate matrix deposition at a number of levels, including fibroblast proliferation and motility, matrix synthesis, and production of collagenases and other proteases. Transforming growth factor–β, for example, is released by activated platelets and macrophages and some T-cell subsets, a well as by somatic renal cells. Its actions include stimulation of transcription of type I collagen and inhibition of collagenase synthesis. T cells activated in experimental interstitial nephritis can also induce fibroblast proliferation, type I collagen secretion, and inhibition of type IV collagen secretion with accompanying tubular atrophy. Platelet-derived growth factor released by renal and inflammatory cells causes fibroblasts to proliferate. Other cytokines involved in regulating the fibrogenic response include interleukin-1, tumor necrosis factor (TNF), and γ-interferon. Since it now appears that fibroblasts derive from epithelium, tubular atrophy and local fibrogenesis are closely linked. The resulting scar is probably irreversible.

ACUTE INTERSTITIAL NEPHRITIS

Acute interstitial nephritis should be considered in the work-up of any patient with acute renal failure (Box 124-1). Although a drug is commonly the offending agent, systemic infections must be considered, particularly in patients with a primarily nonrenal presentation and incidental urinary abnormalities. The latter diagnosis is more likely in the pediatric age-group.

Drugs

Although the list of drugs known to cause acute interstitial nephritis keeps growing, only a small number are common offenders. Drugs frequently implicated include β-lactam antibiotics such as cephalosporins, rifampin (generally in association with tuberculosis), sulfonamides, thiazides, furosemide, and cimetidine. The best-studied cases were described with methicillin, but this drug is no longer in clinical use. It should be noted that acute interstitial nephritis develops in only a minority of patients receiving the preceding drugs. Renal failure develops within days to weeks following initiation of therapy with an average delay of about 2 weeks. Renal dysfunction progresses at a variable rate, the course being more rapid and severe with rifampin and more indolent with diuretics. The extrarenal manifestations of hypersensitivity in this disease have been discussed earlier.

Acute interstitial nephritis attributable to the nonsteroidal antiinflammatory drugs has several distinct features, including an associa-

---

BOX 124-1
Acute interstitial nephritis

Drugs
Antibiotics
  β-Lactams (especially ampicillin, penicillin)
  Rifampin
  Sulfonamides
  Vancomycin
  Ciprofloxacin
  Cotrimoxazole
  Erythromycin
  Tetracycline
Nonsteroidal antiinflammatory drugs
Diuretics
  Thiazides
  Furosemide
  Triamterene
  Ethacrynic acid
Miscellaneous
  Cimetidine
  Phenindione
  Phenytoin
  Allopurinol
  Interferon

Infection
Bacteria
  Legionella sp.
  Brucella sp.
  Diphtheria
  Streptococcus sp.
Viruses
  Epstein-Barr virus
  Cytomegalovirus
  Hantavirus sp.
Other
  Mycoplasma
  Rocky Mountain spotted fever
  Toxoplasma

Idiopathic
Anti–tubular basement membrane disease
Tubulointerstitial nephritis–uveitis syndrome
Other

---

tion with nephrotic syndrome with changes of minimal change disease on pathologic examination, the absence of the typical manifestations of hypersensitivity, and a prolonged delay in onset averaging 5.4 months with a range of 2 weeks to 18 months. Typical allergic interstitial nephritis, perhaps accompanied by papillary necrosis, is only occasionally seen with these agents.

Given the rapidity with which irreversible pathologic changes develop in the tubulointerstitium, prompt therapy is vital. In many patients withdrawal of the offending agent results in improvement in renal function within several days. In the absence of a prompt response, early institution of chemotherapy for patients with biopsy-proven acute interstitial nephritis has been recommended. This consists, first, of a trial of corticosteroids in a dose equivalent to 1 mg/kg per day of prednisone. If improvement in renal function begins within 1 to 2 weeks of initiation of treatment, corticosteroids can be discontinued after 4 to 6 weeks. If no improvement is seen within the first 2 weeks, the addition of a second agent such as cyclophosphamide (2 mg/kg per day) may be considered and, if successful, should be continued for 1 year with appropriate monitoring of the white blood cell count. Both agents should be discontinued if no improvement in renal function is seen after 6 weeks of combined therapy. Although this approach has not been subjected to a randomized prospective trial, retrospective studies have attested to the beneficial effects of corticosteroids and anecdotal reports have supported the use of cytotoxic therapy in some patients. Up to one third of patients with drug-induced acute interstitial nephritis (and more in the case of rifampin) require dialytic therapy before resolution of the disease. Attention must also be paid to the effects of tubular dysfunction during the recovery period.

Infection

Although bacteria may invade the renal interstitium directly, renal dysfunction is a rare sequela of *uncomplicated* pyelonephritis in adults. However, a number of systemic infections can be complicated by acute interstitial nephritis (Box 124-1). Streptococci and diphtheria are the most frequent offenders in the pediatric population. Adults with the pulmonary-renal syndrome attributable to *Legionella* pneumonia and acute interstitial nephritis have been reported. Although the human immunodeficiency virus has not been shown to directly cause an isolated interstitial nephritis, tubulointerstitial lesions from various causes are common in infected patients. These include opportunistic infections (with cytomegalovirus, *Cryptococcus,* or *Histoplasma*), nephrocalcinosis, and acute interstitial nephritis resulting from the sulfa derivatives commonly used. Similarly, renal allograft recipients may be susceptible to such interstitial nephritis as a result of Epstein-Barr virus and cytomegalovirus. The various forms of *Hantavirus* infection that become evident as severe hemorrhagic fever in the Far East and self-limited nephropathia epidemica in northern Europe have also received recent attention because of epidemics in North America. Renal failure in infection-related acute interstitial nephritis generally resolves with treatment of the underlying infection, and corticosteroid therapy is usually not needed.

Idiopathic Causes

In a minority of patients with acute interstitial nephritis no etiologic factor can be identified. In a few of these, circulating anti–tubular basement membrane antibodies have been isolated. Another variety includes the combination of tubulointerstitial nephritis and uveitis (the so-called TINU syndrome), which is usually seen in adolescent females whose biopsies show no granulomas and who have no systemic evidence of sarcoidosis. These patients generally receive treatment with a course of corticosteroids, and many have full recovery of renal function over several weeks.

CHRONIC TUBULOINTERSTITIAL NEPHROPATHY

The various causes of chronic tubulointerstitial disease are listed in Box 124-2. The demographic characteristics may point toward specific etiologic factors such as reflux nephropathy in the young patient, sickle cell disease in the black patient, analgesic nephropathy in the middle-aged woman, and plasma cell dyscrasia in the elderly patient. Obstructive nephropathy is a common diagnosis in any age-group, and occupational exposures must be explored in all patients.

Toxic and Metabolic Disorders

Analgesics. Chronic analgesic ingestion has been recognized as a cause of end-stage renal failure for nearly 40 years. Although the origins and pathogenesis of this complex disease are not fully understood, important epidemiologic observations have been recorded. The prevalence of analgesic nephropathy varies widely and seems to be largely dependent on the composition and frequency of the use of nonprescription analgesics. In Europe in 1986, for instance, the prevalence of analgesic nephropathy among patients with end-stage renal failure varied from 18% in Switzerland to a fraction of 1% in eastern Europe. In the United States the prevalence varies from 5% to 20% of cases of chronic renal failure. There appears to be an inverse relationship between the reported prevalence of analgesic nephropathy and that of nephropathy of unknown origin, suggesting an underestimation of the extent of this problem.

Historically, phenacetin was believed to be a major culprit causing analgesic nephropathy, particularly when ingested in combination with other analgesics. Legislated removal of phenacetin from the market has led to a significant decline in analgesic nephropathy in some European countries. Although it is clear that combination analgesics are nephrotoxic, there has been some controversy over the nephrotoxic potential of monotherapy with analgesics, particularly acetamin-

---

BOX 124-2

Causes of chronic tubulointerstitial nephropathy

Toxic or metabolic disorders
Analgesics
Heavy metals
Other toxins
Uric acid
Oxalic acid
Hypercalcemia
Hypokalemia

Immunologic conditions
Sjögren's syndrome
Transplant rejection
Lupus nephritis

Hematopoietic diseases
Sickle cell disease
Plasma cell dyscrasias
Infiltration

Mechanical disorders
Reflux
Chronic obstruction

Vascular diseases
Radiation
Arteriolar nephrosclerosis

Hereditary diseases
Medullary cystic disease, familial juvenile nephronophthisis
Laurence-Moon-Biedl syndrome
Oculocerebrorenal syndrome

Miscellaneous conditions
Granulomatous nephritis
Balkan endemic nephropathy
Chinese herb nephropathy

---

ophen—a metabolite of phenacetin. At present there is no good evidence that monotherapy with acetaminophen is nephrotoxic.

Eighty percent of patients with analgesic nephropathy are women who consume analgesics for various chronic pain syndromes and often exhibit other addictive behaviors. Renal involvement initially becomes evident as a defect in urinary concentrating ability, which may be accompanied or followed by acidification defects or salt wasting. Azotemia is a late feature and indicates that papillary necrosis, the hallmark of the disease, has already occurred. Radiologic abnormalities include visualization of sloughed papillae (the "ring-shadow" sign) on intravenous pyelography and papillary calcifications detected by computed tomography scanning. Analgesic abuse is also a risk factor for transitional cell carcinoma of the urinary tract, a tumor with a poor prognosis that may be seen more frequently in the coming years as patients with analgesic nephropathy are maintained on dialysis.

Analgesic nephropathy attributable to combination compounds most likely depends on the concentration of phenacetin metabolites in the inner medulla. These moieties are metabolized by the prostaglandin hydroperoxidase pathway to reactive intermediates that bind covalently to interstitial cell macromolecules leading to necrosis. Salicylates and nonsteroidal antiinflammatory drugs may contribute to this process both by reducing glutathione levels (which can prevent covalent binding) and by reducing medullary blood flow through prostaglandin inhibition. The process progresses from the inner medulla to eventually involve the tubulointerstitium of the cortex as well.

Treatment of this disease involves withdrawal of the analgesic responsible, which can result in stabilization or improvement in renal function. The physician must be alert, however, to the continued surreptitious use of these agents. Avoidance of volume depletion may also be protective.

Heavy Metals. Lead can cause both acute, reversible nephrotoxicity and a chronic, irreversible lesion. The acute form, occurring most frequently in children ingesting lead-based paint, results in a Fanconi-like syndrome and is characterized morphologically by the presence of eosinophillic intranuclear inclusion bodies in proximal tubular cells. Chronic, heavy lead exposure is often seen in the setting of occupational exposure (e.g., battery or smelter workers). In the southeastern United States chronic lead exposure may also be seen in "moonshine" whiskey drinkers who process liquor in automobile radiators. In chronic lead nephropathy proximal tubular defects are less prominent, and the picture is one of progressive azotemia, hypertension, and concentrating defects. Saturnine gout, rare in other renal diseases, is common in lead nephropathy. Chronic tubulointerstitial nephritis resulting from lead exposure can be diagnosed by a chelation test revealing urinary excretion of more than 600 μg of lead in the 24 hours following intravenous infusion of 1 g of ethylenediamene tetraacid acid (EDTA). Treatment in the patient without evidence of marked interstitial fibrosis consists of ongoing chelation therapy, although great care must be used in the presence of early renal failure.

Cadmium exposure, usually occupational (although dietary exposure has been documented in some areas of Japan and Belgium), also leads to chronic tubulointerstitial nephritis. This is evident on clinical examination as proximal tubular dysfunction and hypercalciuria with nephrolithiasis. Renal failure is uncommon. No specific therapy other than avoiding exposure is available.

Other Toxins. Several other agents have been associated with chronic interstitial disease. The nitrosourea compounds carmustine and methyl-N-(2-chloroethyl)-N'-cyclohexyl-N-nitrosourea (CCNU) have been demonstrated to cause interstitial fibrosis in cumulative doses of greater than 2000 mg/m². *cis*-Platinum produces interstitial fibrosis and renal magnesium wasting that can be partially prevented by such maneuvers as continuous infusion, vigorous hydration and diuresis, and hypertonic chloride content of the vehicle. Cyclosporine is being used as an immunosuppressive agent in a number of autoimmune diseases, in addition to organ transplantation. Cyclosporine nephrotoxicity may become evident as both short-term reversible injury and chronic, irreversible, and progressive damage characterized by glomerular and vascular abnormalities associated with "stripe" fibrosis of the tubulointerstitium.

Uric Acid. Uric acid can affect the kidney in three ways. Acute urate nephropathy occurs most commonly in the setting of chemotherapy-induced cell lysis in a patient with a large tumor burden (lymphoma, leukemia) but has also been seen during spontaneous lysis of a solid tumor. The ensuing acute oliguric renal failure (associated with a serum uric acid greater than 20 mg/dl and a spot-urine uric acid–to–creatinine ratio greater than 1) results from uric acid crystal deposition in the collecting system. Prophylaxis with allopurinol and hydration in patients receiving chemotherapy may prevent urate nephropathy, but once it is established, dialysis is needed to reduce the uric acid load. Chronic urate nephropathy, previously seen with tophaceous gout, is now an uncommon clinical entity. Medullary urate crystal deposition is a nonspecific finding at autopsy, and any renal dysfunction found in patients with hyperuricemia can be attributed to concurrent disease, usually hypertension or cardiac disease. Uric acid nephrolithiasis, which can occur in the absence of hyperuricemia, produces renal dysfunction through obstructive mechanisms.

Oxalic Acid. Oxalic acid is the metabolic end-product of both endogenous glyoxalic acid and a number of exogenous toxins, so hyperoxaluria leading to oxalate nephropathy occurs in several settings. Primary hyperoxaluria attributable to inherited enzyme deficiencies can cause recurrent calcium oxalate stones, progressive interstitial fibrosis leading to end-stage renal failure, and extrarenal oxalate deposition. Prognosis in patients who are resistant to pyridoxine (a cofactor for the deficient enzyme) is poor, but combined hepatorenal transplant has been successfully used recently as an enzyme replacement strategy. Ethylene glycol, methoxyflurane, and massive ascorbic acid overdose can all result in acute renal failure because of oxalate overproduction and deposition in the kidney. In addition, intestinal hyperabsorption of oxalate can occur in ileal disease or bypass in which luminal calcium, which normally prevents oxalate absorption, is complexed with malabsorbed free fatty acids. Chronic tubulointerstitial nephritis and stone disease can result.

Hypercalcemia. Acute hypercalcemia produces a vasopressin-resistant concentrating defect associated with hypertension, reduced renal plasma flow, and volume depletion, which can result in acute renal failure. Chronic nephrocalcinosis, which is calcium deposition along tubular basement membranes, in tubular epithelial cells, and in the interstitium, can lead to renal insufficiency. Treatment in either case is directed toward lowering the serum calcium level and identifying the underlying cause, most commonly, hyperparathyroidism, malignancy, sarcoidosis, or vitamin D intoxication.

Hypokalemia. Prolonged hypokalemia, often attributable to laxative or diuretic abuse, occasionally causes proximal tubular vacuolization and reversible medullary cyst formation. Functional abnormalities including reduced GFR, impaired concentrating ability, and increased ammoniagenesis have been reported, possibly because of progressive interstitial fibrosis in some cases.

Immunologic Conditions

Sjögren's Syndrome. Sjögren's syndrome becomes evident on clinical examination with dry eyes and mouth (sicca syndrome) and lymphocytic infiltration of other organs. It may be primary or result from another autoimmune disease. Renal involvement occurs in 40% of patients and is characterized by a lymphocytic interstitial infiltrate, a distal tubular acidosis, and a concentrating defect. Azotemia may be seen, but renal failure is rare.

Transplantation. Chronic transplant rejection is a cell-mediated immune process that occurs months to years after transplantation and produces a gradual deterioration in renal function. On pathologic examination a typical chronic interstitial nephritis is accompanied by arteriolosclerosis and glomerular basement membrane thickening. Anti–tubular basement membrane antibodies may be detectable. Enhanced immunosuppressive therapy may reverse the process, but progressive graft failure is not uncommon.

Lupus Nephritis. Lupus nephritis commonly involves the tubulointerstitium, often with immune-complex deposition along the tubular basement membrane, and the severity of interstitial inflammation correlates with renal function. Tubular functional defects may be prominent in some patients, but tubulointerstitial involvement in the absence of glomerular disease is an uncommon occurrence.

Hematopoietic Diseases

Sickle Cell Disease. Patients with sickle cell disease may have several renal manifestations including cortical infarcts, gross hematuria, papillary necrosis, recurrent infections, impaired concentrating ability, impaired acidification, and a glomerulopathy resembling normocomplementemic membranoproliferative glomerulonephritis. Hemoglobin S is particularly susceptible to sickling in the hypoxic, hypertonic, and acidic milieu of the inner medulla. Medullary interstitial fibrosis is a common pathologic finding. A recent study found that in 4.2% of patients with sickle cell anemia and in 2.4% of patients with sickle cell–hemoglobin C disease renal failure developed (which carried a poor prognosis, despite dialysis) and that proteinuria, hematuria, hypertension, and severe anemia were all predictors of this outcome.

Plasma Cell Dyscrasias. Renal involvement in multiple myeloma can take several forms. Although acute renal failure resulting from hypercalcemia, volume depletion, and numerous other factors is common in myeloma, urinary light chain excretion is the primary factor that is responsible for progressive renal failure. Although not detectable by routine dipstick, urinary light chains may be detected by a semiquantitative test involving the addition of an equal volume of 5% sulfosalicylic acid to the urine. Confirmation and further characterization is made by urine immunoelectrophoresis. Urinary light chain excretion in excess of the normal 6 mg/dl causes direct tubular toxicity and obstruction through the formation of intratubular casts with Tamm-Horsfall protein. Proximal tubular dysfunction without azotemia leading to Fanconi's syndrome occurs almost exclusively in association with κ light chains. A plasma cell dyscrasia may be evident. Other tubular manifestations of myeloma include distal tubular acidosis, nephrogenic diabetes insipidus, and combinations of both proximal and distal tubular defects. The diagnosis of myeloma is usually apparent by the time azotemia resulting from urinary light chains occurs. Pathologic findings reveal eosinophillic casts surrounded by a giant cell reaction accompanied by tubular atrophy, interstitial fibrosis, and tubular basement membrane staining for light chains by immunofluorescence, so-called cast nephropathy. Nephrotic-range albuminuria coexistent with urinary light chains suggests possibility of glomerular deposition of either λ or κ light chains, resulting in amyloidosis or light chain glomerulopathy, respectively. Management of these patients includes maintenance of euvolemia and normocalcemia, avoidance of nephrotoxins, and correction of disturbances resulting from tubular defects with the use of sodium bicarbonate administration for distal RTA, and thiazide diuretics for nephrogenic diabetes insipidus. Multiple myeloma is treated with chemotherapy, and dialysis is appropriate in these patients while a response is awaited. Renal function may be recovered in some patients after treatment for the myeloma.

Infiltration. Leukemic and lymphomatous infiltration of the renal interstitium is common, but renal dysfunction and failure are rare.

Mechanical Disorders

Two clinical entities produce chronic renal disease through a primary mechanical mechanism, although complicating factors like superimposed infection may also contribute to the pathogenesis.

Reflux. Reflux nephropathy is a potentially preventable cause of end-stage renal failure in young adults. Typically an adolescent or young adult comes to medical attention with hypertension, renal insufficiency, and a history of urinary tract infections or unexplained fevers in childhood. Proteinuria (>1 g/day) and renal scarring on ultrasonography or intravenous pyelography are common, and progression to end-stage disease is the rule.

The pathogenetic hallmark of reflux nephropathy is intrarenal reflux, which is the retrograde passage of urine past the papilla into the nephron. Since this can rarely be visualized directly, the diagnosis of reflux is generally made by the finding of vesicoureteral reflux on voiding cystourethrography. The incidence of vesicoureteral reflux declines with age from approximately 40% in children under the age of 5 years who have had at least one urinary tract infection to only 5% of adults with urinary tract infection. Whether bacteriuria is required, in addition to reflux, to cause renal scarring is still controversial. Although new scars have been documented in patients receiving antibiotic prophylaxis, this is an uncommon event. It is postulated that bacterial antigens or normal constituents such as Tamm-Horsfall protein in the extravasated urine cause an intense interstitial inflammatory response. The fibrotic healing of these inflamed regions results in the radiologic appearance of the reflux kidney, namely, irregular scarring with areas of cortical thinning overlying blunted calyces. This initial scarring, which occurs early in childhood, leads to an inexorable decline in renal function, usually on the basis of focal glomerulosclerosis and hypertension. Neither surgical correction of reflux nor medical therapy, usually antibiotic prophylaxis, prevents this deterioration once significant scarring has occurred.

Early recognition is crucial in the prevention of reflux nephropathy. This is achieved by the screening of children with urinary tract infections, as well as siblings of children with known vesicoureteral reflux. Medical versus surgical interventions are chosen on an individual basis.

Obstruction. Prolonged obstruction may be the most common cause of chronic tubulointerstitial disease. The causes of obstruction vary with age and include renal calculi, prostatic disease, carcinoma

of the cervix, functional or anatomic abnormalities of the urinary tract, retroperitoneal involvement by tumor, or fibrosis. Regardless of cause, transmission of elevated intratubular pressures to the glomerulus results in a decline in GFR. Prolonged obstruction causes a decline in renal blood flow, probably as a result of local angiotensin II and thromboxane A_2 production. In addition, local release of mediators of inflammation leads to interstitial infiltration, tubular damage, and progressive fibrosis.

Clinical presentation may vary from the asymptomatic patient with insidious obstruction to anuria and flank pain with acute complete obstruction. Urine output may be increased with partial obstruction or may be variable with intermittent obstruction. Distal tubular dysfunction may be evident as hyperkalemia, metabolic acidosis, nephrogenic diabetes insipidus, and occasionally salt wasting. Azotemia is present, and hypertension is common. Renal ultrasonography usually reveals hydronephrosis, but significant obstruction can coexist with a normal ultrasound examination. Alternative imaging studies include diuretic renography, computed tomography scanning, and contrast pyelography. These should be undertaken in the patient with high likelihood of obstruction and normal ultrasonography. Prompt relief of obstruction to minimize long-term renal damage is the goal in treatment of these patients. A postobstructive diuresis often occurs and usually represents an appropriate excretion of retained solute and water, and it is important not to perpetuate the diuresis by excessive volume replacement. Fluid and electrolyte replacement in this setting should be guided by the solute composition of the urine and by clinical assessment of the patient's volume status. Attention to potassium and magnesium losses is also important.

Vascular Diseases

Radiation exposure in excess of 2300 rads leads to injury to the renal vascular endothelium and becomes evident as acute glomerulopathy within 6 to 12 months following exposure and a chronic tubulointerstitial nephritis thereafter. It is commonly seen in bone marrow transplant recipients and can be avoided by shielding the kidneys. Benign arteriolar nephrosclerosis may occur in patients with long-standing hypertension and is characterized by chronic vascular and tubulointerstitial changes followed by glomerulosclerosis. A history of essential hypertension, evidence of other end-organ damage, and mild proteinuria suggest the diagnosis.

Hereditary Diseases

Tubulointerstitial abnormalities occur in a number of hereditary diseases. Juvenile nephronophthisis is an autosomal recessive disorder causing end-stage renal failure in childhood. The gene for this disease has been tentatively localized to chromosome 2. Medullary cystic disease is an autosomal dominant disease in which renal failure is delayed until late middle age. Both diseases are characterized on pathologic study by medullary cyst formation, tubular atrophy, chronic tubulointerstial inflammation, and fibrosis.

Miscellaneous Conditions

Granulomatous Nephritis. As noted earlier, granulomatous nephritis represents a distinct pathologic entity that can exist in chronic form. In a series describing 14 patients with chronic granulomatous interstitial nephritis, sarcoidosis, and tuberculosis were each diagnosed in three patients. In the remaining eight patients there was no evidence of extrarenal granulomas. Four of five of the latter group with idiopathic granulomatous nephritis responded to corticosteroid therapy.

Renal dysfunction in sarcoidosis is usually mediated by hypercalcemia, but granulomatous nephritis with tubular dysfunction and azotemia may occur. Corticosteroid therapy generally leads to improvement in renal function and resolution of granulomas. Tuberculosis can affect the urinary tract at any level and often becomes evident with dysuria, hematuria, and flank pain in the absence of systemic symptoms. Hematuria and pyuria are seen on urinalysis. Intravenous pyelography usually reveals calyceal deformities, calcifications, and cavitation. Complications include secondary bacterial infections, ureteral strictures, and stones. Urine cultures are positive for mycobacterium tuberculosis in 90% of cases, although multiple specimens are usually needed. Azotemia is very unusual in renal tuberculosis, having been described in only 2 of 41 cases in one series. Antituberculous chemotherapy is curative in the majority of cases.

Balkan Endemic Nephropathy The disorder of Balkan endemic neuropathy was first described in the late 1940s, and its origin has remained a mystery. The disease is endemic among farm workers who have lived for at least 20 years in endemic pockets along the Danube River. The disease is characterized by proximal tubular dysfunction, tubular proteinuria (especially β_2 microglobinuria), and slow progression to end-stage renal failure by the fifth or sixth decade of life. An increased incidence of transitional cell carcinoma of the renal pelvis and ureters occurs in the same endemic regions and may also strike patients with the nephropathy. Current opinion suggests that Balkan nephropathy is caused by the interaction between environmental and genetic factors. Candidate environmental factors include selenium deficiency, contaminants in drinking water from nearby coal deposits, and ochratoxin (a mycotoxin) contamination of the food chain.

Chinese Herb Nephropathy. Several recent reports from Europe have described an interstitial nephritis resulting from exposure to Chinese herbs. The disease is characterized by severe interstitial fibrosis and tubular destruction with scant inflammation. The exact pathogenesis of this disease remains unclear, but the herb content of aristolochic acid, a nephrotoxic alkaloid, is thought to be important.

General Approach to Treatment of Chronic Tubular Disease

A variety of specific renal tubular disorders, electrolyte abnormalities, and acid-base disturbances attend the development of chronic interstitial nephritis. Eventually, however, advanced renal failure requires supportive therapy including the treatment of volume overload, hyponatremia, hyperkalemia, hypocalcemia, hyperphosphatemia, and acidosis. Many early forms of progressive renal failure have also been treated expectantly with angiotensin-converting enzyme inhibitors, and the initial results look quite promising. There may also be a role for dietary protein restriction, and one may consider decreasing protein intake to approximately 0.5 to 0.6 g/kg per day in patients with chronic renal insufficiency. Such restriction is typically lifted on initiation of dialysis, if and when it occurs.

BIBLIOGRAPHY

Casella FJ, Allon M: The kidney in sarcoidosis, *J Am Soc Nephrol* 3:1555-1562, 1993.

Garella S: Drug-induced renal disease, *Hosp Pract* 28:129-133, 1993.

Gerding MN, Groen J, Jordans JG, Osterhaus AD: Hantavirus nephropathy in the Netherlands: clinical, histopathological and epidemiological findings, *Neth J Med* 47:106-112, 1995.

Hannedouche T, Albouze G, Chauveau P et al: Effects of blood pressure and antihypertensive treatment on progression of advanced chronic renal failure, *Am J Kidney Dis* 21:131-137, 1993.

Heeger P, Neilson EG, editors: Treatment of interstitial nephritis. In Glassock R, editor: *Current therapy in nephrology and hypertension,* Philadelphia, 1992, BC Decker.

Heeger PS, Neilson EG: Overcoming tolerance in autoimmune renal disease, *Curr Opin Nephrol Hypertension* 3(2):123-132, 1994.

Ishidoya S, Morrissey J, McCracken R, Klahr S: Delayed treatment with enalapril halts tubulointerstitial fibrosis in rats with obstructive nephropathy, *Kidney Int* 49(4):1110-1119, 1996.

Kelly CJ, Neilson EG: Tubulointerstitial diseases. In Brenner B, editor: *The Kidney,* Philadelphia, 1995, WB Saunders.

Kelly CJ, Tomaszewski J, Neilson EG: Immunopathogeneic mechanisms of tubulointerstitial injury. In Tisher CC, Brenner BM, editors: *Renal pathology,* Philadelphia, 1994, WR Saunders.

Murray KM, Keane WR: Review of drug-induced acute interstitial nephritis, *Pharmacotherapy* 12:462-467, 1992.

Neilson EG: Tubulointerstitial injury and its role in progressive renal damage, *Kidney Int* 45:S116-S117, 1994.

Okada HS, Danoff T, Neilson EG: Possible pathogenesis of renal fibrosis, *Kidney Int* 49(554):537-538, 1996.

Riminton S, O'Donnell J: Tubulointerstitial nephritis and uveitis (TINU) syndrome in an adult, *Aust NZ J Med* 23:57, 1993.

Strutz F, Okada H, Lo C et al: Isolation and characterization of a marker for fibroblasts: FSP1, *J Cell Biol* 130:393-405, 1995.

Vanherweghem JL, Depierreux M, Tielemans C et al: Rapidly progressive interstitial renal fibrosis in young women: association with slimming regimen including Chinese herbs, *Lancet* 341:387-391, 1993.

125 Renovascular Diseases

George L. Bakris and S. Luke Kusmirek

RENOVASCULAR HYPERTENSION

Renovascular hypertension (RVH) is the most common form of curable high blood pressure and is estimated to affect 1% of all hypertensive individuals. It occurs when significant unilateral or bilateral renal artery stenosis causes renal ischemia. The ischemic kidney activates the renin-angiotensin-aldosterone (RAA) axis, leading to hypertension. Renal ischemia, when prolonged, results in loss of the kidney function and is one of important causes of end-stage renal disease. Renal artery stenosis is primarily caused by atherosclerosis or fibromuscular dysplasia (FMD). This latter condition is unusual in African-Americans. In most cases renal revascularization can preserve renal function and modify or cure the associated hypertension. Renovascular hypertension remains a retrospective diagnosis; it is established only after hypertension has been permanently cured or improved with the surgical repair of the stenosis of renal artery.

PATHOPHYSIOLOGY

The renin-angiotensin system is pivotal in the genesis of RVH (Fig. 125-1). The initial pathogenesis of renovascular hypertension is associated with high renin production, especially in unilateral renal artery stenosis. Stenosis of unilateral renal artery is associated with a high-renin state that persists. This leads to high angiotensin II and aldosterone levels and usually severe hypertension. Edema is generally absent in this condition unless renal insufficiency is present. This is due to two factors. First, the resultant high arterial pressures result in a "pressure natriuresis" by the contralateral kidney. Second, the nonstenotic kidney "escapes" from the sodium-retaining effect of aldosterone. Prolonged exposure to perfusion pressures elevated above the autoregulatory range commonly causes rapid functional deterioration of the nonstenotic kidney. At that usually late stage of disease, intravascular volume may be expanded, resulting in edema formation.

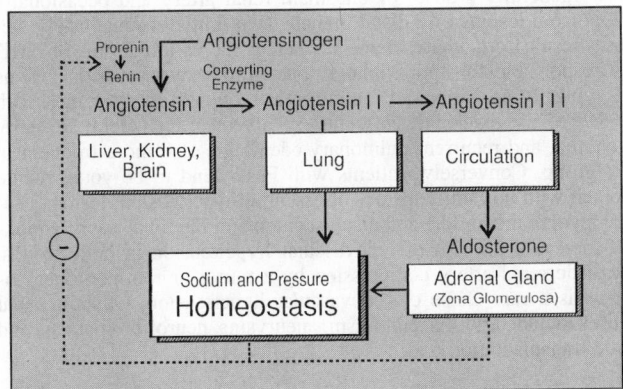

FIGURE 125-1 The generation of the renin-angiotensin-aldosterone (RAA) system and its contribution to salt and blood pressure control. The enclosed boxes represent the areas in the body where the conversions in the RAA system occur.

Table 125-1 Renovascular hypertension versus essential hypertension

CLUES	RENOVASCULAR HYPERTENSION	ESSENTIAL HYPERTENSION
Historical		
Age at onset (years)	<25 (FMD) or >55 (atherosclerosis)	25-55
Family history	Negative	Positive
Refractory HTN	Yes	Uncommon
Smoking	Yes	Equivocal
Atheromatous disease in other vascular territories	Common	Uncommon unless long-standing and poorly controlled
Recent exacerbation of stable HTN	Yes	No
Recent new onset of stage III/IV HTN	Yes	Uncommon
History of recurrent pulmonary edema	Yes	No
Unexplained progressive renal dysfunction, especially precipitated/exacerbated by ACE inhibitors	Yes	No
Blood pressure requiring ≥3 medications to control	Yes	No, unless African-American with history of hypertension
Physical examination		
Abdominal or flank continuous bruit	Yes	No
Advanced retinopathy (grades III, IV by KWB classification)	Yes	Uncommon unless untreated or poorly controlled for >10 years
Laboratory		
Nondiuretic-induced hypokalemia	Yes	No
Hyperreninemia	Yes	Uncommon
Unilateral small kidney detected during workup	Yes	No

ACE, Angiotensin-converting enzyme; *FMD,* fibromuscular dysplasia; *HTN,* hypertension; *KWB,* Keith-Wagener-Barker.

Hypertension associated with bilateral renal artery stenosis is less clearly related to RAA system. More commonly, while both renal arteries are stenosed, one of the two becomes critically narrowed and drives the increase in arterial pressure. Thus with bilateral disease both renal insufficiency and RAA system activation contribute to pressure elevation. In individuals who have long-standing disease of either type, hypertension may persist after revascularization as a result of generalized vascular damage, contralateral nephrosclerosis, or coexisting essential hypertension.

CLINICAL FEATURES

Diagnosis of renovascular disease continues to be a challenge for clinicians. Presentation may vary from a totally asymptomatic patient with varying severity of hypertension and response to medical therapy to a patient with severe hypertension, pulmonary edema, and ischemic nephropathy. Traditionally a group of clinical signs and symptoms, as well as laboratory abnormalities, distinguish RVH from essential hypertension (Table 125-1). The likelihood of renovascular hypertension is 10% to 20% in hypertensive patients who come to medical attention with one or more of these clinical clues.

Renovascular hypertension develops as a result of significant stenosis (generally >60%) of one main renal artery and occasionally arises from lesions of a distal branch. Two thirds of renal artery stenoses result from atherosclerosis, whereas the various forms of FMD are responsible for approximately one third. Atherosclerotic lesions are typically proximal and found more frequently in older men with evidence of extensive vascular involvement. Bilateral disease, azotemia, and recurrent pulmonary edema are also more frequent in this group. Conversely, patients with FMD tend to be young white women with no family history of essential hypertension; lesions usually involve the middle and distal segments of the renal artery. Smoking increases the risk of renovascular hypertension in both groups. Extrinsic renal artery compression by a tumor or retroperitoneal fibrosis is a rare cause of renovascular hypertension. Other unusual causes include arteritis, embolism, aneurysms, neurofibromatosis, and renal transplantation.

DIAGNOSIS

No ideal screening test exists for detecting renovascular hypertension. The positive predictive value of the currently available tests is considered acceptable only when applied to a population with a high probability of renovascular hypertension. Therefore the goal of pa-

tient evaluation for RVH is to assign individuals to low-, moderate-, or high-prevalence groups where the risk-benefit ratio justifies the risk of the next diagnostic or therapeutic intervention. A simple algorithm based on pretest probability and level of clinical suspicion illustrates an approach to the diagnosis of RVH (Fig. 125-2).

In patients with a low level of clinical suspicion, no RVH workup should be pursued apart from studies routinely performed for assessment of essential hypertension.

Currently, angiotensin-converting enzyme (ACE) inhibitor renography is the most popular diagnostic method recommended for patients with moderate pretest probability of RVH. Wide availability and significant experience with this type of nuclear imaging make it the *best* test for initial screening in this group of patients. Sensitivity and specificity vary from 91% to 94% and 95% to 97%, respectively, depending on the series and site where the study was performed. In its simplest form the test consists of two renal scans in a hydrated patient, one before and one after an oral dose of an ACE inhibitor, classically captopril. Some experts advise first performing scans after administration of ACE inhibitor, followed by a "baseline" scan *only* when the initial scan is abnormal. Patients should not be taking any ACE inhibitor for at least 48 to 72 hours before testing. When hemodynamically significant stenosis is present, angiotensin II–dependent filtration is decreased in the presence of the ACE inhibitor. This results in asymmetry of tracer accumulation. Criteria for a positive scan include (1) asymmetric uptake of more than 60% of total activity, (2) unilateral delayed time to peak activity, and (3) prolonged unilateral excretion of tracer. Criteria differ slightly depending on the type of isotope used in the test. No single isotope is clearly superior to the others. Moreover, all of the isotopes may be used with success in patients with preexisting renal insufficiency. Renal scintigraphy also has an additional benefit: it predicts the response to revascularization. A positive scan suggests a high probability of blood pressure normalization with restored blood flow to the stenotic kidney.

Renal artery duplex sonography (RADS) and magnetic resonance angiography (MRA) are two new, promising methods for detecting renal artery stenosis. Neither exposes the patient to the risks of the contrast medium, radiation, or catheters. Both techniques are best employed when screening for proximal arteriosclerotic stenoses. This is because neither method visualizes distal arterial segments adequately. Duplex scanning has a sensitivity and specificity of 88% to 95% and 90% to 99%, respectively, and is highly operator dependent. Additional limitations include obesity, inadequate bowel preparation, unusual anatomic variants of renal vasculature, and lack of experienced personnel. In certain situations (e.g., detection of transplant renal ar-

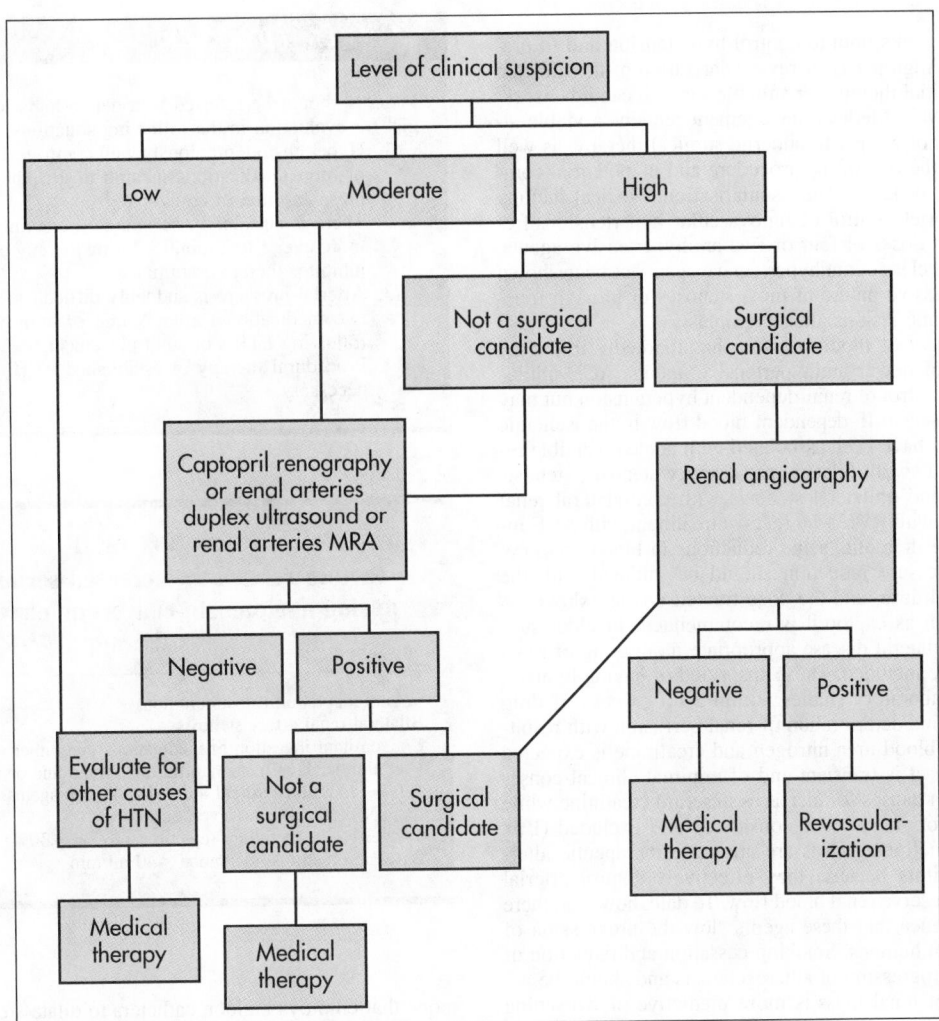

FIGURE 125-2   A simplified approach to the diagnostic assessment of renovascular hypertension. *MRA,* Magnetic resonance angiography.

tery stenosis) it may be the preferred diagnostic method. However, because it is highly operator dependent and technically difficult, it is not recommended for routine use. MRA is also capable of producing high-quality images of proximal renal arteries in completely noninvasive fashion. Sensitivity and specificity vary from 87% to 100% and 92% to 97%, respectively, for detecting a greater than 50% narrowing of the arterial lumen. Limitations are similar to the ones for RADS. In addition, high cost and long duration of image acquisition plague this method. Moreover, neither RADS nor MRA can reliably predict surgical outcome. However, both provide additional anatomic information about kidney size and anatomy to define sites of possible urinary tract obstruction.

Other tests like plasma renin activity with ACE inhibitor (captopril test) or alone, renal vein renin ratio, or intravenous digital subtraction angiography are used rarely and only in selected group of patients. Studies like exercise renography and the aspirin test are only of historical interest and are not commonly used in clinical practice.

Routine *arteriography* of the renal arteries is considered the gold standard for the diagnosis of renal artery stenosis and in patients with strongly suggestive clinical features is sometimes the first and definitive test. Functional tests should be performed before arteriography so that angioplasty of suitable lesions may be performed at the time of arteriography. Blood pressure response to correction of the stenosis determines the significance of the lesion. Patients who have atherosclerotic disease are at increased risk of development of either catheter-related or radiocontrast medium–related renal embolic events. The cost and risk of contrast nephropathy in those patients with renal insuffi-

ciency (i.e., serum creatinine level of 2.5 mg/dl or greater) or increased risk of atheroembolic phenomena (e.g., aneurysms, severe vascular disease) make arteriography an inappropriate screening test. Use of the newer, low-osmotic radiocontrast agents probably is associated with less renal toxicity and therefore is recommended for those at risk. *Intraarterial digital subtraction angiography* provides very similar images of the renal arteries with less contrast medium and is preferred when patients have renal insufficiency or are otherwise at risk for a contrast reaction. Carbon dioxide angiography is a new method for detecting renal arterial stenosis. Although safe, this test is not widely available. Carbon dioxide angiography may be safely used in patients with history of anaphylactic reactions to the radiocontrast media.

Hypertension does not improve with correction of the stenotic lesion in approximately one third of older patients. Functional or physiologic tests can help assign a patient to a group likely to improve with revascularization. The predictive value of available functional tests, however, is less than ideal. Clearly, a young patient with a diastolic flank bruit and severe hypertension of recent onset may be referred directly for arteriogram with immediate angioplasty. In an elderly patient with generalized atherosclerotic disease, moderately severe hypertension, and normal renal function a clinician may wish to increase the certainty of the diagnosis with a noninvasive screening test before exposing the patient to catheter-related and contrast-related risks of arteriography. Similarly, once a stenotic lesion is identified, one should determine whether it is a consequence or a cause of hypertension. Thus individualized evaluation and therapy are essential.

THERAPY

Optimal management seeks both to control hypertension and to preserve renal function. Angioplasty or revascularization of the affected artery is favored as initial therapy for suitable surgical candidates, especially those with FMD. Medical management remains a viable alternative for patients not willing to undergo surgical therapy, as well as in situations when the risk of the procedure and its potential complications exceeds the benefits of revascularisation. Medical therapy often provides only brief control of renovascular hypertension, frequently requiring high doses of four or five antihypertensive agents. Furthermore, no single class of antihypertensive agent has been shown to decrease the progressive nature of most stenoses or prevent reocclusion of atherosclerotic lesions after angioplasty.

Medical management of blood pressure has markedly improved with the availability of newer antihypertensive agents. ACE inhibitors exhibit effective control of renin-dependent hypertension but may compromise the angiotensin II–dependent blood flow in the ischemic kidney. ACE inhibitors have been associated with acute reversible renal failure in individuals with bilateral renal artery stenosis, stenosis of a solitary kidney, and unilateral stenosis with contralateral renal insufficiency. Patients with RVH who receive treatment with ACE inhibitors may also have dramatic, acute reductions in blood pressure. Therapy for blood pressure reduction should be initiated with the smallest recommended dose, and the dose titrated upward slowly. A short-acting agent such as captopril is recommended. In older subjects with suspected bilateral disease appropriate monitoring of renal function should also be included. Those suspected of having bilateral disease should have laboratory studies within 2 to 4 weeks of drug initiation. Although some deterioration of renal perfusion with resulting increase of serum blood urea nitrogen and creatinine is expected in majority of patients, it is transient and of minimal clinical consequence. However, other causes for increases in serum creatinine while receiving ACE inhibitors have to be considered and excluded (Box 125-1). Calcium channel antagonists are attractive therapeutic alternatives to ACE inhibitors because they effectively control arterial pressure and tend to preserve renal blood flow. To date, however, there is no convincing evidence that these agents slow the progression of atheromatous lesions in humans. Smoking cessation and reduction of hyperlipidemia slow progression of atherosclerosis and should be actively pursued. Loss of renal mass is more predictive of worsening perfusion than is blood pressure control. Patients receiving medical treatment should have periodic assessment of renal size and function. No prospective randomized trials have examined the long-term advantages and risks of medical therapy versus surgery or angioplasty.

Surgical revascularisation and percutaneous transluminal renal angioplasty (PTRA) are two invasive strategies employed in the therapy of RVH.

Surgical revascularization yields excellent short-term results for both FMD and atherosclerotic renovascular disease (ARVD). It is the treatment of choice for branch renal artery lesions and most types of atheromatous lesions. Surgical mortality rate is approximately 2% to 6% for patients with atherosclerotic lesions and less than 0.01% for patients with FMD. Use of hepatorenal and splenorenal bypass depending on the site of the stenosis has obviated the need for operating on a badly diseased aorta. In the FMD group approximately 60% of patients are "cured" of hypertension. Cure is defined as a blood pressure of less than 140/90 mm Hg without medications. In addition, 30% show improved control of blood pressure, which is defined by fewer and lower dosages of antihypertensive agents, after surgery. Results for the ARVD group are less favorable because of the nature of the lesion and prevalent comorbidities. Twenty percent to 30% of patients are cured, and 50% to 60% improve with revascularization. The overall failure rate is around 10% in both groups; the same percentage is quoted for the rate of postoperative complications like graft thrombosis or stenosis. Long-term results are encouraging, with 80% of patients remaining cured or improved in long-term follow-up in the atherosclerotic disease group. Results for FMD are even better. Nephrectomy as a mode of therapy is used only when attempts at revascularization are unsuccessful or when the ipsilateral kidney is excessively atrophic and the patient has complications of severe, uncontrollable hypertension.

Percutaneous transluminal renal angioplasty is a nonsurgical technique that employs balloon catheters to dilate stenotic arterial lesions and can be performed at the time of arteriography. In FMD without branch involvement it is the treatment of choice because of a high long-term patency rate. Role of PTRA in the treatment of ARVD is still a subject of controversy. Results of angioplasty vary depending on the localization, type, and complexity of the lesion. PTRA is considered acceptable therapy for discrete midarterial atheromatous lesions and is associated with a 20% to 30% restenosis rate. Repeat dilation is often successful. The majority of lesions (approximately 80%) are proximal to the aorta, involving the ostial portion of renal artery. Angioplasty in this setting is traditionally considered less successful and has very high restenosis rates. With the constant development of the technology used in PTRA and the availability of endovascular stents, further improvement of the angioplasty results can be expected. It must be emphasized that all patients who have PTRA should also be *surgical candidates* because 5% to 6% of patients require emergency surgical repair of the renal artery.

RENAL VEIN THROMBOSIS

See Chapter 108.

RENAL ARTERY THROMBOSIS AND EMBOLISM

Thrombosis of the renal artery is nearly always associated with vascular injury. Most commonly arteriosclerosis is the underlying cause. Other predisposing conditions are summarized in Box 125-2. Interestingly, cyclosporin has been shown to suppress the protein C anticoagulant pathway in cultured endothelial cells and may partially explain the increased risk of renal artery thrombosis in renal transplant patients.

The heart is the source of up to 90% of macroemboli. Cardiac conditions leading to macroemboli formation include atrial fibrillation, valvular vegetations, myocardial infarction, cardiomyopathy, and sep-

---

✔ *WHEN TO REFER*

Patients should be referred to a nephrologist or hypertensionologist for evaluation in the following situations:

1. Hypertension, previously well controlled, now requires three or more medications in high doses, and captopril renography is normal or equivocal.
2. There is sustained rise in serum creatinine level of 30% or more over 1 to 2 months during therapy or shortly after ACE inhibitor therapy is initiated.
3. Arterial pressure is suddenly difficult to control (more than two medications) after "cured or improved" clinical status following PTRA or stent placement.
4. Procedural therapy of established RVH (PTRA, surgery) is necessary.

BOX 125-1

Factors related to increased serum creatinine during angiotensin-converting enzyme inhibitor therapy

Volume depletion (most common)
Bilateral renal artery stenosis
Concomitant ingestion of medications that either alter creatinine secretion such as trimethaprim and cimetidine or reduce renal blood flow, like nonsteroidal antiinflammatory agents
Increased catabolism (fever, burns)
Congestive heart failure (ejection fraction <30%)
Baseline creatinine clearance <40 ml/min

BOX 125-2
Causes of renal artery thrombosis

Aneurysm
Arteriography
Atherosclerosis
Cyclosporin (rare)
Fibromuscular dysplasia
Heparin-induced thrombocytopenia and thrombosis (rare)
Moyamoya syndrome
Polyarteritis nodosum
Syphilis
Thromboangiitis obliterans

tal defects that can allow right-to-left passage of a venous thrombosis. Clinical presentations differ with respect to the abruptness of the occlusion, the number of kidneys involved, and the presence of collateral circulation. Slowly developing disease is often insidious, and hypertension may be the only related manifestation (see the discussion of renovascular hypertension). Acute occlusion can be associated with flank or abdominal pain, fever, nausea, vomiting, leukocytosis, and transient gross or microscopic hematuria. Renal function is usually spared in unilateral occlusion, whereas acute oliguric renal failure is typical of bilateral involvement. Renal infarction generally results in sequential elevation of aspartate aminotransferase, lactic dehydrogenase, and alkaline phosphatase levels. Absence of a nephrogram indicated by intravenous pyelography (IVP), contrast computed tomography (CT), or isotopic renogram is highly suggestive of an acute event. Arteriography is diagnostic. Duplex scanning is commonly used to assess renal circulation in transplantation patients. Anticoagulation with or without thrombolytic agents, angioplasty, and revascularization has been employed with success. No therapeutic consensus has emerged to specify which patients are best treated with which methods. Surgical revascularization, especially in young individuals, is generally advocated within 12 hours of occlusion caused by trauma. Conservative therapy and blood pressure control are the mainstays of management in chronic disease. However, if renal insufficiency is progressive, revascularization should be considered because successful recovery of renal function 1 to 2 months after occlusion has been described in older individuals with collateral circulation.

RENAL ATHEROEMBOLISM

Small to medium renal artery obstruction by microemboli originating from atheromatous plaques of the aorta characterizes atheroembolic renal disease. Microemboli or cholesterol emboli are composed primarily of cholesterol crystals, and their occurrence is usually limited to individuals above the age of 60 years with significant atherosclerotic disease. Showers of cholesterol emboli can be released spontaneously or after arteriography, aortic surgery, trauma, and possibly anticoagulation. Protean clinical features make antemortem diagnosis elusive. Periodic renal microinfarction becomes evident as progressive renal insufficiency and worsening hypertension. A vasculitis-like picture, including pancreatitis, visual disturbances, and painful distal extremities, may be associated with multisystem involvement. Physical features can include livedo reticularis, blue toes, abdominal aneurysm, femoral bruits, and cholesterol emboli of the retinal vasculature. Laboratory findings are transient and nonspecific but can include eosinophiluria (Hansel's stain recommended), proteinuria, eosinophilia, azotemia, hypocomplementemia, and elevated sedimentation rate. Diagnosis is made by tissue biopsy of an affected area. On routine preparation the cholesterol crystals are dissolved, leaving the characteristic "cholesterol clefts" in the material occluding a small artery (Fig. 125-3). Renal biopsy has the highest diagnostic yield, but skin, muscle, and rectal biopsy may also be diagnostic. There is no recognized effective treatment. Anticoagulation may actually prevent stable plaque formation, thereby liberating cholesterol crystals, and worsen the prognosis.

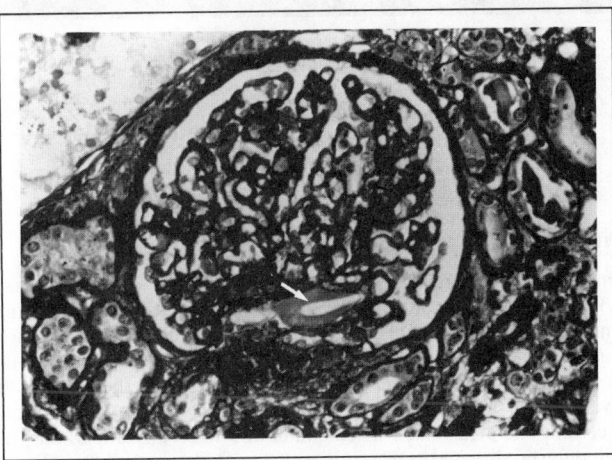

A

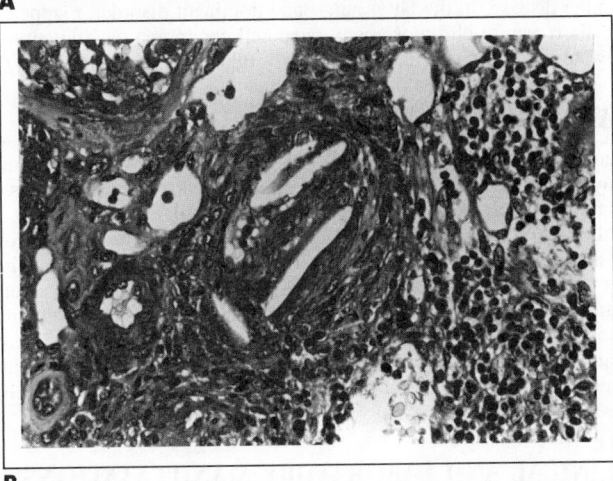

B

FIGURE 125-3   **A,** Glomerulus with cholesterol cleft at the hilus *(arrow)* (magnification ×100). **B,** Atheromatous emboli in interlobular artery (magnification ×100).

Photomicrographs courtesy of Melvin Schwartz, MD.

BIBLIOGRAPHY

Bonelli FS, McKusick MA, Textor SC et al: Renal artery angioplasty: technical results and clinical outcomes in 320 patients, *Mayo Clin Proc* 70:1041, 1995.

Bourgoignie JJ, Rubbert K, Sfakianakis GN: Angiotensin-converting enzyme–inhibited renography for the diagnosis of ischemic kidneys, *Am J Kidney Dis* 24:665, 1994.

Canzanello VJ, Textor SC: Noninvasive diagnosis of renovascular diseases, *Mayo Clin Proc* 69:1172, 1994.

Elliott WJ, Martin WB, Murphy MB: Comparison of two noninvasive screening tests for renovascular hypertension, *Arch Intern Med* 153:755, 1993.

Kent CK et al: Magnetic resonance imaging: a reliable test for the evaluation of proximal atherosclerotic renal artery stenosis, *J Vasc Surg* 13:311, 1991.

Mailloux LU, Napolitano B, Bellucci AG et al: Renal vascular disease causing end-stage renal disease: incidence, clinical correlates and outcomes—a 20-year clinical experience, *Am J Kidney Dis* 24:622, 1994.

Novick AC: Percutaneous transluminal angioplasty and surgery of the renal artery, *Eur J Vasc Surg* 8:1, 1994.

Ploth D, Fitzgibbon W: Pathophysiology of altered renal function in renovascular hypertension, *Am J Kidney Dis* 24,:652, 1994.

Rimmer JM, Gennari FJ: Atherosclerotic renovascular disease and progressive renal failure, *Ann Intern Med* 118:712, 1993.

Schreiber MJ, Pohl MA, Novick AC: The natural history of atherosclerotic and fibrous renal artery diseases, *Urol Clin North Am* 11(3):383, 1984.

Setaro JF, Saddler MC, Chen CC et al: Simplified captopril renography in diagnosis and treatment of renal artery stenosis, *Hypertension* 18:289, 1991.

Slataper RM, Bakris GL: Secondary hypertension. In Taylor RB, editor: *Difficult diagnosis*, ed II, Philadelphia, 1992, WB Saunders.

126 Renal Cell Carcinoma

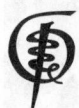

T. Dwight McKinney

INCIDENCE

Renal cell carcinoma is responsible for about 3% of all malignant neoplasms. It occurs at a rate of 7.5 cases per 100,000 population annually and is the most common renal cancer, accounting for more than 80% of renal malignancies in adults. Renal cell carcinoma occurs twice as frequently in men as in women. Risk factors for the development of renal cell carcinoma include tobacco use, exposure to certain chemicals such as cadmium and nitrosohydrocarbons, acquired cystic disease occurring in end-stage kidneys, and von Hippel-Lindau disease. In the latter autosomal dominant disorder, mapped to the short arm of chromosome 3, renal cell carcinoma may develop in 20% to 50% of cases and is frequently bilateral.

PATHOLOGY

Renal cell carcinoma probably arises from proximal tubule cells and may become evident in three main cell types: clear, granular, and sarcomatoid. Both the cell type and degree of cellular differentiation, in addition to the presence or absence of metastases, are important prognostically; nonmetastatic, well-differentiated, clear-cell carcinoma has the most favorable prognosis. Thirty percent of patients have metastatic disease at the time of initial diagnosis. The most frequent sites of metastases are the lung, lymph nodes, liver, bone, and adrenal glands. Extension of tumor into the renal veins or inferior vena cava occurs in more than 20% of cases but, unless there is invasion of the vessel wall, does not affect prognosis.

CLINICAL AND LABORATORY MANIFESTATIONS

Renal cell carcinoma may exhibit a variety of clinical and laboratory abnormalities. Isolated hematuria on microscopic or gross examination is the most common presenting symptom and occurs in 40% to 60% of cases. Other manifestations include abdominal or flank pain (20% to 50%), abdominal mass (20% to 45%), weight loss (25% to 35%), fever (10% to 20%), and varicocele (2% to 10%). Hypertension, which may be mediated through the renin-angiotensin system, is present in 15% to 40% of cases. The classic triad of hematuria, abdominal pain, and abdominal mass occurs in less than 10% of cases at initial presentation. In some patients renal carcinoma is discovered incidentally following radiologic imaging. Approximately 5% to 10% of such asymptomatic lesions are renal cell carcinomas.

Laboratory manifestations include anemia in 20% to 40% of cases. Rarely (3% to 4%), erythrocytosis, presumably as a result of excessive erythropoietin production, occurs. Hypercalcemia, as a result of bone metastasis or humoral mechanisms, is present in 3% to 6% of cases. Abnormal liver function test results, such as elevation of serum alkaline phosphatase activity, occur in 10% to 40% of patients and may be observed in the absence of hepatic metastases.

DIAGNOSIS

Depending on their availability, a variety of diagnostic procedures may be used to make a presumptive diagnosis and to determine the extent of renal cell carcinoma. Intravenous urography, particularly if combined with nephrotomography, is approximately 95% accurate in differentiating renal cancer from benign processes. Renal ultrasonography is a noninvasive procedure that is approximately 95% accurate and is sensitive in diagnosis if tumors are greater than 3 cm in diameter. Ultrasonography may demonstrate a simple cyst; renal cancer occurring in a simple cyst is rare. If ultrasonography demonstrates a complex cyst, percutaneous cyst puncture can be performed and cyst fluid can be analyzed for malignant cells, erythrocytes, and fat con-

tent, which may suggest the diagnosis of renal cancer. In addition, the cyst wall may be further evaluated after injection of air or radiographic contrast medium. Computed tomography with radiographic contrast medium enhancement is currently the most widely available, sensitive, and accurate nonoperative method available for making a presumptive diagnosis of renal cancer and its extent and is the procedure of choice for preoperative staging. If present, involvement of the renal vein, inferior vena cava, regional lymph nodes, and liver by tumor can usually be demonstrated. Nuclear magnetic resonance imaging may be somewhat better than computed tomography in detecting tumor in regional lymph nodes and extension into the renal veins and inferior vena cava. In addition, it is useful in selected patients who have a contraindication to the administration of radiographic contrast medium or if the computed tomography findings are equivocal. Renal arteriography, particularly if performed with epinephrine infusion, which constricts normal arteries but not tumor vessels, is quite accurate in differentiating benign from malignant renal masses but carries certain risks such as bleeding from the arterial puncture site. Angiography has been largely replaced by computed tomography for diagnosis and staging of renal carcinoma and is used only infrequently now to define the vascular anatomy in planning renal-sparing surgery.

TREATMENT

The prognosis for patients who come to medical attention with widespread disease or without metastases but do not have operative intervention is dismal, with less than 5% surviving 5 years. For patients without distant metastases the treatment of choice is radical nephrectomy, which includes resection of the regional lymph nodes, ipsilateral adrenal gland, and perinephric fat and is associated with a higher long-term survival rate than is simple nephrectomy. For patients with bilateral renal cell carcinoma but without tumor elsewhere (approximately 3% of cases), partial bilateral nephrectomies are generally performed. Partial nephrectomy may also be performed in patients with reduced renal function, with a solitary kidney, or with small (<4 cm in diameter) tumors. Selected patients with large symptomatic tumors may be candidates for palliative tumor resection. Postoperative survival depends on the stage of the disease. Five-year survival rates range from 50% to 80% for persons with stage I disease (tumor confined to the kidney) to 25% to 50% for those with stage III disease (tumor locally invasive but without distant metastases). The average survival of patients with metastases at the time of nephrectomy is only 6 to 9 months. There appears to be little benefit from postoperative adjuvant radiation, hormonal therapy, or chemotherapy.

Treatment of patients with metastatic renal cell carcinoma is generally unrewarding. A variety of hormonal and chemotherapeutic agents have been evaluated with only moderate success. One reason many of these tumors are resistant to chemotherapy is the presence of p-glycoprotein 170. Recent studies with biologic response modifiers including interleukin-2 and β-interferon have resulted in objective responses in 30% to 40% of patients with complete remission in some. These results, and ones using other approaches, such as infusion of tumor-infiltrating lymphocytes obtained from resected tumors in combination with biologic response modifiers and chemotherapy, suggest that approaches of this type may lead to more successful therapy of metastatic disease. Patients with metastases confined to the lungs have a more favorable prognosis than those with metastases elsewhere. Solitary metastases may be associated with prolonged survival after irradiation or, in exceptional cases, surgical resection. Very rarely, metastatic renal cell carcinoma may undergo regression either spontaneously or after nephrectomy.

OTHER RENAL TUMORS

Most renal malignancies associated with a sarcomatoid appearance are variants of the usual renal carcinoma. However, primary *sarcomas* of the kidney, although rare, do occur. A variety of cell types may be seen, including leiomyosarcoma, fibrosarcoma, histiocytoma, rhabdomyosarcoma, angiosarcoma, liposarcoma, chondrosarcoma, and osteogenic sarcoma. The most frequent associated findings are abdominal pain, flank mass, and hematuria. In most patients the disease is metastatic at the time of diagnosis, the overall prognosis is poor, and most individuals die within 1 year of diagnosis. For patients without metastatic disease, radical nephrectomy is the treatment of choice. A minority of patients respond to currently employed chemotherapeutic regimens.

Renal chromophobe carcinoma has been described recently and accounts for approximately 4% of renal neoplasms. Findings on electron microscopy are characteristic and consist of cells with numerous cytoplasmic microvesicles. Initial results suggest that this variant is associated with a better prognosis than renal carcinoma of the ordinary type.

Papillary carcinomas, which account for approximately 14% of renal neoplasms, were previously believed to be a variant of usual renal carcinomas. However, these tumors have recently been found to have cytogenetic abnormalities (such as tendency toward loss of the Y chromosome and trisomy of chromosomes 7 and 17) that appear to be unique. The prognosis for these malignancies as compared with the more usual types is not yet resolved.

Renal *adenomas* are small (less than 2 to 3 cm in diameter) benign tumors that are usually asymptomatic and are discovered incidentally at autopsy or during radiographic examination of the kidneys. On histologic examination renal adenomas are quite similar to well-differentiated renal cell carcinoma. Because it may be difficult to exclude renal cell carcinoma, patients with presumed renal adenomas should be followed closely if surgical resection is not performed.

Renal *oncocytoma* is a benign tumor thought to arise from proximal tubular epithelium. In a minority of patients tumors are bilateral. Oncocytoma and renal cell carcinoma can be readily distinguished by histologic examination. However, because these tumors cannot be differentiated by noninvasive means, the diagnosis is usually made at the time of surgery for presumed renal cancer.

Angiomyolipoma of the kidney is a benign tumor (hamartoma) composed of a mixture of blood vessels, smooth muscle, and fatty tissue. The tumor is associated with tuberous sclerosis in 20% to 50% of cases. Angiomyolipomas are generally unilateral and occur more frequently in women, except in association with tuberous sclerosis, when they are usually bilateral and occur equally in both sexes. Characteristically, angiomyolipomas are asymptomatic and are discovered incidentally. However, they may become evident as an abdominal mass or with flank pain and hematuria and, rarely, with massive retroperitoneal bleeding. It is often possible to make a presumptive diagnosis of angiomyolipoma by ultrasonography and computed tomography. However, in some patients surgery may be required to exclude renal cancer.

Other rare renal neoplasms include *collecting duct carcinomas* (Bellini duct carcinoma), which are usually localized to the renal pelvis, and renal neuroendocrine tumors, including both *carcinoid* and *small cell carcinoma. Wilms' tumor* is the most frequent malignant renal tumor in childhood but is exceedingly rare in adults.

TUMORS OF THE UPPER URINARY TRACT

Malignant tumors of the renal pelvis and ureter, usually transitional and less commonly squamous cell carcinomas, account for less than 5% of all adult renal tumors. Malignancies in these locations are much less frequent than those in the urinary bladder. Upper urinary tract tumors are twice as common in men as in women. Predisposing factors include exposure to chemicals such as benzidine and beta naphthylamine, cigarette smoke, chronic analgesic consumption, and Balkan nephropathy.

The most common presenting symptom is painless hematuria, which occurs in 75% of cases. Less frequently, renal colic and urinary urgency and frequency are present. Intravenous urography is generally the first diagnostic procedure performed for the evaluation of hematuria, and its result is almost always abnormal in patients with upper urinary tract tumors. Findings include hydronephrosis, filling defects, decreased or absent excretion of contrast medium by the affected kidney, or a combination of these. Cystoscopy and retrograde pyelograms or ureterorenoscopy are usually performed after intravenous urography. In addition to radiographic or direct visualization of the affected upper urinary tract with these procedures, the bladder and contralateral kidney and ureter can be examined for the presence of simultaneously occurring tumors, and urine and biopsy specimens or brushings can be obtained for cytologic examination. Computed tomography may help to differentiate a radiolucent calculus from a tumor and is useful in determining the extent of tumor. Cytologic examination of voided urine is a useful, noninvasive screening procedure that may be employed at any time in the evaluation of patients suspected of having upper urinary tract tumors but is not sufficiently sensitive by itself to exclude the diagnosis.

Treatment of malignant tumors of the renal pelvis usually consists of radical nephroureterectomy, but local resection of tumor may be appropriate in selected patients, such as those with reduced contralateral renal function. Irradiation and chemotherapy currently appear not to be useful. Close follow-up observation including urinary cytologic evaluation and visualization of the upper tract of the remaining kidney and bladder are mandatory because these tumors are frequently multicentric.

BIBLIOGRAPHY

Levine E: Renal cell carcinoma: clinical aspects, imaging diagnosis, and staging, *Semin Roentgenol* 30:128, 1995.

Nelson JB, Oyasu R, Dalton DP: The clinical and pathological manifestations of renal tumors in von Hippel-Landau disease, *J Urol* 152:2221, 1994.

Novick AG: Management of the incidentally detected solid renal mass, *Semin Nephrol* 14:519, 1994.

Pittman K, Selby P: The management of renal cell carcinoma, *Crit Rev Oncol Hematol* 16:181, 1994.

Stadler WM, Vogelzang NJ: Low-dose interleukin-2 in the treatment of metastatic renal-cell carcinoma, *Semin Oncol* 22:67, 1995.

Taneja SS et al: Management of disseminated kidney cancer, *Urol Clin North Am* 21:625, 1994.

Truong LD et al: Renal neoplasm in acquired cystic kidney disease, *Am J Kidney Dis* 26:1, 1995.

Wagstaff J et al: Renal cell carcinoma and interleukin-1: a review, *Eur J Cancer* 31A:401, 1995.

Weiss LM, Gelb AB, Medeiros J: Adult renal epithelial neoplasms, *Clin Pathol* 103:624, 1995.

Yagoda A, Abi-Rached B, Petrylak D: Chemotherapy for advanced renal-cell carcinoma: 1983-93, *Semin Oncol* 22:42, 1995.

PART SIX

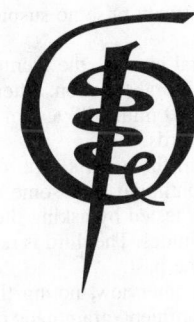

Neurologic Disorders

127 Neurologic History and Examination

Jock Murray

Every patient who has a medical examination should receive a neurologic examination to identify any evidence of abnormality in the nervous system. This should be a practical, efficient survey with high-yield examination techniques that best identify most neurologic abnormalities. A more detailed neurologic examination, if abnormalities are identified, can be found in textbooks of neurology (see Bibliography).

The neurologic examination is aimed at helping the clinician determine whether a neurologic problem is present and, if so, at what level (muscle, myoneural junction, nerve, spinal cord, brainstem, cerebral or cerebellar hemisphere); the likely process involved (pathologic features); the likely cause (etiologic factors); and whether therapy is needed, especially if urgent management is required (therapy). Infrequent application of the neurologic examination results in a disuse atrophy of skills, competence, efficiency, and confidence in assessing neurologic patients. Clinicians must develop a brief, efficient, and reliable examination that can be performed on every patient so that competence and confidence are maintained.

Although the term *neurologic examination* reflects the clinical testing of the patient, the most important diagnostic device is a careful *history*. Experienced clinicians are seldom surprised by the results of a neurologic examination, and they use it to confirm and qualify the conclusions derived from a careful history. Such a detailed interview is not merely the hobbyhorse of an obsessive-compulsive neurologist. It is an important means of developing a relationship with the patient that will be important in subsequent management, and it provides an understanding of the person in the circle of family, fellow workers, and community. Osler taught us that it was more important to know what kind of person has the disease than what kind of disease the person has.

ELEMENTS OF THE NEUROLOGIC EXAMINATION

The elements of the neurologic examination can be divided into the general observation and specific tests. The general observation is often the most informative and sometimes suggests the diagnosis of many disorders before the patient has taken a seat.

The specific tests can be subdivided into the categories of examination of the mental status, cranial nerves, motor and sensory function, and reflexes and the assessment of stance and gait.

Observation

We see what we look for. From the time the patient enters the office, diagnostic observations can be made. The portraits of depression, Parkinson's disease, movement disorders, muscle weakness, myotonic dystrophy, and many other conditions can often be observed. In those initial moments and in the subsequent interview the perceptive, sensitive clinician receives a great deal of information about the patient and the patient's condition.

General observation is best to recognize the patient's emotions and responses, but many specific neurologic signs can be observed during the interview, sometimes better than on the formal examination. These signs include subtle facial weakness, speech difficulties, memory disturbances, and aspects of denial and insight.

Mental Status

Many of the elements of the mental status examination can be observed in the interview, but again, these characteristics may be seen only if the clinician looks for them. In most instances no further detailed assessment is necessary if the person came seeking attention for other symptoms, and the complaint and the clinician's careful assessment of the person on the interview raise no suspicion of mental changes.

If there is a suspicion of mental change, the mental state can be assessed in various domains of cerebral function. Attention and concentration can be tested by the "100 minus 7" test or by asking the patient to name the months backwards.

Memory testing can be done in three parts. The first is orientation, tested by asking the year, month, day, and some current events. The second is immediate memory, tested by asking the person to remember four simple items for 5 minutes. The third is remote memory, tested by asking about events in the past.

Speech is observed during the interview, noting the smoothness of speech; whether it is fluent or nonfluent, grammatic or agrammatic; and if there are any paraphrasic errors.

Comprehension is tested by asking the person to obey commands, and repetition by asking him or her to repeat a sentence. The patient can be asked to name objects, draw a picture, or describe a picture in the office, and to read and show understanding of what was read. Visuospatial function is tested by asking the patient to draw a house or cube, or to copy examples of these, or to draw a clock and put the hands to a specified time.

Frontal system functions are tested by asking for the similarities between an orange and an apple or a fork and knife. Then the person is asked to name as many animals as possible in 1 minute, and to name words starting with a certain letter. Praxis is tested by asking the person to pretend to perform tasks, such as hammering a nail or brushing teeth.

When mental change is suspected, this brief mental status testing gives an assessment of critical cognitive domains, including attention, memory, language, visuospatial function, frontal system tasks, and praxis.

Cranial Nerves

Although there are 12 cranial nerves, a few are particularly important to examine because they are indicators of serious disease or are commonly involved if disease is present. This examination should include assessment of (1) the optic discs, (2) ocular movements and tests for nystagmus, (3) sensory function over the face, (4) motor symmetry of the face, (5) gag reflex, and (6) tongue movements.

Motor System

Is there any weakness and, if so, is it due to a lesion of the upper or lower motor neuron? Also, is there any alteration of muscle tone or coordination, or are there any abnormal movements? By the time the patient has entered the office, shaken hands, and taken a chair, the physician already knows a great deal about the patient's motor system.

On formal testing look for any signs of facial weakness. Test motor power in the shoulder muscles, elbow flexors and extensors, wrists, and grip. In the legs, examine hip, knee, and ankle flexors and extensors and ask the patient to walk on the heels and toes. The two most subtle, high-yield tests for upper motor neuron weakness are to ask the patient, with his or her eyes closed, to hold the hands extended, palms upward, for 1 minute and later to elevate both legs off the bed at the same time. When there is mild weakness, the hand begins to drop and pronate. The weak leg elevates more slowly and to a lower level.

Tone is tested in the arms by shaking the wrists and by gripping the hand and rapidly rotating the forearm. Tone of the legs can be best judged by suddenly lifting the leg from under the knee. In the normal, relaxed limb the heel drags along the examining table, whereas the heel rises off the bed if there is increased quadriceps tone.

Muscle power can be graded on a scale of 1 to 5 that numerically rates total paralysis (0), a flicker of contraction (1), movement only if gravity is eliminated (2), movement against gravity only (3), movement that can be overcome by resistance (4), and full power (5).

Coordination can be observed in the patient's walking and spontaneous movements, and also by the finger-to-nose test, rapid alternating movements of the hand, and heel to shin tests and tandem walking.

Sensory Examination

A scanning survey sensory examination should be made quickly but accurately to identify whether there is any sensory difference on one side of the body from the other, and distal compared with proximal. Pinprick, touch, and temperature can be tested on the arms and legs and compared with those on the opposite side; then the same is done for proximal and distal areas of the limbs. It is much more accurate to compare areas with an area that the physician is satisfied is normal than to use the coarse test of whether the patient feels the pin as sharp or dull. A sensory level (i.e., decreased sensation caudally below a certain body level) should be sought in a patient with a suspected spinal cord lesion. Vibratory sense should be examined over the feet, and the Romberg test is a good measure of proprioception.

If there is any evidence of sensory change on one side, cortical sensation should be tested by two-point discrimination, palm writing, stereognosis, and bilateral simultaneous stimulation.

If there is any complaint suggesting local alteration of sensation, the area should be mapped carefully, seeking a peripheral nerve or root distribution of sensory change.

Reflexes

An examiner becomes reliable and efficient at testing reflexes only by doing the tests often and by thinking about them as they are being done. The major reflexes to be tested are the biceps (C5, C6), brachioradialis (C5, C6), quadriceps (L3, L4), and ankle (S1). The most important superficial reflex is the plantar response, seeking Babinski's sign. If the patient is very sensitive over the feet, use the Chaddock variation by stroking along the lateral side of the foot or gently and repeatedly do both together, using two halves of a broken tongue depressor.

Gait

The patient should be observed walking into the office, but there is often not enough time or distance to allow one to judge the normal stride. Offices are not designed to test gait, although it is one of the most important aspects of the neurologic examination. If necessary, the physician should ask the patient to walk in a hallway after he or she is dressed. Watch for the smoothness, the arm swing, and the pace of gait. Most important, observe the smoothness and balance on quick turning.

CONCLUSION

The skills of neurologic examination can easily be learned, but reliability and confidence come only from continued application to each patient examined. A brief, well-performed, high-yield neurologic examination not only enables the physician to identify and solve neurologic problems but also gives one confidence that the patients do not have neurologic disease.

BIBLIOGRAPHY

Matthews PM, Arnold DL, editors: *Diagnostic tests in neurology,* New York, 1991, Churchill Livingstone.
Mayo Clinic and Mayo Foundation: *Clinical examination in neurology,* St Louis, 1991, Mosby.
Pryse-Phillips W, Murray TJ: *Essential neurology,* ed 4, New York, 1992, Elsevier.

128 Psychologic Testing

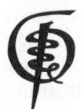

William E. M. Pryse-Phillips

Psychologic (or "psychometric") tests provide valid, reliable data about aspects of a patient's mental status. A variety of psychometric tests can be used to determine whether such personality or cognitive variables are similar to those in a target population. The tests fall under the following main categories:

1. Personality tests. Personality tests provide information about an individual's motives and emotional stability and usually involve completion of a self-administered questionnaire. One such test, the Eysenck Personality Inventory, measures personality along two scales (stability/neuroticism and introversion/extroversion), which allows various patient groups to be characterized. For example, anxiety-neurotics are high on the neuroticism scale and low on the extraversion scale. Many other personality inventories and projective tests are available (e.g., the Minnesota Multiphasic Personal Inventory [MMPI] and the Rorschach test). They are used when information on the presence or degree of depressive illness is sought; in patients with behavioral disturbances, such as suspected conversion reactions; in patients with chronic pain problems; and to assess aspects of personality.
2. Aptitude, interest, and achievement tests. These tests measure global skills or interests in an effort to determine an individual's vocational potential. Again, they compare the performance of an individual with the mean scores of large groups of people who are well established in different careers. The use of this type of test in diagnosis of medical or neurologic states is less common than in counseling.
3. Mood assessment. Tests for depressive illness are most often employed. The best-known short scales are those devised by Hamilton, Zung, or Beck; in each of these the individual is assessed for both psychologic and physical symptoms either by the examiner at interview or by the subject, who completes a self-rating scale. Hamilton's Depression Rating Scale provides both a checklist to help structure the interview and a semiquantitative score to assist in diagnosis.
4. Neuropsychologic tests. These standardized scales are designed to test relatively pure cognitive skills, thus allowing assessment of the presence and site of organic neurologic disease. Various instruments examine, respectively, such items as premorbid ability, overall intellectual endowment, memory (in its many dimensions), calculation, problem solving, alertness and attention, visual or space perception, and constructional skills. The examination of language is another area of interest; the Boston diagnostic aphasia examination and the Western aphasia battery are but two of the complex tools commonly employed in the assessment of spoken language, both to detect the presence of disturbance and to localize the responsible lesion.

A neuropsychologic report can provide much psychometric information, in addition to a detailed interpretation of any particular pattern of results. Such tests refine and deepen the formal bedside examination of higher cerebral functions. Whereas tests in the second group listed earlier describe abilities or skills that are then compared with those of a population of normal individuals, group 4 tests try to determine how specific abilities are being affected by brain disorders in order to localize or characterize such disease. The complex Wechsler Adult Intelligence Scale (WAIS) comprises 11 subtests performing most of the functions listed earlier and provides both a scale of global intellectual ability and values for verbal, performance, and combined (full-scale) intelligence. Subjects with acquired diseases tend to show impairment in performance tests, whereas verbal skills are relatively retained. Some varieties of brain dysfunction, however, result in unique patterns; thus a left-hemisphere stroke lowers verbal rather than performance scores. In the Token Test (widely used to examine receptive language skills) the subject is asked, for example, to ". . . touch a square. . . . In addition to touching the yellow square, touch the blue circle," and is required to follow a simple set of instructions that become progressively more complex; the patient's score suggests to what degree his or her receptive language abilities are impaired.

The tests most likely to be used by internists or neurologists are those that assess the presence, degree, and nature of the dementias. Among these, the mini-mental state examination (MMSE) and its variant, the modified MMS (3MS), are useful screening instruments. They examine orientation, learning capacity, remote memory, attention, calculation, praxis, and aspects of language function and are both valid and reliable, although affected by previous educational standards. The 3MS, although less well validated, nevertheless includes a wider range of cognitive functions than the MMSE and is almost as easy to administer.

The severity of dementing diseases may be determined by using semiquantitative scales such as the Clinical Dementia Rating Scale, which allows the rater to assign scores for memory orientation, judgment and problem solving, community interaction, function in the home, and personal care abilities on the basis of impressions received during interviews of the patient and a caregiver. Thus it acts as a template for the interview, the responses to which may be scored in a defined way, rather than providing a standardized series of questions. Other means of rating disturbance in function include scales for rating a person's ability to perform the usual activities of daily living, both personal (ability to feed, bathe, go to the toilet, dress, transfer, and move about) and instrumental (abilities to use the telephone, shop, handle money, cook, or do housework). Dysfunction in such areas correlates well with cognitive impairment, and since the data are obtained from a caregiver and can be given by telephone, instruments such as these provide a simple, objective assessment of the degree of impairment experienced. Other accepted instruments include the Mattis Dementia Rating Scale, the Brief Cognitive Rating Scale, and the Alzheimer's Disease Assessment Scale, all of which are rather more complex and sometimes require the use of standard test materials but are valid and easily administered after minimal practice by any physician.

Although these assessment procedures are extremely useful, the physician should be aware that whatever technique is used, the outcome represents a probability statement about a given patient's scores resembling those of an identified group of normal subjects or of those with the same disease. But they are not specific; a patient who has chronic organic pain problems could easily score in the same range as a population of hysteria patients on the MMPI. All that can reasonably be concluded in such a case is that the patient has a tendency to focus on somatic complaints to a much greater extent than the normal population. This does not indicate that the patient is malingering. A psychologist would use additional assessment techniques to discriminate between organic and nonorganic components of the patient's reported pain.

Common and appropriate reasons for requesting a neuropsychologic evaluation are (1) assessment of mental status after brain insults such as head injury or stroke; (2) early diagnosis, assessment of severity, follow-up observation, and counseling in patients with suspected dementia; (3) differentiation of the relative part played by functional and by organic components in disease states; (4) detection and evaluation of cognitive deficits in cases of learning disability, mental retardation, and so forth; and (5) counseling of patients and their families regarding the management of acquired cognitive deficits.

BIBLIOGRAPHY

Beck AT et al: An inventory for measuring depression, *Arch Gen Psychiatry* 4:561, 1961.

Berg L: Clinical dementia rating (CDR), *Psychopharmacol Bull* 24:637, 1988.

Boll TJ: The Halstead-Reitan neuropsychological battery. In SB Filskov, TJ Boll, editors: *Handbook of clinical neuropsychology*, New York, 1981, Wiley-Interscience.

Ciplotti L, Warrington EK: Neuropsychological assessment, *J Neurol Neurosurg Psychiatry* 58:655-664, 1995.

Folstein MF, Folstein SE, McHugh PR: "Mini-mental state": a practical method for grading the cognitive state of patients for the clinician, *J Psychiatr Res* 12:189, 1975.

Hamilton M: A rating scale for depression, *J Neurol Neurosurg Psychiatry* 23:56, 1960.

Hamilton M: Development of a rating scale for primary depressive illness, *Br J Soc Clin Psychol* 6:278, 1967.

Lezek MD: *Neuropsychological assessment*, ed 2, New York, 1983, Oxford University.

Mattis S: Mental status examination for organic mental syndrome in the elderly patient.

In Bellck R, Karasu B, editors: *Geriatric psychiatry*, New York, 1976, Grune & Stratton.

Mohs RC, Cohen L: Alzheimer's disease assessment scale (ADAS), *Psychopharmacol Bull* 24:627, 1988.

Reisbert B, Ferris SH: The brief cognitive rating scale (BCRS), *Psychopharmacol Bull* 24:629, 1988.

Teng EL, Chui HC: The modified mini mental state (3MS) examination, *J Clin Psychiatry* 48:314-318, 1987.

Wechsler D: *WAIS-R Manual*, New York, 1981, Psychological Corp.

Wechsler D: Wechsler intelligence scale for children manual, revised ed, New York, 1974, The Psychological Corp.

Zung WWK: A self-rating depression scale, *Arch Gen Psychiatry* 12:63, 1965.

CHAPTER

129 Spinal Fluid Examination

Martin A. Samuels

The introduction of a needle into the lumbar subarachnoid space (lumbar puncture [LP]) allows measurement of the cerebrospinal fluid (CSF) pressure and obtainment of CSF for examination. There is normally free flow of fluid and transmission of pressure between the intracranial and intraspinal subarachnoid spaces. Although some differences exist between the CSF constituents in these two spaces, they are usually minor.

The lumbar puncture is primarily a diagnostic procedure. It is most useful in identifying abnormal intracranial pressure, subarachnoid hemorrhage, and meningeal inflammation and neoplasia. In addition, various abnormal antigens, antibodies, and other abnormal proteins may be present, suggesting specific disease processes (e.g., syphilis, cryptococcosis, and multiple sclerosis).

The patient generally is placed horizontal, in the lateral decubitus position, and a 20-gauge needle is introduced into the L4-5 intervertebral space. A manometer is used to measure the opening pressure after the patient is relaxed. In the first tube, 2 ml of fluid is collected for sugar and protein concentration determinations; 5 ml of fluid is collected in a second tube. This tube should be labeled properly and set aside in the refrigerator; it can be used should any of the determinations require repeating, or unexpected findings in the first sample suggest the need for additional studies. If the circumstances warrant, additional fluid should then be obtained for Gram, India ink, Wright, and Ziehl-Neelsen stains; for bacterial, fungal, or viral cultures; for serologic or special protein studies; and for detection of malignant cells. One milliliter should be collected in the last tube for a cell count. If blood is discovered in the CSF, a cell count on the first tube also should be obtained. The color and clarity of the fluid should be recorded. If low CSF sugar (hypoglycorrhachia) concentration is suspected, and the circumstances warrant, CSF should be collected after the patient has fasted for at least 4 hours. The blood sugar concentration is then stable and "equilibrated" with the CSF sugar concentration; therefore if the concentration is less then 60% of the serum value, hypoglycorrhachia is present.

If the CSF pressure unexpectedly is found to be high (greater than 200 mm H_2O) and the possibility of an intracranial mass lesion exists, only enough fluid to perform the necessary assays should be removed (slowly), and neurologic assistance should be sought. There will be a substantial pressure gradient between the CSF and the extraarachnoid space, and when the needle is removed, fluid will continue to leak from the needle hole in the meninges. In benign intracranial hypertension with papilledema, a lumbar puncture may be therapeutic, and a persistent leak leading to a gradual decompression may be desirable. The risk of brain herniation exists, however, if there are differential pressure gradients within the CSF spaces, caused by either a mass lesion or obstruction of CSF pathways. This risk is greatest when there is a posterior fossa or spinal mass.

Whenever pink or frankly bloody spinal fluid is observed, it is important to distinguish true subarachnoid hemorrhage from a "traumatic tap." Even when the procedure goes smoothly, it is possible for a punctured vessel to bleed and produce a traumatic tap. Usually with a traumatic puncture the CSF clears gradually as it is removed, and the red blood cell count diminishes in each successive tube. One tube should be centrifuged immediately, and the supernatant separated and observed for discoloration. A pink or yellow fluid (provided the CSF protein is less than 150 mg/dl) represents hemoglobin degradation products and indicates that blood has been present for 2 hours or more. If the protein concentration in the CSF is higher than 100 to 150 mg/dl, for any reason, the fluid appears yellow.

The LP procedure should be recorded in the medical record. The recording includes the position of the patient, the type and dose of local anesthetic used, the spine interspace entered, and the size of the needle used. The opening pressure, appearance of the fluid and amount collected in each tube, and tests ordered on each tube should be recorded.

The therapeutic lumbar puncture provides a route of administration for antibiotics, antineoplastic agents, and anesthetics, and a means of relieving the increased pressure in benign intracranial hypertension or subarachnoid hemorrhage.

The main risk in lumbar puncture is brain herniation. This may occur whenever there is an intracranial mass, or obstruction to CSF flow, causing a pressure gradient between two brain compartments. High degrees of obstruction or displacement of the ventricular system are associated with increased risk of brain herniation. All patients with papilledema, focal neurologic signs, or obtundation should be considered for conditions that may cause brain herniation after LP, even though most will not have such conditions. A computed tomography (CT) or magnetic resonance imaging (MRI) brain scan is useful in making this assessment. Other serious risks of LP are less common. Bleeding disorders (including therapeutic anticoagulation) and blood platelet counts below 20,000 to 30,000/mm^3 may lead to intraspinal hemorrhage and cauda equina or spinal cord compression. Infection of skin at the puncture site may result in bacterial meningitis.

The most common complication of lumbar puncture is the post-LP headache. It may appear several hours to a day after the puncture. When a sharp small-bore needle is used (20 gauge or smaller) and a single puncture is successful, the incidence of this complication is approximately 10% to 15%. When a large-bore needle is used or several puncture attempts are necessary, the incidence is probably higher.

The headache is typically bifrontal or generalized, is worse when the patient is upright, and is diminished when he or she lies flat. The headache appears to be due to a loss of CSF that results in intracranial hypotension. Displacement and stretching of pain-sensitive structures then occur when the patient is upright. Maintaining the patient prone (or supine) in the flat, or even in the Trendelenberg position, for 30 to 60 minutes after the procedure diminishes the CSF pressure at the needle puncture site and presumably decreases the persistent leakage of fluid from the subarachnoid space that occurs when the needle is withdrawn.

BIBLIOGRAPHY

Fishman RA: *Cerebrospinal fluid in diseases of the nervous system,* ed 2, Philadelphia, 1992, Saunders.
Marton KI, Gean AD: The spinal tap: a new look at an old test, *Ann Intern Med* 104:840, 1986.
Samuels MA: *Manual of neurologic therapeutics,* ed 5, Boston, 1995, Little, Brown.

CHAPTER

130 Electroencephalography and Evoked Responses

Rodney D. Bell and R. Mañon-Espaillat

ELECTROENCEPHALOGRAPHY

The electroencephalogram (EEG) is a record of the electrical activity of the brain obtained by the standardized placement (International 10-20 system) of recording electrodes on the scalp (Fig. 130-1, *A*). Traditionally the EEG is recorded to paper with a chart recorder; however, newer computer technology has enabled the electrical signals to be digitized and stored on various devices such as optical disks and digital audiotape. With the digitization of the EEG, the potential for

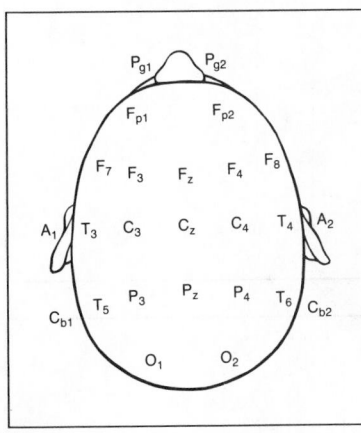

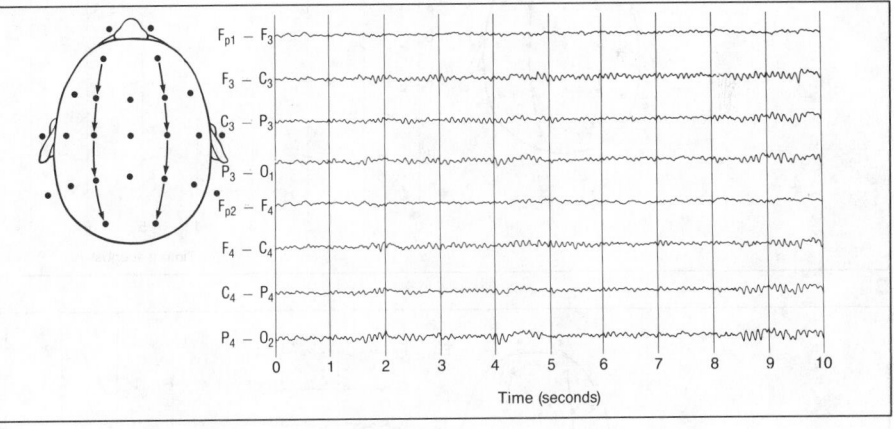

A   **B**

FIGURE 130-1   **A,** The International 10-20 system of electrode placement. Right-sided placements are indicated by even numbers, left-sided placements by odd numbers, and midline placements by z. The C_b notation refers to an electrode placed midway between the posterior temporal and occipital electrodes. C_b was originally part of the International 10-20 system but is seldom used, as it does not accurately reflect cerebellar activity. *A,* Arricular; *C,* central; *F,* frontal; *F_p,* frontal polar; *P,* parietal; *N,* nasopharyngeal; *T,* temporal; *O,* occipital. The electrodes can be connected in various arrays, called montages. The most common montage is straight lines from front to back or transverse across the head. **B,** Eight-channels of normal electroencephalogram. Note the well-organized occipital rhythms (O_1 and O_2) at 8 to 10 Hz; this represents the normal alpha rhythm. The letters and numbers are the standard designations, odd numbers on the left, even on the right. The montages *(electrode connections)* used here are from the front of the head to the back of the head *(occipital).* The first four channels are from the left side of the head, the second four from the right. Current clinical practice of electroencephalography commonly uses 16 to 21 channels of EEG. The distance between each of the vertical lines represents 1 second *(10 seconds for the recording shown).*

developing new ways of viewing the electrical signals of the brain is possible, along with the advantage of decreasing the storage space required for paper (hard copy).

The EEG is obtained by recording from these scalp electrodes in a standard pattern of electrode connections called montages. The montages that are used may vary among individual laboratories (Fig. 130-1, *A* and *B*). The EEG is useful in providing information about the electrical physiologic processes of the brain. Electroencephalography constitutes the most valuable laboratory test in the evaluation of patients with epilepsy. It is a safe, noninvasive, and readily repeated procedure by which patients can be followed up and evaluated during the interictal or ictal periods. It is important to realize that a normal interictal EEG result does not exclude the presence of epilepsy. An initial EEG reveals an epileptiform (suggestive of epilepsy, i.e., containing spikes or sharp waves) abnormality in about 55% of cases. This percentage can be increased to approximately 80% by obtaining serial EEGs over a prolonged time (i.e., a minimum of three EEGs at

intervals of several months). The EEG is also more likely to reveal epileptiform activity in younger patients (below 10 years of age, 80%) than in older patients (above age 40, 30%). Sleep recording and cerebral activation procedures such as hyperventilation and photic stimulation also increase the percentage of "positive" EEG results. Sleep deprivation for 24 hours results in activation (production of an epileptiform abnormality) of the EEG in about 40% of patients. In general, withdrawal of anticonvulsant medication for the purposes of obtaining an abnormal EEG result in a patient with the clinical diagnosis of epilepsy is not warranted because it may precipitate seizures or status epilepticus. Repeating the EEG in a patient with clinical epilepsy is more likely to yield a normal EEG finding and is far less dangerous to the patient. If, however, the diagnosis of epilepsy is in question and the EEG result has been repeatedly normal, it is reasonable to taper and stop anticonvulsant medication and repeat the EEG.

The predominant abnormalities seen in epilepsy are the spike (an evanescent electrical event lasting less than 70 ms) and the sharp wave

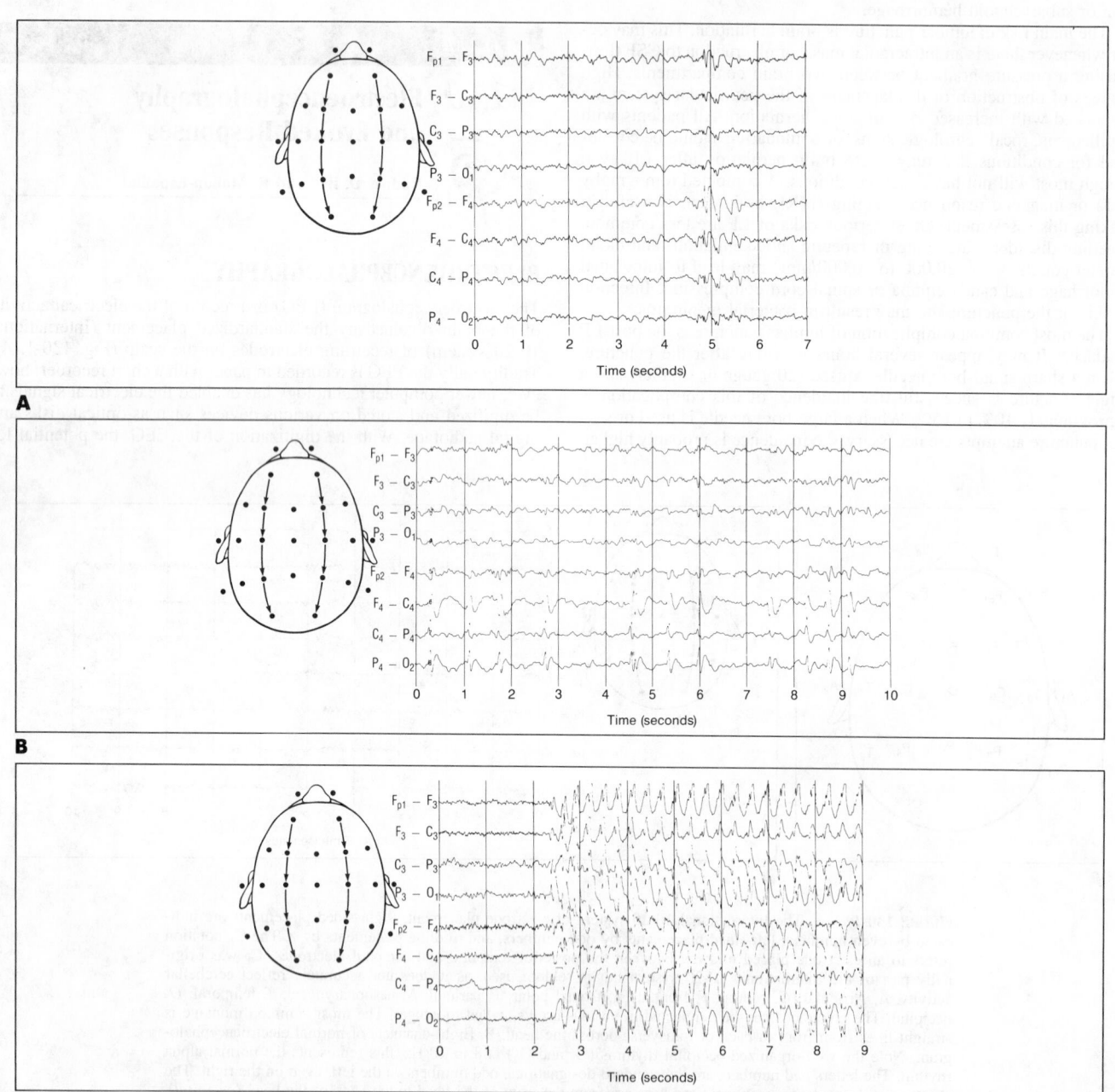

FIGURE 130-2 **A,** Spike and slow wave in a 25-year-old man. **B,** Sharp wave in a 9-year-old boy. **C,** Three-hertz spike and wave in a 1-year-old child with "classic" absence seizures.

(a transient electrical event lasting between 70 and 200 ms). Examples of these events are shown in Fig. 130-2. Spikes and slow waves can occur in adults and children. "Classic" 3-Hz spike- and slow-wave complexes are seen in children with absence seizures. Bursts of multiple spikes followed by a slow wave repeating at rates of every 2 to 3 seconds occur in patients with myoclonic seizures. Paroxysmal rhythmic slow-wave activity (1 to 3 Hz) can also be associated with epilepsy.

When epileptic seizures are poorly controlled, despite adequate therapeutic concentrations of antiepileptic drugs, or when it is necessary to differentiate epileptic seizures from nonepileptic disorders such as pseudoseizures, syncope, movement disorders, or sleep disorders, it is often necessary to admit the patient for prolonged video EEG monitoring to further characterize the nature of the event. With this technology it is possible to record EEG signals continuously for up to several weeks. The EEG signals are synchronized with a videotape of the patient. This allows the clinician to review the clinical and electrographic manifestation of the event as many times as needed. Video EEG can provide information such as the presence and location of interictal epileptiform and nonepileptiform abnormalities, as well as the site of onset and spread of electrographic seizures. Prolonged inpatient video EEG monitoring is very useful, but it can be very expensive and time consuming. At times, no events are recorded, and even when they occur, the absence of abnormalities in the EEG would not rule out epileptic seizures. Prolonged EEG monitoring can also be obtained on an ambulatory basis for up to several days. This allows the recording of interictal epileptiform and nonepileptiform abnormalities. Occasionally electrographic seizures are recorded. The drawback of this technique is the absence of videotape of the clinical behavior to correlate with the abnormalities in the EEG. In some circumstances the presence of much artifact makes interpretation difficult.

In approximately 20% to 40% of patients epilepsy cannot be satisfactorily controlled with the optimal use of antiepileptic drugs. Prolonged inpatient video EEG monitoring with scalp electrodes and at times with intracranial electrodes such as subdural or depth electrodes is necessary to localize the onset and spread of electrographic seizures. This information is used to plan the resection of the epileptogenic zone.

Computed tomography (CT) scanning and magnetic resonance imaging (MRI) have gained widespread acceptance, making the EEG far less important in screening patients for structural disease of the nervous system and in localizing structural brain abnormalities. The EEG is generally not as sensitive as the CT/MRI scan in identifying structural abnormalities. Nevertheless, in certain instances (e.g., herpes simplex encephalitis and strokes), the EEG usually reveals an abnormality long before the CT/MRI scan. This example is particularly relevant because early detection and treatment of this disease are vital. Thus the EEG is complementary to the CT/MRI scan in the identification of structural disease.

Clinical electroencephalography is based on the recognition of electrical patterns. Certain patterns are relatively specific (e.g., spikes for epilepsy), whereas others, such as diffuse slowing (implying diffuse neuronal dysfunction from any cause), are nonspecific. Certain disorders produce patterns that, although nonspecific, help to suggest, support, or establish a diagnosis. Specific patterns with clinical relevance are discussed later.

Hypoxia

Cardiopulmonary arrest is a common clinical problem. The EEG (and serial EEGs) can provide useful physiologic and prognostic information about patients who have experienced cardiopulmonary arrest. The main effects of progressive hypoxia on the EEG are reduction and slowing of the normal background alpha activity (8 to 13 Hz), increased theta activity (4 to 7 Hz), generalized delta slowing (1 to 3 Hz), and suppression of all activity. After a hypoxic insult to the brain several patterns that have prognostic significance can emerge. These patterns have been most thoroughly studied after a minimum of 6 hours has elapsed after the insult. To use the EEG as a prognostic indicator, at least this amount of time should have passed.

An EEG showing a normal background, reactivity to external stimuli, and sleep patterns usually indicates the potential for clinical improvement. Patterns indicating a poor prognosis after a hypoxic insult are (1) alpha coma, which is an EEG pattern that looks very much like a normal awake tracing but is nonreactive to stimulus (alpha coma is also seen with brain stem lesions); (2) burst suppression, a pattern in which the EEG background varies between periods of relative flattening and bursts of higher-voltage slow or sharp activity; (3) periodic spike-wave activity with isoelectric intervals, which is a pattern generally associated with myoclonic jerks; and (4) electrocerebral inactivity, which is present in patients with brain death (Fig. 130-3).

Hepatic Disease

In hepatic stupor or coma, as with any metabolic encephalopathy, the EEG result is generally abnormal by the time there is any alteration of consciousness. In the early stages of hepatic encephalopathy the EEG shows progressive slowing until a triphasic pattern appears. Triphasic waves do not occur in every patient with hepatic coma, nor are they specific for this disease. However, when they do occur, they suggest a hepatic cause of the coma. Triphasic waves consist of medium- to high-voltage broad waves occurring rhythmically or in trains of 1 to 2 Hz in a symmetric fashion over both hemispheres (Fig. 130-4, *A*).

Herpes Simplex Encephalitis

The EEG is frequently the first abnormal laboratory test finding in herpes simplex encephalitis. The earliest changes are focal, temporal slow waves generally in the delta range (1 to 3 Hz). These waves are frequently followed by large, sharp waves, which appear over the affected region and occur with a periodicity of 2 to 4 seconds. These sharp waves can occur bilaterally (Fig. 130-4, *B*).

Creutzfeldt-Jakob Disease

Creutzfeldt-Jakob disease is a rare dementing disease caused by an atypical infectious agent. The classic EEG findings consist of periodic complexes that may be unilateral, are often triphasic, and repeat every 0.5 to 4.0 seconds. In sleep these discharges tend to disappear. The periodic patterns may be associated with myoclonus.

Subacute Sclerosing Panencephalitis

Subacute sclerosing panencephalitis is a rare progressive inflammatory disease in young children and adolescents believed to be caused by a variant of the measles virus. The disease is characterized by progressive intellectual deterioration, a variety of abnormal movements, and a characteristic EEG pattern. The EEG pattern consists of periodic, high-voltage, repetitive polyphasic and sharp- and slow-wave complexes ranging from 0.5 to 2.0 seconds in duration and occurring every 4 to 15 seconds (Fig. 130-4, *C*).

Dementia

Senile dementia and Alzheimer's disease in the early stages cause very little alteration in the EEG. Therefore an abnormal EEG result is more suggestive of a specific structural problem or of a treatable form of dementia, suggesting the need for more extensive clinical investigation. In the late stages of Alzheimer's disease the EEG pattern generally is diffusely slow (Fig. 130-5, *A*).

Metabolic Encephalopathy

Any metabolic derangement, including hypoglycemia or hyperglycemia, hyponatremia or hypernatremia, hypocalcemia or hypercalcemia, uremia, or drug intoxication, that alters sensorium can affect the EEG result. The changes in each of these metabolic derangements are not specific and generally consist in a slowing of the background rhythms from the normal alpha frequency (8 to 13 Hz) to the theta range (4 to 7 Hz). As the derangement becomes more profound, the EEG slows further into the delta range (1 to 3 Hz) (Fig. 130-5, *B*).

In patients with renal failure the slowing of the EEG generally parallels the degree of alteration of consciousness. In patients who have the dialysis disequilibrium syndrome, however, the EEG may reflect the shifts in osmolality with high-voltage paroxysmal activity.

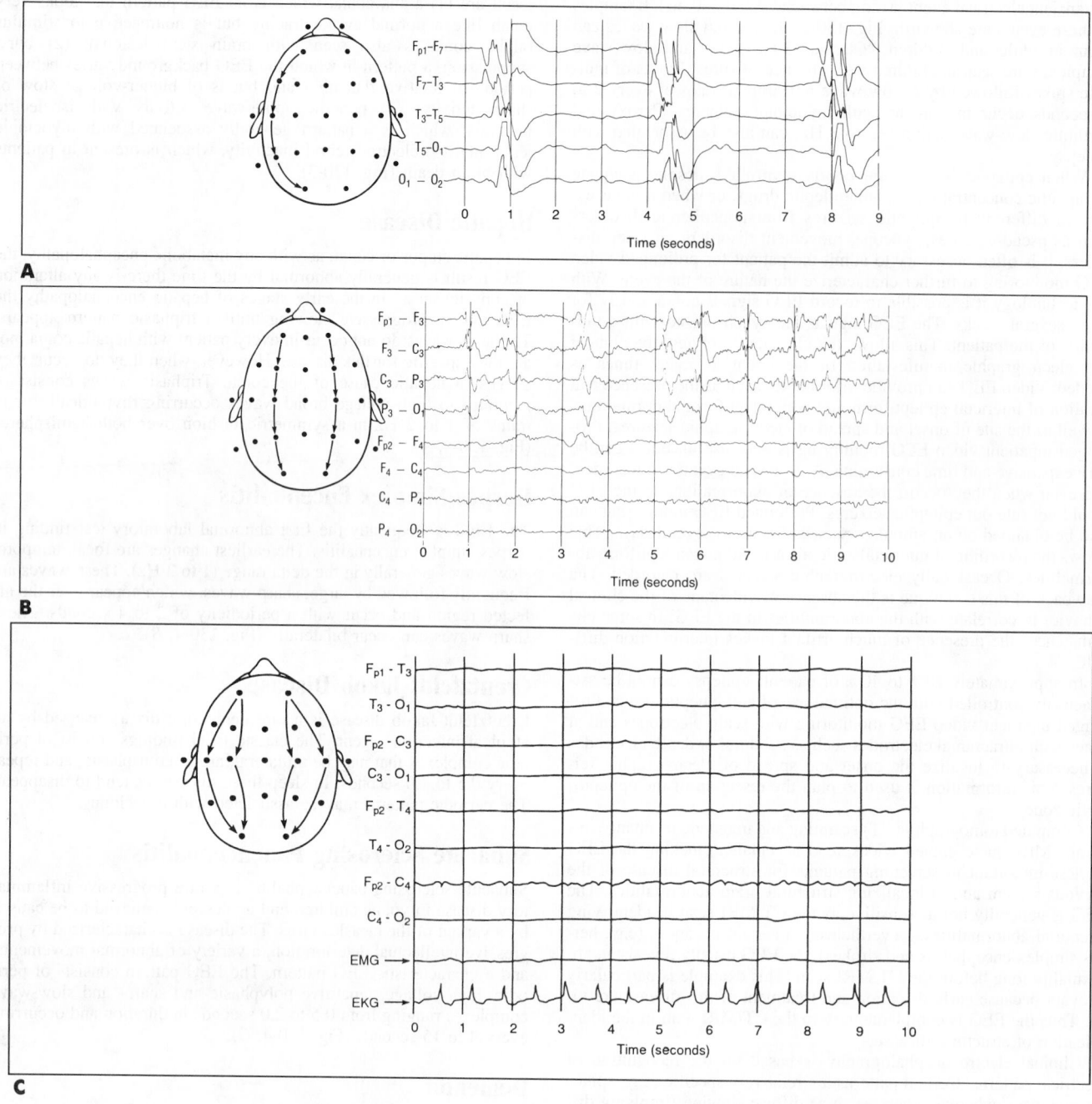

FIGURE 130-3   A, Burst suppression pattern in a 49-year-old man after cardiac arrest. **B,** Periodic spike wave associated with myoclonic jerks of the arm. **C,** Electrocerebral silence in a patient with brain death. Double electrode distance is used, as well as an electromyographic electrode and electrocardiographic monitoring.

Dialysis dementia is a progressively fatal disorder characterized by slowly progressive dementia, speech disturbances, myoclonus, abnormal movements, and convulsions. The EEG can aid in this diagnosis because there is a characteristic pattern of slowing of the background activity with superimposed bursts of high-amplitude slow waves, triphasic contoured waves, sharp waves, or spike- and slow-wave complexes.

Focal Structural Disease

The EEG is neither as specific nor as sensitive as the CT scan in the diagnosis of focal structural disease of the brain. Nevertheless, in either early strokes or small, focal structural disease of the brain the EEG can reveal positive information not available from the CT scan.

EEG features characteristic of focal structural disease include (1) continuous focal delta waves (1 to 3 Hz), which are irregular in waveform; (2) intermittent delta waves, which are regular in waveform; (3) depression or absence of usual background activity in the vicinity of the local slowing; and (4) epileptiform discharges, which remain or begin focally (Fig. 130-5, *C*).

EVOKED RESPONSES

Advances in microprocessing in the early 1970s and commercialization of signal-averaging computers made possible the measurement of small changes in the electrical activity of the brain caused by an external stimulus. These signs, small in voltage as compared with EEG, are not obtainable without the aid of a computer

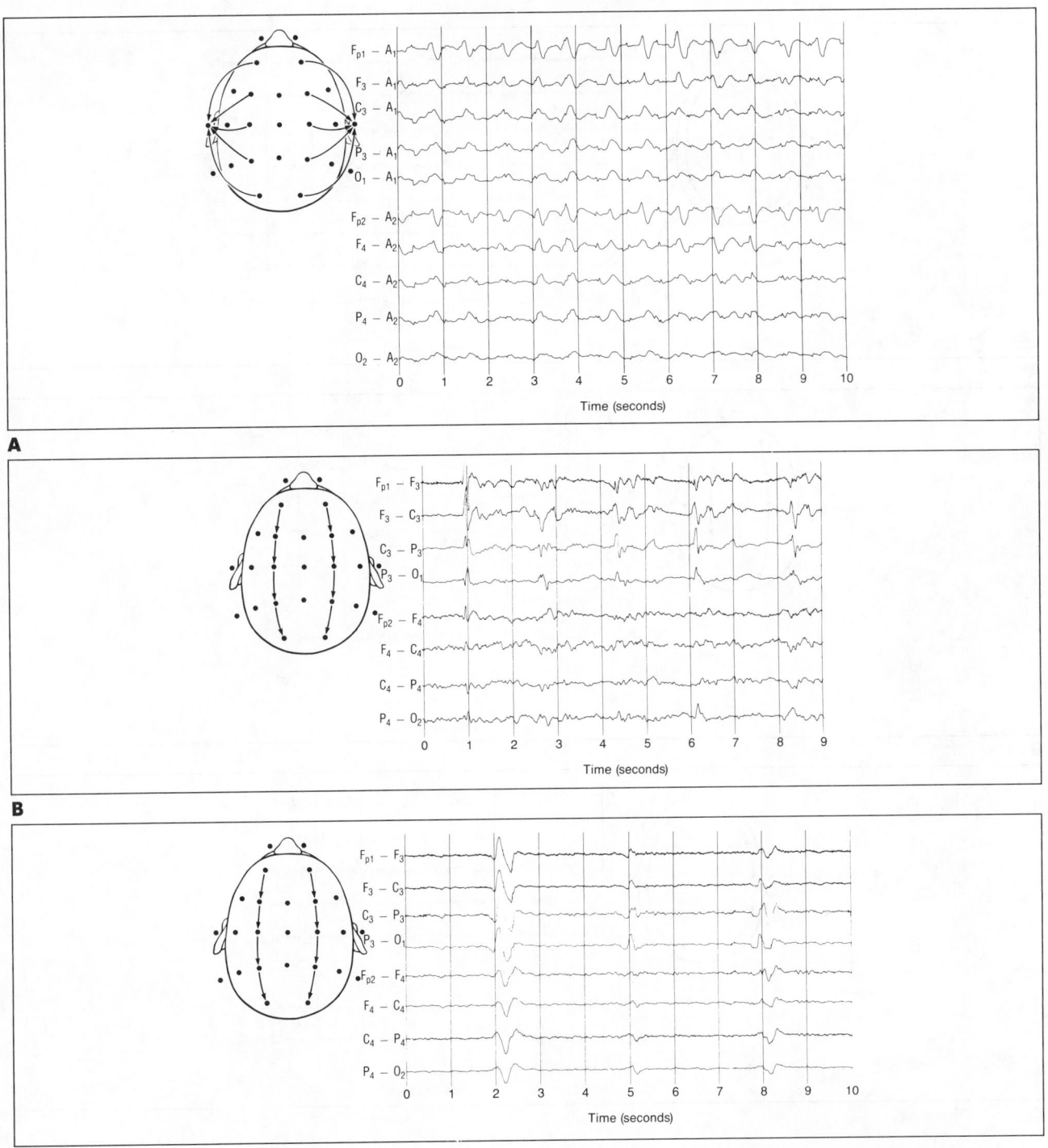

FIGURE 130-4   A, Triphasic waves in a 48-year-old patient with hepatic coma. In this instance all electrodes are referenced to the ear. **B,** Burst of sharp waves in a 29-year-old woman with biopsy-proven herpes simplex encephalitis. **C,** High-voltage periodic complexes in a 6-year-old patient with subacute sclerosing panencephalitis.

that detects and averages the electrical signal and retains it in memory. To average, a sensory stimulus is given that triggers the computer to record a sample of brain electrical activity over a fixed length of time, generally from 10 to 500 ms. The stimulus is repeated several hundred or thousand times, and each evoked potential (or evoked response) is averaged by the computer. The background activity (essentially the EEG) tends to average to a straight line, leaving the recorded evoked potential from the sensory stimulus.

Presently three types of evoked responses are used in clinical medicine: brain stem auditory evoked potentials (BAEPs), visual evoked potentials (VEPs), and somatosensory evoked potentials (SEPs). They are used (1) to demonstrate abnormal sensory system function when the history and neurologic examination findings are equivocal; (2) to reveal the presence of a clinically unsuspected malfunction in the sensory system when demyelinating disease is suggested by symptoms and signs in another area of the nervous system; (3) to help define the anatomic distribution of a disease

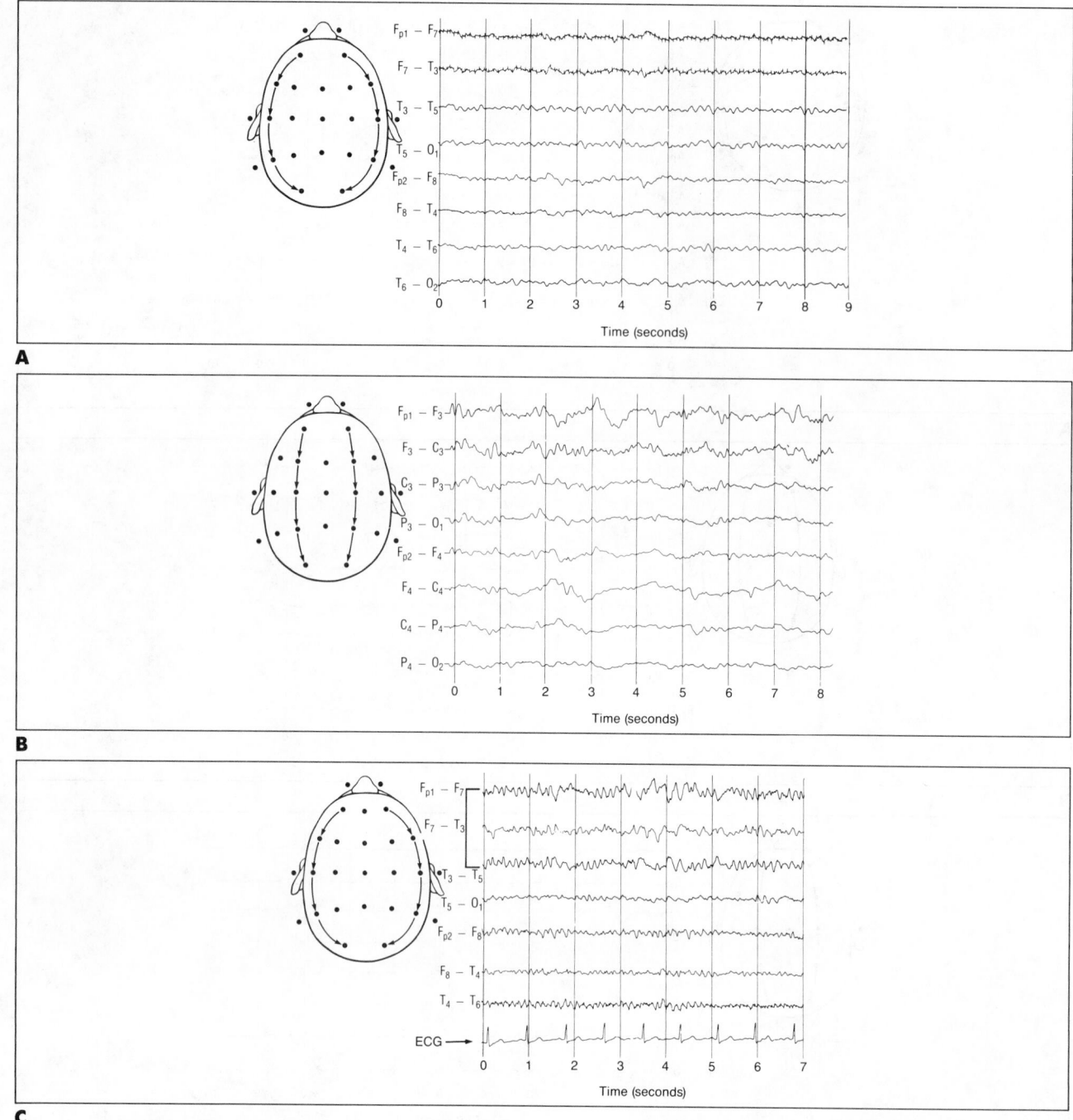

FIGURE 130-5   **A,** An electroencephalogram (EEG) from a 67-year-old patient with senile dementia, Alzheimer's type. The EEG shows mild slowing. **B,** An EEG from a patient with hyponatremia. This type of EEG can be seen in any form of metabolic derangement. **C,** An EEG from a patient with a brain tumor. Focal slowing is indicated by the bracket.

process; and (4) to monitor changes in a patient's status objectively over time.

Visual Evoked Potentials

The pattern-reversal visual evoked potential (PVEP) is a widely used and reproducible response. It is generally performed by using small checks, usually subtending the eye 28 minutes to 1 degree of an arc. These checks appear on a monitor or television screen that has a specific known luminance. The size check fills a 3-degree span of foveal vision and produces a response that is nearly as large as a signal that covers 10 to 20 degrees. The checks are reversed (i.e., black to white) at a specific rate, and the monocular response is recorded over the visual cortex from occipital electrodes O_1, O_z, and O_2. The major potential in this technique is a large positive wave seen at about 100 ms, usually maximally from the midoccipital electrode O_z (Fig. 130-6). This potential is referred to as the P100 response. Measurements usually taken are the (1) absolute latency, (2) interocular absolute latency difference, (3) amplitude, and (4) interocular amplitude difference ratio. Both the shape and the latency of PVEPs are significantly affected by stimulus parameters including luminance, check and pattern size, rate of reversal, and nature of the stimulator, as well as such factors as visual acuity, body temperature, age, and gender.

A prolongation of the latency of the P100 response, an interocular

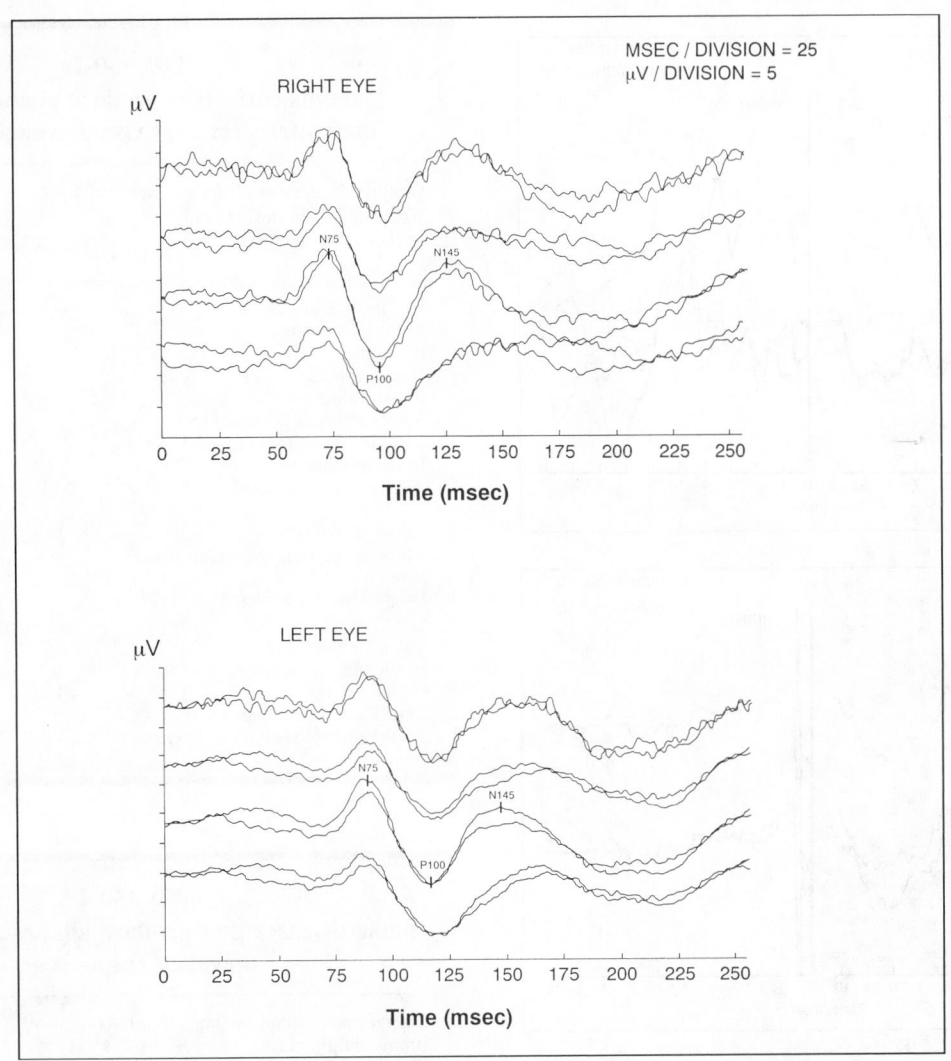

FIGURE 130-6 Normal pattern-reversal visual evoked response (PVEP) with the P100 response at 100 msec in the right eye. The left P100 response is prolonged more than 6 msec as compared with the right. This patient has multiple sclerosis. Microvolts (μV) are in multiples of 5 N75 and N145 indicate the major negative deflections before and after the P100 response with their corresponding approximate latency.

difference of greater than 6 ms (each laboratory must establish its own normal values), and a difference greater than 50% in amplitude of the P100 response are suggestive of an abnormality anterior to the optic chiasm (Fig. 130-6). However, this test is not specific, and the difference between a demyelinating lesion as seen in multiple sclerosis and a compressive lesion involving the optic nerve cannot be ascertained on the basis of this test.

The major clinical use for PVEPs at present is in the diagnosis of subclinical optic neuritis or multiple sclerosis. About 90% of patients who have a clear history of optic neuritis have abnormal PVEPs, regardless of the interval since the clinical episode of neuritis. Abnormalities occur in 75% to 97% of patients with definite multiple sclerosis, including those without visual symptoms.

Abnormalities of the PVEP are not specific for optic neuritis or multiple sclerosis (Box 130-1). Prolonged latencies can occur in diseases that resemble multiple sclerosis on clinical examination, such as the spinocerebellar degenerations.

Brainstem Auditory Evoked Potential

The preferred stimulus for evaluation of the brainstem auditory system is a high-frequency click produced by a high-quality earphone given at a fixed stimulus rate and intensity. Signals generated from this stimulus can be recorded from scalp and ear electrodes. In normal subjects a total of seven short-latency waves can be defined

within 10 msec of the click each measured for absolute latency and compared with that of normal controls (Fig. 130-7, *A*). Wave I arises in the distal portion of the acoustic nerve; wave V is thought to arise near the inferior colliculus. The generators for the other waves are less clearly defined but can be thought of as follows: wave II, cochlear nucleus and proximal acoustic nerve; wave III, superior olivary complex; and wave IV, tract or nuclei of the lateral lemniscus. Many clinicians believe that with the exception of wave I, all waves of the short-latency BAEP originate from a complex interaction of numerous generators in the brainstem and cannot be separated anatomically.

Stimulation rate, click polarity, and intensity are critical parameters in recording the BAEP. Therefore these parameters must be specified in any recording, and normal values defined for each rate, type of click polarity, and intensity above threshold that is used.

BAEPs are the best noninvasive laboratory tests for the detection of acoustic neuromas. The true-positive rate is 98%, and the false-positive rate is about 1%. The BAEP patterns found with acoustic tumors are not specific. Most commonly, wave I is present and all other waves are delayed or absent (Fig. 130-7, *B*). Small lesions produce a prolongation of the wave I to III interpeak latency, and large lesions compressing the brain stem may produce a prolongation of the wave III to V interpeak latency in the contralateral ear.

BAEPs are also useful in the diagnosis of multiple sclerosis. Abnormalities in BAEPs occur in 21% to 55% of patients without brain-

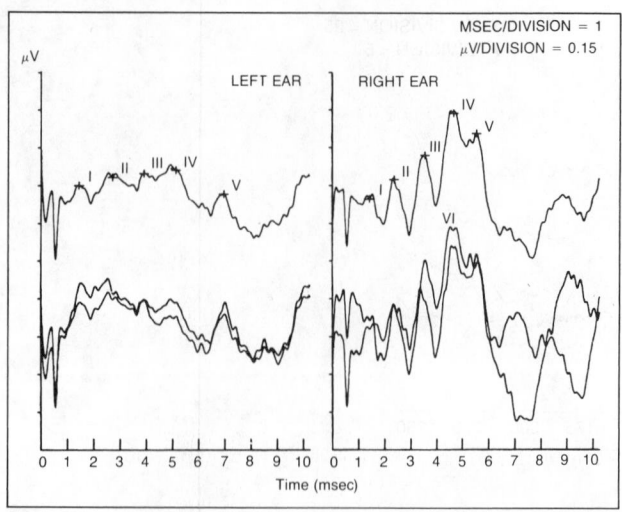

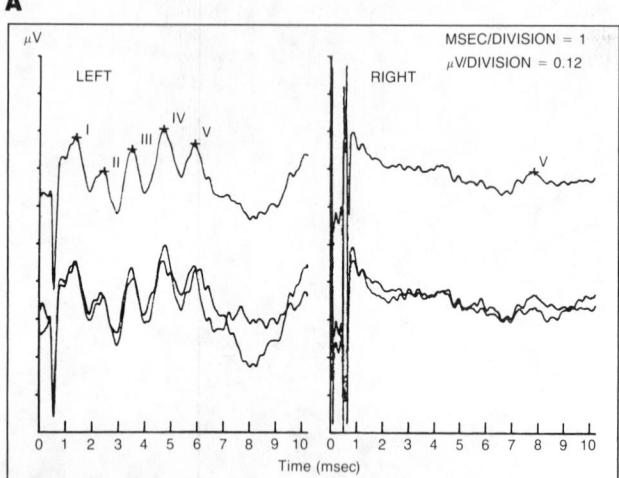

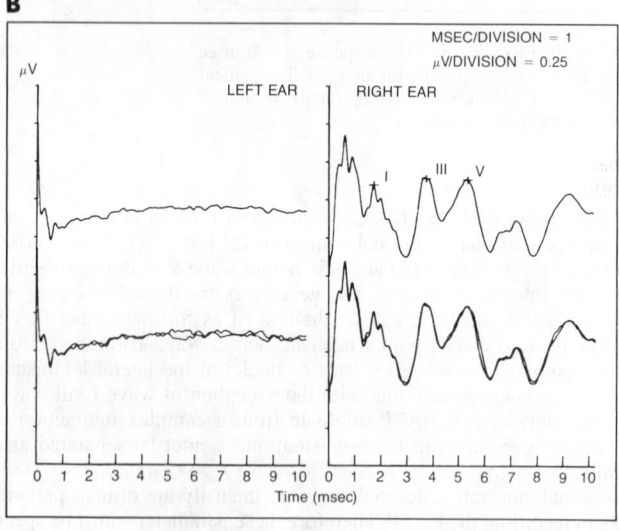

FIGURE 130-7 **A,** A normal brain stem auditory evoked response (BAEP) is shown in the right ear. The left BAEP response is abnormal as a result of the prolongation of left waves I to V and I to III interpeak latencies. This patient has a cerebellopontine angle tumor. Microvolts *(μV)* are in multiples of 0.15. **B,** A BAEP from a patient with an acoustic neuroma on the right. There is essentially no response on the right. Microvolts *(μV)* are in multiples of 0.12. **C,** A BAEP from a child with meningitis. The response is normal on the right ear, and there is lack of response in the left ear, even at high-stimulus intensities, indicating that hearing is impaired on the left. Microvolts *(μV)* are in multiples of 0.25.

BOX 130-1

Some diseases that produce abnormalities in the pattern-reversal visual evoked response

Compressive lesions of the anterior visual pathways
Extrinsic and intrinsic tumors
Pseudotumor cerebri

Generalized central nervous system diseases
Parkinson's disease
Pernicious anemia
Sarcoid
Neurosyphilis
Renal failure
Spinocerebellar degenerations
Charcot-Marie-Tooth disease
Phenylketonuria
Adrenoleukodystrophy

Spinal cord diseases
Chronic progressive myelopathy

Large refractive errors
Glaucoma
Toxic amblyopia
Amblyopia ex anopsia
Hydrocephalus
Central serous retinopathy
Factitious prolongation of latency

BOX 130-2

Some diseases that produce abnormal brain stem evoked responses

Lateral pontomedullary junction infarcts
Brainstem gliomas
Multiple sclerosis
Neonatal hearing loss
Vitamin B_{12} deficiency
Acoustic neuromas
Brain death
Friedreich's ataxia
Charcot-Marie-Tooth disease
Hereditary cerebellar ataxia
Metachromatic leukodystrophy
Adrenoleukodystrophy
Pelizaeus-Merzbacher disease

---

stem symptoms or signs. The most common abnormalities are low-amplitude wave V and prolongation of the III-V interpeak latency. BAEPs are also useful in the early diagnosis of hearing loss in young children who cannot cooperate for formal audiometric testing. They are particularly valuable in evaluating the possibility of hearing loss in children with meningitis (Fig. 130-7, *C*). A partial list of other diseases in which BAEP result has been abnormal is given in Box 130-2.

Somatosensory Evoked Potential

Somatosensory evoked potentials are produced by repetitively stimulating with brief electrical pulses peripheral nerves and recording at various locations along the nervous system to the sensory cortex. Although this technique has been studied for many years, there is lack of uniformity in the recording techniques and the neuroanatomic substrates of the responses obtained with various amounts of stimulation. Therefore in 1985 the American Electroencephalographic Society published guidelines for clinical evoked potentials to help address

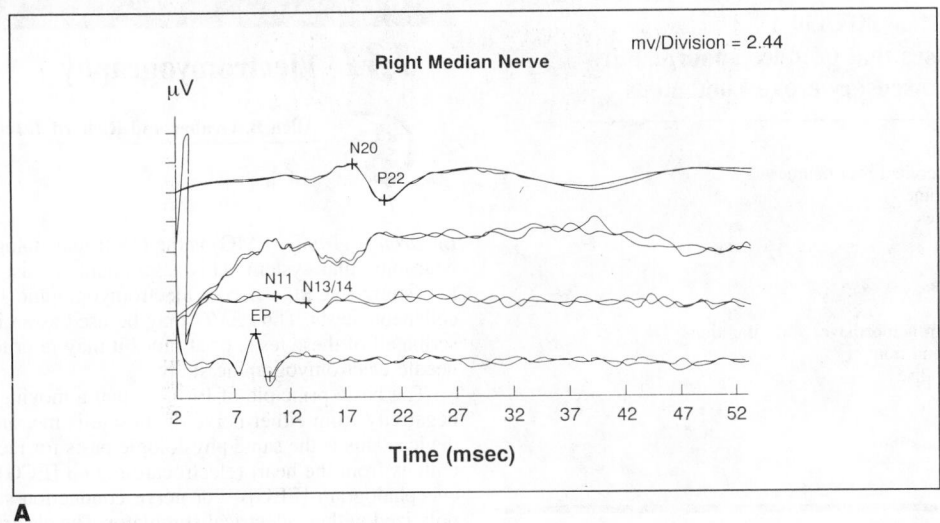

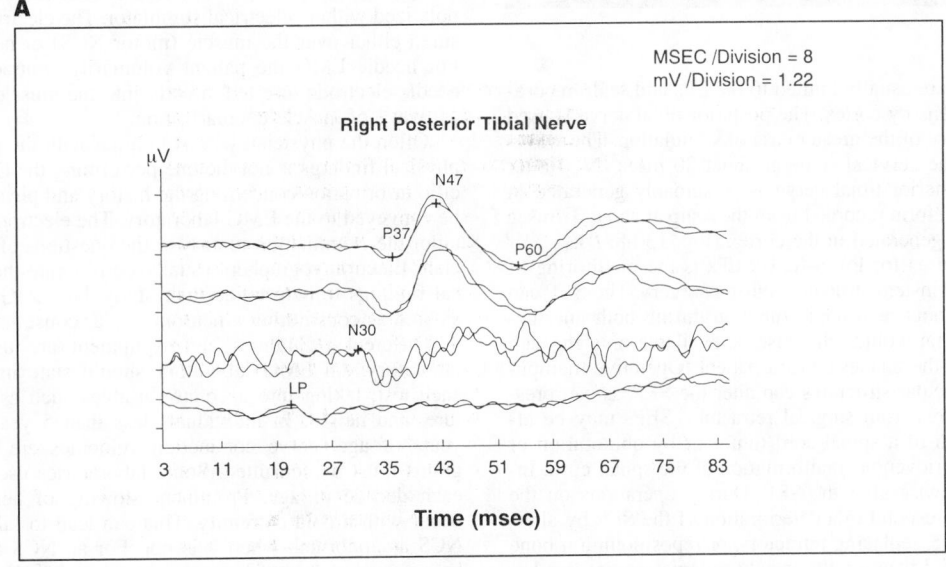

FIGURE 130-8 **A,** A normal median nerve somatosensory evoked potential. The waveforms are thought to represent the following: (1) Erb's point *(EP),* the brachial plexus; (2) N_{11}, cervical cord root entry zone; (3) N_{13-14}, dorsal columns and cuneate nucleus; (4) N_{20}, the thalamus or thalamocortical radiations; and (5) P_{22}, the cortex. **B,** A normal posterior tibial somatosensory evoked potential. The waveforms shown are thought to represent the following: (1) lumbar potential *(LP),* the entry zone for LPs; (2) N_{30}, the thalamus; and (3) P_{37}, cortex.

this issue. The most widely used are the median nerve SEP and posterior tibial nerve SEP. By convention, positive waves are designated with a capital P followed by a number. The number refers to the number of milliseconds following the stimulus where the waveform occurs, for example, P_{38}. Similarly, a negative wave is designated by a capital N followed by a number representing the number of milliseconds following the stimulus, for example, N_{11}.

Median Nerve Somatosensory Evoked Potential. Median nerve SEPs are generally recorded by placing electrodes over Erb's point, the cervical spine over the C5 or C2 process, and over the somatosensory cortex on the scalp. Using a repetitive stimulation rate of 4 to 7/sec, waveforms are generated and represent volleys traversing the posterior columns, medial lemnisci, and spinocerebellar tracts. The waveform recorded over Erb's point is generated from the brachial plexus; the waveform that appears at approximately 11 msec (N_{11}) is generated in the cervical cord root entry zone or posterior columns; the waveform recorded from the C5 or C2 (N_{13-14}) process is generated in the dorsal column and dorsal column nucleus; the scalp-recorded wave at about 20 msec (N_{20}) is generated in the thalamus or thalamocortical radiations; and the waveform occurring at 22 msec (P_{22}) is considered to be of cortical origin (Fig. 130-8, *A*).

SEPs are sensitive to lesions of the dorsal column–medial lemniscus systems and are generally not affected by isolated involvement of the spinothalamic tract. Abnormalities are generally defined by a prolongation of the interpeak wave latency compared with empirically established normal values or by a side-to-side difference of greater than 1 msec. A prolonged interpeak latency between Erb's point and the dorsal column (N_{11}) suggests a lesion located between the proximal portions of the brachial plexus and the dorsal column nuclei. An abnormal latency between the dorsal column and the thalamus and cortex (N_{20}-P_{22} suggests a lesion located between the medulla and the thalamocortical systems. Cerebral lesions usually abolish N_{20} and P_{22} rather than prolonging their latencies. Median nerve short-latency SEPs have been reported to be abnormal in 63% to 87% of patients with definite multiple sclerosis, many of whom appear to lack signs of sensory dysfunction on the appropriate side.

Lower-Limb Somatosensory Evoked Potential. For testing the lower limb (tibial and peroneal nerves) the reference point for latency measurements is the time when the volley of stimuli passes through the cauda equina and lower spinal cord. Activity in these structures is generally referred to as the lumbar potential (LP). Although additional recording sites can be added anywhere along the

BOX 130-3

**Some diseases that produce abnormalities
of somatosensory-evoked potentials**

Peripheral nerve lesions
Brachial plexus and cervical root trauma
Thoracic outlet syndrome
Cervical radiculopathies
Spinal cord trauma
Multiple sclerosis
Lumbar radiculopathies
Thalamic tumors
Cerebral and brainstem hemorrhages and infarctions
Coma secondary to head trauma
Pelizaeus-Merzbacher disease
Adrenoleukodystrophy
Friedreich's ataxia
Spinocerebellar degenerations
Myelodysplasias

neuroaxis, recordings are usually limited to the LPs and scalp recordings over the somatosensory cortex. The posterior tibial nerve is used most frequently because of the greater ease of stimulation. The waveform recorded from the cervical spine at about 30 msec (N_{30}) after stimulation of the posterior tibial nerve is presumably generated in the thalamus. The waveform recorded from the scalp at about 37 msec (P_{37}) is thought to be generated in the cortex (Fig. 130-8, *B*).

One of the major uses for lower-limb SEPs is the monitoring of the spinal cord and brainstem structures during surgery. The SEP can provide information about neurologic function during both anesthesia and an operation that would otherwise be available only through clinical assessment of the unanesthetized patient. Operative manipulation of neural or vascular structures can alter the SEP, as can pressure on neural structures from surgical retractors. SEPs may be affected by manipulation of a spinal cord tumor or by obliteration of vessels feeding an arteriovenous malformation of the spinal cord. Instrumentation can likewise alter the SEP. During operations on the spine the surgeon can respond to a deterioration of the SEP by altering the spinal curvature, replacing retractors, or repositioning a bone graft or Harrington rod. Likewise, the anesthesiologist can reverse hemodilution or raise the arterial blood pressure. Therefore the SEP in the anesthetized patient can provide useful physiologic information about the functional integrity of the nervous system that would otherwise be unavailable.

As with other evoked potentials, an abnormal SEP finding indicates only an anatomic lesion that disrupts the normal physiologic mechanisms of that system, not a specific disease process (Box 130-3).

BIBLIOGRAPHY

American Electroencephalographic Society: Guidelines for clinical evoked potential studies, *J Clin Neurophysiol* 1:3, 1984.

Chiappa KH: Evoked potentials in clinical medicine, ed 2, New York, 1990, Raven.

Daly DD, Pedley TA: *Current practice of clinical encephalopathy*, ed 2, New York, 1990, Raven.

Hecox KE et al: Brainstem auditory evoked response in the diagnosis of pediatric neurologic disease, *Neurology* 31:832, 1981.

Niedermeyer E, Lopes da Silva F, editors: *Electroencephalography: basic principles, clinical applications, and related fields*, ed 2, Baltimore, 1987, Urban & Schwazenberg.

Tyner FS, Knot JR, Myer WB: *Fundamentals of EEG technology*, vol 2, *Clinical correlates*, New York, 1989, Raven.

CHAPTER

131   Electromyography

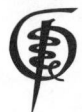

Allen B. Gruber and Richard J. Barohn

Electromyography (EMG) is the electrophysiologic assessment of the neuromuscular system. This assessment consists of a nerve conduction study (NCS), a needle electromyographic study, and other miscellaneous tests. Thus *EMG* may be used as an inclusive term to describe all of these tests, or at times it may refer to the more restricted needle electromyographic study.

The basic principle of EMG is that a moving wave of an electronegativity from either nerve or muscle is measured with a recording device. This is the same physiologic basis for recording electrical potentials from the heart (electrocardiogram [ECG]) and brain (electroencephalogram [EEG]). For nerve conduction studies a nerve is depolarized with an electrical stimulator. The electrical potential is measured either over the muscle (motor NCS) or nerve (sensory NCS). For needle EMG the patient voluntarily contracts a muscle, and a needle electrode inserted directly into the muscle records the electrical wave of muscle depolarization.

Often the physician who is familiar with the patient's history and physical findings is not the one performing the EMG. Therefore specific information concerning the history and physical findings should be conveyed to the EMG laboratory. The electromyographer can then tailor the examination to answer the questions of the referring physician. Electromyographers usually corroborate the history and physical findings to help guide their study, but EMG should not be considered as constituting a neuromuscular consultation.

Different techniques and equipment are used by each EMG laboratory. An EMG laboratory should state its normal values for each test, taking into account variables such as age, skin temperature, and height. In individuals less than 5 years or more than 60 years of age, nerve conduction velocities are slower, and nomograms must be consulted. Some laboratories use normative data for each decade of age. Prominent slowing of nerve conduction can occur with a cold extremity. This can lead to falsely interpreting an NCS as abnormal, when it is not. For an NCS an extremity should be warmed to a surface temperature of 34° C or more. An EMG report should include the raw data and offer an electrodiagnostic interpretation considering technical limitations, such as cooperation of the patient.

For a motor NCS a nerve is supramaximally stimulated with a surface stimulator placed over it at various locations. Electrical activity is recorded with a surface electrode over the belly of a standard muscle innervated by the nerve being studied. For example, in a median motor NCS (Fig. 131-1, *A*), stimulation is typically just above the wrist and at the elbow. The recording electrode is placed over the belly of the abductor pollicus brevis muscle. The evoked muscle potential (also known as the compound motor or muscle action potential [CMAP]) is displayed on an oscilloscope screen and is usually permanently recorded on paper. The amplitude of the CMAP is recorded in millivolts. Amplitudes can be measured either from the peak to the baseline or from the peak to the trough of the potentials, depending on the laboratory convention. For each point of stimulation, a latency is measured (in milliseconds), which represents the time elapsed from the delivery of the stimulus to the appearance of the muscle potential. The latency recorded from the most distal point of stimulation is referred to as the distal latency. In addition to measuring the time of conduction in the distal nerve, the distal latency includes the time of transmission across the neuromuscular junction and the conduction time of the muscle action potential through the muscle. If a standardized distance from the recording electrode is used for the distal stimulation, a normal range for the distal latency is available. A conduction velocity (CV) can be calculated by dividing the distance (in millimeters) between two points of stimulation by the time it takes to travel between these two points. Thus

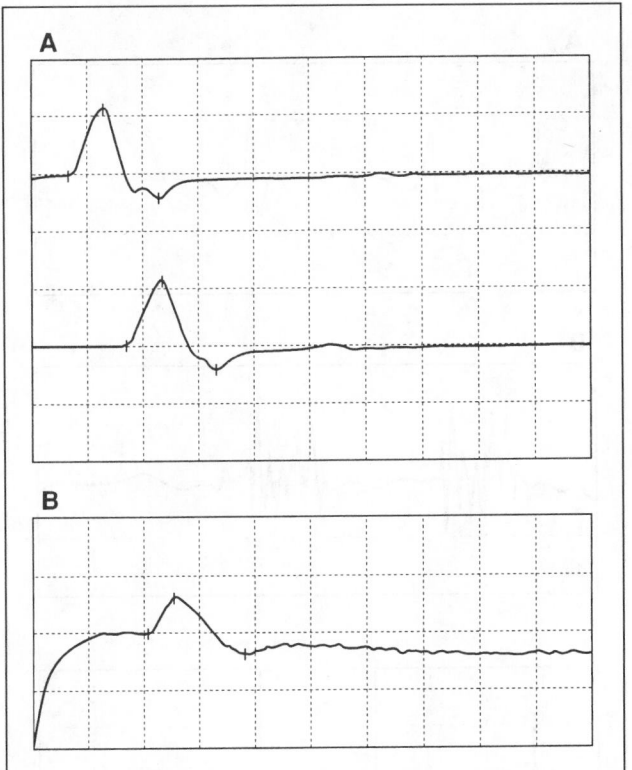

FIGURE 131-1 **A,** Motor nerve conduction study. Median nerve stimulated at the wrist *(top)* and elbow *(bottom).* Recording made over the thenar eminence. Sweep speed: 5 ms/division. Gain: 5 mV/division. **B,** Sensory nerve conduction study. Median nerve stimulated at the wrist and recorded with ring electrode over the index finger. Sweep speed, 1 ms/division; gain, 50 μV/division.

(EQ. 1)

$$CV \ (m/sec) = distance \ (mm) \div (proximal \ latency - distal \ latency \ [msec])$$

In the example of a normal median motor NCS given in Fig. 131-1, *A,* distal latency equals 3.0 msec, proximal latency equals 8.0 msec, and distance from elbow to wrist equals 293 mm. Therefore

(EQ. 2)

$$CV = 293 \div (8.0 - 3.0) = 60.0 \ m/sec$$

The amplitude of the CMAP is 6.0 mV proximally and distally. Commonly measured motor nerves are the median, ulnar, peroneal, and tibial.

For sensory NCSs, either antidromic (opposite to the physiologic direction of current flow; proximal stimulation at different sites and distal recording) or orthodromic (in the physiologic direction of current flow; distal stimulation and proximal recording at different sites) techniques are used. Again, supramaximum surface stimulation is usually employed. The recording is made directly over nerve fibers, with rings around a finger or with disk electrodes taped over the wrist (for median and ulnar nerves) or the lateral ankle (for the sural nerve). For the sensory fibers of the median nerve, stimulation can be given in the palm, at the wrist, and at the elbow, and a recording is typically made over the index finger. For sensory nerves a relatively lower amount of voltage output is needed to reach supramaximum stimulation, the potentials are much smaller than motor potentials (microvolts rather than millivolts), and they usually appear sooner than any volume-conducted motor potential. As with motor nerves, the parameters measured consist of the amplitude, latency, and conduction velocity. Because recordings are made directly over nerves, a conduction velocity can be calculated for the most distal part of the sensory nerve by dividing the distance from stimulation to recording site by the latency. Some laboratories, however, simply report distal laten-

cies without calculating velocity. Latencies can be measured to the onset or to the peak of the potential, depending on the laboratory, and the amplitude is measured either from the peak of the potential to the baseline or from peak to trough. Commonly measured sensory nerves are the median, ulnar, radial, sural, and plantar nerves. In the example given (Fig. 131-1, *B*), this normal median sensory nerve action potential was obtained by wrist stimulation and recording over the index finger. The amplitude (peak to trough) is 49 μV, and the distal latency is 2.6 msec. Because potentials can be quite small, especially in the feet, an average of multiple stimulations may be needed.

In addition to motor and sensory nerve conduction studies, F waves and H reflexes can be helpful. Measurement of these potentials provides some indication of conduction in the proximal portion of the nerve. F waves are small-amplitude, long-latency responses produced by supramaximal stimulation of a motor nerve with the cathode directed antidromically (directed away from the muscle that is being recorded). An F wave represents the muscle potential produced by an alpha motor neuron depolarized by the antidromic stimulus. The latency and shape of the F wave can vary from stimulus to stimulus with a fixed arrangement of stimulating and recording electrodes. Typically, at least 10 F waves are recorded at one stimulus site, and the shortest latency, measured to the onset of the F wave, is recorded. F wave amplitude is not a clinically useful measurement. Some institutions report only the latency of the F waves, using nomograms relating this value to the height of the individual. Others measure the distance over which the F wave travels and calculate a velocity.

An H reflex is a large-amplitude potential produced by submaximum stimulation. Typically, sensory fibers (IA afferents) of the posterior tibial nerve are stimulated in the popliteal fossa, and the muscle potential of the gastrocnemius-soleus muscle, caused by the reflex excitation of anterior horn cells, is recorded. The H reflex is an electrophysiologic correlate of an ankle jerk. The latency is measured to the onset of the H reflex. The absolute latency for the H reflexes is reported, and in most laboratories this value is then compared to the normal range based on the patient's height or leg length.

The interpretation of nerve conduction studies can provide information regarding the location and the pathologic characteristics of a particular neuropathy. Diffuse symmetric NCS abnormalities reflect a generalized polyneuropathy, whereas isolated focal changes indicate a mononeuropathy. The NCS may determine whether the neuropathy is purely motor, only sensory, or mixed. For axonal polyneuropathies the electrophysiologic hallmark is an amplitude reduction of the motor and sensory action potentials, whereas distal latencies and conduction velocities may be only mildly abnormal. This amplitude reduction generally reflects a loss of motor or sensory axons that are available for stimulation. In demyelinating neuropathic conditions, prolonged latencies and very slow conduction velocities are encountered, and the amplitude of potentials is reduced only if there is conduction block (see later discussion). Conduction velocity slowing to greater than 70% of the lower limit of normal is usually attributed to segmental demyelination. For most laboratories motor conduction velocities below 35 m/sec in the arms and 30 m/sec in the legs fulfill this criterion for demyelination. However, often generalized neuropathies do not fit neatly into electrophysiologic demyelinating and axonal paradigms, and other clues from the neurologic examination, spinal fluid analysis, and other laboratory tests (including possibly nerve biopsy) may be needed. Also, results of nerve conduction studies can be normal in small-fiber sensory neuropathy characterized by pure sensory or autonomic symptoms. In a radiculopathy, in which root compression occurs proximal to the dorsal root ganglion cell bodies, the sensory nerve action potentials are always normal. A focal entrapment palsy or mononeuropathy can be manifested by slowing over a particular nerve segment (prolonged latency or slowed velocity) or by a conduction block (failure to conduct above a locus with normal conduction below). Partial motor conduction block may be present if the amplitude of distal stimulation at the wrist or ankle is 50% higher than the amplitude with stimulation above the elbow or knee, respectively. Often, the potentials with proximal stimulation are also prolonged and polyphasic, so-called temporal dispersion, implying a delay in conduction across a focally demyelinated nerve segment. Common examples of entrapment palsies are the carpal tunnel syndrome and the cubital tunnel syndrome (ulnar entrapment at the elbow). In carpal tunnel syndrome the most common NCS finding is a prolonged distal latency of the median nerve motor and sensory potentials with stimulation across the wrist.

F wave and H reflex latencies (long latencies) may complement the routine NCS study. Early in demyelinating polyneuropathies, such as the Guillain-Barré syndrome, F waves may be slowed before there are demonstrable changes in the routine nerve conduction velocities. This indicates that the abnormality is in the proximal nerve segment with relative sparing of the distal nerve. F waves may occasionally be abnormal in focal proximal neuropathic disorders such as a plexopathy. H reflexes can be used to assess conduction over the large sensory fibers of the leg, as well as over proximal nerve fibers, as in an S1 radiculopathy. An H reflex may be prolonged or absent in an S1 radiculopathy, even before the ankle reflex is depressed or lost on the physical examination. Like F waves, the H reflex is often abnormal in demyelinating neuropathies involving the proximal nerve or root.

After appropriate nerve conduction studies a needle EMG examination is done. Electrodes are inserted into various muscles, and electrical discharges are displayed on an oscilloscope screen and simultaneously heard on the speaker. Concentric needle electrodes or monopolar needle electrodes (the latter requiring separate referential surface electrode) are used, depending on the laboratory. Recently, disposable needle electrodes have come into standard use. In a typical examination the initial insertional activity is recorded. The muscle is then observed at rest for spontaneous discharges and then during minimal, moderate, and full contraction. The patient then voluntarily contracts the muscle, and motor units are analyzed for their amplitude, duration, and number of phases (see two normal motor units, Fig. 131-2, *A*). The rate and characteristics of motor unit recruitment and the final interference pattern are noted. All observations must be analyzed in light of the normal range of variation for the muscle being studied. For detailed quantitative motor unit analysis, at least 50 consecutive motor unit potentials are averaged.

Prolonged or increased insertional activity is often a nonspecific finding suggesting irritability of the muscle. In isolation, the finding of prolonged insertional activity should not be overinterpreted. Normally there is no electrical activity at rest. Fibrillations (Fig. 131-2, *C*) and positive sharp waves (Fig. 131-2, *D*) occur at rest when the patient is not voluntarily contracting the muscle and represent spontaneous discharges of individual muscle fibers disconnected from their nerve axons. Fibrillations are stereotyped narrow diphasic or triphasic potentials with a small initial downward slope followed by a larger upward deflection. Positive sharp waves are biphasic potentials with a prominent, sharp initial downward slope, followed by a prolonged phase back to the baseline. The positive sharp wave is believed to represent a fibrillation type of potential that is not propagated directly over the site of the needle recording. Fibrillations and positive sharp waves are typical of a denervating (neuropathic) process but can occur in myopathic disease. In inflammatory myopathy there is often a profusion of fibrillations and positive sharp waves. On the other hand, if these potentials are present in the setting of a neuropathic process, this implies some degree of axonal damage; therefore the neuropathy is not purely demyelinating. These spontaneous potentials have to be distinguished from those normally encountered in the end-plate zone.

Fasciculations are usually large-amplitude potentials that are simple, diphasic, or triphasic, resembling normal motor units, or they are complex large-amplitude polyphasic potentials. They represent the spontaneous discharge of a motor unit, which is a group of muscle fibers of the same histochemical type under control of a single anterior horn cell. Although they do not necessarily imply neuromuscular disease and occur in many normal patients, a profusion of fasciculations in association with other needle EMG abnormalities is suggestive of an anterior horn cell or a nerve disorder. Certain peculiar spontaneous discharges can be observed. One typical pattern occurs with myotonia; it has the sound of a dive bomber, caused by gradually increasing and then decreasing amplitude and frequency of the individual potentials in the discharge. Another pattern is a complex repetitive discharge (or pseudomyotonia) that abruptly starts and stops, and the component potential has a complex waveform. The former pattern usually occurs in the myotonic syndromes (Chapter 149); the latter is less specific and can occur in both chronic neuropathies and myopathies.

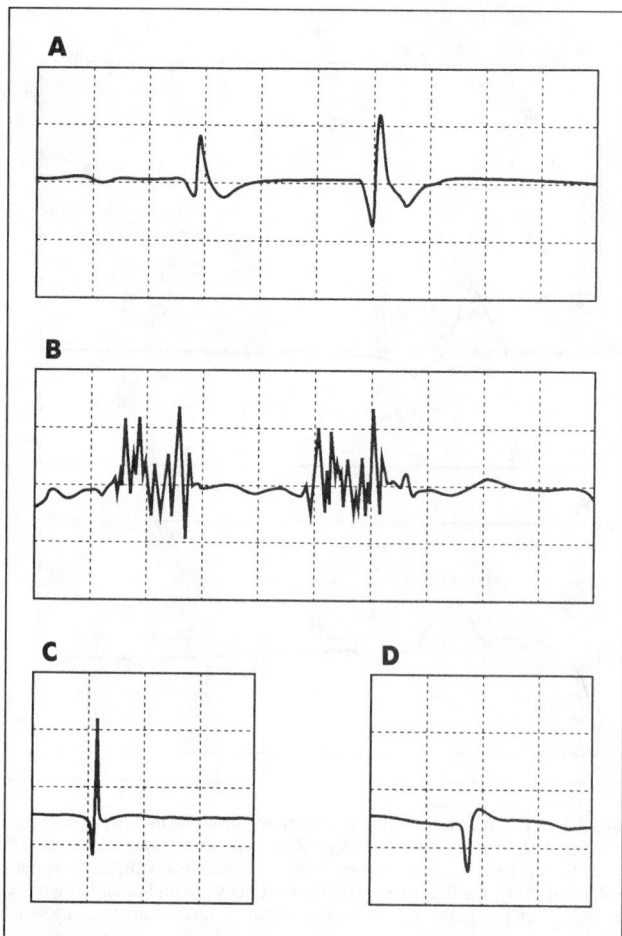

FIGURE 131-2 **A,** Normal motor unit potentials. Gain, 0.5 mV/division. **B,** Polyphasic, long-duration rapidly firing motor unit potential. Gain, 1 mV/division. **C,** Fibrillation potential. Gain, 50 μV/division. **D,** Positive sharp wave. Gain, 50 μV/division. All sweep speeds, 10 msec/division.

In evaluating motor units, the electromyographer evaluates their morphologic features and recruitment. Two morphologic patterns are commonly observed. "Neuropathic" potentials are often increased in amplitude (>5 mV), increased in their phases (polyphasic), and often increased in duration (>10 msec) (Fig. 131-2, *B*). "Myopathic" potentials are small, brief polyphasic potentials (<4 msec). These are generalizations, and there are many examples of denervating illnesses that produce myopathic potentials and vice versa. A mixed pattern is not unusual. In regard to motor unit recruitment, a few patterns emerge. In a neuropathy, rapidly firing motor units are often recruited early, and often a full interference pattern is not accomplished (so-called decreased recruitment). Normally, early recruited motor units fire at less than 10 Hz (Fig. 131-2, *A*); therefore initial units firing faster than 20 Hz are clearly abnormal (Fig. 131-2, *B*). This indicates a loss of motor units with a compensatory increased rate in the remaining units. In a myopathy, multiple motor units are recruited early, and a full interference pattern is obtained at a level of voluntary motor activity lower than normal. A decreased number of motor units without a compensatory increase in the firing rate of remaining units usually indicates lack of effort, or possibly an upper motor neuron lesion, but not a neuropathy. The abnormalities on needle EMG can be interpreted as being due to a generalized myopathy (which predominantly involves proximal muscles); a generalized neuropathy (which predominantly involves distal muscles); a focal process such as radiculopathy, plexopathy, mononeuropathy, or mononeuritis multiplex; or an anterior horn cell disease. The distribution of the findings and the needle EMG findings helps in making the final assessment. For example, anterior horn cell disease (amyotrophic lateral sclerosis) usually produces diffuse needle EMG abnormalities in three or four extremities, but motor and sensory nerve conduction studies are normal.

There are many pitfalls to the interpretation of needle EMG. In acute lesions such as radiculopathy or traumatic palsy, denervation potentials appear only after 1 to 2 weeks, so timing of a study is important. In certain illnesses an EMG is not the most sensitive test, since extensive abnormalities may be necessary to produce electrophysiologic changes clearly outside the normal range. For example, in amyotrophic lateral sclerosis the EMG result for a clinically uninvolved extremity may be normal, whereas the biopsy finding of a muscle in that extremity may show the characteristic changes of the illness, albeit at an early stage. In various forms of muscular dystrophy that are long-standing the electrical changes may be hard to interpret, and a muscle biopsy will give more diagnostic information. In general, for most myopathic disorders, both dystrophic and inflammatory, a muscle biopsy is more specific and sensitive than an EMG. One exception to this are the myotonic disorders, in which the EMG result does nearly always exhibit the typical myotonic discharges, whereas a muscle biopsy result may be only minimally and nonspecifically abnormal. Many electromyographers are hesitant to read changes in small foot muscles such as the toe flexors and extensors because of the large percentage of fibrillations and motor unit changes in these muscles in normal individuals. Some muscles, such as the finger extensor muscles in the forearm and the muscles of facial expression, normally have motor units firing at 20 to 25 Hz. Needle EMG of paraspinal muscles is often rewarding, but most electromyographers restrict their interest to the presence of denervation potentials, since motor units are notoriously difficult to interpret in this muscle. After a laminectomy, fibrillations can persist for years in paraspinous muscles and therefore may not indicate persistent root compression. In trying to distinguish an L5 radiculopathy from a peroneal palsy, it is important to sample the gluteus medius (hip abductor) and the posterior tibial (ankle invertor), which are involved in the former process. Also, the short head of the biceps femoris (a knee flexor supplied by the peroneal nerve above the fibular head) should be sampled to localize the site of a potential peroneal palsy. Despite these potential difficulties, a needle EMG allows several muscles to be sampled, and it can be very helpful in characterizing a neuromuscular illness.

In evaluation of the neuromuscular junction, repetitive stimulation and single-fiber EMG studies are most useful. For repetitive stimulation a series of supramaximal stimuli are given to a nerve (typically at the rate of 3/sec for 2 seconds), and the amount of decrement of the amplitude of the evoked CMAP is recorded. A decrease of greater than 10% of the fourth potential's amplitude as compared with that of the first is considered significant. This test is easiest to perform on distal muscles of the upper extremity, but it can also be performed on facial and proximal arm muscles. If an abnormality is seen, the test of the ability of edrophonium hydrochloride to reverse it is sometimes performed. A standard protocol involves a measurement of baseline responses, a period of 60 seconds of sustained exercise of the relevant muscles, and then a repeat series of stimuli given at 1-minute intervals for up to 5 minutes.

In single-fiber EMG a small needle is inserted into a muscle and, using special techniques, the relationship of two muscle fibers within one motor unit is examined. The fluctuation in the time lag between the excitation of the two fibers can be recorded and is known as the jitter (often reported as a mean value of consecutive differences [MCD]). The muscles most extensively studied are the extensor digitorum communis in the forearm and the orbicularis oculi in the face.

Repetitive stimulation studies and single-fiber EMG are often used to substantiate a diagnosis of myasthenia gravis. In a classic case there is a decrement of the amplitude of the CMAP after repetitive stimulation; the CMAP amplitude increases transiently after exercise (postexercise facilitation) and then progressively decreases (postexercise exhaustion). Some or all of these phenomena may be seen in individual patients, but the most sensitive measurement is that of postexercise exhaustion. However, repetitive stimulation may show a decrement in only 50% to 75% of myasthenia gravis patients. In single-fiber EMG there is an increased jitter suggestive of variable transmission in the neuromuscular junction in an otherwise normal muscle. Blocking, which represents intermittent failure of excitation of the second fiber of the pair, can also occur. This technique is highly sensitive and may yield an abnormal result in 95% of patients with myasthenia gravis. In the Eaton-Lambert syndrome there may be a mild decrement to repetitive stimuli at slow rates (2 to 3 Hz). However, the initial potentials are small and are greatly increased by exercise. Repetitive stimulation at fast rates (20 to 50 Hz) produces an incremental response. The pattern in botulism may be similar, but exercise produces facilitation only at a certain stage of the disease. In organophosphate poisoning and intoxication with antibiotics such as neomycin, there may be a myasthenic pattern. Single-fiber EMG, although a sensitive test for myasthenia gravis and related diseases, is less specific than repetitive stimulation, since it can produce abnormal results in various neuropathies and myopathies.

The blink reflex is obtained by stimulation over the supraorbital nerve, with surface recording over both ipsilateral and contralateral orbicularis oculi. This study is used to assess trigeminal and facial nerve function, including their central connections, and can document lesions in diseases such as Bell's palsy, trigeminal neuropathy, and multiple sclerosis.

BIBLIOGRAPHY

Barry DT: Basic concepts of electricity and electronics in clinical electromyography, *Muscle Nerve* 14:937, 1991.
Brown F, Bolton C: *Clinical electromyography,* Boston, 1987, Butterworth.
Daube JR: *Clinical neurophysiology,* Philadelphia, 1996, FA Davis.
Donofrio PD, Albers JW: Polyneuropathy: classification by nerve conduction studies and electromyography, *Muscle Nerve* 13:889, 1990.
Dumitru D: *Electrodiagnostic medicine,* Philadelphia, 1995, Hanley & Belfus.
Kimura J: *Electrodiagnosis in diseases of nerve and muscle: principles and practice,* Philadelphia, 1989, FA Davis.
Oh SJ: *Clinical electromyography: nerve conduction studies,* Baltimore, 1993, Williams & Wilkins.
Oh SJ: *Electromyography: neuromuscular transmission studies,* Baltimore, 1988, Williams & Wilkins.
Sethi RK, Thompson LL: *The electromyographer's handbook,* Boston, 1989, Little, Brown.
Stewart JD: *Focal peripheral neuropathies,* New York, 1993, Raven.

CHAPTER

132 Neuroradiologic Studies

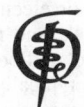

Ashwani Kapila

The practice of neuroradiology began with plain radiography and conventional tomography of the skull and spine to assist in diagnosing neurologic diseases. Angiography, myelography, pneumoencephalography, and ventriculography emerged from the application of standard radiographic techniques during intravascular, subarachnoid, or intraventricular injection of various contrast media. The application of computer-assisted techniques to radiography led to computed tomography, digital radiography, and digital subtraction angiography. Concurrently, imaging techniques using ultrasound, radiopharmaceuticals, and magnetic resonance were developed and applied to the brain and spine. Newer techniques in neuroradiology include functional brain imaging with magnetic resonance, positron emission tomography, transcranial Doppler, local intravascular thrombolysis, and various therapeutic interventional procedures.

COMPUTED TOMOGRAPHY

Computed tomography (CT) is a cross-sectional imaging technique that since its introduction in 1972 has greatly advanced the ability of clinicians to diagnose and manage neurologic diseases. The CT scanner consists of an x-ray tube and an array of movable or fixed x-ray detectors. The body part of interest is exposed to a narrowly collimated x-ray beam of predetermined slice thickness. The transmitted radiation is detected by the radiation detectors. These data are collected in various projections and channeled into a computer, which

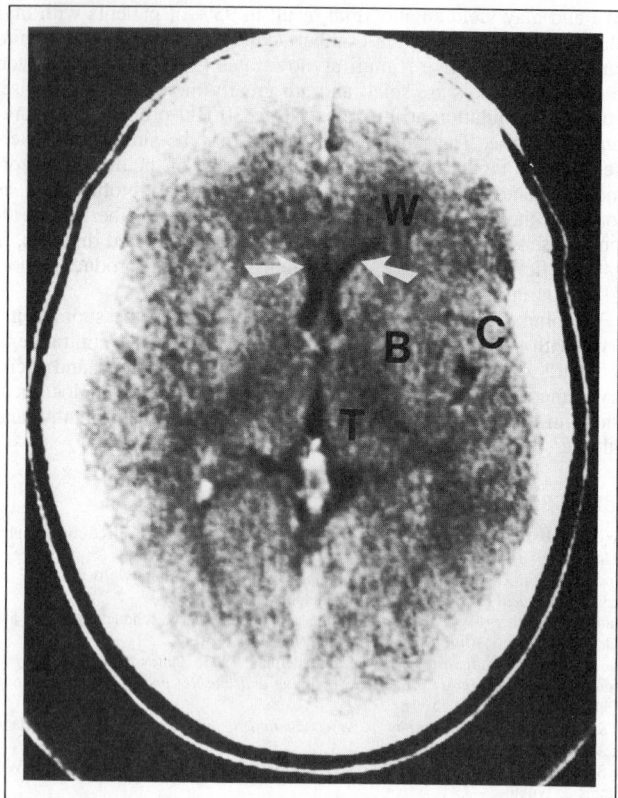

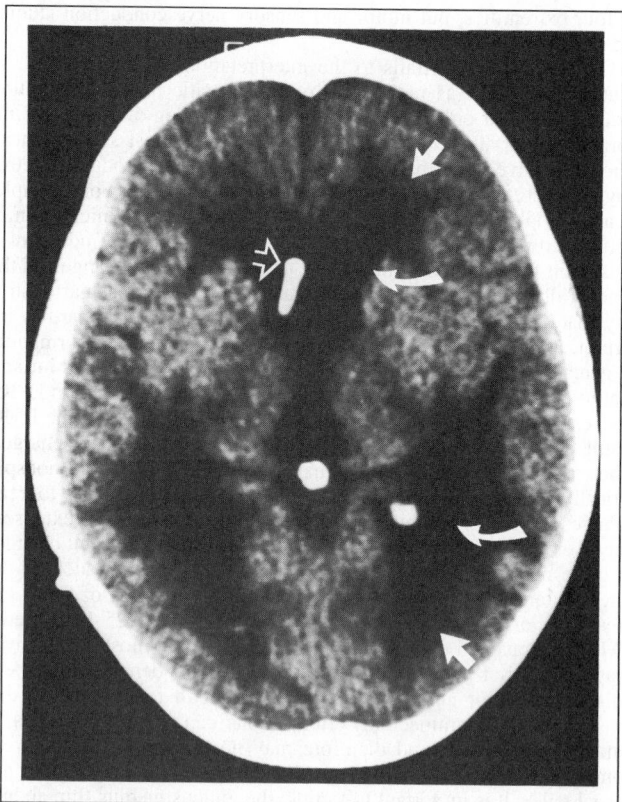

FIGURE 132-1 Computed tomography (CT) scan of the head of a normal individual. The white matter *(W)* is slightly darker shade of gray than the gray matter of the cortex *(C)*, basal ganglia *(B)*, and thalamus *(T)* on this contrast-enhanced scan done at the level of the frontal horns *(arrows)* of the lateral ventricles.

FIGURE 132-2 CT scan showing marked enlargement of the lateral ventricles *(curved arrows)* and periventricular lucency representing cerebrospinal fluid edema *(straight arrows)* in a patient with shunted hydrocephalus in whom shunt failure developed. The ventricular end of the ventriculoperitoneal shunt is identified in the right lateral ventricle *(open arrowhead)*.

by mathematical computation reconstructs the cross-sectional CT image. The various tissues of the head and body are displayed in various shades of gray depending on the x-ray attenuating properties of that particular tissue, which in turn are dependent on their electron density (physical density) and atomic number. Air is black, and fat, cerebrospinal fluid (CSF), white matter, gray matter, blood, and bone are progressively whiter (Fig. 132-1). Brain CT slices are typically 3 to 10 mm thick; spine CT slices are usually 2 to 5 mm thick. Several consecutive slices are obtained to display the entire region of interest. An entire scan of the brain can be obtained in a few seconds to 10 minutes, depending on the type of scanner, slice thickness, and desired resolution. Acquisition time for a CT scan of the spine is somewhat longer and depends on the extent of the spine to be scanned.

CT scanning of the head is usually done without contrast in patients with acute head trauma, in the diagnosis of hydrocephalus and monitoring of ventricular size in shunted patients (Fig. 132-2), in the diagnosis of intracranial hemorrhage (Fig. 132-3), in distinguishing hemorrhagic from bland infarcts, in evaluating diseases of the skull base, and in detecting and displaying complex craniofacial anomalies. Contrast-enhanced CT with intravenously administered iodinated contrast medium is, however, required for adequate evaluation of a number of intracranial diseases. Contrast enhancement has an intravascular component that enhances normal vessels and abnormal vascular structures such as aneurysms and vascular malformations, and an extravascular component where contrast leaks out of vessels into areas of blood-brain barrier disruption such as brain tumors (Fig. 132-4), cerebral infarction, and various inflammatory processes. The need for intravenous contrast enhancement in CT has diminished with the acceptance of magnetic resonance imaging (MRI) as the superior imaging modality for most neurologic disease. Contrast enhancement of CSF in the subarachnoid space or in the ventricles by injection of contrast material by lumbar, cervical, or ventricular puncture was used

for a variety of intracranial abnormalities before the advent of MRI but is rarely used now other than for the evaluation of CSF rhinorrhea.

CT of the spine is used for a large number of spinal disorders including spinal stenosis, degenerative disk disease (Fig. 132-5), vertebral and paraspinal tumors and inflammatory lesions, vertebral fractures, and congenital abnormalities. For detailed evaluation of spinal anatomy and disease CT is often performed with intrathecal contrast enhancement (Fig. 132-6), usually in association with plain film myelography.

MAGNETIC RESONANCE IMAGING

MRI is a cross-sectional imaging modality that has greater sensitivity than CT for detecting pathologic processes and is superior for displaying normal and altered anatomic relations in the brain and spine. MRI has displaced CT as the primary neurodiagnostic imaging modality in most diseases of the brain and spine.

Various elements exhibit nuclear magnetic resonance (NMR) properties; however, current clinical MRI is limited to hydrogen nuclear (proton) imaging. In essence, proton MRI is a hydrogen map of the tissue in the volume of interest that reflects not only the quantitative hydrogen distribution but also the influence of the surrounding physical and chemical environment on these various hydrogen atoms. The process of image generation in MRI is complex, and the scheme that follows is an extreme simplification of basic MRI. In a strong magnetic field, the hydrogen protons, which act like small magnets, are aligned parallel to the main magnetic field and then are energized by applying a radiofrequency pulse of the appropriate energy (resonant frequency). The excited protons return to the ground state or equilibrium (relaxation) by emitting radiofrequency energy, which is recorded by a receiver and constitutes the magnetic resonance signal. Spatial information for image generation is ob-

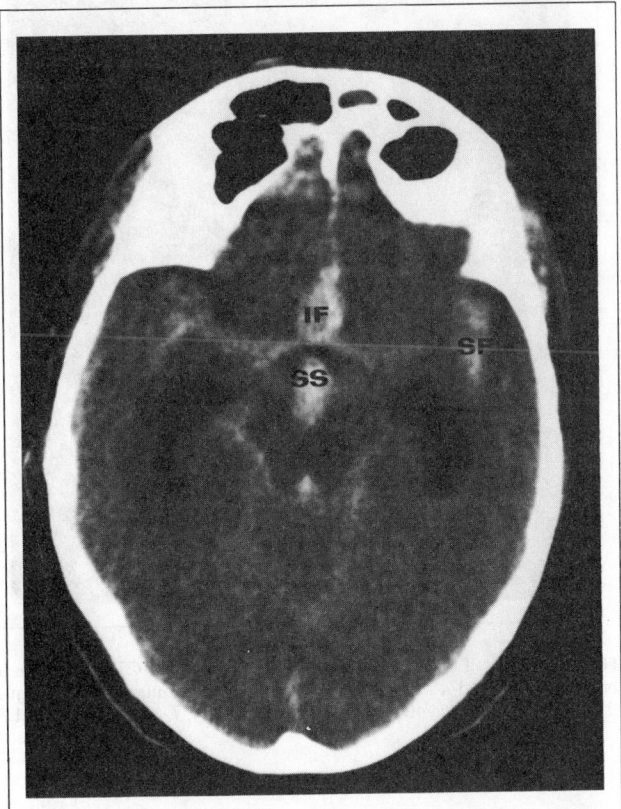

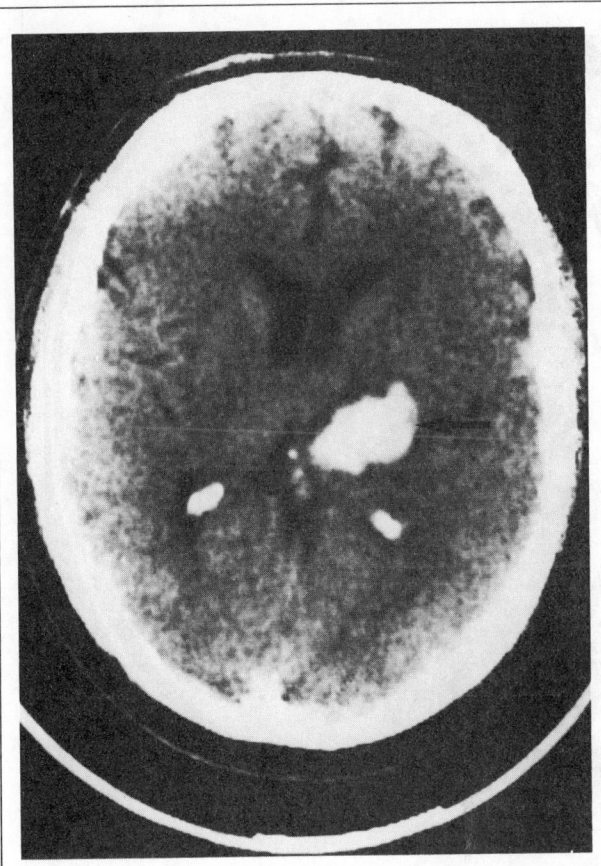

FIGURE 132-3   Intracranial hemorrhage. **A,** CT scan showing a subarachnoid hemorrhage. Rupture of an anterior communicating-artery aneurysm has produced a massive subarachnoid hemorrhage, seen as a high-attenuation *(white)* area in the suprasellar cistern *(SS)*, the anterior interhemispheric fissure *(IF)*, and the sylvian fissures *(SF)*. The aneurysm cannot be seen separately from the hematoma in the interhemispheric fissure. **B,** CT scan showing a hypertensive hemorrhage. A hematoma *(arrow)* is seen in the left thalamus and in the posterior part of the basal ganglia—a classic location for hypertensive hemorrhages.

tained by producing a controlled nonuniformity of the main magnetic field and subsequently determining the source of the various radiofrequency signals by a mathematical process called Fourier transformation.

The strength of the magnetic resonance signal and the appearance of the final image depend on scanner-selectable parameters and on tissue characteristics. Machine selectable parameters are repetition time (TR), echo time (TE), and the angle through which the magnetic vector is deflected by the radiofrequency pulse. Signal from magnetized tissue can be collected by applying a second radiofrequency pulse (spin-echo) or by a process of gradient reversal (gradient-echo). Routine brain imaging is done primarily with spin-echo; spine imaging is done with both spin-echo and gradient-echo. Gradient-echo image formation is used for magnetic resonance angiography (MRA), in detecting blood products, and in examinations where rapid imaging is required. Final image content and contrast can be tailored to the clinical problem by adjusting these basic parameters, changing imaging plane and thickness, and using other options such as fat or water suppression or flow compensation. Tissue characteristics include proton density, the relaxation time constants T1 and T2, and the effects of motion including flow and pulsation of blood and CSF (Fig. 132-7). Tissue relaxation times can be modified with T1-shortening paramagnetic agents that have a pharmacologic distribution similar to conventional iodinated contrast used for CT. Contrast enhancement of tissues with blood-brain barrier disruption and of extracerebral tumors appears on T1-weighted images similar to that on contrast-enhanced CT. Signal changes in vascular structures are governed primarily by intrinsic flow characteristics and are only secondarily affected by paramag-

netic contrast. Agents that modify T2 relaxation are used to evaluate brain perfusion.

MRI has a number of advantages over CT scanning other than its considerably greater capability of displaying anatomic details and superior sensitivity in detecting abnormality: it (1) does not use ionizing radiation and has no apparent adverse biologic effects, (2) is not subject to bone artifact, (3) allows coronal and sagittal imaging with ease and with excellent resolution, (4) requires contrast enhancement less often than CT, and (5) uses contrast agents, which are generally considered safer than agents used for CT scanning. There are also limitations to the use of MRI in its present state of evolution that prohibit it from completely replacing CT. MRI (1) is more expensive than CT; (2) is limited in acutely ill patients on life support because of interactions between the magnetic field and life support equipment; (3) is often unacceptable to claustrophobic patients; (4) cannot be used in patients with ferromagnetic intracranial aneurysm clips, metallic structures in or around the eyes, pacemakers, cochlear implants, or neurostimulator devices; (5) has limited utility when the area of clinical interest is located close to ferromagnetic surgical hardware; and (6) is inferior to CT in detecting acute subarachnoid hemorrhage and in evaluating calcified lesions.

MRI is currently the imaging procedure of choice in the majority of diseases of the brain and spine. It is especially useful in evaluating white matter diseases (Fig. 132-8), cryptic vascular malformations and hemangiomas, neuronal migration anomalies, abnormalities of larger arterial and venous structures, syringomyelia, and intervertebral disk disease. MRI is also the imaging test of choice in most developmental, ischemic, inflammatory, degenerative, neoplastic, and subacute or chronic posttraumatic processes of the brain (Figs. 132-9,

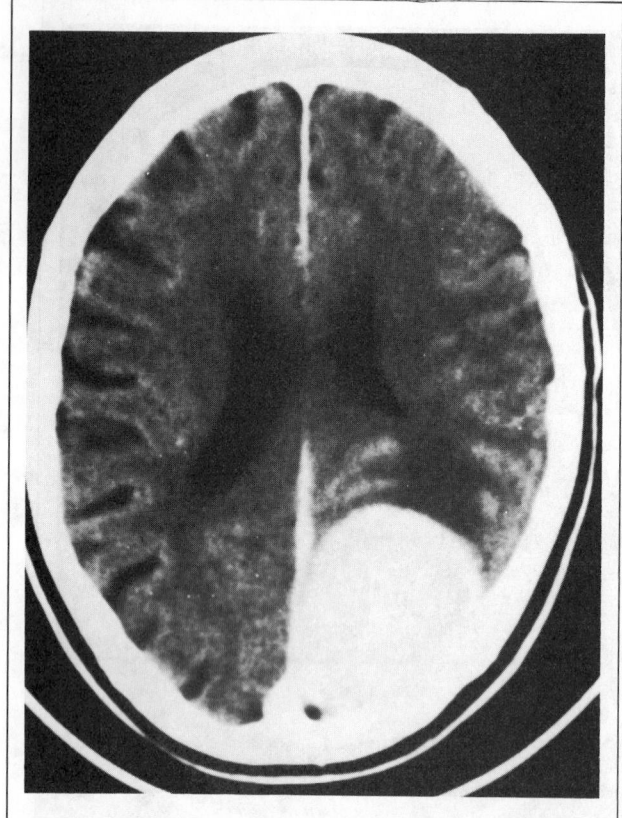

A

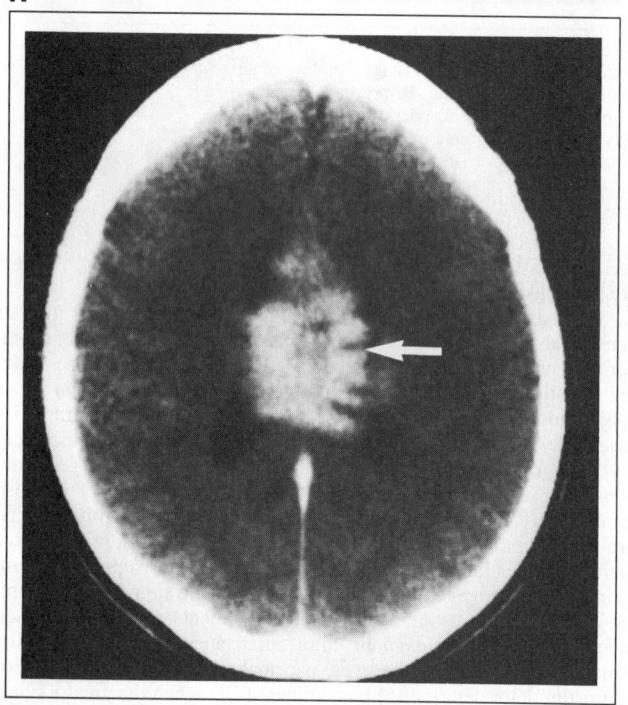

B

FIGURE 132-4 Brain tumors. **A,** Meningioma. Contrast-enhanced CT scan showing a uniform-density, contrast-enhancing meningioma abutting the falx and the calvarium in the left occipital region. **B,** Lymphoma. Contrast-enhanced CT scan showing an enhancing lesion of the corpus callosum *(arrow)*. The location and the absence of surrounding edema or mass effect are characteristic of primary central nervous system lymphoma.

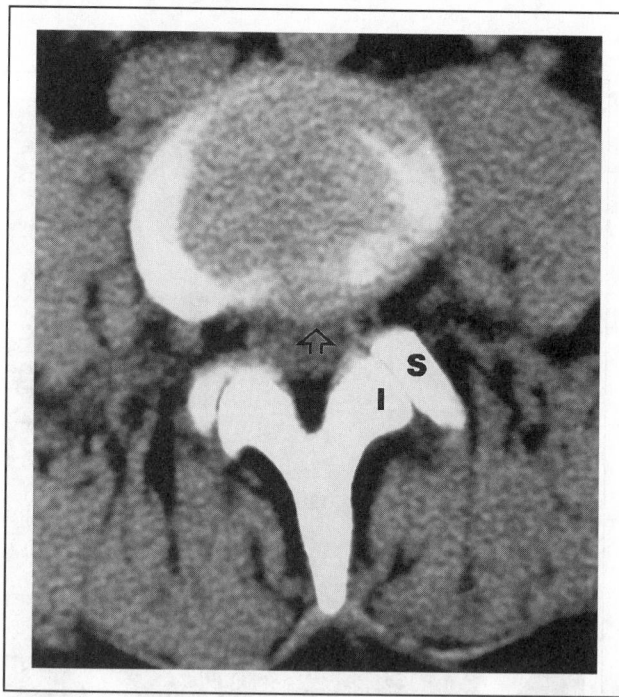

FIGURE 132-5 Lumbar intervertebral disk herniation. CT scan of the lumbar spine at the L3-4 level showing posterior disk herniation centered just to the left of midline *(arrow)*. *S,* superior facet of L4; *I,* inferior facet of L3.

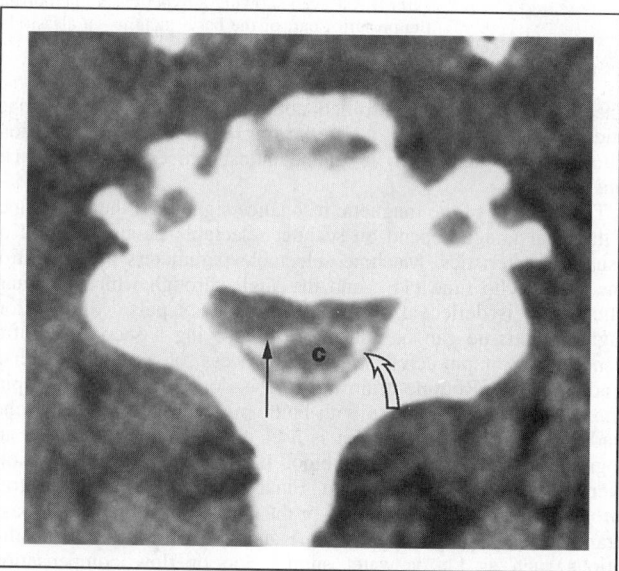

FIGURE 132-6 Cervical epidural abscess. CT scan of the cervical spine at the C5 level after myelography with water-soluble contrast medium showing subarachnoid space opacified with contrast *(curved arrow)* and ventral extradural abscess appearing as a soft tissue mass larger on the right side *(arrow)*. Cord compression is demonstrated as mild degree of flattening of the cervical cord *(C)* at this level.

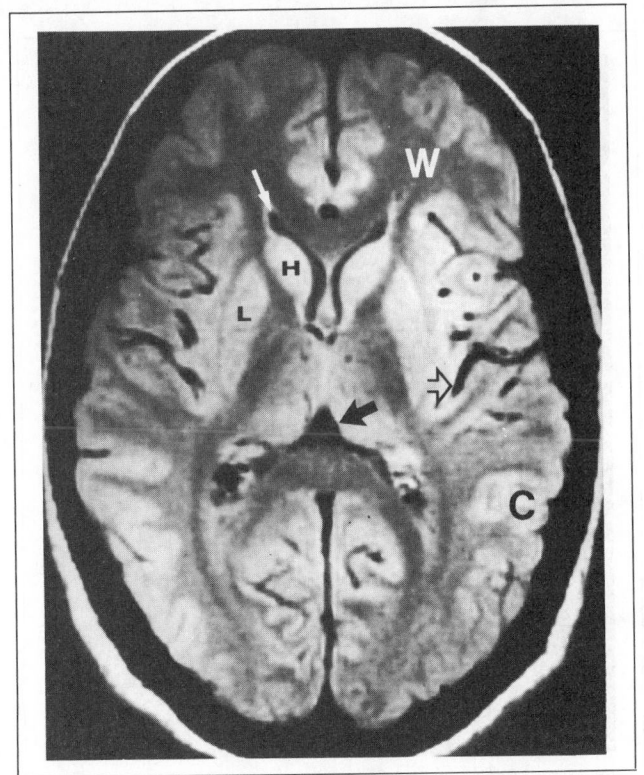
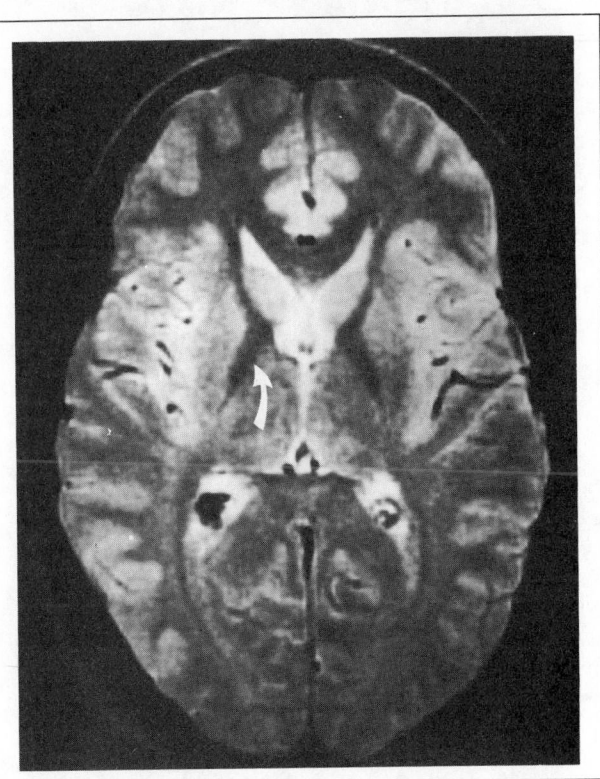

FIGURE 132-7 Normal magnetic resonance imaging (MRI) scan of the head. These two transverse scans are at the same location, done in the same imaging sequence. **A,** The proton density scan *(TR, 2000 ms; TE, 25 ms)* shows relatively high-intensity cortex *(C)*, caudate *(H)*, and lentiform *(L)* nuclei; lower intensity in the white matter *(W);* and low intensity of the cerebrospinal fluid *(CSF)* in the frontal horns *(white arrow)*. There is flow void in the sylvian vessels *(open arrowhead)* and internal cerebral veins *(black arrow)*. **B,** The T2-weighted scan shows high intensity of the CSF. The low intensity evident in the medial part of the globus pallidi *(curved arrow)* is a normal phenomenon caused by increased iron in this region.

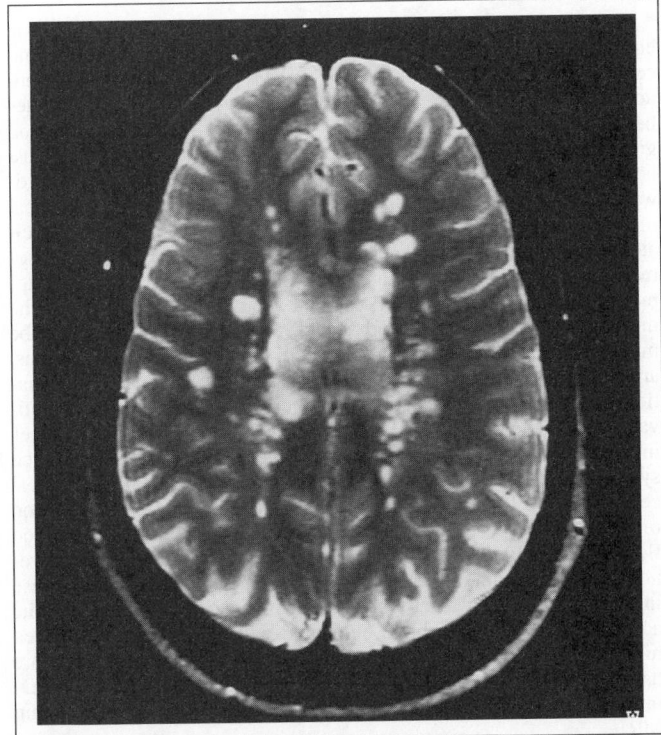
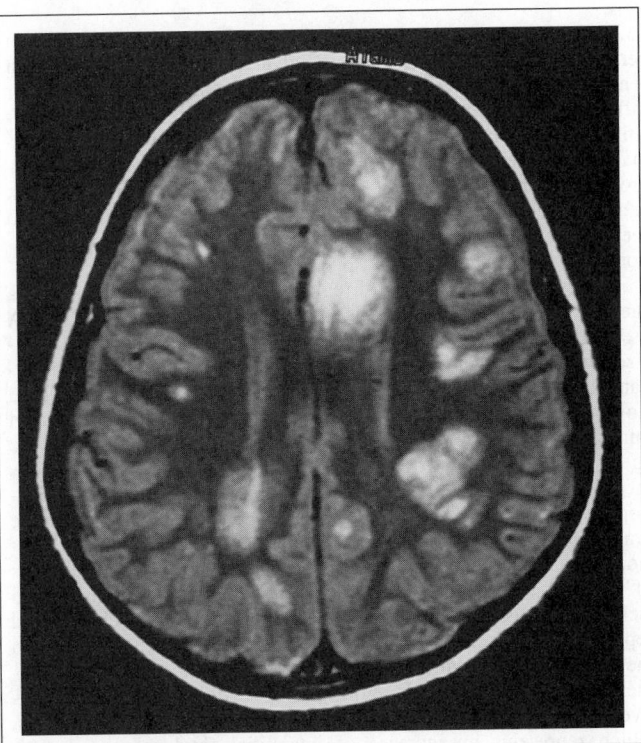

FIGURE 132-8 MRI of the brain in demyelinating disease. **A,** Multiple sclerosis (MS). T2-weighted axial scan shows characteristic periventricular ovoid and horizontal linear plaques of MS. **B,** Acute disseminated encephalomyelitis. Proton-density axial scan in 8-year-old shows subcortical and deep white matter foci of demyelination.

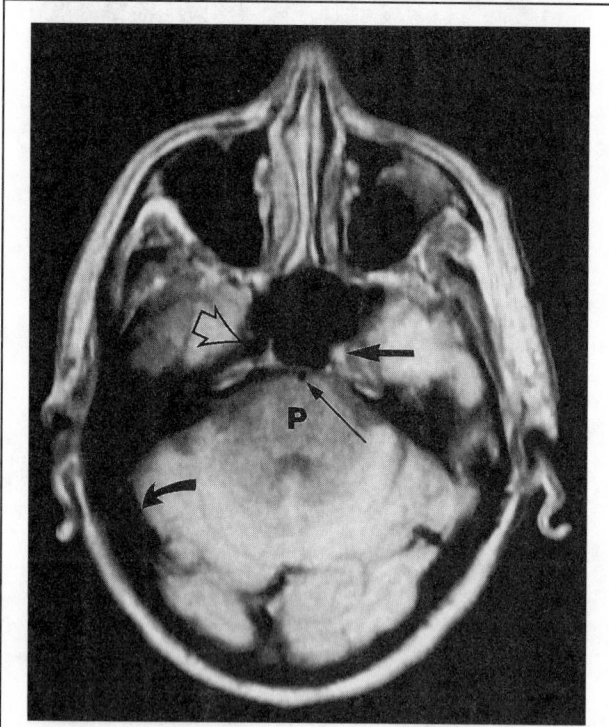

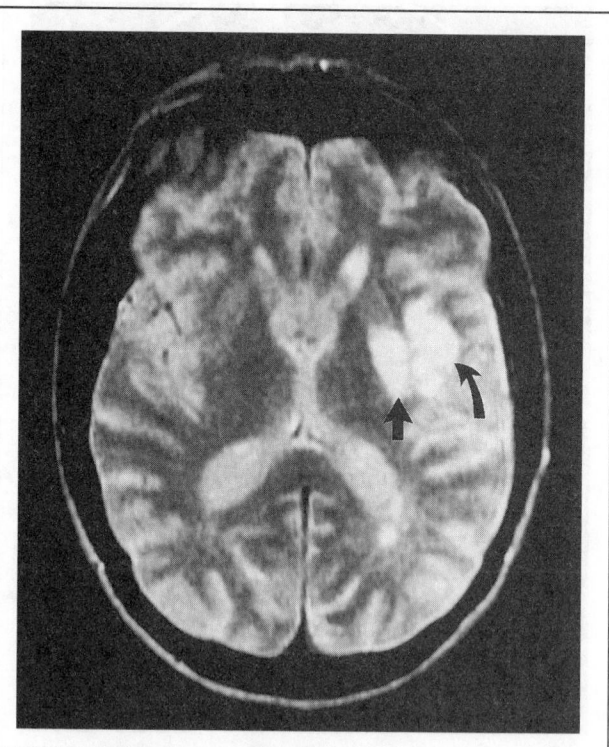

FIGURE 132-9   Cerebral infarction. **A,** MRI scan weighted for proton density *(TR, 2300 ms; TE, 25 msec)* showing slightly increased signal in the left precavernous internal carotid artery *(thick arrow),* a finding representing thrombus in the occluded vascular lumen. Rapidly flowing blood in the right internal carotid artery *(empty arrow),* basilar artery *(thin arrow),* and right transverse sinus *(curved arrow)* appears black, the so-called signal void sign. **B,** MRI scan on the same patient at a higher level using T2 weighting *(TR, 2300 msec; TE, 90 msec)* showing increased signal intensity representing infarction in the left insula *(curved arrow)* and lentiform nucleus *(straight arrow). P,* Pons.

132-10, and 132-11) or spinal cord (Figs. 132-12 and 132-13). When performed with intravenous contrast enhancement, MRI has very high sensitivity in detecting leptomeningeal involvement by neoplastic or inflammatory processes. Contrast enhancement also increases the sensitivity of MRI in detecting small intraparenchymal or extraparenchymal lesions and early cerebral infarction, helps in choosing the appropriate biopsy or resection site for spinal cord and brain tumors, and provides greater diagnostic specificity for lesions that are also seen without contrast such as in distinguishing recurrent disk herniation from epidural fibrosis.

The evaluation with MRI of regional cerebral hemodynamics, tissue metabolism and brain activity constitutes functional MRI. MRA uses special pulse sequences to evaluate flow in large- and medium-sized arteries and veins. Perfusion imaging assesses cerebral hemodynamics at the capillary level and can estimate regional cerebral blood flow and volume by imaging the changes in T2 relaxation induced during first-pass transit of an intravenously injected paramagnetic agent through the microvascular bed. Potential clinical applications include evaluation of stroke and dementia and use in characterization of tumors. Diffusion imaging is done by applying magnetic gradients sensitive to microscopic motion of water protons. Diffusion, or water molecular random motion, appears to reflect the status of cerebral energy metabolism. Diffusion images are sensitive to ischemic change as early as 15 minutes after vascular occlusion and represent the development of cytotoxic edema, which occurs with the shift of water from the extracellular to the intracellular compartment. Routine spin-echo imaging, however, does not become positive until the development several hours later of vasogenic edema, which represents an increase of interstitial fluid associated with breakdown of the blood-brain barrier. In early ischemic stroke the presence of a larger abnormality on perfusion relative to diffusion images suggests the presence of viable tissue in the ischemic penumbra. Identification of this brain at risk is helpful in determining which patients may benefit from thrombolytic therapy.

Cortical mapping of brain function has been done with positron emission tomography (PET) using metabolically active radiopharmaceuticals, magnetoencephalography, and MRI using exogenous or endogenous contrast. MRI has the advantage over the other techniques because of the wide dissemination of magnetic resonance units and greater spatial and temporal resolution compared with PET. It must be noted, however, that most magnetic resonance units require hardware and software modifications for functional imaging. Cortical mapping is the localization of anatomic sites of brain activity associated with specific tasks. Areas of brain associated with various somatosensory and cognitive functions can be mapped by designing appropriate task paradigms, and essential areas of the brain such as the motor strip, visual cortex, and speech and language centers can be mapped before surgical resection of tumors, vascular malformations, and epileptogenic foci. Potential clinical applications include evaluation of dementia and of patients recovering from stroke. Brain activation using functional MRI is measured indirectly through changes in cerebral microvascular perfusion and blood oxygenation. Increased synaptic activity in the brain is accompanied by an increase in local cerebral blood flow and oxygen utilization. The increased utilization of oxygen is proportionately less compared with the increase in blood flow. This leads to a paradoxical increase in oxygen content of venous blood draining the activated cortex. The accompanying decrease in deoxyhemoglobin results in an increase in signal intensity in the activated portion of the brain compared with the resting state when high-speed gradient-echo or echo-planar imaging sequences are used. This is the basis for blood oxygen level–dependent (BOLD) imaging, currently the most common technique for functional brain MRI.

Magnetic resonance spectroscopy is used for biochemically analyzing the brain in vivo. Spectra are currently obtained from hydrogen and phosphorus, both these atoms being abundant in active substrates for brain metabolism. Magnetic resonance spectroscopy provides insight into tissue metabolism in acute and chronic disorders of

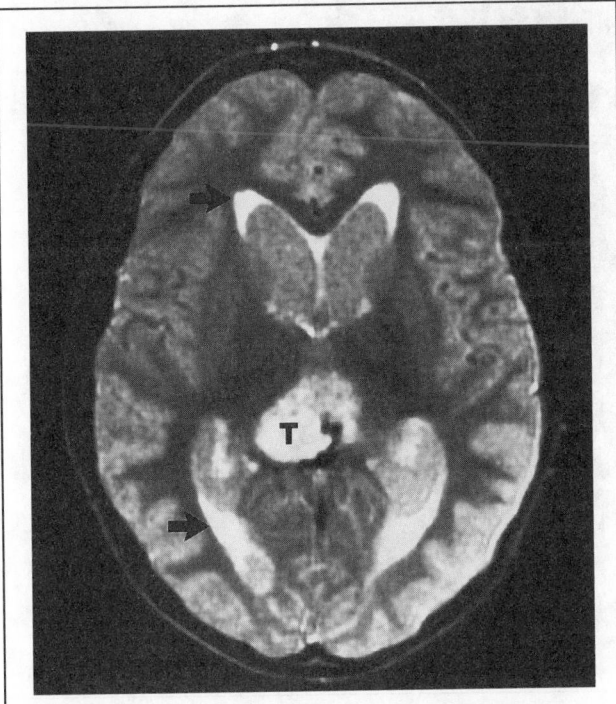

A

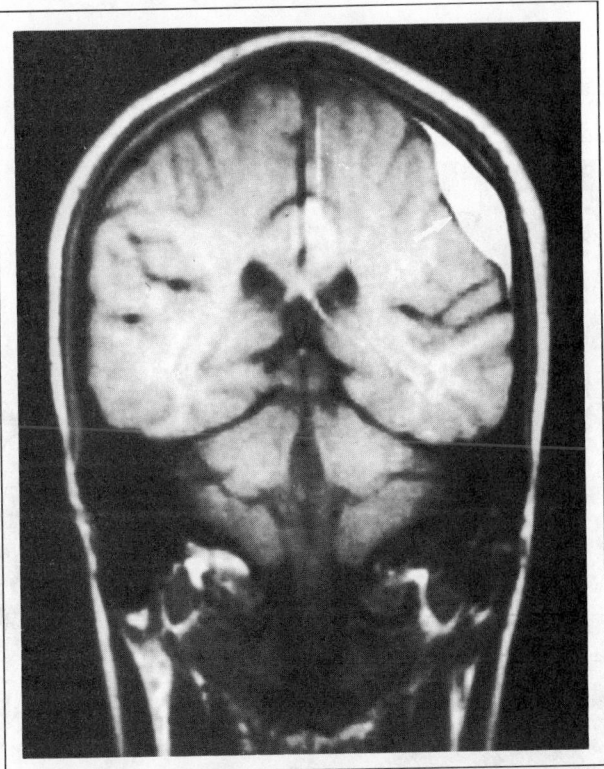

A

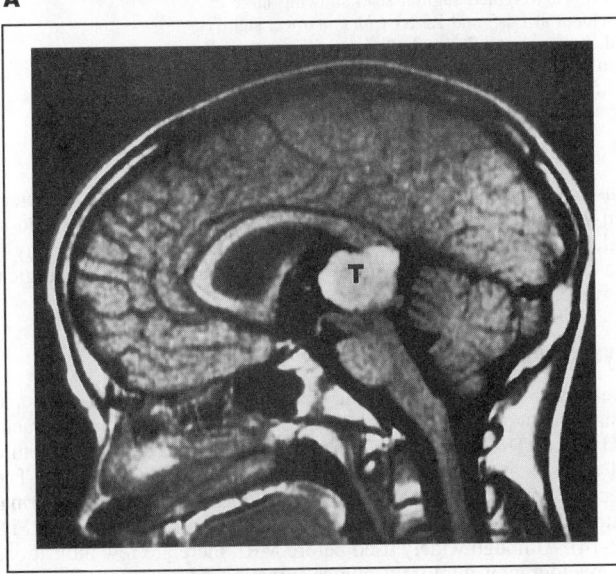

B

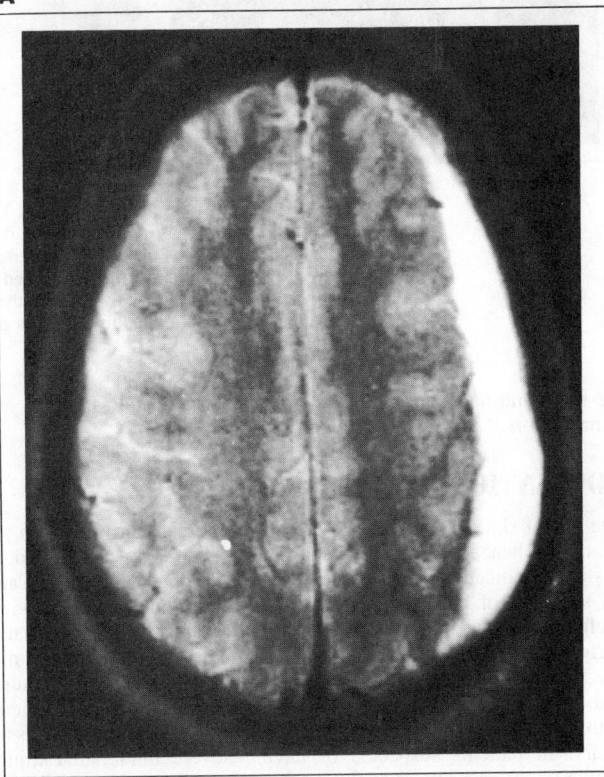

B

FIGURE 132-10   Brain tumor. MRI scan showing pineal tumor in 11-year-old with up-gaze paresis and headache. **A,** T2-weighted *(TR, 2300 msec; TE, 90 msec)* axial scan showing tumor mass *(T)* in region of pineal gland, lateral ventricular enlargement, and an abnormal periventricular rim of high signal *(arrows)* representing cerebrospinal fluid edema attributable to hydrocephalus. **B,** Midsagittal T1-weighted scan after contrast enhancement with Magnevist showing fairly intense but slightly inhomogenous enhancement of the tumor *(T)* clearly delineating its margins.

FIGURE 132-11   MRI of subacute to chronic subdural hematoma. **A,** The coronal T1-weighted scan *(TR, 550 msec; TE, 20 msec)* shows a high-intensity extracerebral biconvex collection over the midconvexity *(arrow).* **B,** The transverse T2-weighted scan *(TR, 2500 msec; TE, 90 msec)* of the same patient shows a large, crescent-shaped, high-intensity abnormality on the same side. These findings are characteristic of a subdural hematoma, estimated to be between 1 week and several months old.

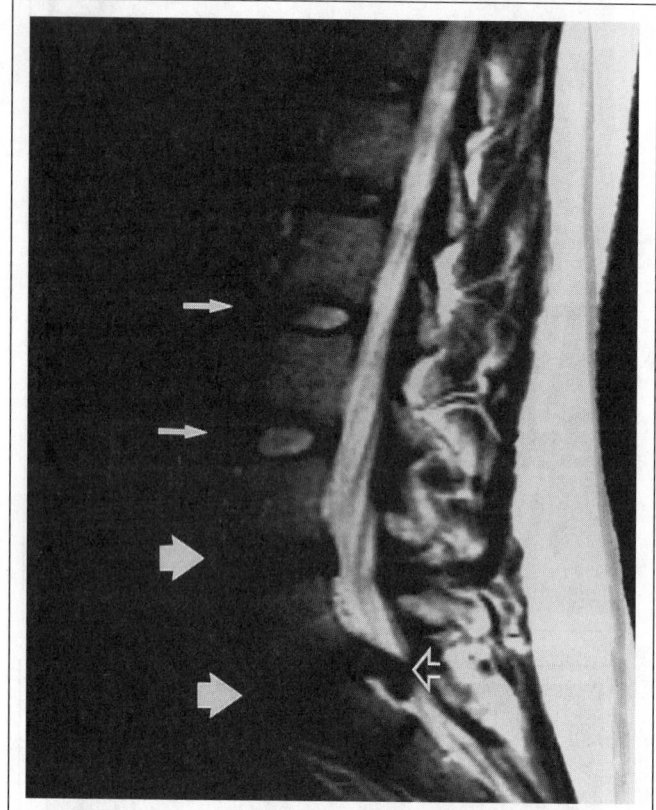

A

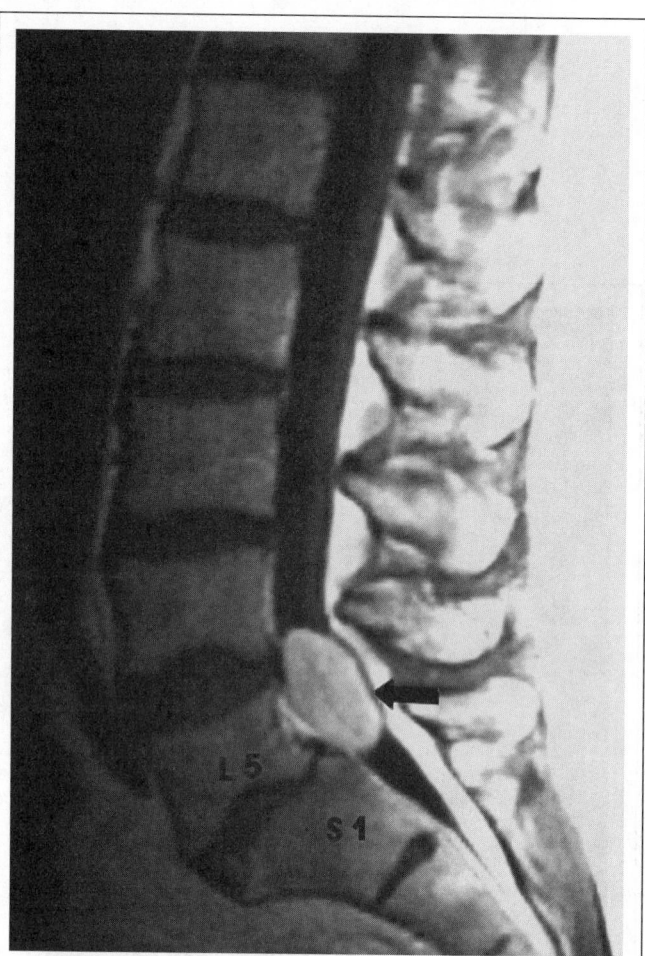

B

FIGURE 132-12 MRI of the lumbar spine. **A,** Disk herniation. T2-weighted sagittal scan showing large extruded disk at the L5-S1 level *(open arrow)*. Dark disks are evident at L4-5 and L5-S1 *(thick arrows)* signifying dessicated or degenerated disks, as opposed to normal disk signal at L2-3 and L3-4 *(small arrows)*. **B,** Intradural tumor. Contrast-enhanced T1-weighted sagittal scan shows an ovoid enhancing intradural schwannoma *(arrow)* at the L5 level. Also evident are the narrowed L5-S1 intervertebral disk and anterior slippage of L5 relative to S1. This anterior subluxation was due to bilateral spondylolysis (not shown on this image).

the brain and has been used to study stroke, neonatal asphyxia, and brain tumors.

CONVENTIONAL RADIOGRAPHY

The use of skull radiographs as a routine screening procedure in patients with headaches, seizures, and transient or fixed neurologic deficits is not indicated, because of extremely low diagnostic yield. Careful selection of patients for skull radiographs, however, may yield useful diagnostic information. Most skull radiographs are currently performed (1) on emergency room patients with relatively mild head trauma and without neurologic findings, to detect fractures and to screen patients for CT examination; and (2) on patients with facial injury, lacerations to the head, or penetrating missile injury. In patients suspected of having severe intracranial injury, skull radiographs are superfluous, and immediate CT is indicated. Skull radiographs can also provide useful information in the assessment of congenital craniofacial abnormalities, palpable lesions in the scalp, and inflammatory conditions of the paranasal sinuses and mastoids.

Plain films of the spine are useful in patients with suspected spinal trauma, and supine lateral cervical spine radiographs should be made in comatose patients with signs of injury to the head and neck before transporting them, to prevent further injury to the spinal cord. Other indications for spine radiographs include scoliosis, congenital anomalies of the spine, back pain, point tenderness, and most condi-

tions for which spine CT or MRI is performed. Flexion and extension views of the spine are often used to diagnose instability and to evaluate adequacy of spinal fusion procedures. Spine radiography is also used to evaluate and follow placement and results of surgical instrumentation.

Myelography

Myelography is the radiographic examination of the spinal canal and spinal cord with nonionic iodinated contrast injected in the subarachnoid space. The injection of contrast is usually via lumbar puncture and occasionally by lateral cervical puncture at the C1-2 level. The injection of contrast is monitored by fluoroscopy, and the normal anatomy and abnormalities are documented with radiographs (Fig. 132-14). Although widely used before MRI, there are few indications for myelography in current clinical practice. Myelography is useful in evaluating spinal vascular malformations, both for diagnosis and to facilitate angiography, and for evaluating spinal malformations when associated with severe scoliosis. In conjunction with CT, myelography can provide more information in cases of cervical spondylosis and in certain postsurgical conditions compared with MRI. Although myelography is relatively safe, side effects do occur and include headache, hypersensitivity reactions, seizures, aseptic meningitis, infection, cardiovascular complications, nausea, vomiting, and vasovagal episodes.

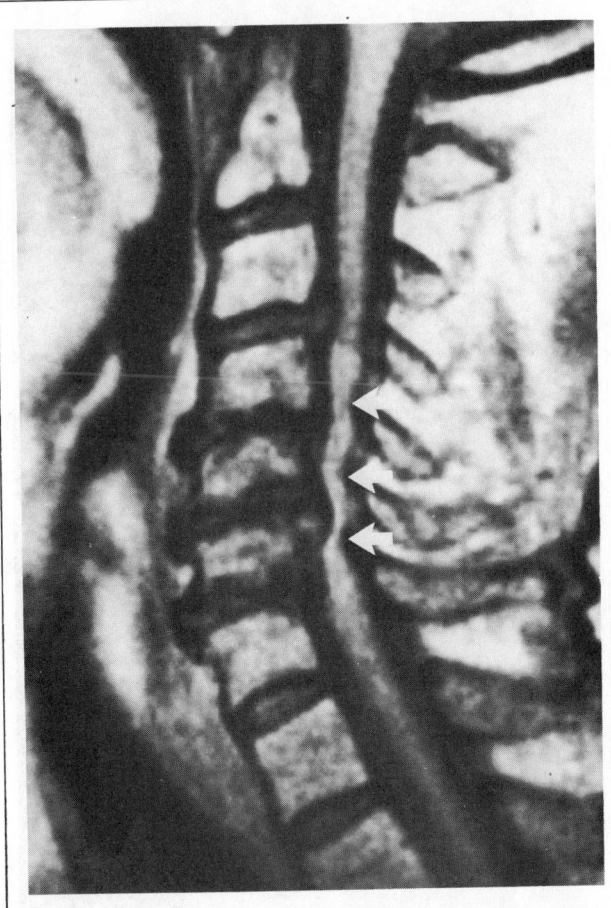

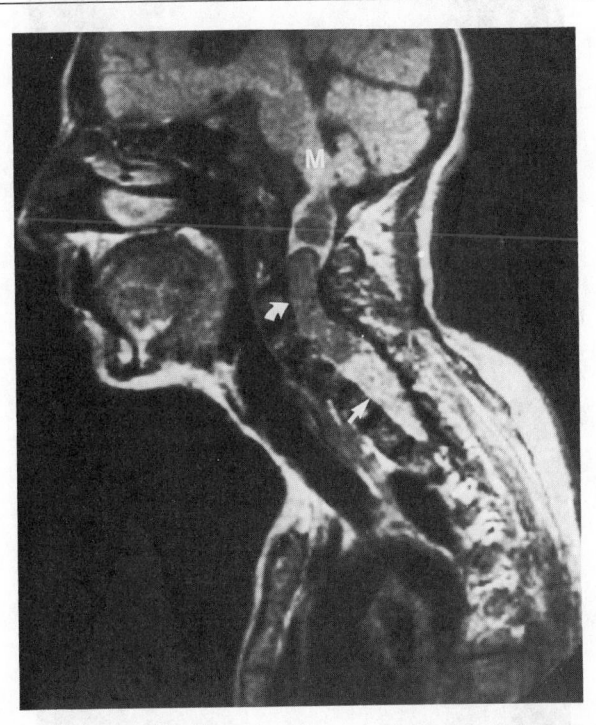

FIGURE 132-13   MRI of cervical spine. **A,** Cervical spondylosis. This sagittal T1-weighted scan shows multiple levels of narrowing of the anteroposterior dimensions of the spinal canal, with compression of the cord at the same levels *(white arrows)*. **B,** Cervical cord astrocytoma. This sagittal proton-density image *(TR, 1500 ms; TE, 40 msec)* shows a cord mass with solid *(straight arrow)* and cystic *(curved arrow)* components extending above the foramen magnum into the medulla *(M)*.

Angiography

Conventional or catheter cerebral angiography is the radiography of intracranial and certain extracranial vascular structures and includes the technical aspects of obtaining vascular access, injection of contrast into the appropriate vessel, recording of information with radiographs, and their interpretation. Access to the vascular tree is usually through the femoral artery; from there a catheter is threaded into the vessel of interest using a guide wire. For carotid or vertebral arteriography the catheter tip is usually placed in the common carotid or vertebral artery. Study of certain tumors and vascular malformations often requires selective internal or external carotid arteriography. Intravascular treatment of vascular malformations, aneurysms, arterial spasm, or thrombolysis generally requires advancing specialized catheters into intracranial branches. Both nonionic and low-osmolality ionic contrast media are used for cerebral angiography. The conventional image recording system using radiographic film screen systems has been almost completely replaced by digital subtraction angiography (DSA). DSA consists of digitization of radiographic information and a process of computer-assisted subtraction and enhancement. DSA is currently used almost synonymously with conventional or catheter angiography. Conventional angiography is used in the diagnosis, presurgical evaluation, and occasionally intraoperative and postsurgical assessment of aneurysms (Fig. 132-15), vascular malformations and fistulas (Fig. 132-16); in the evaluation of cerebrovascular occlusive disease in the grading of carotid stenoses, detecting tandem lesions, assessing the intracranial vasculature for vasculitis and various vasculopathies, and determining the presence and extent of collateral circulation (Fig. 132-17); in confirming the presence and

extent of cerebral venous occlusive disease (Fig. 132-18); and in the evaluation of certain intracranial and skull base tumors, usually for surgical planning. Complications of catheter angiography may be local (hematoma, infection, pseudoaneurysm, fistula, arterial occlusion), systemic (allergic reaction, renal failure), or neurologic (transient neurologic deficit, stroke, cortical blindness). Observation of the patient for several hours afterwards is essential to monitor neurologic status and to prevent serious local complications.

Magnetic resonance angiography is the technique of vascular imaging using magnetic resonance. Two techniques of MRA are currently used. Time-of-flight MRA is obtained by manipulating imaging parameters to enhance magnetization of blood flowing into the imaging volume while simultaneously suppressing signal from stationary tissue. Phase-contrast MRA is generated through a different, more complex mechanism of inducing changes in the phase or spatial orientation of flowing relative to stationary nuclei. MRA is currently widely accepted as a screening technique for extracranial cerebrovascular disease. Screening for intracranial aneurysms can be performed in patients with a family history or in conditions that are associated with aneurysms, such as polycystic kidney disease. Because of a lower sensitivity in detecting aneurysms compared with catheter angiography, MRA is not indicated when aneurysm rupture is suspected, since the consequences of missing an aneurysm in these patients are serious. MRA can be tailored to evaluate the cerebral venous system for occlusive disease or to define venous anatomy before surgery. The primary advantage of MRA relative to catheter angiography is its safety and lower cost. However, MRA requires a relatively high degree of patient cooperation, is subject to artifacts for a

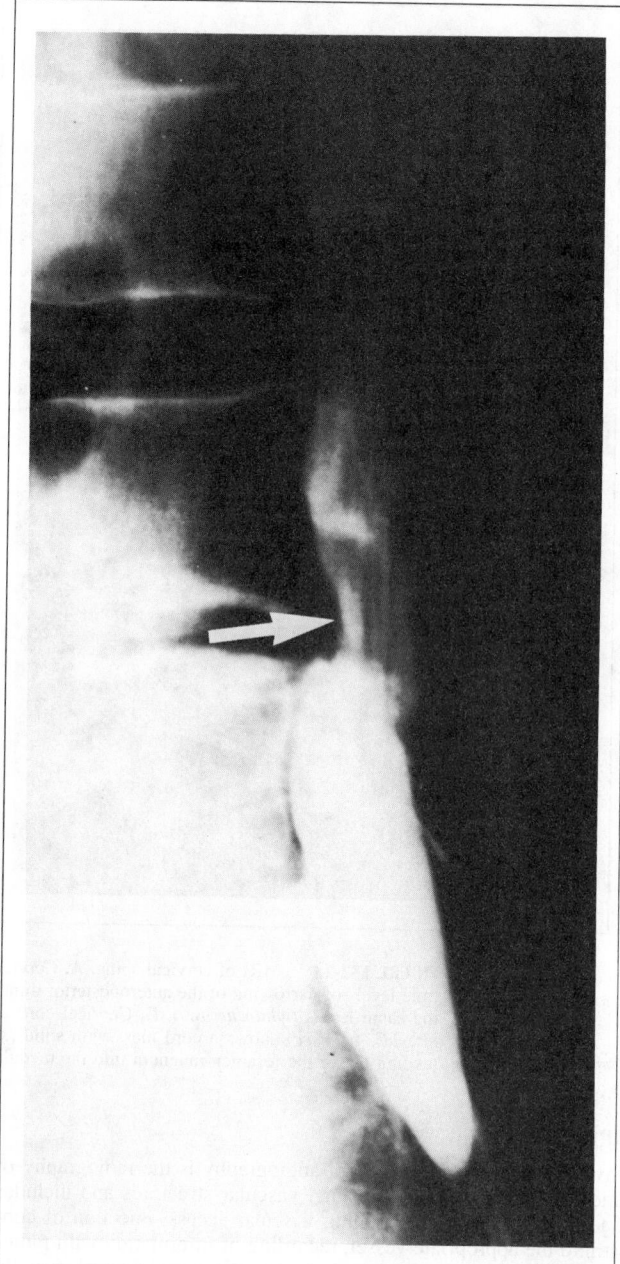

FIGURE 132-14   Lumbar intervertebral disk herniation. **A,** Anteroposterior and, **B,** lateral views of this lumbar myelogram show an extradural defect anteriorly at the L4-5 level on the lateral view *(large arrow)* and on the left side on the anteroposterior view *(large arrow).* The contrast outlines the normal lumbar and sacral nerve roots *(short arrows).* The left-side fifth root does not fill with contrast because of impingement on the root by the herniated disk.

variety of reasons, and provides images of lesser resolution than catheter angiography (Figs. 132-17 and 132-19).

Computed tomographic angiography (CTA) is a relatively recent technique facilitated by the development of high-speed spiral CT scanners. Scans obtained through the extracranial carotid arteries or through the circle of Willis during iodinated contrast infusion can be postprocessed to provide images of the vessels of interest. CTA requires considerable data manipulation to provide useful information and at this time is of limited use in neuroradiology.

RADIONUCLIDE STUDIES

Conventional radionuclide (RN) brain scans were obtained by intravenously administering a radiopharmaceutical that did not cross the blood-brain barrier and recording the gamma emissions from the head with a scintillation camera (gamma camera) to demonstrate areas of blood-brain barrier disruption. This has been replaced by CT and MRI and is only rarely used now other than occasionally to confirm the presence of brain death.

Radionuclide cisternography is performed by injecting a radiopharmaceutical, usually indium-111 diethylene triamine pentaacetic acid (DTPA), into the subarachnoid space via lumbar puncture, then scanning the head to detect its presence and to demonstrate its distribution. Communicating hydrocephalus, commonly called normal pressure hydrocephalus, can be diagnosed by demonstrating intraventricular entry and retention of the radiopharmaceutical (Fig. 132-20). RN cisternography can be used to complement iodinated contrast CT cisternography in the detection and localization of CSF rhinorrhea.

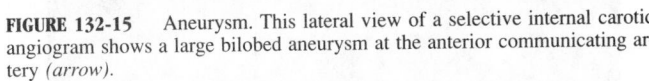

FIGURE 132-15 Aneurysm. This lateral view of a selective internal carotid angiogram shows a large bilobed aneurysm at the anterior communicating artery *(arrow)*.

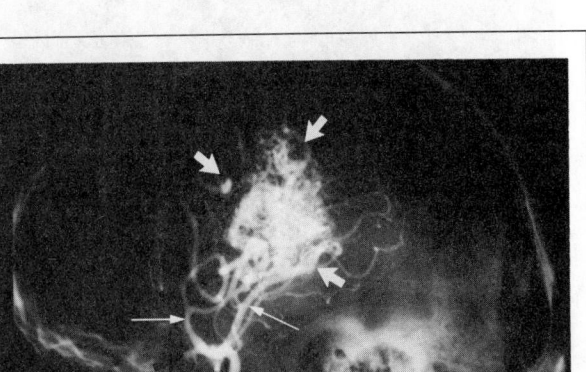

FIGURE 132-16 Vascular malformation. This lateral view of an internal carotid angiogram shows a large arteriovenous malformation *(thick white arrows)* fed by enlarged branches of the middle cerebral artery *(thin white arrows)*. A middle cerebral artery aneurysm is also present *(black arrow)*.

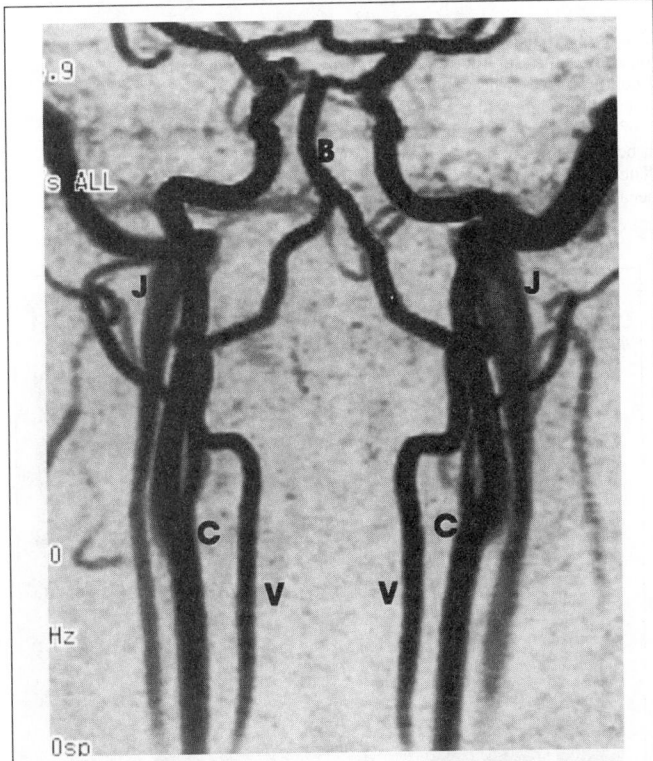

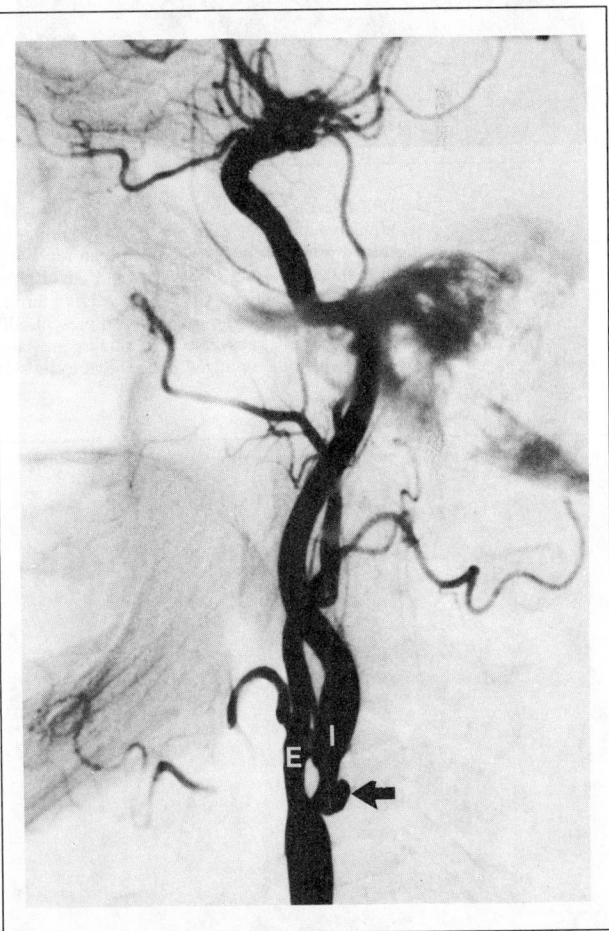

FIGURE 132-17 Extracranial carotid angiography. **A,** Anterior projection from a normal phase-contrast magnetic resonance angiogram (MRA) showing both carotid arteries and bifurcations *(C),* both vertebral *(V)* and the basilar *(B)* arteries, and the jugular veins *(J)*. **B,** Lateral view from a manually subtracted conventional filmscreen arteriogram of one carotid artery shows a large excavated plaque at the origin of the internal carotid artery *(I)*. The external carotid artery *(E)* shows minimal smooth narrowing.

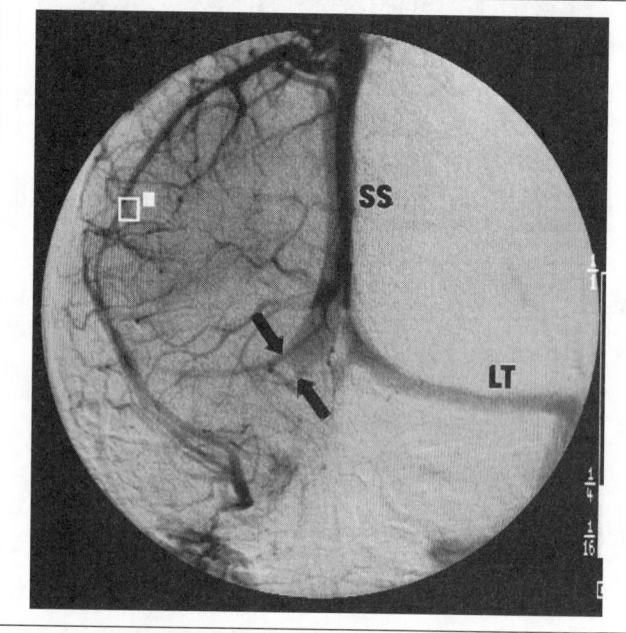

FIGURE 132-18 Dural venous sinus thrombosis. **A,** T2-weighted MRI shows extensive right temporooccipital high-signal lesion *(white arrow)* representing infarction and edema and low signal *(black arrows)* representing blood products in this young woman receiving oral contraceptives who came to medical attention with a seizure and was found to have a field cut. **B,** Anterior view of venous phase of conventional right carotid digital subtraction angiography shows abrupt termination of the larger right transverse sinus *(arrows)* by thrombus. Cortical vein thrombosis was also present, although better seen on other views. The normal superior sagittal *(SS)* and left transverse *(LT)* sinuses are labeled. The white square and box in the image represent the extent to which the digitized images had to be shifted because of patient motion during the injection.

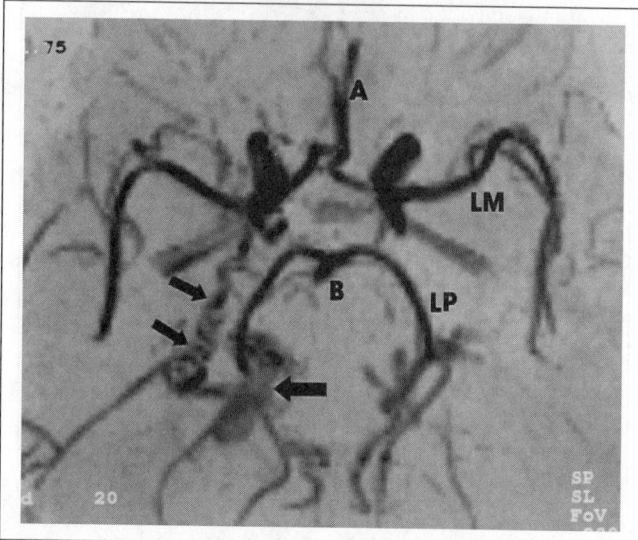
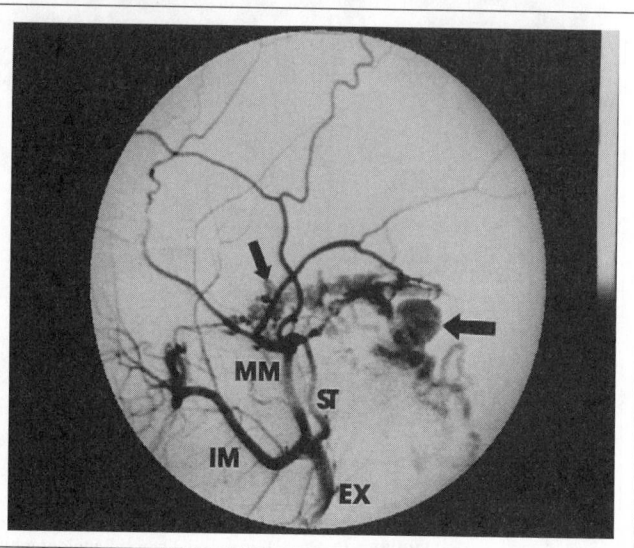

FIGURE 132-19 Dural arteriovenous malformation. **A,** Axial view from time-of-flight MRA shows nidus *(small arrows)*, draining veins, and a varix *(large arrow)* of a dural arteriovenous malformation. Anterior *(A)*, left middle *(LM)*, left posterior *(LP)*, cerebral, and basilar *(B)* arteries are labeled. **B,** Selective right external carotid digital subtraction angiography shows in greater detail the nidus *(small arrow)*, the draining varix *(large arrow)*, and feeding arterial branches from the enlarged middle meningeal *(MM)* and internal maxillary *(IM)* arteries. The external carotid trunk *(EX)* and superficial temporal *(ST)* arteries are labeled.

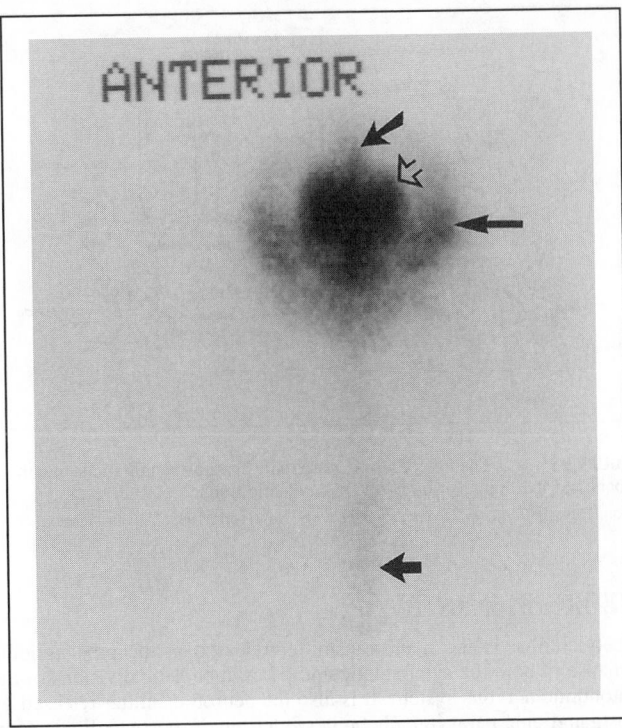

FIGURE 132-20 Communicating hydrocephalus demonstrated by radionuclide cisternogram. Anterior view of the head made 24 hours after radionuclide injection by lumbar puncture showing marked intraventricular reflux of the radionuclide *(open arrow)*. Smaller amounts of radionuclide activity are present in the sylvian fissure *(long straight arrow)*, interhemispheric fissure *(slanted arrow)*, and spinal canal *(short arrow)*.

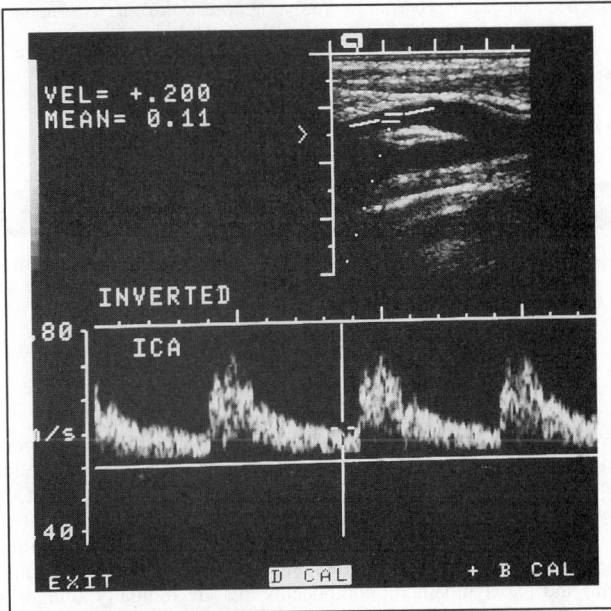

FIGURE 132-21 Carotid sonogram. Duplex sonogram of the carotid bifurcation showing essentially normal carotid bifurcation in the upper right corner of illustration. Pulsed Doppler examination of the proximal internal carotid artery *(short parallel lines over proximal internal carotid artery indicate sample window)* produces normal Doppler tracing shown at bottom of illustration. Maximal measured diastolic velocity of 0.2 m/sec from this tracing, indicated in the upper left corner of illustration, is normal.

Ventriculoperitoneal shunt function can also be assessed by injecting the radiopharmaceutical into the ventricular system or into the shunt reservoir.

Functional imaging of the brain with radiopharmaceuticals can be done with gamma emitters such as technitium-99m labeled hexamethylpropylene amineoxime (HMPAO) using single photon emission computed tomography (SPECT) cameras, or with positron (positively charged electron) emitters using PET. SPECT cameras are widely used but PET scanners are expensive, need cyclotron support, and are available only in large university medical centers. Both these techniques use radionuclides that cross the blood-brain barrier and reflect regional cerebral blood flow or metabolic activity. PET uses synthetic, short-lived, proton-abundant isotopes of biologically active atoms to radiolabel compounds that enter physiologic processes in the brain. PET researchers have used oxygen-15 to measure regional cerebral blood flow, blood volume, and oxygen utilization. Specific levels of mean cerebral blood flow have been correlated with cessation of electrical activity and with cell death. 18F-2 deoxy fluoroglucose is a glucose analog that is used to measure the local glucose utilization. PET and SPECT techniques have been employed in the study of epilepsy, stroke, dementias, brain tumors, Parkinson's disease, and psychiatric disorders. Carbon-11 compounds have been used to study opiate and dopamine receptors in the brain. These are believed to play a role in various neuropsychiatric disorders.

CAROTID ULTRASONOGRAPHY

Duplex scanning, a technique that combines the information provided by high-resolution real-time ultrasonography with the physiologic data obtained by pulse gated Doppler, is used as a screening procedure for extracranial vascular disease primarily at the carotid bifurcation. Real-time sonography is used to detect atherosclerotic plaques and to evaluate plaque morphologic features. Changes in the frequency of the sound wave produced by flowing blood are recorded during the cardiac cycle and constitute the Doppler waveform. The

quantitative frequency shift during the various phases of the cardiac cycle provides a velocity profile of blood flow in the vessel being examined. Stenotic lesions alter the normal velocity profile, and the extent of stenosis can be determined from the Doppler waveform by comparing the systolic and diastolic velocity measurements with known standard values (Fig. 132-21). With color Doppler the velocity-induced frequency shifts in vascular structures are color coded for direction of flow and velocity. This allows easy identification of the flow abnormality and facilitates the examination by letting the sonographer quickly choose the best site for Doppler sampling to determine maximal stenosis. Although totally noninvasive and safe, carotid sonography is an operator-dependent technique requiring a fair amount of skill and experience, is of limited utility for disease above the region of the carotid bifurcations, and is subject to errors of interpretation in cases of high-grade stenoses or complete occlusion.

The role of noninvasive evaluation of cerebrovascular circulation can be expanded with oculoplethysmography, bidirectional periorbital Doppler, and continuous-wave Doppler of the carotid arteries. These techniques have been abandoned by many but can sometimes provide useful information. Transcranial Doppler using low-frequency ultrasonography can not only provide indirect information about extracranial arterial occlusive disease, but can also evaluate the intracranial carotids and the circle of Willis. Transcranial Doppler provides useful information in patients with arterial spasm attributable to subarachnoid hemorrhage and in neonates undergoing extracorporeal membrane oxygenation.

BIBLIOGRAPHY

Carroll BA: Carotid sonography. In *Neuroimaging Clin North Am* 2(3):533, 1992.
Lenkinski RE, Schnall MD: MR spectroscopy and the biochemical basis of neurological disease. In Atlas SW, editor: *Magnetic resonance imaging of the brain and spine,* New York, 1991, Raven.
Modic MT, Masaryk TJ, Ross JS: *Magnetic resonance imaging of the spine,* Chicago, 1989, Mosby–Year Book.
Moseley ME, Glover GH: Functional MR imaging: capabilities and limitations, *Neuroimaging Clin North Am* 5(2):161, 1995.
Newton TH, Potts DG: *Advanced imaging techniques,* San Anselmo, Ca, 1983, Clavadel.
Osborn AG: *Diagnostic neuroradiology,* St Louis, 1994, Mosby.

Rosen BR, Belliveau JW, Fordham JA: The role of dynamic magnetic resonance imaging in stroke, *Neuroimaging Clin North Am* 2(3):559, 1992.

Saloner D: The AAPM/RSNA physics tutorial for residents: an introduction to MR angiography, *Radiographics* 15(2):453, 1995.

CHAPTER

133 Autonomic Nervous System

Roy Freeman

The autonomic nervous system is the principal innervator of visceral and vascular smooth muscle, endocrine and exocrine glands, the immune system, viscera, and certain soft tissues. This division of the neuraxis is almost entirely self-governing and mediates moment-to-moment homeostatic adjustments to the external and internal milieu. The efferent division of the autonomic nervous system has sympathetic and parasympathetic components that are mutually antagonistic in many tissues. The sympathetic nervous system is anatomically widespread and its reactions, best characterized by the "flight or fight response," tend to involve many organ systems simultaneously. In contrast, the parasympathetic nervous system is anatomically more discrete, and its reactions are more localized. The autonomic nervous system also transmits afferent impulses mediating visceral sensation.

The autonomic nervous system is integrally connected to neocortical regions, the limbic system, and somatosensory pathways. It is also subject to neurohumoral influences. Thus such diverse situations as stress, postural change, hypovolemia, pain, fear, and anxiety can activate the appropriate physiologic responses. These reactions are rapid in onset and usually of short duration, in contrast to the longer-lasting effects of the endocrine system.

NEUROANATOMY

The hypothalamus plays a central role in the integration of autonomic function. Projections from the hypothalamus descend to the midbrain and other brain stem structures and then spread in a cascading fashion throughout the spinal cord. The peripheral autonomic nervous system consists of two neurons. The cell body of the first (or preganglionic) neuron, which is found within the central nervous system, sends out an axon that synapses with a ganglion in the periphery. From this ganglion a second (postganglionic) neuron supplies an effector organ. The exception to this scheme is the adrenal gland, where the adrenal medulla functions as a second neuron.

Preganglionic sympathetic neurons extend from the first thoracic (T1) to the second lumbar (L2) levels of the intermediolateral column in the spinal cord. Myelinated sympathetic axons leave the anterior roots as white rami communicantes, forming the paravertebral sympathetic chain and ganglia that extend from the base of the skull to the coccyx. These axons synapse with postganglionic neurons at various segmental levels in the sympathetic chain, and postganglionic axons return to the peripheral nerve as lightly myelinated gray rami communicantes (Fig. 133-1). As an alternative, preganglionic axons may pass through the sympathetic chain, forming the superior, middle, and inferior splanchnic nerves en route to abdominal and pelvic sympathetic ganglia or the adrenal gland. This anatomic arrangement provides the framework for the diffuse, widespread response mediated by the sympathetic nervous system (Fig. 133-2).

The parasympathetic nervous system has its origin in the brain stem and sacral spinal cord. The preganglionic parasympathetic neurons of the brain stem emanate from the cranial nerve nuclei of the oculomotor, facial, glossopharyngeal, and vagus nerves. The sacral division originates in the intermediolateral column of the second, third, and fourth sacral segments of the spinal cord (S2-4) and supplies abdominal and pelvic viscera via the pelvic nerves. These neurons form a postganglionic synapse close to the end-organ, often within the visceral wall (Fig. 133-3).

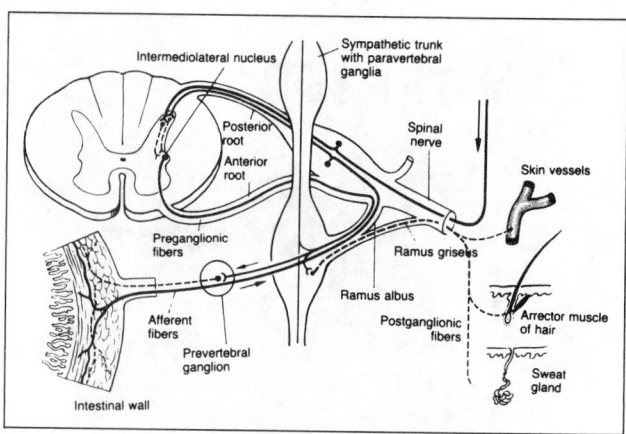

FIGURE 133-1   The course of preganglionic and postganglionic sympathetic fibers and the organization of the sympathetic trunk.

From Duus P: *Topical diagnosis in neurology,* New York, 1983, Thieme-Stratton.

NEUROCHEMISTRY

Acetylcholine is the neurotransmitter released at the preganglionic synapse in both the sympathetic and parasympathetic divisions of the autonomic nervous system. It is also the neurotransmitter released by postganglionic parasympathetic nerve terminals, postganglionic sympathetic nerves to eccrine sweat glands, and possibly nerves to blood vessels supplying skeletal muscle.

Acetylcholine is derived by the enzymatic acetylation of choline with acetylcholine coenzyme A by choline acetyltransferase. Acetylcholine is then stored in vesicles within the axon terminal and, after an action potential, is extruded by exocytosis into the synaptic cleft.

The catecholamine norepinephrine is the neurotransmitter released at the remaining sympathetic postganglionic nerve terminals. The adrenal gland (which is the equivalent in function to a postsynaptic neuron) releases epinephrine and smaller quantities of norepinephrine into the circulation in response to preganglionic nerve impulses.

Norepinephrine is formed within postganglionic nerve terminals by the enzymatic conversion of catecholamine precursors. The aromatic amino acid tyrosine is actively taken up by the nerve terminal and is hydroxylated to dihydroxyphenylalanine (DOPA). This is decarboxylated to form dopamine (DA), which is then converted by dopamine beta hydroxylase (DBH) within the synaptic vesicle to form norepinephrine. Phenylethanolamine-N-methyltransferase, an enzyme in the adrenal gland, allows conversion of norepinephrine to epinephrine (Fig. 133-4).

Norepinephrine is stored within vesicles in the nerve terminals and is released into the synaptic cleft with DBH by exocytosis in response to a nerve impulse. Norepinephrine activates presynaptic or postsynaptic receptors, producing an effect that depends on the nature and site of the receptor.

Released norepinephrine can be actively taken up by the presynaptic neuron (uptake-1), where it is either stored in vesicles ready for rerelease or oxidatively deaminated by intramitochondrial monoamine oxidase (MAO). Norepinephrine can be actively taken up by the postsynaptic cell or (after diffusion into the circulation) by other tissues (uptake-2). Norepinephrine is then degraded by catechol-O-methyltransferase (COMT). The major metabolic end-products of norepinephrine and epinephrine include vanillylmandelic acid (VMA), dihydroxyphenylglycol (DHPG), 3-methoxy-4-hydroxyphenylglycol (MHPG), normetanephrine (NMN), and metanephrine (MN).

Our understanding of autonomic neuroeffector transmission has undergone a major revision in recent years. It is now accepted that most autonomic neurons contain more than one neurotransmitter. These cotransmitters include purines (e.g., adenosine 5'-triphosphate and adenosine), peptides (e.g., neuropeptide Y, vasoactive intestinal peptide, somatostatin, and calcitonin gene-related peptide), amino acids, and nitric oxide. These agents may modify neurotransmission at the neuroeffector junction by prejunctional modulation of the

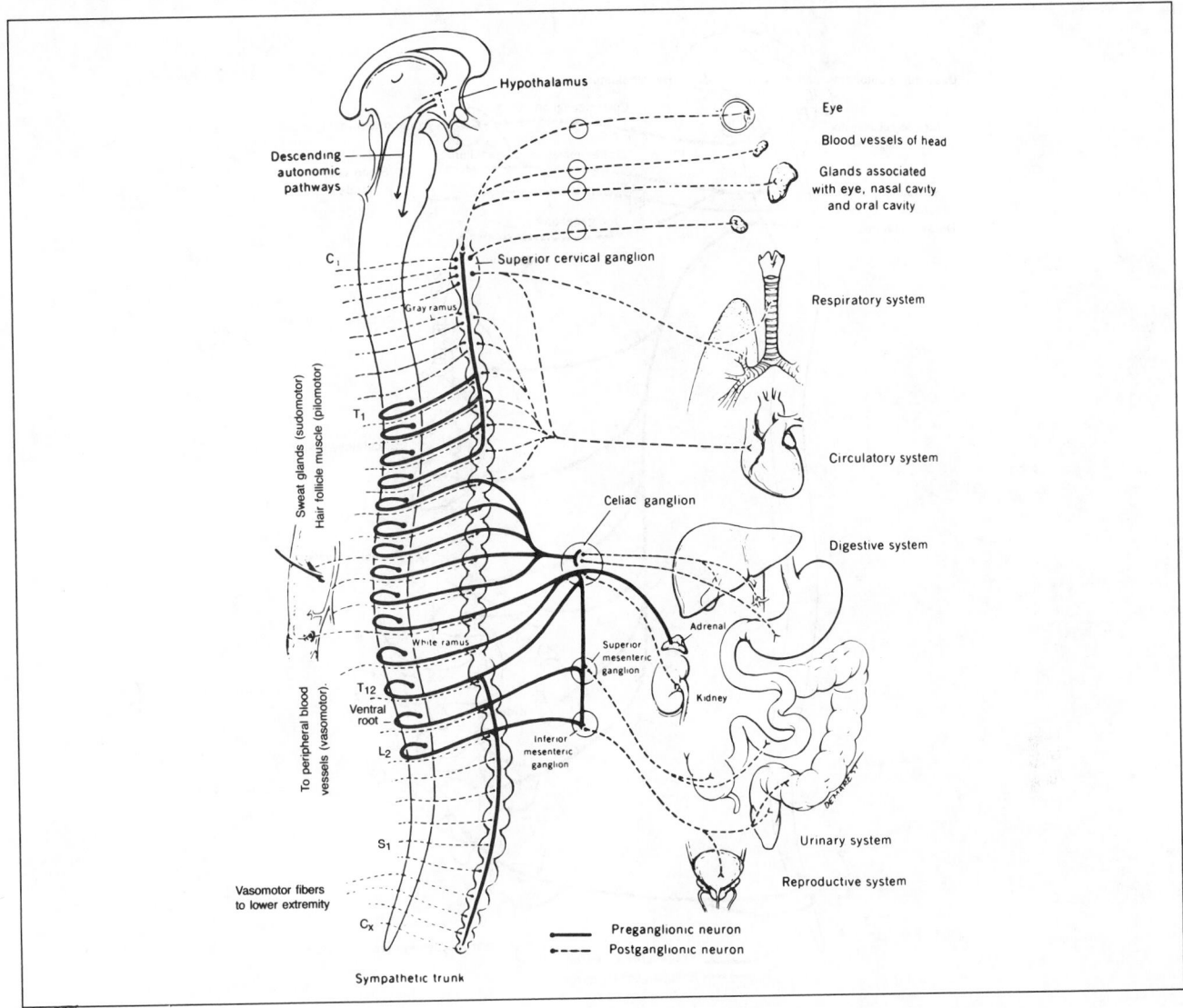

FIGURE 133-2   The sympathetic division of the autonomic nervous system.
From Novak CR, Demarest RJ: *The human nervous system,* ed 2, New York, 1975, McGraw-Hill.

amount of neurotransmitter released or by postjunctional modulation of the duration of action of the neurotransmitter. The process of chemical coding, whereby the specific combinations of different neurotransmitters in autonomic neurons are established, is thus responsible for the remarkable heterogeneity of the human autonomic nervous system.

AUTONOMIC PHYSIOLOGY
Cardiovascular Regulation

The autonomic nervous system mediates immediate cardiovascular homeostatic adjustments, whereas long-term changes are mediated by the endocrine system—in particular, the renin-angiotensin-aldosterone system of the kidney. The short-term changes in cardiac function and vasomotor tone are regulated by a group of brain stem nuclei that integrate information from a variety of neural and humoral sources. Important sites of afferent information for these brain stem centers include the arterial and cardiopulmonary baroreceptors, the cerebral cortex, the limbic cortex, and the hypothalamus.

The baroreceptor reflex arc extends from the cardiopulmonary volume receptors of the great vessels (via the vagus nerve) and the pressure receptors of the carotid sinus and aortic arch (via the glossopharyngeal nerve) to the nucleus of the solitary tract in the ventrolateral medulla. This inhibitory pathway responds to changes in blood pres-

sure. Thus a fall in blood pressure decreases baroreceptor impulses to the nucleus of the solitary tract and other brain stem autonomic nuclei. Parasympathetic pathways extend from the nucleus of the solitary tract to the nucleus ambiguus and dorsal motor nucleus of the vagus. Efferent fibers from these brainstem nuclei then synapse in the heart, and the postganglionic neurons innervate the myocardium, sinoatrial (SA) node, atrioventricular (AV) node, and bundle of His. The nucleus of the solitary tract and associated brainstem autonomic nuclei also give rise to sympathetic fibers passing via the upper thoracic segments of the intermediolateral column to the heart. These mutually antagonistic pathways mediate the changes in heart rate and contractility.

The sympathetic nervous system provides the innervation of the vascular tree. It predominantly supplies the smaller vessels—particularly the small arteries and the arterioles. The most common adrenergic receptor is the α_1 receptor, which causes vasoconstriction when stimulated. Vasodilating β_2-adrenergic receptors and vasoconstricting α_2-adrenergic receptors are also found. Cholinergic axons possibly cause dilation of skeletal muscle blood vessels, and purine derivatives and peptides also play a role in mediating vascular tone.

An important aspect of autonomic circulatory function involves the regulation of the cardiovascular response to postural change. The act of standing, with the resulting gravitational-induced pooling of blood in the lower extremities and splanchnic circulation, produces a

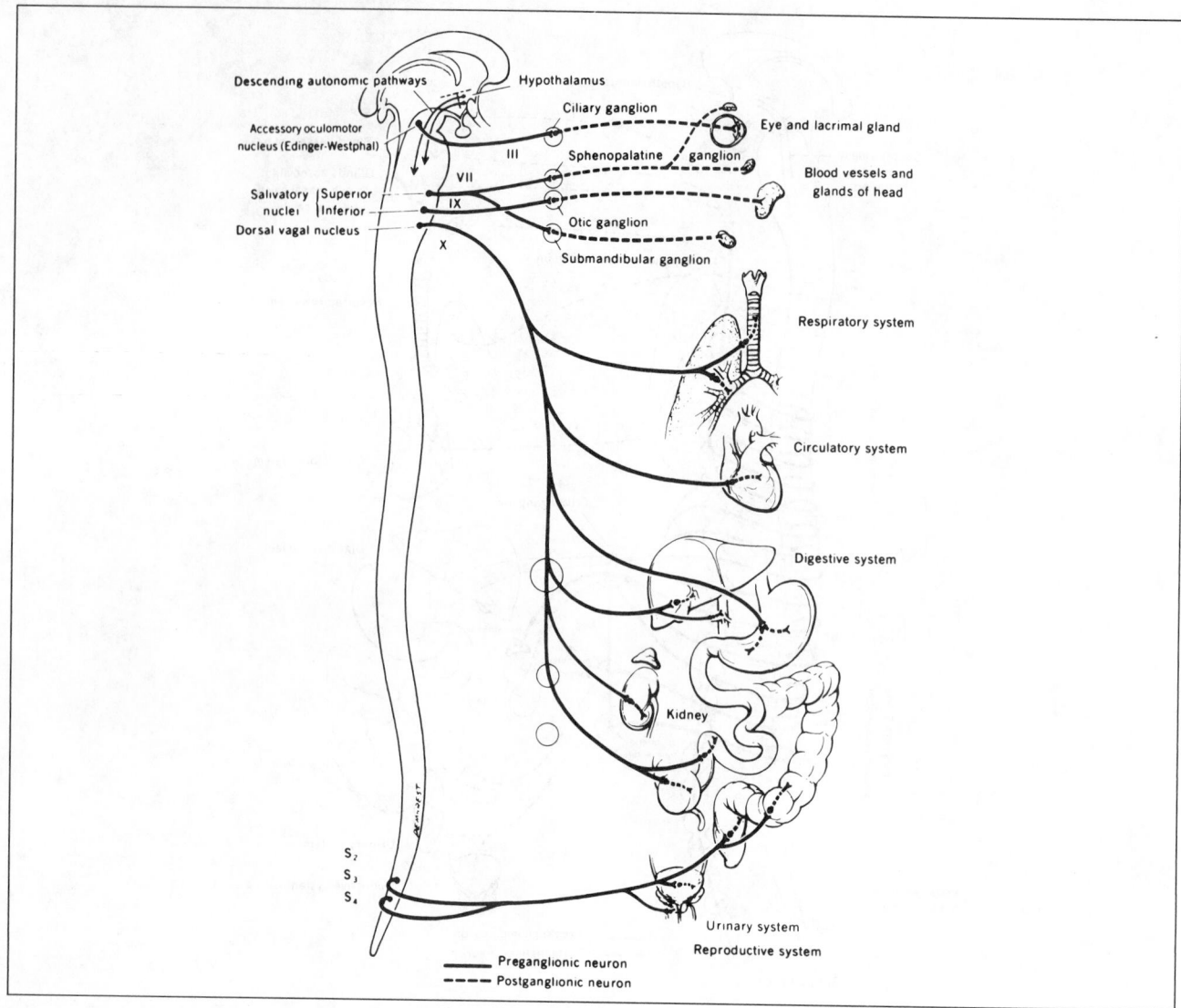

FIGURE 133-3 The parasympathetic division of the autonomic nervous system.
From Novak CR, Demarest RJ: *The human nervous system*, ed 2, New York, 1975, McGraw-Hill.

decrease in the venous return and ventricular filling, with a consequent reduction in stroke volume and cardiac output and thus a fall in blood pressure. The baroreceptors respond by decreasing their inhibitory afferent impulses to the vasomotor centers in the brain stem, provoking immediate adjustments in arterial tone (increasing peripheral vascular resistance) and venular tone (increasing venous return) that occur simultaneously with an increase in heart rate and myocardial contractility. These interrelated physiologic mechanisms maintain blood pressure when the body is in the erect position. When these homeostatic reflexes fail, a postural fall in blood pressure or orthostatic hypotension occurs. As a result of inadequate cerebral perfusion, lightheadedness, fatigue, visual blurring, and syncope may ensue.

Pupil

The pupil best exemplifies the mutual antagonism of the sympathetic and parasympathetic nervous systems—dilating in response to sympathetic impulses and constricting in response to parasympathetic impulses.

Sympathetic fibers en route to the pupil pass through the posterolateral hypothalamus, midbrain, pons, and lateral medulla, descending to the intermediolateral column and leaving the spinal cord after forming a synapse at spinal segments C8-T2. The preganglionic neuron ascends in the sympathetic chain (looping over the subclavian artery and crossing the lung apex) to the superior cervical ganglion located at the bifurcation of the common carotid. The postganglionic neuron extends from the superior cervical ganglion to the eye via a nerve plexus surrounding the internal carotid artery and to the eccrine sweat glands of the face via a plexus surrounding the external carotid artery (Fig. 133-5).

Oculosympathetic paralysis (Horner's syndrome of ptosis, miosis, and anhidrosis) can thus occur with a lesion affecting the primary neuron (e.g., a brainstem stroke, tumor, or syrinx), the preganglionic neuron (e.g., trauma to the brachial plexus, and tumors or infections of the lung apex), or the postganglionic neuron (e.g., a dissecting carotid aneurysm, carotid artery ischemia, migraine, or a middle cranial fossa neoplasm). The lesion site can be determined by pharmacologic testing of the pupil (Table 133-1).

The pupil receives parasympathetic innervation from the third cranial nerve. These parasympathetic pupillomotor fibers originate in the Edinger-Westphal complex of the third cranial nerve nucleus, located in the midbrain, and travel to the ciliary ganglion with the third cranial nerve. The postganglionic short ciliary nerves directly innervate the pupil.

Mydriasis produced by parasympathetic dysfunction can result from a central process affecting the Edinger-Westphal nucleus or third cranial nerve fasciculus (e.g., strokes or tumors of the midbrain), a

Table 133-1   Pharmacologic testing of the pupil

PHARMACOLOGIC AGENT	NORMAL RESPONSE	ABNORMAL RESPONSE	MECHANISM
Cocaine (2%-10%)	Dilation	No response	Blocks presynaptic norepinephrine uptake
Hydroxyamphetamine (1%)	Dilation	No response if lesion is in postganglionic neuron; normal response if postganglionic neuron is intact	Releases norepinephrine from postganglionic neuron
Phenylephrine (1%)	No response or minimal response	Dilates abnormal pupil, especially if postganglionic lesion is present	Pupil supersensitive because of denervation
Pilocarpine (0.125%) (1%)	No response Constriction	Constricts Adie's pupil No response if pupil is pharmacologically dilated	Pupil sensitive because of denervation Pharmacologic blockade
Methacholine (2.5%)	No response	Constricts Adie's pupil	Pupil supersensitive because of denervation

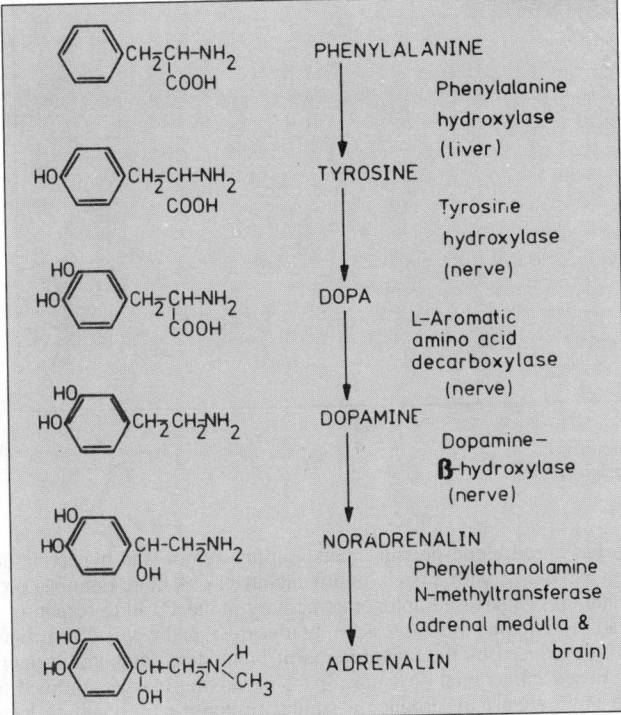

FIGURE 133-4   Catecholamine metabolism.

From Bannister R, editor: *Autonomic failure*, Oxford, 1982, Oxford University Press.

preganglionic lesion affecting the third cranial nerve (e.g., compression by an enlarging posterior communicating artery aneurysm, transtentorial herniation, or a mononeuropathy affecting the third cranial nerve or trauma), or a postganglionic process (e.g., Adie's pupil, a third cranial nerve mononeuropathy, or pharmacologic blockade of the pupil or trauma).

Sweating

Sweating is the thermoregulatory response to an increase in central core temperature and is mediated by heat regulator centers in the anterior hypothalamus. Sweating also occurs in response to gustatory and emotional stimuli. Two types of sweat glands are found. The eccrine glands are innervated by sympathetic nerves with cholinergic synapses at both the preganglionic and postganglionic neuron. The apocrine glands, found in the axilla, the genital region, and the nipples, are not under neurologic control. They respond to circulating humoral factors and produce apocrine secretions, primarily in response to emotional stimuli.

Bladder

The bladder is composed of three layers of interdigitating smooth muscle (the detrusor muscle) and serves as a receptacle for the storage and appropriate evacuation of urine. The detrusor muscle forms the internal sphincter at the junction of the bladder neck and urethra. This sphincter is not anatomically discrete and functions as a physiologic sphincter. In contrast, the external sphincter is formed from the striated muscle of the urogenital diaphragm and is a true anatomic sphincter.

Higher centers involved in bladder control include the anterior and medial frontal lobes, limbic regions, basal ganglia, thalamus, hypothalamus, and brain stem. These regions receive afferent fibers from and send efferent fibers to "micturition centers" in the lower spinal cord.

The bladder has parasympathetic, sympathetic, and somatic innervation. The parasympathetic nerves originate in the intermediolateral column of the second, third, and fourth sacral segments of the spinal cord. Passing through the ventral nerve roots, these fibers form pelvic nerves that synapse with postganglionic neurons on the surface of the bladder. These muscarinic, cholinergic postganglionic nerves produce detrusor muscle contraction. The sympathetic nerve supply to the bladder originates in the intermediolateral column of spinal segments T12-L2. These nerve fibers pass through the sympathetic ganglia and reach the hypogastric plexus via the splanchnic nerves. Postganglionic sympathetic neurons then innervate the dome of the bladder (β-adrenergic receptors) and the internal sphincter (α-adrenergic receptors) via the hypogastric nerves. The striated muscle of the external urethral sphincter is innervated by the pudendal nerves, which originate from the anterior horn cells of the second, third, and fourth sacral segments. This sphincter is under voluntary control but undergoes reflex relaxation during micturition. Afferent fibers mediating bladder sensation and reflex bladder contraction are carried by both the sympathetic and the parasympathetic nerves to the spinal cord (Fig. 133-6).

Normal voluntary micturition is most likely coordinated by pontomesencephalic centers and modulated by higher cerebral regions. This act entails a complex sequence of neural activity, including voluntary relaxation of the striated external sphincter, increased intraabdominal pressure produced by abdominal wall tension, and detrusor muscle contraction with subsequent relaxation and opening of the internal sphincter. Micturition ceases after voluntary contraction of the external sphincter.

Genital System

Normal sexual function involves the integration of several psychologic and physiologic processes. These include appropriate sexual drive (libido) and sexual arousal, penile erection, orgasm, and ejaculation in the male, and genital vascular engorgement in the female. The neurologic control of sexual function thus involves a complex coordination of higher centers with sympathetic, parasympathetic, and somatic nervous activity.

Penile erection is produced by vascular engorgement of the cor-

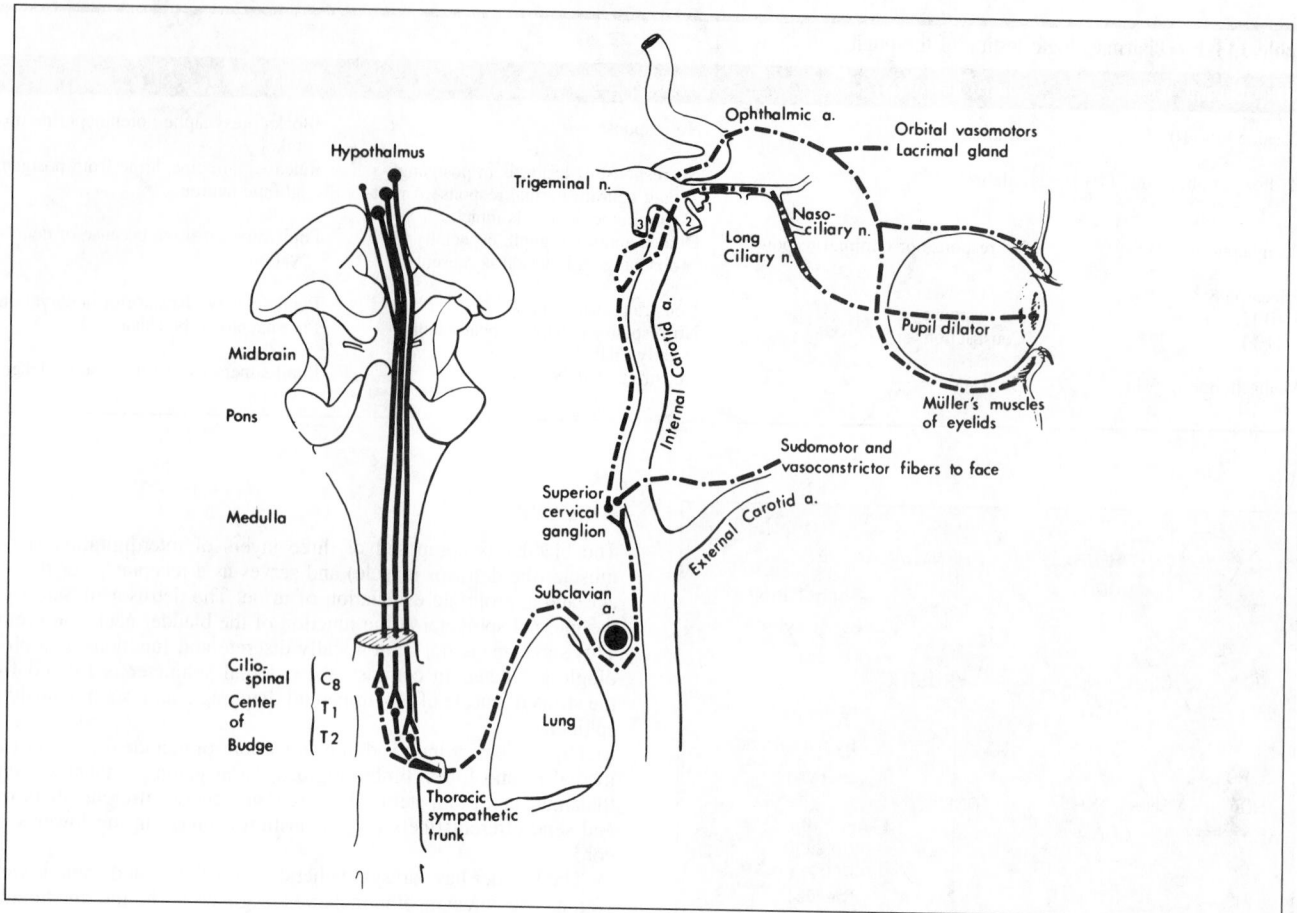

FIGURE 133-5 Ocular sympathetic pathways.
From Glaser JS: *Neuro-ophthalmology,* ed 2, Philadelphia, 1990, Lippincott.

pus spongiosum and corpora cavernosa caused by arterial vasodilation, venous constriction, and closure of arteriovenous shunts. Local stimuli (bowel or bladder distention and tactile stimulation of the external genitalia) provoke this response via a spinal reflex (reflexogenic erections), whereas psychogenic erections are provoked by stimuli to higher centers. Erections are mediated by the parasympathetic pelvic nerves (nervi erigentes) from spinal segments S2-4. The sympathetic nervous system (segments T12-L2) via the hypogastric nerves plays an accessory role, particularly in the production of psychogenic erections. Recent evidence has suggested that nitric oxide, vasoactive intestinal peptide, and neuropeptide Y may also have a role in erectile function.

Ejaculation is a complex reflex mediated by the hypogastric sympathetic nerves (which cause contraction of the smooth muscle of the seminal vesicles, vasa deferentia, epididymides, and ejaculatory ducts) and somatic pudendal nerves (which produce contraction of the ischiocavernosus and bulbocavernosus muscles).

Less is known about the autonomic control of the female genital system. Parasympathetic pelvic nerves stimulate vaginal secretions and mediate vascular engorgement of the vulva, vagina, and clitoris during sexual arousal. The pudendal nerves mediate contraction of the vaginal and pelvic floor muscles during orgasm.

Because sexual function involves vast neural territories and intricate interactions among the sympathetic, parasympathetic, and somatic nervous systems, dysfunction may occur at several levels as a result of diverse psychologic, neurologic, medical, and endocrinologic causes.

GENERALIZED AUTONOMIC DISORDERS
Autonomic Overactivity

A wide range of disorders produces generalized overactivity of the autonomic nervous system. This appears most frequently as tachy-

cardia, raised blood pressure, perspiration, tremor, and hyperventilation associated with anxiety and panic attacks. A more ominous presentation of increased autonomic activity is the Cushing response, a triad of increased blood pressure, bradycardia, and respiratory irregularity produced by the compression of brain stem autonomic centers by raised intracranial pressure. Space-occupying masses confined to the brain stem may produce a similar response as a result of local effects, even in the absence of raised intracranial pressure. In addition, strokes, trauma, subarachnoid hemorrhage, and meningitis can all produce signs of autonomic hyperactivity. The electrocardiographic changes associated with these neurologic diseases are also mediated by autonomic overactivity and may represent microscopic myocardial abnormalities.

Symptoms of autonomic overactivity such as hypertension, sweating, flushing, anxiety, changes in heart and respiratory rates, salivation, abdominal cramps, and pupillomotor responses may occur as manifestations of a seizure. Temporal lobe seizure foci provide the most frequent source of such symptoms. Rarely, central lesions in the region of the third ventricle, thalamus, and hypothalamus also produce this symptom complex. This has been called diencephalic epilepsy. However, rather than a true epileptic phenomenon, it is more likely to be due to pressure on brain stem autonomic centers or release of those centers from cortical and subcortical control. The propensity of seizure foci to affect the autonomic nervous system may well be reflected in the increased incidence of sudden death in patients with epilepsy.

A "mass reflex" of autonomic overactivity, with signs such as hypertension, cardiac arrhythmias, piloerection, and sweating, frequently follows spinal cord injury. Afferent impulses, such as pain or bladder distention, usually provide the provocative stimulus for this response, which most commonly occurs after cervical and high-thoracic–cord lesions.

Sedative or alcohol withdrawal is a common cause of sympathetic

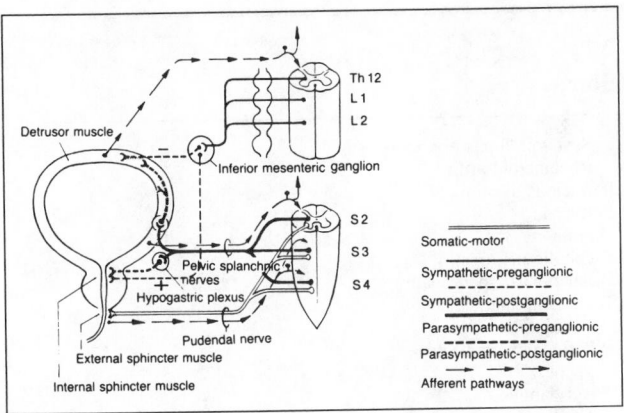

FIGURE 133-6 The innervation of the urinary bladder.

From Duus P: *Topical diagnosis in neurology,* New York, 1983, Thieme-Stratton.

nervous system overactivity. In its most florid form this state consists of agitation, confusion, hypervigilance, hallucinosis, and tremulousness, with autonomic accompaniments such as mydriasis, tachycardia, tachypnea, and sweating. Although these symptoms usually abate gradually after several days, in extreme cases the withdrawal syndrome can be fatal.

Pheochromocytoma and other tumors of chromaffin cell origin produce a picture of autonomic hyperactivity characterized by paroxysmal hypertension, sweating, flushing, tachycardia, and anxiety, generated by intermittent catecholamine release (Chapter 164).

Although peripheral neuropathies customarily produce symptoms of autonomic hypoactivity, acute inflammatory demyelinating neuropathy (Guillain-Barré syndrome) may produce periodic autonomic overactivity, often alternating with symptoms and signs of reduced autonomic function. Acute intermittent porphyria can produce a similar clinical picture of increased autonomic activity associated with an acute progressive neuropathy (Chapters 145 and 147). For a complete list of disorders that produce autonomic overactivity see Box 133-1.

Autonomic Failure

Autonomic failure produces a wide array of symptoms and may be caused by a diverse group of disorders. Orthostatic hypotension, the most debilitating of these symptoms, initially is characterized by occasional lightheadedness or dizziness, usually provoked by sudden standing, a warm environment, or large meals. Patients may also have associated visual disturbances reflecting retinal or occipital lobe ischemia and neck pain caused by ischemia of trapezius and other neck muscles. Eventually, severely afflicted patients are unable to maintain erect posture and may be confined to bed. Frequently, supine hypertension produced by baroreceptor dysfunction accompanies orthostatic hypotension.

Bladder symptoms are a common complaint of patients with autonomic dysfunction. Central nervous system disease usually produces detrusor hyperreflexia, with such symptoms as frequency, urgency, nocturia, and incontinence. This often occurs in conjunction with sphincter dyssynergy—a failure to coordinate bladder contraction with sphincter relaxation. Peripheral nervous system disease, on the other hand, customarily produces detrusor muscle areflexia, with such symptoms as difficulty in initiating urination, failure to maintain an adequate stream of urine, urinary retention, and overflow incontinence. Such patients are often subjected to unnecessary prostatic surgery, which usually exacerbates the clinical condition by producing further incontinence.

Impotence, diminished libido, ejaculatory dysfunction, and failure to attain orgasm may be early symptoms of autonomic dysfunction, although patients often do not seek immediate medical attention for these problems. Depression resulting from the debilitating symptoms of autonomic failure may at times be the primary cause of impotence.

Generalized anhidrosis with attendant thermoregulatory dysfunction occurs late in the clinical course of conditions that produce au-

BOX 133-1
Autonomic overactivity

1. Central nervous system
Raised intracranial pressure
Temporal lobe epilepsy
Diencephalic epilepsy
Cerebrovascular disease
Head trauma
Meningitis
Encephalitis
Spinal cord injury
Tetanus
Familial dysautonomia
Poliomyelitis
Neuroleptic malignant syndrome

2. Peripheral nerve
Acute pandysautonomia
Porphyria
Acute inflammatory demyelinating polyneuropathy
Toxic neuropathies

3. Tumors
Pheochromocytoma
Neuroblastoma
Ganglioneuroblastoma
Ganglioneuroma
Carotid body tumor

4. Drugs
Monoamine oxidase inhibitors
Sympathomimetic agents
Sedative or alcohol withdrawal

Modified from Johnson RH, Lamby DG, Spalding JMK. In Baker AB, Joynt RJ, editors: *Clinical neurology,* vol 4, Philadelphia, 1986, Harper & Row.

tonomic failure. At an early stage, patchy or partial anhidrosis is accompanied by hyperhidrosis in other areas in an attempt to maintain normal thermoregulation. Some patients complain of excess sweating associated with eating.

Gastrointestinal tract complaints of patients with autonomic failure include nausea, vomiting, early satiety caused by gastroparesis, constipation, diarrhea, and incontinence. Symptoms referable to other organ systems include difficulty adapting to changing light conditions because of decreased pupillomotor function and respiratory difficulties caused by paralysis of the abductors of the larynx. Obstructive and central apneic episodes and other disorders of central respiratory control may also occur.

Shy and Drager first described a syndrome of progressive autonomic failure in conjunction with dysfunction in the extrapyramidal, pyramidal, and cerebellar systems. Extraocular movement abnormalities and disturbances in respiratory, bulbar, and peripheral motor neuron function may also occur. This clinical condition, known as the Shy-Drager syndrome or multiple system atrophy, is progressive and culminates in death after several years. When cerebellar features predominate the clinical presentation, this disorder is termed olivoponocerebellar atrophy. When extrapyramidal features are predominate, the clinical presentation of this disorder is termed striatonigral degeneration. The pathologic hallmark of this disorder is extensive loss of the cellular elements in the intermediolateral columns of the spinal cord. Accompanying pathologic changes appear in the striatum, cerebellum, pyramidal system, anterior horn cells, and autonomic nuclei of the brain stem, including the locus ceruleus, nucleus of the tractus solitarius, nucleus ambiguus, and dorsal motor nucleus of the vagus. The norepinephrine content of the basal ganglia, septal nuclei, hypothalamus, locus ceruleus, and nucleus accumbens is reduced. An argyrophilic, intracytoplasmic oligodendriglial inclusion may be a specific pathologic marker for multiple system atrophy. Autonomic failure may also accompany Parkinson's disease and other diseases of the central nervous system (Box 133-2).

BOX 133-2
Autonomic failure

Disorders of the central nervous system

Multiple system atrophy (Shy-Drager syndrome)
    Olivopontocerebellar degeneration
    Striatonigral degeneration
Parkinson's disease
Brain tumors (brain stem, cerebellum, diencephalon)
Wernicke's disease
Multiple infarcts
Syringomyelia and syringobulbia
Hydrocephalus
Multiple sclerosis
Myelopathies

Disorders of the peripheral nervous system

Pure autonomic failure (idiopathic orthostatic hypotension)
Peripheral neuropathies
    Diabetes
    Amyloid
    Guillain-Barré syndrome
    Chronic inflammatory polyneuropathy
    Acute pandysautonomia
    Hereditary neuropathies
        Hereditary sensory and autonomic neuropathies
        Fabry's disease
        Navajo Indian neuropathy
        Hereditary motor and sensory neuropathy
        Tangier disease
    Infectious diseases
        Chagas' disease
        Human immunodeficiency virus neuropathy
        Botulism
        Diphtheria
        Leprosy
    Connective tissue diseases
        Sjögren's syndrome

        Systemic lupus erythematosus
        Rheumatoid arthritis
    Pernicious anemia
    Porphyria
    Uremia
    Alcoholic neuropathy
    Paraneoplastic neuropathy
    Toxic neuropathies
        Vincristine
        Perhexilene maleate
        Vacor
        Acrylamide
        Thallium
        Arsenic
        Mercury
        cis-Platinum
        Taxol
        Organic solvents
    Surgical sympathectomy
    Adie's syndrome
    Dopamine beta hydroxylase deficiency

Miscellaneous disorders

Medications
    Antihypertensive agents
    Tricyclic agents
    Monoamine oxidase inhibitors
    Antipsychotic agents
Aging (?)
Hyperbradykinism
Endocrine
    Adrenocortical deficiencies
    Pheochromocytoma
    Hyperaldosteronism

Various disorders affecting the peripheral nervous system result in autonomic dysfunction. Pure autonomic failure, or idiopathic orthostatic hypotension, is a disorder characterized by progressive autonomic dysfunction that usually occurs without clinical evidence of central nervous system disease or an obvious peripheral neuropathy. This disorder is most likely due to degeneration of the postganglionic peripheral autonomic neuron. Recent investigations have indicated that some pathologic and physiologic preganglionic autonomic nervous system involvement may also occur in this disease.

Acute and subacute presentations of pure autonomic neuropathy occur. Patients with these disorders, which are most likely a form of inflammatory polyneuropathy confined to the autonomic nerves, generally recover autonomic function.

In 20% to 40% of patients with diabetes, evidence of autonomic dysfunction develops as a consequence of small fiber damage (Chapter 168). This usually occurs late in the illness, although subclinical autonomic involvement may be detected in newly diagnosed and teenage diabetics. Cardiovascular autonomic abnormalities associated with diabetes include orthostatic hypotension, resting tachycardia, fixed heart rate, and a tendency to painless myocardial infarction. Insulin may exacerbate the orthostatic hypotension. Other symptoms of autonomic dysfunction include gastroparesis (with nausea, vomiting, early satiety, and postprandial abdominal discomfort), nocturnal diarrhea, constipation, incontinence of feces, sweating abnormalities, bladder dysfunction, and unawareness of hypoglycemia. In one prospective study autonomic dysfunction, as defined by abnormal cardiovascular reflexes, was associated with a mortality rate of 56% at 5 years.

The peripheral neuropathies associated with amyloid, alcoholism, uremia, porphyria, and Fabry's disease are other prominent causes of autonomic dysfunction. Disorders of the peripheral nervous system with autonomic involvement are listed in Box on 133-2.

LOCAL AUTONOMIC DISORDERS

Several diseases are due to or associated with local autonomic nervous system dysfunction. These diseases are listed in Box 133-3. Details of these disorders are covered elsewhere in the text.

TESTING THE AUTONOMIC NERVOUS SYSTEM

The anatomic location of the autonomic nervous system renders it relatively inaccessible for direct clinical testing. Furthermore, because most autonomic fibers are unmyelinated and therefore conduct nerve impulses slowly, conventional neurophysiologic techniques are inadequate means of studying autonomic function. A battery of tests assessing autonomic function and dysfunction has been established to circumvent these problems by measuring end-organ responses to various physiologic and pharmacologic perturbations; by determining the levels of autonomic neurotransmitters and neuromodulators in blood, cerebrospinal fluid, and urine; and by quantifying autonomic receptor density and affinity.

The most frequently used tests are described in the following section.

CARDIOVASCULAR REFLEXES
Reflex-Response Interval Variation

A reflex increase in the heart rate occurs with inspiration and is followed by a reflex decrease in heart rate with expiration. This response is mediated by the vagus nerve and is abolished by atropine. When

---

BOX 133-3
Local autonomic disorders

Head and neck
Baroreceptor denervation
Carotid endarterectomy
Migraine
Cluster headache
Melkersson's syndrome
Spastic dysphonia
Carotid sinus hypersensitivity
Horner's syndrome

Limbs
Raynaud's phenomenon
Acrocyanosis
Angioneurotic edema
Causalgia
Reflex sympathetic dystrophy
Erythromelalgia
Hyperhidrosis
Anhidrosis

Trunk
Cystic fibrosis
Asthma
Spastic colon
Chronic intestinal pseudoobstruction

Modified from Johnson RH, Lamby DG, Spalding JMK: In Baker AB, Joynt RJ, editors: *Clinical neurology,* vol 4, Philadelphia, 1986, Harper & Row.

breathing at a rate of six breaths per minute, normal subjects display a difference between the maximum and minimum heart rates of more than 10 beats per minute. As an alternative, a ratio can be calculated between the sum of the longest reflex-response (R-R) interval occurring on each of six expirations and the sum of the shortest R-R interval occurring on each of six inspirations. This is known as the expiration-inspiration (E-I) ratio. Because there is a progressive decline in the amplitude of heart rate variation (and most other tests of autonomic function) with increasing age, age-based norms should be established. This test provides an index of parasympathetic nervous system function.

Valsalva's Maneuver

The patient is requested to exhale against a resistance of 40 mm Hg for 20 seconds while heart rate and blood pressure are monitored. Four discrete phases occur. In phase 1 the increase in intrathoracic and intraabdominal pressure causes aortic compression and an increase in peripheral resistance that results in a transient increase of blood pressure and decrease in heart rate. In phase 2 the increase in intrathoracic pressure produces decreases in venous return, left ventricular filling pressure, and cardiac output. This causes a fall in pulse pressure, which is terminated after several seconds by reflex vasoconstriction mediated via the baroreceptor reflex pathways. During this phase there is compensatory increase in heart rate. Phase 3 begins with the cessation of forced expiration. In this phase there is a further drop in blood pressure as the aortic compression ceases. In phase 4, blood pressure increases ("the overshoot") as a result of the "postrelease" increase in cardiac output and persisting peripheral vasoconstriction. This blood pressure increase causes a reflex bradycardia.

Valsalva's maneuver tests both the sympathetic and parasympathetic divisions of the nervous system. With sympathetic dysfunction the tachycardia in phase 2 and blood pressure increase at the start of phase 4 are attenuated. The fall in blood pressure occurring in phase 2 may not be terminated by vasoconstriction. With parasympathetic dysfunction the baroreceptor-mediated reflex bradycardic response to the elevated blood pressure in phase 4 does not occur.

Valsalva's maneuver is best tested by measuring blood pressure and heart rate simultaneously; the recent availability of noninvasive beat-to-beat blood pressure recordings permits the direct measurement of this reflex. The Valsalva ratio—a ratio of the longest R-R interval in phase 4 to the shortest R-R interval in phase 2—provides an indirect measure of cardiac vagal function. The blood pressure fall in phase 2 of the maneuver and blood pressure increase in phase 4 of the maneuver provide a measure of sympathetic nervous sytem function.

Heart Rate Response to Standing

On moving from a supine to a standing position, a relative tachycardia occurs, usually maximizing around the fifteenth beat after standing is initiated. This is followed by a relative bradycardia that is maximum at approximately the thirtieth beat. This biphasic response is mediated by afferent impulses from muscle, the vagus nerve, and the baroreflex arc. It does not occur with passive tilting and is blocked by atropine. The ratio of the R-R interval at the thirtieth beat to the R-R interval at the fifteenth beat (the 30:15 ratio) may be used as a measure of this reflex. This test provides an index of parasympathetic nervous system function.

Blood Pressure Response to Standing

On moving from the horizontal to the vertical position, blood pressure is maintained by reflex vasocontriction and an increase in heart rate. A fall in systolic blood pressure of greater than 20 to 30 mm Hg or diastolic blood pressure of 10 to 15 mm Hg is abnormal. This test provides an index of sympathetic nervous system function.

Cold Pressor Test

The patient immerses his or her hand in cold water (4° C) for 60 seconds. A normal response, mediated by afferent sensory pathways and efferent sympathetic pathways that bypass the baroreceptors, is a systolic blood pressure increase of approximately 10 to 15 mm Hg. This test provides an index of sympathetic nervous system function.

Isometric Hand Grip

The patient squeezes a hand grip dynamometer at 30% of his or her maximum strength for 3 minutes. A normal response is a diastolic blood pressure increase of approximately 15 mm Hg or greater. This test provides an index of sympathetic nervous system function.

Other Cardiovascular Reflexes

Other cardiac reflexes include the vagally mediated bradycardic response to apneic facial immersion in cold water, the tachycardia and blood pressure increase in response to mental stress, the blood pressure and heart rate response to passive tilting or lower-body negative pressure, and the bradycardic response to carotid sinus massage.

Power Spectral Analysis

Power spectral analysis of the resting heart rate produces several prominent peaks. A number of animal and human experiments with pharmacologic blockade of the autonomic nervous system have shown that the sympathetic and parasympathetic nervous systems mediate heart rate fluctuations in different frequency bands. Heart rate fluctuations at frequencies greater than 0.15 Hz are mediated by changes in vagal efferent activity alone, whereas heart rate fluctuations at less than 0.15 Hz are mediated by changing levels of both vagal and sympathetic activity. In normal subjects the move from supine to upright position produces a shift in the power spectrum from high to low frequencies. This shift in spectral power, induced by postural change, is reduced by β-receptor blockade and reflects a change in the balance of sympathetic and parasympathetic efferent activity. Indices derived from the power spectrum thus provide a potential measure of both sympathetic and parasympathetic nervous system function.

Pupillometry

The integrity of the autonomic innervation of the pupil can be simply determined by use of pharmacologic agents. The sympathetic supply to the pupil is tested by using cocaine (2% to 10%) and hydroxyamphetamine (1%). The normal pupil dilates after the instillation of cocaine eyedrops, which prevent norepinephrine reuptake by the presynaptic neuron. However, there is no response to cocaine eyedrops if there is a lesion anywhere in the sympathetic pathway to the eye. Both a normal pupil and a miotic pupil (as a result of preganglionic lesion) dilate in response to the instillation of hydroxyamphetamine, which releases intraneuronal norepinephrine from the postganglionic axon terminal. A lesion of the postganglionic neuron distal to the superior cervical ganglion prevents dilation after hydroxyamphetamine instillation. The use of these two agents provides a simple means of diagnosing and localizing the site of neuronal injury responsible for sympathetic ocular paralysis.

Dilute pilocarpine is used to assess parasympathetic postganglionic pupil dysfunction. The normal pupil does not constrict to dilute pilocarpine (0.125%); however, the dilated, denervated supersensitive pupil (e.g., produced by Adie's syndrome or other postganglionic neuronal dysfunction) rapidly becomes miotic. In contrast, pharmacologically induced mydriasis, producing a fixed dilated pupil, can be demonstrated by the use of 1% pilocarpine. This surprisingly frequent clinical phenomenon, which could be confused with imminent transtentorial herniation, is due to the accidental or deliberate contact of sympathomimetic agents with the conjunctival surface. Medication-induced mydriasis does not respond to 1% pilocarpine.

An infrared pupillometer with an attached television camera provides an accurate and sensitive, although expensive, means of assessing a number of aspects of pupil function.

Sweat Testing

Testing the eccrine sweat glands provides a useful means of assessing the sympathetic nervous system. The simplest of the available clinical tests—the thermoregulatory sweat test—entails raising the body temperature with an external thermal source. The sweat response is assessed by measuring the color change in an indicator such as iodine with starch, quinizarin, or alizarin red. Skin bioelectric recordings measuring the electrodermal potential (the sympathetic skin response), skin conductance (the galvanic skin reflex), or skin resistance provide an alternate measure of sweating. These tests examine both central and peripheral aspects of the afferent sympathetic nervous system.

The integrity of the postganglionic sympathetic neuron can be determined by measuring sweat output after iontophoresis or intradermal injection of cholinergic agonists such as pilocarpine or acetylcholine. The response can be quantified by using a sudorometer or by measuring the size of an imprint formed by the sweat droplets.

Catecholamine Measurements

The advent of assays for catecholamines and catecholamine metabolites has provided a quantitative biochemical index of sympathetic nervous system activity. These compounds can now be measured with sensitivity and specificity in plasma, urine, and cerebrospinal fluid.

Plasma norepinephrine level doubles on movement from a supine to an erect position. A substantial further increase occurs after isometric or isotonic exercise. Patients with orthostatic hypotension caused by central nervous system disease have a normal resting norepinephrine level because the postganglionic peripheral sympathetic neuron is intact. The normal norepinephrine increase in response to postural change or other stressful stimuli does not occur because the central nervous system is unable to activate the postganglionic neuron. In contrast, patients with hypotension produced by peripheral nerve injury have a low resting norepinephrine level, which results from the postganglionic peripheral sympathetic nerve dysfunction. These patients also have no postural or stress-induced increase in plasma norepinephrine.

Catecholamines and their metabolites can also be measured in the cerebrospinal fluid (CSF) and urine. Although these determinations are not widely used in clinical practice (with the exception of urinary catecholamine level measurements to diagnose pheochromocytoma),

our understanding of many neurologic, psychiatric, and endocrine diseases has been enhanced by such measurements, which may well have future therapeutic applications.

Pharmacologic Testing

Pharmacologic agents can be used systemically to determine the status of specific regions of the autonomic nervous system. The postsynaptic receptor agonists are generally used to demonstrate the state of enhanced sensitivity that a receptor develops when its presynaptic neuron degenerates (denervation supersensitivity). In this way, norepinephrine and phenylephrine can be used to determine α_1-receptor function, and isoproterenol and epinephrine can be used to determine β_1- and β_2-receptor function. The oral ingestion of yohimbine and clonidine, the respective antagonist and agonist of the α_2-receptor, can be used to assess α_2-adrenoreceptor function. Tyramine, which induces norepinephrine release from the intact postganglionic noradrenergic neuron, provides a useful means of assessing postganglionic neuronal integrity by measuring norepinephrine output. The cholinergic system can be assessed by an intravenous infusion of atropine.

Urodynamic Testing

Current technologies available to most investigators allow for detailed physiologic evaluation of bladder, urethra, and sphincter function. The simplest, yet most important, of these investigations, the measurement of residual urinary volume, entails only transurethral catheterization immediately after micturition. This provides a measure of bladder evacuation and can also gauge the effectiveness of any therapeutic interventions.

The cystometrogram documents intravesical pressure and sensation as the bladder is progressively distended, usually by a transurethral water or carbon dioxide infusion. The perception of bladder filling occurs at 100 to 200 ml, and patients normally feel a strong desire to void at 400 to 500 ml. Patients with detrusor hyperreflexia caused by upper motor neuron disease display inhibited bladder contractions at volumes considerably lower than this. In contrast, the large-capacity atonic bladder produced by lower motor neuron disease shows no increase in intravesical pressure, despite the introduction of large volumes of fluid. The coordination of bladder contraction and sphincter relaxation can be determined by carrying out simultaneous sphincter electromyography.

The voiding cystourethrogram is a radiologic study that provides structural and dynamic measures of bladder function. The patient is requested to void after the introduction of contrast material. Radiography carried out during micturition displays bladder size and shape, sphincter function, and urinary flow.

The selected use of these studies permits accurate diagnosis and appropriate therapy of bladder disturbances.

BIBLIOGRAPHY

Appenzeller O: *The autonomic nervous system: an introduction to basic and clinical concepts,* ed 4, New York, 1990, Elsevier Science.

Bannister R, editor: *Autonomic failure,* ed 3, New York, 1992, Oxford University.

Burnstock G, Hoyle CHV, editors: *Autonomic neuroeffector mechanisms,* Chur, Switzerland, 1992, Harwood Academic.

Ewing DJ, Campbell IW, Clarke BF: The natural history of diabetic autonomic neuropathy, *Q J Med* 49:95, 1980.

Korczyn AD, editor: *Handbook of autonomic nervous system dysfunction,* New York, 1995, Marcel Dekker.

Loewy AD, Spyer KM, editors: *Central regulation of autonomic functions,* New York, 1990, Oxford University Press.

Low PA, editor: *Clinical autonomic disorders: evaluation and management,* Boston, 1993, Little, Brown.

McLeod JG: Autonomic dysfunction in peripheral nerve disease, *Muscle Nerve* 15:3, 1992.

McLeod JG, Tuck RR: Disorders of the autonomic nervous system. I. Pathophysiology and clinical features, *Ann Neurol* 21:419, 1987.

McLeod JG, Tuck RR: Disorders of the autonomic nervous system. II. Investigation and treatment, *Ann Neurol* 21:519, 1987.

Robertson D, Biaggioni I, editors: *Disorders of the autonomic nervous system,* Luxembourg, 1995, Harwood Academic.

Thomas PK: Autonomic involvement in inherited neuropathies, *Clin Autonom Res* 2:51, 1992.

II CLINICAL SYNDROMES

CHAPTER

134 Sleep and Sleep Disorders*

Jean K. Matheson

Sleep is an active, clinically important behavior, during which many physiologic processes of the organism change. These processes are temporally organized under cerebral influence. Sleep abnormality may represent a primary disorder of mechanisms regulating sleep, or failure within a specific organ system that manifests in a unique way during sleep. Thus it is important that sleep complaints are not ignored or treated empirically with pharmacologic agents. More often than not, disordered sleep is a symptom of underlying disease.

PHYSIOLOGY

There are two sleep states, rapid eye movement (REM) and non-REM (NREM) sleep. REM sleep was discovered by Aserinsky and Kleitman in the early 1950s. By waking subjects during REM, they also established that vivid dreaming occurs during this sleep state. Soon thereafter Dement recognized that episodes of REM sleep alternate with NREM sleep, in cycles lasting approximately 90 minutes, throughout the night.

Recordings derived from electroencephalograms (EEG), eye movements (electrooculogram; EOG), and chin tone (electromyogram; EMG) are necessary to distinguish sleep states. Polysomnography is the technique used to record multiple physiologic variables during sleep. In clinical practice several other physiologic measures are typically recorded, including respiratory effort from chest and abdomen, oral and nasal airflow, cardiac rhythm, and electromyographic activity in the anterior tibialis muscles of the legs.

NREM sleep is divided into four sleep stages, numbered I, II, III, and IV. The waking EEG with the eyes closed reveals the characteristic "alpha rhythm," which is a posteriorly predominant 8- to 12-Hz rhythm that attenuates with eye opening. Stage I sleep is characterized by the gradual disappearance of the alpha rhythm, which is replaced by slower, 2- to 7-Hz activity, and some fast 12- to 14-Hz low-voltage activity. Stage II is distinguished by the presence of spindles (bursts of 12- to 14-Hz activity lasting at least 0.5 seconds, with a "spindle" appearance) and K complexes (high-voltage biphasic negative-positive waves best seen at the vertex, usually associated with spindles). Stages III and IV are defined by the presence of high-voltage slow-wave activity of 2 Hz or less. An epoch of 30 seconds is measured: if 20% to 50% of the record shows high-voltage slow activity, it is termed stage III; more than 50% high-voltage slow activity is termed stage IV. Stages III and IV are often described together as *slow wave sleep* or *delta sleep*. Delta sleep can be characterized as "deep sleep," because during this stage subjects are difficult to arouse. Detailed dreaming does not occur, but subjects awakened during this sleep stage have reported "thinking."

The normal subject descends in an orderly progression through the four NREM sleep stages. Delta sleep appears 30 to 45 minutes after sleep onset. The first REM period follows this delta sleep, about 70 to 90 minutes after sleep onset.

The polysomnogram during REM shows dramatic changes. There is a sudden decrease in the EMG reading in the chin muscles, which reflects generalized skeletal muscle atonia. Except for the eye muscles and respiratory muscles, the subject is paralyzed. Rapid eye movements occur in phasic bursts. The EEG shows mixed frequencies similar to those of stage I and waking. Characteristic sawtooth waves sometimes occur during eye movements. Respiration and heart rate are irregular.

The first REM period is short—approximately 10 minutes. The end of the first REM period ends the first sleep cycle. Thereafter NREM continues to alternate with REM; there are four to six cycles in the healthy young adult (Fig. 134-1). Sleep architecture is the organization of sleep stages and cycles. The normal young adult spends approximately 5% of the night in stage I, 50% in stage II, 12% in stage III, 13% in stage IV, and 20% in REM. Delta sleep is concentrated in the first third of the night, whereas REM episodes become progressively longer later in the night. Delta sleep decreases as a function of age, but REM percentage is relatively stable after early childhood. Of the newborn's daily 17 to 18 hours of sleep, 50% is REM. Children and early adolescents sleep 10 to 11 hours. Most adults prefer to sleep 7 to 8 hr/day, but sleep needs vary. Short sleepers are classified as those individuals who feel adequately rested with less than 6 hours of sleep; long sleepers require more than 9 hours.

Sleep efficiency is defined as the time spent asleep divided by the time spent in bed. Sleep efficiency decreases in old age, as both the number of arousals and time spent in bed increase. This does not necessarily represent "normal" aging. Arousals usually have a cause (see Sleep Disorders).

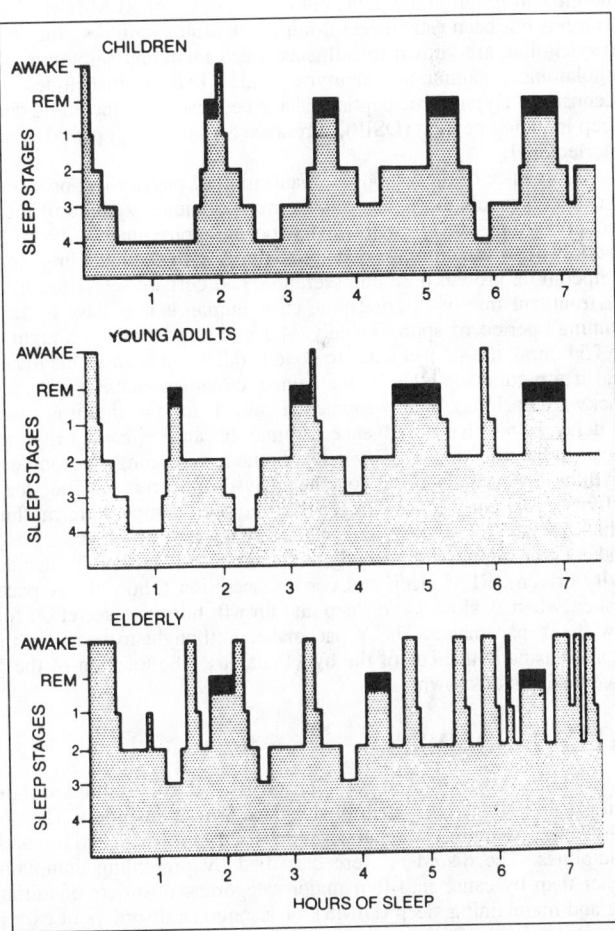

FIGURE 134-1 Sleep architecture. REM sleep alternates with NREM in cycles approximating 90 minutes in all age-groups. Delta sleep is prominent in childhood and decreases in old age as awakenings and wake time increase.
From Kales A, Kales JD: *N Engl J Med* 290:487, 1974.

*Classification and quoted definitions throughout this chapter from Diagnostic Classification Steering Committee, Thorpy MJ, chair: *International classification of sleep disorders: diagnostic and coding manual*, Rochester, Minn, 1990, American Sleep Disorders Association.

If there are frequent external or internal disrupters of sleep, the sleep patterns change. After arousal, the patient develops stage I sleep, followed by stage II sleep, repetitively, and the percentages of delta sleep and REM sleep decrease. Drugs can also inhibit REM and delta sleep. Monoamine oxidase inhibitors and tricyclic antidepressants, for example, decrease the percentage of REM sleep dramatically. Alcohol and caffeine increase arousal. If patients are deprived of either REM or delta sleep, "rebound" is usually seen on recovery nights. REM rebound can be intrusive and frightening, with an abundance of vivid dreams. Chronic partial sleep deprivation results in inattentiveness in monotonous tasks, mood deterioration, irritability, and even mild paranoia.

REM sleep and NREM sleep differ physiologically. REM sleep is characterized by both phasic and tonic changes. The drop in baseline EMG correlates with a tonic change. Rapid eye movements correlate with phasic changes. Tonic physiologic changes also include impaired thermoregulation, hypotension, bradycardia, increased cerebral blood flow and intracranial pressure, increased respiratory rate, and penile erection. Intercostal and upper airway muscles become atonic, but the diaphragm maintains activity. Phasic changes include vasoconstriction, increased blood pressure, tachycardia, and further increases in cerebral blood flow and respiratory rate. During NREM the physiologic state is more stable, but blood pressure, heart rate, cardiac output, and respiratory rate decrease. Growth hormone is secreted during stages III and IV, in the first third of the night. Many other rhythms occur during sleep, but these need not be directly tied to sleep, as discussed later.

Experimentally created lesions of the anterior hypothalamus in animals cause insomnia. Recent evidence suggests that this area is selectively active during sleep and may be important in the initiation of sleep. REM sleep can be abolished by lesions restricted to a cholinergic cell group in the pons, but the generator of REM/NREM cycling has not been established. Multiple neurotransmitters other than acetylcholine are known to influence sleep including serotonin, catecholamines, gamma-aminobutyric acid (GABA), histamine, and adenosine. "Hypnogenic peptides" have been isolated, including delta sleep inducing peptide (DSIP), substance S (a muramyl peptide), and interleukin-1.

The science of the temporal organization of physiologic processes is called chronobiology. Sleep is the most obvious example of a circadian rhythm—body rhythms that occur approximately every 24 hours. There are multiple other circadian rhythms, including body temperature, growth hormone secretion, and cortisol secretion. In an environment free of external time cues, human beings have a "free-running" period of approximately 24.3 hours (previously thought to be 25 hours); the subject tends to go to bed later each day. This means that if a regular schedule is maintained, circadian clocks are "reset" backward each day by environmental cues. It follows that it is easier to delay, rather than to advance bedtime, because circadian rhythms move in the direction of daily delay. In the free-running environment, rhythms that usually occur together may desynchronize. The sleep/activity cycle can become longer than the body temperature rhythm, which remains at slightly longer than 24 hours. Two separate pacemakers emerge, termed X (body temperature–driven) and Y (rest/activity driven). REM sleep and cortisol secretion follow the X pacemaker, whereas slow-wave sleep and growth hormone secretion follow the Y pacemaker. The Y pacemaker is thought to reside in the suprachiasmatic nucleus of the hypothalamus. The location of the X pacemaker is unknown.

SLEEP DISORDERS

In 1972, the Association of Sleep Disorders Centers established a diagnostic classification system of sleep and arousal disorders. The nosology served to unify clinical definitions across medical and research disciplines. The disorders were classified by presenting complaint rather than by cause into four major categories: disorders of initiating and maintaining sleep (DIMS), or insomnias; disorders of excessive somnolence (DOES); disorders of the sleep-wake schedule; and dysfunctions associated with sleep, sleep stages, or partial arousal (parasomnias). This classification is helpful in approaching differential diagnosis. However, for statistical and research purposes it is inadequate because one disorder may be characterized by more than

one symptom. Thus the classification was revised in 1990, as the International Classification of Sleep Disorders (ICSD) (Box 134-1) and is now based on broadly defined pathophysiologic mechanisms rather than presenting symptoms.

The major divisions of the ICSD classification are the (1) dyssomnias, (2) parasomnias, (3) sleep disorders associated with medical and psychiatric disorders, and (4) proposed sleep disorders.

Dyssomnias

The dyssomnias are primary sleep disorders that produce either *difficulty initiating and maintaining sleep* or *excessive daytime sleepiness.*

Difficulty Initiating and Maintaining Sleep (DIMS, Insomnia). Inability to sleep may take the form of prolonged initial latency to sleep, recurrent nocturnal awakenings, or early morning awakening without the ability to return to sleep. Insomnia is an extremely common complaint that causes high levels of frustration and significant misery. For reasons that are inexplicable, insomnia is frequently trivialized by the clinician and treated pharmacologically without attention to the underlying cause of the complaint. Inability to initiate or maintain sleep is a symptom that must be explored with the same approach the clinician uses to assess other medical complaints. As in most disorders, a careful history is the most significant diagnostic tool. Exploring the patient's daily schedule in an orderly fashion is often markedly revealing. A sleep log helps document patterns that suggest specific disease. The schedule of daily activities gives insight into the patient's personality and discloses habits that contribute to poor sleep hygiene. All medical history is relevant, and illnesses that may cause nocturnal arousal are particularly important. A family history of sleep disorder and history of childhood sleep behavior are useful. A review of drug use, including prescription medications, home remedies, caffeine, alcohol, and illicit drugs, is critical.

Excessive Daytime Sleepiness (DOES). Excessive daytime sleepiness is defined as the tendency to fall asleep inappropriately when sedentary. Patients with excessive daytime sleepiness may or may not demonstrate hypersomnolence, that is, excessive sleep during a 24-hour period. Patients with chronic disorders of excessive daytime sleepiness often accept their sleepiness as normal. The clinician should look for a history of excessive daytime sleepiness in any situation presenting as chronically reduced performance, including dementia, or in situations suggesting episodic inattention, such as automobile accidents. Instead of complaining of sleepiness, many patients cite blackouts, forgetfulness, poor concentration, automatic behavior, and amnestic spells. Children may have poor school performance or behavioral problems, including apparent hyperactivity. These situations require the taking of a sleep history that includes questioning the patient as to whether or not sleeping occurs during sedentary activities, social activities, driving, and eating. Sleepiness needs to be distinguished from fatigue and disorders of consciousness secondary to encephalopathy.

Within the classification of the dyssomnias, the sleep abnormalities must be fundamental to the existence of the disorder. Psychiatric and medical disorders that influence sleep, as only one component of the clinical presentation, are not included in the ICSD definition of dyssomnia. The dyssomnias are further divided into three groups: the intrinsic sleep disorders, the extrinsic sleep disorders, and the circadian rhythm sleep disorders. Intrinsic sleep disorders are thought to originate within the body; examples are narcolepsy and obstructive sleep apnea. Extrinsic sleep disorders originate outside the body; these include poor sleep hygiene and environmental disruption. Circadian rhythm sleep disorders represent disorders of the timing of the sleep-wake cycle within the 24-hour day.

Intrinsic Sleep Disorders. "*Psychophysiologic insomnia* is a disorder of somatized tension and learned sleep-preventing associations that results in a complaint of insomnia and associated decreased functioning during wakefulness." These patients usually do not have evidence of underlying psychiatric disease but may be highly focused on their insomnia. Overconcern with the process of going to sleep is alerting, induces increased tension, and becomes a sleep-preventing

BOX 134-1
International classification of sleep disorders
Classification outline

1. Dyssomnias
   A. Intrinsic sleep disorders
   B. Extrinsic sleep disorders
   C. Circadian rhythm sleep disorders
2. Parasomnias
   A. Arousal disorders
   B. Sleep-wake transition disorders
   C. Parasomnias usually associated with REM sleep
   D. Other parasomnias

3. Medical/psychiatric sleep disorders
   A. Associated with mental disorders
   B. Associated with neurologic disorders
   C. Associated with other medical disorders
4. Proposed sleep disorders

---

1. Dyssomnias
   A. Intrinsic sleep disorders
      1. Psychophysiologic insomnia
      2. Sleep state misperception
      3. Idiopathic insomnia
      4. Narcolepsy
      5. Recurrent hypersomnia
      6. Idiopathic hypersomnia
      7. Posttraumatic hypersomnia
      8. Obstructive sleep apnea syndrome
      9. Central sleep apnea syndrome
      10. Central alveolar hypoventilation syndrome
      11. Periodic limb movement disorder
      12. Restless legs syndrome
      13. Intrinsic sleep disorder not otherwise specified (NOS)
   B. Extrinsic sleep disorders
      1. Inadequate sleep hygiene
      2. Environmental sleep disorder
      3. Altitude insomnia
      4. Adjustment sleep disorder
      5. Insufficient sleep syndrome
      6. Limit-setting sleep disorder
      7. Sleep-onset association disorder
      8. Food allergy insomnia
      9. Nocturnal eating (drinking) syndrome
      10. Hypnotic-dependent sleep disorder
      11. Stimulant-dependent sleep disorder
      12. Alcohol-dependent sleep disorder
      13. Toxin-induced sleep disorder
      14. Extrinsic sleep disorder NOS
   C. Circadian rhythm sleep disorders
      1. Time zone change (jet lag) syndrome
      2. Shift work sleep disorder
      3. Irregular sleep-wake pattern
      4. Delayed sleep phase syndrome
      5. Advanced sleep phase syndrome
      6. Non-24-hour sleep-wake disorder
      7. Circadian rhythm sleep disorder NOS
2. Parasomnias
   A. Arousal disorders
      1. Confusional arousals
      2. Sleepwalking
      3. Sleep terrors
   B. Sleep-wake transition disorders
      1. Rhythmic movement disorder
      2. Sleep starts
      3. Sleep talking
      4. Nocturnal leg cramps
   C. Parasomnias usually associated with REM sleep
      1. Nightmares
      2. Sleep paralysis
      3. Impaired sleep-related penile erections
      4. Sleep-related painful erections
      5. REM sleep-related sinus arrest
      6. REM sleep behavior disorder
   D. Other parasomnias
      1. Sleep bruxism
      2. Sleep enuresis
      3. Sleep-related abnormal swallowing syndrome
      4. Nocturnal paroxysmal dystonia
      5. Sudden unexplained nocturnal death syndrome
      6. Primary snoring
      7. Infant sleep apnea
      8. Congenital central hypoventilation syndrome
      9. Sudden infant death syndrome
      10. Benign neonatal sleep myoclonus
      11. Other parasomnia NOS
3. Sleep disorders associated with medical/psychiatric disorders
   A. Associated with mental disorders
      1. Psychoses
      2. Mood disorders
      3. Anxiety disorders
      4. Panic disorder
      5. Alcoholism
   B. Associated with neurologic disorders
      1. Cerebral degenerative disorders
      2. Dementia
      3. Parkinsonism
      4. Fatal familial insomnia
      5. Sleep-related epilepsy
      6. Electrical status epilepticus of sleep
      7. Sleep-related headaches
   C. Associated with other medical disorders
      1. Sleeping sickness
      2. Nocturnal cardiac ischemia
      3. Chronic obstructive pulmonary disease
      4. Sleep-related asthma
      5. Sleep-related gastroesophageal reflux
      6. Peptic ulcer disease
      7. Fibrositis syndrome
4. Proposed sleep disorders
      1. Short sleeper
      2. Long sleeper
      3. Subwakefulness syndrome
      4. Fragmentary myoclonus
      5. Sleep hyperhidrosis
      6. Menstrual-associated sleep disorder
      7. Pregnancy-associated sleep disorder
      8. Terrifying hypnagogic hallucinations
      9. Sleep-related neurogenic tachypnea
      10. Sleep-related laryngospasm
      11. Sleep choking syndrome

From Diagnostic Classification Steering Committee, Thorpy MJ, Chair: *International classification of sleep disorders: diagnostic and coding manual*, Rochester, Minn, 1991, American Sleep Disorders Association.

association. The precipitant for this disorder may be a period of acute insomnia associated with an external stressor (see the discussion of adjustment sleep disorder). A characteristic pattern emerges: inability to obtain satisfactory sleep for a few nights induces fear that another sleepless night will follow. Patients report that they feel alert as soon as they try to initiate sleep. They toss and turn, watch the clock, and

become frustrated and angry that they are unable to sleep. Often sleep improves in a new environment that is free of the usual external sleep-onset associations.

Psychophysiologic insomnia can be treated with relaxation techniques in combination with methods that "decondition" the patient's negative associations with sleep onset. A technique known as *stimulus-control therapy,* proposed by Bootzin, is highly effective. The patient is instructed to (1) go to bed only if sleepy; (2) use the bed only for sleeping and sexual relations, not as a place to read, write, or watch television; (3) get up and leave the bedroom if not asleep within 10 to 15 minutes and engage in a nonstimulating activity until sleepiness is perceived; (4) repeat this step as many times as necessary throughout the night; (5) maintain a fixed schedule of awakening each morning; and (6) take no naps during the day.

"*Sleep state misperception* is a disorder in which a complaint of insomnia or excessive sleepiness occurs without objective evidence of sleep disturbance." There is a small but distinct group of patients who complain of insomnia because of inability to recognize that they have slept. These patients are most clearly identifiable when there is a report of absolute lack of sleep. Polysomnographic recording reveals normal sleep latency, a normal number of arousals and awakenings, and normal sleep duration, but the patient perceives poor or absent sleep. This disorder needs to be distinguished from the phenomenon of paradoxical improvement in sleep during overnight recording in the sleep laboratory, which occurs in patients with psychophysiologic insomnia. In the latter disorder, sleep may improve in a novel environment, such as the sleep laboratory, and this improvement is appreciated by the patient.

Sometimes patients report sleepiness that cannot be verified on objective testing with the multiple sleep latency test (MSLT, discussed later), and this may be a sleep state misperception. Sleepiness, however, is more difficult to measure than presence or absence of sleep.

The underlying pathophysiologic mechanisms of sleep state misperception are not understood. Many patients who report near-absence of sleep are mistakenly treated with hypnotic medications for years without improvement. The existence of this disorder underscores the importance of polysomnographic evaluation of patients with chronic sleep complaints.

"*Idiopathic insomnia* is a lifelong inability to obtain adequate sleep that is presumably due to an abnormality of the neurological control of the sleep-wake system." This disorder may also be termed *childhood-onset insomnia.* Unlike "short sleepers," who feel rested despite short sleep duration, patients with this disorder complain of chronically poor performance caused by poor sleep. Polysomnographic evaluation reveals increased sleep latency, decreased efficiency, and increased arousals, but the cause of the disrupted sleep is not apparent. Because of the chronicity of the disorder, secondary sleep disorders such as psychophysiologic insomnia and hypnotic dependence often develop. There is no effective treatment except directing attention to conditions that may aggravate the underlying insomnia.

"*Narcolepsy* is a disorder of unknown etiology which is characterized by excessive sleepiness that typically is associated with cataplexy and other REM sleep phenomena such as sleep paralysis and hypnogogic hallucinations." Narcolepsy was first defined as a distinct disorder in 1880 by Gelineau, who described the syndrome as a "rare, little known neurosis characterized by imperative need to sleep." It is now known that the disorder is not rare. The prevalence is estimated at between 2 and 16 per 10,000 persons. The onset of symptoms occurs typically in the second or third decade, and both sexes are equally affected. A family history is noted in approximately one third of cases.

The discovery of REM sleep was followed by the finding that patients with narcolepsy have abnormal REM physiology. It is now accepted that the major manifestations of narcolepsy represent a disorder of control mechanisms that regulate REM sleep. Episodes of REM occur at the wrong time, intruding on wakefulness, and the physiologic components of this sleep state dissociate and appear independently. These major symptoms are referred to as the *narcolepsy tetrad:* (1) excessive daytime sleepiness, (2) cataplexy, (3) hypnogogic hallucinations, and (4) sleep paralysis. Few patients report all of these symptoms, especially in the early stages of the disorder, but almost all narcoleptic patients have evidence of excessive daytime sleepiness.

The cardinal symptom of narcolepsy is excessive daytime sleepiness, and approximately 10% of patients complain of this symptom alone. The tendency to sleep inappropriately may have a gradual or an abrupt onset. History taking typically reveals that patients remember brief lapses of attention in sedentary situations years before presentation to a physician. With time, sleepiness is evident in clearly inappropriate situations, such as during driving, holding business conversations, eating, or engaging in sexual intercourse. Patients are frequently able to recognize impending drowsiness and take measures to alert themselves. Irresistible sleep attacks are characteristic, however, and tend to occur when the urge to sleep has been delayed. Two features are unique to the naps of narcoleptics: (1) dreaming during naps is common and (2) brief naps of 5- to 10-minute duration are remarkably refreshing.

Cataplexy is a sudden, usually brief, loss of muscle tone induced by emotion. The presence of cataplexy is considered diagnostic of narcolepsy, but only 60% to 80% of patients experience this symptom, and it may occur years after the onset of sleepiness. Rarely, cataplexy is the presenting symptom of the disorder. Idiopathic cataplexy may exist but is poorly described. Laughter and anger are the most common precipitants, but the emotional trigger may be specific to the patient. The weakness that develops usually involves the muscles of the face or the supporting muscles of the legs; it may be so mild as to give only the sense that the face will not move properly or so profound as to cause a sudden fall. The appearance of facial tremulousness can be confused with seizure activity. Occasionally, patients have difficulty speaking. Consciousness is maintained during a cataplectic episode, but prolonged episodes may be immediately followed by REM sleep. Cataplexy is the result of sudden skeletal muscle atonia, sparing extraocular eye movements and diaphragm motion. Deep tendon reflexes are absent during the episode. This atonia is similar to that which occurs during normal REM sleep. Cataplexy thus seems to represent a dissociation of normal REM phenomena, occurring inappropriately during waking.

In hallucinations occurring at the onset of sleep, referred to as *hypnogogic hallucinations,* the sensory events associated with normal dreaming occur during perceived wakefulness. These hallucinations are a manifestation of the sudden onset of inappropriate and dissociated REM sleep. Hallucinations may involve any sensory system and are frequently visual, auditory, or vestibular.

Sleep paralysis is an inability to move skeletal muscles voluntarily during sleep-wake transitions. Normal subjects may experience the sensation awakening from REM, but narcoleptics typically complain of sleep paralysis at sleep onset. The episodes can be associated with extreme fear, especially when they are accompanied by threatening hypnogogic hallucinations. Sleep paralysis is thought to be another manifestation of REM-related atonia.

Two other symptoms are typical of narcolepsy: automatic behavior and disrupted nighttime sleep. Patients with automatic behavior complain that they perform complex, often routine activities "automatically" with partial amnesia and evidence of inattention during the behavior. *Microsleeps* or poor attentiveness caused by sleepiness may be the cause of this behavior. Just as patients have difficulty maintaining alertness because of intrusion of sleepiness during the day, narcoleptics complain of inability to maintain sleep at night. The narcoleptic's sleep tends to be punctuated by frequent awakenings and vivid dreams. Periodic movements in sleep syndrome and sleep apnea are more common in narcoleptics and contribute to poor-quality sleep.

Cataplexy, hypnogogic hallucinations, and sleep paralysis are episodic symptoms that may resolve. Complaints of automatic behavior, poor memory, and disturbed sleep often worsen with age. The degree of sleepiness remains relatively constant over the years.

The underlying pathogenesis of narcolepsy is not understood. Polysomnographic studies demonstrate two major features: (1) excessive daytime sleepiness, as measured in multiple daytime naps; and (2) the tendency to develop REM sleep within minutes of sleep onset in daytime and nocturnal recordings. Normal patients do not show sleep-onset REM unless they are sleep deprived, on an irregular sleep-wake cycle, or withdrawing from REM-suppressing medication. Recordings during periods of cataplexy and sleep paralysis show the sudden onset of muscle atonia characteristic of REM sleep.

More than 90% of white and Japanese patients with narcolepsy carry antigens HLA-DR2 and HLA-DQw1, specifically the DRw15 subtype of DR2 and the DQw6 subtype of DQw1. Among blacks, only about 30% are DR2 positive, but almost all are DQw6(DQw1)-positive. A specific allele of DQw6, DQB1-0602 is the best marker across ethnic groups, but it need not be present. Patients negative for the DQB1-0602 allele are often familial rather than sporadic cases. Most reported monozygotic narcolepsy twin pairs are discordant for narcolepsy, suggesting an environmental influence independent of the genetic contribution.

Occasionally narcolepsy and/or cataplexy occurs in association with other neurologic disorders, in which case it is called *symptomatic narcolepsy*. Both narcolepsy and cataplexy have been described in patients with tumors in the region of the third ventricle and upper brain stem. Cataplexy has also been described in Niemann-Pick disease. Occasionally narcolepsy is said to follow head trauma and encephalitis. Patients with symptomatic narcolepsy also have been reported to have a high prevalence of the HLA types associated with idiopathic narcolepsy.

The diagnosis of narcolepsy is secure if excessive daytime sleepiness is associated with unequivocal cataplexy. The diagnosis can be confirmed in these patients—and especially in those without a clear history of cataplexy—with polysomnographic studies. The current standard of diagnosis is the multiple sleep latency test (MSLT), which measures the tendency to sleep and the type of sleep the patient obtains in brief naps scheduled throughout the day. The mean latency to sleep is usually less than 5 minutes. The diagnosis of narcolepsy requires that two of five naps include REM sleep. A polysomnogram on the night preceding the multiple sleep latency test is preferred; this will exclude sleep deprivation as a cause of short daytime latencies and to identify other sleep disorders.

The Standards of Practice Committee of the American Sleep Disorders Association (1994) endorsed the effectiveness of the following stimulants for the treatment of sleepiness in patients with narcolepsy: methylphenidate hydrochloride, pemoline, dextroamphetamine sulfate, methamphetamine hydrochloride, and modafinil. Methylphenidate and pemoline have been the mainstay of treatment protocols during the last two decades, with clinicians typically avoiding amphetamines except in the most severe cases. There is recent documentation of liver failure associated with the use of pemoline and, as a result, it is no longer recommended for use as a first-line drug for narcolepsy. Amphetamines are more likely to induce tolerance than nonamphetamines and they have a higher abuse potential; they are also more likely to be associated with psychiatric, cardiovascular, and cerebrovascular complications. Modafinil has been shown to be effective in narcolepsy but is not yet available in the United States. The mechanism of action of modafinil has not been determined. The drug has a very low abuse potential and fewer cardiovascular side effects than other stimulants. Efficacy thus far appears to be similar to that of methylphenidate. In general, the goal of treatment is to use the lowest effective doses of stimulant medication that will maintain adequate alertness to perform day-to-day activities. A stable daily dose of stimulant medication is more efficacious than relying on as-needed dosing. High doses of stimulants or stimulants used late in the day may increase nocturnal sleep deprivation and, paradoxically, increase excessive daytime sleepiness.

Cataplexy is most effectively treated with tricyclic antidepressant drugs, particularly those with prominent anticholinergic properties. This treatment effect takes advantage of the REM-inhibiting effects of these drugs. Clomipramine is the most effective anticataplectic drug currently available. Protriptyline is also highly effective, widely used, and frequently better tolerated than clomipramine. Selective serotonin uptake inhibitors are less effective in treating cataplexy than tricyclic antidepressants but can be especially useful in patients who cannot tolerate the anticholinergic side effects of the tricyclic drugs.

Nonpharmacologic treatment techniques include the use of "strategic napping." Brief naps during the day, during periods of maximum fatigue, or before periods of required alertness result in decreased sleepiness and decreased total daily dose of stimulant medication. Attention is directed to maintenance of nocturnal sleep by avoidance of stimulant drugs, caffeine, and alcohol in the evening. Lack of response to treatment should raise the suspicion of coexistent sleep apnea and/or periodic movements in sleep syndrome.

"*Recurrent hypersomnia* is a disorder characterized by recurrent episodes of hypersomnia that typically occur weeks or months apart." Kleine-Levin syndrome is the prototype of these disorders. This is usually thought of as a disorder of young men, but young women are also affected in a male/female ratio of 3:1. In a large series, median age at onset was 16.0 for males and 19.5 for females. Daily sleep durations of 18 to 20 hours are associated with behavioral abnormalities including hyperphagia and lack of sexual inhibition. During periods of wakefulness, the patient appears apathetic and irritable. Delusions and hallucinations occasionally occur. Electroencephalograms (EEGs) may show background slowing and bursts of high-voltage slow waves. Spontaneous remission is typical. A thorough neurologic evaluation is appropriate to exclude structural abnormalities of the brain.

"*Idiopathic hypersomnia* is a disorder of presumed central nervous system cause that is associated with a normal or prolonged major sleep episode and excessive sleepiness consisting of prolonged (1-2 hours) sleep episodes of non-REM sleep." This disorder has also been termed *non-REM narcolepsy* and *CNS hypersomnolence*. Patients demonstrate excessive sleepiness on the MSLT, but there is no evidence of sleep-onset REM. The all-night polysomnogram should not show nocturnal disruption induced by sleep-disordered breathing, leg movements, or other causes. Psychiatric and medical conditions that might contribute to sleepiness are absent. Thus the diagnosis is one of exclusion. However, a group of these patients, when restudied, have been shown to demonstrate subtle evidence of sleep-disordered breathing (discussed later), which has been termed *upper airway resistance syndrome*. Brain tumors, especially those in the region of the third ventricle, may induce sleepiness as a primary symptom. Magnetic resonance imaging (MRI) or computed tomography (CT) of the brain is an appropriate screening technique in patients whose hypersomnia is unexplained.

"*Posttraumatic hypersomnia* is excessive sleepiness that occurs as a result of a traumatic event involving the central nervous system." Subtle derangements of neurologic function often follow head trauma, and there may be disruption of usual sleep patterns. It is critical, however, to exclude life-threatening conditions such as subdural hematoma and atlantoaxial dislocation. The latter condition has been associated with sleep attacks that may be secondary to brain stem ischemia or involvement of medullary respiratory centers.

"*Obstructive sleep apnea syndrome* is characterized by repetitive episodes of upper airway obstruction that occur during sleep, usually associated with a reduction in blood oxygen saturation."

"*Central sleep apnea syndrome* is characterized by a cessation or decrease of ventilatory effort during sleep usually with associated oxygen desaturation."

"*Central alveolar hypoventilation syndrome* is characterized by ventilatory impairment, resulting in arterial oxygen desaturation that is worsened by sleep, which occurs in patients with normal properties of the lung."

When decreased ventilation and irregular breathing patterns result in sleep disruption and/or hypoxemia, the patient may be said to have sleep-disordered breathing. These syndromes are discussed in detail in Chapter 36. Most of these patients, particularly those with obstructive sleep apnea, demonstrate excessive daytime sleepiness as the primary complaint. Others, especially those with central sleep apnea, including Cheyne-Stokes respirations, complain of insomnia—usually difficulty maintaining sleep.

In patients with sleep-disordered breathing, treatment of the insomnia symptomatically with hypnotic medications can be life-threatening because of respiratory depression and increased atonia of the upper airway muscles. Sleep-disordered breathing is a ubiquitous problem. The important risk factors are listed in Box 134-2. Patients who have any of these risk factors should never receive hypnotic drugs for symptomatic treatment of insomnia. In this group, a polysomnogram should be used for diagnosis of the underlying sleep dis-

---

BOX 134-2
Risk factors for sleep-disordered breathing

Advanced age
Loud snoring
Obesity
Upper-airway abnormality (tonsillar hypertrophy, micrognathia, macroglossia, nasal obstruction)
Pulmonary disease
Muscular weakness (muscular dystrophy, myasthenia, polymyositis, Guillain-Barré syndrome)
Brain stem lesions (Shy-Drager syndrome, infarct)
Cheyne-Stokes respiratory pattern (congestive heart failure, bihemispheric cerebral disease)

order. Oximetry alone may be helpful. Even bedside observation, although not ideal, may be diagnostic.

"*Periodic limb movement disorder* is characterized by periodic episodes of repetitive and highly stereotyped limb movements that occur during sleep."

"*Restless legs syndrome* is a disorder characterized by disagreeable leg sensations, usually prior to sleep onset, that cause an almost irresistible urge to move the legs." It is an extremely annoying, aching, crawling sensation affecting predominantly the legs when sedentary, especially when trying to initiate sleep. The subject feels the overwhelming urge to move the legs continually to abort the sensation. All patients with restless legs syndrome have another disorder, periodic limb movement disorder (also termed *periodic leg movements* or *nocturnal myoclonus*). Periodic limb movement disorder may also occur without restless legs. Patients show recurrent, periodic leg jerks involving flexor muscles of the legs, analogous to the withdrawal reflex. Upper extremity movements may also occur. Leg twitches occur approximately every 20 to 40 seconds episodically throughout the night. Hundreds of leg jerks may occur, unknown to the patient but often witnessed by the bed partner. The repetitive movements result in arousal. Patients with these disorders may have difficulty initiating and maintaining sleep or experience excessive daytime sleepiness. Restless legs syndrome is sometimes familial. Periodic limb movements can be exacerbated and possibly induced by drugs, especially tricyclic antidepressants. Both disorders may be intermittent or may be related to an underlying metabolic abnormality, especially iron deficiency, uremia, or and chronic alcohol use. Symptoms may be worse during pregnancy. Peripheral neuropathy with or without apparent systemic metabolic abnormality is another important risk factor. Periodic limb movements may also accompany other primary sleep disorders, including sleep apnea and narcolepsy. Often no cause is discovered. The treatment of restless legs and periodic movements in sleep represents a difficult clinical challenge. In the late 1980s it was discovered that carbidopa-levodopa and dopaminergic agonists dramatically improve both the restless sensation and leg movements. Many patients report long-lasting results with small doses of carbidopa-levodopa in the evening. In others, a clear syndrome of augmentation of the symptoms occurs, with paresthesias occurring progressively earlier in the day, increasing in severity and anatomic distribution. This augmentation worsens as the carbidopa-levodopa dosage is increased. Once augmentation is recognized, it is prudent to taper carbidopa-levodopa and substitute another drug. Pergolide, a dopaminergic agonist, can be particularly useful in patients who demonstrate augmentation on carbidopa-levodopa. Clonazepam was one of earliest reported drugs for these disorders and tends to be more effective for leg movements than paresthesias; the development of tolerance and only moderate effectiveness limit its usefulness in this setting. Codeine may be remarkably successful in small nightly doses, suggesting an effect other than analgesia alone. Gabapentin has recently been used with moderate success, especially in patients with painful paresthesias associated with restless legs.

Extrinsic Sleep Disorders. "*Inadequate sleep hygiene* is a sleep disorder due to the performance of daily activities that are inconsistent with the maintenance of good quality sleep and full daytime alertness." Many types of daily behavior are inconsistent with obtaining good-quality sleep. Frequent daytime napping, inattention to maintenance of regular sleeping hours, and use of caffeine, nicotine, or alcohol are the most common offenders. Poor sleep secondary to this or another disorder may perpetuate the maladaptive habits. For example, insomniacs frequently insist on maintaining caffeine intake or daytime naps to counteract the effects of sleep deprivation.

The presence of at least one of the following is necessary for the diagnosis of inadequate sleep hygiene by ICSD standards: "(1) daytime napping at least two times each week; (2) variable wake-up times or bedtimes; (3) frequent periods (two to three times per week) of extended amounts of time spent in bed; (4) routine use of products containing alcohol, tobacco, or caffeine in the period preceding bedtime; (5) scheduling of exercise too close to bedtime; (6) engaging in exciting or emotionally upsetting activities too close to bedtime; (7) frequent use of the bed for nonrelated activities (e.g., television watching, studying); (8) sleeping on an uncomfortable bed (poor mattress, inadequate blankets, etc.); (9) bedroom that is too bright, too stuffy,

too cluttered, too hot, too cold, or in some way nonconducive to sleep; (10) performance of activities demanding high levels of concentration shortly before bed; (11) occurrence in bed of such mental activities as thinking, planning, or reminiscing."

"*Environmental sleep disorder* is a sleep disturbance due to a disturbing environmental factor that causes a complaint of either insomnia or excessive sleepiness." External physical factors are temporally associated with the development and resolution of the sleep complaint. The elderly appear to be at more risk for this disorder. Attention to the quality of the sleep environment may prevent needless trials of hypnotic medication. Perhaps nowhere is this more apparent than in the hospital setting.

"*Altitude insomnia* is an acute insomnia, usually accompanied by headaches, loss of appetite, and fatigue, that occurs following ascent to high altitudes." This insomnia is associated with a periodic (Cheyne-Stokes) respiratory pattern caused by low inspired oxygen pressure. Arousals are associated with the hyperventilatory phase of the periodic breathing (Chapter 36).

"*Adjustment sleep disorder* represents sleep disturbance temporally related to acute stress, conflict, or environmental change causing emotional arousal." Inability to initiate sleep in the presence of an acute stressor is a nearly universal experience. Occasionally the opposite is true: patients note excessive sleepiness in response to a stressful situation. Symptoms are generally short lived and resolve with removal of the stressor.

"*Insufficient sleep syndrome* is a disorder that occurs in an individual who persistently fails to obtain sufficient nocturnal sleep required to support normally alert wakefulness." A large percentage of the population suffers from self-imposed sleep deprivation. Sleep logs help document the disorder for the patient who is unwilling to recognize the problem. A history reveals that symptoms resolve during vacations and weekends when sleep duration increases. Symptoms resolve if the patient chooses to prolong nocturnal sleep.

"*Limit setting disorder* is a predominantly childhood disorder that is characterized by the inadequate enforcement of bedtimes by a caretaker, with resultant stalling or refusal to go to bed at an appropriate time." The disorder is characterized by persistent struggle between the caretaker and child, with sleep disruption for both. Irregular sleep-wake cycles may develop. The disorder resolves with the institution of firm limits. The underlying psychosocial factors that may foster the lack of limit setting are several, and deserve exploration.

"*Sleep onset association disorder* occurs when sleep onset is impaired by the absence of a certain object or set of circumstances."

"*Food allergy insomnia* is a disorder of initiating and maintaining sleep due to an allergic response to food allergens." Onset of this disorder is usually within the first 2 years of life, especially after the introduction of cow's milk into the diet. The disorder may also occur in adults. Sleep is characterized by frequent arousals and awakenings. Symptoms of allergy, such as wheezing, abdominal pain, or itching, need not be present.

"*Nocturnal eating (drinking) syndrome* is characterized by recurrent awakenings with the inability to return to sleep without eating or drinking." This disorder occurs predominantly in early childhood in association with breast or bottle feeding. Large amounts of fluid consumed during the night contribute to repeated awakenings and excessive urination. An adult variant of this disorder is unusual but striking in its presentation. Patients wake fully and engage in uncontrolled binge eating without evidence of similar behavior during daytime hours.

"*Hypnotic-dependent sleep disorder* is characterized by insomnia or excessive sleepiness that is associated with tolerance to or withdrawal from hypnotic medications." Hypnotic medications are to be avoided whenever possible. The benzodiazepines are the safest sleep-inducing medications but should be reserved for short-term use in patients with transient, usually situationally induced insomnia. Hypnotics are discouraged for several reasons. The underlying cause of the insomnia may be masked or exacerbated, as in sleep-disordered breathing. Tolerance to the benzodiazepines develops with regular use, and the medication becomes ineffective, resulting in escalation of dose. Half-lives of the benzodiazepines and their active metabolites vary widely. Drugs with long half-lives accumulate and impair performance during waking, especially in the elderly. Withdrawal effects are more evident with shorter-acting drugs. Rebound insomnia follows withdrawal, leading the patient to overestimate the underlying sleep disorder.

"*Stimulant-dependent sleep disorder* is characterized by a reduction of sleepiness or suppression of sleep by central stimulants and resultant alterations in wakefulness following drug abstinence." Use of stimulants is an obvious cause of difficulty initiating and maintaining sleep but can be easily overlooked in the history. Caffeine is the most common stimulant, in the form of coffee, tea, soft drinks, or chocolate. Decongestants and bronchodilators are often-forgotten offenders. Nonamphetamine stimulants prescribed for attention deficit disorder and narcolepsy, such as pemoline and methylphenidate, may produce insomnia as a major side-effect, usually because of dosage taken too late in the day. Prolonged periods of sleeplessness followed by excessive sleep are seen with amphetamine and cocaine abuse.

"*Alcohol-dependent sleep disorder* is characterized by the assisted initiation of sleep onset by the sustained ingestion of ethanol that is used for its hypnotic effect." Alcohol usually causes fragmentation of sleep and frequent arousal, contrary to the popular belief that it helps induce sleep. It also exacerbates sleep-disordered breathing. Many patients become alcohol dependent in attempting to treat insomnia from other causes with nocturnal use of alcohol; in fact it exacerbates the problem.

"*Toxin-induced sleep disorder* is characterized by either insomnia or excessive sleepiness produced by poisoning with heavy metals or organic toxins."

Circadian Rhythm Sleep Disorders. The activities of modern society allow for marked variations in the patterns of day-to-day activity. Air travel and shift work are common, and nighttime activities are no longer limited by darkness. Continuous activity with the potential for disrupting sleep-wake cycles is particularly evident in the hospital setting. When the timing of sleep is disrupted, the patient is said to have a circadian rhythm sleep disorder.

"*Time zone change (jet lag) syndrome* consists of varying degrees of difficulties in initiating or maintaining sleep, excessive sleepiness, decrements in subjective daytime alertness and performance, and somatic symptoms (largely related to gastrointestinal function) following rapid travel across multiple time zones."

"*Shift work sleep disorder* consists of symptoms of insomnia or excessive sleepiness that occur as transient phenomena in relation to work schedules."

An abrupt change in the sleep schedule induced by travel across time zones or a change in work shift results in transient disorders of the sleep-wake cycle. Circadian rhythms are out of phase with the imposed sleep schedule. Subjects note difficulty in both initiating and maintaining sleep, as well as experiencing sleepiness during waking hours. Schedules that result in an "advance" of the sleep cycle, as in eastward flight, are more poorly tolerated. An endogenous rhythm of slightly longer than 24 hours makes it easier to delay, rather than advance, bedtime. Symptoms resolve after circadian rhythms entrain to the new schedule, which may take more than a week.

If the sleep-wake cycle changes constantly, because of either travel or shift work, no entrainment occurs and the circadian rhythm disorder becomes persistent.

"*Irregular sleep-wake pattern* consists of temporally disorganized and variable episodes of sleep and waking behavior." The sleep pattern of the patient with irregular sleep-wake cycle is erratic. Unlike those of patients with non–24 hour sleep-wake syndrome (discussed later), sleep logs reveal no underlying periodicity. This disorder usually occurs in patients with developmental or degenerative abnormalities of the brain. Prolonged illness with enforced bed rest and absence of attention to daily routines may be precipitating factors. Patients complain of chronic fatigue, and neither sleep nor wakefulness is well maintained. This disorder is treated by external reinforcement of a normal sleep-wake cycle but usually recurs.

"*Delayed sleep phase syndrome* is a disorder in which the major sleep episode is delayed in relation to the desired clock time that results in symptoms of sleep-onset insomnia or difficulty in waking at the desired time." Patients habitually adopt a late bedtime and wake late in the day. The amount of sleep and its quality are normal. The patient is symptomatic when attempts to advance the bedtime to an earlier hour fail. These patients appear to be less able to advance their

circadian rhythms to reset the body's natural tendency to delay endogenous rhythms or to compensate for occasional schedule changes. Bright-light therapy is the most effective treatment. Patients are exposed to bright light in the range of 2500 to 10,000 lux during morning hours, which serves to advance endogenous rhythms and allows earlier sleep onset.

"*Advanced sleep phase syndrome* is a disorder in which the major sleep episode is advanced in relation to the desired clock time, that results in symptoms of compelling evening sleepiness, an early sleep onset, and an awakening that is earlier than desired." This disorder is commonly seen in the elderly. Advanced sleep phase may explain the physiologic changes seen in endogenous depression, including early REM latency and early morning awakenings. Patients with advanced sleep phase syndrome alone generally do not complain of the disorder. When symptoms are bothersome, patients can be treated with progressive delay of bedtime or bright-light therapy in the evening.

"*Non–24 hour sleep-wake syndrome* consists of a chronic steady pattern comprised of 1- to 2-hour daily delays in sleep onset and wake times in an individual living in society." Patients with this disorder have what appears to be an erratic sleep-wake cycle. However, sleep logs demonstrate a non–24 hour periodicity in the sleep-wake cycle. This disorder mimics the prolongation of the sleep cycle that can be seen in experimental environments in which subjects are isolated from time cues and are said to be "free-running." In patients who do not attend to environmental cues, including the blind, this syndrome may develop. Exogenous melatonin has been shown to be useful in entraining normal rhythms in blind patients without adequate light perception.

Parasomnias

The term *parasomnia* refers to undesirable physical events that occur during sleep or are exacerbated by sleep. These phenomena are often sleep-stage specific. Subdivisions of the parasomnias are (1) the arousal disorders, (2) the sleep-wake transition disorders, (3) the parasomnias usually associated with REM sleep, and (4) the other parasomnias.

Arousal Disorders. Arousal disorders are characterized by confusion and automatic behavior after sudden arousal from delta sleep. The tendency to arouse from delta sleep spontaneously is a familial trait unrelated to epilepsy. Most patients have an affected first-degree relative; the cooccurrence of these disorders in the same patient is common. Onset in childhood and resolution by adolescence are typical, but episodes may recur or occur for the first time with greater severity in adolescence and adulthood. Stress, sleep deprivation, and any factors that may contribute to sleep disruption are clear exacerbants. Sleep-disordered breathing and nocturnal alcohol consumption are common precipitants of arousal in the predisposed adult population. Psychopathologic abnormality—especially anxiety, depression, obsessive compulsive behavior, and phobia—is said to be more common in the symptomatic adult.

"*Confusional arousals* consist of confusion during and following arousals from sleep, most typically from deep sleep in the first part of the night." These episodes are most commonly seen in forced arousals from delta sleep, particularly in individuals with a family or personal history of sleepwalking or sleeptalking, and in children younger than the age of 5. Amnesia for the events during the arousal is typical. This is predominantly a problem for individuals, such as physicians, who are called at night and must react appropriately.

"*Sleepwalking* consists of a series of complex behaviors that are initiated during slow wave sleep and result in walking during sleep." Sleepwalkers characteristically arouse during the first third of the night from delta sleep, leave the bed in a confused state, and perform complex, automatic acts. Some episodes of sleepwalking are initiated by sleep terror (discussed later), in which case the behavior exhibited may be violent, as the subject tries to combat a perceived threat. More routine behavior, such as eating and urinating, may be performed in a remarkably stereotyped fashion idiosyncratic to the subject. The patient may awaken during the behavior feeling embarrassed and bewildered. Most often the patient returns to bed and has no memory of the episode. Patients with this disorder are at risk of injuring themselves and their bed partners. Care must be taken to secure the sleep environment to prevent falling from heights. Occasionally, dangerous objects such as knives and guns need to be made inaccessible. Although sleepwalking is frequently perceived as amusing, it may entail social stigma, especially when there is associated violence. Murders have been committed during apparent sleepwalking, and serious personal injury occurs frequently.

"*Sleep terrors* are characterized by a sudden arousal from slow wave sleep with a piercing scream or cry, accompanied by automatic and behavioral manifestations of intense fear." Typically, the individual arouses within the first 2 hours of sleep, sits bolt upright, and screams. Marked tachycardia, mydriasis, and sweating may be evident. The subject is agitated, confused, and difficult to console or arouse fully. There is no detailed dream recall, but a single terrifying image, such as a demon, insect, or intruder, may be reported. Generally sleep is resumed in a few minutes, with amnesia for the entire episode the next morning.

In patients with arousals from delta sleep, polysomnography may show characteristic high-voltage synchronous delta activity followed by arousal, even in the absence of a clinical episode. Most patients can recognize factors that tend to exacerbate their sleep terrors or sleepwalking. If episodes persist after attempts to control the underlying precipitants, a small nightly dose of clonazepam is usually effective.

Sleep-Wake Transition Disorders. "*Rhythmic movement disorder* comprises a group of stereotyped, repetitive movements involving large muscles, usually of the head and neck, which typically occur immediately prior to sleep onset and are sustained into light sleep." This disorder is predominantly recognized as headbanging or rocking in children, with onset at about 6 months, and resolution, in most cases, by the age of 4. Persistence into adulthood is sometimes seen.

"*Sleep starts* are sudden, brief contractions of the legs, sometimes also involving the arms and head, which occur at sleep onset." Also called *hypnic jerks,* these episodes are often associated with the sensation of falling and are considered normal unless they occur so frequently as to interfere with sleep onset. When episodes are disruptive, sleep-onset epilepsy should be considered. Periodic limb movement disorder may induce arousal at sleep onset, but the movements are less generalized, and polysomnographic study reveals persistent movements during sleep.

Parasomnias Usually Associated With REM Sleep. "*Nightmares* are frightening dreams that usually awaken the sleeper from REM sleep." Because nightmares occur during REM sleep, the subject arouses easily and has detailed dream recall. Episodes typically occur later in the night, when REM is more predominant. Autonomic activation and confusion are not characteristic features of the nightmare. Commonly, the episodes are recurrent in the same night during each REM period. Nightmares occur normally in childhood. In adults, recurrent nightmares may represent underlying psychiatric disorders, especially anxiety and depression, or REM rebound secondary to drug withdrawal. Sometimes, recurrent nightmares seem to be induced by physiologic disruptions occurring during REM sleep, such as sleep-disordered breathing or arrhythmia.

"*Sleep paralysis* consists of a period of inability to perform voluntary movements either at sleep onset (hypnogogic or predormital form) or upon awakening either during the night or in the morning (hypnopompic or postdormital form)." Sleep paralysis represents a partial arousal or entry into REM sleep such that the atonia of REM sleep is present but the cerebral cortex is awake. This is a common symptom of narcolepsy (discussed earlier), especially at sleep onset. Normal subjects may have occasional episodes of sleep paralysis on awakening. A familial disorder characterized by sleep-onset sleep paralysis without other features of narcolepsy has been described. Sleep paralysis is particularly common in patients taking REM-modifying drugs, especially MAO inhibitors.

"*REM sleep–related sinus arrest* is a cardiac rhythm disorder that is characterized by sinus arrest during REM sleep in otherwise healthy individuals." Asystole may be prolonged, lasting as long as 9 seconds. This arrhythmia responds to atropinergic drugs. Most patients have been treated with artificial pacemakers, because the natural history of the disorder and the risk of sudden death are unknown.

"*REM sleep behavior disorder* is characterized by the intermittent loss of REM sleep electromyographic (EMG) atonia and by the appearance of elaborate motor activity associated with dream mentation." Lack of the usual atonia of REM sleep allows the patient to enact dreams. Patients typically run, punch, kick, or leap from bed. Vocalization consistent with the dream activity is usual. This disorder predominantly affects men in late middle age. Forty percent of cases have been associated with neurologic disease, most commonly dementing illnesses of unknown cause, as well as olivopontocerebellar degeneration, Parkinson's disease, and subarachnoid hemorrhage. A familial predisposition may exist. Diagnosis is made by polysomnography, which shows excessive EMG tone during REM associated with dream enactment. Treatment with a nightly dose of clonazepam is highly effective.

Other Parasomnias. "*Sleep bruxism* is a stereotyped movement disorder characterized by grinding or clenching of teeth during sleep." This is a common disorder that is sometimes correlated with stress. It results in disrupted nocturnal sleep, temporomandibular joint dysfunction, damage to teeth, and morning headache. Bruxism is inhibited by the use of a nocturnal tooth guard.

"*Sleep enuresis* is characterized by recurrent involuntary micturition that occurs during sleep." Bedwetting after the age of 5 years is considered abnormal. There may be a delay in toilet training without the development of continence during sleep, termed *primary enuresis.* Secondary enuresis refers to the development of bedwetting after toilet training is complete. Symptomatic enuresis is secondary to underlying medical disease—for example, urogenital disorder or nocturnal seizure. Some cases of enuresis follow arousal from delta sleep, but enuresis may occur in any sleep stage. If no underlying medical cause is identified, the disorder is treated with behavioral techniques that incorporate bladder capacity training and a wetness alarm. When behavioral techniques fail, medications may be used, including nocturnal nasal desmopressin (DDAVP) or imipramine.

"*Nocturnal paroxysmal dystonia* is characterized by repeated dystonia or dyskinetic (ballistic, choreo-athetoid) episodes that are stereotyped and occur during NREM sleep." Both short- and long-lasting episodes have been described and appear to have different mechanisms. Short episodes often respond to carbamazepine, and there has been debate as to whether these episodes may represent seizure activity that is difficult to record with surface electrodes. Most evidence suggests that nocturnal paroxysmal dystonia of short duration represents nocturnal seizures of frontal lobe origin. Long-duration episodes have been observed in only a few patients; in one patient Huntington's disease later developed.

"*Sudden unexplained nocturnal death syndrome (SUND)* is characterized by sudden death during sleep in healthy young adults, particularly of Southeast Asian descent."

Medical and Psychiatric Sleep Disorders

Associated With Mental Disorders. Disordered sleep is typical of most psychiatric disorders. Unipolar depression is characteristically associated with a disorder of initiating and maintaining sleep, most commonly early morning awakening. The patient may fall asleep easily but wake a few hours later, alert and unable to return to sleep. This can be the earliest symptom apparent to the patient. Sleep studies in some of these patients demonstrate an earlier-than-normal REM latency and increased phasic REM activity early in the night. In contrast, the sleep in bipolar depressive disease is characterized by prolonged periods of inability to sleep during the manic phase and excessive sleep during the depressive phase. Most actively psychotic patients have difficulty maintaining sleep, but some may be hypersomnolent at the onset of their psychosis. Patients with panic disorder may wake suddenly at night with panic; polysomnographic evaluation is sometimes useful to distinguish these episodes from sleep terror or seizure. The treatment of sleep disorders of psychiatric cause is directed to treatment of the underlying illness. Improvement in sleep is often a sensitive measure of the effectiveness of treatment.

Associated With Neurologic Disorders
Cerebral degenerative disorders, dementia, parkinsonism.
Sleep disruption is a prominent, but not well studied, symptom in all of the degenerative diseases of the brain. Patients with degenerative

disease of the brain are at particular risk for sleep-disordered breathing produced by Cheyne-Stokes respirations, abnormal chest wall and upper airway muscle tone, brain stem dysfunction, and use of sedating medications. The resulting hypoxemia can contribute to episodes of nocturnal confusion. In the disorders involving motor systems, sleep fragmentation also occurs secondary to rigidity, tremor, myoclonus, and periodic limb movements. Brain stem involvement induces REM sleep abnormalities, including REM sleep behavior disorder. REM behavior disorder may be the presenting symptom of Parkinson's disease and Shy-Drager syndrome (multisystem atrophy) years before other abnormalities are detected. Circadian rhythm disorders in the degenerative diseases are frequent and probably represent derangement of neurologic control mechanisms, coupled with the secondary effects of disrupted sleep and medication.

Sleep-related epileptic seizures are facilitated by sleep, particularly stage II sleep. Hypoxia secondary to sleep apnea also precipitates seizures. Some types of seizure disorders, especially complex partial seizures with temporolimbic symptoms, closely mimic sleep terrors and sleepwalking. Usually the clinician is alerted by features that would be atypical of delta sleep arousals, including recurrent episodes during the same night, history of seizures, or abnormal neurologic examination. Nocturnal wandering secondary to epilepsy tends to be less well organized and goal directed. Grand mal seizures are suggested by falls from bed, incontinence, bitten tongue, and morning confusion.

Sleep-related headaches are of various types. Cluster headache is a severe unilateral orbital headache associated with ipsilateral rhinorrhea and tearing. The headache is frequently nocturnal and appears to be exacerbated specifically by REM sleep. Chronic paroxysmal hemicrania, a similar headache disorder that occurs more frequently in women and is responsive to indomethicin, is also REM related. Increased blood flow and hypoxemia during REM may be etiologic factors. Most patients note that migraine is improved by sleep, but occasionally the reverse is true. Sleep-related headache may be the presentation of increased intracranial pressure, which is exacerbated by the supine posture and episodic elevation in intracranial pressure during REM sleep. Morning headache is typical of sleep apnea syndrome and bruxism.

Associated With Other Medical Disorders. Just as medical illness disrupts the quality of life during the day, it also affects the maintenance of sleep. A careful consideration of possible systemic disease is important in every patient with a sleep disorder. Almost every disease, at some point in its course, may disrupt sleep. Most painful disorders cause nocturnal arousal, especially arthritis and peptic ulcer disease. Insomnia may be the presenting complaint of congestive heart failure with nocturia, paroxysmal nocturnal dyspnea, or arousal secondary to Cheyne-Stokes respirations. Pulmonary dysfunction is exacerbated during sleep and predisposes patients to sleep-disordered breathing. Sleep disruption is particularly prominent in hyperthyroidism and uremia.

Proposed Sleep Disorders

"Menstrual-associated sleep disorder is a disorder of unknown cause, characterized by a complaint of either insomnia or excessive sleepiness, that is temporally related to the menses or menopause." Premenstrual excessive sleepiness is a sometimes dramatic disorder that appears within the first 2 years after the onset of menstruation. Periodic episodes of hypersomnolence tend to occur 6 to 10 days before the onset of menses. The disorder is treated successfully with birth control pills. Menopausal insomnia is characterized by recurrent awakenings, often associated with hot flashes or night sweats. Premenstrual insomnia is common, characterized by difficulty both initiating and maintaining sleep, and is often associated with other symptoms attributed to the premenstrual syndrome.

"Sleep-related laryngospasm refers to episodes of abrupt awakenings from sleep with an intense sensation of inability to breathe, and stridor." The disorder is frightening but apparently benign. Otolaryngologic examination reveals no abnormality. The disorder usually recurs several times and then resolves. It is more common in smokers and patients with esophageal reflux. Sleep apnea and upper-airway abnormality need to be considered.

BIBLIOGRAPHY

Bootzin RR, Engle-Friedman M, Hazelwood L: Insomnia. In Lewinsohn PM, Teri L, editors: *Clinical geropsychology: new directions in assessment and treatment*, New York, 1983, Pergamon Press.

Broughton RJ: Sleep disorders: disorders of arousal? *Science* 159:1070, 1968.

Diagnostic Classification Steering Committee, Thorpy MJ, chair: *International classification of sleep disorders: diagnostic and coding manual*, Rochester, Minn, 1990, American Sleep Disorders Association.

Guilleminault C et al: Sinus arrest during REM sleep in young adults, *N Engl J Med* 311:1006, 1984.

Kryger MH et al, editors: *Principles and practice of sleep medicine*, ed 2, Philadelphia, 1994, Saunders.

Lewy AJ et al: Antidepressant and circadian phase-shifting effects of light, *Science* 235:352, 1987.

Mignot E et al: DQB1*0602 and DQA1*0102(DQ1) are better markers than DR2 for narcolepsy in Caucasian and Black Americans, *Sleep* 17:S60-S67, 1994.

Mitler M et al: ASDA standards of practice: narcolepsy and its treatment with stimulants, *Sleep* 17:352, 1994.

Moore-Ede MC et al: Medical progress: circadian timekeeping in health and disease, *N Engl J Med* 309:469, 530, 1983.

Schenck CH et al: Rapid eye movement behavior disorder, *JAMA* 57:1786, 1987.

Sherin JE et al: Activation of ventrolateral preoptic neurons during sleep, *Science* 271:216, 1996.

Thorpy MJ, editor: *Handbook of sleep disorders*, New York, 1990, Marcel Dekker.

CHAPTER

135 Coma and Related Disorders

Martin A. Samuels

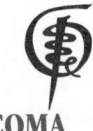

COMA

Coma is a clinical state of total unresponsiveness to all external stimuli; only residual reflex activity remains. It represents the final stage of brain failure in the continuum of consciousness from alert, confusion and delirium, drowsiness, stupor, and finally coma. Since many of these terms have imprecise meanings, it is best to describe the patient's behavior in terms of spontaneous activity and response to spoken words or noxious stimulation.

A large number of structural and metabolic conditions may disrupt brain function and impair consciousness. Consciousness consists of two components: arousal or wakefulness due to function of the ascending reticular activating system in the brain stem and thalamus, and awareness mediated by the integrated function of the cerebral cortex. Disorders of consciousness are therefore all due to metabolic or structural dysfunction of either or both of these anatomic substrates. The causes of coma may be divided into four basic categories (Box 135-1) according to a classification modified from Plum and Posner. The first diagnostic objective of the physician confronted with a comatose patient is to determine which of the four fundamental types of coma is operant, as this will have implications for both diagnosis and treatment. By evaluating five important physical findings (state of consciousness, pupillary responses, oculocephalic responses, motor responses, and respiratory pattern), it is usually possible to determine which pathophysiologic type of coma the patient is experiencing (Box 135-2 and Table 135-1).

The state of consciousness is characterized best by describing the examiner's stimulus (e.g., a quiet question, a shout, a gentle shake, a painful compression of the sternum) and the patient's response (e.g., eye opening and meaningful speech, a semipurposeful attempt to remove the painful stimulus, decorticate posturing, no response). The pupillary response is best elicited by a very bright light. Small constrictions are especially difficult to visualize when the pupils are small, and small reactive pupils are commonly mistaken for unreactive ones. Such a mistake may be very important.

The vestibulocular reflex (VOR) may be tested in two ways. The oculocephalic reflex (doll's eye response, doll's head eye phenomenon) is elicited by holding the patient's eyelids open and gently rocking the head briskly from side to side. If the reflex is intact, the eyes deviate conjugately to the side opposite that to which the head is ro-

BOX 135-1
Pathophysiologic and etiologic classification of coma

I. Supratentorial mass lesions
  A. Intracranial hemorrhage
    1. Epidural
    2. Subdural
    3. Intracerebral
  B. Neoplasm
  C. Infarct plus edema
  D. Abscess
II. Subtentorial structural lesions
  A. Hemorrhage
    1. Pontine
    2. Cerebellar
  B. Infarction
    1. Brainstem
    2. Cerebellar plus edema
  C. Tumor
  D. Abscess, cerebellar
III. Metabolic (diffuse)
  A. Poisoning
  B. Hypoxia
  C. Hypoglycemia
  D. Diffuse ischemia
  E. Concussion-contusion
  F. Meningoencephalitis
  G. Primary organ failure
    1. Lung
    2. Kidney
    3. Liver
  H. Acid-base, electrolyte disorders
IV. Psychogenic

BOX 135-2
Evaluation of the comatose patient

Is the cause:
  1. Supratentorial structural disease (mass)?
  2. Infratentorial structural disease?
  3. Diffuse brain disease (metabolic)?
  4. Psychogenic?
Physical examination emphasizing five key findings will determine the cause.
  1. Five key physical findings*
    a. Level of consciousness
    b. Pupils
    c. Oculocephalic reflex
    d. Respiratory pattern
    e. Motor tone and responses
  2. Simplified brainstem schema*

*See Table 135-1.

tated and then drift quickly back to the resting position. An intact reflex indicates that the tegmentum of the midbrain, pons, and medulla is largely intact structurally. This maneuver should not be done when there is a possibility of neck injury. Rather, the caloric test is done by infusing 20 to 50 ml ice water into the external auditory canal. The slow phase of the resulting nystagmos is mediated by the brain stem, whereas the fast phase is generated by the cortex.

Motor responses may occur spontaneously (e.g., purposeless thrashing of the limbs on one or both sides of the body, decerebrate posturing) or only with voice or painful stimulation. Spontaneous respiratory patterns should be observed first before stimuli are applied by the examiner.

PATHOPHYSIOLOGY

Supratentorial mass lesions impair consciousness by compressing the diencephalic ascending reticular activating system. If the mass expands sufficiently, the brain may herniate downward through the tentorial notch. The rostral brain-stem may be displaced caudally and be associated with hemorrhagic infarction of the central brainstem, which results in irreparable injury. Initially, the focal hemispheric lesion generally produces focal symptoms such as aphasia, hemiparesis, or homonymous hemianopia. As the mass grows, headache and altered consciousness often occur. If the hemispheric mass is located laterally rather than medially, the uncus of the temporal lobe may be squeezed over the notch of the tentorium; this compresses the ipsilateral oculomotor nerve and cerebral peduncle and produces an ipsilateral dilated pupil and a contralateral hemiparesis (uncal, or lateral, herniation syndrome). Sometimes the contralateral cerebral peduncle is compressed against the opposite notch of the tentorium, causing a hemiparesis ipsilateral to the hemispheric mass. With more centrally placed masses, as the diencephalon becomes compressed, brain function is impaired just as though the diencephalon were functionally transected (central herniation syndrome). The patient becomes stuporous; pupils are small but reactive; the oculocephalic responses are brisk; generalized paratonia (also called *gegenhalten*) or decorticate posturing occurs; and Cheyne-Stokes respiration becomes apparent (see Table 135-1). It is imperative that this constellation of physical findings resulting from transtentorial herniation be recognized and that the patient be treated urgently for intracranial hypertension. Otherwise, hemorrhagic infarction of the brainstem results if further herniation occurs. As caudal deterioration to the midbrain level evolves, with both the uncal and central syndromes, coma supervenes; the pupils become 4 to 5 mm in diameter, without reaction to light; oculocephalic and vestibuloocular (caloric) responses disappear; decorticate posturing becomes decerebrate; and transient hyperventilation appears. With further decompensation, the patient remains comatose, with unreactive midposition pupils and absent vestibuloocular responses. Tone becomes flaccid, and respiration becomes eupnea-like at the pontine level. Ataxic respiration follows as the medullary level of function is reached. Hypotension and death typically follow. Except for the pupillary and motor asymmetry that occurs early in the herniation process with a laterally placed supratentorial mass (uncal herniation syndrome), neurologic function deteriorates symmetrically and in an orderly rostral-to-caudal sequence from diencephalon, to midbrain, to pons, and to medulla (central herniation syndrome).

In subtentorial structural disease, coma is commonly preceded by nausea, vomiting, vertigo, diplopia, nystagmus, ataxia, and occipital headache. The coma is produced by destruction or compression of the reticular formation. It is uncommon for the brainstem to be transected in a single plane as it is with transtentorial herniation, and asymmetric dysfunction is common (e.g., unilateral oculomotor, gag, pharynx, tongue or sympathetic palsies, hemiparesis, and hemianesthesia). Often the dysfunction is focal and can be localized to a specific area such as the right midbrain or left pons.

Metabolic encephalopathy is a diffuse disorder of cerebral function resulting from impaired neuronal metabolism. It is caused by (1) systemic disorders that result in inadequate delivery of nutrients to the brain, (2) endogenous or exogenous systemic poisons, (3) electrolyte disturbances, or (4) the products of intracranial infection or hemorrhage (Box 135-3). In its mildest form, it is manifested by inattention, indifference to the surroundings, and mild intellectual impairment. As confusion worsens, there may be irritability, agitation, hallucinations, aberrant perception, and other signs of delirium before brain function is more severely impaired and stupor and coma supervene. Asterixis, tremulousness, myoclonus, and convulsions may also occur. Although neurologic dysfunction is generally symmetric, multiple levels of brainstem function may be impaired simultaneously. For example, in opiate poisoning, the patient may be conscious and have "thalamic" (small, minimally reactive) pupils, purposeful movements, and near apnea. It is not known why certain functions are selectively vulnerable to the effects of specific metabolic disturbances, but the "liver flap" (asterixis), multifocal myoclonus of uremia, posthypoxic action myoclonus, and opiate-induced miosis-hypopnea are characteristic enough to suggest a specific cause for the encephalopathy. Unless the patient has ingested substances that directly affect the autonomic nervous system, the pupils are nearly always symmet-

Table 135-1   Neurologic signs in central transtentorial herniation

STAGE	LEVEL OF CONSCIOUSNESS	PUPILS	OCULOCEPHALIC REFLEX	RESPIRATORY PATTERN	MOTOR TONE AND RESPONSES
Diencephalon	Lethargy to stupor	Small and reactive	Brisk	Sighs and yawns to C-S*	Semipurposeful to decorticate
Midbrain	Coma	MPF†	Decreased to absent	Tachypneic hyperpnea	Decerebrate
Pons	Coma	MPF	Absent	"Eupnea"‡	Decerebrate to flaccid
Medulla	Coma	MPF	Absent	Ataxic	Flaccid

Modified from Plum F, Posner JB: *The diagnosis of stupor and coma,* ed 3, Philadelphia, 1980, FA Davis.
*Cheyenne-Stokes respiration.
†Midposition and fixed: i.e., 4-5 mm in diameter and unresponsive to light.
‡Regular respiration, often shallow; rate of 25-40 per minute.

BOX 135-3
Common causes of metabolic encephalopathy

Substrate deprivation
  Hypoxia
  Diffuse ischemia
  Hypoglycemia
  Vitamin deficiency
Systemic diseases
  Respiratory failure (hypercapnia)
  Kidney failure (uremia)
  Liver failure
  Endocrine dysfunction
    Thyroid
    Parathyroid
    Adrenal
    Pancreas
  Hypertensive encephalopathy
  Fever
  Sepsis
  Porphyria
Poisoning
  Alcohol
  Prescribed drugs
  Poisons
  Drug withdrawal
Meningitis
Encephalitis
Subarachnoid hemorrhage
Electrolyte disorders
  Water, sodium, calcium, magnesium, possibly aluminum
Acid-base disorders
Concussion-contusion
Seizures plus postictal states
Mixed metabolic encephalopathy
Intensive care unit delirium

BOX 135-4
High-yield laboratory studies

Blood glucose
Blood Po_2, Pco_2, pH, NH_3
Na^+, Ca^{2+}, Mg^{2+}, BUN
Liver function tests
Sedative drug screen
Lumbar puncture
Blood and CSF cultures
EEG

BOX 135-5
Diagnostic studies in coma patients

Supratentorial mass lesions
  Primary
    CT scan
    MR scan
  Secondary
    Angiography
Subtentorial structural lesions
  Primary
    CT scan
    MR scan
    Angiography
Metabolic diffuse*
Psychogenic
  Opticokinetic nystagmus
  Calorics
  EEG
  Amobarbital (Amytal) interview

*See Box 135-3.

---

ric and reactive in metabolic brain disease, even in deep coma. Many of these metabolic disorders can be treated, and cerebral function may fully recover. However, some of them can produce irreparable brain injury. Consequently, the physician must proceed quickly, with an orderly and thorough consideration of the conditions known to produce this clinical syndrome, and should obtain appropriate laboratory confirmation (Box 135-4).

In psychogenic coma, the neurologic examination is normal except for the patient's unresponsiveness. Response to visual threat is normal, and the corneal, pharyngeal, abdominal, and other reflexes are also normal. Opticokinetic nystagmus, caloric-induced nystagmus, and the electroencephalogram (EEG) are normal. The fast phase of opticokinetic and caloric-induced nystagmus is absent in neurogenic coma. Covering the nose and mouth asphyxiates the patient and often induces immediate "awakening." This practice is discouraged, however, since some catatonic schizophrenic and hysterical patients have failed to arouse in this setting and have experienced hypoxic seizures and circulatory collapse. However, inhaled ammonia is a

powerful noxious stimulus, and ammonia capsules often induce awakening.

The neurologic examination usually establishes the pathophysiology of the coma. When this information is coupled with the history of how the unresponsiveness came about, and in what setting, it is often possible to limit the diagnostic possibilities to just one or two. Selected laboratory studies then may provide definitive diagnostic information.

LABORATORY STUDIES

Box 135-5 lists the most useful diagnostic studies. Computed tomography (CT) has contributed immeasurably in the evaluation of the comatose patient (Chapter 132). It demonstrates intracranial mass effects and often provides specific information about the pathologic lesion and its precise location. Consequently the CT scan is especially valuable in patients with suspected structural or mass lesions. MR scanning is extremely precise in the information its images provide but the technique is expensive, time consuming, and difficult to utilize in patients on ventilators. Cerebral angiography is more cumbersome and generally provides less precise information than does CT scanning. However, angiography may provide definitive information regarding aneurysms, arteriovenous malformations, vascular occlusions, and other lesions. In addition, angiography often provides information about abnormal vasculature that is important for the neurosurgeon in planning an operation. The EEG may demonstrate a focal or epileptic disturbance, but it is considerably less helpful than CT and MR scanning. The EEG can demonstrate diffuse physiologic disturbances and is helpful in diagnosing metabolic brain disease and brain death.

Lumbar puncture should be avoided in any patient suspected of having an intracranial mass lesion or noncommunicating hydrocephalus, because it may accentuate an intracranial pressure gradient and facilitate herniation of the intracranial contents from one compartment to another. Obtundation, focal signs, and papilledema are warning signs of a possible intracranial mass and suggest that other studies may be indicated before lumbar puncture. If treatable causes of meningitis (e.g., bacteria, fungi) are considerations, however, immediate examination of the spinal fluid may be mandatory, even if there is some risk of harm.

MANAGEMENT

The first step in managing the comatose patient is to protect the airway. Often, this simply requires gentle oropharyngeal suction and an oral airway, while at other times intubation and assisted ventilation are required. To prevent detrimental vasovagal effects of pharyngeal stimulation, atropine, 1.0 mg IV, should be given to any obtunded patient whose oropharynx will be stimulated by suctioning or by endotracheal or nasogastric intubation. The circulation must be maintained simultaneously. Hypotension in the coma patient is often caused by systemic acidosis, and correcting coexisting respiratory failure corrects the hypotension. Unless it is virtually certain that hypoglycemia is not playing a role in the patient's unresponsiveness, a sample of blood should be obtained for glucose determination, and 50 ml of 50% glucose should be given intravenously. Thiamin, 50 mg, can be given intravenously at the same time to any patient in whom Wernicke's encephalopathy is a consideration. If there is any possibility of a narcotic overdose, naloxone, 0.4 mg, should be given

intravenously one or more times. It must be used cautiously, however, in persons suspected to be physically dependent on opioids, because it may precipitate an acute abstinence syndrome. Once these supportive measures have been carried out to protect the patient from anoxia, ischemia, and hypoglycemia, a history can be obtained and the nervous system examined, paying particular attention to the aforementioned five physical findings.

HYPOXIC-ISCHEMIC ENCEPHALOPATHY AND PERSISTENT VEGETATIVE STATE

Hypoxic-ischemic encephalopathy after cardiopulmonary arrest is a frequent cause of prolonged coma. Survivors of cardiopulmonary arrest can experience a wide range of brain injury, varying from full recovery to brain death. In patients who have neurologic damage but whose brainstem functions are intact, management is often an ethical and medicolegal dilemma, especially since the extent of cortical damage may be severe, moderate, or mild.

Patients with prolonged survival who have intact brainstem function but virtually no cortical function are said to be in a *persistent vegetative state*. During hypoxiaischemia, neocortical neurons are especially susceptible to anoxic injury and can be irreversibly damaged while the brainstem remains largely intact. After 1 to 2 weeks of sleeplike coma with brainstem reflexes present, patients in the persistent vegetative state resume periods of "wakefulness" in which the eyes are open and moving, but responsiveness is limited to primitive reflexes. The return of spontaneous eye opening often gives false hope to families because patients in a persistent vegetative state remain mindless, devoid of thought or emotion.

Predicting which survivors of cardiopulmonary arrest will remain in a permanent vegetative state is a frequent problem. Reliable clinical predictors of long-term neurologic outcome have been developed (Table 135-2), but none are absolute. Rare instances of remarkable recoveries belying these predictors have occurred, especially in young patients. The decision to either limit or terminate intensive supportive treatment in patients with severe neurologic deficits who have only a small chance of functional recovery is difficult for both physicians and families. Each clinical situation must be dealt with individually when considering limitation of care in this setting. However, several general principles apply to this ethical and medicolegal dilemma: (1) an adequate period of observation must occur, during which careful neurologic examinations should be recorded; (2) the prognosis, if maximal care is provided, should be clearly stated; (3)

Table 135-2   Features predictive of neurologic recovery in hypoxic-ischemic coma patients in accordance with their best functional state within the first year*

	NO RECOVERY OR VEGETATIVE STATE	SEVERE DISABILITY	GOOD RECOVERY
Third-day examination No———————→	93%	7%	0%
Motor response: withdrawal or better ↓ No———————→	61%	21%	18%

Yes→ Spontaneous eye movements with fixation
          ↓
          Yes———————→
	8%	15%	77%

Seventh-day examination No———————→	100%	0%	0%

No———→
                   ↑   Spontaneous eye
                            opening at 3 days
                            ↓
                            Yes———————→
	58%	42%	0%

No→ Initial eye movements roving and conjugate ↑ Yes———————→	67%	17%	16%

Obeys commands
  ↓
  Yes———————→
	6%	22%	72%

Modified from Levy DE et al: Predicting outcome from hypoxic-ischemic coma, *JAMA* 253:1420, 1985.
*Residual anesthetics, anticonvulsants, or metabolic derangements may be confounding.

the wishes of the patient, if previously expressed, and of the patinet's family, should be considered; and (4) a second neurologic consultation is often advisable. In cases deemed hopeless, withdrawal or limitation of supportive treatment is not mandatory but may be permissible, if the family agrees.

Other neurologic syndromes can follow less severe hypoxic-ischemic encephalopathy. In the "man-in-the-barrel" syndrome, patients recovering from hypoxic-ischemic brain injury can move their face and lower limbs spontaneously, or in response to pain, but not their upper limbs. Hypoperfusion of the distal branches of the middle cerebral artery causes selective damage to cortical motor neurons subserving the upper extremities. This syndrome is often transient and, when prolonged, is often associated with substantial cognitive impairment. Isolated cortical blindness caused by occipital lobe ischemia may also be seen following hypotension, presumably by a similar mechanism. Spinal cord ischemia, action myoclonus, and delayed, postanoxic leukoencephalopathy are uncommon neurologic sequelae of hypoxia-ischemia.

DEATH BY BRAIN CRITERIA

Since the late 1950s, it has been possible to keep patients alive who have irreversibly lost all brain function, by using mechanical ventilation and vasopressors. In these patients who are brain dead, the heart and peripheral circulation continue to function in the absence of brain activity. *Brain death* implies irreversible damage to the entire brain, including the brain stem. This state is to be clearly distinguished from the persistent vegetative state, in which partial preservation of brain stem function occurs. The growing importance of organ donation for human transplantation has been a major impetus for the generation of reliable clinical criteria for brain death.

The medicolegal criteria for brain death vary widely, according to local laws and medical customs. The recommendations of the President's Commission (1981) are guidelines widely accepted in the United States for defining brain death in adults (Box 135-6). Criteria often differ for adults and children, the latter usually requiring more prolonged observation. The criteria may seem needlessly complex because no false-positive determinations are allowable. False-negative conclusions are more acceptable. The diagnosis of brain death should be made only by clinicians who are experienced in evaluating comatose patients, and documentation should be meticulously recorded in the medical record.

A patient with reactive pupils, a corneal or gag reflex, or any respiratory activity is not brain dead. Any type of decerebrate or decorticate posturing, even though nonpurposeful, reflects brain stem activity and also precludes the diagnosis of brain death. The pupils in brain death are usually midposition or dilated, and unreactive. Small pupils are uncommon and should be carefully checked for reactivity; they indicate possible drug intoxication. The preservation of purely spinal reflexes (e.g., tendon stretch reflexes, Babinski's response) is consistent with brain death in most criteria. A general drug screen is usually required to exclude the occult presence of central nervous system depressants. Hypothermia and occult drug ingestion are the two conditions most often producing a reversible loss of brain function that is misdiagnosed as brain death. Neuromuscular blocking agents may also abolish motor and respiratory activity.

Apnea testing is an important measure of brain stem function. It should be carried out in a standardized manner to prevent hypoxemia and to ensure that the partial pressure of carbon dioxide (PCO_2) reaches the critical level to stimulate medullary respiratory centers. The patient is given 100% oxygen for 10 minutes; then oxygen is delivered at 6 L/min by a catheter placed in the trachea to maintain tissue oxygenation during apnea testing. Arterial blood gases are initially obtained and are then repeated after 8 to 10 minutes. The PCO_2 usually increases at a rate of 2.0 to 2.5 mm Hg/min in immobile, comatose patients. If no respiratory activity is associated with a PCO_2 of more than 60 mm Hg, apnea compatible with brain stem death exists. This test is invalid in patients with severe pulmonary disease who are carbon dioxide retainers and who have hypoxemia as the driving mechanism for respiration.

An isoelectric EEG is not synonymous with brain death, but only reflects electrical silence of the cerebral cortex. Drug intoxication, hypothermia, and viral encephalitis are well-known causes of an isoelectric EEG, and each is associated with a high probability of complete or partial neurologic recovery. An isoelectric EEG is a necessary but not sufficient requirement for brain death in many of the published criteria, although other criteria do not require EEG testing.

All reversible metabolic derangements that might contribute to central nervous system dysfunction must be absent to strictly meet most criteria of brain death, although the degree of allowable derangement is largely a matter of clinical judgment in individual patients. The potential importance of contributing metabolic derangements requires careful clinical consideration. In equivocal cases, confirmatory tests to document the absence of blood flow to the brain (e.g., angiography) may be considered.

Once brain death has been diagnosed according to local medical and legal standards, withdrawal of supportive treatment is legally and ethically justified. In the opinion of many experts, it is actually indicated. In patients with suspected brain death in whom the criteria are incompletely met, or in whom other uncertainties exist, observation with continued support is proper. Most patients who are brain dead experience somatic death from cardiovascular collapse within 48 to 72 hours despite supportive treatment, and prolonged somatic survival is rare, in contrast to patients in a persistent vegetative state.

Unusual movements of the extremities can occur for 15 to 30 minutes after ventilatory assistance is withdrawn in brain dead patients and are presumably a manifestation of terminal spinal cord ischemia. Families of patients should be discouraged from remaining at the bedside during this period.

BOX 135-6
Death by brain criteria in adults*

I. Cessation of all function of the entire brain
  A. Unresponsive coma
  B. Absent brain stem reflexes
    1. Pupillary light reflex
    2. Corneal reflex
    3. Cephalic (caloric) reflexes
    4. Oropharyngeal (gag) reflex
    5. Respiration (apnea testing)
II. Irreversibility
  A. Coma of known cause without potential for reversibility
  B. Exclusion of contributory, reversible conditions
    1. Drug intoxication
    2. Neuromuscular blockade
    3. Hypothermia (<32.2° C, 90° F)
    4. Shock
    5. Major metabolic disturbance
  C. Persistence for an appropriate period of observation (6-24 hours, depending on cause of coma and local practice)
III. Confirmatory investigations (optional)
  A. Electrocerebral silence (isoelectric EEG)
  B. Absence of circulation to the brain

Modified from Guidelines for the determination of death: report of the medical consultants on the diagnosis of death to the President's Commission for the Study of Ethical Problems in Medicine and Biomedical and Behavioral Research, *JAMA* 246:2184, 1981.
*Note: Local and institutional rules are superseding.

BIBLIOGRAPHY

Bates D: The management of medical coma, *J Neurol Neurosurg Psychiatry* 56:589-598, 1993.

Council on Scientific Affairs and Council on Ethical and Judicial Affairs: Persistent vegetative state and the decision to withdraw or withhold life support, *JAMA* 263:426, 1990.

Jennett B, Bond M: Assessment of outcome after severe brain damage: a practical scale, *Lancet* 1:480, 1975.

Kinney HC, Samuels MA: Neuropathy of the persistent vegetative state: a review, *J Neuropath Exp Neuro* 53:548-558, 1994.

Kinney HC, Korein J, Panigraphy A et al: Neuropathologic findings in the brain of Karen Ann Quinlan: the role of the thalamus in the persistent vegetative state, *N Engl J Med* 330:1469-1475, 1994.

Kinomura S, Larsson J, Gulyas B, Roland PE: Activation by attention of the human reticular formation and thalamic intralaminar nuclei, *Science* 271:512-514, 1996.

Levy DE et al: Predicting outcome from hypoxic-ischemic coma, *JAMA* 246:2184, 1981.

Medical Consultants on the Diagnosis of Death: Guidelines for the determination of death, *JAMA* 246:2184, 1981.

Plum F, Posner JP: *The diagnosis of stupor and coma,* ed 3, Philadelphia, 1980, Davis.

Spudis EV: The persistent vegetative state—1990, *J Neurol Sci* 102:128, 1991.

Teasdale G, Jennett B: Assessment of coma and impaired consciousness: a practical scale, *Lancet* 2:81, 1974.

CHAPTER

136   Faintness and Syncope

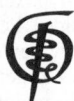

Sumanth D. Prabhu, Robert A. O'Rourke, and J. Donald Easton

Syncope (fainting) is a transient loss of consciousness and postural tone with spontaneous recovery caused by generalized cerebral hypoperfusion. *Presyncope* (faintness) is the sensation of impending loss of consciousness that usually precedes full syncope. This symptom is manifested by light-headedness, weakness, nausea, visual spots or vision dimming, ringing or roaring in the ears, diaphoresis, and skin pallor. Presyncope is often confused with the more general sensation of dizziness, variably described by the patient as giddiness, disequilibrium, vertigo, imbalance, fuzziness in the head, or a floating feeling (Chapter 139). Presyncope usually manifests over several seconds. Unless the episode is caused by cardiac arrhythmias, the patient is usually in an upright position. If there is progression to complete syncope, the patient usually slumps, with minimal injury, and remains unconscious for a few seconds, sometimes for 1 to 2 minutes and, rarely, for 5 to 10 minutes or longer. Usually the patient lies motionless, although a few clonic jerks can occur. Rhythmic, clonic convulsions and fecal or urinary incontinence are rare. The patient usually awakens feeling weak but mentally clear, without headache or drowsiness. If he or she is prevented from falling to a recumbent position, the unconsciousness may be prolonged, resulting in ischemic cerebral injury. Presyncope often aborts before progressing to a full faint, but most faints are preceded by presyncope.

PATHOPHYSIOLOGY

Syncope results from a temporary and significant reduction in cerebral blood flow, which is largely determined by arterial blood pressure and cerebrovascular resistance. *Cerebral blood flow autoregulation* refers to the reflex constriction or dilation of cerebral blood vessels in response to rising or falling systemic blood pressure. This intrinsic control mechanism maintains a virtually constant cerebral blood flow in the face of significant fluctuations in arterial blood pressure. In healthy young adults in the upright position, the systolic blood pressure may fall to 60 to 70 mm Hg without significant cerebral ischemia. Below that, resistance vessels become maximally dilated, and further decreases in blood pressure result in progressive decreases in blood flow. In older patients with diminished cerebral autoregulatory capacity, there may be significant cerebral ischemia with much smaller reductions in arterial blood pressure.

Reductions in cerebral blood flow can also result from increased cerebrovascular resistance (e.g., hyperventilation, with its fall in arterial P_{CO_2}, induces $[H^+]$ changes in the interstitium around arteriolar resistance vessels, mediating vasoconstriction). However, syncope usually is caused by a fall in systemic blood pressure, either from peripheral vasodilation or from a decrease in cardiac output. With most causes of syncope, blood pressure returns to the critical cerebral perfusion level as soon as the recumbent position is assumed.

CLASSIFICATION OF SYNCOPE

Syncope may be broadly classified as neurally mediated (circulatory) or cardiogenic. The underlying causes range from benign conditions to potentially life-threatening illnesses (Box 136-1).

Neurally Mediated (Circulatory) Syncope

Vasodepressor (Vasovagal) Syncope. Also known as neurocardiogenic or vasovagal syncope, vasodepressor syncope occurs from sudden hypotension due to an acute failure of autonomic cardiovascular control mechanisms. Patients with vasodepressor syncope usually display normal cardiovascular regulation between syncopal episodes, indicating a transient alteration of autonomic function during syncope. This is the most common type of syncope and is generically referred to as the *common faint*. It occurs frequently in the young adult population, but it may occur at any age. It is often precipitated by sudden emotional stress, pain, or threat of injury and aggravated by situations that decrease central venous volume or increase cardiovascular adrenergic tone (e.g., fasting, poor physical condition, warm environment, and excessive fatigue). For example, the sight of a shocking accident, a hypodermic needle, or blood withdrawal may evoke an attack. Conversely, a syncopal attack may occur without any obvious precipitating factors after a person has been standing for a prolonged time.

BOX 136-1
Classification of syncope

I. Neurally mediated (circulatory) syncope
  A. Vasodepressor (vasovagal)
  B. Reflex
    1. Cough
    2. Micturition
    3. Defecation
    4. Swallow
    5. Acute pain states (e.g., neuralgias)
    6. Carotid sinus syncope
  C. Orthostatic hypotension
    1. Autonomic failure
      a. Primary
      b. Secondary
      c. Drug-induced
    2. Intravascular volume depletion
II. Cardiogenic syncope
  A. Mechanical
    1. Left ventricular outflow obstruction
      a. Aortic stenosis
      b. Hypertrophic cardiomyopathy
      c. Left atrial myxoma
      d. Prosthetic valve thrombosis
    2. Right ventricular outflow obstruction
      a. Primary pulmonary hypertension
      b. Severe pulmonic stenosis
      c. Pulmonary embolism
      d. Tetralogy of Fallot
      e. Right atrial myxoma
    3. Cyanotic congenital heart disease
    4. Myocardial disease
      a. Massive myocardial infarction
      b. Pump failure
    5. Cardiac tamponade
    6. Subclavian steal syndrome
  B. Electrical
    1. Bradyarrhythmias
      a. His-Purkinje system heart block
      b. Sick sinus syndrome
      c. Atrioventricular nodal heart block
      d. Vagotonic heart block
    2. Tachyarrhythmias
      a. Ventricular tachycardia
      b. Q-T interval prolongation
      c. Paroxysmal atrial tachyarrhythmias

The upright posture results in lower extremity pooling of blood, reducing venous return. The normal physiologic response via arterial and cardiopulmonary baroreceptors is to decrease receptor firing, resulting in increased sympathetic outflow and reduced parasympathetic outflow, increasing heart rate, contractility, vascular tone, and blood pressure. Patients susceptible to vasodepressor syncope display an initial exaggerated sympathetic response with a hypercontractile ventricle and reduced chamber volume. This is believed to paradoxically activate left ventricular mechanoreceptor (C-fiber) afferents, which travel via the glossopharyngeal and vagus nerves to the brain stem. These afferent signals then excite medullary neuronal centers and efferent pathways, resulting in sympathetic withdrawal and parasympathetic activation and producing profound vasodilation, bradycardia, and hypotension. Ischemia of the mechanoreceptors themselves can also trigger this reflex arc, as evidenced by the classic Bezold-Jarish reflex in patients with inferoposterior myocardial infarction. Similarly, this pathway may be partially responsible for exertional syncope in patients with severe aortic stenosis because mechanoreceptor stimulation can occur from excessive left ventricular pressure resulting in inappropriate vasodilation.

This mechanism can also be activated by stimuli other than changes in blood volume and afferent pathways distinct from ventricular mechanoreceptors. Afferent signals from the carotid sinus baroreceptors (carotid sinus syncope), urinary bladder mechanoreceptors (micturition syncope), and gastrointestinal tract mechanoreceptors (swallow syncope) can all act via this pathway. As described previously, acute pain, strong emotions, or fear of injury can also serve as triggers, especially in the setting of volume depletion. Regardless of whether vasodepressor syncope is triggered by arterial, ventricular, or visceral afferents, the efferent pathway is similar, resulting in vasodilation and bradycardia due to sympathetic withdrawal and parasympathetic stimulation. The clinical response may be primarily *cardioinhibitory* (bradycardia predominance), primarily *vasodepressor* (dysautonomic response), or *mixed* (both elements present). Centrally acting serotonin and endogenous nitric oxide have been implicated in the pathogenesis of neurocardiogenic syncope. In addition, there is some evidence for paradoxical cerebral vasoconstriction during hypotension in these patients, suggesting abnormalities in cerebral blood flow autoregulation. The pathogenesis is summarized in Fig. 136-1.

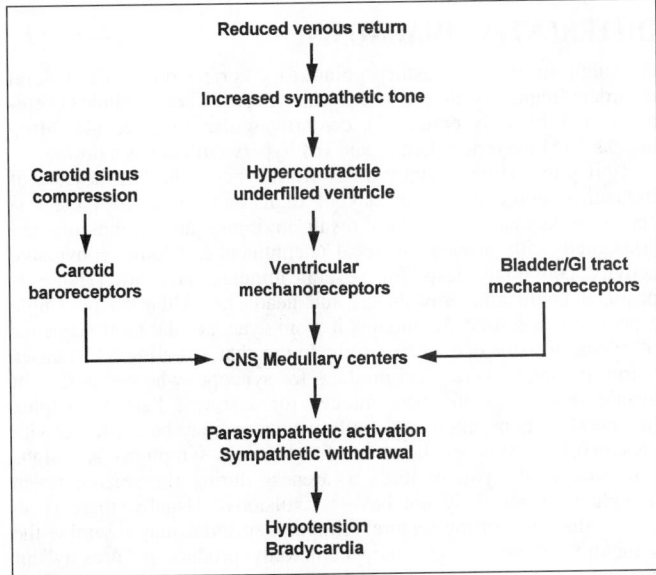

FIGURE 136-1 Pathophysiology underlying vasodepressor (vasovagal) syncope. Arterial, ventricular, and visceral afferents can all activate brain stem centers, predominantly via the glossopharyngeal and vagus nerves. This leads to the stimulation of an efferent pathway, producing parasympathetic activation and sympathetic withdrawal. The end result is hypotension, bradycardia, and syncope. *CNS,* Central nervous system; *GI,* gastrointestinal.

Reflex Syncope. *Cough syncope* usually occurs after vigorous paroxysms of coughing in men with chronic obstructive lung disease. It may be caused by the sudden increase in intrathoracic and intraabdominal pressure, which decreases venous return and cardiac output. There also may be severe, secondary increases in intracranial pressure because of the cough paroxysm, which reduces cerebral blood flow. A prolonged Valsalva maneuver in association with hyperventilation certainly appears to produce syncope in breath-holding spells of infancy and weight-lifter's blackout.

Micturition syncope is usually seen in males who arise from sleep to urinate and faint during or immediately after voiding. The cause is likely multifactorial and includes orthostatic hypotension, reduced peripheral resistance and heart rate during sleep, vasodepressor reflex stimulation with sudden decompression of the distended bladder, vagal stimulation with micturition, and Valsalva effects with decreased venous return.

Defecation syncope has also been described in patients who were either recumbent or asleep before defecation, many of whom had underlying gastrointestinal and cardiovascular illnesses. The underlying mechanisms of defecation syncope are not well elucidated but may be similar to those producing micturition syncope.

Swallow syncope has been reported in patients with underlying esophageal disease. Syncope occurs during or immediately following deglutition and is associated with bradycardia, asystole, and hypotension. An exaggerated vasodepressor reflex arc originating from esophageal afferents is thought to be the underlying mechanism (see previous discussion).

Similar neurally mediated vasodepressor reflexes underlie syncope associated with acute pain states (e.g., vagal and glossopharyngeal neuralgia, gallbladder colic, perforation of a viscus, needling of body cavities), intense vertigo and migraine headaches, and carotid sinus hypersensitivity. The diagnosis of glossopharyngeal neuralgia is suggested by the invariable sequence of severe unilateral pain in the posterior oropharynx or ear, followed by loss of consciousness caused by profound sinus bradycardia or asystole. A history of syncope while shaving the neck, wearing tight collars, or during sudden head movements suggests a diagnosis of carotid sinus hypersensitivity.

Orthostatic Hypotension with Syncope. Orthostatic hypotension, defined as a drop in systolic blood pressure of 20 mm Hg or more upon standing, occurs in individuals who have either chronic or transient vasomotor instability, or intravascular volume depletion. Sudden rising from the recumbent or sitting position to a sitting or standing position or standing still for several minutes results in the pooling of blood in the lower extremities and viscera as a result of the loss of compensatory reflex peripheral vasoconstriction, producing hypotension and syncope.

Orthostatic hypotension can result from the following, either singly or in combination: (1) impaired autonomic reflex control, which may be primary or secondary; (2) depletion of central or total blood volume; (3) circulating vasodilators (e.g., carcinoid syndrome); and (4) pharmacologic agents (e.g., nitrates and calcium blockers). Orthostatic hypotension can occur in otherwise normal people after physical deconditioning, prolonged bed rest, fasting, and alcohol use. Varicose veins and normal pregnancy may also be implicated.

Primary autonomic failure may be caused by several degenerative diseases of the autonomic nervous system, including idiopathic orthostatic hypotension, Shy-Drager syndrome, and Parkinson's disease. Secondary autonomic failure can occur from involvement of sympathetic and parasympathetic fibers by systemic diseases such as diabetes, amyloidosis, alcoholism, and pernicious anemia. These and other neuropathies can affect the autonomic nervous system and cause sexual impotence, impaired sweating, and paralysis of vasomotor reflexes. Diminished ankle jerk reflexes and diminished sensation in the feet should be sought on examination as evidence of a peripheral neuropathy and should suggest the possibility of concomitant autonomic involvement.

Intravascular volume depletion and side effects of pharmacologic agents are the most common causes of orthostatic hypotension with syncope in adults. The elderly are especially susceptible. Antihypertensive, antidepressant, and other medications commonly cause orthostatic hypotension by plasma volume depletion or sympatholytic vasomotor effects. Bleeding and persistent vomiting and diarrhea also may cause volume depletion.

Cardiogenic Syncope

Syncope of cardiac origin involves loss of consciousness produced by a sudden, marked reduction in effective cardiac output. Etiologic classification of these disorders may be divided broadly into mechanical and electrical (arrhythmic) causes.

Mechanical Causes. Left ventricular outflow obstruction is the most frequently encountered cause of mechanical cardiac syncope in adults. Obstruction may occur at the valvular, subvalvular, or supravalvular level and may be fixed (e.g., aortic stenosis) or dynamic (e.g., hypertrophic cardiomyopathy). In these conditions, cardiac output may not increase sufficiently during skeletal muscle exercise to meet peripheral oxygen demands. Blood preferentially flows to the exercising muscle, and this results in systemic arterial hypotension, cerebral anoxia, and effort-related syncope. Inappropriate vasodilation may also be secondary to discharge of left ventricular mechanoreceptors due to high chamber pressure. In hypertrophic obstructive cardiomyopathy, the dynamic obstruction is worsened by conditions that increase contractility, decrease preload, or decrease afterload. Left atrial myxomas are an uncommon but definite cause of mechanical cardiac syncope (Chapter 25). The patient may have clinical findings suggestive of mitral stenosis but will complain of faintness or syncope, which occurs with change of position as the tumor mass suddenly obstructs the mitral orifice. Thrombosis or prosthetic valve malfunction also may produce sudden mechanical obstruction of the circulation and syncope.

Right ventricular outflow obstruction, such as occurs with primary pulmonary hypertension, severe pulmonic stenosis, pulmonary embolism, right atrial myxomas, and tetralogy of Fallot, can also be associated with effort syncope because of insufficient increases in cardiac output with exercise. Cyanotic congenital heart defects characterized by right-to-left shunting and either pulmonary hypertension or right ventricular outflow obstruction can occasionally produce exertional syncope. Decreased peripheral resistance with exercise increases right-to-left shunting, which maintains cardiac output but results in further reduction of systemic arterial oxygen saturation and cerebral hypoxia, causing faintness or syncope. Vagal reflexes, however, may be involved in these conditions as well as in the syncope that occurs with massive pulmonary embolism.

Syncope at rest may occur in any of these disease states resulting from arrhythmias (see Electrical Causes). Cardiac syncope also may result from acute massive myocardial infarction on the basis of low cardiac output or transient severe arrhythmias, or cardiac tamponade resulting from reductions in cardiac output. Syncope in the setting of upper extremity exercise should raise the possibility of subclavian artery stenosis and reversal of flow in the vertebral artery (subclavian steal syndrome).

Electrical Causes. Electrical (arrhythmia) disorders are more frequent causes of cardiac syncope than mechanical abnormalities. Cerebral blood flow is maintained in supine healthy individuals over a wide range of heart rates from approximately 40 to 185 beats per minute. Alterations in pulse rate outside these limits may reduce cerebral circulation and function. In addition, cerebrovascular disease, upright posture, and coronary artery, valvular, or myocardial dysfunction of any etiology may diminish tolerance to even more modest alterations in heart rate.

Advanced degrees of atrioventricular (A-V) block are the most frequent arrhythmic causes of faintness or syncope (the Stokes-Adams-Morgagni syndrome). Stokes-Adams syncope is characterized by its abrupt onset and lack of relation to posture, position, or effort. Like seizures, it may occur in the recumbent position. Sometimes, as a result of prolonged cardiac asystole and attendant severe cerebral anoxia, seizurelike activity and sphincter incontinence may occur and be misdiagnosed as epilepsy.

Symptomatic chronic or acute forms of heart block usually involve the distal conduction system (His-Purkinje system), occur in the elderly or postinfarction patient, and may be persistent or episodic. The resting electrocardiogram may provide evidence of impaired conduction in one or any combination of the three fascicles through which the ventricles are normally activated (Chapter 9). Heart block involving the proximal conduction system (A-V node) is less often symptomatic and is most frequently congenital, drug-induced (e.g., digitalis, β-blockers, calcium blockers), or ischemic in origin. Syncope is often reported in patients with sick sinus syndrome, which is characterized by impaired sinoatrial impulse formation or conduction, manifested as inappropriate sinus bradycardia, sinus pauses, or sinus exit block. These patients may also have paroxysms of rapid atrial tachyarrhythmias alternating with periods of slow sinus rates (tachycardia-bradycardia syndrome). This disorder is being recognized increasingly in the elderly and in the postoperative patient with congenital heart disease. Vagally mediated heart block or ventricular asystole (vagotonic block) has been observed in many disease states (carotid sinus or mediastinal tumors, esophageal diverticula, peritoneal or pleural irritation) and during a variety of diagnostic procedures (e.g., endoscopy and cardiac catheterization). Vagal and glossopharyngeal neuralgia may induce a similar reflex form of syncope.

Self-limited, malignant ventricular arrhythmias (fibrillation or tachycardia) constitute another important cause of cardiac syncope. Ventricular tachycardia usually occurs in patients with structural heart disease and ventricular dysfunction. Polymorphic ventricular tachycardia, occurring in patients with a prolonged Q-T interval (torsades de pointes), may result from sympathetic autonomic imbalance of ventricular innervation as a genetically determined cause of prolonged syncope and sudden death. This familial condition may occur alone (Romano-Ward syndrome) or may be associated with congenital deafness (Jervell-Lange-Nielsen syndrome). Acquired forms of Q-T interval prolongation with torsades de pointes can occur with type IA and IC antiarrhythmic drugs, nonsedating antihistamines (e.g., terfenadine, astemizole), phenothiazines, tricyclic antidepressants, liquid protein diets, hypokalemia, hypomagnesemia, severe bradycardia, and central nervous system disorders. Paroxysmal atrial tachyarrhythmias can also be associated with frank syncope, usually in the elderly patient with underlying cerebrovascular disease.

Ambulatory electrocardiogram (ECG) recordings, atrial pacing studies, and bundle of His recordings, alone or in combination, are often necessary to define the presence or absence of a responsible cardiac arrhythmia in patients with dizziness or syncope. In patients with arrhythmia-induced syncope, appropriate pacemaker or drug therapy depends on demonstrating the causative rhythm disturbance (Chapter 9).

DIFFERENTIAL DIAGNOSIS

Although an accurate history points to a correct diagnosis, several disorders frequently are confused with syncope. These include (1) epilepsy, (2) hypoglycemia, (3) cerebrovascular disease, (4) "drop attacks," (5) hysterical faints, and (6) hyperventilation syndrome.

Epileptic seizures usually differ from syncope in that they are of immediate onset and occur day or night and while the patient is active or supine. They often result in injury and commonly are associated with urinary or fecal incontinence. Clonic convulsive activity commonly lasts for several minutes, and often there is postictal confusion, drowsiness, and headache. Although no single aspect of a seizure differentiates it from syncope, the total sequence of events usually does. One study found that sweating and nausea before the event were good markers for syncope, whereas postevent disorientation was the best marker for seizures. Partial complex (temporal lobe, psychomotor, limbic) seizures may be confused with presyncope or syncope because of autonomic symptoms and signs and because the patient loses awareness during the seizure (even though he or she may not have convulsions). Usually, there is an aura at the onset of the seizure. Although episodes may resemble the symptoms of presyncope, they commonly produce a "dreamy" or confused state; patients often experience hallucinations, illusions involving themselves or their environment, or unusual feelings of déjà vu. During the ictus, the patient frequently carries out automatic activity that is generally stereotypic for that patient. *Akinetic seizures* are brief attacks of unconsciousness with loss of muscle tone; they are uncommon, occur primarily in children and may be confused with syncope.

Hypoglycemia typically produces confusion or behavioral abnormalities and then hunger and salivation. This is followed by sympathetic hyperactivity manifested by sweating, tachycardia, and nervousness. Obtundation progressing to coma and seizures may ensue. It is unusual for hypoglycemia to produce a relatively abrupt and transient loss of consciousness; thus this condition generally is not confused with syncope.

Cerebrovascular disease rarely causes transient loss of consciousness. Subarachnoid hemorrhage may cause temporary unconsciousness, but it usually has an explosive onset, with severe headache, and the patient is typically left with obtundation, often prominent neurologic deficits, and neck stiffness after several hours. A major cerebral embolism or thrombosis may produce transient unconsciousness, but residual neurologic deficits are present. Transient cerebral ischemic attacks involving the carotid artery distribution almost never produce transient unconsciousness. Whereas dizziness is one of the cardinal signs of brain stem ischemia, true syncope is uncommon. When dizziness results from brain stem ischemia, it usually is associated with tinnitus, deafness, diplopia, dysarthria, extremity paralysis or numbness, or other symptoms of brain stem ischemia. Therefore cerebrovascular disease usually produces many associated symptoms of focal cerebral dysfunction that readily distinguish it from syncope.

The drop attack is a puzzling phenomenon. It usually occurs after the sixth decade and is characterized by a sudden drop to the ground with no apparent loss of consciousness. The patients may bruise their knees but usually are otherwise unhurt and able to stand immediately. Although the cause of this disorder is unknown, it has been attributed to basilar artery insufficiency producing transient ischemia to the part of the reticular formation that regulates postural tone. Because these patients often have attacks for many years without other evidence of brain stem ischemia, many physicians believe that a diagnosis of vertebral-basilar insufficiency cannot be made with confidence.

Hysterical faints or swoons must be differentiated from syncope, particularly emotion-induced vasovagal syncope. Hysterical faints occur dramatically and in the presence of others; they are not associated with pallor, diaphoresis, or weakening or slowing of the pulse. They draw attention to the hysterical personality who may be seeking secondary gain through this and other physical complaints. There may be prolonged periods of "unresponsiveness," with resistance to passive opening of the eyelids, bizarre posturing, or resistance to movement of the limbs.

Hyperventilation rarely causes syncope; however, it does cause presyncope. This faintness, together with anxiety, dyspnea, palpitations, and paresthesias of the distal extremities and perioral area in a setting of overventilation, constitutes the hyperventilation syndrome. It is usually caused by acute anxiety. Sometimes, vasodepressor mechanisms are superimposed, and syncope results.

DIAGNOSTIC EVALUATION

The cornerstone of the diagnostic evaluation of syncope is the history, followed by the physical examination and the electrocardiogram (ECG) (Fig. 136-2). A detailed history and physical examination will identify the majority of syncopal etiologies. Prior studies have shown that in patients with syncope of known origin, the history and physical lead to the identification of up to 85% of the underlying causes. The physician needs a detailed, chronologic account of precisely what the patient was doing, what his or her position or posture was, and the first thing that appeared to the patient to be wrong, in addition to other details (Box 136-2). The physician who can visualize the precise clinical picture at the completion of the history taking usually has considerable confidence in his or her diagnosis of syncope or its exclusion. In reflex syncope induced, for example, by cough, micturition, or acute pain states, the history is virtually diagnostic. The same can be said of vasodepressor syncope, although a search should be made for factors contributing to orthostatic hypotension. The medication history is especially important in this regard. In addition, inquiry should be made regarding the association of the syncope with exertion, dyspnea, palpitations, chest pain, or other symptoms of cardiac awareness. A history of rheumatic heart disease, coronary artery disease, or hypertension may be important.

The physical examination also provides important clues. Particu-

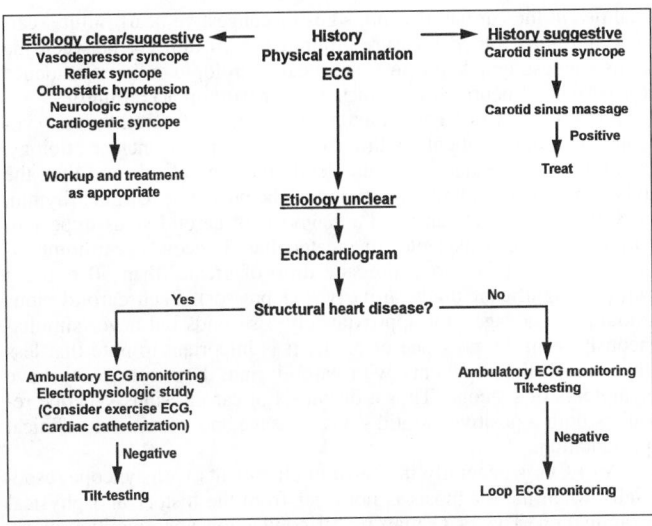

FIGURE 136-2 Approach to evaluation of syncope, beginning with the history, physical examination, and electrocardiogram (ECG).

BOX 136-2

Questions to ask the patient and observers in the evaluation of syncope

Questions for the patient

1. What were you doing during the hours and minutes preceding the blackout?
2. What was your situation regarding loss of sleep, ingestion of food and alcohol, and use of drugs or medications before the blackout?
3. What was your body position or posture?
4. What was the first thing you noticed to be wrong?
5. What symptoms did you experience next, in what order, and for how long?
6. Do you remember slumping or striking the floor?
7. What was the next thing you remember, and what position were you in when you regained awareness?
8. Did you hurt yourself in the fall?
   a. Did you injure your tongue or mouth?
   b. Did your back or muscles ache?
   c. Did you have a headache?
   d. Did you lose control of your bladder or bowels?
   e. How did you feel on awakening, and how long did it take for you to feel entirely normal again—seconds, minutes, or longer?

Questions for the observers

1. Ask the observers to answer the preceding questions when appropriate.
2. Was there any turning of the eyes or head?
3. Was there any twitching or jerking of the face or extremities?
4. Was the skin sweaty, pale, flushed, or blue?
5. Did the patient respond to observers in any way during the apparent unconsciousness?

---

lar attention should be given to the presence of orthostatic hypotension, cardiovascular findings, and neurologic signs. Orthostatic hypotension is demonstrated by obtaining the blood pressure in the supine and standing positions. In some patients, vasomotor tone will not fall immediately, so it is important to record the blood pressure immediately after standing and then at 1, 3, and 5 minutes or longer. Because orthostasis is relatively common in the absence of syncope, especially in the elderly, orthostatic hypotension as the etiology of syncope is suggested if symptoms are reproduced or if there is severe hypotension during standing. The presence of objective cardiovascular or neurologic physical findings (e.g., hypertension, abnormalities in the cardiac rhythm, signs of congestive heart failure, cardiac murmurs, blood pressure difference >20 mm Hg between the arms suggesting subclavian steal, focal neurologic deficits, evidence for peripheral neuropathy) directs further workup accordingly.

In patients who have symptoms suggestive of carotid sinus syncope or in older patients with recurrent syncope of unclear etiology, carotid sinus massage is useful. Gentle massage of one and then the other carotid sinus, with monitoring of the pulse rate, cardiac rhythm, and blood pressure, can yield a diagnosis of carotid sinus hypersensitivity if there is asystole for greater than 3 seconds (cardioinhibitory), or a systolic blood pressure drop of greater than 50 mm Hg without significant bradycardia (vasodepressor). Each carotid sinus should be massaged for approximately 5 seconds but never simultaneously or in the presence of bruits. It is important to note that less than one fifth of patients with carotid sinus hypersensitivity have symptoms of syncope. Thus a diagnosis of carotid sinus syncope requires both a positive carotid sinus massage and a consistent clinical presentation.

An ECG is generally indicated in all patients with syncope, especially when the diagnosis is not clear from the history and physical examination. The ECG may reveal conduction abnormalities or arrhythmias, which establish the etiology (e.g., complete heart block, ventricular or supraventricular tachycardia) or direct further diagnostic evaluation (e.g., preexcitation, old myocardial infarction, prolonged Q-T interval). A normal ECG in the setting of syncope indicates a low likelihood of arrhythmia and a favorable prognosis.

If a detailed history, physical examination, and ECG are not diagnostic or suggestive of an underlying cause, further workup is directed by the presence or absence of structural heart disease. Echocardiography is the diagnostic test of most yield in this regard and may point to the cause of syncope. In the presence of structural heart disease, ambulatory ECG monitoring (for arrhythmia detection), exercise ECG (for arrhythmias and/or ischemia), electrophysiologic studies (EPS), and cardiac catheterization are indicated in specific patient subsets depending on the history, ECG, and results of echocardiography (Chapter 10; Fig. 136-2). Passive head-up tilt-testing to evaluate for vasodepressor syncope (see later discussion) should be considered if specialized cardiac testing is negative in this subgroup. In the absence of structural heart disease on echocardiography, tilt-testing and ambulatory ECG monitoring are indicated.

Passive head-up tilt-testing with hemodynamic monitoring has been identified as a modality for detecting vasodepressor and orthostatic syncope. In susceptible patients, prolonged upright tilt at 60 to 70 degrees can result in venous pooling, reduced venous return, and stimulation of the vasodepressor reflex arc described previously, producing syncope or near-syncope in association with hypotension, bradycardia, or both. Positive responses in less than 15 minutes appear to be most specific. Positive responses occurring after longer periods of tilt (>30 minutes) with isoproterenol infusion are somewhat less specific and can yield false-positive responses.

The role of electrophysiologic study (EPS) in the evaluation of syncope has not been rigorously defined but is best reserved for patients with structural heart disease, left ventricular dysfunction (ejection fraction <40%), abnormal baseline ECG, or abnormal ambulatory monitoring. EPS findings of greatest specificity in bradycardic rhythms include a sinus node recovery time of >3 seconds, pacing induced infranodal block, and a His-to-ventricle (H-V) conduction time of >100 msec. These findings would support pacemaker implantation in these patients. EPS findings in tachycardic rhythms of greatest specificity include sustained monomorphic ventricular tachycardia and supraventricular tachycardia reproducing symptoms. A negative EPS confers a good prognosis.

The prognosis in patients with syncope in the absence of heart disease is excellent. With a cardiac cause, however, the 1-year mortality rate is 20% to 30%. Thus most patients of middle age or older who have a syncopal episode without an easily identifiable benign cause probably should be hospitalized. In as many as 40% of patients, no cause for syncope can be found despite extensive evaluation. Most of these probably have vasodepressor syncope or psychiatric illness and are more likely to have multiple recurrences. Tilt-testing and transtelephonic loop ECG recordings may be useful in this subgroup of patients, especially those with disabling symptoms.

A glucose tolerance test, prolonged fasting, or other provocative tests for hypoglycemia; tests for autonomic failure; and electroencephalography for epilepsy should be reserved for patients in whom the diagnosis of syncope is uncertain. Aortic arch and cerebral angiography rarely need to be considered. Even if vascular abnormalities are found in elderly patients, they will not necessarily be diagnostically meaningful. An electroencephalogram (EEG) and cerebral computed tomography (CT) scan often provide important information when a neurologic cause for the patient's symptoms is suspected.

MANAGEMENT

The treatment of syncope should be directed toward preventing or correcting the cause of the decreased cerebral perfusion.

Vasodepressor syncope is best treated by eliminating such precipitating factors as emotional excitement, fatigue, hunger, inactivity, or sedative drugs. These patients should be instructed to assume a sitting or recumbent position with the first presyncopal symptom. The management of recurrent vasodepressor syncope often is very challenging. Several pharmacologic therapies have been reported to prevent recurrences. Fludrocortisone acetate is thought to exert a beneficial effect through volume expansion and sensitization of α-adrenergic receptors. Beta-adrenergic blockade can theoretically act via several mechanisms, including preventing the exaggerated sympathetic response and excessive stimulation of ventricular mechanoreceptors, reducing the activation of mechanoreceptors directly, and allowing unopposed peripheral α-adrenergic stimulation. Disopyramide may be effective because of its anticholinergic, negative inotropic, and vasoconstrictive properties. Anticholinergic agents, theophylline, α-agonists, and the serotonin reuptake blocker fluoxetine have also been reported to have beneficial effects. However, pharmacologic therapy of vasodepressor syncope should be used highly selectively, as most trials reporting effectiveness have been small. Larger scale, more rigorous testing is needed before widespread use of these drugs can be recommended. The role of dual-chamber cardiac pacing in this disorder is controversial. Although this modality restores near-normal heart rate during the syncopal episode, it is often not fully effective in preventing recurrent syncope because of the untreated peripheral vasodilation. Thus this therapy is most beneficial in those with a predominant cardioinhibitory response.

Reflex syncope associated with micturition or coughing may be improved by having the patient avoid standing at the time of these activities. Orthostatic hypotension is treated by addressing the underlying cause. Neurologic consultation is prudent in a patient with any of the widespread neurologic abnormalities, suggesting one of the primary nervous system diseases associated with degeneration of the preganglionic or postganglionic autonomic nervous system (e.g., Parkinson's disease, Shy-Drager syndrome).

Treatment of cardiogenic syncope depends on making the correct pathophysiologic diagnosis. Tachyarrhythmias may be treated in various ways, depending on the seriousness of the arrhythmias (Chapter 9). Maneuvers such as breath-holding or Valsalva or carotid sinus massage may abort supraventricular tachyarrhythmias. More serious arrhythmias may be controlled by the use of such drugs as quinidine, procainamide, digitalis, or propranolol. Electrocardioversion or insertion of a pacemaker may be necessary in other patients. Syncope caused by a valvular lesion may not be relieved without surgical correction.

BIBLIOGRAPHY

Abboud FM: Neurocardiogenic syncope, *N Engl J Med* 328:1117, 1993.

Almquist A et al: Provocation of bradycardia and hypotension by isoproterenol and upright posture in patients with unexplained syncope, *New Engl J Med* 320:346, 1989.

Benditt DG, Petersen M, Lurie KG et al: Cardiac pacing for the prevention of recurrent vasovagal syncope, *Ann Intern Med* 122:204, 1995.

Hoeffnagels WAJ, Padberg GW, Overweg J et al: Transient loss of consciousness: the value of the history for distinguishing seizure from syncope, *J Neurol* 238:39, 1991.

Kapoor WN: Evaluation and management of the patient with syncope, *JAMA* 268:2553, 1992.

Kapoor WN: Hypotension and syncope. In Braunwald EB, editor: *Heart disease: a textbook of cardiovascular medicine*, ed 4, Philadelphia, 1992, WB Saunders.

Kapoor WN: Upright tilt testing in evaluating syncope: a comprehensive literature review, *Am J Med* 97:78, 1994.

Kaufmann H: Neurally mediated syncope: pathogenesis, diagnosis, and treatment, *Neurology* 45(suppl 5):S12, 1995.

Klein GJ, Gersh BJ, Yee R: Electrophysiological testing: the final court of appeal for diagnosis of syncope? *Circulation* 92:1332, 1995.

Kosinski D, Grubb BP, Temesy-Armos P: Pathophysiological aspects of neurocardiogenic syncope: current concepts and new perspectives, *PACE* 18:716, 1995.

Maloney JD, Jaeger FJ, Rizo-Patron C, Zhu DWX: The role of pacing for the management of neurally mediated syncope: carotid sinus syndrome and vasovagal syncope, *Am Heart J* 127:1030, 1994.

Rubenstein LZ et al: The value of assessing falls in an elderly population: a randomized clinical trial, *Ann Intern Med* 113:308, 1990.

Schaal SF et al: Syncope, *Curr Prob Cardiol* 17:211, 1992.

Sra JS, Jazayeri MR, Avitall B, et al: Comparison of cardiac pacing with drug therapy in the treatment of neurocardiogenic (vasovagal) syncope with bradycardia or asystole, *N Engl J Med* 328:1085, 1993.

CHAPTER

137   Headache and Facial Pain

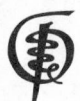

John Edmeads

HEADACHE
Mechanisms of Headache

The brain itself is not sensitive to pain. When lesions of the brain cause headache, they do so by involving pain-sensitive structures inside the skull, such as the arteries at the base of the brain, the dural venous sinuses, some other portions of the dura, and cranial nerves that carry pain fibers (i.e., cranial nerves V, VII, IX, and X). The external structures of the head are all pain-sensitive and give rise to a variety of headaches (Table 137-1).

The richly innervated superficial structures tend to localize the headache fairly precisely. For example, inflammation of the right temporal artery (temporal arteritis) produces right temporal headache, and purulent left frontal sinusitis causes left frontal headache. Involvement of deeper structures leads to less precise localization (e.g., although sphenoidal sinusitis may cause pain between the eyes, it may also refer pain to the vertex of the skull). Intracranially, pain localization is quite imprecise, and headache often is felt in an area distant from the lesion. A right occipital lobe tumor may cause frontal headache because the structures of the anterior and middle cranial fossae are innervated by the first division of the trigeminal nerve (V1). Stimulation of any of these structures produces pain referred to the superficial distribution of V1, which is the front half of the head. Posterior cranial fossa structures are innervated mostly by pain fibers from the second cervical cord segment. Disease of these structures generally causes pain that is referred to the back of the head or the neck. Thus a left cerebellar abscess usually causes a left occipital headache. Lesions at the craniocervical junction or in the upper part of the neck, however, may produce pain felt in the front of the head. This occurs because the descending portion (nucleus caudalis) of the trigeminal nucleus extends down to the third or fourth cervical segments (C3-C4), becoming confluent there with the dorsal horn of the cervical cord, so that pain impulses from the upper cervical segments can gain access to the trigeminal system and be referred anteriorly.

Headache Syndromes

Although ideally headaches should be understood in terms of what structures they arise from, this information is not always clear (see Table 137-1). Therefore the International Headache Society (IHS) has devised a classification of headaches and facial pains, with diagnostic criteria, based entirely on clinical attributes. Intended primarily to ensure uniformity of terminology for researchers, the IHS classification is quite lengthy and thus unwieldy for clinical use. Box 137-1 is a simpler, much shorter classification. It incorporates some of the new IHS terminology (in italics) but is not entirely consistent with the groupings used by the IHS.

Migraine. Migraine affects 10% to 20% of the population. It is the second most common headache syndrome, next to tension-type headache (Table 137-2). Migraine is not a single entity but a group of disorders sharing the following characteristics: (1) a constitutional predisposition (about 70% of patients with migraine have a first-order relative with a history of migraine); (2) a pattern of repeated unilateral or bilateral headaches of a vascular type (see later discussion), with freedom from pain between attacks; and (3) association of the headaches with autonomic and/or neurologic features that may vary in type and prominence from person to person and from attack to attack.

Most migraine sufferers have their first attack in childhood or adolescence. Although migraine can begin at any age, its commencement after the age of 50 years is uncommon, so another diagnosis should be sought in those who begin to have headaches for the first time after middle age. Women are affected more often than men, in a ratio of 3:2, possibly because hormonal factors such as menstruation may play a prominent role in precipitating attacks.

Migraine without aura (formerly called "common migraine") is the most frequently encountered form. Criteria for diagnoses are multiple attacks of headaches that last, untreated, for a few hours to a few days and that have at least two of the following characteristics: unilaterality, pulsatility, moderate to severe intensity, and aggravation by activity. The headaches should be accompanied by aversion to noise and light (phonophotophobia) and/or by nausea or vomiting.

Migraine with aura (formerly called "classic migraine") is much less frequent and is characterized by the occurrence of a neurologic aura before or in the early part of a headache that meets the preceding criteria. Typically, the aura consists of bright shimmering visual manifestations of crude or well-formed configuration, beginning in one part of the visual field and slowly spreading and expanding to involve other portions of it. Various types of visual auras include fortification spectra, flickering photopsias, heatwavelike distortions, and less frequently, negative phenomena such as hemianopia. Occasionally, the visual symptoms may be succeeded by transient paresthesias in the mouth or face, or in one upper limb. These neurologic features fade after 15 to 30 minutes to be replaced by a throbbing headache, often associated with nausea and vomiting.

Many attacks of migraine appear out of the blue, but some seem to be precipitated by stress, excitement, bright lights, menstruation, alcohol, or food such as chocolate or cheese. Oral contraceptive medication may increase the frequency of migraine attacks, and some evidence suggests that it increases the risk of permanent neurologic deficits such as hemianopia and hemiparesis occurring in the wake of attacks of migraine with aura.

A few hours to a day or so before the onset of headache, some people experience behavioral alterations such as depression, elation, hyperactivity, or craving for specific foods. These prodromal syndromes suggest hypothalamic or limbic complicity in the pathogenesis of migraine.

The pathophysiology of migraine is complex and obscure, with neurologic, vascular, and chemical aspects. Most believe that the pain of migraine headache comes from dilation and sterile inflammation of cranial blood vessels, mostly inside but sometimes outside the skull. These vascular changes may be produced by fluctuations in various bloodborne substances such as serotonin (5HT) and estrogens, or by exogenous agents such as alcohol. A purely vascular pathogenesis, however, is insufficient to account for all the phenomena of migraine, including the aura; the brain must be involved. The aura of migraine is associated with a wave of oligemia that begins at the occipital pole and spreads anteriorly across the cortex; this spreading oligemia likely results from primary alterations in cortical metabolism and function.

The trigeminal nerve links brain and blood vessel. It is more than just a passive conductor of pain impulses from vessel to brain stem. Neural traffic in the trigeminal nerve may also be in the opposite direction, with impulses from the brain stem impinging on the blood vessels and, via release of substance P and other peptides from the trigeminal axon terminals, producing dilation and inflammation of the vessels. These neurogenic changes in the vessel may themselves generate pain, which ascends the trigeminal nerve to the brain stem. The painful aspects of the migraine attack may thus originate in or be perpetuated by reverberations up and down this trigeminovascular system.

BOX 137-1
A classification of headaches and facial pain

I. Vascular headaches
  A. Migraine
    1. Migraine with headaches and inconspicuous neurologic features
      a. *Migraine without aura* ("common migraine")
    2. Migraine with headaches and conspicuous neurologic features
      a. With transient neurologic symptoms
        (1) *Migraine with typical aura* ("classic migraine")
        (2) *Sensory, basilar,* and *hemiplegic migraine*
      b. With prolonged or permanent neurologic features ("complicated migraine")
        (1) *Ophthalmoplegic migraine*
        (2) *Migrainous infarction*
    3. Migraine without headaches but with conspicuous neurologic features ("migraine equivalents")
      a. *Abdominal migraine*
      b. *Benign paroxysmal vertigo of childhood*
      c. *Migraine aura without headache* ("isolated auras," transient migrainous accompaniments)
  B. Cluster headaches
    1. *Episodic cluster headache* ("cyclic cluster headaches")
    2. *Chronic cluster headaches*
    3. *Chronic paroxysmal hemicrania*
  C. Other vascular headaches
    1. Headaches of reactive vasodilation (fever, drug-induced, postictal, hypoglycemia, hypoxia, hypercarbia, hyperthyroidism)
    2. *Headaches associated with arterial hypertension*
      a. Chronic severe hypertension (diastolic >120 mm Hg)
      b. Paroxysmal severe hypertension (pheochromocytoma, some coital headaches)
    3. Headaches caused by cranial arteritis
      a. *Giant cell arteritis* ("temporal arteritis")
      b. Other vasculitides
II. Headache associated with demonstrable muscle spasm
  A. Headaches caused by posturally induced or paralesional muscle spasm
    1. Headaches of sustained or impaired posture (e.g., prolonged close work, driving)
    2. Headaches associated with cervical spondylosis and other diseases of cervical spine
    3. Myofascial pain dysfunction syndrome (*headache or facial pain associated with disorders of teeth, jaws, and related structures, or "TMJ syndrome"*)
  B. Headaches caused by psychophysiologic muscular contraction ("muscle contraction headaches," or *tension-type headache associated with disorder of pericranial muscles*)

III. Headaches and facial pain without demonstrable physical substrate
  A. Headaches of uncertain etiology
    1. "Tension headaches" (*tension-type headache unassociated with disorder of pericranial muscles*)
    2. Some forms of posttraumatic headache
  B. Psychogenic headaches (e.g., hypochondriacal, conversional, delusional, malingered)
  C. Facial pain of uncertain etiology ("atypical facial pain")
IV. Combined tension-migraine headaches
  A. Episodic migraine superimposed on chronic tension headaches
  B. Chronic daily headaches
    1. Associated with analgesic and/or ergotamine overuse ("rebound headaches")
    2. Not associated with drug overuse
V. Headaches and head pains caused by diseases of eyes, ears, nose, sinuses, teeth, or skull
VI. Headaches caused by meningeal inflammation
  A. Subarachnoid hemorrhage
  B. Meningitis and meningoencephalitis
  C. Others (e.g., meningeal carcinomatosis)
VII. Headaches associated with altered intracranial pressure ("traction headaches")
  A. Increased intracranial pressure
    1. Intracranial mass lesions (e.g., neoplasm, hematoma, abscess)
    2. Hydrocephalus
    3. Benign intracranial hypertension
    4. Venous sinus thrombosis
  B. Decreased intracranial pressure
    1. Post–lumbar-puncture headaches
    2. Spontaneous hypoliquorrheic headaches
VIII. Headaches and head pains caused by cranial neuralgias
  A. Presumed irritation of superficial nerves
    1. Occipital neuralgia
    2. Supraorbital neuralgia
  B. Presumed irritation of intracranial nerves
    1. Trigeminal neuralgia ("tic douloureux")
    2. Glossopharyngeal neuralgia

Table 137-1 Mechanism of headaches

STRUCTURE INVOLVED	MECHANISM	HEADACHE SYNDROME
Cranial blood vessels		
Intra- and extracranial	Neurogenic and humorally induced vasodilation and inflammation	Migraine, cluster headache
	Immunogenic inflammation	Vasculitis, including temporal arteritis*
Intracranial	Chemically induced vasodilation	Hunger, fever, medications, hangover, hypoxia, hyperthyroidism
	Pyogenic inflammation	Meningitis
	Chemical inflammation	Subarachnoid hemorrhage
	Mechanical dilation	Severe hypertension, postpuncture headaches†
	Traction (displacement)	Postpuncture headaches, mass lesions (tumors, hydrocephalus, etc)
Mucosa of sinuses	Inflammation, pressure changes	Sinus headaches
Eyes	Inflammation, increased pressure	Iritis, glaucoma
Muscles		
Face and jaw	Mechanical strain, inflammation	Myofascial pain dysfunction syndrome ("TMJ headache")
Neck and scalp	Sustained contraction	Some tension-type headaches
Unknown	Unknown	Most tension-type headaches

*The headache of temporal arteritis comes mainly from extracranial arteries.
†Postpuncture headaches are caused by a combination of traction and vasodilation.

Further linking the brain and the cranial blood vessels is the action of serotonin (5HT) in migraine. The concentration of this neurotransmitter declines during an attack, and restitution to normal levels by intravenous injection of serotonin may abort an attack. Substances that stimulate the 5HT-1D receptors located presynaptically on the terminals of the trigeminal nerve can inhibit the release of peptides from the terminals and prevent or reverse the dilation and inflammation of the blood vessels. This effect has been demonstrated with the selective 5HT-1D agonist sumatriptan and the nonselective 5HT-1D agonist dihydroergotamine (DHE). Both these substances have clear efficacy in terminating acute attacks of migraine.

Other agonists of the 5HT-1D receptors are under development. Some of these new drugs can cross the blood-brain barrier to gain access to receptors near the proximal synapse of the trigeminal nerve with the brain stem, thus perhaps influencing some of the central neurogenic mechanisms of migraine. Other receptors have been identified at the central and peripheral termini of the trigeminal system—for example, mu opioid and somatostatin receptors—and study of the role of these may accelerate what are already rapid advances in our understanding and treatment of migraine.

Cluster Headache. Unlike migraine, with its predilection for young females, the much less common condition of cluster headache affects males almost exclusively. It usually begins in the third or fourth decades. Cluster headaches take their name from their tendency to cluster in time. An affected individual typically suffers up to eight headaches every day for a few weeks or months, and then the headaches cease, only to reappear in successive clusters months or years later (episodic cluster headache). Occasionally, the headaches recur daily and the cluster never ends (chronic cluster headaches).

Each cluster headache lasts 0.25 to 3 hours, commonly 45 minutes. Typically, they come on during sleep, rousing the patient and forcing him to pace the floor moaning, unlike the migraine sufferer, who prefers to lie quietly in bed. The headache is a deep, agonizing, nonthrobbing pain that involves the same part of the head or face in every headache. It usually involves one eye and the adjacent temple, cheek, or forehead. It is associated with watering and redness of the affected eye, drooping of the ipsilateral lid, sometimes miosis of that eye (i.e., a partial Horner's syndrome), and congestion or running of the ipsilateral nostril. Nausea is uncommon, and vomiting is rare. After the headache disappears, the patient typically sinks into exhausted sleep, only to be awakened hours later by another headache. Although night is the time of predilection, some cluster headaches occur during the daylight hours, particularly if the patient drinks alcohol, which can be a powerful trigger. The pathophysiology of cluster headaches is unknown, but they may arise from periodic spasm, edema, or inflammation of the internal carotid artery near the skull base, probably driven by chronobiologic input from the brain. Little is known about the biochemical concomitants of cluster headache.

Tension-Type Headache. Physicians once believed that these headaches, the most common type of headache, were caused by sustained, painful contraction of the muscles of the scalp and neck occurring as a somatic manifestation of psychic tension. The evidence for this is flimsy. Electromyography may show increased activity of these muscles during a so-called muscle contraction headache, but equally as often it does not. Sometimes more electromyographic activity is present in people with migraine headaches than in those believed to have tension-type headaches. All in all, the pathogenesis of tension-type headaches is obscure. Very likely some headaches, particularly those incurred during prolonged close work or associated with fatigue, are caused at least in part by painful neck or scalp muscle spasm. Other headaches, perhaps those more overtly connected with depression or other forms of emotional stress, may have no organic substrate but rather represent a referral of psychic pain to the soma. The IHS classification avoids controversy by coining a new term, *tension-type headache,* which makes no statement about pathogenesis.

Tension-type headaches tend to be bilateral, dull, nonpulsatile, and from the point of view of the observer, not very intense. They may be bifrontal or nuchal-occipital and are often described as "like a weight on top of the head," "like a tight band around the head," or "like a feeling of expansion within the head." Nothing seems to aggravate these headaches except more stress or fatigue, and nothing seems to benefit them except removal of stress and, in the milder and less entrenched cases, analgesics and antidepressants.

Nausea is uncommon, unless it occurs as a side effect from medication, and vomiting is not seen. Neurologic accompaniments do not occur.

These headaches run a spectrum of seriousness. At one end is most of the normal population who have occasional mild to moderate headaches in response to easily recognized transient stress or fatigue. These headaches respond promptly to simple analgesics and to removal of stress. Further along the spectrum are patients who are habitually somewhat tense and worried or depressed, who have more frequently recurring headaches, but who are well most of the time. These people usually have some insight into the relationship between their symptoms and their life and feelings, and usually show some response to counseling, to antidepressant medication, and to analgesics.

At the far end of the spectrum are the patients with "chronic daily headaches." They have headaches all day, every day and have had them for months or years. In these patients, the admixture of migraine is most apparent. They often have, superimposed on their constant dull background headaches, recurrent severe hemicranial throbbing headaches associated with nausea and vomiting. These patients often organize their entire lives, and those of their family, around their headaches and complain bitterly of the pain. Nevertheless, they do not appear to be in physical distress. Their headaches are "worsened by everything and helped by nothing." They have been unresponsive to, or have developed side effects from, a wide range of medications. Though adamant that analgesics are "useless," they frequently overuse them. When informed that analgesic overuse may be perpetuating their headaches (see later discussion), they often are either unreceptive or profess their inability to discontinue these medications. Their insight is defective, and they are resistant to and resentful of any suggestion that their intractable headaches may be related to psychologic disequilibrium. Convinced that organic disease is being missed, they demand and receive repeated investigations, all of which render normal findings.

Temporal Arteritis. Unlike the foregoing headache syndromes, temporal arteritis characteristically begins after the age of 50 years, is caused by visible pathology, and is dangerous.

This progressively obliterative giant-cell arteritis involves not only the arteries of the scalp, causing headache, but also other vessels, including those supplying the eyes and occasionally the brain. About half of those with the headache of temporal arteritis who are not treated go on to develop blindness. The syndrome of temporal arteritis is recognizable, and treatment is effective. The headaches are but part of a generalized arteritis. They occur in individuals who feel and look ill with malaise, fever, sweating, weight loss, arthralgias, and aching in the back and shoulders (polymyalgia rheumatica). Claudication of the jaw is uncommon but virtually pathognomonic. It is produced by narrowing of the arteries supplying the muscles of mastication. Typically the headache involves one temple, although any part of the scalp can be involved, depending on which branches of the external carotid artery are inflamed. The headache is often described as head soreness rather than headache. It typically begins as an intermittent soreness or burning discomfort and steadily escalates over several weeks or months to become a constant, well-localized pain. Sometimes the affected scalp artery is prominent, tender, incompressible, and pulseless. Rarely there may be a red streak in the overlying skin.

The diagnosis is suspected with the occurrence of a localized, progressively worsening "sore" headache in an elderly individual. Suspicion is heightened by other complaints suggesting a more generalized illness, by the finding of an abnormal scalp artery, and by the demonstration of an elevated erythrocyte sedimentation rate present in about 90% of cases. The diagnosis is confirmed by biopsy of the affected artery.

Corticosteroids are effective in relieving the headache and preventing complications. They should be started in a dose of 80 to 100 mg/day (prednisone equivalent) and be continued at that dose until symptoms resolve and the erythrocyte sedimentation rate normalizes. The dose is then tapered to the smallest dose that keeps the patient asymptomatic and the erythrocyte sedimentation rate normal.

Table 137-2 Important headache syndromes

| | MIGRAINE | | CLUSTER HEADACHE | TENSION-TYPE HEADACHE |
	WITHOUT AURA	WITH AURA		
Incidence	Common	Uncommon	Uncommon	Very common
Age of onset	Childhood, adolescence, or young adulthood	Childhood, adolescence, or young adulthood	Young adulthood, middle age	Young adulthood, middle age
Sex bias	Female	Female	Male	No
Family history of headaches	Yes	Yes	No	Yes
Onset and evolution of headache	Slow to rapid	Slow to rapid	Rapid	Slow to rapid
Time course of headache	Episodic	Episodic	Clusters in time	Episodic, may become constant
Quality	Usually throbbing	Usually throbbing	Steady	Steady
Location	Variable, often unilateral	Variable, generally unilateral	Orbit, temple cheek	Variable
Exacerbators	Head-low position, exertion	Head-low position, exertion	None	Stress
Associated features	Prodrome, vomiting	Prodrome, aura, vomiting	Lacrimation, rhinorrhea, Horner's syndrome	None
Physical signs	No	No	Partial Horner's syndrome	No

Subarachnoid Hemorrhage. The headache of subarachnoid hemorrhage is one of the most dramatic events in clinical medicine. It is usually abrupt in onset and incapacitating in severity. The headache usually involves the entire head and often radiates into the neck and even into the back. It is often accompanied by some blunting of consciousness, and vomiting is common. The headache remains severe for several days and then gradually abates. On examination the patient is typically in severe pain. There are signs of meningeal irritation, such as nuchal rigidity and sometimes limitation of straight-leg raising, and occasionally subhyaloid hemorrhages in the optic fundus. Often there are no focal neurologic deficits; however, if the hemorrhage or associated infarction involves the brain parenchyma, hemiparesis, aphasia, or visual field abnormalities may occur. Subarachnoid hemorrhage is most often caused by rupture of a berry aneurysm, and the majority occur in middle age.

The initial pain of subarachnoid hemorrhage is probably produced by tearing and distortion of the blood vessel and its adjacent arachnoid membrane, with the pain perpetuated through chemical irritation by blood of the pain-sensitive vessels and perivascular meninges. Increased intracranial pressure may contribute to the headache.

A full-blown subarachnoid hemorrhage is difficult to misdiagnose. Sometimes, however, an aneurysm or arteriovenous malformation bleeds only a little, causing a moderate or severe headache of sudden onset but without signs of meningeal irritation or neurologic injury. These patients are worrisome. Is this headache a migraine, or is it a "minibleed" that may precede by a few hours or days a massive subarachnoid hemorrhage? In general, young people who have a previous history of similar headaches, whose present headache is easing, who did not have the headache come on during exertion, who are alert and oriented, and who on repeated examinations have no neurologic abnormalities or neck stiffness, probably do not have a subarachnoid hemorrhage. All others are suspect for subarachnoid hemorrhage and need a computed tomography (CT) scan to demonstrate or exclude a parenchymal hemorrhage or obvious subarachnoid blood. If the CT scan is normal, a lumbar puncture should be obtained to detect small amounts of blood in the cerebrospinal fluid (CSF). A normal CT scan does not exclude a small subarachnoid hemorrhage. Magnetic resonance imaging (MRI) is not useful for showing early hemorrhage.

Meningoencephalitis. The headache of meningoencephalitis is also caused by meningeal irritation. The onset is usually over several minutes to an hour or so. The headache of meningitis may ultimately become as intense as that of a subarachnoid hemorrhage and may similarly be associated with blunted consciousness and vomiting, especially in children. While meningitis is usually associated with signs of meningeal irritation (e.g., nuchal rigidity, limited straight leg raising), these may be absent in the very young, the very old, and the very sick. The slower onset of meningitis pain and its association with

symptoms and signs of infection (especially fever) usually distinguish it from the headache of subarachnoid hemorrhage.

Headaches caused by meningeal irritation—subarachnoid hemorrhage and meningitis—are intense and serious. Failure to recognize them and to institute immediate appropriate treatment is often fatal.

Brain Tumor (Increased Intracranial Pressure). In this syndrome a progressively enlarging mass, such as a neoplasm or subdural hematoma, causes progressive displacement of, or traction on, pain-sensitive intracranial structures, producing a progressively worsening headache. Initially, the headache is mild and intermittent, but over a period of days, weeks, or months it becomes more persistent and more intense. It is aggravated by factors that increase intracranial pressure such as the head-low position (the headache is typically worse in the morning and improves as the patient gets up and about), coughing and straining, or by transient displacement of the intracranial contents such as with jarring the head. The headache location is constant.

Not everyone with a brain tumor develops headaches. When headaches do occur, they exhibit the previously noted "textbook picture" in fewer than half the cases; the remainder resemble banal tension-type headaches. In these cases, the company that the headaches keep may be a clue to their ominous origin. By the time an intracranial mass lesion is big enough to produce headaches, it generally produces other neurologic symptoms and signs that may be subtle. There may be vague dizziness, slight difficulty in thinking, or changes in the personality. There may be "soft" signs such as a droop of one corner of the mouth or a reflex abnormality. Sometimes more flagrant features, such as seizures, supervene to reveal the diagnosis.

The syndrome of a recent-onset, progressively worsening headache, especially if associated with other neurologic symptoms and signs, should prompt immediate investigation for an intracranial mass lesion.

Hypertension. High blood pressure is an infrequent cause of headache. Most people with hypertension either have no headaches or have the same migraine or tension headaches experienced by the normotensive population. However, moderately severe hypertension (diastolic >120 mm Hg) may produce headaches that appear in the morning, sometimes awakening the patient. This dull, sometimes throbbing ache, either diffuse or occipital, eases as the patient gets up and about. Paroxysmal very severe hypertension, as sometimes seen in pheochromocytoma or drug reactions, may also be associated with paroxysmal headaches.

Evaluation

The key to the diagnosis of headache is in the patient's history. Important factors include the duration of the complaint, the age at on-

Table 137-2 Important headache syndromes—cont'd

TEMPORAL ARTERITIS	SUBARACHNOID HEMORRHAGE	MENINGITIS	BRAIN TUMOR
Uncommon	Uncommon	Uncommon	Uncommon
Over 50	Over 35	Any age	Any age
No	No	No	No
No	No	No	No
Slow	Abrupt	Rapid	Slow
Increasing, becoming constant	Persists for days	Persists for days	Duration steadily increases
Constant	Steady	Steady	Steady
Localized	Diffuse	Diffuse	Localized, then diffuse
None	None	None	Head-low position, exertion
Generally ill	Altered consciousness, sometimes vomiting	Altered consciousness, sometimes vomiting	Altered consciousness, sometimes vomiting
Arterial changes	Meningeal irritation, sometimes focal signs	Meningeal irritation, sometimes focal signs, fever	Focal signs common, sometimes papilledema

set, the time course pursued by the headache, factors that exacerbate and relieve it, and the constancy and location of the headache. The physical examination is normal in most of the benign headache syndromes but gives crucial information regarding the serious ones (see Table 137-2).

Features of the history and examination suggesting that a particular headache may be ominous are shown in Box 137-2. When any of these danger signals are recognized, investigation is mandatory. Conversely, studies have demonstrated that "routine" neuroimaging (CT or MRI) of people with headaches conforming to the profiles of migraine or tension-type headaches, with normal physical examinations, has a very low yield, and is not cost-effective in detecting lesions.

A contrast-enhanced CT scan is an effective test for identifying serious lesions causing headache. This scan detects most space-occupying lesions (e.g., brain tumors, subdural hematomas, abscesses), reveals hydrocephalus and cerebral edema, and shows some arteriovenous malformations. CT scanning can miss aneurysms. However, aneurysms seldom produce headaches unless they rupture or leak, and when they do, the blood in the brain parenchyma or in the cerebrospinal fluid is commonly visible on the CT scan. If there is still suspicion of a subarachnoid hemorrhage in the presence of a normal CT scan or if there is suspicion of meningitis, a lumbar puncture should be performed.

MRI is a more sensitive test for detecting lesions within the posterior fossa and for identifying some otherwise occult tumors and infarcts, but it tends to be not as sensitive as CT in revealing early subarachnoid bleeding.

The erythrocyte sedimentation rate should be checked in all patients with new onset of headache after the age of 50 years to help identify temporal arteritis.

Treatment

Migraine. A careful history may elicit dietary, environmental or behavioral triggers of the migraine attacks. These may include habitual overwork and fatigue, caffeine, monosodium glutamate (MSG), nitrates in smoked meats, alcohol, cheese, sleep deprivation or excess, oral contraceptives and other estrogenic hormones, and poorly handled anxiety. Sometimes the patient is unaware of these triggers until asked about them. Avoidance of the triggers, if feasible, may substantially improve the migraine and reduce the need for medication.

Most migraine sufferers of acute attacks simply take over-the-counter (OTC) analgesics such as aspirin or acetaminophen, usually with adequate results. The efficacy of these OTC analgesics can be improved by taking them in a large dose (1000 mg rather than the 650 mg usually advised) and, if possible, in a liquid or effervescent form to enhance absorption. Many physicians prescribe analgesic

BOX 137-2
Danger signals of an ominous headache

1. Failure to conform *readily* to an innocuous pattern such as migraine, tension headache, or cluster headache
2. Onset in or after middle age
3. Recent onset and progressive course
4. Association with other neurologic or systemic symptoms
5. The presence of abnormal physical signs

compounds containing codeine and/or a barbiturate, and these can be quite effective *when taken properly*. However, they have a high potential for abuse; taking them too frequently (that is, on more than 3 days in any one week) may establish a rebound headache cycle. In this cycle some hours after the last dose of analgesic, withdrawal symptoms including headache may occur; the patient takes more analgesic for the headache, raising the tissue level of the analgesic and lessening or abolishing the headache until withdrawal from that dose occurs some hours later. In this fashion a patient can be lured into taking narcotic or barbiturate analgesics every day, often many times a day. Some authorities believe that these rebound headaches may occur from overuse of even plain aspirin or acetaminophen. All agree that rebound headaches can result from the overuse of caffeine, codeine, barbiturates, and ergotamine. Contributing to the development of rebound are the prescribing habits of some physicians, who issue almost infinitely repeatable prescriptions for habituating analgesics to patients who have no idea of the potential of these agents to produce perpetual headaches. Another factor is the tendency of some physicians to prescribe only analgesics for migraine, allowing their patients no access to the generally more effective specific antimigraine drugs, ergot and sumatriptan, for their more intense headaches; use of less effective agents for intense headaches leads to overuse and rebound.

Properly prescribed and taken, ergotamine tartrate, 1 to 2 mg, taken orally very early in an attack aborts about 50% of migraine episodes. In some of the remainder, poor absorption may be a factor; ergotamine could then be tried in subsequent attacks by other routes, such as 2 mg rectally or sublingually. Some patients can be taught to self-inject DHE subcutaneously or intramuscularly in a dose of 0.5 to 1.0 mg; DHE nasal spray may soon be available in the United States and Canada. To minimize the risk of habituation and of rebound headaches, ergotamine should not be given more often than 2 days a week.

Ergotamine and DHE are believed to exert their antimigraine effects by stimulating the presynaptic 5HT-1D receptors in the trigeminovascular system, thus reducing neurogenic inflammation and facilitating vasoconstriction. Because they combine with other receptors, including dopaminergic and adrenergic receptors, side effects such as nausea, vomiting, and peripheral vasoconstriction may occur; administration of an antinauseant before or with the ergotamine or DHE may be helpful in lessening gastrointestinal side effects.

Sumatriptan is believed to combine only with the 5HT-1D receptor and thus has a more specific action with fewer side effects. It can be given in a dose of 25 to 100 mg orally or 6 mg subcutaneously using a self-injector. Rebound cycles from sumatriptan have recently been reported.

Status migrainosus occurs when, as a result of a severe prolonged (>72 hours) attack of migraine unresponsive to self-administered medications, the patient has decompensated emotionally and physically and has approached a physician for emergency treatment. After ensuring through history, examination, and appropriate investigations (sometimes a CT scan and a lumbar puncture) that the diagnosis truly is status migrainosus and not a leaking aneurysm or early meningitis, treatment is intravenous rehydration of the patient followed by the use of *one* of the following regimens:

1. Antiemetic (e.g., promethazine 25 mg) by slow IV push followed by narcotic (e.g., meperidine 75 to 100 mg) by slow IV push.
2. Antiemetic (e.g., promethazine 25 mg or metoclopramide 10 mg) by slow IV push followed by DHE (0.5 to 1.0 mg) by slow IV push; DHE 0.5 mg may be repeated if necessary in 1 hour.
3. Double-check that the patient is adequately rehydrated and then give chlorpromazine by repeated miniboluses of 5 mg every 5 minutes until either the headache is relieved or a maximum of 25 mg have been given; watch for hypotension. Other neuroleptics also have been used intravenously to terminate status migrainosus. These include prochlorperazine (2 mg every 5 minutes to a maximum of 10 mg) and haloperidol (5 mg in a minibag over 3 minutes). Dyskinesias are uncommon, and may be reversed with benztropine 1 mg intramuscularly.
4. Sumatriptan 6 mg subcutaneously (note: sumatriptan should not be given within 24 hours of the last dose of ergotamine or DHE, and DHE should not be given within 6 hours of the last dose of sumatriptan).

Prevention of migraine attacks. Prophylactic medications are used when ergotamine, analgesics, or sumatriptan do not abort attacks or, if they do, are consumed so regularly as to risk habituation, abuse, or toxicity. Medications useful in the prophylaxis of migraine include propranolol, 80 to 240 mg/day (and other β-blockers: atenolol, metoprolol, nadolol, timolol); verapamil, 240 mg/day, or nifedipine, 60 mg/day; amitriptyline or nortriptyline 50 to 125 mg/day; valproate 750 to 2000 mg/day; and methysergide, 4 to 12 mg/day for no more than 5 consecutive months.

All medications mentioned should be started in low doses and gradually increased. Other agents occasionally useful in the prophylaxis of certain types of migraine include nonsteroidal antiinflammatory drugs, lithium, and monoamine oxidase inhibitors. Nonpharmacologic modalities such as biofeedback and hypnotherapy are occasionally useful.

Cluster Headaches. Treatment of the acute attack with medication is often not feasible because of the sudden nocturnal onset. Self-injected dihydroergotamine or sumatriptan may be helpful. Oxygen inhalation shortens attacks in about half of patients. Prophylaxis is preferable, using any of the following regimens for the expected duration of the headache cluster: (1) methysergide, 4 to 12 mg/day; (2) lithium carbonate, 600 to 1200 mg/day; (3) prednisone, 15 to 60 mg/day; (4) verapamil, 240 mg/day; or (5) valproic acid, 750 to 2000 mg/day. WARNING: Methysergide and prednisone must not be used on a long-term basis, as in *chronic* cluster headache.

Tension-Type Headaches. Occasional tension-type headaches respond well to OTC analgesics and are seldom a medical problem. More frequent headaches may improve with explanation and reassurance, although, as a rule, the more frequent and prolonged the head-

---

✔ **WHEN TO REFER**

Most patients with benign dysfunctional headaches (migraine, tension-type headaches, and cluster headaches) can be managed well by primary care physicians. Failure to respond to appropriate treatment, and/or the development of rebound cycles, are indications for referral to a specialist, usually a neurologist or an internist. Not all neurologists or internists are interested or well versed in headache treatment; a useful indicator is whether they are involved with organizations such as the American Association for the Study of Headache or the International Headache Society.

When a primary care physician recognizes features in a headache pattern inconsistent with a benign dysfunctional etiology or detects any abnormality on physical examination, investigation is mandatory and is often facilitated by referral to a specialist.

---

aches, the less the patient's insight and the less likely the benefit from this brief, informal psychotherapy. Antidepressant medication (e.g., amitriptyline) alone or in combination with a short-term neuroleptic or benzodiazepine can be useful in some cases of chronic, recurrent tension-type headaches. If there is a vascular component, the addition of a migraine prophylactic agent can be helpful.

Chronic Daily Headaches. At least half these patients develop headaches as a result of analgesic and/or ergotamine rebound cycles; in the others the chronic daily headaches are fueled by psychologic disturbances or, very rarely, by undetected disease. If the headaches are drug induced, the only treatment likely to work is to withdraw all analgesics and ergotamine, a daunting task that can be accomplished by a motivated patient and a determined physician, usually on an outpatient basis. In rare cases it requires hospitalization. Protocols have been developed for the use of repetitive intravenous DHE to assist in managing resistant headaches. Close, prolonged follow-up of these patients is essential; they have a tendency to slip back into overuse of medications and once again develop chronic daily headaches.

FACIAL PAIN

Facial pain frequently is caused by easily diagnosed local diseases, such as a tooth abscess, sinusitis, or parotitis. Diagnosis is a problem only with certain neuralgic, vascular, and psychogenic syndromes (Table 137-3). *Tic douloureux,* or trigeminal neuralgia, is the most common neuralgic facial pain. It typically affects the elderly and presents as recurrent 1 or 2 second jabs of sharp, severe, unilateral pain most often located in the V2 or combined V2-V3 distribution of the trigeminal nerve. Pathognomonic of tic douloureux is the ability of the patient to trigger the pains by stimulating the face or the buccal mucosa (e.g., washing the face, eating, or brushing the teeth). Although the cause is unknown, some cases may be caused by irritation of the root of the trigeminal nerve by a pulsating loop of an elongated arteriosclerotic vessel. When typical tic douloureux appears in a young person, multiple sclerosis should be suspected. Carbamazepine, 200 to 800 mg/day, is effective treatment in the majority of patients. When carbamazepine fails, a percutaneous radiofrequency lesion of the ipsilateral trigeminal ganglion or surgical decompression of the trigeminal root in the posterior fossa can be helpful.

Cluster headache is the most common vascular cause of facial pain. Diagnosis is rarely a problem, except for cases in which the pain is primarily in the cheek. Several other facial pain syndromes (e.g., Sluder's syndrome, lower-half headache, Vail's neuralgia) have been described, but they may be unusual variants of cluster headache.

Atypical facial pain is a poorly understood and uncommon syndrome in which constant deep aching pain affects one side of the face or, rarely, both sides. It affects patients who have no abnormal physical signs but who usually manifest prominent psychologic disability. There is no evidence that the pain is neuralgic, and considerable evidence that it is psychogenic. Treatment is difficult, but psychotherapy and antidepressant medication may help.

Table 137-3   Facial pain

	LOCATION	NATURE	TIMING	ASSOCIATED PHYSICAL FINDINGS
Tic douloureux	V2, then V2-V3; rarely V1	Triggered	Brief jabs	None
Geniculate neuralgia	Ear	Not often triggered	Brief jabs, or long duration	Vesicles in ear, VII palsy, ± VIII findings
Glossopharyngeal neuralgia	Tonsillar fossa, ear	Triggered	Brief jabs	Episodes of syncope
Postherpetic neuralgia	One or more adjacent cranial or cervical nerves	Burning	Constant	Healed skin lesions, sensory loss, or hyperpathia
Posttraumatic neuralgia	Usually one cranial or cervical nerve	Burning, aching	Constant	Sensory disturbances
Cluster headache	Retroorbital, cheek, temple	Boring, deep, intense	Attacks of 30-120 min	Lacrimation, ptosis, rhinorrhea
"Lower-half headache"	Orbit, nose, cheek, mastoid; may spread to neck and arm	Boring, deep, intense	Attacks lasting one or more hours	Sometimes flushing, lacrimation, rhinorrhea
Carotidynia	One side of neck	Deep, aching	Several days	Tender carotid in neck
Atypical facial pain	Cheek, jaw, entire face	Aching, may be bizarre	Constant	Emotional disturbance

BIBLIOGRAPHY

Headache Classification Committee of the International Headache Society: Classification and diagnostic criteria for headache disorders. Cranial neuralgias and facial pain, *Cephalalgia* 8(suppl 7):1, 1988.

Ferrari MD, Haan AB: Acute treatment of migraine attacks, *Curr Opin Neurol* 8:237, 1995.

Forsyth PA, Posner JB: Headaches in patients with brain tumors: a study of 111 patients, *Neurology* 43:1678, 1993.

Frishberg BM: The utility of neuroimaging in the evaluation of headache in patients with normal neurological examinations, (Views and reviews), *Neurology* 44:1191, 1994.

Moskowitz MA, Buzzi MG: Neuroeffector functions of sensory fibres: implications for headache mechanisms and drug actions, *J Neurol* 238:S18, 1991.

Silberstein SD, Schulman EA, Hopkins MM: Repetitive intravenous DHE in the treatment of refractory headache, *Headache* 30:334, 1990.

CHAPTER

138 Neck and Back Pain

Kenneth K. Nakano

Every physician will encounter the common clinical problem of patients complaining of both neck and back pain. Pain is an evolutionary protective mechanism; by creating anxiety and by limiting activity, it serves to forewarn of physiologic excess and to prevent tissue damage and organ dysfunction. The physiologic production of pain depends on the stimulation of a variety of specialized nerve endings, and the pathologic production of pain depends on damage or irritation of the nerve fibers or cell bodies. Nerve endings of pain fibers vary in density and in stimulus sensitivity from tissue to tissue, so that areas supplied with sensitive endings in high density will normally be more sensitive to pain than areas poorly supplied in low density. Moreover, the endings tend to be sensitive to different stimuli and evoke in the central nervous system different sensations, all of which can be called painful.

Pain in the neck and/or back is normally limited in duration and responsive to rest, local measures (ice, heat, massage), analgesics, and muscle relaxants. The pathophysiologic basis for episodes of neck and/or back pain includes inflammatory, degenerative, and traumatic changes of the fascia, ligaments, apophyseal joints of the spine, and paraspinal muscles. Strain of the muscle or ligaments produces inflammation, edema, and spasm, resulting in pain and stiffness. Irritation of spinal nerve roots from a herniated disk (nucleus pulposus), an osteophytic spur, or less likely, a malignancy, may produce diffuse spasm and discomfort, and radicular pain, sensory loss, and weakness in the distribution of the affected nerve root (dermatome pattern). Disc herniation in either the neck or back occurs when the annulus fibrosus encircling the soft nucleus pulposus becomes weakened or torn, allowing the central disk material to extrude into the spinal canal to compress nerve roots or the spinal cord. Degenerative disk changes and adjacent vertebrae (spondylosis) occur in people older than age 40, are seen on radiographs of the spine, and generally do not produce symptoms unless the spondylitic changes encroach on the intervertebral foramina (IVF) (and produce symptoms of nerve root irritation). In persons with congenitally narrow spinal canals, degenerative disk changes compromise the spinal canal and IVF and may produce symptomatic spinal stenosis, a condition now much more easily diagnosed with the use of magnetic resonance imaging (MRI).

A clinician must possess the knowledge of the dermatome, sclerotome, and myotome distribution patterns for the cervical and lumbosacral nerves (Table 138-1). Moreover, it is important to confirm the source of dysfunction in the neck and low back, understand the mechanism by which the symptoms occur, and recognize the tissues capable of eliciting clinical signs. A thorough history and complete physical and neurologic examination will reveal the problem clearly; only after the physician recognizes certain conditions and arrives at a diagnosis can he or she direct effective therapy.

LOW BACK PAIN

Low back pain is one of the most frequent reasons that patients visit health care providers; in fact, low back pain is second only to upper respiratory infection as a symptom-related reason for office visits to physicians. Furthermore, an estimated 90% of adults experience an episode of low back pain at some point in their lives; in addition, in people younger than age 45, it is the most common impairment that limits physical activity. Thus low back pain is enormously costly to society in both human and monetary terms. In the United States in 1990 the direct costs of diagnosing and treating low back pain approximated $23.5 billion, whereas the indirect costs neared $35 billion, resulting in total costs of more than $50 billion.

Many disorders cause low back pain (Box 138-1); as a result, various modes of diagnosis and treatment will challenge the clinical acumen of health care providers. Medical management can be complicated by the absence of consistent, commonly accepted diagnostic terminology and variation in the use of diagnostic procedures and therapies among clinicians from various specialties. A precise anatomic explanation of the patient's low back pain can be identified objectively in less than 25% of patients, and only 1% to 2% of individuals with low back pain have lumbar disk herniation with radiculopathy. However, the focus of the clinical evaluation and the patient's concerns is often on a possible disk "rupture" and "nerve" involvement.

The fundamental questions of what makes a lumbar spine painful remain open to discussion and research. In the past the principal focus of lumbar spinal pain research has been mainly biomechanical and structural; the low back was viewed as a structural entity that was capable of suffering from a variety of mechanical deficiencies. Lumbar disk herniation has been viewed as causing compression of neural structures, spinal stenosis as a compressive lesion of the nerve root canals, and degenerative disk disease as segmental instability.

Table 138-1 Relation of reflexes to peripheral nerves and spinal cord segments

REFLEX	SITE AND MODE OF ELICITATION	RESPONSE	MUSCLE(S)	PERIPHERAL NERVE(S)	CORD SEGMENT
Scapulohumeral reflex	Tap on lower end of medial border of scapula	Adduction and lateral rotation of dependent arm	Infraspinatus and teres minor	Suprascapular (axillary)	C4 to C6
Biceps jerk	Tap on tendon of biceps brachii	Flexion at elbow	Biceps brachii	Musculocutaneous	C5 and C6
Supinator jerk (also called *radial reflex*)	Tap on distal end of radius	Flexion at elbow	Brachioradialis (and biceps brachii and brachialis)	Radial (musculocutaneous)	C5 and C6
Triceps jerk	Tap on tendon of triceps brachii above olecranon, with elbow flexed	Extension at elbow	Triceps brachii	Radial	C7 and C8
Thumb reflex	Tap on tendon of flexor pollicis longus in distal third of forearm	Flexion of terminal phalanx of thumb	Flexor pollices longus	Median	C6 to C8
Extensor finger and hand jerk	Tap on posterior aspect of wrist just proximal to radiocarpal joint	Extension of hand and fingers (inconstant)	Extensors of hand and fingers	Radial	C6 to C8
Flexor finger jerk	Tap on examiner's thumb placed on palm of hand; sharp tap on tips of flexed fingers (Tromner's sign)	Flexion of fingers	Flexor digitorum superficialis (and profundus)	Median	C7 and C8 (T1)
Epigastric reflex (exteroceptive)	Brisk stroking of skin downwards from nipple in mammillary line	Retraction of epigastrium	Transversus abdominis	Intercostal	T5 and T6
Abdominal skin reflex (exteroceptive)	Brisk stroking of skin of abdominal wall in lateromedial direction	Shift of skin of abdomen and displacement of umbilicus	Muscles of abdominal wall	Intercostal, hypogastric, and ilioinguinal	T6 and T12
Cremasteric reflex (exteroceptive)	Stroking skin on medial aspect of thigh (pinching adductor muscles)	Elevation of testis	Cremaster	Genital branch of genitofemoral	L2 and L3 (L1)
Adductor reflex	Tap on medial condyle of femur	Adduction of leg	Adductors of thigh	Obturator	L2, L3, and L4
Knee jerk	Tap on tendon of quadriceps femoris below patella	Extension at knee	Quadriceps femoris	Femoral	(L2), L3, and L4
Gluteal reflex (exteroceptive)	Stroking skin over gluteal region	Tightening of buttock (inconstant)	Gluteus medius and gluteus maximus	Superior and inferior gluteal	L4, L5, and S1
Posterior tibial reflex	Tap on tendon of tibialis posterior behind medial malleolus	Supination of foot (inconstant)	Tibialis posterior	Tibial	L5
Semimembranosus and semitendinosus reflex	Tap on medial hamstring tendons (patient prone and knee slightly flexed)	Contraction of semimembranosus and semitendinosus muscles	Semimembranosus and semitendinosus	Sciatic	S1
Biceps femoris reflex	Tap on lateral hamstring tendon (patient prone and knee slightly flexed)	Contraction of biceps femoris	Biceps femoris	Sciatic	S1 and S2
Ankle jerk	Tap on tendo calcaneus	Plantar flexion of foot	Triceps surae and other flexors of foot	Tibial	S1 and S2
Bulbocavernosus reflex (exteroceptive)	Gentle squeezing of glans penis or pinching of skin of dorsum of penis	Contraction of bulbocavernosus muscle, palpable at root of penis	Bulbocavernosus	Pundendal	S3 and S4
Anal reflex (exteroceptive)	Scratch or prick of perianal skin (patient lying on side)	Visible contraction of anus	Sphincter ani externus	Pudendal	S5

From Nakano KK: Neck pain. In Kelley WN et al, editors: *Textbook of rheumatology,* Philadelphia, 1985, WB Saunders.

This "structural" explanation led to "structural" therapies designed to relieve compression and stabilize the unstable spine. Biomechanical testing was used to evaluate structural integrity. However, large but asymptomatic lumbar herniations that display structural signs of neural compression have been documented. Moreover, symptom changes following lumbar laminectomy, diskectomy, or chemonucleolysis have not been correlated with the abolition of the compressive lesion. Some patients with excellent postprocedure relief demonstrate a high degree of mass effect, whereas others with persistent symptoms show the absence of postinterventional compressive mass effect. Likewise, patients with severe nerve root canal narrowing may be asymptomatic, whereas others have severe pain. Furthermore, the patient response after decompression is mixed and cannot be entirely correlated with the degree of compressive relief. The complex interactions between inflammatory enzymes, degratory enzymes, neurotransmitters, and vascular responses may also be involved in the processes that cause back pain.

Clinical Evaluation

Documentation of the history becomes a vital aspect of the examination. Three clinical features assist to direct the medical diagnosis and management of back pain: (1) duration of the symptoms, (2) distribution of the pain, and (3) age of the patient.

BOX 138-1
Classification of disorders causing low back pain

Lumbar disk syndromes
  L4 nerve root compression
  L5 nerve root compression
  S1 nerve root compression
  Large midline disk herniation
Congenital abnormalities
  Facet asymmetry
  Transitional vertebral (Bertolloti's syndrome)
  Spondylolisthesis-spondylolysis
  Scheuermann's disease
  Achondroplasia
Arthritic conditions
  Hypertrophic arthritis
  Osteoarthritis
  Ankylosing spondylitis
  Rheumatoid arthritis
  Osteitis condensans ilii
Infections
  Acute bacterial disk space infection
  Tuberculous spondylitis
  Sacroiliac infection
Tumors
  Benign
    Meningioma or neurinoma
    Osteoid osteoma
    Osteoblastoma
  Malignant
    Metastatic cancer (breast, lung, prostate, etc.)
    Primary neural tumors
    Myelogenous diseases
      Multiple myeloma
      Hodgkin's disease
      Lymphoma
      Eosinophilic granuloma
      Hand-Schüller-Christian syndrome
Metabolic disease
  Osteoporosis
  Ochronosis
  Paget's disease
  Sickle cell disease
Trauma
  Lumbar strain
  Compression fracture
  Subluxation of facet joint
Nonskeletal disorders
  Myofascial pain
  Pelvic disorders (pelvic inflammatory disease, uterine fibroids, tumors)
  Ectopic pregnancy
  Retroperitoneal tumors or hematoma
  Prostatitis
  Abdominal aortic aneurysm
  Kidney stones
  Pyelonephritis
  Pancreatitis
  Peptic ulcer
  Large bowel obstruction

BOX 138-2
Differential diagnosis of true sciatica versus pseudosciatica

Pseudosciatica
Meralgia paresthetica
Hip disease (e.g., osteoarthritis)
Trochanteric bursitis
Diabetic amyotrophy
Vascular claudication

True sciatica
Herniated disc (nucleus pulposus)
Lateral and/or foraminal stenosis
Intraspinal infection or tumor
Piriformis syndrome
Lumbar canal stenosis

patients with chronic pain, especially when litigation or compensation becomes an issue.

In the clinical evaluation of a patient with low back pain, the distribution of the pain (i.e., the back pain/leg pain ratio) is important in establishing the differential diagnosis. Leg pain as a primary symptom, especially below the knee and involving the foot, is characteristic of true sciatica. Absence of leg pain raises a different set of possibilities. True sciatica refers to symptoms (e.g., paresthesia, weakness, pain) related to nerve-root impingement and inflammation; leg pain becomes the predominant symptom, as opposed to low back pain. Pseudosciatica refers to a similar set of symptoms with a nonradicular etiology. Sciatica has several causes, the most common being lumbar disk herniation with nerve-root involvement (Box 138-2). More than 95% of lumbar disk herniations occur at the L4-L5 or L5-S1 level, producing L5 or S1 radiculopathy, respectively. Typically, the leg pain extends below the knee and into the foot; this will be useful for discriminating sciatica from other nonsciatic entities. An additional clinical feature of sciatica is greater pain when seated, when intradiskal pressure is highest. Pain is often relieved in the supine position and increases with coughing or the Valsalva maneuver. A positive straight leg raising (SLR) test (sciatic pain when the straight leg is passively raised between 30 and 60 degrees while the patient is supine) is more than 80% sensitive for disk herniation in patients with L5 or S1 radiculopathy; and a positive SLR test is more common in lumbar disk herniation than spinal stenosis.

The piriformis syndrome (PS) is characterized by buttock and leg pain; low back pain and difficulty sitting and walking occur in more than half of patients. The piriformis muscle arises from the inside of the pelvis over the sacrum and courses laterally through the sciatic notch, and trauma to the piriformis muscle with spasm and inflammation may produce sciatic nerve impingement. Patients with the PS demonstrate muscle tenderness, which may require a rectal examination to demonstrate. In patients with lumbar spinal stenosis, the patient will complain of pseudoclaudication characterized by buttock, thigh, or leg pain and paresthesia or weakness on standing or walking; pain will be relieved with spinal flexion. The majority of patients with spinal stenosis complain of bilateral symptoms, in contrast to the unilateral symptoms of lumbar disk herniation and sciatica. Lateral recess or foraminal stenosis may cause more unilateral symptoms, but unlike those of sciatica related to lumbar disk herniation, symptoms will not be relieved by supine posture and sciatic pain on SLR will be less common.

Individuals older than age 50 years will be at greater risk for serious nonmechanical sources of subacute and chronic low back pain (e.g., malignancy or infections). In addition, degenerative disk and joint disease, often at multiple levels, will be another frequent cause of low back pain in this age-group. The peak age for lumbar disk herniation and sciatica is 30 to 50 years; similarly, fibromyalgia is more common in patients younger than age 50. Subacute or chronic low back pain in younger patients should make the clinician suspicious of a spondyloarthropathy, such as ankylosing spondylitis or Reiter's syndrome.

Low back pain can be classified according to its duration. Acute low back pain has lasted less than 4 weeks, subacute pain 5 to 12 weeks, and chronic pain more than 12 weeks. The duration of back pain has diagnostic and prognostic implications. The majority of acute low back pain resolves quickly with little medical intervention; at least 60% of patients suffering with acute low back pain return to work within 1 month, and 90% return within 3 months. In the early diagnostic evaluation of a patient with low back pain, the physician should focus on recognizing the rare individual with a visceral or inflammatory cause of the pain. If symptoms fail to resolve as expected, the physician needs to reevaluate the patient and to identify complicating issues (e.g., nonorganic and/or psychosocial factors) delaying recovery. Nonorganic psychosocial barriers need to be evaluated in

Table 138-2   Neurologic findings in lumbosacral nerve root disorders

NERVE ROOT	PAIN DISTRIBUTION	WEAKNESS	SENSORY FINDINGS		REFLEXES
L3	Anterior thigh	Paresis of quadriceps, psoas, and adductors	L3		Knee jerk reduced or absent
L4	Upper gluteal region to anterior and medial thigh and to knee	Mild paresis of adductor and quad-riceps	L4		Knee jerk reduced or absent
L5	Lateral gluteal area to posterior, lateral thigh, lateral calf, lateral malleolus, dorsum of foot, and into big toe	Paresis of extensors of big toe; with severe weakness, toe and foot extensors weaken	L5		Posterior tibial reflex reduced or absent (significant if unaffected side is normal)
S1	Gluteus maximus to lateral posterior thigh, leg, and into heel and lateral foot	Paresis of plantar flexion muscles of foot	S1		Ankle jerk reduced or absent
S2	Gluteus maximus to posterior medial side of thigh and medial posterior calf; pelvic pain	Slight weakness plantar flexion; occasional bladder dysfunction	S2		Ankle jerk may be slightly reduced

Physical and Neurologic Examination

The physical examination is aimed at determining the presence of systemic or vascular disease, and the neurologic evaluation seeks nerve root compression, instability, and a nonmusculoskeletal origin for the symptoms. In patients with acute lumbar pain, lumbar muscle spasm straightens the normal lumbar lordosis (this can be both seen and palpated). Most often, the muscle in spasm is tender. When only one side is involved with low back pain, there is compensatory scoliosis (scoliosis concave to that side; this shortens one leg by lifting the pelvis). Motor examination should test the flexion and dorsiflexion strength of the foot and toes. The ability of the patient to flex and extend the leg at the knee should be assessed, and the ankle and knee deep tendon reflexes should be recorded (Table 138-2). SLR testing should be done with the patient supine and each extended leg lifted from the bed. If this produces sciatic pain in either leg, nerve root compression can be assumed. With L4 nerve root compression, there is diminution of the knee jerk and altered sensation of the medial side of the leg. There is also some weakness of the quadriceps, but this can be inconstant since L3 also contributes to these muscles. L5 nerve root compression produces reduced sensation of the lateral leg, dorsum of the foot, and around the base of the large toe. There is weakness of dorsiflexion of the foot and toes but no deep tendon reflex change. Root compression of S1 shows a loss or diminution of the ankle reflex and sensory loss on the lateral side of the foot and sole. In addition, there will be weakness of plantar flexion (often brought out by the patient walking on the toes). The majority of lumbar disc herniations occur at L4-L5 and L5-S1, and only a small minority affect L3-L4. Lumbar disc herniations at higher levels will be unusual. Lumbar facet degeneration or injury may cause both low back pain and nonradicular leg pain. Leg pain may occur without nerve root compression. Referral of pain by facet syndromes will be diffuse: into the hip and coccyx from L5 to S1, down the back of the thigh from L4 to L5, and into the anterior thigh from L3 to L4.

Diagnostic Evaluation

In most cases of lumbar disk herniation, the history and physical/neurologic examinations will provide the diagnosis. Because most patients with lumbar disk herniation and sciatica improve with nonoperative care, and the results of imaging studies will not affect initial management in most cases, imaging should be considered only in cases of diagnostic uncertainty, failure of nonoperative care (symptoms persisting 6 to 12 weeks, suggesting the need for surgical consultation and intervention), or suspected cauda equina syndrome (the usual presentation being the triad of saddle anesthesia, leg weakness, and loss of bowel and bladder control) (Fig. 138-1).

Electrodiagnostic studies (electromyography [EMG], nerve conduction studies [NCS], and somatosensory evoked responses [SER]) have the greatest diagnostic value in atypical sciatic syndromes (e.g., PS) or in patients who have had prior lumbosacral surgery. The purpose of the electrodiagnostic studies is to define the nerve roots or peripheral nerves involved (as well as the level—paraspinal or distal) in the pain syndrome.

BOX 138-3
Indications for spine radiographic study

History of significant trauma
Unexplained weight loss (>10 pounds in past year)
Age greater than 50 years at onset of back pain
Substance (drug) and alcohol abuse
History of malignancy
Chronic temperature elevations (>100° F)
Corticosteroid use
Administrative (occupation and other screening) or legal requirements

---

MRI and computed tomography (CT)/myelography have comparable sensitivity and specificity in identifying disk herniation. Gadolinium contrast allows MRI to distinguish scar formation from disk material as the source of radicular symptoms. Approximately 20% of subjects younger than age 60 without symptoms are found to have herniated disks by MRI or CT. In addition, spinal stenosis or lumbar disk degeneration is frequently found in asymptomatic persons, particularly after age 60. These imaging findings must be integrated with the clinical picture for appropriate interpretation.

Plain radiographs of the lumbar spine infrequently provide clinically useful information in the initial evaluation; in more than 75% of patients lumbar spine radiographs are normal or of questionable clinical significance, and oblique views add useful information in less than 3% of patients. Owing to the benign natural history of acute low back pain and the low yield of radiographic studies, selective criteria for ordering a lumbar spine radiographic series should be considered on a patient's first visit for acute back pain (Box 138-3).

Treatment

Nonnarcotic and/or nonsteroidal antiinflammatory drugs (NSAIDS) often ease the acute low back pain, and muscle relaxants can curtail the spasm, with the goal of permitting the patient to resume normal physical activity. In cases of severe acute low back pain, narcotic drugs may be necessary, although only on a short-term basis to minimize the possibility of addiction. Passive modalities such as ultrasound, message, or heat may be used briefly for early symptom relief. Prolonged bed rest often prolongs disability; patients told to rest for 2 days had similar clinical outcomes compared with those for whom 7 days of rest were prescribed, but the latter group missed 45% more work days. Excessive bed rest may result in deconditioning and reinforcement of sick-role behavior.

Often in both acute and chronic musculoskeletal disorders, the physician finds "trigger points." There are two approaches to the management of focal myositis. The traditional technique is to identify the area of focal spasm and pain by palpation and then inject it with a

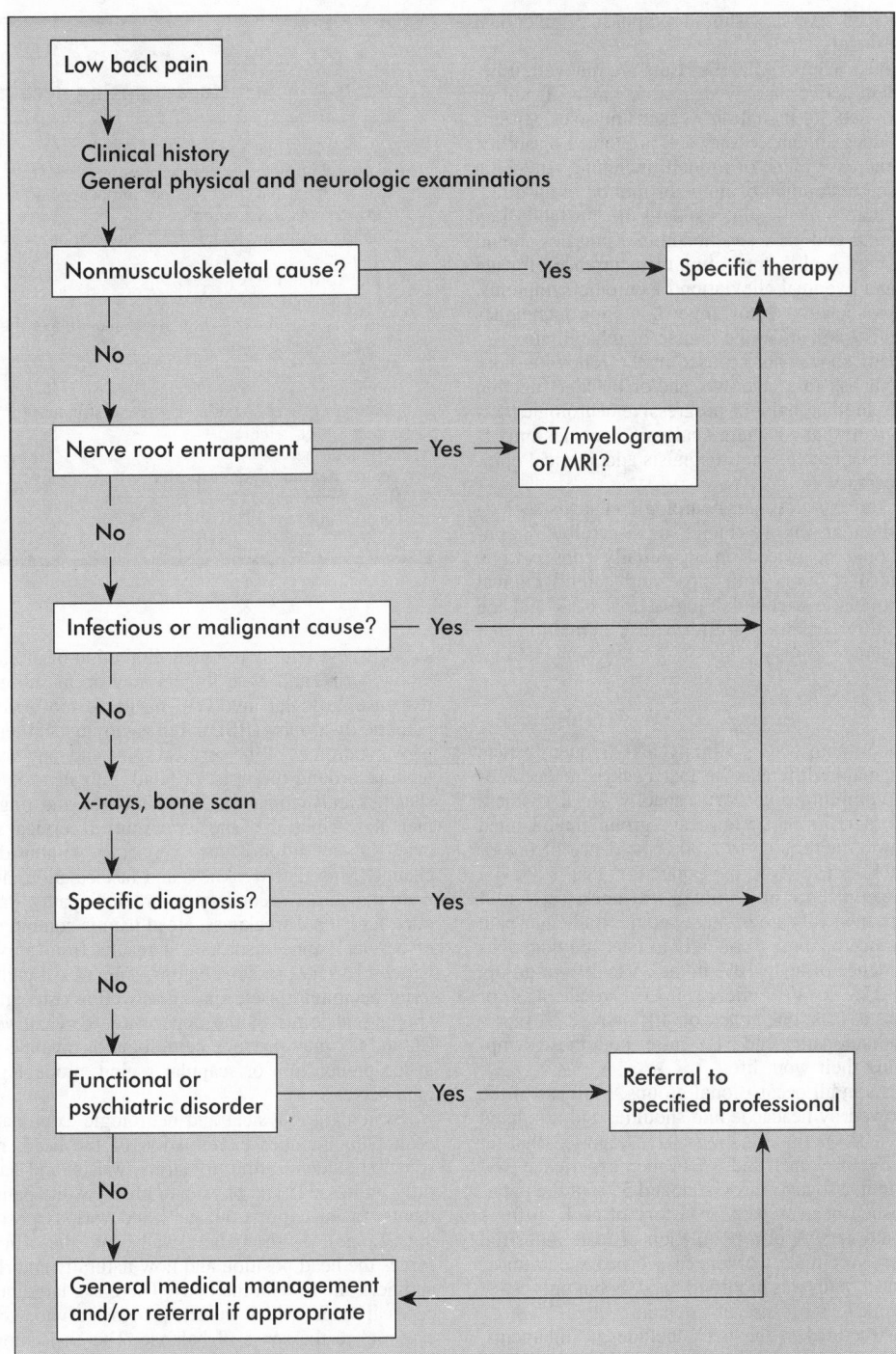

FIGURE 138-1 Algorithm for the evaluation of a patient with low back pain.

local anesthetic combined with steroids. An alternative method of eliminating the trigger point, especially in the acute phase, is the use of local electrical stimulation, which also provides local analgesia. Repeated injection of these areas often provides long-lasting pain relief. These techniques should provide more than temporary relief. Active physical therapy emphasizing range of motion and exercise must supplement trigger point injection and stimulation.

Spinal manipulation may provide marginal short-term benefit; at 3 weeks, 67% of patients with acute low back pain treated with manipulation improved, compared with 50% of those treated without manipulation. However, presently no conclusions regarding the efficacy of spinal manipulation for chronic low back pain can be made.

Most patients with acute low back pain improve within 4 to 6 weeks; however, if the patient does not show the expected improve-

ment, the clinician should consider three questions: (1) Was the initial diagnosis accurate? (2) Do psychophysiologic/social factors hinder recovery? and (3) Was the original therapy appropriate? In regard to the first question, if a patient with acute low back pain fails to improve within 6 weeks, the examiner should expand the differential diagnosis and order additional diagnostic studies such as imaging studies. To address the second question, a clinical history and physical findings assist in identifying patients in whom nonorganic factors are present (e.g., compensation, job dissatisfaction, anxiety or depression, substance abuse, nonanatomic distribution of pain symptoms, and sensory reports). In answer to the third question, the physician must ascertain whether the therapy was too passive for too long, resulting in deconditioning, depression, pain behavior, and anxiety of reinjury. In this situation, aggressive physical rehabilitation and exercise should emphasize functional restoration to a normal level.

As soon as the patient's acute pain and spasms are relieved, it becomes important to begin active therapy to restore range of motion and function. Long-term activity limitation weakens muscles, stiffens ligaments, and may produce an unnecessary and prolonged disability. Exercises designed to increase range of motion, including stretching at the knees and hips and restoration of range of motion in all directions of bending for the lumbar spine, should be pursued. Leg strengthening is important, and back and abdominal muscles should be exercised regularly. One goal is prevention of recurrence of acute back pain syndromes and eventual alleviation of chronic symptoms. Isometric exercises in association with range of motion techniques are tolerated well by most patients in the course of rehabilitation.

Conservative regimens should not be used in the following conditions: (1) if the patient has loss of bowel and/or bladder function and (2) if the patient has another major or progressive neurologic deficit, or such intractable pain that adequate analgesia becomes impossible. In these clinical situations, prompt diagnosis and surgical opinion(s) may become necessary.

Most patients, even those with minor neurologic changes such as a reflex abnormality, radicular sensory change, or discernible but unimportant weakness should be placed on an initially conservative, noninterventional medical regimen with close and careful clinical monitoring. In those populations complaining of low back and leg pain, only 1% to 2% suffer from a significant disk herniation that requires low back surgery.

NECK PAIN

In clinical medicine, neck pain occurs slightly less frequently than does low back pain; a major difference is that neck pain becomes less disabling, seldom compromising work capacity. Neck stiffness exists as a common disorder. For the 25 to 29 age-group in the United States working population, there is up to a 30% incidence of one or more attacks of stiff neck. For the working population that is age 45, this figure rises to 50%. Episodes of "simple" stiff neck last 1 to 4 days and seldom require medical care in most people. Radicular pain to the shoulder and arm occurs more frequently in later life than does stiff neck; it has an incidence of up to 10% in the 25 to 29 age-group, subsequently rising to 25% to 40% after age 45. Overall, 45% of working men experience at least one attack of stiff neck, 23% report at least one attack of radiculopathy, and 51% suffer both these symptoms at some time during their work life.

Pain in the neck exists in all occupational groups. Stiffness of the neck appears first, followed by headache and shoulder and arm/hand pain (brachial neuralgia; BN). Investigations have reported that, at any time, as many as 12% of women and 9% of men experience pain in the neck with or without associated arm pain, and 35% of the population can recall an episode of neck pain. A history of neck stiffness and arm pain was elicited in 80% of a population of male industrial forest workers. In a series of male workers in a broad spectrum of jobs, the number with neck pain was modified to 51%, but only 5.4% had experienced any work loss because of the pain.

The pain-sensitive structures of the neck include the ligaments, nerve roots, articular facets and capsules, muscles, and the dura. Pain in the neck area can originate from several tissue sites and result from several mechanisms (Box 138-4). Neck pain can originate from the involved cervical anatomic structures, or it may seem to do so but may actually be due to referral from another site (Box 138-5). Musculoskeletal conditions involve neurologic anatomy, and the converse also seems to be true. The frequency of BN is approximately three times higher in those who complain of stiff neck, suggesting common factors in the pathogenesis.

Clinical Evaluation

The essential means of diagnosis and management of neck pain include elicitation of the history and the physical and neurologic examinations. The most common symptom of cervical spine disorders is pain. Cervical nerve root irritation causes a well-localized area of pain, whereas poorly defined areas of pain arise from deep connective tissue structures, muscle, joint, bone, or disk. The patient's ability to describe the pain gives the clinician essential clues to diagno-

---

BOX 138-4
Structures causing neck pain

Acromioclavicular joint
Heart and coronary artery disease
Apex of lung, Pancoast's tumor, bronchogenic cancer (C3, C4, C5 nerve roots in common)
Diaphragm muscle (C3, C4, C5 innervation)
Gallbladder
Spinal cord tumor
Temporomandibular joint
Fibrositis and fibromyositis syndromes (upper thoracic spine, proximal arm, and shoulder)
Aorta
Pancreas
Disorders of any somatic or visceral structure (produces cervical nerve root irritation)
Peripheral nerves
Central nervous system (posterior fossa lesions)
Hiatus hernia (C3, C4, C5)
Gastric ulcer

---

sis. Stiffness with consequent limitation of motion of neck, shoulder, elbow, wrist, and even fingers may occur subsequent to prior injury response, articular involvement, nerve root irritation, or reflex sympathetic dystrophy (RSD). Tenosynovitis and tendinitis often accompany syndromes of the cervical spine and may involve the rotator cuff, tendons around the wrist or hand with stenosis or fibrosis of tendon sheaths, and palmar fascia. Numbness and tingling follow the segmental distribution of the nerve roots in cervical spine disorders; however, this condition occurs frequently without demonstrable sensory change. Muscular weakness and fasciculation indicate a lower motor neuron disorder secondary to a radiculopathy. Pain and guarding produce functional weakness. Head pain is common and is characteristic of cervical spine disorders; it results from nerve root compression, vertebral artery pressure, compression of sympathetic nerves, and posterior occipital muscle spasm, as well as osteoarthritic changes of the apophyseal joints of the upper three cervical vertebrae. A lesion of C6 and C7 may produce neurologic or myalgic pain with tenderness in the precordium or scapular region, producing confusion with angina pectoris.

Systematic physical and neurologic examination of patients with neck pain includes examination of the head, neck, upper thoracic spine, shoulders, arms, forearms, wrists, and hands with the patient fully undressed. The physician observes the patient's posture, movements, facial expression, gait, and various positions (sitting, standing, supine). As the patient walks into the office, the physician observes the head position and how naturally and rhythmically the head and neck move with the body. There is a large range of motion of the cervical spine, which in turn provides a wide scope of vision and is essential to the sense of balance. The basic movements of the neck include flexion, extension, lateral flexion to the right and left, and rotation to the right and left. A decrease in specific motion may occur with blocking at a joint, pain, fibrous contracture, bony ankylosis, muscle spasm, mechanical alteration in joint and skeletal structures, or a tense and uncooperative patient. Other causes of muscle spasm include injury to muscle, involuntary splinting over painful joints or skeletal structure, and irritation or compression of nerve roots of the spinal cord. Reflexes indicate the state of the nervous system and its afferent pathways (see Table 138-1). Certain abnormal reflexes appear only with spasticity and paralysis; these indicate injury to the corticospinal tract. The primary deep tendon reflexes and plantar responses should be routinely examined.

Differential Diagnosis

Several medical conditions arising outside the cervical spine but perceived in or around the neck area mimic cervical nerve root irritation, muscle spasm, ligament strain, bone disease, and joint disorders (see Box 138-5). Peripheral neuropathy may produce pain both proxi-

BOX 138-5
Cervical spine syndromes

Localized neck disorders

Osteoarthritis (apophyseal joints, C1-C2-C3 levels most often)
Rheumatoid arthritis (atlantoaxial)
Juvenile rheumatoid arthritis
Sternocleidomastoid tendinitis
Acute posterior cervical strain
Pharyngeal infections
Cervical lymphadenitis
Osteomyelitis (staphylococcal, tuberculosis)
Meningitis
Ankylosing spondylitis
Paget's disease
Torticollis (congenital, spasmodic, hysterical)
Neoplasms (primary or metastatic)
Occipital neuralgia (greater and lesser occipital nerves)
Diffuse idiopathic skeletal hyperostosis
Rheumatic fever (infrequently)
Gout (infrequently)

Lesions producing neck and shoulder pain

Postural disorders
Rheumatoid arthritis
Fibrositis syndromes
Musculoligamentous injuries to neck and shoulder
Osteoarthritis (apophyseal and Luschka)
Cervical spondylosis
Intervertebral osteoarthritis
Thoracic outlet syndromes
Nerve injuries (serratus anterior, C3-C4 nerve root, long thoracic nerve)

Lesions producing predominantly shoulder pain

Rotator cuff tears and tendinitis
Calcareous tendinitis
Subacromial bursitis
Bicipital tendinitis
Adhesive capsulitis
Reflex sympathetic dystrophy
Frozen shoulder syndromes
Acromioclavicular secondary osteoarthritis
Glenohumeral arthritis
Septic arthritis
Tumors of the shoulder

Lesions producing neck and head pain with radiation

Cervical spondylosis
Rheumatoid arthritis
Intervertebral disk protrusion
Osteoarthritis (apophyseal and Luschka joints; intervertebra disk osteoarthritis)
Spinal cord tumors
Cervical neurovascular syndromes
Thoracic outlet and associated syndromes

relieve) the pain, one then looks at potential visceral or somatic structures having the same segmental neural supply.

Neck pain occurs in malingerers, depressed persons, people seeking compensation, and hysterical and psychoneurotic individuals. These patients possess no concomitant nerve root irritation and derive no relief from local anesthetic injections. Furthermore, absence of muscle spasm, an antalgic position, and feigning of limitation of neck motion should arouse the physician's suspicion. Skilled clinical elicitation of historical data and the physical and neurologic examinations constitute the principal reproducible means of making a differential diagnosis (Fig. 138-2).

Diagnostic Evaluation

The investigation of patients experiencing neck pain is constructed to evaluate the origin of the symptoms and signs, the extent of the lesion, and whether medical or surgical treatment is required. Components of the investigation are radiographic, neuroimaging, neurophysiologic and laboratory studies. If the clinical history or general physical and neurologic examinations suggest an abnormality, then cautious laboratory studies, electrodiagnostic (EMG, NCS, SER) and neuroimaging (MRI, CT, myelography) assessment may be required for an accurate diagnosis and appropriate therapy (Fig. 138-2).

When ordering radiographs of their patients, physicians should not rely solely on the radiologist; clinical correlation is necessary because gross radiologic signs and abnormalities may be associated with minimal or no clinical disturbance, whereas the reverse situation (minimal radiographic change with the patient demonstrating neurologic signs) may also occur. Routine cervical radiographic views include (1) anteroposterior of the atlas and axis through the open mouth; (2) anteroposterior of the lower five vertebrae; (3) lateral views in flexion, neutral, and extension; and (4) both right and left oblique. The bones should be particularly examined for osteoporosis. The joints might reveal osteophytes with or without foramina encroachment or even the erosions of systemic arthritis. Congenital abnormalities such as vertebral fusion should be sought. Ligamentous calcification might indicate degeneration, trauma, ankylosing spondylitis, or diffuse idiopathic skeletal hyperostosis (DISH). Instability in the action views might be due to trauma (such as an athletic injury or automobile crash) but is far more often due to constitutional ligament laxity in a person who is not physically fit. Signs of previous surgery might give a clue as to the nature of the problem.

Neuroimaging studies include MRI, CT myelography, and radionuclide bone scans. MRI combines the best features of these conventional techniques; it can display vertebrae, intervertebral discs, the thecal space, neural elements, blood vessels, and paraspinal structures without the use of radiographic or intravenous or intrathecal contrast agents or both. Furthermore, MRI is the preferred modality for the evaluation of suspected cervical radiculopathy, spinal stenosis, congenital anomalies (particularly Chiari malformations), syringomyelia, spinal cord neoplasm, multiple sclerosis, and early disk degeneration. CT and MRI are approximately equivalent for evaluation of extramedullary spinal tumors and trauma; certain acutely traumatized patients must be excluded from MRI owing to accompanying life support apparatus. Radioisotope bone scans are best used for the evaluation of possible inflammatory joint disease or metabolic disorder of the bone. At times it is helpful to do a full-body bone scan and obtain radiographs (and at times CT) of those areas of increased uptake that might help in the overall assessment. Three-phase studies can be helpful in the diagnosis and follow-up of reflex sympathetic vasomotor disorder and RSD.

Neurophysiologic tests can be used to document sensory and motor dysfunction of the peripheral nerves. It can also be used to distinguish between a lesion in the peripheral nervous system and one in the central nervous system. EMG-NCS can also be used to differentiate between a nerve and a muscle disorder.

The clinical laboratory offers some help in the diagnosis and management of neck pain in specific diseases (e.g., rheumatoid arthritis, hyperparathyroidism, HIV infection, multiple myeloma, ankylosing spondylosis, or certain metastatic malignant cancers). Cerebrospinal fluid (CSF) should be evaluated in patients with neck pain suspected of having infection (meningitis, meningismus) or subarachnoid hemorrhage; in the latter conditions, the CSF becomes diagnostic.

mal and distal to the irritative site. Muscle spasm is not associated with peripheral neuropathy. Spinal cord tumors produce a poorly localized and ill-defined neck pain, hyperreflexia, and spasticity. Immobilization does not relieve the pain, and deep tenderness and local muscle spasms are absent. Cerebral or subarachnoid hemorrhage, meningitis, head and neck trauma, or a central tumor can produce neck pain, mimicking cervical spine syndromes. In these instances, clinical examination, MRI, CT scan, and spinal fluid evaluation may be used to differentiate the various conditions.

An important clinical fact in the differential diagnosis of neck pain is that compression or irritation of cervical nerve roots with radiation of pain is associated with deep tenderness at the site of pain. Segmental areas of deep tenderness that are not painful until palpated indicate nerve root involvement. A 1% injection of lidocaine into the painful area results in transient reproduction of the radicular pain, followed by relief of pain for days or weeks in the patient with nerve root involvement. If local anesthetic injection fails to reproduce (and

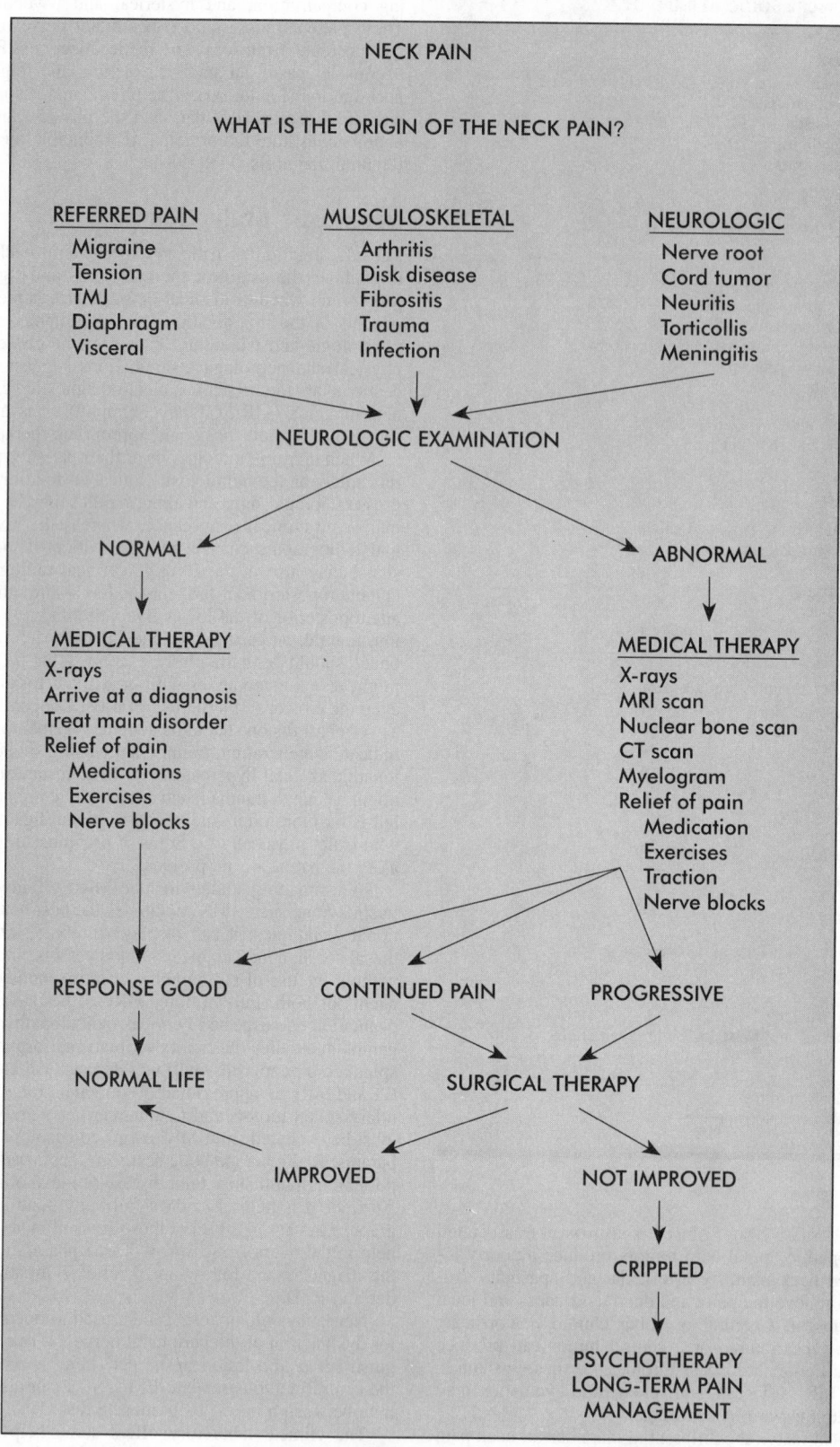

FIGURE 138-2   Neck pain algorithm for diagnosis and therapy.

Treatment

In the treatment regimen of neck pain, the physician considers the following: (1) severity of symptoms, (2) presence or absence of neurologic findings, and (3) severity of the condition as seen by radiologic imaging and neuroimaging and electrodiagnostic studies (when indicated) (Fig. 138-2).

Medical therapy aims at the relief of pain and stiffness in the neck and upper limbs. Early mobilization exercises in patients with acute sprains often improve outcome. For relief of pain, NSAIDs and muscle relaxant medications suffice, and most acute neck pain subsides within 7 to 10 days. When the acute pain subsides, the patient may commence therapeutic exercises: anterior-neck mobilizing, shoulder raising, and muscle strengthening. Shoulder exercises, aimed at elevating the shoulder girdle and relieving drag on the nerve roots, can be combined with the use of a cervical collar. Head positioning may be used to relieve symptoms because placing the head in certain positions relieves pain. The head should be carried at all times in its optimal position of slight flexion with chin drawn in. Traction, either continuous or intermittent, should be considered when rest fails. Continuous cervical traction should be reserved for more severe cases with symptoms of nerve root compression. However, traction will be unsuitable for patients with gross radiographic-visible changes of the cervical spine because of danger of spinal cord compression or pressure on the vertebral arteries; occasionally side effects of traction are seen, and rarely hemianopic visual field defects develop. Cervical collars may prove helpful, in part because they also help correct posture faults. These should fit well and maintain the neck in the most comfortable position. Collars should not be worn continuously for more than 2 months to prevent weakness and wasting of neck muscles.

Physical therapy benefits most patients with neck pain; some persons are helped by cryotherapy; others benefit from heat (both superficial and deep). Mechanical therapy (e.g., therapeutic message) may also help relieve symptoms. In certain cases, electrotherapy and transcutaneous nerve stimulation may be beneficial. Still other patients may respond to biofeedback and relaxation techniques.

Surgery appears appropriate for two groups of patients. In the first group, symptoms relate principally to the nerve roots emerging from the cervical spine, and the condition is manifested with either neck or arm pain. In the second group, a slowly progressive spinal cord syndrome involves the legs first and then the arms. One of the primary factors in the pathogenesis of radiculopathy and myelopathy is compression. Treatment is aimed at the elimination of this pressure. The most definite indication for surgery is the presence of a neurologic deficit related to compression that is unrelieved by medical treatment. Formerly, the initial surgical approach was from the posterior midline, but recently many surgeons have advocated an anterior approach. In patients with defined neurologic deficits, results have been excellent in 80% to 90% of cases, irrespective of surgical approach. Success is especially likely with a centrally herniated disc. In cases of myelopathy, the surgical approach may be either anterior or posterior. However, surgical repair of cervical myelopathies is less effective than in cases of acute radiculopathy, with approximately 60% to 70% of treated patients remaining stable or improving. In patients with cervical boney canal diameter of 11 mm or less at several levels, a long posterior decompression may be necessary. In those with a diffuse bulging disk or an osteophytic ridge, and when the boney elements are normal (or slightly small), the site of compression and approach may be anterior (several levels may be operated on at the same time). In patients with a large, centrally herniated cervical disc, the surgeon may have difficulty deciding on the appropriate approach. It should be emphasized that opinions differ as to the optimal surgical technique in these cases.

CONCLUSIONS

In the clinical evaluation and treatment of an individual with neck and low back pain, the physician should answer the following questions: (1) Am I treating the right condition? (2) Am I using therapy that is correct for the cause of the pain in this particular patient at this particular time? (3) Is the patient's account of nonimprovement in keeping with observed changes in mobility, ability to carry out daily activities, and analgesic consumption? (4) Are there mechanical perpetuating factors? (5) Is neurologic injury present? (6) Is an underlying systemic or metabolic disease present? (7) Does the patient have a space-occupying lesion? and (8) Are secondary gain and/or motivational factors at work?

Many medical conditions produce neck and low back pain both locally and referred. Confirming the source of dysfunction in the neck, understanding the mechanism by which the symptoms occur, and recognizing the tissues capable of eliciting clinical signs assume importance. A careful, thorough history and complete physical and neurologic examination usually reveal the problem clearly. When physicians recognize which symptoms can be reproduced and which movements and positions produce them, they can make a working diagnosis and direct effective therapy. The principles established on that basis reaffirm the fact that the diagnosis need not be one of exclusion.

BIBLIOGRAPHY

Anderson GJ, Svensson HO, Oden A: The intensity of work recovery in low back pain, *Spine* 8:880, 1983.

Cherkin DC, Deyo RA, Loeser JD et al: An International comparison of back surgery rates, *Spine* 19:1201, 1994.

Cypress BK: Characteristics of physician visits for back symptoms: a national perspective, *Am J Public Health* 73:389, 1983.

Deyo RA, Diehl AK, Rosenthal M: How many days of bed rest for acute low back pain? A randomized clinical trial, *N Engl J Med* 15:1064, 1986.

Frymoyer JD: Back pain and sciatica, *N Engl J Med* 318:291, 1988.

Frymoyer JW: Quality: an international challenge to the diagnosis and treatment of the lumbar spine, *Spine* 18:2147, 1993.

Hold L: Frequency of symptoms for different age groups- and professions. In Hirsch C, Sotterman Y, editors: *Cervical pain,* New York, 1971, Pergamaon Press.

Hult L: The Munkfors investigation, *Acta Orthop Scand* 16(suppl):1, 1954.

Jacchia GE, Innocenti M, Pavolini B et al: Indications and results of surgical treatment of cervical disc disease by anterior and posterior approach, *Chir Organi Mov* 77:111, 1992.

Jensen MC, Brant-Zawadzki MN, Obuchowski N et al: Magnetic resonance imaging of the lumbar spine in people without back pain, *N Engl J Med* 331:69, 1994.

Jonsson B, Stromqvist B: The straight leg raising test and the severity of symptoms of in lumbar disc herniation: a preoperative and postoperative evaluation, *Spine* 20:27, 1995.

Kelsey JL, Pastides H, Bisbee GE: Musculoskeletal disorders: their frequency of occurrence and their impact on the population of the United States, New York, 1978, Watson Academic Publications.

Lunsford LN, Bassonett DJ, Jannetta PJ, et al: Anterior surgery for cervical disc disease, *J Neurosurg* 53:1, 1980.

Nakano KK: Neck pain. In Kelley WN, Harris ED Jr, Ruddy S, Sledge CB, editors: *Text of rheumatology,* ed 4, Philadelphia, 1993, WB Saunders.

Nakano KK: *Neurology of musculoskeletal and rheumatic disorder,* Boston, 1979, Houghton Mifflin.

Nakstad PH, Hald JK, Bakke SJ et al: MRI in cervical disc herniation, *Neuroradiology* 31:382, 1989.

Scavone JG, Latshaw RF, Rohrer GV: Use of lumbar spine films: statistical evaluation at a university teaching hospital, *JAMA* 246:1105, 1981.

Scavone JG, Latshaw RF, Weidner WA: Anteroposterior and lateral radiographs: an adequate lumbar spine examination, *Am J Roentgenol* 136:715, 1981.

Shekelle PG, Adams AH, Chassin MR et al: Spinal manipulation for low-back pain, *Ann Intern Med* 117:590, 1992.

Simeone FA, Rothman RH: Cervical disc disease. In Simeone FA, Rothman RH, editors: *The spine,* Philadelphia, 1992, WB Saunders.

CHAPTER

139 Otoneurology

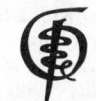

Stephen W. Parker

ANATOMIC SUBSTRATE OF BALANCE

Balance is controlled by sensory systems in the central and peripheral nervous systems. These are organized so that an individual can still function after damage to one system; if more than one is damaged, the individual is unstable. Sensory receptors of the vestibular system reside in the inner ear. The semicircular canals respond to angular acceleration and the utricle and saccule to movements in relation to gravity (linear acceleration). These structures are connected to the vestibular nuclei in the brain stem via the eighth nerve. The midline cerebellar structures, including the flocculus, nodulus, and vermis, are integral parts of the vestibular system and have a powerful inhibitory effect on the vestibular nuclei. The cerebellar hemispheres are not part of the vestibular system, but they play an important role in balance by modulating motor activity and coordination. Vision also plays a major role in balance and in normal individuals often overrides other balance modalities. The final major sensory modality contributing to balance is proprioception mediated by peripheral nerves. Disease processes that impair one or more of these modalities impair the individual's ability to balance. If multiple systems are not functioning, balance is severely impaired. A syndrome of multiple sensory deficits may be seen in elderly patients with degenerative central nervous system or labyrinthine changes, plus neuropathy, retinopathy, or arthropathy.

DISEASES AND THEIR LOCI
Systemic

Systemic or distant causes of dizziness include postural hypotension, which is a frequent cause of a lightheaded type of dizziness that occurs on standing from a supine or sitting position, although there may be a delay in the onset of symptoms. Anemias often produce dizziness on standing. Pernicious anemia has been associated with episodes of spinning dizziness and positional dizziness. Cardiac arrhythmias can produce a lightheaded type of dizziness and episodes of spinning dizziness, which suggest ear rather than cardiac disease. Aortic stenosis may be associated with a lightheaded or faint feeling that occurs after limited exercise. Hypothyroid patients may have a Ménière's-like picture, with bilateral hearing loss and episodes of spinning dizziness. The dizziness usually resolves with treatment, but the hearing loss may not improve. Hyperthyroid patients rarely have hearing loss but may complain of tinnitus. They may have spinning dizziness, but more frequently they complain of a lightheaded, off-balance sensation. Hypoglycemia may produce a lightheaded type of dizziness and, less frequently, spinning.

Inner Ear

The relatively few diseases that affect the inner ear are among the most common causes of dizziness. Labyrinthitis is an inflammation of the inner ear that most typically affects both auditory and vestibular portions of the inner ear. Symptoms are the sudden onset of hearing loss and dizziness. The hearing loss may resolve or persist. The dizziness may be quite intense at the onset but gradually resolves. The resolution of symptoms may take hours, days, weeks, or months. This illness is a monophasic one with the possibility of some fluctuation. Labyrinthitis has been classified in three types. The most severe is bacterial labyrinthitis, which occurs in the setting of a meningitis. Often these patients are so sick that the initial dizziness and hearing loss are not clinically apparent, and instability and hearing loss are appreciated after the patient has recovered from the acute effects of the meningitis. Serous labyrinthitis is seen in patients with middle ear infections. Bacteria do not appear to enter the inner ear, but toxic substances apparently do. On pathologic examination, mononuclear cells in the inner ear and damage to the hair cells of the basal turn of the cochlea adjacent to the round window can be seen. There may be high frequency hearing loss as well as dizziness. The most common type of labyrinthitis is viral, the prototypes of which are measles and mumps. The clinical entity of vestibular neuronitis is used to explain the sudden onset of dizziness associated with a decrease in vestibular function on one side without auditory symptoms. Thus it is characterized by the sudden onset of severe dizziness with no auditory symptoms. Examination reveals instability with a tendency to fall to one side. There may be spontaneous or gaze nystagmus with the fast-phase beating to the side opposite that to which the patient is falling. No other neurologic signs or symptoms are present. Testing reveals a reduced response to caloric stimulation on the side to which the patient is falling and the side opposite spontaneous and gaze nystagmus fast phase. Ménière's syndrome is a multiphasic illness characterized by repeated episodes of spinning dizziness, fluctuating hearing with gradual deterioration, a feeling of pressure in the affected ear, and tinnitus in the affected ear. The etiology of this process is unclear, but the pathophysiology appears to be an

overproduction of endolymph or a problem with absorption of endolymph that results in swelling of the endolymphatic space (endolymphatic hydrops) with episodes of dizziness and hearing loss, possibly occurring at the time of repeated rupture of membranes in the inner ear. The process has a variable course and may resolve spontaneously. Many forms of medical treatment have been tried without well-documented success. Sometimes vestibular suppressant medication helps to decrease the severity of symptoms. If symptoms persist in a severe form, surgical treatment may be helpful. Operations to change the abnormal pathophysiology have had limited success in relieving symptoms (66% with improvement). Destructive procedures, such as labyrinthectomy or selective sectioning of the vestibular portion of the eighth nerve, have had a higher incidence of success if patients are carefully selected to include only those with documented unilateral inner ear dysfunction. Over a period of 5 years, 15% to 30% of patients may have involvement of both inner ears. There may be systemic causes of Ménière's-like symptoms, especially with bilateral involvement. This can be seen with hypothyroidism, lues, and vasculitis. Positional vertigo and nystagmus are common symptoms that often come from the inner ear. The most common type is benign paroxysmal positional vertigo (BPPV), which is characterized by spinning dizziness on lying down as well as on sitting up. There may be dizziness on turning the head from side to side or on flexing and extending the neck. The classic finding on examination is a burst of rotary nystagmus when the patient is rapidly placed in the right- or left-ear-down position. This nystagmus has a brief latency and a duration of less than 60 seconds, and it is associated with dizziness. The nystagmus and dizziness fatigue (decrease) on repeated movements into the provoking ear-down position. On sitting up from the provoking ear-down position, there are similar symptoms of nystagmus and dizziness, but the nystagmus reverses direction so that it has a downward rather than upward vertical component. Other features—latency, brief duration, dizziness, and fatiguing—are unchanged. BPPV most frequently comes from the posterior semicircular canal of the inner ear on the side from which the symptoms may be provoked. A horizontal canal variant with horizontal rather than rotary nystagmus has been described but not documented pathologically as has the posterior canal variant. This is a self-limited process that most frequently occurs spontaneously but can occur after trauma and usually resolves spontaneously after weeks to months. It is secondary to debris, possibly detached from the otolith, in the endolymph of the affected semicircular canal. Patients learn to deal with the symptoms or to avoid the provoking positions. Repositioning maneuvers (Epley and Semont liberatory) are often effective in immediately relieving the symptoms, presumably by removing debris from the affected semicircular canal. Exercises in which the patient repeatedly attempts to provoke the symptoms (Brandt-Daroff exercises) may also be effective in relieving symptoms, over a period of days to weeks. There are other forms of positional vertigo and nystagmus that originate in the central nervous system. Central nervous system lesions are characterized by purely vertical nystagmus, persistent nystagmus (lasting more than 60 seconds), and nystagmus occurring without dizziness. Head trauma frequently causes dizziness secondary to concussive effects on the labyrinth. This is frequently a positional dizziness that may be a variant of BPPV. The most common causes of serious ototoxicity in the United States are aminoglycoside antibiotics, which may produce vestibular and auditory damage in the inner ear by damaging hair cells. The incidence of this damage may be decreased but not eliminated by careful attention to blood levels and renal function. The relative amount of auditory and vestibular dysfunction caused varies among the different members of this group. Neomycin and kanamycin have mainly auditory effects. Gentamicin and tobramycin affect vestibular function more than auditory function, and streptomycin affects vestibular function much more than auditory function. Damage to hearing occurs initially in the higher frequencies, and there is relative preservation of speech discrimination. Eventually a profound hearing loss may occur. The vestibular dysfunction may be insidious and often is initially not appreciated in critically ill patients. It becomes apparent as an instability on attempting to walk and as an instability of the environment when sitting in a bouncing car or wheelchair. The patient finds it difficult to read when the head is moving. Although there may be some improvement in the damage to the vestibular system, most of the functional improvement comes from central nervous system adaptation and the ability to use information from other sensory systems, such as the visual and the proprioceptive. Thus patients with multiple sensory deficits may not be able to compensate for the loss of inner ear vestibular information and may remain unstable. Perilymph fistulas between the inner and middle ear occur with erosive tumors and after barotrauma, such as explosions or rapid pressure changes in scuba diving. With classic barotrauma there is sudden onset of hearing loss and dizziness. Over the past several years, the possibility of chronic perilymph fistulas being responsible for unexplained dizziness and hearing loss has been raised. This issue is still controversial.

Eighth Nerve

Abnormalities of the eighth nerve are less frequent than those of the inner ear. Acoustic neuromas constitute 2% of intracranial tumors and are the most common tumor of the cerebellopontine angle. These Schwann's cell tumors of the vestibular portion of the eighth nerve originate in the internal auditory canal, because it is at this point that the eighth nerve changes its sheath from glial to Schwann's cell. Symptoms are produced by compression of the neurovascular bundle in the internal auditory canal. The most common symptom is a slowly progressive unilateral hearing loss. Dizziness is less common and may be only a mild instability as the central nervous system adapts to the slow loss of peripheral vestibular function. Although the seventh nerve is compressed in the internal auditory canal, facial paralysis is relatively rare, because motor function is resistant to the compressive effects of this type of tumor. Other symptoms appear as the tumors grow out of the internal auditory canal and fill the cerebellopontine angle. The next most common finding is decreased facial sensation from compression of the fifth nerve or fifth-nerve nucleus, but tumors must be at least 2 cm in posterior fossa extension to symptomatically compress the fifth nerve. Other late symptoms from compression of the brain stem and cerebellum include limb ataxia, gait ataxia, headache, and memory loss from hydrocephalus. Approximately one fourth as common are cerebellopontine angle meningiomas. These tumors tend to be larger at the time of presentation, since they originate on the dura of the posterior fossa and often must fill the cerebellopontine angle before causing symptoms.

Brain Stem

Although diseases of the brain stem that cause dizziness are less common than diseases of the inner ear, they are often more dangerous. These include strokes, tumors, and demyelinating and degenerative diseases. Strokes are the most worrisome, because they can progress to irreversible loss of function in a matter of hours. Two well-defined stroke syndromes are the lateral medullary stroke and the anterior inferior cerebellar artery (AICA) stroke. The presenting symptoms of the lateral medullary stroke are dizziness with veering (lateral pulsion) toward the side of the lesion, nystagmus beating toward the side of the lesion, ipsilateral limb ataxia, loss of pin and temperature response on the contralateral foot, and decreased sensation on the ipsilateral side of the face. In the AICA syndrome, there is dizziness with severe ipsilateral hearing loss, ipsilateral peripheral-type facial paralysis, ipsilateral decreased facial sensation, contralateral decreased limb sensation, and, sometimes, ipsilateral limb ataxia. The AICA syndrome is much less common than the lateral medullary syndrome. Other basilar branch occlusions and lacunae may produce dizziness. Cerebellar hemorrhages may present with symptoms similar to those of vestibular neuronitis. There may be sudden onset of dizziness, which may be spinning and made worse by movement. Limb ataxia and headache are often absent, and unassisted walking is impossible. That there usually is no nystagmus is an important differential point, since patients with acute peripheral vestibular lesions who are unable to walk usually have nystagmus. The diagnosis of cerebellar hemorrhage can be made with a computed tomography (CT) scan without contrast enhancement. If cerebellar hemorrhage is suspected, it is imperative that a CT scan be performed without delay, because once these patients become obtunded from brain stem compression, the prognosis is poor. Cerebellar infarction in the distribution of the distal posterior inferior cerebellar artery (PICA) is important, because with intravenous free water these infarcts often swell and result in

brain stem compression. Infarction in this distribution spares the brain stem and damages the inferior and medial ipsilateral cerebellar hemisphere. Patients are dizzy and unsteady; there is no limb ataxia. The clinical clue is nystagmus beating to the left on left lateral gaze and to the right on right lateral gaze, whereas in acute labyrinthine disease the nystagmus should beat only in one direction whatever the direction of gaze. Tumors involving the brain stem may affect both balance and hearing. Usually there are other neurologic signs and symptoms suggestive of brain stem disease. Demyelinating disease may present with dizziness as the initial symptom; with time, other signs and symptoms suggestive of central nervous system abnormality appear. In many degenerative diseases of the central nervous system, dizziness and instability of gait and posture are prominent symptoms. These disorders include cerebellar and spinocerebellar degenerative diseases and progressive supranuclear palsy.

Cerebral Cortex

The sensation of dizziness can occasionally come from the cerebral cortex. Penfield demonstrated that stimulation of the parietal cortex provoked sensations of dizziness. Vestibular epilepsy occurs with two types of presentation. In the more common type, spinning dizziness is an ictal phenomenon of a partial seizure disorder. The less common type is a generalized seizure disorder provoked by a vestibular stimulus such as rotation or caloric stimulation. Hydrocephalus may produce problems with balance and stability. Patients complain of unsteady gait and instability of balance. They have a shuffling, small-stepped gait and, often, difficulty initiating gait, which is called *apraxia of gait*. Memory loss and urinary urgency or incontinence are often part of this syndrome.

DIFFERENTIATION OF CENTRAL (BRAIN STEM) AND PERIPHERAL (EIGHTH NERVE AND INNER EAR DISEASE)

Dizziness

The sensation of motion alone does not permit a differentiation between ear and central nervous system disease. Spinning dizziness can come from the ear or the brain. Only the associated symptoms and signs allow the differential diagnosis. Headache at the back of the head or between the ears can come from ear or brain disease. Pain perceived on the forehead, in the eye, or at the root of the nose is suggestive of disease in the posterior fossa. Facial or extremity numbness is consistent with disease in the brain, as is limb ataxia, focal weakness, double vision, trouble with speech, and trouble swallowing. In acute situations, close attention must be given to disturbances of consciousness. Differentiation must be made between the vertiginous patient who wants to lie still and the patient who is unable to maintain alertness. The combination of dizziness and impairment of consciousness suggests widespread involvement of the brain stem consistent with a tumor or basilar artery occlusion. It is important to recognize basilar artery disease, because relatively mild symptoms can rapidly progress to devastating and irreversible deficits. The clues to the identification of brain stem disease are the associated neurologic symptoms and signs; it is not possible to make the diagnosis of brain stem disease on the basis of dizziness alone. Although as many as 25% of patients who subsequently develop clear basilar transient ischemic attacks initially present with unaccompanied dizziness, the diagnosis cannot be made at that time from the symptoms. Fortunately these patients usually demonstrate other signs and symptoms before a permanent deficit occurs. Hearing loss and positional dizziness are more common with inner ear disease but can be seen with diseases of the brainstem.

Spontaneous and Gaze Nystagmus

The characteristics of nystagmus can sometimes help localize an abnormality. The usual inner ear nystagmus is horizontal or rotary and beats in only one direction. The components of the nystagmus may vary as the eyes are moved in different positions. Thus in one position the nystagmus may be mainly horizontal and in another position more vertical. After acute severe damage to one inner ear or eighth nerve, there may be nystagmus with the fast-phase beating to the side opposite the lesion in all directions of gaze. Nystagmus beating to the right on right lateral gaze and to the left on left lateral gaze is characteristic of nystagmus from the central nervous system. The most common cause of this type of nystagmus is drug effect. Nystagmus that is different in the two eyes (dissociated), pure vertical nystagmus, and direction-changing nystagmus all are from the central nervous system. If nystagmus is present for days or weeks without accompanying dizziness, it is from the central nervous system. Nystagmus that does not change its components as the eyes are moved around is consistent with a central nervous system lesion.

HEARING

Disorders of the auditory system are manifested by reduced ability to hear, distortion of the ability to hear, increased sensitivity to sound, and the production of sound or the perception of sound when it is not present (tinnitus). A conductive hearing loss occurs when sound is better conducted through the bone of the skull than through the air and the ossicles in the middle ear to the inner ear. Fluid, infection, tumor, and fixation of the ossicles (as in otosclerosis) result in a conductive hearing loss. Damage to the cochlea results in a sensory neural hearing loss characterized by a decrease in the ability to hear pure tones and a proportionate decrease in the ability to understand speech. There also may be distortion of perceived sounds. Lesions affecting the eighth nerve, such as acoustic neuromas, produce hearing losses that may vary. Typically, there is a high frequency hearing loss, and speech discrimination is more severely affected than would be expected from the pure tone loss. Damage to the auditory pathways in the brain stem often does not produce hearing loss, because there is so much crossing of the auditory pathways that large bilateral lesions are required to produce hearing loss. However, there may be difficulty with complicated or competing auditory stimuli or with localization of sound. Lesions in the temporal lobe may produce impairment of the ability to understand speech, with competing background words in the ear contralateral to the lesion. Testing of hearing is precise and standardized in the audiogram. This test investigates behavioral hearing by presenting pure tones or words at different frequencies, by either air or bone conduction, to determine the thresholds for pure tone hearing at frequencies from 250 to 8000 Hz. The ability to understand speech is an important function of the auditory apparatus and can sometimes help localize the site of an auditory lesion. Speech discrimination is tested by giving phonetically balanced words at an intensity 40 Db above threshold and recording the percentage of correct responses. The audiogram is most helpful in documenting behavioral hearing and in identifying and localizing hearing loss from the middle and inner ear. At times, it can help differentiate inner ear from eighth nerve disease. A more sensitive test of abnormalities of the eighth nerve or brain stem is that for short-latency auditory-evoked potentials. These are submicrovolt potentials that can be recorded in the first 7 msec after an auditory stimulus such as a broadband click with surface electrodes at the scalp and the ear lobe. A series of reproducible waves at constant interwave latencies is found in normal individuals. With conductive or cochlear hearing loss, all waves are delayed. With damage to the auditory pathways in the eighth nerve or brain stem, there may be interwave latency prolongations, loss of waves, or distortion of waves. This test is extremely sensitive in the diagnosis of acoustic neuromas, with a false-negative rate of between 4% and 8%, and may show abnormalities in brain stem lesions when hearing is normal, as is often the case in multiple sclerosis.

CLINICAL EVALUATION

The clinical evaluation of patients with balance and hearing problems should begin with a thorough and careful history and a physical examination focused especially on hearing loss and dizziness, as well as possible associated neurologic symptoms and signs. The audiogram should often be the initial test for patients with hearing loss or auditory symptoms, and it should be performed on most patients with balance problems. If there is a unilateral hearing loss, the next test should be for auditory-evoked potentials, to search for a possible retroco-

chlear locus of abnormality. If the evoked potentials are abnormal and consistent with an eighth-nerve lesion, an imaging study must be performed. The most sensitive technique for looking at the posterior fossa, and especially the internal auditory canal, is contrast-enhanced magnetic resonance imaging (MRI) scan. This imaging method permits the identification of intracanalicular acoustic neuromas and small brain stem lesions, as well as large cerebellopontine angle lesions. The CT scan is still a good way to look at the posterior fossa. It is superior to the MRI scan for acute hemorrhages, but it does not visualize intracanalicular acoustic neuromas or tumors extending less than 1 cm into the posterior fossa. It is necessary to use intravenous contrast enhancement to visualize acoustic neuromas on the CT scan. If vertebrobasilar ischemia is thought to be causing symptoms, noninvasive vascular studies including duplex Doppler, transcranial Doppler, and magnetic resonance angiography can demonstrate blood flow and the status of large blood vessels. The MRI scan identifies areas of infarction. If the symptom of concern is dizziness or imbalance, it is often helpful to obtain tests of vestibular and balance function. Among the battery of tests of balance that can help localize and characterize abnormalities are the electronystagmogram (ENG), sinusoidal vertical axis rotation, visual-vestibular interaction rotation testing, and posturography. The ENG is a battery of tests in which eye movements are recorded under conditions designed to demonstrate different functions of the vestibular system. Eye movements are recorded with eyes open in the light, eyes open in the dark, and eyes closed. Spontaneous, gaze, optokinetic, positional, and caloric nystagmus are recorded, as well as saccades and pursuit eye movements. These tests give information about the brain stem control of eye movements, the brain stem vestibular system, and the inner ear and eighth nerve vestibular system. Sinusoidal vertical axis rotation is a sensitive computerized test of the vestibuloocular reflex of the horizontal semicircular canals that is complementary to caloric stimulation but more sensitive and more reliable. Visual-vestibular interaction testing gives information about the relationships among the inner ear vestibular system, the brain stem, the cerebellum, and the visual systems by rotating the patient with eyes open in the dark, with visual fixation, and with optokinetic stimulation. Dynamic posturography permits a different and more direct investigation of balance than has been previously available. Patients stand on a platform that can measure sway with strain gauges and computer control. The platform can be moved in different directions, as can a visual surround, to make the task more difficult and to selectively abolish or distort sensory inputs such as vision and proprioception. These tests permit an objective characterization of standing balance under a variety of conditions and may give functional information about an individual's difficulty with balance.

TREATMENT

Choice of treatment depends on the cause of symptoms and the type of symptoms. Acoustic neuromas are usually surgically resected. Dizziness associated with hypothyroidism often resolves on treatment with thyroid hormones, and dizziness from partial seizures resolves with anticonvulsant treatment. Episodes of spinning dizziness from inner ear dysfunction may be treated with vestibular suppressant medications such as meclizine, dimenhydrate, and promethazine. The disadvantages of these medications are that they often cause drowsiness and that they may make some patients' balance worse by suppressing a damaged vestibular system. Diphenidol is an effective vestibular suppressant that does not cause drowsiness, but in a small percentage of patients it causes visual hallucinations. Some physicians advocate treatment with low-salt diets, diuretics, and the avoidance of caffeine. These treatments have not been proven to be effective. Lightheaded unsteady dizziness often decreases when patients are treated with small doses of benzodiazepines. There is evidence from animal experiments that diazepam suppresses vestibular nucleus firing rates and therefore acts as a vestibular suppressant as well as having a tranquilizing effect. This class of medication usually only partially suppresses symptoms and may be habituating, so stopping medication can exacerbate symptoms. Persistent episodes of spinning dizziness that do not stop with medication and can be proven to come from one ear can usually be stopped with a labyrinthectomy or selective vestibular nerve section.

✔ *WHEN TO REFER*

Patients with benign positional vertigo and nystagmus can often rapidly be relieved of symptoms. Therefore if symptoms do not resolve within a short time, referral to a physician who knows how to perform the repositioning maneuvers can be helpful. If there is a question of brain stem vascular disease causing symptoms and the physican is not familiar with the evaluation and treatment of vertebrobasilar insufficiency, there should be an urgent referral to a neurologist or otoneurologist because this type of symptom can rapidly result in severe brain stem strokes. If patients have persistent dizziness that is interfering with function, referral to a physician familiar with the diagnosis and treatment of this symptom (otoneurologist, neurootologist, neurologist, otolaryngologist) may be helpful.

The nerve section is designed to preserve hearing. The labyrinthectomy completely destroys hearing. Transtympanic gentamicin, endolymphatic shunting, and endolymphatic saculotomy procedures are less destructive, but are successful in a smaller percentage of patients. Patients with positional dizziness often benefit from repositioning maneuvers (Epley and Semont liberatory) designed to remove debris from the affected semicircular canal. Patients with persistent (rather than episodic) dizziness or instability are often able to decrease their symptoms by performing exercises designed to produce central nervous system adaptation or compensation. These exercises (vestibular physical therapy) are most effective when they are tailored to the patient's deficit and modified by interaction between a trained therapist and the patient. Data from several groups suggest that vestibular physical therapy is very helpful in decreasing symptoms of dizziness and imbalance.

BIBLIOGRAPHY

Baloh RW, Halmagyi GM, editors: *Disorders of the vestibular system,* Oxford, 1996, Oxford University Press.

Baloh RW, Honrubia V: *Clinical neurophysiology of the vestibular system,* ed 2, Philadelphia, 1990, Davis.

Baloh RW et al: Recent advances in clinical neurotology, *J Vestibular Res* 5:231, 1995.

Brandt T, Steddin S, Daroff RB: Therapy for benign paroxysmal positioning vertigo, revisited, *Neurol* 44:796, 1994.

Honrubia V, Brazier MAB, editors: *Nystagmus and vertigo: clinical approaches to the patient with dizziness,* Orlando, Fla, 1982, Academic.

CHAPTER

140   Disorders of Speech and Language

 Daniel B. Hier

Disordered speech and language are among the most important signs of neurologic disease. Careful evaluation of the speech-disordered patient gives clues to the etiology and anatomic site of neurologic illness. A disorder of language always implies disease of the brain. A language disorder is a defect in the ability to understand linguistic symbols or a defect in the ability to express meaning using linguistic symbols. Language disorders can disrupt either spoken language (aphasia) or written language (alexia or agraphia). These language disorders are usually caused by injury to language-related structures in the frontal, temporal, parietal, and occipital lobes of the dominant hemisphere or their underlying subcortical connections. In addition to aphasia, a variety of other speech disorders may result from injury elsewhere in the nervous system (the nondominant hemisphere, the frontal lobes, the cerebellum and its connections, the basal ganglia and their connections, the corticospinal tract and its connections, the peripheral nerves innervating respiratory and oropharyngeal muscles) or dysfunction outside the nervous system, including the respiratory apparatus, the oropharynx, and the tongue.

APHASIA
Testing for Aphasia

Aphasia is tested at the bedside by examining the patient for defects in repetition of speech, impairment in comprehension, abnormalities in speech fluency, and difficulties in word retrieval.

Repetition. Repetition is tested by having the patient repeat short phrases (e.g., "I am here"; "no ifs, ands, or buts"). Repetition is normal or near-normal in anomic aphasia and the transcortical aphasias. Repetition is abnormal in conduction aphasia, Broca's aphasia, Wernicke's aphasia, and global aphasia.

Comprehension. Comprehension is tested by having the patient follow one-step, two-step, and three-step spoken commands. Patients who can follow simple two-step or three-step commands are considered to have grossly intact comprehension for the purposes of aphasia classification. Although gross comprehension is generally impaired in Wernicke's aphasia, patients with milder degrees of aphasia show a less severe pattern of comprehension defects. Even aphasic patients without gross comprehension deficits have trouble comprehending complex logicogrammatical constructions (e.g., "Put the red chip in front of the white chip," "What relation to you is your mother's brother?," or "Does summer come before spring?").

Fluency. Fluency encompasses two somewhat different concepts: quantity of speech output and ease of speech output. Patients with fluent aphasia produce utterances of longer length (usually five or more words) and produce more words per unit time than do patients with nonfluent aphasia (normal speakers produce more than 100 words per minute). Furthermore, fluent aphasics speak easily and without effort. Nonfluent aphasics produce sparse speech that is hesitant, labored, and effortful. Problems in classification occur with aphasics who speak their utterances effortlessly, but generate little output because of severe word-retrieval problems. This often occurs in Wernicke's aphasia, in which speech output (quantity of words per minute) is reduced as a result of severe anomia. Because utterances are easily articulated, these aphasics should still be classified as fluent despite sparse speech output. Wernicke's, conduction, anomic, and transcortical sensory aphasias are classified as fluent aphasias. Broca's, transcortical motor, transcortical mixed, and global aphasias are nonfluent aphasias.

Word Retrieval. Word retrieval problems can be elicited by asking the patient to name commonplace objects, or they may become apparent during spontaneous speech. Word retrieval deficits are called *anomia*. Anomia is a central feature of all aphasias but also occurs in dementia, encephalopathy, and delirium. Anomia may occur on confrontation naming of objects or in running speech. Among aphasic and demented subjects, speech is altered in predictable ways by word-retrieval problems. Lexical access is generally more difficult for nouns than for verbs and adjectives. Prepositions and conjunctions are least affected. High-frequency nouns (e.g., *cat*) are easier to retrieve than low-frequency nouns (e.g., *gyroscope*). Picturable nouns are easier to retrieve than abstract nouns. Indicators of anomia are numerous. *Circumlocutions* are attempts by patients with anomia to substitute a description of a word for the unretrievable word (e.g., a watch is called "something I tell time with"). Excessive use of circumlocutions makes the speech verbose. Empty words (*thing, one, those,* etc.) and pronouns are used in place of nouns. This gives anomic speech an empty quality. Other manifestations of word retrieval difficulties include verbal paraphasia (substitution of one word for another, such as *clock* for *watch*) and neologisms (invented words).

Classification of Aphasia

Controversy exists about the validity of aphasia syndromes. Although patients with aphasia are routinely assigned a diagnostic category, one third of aphasics cannot be easily categorized. Discrepancies in classification of aphasics are commonplace even among experienced raters. Within a given aphasia category (e.g., Wernicke's aphasia), heterogeneity exists among aphasic patients. Furthermore, there is not an exact relationship between areas of cerebral injury and any given aphasia syndrome. Despite these problems, aphasia categorization is a routine and often useful exercise. The most widely accepted classification scheme is that of the Boston Diagnostic Aphasia Examination. Most aphasiologists recognize eight forms of aphasia: anomic, conduction, Broca's, Wernicke's, global, transcortical motor sensory, transcortical mixed, and transcortical sensory.

Wernicke's Aphasia. The speech of patients with Wernicke's aphasia is well articulated with normal melody, rhythm, and inflection. Fluency (as measured by both ease of articulation and quantity of output) is often normal. Some patients with Wernicke's aphasia are laconic with sparse output, reflecting severe word-retrieval problems. Others with Wernicke's aphasia are verbose with sometimes uncontrollable verbal output (logorrhea). Although grammatical structure is often intact, the information conveyed is diminished. An excess of words is used to convey little meaning (circumlocution), reflecting the limited use of substantive words. Nonspecific or empty words (e.g., *it, thing, this*) are used excessively. In Wernicke's aphasia, verbal paraphasic errors (word substitutions) predominate over phonemic paraphasic errors (sound substitutions). Some word substitutions are invented words; these are termed *neologisms*. Frequent use of neologisms creates jargon. Reading comprehension, auditory comprehension, naming, and repetition of speech are impaired. Oral reading is occasionally relatively spared. Elementary neurologic findings such as hemiparesis and sensory loss are generally not present. A right superior quadrantanopia is present when the lesion injures optic radiations in the left temporal lobe. The responsible lesion is usually in the posterior superior temporal lobe.

Broca's Aphasia. Broca's aphasia is a syndrome of nonfluent speech associated with relatively spared comprehension. Speech is laconic and hesitant, giving it a telegraphic quality. Speech is uttered effortfully and lacks normal melody (*dysprosody*). Repetition is severely impaired. Confrontation naming deficits are variable. Articulatory disturbances are often prominent, and a marked dysarthria is usually present. Although commonly associated with Broca's aphasia, these articulatory disturbances are not a true aphasic disorder. Phonemic paraphasias (sound substitution errors) abound in Broca's aphasia. Agrammatism is a hallmark of Broca's aphasia. Agrammatic speech is characterized by an abundance of substantive words (e.g., nouns, verbs) and few functor words (prepositions, conjunctions, articles). The failure to utilize functors leads to speech that is economical but violates the rules of syntax (telegraphic speech). Broca's aphasia is usually associated with a dense right hemiparesis. However, rare instances of Broca's aphasia without hemiparesis have been reported. Visual fields and sensation are usually normal. Oral-buccal-lingual apraxia (inability to protrude tongue, pucker lips, whistle, etc.) frequently accompanies Broca's aphasia, reflecting injury to the prefrontal motor cortex. Ideomotor apraxia of the left upper extremity may also accompany Broca's aphasia. These patients pantomime the acts of waving good-bye, hammering, dealing cards, or saluting clumsily with their nonparetic left arm, reflecting interruption of crossing callosal fibers from the left premotor cortex. The ideomotor apraxia can be demonstrated only in the nonparetic left arm that has been disconnected from motor programs in the left parietal lobe (callosal apraxia). The lesion responsible for Broca's aphasia is a large left frontal lesion extending backward to the rolandic fissure. Lesions limited anatomically to Broca's area produce a transient syndrome of muteness followed by effortful speech that rapidly resolves.

Conduction Aphasia. Conduction aphasia is a less common aphasic disorder. Comprehension is well preserved. Spontaneous speech is usually fluent, although it may be contaminated by both phonemic (sound substitution) and verbal (word substitution) paraphasic errors. The hallmark of the disorder is repeated speech that is impaired as compared with spontaneous speech. Writing and spelling are impaired. Anomia of varying degrees accompanies conduction aphasia, although the anomia may be mild. Anatomic site of injury

in conduction aphasia may be the superior left temporal lobe, the inferior parietal lobe, or the insula and underlying arcuate fasciculus.

Global Aphasia. Global aphasia is a common aphasic syndrome characterized by disruption of all language functions including spontaneous speech, naming, repetition, reading, writing, and comprehension. Patients are nonfluent, with little or no speech output. Marked deficits in repetition and comprehension of spoken language are present. Reading comprehension and writing are severely impaired. Global aphasia is often associated with a dense right hemiplegia, right hemisensory loss, and right hemianopia. Uncommon instances of global aphasia without hemiparesis have been reported. The responsible lesion is usually large and encompasses both Wernicke's area in the temporal lobe and Broca's area in the frontal lobe. Global aphasia may follow left carotid occlusion, embolism to the stem of the left middle cerebral artery, or large left basal ganglionic hemorrhages.

Anomic Aphasia. Anomic aphasia or amnestic aphasia is a common form of aphasia but one with little localizing significance. In its purest form, it is characterized by normal comprehension and fluent speech complicated by word-finding difficulties. Repetition is normal. Speech may be circumlocutory, with verbal paraphasic errors. Confrontation naming is impaired. In its less pure (and more common) form, anomic aphasia is associated with a mild reduction in comprehension of spoken and written language. Characteristically, articulation, prosody, oral reading, repetition, and writing from dictation are normal. Etiologies of anomic aphasia include raised intracranial pressure, brain tumors, toxic and metabolic disorders, head injury, and Alzheimer's disease. In cases of cerebral infarction, anomic aphasia is of little anatomic localizing value (lesions may be left frontal, occipital, parietal, temporal, or deep). Some cases of Wernicke's aphasia resolve into an anomic aphasia during recovery.

Transcortical Aphasia. In transcortical aphasia, repetition of speech is markedly superior to spontaneous speech. In a few patients with transcortical aphasia the tendency to indiscriminately repeat all heard speech constitutes *echolalia*. However, echolalia is not an essential feature of transcortical aphasia. Transcortical aphasia contrasts with conduction aphasia, which is characterized by spontaneous speech that is superior to repetition. The major forms of transcortical aphasia are transcortical motor aphasia, transcortical sensory aphasia, transcortical mixed aphasia, and isolation of the speech area. Transcortical motor aphasia resembles Broca's aphasia, but repetition is relatively intact. The lesion is often in the deep subcortical structures of the left frontal lobe. Transcortical sensory aphasia resembles Wernicke's aphasia except that repetition is intact. Transcortical sensory aphasia may occur after the development of posterior temporal or parietal lobe lesions or subcortical lesions that undercut parietal or temporal cortex. Marked deficits in naming, comprehension, and spontaneous speech characterize transcortical mixed aphasia. Repetition is disproportionately spared. Some patients are echolalic and lack spontaneous speech. These severe instances of transcortical mixed aphasia have been termed *isolation of the speech area.*

Thalamic Aphasia. The aphasia that follows left thalamic hemorrhage or infarction often has "transcortical" features. Repetition is usually spared. Voice volume is low. Variable word access and comprehension problems occur. When speech output is reduced, the aphasia of left thalamic infarction or hemorrhage resembles transcortical mixed aphasia. Echolalia may occur. When speech output is greater, the aphasia that follows left thalamic stroke resembles transcortical sensory aphasia.

Crossed Aphasia. Because the left hemisphere is dominant for language in nearly all right-handed individuals and as many as 60% of left-handed people, aphasia after right hemisphere injury is unusual. Crossed aphasia is the combination of right hemisphere injury with aphasia in a right-handed patient. With regard to left-handed patients, the concept of crossed aphasia is moot since their hemispheric dominance for language is unpredictable. The frequency of crossed aphasia in right-handed individuals after right hemisphere injury ranges from 0.4% to 1.8%. Crossed aphasia may be either fluent or nonfluent. The pattern of anatomic localization of aphasia in cases of crossed aphasia resembles the left hemisphere pattern. Anterior (frontal) lesions are associated with Broca's aphasia and posterior (temporal) lesions with Wernicke's aphasia.

SPEECH DISORDERS

In addition to aphasia, a variety of speech disorders are frequently encountered, including impaired articulation (dysarthria), impaired melody of speech, impaired voice volume, mutism, and perseveration.

Hypophonia

Decreased voice volume *(hypophonia)* may reflect respiratory or airway difficulties, diseases of the basal ganglia such as Parkinson's disease, or psychiatric disease (hysteria, malingering, depression, or schizophrenia). *Aphonia* is a complete loss of voice. Aphonic patients may be unable to phonate for a variety of reasons, including respiratory difficulties; paralysis of respiratory muscles; abnormalities of the tongue, larynx, and oropharynx; bulbar paralysis; and pseudobulbar palsy.

Dysarthria

Dysarthria is a broad term that encompasses a variety of disorders of speech articulation. Dysarthria is a disorder of speech, not language. Dysarthric patients need not be aphasic, although many patients with aphasia (especially motor or Broca's aphasia) are dysarthric. Dysarthria can arise from structural lesions of the pharynx, tongue, palate, or lips; from dysfunction of muscles that control the vocal apparatus; or from neurologic dysfunction of the peripheral and cranial nerves, brain stem nuclei, or cortical centers and pathways controlling the vocal apparatus. Three major types of dysarthria are recognized.

Paretic dysarthria or *flaccid dysarthria* is characterized by weakness of the muscles of articulation. The responsible lesion disrupts the function of the lower motor neuron, with paralysis of the lips, tongue, or soft palate. Paretic dysarthria may complicate bulbar poliomyelitis, progressive bulbar palsy, brain stem stroke, or idiopathic polyneuritis. The flaccid state of the musculature of both respiratory apparatus and oropharynx produces speech that is of low volume, hypernasal, and poorly articulated.

Spastic dysarthria or *rigid dysarthria* occurs with lesions of the upper motor neuron. The most common cause of spastic dysarthria is single or multiple strokes. Voice volume may be good, but the voice has a harsh, sometimes strangled quality. Melody and rhythm of speech are choppy *(dysprosody).* Articulation is impaired.

Ataxic dysarthria occurs with cerebellar disease. It is seen most commonly with cerebellar degeneration (hereditary or alcoholic) or multiple sclerosis. The speech of these patients is characterized by the inappropriate stress on unstressed syllables (scanning speech) that is one hallmark of cerebellar disease. Voice volume may vary excessively. Speaking rate is decreased. At times poorly controlled expirations of air betray the ataxic quality of the speech.

Hypokinetic dysarthria is typical of Parkinson's disease and multiinfarct dementia. Voice volume is low, and there is marked hypoprosody.

Hyperkinetic dysarthrias occur with certain other basal ganglia diseases such as Huntington's chorea and torsion dystonia. The speech disorder tends to parallel the hyperkinetic movements found in the limbs. There may be excessive variations in speaking rate, voice tremor, excessive variation in voice volume, and impaired articulation.

Mutism

Mutism is failure to speak. Mutism may occur for a variety of reasons. *Pure word mutism* (also known as *cortical anarthria* or *aphemia*) is inability to speak caused by cerebral injury. Auditory and reading comprehension are intact. Written expression is usually normal. Recovery from initial mutism is the rule. The cerebral lesion is usually in the area of the left frontal lobe responsible for articulation. Loss of language (aphasia) is an important cause of mutism. Patients with global aphasia or severe Wernicke's aphasia may be mute because they cannot formulate any language. Similarly, mutism may complicate the late phases of the degenerative dementias (Pick's disease and Alzheimer's disease) when profound aphasia deprives the patient of spontaneous speech.

Mutism may be a complication of certain psychiatric conditions, including catatonic schizophrenia, severe depression, malingering, and conversion reaction. Mutism also occurs with akinetic mutism, chronic vegetative state, and "locked-in" state. *In akinetic mutism* there is a profound abulia (usually resulting from hydrocephalus or bifrontal damage). Patients fail to speak as a result of profound lack of motivation and mental inertia. Patients in a *chronic vegetative state* have sustained massive brain damage and are severely demented. Although these patients go through sleep-wake cycles, they show little evidence of intellectual activity. They may gaze purposfully about the room but never speak. Chronic vegetative state may follow severe anoxia, hypotension, hypoglycemia, or head trauma with diffuse brain injury. In chronic vegetative state the electroencephalogram is abnormal, with severe slowing and low voltage. *Locked-in* patients are alert but are unable to move or speak as a result of a brain stem lesion, usually in the mid or low pons. The lesion is low enough in the pons to spare the reticular activating system in the upper pons and midbrain, so alertness is preserved. Locked-in patients are quadriplegic and unable to move most oral-facial musculature. The electroencephalogram shows relatively normal activity, and the patient can understand speech and writing. Vertical eye movements and eyelid blinking (which are controlled by midbrain structures) are preserved as the only communication system available to the locked-in patient.

Perserverative Speech Disorders

Cortical Stuttering. Although stuttering is a common developmental disorder of childhood, it also occurs in some adults after brain injury. *Stuttering* is characterized by the abnormal repetition of individual syllables. Most cases of cortical stuttering are associated with aphasia and left hemisphere damage.

Palilalia. *Palilalia* is abnormal repetition of syllables, words, or short phrases. It may be difficult to distinguish palilalia from cortical stuttering, which involves the involuntary repetition of an initial syllable. Palilalia occurs in Parkinson's disease and other diseases of the basal ganglia. Palilalia may also complicate aphasia or dementia.

Echolalia. *Echolalia* is the abnormal tendency to echo words and phrases. In striking cases the patient may fail to comprehend the request but accurately repeat it (e.g., when asked "Tell me your name?" the patient may simply reply "Tell me your name.") Echolalia may occur in a variety of disorders, including advanced Alzheimer's disease, infantile autism, schizophrenia, and transcortical aphasia.

Disordered Speech Melody

Prosody is the musical quality of speech produced by variations in pitch, rhythm, and stress of pronunciation. In *hyperprosody,* normal prosodic variations are exaggerated. Hyperprosody sometimes occurs in manic psychiatric states. *Dysprosody* is the loss of normal melody of speech that occurs after left frontal lobe damage. The speech is halting, dysarthric, and lacks normal rhythm and melody. Dysprosody is characteristic of Broca's aphasia and other motor aphasias. In hypoprosody, normal prosodic variations are lost. Speech has a dull and monotonous quality. Hypoprosody is characteristic of Parkinson's disease and is often accompanied by low voice volume. After right hemisphere damage, some patients are unable to intone affect into their speech. Their speech has a flat, unemotional quality. This deficit is known as *aprosody.* In practice, it is difficult to distinguish aprosody from hypoprosody. However, the term *aprosody* is usually reserved for the prosodic disturbance that follows right hemisphere damage, whereas *hypoprosody* is used to describe the prosodic disturbance of Parkinson's disease and other basal ganglionic disorders.

DISORDERS OF WRITTEN LANGUAGE
Agraphia

Agraphia is a disorder of written language caused by brain disease. Writing may be disrupted by several mechanisms: words may be misspelled (a disorder of language), letters may be malformed (dysmorphic letters suggest either constructional or ideomotor apraxia), or words may be misplaced on the page (a spatial disorder). *Pure agraphia* is the misspelling of words in the absence of gross aphasia, apraxia, or alexia. It is usually associated with focal left parietal lobe disease. It may occur in association with the other elements of Gerstmann's syndrome (dyscalculia, right-left confusion, and finger agnosia). *Aphasic agraphia* is impaired writing found in association with aphasia. Agraphia may occur with either fluent aphasia (e.g., Wernicke's) or nonfluent aphasia (e.g., Broca's). The writing deficit is at least as severe as the oral language deficit, although exceptions have been reported. *Apraxic agraphia* results from loss of the skilled motor programs necessary for writing. Handwriting is performed clumsily, and the letters are poorly formed. Other signs of ideomotor apraxia are usually present. Apraxic agraphia may follow damage to the left parietal lobe. Spatial agraphia may occur after right hemisphere injury. There is no aphasic deficit and words are properly spelled. However, left unilateral spatial neglect interferes with the correct placement of letters and words on the page. Constructional apraxia is often present as well.

Alexia

Pure alexia or *alexia without agraphia* is an acquired disorder of reading with preserved writing. Pure alexia is also known as *occipital alexia, posterior alexia, pure word blindness, verbal alexia,* and *receptive* or *sensory alexia.* Gross aphasia is absent, although mild degrees of anomia may be present. A right homonymous hemianopia regularly accompanies pure alexia, although rare cases without hemianopia have been reported. Color agnosia (the inability to name colors presented visually) frequently accompanies pure alexia. Typically, the lesion responsible for pure alexia is in the left occipital lobe and is large enough to involve both the left visual cortex and fibers crossing the splenium of the corpus callosum from the right visual cortex. Pure alexia may also occur after deep lesions near the angular gyrus. These subangular lesions presumably disconnect the angular gyrus from visual input. *Alexia with agraphia* is most commonly associated with lesions in the angular gyrus region. It is also known as *parietal alexia* or *aphasic alexia.* Both reading and writing are disturbed. A mild fluent aphasia often accompanies alexia with agraphia. Anomia and verbal paraphasias are often present. Visual field disturbances (either a right homonymous hemianopia or a right inferior quadrantanopia) are variably present. Elements of Gerstmann's syndrome and constructional apraxia often accompany alexia with agraphia. *Frontal alexia* is the alexia that occurs with frontal lobe damage and Broca's aphasia. Oral reading and reading comprehension are often limited to single substantive words, with little ability to read paragraph-length material aloud or for comprehension.

MANAGEMENT

Because aphasia, alexia, and agraphia reflect a brain disorder, definitive management depends on diagnosis of the underlying brain lesion. The efficacy of speech therapy for aphasia has been controversial. Evaluation of the efficacy of speech therapy requires controlling for many variables that influence recovery from aphasia, including age at onset (younger aphasic patients do better than older ones), size and site of lesion (patients with smaller lesions away from the central language zone do better than patients with larger lesions in the central language zone), etiology (those with hemorrhages tend to do better than those with infarctions), handedness (some studies have found that left-handed patients do better than right-handed ones), educational and socioeconomic backgrounds, neurobehavioral complications, motivation, insight into language deficits (patients with better insight into their deficits tend to do better), general health of the patient, quality of therapy available, and time elapsed before the onset of therapy. Within 1 to 2 weeks after a stroke or other brain injury, spontaneous recovery begins because of resolution of acute ischemia,

✔ *WHEN TO REFER*

With few exceptions, disordered spoken language (aphasia), disordered written language (alexia or agraphia), and nonlinguistic speech disorders (disordered articulation, disordered volume, and disordered melody) imply a disorder of the nervous system. Neurologic consultation is routinely sought to assist in determination of underlying lesion location, etiology, and management. Speech pathologists are consulted to assist in diagnosis and management of the aphasia, alexia, agraphia, or dysarthria. In some specialized centers, behavioral neurologists and cognitive neuropsychologists are available to assist in the diagnosis and management of these patients.

hemorrhage, or mass effect. A concomitant improvement in language function also occurs spontaneously. However, the mechanisms governing improvement in aphasia over the long term (months to years) are not understood. Many approaches to therapy have been taken, including both traditional approaches based on principles of education (reteaching language) and techniques aimed at facilitating recovery for specific types of linguistic deficits. In addition to providing therapy, the therapist accurately assesses the speech status of the patient and the psychologic support needed. Recent controlled studies have suggested that speech therapy may be efficacious in the recovery from aphasia, especially when motivation, insight, and comprehension are spared.

Language retraining is often attempted in instances of alexia or agraphia. Controlled studies of its usefulness are not available. A trial of speech therapy is useful for assessing its efficacy in instances of dysarthria or other nonlinguistic speech disorders.

BIBLIOGRAPHY

Albert ML, Helm-Estabrooks N: Diagnosis and treatment of aphasia. Parts I and II, *JAMA* 259:1043, 1205, 1988.
Damasio AR: Aphasia, *N Engl J Med* 326:531, 1992.
Hier DB, Gorelick PB, Shindler AG: *Topics in behavioral neurology and neuropsychology,* Stoneham, Mass, 1987, Butterworths.
Kirshner HS (editor): *Handbook of neurological speech and language disorders,* New York, 1995, Marcel Dekker.

III NEUROLOGIC DISEASES

CHAPTER

141 Epilepsy

John Davenport

PATHOPHYSIOLOGY

The term *epilepsy,* or *seizure disorder,* broadly denotes recurrent episodes of disturbed behavior caused by paroxysmal, uncontrolled, hypersynchronous discharges of cerebral neurons. Clinical seizure events are symptoms of intrinsic cerebral disease or of alteration of cerebral function by systemic conditions.

Epileptic hyperactivity arises in the complex circuitry of cerebral gray matter. The normal asynchronous activity of cerebral neurons becomes abnormally synchronized, and the firing characteristics of individual cells take on various stereotyped features, especially bursting patterns. When restricted to only a small portion of cerebral gray matter, this pathologic electrical activity is termed an *epileptogenic focus.* Such asymptomatic localized disturbances may spread by physiologic mechanisms to recruit anatomically contiguous gray matter, creating a larger abnormality and causing focal cerebral symptoms. They may also include more widely projecting connections within or between the hemispheres. When conditions are suitable, subcortical integrating mechanisms may become involved in the overall hyperactivity, resulting in a generalized discharge of the cerebral cortex and its downstream connections.

The great variety of clinical seizure symptoms and signs thus is derived from the interaction of several possible disturbances: (1) local alterations of cerebral cortex structure, either congenital or acquired, resulting in a tendency to abnormal synchronization; (2) metabolic factors that alter the firing characteristics of cortical cells; (3) individual variations of the interconnections between cortical and subcortical regions that integrate normal cerebral function; and (4) the maturation, evolution, and degeneration of brain tissues during childhood, adolescence, and adulthood. These multiple factors influence the threshold for seizure discharge, the route and speed of spread from a focal abnormality, the presence or absence of generalized convulsions, and the likelihood of recurrent attacks. The clinical patterns of individual seizures are determined by the physiologic functions of the brain areas where the discharge begins and through which it spreads.

CLINICAL SEIZURE PATTERNS

The archetype of epileptic seizures, the generalized tonic-clonic (GTC) convulsion (major motor, or grand mal seizure) (Box 141-1), is an impressive and frightening experience for both patient and observer. The patient abruptly ceases ongoing behavior and falls. There is rigid stiffening of the muscles, including those of the chest and abdomen, which causes cyanosis; garbled cry or groan occurs, and often the patient is incontinent of urine. This tonic phase gradually becomes interrupted by rhythmic clonic muscular jerking that gradually decreases in frequency and dies away. The ictal convulsion rarely lasts more than 2 or 3 minutes and leaves the patient in a limp, unresponsive state. Progressive recovery occurs in a postictal phase characterized by confusion, lethargy, headache, and diffuse myalgia, which lasts several hours or, less often, up to several days, until full baseline function is restored. The patient has only vague or no recall of the onset and no memory of the ictal events or of a portion of the postictal period.

A second common pattern is the *absence seizure (petit mal seizure),* wherein the patient, almost always a child, abruptly stops activity and stares vacantly, perhaps with a fluttering of the eyelids or minor changes in muscle tone or posture. A motor convulsion does not occur, and after only 5 to 10 seconds, the child quite abruptly

recovers to a completely normal state, with partial or complete amnesia of the period of staring.

Other less common generalized seizure types also occur primarily in infants and children, including *tonic seizures,* a sudden stiffening of trunk or limb muscles with loss of consciousness lasting 10 to 60 seconds; *myoclonic seizures,* manifested by single or multiple sudden jerks of limb muscles without altered consciousness; *clonic seizures,* with impaired consciousness and jerking lasting for several minutes and demonstrating quite variable distribution and symmetry; and *akinetic seizures,* with brief loss of tone with intact awareness, producing head nodding if involving only the neck muscles but, with more diffuse distribution, leading to falling and possible injury.

All these various types of *generalized seizures* are due to more or less widespread involvement of both hemispheres. In many attacks, however, restricted electrical discharge leads to a wide range of focal symptoms and signs, termed *partial seizures.*

Simple partial seizures may occur in the form of isolated, self-limited motor or sensory features. There can be rhythmic jerking of the hand or part of the face, turning of the head or eyes, speech arrest, or inarticulate vocalization when the precentral cortex is involved. Unpleasant paresthesias of limbs or face, clicking or buzzing sounds, flickering unformed light patterns, or foul smell or taste sensations may result from discharges in the various primary sensory cortical areas. More often, partial seizures are composed of a series of symptoms caused by a "march" of epileptic neuronal activity sequentially involving different cortical areas. *Jacksonian seizure* is the eponym applied to clonic movements gradually migrating from face to hand or the reverse, but this is only one of many diverse patterns of involvement of multiple cortical functions.

Extremely varied and complicated experiences result from activation of temporal-parietal association areas, with psychic symptoms of inappropriate familiarity (déjà vu) or unfamiliarity, detailed sensory distortions or hallucinations, intricate memory experiences, and "dreamy states." Emotions of anxiety, fear, or, less commonly, euphoria or ecstasy may be produced by activation of medial temporal areas. Any of these may be reported by the patient with intact consciousness and complete memory for the event, an essential criterion for *simple partial seizures* (SPS).

Complex partial seizures (CPSs), on the other hand, by definition have total or partial interruption of memory and consciousness. Patients usually have absent or inappropriate responsiveness to the environment during the ictus. These deficits correlate with discharge within the limbic system circuits in the medial temporal and frontal lobes of one or both hemispheres, including cingulate gyrus, hippocampus, and septal area.

CPS attacks often begin with a motionless stare that abruptly interrupts previous behavior. After only a few seconds, a second phase occurs, with stereotyped nonpurposeful movements, or *automatisms,* such as swallowing, lip-smacking, chewing, pacing, repetitive or fumbling hand movements, humming, or mumbling. This phase lasts a minute or so, during which the patient is amnestic and apparently unaware of the environment. After this there is a subtle transition to more environmental responsiveness, with more coordinated and purposeful activity, including intelligible verbalization, but with persistent amnesia. The ictal phase usually lasts 2 or 3 minutes—rarely more than 5 minutes—and is difficult to clearly distinguish from the period of postictal confusion. The stereotypic ictal automatisms have been related to discharge in the anteromedial temporal areas, near the amygdala nucleus, and are common and objective features of CPS attacks. Although CPSs usually arise from lesions in the temporal lobe (*temporal lobe epilepsy, psychomotor seizures),* they may be manifestations of pathology in the frontal or parietal lobes.

An *aura* is a brief sensation remembered by the patient before loss of consciousness occurs in a complex partial or generalized seizure. An aura indicates that the seizure began focally and, by its specific quality, suggests the seizure's anatomic focus. An aura lasting more than a few seconds is classified as an SPS; if it evolved to other stereotyped ictal signs without responsiveness or memory, it then would become a CPS, especially if an automatism occurs. A common example of a CPS would be a feeling of strange, fearful uneasiness, followed in a few seconds by an involuntary turning of the head to the side; then with lapse of memory, a smacking of lips and staring

---

BOX 141-1
Classification of epileptic seizures

Generalized (no detectable focus)
  Tonic-clonic (grand mal)
  Absence (petit mal)
  Tonic
  Myoclonic
  Clonic
  Akinetic
Partial (focal onset)
  Simple (consciousness intact)
    Motor
    Sensory
    Autonomic
    Psychic
  Complex (consciousness impaired)
    Simple onset, with later impairment of consciousness
    Impaired consciousness at onset
  Partial, evolving to secondarily generalized convulsion

BOX 141-2

Common causes of seizure

Metabolic factors, especially
  Hypoglycemia
  Hypoxia
  Hyponatremia
  Hypocalcemia
  Acid-base disturbances
  Organ failure: renal, hepatic
  Drug withdrawal: alcohol, sedatives
  Drug intoxication: aminophylline, lidocaine
Focal cortex lesions, including
  Infarction
  Contusion
  Tumor
  Abscess
  Meningitis
  Encephalitis
Congenital: hereditary or acquired
  Idiopathic
    Grand mal
    Petit mal
  Perinatal injury
  Maldevelopment
  Degenerations

---

lasting 2 minutes; and finally, a dazed and confused feeling for a period of 20 minutes.

Attacks of amnesia or staring spells occurring with other simple or complex patterns but without convulsion are often erroneously called "petit mal." Particularly in adulthood, such attacks are usually CPSs and imply a need for investigation of the responsible focal lesion. Similarly, seizures that appear to be classic nonfocal grand mal attacks may result from the rapid generalization of an initially focal discharge.

In childhood and early adolescence, approximately two thirds of patients with recurrent seizures have no detectable epileptic focus. In late adolescence and adulthood, the distribution inverts, and late-onset seizures are usually the result of acquired localized cerebral damage.

ETIOLOGY
Metabolic Causes

Cerebral neuronal function depends on critical supplies of glucose and oxygen, on electrolyte distribution across cell membranes, and on the detoxifying processes of visceral organs. In general, the more rapid the metabolic change, either from normality or back toward normality during therapeutic procedures, the more likely a seizure is to occur (Box 141-2). Seizures caused by metabolic disturbances are usually generalized motor convulsions, although partial seizures may result from hypoglycemia, and from hypocalcemia in neonates. Focal features appearing in these and other systemic derangements should be considered to have an underlying structural cause until it is reasonably demonstrated otherwise.

Single or even multiple seizures occurring in the context of an acute illness, with metabolic derangement, fever, and possible medication side effects, are not considered to be epilepsy. They are regarded as *provoked* or *symptomatic seizures*. With resolution of the illness the prognosis is usually good unless structural damage has occurred, and chronic antiepileptic drug treatment is unnecessary.

Focal Cortex Lesions

Any disease that results in damage to cortical tissue may cause a seizure and lead to a chronic epileptic disorder. Determining factors include the magnitude and acuteness of the derangement and the specific site of injury. The temporal and basal frontal lobes and the primary motor and sensory areas of the cortex are more likely to support epileptic dysrhythmias than are the parietal and occipital lobes, in part because of their extensive limbic and thalamic connections. A partial or generalized seizure may occur at the time of an ischemic stroke, or brain hemorrhage. Some patients may first have seizures several months after the acute event, following evolution of the cortical scar. Seizures occur rarely in transient ischemic attacks (TIAs).

Head trauma may cause epileptogenic cortical scarring as a result of brain laceration by depressed fracture or penetrating wounds. More frequently, closed head injuries are associated with contusions of the frontal or temporal lobes. There is usually delayed onset of partial or secondarily generalized seizures; they may occur 6 months to a few years after the traumatic incident. The risk of late epilepsy is directly related to the duration of posttraumatic stupor and identifiable local brain contusion, hematoma, or direct penetration.

A partial or generalized seizure may be the first symptom of brain tumor, either primary or metastatic. Seizures occur in about one third of tumor patients sometime during the course of illness; low-grade primary neoplasms occasionally are discovered after many years of follow-up for idiopathic epilepsy. The highest incidence of epilepsy caused by cerebral tumors occurs in middle-aged or elderly adults, particularly those with partial seizure patterns.

Acute bacterial and viral infections may be complicated by partial or generalized seizures precipitated by multiple pathophysiologic factors, including fever, dehydration, cerebritis, and abscess formation. The seizure may be one of the earliest clinical manifestations of the illness, but an infectious process can usually be determined easily by physical and cerebrospinal fluid (CSF) examination. A chronic seizure disorder may follow successful medical treatment of the infection.

Congenital Causes

The importance of genetic factors has been demonstrated for certain childhood epilepsies. For example, the 3/s spike-wave electroencephalogram (EEG) abnormality of petit mal appears to be inherited as an autosomal dominant trait. A family history of seizures is statistically more likely to be obtained from patients with epilepsy beginning in childhood (7.5%) than in adulthood (1.5%) but still does not define the individual patient's condition as familial or idiopathic. Rather, it indicates a possible contribution of lowered seizure threshold for physiologic stresses such as sleep deprivation, fever, hyperventilation, certain repetitive stimuli (e.g., light flashes), and psychic turmoil. Maturation of the infant brain that is maldeveloped or has been damaged in the perinatal period may produce seizures at any time during later life but most commonly in the first decade. Any of the rare hereditary cerebral degenerations may manifest seizures at some point in the clinical course.

Statistically, the most common seizure disorders are the idiopathic petit mal and grand mal types in which no structural lesion is apparent. It is common that patients with no epileptic EEG focus or defined lesion by computed tomography (CT) or magnetic resonance imaging (MRI) are said to have idiopathic epilepsy. There is some danger in this description, in that an erroneous presumption arises that no focus ever will be found, and that a hereditary condition that may be transmittable to offspring is present. It is preferable to maintain an uncommitted position and regard such cases as cryptogenic; only after many years may some neoplastic or degenerative process show other unmistakable signs of its presence.

DIAGNOSIS AND LABORATORY EVALUATION

The proper management of seizure disorders rests on a complete and accurate characterization of the patient's symptoms and confidence that they are epileptic events. Because the physician rarely sees the patient during the attack itself, the usual evaluation during the postictal or interictal period depends on reports of other observers and on the patient's recollection, compromised as that may be by amnesia for ictal and postictal periods. Occasionally, the epileptic nature of the event may be obscured by the failure to elicit a description of a familiar seizure pattern. In dealing with such unusual and occasionally bizarre episodes, one should remember that diagnostic characteristics of seizure events include the following:
1. *A sudden alteration of behavior.* Typically, a seizure abruptly and unpredictably interrupts the normal flow of subjective and objec-

Table 141-1   Differential diagnosis of epilepsy

DISORDER	UNLIKE EPILEPSY	LIKE EPILEPSY
Syncope	Premonitory symptoms Precipitating factors Diffuse fading vision	Myoclonic jerks or tonic stiffening, on occasion
Transient ischemic attack	No "march" of symptoms No jerks, twitches No loss of consciousness, amnesia Brain stem symptoms	Focal EEG slowing Normal examination between attacks
Migraine	Prominent headache Preserved consciousness	Focal symptoms Focal EEG slowing
Hypoglycemia	Temporal relationship to fasting Initial sympathetic discharge	Focal symptoms and EEG slowing Loss of consciousness Postictal headache, confusion
Paroxysmal vertigo	Preserved consciousness Monosymptomatic spells Auditory, vestibular abnormalities	Severe temporary disability
Narcolepsy	Cataplexy Appropriate sleep behavior with attacks	Hallucinations Inappropriate, unpredictable timing of attacks
Psychogenic spells	Event-related Stressful context Lack of autonomic features Lack of incontinence	Dramatic convulsive behavior

tive brain function. Only infrequently do patients have seizures precipitated by specific external events or stimuli or characterized by a slow crescendo of symptoms.

2. *Stereotyped patterns.* Although almost any human behavior can be produced by a seizure, the epileptic attacks of a given patient have only one or a few recurring patterns. The march of symptoms is predictable from one attack to the next. The occurrence of a tonic-clonic convulsion as the cause of a brief unwitnessed amnestic period may reasonably be inferred from the strong circumstantial evidence of headache, myalgia, sluggish mentation, lethargy, sleep craving, and gingival-labial contusions.

3. *Alteration of consciousness.* Loss of awareness, ranging from mild confusion to coma during the attack and various degrees of amnesia after it, should suggest epilepsy. If memory is preserved, the patient's recollected description should be consistent and clear.

4. *Brief duration.* The ictal period rarely lasts more than 4 or 5 minutes. The postictal period may be prolonged but has the characteristics of progressive normalization of function.

Careful history taking from the patient and all potential witnesses is of central importance in the diagnosis of seizures and deserves the utmost respect. Without this salient information, mistakes in evaluation and management are frequently made and are seldom adequately corrected by resort to laboratory testing. Even sophisticated computerized imaging and electrophysiologic technologies are limited in their diagnostic power by the context of the clinical problem at hand.

Table 141-1 lists other common disorders often considered in the differential diagnosis of epilepsy.

Once a seizure disorder is suspected or proved on clinical grounds, prompt medical evaluation is indicated to assess the clinical implication of the epileptic symptoms and to set a course of management. The neurologic examination is usually normal in patients with a seizure disorder, even in those with structural lesions. If focal neurologic abnormalities are present, however, they are often enhanced immediately after a seizure. The cortical anatomic correlation of the postictal focal signs is a clue to the site of the epileptogenic focus. Postictal focal abnormalities can be of any type (e.g., aphasia, hemianopsia, sensory deficit, conjugate gaze preference). Transient localized weakness that follows a convulsion is called *Todd's paralysis.*

The EEG holds special prominence in the diagnosis of epilepsy because of its exclusive ability to record and characterize the pathophysiologic electrical events. The EEG abnormalities that confirm a clinical diagnosis of epilepsy include sharp or spike discharges, spike-and-slow-wave patterns, and other paroxysmal rhythmic activity having anomalous location or form, all of which are evidence of pathologic hypersynchrony. In addition, the EEG may demonstrate a nonspecific localized slow-wave pattern that indicates the presence of a

focal lesion, of which the seizure itself is a symptom. Because both slow and sharp abnormalities may be more prominent immediately after a seizure, *early postictal recording of the EEG is highly desirable.* Finally, EEG abnormalities roughly parallel the frequency and severity of clinical manifestations. A repeatedly normal EEG in the presence of frequent clinical attacks should suggest another pathophysiologic diagnosis.

The diagnostic yield of epileptic EEG abnormalities may be increased with hyperventilation or photic stimulation, or by recording the EEG during sleep, as it may occur in a routine session, by induction with mild sedation, or by recording in the morning after overnight sleep deprivation. A potential pitfall is that an epileptic discharge on EEG may mislocalize a structural abnormality. Specific localization must be made with other clinical and imaging techniques.

Limitations of the EEG should be recognized. Because it is a short temporal sampling of relatively brief episodic events, a single interictal EEG recording may fail to disclose any abnormality in an epileptic patient. As a consequence, *a normal EEG does not rule out epilepsy.* Of course, a specific EEG pattern is not required for diagnosis if epilepsy is undeniably present on clinical grounds. In this situation a normal study reduces the likelihood of serious pathology and can serve as documentation of cerebral electrical status for future comparison.

It should be emphasized that the diagnosis of epilepsy is primarily clinical, by the characterization of the attacks, supported by EEG evidence. One should therefore insist that EEG support be very convincing if the clinical information is incomplete, and be wary of overreading EEG studies that may be "compatible with epilepsy."

Although systemic metabolic derangements may be more or less obvious, specific investigation for occult abnormalities may substantially alter the diagnostic and therapeutic approach to the patient. Successful treatment of a systemic disturbance may control all seizures without antiepileptic drug therapy. Conversely, if metabolic disturbances are not corrected, attempts to suppress seizures with drugs will be unsatisfactory.

Evaluation of a partial seizure logically begins with clinical consideration of potential sources of cerebral pathology: a history of strokelike events, incidents of head trauma, or symptoms suggestive of progressing malignancy. Standard CT scanning, with or without contrast enhancement, is recommended in every patient to identify treatable structural conditions, especially neoplasms. The great majority of these scans are normal or show nonspecific abnormalities, such as atrophy. MRI (see Chapter 132) is more sensitive than CT in documenting epileptogenic lesions in temporal or frontal lobes, especially for the small atrophic scars resulting from cortical contusion and subtle white matter intensities after infection or concussion. The relatively high cost of MRI makes routine use inadvisable; rather,

---

BOX 141-3
Seizure diagnosis

Detailed history: outside observers
General and neurologic examinations
EEG: waking, sleeping
Metabolic evaluation
    Electrolytes, calcium
    Glucose
    Acid-base status
    BUN, liver function tests
    Serum (or urine) drug screen
Structural lesion evaluation
    CT scan, MRI
    Lumbar puncture
    Angiography

MRI should be considered in patients with suboptimal control from medical therapy, especially those being evaluated for surgery.

Cerebral angiography is reserved for detailed evaluation of suspected vascular lesions, especially arteriovenous malformations, suspected embolic stroke in young patients, and some neoplasms. After a focal mass has been excluded by CT, lumbar puncture and CSF analysis may help resolve suspicions of bleeding, inflammation, and infection in the pertinent setting. Routine CSF study is not advised.

The extent and urgency of the diagnostic evaluation depend on the clinical status of the patient. In all cases, initial seizures must be investigated promptly. It is advisable to hospitalize the patient so that complete and perhaps repeated assessment can be made of the neurologic status. A careful search for a structural lesion—occult in the case of a generalized convulsion—should be completed soon after the first patient contact. This should include a CT scan, a metabolic screen, and, in certain cases, a lumbar puncture (Box 141-3). In addition, the potential seriousness of the incident can be communicated to the patient, and a plan for antiepileptic drug treatment can be formulated.

Two common types of metabolic seizures deserve special discussion. In *febrile seizures,* there is hereditary predisposition to experience brief generalized convulsions with sudden elevation of body temperature. This condition is essentially confined to children between 6 months and 5 years of age. With a relatively brief history of illness caused by a nonspecific viral infection, the child abruptly has a convulsion that lasts only a few minutes. There are no focal components, the neurologic examination discloses no sign of cerebral disease, and routine metabolic studies are normal. There is often a family history of epilepsy, including other febrile episodes. A lumbar puncture is usually advisable at the time of the first seizure, to be certain there is no CNS infection, and in other circumstances when the convulsion is prolonged beyond 10 minutes, focal or lateralized ictal or postictal features are present, or if there are other clues of suboptimal cerebral function. Although febrile seizures can recur, prophylactic antiepileptic drug therapy is usually not required unless the seizures are atypical or neurologic impairment is present.

Alcohol withdrawal seizures are encountered in patients with chronic alcoholism. In the setting of an alcoholic debauch, often with nutritional impairment, the patient has a generalized convulsion and is brought to the hospital. There is a history of relative abstinence, although the blood alcohol level may still be elevated. The patient recovers from the convulsion rapidly, with normal neurologic function and early signs of the abstinence syndrome of mild anxiety, tachycardia, and tremulousness. Several brief seizures may occur while the patient is being evaluated, but the attacks are essentially self-limited. If focal signs are present during the attack or in the postictal period, CT scanning is recommended because these patients often are self-neglectful and have poor memory, and they may sustain head injury. If the convulsions are prolonged, acute loading with phenobarbital is indicated. Hospitalization and treatment for the abstinence syndrome are advisable, since many patients proceed to develop delirium tremens. Chronic antiepileptic drug therapy is not indicated.

TREATMENT

Once systemic diseases, acute metabolic derangements, and progressive cerebral diseases have been excluded by appropriate testing, the patient can be assured that the attacks will probably be successfully suppressed with antiepileptic drugs (AEDs) (Tables 141-2 and 141-3). Three fourths of adults with recurring seizures have a major reduction of seizure frequency, and more than half achieve complete control.

Primary generalized seizures, both grand mal and petit mal types, are most easily suppressed; partial attacks—particularly complex partial seizures—are less successfully handled. Patients with multiple seizure types or progressive lesions usually experience more difficulty.

Effective AED treatment is promoted by attention to the following considerations.

1. Treatment with a single AED (monotherapy) is the ideal strategy to maximize control and minimize side effects. Start with an effective dose and increase the dose until seizure control is achieved or clinical toxicity occurs.
2. Use blood AED concentrations judiciously in assessing both undertreatment and overtreatment. If there are no recurrent seizures or overt clinical toxicity, one or two samples in the first 2 months of therapy confirm compliance and allow early revision of the dose schedule. After any change of dose, four or five drug half-lives must elapse before stable blood concentrations are achieved. The local laboratory values for the "therapeutic range" should be considered as an initial target. Some patients require high doses and plasma levels for suppression of clinical seizures.
3. If the first-choice drug is inadequate or not tolerated, it should be stopped and another agent established. Some simultaneous treatment with both drugs may be appropriate temporarily to avoid seizure recurrence.
4. Subjective neurotoxicity is the most common factor causing discontinuation of AED agents. Laboratory evidence of systemic toxicity is less common. *Minor and temporary alterations in blood cell counts and hepatic enzyme levels are frequent and should not prompt AED discontinuation unless associated clinical symptoms appear or values progressively worsen.*

After lengthy development and clinical trials, several new AEDs have become available in the last few years. They show promise for improving seizure control for those patients in whom standard AEDs fail (see Table 141-2). Because of their novelty, their use should be accompanied by increased surveillance for systemic and neurologic toxicity, beyond the caution exercised with established AEDs. With more widespread experience, their overall role in medical seizure management will become established.

Status Epilepticus

In generalized tonic-clonic status epilepticus, there are continuous or frequent and repeated convulsions without recovery of full consciousness. It requires prompt and vigorous treatment to prevent major morbidity and mortality from hypoxia, hyperthermia, hypoglycemia, and acidosis. Mortality increases proportionately with the duration of the convulsions. In the emergency room or intensive care setting, pathogenic mechanisms must be defined and treatment instituted simultaneously (Box 141-4). The airway and ventilation must be ensured, intravenous lines established, and blood obtained for glucose and electrolyte levels and antiepileptic and toxic drug determinations. Arterial blood gases and pH also should be measured. The patient then should be given 25 g glucose intravenously, as well as 50 mg thiamine. Acidosis should be treated with intravenous bicarbonate.

These maneuvers may be facilitated by temporarily suppressing active convulsions with diazepam, 5 to 10 mg given intravenously over 1 to 2 minutes.

The history of illness must be obtained simultaneously. Anticonvulsant drug withdrawal or noncompliance in treated epileptics is often at fault. Other common causes are brain trauma, neoplasms, infections, and major metabolic derangements.

In addition to terminating the seizures, it is important to prevent

Table 141-2 Antiepileptic drugs in common use

GENERIC NAME	TRADE NAME	TYPICAL ADULT DOSE RANGE (MG/DAY)	TARGET PLASMA LEVEL (μg/ml)	SERUM HALF-LIFE (H)	SIDE EFFECTS DOSE-DEPENDENT	SIDE EFFECTS IDIOSYNCRATIC
Carbamazepine	Tegretol	600-1200	4-12	15	Ataxia, diplopia, nystagmus	Hyponatremia, rash, aplastic anemia
Phenytoin	Dilantin	300-400	10-20	24	Ataxia, nystagmus, gingival hyperplasia	Rash, lymphadenopathy
Valproate	Depakote	1000-2500	50-100	12	Gastric distress, alopecia, weight gain	Tremor, hepatic failure, decreased platelets
Phenobarbital	Luminal	60-180	15-40	96	Sedation, ataxia, blurred vision	Hyperactivity
Primidone	Mysoline	500-1500	5-10	16	Sedation, ataxia, blurred vision	
Ethosuximide	Zarontin	750-1500	40-100	36	Ataxia, sedation, gastric distress, headache	Rash
Clonazepam	Klonopin	1-4	None	30	Sedation, ataxia	

Table 141-3 Seizure types and preferred drug treatment

SEIZURE TYPE	PREFERRED AGENTS
Generalized tonic-clonic	Carbamazepine Phenytoin Valproate
Simple and complex partial	Carbamazepine Phenytoin
Absence	Ethosuximide Valproate
Myoclonic	Valproate Clonazepam
Status epilepticus (generalized)	Diazepam/phenytoin Phenobarbital Lorazepam

BOX 141-4

Management of generalized status epilepticus in adults

1. Observe seizures briefly while getting history: consider pseudoseizures.
2. Give diazepam, 10 mg IV, to arrest convulsion.
3. Start IVs; intubate trachea; draw blood samples; give glucose 25 g, thiamine 50 mg, calcium gluconate 100 mg IV. Reexamine briefly.
4. Begin phenytoin infusion, 18 mg/kg, 50 mg/min maximum rate, with ECG and BP monitoring: expect convulsions to subside during or soon after phenytoin loading.
5. If seizures are uncontrolled, give phenobarbital 3-5 mg/kg IV over 5-10 min; expect prompt control.
6. If seizures are uncontrolled, assess plasma AED levels (phenytoin >30, phenobarbital >45), plasma glucose, oxygenation, and acidosis; give bicarbonate; get experienced neurologic advice.
7. If seizures are controlled, give maintenance AED.

their recurrence. This is accomplished by treating the underlying pathogenic abnormality (an important point often neglected) and by administering antiepileptic drugs that rapidly penetrate brain tissue and also have long-lasting effects. Careful monitoring of the patient is required to avoid respiratory and circulatory failure and other complications of coma.

Many methods of drug treatment have been recommended for status epilepticus. Occasionally, two or three 5- to 10-mg doses of diazepam given intravenously permanently terminate the seizures. More often, the rapid redistribution of diazepam to noncerebral tissue allows seizures to recur, and repeated doses lead to undesirable sedative toxicity without achieving lasting seizure control.

Intravenous phenytoin is the drug of choice for adult status epilepticus. The usual loading dose is 15 to 20 mg/kg body weight. It should be given no faster than 50 mg/min, while respiration, blood pressure, and the electrocardiogram (ECG) are monitored. Attempts to give phenytoin more rapidly may cause hypotension or cardiac arrest, especially in the elderly. Phenytoin loading takes 30 to 60 minutes, and seizures should come under lasting control within another 30 minutes. The plasma concentration can then be maintained either intravenously or orally. Phenobarbital likewise can be given intravenously rapidly enough to control seizures and also can provide long-term maintenance. It is limited primarily by its sedative side effects but is the drug of first choice in patients known to be intolerant of phenytoin and in children under 15 years old. Phenobarbital can be given secondarily to patients who have not been controlled by phenytoin as described previously. The recommended loading dose is 3 to 5 mg/kg body weight for adults, given over 1 to 2 minutes. Up to 10 to 15 mg/kg may be given to children. Phenobarbital may interact with previously administered diazepam to cause respiratory arrest during the infusion. If seizures continue after another 30 minutes, a second dose of the same size may be administered, and maintenance doses are given after seizures are controlled.

Intravenous lorazepam (Ativan) is an alternative to diazepam for

initial seizure control. Its longer duration of antiepileptic action, related to distribution kinetics, reduces the occurrence of early seizure relapse and is thus an advantage in the acute situation. It may avoid the complications of high-dose rapid phenytoin or phenobarbital loading. This use of lorazepam has not yet been approved for general application and is now undergoing controlled clinical study.

Status epilepticus refractory to both phenytoin and phenobarbital usually is caused by unresolved serious metabolic disturbances, drug toxicity, cerebral trauma, or infection. Experienced neurologic advice is recommended at that point to help choose between several less well-established and controversial treatments.

In general, status epilepticus is best controlled by adequate drug dosage given intravenously so that effective brain concentrations are reached as rapidly as possible. Intramuscular or rectal administration may avoid some intravenous toxicity but because of delayed absorption and low plasma levels fails to attain the primary therapeutic goal. A leisurely approach is likely to fall short, and the physician should remain immediately available until seizure control is achieved.

Partial seizures may also be persistent, typically as focal motor status (continuous partial epilepsy, epilepsia partialis continua), most commonly with repetitive arm or face jerking, or psychomotor status, consisting of frequent behavioral automatisms with partial or complete amnesia. Although assessment and prompt AED management are desirable to avoid generalized status, these conditions are less hazardous to life and cerebral function and are often considerably more difficult to control. The aggressive protocol outlined previously should be tempered to avoid AED overdosage, particularly when consciousness is minimally disturbed. If plasma levels of phenytoin are 25 to 30 µg/ml and of phenobarbital are 35 to 40 µg/ml, further increases are unlikely to improve the situation.

Relatively uncommon is the syndrome of nonconvulsive status epilepticus. A patient, usually with a seizure history, becomes stuporous or confused for hours or days but has had no obvious convulsion. Subtle nystagmoid conjugate ocular movements and random facial twitches or limb myoclonic jerks may indicate the true pathophysiology. An urgent bedside EEG shows a chaotic pattern with hypersynchrony or spike discharges, which can be suppressed easily with small quantities of diazepam, 1 to 2 mg intravenously, occasionally with prompt arousal of the subject as well.

Pseudoseizures

In some patients, episodes of convulsive or nonconvulsive seizure-like behavior can result from psychogenic influences. Pseudoseizure attacks have a superficial resemblance to true epilepsy but characteristically occur in a provocative or emotionally charged setting, have unusual convulsions consisting of alternating "thrashing" limb movements without bilateral symmetric features, and lack the autonomic discharge and pathologic reflex findings characteristic of organic epilepsy. Nonconvulsive, CPS-like attacks may present as episodes of amnesia, rage, or aggressive outbursts, staring spells, or any kind of "funny feeling" that may be misinterpreted by the patient as being of epileptic origin. The EEG is normal during the ictus, although it is often obscured and rendered unreliable by movement artifact, and normal waking EEG patterns are present immediately afterward, with no postictal slowing. Although in some instances the attacks may be under full voluntary control (malingering), it is more likely that the patient suffers from a psychiatric disorder, including but not limited to classic hysteria or conversion disorder following the usual psychiatric criteria.

Many patients with pseudoseizures have an organic seizure disorder as well, and a confident differential diagnosis may be difficult even for an experienced observer. Evaluation should include careful clinical observation of the attacks, including provocation of one or more spells by suggestion, preferably with the patient in the EEG laboratory.

An additional objective test is measurement of serum prolactin, which is temporarily elevated after GTC or CPS events. To use this test to identify true seizures, the blood sample must be obtained within 20 minutes of the episode and compared to a control sample drawn exactly 24 hours later to account for normal diurnal variation of the hormone.

The suspicion of pseudoseizures in an epileptic patient demands a careful assessment of both AED and nondrug management. AEDs may have been increased in number or dosage in an attempt to stop the attacks, and reduction of dosage may be followed by improvement. It is essential to view pseudoseizures as psychiatric symptoms, requiring evaluation of the emotional and interpersonal stresses generating them. Although formal psychologic or psychiatric referral is usually helpful and sometimes necessary, the primary physician has a great advantage in defining the medical and epileptic context of the spells and in providing the patient with emotional support.

PSYCHOLOGIC ISSUES AND BEHAVIOR CHANGES

In some cases, the presence of epilepsy is associated with long-term changes in behavior and personality. This phenomenon is extremely variable among patients. It is at least multifactorial, the result of underlying personality traits, the effects of any structural lesions on cerebral function, the frequency and type of seizures, medication side effects, and ill-defined factors of self-perception and esteem. The relative contribution of these components is often difficult to resolve and considerable controversy has arisen regarding many practical and theoretic details, such as whether certain seizure foci lead to specific emotional reactions, or how much effect some medications have on cognition.

Prognosis

The natural history of seizure disorders is extremely varied and is influenced by heredity, age at onset, frequency of attacks and multi-

plicity of patterns, permanent brain injury, and perhaps promptness and adequacy of AED seizure control. The initial diagnostic uncertainties and many possible seizure factors make calculation of the future of a single patient unreliable. After a single unprovoked seizure (i.e., one not related to acute and transient metabolic stress), the risk of further attacks is a matter of some controversy, recurrence within 2 years being reported to vary in prevalence between 30% and 70%. Because of this uncertainty, many neurologists recommend no AED treatment until a second seizure occurs, unless a higher risk of recurrence can be presumed on the basis of clinical, EEG, or CT scan evidence that a structural lesion is present. This is especially true for children, in whom brain maturation may reduce future risks. If seizures occur after age 30, on the other hand, a structural lesion is highly probable even without independent evidence, and the social morbidity of even one more seizure may justify a more aggressive approach, with single-drug AED therapy given for 2 to 5 years.

After an appropriate (but admittedly arbitrary) seizure-free period, consideration may be given to AED withdrawal, accomplished by slow reduction of daily doses, changes being made at monthly or even longer intervals. Rapid discontinuation may precipitate status epilepticus. The patient must be counseled about the possibility of future seizures even if the withdrawal period is uneventful, particularly with adults, who must decide whether the disruption of life attendant with seizure recurrence is worth risking.

Intractable Seizures

Some patients continue to have seizures despite therapeutic efforts— always a frustrating experience for both physician and patient. In this situation, several possibilities should be considered.

1. The patient is receiving inadequate drug treatment, because of either noncompliance, as assessed by blood levels, or the physician's failure to press dosages to clinical toxicity.
2. The specific seizure type has been incorrectly diagnosed and inappropriate AEDs prescribed (e.g., ethosuximide for petit mal when the problem is in fact a CPS atypical absence).
3. The patient is receiving multidrug therapy with sedative side effects that increase the tendency for seizures to occur.
4. Some or all of the attacks are pseudoseizures.
5. The epilepsy truly is medically refractory.

Surgery for Epilepsy

Specific excision of cortex proven to be the source of the patient's typical seizures can be considered for medically refractory patients who have definitively localized seizure foci lying in anterior temporal lobes, the most common site, or in other locations where resection will not cause neurologic handicap. Other patient selection factors include lack of progressive pathology (e.g., tumor), relative youth, preserved intelligence, and psychologic stability. Both noninvasive and invasive techniques of localization have been considerably refined in recent years, and reliable prognosis for improved seizure control can be given to most patients after intensive evaluation.

Chronic Care

Despite the statistically good prognosis for AED control of seizures, there is considerable need for the physician to maintain continuous and constructive contact with the patient with epilepsy. The unpredictability and dramatic appearance of the seizures often have serious consequences for the patient's personal and social life. Some occupations involving hazardous working conditions may no longer be possible, and the patient may require vocational rehabilitation. Life and health insurance policies may have to be renegotiated. Driving motor vehicles must be interdicted, except for individuals with significant warning or restricted partial symptoms. The emotional stress of having such a potentially serious and often mysterious illness can cause important psychologic effects that may be more difficult to manage than the seizures themselves. The need for conscientious daily drug treatment requires full understanding and acceptance of the condition by the patient. Supportive physician-patient interaction is the key to effective use of all available resources.

✔ *WHEN TO REFER*

In cases in which the differential diagnosis of epilepsy is undecided (see Table 141-1), one should seek diagnostic help from a neurologist before committing a patient to expectant AED treatment for even a short time. Because seizures beginning in adulthood are usually symptoms of acquired cerebral disease, neurologic consultation is valuable when the underlying condition is not clearly characterized. When seizures are not promptly controlled by one or a second AED, and in cases of status epilepticus, neurologic advice should be obtained. When there are ongoing difficulties with family, workplace, or other psychosocial matters, referral to both psychology or psychiatry and neurology consultants is highly desirable, with a full discussion between them of all interrelated medical and nonmedical issues.

Patients with uncontrolled seizures of any type should be referred to special inpatient units for intensive monitoring. The basic technology available is continuous simultaneous recording of EEG and patient activity on videotape for up to 2 to 3 weeks. Both seizure events and interictal EEG patterns can be evaluated by a multidisciplinary team with neurologic, neurosurgical, pharmacologic, and psychologic expertise. Special procedures such as cerebral metabolic studies and intracranial electrode placements can be performed to document and critically define seizure types and their anatomic origins. For patients without a defined focus or with diffuse or otherwise unresectable disease, enrollment in protocols investigating new AED agents may be an option.

BIBLIOGRAPHY

Brodie MJ, Dichter MA: Antiepileptic drugs, *N Engl J Med* 334:168-175, 1996.
Delgado-Escueta AV, Bacsal FE, Treiman DM: Complex partial seizures on closed-circuit television and EEG: a study of 691 attacks in 79 patients, *Ann Neurol* 11:292, 1982.
Engel J: *Seizures and epilepsy,* Philadelphia, 1989, FA Davis.
Engel J: Surgery for seizures, *N Engl J Med* 334:647-652, 1996.
Porter RJ: *Epilepsy: 100 elementary principles,* ed 2, Philadelphia, 1989, WB Saunders.
Working Group on Status Epilepticus: Treatment of convulsive status epilepticus, *JAMA* 270:854-859, 1993.

CHAPTER

142 Cognitive Failure Dementia

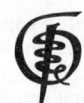

Thomas M. Walshe III

SYNDROMES OF MENTAL FAILURE

When a human being loses the traits that control behavior and the ability to process information adequately, the cause is a failure in cerebral function. The general concept of brain failure is akin to that of heart failure: either can arise from many causes, can be transient or progressive, can be of several types, and can vary in the localization of pathologic effects. Cerebral failure causes the human being to deviate from his or her established character, personality, bearing, and intellect. Specific losses of language and praxis may also accompany the changes in behavior. In the most general sense, cerebral failure may produce disorders of thought and mood (psychiatric diseases) or disorders of memory and cognition (neurologic diseases). The mind, however, is not compartmentalized by medical specialty, so a person having a thought disorder (e.g., schizophrenia) may have signs of cognitive failure, and a patient with dementia (e.g., Alzheimer's disease) may have signs of a mood disorder. The overlap of clinical signs is a pervasive theme in the description of disorders that alter mental function. Abnormality of cerebral function alters the relationships between language, memory, affect, and the innumerable other aspects that underlie human performance. Specific lesions of the system produce expected mental status changes but always in context of the system as a whole.

When the brain first begins to fail, the deficit may disrupt only subtle personal relationships or may interfere with the execution of complex tasks. Such changes are hardly measurable by clinical methods and are often reported not as failures in cognition, but as vague medical or emotional complaints. If the deficit becomes worse, the patient fails at home, at work, and in other social interactions, making the source of the problem obvious. There are several signs of cognitive failure, each with its own neurologic features and underlying pathologic causes.

Dementia

The neurologic sign of dementia comprises failure of learning, loss of memory, and loss of analytical ability. Patients are alert (when not treated with drugs) and attentive to the given task but fail because of memory deficits. In most cases dementia is recognized as existing over months or years. Dementia seldom occurs acutely and then it is usually overshadowed by other medical or neurologic deficits that delay its diagnosis. Dementia associated with stroke and HIV-associated dementia are notable examples. In focal neurologic diseases, dementia coexists with other signs, such as aphasia (failure of language) and apraxia (failure to execute learned tasks). When memory alone is lost and other cognitive powers remain largely intact, the mental state is described as *amnesia*. Amnesia is a neurologic sign associated with specific brain lesions and may occur in neurotic patients who have no gross brain lesions. The causes of dementia are usually diseases of the brain itself.

Confusional States

The neurologic sign of confusion combines inattention, apathy, and somnolence. Poor organization of information prevents a coherent sequence of thought. Specific memories may be preserved, although they appear out of context and so distorted that the patient cannot answer questions correctly. Language is preserved. Confusional states occur over short periods (hours or days). The causes of confusion are usually found outside the skull, and the cerebral failure often is reversible. Delirium is a confusional state in which hyperactivity replaces apathy. The archetype for delirium is the syndrome of acute alcohol withdrawal, *delirium tremens.* The quiet confusional state may lead to coma, whereas it is unusual for the delirious patient to progress to coma.

The neurologic signs dementia, amnesia, confusion, and delirium are caused by specific disorders. They may coexist, and because they are similar in many ways, they may not always be clearly separated. However, it is worth attempting to determine by the history and physical examination which sign is dominant in the case, so that one can focus on the most likely diagnostic possibilities. When the dominant sign is dementia, an organized approach often leads to the diagnosis.

APPROACH TO THE DEMENTED PATIENT

Dementia, as any clinical sign, requires an evaluation to determine which of the several possible disorders is the cause. The character of the dementia and its natural history as determined by the clinical history help to narrow the possibilities. History taken from the patient and the family reveals the mode of onset, the speed of progression (if any), drug history, and associated illnesses or complaints. The physical examination discloses the severity of the cognitive failure, the presence of other neurologic signs, and clues to underlying medical illness. Using this data a clinical picture takes shape so that the syndrome begins to fit broadly into the several groups of disease in which dementia is the primary sign: dementia alone, dementia with medical signs, dementia with variable neurologic signs, and dementia as part of a neurologic syndrome. Epidemiologic data also help. The most prevalent dementia, especially among the elderly seen in the outpatient setting, is Alzheimer's disease (AD). In inpatient populations the frequency of vascular dementia is very high. Among patients older than 65 years, however, the diagnostic imperative is to separate other disorders, some of which can be cured, from AD.

Brain imaging technology (magnetic resonance imaging [MRI], single photon emission computed tomography [SPECT], positron-emission tomography [PET]) simplifies the identification of obvious anatomic lesions that cause dementia. When the image fails to show a lesion, analysis of the history and physical signs, properly construed, provide the basis for a diagnosis. Much more important, the clinical data must be coupled with the anatomic abnormalities on the images lest the naive clinician be seduced by the sirens of technology from the true course.

DEMENTIA WITHOUT OTHER NEUROLOGIC OR MEDICAL SIGNS

Alzheimer's disease is an age-related disorder. In a community study in East Boston, Massachusetts, the prevalence of dementia was 10%. The prevalence rose steeply with age so that in persons older than 85 years, the rate was 47%. In that community 84% of the demented persons were diagnosed to have AD. Other community studies estimate the prevalence of dementia somewhat lower. AD is estimated to have a 6% to 10% prevalence in patients over age 65 years. Because it is so common, AD must enter into the differential diagnosis of any adult patient who is found to have dementia. By knowing the clinical features of AD and the disorders that resemble it, the clinician can usually make the diagnosis. AD occurs in patients as young as 40, but is extremely rare in younger patients. AD occurs in some families as an autosomal dominant trait, and the onset is early.

In AD the cortical neurons degenerate along with their axons, so the white matter of the brain shrinks and the cerebral ventricles enlarge. The temporal, frontal, and parietal lobes bear the brunt of the disease. The occipital lobes show fewer changes, and the posterior fossa contents are usually not affected. Microscopic examination shows neuronal loss with neurofibrillary and granulovacuolar degeneration.

The pathogenesis of the underlying lesions in AD is a target of active research. The hallmarks of the disease are the β-amyloid plaques in the neuropil and the neurofibrillary tangles in the neurons. β-amyloid deposition is of two types. In one type there is a diffuse noncompacted amyloid deposition, which is not associated with dystrophic neurites or neurofibrillary changes. This type of deposition occurs often in the brains of old persons without overt dementia. The other type of plaque is a compacted β-amyloid deposit with a dense core. The dense plaques are associated with neurofibrillary changes in the neurons, and they are numerous in patients with AD. The total number of amyloid plaques is not as important as the number of the dense plaques, which relates to the degree of dementia. The β-amyloid has been identified at least in tissue culture to be toxic to mature neurons. The exact mechanism of cell death remains unclear.

Neurochemical studies show that the cholinergic system is affected more than other neurotransmitter systems in AD. Reduced acetylcholine and choline acetyltransferase in the cortex and deep nuclei such as the nucleus basalis suggest that the loss of cholinergic transmission plays a part in the syndrome. It has become increasingly clear that AD causes much more than cholinergic failure. The noradrenergic system is also affected, and there is cell loss in the locus ceruleus and decreased norepinephrine in many brain regions. Cell loss, nucleolar volume loss, and neurofibrillary tangles in the raphe nuclei implicate the serotonergic systems as a target of AD. Low serotonin levels in the caudate, hippocampus, and other nuclei are present and fit with the cellular losses.

AD occurs sporadically in most cases, but there are familial forms of the disease that may have an earlier age of onset. AD seems to be genetically heterogeneous; in the familial cases, several genetic loci have been identified. Familial AD is related to the amyloid protein precursor (APP) gene on chromosome 21 and to another locus (AD3 gene) on chromosome 14. Chromosome 1 also has a genetic locus related to familial AD. The effects of the abnormal genes is not yet fully known. Another genetic lesion is associated with increased risk of AD both in familial and sporadic disease. About two thirds of AD patients have repeats of the apolipoprotein E (APOE) gene located on chromosome 19. The presence and quantity of the APOE4 allele are related to the age at onset of familial AD and to the incidence in nonfamilial cases. Testing for the abnormal gene may predict the risk for AD; however, the gene is absent in a third of AD cases and is

present in persons without AD. It is not specific nor sensitive enough to be used as a difinitive diagnostic test. There is a suggestion that the APOE4 interferes with the cholinergic mechanism of memory, and patients without the APOE4 gene may respond to cholinergic treatment more robustly than others. Although available to patients and their families, the APOE test is not used in routine clinical practice because of the current ambiguity of its meaning.

The clinical syndrome of AD begins in midlife or late life and is usually unnoticed or ignored for several years. Patients change their habits and often lose interest in their usual pursuits before it becomes obvious what is happening. Some develop psychotic symptoms or appear depressed. Most patients present to the generalist with complaints not obviously associated with decreased mental functions. At that early stage, the disease is clinically undiagnosable. Most patients with AD worsen over 6 to 12 months; the younger patients seem to progress more quickly than the older ones. By the time the patient is clearly demented, there is often a history of 2 or 3 years of gradually increasing dysfunction. Impairment of learning, loss of recent and remote memory, and failure to analyze information follow the initial behavioral symptoms. Language is almost always affected, so patients have a striking dysnomia. Losses in calculation, praxis, and other functions add to the global mental failure. The dementia is usually moderately severe by the time the patient appears at the neurologist's office. Patients with moderately severe AD sometimes have bradykinesia and gegenhalten. The disease progresses smoothly over 5 to 10 years, eventually leaving the patient bedridden, immobile, mute, and in a persistent vegetative state. Intermittent illness may cause transient worsening, but the dementia does not improve. Death intervenes from repeated aspiration pneumonia and recurrent infectious diseases. In the late stages, myoclonus or seizures occur in about 25% of cases. The gait is usually preserved until very late in the illness.

AD that begins late in life causes less severe aphasia, enabling the patient to maintain communication that reveals a rambling, incoherent stream of thought similar to that seen in acutely confused patients. Some elderly patients with AD become unable to walk but have no clear motor deficit to explain the gait failure.

Most patients with AD require chronic hospitalization in the last several years of their illness because of uncontrolled aggressive behavior, wandering, urinary and fecal incontinence, and the need for constant supervision in all aspects of life.

There is no cure for AD. During the early stages the family can manage the patient's failure by reducing their expectations and simplifying the household routine. Sleep disorders can be treated with mild sedatives (diphenhydramine, chloral hydrate) at night. Incontinence can sometimes be reduced by toileting the patient on a time schedule and monitoring fluid intake. Wandering, incontinence, and general nuisance behaviors are rarely controlled with drugs unless the patient is heavily sedated.

Emphasis on the cholinergic deficit in AD has directed therapeutic trials of anticholinesterase drugs. Donepezil is an anticholinesterase drug approved for treatment of mild to moderate AD. Clinical trials show that it has an efficacy similar to Tacrine, the first anticholinesterase drug available for AD. Donepezil does not cause liver toxicity and has fewer cholinergic side effects than Tacrine. Anticholinesterase drugs improve performance on neuropsychologic tests, but there is not always an improvement in the patient's performance in the activities of daily living. The drugs act specifically to increase the activity of acetylcholine in the synapse; they have no direct effect on the health of the neuron. It is not likely that treatment with Tacrine or donepezil retards the death of cells in AD although it may improve some aspects of cognition in some patients. The drugs are not indicated in patients with severe AD or in other types of dementia. Other strategies include attempts to slow the progress of the disorder or to interfere with the amyloid deposition.

Management of the behavioral symptoms of the dementia is crucial to the treatment of the demented patient. Aggressive and assaultive behavior responds in some cases to short-acting benzodiazepines (lorazepam, oxazepam) used only when the unwanted behavior is a problem. Continued use of sedatives sometimes reduces function in demented patients or may cause paradoxical agitation. Intermittent use of the drugs avoids oversedation and allows optimal function. If behavior is unacceptable and no other treatment works, neuroleptics (chlorpromazine, haloperidol) are useful in curtailing assaultiveness.

Table 142-1 Nonneurologic diseases sometimes presenting as dementia

DISEASE	DIAGNOSTIC INDICATORS
Thyroid disease	T_3, T_4, TRH
Adrenal disease	Serum cortisol
Hypoparathyroidism	Serum calcium (parathormone levels)
Chronic renal disease	History of renal disease, BUN, creatinine
Chronic liver disease, hepatocerebral degeneration	History of liver disease, ammonia, LFTs acquired
Chronic drug toxicity	History of drug use, screens
Thiamine deficiency	History of alcoholism or other cause of thamine deprivation; purely amnestic dementia, Wernicke-Korsakoff syndrome
Pernicious anemia	CBC, vitamin B_{12} level, gastric analysis, dietary history, loss of vibratory sensation
Niacin deficiency	Dermatitis, history of malnutrition
Neurosyphilis	FTA-ABS of CSF, other neurologic signs
Acquired immunodeficiency syndrome (AIDS)	HIV antibodies, other neurologic signs
Paraneoplastic syndromes	Chest radiograph, signs and symptoms of cancer
Whipple's disease	Malabsorption, arthritis, gaze palsy, amnestic dementia
Chronic dehydration	Elderly patients, elevated serum and urine osmolality

BUN, Blood urea nitrogen; *LFTs,* liver function tests; *TRH,* thyrotropin-releasing hormone; *FTA-ABS,* fluorescent treponemal antibody absorption test.

Neuroleptics used in doses that control the unwanted behavior reduce function in demented patients and also cause tardive dyskinesia and parkinsonism. Neuroleptic-induced dysphagia and immobility increase the chances of aspiration pneumonia.

The chronic care of patients with progressive dementia depends on an understanding of the natural progression of the disease. The physician and family can agree on appropriate levels of care as the patient moves from stage to stage toward the inevitable end of the disease. Counseling the caregiver and family so that they understand the progressive limitations of the patient helps reduce the strife generated by the disease.

Other entities cause a clinical picture almost identical to that of AD. Lobar atrophy, or Pick's disease, is clinically indistinguishable from AD but has few neurofibrillary tangles or amyloid plaques. The neurons swell and contain cytoplasmic inclusions. The atrophy is particularly severe in the temporal and frontal lobes. Some patients with severe chronic dementia have a pathology unlike either Pick's or Alzheimer's disease yet have a similar clinical course. The course and management of the other progressive degenerative dementias are similar to those of AD. Treatable disorders almost never cause the isolated, chronic, severe, global dementia seen in advanced AD.

SYSTEMIC MEDICAL ILLNESS CAUSING DEMENTIA

Systemic illness affecting mental status usually causes a confusional state rather than dementia, but a few medical disorders cause a dementia that might be confused with early AD. Most of the time in systemic illness, the altered cognition is a secondary diagnostic clue rather than the major clinical feature. Elderly patients are more likely than young patients to present with dementia as the major sign of non-neurologic illness. The dementia is reversible when there is treatment for the underlying disease and the disease has not permanently damaged the brain.

The history of the dementia is usually short, decline almost always being reported in less than a year. The onset is rapid, with stabilization over a few months, and there is often a clear beginning, unlike in the progressive degenerative cases. The dementia is almost always mild or moderate, and language is often spared. The memory deficit is likely to fluctuate more widely than in AD. There may be elements of inattention and obtundation that make the separation between dementia and confusion difficult.

The major systemic medical causes of dementia are listed in Table 142-1. The details of their clinical profiles can be found elsewhere in this book. Many other medical disorders are associated with mental failure, but they usually cause delirium or confusional state and thus can be distinguished from AD. They are not listed.

Almost any systemic medical perturbation can cause an elderly patient, especially one with mild dementia, to decompensate and appear acutely confused. When the underlying dementia has gone unrecognized, there may be an illusion of an acute onset of the dementia that persists after the confusion abates. The progressive degenerative disorders do not begin acutely.

As a rule, the reversible medical causes of dementia do not cause specific neuropathologic changes. There are, however, systemic disorders that attack the brain directly and create their own neuropathologic change. Patients with Whipple's disease have neuropathologic changes of the brain and may have neurologic signs other than the dementia.

The most common cause of dementia in young patients is the AIDS dementia complex or HIV-associated dementia complex (HADC). The pathology remains unknown, but there is suggestion that the virus itself or toxins emanating from the virus cause the neurologic deficits. HADC occurs in 7% of patients with AIDS within 12 months of diagnosis and in 14% within 24 months; 3% to 4% of patients present with dementia as the first sign of AIDS. HADC bodes ill since the average time until death is about 5 months after the diagnosis. HADC does not occur in patients who are HIV positive without AIDS. Patients with HADC lose the ability to perform complex sequencing tasks, develop a slowness of thinking, and become inattentive. The memory loss is mild in the beginning but becomes severe as the syndrome progresses. The dementia is usually accompanied by slowness of motor function, including the eye movements, and by hyperreflexia, Babinski signs, and ataxia. There are changes in personality and affect. The earliest sign is sometimes psychosis. Myelopathy and neuropathy are also found in patients with HADC. The diagnosis is made by observing the neurologic signs and excluding other brain lesions. Toxoplasmosis, cryptococcal meningitis, progressive multifocal leukoencephalopathy (PML), and central nervous system lymphoma are frequent complications, which can be separated using CSF analysis and imaging. Cytomegalovirus (CMV) encephalitis may pose as primary HIV infection, but assay for traces of the CMV genome in CSF, systemic CMV infection, hyponatremia, and other factors help make the distinction. Some patients with AIDS have focal signs on clinical examination (e.g., aphasia) but have no specific abnormality on MRI, SPECT, or in the CSF.

DEMENTIA IN DISORDERS WITH VARIABLE NEUROLOGIC FEATURES

Several neurologic disorders feature dementia that may be confused with AD but have neurologic signs or histories that help the clinician make the diagnosis. Table 142-2 enumerates the various diagnostic tests that help distinguish the major disorders in which dementia is a key feature.

Subacute spongiform encephalopathy (Creutzfeldt-Jakob disease) is a dementing disease caused by a transmissible agent thought to be a virus. It is an unusual cause of dementia, with an incidence of approximately one case per 1 million population. The disorder causes gliosis and cell loss in the cerebral and cerebellar cortices. A characteristic vacuolated (spongy) appearance of the tissues and the lack of inflammatory cells give it a distinct neuropathologic picture.

Table 142-2 Neurologic tests that help to diagnose causes of dementia*

CAUSE	EEG	CT/MRI	LP
Trauma	Asymmetric waveforms, paroxysmal activity	Shows areas of damage	Normal
Tumor	Asymmetric waveforms, paroxysmal activity	Shows lesion	Abnormal
Chronic subdural hematoma	Normal or slow, low amplitude on side of lesion	Shows lesion	Normal in half
Multiple sclerosis	Normal	MRI shows lesion	Elevated gamma globulin
Hydrocephalus	Generalized slowing	Enlarged ventricles	Pressure high "normal" or above
Progressive degenerative dementia	Nonspecific slowing or normal	Normal or general atrophy	Normal
Vascular dementia	Asymmetric changes, slowing, paroxysmal activity; may be normal	Shows lesions in many cases	Normal
Creutzfeldt-Jakob disease	"Burst suppression" late in disease	Atrophy	Normal
Medical causes	Nonspecific slowing or normal	Normal	Normal
Syphilis	Nonspecific slowing or normal	Normal or focal defects, atrophy	FTS-ABS+, cells in active cases
Depression	Normal	Normal	Normal

*A normal laboratory test almost never rules out the possibility of a disease.
FTS-ABS, Fluorescent treponemal antibody absorption test.

Creutzfeldt-Jakob disease usually affects patients beyond middle age and begins with altered behavior. Dementia develops rapidly and devastates the patient within a year in almost all cases. Ataxia, gait disorder, and other signs of cerebellar dysfunction are frequent and may precede the mental decline. Visual complaints occur in some patients. Myoclonus occurs in most cases. The electroencephalogram (EEG) shows synchronous bursts of high-voltage sharp waves with intervals of low voltage.

The diagnosis can be suggested by brain biopsy, but for absolute certainty, diagnosis requires the transmission of the disorder by the inoculation of suspected tissue into brains of chimpanzees.

Creutzfeldt-Jakob disease is not contagious in the usual sense, but infected blood and other body fluids should be kept isolated. There is no treatment for the disease.

Patients with head trauma have residual abnormalities in mental function, often with failure of memory. The degree of the trauma determines the degree of dementia. Almost invariably, there are other signs and a clear history of trauma with a period of coma. As they age, patients with repeated head trauma, such as professional boxers, exhibit a mental decline that resembles AD. The dementia can be moderate or (sometimes) severe, but language is usually spared. Many head trauma patients are abulic and may have extrapyramidal features. Survivors of heat stroke also are sometimes left with a dementia, although the details of the syndrome are not well established.

A slowly growing brain tumor may present as dementia and be confused with progressive degenerative dementia. The onset is subacute, over weeks or months; there are almost always other signs of neurologic dysfunction, and in metastatic tumor a primary lesion may be identified. The dementia is mild or moderate. In many cases the patient suffers from increased intracranial pressure, causing somnolence and a confusional state instead of (or in addition to) dementia. Tumors of the diencephalon or the medial temporal lobe may cause an amnestic state. Frontal lobe tumors cause a failure of analytic thought, abulia, and increased intracranial pressure.

Chronic subdural hematoma (SDH) in elderly patients can cause an insidiously progressive dementia occurring over several days or weeks. The syndrome may mimic AD, except that most elderly patients with SDH are lethargic. Patients may not have other neurologic signs, but most have at least traces of motor dysfunction. Seizures and headache are also associated with chronic SDH. The CSF may be normal, but in one half of patients there is xanthochromia, pleocytosis, and elevated opening pressure. The EEG is abnormally slow, with reduced amplitude on the side of the lesion. The hematoma is almost always identified by computed tomography (CT) or MRI scan. Subdural hematoma is one cause of acute neurologic change in patients with AD.

Hydrocephalus causes lethargy and a variety of neurologic signs, along with changes in mental function. The CSF pressure in some cases may not be elevated but is almost always above 100 cm H$_2$O and usually at the upper normal limit. Normal pressure hydrocepha-

lus is an unusual cause of dementia occurring as a late complication of intracerebral infection or subarachnoid hemorrhage. In a few patients no predisposing reason is identified. The syndrome develops subacutely over a few weeks, causing lethargy and mental failure accompanied by a gait disorder and incontinence. Frequent falls and failure in the pursuit of usual activity are the chief complaints. The dementia is moderate, and language is usually minimally affected. The patient is slow to respond (abulic) but, when given time, often produces the correct answer. The EEG is slow in most cases, and the CT or MRI shows dilated ventricles. Placement of a ventricular shunt to relieve the pressure improves the patient's condition when hydrocephalus is the problem.

Dilated ventricles also occur in progressive degenerative dementia, in vascular dementia (see later discussion), and in normal elderly persons. One must relate all the laboratory and clinical data to make the diagnosis of normal pressure hydrocephalus. Acute subdural hematoma is a complication of ventricular shunt in hydrocephalus.

VASCULAR DEMENTIA

Vascular dementia results from stroke and accounts for approximately 15% of patients who present with dementia as the primary complaint. Cerebrovascular disease, however, produces dementia in a larger number of patients who are not counted among those who present with dementia as the major complaint. One of the chief factors that prevents stroke patients from returning to their prestroke ability is failure of mental function. Many patients have specific cerebral syndromes (aphasia, apraxia), but less obvious mental syndromes of inattention, failure of planning, poor memory, and other mental deficits also occur. The dementia occurs in most strokes along with other signs, but in some cases multiple recurrent strokes accumulate over years to cause a gradual decline in ability. There is often a clear history of at least one stroke in the past, and there is a stepwise deterioration in which the patient or family can mark plateaus and declines. The onset of the dementia can usually be dated within a few months. Risk factors for stroke (hypertension, atherosclerosis, family history) can also be found. Focal neurologic signs are the rule but may be only subtle reflex changes or changes in motor tone.

Multiple Cerebral Infarct

Several vascular syndromes cause a progressive dementia that may mimic AD. Multiple cortical strokes occur in patients with cardiac arrhythmias, valvular disease, cardiomyopathy, and other sources for embolism. The CT scan shows medium-sized lesions in the distribution of the middle cerebral artery (MCA) involving the cortex. Thrombotic vascular disease of the carotid or cerebral arteries that causes multiple infarction can also produce dementia. Moya moya, a slowly progressive thrombosis of the large arteries at the base of the brain, may cause a dementia with few other neurologic signs.

Multiple lacunar strokes occur in the setting of chronic hypertension. The syndrome of multiple lacunar infarction from small vessel thrombosis sometimes is more indolent than multiple embolism, because the lesions are smaller and may go unnoticed longer. The CT scan shows enlarged ventricles and areas of damage in the deep white matter, basal ganglia, and brain stem. Dysarthria, dysphagia, and pseudobulbar palsy are frequently part of the picture. The dementia in these cases is not as severe as that seen in AD of equal duration, and there is usually no aphasia, apraxia, or hemianopia. Systemic lupus erythematosus (SLE) sometimes causes multiple cerebral infarctions. In SLE patients, mental failure occurs along with variable neurologic signs, but the finding is usually psychosis rather than dementia.

Single Cerebral Infarct

Occlusion of the posterior cerebral artery is a single-stroke syndrome that causes amnesia. The deficit occurs with a hemianopia and may be transient. Anoxia and hypotension after cardiac arrest may leave the resuscitated patient with an amnestic dementia. Recurrent severe hypoglycemia may produce a dementia with abulia, memory loss, and other signs. Right middle cerebral artery occlusions are sometimes associated with depression and a chronic inattention, failure to form a coherent line of reasoning, and failure to analyze information properly. The syndrome resembles the confusional state except that the patient is fully alert and the state is chronic. The vascular dementias do not progress unless strokes continue to accumulate.

NEUROLOGIC SYNDROMES WITH DEMENTIA

Several neurologic disorders combine dementia with specific neurologic findings. The dementia occurs as a part of a rather stereotyped syndrome. Huntington's disease, Parkinson's disease, and progressive supranuclear palsy are the best known. These disorders are discussed elsewhere in this book.

BIBLIOGRAPHY

Boller F, Lopez OL, Moossy J: Diagnosis of dementia: clinicopathologic correlations, *Neurology* 39:76, 1989.

Evans DA et al: Prevalence of Alzheimer's disease and other dementing diseases in a community population of older persons higher than previously reported, *JAMA* 262:2551, 1989.

Farrer LA, Cupples LA, van Duijn CM, et al: Apolipoprotein E genotype in patients with Alzheimer's disease: implications of the risk among relatives, *Ann Neurol* 38:797, 1995.

Joachim CL, Morris JH, Selkoe D: Clinically diagnosed Alzheimer's disease: autopsy neuropathological results in 150 cases, *Ann Neurol* 24:50, 1988.

Power, C, Johnson, RT: HIV-1 associated dementia: clinical features and pathogenesis, *Can J Neurol Sci* 22:92, 1995.

Yankner BA, Mesulam M-M: β-Amyloid and the pathogenesis of Alzheimer's disease, *N Engl J Med* 325:1849, 1991.

143 Parkinsonism and Movement Disorders

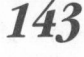

Lewis Sudarsky

Disorders of motor control, once considered the exclusive province of the neurologic specialist, are common in general medical practice. The prevalence of Parkinson's disease exceeds 1% after age 65, affecting a growing segment of the population. Many more patients have essential tremor, and there is a greater sophistication among patients and physicians about available treatment options. Focal dystonias such as torticollis and writer's cramp are more often recognized and can be treated with focal injection of botulinum toxin. The deinstitutionalization of chronic psychiatric patients over the last decade has created important changes in Western societies. As these patients

---

BOX 143-1
Motor control disorders

Parkinson's and related disorders
Parkinson's disease
Atypical parkinsonism
Secondary parkinsonism

Hyperkinetic movement disorders
Tremor
Chorea
Athetosis
Dyskinesia
Dystonia
Myoclonus
Tic

Other disorders with increased tone
Spasticity
Stiff-man syndrome

---

have hit the streets and shelters in growing numbers, phenothiazine-induced dyskinesias have become commonplace in office and hospital practice.

An established approach to the disorders of motor control is to divide manifestations into negative and positive symptoms: parkinsonism and the hyperkinetic movement disorders (Box 143-1). This approach provides a descriptive framework for systematic review of a rather diverse group of disorders. In some cases, particularly with tremor, dystonia, and myoclonus, the underlying physiology has been only partially characterized. With Parkinson's disease, the pathophysiology is understood at the level of the synapse, and the cell biology is under active study. Genetic mutations have been identified for Huntington's disease, Wilson's disease, and several forms of inherited ataxias; and investigations are focusing on disease mechanisms at the molecular level.

PARKINSON'S DISEASE

Parkinson's disease was described by James Parkinson in 1817, but the neurochemical basis of the disorder was never really understood until the advent of levodopa. Incidence increases with age. Parkinson's disease is relatively uncommon before age 40; the prevalence approaches 2.5% at age 85. Familial cases are described, but the condition is generally not considered to be heritable.

Clinical Features

Parkinson's disease is a clinical diagnosis that relies on the recognition of four cardinal clinical features: bradykinesia, rigidity, tremor, and a characteristic disorder of posture and gait. Bradykinesia (slowness and difficulty in initiating movement) is the most disabling feature. It is commonly reported by patients as weakness or increased difficulty at daily activities, such as washing and dressing. Extrapyramidal rigidity with "cogwheeling" is most easily appreciated in passive movement of the neck and limbs. The most typical case begins asymmetrically in the limbs with a resting tremor. The tremor, which lasts 3 to 5 seconds, is present at rest and subsides during limb movement. It is most evident in pronation/supination of the forearm and flexion of the fingers ("pill rolling"). The jaw and perioral area may be involved. Posture and gait disorders are the least specific of the major presenting features. A flexed posture is observed, and the gait is shuffling, with a tendency to turn "en bloc." Patients may experience a tendency to accelerate (festination). Later in the illness, there is loss of postural stability and a tendency to fall. This is seldom an early feature in idiopathic Parkinson's disease, and early postural instability may be a clue to another akinetic/rigid disorder.

Associated features are also helpful in recognition and diagnosis. Facial expression is diminished; seborrhea and blepharospasm are often observed. There may be dysarthria (monotonous, hypophonic

---

BOX 143-2
Differential diagnosis of parkinsonism

Idiopathic Parkinson's disease

Systems degeneration (Parkinson's-plus syndromes)
Progressive supranuclear palsy
Shy-Drager syndrome
Olivopontocerebellar atrophy
Striatonigral degeneration
Cortical-basal ganglionic degeneration
Huntington's disease (rigid variant)
Wilson's disease
Alzheimer's disease with extrapyramidal rigidity

Secondary parkinsonism
Postencephalitic parkinsonism
  Drug-induced parkinsonism
  Cerebrovascular disease
    Binswanger's disease
    Basal ganglia lacunes
  Normal pressure hydrocephalus
  Trauma, midbrain injury
  Tumor, vascular malformation (rare)
  Toxic or metabolic causes
    N-methyl-4-phenyl-tetrahydropyridine (MPTP)
    Manganese
    Carbon monoxide poisoning
    Non-Wilsonian hepatocerebral degeneration
    Hyperparathyroidism

---

speech) or drooling. The patient's handwriting may degenerate into a micrographic scrawl. The differential diagnosis relies on distinguishing idiopathic Parkinson's disease from other causes of a parkinsonian syndrome (Box 143-2). In the London Brain Bank study, 24% of patients thought to have Parkinson's disease during life did not meet accepted pathologic criteria at autopsy. Associated pyramidal, autonomic, or cerebellar features are usually caused by a systems degeneration, a presentation sometimes referred to as *Parkinson's-plus*.

Parkinson's remains a clinical diagnosis, often based on impressions rather than formal diagnostic criteria. No laboratory tests are used routinely. Of patients who present with an akinetic/rigid disorder, 10% to 30% ultimately turn out to have another illness, so magnetic resonance imaging (MRI) is sometimes used to screen patients with atypical parkinsonism. Parkinson's disease can be detected in a preclinical phase using positron emission tomography (PET) with fluoro-DOPA.

The natural history is one of gradual progression. In the pre-levodopa era, the median survival was on the order of 10 to 15 years. Death was from the complications of immobility: inanition and pneumonia. Patients today live longer. There is some suggestion that those who present with tremor have a more benign course. As levodopa has improved survival, it has also had an impact on the clinical spectrum of disease. More refractory late-stage patients are seen, and there is a greater awareness of mental status changes.

Etiology and Pathogenesis

There are approximately 500,000 specialized dopamine cells in the midbrain at birth, most of which lie in the pars compacta of the substantia nigra. These cells contain neuromelanin and manufacture the neurotransmitter dopamine. Together with the pigmented cells in the adjacent ventral tegmental area, they supply virtually all of the dopamine innervation of the forebrain. The striatopallidal loop (Fig. 143-1) participates in the planning and automatic execution of learned movement. The dopamine pathway to the striatum is thought to have a modulatory role in this processing. The small population of substantia nigra neurons thus influences the entire motor production of the basal ganglia and the cortical motor system.

The substantia nigra is the principal site of pathology in Parkinson's disease. The large, pigmented cells in the midbrain degenerate,

and pallor can be observed by gross inspection at postmortem examination. Intraneuronal inclusion bodies (Lewy bodies) are a biologic marker for the disease process. Symptoms and signs of parkinsonism emerge when 60% to 80% of the dopamine innervation is gone. With steady progression past this point, the clinical disorder grows more severe.

The etiology of Parkinson's disease is still not understood. Incidence increases sharply with age, as noted previously. Twin studies argue against inheritance and suggest that Parkinson's disease is somehow acquired in postnatal life. The experience in the 1970s with MPTP-induced parkinsonism has emphasized the biologic vulnerabilities of the nigral cell population. There is considerable interest in the possibility that idiopathic Parkinson's disease may be caused by exposure to an environmental toxin or to free radical by-products of dopamine oxidation. Limited postmortem studies on brain tissue demonstrate evidence of oxidant injury, but it is not clear whether oxidant stress is the cause or effect.

If oxidative damage is important in the pathogenesis of Parkinson's disease, it might be possible to retard the progression of the illness with antioxidants or inhibitors of the monoamine oxidase enzyme. Early diagnosis and institution of treatment might then become important. This strategy of neuroprotective therapy was examined in a large multicenter clinical trial (DATATOP study), the results of which were published in 1989. Daily use of selegeline, a monoamine oxidase (MAO) B-isoenzyme inhibitor, significantly slowed the evolution of disability in early patients. The study does not establish a neuroprotective mechanism for the drug effect, however, and its interpretation has been controversial. A more recent study from the United Kingdom did not suggest any neuroprotective benefit.

Management

It is important for all patients with parkinsonism to remain physically active. Physical therapy and exercise are often as helpful as medication in the early stages. For consideration of drug treatment, patients are divided into three groups: early, moderate, and advanced disease. The patient with early disease, often newly diagnosed, is easily able to work and perform daily activities. Such patients experience symptoms primarily at a nuisance level, with some social embarrassment, and a great deal of anxiety about the outlook. Moderate parkinsonism begins to impinge on function as the patient shows a change in mobility. Daily activities require more time. Advanced disease is marked by limitations in daily activities despite drug treatment. Such patients may develop fluctuations, treatment-limiting side effects, and a loss of independence in activities of daily living.

There is controversy regarding the use of selegeline, which appears to provide no measurable long-term benefits. In one British study, patients taking selegeline and levodopa had excess mortality compared with patients on levodopa only. Selegeline can cause confusion in older, demented patients. It also aggravates postural hypotension when used with other antiparkinsonian medications. There is a distinct symptomatic benefit of selegeline in some patients, who report modest improvements in motor function and mood elevation.

Moderate Disease

Symptomatic therapy (some form of dopamine replacement) is added as soon as slowness or stiffness has begun to interfere with the patient's occupation or daily activities. Large studies have not demonstrated any advantage to withholding levodopa at this stage, although the best results are generally achieved in the first 5 or 6 years of its use. It is interesting to note that one can influence the function of the brain by the oral loading (by feeding) of neurotransmitter precursors, yet this is precisely the mechanism of action of levodopa. Levodopa enters the nervous system by facilitated transport and is converted directly into neurotransmitter dopamine. The regulatory step in catecholamine synthesis is bypassed, so large quantities of neurotransmitter dopamine can be made and stored presynaptically. Peripheral inhibitors of dopa decarboxylase enhance the central accumulation of transmitter and diminish side effects caused by receptors in the periphery. For this reason, levodopa is usually given in combination with 75 to 150 mg/24 hours of carbidopa (Table 143-1). It is best to begin with a small dose (half a 25/100 Sinemet tablet, twice a day; or half

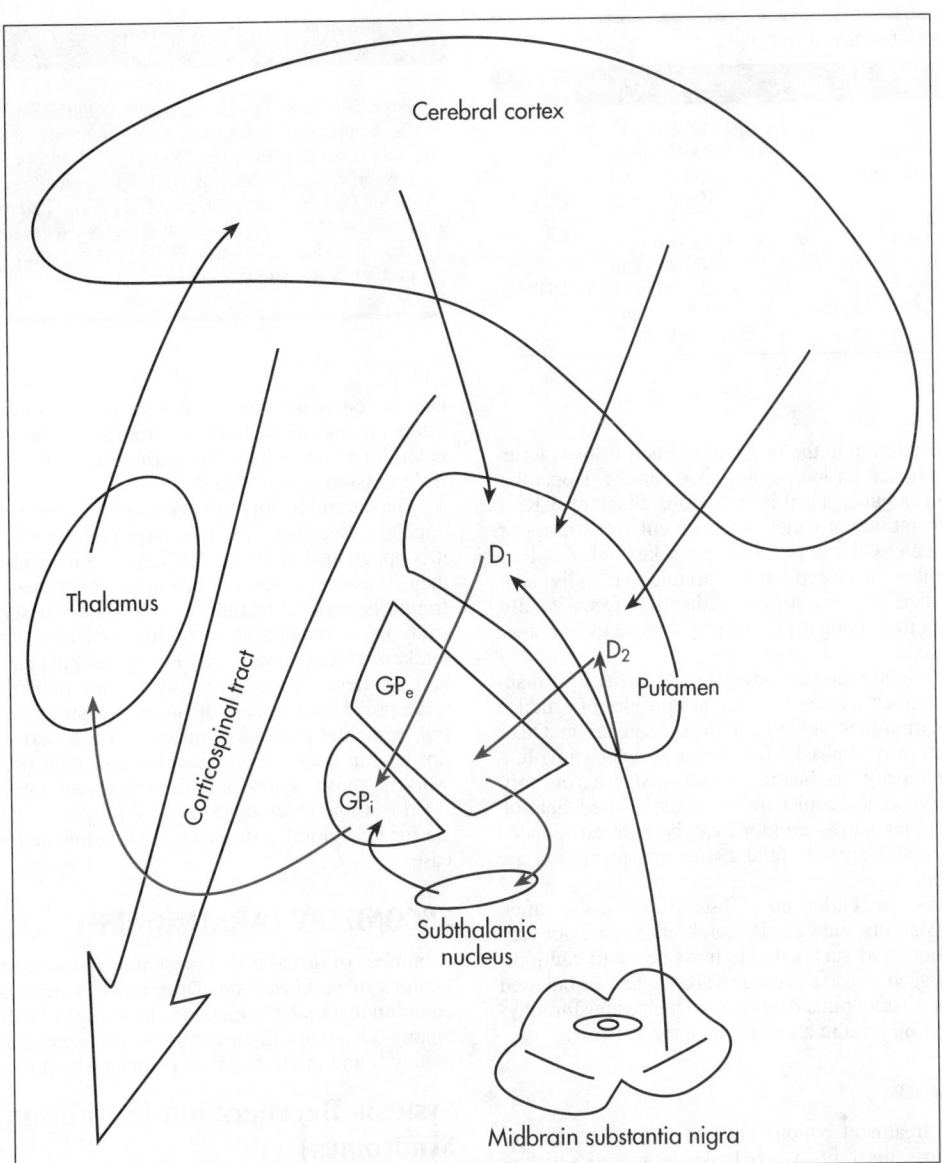

FIGURE 143-1 The striatopallidal loop is involved in the production of voluntary movement through the corticospinal tract. Afferents to the striatum (caudate and putamen) come from the cerebral cortex. Direct and indirect pathways through the basal ganglia influence the inhibitory output of the internal globus pallidus. Projections from the dopamine neurons in the midbrain substantia nigra modulate the motor production of the basal ganglia circuits. (Excitatory pathways are drawn in black, inhibitory pathways in green).

a Sinemet CR). If nausea is a problem, options include reducing the selegeline dose to 5 mg, adding extra carbidopa (available from the manufacturer), or adding an antiemetic. There is less nausea with Sinemet CR, which does not cause a rapid surge in the plasma levodopa level.

Authorities on the treatment of Parkinson's disease increasingly advocate early introduction of a dopamine receptor agonist drug, such as bromocriptine (7.5 to 25 mg) or pergolide (1.0 to 4 mg), together with levodopa. The principal advantage of this approach is that it allows the levodopa dose to remain in the low range (300 to 500 mg/day) for most patients. (For theoretical reasons, smaller doses of levodopa may be preferable.) In one commonly cited study, patients treated with bromocriptine from the outset had less difficulty in subsequent years with response fluctuations and dyskinesias.

One point against this strategy is the greater toxicity and expense of the dopamine agonists, which are generally less potent therapeutic agents than levodopa-carbidopa. Synthetic dopamine agonists can cause nausea, dizziness, leg edema, orthostatic hypotension, confusion, and dyskinesias. In large doses, they can even produce symp-

toms of ergotism, including digital vasospasm and chest pain. Best results are obtained by starting with a small dose (1.25 mg bromocriptine, 0.05 mg pergolide) and gradually increasing over 2 to 3 weeks into the desired dose range. The agonist drugs have the advantage of a longer half-life and, used together with levodopa, they provide a smoother response. Few patients succeed with these drugs alone as primary therapy.

Advanced Disease

The transition to advanced Parkinson's disease is often marked by the development of response fluctuations. Patients have trouble maintaining an even response to levodopa after 5 or 6 years of therapy. The half-life of levodopa is short (90 to 120 minutes), and many late-stage patients experience "wearing off" of its effect 2 to 3 hours after a dose. At the same time, they may be more sensitive to central nervous system toxicity at the peak dose. Because of the narrow therapeutic window, replacement of neurotransmitter dopamine by interval administration of precursor is unphysiologic and unsatisfactory

Table 143-1   Antiparkinsonian drugs

PREPARATION	AVERAGE DAILY DOSE
Levodopa	1.5-8.0 g
Levodopa-carbidopa (Sinemet)	300-1200 mg
Levodopa-benserazide (Madopa)	300-1200 mg
Amantadine (Symmetrel)	100-300 mg
Trihexyphenidyl (Artane)	2-15 mg
Benztropine (Cogentin)	1.0-6.0 mg
Ethopropazide (Parsidol)	100-400 mg
Bromocriptine (Parlodel)	7.5-30 mg (with DOPA)
Pergolide (Permax)	1.5-4.0 mg
Selegeline (Eldepryl)	5-10 mg

✔ *WHEN TO REFER*

Parkinson's is a common disease, and medication-responsive patients with mild symptoms are often managed by primary care physicians for several years. Referral is appropriate for initial confirmation of diagnosis, especially in atypical cases, since misdiagnosis of Parkinson's is relatively common. Patients with complicated Parkinson's (fluctuations, dyskinesias, mental change, postural instability, and falls) generally do better with a neurologist with expertise in movement disorders.

for these patients. The solution to the problem of end-of-dose "wearing off" is a greater reliance on long-acting medications. Dopamine agonists are a useful adjunct in this situation. Sinemet CR, a sustained-release preparation, provides delayed enteric absorption over 4 to 6 hours. Sinemet CR can be expected to last twice as long as regular Sinemet, although absorption is variable and individuals differ with respect to their response to this medication. Occasionally, selegeline can be useful to prolong the effect of levodopa in late-stage patients.

Other patterns of response fluctuation are more difficult to manage. Some patients describe transient freezing or episodes of "sudden off," which resolve over minutes without additional medication. Other patients develop a pattern of diphasic dyskinesia, in which involuntary movements accompany medication onset and wearing off. Greater reliance on dopamine agonist medications is often helpful, especially if the dose of levodopa-carbidopa can be reduced. Experimental treatment modalities such as fetal tissue transplantation are still under investigation.

Patients with late-stage Parkinson's disease are quite often disabled by postural instability and falls. Postural reflexes are not very responsive to medication, and such patients must be more cautious. They should be encouraged to use a cane or walker when ambulation is unstable. Symptoms of autonomic dysfunction such as postural hypotension and constipation require attention in some patients.

Surgical Treatment

A number of surgical treatment options are under development for late-stage patients whose disability is no longer managed satisfactorily with mediations. Posteroventral medial pallidotomy, done properly with microelectrode recording and physiologic mapping of the target area, has reduced primary symptoms (bradykinesia, rigidity, tremor) in the contralateral limbs and improved dyskinesia. The procedure reduces excess inhibitory output through the pallidothalamic pathway, which is the principal physiologic abnormality of basal ganglia circuits in Parkinson's disease. Fluctuations are sometimes less severe after pallidotomy, although off times persist and patients continue to require levodopa therapy. Tremor alone can be controlled with high-frequency electrical stimulation of the ventral intermediate thalamic nucleus. Implantation of fetal mesencephalic tissue or dopamine-producing cultured cell lines are still investigational.

Mental Status Changes

Although James Parkinson described a pure motor disorder, it is now apparent that a subgroup of patients with Parkinson's disease suffer mental change (delirium, depression, dementia). Delirium is generally transient and reversible and is related to medications. All the commonly used antiparkinsonian medications have the potential to cause delirium, even transient psychosis. Anticholinergic drugs are the worst offenders; it may be best to avoid them altogether in patients older than 70 years old. In patients prone to confusion the preferred strategy is to avoid polytherapy and focus on the single drug with the greatest therapeutic index (e.g., levodopa-corbidopa).

Depression occurs in a substantial number of patients. It is generally mild to moderate but can be a difficult management problem.

Depression is not correlated with the magnitude of disability and is often a feature in early-stage Parkinson's disease. Selegeline elevates mood for some patients, but a tricyclic antidepressant may be required if depression is significant.

The natural history of Parkinson's disease has changed in the levodopa era. Because more late-stage patients are alive and functioning, it is apparent that 10% to 20% have a dementia syndrome as part of their illness. Episodic confusion (even off medication), slowness, and frontal behavioral features are most often observed. Neuropathologic study of such cases at postmortem examination reveals cytoskeletal markers of Alzheimer's disease (cortical plaques and tangles) in about half of them. Some have only lesions of Parkinson's disease, with widespread involvement of subcortical structures (locus ceruleus, ventral tegmental area, basal nucleus of Meynert). It is best to avoid antipsychotic drugs, if possible, because their prolonged use inevitably worsens motor symptoms. Clozapine, an antagonist specific for the D4 dopamine receptor in the limbic system, has shown some promise for behavioral disturbances and hallucinations in Parkinson's disease.

SECONDARY PARKINSONISM

A number of diseases can present as an akinetic/rigid syndrome with features of parkinsonism. Drug-induced parkinsonism is particularly common in nursing homes and chronic care facilities, but it is also seen among outpatients in the community. A degeneration of systems is ultimately found in 4% to 6% of patients who present with parkinsonism.

Systems Degeneration (Parkinson's-Plus Syndromes)

Of patients initially thought to have Parkinson's disease, 3% to 4% evolve to the typical clinical picture of progressive supranuclear palsy (PSP) (Steele-Richardson-Olszewski syndrome). It is distinguished clinically by axial dystonia (especially extension of the head), a characteristic facial expression (suggesting horror or astonishment), and supranuclear gaze palsy. Postural instability and mental change are often prominent findings. Ocular signs may not be present initially, but the emergence of downward gaze palsy is pathognomonic. PSP is associated with nerve cell loss, gliosis, and globose neurofibrillary tangles in the substantia nigra, the subthalamic region, and the periaqueductal gray matter. Response is partial, at best, to antiparkinsonian medications.

A disorder known as cortical-basal ganglionic degeneration has poor response to levodopa and shows additional motor signs not typical in idiopathic PD. Rigidity is often unilateral or highly asymmetric, and patients have apraxia or the "alien hand" phenomenon (in which the limb appears to wander without full volitional control). Dementia is sometimes a feature of this disorder as well.

In the Shy-Drager syndrome, parkinsonism is associated with progressive autonomic failure. Sleep apnea and vocal cord paralysis are frequently associated. Mild orthostatic hypotension is not unusual in idiopathic Parkinson's disease, but hypotension is severe in these patients and may be made worse by levodopa. Olivopontocerebellar atrophy (OPCA) is characterized by parkinsonism and cerebellar dysfunction, with gross atrophy of the pons and cerebellum on imaging studies. Dysarthria is a prominent feature. Some cases are familial, and some are sporadic. A wide range of heterogeneity is observed,

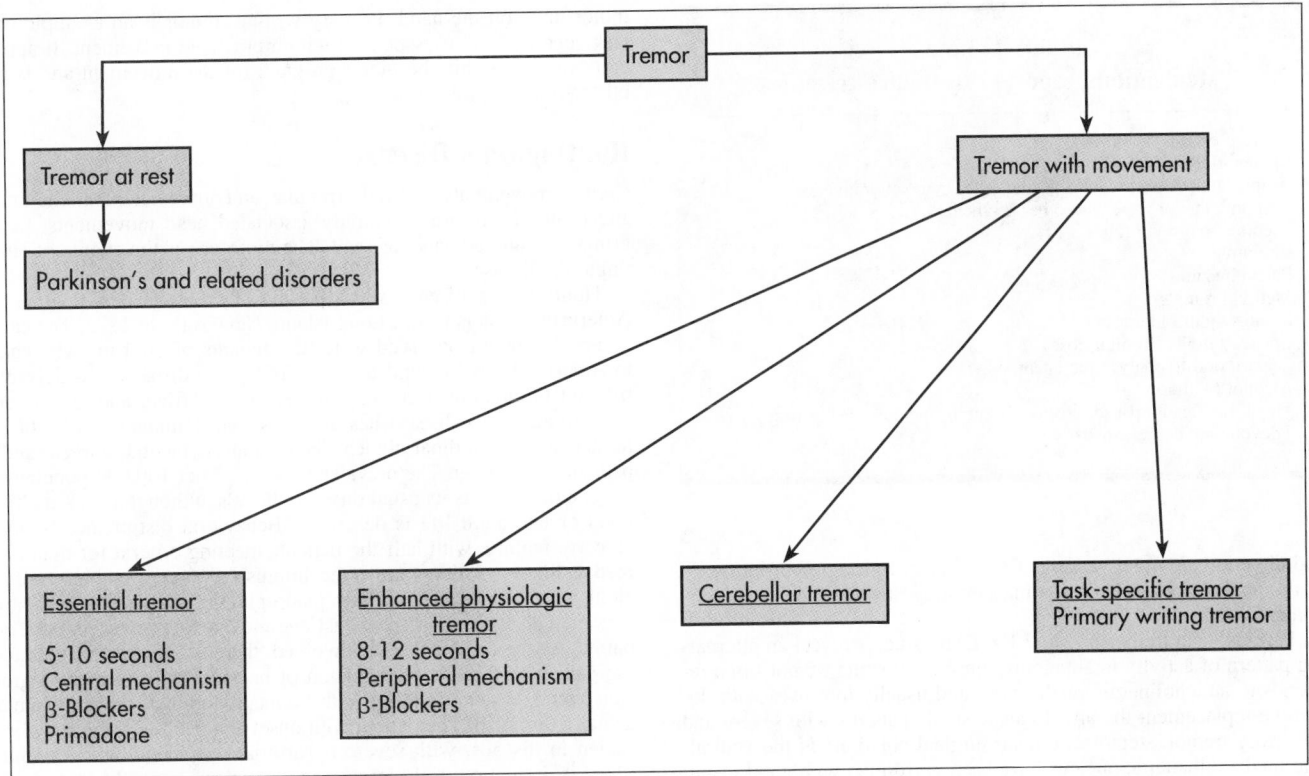

FIGURE 143-2 Classification of common tremors.

even within an affected family. Bannister and Oppenheimer have suggested that OPCA, Shy-Drager syndrome, and striatonigral degeneration be lumped together under the heading *multiple system atrophy,* since the range of syndrome variability and overlap is substantial.

Drug-Induced Parkinsonism

Chronic administration of drugs that depress dopamine synaptic function can cause a form of parkinsonism. Reserpine, which depletes catecholamines presynaptically, and the dopamine receptor antagonists (including haloperidol, prochlorperazine, and metaclopramide) have motor "neuroleptic" effects. Drug-induced parkinsonism is endemic in chronic psychiatric hospitals and common in nursing homes. It is difficult to distinguish clinically from idiopathic Parkinson's disease. Perioral tremor is somewhat more common, with gait impairment being somewhat less severe. Coexistent tardive dyskinesia may be an important clue. The diagnosis is usually made after a review of the patient's medications. The disorder persists for 1 to 3 months (median duration, 7 weeks) after discontinuation of neuroleptic drug treatment. Anticholinergic drugs are commonly used to improve function pending recovery; most neurologists prefer not to use levodopa in this context.

Destructive Lesions of the Midbrain or Corpus Striatum

Strokes in the basal ganglia have long been recognized as the occasional cause of a parkinsonian syndrome. In these cases—often in hypertensive patients with multiple subcortical infarcts—there are usually pyramidal signs, frontal gait disorder ("gait apraxia"), and abnormal mental state. Rarely, late-life hydrocephalus presents a somewhat parkinsonian appearance. Other structural pathology in the midbrain or striatum is occasionally encountered in patients with parkinsonism. Trauma to the midbrain is a rare cause of a parkinsonian syndrome.

Postencephalitic Parkinsonism

Encephalitis was once a common cause of parkinsonism. Most cases occurred in the wake of von Economo's encephalitis, an epidemic illness from 1916 to 1927. Today the condition is quite rare. Many of the patients are younger. An acute encephalitic illness progresses over days to akinetic mutism or coma. Features of the acute illness include external ophthalmoplegia, sleep, and respiratory disorder. A severe behavioral disturbance is often observed. Residua include chronic parkinsonism with dystonic features and oculogyric crises.

Toxic or Metabolic Etiology

A toxic parkinsonian syndrome was first recognized by Cotzias among workers in the manganese mines of South America. Carbon monoxide poisoning can produce a striking clinical picture, with necrosis in the globus pallidus, extrapyramidal rigidity, and dystonia. Such patients are rarely normal mentally. MPTP toxicity is a more recent phenomenon. Patients have an apparently normal mental state and a rather pure parkinsonism. The toxin was a by-product in the manufacture of "designer drugs" for recreational use. Asymptomatic patients known to be exposed should be followed closely for signs of emergent parkinsonism.

HYPERKINETIC MOVEMENT DISORDERS
Tremor

Tremor is an oscillating involuntary movement about a joint. Its recognition usually poses little problem. Contractions of reciprocally innervated antagonist muscles produce the movement. Tremor is divided into resting tremor and tremor with movement (action tremor). The latter category includes essential tremor, enhanced physiologic tremor, cerebellar intention tremor, and task-specific tremor, such as primary writing tremor (Fig. 143-2). Essential tremor is sometimes mistaken for Parkinson's disease. Parkinsonian tremor subsides with movement, while movement brings out essential tremor. The topography of the tremor is also a clue. Involvement of the legs or jaw favors Parkinson's disease, whereas a whole-head or pure vocal tremor is rarely due to Parkinson's disease. Surface electromyography (EMG) or accelerometric recording can be used to resolve difficult cases. Distinguishing cerebellar intention tremor from essential tremor is often more difficult. In essential tremor, tremor amplitude

---

BOX 143-3
Medications reported to induce tremor

Thyroid extract, synthroid
Epinephrine
Amphetamine, phenylephrine, and other sympathomimetics
Caffeine, theophyline, and other xanthenes
Nicotine, oxytremorine
Lithium
Phenothiazines
Methyl bromide
Monosodium glutamate
Corticosteroids (in high dose)
Insulin, oral hypoglycemic agents
Alcohol (withdrawal)
Metal intoxication (lead, arsenic, bismuth, mercury, manganese)
Tricyclic antidepressants

---

and direction are more variable. Cerebellar intention tremor increases as the goal is approached, in a manner suggestive of a defective servomechanism.

Parkinsonian tremor is 3 to 7 Hz. EMG studies reveal an alternating pattern of activity in antagonist muscles. Resting tremor often responds to anticholinergic medications and usually improves with dopamine replacement therapy. In some stable patients with severe and refractory tremor, stereotactic neurosurgical ablations of the ventral-intermediate thalamic nucleus have been performed with good result. For the vast majority of patients with longstanding Parkinson's disease, tremor is not the limiting feature.

Essential tremor is a 5 to 10 Hz action tremor, often large enough in amplitude to interfere with eating, writing, and activities of daily living. Its prevalence (380 in 100,000 population) makes it the most common movement disorder in adult patients. Physiologic studies show co-contraction of agonist and antagonist muscles (a synchronous pattern) in most cases. Sixty percent of patients have a positive family history, most typically an autosomal dominant pattern of inheritance. Sporadic cases are sometimes associated with another neurologic disease, such as Parkinson's disease or focal dystonia. In some cases, an action tremor can be the heralding feature of Parkinson's disease, making differential diagnosis difficult. Some patients discover for themselves the beneficial effects of alcohol on essential tremor. Beta-adrenergic blockers are often used for treatment; a central mechanism has been proposed. Sustained trials of high doses (up to 320 mg/day of propranolol, or its equivalent) are sometimes required. Primadone in doses of 50 to 250 mg/day has also been used. Tremors with lower frequency and head tremors in the elderly are sometimes refractory to treatment.

A low-amplitude, high-frequency tremor (8 to 12 Hz) is present among asymptomatic normal persons. It can be amplified by catecholamines, stress, fatigue, drug or alcohol withdrawal, thyroid hormone, caffeine, nicotine, or numerous other medications (Box 143-3). It is difficult to study physiologically because the tremor is buried in the normal interference pattern of the muscle. Young and Shahani suggest a peripheral mechanism, because intraarterial injection of β-blockers can often quiet this tremor in a single limb. The use of small doses of β-blockers has become a common practice among performing artists. The preferred management of the symptomatic patient with enhanced physiologic tremor is treatment of the underlying disorder, commonly anxiety, thyroid disease, or substance abuse.

Intention tremor is a part of a cerebellar syndrome. It is characterized by rhythmic oscillation about the target of movement. Dysmetria, a tendency toward erratic movement, and gait ataxia are often more disabling to the patient than the tremor. Patients with cerebellar disease may have both intention tremor and a postural tremor. Limb weighting may be helpful; mechanical damping has been used to design assistive devices.

Patients with neuropathy may have a tremor, the mechanism for which is ill understood. Patients with motor neuron disease appear to have tremor caused by the irregular action of a small pool of giant motor units on the hand. Primary writing tremor is an example of a task-specific tremor associated with a practiced movement. It apparently resides within the motor program for the movement and is not otherwise expressed.

Huntington's Disease

Choreic movements are brief, irregular, and unpredictable in the limbs and trunk. There are commonly associated head movements, facial grimacing, and a "dancing" gait. The prototype is the chorea of Huntington's disease.

Huntington's disease was described by George Huntington, an American physician from Long Island, New York, in 1872. The cases he and his father observed were descendants of pilgrims who came to America from England in 1649. Today the disease is widely distributed throughout northern Europe, South Africa, and the Americas. Huntington's disease has an autosomal dominant pattern of inheritance. The cardinal clinical features are dementia, chorea, and a behavioral disorder. The prevalence is 4 to 7 per 100,000 population.

The disease has its usual onset in the 30s, although onset in childhood or late adult life is described. Behavioral disturbance is often an early feature, with half the patients meeting criteria for major affective illness. Patients are often impulsive, erratic, or "hard to get along with." Chorea begins with piano-playing movements of the fingers or with facial grimaces. Fast eye movements (saccades) are impaired. As the trunk becomes involved, there is a characteristic dancing gait, with relative preservation of balance. With further progression over a decade, rigidity and dystonia predominate and chorea may actually diminish. The patient with onset at age 35 is commonly bedridden in his 50s, with severe dysarthria, dysphagia, and dementia. There is dramatic weight loss caused by caloric expenditure from the movements. Childhood-onset cases are predominantly rigid, rather than choreic, and may include seizures.

Pathologic examination reveals gross atrophy and neuronal loss in the caudate, with lesser changes in the putamen and globus pallidus and mild change in the frontal cortex. Caudate atrophy can often be appreciated by the loss of the caudate impression on the lateral ventricle by computed tomography (CT) or MRI. Microscopic examination reveals gliosis and loss of intrinsic neurons, especially the spiny striatal cells, which are the principal projection neurons. Cell loss in the striatum results in excess inhibition of the subthalamic nucleus and disinhibition of thalamocortical afferents. The genetic defect has been localized to the short arm of chromosome 4, where there is an expanded cytosine-adenine-guanine (CAG) trinucleotide repeat in the code for a 348 kD protein. Protein expression is not restricted to the nervous system or within it to areas that show pathologic injury. The selectivity of the disease process is not presently understood.

A neurologist familiar with the disorder can diagnose Huntington's disease in a symptomatic individual with a known family history. Alternately, the diagnosis can be established by a genetic test, demonstration of the Huntington's disease mutation in white cells from the patient's blood. Screening for an expanded CAG repeat in the relevant part of chromosome 4 has a sensitivity greater than 98% and a specificity approaching 100%. It is also possible to identify the Huntington's disease mutation in presymptomatic patients known to be at risk. Presymptomatic testing and management of affected individuals should be referred to a center with expertise in the disorder and related issues of genetic counseling. A treatment to alter the progression of the disease is not yet available. Haloperidol and diazepam are used in small doses by many patients to reduce involuntary choreic movements.

Non-Huntington Choreas

Box 143-4 provides a list of rather diverse disorders that have in common the tendency to cause choreic movements. These diseases all affect the basal ganglia and produce a disorder of striatopallidal output.

Sydenham's chorea is the neurologic manifestation of acute rheumatic fever. It is a self-limited condition, seen primarily in childhood. It is now uncommon in the United States. Neuroacanthocytosis, a genetic disorder, is characterized by involuntary movements and acanthocytosis in the peripheral blood, presumably a manifestation of an

BOX 143-4

Differential diagnosis of choreic disorders

Huntington's disease
Acute rheumatic (Sydenham's) chorea
Chorea gravidarum
Systemic lupus erythematosus
Neuroacanthocytosis
Dentato-rubro-pallido-luysian atrophy (DRPLA)
Glutaric acidemia
Methylmalonic aciduria
Familial calcification of the basal ganglia
Acute vascular hemichorea
Senile chorea
Spontaneous oral dyskinesia in the edentulous patient
Drug-induced dyskinesias
    Levodopa, bromocriptine
    Anticholinergics
    Antihistamines
    Oral contraceptives
    Neuroleptics

BOX 143-5

Causes of acquired (secondary) dystonia

Cerebral palsy
    Kernicterus
    Asphyxia (hypoxic/ischemic encephalopathy)
Posthemiplegic dystonia
Dystonia resulting from encephalitis or trauma
Acute drug-induced dystonia
Chronic tardive dystonia
Huntington's disease
Progressive supranuclear palsy
Wilson's disease
Hallervorden-Spatz disease
Neuronal ceroid lipofuscinosis
GM_1, GM_2 gangliosidosis
Lipidosis with sea-blue histiocytes
Lesch-Nyhan syndrome
Machado-Joseph disease
Leigh's disease

inherited membrane defect. Central nervous system lupus (lupus cerebritis) may have chorea as a symptomatic manifestation when immunologic injury involves the basal ganglia. Transient chorea has been associated with pregnancy in some patients and with the use of oral contraceptives. It is unclear whether such patients have an underlying structural injury.

Stroke in the region of the subthalamic nucleus can cause severe flinging movements on the contralateral side. These violent movements (hemiballismus) improve over days but may leave a residual hemichorea. Patients have been described with basal ganglia lacunes and generalized chorea, although it is striking how rarely small strokes in this region produce any involuntary movements. Spontaneous oral dyskinesias are found occasionally among older patients (senile chorea). Many of these cases occur among edentulous patients or are related to medications. Choreoathetosis (a slower, somewhat writhing movement disorder) is commonly caused by perinatal injury to the basal ganglia from ischemia or kernicterus. Athetosis has been described following hemiplegia when the injury occurs early in life.

Drug-Induced Dyskinesias

Dyskinesias related to medication can be acute or chronic. Unlike the chorea of Huntington's disease, movements are repetitive and stereotyped. Involvement of the perioral area (oral-buccal-lingual syndrome) is most typical although not universally present. Acute dyskinesias have been reported with anticholinergics, dopaminergic agonists, antihistamines, and a variety of other drugs.

Chronic tardive dyskinesia is an array of dyskinetic and dystonic disorders, delayed in appearance, related to long-term administration of neuroleptic drugs. Three months' exposure is probably the minimum necessary to produce a persistent dyskinesia. The problem is by no means universal in patients at risk. The prevalence of persistent dyskinesias in neuroleptic-treated patients (15% to 40%) increases with age and is greater among women. Tardive dyskinesia is thought to be a disorder of regulation at the postsynaptic dopamine receptor caused by chronic exposure to neuroleptic drugs. Postsynaptic suprasensitivity to dopamine has been demonstrated in an animal model. Tardive dyskinesia and drug-induced parkinsonism may coexist in the same patient. The movements are not always permanent. If the offending agent is discontinued, spontaneous improvement may occur within 18 months, particularly in younger patients. Otherwise, treatment of tardive dyskinesia is not entirely satisfactory. The most successful approach has utilized drugs that deplete dopamine from the nerve terminal presynaptically (reserpine, tetrabenazine). In patients who require long-term antipsychotic medication, a change to clozapine may be associated with an improvement in dyskinesia.

Dystonia

The term *dystonia* means sustained abnormal fixed posture and also refers to the spasms associated with dysfunctional posture. Dystonia may be generalized or restricted (focal or segmental). It is important to distinguish primary dystonia from secondary dystonia, for which a number of causes have been described (Box 143-5).

Primary generalized dystonia (idiopathic torsion dystonia, dystonia musculorum deformans) is a disorder with autosomal dominant inheritance and variable penetrance. It is particularly prevalent among families of Ashkenazic Jewish extraction, where the disorder has been localized to the long arm of chromosome 9. There are no consistent neuropathologic findings at the light microscope level, and the pathophysiology is not well understood. Changes in norepinephrine levels have been found in the hypothalamus, subthalamus, and locus ceruleus in postmortem study of the brain, but the number of cases studied to date is small.

The disorder begins in childhood, usually with an inturned foot or torsion of the trunk. The mental state and deep tendon reflexes are normal. The postural distortions may be quite extreme, and distinguishing true dystonia from a psychogenic dystonia may be difficult. Periods of remission may occur, especially early. Successful treatment with high doses of anticholinergic drugs has been described. Another form of generalized dystonia with young-adult onset and marked diurnal variation (fluctuations) is exquisitely responsive to levodopa. Levodopa should thus be tried in children and young adults with generalized dystonia, particularly in those whose family history is unclear. The genetic mutation for dopa-responsive dystonia has been identified on chromosome 14, within the gene for GTP cyclohydrolase 1.

In patients with generalized dystonia, it is always necessary to exclude Wilson's disease and the other listed causes of secondary dystonia. Dystonic symptoms are very common in patients with cerebral palsy and patients with neurodegenerative diseases involving the basal ganglia. Neuroleptic drugs can cause an acute dystonic reaction. Animal studies suggest that acute dystonic reactions to neuroleptic drugs result from a transient disorder of regulation at the dopamine synapse. They respond dramatically to anticholinergic drugs. A chronic, persistent dystonia sometimes occurs within the clinical spectrum of tardive dyskinesia (tardive dystonia).

Focal Dystonias

Focal dystonias, such as blepharospasm, torticollis, laryngeal dystonia (spasmodic dysphonia), and writer's cramp, have been increasingly recognized during the last decade. Dystonias involving the hand are particularly common among certain occupational groups, such as keyboard operators and musicians. Focal hand dystonias sometimes occur in relation to peripheral nerve injury. Response to systemic pharmacotherapy in these disorders has generally been disappointing, and focal intramuscular injection of botulinum toxin has rapidly become the treatment of choice. The pathophysiology of focal dystonia and the rationale for the therapeutic effect of botulinum toxin are not well understood. The toxin produces a chemical denervation at the neuromuscular junction, which persists for 3 to 4 months, and may have an effect also at the muscle spindle. Patients require repeated treatments.

Idiopathic cervical dystonia (spasmodic torticollis) has its usual onset in middle adult life. There is sometimes a brief remission in the first year, after which the disorder tends to persist. A positive family history is found in 10% to 15% of patients. Head turning may be mixed with retrocollis or head tilt. In one large series, 75% of patients had neck pain. Attempts at treatment with anticholinergic drugs, carbamazepine, or baclofen rarely succeed for very long. Surgical procedures may weaken the support of the head, and the disorder usually recruits other muscles to express itself. Experience with botulinum toxin has been highly successful. Neck motion is substantially improved in 60% to 80% of patients, and 90% get good relief of pain. Use of EMG to localize the posterior neck muscles may be required to achieve the best result.

Myoclonus

Myoclonus is a brief muscle jerk originating from the central nervous system. It can be spontaneous, or it may be evoked by voluntary movement (action myoclonus), or triggered by sensory stimuli (reflex myoclonus). Myoclonus should be distinguished from asterixis, a brief lapse in tonic muscle activation. Both myoclonus and asterixis are seen together in certain metabolic encephalopathies. Sporadic myoclonus may be related to cortical epileptic activity. Long-duration jerks (50 to 300 msec) are sometimes caused by a disorder of the brain stem or spinal segmental mechanism. Spinal myoclonus is typically rhythmic. The physiology of myoclonus can be studied by recording the muscle jerk (using surface EMG), and by back-averaging the electroencephalogram (EEG) to derive the related cerebral potential. Box 143-6 adopts the etiologic classification proposed by Marsden, Hallett, and Fahn. Under some circumstances (transition to sleep, hiccup), myoclonus can be a physiologic phenomenon.

Essential myoclonus is often a familial disorder, with onset in the first or second decade, a benign course, and a normal EEG. Otherwise typical cases are commonly seen with no family history. Based on the success with posthypoxic myoclonus, 5-hydroxytryptophan has been used to treat other patients. Many respond as well to clonazepam and some to valproate.

Quite frequently, myoclonus is observed as a fragment of an epileptic disorder. It may occur in relation to partial epilepsy or with some of the generalized epilepsies. In these cases, EEG is often diagnostic, and therapy is directed at the underlying seizure disorder. Valproate is preferred over phenytoin in predominately myoclonic generalized epilepsies.

Attention has recently been focused on the syndrome of progressive myoclonus epilepsy. Usually familial, these cases combine myoclonic seizures, tonic-clonic seizures, progressive ataxia, and dementia. The differential diagnosis includes Lafora body disease, several of the storage diseases, and the recently characterized mitochondrial encephalopathies. The clinical syndrome known as MERRF (myoclonus epilepsy, ragged-red fibers) caused by a mitochondrial disorder may have onset in middle adult life.

In hospital practice, myoclonus is most often the marker of a metabolic encephalopathy caused by hepatic disease, CO_2 retention, or chronic renal failure. Other causes of symptomatic myoclonus (myoclonus as a feature of a more generalized neurologic disorder) are listed. Myoclonus may be seen with late-stage Alzheimer's disease. Reflex myoclonus with periodic discharge on the EEG is characteristic of Creutzfeldt-Jakob disease. Segmental syndromes have been described that are restricted to the brain stem (palatal myoclonus) or the spinal cord. Spinal myoclonus has been described in association with tumor, infection and, rarely, as a complication of spinal anesthesia or lumbar disc surgery.

BOX 143-6
Etiologic classification of myoclonus

Physiologic
Sleep jerks
Hiccup

Essential
Familial essential myoclonus
Sporadic essential myoclonus
Startle syndromes

Epileptic myoclonus (fragments of epilepsy)
Partial continuous epilepsy
Photomyoclonic response
Primary generalized epileptic myoclonus
Juvenile atonic-myoclonic epilepsy (Lennox-Gastaut)
Infantile spasms
Benign myoclonus of infancy
Baltic myoclonus (Unverricht-Lundborg)

Symptomatic myoclonus
Storage disease with progressive myoclonus epilepsy
  Lafora body disease
  Neuronal ceroid lipofuscinosis
  Sialidosis
  Gaucher's disease
  GM_2 gangliosidosis
  Mitochondrial encephalomyopathy (MERRF)
Toxic/metabolic encephalopathy
Spinocerebellar, basal ganglia degenerations
  Friedreich's ataxia
  Wilson's disease
  Progressive supranuclear palsy
  Huntington's disease
Alzheimer's disease
Creutzfeldt-Jacob disease
Viral encephalitis
Posthypoxic (Lance-Adams)
Focal CNS damage
  Palatal myoclonus
  Spinal myoclonus

Modified from Marsden CD, Hallett M, Fahn S: In Marsden CD, Fahn S, editors: *Movement disorders*, London, 1982, Butterworth.

Tics and Tourette's Syndrome

A tic is a brief involuntary movement, that is abrupt and occurs out of a background of normal motor activity. Simple tics are isolated movements involving a small group of related muscles, such as a shoulder shrug or facial grimace. Complex tics are more widespread, often a caricature of a voluntary movement that has taken on a life of its own. Patients describe a subjective aspect to the movement, an urge to tic. Tics may be suppressed for a time by act of will, but tend to reemerge when voluntary control is released.

Diagnostic criteria for Tourette's syndrome (TS) include the presence of multiple motor tics, vocal tics, onset before age 21, and a persistence of the disorder for more than a year, although individual tics wax and wane over time. Coprolalia (phonic tics with profanity) is present in one third to one half of patients, and is not required for diagnosis. Tourette's Syndrome is a spectrum disorder, including involuntary movements and behavioral features. Compulsive behavior is quite common, and many patients have associated obsessive compulsive disorder (OCD). Many patients have a family history of TS or OCD in a first-rank relative, and a common genetic basis is suspected for this symptom complex. The prevalence of the disorder is estimated at 30 to 1600 per 100,000 population, but it may be higher when the full range of expression of the TS gene is considered.

Treatment for TS and related tic disorders must be individualized. Neuroleptics such as haloperidol or pimozide have been used to supress the movements, but many patients prefer not to take them. Small doses are recommended to reduce the risk of tardive dyskinesia. Clonazepam has also been used for tics, and fluoxetine or clomipramine can be helpful in treating associated symptoms of OCD.

OTHER DISORDERS WITH INCREASED TONE
Spasticity

The term *spasticity* describes a range of phenomena associated with the upper motor neuron syndrome. The principal characteristics are (1) increased muscle tone, (2) velocity-dependent increase in tonic stretch reflexes, and (3) increased tendon jerks with clonus. The "clasp-knife" phenomenon is appreciated during passive movement. There is an initial resistance, followed by a collapse of tension, a response mediated by stretch receptors in the Golgi tendon organ. Clinically, spinal spasticity differs somewhat from spasticity seen with cerebral disorders.

The muscle spindle supports the tonic stretch reflex. Specialized receptors are found in the spindle within the intrafusal fibers for both static and dynamic stretch. Ia afferents convey this information to the gray matter of the spinal cord. Alpha and gamma efferents maintain contraction in the muscle. In spastic disorders, the spinal segment is released from inhibitory influences deriving from the upper motor neurons (the corticospinal tract). A cerebral lesion also facilitates excitatory influences from the vestibulospinal and pontine reticulospinal tracts. The end result is increased activation of both alpha and gamma efferents, an increase in tone and intrinsic spinal motor activity.

A number of medications are used to treat spasticity, which may be a substantial problem for patients with spinal injury. Baclofen, a GABA$_B$ agonist, promotes inhibition in multisynaptic spinal reflex pathways and is remarkably effective for painful flexor spasms in spinal patients. Diazepam promotes intrinsic inhibition but is sometimes sedating. These two medications are often used in combination. The benefits are sometimes disappointing in ambulatory patients, as the drugs cause some degree of weakness. Dantrolene acts primarily on skeletal muscle, decreasing excitation-contraction coupling. It is preferred by many patients with cerebral palsy. Cutaneous toxicity is common, and hepatotoxicity must be monitored. Tizanidine, an α_2-adrenergic agonist, is increasingly popular for treatment of spasticity in Europe. For severe spasticity refractory to oral agents, intrathecal administration of baclofen using a catheter and infusion pump has been quite successful. A variety of surgical procedures have been used to reduce dysfunctional muscle contraction, ranging from nerve block to section of tendons or nerve roots.

Stiff-Man Syndrome

Originally described by Moersch and Woltman at the Mayo Clinic in 1956, stiff-man syndrome has reemerged as a clinical entity with the discovery of associated autoantibodies to glutamic acid decarboxylase (GAD) in 85% of patients. Other immune-mediated disorders such as diabetes, vitiligo, and thyroiditis are frequently associated. Painful muscle spasms occur in the lower back and legs, with hyperlordosis of the spine and hypertrophy of the paraspinal muscles. This spinal deformity is the most characteristic feature of described cases. The disorder is quite uncommon. The spasms respond to benzodiazepines (often large doses are required). Immunotherapy with plasmapheresis and the use of corticosteroids are of less consistent benefit.

BIBLIOGRAPHY

Albin RL, Young AB, Penny JB: The functional anatomy of basal ganglia disorders, *Trends Neurosci* 12:366, 1989.

Burke R: Tardive dyskinesia: current clinical issues, *Neurology* 34:1348, 1984.

Calne DB: Treatment of Parkinson's disease, *N Engl J Med* 329:1021-1027, 1993.

Fahn S: Clinical variants of idiopathic torsion dystonia, *J Neurol Neurosurg Psychiatry* 52(suppl):96, 1989.

Jankovic J, Brin M: Therapeutic uses of botulinum toxin, *N Engl J Med* 324:1186, 1991.

Kremer B, Goldberg P, Andrew SE, et al: A worldwide study of the Huntington's disease mutation, *N Engl J Med* 330:1401-1406, 1994.

Lees AJ: Comparison of therapeutic effects and mortality data of levodopa and levodopa combined with selegiline in patients with early, mild Parkinson's disease, *Br Med J* 311:1602-1607, 1995.

Marsden CD: Parkinson's disease, *J Neurol Neurosurg Psychiatry* 57:672-681, 1994.

Marsden CD, Hallett M, Fahn S: The nosology and pathophysiology of myoclonus. In Marsden CD, Fahn S, editors: *Movement disorders,* London, 1982, Butterworth.

Martin JB, Gusella JF: Huntington's disease: pathogenesis and management, *N Engl J Med* 315:1267, 1986.

Parkinson Study Group: Effect of deprenyl on the progression of disability in early Parkinson's disease, *N Engl J Med* 321:1364, 1989.

Singer HS, Walkup JT: Tourette syndrome and other tic disorders: diagnosis, pathophysiology and treatment, *Medicine* 70:15, 1991.

144 Cerebrovascular Disease (Stroke)

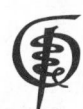 **Louis R. Caplan**

Stroke is a simple term, yet it describes a group of heterogeneous conditions that have in common death of brain tissue caused by disease of its vascular supply. The causes of stroke can be conveniently divided into two large categories: hemorrhage and ischemia. Bleeding and lack of blood are diametrically opposite conditions requiring quite different diagnostic and treatment strategies.

STROKE SUBTYPES
Hemorrhagic Stroke

Hemorrhage injures tissues by exerting local pressure on brain structures, by interrupting and disconnecting vital brain pathways, and by increasing intracranial pressure, causing pressure shifts and herniations of brain tissue, with brain stem compression. There are two large subcategories of hemorrhage: subarachnoid hemorrhage (SAH), in which bleeding is into the spaces surrounding the brain, and intracerebral hemorrhage (ICH), in which bleeding is directly into brain parenchyma. SAH and ICH are important to distinguish because they have different causes, outcomes, and treatments.

SAH is most often caused by leakage of blood from abnormal blood vessels on the surface of the brain—either aneurysms or vascular malformations. Aneurysms, often referred to as *berry* or *congenital,* are outpouchings on arteries, probably caused by a combination of congenital defects in the vascular wall and degenerative changes. Aneurysms usually occur at branching sites on the large arteries of the circle of Willis at the base of the brain (Table 144-1). When an aneurysm ruptures, blood is released under arterial pressure into the subarachnoid space and quickly spreads through the cerebrospinal fluid around the brain and spinal cord. The abrupt increase in intracranial pressure and the meningeal irritation cause sudden headache, at least temporary cessation of physical and intellectual activity and, often, vomiting and alteration in the state of alertness. Drowsi-

Table 144-1 Most common aneurysm sites and clinical signs

LOCATION	SIGNS
ICA–posterior communicating artery junction	Ipsilateral third-nerve palsy
Anterior communicating artery	Bilateral leg weakness, numbness, and extensor plantar signs
MCA bifurcation	Contralateral face weakness, aphasia ([L] lesion) or visual neglect ([R] lesion)
Basilar bifurcation	Bilateral third-nerve palsies, extensor plantar reflexes, coma
Vert–PICA junction	Dizziness, lateral medullary infarct

MCA, Middle cerebral artery; *ICA,* inferior cerebral artery; *vert,* vertebral; *PICA,* posterior inferior cerebellar artery.

Table 144-2   Most common loci of hypertensive ICH and signs

LOCATION (FREQUENCY)	MOTOR/SENSORY	PUPILS	EYE MOVEMENTS
Putamen (40%)	Contralateral hemiparesia and hemisensory loss	Normal	Conjugate gaze paresis to opposite side
Caudate (8%)	Transient contralateral hemiparesis	Sometimes ipsilateral Horner's	Sometimes conjugate gaze paresis to opposite side
Lobar (15%)	Sometimes contralateral hemiparesis (aphasia, hemianopia, etc., varying with lobe)	Normal	Sometimes conjugate gaze paresis to opposite side, depending on lobe
Thalamus (20%)	Contralateral sensory loss greater than motor	Small, poorly reactive, unilateral or bilateral	Eyes down and in, upgaze paralysis, sometimes ipsilateral conjugate gaze paresis
Pons (8%)	Quadraparesis	Small, reactive	Absent, horizontal gaze, ocular bobbing
Cerebellum (8%)	Ipsilateral ataxia, no paralysis	Sometimes ipsilateral pupil smaller	Ipsilateral sixth nerve or conjugate gaze paresis

ness and restlessness with agitation are especially common. Most often, there is no associated bleeding into the brain, so severe focal neurologic signs such as hemiplegia and hemianopia are unusual. The expanding aneurysm or focal surrounding collections of blood within the cisterns and subarachnoid space can affect the cranial nerves and adjacent brain structures, causing characteristic focal features that depend on the location of the aneurysm (see Table 144-1). In some cases the initial bleeding is so severe that death or irreversible brain damage occurs. If the bleeding is limited, the patient survives but is at risk of rebleeding in the days and weeks after the initial SAH. The arteries bathed by subarachnoid blood collections often become constricted, leading to delayed brain ischemia. Breakdown products of blood affect the vascular endothelia, leading to transient, and later, persistent, luminal narrowing. Less often, aneurysms are caused by dissection (traumatic or spontaneous) through the adventitia of arterial walls, embolism of infected or myxomatous material to the vasa vasorum of distal cerebral arteries ("mycotic aneurysms"), or degenerative elongation and tortuosity of arteries ("dolichoectatic"). Vascular malformations (AVMs) contain abnormal capillary, venous, or arteriovenous channels. Bleeding from AVMs is mostly into the brain and/or into the subarachnoid space on the surface of the brain, and it is usually less vigorous and under less pressure than is hemorrhage from aneurysmal rupture. Less frequent causes of SAH include bleeding diatheses, trauma, amyloid angiopathy, bleeding into meningeal tumors, and the use of drugs that precipitously raise systemic blood pressure, such as methamphetamine and cocaine. Some patients who fall or hit their heads have concussions and so are amnestic and may not recall the trauma. Amyloid angiopathy is an important cause of SAH during the geriatric years.

Intracerebral hemorrhage is most often caused by hypertension. Chronic hypertension causes degenerative changes in penetrating and subcortical arteries and arterioles with weakening of the arterial walls and small aneurysmal outpouchings (usually called *Charcot-Bouchard microaneurysms*). Acute increases in blood pressure and blood flow can also cause leakage from the same arteries. The affected penetrating arteries lie deep within the brain. Hypertensive ICH is most often located in the basal ganglia (putamen or caudate nucleus), thalamus, cerebral white matter, pons, and cerebellar white matter (Table 144-2). Bleeding is under arteriolar pressure and is cushioned by the resistance of tissue pressure in the surrounding brain structures. The initial release of blood into brain parenchyma causes pressure damage to local tissues and surrounding small vessels. The surrounding capillaries and arterioles break, leading to enlargement of the hematoma. The first signs of the hemorrhage are caused by dysfunction at the site of the bleeding: for example, in putamenal hemorrhage, weakness of the face, arm, or leg on the opposite side of the body; and in cerebellar hemorrhage, gait ataxia (see Table 144-2). If the hemorrhage is large, distortion of structures and increased intracranial pressure cause headache, vomiting, and decreased alertness. The cranial cavity is a closed system, and the bony skull and dura mater act as a fortress that protects the brain from outside injury. When swelling or hemorrhage arises inside the fortress, these structures may constitute a prison, restricting and strangulating their enclosed contents and forcing herniation of tissue from one com-

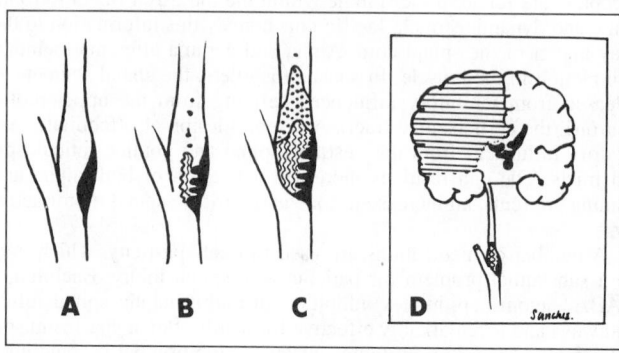

FIGURE 144-1   Internal carotid artery atherosclerotic lesions. **A,** Flat plaque on the posterior wall. **B,** Plaque with platelet-fibrin emboli. **C,** Plaque with occlusive thrombus. **D,** Recent ischemic cerebral infarct in anterior and middle cerebral artery territories caused by internal carotid artery occlusion.

partment to another. Survival depends on the size and rapidity of development of the hematoma and the extent of the surrounding edema. ICHs are at first soft and dissect along white-matter fiber tracts. If the patient survives the initial pressure changes, blood is absorbed, and after macrophage clearing of the debris, a cavity or slit forms that may disconnect brain pathways. ICH can also be caused by bleeding from arteriovenous malformations (AVMs); trauma; bleeding diatheses, especially with the prescription of anticoagulants; amyloid angiopathy; bleeding into brain tumors or granulomas; and sympathomimetic drugs such as cocaine and methamphetamine. Aneurysms rarely bleed only into the brain.

Ischemic Stroke

Deprivation of blood flow can be attributed to one of three different processes: *thrombosis,* defined as local in situ narrowing or occlusion of an artery obstructing or impeding distal blood flow; *embolism,* defined as blockage of an artery by material arising more proximally in the heart, venous system, or proximal arteries; and *systemic hypoperfusion,* which denotes a global decrease in brain blood flow caused by hypotension, cardiac pump failure, or hypovolemia. In thrombosis and embolism, ischemia exists in a local region of the brain fed by the affected artery, but in systemic hypoperfusion the decrease in blood flow and ischemia is more widespread.

Thrombosis implies obstruction of blood flow caused by a localized occlusive process within one or more blood vessels. The lumen of the vessel is narrowed or occluded by an alteration in the vessel wall or by superimposed clot formation (Fig. 144-1). The most common type of vascular pathology is atherosclerosis. Fibrous and muscular tissues overgrow in the subintima, and fatty materials form plaques that can encroach on the lumen. Platelets adhere to the crevices in the plaques and form clumps that serve as nidi for the deposition of fibrin, thrombin, and clot. Plaques and ulcers are associated

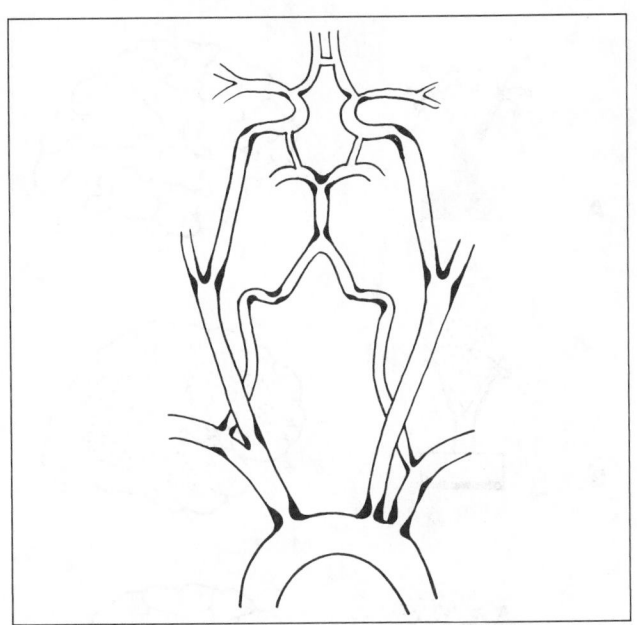

FIGURE 144-2   Sites of predilection for atherosclerotic narrowing. Black areas represent plaques.

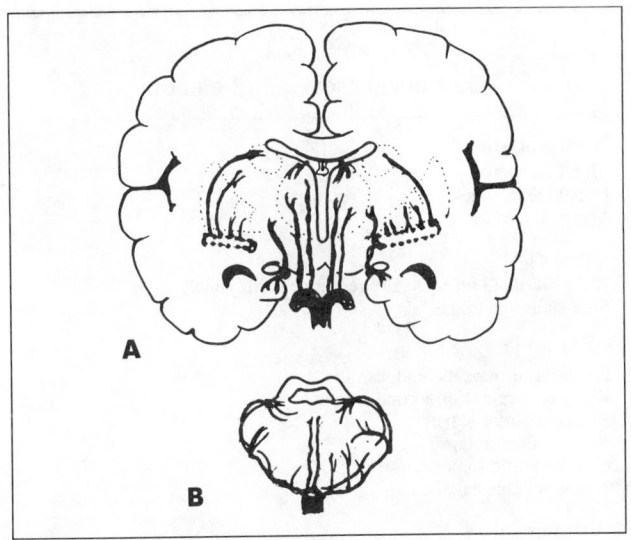

FIGURE 144-3   Penetrating arteries prone to lipohyalinosis and microaneurysms. **A,** the lenticulostriate and thalmogeniculate arteries, and **B,** penetrating arteries to the pons.

From Caplan LR, Stein RW: *Stroke: a clinical approach,* Boston, 1986, Butterworth.

with denudation of the endothelium and decreased release of endothelial relaxing factors (EDRF). Endothelins can promote platelet activation and thrombus formation. Intraluminal thrombi are of different types: so-called *white clots,* which comprise mostly platelets and fibrin, and *red thrombi,* which are red blood cells enmeshed in fibrin. White platelet clumps form most often in fast-moving streams, adhering to crevices and irregularities along the intimal surface. Fibrin-dependent red thrombi develop in slow-moving streams, for example, arteries with severe luminal narrowing. Atherosclerosis affects chiefly the large extracranial and intracranial arteries (Fig. 144-2), but there are important sex and racial differences in the distribution and incidence of lesions at these sites. White patients and men have more disease of the extracranial arteries, especially the internal carotid and vertebral artery origins; blacks, persons of Asian origin, and women have a predilection for narrowing of intracranial arteries, especially the middle and posterior cerebral arteries.

Narrowing of arteries decreases blood flow, leading to stagnation and altered dynamics of the blood column and activation of clotting factors. Clot and fibrin-platelet clumps form and break off, blocking distal arteries and further impeding flow in the parent affected artery. Less often, "thrombosis" is caused by a primary disorder of blood coagulation and not by abnormalities of the arterial wall. Deficiencies of natural coagulation-inhibiting factors (antithrombin III, protein C, protein S), abnormal fibrinolytic activity, acquired and inherited qualitative and quantitative abnormalities in serologic coagulation factors, acquired immunologically mediated syndromes such as antiphospholipid antibodies, and systemic diseases such as cancer, inflammatory bowel diseases, and infections can all cause hypercoagulable states. Less common vascular pathologies leading to occlusive disease include fibromuscular dysplasia, an overgrowth of medial and intimal elements that compromise vessel contractility and the size of the luminal opening; "arteritis," especially caused by temporal arteritis; Takayasu's disease; injection of illicit drugs; dissection of the arterial wall with luminal or extraluminal clot temporarily obstructing the lumen; and dilative arteriopathy, also called dolichoectasia, in which blood flow through dilated arteries is very abnormal.

The small penetrating arteries deep within the brain substance are the sites of a different type of occlusive process from that of the larger extracranial and intracranial arteries. Variously called *lipohyalinosis* or *fibrinoid degeneration,* the changes in the penetrating arteries are mostly caused by hypertension. Subintimal lipid-laden foam cells and pink-staining fibrinoid material thicken the arterial walls, sometimes compressing the lumens. In places the arteries are replaced by tangles

and wisps of connective tissue that obliterate the usual vascular layers. The arteries affected are the lenticulostriate branches of the middle cerebral arteries (MCA), the thalamoperforating and thalamogeniculate branches of the posterior cerebral arteries (PCA), and the midline and paramedian penetrating branches of the vertebral and basilar arteries (Fig. 144-3). The small, deep infarcts that result from occlusion of these penetrating arteries are usually called *lacunes.*

Small, deep infarcts can also result from miniature atheromas (microatheromas) that form at the origin of penetrating arteries, and by plaques within the parent arteries that obstruct or extend into the branches.

Embolism is of two major types, cardiogenic and intraarterial. Improved technology for evaluating cardiac disease has led to identification of previously unrecognized potential embolic sources and has documented that a higher proportion of ischemic strokes than previously suspected are caused by emboli of cardiac origin. At least 30% of ischemic strokes are caused by embolism from the heart, a figure close to that derived from the Harvard Stroke Registry before sophisticated cardiac testing. Cardiac sources include endocardial and valve disease, myocardial infarcts and myocardopathies, arrhythmias, and intracardiac lesions such as tumors and clots (Box 144-1). Recently, transesophageal echocardiography has shown that protruding, often mobile and pedunculated atheromas and clots can be found in the thoracic aorta and are a relatively common source of embolism. Angiography and cardiac surgery with clamping of the aorta promote embolism from aortic lesions. A less common form of cardiac embolism occurs when the heart serves as a conduit for emboli arising from clots in systemic veins; these clots pass through interatrial septal defects or patent foramen ovale to reach the brain and systemic circulation (so-called *paradoxical emboli*). Artery-to-artery emboli are composed most often of clot, platelet clumps, or fragments of plaques that break off from atherosclerotic lesions in proximal arteries. The most common sources of intraarterial emboli are stenotic lesions in the carotid and vertebral arteries in the neck. Embolism is especially apt to occur just after a clot is formed, before it organizes and adheres to the arterial wall. Cholesterol crystals, fat, tumor, and foreign body material, particularly talc and cornstarch injected by drug abusers, are less frequent intraarterial embolic materials. Embolic fragments, no matter what the source, tend to arrest in a recipient artery, depending on the location of branch points and the size of the embolic matter. Once lodged, the embolic matter often moves on and breaks into fragments within 48 hours, allowing reperfusion of the previously ischemic zone.

Blockage of arteries, whether caused by thrombi or emboli, sets

BOX 144-1
Cardiogenic sources of emboli

Myocardial ischemia
Mural thrombi
Hypokinetic zones
Ventricular aneurysms

Arrhythmia
Atrial fibrillation (especially recent or paroxysmal)
Sick sinus syndrome

Valvular
Bacterial or marantic endocarditis
Rheumatic mitral or aortic stenosis
Bicuspid aortic valve
Mitral valve prolapse
Calcific aortic stenosis
Mitral annulus calcification

Cardiomyopathies
Endocardial fibroelactosis
Alcoholic cardiomyopathy
Myocarditis
Amyloid

Intracardiac lesions
Myxomas
Primary or metastatic cardiac malignancies
Ball valve thrombi

Intracardiac defects with paradoxical emboli
Atrial septal defects
Patent foramen ovale

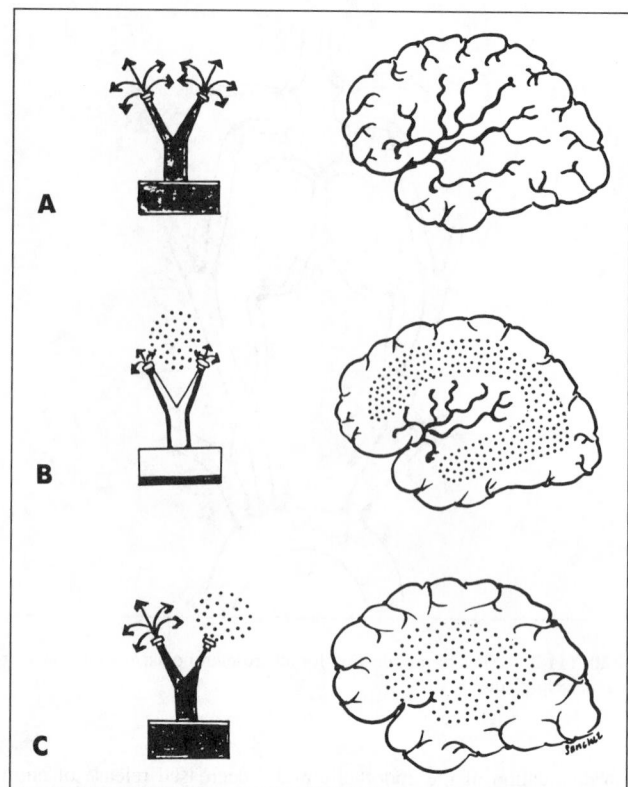

FIGURE 144-4   Heart (pump) failure and watershed infarction. On the left is a diagrammatic schema of a water pump and two hoses. On the right are lateral surfaces of the brain. **A,** Normal pump and arterial circulation. **B,** Low pump pressure and border-zone ischemia: water goes to center of hoses (arteries); stippled areas are those of poor flow. **C,** "Blocked hose" and middle cerebral artery infarction. Water is deficient in center of supply *(stippled areas).*

From Caplan LR, Stein RW: *Stroke: a clinical approach,* Boston, 1986, Butterworth.

in motion a series of events. Perfusion pressure distal to the occlusion drops, and the part of the brain supplied by that artery is deprived of blood. Decreased blood flow in turn activates protective mechanisms that help restore blood flow to that ischemic region. Low pressure and release of lactic acid and other metabolites help open collateral channels, bringing blood to the ischemic zone. At the same time, the process in the artery is not static; emboli pass, thrombolysis and fibrinolytic factors help lyse clots, and some clots propagate and embolize. These pathophysiologic events explain the clinical signature of thromboembolic stroke: that is, transient ischemic attacks (TIAs) and clinical fluctuations with progressive, stepwise, and fluctuating deficits. Thrombosis is most frequent in the morning after arising from sleep. Emboli occur more often with activity, and the deficit often develops more abruptly than it does in thrombosis. Fluctuations, improvements, and stepwise and progressive changes in signs result from changes in the clot, emboli, and altered flow in collateral channels. During a period of 7 to 10 days, the clot in the vessel and the collateral channels stabilize. The clinical signs depend on the part of the brain that is ischemic, but in thromboembolic stroke there are always prominent focal signs and not global neurologic dysfunction.

Systemic hypoperfusion is mainly caused by inadequate pumping of blood to the head. This occurs when there is too little blood in the system (shock, hypovolemia), when the pump itself fails (myocardial failure or severe arrhythmia), or when there is systemic hypotension. Faintness, pallor, sweating, dim vision, dim hearing and lightheadedness, dizziness, and lack of thought clarity are commonly noticed. The patient is worse when sitting or standing, and the blood pressure is low. In contrast to thromboembolic stroke, hypoperfusion is global but favors the so-called border zones or watershed areas between the major regions of vascular supply (Fig. 144-4).

CLINICAL SEPARATION OF STROKE SUBTYPES

The first question to ask is whether the patient has a stroke or a vascular lesion rather than another disease process. Although most abrupt-onset focal neurologic disorders are caused by cerebrovascu-

lar disease, sometimes other disorders can mimic or be confused with stroke (Box 144-2). These disorders should be considered. In patients with vascular disease, the next step is to classify the patient in one of the stroke subtype categories discussed: that is, subarachnoid hemorrhage, intracerebral hemorrhage, thrombosis, embolism, or systemic hypoperfusion. Clinical data are often sufficient to arrive at a differential diagnosis in which some subtypes are considered more likely than others and some are excluded. Assigning probabilities is important, because a single diagnosis is seldom 100% certain. In a given patient, a single diagnosis—for example, thrombosis—usually is most likely (perhaps 70% probability), but embolic occlusion requires consideration (perhaps 20% probability), and ICH, although unlikely, is still possible (10% probability). SAH and systemic hypoperfusion can be excluded in this patient. Most of the data used to estimate probabilities come from the history of the development of the stroke. When the history is meager (for example, if the patient is stuporous or aphasic or cannot recall what happened), the likelihood of an accurate clinical diagnosis diminishes. The clinical diagnosis can be checked, modified, and amplified by laboratory data.

Demographics and Past Medical Illnesses

The patient's age, sex, race, family history, and personal medical history strongly affect the probability of given stroke mechanisms. For example, if a young hypertensive black man without known heart disease had a stroke, ICH would be highly probable. In a 65-year-old diabetic man with coronary and peripheral vascular disease, there is a high probability of associated extracranial occlusive disease and thrombotic stroke or intraarterial embolism. Of course, some diseases, such as hypertension, predispose to more than one stroke subtype. Hypertension can cause ICH, but it also strongly increases the fre-

Table 144-3 Weighting of risk factors

	THROMBOSIS	LACUNAE	EMBOLISM	ICH	SAH
Hypertension	++	+++		++	+
Severe hypertension		+		++++	+
Coronary artery disease	+++		++		
Claudication	+++		+		
Atrial fibrillation			+++		
Sick sinus syndrome			++		
Valvular heart disease			+++		
Diabetes	+++	+	+		
Bleeding diathesis				++++	+
Hyperlipidemia	+++	+	+		
Cancer			++	+	+
Old age	+++	+		+	−
Black or Japanese origin	+	+		++	

Adapted from Caplan L, Stein R: *Stroke: a clinical approach,* Boston, 1986, Butterworth.

BOX 144-2
Differential diagnosis of stroke

Migraine
Syncope
Hyperventilation
Metabolic encephalopathy
Drug overdose or intoxication
Transient global amnesia
Vestibular vertigo
Seizures
Hypoglycemia
Hysterical conversion reaction

---

quency of atherosclerosis of the extracranial arteries and thrombotic stroke and of penetrating artery disease. Patients with coronary artery disease have a predilection for associated extracranial vascular disease but also may have myocardial ischemic lesions that can lead to cardiogenic cerebral embolism. The racial and sex differences in the distribution of occlusive lesions have already been noted. Table 144-3 depicts relative weighting of various risk factors.

Prior Cerebrovascular Events

Past strokes and transient ischemic attacks are especially important clues to stroke subtype. As an artery gradually becomes occluded, intermittent decreased distal flow or intraarterial emboli, consisting of clot, fibrin platelet clumps, or plaque, are common. Approximately 50% of patients with infarcts caused by thrombosis of large extracranial or intracranial arteries have TIAs before their stroke, and about 25% of patients with small-artery occlusion (lacunes) have premonitory TIAs. However, patients sometimes do not volunteer the occurrence of a prior attack, not recognizing the relationship. A patient with a left hemiparesis may not volunteer that 1 month ago he had temporary visual loss characterized by a shade descending over his right eye for 2 minutes, because to him the eye has no relation to the weak limbs. A patient with arm weakness may not tell the physician about attacks of previous transient leg numbness, believing them to be unrelated. The physician must *repeatedly* ask about prior transient spells, asking about specific symptoms (e.g., Have you ever had temporary weakness, numbness, or shaking of a leg or a limp? Temporary weakness of an arm? Temporary speech trouble? A shade over your eye?). The presence of a TIA in the same vascular territory as a stroke very heavily weights the probabilities to a thrombotic stroke. A past TIA or stroke in a different vascular territory makes cardiogenic embolism more likely.

Activity at Stroke Onset and Early Course of Development of the Signs

Thrombotic stroke sometimes develops when the circulation is quiet, for example, during nocturnal sleep or a nap. Recent studies show that the hours between 8 and 12 A.M. are the most frequent time for ischemic stroke to develop. Embolism, ICH, and SAH more often develop during physical activity. Exceptions to this rule are common, and in practice most strokes begin during activities of daily living. The early course of the signs is very helpful in predicting stroke mechanism. Embolic strokes most often produce a neurologic deficit that develops abruptly and is maximal at onset (80%). Thrombotic strokes, in contrast, more often cause stuttering or stepwise signs (33%), gradual progression (13%), or signs that fluctuate from abnormal to normal (12%). Improvement or fluctuations early in the course of illness is virtually never found in ICH, which most often progresses gradually during minutes or hours (60%) or causes a deficit that appears to be maximal at onset (35%). Patients and family members are often not good at describing the progression of signs, but "walking through the events" by having the patient describe in detail his or her activities and observations near the time of the stroke can be very helpful. For example, a 63-year-old woman notes weakness of the left hand while fixing breakfast. Alarmed, she walks normally to her bed upstairs and lies down. Arising an hour later, she is happy to find that her hand works well. Later in the morning she has a notable limp as she ascends the stairs. In the afternoon she cannot climb the stairs, and her hand is weak. This course of illness with fluctuations and temporary improvement is characteristic of a thrombotic stroke.

Symptoms Accompanying the Neurologic Deficit

Headache, loss of consciousness, vomiting, seizures, chest pain, and systemic symptoms such as fever are also important clues that help identify stroke mechanisms. All patients with SAH who are able to give a history have headache at the onset of the stroke. The absence of headache virtually excludes the diagnosis of SAH. Seizures are most common in patients with ICH or embolism. Vomiting is most often caused by increased intracranial pressure related to SAH or ICH or to ischemia within the posterior circulation. It is rare for a patient with thrombotic stroke other than basilar artery occlusion or embolism to lose consciousness at the onset of the stroke. Chest pain or arrhythmia before the stroke increases the possibility of cardiogenic embolism, and fever and malaise raise the possibility of bacterial endocarditis and temporal arteritis.

Findings from the Neurologic and General Examinations

Many nonneurologists, wary about the complexities of the neurologic examination, shy away from the stroke patient. The diagnosis of stroke subtype rests primarily on the items discussed so far—the back-

Table 144-4   Common localization patterns

BRAIN LOCALE OR SYNDROME	VESSELS	FINDINGS
Left hemisphere anterior circulation	Left ICA, MCA, ACA	Aphasia, right-limb and right-face weakness and/or sensory loss, right visual inattention
Right hemisphere anterior circulation	Right ICA, MCA, ACA	Left visual neglect, left-limb and left-face weakness and/or numbness, poor drawing and copying, lack of recognition of deficit
Left occipitotemporal	Left PCA	Right hemianopsia, inability to read but not write and spell, no limb weakness, occasional right hemisensory loss
Right occipitotemporal	Right PCA	Left hemianopsia, occasional left hemisensory loss, occasional left neglect
Brain stem-cerebellum	Vertebral and basilar arteries	Vertigo, bilateral visual loss, quadraparesis, ataxia, crossed signs (cranial nerves on one side, limb weakness or sensory loss on other side), nystagmus
Pure motor stroke (internal capsule in pons)	Penetrating artery	Hemiparesis without cognitive, sensory, or visual loss
Pure sensory stroke (thalamus or postlimb internal capsule)	Penetrating artery	Hemisensory symptoms without motor, cognitive, or visual abnormalities

ICA, Internal carotid artery; *MCA,* middle cerebral artery; *ACA,* anterior cerebral artery; *PCA,* posterior cerebral artery.

ground history and historical data about the stroke. The neurologic findings tell more about *where* the lesion is than *what* it is. At times the location of a lesion can heavily influence etiology: for example, a small deep lesion in the internal capsule or basal ganglia is likely to be a small ICH or a lacunar thrombotic infarct, whereas a superficial lesion in the left temporal lobe cortex is most likely an embolic infarct. Table 144-4 lists common localization patterns. Stroke localization heavily influences investigation of the vascular cause. For example, posterior circulation ischemic events are not clarified by noninvasive or angiographic studies of the carotid artery.

Examination of the heart and arteries in the head, neck, and arms can also provide evidence of occlusive disease by the presence of delayed or absent pulses, collateral circulation, or bruits. The ocular fundus also gives important information about the arterial pressure and the carotid-ophthalmic circulation.

After acquiring the data items discussed, the physician, following the clinical encounter, should be able to construct a probability-oriented differential diagnosis of stroke mechanism and locale. These hypotheses can then be tested and amplified by eclectically chosen investigations.

LABORATORY DIAGNOSIS: AMPLIFICATION OF THE CLINICAL DIAGNOSIS

The choice of laboratory tests should depend on the question to be answered. Technology has vastly improved recently and is capable of determining where the brain lesion is, whether it is ischemic or hemorrhagic, how big it is, where lesion/s are within the vessels, how severe the vascular lesions are, whether there is a cardioembolic source, and whether there is a hematologic problem causing hypercoaguability or excess bleeding. Box 144-3 lists the various tests commonly available.

The most important first step is to determine whether the brain lesion is caused by hemorrhage or ischemia. In some patients, this will be obvious clinically. For example, a patient with a transient or rapidly improving neurologic deficit and no headache does not have a hemorrhagic process. The single best test to determine if a lesion is an ICH or an infarct is computed tomography (CT) scanning. CT or magnetic resonance imaging (MRI) should be used in every patient with a stroke or transient ischemic attack because of the overwhelming amount of information gained and the safety of the procedure. Clinicians should not be swayed in this regard by those who, however appropriately, urge economy. Stroke is such an important, serious, and expensive disease that each case deserves careful investigation aimed at minimizing deficits and logically treating the causative process. CT not only differentiates hemorrhages from infarcts; it also shows the extent of ICH and documents the size and location of the lesion, drainage into the cerebrospinal fluid (CSF) or surface, pressure effects on secondary structures, and the presence of edema surrounding the lesion. CT also accurately images the size and location of infarcts. In a highly significant number of patients, CT uncovers

---

BOX 144-3

Laboratory procedures to evaluate cerebrovascular disease

Brain imaging
Computed tomography (CT)
Magnetic resonance imaging (MRI)
Positron emission tomography (PET)
Single photon emission computed tomography (SPECT)
Xenon-enhanced CT

Functional brain tests
Diffusion-weighted MRI
Electroencephalography (EEG)
Topographic EEG
Evoked responses
PET
SPECT
Xenon cerebral blood flow (XeCBF)
Xenon-enhanced CT
Perfusion MRI

Vascular lesion
B-mode ultrasound
Continuous-wave (CW) or pulsed Doppler ultrasound
Color-flow Doppler
Transcranial Doppler ultrasound (TCD)
Magnetic resonance angiography
CT angiography
Catheter dye angiography

Spinal fluid analysis
Lumbar puncture

Hematologic tests
Hemoglobin
Platelet count
Prothrombin time (PT)
Partial thromboplastin time (PTT)
Antithrombin III
Protein C and S levels
Antiphospholipid antibodies

Cardiac tests
Electrocardiography
Echocardiography
Ambulatory rhythm monitoring
Doppler
Multiple-gated acquisition (MUGA) scan

clinically unsuspected past vascular lesions and lesions that mimic stroke such as meningiomas and subdural hematomas.

MRI is probably more sensitive but less specific than CT; it does not readily separate ischemia or edema or wallerian degeneration from the primary infarct or hemorrhage. Casual inspection of an MRI scan usually does not allow easy distinction between ICH and infarction, but these two can be distinguished by analysis of the characteristics of different spin echo techniques, that is, the T1 and T2 weighting of images. MRI is more accurate in detecting posterior fossa lesions and lesions at the base of the brain. The MRI capability of imaging lesions in sagittal, horizontal, and coronal planes is a distinct advantage in localizing some lesions. Large and very recent (within 48 hours) subarachnoid hemorrhages are usually seen on CT but not imaged by MRI. Lumbar puncture with careful analysis of the CSF is a key diagnostic test for SAH.

The next question to settle is the *location* of the brain dysfunction, which not only helps in understanding and interpreting the symptoms but is crucial for planning investigations of the causative vascular lesion. Most often, neurologic examination, CT, and/or MRI allows accurate definition of the brain localization and vascular territory involved. Some patients with transient or reversible neurologic deficits have normal examinations or findings that cannot be definitively localized to a brain region. For example, weakness of an arm could occur with lesions in the precentral cortex, cerebral white matter, or brain stem, whereas a patient with aphasia plus weakness and numbness of the right face and hand definitely has a left paracentral cortical lesion. Most patients with normal neurologic examinations have nondiagnostic brain imaging tests, and some patients with abnormal examinations also have normal images on CT and MRI. In these patients, brain tissue, although not functioning normally, has not been anatomically altered and so does not show abnormal findings on brain imaging. A number of "functional tests" can give evidence of abnormal brain function or abnormal blood flow. In some patients, electroencephalogram (EEG), evoked-response tests after visual, somatosensory, or auditory stimuli, and topographic EEG mapping can indicate the brain regions not showing normal electrical function. Positron emission tomography (PET) gives even more data about local brain metabolic and blood flow abnormalities. In practice, PET is seldom available clinically, and electrical testing is very infrequently of practical help. Some tests such as single photon emission computed tomography (SPECT) scanning, xenon cerebral blood flow (Xe-CBF), and xenon-enhanced CT provide functional information about blood flow, but these data tell more about the vascular lesions than about the brain lesion.

Once the localization and mechanism (ischemia or hemorrhage) have been determined, the clinician should turn to analysis of the *causative vascular lesion*. The investigations chosen differ depending on whether hemorrhage or ischemia is present. If SAH is present, CT with contrast occasionally images an aneurysm or AVM, but angiography is the method of choice for opacifying these causative vascular lesions. The blood should also be screened for a bleeding diathesis. If an ICH is present on CT in a common location for hypertensive hemorrhage (see Table 144-2) and the patient is hypertensive, no further evaluation usually is needed to diagnose a hypertensive ICH. If the location or morphology is atypical, contrast enhancement of CT or angiography (magnetic resonance angiography [MRA], spiral CT angiography [CTA], or standard catheter angiography) sometimes is used to diagnose AVMs, aneurysms, or tumors that could have precipitated bleeding. Blood screening for a bleeding diathesis is also important.

When an infarct is found on CT or when no hemorrhage is seen in a patient with stroke or TIA, an ischemic etiology is inferred. Tests chosen to document and define the vascular lesion depend on the location of the lesion (anterior or posterior circulation) and the patient's demographics and risk factors. B-mode ultrasound and Doppler examination of the carotid arteries are both excellent techniques for studying internal carotid artery occlusive lesions in the neck. These two techniques are now usually combined in a duplex system that improves the diagnostic yield of the examination. Transcranial Doppler (TCD) ultrasound is a good technique for quantifying intracranial occlusive disease of the internal carotid artery siphon, middle cerebral artery, and anterior cerebral artery, as well as the intracranial vertebral and basilar arteries. Doppler is also a good technique for

diagnosing vertebral artery disease in the neck. Ultrasound and functional tests do not substitute for angiography, which shows the full extent of the major extracranial and intracranial arteries. MRA and spiral CTA are important and useful noninvasive techniques for showing the cervical-cranial circulation of the brain. MRA films are images of the blood vessels created by the capability of the technique to show pictures of moving blood columns. These are functional representations of blood flow rather than anatomically accurate images. For example, dolichoectatic dilated arteries with to-and-fro antegrade and retrograde flow regions may fail to image well by MRA, but the artery is fully patent when opacified with dye. Separate films are taken of the neck arteries and the intracranial large arteries. It is also possible to create images of blood flowing in the cranial dural sinuses and veins, which is helpful in assessing patients with suspected dural sinus occlusions. MRA shows good images of the extracranial internal carotid origins and can accurately separate patients with serious occlusive disease from those with minor or normal arteries. The extracranial vertebral arteries are also imaged, but the origins of these arteries from the subclavian arteries are usually not well seen. The major intracranial arteries (internal carotid, middle, anterior, posterior, and vertebral and basilar arteries) are usually well shown on cranial MRA images, but the branches are not reliably seen. MRA has the significant advantage of being performed at the same time as MRI so that both brain and vascular images are created. MRA and ultrasound (extracranial Duplex and TCD) are complementary studies. The two tests used together are more effective in detecting important occlusive disease than either test alone. CTA is a newer diagnostic technique that is performed by using spiral CT to create images of the arteries after the intravenous introduction of dye. This technique is useful in focusing on particular arteries and segments (e.g., the right carotid and middle cerebral arteries in a patient with a left hemiparesis and brain imaging that shows a right MCA territory infarct).

At times, aneurysms, dissections, and dolichoectatic arteries are suspected based on brain imaging films; in that circumstance CTA focused on the abnormal regions can help establish and clarify the vascular abnormality. Films of the vessels are reconstructed by cross-sectional images and are not usually available on-line. CTA is not as effective as a screening test as MRA or ultrasound but has the advantage of being able to be performed concurrently with cranial CT images of the brain. Catheter angiography by femoral artery catheterization remains the most precise way of imaging the arterial tree, but it carries a small risk (1% to 2% morbidity and mortality). Catheter angiography should be performed if the diagnosis is still unclear after the screening vascular tests, a primary vascular lesion is strongly suspected, and identification of the nature of the vascular lesion will guide treatment. All patients with ischemia should have at least screening studies of blood coagulation to exclude a hypercoagulable state.

Cardiogenic embolism should be suspected strongly in patients with (1) infarcts in different vascular territories, (2) known cardiac disease, (3) sudden-onset neurologic deficits without premonitory TIAs, (4) relative youth (<40 years old), and (5) no occlusive vascular lesion. Cardiac investigations usually include an electrocardiogram, echocardiogram, and ambulatory cardiac rhythm monitoring. Doppler study of the septum during echocardiography and after injection of a few bubbles of air helps detect septal defects and paradoxical embolism. As an alternative, monitoring of the intracranial arteries after intravenous injection of air bubbles also identifies passage of the bubbles across the septum. Transesophageal echocardiography (TEE) is more accurate in detecting atrial septal pathology, atrial clots, and aortic plaques. Large-vessel occlusive disease and cardiogenic embolism are especially likely if the brain lesion is superficial and affects the cerebral cortex. Small, deep lacunes are sometimes imaged by CT and MRI, thus defining the lesion and making further evaluation unnecessary if the risk factor profile and clinical picture are typical for lacunar disease. Border-zone bilateral infarction suggests cardiac disease or hypotension and should stimulate cardiac investigations. Tests of cerebral blood flow are useful only when the causative vascular lesions are known. PET, SPECT, xenon-enhanced CT, perfusion- and diffusion-weighted MRI, and xenon-inhalation cerebral blood flow (CBF) studies all can show regions of relatively decreased blood flow. When these regions of abnormal CBF are superimposed on the infarct, the physician can tell whether collateral flow is good or there are important or large areas of brain tissue that, although not yet infarcted, are tenuously supplied with blood. Knowing the causative vascular lesion, the state of the blood, and the extent of the brain damage, the clinician can logically tailor therapy to the patient.

THROMBOTIC STROKE

Treatment of patients with thrombotic lesions should be guided by (1) the severity and reversibility of the brain damage; (2) the nature, location, and severity of the vascular occlusive lesion; and (3) the state of the blood. In general, the more severe and irreversible the brain lesion, the more remote the possibility of effective reperfusion and restoration of function. Another aim of treatment is prevention of further damage. To judge the brain tissue still "at risk" for further ischemia, the physician must know the vascular lesion and mechanism of stroke. An example would be a patient with a small lesion in the white matter of the frontal lobe. If the damage is caused by a lacune, the entire territory of the lipohyalinotic disorganized artery may be infarcted, so no further tissue is at immediate risk. If the vascular process was occlusion of the internal carotid artery in the neck or in the siphon, however, then nearly the entire hemisphere is still at risk. In another patient with a large right-anterior cerebral and middle cerebral territory infarct, if the causative vascular lesion was occlusion of the internal carotid artery, then the entire territory of that vessel has been infarcted and little tissue is at further risk. If the cause was an embolus from a cardiac mural thrombus, however, then the posterior circulation and entire opposite hemisphere are at risk. The less the cerebral damage, the higher the benefit/risk ratio. Especially likely to benefit from treatment are patients with TIAs but no brain damage.

In each series of ischemic stroke patients with a given vascular lesion, for example, stenosis of the internal carotid artery, the likelihood of stroke increases with increasing severity of stenosis. As stenosis becomes more severe, platelet fibrin deposits tend to form and embolize, and decreased flow through the stenotic vessel leads to the formation of fibrin-dependent "red clots." Red clots form in areas promoting stasis, such as leg veins and dilated cardiac atria, whereas "white platelet clumps" tend to form on rough areas in fast-moving arterial streams, such as the internal carotid artery. Theoretically, red clots would respond more to warfarin anticoagulants and heparin, and white clots would be prevented better with platelet antiaggregants, such as aspirin. Surgery (endarterectomy) or warfarin therapy may be indicated for patients with tight stenotic lesions and important tissue at risk for further ischemia. The choice of warfarin or surgery depends on the accessibility of the lesions to the surgeons, the risk of surgery, the patient's wishes, the likelihood the patient will be compliant with anticoagulant therapy, and any contraindication to the use of anticoagulants. Heparin and later warfarin should be used for 3 to 6 weeks when there is an acute occlusion of an artery to prevent propagation and embolization of clot. Usually, long-term warfarin is not needed after the clot organizes and adheres to the vessel wall. Aspirin, 325 mg/day, can prevent platelet-fibrin emboli in patients with minor or moderate stenosis. Increasing the dose of aspirin (especially if an in vitro aspirin effect is not shown at the lower dose) or use of ticlopidine should be tried if symptoms recur. Neither warfarin nor surgery is recommended in patients with slight to moderate stenosis. Obviously, if the patient has a primary coagulopathy, polycythemia, or thrombocytosis, these disorders should be treated more specifically.

Anterior Circulation Large-Vessel Occlusive Disease

Internal Carotid Artery Origin. The distal common carotid artery (CCA) and first 3 cm of the internal carotid artery (ICA), especially along the posterior wall directly opposite the flow divider between the external carotid artery (ECA) and the internal carotid artery, is the most common site of plaque formation in the cerebrovascular system. Symptoms correlate with the severity of stenosis. The most common presentations are (1) TIA, (2) transient monocular blindness (TMB), and (3) sudden-onset stroke. TIAs are usually multiple. Temporary weakness and/or numbness of the limbs on the opposite side of the body is the most common symptom, and the hand and the arm are the most frequently affected body parts. Dysphasia is also common. Spells are often not stereotyped; a patient with right-ICA stenosis might have numbness of the left hand and foot in one spell, numbness and weakness of the left arm and hand in another, and sudden giving way of the left leg in a third spell. TMB is common and especially important to recognize, because it identifies the ICA–ophthalmic artery circuit as the location of the causative vascular lesion. The visual symptoms are usually described in terms of a dark shade or curtain descending over vision in the eye ipsilateral to the occlusive process. The shade may descend only halfway or, occasionally, may block vision from the side, like a curtain closing. The visual loss lasts seconds to minutes, then recedes, usually with no residual loss of vision. Attacks can be precipitated by bending, sudden rising, or straining. Some patients with chronic ocular ischemia note loss of vision in the ischemic eye when exposed to bright light, a kind of "visual claudication." Sudden-onset strokes are usually caused by embolism of plaque or clot from an occluded or tightly stenotic internal carotid artery origin (ICAO) lesion. Less often, embolism can arise from a seemingly minor plaque, a clot loosely attached to the vessel wall, or carotid artery dissection.

Noninvasive tests are usually adequate to reflect the severity of ICA stenosis but not to predict ulceration. Duplex scans (B-mode and Doppler combined) give an accurate image of the CCA and its ICA and ECA branches. TCD ultrasound, by measuring blood flow velocities in carotid artery tributaries, adds information about the functional severity of the proximal lesion. When the ICAO lesion is severe (>70% stenosis), angiography, MRA, CTA, or standard femoral artery catheterization is usually needed to further define the ICA lesion and to show the important ICA intracranial branches.

Internal Carotid Artery Siphon (ICAS). The tortuous S-shaped portion of the ICA, from where it enters the bony skull to where it emerges from bone at the clinoid process to enter the cranial cavity, is usually called the *siphon*. When narrowing occurs before the ophthalmic artery branch, the symptoms are indistinguishable from those of ICAO disease except for the absence in ICAS disease of physical signs of disease in the neck, such as a bruit. When the occlusive lesion is above the ophthalmic artery branch, TMB does not occur. ICAS disease causes TIAs or strokes with ischemia in the territories of the MCA and anterior cerebral artery (ACA). Weakness and/or numbness of the leg and face are most common. Because ICAS lesions have a much higher stroke/TIA ratio than ICAO disease, the former have a poorer prognosis.

Tests used to directly image the ICA in the neck, such as duplex scans and Doppler, are not helpful in ICAS disease. Ocular pneumoplethysmography (OPG) can show reduced flow when the ICAS lesion is proximal to the ophthalmic artery. TCD is effective in studying ICAS disease, but only an experienced technician can provide accurate interpretation. Angiography is the preferred method for showing the lesion. ICAS disease is not surgically accessible, so treatment is usually platelet antiaggregants or warfarin therapy, depending on the degree of stenosis, the severity of the stroke, and the presence of still-at-risk brain.

Middle Cerebral Artery. Intrinsic lesions of the MCA are less common than emboli to this vessel that arise from either the heart or the vascular system. In situ narrowing usually affects the proximal portion of the artery before the lenticulostriate branches and is most common in blacks, individuals of Asian origin, and women. Strokes are caused by blockage of flow to the MCA territory or by embolization of material to MCA branches. Common symptoms are hemiparesis, aphasia, and neglect of the contralateral visual field. Weakness or numbness of one limb is less common than in ICAO disease. Compared with ICAO disease, strokes usually are more frequent but less severe. On CT scans, infarcts caused by MCA disease are usually deep, imaging greater than 2 cm in the striatum and capsule (so-called striatocapsular infarcts) or wedge-shaped sylvian infarcts in the distribution of a branch of the MCA. TCD can give accurate data about pressure and flow in the MCA. MRA, CTA, and catheter angiography are the only procedures that provide an image of the lesions, but lack of distal flow in the MCA can sometimes be suspected on contrast-enhanced CT scans and MRI.

Anterior Cerebral Artery. This vessel supplies the paramedian frontal lobes. Symptoms of ischemia include weakness of the contralateral foot, leg, and thigh; incontinence; and abulia (lack of spontaneity and increased latency of responses). Embolism, especially from the ICA, is a more common cause of ACA occlusion than is intrinsic disease. Diagnosis usually depends on angiography.

Posterior Circulation Large Artery Occlusive Disease

Subclavian Artery and Vertebral Artery Origin. Plaques most often occur within the subclavian artery before the vertebral artery origin (VAO); plaques can extend into the VAO or originate within the first 2 to 3 cm of the proximal vertebral artery. When the subclavian artery is very stenotic or occluded, the most common symptoms relate to the ischemic arm: fatigue, coolness, and lack of power or endurance, along with a small, delayed pulse; cool hand; and asymmetrically reduced blood pressure. Less often, patients report TIAs, with dizziness, staggering, or double vision occasionally precipitated by exercise of the ischemic arm. When the lesion is within the VAO and the subclavian artery is not narrowed, identical attacks of vertigo, imbalance, and transient double vision or visual blurring occur, but the arm is not symptomatic.

Diagnosis of subclavian stenosis is usually possible clinically by detection of a supraclavicular bruit, careful palpation of the wrist and arm pulses, and measurement of blood pressure in the two arms. Noninvasive tests of arm blood flow and Doppler studies of the vertebral arteries can usually identify obstruction of subclavian or vertebral flow and detect retrograde flow down the vertebral artery. Angiography with delayed films can identify the vascular lesion and the presence of retrograde flow ("subclavian steal"). Disease of the subclavian artery and vertebral artery origins is usually benign and occurs most often on the left. Usually, adequate collateral vessels develop to prevent serious arm or posterior circulation ischemia. When the proximal vertebral artery occludes, the clot can embolize to the intracranial posterior circulation; heparin and later warfarin should be used for 3 to 6 weeks in such a situation. Right-sided subclavian or innominate artery disease is more serious, since the clot can extend into or embolize to the right carotid artery. Occlusive disease of the remainder of the extracranial vertebral arteries is infrequent, but the distal extracranial vertebral artery, where the artery loops around the atlas, is a vulnerable place for injury or dissection during sudden movements or neck manipulation.

Vertebral Artery Intracranially. The intracranial vertebral artery supplies the medulla oblongata and the inferior surface of the cerebellum. Stenosis or occlusion causes (1) lateral medullary infarction, for which symptoms and signs are noted in Table 144-5; (2) ischemia of the lateral and medial medulla, in which hemiparesis of the limbs opposite to the lesion is often found with symptoms of lateral medullary ischemia; and (3) cerebellar infarction, characterized by gait ataxia, dizziness, and vomiting. Sometimes, occlusion of the intracranial vertebral artery is detected asymptomatically when the patient is studied because of a sudden hemianopia caused by posterior cerebral artery territory infarction; the distal occlusion has been caused by intraarterial embolization of clot from the vertebral artery

intracranially (VAIC). TCD and continuous-wave Doppler can detect decreased flow in the VAICs. Bilateral occlusion or stenosis of the VAICs is particularly serious and can cause frequent posturally related TIAs and chronic medullary and cerebellar ischemia with posturally induced dizziness and visual blurring, as well as progressive weakness and ataxia of the limbs.

Basilar Artery Disease. The basilar artery supplies the pons. Occlusion develops because of in situ atherosclerosis of the basilar artery or extension of clot from the distal VAIC. The most common symptoms are weakness of the limbs—often both legs. At times, weakness is crossed (that is, one side of the face and opposite side of the body) or affects only one side of the body, sometimes alternating sides in different attacks. Double vision, dysarthria, and dizziness are also common. The most severe risk of serious brain stem infarction occurs shortly after the basilar artery occludes. In some patients, collateral circulation develops quickly, and slight or no brain damage results despite basilar artery occlusion. Maintenance of blood volume and blood pressure during the crisis helps as collateral circulation develops, and heparin probably is useful in preventing clot extension and embolization. Long-term warfarin therapy is probably not needed unless the basilar artery is tightly stenotic or harbors clot and is not yet occluded. Diagnosis is by MRA, CTA or catheter angiography, or TCD. CT with contrast can identify tortuous dolichoctatic basilar artery aneurysms and can occasionally image a fresh basilar artery clot. MRI is the preferred technique for identifying brain stem and cerebellar infarction.

Occlusion of the rostral basilar artery is most often embolic, with clot arising from the heart or proximal vertebral basilar system. Symptoms include visual loss—hemianopia or bilateral visual loss—loss of memory, and various oculomotor signs. Ischemia is in the territories of the arteries penetrating from the basilar artery apex to the medial midbrain and thalamus and in the territories of the PCAs.

Posterior Cerebral Arteries. These vessels supply the occipital lobes and the undersurfaces of the temporal lobes. Occlusion of a PCA is most often embolic, arising from the heart or proximal vertebral basilar system. When intrinsic stenosis of the PCA is present, the lesion almost always involves the proximal perimesencephalic or ambient segments. The most common symptom is loss of vision to one side. Patients describe a void or lack of ability to see to the side. Despite the hemianopia, and unlike visual loss in lesions of the MCA territory, patients usually do not neglect or ignore the hemianopic side. Some patients with left PCA occlusion have alexia without agraphia: that is, they can write and spell but cannot read. They usually also cannot identify colors. Patients with right PCA territory infarction, especially if it is extensive and includes the temporal and parietal lobes, have left visual neglect. Hemisensory loss on the side contralateral to the lesion may accompany hemianopia, but paralysis is not common.

Penetrating Artery Disease

Treatment consists primarily of controlling the underlying causative process, hypertension. Hyperlipidemia and polycythemia may be contributory factors and should also be treated. During the acute phase,

Table 144-5 Signs and symptoms in lateral medullary infarction

ANATOMIC STRUCTURE	IPSILATERAL FINDINGS	CONTRALATERAL FINDINGS
Descending tract and nucleus of V	Jabs of pain in the face, loss of pain and temperature sensation in the face, loss of corneal reflex	
Vestibular nuclei	Whirling dizziness, nystagmus	
Restiform body and cerebellum	Clumsiness and inability to stand or walk; gait ataxia, leaning to the affected side; ataxia on finger-to-nose and toe-to-object testing	
Descending sympathetic fibers	Horner's syndrome	
Nucleus ambiguous	Dysphagia and hoarseness, decreased pharyngeal movement, paralysis of the vocal cord	
Spinothalamic tract		Loss of pain and temperature sensation on the body and limbs, sometimes with a "level" on the trunk

blood pressure should *not* be extensively lowered, since this decreases pressure in collateral channels and may extend the infarct. The patient should be kept supine and blood volume and flow maximized during the acute phase of the infarct; only during convalescence, 2 to 3 weeks later, should vigorous antihypertensive treatment be prescribed.

Neurologic deficit in patients with lacunar infarction can progress gradually or stepwise for 1 to 7 days. Evidence for a lacunar (i.e., penetrating artery) etiology includes hypertension, past or present; short clinical history of TIAs or stroke progression; purely motor or purely sensory nature of clinical signs affecting face, arm, and leg; CT or MRI that images a small deep infarct or no lesion; a normal or symmetric electroencephalogam (EEG); and no occlusive large artery lesions.

EMBOLISM

The major treatment of cerebral embolism is prophylactic prevention of the next embolus. When the source is intraarterial, treatment depends on the nature of the arterial lesion and the severity of the resulting brain damage, and one should follow the guidelines given under thrombotic stroke. Heparin, followed by warfarin for 3 to 6 weeks, should be used when an acute occlusion of a proximal artery has occurred. When the proximal arterial embolic source is a tightly stenotic artery, either surgery (if feasible) or longer-term warfarin therapy is indicated. When the proximal source is plaque without severe stenosis, platelet antiaggregants, such as aspirin, should be used. Recent studies have shown that warfarin prophylaxis is very effective in preventing cardiogenic embolism in patients with atrial fibrillation. Treatment of other cardiac sources has not been as well studied. Some cardiac sources require direct treatment of the heart lesion, which may eliminate or reduce their embologenic potential, for example, surgery for valvular disease or a ventricular aneurysm or interatrial septal defect, and the use of cardioversion and antiarrhythmic drugs to convert atrial fibrillation to normal rhythm.

Because it has been demonstrated that warfarin anticoagulants decrease the incidence of embolism in patients with rheumatic mitral stenosis and atrial fibrillation and those with recent myocardial infarction, many physicians prophylactically use warfarin in any patient with cardiogenic embolism. When warfarin anticoagulation is used, it is advisable to keep the prothrombin time at approximately 1.5 times the control value (international normalized ratio [INR] 2-3) and no higher. Many cardiac lesions occur in older patients in whom long-term anticoagulation poses important risks and problems. Some cardiac lesions known to be potential embolic sources probably have a relatively low frequency of embolism: for example, mitral valve prolapse and porcine valves. In elderly patients and in cases in which there is a low frequency of embolism, the risk/benefit ratio of anticoagulants is not known. Aspirin may also be effective prophylaxis in some patients with potential cardiac sources of embolism. Dipyridamole in high doses (400 mg/day) seems to add protection when used with warfarin in patients with prosthetic valves. Despite the lack of data, aspirin may be useful for prophylaxis in some patients with cardiac lesions of low embolic potential and in patients with absolute or relative contraindications to warfarin use.

The onset of neurologic signs in patients with cerebral embolism is usually abrupt, and most often the deficit is maximal at or near onset. Fluctuations or worsenings and sudden improvement are common during the first 24 to 48 hours, probably because of the passage of emboli distally. Angiography within the first 12 hours has a high yield of showing emboli, but after 48 hours most emboli are no longer detectable. The most common recipient arteries are the MCA and ACA in the anterior circulation and the vertebral, distal basilar artery, and PCA in the posterior circulation. The clinical signs and imaging findings are the same as those described in the discussion of these vessels in the section on thrombotic stroke.

HEMORRHAGIC STROKE

Treatment of patients with ICH depends on the size and location of the hematoma, the severity of the clinical neurologic deficit, and the etiology of the bleeding. Bleeding diatheses, such as hypoprothrombinemia caused by warfarin prescription, hemophilia, or thrombocy-

topenia, should be reversed when possible, and hypertension should be controlled. Some advocate surgical drainage of hematomas to relieve mass effect and accelerate recovery. Surgery can be life saving in patients with increasing mass effect, but it should be remembered that surgical drainage does not remove the lesion; it merely replaces the hematoma with a hole or cavity more quickly than nature will. Small lesions (<1 cm) usually heal well by themselves and do not require drainage. Large lesions (>4 to 5 cm) are invariably fatal, and usually the patient is devastated even before reaching a medical facility; drainage of these large lesions may allow survival in a very poor vegetative state. Surgery probably is most useful for moderate-sized (>2 cm) hematomas in surgically accessible sites, such as the cerebellum, cerebral lobes, and right putamen, in patients who are worsening while under observation, who are developing signs of increased intracranial pressure (e.g., increased stupor, headache, a dilated pupil), and in whom CT or MRI shows shifts of intracranial contents. Without surgery, the prognosis for such patients is poor.

In SAH the aim is to treat the source of the hemorrhage, usually an aneurysm or AVM, before it can bleed again. Most often, this involves surgical clipping or coating of an aneurysm and surgical removal of an AVM. In the acute stage after the bleed, brain swelling and the presence of blood make the surgery more difficult and the outcome of surgery more tenuous. Generally, the surgeon waits until the patient is in good clinical condition. Prevention of ischemia caused by vasoconstriction is also an important consideration while waiting for surgery and during the postoperative period. Calcium channel blockers such as nimodipine and nicardipine may help decrease vasoconstriction. Hypovolemia and hyponatremia are common after SAH, and volume depletion can augment ischemia caused by vasoconstriction. Volume replacement is an important treatment in patients with delayed cerebral ischemia after SAH.

STROKE PREVENTION, PREVENTION AND TREATMENT OF STROKE COMPLICATIONS, AND REHABILITATION

Prevention of cerebrovascular disease and stroke is clearly better than treatment after stroke has occurred. Several conditions (e.g., hypertension, smoking, hyperlipidemia) are definite risk factors for stroke and heart disease. Others, such as taking birth control pills, excessive alcohol and coffee consumption, elevated hematocrit, obesity, chronic emotional stress, and lack of exercise, are possible risk factors, but the epidemiologic data are not definitive or sufficient. The earlier these risk factors are corrected or treated, the more likely is prevention or delay in the development of occlusive vascular disease. The presence of atherosclerosis (symptomatic coronary or peripheral vascular occlusive disease and extracranial carotid artery disease detected by noninvasive testing) carries a more immediate risk. The most immediate risk is the presence of a transient ischemic attack, which requires urgent evaluation, accurate diagnosis of mechanism, and treatment. Prevention is the job of every general physician who sees patients. Often forgotten is the duty of the specialist who cares for the patient during the acute stroke or ischemic attack. In the haste to deliver specific therapy to treat the lesion causing the present symptoms, specialists often overlook their responsibility to treat or moderate risk factors, in the hope of preventing further progression of any underlying atherosclerosis. If prevention is not begun early in treatment, it is often neglected.

Death, disability, and prolongation of hospitalization are most often caused by complications of stroke and its treatment, rather than by the stroke itself. Some of these complications are readily predictable and preventable with good medical and nursing care. Table 144-6 contains a brief list of these complications, the most important of which are pneumonia, phlebothrombosis, pulmonary embolism, nutritional deprivation, and depression.

In the United States, unfortunately, rehabilitation, prevention, and acute stroke care are generally managed at different sites and by different physicians. Yet all three form a continuum of care for patients with cerebrovascular disease. Rehabilitation, which emphasizes recovery and readaptation strategies, should begin very soon after the stroke, while the patient is in the acute care unit. Passive movement of weak limbs, use of ancillary devices to help maintain function, and

Table 144-6   Common stroke complications and causes

COMPLICATION	CAUSES
Pneumonia	Aspiration and hypoventilation
Phlebothrombosis	Immobility of paretic lower extremities
Hypovolemia	Lack of fluid intake, often because of dysphagia
Hyponatremia	Inappropriate ADH, diuretics, poor intake
Seizures	Excitable partially injured cerebral tissue
Depression	Organic mental changes, discouragement
Shoulder dislocation	Lack of proper care of paralyzed arm
Peripheral nerve injuries	Improper positioning of paretic limbs
Decubiti	Immobility, lack of turning and movement, inanition
Urinary tract infection	Indwelling urinary catheter, bladder distention
Bleeding, brain or systemic	Excessive anticoagulation
Congestive heart failure	Fluid overload
Hypotension	Excessive use of antihypertensives

ADH, Antidiuretic hormone.

education about specific neurologic deficits can be performed by the ward medical and nursing staff and should not be relegated solely to the therapist and physiatrist, who see the patient for only a small fraction of the day. If and when the patient is transferred to a rehabilitation unit, acute or preventive medical treatment begun in the acute unit should be vigorously pursued. All too often the patient is appropriately educated about treatment of hypertension, the need for avoidance of salt, and the value of a low-cholesterol, low-fat diet, only to be given free salt, butter, cream, and ice cream on the rehabilitation service.

Rehabilitation can also be overdone. The aim of rehabilitation is to allow readaptation to life's daily activities and full reintegration into home and community life. During rehabilitation, however, therapy for specific deficits, such as weakness of the left arm and hand, may be emphasized. After returning home, patients may be so centered around exercising and improving left-arm strength and dexterity that they lose sight of the major aim—a return to full living. Most people's activities do not depend on having a "normal" left hand, normal gait, or normal visual fields. Despite a residual deficit, many patients are able to live full lives. Continued intense attention to deficits detracts from recovery instead of promoting it. Rehabilitation and acute care must be integrated. Each must come to appropriate closure.

BIBLIOGRAPHY

Albers G et al: Stroke prevention in nonvalvular atrial fibrillation: a review of prospective randomized trials, *Ann Neurol* 30:511, 1991.
Barnett HJ et al: *Stroke: pathophysiology, diagnosis, and management,* ed 2, New York, 1992, Churchill Livingstone.
Bogousslavsky J, Caplan LR: *Stroke syndromes,* New York, 1995, Cambridge University Press.
Caplan LR: Diagnosis and treatment of ischemic stroke, *JAMA* 266:2413, 1991.
Caplan LR: *Stroke: a clinical approach,* ed 2, Boston, 1993, Butterworth-Heinemann.
Caplan LR et al: Race, sex, and occlusive vascular disease: a review, *Stroke* 17:648, 1986.
Caplan LR et al: Lumbar puncture and stroke, *Stroke* 18:540A, 1987.
Caplan LR et al: Transcranial Doppler ultrasound: present status, *Neurology* 40:696, 1990.
Kase CS, Caplan LR: *Intracerebral hemorrhage,* Boston, 1994, Butterworth-Heinemann.
Mohr J et al: The Harvard Cooperative Stroke Registry: a prospective registry, *Neurology* 28:745, 1978.
Mohr JP: Lacunes, *Stroke* 13:3, 1982.
Wolf P, Dyken M, Barnett HJM: Risk factors in stroke, *Stroke* 15:1105, 1984.

145 Demyelinating Diseases

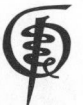

David M. Dawson

The demyelinating diseases (Box 145-1) are illnesses in which the primary site of histopathologic change is in the myelin sheath covering axons. By convention, the term is restricted to disorders of central nervous system myelin. Other illnesses, comparable in many respects, attack peripheral myelin, a product of the Schwann cell rather than the oligodendrocyte. These peripheral illnesses include acute Guillain-Barré syndrome and chronic inflammatory demyelinating polyneuropathy. *Dysmyelination,* or *leukodystrophy,* is a disease in which myelin degenerates, presumably because it is formed abnormally. A final category comprises illnesses involving subtotal necrosis of portions of the brain, primarily the white matter of the cerebral hemisphere, such as methotrexate leukoencephalopathy and subcortical arteriosclerotic encephalopathy.

Although demyelinating diseases share certain histologic features, including infiltration by lymphocytes and plasma cells, some tendency for perivascular localization of cells, and a variable degree of infiltration by macrophages that remove the damaged myelin fragments, they are clinically quite distinct, and this discussion is based on the clinical features.

MULTIPLE SCLEROSIS

Multiple sclerosis (MS) is the most common demyelinating illness. It is far more common in the temperate zones of the world, and particularly in the more highly developed countries, where in some instances the prevalence approaches 100 cases per 100,000 population. In Southeast Asia, in contrast, the illness is practically unknown in the native-born population. Population migration studies indicate that the risk of developing MS is carried with an individual if migration occurs after adolescence. All races are affected, but the illness is twice as common in whites as in blacks in the U.S. population. The female/male ratio is approximately 3:2.

Course and Prognosis

MS is a disease of middle life. It is common for the first symptoms to occur in the third or fourth decade of life, and onset of illness before adolescence is extremely rare. There are only a few documented cases of typical MS occurring in childhood. Onset after age 60 is rare. The illness is extremely variable in its course. About 20% of patients have benign illness, consisting of brief relapses of symptoms and signs (described later), with no accumulated deficit over the course of many years. Another 10% of patients have severe illness from the onset, with rapidly developing dementia, severe weakness, ataxia, and visual disorder within a few months. The majority of patients pursue an intermediate course, often beginning with attacks of illness (relapsing-remitting MS) and continuing with a chronic, progressive phase in later years. Some patients, particularly those with onset after age of 35, are in the progressive phase of the illness from the outset. Although there are no fully reliable guidelines as to the particular course an individual patient's illness will take, the pace of the disease is usually apparent within the first 5 years. MS has only a slight effect on overall life span, which is primarily attributable to those few patients who have highly aggressive forms of the illness.

Common Clinical Signs and Symptoms

Although MS can attack almost any portion of the central nervous system, certain locations are especially characteristic (Table 145-1).

The first symptom often is acute optic neuritis, which presents as loss of central vision in one eye, impaired pupillary reflex, and pain on ocular movement. The symptoms often develop over the course

Table 145-1 Differential diagnosis of common multiple sclerosis syndromes

CLINICAL SYNDROME	ALTERNATE DIAGNOSIS	DISTINCTIVE FINDINGS	LABORATORY EXAMINATION
Optic neuritis	Ischemic optic neuropathy	Edema of disc margin, older age	Elevated ESR
	Serous retinopathy	Abnormal macula	
	Retroorbital tumor	Slow progression	Visualization by CT or MRI scan
Brainstem disorder	Tumor	Slow progression	Visualization by CT or MRI scan
	Infarction	Older age, history of TIA	
Spinal cord syndrome	Cervical spondylosis	Neck pain, loss of some reflexes	Cervical radiograph
	Motor neuron disease	No sensory loss	EMG
	Cervical tumor	Progressive course	Spinal MRI scan
Neurogenic bladder	Lumbosacral tumor	Pain, slow progression	Myelogram, spinal CT
	Subacute myelitis	Painful, atrophy, weakness	Spinal angiograph shows dural AVM

ALS, Acute lateral sclerosis; *TIA,* transient ischemic attack; *ESR,* erythrocyte sedimentation rate; *CT,* computed tomography; *MRI,* magnetic resonance imaging; *EMG,* electromyography; *AVM,* arteriovenous malformation.

BOX 145-1
Disorders of central nervous system myelin

Demyelinating diseases
Unknown etiology, possible immune etiology
Multiple sclerosis
Transverse myelitis
Neuromyelitis optica (Devic's disease)
Acute disseminated encephalomyelitis
Acute hemorrhagic leukoencephalitis
Postviral, postvaccinial encephalomyelitis

Viral etiology
Progressive multifocal leukoencephalopathy
Subacute sclerosing panencephalitis
Necrosis of white matter

Systemic toxic, nutritional disorders
Anoxia
Nutritional deprivation
Vitamin B_{12} deficiency
Central pontine myelinolysis
Marchiafava-Bignami disease
Methotrexate poisoning
Cranial irradiation
Lead poisoning
Organic mercury poisoning
Triethyl tin poisoning

Dysmyelinating diseases
Leukodystrophies
Lipidoses
Aminoacidurias
Congenital hypothyroidism

---

of a few days to a week, stabilize for a month or two, and then improve. In the majority of instances, optic neuritis resolves, leaving only some pallor of the disk and impaired appreciation of bright colors. About 40% of patients with acute optic neuritis go on to develop clinically apparent MS. Whether the others represent a *forme fruste* is not known.

An acute attack of MS affecting the brain stem or pons may produce double vision, dizziness, unsteady gait, numbness of one side of the face, and cerebellar ataxia. A highly characteristic finding is the internuclear ophthalmoplegia (INO) caused by a lesion of the medial longitudinal fasciculus. It consists of delay of adduction of one eye, with nystagmus of the abducting eye on lateral gaze.

An acute attack of MS affecting the cervical spinal cord may produce numbness of one or both hands; weakness of gait; brisk reflexes in the lower extremities, with extensor plantar responses; and the highly characteristic Lhermitte's phenomenon, in which flexion of the neck produces tingling and paresthesias into the legs.

MS may attack the most caudal portions of the spinal cord, in which case the patient may complain of atonic bladder, constipation, impotence, and loss of sensation in the saddle region. Lesions of the thoracic spinal cord often affect the sensory tracts or entering sensory fibers, so that patients complain of numbness of an area of skin or numbness from the waist or rib cage downward. A few patients present with primarily cerebral symptoms, such as depression, difficulty in concentration, defective memory, or speech disorder. Such symptoms are far more common in patients with well-advanced, chronic, severe MS, but in rare instances they may occur at an early stage.

At all stages of the illness, fatigue is a recognizable and common symptom that may produce a specific type of disability in addition to the disability produced by the neurologic deficit. All symptoms of MS, particularly the milder symptoms, tend to fluctuate with levels of fatigue, excitement, and body temperature. Patients report a change in visual acuity as the day progresses or report that they can walk a certain distance and then their legs tire. This day-to-day and hour-to-hour variability of symptoms is quite characteristic.

Etiology and Pathogenesis

The cause of MS remains unknown. Recent evidence indicates an autoimmune attack on the central nervous system by activated lymphocytes, followed by macrophages. Why this attack occurs is unknown. Certain epidemiologic evidence suggests that MS is acquired, and that there is a long latency between exposure to an unknown agent and the development of clinically apparent symptoms. The incidence in close family members (parents and siblings) is at least five times what it is in the population at large. It is not settled whether this represents a common exposure to a pathogenetic agent or an inherited disorder of immune regulation; the latter explanation seems more likely. If one identical twin has MS, in 50% of instances the other twin will have clinical or laboratory evidence of MS. Many unsuccessful efforts to isolate a virus from patients with MS have been made.

Unlike patients with other autoimmune diseases, such as lupus erythematosus and myasthenia gravis, patients with MS are singularly free of coexisting illness. Rare instances of chronic demyelinating neuropathy with MS are known. Bipolar manic-depressive illness is overrepresented among the MS population compared with other psychiatric illnesses.

The histopathologic lesions in the brain suggest a cell-mediated autoimmune disease. Studies of populations of lymphocytes in the brain have indicated that the lymphocytes show an overrepresentation of $T8^+$ (suppressor/cytotoxic) cells. Studies of the immunoglobulin G (IgG) that is present in the spinal fluid in patients with MS indicate a polyclonal response.

Many patients with chronic, active, progressive MS will show a reduction of $T8^+$ cells in the peripheral blood. Current efforts at many laboratories to define a regulatory defect in the immune system of MS patients, particularly a defect correlating with disease activity, have thus far proved unsuccessful.

Recent data indicate a role for circulating lymphocytes that are reactive to immunologically dominant peptides of myelin basic protein.

Diagnosis

Although several laboratory investigations are now available to assist in the diagnosis of MS, the diagnosis remains a clinical one. It must be based on the observation of a chronic recurring or chronic progressive disease of the central nervous system, affecting more than one location in the nervous system and dispersed over time. Mistakes in diagnosis usually can be traced to failure to observe these simple rules, or to overreliance on laboratory tests. There is commonly a delay of several years between the onset of the first symptoms and the confirmed diagnosis of MS.

Laboratory Tests. Diagnostic aid from the laboratory allows earlier diagnosis in many instances. The five specific areas of laboratory investigation are described.

Examination of the cerebrospinal fluid. The cerebrospinal fluid (CSF) of a patient with MS commonly contains 5 to 100 lymphocytes/mm^3 at any stage of the illness. The total protein is usually normal or mildly elevated. CSF protein over 100 mg/dl is distinctly unusual in MS and should immediately raise suspicion of some other process. Spinal fluid IgG is elevated, particularly in the middle or later stages of the illness. Elevation of CSF IgG can be measured as the total IgG in mg/dl (normally less than 5 mg/dl), ratio of IgG to albumin (normally less than 12%), or as an index relating the ratio of CSF IgG synthesized within the nervous system to systemic IgG. All of these are satisfactory and give equivalent results, being positive in approximately 80% of patients with chronic relapsing or chronic progressive MS. Patients in the early phases of the illness are the most likely to have a normal CSF IgG.

If subjected to electrophoresis, the IgG is seen to form into one or more distinct bands (oligoclonal bands). This is characteristic of MS, although it is also observed in other illnesses in which IgG is synthesized within the nervous system, such as syphilis, subacute sclerosing panencephalitis, and, occasionally, lupus erythematosus.

Evoked-potential testing. These are electrophysiologic measurements in which a stimulus is delivered and its transit through the nervous system is timed. The commonly used tests include visual-evoked response, brain stem auditory-evoked response, and somatosensory-evoked response. It is characteristic of demyelination of the central nervous system to produce electrophysiologic delay in these measurements. Evoked-response testing is abnormal in more than 80% of patients with chronic relapsing or chronic progressive MS. The visual-evoked response is the most likely to be abnormal and is the most clinically relevant test. In patients who have only chronic progressive myelopathy on clinical examination, the discovery of delay, particularly an asymmetric delay, of visual-evoked response is clear evidence of a second lesion of the nervous system and thus helps to confirm the diagnosis.

Computed tomography scanning. A minority of patients with MS show lesions on computed tomography (CT) scan. Such lesions are often hypodense and may enhance with contrast material, particularly when they are acute. Patients with chronic MS may show nonenhancing hypodense lesions, as well as signs of cerebral atrophy. Diagnostic changes on CT scan occur in no more than 15% of all patients with MS.

Magnetic resonance imaging. Magnetic resonance imaging (MRI) scans show lesions within the brain in more than 90% of patients and in the spinal cord in a smaller percentage. Patients with relapsing disease or with secondary progressive MS show more lesions than do those with primary progressive MS. The lesions appear as high-intensity bright lesions in the central white matter; they are bright on T2-weighted images owing to high water content (Figs. 145-1 and 145-2). Newly developed lesions can be distinguished by their enhancement with gadolinium, an ionized compound that will traverse a disrupted blood-brain barrier.

Recent serial studies of MRI in MS patients have shown that (1) the disease is much more continuously active than the clinical course will show, (2) most lesions are asymptomatic, and (3) there is a correlation between new, enhancing, or enlarging lesions and overall clinical course.

Other illnesses cause comparable MRI appearances. The diagnosis of MS should never be based on MRI data alone. Small vascular lesions, infarctions due to migraine, Sjögren's syndrome, and AIDS encephalopathy are examples of illnesses that may resemble MS by

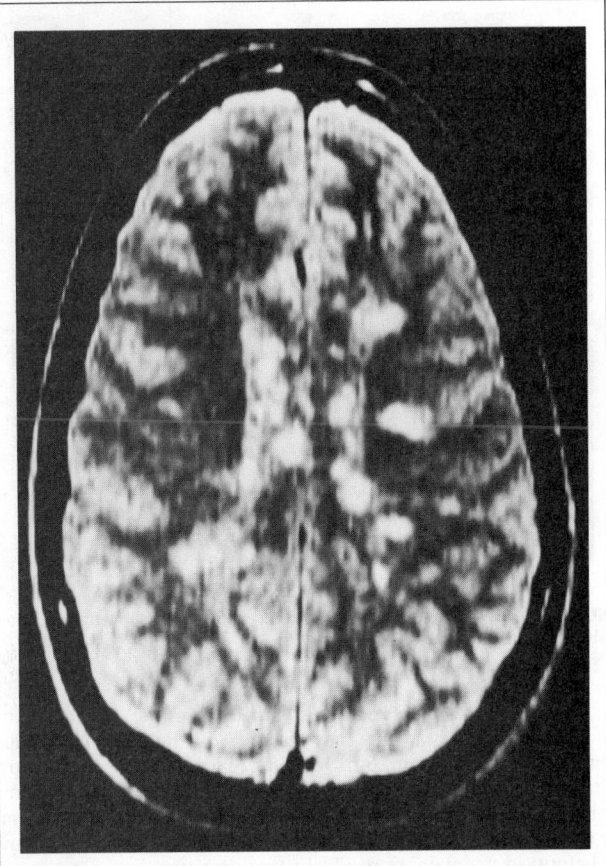

FIGURE 145-1   MRI scan of cerebral hemispheres in a patient with early relapsing-remitting multiple sclerosis. The bright periventricular lesions are characteristic; in this patient they were asymptomatic.

MRI criteria. Very small T2-weighted bright lesions in white matter can be seen in patients who appear to be clinically normal.

Informing the Patient. Under which circumstances a patient should be advised of the diagnosis of MS is often a difficult decision. The great majority of patients prefer to be told of the diagnosis at the early stage. Only if there are specific contraindications, such as emotional instability, depression, or turmoil within the family, should a diagnosis be withheld. Once a decision has been made to impart the diagnosis, the illness should be explained in a clear and easily comprehensible fashion, avoiding euphemisms and stressing the possibilities of treatment. At all stages of illness, alternate diagnoses should be considered. These possibilities are listed in Table 145-1.

TREATMENT

Myriad treatments have been proposed for this long-term, variable illness. The list of proposed treatments encompasses everything from diet to electrical stimulation to acupuncture, emotional support, bee stings, and various forms of immunosuppressive therapy. Patients and families frequently seek guidance as to the veracity of such treatments. General supportive psychologic and medical care is important. Specific symptoms can often be treated quite effectively, even when the overall course of the illness cannot be altered. Patients with significant degrees of depression may benefit from antidepressant medications, counseling, or formal psychotherapy. Flexor spasms of the limbs, spasticity when walking, and other symptoms of pyramidal tract dysfunction may respond to antispasticity medications such as baclofen, 20 to 60 mg/day. Benzodiazepines may be used for the same purpose but pose a significant risk of addiction. Patients with MS frequently have bladder dysfunction, either atonic bladder or neurogenic bladder with early urgency and rapid voiding, or various com-

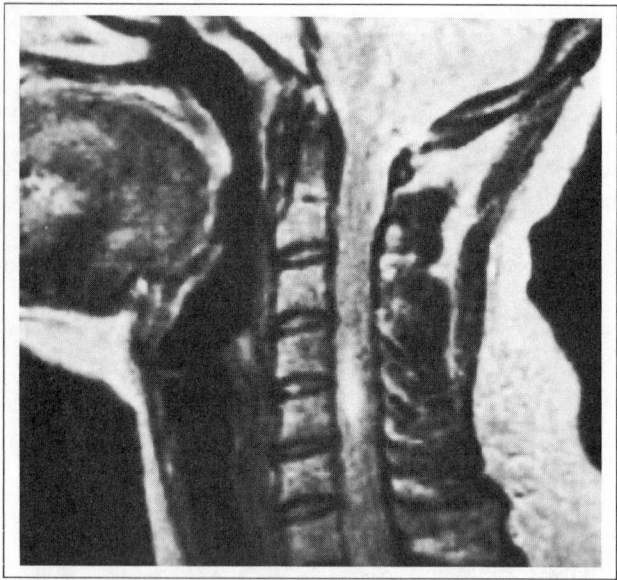

FIGURE 145-2   MRI scan through the cervical region showing a lesion of multiple sclerosis in the C4-5 region.

binations of these two syndromes with dyssynergic contractions of the sphincter. Some patients may respond to anticholinergic medications such as oxybutynin, 5 mg once or twice a day, or to low doses of tricyclic antidepressants. Tonic spasms or trigeminal neuralgia may be treated by carbamazepine. For patients with specific types of motor disorders, particularly spasticity and weakness, physiotherapy may be helpful in maintaining residual neurologic function.

For individual attacks of MS that occur in the setting of the relapsing/remitting disease, many neurologists use brief courses of corticosteroids. ACTH (adrenocorticotrophic hormone) has been demonstrated to have some slight but definite effect in shortening the course of attacks of MS but is now rarely used.

Intravenous steroids, in the form of 1000 mg/day of methylprednisolone given over 1 to 2 hours for 5 to 7 days, are now commonly used. Preliminary data indicate a better response in acute relapses than other forms of treatment. An important trial of therapy for optic neuritis showed a better response to intravenous steroids than to placebo or oral prednisone and demonstrated a higher subsequent relapse rate after oral steroids. This may serve to further limit the use of oral steroids for relapses of MS, as well as for optic neuritis.

To influence the long-term course of the illness, many immunosuppressive regimens have been advocated. At present, only one agent, β-interferon, has Food and Drug Administration (FDA) approval for use in MS to control the course of illness. A trial of this agent, given every other day by subcutaneous injection, as Betaseron, showed a reduction in attack rate and a reduction in development of new lesions on MRI. A different β-interferon preparation (Avmex) is given as weekly intramuscular injections; trials have shown comparible efficacy. Beta-interferon is approved for use in relapsing-remitting ambulatory MS patients.

Another immunomodulating agent, Copolymer I, has produced comparable results in trials in comparable patients and has been released for general use. All these agents reduce attack frequency by approximately 30% in trials.

No effective treatment is available for patients with progressive MS, with either primary or secondary progression. At present, this is a field of intense interest, and new protocols are being tried at many institutions. Long-term oral azathioprine accompanied by steroids and high-dose intravenous cyclophosphamide are the immunosuppressive therapies that have the best supporting data at present.

Limitations of azathioprine, as judged by metaanalysis of many trials, apparently derive from toxicity associated with its use. Limitations of effectiveness of cyclophosphamide seem to derive from lack of effect in patients age 40 or older.

More specific treatments (anti–T-cell monoclonal antibodies, oral myelin desensitization, β-interferon) may be more useful but remain experimental.

The unpredictable course of MS requires great care in the choice of treatment. Patients should not begin ill-advised and dangerous treatments when it is possible that the overall nature of the illness may remain benign throughout. However, patients who enter an active progressive phase of the illness can expect that deterioration will, in all likelihood, continue, and such patients may be candidates for aggressive treatment.

ACUTE DISSEMINATED ENCEPHALOMYELITIS

This rare illness occurs in all age-groups but is more commonly recognized in the pediatric and young adult age-groups. It is a monophasic illness, consisting pathologically of a multitude of small perivenous demyelinating lesions throughout the nervous system. The symptoms frequently develop after a prior viral illness, such as the exanthems of childhood; they have also been reported following vaccinations, such as diphtheria-pertussis-tetanus (DPT), smallpox, and rabies. Unlike in MS, both the central and peripheral nervous systems characteristically are involved. Symptoms may consist of confusion, stupor, blindness, transverse myelitis, weakness of the extremities, ataxia, and incontinence—all occurring at approximately the same time.

Rarely, the CSF is normal; usually, it contains a mild-to-moderate elevation of total protein and several hundred lymphocytes/mm^3.

ACUTE HEMORRHAGIC LEUKOENCEPHALOPATHY

This very rare illness presents as a large patch of demyelination affecting one hemisphere, frequently tracking down within the cerebral peduncles into the corresponding brain stem and cerebellum. The CSF may contain blood. It has a very high mortality rate. In all likelihood, this entity represents an acute and severe version of the preceding illness, although in a few cases that have been well studied, no prior exanthem or prior illness was recognized.

PROGRESSIVE MULTIFOCAL LEUKOENCEPHALOPATHY

Although still classified as a demyelinating illness, this rare disease is now known to be a chronic viral infection. It occurs in patients in whom the immune system is suppressed, particularly those with leukemia, lymphoma, or AIDS, and also in rare patients receiving immunosuppressive drugs for renal transplantation or rheumatoid arthritis. The plaques of viral infection usually begin in one hemisphere and spread over the course of weeks or months throughout the nervous system. The plaques are normally visible by CT scan at a time when clinical symptoms appear. The CSF is characteristically normal. At biopsy or autopsy the lesions are shown to contain Jakob-Creutzfeldt (JC) virus, a papovavirus. No effective therapy is known, and the disease is uniformly fatal.

TRANSVERSE MYELITIS

This term refers to a clinical syndrome in which a patient suffers a total or near-total spinal cord lesion, usually over the course of a few days. On pathologic examination, the lesion not only is demyelinating but also may include necrosis of neurons or axons. Thoracic and lumbar segments of the cord are usually affected. Recovery is often incomplete, with significant residual disability. About 10% of patients with acute transverse myelitis are later found to have MS on the basis of later-developing lesions.

BIBLIOGRAPHY

Beck RW, Cleary PA, Trobe JD et al: The effect of corticosteroids for acute optic neuritis on the subsequent development of multiple sclerosis, *N Engl J Med* 329:1764-1769, 1993.

Hafler DA, Weiner HL: Immunologic mechanisms and therapy in multiple sclerosis, *Immunol Rev* 144:75-105, 1995.

IFNB Multiple Sclerosis Study Group: Interferon beta-1b is effective in relapsing-remitting multiple sclerosis. I. Clinical results of a multicenter, randomized, double-blind, placebo-controlled trial, *Neurology* 43:655-661, 1993.

Johnson KP, Brooks BR, Cohen JA et al: Copolymer 1 reduces relapse rate and improves disability in relapsing-remitting multiple sclerosis: results of a phase III multicenter, double-blind, placebo-controlled trial, *Neurology* 45:1268-1276, 1995.

Miller DH, McDonald WI: Neuroimaging in multiple sclerosis, *Clin Neurosci* 2:215-224, 1994.

Minden SL, Scheffer RB: Affective disorders in multiple sclerosis, *Arch Neurol* 47:98-104, 1990.

Quality Standards Subcommittee of the American Academy of Neurology: Practice advisory on selection of patients with multiple sclerosis for treatment with Betaseron, *Neurology* 44:1537-1540, 1994.

CHAPTER

146   Myelopathies

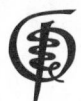

Frisso A. Potts

Myelopathy is the term used to designate disease in the spinal cord. When there is evidence of inflammation, the term *myelitis* is preferred. The disease may involve one or many segments and may extend partially or completely across the transverse diameter of the cord. Lesions may arise within the cord *(intramedullary)* or be caused by pressure by an external mass *(extramedullary)*. The clinical presentation varies depending on the level and extent of the pathologic process. Box 146-1 lists a few of the more commonly encountered causes of myelopathy.

RELEVANT PHYSIOLOGY AND PATHOPHYSIOLOGY
Anatomic Aspects

The spinal cord is composed of longitudinal tracts subserving motor and sensory functions. Motor tracts carry descending impulses from higher centers to the appropriate anterior horn cells, and from there, motor axons exit the cord by way of anterior roots into peripheral nerves to innervate specific muscle groups. Conversely, sensory input carried by peripheral nerves enters the cord through posterior roots at discrete levels before forming ascending tracts. This segmental arrangement allows the clinician to localize precisely the rostral extent of a lesion. In addition, its anteroposterior and transverse extent can be inferred with some knowledge of the arrangement of these tracts. Figure 146-1 diagrams the essential anatomy of the spinal cord.

The most diagnostically useful tracts are the following:

1. *Corticospinal tract.* The corticospinal tract carries motor input from the contralateral cerebral cortex to the anterior horn cells. It decussates in the medulla and remains ipsilateral to the point of exit of the motor roots. Fibers descending to sacral levels are laterally placed; those reaching the cervical segments are more medially placed.
2. *Dorsal columns.* The dorsal columns carry the sensations of discriminative touch, position, and vibration to the contralateral cerebral cortex. In the cord they remain ipsilateral to the side of entry of the posterior roots because they do not decussate until they reach the medulla. The sacral segments are located medially and the cervical, laterally.
3. *Lateral spinothalamic tract.* The lateral spinothalamic tract carries crude touch, pain, and temperature sensation from the contralateral side of the body. Fibers carrying these modalities from the periphery enter the spinal cord through posterior roots, synapse, and decussate within a segment or two. The resulting tract has sacral input outermost and cervical innermost.
4. *Autonomic fibers.* Autonomic fibers run in the white matter of the cord near the central canal and carry sympathetic outflow to the thoracic cord, whence motor fibers exit to provide sympathetic innervation to various organs. These tracts also carry input to sacral centers concerned with voluntary bowel and bladder function, as well as penile erectile function in the male.

> ### BOX 146-1
> ### Causes of myelopathy and myelitis
>
> **Inflammatory**
> Infectious
>   Bacterial: Spirochetal, tuberculous
>   Viral: Poliomyelitis; herpes HTLV, HIV, zoster; rabies
>   Other: Rickettsial, fungal, parasitic
> Noninfectious
>   Idiopathic transverse myelitis, multiple sclerosis
>
> **Toxic/metabolic**
> Arsenic
> Pernicious anemia
> Pellagra
> Diabetes mellitus
> Chronic liver disease
>
> **Trauma**
> Spinal fracture/dislocation
> Stab/bullet wound
> Herniated nucleus pulposus
>
> **Compression**
> Spinal neoplasm
> Cervical spondylosis
> Extramedullary hematopoiesis
> Epidural abscess
> Epidural hematoma
>
> **Vascular**
> Arteriovenous malformation
> Periarteritis nodosa
> Lupus erythematosus
> Dissecting aortic aneurysm
>
> **Physical agents**
> Electrical injury
> Irradiation
>
> **Neoplastic**
> Spinal cord tumors
> Paraneoplastic myelopathy
>
> ---
> *HTLV,* Human T-cell leukemia virus; *HIV,* human immunodeficiency virus.

The following basic principles are helpful in defining the location and extent of cord disease:

1. Transverse spinal cord lesions give signs and symptoms below the level of the lesion.
2. Lesions in the region of the central canal affect primarily decussating pain and temperature fibers, giving signs and symptoms at the level of the lesion. However, if the transverse extent of the lesion is large, the longitudinal tracts and even the motor neurons in the anterior horn may be affected. When spinothalamic fibers are involved by an expanding central lesion, the sacral fibers tend to be spared.
3. Intrinsic cord lesions are usually painless and affect autonomic function early. Extrinsic compression is usually accompanied by focal pain in the affected segment of the spine, and autonomic involvement is late.

Clinical Aspects

Acute Spinal Cord Compression or Transection. The acute spinal cord compression or transection syndrome is most commonly the result of trauma, such as vertebral fracture or gunshot wound. Rarely, it may be seen as a result of intervertebral disk herniation or as a result of intramedullary spinal cord disease (hemorrhage or infarction). Complete spinal cord transections give rise to *spinal shock.* There is complete flaccid paralysis and sensory loss below the level of the lesion, and urinary and fecal retention occur. If the lesion is

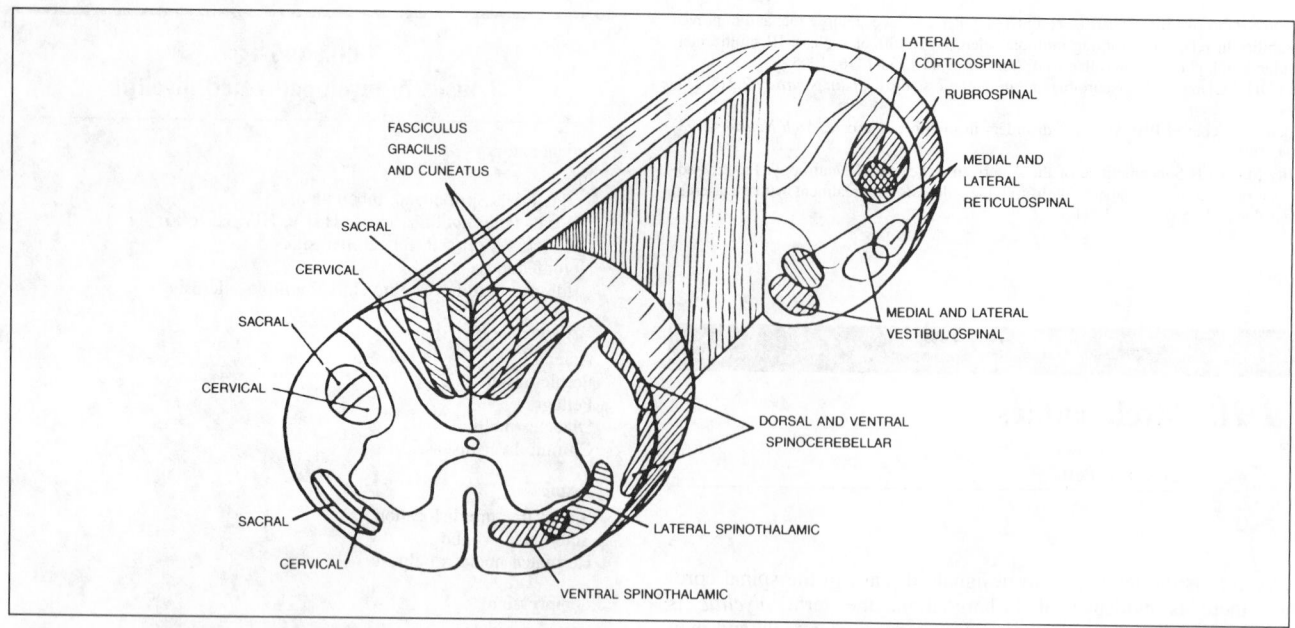

FIGURE 146-1   Principal tracts of the spinal cord. Lamination in the posterior columns and corticospinal and spinothalamic tracts is shown in the left half of the diagram. The location of the sensory pathways is shown at the same level on the right, and the location of the motor pathways is shown at another level on the far right.
Modified from Daube JR, Sandok BA: *Medical neurosciences,* Boston, 1978, Little, Brown.

above the midthoracic level, interference with descending sympathetic tracts gives rise to failure of the sympathetic nervous system with attendant hypotension, and anhydrosis is evident below the level of the lesion. With high cervical lesions, severe respiratory embarrassment is the rule. If the patient does not succumb to respiratory failure or urinary tract infection, recovery from spinal shock starts in several days to weeks, with return of stretch reflexes and the beginning of reflex micturition. As weeks and months progress, increasing spastic rigidity of previously flaccid muscles occurs, and patients usually have involuntary muscle spasms (flexor spasms).

Subacute Spinal Cord Compression. The subacute spinal cord compression syndrome is most likely to occur as a result of extrinsic cord lesions; tumors and degenerative joint disease of the spine are the leading causes. It is imperative for the physician to make an early diagnosis of spinal compression, since in many instances decompression is feasible and permanent loss of function may be avoided. Early signs of spinal compression include paresthesia and sensory loss below the level of the lesion. Stiffness and weakness of the legs are common. In more advanced cases, urinary frequency with urgency and flexor spasms of the lower extremities are seen.

Brown-Séquard Syndrome. The Brown-Séquard syndrome of hemisection of the cord may be seen with intrinsic or extrinsic lesions and consists of motor weakness and spasticity in segments below and ipsilateral to the lesion. Loss of vibratory and position sense also occurs ipsilateral to the lesion (undecussated tracts), whereas loss of pain and temperature sensation (decussated tracts) is found contralateral to the lesion.

Central Cord Syndrome. The term *central cord syndrome* is applied to myelopathies that affect the most central region of the cord. They give rise to deficits in pain and temperature sensation at the level of the lesion (since the incoming fibers decussate through the center of the cord) with sparing of vibratory and position sense—the so-called *dissociated sensory loss.* By the same token, stretch reflexes at the level of the lesion are impaired, and if the lesion is large enough to involve the more laterally placed tracts, there is spasticity and sensory loss to temperature and pain below the level of the lesion. Sacral sparing is the rule, since these segments are represented by lat-

erally placed fibers. A classic example is the developmental anomaly known as *syringomyelia.* Hyperextension injuries of the neck have also been known to give rise to the central cord syndrome.

Syndrome of the Anterior Spinal Artery. As its name implies, this myelopathy occurs as a result of ischemia in the territory of the anterior spinal artery. It causes a functional transection of the cord involving the spinothalamic and corticospinal tracts, as well as the anterior horn cells in the affected region. The posterior columns are spared, since they derive their blood supply from the posterior spinal artery.

Laboratory and Other Diagnostic Tests

Once the lesion is localized on clinical examination, plain x-rays of the spine may reveal bony abnormalities such as fractures, bony spurs impinging on the spinal canal, or bone erosion by neoplasm. Abnormal uptake in bone scans also aids in identifying bony abnormalities and extramedullary masses. Myelography, particularly when combined with computed tomography (CT) of the spine, is an excellent way of defining extramedullary and intramedullary lesions. However, the best method for defining spinal cord disease is magnetic resonance imaging (MRI), which provides excellent resolution of intrinsic as well as extrinsic lesions (see Chapter 132). As an adjunct to these procedures, examination of cerebrospinal fluid (CSF) may demonstrate the presence of hemorrhage, of inflammatory or malignant cells, and of abnormal proteins, thus giving clues to etiologic factors.

Differential Diagnosis

Cervical Spondylosis. Cervical spondylosis is the most common cause of myelopathy. In its earliest or simplest form, it becomes evident with neck pain that may radiate into the arms. Babinski's sign is usually present early in the course and may be the only sign of cord involvement. Indeed, it is thought that cervical spondylosis with asymptomatic cord compression is the underlying reason for the high incidence of extensor plantar responses in the elderly. The course is extremely variable, but in its progressive form it gives rise to the syndrome of subacute cord compression (see earlier discussion). A coexistent radiculopathy may decrease or obliterate stretch reflexes in the upper extremities. Treatment of mild, slowly progressive cases consists of immobilization of the neck with a collar. If progression occurs, cervical laminectomy for cord decompression may be necessary. An anterior cervical approach with intervertebral disk removal and spinal fusion has also been used.

Transverse Myelitis. The term *transverse myelitis* is used to describe a rapidly progressive (hours or days) myelopathy characterized by necrosis of the spinal cord in one or several segments. The clinical picture is as described earlier for acute spinal cord compression. The CSF may show an inflammatory pleocytosis with or without evidence of a hemorrhagic component. Protein elevation is the rule. MRI may show a swollen cord at the involved level. The syndrome may be temporally related to a number of viral illnesses or to vaccinations (notably influenza and smallpox vaccines). In these cases recovery does not often occur and no successful therapy is available, although treatment with steroids or adrenocorticotropic hormone (ACTH) may be palliative. When this condition is associated with multiple sclerosis (MS), there usually are signs of involvement elsewhere in the central nervous system and remissions and exacerbations are the rule. The presence of monoclonal bands on CSF protein electrophoresis would suggest that a transverse myelopathy is caused by MS, although it would not prove this unequivocally.

Epidural Abscess. Epidural abscesses usually occur in the lumbar region and are rarely the cause of spinal cord compression. When they occur in the thoracic or cervical cord, they give rise to subacute spinal cord compression (see earlier discussion) with early involvement of posterior columns, since the usual site for the abscess is posterior to the cord. Frequently there is pain at the site of involvement. In their more common location, the abscesses give rise to cauda equina syndrome, which is characterized by focal pain, development of hyporeflexia in the lower extremities, and in the most severe cases, progressive sensory loss, motor weakness, and, eventually, sphincter paralysis. Although not every case develops in this inexorable, devastating fashion, a high index of suspicion is necessary to prevent worsening in mild cases. Radiologic studies easily demonstrate the abscess, and progression may be arrested with antibiotic therapy; however, surgical decompression is usually necessary.

Retrovirus Infection. A slowly progressive, nonhemorrhagic, usually noninflammatory myelopathy has been associated with systemic infection by the viruses human T-cell leukemia virus-I (HTLV-I) and human immunodeficiency virus (HIV) (formerly known as HTLV-III). The former may occur in familial form and accounts for many cases of tropical spastic paraparesis. Spastic lower-extremity weakness with variable sensory loss develops over a period of months. The spinal level of the lesion may "ascend," originally starting in the thoracic cord but eventually involving the high cervical cord. Autonomic function may be spared. The CSF is usually acellular with only mild protein level elevations and in most cases contains antibodies against the offending virus.

Metabolic Myelopathies. The most notorious example of these disorders (although rarely seen today) is combined systems degeneration, the myelopathy associated with pernicious anemia (see Chapter 80) that consists of progressive lower-extremity spastic paraparesis resulting from corticospinal tract disease with superimposed ataxia caused by posterior column involvement. There usually is a fairly well-defined sensory cord level to vibratory sense. A peripheral neuropathy of vitamin B_{12} deficiency is invariably present. A similar myelopathy has been described with folate deficiency. Chronic liver failure is also associated with a myelopathy—a slowly progressive spastic paraparesis or quadriparesis with a poorly defined sensory level. Autonomic sparing is the rule. Its origin is not clear, although it is thought that nutritional factors may play a role.

Paraneoplastic Myelopathies. Spastic paraparesis or quadriparesis with a relatively well-defined sensory level may occur in the setting of systemic malignancy, such as lymphoma or various other tumors. When no evidence of concurrent retrovirus infection or direct involvement of the cord by tumor is evident, the term *paraneo-*

plastic may be applied. This is an uncommon manifestation of systemic malignancy, and its pathophysiologic and etiologic features are not clear.

Radiation-Induced Myelopathy. This complication of radiation treatment may occur in as many as 4% of patients who have received radiation therapy for spinal or body cavity tumors. It occurs most often when the location makes incidental irradiation of the cord possible, and its onset usually occurs between 12 and 15 months after completion of treatment, although it has been reported as early as 6 months and as late as 60 months. The process is a slowly progressive one, involving the cord levels subjected to the irradiation. Initial minor symptoms usually progress over a period of months to a full-blown spinal transection syndrome with severe motor, sensory, and autonomic impairment. No form of treatment has been successful, although steroids may have a transient beneficial effect. This complication is clearly related to radiation dose, and it is rarely seen when the cord has received less than 3300 rad.

Spinal Tumors. About half of spinal tumors are metastatic to the extramedullary structures and invade locally to produce the subacute spinal cord compression as described earlier. Bone involvement is usually heralded by focal pain and easily detected by plain radiographic films and bone scan. More subtly invasive tumors such as the lymphomas and sarcomas spread through the meninges and cause spinal compression with little bony evidence of their presence. Identification must rely on CT scanning or MRI. Once the tumor has been identified, irradiation and chemotherapy are the treatments of choice. The second most common spinal tumor is the meningioma that arises outside the cord but within the dural sac; these tumors are amenable to surgical excision. Primary intraspinal tumors are the rarest of the lot, and they consist mainly of gliomas. The myelopathies produced by primary intraspinal tumors (unlike those produced by metastatic tumors) generally are slowly progressive.

Complications of Vascular Surgery. Ischemic infarction of the spinal cord can complicate aortic surgery. The incidence of this complication is highest (28%) in procedures involving the thoracic and abdominal aorta. A much higher incidence of myelopathy (48%) has been reported in aneurysmal repair after dissection or rupture of the aneurysm. However, aortic surgery below the level of the renal arteries carries little or no danger of ischemic myelopathy. The clinical presentation in most cases is that of acute spinal transection at a middle or lower thoracic cord level. Hypotension that is caused by spinal shock may further complicate the clinical picture. Full recovery is the exception rather than the rule. Many procedures have been used in an attempt to prevent this surgical complication. Among these are artery-to-artery shunting, pretreatment with steroids, free-radical scavengers, thiopental, papaverine, and hypothermia. Of these, only the last seems to have a beneficial effect.

Management

Successful management of myelopathy depends on the rapid identification and treatment of its cause. When faced with an acute myelopathy, the clinician must make every effort to find a reversible cause. Speed is of the essence, in order to prevent permanent damage. There is evidence to show that patients with acute myelopathies, regardless of origin, may benefit from early treatment with methylprednisolone. Present recommendation is for a bolus of 30 mg/kg to be administered as early as possible, preferably within 8 hours of onset. Continuing treatment with methylprednisolone may be helpful in some cases, and the reader is referred to the bibliography at the end of the chapter for further reading. The specific mode of therapy is mandated by the nature of the lesion. Surgical intervention may be appropriate in cases of compression resulting from masses extrinsic to the cord. Some metastatic implants, however, may be best treated by irradiation. As a general rule, acute intramedullary lesions, whether vascular, neoplastic, or inflammatory, are not as amenable to the surgical approach as extramedullary ones. Other agents such as naloxone, N-methyl-D-aspartate receptor antagonist, and GM$_1$ ganglioside are under investigation.

✔ *WHEN TO REFER*

Management of acute or chronic myelopathies is best left to experts in this field. The mere suspicion of myelopathy should prompt the general internist to seek consultation from a specialist well versed in spinal cord injury. Little resistance will be encountered by the referring physician. Specialists in this area, be they neurologic surgeons, orthopedic surgeons, neurologists, or spinal cord injury specialists, are well aware of the disastrous consequences resulting from delay in diagnosis or treatment.

Treatment of subacute myelopathies, which are commonly encountered in cervical spondylosis and slowly growing spinal tumors, is, again, dictated by the nature of the lesion and the speed of progression. Methylprednisolone as a sole agent is probably not useful in these cases, although it may be a useful adjunct to surgical or radiation treatment.

BIBLIOGRAPHY

Bracken MB: Pharmacological treatment of acute spinal cord injury: current status and future prospects, *Paraplegia* 30:102, 1992.

Dawson DM, Potts FA: Acute nontraumatic myelopathies. In Woolsey RM, Young RR, editors: *Diagnosis and management of disorders of the spinal cord,* Philadelphia, 1995, WB Saunders.

Helweg-Larsen SJ et al: Myelopathy in AIDS: a clinical, neuroradiological and electrophysiological study of 23 Danish patients, *Acta Neurol Scand* 77:64, 1988.

Nussbaum E et al: Spinal epidural abscess: a report of 40 cases and review, *Surg Neurol* 38:225, 1992.

Plum F, Olson ME: Myelitis and myelopathy. In Baker AB, Baker LH, editors: *Clinical neurology,* Hagerstown, Md, 1984, Harper & Row.

Salazar-Grueso EF et al: Familial spastic paraparesis syndrome associated with HTLV-I infection, *N Engl J Med* 323:732, 1990.

Yu YL et al: Cervical spondylotic myelopathy and radiculopathy, *Acta Neurol Scand* 75:367, 1987.

CHAPTER

147   Diseases of Peripheral Nerve and Motor Neurons

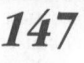

Eric L. Logigian

Signs and symptoms of a peripheral nerve disorder depend on the fiber composition (sensory, motor, and autonomic) of the affected nerves, the selectivity of the disease process (which fiber types are affected), the part of the body they innervate, and the patient's sensitivity to dysfunction of the affected fibers. For example, mild entrapment of the median nerve at the wrist may spare motor and autonomic fibers and affect the sensory fibers alone, resulting in sensory symptoms, sometimes without signs, in the median nerve distribution of the hand. Such symptoms may be more disturbing to a musician than to someone whose livelihood is not so dependent on optimal hand function.

Disorders of peripheral nerve result in "negative" and "positive" symptoms and signs, many of which are listed in Table 147-1. Not listed are functional problems that the patient may notice, such as dropping things from the hand, which may signify finger weakness or sensory loss. Similarly, falling or unsteadiness when walking may be caused by polyneuropathy affecting the sensory or motor fibers in the lower extremities. Inquiry about what the patient can and cannot do is often useful in characterizing muscle weakness. Oculobulbar weakness becomes evident as ptosis, diplopia, swallowing or chewing trouble, nasal regurgitation of fluids, and drooling. Proximal limb weakness typically causes trouble with reaching above the head, getting out of a chair, or going upstairs, or a waddling gait, whereas

Table 147-1   Signs and symptoms of peripheral nerve disease

FIBER TYPE	NEGATIVE	POSITIVE
Motor	Weakness, atrophy, fatigability, clumsiness, areflexia, hypotonia, deformities (pes cavus, kyphoscoliosis)	Muscle twitches (fasciculations, myokymia), cramps
Sensory	Sensory loss, ataxia, clumsiness, areflexia, hypotonia	"Tingling," "pins and needles," "burning"
Autonomic	Postural hypotension, loss of sweating, impotence, bowel and bladder symptoms	Hyperhidrosis, gustatory sweating
Trophic		Foot ulceration, Charcot's arthropathy

Table 147-2   Large- and small-fiber sensory symptoms and signs

	LARGER FIBER	SMALL FIBER
Symptoms	"Tingling," "pins and needles"	"Burning," "aching," "jabbing"
Signs	Loss of vibratory and joint position sense, areflexia, ataxia	Loss of sharp-dull or temperature discrimination

distal limb weakness results in trouble with unscrewing jar lids, buttoning, zipping, holding a pen or eating utensils, or tripping.

Peripheral nerve disease may not only selectively affect motor, sensory, or autonomic fibers, but it also may affect nerve fibers according to size. Table 147-2 lists the sensory symptoms and signs referable to nerve fibers of large and small diameter. Not listed is autonomic dysfunction, which, if on a peripheral basis, is evidence for small-fiber neuropathy, whereas motor dysfunction from disease of motoneuron axons represents a disorder of medium to large fibers. Since large fibers are more thickly myelinated than are thinly myelinated or unmyelinated small axons, "large fiber" dysfunction may result from disorders predominantly affecting myelin (i.e., demyelinative neuropathy) or larger axons (i.e., axonal neuropathy). The two can frequently be differentiated with electrophysiologic studies.

DIFFERENTIAL DIAGNOSIS
Peripheral Nervous System Versus Central Nervous System

Before ascribing weakness or sensory loss to the peripheral nervous system, the physician should be certain there are no central nervous system (CNS) signs (Table 147-3). Ordinarily, hyporeflexia, hypotonia, and muscle wasting are indicative of peripheral nerve disease, although acute lesions of the CNS can result in hyporeflexia and hypotonia, and a chronic lesion of the CNS can lead to "disuse" atrophy. In addition, several diseases affect both the CNS and the peripheral nervous system (PNS). Therefore CNS signs in a patient with peripheral neuropathy are important clues.

Nerve Versus Neuromuscular Junction and Muscle Weakness

Muscle weakness without any sensory signs or symptoms is rarely caused by peripheral nerve disease and should suggest disease of motor neurons, neuromuscular junction (NMJ), or muscle. Patients with myasthenia gravis typically have prominent oculobulbar weakness with or without proximal limb weakness. Patients with Lambert-Eaton myasthenic syndrome (LEMS) may cause some diagnostic confusion, since they are usually areflexic. In both these conditions, electrophysiologic evaluation and autoantibody studies can localize the disease to the NMJ rather than the nerve. In contrast to most polyneuropa-

Table 147-3 Central nervous system signs and possible implications

SIGN	POSSIBLE IMPLICATION
Extensor plantar response	Lesion of the upper motor neuron
Hyperreflexia, hypertonus	Lesion of the upper motor neuron
Sensory or motor level	Spinal cord lesion
Loss of sharp-dull discrimination contralateral to limb weakness	Spinal cord lesion

Table 147-4 Clinicopathologic syndromes in peripheral neuropathy and neuronopathy

SYNDROMES	PRIMARY DISEASE OR DISORDER
Neuronopathy	
Motoneuronopathy	Lower motoneurons in spinal cord, brain stem, and/or upper motoneurons
Sensory neuronopathy	Dorsal root ganglia
Autonomic neuronopathy	Autonomic ganglia
Radiculopathy	Dorsal and/or ventral roots, or both
Polyradiculopathy, cranial neuropathy, meningitis	Roots, cranial nerves, meninges
Polyradiculoneuropathy	Roots, plexus, and nerves
Plexopathy	Plexus
Mononeuropathy	One nerve (sensory, motor, or mixed)
Mononeuropathy multiplex	Two or more nerves
Polyneuropathy	Many or all nerves
Demyelinative neuropathy	Myelin
Axonal neuropathy	Axon
Polyneuropathy or mononeuritis multiplex with central nervous system involvement	Peripheral and central nervous system

thies, muscle disease more frequently affects proximal muscles and is associated with preserved tendon jerks, elevated levels of muscle enzymes, and "myopathic" abnormalities on electromyography (EMG). However, proximal weakness is evident in some of the spinal muscular atrophies and in selected polyneuropathies, sometimes with minimal sensory involvement, such as acute or chronic inflammatory demyelinating polyradiculoneuropathy (AIDP or CIDP) and porphyric neuropathy.

Clinicopathologic Syndromes of Nerve Disease

Peripheral nerve disease results in several clinicopathologic syndromes (Table 147-4) that should be recognized as a first step in making an etiologic diagnosis. The following discussion is organized according to the clinical presentation, which usually allows the physician to predict the site of disease and, subsequently, the cause or origin on which treatment is based. This is occasionally complicated because the same etiologic factors can result in different clinicopathologic syndromes (Table 147-5), and vice versa (see Table 147-10).

CLINICAL SYNDROMES
Progressive Lower Motor Neuron Deficit With or Without Upper Motor Neuron Deficit

Progressive loss of lower motor neurons (LMNs) (muscle wasting, weakness, fasciculations) or upper motor neurons (UMNs) (brisk tendon jerks, increased muscle tone) with relative sparing of those innervating extraocular and sphincter muscles occurs in several forms throughout life; collectively, these disorders are referred to as the motor neuron diseases. Inherited or sporadic forms with relatively symmetric proximal or distal muscle weakness caused by loss of LMNs are referred to as the spiral muscular atrophies (SMAs). With the exception of infantile Werdig-Hoffman disease, type I, and progressive

bulbar palsy of childhood (Fazio-Londe disease), which lead to death within 18 months of onset, SMA is compatible with long survival. There are even sporadic cases limited to one extremity (benign focal amyotrophy). The workup in suspected SMA should exclude muscle disease; myasthenia gravis; postpolio syndrome; and various forms of neuropathy such as diabetic motor neuropathy, CIDP, multifocal motor neuropathy, and neuropathy caused by porphyria, lead, dapsone, or nitrofurantoin; and hexosaminidase deficiency. The diagnosis of SMA can usually be established through the history and examination supplemented by electrophysiologic testing and various laboratory tests; muscle biopsy may also be required.

In the adult, forms of pure UMN deficit (primary lateral sclerosis) and LMN deficit (spinal muscular atrophy, benign focal amyotrophy) exist, but *amyotrophic lateral sclerosis (ALS)* is the most common form, with both UMN and LMN involvement. The findings usually are asymmetric initially, resulting in progressive skeletal muscle wasting, weakness, fasciculations, and cramping, often beginning in one limb but then becoming generalized. Tendon jerks may remain brisk, despite muscle atrophy. Some cases have predominant involvement of brain stem motor neurons (progressive bulbar palsy). Mean disease duration is about 4 years, but survival in a given patient depends mainly on maintenance of bellows function (i.e., diaphragm and intercostal muscles) and airway protection (i.e., cough reflex and swallowing). Among the most important clinical signs in ALS are those originating from disease above the foramen magnum (atrophy or fasciculation of the tongue, palate, or face and a brisk jaw jerk). If these signs are absent, the diagnostic workup must exclude disease of the spinal cord and nerve roots, as in cervical spondylosis; such diseases can cause multiple root compressions with LMN findings and spinal cord compression with UMN findings and thereby simulate ALS. The diagnosis of ALS is confirmed with electrophysiologic testing and occasionally with spine magnetic resonance imaging (MRI) to exclude significant cervical spondylosis.

Because of vaccination, poliomyelitis, resulting in a flulike illness followed by rapid asymmetric paralysis, is now rare. However, some polio survivors from the epidemics of 30 to 40 years ago are now beginning to have pain, muscle fatigue, and weakness (postpolio syndrome). Some have progressive weakness and wasting in muscles that were not necessarily weak at the onset of polio (postpolio muscular atrophy). A reduced motor neuron pool resulting from the original illness, further depleted by progressive loss of anterior horn cells that occurs with aging and by the increased metabolic demand placed on the residual cells, may be the cause. The workup should exclude other causes of muscle weakness, such as radiculopathy or entrapment neuropathy.

Treatment of motor neuron and related diseases is largely supportive at this time. Decisions regarding respiratory support and hyperalimentation should be discussed early in the course. Rehabilitative techniques (discussed later) and individual or group psychiatric support for both the patient and the family are often helpful.

Proximal Pain in One Limb, With Sensory, Motor, or Reflex Abnormalities

The constellation discussed here suggests radiculopathy, plexopathy, or proximal mononeuropathy (i.e., spinal accessory nerve palsy or femoral neuropathy; see Table 147-7) but can be simulated by a primary rheumatologic disorder affecting the shoulder or hip joint, as well as adjacent bursae or tendons. Although in the latter case patients may be weak from guarding or disuse atrophy, the correct diagnosis is suggested by limited range of motion, localized tenderness, and a normal EMG examination.

Cervical radiculopathy usually becomes evident with sensory symptoms, which often worsen with neck movement. These include a nonspecific neck, shoulder, or scapular pain and, occasionally, a more "localizing" sensation that radiates into the dermatome of the specific nerve roots involved. Similarly, side-to-side asymmetries in muscle strength, sensation, or tendon jerks depend on the involved roots (Table 147-6). The most common causes of cervical radiculopathy are nerve root compression from intervertebral foraminal stenosis or disk herniation and, rarely, extramedullary or intramedullary tumors. Signs of cervical myelopathy (i.e., hyperactive tendon jerks or extensor plantar response), which can occur in addition to cervical

Table 147-5   Diseases associated with different types of neuropathy

	AIDP	CIDP	AXONAL SMP	MN	MNMP	PLEX	SMALL
Metabolic							
Diabetes			+	+	+	+	+
Acromegaly*			+	+ (CTS)			
Hypothyroidism*		+	+	+ (CTS)			
Infectious							
AIDS*	+	+	+		+		
Leprosy			+		+		
Lyme disease*	+		+	+	+		
Connective tissue							
SLE*	+		+		+		
Rheumatoid arthritis			+	+	+		
Sjögren's syndrome			+		+		
Periarteritis nodosa*			+		+		
Wegener's granulomatosis*			+		+		
Cranial arteritis*			+		+		
Churg-Strauss syndrome			+		+		
Cryoglobulinemia			+		+		
Hypersensitivity angiitis			+		+		
Idiopathic							
Sarcoidosis*			+		+		

AIDP, Acute inflammatory demyelinating polyneuropathy; *CIDP*, chronic idiopathic demyelinating polyradiculoneuropathy; axonal *SMP*, axonal sensorimotor polyneuropathy; *MN*, mononeuropathy; *MNMP*, mononeuropathy multiplex; *plex*, plexopathy; *small*, small-fiber polyneuropathy; *CTS*, carpal tunnel syndrome; *AIDS*, acquired immunodeficiency syndrome; *SLE*, systemic lupus erythematosus.
*Central nervous system manifestations may be present.

Table 147-6   Spinal root signs and symptoms

SPINAL ROOT	DISTRIBUTION OF PAIN, PARESTHESIAS, OR SENSORY LOSS	WEAK MUSCLES	DIMINISHED REFLEXES
C5	Shoulder, anterolateral arm and forearm	Deltoids, infraspinatus and supraspinatus, biceps	Pectoralis, biceps
C6	Shoulder, radial forearm, thumb	Biceps and brachioradialis, pronator teres	Biceps, brachioradialis
C7	Pectoral area, axilla, posterolateral forearm, 2nd and 3rd digits	Triceps, wrist extensors	Triceps
C8	Axilla, posteromedial arm, 4th and 5th digits	Hand interossei (ulnar nerve), abductor pollicis brevis (median nerve)	Finger flexors
L4	Hip, anterior thigh, anteromedial leg, great toe	Knee extensors, hip flexors	Knee
L5	Hip, posterolateral thigh, anterolateral leg, middle of foot	Foot extensors, great toe extensor, knee flexors	Medial hamstring
S1	Gluteal area, posterior thigh and leg, lateral foot	Foot flexors	Ankle
S2	Posterior thigh and leg	Toe flexors	—
S3-5	Sacral area	Sphincters	Bulbo cavernosus, anal wink

C, Cervical; *L*, lumbar; *S*, sacral.

root compression (i.e., cervical spondylosis), should be sought in the legs.

Lumbosacral radiculopathy becomes evident with low back, hip, or buttock pain and occasional "dermatomal radiation" and sensory, motor, and reflex changes, depending on the involved root or roots (Table 147-6). The pain may begin after heavy lifting and is generally worse in the sitting position or when coughing, sneezing, or straining at stool. Pressure over the sciatic notch and straight-leg raising may reproduce the pain somewhat. Common causes are compression by a laterally herniated intervertebral disk (most commonly, L4-5 or L5-S1) followed by tumor and herpes zoster. A midline herniated disk, lumbar spondylosis, and arachnoiditis are other causes, but these usually produce bilateral lumbosacral polyradiculopathy.

The diagnosis of unilateral cervical or lumbar radiculopathy may be supported by spine films and EMG. Metrizamide myelogram, computed tomography (CT) scan, or MRI may be needed to determine the cause of root compression in cases without clear cause and to visualize (1) the cervical cord in patients with myelopathy or (2) the cauda equina/conus medullaris in patients with bilateral lumbosacral radiculopathy with bladder dysfunction or symptoms of spinal claudication. Conservative treatment (cervical collar, traction in cervical radiculopathy, or bed rest in lumbosacral radiculopathy) is usually successful. Patients may benefit from a course of nonsteroidal anti-inflammatory drugs and, if necessary, a short course of narcotic analgesics. Some cases may require surgery to decompress roots, the spinal cord, or the cauda equina. Although comprehensive therapy of chronic low back pain in patients with lumbosacral radiculopathy is beyond the scope of this chapter, some of the simpler measures are discussed later.

A form of radiculopathy that is occasionally seen is thoracic or thoracolumbar radiculopathy. It is most commonly caused by reactivation of herpes zoster and produces dermatomal pain and skin rash with little sensory loss; it can also be caused by diabetes, Lyme disease, and thoracic disk herniation. Pain control is the main problem (discussed later).

The diagnosis of plexopathy is suggested when the sensorimotor deficit is not limited to or affects more than one nerve or two roots. Proximal limb or girdle pain is often present. In the arm, brachial plexopathy occurs as a result of traction injury from two-wheeled vehicle accidents, tumor infiltration, or radiation and immunologic causes (postinfection or postvaccination). A recurrent, autosomal dominantly inherited form has also been described. In the lower ex-

Table 147-7 Common mononeuropathies

NERVE	CLINICAL PRESENTATION	CAUSES
Spinal accessory	Shoulder pain, drop and weakness of abduction, trapezius wasting	Nerve trauma
Long thoracic	"Winging" of scapula	Backpacking, idiopathic
Axillary	Deltoid weakness, sensory loss over lateral upper arm	Trauma
Radial at the spiral groove (Saturday-night palsy)	Wrist and finger drop, weakness and areflexia of brachioradialis, sensory loss over dorsum of first web space	Acute compression
Musculocutaneous	Weakness of elbow flexion, sensory loss over radial aspect of forearm	Trauma, elbow hyperextension
Ulnar at the elbow	Wasting, weakness of interossei; sensory loss over palmar and dorsal surface of the ulnar aspect of the hand	Chronic compression
Median in the forearm (pronator syndrome)	Forearm ache, weakness of intrinsic and extrinsic median muscles, sensory loss over the palmar, radial aspect of the hand	Chronic compression
Radial in the forearm (posterior interosseous palsy)	Forearm pain, finger drop, radial deviation of the extended wrist	Mass lesion, trauma, idiopathic
Median at the wrist (carpal tunnel syndrome)	Nocturnal hand "tingling"; weakness, wasting of abductor pollicis brevis; sensory loss over volar aspect of fingers 1 to 3	Chronic compression
Ulnar at the wrist	Weakness, wasting of interossei; variable sensory loss over 4th and 5th fingers	Occupational trauma
Femoral	Hip, groin pain; knee buckling; knee extensor weakness; absent knee jerk; sensory loss over anteromedial thigh and medial calf	Diabetes, retroperitoneal hemorrhage or tumor, postsurgical
Lateral femoral cutaneous at inguinal ligament	Thigh pain, sensory loss over lateral thigh, Tinel's sign lateral inguinal ligament	Chronic compression
Sciatic	Weakness of dorsiflexion plantar flexion, foot eversion and inversion, sensory loss over dorsum and sole of foot	Hip surgery, prolonged bed rest
Peroneal at the fibular head (peroneal palsy)	Tripping; foot drop; sensory loss over lateral calf and dorsum of foot; normal foot eversion and inversion	Acute compression (i.e., leg crossing)
Posterior tibial at ankle (tarsal tunnel syndrome)	Nocturnal foot pain and tingling, Tinel's sign posterior to medial malleolus	Chronic compression, trauma

tremity common causes of lumbosacral plexopathy are retroperitoneal tumor or hemorrhage and irradiation. In addition, in elderly individuals with type II diabetes, asymmetric, painful lower extremity weakness and wasting associated with weight loss sometimes develop, often with minimal sensory findings. Although becoming evident as plexopathies, such cases probably represent a localized lumbosacral radiculoneuropathy. They are sometimes referred to as *diabetic amyotrophy, diabetic motor neuropathy,* or *proximal diabetic neuropathy.*

Electromyography can be helpful in the diagnosis of plexopathy. Computed tomography or MRI scan of the plexi can be performed to rule out tumor infiltration or hemorrhage. The therapeutic aims are pain control and treatment of the underlying disease.

The mononeuropathies are among the simplest neurologic lesions, and each has its own clinical presentation (Table 147-7). Single-cranial-nerve palsies are occasionally seen in diseases that produce mononeuritis multiplex or in those which simultaneously infiltrate nerve and the leptomeninges (see later discussion), but the most common cranial mononeuropathies are diabetic third- or sixth-nerve palsies, trigeminal neuropathy attributable to herpes zoster, and Bell's (seventh cranial nerve) palsy. Isolated seventh-nerve palsy is usually idiopathic but can be caused by herpes zoster (with vesicles in ear, palate, or tongue), trauma, sarcoidosis, or Lyme disease. Patients come to medical attention with acute onset of panfacial weakness of varying severity with prominent affection of the frontalis muscle, indicating that the facial weakness is of LMN rather than UMN type. Hyperacusis and abnormalities of tearing, taste, and even sensation (pain, sensory loss) may also occur. In idiopathic cases some authors recommend an early course of prednisone (1 mg/kg per day) for 5 to 16 days, depending on the severity of facial paresis, followed by a 5-day taper. In cases with incomplete eye closure, the eye should be protected with artificial tears during the day and an ointment during sleep. Mononeuropathies of the extremities (Table 147-7) are most often caused by chronic compression, stretch, or angulation as nerves pass through bony or ligamentous canals (e.g., carpal or tarsal tunnel syndrome, ulnar neuropathy at the elbow or wrist, meralgia paresthetica). Nerves that pass around bony or ligamentous structures are also vulnerable to acute compression from external pressure (e.g., peroneal or radial nerve palsy). The predominant early pathologic substrate of these so-called entrapment neuropathies is focal demyelination, but later or in more severe cases axonal injury occurs as well.

Electromyography and nerve conduction studies confirm the diagnosis, rule out other causes for the clinical deficit, and determine the degree of axonal injury. In cases of acute compression and in mild to moderate chronic nerve compression, treatment is usually conservative: splinting, pain control, and prevention of further injury. In refractory cases with severe pain or significant axonal degeneration, surgical therapy aimed at decompressing or transposing the nerve may be required.

Stepwise, Asymmetric Neuropathic Symptoms, Signs, or Electromyographic Findings Over Days to Weeks

The constellation discussed here suggests *mononeuropathy multiplex,* a term indicating discrete disease of two or more named nerves in more than one limb. Nerve disease usually is outside areas where entrapment commonly occurs—a feature that distinguishes mononeuritis multiplex from the more chronic condition of hereditary predisposition to pressure palsy. Most commonly this syndrome is caused by systemic vasculitis with nerve infarction. It is important to remember that this syndrome can sometimes present as a symmetric polyneuropathy (see Table 147-5). Workup and therapy should be directed to the underlying illness. Biopsy of an involved nerve may be diagnostic.

Headache, Back Pain, Multiple-Cranial-Nerve Palsies, and Polyradiculopathy

Because the nerve roots and cranial nerves traverse the subarachnoid space, they are sometimes affected by disease processes that also affect the meninges. This syndrome can be caused by tumor infiltration from carcinomatous meningitis, leptomeningeal inflammation from neurosarcoidosis, or infectious causes such as chronic meningitis (e.g., tuberculosis, cryptococcosis, neurosyphilis, or Lyme disease). Cerebrospinal fluid (CSF) examination is crucial to the diagnosis.

Polyneuropathy

The first step in narrowing the differential diagnosis of polyneuropathy is to note its time course and tempo. Other important issues in the diagnosis and treatment of polyneuropathies are shown in Box 147-1.

Acute Symmetric, Generalized Weakness With Sensory Complaints Progressing Over 1 to 4 Weeks. Today the presentation discussed here is almost always an acute inflammatory demyelinating polyradiculoneuropathy (AIDP), often referred to as the Guillain-Barré syndrome. However, other causes should be considered (Box 147-2). AIDP is usually preceded by an infectious illness, vaccination, or surgery. Ataxia of gait or limbs is often an early symptom, followed by weakness of proximal and then distal muscles; sometimes, facial, extraocular, and respiratory muscles are eventually involved. Sensory loss occurs but is generally exceeded by sensory symptoms. Autonomic abnormalities affecting the cardiac rhythm, thermoregulation, and the pupils or sphincters may develop, presumably as a result of involvement of the white rami communicantes. After several days the CSF reveals an elevated protein level with little or no cellular response, and electrical studies can often demonstrate a demyelinating neuropathy. An axonal form of the disease has also been recognized, particularly in patients with a diarrheal illness attributable to infection with *Campylobacter jejuni*. Intensive care unit (ICU) monitoring of respiratory function and cardiac rhythm is required for progressive cases, with timely intubation if necessary, prophylaxis of venous thrombosis, frequent turning to prevent decubiti,

intermittent catheterization for urinary retention, pain control, and emotional support. Early plasmapheresis has been shown to shorten the course in AIDP patients with significant weakness. Intravenous immunoglobulin (IVIG) also appears to be effective.

Stepwise, Relapsing, or Slowly Progressive Symmetric Motor and Sensory Polyneuropathy With Slow Nerve Conduction Velocities. Most commonly the presentation discussed here is caused by CIDP, which has features in common with AIDP (proximal muscle weakness, motor greater than sensory deficit, elevated CSF protein levels, and similar disease) but has a different time course (from onset to peak deficit, longer than 6 weeks) and less autonomic involvement. The demyelinating forms of hereditary motor and sensory polyneuropathy (HMSN), such as HMSN types I, III, and IV, should be considered in cases of childhood onset, along with other acquired disorders simulating CIDP, such as some of the paraproteinemias and acquired immunodeficiency syndrome (AIDS) (Box 147-3). Immunosuppressive agents, plasmapheresis, and IVIg are useful in treating idiopathic CIDP and the paraproteinemias. Plasmapheresis may be used to treat AIDS-related CIDP.

Chronic, Symmetric, Slowly Progressive Sensorimotor Polyneuropathy Affecting Legs More Than Arms (From Onset to Peak Deficit, Months to Years). The majority of chronic polyneuropathies are axonopathies, predominantly affecting large- or medium-sized fibers and initially affecting the longest ax-

---

BOX 147-1

Important factors in the evaluation and therapy of polyneuropathy

1. Tempo
2. Symmetry of signs and symptoms
3. Physiology: axonal versus demyelinative
4. Clues to origin: family history, drugs, occupational exposure, nutrition, systemic disease, vaccination
5. Functional impairment
6. Efficacy, risks, cost of treatment

BOX 147-2

Acute neurologic diseases in the differential diagnosis of acute inflammatory demyelinating polyradiculoneuropathy

Central nervous system

Acute cervical myelopathy
Basilar artery thrombosis

Anterior horn cell poliomyelitis
Nerve

Acute inflammatory demyelinating polyradiculoneuropathy (AIDP)
Porphyric neuropathy
Diphtheritic neuropathy
Drugs: dapsone, nitrofurantoin (occasionally)
Toxins: organophosphate, arsenic (single exposure), thallium (single exposure)
Tick paralysis

Neuromuscular junction

Botulism
Myasthenia gravis

Muscle membrane

Hypokalemic, hyperkalemic, and normokalemic periodic paralysis

Muscle

Acute polymyositis

Table 147-8 Small-fiber neuropathies

	DIAGNOSIS MADE BY

Amyloidosis
  Hereditary types I-IV
  Nonhereditary
	Positive family history in some cases; mucous membrane, nerve biopsy

Diabetes (sometimes)	Fasting and postprandial blood glucose levels, hemoglobin AlC
Dimethylpropionitrile (DMAPN)	History of exposure
Fabry's disease* (alpha-galactosidase A deficiency)	Family history, tissue biopsy
Hereditary sensory neuropathy types I, III, IV	Family history, clinical presentation
Tangier's disease (hereditary high-density lipoprotein deficiency)	Reduced levels of high-density alpha lipoproteins and cholesterol

*Central nervous system manifestations.

BOX 147-3

Causes of demyelinative neuropathy

I. Hereditary conditions
  A. Hereditary motor sensory neuropathy
    1. Type I (Charcot-Marie-Tooth disease)
    2. Type III (Dejerine-Sottas disease)
    3. Type IV (Refsum's disease)
  B. Hereditary predisposition to entrapment neuropathy
  C. Metachromatic leukodystrophy*
  D. Globoid cell leukodystrophy (Krabbe's disease)*
  E. Adrenoleukodystrophy or adrenomyeloneuropathy*
  F. Cockayne syndrome*
II. Acquired conditions
  A. Chronic inflammatory demyelinating polyradiculoneuropathy
  B. "Benign" monoclonal gammopathies, particularly immunoglobulin M
  C. Osteosclerotic myeloma
  D. Waldenström's macroglobulinemia
  E. Perhexiline therapy
  F. Acquired immunodeficiency syndrome*

*Central nervous system manifestations.

Table 147-9 Causes of chronic axonopathy

CAUSE	DIAGNOSIS CONFIRMED BY
I. Malnutrition or malabsorption	
A. Thiamine deficiency (beriberi)*	Erythrocyte transkelolase assay
B. Pyridoxine deficiency	Measurement of tryptophan metabolites after tryptophan loading
C. Pantothenic acid	Clinical presentation
D. Vitamin B_{12} deficiency*	Schilling's test, vitamin B_{12} level
E. Pellagra* (deficiency of niacin and other B vitamins)	Clinical presentation
F. Vitamin E deficiency*	Clinical presentation, vitamin E levels
II. Metabolic disease	
A. Diabetes	Fasting and postprandial blood glucose levels
B. Renal failure	Blood urea nitrogen, creatinine levels
C. Hypothyroidism, hyperthyroidism	Thyroid function tests
D. Acromegaly	Growth hormone studies
III. Infection	
A. Acquired immune deficiency syndrome	Human immunodeficiency virus
B. Leprosy	Nerve biopsy
IV. Neuropathy associated with malignancy	
A. Paraproteinemia or dysproteinemia	
1. "Benign" monoclonal gammopathy	Serum and urine protein and immunoelectrophoresis
2. Multiple myeloma	Bone films, bone marrow aspirate, serum and urine protein and immuno-electrophoresis
3. Cryoglobulinemia	Serum for cryoglobulins
B. Carcinoma	
1. Lung carcinoma	Thorough physical examination, chest x-ray, etc.
2. Gastrointestinal tract malignancy	Thorough physical examination, stool guaiacs, etc.
3. Breast cancer	Thorough physical examination, mammography
4. Genitourinary tract carcinoma	Pelvic examination, urinalysis, etc.
C. Lymphoma, Hodgkin's disease	Biopsy of lymph node, etc.
V. Connective tissue diseases (see Table 147-5)	Antinuclear antibodies, rheumatoid factor, erythrocyte sedimentation rate, etc.
VI. Hereditary axonopathies	
A. Hereditary sensorimotor polyneuropathy, type II (Charcot-Marie-Tooth)	Clinical presentation, including electrophysiologic testing
B. Hereditary sensory neuropathy, type II	Clinical presentation, including electrophysiologic testing, nerve biopsy
C. Neuropathy associated with the hereditary ataxias*	Clinical presentation, including presence of ataxia
D. Ataxia telangiectasia*	Clinical presentation
E. Xeroderma pigmentosa	Genetic studies, clinical presentation, electrophysiolgic testing
F. Abetalipoproteinemia* (Bassen-Kornzweig disease)	Diminished vitamin E level, cholesterol, and low-density lipoproteins
G. Porphyric neuropathy*	
1. Acute intermittent	Elevated levels of urinary porphyrin precursors, erythrocyte assay of uropor-phyrinogen synthetase I
2. Coproporphyria	Elevated fecal porphyrin level
3. Variegate	Elevated levels of fecal and urinary porphyrins and urinary porphyrin precursors
VII. Idiopathic	Absence of peripheral neuropathy in family members, negative workup

*Central nervous system involvement.

ons, which subsequently "die back," with progressive involvement of shorter axons. Hence sensory dysfunction, weakness, and areflexia begin in the toes and, depending on the severity of the neuropathy, ascend, in order, to the lower legs, fingertips, upper legs, forearms, midline trunk, upper arms, and top of the head. Far less frequent are chronic small-fiber axonopathies (Table 147-8), whose signs and symptoms (discussed earlier) can often be recognized at the bedside, and the chronic demyelinative neuropathies (Box 147-3), which can be distinguished from axonopathies by nerve conduction studies and electromyography. In addition, the diagnosis of several of the hereditary demyelinative neuropathies (types IA, IB, IX, and hereditary predisposition to pressure palsy) can now be confirmed with commercially available genetic tests.

Clues to the origin of chronic axonopathy primarily affecting large and medium fibers are the presence of systemic illness, hereditary predisposition (Table 147-9), and exposure to drugs or toxins (Table 147-10). To elicit a family history of neuropathy, one should determine whether family members have deformity of foot, spine, or hand or can walk only with the use of assistive devices. In cases without a known cause examination of family members is necessary to rule out hereditary neuropathy.

The most common cause of polyneuropathy in Western civilization is diabetes, which, in addition to chronic symmetric sensorimotor or small-fiber polyneuropathy, also produces several asymmetric forms: cranial or limb mononeuropathy, thoracolumbar radiculopathy, lumbosacral plexopathy, and mononeuritis multiplex. Whereas the asymmetric forms are probably ischemic in origin, the symmetric forms may have either an ischemic or a metabolic cause (i.e., abnormalities of sorbitol metabolism). Treatment of diabetic neuropathy should include tight glucose control, control of pain and autonomic symptoms, and good foot care (discussed later).

In Western society neuropathy caused by vitamin deficiency occurs in malnourished, alcoholic patients, in patients treated with isoniazid or hydralazine, and rarely, in malabsorption syndromes. In alcoholics the neuropathy becomes evident as a subacute or chronic, symmetric, painful sensorimotor axonopathy and represents the result of months to years of inadequate nutrition with deficiency of B vitamins, particularly thiamine. Treatment of alcoholic neuropathy consists of adequate nutrition, thiamine and other B vitamin supplementation, and pain control. Isoniazid (INH) and hydralazine appear to interfere with pyridoxine metabolism and can produce an axonal sensorimotor polyneuropathy. Administration of oral pyridoxine (50 mg two times a day) prevents INH neuropathy. (Higher doses, i.e., 500 mg per day, can result in a sensory neuronopathy.) Vitamin B_{12} deficiency is among the most important of the diseases that can affect both the peripheral and the central nervous systems (see diseases with asterisk in Tables 147-5 and 147-8 to 147-10; Box 147-3), because replacement therapy is curative if begun early. Although peripheral nerves are often mildly affected in vitamin B_{12} deficiency, the predominant disease or disorder tends to be in the posterior and

Table 147-10   Sensorimotor neuropathy caused by drugs and toxins

Drugs

Anesthetics/hypnotics
  Glutethimide
  Nitrous oxide
  Thalidomide
Antibiotics: Chloramphenicol, clioquinol,* dapsone,† ethambutol,* ethionamide, isoniazid, metronidazole,* nitrofurantoin†
Anticonvulsants: Phenytoin
Cardiovascular medicines: Amiodarone, hydralazine, perhexilene maleate
Cancer chemotherapeutic agents: Cisplatin,* doxorubicin, misonidazole,* suramin, vincristine
Rheumatoid medicines
  Gold
  Colchicine

Toxins	Associations
Acrylamide	Used in production of grouting and flocculating agents
Arsenic†	Smelting, mining
Carbon disulfide	Used in production of rubber, rayon, or cellophane
Cyanide*	Consumption of stone fruits, cassava plants
Dichlorophenoxyacetic acid (2,4 D)	Used as a herbicide
Dimethylpropionitrile (DMAPN)	Used in production of polyurethane grouting agents
Ethylene oxide	Used in chemical sterilization
Hexacarbons (i.e., h-hexane methyl n-butyl ketone)	Industrial solvents, glue sniffing
Lead	Smelting, battery production, repair of automobile radiators, moonshine whiskey
Mercury*	Used in a number of industries, fungicide
Methyl bromide	Used as insecticide, fire extinguisher, refrigerant, fumigant
Organophosphorus esters*: Leptophos, mipafax, trichlorfon, triorthocresyl phosphate	Used as insecticides and petroleum or plastic additives
Polychlorinated biphenyls	Used as plasticizers, electrical insulators, fungistatic agents
Thallium*†	Rodenticides, insecticides

*Central nervous system manifestations.
†Sometimes associated with acute polyneuropathy.

lateral columns of the spinal cord. Indeed, the initial symptoms and signs appear to be all peripheral, but the distal limb paresthesias (e.g., tingling), followed by vibratory and joint position sense loss, sometimes loss of ankle jerks, and, subsequently, gait ataxia, can all be caused by dorsal column with little or no peripheral nerve disease. In addition, pyramidal signs eventually develop. The usual cause is pernicious anemia; rarely, other causes of malabsorption may be involved.

Peripheral neuropathy frequently results from cancer or its treatment. Direct invasion of spinal roots, cranial nerves, or plexi occurs, as does sensorimotor polyneuropathy, a "remote effect" of cancer. The latter, sometimes referred to as *paracarcinomatous neuropathy,* has several forms: AIDP, CIDP (see Box 147-3), motor or sensory neuronopathy, and most commonly sensorimotor axonopathy. Patients with significant polyneuropathy without obvious cause should be screened with a careful examination, electrophysiologic studies and judicious laboratory testing (Table 147-9; Box 147-3) to rule out an underlying malignancy. However, without some clue from the history, the examination, and screening laboratory studies, extensive evaluation for occult malignancy is generally fruitless and not recommended. Of the several chemotherapeutic drugs that produce sensorimotor polyneuropathy (Table 147-10), the most common is vincristine, and the neuropathy improves when the drug is stopped. Radiation therapy can result in plexopathy, which can usually be distinguished from tumor invasion of the plexus by slower progression,

little or no pain, a tendency to involve the upper or whole brachial or the lower or whole lumbosacral plexus, and myokymic discharges on EMG of affected muscles. However, CT scanning, MRI, or even biopsy of the plexus may be required to be certain of tumor invasion, since its treatment usually includes radiation therapy.

MANAGEMENT

Therapy of peripheral nerve disorders includes specific treatment of the underlying disease process and general supportive measures. The latter consists of preventive care, such as (1) good foot care for all with insensate feet, particularly for the diabetic (competent podiatry, properly fitting shoes, prompt treatment of infection), and (2) avoidance of nerve trauma, as in leaning on elbows or crossing legs, since polyneuropathy predisposes to compressive mononeuropathy. The following rehabilitative techniques are important: (1) range-of-motion exercises to prevent contractures and subsequent disability in the event of nerve recovery, (2) strengthening exercises, and (3) proper selection of orthoses (such as a lightweight plastic ankle foot orthosis to prevent foot drop while walking), wrist splints for carpal tunnel syndrome or radial nerve palsy, and assistive devices for ambulation (such as canes, crutches, and wheelchairs). Pain can sometimes be controlled with nonsteroidal antiinflammatory medicines, but narcotics may be required in acute circumstances. In chronic neuropathy, anticonvulsants (carbamazepine, phenytoin) or tricyclic antidepressants (amitriptyline), sometimes in conjunction with phenothiazines (fluphenazine), may be required. Occasionally, pain results from altered biomechanics (i.e., knee or back hyperextension in postpolio patients) and may be amenable to rehabilitative therapy (e.g., bracing). Autonomic dysfunction, such as orthostatic hypotension, can be treated by (1) "dangling" the legs before standing up, (2) avoidance of prolonged bed rest and elevating the head of the bed, (3) the use of made-to-measure elastic stockings, and (4) fludrocortisone therapy. Cholinergic therapy may be useful in treating gastroparesis (metoclopramide) or cystopathy (bethanechol).

BIBLIOGRAPHY

Asbury AK, Gilliat RW, editors: *Peripheral nerve disorders,* London, 1984, Butterworth.
Dawson DM, Hallett M, Millender LH: *Entrapment neuropathies,* ed 2, Boston, 1990, Little, Brown.
Dyck PJ et al, editors: *Peripheral neuropathy,* ed 3, Philadelphia, 1993, WB Saunders.
Schaumberg HH, Berger AR, Thomas PK: *Disorders of peripheral nerves,* ed 2, Philadelphia, 1991, FA Davis.

CHAPTER

148   Diseases of the Neuromuscular Junction

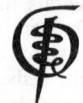

Marjorie E. Seybold

MYASTHENIA GRAVIS

Myasthenia gravis (MG) is a disorder of neuromuscular transmission that affects approximately 1 in 10,000 persons. It has an autoimmune basis characterized by a 7 S gamma globulin antibody (AChR-ab) directed against the nicotinic acetylcholine receptor (AChR) of the neuromuscular junction. There is no racial or geographic predilection, and the disorder can occur at any age. It most commonly begins in young adulthood, and women are affected more often than men in this age-group. Among the elderly, men are affected at least as frequently as women. Familial cases are rare. Human leukocyte antigen (HLA) typing has revealed a frequent association of MG with HLA-A1, HLA-B8, and HLA-DR3 in patients without thymoma with onset of the disease in young adulthood, but these HLA types are inconsistently present, even in familial cases.

Two other disorders of neuromuscular transmission that are simi-

✔ *WHEN TO REFER*

Ascending or progressive multifocal paralysis

Rapidly progressive neuropathies as in Guillain-Barré syndrome or severe systemic vasculitis can quickly impair limb, trunk, bulbar, and respiratory function. Since appropriate therapy for these conditions can prevent progression if initiated early, patients with this syndrome should be referred on an emergency basis.

Diagnostic dilemmas

Any neuropathy of clinical significance in which the origin or cause is uncertain should be referred for detailed evaluation. Determination of the cause may lead to effective therapy.

If nerve biopsy is being considered, referral to a specialist is probably warranted, since biopsy is almost never employed to confirm the presence of neuropathy. Rather, it is indicated in the infrequent patients with suspected inflammatory or metabolic neuropathies such as vasculitis, sarcoidosis, leprosy, or amyloidosis.

In patients with atypical mononeuropathies or radiculopathies who are being considered for decompressive surgery, input from an experienced clinician is often helpful. Such patients may have other conditions (e.g., brachial plexus neuropathy that is not cervical radiculopathy, proximal diabetic neuropathy that is not lumbosacral radiculopathy, or ALS that is not ulnar neuropathy) that do not benefit from surgery.

Therapeutic dilemmas

Even when the cause is known, the generalist may not be experienced in treatment options. This is often the case in the immune-mediated neuropathies such as AIDP, CIDP, monoclonal gammopathies of undetermined significance, or multifocal motor neuropathy. These disorders are often amenable to immunomodulatory therapy, but input from an experienced clinician is required because the treatment options are complex and manifold. Other examples are autonomic and hereditary neuropathies.

Amyotropic lateral sclerosis

Patients with the fatal condition of ALS usually benefit from a specialist's input for confirmation of the diagnosis, family counseling, neurorehabilitation, and discussion of the terminal life-support decisions and of the emerging therapies for this condition.

lar to MG on clinical examination are recognized. Neonatal MG is the development of transient weakness in an infant born to a myasthenic mother. It occurs in only 15% of at-risk infants, despite the transplacental transfer of AChR-ab from the mother to her infant in almost all pregnancies involving a mother with MG. The possibility of brief autonomous infant production of AChR-ab in the affected cases has been suggested. Another possibility is that the affected infants share histocompatibility antigens with their mothers, which predispose them to the development of neonatal MG. There is no correlation between maternal disease severity and occurrence of MG symptoms in the neonate. Treatment with anticholinesterase medication is necessary if weakness is severe. Spontaneous recovery occurs, usually within 3 to 4 weeks after birth. Reoccurrence of MG in later life is very unlikely.

Penicillamine-induced MG (PEN-MG) describes the development of MG symptoms in patients who receive treatment with the drug D-penicillamine. It occurs in patients with a variety of underlying disorders, including rheumatoid arthritis, Wilson's disease, biliary cirrhosis, and systemic sclerosis. Preliminary HLA studies have raised the possibility of association between B35/DR1 and the development of PEN-MG. This differs from the increased prevalence of B8/DR3 reported in spontaneous MG. PEN-MG appears to be clinically identical to spontaneous MG, and AChR-ab is characteristically present. The symptoms usually are predominantly ocular, but generalized weakness may occur. The disorder responds to treatment with anticholinesterase medications and usually remits spontaneously within 1 year of the discontinuation of penicillamine therapy. However, occasional cases of persistent MG have been reported.

Pathophysiology

The autoimmune form of MG is characterized by the presence of AChR-ab and a reduction in the number of AChRs on the postsynaptic portion of the neuromuscular junction. These changes result in reduction in postsynaptic response to acetylcholine (ACh). Acetylcholine, although released in normal amounts from the nerve terminal, is at times unable to induce sufficient depolarization of the postsynaptic membrane to initiate muscle excitation. Muscle weakness and fatigability result.

The mechanisms responsible for AChR-ab induction of MG in humans are poorly understood. Some information regarding MG has been extrapolated from studies of experimental autoimmune myasthenia gravis (EAMG) in animals. This disease, induced by injecting animals with adjuvant and purified AChR, mimics MG on pharmacologic, histologic, physiologic, and clinical examination. The animals develop AChR-ab and appear to represent a valid immunologic model for MG in humans.

Studies of EAMG have implicated humoral, cellular, and complement factors in the disease. The disease may be transferred from animal to animal or from MG patient to animal by antibodies. However, this passive transfer of disease is blocked in animals depleted of complement (C3). EAMG also may be transferred by lymph node cells from immunized animals. Production of AChR-ab and EAMG in animals treated with AChR and adjuvant can be prevented in animals depleted of T cells.

In MG, immunoglobulin G and complement have been identified on the postsynaptic folds of the neuromuscular junction, and a prominent reduction in AChR has been documented. The reduction in receptors is presumed to be induced by the AChR-ab, both by enhancing receptor degradation and by complement-mediated destruction of the end-plate. AChR-ab enhances destruction of AChR by crosslinking receptors, which, in turn, accelerates internalization and degradation of AChR. Complement-mediated injury of the postsynaptic membrane reduces the numbers of receptors by direct destruction and probably also by interference with proper insertion of the new AChR into the membrane.

Almost 90% of MG patients with generalized weakness, but only 50% to 60% of those with purely ocular findings, have detectable AChR-ab in their sera. The concentration of antibody does not correlate well with clinical symptoms, although patients with only ocular symptoms usually have relatively low levels of AChR-ab. AChR-ab response in MG is polyclonal, being directed against the various subunits of the AChR. No specific subunit antibodies appear to be linked to clinical severity or to the presence of thymoma. In most patients the majority of the AChR-ab are directed against a specific region of the alpha subunit separate from the ACh binding site on that subunit.

Evidence of altered cellular immunity in MG has been reported, but no specific defect has yet been identified. Peripheral blood lymphocytes (PBLs) undergo antigen-specific transformation when exposed to AChR. This increased PBL responsiveness appears to occur in helper T cells and, although proportional to disease severity in EAMG in rats, has not been correlated consistently with disease activity or patient age in MG.

Either hypothyroidism or hyperthyroidism occurs in approximately 10% of MG patients. Other presumed autoimmune diseases, such as lupus erythematosus, rheumatoid arthritis, pernicious anemia, and polymyositis, occur in MG patients more often than expected by chance. Myasthenic patients, even those without overt symptoms of other disease, often produce antinuclear, antithyroid, and antistriated muscle antibodies. The latter are particularly common in MG patients who also have thymomas.

Pathologic Features

The most striking pathologic change observed in MG is the "simplification" of the postsynaptic portion of the neuromuscular junction. AChR, which is concentrated at the tips of the postsynaptic membrane folds, is frequently reduced to less than half the normal amount, and much of the remaining AChR has antibody bound to its surface. Complement components C3 and C9 are localized to the AChR area, and fragments containing AChR, antibody, and complement are detected in the synaptic cleft. The cleft itself is wider than normal.

Pathologic changes in the muscle itself are not prominent. Local collections of lymphocytes ("lymphorrhages") are sometimes seen within the muscle, but the role and origin of these cells are not clear.

Thymus gland abnormalities are usually present in MG patients. At least 10% have a thymoma, and most of these patients are 30 years of age or older at the time of MG onset. The distinction of malignant, as opposed to benign, thymoma is based on the presence of tumor invasion of the surrounding tissue rather than on cell type. Thymomas rarely metastasize outside the thoracic cavity.

Patients without thymoma frequently have germinal centers in the thymic medulla, often called *thymic hyperplasia.* Hyperplasia is common in young patients, whereas those over 60 years old often have little remaining thymic tissue. Thymic cells from MG patients often spontaneously produce AChR-ab in vitro and, after irradiation, stimulate peripheral blood lymphocytes to produce AChR-ab, suggesting the presence of both specific B cells and helper T cells in thymic tissue.

Clinical and Laboratory Findings

The hallmark of MG is weakness that is made worse with exercise and improved with rest. Other factors, such as heat, menses, emotional stress, and intercurrent illness, frequently exacerbate the weakness. The onset of symptoms may be gradual or abrupt. Any skeletal muscle can be affected, but ocular symptoms are the most frequent initial complaint. Ptosis or ocular muscle weakness, or both, may occur. Dysarthria, chewing fatigue, and dysphagia are also common. Involvement of the muscles of respiration may be sufficiently severe to require assisted ventilation. The extremities are often more weak proximally than distally, but either or both muscle groups may be involved. Arm weakness may result in an inability to shave or comb the hair, and leg weakness may result in sudden falls. Fluctuations in severity usually occur during the day, and asymmetry is common. Pain may occur in a fatigued muscle and is common in weakened neck muscles after prolonged head support. Paresthesias and sensory loss do not occur.

Muscle examination may be normal in rested patients, but weakness usually can be brought out with exercise. Patients with more severe disease are weak even at rest. Muscle atrophy is uncommon, and tendon reflexes and sensory examination are normal.

Myasthenia gravis can be remitting, static, or progressive. Some patients have only ocular symptoms, although the majority develop generalized disease. Rapid development of severe symptoms refractory to anticholinesterase medications is called a *myasthenic crisis.*

Laboratory testing reveals an elevated level of AChR-ab in as many as 90% of patients, depending on the laboratory method used. Repetitive nerve stimulation shows a decrement of the compound motor action potential of muscle in approximately 90% of patients if three or more muscles, especially proximal ones, are studied. Individual motor units also show an abnormal fluctuation in amplitude from moment to moment on electromyographic needle examination and reflect the fatigue of individual muscle fibers. More sophisticated electromyographic testing, such as single-fiber electromyography, can detect abnormalities when conventional repetitive stimulation is normal.

Because of the increased incidence of thyroid disease in MG patients, thyroid test results may be abnormal. Likewise, vitamin B_{12} levels may be low because of associated pernicious anemia. Autoantibodies such as antinuclear antibody, antithyroid, rheumatoid factor, antistriated muscle, and antiparietal cell antibody are often present.

Chest x-ray or CT may demonstrate a thymoma or a prominent thymus gland.

Pulmonary function test results may be abnormal in patients with respiratory muscle weakness or impaired clearing of pulmonary secretions. Falling respiratory capacity indicates the need for consideration of intubation and ventilator support.

Diagnosis

People with MG commonly see several doctors before the disease is recognized. The patient may be considered to be hysterical or malingering for a time before the correct diagnosis is suspected.

The clinical diagnosis is based on the history of fluctuating weakness and on the demonstration of skeletal muscle weakness. Confirmation is obtained by demonstrating improvement after injection of anticholinesterase medication, either in the short-acting (edrophonium) or long-acting (neostigmine) form. A decrementing response of the muscle potential to repetitive nerve stimulation and demonstration of AChR-ab in the serum are further confirmatory evidence of MG. In patients in clinical remission AChR-ab may still be present. The use of minimal doses of curare as a diagnostic test to bring out weakness should be discouraged, since respiratory failure may occur.

Other disorders of neuromuscular transmission, such as the Lambert-Eaton myasthenic syndrome (frequently associated with oat cell carcinoma of the lung), botulism, organophosphate poisoning, and antibiotic-induced neuromuscular block, usually can be distinguished by their mode of clinical presentation, poor response to anticholinesterase drugs, differing electrical characteristics, and the absence of AChR-ab. Dysthyroid ocular disease, dystrophies of ocular muscles, and brain stem–induced eye movement abnormalities must be distinguished from MG in the patient with only ocular symptoms. Easy fatigue as the result of metabolic imbalance, drug abuse, depression, or systemic disease also must be considered in the differential diagnosis of generalized MG.

Treatment

Treatment usually begins with anticholinesterase medications. The dosage varies widely, depending on the patient's symptomatic response and sensitivity to side effects. The most commonly used drug, pyridostigmine, is given in divided doses as needed during the day. Its onset of effect is about 30 minutes, and it lasts up to 4 hours. A long-acting form (Timespan) is available for bedtime use if bulbar or respiratory weakness occurs throughout the night or on awakening in the morning. The uneven Timespan release makes it less popular than the shorter-acting form for daytime use. Muscarinic side effects of the anticholinesterase medications may be reduced by the use of low doses of atropine. Excessive anticholinesterase medication can induce muscle weakness by depolarizing or desensitizing available AChR and may lead to severe distress, termed *cholinergic crisis.* This crisis is treated by withdrawal of all anticholinesterase drugs for 24 to 48 hours and provision of ventilator support as needed. Supplementary medications such as ephedrine, potassium, and calcium are of uncertain value.

Additional therapy for MG includes thymectomy, adrenal corticosteroids, other immunosuppressant drugs, plasmapheresis, and intravenous gamma globulin (intravenous immune globulin [IVIG]), although each of these modalities is controversial.

Thymectomy is accepted treatment for thymoma. Radiation therapy also has been used, especially if a contraindication to surgery exists. Thymectomy in the absence of evidence for thymoma is more controversial. Many authorities propose thymectomy for all adult patients with generalized MG, except very elderly individuals. Others favor thymectomy only in patients who are not responding well to medical treatment. The likelihood of improvement or remission after thymectomy is thought by some to be greater in younger patients with recent onset of the disease. Sustained improvement, when it occurs, may begin months or up to several years after the surgery.

Steroid therapy is used frequently. Many different regimens have been suggested, including high (e.g., 60 to 100 mg prednisone) and low (e.g., 20 mg prednisone) doses for initial treatment and daily and alternate-day schedules. Low-dose, alternate-day prednisone is generally preferred for maintenance therapy. Exacerbations of weakness may occur when therapy is initiated, especially if large doses are given. Frequently, when alternate-day prednisone is used, more weakness is experienced on the steroid off-days during the early stages of therapy. The course usually becomes smoother with prolonged use of the drug. Most patients require steroids indefinitely. Cataracts, osteoporosis, aseptic necrosis of bone, and decreased resistance to infection are long-term side effects.

Immunosuppressant drug therapy with azathioprine is now being used more commonly, especially in patients with severe disease who are poorly responsive or refractory to corticosteroids. Azathioprine may be given in conjunction with steroids or as the only immunosuppressant therapy. Side effects such as bone marrow suppression

✔ *WHEN TO REFER*

Myasthenia gravis is a relatively uncommon disease. Since few physicians see more than one or two MG patients in the course of their medical careers, consultation with physicians specializing in MG is often obtained.

The diagnosis of MG is sometimes difficult to confirm, particularly in patients with only ocular complaints. Referral to a physician who is experienced in the various diagnostic tests should be considered.

Management decisions should be made by the physician and patient after consideration of the condition's severity, the expectations of the patient, and the potential benefits, risks, and costs of the various treatment options. For the physician who has limited experience with MG, consultation with an authority in the field is often helpful.

Any operative procedure on a patient with MG requires the anesthesiologist to be alerted in advance to the patient's MG condition to allow appropriate selection of medications. If possible, the surgeon and anesthesiologist would both be familiar with the care of MG patients.

✔ *WHEN TO REFER*

The congenital MG syndromes are very rare and are separable from one another only by sophisticated electrophysiologic and muscle biopsy studies. Referral to a center having such expertise is necessary for accurate diagnosis and recommendations for management.

and the late development of neoplasms must be considered. Discussion of azathioprine's potential for injury to the fetus is required before it is used in patients of childbearing age.

Other immunosuppressant therapies such as cyclophosphamide and cyclosporine have been used in a small number of MG patients. The toxicity of these medications discourages their frequent use in this disease.

Plasmapheresis has been used successfully in seriously ill patients to avoid or relieve respirator dependency. It has also been used to improve patients' clinical status before thymectomy. Improvement typically occurs within days and is usually temporary, rarely persisting for longer than 3 months. Although repeated plasmapheresis is occasionally used for long-term care, its routine application for less severely involved patients is not widely accepted.

Like plasmapheresis, IVIG is reported to have a temporary beneficial effect in MG, although controlled clinical trials have not been carried out. It is sometimes favored over plasmapheresis because it does not require special equipment and vascular access is easier to accomplish. Duration of effectiveness and cost are generally similar to plasmapheresis. Side effects include headache, aseptic meningitis and, rarely, renal failure. Immunoglobulin A–deficient patients are at risk for a severe allergic reaction.

CONGENITAL MYASTHENIA

Congenital myasthenia is a general term used to designate several different developmental defects in neuromuscular structure and function, including a presynaptic disorder characterized by impairment of acetylcholine resynthesis or storage (familial infantile myasthenia) and one associated with a paucity of synaptic vesicles and reduced quanta release. Presynaptic and postsynaptic defects may occur with impaired ACh breakdown (congenital end-plate acetylcholinesterase [AChE] deficiency). The several postsynaptic defects include slow ACh receptor ion channel closure (slow-channel syndrome), inadequate AChR production (congenital end-plate AChR deficiency), abnormal interaction of ACh and AChR, high AChR channel conductance and shorter-than-normal channel open time (high-conductance fast-channel syndrome), and prolonged channel open time with mutation of the epsilon subunit of the AChR. Autosomal recessive inheritance has been described or suspected in familial infantile myasthenia, congenital end-plate AChR deficiency, AChE deficiency, abnormal ACh-AChR interaction, and high-conductance fast-channel syndrome. Slow-channel syndrome is an autosomal dominant or sporadic disorder. AChR-ab has not been detected in congenital myasthenia, and there is no evidence linking it with an abnormality in the immune system.

Ptosis, ocular movement abnormalities, poor suck and cry, weakness, and easy fatigue may all occur in congenital myasthenia and

may be clinically indistinguishable from autoimmune myasthenia gravis. Symptoms are usually present at birth, but particularly with slow-channel syndrome, later onset may occur. Edrophonium test results may be positive or negative. All of the disorders are reported to display a decremental response to 2-Hz stimulation, at least in muscles that are clinically weak. A repetitive response to a single-nerve stimulus occurs with slow-channel syndrome and end-plate AChE deficiency.

Familial infantile myasthenia, end-plate AChR deficiency, abnormal ACh-AChR interaction syndrome, and the syndrome associated with a paucity of synaptic vesicles have all been reported to respond to anticholinesterase medication. Because there is no evidence of immune abnormality, thymectomy, corticosteroids, and other immunosuppressant drugs are not recommended.

LAMBERT-EATON MYASTHENIC SYNDROME

Lambert-Eaton myasthenic syndrome (LEMS) is a disorder of neuromuscular transmission resulting from defective release of ACh by the nerve terminal after nerve stimulation. It is frequently seen in association with malignancy and is autoimmune in origin.

The disorder is most often seen in adults, usually over the age of 40. Men are affected more often than women in most series, especially among patients with coexisting carcinoma of the lung. Gender bias is less clear in patients without tumor. The association with underlying malignancy approaches 60%; the majority of tumors are oat cell carcinomas of the lung.

Pathophysiology

Lambert-Eaton myasthenic syndrome is an autoimmune disorder directed against the presynaptic nerve terminal. Exocytosis of synaptic vesicles containing ACh occurs at the active zones on the presynaptic membrane by a calcium-dependent process. Antibody-induced disruption of these active zones is believed to hinder calcium uptake and thus impair ACh release. As a result, both skeletal muscle and autonomic cholinergic responses are impaired.

In favor of an autoimmune origin for LEMS is the observation that mice injected with immunoglobulin G from LEMS patients develop a loss of active zones and active zone particles and display electrophysiologic abnormalities characteristic of LEMS. The responsible antibodies are thought to be directed against voltage-gated calcium channels (VGCCs), and antibodies specific for the P/Q type of neuronal calcium channels were detected in 95% of LEMS patients by Lennon and others. The response of LEMS patients to plasmapheresis and immunosuppressant therapy also favors an autoimmune basis for the disease.

Pathologic Features

In humans morphologic studies show both presynaptic and postsynaptic abnormalities. Freeze-fracture electron microscopy shows a decrease in and disorganization of the active zones. Postsynaptic studies reveal reduplication of end-plate folds. Whether this change is caused by the disease process or is a result of presynaptic events is not known.

Clinical and Laboratory Findings

Clinical signs of LEMS include weakness and fatigability. Proximal muscles, especially those of the pelvic girdle, are often affected, and

✔ *WHEN TO REFER*

The electrical testing necessary to confirm the diagnosis of LEMS should be performed by an experienced electromyographer.

Management of LEMS is often improved by the use of 3,4 diaminopyridine, which may be available under "compassionate use" approval. Physicians specializing in neuromuscular junction disorders should be contacted regarding drug availability and selection.

gait difficulty is a frequent presenting complaint. Ptosis and diplopia are often present, but bulbar weakness, common in myasthenia gravis, is infrequently present in LEMS. Autonomic nervous system involvement occurs in LEMS, and complaints of dry mouth and impotence may result. Paresthesias are frequently reported, but detectable sensory loss is rare. Despite patient complaints of severe disability, it is common to find only mild weakness on examination. Tendon reflexes are usually depressed or absent.

The most readily available laboratory test for LEMS is repetitive nerve stimulation. At low rates of stimulation (2 to 3 Hz), a small motor response is detected that further diminishes between the first and fifth response. Brief exercise (10 to 20 seconds) results in an improvement in the amplitude of muscle response toward the normal range. Two minutes later, the defects seen in the rested muscle have recurred, and the amplitude of response is once again small. Repetitive stimulation of rested muscle at rapid (20 to 50 Hz) rates of stimulation produces an increasing amplitude of response that may reach 2 to 20 times the amplitude of the initial response.

Microelectrode studies of the neuromuscular function in LEMS patients show that the number of quanta of ACh released by a nerve impulse is small. Rapid repetitive stimulation or voluntary activation briefly facilitates the release of quanta, enhancing the depolarization of the postsynaptic membrane and improving neuromuscular transmission.

Calcium channel antibody detection is now commercially available as a diagnostic aid.

Associated Disorders

Lambert-Eaton myasthenic syndrome frequently occurs in association with tumors, usually oat cell carcinoma of the lung. In these cases it is suspected that antibodies made to tumor determinants cross-react with the active sites on the nerve terminals. Symptoms usually precede recognition of the tumor, at times by as long as several years. Treatment of the underlying tumor sometimes results in improvement in LEMS symptoms as well.

Patients with LEMS may have evidence of other autoimmune disorders, especially those that are organ specific. Organ-specific autoantibodies, (thyroid, gastric, and/or skeletal) are present in up to 45% of LEMS patients. Thyroid disease, vitiligo, and pernicious anemia have been clinically observed. Over 10% of LEMS patients also have detectable antibodies to ACh receptors. In these cases differentiation between LEMS and myasthenia gravis should be based on clinical and electrophysiologic markers.

Treatment

Anticholinesterase medications usually produce modest improvement. Drugs that enhance ACh release, such as guanidine hydrochloride, are more effective. However, side effects such as paresthesias and toxicity, including aplastic anemic and renal failure, limit prolonged use. 3,4, diaminopyridine, a drug that promotes ACh release from presynaptic vesicles, has shown encouraging beneficial effects in patients with LEMS but is not yet approved for general use. Corticosteroids, azathioprine, intravenous gamma globulin, and plasmapheresis have been used with success in LEMS. As far as is known, the use of immunosuppressive therapy does not impair the body's ability to suppress an as yet undiscovered tumor.

BIBLIOGRAPHY

Myasthenia Gravis

DeBaets MH, Oosterhuis HJGH, editors: *Myasthenia gravis*, Boca Raton, Fla, 1993, CRC.

Drachman DB: Medical progress: myasthenia gravis, *N Engl J Med* 330:1797, 1994.

Lisak RP, editor: *Handbook of myasthenia gravis and myasthenic syndromes*, Neurological disease and therapy series, vol 23, New York, 1994, Marcel Dekker.

Penn AS et al, editors: Myasthenia gravis and related disorders: experimental and clinical aspects, *Ann N Y Acad Sci* 681, 1993.

Seybold ME: Myasthenia gravis: diagnostic and therapeutic perspectives in the 1990s, *Neurologist* 1:345, 1995.

Congenital Myasthenia

Engel AG: Congenital myasthenic syndromes. In Lisak RP, editor: *Handbook of myasthenia gravis and myasthenic syndromes*, New York, 1994, Marcel Dekker.

Engel AG: Myasthenic syndromes. In Engel AG, Franzini-Armstrong C, editors: *Myology*, New York, 1994, McGraw-Hill.

Penn AS et al, editors: Myasthenia gravis and related disorders: experimental and clinical aspects, *Ann N Y Acad Sci* 681, 1993.

Lambert-Eaton Myasthenic Syndrome

Bird SJ: Clinical and electrophysiologic improvement in Lambert-Eaton syndrome with intravenous immunoglobulin therapy, *Neurology* 42:1422, 1992.

Chalk CH et al: Response of the Lambert-Eaton myasthenic syndrome to treatment of associated small-cell lung carcinoma, *Neurology* 40:1552, 1990.

Elrington G, Newsom-Davis J: Clinical presentation and current immunology of the Lambert-Eaton myasthenic syndrome. In Lisak RP, editor: *Handbook of myasthenia gravis and myasthenic syndromes*, New York, 1994, Marcel Dekker.

Lennon VA et al: Autoimmunity in the Lambert-Eaton myasthenic syndrome, *Muscle Nerve* 5:S21, 1982.

Lennon VA et al: Calcium-channel antibodies in the Lambert-Eaton syndrome and other paraneoplastic syndromes, *N Engl J Med* 332:1467, 1995.

McEvoy KM: Diagnosis and treatment of Lambert-Eaton myasthenic syndrome, *Neurol Clin* 12:387, 1994.

Penn AS et al, editors: Myasthenia gravis and related disorders: experimental and clinical aspects, Ann N Y Acad Sci 681, 1993.

CHAPTER

149 Muscle Disease

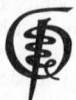

Robert H. Brown, Jr.

The cardinal symptom of muscle disease is weakness. A careful clinical analysis usually distinguishes the weakness of primary muscle disease from that caused by problems elsewhere in the motor unit or central nervous system. Distinguishing diagnostic features are outlined in Table 149-1. Most primary muscle diseases preferentially affect the proximal muscles. Thus there may be difficulty lifting the arms to comb the hair or rising from a low chair, while fine finger movements, removing a lid from a jar, and walking on tiptoes may be normal. Weakness is sometimes described as fatigue. In primary myopathies, weakness and fatigue symptoms usually significantly disrupt normal daily activities, whereas this may not be the case in systemic or psychiatric illnesses that produce fatigue. By the same token, in the primary myopathies the actual signs of muscle dysfunction may be more severe than the symptoms. Patients with primary myopathies such as disorders of muscle metabolism may complain of muscle cramping and pains. Myalgias induced by brief bursts of intense activity such as sprinting may occur in disorders of glycogen utilization; such activity depends primarily on recruitment of anaerobic type II muscle fibers that are glycogen-dependent. Conversely, in disorders of lipid metabolism, muscle pain may be most severe after sustained, low-level activities such as hiking that recruit oxidative, lipid-dependent type I fibers. Indeed, the lipid myopathies may be associated with episodic dark urine after chronic muscle exercise, indicating frank muscle breakdown and myoglobinuria. Weakness in primary myopathies is generally constant from day to day, perhaps with some worsening with sustained exercise; this is in marked contrast to the weakness in neuromuscular junction disorders such as myasthenia gravis or Eaton-Lambert syndrome, which may be highly

Table 149-1 Differential diagnosis of disorders of the motor unit

FINDING	NERVE	NEUROMUSCULAR JUNCTION	MUSCLE
Clinical			
Weakness, wasting	+	±	+
Fasciculations	+	−	+
Cramps	+	−	−
Sensory loss	±	−	−
Hyperreflexia	±	−	−
Laboratory			
Elevated CPK	−	−	+
Elevated myoglobin	−	−	+
High CSF protein	+	−	±
EMG-NCT			
Slowed conduction	+	−	−
MUAP amplitude	Increased	Normal	Decreased
MUAP duration	Increased	Normal	Decreased
Fasciculations	+	−	−
Decremental response	−	+	−
Muscle biopsy	Grouped atrophy	Normal	Degeneration-Regeneration

+, Positive; −, negative; *CPK*, creatine phosphokinase; *CSF*, cerebrospinal fluid; *MUAP*, motor unit action potential.

variable over the course of only a few hours. It is axiomatic that the primary myopathies, in contrast with peripheral neuropathies or central nervous system diseases, do not produce numbness or sensory loss.

It is useful to begin the muscle examination by observing the exposed torso and extremities. The hallmark of long-standing muscle disease is muscle wasting, which is often symmetric and proximal. Myopathic weakness and wasting of the facial and eyelid muscles is prominent in facioscapulohumeral, myotonic, and oculopharyngeal dystrophies; in the latter two there may also be pharyngeal weakness. Focal atrophy may be evident after muscle trauma or focal denervation. There is generally little visible spontaneous twitching of myopathic muscles; by contrast, muscles atrophied by denervation often reveal fasciculations. In some disorders there is infiltration of muscle with connective tissue and fat, which increases muscle bulk. Such pseudohypertrophy is particularly prominent in the calves in patients with Duchenne's and Becker's dystrophies. Muscle swelling with tenderness may be evident in focal or diffuse inflammatory muscle diseases.

It is conventional to rate muscle strength on a scale of 0 to 5 as follows: 5, full power; 4, nearly full power against both resistance and gravity; 3, moves against gravity but not resistance; 2, moves but not against gravity or resistance; 1, trace of movement; 0, no movement. In practice, rating muscle strength numerically is less important than describing performance of standard tests of muscle function such as lifting the head from a position of hyperextension or flexion over the edge of a bed; doing a sit-up; holding the arms overhead; rising from a chair or a squat without using the arms; walking; stepping up onto a stool; hopping on either foot alone; or pursing the lips to blow.

LABORATORY EVALUATION

Several laboratory tests assist in the diagnosis of neuromuscular disorders. Particularly helpful are serum levels of muscle enzymes released with muscle injury such as aldolase or the MM isoform of creatine kinase (CK). In fulminant myopathies such as Duchenne's dystrophy, CK may be elevated as much as a hundredfold. By contrast, in slowly progressive disorders it may be normal or elevated no more than twofold to threefold. Increases in CK are not specific to primary myopathies; the enzyme may be mildly elevated in active denervating disease such as amyotrophic lateral sclerosis. Levels may also rise after incidental trauma or intramuscular injections. Like muscle enzyme levels, serum and urine creatine and myoglobin are elevated when active muscle breakdown occurs. Myoglobin release does not

necessarily correlate with CK elevations; indeed, myoglobinuria is rare in Duchenne's dystrophy. Systemic and muscle-specific carnitine deficiencies produce lipid myopathies that may be diagnosed by assaying serum and muscle levels of this substance. Abnormalities in the major pathways of muscle energy production may be detected with two simple clinical tests. In the ischemic forearm lactate test, the forearm is exercised vigorously for one minute under ischemic conditions, which effectively disables mitochondria, rendering the muscle dependent on glycolysis for ATP production. Normally there is at least a twofold rise in serum lactate by about 6 minutes after the ischemic exercise. A flat lactate response is typical of glycolytic enzyme disorders such as myophosphorylase deficiency (McArdle's disease). By obtaining pyruvate and ammonia levels simultaneously, one may also screen for deficiencies of lactate dehydrogenase, or myoadenylate deaminase. To test muscle for ATP generation from lipids, the patient fasts until glycogen stores are depleted, usually more than 24 hours, while serum glucose and urinary ketone levels are monitored. In normal glycogen-depleted muscle, glucose levels are maintained by fatty acid metabolism, which secondarily produces urinary ketones. In disorders such as deficiencies of carnitine or carnitine palmityl-transferase, blood glucose may fall precipitously without ketonuria. Fasting serum lactate and pyruvate levels may be elevated in mitochondrial disorders. Finally, it is increasingly possible to diagnosis specific muscle gene defects using small quantities of blood lymphocyte DNA and polymerase chain reaction methods. Thus blood-based diagnosis is now possible for most cases of Duchenne's and Becker's dystrophies and the respective carrier states, myotonic dystrophy, hyperkalemic periodic paralysis, some mitochondrial muscle diseases, and some neuropathies such as Charcot-Marie-Tooth disease and familial amyloidosis.

ELECTROMYOGRAPHY

Analysis of the electrophysiological properties of muscle by electromyography (EMG) helps distinguish primary myopathies from other disorders that produce weakness. The first major diagnostic EMG parameter is *spontaneous activity*. When muscle undergoes active denervation, spontaneous twitches of single muscle cells or fibrillations occur, reflecting electrical irritability. *Fasciculations*—spontaneous discharges of an intact motor unit—may be seen in normal or denervated muscle. The second major parameter is *amplitude and shape of the motor unit action potential (MUAP)*. In primary myopathies the MUAP is often brief and reduced in amplitude; in denervating diseases with chronic reinnervation and motor unit enlargement the MUAP may be enlarged and prolonged. *Electrical irritability of the muscle membrane* is the third parameter. In myotonic disorders, the muscle membrane or sarcolemma shows sustained high but variable frequency discharges after needle insertion and after volitional contraction of muscle fibers (the "dive-bomber" sound heard on audio analysis of the EMG). In contrast, the sustained muscle contraction caused by energy deficiency, as seen in McArdle's disease, is electrically silent. The final parameter is a *pattern of recruitment of fibers* with voluntary muscle contraction. In primary muscle disease, the number of recruitable motor units is normal; however, the number of fibers per unit may be decreased, resulting in a pattern of low amplitude on recruitment. In contrast, denervating diseases such as poliomyelitis or motor neuron disease may reduce the number of recruitable motor units although the actual recruited compound muscle action potentials may be of normal or increased amplitude. Nerve conduction studies should be normal in primary muscle disease.

PATHOLOGY

Muscle biopsy may distinguish myopathic from neurogenic disease and may lead to specific morphologic diagnoses. In primary myopathies, muscle is characterized by fiber size variation and evidence of degeneration (fiber necrosis and phagocytosis; possibly inflammation) and regeneration (basophilia; central nucleation; fiber splitting). In chronic myopathies there may be extensive connective tissue proliferation and fatty infiltration. By contrast, in denervating diseases there may be evidence of active (small, angulated fibers) and chronic (fiber type grouping and grouped atrophy) denervation. Other features may suggest specific diagnoses such as the presence of fibers with a ragged red appearance in mitochondrial myopathies; marked lymphocytic infiltration of interstitium in polymyositis; glycogen-rich vacuoles in some glycolytic enzyme deficiency states (e.g., Pompe's disease or acid maltase deficiency); or lipid inclusions in the lipid myopathies. Muscle tissue from biopsy specimens is also useful for direct muscle biochemical assay or protein analysis using Western immunoblotting or immunofluorescence techniques.

SPECIFIC CATEGORIES OF MUSCLE DISORDERS

Box 149-1 lists the major categories of muscle diseases. The inflammatory myopathies are discussed in detail elsewhere. Several categories of myopathies are inherited, as outlined in Table 149-2; the largest group is the muscular dystrophies, a diverse group of disorders whose common feature is a period of relatively normal muscle function early in life followed by deterioration in strength in selected muscle groups. Despite recent dramatic research progress, these disorders remain untreatable.

Duchenne Muscular Dystrophy

This is the most common muscular dystrophy, affecting about 1 in 3000 boys. It is an X-linked disorder that frequently arises as a spontaneous mutation. Boys with DMD often have some delay in motor milestones and generally do not run normally. By the age of about 4 they may have difficulty walking up stairs and may fall easily. They are unable to rise from a squatting position unless they use the hands and arms to push off on the legs (Gowers' maneuver). Early in the course the calves show pseudohypertrophy. Before about the eighth year, most boys with DMD experience heel cord tightening and tend to walk on their toes. Most use wheelchairs by about the twelfth year. The myocardium may be involved, as indicated by persistent tachycardia, ectopic rhythms, subtle conduction defects, and ECG abnormalities (tall R waves and deep Q waves respectively over the right and left precordium). Death is usually from pulmonary failure with recurrent pneumonias. Becker's muscular dystrophy (BMD) is a less severe variant of DMD; it is usually also characterized by calf pseudohypertrophy and progressive proximal muscle weakness; BMD and DMD do not occur within the same family. Patients with BMD remain ambulatory beyond the age of 15 and often well into adult life.

Recent studies have identified both the DMD/BMD gene on the X chromosome and its product dystrophin. This is a large, muscle-specific protein, which has a rodlike structure and is membrane as-

---

BOX 149-1
Classification of primary myopathies

I. Hereditary
  A. Muscular dystrophies
  B. Congenital myopathies
  C. Metabolic myopathies
    1. Glycogenolysis and glycolysis
    2. Lipid metabolism
    3. Mitochondria
      a. Defects in substrate transport (e.g., CPT deficiency)
      b. Defects in substrate utilization (e.g., b-oxidation)
      c. Defects in Krebs cycle enzymes
      d. Defects in respiratory chain and ox-phos coupling
      e. mtDNA defects
        (i) large deletions (PEO, KSS)
        (ii) missense mutations (e.g. MELAS, MERRF, NARP, LHON, PEO)
  D. Membrane excitability disorders
    1. Dystrophic: myotonic dystrophy
    2. Nondystrophic
      a. Sodium channel mutations
        (i) Hyperkalemic periodic paralysis
        (ii) Normokalemic periodic paralysis
        (iii) Sodium channel myotonia
      b. Muscle calcium channel mutations—hypokalemic periodic paralysis
      c. Muscle chloride channel mutations—myotonia congenita
II. Inflammatory
  A. Polymyositis with dermatomyositis
  B. Polymyositis
  C. Inclusion body myositis
  D. Infectious
    1. Bacterial (e.g., clostridia)
    2. Viral and retroviral
    3. Parasitic (e.g., toxoplasmosis)
  E. Drug induced
  F. Miscellaneous (e.g., sarcoidosis, paraneoplastic)
III. Endocrine metabolic
  A. Electrolyte disturbances (including calcium, magnesium)
  B. Endocrine disturbances
    1. Hypothyroidism and hyperthyroidism
    2. Cushing's disease
    3. Hypoparathyroidism and hyperparathyroidism
IV. Toxic (e.g., alcohol, steroids, halothane, vincristine, chloroquine)
V. Primary muscle tumors
VI. Miscellaneous (e.g., malignant hyperthermia)

CPT, Ciliary particle transport; *mtDNA*, mitochondrial deoxyribonucleic acid; *PEO*, progressive external ophthalmoplegia; *KSS*, Kearns-Sayre syndrome; *MELAS*, mitochondrial encephalopathy, lactic acidosis and stroke-like episodes; *MERRF*, myoclonic epilepsy with ragged red fibers; *NARP*, neurogenic atrophy, ataxia and retinitis pigmentosa; *LHON*, Leber's hereditary optic neuropathy.

---

sociated. It is almost uniformly absent in DMD biopsies; in BMD muscle it is usually present but abnormal in size. The laboratory diagnosis of BMD and DMD has conventionally relied on elevation of serum CK levels and the presence of myopathic findings on EMG and muscle biopsy. It is now possible to assay muscle directly for dystrophin with immunoblotting and immunofluorescence techniques. One may also use polymerase chain reaction to diagnose deletions characteristic of DMD/BMD in blood DNA; this can assist in prenatal and preclinical diagnosis as well as carrier detection for genetic counseling.

Limb Girdle Muscular Dystrophy

The limb girdle muscular dystrophies (LGMDs) are a group of disorders that share several common features: (1) slowly progressive, proximal muscle weakness; (2) variable onset, ranging from childhood in some families to early adulthood in others; (3) a tendency to spare nonskeletal muscle tissues; and (4) generally long-term survival. In these disorders the CPK is elevated, sometimes as much as 50-

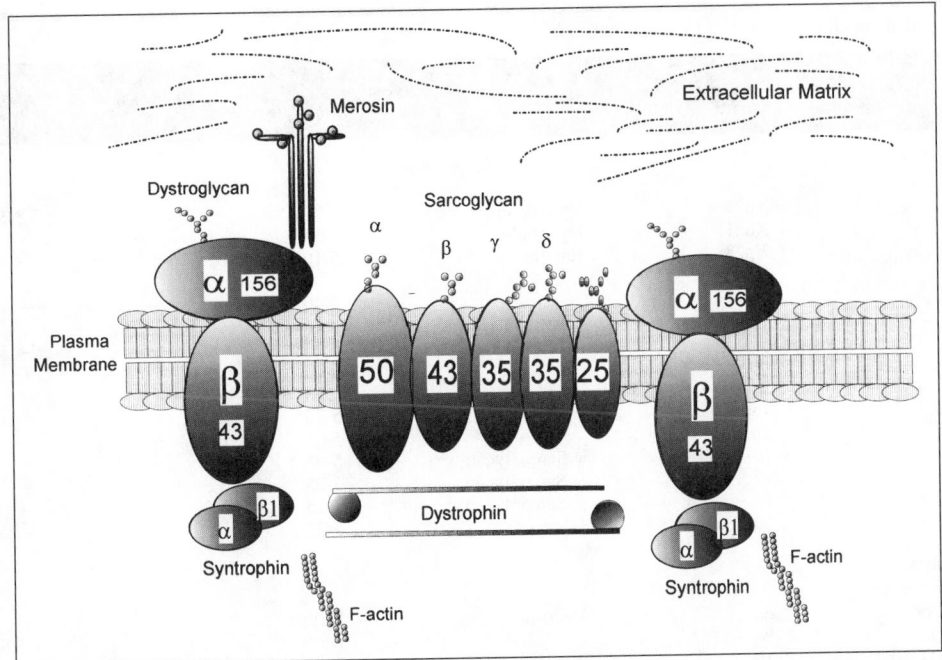

FIGURE 149-1 The dystrophin-associated glycoproteins (DAG) include merosin (extracellular), α-dystroglycan and β-dystroglycan, and the complex of sarcoglycan proteins (transmembrane) and dystrophin (submembrane). Dystrophin is also associated with F-actin, as well as α-syntrophin and β1-syntrophin. Merosin is a component of the extracellular matrix. The DAGs thus define a complex of proteins that potentially allows events in the milieu of the extracellular matrix to signal responses within the intracellular compartment and vice versa.

fold to 100-fold. Molecular analyses of patients with LGMD have defined subgroupings of these diseases, but they are often clinically difficult to distinguish. It was recognized at least 10 years ago that some cases of acid-maltase deficiency might be mistaken for LGMD, although the presence of glycogen-rich vacuoles usually distinguishes this disease from the limb-girdle dystrophies. More recently, a complex array of dystrophin-associated muscle glycoproteins has been delineated (Fig. 149-1). These form a potential link between the extracellular matrix and intracellular actin, via merosin at the extracellular surface, α- and β-dystroglycan spanning the muscle membrane, and dystrophin at the inner membrane face. Associated with the dystroglycans within the membrane are five distinct sarcoglycan proteins. Mutations that prevent expression of the dystroglycans cause recessively inherited forms of LGMD (Table 149-2). Loss of merosin causes a severe, lethal form of congenital muscular dystrophy. Recent investigations have also shown that one form of dominantly inherited LGMD arises from mutations in the gene encoding calpain.

Given these recent developments, the full analysis of LGMD entails screening for sarcoglycanopathies and calpain mutations. In theory, this is possible using genomic DNA from blood, although the testing is cumbersome and not yet commercially available. Muscle biopsy is potentially helpful, as one can screen for expression of dystrophin and the dystrophin-associated proteins using immunofluorescence. In general, when one sarcoglycan protein is absent, none are able to assemble in the membrane and associate with dystroglycan and dystrophin. In evaluating LGMD, muscle biopsy and electrophysiologic studies are also essential to exclude polymyositis and spinal muscular atrophy of the Kugelberg-Welander type. Without EMG the latter may be clinically indistinguishable from limb girdle dystrophy. Indeed, in chronic denervating diseases, biopsied muscle may acquire a "myopathic" histopathologic appearance, although fiber type grouping should point to denervating disorders.

Facioscapulohumeral Dystrophy

Facioscapulohumeral dystrophy typically affects muscles of the face and proximal upper extremities; weakness of the peronei and anterior tibial muscles may produce footdrop as well. The disorder is usually autosomal dominant; most cases of FSH dystrophy are genetically linked to the distal long arm of chromosome 4. There is considerable variation in the onset and severity of the illness. Most patients come to medical attention in the third decade, some never do, and some are diagnosed as children. In infants the earliest manifestation may be a tendency to get soap in the eyes while bathing. In children it may be an inability to purse the lips to whistle. In affected individuals there is prominent scapular winging. Abduction of the arms produces scapular elevation, which appears anteriorly as a step between the neck and shoulders. Weakness of the trapezeium and rhomboid muscles may produce extreme shoulder sagging and even, in rare cases, brachial plexopathies.

Myotonic Dystrophy

Myotonic dystrophy is an autosomal-dominant, multisystem disorder whose muscle features include myotonia (prolongation of muscle contraction caused by sustained firing of the muscle membrane) and progressive wasting of the facial (eyelids, masseters, temporalis), neck, and distal limb muscles. The myotonia is painless; individuals first diagnosed in adulthood often describe lifelong difficulty letting go of a doorknob. Nonmuscle features include frontal balding, cataracts (posterior, subcapsular, stellate), testicular atrophy and infertility, diminished insulin sensitivity, cardiac disease (particularly conduction system defects), and mental retardation. Facial muscle involvement produces a pathognomonic "hatchet" face with ptosis, prominent temporal and masseter wasting, and jaw slackness. In adults the onset of the illness is insidious in the second or third decade. In babies of mothers with myotonic dystrophy, there may be severe hypotonia and floppiness with weak respiration and sucking but no myotonia. The most useful laboratory investigation of any myotonia is the EMG, which demonstrates the typical myotonic dive-bomber bursts as mentioned previously. Muscle biopsy shows typically myopathic features and prominent type I fiber atrophy, increased central nucleation, chains of nuclei, and ring fibers. Phenytoin or mexilitine may improve the myotonia; other membrane active medications such as quinine may be hazardous because of potential cardiac conduction defects. The genetic defect in myotonic dystrophy appears to be an ex-

Table 149-2 Inherited myopathies*

DISEASE	CHROMOSOME	GENE	ONSET (YRS)	CLINICAL FEATURES		
				HEART	OTHER	COURSE
Major muscular dystrophies						
X-linked						
Duchenne	Xp21	Dystrophin	2-3	+	CNS	
Becker	Xp21	Dystrophin	5-15	±	−	Rapid
Emery-Dreifuss	Xp28	Emerin	5-10	±	−	Slow
Autosomal dominant						Slow
Facioscapulohumeral	4q	—	5-40	−	−	Slow
Myotonic dystrophy	19q	Myotonin	Any	+	+++	Slow
LGMD-1A	—	—	5-15	−	−	Slow
LGMD-1B	—	—	5-15	−	−	Slow
Autosomal recessive						
LGMD-2A	15q	Calpain	5-25	−	−	Slow
LGMD-2B	2p	—	5-25	−	−	Slow
LGMD-2C	13	γ-Sarcoglycan	5-25	−	−	Slow
LGMD-2D	17q	α-Sarcoglycan	5-25	−	−	Slow
LGMD-2E	4	β-Sarcoglycan	5-25	−	−	Slow
LGMD-2F	5q	δ-Sarcoglycan	5-25	−	−	Slow
Other inherited myopathies						
Congenital dystrophies						
Congenital dystrophy (AR)	6q	Merosin	Birth			Fulminant
Fukuyama disease (AR)	9q	—	Birth		CNS	Fulminant
Central core disease (AD, AR)	19	Ryanodine receptor	Birth	−	−	Slow
Nemaline rod disease (AD, AR)	1	Tropomyosin	Birth	−	−	Slow
Nondystrophic myotonias						
Hyperkalemic paralysis (AD)	17	Sodium channel	3-5	−	−	
Sodium channel myotonia						Slow
Paramyotonia congenita						
Hypokalemic paralysis (AD)	1	Calcium channel	10-15	−	−	Slow
Myotonia congenita (AD, AR)	7q	Chloride channel	3-5	−	−	Slow
Miscellaneous						
Oculopharyngeal dystrophy (AD)	14	—	50-60	−	−	Slow

*Excludes biochemically defined metabolic myopathies.
AD, Autosomal dominant; *AR,* autosomal recessive; *CNS,* central nervous system; +, positive; −, negative.

panded CTG trinucleotide repeat arising in a protein kinase encoded on chromosome 19.

In contrast to myotonic dystrophy, *myotonia congenita* (MC) is a muscle-specific disorder that begins in early childhood and produces profound, sometimes disabling muscle stiffness. Strictly speaking, this is not a dystrophy. Most MC patients have a "herculean" appearance with muscle hypertrophy and unusually distinct definition of muscle bulk; as a rule there is no muscle wasting. *Paramyotonia congenita* (PMC) is a related disorder in which there occurs cold-provoked muscle stiffness, particularly of the eyes and hands, and in severe instances, paralysis. PMC is caused by mutations in a skeletal muscle sodium channel, as are hyperkalemic periodic paralysis and some forms of MC. It is thus not surprising that the muscle stiffness in these diseases may respond to the sodium channel blocking agent mexiletine.

Oculopharyngeal Dystrophy

Oculopharyngeal dystrophy is a late-life, dominantly inherited disorder characterized by ptosis and difficulty swallowing leading to recurrent aspiration pneumonia and cachexia. In large families from French Canada, relative sparing of the extraocular muscles is reported. By contrast, in families of Italian origin external ophthalmoplegia may be profound.

The classification in Table 149-2 includes several other inherited myopathies; most are uncommon. The congenital dystrophies are somewhat arbitrarily grouped because they are clinically evident at birth or very early in life and because they lack distinguishing pathologic features. For example, in Fukuyama congenital muscular dystrophy, hypotonia and weakness of the face and proximal limbs occur with severe myopathy and developmental abnormalities in the central nervous system. Some of the congenital myopathies are characterized by distinctive myopathological features. They often produce

hypotonic weakness at birth followed by a nonprogressive or even an improving course; patients may show skeletal abnormalities, minimal CK elevations, and only mildly myopathic findings on EMG. In central core disease, weakness of the eyelids and face is also found. Muscle biopsy reveals long, centrally located cores lacking oxidative enzymes. It is now established that central core disease is sometimes triggered by defects in a protein (the ryanodine receptor) that governs release of calcium into the muscle cytosol following electrical stimulation. In nemaline rod myopathy, clumps of bacilliform rods or threads are seen in the subsarcolemmal space predominantly in type I fibers. Their ultrastructure is composed of enlarged Z bands. It is therefore not entirely unexpected that, in some kindreds, this disorder arises from defects in α-tropomyosin, a component of the thin filaments that insert on the Z band.

Metabolic Myopathies

Numerous inherited disorders alter muscle metabolism. It is convenient to group the familial metabolic myopathies into three categories: those affecting glycogen and glucose metabolism, lipid metabolism, and mitochondrial function (see Fig. 149-1). Defective glucose metabolism may arise from defects in enzymes either of glycogenolysis or glycolysis; not all of the enzyme disorders are muscle-specific. Deficiency of the lysosomal enzyme acid maltase results in abnormal glycogen accumulation in multiple tissues. In its infantile form, Pornpe's disease, absence of acid maltase, is characterized by myopathy, dysfunction of CNS neurons, cardiomegaly, hepatosplenomegaly, and macroglossia. Muscle weakness is a consequence both of myopathy and denervation. By contrast, in adult acid maltase disease, myopathy is the primary manifestation. Slowly progressive proximal weakness and in some instances respiratory failure occur with mild elevation of serum CK. The EMG is myopathic and may show high-frequency discharges. The enzyme deficiency may be measured in lysosomal preparations from fibroblasts and lymphoblasts as well as muscle.

Myophosphorylase deficiency (McArdle's disease) and *phosphofructokinase deficiency* impair glycolysis and cause painful muscle cramping after intense exercise, which preferentially uses glycogen-rich type II fibers. Patients may develop a "second wind" with sustained, submaximal exercise. Prolonged exertion may induce rhabdomyolysis, myoglobinuria, and even renal failure. Muscle microscopy demonstrates subsarcolemmal glycogen accumulation. As described previously, the absence of a rise in lactate after ischemic forearm exercise is a useful screening test for these disorders. Because the enzymes are muscle-specific, definitive diagnosis requires enzyme assay of muscle tissue. Deficiencies of *distal glycolytic enzymes* (phosphoglycerate kinase, phosphoglycerate mutase, and lactate dehydrogenase) are associated with exercise-induced muscle pain and myoglobinuria. In these diseases, lactate elevations after ischemic forearm exercise are subnormal. Muscle biopsy is required for definitive diagnosis.

Several disorders of *muscle lipid metabolism* have been defined. With sustained muscle exercise, muscle glycogen stores are depleted and lipid becomes essential for generation of energy in muscle. Carnitine, an essential factor in the breakdown of muscle lipids, may be deficient either systemically or selectively in muscle. In the former case, a progressive myopathy develops early in life in association with recurrent hepatic encephalopathy and even coma; the systemic features are absent in selective muscle carnitine deficiency. Some patients in both categories respond to treatment with oral carnitine. Recurrent crises of rhabdomyolysis and myoglobinuria may occur when either form of the enzyme carnitine palmityl-transferase is deficient. Once palmitate enters the mitochondrion, it is degraded to acetyl-CoA by sequential steps of beta oxidation; defective beta oxidation may also be associated with aberrant muscle lipid metabolism (Fig. 149-2). As described previously, screening for defective lipid metabolism is performed by having a patient fast and then monitoring for maintenance of normal blood glucose by gluconeogenesis as indicated by production of urinary ketones. Confirmation of the diagnosis requires assay of levels of carnitine palmityl-transferase or beta-oxidation activity in muscle. Some patients may improve with increased intake of carbohydrates or medium-chain triglyceride diets.

A syndrome of diffuse, postexertional muscle pain has been ascribed to deficiency of the enzyme myoadenylate deaminase. However, inasmuch as the deficiency is common even in asymptomatic individuals, the significance of this entity remains uncertain. The enzyme deficiency causes a subnormal rise in ammonia after ischemic forearm exercise; it must be confirmed by direct histochemical or enzymatic assay in muscle.

Mitochondrial abnormalities underlie a disparate group of myopathies whose most common feature is their multi-systemic character. In many the muscle is characterized by peripheral, submembrane accumulations of mitochondria described as ragged red fibers because of their irregular, reddish appearance on trichrome staining. Ultrastructural examination of the mitochondria may reveal enlargement, crystalline inclusions, and morphologic abnormalities of cristae such as elongation, flattening, or concentric duplication. In many instances, specific biochemical defects or mutations in mitochondrial DNA (mtDNA) have been defined. Although some patients have isolated myopathies, in most there is additional involvement of other tissues. In many adults the major clinical manifestation is chronic progressive external ophthalmoplegia (PEO), which develops symmetrically and insidiously with ptosis and sometimes proximal muscle weakness. This may be inherited (see later discussion) but is often sporadic. Individuals with this disorder may eventually be afflicted with dementia, epilepsy, retinal pigmentary degeneration, pyramidal and extrapyramidal signs, cerebellar ataxia, cardiomyopathy and heart block, neuropathy, diabetes, and hypoparathyroidism. When these features develop sporadically in childhood or adolescence in individuals with abundant ragged red fibers, the term *Kearns-Sayre syndrome* (KSS) may be applied. KSS is caused by large deletions in mtDNA; these are described as heteroplasmic because not all species of mtDNA in a given tissue are mutated in KSS. Other categories of mitochondrial disorders include those with myoclonic epilepsy and ragged red fibers (or MERRF) and mitochondrial encephalopathy, lactic acidosis, and stroke (or MELAS). In MERRF, MELAS, and Leb-

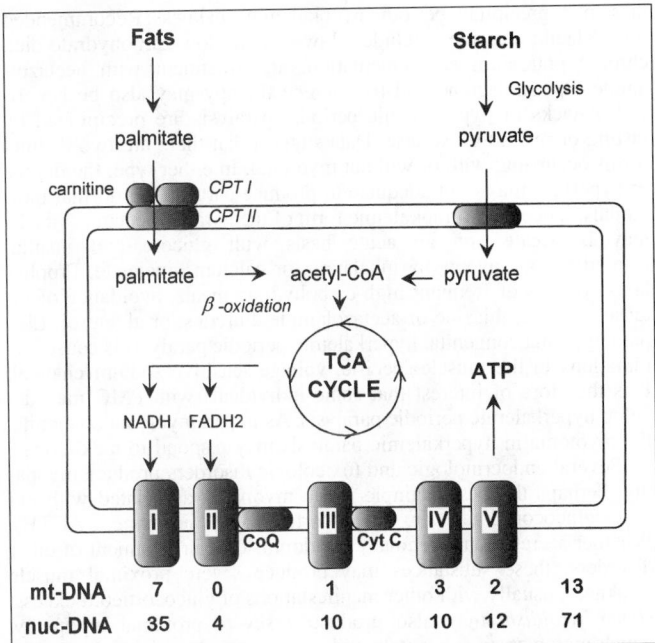

FIGURE 149-2   Overview of energy production in muscle. CPT I and II respectively designate forms I and II of the enzyme carnitine palmityltransferase, located in the membrane of the mitochondrion. The major pathways in the generation of adenosine triphosphate *(ATP)* entail breakdown of either carbohydrates or lipids, respectively producing pyruvate or palmitate as substrates to be transported in the mitochondrion. Palmitate is converted to acetyl-CoA following beta oxidation. Acetyl-coA is metabolized via the tricarboxylic acid (TCA, Krebs) cycle; TCA cycle enzymes are soluble within the mitochondrial matrix. The final common pathway in the process of ATP generation is the respiratory chain, located within the mitochondrial inner membrane. The respiratory chain complexes are composed of approximately 84 proteins, of which 13 are encoded by mitochondrial DNA *(mtDNA)*. The other 71 or so proteins are encoded by nuclear DNA *(nucDNA)*. *CoQ*, Coenzyme Q; *Cyt C*, cytochrome C.

er's hereditary optic neuropathy (LHON), the primary defect appears to be a point mutation affecting regions of mitochondrial DNA encoding tRNAs or respiratory complex proteins (see Box 149-1). As in LHON, many of the point mutations are homoplasmic; the mtDNA mutation is uniformly present in all mitochondria. In some cases, pedigree analysis indicates maternal inheritance of the disease trait; this pattern is expected for a mutation in mitochondrial DNA, which at conception is transmitted to the fetus via the egg cytoplasm. Another recently defined category of mtDNA diseases is characterized by tissue-specific depletion of mtDNA. This may arise either as an inherited condition or secondary to exposure to drugs such as azidothymidine (AZT) or nucleoside analogs used in HIV therapy.

Several inherited myopathies are characterized by abnormal electrical excitability of the muscle cell. Those with heightened electrical discharges, or myotonia, were mentioned previously. A second subgroup has intermittently diminished electrical activity arising with either diminished or elevated serum potassium levels. Thus these disorders are designated hypokalemic and hyperkalemic periodic paralyses. Hypokalemic paralysis is dominantly inherited, typically begins in adolescence, and affects males more commonly than females. In hypokalemic periodic paralysis, episodes are provoked by diets high in sodium and carbohydrates and rest or sleep after intense exertion. The attacks may last several hours and may eventually lead to permanent muscle weakness. If hypokalemia is severe, life-threatening arrythmias may ensue. Attacks may respond to oral potassium or intravenous potassium administered in mannitol (to avoid intracellular shifts in potassium caused by sodium- or glucose-containing solutions). Diagnostic measures provoking hypokalemia include the administration of glucose with or without insulin and infusion of intravenous epinephrine. When considering the diagnosis of hypokalemic paralysis, one must exclude thyrotoxicosis and barium toxicity, as these may precipitate periodic hypokalemic weakness. Recommended prophylactic measures include a low-sodium, low-carbohydrate diet, chronic potassium supplementation, and treatment with acetazolamide. Spironolactone and triamterene therapy may also be beneficial. Attacks of hyperkalemic periodic paralysis are precipitated by fasting or rest after exercise. Data suggest that there are two distinct forms occurring: with or without myotonia. In either type, the degree of hyperkalemia is not adequate to produce paralysis in normal individuals; indeed, a normokalemic form of the paralysis occurs. Attacks may be treated on an acute basis with glucose and insulin, beta-adrenergic agents by inhalation, or calcium gluconate. Prophylaxis consists of frequent high-carbohydrate meals, avoidance of intense exercise, thiazide or acetazolamide diuretics, or albuterol. Like paramyotonia congenita, hyperkalemic periodic paralysis is caused by mutations in the muscle-specific, voltage-sensitive sodium channel. It is therefore of interest that some individuals with PMC may develop hyperkalemic periodic paralysis. As in paramyotonia congenita, the myotonia in hyperkalemic paralysis may respond to mexiletine.

Several endocrinologic and toxicologic disorders produce myopathy. Perhaps the best example is the myopathy associated with excess glucocorticoids or adrenocorticotropic hormone (ACTH). Whether secreted endogenously or administered in treatment of other disorders, these substances may produce severe proximal muscle weakness, usually with other manifestations of glucocorticoid excess. *Hyperthyroidism* may also produce a severe proximal myopathy, which may worsen subacutely and mimic polymyositis. Unlike polymyositis, thyrotoxic myopathy does not elevate the serum CK. It should be recalled that thyrotoxicosis may be associated with an increased incidence of myasthenia gravis and may in some individuals produce periodic weakness with hypokalemia closely resembling familial hypokalemic periodic paralysis. Thyrotoxic patients may also demonstrate selective dysfunction of the eye muscles occurring in association with exophthalmos, or thyrotoxic ophthalmopathy. *Hypothyroidism* may produce proximal weakness and fatigue with muscle stiffness and hyporeflexia; in these patients the serum CK may be elevated as much as 10 to 100 times greater than normal. Pituitary disorders may impair muscle function. Proximal weakness may be evident in as many as 50% of patients with acromegaly and may also result from pituitary failure. Disorders of *calcium metabolism* may mimic myopathies. A syndrome of proximal muscle wasting and easy fatiguability has been described with both primary and secondary hypoparathyroidism, usually with a normal serum CK. Hypoparathyroidism may produce hyperexcitability of nerve and muscle and even frank tetany. In some patients this is latent but may be provoked by metabolic or respiratory alkalosis or by percussing the facial nerve (Cvostek's sign). A chronic myopathy has been described with calcium deficiency, responding to treatment with calcium and vitamin D. Pathologic evaluation of muscle is not specifically diagnostic in any of the endocrine myopathies; some may show selective type II fiber atrophy.

A variety of substances are directly or indirectly toxic to muscle. Alcohol may produce a skeletal and cardiac myopathy, although it remains unclear whether this is direct toxicity of ethanol or secondary to nutritional deficiencies. There is clearly an alcoholic, hypokalemic myopathy characterized by subacute evolution of profound muscle weakness in conjunction with elevated serum CK values and vacuolar changes on muscle biopsy. Several drugs cause rhabdomyolysis and myoglobinuria, including heroin, amphetamines, phenformin, fenfluramine, clofibrate, phencyclidine, barbiturates, and azathioprine. There is evidence that myopathy without rhabdomyolysis may be caused by chloroquine, emetine, vincristine, colchicine, and the β-blockers labetalol and propranolol. Rarely, intramuscular injections of certain agents may cause local fibrosis and contracture; offending substances include pentazocine, meperidine, and the antibiotics penicillin, streptomycin, and chloramphenicol. Selected drugs such as cimetidine, d-penicillamine, and procainamide may produce muscle inflammation.

One other muscle disorder with which the general clinician should be familiar is malignant hyperthermia (MH), a clinical syndrome induced by certain anesthetic agents and characterized by acute development of severe, diffuse muscle rigidity, acidosis, tachycardia, and fulminant life-threatening fever. MH may be inherited as an autosomal dominant trait caused by a mutation in the gene for the ryanodine receptor, a protein that triggers muscle contraction by releasing calcium from the sarcoplasmic reticulum. MH may be more common in individuals with certain myopathies such as Duchenne dystrophy and central core disease. Hyperthermic crises are triggered by multiple agents including depolarizing cholinergic agonists such as succinylcholine, volatile anesthetics such as halothane, or membrane-active agents such as lidocaine. Fortunately, if recognized, the disorder may be treated specifically with dantrolene and symptomatic measures.

BIBLIOGRAPHY

Brooke M: *A clinician's view of neuromuscular disease,* ed 2, Baltimore, 1986, Williams & Wilkins.

DiMauro S, Tonin P, Servidei S: Metabolic myopathies. In Rowland LP, DiMauro S, editors: *Handbook of clinical neurology,* vol 18, Myopathies, 1992, Elsevier Science Publishers.

DiMauro S, Bonilla E: Mitochondrial encephalomyopathies. In Rosenberg RN, Prusiner SB, DiMauro S, Barchi RL, editors: *The molecular and genetic basis of neurological disease,* ed 2, Boston, 1997, Butterworth-Heinemann.

Dubowitz V: *Muscle disorders in childhood,* ed 2, London, 1995, WB Saunders.

Engel AG, Banker BQ: *Myology,* New York, 1986, McGraw-Hill.

Griggs RC, Mendell JR, Miller RG: *Evaluation and treatment of myopathies,* 1995, FA Davis.

Schon EA: The mitochondrial genome. In Rosenberg RN, Prusiner SB, DiMauro S, Barchi RL, editors: *The molecular and genetic basis of neurological disease,* ed 2, 1997, Boston, Butterworth-Heinemann.

IV NEUROLOGY OF BEHAVIOR

CHAPTER

150 Behavioral Neurology

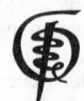

Roy Freeman

Cognition, language, personality, and the emotions, the traditional province of psychologists, psychiatrists, and philosophers, were for decades of only cursory interest to the neurologist. The past 30 years, however, have seen a movement, spearheaded by Dr. Norman Geschwind, built on the careful European clinicopathologic correlations of the nineteenth and early twentieth centuries and furthered by modern anatomic and neuroradiologic techniques, which has culminated in the legitimate establishment of the study of behavior within the realms of neurology.

The traditional approach to lesion localization, based on a careful examination of the patient's mental status, is as much a part of this dimension of clinical neurology as it is in examination of the cranial nerves, motor system, or sensory system.

This chapter discusses the most common derangements of cognition, emotion, and behavior that are seen in clinical practice. Knowledge of these behavioral syndromes is of more than theoretic importance. A detailed neurobehavioral evaluation in conjunction with the motor and sensory examination often enables the examiner to accurately localize the site of disease or identify a clinical syndrome before any abnormality becomes evident on computed tomography (CT) or magnetic resonance imaging (MRI) scan. Furthermore, attention to this aspect of the neurologic examination permits the early diagnosis of neurobehavioral disorders that occur in the absence of any abnormality on the general neurologic examination. Early recognition that the personality change occurring as a consequence of an occult frontal lobe tumor or that the confusion that is evident as a result of a right parietal lobe stroke is caused by neurologic disease is of obvious clinical importance.

ACUTE CONFUSIONAL STATE

The acute confusional state is unquestionably the most common cause of mental status change and probably the most frequent reason for neurologic consultation in any general hospital. The hallmark and salient deficit in this condition is the inability to maintain attention. Confused or inattentive patients have difficulty focusing their cognitive faculties on relevant environmental stimuli and, of equal importance, fail to exclude irrelevant stimuli from consciousness. The wide spectrum of mental states accompanying this inattention range from apathy and lethargy to agitation and hypervigilance. The confused patient may also display inappropriate jocularity and facetiousness. Confusion associated with agitation that is frequently accompanied by autonomic overactivity, such as mydriasis, tachycardia, diaphoresis, and tachypnea, is called *delirium*.

Disorientation is a frequent accompaniment to an acute confusional state, although it is not essential to the diagnosis. A peculiar form of disorientation known as *reduplicative paramnesia* or reduplication for place is occasionally seen. In this case the patient places himself or herself appropriately in the hospital environment and simultaneously believes he or she is in a second environment, usually closer to home.

On mental status testing, the patient in a confusional state may be disoriented and has difficulty with tests of attention. Such tests include the digit span (most patients normally are able to repeat seven digits forward and five digits backward), continuous performance tests (such as the serial subtractions of 7 or the recitation of the months of the year backward), and tests of vigilance (such as the recognition of the letter *A* from a list of letters randomly recited by the examiner). Spontaneous speech may be mildly aphasic, typically displaying word-finding difficulties and verbal paraphasias. There is often agraphia that is characterized by poor penmanship, as well as by spelling and grammatic errors. Further cognitive testing is usually limited by inattention.

On physical examination the patient may appear tremulous, with asterixis, myoclonus, and picking behavior. Autonomic overactivity as mentioned earlier is sometimes seen. The electroencephalogram usually shows generalized slowing.

The acute confusional state is most frequently a result of a primary disorder outside the central nervous system. In the evaluation of the confused patient careful attention should be paid to the possibility of metabolic dysfunction, drug and toxin ingestion or withdrawal, and infection both in and out of the central nervous system (Box 150-1).

Focal cerebral lesions at several sites—usually occurring as a consequence of a cerebrovascular event—can result in an acute confusional state. Nondominant parietal lobe lesions frequently produce this syndrome. In this case the neurologic examination may reveal denial of illness (anosognosia), a left homonymous hemianopsia or neglect, spatial or constructional difficulties, and contralateral cortical somatosensory loss or extinction.

Infarcts in the distribution of the posterior cerebral artery resulting in lesions affecting the fusiform and parahippocampal gyri (right or left) may also produce an agitated confusional state. Cortical blindness and short-term memory loss may be present, although a tendency to deny these deficits (Anton's syndrome) or amnestic confabulation sometimes confounds the examination.

Right frontal lobe lesions, particularly those involving the medial orbital cortex, are another focal cause of an acute confusional state. Hemorrhage resulting from a cerebral aneurysm or an arteriovenous malformation is a frequent cause of such lesions.

AMNESIC SYNDROME

The salient feature of the amnesic syndrome is memory loss with grossly normal attention, language, motivation, and cognition. Typically there are several aspects to this syndrome, including an anterograde memory loss (the inability to acquire new information since the onset of the responsible illness), a retrograde memory loss (the inability to recall information and events memorized before the onset of the illness), and confabulation (a tendency to fabricate, or "fill in," the memory hiatus). The latter, when present, occurs early in the course of an amnesic syndrome and is invariably accompanied by confusion.

BOX 150-1
Causes of acute confusional state

Metabolic dysfunction
Electrolyte abnormalities
Hepatic failure
Renal failure
Hypoxia
Hypercarbia
Endocrinopathies (e.g., thyroid, parathyroid, and adrenal dysfunction)
Blood glucose abnormalities
Acidosis
Alkalosis
Porphyria
Vitamin deficiencies

Drugs and toxins
Psychoactive medications
Alcohol
Toxic ingestions
Drug and alcohol withdrawal

Infections
Systemic infections
Central nervous system infections (meningitis, encephalitis)

Seizures
Complex partial seizures
Psychomotor and absence status epilepticus
Postictal states

Brain disease
Focal brain lesions
  Right parietal lobe
  Medial occipital lobes
  Right frontal lobe
Generalized brain lesions
  Head trauma
  Hypertensive encephalopathy
  Subdural hematoma
  Space-occupying masses
  Vasculitis
  Petechial hemorrhages

Because a reciprocally connecting circuit of limbic structures involving medial temporal lobes, specific diencephalic structures, and the basal forebrain is responsible for memory function, a variety of clinical conditions that produce lesions in diverse anatomic sites may cause an amnestic syndrome. Specific structures in this circuit include the hippocampus, the fornix, the mammillary bodies, the anterior and dorsomedial thalamic nuclei, the septal area, the cingulum, and the amygdala.

Researchers have delineated several phases in the process of memorization and recall. A useful clinical approach divides memory into registration (the reception of information), retention (the storage of information), and retrieval (the recall of stored information). Recent evidence suggests that different diseases that produce different neuroanatomic and neurochemical lesions cause specific patterns of memory loss. For example, disease processes affecting structures in the medial temporal, diencephalic, and basal frontal regions produce deficits in declarative memory (the recall and recognition of events and facts) while sparing procedural memory (skill learning). In contrast, diseases such as Huntington's disease that involve the basal ganglia produce procedural memory deficits.

Memory is best tested at the bedside by considering the somewhat artificial division of immediate, recent, and remote memory. Clinical tests for immediate memory are identical to those used to test attention and were described earlier. Recent memory is tested by asking the patient to recall events that took place in the preceding minutes, hours, or days. As an alternative, the patient can be asked to recount presented material (both visual and verbal) after a similar interval. Remote memory is tested by asking the patient to recall personal and historical events of the preceding years.

Several focal cerebrovascular lesions produce an amnestic syndrome. The best-described syndrome occurs as a result of a medial temporal lobe infarct in the distribution of the posterior cerebral artery, resulting in injury of the hippocampal and parahippocampal region. Coincident neurologic findings include alexia with or without agraphia, color anomia, hemianopsia, and, less frequently, central achromatopsia and prosopagnosia. Bilateral lesions are probably necessary to produce a permanent amnestic syndrome.

Strokes in the distribution of the thalamoperforate and tuberothalamic arteries, which supply diencephalic structures, also produce an amnestic syndrome. The neurologic examination in this case may reveal apathy and akinesia, as well as supranuclear paralysis of vertical gaze and other motor deficits.

Vascular lesions (such as ruptured arteriovenous malformations and anterior communicating aneurysms) of the basal forebrain (septal area) also produce memory loss. Amnesia attributable to basal forebrain injury is often accompanied by confabulation and may be improved with cueing.

The term *transient global amnesia* is used to describe a syndrome of uncertain cause in which there is a sudden loss of recent and remote memory. This condition is sometimes preceded by an emotionally charged situation, exertion, pain, or sexual intercourse. An anterograde amnesia develops that is characterized by bewilderment and mild agitation. The patients ask questions repeatedly and are not placated by appropriate replies. There is a retrograde amnesia of variable extent in which the patients have difficulty recalling events ranging from the preceding hours to past years. Intellectual function remains otherwise intact. The amnesia terminates abruptly and the entire episode usually lasts less than 24 hours. There remains, however, a permanent memory hiatus for the duration of the spell. Some authors have suggested a recurrence rate of 10% to 20%. Migraine, transient vertebrobasilar ischemia, epileptiform discharges, medication reactions, occult head trauma, and conversion hysteria have been reported as etiologic factors in this restricted disorder of registration and recall, but most cases remain unexplained.

Korsakoff's syndrome is another frequently encountered cause of the amnestic syndrome. Wernicke's encephalopathy, a clinical triad of confusion, ataxia, and ophthalmoplegia, frequently precedes the development of this chronic amnestic state. Thiamine deficiency associated with the malnutrition of alcoholism is the most common cause of the Wernicke-Korsakoff syndrome, but hemodialysis, hyperalimentation, hyperemesis gravidarum, gastric plication, and other causes of malnutrition may also produce this devastating clinical picture. Symmetric lesions are present at the base of the third and fourth ventricles and the aqueduct of Sylvius. Mammillary body and thalamic (in particular, the dorsomedial thalamic nuclei) lesions appear critical for the development of the amnestic syndrome.

Further causes of an amnestic syndrome are listed in Box 150-2.

FRONTAL LOBE SYNDROME

The frontal lobes encompass more than one third of the cerebral hemispheres and are divided into motor, premotor, and prefrontal regions. Injury to the prefrontal region, which makes up half of the frontal lobe, produces the so-called frontal lobe syndrome. This syndrome manifests as a disorder of behavior and personality, producing only subtle deficits in cognitive and intellectual function.

Patients with frontal lobe lesions do not adequately regulate or monitor their behavior, and thus language, conduct, and demeanor may be profane, childish, exhibitionistic, and socially inappropriate. Such patients appear thoughtless, impulsive, and unable to delay gratification. Their behavior lacks reverence for prevailing environmental and social conventions, and their actions are poorly planned and executed with limited insight into possible consequences. It is as if frontal lobe injury allows previously latent thoughts and actions to become manifest.

Disorders of mood and affect also occur with frontal lobe injury. Patients can display depression (particularly with left frontal lobe damage), as well as euphoria or elation (perhaps more commonly with right frontal lobe damage). Anger and irritability also are commonly

---

BOX 150-2
Causes of amnesia

Cerebrovascular events
  Hippocampal lesions
  Thalamic lesions
  Basal forebrain lesions
Wernicke-Korsakoff syndrome
Head trauma
Hypoxia
Hypoglycemia
Herpes simplex encephalitis
Degenerative diseases
  Alzheimer's disease
  Pick's disease
  Huntington's disease
Creutzfeldt-Jakob disease
Transient global amnesia
Neoplasms
Limbic encephalitis
Postsurgery
  Bilateral temporal lobectomy
  Bilateral fornix section
  Mammillary body surgery
  Cingulectomy

---

seen. Characteristically these moods are shallow and superficial, with labile and easily elicited shifts from one emotional state to another.

Apathy, indifference, and diminished arousal with lack of spontaneity and motivation are known as *abulia* and may also be seen as a consequence of frontal lobe injury. An extreme form of this behavior, in which there is an absence of self-generated or stimulus-elicited speech or movement, is referred to as *akinetic mutism,* or *coma vigil.* The akinetic mute patient neither speaks nor moves spontaneously, is only minimally responsive to the environment, and yet appears alert and is able to track objects within his or her visual field.

Patients with frontal lobe lesions may also display reduced cognitive flexibility, diminished creativity and capacity for abstract thought, and disordered regulation of motor skills such as motor sequencing. These dysfunctions manifest as perseveration, impersistence, imitative behavior, and lack of personal autonomy, particularly in an unstructured environment.

These abnormalities of mental status are sometimes associated with gait disturbance, alterations in muscle tone, incontinence, and grasp or other primitive reflexes.

A similar constellation of symptoms and signs that includes deficits in planning, abulia, loss of initiative and drive, anxiety with agitation, and obsessive-compulsive behaviors occurs with lesions of the basal ganglia. This may reflect interruption of the circuits that link the striatum to the frontal cortex.

This clinical profile can be produced by head injury, brain tumors (including gliomas, meningiomas, and metastases), hydrocephalus, demyelinating disease, degenerative disease (such as Alzheimer's and Pick's diseases), and cerebrovascular lesions (such as strokes in the distribution of the anterior cerebral artery and rupture of arteriovenous malformations or anterior communicating artery aneurysms).

Researchers have attempted to correlate specific features of the frontal lobe syndrome with certain anatomic regions. In this regard, it has been suggested that lesions of the orbitofrontal surface of the frontal lobe result in behavioral and emotional abnormalities, medial frontal lesions result in disorders of arousal, and dorsolateral lesions result in disorders of cognitive and motor flexibility and abstract reasoning. The concurrence of various signs and symptoms, the close anatomic juxtaposition of the various anatomic regions, and the failure of the various clinical conditions to respect anatomic boundaries, has rendered such an approach merely a hypothetical model at this point.

VISUAL AND VISUOSPATIAL BEHAVIORAL DISTURBANCES

The visual system is arguably the most complex sensory network in the primate brain. Lesions within this system and its connections produce a variety of perceptual and behavioral disorders. The disorders of perception primarily reflect damage in the visual and visual association cortex, whereas the more complex neurobehavioral disorders associated with visual dysfunction are most commonly caused by the disconnection of visual cortex from other cerebral regions.

The most frequent disturbance of visuospatial behavior is the hemiinattention or hemineglect syndrome. Such patients fail to report, respond to, or orient to stimuli contralateral to a brain lesion. In the most severe form of this disorder the patient fails to respond to all contralateral sensory modalities; dresses, shaves, and grooms only half of the body; eats only from half of the plate; and visually and motorically ignores half of the environment. In milder forms this abnormality can be demonstrated only by simultaneously providing a rival perceptual stimulus.

Several other behavioral disorders may accompany the syndrome of hemineglect. Patients may minimize the neurologic deficit (anosodiaphoria) or even refuse to acknowledge it (anosognosia). The patient may even deny ownership of a limb or express hatred of it.

Hemispatial neglect may be demonstrated by tests of line bisection (the patient divides the line closer to his or her intact hemifield), cancellation tests (the patient fails to cross out all letters or lines in the affected hemifield), and tests of drawing (the patient fails to complete the drawing of a clock or flower in the affected hemifield). Hemispatial neglect can result in a "paralexia." In this circumstance the patient neglects half of a word: for example, a word such as *greenhouse* would be read as *house.*

Typical neglect syndromes have been described with lesions involving the frontal lobe, parietal lobe, basal ganglia, and reticular formation. The neglect syndrome occurs more commonly, is more severe, and is of greater duration with right hemisphere lesions. This observation, together with the proclivity of right hemisphere lesions to produce global disorders of inattention (see earlier discussion), lends credence to the notion that the right hemisphere is dominant for attention.

Numerous disorders of perception have been associated with diseases within the visual system. These include illusions of size (micropsia and macropsia), shape (metamorphopsia), and number (monocular diplopia, triplopia, or polyopia). Patients have described a visual image shifting to another part of their visual fields (visual allesthesia), the persistence or recurrence of visual images after the removal of the visual stimulus (palinopsia), unpleasant visual sensations upon looking at an object in the hemianopic hemifield (visual dysesthesia), and a visual illusions induced by a nonvisual sensory stimulus (visual synesthesia).

Visual hallucinations may be simple (flashes of light, dots, colors, lines, and geometric forms) or complex (objects, animals, persons, and landscapes). Simple visual hallucinations are usually associated with local ocular disease, but occipital lobe lesions, occipital epilepsy, migraine, and, occasionally, toxic metabolic states can produce these phenomena.

Complex hallucinations are most frequently associated with a state of agitated confusion or delirium (see earlier discussion). Other causes include the Charles-Bonnet syndrome, which is the appearance of hallucinations caused by eye disease in elderly individuals, as well as hemianopsias and seizure foci involving the temporoparietal cortex. Brain stem and diencephalic lesions have also been associated with characteristically vivid, often pleasant hallucinations, a condition known as *peduncular hallucinosis.* Peduncular hallucinosis is frequently associated with and may be caused by a disturbance of the sleep-wake cycle.

The cortically blind patient is unable to perceive visual stimuli throughout the visual field while maintaining normal pupillary light reflexes and extraocular movements. This state is often accompanied by other disturbances of higher function, and the patient is frequently amnestic or confused. Such patients may fail to acknowledge their lack of vision and confabulate when asked to describe their visual world (Anton's syndrome). They typically rationalize their errors by attributing them to an environmental cause, such as dim light or the wrong pair of spectacles. Bilateral lesions of the geniculocalcarine tract are necessary to produce this syndrome and may occur as the result of a single embolus to the basilar artery bifurcation or a posterior circulation cerebrovascular accident in a patient with a preexisting contralateral hemianopsia, following vertebral angiography, with arrested transtentorial herniation, after hypoxic or ischemic events, and, rarely, with brain tumors and demyelinating disease.

Balint described a curious constellation of abnormal visuospatial behavior. In this syndrome the patient is unable to direct his or her gaze on command or in response to an orientating stimulus (apraxia of gaze), manual reaching under visual guidance is impaired (optic ataxia), and the patient cannot willfully direct his or her gaze appropriately (psychic paralysis of gaze). The patient is unable to perceive the visual field as a whole (simultanagnosia) and tends to focus on small, often irrelevant, peripheral aspects of the visual panorama. This syndrome is most frequently associated with bilateral occipitoparietal disease (i.e., dorsal cerebral regions) resulting in disconnection of the visual cortex from those cerebral areas mediating visuomotor exploration.

In contrast to this, visual agnosias—such as visual object agnosia, prosopagnosia (the failure to identify familiar faces), environmental agnosia, and color agnosia—have all been associated with bilateral inferotemporal and medial occipital damage (i.e., ventral cerebral regions). These disorders of recognition probably reflect the disconnection of the visual cortex from those regions of the brain subserving memory.

DISORDERS OF EMOTIONAL EXPRESSION

Disorders of affect, mood, and emotion associated with brain disease have been mentioned earlier. In this section, two commonly seen disturbances of emotional expression are discussed—pseudobulbar affect and aprosodia.

Pseudobulbar affect refers to brief, inappropriate, uncontrollable outbursts of laughing and/or crying that occur spontaneously or with minimal provocation. The observation that the laughing or crying lacks congruence with the mood state of the patient has led to terms such as *forced, released,* or *inappropriate* laughter and crying. The laughter or crying fails to elicit a similar response among observers, and the patient usually becomes distraught and embarrassed at the lack of control over his or her demeanor.

Pseudobulbar affect is usually associated with other stigmata of pseudobulbar palsy, such as dysarthria, dysphagia, a brisk jaw jerk, and hyperactive gag reflex, as well as with bilateral motor and sensory findings. Bilateral lesions caused by vascular disease, trauma, and demyelinating and degenerative disease that involve cortical, subcortical, or upper brainstem structures are responsible. Although the exact mechanism for producing inappropriate laughter and crying is unknown, the phenomenon is thought to result from the release of brainstem regions from inhibitory hemispheric control. Pharmacotherapy directed at central catecholamine and seratonergic pathways with agents such as amitriptyline, methylphenidate, levodopa, amantadine, and fluoxetine may attenuate these episodes.

Involuntary laughing and crying may also occur as an ictal manifestation, as in gelastic and dacrystic epilepsy, respectively. The emotional response is stereotyped, unprovoked, and usually unaccompanied by the appropriate mood state. This symptom is most frequently associated with epileptic foci in limbic regions and thus may be accompanied by other characteristic complex partial seizures and lead to secondary generalized seizures.

A common disorder of emotional expression is the inability to impart emotion to spoken language. This disruption in the production of prosody—the pitch, tempo, rhythm, and melody of speech—is most frequently seen with lesions occurring in the right hemisphere. The loss of prosody, called *aprosodia,* results in monotonous, expressionless speech and may be mistaken for depression. This disturbance in the production of prosody may be accompanied by a disturbance in the interpretation of prosody. Aprosody, a disorder of the emotional aspects of language, should be seen in contrast to aphasia, which is a disruption in the semantic, syntactic, and grammatic components of language.

CONCLUSION

This chapter has covered the neurobehavioral syndromes most frequently encountered in the clinical environment. Our knowledge of the relationship between brain and behavior is rapidly expanding as a consequence of more sophisticated neuropsychological research methods, neurochemical techniques, and brain metabolic and blood-flow imaging studies. The reader desiring a more detailed review of this rapidly growing area should consult the references listed in the bibliography.

BIBLIOGRAPHY

Balint R: Seelenlähmung des "schauens," optische Ataxie, räumliche Störung der Aufmersamkeit mschr, *Psychiatr Neurol* 25:51-81, 1909.
Cummings JL, editor: *Clinical neuropsychiatry,* New York, 1985, Grune & Stratton.
Cummings JL, editor: *Subcortical dementia,* New York, 1990, Oxford University.
Freeman R, Bear D, Greenberg MS: Behavioral disturbances in cerebrovascular disease. In Vinken PJ, Bruyn GW, Klawans HL, editors: *Handbook of clinical neurology,* vol 11, (S5) Amsterdam, 1985, Elsevier.
Geschwind J: Disorders of attention: a frontier in neuropsychology, *Philos Trans R Soc Lond (Biol)* 298:173, 1982.
Heilman KM, Valenstein E, editors: *Clinical neuropsychology,* ed 3, New York, 1993, Oxford University.
Levin HS, Eisenberg HM, Benton AL: *Frontal lobe function and dysfunction,* New York, 1991, Oxford University.
Lezak MD: *Neuropsychological assessment,* ed 3, New York, 1995, Oxford University.
Mesulam MM, editor: *Principles of behavioral neurology,* Philadelphia, 1985, FA Davis.
Squire LR, Zola-Morgan S: The medial temporal lobe memory system, *Science* 253:1380, 1990.
Whitehouse PJ: *Dementia,* Philadelphia, 1993, FA Davis.

151 Anxiety

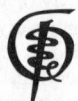

Barry S. Fogel

Anxiety may be a transient mood, a persistent or recurrent dysfunctional mood, or a rigorously defined psychiatric illness—an anxiety disorder. Anxiety disorders include panic disorder (recurrent stereotyped panic attacks), generalized anxiety disorder (persistent unrealistic or excessive worry for 6 months or more), phobias, obsessive-compulsive disorder, and posttraumatic stress disorder. These disorders are the most common psychiatric disorders in the United States, with a combined lifetime prevalence approaching 15%. They are even more prevalent in medical practice, because of the frequent presentation of anxiety with somatic symptoms. Panic disorder and generalized anxiety disorder usually present with multiple somatic symptoms, including dyspnea, dizziness, numbness and tingling, palpitations, trembling, sweating, choking, dysphagia, nausea, flushing, and chills. Panic attacks frequently include fears of dying or "going crazy," feelings of unreality, or chest discomfort. Chronically anxious people may complain of fatigue, tension, impaired concentration, irritability, or insomnia. Typically, anxious patients complain of difficulty falling asleep. Although each of the somatic symptoms of panic disorder and generalized anxiety disorder has a wide differential diagnosis, the simultaneous occurrence of multiple somatic symptoms of anxiety favors a psychiatric diagnosis, particularly if the onset occurs prior to age 35, symptoms have been long standing, and the physical examination and laboratory screening are negative.

Patients with anxiety disorders often offer a chief complaint appropriate to the internist's subspecialty: chest pain to the cardiologist, dyspnea to the pulmonologist, numbness and tingling to the neurologist. If multiple additional symptoms are elicited, the diagnosis of an anxiety disorder is supported. If not, anxiety can still be the cause of the symptoms. Anxiety should remain in the differential diagnosis, and a trial of antianxiety treatment should be undertaken if the complaint is not explained sufficiently by other medical findings. In this situation, monosymptomatic anxiety with definite recurrent attacks would be treated as panic disorder, and monosymptomatic anxi-

ety with continual symptoms would be treated as generalized anxiety disorder.

The differential diagnosis of anxiety includes medical disorders, drug-induced anxiety, and anxiety as a manifestation of depression. Severe anxiety beginning after age 40 usually implies one of these possibilities. Common medical conditions in which anxiety can be a prominent presenting feature include alcoholism, angina pectoris, cardiac arrhythmias, recurrent pulmonary emboli, asthma, congestive heart failure, hypoglycemia, hyperthyroidism, limbic (temporal lobe) epilepsy, Parkinson's disease, and hypercalcemia. Pheochromocytoma and carcinoid are very rare causes of anxiety, and assessment for their presence is not part of the ordinary medical evaluation of the anxious patient. Drugs frequently associated with anxiety include psychostimulants (including amphetamines and cocaine), sympathomimetic agents including barbiturates and nonprescription decongestants, theophylline, and indomethacin. Severe anxiety accompanies akathisia, a movement disorder in which the patient has an irresistible impulse to move and may complain of "jumping out of my skin." The most common causes of this disorder are antipsychotic medications and related drugs such as metoclopramide and prochlorperazine. Withdrawal from sedative-hypnotic drugs, benzodiazepines, opiates, tricyclic antidepressants, neuroleptics, or alcohol is an even more frequent precipitant of anxiety symptoms. Caffeine, at levels as low as 250 mg/day (two to three cups of brewed coffee) can cause or aggravate anxiety symptoms. Thus the diagnostic evaluation of the anxious patient includes a careful cardiopulmonary and neurologic history and examination, an alcohol and drug history, and a detailed inquiry about the symptoms of depression. Patients seeking medical treatment for anxiety require tests of thyroid function, a calcium level, and laboratory screening appropriate to their age and epidemiologic setting, including an electrocardiogram for patients older than 40 and those who complain of chest pain or palpitations in connection with their anxiety. An electroencephalogram (EEG) should be considered in patients with prominent episodic neurologic symptoms or panic attacks resistant to usual treatment.

The psychiatric history focuses on data especially relevant to treatment selection. Past history should include inquiry about prior psychiatric illness, treatment and response, prior substance abuse, and the occurrence of major traumatic life events. The last may include negative experiences with hospitalization or surgery and domestic violence.

In patients with significant family problems, unexplained injuries, or a history that seems inconsistent or puzzling, physical abuse by a spouse or other relation should be considered. Relevant history may be elicited by tactful inquiry without family members present; patients who do not volunteer a history of abuse may acknowledge it on direct and confidential questioning.

The review of current symptoms should cover symptoms that distinguish one anxiety disorder from another. These include obsessions and compulsive rituals, phobic avoidance of particular situations, and "flashbacks" that suggest a posttraumatic stress disorder.

Patients with anxiety disorders usually require both psychologic management and drug therapy. Regarding the former, patients definitely should not be given bland reassurance that they are "just anxious." Instead, their physical complaints should be acknowledged as "real" and attributed to a benign disturbance of nervous system function that produces frightening physical symptoms. Patients should be advised to avoid caffeine and other stimulants, and should be taught some formal method of relaxation. Self-help books and instructional tapes on meditation and other methods for dealing with stress are widely available; patients should be encouraged to find one compatible with their own beliefs and personal style. Books and tapes found helpful by patients in one's practice might be recommended to other patients.

Drug therapy should be offered in all cases and strongly encouraged in cases in which the patient has begun to avoid work or usual life activities, or when anxiety aggravates a chronic disease such as asthma or angina pectoris. Patients with specific interpersonal difficulties, posttraumatic stress disorder, or poor adjustment to a current life situation should be referred to a mental health professional for psychotherapy.

Patients with significant phobic avoidance require systematic exposure to the situations they fear. In milder cases this can be accomplished with informal support from the physician and family or friends. In more severe cases, formal behavior therapy is necessary. Patients who perform compulsive rituals such as hand washing or checking are best treated with serotonergic drugs (e.g., fluoxetine, fluvoxamine, sertraline, or paroxetine). Behavior therapy that prevents their rituals is a useful adjunct and may be adequate by itself in patients who reject drug therapy. Psychotherapy for posttraumatic stress disorder usually involves reviewing the traumatic event in a safe and confidential environment. Support groups are particularly useful for homogeneous groups such as incest survivors, victims of domestic abuse, and veterans with combat-related trauma.

Benzodiazepines are the most common treatment for anxiety in general medical practice. They are most valuable in the treatment of transient anxiety caused by life stresses or medical procedures. In these situations they offer the advantages of rapid action and low toxicity.

Long-term use of benzodiazepines often leads to pharmacologic and psychologic dependence. In elderly patients and those with impaired brain function, the drugs often cause cognitive impairment or gait disturbance. Also, the drugs can be abused by patients with addictive tendencies. For these reasons, long-term benzodiazepine therapy usually should not be instituted without consultation with a specialist. However, patients who have a long and continuing history of appropriate benzodiazepine use, a known or probable diagnosis of an anxiety disorder, and no evidence of side effects, may continue to take them.

Drug treatment for a newly diagnosed anxiety disorder may start with a benzodiazepine. After benzodiazepines have provided quick relief and have promoted cooperation, longer-term treatment with psychotherapy, behavior therapy, or other medications can be initiated. A consultation with a specialist to confirm the diagnosis and recommend treatment strategy is advisable before committing to long-term benzodiazepine therapy.

For generalized anxiety without panic, drugs of choice include the tricyclic antidepressants imipramine and nortriptyline, and buspirone. In patients with prominent insomnia, and those expected to be especially sensitive to the anticholinergic or quinidine-like effects of the tricyclics, trazodone and nefazodone are possibilities. However, daytime sedation and hypotension can be significant. Tricyclics should be started at 10 mg/day and increased gradually until symptoms are relieved, side effects develop, or a full antidepressant dose is reached (Chapter 152). Buspirone should be started at 5 mg t.i.d. and increased every few days as tolerated to a maximum of 20 mg t.i.d. if necessary for control of symptoms. Trazodone or nefazodone should be started at doses of 50 mg at bedtime and increased gradually if necessary to a full antidepressant dose.

Patients with panic attacks respond best to tricyclic antidepressants or to the monoamine oxidase inhibitor (MAOI) phenelzine given at a dose of 45 to 90 mg/day. Although phenelzine use involves the inconvenience of dietary restrictions, it may have specific benefits for patients whose anxiety is associated with social phobia. Phenelzine may also relieve phobic avoidant behaviors more rapidly and completely than other drugs. Both anxious patients and their physicians have avoided MAOIs because of the perception that the dietary restrictions are burdensome and the risks of hypertension high. However, if patients avoid cheese and over-the-counter decongestants, the risk of hypertension is small. Consultation with a psychiatrist is usual before starting MAOIs. However, nonpsychiatrists can safely manage ongoing MAOI therapy using guidelines provided by the psychiatrist.

Patients with obsessions and compulsions should be treated with either fluoxetine, fluvoxamine, sertraline, paroxetine, or clomipramine in full antidepressant dosages, building up gradually to minimize side effects. For posttraumatic stress disorder there is no specific pharmacologic treatment, but antidepressants are helpful in patients with prominent depressive symptoms. Mood-stabilizing drugs, described in Chapter 152, should be considered when mood swings are prominent and disabling.

The prognosis of anxiety disorders is variable; both chronic and relapsing-remitting courses are common. Patients with mild disorders often discontinue treatment on their own. For those who have more severe symptoms that have remitted on medication, gradual withdrawal of medication should be attempted every 3 to 6 months. After two or three unsuccessful trials of tapering medication, the patient

should receive long-term maintenance treatment. Dosage of medications for long-term treatment generally is the same as the dose that induced the remission of symptoms.

Rational benzodiazepine selection is based on the expected duration of treatment, the patient's hepatic status, and the specific indication and route of administration. For very short-term treatment, as for preoperative anxiety, virtually any drug except triazolam is acceptable. For longer-term treatment, the most important concern is pharmacokinetics. The short-acting benzodiazepines oxazepam and lorazepam do not have persistent active metabolites that accumulate if hepatic function is decreased by age or disease. Longer-acting agents, such as diazepam and chlordiazepoxide, do have persistent active metabolites; however, these agents offer the advantage of once-a-day dosage and a milder withdrawal syndrome on abrupt discontinuation. Lorazepam is reliably absorbed with intramuscular injection and is the preferred agent when this route is to be used. Acute panic attacks respond to almost any benzodiazepine if the dosage is sufficient; alprazolam and clonazepam are more effective than other benzodiazepines for recurrent panic attacks. Alprazolam is associated with rebound anxiety, so it should be given three or four times daily. Clonazepam has a long half-life and can be given once or twice daily, but a week or more should be allowed between dosage increases. Patients vary greatly in their sensitivity to benzodiazepines; dosage should be individualized according to clinical response.

In the elderly, shorter-acting benzodiazepines generally are preferable because of an increased risk of falls and fractures associated with longer-acting agents. When the latter are prescribed, the long half-life of active metabolites implies that the drug may not be in steady state for weeks following initiation or change in dosage. Thus frequent monitoring for ataxia is necessary, and dosage increases must be spaced several weeks apart.

BIBLIOGRAPHY

American Psychiatric Association: *Diagnostic and statistical manual of mental disorders,* ed 4, Washington, DC, 1994, The Association.

Bloom FE, Kupfer DJ, editors: *Psychopharmacology: the fourth generation of progress,* New York, 1995, Raven Press.

Charney DS, Nagy LM, Bremer D et al: Neurobiological mechanisms of human anxiety. In Fogel BS, Schiffer RB, Rao SM, editors: *Neuropsychiatry,* Baltimore, 1996, Williams & Wilkins.

Sheikh JI: Anxiety disorders. In: Sadavoy J, Lazarus LW, Jarvik LF et al: *Comprehensive review of geriatric psychiatry.* II. Washington, DC, 1996, American Psychiatric Press.

Spiegel D, Liebowitz M, Nemiah JC: Anxiety disorders, dissociative disorders, and adjustment disorders. In Gabbard GO, editor: *Treatments of psychiatric disorders,* Washington, DC, 1995, American Psychiatric Press.

CHAPTER

152 Mood Disorders

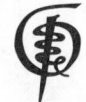

Barry S. Fogel

Mood disorders are widespread in the general population. The lifetime prevalence of major depression in the United States is approximately 10%. In patients who seek medical treatment, the prevalence is especially high, both because illness and trauma can precipitate depression and because major depression frequently presents with primarily physical symptoms.

The mood disorders comprise depression in its various forms, and bipolar (manic-depressive) disorders. The term *depression* in common usage may refer to a transient mood, a persistent and dysfunctional mood, or a mood disorder with physical and mental symptoms of sufficient severity, multiplicity, and duration to warrant formal diagnosis as an illness. Patients with depressive symptoms seemingly explained by a life stress or a physical illness still qualify for a psychiatric diagnosis if the symptoms are persistent and cause dysfunction. An exception is made for bereavement: physical and mental symptoms of grief are not diagnosed as a mental disorder unless they exceed cultural norms for severity, duration, or degree of impairment.

Medical illness and mood disorder usually have a circular relationship. Medical illness is a stress that can precipitate or aggravate depression, and depression can produce or intensify physical symptoms and impair a patient's ability to participate fully in treatment and rehabilitation. Major depression impairs cognitive efficiency with potential consequences of memory impairment and poor judgment. It also can alter immune functions; this possibly influences prognosis in infectious, autoimmune, and neoplastic diseases.

The presentation of depressive disorders varies with the patient's age. Young and middle-aged adults complain primarily of sad, depressed, or irritable moods, and their emotional symptoms usually are prominent. Children and adolescents often have changes in behavior, such as withdrawing from or displaying a negative attitude toward friends, school, and hobbies. Elderly patients often focus on the somatic or cognitive accompaniments of depression such as insomnia, anorexia, constipation, memory loss, or difficulty concentrating. They may fear they have Alzheimer's disease or cancer. They may deny depressed mood altogether or may attribute their mood changes entirely to physical symptoms and steadfastly resist the diagnosis of a mental disorder. When elderly patients suffer from dementia, they may deny depressive symptoms that are blatantly obvious to their caregivers. A common feature of major depression in all age-groups is loss of pleasure or interest in activities that the patient usually enjoys.

Major depression is diagnosed when the entire syndrome lasts at least 2 weeks and a change of mood or interest is accompanied by four or more of the following symptoms:

1. Changes in appetite or weight;
2. Insomnia or hypersomnia;
3. Psychomotor agitation, retardation, or both;
4. Fatigue or loss of energy;
5. Feelings of worthlessness or excessive guilt;
6. Impaired concentration or indecisiveness;
7. Recurrent thoughts of death, death wishes, or suicidal ideas, plans, or actions.

Only three of the symptoms are needed if the patient has both a mood change *and* a loss of interest or pleasure in activities.

Physical signs of depression include a persistently sad or pained affect, slowed speech or movement (psychomotor retardation), and agitation. A severe depression may be accompanied by thought disorder, as discussed in Chapter 154.

Depressed mood with fewer associated symptoms and a close temporal association with a life stress is termed an *adjustment disorder with depressed mood;* a long-standing persistent depression with less than the full major depressive syndrome is called *dysthymia.* Dysthymia produces as much disability as many other common chronic diseases, such as arthritis. It *can* be treated.

At least 20% of patients with major depression also have some history of distinct periods of elevated, expansive, or irritable mood. These periods may be accompanied by the following:

1. Inflated self-esteem or grandiosity,
2. Decreased need for sleep,
3. Excessive talking,
4. Racing thoughts,
5. Distractibility,
6. Increased goal-directed activity,
7. Excessive involvement in pleasurable activities with potentially painful consequences, such as sexual indiscretions or spending sprees.

Hypomania is diagnosed if an elevated or expansive mood is accompanied by at least three of these features or if an irritable mood is accompanied by four of these features. Mania is diagnosed when hypomania is accompanied by marked impairment in social or occupational function, by signs of psychosis such as delusions, hallucinations, or paranoia, or by psychiatric hospitalization.

Mania and hypomania usually develop before the patient reaches age 40, unless the patient has had prior depressive episodes. The differential diagnosis of new-onset mania in a younger person should include drug-induced mental disorders and brief reactive psychosis. If thought disorder is prominent, a primary thought disorder in the schizophrenic spectrum must be considered. If the patient is confused or disoriented, agitated delirium is a relevant consideration.

The new onset of manic symptoms in a patient older than 40 years of age without a prior history of depression strongly suggests secondary mania caused by a specific organic disorder such as hyperthyroidism or right hemisphere stroke. Other relatively common causes of secondary mania include multiple sclerosis, head injury, and medications such as stimulants, antidepressant drugs, dopamine agonist antiparkinson drugs, corticosteroids, cimetidine, procarbazine, and baclofen.

Patients with a mood disorder who have had any episodes of mania or hypomania carry the diagnosis of *bipolar disorder;* major depression without mania is called *unipolar depression.*

ORGANIC FACTORS

Organic factors frequently precipitate or aggravate mood disorders. On occasion, they are causal. Treatment or elimination of relevant organic factors is a usually necessary but not always sufficient step in treating the mood disorder. Specific investigations for organic factors should be based on the medical history and the epidemiologic setting. Comprehensive lists of medical disorders associated with depression can be found in the standard psychiatric textbooks. The key to rapid diagnosis of organic factors in clinical settings is generating a short list of medical conditions that have a relatively high probability given the patient's unique circumstances. For example, depression in a patient with known HIV infection immediately raises a concern of cerebral infection.

Substance abuse can be associated with either major depressive or manic episodes. Major depression can occur in the context of alcohol abuse; usually, the patient's mood will improve with 1 month of abstinence. Depression persisting beyond that time requires specific treatment. Alcohol abuse can precipitate manic episodes in individuals with a previous history of bipolar disorder, but more commonly, excessive drinking is a *symptom* of hypomania rather than its cause. Sympathomimetic drugs, including cocaine and amphetamines, can produce mania. After prolonged use, and especially after withdrawal, they may precipitate a major depression. Depression after stimulant withdrawal usually resolves spontaneously with abstinence. If it does not, it usually will respond to treatment with a stimulating tricyclic antidepressant such as desipramine.

Prescription drugs can provoke depression. Some well-known offenders are reserpine, methyldopa, propranolol, cimetidine, corticosteroids, and barbiturates. Even when a drug is not known to commonly provoke depression, the new onset of depression shortly after a new drug is started or its dosage is increased should raise the suspicion that the drug is an aggravating factor. The prescribed drugs that most commonly precipitate mania are stimulants, antidepressants, and corticosteroids. Drug-induced depressions more commonly affect patients with a prior history or family history of primary depression (i.e., depression *not* due to medication).

Thyroid disorders commonly are associated with mood disorders. Hypothyroidism may present with depression, or depression may supervene later in the course of hypothyroidism. Depression caused by hypothyroidism can occur with a normal or low-normal T4 level. In this situation, the thyroid-stimulating hormone (TSH) level is elevated; a thyrotropin-releasing hormone (TRH) stimulation test, if performed, would show an exaggerated response. Hyperthyroidism can present as either depression or mania, but care should be taken not to over-diagnose this condition, because the T4 level may be transiently elevated by the stress of any acute mental illness. Cushing's disease usually produces depression. Adrenal insufficiency causes fatigue, which usually is not confused with depression, because physical signs normally are evident by the time mood symptoms develop.

Neurologic diseases associated with a high prevalence of depression include Parkinson's disease, multiple sclerosis, temporal lobe epilepsy, and stroke. All but the last can present with depression alone. In this case, the neurologic diagnosis requires a detailed history, and often requires ancillary tests such as an electroencephalogram (EEG) or brain imaging. Sometimes the initial neurologic evaluation is negative but the brain disease becomes evident as the patient is followed. For this reason, the possibility of an emerging organic problem should be considered in any depressed patient who does not improve with treatment.

Tumors and infections of the central nervous system (CNS) may present with depression before unequivocal neurologic signs are manifest. Therefore neurodiagnostic tests are indicated when a patient in a high-risk group for CNS infection, malignancy, or stroke develops a new depressive illness. Both multiple sclerosis and stroke, particularly in the right hemisphere, can precipitate mania or hypomania.

Patients who reside in or have recently traveled to less developed countries may be at risk for depression caused by parasitic disease. Parasitic diseases with CNS involvement (e.g., trypanosomiasis) or with hepatic involvement (e.g., schistosomiasis) are most likely to present with depression. Lyme disease and HIV-associated illness can present with mood changes; serologic tests are indicated in patients at risk.

Depression, but usually not mania, can be a presenting symptom of occult malignancy; cancer of the pancreas is particularly notorious for presenting with depression. New-onset depression in later life, particularly if accompanied by weight loss, anemia, elevated ESR, or other signs of internal disease, should trigger a thorough search for occult cancer.

Finally, chronic pain both causes depression and is aggravated by it. After thorough assessment of the cause of the pain, patients with chronic pain and depression should be treated simultaneously for both conditions.

TREATMENT

Treatment of mood disorders begins with establishing the diagnosis and treating relevant organic factors, including those related to substance abuse. Hospitalization is considered if the patient poses a significant threat to self or others because of suicidal, self-destructive, or violent behavior, or if outpatient treatment is not feasible. Common impediments to outpatient treatment include cognitive impairment; lack of insight into the illness; lack of an informed, supportive family member; and unstable medical conditions that increase the risks associated with antidepressant drug treatment.

Patients with severe thought disorders, and particularly those with delusions and hallucinations, initially are treated with neuroleptic drugs while specific treatment for their mood disorder is begun. Such patients, like all those with severe depression, should be evaluated by a psychiatrist whenever it is feasible.

Major depression is treated with a combination of psychologic and pharmacologic modalities. Psychologic treatment for depression may be either educational and supportive or more formally psychotherapeutic. Formal psychotherapeutic treatment is indicated when interpersonal conflicts, unresolved grief, or habitual self-defeating thinking and behavior contribute to the illness. Most patients with dysthymia improve when their treatment includes psychotherapy. Patients with fewer psychologic symptoms and more physical symptoms often respond to informal supportive counseling, education about the disorder, and reassurance that medical treatment is likely to be effective in relieving symptoms.

The principal drug therapies for depression are the tricyclic antidepressants, the selective serotonin reuptake inhibitors (SSRIs) (fluoxetine, sertraline, paroxetine, and fluvoxamine), bupropion, venlafaxine, trazodone, nefazodone, and the monoamine oxidase inhibitors (MAOIs). A list of antidepressant drugs with usual and extreme dosages is presented in Table 152-1. Different antidepressants are comparable in efficacy if given at appropriate dosages, so initial drug choice should aim at minimizing those side effects to which the patient would be especially vulnerable or would be unlikely to tolerate. For example, the tricyclic antidepressants have significant anticholinergic and quinidine-like effects, and should be avoided in patients with narrow-angle glaucoma, heart block, or obstructive uropathy.

Table 152-1   Antidepressant drugs

DRUG	TYPICAL DAILY DOSE (MG)	DOSAGE RANGE (MG)	NOTES
Tertiary amine tricyclic:			1 2 3 4
Amitriptyline	100-200	10-300	1 2 3 4
Doxepin	100-200	10-300	1 2 3 4
Imipramine	100-200	10-300	1 2 3 4
Trimipramine	100-200	25-300	1 2 3 4
Clomipramine	100-200	25-250	1 2 3 4
Secondary amine tricyclic:			
Desipramine	100-200	10-300	3 4
Nortriptyline	50-100	10-150	4
Protriptyline	20-30	10-60	1 4 5
Venlafaxine	150-300	75-450	5 6
Amoxapine	100-200	25-300	3 4 5 7
Maprotiline	100-200	25-225	2 3 4 8
Phenylpiperazines:			
Trazodone	200-400	50-600	2 3
Nefazodone	200-400	50-600	2
Bupropion	300-400	150-450	5 8
Serotonin reuptake inhibitors:			
Fluoxetine	20-60	5-80	5
Sertraline	50-150	25-200	9
Paroxetine	20-60	10-60	
Fluvoxamine	50-150	25-200	2 9
MAO inhibitors:			
Phenelzine	45-60	30-90	3 5 10
Tranylcypromine	30-40	20-60	3 5 10

NOTES
1. Relatively high anticholinergic effects.
2. Relatively high sedation.
3. Relatively high rate of orthostatic hypotension.
4. Quinidine-like effects on cardiac conduction.
5. Prominent stimulating effect; may cause agitation.
6. Similar efficacy to tricyclics but may cause hypertension.
7. Tricyclic with neuroleptic effects—risk of parkinsonism, akathisia, and tardive dyskinesia.
8. Relatively high seizure risk; raise dosage slowly and avoid single bupropion doses >150 mg and single maprotiline doses >100 mg.
9. Frequent nausea or diarrhea.
10. Special dietary and drug interaction precautions needed.

A second consideration is whether the drug is sedating or stimulating. Fluoxetine, bupropion, protriptyline, and MAOIs are the most stimulating; trazodone, nefazodone, and amitriptyline are the most sedating. Finally, drug choice can take into account additional features of the patient's mental illness. The serotonin reuptake inhibitors may be particularly useful for patients with dysthymia, or with depression accompanied by obsessive-compulsive symptoms. Imipramine, nortriptyline, and the MAOIs are simultaneously effective for depression, panic attacks, and phobias. Clomipramine, venlafaxine, and the MAOIs may help patients unresponsive to other drug treatments.

Successful drug therapy for depression is based on several principles. First, the patient must understand the diagnosis and be aware that full antidepressant response to a drug may take several weeks. This sometimes requires tolerating side effects before the depression lifts. During this period, the physician or other clinical staff must be available to respond to the patient's questions and concerns, and frequent appointments should be scheduled if the patient is physically frail, anxious, or ambivalent about treatment, or if the patient has significant suicidal thoughts. Brief, scheduled follow-ups by telephone, fax, or electronic mail help promote treatment adherence and may detect side effects or worsening symptoms at an earlier stage.

Second, initial dosages should be relatively low in all patients and especially low in patients who are physically frail, neurologically impaired, very anxious, or have a history of tolerating medications poorly. Dosage should be advanced every few days as tolerated until symptoms remit, a full therapeutic dose is reached, or treatment is limited by dose-related side effects. Further increases in dosage beyond the average range are justified if the patient has responded partially and side effects are not too severe. A blood level determination and an electrocardiogram are reasonable precautions when tricyclic antidepressants are used at high dosages. Blood levels also should be considered when a patient has severe side effects on a low dose of medication. There is great variation in antidepressant pharmacokinetics among individuals. Therefore a response to a low dose does not imply a placebo effect, nor do side effects at a low dose imply hypersensitivity to the drug.

Third, side effects should be managed *actively*. Transient worsening of insomnia and anxiety on stimulating antidepressants responds to benzodiazepines. Constipation is helped by stool softeners and bulk supplements. Orthostatic hypotension on tricyclics is helped by stopping diuretics, liberalizing fluids, elevating the head of the bed at night, and using fludrocortisone if necessary.

Fourth, difficulty in drug treatment of a disabling major depression should lead to psychiatric consultation rather than abandonment of treatment. Timely consultation is preferable to many months of unsuccessful drug trials that exhaust the patient and family while function and morale decline further.

Patients with major depression unresponsive to medications usually remit with electroconvulsive therapy (ECT). Approximately 60% of patients with delusional depression do not improve with antidepressant drugs alone. Either antidepressant-neuroleptic combinations or ECT are required to induce remission. Patients with bipolar depression may respond less well to tricyclics than patients with unipolar depression and may do better with MAOIs or ECT, or when their antidepressant drug is augmented with lithium therapy. Most patients with bipolar disorder require maintenance therapy with a mood-stabilizing drug.

Patients with depression complicating severe medical illness or physical frailty usually cannot tolerate full doses of antidepressant drugs. Many will respond to a low dose of a conventional antidepressant drug. Others, particularly those with prominent apathy or lethargy, will respond to a psychostimulant. Methylphenidate or dextroamphetamine, beginning with 5 to 10 mg once or twice a day, can be used in the short term to help mobilize a lethargic, depressed patient. Since stimulants have not been proved to be an effective treatment for major depression, patients who respond to stimulants should be switched to conventional antidepressants if continued drug therapy appears necessary once the patient is mobilized. Long-term stimulant use would be considered if this switch led to significant apathy.

Major depression remits with the first drug therapy chosen in about 70% of cases; ECT is effective in 80% to 90% of cases. More than 90% of patients eventually will respond to some biologic treatment. Regardless of what treatment is used to induce a remission, contin-

ued treatment with antidepressant drugs for at least 6 to 12 months is advisable to reduce the risk of early relapse. The maintenance dose is the same as the dose used to induce a remission of symptoms.

The primary treatment for mania or hypomania is therapy with a mood-stabilizing drug, of which lithium was the first and is the best-studied. Patients who do not respond to lithium, those with rapid cycles between depression and mania, and those with a mixture of manic and depressive symptoms may respond well to a mood-stabilizing antiepileptic drug. These drugs are given at typical antiepileptic dosages. The effects of valproate and carbamazepine are well-established by clinical trials; gabapentin has shown mood-stabilizing effects when used as an anticonvulsant and may eventually be used as a psychiatric drug. Functionally impaired patients with prominent paranoid features, and those who fail to respond to both lithium and antiepileptic drugs, should be treated with neuroleptics.

Patients with bipolar disorder usually require long-term, or even lifetime, treatment with mood-stabilizing drugs to minimize relapses. Psychologic therapy begins with an educational and supportive approach to the patient and family; selected patients profit from formal psychotherapy once their mood has been stabilized. Because of the chronicity of the illness, the frequency with which it causes disability, and the complexity of its treatment, patients with bipolar disorder should be evaluated by psychiatrists. Stable patients may do well receiving maintenance drug therapy from a nonpsychiatric physician, with periodic specialist reassessments and backup consultation as needed. Those with more active or unstable symptoms require primary care by a psychiatrist.

REFERENCES

Alexopoulos GS: Affective disorders. In Sadavoy J, Lazarus LW, Jarvik LF et al: *Comprehensive review of geriatric psychiatry*. II. Washington, DC, 1996, American Psychiatric Press.

American Psychiatric Association: *Diagnostic and statistical manual of mental disorders*, ed 4, Washington, DC, 1994, The Association.

Bloom FE, Kupfer DJ: *Psychopharmacology: the fourth generation of progress*, New York, 1995, Raven Press.

Cohen-Cole SA, Brown FW, McDaniel S: Diagnostic assessment of depression in the medically ill. In Stoudemire A, Fogel B, editors: *Psychiatric care of the medical patient*, New York, 1993, Oxford University Press.

Fogel BS, Stone AB: Practical pathophysiology in neuropsychiatry: a clinical approach to depression and impulsive behavior in neurologic patients. In Yudofsky SC, Hales RE, editors: *American psychiatric press textbook of neuropsychiatry*, ed 2, Washington, DC, 1992, American Psychiatric Press.

Robinson RG, Travella JI: Neuropsychiatry of mood disorders. In Fogel BS, Schiffer RB, Rao SM, editors: *Neuropsychiatry*, Baltimore, 1996, Williams & Wilkins.

Rush AJ: Mood disorders. In Gabbard GO, editor: *Treatments of psychiatric disorders*, Washington, DC, 1995, American Psychiatric Press.

Stoudemire A et al: Psychopharmacology in the medically ill. In Stoudemire A, Fogel BS, editors: *Psychiatric care of the medical patient*, New York, 1993, Oxford University Press.

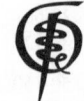

CHAPTER

153 Personality Disorders, Maladaptive Illness Behavior, and Somatization

Barry S. Fogel

Physicians most often encounter disturbances of personality in the form of noncompliance with treatment, inappropriate behavior in medical settings, self-defeating health habits, litigious behavior, doctor shopping, or apparent attachment to physical symptoms and the sick role. Personality traits are called *disorders* when they are inflexible, maladaptive, and lead to functional impairment, subjective distress, or both. Personality traits and personality disorders form a continuum, as do most behavioral phenomena. However, certain constellations of maladaptive traits occur with sufficient frequency to become classified as mental disorders with widely accepted diagnostic criteria. The obsessive-compulsive personality and the antisocial personality are two well-known examples.

PERSONALITY DISORDERS

A personality disorder should not be diagnosed unless the patient's maladaptive traits *persistently* affect function or well-being. Thus individuals who show inflexible, maladaptive behavior patterns only at times of acute stress, pain, or physical illness would not receive a personality disorder diagnosis. Such patients present more frequently in medical practice than do those with definite personality disorders. The same principles of assessment and management can be applied to both groups of patients, but definite diagnoses of personality disorders should be deferred until patients have recovered from acute physical illness.

The common personality disorders have been grouped into three clusters; within each cluster, the disorders have a common feature. Diagnostic assignment to a given cluster is much more reliable than is assignment to a particular disorder within the cluster. The three clusters of personality disorders are presented in Box 153-1.

The cluster of greatest interest to most nonpsychiatric physicians is the dramatic cluster, which consists of the antisocial, borderline, histrionic, and narcissistic personality disorders. These disorders have the common feature of dramatic, erratic, or overly emotional behavior. The specific criteria for each disorder can be found in the *Diagnostic and Statistical Manual of Mental Disorders* (DSM-IV-R), the standard reference on American psychiatric nosology. The disorders overlap, and it is not uncommon for patients to simultaneously meet criteria for two or three disorders within this cluster. Patients with these disorders come to their physicians' attention by displaying behavior that is overly dramatic, unstable, or unreasonable—such as threatening suicide, self-injury, or litigation; misusing medications; or abruptly terminating medical treatment, as by signing out of the hospital against medical advice. In addition, patients with antisocial personalities may engage in overtly criminal acts, such as stealing drugs or forging prescriptions, or may violate others' rights by assaultive or disruptive behavior in hospitals, clinics, or physicians' offices.

Another cluster, the *anxious* cluster, consists of avoidant, dependent, obsessive-compulsive, and passive-aggressive personality disorders. Patients with these disorders have the common feature of anxiety or fearfulness, although these feelings may be more implicit in patients' behavior than directly expressed. Patients with these disorders come to their physicians' attention through noncompliance with treatment; difficulties participating fully in self-care; and trouble making adjustments in their personal habits when required for medical treatment, rehabilitation, or disease prevention. Thus dependent personalities may excessively request advice and reassurance from the physician while clinging to a sick role that gives them a claim on their relatives' attention. Passive-aggressive personalities may forget appointments, miss doses of medications, and "misunderstand"

instructions, all the while denying responsibility for the lack of success of medical treatment.

The third cluster—the *odd* group—consists of paranoid, schizoid, and schizotypal personality disorders. These disorders feature odd or eccentric behavior. Patients with these disorders have difficulties in *all* personal relationships, including the relationship between physician and patient. Patients may fail to confide in the physician or fail to accept medical advice because of mistrust, suspicion, or social discomfort. Some have unusual and strongly held ideas that conflict with medical recommendations and are not open to reconsideration.

Personality disorders are diagnosed on the basis of a detailed personal and social history, ideally corroborated by a third party. A social history must show that the patient's maladaptive traits have been continually present since early adulthood. In the case of antisocial personality, the history of antisocial conduct must begin in childhood, with truancy, running away, cruelty to animals, lying, stealing, or other evidence of irresponsible or heedless behavior.

The social history usually accumulates over the course of medical diagnosis and treatment. Occupational and educational history, marital history, military history, and history of involvement in litigation, if explored systematically, usually permit a diagnosis. For example, a dishonorable discharge from military service raises a suspicion of antisocial personality; apparently frivolous lawsuits suggest a paranoid personality.

Antisocial and borderline personalities are common among drug addicts. Alcoholics are more likely than nonalcoholics to have some form of personality disorder, although there is no unique personality common to all alcoholics. Survivors of childhood abuse or incest have an increased prevalence of borderline personality, and the perpetrators of abuse and incest almost always have a personality disorder, often antisocial, borderline, or narcissistic.

Personality disorders usually are seen as behavioral phenomena caused by a patient's development and life circumstances. However, biologic influences, including variations in inborn temperament, also are relevant. Schizotypal personalities share biochemical, brain imaging, and neurophysiologic features with schizophrenic patients. Personality disorders of the anxious cluster occur more frequently in families of patients with anxiety disorders than in the general population; for example, obsessive-compulsive *personality* disorder is associated with obsessive-compulsive disorder, one of the anxiety disorders. Patients with personality disorders of the dramatic cluster who display irritability and impulsive aggression may show decreased central serotonergic function. Observations of this kind form the basis for attempts at drug treatment of personality disorders.

Any maladaptive personality trait can be aggravated by anxiety, depression, pain, stress, or mild delirium. Thus any patient who has maladaptive behavior in a medical setting deserves evaluation for anxiety, depression, and adequacy of pain relief, and a cognitive mental status examination specifically screening for a confusional state. The stress of illness and its treatment often can be reduced by careful explanation of the illness and its treatment and by informed consent procedures tailored to the patient's intelligence and cognitive style. For example, obsessive-compulsive patients may benefit greatly from detailed, formal patient education, whereas dependent patients may do better with less information and more reassurance. Patients at risk for noncompliance due to personality conflicts will profit from an especially careful and deliberate explanation of what they can expect from their treatment and what the physician expects from them with regard to cooperation.

Patients with more severe personality disorders, such as antisocial and borderline, may be manipulative, threatening, or dishonest. At times they may put themselves or others at risk of physical harm. In these situations, the patient must be told firmly *but without anger* what limits must be respected if medical treatment is to continue. Violation of these limits should imply termination of the physician-patient relationship. If a patient is too physically ill to be discharged from treatment, psychiatric consultation should be obtained. Security personnel or police should be called without hesitation if the patient is endangering others or violating the law.

Frequently, patients with severe personality disorders will employ charm, manipulation, or threats to enlist the support of a health professional for bending or violating accepted behavioral limits or rules of medical practice. A patient might request unreasonable quantities

---

BOX 153-1
Personality disorder clusters

"Dramatic"
  Antisocial
  Borderline
  Histrionic
  Narcissistic
"Anxious"
  Avoidant
  Obsessive-compulsive
  Dependent
  Passive-aggressive
"Odd"
  Schizoid
  Schizotypal
  Paranoid

of narcotics, convincing at least one physician that all other physicians and nurses are unfairly denying appropriate relief from pain. In such situations, the physician primarily responsible for the patient's medical treatment must bring together all involved health professionals to review the case and reach consensus on a single, consistent policy. The group's decision should be put in writing and made available to all members of the treatment team.

When medical treatment is significantly compromised by a personality disorder or maladaptive personality traits, formal psychiatric consultation should be obtained. It is generally best not to wait for a crisis, such as a suicide attempt, violence, or self-injury. The psychiatrist should be asked to help develop a written management strategy, or, when appropriate, to arrange the patient's transfer to a different treatment setting. If the patient is not to be referred elsewhere, the primary physician should maintain the same frequency of patient contact after psychiatric consultation, to avoid evoking feelings of abandonment in the patient.

There is not yet any well-established drug treatment for any personality disorder. Therefore nonspecialists generally should initiate drug treatment of patients with personality disorder only when there is a clearly treatable acute condition such as major depression. The treatment of personality disorders as such is a psychiatric specialty. Psychotherapy and behavioral therapies are the most commonly used treatments. In recent years, these have been supplemented by drug treatment for specific symptoms, such as mood instability and irritability.

SOMATIZATION

Many patients present with multiple somatic complaints affecting several organ systems and interfering with function, the symptoms of which are out of proportion to physical findings and laboratory values. Others have single symptoms or signs with no demonstrable organic basis. These patients, whose behavior is called *somatization,* fall into several distinct groups.

1. Patients with multiple physical complaints beginning before age 30 and a lifelong conviction that they are sickly. These patients suffer from *somatization disorder,* a psychiatric condition of unknown cause. They tend to have continual medical complaints that fluctuate in intensity throughout life, despite medical or psychiatric treatment. They often abuse prescribed medications and many also have a personality disorder of the dramatic cluster.
2. Patients with personality disorders, usually in the dramatic cluster, who somatize at times of stress, to either dramatize their plight, attract attention, obtain compensation, or avoid responsibility.
3. Patients with primary psychiatric disorders, such as panic disorder, major depression, or schizophrenia, in whom the multiple somatic complaints are symptoms of the psychiatric illness and remit with its effective treatment.
4. Patients with chronic physical disorders such as multiple sclerosis, Lyme disease, HIV, or systemic lupus erythematosus that may present with multiple physical symptoms before unequivocal diagnostic signs are evident.
5. Patients with specific physical symptoms or signs, without a demonstrable organic cause, that have an evident emotional significance of which the patient is unaware. For example, a patient may become blind after witnessing a gruesome scene or become paraplegic on the eve of an athletic contest he or she fears losing. These patients suffer from *conversion disorder,* a condition formerly known as *hysteria.* Their symptoms are not consciously feigned, and the patients consider themselves to be ill.
6. Patients who consciously feign illness or deliberately cause themselves to be sick, for example, by covert injection of drugs or toxins. The former are *malingerers,* the latter have *factitious illness.* The former always have the motive of personal gain of some kind; the latter may be motivated either by external reward or by an emotional need to be ill, to receive care, or to deceive others. Most patients with factitious illness have personality disorders of the dramatic cluster.

Patients with somatization disorder should be managed by their primary physician, with a conservative approach to laboratory tests and invasive procedures and with regular visits not contingent on new or increased symptoms. Patients with somatic complaints caused by

other psychiatric disorders or resulting from disordered personality will benefit from psychiatric consultation and treatment appropriate to the diagnosis.

Physical disorders with multiple somatic complaints are most often misdiagnosed as psychiatric when the patient also shows dramatic or abnormal behavior. Simultaneous and comprehensive medical, neurologic, and psychiatric evaluation helps avoid error. When apparent somatization develops in middle age or later and without definite evidence of a personality disorder or a major mental illness, occult medical illness is the most likely possibility.

Conversion disorder usually has a good prognosis. It is treated either with formal psychotherapy or with support and reassurance by the primary physician that there is an excellent chance of recovery. Gross malingering is a legal and administrative issue, although its confrontation may precipitate dramatic or threatening behavior that requires psychiatric assessment. Factitious illness indicates psychiatric consultation because it is a form of self-injury. However, the results of psychiatric treatment of factitious illness usually are disappointing.

MALADAPTIVE ILLNESS BEHAVIOR

Patients without psychiatric illness or personality disturbance may respond behaviorally to medical illness in ways that impede a good outcome. Two common forms of maladaptive illness behavior are amplification of pain or disability, and denial phenomena.

Emotional factors that cause excess pain or disability can be internal, such as a need to suffer or identification with a loved one who had similar pain or disability, or interpersonal, such as receiving more attention from a spouse when in pain. These factors are best identified by structured psychosocial assessment, including a conjoint interview with the patient and the spouse or family. Treatment is by individual or family therapy, which may focus on either the emotions or the overt behavior, depending on the apparent reason for symptom amplification.

Denial phenomena include gross denial of illness ("There is nothing wrong with me") or denial of the implications of illness ("It's cancer, but I've got it licked"). Denial phenomena are common in acute myocardial infarction and when a severe chronic or life-threatening illness like cancer or HIV infection is first diagnosed. Denial is maladaptive when it interferes with treatment or rehabilitation. Appropriate management consists of gentle but repeated confrontation in the context of support and empathy. Attempts to frighten the patient into compliance usually are unsuccessful.

In elderly patients, difficulties coping with illness can be either long standing or recent. Newly acquired coping difficulties raise a question of cognitive impairment, because memory, reasoning, and judgment are all needed for effective coping with illness, and dementia is common in old age. Screening for dementia and delirium is warranted in this situation.

REFERENCES

American Psychiatric Association: *Diagnostic and statistical manual of mental disorders,* ed 4, Washington, DC, 1994, The Association.

Coccaro EF, Siever LJ: The neuropharmacology of personality disorders. In Bloom FE, Kupfer DJ, editors: *Psychopharmacology: the fourth generation of progress,* New York, 1995, Raven Press.

Fogel BS: Personality disorders in the medical setting. In Stoudemire A, Fogel BS, editors: *Psychiatric care of the medical patient,* New York, 1993, Oxford University Press.

Fogel BS, Sadavoy J: Somatoform and personality disorders. In Sadavoy J, Lazarus LW, Jarvik LF et al, editors: *Comprehensive review of geriatric psychiatry.* II. Washington, DC, 1996, American Psychiatric Press.

Folks DG, Houck CA: Somatoform disorders, factitious disorder, and malingering. In Stoudemire A, Fogel BS, editors: *Psychiatric care of the medical patient.* New York, 1993, Oxford University Press.

Ford CV: Somatoform and factitious disorders. In Gabbard GO, editor: *Treatments of psychiatric disorders,* ed 2, Washington, DC, 1995, American Psychiatric Press.

Gunderson JG, Gabbard GO: Personality disorders. In Gabbard GO, editor: *Treatments of psychiatric disorders,* ed 2, Washington, DC, 1995, American Psychiatric Press.

Ratey JJ: *Neuropsychiatry of personality disorders,* Cambridge, Mass, 1995, Blackwell Scientific.

Ron M: Somatization and conversion disorders. In Fogel RS, Schiffer RB, Rao SM: *Neuropsychiatry,* Baltimore, 1996, Williams & Wilkins.

Tyrer P, editor: *Personality disorders: diagnosis, management and course,* London, 1988, Wright.

154 Thought Disorders

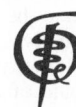

Barry S. Fogel

Disordered thinking can be either a disorder of thought content, such as false beliefs or hallucinated experiences, or a disorder of thought process, as reflected by incoherence of speech, illogical thinking, or disorganized behavior. Disordered thinking is remarkably common in acutely ill medical patients. Delirium and dementia are the most common causes. Other causes of thought disorder are listed in Box 154-1 and are discussed later.

Patients with impaired attention and orientation, and with disorders of higher cortical function caused by metabolic disturbance or degenerative disease, may misperceive their environment, have difficulty producing coherent speech, and produce logical inconsistencies of which they are unaware. Actual delusions or specific false beliefs can occur in delirious or demented patients, but they are rarely elaborate or systematized. General suspiciousness and hyperarousal are much more common in organic disorders than are specific and detailed delusions. Any patient showing a new onset of conspicuous suspiciousness in the context of medical illness deserves careful evaluation of cognitive mental status and screening for toxic, metabolic, and primary neurologic disorders if there are cognitive abnormalities suggesting delirium.

A second common cause of disordered thinking in medical settings is brief reactive psychosis. This disorder is diagnosed when a patient without any conspicuous prior abnormality of thinking and behavior develops florid psychotic symptoms after a major life stress, such as a life-threatening illness, major physical trauma, or the sudden or unexpected loss of a significant person.

Personality disorders, particularly those of the dramatic and odd clusters, are predisposing factors, as are mild organic cognitive disorders of insufficient severity or generality to warrant a diagnosis of delirium. A social history and a cognitive mental status examination therefore are necessary for accurate diagnosis. Drugs, both prescribed and self-administered, also can produce brief psychotic experiences of acute onset; an appropriately targeted drug history should be obtained from all psychotic patients. Laboratory screening for toxins and drugs of abuse should be targeted toward the most likely agents for the setting and should be performed on specimens appropriate to the suspected time of ingestion or injection (e.g., blood screening for exposure a few hours ago, urine screening for exposure 2 days ago).

Both delirium with thought disorder and brief reactive psychosis can be accompanied by agitation, uncooperative behavior, insomnia, and paranoid thinking. These symptoms can interfere significantly with medical diagnosis and treatment and can cause considerable suffering for the patient and family. Therefore both disorders usually are treated with neuroleptic medication. High-potency neuroleptics generally are preferable because of their lesser autonomic and anticho-

linergic side effects. The dose range used is wide; elderly or debilitated patients or those with brain damage may need a considerably smaller dose than young, large, physically healthy, and severely agitated men with histories of violent assaults. The lower end of the dose range is 1 mg/day of haloperidol or 2 mg/day of thiothixene; at the upper end, 5 mg of haloperidol or 10 mg of thiothixene can be used every half hour until the patient is calm. Combining haloperidol with lorazepam at the ratio of 5:1 controls agitated behavior more rapidly, and the lorazepam mitigates the side effects of muscle stiffness and motor restlessness that can be caused by haloperidol. The drugs can be mixed and given by intravenous or intramuscular route in patients unable or unwilling to take oral medication. The total dose needed for initial behavioral control can be repeated every 24 hours thereafter until the disorder causing the agitation has begun to resolve.

When haloperidol is given alone, extrapyramidal side effects such as dystonia, rigidity, and tremor are not unusual. Antiparkinson medication should be given promptly if these side effects develop, and prophylactic antiparkinson medication should be strongly considered for older patients, brain-damaged patients, and patients with a past history of extrapyramidal reactions to neuroleptics. Typical antiparkinson drug dosages are amantadine, 100 mg two to three times a day, or benztropine, 2 mg two or three times a day. Lower doses are appropriate for elderly or debilitated patients and for individuals with impaired renal function.

In addition to drug therapy, patients with acute psychoses are aided by a calm, consistent environment with a minimum number of different caretakers, frequent reorientation to place and situation, and minimal the use of medications that frequently cause mental side effects. Examples of the latter include pentazocine, meperidine, cimetidine, methyldopa, corticosteroids, indomethacin, and procainamide. Thought disorder can accompany the more severe forms of depression and invariably accompanies mania. Severely depressed patients usually are preoccupied with negative ideas that may relate to guilt, physical illness or incapacity, persecution, poverty, or regret. These ideas can assume delusional proportions—a development that implies a poorer prognosis and a less satisfactory response to antidepressant drugs. Auditory hallucinations ("voices") may deprecate the patient or command the patient to commit suicide. Patients with mania overvalue themselves and their projects and frequently have delusions of grandeur and importance. Auditory hallucinations usually are in keeping with the patient's exalted ideas—he may hear the voice of God or take direct orders from powerful figures. Both in severe depression and in mania, thought *process* is also disturbed. Depressed patients experience a slowing of thought that at times produces the impression of dementia or an apathetic confusional state. Manic patients have a rapid stream of thought that can degenerate into a confusing flight of ideas or even into total incoherence and confusion, suggesting an agitated confusional state.

Disordered thought content not compatible with the patient's mood also can occur. Such mood-incongruent delusions imply a worse long-term prognosis, even with appropriate treatment.

The treatment of thought disorder associated with mood disorder begins with neuroleptic medication and provision of a stable, calm environment, as in the treatment of brief reactive psychosis. Once the patient is more cooperative and less agitated, specific treatment is directed toward the mood disorder. Lithium or mood-stabilizing antiepileptic drugs are used for mania, whereas antidepressant drugs or electroconvulsive therapy is used for depression. Long-term use of neuroleptics usually is unnecessary in patients with mood disorders and should be avoided whenever possible because of the risk of tardive dyskinesia.

Chronic, persistent, or recurrent thought disorder not associated with a mood disorder usually is caused by one of the schizophrenic disorders. Schizophreniform disorder is diagnosed when the illness lasts less than 6 months; schizophrenia is diagnosed when the illness lasts 6 months or more. Both conditions involve active symptoms associated with overt behavioral changes and prodromal or residual symptoms that precede and follow episodes of active symptoms. The active symptoms include delusions, hallucinations, incoherence, markedly abnormal motor behavior (catatonia), and inappropriate or markedly unreactive affect. The delusions tend to be bizarre, such as the belief that the patient's thoughts are being controlled by occult forces or creatures from another planet. Hallucinations, usually audi-

---

BOX 154-1
Causes of thought disorders

Gross brain dysfunction
    Delirium
    Dementia
    Neurologic diseases, for example, Huntington's chorea
Brief reactive psychosis
Mood disorders
    Depression with delusions
    Mania
Schizophrenic disorders
Drug induced

tory, can consist of a running commentary on the patient's actions or a dialogue between different voices. Visual hallucinations are not rare but occur less often than do auditory hallucinations; their presence should suggest delirium or drug intoxication.

The prodromal or residual symptoms include social isolation or withdrawal, impaired occupational function, impaired hygiene and grooming, inappropriate or flat affect, abnormal speech, odd beliefs, unusual perceptual experiences, and peculiar behavior such as talking to oneself in public. The abnormal speech may be vague or lacking in content, or, alternatively, overelaborate and circumstantial.

Schizophrenia is a chronic brain disease of multifactorial causation that affects 1% of the world's population. Genetic factors are known to be a significant cause of schizophrenia, with monozygotic twins having a 65% concordance rate. Overwhelming evidence exists that brain structure and function differ between schizophrenic patients and controls. People with schizoid or schizotypal personality disorders are more vulnerable to the disease. Hallucinogens or psychostimulants, such as amphetamines and cocaine, can precipitate psychoses clinically indistinguishable from schizophrenia, although most drug-induced psychoses are of relatively short duration. A chronic thought disorder resembling schizophrenia occurs in a minority of patients with limbic (temporal lobe) epilepsy.

Since schizophrenia is a subacute or chronic disease with blatant psychologic symptoms, the diagnosis of a major mental illness usually is obvious by the time a patient sees a physician. Alternate, less common presentations include obscure or bizarre somatic complaints representing somatic delusions, serious organic disease neglected because of apathy or delusional beliefs, or unexplained academic or occupational failure. Because patients with schizophrenia often avoid medical care or neglect physical problems, the newly presenting schizophrenic patient requires a thorough physical evaluation and laboratory screening. The evaluation should be modified to take into account any positive physical findings, the patient's nutritional status, any history of alcohol or drug use, and risks associated with the patient's family history, travel history, environment, and life-style.

Treatment of schizophrenia combines drug treatment with psychosocial interventions. Drug treatment is based on the long-term use of neuroleptic drugs. Drug treatment is more effective for the positive symptoms of schizophrenia, such as delusions and hallucinations, than for its negative symptoms, such as flat affect or social withdrawal. However, the atypical neuroleptic agents—clozapine, olanzapine, and risperidone—appear to be more helpful for negative symptoms than the conventional neuroleptics that preceded them to market.

The approach to initiating neuroleptic treatment depends on whether the patient is acutely agitated. Agitated patients usually are calmed with frequent doses of a high-potency neuroleptic, as described earlier. Other patients, including patients now controlled with high-potency neuroleptics, should be started more slowly on one of the atypical neuroleptics, since these are the drugs of choice for long-term treatment. Risperidone or olanzapine should be used, because they have lesser extrapyramidal side effects than the typical agents but lack the hematologic toxicity of clozapine.

A typical daily maintenance dose of a high-potency neuroleptic is 5 to 10 mg of haloperidol or 10 to 20 mg of thiothixene. Comparable doses for the atypical agents are 10 to 20 mg for olanzapine, 3 to 6 mg of risperidone, and 300 to 500 mg of clozapine. The range of doses used in practice is wide because there is marked variation among individuals, both in clinical response and in sensitivity to side effects. Pharmacokinetics vary widely also.

Antiparkinson drugs often are necessary when high-potency agents are used. They are indicated not only for gross tremor and rigidity but also for apathy or markedly diminished voluntary activity. Tardive dyskinesia, a persistent and often permanent movement disorder involving involuntary facial movements, choreoathetosis, or dystonia, is the most common complication of long-term neuroleptic treatment, occurring in approximately one fourth of patients receiving long-term treatment. Informing the patient (or guardian) about the risk of tardive dyskinesia is an ethical and legal necessity if neuroleptic therapy is to be long-term. The atypical agents have a lesser risk of tardive dyskinesia; clozapine may actually alleviate the symptoms of this movement disorder.

Probably the most disturbing acute side effect of neuroleptics is akathisia. This is a motor disorder characterized by subjective restlessness and continual motor activity, such as rocking or pacing. Patients describe an almost unbearable discomfort if they attempt to hold still. Treatment begins with reducing the dosage of the neuroleptic if feasible. Drug treatments include propranolol 20 mg tid, diazepam 5 to 10 mg as needed, or typical doses of antiparkinson medication. Propranolol probably is the best initial choice; the dose may be increased if the drug is tolerated and relieves symptoms partially.

Neuroleptics are usually classified as typical or atypical; the typical neuroleptics usually are classified by potency and route of administration. The atypical agents have become the drugs of first choice in the treatment of schizophrenia because they reduce disability more than the typical agents. Several studies have shown that drugs with equal effects on psychotic symptoms may have differing effects on everyday functioning. Among the atypical neuroleptics, risperidone is the least sedating but the most likely to cause parkinsonian symptoms or orthostatic hypotension. Olanzapine is more sedating but has fewer motor side effects and may be somewhat better for control of residual symptoms.

Clozapine is the "gold standard" neuroleptic. It can be dramatically effective in patients unresponsive to other neuroleptics, and it rarely causes extrapyramidal side effects. Its use is limited by a risk of life-threatening agranulocytosis in 1% to 2% of patients. Clozapine also causes seizures in 3% to 4% of patients, can cause fever up to 103° F during the first 6 weeks of treatment, and can produce numerous other side effects including sedation, tachycardia, hypotension, ECG changes, and hypersalivation. Side effects require drug discontinuation in about 6% of cases. For these reasons, its use is reserved for patients who have not responded to two other agents, including at least one of the other atypical neuroleptics. Clozapine should be started at a dosage of 25 to 50 mg/day and increased gradually to an average dosage of 300 to 500 mg/day. Weekly blood cell counts are mandatory for the duration of therapy; the drug should be stopped immediately if neutropenia develops.

Typical agents are used in acute situations, when the drug must be given parenterally, and when the patient is currently in remission while taking one of them without troublesome side effects. Among the typical agents, the high-potency drugs such as haloperidol and fluphenazine have the fewest anticholinergic and cardiovascular side effects but cause the most extrapyramidal reactions. The low-potency drugs, such as chlorpromazine and thioridazine, have the opposite profile and are substantially more sedating. Thioridazine and perphenazine have substantial antianxiety effects that sometimes are desirable. Two high-potency drugs, haloperidol and perphenazine, come in a depot intramuscular preparation that permits treatment by biweekly or even monthly injections in patients unable to comply with daily oral medication.

In patients receiving neuroleptics, adverse effects can be minimized by keeping the dose at the minimum level necessary to control major positive symptoms such as hallucinations and delusions. If additional mental symptoms require drug treatment, these should be handled with specific nonneuroleptic adjuncts. Depression should be treated with antidepressants, anxiety with benzodiazepines or buspirone, and fluctuating moods with lithium or a mood-stabilizing antiepileptic drug.

Psychosocial measures are directed at preserving and enhancing social function. Individual, group, and family psychotherapy all have a place, but the last has the greatest proven benefit and is usually the treatment of choice for patients who live with their families. Formal training in social skills is valuable when those skills are lacking, as is vocational rehabilitation for the unemployed. Employment, when the patient is able to work, is particularly valuable in preserving social skills and function. With treatment, 60% of people with schizophrenia have a social recovery within 5 years and about one third are able to work.

REFERENCES

American Psychiatric Association: *Diagnostic and statistical manual of mental disorders,* ed 4, Washington, DC, 1994, The Association.

Bloom FE, Kupfer DJ: *Psychopharmacology: the fourth generation of progress,* New York, 1995, Raven Press.

Hirsch SR, Weinberger DR: *Schizophrenia,* Cambridge, Mass, 1995, Blackwell Scientific.

Jeste DV, Harris MJ, Paulsen J: Psychoses. In Sadavoy J, Lazarus LW, Jarvik LF et al:

Comprehensive review of geriatric psychiatry. II. Washington, DC, 1996, American Psychiatric Press.

Jeste DV, Galasko D, Corey-Bloom J et al: Neuropsychiatric aspects of the schizophrenias. In Fogel BS, Schiffer RB, Rao SM: *Neuropsychiatry,* Baltimore, 1996, Williams & Wilkins.

Lipowski ZJ: *Delirium: acute confusional states,* New York, 1990, Oxford University Press.

V Neurology in General Medicine and Surgery

CHAPTER

155 Head Trauma

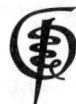

Peter M. Black

Head trauma is an important medical problem both in its acute management and its long-term sequelae. This chapter discusses the pathology, clinical presentation, differential diagnosis, management, and possible complications of patients with head injuries.

PATHOPHYSIOLOGY

The skull acts as a rigid container that does not allow expansion of masses within it. Intracranial pressure (ICP) rises exponentially as volume increases. Cerebral perfusion pressure (CPP), defined as mean arterial pressure minus mean intracranial pressure, is a measure of the effect of increasing brain pressure on cerebral blood flow: it should be kept at 40 mm Hg or higher to assure adequate brain perfusion.

Head injuries can be divided into three categories: skull fractures, which may be linear, basilar, or depressed; focal brain injuries, including contusions, intracranial hematomas, and missile wounds; and diffuse injuries, including concussion and diffuse axonal injury.

Skull fractures may be associated with underlying brain injury, such as epidural or subdural hematoma, or may be silent with respect to the brain.

Focal injuries include epidural, subdural, and intracerebral hematomas; and cerebral contusions. Epidural hematomas occur between dura and skull and separate the dura from the skull at the inner table of the bone; they have a characteristic lenticular shape and are associated with skull fractures in 75% to 90% of cases. Subdural hematomas occur between the surface of the brain and the dura. Hematomas of this type have major mass effect on the whole hemisphere because of the continuous nature of the subdural space. Intracerebral hematomas are surrounded by brain parenchyma; they may be difficult to separate from contusions. Brain contusions may occur adjacent to prominences such as the frontal or middle fossa or may occur in the brainstem. They are usually mottled in computed tomography (CT) appearance and contain pulped brain. They may be "coup," (under the impact site) or "contrecoup" (on the opposite side of the brain from impact). The coalescence of brain contusions after the initial injury is an important cause of delayed neurologic deterioration. Diffuse injuries include subarachnoid hemorrhage and shear lesions. Subarachnoid hemorrhage is the most common hemorrhage in head injury and may be responsible for delayed hydrocephalus as well as diffuse brain dysfunction. Shear lesions of white matter involve axonal tearing and may be devastating despite minimal CT evidence of injury.

Intracranial hemorrhage may precede rather than follow a head injury; an example is a middle cerebral aneurysm that ruptures and creates a subdural hematoma that results in loss of consciousness, lead-

ing to an automobile accident and subsequent head injury. This possibility should always be considered when evaluating unusually placed hematomas.

CLINICAL PRESENTATION

Head injury presentations can be classified as acute or chronic, and in the acute phase can be classified as severe, moderate, or mild. For the patient with acute head injury, the problem is appropriate management. For the patient with chronic head injury, the problem is often recognizing the diagnosis.

Acute Head Injury

The patient with a significant acute head injury may have findings ranging from full alertness to deep coma. The Glasgow Coma Scale is useful in classifying and following severity in the acute case (Table 155-1). A mild injury has a coma score of 13 to 16; a moderate injury, 8 to 15; and a severe injury, less than 8.

Evaluation of Patients With Severe Head Injury

The evaluation and management of patients with severe head injury should proceed together. In the evaluation, four important questions must be answered.

1. *How severe is the injury?* The most widely used mechanism for evaluating severity of injury is the Glasgow Coma Scale (summarized in Table 155-1). Three features are examined: the best verbal response; best motor response, usually in the best limb; and what is required for eye opening. The coma score is important for initial grading and also for follow-up of the patient. Patients with a coma score of less than 8 have a 40% likelihood of requiring immediate surgery.

2. *What brain structures are affected?* This question has importance both for prognosis and for therapy. The major structures potentially affected are the cerebral hemispheres, brainstem, and cerebellum. Aphasia, cortical sensory loss, or visual field loss suggests focal cortical injury. Ataxia is an important sign of a cerebellar mass. Pupillary or eye movement abnormality suggests a brainstem lesion. Most comatose states after head injury appear to result from shear injury to the white matter of the cerebral hemispheres rather than to brainstem injury.

3. *Is there evidence of a lateralizing mass?* Lateralization of signs is an important physical finding in head injury evaluation. The lateral tentorial herniation syndrome, discussed later, is especially important and should be recognized by every physician.

4. *Is the patient's condition worsening?* This question is best answered by sequential examinations using the Glasgow Coma Scale.

Table 155-1   Glasgow Coma Scale

FUNCTION TESTED	RESPONSE	GRADE
1. Eye opening (E)	Spontaneously	E4
	To voice	3
	To pain	2
	None	1
C = eyes closed by swelling		
2. Best motor response (M)	Obeys commands	M6
	Localizes pain	5
	Withdraws	4
	Decorticate to pain	3
	Decerebrate to pain	2
	None	1
3. Best verbal response (V)	Oriented, appropriate	V5
	Confused conversation	4
	Inappropriate words	3
	Incomprehensible sounds	2
	None	1
T = intubated or tracheostomy		

Herniation Syndromes

The most important syndromes to recognize after head injury are the lateral tentorial herniation syndrome, central herniation, and tonsillar herniation. These all indicate imminent brainstem damage and death.

Lateral tentorial herniation is characterized by increasing restlessness or drowsiness, followed by weakness of the limb opposite the mass (pyramidal tract compression at the tentorial notch), pupillary dilation on the side of the lesion (oculomotor nerve and therefore parasympathetic compression), and, ultimately, central herniation.

Central tentorial herniation occurs with bilateral compression through the tentorial notch: small pupils, increasing obtundation, and decorticate or decerebrate posturing are its findings. It is usually caused by bilateral subdural hematomas, but acute hydrocephalus may also give this appearance.

Tonsillar herniation is heralded by headache and ataxia, with sudden subsequent respiratory arrest. It is the most treacherous form of herniation, because a patient may be well one moment and moribund the next; it is caused by an expanding cerebellar mass.

LABORATORY AND OTHER DIAGNOSTIC TESTS
Radiologic Diagnosis

The CT scan has made an enormous difference in the management of head injury. In the acute injury, four patterns should be recognized by the physician: epidural hematoma, subdural hematoma, intracerebral hematoma, and contusion. All are best evaluated in an unenhanced scan. Magnetic resonance imaging (MRI) is less useful than CT in the acute head injury.

An epidural hematoma has a characteristic white lenticular shape adjacent to bone. It tends not to traverse sutures, as the dura is fixed at these sites. An associated skull fracture may be seen on bone windows. A *subdural hematoma* tracks over the entire convexity. There is often greater shift associated with it than the hematoma itself would suggest, because of its distribution over the entire hemisphere. An *intracerebral hematoma* is a high-absorption mass within parenchyma. Mass effect may not be associated with this injury initially. A *cerebral contusion* is a mottled pattern of high and low absorption representing both axonal shearing and hemorrhage. *Edema,* characterized by diffuse low absorption on CT, is also present after head injury in some patients. These patterns, especially in the acute phase, are much better seen on the CT than on the MRI, which may not demonstrate an acute hematoma.

On CT scans three brain regions are particularly treacherous in the acute stage. The first is the temporal fossa, where bony artifact may obscure an epidural hematoma. The second is the vertex of the brain; because CT sections pass transversely through brain tissue, a high subdural hematoma may be missed, and coronal scans may be necessary to detect it. The third is the posterior fossa, where bony artifact may obscure a hematoma; 4-mm sections may be necessary to achieve good resolution.

DIFFERENTIAL DIAGNOSIS

The diagnosis of acute head injury is usually straightforward. One problem is to establish whether a preexisting neurologic condition led to the head injury. Potential problems of this kind include aneurysm rupture with intracerebral hemorrhage, hypertensive intracerebral hemorrhage, and carotid occlusion or dissection.

Drug overdosage may make the head injury appear worse than it is. A toxic screen should be obtained if there is any question of drug usage.

MANAGEMENT
Severe Head Injury

Evaluation and management of acute severe head injury should proceed simultaneously. A history of the injury should be obtained as quickly as possible from ambulance drivers or other witnesses while initial neurologic evaluation is proceeding. This evaluation, as noted previously, should include the Glasgow Coma Scale, assessment of degree and level of injury, possible asymmetries in examination, and assessment of whether the patient's condition is worsening.

In the initial management, three steps are of paramount impor-

tance: first, ensuring that airway and ventilation are adequate; second, ensuring that there is no bleeding elsewhere that might lead to death during the neurologic evaluation; and third, excluding cervical spine injury.

A good rule for head injury management is to intubate in patients who will tolerate intubation, since considerable hypoxic brain damage may accompany an acute injury. Intubation should be nasotracheal if there is any cervical injury. Bleeding elsewhere can be excluded by chest film and physical examination, as well as by evaluation of the extremities. Cervical spine injury is best assessed by a lateral cervical spine film obtained portably in the emergency room.

In the triage of acute head injury, three levels can be distinguished: the first is the patient with a Glasgow Coma Scale of less than 8 who does not respond purposefully to commands. This patient requires immediate CT scanning. If this cannot be done expeditiously in the institution, the patient should be transferred to a larger center where CT scanning facilities and neurosurgical help are available. The second is the patient who is drowsy but is still following commands: this patient requires CT scanning to be performed within 4 to 6 hours; if the neurologic status is changing, immediate scanning is necessary. Third, patients who have evidence of a significant injury by history or examination but are now clinically well require observation for 12 to 24 hours or CT scanning.

Nonoperative management of patients with severe head injury includes support of ventilation and blood pressure, limitation of intravenous fluids, use of phenytoin or another anticonvulsant if there is a discrete mass, and intensive-care neurologic monitoring. An ICP monitor may be used—usually a fiberoptic catheter—which facilitates maintenance of cerebral perfusion pressure above 40 torr. Intracranial pressure ICP itself should be maintained below 20 torr. Methods used to decrease ICP include mannitol intravenously to keep osmolarity at 300 to 310 mOsm/L and hyperventilation to sustain partial pressure of carbon dioxide (PCO_2) at 30 to 35 mm Hg. Corticosteroids are of uncertain efficacy in posttraumatic edema, although they are used in many centers. The use of high-dose barbiturates has also diminished, as it may lead to increased incidence of a chronic vegetative state. However, pentobarbital in boluses, 50 mg intravenously to maintain ICP less than 25 mm Hg, may be a useful adjunct to keep ICP under control.

Chronic Sequelae of Head Injury

Several patterns should be recognized as sequelae of head injury. The first is global deterioration in an elderly patient, characterized by increasing memory loss, gait trouble, and slowing of activity. Even without an antecedent history of head injury, this presentation deserves CT scanning; chronic subdural hematoma and hydrocephalus are two head injury sequelae that may be found. A second pattern is loss of mental acuity and ambition in a young patient with a normal CT scan after mild head injury. This posttraumatic/postconcussive syndrome is very subtle but is increasingly being recognized. Seizure disorder and cerebrospinal fluid (CSF) leak may also be late sequelae of head injury; anticonvulsants are used by many centers for at least 6 months after injury.

For the patient with chronic head injury, management decisions are less emergent but are sometimes quite difficult. They include how long the patient should stay away from work or school and to what extent difficulties with work or school are a result of the head injury. There are few good guidelines for these decisions.

Minor Head Injury

A minor head injury can be defined as one with a Glasgow Coma Scale of 13 to 15. There are several recurring questions with such patients.

1. *Should a patient with a mild head injury be admitted for observation?* Patients who are feeling unwell following head injury require observation by a competent observer. Whether this is done in the hospital or in the home depends on the circumstances. A CT scan is an important initial step in anyone with symptoms after a head injury. Admission, in the author's opinion, is necessary if there is evidence of contusion on the CT scan, if the patient is

drowsy or confused at the time of examination, or if a fracture crosses a venous sinus. Children under age 5 years should also usually be admitted if they have been at all unresponsive. For other patients, observation at home may be adequate if another adult is continuously present and the patient has only signs of mild discomfort with a normal CT. A set of head injury instructions should be given to each patient.

2. *Should every patient with a head injury have skull films?* Obtundation, CSF leak, asymmetric neurologic findings, and an obvious depressed fracture are accepted guidelines for skull films. However, routine skull films are being used less and less, as CT scanning becomes more prevalent. Any patient who had a loss of consciousness and who is not feeling well should be given a CT scan.

3. *What should be done if a patient's condition is deteriorating?* In most institutions a CT scan can be obtained quickly enough that an emergency room burr hole is not indicated. Mannitol, 100 g, can be given intravenously during a brief sojourn at the CT scan for rapid-sequence examination of the temporal fossa or any other area where there is a contusion. However, if the patient's status is changing rapidly, with evidence of increasing hemiparesis, obtundation, and pupillary dilation, serious consideration must be given to emergency evacuation of a presumed epidural hematoma. This is best done in the operating room with a burr hole on the side with the dilating pupil, although in exceptional circumstances it may be necessary to proceed in the emergency room. Surgical help should be obtained for this.

Emergent Management of Specific Clinical Entities

Epidural hematomas are the most reversible intracranial hematomas. They usually occur in the temporal fossa from middle cerebral artery tears or in the posterior fossa from transverse sinus tears. In 75% to 90% of cases there is an associated fracture. The clinical presentation is often a transient loss of consciousness with recovery (the "lucid interval"), followed by increasing drowsiness, headache, weakness on the side of the body opposite the epidural hematoma, and pupillary dilation on the same side. Treatment is emergency evacuation of the clot; overall mortality is 15% to 43%.

Subdural hematomas are often associated with underlying brain contusions. They are more common after automobile injuries and may appear initially in patients with coma or as the herniation syndromes noted previously. Mortality is 35% to 50% despite CT scanning; younger patients have better outcomes, as do patients operated on within 3 hours of injury.

Intraparenchymal hematomas occur in 2% of severe injuries. They should be removed if there is more than a 1-cm associated CT shift or unless they are in an important area of brain, such as the speech or motor areas: mortality varies from 25% to 72%, depending primarily on the level of consciousness prior to surgery.

Missile wounds are generally treated by debridement of the missile track in the operating room. Deep fragments of bullet need not be removed.

Linear skull fractures require no treatment except observation for potential hematomas.

Depressed skull fractures should be elevated if the depression is deeper than the inner table of the skull; if there is an associated CSF leak; or if there is intracranial air on CT, which suggests a dural tear.

COMPLICATIONS

Acute head injury may be complicated by delayed intracerebral hematoma formation, increasing brain edema, or disseminated intravascular coagulation (DIC). A delayed cerebral hematoma is diagnosed by a high index of suspicion in the setting of cerebral contusion using sequential CT scans. It should be removed if it is symptomatic. Increasing brain edema is treated by steroids, mannitol, and lasix, DIC is treated with the help of a hematologist. Other complications include the following.

Posttraumatic epilepsy may be early (within 1 week) or delayed: early seizures occur in 2.5% to 7% of patients, delayed seizures in 7.1%. Prophylactic anticonvulsants may diminish the incidence of

✔ **WHEN TO REFER**

Patients with an abnormal CT scan, with a normal CT scan but incapacitating symptoms, or with external signs of trauma, especially a laceration or CSF leak, should be referred to a neurosurgeon. In the posttraumatic period patients with the syndromes noted earlier should be referred.

later seizures. Parenchymal hemorrhage or dural lacerations appear to be associated with a greater likelihood of late seizures.

Posttraumatic hydrocephalus mainly results from subarachnoid hemorrhage at the time of injury but may also be contributed to by shearing of white matter fibers and subsequent dilation *ex vacuo*. There is progressive enlargement of ventricles, along with gait disturbances, memory difficulty, and urinary incontinence. Shunting may help; however, distinguishing patients in whom shunts are not helpful is sometimes quite difficult with posttraumatic syndrome.

Chronic subdural hematoma is an important and sometimes overlooked sequela of even minor injury in the elderly. The hematoma increases in size by continued oozing of blood from subdural membranes. Surgical evacuation is necessary, often by drainage.

Posttraumatic syndrome is a poorly characterized condition marked by loss of concentration, memory difficulty, headache, and difficulty with work. Over 50% of patients with minor head injury have one or more of these complications 3 months after injury. Psychometric tests may help in the evaluation. There is no specific treatment at present, but there is increasing recognition of this important problem.

BIBLIOGRAPHY

Becker DP et al: The outcome from severe head injury with early diagnosis and intensive management, *J Neurosurg* 47:491, 1977.
Gennarelli TA, Timbault LE: Biomechanics of head injury. In Wilkins RH, Rengachary SS, editors: *Neurosurgery,* New York, 1995, McGraw-Hill.
Rimel RW et al: Disability caused by minor head injury, *Neurosurgery* 9:221, 1981.
Seeling JM et al: Traumatic acute subdural hematoma: major mortality reductions in comatose patients treated within 4 hours, *N Engl J Med* 304:1511, 1981. $msp;1

CHAPTER

156 Spinal Cord Injury

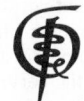

Paul A. Gutierrez and Robert R. Young

Until the middle of this century, spinal cord injury (SCI) was considered a malady with little hope for successful treatment. The oldest known description of the symptoms of spinal cord injury was recorded 5000 years ago in what has become known as the Edwin Smith Surgical Papyrus. Hippocrates described the complications of chronic paraplegia, including pressure sores, disorders of bowel motility, urinary tract infections, and lower extremity dependent edema. Galen introduced the concept of surgical treatment for spinal cord injuries, but it would be centuries before surgical interventions, antibiotic therapies, and comprehensive rehabilitation programs made significant impacts on outcome of patients with spinal cord injuries.

Ernest Bors, Sir Ludwig Guttman, and Donald Munro were leaders in the development of specialized centers dedicated to the care and rehabilitation of patients with spinal cord injuries. They demonstrated that these patients could be successfully managed and could return to the community as productive, contributing members of society. The modern era of treatment of persons with spinal cord injuries began with the development of special spinal injury centers during World War II. Sir Ludwig Guttman, a neurosurgeon, was responsible for the National Spinal Injuries Centre at the Ministry of Pensions Hospital, Stoke Mandeville, Aylesbury, England. Ernest Bors, a urologist, was a key figure in the development of Veterans Administration specialized Spinal Cord Injury Centers in the United States. Donald Munro, a neurosurgeon at Boston City Hospital, pioneered the use of tidal drainage for initial management of the paralyzed bladder. The advent of antibiotic therapy and rational management of the neurogenic bladder have significantly decreased mortality from urosepsis, which was previously the major cause of death in these patients.

It is now well established that, with an organized and comprehensive management plan, most spinal cord–injured patients can be successfully returned to a functional status as valuable, productive members of society. This plan must include rapid identification of the degree of neurologic impairment and protection of the spinal cord from further primary damage or from secondary damage. In addition, early treatment of associated injuries to other parts of the body should be a top priority. Once the patient's other injuries have been stabilized, a comprehensive neurorehabilitation program must be started to enhance the return of function and reduce the incidence of secondary complications.

An important concept to remember is that much of what follows in this chapter is applicable to the management of spinal cord impairment produced by nontraumatic disorders. These include cord infarction (caused by atherosclerosis, hypotensive episodes, dural arteriovenous malformations, or surgery for abdominal aortic aneurysm), cord compression from tumor or abscess, Foix-Alajouanine syndrome, multiple sclerosis, and the end-stage degenerative diseases and amyotrophic lateral sclerosis. The management of spinal cord injury or impairment constitutes a particularly well-developed area within neurologic rehabilitation and provides us with paradigms for similar approaches to patients with other neurologic impairments.

EPIDEMIOLOGY

Spinal cord injury predominantly affects males, who constitute 85% to 90% of the patients. Most are single and young; 60% of injuries occur in individuals between the ages of 16 and 30 years.

The incidence of spinal cord injuries in the United States is estimated at 8000 to 10,000 new cases annually. These are roughly equally distributed between incomplete tetraplegics, complete tetraplegics, incomplete paraplegics, and complete paraplegics. There is an increased incidence of spinal cord injury in the summer months, in the early hours of the morning, and on weekends; alcohol and drug use are frequently involved. Causes include motor vehicle accidents (50%), falls (20%), sports (15%), and violence (15%). Approximately two thirds of sports-related spinal cord injuries occur in diving accidents. Two particularly common causes are motor vehicle accidents in 16- to 30-year-olds and falls in 61- to 75-year-olds.

Most spine injuries occur at levels where there is relatively increased mobility. The midcervical region and the thoracolumbar junction are the sites in the spine with the greatest mobility, in contrast to the thoracic spine, which is stabilized by the rib cage. In the cervical region, movement of the relatively massive head produces large forces that are apt to cause fractures during rapid deceleration such as occurs with motor vehicle and diving accidents and falls. The pelvic girdle and legs inferiorly and the thorax superiorly act as large masses producing stress at the thoracolumbar junction during deceleration.

Spinal cord injuries rarely occur in isolation. Associated trauma includes head injuries, closed or open, in 15% of patients. Limb fractures are seen in approximately 10% of patients with acute spinal cord injuries, with fractures of some portion of the trunk in about 20% and significant chest or thoracic injuries in 15%. Associated operations after an acute spinal cord injury include spinal fusion in 35%, halo traction in 20%, open reduction of fractures in 20%, and tracheotomy in 10%.

CLASSIFICATION

Spinal cord injuries can be classified according to anatomic or functional schemes. The skeletal level of injury (SLI), determined by radiologic examination, is named after the vertebra with the greatest

---

BOX 156-1
Key muscles determining motor level

C1-4	Diaphragm
C5	Elbow flexors (biceps)
C6	Wrist extensors
C7	Elbow extensors (triceps)
C8	Finger flexors, distal phalanx
T1	Hand intrinsics (interossei)
T2-L1	Use sensory level and Beevor's sign
L2	Hip flexors (iliopsoas)
L3	Knee extensors (quadriceps)
L4	Ankle dorsiflexors (tibialis anterior)
L5	Long toe extensors (extensor hallucis longus)
S1	Ankle plantar flexors (gastrocnemius)
S2-5	Use sensory level and sphincter ani

BOX 156-2
Key areas determining sensory level

C2	Occipital protuberance
C3	Supraclavicular fossa
C4	Top of the acromioclavicular joint
C5	Lateral side of the antecubital fossa
C6	Thumb
C7	Middle finger
C8	Little finger
T1	Medial side of the antecubital fossa
T2	Apex of the axilla
T3	Third intercostal space
T4	Fourth intercostal space, nipple line
T5	Fifth intercostal space
T6	Sixth intercostal space, xiphisternum
T7-9	Intercostal spaces
T10	Umbilicus
T11	Intercostal space
T12	Inguinal ligament
L1	Upper anterior thigh
L2	Midanterior thigh
L3	Medial femoral condyle
L4	Medial malleolus
L5	Dorsum of the foot at the third metatarsophalangeal joint
S1	Lateral heel
S2	Popliteal fossa in the midline
S3	Ischial tuberosity
S4-5	Perianal area

---

damage or the two adjacent vertebrae with the greatest damage. This is often referred to as the *motion segment.*

The neurologic level of injury (NLI) is determined by the neurologic examination. The NLI is defined as the most caudal segment with good motor and sensory function. The motor level of injury should be determined independently from the sensory level of injury on each side of the body. Good motor function is defined by the most caudal myotome with at least enough power to overcome gravity, a grade of 3 of 5, as follows: 0 of 5, no movement; 1 of 5, only trace movement; 2 of 5, movement through full range with gravity eliminated; 3 of 5, movement through full range against gravity; 4 of 5, movement through full range against some resistance; 5 of 5, normal power. Key muscles used to determine the motor level for classification are listed in Box 156-1. Normal sensory function is determined according to dermatomal testing. Key sensory areas recommended for testing the dermatomes are listed in Box 156-2 and shown in Fig. 156-1.

When the most caudal segments with good function are the same on both sides of the body, the NLI may be identified as one segment.

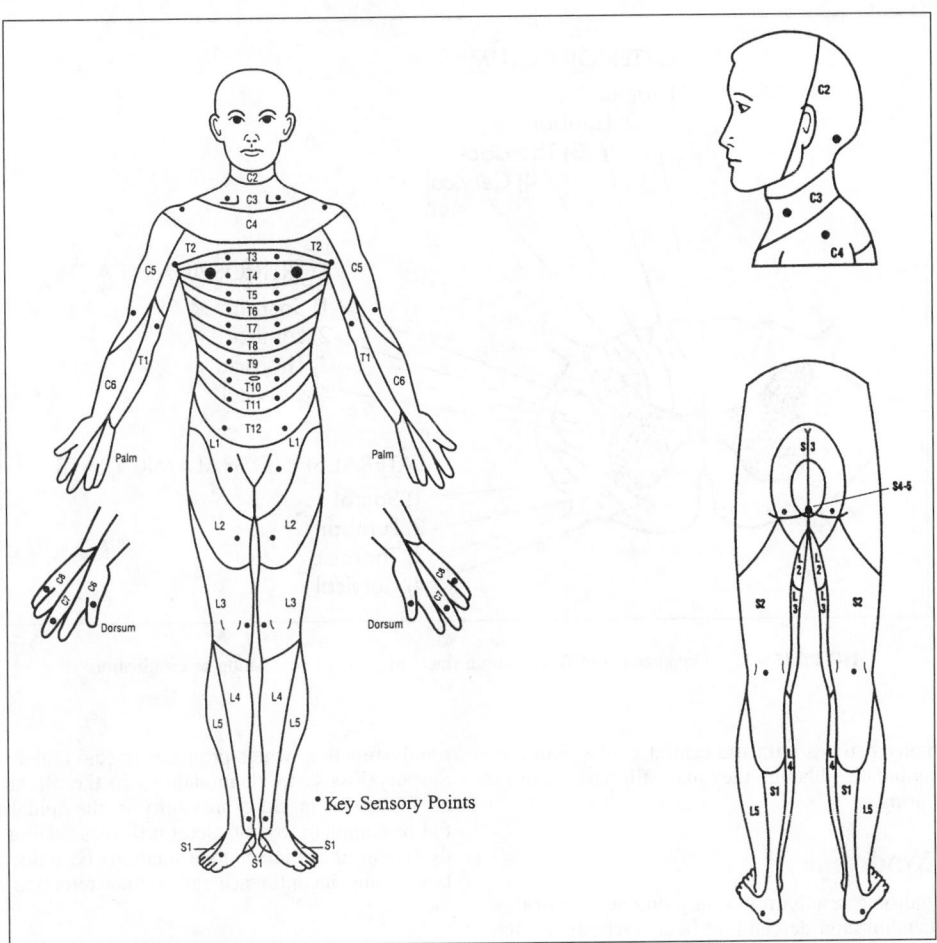

FIGURE 156-1   Areas to test in determining sensory level of injury.

From Maynard FM, editor: *International standards for neurological and functional classification of spinal cord injury,* Chicago, 1996, American Spinal Injury Association.

When they are different, each side's NLI should be described independently. The zone of partial preservation (ZPP) is the region of the cord immediately below the NLI with some remaining sensation or motor function. If it includes up to three consecutive segments caudal to the NLI, the injury is still considered complete. If any nonreflex neurologic function is found below the ZPP, the injury is considered incomplete.

The Frankel classification system describes the degree of preservation of function below the NLI. Frankel A lesions are complete, with no preservation of motor or sensory function below the ZPP. Frankel B lesions are incomplete but with only preserved sensation below the ZPP. Frankel C lesions are those with preserved but useless voluntary motor function below the ZPP. Frankel D lesions are those with preserved, useful, voluntary motor function below the ZPP. This is defined as preserved voluntary motor ability below the NLI with most of the key muscles having at least grade 3 power. Frankel E denotes return of normal motor and sensory function, although reflexes may remain abnormal.

The Frankel classification system can be used as a prognostic indicator for functional recovery. This makes it imperative that a careful, complete neurologic evaluation be made as soon as possible after a spinal injury. Of all patients with spine fractures from C1 to S5, 50% arrive at the hospital as Frankel A, 10% as Frankel B, 10% as Frankel C, and 30% as Frankel D. Of all patients who arrive as Frankel A, 94% are still Frankel A (complete lesions) on discharge from the hospital,

despite all therapeutic efforts. The remaining 6% are Frankel B (50%) or Frankel C or D. None have complete recovery. Of patients who arrive as Frankel B, 62% are unchanged at the time of discharge. Fifty percent of those who come to medical attention with Frankel C injuries and 94% of those who arrive at the hospital with Frankel D injuries are unchanged or improved at the time of discharge.

SPINAL CORD INJURY SYNDROMES
Central Cord Syndrome

Incomplete spinal cord injuries can be further classified into clinical syndromes based on the anatomic location of damage within the cord. The central cord syndrome is seen most commonly with hyperextension injuries of the cervical spine. This syndrome is particularly common in the elderly and in individuals with congenital or acquired cervical stenosis. As a result of the trauma, they develop hemorrhagic necrosis of the central gray matter and the more medial white matter. With the central cord syndrome, patients have greater weakness in the arms than the legs. Thus the term "upside-down tetraplegia" is used to describe the physical findings. On anatomic study this can be explained by the fact that the corticospinal and spinothalamic tracts are organized such that the sacral fibers are more lateral and the cervical fibers are more medial (Fig. 156-2). The more caudal fibers are protected from central cord necrosis and have a greater chance of surviving damage in this type of cervical cord injury. The significance

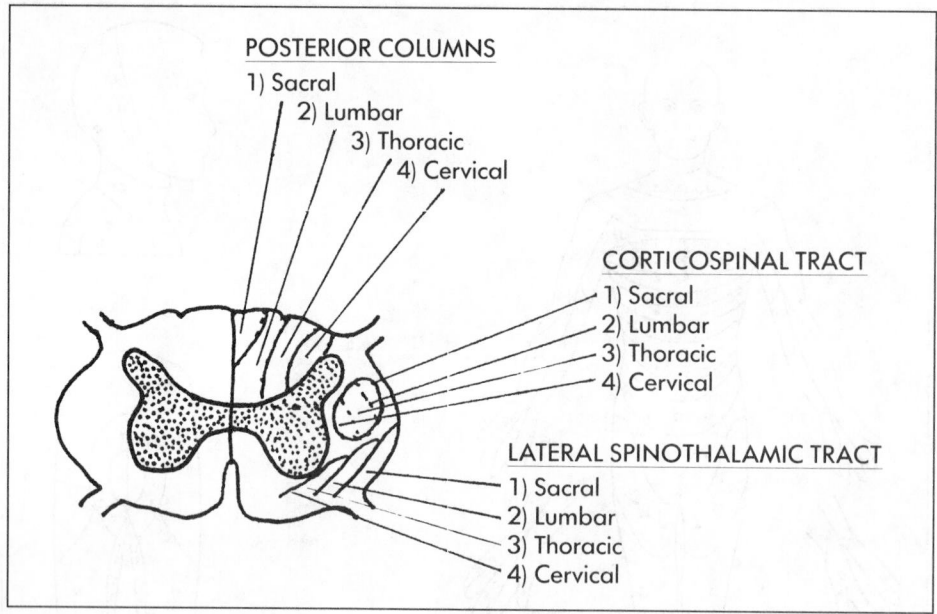

FIGURE 156-2.   Organization of fibers within tracts by level of origination or termination.

of these facts is that many patients with the central cord syndrome are eventually able to ambulate, although they may still have significant weakness in their arms.

Brown-Séquard Syndrome

The Brown-Séquard syndrome results from injury on one side of the cord that interrupts ascending and descending fiber tracts. It results in ipsilateral motor weakness, loss of fine touch and position sense, and contralateral sensory deficits in pain and temperature. At the NLI there is also ipsilateral flaccid weakness and anesthesia caused by damage to the nerve roots and motor and sensory neurons in that area. This syndrome can result from any spinal injury but is more common with penetrating injuries and asymmetric herniations of the nucleus pulposus. A pure Brown-Séquard syndrome is rare; usually one finds the two major features to be predominantly ipsilateral spastic weakness and contralateral loss of pain and temperature sensation.

Anterior Cord Syndrome

The anterior cord syndrome is rare in its pure form. It may be seen with flexion injuries, acute central herniations of the nucleus pulposus, and some vascular insults to the spinal cord. The regions of the cord involved are those supplied by the anterior spinal artery. The areas spared include the posterior columns and dorsal horns. Thus below the level of injury there is weakness and loss of pain and temperature sensation.

Posterior Column Syndrome

The posterior column syndrome is the rarest syndrome in its pure form. It has been associated with hyperextension injuries. The clinical manifestations are those of loss of posterior column function: vibratory and fine touch sensations and proprioception. Power and gross sensation are preserved, so these patients have a chance for useful functional recovery after rehabilitation.

Cauda Equina and Conus Medullaris Syndrome

The cauda equina syndrome results from low-level spine injuries, those at or below the thoracolumbar junction. This differs from the other syndromes mentioned earlier, since there is no intact caudal spinal cord and the damage is primarily to spinal nerve roots and perhaps the conus. Loss of motor power results from lower motor neu-

ron dysfunction, which produces flaccid rather than spastic weakness. Sensory loss is to all modalities in the affected dermatomes, since all fibers run in close proximity in the spinal nerves. There is partial or complete loss of sacral reflexes, leading to bladder and bowel dysfunction. Sphincter tone tends to be reduced in the bladder and bowel, and incontinence rather than retention of urine and feces is the rule.

Immediate Management of Spinal Cord Injury

In the last decade the eventual outcome from spinal trauma has improved significantly. A major emphasis has been placed on spine stabilization in the field to prevent further neurologic injury during transport to the trauma center. This has involved well-trained emergency medical technicians and paramedics and has resulted in a shift from the majority of injuries being complete (Frankel A) to incomplete (Frankel B to E) lesions. At the accident scene the priorities remain the ABCs (airway, breathing, and circulation), but spinal column stabilization on a spine board or splint is the next greatest priority. More sophisticated stretchers have been developed, including some that can be used during x-ray and other imaging studies. Intravenous fluids should be administered, and transport in Trendelenburg's position may decrease the risk of shock and aspiration.

On arrival at the hospital, a reassessment of the patient should include a brief history, physical examination, and neurologic evaluation. Spinal column immobilization and cardiopulmonary stabilization must be maintained. The latter must emphasize prevention of hypoxia and hypotension. A Foley catheter should be inserted into the bladder, and urinalysis performed to look for hematuria. Sources of internal bleeding in the abdomen, chest, and pelvis must be identified and treated. The National Acute Spinal Cord Injury Study II (NASCI II) demonstrated that intravenous megadose methylprednisolone therapy that is instituted within 8 hours of the initial injury decreases the neurologic deficits resulting from spinal cord injury. The dose used in that study was an initial bolus of 30 mg/kg body weight, followed by a continuous intravenous infusion of 5.4 mg/kg per hour over the next 23 hours. Patients receiving that therapy had statistically significant improvement in recovery of motor and sensory function at 6-month follow-up compared with those given placebo or naloxone. It should be emphasized, however, that this treatment has not been shown to produce dramatic functional recovery and should not replace surgical decompression if that is indicated by radiologic examination.

Patients with cervical spinal cord injuries often have bradycardia caused by the unopposed action of the parasympathetic nervous system on the heart. Parasympathetic inputs to the heart are from the vagus nerve, which reaches this organ via an extraspinal pathway. It is rarely damaged in cervical spine trauma, whereas sympathetic function may be impaired. The vagal outflow can be increased by tracheal suction, which may lead to serious bradycardia or even asystole with sudden death. Therefore in patients the lungs should be fully oxygenated before secretions are suctioned. Atropine should be readily available in the event of a sudden bradycardic episode or cardiac arrest. In addition, patients with head injuries as well as those with spinal cord injuries can have loss of autoregulation of cerebral blood flow for weeks or several months after the initial trauma. In the early stages this can lead to or extend ischemic injuries in the cord or cerebrum should hypotension occur.

Once the patient's cardiovascular status is stable, radiographic evaluation should be performed. Continued caution is needed to prevent further neurologic injury. Fractures of the cervicothoracic junction, thoracic spine, and thoracolumbar junction can easily be missed unless roentgenograms, including computed tomography (CT) scans, of these regions are obtained. The highest level of neurologic injury may mask a second, lower level of injury on a clinical but not on a radiologic examination. If there is no radiographic evidence of compression of neural elements or spinal column instability, management should be medical in the intensive care unit. When there is recognition of mechanical neural compression or stretch in patients with *incomplete* injuries, this should be relieved as soon as possible by restoring spinal alignment, removing bony or disk fragments or blood from the neural canal, or providing spinal stability by the appropriate technique. In patients who present with *complete* (Frankel A) injuries, emergency decompression or stabilization is not warranted, since recovery of useful neurologic function in such patients is virtually nil, even with surgery. Spinal alignment in cervical spine fractures is best restored through spinal traction. This may require application of hardware such as Garner-Wells tongs by a surgical trauma team and placement of the patient on a fracture bed or frame. Closed reduction can then be achieved by the application of weights. Careful monitoring of the neurologic examination and serial radiographs are essential to avoid overdistraction. Traction is generally not effective in lower level fractures.

Surgical management of spinal cord injury may be necessary when closed reduction cannot be achieved (some fracture dislocations), when decompression of the spinal cord from bone fragments or blood is needed (some burst fractures), or for definitive stabilization of any unstable fracture of the spine. Many of these last injuries would eventually heal with bed rest, but surgical stabilization permits the patient to be out of bed sooner, thus accelerating the rehabilitation process. Again, it must be emphasized that timing of any surgical procedure depends on findings on the neurologic examination. Acute surgery is not indicated for patients with complete (Frankel A) spinal cord injuries. In patients with incomplete injuries, including sacral sparing, stabilization may be anterior, posterior, or both, depending on the site and type of fracture. Bone grafts, metal plates or rods, or wires can be used; a discussion of the type of surgery for a given injury is beyond the scope of this chapter. It is essential to remember that spinal fusion does not provide immediate, complete stabilization, and care should be taken to avoid destabilization when the patient is moved after surgery. It may take 12 to 24 weeks for bony fusion to mature, and during this time the patient needs to be protected with external bracing such as a halo device, rigid collar, or thoracolumbar jacket.

SUBACUTE MANAGEMENT OF SPINAL CORD INJURY
Cardiovascular System

Homeostasis is interrupted by a spinal cord lesion; therefore once immediate stabilization of the patient is achieved it is essential that the care team address multiple other systems affected by the altered nervous system function. As previously mentioned, the cardiovascular system is compromised in its ability to regulate blood pressure. Hypotension may be particularly prominent after meals. This results from increased blood volume in the splanchnic bed, secretion of intestinal vasoactive peptides, and vasodilation caused by insulin release. These patients should be raised to a sitting position slowly and may require ephedrine to maintain adequate blood pressure. Eventually the renin-angiotensin system usually compensates for loss of autonomic nervous system control. Patients may maintain a greater intravascular volume and better orthostatic blood pressure if they do not lie absolutely horizontal; the bed may need to be tilted in the head-up position. Angiotensin-converting enzyme (ACE) inhibitors are usually not well tolerated in the treatment of hypertension in chronic spinal cord injury patients.

Peripheral cardiovascular consequences of spinal cord injury include potentially life-threatening deep venous thrombosis (DVT). In the first few weeks, patients with spinal cord injury are especially susceptible to DVT as a result of immobilization, lack of muscle tone, and altered vascular tone. Subcutaneous heparin, pneumatic stockings, or almost continuous electrical stimulation of the calves can help prevent development of DVT and its most dangerous consequence, pulmonary embolism. Once an acutely injured patient is able to get out of bed and into a wheelchair, the risk of DVT begins to diminish. In patients with chronic spinal cord injury, arterial atrophy and distal ischemia, especially in the legs, may lead to the need for amputations. Tetraplegics have difficulty with thermoregulation because of altered peripheral vascular control. They have lost normal mechanisms to prevent hypothermia (such as cutaneous vasoconstriction and shivering) or hyperthermia (vasodilation and sweating).

Autonomic dysreflexia, a condition equivalent to "spasticity" of the sympathetic nervous system, should be treated as a life-threatening emergency. It is generally seen in patients with neurologic levels of injury at T6 and higher because most of the spinal sympathetic system is below this level. It results from massive discharge of a relatively intact sympathetic nervous system triggered reflexly by a noxious stimulus below the level of injury, most commonly urinary bladder distention but possibly fecal impaction, skin lesions, or any noxious stimulus that would produce discomfort if its effects could reach the cerebrum. Because of the spinal cord injury, the sympathetic outflow, once begun, cannot be turned off by descending outflow from higher brain centers. Blood pressure rises dramatically, and bradycardia is common, in contrast to most other causes of hypertension. The patient has a pounding headache, piloerection and sweating below the NLI, nasal congestion, flushing, or even simple malaise (one cause of the "feel-terrible syndrome"). Although severe hypertension is the most dangerous of the consequences of dysreflexia (because of the risk of intracerebral hemorrhage), it can be missed if the patient is not examined early in the course of an episode. Sometimes reactive hypotension occurs if the noxious stimulus is removed before the blood pressure is taken.

The most important immediate management for autonomic dysreflexia involves removing the source of the noxious stimulus. The patient should be sat up in bed to help decrease intracerebral pressure, and the urinary bladder should be drained. Topical anesthetic jelly can be used for catheterization, and the bladder can be irrigated with topical anesthetic. If this does not relieve the symptoms or control the blood pressure, the rectum should be checked for fecal impaction after topical anesthetic jelly is applied. If these measures fail to bring the blood pressure down within a few minutes, nifedipine should be given. A 10-mg capsule should be bitten and swallowed by the patient. This dose of nifedipine can be repeated in 15 minutes if needed. As an alternative, hydralazine, 5 mg, can be given intravenously and repeated every 5 to 10 minutes as necessary, but the total dose should not exceed 20 mg. Blood pressure should then be monitored every 5 minutes until it is back to normal and then every 30 minutes for 4 hours. Should the hypertension prove to be refractory to the previously described measures, the patient should be transferred to an intensive care unit for more definitive treatment including intravenous hypotensive agents and, if all else fails, spinal anesthesia.

Respiratory System

The respiratory system is compromised to varying degrees in almost all patients with spinal cord injury, depending on the NLI. Injuries at or above C4 can paralyze the phrenic nerves and compromise function of the diaphragm and other muscles responsible for inhalation. This may result in ventilator dependence, although the patient may be able to compensate during short periods by using accessory muscles in the neck. The ventilator must be adjusted, not only to produce physiologic levels of partial pressure of oxygen (PO_2) and partial pressure of carbon dioxide (PCO_2) but also to avoid prolonged increased intrathoracic pressure, which would reduce venous return to the heart. Spinal cord–injured patients also have compromise of the thoracic and abdominal muscles of exhalation, which results in a poor cough. This, along with the production of abnormally viscous mucous, makes spinal cord patients particularly susceptible to mucous plugging, atelectasis, and pneumonia. Patients with high-level lesions are also at great risk for aspiration.

Gastrointestinal System

Gastrointestinal tract manifestations of spinal cord injury are predominantly those of hypomotility. Gastric hypomotility can lead to nausea, dyspepsia, and reflux, with eventual esophagitis and aspiration pneumonitis. Stress gastritis and upper gastrointestinal tract hemorrhage are additional problems, especially early after the injury. Gallstones develop frequently, even in young men, perhaps as a result of gallbladder hypomotility and hypercalcemia. Colonic hypomotility and anal sphincter spasticity lead to chronic constipation and megacolon. Patients must be placed on a bowel training program with digital rectal stimulation performed every other day to help promote regular evacuation of the bowel. Stool softeners and dietary fiber supplements can be helpful in avoiding fecal impaction. Suppositories and enemas should be avoided if possible. Hemorrhoids, anal fissures, and fistulas may further complicate the care of spinal cord–injured patients.

Genitourinary System

Genitourinary tract complications of spinal cord injury were once a major factor in the early demise of these patients. Although great advancements have been made in urologic management and antibiotic therapy, renal failure is still an important cause of morbidity and mortality. The primary goal in management of the urinary system is to maintain renal function. Once the new patient's condition has been stabilized, initiation of intermittent catheterization is a major priority. Prolonged management with an indwelling catheter can lead to refractory urinary tract infections, bladder stones, neoplasms, and in males, urethritis and epididymitis. Intermittent catheterization can be started at intervals of 4 to 6 hours, depending on fluid intake. The frequency of catheterization can then be adjusted to allow the accumulation of no more than 300 to 350 ml of urine at a time. The achievement of a "balanced bladder" is the goal, which is defined as a bladder with sufficient capacity to store urine reliably and the ability to empty sufficiently without excessively high pressure or vesicoureteral reflux.

Spontaneous voiding develops in many patients after the initial period of spinal shock. Urodynamic studies to assess intravesicular pressures should be made on all patients. Those who are voiding should have a simultaneous uroflow and electromyogram (EMG) of the external sphincter. The findings of increased EMG activity and excessive intravesicular pressure with decreased flow suggest that there is detrusor-sphincter dyssynergia. This occurs when there is simultaneous contraction of the detrusor muscle (which decreases the size of the bladder) and external sphincter (which obstructs outflow through the urethra). It occurs most commonly in patients with suprasacral injuries and is accompanied by bladder hyperreflexia. These patients tend to have urinary retention, and vesicoureteral reflux of varying degrees can develop. If the bladder pressure is less than 60 to 70 cm H_2O and the residual urine is less than 75 ml, spontaneous or stimulated voiding can be used. Otherwise, action must be taken to lower bladder pressure and residual volume. In patients with outflow obstruction resulting from dyssynergia the external sphincter can sometimes be successfully relaxed with alpha sympatholytics such as phentolamine, phenoxybenzamine, or prazosin. Transurethral external sphincterotomy can also be used to relieve the obstruction. In addition, some patients require transurethral resection of the prostate and bladder neck. An external urine collection device can be used for incontinent in men, and high-absorbency pads can be used by women. Patients with hyperreflexia and high intravesicular pressures can

sometimes be managed with detrusor-relaxing agents such as oxybutynin or propantheline and intermittent catheterization.

Patients with areflexic bladders who are unable to empty the bladder by abdominal straining should be managed with intermittent catheterization. Areflexic bladders are most commonly seen in patients with low-level paraplegia or those with the cauda equina syndrome. They should be instructed in the methods of clean intermittent self-catheterization and urinary acidification. Fluid intake should be regulated to avoid rapid filling of the bladder so that a regular schedule of self-catheterization can be followed. Some patients are unable or unwilling to perform self-catheterization. In patients with hyperreflexic bladders, sometimes the bladder can be stimulated to empty reflexively by tapping the suprapubic region, stimulating the anal sphincter, or by pulling the pubic hair. Every possible effort should be made to avoid using a chronic indwelling catheter because of the long-term complications mentioned previously.

Urinary tract infections are a common problem in spinal cord–injured patients. In general, prophylactic antibiotics have not proven to be useful in either catheter-free or catheter-dependent individuals. Most patients have bacteriuria, but this should be considered only colonization of the urine, not a tissue infection. Bacteriuria should not be treated unless there is significant pyuria (at least 50 white blood cells per high-power field) or other symptoms such as fever, bladder spasms, and malaise.

Bladder and renal calculi are another important long-term complication of spinal cord injury. Bladder calculi are usually infected and can cause severe irritation to the bladder. If detected early, they can sometimes be flushed out through a catheter. Larger stones can be crushed during cystoscopy or with transurethral electrohydraulic lithotripsy. Renal calculi are most common in the first year after injury. Calcified stones are common because impaired mobility leads to bone resorption, hypercalcemia, and hypercalciuria. Struvite stones also occur much more frequently than in the general population. In fact, up to 98% of stones in patients with spinal cord injury include struvite in their composition, whereas only 15% of stones in the general population have struvite. Struvite stones are frequently infected with urease-producing bacteria, which cause chronic urinary tract infections. Also, urease-producing bacteria release ammonia, which alkalinizes the urine and promotes stone formation in the kidneys and urinary tract.

Sexual dysfunction is another major source of concern for spinal cord–injured patients. Approximately two thirds of male patients regain some erectile function within 6 months of injury, but only 10% ejaculate normally. Sexual function depends on the level and completeness of the neurologic injury. Patients with suprasacral lesions can have reflexively induced erections, but those with complete lesions cannot have psychologically induced erections. Patients with conus or cauda equina injuries are less likely to have any erections, but some with incomplete lesions may have only psychogenic erections. Electroejaculation, vacuum tumescence, injection of prostaglandins or other medications into the penis, and vibratory stimulation are methods that have been developed to aid in the generation of erection and ejaculation. Those with retrograde ejaculations who desire to have children can have the ejaculate retrieved from the bladder.

Musculoskeletal System

Bone demineralization occurs rapidly and irreversibly after spinal cord injury. The elimination of gravitational load or stress of bone caused by immobilization is probably the major cause. The resultant hypercalcemia and hyperphosphatemia may lead to nausea and vomiting in the first few weeks after spinal cord injury. Inactivity may also lead to rapid muscle atrophy below the neurologic level of injury, even if lower motor neurons remain intact. Eventually demineralization leads to fragility and an increased tendency for fractures of long bones and compression fractures of vertebral bodies. Any fall or trauma should be considered a potential cause of fractures, and radiographs may be necessary, despite lack of pain or immediate swelling. A more comprehensive review of this subject is cited in the bibliography.

Heterotopic ossification (HO) is bone formation in abnormal locations, most commonly around the hips and knees after spinal cord injury. The clinical presentation varies, and it can be asymptomatic.

Heterotopic ossification may become evident as swelling around the joint or decreased range of motion. It can also cause distal extremity swelling as a result of vascular compression and in this presentation must be distinguished from DVT. Diagnosis is usually possible with plain radiographs, but radionuclide triphasic bone scans may be necessary early in the development of HO. Etidronate disodium (Didronel) is the treatment of choice with an initial dose of 20 mg/kg per day for 2 weeks followed by 10 mg/kg per day for 10 weeks. If gastrointestinal tract side effects such as diarrhea occur, the dosage can be divided. For more severe cases the treatment can be continued up to 6 months. Surgical removal of HO should not be undertaken until nuclide scans show that it is no longer active (i.e., bone is no longer being formed).

Integumentary System

Skin integrity can be difficult to maintain in any immobilized or paralyzed patient. A pressure sore is an area of skin that has become necrotic because unrelieved pressure causes ischemia and mechanical damage. This occurs most commonly over a bony prominence such as the ischium, greater trochanter, or heel or in the sacrococcygeal region. Other factors that can contribute to the development of pressure sores include fecal and urinary incontinence, friction, shear forces, elevated body temperature, sepsis, accumulation of metabolic waste products, altered lymph drainage, hypoalbuminemia, advanced age of the patient, and fractures. Persons with normal sensation and mobility subconsciously detect prolonged pressure in tissues and periodically shift their position to relieve this pressure. Patients with impaired sensation and mobility must consciously move or rely on others to move them to relieve pressure on skin and subcutaneous structures.

Prevention of pressure sores should be given a high priority for spinal cord–injured patients. The goal can best be met if the patient can be regularly turned in bed at least every 2 hours without generating excessive shear forces. In addition, many cushions and beds have been designed to spread out pressure over as great an area as possible. Flotation beds of various types (air, water, or silicon beads and air) have generally proven to be the most useful. Wheelchair cushions with cutouts to relieve pressure in one area must be carefully designed to avoid causing excessive shear forces in surrounding skin. Controlling flexor spasms with medications or nerve blocks can also help prevent sores resulting from friction. In addition, patients can be trained in methods to provide pressure relief in their chairs every 20 to 30 minutes.

Treatment of pressure sores can involve surgery or more conservative approaches. In general, local therapy of wounds should include removal of pressure and regular debridement of necrotic tissue, control of infection, and promotion of epithelialization. Traditionally, gauze soaked with Dakin's solution, sterile saline, hydrogen peroxide, or silver nitrate has been used to pack the wound in a wet-to-dry manner. As the dried dressings are removed, debridement takes place. It is now generally accepted that drainage from wounds should be absorbed with hydroactive dressings and granules. Hyperbaric oxygen treatments have been used to promote wound healing and decrease recovery time. Promising new approaches such as the use of calcium alginate preparations are currently under study. Another innovative approach to the treatment of pressure sores has been the reintroduction of maggot-debridement therapy, which had previously fallen out of favor with those treating pressure sores in this country. It is promising in that sterile maggots can be used safely in debridement of dirty wounds in fragile patients to promote epithelialization of those wounds.

Surgical therapy can include split-thickness skin grafts over a well-granulated superficial wound. Larger, deeper sores may need to be excised and underlying bony prominences reduced, with the wound then being closed with a myocutaneous flap, the muscles serving as padding. After surgery, pressure must be kept off the wound, so the patient should be placed in a flotation bed.

Nervous System

Initially after spinal cord trauma, there may be a period during which there appears to be no function in any portion of the caudal spinal cord. This period of areflexia and flaccid paralysis has been termed *spinal shock* and may last for a few weeks. Eventually, however, function begins to return to the areas of the cord not directly damaged in the trauma. First is the bulbocavernosus reflex, which returns almost immediately, followed by deep-tendon reflex activity. This is followed shortly by enhancement of sacral parasympathetics and the strengthening of anal and bladder sphincter reflexes. Primitive withdrawal responses from noxious stimuli such as an extensor plantar response or a triple flexion response in the leg may then soon appear. Exaggerated flexor spasms can be seen in response to tactile stimuli. An extreme "mass response" may involve bilateral flexion at the knee and flexion and adduction at the hip. Abdominal contractions may result in evacuation of the bowel and bladder. Reflex diaphoresis may also be seen.

Spasticity after spinal cord injury is a result of loss of descending inhibitory input from motor systems that normally control and coordinate movement and muscle activity. Below the neurologic level of injury, segmental reflex arcs remain intact so that sensory inputs can still trigger motor and autonomic outflow. Spasticity can interfere with functional activities, personal care, and positioning and can cause discomfort for the patient. It can sometimes be controlled with range-of-motion exercises, which stretch muscles. Spasticity can be exacerbated by a noxious stimulus such as a urinary tract infection, pressure sore, fecal impaction, or other intraabdominal process; it may improve when these conditions are treated.

Pharmacologic control of spasticity should be instituted with specific treatment goals defined; for example, paresis or inability to use the upper limb is rarely improved. These goals would include a noticeable increase in a few restricted functional abilities, a decrease in the need for intensive nursing care, or relief of pain and discomfort. Baclofen is generally considered the medication of choice because of its effectiveness and relatively low incidence of adverse reactions. It is thought to be an agonist of the inhibitory neurotransmitter gamma-aminobutyric acid (GABA). Baclofen's primary site of action is believed to be in the spinal cord, where it presumably mimics some of the descending inhibitory actions lost after spinal cord injury. It apparently also has actions on higher centers, since it can cause sedation in some patients early in treatment. The treatment usually recommended is 15 to 80 mg per day in divided doses, starting at a minimum and increasing to the dose needed to achieve the desired response without intolerable adverse effects. Some authors have had better success with higher doses than those recommended by the manufacturer (e.g., 240 to 300 mg per day) without producing intolerable adverse reactions.

Tizanidine, an α_2-adrenergic agonist, is now available in the United States for treatment of spinal spasticity. It is well tolerated and, apart from dry mouth, causes few adverse reactions. Treatment begins with 4mg at bedtime, increased slowly to a maximum dosage of 36mg per day in three divided doses.

Diazepam is another medication that acts centrally to mimic the action of descending inhibitory motor systems. Diazepam is effective in the control of spasticity, but it has prominent actions on the limbic system, thalamus, and hypothalamus and can cause sedation and other cognitive adverse reactions that may limit its usefulness. Dosage should be started at 2 mg twice per day and titrated upward to a maximum of 20 mg per day, although some patients can tolerate at least 10 mg four times per day. Clonazepam is another benzodiazepine that can be effective for the control of myoclonus. These are brief jerks of predominantly flexor groups and can interfere with functional abilities and annoy the patient. Sometimes as little as 1 mg per day can decrease these myoclonic jerks, but usually higher doses are needed. Clonidine is a centrally acting α_2-adrenergic agonist that has also been shown to be effective in the control of spinal spasticity. It may be given orally or through a transdermal patch at dosages of 0.1 to 0.5 mg per day. The limiting adverse reactions include hypotension (rare in patients with complete spinal cord injury) and sedation. Dry eyes and mouth generally are transient problems.

Dantrolene works peripherally to inhibit the release of calcium from the sarcoplasmic reticulum and thus decreases the contractility of skeletal muscle. Its use is limited by adverse reactions including drowsiness, lethargy, light-headedness, and a potentially serious hepatotoxicity. Hepatotoxicity is more common in the elderly, in women, and in anyone receiving estrogen therapy. Liver enzyme values must be checked regularly, especially in these groups. Dosage should start at 25 mg twice per day and be titrated upward slowly to a maximum of 100 mg four times per day.

Medical therapy has varying effectiveness, and some patients may require more aggressive therapy to control spasticity. Motor point blocks with phenol may be used to selectively decrease spasticity in desired muscle groups. Surgical procedures, including tendon lengthening and peripheral neurectomy, should be used only as a last resort, and never in the first year after injury. Dorsal rhizotomies, either open surgical or percutaneous radiofrequency procedures, and myelotomies restricted to the dorsal root entry zone can be effective. Recurrence of spasticity has been seen even after these destructive procedures. The latest developments in the treatment of spasticity include the use of a small, implantable pump to deliver a continuous infusion of baclofen to the intrathecal space. This procedure is very effective. Botulinum toxin may be injected into spastic muscles to weaken them for periods of approximately 3 months.

Syringomyelia is a condition in which cavitation develops in the central region of the spinal cord. It is seen commonly as a posttraumatic phenomenon in spinal cord injury but can be associated with Arnold-Chiari malformation and can be idiopathic. These cavitations may be single or multiloculated, and they may have both caudal and rostral extension from the site of the initial trauma. Fluid with a composition similar to cerebrospinal fluid fills these cavities, although extensive analysis of the cyst contents has not yet been carried out. Clinical manifestations include loss of pain and temperature sensation (classically in a capelike distribution over the shoulders and neck), muscle atrophy and loss of motor power, respiratory insufficiency, pain, and changes in the degree of spasticity. The presentation is highly variable depending on the location and extent of the cyst, but increased pain and deterioration of function, especially above the original level, are serious complications of spinal cord injury. Diagnosis is best made with magnetic resonance imaging (MRI), but a delayed CT scan after myelography may show the water-soluble contrast collected in the cavity after it has cleared the subarachnoid space.

The exact origin and pathogenesis of syringomyelia is not known. Tethering of the cord from adhesions is a commonly associated finding on MRI. Some authors speculate that increases in pressure within the cysts during Valsalva's maneuvers may lead to further breakdown of tissue and extension of the cyst. Another possible mechanism is that an as-yet-unknown substance in the cyst fluid acts as a destructive agent leading to further tissue breakdown. Treatments for syringomyelia include spine stabilization, release of the tethered cord, and shunting or fenestration of the cyst cavity to allow drainage of the fluid into the subarachnoid space. Results are variable and are generally limited to halting progression of the cystic degeneration of the spinal cord and maintaining function rather than restoring it.

SPINAL CORD INJURY REHABILITATION

Rehabilitation after spinal cord injury is best provided by an interdisciplinary team at a specialized facility. A comprehensive program encompassing therapies for both physical handicaps and psychological adjustments is essential and should include peers and other patients. It should encourage patient participation, which is vital to promote the resumption of meaningful integration into society.

Rehabilitation can and should begin even in the acute phase of the injury. Prevention of pressure sores should be an important part of care given from the onset of medical therapy. As previously discussed, frequent turning of the patient, flotation beds, and constant inspection of the skin are essential to protect the skin of the immobile patient. Prevention of joint contractures should include range-of-motion exercises and splinting as soon as the patient's condition is medically stable. This is especially true if associated trauma has occurred to any limb or joint. These measures, applied early in the treatment of a spinal cord–injured patient, can reduce the time needed for rehabilitation; if contractures are allowed to develop, they are difficult to overcome. As spasticity develops, the frequency of range-of-motion exercises must to be increased. These can be performed by both therapists and nurses, and in some selected cases can be a way to involve family members in the rehabilitation and healing process.

Once the patient's condition is medically and surgically stable, the neurorehabilitation team should be actively involved in primary care of the patient. The physician coordinates the activities of the team

and manages the medical complications. He or she obtains the appropriate consultations from other physicians and surgeons for assistance in the complex care of the spinal cord–injured patient.

The rehabilitation nurse in a center specializing in spinal cord injury or impairment has multiple responsibilities. These include basic nursing care, skin care, bowel and bladder care, patient and family education, and ensuring that skills learned in therapies are put to use on the nursing unit. The nursing team member is also most involved in the prevention and management of complications such as autonomic dysreflexia, DVT, and urinary tract infection.

The occupational therapist provides training in activities of daily living and works with the patient on improving upper extremity function. This includes training in dressing, feeding, grooming and personal hygiene, and homemaking. It also includes maintenance of range of motion, which may require the construction of splints for some patients. The occupational therapist may also be involved in providing environmental control devices and in electric wheelchair training with chin controls or sip-and-puff controls.

Physical therapists (and kinesiotherapists in Department of Veterans Affairs [VA] hospitals) work with the patient to develop a reconditioning and strengthening program. Physical therapists are also highly involved in mobility skills such as training in safe wheelchair operation, sitting balance, and turning in bed. They are most involved with lower extremity function including range of motion and, if applicable, gait training with walkers, braces, canes, or crutches. They also are involved in training paraplegics and some patients with low-level tetraplegia to do transfers from bed to wheelchair and back and into shower chairs or automobiles. Another function of these therapists is to help in the ordering of appropriate adaptive devices for the home and evaluation of the patient for an appropriate wheelchair. They also may assist with adaptive devices for an automobile and driver training and may be involved in treating pain with physical modalities such as heat, cold, stretching, ethyl chloride sprays, and transcutaneous electrical nerve stimulation devices.

Social workers are important members of the rehabilitation team whose responsibilities involve coordination of discharge planning and reentry into the community. They provide important support to the patient and family members to help find means for financing the hospitalization and equipment or attendant care that may be needed after hospitalization. They help apply for government benefits that may be available for the physically disabled. They also coordinate linking the patient with peer support groups who may be able to provide additional assistance in coping with the challenges of life after a spinal cord injury. This peer counseling can be both formal and informal (i.e., newly injured patients talking with and watching other inpatients at the spinal cord injury center). Social workers work closely with clinical psychologists to anticipate and manage any psychosocial problems that may arise.

The clinical psychologist provides counseling services to both the patient and family members to assist in their adaptation to the physical and psychological stresses of a spinal cord injury. Depression and grieving for the loss of abilities are natural parts of the rehabilitation process. Many patients go through a period of denial before they are ready to begin active participation in rehabilitation. Neuropsychologic testing may also have to be performed to identify any subtle cognitive deficits that may have resulted from either traumatic or ischemic brain injuries. This can be crucial in planning for vocational rehabilitation and directing interventions that may be necessary for maximizing rehabilitation outcome.

Vocational rehabilitation counselors help patients return to work or obtain training or schooling so that they can find a new career. They work with representatives of the state offices of rehabilitation services and other community organizations to give the patient opportunities to reenter the work force if at all possible. They may also be involved in evaluations of the patient's capabilities and aptitudes so that a wise career choice can be made.

Rehabilitation engineering is another important aspect of the team approach to treatment of the spinal cord–injured patient. Rehabilitation engineers help design and construct various prosthetic and orthotic devices that are used to improve a patient's abilities. They modify wheelchairs to improve a patient's posture and prevent pressure sores. They may also supervise modifications to the patient's home or automobile and construct environmental control devices that allow the paralyzed patient to control telephones, lights, televisions,

---
✔ *WHEN TO REFER*

All patients with a new spinal cord injury should be given mega-dose steroid therapy as noted earlier while being transported by emergency medical personnel directly to a trauma center with surgeons who are experienced in the evaluation of such patients and in emergency decompression of the cord when it is indicated. Prompt decompression may reduce the extent of permanent neurologic dysfunction for some patients. Rehabilitation for a patient with spinal cord injury is most effective when the patient is referred to a specialized multidisciplinary center with expertise in this particular condition. Such patients also benefit, both psychologically and practically, from the peer interactions that are more readily available at a spinal cord injury center. Many authors also now advocate the concept that primary care for persons with spinal cord injury should be provided by health care providers with additional training in the special care needs and medical problems of individuals with disorders affecting the spinal cord.

radios, heating and air-conditioning systems, and other appliances in the home.

Functional outcomes for patients after rehabilitation for spinal cord injury differ according to many factors, but the most important is the NLI. If the NLI is C4 or higher, the patient requires assistance for virtually everything, including assisted coughing, feeding, grooming, dressing, bathing, bowel and bladder care, and ambulation. Patients with a C5 NLI are totally dependent for bowel and bladder care, lower extremity dressing, and bathing. They usually need assistance with coughing and upper extremity dressing. With special adaptive devices, patients with C5 tetraplegia can be independent after setup for electric wheelchair ambulation, feeding, and grooming. A patient with C6 tetraplegia usually needs assistance for bladder management, coughing in the supine position, and lower extremity dressing. These patients can be independent with adaptive equipment in their bowel care, bathing, upper extremity dressing, grooming, and feeding. Some of these patients can safely operate an adapted van, driving with specially designed hand controls.

The addition of elbow extension that comes with a C7 NLI is extremely important for enhancing transfer and mobility skills. These patients can be nearly independent if they are highly motivated and are provided proper adaptive equipment. Wheelchair propulsion may be strong enough to negotiate slopes and uneven terrain, but curbs and stairs remain a barrier. Feeding, grooming, bathing, bowel and bladder care, bed mobility, and pressure relief can all be managed with equipment without the assistance of an attendant. Driving can be independent with hand controls, and some patients may be able to transfer themselves and then independently place their wheelchair into the car. Patients with C8-T1 NLI, in addition, are totally independent for all grooming, bathing, and so forth and have significantly better control of fine movements with the hands.

Patients with NLI below T6 need no assistance with cough or pulmonary hygiene. Some can ambulate to a limited degree with a physical assist or guarding and orthoses and walkers. Those with injuries below T10 through L2 have the potential for independent functional ambulation for short distances with orthoses such as long leg braces, ankle or foot orthoses, and forearm crutches. Patients with hip extension (L3 NLI), have potential for community ambulation. The Vannini-Rizzoli boot is a custom-fitted device that patients with NLIs at or below T6 can be trained to use for community ambulation. Current research is ongoing to develop elaborate systems of microprocessor-controlled electrodes (functional electrical stimulation [FES]), which can be used for stimulation of lower extremity muscles in a pattern that allows ambulation with walkers and braces. These systems are not yet practical because of their bulk and inefficiency and the difficulty of activating small, nonfatigable motor units. However, FES in the form of phrenic nerve pacemakers is very successful in providing respiration for tetraplegics with injuries above C4 that spare phrenic motor neurons. Functional electrical stimulation (FES) is also increasingly useful in restoring upper-limb function in patients with good biceps function but paralysis of muscles controlling the hand.

SUMMARY

Spinal cord injury or impairment remains a devastating lesion of the nervous system. Previous and current therapies have not proven to be particularly effective in preventing or reversing damage to the spinal cord. Nevertheless, every effort should be made to preserve remaining function and prevent complications. The care of these patients has been significantly improved by the development of specialized multidisciplinary centers. The emphasis in current treatment focuses on rehabilitation and adaptation to the disability and prevention of secondary disabilities.

Research activities directed at finding a cure or more effective treatment for spinal cord injury are receiving greater attention than ever. In addition to the megadose steroid therapy for acute injuries mentioned earlier, several other medications are currently under investigation. These include 4-aminopyridine (which promotes transmission of impulses in the few remaining, poorly myelinated axons), GM-1 ganglioside and compounds to reduce these trauma-induced effects: production of free radicals, liberation of other cytotoxic components of the inflammatory response, and accumulation of edema. Others block N-methyl-D-aspartate receptors and reduce secondary damage resulting from excitotoxic cascades. If these reactions can be controlled, secondary injury to neurons and axons that survive the initial injury, which then leads to greater loss of function, may be limited.

Another area of exciting progress focuses on attempts to promote regeneration and redirection of axons damaged by the injury and reconstitution of synaptic function. These involve various nerve growth factors and, because mature human nervous tissue inhibits spontaneous growth, agents to disinhibit axon growth and ensure that regenerating axons reach their appropriate targets.

Nevertheless, even when these new developments become practically implemented, the neurorehabilitation team will still be essential for the care of these patients. It is important that ongoing efforts continue to be made to integrate people with disabilities into society so that they may lead full and productive lives.

BIBLIOGRAPHY

Bodner DR, editor: Spinal cord injury, *Urol Clin North Am* 20:373, 1993.
Bracken MB et al: A randomized controlled trial of methylprednisolone or naloxone in the treatment of acute spinal cord injury, *N Engl J Med* 322(20):1405, 1990.
Care and treatment of spinal cord injury patients, IB 141-85, Washington, DC 1991, Pub no Department of Veterans Affairs, *J Am Paraplegia Soc* 15:295, 1992.
Elias AN, Gwinup G: Immobilization osteoporosis in paraplegics, *J Am Paraplegia Soc* 15:163, 1992.
Hammell KW: *Spinal cord injury rehabilitation*, London, 1995, Chapman & Hall.
Lee BY et al, editors: *The spinal cord injured patient: comprehensive management*, Philadelphia, 1991, WB Saunders.
NIDRR consensus statement: The prevention and management of urinary tract infections among people with spinal cord injury, *J Am Paraplegia Soc* 15:194, 1992.
Yarkony GM, editor: *Spinal cord injury: medical management and rehabilitation*, Gaithersburg, Md 1994, Aspen.
Young RR, Woolsey RM, editors: *Diagnosis and management of disorders of the spinal cord*, Philadelphia, 1995, WB Saunders.
Zejdlik CP: *Management of spinal cord injury*, Boston, 1992, Jones & Bartlett.

157 Principles of Neurorehabilitation

Bhagwan T. Shahani

NEUROLOGIC REHABILITATION

Neurologic rehabilitation is a relatively new area of specialization for neurologists and physiatrists. The concept of medical rehabilitation arose from the belief that a physician's responsibility does not end when the patient's acute injury or illness has been treated. Development of new therapies and better medical management have resulted in greater survival of patients with disabling neurologic diseases and neurotrauma. Rehabilitation is particularly important in neurologic disorders, since neurologic impairment often causes severe disability that produces a wide variety of deficits.

Therefore it is not surprising that increasing numbers of neurologists, who were formerly interested primarily in the intellectual exercise of making the diagnosis and pinpointing a lesion in the central nervous system (CNS), are now focusing their attention on long-term management using principles of rehabilitation medicine.

Technologic advances in diagnostic techniques, understanding of pathogenetic mechanisms, development of newer medications, and evidence of CNS plasticity are making a great impact on the acute and long-term management of neurologic diseases. In recent years new research techniques in cellular and molecular biology have resulted in awareness of the growth potential of neurons in the CNS of human subjects. Studies are being performed to evaluate mechanisms responsible for the increasing or decreasing nerve fiber growth in the adult CNS. It has been documented that fetal neuronal transplants in adult mammalian brain result in synaptogenesis with beneficial functional effects. These findings, as well as experiments documenting CNS regeneration with evidence of plasticity, have brought new hope to the field of rehabilitation medicine.

Rehabilitation medicine, as practiced today, uses a team approach, drawing on the specialized skills of the physician, physical therapist, occupational therapist, social worker, psychologist, speech and hearing therapist, nurse, vocational counselor, and specialists in orthotics and prosthetics. In addition, a biomedical engineer can play an important role on the rehabilitation team. This interdisciplinary approach is usually available at specialized centers for rehabilitation. However, as Rusk points out:

> If patients are to benefit from present-day developments in rehabilitation, the concept of rehabilitation and the basic technics must be made a part of the medical programmes of all our hospitals. The concept of rehabilitation and the basic technics must also be made a part of the armamentarium of all physicians: for, regardless of the type of disability, the responsibility of the physician to his patient cannot end when the acute injury or illness has been cared for. Medical care is not complete until the patient has been trained to live and work with what he has left.

Important topics in neurorehabilitation are discussed in the following sections. The principles of rehabilitation of the patient with stroke can also be applied to other neurologic disorders of the CNS.

STROKE REHABILITATION

The estimated prevalence of stroke in the United States population is 1.4 million. Approximately 500,000 people in the United States have a stroke each year, of whom about 150,000 die within the first month. Several studies have shown that comprehensive rehabilitation programs improve the functional outcome of stroke patients. Comprehensive stroke rehabilitation is individualized for every patient and includes various methods such as medication, proper positioning, casting, orthotics, nerve blocks, therapeutic exercise, functional training, neuromuscular facilitation, audiovisual biofeedback, and functional electrical stimulation. Patients receiving such treatment do better in ambulation, activities of daily living (ADLs) and transfer function. Furthermore, rehabilitation methods help patients (and their families) to cope with their deficits much better.

After determining the origin or cause of the stroke, emphasis is placed on managing fluid and electrolyte balance, dysphagia, and during the acute phase, bowel and bladder control. In some instances when dysphagia is a prominent feature, a gastroenterologist and/or speech therapy consultant interested in dysphagia can be helpful in organizing the feeding program for the patient. It may be necessary to perform a modified barium swallow videofluoroscopic examination to evaluate the patient's ability to swallow liquids and solid foods. Many patients may find that a pureed diet of puddings or custards is easier to swallow than a liquid diet. Patients with dysphagia can be trained to produce compensating head and neck movements and perform specific exercises with the help of the speech therapist. Dietitians are helpful in recommending foods with proper consistency that can provide sufficient caloric input. In severe cases of dysphagia it may be necessary to use nasogastric feeding or to perform gastrostomy to provide adequate nutrition for the patient.

To prevent pressure sores, the patient must be turned once every 2 hours and the limbs should be positioned properly. The two most vulnerable areas for development of pressure sores are the ankle and the lateral malleolus. The other areas where pressure sores may develop are over the greater trochanter of the femur, the sacrum, and the coccyx. Once the pressure sore develops, the treatment consists of removal of pressure over the area where the sore has developed, high-protein diet, heat-lamp application, and cleansing of the area with an antiseptic solution. The application of povidone-iodine is controversial. Plastic surgery with a skin-muscle flap is rarely needed if proper precautions are taken to prevent pressure sores.

Bowel and bladder management is of utmost importance in the acute phase after stroke. For proper bowel management the patient must receive sufficient fiber or stool softener (e.g., docusate sodium [Colace] 100 mg three times a day). If spontaneous bowel movements do not take place, bisacodyl (Dulcolax) suppositories may be used every other day to regulate bowel evacuation. For proper bladder management it may be necessary to use intermittent catheterization if the residual urine is greater than 100 ml.

If preventive measures with anticoagulant agents are not taken, up to 75% of patients may show evidence of deep vein thrombosis. The risk of venous thrombosis persists as long as the patient is nonambulatory.

Physical and occupational therapy must be started immediately during the acute phase of stroke. Every joint must be given a full range of motion at least once a day. Active assistive exercises should be given whenever possible. If the patient is able to cooperate, an occupational therapist can train the patient to use the unaffected limb (as much as possible) for ADL. Speech therapists are helpful for teaching proper methods for communication with the patient and management of dysphagia.

In the subacute phase the patient can be transported to physical therapy, occupational therapy, speech therapy, and cognitive rehabilitation therapy programs for the rehabilitation treatment. Starting with mat exercises, physical therapists gradually use different forms of therapies based on established techniques (e.g., Bobath, Rood, Brunnstrom, Knott, and Voss) either to increase or decrease tone in appropriate muscles or to suppress and/or enhance associated movements. Although different proprioceptive neuromuscular techniques are used, no one particular method of treatment has been proved to be superior to others. A skilled physical therapist usually uses a combination of these techniques to develop the best possible motor performance in the hemiparetic upper and lower extremity. Once the patient is able to develop good sitting balance and turn on the mat, it is usually possible to start ambulation training at the fixed hemibar or parallel bars. The patient progresses from periods of standing with the help of parallel bars or a hemibar to walking with the help of a cane. During this phase the patient is evaluated for bracing as necessary. By the time of discharge most patients need no more than a light polypropylene ankle brace. While the patient is progressing in ambulation, it is important to teach the patient simple transfers. The patient should be allowed to go home on a day pass so that family members can adjust to and participate in the patient's rehabilitation program.

In addition to receiving physical therapy, the patient is regularly sent to an occupational therapy clinic where he or she receives cognitive and ADL retraining and training in transfer techniques and wheelchair use, if indicated. Computer-based technology can be used for cognitive rehabilitation for patient's wtih higher-level needs. Dressing using clothing adaptations such as Velcro closure, feeding using special devices such as friction plates, and grooming are taught by occupational therapists. Wheelchair assessment and training can also be performed in the occupational therapy department under supervision of a physiatrist. To prevent shoulder subluxation, occupational therapists provide shoulder support in the form of figure-eight support, a Bobath sling, a Brunnstrom support, or modifications of these. It is essential that the patient receive full range of motion of upper extremity joints during these sessions; this is provided by occupational therapists as well as members of the patient's family.

Although controlled scientific studies have produced uncertain results, every patient with dysarthria and dysphasia deserves to receive evaluation and treatment by a speech therapist. In addition to teaching patients to respond to simple questions, speech therapists can help train the family to cope with the patient's language deficit. As mentioned earlier, speech therapists also contribute significantly to management of dysphagia in patients with stroke. Among the treatment options are individual and group speech therapy and the use of communication devices.

Some patients are severely troubled by visual-spatial perceptual deficits. Special training and the prescription of prism glasses to compensate for these deficits may be necessary.

Patients and their family members may also have emotional problems and mood disorders such as depression. Apart from being troublesome by themselves, these problems also interfere with the progression of the rehabilitation treatment. Appropriate psychologic therapy should be provided.

Shoulder-Hand Syndrome

Shoulder-hand pain syndrome or reflex sympathetic dystrophy is common in patients with stroke. Many of these patients have proprioceptive sensory loss in the affected upper extremity. The main treatment aims to reduce pain and provide active range of motion to joints of the affected upper extremity. Initially pain medication consists of nonsteroidal anti-inflammatory agents. Some patients respond to treatment with prednisone, 30 to 40 mg per day. It is usually not necessary to subject the patient to stellate ganglion blocks, which are recommended by some authors.

In recent years calcitonin has been used extensively in Europe for the management of patients with reflex synpathetic dystrophy.

Brachial Plexus and Peripheral Nerve Injuries

Brachial plexus and other types of peripheral nerve injuries such as entrapments at wrist, elbow and fibular head are not uncommon in stroke patients. Detailed electrophysiologic studies performed in the electrodiagnostic laboratory can provide useful information to document lower motor neuron involvement. One should especially suspect associated peripheral nerve lesions in cases of atypical recovery from stroke.

Electromyographic Biofeedback

Biofeedback is based on the rationale that after receiving instantaneous information of a physiologic parameter (e.g., electromyographic activity) in the form of audiovisual signals, a person can be trained to change the given parameter. In a controlled study we have found that eletromyographic biofeedback hastens recovery of function of dorsiflexion of the foot, significantly improving the strength, repetitive activity, and active range of motion. However, biofeedback does not affect the course of recovery of function in proximal muscles, such as quadriceps and hamstrings. Biofeedback has also not been useful for treating the control of distal musculature in the upper extremity.

Functional Electrical Stimulation

In upper motor neuron syndromes the lower motor neuron and the spinal segmental reflex arc are intact. Functional electrical stimulation (FES) utilizes the motor activity in response to reflex stimulation of proprioceptive and musculocutaneous reflex mechanisms. Functional electrical stimulation has been used to alleviate spasticity and also to improve control of movement. The results of FES are still controversial. Further studies are needed to evaluate its role in patients with stroke.

SPASTICITY

The strict physiologic definition of spasticity describes it as a motor disorder characterized by a velocity-dependent increase in tonic stretch reflexes ("muscle tone") with exaggerated tendon reflexes, resulting from hyperexcitability of the stretch reflex as one component of the upper motor neuron syndrome. This definition has many limitations. The vast majority of patients who have lesions in the spinal cord (e.g., multiple sclerosis) have abnormalities of polysynaptic re-

flexes resulting in spontaneous flexor spasms and flexor dystonia. This group of patients, who can be successfully treated with pharmacologic agents, are excluded from the definition if spasticity is considered an abnormality only of the stretch reflex arc.

Baclofen (Lioresal) has been found to be the drug of choice for the treatment of spontaneous flexor spasms. Sometimes a combination of lower doses of baclofen and diazepam (Valium) may be more effective than either drug alone. Dantrolene sodium (Dantrium) is reserved for some bedridden patients with severe spasticity, when the goal is to "weaken" the muscles to reduce spasticity and help in the nursing care.

Approximately 2 to 3 months after stroke, patients are ready to be discharged home. The social worker, who works with the family and the patient throughout the inpatient stroke rehabilitation, assesses the structure of family support and financial needs for proper care of the patient at home. During the transition period it is useful to arrange for a visiting nurse to be with the patient three or four times a week. If indicated, the patient can be followed up in the outpatient rehabilitation clinic, where he or she can receive physical, occupational, and speech therapy. However, it must be recognized that the goal of stroke rehabilitation is to make the patient and his or her family fully responsible for the care of the patient.

MANAGEMENT OF PATIENTS WITH MULTIPLE SCLEROSIS

There are approximately 200,000 to 500,000 people with multiple sclerosis (MS) in the United States; it is one of the most common causes of severe disability during the young, productive years of life. Since no pharmacologic agent can cure MS, the best that can be done for these patients is symptomatic treatment with techniques that are used in rehabilitation medicine. The principles of rehabilitation are similar to those described for stroke rehabilitation; the neurologist, physiatrist, physical therapist, occupational therapist, speech therapist, social worker, rehabilitation nurse, and neuropsychologist all play important parts in the team effort to rehabilitate the patient with MS.

Most patients with MS complain of gait disturbance as a major primary symptom. Gait disturbance is produced by a variety of underlying causes, including weakness (usually upper motor neuron type), spasticity, cerebellar or sensory ataxia, or a combination of these factors. As mentioned earlier, spinal spasticity in patients with MS responds well to treatment with baclofen. There is no specific treatment for weakness; patients are advised to exercise regularly within the limits of their tolerance to improve endurance. In some instances assistive devices are necessary to improve gait.

There are no pharmacologic agents for the treatment of cerebellar ataxia. Some patients improve by performing specific exercises in front of mirrors to provide visual feedback. Some evidence suggests that attaching weights to appropriate parts of the body may improve motor performance in patients with cerebellar ataxia. If none of these methods works, it may be necessary to train the patient to walk with a cane, crutch, or walker. Patients who are unable to ambulate safely may have to use a wheelchair.

One of the most disabling symptoms of MS patients is related to bladder dysfunction. The detailed diagnosis and management of the bladder dysfunction is beyond the scope of this chapter but has been well described in reviews of neurorehabilitation (Scheinberg and Shahani, 1987). Not infrequently, urinary tract symptoms are accompanied by bowel dysfunction in these patients. Most patients complain of constipation as the primary symptom. Principles of management of bowel dysfunction are similar to those described for stroke rehabilitation.

In some patients with severe neurologic impairment, dysarthria and dysphagia may require treatment by a speech pathologist. These symptoms frequently are not severe enough to cause a major disability for MS patients. Pressure sores develop in approximately 15% of the patients with MS, and every effort should be made to prevent their occurrence as described previously in this chapter.

BRAIN INJURY REHABILITATION

Whereas at one time physical restoration was the emphasis in brain injury rehabilitation, in recent years the focus has been on cognitive and behavioral aspects as well. However, it should be recognized that it is not possible to treat cognitive deficits without influencing the patient's behavioral, social, and motor functions. Cognitive remediation after brain injury, along with new pharmacologic therapies, has become one of the most exciting areas in neurorehabilitation.

BIBLIOGRAPHY

Braddom RL, editor: *Physical medicine and rehabilitation,* Philadelphia, 1996, WB Saunders.

DeLisa JA et al: *Rehabilitation medicine: principles and practice,* Philadelphia, 1993, JB Lippincott.

Rusk HA: Philosophy and need of rehabilitation. In Rusk HA, editor: *Rehabilitation medicine,* St Louis, 1977, Mosby.

Shahani BT, editor: *Electromyography in CNS disorders: central EMG,* Boston, 1984, Butterworth.

Scheinberg L, Shahani BT, editors: Neurologic rehabilitation, *Neurol Clin* 5:4, 1987.

Shahani BT, editor: Motor control disorders, *Physical Med Rehabil Clin North Am* 4:4, 1993.

CHAPTER

158 Ocular Manifestations of Neurologic Disorders

John E. Carter

ABNORMALITIES OF VISION

The neural networks involved in processing vision and eye movements are complex and involve multiple areas of the nervous system, including the retina, several cranial nerves and many regions of the cortex, hemispheric white matter, and brainstem. The basic anatomy and physiology of the visual and ocular motor system are clearly understood. Consequently, the physician who learns the anatomy and common diseases of these systems has invaluable knowledge for understanding many neurologic disease processes.

Many instances of visual loss are caused by local ocular disease. Other visual disturbances, some with visible funduscopic changes and some with normal-appearing eyes, are only one part of a larger neurologic condition. The temporal profile of the visual loss, the characteristics of the visual deficit, and the funduscopic appearance are all important in establishing a diagnosis.

Patient's History

The nature of a lesion causing visual loss is most likely to be indicated by an accurate history. What did the patient first notice—a film over the eye, dirty glasses, looking through a fog? An observant patient may report changes in the color of objects or difficulty with tuning a color television. Bumping into objects on one side may lead to awareness of a visual field defect. Is the disturbance throughout the visual field or in one specific area? Are the symptoms in one eye or both eyes? What happens when each eye is covered individually? Both formed and unformed visual hallucinations are common in patients with visual loss, but these patients may be reluctant to mention them unless specifically questioned.

The temporal profile of the visual loss is most important. When did the patient first become aware of the problem? Difficulty in establishing this point often means that a slowly progressive lesion is present. Sudden onset, on the other hand, suggests a vascular cause. It is important, however, to determine how the patient first noticed the visual loss. If the patient happened to cover one eye and suddenly became aware of visual loss in the other eye, the loss is often interpreted as an acute change by the patient when it may have been present for some time. How long did it take the deficit to become maximal? Is it improving, stable, or continuing to worsen? If the visual loss is intermittent, how often does it occur and are there any factors that seem to precipitate it? Figure 158-1 provides a graphic representation of the temporal profile of the major processes causing visual loss.

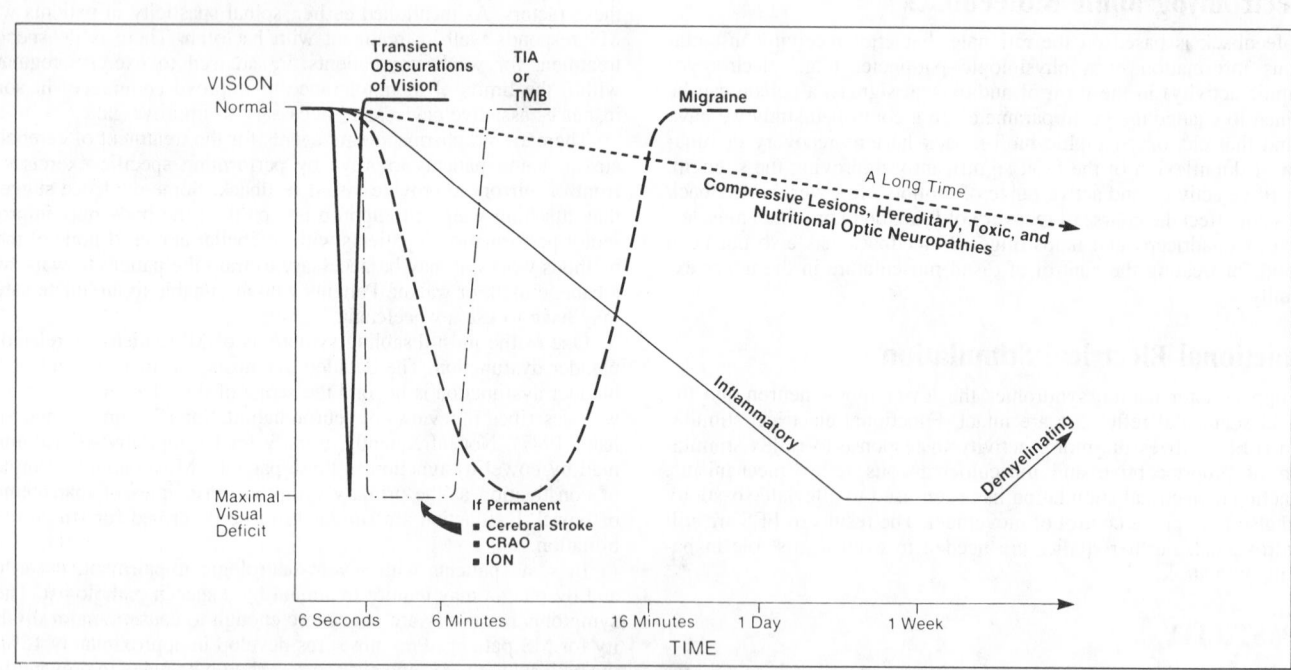

FIGURE 158-1   Temporal profile of visual loss caused by different disease processes. *TIA,* transient ischemic attack; *TMB,* transient monocular blindness; *CRAO,* central retinal artery occlusion (retinal infarction); *ION,* ischemic optic neuropathy. Idiopathic demyelinating optic neuritis is the most common inflammatory optic neuropathy and has a good prognosis for recovery, whereas more specific inflammatory processes such as infections or systemic arteritis are less likely to be associated with good recovery.

From Carter JE. In Taylor RB, editor: *Difficult diagnosis,* Philadelphia, 1985, WB Saunders.

Clinical Evaluation

The patient's best acuity should be obtained with glasses on, and if not 20/20, the acuity may be further tested by having the patient look through a pinhole in a card. If there is no ocular disease or disorder and the best corrected acuity is less than 20/20, a neurologic cause must be sought.

Color vision is tested with Ishihara or American Optical color plates and is most useful in diagnosing an optic neuropathy. With lesions of the optic nerve, color vision becomes abnormal before there is any loss of visual acuity or is abnormal out of proportion to the acuity loss.

The pupillary reaction to light may be abnormal as a result of a lesion of the efferent limb of the reflex in the third cranial nerve, in which case the consensual reaction is still present and normal. An afferent limb pupillary defect indicates a lesion of the optic nerve; the response to light is smaller, less brisk, and often unsustained.

Confrontation visual field testing is performed with the examiner seated in front of the patient. The important areas to explore are the horizontal and vertical meridians (Fig. 158-2). The left and right sides of the vertical meridian are compared superiorly and inferiorly; then superior and inferior areas are compared along the horizontal meridian. These comparisons should allow the examiner to detect a qualitative difference in function in the two eyes (e.g., a central scotoma or optic nerve lesion), in the superior and inferior fields of an individual eye (altitudinal defect), or in the left and right hemifields of each eye (either bitemporal or homonymous hemianopia).

Examination of the fundus with the direct ophthalmoscope should be performed after dilating the pupils. Tropicamide 1% provides good dilation for a short duration.

OCULAR VASCULAR DISEASE IN NEUROLOGY

Three syndromes reflecting ocular circulatory insufficiency have neurologic implications: amaurosis fugax (or transient monocular blindness), retinal artery occlusion, and ischemic optic neuropathy. Retinal arterial emboli may be found in association with any of these syndromes or may be an incidental finding.

Retinal arterial emboli occur in three common compositions: platelet-fibrin aggregates, cholesterol crystals (Hollenhorst plaques), and calcific emboli. Platelet-fibrin aggregates disintegrate within a few minutes or less and therefore are seen only when the patient has an episode of amaurosis fugax while being examined. A column of white material is seen in the retinal arterial tree, where it stops briefly at an arterial bifurcation, pulsating with the heart, and then breaks up into smaller columns and moves along the arteries to the next bifurcation. Shortly after this material disappears, the vision begins to return, and the retina and optic disc become hyperemic.

Cholesterol crystals are the most common arterial emboli observed in the eye (Fig. 158-3). They can occlude the artery and cause retinal infarction. However, they are flat crystals and typically lodge at arterial bifurcations that are too narrow for their width, but blood is able to flow over the top and bottom surfaces without causing symptoms. Cholesterol crystals are highly refractile and yellow. They often appear to be larger than the vessel in which they lie, reflecting the fact that the vessel walls themselves are not visible; rather, it is the column of blood that is observed during fundoscopy. Cholesterol emboli may lodge at one location permanently or may disappear between examinations; they are an important indicator of risk for future stroke and for future coronary artery disease and death. In a study of 70 patients with asymptomatic cholesterol emboli the annual stroke rate was 8.5% compared with 0.8% for controls. Strokes occurred in the ipsilateral carotid territory two thirds of the time, that is, about 6% per year. This compares with studies of asymptomatic carotid stenosis where patients with carotid stenosis equal to or greater than 60% have an annual stroke risk of 2% per year and patients with no carotid stenosis have an annual stroke risk of 1% per year.

Calcific emboli are much less common and consist of whitish-gray clumps of material (Fig. 158-4) that usually lodge in the retinal arteries between bifurcations. They are often the product of calcific cardiac valvular disease but may be seen associated with carotid atherosclerosis. All forms of retinal emboli are serious indicators of potential stroke.

Transient monocular blindness, or amaurosis fugax, consists of sudden loss of vision in one eye. Vision may simply fade out, or there may be the sensation of a shade being drawn across the eye, usually from top to bottom. The visual loss usually lasts for 2 to 10 minutes and either fades back in or resolves in a manner similar to a shade

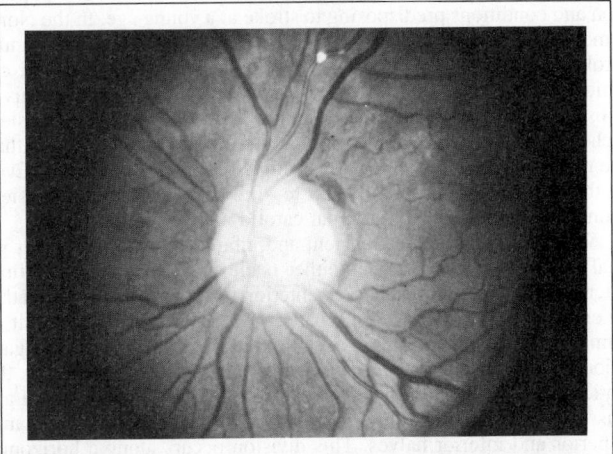

A

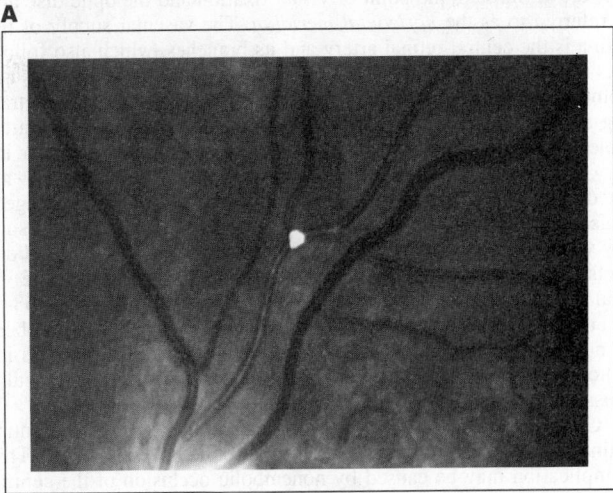

B

FIGURE 158-3 A and B, A cholesterol crystal embolus lodged at an arterial bifurcation.

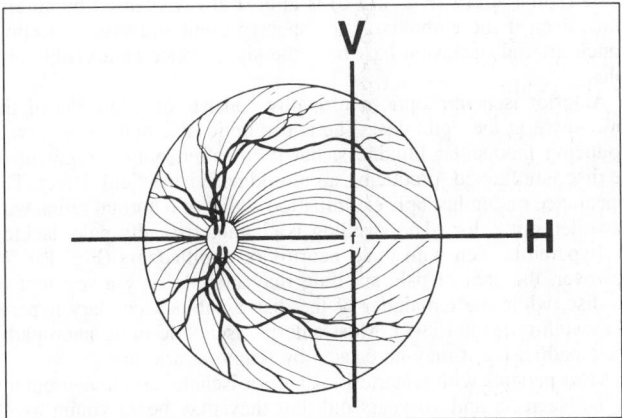

FIGURE 158-2 The pattern of the retinal circulation and the relationship of the circulation, optic disc, and fovea *(f)* to the vertical *(V)* and horizontal *(H)* meridians of the visual field.

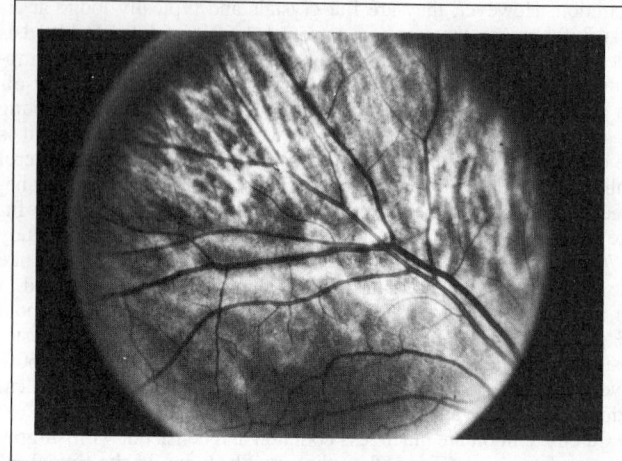

FIGURE 158-4   An amorphous clump of calcific material that has lodged at an arterial bifurcation.

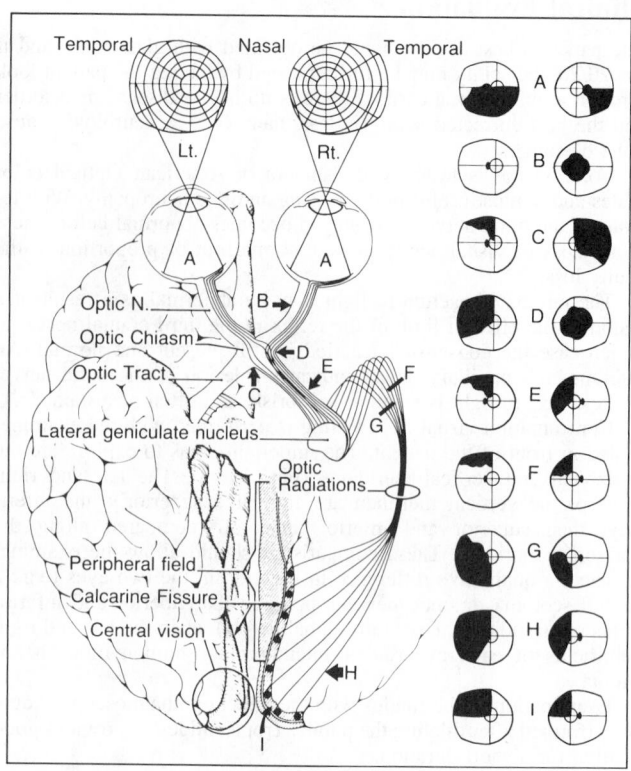

FIGURE 158-5   *A*, Two examples of altitudinal visual field defects that could be caused either by occlusion of a superior branch of the central retinal artery or by an episode of ischemic optic neuropathy involving the superior optic disc. On the left is a large field defect involving both lower quadrants. On the right the injury is more limited and the defect involves only the temporal quadrant, but it connects with the blind spot and does not go to fixation or have a border at the vertical meridian. *B*, A central scotoma in the visual field of the right eye caused by a lesion of the right optic nerve. *C*, Bitemporal hemianopia caused by a lesion of the optic chiasm. The asymmetry is typical of chiasmal field defects until a late stage, when the hemianopia may be complete in both eyes. *D*, Junctional scotoma, that is, a central scotoma on the side of a lateral chiasmal lesion with a temporal hemianopia in the visual field of the opposite eye. *E*, Markedly incongruous homonymous hemianopia seen with a lesion of the optic tract. *F*, Homonymous superior quadrantanopia seen with lesions of the optic radiations in the temporal lobe. *G*, Homonymous inferior quadrantanopia seen with lesions of the superior optic radiations in the low parietal or parietotemporal lobe junction. *H*, Congruous homonymous hemianopia seen with lesions either of the optic radiations close to their termination or of the calcarine cortex itself. *I*, Precise inferior quadrantanopia seen if an occipital lobe lesion involves just the superior bank of the calcarine cortex.

being pulled up. Transient monocular blindness is the ocular equivalent of transient ischemic attack. Since the fundus is usually normal between episodes, diagnosis of transient monocular blindness is made from history alone. Identical symptoms have been described in migraine, with Raynaud's phenomenon, and in young patients with no known cause. Therefore, transient monocular blindness as an indicator of carotid system ischemia is limited to the stroke-aged population and conditions predisposing to stroke at a young age. In the North American Symptomatic Carotid Endarterectomy Trial the annual stroke rate for patients with transient monocular blindness and carotid stenosis equal to or greater than 70% was 8% per year. This is substantially less that the annual stroke rate for hemispheric transient ischemic attacks (22% per year) but is still substantially worse than the risk of stroke in patients with asymptomatic carotid stenosis. Even in the stroke-aged population, up to 40% of patients with transient monocular blindness have normal carotid angiograms.

When ischemia is not transient and infarction with permanent visual loss occurs, the cause is either occlusion of the central retinal artery or one of its branches or anterior ischemic optic neuropathy. In either case the characteristic pattern of visual loss is the result of damage to the retinal ganglion cell axons. Within the eye the ganglion cell axons must swing above and below the fovea to reach the optic nerve (Fig. 158-2). This arcuate pattern of the ganglion cell axons effectively divides the retina and its respective visual field into superior and inferior halves. This division occurs along a horizontal line drawn through the point of visual fixation and the optic disc and is referred to as the *horizontal meridian*. The vascular supply of the retina is the central retinal artery and its branches, which also follow this arcuate pattern. The blood supply of the optic disc itself does not come from the central retinal artery but rather from short, penetrating arterioles derived from the posterior ciliary arteries. These arterioles supply individual segments of the optic disc, and vascular injury here produces a discrete visual field defect whose location is related to the group of nerve fiber bundles that have been damaged. This characteristic distribution of the nerve fibers and the blood supply within the eye provides localization of altitudinal visual field defects (i.e., visual field defects that lie in one vertical half of the visual field with a sharp border at the horizontal meridian [Fig. 158-5, *A*]) to the eye itself. The other disease that can destroy large numbers of nerve fibers at the optic disc is glaucoma, which may progress insidiously to produce a large altitudinal field defect. The intraocular pressure must be determined to exclude glaucoma.

Central retinal artery occlusion produces infarction of the entire retina. The arteries are attenuated, and the retina is a milky color. This complication may be caused by nonembolic occlusion of the central retinal artery as it enters the eye through the lamina cribrosa, or it may be associated with emboli from the carotid arteries or heart. When emboli are in the fundus, the likelihood of finding major occlusive disease in the carotid system is higher. Occlusion of a branch

of the retinal artery (Fig. 158-6) is almost always caused by an embolus, even if the embolus is no longer present and visible. Retinal branch arterial occlusion has the same significance as a visible embolus.

Anterior ischemic optic neuropathy consists of infarction of the optic nerve at the optic disc. The entire optic disc may be involved, producing monocular blindness, but more often only a segment of the disc is infarcted, producing an altitudinal visual field defect. The appearance on funduscopic examination is that of a normal retina with a swollen optic disc. The swelling is characteristically pale, lacking the hyperemia seen with optic neuritis or papilledema (Fig. 158-7). However, the area of pale swelling may include only a segment of the disc, while the remainder of the disc exhibits secondary hyperemic swelling (Fig. 158-8). Most anterior ischemic optic neuropathy is idiopathic, but it may be caused by temporal arteritis.

Most patients with nonarteritic anterior ischemic optic neuropathy are between 55 and 70 years old, but they may be as young as 40 years of age. These patients are generally healthy, although hypertension and diabetes are common findings. Anterior ischemic optic neuropathy occasionally occurs in association either with occlusion of the internal carotid artery or with multiple cholesterol emboli in the

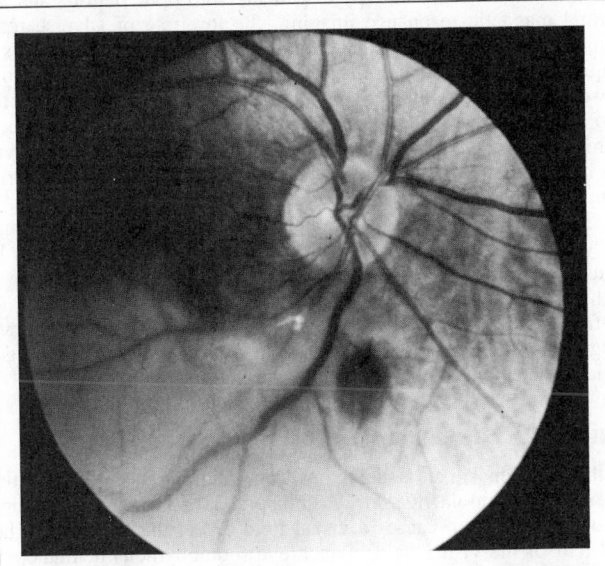

A

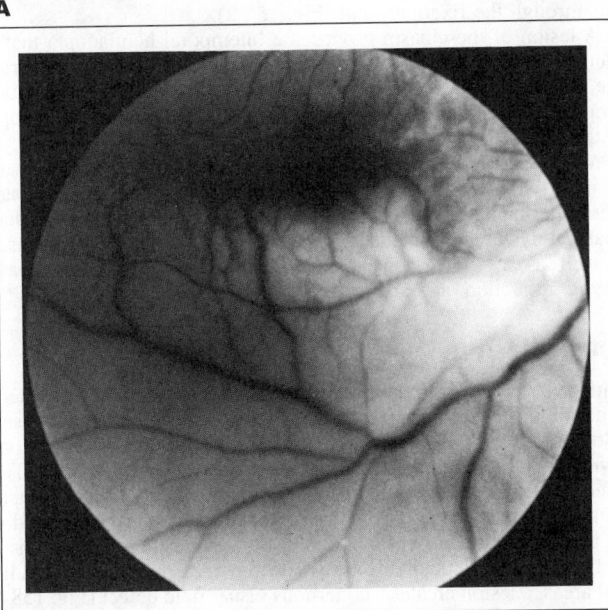

B

FIGURE 158-6   **A,** An embolus at an arterial bifurcation. The resulting isch-emia has produced an intraretinal hemorrhage below the optic disc and a pale, infarcted retina distal to the embolus and extending across the inferior retina below the fovea in **B.**

From Carter JE. In Taylor RB, editor: *Difficult diagnosis,* Philadelphia, 1985, WB Saun-ders.

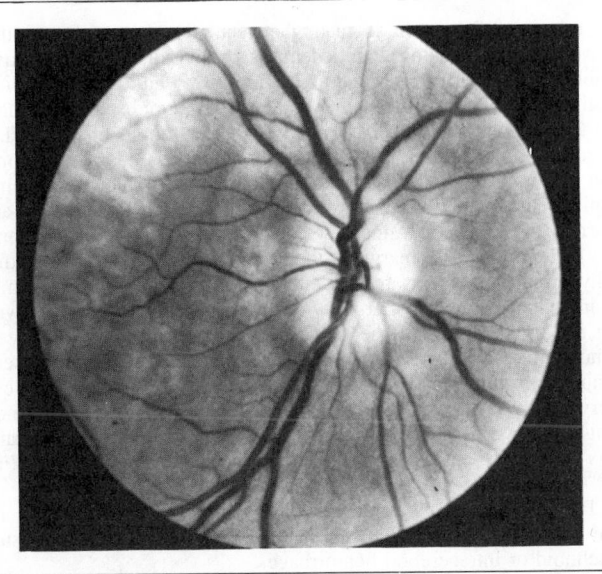

FIGURE 158-7   Pallor and swelling of the entire optic disc in an elderly woman with sudden total visual loss and ischemic optic neuropathy caused by temporal arteritis. Compare the inner area of this optic disc with the hy-peremic central area optic disc swelling caused by papilledema or optic neu-ritis in Fig. 158-9.

From Carter JE. In Packard RC, editor: *Neurologic clinics,* vol 1, Philadelphia, 1983, WB Saunders.

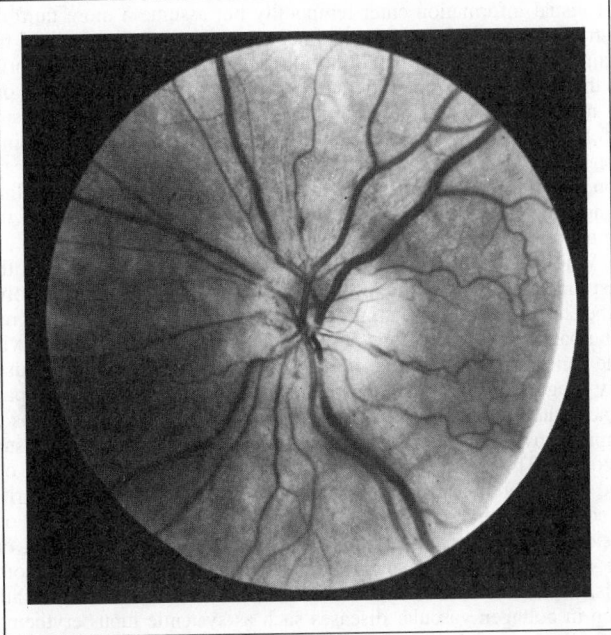

FIGURE 158-8   Ischemic optic neuropathy with loss of the superior visual field. The inferior aspect of the optic disc is pale, while superiorly the disc is also swollen but remains adequately perfused and does not exhibit pallor.

From Carter JE. In Taylor RB, editor: *Difficult diagnosis,* Philadelphia, 1985, WB Saunders.

retinal arterioles. Emphasis should be on control of hypertension. Nonarteritic anterior ischemic optic neuropathy seldom occurs a sec-ond time in the same eye, but up to half of patients have a subse-quent episode in the other eye in the next 10 years.

Temporal arteritis is commonly diagnosed because of an episode of anterior ischemic optic neuropathy. Most patients are over 70 years old. Other symptoms of temporal arteritis, such as progressively wors-ening headaches, jaw claudication, polymyalgia rheumatica, night sweats, anemia, or fever of unknown origin, may be relatively mild. As many as 40% of patients with temporal arteritis may have visual loss. Sixty-five percent of patients who come to medical attention with ischemic optic neuropathy caused by temporal arteritis in one eye have visual loss in the other eye, often within 24 hours and usually within the first week, if they do not receive treatment. A history sug-gestive of this disorder should prompt therapy with corticosteroids

pending a temporal artery biopsy. In a patient with ischemic optic neuropathy but no other symptoms of temporal arteritis the erythro-cyte sedimentation rate should be determined. A value above 40 mm per hour justifies the use of corticosteroids until a temporal artery biopsy is performed.

Papilledema

An arbitrary distinction is made between disc edema from other causes and papilledema. Papilledema is passive disc swelling attributable to increased intracranial pressure transmitted to the optic discs by the cerebrospinal fluid (CSF) in the subarachnoid space surrounding the optic nerves. Except for transient obscurations of vision (i.e., episodes of monocular visual loss lasting a few seconds), visual function is normal until the late stages of chronic atrophic papilledema. Papilledema is often asymmetric but seldom unilateral. Elevation and blurring of the disc margins is seen earliest superiorly and inferiorly, and the temporal disc margin is the last to be affected. The optic disc is hyperemic. The veins are dilated and tortuous, and the vessels may be indistinct at the disc margin where they are obscured by the swollen nerve fiber layer of the retina. Venous pulsations are not seen, although they are also absent in 20% of normal individuals. If present, venous pulsations usually indicate a CSF pressure of 220 mm or less. Nerve fiber layer hemorrhages (splinter and flame-shaped hemorrhages), nerve fiber layer infarcts (cotton-wool spots), and exudates may all be present as the papilledema becomes more severe (Fig. 158-9).

Papilledema is usually the result of chronic elevation of intracranial pressure, although it may develop within a few hours after subarachnoid or intracerebral hemorrhage.

Idiopathic intracranial hypertension, also referred to as benign intracranial hypertension or pseudotumor cerebri, typically causes papilledema (see Chapter 160) and is probably the most common cause of papilledema since the development of computerized tomography and magnetic resonance imaging has resulted in early diagnosis of most intracranial neoplasms.

Optic Neuritis and Optic Neuropathies

Retinal ganglion cell axons enter the optic nerve in an orderly fashion. Those from the papillomacular bundle carrying macular or central visual information enter temporally but assume a more uniform distribution throughout the optic nerve as they progress toward the brain. Axons from the papillomacular bundle make up the majority of the axons within the optic nerve. On clinical examination the optic nerve behaves as though it were primarily carrying central visual information. Therefore lesions of the optic nerve produce a combination of the following: loss of visual acuity, diminished color perception, diminished brightness of the visual environment (visual dimming), defective pupillary reaction to light, and a depression of the central visual field in a central scotoma (Fig. 158-5, *B*).

When the findings indicate an optic neuropathy, the history is the best indicator of the nature of the process. Optic neuritis may involve either the optic nerve head, producing visible disc edema, or the retrobulbar portion of the optic nerve, producing visual loss without visible fundus changes. Visual loss may develop very rapidly but usually progresses for several days to a week, and an aching orbital pain exacerbated by eye movements is common. Vision usually begins to improve by the end of 2 weeks, and most patients have good visual recovery. The majority of cases occur in patients 20 to 40 years old and are unilateral. In patients less than 20 years of age optic neuritis is commonly bilateral. Optic neuritis is usually idiopathic but is occasionally caused by contiguous inflammation of the meninges, orbit, or paranasal sinuses and may also be caused by syphilis, sarcoidosis, tuberculosis, and cryptococcosis. Optic neuritis is occasionally seen in collagen vascular diseases such as systemic lupus erythematosus. If there is no evidence of a systemic inflammatory disease or inflammation in structures along the course of the optic nerve, the patient may be followed up expectantly or consideration may be given to treatment with high-dose intravenous steroids. Traditional doses of steroids (60 mg per day) have no benefit and may be harmful. High doses (1 g methylprednisolone intravenously for 3 days followed by 11 days of 1 mg/kg prednisone by mouth and a 3-day taper) hasten recovery but do not affect the final visual recovery. This regimen, however, decreased the rate at which additional symptoms and signs of demyelinating disease developed in the 2 years following the initial attack of optic neuritis. This effect was most pronounced in patients whose magnetic resonance imaging showed at least two white matter lesions, which were either located in the periventricular region or were at least 3 mm in diameter and ovoid. Kupersmith reviewed

data that might justify therapy in patients with optic neuritis and abnormal magnetic resonance imaging; the low rate of adverse reactions in the trial may justify treating optic neuritis in all patients if magnetic resonance imaging is not undertaken routinely. It is notable, however, that the number of patients equalized after 3 years in the two groups in the study in whom multiple sclerosis had developed. Care must be taken in discussing multiple sclerosis in patients who are having their first episode of optic neuritis. The diagnosis carries a high psychological morbidity and requires sensitive counseling.

Optic nerve compression may be caused by neoplastic, aneurysmal, or cystic mass lesions and is usually unilateral. Diffuse infiltrative lesions such as sarcoidosis, lymphoma, or leukemia may affect one or both optic nerves in the orbit or intracranially. Meningeal carcinomatosis frequently affects the optic nerves bilaterally. Insidious and slowly progressive bilateral loss of vision with central scotomas suggests a toxic or nutritional optic neuropathy or hereditary optic atrophy.

Chiasmal Disease

At the optic chiasm all visual axons from the nasal half of each retina cross to the contralateral side. A unilateral visual system lesion posterior to the chiasm causes a visual field defect that affects one lateral half of the visual field in each eye (homonymous hemianopia). These visual field defects should not cross the vertical meridian that runs through the fixation point (Fig. 158-2).

A lesion of the chiasm produces a bitemporal hemianopia that is often asymmetric (Fig. 158-5, *C*). The chiasm is not an isolated structure, however, and a laterally placed lesion may give a combination of optic nerve deficit on the ipsilateral side and a temporal hemianopia on the other (Fig. 158-5, *D*).

Most chiasmal visual disturbances are caused by compression and are usually the result of pituitary adenomas, craniopharyngiomas, and suprasellar meningiomas. Other neoplastic processes that can produce chiasmal dysfunction include optic glioma, teratoma, and metastases, as well as cysts, vascular malformations, demyelinating disease, trauma, infarction, and arachnoiditis.

Retrochiasmic Disease

Behind the chiasm all visual information relates to the contralateral visual field. Lesions behind the chiasm produce homonymous visual field defects (Fig. 158-5, *E* to *I*). Incongruous field defects are homonymous but of different degree in the two eyes (Fig. 158-5, *E*). This defect indicates a lesion either of the optic tract or of anterior optic radiations where the axons from the same area of the visual field of the two eyes have not yet moved close to each other. Farther posteriorly, and in the occipital lobe where these fibers synapse in adjacent areas, a lesion creates a congruous visual field defect (Fig. 158-5, *H*). Since the vertical meridian splits the fixation point, and since either half of the fovea is capable of maximal visual resolution, visual acuity is normal even with a complete, unilateral homonymous hemianopia.

Lesions of the optic tract cause incongruous homonymous visual field defects. Since the optic tracts encircle the midbrain, associated brainstem abnormalities are expected. After leaving the lateral geniculate nucleus, the most inferior fibers of the optic radiations run forward around the temporal horn of the lateral ventricle before continuing posteriorly to the occipital lobe. Lesions here create a homonymous superior quadrantanopia (Fig. 158-5, *F*). The most superior fibers of the optic radiations run in the inferior parietal lobe, where lesions produce a homonymous inferior quadrantanopia (Fig. 158-5, *G*). A discrete lesion in the occipital lobe produces a homonymous visual field defect that is identical in the two eyes (Fig. 158-5, *H*). The optic radiations synapse in the calcarine cortex, which lies on the medial surface of the occipital lobe and is split into superior and inferior banks by the calcarine fissure. The superior bank receives all information originating in the inferior half of the visual field, and the inferior bank receives information from the superior field. A lesion limited to one of the banks is the only lesion likely to produce a visual field defect that occupies exactly one quadrant of the homonymous visual fields (Fig. 158-5, *I*).

The majority of patients with symptomatic homonymous visual field defects have vascular lesions, usually within the occipital lobe.

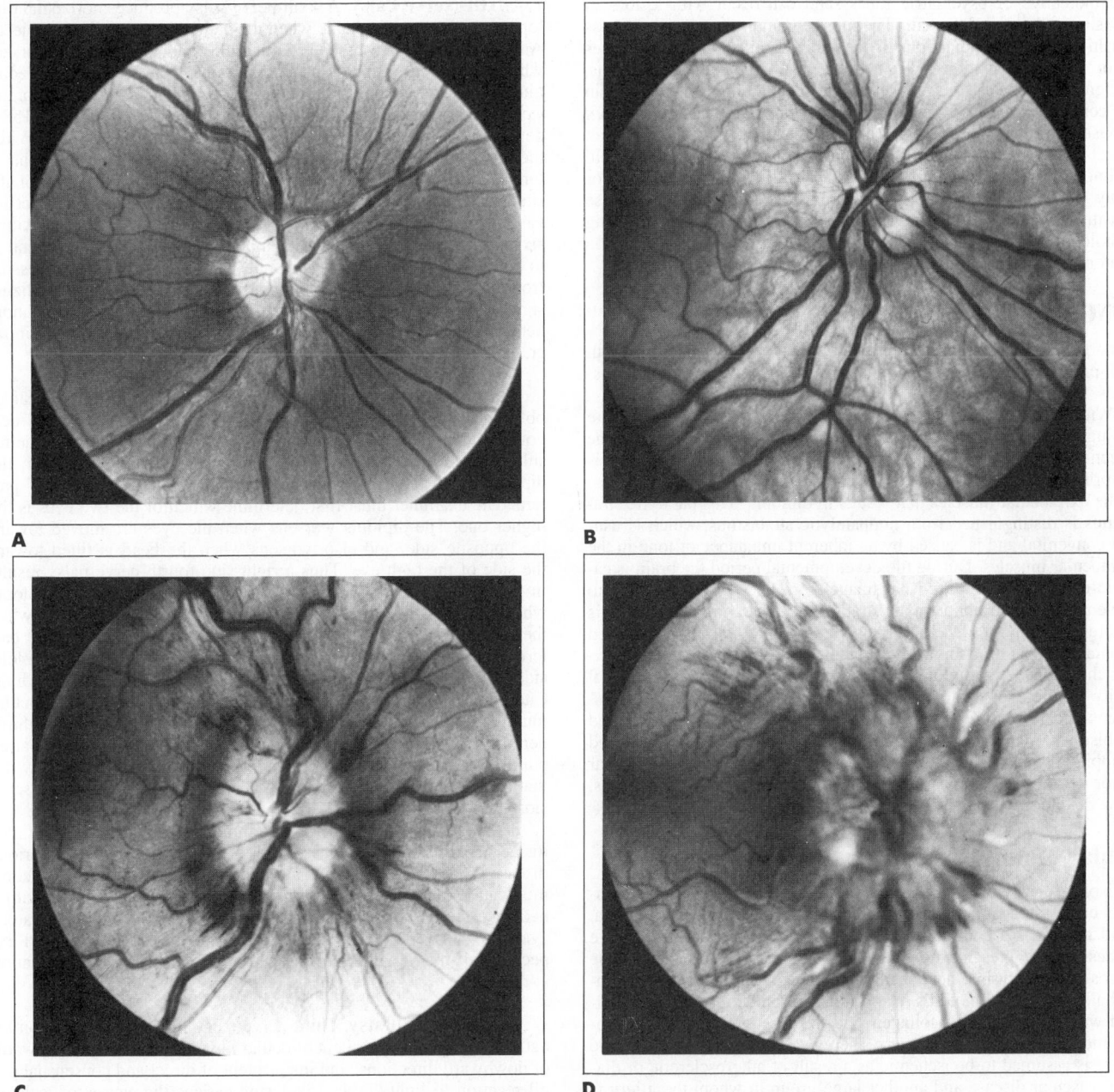

FIGURE 158-9 **A,** A normal optic disc with the macula to the left of the disc. The arcuate fibers enter the disc superiorly and inferiorly and make the nerve fiber layer thicker and the disc margins less clearly visualized in these two quadrants. The earliest changes in papilledema will be seen in these quadrants. The nerve fiber layer at the nasal quadrant on the right in the picture is intermediate in thickness, and the disc margin is more clearly seen, but not as sharply as the temporal quadrant on the left where the nerve fiber layer is thinnest. **B,** Mild disc edema in a patient with pseudotumor cerebri. There is marked hyperemia and opacification of the peripapillary nerve fiber layer. **C** and **D,** Progressively more severe swelling of the optic disc, with splinter hemorrhages located in the nerve fiber layer and cotton-wool spots, which are microinfarctions of the nerve fiber layer.

From Carter JE. In Packard RC, editor: *Neurologic clinics,* vol 1, Philadelphia, 1983, WB Saunders.

Other patients may have substantial visual field defects without being aware of them and may have vascular or neoplastic lesions anywhere along the visual pathways. Because both left and right posterior cerebral arteries have a common origin from the basilar artery, bilateral infarction of the occipital lobes may occur. The resulting visual loss affecting both visual fields in both eyes may resemble bilateral optic nerve lesions. However, the pupil reactions to light are normal.

Lesions of the dominant hemisphere that disrupt projections from the occipital lobe to the parietal and temporal lobes may create an inability to read while writing is preserved (alexia without agraphia), or an inability to recognize objects visually, despite the preserved ability to identify them by sound or feel (visual agnosia). Similar lesions of the nondominant hemisphere may produce an inability to recognize familiar faces, despite the ability to identify the persons by their voices (prosopagnosia). These conditions are accompanied by a homonymous hemianopia.

Unlike auditory hallucinations, visual hallucinations are not usually indicative of psychiatric illness and can occur with lesions at any site in the visual system. The most common neurologic process causing visual hallucinations is classic migraine, which produces unformed hallucinations. Formed visual hallucinations, that is, recognizable objects, places, or people, occur only with lesions in the central nervous system, usually anterior to the calcarine cortex in visual association areas. Occasionally patients complain that an object or a face they have just seen persists in the visual field (palinopia), or that when an object is seen it is reduplicated once or many times, creating a cerebral diplopia or polyopia. All of these "positive" visual phenomena are usually indicative of an ongoing pathologic process and are almost always accompanied by a homonymous hemianopia.

ABNORMALITIES OF EYE MOVEMENT

Abnormal eye movements often provide localizing information about both primary disease of the nervous system and various systemic diseases.

With the exception of convergence, all normal eye movements are conjugate, that is, the two eyes move an equal distance in the same direction. Most cases in which an abnormality of eye movement is the primary neurologic problem involve an acquired weakness of one of the extraocular muscles that results in diplopia. This paralytic strabismus is distinguished from nonparalytic strabismus, which is usually congenital and is caused by an inherent imbalance of tone in the extraocular muscles. During the developmental period the brain is capable of suppressing the visual image from one of the two eyes to prevent diplopia. If nonparalytic strabismus is not corrected early, this suppression may produce a permanent loss of visual acuity referred to as amblyopia ex anopia. In the adult with disconjugate eye position the absence of diplopia and the presence of diminished visual acuity in one eye, without other signs of retinal or optic nerve disease, indicate the presence of a congenital rather than an acquired strabismus. Acquired disconjugate eye movements with associated diplopia are most likely to be caused by injury to one of the ocular motor nerves (i.e., cranial nerves III, IV, and VI), myasthenia gravis, skew deviation, or dysthyroid myopathy.

Ocular Motor Nerve Disorders

An isolated palsy of one of the ocular motor nerves is the most common cause of acquired disconjugate eye movements and diplopia. Head trauma is a common cause of third-, fourth-, and sixth-nerve palsies, and it presents no diagnostic difficulty. Other identifiable causes are aneurysms; neoplasms; infections such as meningitis, encephalitis, otitis, ethmoiditis, or syphilis; postinfectious cases associated with a viral illness; collagen vascular diseases; multiple sclerosis; and complications of surgery. There is a large group in whom the injury is assumed to be ischemic as a result of atherosclerotic or diabetic vascular disease and another large group in whom the injury is idiopathic. The primary concern is to distinguish between patients in these latter two groups, who generally recover in 2 or 3 months, and those in whom ocular motor palsy is the presenting sign of a neoplasm or an intracranial aneurysm. Pain may be a prominent complaint in all of these conditions, but the pain should resolve within a few days in patients with benign etiologic factors. Table 158-1 shows the frequency of the various causes of ocular motor palsies.

Sixth-Nerve Palsy. A sixth-nerve palsy produces horizontal diplopia, which is most notable when the patient looks at distant objects. An esotropia is present on examination, and the diplopia worsens when the eyes are moved in the direction of the weak lateral rectus muscle. A lesion of the sixth-nerve nucleus or its axons in the brainstem is associated with other neurologic abnormalities. Table 158-1 details the most common causes of isolated sixth-nerve palsies. While the majority of sixth-nerve palsies are benign, the sixth nerve has a long course next to bony structures as it travels up the base of the skull, and involvement by metastatic tumor, especially by direct invasion from the nasopharynx, is common enough that patients with a sixth-nerve palsy should have computed tomography with attention to bony detail at the base of the skull. Increased intracranial pressure from any cause can produce a sixth-nerve palsy as a false localizing sign. Sixth-nerve palsies can occur as the result of a subarachnoid hemorrhage but are rarely the presenting sign of an unruptured intracranial aneurysm.

Fourth-Nerve Palsy. Fourth-nerve palsy produces vertical or oblique diplopia that is worse when looking down. The central nervous system attempts to compensate for this abnormality, and the resulting pattern of eye movements may be confusing. However, the diplopia of the fourth-nerve palsy should follow a "marching" pattern. The examiner must first determine which of the two eyes is the higher one. The diplopia worsens when the eyes are moved toward the opposite side, and also worsens when the head is tilted toward the side of the high eye. Thus a right-side fourth-nerve palsy results in the right eye being higher than the left eye, worsening diplopia when the eyes move to the left side, and worsening diplopia when the patient tilts his or her head to the right side. A left-right-left pattern when the left eye is the higher of the two eyes indicates a left-side fourth-nerve palsy. Any other pattern in this three-step test indicates a weakness of one of the other vertically active extraocular muscles. If this is the case, and if there are no other signs of third-nerve dysfunction, such as impaired adduction, ptosis, or impaired pupillary reaction to light, the patient most probably has a skew deviation, myasthenia gravis, or dysthyroid myopathy (see later discussion).

Fourth-nerve palsy is the least commonly encountered ocular motor nerve palsy and is the least likely to be associated with a serious disease process (Table 158-1). Intracranial aneurysm is a very uncommon cause. Neoplasm is also not common, and most patients with a neoplasm have other neurologic signs early. A limited laboratory evaluation may be undertaken, and the patient can be observed expectantly if the remainder of the neurologic history and examination is normal.

Third-Nerve Palsy. Third-nerve palsy is recognized by combinations of ptosis; impairment of ocular movements in medial, upward, or downward directions; and impairment of direct and consensual pupil reaction to light. Table 158-1 summarizes the causes of isolated third-nerve palsy. The third nerve is the only ocular motor nerve that is commonly affected by an expanding intracranial aneurysm before its rupture, so consideration must be given to performing cerebral arteriography even if computed tomography is normal. The pupillomotor fibers travel superficially in the third nerve and are susceptible to external compressive lesions. Ischemic damage to the third nerve tends to involve the substance of the nerve, sparing the most superficial fibers. Three fourths of patients with ischemic third-nerve palsy have a normal pupillary reaction to light, and less than 5% of patients with an aneurysmal third-nerve palsy have spared pupillary function. Therefore a patient with diabetes or an older patient with hypertension or atherosclerotic disease and a pupil-sparing third-nerve palsy is unlikely to have an aneurysm. Even if such a patient has a third-nerve palsy with the pupil involved, the frequency of ischemic third-nerve palsy is high enough that the morbidity of cerebral arteriography justifies a period of observation if magnetic resonance imaging is normal with no evidence of aneurysm or other mass and no evidence of subarachnoid hemorrhage is seen. Magnetic resonance angiography is ineffective in performing a general search for aneurysms following a subarachnoid hemorrhage. If, however, the clinician can direct the radiologist to a specific site such as the posterior communicating artery–internal carotid artery junction in a case with a third-

Table 158-1 Frequency of causes of impaired function of the ocular motor nerves

CAUSE	SIXTH CRANIAL NERVE (%)	FOURTH CRANIAL NERVE (%)	THIRD CRANIAL NERVE (%)
Undetermined	24	31	24
Head trauma	14	31	14
Neoplasm	21	5	13
Ischemic	15	22	20
Intracranial aneurysm	3	1	17
Other	23	10	12

nerve palsy, magnetic resonance imaging may be adequate to exclude an aneurysm.

Combined Injury to the Ocular Motor Nerves. Dysfunction of a combination of the third, fourth, and sixth cranial nerves can occur. In general, this parasellar syndrome indicates disease in the region of the cavernous sinus. Since the ophthalmic division of the trigeminal nerve also runs in the wall of the cavernous sinus, sensory disturbances of the upper face may be seen. Primary neoplasms sometimes occur in this region, but metastatic lesions are more common. Other processes producing the parasellar syndrome include cavernous sinus thrombosis, carotid-cavernous sinus fistula, and aneurysm of the intracavernous carotid artery. If a specific cause cannot be found, the diagnosis of Tolosa-Hunt syndrome may be considered. Tolosa-Hunt syndrome is a nonspecific inflammation of the cavernous sinus that responds dramatically to corticosteroids.

Skew Deviation. Skew deviation is an acquired, vertical strabismus caused by a disturbance of vertical eye movement pathways proximal to the ocular motor nerve nuclei. Patients complain of vertical diplopia, but examination demonstrates a pattern of extraocular muscle weakness that is not consistent with weakness of the superior oblique muscle (fourth cranial nerve), and the remaining function of the third nerve is intact, making a lesion of the third cranial nerve unlikely. Skew deviation always indicates a lesion in the posterior fossa and is almost always caused by disease within the substance of the brainstem or cerebellum rather than by an external, compressive lesion. Skew deviation is frequently associated with an internuclear ophthalmoplegia. In younger patients a skew deviation is most commonly seen in multiple sclerosis, whereas in older patients it is probably caused by a stroke.

Myasthenia Gravis. Myasthenia gravis may be the most commonly missed diagnosis in patients who come to medical attention with abnormal eye movements. Eighty percent of patients with myasthenia gravis present with symptoms and signs of ocular motor dysfunction. Myasthenia may mimic an internuclear ophthalmoplegia, a sixth-nerve palsy, or a fourth-nerve palsy, or it may present any of the features of a third-nerve palsy except a dilated pupil. The hallmark of myasthenia gravis is ocular ptosis or diplopia, which varies from hour to hour and day to day, typically being variable on successive examinations. Myasthenia gravis should be considered in any patient with disconjugate eye movements.

Dysthyroid Ophthalmopathy. Thyroid eye disease, or dysthyroid ophthalmopathy, consists of an infiltration of the extraocular muscles and other orbital contents by inflammatory cells and a mucilaginous ground substance, followed later by fibrosis of orbital tissues. Patients often have diplopia caused by restriction of the extraocular muscles, most commonly the inferior rectus. Forced ductions in which the examiner attempts to manually rotate the eye show that the passive movement of the eye is limited by the involved muscle. Other findings include proptosis, vascular congestion seen over the insertion of the lateral or medial rectus muscle on the globe, lid retraction or lid lag, and edema of the eyelids. Dysthyroid ophthalmopathy can occur in a patient who has hyperthyroidism but can also occur in patients who have received treatment for hyperthyroidism and have euthyroidism or even hypothyroidism. It may even occur in patients who have not yet developed other evidence of thyroid disease. Therefore it is a clinical diagnosis based on the findings of the eyes rather than on laboratory evidence of thyroid dysfunction. Dysthyroid ophthalmopathy is probably the leading cause of unilateral exophthalmos and is the leading cause of bilateral exophthalmos in adults.

Lid retraction, when seen with exophthalmos, is diagnostic of dysthyroid myopathy. Lid retraction by itself, without signs of parkinsonism or dorsal midbrain disease, is also probably caused by dysthyroid myopathy. Computed tomography or magnetic resonance imaging is often used to demonstrate the enlarged extraocular muscles, but orbital echography is more sensitive. Even if these studies do not demonstrate muscle enlargement, they do not exclude the clinical diagnosis of dysthyroid myopathy.

DISTURBANCES OF CONJUGATE EYE MOVEMENTS

Patients with a disturbance of conjugate eye movements commonly do not have symptoms, in contrast to patients with disconjugate eye movements that produce diplopia. Conjugate eye movement abnormalities are more often recognized by abnormal signs on examination.

There are three types of conjugate eye movement: saccadic, pursuit, and vestibular. Fast eye movements, or saccades, are refixation eye movements that shift the eyes from one object to another. Saccadic eye movements are modulated by a pathway arising in the frontal lobes anterior to the primary motor cortex. The pathway for rightward gaze arises in the left frontal lobe, descends through the internal capsule to the midbrain reticular formation, decussates in the caudal midbrain at the level of the fourth cranial nerve nucleus, and synapses in the right pontine paramedian reticular formation (PPRF). The PPRF is also known as the paraabducens nucleus or the pontine gaze center. The PPRF is the brainstem integrator or the final common pathway for all conjugate horizontal eye movements. From the right-side PPRF the same eye movement output is delivered to the right sixth-nerve nucleus to move the right eye to the right, and, via the medial longitudinal fasciculus, to the medial rectus subnucleus of the left third-nerve nucleus to move the left eye to the right. Thus impulses arising in the left frontal lobe ultimately move the eyes conjugately to the right. Lesions of the frontopontine pathway for saccadic eye movements are common and in the acute phase produce a gaze paresis in which the patient's gaze tends to be tonically deviated in the direction of normal gaze. That is, damage to the left frontal lobe causes a right-side gaze paresis. The patient cannot voluntarily look to the right, and the eyes spontaneously deviate to the left (toward the injured frontal lobe). Although the patient may be able to voluntarily return his or her gaze to the midline, he or she is unable to move the eyes past the midline into the paretic field of gaze. If a single, unilateral lesion is responsible, recovery occurs in a few days or weeks. Consequently, gaze paresis is seen predominantly with acute lesions. During recovery the patient's relaxed gaze returns to the primary position. The eyes can be moved voluntarily in the paretic direction, but this movement often cannot be sustained, and there may be a gaze-evoked nystagmus. Optokinetic nystagmus with the target moving toward the opposite side produces the slow component but no return fast phase. When associated with a hemiparesis, a gaze paresis may be either ipsilateral, indicating a hemispheric lesion, or contralateral, indicating a lesion in the brainstem where the pathway has crossed to the contralateral side.

Pursuit eye movements are modulated by a pathway descending from the occipital cortex close to the lateral ventricle into the midbrain reticular formation to the PPRF. This pathway appears to be uncrossed. A lesion in this pathway produces an absence of optokinetic nystagmus when the target is moving toward the side of the lesion. The lesion may be associated with a homonymous hemianopia on the opposite side. When no homonymous hemianopia is present, the lesion is usually deep in the hemispheric white matter and is more likely to be neoplastic than ischemic.

Conjugate vertical eye movements are bilaterally modulated. They are not usually affected by hemispheric disease unless the disease is bilateral and fairly extensive. Lesions of the pretectum or rostral midbrain tectum produce Parinaud's syndrome (dorsal midbrain syndrome, or Sylvian aqueduct syndrome), consisting of impaired vertical gaze, lid retraction, light-near dissociation of the pupillary reaction, and convergence-retractory nystagmus. Upward gaze progressively diminishes with increasing age, but downward gaze is not affected. Impaired downgaze combined with features of Parkinson's disease is characteristic of progressive supranuclear palsy in which diffuse neuronal degeneration occurs in brainstem motor nuclei.

Impaired vertical movement of a single eye caused by a supranuclear lesion is very uncommon, because of the bilaterality of vertical gaze mechanisms and because of the close anatomic association of the vertical gaze centers in the pretectum and rostral midbrain and the third-nerve nuclei in the rostral midbrain.

Interruption of the medial longitudinal fasciculus between the sixth-nerve nucleus and the contralateral third-nerve nucleus produces an internuclear ophthalmoplegia. On attempted horizontal gaze the ad-

Table 158-2   Types of nystagmus with localizing value and the common location and cause of the responsible lesions

TYPE	COMMON LOCATION	COMMON CAUSES
Up-beat nystagmus	Cerebellar vermis or brainstem, especially cervicomedullary junction	Alcoholic cerebellar degeneration, multiple sclerosis, neoplasm, anticonvulsants and sedatives
Down-beat nystagmus	Cervicomedullary junction, cerebellar vermis	Cranial malformation (Arnold-Chiari), multiple sclerosis, lithium toxicity, anticonvulsants and sedatives, infarction, alcoholic cerebellar degeneration
Periodic alternating nystagmus	Cervicomedullary junction	Cranial malformation, multiple sclerosis
Seesaw nystagmus	Anterior third ventricle	Neoplasm
Convergence-retractory nystagmus	Dorsal midbrain	Neoplasm, multiple sclerosis
Ocular myoclonus	Dentatorubroolivary triangle	Infarction, multiple sclerosis
Ocular flutter and opsoclonus	Cerebellum	Immunologically mediated cerebellar encephalitis, postinfectious, or as a remote effect of neoplasia
Ocular bobbing	Pons	Infarction, toxic or metabolic encephalopathy

ducting eye remains in the primary position or adducts poorly, and the abducting eye exhibits horizontal nystagmus. Since the medial longitudinal fasciculus crosses just rostral to the sixth-nerve nucleus, the interruption is on the side of the eye that fails to adduct. Patients with internuclear ophthalmoplegia may have preserved convergence, demonstrating intact function of the third-nerve nucleus input to the medial rectus. The eyes are usually aligned normally in the primary position, so the patient does not complain of diplopia, although in bilateral cases an exotropia may become evident in the acute stage. The absence of ptosis, with normal pupillary action and vertical eye movements, distinguishes these cases from medial rectus weakness caused by a third-nerve palsy. Unilateral or bilateral internuclear ophthalmoplegia in younger adults is a common manifestation of multiple sclerosis.

Nystagmus and Other Ocular Oscillations

Nystagmus (Table 158-2) is a rhythmic, to-and-fro oscillation of the eyes. Jerk nystagmus has clearly defined slow and fast phases and is named for the fast phase. Pendular nystagmus appears to have equally rapid to-and-fro components. Most cases of pendular nystagmus are congenital. Congenital nystagmus is horizontal in the primary position, remains horizontal in vertical gaze positions, appears to convert to jerk nystagmus on lateral gaze, and is decreased by convergence. Congenital nystagmus produces some decrease in visual acuity but does not produce oscillopsia, the sensation of movement of the environment.

The most common nystagmus is gaze-evoked nystagmus. It is seen when the gaze is sustained in an eccentric position. The slow phase is back toward the primary position, and the fast phase is in the direction of gaze. Gaze-evoked nystagmus may be present on lateral gaze only or also on upgaze. It is seldom present on downgaze. Gaze-evoked nystagmus is a physiologic nystagmus that is more likely to be seen when the patient is subjected to external factors such as fatigue, drugs, and head trauma. This type of nystagmus has no localizing significance unless it is markedly asymmetric, in which case a brainstem lesion may be suspected.

Vestibular nystagmus may be the result of injury to the peripheral vestibular apparatus or nerve or injury to the central vestibular pathways. Vestibular nystagmus is present in the primary position and is increased in amplitude when the eyes are moved in the direction of the fast component. This nystagmus is usually horizontal but always has some torsional component, and it remains horizontal even on upgaze. If the lesion is peripheral, the direction of apparent environmental spin is the same as the fast phase of the nystagmus, while the patient past-points and falls toward the side of the slow component. These relationships may not be maintained when the lesion is in the brainstem. Peripheral lesions are more likely to be associated with tinnitus and hearing loss and are more likely to produce acute symptoms and associated nausea and vomiting.

Several varieties of nystagmus are less common but are more important because they provide specific localizing information and are very likely to be associated with an active process producing acquired changes in the central nervous system. These varieties of nystagmus all exhibit nystagmus in the primary position and are often associated with oscillopsia. Although most of these cases occur with injury anywhere in the brainstem or cerebellum, each is most commonly associated with a lesion in one specific location.

Down-beat nystagmus is present in the primary position. It may be accentuated by downgaze but is most accentuated by moving the eyes to the side and down. Down-beat nystagmus is most commonly associated with a disturbance at the cervicomedullary junction, for example, Arnold-Chiari malformation.

Up-beat nystagmus occurs in two varieties. The first type is a relatively fine up-beating nystagmus in the primary position that increases on downgaze. Like down-beating nystagmus, it is most often associated with a lesion of the medulla. A more coarse up-beating nystagmus that increases on upgaze is seen in association with injury to the anterior vermis of the cerebellum and is commonly seen with alcoholic cerebellar degeneration.

Periodic alternating nystagmus is a horizontal jerk nystagmus that periodically changes direction. It begins with a brief period of no nystagmus lasting a few seconds. Then there is beating to one side, with increasing amplitude followed by decreasing amplitude, until the nystagmus ceases for a few seconds, followed by the same crescendo-decrescendo pattern beating in the other direction. The entire cycle typically lasts 3 to 4 minutes. Periodic alternating nystagmus is also most commonly associated with injury to the medulla.

Convergence-retractory nystagmus is a feature of the dorsal midbrain syndrome; thus there is associated impaired upgaze. With attempts to look up, especially attempted saccadic upward eye movements, there is a cocontraction of all the extraocular muscles, producing convergence of the two eyes and retraction of the eyes into the orbit. This nystagmus is best elicited with an optokinetic nystagmus target moving downward, which induces downward pursuit movements and repetitive upward saccades that evoke convergence-retractory nystagmus.

Ocular myoclonus describes rhythmic, pendular vertical eye movements, which sometimes accompany palatal myoclonus. These findings indicate disruption of the pathway between the red nucleus, the ipsilateral inferior olivary nucleus, the contralateral dentate nucleus of the cerebellum, and the red nucleus again.

Ocular flutter and opsoclonus are saccadic intrusions during which saccades interrupt fixation. Ocular flutter is a brief flurry of horizontal saccades around fixation; opsoclonus is a burst of conjugate saccadic eye movements in random directions. Both findings are indicative of a lesion in the cerebellar pathways within the cerebellum or brainstem.

Ocular bobbing describes a rapid downward movement of the eyes, followed after a short, variable delay by a slow drift of the eyes back to the primary position. This is most often seen in comatose patients with extensive pontine damage. Similar movements with different patterns have been called reverse bobbing when the eyes have a quick movement upward and a slow movement back to the primary position or inverse bobbing when the eyes drift downward followed by a quick movement upward. Inverse bobbing is associated with metabolic encephalopathy.

BIBLIOGRAPHY

Beck RW, Cleary PA, Anderson MMJ et al: A randomized, controlled trial of corticosteroids in the treatment of acute optic neuritis, *N Engl J Med* 326:581-588, 1992.

Beck RW, Cleary PA, Trobe JD et al: The effect of corticosteroids for acute optic neuritis on the subsequent development of multiple sclerosis, *N Engl J Med* 329:1764-1769, 1993.

Beck RW, Trobe JD, for the Optic Neuritis Study Group: What we have learned from the optic neuritis treatment trial, *Ophthalmology* 102:1504-1508, 1995.

Bruno A, Jones WL, Austin JK et al: Vascular outcome in men with asymptomatic retinal cholesterol emboli: a cohort study, *Ann Intern Med* 122:249-253, 1995.

Burde RM, Savino PJ, Trobe JD: *Clinical decisions in neuro-ophthalmology*, St Louis, 1993, Mosby.

Chrousos G, Kattah J, Beck R et al: Side effects of glucocorticoid treatment: experience of the Optic Neuritis Treatment Trial, *JAMA* 269:2110-2112, 1993.

Kupersmith MJ et al: Megadose corticosteroids in multiple sclerosis, *Neurology* 44:1-4, 1994.

Leigh RJ, Zee DS: *The neurology of eye movement*, Philadelphia, 1991, FA Davis.

Paton D, Hyman BN, Justice J Jr: *Introduction to ophthalmoscopy*, Kalamazoo, Mich, 1976, The Upjohn Company.

Slamovits TL, Burde R: *Neuro-ophthalmology*, London, 1994, Mosby-Year Book.

Streifler JY, Eliasziw M, Benavente OR et al: The risk of stroke in patients with first-ever retinal vs. hemispheric transient ischemic attacks and high-grade carotid stenosis, *Arch Neurol* 52:246-249, 1995.

CHAPTER

159 Neurology of the Lower Urinary Tract

Frances M. Dyro

INNERVATION OF THE LOWER URINARY TRACT

Bladder function depends on the interplay of sacral parasympathetics, thoracic sympathetics, motor neurons in Onuf's nucleus, and pontine micturition centers. Cortical regions 6 and 9 of the frontal lobes impose voluntary control over voiding reflexes. The peripheral innervation of the lower urinary tract consists of preganglionic parasympathetic fibers that travel with the pelvic nerves through the inferior hypogastric plexus, then synapse with postganglionic neurons distributed in ganglionic clumps in the adventitia of the detrusor and internal sphincter. Sympathetic fibers originating in the lower thoracic and upper lumbar segments descend along the aorta to form the superior hypogastric plexus. These act to contract the internal sphincter during ejaculation, preventing retrograde ejaculation. The pudendal nerve, supplying the external rhabdosphincter, arises from the anterior primary rami of S2, S3, and S4, with pelvic floor efferents deriving mainly from the S3 and S4 motor roots. The nerve also carries afferents from the posterior urethra. Sensation of bladder fullness as well as painful impulses from the bladder dome and trigone travel along the pelvic nerve.

BLADDER ANATOMY

The bladder is composed of a meshwork of smooth-muscle fibers forming the detrusor and the internal sphincter. The contractile properties of smooth and striated muscle are similar, but the velocity of shortening and rate of relaxation are much slower in smooth muscles. The smooth-muscle cells form "tight junctions" representing low-resistance extrasynaptic pathways of excitation (electrical rather than pharmacologic). Distention and stretch of the smooth muscle lowers its transmembrane potential, rendering the muscle cells hyperexcitable as the bladder fills. There is also a nonneural component of bladder tonus attributable to the elastic properties of smooth muscle and collagen.

BLADDER FILLING

Urination is a phenomenon that can be considered in two phases. During the filling phase the detrusor muscle of the bladder is relaxed, and the internal and external sphincters are contracted. The detrusor is kept relaxed by inhibition by parasympathetic cholinergic nerve impulses and stimulation of sympathetic β-adrenergic impulses. Sphincter and pelvic floor muscle contraction is a function of somatic nerves and sympathetic α-adrenergic receptors in the proximal urethra and bladder neck.

Filling of the bladder stimulates the stretch receptors in the detrusor muscle. Afferent information from the stretch receptors is conveyed to the central nervous system via pelvic nerves. This may produce increased efferent discharges in the preganglionic nerves of the thoracolumbar sympathetic outflow, which inhibits efferent transmission across pelvic ganglia. This promotes bladder filling by β-adrenergically mediated relaxation of the detrusor. α-Adrenergic effects increase tone in the proximal urethra.

BLADDER EMPTYING

The normal emptying, or micturition, phase begins when the bladder neck smooth muscle and the striated external sphincter relax in response to inhibition of α-adrenergic impulses. Contraction of the detrusor smooth muscle then occurs in response to parasympathetic cholinergic stimulation. This sequence is coordinated by nuclei in the dorsal tegmentum of the pons. Failure of the sphincters to relax as the detrusor contracts is called *dyssynergia*. Continence has active and passive components. Passive continence is a result of resting tonus of the somatic innervated striated sphincters, α-adrenergic innervated smooth muscle, and the elastin and collagen of the urethra and pelvic floor. Active continence is the result of voluntary contraction of the sphincter and pelvic floor muscles. Key features and treatment of the major categories of bladder-emptying dysfunction are summarized in Table 159-1.

Reflexes

The baseline activity of muscles of the pelvic floor and the striated sphincter mechanism increases during rises in intraabdominal pressure (Valsalva's maneuver or cough), with stimulation of the perineum, and with bladder filling. During micturition this reflex activity is inhibited. In lesions below the pons but above the sacral segments there is dyssynergia or inappropriate contraction of the sphincter.

PHARMACOLOGY

Anticholinergic agents such as propantheline, imipramine, atropine, and hyoscyamine block muscarinic receptors and inhibit detrusor contractions. These may be used therapeutically to control the urgency and frequency resulting from uninhibited contractions of the bladder. Anticholinergic agents used in the treatment of Parkinson's disease may produce urinary retention by inhibiting detrusor contractions; cholinergics such as bethanechol stimulate muscarinic receptors, increasing detrusor tone and contractile force in cases in which poor detrusor contraction results in incomplete emptying.

Adrenergic agents such as levarterenol, ephedrine, and phenylephrine stimulate α- and β-adrenergic receptors, causing relaxation of detrusor but tightening of the bladder neck.

Oxybutynin is a smooth-muscle relaxant with adrenergic properties that increases bladder capacity and decreases uninhibited contractions. Drugs used for other reasons may produce bladder dysfunction. Tricyclic antidepressants with anticholinergic properties and calcium channel blockers may produce urinary retention by decreasing detrusor contractibility. Some sympathomimetic agents such as pseudoephedrine and phenylpropanolamine, which are found in cough remedies, can increase urethral resistance. α-Adrenergic antagonists such as prazosin may be used to lower urethral resistance in prostatic obstruction.

VOIDING DYSFUNCTION
Aging

Voiding dysfunction, incontinence, or inability to empty the bladder may result from neurologic, structural, or mechanical abnormalities (Chapter 123). Many structural changes occur with aging. Bladder capacity may be reduced below the lower limit of normal (400 ml).

Table 159-1   Key features and treatment of the major categories of bladder-emptying dysfunction

DYSFUNCTION	SITE OF LESION	VOIDING PATTERN	TREATMENT
Detrusor hyperactivity			
Coordinated sphincter	Cerebrum or basal ganglia, dementia, Parkinson's, cerebrovascular accident, multiple sclerosis	Urgency, urge incontinence voiding without awareness	Anticholinergics
External sphincter dyssynergia	Suprasacral spinal cord	Incomplete emptying, low volume, uninhibited contractions	Anticholinergics, intermittent catheterization
Internal sphincter dyssynergia	Cord lesion above T6-12	Incomplete emptying, autonomic dysreflexia	Phenoxybenzamine, anticholinergics
Detrusor areflexia			
Coordinated sphincter	Sacral cord or cauda equina	Interrupted flow, voiding by straining	Bethanechol, intermittent catheterization, credé
External sphincter overactivity	Sacral cord	Decreased sensation of fullness, voiding by straining	Bethanechol, diazepam, intermittent catheterization
External sphincter denervation	Sacral cord, peripheral nerves, cauda equina	Incontinence, large residual urine	Intermittent catheterization
Poor relaxation of smooth-muscle sphincter	Sacral cord	High capacity	Phenoxybenzamine, bethanechol

Uninhibited contractions may occur, giving a sense of urgency and uncontrollable loss of varying amounts of urine. This phenomenon is often accompanied by inefficient detrusor contractions, resulting in incomplete emptying and frequent urinary tract infections because of high residual urine volumes.

The outflow obstruction caused by benign prostatic hypertrophy in turn can produce supersensitivity to a range of different agonists of the smooth muscle, analogous to denervation supersensitivity. The patient reports urgency and frequency but a decreased stream and incomplete emptying as a result of the detrusor instability and poor contractions. Following prostatic surgery, incontinence may result from injury to striated or smooth-muscle sphincters and continued detrusor irritability.

In elderly women weakened pelvic musculature, damage to the striated sphincter during childbirth, or tissue changes attributable to estrogen deficiency result in incontinence during any activity that increases intraabdominal pressure (stress incontinence).

Cortical Disease

In cortical disease (cerebrovascular accident, Parkinson's disease, diffuse atherosclerotic disease or dementias) there may be loss of cortical inhibitory impulses to the bladder. The patient feels the desire to void but is unable to prevent voiding by inhibiting reflex contractions.

ABNORMALITIES OF INNERVATION
Neuropathic Bladder

If sensory pathways are interrupted between sacral spinal neurons and cortical centers, there may be loss of sensation of bladder fullness. If the sphincters are functioning, overflow incontinence results when bladder pressure exceeds pressure generated by sphincter contraction. This results in chronic infection because there is always a high residual urine volume. Intermittent catheterization usually results in a reduction in urinary tract infections and dryness.

Motor Paralytic Bladder

The atonic neurogenic bladder is often caused by the peripheral neuropathy of diabetes or alcoholism but may be the result of trauma or pelvic surgery. Sphincter weakness may be caused by damage to pudendal nerves or sacral roots or by trauma during childbirth or with perineal injuries. Myasthenia gravis and Shy-Drager syndrome have been reported to cause striated sphincter weakness.

Dyssynergia

Outflow obstruction occurs when the detrusor contraction fails to inhibit sphincter contraction. This dyssynergia is seen in spinal cord and bilateral cortical lesions. The simultaneous contraction of the de-

✔ **WHEN TO REFER**

Function of the lower urinary tract is the result of a complex interplay between physical and neurologic factors. Malfunction can occur at many levels. Treatment depends on the type of abnormality. A review of the patient's medications may reveal iatrogenic voiding dysfunction that is correctible. Management of stress incontinence of mild degree may involve Kegel exercises to improve pelvic muscle tone, estrogen replacement, or simply the use of absorbant pads. More severe incontinence may require surgical treatment, as does medication-unresponsive prostatic disease.

Voiding dysfunction in association with spinal cord injury, demyelinating disease, or degenerative disorders should be managed by using a team approach that incorporates the input of the internist, neurologist, and urologist. Adult onset of urinary or fecal incontinence can be devastating to the patient and his or her family but, when understood, may be corrected or improved with treatment.

trusor and sphincters gives rise to incomplete emptying and reflux. If it is not detected, hydroureter and hydronephrosis with renal damage may result.

Autonomic dysreflexia is seen in complete neurologic lesions above the T5 level and is usually a result of bladder overdistention or urethral instrumentation. The exaggerated sympathetic response gives a huge rise in diastolic and systolic blood pressure, producing headache and even intracranial bleeding. Minor symptoms of autonomic dysreflexia such as sweating in normally innervated areas may be helped by an adrenergic blockade.

Neurourologic techniques are available for the study of the voiding mechanism. A urodynamic study begins with uroflowmetry, in which the patient urinates into a commode fitted with a sensor that measures rate and volume of urine flow. The bladder is then catheterized to measure the amount of residual urine. An electromyographic needle electrode is placed in the sphincter to give information about the presence or absence of denervation and to monitor the level of muscle activity. The catheter is slowly moved through the urethra while measurements of pressure are made. This procedure indicates the length of the active sphincter mechanism ("the continence zone") and the maximum resistance. During bladder filling, pressure within the bladder and sphincter activity are monitored. At capacity the sphincter should relax completely as the detrusor contracts, emptying the bladder smoothly and completely. Measurements may also be made of the sacral reflex arc. This measurement is obtained by electrically stimulating the perineum and measuring a two-component response from the sphincter. This analog of the blink reflex is a measure of the integrity of the sacral cord and roots. Somatosensory evoked potentials may be obtained by stimulating the pudendal nerve and recording over the cortex or by magnetic stimulation of the cortex while recording from the external sphincter in suspected cord injury or demyelinating disease. Sensory conduction velocity of the pudendal nerve may be measured to evaluate neuropathy. Magnetic resonance imaging of the lumbosacral spinal cord is helpful when an occult dysraphism or degenerative process is suspected.

BIBLIOGRAPHY

Berger AR et al: Myasthenia gravis presenting as uncontrollable flatus and urinary/fecal incontinence, *Muscle Nerve* 19:113-114, 1996.

Dyro FM: Electrophysiology of the lower urinary tract. In Yalla SV et al, editors: *Neurourology and urodynamics*, New York, 1988, Macmillan.

Ertekin C et al: Examination of the descending pathway to the external anal sphincter and pelvic floor muscles by transcranial cortical stimulation. *Electroencephalogr Clin Neurophysiol* 75:500, 1990.

Fowler CJ: Bladder dysfunction in multiple sclerosis: causes and treatment, *Int Multiple Sclerosis J* 1:99-107, 1994.

Grand Round: Science of urinary incontinence: University College London, *Lancet* 344:311-314, 1994.

Resnick NM, Yalla SV, Laurino E: The pathophysiology of urinary incontinence among institutionalized elderly persons, *N Eng J Med* 320:1, 1989.

Thind P: The significance of smooth and striated muscles in the sphincter function of the urethra in healthy women, *Neurourol Urodyn* 14:585-618, 1995.

CHAPTER

160 Neurooncology

Amy A. Pruitt

INTRACRANIAL NEOPLASMS
Incidence

Intracranial neoplasms are the second most common neurologic cause of death, next to stroke. In 1993, 17,500 new primary brain tumors were reported in the United States. Since a high percentage of primary brain tumors are malignant and since most metastatic tumors are unresectable, inexorable clinical deterioration is the course for most patients. Both neurologists and internists are asked to treat increasing numbers of neurologic cancers because of more successful treatment of systemic malignancies. Recent advances in diagnostic techniques and in perioperative management of cerebral edema have resulted in valuable palliative therapy for these tumors.

Adequate clinical management of neurologic cancer requires (1) recognition of signs and symptoms suggesting intracranial neoplasm; (2) early use of appropriate diagnostic tests to distinguish tumor from other causes of progressive neurologic dysfunction, such as metabolic derangement, infection, and subdural hematoma; (3) efficient exclusion of systemic malignancy prior to directing the patient to a neurosurgeon for biopsy; (4) appropriate use of medication to control cerebral edema and seizures; and (5) recognition of the medical problems to which these patients are prone both from their tumor and from its treatment.

Pathophysiology

The symptoms and signs caused by brain tumors are determined by their size, location, invasiveness, and rate of growth. Brain tumors produce focal disturbances of function by infiltrating or compressing brain tissue. When the tumor becomes large enough, the mass and its associated edema may result in more generalized neurologic dysfunction from raised intracranial pressure. Symptoms of tumor masses reflect expansion within a fixed bony vault into space normally occupied by brain, blood, and cerebrospinal fluid (CSF). Although the brain can accommodate the presence of slow-growing tumors, both benign and malignant masses larger than 3 cm in diameter increase the intracranial pressure. The increased pressure in the subarachnoid space surrounding the optic nerves impairs venous and lymphatic drainage and causes papilledema. Vessels associated with a growing tumor contain gaps or fenestrations through which a plasma filtrate escapes, producing "vasogenic cerebral edema" and greatly increasing the effective tumor volume. If brainstem structures become distorted or if the pressure becomes high enough to impair cerebral blood flow, stupor and coma result.

As brain tissue is compressed, it may herniate under the falx cerebri or through the tentorium that forms immobile divisions between the various intracranial compartments. Decompression of the spinal subarachnoid space by lumbar puncture accentuates the pressure gradient and may precipitate brain herniation.

Clinical Findings

Based on the mechanisms discussed earlier, brain tumors may produce both focal deficits and more generalized, or "nonlocalizing," disturbances in brain function. Headache, the initial symptom in 50% of patients with brain tumors, results from traction on pain-sensitive dura, blood vessels, or cranial nerves caused by edema, intracranial hypertension, hydrocephalus, or local compression. In most patients with supratentorial tumor, this pain radiates to the side of the tumor, while posterior fossa masses elicit retroorbital or nuchal pain. Tumors of the frontal and temporal lobes can grow very large before producing symptoms, and such symptoms may be quite nonspecific. Subtle, progressive disturbances of mentation and memory, or simply apathy and drowsiness, may be noted.

Seizures are the initial symptom in 20% of patients with brain tumors. Any adult with a first seizure that is not readily explainable on other grounds is a brain tumor suspect. Occasionally the first symptom is an event simulating a transient ischemic attack.

Tumors of the posterior fossa produce specific, progressive signs and symptoms. Rapidly growing tumors may cause obstructive hydrocephalus, resulting in headache, vomiting, lethargy, abducens nerve palsies, and papilledema. More slowly growing tumors give rise to a unilateral sixth-nerve deficit along with a combination of progressive unilateral hearing loss, facial weakness, and facial pain or numbness, a symptom complex suggestive of a lesion in the cerebellopontine angle. Gait ataxia results from cerebellar tumor, and nuchal or occipital head pain along with corticospinal signs develop with further tumor enlargement and encroachment on brainstem connections.

Tumors typically produce a gradual, progressive loss of function. Metastatic tumors are more likely to produce symptoms that evolve in days to weeks, or even in minutes as in the case of such hemorrhagic tumors as melanoma, hypernephroma, lung carcinoma, and choriocarcinoma. In contrast, a careful history in patients with primary brain tumors may disclose subtle personality changes or partial seizures that antedate the diagnosis by months or years.

Laboratory Evaluation

Contrast-enhanced computed tomography (CT) and magnetic resonance imaging (MRI) have largely replaced the combination of skull radiograph, electroencephalogram, radionuclide brain scan, and arteriography as the principal diagnostic tests for the evaluation of patients with suspected brain tumor.

CT scan without contrast enhancement detects tumors whose density exceeds that of normal brain parenchyma, including meningioma, melanoma, and primary cerebral lymphoma; tumors with spontaneous hemorrhage; and hydrocephalus produced by masses obstructing the ventricular system. The use of iodinated contrast is essential in detecting intracranial neoplasms and outlines the tumors as homogeneous or ring-enhancing masses surrounded by variable amounts of edema. Ringlike enhancement can occur in conditions other than tumor such as abscesses, recent cerebral infarctions, the plaques of multiple sclerosis, and certain vascular malformations. An initially negative CT scan is sometimes found in patients with glial tumors, meningeal carcinomatosis, metastases, and primary brain lymphoma, but repetition of the scan 4 to 6 weeks later, when the clinical circumstances remain highly suspicious for tumor, usually detects the lesion. An MRI should be obtained as well.

MRI usually is more sensitive than CT for evaluating central nervous (CNS) neoplasms. In situations in which only nonspe-

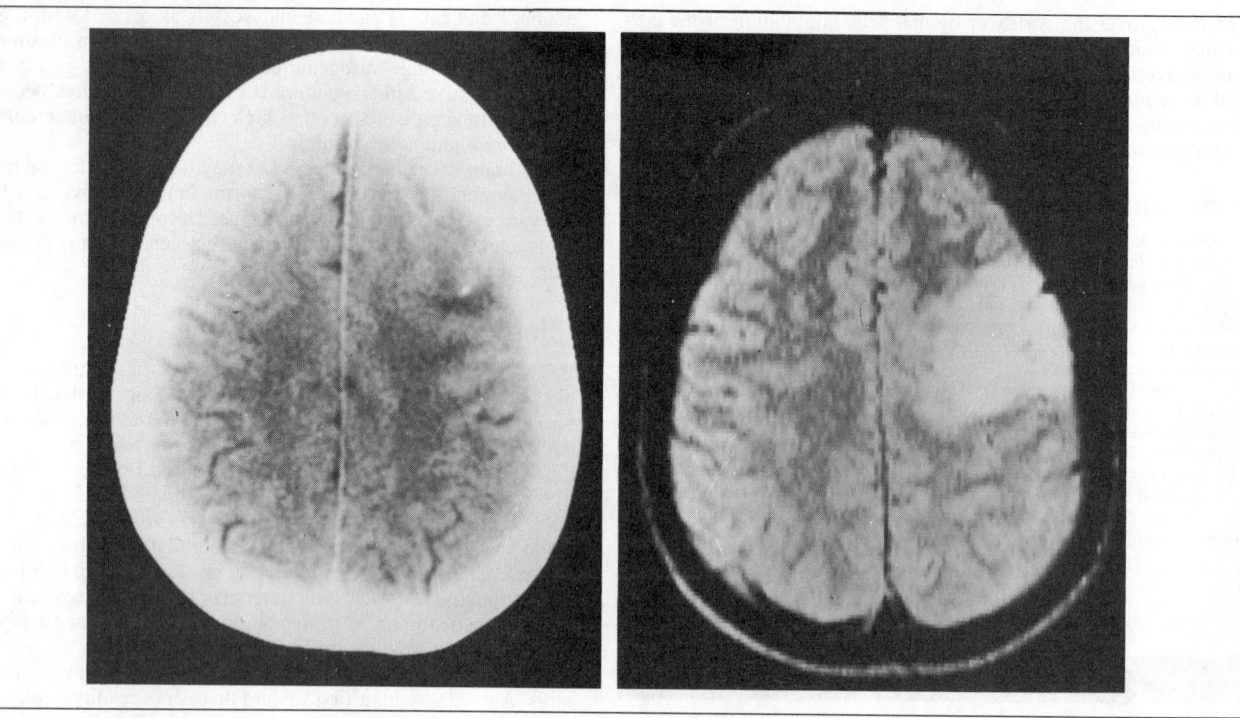

FIGURE 160-1 This oligodendroglioma appears as a small area of hypodensity with calcium on computed tomography (CT) *(left)* but as a much larger area of T2-weighted signal abnormality on magnetic resonance imaging (MRI) *(right)*. Contrast images (not shown) showed no enhancement on either CT or MRI that was consistent with the low-grade histologic findings on biopsy.

cific mass effect can be discerned on CT, MRI can more fully define the extent of infiltrating tumor. The ability of MRI to detect small amounts of increased brain water content allows assessment of the full extent of tumor and its surrounding edema. High-resolution, high-contrast images of the brain in axial, coronal, and sagittal planes allow for three-dimensional assessment of tumor volume and location for surgical and radiation therapy planning (Fig. 160-1). Administration of the paramagnetic contrast agent gadolinium diethylene-triamine pentaacetic acid (gadolinium DTPA) further defines tumor vascularity and the degree of blood-brain barrier breakdown, which often correlates with histologic malignancy (Fig. 160-2).

MRI specifically may be better than CT for the assessment of tumors at the skull base, pineal region, posterior fossa, and spinal cord. Large arteries and veins associated with the tumor may be well demonstrated, obviating arteriography in some cases. Subacute or remote hemorrhage has a characteristic MRI appearance (shortened T1 signal; see Chapter 108), allowing distinction between tumor and arteriovenous malformations and suggesting tumor histology in those tumors prone to hemorrhage, such as melanoma, choriocarcinoma, and metastases of lung and renal origin. Fat-containing tumors, such as epidermoids and lipomas, may be well outlined. Cysts can be evaluated to determine if their characteristics match those of CSF (arachnoid cyst, porencephalic region) or differ from those of CSF (cystic astrocytoma).

Arteriography provides selective visualization of intracranial arteries. Some malignant tumors are characterized by an angiographic "blush" with early draining veins. Demonstration of the vascular anatomy aids in neurosurgical planning, but the accuracy of MRI, and more recently magnetic resonance angiography (MRA), in defining tumor vascularity has reduced the use of arteriography for this purpose.

Surgery produces specific tissue diagnosis in patients with solitary or multiple intracranial masses. In general, brain masses should be biopsied even if they cannot be excised when the clinical diagnosis is in doubt. In the setting of multiple intracranial masses, a biopsy often follows an unrewarding systemic search for malignancy. This evaluation should include a hemogram, chest x-ray, CT scan of the chest, sputum cytologic studies in a smoker, liver function stud-

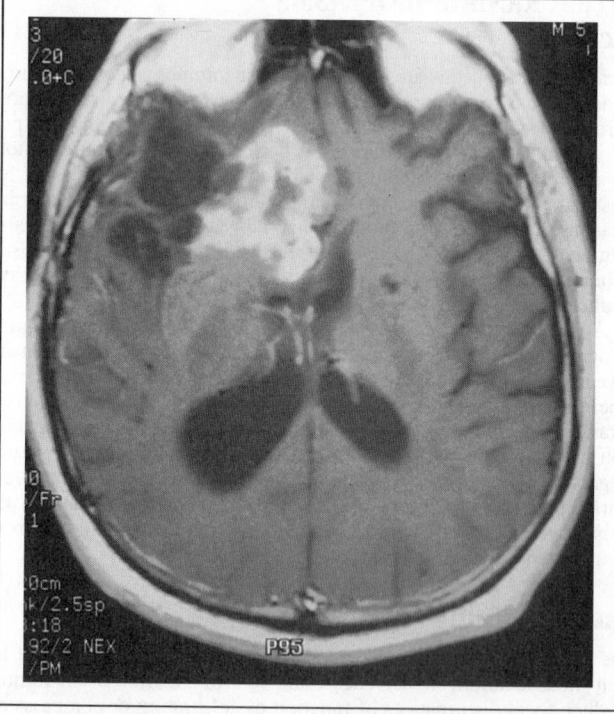

FIGURE 160-2 MRI of a glioblastoma multiforme arising at a site of previously resected low-grade glial neoplasm shows pronounced enhancement of the tumor when gadolinium is administered. The tumor now extends into the corpus callosum.

ies, and carcinoembryonic antigen (CEA) testing. Biopsy is performed through an open craniotomy or by using CT- or MRI-guided stereotactic techniques. Resection may be curative for histologically benign tumors that are surgically accessible, including meningiomas, acoustic neuromas, ependymomas, oligodendrogliomas, pituitary adenomas, and some astrocytomas. Partial resection improves symptoms and seizure control and reduces dependence on corticosteroids.

Preoperative surgical management is based on the need to control cerebral edema and seizures. Corticosteroids may relieve symptoms dramatically within 48 hours of their initiation. Dexamethasone, 10 mg intravenously followed by 4 to 6 mg orally or intramuscularly every 6 hours, is the initial therapy usually recommended. Steroids may not suffice to control symptoms caused by tumors blocking the ventricular system, and emergency ventriculoperitoneal shunting may be required. Anticonvulsants are usually prescribed only for patients who have already had a seizure, but many physicians choose to treat prophylactically.

Management of Primary Brain Tumors

Common primary brain tumors are listed in Table 160-1. In all adult age-groups, malignant astrocytoma or glioblastoma is the most common type of primary tumor. Metastases account for nearly two thirds of intracranial neoplasms treated in general hospitals and are discussed under Systemic Cancer and the Nervous System, later in this chapter.

Anaplastic astrocytoma and *glioblastoma multiforme* represent three fourths of the glial tumors diagnosed yearly in adults in the United States. These highly invasive, rapidly growing tumors commonly occur in the corpus callosum; the frontal, parietal, and temporal lobes; and the thalamus. Peak age of tumor development is between 40 and 70 years, and the tumor is somewhat more common in males. The tumor may be vascular, and CT scan reveals a usually solitary, heterogeneously enhancing lesion. Clinical history may reveal symptomatic changes for several months; however, the clinical history is much shorter if seizures are the presenting feature. If untreated, patients survive only 17 weeks. Surgery is the first line of treatment with an extensive debulking of surgically accessible lesions and biopsy of critically located ones. Recent data suggest that biopsy alone may underestimate the grade of malignancy in glial tumors. Despite refinement in radiotherapeutic schedules, aggressive surgery, and recent chemotherapy, median survival after all available therapeutic modalities is only 62 weeks. Nineteen percent of patients are alive at 18 months from the time of diagnosis. Current chemotherapeutic programs include single-agent chemotherapy (BCNU, CCNU, and cisplatin) and multiagent programs (CCNU, vincristine, and procarbazine). Anaplastic oligodendrogliomas respond particularly well to chemotherapy. Interstitial implantation of tumor with radioactive seeds containing iodine or iridium is also being studied but is applicable only to a small subset of patients with tumor volumes small enough for implantation and with a possibly better prognosis because of small size alone.

Several reports suggest that stereotactic radiosurgery using a gamma knife or modified linear accelerator more than doubles survival time for patients with anaplastic astrocytoma or glioblastoma multiforme. Tumors must be volumetrically appropriate for this therapy, and a high percentage of patients require reoperation for radiation necrosis. Patients with recurrent malignant glial tumors also may benefit from stereotactic radiosurgery.

Well-differentiated astrocytomas (formerly grades I and II) occur throughout the brain and spinal cord and slowly infiltrate the white matter of these areas. Subcortical white matter of the hemispheres is the most common location in adults, while optic nerve, cerebellum, and brainstem are the usual locations in children. These tumors are avascular and on CT or MRI appear as indistinct masses with little or no contrast enhancement. The tumors may evolve over several years. Excision is curative for some cerebellar, optic nerve, and lobar astrocytomas. Biopsy is recommended for all suspected low-grade astrocytomas with surgical resection if the tumor is favorably located. Biopsy confirms diagnosis and identifies patients with anaplastic tumors that do not enhance on CT or MRI. Cyst drainage and partial resection are feasible for many supratentorial tumors. Median life expectancy is 67 months with tumors in supratentorial locations and 89

Table 160-1 Adult primary brain tumors: Distribution of tumor types

TUMOR	PATIENTS (%)	MEAN AGE AT DIAGNOSIS (YEARS)
Glioblastoma	40	54
Astrocytoma	16	37
Meningioma	18	55
Schwannoma	2	57
Pituitary adenoma	12	39
Lymphoma	2	46
Other	10	—

From Continuum. In *Neuro-oncology*, vol 1, no 2, Cleveland, 1994, Advanstar Communications.
Data from Laws ER, Thapar K: *CA Cancer J Clin* 43:263, 1993; Boring CC, Squires TS, Tong T: *CA Cancer J Clin* 43:7, 1993.

months when the growth is in the cerebellum. Chemotherapy has no established role. The timing of radiation therapy of low-grade astrocytomas remains controversial and is under investigation in multicenter protocols that also address long-term cognitive effects of radiation therapy.

Meningioma is the only brain tumor more common in women and represents 20% of intracranial masses. These tumors are generally benign histologically, although they can invade adjacent skull; since meningiomas may involve critical brain structures or blood vessels, they sometimes cannot be completely removed. The mass is frequently quite round and hyperdense with respect to surrounding brain tissue on the unenhanced CT scan with homogeneous enhancement after contrast administration. An arteriogram may reveal striking vascularity, with some of the blood supply coming from external carotid artery branches. Common sites are in the midline along the falx, the olfactory groove, the tuberculum sellae, the foramen magnum, the sphenoid ridge, and along the lateral cerebral convexity and tentorium of the cerebellum. Resection is both diagnostic and curative for subfrontal, intraventricular, and parasagittal tumors. Incompletely excised tumors and those with more invasive histologic features are sometimes irradiated.

Recent data suggest an increased incidence of *primary central nervous system lymphoma* (PCNSL), in part because of the increased frequency of PCNSL in patients with the acquired immunodeficiency syndrome, but the incidence is also increased in apparently immunocompetent individuals. Patients with PCNSL may present with symptoms resulting from intracranial mass lesions, or with symptomatic uveal/vitreal deposits, diffuse meningeal seeding (lymphomatous meningitis), or intradural spinal masses.

PCNSL has a distinctive radiographic appearance with diffusely enhancing lesions, often in a periventricular location. In about 50% of patients the lesions are multifocal. These lesions are highly sensitive to the administration of high-dose glucocorticoids and may disappear entirely. Since lysis of lesions by corticosteroid may result in non-diagnostic biopsy results and since other processes such as multiple sclerosis and sarcoidosis can be improved by steroid administration, steroid use should be deferred, if possible, until histologic confirmation of the diagnosis is obtained.

The surgical approach to PCNSL is different from that used for most primary brain tumors. Surgical resection does not contribute to overall survival with this disease, and patients should have a stereotactic biopsy. At times, the diagnosis can be established by CSF cytologic study or vitreous biopsy. Recent studies have strongly suggested improved survival in patients receiving chemotherapy in addition to cranial irradiation. The chemotherapy is usually administered before radiation therapy, but chemotherapy has been used as the sole therapy for some patients over age 50 years to reduce the high frequency of leukoencephalopathy that occurs when radiation and chemotherapy are used together. Various combinations of methotrexate and high-dose cytosine arabinoside have been roughly comparable in extending median survival to 42 months, compared with 15- to 18-month survival in patients receiving radiation therapy alone.

Tumors of the pineal region include germ cell neoplasms, true tumors of the pineal body (pineocytoma and pineoblastoma), and uncommon presentations of metastatic, glial, and meningeal growths. Recent surgical advances allow more specific histologic diagnosis than previously was possible. Since the prognosis is quite variable and since treatment depends heavily on histology, every effort should be made to refer the patient to a surgeon experienced with surgery in this site. Germ cell tumors include germinomas, endodermal sinus tumors, teratoma, embryonal carcinoma, and choriocarcinoma. Symptoms of such tumors may involve diabetes insipidus, bitemporal visual field defects, headache caused by hydrocephalus, failure of upward gaze, and pupillary abnormalities. Germinomas may be very sensitive to relatively small amounts of radiation, but other histologic types have worse prognoses and may seed the cranial and spinal nerves. Pineocytoma and the more primitive pineoblastoma are treated with radical surgical excision. Both tend to recur, and some recent successes with chemotherapy have been reported.

Most previously discussed types of tumor can occur in the posterior fossa. However, several histologic types are specific to this region. *Medulloblastoma,* one type of primitive neuroectodermal tumor, is commonly located in the midline cerebellum and presents with headache and ataxia. Removal of the tumor is the first step in treatment, followed by lumbar puncture and gadolinium-enhanced MRI of the spinal cord to detect spinal seeding. Radiation is given to the posterior fossa and to the neuraxis. Chemotherapy has been somewhat successful in controlling recurrent tumors. Commonly used regimens include nitrogen mustard, vincristine, procarbazine, and prednisone (MOPP); and lomustine, vincristine, and methotrexate. *Ependymomas* are glial tumors occurring largely in childhood and young adulthood; their typical intracranial location is at the fourth ventricle. After resection of tumor, sampling of spinal fluid, and radiation to the cranium or whole neuraxis (depending on CSF results), 5-year survival is nearly 70%.

Acoustic neuroma is a benign tumor composed of the cells covering the acoustic nerve as it leaves the brain through the internal auditory meatus. When bilateral, these tumors suggest the central form of neurofibromatosis. Early detection is essential, as hearing may be spared when the tumor is removed while it is still confined to the canal. Brainstem auditory-evoked potentials, CT, MRI, and metrizamide or air cisternography have greatly accelerated diagnosis of such tumors. Patients with progressive unilateral hearing loss should be referred to a neurologist for further investigation.

Benign Intracranial Hypertension (Pseudotumor Cerebri)

Benign intracranial hypertension is an idiopathic syndrome of increased intracranial pressure manifested by headache, papilledema, sixth-nerve palsies, and progressive visual loss. The syndrome is most often seen in obese adolescent females. Although the majority of cases are of unknown cause, associated clinical settings include pregnancy, corticosteroid administration, sex hormone use, adrenal and parathyroid disorders, venous sinus thrombosis, and use of vitamin A, tetracycline, or nalidixic acid.

The CT or MRI scan commonly shows small, "slitlike" lateral ventricles, and the CSF is found to be under elevated pressure, often with a low spinal fluid protein level. The syndrome may resolve spontaneously over several months, although it may take as long as 2 years. However, the pressure on the optic nerve can lead to permanent visual loss.

Repeated lumbar punctures, initially at daily intervals, to lower the pressure to less than 180 mm Hg are the appropriate treatment. This treatment provides symptomatic relief, although lumbar-peritoneal shunting may be required when vision is seriously threatened. Adrenal corticosteroids, acetazolamide, furosemide, and oral glycerol have all been advocated, but their efficacy has not been proved.

SYSTEMIC CANCER AND THE NERVOUS SYSTEM

Neurologic complications are common in patients with systemic cancer, largely because improved therapy has resulted in longer survival. Metastatic complications have increased along with adverse effects of the therapy itself. One third of cancer patients are found at autopsy to have metastatic, infectious, or vascular complications affecting the nervous system.

Clinical Findings

Metastatic Complications. The clinical findings arising from metastasis to various elements of the nervous system are outlined in Table 160-2 and have, in large part, been discussed earlier. The hallmarks of cerebral metastasis are headache, mental status changes, seizures, focal motor or sensory signs, and papilledema.

Table 160-2   Metastatic complications of cancer

	INTRACRANIAL	SPINAL	MENINGEAL	NERVES, ROOTS, PLEXUS
Clinical findings	Headache Seizures Mental status changes Focal signs Papilledema	Back pain Weakness Bladder dysfunction Sensory loss Increased DTRs Babinski's signs	Cranial nerve findings: Diplopia, bulbar palsy Spinal root findings: Weakness, areflexia, bladder dysfunction Hydrocephalus: Headache, mental status changes	Pain Cranial nerve palsies Brachial plexus: C7, C8, T1 palsy; Horner's syndrome; extremity edema Lumbosacral plexus: Extremity pain with weakness and sensory loss in multiple segmental pattern; unilateral
Radiographic and laboratory findings	CT, MRI	Spine x-ray Bone scan Myelogram: block MRI: block	MRI, CT: Hydrocephalus CSF: Low glucose, elevated protein levels Cytology: Malignant cells Myelogram: Nodules	Skull x-ray: Erosion Tomography: Erosion MRI, CT: Mass lesion
Differential diagnosis	Primary CNS tumor Cerebral hemorrhage Cerebral infarction Cerebral abscess	Primary cord tumor Radiation myelopathy Herniated disk Epidural hematoma	Peripheral neuropathy Myopathy Chronic fungal meningitis	Radiation effects Radiation-induced neoplasm Surgical trauma
Common primary tumors	Lung Breast Melanoma Genitourinary Leukemia Lymphoma Gastrointestinal	Breast Lung Prostate Kidney Lymphoma Myeloma Melanoma	Leukemia Breast Lymphoma Lung Melanoma	Breast Lung Lymphoma Prostate Head and neck

CSF, Cerebrospinal fluid; *CT,* computed tomogram; *DTRs,* deep tendon reflexes; *MRI,* magnetic resonance imaging.

Pathophysiology

The nervous system complications of cancer can be classified as metastatic or nonmetastatic (Box 160-1). Direct neoplastic invasion of the brain, meninges, spinal roots, or peripheral nerves causes most of the neurologic symptoms. Spinal epidural metastases are also common and are manifested as a myelopathy (see Chapter 146). Metabolic effects occur owing to the failure of other organs (e.g., liver, lungs). Increased susceptibility to nervous system infections results from altered host resistance as a consequence of either the tumor itself or its treatment. Cerebrovascular disorders are common in cancer patients. Multiple cerebral infarctions are the most common pathology and may result from septic embolization or nonbacterial thrombotic endocarditis. Disseminated intravascular coagulation (DIC) and intracerebral hemorrhage are more common in patients with leukemia or lymphoma than in those with solid tumors, coagulopathies being the major risk factor for these patients. Like DIC, multiple cerebral infarctions may present either in a focal, strokelike series of events or with diffuse, progressive encephalopathy. Moreover, direct toxic effects of chemotherapeutic agents and radiation therapy may cause persistent neurologic disability, even in the patient who has no residual tumor. Finally, occasional patients manifest one of the "remote" effects of cancer that are presumably caused by toxic or metabolic influences of the primary neoplasm (Box 160-2).

Sixty percent of cerebral metastases occur in the setting of previously diagnosed systemic cancer. Cancers of lung in men and breast in women account for the largest absolute number of metastases, although melanoma is the tumor with the highest likelihood of spread to the central nervous system. Twenty percent of patients with cerebral metastasis have neurologic symptoms predating the diagnosis of the primary malignancy, which is most often in the lung. Multiple metastases are present in half of all cases.

Contrast-enhanced MRI is the procedure of choice for the diagnosis of cerebral metastases. MRI should be done as part of the initial or pretreatment evaluation for three groups of patients. (1) Patients with lung carcinoma for whom curative lobectomy is planned require a preoperative MRI. (2) Patients with small-cell lung carcinoma should have scanning before prophylactic cranial radiation. (3) Patients with widely disseminated melanoma, breast, or testicular tumors about to undertake an aggressive chemotherapy regimen should have MRI as part of their staging evaluation. Patients for whom MRI is contraindicated because of surgical clips or cardiac pacemakers should have a contrast-enhanced CT scan.

An apoplectic onset occurs 5% to 10% of the time and is often caused by hemorrhage into a metastatic lesion. Intracerebral hemorrhages are particularly common in metastasis of choriocarcinoma and melanoma. Occasionally, multiple small metastases to the cerebral hemispheres or a small metastasis to the brainstem reticular formation may present as an encephalopathy.

Metastasis to the base of the skull produces a number of "syndromes" depending on the area involved. The orbital syndrome presents as painful ophthalmoplegia or diplopia, with visual acuity preserved until late in the course of the disease. A CT scan typically identifies a metastasis to the orbit and adjacent bone. The parasellar syndrome results from metastasis to the petrous apex and sellar region, with compression of the structures within the cavernous sinus. The patient complains of a dull, aching, ipsilateral frontal or temporal headache accompanied by diplopia. Proptosis is not present, and there is impairment of the oculomotor, abducens, or trochlear nerves and the ophthalmic division of the trigeminal nerve. The middle fossa, or gasserian ganglion, syndrome is characterized by progressive facial numbness caused by metastasis to the gasserian ganglion. Occasionally the tumor may extend laterally to involve either the abducens or facial nerves. The tumor may be confined to the ganglion and therefore may not be readily seen by CT or plain radiographs. The jugular foramen syndrome is characterized by retroauricular pain, hoarseness, and dysphagia, which are manifestations of glossopharyngeal, vagus, and accessory nerve dysfunction. Bony erosion adjacent to the jugular foramen can usually be demonstrated by CT scan. The occipital condyle syndrome is characterized by severe, unremitting, ipsilateral occipital headache accompanied by dysphagia and dysarthria from a hypoglossal nerve paralysis.

Spinal cord compression from metastatic tumor is most commonly the result of vertebral body metastasis with extension into the adjacent epidural space causing compression of the spinal cord, roots, or cauda equina. Back pain is the first symptom in over 95% of these patients, often preceding other neurologic symptoms or signs by several weeks, and local spine tenderness is common. Spine x-rays, bone scan, and myelography are the most important methods for establishing the diagnosis. MRI has begun to play an increasing role in the emergency diagnosis of epidural spinal cord compression and is particularly valuable for those patients whose coexisting intracranial metastases preclude lumbar puncture.

Meningeal carcinomatosis is manifested clinically by cranial nerve and spinal root palsies that often are accompanied by localized pain. Communicating hydrocephalus may result from impaired CSF flow and cause increased intracranial pressure, with headache and mental status changes. CSF pleocytosis and hypoglycorrhachia are common.

BOX 160-1
Neurologic complications of systemic cancer

Metastatic
Intracranial
Intraspinal
Meningeal
Nerves, plexuses, roots

Nonmetastatic
Metabolic encephalopathy
Infections
Vascular disorders
Complications of therapy
Remote effects of cancer

BOX 160-2
Neurologic paraneoplastic syndromes

Brain/cranial nerves
Limbic encephalitis
Brainstem encephalitis
Retinal degeneration
Optic neuritis

Cerebellum
Paraneoplastic cerebellar degeneration
Opsoclonus/myoclonus

Spinal cord/dorsal root ganglia
Myelitis
Necrotizing myelopathy
Subacute motor neuropathy
Motor neuron disease
Subacute sensory neuropathy

Peripheral nerve
Subacute or chronic peripheral neuropathy
Acute polyradiculopathy (Guillain-Barré)
Chronic inflammatory neuropathy
Mononeuritis multiplex
Brachial neuritis
Acute or subacute autonomic neuropathy
Peripheral neuropathy associated with paraproteinemia

Neuromuscular junction and muscle
Lambert-Eaton myasthenic syndrome
Myasthenia gravis
Dermatomyositis/polymyositis

Table 160-3 Neurologic complications of chemotherapy

NEUROLOGIC PROBLEM	DRUG	ROUTE OF ADMINISTRATION
Encephalopathy (including cerebral edema and leukoencephalopathy)	Corticosteroids	Oral/intramuscular/intravenous
	L-Asparaginase	Intravenous
	Procarbazine	Oral/intravenous
	Nitrosoureas	Oral/intravenous/intra-arterial/high-dose intravenous
	Cytosine arabinoside	High-dose intravenous
Optic nerve damage	Nitrosoureas	Intraarterial/high-dose intravenous
Cerebellar ataxia	5-Fluorouracil	Intravenous
	Cytosine arabinoside	Intrathecal
Cranial neuropathy	Vincristine	Intravenous
	Cisplatin	Intravenous/intra-arterial
Myelopathy/radiculopathy	Thiotepa	Intrathecal
	Methotrexate	High-dose intravenous/intrathecal
	Cytosine arabinoside	High-dose intravenous/intrathecal
Peripheral neuropathy	Vincristine	Intravenous
	Cisplatin	Intravenous
	Paclitaxel	Intravenous
Myopathy	Corticosteroids	Oral/intramuscular/intravenous
	Vincristine	Intravenous

Modified from Young DF. In Silverstein A, editor: *Neurological complications of therapy,* Mt Kisco, NY, 1982, Futura.

Repeat CSF cytologies may be necessary before malignant cells are identified and the diagnosis is established.

MRI of the head and spine is superior to CT for the diagnosis of carcinomatosis of the meninges. Some of the findings suggestive of this complication include ventricular enlargement, sulcal and/or cisternal obliteration, enhancing cortical nodules, and leptomeningeal enhancement. These changes may be seen before clinical evidence of meningeal metastasis; at other times changes may be noted only after serial scans are performed.

Metastatic involvement of peripheral nerves or plexuses may be difficult to differentiate from dysfunction resulting from prior surgical or radiation therapy. If weakness and sensory symptoms in the arm are the result of neoplastic infiltration of the cervical roots or brachial plexus, there is often pain in the shoulder, Horner's syndrome, and a pattern of weakness suggesting involvement of C7, C8, and T1 roots. Patients who have received previous radiation therapy to the area and have a radiation-induced brachial plexopathy less often have shoulder pain or Horner's syndrome, and their pattern of weakness suggests C5 and C6 root involvement.

Nonmetastatic Complications

Vascular disorders. Certain cancer patients are predisposed to ischemic and hemorrhagic cerebrovascular complications. DIC and septic embolization are more common in patients with leukemia and lymphoma than in patients with solid tumors. Like DIC, nonbacterial thrombotic endocarditis with cerebral embolization may manifest itself either in a focal, strokelike event or in diffuse, progressive encephalopathy. Intracerebral hemorrhage may occur because of bleeding into a parenchymal metastasis; it is particularly common in melanoma and choriocarcinoma. Spontaneous intracerebral and subarachnoid hemorrhages are common in acute myelogenous leukemia and treatment-induced thrombocytopenia.

Complications of therapy. The successful treatment of many tumors is accomplished at the cost of injury to normal tissue.

A therapy-related complication can mimic recurrent tumor, infection vascular disease, metabolic derangement, or paraneoplastic process, all of which must be excluded before ascribing the new problem to therapy. Familiarity with the more commonly occurring therapy complications and their temporal relationship to treatment spares the patient unnecessary diagnostic studies.

Chronic corticosteroid therapy may induce insulin-dependent diabetes in some patients. At doses of greater than 8 mg dexamethasone, or its equivalent, for more than a few weeks, myopathic changes are often seen. Painless symmetric weakness of the proximal arm and leg muscles responds to tapering of the steroids and to vigorous physical therapy. The combination of corticosteroids, relative immobility, and perhaps a hypercoagulable state caused by the underlying tumor leads to a high incidence of thrombophlebitis. Patients with primary brain tumors and with cerebral metastases attributable to primary neoplasms other than melanoma, choriocarcinoma, and hypernephroma can have safe anticoagulation with heparin and warfarin. Anticoagulation for thrombophlebitis is feasible 2 or more weeks after any neurosurgical procedure. International normalized ratio (INR) should be kept at about 1.3.

The second most commonly used type of medication in these patients, anticonvulsants, is associated with rashes and altered steroid metabolism. Allergy to an anticonvulsant may be masked by the corticosteroid and revealed later when the steroid is tapered off.

Many chemotherapeutic agents adversely affect several parts of the nervous system (Table 160-3). The introduction of granulocyte colony-stimulating factors has permitted the use of higher doses of chemotherapeutic agents resulting in a higher incidence of some neurologic complications. The clinician should be familiar with commonly prescribed chemotherapeutic agents and their complications to avoid misdiagnosing neurologic conditions resulting from cancer chemotherapy. For example, the combination of 5-fluorouracil and levamisole, frequently used for the treatment of colon cancer, has produced a multifocal demyelinating disease that resembles multiple sclerosis on clinical and radiographic examination and responds to chemotherapy cessation and corticosteroids. Paclitaxel (Taxol), a mitotic inhibitor that enhances microtubular assembly, is very active against ovarian cancers. It produces an acute myalgia and a peripheral neuropathy. Since it is frequently used in combination with cisplatin, another agent with peripheral neuropathic toxicity, an often quite severe, predominantly sensory neuropathy often occurs and appears to be related both to the cumulative dose of chemotherapeutic agent and to the dose given at each course. Rapid onset in some patients of symptoms in arms, legs, and even face with more severe involvement of large-fiber function and diffuse areflexia suggests that some of the toxicity is at the neuronal level.

Radiation therapy to the nervous system may be associated with acute (1 to 2 days), subacute (10 to 13 weeks), or chronic (4 to 30+ months) complications. Acute effects take the form of headache, nausea, lethargy, and transient worsening of focal symptoms and signs, apparently resulting from edema. These acute symptoms are more likely to occur with high initial radiation doses. The subacute injury occurs 10 to 13 weeks after radiation, at which time demyelination occurs, accompanied by attendant cerebral, cerebellar, or spinal cord findings that may resolve spontaneously in 6 to 8 weeks.

Late, chronic irradiation injury is accompanied by pathologic changes of small-vessel occlusion with infarction and glial proliferation in the white matter. These patients may present with either an insidiously progressive multifocal encephalopathy or a sudden strokelike onset. The CT scan shows single or multiple low-density lesions predominantly in the white matter. MRI reveals widespread areas of prolonged T2-weighted signal both at the site of the original tumor and remote from it. Foci may coalesce into a large necrotic mass. MRI does not clearly differentiate radiation necrosis from recurrent tumor. The problem of mass effect may become significant enough to justify surgical removal both for diagnosis and for therapy if the lesion is located in an accessible area. This situation is more likely to arise after radiation therapy of primary tumors, in which the radiation doses used are usually larger than are those employed for metastatic tumors.

Stereotactic radiosurgery particularly is associated with a high incidence of radiation necrosis. In some series nearly half of the patients required surgical resection of a necrotic mass lesion weeks to months following radiosurgery. MRI and CT are unable reliably to distinguish radiation necrosis from viable brain tumor. Positron emission tomographic (PET) studies have demonstrated differences between viable tumor and radiation necrosis with respect to glucose metabolism but are often difficult to interprete when patients have had antecedent brachytherapy or stereotactic radiosurgery. Symptoms resulting from necrotic masses may respond to corticosteroids, which usually are required for several months. A recent study suggests that radiation necrosis, whose pathogenesis is believed to relate in part to arterial ischemic injury, may respond to anticoagulation with heparin and warfarin. Cognitive dysfunction, hypothalamic-pituitary insufficiency, and secondary neoplasms are other late sequelae of radiation therapy.

Late radiation injury to the spinal cord results in progressive weakness and sensory loss below the level of treatment, often with prominent painful paresthesias. MRI is useful for excluding recurrent tumor and demonstrates prolonged T2-weighted signal in the radiation-injured cord. Spinal radiation injury does not respond to corticosteroids or any other form of treatment.

Radiation-induced brachial or lumbar plexopathies and peripheral neuropathies may develop months or years following radiation to these structures. Weakness and atrophy insidiously develop in the innervated muscles, with pain and sensory loss absent or late. If pain and sensory loss are early findings, the possibility of tumor infiltration of the nerve or plexus increases. Radiation-induced tumors of the plexus or peripheral nerves may develop many years after high-dose irradiation to the nerve. The typical clinical findings are painful, progressive, asymmetric motor and sensory dysfunction in regions innervated by the irradiated plexus or nerve, with enlargement of the nerve or plexus demonstrated on clinical examination, CT scan, or MRI.

In patients with cancer previously treated with radiation therapy to ports encompassing the brachial plexus, it may be difficult to differentiate tumor invasion of the plexus from radiation effects when shoulder and arm symptoms occur. Lung and breast cancer are the commonest neoplasms to invade the brachial plexus. Pain in the shoulder and arm is the major initial complaint in 90% of these patients. Weakness and atrophy are present in over two thirds and typically involve muscles innervated by the lower portions of the brachial plexus (C7, C8, T1). This portion of the plexus is in closest proximity to the lymphatic channels from the chest and breast. Horner's syndrome is present in half of the patients with plexus metastasis and is especially useful in predicting those patients with brachial plexus metastasis who will have cervical epidural metastasis found at myelography. Arm symptoms caused by the effects of radiation to the brachial plexus typically have their onset 4 to 5 years after radiation therapy. Symptoms may, however, begin as soon as a few months after therapy. Surprisingly, the dose of radiation seems to correlate poorly with the likelihood of developing radiation-induced changes. Pain is not a prominent complaint but it does occur in 20% of patients. Compared with the patients who have brachial plexus metastasis, these patients more often have a swollen limb, weakness and atrophy occur in the upper plexus (C5, C6), and Horner's syndrome is uncommon.

At times it may be difficult to differentiate tumor infiltration of the lumbosacral plexus from the delayed effects of prior radiation to the pelvis. Tumor infiltration of the plexus is typically first manifested by an ever-increasing pain in the hip, back, and leg, which is often worse at night. A radiation-induced plexopathy normally presents with the slow progression over months or years of hip and leg weakness, and numbness. The symptoms frequently are bilateral. An electromyogram (EMG) may show myokymic discharges not generally present

with metastasis. A CT or MRI scan of the pelvis is unremarkable in radiation damage but often confirms the presence of a tumor mass or adenopathy in the patient with recurrent tumor.

Vascular complications of remote radiation have been reported, particularly in patients who have received cervical and mediastinal irradiation for Hodgkin's disease or high-dose (6000 cGy) cervical radiation for head and neck primary tumors. The neurologic presentation of these problems mimics naturally occurring atheromatous stroke or transient ischemic attack. Angiographic findings in these patients include disproportionate involvement of the distal common carotid artery and unusually long carotid lesions. Surgical reconstruction of these vessels is difficult, and the vessels demonstrate destruction of the internal elastic lamina and replacement of the normal intima and media with fibrous tissue.

Neurologic paraneoplastic syndromes. Several neurologic syndromes associated with systemic cancer but not the result of direct invasion of the CNS by tumor are summarized in Box 160-2. General clinical characteristics of paraneoplastic processes involving the nervous system include acute or subacute onset, severe disability at peak, stereotypical syndromes irrespective of the type of underlying neoplasm, modest CSF pleocytosis, elevation of CSF protein, IgG elevation, oligoclonal bands, frequent involvement of more than one type of neural cell, and low incidence (less than 1%) in patients with cancer despite the relative frequency of cancers associated with paraneoplastic syndromes such as small cell lung cancer, lymphomas, and breast carcinoma/gynecologic malignancies.

Though rare, these syndromes assume an importance out of proportion to their incidence, for several reasons. From half to two thirds of patients develop the paraneoplastic syndrome prior to the diagnosis of systemic neoplasm. Paraneoplastic syndromes may be mimicked by many other processes, leading to inappropriate diagnostic tests or treatments. Symptoms of the paraneoplastic disease, which is often acute or subacute in onset, are often more disabling than the symptoms of the tumor, and though usually unaffected by treatment directed at the tumor, occasionally can be ameliorated by treatment of the systemic neoplasm. Anecdotal evidence suggests that the cancer of patients with paraneoplastic syndromes often runs a more benign course.

The recent demonstration of circulating antibodies and antigens identified by these antibodies in both the nervous system and in the tumor tissue of some patients with paraneoplastic syndromes offers clues about the body's immunologic response to neoplasms. The identification of specific antibodies (summarized in Table 160-4) in a patient without known cancer may focus the search on one or a few malignancies. Various therapies, including plasmapheresis, steroids, and cyclophosphamide have been largely unsuccessful.

Treatment of Metastatic Cancer

The treatment of nervous system metastasis primarily involves radiation therapy, surgery, glucocorticoids, and chemotherapeutic agents. The therapeutic plan for a patient with cerebral metastasis is dictated by the clinical status. Patients with solitary, accessible lesions and little or no active systemic disease may be considered for surgery with postoperative radiation. *Stereotactic radiosurgery* appears to be an equally effective treatment option for solitary metastases, offering local disease control for at least 80% of patients. It is usually followed by whole brain radiation therapy. Patients with advanced, widespread systemic cancer may be treated with corticosteroids alone to maximize neurologic function and to reduce headache. Most patients with multiple metastases or unresectable solitary lesions are referred for radiation therapy. Three fourths of patients treated with any of the various radiation schedules in common use improve both clinically and by CT or MRI. Over half are able to discontinue steroid medication. While treatment failure for primary brain tumors is caused by local recurrence or attributable to spinal dissemination of tumor, for two thirds of patients with cerebral metastases the cause of death is recurrent systemic tumor at a time of neurologic remission.

Upon demonstration of a block caused by spinal epidural cancer, high doses of corticosteroids (dexamethasone, 10 to 20 mg intravenously, followed by 16 to 24 mg per day in divided doses orally or parenterally) are administered, and radiation therapy is recommended. Recently, reconsideration has been given to surgical therapy as a pri-

Table 160-4   Autoantibodies in neurologic paraneoplastic syndromes

SYNDROME	TUMOR	ANTIBODY	SPECIFICITY	ANTIGEN (WESTERN BLOT)
PCD	Ovary Breast	Anti-Yo	Purkinje cell cytoplasm	34 and 62 kd band from Purkinje cells and breast and ovary tumors
	Lung	Anti-Hu (one case)	Nuclei of CNS neurons	35-40 kd band from neurons and sclc
	Hodgkin's	No antibody		
SSN limbic encephalopathy	Sclc ? Prostate	Anti-Hu	Nuclei of CNS neurons	35-40 kd band from neurons and sclerosing tumors
Retinal degeneration	Sclc	Antiretinal	Ganglion cells	20-24, 65, 145, 205 kd band from retina
Opsoclonus/myoclonus	Breast	Anti-Ri	Neuronal nuclei	55 and 80 kd band from neurons
Lambert-Eaton myasthenic syndrome	Lung (sclc) No tumor	Antivoltage sensitive Ca^{++} channels	L-Ca^{++} channels (particles in presynaptic active zones)	Voltage-gated calcium channels

Modified from Posner JB: *Curr Neurol* 9:245, 1989.
PCD, Paraneoplastic cerebellar degeneration; *SSN,* subacute sensory neuropathy; *Sclc,* small cell lung cancer.

✔ WHEN TO REFER

Within the purview of neurooncology are patients with primary tumors of the nervous system and those with neurologic complications of systemic cancer. Neurooncology also deals with medical complications of nervous system cancers and their treatment. These include infectious, vascular, toxic, metabolic, and degenerative diseases whose prompt recognition is essential appropriate management. The psychosocial sequelae of these devastating disorders dictate that the patient and family be offered access to support services.

Neurooncologic patients often require management by a team consisting of medical oncologists, radiation oncologists, surgeons, and neurologists. The discovery of a nervous system tumor or related illness should occasion referral to a specialized center. A survey of patterns of care for brain tumor patients in the 1980s found that only 7.6% of potentially eligible patients were entered into investigational clinical protocols. Implementation of clinical trials is likely to continue to be problematic in a cost-conscious health care environment, since the 5-year survival of the most common adult primary brain tumor, glioblastoma multiforme, is under 5%. Despite their relative infrequency, however, brain tumors represent extremely costly diseases and provide a fertile territory for the investigation of new therapies such as gene therapy. Failure to attempt to improve survival statistics results in enormous societal costs both in patient care and in the understanding of the basic biology of brain neoplasia.

Clouston PD: The spectrum of neurological disease in patients with systemic cancer, *Ann Neurol* 31:628, 1992.

DeAngelis LM, Yahalom J, Thaler HT et al: Combined modality therapy for primary CNS lymphoma, *J Clin Oncol* 10:635, 1992.

Dropcho EJ: Autoimmune CNS paraneoplastic disorders: mechanisms, diagnosis, and therapeutic options, *Ann Neurol* 37(suppl 1):S102, 1995.

Fine HA, Dear KB, Loeffler JS et al: Meta-analysis of radiotherapy with and without adjuvant chemotherapy for malignant gliomas in adults, *Cancer* 71:2585, 1993.

Flickinger JC, Kondziola D, Lundsford LD et al: A multi-institutional experience with stereotactic radiosurgery for solitary brain metastasis, *Int J Radiat Oncol Biol Phys* 28(4):797, 1994.

Florell RC, MacDonald DR, Irish WD et al: Selection bias, survival, and brachytherapy for glioma, *J Neurosurg* 76:179, 1992.

Freilich RJ, Delattre JYU, Monjour A et al: Chemotherapy without radiation therapy as initial treatment for primary CNS lymphoma in older patients, *Neurology* 46:435, 1996.

Glantz MJ, Burger PC, Friedman AH et al: Influence of the type of surgery on the histologic diagnosis in patients with anaplastic gliomas, *Neurology* 41:1741, 1991.

Glantz MJ, Burger PC, Friedman AH et al: Treatment of radiation-induced nervous system injury with heparin and warfarin, *Neurology* 44:2020, 1994.

Horowitz D: Central nervous system germinomas: a review, *Arch Neurol* 48:652, 1991.

Loeffler JS, Kooy HM, Wen PY et al: The treatment of recurrent brain metastases with stereotactic radiosurgery, *J Clin Oncol* 8(4):576, 1990.

Mahaley MS Jr, Mettlin C, Natarajan N et al: National survey of patterns of care for brain-tumor patients, *J Neurosurg* 71:826, 1989.

Norris LK, Grossman SA: Treatment of thromboembolic complications in patients with brain tumors, *J Neurooncol* 22:127, 1994.

Patchell RA, Tibbs PA, Walsh JW et al: A randomized trial of surgery in the treatment of single metastases of the brain, *N Engl J Med* 322:494, 1990.

Portenoy RK, Galer BS, Salamon O et al: Identification of epidural neoplasm: radiography and bone scintigraphy in the symptomatic and asymptomatic spine, *Cancer* 64:2207, 1989.

Recht LD, Lew R, Smith TW: Suspected low-grade glioma: is deferring treatment safe? *Ann Neurol* 31:437, 1992.

Shaw E, Daumas-Duport C, Scheithauer B et al: Radiation therapy in the management of low-grade supratentorial astrocytomas, *J Neurosurg* 70:853, 1989.

Siegal T, Lossos A, Pfeffer MR: Leptomeningeal metastases: analysis of 31 patients with sustained off-therapy response following combined-modality therapy, *Neurology* 44:1463, 1994.

Siegal T, Siegal T: Surgical decompression of anterior and posterior malignant epidural tumors compressing the spinal cord: a prospective study, *Neurosurgery* 17:424, 1985.

Sorensen PS, Borgesen SE, Rohide K et al: Metastatic epidural spinal cord compression: results of treatment and survival, *Cancer* 65:1502, 1990.

Thyagarajan D, Cascino T, Harms G: Magnetic resonance imaging in brachial plexopathy of cancer, *Neurology* 45:421, 1995.

mary mode of treatment for radioresistant malignancies such as prostate, lung, and colon cancers. The clinical condition of the patient at the time of treatment appears to be the most important factor in outcome. Only 3% of patients who are paraplegic at the time of diagnosis regain the ability to walk, regardless of type of therapy, while nearly 50% of those with only mild weakness are ambulatory after surgery or radiation therapy. Meningeal carcinomatosis is managed with combined irradiation and intrathecal chemotherapy (e.g., methotrexate, thiopeta, or cytosine arabinoside, often instilled through an indwelling ventricular reservoir). Meningeal tumor caused by leukemia, lymphoma, or breast carcinoma is more likely to respond to treatment, whereas leptomeningeal metastases of lung or melanoma origin are resistant to currently available intrathecal chemotherapeutic agents.

BIBLIOGRAPHY

Black PM: Brain tumors, *N Engl J Med* 324:1471, 1991.

Chaudhry V, Rowinsky EK, Sartorius SE et al: Peripheral neuropathy from Taxol and cisplatin combination chemotherapy: clinical and electrophysiological studies, *Ann Neurol* 35:304, 1994.

CHAPTER

161 Neuroendocrinology

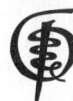

David Borsook and Steven E. Hyman

Hormonal regulation of central nervous system (CNS) activities provides a mechanism by which circulating hormones can regulate behavior and the short- and long-term neural adaptation to the environment. Neuroendocrinology is the field that deals with the relationship between the nervous system and the endocrine system. Tremendous advances in neurobiology and molecular biology have provided new insights into the complex nature of neuroendocrine physiology. The classic neural systems that regulate hormone secretion, namely, the hypothalamic-pituitary-endocrine gland system, have been well described. More complex interneural systems, for example, regulation of the hypothalamus by the amygdala, hippocampus or other limbic structures, are now more completely understood. Thus, although hormone secretion is controlled via hypothalamic neurons, these in turn are influenced by other neural systems. Responses to environmental influences act via these pathways. Furthermore, while hormones act on tissues and cells they also act directly or via feedback loops on neuronal systems (i.e., communication between the nervous system and the endocrine system travels in both directions). Neuroendocrine systems are critical for homeostatic maintenance; responses to environmental stimuli (e.g., danger), control of reproductive function, and the stress response and for many other behaviors including parental, memory, aggression and social behavior and mood. Some of these responses are cyclic or reversible (e.g., gonadal hormonal secretion); others are permanent (e.g., growth and development, sexual differentiation or behavior). Although the neuroendocrine system usually acts to preserve the *milieu interieur,* altered regulation may be deleterious to the organism. Chronic stress, for example, has been shown to produce neuronal loss in the hippocampus.

REGIONS OF CENTRAL NERVOUS SYSTEM INVOLVEMENT IN NEUROENDOCRINE REGULATION

The major anatomic substrates of neuroendocrine regulation (Table 161-1) are the basal forebrain, limbic system, and midbrain, all of which have major inputs to the hypothalamus; the hypothalamus itself, with its median eminence-portal capillary system; and the anterior and posterior pituitary. Neurons from the higher centers projecting to the hypothalamus regulate hormone synthesis and release by the hypophysiotropic neurosecretory cells.

NEUROSECRETION

The CNS, acting throughout the hypothalamus, controls hormonal secretion. Circulating hormones coordinate responses in physiologic processes such as reproduction, stress, and growth. The result of hormonal secretion is not dependent on neuronal connections, since as long are there are specific hormonal receptors on neuronal cells, hormones may produce effects on tissue. These effects are longer lasting than those seen following classic neurotransmitter release. The brain, however, also produces some hormones (e.g., neurosteroids).

NEUROPEPTIDES

A large number of peptides, many of them originally defined as hormones, have been found to act as neurotransmitters in the nervous system. Recent cloning of various peptide hormone receptors have allowed for regional localization of various receptors in the CNS using in situ hybridization techniques for localizing receptor mRNAs. Box 161-1 lists neuroendocrine receptors that have been cloned.

BOX 161-1

Neuropeptide receptors that have been cloned and are known to be involved in neuroendocrine regulation

Adrenocroticotropic hormone
Arginine vasporessin
Corticotrophin-releasing hormone
Cholecyctokinin a
Cholecystokinin b
Gastrin
Gonatadropin-releasing hormone
Melanocyte-stimulating hormone
Neuromedin B
Neuromedin K
Neurotensin
Neuropeptide Y
Melatonin
Opioid (δ)
Opioid (μ)
Opioid (κ)
Oxytocin
Somatostatin
Substance P
Substance K
Thyrotropin-releasing hormone
Vasoactive intestinal peptide

Table 161-1   Anatomic substrates of neuroendocrine regulation

CNS REGION	NEUROENDOCRINE FUNCTION
Hypothalamus	
Preoptic behavior	Fluid homeostasis; cardiovascular responses, gonadotropin secretion; maternal diurnal rhythms
Suprachiasmatic	Sex hormone regulation (gonadotropin secretion somatostatin)
Periventricular	Fluid homeostasis (vasopressin, oxytocin)
Supraoptic	Stress response, control of pituitary hormone release (corticotrophin-releasing hormone, thyrotropin-releasing hormone,
Paraventricular	Prolactin-releasing hormone, somatostatin)
Dorsomedial	Ingestive behavior
Ventromedial	Appetitive, reproductive, complex motivated behaviors
Arcuate	Gonadotropin secretion, melatonin inhibitory factor, prolactin inhibitory factor
Lateral	Feeding
Hippocampus	Feedback control of glucocorticoid release in hypothalamus
Septum	Feedback control of glucocorticoid release in hypothalamus
Amygdala	Integrates stressful stimuli, fear, control of hypothalamic release
Cingulate gyrus	Integrates stressful stimuli, fear, control of hypothalamic release
Pineal gland	Melatonin (circadian timekeeping)

HORMONES AS NEUROTRANSMITTERS

In recent years the purview of neuroendocrinology has been broadened to include all of neurosecretion, because of the realization that many of the classic distinctions between the nervous system and the endocrine system had been too simplistically drawn. In retrospect, it is not surprising that the two major systems responsible for intercellular communication may share many physiologic mechanisms and even the molecules they use for signaling. For example, by definition, endocrine glands secrete directly into the bloodstream; neurons, on the other hand, were initially thought to secrete their transmitters only at specialized structures called synapses. More recently, it has been found that the mechanisms of neurosecretion are quite varied. Within the nervous system many transmitters appear to be released not at classic synapses, but into the intercellular space between neurons, and to diffuse over relatively large distances before reaching postsynaptic receptors. In addition, certain hypothalamic neurons secrete hormones directly into the blood; not only are these secreting cells in morphologic appearance neurons, but their secretion is caused by depolarization. This latter type of release, often called neuroendocrine secretion, is the mode of secretion of the hypophysiotropic-releasing hormones and the posterior pituitary hormones, oxytocin and vasopressin. Another initially unsuspected similarity between the nervous and endocrine systems has been the discovery that peptides, many of which act as classic hormones, may also serve as transmitters within the CNS; indeed, almost all of the traditional peptide hormones and receptors of the endocrine system have now been found in the CNS.

Peptides have extremely irregular distribution in the CNS, with individual peptides being represented in some areas but not in others. Where present, they often occur in very low concentrations in comparison to other neurotransmitters (about 10^{-9} mol/L). Like the biogenic amines, they appear to function as modulators of other neural circuits but appear to act more locally. However, there is also good evidence to show that these hormones act as neurotransmitters. These hormones are present in axon terminals that synapse onto dendrites and may be released in a Ca^{++}- or K^+-dependent manner, and microinjections produce activity in responsive neurons in a dose-dependent, receptor-mediated manner.

NEUROTRANSMITTER REGULATION OF HORMONES

The major inputs from higher centers probably utilize the excitatory neurotransmitter glutamate to evoke hormone release (while local circuits transmitting or secreting γ-aminobutyric acid [GABAergic circuits] generally are inhibitory), but these effects are powerfully modulated by noradrenergic and serotonergic afferents from the brainstem by dopaminergic and opioid peptide-containing afferents from within the hypothalamus and by inputs from other hypothalamic regions including the circadian pacemaker (suprachiasmatic nucleus). In addition to these regulatory systems within the brain, there are inhibitory feedback loops mediated by peripheral hormones. What results are complex patterns of hormone release required for optimal end-organ effects of each hormone. These patterns include basal release, pulsatile release (e.g., gonadotropin-releasing hormone), circadian patterns of release (e.g., growth hormone–releasing hormone and corticotropin-releasing hormone [CRH]), and evoked release following stress (e.g., CRH and opioid peptides).

Neurotransmitter regulation of the releasing hormones may involve both single and multisynaptic pathways. The *dopaminergic pathways* involved in neuroendocrine regulation arise mainly in the arcuate nucleus of the hypothalamus and descend into the median eminence (the tuberohypophyseal system), where they are involved in the control of anterior pituitary secretion, most prominently the inhibition of prolactin release. The *noradrenergic pathways* that affect pituitary secretion ascend to the hypothalamus from their nuclei of origin in the pons, which are adjacent to the major noradrenergic nucleus of the brain, the locus coeruleus. *Serotinergic projections* to the hypothalamus ascend from the brainstem raphe nuclei.

Brain as a Target for Circulating Hormones

As stated earlier, hormones have direct effects on CNS neurons. These effects are mediated via membrane-bound receptors (e.g., CRH) or intracellular receptors (e.g., steroid or thyroid hormones). Hormones that act at the membrane may be specific or act on different types of receptors. For example, steroid hormones may have direct or facilitatory effects on membrane-bound receptors (e.g., at the GABA-A receptors, directly on corticosterone receptors, or facilitating certain types of excitatory amino acid effects).

Circulating hormones or endogenous (neurohormone) release may have the following effects.

Altered Cellular Processing. There may be rapid increases in mRNA synthesis (e.g., following stress, estradiol, or glucocorticoids). Glucocorticosteroids are known to promote enhanced cognitive function including processes thought to be important in memory such as long-term potentiation.

Altered Structural Effects. Gonadal steroids exert a significant influence over structure of sex-steroid responsive regions in the CNS. Glia also have sex steroid receptors and may produce other neurotrophic factors, which may then affect neuronal populations (i.e., produce sexual dimorphism). Synaptic density is also regulated by estradiol and progesterone during the estrous cycle of the rat. New synaptic contacts may form and disappear within a very short time (approximately 24 hours). Furthermore, there may also be induction of various receptors. Examples include changes in the number of corticotropin-releasing factor (CRF) receptors following stress or in oxytocin receptors following estradiol treatment. Some hormonal effects may promote neuronal loss (e.g., pyramidal neurons during aging or following chronic stress).

Altered Neuronal Survival. Adrenal steroid can cause damage to pyrimadal neurons, including neuronal death.

Altered Long-term Adaptation. Prenatal stress, for example, alters the stress response in the adult. Recent evidence has shown that long-term changes in the hypothalamic-pituitary-adrenal axis can be produced following certain environmental stressors. For example, the cytokine interleukin-1 (IL-1), when given as a single systemic dose, can produce alteration in the stress axis as measured by cortisol output, as well as morphologic changes in the staining of certain neurohormones (e.g., vasopressin) in the hypothalamus. Long-term potentiation in the hippocampus is regulated by adrenal steroids.

Altered Behavior. Numerous behaviors are produced by alteration of the hormonal milieu. Gender and sexual orientation are perhaps the best-studied behaviors that result from alterations in hypothalamic structure, based on the neurotrophic effects of circulating hormones. Reproductive behavior is complex, requiring regulation of reproductive behavior (female cycles) including the response to the sexual act itself and preparing the uterus for pregnancy, gender identity, and of a more controversial nature, sexual orientation. Such cycles can be disrupted by altered circadian timekeeping. The ventromedial hypothalamic nuclei, found in the posterior hypothalamus, play a significant role in female reproductive behavior. Other behaviors are discussed later.

NEUROENDOCRINOLOGY IN HEALTH AND DISEASE

Clinical examples of altered neuroendocrine regulation (although not an exhaustive list of these) are described in this section.

Aging

Studies have clearly shown that the aged CNS acts differently to circulating hormones. This is significant in terms of pharmacotherapy for elderly individuals that might influence the neuroendocrine system. Several studies have shown that there is a decrease in CRF content and increases in CRF receptors in Alzheimer's disease. Clinical and basic research has shown that certain hormones, including oxytocin, vasopressin, adrenocorticotropic hormone (ACTH), opioids or cholecystokin, (CCK) may have effects on memory.

Psychiatric Disease

Neurohormonal regulation of a number of psychiatric problems has been shown, including perimenstrual syndrome, depression, and the steroid rage that occurs among anabolic steroid abusers. Glucocorticoids, however, are generally anxiolytic. Because monoamine neurotransmitters have critical effects on neuroendocrine secretion, hormone regulation can possibly serve as a window on the brain. For example, although the pathophysiology of major depressive disorders is unknown, it is believed to involve dysfunction of monoamine neuronal systems, including noradrenergic and possibly serotonergic projections, and it has been found that nearly 50% of patients with major depression have a strikingly abnormal pattern of cortisol secretion, with hypersecretion and loss of normal diurnal variation. Anorexic patients, as is the case with depressed patients, have hypercortisolism. The role of neuroendocrine regulation in affective disorders is not well understood, but it is clear that seasonal affective disorders and depressed mood may result from altered neuroendocrine regulation. Violent or antisocial behavior may be mediated by androgen effects on the CNS.

There are altered ratios of males to females in specific psychiatric diseases: the incidence of anorexia, bulimia, anxiety disorder, and depression have been reported to be higher in women. The specific causes or origins of these disorders and the contribution of neuroendocrine pathophysiology remain to be fully elucidated.

Drugs

Understanding the neurobiology of the neuroendocrine system has been helpful in determining the effectiveness or clinical use of certain drugs. For example, the use of melatonin in shift work or for jet lag has been promoted in popular journals and books, yet our understanding of the long-term effects of this peptide is still unknown.

Significantly, an understanding of the neurotransmitter inputs into neuroendocrine regulation can lead to important clinical implications. Since hypophysiotropic-releasing hormones are under neuronal control, drugs that affect neurotransmitters or their receptors can alter endocrine function. For example, because dopamine has inhibitory effects on prolactin synthesis and release, dopamine receptor agonists such as bromocriptine have been used successfully in the treatment of prolactinomas. Drugs that affect neurotransmitters can also result in significant side effects. For example, antipsychotic drugs are dopamine antagonists, and they may result in hyperprolactinemia.

Sexual Differences

Sexual differentiation of the CNS is determined in part by genetic factors. However, neurohormonal regulation is known to play a significant role. Testosterone is critical in producing masculinization of the reproductive system but also CNS structures such as the hypothalamus. Sex differences in brains of humans and other species have been clearly demonstrated. These differences are thought to arise from the effects of testosterone on intracellular androgen receptors in neurons. In what is still a controversial finding, there may even be differences in the morphologic features of brains derived from homosexual and heterosexual males.

Stress

Significant stressors in the human experience may produce profound disease. Whether a result of war, natural disaster, or stressful personal events such as divorce, these environmental issues can produce a significant alteration in behavior. This has been commonly termed the posttraumatic stress disorder. Some stressors are not obvious but may produce significant morbidity, for example, the stress from shift work, in which an increase in cardiovascular disease has been demonstrated. The evidence is quite good that biologic rhythms synchronize the activity of the individual to the environment to provide optimal adaptation. Altered sleep-wake cycles can be produced by hormones (e.g., estrogen or progesterone).

Feeding Disorders

Hormones affect feeding by altering neuronal signals related to regions of the CNS involved in feeding and the control of food intake. Feeding disorders such as anorexia, bulimia, or excessive feeding are well known. The biologic basis has been extensively studied in animal models in which neuroendocrine regulation plays an all-important role. For example, hormones (e.g., CCK) can inhibit feeding.

BOX 161-2

Classification of CNS peptides by other tissues and functions in which they are prominent

Neurohypophyseal hormones
Vasopressin
Oxytocin
Neurophysins

Hypophysiotropic-releasing hormones
Thyrotropin-releasing hormone
Gonadotropin-releasing hormone
Somatostatin
Corticotropin-releasing hormone
Growth hormone–releasing hormone
Prolactin inhibitory factor

Pituitary hormones
Corticotropin
β-Lipotropic pituitary hormone, β-endorphin
Prolactin
Growth hormone
Luteinizing hormone
Thyrotropin

Opioid peptides
β-Endorphin
Methionine enkephalin
Leucine enkephalin
Dynorphin

Gastrointestinal peptides
Vasoactive intestinal polypeptide
Cholecystokinin
Gastrin
Neurotensin
Insulin
Glucagon
Secretin
Motilin
Pancreatic polypeptide

Tachykinins
Substance P
Substance K

Invertebrate peptides
Hydra head activator
FMRF amide

Other peptides
Angiotensin
Bradykinin
Calcitonin
Calcitonin gene–related peptide
Carnosine
Neuropeptide Y
Atrionatriuretic peptide
Bombesin

CONCLUSION

Because of rapid progress in application of radioimmunoassay, immunohistochemistry, and molecular cloning techniques, the identification of peptide transmitters has proceeded rapidly. Indeed, in the last 3 to 5 years numerous peptide receptors have been cloned (Box 161-2). Understanding their particular functions, however, has remained a difficult problem. Nevertheless, future research involved in neuroendocrine biology will undoubtedly contribute to a more complete understanding of the intricate mechanisms and interactions of the hormone effects on neurobiology and behavior. Recent examples of the discovery of new peptides in the hypothalamus, including the opioid-orphan–like peptide that produces hyperalgesia, the discovery of melanin-concentrating hormone in central regulation of feeding behavior, or the discovery of a new neurotensin receptor, have already provided new insights into the complexities of neuroendocrine regulation. One of the most surprising results has come from the use of knockout technology in which the CRH gene was deleted from mice lines where glucocorticoid requirements were essential in fetal development but did not seem essential in postnatal life. The results showed that glucocorticoids are a critical requirement for lung maturation and do not seem essential after birth. It is hoped that our understanding of transduction and transcription regulation of different genes will allow us to regulate gene expression in a therapeutic manner.

BIBLIOGRAPHY

Abelson JL, Nesse RM, Vinik AI: Pentagastrin infusions in patients with panic disorder. II. Neuroendocrinology, *Biol Psychiatry* 36:84-96, 1994.

Berbel P, Guadano-Ferraz A, Angulo A, Ramon Cerezo J: Role of thyroid hormones in the maturation of interhemispheric connections in rats, *Behav Brain Res* 64:9-14, 1994.

Bernardis LL, Bellinger LL: The lateral hypothalamic area revisited: neuroanatomy, body weight regulation, neuroendocrinology and metabolism, *Neurosci Biobehav Rev* 17:141-193, 1993.

Borsook D, Hyman SE: Proenkephalin gene regulation in the neuroendocrine hypothalamus: a model of gene regulation in the CNS, *Am J Physiol* 269:E393-408, 1995.

Decavel C, van den Pol AN: Converging GABA- and glutamate-immunoreactive axons make synaptic contact with identified hypothalamic neurosecretory neurons, *J Comp Neurol* 316:104-116, 1992.

de Wied D, Diamant M, Fodor M: Central nervous system effects of the neurohypophyseal hormones and related peptides, *Front Neuroendocrinol* 14:251-302, 1993.

Epelbaum J, Dournaud P, Fodor M, Viollet C: The neurobiology of somatostatin, *Crit Rev Neurobiol* 8:25-44, 1994.

Feldman S, Conforti N, Weidenfeld J: Limbic pathways and hypothalamic neurotransmitters mediating adrenocortical responses to neural stimuli, *Neurosci Biobehav Rev* 19:235-240, 1995.

Garcia-Segura LM, Chowen JA, Parducz A, Naftolin F: Gonadal hormones as promoters of structural synaptic plasticity: cellular mechanisms, *Prog Neurobiol* 44:279-307, 1994.

Garfinkel D, Laudon M, Nof D, Zisapel N: Improvement of sleep quality in elderly people by controlled-release melatonin, *Lancet* 346:541-544, 1995.

Heilig M, Koob GF, Ekman R, Britton KT: Corticotropin-releasing factor and neuropeptide Y: role in emotional integration, *Trends Neurosci* 17:80-85, 1994.

Kalra SP, Crowley WR: Neuropeptide Y: a novel neuroendocrine peptide in the control of pituitary hormone secretion, and its relation to luteinizing hormone, *Front Neuroendocrinol* 13:1-46, 1992.

Knapp RJ, Malatynska E, Collins N et al: Molecular biology and pharmacology of cloned opioid receptors, *FASEB J* 9:516-525, 1995.

LeVay S: A difference in hypothalamic structure between heterosexual and homosexual men, *Science* 253:1036-1038, 1991.

Lindholm D, Castren E, Berzaghi M et al: Activity-dependent and hormonal regulation of neurotrophin mRNA levels in the brain: implications for neuronal plasticity, *J Neurobiol* 25:1362-1372, 1994.

McEwen BS, Stellar E: Stress and the individual: mechanisms leading to disease, *Arch Intern Med* 153:2093-2101, 1993.

McEwen BS: Corticosteroids and hippocampal plasticity, *Ann N Y Acad Sci* 746:134-142, 1994.

Molis TM, Spriggs LL, Hill SM: Modulation of estrogen receptor mRNA expression by melatonin in MCF-7 human breast cancer cells, *Mol Endocrinol* 8:1681-1690, 1994.

Muglia IJ, Jacobson L, Majzoub JA: Corticotropin-releasing hormone deficiency reveals major fetal but not adult glucocorticoid need, *Nature* 373:427-432, 1995.

Naftolin F, Leranth C, Perez J, Garcia-Segura LM: Estrogen induces synaptic plasticity in adult primate neurons, *Neuroendocrinol* 57:935-939, 1993.

Paul S, Purdy R: Neuroactive steroids, *FASEB J* 6:2311-2322, 1992.

Potter E, Sutton S, Donaldson C et al: Distribution of corticotropin-releasing factor receptor mRNA expression in the rat brain and pituitary, *Proc Natl Acad Sci U S A* 91(19):8777-8781, 1994.

Qu D, Ludwig DS, Gammeltoft S et al: A role for melanin-concentrating hormone in the central regulation of feeding behavior, *Nature* 380:243-247, 1996.

Reppert SM, Godson C, Mahle CD et al: Molecular characterization of a second melatonin receptor expressed in human retina and brain: the Mel1b melatonin receptor, *Proc Natl Acad Sci U S A* 92:8734-8738, 1995.

Rossmanith WG, Reichelt C, Scherbaum WA: Neuroendocrinology of aging in humans: attenuated sensitivity to sex steroid feedback in elderly postmenopausal women, *Neuroendocrinol* 59:355-362, 1994.

Schally AV: Hypothalamic hormones: from neuroendocrinology to cancer therapy, *Anticancer Drugs* 5:115-130, 1994.

Schumacher M, Coirini H, Pfaff DW, McEwen BS: Behavioral effects of progesterone associated with rapid modulation of oxytocin receptors, *Science* 250:691-694, 1990.

South SA, Yankov VI, Evans WS: Normal reproductive neuroendocrinology in the female, *Endocrinol Metab Clin North Am* 22:1-28, 1993.

Svanborg A: Clinical problems in the neuroendocrinology of aging, *Neurobiol Aging* 15:485-487, 1994.

Swaab DF, Hofman MA: Sexual differentiation of the human hypothalamus in relation to gender and sexual orientation, *Trends Neurosci* 18:264-270, 1995.

van den Pol AN, Wuarin JP, Dudek FE: Glutamate: the dominant excitatory transmitter in neuroendocrine regulation, *Science* 250:1276-1278, 1990.

Verkhratsky NS: Limbic control of endocrine glands in aged rats, *Exper Gerontol* 30:415-421, 1995.

Witt DM: Oxytocin and rodent sociosexual responses: from behavior to gene expression, *Neurosci Biobehav Rev* 19(2):315-324, 1995.

Wooley C, McEwen BS: Roles of estradiol and progesterone in regulation of hippocampal dendritic spine density during the estrous cycle in the rat, *J Comp Neurol* 336:293-306, 1993.

Zhong P, Ciaranello RD: Transcriptional regulation of hippocampal 5-HT1a receptors by corticosteroid hormones, *Brain Res Mol Brain Res* 29(1):23-34, 1995.

CHAPTER

162 Metabolic and Toxic Disorders

Stephen M. Sagar

METABOLIC ENCEPHALOPATHY

A wide variety of toxins and metabolic derangements depresses CNS function and produces metabolic encephalopathy (Box 162-1). The clinical signs are relatively stereotyped and reflect a rostral-to-caudal gradient of sensitivity to metabolic and toxic insults. The cerebral cortex is affected earliest. As the degree of abnormality progresses, there is successive involvement of basal ganglia, diencephalon, and brain stem. Consequently, the earliest signs of metabolic encephalopathy are those of diffuse depression of cerebral cortical activity. There is impairment of attention and of higher intellectual function. The patient has difficulty with abstractions and constructional problems, such as drawing a clock, and may become dysarthric, have word-finding difficulty (anomia), and make paraphasic errors. As the encephalopathy progresses, the patient becomes confused and then delirious and progressively drowsy. Periodic (Cheyne-Stokes) respiration is common in the early stages of metabolic encephalopathy. Asterixis, a flapping tremor of the outstretched hands caused by brief lapses in postural muscle tone, is a nonspecific sign of metabolic encephalopathy that helps distinguish the condition from focal lesions.

The patient becomes stuporous and responsive only to noxious stimuli. There may be extrapyramidal rigidity, or, unusually, posturing of the extremities. However, the brain stem reflexes, including pupillary responses and extraocular movements, are intact.

Metabolic encephalopathy in its early stages must be distinguished from focal deficits of higher cortical function and in its later stages from the syndrome of central herniation, in which the patient becomes stuporous and may not have lateralizing neurologic signs but has sluggish or absent pupillary reflexes and decorticate or decerebrate posturing of the extremities. A more complex picture may be presented by overdoses of drugs that have direct autonomic actions (e.g., tricyclic antidepressants, neuroleptics, atropine-like drugs, and sympathomimetic agents) that may impair pupillary light responses early in the course of encephalopathy.

With progressive involvement of more caudal brain regions by metabolic encephalopathy, the patient becomes unresponsive to even noxious stimuli. The extraocular movements become progressively more difficult to elicit, but pupillary light reflexes are typically maintained. Medullary respiratory centers are affected, leading to respiratory arrest and death unless the patient receives ventilator support.

BOX 162-1
Causes of acute metabolic encephalopathy

Substrate deficiency
Hypoxia/ischemia
Carbon monoxide poisoning
Hypoglycemia

Cofactor deficiency
Thiamin
Vitamin B$_{12}$
Pyridoxine (isoniazid administration)

Electrolyte disorders
Hyponatremia
Hypercalcemia
Carbon dioxide narcosis
Dialysis disequilibrium syndrome

Endocrinopathies
Hyperglycemia
    Diabetic ketoacidosis
    Nonketotic hyperglycemic hyperosmolar coma
Hypothyroidism
Hyperadrenocorticism
Hyperparathyroidism

Endogenous toxins
Liver disease
    Portal-systemic shunting
    Liver failure
Uremia
Porphyria

Exogenous toxins
Drug overdose
    Sedative/hypnotics
    Ethanol
    Narcotics
    Salicylates
    Tricyclic antidepressants
Drug withdrawal
Toxicity of therapeutic medications
Industrial toxins (e.g., organophosphorus insecticides, heavy metals)
Sepsis

Heat stroke
Epilepsy (postictal)

This entire sequence of events may occur over minutes in the case of hypoglycemia, over about an hour if rapidly absorbed sedative-hypnotic drugs such as pentobarbital are ingested, or over weeks for slowly developing metabolic conditions.

With certain causes of metabolic encephalopathy, particularly hyponatremia, uremia, and porphyria, generalized major motor seizures may intervene. These may occur at any stage of the encephalopathy but are usually seen at the point when the patient enters the delirious phase or later. In withdrawal syndromes from alcohol and short-acting barbiturates, seizures may occur before signs of encephalopathy appear.

Laboratory and radiographic data are helpful in defining the cause of encephalopathy and excluding structural causes of altered mental status. The electroencephalogram (EEG) is sensitive to metabolic derangements of the cortex and demonstrates symmetric slowing of background rhythms. Therefore the EEG is helpful in excluding focal cortical disease and in following the progression and resolution of encephalopathy. Computed tomography (CT) and magnetic resonance imaging (MRI) scans are normal in uncomplicated metabolic encephalopathy; in severe cases and cases complicated by global hypoxia or ischemia there may be diffuse brain swelling.

Other specific laboratory abnormalities relate to the origins or causes of individual cases. Endocrine and electrolyte abnormalities, abnormal liver or renal function, abnormalities of blood gas values, and the presence of toxic levels of drugs may be diagnostic in cases of obscure origin.

SPECIFIC CAUSES OF METABOLIC ENCEPHALOPATHY
Hypoglycemia

Since glucose is the major fuel for brain metabolism and brain neurons contain only minimal glycogen stores, a rapid fall in blood glucose level can produce severe impairment of central nervous system (CNS) function. The level of blood glucose at which encephalopathy occurs depends on the rapidity with which the glucose level falls. In diabetics whose glucose level drops rapidly in response to an insulin injection, symptoms may develop at levels of blood sugar that are well tolerated by a nondiabetic, starved person. With rapidly falling glucose level, the encephalopathy may progress over minutes. Seizures, usually major motor, may occur. Unlike other causes of metabolic encephalopathy, hypoglycemia may cause focal neurologic signs, including aphasias and hemiparesis, in the absence of an underlying brain lesion.

These deficits are rapidly correctable with the administration of glucose. Because the administration of glucose to thiamin-deficient patients can precipitate Wernicke's encephalopathy, it is standard practice to administer thiamin along with the glucose if the patient's history is unknown or if there is a question of malnutrition or alcoholism. The routine administration of glucose in cases of acute encephalopathies of unknown cause is standard practice in the emergency room setting.

Hyponatremia

Hyponatremia causes water to enter cells, including cells of the CNS. This results in brain edema and disruption of neuronal physiology. Serum sodium levels below 125 mEq/L are frequently associated with seizures and encephalopathy. Chronic hyponatremia is better tolerated than a rapid decrease in the serum sodium level.

Hyponatremia is common in three settings (Chapter 112): when dehydrated patients are given hypotonic fluids intravenously; with the syndrome of inappropriate antidiuretic hormone (vasopressin) secretion (SIADH); and with the ectopic secretion of vasopressin-like substances by tumors, most commonly small cell carcinoma of the lung. A syndrome of cerebral salt wasting has also been described in association with subarachnoid hemorrhage. This condition produces hyponatremia with elevated circulating levels of both atrial natriuretic peptide and vasopressin, but it responds to salt repletion rather than fluid restriction.

The treatment of hyponatremia is detailed in Chapter 112. The rapidity with which symptomatic hyponatremia should be corrected is a matter of controversy. It is generally agreed that in severe hyponatremia the serum sodium level should be raised rapidly to about 125 mEq/L to prevent seizures. The rate at which the serum sodium level should be corrected from that point to normal depends on the underlying cause and the rate at which the hyponatremia developed. Rapidly developing hyponatremia, as in postoperative patients, is probably best corrected to nearly normal sodium levels over about 24 hours. Chronic hyponatremia should probably be more slowly corrected over several days to avoid central pontine myelinolysis.

Acute Hepatic Encephalopathy

The clinical manifestations of portal-systemic shunting are discussed in Chapter 56. Acute hepatic encephalopathy is of neurologic interest because tremor and other extrapyramidal movement disorders, including chorea and parkinsonian-like rigidity, are more common in hepatic encephalopathy than in other metabolic encephalopathies. Hyperventilation with respiratory alkalosis is also characteristic. The EEG may show triphasic waves, waveforms in the delta frequency range with characteristic appearance. Triphasic waves can occur in other encephalopathies but are typical of hepatic disease. Laboratory confirmation of the diagnosis of hepatic encephalopathy may be difficult, since liver enzyme and bilirubin levels are not necessarily abnormal in portal-systemic shunting. Arterial ammonia concentration is difficult to measure in a standardized fashion and is highly variable in normal patients. Cerebrospinal fluid glutamine concentration is a more reliable indicator and is now readily available, but it requires a lumbar puncture, which is contraindicated in the presence of clotting abnormalities.

The treatment of hepatic encephalopathy is based on reducing the ammonia levels in the brain, although ammonia is probably only one of several toxins responsible for the encephalopathy. Protein restriction plus lactulose and nonabsorbable antibiotics administered orally or by enema are the mainstays of treatment. Overactivity of neuronal systems that employ γ-aminobutyric acid (GABA) may play a role in hepatic encephalopathy. Flumazenil, a benzodiazepine antagonist that inhibits GABAergic transmission, is quite effective in animal models of hepatic encephalopathy. Human trials, however, have yielded conflicting results. Flumazenil may produce a modest and, at best, short-term improvement in some patients with hepatic encephalopathy. No benefit of flumazenil on the long-term outcome has been demonstrated. Fever of any cause and bleeding into the gut may exacerbate hepatic encephalopathy.

Patients with portal-systemic shunting may have subclinical neuropsychiatric abnormalities without overt encephalopathy. It is possible that their daily functioning can be improved by dietary protein restriction and lactulose therapy.

The neurologic syndrome of acute liver failure is indistinguishable from that of portal-systemic shunting but generally develops rapidly. The same treatment modalities are employed for both conditions.

CHRONIC EFFECTS OF METABOLIC DERANGEMENT
Chronic Acquired Hepatocerebral Degeneration

In patients who undergo repeated bouts of hepatic encephalopathy a chronic and irreversible neurologic syndrome develops that is characterized by dysarthria, tremor, and ataxia. A rigid extrapyramidal movement disorder may develop as well. There is no specific therapy for this condition except avoidance of acute hepatic encephalopathy.

Central Pontine Myelinolysis (Osmotic Demyelination Syndrome)

Since the advent of intravenous fluid therapy, a new disease has appeared marked by quadraparesis, ataxia, and abnormalities of extraocular movements. The disease occurs most commonly in patients with severe liver disease and electrolyte imbalance. The neuropathologic features consist of a focus of demyelination in the basis pontis, without inflammation, hemorrhage, or necrosis. There may be other foci of demyelination in the thalamus or centrum semiovale. The condition is associated with the rapid correction of hyponatremia. Other factors, including liver disease and alcoholism, also play an important role, since the condition occurs in liver transplant recipients, some of whom have no documented hyponatremia. Coexisting hypokalemia may predispose to the condition. The diagnosis may be confirmed by MRI. Aside from preventing rapid electrolye shifts, there is no known treatment, and recovery of neurologic function is variable.

Cobalamin (Vitamin B$_{12}$) Deficiency

Cobalamin deficiency, generally a result of impaired ileal absorption resulting from intrinsic factor deficiency (pernicious anemia), may lead to a demyelinating disease of the spinal cord known as *subacute combined degeneration* (Chapter 87). Moreover, deficits of higher cortical function and a variety of psychiatric disorders, including delirium, psychosis, or dementia, may occur either in association with or in the absence of myelopathy or hematologic abnormalities. Exposure to the anesthetic gas nitrous oxide may precipitate neurologic disease in patients with borderline cobalamin stores. Cobalamin levels in the blood may be low or in the low-normal range. The diagnosis may be confirmed biochemically by elevated serum methylma-

lonic acid and total homocysteine levels. The presence of achlorhydria, low serum gastrin levels, or antiparietal cell antibodies supports the diagnosis of pernicious anemia.

ALCOHOL-RELATED DISORDERS
Acute Intoxication

Ataxia usually occurs at blood ethanol levels of 50 to 100 mg/dl, confusion at levels over 200 mg/dl, and stupor and coma at levels above 300 mg/dl. Chronic alcoholics demonstrate tolerance to the neurologic effects of ethanol.

The neurologic manifestations of acute ethanol intoxication are reversible. Therefore the treatment is medical support as necessitated by the level of intoxication. There is no benefit from the administration of CNS stimulants or flumazenil. Rarely, individuals exhibit pathologic intoxication after ingestion of even small amounts of ethanol. They display bizarre, aggressive behavior and delusional thinking; they are usually amnestic for the episode. The condition resolves after a few hours but may require observation in a protected and supervised setting.

Ethanol Withdrawal

The mildest manifestation of withdrawal from chronic ethanol ingestion is tremulousness, which appears within 36 hours of abstinence and may persist for several days. The tremor responds to propranolol, benzodiazepines, and renewed ethanol ingestion but is self-limited and does not require specific therapy.

Withdrawal seizures characteristically occur 18 to 48 hours after cessation of heavy drinking and are major motor in type. They are usually brief, few in number, and self-limited, but prolonged seizures and even status epilepticus can occur. Whether alcohol withdrawal seizures can be prevented by prophylactic anticonvulsants is unclear.

Alcohol withdrawal may also precipitate seizures in patients with underlying epilepsy, but the occurrence of a generalized, uncomplicated major motor seizure during ethanol withdrawal does not imply the presence of epilepsy. Since alcoholics are susceptible to head trauma, infections, and other causes of epilepsy, it may be difficult to decide in an individual case whether the patient's seizures are purely withdrawal seizures or whether chronic anticonvulsant therapy is indicated.

Delirium tremens is the most dramatic and potentially life-threatening result of acute ethanol withdrawal. The syndrome begins within 5 days after abstinence and persists for 1 to 5 days, depending on severity. It is heralded by increasing tremulousness, agitation, and signs of sympathetic overactivity, including diaphoresis, tachycardia, hypertension, and hyperthermia. The patient becomes confused, then delirious. Visual hallucinations, characteristically vivid and disturbing, are a prominent feature. These agitated, delirious patients are challenging management problems. Cardiac arrhythmias, dehydration, and complications of intercurrent illnesses, such as pancreatitis, liver disease, and infection, may be life threatening.

Treatment consists of careful hydration and electrolyte management, sedation with benzodiazepines, cardiac monitoring and treatment of arrhythmias, and fever reduction with antipyretics. Because of sympathetic overactivity and resulting cardiac arrhythmias, particular care must be taken with the intravenous administration of potassium to correct hypokalemia. If possible, potassium should be supplemented orally.

Sedation is best carried out with benzodiazepines. On presentation the patient may be given diazepam intravenously in increments of 5 mg every 10 to 20 minutes until the patient is sedate but still easily arousable. The patient must then be monitored frequently and supplemental doses given intravenously or intramuscularly as needed. It is important to recognize the long-acting nature of diazepam, which frequently results in oversedation when used in a fixed schedule of doses.

Alcoholic hallucinosis is a relatively benign withdrawal syndrome during which patients have recurrent hallucinations that are typically auditory and may be threatening and disturbing. This syndrome usually lasts a few days and is self-limited; rarely it runs a prolonged course.

Nutritional Deficiency

Chronic alcoholics may obtain much of their daily caloric intake from ethanol. Therefore they are subject to nutritional deficiency, especially of folate and thiamin. The cardinal manifestation of folate deficiency is a macrocytic anemia, but a peripheral neuropathy may also result. The CNS bears the brunt of thiamin deficiency. Wernicke's encephalopathy is an acute neurologic emergency. The disease is most common in alcoholics but occurs in other malnourished individuals as well. The neuropathologic features consist of focal hemorrhagic necrosis, especially in sites surrounding the third ventricle and aqueduct. The mammillary bodies are the most vulnerable regions, but thalamus, hypothalamus, the periaqueductal gray matter, the floor of the fourth ventricle, and the cerebellar cortex are affected as well.

The clinical syndrome has three cardinal manifestations: an acute confusional state with loss of ability to form new memories, ophthalmoplegia, and ataxia. Rarely, the patient may be stuporous or comatose. Immediate therapy with thiamin is undertaken whenever the disease is suspected. Ophthalmoplegia responds best to therapy, ataxia less well. The loss of recent memory shows the least improvement.

Patients may be left with Korsakoff's psychosis, the chronic inability to form new memories. Typically these patients confabulate; that is, they manufacture untruthful stories in response to questions. When presented with verbal material in memory testing, they register the information correctly but retain it for less than 1 minute.

Chronic Ethanol Toxicity

Chronic ethanol ingestion is directly toxic to the nervous system. It commonly produces a distal, symmetric sensory-motor peripheral neuropathy that can be painful. The neuropathy is primarily axonal, and recovery is slow if ethanol ingestion ceases. Cerebellar degeneration also occurs, both in association with acute Wernicke's encephalopathy and as an isolated disease. The anterior vermis is the most vulnerable region, producing trunkal ataxia as the major manifestation. Cerebellar atrophy can be seen on CT or MRI scans; on pathologic examination there is loss of Purkinje's cells in the regions affected.

Myopathy may result from chronic ethanol abuse and may be acute or chronic. Binge drinking may result in acute rhabdomyolysis, with generalized muscle weakness and soreness, serum creatine phosphokinase (CPK) values in the thousands, and myoglobinuria. Hydration to prevent renal failure is required. The chronic form of alcoholic myopathy produces progressive proximal muscle weakness with only modest elevation of serum CPK. The muscles are not tender. The electromyogram and muscle biopsy show a myopathic picture, and peripheral neuropathy frequently coexists.

Two rare conditions associated with chronic alcoholism are optic neuropathy, a subacute demyelinating lesion of the optic nerves sometimes called alcohol-tobacco amblyopia, and Marchiafava-Bignami disease, a demyelinating disease beginning in the corpus callosum and spreading bilaterally into centrum semiovale. Mild, asymptomatic cases of this illness are being recognized by MRI scanning, but the disease can be devastating, with the subacute development of dementia, paralysis, and even coma and death possible. The pathophysiology of these uncommon demyelinating diseases is unknown.

BIBLIOGRAPHY

Basile AS, Jones EA, Skolnick P: The pathogenesis and treatment of hepatic encephalopathy: evidence for the involvement of benzodiazepine receptor ligands, *Pharmacol Rev* 43:27, 1991.

Diamond I, Messing RO: Neurologic effects of alcoholism, *West J Med* 161:279, 1994.

Estol CJ et al: Central pontine myelinolysis after liver transplantation, *Ann Neurol* 39:493, 1989.

Green R, Kinsella LJ: Current concepts in the diagnosis of cobalamin deficiency, *Neurology* 45:1435, 1995.

Greenberg DA: Ethanol and sedatives, *Neurol Clin* 11:523, 1993.

Healton EB et al: Neurologic aspects of cobalamin deficiency, *Medicine* 70:229, 1991.

Jones DB: Hepatic encephalopathy, *J Gastroenterol Hepatol* 8:363, 1993.

Oster JR, Singer I: Hyponatremia: focus on therapy, *South Med J* 87:1195, 1994.

Plum F, Posner JB: *The diagnosis of stupor and coma,* Philadelphia, 1980, FA Davis.

Victor M, Adams RD, Collins GH: *The Wernicke-Korsakoff syndrome and related neurological disorders due to alcoholism and malnutrition,* ed 2, Philadelphia, 1989, FA Davis.

Wijdicks EFM et al: Atrial natriuretic factor and salt wasting after aneurysmal subarachnoid hemorrhage, *Stroke* 22:1519, 1991.

CHAPTER

163 Principles of Coma and Neurologic Emergencies

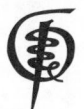

Allan H. Ropper

Certain neurologic problems cause catastrophic, usually abrupt, brain damage and coma. The most prominent of these are trauma, subarachnoid hemorrhage, cerebral hemorrhage, encephalitis, meningitis, brain tumor, brain edema after large cerebral infarctions, and basilar artery occlusion. All except the last have in common an increase in the volume of the intracranial contents and associated rise in intracranial pressure (ICP) that itself may cause additional damage. Another category of neurologic diseases requires emergency or intensive care because the diseases produce generalized weakness and respiratory failure; foremost are the Guillain-Barré syndrome, myasthenia gravis, and upper cervical spinal cord injury. These disparate problems, representing the extremes of otherwise less severe neurologic diseases, require immediate diagnosis and management, frequent nursing attention, and the ability to respond quickly to clinical and pathophysiologic changes. There has also been increased appreciation of the frequency and importance of the neurologic complications that accompany severe systemic diseases in medical and surgical intensive care units. These complications include encephalopathy, polyneuropathy, and seizures. Therefore the main clinical problems of neurologic emergency and intensive care are (1) increased ICP, (2) respiratory failure, and (3) the neurologic complications of critical illness.

A related field of cerebral resuscitation and brain sparing is concerned with minimizing neuronal damage after cardiac arrest and stroke. Despite interesting scientific advances, cerebral resuscitation has not yet achieved great clinical success. For example, a controlled study of use of high-dose barbiturates after cardiac arrest, used for their ability to reduce cerebral metabolic requirements, has shown no benefit. Similar attempts to improve the outcome of stroke by thrombolysis or by blocking the entry of calcium into ischemic cells have given mixed results. Nonetheless, there is an expectation that these approaches will change neurologic medicine over the coming years.

PATHOPHYSIOLOGY OF RAISED INTRACRANIAL PRESSURE

Intracranial masses produce brain death or brain ischemia by raising the pressure within the skull to levels near arterial pressure. This reduces the difference between systemic blood pressure (BP) and ICP, called *cerebral perfusion pressure* (CPP = BP − ICP). Reduced CPP that results from systemic hypotension, as from cardiac arrest, appears to cause more neural damage than an identical reduction in cerebral perfusion from raised ICP. In both circumstances the duration and rapidity of onset of ischemia, as well as the absolute level of cerebral blood flow (CBF), determine the extent of brain damage. Intracranial pressure is normally below 10 mm Hg. Persistent elevation above approximately 15 mm Hg indicates that the mechanisms that compensate for the addition of volume to the brain, specifically a shifting of cerebrospinal fluid (CSF) and of brain tissue away from a mass, are failing. Despite the imprecise methods available for measuring ICP and the uncertainty of blood pressure within cerebral vessels, an ICP greater than approximately 40 mm Hg, with normal systemic blood pressure, causes ischemic damage to neurons. Although an ICP between 15 and 40 mm Hg is not itself harmful, these levels indicate that precipitous further rises are about to occur, thus reducing the margin of safety before ischemia and brain death. Because the relationship between ICP and volume, termed *compliance,* approximates an exponential function (Fig. 163-1), the risk of deterioration increases greatly as ICP or intracranial volume increases. Therefore the aim of therapy is to keep the ICP below or near 15 to 20 mm Hg in order to prevent sudden deterioration resulting from critically low CPP.

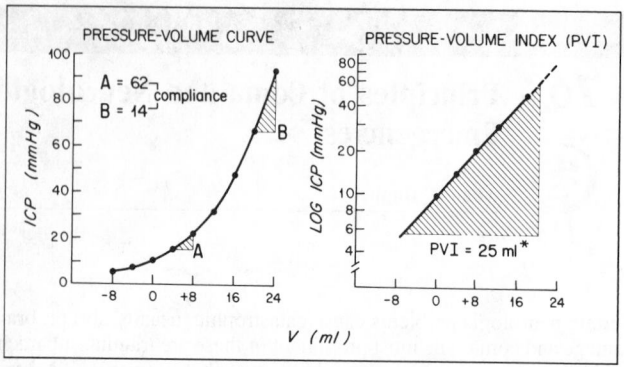

FIGURE 163-1   Intracranial compliance curve showing the exponential relationship between intracranial pressure (ICP) and increments of volume in the cranial cavity of a normal adult. The steepness of the curve changes with age, mannitol, and other factors.
*Calculated volume to raise ICP times 10.
From Ropper AH: *Semin Neurol* 4:397, 1984.

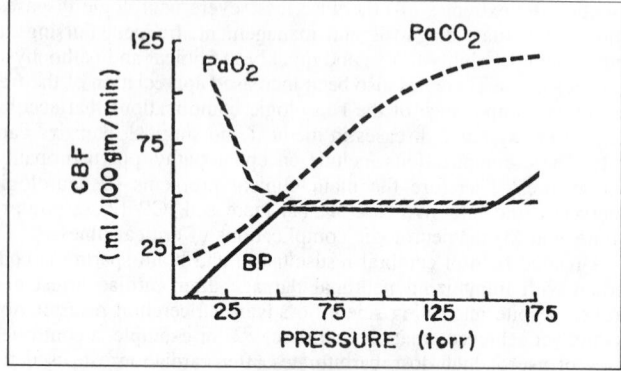

FIGURE 163-2   Relationship between blood pressure, partial pressure of carbon dioxide ($PaCO_2$), and cerebral blood flow (CBF). The cerebral circulation autoregulates over a wide range of blood pressures.
From Shapiro HM: *Anesthesia* 43:445, 1975.

Blood Pressure and Autoregulation

Systemic blood pressure has an important but complex relationship to ICP and cerebral perfusion. In undamaged areas of the brain a constant CBF is maintained by an intrinsic mechanism that regulates vessel caliber. This autoregulation is effective as systemic systolic blood pressure varies from approximately 80 to 170 mm Hg, but it fails under circumstances of mean blood pressure less than approximately 60 mm Hg or above 180 mm Hg. At the lower end of autoregulatory compensation, perfusion pressure drops in parallel with blood pressure (Fig. 163-2). Furthermore, inadequate blood flow occurs even earlier in regions subject to raised pressure from an adjacent mass. Simply elevating blood pressure to match raised ICP does not ensure adequate CPP, since elevated blood pressure worsens edema in damaged regions, eventually itself acting as an enlarging mass. The edema associated with trauma, hemorrhages, or infarctions—all associated with acute spontaneous hypertension—are particularly prone to progress in this manner if there exists even moderate systemic hypertension. Above the upper limits of autoregulatory ability (exemplified by malignant hypertension) the blood-brain barrier is disrupted in such a way that brain edema results. The edema, which is concentrated in the occipital lobe white matter on computed tomography (CT) or magnetic resonance imaging (MRI) scans, is apparently the result of enhanced pinocytosis across vascular walls, in addition to a true leakage of fluid and protein through disrupted tight junctions in the endothelium.

The cerebral vasculature normally responds to changes in arterial carbon dioxide and oxygen tension in a predictable way (Fig. 163-2).

Lowering the partial pressure of arterial carbon dioxide causes vasoconstriction and reduction in CBF. This response may be used as a therapeutic method of lowering ICP (see later discussion); conversely, hypercarbia causes increased CBF and raised ICP. Arterial oxygen has less effect on CBF and ICP, but severe hypoxia causes cerebral vasodilation and increased ICP. All these relationships of systemic physiology, that is, blood pressure, carbon dioxide, and oxygen, to CBF and ICP are altered in damaged regions of brain, particularly in the region of ischemic, hemorrhagic, traumatized, or electrically discharging lesions.

Plateau Waves

Patients with raised ICP have spontaneous or iatrogenically induced elevations in ICP that are caused by cerebrovascular dilation. Cerebral blood volume generally parallels CBF, so increases in flow result in elevated ICP, particularly if compliance is poor. These episodes, termed plateau waves, cause high elevations in ICP for up to 30 minutes, often accompanied by clinical deterioration or brain death.

Other derangements that exaggerate cerebral edema include serum hypoosmolarity relative to brain that creates a gradient for water into brain tissue; increased cerebral venous pressures, as from sagittal sinus thrombosis, jugular vein compression, or congestive heart failure; and increased CBF from fever or seizure.

COMA AND THE PATHOANATOMY OF INTRACRANIAL MASS EFFECT

The clinical features associated with an intracranial mass are the result of both direct damage to brain regions around a lesion (hemiplegia is most common) and signs caused by secondary distortion of the diencephalon and upper brain stem that contain the reticular activating system. The latter is a loosely grouped chain of neurons that are responsible for maintaining alertness. It follows that compression or direct destruction of this region leads to a diminished level of consciousness, and in extreme form, to coma. The falx, a thick fold of dura separating the cerebral hemispheres, and the tentorium, the dural barrier that separates the posterior fossa from the hemispheres, create structural limitations to the tissue displacements created by a hemispheric mass. The classic literature attributes the clinical signs that are caused by a mass lesion to movements of tissue downward through the tentorial opening or across the falx. These displacements, called *herniations*, are seen commonly in pathologic specimens and are associated with obvious compression and deformation of the upper midbrain, either laterally, from parahippocampal and uncal herniation, or more symmetrically, from downward transtentorial central herniation. Each of these distortions has been associated with a relatively sterotyped clinical syndrome that reflects brain dysfunction that progresses from rostral to caudal regions of the brain stem. The central syndrome begins with drowsiness and pupils that are bilaterally miotic, 1 to 2 mm in diameter, and light-reactive, and proceeds to stupor and enlarging, 4- to 6-mm diameter pupils that eventually become unreactive to light. The uncal syndrome has as its main feature a unilaterally enlarged pupil (on the side of the mass in over 90% of cases, or paradoxically, on the other side in the remainder), followed by progressively diminished alertness. Both syndromes then converge with loss of horizontal eye movements (a sign of pontine damage), abnormalities of respiratory rhythmicity (reflecting medullary dysfunction), and eventual loss of all clinically testable brain function.

The central syndrome has been interpreted as the clinical result of symmetric downward compression of the upper midbrain as it is displaced centrally through the tentorial opening. The inital stage of the uncal syndrome represents compression by the medial temporal lobe of the upper midbrain and the third cranial nerve as it is pushed over the edge of the tentorium, or in some cases by the downward movement of the posterior cerebral artery. Other well-described phenomena related to herniations in other regions are compressions of the posterior or anterior cerebral arteries against the dura causing infarction of the occipital lobe or frontal lobes; hemorrhages within the brain stem caused by distortion and rupture of small arteries (multiple small hemorrhages in the medulla, near the lower fourth ventricle are properly called *Duret hemorrhages*, although this term is in

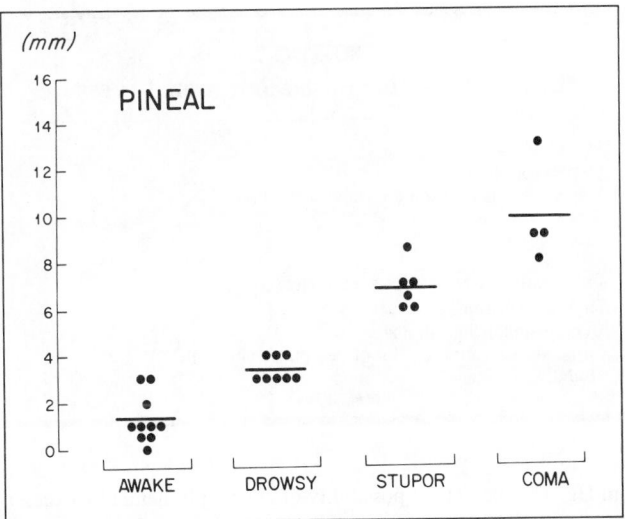

FIGURE 163-3   Horizontal displacement of the pineal calcification from the midline and the corresponding clinical state in patients with an acute hemispheric mass (hemorrhage, edema with middle cerebral artery infarction, or subdural hematoma).
Ropper AH: *N Engl J Med* 314:953, 1986.

BOX 163-1
Clinical features of brain death

Hemisphere death
Deep coma
Absence of purposeful movement, well-defined posturing, or convulsions
Can be corroborated by electroencephalogram, brain scan, or angiography*

Brainstem death
Unreactive midposition or enlarged pupils
Absent eye movements with oculocephalic ("doll's eyes") and oculovestibular (caloric) stimulation
Absent corneal responses
Absence of spontaneous breathing with apnea testing

Exclusions
Sedative drugs, neuromuscular blockade
Severe hypothermia
Immediately preceding circulatory arrest

*Brain death is a clinical diagnosis; laboratory confirmation may be used in special circumstances.

---

common use for all secondary brain stem hemorrhages); and damage to the pituitary stalk. Downward impaction of the cerebellar tonsils (inferiorly and medially lying structures) into the foramen magnum causes direct medullary compression, apnea, and death; upward herniation of the superior cerebellum through the tentorial opening, produces a syndrome that involves early pupillary abnormalities; and horizontal herniation of the medial cingulate gyrus of the frontal lobe under the falx, is associated with frontal lobe dysfunction. With the advent of CT scanning and MRI, other features of secondary tissue distortion from an acute hemispheric mass have been emphasized—most commonly, enlargement of all or the posterior portion of the lateral ventricle on the side opposite a mass.

The relationship between a mass, herniation, and clinical signs depends on the size and location of the mass, its speed of evolution, and the shape and size of the tentorial opening. The brain tolerates large masses in the frontal and occipital lobes, distant from the tentorial aperture, better than central or parietal lesions, and accomodates slowly evolving masses such as tumors better than acute lesions, such as hemorrhages. The shape and size of the spaces surrounding the upper midbrain at the level of the tentorial opening vary greatly among individuals, which may account for some of the variation in clinical signs with herniation syndromes.

There is an inconsistent relationship between the various herniations, coma, and the other clinical signs that have been traditionally associated with an intracranial mass. In cases of an acute unilateral mass, however, there is a relatively constant relationship between the horizontal displacement of the deep portions of the hemispheres and the level of consciousness. The pineal calcification serves as an approximate but easily identifiable marker of midline displacement of the lower thalamic and upper midbrain region, where the important reticular nuclei reside. Alertness is maintained with horizontal displacement of the pineal gland less than 3 mm from the midline, drowsiness occurs with 4 to 6 mm displacement, stupor with 6 to 8 mm displacement, and coma with greater than 8 mm displacement (Fig. 163-3). These may occur without evident downward herniation, although most displacements are associated with so much tissue distortion that both vertical and horizontal herniations are seen. On occasion, substantial displacement of more anterior portions of the hemispheres—greater than a 12-mm horizontal shift of the septum pellucidum—is associated with stupor.

It has also been suggested that acute large hemispheric lesions cause drowsiness or stupor by a mechanism of reticular activating system "shock." Plum has proposed that acute damage in the reticular system at any level disrupts the system temporarily and gives rise to

a decreased level of consciousness. This view is corroborated by acute drowsiness that occurs after large middle cerebral artery infarctions, at which time there is no mass effect (edema generally takes 24 to 72 hours to develop).

It is often not possible to separate the effects of herniations or large displacements from the damage caused by hypotension, hypoxia, or unseen traumatic damage at the time of many intracranial catastrophes. A clinical state worse than expected from the degree of horizontal shift is usually due to one of these simultaneous injuries.

BRAIN DEATH

Brain death has become increasingly important as progress in the field of transplantation advances and public awareness increases. Most legal jurisdictions in the United States have determined that there is no difference between cessation of heart activity and the entity of brain death. The pathologic state is characterized by progressive softening of the entire brain and the histologic changes of early cell death ("respirator brain"). This is reflected clinically by cessation of all function of the hemispheres and brain stem. Bedside testing to demonstrate brain death includes the observation of deep coma with no purposeful movements and the absence of classic posturing (segmental spinal reflexes and unusual limb movements do occur); light-unreactive pupils that should be midposition or dilated, but not small; the absence of spontaneous or caloric-induced eye movements; no facial movement or corneal reaction; and apnea when the ventilator is removed (Box 163-1). Apnea for these purposes has been defined in various ways, and standardized tests are therefore utilized to demonstrate that the arterial partial pressure of carbon dioxide ($Paco_2$) has risen above 50 or 60 mm Hg without stimulating breathing. An isoelectric electroencephalogram (EEG) is often used as a confirmatory test to demonstrate massive cortical dysfunction but is not always necessary. In all circumstances, drug overdose and the influence of neuromuscular blocking drugs that are administered in intensive care units must be excluded by history and laboratory testing. This constellation of clinical signs is only an indirect reflection of severe underlying brain damage, but it serves well as an operational definition for brain death. Another approach has been to equate brain death with the cessation of CBF that can be demonstrated with angiographic or radionuclide brain scan techniques. Some nuances of the clinical state, criteria for its demonstration, and the appropriate approach to the family and to transplantation are established at the local hospital level.

RELATIONSHIP OF INTRACRANIAL PRESSURE TO OUTCOME

A number of studies have demonstrated an association between raised ICP and poor outcome in head trauma. The most important lesson learned from this work was that at least half of hospital deaths in head-injured patients were caused by uncontrolled elevation in ICP that eventually led to global ischemia and brain death; the remainder were caused largely by sepsis and other medical complications. There has always been a strong but unproved belief that aggressive therapy for raised ICP would improve clinical outcome. Skeptics have begun to question this premise, instead contending that uncontrollable ICP reflects severe, widespread damage that cannot be ameliorated. However, there remains a consensus that careful attention to the control of ICP prevents death from reduced cerebral perfusion.

Several small series of nontraumatic intracranial lesions—including cerebral hemorrhage, large strokes accompanied by progressive edema, encephalitis, hepatic encephalopathy with brain swelling, and some cases of massive brain swelling after cardiac arrest—suggest that there is also a relationship between raised ICP and poor outcome in these diseases, particularly because of the absence of associated systemic injuries that cloud the issue in head trauma. Nevertheless, uncertainty exists about the beneficial effects of aggressive ICP therapy, and many neurologic practitioners currently favor an approach that stops short of monitoring ICP directly. In some experienced units, therapy is guided by ICP measurements, and there is the clinical impression that a few patients are salvaged who would otherwise have died from severe rises in ICP. The alternative to using ICP measurements to guide therapy is to treat all comatose patients with cerebral masses with moderate doses of mannitol and with hyperventilation as described later.

MEDICAL TREATMENT OF RAISED INTRACRANIAL PRESSURE

Medical treatment of raised ICP reduces intracranial volume by (1) extracting extracellular water from brain tissue with osmotic agents, (2) reducing cerebral blood volume by constricting capacitance vessels with hypocarbia (hyperventilation) or barbiturates, and (3) preventing avoidable elevations of CBF and edema caused by reversible entities such as fever, hypoxia, hypercarbia, inhaled anesthetics, and, especially, hypertension, or by reductions in perfusion pressure from hypotension (Box 163-2).

Mannitol, given in bolus infusions, is the most commonly used hyperosmolar therapy for raised ICP, although glycerol or hypertonic saline is favored by some authors, and renal loop diuretics may produce a similar effect. The major effect of osmotic agents is thought to be the creation of an osmotic gradient between brain and blood in undamaged brain, extracting water that is subsequently excreted in a diuresis. There may also be a more acute effect from a brief but rapid cerebral vasoconstriction in response to extreme serum hyperosmolarity. Contributions to serum osmolarity from sodium or glucose alone are ineffective in reducing brain volume. Like hyperventilation, hyperosmolar therapy is effective mainly in undamaged regions of brain. Although free water administration is avoided by restricting fluids and giving only normal saline intravenously (all other standard intravenous fluids are hypoosmolar), intravascular hypovolemia resulting from "fluid restriction" must be avoided, to prevent hypotension. In other words, the ideal state is euvolemic hyperosmolarity. Intravascular volume support with crystalloid, colloid, or, least desirable, pressors, is necessary in some cases. A "rebound" from treatment is rarely seen.

Hyperventilation, by reducing arterial carbon dioxide pressure, causes a serum and cerebrospinal fluid (CSF) alkalosis that leads to cerebral vasoconstriction and begins to reduce ICP within 15 seconds. Hypocarbia continues to be effective for minutes to an hour or more in most cases. The CSF pH gradually returns to normal, and the beneficial effect then ceases. The precise level of hypocarbia that is necessary to reduce ICP and its effective duration varies; little additional benefit occurs from $Paco_2$ levels below approximately 24 mm Hg; young children may continue to respond down to $Paco_2$ of 17 to 19

BOX 163-2

Main therapies for raised intracranial pressure

Conventional
Hyperventilation
Hyperosmolar infusion and fluid restriction
Blood pressure control
Craniectomy

Unconventional or used in special circumstances
High-dose barbiturates
Cerebrospinal fluid drainage
Surgical evacuation of clot or necrotic brain tissue
Diuretics

---

mm Hg. The theoretical possibility of creating ischemia by excessive hyperventilation seems to be rare or minimal in clinical practice. The benefits of hyperventilation have recently been questioned; a small group of head-injured patients had better outcomes without hyperventilation, and it has been suggested that the duration of effect of hyperventilation is prolonged by the administration of buffers such as tris (hydroxymethyl) aminomethane (THAM) that delay the equilibration of CSF pH. As with most other ICP therapies, hypocarbia is effective only in undamaged areas of brain where vessels remain reactive to physiologic stimuli.

Hypertension may exaggerate edema more than almost any other physiologic abnormality in patients with raised ICP that is attributable to a focal mass lesion that disrupts the blood-brain barrier. Since most patients with intracranial masses become acutely hypertensive (especially those with hemorrhages or trauma), blood pressure control is a prime objective in ICP therapy. Normal areas of brain autoregulate to keep perfusion pressure approximately normal while damaged areas leak edema fluid that cannot be extracted. Therefore raising blood pressure is not a viable way of maintaining CPP. Conversely, excessive reduction in blood pressure creates a risk of hypoperfusing brain regions that are subject to raised ICP.

Antihypertensive drugs that cause vasodilation, such as nitroglycerin and most calcium channel blockers, are generally eschewed in order to avoid increased cerebral blood volume and raised ICP.

The traditional approach of aggressively treating hypertension has been questioned because of the finding that mild reductions in blood pressure are prone to elicit plateau waves. For this reason a balanced strategy is recommended in which extremes of either hypertension (>200/100 mm Hg) or hypotension are both avoided.

High-dose barbiturates dependably reduce raised ICP, but their use has gone through cycles of popularity and, more recently, decline. Although the addition of high-dose barbiturates does not improve outcome in head trauma, they remain useful adjuncts for controlling ICP, particularly by muting the blood pressure and ICP elevations associated with endotracheal intubation or suctioning, chest physical therapy, and other intensive care unit treatments. Some clinicians believe that the judicious use of barbiturates after conventional measures have failed salvages a few patients who would otherwise become brain dead. The major risk in the use of high-dose barbiturates is hypotension, particularly when there is also dehydration and positive pressure ventilation—all of which conspire to reduce cardiac output. Should ICP fail to be controlled, barbiturates also confound the clinical diagnosis of brain death.

Surgical therapies, including ventricular CSF drainage, removal of blood clots or necrotic brain tissue, and hemicraniectomy, are dictated by the CT scan and the clinical state. It has become clear that removal of the skull overlying a massive stroke with brain edema (hemicraniectomy) is a lifesaving option for appropriate patients, generally those who are younger and have an infarction on the nondominant side, but the technique has been extended with success to others in less favorable circumstances. There is no evidence that surgery improves the ultimate deficit caused by traumatic or spontaneous hemorrhages, but removal of clot and drainage of hydrocephalus, by reducing intracranial volume, do lower ICP and in the opinion of many clinicians save some patients from death. When hydrocephalus is thought to be the cause of stupor or coma, as it is after subarachnoid hemorrhage, ventricular drainage is the treatment of choice.

CEREBRAL BLOOD FLOW, METABOLISM, AND BRAIN RESUSCITATION

Normal function of neurons depends on the delivery of oxygen and glucose by adequate blood flow. Cerebral blood flow in the hemisphere is normally approximately 60 ml/100 g per minute (75 ml/100 g per minute in gray matter, 45 ml/100 g per minute in white matter, and 15 to 30 ml/100 g per minute in the brainstem). The vasculature of the brain has the capacity to alter regional flow through autoregulation by at least 50% in response to the metabolic demands of neurons. Because cortical neurons have a very limited anaerobic capacity, cortical electrical activity as detected by EEG stops several seconds after the onset of severe cerebral ischemia. The cortex becomes dysfunctional when CBF falls to 23 ml/100 g per minute and prolonged ischemia at this level leads to neuronal damage. Neurons are irrevocably damaged if CBF is reduced even momentarily below 15 ml/100 g per minute; at that level, energy processes that maintain membrane and mitochondrial stability are disrupted. In all cases abrupt CBF reduction is less well tolerated than is subacute or chronic ischemia.

The observation that barbiturates can reduce the cerebral damage caused by experimental hypoxia or ischemia has led to clinical attempts at brain sparing, or "brain resuscitation," that aims to optimize substrate delivery and reduce neuronal metabolic demands after cardiac arrest and stroke. Despite success with the administration of barbiturates before or soon after cardiac arrest in animals, a large randomized trial with these drugs has failed to show benefit in clinical circumstances. Modifications of CPR to improve CBF by increasing cerebral venous pressure through increases in intrathoracic venous pressure have also been suggested. Some research, still not fully corroborated, suggests that the lactic acidemia attributable to hyperglycemia may be harmful during ischemia.

The most recent interest in brain resuscitation derives from the observation that several excitatory neurotransmitters in the cortex, especially glutamate, are neurotoxic. Their release in large quantities after arrest of circulation is thought to lead to ongoing but reversible neuronal damage. Glutamate may act as a neurotoxin by opening channels that allow calcium influx, thus causing mitochondrial and cell death, and by modifying sodium channels and causing cell swelling. Calcium channel blockers and specific glutamate-binding antagonists are being studied as brain protectors, with mixed success.

Generalized brain ischemia causes one of three types of anatomic brain injury. A limited hypoxic state coupled with a lesser degree of ischemia causes loss of neurons predominantly in Sommer's sector of the hippocampus, with subsequent shrinkage and gliosis of the hippocampal gyri. This is evident in patients after cardiac arrest as a Korsakoff's type of memory loss with sparing of other mental performance. The dense distribution of glutamate receptors in the hippocampus may be a factor in the region's preferential susceptibility to hypoxic ischemia. More severe, widespread cortical neuronal damage results from greater degrees of ischemia after arrest of the circulation. Virtually all regions of the cortex are affected, with most neuronal loss being found in layers 2 and 5 of the cortex, in Purkinje's cells of the cerebellum, and in the hippocampus. The corresponding clinical state varies from dementia with apathy to a virtually functionless vegetative or so-called apallic state that becomes evident as "neocortical death" in which only brain stem function persists. Even more severe degrees of generalized ischemia can lead to necrosis of the basal ganglia as well. The third type of anatomic lesion results from a more brief and predominantly ischemic insult that produces infarction in the watershed or low-flow border-zone regions that lie between the main large arterial territories. The resulting ischemic lesions are situated in the high frontoparietal cortex between the territories of supply of the middle and anterior cerebral arteries, or in the posteroinferior parietal cortex between the middle and posterior cerebral artery territories. The first watershed stroke produces shoulder and proximal arm weakness; the second, cortical blindness and related visual difficulties.

BOX 163-3
Neurologic complications of critical medical illness

Cerebral
Encephalopathy
  Septic
  Hepatic
  Uremic
  Anoxic
  Hyponatremic
  Hypoglycemic or hyperglycemic
  Medication induced
Seizures
  From underlying brain lesion
  From metabolic derangement
  Medication induced
Stroke

Polyneuropathy and paralysis
Septic, multiorgan failure
Guillain-Barré syndrome
Uremic
Prolonged effect of neuromuscular blockers
Malnutrition
Profound hypokalemia or hypophosphatemia

Status Epilepticus

Status epilepticus, defined as repeated seizures without regaining consciousness, represents a special derangement of neuronal function in which the metabolic demands of neurons are greatly increased. Blood flow also rises proportionately. In the presence of an intracranial mass the increased flow and, consequently, increased blood volume cause dangerous elevations of ICP. In addition to the systemic risks associated with status epilepticus, including aspiration, hypoxia, cardiac stress, and self-injury, prolonged and continued seizures, even without convulsions, lead to cortical damage that is similar to generalized ischemic injury.

NEUROLOGIC COMPLICATIONS OF CRITICAL ILLNESS

Approximately 20% of patients with acute illnesses in medical intensive care units have major neurologic complications (Box 163-3) mainly encephalopathy resulting from hepatic or renal failure or ischemia-hypoxia, seizures, polyneuropathy, or stroke. All of these substantially worsen the prognosis. A special syndrome of encephalopathy and polyneuropathy has been found to follow sepsis or multiorgan failure. The neuropathy (termed *critical-illness polyneuropathy*) is now appreciated as perhaps the most important cause of difficulty in weaning mechanical ventilation in critical care or postoperative settings. Seizures in critically ill medical patients are often clinically inevident and may be apparent only as periods of confusion or unresponsiveness. An EEG is required for detection.

Many neurologic conditions that lead to consultation in an intensive care unit are the result of medications, particularly sedatives, corticosteroids, and neuromuscular blocking drugs. High-dose steroids have been associated with a severe myopathy that has the unusual characteristic of myosin loss. The concomitant administration of neuromuscular blockers is thought to enhance the likelihood of this complication.

RESPIRATORY FAILURE IN NEUROLOGIC DISEASES

Several important neurologic diseases cause diaphragmatic weakness and require intensive care, foremost among them Guillain-Barré syndrome, but also myasthenia gravis, critical-illness polyneuropathy, amyotrophic lateral sclerosis, and spinal cord injuries. A few of these illnesses can (rarely) become evident as primary respiratory failure. Coma from any source also creates a special situation of combined failure of airway protection and central respiratory drive. The neurologic aspects of these diseases are discussed elsewhere in the text, but the management of mechanical respiratory failure is common to all of them.

Diaphragmatic weakness becomes evident first, by reduced airflow rates that result in poor coughing and airway clearing. As weakness progresses, the maximum volume of breathing is diminished, resulting in atelectasis and mild hypoxemia. Because the diaphragm has special physiologic properties that cause it to fatigue and fail when muscle contraction exceeds narrow limits of the rate and the tension of contraction, respiratory arrest can occur rapidly and may not reflect weakness in other muscles. Most peripheral neurologic diseases also affect oropharyngeal muscles and impair airway protection, compounding the risk of aspiration and poor airway clearing. Chest physical therapy and deep breathing are mainstays for assisting airway clearing. Once the diaphragm fatigues, air exchange is compromised and hypercarbia occurs, but this is a late feature. The complications of mechanical neuromuscular respiratory failure can be anticipated and are ultimately treated by endotracheal intubation and mechanical ventilation.

BIBLIOGRAPHY

Ivan B, editor: *Coma: physiopathology, diagnosis and management,* Springfield, Mass, 1982, Charles C Thomas.

Plum F, Posner JB: *Diagnosis of stupor and coma,* ed 3, Philadelphia, 1980, FA Davis.

Ropper AH: Acute increased intracranial pressure. In Asbury AK, McKhann GM, McDonald WI, editors: *Diseases of the nervous system,* ed 2, Philadelphia, 1991, WB Saunders.

Ropper AH, editor: *Neurological and neurosurgical intensive care,* ed 3, New York, 1993, Raven.

CHAPTER

164 Neurocardiology

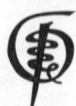

Martin A. Samuels

CARDIAC MANIFESTATIONS OF NEUROLOGIC DISEASE
Duchenne's Muscular Dystrophy

Boys with progressive, fatal, sex-linked Duchenne's dystrophy rarely have clinical evidence of myocardial dysfunction before the age of 10 years, but by age 18 all patients have clinically detectable cardiomyopathy. Congestive heart failure is a frequent terminal event, and autopsy invariably shows dystrophic myocardial involvement. Early dystrophy is characterized by tachycardia, large electrocardiogram (ECG) R/S ratios in chest lead V_1, diminished systolic function of the left ventricular posterior wall and septum, and decreased rate of relaxation of the posterior wall. With the development of a dilated cardiomyopathy in late dystrophy, additional cardiac abnormalities appear, including enlarged heart volume by x-ray; reduced left ventricular ejection fraction; diminished left ventricular diameter; and a decreased rate of circumferential fiber shortening, as detected in the echocardiogram (Chapter 13). The ECG in a patient with Duchenne's dystrophy characteristically indicates posterior wall fibrosis and is abnormal in nearly every case. It consists of tall, upright, precordial R waves with increased R/S amplitude ratios, often with deep limb lead and lateral precordial Q waves. Similar ECG abnormalities are regularly seen in affected siblings and even in female carriers. Sudden death may be more common in patients with Duchenne's dystrophy, but this has not been as well documented as it has been in the case of myotonic dystrophy.

The cardiac disease is distinctive. It consists of dilation of both ventricles and patchy but fairly extensive scarring in both subendo-

cardial and subepicardial locations within the posterolateral left ventricular free wall, without narrowing of the extramural coronary arteries. The classic histologic changes in skeletal muscle are basically the same as those in cardiac muscle, that is, degeneration and subsequent loss of fibers, variation in fiber size, abnormal enlargement and atrophy of some fibers, concomitant proliferation of endomysial and perimysial connective tissue, and subsequent replacement with adipose tissue. The distinctive ECG pattern associated with Duchenne's dystrophy probably results from multifocal myocardial degenerative changes involving predominantly the posterobasal left ventricle and the posterior papillary muscle.

Facioscapulohumeral (Landouzy-Dejerine) Dystrophy

Facioscapulohumeral muscular dystrophy is consistent with a normal life expectancy and is usually transmitted as an autosomal dominant trait. Most patients do not have congestive heart failure during life, although rare cases have been reported in which cardiac involvement was predominant.

Limb-Girdle (Erb's) Muscular Dystrophy

Little is known about the cardiac disease in limb-girdle dystrophy. It may be frequent on pathological study but is rarely of clinical importance.

Myotonic Dystrophy and Myotonia Congenita

Approximately two thirds of patients with myotonic dystrophy have cardiac involvement with conduction disturbances, including prolonged PR and QRS intervals and left bundle branch block, frequent cardiomegaly, and congestive heart failure. On pathologic examination there is fatty infiltration and replacement of myocardium, interstitial fibrosis, and destruction of muscle fibers. Many patients with myotonic dystrophy have symptomatic congestive heart failure and rhythm disturbances; sudden death is not at all unusual, probably as a result of cardiac arrhythmias. Even patients with congenital myotonic dystrophy have evidence of myocardial involvement as manifested by conduction defects and, sometimes, impaired systolic function.

Myotonia congenita (Thomsen's disease) is not a progressive disorder and may actually improve in adult life. Although there is often no cardiac involvement, cases have been reported with findings identical to those seen in myotonic dystrophy.

Other Rare Dystrophies

Cardiac involvement has been reported in isolated instances of nearly every type of the less common muscular dystrophies, including X-linked benign Becker's dystrophy and humeroperoneal dystrophy. Abnormalities in common include frequent atrial arrhythmia and conduction disturbances that range from P-R interval prolongation and abnormal P waves to sinus node arrest. Congestive heart failure is rare during life, but arrhythmias seem to be a common cause of death.

Metabolic Myopathies

A myopathic illness caused by abnormal glucose metabolism is called a *metabolic myopathy.* Many of these illnesses result from abnormal mitochondrial function in various parts of the nervous system and sometimes in other organs. These illnesses are unique because they are inherited in a nonmendelian fashion—the mitochondrion is the only subcellular organelle that possesses its own DNA. These mitochondrial illnesses are divided into the following types:

1. Deficits of transport (e.g., carnitine deficiency)
2. Defects in substrate utilization (e.g., pyruvate carboxylase deficiency, pyruvate dehydrogenase complex deficiency)
3. Defects of the Krebs cycle (e.g., fumarase deficiency, α-ketoglutarate deficiency)
4. Defects of oxidation-phosphorylation coupling
5. Defects in the respiratory chain (e.g., complex I, II, III, IV, or V deficiency).

On clinical examination, many disorders in this group include a cardiomyopathy, the manifestations of which vary from asymptomatic cardiac enlargement to severe cardiac arrhythmias (e.g., complete heart block) and occasionally even overt heart failure. Two well-recognized clinical syndromes with cardiomyopathy are carnitive deficiency and the Kearns-Sayre syndrome. The former is characterized by attacks of hypoketotic hypoglycemia and progressive dilated cardiomyopathy resulting from a lipid storage myopathy, which is usually inherited as an autosomal recessive trait. The latter is a triad of progressive external ophthalmoplegia, retinal pigmentary degeneration, and heart block, apparently occurring as a sporadic condition. Most of the other mitochondrial myopathies, such as myoclonus epilepsy with ragged red fibers (MERRF); mitochondrial encephalomyopathy, lactic acidosis, and strokelike episodes (MELAS); Leigh's subacute necrotizing encephalomyelopathy; and Menke's trichopoliodystrophy, have little or no effect on cardiac muscle.

Polymyositis and Dermatomyositis

The group of disorders discussed here is divided into several subgroups: polymyositis, dermatomyositis, childhood myositis, myositis with malignancy, and overlap syndromes.

Approximately half of patients with polymyositis and dermatomyositis have ECG abnormalities. These changes are rare in patients with myositis with malignancy and in childhood myositis.

Approximately one third of patients with polymyositis have laboratory abnormalities indicating left ventricular dysfunction. Thus subclinical cardiac dysfunction is a fairly common manifestation of polymyositis but rarely requires specific therapy.

Myasthenia Gravis

Cardiac abnormalities clearly exist in myasthenia gravis. Prolonged Q-T intervals, sinus tachycardia, sinus arrhythmias, right bundle branch block, and nonspecific ST-T wave changes occur more frequently among myasthenic patients. The incidence of congestive heart failure is not greater among myasthenic patients, and these ECG changes probably do not represent myasthenic disease of cardiac neuromuscular junctions.

Neuropathic Diseases

Neuropathies affect the heart only through the mechanism of autonomic neuropathy. The most common autonomic polyneuropathy is diabetes mellitus. The specific cellular mechanism is unknown, but patients with diabetes are known to have significant orthostatic instability without the normal heart rate increase and maintenance of blood pressure on standing, to have abnormal sweating patterns, and frequently to complain of bowel, bladder, and sexual dysfunction. There is no specific therapy for this orthostatic instability except control of the diabetes and mechanical assistance, such as elastic stockings or body suits. Amyloidosis may produce a similar circumstance but much more rarely.

In familial dysautonomia (Riley-Day syndrome) there is gross dysfunction of the autonomic nervous system with severe orthostatic hypotension.

Blood pressure control may be a major problem in patients with acute idiopathic polyradiculoneuritis (Guillain-Barré syndrome). Hypotension, labile hypertension, and persistent hypertension have all been seen in this disease. Several mechanisms have been considered. Some authors believe that the hypertensive episodes are caused by denervation hypersensitivity of vessels to circulating catecholamines because of an autonomic neuropathy. Denervation of baroreceptors could also theoretically produce hypertension, as has been proved experimentally. In most cases the clinically significant problems are orthostatic hypotension and labile blood pressure in the acute phase of the illness. Because of the extreme sensitivity of the blood pressure to posture, blood pressure control can usually be obtained merely by adjusting the head of the patient's bed. Antihypertensive agents and pressors should be avoided if possible, because of their probable excessive effect, probably from denervation hypersensitivity. It is rare for the problem to persist after the illness has reached its improvement phase.

Electrocardiography and Myocardial Abnormalities in Neurologic Disease

Many different ECG abnormalities have been seen in the setting of acute neurologic illness (see Chapter 12). The classic clinical setting is that of a subarachnoid hemorrhage, and the most characteristic ECG changes are tall, peaked, or inverted T waves, sometimes referred to as *cerebral T waves*. More worrisome are prolonged Q-T intervals and S-T segment changes suggestive of anterior wall myocardial ischemia. These and other, less dramatic abnormalities are seen in as many as half of patients with subarachnoid hemorrhages and in as many as 90% of patients with ischemic strokes, many of whom have hypertension. Head injury and psychologic stress have also been associated with arrhythmias.

Cardiac arrhythmias have been produced by electrical stimulation of several structures in the brains of experimental animals. Insular and posterior hypothalamic stimulation are particularly effective, but subthalamic, hippocampal, and midbrain stimulation have also produced abnormalities. The most consistent and dramatic ECG abnormalities are produced by stimulation of the stellate ganglia in the neck. Lengthening of the Q-T interval (and thus susceptibility to ventricular arrhythmias) is relatively easily effected by stimulation of the left stellate ganglion, but ablation of the right stellate ganglion can produce the same result.

The asymmetry of autonomic innervation of the heart is striking. Sympathetic fibers from the left stellate ganglion are dominant over the posterior aspect of the left ventricle, whereas the right stellate ganglion supplies the anterior wall. Similarly, the right vagus nerve supplies the sinoatrial (SA) nodes and has a dominant role in setting heart rate, whereas the left vagus nerve supplies the atrioventricular (AV) node, and its stimulation can lead to atrioventricular block.

For many years the ECG changes found in acute neurologic illness were thought to represent some noncardiac electrical disturbance, partly because autopsy studies showed no clear abnormalities in the myocardium. However, histopathologic abnormalities in heart muscle have been repeatedly demonstrated in cases of acute neurologic illness with ECG changes but no preexisting cardiac disease.

Endocardial hemorrhages have followed head trauma, seizures, and subarachnoid or other intracranial hemorrhages, particularly those involving the insular and orbitofrontal areas, which appear to be part of the cortical representation of the autonomic nervous system. In acute neurologic illness with cardiac changes, the characteristic abnormality is myocardial contraction band necrosis (MCBN). This cardiac abnormality can also be seen with marked catecholamine excess, with reperfusion of the myocardium (such as after bypass surgery), and in sudden death attributed to stress. These cardiac changes are distinctly different from the coagulative necrosis seen in cases of coronary artery disease and myocardial infarction. Similar focal cardiac necrosis has been found in as many as one third of patients with raised intracranial pressure and in victims of sudden death.

It is clear that ECG abnormalities in the setting of acute neurologic illness are "cerebral" only in the sense of cause or origin. It is a threatened or damaged myocardium that produces the abnormal ECG. Of course, hypoxia and other metabolic stresses can be synergistic with the nervous system input in the induction of cardiac lesions. Experimentally, hypoxia and steroids potentiate catecholamines in the generation of cardiac lesions. The incidence of sudden death increases dramatically around the time of a natural catastrophe. These deaths, which are probably cardiac in origin, may be due to myocardial ischemia induced by stress via mechanisms involving coronary vasospasm or a hypercoagulable state. However, it is also possible that cardiac damage and lethal arrhythmias may be caused by cardiotoxic effects of catecholamines.

On experimental study the subendocardial hemorrhages that follow hypothalamic stimulation can be prevented by section of the cervical spinal cord. Lack of a similar benefit from vagotomy again suggests that the cardiac lesions are mediated by the sympathetic nervous system. Prevention of central nervous system (CNS) stimulation–induced arrhythmias by treatment with sympathetic antagonists or by reserpine also implicates the sympathetic nervous system. The effects of stellate ganglia stimulation and lesions suggest the same.

Several preventive therapies are possible. Sympathetic nervous system blockade by β-adrenergic antagonists may provide protection against arrhythmias. More speculative treatment includes the use of calcium channel blockers. Left stellate ganglion block has been employed successfully in cases of refractory cardiac arrhythmias after subarachnoid hemorrhage.

Specific Neurocardiac Syndromes

Friedreich's Ataxia. Cardiac involvement has long been recognized in the familial neurologic disorder of Friedreich's ataxia. Three of Friedreich's original six cases showed severe fatty degeneration of the heart. This incidence of 50% has remained constant, although ECG changes that are not necessarily associated with cardiac symptoms occur in more than 90% of patients. In rare cases the cardiac disease may be much more severe than the neurologic disease and may even be the presenting symptom.

In the typical patient the cardiac symptoms are progressive congestive heart failure and angina pectoris. ECG changes include arrhythmias, heart block, and Q waves in limb leads I and II and chest leads V_1, V_5, and V_6. On pathological study the heart is large, with fatty infiltration and fibrous replacement of myocardium. The fibers are hypertrophied, and the pathologic picture is often that of a hypertrophic cardiomyopathy.

The prognosis is poor, and most patients die of congestive heart failure. The importance of the cardiac aspect of the disease is clear, but there is no evidence at this time that any treatment alters the course of this hypertrophic cardiomyopathy.

External Ophthalmoplegia With Cardiac Conduction Disorders (Kearns-Sayre Syndrome). One of the many "ophthalmoplegia plus" syndromes includes pigmentary degeneration of the retina and disorders of cardiac conduction. Most of these patients have severe disease of the conduction system with propensity to complete heart block. These patients are often young, and insertion of a permanent (lifelong) pacemaker is required to prevent sudden death.

NEUROLOGIC ASPECTS OF CARDIAC DISEASE
Arrhythmias

Atrial Fibrillation. Atrial fibrillation (see Chapter 18) greatly increases the risk of systemic embolism in patients with mitral valve disease, and anticoagulation therapy for life has been common practice in all such reliable patients to prevent systemic emboli, including cerebral emboli. In the past, however, patients with atrial fibrillation in the absence of mitral valve disease did not receive anticoagulation therapy, since they were said not to have the same risk for systemic embolism as patients with mitral valve disease. It is now known that atrial fibrillation, regardless of its origin, imparts a high risk for stroke. Although mitral disease plus atrial fibrillation does, indeed, produce the highest risk group, atrial fibrillation in other settings also produces a greatly increased risk, many times that of the control group.

Several large prospective studies have now shown conclusively that low-intensity anticoagulation therapy with warfarin reduces the risk of stroke in patients with nonrheumatic atrial fibrillation. The lowest effective dose of warfarin thus far demonstrated in a well-done trial is an amount capable of increasing the prothrombin time to 1.2 to 1.5 times the control (i.e., international normalized ratio [INR] 2 to 3). Aspirin, approximately 500 mg daily, has been shown to reduce the risk of stroke in people with nonrheumatic atrial fibrillation but not as effectively as is accomplished with warfarin.

A further dilemma arises when a patient with atrial fibrillation has an embolic stroke. Such infarctions often are hemorrhagic, presumably because of lysis of the embolic material and reflow of blood under arterial pressure into necrotic vessels. The amount of hemorrhage is usually small and is not sufficient to be seen on the computed tomography (CT) scan, so the clinician is often faced with the problem of treating an embolic source with an anticoagulant that theoretically could convert a relatively benign hemorrhagic infarction into a full-blown intracerebral hemorrhage. Indeed, anecdotal cases have been reported in which a very atypical intracerebral hemorrhage was seen to develop after an embolic stroke in a patient receiving an anticoagulant. It is common practice to maintain anticoagulation therapy in patients who have small embolic strokes and to temporarily discontinue anticoagulation therapy in patients with large embolic strokes.

Ventricular Arrhythmias and Heart Block. Ventricular arrhythmias (particularly ventricular tachycardia) and heart block (Chapter 18) with bradycardia may produce transient or permanent neurologic syndromes. Whether the deficit is transient or permanent is determined primarily by the duration of the arrhythmia with the consequent decreased cerebral blood flow. Additional factors, such as fixed arterial lesions in the carotid or vertebrobasilar arterial system, probably modulate the degree and distribution of deficit, but firm data are lacking.

Transient deficits from brief periods of generalized decreased cerebral blood flow are probably extremely common, particularly in elderly individuals. Often, these arrhythmias are sufficiently brief and infrequent to elude detection by routine ECG examination. Ambulatory ECG recording techniques have permitted the diagnosis of many brief arrhythmias and clarified their clinical correlates (Chapter 12).

Cardiac Arrest

Cardiac arrest refers to absent cardiac output resulting from any cause, but its most common origin is probably ventricular tachyarrhythmia (ventricular tachycardia and fibrillation). The patient loses consciousness promptly when cardiac output ceases, and the degree of recovery of neurologic function after resuscitation depends on the efficiency and speed with which cerebral circulation is restored. Clearly there is a great deal of individual variation in the amount of time that must elapse before irreversible damage has occurred. In clinical practice it is extremely difficult to weigh the efficiency of a cardiac resuscitation. Its true effectiveness is, after all, reflected most accurately in the residual state of the patient's nervous system.

Until recently the clinician had very little information on which to estimate the prognosis for useful life after cardiac arrest. Only the syndrome of brain death was clearly identified and defined as apnea, unresponsiveness, and absence of cranial reflexes on an isoelectric electroencephalogram. This circumstance is rare after a cardiac arrest. Most often, the physician is faced with a patient who is severely impaired but does not meet all the criteria for brain death. In this circumstance additional guidelines are needed. Briefly stated, the absence of eye movements after cardiac arrest is a bad prognostic sign, despite other intact brain stem functions, including respiratory and blood pressure control mechanisms. Few patients without eye movements after cardiac arrest recover to a level of useful neurologic function. In other words, these patients, although not meeting the strict definition of death by brain criteria, are left in a permanent vegetative state. It should be clearly understood, however, that these guidelines are purely medical and do not necessarily reflect the prevalent legal or social attitudes toward death and vegetative states.

Between the extremes of death and persistent vegetative state, on the one hand, and full recovery, on the other, is a wide spectrum of neurologic abnormalities consequent to cardiac arrest. These fall into two major categories: cases in which the return of blood flow occurs promptly but with a prolonged period of hypoxia (nonischemic anoxia) and cases in which the return of blood flow is delayed (ischemic anoxia). In the former case, damage occurs in areas of the brain known to be particularly sensitive to hypoxemia, despite adequate blood flow. These areas include layers three and five of the cerebral cortex (laminar necrosis), the Sommer sector of Ammon's horn, the basal ganglia (particularly the globus pallidus), and Purkinje's cells of the cerebellum. The dentate nucleus of the cerebellum and the inferior olivary nucleus of the medulla also are particularly vulnerable to anoxia. The prototypic form of nonischemic anoxia is carbon monoxide poisoning, in which cerebral blood flow is normal but with a very low oxygen content. From the distribution of cerebral damage described earlier, one might predict the types of syndromes that are commonly seen. These include epilepsy and myoclonus, particularly intention myoclonus (Lance-Adams syndrome); various degrees of cortical dysfunction, including aphasia, apraxia, visual disturbance, and behavioral and intellectual dysfunction; movement disorders, including dystonias, choreoathetosis, and tremors; memory loss; and cerebellar ataxia.

Ischemic anoxia entails both decreased blood flow and anoxia. The lesions of nonischemic anoxia are often seen but frequently are more severe and widespread. Furthermore, there may be additional lesions in the distribution of stenotic arterial circulations (e.g., a middle cerebral distribution infarction distal to a high-grade carotid stenosis) or in the border zones between major arterial circulations. The circumstance of cardiac arrest most resembles that of ischemic anoxia. When the underlying cerebral circulation is normal and the period of anoxia relatively brief, the syndrome more approaches the circumstance of nonischemic anoxia. The more prolonged the period of ischemia, the more the syndrome approaches that of ischemic anoxia.

Patients must be approached individually. Maximal recovery may take many months, but the majority of the improvement occurs within 72 hours of the insult. A few of the postanoxic syndromes can be treated with some success—for example, anticonvulsants, diazepam, clonazepam, or tryptophan for postanoxic myoclonus—but many are best managed with patience and physical rehabilitation.

Ischemic Heart Disease: Acute Myocardial Infarction

It is logical to assume a relationship between myocardial (Chapter 23) and cerebral infarction, since the underlying process in both conditions is atherosclerosis, a systemic disease. Obviously, if the acute myocardial infarction is attended by cardiogenic shock with severe systemic hypotension, the patient may show some or all of the manifestations of ischemic anoxia mentioned in the previous section.

Aside from the problem of systemic hypotension or cardiac arrhythmias, there is a definite correlation between cerebral infarction and recent myocardial infarction. Of all patients admitted to a hospital with stroke, about one in eight are found to have had recent myocardial infarctions, three quarters of which are asymptomatic. The 1-year mortality rate for patients with both heart and brain infarct is about 50%—twice that of patients with only stroke.

Several possible explanations for the preceding association are possible. The first is that the myocardial infarction predated the cerebral infarction and led to the stroke by acting as a source for systemic emboli, perhaps arising from a mural thrombus on a dyskinetic ventricular wall. The second, less likely hypothesis is that an unknown source produced both cerebral and coronary emboli. The third possible explanation would be that the cerebral infarction predated and somehow caused the myocardial infarction. This may seem an unlikely sequence, but suggestive evidence was provided by Feibel and others, who studied 27 patients with various types of stroke (14 with hemisphere infarction, 5 with brain stem infarction, and 8 with subarachnoid hemorrhage) with serial ECGs and systemic catecholamine determinations. Nine patients showed severe myocardial ischemia or infarction and had elevated catecholamine levels; of these, five who had myocardial infarction had the most elevated levels and the worst prognosis (four died). Twelve patients showed mild or possible ischemia, had mild elevations of catecholamines, and survived, and six others with normal ECGs and cardiac enzymes had normal catecholamine levels and survived as well. The criteria for myocardial infarction were not only ECG changes, but also characteristic cardiac enzyme elevations. These data suggest that central nervous system disease may actually cause myocardial ischemia and infarction, possibly mediated via catecholamine release.

In general, it appears that there is a positive association between myocardial infarction and cerebral infarction. This population may contain some cases of myocardial infarction causing embolic stroke, some cases of cerebral infarction precipitating cardiac ischemia, and a few cases of concomitant cerebral and coronary ischemia, possibly from another embolic source or generalized hypotension.

Concomitant Coronary and Carotid Occlusive Disease

It is not surprising to find a high incidence of cerebral occlusive vascular disease in a population of patients with coronary occlusive vascular disease, since the underlying process is systemic. The frequent coexistence of these two disorders leads to a number of difficult problems in the management of patients who are to undergo coronary artery bypass surgery. In this circumstance most vascular surgeons would recommend combined surgical management of the carotid and coronary disease, either simultaneously or in a staged procedure. In the circumstance of impending coronary artery bypass surgery, most neurologists would demand the occurrence of hemispheric transient ischemic attacks, with or without transient monocular blindness or submaximal cerebral hemisphere infarction in the distribution of a stenotic carotid artery, before recommending carotid endarterectomy.

Endocarditis

The modern spectrum of neurologic complications of infective endocarditis has been well analyzed in two large retrospective studies, one from the Massachusetts General Hospital, analyzing 218 patients between 1964 and 1973, and a second from the University of Texas at San Antonio–affiliated hospitals, studying 166 patients between 1978 and 1986. The results of these two studies are remarkably similar and may be summarized as follows.

Neurologic complications were common (see Chapter 24), and they were recognized on clinical examination in 35% to 39% of the patients. These neurologic complications were important (40% to 58% of these patients died), whereas only 20% of patients without neurologic complications died. The frequency of neurologic complications is clearly related to the infecting organism. The more virulent organisms, such as *Staphylococcus aureus, Streptococcus pneumoniae,* anaerobic streptococci, or enterobacteriaceae, have a higher incidence (53% to 90%), whereas infection with a less virulent organism, such as *Streptococcus viridans,* shows a much lower incidence (28%). Furthermore, the major valve involved is related to the frequency of neurologic complications, with mitral valve disease carrying nearly twice the risk of either aortic or tricuspid valve involvement.

By far the most frequent neurologic complication in bacterial endocarditis is major cerebral embolic infarction, which occurred in 17% to 20% of the 218 patients. In the vast majority of cases the middle cerebral artery or one of its branches was involved, with an appropriate clinical syndrome. The majority of these patients died, and postmortem examination showed a characteristic hemorrhagic infarction. An occluded vessel was sometimes found, but microorganisms were very rarely found in the brain parenchyma. Thus most emboli arising from cardiac vegetations in this situation are bland and produce typical embolic hemorrhagic infarction of the brain. The very high mortality probably reflects merely the combined mortality of stroke and infective endocarditis.

Microscopic (i.e., less than 1 cm^3) brain abscesses are seen rarely (8 of 218 Massachusetts General Hospital patients) and almost certainly result from miliary spread of infected emboli arising from cardiac vegetations (see Chapter 15). However, this is quite rare compared with the relatively common event of major bland cerebral emboli. Macroscopic brain abscess is practically unknown in pure bacterial endocarditis. The treatment of microscopic abscesses requires antibiotic therapy alone, and macroscopic abscess requires surgical drainage plus antibiotic therapy. The latter should not be considered a manifestation of pure bacterial endocarditis, regardless of the infecting organism.

Cerebral mycotic aneurysm, another rare complication of endocarditis, is presumably caused by infected emboli from cardiac vegetations. Most occur with *S. aureus* infection and are found in branches of the middle cerebral artery. The characteristic clinical picture is sudden onset of middle cerebral artery syndrome followed by an intracerebral hemorrhage.

Whether to use anticoagulant or antiplatelet therapy to prevent cerebral emboli in endocarditis patients is an extremely difficult question. The crucial issue is whether the increased risk of intracerebral hemorrhage produced by anticoagulants is greater or less than the decrement in cerebral emboli prevented by the anticoagulant. Most data remain anecdotal.

Seizures occur in approximately 10% of patients with endocarditis. Focal seizures, which occur in approximately half of this 10%, usually represent cerebral infarction from embolus, whereas generalized seizures may be a sign of numerous metabolic disturbances, including uremia, hypoxemia, electrolyte disturbances, and penicillin toxicity but usually do not indicate focal neurologic disease.

Spinal fluid examination is not particularly useful in clinical practice in the setting of endocarditis, and findings generally depend on the virulence of the infecting organism rather than on any specific neurologic complications.

Nonbacterial (marantic) thrombotic endocarditis (NBTE) is a paraneoplastic syndrome most often associated with mucin-secreting adenocarcinoma. In about one fifth of the cases there is evidence of some degree of disseminated intravascular coagulation (DIC), suggesting that at least in some cases NBTE is part of a generalized hypercoagulable state. Arterial thrombosis and/or embolism may occur in many peripheral organs, including the brain, but much less is known about the detailed neurologic syndromes that occur in this entity than about those in bacterial endocarditis, primarily because of the former's relative rarity. In cancer patients NBTE may be a more common cause of stroke than previously recognized. The treatment is that of the underlying tumor. Anticoagulants are contraindicated because of the fear of hemorrhagic complications from disseminated tumor.

CARDIAC TRANSPLANTATION

Cardiac transplantation (Chapter 34) is used in the treatment of medically intractable dilated, hypertrophic, restrictive and ischemic cardiomyopathies, as well as rheumatic heart disease in some patients. Neurologic complications are very common, occurring in 50% to 60% of patients, and may be divided into those attributable to the use of immunosuppressive drugs and those peculiar to the cardiac transplantation procedure itself.

Cyclosporine, the most commonly used antirejection drug, works by inhibiting lymphokine release. Although its major toxic effect is renal, the hypertension that nearly always complicates its use results, to a large extent, from its direct stimulation of the sympathetic nervous system. Most of its neurologic toxicity is due to its tendency to produce hypertension. The encephalopathy of cyclosporine is roughly correlated with blood levels (therapeutic level, 250 to 500 mg/ml of whole blood or 50 to 300 ng/ml of plasma), but it is much better correlated with the rate of change in blood pressure from the patient's baseline level. Cyclosporine toxicity may be considered a *forme fruste* of hypertensive encephalopathy and as such is due to failure of cerebral autoregulation most prominent in the border zone between the posterior and middle cerebral artery territories. Therefore it is characterized on clinical examination by tremor, abnormalities in mental state ranging from mild inattention to coma, seizures, and various syndromes referable to the parietooccipital junction including visual field defects, visual agnosias, Balint's syndrome (i.e., the triad of simultanagnosia, abnormalities in visually directed reaching, and difficulties with voluntary eye movements), and cortical blindness, sometimes with denial of deficit (i.e., Anton's syndrome). Magnetic resonance imaging (MRI) shows increased signal on T2-weighted images in the parietooccipital white matter, a finding that may be quite evanescent and does not represent stroke. Flow studies such as single photon emission computed tomography (SPECT) demonstrate that this is due to increased flow with extravasation of water. These findings are identical to those found in patients with hypertensive encephalopathy, including the syndrome of toxemia of pregnancy. It should be emphasized that the blood pressure need not be very high (i.e., in the range of malignant hypertension) for this to occur. Lowering of blood pressure by any means including, but not limited to, lowering the blood level of cyclosporine results in resolution of the clinical syndrome and the imaging abnormalities. FK 506, a newer antirejection drug, works by a mechanism similar to that of cyclosporine. Although there is less experience with the new agent, the spectrum of neurologic abnormalities appears to be the same.

OKT3 is a monoclonal antibody directed against T cells. Its major neurologic side effect is aseptic meningitis, which occurs in about 1 in 20 patients during the first 3 days of exposure to the drug. Cerebrospinal fluid analysis shows a lymphocytic pleocytosis with normal glucose and normal or slightly elevated protein levels. The syndrome is self-limited and benign, but one should be certain to perform a lumbar puncture and culture the spinal fluid to exclude a bacterial or fungal meningitis before settling on the more benign diagnosis of OKT3-induced aseptic meningitis. The mechanism of the meningeal inflammation is probably allergic and similar to that seen in some patients receiving nonsteroidal antiinflammatory drugs such as ibuprofen or in some patients who receive treatment with intravenous immunoglobulin (IVIG). The ibuprofen syndrome appears to be

more common in patients with rheumatic diseases such as lupus erythematosus. Whether this is also true for the IVIG- and OKT3-induced meningitis is unknown. A more severe syndrome that includes variable degrees of mental status derangement such as seizures may occur even more rarely. It is associated with neuroimaging evidence of cerebral edema but is also self-limited and benign, even if the OKT3 is continued. The long-term, serious side effect of OKT3 use is the development of lymphoma, which appears to be dose related.

Antithymocyte globin (ATG) and *antilymphoblast globulin* (ALG) are antisera directed against thymocytes or lymphocytes. Rarely, a picture of aseptic meningitis similar to that seen with OKT3 develops, which is also self-limited and benign.

Corticosteroids, the oldest immunosuppressive drugs, are less specific in their actions than the newer agents listed earlier. Neurologic complications include psychosis and mania, a proximal myopathy and, rarely, spinal cord compression as a result of epidural lipomatosis. Long-term use of steroids also predisposes to glucose intolerance, gastrointestinal tract bleeding, and osteoporosis, all of which have their own secondary neurologic effects. These are well known to most generalists and are discussed in other sections of this text.

Neurologic infections occurs in about 10% of all transplant recipients but is more important in clinical practice than that number implies, since about half of the central nervous system infections that occur in immunocompromised patients result in death. Nearly every conceivable organism has been reported to infect transplant recipients, but about 80% of the cases are due to infection with *Listeria monocytogenes, Cryptococcus neoformans,* and *Aspergillus fumigatus.* Central nervous system infections in immunocompromised hosts may be difficult to recognize because the usual signs of infection such as fever and meningismus may be minimally present or absent in such patients, since these signs depend in part on a vigorous immune response to the infection. Since the expected signs of central nervous system infection may be absent and since nearly any organism (bacterium, fungus, parasite, or virus) may be responsible, the clinician should have a high index of suspicion for infectious causes of neurologic deterioration in any transplant recipient. A few clues may be of help in determining the most likely predominant organism.

An infection outside the nervous system should alert the clinician to a possible neurologic infection. Skin lesions may be found to harbor cryptococci, and lung infection suggests *Aspergillus, Nocardia,* or *Cryptococcus* organisms.

Acute meningitis is often due to L. *monocytogenes,* whereas chronic meningitis, often with cranial nerve palsies, suggests tuberculosis or fungal organisms. A progressive multifocal syndrome with hemiparesis, visual symptoms, ataxia, dysarthria, and dementia should raise the specter of progressive multifocal leukoencephalopathy caused by the Creutzfeldt-Jakob (JC) polyomavirus. A localized mass lesion (e.g., a brain abscess) is often due to multiple organisms, including anaerobes, but the predominant organism in the immunocompromised patient is usually *Aspergillus, Nocardia,* or *Toxoplasma.*

Another clue to the causative organism comes from the time period after transplantation. In the early period (i.e., up to 1 month) infections are due to organisms common in the nonimmunocompromised patient. In the intermediate period (i.e., between 1 and 6 months after transplantation), the risk of neurologic infection peaks, usually as a result of either virus (e.g., cytomegalovirus, Epstein-Barr virus) or opportunistic bacteria and fungi (e.g., *Listeria, Aspergillus,* and *Nocardia* organisms). Late infections (i.e., more than 6 months after transplantation) are related to the chronic use of potent antirejection medications such as steroids, monoclonal antibodies, and cyclosporine. The most common organisms are *Cryptococcus, Listeria,* and *Nocardia.*

Lymphoproliferative syndromes occur after prolonged immunosuppression, ranging from apparently benign polyclonal lymphoid hyperplasia to monoclonal lymphoma. The nervous system is involved in about 20% of such patients. When the central nervous system is involved, it is the only apparent site of involvement in 85% of the cases. Posttransplantation lymphoproliferatiave syndromes are strongly associated with Epstein-Barr virus infection, whereas primary central nervous system lymphomas in immunocompetent people are not associated with Epstein-Barr virus infection. These B-cell lymphomas arise deep in the brain, with a propensity for the perivascular spaces. Central nervous system lymphoma is distinguished from progressive multifocal leukoencephalopathy by the fact that the former produces mass effect and enhances with gadolinium.

The cardiac transplantation procedure itself is associated with variable periods of extracorporeal circulation, which may result in diffuse hypoxic-ischemic injury or focal cerebral infarction related to thromboembolism or air embolism. Damage to the brachial plexus is also commonly seen as a result of retraction of the chest wall, and the phrenic nerve may be damaged when the heart is packed in ice during the procedure.

BIBLIOGRAPHY

Boston Area Anticoagulation Trial for Atrial Fibrillation Investigators: The effect of low-dose warfarin on the risk of stroke in patients with non-rheumatic atrial fibrillation, *N Engl J Med* 323:1505, 1990.

DiMauro S et al: Mitochondrial encephalomyopathies, *Neurol Clin* 8:483, 1990.

Drislane FW et al: Myocardial contraction band lesions in patients with fatal asthma: possible neurocardiologic mechanisms, *Am Rev Respir Dis* 135:498, 1987.

Forsberg H, Ologsson B-O, Eriksson A: Cardiac involvement in congenital myotonic dystrophy, *Br Heart J* 63:119, 1990.

Hotson JR, Enzmann DR: Neurologic complications of cardiac transplantation, *Neurol Clin* 6:349, 1988.

Kanter MC, Hart RG: Neurologic complications of infective endocarditis, *Neurology* 41:1015, 1991.

Karch SB, Billingham ME: Myocardial contraction bands revisited, *Hum Pathol* 17:9, 1986.

Leor J, Poole K, Kloner RA: Sudden cardiac death triggered by an earthquake, *N Engl J Med* 334:413, 1996.

Levy DE et al: Predicting outcome from hypoxic-ischemic coma, *JAMA* 253:1420, 1985.

Nigro G, Comi LI, Vain RJI: The incidence and evolution of cardiomyopathy in Duchenne muscular dystrophy, *Int J Cardiol* 26:271, 1990.

Pruit AA, Rubin RH, Karchmer AW: Neurologic complications of bacterial endocarditis, *Medicine (Baltimore)* 57:329, 1978.

Rudehill A et al: ECG abnormalities in patients with subarachnoid haemorrhage and intracranial tumors, *J Neurol Neurosurg Psychiatry* 50:1375, 1987.

Samuels MA: The heart and neurologic disorders. In Tyler HR, Dawson DM, editors: *Current neurology,* Boston, 1979, Houghton Mifflin.

Samuels MA: Neurogenic heart disease: a unifying hypothesis, *Am J Cardiol* 60:15J, 1987.

Samuels MA: Cardiopulmonary aspects of neurological catastrophes. In Ropper AH, Kennedy S, editors: *Neurological and neurosurgical intensive care,* ed 2, Rockville, Md, 1988, Aspen.

Samuels MA: Unexpected demise: sudden death in neurology. In Hachinski V, editor: *Challenges in neurology,* Philadelphia, 1992, FA Davis.

Samuels MA, Patchell RA: The neurologic complications of organ transplantation. In Samuels MA, Feske S, editors: *Office practice of neurology,* New York, 1996, Churchill Livingstone.

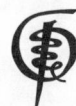

CHAPTER

165 Neurorheumatology

Kenneth K. Nakano

Rheumatologic and connective tissue (CT) disease may become evident as a neurologic disorder, with the primary diagnosis of an underlying disease or condition being made during the course of the neurologic assessment. The possibility of a CT or rheumatologic disease (i.e., systemic lupus erythematosus [SLE], antiphospholipid antibody syndrome [AAS], rheumatoid arthritis [RA], Takayasu's arteritis [TKA], granulomatous giant-cell arteritis [GGA], periarteritis nodosa [PN], Wegener's granulomatosis [WG], polymyositis [PM], dermatomyositis [DM], polymyalgia rheumatica [PMR], scleroderma [systemic sclerosis, SS], Sjögren's syndrome, mixed connective tissue disease [MCTD], and temporal arteritis [TA]) should be kept in mind with the new onset of neurologic symptoms and/or signs in young persons, particularly women. The neurologic manifestations of the rheumatologic and CT disorders are listed and categorized in Table 165-1.

Rheumatologic and CT disorders are autoimmune diseases; both humoral and cell-mediated immune responses are increased in premenopausal women as compared with men, and CT diseases are rela-

tively frequent in women of childbearing age. Both the presence of testosterone and the postmenopausal loss of estrogen production reduce the immune response, lowering the risk of many of these disorders in men and women with aging.

The individual rheumatologic and CT disorders are discussed as diseases elsewhere in this textbook; this chapter emphasizes the neurologic complications of these diseases. Because these CT disorders are multiple system diseases, it is recommended that an interdisciplinary medical team approach be used for management in these patients.

CONNECTIVE TISSUE DISORDERS

The symptoms and signs resulting from CT disorders (Table 165-1) include those resulting from systemic reaction to the disease and involvement of the viscera. Disorders of the peripheral nerve that develop in association with CT diseases are a medical challenge (Box 165-1). First, a patient with known CT disease may have more than one type of peripheral neuropathy. Second, certain types of peripheral neuropathy may represent the initial manifestation of an undiagnosed CT disease.

Vasculitis can be defined as inflammation of blood vessels and is associated with necrosis causing compromise of vessel lumen and secondary ischemia in involved tissues. Vasculitis appears often in the differential diagnosis of nearly all neurologic disorders because it can closely mimic most central nervous system (CNS) and peripheral nervous system (PNS) diseases. However, certain clinical symptoms and signs, alone or in combination, can be suggestive of a vasculitic disorder.

The following basic types of peripheral neuropathy appear when vasculitis affects the PNS: (1) mononeuritis multiplex (MM), (2) distal symmetric "stocking-glove" sensorimotor peripheral neuropathy, and (3) overlapping, extensive MM. Regardless of the type of peripheral neuropathy seen in the vasculitis syndromes, the symptoms include a severe, burning paresthesia in the distribution of the involved nerve or nerves.

When skeletal muscle becomes involved with vasculitis, patients demonstrate symmetric proximal muscle weakness that appears indistinguishable on clinical examination from that seen in PM or DM. In patients with an underlying collagen vascular disease (i.e., SLE, RA, Sjögren's syndrome, or SS), the skeletal muscle involvement is often caused by a primary inflammatory involvement of the muscle itself rather than vasculitis.

Two primary patterns of clinical involvement occur for CNS vasculitis, depending on whether the vasculitis is predominantly diffuse or focal. With diffuse involvement the patient complains of acute or subacute headache, psychiatric impairment (personality, behavioral, and affective disturbances), and cognitive impairment (memory and mental status changes). Generalized seizures may occur in association with an encephalopathy. On the other hand, focal CNS vasculitis causes focal cerebral deficits. Any strokelike event, especially in a young person without risk factors of stroke, should alert the clinician about vasculitis. Furthermore, single or multiple cranial nerve palsies (visual loss, diplopia, facial paresthesia or weakness, vertigo, tinnitus, dysphagia) can be manifestations of focal CNS vasculitis. Less commonly, focal CNS vasculitis causes intracerebral or subarachnoid hemorrhage, movement disorder (e.g., chorea), and an isolated myelopathy (e.g., isolated granulomatous angiitis). Overlap in the symptoms of these two patterns occurs because all of the vasculitides can produce either diffuse or focal CNS disease.

Most of the vasculitic syndromes can produce disease in both the CNS and PNS, often simultaneously. Atypical cases that do not fit neatly into any of the diagnostic categories occur frequently and are suggestive that there is some overlap in clinical syndromes (e.g., SLE and RA). The institution of therapy (including immunosuppressive therapy) can alter the natural history of many forms of vasculitis that were previously untreatable and often fatal. Therefore it becomes vital that the clinician arrive at an early diagnosis and classification to prevent the development or progression of CNS and PNS manifestations of the CT disorders, including the various vasculitides.

Table 165-1   Neurologic manifestations of the collagen vascular diseases

ENTITY	PREVALENCE RATE	GENETICS	AGE AT ONSET	M:F	CLINICAL FEATURES	PATHOLOGIC FEATURES	THERAPY
Systemic lupus erythematosus (SLE)	Rare in general population, CNS complications in 30%-75%	Sporadic	24 months after diagnosis	1:9	Seizures 54%, CNS 42%, mental change 33%, hemiparesis 12%, paraparesis 4%, movement disorder 4%, polyneuropathy 8%	Microinfarcts in the CNS; globulin in choroid plexus; fibrinoid degeneration	Probably steroids and/or immunosuppressive therapy
Temporal arteritis (TA)	Rare	Sporadic	60-80 years of age	M = F	Headache (temporal more than occipital), fever, weight loss, ESR >50 mm; prominent temporal artery; 30% can go blind; CNS involved	Giant-cell arteritis in media of vessels	Temporal artery biopsy, steroids for at least 6 mos
Polymyalgia rheumatica (PMR)	Rare	Sporadic	60-80 years of age	M = F	Malaise, weight loss, ESR >50 mm; brainstem strokes occasionally; normal enzymes, EMG; not much weakness	Can show similar pathology as TA or nothing	Steroids until ESR remains low
Granulomatous giant-cell arteritis (GGA); Wegener's granulomatosis (WG)	Rare	Sporadic	30-60 years of age (but any age)	M < F	CNS: seizures, hemiparesis, SAH, infarcts, MS change; PNS: mononeuritis multiplex, neuropathy	Granulomatous lesions in respiratory tract, kidneys; vasculitis in nerves and CNS	Steroids and/or immunosuppressives (especially cyclophosphamide)
Periarteritis (P)	Rare	Sporadic	30-40 years of age in 50%	M = F	Acute or insidious; fever, malaise, weakness, arthralgias, visceral involvement; PNS: neuropathies 50%; CNS: Sz, HA, psychosis	Inflammatory arteritis of medium-sized arteries, vasonervorum ischemia; progressive	Steroids
Polymyositis (PM)	6.3/10^5	Sporadic	40-70 years of age	5:1	Subacute girdle muscle weakness 98%; dysphagia 51%; muscle pain 58%; ESR, CPK, EMG abnormalities in the majority	?Sensitized lymphocytes; ?virus; degenerative and inflammatory changes in muscle with perivascular lymphs and plasma cells Skin DM involved	Steroids; for severe, relapsing cases immunosuppressives may be of benefit
Dermatomyositis (DM)		Sporadic	Child, adult	M = F	Skin findings in DM; often associated with cancer		
Takayasu's arteritis (TKA)	Rare	Sporadic	10-30 years of age	1:9	Headache, claudication, visual disturbance, reduced or absent pulses	Vasculitis of large arteries, especially the aorta	Steroids with or without cytotoxics
Periarteritis nodosa (PN)	0.7/10^5	Sporadic	40-60 years of age	2:1	Mononeuritis multiplex, muscle disease, stroke, inflammation of orbit	Vasculitis of small and medium-sized vessels	Steroids and immunosuppressive
Scleroderma (systemic sclerosis [SSI])	20/10^6	Sporadic	Peaks over 60 years of age	1:3	Peripheral nerve, trigeminal neuralgia, Raynaud's, skin and esophageal dysfunction, trigeminal sensory neuropathy	Skin fibroblasts synthesize excessive quantities of collagen precursors	D-penicillamine, but no truly effective drug has been shown
Mixed connective tissues disease (MCTD)		Sporadic			Overlapping features with SLE, SS, PM	High antiribonucleoprotein (RNP) level	

CNS, Central nervous system; ESR, erythrocyte sedimentation rate; EMG, electromyogram; SAH, subarachnoid hemorrhage; MS, mental status; PNS, peripheral nervous system; Sz, seizure; HA, headache; CPK, creatine phosphokinase.

BOX 165-1
Neuropathies associated with connective tissue disease

Distal axonal polyneuropathy, not clearly vasculitic
Compression neuropathy (e.g., carpal tunnel syndrome)
Sensory neuropathy
Trigeminal sensory neuropathy
Vasculitic neuropathy
    Mononeuropathy multiplex or overtly multifocal mononeuropathies
    Asymmetric polyneuropathy or multiple mononeuropathies with partial confluence
    Distal symmetric polyneuropathy or confluent multifocal mononeuropathies
Other neuropathies that may be associated with connective tissue disease
    Acute demyelinating polyneuropathy
    Chronic demyelinating polyneuropathy
    Brachial plexus neuropathy

Table 165-2 Frequency of neurologic manifestations of systemic lupus erythematosus

NEUROLOGIC MANIFESTATIONS	REPORTED FREQUENCY RANGE (%)
Peripheral nervous system	
Peripheral neuropathy	5-10
Inflammatory myopathy	2-12
Central nervous system (CNS)	
Seizures	18-70
Thrombotic stroke	32-43
CNS hemorrhage	10-40
Altered consciousness	4-20
Behavioral change	8-15
Psychosis	
Confusion	
Dementia	
Headache	5-16
Cranial nerve palsies	5-12
Myelopathy	2-8
Chorea	1-3

Systemic Lupus Erythematosus

The diagnosis of SLE can be made on combined clinical and laboratory criteria; neurologic manifestations or symptoms occur in about half of these patients (Table 165-2). The differences in the reported frequencies of specific neurologic manifestations or complications represent variable severity of the systemic disease between series, along with a variance in the ascertainment of a particular neurologic disorder (e.g., diagnosis of stroke with changing clinical levels of diagnosis and technologic neuroimaging).

Stroke is a recognized complication of SLE; predisposing factors appear to be a prothrombotic state produced by antiphospholipid antibodies or the lupus anticoagulant or by cardiac embolism, often related to Libman-Sacks endocarditis. Owing to the high frequency of stroke recurrence, recommendation for stroke prevention is long-term anticoagulation if there are no contraindications. In patients with continued cerebrovascular ischemic events, despite therapeutic anticoagulation, brief corticosteroid therapy may be considered (steroids do not have a reliable effect on titers of antiphospholipid antibodies, and the side effects make this treatment impractical for the long-term prevention of stroke). Ticlopidine, a platelet inhibitor, may be useful but has not been studied in SLE patients and stroke prevention.

Central nervous system SLE consists of a spectrum of neurologic disorders and does not represent a single disease. An immune mechanism for cerebral symptoms in SLE patients has never been proven and raises question of whether to treat neurologic signs and/or symptoms with corticosteroids.

The most frequent neurologic manifestation of SLE is seizures (frequency varying from 18% to as high as 70%), and the reported association of seizures with a history of stroke varies from 30% to 60%, raising the possible association of the seizure disorder resulting from older stroke(s). In addition, seizures occur during exacerbation of the SLE or during infections, requiring treatment of the underlying systemic process as well as appropriate anticonvulsant medications. There has been no systematic study to determine which anticonvulsants are the safest and/or most effective in SLE, and anticonvulsant complications (such as allergic reactions or leukopenia) appear to be more frequent in patients with SLE than in general.

Headaches, often with migrainous features, are common in SLE. In cases refractory to medical antimigraine therapy the clinician should exclude headache resulting from venous thrombosis and/or the underlying systemic disease, directing therapy accordingly. Ergots should be avoided in treating patients with SLE, since this class of medications may enhance the risk of strokes; beta blockers or tricyclic medications may be effective in headache prophylaxis.

Behavioral changes, including psychosis and depression, are common in patients with SLE and may be associated with elevated levels of antiribosomal P protein antibodies, suggesting responsiveness to steroid. At times, systemic infections are associated with behavioral changes, especially if consciousness is impaired, and a careful evaluation for infections should be performed (e.g., cerebrospinal fluid [CSF] assessment). Chorea infrequently occurs with SLE and, rarely, confusion can arise during pregnancy (chorea gravidum), with the onset of definite SLE occurring months or years later. This may be related to antiphospholipid antibodies, since a similar disorder has been seen in primary AAS.

Antiphospholipid Antibody Syndrome

The AAS syndrome consists of recurrent episodes of venous and arterial thrombosis. Although patients with AAS by definition do not have SLE, many have positive antiphospholipid antibodies and some features of SLE, raising the possibility that the primary AAS could be a variant of SLE. The major neurologic complication of AAS is stroke with a recurrence of about 50% (similar to stroke patients with SLE) and the risk of other thrombotic events (deep venous thrombosis or pulmonary embolus), is also high. Additional neurologic manifestations of AAS include migraine, retinal infarction, and chorea.

Rheumatoid Arthritis

Approximately 75% of patients with RA who have had symptoms of the disease for less than a year improve, and approximately 15% to 20% show complete remission. However, when the disease becomes recurrent or is sustained over years, increasingly serious and permanent disturbance in joint function develops. Neurologic complications become evident with moderate and severe forms of the disease. The neurologic manifestations of RA can be divided into articular and extraarticular disorders (Box 165-2).

Articular Involvement. Approximately 30% to 40% of all patients with chronic RA and severe peripheral joint disease who are hospitalized have radiologic evidence of cervical spine subluxation. Often, these x-ray findings are not associated with neurologic symptoms. However, in 2% to 5% of all patients with significant cervical subluxation, pyramidal tract signs or vague subjective sensory findings are evident on neurologic examination. Usually RA affects the upper levels of the cervical spine and produces different clinical features at different ages. In children with RA, growth is deficient and apophyseal joints often fuse, with resultant limitation of neck movement. In adults the main change in the cervical spine is subluxation, which can take the following forms: (1) C1 moves anteriorly on C2 (this is the most common form and results from insufficiency of the transverse ligament or from erosion or fracture of the odontoid); (2) C1 moves posteriorly on C2 (this results from severe erosion or frac-

---

BOX 165-2

Neurologic manifestations of rheumatoid arthritis

Articular-cervical spine disease
Cervical subluxations (four types)
   C1 moves anteriorly on C2
   C1 moves posteriorly on C2
   Vertical subluxation of odontoid
   "Staircase" or multiple lower-level subluxations
Radiologic findings often with clinical symptoms
   Double-crush syndrome
   Narrowed disk spaces above C5
Radiologic findings without clinical symptoms
   Vertebral plate erosion
   Apophyseal joint erosion
   Basilar impression of the skull

Extraarticular
Peripheral neuropathies
   Compression leading to entrapment
   Mild sensory neuropathy with a good prognosis
   Diffuse sensorimotor neuropathy
   Fulminant sensorimotor neuropathy
Diffuse myopathy and focal myositis
Polymyositis-dermatomyositis
Vasculitis—often with other connective tissue disorders
   Mononeuritis complex
   "Cerebral vasculitis"—often with lupus erythematosus and rheumatoid arthritis
Dural rheumatoid nodules causing brain and spinal cord compression
Progressive multifocal leukoencephalopathy

---

ture of the odontoid); (3) vertical subluxation of the odontoid and body of C2 (a result of destruction of the lateral atlantoaxial joints or of the bone around the foramen magnum, the rarest form of cervical subluxation in RA); and (4) "staircase" subluxation of one vertebra on another, often multiple and below the C2 level (second most common cervical subluxation in RA; depends on destruction of the apophyseal joints rather than on loss of ligamentous connections).

Characteristic neuritic pain radiating up to the occiput is frequently present in patients with RA. Crepitation and instability of the cervical spine can cause alarm. Paresthesia can be caused by head or neck movement and Lhermitte's sign may be elicited by sudden flexion of the neck. Rarely the complaints reflect transient ischemic attacks (TIAs) in the posterior cerebral circulation (transient visual disturbances, such as diplopia, vertigo, paresthesia, or paresis). Early spinal cord compression or ischemia may produce subtle spastic quadriparesis and hyperreflexia, which may be especially unwelcome when a patient is already debilitated. Pyramidal tract signs (increased reflexes and Babinski's responses) or early proprioceptive loss in the hands represent early signs of impending spinal cord compression. The classic spinal cord compression picture, including an altered sensory level to all modalities, bladder and bowel dysfunction, and flaccid quadriplegia, is a late development. To make a clinical diagnosis of cervical subluxation in RA, radiologic confirmation becomes necessary. Lateral views of the cervical spine in extension and flexion to open the gap between the odontoid and the arch of C1 are helpful. Tomography, computed tomography (CT), and magnetic resonance imaging (MRI) may become necessary for detailed anatomic study and precise measurement of the spinal cord and canal.

Treatment for the less severe and neurologically asymptomatic cases of cervical subluxation includes firm cervical collars aimed at improving stability and easing pain. Neurosurgical and orthopedic surgical immobilization of the neck and halo traction should be considered in the patient with progressive spinal cord signs. Stabilization becomes most useful before permanent neurologic or vascular damage occurs to the spinal cord. If surgery is considered, it should be performed before the patient has had permanent cord injury and at a center familiar with chronic RA and techniques of cervical and occipitocervical fusion.

Extraarticular Manifestations

Peripheral neuropathies. Various types of neuropathies have been reported in RA: compression leading to entrapment (e.g., carpal tunnel syndrome (CTS), ulnar nerve compression at the elbow, posterior interosse- ous nerve syndrome, tarsal tunnel syndrome), mild sensory neuropathies with a good prognosis, diffuse sensorimotor polyneuropathy, and a fulminant sensorimotor disorder often related to a generalized vas culitis. Proposed causes of the neuropathy in RA include vascular disturbances, nutritional deficiencies, and demyelination. The neuropa- thy most commonly encountered, however, is a mild sensory one, primarily of the feet and legs. Patients often complain of varying degrees of paresthesia, dysesthesia, or "burning feet" for varying periods. Often when the RA stabilizes, the symptoms of the peripheral neuropathy subside over weeks. Optimal nutrition, additional vitamins, and carbamazepine have offered some relief of the subjective dysesthesia and burning feet. A more severe sensorimotor polyneuropathy can be seen occasionally in patients with acute joint disease, in which the patient has some objective weakness, in addition to the sensory symptoms. Vasculitis is not present on clinical examination, and the patient may show symmetric distal weakness of the limbs, as well as diminished vibration and touch sensations in the feet and legs, more than in the hands and arm. Often, the patients in this category have neglected the RA, or there has been an acute recurrence of the disease. The aim of therapy should be to effect remission of the RA. One must rule out other possible causes of peripheral neuropathy (e.g., diabetes, toxins, alcohol excess, and drugs). Subjective relief of pain can be achieved with phenytoin or carbamazepine. Generally the patient recovers most of the neurologic function independent of therapy, and the neuropathy improves. A small number of patients may be left with chronic neuropathy, as evidenced by neurologic examination and nerve conduction studies. In a small percentage of cases malignant rheumatoid vasculitis becomes evident with a fulminant sensorimotor disorder, often with a mononeuritic component. Often, these patients have been treated with steroids or their disease has followed an unremitting course. Evidence of vasculitis is seen on the skin, and the neurologic picture can be similar to that in periarteritis (PA). These patients may have concomitant CT disease, or their symptoms may represent a spectrum of diseases (e.g., a patient can have RA and features of SLE). Medical therapy should be directed at control of the vasculitis and the RA. Even with optimal therapy, most of these patients are left with severe neuropathies.

Myopathy and focal myositis. Seventy to 80% of patients with chronic and recurrent RA have some muscle weakness, usually around the areas of joint involvement. These patients report diminished proximal strength and peripheral joint disability. RA myopathy is independent of steroid therapy, and these patients do not progress to diffuse, severe muscle necrosis if the RA remains controlled with medications and physical therapy. Although there is a combination of muscle and joint inflammation, the prognosis depends more on the joint disease than on the muscle involvement.

Vasculitis. Generalized RA vasculitis is rare. In a severe case of RA with multiple neurologic findings suggesting CNS involvement or a mononeuritis complex, a complete neurologic evaluation includes electroencephalogram, MRI, and CSF examination. Short-term steroid therapy and/or immunosuppressive drugs may be indicated in the acute condition.

Dural rheumatoid nodules. If the patient with RA has severe subcutaneous nodules, dural nodules may rarely develop, which can compress the brain or spinal cord. Dural nodules cannot be clinically separated from other disorders causing compression either of the brain or spinal cord (i.e., subdural hematoma, metastatic cancer, or neurofibroma). When a compressive syndrome within the CNS is suspected, MRI of the brain and spine should be performed to make a diagnosis.

Progressive multifocal leukoencephalopathy. Progressive multifocal leukoencephalopathy (PML), a rare complication of RA, is an asymmetrically diffuse CNS disorder evidenced by multifocal areas of demyelination. It is an infection by the papovaviruses that overwhelms an immunologically suppressed host. No known therapy exists, and the patient's course is rapidly fatal.

Ankylosing Spondylitis

Ankylosing spondylitis (AS) represents a chronic progressive form of arthritis involving the sacroiliac joints, the spinal apophyseal (synovial) joints, and the paravertebral soft tissues. Characteristically this disease produces ossification of the annulus fibrosus of the intervertebral disks and of the connective tissue immediately adjacent to the annulus and changes in the intervertebral diarthrodial joints similar to those occurring in RA. Over a period of 10 to 20 years the patient with AS develops the poker-type deformity or cervicodorsal kyphosis. Both atlantoaxial and atlantooccipital subluxations occur. External bracing may provide relief of bulbar symptoms from vascular ischemia in the latter situation. Other neurologic involvement in AS includes the cauda equina syndrome, vertebrovasilar insufficiency, and peripheral nerve lesions. Therapy should be directed at controlling the AS. In the event of the cauda equina syndrome, neurosurgical decompression of the lower spine may be necessary.

Takayasu's Arteritis

Takayasu's arteritis is a rare vasculitis that involves large arteries, primarily the aortic arch and its branches, and becomes evident with headache, decreased or absent pulses, visual disturbances, and claudication. Stroke is a potential complication, and treatment with steroids (with or without cytotoxic agents) may become necessary.

Periarteritis Nodosa

Periarteritis nodosa is a serious systemic disorder, producing necrotizing vasculitis with hyaline degeneration in small and medium-sized blood vessels. This condition may become evident with cardiac or renal manifestations or with MM; and neurologic complications include MM, muscle disease, stroke, and inflammation of the orbit, generally caused by necrotizing vasculitis producing tissue infarction. Stroke may occur if cardiac function becomes impaired, again as a result of vasculitis and infarction, producing cardiomyopathy. Steroids may be used for treatment, but cyclophosphamide is often necessary. Because the vascular disease is inflammatory rather than thrombotic, steroids or immunosuppressive drugs may be effective in stroke prevention. Since cardiomyopathy is relatively common in patients with PN, the treatment for stroke prevention is anticoagulation therapy.

Wegener's Granulomatosis

Wegener's granulomatosis is a systemic vasculitic disease, that presents with granulomas involving the kidneys, sinuses, and lung and occurs most often in men 40 to 50 years of age. Neurologic complications occur in about 22% of patients with WG and are equally distributed between cranial nerve palsies and MM. Loss of anterior pituitary hormones as a result of vasculitis, often leading to thrombosis, has also been reported. Steroid treatment increases average survival to 12.5 months, and without treatment WG is usually rapidly fatal. Standard treatment with cyclophosphamide produces remissions in about 90% of patients.

Scleroderma

The common systemic manifestations of scleroderma or systemic sclerosis (SS) include Raynaud's phenomenon, esophageal dysfunction, atrophic skin, pulmonary dysfunction, and renal failure. Although neurologic problems of SS are infrequent, mild peripheral nerve disorders, particularly CTS and trigeminal neuralgia, are not uncommon. Disorders of muscle with weakness and elevated creatine phosphokinase (CPK) levels occur in approximately 20% of patients, and trigeminal sensory neuropathy has occurred in some. Stroke occurred in 3 of 50 patients in one series; however, all of these patients were between 50 and 60 years of age.

Sjögren's Syndrome

Sjögren's syndrome is characterized by keratoconjunctivitis sicca and xerostomia and is often associated with another CT disease. Neuro-

logic manifestations include peripheral neuropathy and trigeminal sensory neuropathy, along with inclusion body myositis.

Mixed Connective Tissue Disease

Mixed connective tissue disease (MCTD) is a multiple system disease that has overlapping features with SLE, SS, and PM. High antiribonucleoprotein (anti-RNP) levels assist in the diagnosis. The neurologic complications of MCTD are similar to SS, with trigeminal neuralgia and trigeminal sensory neuropathy.

SUMMARY

Neurorheumatology encompasses the neurologic syndromes and complications that occur in RA, AS, and the various CT disorders. Although the involvement of the PNS and CNS may be infrequent with the rheumatologic diseases, they represent well-defined clinical entities that require a keen clinical awareness and medical (and at times surgical) treatment.

BIBLIOGRAPHY

Arkin A: A clinical and pathological study of periarteritis nodosa, *Am J Pathol* 6:401, 1930.

Asherson RA, Khamashta MA, Ordi-Ros J et al: The "primary" antiphospholipid syndrome: major clinical and serological features, *Medicine* 68:366, 1989.

Averbuch-Heller L, Steiner I, Abramsky O: Neurologic manifestations of progressive systemic sclerosis, *Arch Neurol* 49:1292, 1992.

Bathon JM, Moreland LW, DiBartolomeo AG: Inflammatory central nervous system involvement in rheumatoid arthritis, *Semin Arthritis Rheum* 18:258, 1989.

Briley DP, Coull BM, Goodnight SH Jr: Neurological disease associated with antiphospholipid antibodies, *Ann Neurol* 25:221, 1989.

Drachman DA: Neurological complications of Wegener's granulomatosis, *Arch Neurol* 8:45, 1963.

Fahey JL, Leonard E, Churg J et al: Wegener's granulomatosis, *Am J Med* 17:168, 1954.

Fauci AS, Haynes BF, Katz P et al: Wegener's granulomatosis: prospective clinical and therapeutic experience with 85 patients for 21 years, *Ann Intern Med* 98:76, 1983.

Futrell N, Millikan C: Frequency, etiology, and prevention of stroke in patients with systemic lupus erythematosus or lupus anticoagulant, *Stroke* 20:583, 1989.

Futrell N, Schultz LR, Millikan C: Central nervous system disease in patients with systemic lupus erythematosus, *Neurology* 42:1649, 1992.

Gutmann L, Govindan S, Riggs JE et al: Inclusion body myositis and Sjögren's syndrome, *Arch Neurol* 42:1021, 1985.

Ishikawa K, Maksuura S: Occlusive thromboarthropathy (Takayasu's disease), *Am J Cardiol* 50:1293, 1982.

Mauch E, Volk C, Kratzsch G et al: Neurological and neuropsychiatric dysfunction in primary Sjögren's syndrome, *Acta Neurol Scand* 89:31, 1994.

Mills JA: Systemic lupus erythematosus, *N Engl J Med* 330:1871, 1994.

Nakano KK: The neurological complications of rheumatoid arthritis, *Orthop Clin North Am* 6:861, 1975.

O'Connor JF, Musher DM: Central nervous system involvement in systemic lupus erythematosus, *Arch Neurol* 14:157, 1966.

Omdal R, Roalso S: Chorea gravidarum and chorea associated with oral contraceptives: diseases due to antiphospholipid antibodies? *Acta Neurol Scand* 86:219, 1992.

Schady W, Sheard A, Hassell A et al: Peripheral nerve dysfunction in scleroderma, *Q J Med* 80:661, 1991.

Sibley JT, Olszynski WP, Decoteau WE et al: The incidence and prognosis of central nervous system disease in systemic lupus erythematosus, *J Rheumatol* 19:47, 1991.

Tan EM, Cohen AS, Fries JF et al: The 1982 revised criteria for the classification of systemic lupus erythematosus, *Arthritis Rheum* 25:1271, 1982.

Teasdall RD, Frayha RA, Shulman LE: Cranial nerve involvement in systemic sclerosis (scleroderma): a report of 10 cases, *J Med* 59:149, 1980.

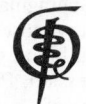

CHAPTER

166 Neuropulmonology

Frank W. Drislane and Martin A. Samuels

Interactions of central and peripheral nervous system diseases and respiratory function are numerous. The most important is probably ventilatory failure attributable to neurologic illness ("neurogenic respiratory failure"). There are also interesting and potentially critical alterations of respiratory rhythm without necessary impairment of ventilation; these arrhythmias can be important, useful signs both in patients with impaired consciousness and in those who remain awake. This chapter also includes a discussion of neurogenic pulmonary edema, a less common syndrome in which oxygenation may be impaired.

NEUROGENIC RESPIRATORY FAILURE

In physiologic terms, respiration begins in the brain. Voluntary respiration (used in speaking, singing, laughing, and intentional ventilatory movements) begins with corticospinal tract control of the diaphragm and accessory muscles of respiration. These tracts descend from the medulla in the lateral spinal cord to innervate the alpha motor neurons in the anterior horn of the spinal cord at the C3-5 level, where they compose the origins of the phrenic nerve to the diaphragm. The scalene, sternocleidomastoid, trapezius, and pectoral muscles are innervated by the eleventh cranial nerve and cervical spinal roots. Intercostal muscles are innervated by all of the thoracic roots, and deficits may affect the strength of cough. Voluntary breathing can be impaired by strokes and other central lesions. For example, a stroke can diminish respiratory movements on the affected side of the body during wakefulness but leave automatic breathing symmetric during sleep. Bilateral damage can lead to "respiratory apraxias," sometimes in association with a pseudobulbar palsy. Strokes and other central lesions may also cause altered respiratory rhythms and are discussed later.

Most respiration, however, is automatic and occurs in response to metabolic demands. This is controlled by respiratory centers in the brain stem. In the medulla the nucleus of the solitary tract (NTS) receives afferent information through the vagus (tenth) and glossopharyngeal (ninth) nerves from receptors in the carotid body that sense oxygen tension and from chemosensors in the aorta. Afferent firing in these receptors increases with a decline in oxygen pressure (Po_2) or increased carbon dioxide pressure (Pco_2). Hypotension in the carotid sinus also increases the frequency of afferent volleys through cranial nerve IX and stimulates respiration. There are also chemoreceptors sensing pH and CO_2 in the medulla itself. Stretch receptors in the lung provide additional information to the medulla through the vagus nerve; these generally inhibit respiration.

A more dorsal respiratory group (DRG) near the NTS stimulates the phrenic nerve to drive inspiration but projects through a more ventral respiratory group (VRG) of neurons in the nucleus ambiguus (NA) and nucleus retroambigualis (NRA); this center prompts coordinated expiration as well. From these respiratory centers, reticulospinal fibers descend along the anterolateral surface of the cervical spinal cord to the phrenic nerve alpha motor neurons at C3-5. Higher respiratory centers in the pons modulate these rhythms and superimpose more regularity. Corticospinal control of alpha motor neurons in the cervical spinal cord can override automatic respiration. Lesions causing respiratory failure can occur in these central nervous system structures or more distally in the peripheral nervous system.

Cardiopulmonary diseases often cause damage to the lung parenchyma and vasculature, impairing oxygenation. Patients with neurogenic-based failure of respiratory muscles, or failure to stimulate them adequately, tend to have normal circulation, lung structures, and compliance. In neurologic dysfunction, ventilation is usually impaired more than oxygenation. When neurologic dysfunction begins to threaten ventilation, patients may compensate, at least initially, by increasing respiratory rate, often without dyspnea. Impending respiratory failure may be subtle at first. A sign of progression is paradoxical movement of the abdomen (i.e., inward movement during inspiration, as opposed to the usual outward movement prompted by a downward excursion of the diaphragm, all resulting from the excessive use of accessory muscles of respiration taking over diaphragmatic work and thus pulling the abdomen inward). Use of accessory muscles is a sign of diaphragmatic and respiratory failure. Arterial blood gas levels may remain normal until relatively late in a progression. Pulmonary function tests can provide more quantitative signs of neurogenic respiratory failure. A decline in vital capacity by 40% may impair the handling of secretions, and at 10 to 15 ml/kg (usually a 70% decline) ventilatory failure occurs. Maximal inspiratory pressures may be an even more sensitive guide to ventilatory sufficiency. Normal

---

BOX 166-1

Neurogenic causes of ventilatory failure

Common causes

1. Encephalopathy: Metabolic, drugs
2. Critical illness polyneuropathy
3. Prolonged paralyzing agent with or without steroids
4. Strokes

Occasionally missed diagnoses of less common illnesses

5. Guillain-Barré syndrome
6. Motor neuron disease (amyotrophic lateral sclerosis)
7. Myasthenia gravis
8. Basal ganglia disease
9. Myopathies
10. Other spinal cord, peripheral nerve disease

---

subjects can usually generate -70 cm of water pressure on inspiration and may fail to clear CO_2 production at -20 cm H_2O. Airway occlusion pressure (the pressure drop in the first 100 milliseconds of inspiration against an occluded airway) may be an even better measure of neurologic "drive." Pulmonary function tests are described in greater detail in Chapter 41.

Neurogenic respiratory failure (Box 166-1) may occur in structures anywhere from the cortex to the respiratory muscles, and a diagnostic search can be organized in the same geographic pattern. Beginning with the cerebrum, one finds that severe encephalopathies are a relatively common cause of ventilatory failure in severely ill patients. Sedatives, alcohol, and narcotics are common contributors, although severe metabolic derangement can produce the same failure. Most of these causes of ventilatory failure are reversible. Strokes can impair respiration in many ways.

Failure of automatic breathing (Ondine's curse) is readily understood on consideration of the two independent systems of neural control of respiration. Whereas cortical and other lesions above the pons can alter voluntary breathing without disturbing automatic respiration, medullary and cervical spinal cord lesions can interrupt automatic breathing, leaving voluntary respiration intact. Failure of automatic breathing is uncommon and usually acquired rather than congenital. It is usually caused by bilateral interruption of the fibers from respiratory centers in the paramedian reticular formation of the medulla descending to the anterolateral cervical spinal cord, where the phrenic nerves and other nerves to respiratory muscles originate. These fibers are separate from the corticospinal tract and can be interrupted by bilateral infarctions in the medullary tegmentum, leaving the more lateral corticospinal fibers untouched. These are rare infarctions, given the bilateral blood supply of the medulla. Patients with failure of automatic respiration breathe adequately while awake, but hypocapnia, hypoxia, and pulmonary hypertension caused by respiratory failure may develop during sleep.

Hypoventilation can also be seen after encephalitis, presumably caused by medullary failure and insensitivity of medullary receptors to the usual chemical stimuli. A diminished responsiveness to CO_2 can also be demonstrated even years after recovery from acute poliomyelitis. Such chronic medullary failure is generally irreversible. Attempts at treatment of primary hypoventilation have included the use of progesterone as a respiratory stimulant and the use of phrenic nerve pacers.

Rare patients with a history and symptoms suggestive of failure of automatic breathing usually must be studied during sleep to reach a diagnosis. The far more common cases of sleep apnea syndromes are diagnosed in the same studies. Interestingly, rapid eye movement (REM) sleep can lead to more precipitous apnea in cases of Ondine's curse, possibly because of the inhibition of muscular tone that REM produces.

Ondine's curse has occurred in several cases of bilateral cervical cordotomy performed to sever the spinothalamic tracts for treatment of intractable pain. Nearby reticulospinal fibers can be damaged in this procedure, leading to a failure of automatic respiration while leaving voluntary respiration intact. Such complications are rare with unilateral lesioning but may occur in 5% to 20% of patients with bilateral cordotomies. These patients may appear to be healthy but have subsequent fatal apnea during sleep. Barbiturate and narcotic medications may precipitate declines. Permanent bilateral phrenic nerve stimulation may prevent sudden death. Failure of automatic respiration can be seen rarely after bilateral carotid endarterectomy, caused by the loss of chemosensitivity in the carotid bodies.

Spinal cord injuries above the C5 level may impair respiration substantially, and complete transection above C3 prevents respiration altogether. In most of these patients diagnosis is made at the time of major trauma, but others may have bone or disk disease and a deterioration through sudden neck movement. Diaphragmatic pacing may be the treatment of choice for patients with upper cervical spinal cord lesions. Similar problems may occur with acute myelopathies, including multiple sclerosis or transverse myelitis.

With both central and peripheral disease based in the spinal cord itself, amyotrophic lateral sclerosis (ALS) can also lead to ventilatory failure, usually long after the diagnosis. Respiratory and pulmonary complications are frequent, particularly aspiration pneumonias. Although weakness is often present in other areas, many ALS patients come to medical attention with respiratory symptoms. The neurologic examination and neurophysiologic testing are often characteristic (see Chapter 127), but there are many mimicking diseases that must be excluded, including multifocal conduction block and combined cervical and lumbar radiculopathies. Although specific treatment for ALS is still in experimental stages, many patients can obtain symptomatic benefit from respiratory support even short of intubation and full mechanical ventilation (e.g., through intermittent positive pressure ventilation or external assistive devices). Other diseases affecting the anterior horn cells, such as poliomyelitis, rabies, and spinal muscular atrophies, can produce similar problems.

Guillain-Barré syndrome (GBS) has about twice the incidence of ALS and prompts even more mechanical ventilation. Sometimes the diagnosis is less obvious, and patients can come to medical attention with respiratory failure. Weakness may ascend or progress gradually, but some patients may have precipitous ventilatory failure. There are less common axonal and primarily autonomic forms, and the autonomic instability may include marked blood pressure, temperature, and cardiac rhythm disturbances. The latter may be one of the most frequent causes of death in GBS. Patients with vital capacity of less than 20 ml/kg require intensive observation, and most of these patients progress to require mechanical ventilation, with a mean duration of mechanical ventilation of more than a month. Many illnesses can mimic GBS, including those with symmetric polyneuropathies and spinal fluid pleocytosis, such as Lyme disease, human immunodeficiency virus (HIV), sarcoidosis, and cytomegalovirus (CMV). Porphyria, diphtheria, and toxins, including vincristine, amiodarone, and dapsone, may cause severe neuropathies with respiratory complications similar to GBS. Botulism can appear similar in later stages, although it often begins with cranial nerve weakness and with descending symptoms, often after gastrointestinal tract illness. Many other diseases mimic GBS (Ropper, 1992).

Critical illness polyneuropathy is a more recently recognized syndrome (Chapter 147) occurring in patients with sepsis and multiorgan failure. It may be the most common neurologic explanation of failure to gain independence from mechanical ventilation. It occurs in a large percentage of patients who are in intensive care units for more than 2 weeks, with the most prominent feature being a severe axonal neuropathy, usually attributed to the toxins of sepsis. Neurophysiologic studies are crucial, although often difficult to perform in an intensive care unit, and they demonstrate widespread motor and sensory axonal neuropathy with denervation. Mortality is high because of the underlying illnesses, but the neuropathy tends to abate over 3 to 6 months in survivors. The neuropathy does not appear to be due to aminoglycosides or other medications, nutritional factors, metabolic disorders, or any specific infection.

Ventilatory failure is an ominous sign in myasthenia gravis, a relatively common cause of neurogenic respiratory failure (although less common than GBS). Ventilatory failure may occur at the time of exacerbations of myasthenia because of decreased anticholinesterase or steroid treatment of the disease, occasionally following edrophonium testing, occasionally at the beginning of corticosteroid treatment, fol-

lowing surgery, or with acute medical illness such as infection, hyperthyroidism, or medication use, including that of penicillamine, neuromuscular blocking agents, aminoglycosides, other antibiotics and antiarrhythmics, and several other medications. Tic paralysis, botulism, and Lambert-Eaton myasthenic syndrome can also cause severe weakness through actions at the neuromuscular junction.

Myopathies are relatively rare causes of ventilatory failure. Chronic respiratory disease is the most important problem in muscular dystrophies, including the chest wall deformities caused by kyphoscoliosis with its restrictive lung disease. Duchenne's muscular dystrophy is primary here and often ends in pulmonary infections and ventilatory failure in the third decade of life. Acid maltase deficiency and carnitine palmityl transferase deficiency are hereditary myopathies and very rare causes of ventilatory failure. Mitochondrial disease may cause myopathy and ventilatory failure as well. Metabolic myopathies can cause proximal weakness and, when particularly severe, respiratory compromise. Corticosteroids, thyroid disease, hypokalemia, and hypophosphatemia are among the more common causes. Medications such as chloroquine, amiodarone, clofibrate, and azidothymidine (AZT) are occasional culprits. Muscle paralyzing agents, with or without corticosteroids, may lead to severe weakness, including ventilatory failure, sometimes long outlasting their usual pharmacologic effects.

ABNORMAL RESPIRATORY RHYTHMS IN PATIENTS WITH ALTERED STATES OF CONSCIOUSNESS

In altered states of consciousness the most common (but least specific) respiratory abnormality is periodic breathing, most often Cheyne-Stokes respiration (CSR): that is, a regular waxing and waning of respiratory rate and volume, with apneic periods at the low points. CSR represents an increased sensitivity of the respiratory drive in response to CO_2. This is usually the result of bilateral cerebral dysfunction, although other factors contributing to an aberrant modulation of respiratory rhythms (such as hypoxia, other metabolic derangements, or prolonged circulation time, as in congestive heart failure) can lead to CSR.

The pneumotaxic center in the upper pons modulates inspiratory and expiratory centers lower in the brain stem. Bilateral abnormalities anywhere above this center can disrupt descending influences from forebrain structures and lead to CSR.

Ventilation persists in CSR, and patients do not become hypoxic: indeed, respiratory alkalosis may even develop. While periodic breathing is of limited localizing value in neurologic illness, its appearance may be the only sign of deterioration in a patient with known disease—for example, a mass lesion.

CSR may also be the primary respiratory abnormality in sleep apnea syndrome (rather than the more sudden apneas usually associated with this syndrome). In this case, CSR, possibly along with increased upper airway resistance, can lead to sleep fragmentation, increased arousals, and diminished oxygen saturation. In these patients (though not in sleep apnea in general), theophylline has been helpful in reversing the hypoxemia.

Posthyperventilation apnea (PHVA) also signifies an abnormal responsiveness to CO_2. Apnea of more than 10 seconds after five deep breaths is considered abnormal and can be seen with bilateral hemispheric dysfunction (including that caused by metabolic abnormalities or drugs). Most individuals with CSR or PHVA have neurologic illness, although each is seen occasionally in normals, especially during sleep.

Central neurogenic hyperventilation (CNH) is often discussed but rarely seen. To be certain of the diagnosis of CNH, one should demonstrate a low arterial P_{CO_2} and a high P_{O_2} on room air; the hyperventilation should persist during sleep and in the absence of stimulant medications. Respirations are very large in volume, with equal phases of inspiration and expiration. CNH has been seen in a few cases of anterior and medial pontine lesions, sparing the lateral pontine regulatory centers. Even in comatose patients, however, CNH is far less frequent than is pulmonary disease (especially congestive failure), which should always be sought. It is most prudent to look for metabolic and pulmonary causes of deep regular respiration, even in stuporous and comatose patients. An elevated respiratory rate, if associated with actual hyperventilation, is a poor prognostic sign.

Apneustic breathing (or failure of normal expiration) is similarly rare but of greater localizing value. These prolonged inspiratory cramps signify neurologic damage in the lower pons, often the result of a pontine stroke, though they can also be seen with hemorrhage and meningitis. Often, these strokes are extensive and produce near transection of the pons. An apneustic (inspiratory) center at the pontomedullary junction is presumably released from higher controls by these lesions.

Ataxic breathing is completely irregular respiration and is a clear marker of disease in the medulla. Respirations have no discernible pattern and consist of unpredictable gasps. This is most characteristically seen with compression of the medulla caused by mass lesions, such as cerebellar tumors and hemorrhages; less often, it is seen in demyelination and in strokes (less common because of the bilateral blood supply of the medulla). It may be seen in poliomyelitis as part of a spectrum of hyporesponsiveness of the respiratory centers to chemical stimuli such as hypoxia. This loss of rhythmicity in respiration denotes a failure of the most fundamental (and essential) respiratory centers, as opposed to an interruption of higher centers that modulate respiratory rhythms. It is in such cases that the basic inspiratory and expiratory centers in the medulla are most imperiled. Not surprisingly, when there is ataxic breathing, even the mildest sedation can lead to complete respiratory failure.

As a general rule, rapidity of respiration suggests pulmonary or metabolic disease, whereas loss of regularity is more suggestive of brain stem dysfunction.

RESPIRATORY RHYTHM ABNORMALITIES IN CONSCIOUS PATIENTS

The most important respiratory rhythm abnormality in conscious patients is hypoventilation, as discussed earlier. This section, however, concentrates on respiratory irregularities in waking patients without more widespread weakness.

Strokes may affect respiration in several ways. Large hemispheric strokes impair corticospinal input to respiration and limit contralateral diaphragmatic and chest wall movement during voluntary respiratory activity. Unless there are additional lesions, automatic breathing will continue unaffected on both sides. Bilateral strokes affecting corticobulbar fibers can produce a pseudobulbar palsy with difficulty in swallowing, coughing, and other respiratory functions. Concomitant bulbar weakness may complicate respiratory failure through upper airway obstruction.

Seizures are a rare cause of respiratory dysrhythmia. Seizures and cortical stimulation can cause respiratory arrest, often with a focus in the temporal lobe or other limbic areas. Most episodes cease in less than a minute. Of more concern in hospitalized patients are nonconvulsive seizures or status epilepticus, contributing to an encephalopathy and prompting the use of medications that can impair ventilation and even prevent a patient's weaning from a ventilator.

Basal ganglia disorders such as Parkinson's disease may include dysfunction of bulbar musculature as a result of degeneration of brain stem nuclei. Such disorders have been overlooked frequently as causes of respiratory and upper airway dysfunction. Obstructive airway disease may occur in one third of Parkinsonian patients. Respiratory failure is more likely to be due to pneumonia, but involuntary movements can cause dyspnea or discomfort, and upper airway obstruction can be severe enough to impair ventilation. Patients may complain of dyspnea and chest pain caused by bulbar dyskinesias. Tardive dyskinesias and postencephalitic Parkinsonism may also cause respiratory irregularities. A more pervasive disorder, multiple system atrophy (MSA), can include severe autonomic failure, variable respiration, and intermittent airway obstruction. Such patients are occasionally reported to have fatal apnea during sleep, suggesting that MSA patients with autonomic failure should be considered for tracheotomies.

Tic syndromes, especially Gilles de la Tourette's syndrome, commonly become evident with respiratory symptoms and signs. They are often mistaken for respiratory ailments and misdiagnosed for years. Indeed, repetitive throat clearing may be the most frequent symptom in Tourette's syndrome (TS). The diagnosis of TS rests on the presence of vocal tics, as well as multiple motor tics, both present for at least a year and with onset before age 21 years. Simple vocal tics involve individual noises without verbal meaning, such as barking, coughing, snorting, sniffing, shrieking, grunting, and sneezing. Complex vocal tics are words and longer phrases and can include echolalia and palilalia. Often the diagnosis is not made until the patient displays involuntary shouting of obscenities (coprolalia), but this occurs only in a minority of TS patients and may follow the initial symptoms by years. Eye blinking, facial grimacing, and tics of the limbs are common, but vocalizations are the most common presenting symptom. Sensory tics are unpleasant somatic sensations, often localized to a specific part of the body, occurring in about 40% of patients with TS. Often, tics can be suppressed, at least temporarily, but they may increase during stress. Tics must be differentiated from other causes of movement disorders, such as Wilson's disease, Huntington's disease, various dystonias, and late effects of neuroleptics. Tics may also occur as a result of neuroacanthocytosis, encephalitis, and drug toxicity.

As many as one fourth of all children may have tics at some time. Most, however, are transient and last weeks to months. The more persistent tics of TS appear at an average age of 7 years, but the diagnosis may be delayed for decades. TS is not rare, occurring in up to 1% of the population. There is increasing evidence that TS is transmitted genetically in an autosomal dominant manner, although with variable penetrance and expression. Penetrance is higher in males, who make up more than three fourths of the patients. Chronic multiple tic disorder includes motor or vocal tics, but not both. This is differentiated from TS, but genetic studies suggest that this (and transient tic disorders) are part of the same genetic syndrome with different expression. TS is strongly associated with obsessive-compulsive disorder (OCD), occurring in as many as 50% of TS patients. Many consider OCD and TS as different expressions of the same genetic trait. Attention-deficit hyperactivity disorder is also found in about 50% of TS patients.

Pharmacologic evidence argues for an abnormality in dopamine neurotransmitter function in TS. Amphetamines (often used in cases of attention-deficit disorder) and levodopa have led to the exacerbation or beginning of TS, and TS has been seen after phenothiazine withdrawal. More recently, serotonergic and endogenous opioid system abnormalities have been considered important, as well. Anatomically there is evidence for basal ganglia dysfunction, particularly in the left hemisphere. Dopamine receptor blockade with haloperidol or pimozide has been the mainstay of therapy and is effective in more than three fourths of patients. Pimozide can lead to a prolonged QT cardiogram interval and requires electrocardiographic monitoring; it may produce less sedation than haloperidol, but one controlled trial found no difference in efficacy or side effects. Clonidine (thought to act on the norepinephrine system) appears helpful in a smaller percentage of patients and possibly for a shorter duration, but it is often the first choice because of lessened concern about serious long-term side effects and for possible help with the attention-deficit disorder. Others have reported success with reserpine, tetrabenazine (available through protocols only), calcium channel blockers, and other medications. Selective serotonin reuptake inhibitors such as fluoxetine have also been reported beneficial, possibly even more for the OCD. It is important to tailor the treatment to a target symptom, and many patients require no medication. For others, it is the associated OCD or attention-deficit disorder that is most troublesome. Some patients benefit from a combination of haloperidol and stimulants to treat both the TS and attention-deficit disorder. A taper of medications is appropriate if tics have been under control for many months.

Diaphragmatic flutter can be caused by thoracoabdominal or neurologic disease. This rare condition may present with chest pain and is often caused by irritation of the phrenic nerve or abnormalities in the pleura, such as adhesions. On examination, it is realized readily that the diaphragmatic movement (often 100 to 150 times per minute) is independent of the heartbeat. It usually does not lead to hypoventilation or hyperventilation, because voluntary respiration continues to be superimposed, but it can be very distressing. Most cases improve with sleep and are intermittent. Individual episodes may last from seconds to months and may recur. Medications are usually of no help. Phrenic nerve section has been used as a treatment in some patients, but the disease is often bilateral.

In some patients, electromyographic studies have demonstrated synchronous contractions of the diaphragm and intercostal muscles, suggesting a central neurologic basis for the "respiratory myoclonus." Thus the syndrome can be considered analogous to palatal myoclonus, seen with lesions in the lower brain stem caused by stroke, tumor, demyelination, or encephalitis. Some of these patients have responded to treatment with phenytoin.

Hiccups are extremely common, are almost always benign, and are usually caused by problems in the chest or abdomen. Their central component is shown by the simultaneous involvement of all inspiratory muscles. They are inhibited by breath holding and hypercarbia, whereas hyperventilation can lead to an exacerbation of bursts of hiccups. Rarely, they are manifestations of primary neurologic disease, such as syringomyelia, strokes, tumors, or medullary compression. Similarly, yawning may be a sign of medullary compression from a posterior fossa mass or a sign of raised intracranial pressure, and it may be a useful sign in comatose patients.

NEUROGENIC PULMONARY EDEMA

Neurogenic pulmonary edema (NPE) is characterized by the rapidity with which it may develop and by the high protein content of the pulmonary edema fluid. The most characteristic causes are head injury, prolonged seizures, and subarachnoid hemorrhage, although many causes have been identified. In its rare, most severe form it has a grim prognosis, but a less severe, more gradual and unrecognized form of NPE may be relatively common. The pathophysiology of NPE is complex and controversial and is expertly summarized by Malik (1985).

Hypothalamic lesions provided some of the earliest experimental models of NPE. Bilateral preoptic lesions in rats have led to hemorrhagic and fatal pulmonary edema. The observation that prior midline lesions more caudal in the hypothalamus prevent this effect led to the concept of NPE as a "release phenomenon" caused by failure of inhibition of posterior hypothalamic structures, which produce an intense sympathetic nervous system discharge. Subsequent experiments have suggested that the preoptic lesions were actually irritative and that purer ablations give different results—thus putting into question the idea of a release phenomenon. The hypothalamus, however, is not *the* essential structure involved in NPE, since transection of the brain below the hypothalamus does not prevent the NPE produced by abnormalities in the brain stem below.

The medulla oblongata is the crucial brain structure involved in the genesis of NPE. Exquisite physiologic studies done by Chen and Chai (1976) have detailed the interactions of the nucleus of the solitary tract (NTS), the dorsal motor nucleus of the vagus nerve, and the nucleus ambiguus, as well as their roles in mediating the autonomic dysfunction that leads to pulmonary and systemic hypertension and pulmonary edema. Cardiopulmonary abnormalities can be produced by ischemia in the medulla. More common than ischemia, however, is the presumed compression (or distortion) of the brainstem found in raised intracranial pressure (ICP), head injury, and hemorrhage. Medullary lesions may cause an interruption of the baroreceptor reflex arc, leading to an intense sympathetic vasomotor activation. This is mediated through circulating catecholamines and, more powerfully, through direct sympathetic innervation. That NPE produced by cerebral compression is prevented by spinal transection at the C7 level (but not by vagotomy, adrenalectomy, or decerebration) implicates the sympathetic outflow tracts in the generation of NPE. NPE produced by cerebral compression or by NTS lesions can be prevented by pretreatment with phentolamine, which demonstrates mediation by alpha-adrenergic receptors. Stellate ganglion stimulation can produce the same rise in pulmonary vascular resistance, also preventable with alpha-adrenergic blockade.

Vagotomy prevents some of the bradycardia and gastric erosions seen with CNS lesions but does not prevent the systemic and pulmonary hypertension and NPE produced by raised intracranial pressure and medullary lesions. The bradycardia seen in the Cushing response to raised ICP is effected through the vagus nerves, but this appears to be separable from the hypertension and NPE. Vagotomy has produced pulmonary edema in some species, but it is unclear whether respiratory obstruction and airway constriction lead to some of this effect.

Autonomic innervation of the lungs is extensive. Nerves to the lung enter through the anterior and posterior pulmonary plexus from the sympathetic trunks and vagus nerves. At the hila the nerves follow the airway and blood vessels to smaller branches. Sympathetic fibers extend to pulmonary vessels as small as 30 μm in diameter. Although innervation is less extensive than that in the systemic circulation, central nervous system (CNS) insults can lead to a reduction in pulmonary vascular compliance and a dramatic rise in both systemic and pulmonary pressures.

Adrenal catecholamines may contribute to pulmonary vasoconstriction (catecholamine concentrations can increase by up to 1000 times their baseline value with raised ICP!), but adrenalectomy does not abolish the NPE that follows raised ICP. The local effect of splanchnic sympathetic innervation appears to be primary, as section of these splanchnic nerves prevents development of NPE.

Systemic hypertension is often found with raised ICP or other neurologic catastrophe. Some have postulated that systemic vasoconstriction causes a shift of blood volume toward the lower resistance pulmonary vasculature, thus causing NPE. At the same time, the sympathetic stimulation of vessels in the pulmonary circulation leads to elevated resistance. In the lung, alpha receptors (vasoconstricting) predominate over beta receptors (dilating), so vasoconstriction is the predominant sympathetic response. The effect of the adrenergic receptor appears to be greater in the pulmonary venous circulation than in the arterial, thus leading to a marked rise in the pulmonary capillary hydrostatic pressure.

Pulmonary vascular hypertension has been thought to be important in NPE, but it may be neither sufficient nor necessary. Experimentally, NPE can be produced by raised ICP even with control of the systemic blood pressure. Also, the pressure produced even with the most intense sympathetic vasoconstriction seems insufficient to lead to the pulmonary dysfunction seen in NPE. Finally, the high protein content of the pulmonary fluid in NPE clearly implies an alteration of vascular permeability.

This alteration in pulmonary vascular permeability appears necessary for the development of NPE, but its origin is unclear. Its rapid development and the frequent accompanying pulmonary hypertension have led to the theory that a pulse, or "blast," of hypertension leads to structural damage of the vascular endothelium. Other studies, however, have shown increased permeability with no alteration whatsoever in vascular pressure. Conversely, no alteration in permeability was seen when a rapid pulse of pulmonary hypertension was applied experimentally.

Direct changes in the vascular endothelium with loosening of tight junctions have been produced by CNS lesions. This may be even more damaging when superimposed upon vascular hypertension. The permeability changes seem to be mediated by the sympathetic nervous system, but additional "second messengers," such as histamines, opioids, or prostaglandins, could be involved locally. Increased permeability may be the result of a distortion in the contractility of the endothelial cells or pericytes by bradykinin or histamine. This may explain the mechanism of opiate-induced and other noncardiac forms of pulmonary edema.

In summary, despite the frequent occurrence of systemic and pulmonary vascular hypertension following CNS lesions, a direct, probably sympathetic-mediated, alteration in pulmonary vascular permeability appears to be essential in the production of NPE.

In clinical practice the most important aid to therapy is making the proper diagnosis promptly. Suspicion should be particularly high in relatively few situations (Box 166-2). Head injury with raised ICP is the classic experimental paradigm for NPE. In these models and in humans NPE can develop with extreme rapidity. It may occur to a lesser degree in many serious head injuries. Epilepsy, on the other hand, is certainly the most common precipitant. NPE is particularly to be suspected with status epilepticus, and it may help to explain some cases of sudden, unexpected death occurring in epilepsy patients. Often, pulmonary dysfunction following seizures is attributed to aspiration pneumonia, and it can be difficult to tell these conditions apart. Aspiration is more likely to be associated with focal pneumonias and other signs of infection, whereas NPE may develop much more rapidly and may resolve more rapidly, as well. Cerebral hemorrhage is a relatively common precipitant of NPE, and NPE may contribute substantially to mortality in subarachnoid hemorrhage. Other causes of NPE

BOX 166-2

Causes of neurogenic pulmonary edema

Major causes
Head injury
Epileptic seizures
Cerebral hemorrhage

Rare causes
Brain stem strokes, hemorrhages and trauma
Multiple sclerosis, with plaques near the nucleus of the solitary tract
Medullary edema after surgery (with brain stem arteriovenous malformation)
Bulbar poliomyelitis
Vertebral artery ligation
Trigeminal nerve block
Air emboli
Brain tumors
Ruptured thoracic spinal cord arteriovenous malformation

---

are far less common and should be considered with skepticism. Many true cases involve acute lesions in the medulla. Most other cases of pulmonary edema are cardiogenic or related to sepsis. NPE typically occurs within minutes of the major neurologic insult. The physical examination suggests pulmonary edema, although cardiac and pulmonary wedge pressures tend to be normal by the time of measurement.

Treatment of NPE depends on recognition of the syndrome in the appropriate setting and differentiation from other illnesses common in the same settings, such as aspiration pneumonia. Ensurance of a good airway, oxygenation, and diuresis is appropriate, as in other forms of pulmonary edema. Treatment is generally supportive and conservative, since much of the morbidity depends on the underlying illness and many milder cases resolve in hours to days without intervention. Many authorities recommend positive end-expiratory pressure (PEEP) ventilation, while cautioning that it can decrease venous return to the heart, cardiac output, and cerebral venous drainage, all contributing to raised ICP. In these patients cerebral pressure monitoring may be appropriate.

Especially when cerebral edema is involved, diuresis with osmotic agents such as mannitol may be helpful. Alpha-adrenergic receptor blocking agents such as phentolamine may be useful in treating NPE, assuming that systemic blood pressure tolerates these medications, but they have not had clinical trials in humans. Beta blockers could theoretically ameliorate the permeability defect postulated in NPE but would appear ill-advised, given the possibility of concomitant heart disease and cardiogenic pulmonary edema. Dobutamine has been suggested as an alpha- and beta-adrenergic agonist that can increase cardiac output and cerebral perfusion. Steroids have been helpful in one experimental model, although higher doses were more harmful than helpful; applicability to humans is untested as yet. When NPE is the result of status epilepticus, anticonvulsants are obviously indicated, and some have suggested that phenytoin may be useful in NPE, even without overt seizures. Naloxone has been helpful in animal experiments in NPE, although its use in clinical settings has not yet been determined. Considering the physiology postulated earlier, some authors have suggested the use of antihistamines in treatment of NPE. Rapid recognition and understanding of the implications of NPE are the keys to treatment, as are the institution of supportive measures and avoidance of treatments potentially exacerbating the NPE or underlying disease.

BIBLIOGRAPHY

Berger AJ, Mitchell RA, Severinghaus JW: Regulation of respiration, *N Engl J Med* 295:92, 138, 194, 1977.

Bolton CF et al: Critically ill polyneuropathy: electrophysiological studies and differentiation from Guillain-Barré syndrome, *J Neurol Neurosurg Psychiatry* 49:563, 1986.

Chen HI, Chai CY: Integration of the cardiovagal mechanism in the medulla oblongata of the cat, *Am J Physiol* 231:454, 1976.

Knudsen F, Jensen HP, Petersen PL: Neurogenic pulmonary edema: treatment with dobutamine, *Neurosurgery* 29:269, 1991.

Kurlan R: Tourette's syndrome: current concepts, *Neurology* 39:1625, 1989.

Malik AB: Mechanisms of neurogenic pulmonary edema, *Circ Res* 57:1, 1985.

Plum F, Posner JB: The diagnosis of stupor and coma, ed 3, Philadelphia, 1982, FA Davis.

Ropper AH: The Guillain-Barré syndrome, *N Engl J Med* 326:1130, 1992.

Terrence CF, Rao GR, Perper JA: Neurogenic pulmonary edema in unexpected, unexplained death of epileptic patients, *Ann Neurol* 9:458, 1981.

Tranmer BI, Tucker WS, Bilbao JM: Sleep apnea following percutaneous cervical cordotomy, *Can J Neurol Sci* 14:262, 1987.

CHAPTER

167 Neurogastroenterology

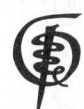

Martin A. Samuels

MALABSORPTION AND DEFICIENCY STATES

The neurology of gastrointestinal tract diseases is largely related to maldigestion, malabsorption, and malnutrition (Chapters 326, 340, and 347). It stands to reason that the developing nervous system is particularly sensitive to deprivation of protein, carbohydrate, fat, minerals, and vitamins. As a consequence, it is generally true that inherited defects that lead to a deficiency of one or more of these critical elements cause dramatic, often devastating neurologic disease. Acquired deficiencies, on the other hand, lead to more circumscribed, often reversible syndromes. In general, neuronal systems that use long axons are the most susceptible to defects that disable energy metabolism. Thus polyneuropathy and focal encephalopathies (e.g., spastic paraparesis caused by dying back of corticospinal axons or blindness caused by dying back of retinal ganglion cell axons) are the most common manifestations of many of the dietary deficiency or malabsorption syndromes. For a detailed description of the neurologic consequences of the many deficiency states, the interested reader should refer to the excellent textbook by Pallis and Lewis.

Most substances of neurologic significance in adults are absorbed from the proximal and middle thirds of the small bowel. Vitamin B_{12}, the notable exception, is absorbed with its gastric-derived intrinsic factor in the terminal ileum. Deficiencies of nearly all of the water-soluble vitamins (i.e., thiamine, riboflavin, nicotinic acid, pyridoxine, pantothenic acid, vitamin B_{12}, folic acid, and ascorbic acid) are known to be associated with a polyneuropathy in which sensory symptoms (e.g., burning feet and paresthesias) overshadow motor difficulties. Since in real life patients usually have multiple water-soluble vitamin deficiencies, it is difficult to know precisely which one causes a particular symptom. For example, pure folate deficiency does not cause a neurologic syndrome in animals, whereas patients with folate deficiency almost invariably have a polyneuropathy, possibly as a result of the associated deficiency of other vitamins or other dietary substances.

Above and beyond the neuropathy, several of the water-soluble vitamin deficiencies produce specific neurologic syndromes that deserve mention. Thiamine (vitamin B_1) deficiency causes Wernicke's encephalopathy, an acute syndrome characterized by a mental abnormality (usually confusion and amnesia), ataxia, and various oculomotor problems (e.g., nystagmus or bilateral abducens palsies). All of the clinical syndromes are caused by biochemical (and ultimately pathologic) lesions in central nervous system nuclei (paraventricular regions of the thalamus and hypothalamus mammillary bodies, periaqueductal gray, floor of the fourth ventricle, vestibular nuclei, and superior cerebellar vermis), which presumably are particularly dependent on thiamine-mediated reactions. Most severe thiamine deficiency is caused by malnutrition, often associated with alcoholism, although any cause of malnutrition (e.g., nausea and vomiting caused by chemotherapy) can result in enough thiamine deficiency to cause clinically evident Wernicke's encephalopathy. Multiple clinical or subclinical attacks of Wernicke's encephalopathy may result in a chronic state of amnestic dementia (Korsakoff's disease). Severe untreated Wernicke's encephalopathy may be fatal or result in irreversible amnestic dementia, so all patients who may be affected (e.g., alcoholics, severely malnourished people, comatose patients) should be treated with parenteral (intravenous or intramuscular) thiamine, 100 mg initially followed by 50 mg per day for 5 days or until a normal diet can be reestablished. Carbohydrates should never be given to severely malnourished patients until thiamine has been infused because thiamine-dependent cells become more acidotic as a result of anaerobic metabolism of the carbohydrate.

Nicotinic acid deficiency (pellagra) produces a dementia, in addition to its classic effects on the skin and gastrointestinal tract (dermatitis and diarrhea). The dementia is characterized by memory loss and attentional defects similar to those seen in vitamin B_{12} deficiency and therefore is nonspecific in and of itself. Whether nicotinic acid deficiency can cause an acute encephalopathy progressing rapidly to coma (Jolliffe's disease) is unsettled, since most patients in this circumstance have unequivocal signs of Wernicke's encephalopathy as well. Pellagra is now rare, probably because bread is enriched with niacin (nicotinic acid); however, it can be seen in severely malnourished patients.

Pyridoxine (vitamin B_6) deficiency is known to result in seizures, particularly in infancy. Some infants require large nonphysiologic doses of pyridoxine (i.e., 50 to 100 mg per day) to terminate neonatal seizures. This disorder, which is inherited as an autosomal recessive trait, is known as pyridoxine dependency. Most pyridoxine deficiency in adults is caused by the use of pyridoxine antagonists, such as isonicotinic acid hydrazide (INH) for the treatment of tuberculosis. It is recommended that patients receiving INH be given pyridoxine, 50 mg daily, to prevent the polyneuropathy and seizures caused by vitamin B_6 deficiency. Patients with various malabsorption disorders, such as sprue and celiac disease, may also become pyridoxine deficient.

Vitamin B_{12} deficiency also causes neurologic syndromes beyond neuropathy. This subject is covered in Chapter 87.

The fat-soluble vitamin deficiencies do not produce polyneuropathies but have other characteristic neurologic manifestations.

Vitamin A (retinol) deficiency results in impaired dark adaptation (night blindness).

Vitamin D deficiency causes osteomalacia, which may be associated with a proximal myopathy similar on clinical examination to that seen in thyroid disease.

Vitamin E deficiency is known to be associated with abetalipoproteinemia (Bassen-Kornzwieg disease), a disorder characterized by retinitis pigmentosa, ataxia, pes cavus, areflexia, red blood cells with spikelike processes, and fat malabsorption. Beta lipoprotein and vitamin E are both totally absent from the blood, but the relationship of vitamin E deficiency to the pathogenesis of the Friedreich's ataxia–like neurologic illness remains obscure.

Vitamin K deficiency results in a bleeding diathesis that may result in hemorrhages in or around neurologic structures.

WHIPPLE'S DISEASE

Whipple's disease is a multisystemic chronic disease that regularly affects both the nervous system and the gastrointestinal tract. It is characterized by weight loss with steatorrhea, arthralgias, and abdominal pain. The patients may be asymptomatic on neurologic examination or may show visual disturbances, amnestic dementia, ophthalmoplegia, myoclonus, and a relatively specific movement disorder called *oculomasticatory myorhythmias,* in which rhythmic convergence or vertical pendular eye movements are combined with synchronous opening and closing of the jaw. On neuropathologic study the same macrophages that are positive on periodic acid–Schiff stain (PAS) can be found in the brain as are found in other tissues of the body. This PAS-positive material stains a bacterium, which is a β-hemolytic streptococcus now designated *Tropheryma whippelli.* The diagnosis is usually made by intestinal biopsy, but in pure central nervous system cases brain biopsy may be required. If an organism can be identified in the biopsy specimen, the diagnosis is considered certain. If no organism can be found, empiric treatment with tetracycline, erythromycin, or trimethoprim-sulfamethoxazole is usually tried. Some patients respond well to therapy, their condition stabilizing and even dramatically improving in some

circumstances. The role of altered immunity is uncertain, but the condition has been seen in patients with acquired immunodeficiency syndrome (AIDS).

PANCREATIC DISEASE

Patients with pancreatic disease (Chapter 366) often have episodes of hypoglycemia. It is unlikely that mild degrees of hypoglycemia (i.e., greater than 50 mg/dL) have any transient or lasting effect on neurologic function. However, severe hypoglycemia has clear neurologic and neuropathologic correlates. This is obvious when one considers how dependent the brain is on a constant supply of glucose, being virtually unable to use any other energy substrate. Acute hypoglycemia results in a massive effort by the autonomic nervous system to mobilize sugar from stored carbohydrate. This results in tachycardia and sweating. If this effort fails to maintain an adequate blood sugar, the level of consciousness rapidly falls, descending from confusion through drowsiness and stupor to coma. The cellular structures most susceptible to the ravages of hypoglycemia are similar to those that fail in circumstances of anoxia. These include the deep layers of the cerebral cortex, the basal ganglia (particularly the globus pallidus), the hippocampal formation (particularly the Sommer sector), and cerebellar Purkinje's cells. With repeated attacks of hypoglycemia, a clinical syndrome develops that probably relates to the cell loss in these and other regions of the brain, that is, an amnestic dementia (the hippocampal lesion); myoclonus, often worse on action or intention (the cortical lesions); various movement disorders, such as myoclonus, chorea, and dystonia (the basal ganglia lesion); and ataxia (the cerebellar lesion). This syndrome progresses if the episodes of hypoglycemia continue to occur, as frequently happens in severe insulin-dependent type I diabetics or in alcoholics with severe pancreatic insufficiency and liver disease.

Pancreatic encephalopathy refers to a vaguely characterized disorder that is seen in the course of acute pancreatitis and consists of an abnormality in the level of consciousness ranging from confusion to coma, slowing of the electroencephalogram and, sometimes, motor disorders such as tetraparesis and increased tendon reflexes. It is difficult to be certain that the neurologic disorder in such acutely ill patients is, in fact, caused by the pancreatic failure rather than by commonly associated conditions such as shock, sepsis, alcohol withdrawal, Wernicke's encephalopathy, metabolic acidosis, hepatic failure, and electrolyte disturbances. It is clear that some of the pathologic reports of so-called pancreatic encephalopathy are examples of central pontine myelinolysis, a condition now thought to be associated with hyponatremia or its rapid correction.

PARASITIC INFESTATIONS

A number of intestinal parasitic diseases affect the nervous system. These include protozoan diseases (e.g., *Entamoeba histolytica* causes meningoencephalitis) and platyhelminth-caused diseases, the most important and frequent of which is cysticercosis, the larval phase of the human tapeworm, *Taenia solium.* The life cycles and clinical manifestations of these parasitic diseases are discussed in Chapters 279 and 281.

INFECTIOUS DIARRHEAS

The infectious diarrheas, such as shigellosis and salmonellosis, may cause profound neurologic disturbances, but these are almost certainly caused by the electrolyte disturbances, fever, and generalized illness produced by these pathogens, rather than attributable to any direct effect on the nervous system.

PANCREAS TRANSPLANTATION

Pancreas transplantation is used to treat patients with type I diabetes who have severe end-organ damage. Many times it is performed in conjunction with renal transplants with the aim of making the patient insulin independent and reversing some of the end-organ damage. Neurologic complications are very common, occurring in perhaps as many as two thirds of the patients. Much of the neurologic difficulty is related to the fact that all pancreas transplant recipients have retinopathy and neuropathy at the time of the transplant. In addition, nearly all patients have cerebrovascular disease related to the premature atherosclerosis associated with type I diabetes.

The procedure involves either transplanting the whole pancreas into the abdomen or transplanting free islet cells. The former is thus far the most successful in correcting the diabetes and reversing or retarding damage to end-organs. There are no unique neurologic complications as a result of the procedure itself.

BIBLIOGRAPHY

Pallis CA, Lewis PD, editors: *The neurology of gastrointestinal disease,* Philadelphia, 1974, WB Saunders.
Sharf B, Bental E: Pancreatic encephalopathy, *J Neurol Neurosurg Psychiatry* 34:357, 1971.
Victor M, Adams RD, Collins GH: *The Wernicke-Korsakoff syndrome,* ed 2, Contemporary neurology series, vol 30, Philadelphia, 1989, FA Davis.
Wroe SJ et al: Whipple's disease confined to the CNS presenting with multiple intracerebral mass lesions, *Neurol Neurosurg Psychiatry* 54:989, 1991.

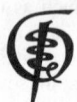

CHAPTER

168 Neurohepatology

Martin A. Samuels

The neurologic aspects of liver disease can be divided into two major categories: the reversible portosystemic encephalopathies (also known as hepatic encephalopathy) and the irreversible portosystemic encephalopathies (i.e., Wilson's disease and acquired non-Wilsonian hepatocerebral degeneration).

Reversible means that the neurologic aspects of the illness will disappear, assuming the underlying process causing the liver failure can be treated successfully. Many patients with potentially reversible neurologic complications of liver disease die of the hepatic failure before the nervous system can recover. On pathologic examination of brains of patients who die of acute hepatic failure, one finds only cerebral edema and an increase in the size and number of the protoplasmic astrocytes. These so-called Alzheimer type II glia are nearly pathognomonic of liver failure.

REVERSIBLE PORTOSYSTEMIC SYNDROMES

Reversible portosystemic encephalopathy (PSE) may be acute (e.g., acute yellow atrophy or Reye's syndrome) or chronic and recurrent (episodes of acute PSE superimposed on stable liver disease, such as alcoholic cirrhosis).

When symptoms are evident, patients with reversible PSE show a mental disorder ranging from slight inattention to coma, prominent motor abnormalities (e.g., tremor, asterixis, myoclonus, or hyperreflexia), and fairly consistent laboratory abnormalities (e.g., hyperammonemia, mild hypoxemia, respiratory alkalosis, elevated cerebrospinal fluid glutamine levels, and high-voltage, sharp triphasic delta waves on the electroencephalogram). The neurotoxin is still not definitely known. False neurotransmitters, such as octapamine, and other potential toxins, such as fatty acids, mercaptans, and amino acids, have all had advocates. The original idea that ammonia is the toxin is probably as accurate as any hypothesis. It may be true that the glutamate-glutamine detoxification system for ammonia is compartmentalized to the glial cells and that the Alzheimer's type II glia are a reflection of brain efforts to detoxify high levels of ammonia. When this system becomes saturated, the nervous system is no longer capable of removing ammonia, which then produces its toxic effects on neuronal function.

The other prevalent hypothesis is that liver disease somehow results in the elaboration of a substance that activates the γ-aminobutyric acid receptor, type A ($GABA_A$). This $GABA_A$ receptor is modulated allosterically by benzodiazepines, barbiturates, and

the endogenous family of peptides derived from the precursor polypeptide, diazepam-binding inhibitor (DBI). It is possible that endogenous benzodiazepine-like substances may be synthesized by animals or ingested from dietary sources and that these substances may reach the brain in larger-than-normal amounts when there is portosystemic shunting, thereby activating the inhibitory action of the $GABA_A$ receptor and producing coma. The major argument supporting this hypothesis is that the benzodiazepine antagonist flumazenil ameliorates portosystemic encephalopathy in animals and humans.

Whatever the mechanism of the neurotoxic effects of liver failure, it can be treated by reducing the production and absorption of nitrogenous products from the gastrointestinal tract. This can be accomplished by using protein restriction, antibiotics, catharsis, and lactulose.

IRREVERSIBLE PORTOSYSTEMIC SYNDROMES

There are two major chronic, progressive, irreversible portosystemic encephalopathies: hepatolenticular degeneration (Wilson's disease) and acquired hepatocerebral degeneration. Wilson's disease is an autosomal-dominantly inherited illness in which there is an inability to synthesize ceruloplasmin, the copper-carrying enzyme. Copper is deposited in many tissues, including the liver (leading to cirrhosis) and the cornea (the pathognomonic Kayser-Fleischer ring). Neuropathologic examination shows cavitation of the lenticular nuclei (putamen and globus pallidus), laminar cortical necrosis, and widespread Alzheimer's type II glial cells—findings that imply that the chronic liver disease produces many of the neurologic and neuropathologic features of the illness. The treatment is copper chelation with D-penicillamine (see Chapter 359).

In some patients with chronic liver disease there develops a relentlessly progressive neurologic illness, similar on neurologic study in many ways to Wilson's disease. These patients show prominent dysarthria and akinesia, often with tremor. Tendon reflexes are increased and Babinski's sign is present. In some patients there develops a pure motor spastic paraparesis that, rarely, can dominate the clinical picture (the so-called hepatic paraplegia). Superimposed on this degenerative process are often episodes of acute reversible PSE with worsening confusion and asterixis. Pathologic examination reveals laminar cortical necrosis and Alzheimer's type II glial cells, reminiscent of those seen in acute PSE and in Wilson's disease. There is no abnormality in copper metabolism or deposition of copper in the brain, and there are no Kayser-Fleischer rings. It appears that the sine qua non in the development of this syndrome in the context of liver disease is the existence of a portosystemic shunt. This shunt may be produced surgically (e.g., splenorenal shunt or portocaval shunt) in an effort to reduce portal pressures or may happen spontaneously within the liver itself (intrahepatic portosystemic shunts) in the course of hepatic cirrhosis. Some of these patients seem to respond transiently to levodopa or dopamine-receptor agonists (e.g., bromocriptine), implying that neurotransmitter failure is part of the pathogenesis of the illness (Chapters 348 and 354).

Neurologic Effects of Liver Transplantation

Orthotopic liver transplants are associated with a variety of neurologic complications, which fall into several major categories. About 10% of patients have seizures, 90% of which are single. The remaining 10% with recurrent seizures can usually be managed with phenobarbital. However, some of these patients have a prolonged period of unconsciousness followed by a persistent or slowly resolving cerebrocerebellar syndrome characterized by ataxia, dysarthria, and weakness. It is probable that this is caused by cyclosporine toxicity (Chapter 164.) In approximately 2.5% of patients the diagnosis on clinical examination is stroke. Infarctions are possible, but most are subarachnoid and/or intracerebral hemorrhages, probably related to the coagulopathy of the liver disease. In some cases hemorrhagic infarction is related to infection with an organism known to produce a vasculitis (e.g., *Aspergillus* species). In the immediate postoperative period these patients are nearly all encephalopathic as a result of infections, metabolic imbalance, drug toxicity, and the effects of graft malfunction.

BIBLIOGRAPHY

Belle SH, Detre KM: Report of the Pitt-UNOS liver transplant registry, *Transplant Proc* 25:1137, 1993.

Estol CJ, Pessin MS, Martinez AJ: Cerebrovascular complications after orthotopic liver transplantation, *Neurology* 41:815, 1991.

Moreno E, Gomez SR, Gonzalez I et al: Neurologic complications in liver transplantation, *Acta Neurol Scand* 87:25, 1993.

Morgan MY et al: Successful use of bromocriptine in the treatment of chronic hepatic encephalopathy, *Gastroenterology* 78:663, 1980.

Mousseau R, Reynolds T: Hepatic paraplegia, *Am J Gastroenterol* 66:343, 1976.

Plum F, Hindfelt B: The neurological complications of liver disease. In Vinken PJ, Bruyn GW, editors: *Handbook of clinical neurology,* vol 27, Amsterdam, 1976, Elsevier.

Stein DP, Lederman RJ, Vogt DP et al: Neurological complications following liver transplantation, *Ann Neurol* 31:644, 1992.

Victor M, Adams RD, Cole N: The acquired (non-Wilsonian) type of chronic hepatocerebral degeneration, *Medicine (Baltimore)* 44:345, 1965.

Victor M, Rothstein JD: Neurologic manifestations of hepatic and gastrointestinal disease. In Asbury AK, Mcdonald WI, McKhann CM, editors: *Diseases of the nervous system,* ed 2, Philadelphia, 1992, WB Saunders.

Vogt DD et al: Neurologic complications of liver transplantation, *Ann Neurol* 31:644, 1992.

Wilson SAK: Progressive lenticular degeneration: a familial nervous system disease associated with cirrhosis of the liver, *Brain* 34:295, 1912.

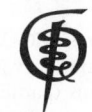

CHAPTER

169 Neurohematology

Martin A. Samuels

ANEMIA

Anemia (Chapter 79) in its own right rarely produces neurologic symptoms. When severe, it can result in a generalized dull headache, and, occasionally, retinal hemorrhages may occur. Iron-deficiency anemia is, for unknown reasons, associated with obsessive-compulsive behaviors that fall into two categories: compulsive eating (pica) and compulsive moving of the limbs, usually the legs (restless legs syndrome). Common pica behaviors include the eating of starch, paint chips, clay, earth (geophagia), or ice (pagophagia). It is clear that the pica does not represent replacement of iron, since eating ice, the most common pica behavior, usually does nothing in this regard and many clays actually contain substances that chelate iron. The restless legs syndrome is a common cause of insomnia. It consists of an unpleasant creeping sensation deep in the legs (and occasionally in the arms) when the person is at rest. The person feels compelled to move the legs. Most frequently affected are women who pace the floors at night and complain of insomnia. The syndrome may progress to severe motor restlessness (akathisia), which in its most severe form occurs throughout the day (Ekbom syndrome). Serum iron levels and total iron-binding capacity should be measured in all patients complaining of pica or restless legs syndrome. If iron replacements fail to relieve the symptoms, the patient may respond to low-dose benzodiazepines (particularly clonazepam) at bedtime, or dopamine agonists (e.g., levodopa-carbidopa [Sinemet] or bromocriptine). The megaloblastic anemias are associated with very specific neurologic syndromes. Vitamin B_{12} deficiency, once a common and dreaded illness, now is relatively rare, although sporadic cases of pernicious anemia, dietary deficiency of vitamin B_{12}, malabsorption, and infestation with the fish tapeworm *(Diphyllobothrium latum)* are still seen (Chapter 87). It is probably true that all forms of vitamin B_{12} deficiency produce the same array of neurologic complications, although most of the experience is with patients who have pernicious anemia. The neurologic manifestations of vitamin B_{12} deficiency span nearly the entire nervous system. There is a myelopathy (subacute combined degeneration of the spinal cord), an encephalopathy, and an optic neuropathy. The myelopathy produces a spastic weakness of the legs (and sometimes arms), a profound loss of vibration sense out of proportion to the severity of the neuropathy, and a positive Romberg's sign. The encephalopathy produces a dementia best characterized in modern terms as a chronic confusional state with poor memory and a severe attentional deficit but little or no aphasia or apraxia—thus distinguishing it from typical Alzheimer's disease. The optic neuropathy may produce anything from red desaturation to severe loss of visual acuity with a deafferented pupil in one eye or both eyes.

Despite its once-high prevalence and intense interest by generations of physicians, the precise mechanism by which vitamin B_{12} deficiency produces neurologic problems remains a mystery. The fact that vitamin B_{12} is necessary for DNA synthesis may explain the megaloblastic anemia, leukopenia, and glossitis seen in patients with B_{12} deficiency, but this does not explain the effects on neurons of the adult nervous system, which do not divide. Oligodendrocytes, which do divide, may be affected by deficiency of methylcobalamin, thus leading to the demyelination that is so characteristic of the neuropathology of vitamin B_{12} deficiency. The fact that nitrous oxide, an inhibitor of methyl transferase activity, also causes subacute combined degeneration of the nervous system lends support to this hypothesis. The role of vitamin B_{12} in other enzymatic reactions (i.e., the conversion of 1-methylmalonyl coenzyme A [CoA] to succinyl CoA may explain many of the neurologic complications of cobalamin deficiencies. Accumulation of methylmalonic acid may result in the formation of unstable myelin containing long-chain fatty acids with an odd number of carbon atoms).

Folate deficiency, another cause of megaloblastic anemia usually produced by malnutrition, is often part of a multiple vitamin deficiency syndrome. For this reason, it is not clear whether folate deficiency itself causes any neurologic disorder. Many patients with folate deficiency have a polyneuropathy, but this may be caused by deficiencies in other elements in the diet (see Chapter 147).

HEMOGLOBINOPATHIES AND THALASSEMIA

The hemoglobinopathies and thalassemia (Chapter 88) often are associated with neurologic complications. Patients with sickle cell anemia have painful crises and may have small-vessel occlusions involving the brain or spinal cord. These small-vessel occlusions produce infarctions, hemorrhagic infarctions, and, occasionally, intracerebral hemorrhages. The supraclinoid carotid is a location that seems predisposed to occlude in patients with sickle cell anemia. The precise mechanism for this predisposition is not known, but it is possible to noninvasively predict an impending occlusion using transcranial Doppler technology. Seizures may also occur, probably as a result of small-vessel–distribution infarcts of various ages. These patients are also subject to recurrent attacks of bacterial meningitis, possibly related to functional or surgical asplenism. Although the incidence of these neurologic problems is higher in the patients with homozygous sickle cell anemia, they may all be seen occasionally in patients with various heterozygous hemoglobinopathies, including SC, SD, SF, and S thalassemia syndromes. Patients with thalassemia may also have recurrent episodes of meningitis, particularly after surgical splenectomy. They also may have extramedullary hematopoiesis (see later discussion) and an array of vaguely described neuromuscular disorders that may be coinherited with the thalassemia, rather than caused by the thalassemia per se.

EXTRAMEDULLARY HEMATOPOIESIS

Extramedullary hematopoiesis is the production of blood cells outside of the usual bone marrow compartments. This usually occurs in reticuloendothelial organs, such as liver and lymph nodes, but can occasionally be found near the nervous system—usually in the thoracic epidural space, rarely in the intracranial subdural space. These masses can compress the spinal cord or brain, producing a myelopathy or an encephalopathy. Approximately half of the patients with dural extramedullary hematopoiesis have had thalassemia, and a fourth of them have had myelofibrosis. The other fourth comprises a potpourri of diagnoses, including polycythemia, sickle cell anemia, pyruvate-kinase deficiency, and Paget's disease of bone. Extramedullary hematopoiesis can be treated very effectively with radiation therapy.

HEMORRHAGIC DIATHESIS

Hematologic disorders associated with a hemorrhagic diathesis may produce neurologic complications resulting from bleeding into or around the brain, spinal cord, roots, plexuses, or nerves. Until quite recently hemophiliacs often died of neurologic complications; however, modern replacement therapy has made these problems quite rare. Patients with hemophilia still are more prone than normal people to the development of intramuscular or retroperitoneal hemorrhages, particularly when there is a history of trauma. Retroperitoneal hemorrhages may produce a compressive sacral plexopathy that usually recovers slowly with resolution of the blood. Intracranial and interspinal hemorrhages (epidural, subdural, subarachnoid, or parenchymal) are still more common in patients with hemophilia than in normal individuals, but only slightly so. Thrombocytopenia of any cause may result in intracranial or spinal hemorrhages. In conditions in which the few remaining platelets are presumed normal (e.g., immune-ediated idiopathic thrombocytopenic purpura), patients usually do not have serious neurologic hemorrhages until the platelet count approaches 10,000 cells/mm^3. However, when platelets are both abnormal and reduced in number (e.g., in patients receiving chemotherapy), one can expect neurologic hemorrhages when the platelet count reaches about 50,000 cells/mm^3. Thrombotic thrombocytopenic purpura (TTP) is a particular neurohematologic syndrome consisting of thrombocytopenic purpura, hemolytic anemia, and various neurologic symptoms and signs (e.g., headache, confusion, aphasia, seizures, cranial neuropathies, weakness, and sensory loss), which are now known to be caused by small-vessel occlusions in the brain and spinal cord. Renal failure and fever are also frequently seen. Various therapies (e.g., heparin, antiplatelet drugs, steroids) in the past have shown equivocal results. It now appears that plasma exchange provides the best chance for the patient; despite this, the prognosis for this cryptogenic syndrome remains poor.

Disseminated intravascular coagulation (DIC) of any origin rarely causes gross neurologic hemorrhage. In a few patients with DIC, multiple cerebral infarctions may occur, and autopsy may show multiple small petechial hemorrhages. It is likely that these findings would produce little persistent neurologic deficit should the patient survive the episode of DIC and not die of the underlying cause (e.g., sepsis). Hypoprothrombinemia is usually iatrogenic, caused by the various anticoagulant drugs used to prevent thromboembolism. It is now clear that anticoagulation to prothrombin times longer than 18 seconds carries an increased risk of nervous system hemorrhages. It is probable (but not yet proved) that antithrombotic therapy aiming for a prothrombin time of 15 to 18 seconds ("Coumadin light") can produce the same protection without the associated risk of hemorrhage.

HYPERCOAGULABLE STATES

A patient is said to be in a hypercoagulable state (Chapters 75 and 82) if he or she has laboratory or clinical conditions related to an increased risk for thrombosis. Hypercoagulable states are divided into a primary (usually inherited) type (e.g., antithrombin IV deficiency, protein C and protein S deficiencies) and a secondary (acquired) type (e.g., malignancy, pregnancy, use of oral contraceptives, or antiphospholipid antibodies). In both types, cerebral vessels may have thrombosis in situ with consequent infarction. Most standard hematologic tests do not reveal the presence of a hypercoagulative state, but specialized studies can be obtained if one suspects that such a state exists based on arterial or venous thrombosis in otherwise risk-free patients. Young women with stroke represent a group of patients in whom a hypercoagulable state should be sought. In one circumstance a standard hematologic test valve, the partial thromboplastin time (PTT), may be found to be prolonged in a patient having a thrombotic event. This artifactual prolongation of the PTT is caused by the presence of an acquired immunoglobulin, usually directed against phospholipids (the so-called lupus anticoagulant). The prolongation of the PTT results from the fact that the antibody inhibits the activity of phospholipid in the in vitro clotting reaction. It is not really an anticoagulant and is, in fact, a cause of a hypercoagulable state that can result in thrombosis of cerebral veins or arteries. The lupus anticoagulant is found in some patients with systemic lupus erythematosus, as well as in patients receiving neuroleptic drugs and patients with other autoimmune disorders. It is common practice to screen for the hypercoagulable state in young stroke patients.

HYPERVISCOSITY

Hyperviscosity is a clinical syndrome characterized by confusion, headache, blurred vision, and specific retinal funduscopic findings (i.e., venous engorgement [sausage veins] and retinal hemorrhages). It is caused by sludging of blood in brain vessels as a result of increased viscosity and is seen in polycythemia (particularly when associated with iron deficiency) and paraproteinemias. Among the paraproteinemias, macroglobulinemia has the greatest propensity for the production of hyperviscosity. The presence of cryoglobulins and cold agglutinins is also associated with hyperviscosity. The treatment for the hyperviscosity syndrome is plasma exchange.

PARAPROTEINEMIAS

Paraproteinemias (Chapters 74 and 94) cause an array of neurologic complications above and beyond their tendency to produce hyperviscosity. This may be a result of the fact that immunoglobulins produced by the neoplastic clone of cells may be directed against components of the normal nervous system (e.g., myelin-associated globulin [MAG]) or to the production of amyloid that infiltrates nervous tissue. Thus multiple myeloma is commonly associated with many different types of peripheral neuropathy (e.g., polyneuropathy and mononeuropathy multiplex). In addition, in some patients with paraproteinemias, plasma cells emanating from cerebral veins may infiltrate the brain, producing a clinical syndrome (the Bing-Neel syndrome) characterized by cerebrospinal fluid pleocytosis, multifocal neurologic signs with a downhill course, and sometimes the appearance of a histiocytic lymphoma in the brain. The disorder is unresponsive to plasma exchange and probably represents a widespread neoplastic infiltration of the nervous system.

Monoclonal gammopathy of undetermined significance (MGUS) is associated with various peripheral and sometimes central nervous system manifestations. It is probable that these paraproteins (particularly the immunoglobulin M type) are directed against components of the peripheral and, rarely, central nervous system, thereby producing polyneuropathies, mononeuropathies, and possibly even multifocal central nervous system demyelination, which may on clinical examination and by imaging techniques look like multiple sclerosis. There is some evidence that the neurologic manifestations of MGUS respond partially to plasmapheresis.

BONE MARROW TRANSPLANTATION

Bone marrow transplantations are performed for two major indications: (1) abnormal or absent marrow (e.g. aplastic anemia, genetic diseases such as lysosomal storage diseases or thalassemia major; acute leukemia such as acute myelocytic, acute lymphoblastic or chronic lymphocytic; or combined immunodeficiency disease) and (2) hazard to the marrow, which is the limiting factor in aggressive treatment of a disease (e.g. lymphoma, solid tumor autologous marrow programs for breast cancer, glioblastoma multiforme, and neuroblastoma). Three kinds of transplants exist: syngenic (identical twins), allogenic (different genetic origins), and autologous (patient's own tissue.)

Neurologic complications occur in about 70% of bone marrow transplant recipients and are the cause of death in 6%. The most common problem is metabolic encephalopathy caused by respiratory failure, hepatic failure, electrolyte disorders, or renal failure. The drugs used to prepare patients for the transplantation including intrathecal methotrexate, busulfan, cyclophosphamide, and adriamycin may also contribute to the metabolic encephalopathy. Total body irradiation is often used (2000 cGy or less), which can lead to long-term cognitive dysfunction, particularly in children.

Graft-versus-host disease (GVHD) occurs in about a third of human leukocyte antigen (HLA)–matched and two thirds of HLA-mismatched transplantations. Acute GVHD, which occurs within 3 months of transplantation, consists of rash, diarrhea, and hepatic dysfunction, but no neurologic complications have been reported. Chronic GVHD occurs in about a third of patients who survive more than 3 months after transplantation. It may have an autoimmune pathogenesis and has been associated with polymyositis, myasthenia gravis, and chronic inflammatory demyelinating neuropathy (CIDP).

A leukoencephalopathy occurs in bone marrow transplant recipients who have received treatment with methotrexate and total body irradiation. It appears that either high-dose intravenous or intrathecal methotrexate must be combined with radiation therapy to produce the leukoencephalopathy. Hemorrhages are usually related to severe thrombocytopenia (i.e., platelets fewer than 20,000 cells/mm³). Cerebral infarcts are largely caused by emboli from endocarditis, either infective or nonbacterial thrombotic endocarditis (NBTE), which can occur as part of a generalized hypercoagulable state in bone marrow transplant recipients.

REFERENCES

Adams R et al: The use of transcranial ultrasonography to predict stroke in sickle cell disease, *N Engl J Med* 326:605, 1992.

Beck WS: Neuropsychiatric consequences of cobalamin deficiency, *Adv Intern Med* 36:33, 1991.

Dyck PJ et al: Plasma exchange in polyneuropathy with monoclonal gammopathy of undetermined significance, *N Engl J Med* 325:1482, 1991.

Feldman E, editor: The antiphospholipid antibody and stroke symposium (APASS), *Stroke* 23:II, 1992.

Grotta JC et al: Red blood cell disorders and stroke, *Stroke* 17:811, 1985.

Openshaw H, Slatkin NE: Differential diagnosis of neurological complications in bone marrow transplantation, *Neurologist* 1:191, 1995.

Petty GW et al: Complications of long-term anticoagulation, *Ann Neurol* 23:578, 1988.

Samuels MA: Neurologic manifestations of hematologic diseases. In Asbury AK, McKhann GM, Mcdonald WI, editors: *Diseases of the nervous system: clinical neurology,* ed 2, Philadelphia, 1992, WB Saunders.

Schafer AI: The hypercoagulable states, *Ann Intern Med* 102:814, 1985.

CHAPTER

170 Neuronephrology

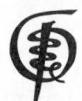

Martin A. Samuels

Patients with renal failure are subject to several major classes of neurologic disease (Chapters 109 and 110), which are caused by either the uremia itself or its treatment (e.g., dialysis transplantation).

NEUROLOGIC COMPLICATIONS OF UREMIA

Uremic encephalopathy occurs in the course of renal failure when the glomerular filtration rate falls below 10% of normal and usually is dramatically relieved by dialysis or renal transplantation. Its neurologic characteristics are nonspecific, consisting of an abnormality in the level of consciousness ranging from inattention to coma, with variable numbers of motor signs, such as asterixis, myoclonus, tremor, and seizures. When an encephalopathy develops in a patient with uremia, other contributing factors, such as drugs or concomitant hepatic failure, should be identified and treated. It is important to bear in mind that drugs that are cleared by the kidney may reach toxic levels in uremic patients, even when taken in normal doses.

There is no absolute relationship between the degree of renal failure, as measured by any of the usual blood chemistry tests, and the severity of the encephalopathy. The most consistent abnormality found in brains of animals and humans who have died of uremia is a dramatic increase in calcium content. Furthermore, some of the encephalopathy can be reversed with parathyroidectomy or medical suppression of parathyroid hormone (PTH). Since calcium is important in neurotransmitter release and action, it is possible that PTH-mediated changes in calcium metabolism may underlie some of the encephalopathy seen in uremic patients. In addition, there is evidence that PTH may, itself, be toxic to the nervous system, above and beyond its effect on calcium metabolism.

At present, the best treatment for uremic encephalopathy is improvement in the uremic state.

Uremic neuropathy is common in patients with chronic renal failure but is a significant clinical problem in only about 10% of patients receiving long-term renal dialysis. Most of these patients also have diabetes mellitus (diabetics compose about one third of patients receiving long-term renal dialysis), which is well known to produce a similar neuropathy, so it is usually difficult in practice to separate the true uremic neuropathy from the diabetic neuropathy. However, it is clear that in a small number of nondiabetic patients there is a neuropathy severe enough to become a significant clinical problem.

The most common uremic neuropathy is a symmetric sensorimotor polyneuropathy affecting the longest nerves first and then dying back toward the spinal cord. The clinical phenomena (i.e., burning feet, tender feet and calves, "restless legs," and, rarely, distal weakness) are indistinguishable from those in any other metabolic axonopathy (e.g., diabetes mellitus, alcohol abuse, vitamin deficiency, and cancer). Electrophysiologic studies are rarely helpful, since they invariably show mild slowing of the nerve conduction velocities and widespread denervation but nothing pathognomonic of the uremic neuropathy. The neurotoxic substance(s) in renal failure have not been convincingly identified.

Another neuropathy that occurs in uremic patients is the mononeuropathy syndrome, which is caused by compression of metabolically deranged nerves. Compression in bedridden patients of the ulnar, radial, femoral, or peroneal nerves can produce neuropathies in uremic patients more readily than in normal people.

Carpal tunnel syndrome is particularly common in uremic patients, and some of these patients have been shown to have secondary amyloidosis with accumulation of the amyloid in the carpal tunnel. The amyloid in this circumstance is made from a β_2 microglobulin that normally is cleared by the kidney. Being a large molecule with a molecular weight of about 12,000 daltons, β_2 microglobulin is not cleared by hemodialysis. Therefore it can accumulate and be incorporated into a beta-pleated sheet (i.e., amyloid) and be deposited in soft tissue or the heart, producing clinical syndromes such as carpal tunnel syndrome.

NEUROLOGIC COMPLICATIONS OF THE TREATMENT OF UREMIA

Hemodialysis is associated with two distinct neurologic conditions: the dialysis dysequilibrium syndrome (DDS) and dialysis dementia (also known as dialysis encephalopathy) (Chapter 110).

The dialysis dysequilibrium syndrome consists of a spectrum of neurologic abnormalities ranging from headache and muscle cramps to coma. The severe form (i.e., severe encephalopathy, stupor, or coma) is very rare in modern practice, probably because patients receive dialysis at much higher levels of renal function than in prior eras. It may be inferred from this fact that severe DDS is caused by rapid correction of extreme hyperosmolarity. This probably explains the fact that patients receiving long-term dialysis or in whom the blood urea nitrogen (BUN) level is allowed to slowly drift downward over many days or weeks rarely have severe DDS. Mild forms of DDS (i.e., headache, muscle cramps, and mild confusion) still are seen and usually respond favorably to infusions of hypertonic saline, glucose, or mannitol.

It was originally hypothesized that DDS was caused by the so-called reverse urea effect: urea was thought to be cleared less rapidly from the brain than from the blood during hemodialysis, thereby leading to a movement of water into the brain and resulting in cerebral edema, which was said to cause the symptoms. It has subsequently been shown that urea is cleared from the brain and blood at the same rate, making the reverse-urea-effect hypothesis untenable. Currently it is theorized that a cerebral intracellular acidosis is caused by the production of organic acids (so-called idiogenic osmoles) by the brain and that this pH disturbance produces the neurologic symptoms. The precise stimulus for the production of these organic acids remains obscure.

Dialysis dementia (or dialysis encephalopathy) is a progressive, usually lethal disease characterized by dysarthria, with a rather characteristic stuttering quality, polymyoclonus, and rapidly progressive dementia. The electroencephalogram (EEG) is usually quite abnormal, often showing rhythmic bursts of high-voltage, sharp activity. Early in the course of the disease intravenous diazepam infusion often strikingly improves the EEG and the speech disorder. The brain pathologic findings are usually unimpressive but may show a spongioform encephalopathy, reminiscent in many ways of the pathologic findings of Jakob-Creutzfeld disease. This disease has not been transmitted to subhuman primates by intracerebral injection of brain material from affected patients. There is some evidence that high levels of aluminum in the dialysate are associated with this illness, and most dialysis units now employ routine deionization of water that is used to prepare dialysate. It is known that high levels of aluminum are neurotoxic and that aluminum can produce neurofibrillary tangles in animals; however, the pathologic features of the dialysis dementia syndrome are not reminiscent of Alzheimer's disease and there is very little direct evidence that aluminum causes this disease in animal models.

It had been argued that elevated aluminum levels decrease the activity of an enzyme, dihydropteridine reductase, which in turn is involved in neurotransmitter synthesis. This neurotransmitter deficiency would then cause the dialysis encephalopathy. However, recent studies have failed to show any relationship between this enzyme's activity and either aluminum levels or cognitive function. Thus the origin of dialysis encephalopathy remains obscure.

RENAL TRANSPLANTATION

Renal transplantation is most often performed in patients with glomerulonephritis (membranous or membranoproliferative), diabetes mellitus, and hypertensive renal disease. Other underlying diseases include polycystic kidney disease, lupus erythematosus, amyloidosis, analgesic nephropathy, and obstructive nephropathy.

Most of the neurologic complications of renal transplantation are due to the underlying disease for which the transplantation was performed. For example, polycystic kidney disease may be associated with multiple cerebral berry aneurysms, hypertension with ischemic and hemorrhagic stroke, lupus erythematosus with antineuronal antibodies, and mental status changes and uremic encephalopathy with hepatorenal syndrome. Rapid correction of hyponatremia may lead to central pontine myelinolysis, a syndrome that can range in severity from mild tetraparesis to deep coma or even death and can now be easily demonstrated in the pons or extrapontine sites by magnetic resonance imaging.

The renal transplantation procedure itself is the oldest of all the organ transplantations and now rarely causes any neurologic problems. Occasionally peripheral nerve injuries (e.g., of the lateral femoral cutaneous nerve of the thigh) may be caused by retractors or patient positioning during the surgical procedure, but these are usually reversible without specific treatment.

The most common neurologic complication after renal transplantation is stroke that is related to underlying cerebrovascular and/or cardiac disease as a result of the risk factors of hypertension and diabetes, which are so often present in renal transplant recipients.

BIBLIOGRAPHY

Adams HP, Dawson G, Coffman TJ, Corry MD: Stroke in renal transplant recipients, *Arch Neurol* 43:13, 1986.
Bolla KI et al: Dihydropteridine reductase activity: lack of association with serum aluminum levels and cognitive functioning in patients with end-stage renal disease, *Neurology* 41:1806, 1991.
Fraser CL, Arieff AI: Nervous system complications of uremia, *Ann Intern Med* 109:143, 1988.
Junaid I, Kwan JTC, Lord RHH: Femoral neuropathy in renal transplantation, *Transplantation* 56:240, 1993.

PART SEVEN

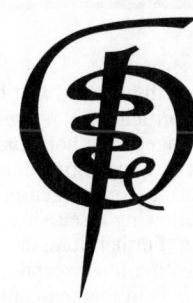

Clinical Immunology, Rheumatology, and Dermatology

The immune response has developed through evolution to protect against environmental pathogens *(nonself),* while at the same time discriminating against the host's own tissues (noninfectious *self).* The two main phases of the response are an initial recognition event, followed by an effector phase. Immune recognition is critical in the normal functioning of the system and is accomplished by three sets of antigen-binding molecules: the T-cell antigen receptor, the class I and class II molecules of the major histocompatibility complex (MHC), and the B-cell antigen receptor (immunoglobulin). The effector phase is designed to block, isolate, or eliminate environmental pathogens and is mediated by a variety of cells and soluble factors. Occasionally the immune response is defective. Failure in "self" recognition can result in autoimmune diseases, whereas misdirected effector systems can induce tissue injury and hypersensitivity diseases. Chapter 171 is an excellent starting point for the uninitiated or those wishing an overview of the human immune response. The subsequent chapters detail the various elements of the recognition and effector systems.

CHAPTER

171 Human Immune Response

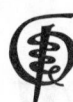

Robert R. Rich

IMMUNE FUNCTION AND SELF/NONSELF DISCRIMINATION

The vertebrate immune system is a complex, sophisticated mechanism of defense against invasion by infectious organisms. The system is multidispersed with cellular elements resident in or accessible to virtually every organ system. Organized tissues specialized for immune function are designated as primary or secondary. The *primary* lymphoid organs (bone marrow, thymus) are the sites of differentiation of lymphoid progenitors; the *secondary* lymphoid organs (lymph nodes, spleen, submucosal lymphoid tissues) are sites from which immune responses are mounted. The cells and tissues of the immune system are interconnected by a complex vascular system of lymphatic and blood vessels. This system delivers lymphoid cells and antigen from peripheral sites and transports cells between organs of the immune system and to inflammatory loci.

Microbial targets of an immune response include the entire range of infectious agents, from viruses to multicellular parasites. The specific defense may differ, however, based on the nature of the infecting organism and its physical location within the body. For example, defense against infections with intracellular organisms often depends predominantly on cytolytic T-cell responses, whereas antibodies and granulocytes more frequently have principal roles as effectors against extracellular microbes. Regardless, one consequence of immune recognition is an inflammatory response, which attacks the invading organism, leading to its destruction. A secondary consequence of this attack may be significant damage to host cells, either as sites of microbial residence or as "innocent bystanders" that do not express the inducing antigen. Depending on the reaction's site and severity, it may be accompanied by the classic local and systemic symptoms and signs of inflammation.

The essence of immune system function is its capacity for molecular discrimination between "self" and "nonself." Such discrimination is primarily the responsibility of T-lymphocytes. It reflects the

BOX 171-1

Pathogenetic processes in immunologic diseases

Immunologic deficiencies (congenital or acquired)
Malignant transformation
Immunologic dysregulation
Ambiguity of self/nonself discrimination
Inflammatory consequences of normal immune function

selection within the thymus of those thymocytes that have generated antigen receptors with binding specificity for nonself. In simplest terms, T-lymphocytes recognize antigens as short linear peptides (8 to 18 amino acids) that are bound to major histocompatibility complex (MHC) molecules on the surface of antigen-presenting cells. With the exception noted in the following discussion, T-cells do not bind antigen in native configuration. Furthermore, they do not recognize antigen in soluble form and, with a few exceptions, they do not recognize nonpeptide antigens. This is in marked contrast to antigen recognition by antibody molecules. B-cells are not selected for self/nonself discrimination. On the other hand, antibodies, unlike T-cells, can bind specifically to complex macromolecules, which are encountered either at cell surfaces or in solution. Moreover, antigens reactive with antibodies include not only proteins, but also carbohydrates, nucleic acids, and lipids.

An essential element of self/nonself discrimination is the clonal specificity of recognition that targets potential invaders. Although the immune system can recognize a vast array of distinct antigens, all the receptors of a single T-cell or B-cell have identical antigen-binding sites and thus a particular specificity. An additional feature that enhances the effectiveness of the response is antigen-driven *immunologic memory.* This memory derives from the fact that, after an initial encounter with antigen, those clones of lymphocytes of appropriate specificity replicate, resulting in a greater and more rapid response on a subsequent antigen encounter. These features, clonal specificity and immunologic memory, provide a conceptual foundation for use of vaccines in the prevention of infectious diseases. Immunologic memory involves not only the T-cells charged with initial discrimination between self and nonself, but also those effector cells that mediate the efferent limb of an inflammatory response. These include both T-cells and B-cells. On the efferent side the immune response may display exquisite *specificity,* such as the lysis of virus-infected target cells by cytolytic T-cells, or *nonspecificity,* such as the response of macrophages to inflammatory mediators.

Implications for Disease Pathogenesis

The features of the immune system just described are important to understanding pathogenic mechanisms of immunologic diseases. Five distinct pathways to pathogenesis can be identified (Box 171-1). First, immunologic disease may represent a failure or deficiency of the immune system. This mechanism is similar to that which accounts for most diseases of other organ systems. Failure may be congenital (e.g., x-linked agammaglobulinemia) or acquired (e.g., acquired immunodeficiency syndrome [AIDS]). It may be global (e.g., severe combined immunodeficiency) or quite specific, involving only a particular component of the immune system (e.g., selective immunoglobulin A [IgA] deficiency). Such failures are usually identified by increased susceptibility to infection, which may range from subtle to profound.

Malignant transformation of its various cellular constituents represents a second pathogenetic pathway that the immune system shares with other organ systems. By infiltrating other organs, leukemias, lymphomas, myelomas, and related malignancies can present a remarkable array of clinical problems. However, the most commonly encountered problems are direct complications of the malignant process on hematopoietic differentiation, secondary effects of infiltrating bone marrow and lymphoid organs, or both.

Dysregulation of an essentially intact immune system provides a third pathway to immune pathogenesis. Features of an optimal immune response include antigen recognition and elimination with little if any adverse consequence to the host. Both initiation and termination of the response involve complex regulatory interactions that may go awry when challenged by antigens of a particular structure or in a particular mode of presentation. Diseases of immune dysregulation typically reflect a combination of genetic and environmental factors that, acting together, subvert a normal immune response to some pathologic end. The acute allergic diseases are typical of these disorders. For example, the pathogenesis of allergic asthma may involve a genetically determined excessive response to some environmental antigen, such as the immunoglobulin E (IgE) response to animal danders, as well as an abnormality in effector responses to inflammatory signals.

The fourth and fifth pathways to pathogenesis are more specific to the immune system. The fourth lies at the heart of specific immune system function, that is, the molecular discrimination between self and nonself. An untoward consequence of ambiguity in this discrimination is the development of autoimmune tissue damage. Although such damage may be mediated either by antibodies or T-cells, the basic pathogenesis of autoimmune diseases usually represents a failure of T-cell function because of these cells' central responsibility for self/nonself discrimination. Failures may be general, leading to development of systemic autoimmune diseases, such as lupus erythematosus, or local, as in organ-specific autoimmune diseases. With local failure the attack is directed against specific cells and usually particular cell surface molecules expressed by such cells. Pathology is usually a consequence of target tissue destruction (e.g., multiple sclerosis, rheumatoid arthritis, insulin-dependent diabetes mellitus). However, it may also reflect hormone receptor blockade (e.g., type B insulin-resistant diabetes) or hormone receptor stimulation (e.g., Graves' disease). Autoimmune disease may represent the consequence of an ambiguity in self/nonself discrimination resulting from an encounter with an infectious organism. In most cases the infectious episode is unidentified and merely postulated; in some cases, however, it may be associated with a clearly identified infectious event (e.g., rheumatic fever, Reiter's disease). The result in either case may be secondary autoimmune attack on a particular cell type, based on cross-reactivity of antigenic determinants between the infectious agent and the target tissue.

A fifth important pathogenetic mechanism is disease development as a consequence of physiologic rather than pathologic function. These are diseases in which the development of an inflammatory lesion represents nothing more than normal functioning of the system. Typical of such diseases is allergic contact dermatitis to such potent skin sensitizers as urushiol, the causative agent of poison ivy dermatitis. These diseases may also have an iatrogenic etiology; they may range from benign (e.g., delayed hypersensitivity skin test reactions) to life threatening (e.g., graft-versus-host disease, in which the physiologic immune function of an engrafting bone marrow threatens the viability of an immunologically incompetent host). Furthermore, studies in experimental animals have shown that diseases resulting from an encounter with certain infectious agents may reflect secondary consequences of a physiologic immune response to the infectious organism. Classic examples with probable implications for human diseases include coxsackie myocarditis and lymphocytic choriomeningitis in mice.

CONSTITUENTS OF IMMUNE SYSTEM

Immune responses are traditionally categorized as *humoral* or *cellular.* The first refers to those carried out by circulating antibodies and the latter to those mediated by specifically sensitized T-lymphocytes. The system actually is far more complex; it includes cellular interactions that control the development of antibody responses and the effects of short-range soluble mediators, termed *cytokines,* in the induction and regulation of both T cell–mediated and B cell–mediated immune responses.

Cellular Components

The cellular constituents of the immune system are leukocytes and related cells with common precursors resident in solid organs. These cells arise from pluripotent stem cells present throughout life in the bone marrow. Components not derived from bone marrow include stromal elements of the solid lymphoid organs and certain specialized epithelial cells that are important in antigen presentation and lymphocyte differentiation, such as in the thymus and the intestinal mucosa.

The lymphocytes capable of specific immune recognition, based on their clonally specific cell surface display of antigen receptors, are T-cells and B-cells. Arising from bone marrow precursors, *T-cells* are selected in the thymus based on the expression of T-cell receptors (TCRs) useful in self/nonself discrimination. Mature T-cells emerging from this differentiative process are found in T cell–dependent areas of solid lymphoid organs and normally constitute 60% to 85% of the lymphocyte population in the peripheral blood of adults. *B-cells* mature in the bone marrow. On emigration, they reside within lymphoid follicles and germinal centers of solid lymphoid organs; they represent 7% to 20% of lymphocytes in peripheral blood. When stimulated with antigen, B-cells undergo terminal differentiation to nondividing, antibody-producing plasma cells. Plasma cells are resident within lymphoid tissues but do not normally circulate in the peripheral blood.

A third class of lymphocytes is comprised of those identified functionally as *natural killer* (NK) *cells* and morphologically as *large granular lymphocytes* (LGLs). Such cells, representing 10% to 30% of circulating lymphocytes, are clearly distinct from T-cells and B-cells because they do not rearrange the genes encoding the antigen receptors of either. They are nevertheless capable of a less specific type of recognition that is likely important during primary encounter with certain cell-associated antigens, such as those expressed on tumor cells or virus-infected cells. The molecular basis of this recognition is not well understood, but NK cell receptors for polymorphic determinants of MHC class I molecules on target cells have been identified. Interestingly, engagement of such receptors *downregulates* NK cytolytic activity. Hence, susceptibility of targets in NK cell–mediated cytolysis is inversely correlated with their expression of MHC class I molecules.

The remaining mononuclear cell type present in peripheral blood is the *monocyte,* normally constituting 4% to 15% of total leukocytes. Monocytes and their relatives are important in antigen processing and presentation, particularly to T-cells. Although apparently derived from a common monocytoid precursor in the bone marrow, such cells may exhibit a wide variety of morphologic features and specialized functions within solid organs, where they include macrophages and dendritic cells in lymph nodes, Kupffer's cells in the liver, Langerhans' cells in skin, and microglial cells in brain.

Discussions of the specific immune system often overlook the *polymorphonuclear leukocytes* (PMNs). Nevertheless, these cells are essential to most antibody-mediated defenses. Derived from granulocyte precursors in the bone marrow, PMNs undergo terminal differentiation along three general pathways, as neutrophils (35% to 75% of total leukocytes in the circulation of adults), eosinophils (0% to 5%), and basophils (0% to 1%). *Neutrophils* are the principal effectors of responses to pyogenic infections. They phagocytose foreign particles coated (opsonized) with antibodies and/or complement components. This process largely depends upon their cell surface display of immunoglobulin (Ig) Fc receptors and receptors for complement components, particularly C3b. Phagocytized particles are degraded within granules of PMNs; living organisms are killed by various cellular mechanisms, including generation of oxygen radicals and halogenation. In addition to their central importance in phagocytosis and killing of microorganisms, neutrophils may function as immunoregulators capable of synthesis and release of cytokines such as interleukin 1 (IL-1), IL-6, and tumor necrosis factor α (TNF-α).

Eosinophils and *basophils,* identified by the morphology and staining properties of their intracellular granules, are particularly important in host defenses to multicellular parasites. *Mast cells* are fixed tissue relatives of basophils; they are further divided into subtypes, mucosal and epithelial mast cells, based on tissue location and differences in morphology and function. Eosinophils, basophils, and mast cells are also prominent participants in acute allergic reactions, a secondary reflection of the shared role of IgE molecules in parasite defenses and the immune reactions of immediate hypersensitivity.

Soluble Factors

Immunoglobulins (Ig) or antibodies, produced by plasma cells, are the soluble effectors of immune responses with specific antigen-binding activity. As such, they differ importantly from the other humoral constituents of immunity, which may be critical to genesis of an inflammatory response, but do not bind antigen. The five major Ig classes (isotypes) are IgM, IgG, IgA, IgD, and IgE. The IgG class is further divided into four subclasses, and the IgA class into two subclasses. Antibody molecules are comprised of heavy and light chains, each of which has a *variable region* of 108 to 120 amino acids at the amino-terminal end connected to a carboxy-terminal *constant region* of approximately equal length for light chains and three-fold or four-fold longer for heavy chains. The chains are connected to one another by interchain disulfide bonds. The major classes of antibody *(isotypes)* are defined by the heavy chain, the genes for which map to human chromosome 14q32.

During the course of an antibody response, a given B-cell may change the class of antibody that it synthesizes *(isotype switching)* without affecting the antigen specificity. This is accomplished by differential ribonucleic acid (RNA) splicing or deoxyribonucleic acid (DNA) rearrangements, both of which have the effect of bringing the gene segments encoding a particular variable region into immediate proximity with one or another of the genes encoding constant region segments of the heavy chain (Chapter 173). Light chains are of two types, κ and λ, encoded on chromosomes 2 and 22, respectively. Either light chain can associate with heavy chains of any class, but any particular B-cell or plasma cell synthesizes antibody molecules of a single light chain isotype. All the antibodies synthesized by a particular cell have identical variable regions, a feature that is essential to the principle of clonal specificity of an immune response. This reflects that the genes on only one member of the pair of chromosomes encoding a heavy chain and only one of the pairs of either κ or λ light chain genes are active in any B-cell. This process, termed *allelic exclusion,* also applies to the synthesis of T-cell receptors.

Although the isotype of an antibody molecule does not affect its antigen-binding specificity, it largely determines the particular biologic activity and physical characteristics of the molecule. Serum IgM is a pentameric structure, each subunit of which is comprised of two μ-heavy chains and two light chains (either κ or λ). It is the principal antibody of a primary immune response. Because of its large molecular mass (about 900 kilodaltons [kD]), IgM distribution is essentially limited to the vascular compartment. Monomeric IgM molecules are expressed as antigen receptors on the surface of B-cells; RNA encoding the carboxy-terminal segment of the μ-chains is differentially spliced to provide the transmembrane and intracytoplasmic domains absent from the secreted form of the molecule. IgG antibodies are the most abundant in the serum and are the principal antibodies of a memory (secondary) response. IgG is comprised of two light chains and two γ-heavy chains. It is the only antibody isotype that is transported by an active process across the placenta from mother to fetus. IgA molecules are the principal antibodies in secretions across mucous membranes. In secretions, IgA is present as dimers connected by a joining chain; secretion is an active process promoted by the addition of *secretory component,* an epithelial cell product. Appropriate to its function, secretory IgA is relatively resistant to digestion by proteolytic enzymes. IgA is found in serum in monomeric or dimeric form, but without secretory component attached. IgD molecules are primarily expressed as antigen receptors on B-cells, particularly memory B-cells, either with or without cell surface IgM molecules of the same antigen-binding specificity. Only small amounts of IgD are found in serum, and the biologic function of soluble IgD is unknown. IgE is present in the serum in the lowest concentration of the five isotypes (about 1/120,000 of the IgG concentration). IgE molecules, however, may have profound biologic effects based on their specific binding to the surfaces of mast cells and basophils, which are induced to degranulate on cross-linking of surface IgE by antigen. This process is important in defenses against parasitic infestation and is also a critical pathogenetic event in the diseases of immediate hypersensitivity.

It is the variable portion of an Ig molecule, termed the *Fab fragment,* that contains the antigen-binding site. The biologic effector functions, on the other hand, are provided by distinct sites on the constant region of the heavy chains *(Fc fragment).* These include sites that bind and activate the first component of complement (IgM, IgG), that bind to the surface of phagocytic cells (IgM, IgG) or mast cells and basophils (IgE), and that account for the active transport of IgG across the placenta.

The biologic functions of IgG and IgM are largely reflections of their capacities to activate the complement cascade (Chapter 175). Through a series of sequential substrate-enzyme interactions, the 11 principal components of the classical complement system (C1q, C1r, C1s, C2 to C9) effect many of the consequences of an antigen-antibody interaction. These include the establishment of pores in a target membrane by the terminal components (C5 to C9), leading to osmotic lysis; opsonization by C3b, promoting phagocytosis; the production of factors with chemotactic activity (C5a); and the ability to induce mast cell degranulation (C3a, C5a). It is important to recognize that although complement activation is accomplished by the interaction between IgG or IgM and C1q (the *classical pathway*), many substances, including certain bacterial products, can directly activate the cascade through the central C3 component. This bypasses involvement of C1, C4, and C2 but leads to all the biologic consequences of C3 to C9 activation. Non–antibody-induced activation of C3 is referred to as the *alternative,* or *properdin, pathway.*

In contrast to the abundance of Ig molecules (up to 15 mg/ml or 0.1 M for IgG), the soluble products of T-cells and antigen-presenting cells (APCs) are present at the sites of an immune response in extremely low concentration (e.g., approximately 10^{-10} M). These factors are a diverse group of generally small protein hormones (8 to 35 kD) that do not bind antigen and are collectively referred to as *cytokines* (Chapter 174). Among others, they include IL-1 through IL-17, interferon γ (IFN-γ), TNF, transforming growth factor β (TGF-β), and the colony-stimulating factors (CSFs). Some cytokines are produced predominantly by T-cells (or T-cells and mast cells). Others are produced by many cell types, including APCs and cells of other organ systems. A characteristic feature of cytokines is their pleiotropy of function. Within the immune system this can include promotion of proliferation of specific subsets, control of the differentiation of B-cell and T-cell effector functions, and the regulation of immunoglobulin production and isotype switching. Certain cytokines, particularly IL-10, IL-13, and TGF-β are particularly important in downregulation of immunologic responses. Others, such as IL-3, IL-5, and the CSFs, are important as regulators of the differentiation of hematopoietic cells in the bone marrow. It is through the action of cytokines produced by T-cells that their capacity for self/nonself discrimination is translated to control of antibody responses.

MOLECULAR IMMUNOLOGY AND IMMUNOGLOBULIN SUPERFAMILY

Many of the principal molecules involved in activation, regulation, cell-to-cell contact, and effector function in immune responses share structural features indicative of a common evolutionary origin. These molecules and the genes that encode them are collectively referred to as the *Ig superfamily.* The family includes more than 35 distinct members that exhibit significant sequence homology to one another. An essential feature is a *domain* subunit structure of approximately 100 amino acids, usually including a single intrachain disulfide bond. Protein organization generally correlates well with genomic structure, with separate protein domains typically encoded by distinct exons. Functions of the Ig superfamily are related principally to antigen binding (Ig, TCR, MHC molecules) and to cell-cell interaction and recognition (e.g., CD4$^+$, CD8, lymphocyte function–associated [LFA] molecules, intercellular adhesion molecules [ICAMs]). A frequent feature of Ig superfamily interactions is that different members expressed on different cells function as ligand-receptor pairs for one another, often to increase adhesiveness of a cell-cell interaction (e.g., CD2 and LFA-3; LFA-1 and ICAM-1; CD8 and MHC class I; CD4 and MHC class II).

An understanding of molecular specificity of an immune response requires some appreciation of the structural basis of antigen binding. The three types of molecules with this capability, MHC, Ig, and TCR, all construct an antigen-binding groove, with side chains and pockets that accommodate specific structural features of the ligand. For Ig molecules the ligand (an antigenic determinant, or *epitope*) may be present as a specific chemical moiety or conformational site on the surface of a molecule that varies in complexity from a simple substituted aromatic ring to a macromolecule. Binding by antibody is of relatively high specificity and high affinity. The TCR antigen-binding site is also of high specificity but of relatively low affinity, reflecting the process by which it is selected for self/nonself discrimination. The TCR binds, within a single complex site, both to a foreign peptide and the surrounding α-helices of the MHC molecule that presents it. MHC molecules are the third members of the antigen-binding team. They bind short peptides, derived from either self or nonself proteins, with low specificity and medium to high affinity. Ig and TCR share a strategy for achieving specificity of the antigen-binding pocket that differs fundamentally from that of MHC molecules. Ig and TCR use families of rearranging gene segments to construct variable regions particular to specific T-cells or B-cells and their clonal progeny. MHC molecules, on the other hand, do not rearrange; they do not undergo allelic exclusion and are codominantly expressed. Thus a particular APC may display a full complement of MHC molecules, with capacity to bind numerous distinct antigen peptides in a nonclonally specific manner.

Immunoglobulin and T-Cell Receptor Diversity

Antigen-binding specificity of both Ig and TCR reflects the random joining by DNA rearrangement and splicing of two or three segments selected from a "gene library" encoding each chain of the variable domain of the molecule. For Ig heavy chains this involves the joining of one particular V segment (of more than 100 available) to one D segment (of at least 20) and a J segment (of six) (Chapter 173). The particular V-D-J unit is then joined (by RNA splicing or DNA rearrangement) to a C region, one of a series of tandemly arrayed genes encoding isotype-specific heavy chain constant regions, leading to transcription of a specific Ig heavy chain. For κ- and λ-light chains, only two segments, V and J, are used to encode the variable portion of the molecule.

The structure of TCR is highly homologous to that of Ig molecules. Four distinct rearranging gene families have been identified: α, β, γ, and δ. Two isoforms of TCR are expressed; both are heterodimers of integral membrane proteins, comprised of α- and β-chains or γ- and δ-chains. In the circulation, 97% or more of T-cells display the αβ-receptor, whereas in some tissue sites, such as the intestinal mucosa, γδ-bearing T-cells may predominate. The αβ-heterodimer is invariably bonded by an interchain disulfide link; γδ-TCR may be disulfide linked or unlinked. Functional differences between T-cells expressing αβ- and γδ-receptors are a matter of current study; they may reflect responses to antigens of differing origin or the use of distinct subsets of MHC class I molecules for presentation. For example, recent data suggest that T-cells expressing γδ-TCR may have specialized functions in responses to nonconventional (class I-b) MHC molecules and to nonpeptide antigens such as lipid components of bacterial cell walls.

The general strategy for assembly of TCR variable regions is the same as that for Ig, with some differences in gene organization that allow additional variability in rearrangement. The variable segments of β- and δ-chains are assembled from V, D, and J segments randomly selected and joined to the C region gene; α- and γ-chains, as with Ig light chains, are assembled only from V and J segments. Interestingly, genes for δ-chains are imbedded within the chromosomal segment encoding α-chains, between the Vα- and Jα-regions. Both TCR isotypes are associated with a multimeric structure, CD3, that is required for TCR cell surface expression and for signal transduction. In contrast to the TCR heterodimer, the CD3 components do not rearrange and do not exhibit clonal variability.

Extraordinary diversity is achieved, both for TCR and Ig molecules, by the random selection of segments encoding the variable regions plus the additional *"combinatorial" diversification* accomplished by the pairing of particular chains with one another in construction of the complete Ig or TCR molecule. Further diversification is achieved by a mechanism termed *N-nucleotide addition,* in which one or more individual nucleotides, not encoded within the genome, are frequently added concomitantly with gene rearrangement at the junctions between variable region segments. The addition of nucleotides results in a high likelihood of frame-shift mutations and in-

creases the probability that any given rearrangement will be nonproductive.

One molecular mechanism in antigen receptor construction is unique to Ig genes. This is a process of *somatic mutation* that continues within the rearranged V-D-J gene throughout the lifetime of a particular B-cell and its clonal progeny. Such mutations within the antibody-combining site occasionally result in production of an antibody with increased affinity for the antigen that originally induced its production. Because clonal proliferation of lymphocytes is driven by contact with antigen, B-cells expressing surface Ig molecules with higher affinity for a particular antigen than parent or sibling cells will be preferentially selected and stimulated to divide. Consequently, over generations of the B-cell response to antigen, antibodies of progressively higher affinity are produced. This process, termed *affinity maturation,* contributes significantly to the much higher antigen-binding affinity of Ig than TCR molecules. The difference, however, is at the core of the capacity for self/nonself discrimination uniquely possessed by T-cells. Such discrimination requires that TCR affinity be fixed within the thymus before an encounter with foreign antigen. Thus somatic mutation of TCR does not occur during antigen-driven T-cell clonal proliferation.

Major Histocompatibility Complex

The third family of antigen-binding molecules is the products of the MHC (Chapter 172). The MHC, termed *human lymphocyte antigen* (HLA) in humans and encoded on chromosome 6p, represents a highly duplicated system of genes of two basic types, class I and class II. Products of the three principal MHC class I genes, designated HLA-A, HLA-B, and HLA-C, are involved in antigen presentation. An as yet unknown number of additional "nonclassic" class I-b gene products may have more specialized roles in antigen presentation or cell-cell interaction. Three principal class II genes and gene products also exist, HLA-DR, HLA-DQ, and HLA-DP. Both class I and class II molecules possess a peptide-binding (antigen-binding) groove with walls of α-helices and a floor of antiparallel β-pleated strands. The class I groove accommodates peptides 8 to 10 amino acids in length; the class II groove allows peptides of 12 to 18 amino acids. Although highly homologous to one another, the class I and class II molecules have substantial structural differences. Class I molecules are comprised of a polymorphic HLA-A, HLA-B, or HLA-C heavy chain of approximately 45 kD that is noncovalently associated with a nonpolymorphic non-MHC product, β_2 microglobulin (β_2m). The class I heavy chain is an integral membrane protein; β_2m is not. In contrast, both chains of class II molecules are encoded within the MHC, and both are integral membrane proteins. The class II polypeptides are of similar molecular size (28 to 32 kD). For HLA-DQ, both chains, designated α and β, are polymorphic, whereas for HLA-DR, polymorphism is essentially limited to the β-chain. Because the MHC genes do not rearrange, they are far less diverse within an individual than the Ig and TCR products. Specificity of the peptide-binding groove is determined by "pockets" within the binding groove capable of accepting particular amino acids of a peptide antigen. These pockets define a "motif" that characterizes the binding specificity of any particular class I or class II molecule. Moreover, the multiplicity of MHC genes coupled with their extraordinary population polymorphism ensures that an array of different MHC molecules, with different binding specificities, is expressed on the surface of an APC.

ANTIGENS AND ANTIGEN PROCESSING

The process by which proteins are partially digested and represented to T cells as oligopeptides in an appropriate MHC context is termed *antigen processing.* Two distinct pathways can be distinguished, depending on the source of the antigen (Fig. 171-1). These pathways largely, but not exclusively, determine the subset of T-cells that will recognize a particular antigen.

Antigens that are synthesized within the antigen-presenting cell (APC) itself (termed *endogenous* antigens, e.g., viral and tumor antigens) undergo hydrolysis to peptides of 8 to 10 amino acids within the cytoplasm. Components of the proteosomes that mediate this digestion and the transporter (TAP) proteins with which the peptide fragments are then associated are also encoded within the MHC. TAP-

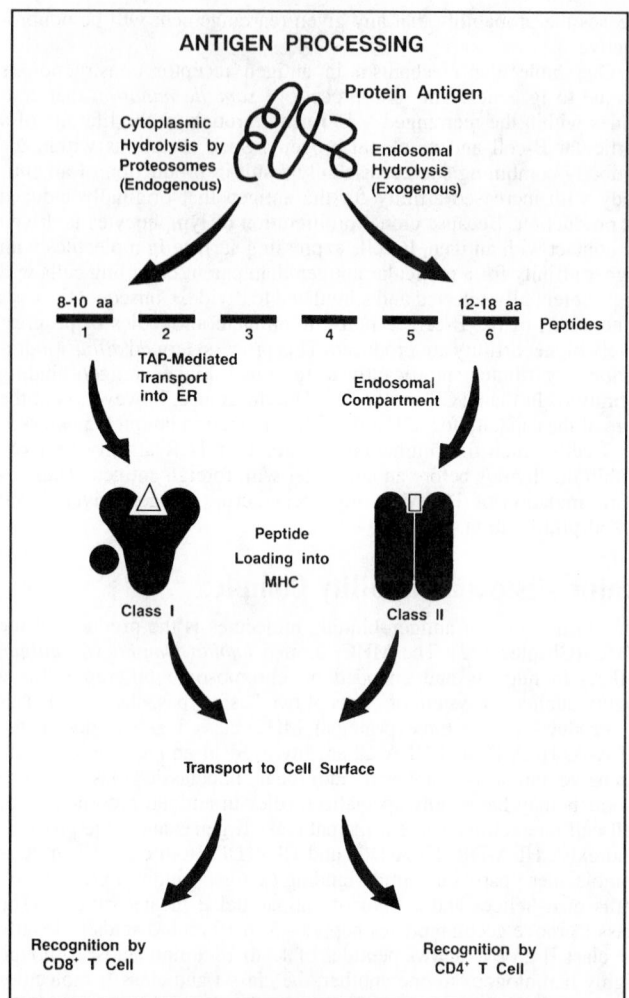

ANTIGEN PROCESSING

FIGURE 171-1 Distinct pathways for processing (hydrolytic digestion) of endogenous and exogenous protein antigens and peptide loading into antigen-binding clefts of major histocompatibility complex (MHC) class I and class II molecules, respectively.

associated antigen peptides are then transported into the lumen of the endoplasmic reticulum (ER), where they are loaded into the binding groove of newly synthesized MHC class I proteins. It is this complex of peptide, class I heavy chain, and β_2m that is then expressed at the cell surface, where it can be recognized by T-cells of the CD8$^+$ subset.

In contrast, antigens synthesized outside the APC (termed *exogenous* antigens) enter the cell by phagocytosis (e.g., monocytes, macrophages) or receptor-mediated endocytosis (e.g., B-cells functioning as APCs). They are then hydrolyzed by lysosomal enzymes and, within endosomes, peptides of 12 to 18 amino acids are loaded into binding grooves of MHC class II molecules. Class II–peptide complexes are then transported to the cell surface for recognition by T-cells of the CD4$^+$ subpopulation. Two additional molecules that interact with class II molecules to ensure the loading of exogenous peptide are invariant (or Ii) chain and HLA-DM. Invariant chain (so-called because, in contrast to MHC molecules, it is nonpolymorphic) binds to newly synthesized class II complexes within the endoplasmic reticulum and prevents loading by antigenic peptides until the complex has been transported to the endosomal compartment. Within endosomes, invariant chain is then removed by the catalytic activity of a class II–like MHC heterodimer, HLA-DM.

The tissue distributions of class I and class II MHC molecules differ significantly. Class I molecules are expressed on almost all nucleated cells. Consequently, many cells that are not components of the immune system may be capable of presenting an endogenous antigen and may serve as targets of a CD8$^+$ T-cell immune attack. In con-

trast, the tissue distribution of MHC class II molecules is quite restricted, being limited primarily to those cells of the immune system that have differentiated specifically to function as APCs. Because the initial activation of an immune response is controlled by CD4$^+$ T-cells, it consequently depends on appropriate processing and presentation of antigen by MHC class II–expressing cells.

Recently recognized exceptions to these principles of antigen presentation and recognition are the so-called *superantigens*. They are exemplified by the staphylococcal enterotoxins and related exotoxins produced by gram-positive cocci. The superantigens are proteins of about 30 kD that do not require processing but bind in native form to class II MHC molecules outside the antigen-binding groove. Moreover, they activate both CD4$^+$ and CD8$^+$ T-cells when bound to class II molecules. Superantigens' capacity to stimulate T-cells is determined primarily by the V segment of the TCR β-chain; it is less dependent on the other TCR components that define binding specificity for conventional peptide antigens. This results in a much higher frequency of T-cells responsive to superantigens than to conventional antigens, thus their name. In the mouse, not only bacterial exotoxins but also certain retroviral products have been shown to exhibit superantigen properties, indicating considerable diversity in the origin of such antigens. Bacterial superantigens are etiologic agents of various important diseases, including staphylococcal food poisoning, toxic shock syndrome, and scarlet fever. Superantigens of undetermined origin have also been implicated indirectly in the pathogenesis of several autoimmune diseases, including guttate psoriasis and Kawasaki's disease.

LYMPHOCYTE DIFFERENTIATION AND ACTIVATION
Thymocyte Education

The extraordinary process of T-cell education for self/nonself discrimination occurs during differentiation in the thymus; it reflects selection based on contact with self MHC molecules (plus peptide) in the thymic microenvironment. Prothymocytes, which enter the thymic cortex from the bone marrow, display CD2 (sheep erythrocyte receptor) and CD7; CD4 and CD8 have not yet been expressed, and TCR genes are in a germline (unrearranged) configuration. Soon thereafter the early thymocytes begin rearrangement of TCR genes and coexpress CD4 and CD8. TCR with randomly generated V regions, either αβ or γδ, are then coexpressed with CD3 at the thymocyte surface, where they encounter an array of self MHC class I and class II molecules on the surfaces of cortical epithelial cells. For most thymocytes the nascent TCR does not have appreciable affinity for any available self MHC molecule. In such cases, in the absence of TCR activation, the cell undergoes programmed death by a process termed *apoptosis* involving DNA fragmentation.

A few cells display appreciable affinity for one particular self MHC class I or class II molecule and are *positively selected* for further differentiation based on this property (Fig. 171-2, *A*). If the MHC molecule chosen is class II, the thymocyte downregulates its expression of CD8 and increases expression of CD4, becoming a *single-positive* CD4$^+$ thymocyte. Similarly, binding to a class I MHC molecule leads to development of a single-positive CD8$^+$ thymocyte. At this stage, those thymocytes that have survived the round of positive selection undergo a second round of *negative selection* (Fig. 171-2, *B*). The objective of negative selection is the opposite of the first round, that is, to eliminate those thymocytes that possess receptors of very high affinity for self MHC plus the self peptide (derived from autologous proteins) within the MHC antigen-binding groove. Elimination of such cells is essential to the process of self/nonself discrimination, since their emigration from the thymus would permit terminal differentiation of cells capable of autoimmune attack. Thus clones of cells with high-affinity receptors for self MHC plus peptide are similarly deleted by an apoptotic process. In the end, fewer than 5% of the prothymocytes that enter the thymus survive the education/selection process. Those that do survive emerge several days later as mature T-cells for distribution in the periphery. Such cells have low-affinity receptors for self-MHC plus self peptide but may have increased affinity for the complex of MHC plus some undefined nonself peptide that may be subsequently encountered.

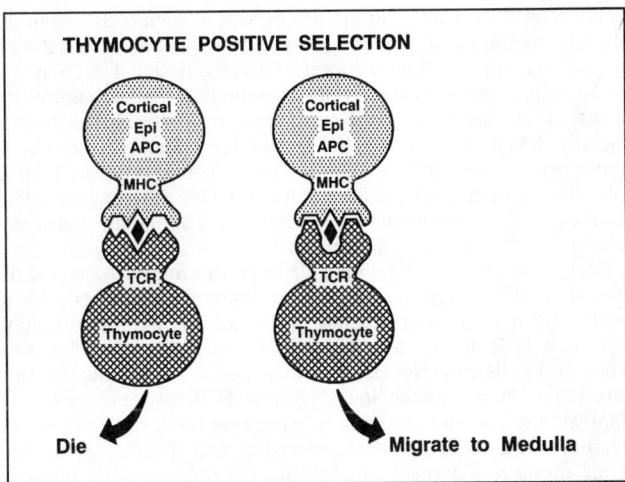

A

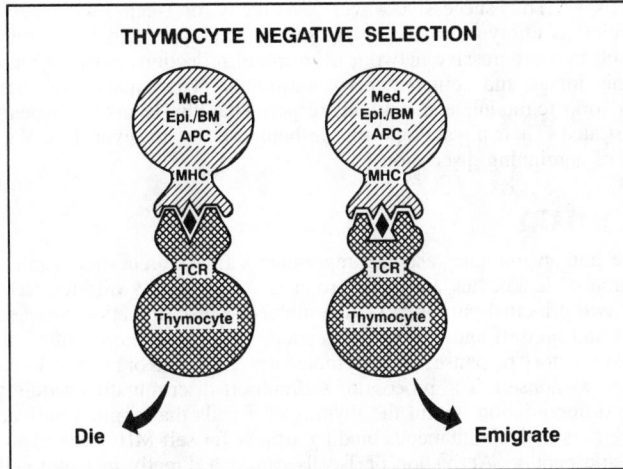

B

FIGURE 171-2   Two-stage selection of thymocytes based on binding characteristics of randomly generated T-cell responses (TCRs). **A,** Positive selection. *Double-positive* (CD4$^+$, CD8$^+$) thymocytes with TCR capable of *low* affinity binding to some specific self MHC molecule (either class I or class II) expressed by thymic cortical epithelial cells are positively selected; all other thymocytes die by apoptosis. The solid diamond represents a self peptide derived from hydrolysis of an autologous protein present in the thymus microenvironment or synthesized within the thymic antigen-processing cell *(APC)* itself. **B,** Negative selection. *Single-positive* (CD4$^+$ or CD8$^+$) thymocytes, positively selected in stage one, that display TCR with *high* affinity for the combination of self MHC plus some self (autologous) peptide present in the thymus are negatively selected (i.e., die). Those few thymocytes that have survived both positive and negative selection emigrate as mature T-cells to the secondary lymphoid tissues.

CD4 and CD8*

Throughout the differentiative process, as well as in the peripheral tissues, CD4 and CD8 molecules are importantly involved in T-cell activation. CD4 is a monomeric integral membrane protein with four extracellular domains, three of which share membership in the Ig superfamily. In contrast, CD8 is a dimeric structure, either a homodimer or heterodimer, both chains of which are transmembrane and both of which have a single Ig-like external domain. The contributions of CD4 and CD8 to T-cell differentiation and function are two-fold. First, CD8 molecules display a specific contact point for binding to a nonpolymorphic site on MHC class I molecules, thereby increasing the

---

*CD designates *cluster of differentiation,* an official international nomenclature for designation of cell surface molecules expressed on leukocyte surfaces that vary with cell type. Thus they are useful in characterization of phenotypic subpopulations.

avidity of the CD8$^+$ T cell–APC interaction. Similarly, CD4 molecules bind to MHC class II molecules, enhancing the adhesiveness of that interaction. Because the TCR was specifically selected for its relatively low affinity for self MHC, the development of adhesion-strengthening interactions of this type is important to effective engagement of T-cell and APC; other non–TCR-associated interactions, such as CD2 and LFA-1 on T-cells with LFA-3 and ICAM-1 on APC, respectively, also contribute significantly in this respect. A second function of CD4 or CD8 is in signal transduction. These molecules interact with other membrane constituents (members of the *src* family of cellular oncogenes), resulting in protein phosphorylation associated with cell activation (Chapter 185). Because the intracytoplasmic tail of the TCR heterodimer lacks sites for phosphorylation, perturbations of TCR-associated molecules, including CD3 and CD4 or CD8, are essential in transmitting the signal of antigen interaction to the cell's interior.

B-Cell Differentiation

Progenitors of B-cells are derived from lymphoid stem cells and are first identified by rearrangement of Ig heavy chain genes. As these cells differentiate into pre–B cells, they are distinguished by the expression of isolated μ-chains within the cytoplasm. These represent the protein products of one of the two Ig heavy chain gene complexes that have undergone a productive genetic rearrangement. At the pre–B cell stage, the cells are devoid of membrane Ig (mIg). As they differentiate into immature B-cells, light chain genes are also rearranged, and their products (κ- or λ-chains) are combined with cytoplasmic μ-chains, leading to the cell surface expression of monomeric mIgM. Expression of mIg is in association with a nonpolymorphic heterodimeric molecule Igαβ (CD79). Like CD3 on T-cells, Igαβ is required for both receptor (i.e., mIg) expression and for antigen-induced signal transduction and cell activation. The B cell–specific differentiation markers CD19, C20, and CD21 are also sequentially expressed during the pre-B and immature B-cell stages of differentiation.

By a process of differential RNA splicing, immature B-cells undergo their first Ig isotype switch, leading to the coexpression of IgM and IgD as antigen receptors at the B-cell surface. On expression of mIg, B-cells may emigrate from the bone marrow to the periphery and the solid lymphoid organs, where they undergo further antigen-driven differentiation. On encounter with antigen in the periphery, B-cell clones proliferate; this leads to development of memory B-cells or to terminal differentiation into nondividing, Ig-secreting plasma cells. Reflecting secondary DNA rearrangements, memory B-cells may lose expression of membrane IgD and acquire instead mIgG, mIgA, or mIgE. On antigen stimulation, plasma cells cease cell surface expression of mIg as synthesis of Ig molecules switches from the membrane-bound to the secreted form. Although not selected for recognition of foreignness in the context of self, maturing pre–B cells in the bone marrow also are subject to negative selection upon encounter with self soluble or particulate antigen, and B-cells in peripheral tissues may be rescued by ligand engagement in a process resembling positive selection. Recent studies in transgenic mice suggest that when an initial pre–B cell mIg is cross-linked by encounter with self antigen in the bone marrow, secondary light chain rearrangements can occur. This process, which can generate a new receptor lacking self reactivity, has been termed *receptor editing.*

Lymphocyte Activation

For both T-cells and B-cells, activation is a two-signal process. In both cases the first signal is supplied by antigen and the second by engagement of an accessory cell surface molecule. For T-cells the best understood accessory pathway involves binding of the costimulatory receptor CD28 by its ligand on an APC, CD80 or CD86. B-cell triggering similarly involves engagement of a costimulatory receptor CD40 by its ligand, CD40L. CD40L is expressed by activated T-cells, thereby establishing T-cell control over B-cell activation. As noted in later discussion, various cytokines produced by APC and/or activated T-cells also regulate proliferation and differentiation of antigen-stimulated T-cells and B-cells (Chapter 174).

If cells are stimulated only with signal one, in the absence of signal two the usual effect is to render the cell tolerant *(anergic)* and refractory to subsequent activation. Cells stimulated in this manner may subsequently undergo apoptosis, which, in the intact animal, may lead to long-term unresponsiveness to a particular antigen and may be important as a secondary mechanism for self tolerance.

Encounter with antigen in the context of an appropriate accessory signal leads to complex biochemical cascades that transmit the activation signal to the nucleus. Cellular receptors transduce signals by a process that involves membrane G proteins and cyclic nucleotides, Ca^{2+} flux, and membrane phospholipid metabolism. Protein kinases are activated and cellular oncogene products are phosphorylated. This results in transduction of transcription factors such as NF-AT and NF-κB to the nucleus, where they bind to the 5′ regulatory regions of genes critical to lymphocyte activation.

A possible exception to the generalization regarding two-signal activation of lymphocytes is seen with antigens with multiple repeating subunit structure that can directly stimulate B-cells. Such antigens, the prototypes of which are complex carbohydrates, can cause extensive cross-linking of mIg, leading to *thymus-independent* (TI) B-cell activation. Although antibody production by TI antigens does not require T-cells, it may depend upon cytokines elaborated by other accessory cells. IFN-γ and granulocyte-macrophage CSF (GM-CSF) produced by NK cells enhance Ig production and promote Ig isotype switching by TI antigen–activated B-cells. Nevertheless, B-cells stimulated by TI antigens exhibit relatively little isotype switching and little if any clonal proliferation. Consequently, antibody responses to TI antigens are predominantly of the IgM class and do not exhibit immunologic memory.

T-CELL SUBSETS AND IMMUNOREGULATION

The essence of an immune response is defense and homeostasis. Several phenotypically distinct subpopulations of T-cells have roles as the effectors and regulators of these processes. CD8$^+$ T-cells, approximately one third of T-cells normally present in peripheral blood, include the primary effectors of cytotoxic T-lymphocyte (CTL) responses. Recognizing foreign peptides bound to class I MHC cells, CTLs directly transmit a unidirectional lethal signal to target cells. Neither the CTLs themselves nor any non–antigen-expressing "innocent bystander" cells are damaged in the process. In an experimental setting, CD4$^+$ T-cells are also capable of differentiating into CTLs; in this case, however, target cell recognition is in the context of a class II MHC molecule.

Two subsets of CD4$^+$ T-cells can be distinguished based on the pattern of cytokines that they elaborate when appropriately stimulated. Since both subsets exhibit helper function for B-cells and other T-cells, they have been designated Th1 and Th2 cells. The pattern of cytokine production of Th1 cells is skewed to so-called inflammatory cytokines such as IL-2 and IFN-γ. IL-2 is the major growth factor for both CD4$^+$ and CD8$^+$ cells. IFN-γ is an inflammatory mediator that is a potent activator of APC and contributes to the differentiation of cytolytic activity by CD8$^+$ T-cells; it also has reciprocal effects with IL-4 in regulation of Ig isotype synthesis. Th2 T-cells produce cytokines (e.g., IL-4 and IL-13) that are essential to proliferation and differentiation of B-cells into antibody-producing cells. Although the identification of Th1 and Th2 subsets provides a useful paradigm, particularly in understanding susceptibility or resistance to infectious agents, it should be appreciated that it represents an oversimplification. Thus T-cell clones producing both inflammatory and helper cytokines are not uncommon. Moreover, some cytokines (e.g., IL-3) are generally produced in approximately equal quantity by Th1 and Th2 cells.

An important element of immune homeostasis is the production of cytokines that downregulate the response when appropriate. Two cytokines are particularly important in this regard. IL-10 and TGF-β inhibit production of IL-2 and IL-4. TGF-β also inhibits the synthesis of antibodies, the proliferation of B-cells and CD4$^+$ T-cells, and the differentiation of CD8$^+$ cytotoxic T-lymphocytes. Interestingly, TGF-β does act as a costimulator to promote the proliferation of a specific subset of CD8$^+$ T-cells, possibly with suppressor cell function.

A role for *suppressor T-cells* in control of physiologic immune responses and prevention of undesired responses has been controver-

sial because of difficulties in in vitro growth of such cells and in the molecular definition of their antigen receptors. Nevertheless, substantial evidence suggests that a subset of T-cells, designated *Ts,* is important in preventing synthesis of autoantibodies and in controlling the magnitude and duration of an immune response. Such cells are generally thought to be CD8$^+$ but are lacking in cytolytic activity. It is not clear whether they recognize antigen bound by class I MHC molecules or in another mode. Failure of CD8$^+$ immunoregulatory activity may be important in the pathogenesis of autoimmune diseases such as systemic lupus erythematosus.

Regulation of physiologic immune responses may also involve the generation of *anti-idiotypic networks,* both of antibodies and of T-cells. The uniqueness of structure of the variable portions of Ig molecules and TCR implies that they may be recognized by other antibodies or T-cells as antigenic determinants. Such antigenic determinants within the variable region of an Ig or TCR molecule are termed *idiotopes;* the complete molecules expressing them (Ig or TCR) are *idiotypes.* An immune response induced by and specific for variable region idiotopes is termed an *anti-idiotypic response.* The phenomenology of such complex and potentially endless circuitry is well established. Thus successive waves of antibody (or T-cells) with specificities as idiotype, anti-idiotype, anti-anti-idiotype, and so on may result in a progressive network of mirrored reflections between antigenic image and complementary anti-image. The capacity of such networks to modulate an antibody response has also been clearly demonstrated. Their physiologic role in homeostasis, however, is a matter of continuing discussion.

SUMMARY

The human immune response represents a finely orchestrated interaction of leukocytes and their products that is highly differentiated for two principal purposes: (1) the molecular discrimination between self and nonself and (2) the destruction, through development of an inflammatory response, of those molecules, cells, and organisms identified as nonself. The process of self/nonself discrimination requires the differentiation within the thymus of T-cells that express surface receptors with simultaneous binding affinity for self MHC and an antigenic peptide. Activation of T-cells can lead directly to target cell destruction or, through the elaboration of cytokines, can stimulate (or suppress) antigen-driven B-cell activation. Antibodies, the products of antigen-activated B-cells, enhance the phagocytosis and digestion of antigenic particles (or cells) by exposure of binding sites to surface receptors on phagocytes and/or activation of the complement cascade. Damage to host tissues may be a secondary consequence of the inflammatory response that follows from T-cell or B-cell activation. This may result in local and/or systemic signs and symptoms of inflammation and may cause damage to host tissues that is disproportionate to that induced by the microbe (i.e., antigen) itself. Finally, the very sophistication of the immune response offers considerable opportunity for error. Those errors that lead to disease are primarily of two types, dysregulation and ambiguity in self/nonself discrimination, the consequences of which are a pathologically excessive immune response or autoimmunity.

BIBLIOGRAPHY

Ashwell JD, Weissman AM: T-cell antigen receptor genes, gene products, and coreceptors. In Rich RR et al, editors: *Clinical immunology principles and practice,* St Louis, 1996, Mosby.

Cambier JC, Pleiman CM, Clark MR: Signal transduction by the B-cell antigen receptor and its coreceptors, *Annu Rev Immunol* 12:457, 1994.

Germain RN: MHC-dependent antigen processing and peptide presentation: providing ligands for T lymphocyte activation, *Cell* 76:287, 1994.

Gumperz JE, Parham P: The enigma of the natural killer cell, *Nature* 378:245, 1995.

Janeway CA Jr: The immune system evolved to discriminate infectious nonself from noninfectious self, *Immunol Today* 13:11, 1992.

Janeway CA Jr, Bottomly K: Signals and signs for lymphocyte responses, *Cell* 76:275, 1994.

Marrack P, Kappler J: Subversion of the immune system by pathogens, *Cell* 76:323, 1994.

Mond JJ et al: T-cell independent antigens, *Curr Opinion Immunol* 7:349, 1995.

Paul WE, Seder RA: Lymphocyte responses and cytokines, *Cell* 76:241, 1994.

Potter KN, Capra JD: Immunoglobulin genes and proteins. In Rich RR et al, editors: *Clinical immunology principles and practice,* St Louis, 1996, Mosby.

Reda KB, Rich RR: Superantigens. In Rich RR et al, editors: *Clinical immunology prin-ciples and practice,* St Louis, 1996, Mosby.

Roche PA: HLA-DM: an in vivo facilitator of MHC class II peptide loading, *Immunity* 3:259, 1995.

Siegel JN, June CH: Signal transduction and T lymphocyte activation. In Rich RR et al, editors: *Clinical immunology principles and practice,* St Louis, 1996, Mosby.

Theofilopoulos AN: The basis of autoimmunity, *Immunol Today* 16:90, 1995.

CHAPTER

172 Human Leukocyte Antigen Complex

Benjamin D. Schwartz

The human leukocyte antigen (HLA) complex is the major histocompatibility complex of humans. It was originally discovered as a result of the analysis of reactions of antibodies found in the sera of multiply transfused patients and multiparous women. Subsequently the complex became the object of study because of its roles in the rejection of tissue and organ transplants and in predisposition to certain diseases. The molecules determined by the HLA complex are now known to be critical to the regulation of several aspects of the immune response.

HLA GENETICS

The HLA complex is located on the short arm of chromosome 6 and contains multiple loci that determine several different types of molecules. The HLA-A, HLA-B, and HLA-C genes determine the classical class I, or class I-a histocompatibility molecules, and the HLA-E, HLA-F, and HLA-G genes determine the nonclassical class I, or class I-b molecules; all are located within the class I region. The HLA-DR, HLA-DQ, and HLA-DP genes determine the respective class II molecules, and are found within the class II region. In addition, the HLA-DM class II genes, the transporter associated with antigen processing (TAP)-1 and TAP-2 genes and the large multifunctional protease (LMP)-2 and LMP-7 genes, all of which determine proteins that are involved in antigen processing, are located within the class II region. Finally, the BF, C2, C4A, and C4B genes, which determine the second, fourth, and factor B components of the complement system; the 21-hydroxylase genes determining 21-hydroxylase; the heat shock protein (HSP)-70 genes; and the tumor necrosis factor (TNF)-A and TNF-B genes determining TNF-α and TNF-β are found within the class III region. The relative location of these loci within the HLA complex is shown in Fig. 172-1.

The HLA complex is one of the most polymorphic genetic complexes known. Multiple alleles (alternative forms of a gene) at each locus have been identified in population studies. For example, 149 distinct alleles are present at the HLA-B locus. A complete listing of the currently recognized class I and class II alleles and the antigenic determinants they encode is given in Tables 172-1 to 172-4. Each allele is designated by the letter of the locus at which it is found and a four-digit number, for example, HLA-B*2701. The first two digits in

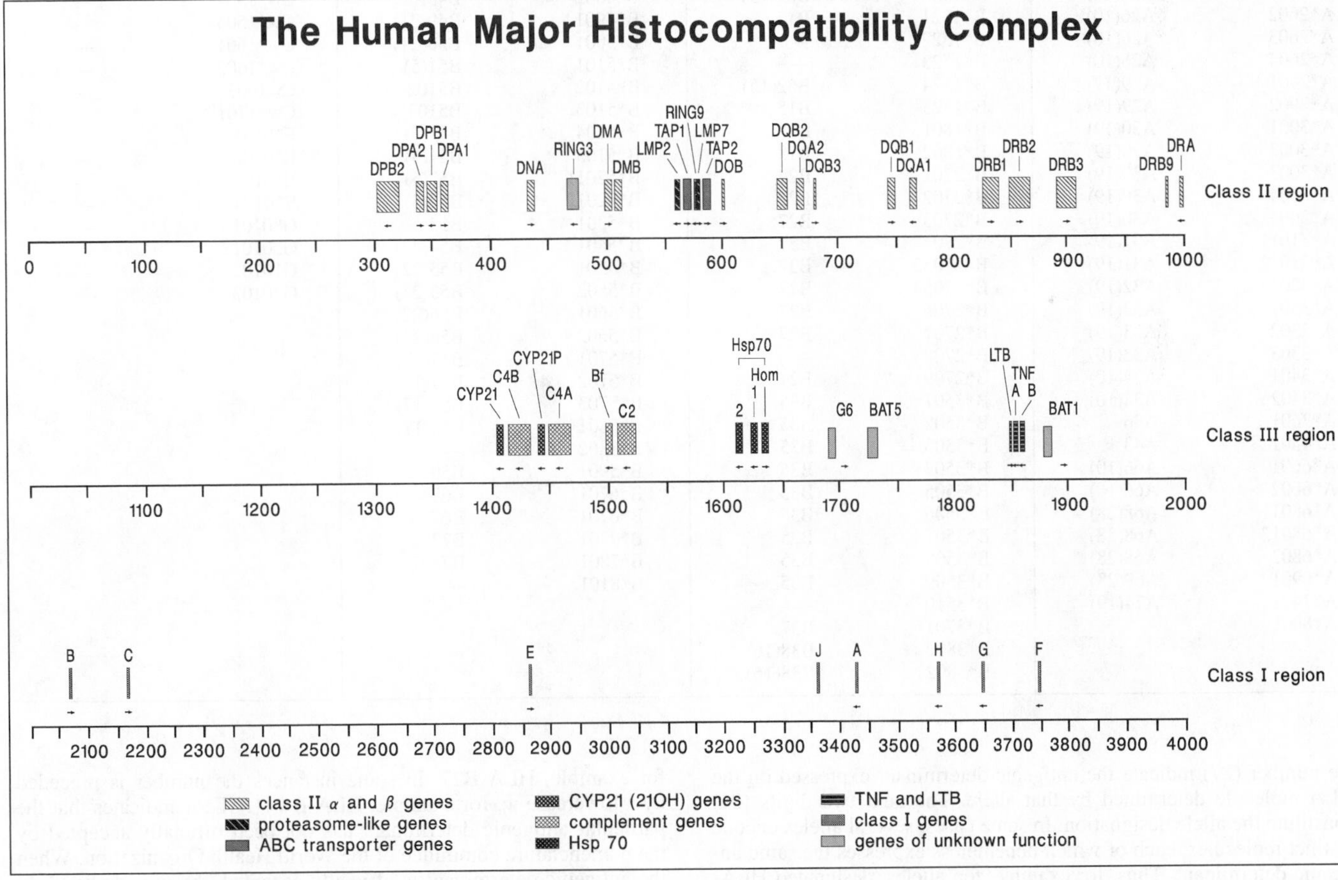

The Human Major Histocompatibility Complex

FIGURE 172-1 HLA complex. The entire HLA complex spans approximately 4000 kilobases, and is divided into three regions, termed (in order from the centromere) *class II, class III,* and *class I.* Each of the regions was named for the class of HLA molecules that was first mapped to it. The types of loci are shown by different shadings.

Modified from Campbell RD, Trowsdale J: *Immunol Today* 14:349, 1993.

Table 172-1   Recognized HLA class I alleles and their related antigens.

HLA ALLELE	HLA ANTIGEN	HLA ALLELE	HLA ANTIGEN	HLA ALLELE	HLA ANTIGEN	HLA ALLELE	HLA ANTIGEN
A*0101	A1	B*0702	B7	B*39011	B3901	Cw*0101	Cw1
A*0102	A1	B*0703	B703	B*39013	B3901	Cw*0102	Cw1
A*0201	A2	B*0704	B7	B*39021	B3902	Cw*0201	Cw2
A*0202	A2	B*0705	B7	B*39022	B3902	Cw*02021	Cw2
A*0203	A203	B*0801	B8	B*3903	B39(16)	Cw*02022	Cw2
A*0204	A2	B*0802	B8	B*3904	B39(16)	Cw*0302	Cw3
A*0205	A2	B*1301	B13	B*3905	—	Cw*0303	Cw3
A*0206	A2	B*1302	B13	B*39061	B39(16)	Cw*0304	Cw3
A*0207	A2	B*1303	—	B*39062	B39(16)	Cw*0401	Cw4
A*0208	A2	B*1401	B64(14)	B*3907	—	Cw*0402	Cw4
A*0209	A2	B*1402	B65(14)	B*40011	B60(40)	Cw*0501	Cw5
A*0210	A210	B*1501	B62(15)	B*40012	B60(40)	Cw*0602	Cw6
A*0211	A2	B*1502	B75(15)	B*4002	B60(40)	Cw*0701	Cw7
A*0212	A2	B*1503	B72(70)	B*4003	B40	Cw*0702	Cw7
A*0213	A2	B*1504	B62(15)	B*4004	B40	Cw*0703	Cw7
A*0214	A2	B*1505	B62(15)	B*4005	B4005	Cw*0704	Cw7
A*0215N	—	B*1506	B62(15)	B*4006	B61(40)	Cw*0801	Cw8
A*0216	A2	B*1507	B62(15)	B*4007	—	Cw*0802	Cw8
A*0217	A2	B*1508	B62(15)	B*4101	B41	Cw*0803	Cw8
A*0301	A3	B*1509	B70	B*4102	B41	Cw*1201	—
A*0302	A3	B*1510	B71(70)	B*4201	B42	Cw*12021	—
A*1101	A11	B*1511	B15	B*4402	B44(12)	Cw*12022	—
A*1102	A11	B*1512	B76(15)	B*4403	B44(12)	Cw*1203	—
A*2301	A23(9)	B*1513	B77(15)	B*4404	B44(12)	Cw*1301	—
A*2401	A24(9)	B*1514	B76(15)	B*4405	B44(12)	Cw*1401	—
A*2402	A24(9)	B*1515	B62(15)	B*4406	B44(12)	Cw*1402	—
A*2403	A2403	B*1516	B63(15)	B*4501	B45(12)	Cw*1403	—
A*2404	A24(9)	B*1517	B63(15)	B*4601	B46	Cw*1501	—
A*2406	A24(9)	B*1518	—	B*4701	B47	Cw*1502	—
A*2501	A25(10)	B*1519	B76(15)	B*4801	B48	Cw*1503	—
A*2601	A26(10)	B*1520	B62(15)	B*4802	B48	Cw*1504	—
A*2602	A26(10)	B*1521	B15	B*4901	B49(21)	Cw*1505	—
A*2603	A26(10)	B*1522	—	B*5001	B50(21)	Cw*1601	—
A*2604	A26(10)	B*1523	—	B*5101	B51(5)	Cw*1602	—
A*2901	A29(19)	B*1524	B62(15)	B*5102	B5102	Cw1603	—
A*2902	A29(19)	B*1525	B15	B*5103	B5103	Cw*1701	—
A*3001	A30(19)	B*1801	B18	B*5104	B51(5)	E*0101	—
A*3002	A30(19)	B*1802	B18	B*5105	B51(5)	E*0102	—
A*3003	A30(19)	B*2701	B27	B*52011	B52(5)	E*0103	—
A*3004	A30(19)	B*2702	B27	B*52012	B52(5)	E*0104	—
A*3005	A30(19)	B*2703	B27	B*5301	B53	G*01011	—
A*31011	A31(19)	B*2704	B27	B*5401	B54(22)	G*01012	—
A*31012	A31(19)	B*27052	B27	B*5501	B55(22)	G*0102	—
A*3201	A32(19)	B*27053	B27	B*5502	B55(22)	G*0103	—
A*3301	A33(19)	B*2706	B27	B*5601	B56(22)		
A*3302	A33(19)	B*2707	B27	B*5602	B56(22)		
A*3303	A33(19)	B*2708	—	B*5701	B57(17)		
A*3401	A34(10)	B*2709	B27	B*5702	B57(17)		
A*3402	A34(10)	B*3501	B35	B*5703	B57(17)		
A*3601	A36	B*3502	B35	B*5801	B58(17)		
A*4301	A43	B*3503	B35	B*5802	—		
A*6601	A66(10)	B*3504	B35	B*5901	B59		
A*6602	A66(10)	B*3505	B35	B*67011	B67		
A*68011	A68(28)	B*3506	B35	B*67013	B67		
A*68012	A68(28)	B*3507	B35	B*7301	B73		
A*6802	A68(28)	B*3508	B35	B*7801	B7801		
A*6901	A69(28)	B*3509	B35	B*8101	—		
A*7401	A74(19)	B*3510	—				
A*8001	—	B*3701	B37				
		B*3802	B38(16)				
		B*3802	B38(16)				

the number (27) indicate the antigenic determinant expressed on the HLA molecule determined by that allele. The next two digits (01) constitute the allele designation. In some cases, several alleles encode distinct molecules, each of which nonetheless expresses the same antigenic determinant. Thus, for example, ten alleles, designated HLA-B*2701 through HLA-B*2709, determine distinct HLA molecules, all of which express the HLA-B27 antigenic determinant. (HLA-B*27052 and HLA-B*27053 differ by one codon change, which is silent, i.e., the two different codons specify the same amino acid.)

The antigenic determinants on the HLA molecules are recognized by antibodies and are designated by the locus letter and a number,

for example, HLA-B27. In some instances the number is preceded by a lowercase *w;* for example, HLA-Bw41. The *w* indicates that the particular antigenic determinant has not been officially accepted by the nomenclature committee of the World Health Organization. When the antigenic determinant is officially accepted, the *w* is dropped. In other instances the number is followed by a second number in parentheses, for example, HLA-A25(10). This designation indicates that the antigenic determinant given by the first number is a "split" of the antigenic determinant designated in parentheses. In our example, HLA-A10 was originally thought to be a single antigenic entity, but subsequent analysis indicated that HLA-A10 is a determinant present

Table 172-2 Designations of HLA-DR alleles

HLA ALLELE	HLA-DR SEROLOGIC ANTIGEN	HLA D–ASSOCIATED (T CELL–DEFINED) ANTIGEN	HLA ALLELE	HLA-DR SEROLOGIC ANTIGEN	HLA D–ASSOCIATED (T CELL–DEFINED) ANTIGEN	HLA ALLELE	HLA-DR SEROLOGIC ANTIGEN	HLA D–ASSOCIATED (T CELL–DEFINED) ANTIGEN
DRA*0101	—	—	DRB1*1112	—	—	DRB1*0808	DR8	—
DRA*0102	—	—	DRB1*1113	DR11(15)	—	DRB1*0809	DR8	—
DRB1*0101	DR1	Dw1	DRB1*1114	—	—	DRB1*0810	DR8	—
DRB1*0102	DR1	Dw20	DRB1*1115	DR11(15)	—	DRB1*0811	DR8	—
DRB1*0103	DR103	Dw'BON'	DRB1*1116	—	—	DRB1*09011	DR9	Dw23
DRB1*0104	DR1	—	DRB1*1117	—	—	DRB1*09012	DR9	Dw23
DRB1*1501	DR15(2)	Dw2	DRB1*1118	—	—	DRB1*1001	DR10	—
DRB1*15021	DR15(2)	Dw12	DRB1*1119	—	—	DRB3*0101	DR52	Dw24
DRB1*15022	DR15(2)	Dw12	DRB1*1201	DR12(5)	Dw'DB6'	DRB3*0201	DR52	Dw25
DRB1*1503	DR15(2)	—	DRB1*12021	DR12(5)	—	DRB3*0202	DR52	Dw25
DRB1*1504	DR15(2)	—	DRB1*12022	DR12(5)	—	DRB3*0301	DR52	Dw26
DRB1*1601	DR16(2)	Dw21	DRB1*12031	DR12(5)	—	DRB4*01	DR53	Dw4, Dw10, Dw13,
DRB1*1602	DR16(2)	Dw22	DRB1*12032	DR12(15)	—			Dw14, Dw15,
DRB1*1603	—	—	DRB1*1301	DR13(6)	Dw18			Dw17, Dw23
DRB1*1604	DR16(2)	—	DRB1*1302	DR13(6)	Dw19	DRB4*01011	DR53	Dw17
DRB1*1605	—	—	DRB1*1303	DR13(6)	Dw'HAG'	DRB4*01012N	—	Dw11
DRB1*1606	DR2	—	DRB1*1304	DR13(6)	—	DRB4*0102	DR53	—
DRB1*03011	DR17(3)	Dw3	DRB1*1305	DR13(6)	—	DRB4*0103	DR53	Dw4
DRB1*03012	DR17(3)	Dw3	DRB1*1306	DR13(6)	—	DRB5*0101	DR51	Dw2
DRB1*0302	DR18(3)	Dw'RSH'	DRB1*1307	—	—	DRB5*0102	DR51	Dw12
DRB1*0303	DR18(3)	—	DRB1*1308	DR13(6)	—	DRB5*0201	DR51	Dw21
DRB1*0304	DR3	—	DRB1*1309	—	—	DRB5*0202	DR51	Dw22
DRB1*0305	DR3	—	DRB1*1310	DR13(6)	—	DRB5*0203	DR51	—
DRB1*0401	DR4	Dw4	DRB1*1311	DR13(6)	—	DRB6*0101	—	—
DRB1*0402	DR4	Dw10	DRB1*1312	—	—	DRB6*0201	—	—
DRB1*0403	DR4	Dw13	DRB1*1314	DR13(6)	—	DRB6*0202	—	—
DRB1*0404	DR4	Dw14	DRB1*1315	—	—	DRB7*01011	—	—
DRB1*0405	DR4	Dw15	DRB1*1316	—	—	DRB7*01012	—	—
DRB1*0406	DR4	Dw'KT2'	DRB1*1317	—	—			
DRB1*0407	DR4	Dw13	DRB1*1318	—	—			
DRB1*0408	DR4	Dw14	DRB1*1319	—	—			
DRB1*0409	DR4	—	DRB1*1401	DR14(6)	Dw9			
DRB1*0410	DR4	—	DRB1*1402	DR14(6)	Dw16			
DRB1*0411	DR4	—	DRB1*1403	DR1403	—			
DRB1*0412	DR4	—	DRB1*1404	DR1404	—			
DRB1*0413	DR4	—	DRB1*1405	DR14(6)	—			
DRB1*0414	DR4	—	DRB1*1406	DR14(6)	—			
DRB1*0415	DR4	—	DRB1*1407	DR14(6)	—			
DRB1*0416	DR4	—	DRB1*1408	DR14(6)	—			
DRB1*0417	DR4	—	DRB1*1409	DR14(6)	—			
DRB1*0418	DR4	—	DRB1*1410	—	—			
DRB1*0419	DR4	—	DRB1*1411	—	—			
DRB1*0420	DR4	—	DRB1*1412	—	—			
DRB1*0421	DR4	—	DRB1*1413	—	—			
DRB1*0422	DR4	—	DRB1*1414	—	—			
DRB1*11011	DR11(5)	Dw5	DRB1*1415	—	—			
DRB1*11012	DR11(5)	Dw5	DRB1*1416	—	—			
DRB1*1102	DR11(5)	Dw'JVM'	DRB1*1417	—	—			
DRB1*1103	DR11(5)	—	DRB1*1418	—	—			
DRB1*11041	DR11(5)	Dw'FS'	DRB1*0701	DR7	Dw17, Dw'DB1'			
DRB1*11042	DR11(5)	—	DRB1*0801	DR8	Dw8.1			
DRB1*1105	DR11(5)	—	DRB1*08021	DR8	Dw8.2			
DRB1*1106	DR11(5)	—	DRB1*08022	DR8	Dw8.2			
DRB1*1107	—	—	DRB1*08031	DR8	Dw8.3			
DRB1*11081	DR11(5)	—	DRB1*08032	DR8	Dw8.3			
DRB1*11082	DR11(5)	—	DRB1*08041	DR8	—			
DRB1*1109	DR11(5)	—	DRB1*08042	DR8	—			
DRB1*1110	—	—	DRB1*0805	DR8	—			
DRB1*1111	—	—	DRB1*0806	DR8	—			
			DRB1*0807	DR8	—			

on two distinct molecules, which bear the distinct antigenic determinants HLA-A25 and HLA-A26. Thus HLA-A25 and HLA-A26 are said to be splits of HLA-A10.

Because of the presumed extensive interbreeding that has occurred throughout the existence of the human species, the chance of finding a particular allele at one locus together with a particular allele at a second locus should be the product of the frequencies of each of the alleles in a given population. However, particular combinations of alleles are found with an observed frequency greater than expected. This phenomenon, termed *linkage disequilibrium,* has been attributed both

to a selective advantage of a particular combination of alleles and to the admixture of inbred populations. However, both these hypotheses remain speculative.

The combination of alleles at each locus on a given chromosome is termed the *haplotype.* Thus each individual inherits one haplotype from the mother and one from the father. Haplotypes are inherited in a simple mendelian fashion. Two siblings from the same parents have a 25% chance of being HLA identical, a 50% chance of being HLA haplo-identical (i.e., sharing one haplotype), and a 25% chance of being totally HLA nonidentical. HLA molecules are expressed codomi-

Table 172-3   Designations of HLA-DQ alleles

HLA ALLELE	HLA-DQ SEROLOGIC ANTIGEN	HLA D–ASSOCIATED (T CELL–DEFINED) ANTIGEN
DQA1*0101	—	Dw1
DQA1*01021	—	Dw2, w21, w19
DQA1*01022	—	Dw21
DQA1*0103	—	Dw18, w12, w8, Dw'FS'
DQA1*0104	—	Dw9
DQA1*0201	—	Dw7, w11
DQA1*03011	—	Dw4, w10, w13, w14, w15
DQA1*0302	—	Dw23
DQA1*0401	—	Dw8, DW'RSH'
DQA1*0501	—	Dw3, w5, w22
DQA1*05011	—	Dw3
DQA1*05012	—	Dw5
DQA1*05013	—	Dw22
DQA1*0502	—	—
DQA1*0601	—	Dw8
DQB1*0501	DQ5(1)	Dw1
DQB1*0502	DQ5(1)	Dw21
DQB1*05031	DQ5(1)	Dw9
DQB1*05032	DQ5(1)	Dw9
DQB1*0504	—	—
DQB1*06011	DQ6(1)	Dw12, w8
DQB1*06012	DQ6(1)	Dw12, w8
DQB1*0602	DQ6(1)	Dw2
DQB1*0603	DQ6(1)	Dw18, Dw'FS'
DQB1*0604	DQ6(1)	Dw19
DQB1*06051	DQ6(1)	Dw19
DQB1*06052	DQ6(1)	Dw19
DQB1*0606	—	—
DQB1*0607	—	—
DQB1*0608	—	—
DQB1*0609	—	—
DQB1*0201	DQ2	Dw3
DQB1*0202	DQ2	Dw7
DQB1*0301	DQ7(3)	Dw4, w5, w8, w13
DQB1*0302	DQ8(3)	Dw4, w10, w13, w14
DQB1*03032	DQ9(3)	Dw23, w11
DQB1*0304	DQ7(3)	—
DQB1*0305	—	—
DQB1*0401	DQ4	Dw15
DQB1*0402	DQ4	Dw8, Dw'RSH'

Table 172-4   Designations of HLA-DP alleles

HLA ALLELE	ASSOCIATED HLA-DP ANTIGEN	HLA ALLELE	ASSOCIATED HLA-DP ANTIGEN
DPA1*0103	—	DPB1*3001	—
DPA1*0104	—	DPB1*3101	—
DPA1*02011	—	DPB1*3201	—
DPA1*02012	—	DPB1*3301	—
DPA1*02021	—	DPB1*3401	—
DPA1*02022	—	DPB1*3501	—
DPA1*0301	—	DPB1*3601	—
DPA1*0401	—	DPB1*3701	—
DPB1*01011	DPw1	DPB1*3801	—
DPB1*01012	DPw1	DPB1*3901	—
DPB1*0201	DPw2	DPB1*4001	—
DPB1*02011	DPw2	DPB1*4101	—
DPB1*02012	DPw2	DPB1*4401	—
DPB1*0202	DPw2	DPB1*4501	—
DPB1*0301	DPw3	DPB1*4601	—
DPB1*0401	DPw4	DPB1*4701	—
DPB1*0402	DPw4	DPB1*4801	—
DPB1*0501	DPw5	DPB1*4901	—
DPB1*0601	DPw6	DPB1*5001	—
DPB1*0801	—	DPB1*5101	—
DPB1*0901	—	DPB1*5201	—
DPB1*1001	—	DPB1*5301	—
DPB1*11011	—	DPB1*5401	—
DPB1*11012	—	DPB1*5501	—
DPB1*1301	—	DPB1*5601	—
DPB1*1401	—	DPB1*5801	
DPB1*1501	—		
DPB1*1601	—		
DPB1*1701	—		
DPB1*1801	—		
DPB1*1901	—		
DPB1*20011	—		
DPB1*20012	—		
DPB1*2101	—		
DPB1*2201	—		
DPB1*2301	—		
DPB1*2401	—		
DPB1*2501	—		
DPB1*26011	—		
DPB1*26012	—		
DPB1*2701	—		
DPB1*2801	—		
DPB1*2901	—		

nantly; that is, the HLA molecules determined by both maternal and paternal haplotypes are expressed in each individual. For example, each individual expresses two HLA-A molecules, one determined by each haplotype.

TISSUE DISTRIBUTION, STRUCTURE, AND FUNCTION
HLA Class I Molecules

Classical HLA class I-a molecules are widely expressed on tissues, though the level of expression varies by the particular class I-a molecule and the tissue. For example, HLA-C molecules are expressed at approximately 10% of the level of HLA-A and HLA-B molecules, and little if any class I-a expression occurs on neurons of the central nervous system. The wide tissue distribution subserves the physiologic role of the classical class I-a molecules. For a cell infected with virus to be killed by a cytotoxic $CD8^+$ T-cell, the T-cell must recognize a processed viral antigenic peptide in conjunction with a class I molecule. This phenomenon is known as *HLA restriction of T-cell recognition* and is thought to be important in the distinction of nonself from self. A given T-cell, specific for a given viral antigenic peptide, can recognize this peptide only when the peptide is associated with a particular class I molecule. It cannot recognize this viral antigenic peptide associated with a different class I molecule, it cannot recognize a different antigenic peptide associated with the same class I molecule, and it cannot recognize the class I molecule by itself.

This restriction phenomenon can perhaps best be appreciated through an understanding of the structure of the class I molecule (Fig. 172-2). The class I molecule consists of a 44,000 dalton glycoprotein chain designated the heavy chain, or α-chain, determined by an HLA class I allele, in noncovalent association with the 12,000-dalton β_2 microglobulin (β_2m) determined by a nonpolymorphic gene on chromosome 15. The HLA class I heavy chain consists of several domains. Three extracellular domains exist, designated α_1, α_2, and α_3, each consisting of approximately 90 amino acids, a transmembrane domain, and an intracytoplasmic domain. β_2m and the α_3 domain of the heavy chain have structural homology to the constant regions of the immunoglobulin (Ig) molecule, making the class I molecule a member of the Ig supergene family, and are essentially nonpolymorphic. In contrast, the α_1- and α_2-domains contain most of the polymorphism of the HLA molecule. X-ray crystallographic analysis of the structure of the class I molecule (see Fig. 172-2) indicates that the α_3-domain and β_2m form a base that supports an interactive structure formed by the α_1- and α_2-domains. This structure is composed of a platform consisting of a β-pleated sheet (formed by eight β-strands), on which rest two α-helices that form a cleft into which a foreign (viral) antigenic peptide can fit. (The α-helix should not be confused with the α-chain or α_1- or α_2-domains, and the β sheet and the β strands should not be confused with β_2m.) These two α-helices and the foreign antigenic peptide make up the ligand that is recognized by the T-cell receptor on the $CD8^+$ T-cells.

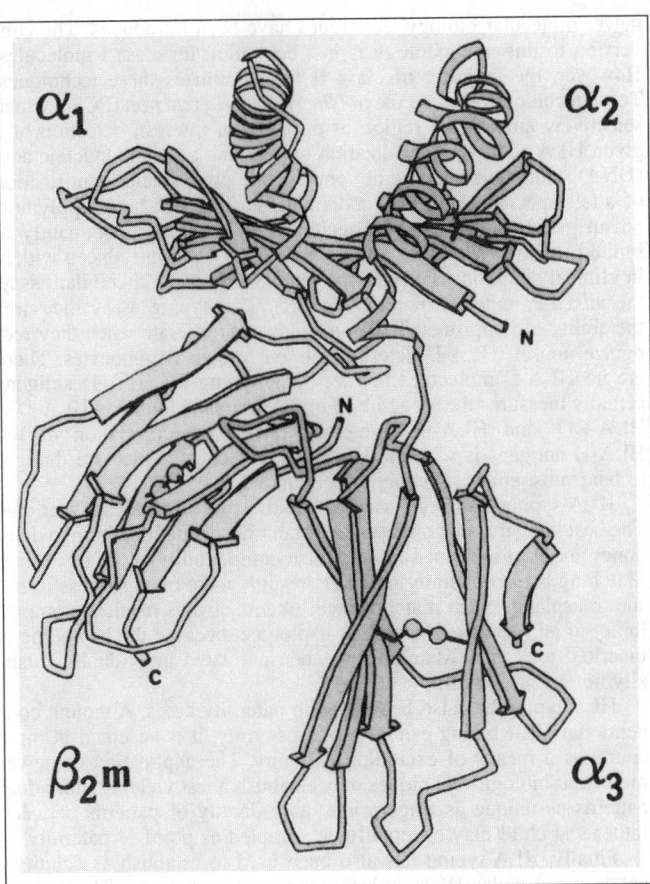

FIGURE 172-2 Crystal structure of an HLA class I molecule. The extracellular portion of the molecule is depicted in side view, with the distal end on top and the proximal end at the bottom. The transmembrane and intracytoplasmic domains are not shown. The α_1-, α_2-, and α_3-domains are labeled, as is the β_2-microglobulin *(β_2m)*. β_2m and the α_3-domain form a base supporting the interactive structure formed by the α_1- and α_2-domains. This interactive structure consists of a platform of a β-pleated sheet supporting two α-helices that form a cleft that binds foreign antigenic fragments. *N*, Amino terminus; *C*, carboxy terminus.
From *Nature* 329:506, 1987.

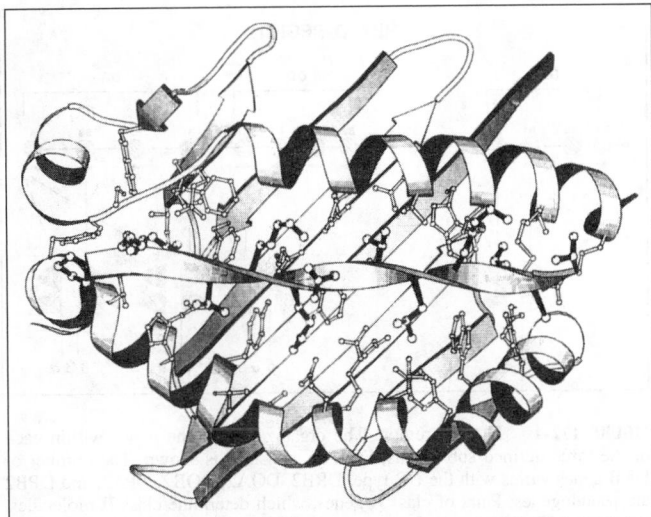

FIGURE 172-3 Crystal structure of an HLA class II molecule. The molecule is depicted in the top view, as a T-cell receptor might view it. The α_1- and β_1-domains are seen from above, looking down into the groove. The α-helices and a portion of the β-pleated sheet from the groove in which the peptide, shown as a twisted ribbon, binds.
From *Nature* 368:215, 1994.

HLA Class II Molecules

Recent evidence suggests that HLA-C and HLA-B molecules are also recognized by receptors on NK cells, and that this recognition event generates a negative signal that inhibits NK cell–mediated cytotoxicity. Of note, HLA-C molecules have recently been found on first trimester human placenta, suggesting a way by which maternal NK cells might recognize the implanting placenta.

The nonclassical HLA class I-b molecules have structural features similar to that of class I-a molecules but have limited polymorphism and a different tissue distribution and function. HLA-G molecules are present on the trophoblast during pregnancy and have been postulated to play a role in maternal-fetal interactions. In addition, recent data suggest that HLA-G molecules may be on the brain, thymus, testis, skin, and fetal liver. Other recent findings indicate that other class I-b molecules can bind *N*-formylated peptides, suggesting that these molecules may be involved in host defenses against prokaryotes.

In contrast to the class I molecules, the class II molecules have a restricted tissue distribution. They are found predominantly on immunocompetent cells, including B-lymphocytes, activated T-lymphocytes, and antigen-presenting cells (macrophages and dendritic cells). In addition, class II molecules can be induced on cells that do not normally express them. It has been speculated that this anomalous expression may contribute to the predisposition to certain autoimmune diseases (see later discussion). Foreign antigenic peptide is thought to be recognized in association with class II molecules by CD4$^+$ (predominantly helper) T-lymphocytes, just as it is recognized in association with class I molecules by CD8$^+$ cytotoxic T-cells.

HLA class II molecules are composed of two glycoprotein transmembrane chains, both encoded by the HLA complex (Fig. 172-3). The α-chain is approximately 34,000 daltons, and the β-chain is approximately 29,000 daltons. Each of these chains contains two extracellular domains, designated α_1 and α_2 or β_1 and β_2, respectively, a transmembrane domain, and an intracytoplasmic domain. The α_2- and β_2-domains have homology to the constant region domains of Ig, indicating class II molecules are also members of the Ig supergene family. Crystallographic analysis of the HLA-DR1 molecule indicates that the structure is very similar to that of the class I molecule. Thus the α_2- and β_2-domains are closest to the cell membrane and form a base for the interactive structure formed by the α_1- and β_1-domains. The α_1- and particularly the β_1-domains are responsible for the most polymorphism seen within the class II system. These two domains make up a structure that also consists of a platform of a β-pleated sheet, on which rest two α helices, forming a cleft for foreign antigenic peptide.

Other HLA Molecules Involved in Antigen Processing

There are two pathways by which the immune system processes respectively predominantly extracellular antigens, such as bacteria and soluble toxins, and predominantly intracellular antigens, such as viruses and other intracellular parasites (Chapter 171). Antigens derived from extracellular sources are processed through the *exogenous* pathway, and the processed peptides are recognized in conjunction with class II molecules. In contrast, antigens derived from intracellular sources are processed predominantly through the *endogenous* pathway, and the processed peptides are recognized in association with class I molecules. Proteins encoded within the HLA complex are involved in both pathways. HLA-DM molecules, which are class II–like, are found in the endosomal compartment where antigen processing of the exogenous pathway takes place, and facilitate the binding of antigenic peptides to HLA-DR, HLA-DQ, and HLA-DP molecules. The LMP-2 and LMP-7 proteins are two components of a cytoplasmic proteasome that processes proteins to peptides in the *endogenous* antigen processing pathway. The TAP-1 and TAP-2 proteins then transport these peptides into the endoplasmic reticulum, where

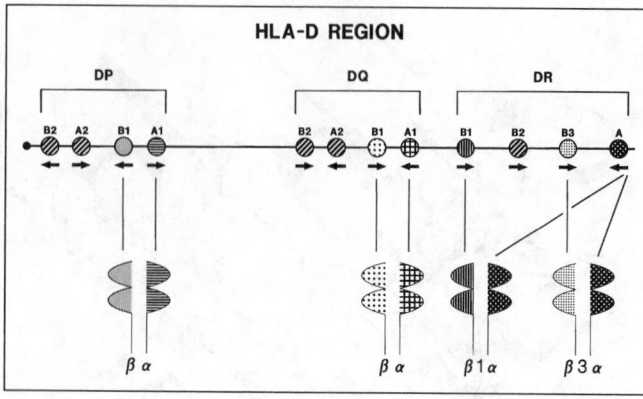

FIGURE 172-4   HLA-D region. The organization of the genes within each of the three defined subregions, DP, DQ, and DR, is shown. The number of DRB genes varies with the DR type. DRB2, DQA2, DQB2, DPA2, and DPB2 are pseudogenes. Pairs of class II genes, which determine class II molecules, are shown. The direction of transcription (5' to 3') is given below the genes.

the peptides can bind to and stabilize newly synthesized class I molecules.

HLA Class II Genes

As already indicated, three distinct sets of HLA class II molecules exist: DR, DQ, and DP. Although each consists of the αβ-chain structural unit just described, the organization and polymorphism of the genes determining this unit vary for each type of class II molecule (Fig. 172-4). The HLA-DR subregion contains one α-chain locus, designated DRA. The DRA gene is essentially nonpolymorphic. The DR subregion also usually contains three β-chain loci, designated DRB1, DRB2, and DRB3 (or DRB4 or DRB5). The DRB genes are highly polymorphic and encode the DRβ-chains, which are responsible for the different DR types. Alleles at the DRB1 locus encode the DRβ1 chains responsible for DR types DR1 through DR18. DRB2 is a pseudogene; that is, it is not expressed. The DRB3 gene encodes the DRβ3 chain bearing DR52, the DRB4 gene encodes the DRβ4 chain bearing DR53, and DRB5 alleles encode the DRβ5 chains bearing DR15 or DR16. DRB3, DRB4, and DRB5 appear to be mutually exclusive within a single haplotype. Both the DRβ1 chain and the DRβ3 (or DRβ4 or DRβ5) chains can combine with the DRα-chain to form a DRαβ-molecule. Thus in most haplotypes, there are two distinct DR molecules: DRαβ1 and DRαβ3 (or DRαβ4 or DRαβ5).

The HLA-DQ subregion contains two pairs of α-chain and β-chain genes. One pair, designated DQA2 and DQB2, is a pair of pseudogenes and is not expressed. The other pair, DQA1 and DQB1, encodes the DQα- and DQβ-chains. In contrast to the DR molecules, in which the α-chain shows no polymorphism, both the DQα- and DQβ-chains are polymorphic. This polymorphism may be important, in that the DQα-chain encoded by one chromosome can combine not only with the DQβ-chain encoded by the same chromosome, but also with the DQβ-chain encoded by the second chromosome. If this proves to be true, HLA heterozygotes may have DQ "hybrid" molecules that would be unique to the heterozygotes and not found in either parent. These hybrid molecules could conceivably be important in terms of predisposition to disease (see later discussion).

As with the DQ subregion, the DP subregion also contains two pairs of α-chain and β-chain genes. One pair, designated DPA2 and DPB2, is a set of pseudogenes; the expressed pair is designated DPA1 and DPB1. The DPα-chain displays limited polymorphism, whereas the DPβ-chain displays moderate polymorphism.

HLA TYPING

HLA typing has traditionally been done serologically, utilizing the microlymphocytotoxicity assay, which determines the HLA type by the ability of a given cell to be lysed by an antibody of known specificity. However, this assay does not allow delineation of all alleles, and

newer molecular biology techniques have been introduced. The conversion to this methodology is just beginning for class I molecules. However, the majority of class II typing utilizes these techniques. These techniques include the *polymerase chain reaction* (PCR), which selectively amplifies a region of the gene of interest; detection of a given HLA allele by hybridization of genomic deoxyribonucleic acid (DNA) with allele-specific oligonucleotide probes; and identification of allele-specific restriction endonuclease fragment length polymorphism patterns. These typing techniques are used predominantly in limited research situations and have recently been introduced widely in clinical situations. HLA-D antigens are typed by a cellular assay, the *mixed lymphocyte reaction* (MLR). This typing assay measures the ability of nonprimed T-lymphocytes to proliferate when they recognize nonself HLA-D determinants on foreign lymphocytes. There are no HLA-D molecules per se; MLR typing for HLA-D antigens actually measures the recognition of determinants found on HLA-DR, HLA-DQ, and HLA-DP molecules. The best correlation of the HLA-D antigens is with the HLA-DR molecules, which are thought to bear most epitopes recognized in an MLR.

HLA typing has been used in a variety of clinical applications. The best known is that of tissue or organ transplantation, during which donor and host are typed to maximize compatibility at the HLA loci. Matching between family members results in the most successful tissue transplants. Such matching will almost always result in compatibility at all loci of a given HLA haplotype, because the haplotype is inherited as a unit. Matching between unrelated individuals is usually not so successful.

HLA typing has also been used in paternity cases. Although conventional HLA typing cannot prove paternity, it is accepted in most courts as a means of excluding paternity. The application of newer molecular biologic techniques may establish a test yielding individual patterns as unique as fingerprints, and identity of patterns between father and child may eventually be accepted as proof of paternity.

Finally, HLA typing has also been used to establish associations between particular HLA antigens and certain diseases. These associations and their possible basis are described further in the following section.

HLA AND DISEASE

In 1973, HLA-B27 was found to be highly associated with ankylosing spondylitis. Among Caucasian patients with ankylosing spondylitis, 90% were found to possess HLA-B27, compared with only 8% of the normal Caucasian population. HLA disease associations within a population are quantified by an entity termed the *relative risk* (RR), which indicates the strength of the association. The higher the relative risk greater than 1, the greater is the association of the given HLA antigen with disease. A relative risk between 0 and 1 indicates a negative association between the given HLA and a disease and suggests the given HLA antigen may be protective. For ankylosing spondylitis the relative risk is approximately 80; that is, an individual who possesses HLA-B27 is 80 times more likely to develop ankylosing spondylitis than is an individual who lacks HLA-B27. However, the absence of HLA-B27 does not guarantee that an individual will not develop the disease, and the presence of HLA-B27 does not suggest that an individual will definitely contract the disease. In fact, the absolute risk of developing ankylosing spondylitis if an individual possesses HLA-B27 is only 4%; that is, of 100 individuals who possess HLA-B27, only four will develop clinically significant and apparent ankylosing spondylitis.

Only a few diseases are associated with HLA class I antigens; most HLA-associated diseases are associated with HLA class II antigens (Table 172-5). This association may well reflect the physiologic role of class II molecules in initiating the immune response by presenting processed antigenic peptide to helper CD4+ T-cells. Indeed, it has been proposed that anomalous expression of class II molecules on certain tissues, such as thyroid, pancreas, synovium, and others, may allow the presentation of otherwise nonimmunogenic tissue-specific antigens to helper T-cells, resulting in an autoimmune response. In this context it should be noted that most HLA-associated diseases do show some manifestation of autoimmunity.

Comparisons of the HLA-DQ molecules possessed by normal and insulin-dependent diabetic individuals have allowed specific correla-

Table 172-5   Selected HLA and disease associations in Caucasian patients

DISEASE	HLA ALLELE OR ANTIGEN	APPROXIMATE RLEATIVE RISK
Ankylosing spondylitis	B27	82
Reiter's syndrome	B27	41
Acute anterior uveitis	B27	8
Rheumatoid arthritis	DR4	6
Juvenile rheumatoid arthritis		
Seropositive	DR4	7.2
	DRB1*0401	25.8
	DRB1*0404	47
	DRB1*0401/DRB1*0404	116
Pauciarticular	DR5	3
Systemic lupus erythematosis	DR2	3.5
	DR3	2.7
	C4A*Q0	5.5
Behçet's disease	B51	3.3
Sjögren's syndrome	DR3	5.6
Graves' disease	DQA1*0102	9
Insulin-dependent diabetes mellitus	DQA1*0301-DQB*0302/ DQA1*0501-DQB*0201	35
	DQβAsp^{57}/DQβAsp^{57}	0.1
Celiac disease	DQA1*0501-DQB1*0201	40
Psoriasis vulgaris	B13	4.5
	B17	3.1
	Cw6	7.2
Pemphigus vulgaris	DR4	21
Dermatitis hepetiformis	DR3	18
Idiopathic hemachromatosis	A3	6.6
Goodpasture's syndrome	DR2	20
Multiple sclerosis	DQA1*0102-DQB1*0602- DRB1*1502	3
Narcolepsy	DR2	129
Tuberculoid leprosy	DRβ1Arg$^{13 \text{ or } 70\text{-}71}$	8.8

tions to be established for predisposition to insulin-dependent diabetes mellitus. It appears as if the presence of a non–aspartic acid residue at amino acid position number 57 of the DQβ-chain (as in DQ8) predisposes an individual to diabetes, whereas the presence of aspartic acid in this position protects an individual from this disease. For example, if both the HLA-DQβ-chains possessed by an individual have an aspartic acid at position 57, the individual is highly protected from insulin-dependent diabetes mellitus (RR, 0.1).

In certain diseases, it appears as if gene complementation between two different class II genes may play a role in disease predisposition. In insulin-dependent diabetes, for example, the DR3/DR4 (RR, 25) and more recently the DQA1*0301-DQB1*0302/DQA1*0501-DQB*201 (RR, 35) heterozygous states occur more frequently than any antigen or allele in the homozygous state. Similarly, the antibody response to Ro (SS-A) and La (SS-B) antigens in Sjögren's syndrome and systemic lupus erythematosus is highest in patients who are DQ1/DQ2 heterozygotes. The molecular basis for these phenomena has not yet been clearly delineated, but may involve "hybrid" DQ molecules formed by the α-chain encoded by one haplotype and the β-chain encoded by the opposite haplotype, which cannot occur in DQ homozygotes.

Proposed Mechanisms for HLA Disease Associations

Several hypotheses have been put forth to explain HLA disease associations. First, HLA molecules may serve as specific receptors for putative etiologic agents. If only a certain HLA antigen can act as such a receptor for an agent that causes a particular disease, the HLA disease association would be seen. The second hypothesis, designated the *molecular mimicry hypothesis,* suggests that a particular HLA antigen is immunologically similar to the etiologic agent that causes the disease and further suggests one of two alternatives. First, because of the similarity of the etiologic agent and the HLA antigen, the etio-

logic agent is not recognized as foreign, no immune response is elicited, and the disease caused by the etiologic agent proceeds without interference. The second alternative postulates that the etiologic agent is recognized as foreign, and a vigorous immune response is elicited. Because of the immunologic similarities between the etiologic agent and the HLA antigen, the HLA antigen becomes the target of the immune response, and an autoimmune disease is eventually manifest.

The third hypothesis states that the actual disease-susceptibility genes are not the HLA genes per se, but rather the T-cell receptor α-chain and β-chain genes. This hypothesis holds that a particular T-cell receptor α-chain and β-chain combination that predisposes to disease can only recognize a particular HLA antigen, or a processed foreign antigenic peptide in association with that particular HLA antigen. Because of this constraint on T-cell receptor recognition, an apparent association with the HLA antigen is observed. The fourth hypothesis is based on the physiologic role of the class I and class II molecules in presenting foreign antigenic peptides to cytotoxic and helper T-cells, respectively. This hypothesis holds that only certain class I and class II molecules can bind and present particular processed antigenic peptides. Depending on the pathogenesis of disease, the ability or inability of a given HLA molecule to bind and present a particular antigenic peptide may either predispose to or protect from disease.

Other mechanisms besides these have also been postulated. It should be noted that different mechanisms may apply in the predisposition to different diseases and that more than one mechanism may operate concurrently to predispose to a given disease.

As our understanding of the structure and function of the HLA complex increases, the role of the HLA molecules in predisposing to disease will become elucidated and eventually may allow therapeutic intervention.

BIBLIOGRAPHY

Bjorkman PJ et al: Structure of the human class I histocompatibility antigen HLA-A2, *Nature* 329:506, 1987.

Bodmer JG et al: Nomenclature for factors of the HLA system, *Hum Immunol* 43:149, 1995.

Bottino C et al: Receptors for HLA class I molecules in human NK cells, *Semin Immunol* 7:67, 1995.

Campbell RD, Trowsdale J: Map of the human MHC, *Immunol Today* 14:349, 1993.

Heimberg H et al: Complementation of HLA-DQA and DQB genes confers susceptibility and protection to insulin-dependent diabetes mellitus, *Hum Immunol* 33:10, 1992.

King A et al: Evidence for the expression of HLA-C class I mRNA and protein by human first trimester trophoblasts, *J Immunol* 156:2068, 1996.

Le Bouteiller P: HLA class I chromosomal region, genes, and products: facts and questions, *Crit Rev Immunol* 14:89, 1994.

Nepom GT: Class II antigens and disease susceptibility, *Ann Rev Med* 46:17, 1995.

Parham P, Ohta T: Population biology of antigen presentation by MHC class I molecules, *Science* 272:67, 1996.

Roche PA: HLA-DM: an in vivo facilitator of MHC class II peptide loading, *Immunity* 3:259, 1995.

Schwartz BD: Infectious agents, immunity, and rheumatic diseases, *Arthritis Rheum* 33:457, 1990.

Stern LJ et al: Crystal structure of the human class II MHC protein HLA-DR1 complexed with an influenza virus peptide, *Nature* 368:215, 1994.

Tiwari JL, Terasaki PI, editors: *HLA and disease associations,* New York, 1985, Springer-Verlag.

CHAPTER

173 Antibodies: Structure and Genetics

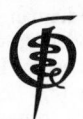

Roger M. Perlmutter

The antibodies constitute an extremely diverse set of closely related serum glycoproteins (immunoglobulins) that mediate humoral immunity. During the past decade, advances in molecular biology have provided a detailed description of mechanisms that permit the somatic generation of more than 10^8 chemically distinct antibody molecules from a germline repertoire of fewer than 1000 genetic elements. Defects in this diversification process result in heightened susceptibility to infection and may also predispose to autoimmune disease.

STRUCTURE OF ANTIBODIES

Antibodies are polymeric molecules composed of paired disulfide-bonded heavy and light polypeptide chains in the general form $[(HL)_2]_n$. A typical serum antibody (immunoglobulin G, or IgG) consists of two identical heavy and two identical light chains (Fig. 173-1). The heavy and light chains are composed of a series of Ig domains, or *homology units,* each of which is about 110 amino acids in length and contains a centrally placed intrachain disulfide bond. The light chain contains two such domains, an amino-terminal variable domain (V_L) that participates in antigen binding and a carboxy-terminal constant domain (C_L) that assists in interactions with the heavy chain. Similarly, each heavy chain contains an amino-terminal variable domain (V_H) joined by a "hinge" region to a series of three constant domains designated C_H1, C_H2, and C_H3 (see Fig. 173-1). The hinge region can be cleaved by enzymatic digestion to yield two antigen-binding, or *Fab,* fragments, containing the V_L and C_L domains of the light chain and the V_H and C_H1 domains of the heavy chain, and a third fragment, the *Fc* fragment, containing the remaining heavy-chain constant domains. Although all antigen-binding activity resides in the Fab fragments, the Fc fragment mediates important effector functions of antibody molecules, such as complement fixation and mast cell sensitization. Moreover, these functions can be localized to specific domains; for example, the C_H3 domain is principally responsible for binding to Fc receptors on macrophages and monocytes, and the C_H2 domain interacts with the C1q component of complement. Thus Ig domains are the structural and functional (and genetic) subunits of antibody molecules. Binding of antigen near the amino terminus of an antibody can alter the properties of the carboxy-terminal effector region, thus transducing a recognition signal.

In humans, as in all mammalian species, five classes of immunoglobulins exist: IgA, IgD, IgE, IgG, and IgM. There are also two subclasses of IgA (IgA1, IgA2) and four subclasses of IgG (IgG1, IgG2, IgG3, IgG4). These distinctions reflect variation in the structures of the constant domains and hinge regions of the heavy chains. Thus nine different heavy chain types exist, which are identified using Greek letters: $\alpha1$, $\alpha2$, δ, ϵ, $\gamma1$, $\gamma2$, $\gamma3$, $\gamma4$, and μ. Each of these heavy chains mediates slightly different functions after antigen binding. In addition, there are two classes of light chains, κ and λ. About 70% of human antibodies contain κ light chains.

The classes and subclasses of immunoglobulins can be defined serologically and are collectively referred to as *isotypes.* All normal individuals are capable of generating antibodies of all isotypes. Serologic methods also permit the definition of determinants that are present on the antibody molecules of some individuals but not on those of others. These *allotypic* determinants are usually localized within the constant domains and behave as mendelian genetic markers. Finally, some serologic determinants are found in the variable regions and thus are associated with a specific antigen-binding structure. These are the *idiotypic* determinants of the antibody.

Importance of Antibody Class

The structural and functional properties of each antibody (Ig) class are summarized in Table 173-1 and are discussed next.

IgG. More than 70% of serum immunoglobulin is IgG, the dominant species induced by secondary immunization. IgG is always a four-chain molecule (see Fig. 173-1), containing variable amounts of carbohydrate linked to the C_H2 domain. The human IgG subclasses are named in order of relative serum abundance, with IgG1 typically making up about three fourths of the total serum IgG. Although functionally distinguishable, the $\gamma1$, $\gamma2$, $\gamma3$, and $\gamma4$ heavy chains are more than 90% identical in structure. The principal differences between the subclasses are found in the hinge regions and probably affect the flexibility of the molecule and its susceptibility to proteolysis. Certain immunogens recruit antibodies of particular subclasses; for example, bacterial carbohydrates elicit

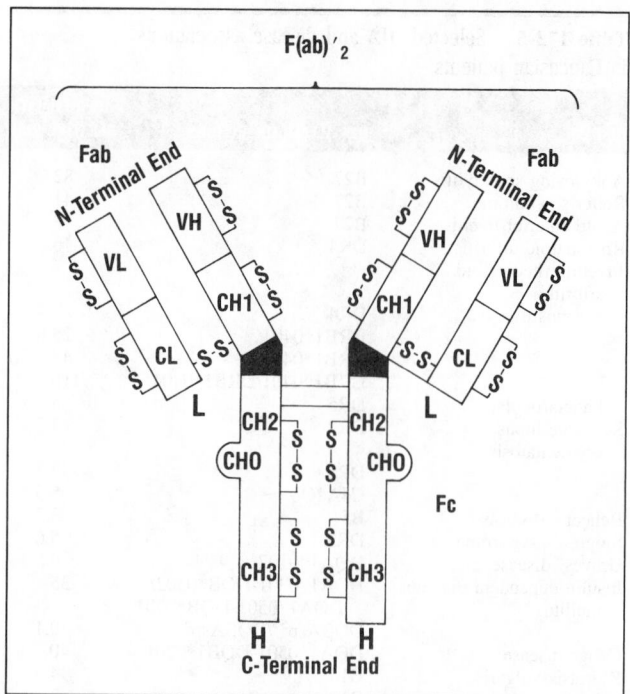

FIGURE 173-1   Schematic diagram of immunoglobulin G1 (IgG1) molecule. *H* and *L* designate heavy and light polypeptide chains. Disulfide bonds are indicated by S-S links. The principal site of asparagine-linked carbohydrate is designated *CHO.* See text for descriptions of the domain organization and the Fc and Fab fragments.

predominantly IgG2 responses. This fact may explain the heightened susceptibility to pyogenic infection seen in individuals with selective IgG2 or combined IgG2 and IgG4 deficiency. The Fc portions of IgG molecules, particularly IgG1 and IgG3, bear the determinants recognized by rheumatoid factors.

IgM. Primary immunization initially elicits an IgM response. IgM is the first antibody formed in the neonate and is the most evolutionarily conserved Ig class. The μ-chain contains an additional C_H4 domain that appears to assist in complement fixation. In serum, IgM consists of five disulfide-linked μ_2L_2 units that form a circular array, with the 10 antigen-binding sites oriented outward. Another B-lymphocyte product, the J chain, is required for the initiation of IgM polymerization. The J chain is 129 amino acids in length and joins two of the μ heavy chains through their carboxy-terminal cystine residues. Circulating IgM molecules are particularly important as rheumatoid factors, cold agglutinins, and isoagglutinins. IgM is also produced as a membrane-associated μ_2L_2 monomer in B-lymphocytes, and this form serves as an antigen receptor (see later discussion).

IgA. Only about 10% of circulating immunoglobulin is IgA; however, it is the predominant Ig class in extravascular secretions, such as mucus, prostatic fluid, saliva, tears, and milk. Although IgA may circulate as an α_2L_2 monomer, it is most frequently encountered as a polymer of two or three such units joined with one molecule of J chain. Secretory IgA is a dimer associated with one molecule of J chain and a second polypeptide called the *secretory component* that is synthesized by epithelial cells. The secretory component is a fragment of the epithelial cell IgA receptor that permits the uptake of dimerized IgA from the serum and its subsequent transport and secretion. In humans, IgA1 is the principal subclass found in serum, whereas IgA2 is slightly more abundant than IgA1 in secretions. IgA in milk is extremely important in providing maternal immunity to the neonate. It is also extremely important in maintaining local immune defense in adults. Selective

Table 173-1 Properties of immunoglobulin (Ig) classes

ISOTYPE	H CHAIN DESIGNATION	MOLECULAR FORMULA	MOLECULAR WEIGHT ($\times 10^3$ DALTONS)	NO. OF DOMAINS IN H CHAINS	NORMAL SERUM CONCENTRATION (MG/ML)	HALF-LIFE DAYS	COMOPLEMENT FIXATION	PLACENTAL TRANSFER
IgG1	$\gamma 1$	$(\gamma_1)_2 L_2$	145	4	9	21	++	+
IgG2	$\gamma 2$	$(\gamma_2)_2 L_2$	145	4	3	20	+	+/−
IgG3	$\gamma 3$	$(\gamma_3)_2 L_2$	165	4	1	7	+++	+
IgG4	$\gamma 4$	$(\gamma_4)_2 L_2$	145	4	0.5	21	+/−	+
IgM	μ	$(\mu_2 L_2)_5$-J	970	5	1.2	5	++++	−
IgA1	$\alpha 1$	$[(\alpha_1)_2 L_2]_n$	160	4	2.0	6	−	−
IgA2	$\alpha 2$	$[(\alpha_2)_2 L_2]_n$	160	4	0.5	?	−	−
sIgA	$\alpha 1$ or $\alpha 2$	$[(\alpha_1$ or $\alpha_2)_2 L_2]_2$-J-SC	400	4	0-0.05	−	−	−
IgD	δ	$\delta_2 L_2$	170	4	0.06	3	−	−
IgE	ϵ	$\epsilon_2 L_2$	190	5	0.0002	2.5-4.0	−	−

H chain, Heavy chain; *SC,* secretory component; *sIgA,* secretory IgA.

IgA deficiency occurs in about 1 in 700 persons and in some is associated with an increased frequency of autoimmune disorders, infections, and malabsorption syndromes.

IgE. Although only a minor component of serum immunoglobulin, IgE is the principal Ig class involved in allergic reactions. IgE exists only in a monomer $\epsilon_2 L_2$ form. The ϵ heavy chain, as with μ, contains an extra constant domain but lacks the cystine involved in polymerization. After secretion by B-lymphocytes, IgE adheres to mast cells and basophils through their high-affinity ϵ-specific Fc receptors. Binding of antigen by IgE provokes the release of vasoactive amines from these cells. IgE production is stimulated by parasitic infection, and it is believed that IgE antibodies assist in protection against parasitic disease.

IgD. Little is known about the function of IgD, which is principally a cell surface immunoglobulin. It exists only in the monomer form and is present at quite low levels in normal serum. B-lymphocytes able to be stimulated usually possess both IgM and IgD antigen receptors. IgD does not fix complement and is not known to sensitize any phagocytic cell populations.

Immunoglobulins as B-Cell Receptors

Although all antibody classes are secreted by B-lymphocytes into the serum to some extent, they also serve as cell surface receptors. Each B-lymphocyte synthesizes 7S antibody of a single specificity and displays this antibody on its surface. Interaction of antigen with the membrane-bound antibody triggers proliferation of the B-lymphocyte and also induces increased secretion of the antibody. Thus antigen selectively expands individual clones of B-lymphocytes by triggering B-cell proliferation. The difference between the membrane-bound and secreted forms of antibodies lies at the carboxy-terminal end of the heavy chain. The membrane form terminates in a series of hydrophobic residues that anchor the entire protein in the lipid bilayer.

ANTIBODY GENES

The existence of variable and constant regions on the same polypeptide poses a genetic paradox: how is it possible to maintain hundreds of different heavy chain genes with identical constant regions? Over evolutionary time, these constant regions would be expected to accumulate mutations. Worse yet, individual variable regions are found associated with more than one type of constant region. How can this be explained? Dreyer and Bennett were the first to propose that some type of deoxyribonucleic acid (DNA) rearrangement mechanism might be responsible for the juxtaposition of variable and constant regions. Almost 10 years later, Tonegawa demonstrated that the variable region and constant region genes undergo specific gene rearrangements in lymphocytes. The organization and reorganization of antibody genes is now understood in considerable detail.

Light Chain Genes

Antibodies are encoded by three unlinked gene families, κ (chromosome 2), λ (chromosome 22), and heavy (chromosome 14). In each gene family, multiple gene segments positioned discontinuously on germline DNA are juxtaposed through DNA rearrangement events during B-cell development. Figure 173-2 diagrams the organization and reorganization of the κ locus. About 70 germline κ–variable region gene segments (V_κ) exist, all of which include a first exon encoding 5' untranslated region and leader peptide sequences, a single intron of about 100 base pairs (bp), and a 300 bp second exon encoding most of the variable region. Immediately 3' to this variable region are short sequences that are recognition sites for the DNA recombinase that catalyzes Ig gene rearrangement. In all, these variable region segments span more than 2 million bp of germline DNA. About 23 kilobases (kb) 3' to the last V_κ gene segment is a series of five J_κ (for joining region) gene segments arrayed in a region of 2 kb. Each of these extremely short (13 codons) gene segments is preceded by rearrangement recognition sequences and ends in a typical eukaryotic splice donor sequence. The C_κ gene segment is represented on a single exon that is separated by a 2 kb intron from the J_κ gene segments. The intron contains an *immunoglobulin enhancer* sequence that is necessary for appropriate lymphocyte-specific transcription of the rearranged κ–light chain gene.

During B-lymphocyte development, which occurs in the bone marrow in adults, a germline V_κ gene segment is juxtaposed to one of the five J_κ gene segments. This rearrangement is imperfect and may delete one or a few bases at the 3' end of the V and at the 5' end of the J. Although the enzymatic machinery responsible for catalyzing rearrangement of antibody gene segments remains incompletely characterized, details of the process have recently emerged. First, the same "recombinase" appears to regulate assembly of both heavy chain and light chain variable regions, as well as catalyzing rearrangment of the analogous gene segments that encode T-cell receptor variable regions. In the majority of cases, formation of a complete variable region–encoding sequence is achieved through somatic deletion of intervening DNA, even when many hundreds of kilobases of DNA must be excised. In all cases, juxtaposition of antibody gene segments requires recognition of the recombination signal sequences positioned adjacent to each gene segment. This recognition is mediated by the products of the *RAG-1* and *RAG-2* genes, which also act to incise the DNA, thereby initiating recombination. Several other proteins, for example, the multicomponent DNA-dependent protein kinase, participate in completing the correct religation of this incised DNA. These latter enzymes catalyze DNA repair in all cells, while RAG-1 and RAG-2 are expressed exclusively in immature lymphocytes.

Gene rearrangement permits formation of a complete transcriptional unit, since a promoter located upstream of the V gene segment is now in proximity with the enhancer element located within the intron between J and C. The primary transcript from this

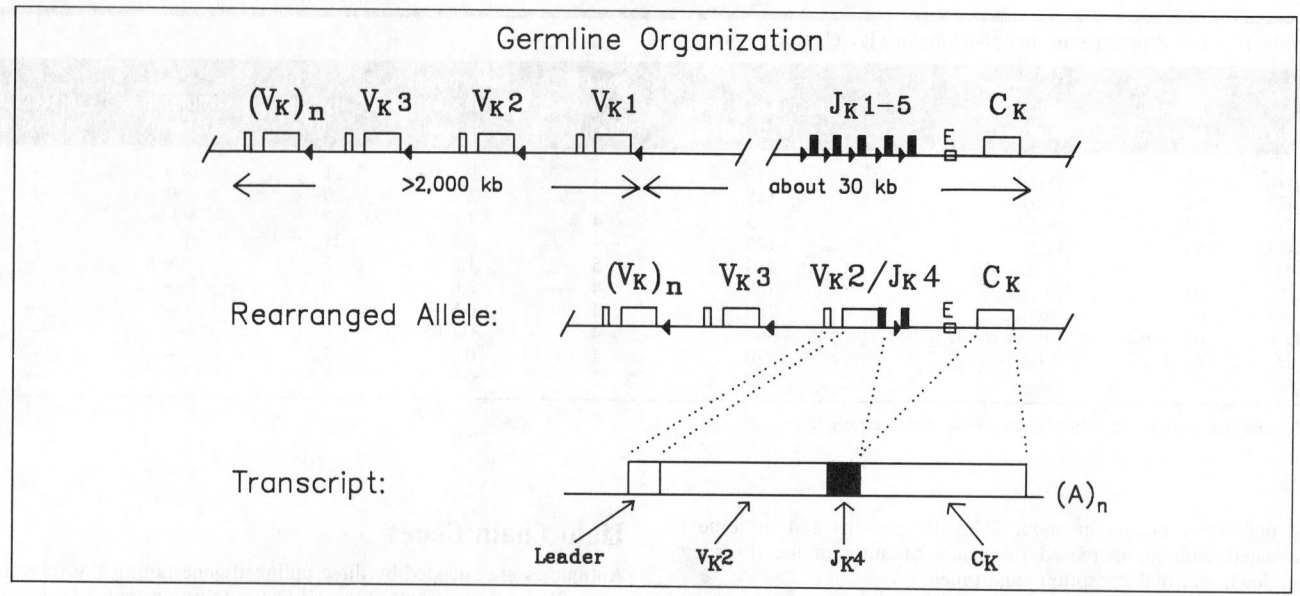

FIGURE 173-2   Germline organization and reorganization of the κ–light chain locus in humans. Boxes represent coding exons. The J gene segments are shaded for emphasis. The box designated *E* represents the transcriptional enhancer. Shaded triangles denote recognition sequences for the antibody gene recombinase. The middle diagram shows the structure of the locus after joining of V and J (arbitrarily V$_κ$2 and J$_κ$4) gene segments. The bottom diagram illustrates the configuration of the mature messenger ribonucleic acid (mRNA) encoding the light chain polypeptide. See the text for details.

rearranged gene is spliced to produce mature κ–light chain messenger ribonucleic acid (mRNA). These events are diagrammed in Fig. 173-2.

Heavy Chain Genes

Rearrangements in the heavy chain locus resemble those in the light chain locus, except that an additional gene segment, the *diversity* (D) gene segment, contributes to the formation of the variable region. Approximately 80 V$_H$ gene segments span several million base pairs of germline DNA near the telomere of chromosome 14. Each has a leader exon and a 300 bp variable-region exon, followed by rearrangement recognition sequences. More than 50 D$_H$ gene segments may be present, varying in length from as few as 9 to perhaps 30 bp, positioned at some distance from the V elements. Each of these D gene segments is flanked by recombination recognition sequences. In humans, six functional J$_H$ gene segments are positioned 70 kb 3′ to the first V$_H$ gene segment and about 3 kb 5′ to the first exon of the C$_μ$ gene. The pattern of rearrangement of these elements is diagrammed in Fig. 173-3. As with the κ light chain, important transcriptional regulatory elements are located in the intron between the J$_H$ and C$_μ$ sequences. During B-cell development, heavy chain rearrangement precedes light chain rearrangement and usually occurs on both alleles. Once again, rearrangement is often imperfect. With the heavy chain, bases may be truncated from the sites of V-D or D-J joining. In addition, bases are frequently added at the sites of joining through the action of the enzyme terminal transferase. These added bases are called *N regions* and are less frequently seen in rearranged light chain genes.

Alternative Processing

Each domain of the heavy chain constant region is encoded by a separate exon. This observation is in accord with the view that the Ig domain is the principal functional, and thus selective, unit in antibody molecules. In addition, differential processing of the heavy chain mRNA can produce mature proteins that have either a secreted type or a membrane type of carboxy terminus. The membrane exon is positioned 3′ to the constant region gene (see Fig. 173-3). Alternative polyadenylation yields a product that either is spliced to include the membrane exon or lacks the membrane exon entirely. The ratio of membrane-type to secreted-type heavy chain mRNA can be altered

in response to stimulation. Thus cross-linking of surface Ig in B-lymphocytes triggers increased expression of mRNA encoding the secreted form of the heavy chain.

Isotype Switching

Different antibody heavy chain classes are encoded by linked genes on chromosome 14. This arrangement explains how a single variable region sequence can be associated with many different constant region sequences. Immediately after rearrangement, B-lymphocytes first express IgM and later both IgM and IgD. This dual expression is achieved by alternative splicing of a long primary transcript. The δ-constant region sequences are positioned adjacent to the μ-constant region sequences. Subsequent expression of other isotypes may occasionally occur by differential processing of an exceedingly long (more than 250 kb) primary transcript but more frequently results from a second type of gene rearrangement event called *isotype switching*. As shown in Fig. 173-4, the isotype switching process occurs through the juxtaposition of specialized "switch" regions located 5′ to each constant region gene and results in the deletion of intervening constant region exons. This process permits the expression of an already rearranged V$_H$ gene segment with a different constant region isotype.

Five Mechanisms Contributing to Antibody Diversity

Detailed characterization of antibody molecules produced in response to immunization has delineated five important mechanisms responsible for antibody diversification.

1. The germline repertoire includes hundreds of tandemly linked variable-region gene segments. (The actual complement of variable regions inherited by each individual varies somewhat, which may contribute to susceptibility to both infectious and autoimmune diseases.)
2. "Combinatorial" joining of germline V, D, and J gene segments produces a repertoire of more than 10,000 different heavy chains. Joining of V and J gene sequences yields at least 1000 different κ light chains. The human λ light chain repertoire includes four different constant-region gene segments, each with its own J and at least 30 different V$_λ$ gene segments.

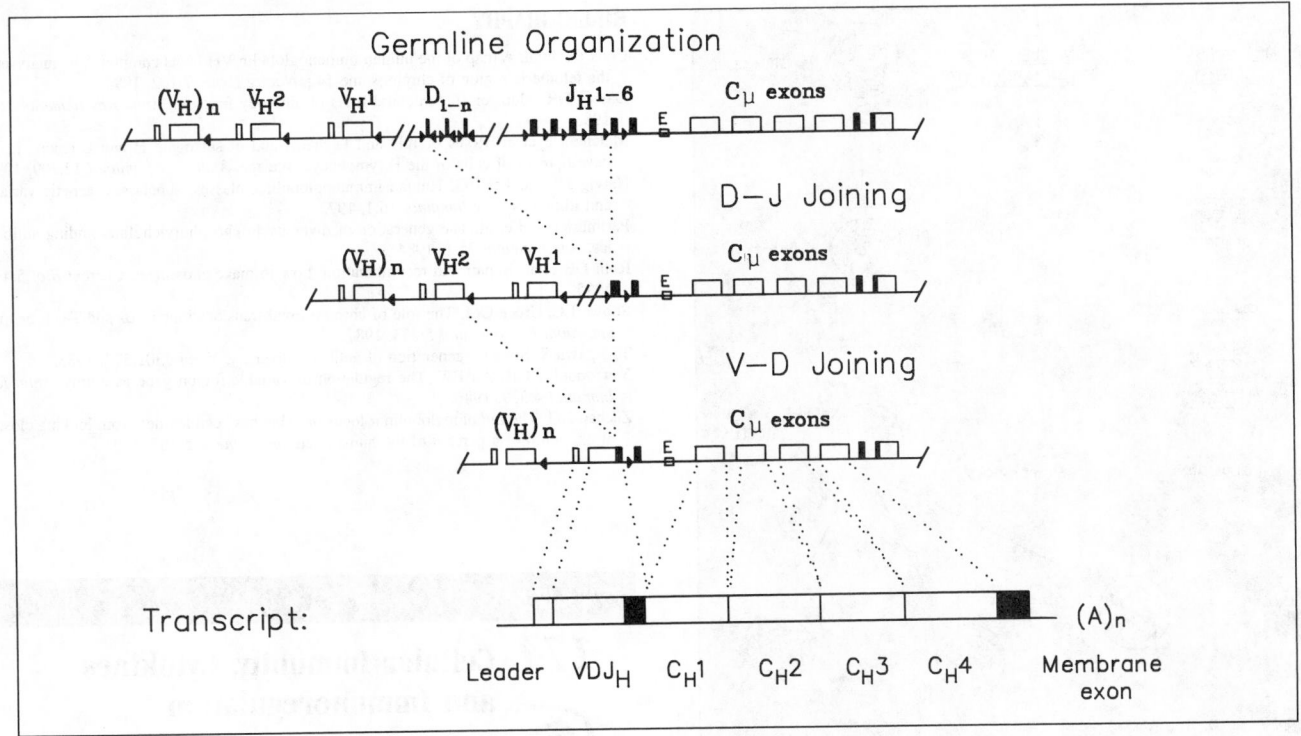

FIGURE 173-3 Germline organization and reorganization of the human heavy chain locus. The D and J gene segments and the membrane exons are shaded. V-D joining follows D-J joining and yields a functional transcriptional unit, the mature product of which encodes a membrane-associated μ-chain. See legend for Figure 173-2 for additional description.

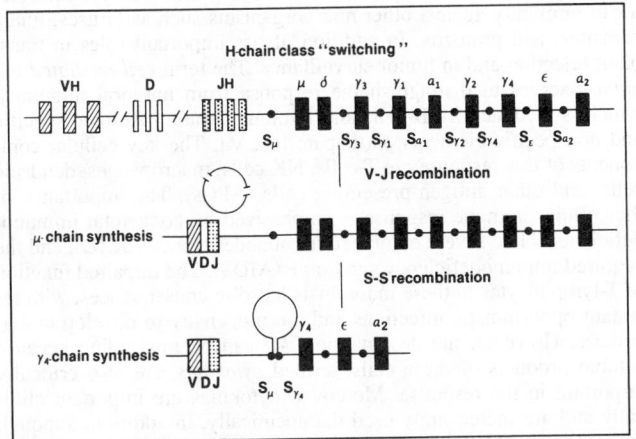

FIGURE 173-4 Mechanism of isotype switching. V-D-J recombination permits μ-chain synthesis. Juxtaposition of the γ4 gene is achieved through a deletion mechanism involving recombination at specialized "switch" sequences (S). See text for description.

3. Flexibility in the joining process adds increased variability at the sites of joining. Although two thirds of the flexibility at the site of J region joining will yield out-of-frame (and thus nontranslatable) antibody chains, flexibility in joining probably increases the overall size of the repertoire by at least a factor of 10. Included in this description of flexibility is the phenomenon of N-region addition by terminal transferase.

4. Combinatorial association of heavy and light chains yields many different combining sites. Thus if 10,000 different heavy chains pair randomly with 1000 different light chains, 10^7 different antibodies are produced. If flexibility in the joining process increases the potential repertoire of heavy and light chains by tenfold, at least 10^8 different binding sites can be generated through gene rearrangement.

5. Superimposed on these combinatorial mechanisms is a process of somatic hypermutation that introduces deletions, insertions, and substitutions into the rearranged V gene segment. Hypermutation is quite specific in that it targets a region of only about 1000 bases centered around the rearranged V element and operates for a limited time during the life of an individual B-lymphocyte. The hypermutation process is partially responsible for the phenomenon of *affinity maturation:* antibodies synthesized late in a response have higher overall affinity for antigen than do antibodies synthesized early in the response. The rate of hypermutation is extremely high, greater than 10^{-3}/bp/generation (at least four orders of magnitude higher than rates for other non-Ig genes). Thus the extent of antibody diversity may be essentially unlimited.

Developmental Order of Antibody Gene Rearrangements

The rearrangement of antibody genes follows a precisely regulated developmental sequence. In B-lymphoid progenitors, joining of D_H to J_H gene segments occurs first and typically on both alleles. Thereafter, V_H-D_H joining produces a functional transcriptional unit. If a first rearrangement produces a nonfunctional product, rearrangement continues using the allelic chromosome. Synthesis of a heavy chain polypeptide permits assembly of a "pre-B receptor," which includes membrane-spanning components of the antigen receptor complex (the Igα and Igβ polypeptides) and a "surrogate light chain" comprising two small proteins, the V-pre-B and λ5 molecules, together with the heavy chain itself. Signals derived from this pre–B cell receptor stimulate B-cell maturation and suppress further heavy chain gene rearrangement. This process ensures that indivudal B-cells express the products of only a single set of heavy chain gene alleles, a phenomenon referred to as *allelic exclusion.* Light chain rearrangement occurs next and also follows a specific order. The κ-genes rearrange first, one allele at a time, until a functional product is obtained. If

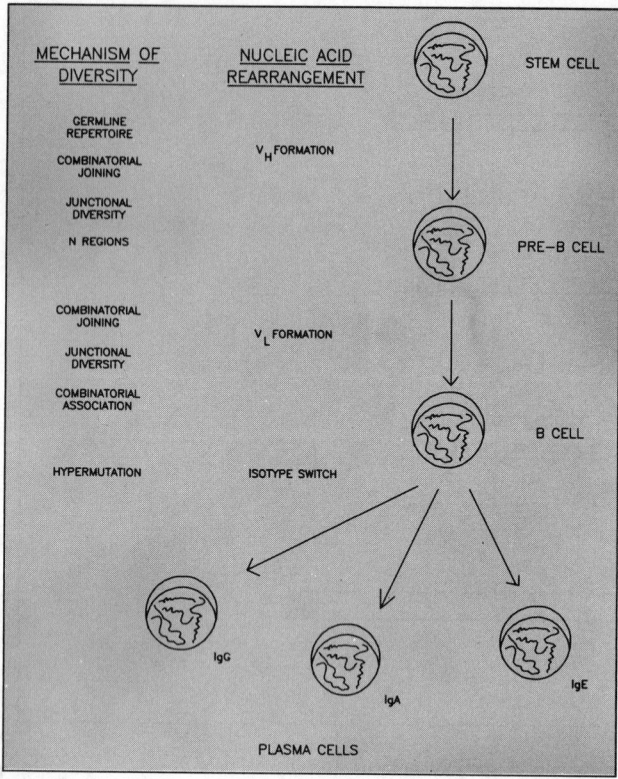

FIGURE 173-5 Generation of antibody diversity. Each of the mechanisms of antibody diversification *(left)* is associated with specific nucleic acid rearrangements *(center)* and occurs at defined points along the time line of B-cell development *(right)*.

From Perlmutter RM et al: *Adv Immunol* 35:1, 1984.

neither allele yields a functional product, λ–light chain gene rearrangement occurs. Thus λ-secreting B-lymphocytes contain rearranged (or in some cases deleted) κ-loci, whereas κ-secreting B-lymphocytes generally retain their λ-genes in germline configuration. Somatic hypermutation occurs to the greatest extent in mature B-lymphocytes. Isotype switching occurs last and is often associated with terminal differentiation into plasma cells. Some IgG B-lymphocytes differentiate into *memory cells,* which may remain in the peripheral lymphoid organs for many years. This explains the long-lasting serologic immunity achieved by vaccination.

Figure 173-5 outlines the major events in B-cell differentiation from the perspective of antibody genes.

Pathologic Gene Rearrangements in Lymphoid Cells

Rearrangement of antibody genes (and of T-cell antigen receptor genes, which are similarly organized) occurs uniquely in lymphoid cells. This rearrangement process occasionally operates on inappropriate substrates, resulting in pathologic changes in DNA content. For example, virtually all examples of Burkitt's lymphoma in humans contain an 8;14 chromosomal translocation that juxtaposes antibody heavy chain genes with the protooncogene c-*myc*. Similarly, a large percentage of follicular B-cell lymphomas contain a 14;18 translocation, resulting in juxtaposition of the antibody genes with the protooncogene *bcl*-2. In each case, good reason exists to believe that activation of the translocated oncogene makes an important contribution to the expansion of the malignant clone. Thus the process of gene rearrangement, although a spectacularly effective mechanism for diversifying the repertoire of antigen receptors, represents a form of mutagenesis that can predispose persons to the development of neoplastic disease.

BIBLIOGRAPHY

Cook GP et al: A map of the human immunoglobulin VH locus completed by analysis of the telomeric region of chromosome 14q, *Nature Genet* 7:162, 1994.
Davies DR, Metzger H: Structural basis of antibody function, *Annu Rev Immunol* 1:87, 1983.
Melchers F et al: Roles of IgH and L chains and of surrogate H and L chains in the development of cells of the B lymphocyte lineage, *Annu Rev Immunol* 12:209, 1994.
Natvig JB, Kunkel HG: Human immunoglobulins: classes, subclasses, genetic variants and idiotypes, *Adv Immunol* 16:1, 1973.
Perlmutter RM et al: The generation of diversity in phosphorylcholine-binding antibodies, *Adv Immunol* 35:1, 1984.
Roth DB et al: Repair and recombination: how to make ends meet, *Current Biol* 5:496, 1995.
Showe LC, Croce CM: The role of chromosomal translocations in B- and T-cell neoplasia, *Annu Rev Immunol* 5:253, 1987.
Tonegawa S: Somatic generation of antibody diversity, *Nature* 302:575, 1983.
Yancopoulos GD, Alt FW: The regulation of variable region gene assembly, *Annu Rev Immunol* 4:339, 1986.
Zachau HG: The immunoglobulin κ locus or, what has been learned from looking closely at one-tenth of a percent of the human genome, *Gene* 135:167, 1993.

CHAPTER

174 Cellular Immunity, Cytokines, and Immunoregulation

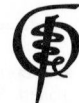

John J. O'Shea and Thomas B. Nutman

Cell-mediated immunity (CMI) is the primary defense against intracellular pathogens like *Mycobacterium* and is also a major contributor to immunity against other microorganisms such as viruses, fungi, parasites, and protozoa. In addition, it has important roles in transplant rejection and in tumor surveillance. The term *cell-mediated immunity* serves to distinguish the response from humoral immunity, which is mediated by B-cells and immunoglobulin. Antigen-specific and nonspecific elements participate in CMI. The key cellular components of this response are T-cells, NK cells, macrophages, dendritic cells, and other antigen-presenting cells (APCs). The importance of the cellular immune response is emphasized by congenital immunodeficiencies like severe combined immunodeficiency (SCID), and the acquired immunodeficiency syndrome (AIDS). The impaired function of T-lymphocytes in these individuals has dire consequences, with resultant opportunistic infections and the propensity to develop malignancies. However, the designation *CMI* can be misleading because soluble products of these cells, termed *cytokines,* are also critically important in the response. Moreover, cytokines are important clinically and are increasingly used therapeutically. In addition, although the cellular and humoral responses are distinguished from one another, T-cells play a major role in regulating B-cell function, and conversely, B-cells are important APCs. Therefore the distinction between the two limbs of the immune system is not a sharp one. It should also be stated that although the cell-mediated immune system has evolved to a remarkable state of efficiency and sophistication, it is still rather imperfect. In a vigorous response to pathogens, significant damage to normal tissue can occur. Indeed, there are many circumstances in which the host's response to an invading microorganism is more destructive than the organism itself. The consequence of immunologic diseases following various infectious diseases is well documented. In addition, it is now very clear from animal models that immune-mediated tissue damage can occur as a consequence of mutations of many different genes. So although the complexity of the immune response provides a remarkably orchestrated response to pathogenic organisms, there are many steps at which dysregulation can lead to disease. The major cells that participate in cell-mediated immunity are discussed in Chapter 171; however, it is useful to briefly review the function of these cells in the context of this aspect of the immune response.

CELLULAR CONSTITUENTS
T-Cells

As discussed, T-cells and the cytokines they produce are the major regulatory elements in the cellular and humoral immune responses. T-cells arise in the bone marrow and develop in the thymus. These lymphocytes recognize processed peptide antigens that are displayed on the surface of APCs. A subset of T-cells (about 25% to 40%) express the CD8 molecule, a co-receptor that binds MHC class I. CD8$^+$ T-cells recognize endogenously produced peptide antigens including foreign antigens like viral products that are presented by class I molecules. Most cells express MHC class I molecules and so participate in antigen presentation of endogenous antigens. CD8$^+$ T-cells are a major component of the immune response against virally infected cells; MHC class I expression is upregulated by interferon (IFN) α/β produced in response to viral infection. Upon activation with cytokines like interleukin (IL)-2 and IL-12, CD8$^+$ T-cells acquire the ability to lyse infected cells. Previously, the CD8 molecule was thought to be a marker for T-cells that possessed suppressor activity, that is, they were responsible for downmodulating the immune response. However, present evidence for a unique population of cells with such a defined surface marker is lacking. "Suppressor cell" activity can also be due to the secretion of cytokines.

The CD4 molecule is a co-receptor for MHC class II, thus enabling CD4$^+$ T-cells (55% to 70% of T-cells) to recognize antigen presented by class II. In contrast to MHC class I molecules, MHC class II molecules are expressed by a limited number of cells including: macrophages, B-cells, dendritic cells, Langerhans' cells, activated T-cells, and activated endothelial cells. These cells endocytose and process extracellular antigens, and then present these exogenously derived peptide antigens to CD4$^+$ T-cells. CD4$^+$ T-cells are termed *helper T-cells* and they function to regulate cellular and humoral responses. Helper T-cells themselves can be divided into one of two classes, denoted T-helper 1 (Th1) and T helper 2 (Th2) subsets, which drive the immune response toward a cell-mediated response (Th1) versus an allergic-type response (Th2). The cellular response is characterized by the recruitment and activation of macrophages and termed *delayed type hypersensitivity* (DTH). In contrast, in the allergic response IgE is produced, which binds to receptors on mast cells and basophils. Following cross-linking of these receptors with antigen, the cells are activated and release a variety of mediators and cytokines. Eosinophils are also recruited and activated. The means by which this differentiation occurs will be discussed, but cytokines like IL-12 and IL-4 play a key role.

While the majority of T-cells (greater than 90%) co-express either CD4 or CD8 and heterodimeric T-cell receptors (TCR) consisting of $\alpha\beta$-subunits, a subset of T-cells expresses a different receptor consisting of $\gamma\delta$-subunits and typically does not express either CD4 or CD8. While $\alpha\beta$–T cells only recognize peptide antigens, this is not exclusively the case for $\gamma\delta$–T cells. Some $\gamma\delta$–T cells do respond to peptide antigens, but others recognize nonpeptide antigens like mycobacterially derived prenyl pyrophosphate derivatives and perhaps other nonpeptide antigens.

Each clone of T-cells expresses a genetically determined immunoglobulin-like antigen receptor, the product of rearranged α and β or γ and δ genes, which confers the ability to recognize antigen. Large numbers of different T-cell clones can also be activated by molecules that directly bind T-cell receptors and MHC molecules. Such molecules are called *superantigens*. They are produced by bacteria and the response to superantigen is an important aspect of the pathogenicity of these bacteria.

Engagement of the antigen receptor results in activation of the protein tyrosine kinases, Lck and Zap-70 (ζ-associated protein of 70 kD); deficiency of Zap-70 is a cause of severe combined immunodeficiency disease [SCID] (Chapter 185). With the appropriate costimulatory stimulus (such as that provided by the CD28 molecule), signals are generated that lead to activation of T-cells. Interfering with TCR-mediated signals, with drugs like cyclosporin and FK506, is an important means of inducing immunosuppression. Likewise, interfering with the costimulatory signal also appears to be an efficacious means of ameliorating autoimmune disease in animal models. However, these signals represent only the first level of activation. The second phase of T-cell activation occurs in response to the cytokines that T-cells produce. Without the signal provided by cytokines (like IL-2), activated T-cells do not enter the S phase of the cell cycle and so do not proliferate. In fact, preventing T-cells from responding to cytokines can lead to a state of unresponsiveness of the T-cells, termed *anergy*. The major cytokines produced by T-cells include IFN γ, IL-2, IL-3, IL-4, IL-5, IL-9, IL-10, GM-CSF, and a variety of *chemo*tactic *cytokines* that are known as *chemokines*.

Natural Killer Cells

Natural killer (NK) cells or large granular lymphocytes are a cytolytic lymphocyte subset that lacks rearranged antigen receptors as seen with T- and B-cells. Nonetheless, these cells very efficiently kill tumor cells and virally infected cells. Rare individuals have been described who lack NK cells and they are highly susceptible to viral infections. Interestingly, NK cells recognize MHC molecules by a recently identified class of receptors. If a cell, such as a tumor cell, lacks the appropriate MHC molecule, NK cells will recognize and kill it. The NK cells also have receptors for immunoglobulin (Fc receptors) and so can lyse antibody-coated particles (antibody-dependent cellular cytotoxicity or ADCC). NK cells produce IFNγ and tumor necrosis factor (TNF) and so participate in cell-mediated immunity and inflammation. NK cells also are an important component of graft-versus-host disease. NK cells respond strongly to cytokines like IL-2, IL-12, IFNα/β and IFNγ. Such treatment greatly increases the cytolytic function of these cells and they are therefore called *lymphokine activated killer* (LAK) cells. This capacity has been capitalized upon in the treatment of certain malignancies. The majority of the peripheral blood lymphocytes in patients treated with IL-2 are NK cells. This approach has been successful in some but not all tumors and efforts are underway to optimize this therapy. Additionally, IL-12, which has similar effects on lymphocyte cytotoxicity as IL-2, is also being used experimentally in the treatment of malignancy.

Mononuclear Phagocytes

Mononuclear phagocytes are an essential component of CMI. They have a number of important effector functions in host defense and also serve as APCs for T-cells. They constantly sample the environment by pinocytosis and phagocytosis of foreign particles, microbes, tissue debris, and senescent cells. They can kill microorganisms and tumor cells. Moreover, mononuclear cells synthesize and secrete a large number of products that are important in host defense. Their participation in CMI comes from cooperation with T-cells in the generation of specific immunity.

Mononuclear phagocytes originate and develop in the bone marrow. They emerge in peripheral blood as monocytes that are incompletely differentiated. However, once they migrate into tissues, they further differentiate to macrophages. Several colony-stimulating factors (CSFs) are involved in the growth and differentiation of these cells but the only macrophage-specific CSF is macrophage-CSF or CSF-1. Macrophages in different tissues are given different names, for example, in neural tissue, they are termed *microglia;* in the liver, *Kupfer's cells;* in the lung, *alveolar macrophages;* and in bone, *osteoclasts.* Macrophages are also present in other tissues like the kidney glomerulus, the lining of the joint, and various endocrine organs.

Macrophages have a number of membrane receptors of immunologic importance. They have receptors for immunoglobulin (Fc receptors) and complement receptors. This allows them to phagocytose opsonized particles and to mediate ADCC. Macrophages have receptors for many different cytokines and are activated by granulocyte-macrophage-CSF (GM-CSF), IFNγ, and IL-2, whereas IL-4 inhibits their function. They are efficient APCs for T-cells because they express both class I and class II MHC molecules; adhesion molecules like ICAM-1 and LFA-3 that bind LFA-1 and CD2, respectively, on T-cells; and the key costimulatory molecules B7-1 and B7-2 that provide a critical activation signal for T-cells via CD28.

It is important to note that macrophages also secrete a wide range of products. These include enzymes such as elastase, collagenase, lysosomal enzymes, plasminogen activator, tissue procoagulant, angiotensin converting enzyme, and lysozyme. In addition, they produce extracellular matrix components like fibronectin and complement components including C2, C3, C4, C5, factors B, D, H, and I. They also generate proinflammatory lipid mediators like prostaglandins, leukotrienes, and platelet activating factor. As part of their microbicidal apparatus they produce reactive oxygen species and nitric oxide.

Macrophages produce a large number of cytokines including: granulocyte (G)-CSF, GM-CSF, M-CSF, IL-1, IL-6, TNFα, TNFβ, IL-8, and interferon α/β as well as chemokines. One of their most important products is IL-12, which has critical functions in regulating CMI and Th1 cell development. They also synthesize antiinflammatory cytokines like IL-10, TGFβ-1, and IL-1 receptor antagonist (IL-1RA), and growth factors such as platelet derived growth factor (PDGF) and fibroblast growth factor (FGF), factors that promote the proliferation of fibroblasts and vascular endothelium. Therefore in addition to being simply "big eaters" of microorganisms, macrophages are major contributors to tissue inflammation and repair. Importantly though, they are also critical elements in specific immunity and immunoregulation.

Dendritic Cells

Dendritic cells (DC) are morphologically distinguishable cells of two types with different functions. Interdigitating dendritic cells are abundant in T cell–rich areas of lymph nodes and spleen. In the skin, these cells are called Langerhans' cells and represent about 5% of the epidermal cells. DC are mobile; they ingest antigens and then migrate to the regional lymph node. Because they express MHC class II at high levels, DC are extremely efficient in presenting antigen. DC are bone marrow derived but appear to be distinct from typical mononuclear phagocytes. Follicular dendritic cells (FDC) are not of bone marrow origin. FDC are present in germinal centers of lymphoid follicles in lymph nodes and spleen where they trap antigens for presentation to B-cells.

CYTOKINES AND IMMUNOREGULATION

Many factors can regulate the immune response, including genetic determinants like MHC or TCR molecules. While these structures determine what is seen as an antigen, other factors are of great importance in regulating the magnitude and character of the immune response. Predictably these factors are clinically very relevant. For example, an important mechanism of dampening the immune response is mediated by the interaction of the membrane molecules Fas and Fas ligand, which induces T-cells to undergo programmed cell death or apoptosis. Fas mediated death is clearly an important means of regulating lymphocyte proliferation because mutations of Fas in mice and humans cause a severe lymphoproliferative disease that is associated with autoimmunity (Chapter 177). In humans, the disease is termed *autoimmune lymphoproliferative syndrome* (ALPS). Other factors that are important in regulating the immune response include the nature, route of exposure, and quantity of antigen. Coadministration of an adjuvant also increases the immunogenicity of substances by nonspecifically activating APCs. The mechanisms by which these different variables influence the immune response are not entirely understood, however, it is clear that a major component of immunoregulation is mediated by soluble factors termed *cytokines*.

Unfortunately, the term *cytokine* is not very specific. It does not denote a specific class of factors that are structurally or functionally related. Rather it encompasses many different factors that are made by lymphoid and nonlymphoid cells that mediate intracellular communication. Many types of nonimmunologic cells produce cytokines; those made by lymphocytes (principally T-cells) are called *lymphokines,* those made by mononuclear phagocytes have been called *monokines.* Cytokines that are produced by and act on leukocytes are termed *interleukins* (IL). Cytokines can act on cells in an autocrine or paracrine fashion, but can also enter the bloodstream and act in a typical endocrine fashion. In fact, the boundary between cytokines and hormones is rather indistinct.

There are several ways that cytokines can be classified. One way is to group the factors by the type of receptor that they bind. A large group of cytokines bind a class of receptors termed the *hematopoietic cytokine receptor superfamily.* These cytokines include hormones such as growth hormone, erythropoietin, thrombopoietin and prolactin; colony-stimulating seting factors such as GM-CSF, G-CSF; the interferons; and various interleukins (Table 174-1). The newest member of this family is the factor leptin, which regulates obesity. As a group

they are related structurally, bind to structurally related receptors, and use related molecules for signal transduction (see later discussion). Another large class of factors that bind a different class of receptor are the growth factors like stem cell factor, M-CSF or CSF-1, platelet derived growth factor (PDGF), and fibroblast growth factor (FGF). These ligands bind to receptors with intrinsic enzymatic activity, the receptor tyrosine kinase family. Tumor necrosis factor α (TNFα) binds to a receptor that has homology to a number of other molecules including Fas and CD40. In contrast, the chemokines bind to receptors that are members of a seven transmembrane receptor superfamily. Other cytokines that bind to structurally distinct receptors include interleukin-1 and transforming growth factor β (TGFβ). For the purposes of this chapter, however, it is most useful to classify cytokines functionally, keeping in mind that these factors are often pleiotropic and redundant in their effects. That is, each cytokine has multiple functions and a given effect is often mediated by several different cytokines. In addition, cytokines frequently induce or influence the action of other cytokines.

The critical functions of individual cytokines have been delineated in knockout mice, that is, mice that have been genetically engineered to lack specific cytokines through homologous gene recombination. In these mice, the nonredundant effects of cytokines become apparent. Cytokines can be grouped functionally as factors that either regulate hematopoiesis; mediate inflammation and natural immunity; and/or function in the regulation of the immune response. In the interest of brevity, hormones like growth hormone and prolactin are not discussed here (Chapter 147). Information on growth factors for nonlymphoid cells, like PDGF, is included as they contribute to fibrosis seen in immunologic disease. Because it is beyond the scope of this chapter to adequately cover all cytokines, the focus will be on those that regulate the immune and inflammatory responses.

Cytokines That Regulate Hematopoiesis

These cytokines are important in CMI because they are responsible for the growth and development of many of the cells that contribute to this arm of the immune system. Stem cell factor (c-kit ligand) is synthesized by bone marrow stromal cells as a secreted and transmembrane protein and is needed to make stem cells responsive to other CSFs. IL-3 stimulates the growth of immature progenitor cells of all lineages and is therefore a multilineage CSF as is granulocyte-macrophage-CSF. The latter also supports myelomonocytic differentiation and activates mature leukocytes. IL-3, GM-CSF, and IL-5 have a shared receptor subunit (the common β-subunit, βc), which explains some of their common effects. Also they are all produced by activated CD4$^+$ T-cells. Granulocyte-CSF acts on committed progenitor cells in the marrow and promotes granulocytic differentiation. Monocyte-macrophage-CSF (CSF-1) acts on committed progenitors to drive mononuclear phagocyte differentiation. Erythropoietin is required for erythrocyte growth and development, as thrombopoietin is for megakaryocytic development. IL-11 also stimulates megakaryocytopoiesis. Analogously, IL-7 is absolutely required for proper growth and development of T- and B-lymphocytes as illustrated by IL-7 and IL-7R knockout mice, which have severe impairment of T-cell and B-cell development. IL-7 is produced by marrow stromal cells and perhaps thymic stromal cells. Some of the aforementioned cytokines including erythropoietin, G-CSF, and GM-CSF are widely used clinically for their prohematopoietic properties (Chapter 69). It is anticipated that others, like thrombopoietin, will be available in the near future.

Cytokines Involved in Natural Immunity and Inflammation

A number of cytokines appear to have important roles in producing inflammation. Many of these cytokines are made by mononuclear phagocytes, two of the most important are TNFα and IL-1.

A principal function of IL-1 is the induction of fever, acute phase protein synthesis, and cachexia. It induces production of IL-6 and chemokines, promotes leukocyte adhesion to endothelium, and has procoagulant effects. Unlike TNFα it does not induce cell death and does not augment expression of MHC class I. IL-1 also enhances hematopoiesis. The major source of IL-1 is the mononuclear phagocyte but

Table 174-1   Major cytokines of importance in immunity and inflammation*

CYTOKINE	PRODUCED BY	TARGET CELLS	EFFECT
Prohematopoietic			
Granulocyte-macrophage CSF	T-cell Macrophage Endothelium Fibroblast	Immature and committed progenitors Macrophages	Growth and differentiation Activation
Granulocyte-CSF	Macrophage Endothelium Fibroblast	Committed progenitors	Differentiation
Macrophage CSF	Macrophage Endothelium Fibroblast	Committed progenitors	Differentiation
Erythropoietin	Kidney, liver	Erythroid precursors	Erythroid differentiation
Thrombopoietin	Liver, kidney	Committed stem cells and megakaryocytes	Platelet growth and differentiation
Stem cell factor	Bone marrow Stromal cell	Pluripotent stem cell	Activation, growth
Interleukin-3	T-cell	Immature progenitors	Growth and differentiation of all lineages
Interleukin-7	Bone marrow, thymic stromal cells, spleen	T-cells B-cells	Growth and differentiation Growth and differentiation
Proinflammatory			
Interleukin-1	Many cells, especially macrophages	CNS Endothelial cells Liver Thymocyte Macrophage	Fever, anorexia Activation Acute phase reactants Costimulation Activation, cytokine production
Tumor necrosis factor α	Macrophages T-cell	Neutrophil Macrophage Endothelium CNS Muscle, fat Many cells	Secretion Adhesion Activation, cytokine production Adhesion Coagulation Fever, cachexia Catabolism Cytolysis
Lymphotoxin (Tumor necrosis factor β)	T-cell	Lymph node Endothelial cell	Structure Activation
Interleukin-6	Macrophage, endothelium, T-cell	Liver B-cell Thymocyte	Acute phase reactants Proliferation, differentiation Co-stimulation
Chemokines: IL-8, others	Macrophages, endothelium, T-cells, platelets	Leukocytes	Chemotaxis, activation
Natural immunity			
Interferon α/β	Macrophages Fibroblasts Other	All NK cell T-cell	Antiviral, antiproliferative Increased MHC class I Activation Upregulates IL-12RB$_2$ expression
Immunoregulatory			
Interferon γ	Th1 T-cells NK cells	Macrophages Endothelium NK cells	Activation, increased MHC class II Activation, increased MHC class II Activation
Interleukin-2	T-cells	T-cells NK cell B-cell	Proliferation, cytotoxicity IFNγ secretion, cytotoxicity Proliferation, antibody production
Interleukin-4	Th2 T-cells Mast cells Basophils Eosinophils	T-cell B-cell Macrophage	Proliferation, Th2 differentiation IgE production Inhibition
Interleukin-5	Th2 T-cells	Eosinophil B-cell	Proliferation, activation Proliferation, activation
Interleukin-9	Th2 T-cells	T-cells Mast cell precursors	Proliferation Proliferation
Interleukin-10	Th2 T-cells, other cells	Macrophages T-cells	Decreased MHC class II Decreased antigen presentation Th1 differentiation, proliferation
Interleukin-12	Macrophages B-cells	T-cells NK cells	Th1 differentiation, proliferation Proliferation, cytotoxicity
Interleukin-13	Activated T-cells	B-cells Macrophages	Costimulator of proliferation, IgE Increased CD23 and class II, inhibits cytokine secretion
Interleukin-15	Nonlymphoid cells, muscle	T-cells NK cells	Growth, cytotoxicity Growth, cytotoxicity
Transforming growth factor β	T-cells Macrophages Other	T-cell Macrophage Other	Inhibit growth and activation Inhibit activation Growth regulation

*The major proinflammatory, immunoregulatory, and prohematopoietic cytokines are shown along with their major cellular producers and targets. The list does not include many other cytokines like growth hormone, prolactin, or leptin, and growth factors like platelet-derived growth factor, but rather focuses on those cytokines that are important in immunity and inflammation.

it is produced by other cells too. It is induced by lipopolysaccharide, TNFα, and IL-1 itself. There are two forms, IL-1α and IL-1β, but most circulating IL-1 is the latter and IL-1β knockout mice have impaired febrile responses. IL-1 β is processed to an active form that can be secreted by IL-1 converting enzyme (ICE).

An endogenous antagonist is also produced by a variety of cells. The IL-1 receptor antagonist, which is homologous to IL-1, binds to IL-1 receptors but does not transmit signals and therefore limits IL-1 action. In addition, IL-1 receptors are shed and can also inhibit IL-1 activity.

TNFα is the principal mediator of the response to gram-negative bacteria that produce lipopolysaccharide (LPS). IFNγ also induces TNFα and augments its effects. The actions of TNFα are multiple: it induces fever, activates the coagulation system, induces hypoglycemia, depresses cardiac contractility, reduces vascular resistance, and induces cachexia and the production of acute phase proteins in the liver. TNFα is the major mediator of septic shock. It also upregulates class I, activates phagocytes, and induces mononuclear phagocytes to produce cytokines such as IL-1, IL-6, chemokines, and TNFα itself and increases adhesion molecules on vascular endothelium. TNFα is also cytotoxic to certain cells. The receptor for TNF has homology to Fas, another inducer of apoptosis. The multiple actions of TNFα emphasize the point that although the goal of the immune response is to eliminate invading microorganisms, the response itself may be injurious to normal host tissue, septic shock being a particularly graphic example. The primary source of TNFα is the mononuclear phagocyte, but it is also produced by T, NK, and other cells. Interestingly, the TNFα gene is encoded within the MHC locus.

Lymphotoxin (LT), also termed *TNFβ,* is homologous to and competes with TNFα for binding to the same receptors. LT has many of the same effects as TNFα but LT also binds to another protein, LTβ, which forms a cell surface complex. LTβ knockout mice have severe disruption of lymph node architecture indicating that both LT and LTβ have important functions in regulating the structure of this organ, though the mechanism is not understood. LT like TNFα is encoded within the MHC. LT is produced by activated T-cells.

IL-6 acts on liver to induce hepatic synthesis of C-reactive protein, serum amyloid A, α2 macroglobulin, and fibrinogen, together known as the *acute phase response.* The elevation of the erythrocyte sedimentation rate in inflammatory disease largely reflects the accelerated synthesis of these proteins. In response to IL-6, the liver also decreases synthesis of albumin and transferrin. In addition, IL-6 is a growth and differentiation factor for B-cells. The IL-6 receptor is composed of the gp130 protein, a subunit that is shared by other cytokines including IL-11 (see Fig. 174-2). IL-6 is produced by a variety of cells including mononuclear phagocytes in response to IL-1 and TNFα.

Chemokines are a large family of *chemo*tactic cyto*kines* that attract various types of leukocytes. The term comprises two families of factors that differ in their amino acid sequence (Cys-Cys vs. Cys-X-Cys). The Cys-Cys family of chemokines, such as Rantes, MIP1α, and MIP1β are made by T-cells, whereas the Cys-X-Cys subgroup, like IL-8, are made by mononuclear phagocytes and other cells. Chemokines recruit T-cells, granulocytes, and mononuclear cells.

The major effect of IFNα/β or type I interferons is antiviral action. These interferons comprise a family of factors, the products of distinct genes, which act on all cells to inhibit viral replication and inhibit cellular proliferation. They upregulate MHC class I and downregulate class II expression. IFNα/β also increases the cytolytic activity of NK cells. INFα/β also upregulates the IL-12 receptor beta 2 (IL-12 Rβ₂) subunit or T cells making them responsive to IL-12. A major source is the mononuclear phagocyte, but these interferons are ubiquitously produced. IFNα/β is used clinically in the treatment of viral hepatitis (Chapter 57). In addition, it is also used in the treatment of certain malignancies, such as hairy cell leukemia, because of its antiproliferative effects.

Cytokines That Regulate Lymphoid Growth and Differentiation

These cytokines include: interleukin (IL)-2, IL-4, IL-7, IL-9, IL-10, IL-12, IL-13, IL-15. Each in its own way can dramatically affect not only the strength of the immune response but also its form.

Th1 Versus Th2 Differentiation. An important concept that has recently emerged is that precursor CD4⁺ or helper T-cells differentiate into one of two phenotypes (Fig. 174-1) (Chapter 171). T helper 1 (Th1) cells drive the immune response towards cell-mediated immune responses whereas T helper 2 (Th2) cells promote a humoral or allergic response. Th1 cells produce IL-2, TNFβ, and IFNγ, whereas Th2 cells produce IL-4, IL-5, and IL-10. Both subsets of helper T-cells produce IL-3.

All the mechanisms underlying the regulation of Th1 versus Th2 development have not been elucidated, but a major factor that drives Th1 differentiation is IL-12. It is produced by B-cells and monocytes in response to pathogenic organisms. It is a very potent activator of NK cells, inducing proliferation, IFNγ secretion, and augmenting cytolytic activity. IL-12 also stimulates the differentiation of precursor CD4⁺ cells to Th1 cells and augments the cytolytic function of CD8⁺ T-cells. Because of these effects, IL-12 may be very useful clinically. IFNα/β regulates IL-12 R expression. IL-2, an autocrine T-cell growth factor, is an important factor in determining the magnitude of T-cell and NK cell responses. It is made by uncommitted T helper cells as well as Th1 cells and is a T-cell growth factor that is required for progression from the G1 to S phase of the cell cycle. In addition, it augments the cytolytic activity of T and NK cells and induces IFNγ secretion by NK cells. IL-2 is a growth factor for B cells and induces immunoglobulin class switching (Chapter 173). It also activates macrophages. Surprisingly, IL-2 knockout mice do not have the impairments expected. In particular, they do not die as a result of immunodeficiency. On the contrary; they succumb to autoimmune disease! The reasons for this are not yet clear. One explanation for their lack of immunodeficiency is that another cytokine, IL-15, also binds to the IL-2R β and γ subunits and has effects similar to IL-2. However, it is made by nonlymphoid cells and may be of importance in immunologically mediated diseases. IL-2 also has important actions in constraining lymphocyte growth by enhancing apoptotic death of activated lymphocytes.

IFNγ is the principal activator of macrophages. It enhances their ability to kill microorganisms, upregulates class II expression, and suppresses Th2 responses. IFNγ also activates endothelial cells and neutrophils. Furthermore, it acts on CD4⁺ T-cells to promote Th1 differentiation and acts on CD8⁺ T-cells to promote their maturation as cytotoxic cells. IFNγ also augments NK cytolytic activity. It also acts on B-cells to promote switching to IgG2a and IgG3 and inhibits switching to IgG1 and IgE. IFNγ knockout mice have increased sus-

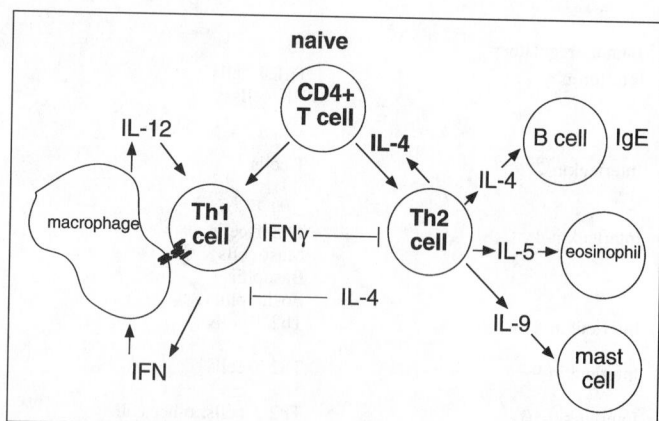

FIGURE 174-1 Regulation of the immune response by cytokines: Th1 versus Th2 differentiation. Naive CD4⁺ T helper cells can be differentiated to T helper 1 cells that produce interferon (IFN)γ, tumor necrosis factor, and IL-2. IFN γ, in particular, is a potent macrophage activator that upregulates class II MHC expression, macrophage cytolytic, and microbicidal activity, and suppresses Th2 responses. Th1 cells therefore promote cellular immune responses, and IL-12, a cytokine produced by macrophages in response to pathogenic organisms, is an important regulator of Th1 differentiation. Naive helper cells can also differentiate to Th2 cells that produce IL-4, IL-5, IL-9, and IL-10. IL-4 is a critically important cytokine as it induces B-cell class switching to IgE production and drives Th2 differentiation itself. IL-5 is an activator of eosinophils whereas IL-9 is growth factor for mast cells. IL-10 is a critical negative regulator of macrophage function.

ceptibility to pathogens, especially intracellular microbes, diminished macrophage class II expression, and decreased NK function.

In contrast to Th1 cells, Th2 cells promote an allergic type response. IL-4 is made by $CD4^+$ Th2 cells and promotes differentiation of naive $CD4^+$ cells to a Th2 phenotype. It is also a growth factor for mast cells, is required for class switching of B-cells to produce IgE, inhibits macrophage activation, and blocks the effects of IFNγ. The critical importance of IL-4 in directing the Th2 response is supported by IL-4 knockout mice, which cannot produce IgE or eosinophilia in response to helminthic (worm) challenge. IL-13 has many of the same effects as IL-4 and even shares a receptor subunit(s) with IL-4; however, based on the IL-4 knockout mice, it cannot fully compensate for the lack of IL-4. Th2 cells also generate IL-5, which promotes the growth, differentiation, and activation of eosinophils and IL-9, which supports growth of T-cells and bone marrow–derived mast cell precursors.

IL-10 is an important cytokine that impedes cell-mediated immunity. It inhibits macrophage antigen presentation and decreases MHC class II expression. It is made by Th2 $CD4^+$ T-cells and also made by some Th1 cells, activated B-cells, macrophages, and keratinocytes. The importance of IL-10 as an endogenous inhibitor of cell-mediated immunity is underscored by the finding that IL-10 knockout mice develop autoimmune disease. Therefore IL-10 is now being used experimentally in the treatment of autoimmune disease.

The differentiation of helper T-cells has extremely important implications for disease in humans. In animal models of helminthic diseases, the failure of some strains to mount a Th1 response results in the majority of the mice succumbing to the infection. Conversely, in other disease models production of a Th2 response results in enhanced survival whereas a Th1 response causes more damage to the host.

The TGFβ family is an important group of cytokines with diverse effects and consists of TGFβ1, β2 and β3. T-cells and monocytes mainly synthesis TGFβ1, a critical function of which is to antagonize lymphocyte responses as evidenced by TGFβ1 knockout mice. These mice die soon after birth from overwhelming immunologic disease. The disease is characterized by lymphoid and mononuclear infiltration of the heart, lung, and other tissues. They also develop infiltrates in salivary glands, pseudolymphoma, and have elevated antibody levels to dsDNA, ssDNA, and Sm ribonucleoprotein, indicating that TGFβ1 is a critical inhibitor of autoimmunity. Despite the name, TGFβs inhibit growth of many other cells, though in combination with other cytokines and growth factors they may also induce growth. TGFβs also induce collagen and fibronectin production by fibroblasts and are thought to be responsible in part for diseases characterized by fibrosis such as systemic sclerosis and pulmonary fibrosis.

Several new cytokines have been identified, but their functions are less clear. IL-14 is also known as high molecular weight B-cell growth factor and is produced by T-cells and some B-cell tumors. It is unrelated to other cytokines but shares homology with complement factor Bb. IL-16 is a lymphocyte chemoattractant factor produced by $CD8^+$ T-cells that recruits $CD4^+$ T-cells. It also inhibits HIV replication. IL-17 is a very recently identified cytokine, whose function is incompletely understood. It induces IL-6 secretion in fibroblasts, costimulates T-cell proliferation, and induces the transcription factor NFκB; a homolog of IL-17 is produced by *Herpesvirus saimiri*. Its receptor is distinct from other cytokine receptors. IL-18 induces INFγ production.

Growth and Differentiation Factors for Nonlymphoid Cells

PDGF is generated primarily by platelets, but is also made by macrophages, endothelial cells, and other cells. Epidermal growth factor (EGF) and fibroblast growth factors (FGF) are also factors that are produced by many different cells. PDGF, EGF, and FGF have diverse effects but all contribute to fibrosis and angiogenesis. The proliferation of synovial cells in rheumatoid arthritis is mediated to a large extent by these growth factors. They may also contribute to the pathogenesis of some fibrotic diseases.

Cytokine Signal Transduction

As delineated earlier, cytokines have critical functions in many aspects of the immune response. Understanding precisely how these cy-

tokines regulate cell function is important for a variety of reasons, not the least of which is that pharmacologic compounds might ultimately be devised that could manipulate the immune response in a therapeutically desirable manner.

Though cytokine signaling is still incompletely understood, we do know that ligands that bind receptors belonging to the hematopoietic cytokine receptor superfamily have several common features in signaling. One is that engagement of their receptors results in activation of a family of cytoplasmic protein tyrosine kinases known as *Janus kinases* (JAKs). Named after the two-headed Roman god because of their distinctive structure, that is, tandem kinase and pseudokinase domains, JAKs bind to cytokine receptors and become activated following cytokine binding to the receptor; different cytokines activate different JAKs (Fig. 174-2). The JAKs phosphorylate the receptor subunits on tyrosine residues and these sites can recruit proteins that have molecules termed SH2 (Src homology 2) domains, which bind phosphorylated tyrosines. A variety of adapter and signaling molecules have such domains. One such class of signaling molecules is the STAT (signal transducers and activators of transcription) family of transcription factors. These proteins bind the phosphorylated receptor subunits, become phosphorylated themselves, and then translocate to the nucleus where they regulate gene expression. Different cytokines activate different STAT proteins.

The importance of the receptors and kinases responsible for trans-

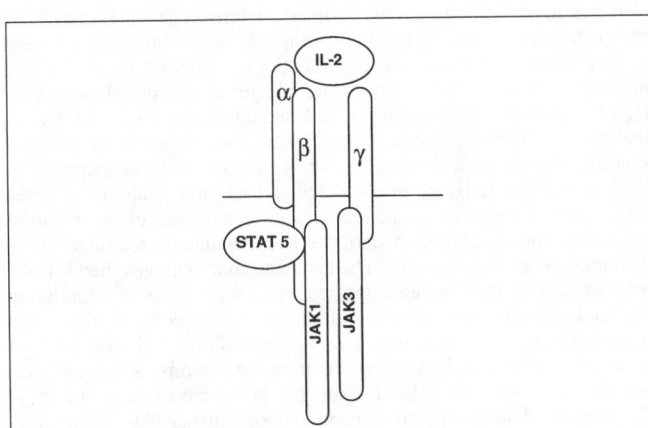

Cytokine Receptor	JAK	STAT
Hormones		
EPO, TPO, GH	JAK2	STAT5, STAT3, STAT1
βc receptors		
IL-3, IL-5, GM-CSF	JAK2	STAT5, STAT1
gp 130 receptors		
IL-6, IL-11 others	JAK1, JAK2, TYK2	STAT3, STAT1
γc receptors		
IL-2, IL-7, IL-9, IL-15	JAK3, JAK1	STAT5, STAT3, STAT1
IL-4	JAK3, JAK1	STAT6, STAT3
INF receptors		
INF α/β	TYK2 JAK1	STAT1, STAT2, STAT3, STAT4
INF γ	JAK1, JAK2	STAT1, STAT3
IL-10	JAK1, TYK2	STAT1, STAT3
other		
IL-12	JAK2, TYK2	STAT4, STAT3
IL-13	JAK1	STAT6

FIGURE 174-2 Role of JAKs and STATs in cytokine signal transduction. Cytokine receptors may be homodimeric or heterodimeric. In the case of the latter, they comprise subunits that are the products of different genes. This is the case for IL-2 receptors, which are composed of the IL-2Rb and γ subunits. These subunits are members of the hematopoietic cytokine receptor superfamily. In contrast, the IL-2Ra subunit is not. The b and γ subunits each bind a different Janus family protein tyrosine kinase or JAK, which, following cytokine binding to the receptor, becomes activated and phosphorylates the receptor. STAT family transcription factors then bind to the receptor and become phosphorylated. These in turn become activated and translocate to the nucleus and regulate gene expression. The various JAKs and STATs activated by different cytokines are listed. *EPO*, Erythropoietin; *TPO*, thrombopoietin; *GH*, growth hormone.

mitting signals from cytokine binding is underscored by two forms of severe combined immunodeficiency (SCID)(Chapter 185). One form is due to mutation of the common γ-subunit (γc), a constituent of the receptors for IL-2, IL-4, IL-7, IL-9, and IL-15. In γc deficiency, signaling via all these cytokines is disrupted, resulting in the failure of the immune system to develop and function properly. The γc subunit is found on the X chromosome and the immunodeficiency is termed XSCID. It accounts for roughly half of the cases of SCID. The γc subunit binds JAK3 and the γc cytokines (IL-2, IL-4, IL-7, IL-9, and IL-15) all activate this JAK. Deficiency of the JAK3 also leads to a form of SCID that is identical to XSCID except that girls and boys are both affected since JAK3 is not on the X chromosome.

Other cytokine receptors have different means of signal transduction. Factors like M-CSF (CSF-1), stem cell factor, PDGF, EGF, and FGF bind to receptors that are themselves tyrosine kinases (receptor tyrosine kinases). Activation of the intrinsic kinase activity is the mechanism through which signaling is initiated. The TNF receptor is structurally similar to the Fas receptor molecule and the CD40. Signaling by TNF and Fas are incompletely understood; however, both molecules have similar motifs in their intracellular domains known as "death domains." These motifs are also expressed on other molecules, some of which associate with these molecules.

FUNCTIONS OF CELL-MEDIATED IMMUNITY
Delayed Type Hypersensitivity

Cell-mediated immunity is the primary defense against intracellular pathogens and occurs as follows: at the site of the infection antigen-specific T-cells recognize foreign peptides expressed by APCs like macrophages or dendritic cells. Macrophages at this site also produce IL-12, which promotes a Th1 or cell-mediated response. The T-cells that are activated produce IL-2, IFNγ, and chemokines. Non–antigen-specific T-cells are called to the site and proliferate in response to IL-2, and IFNγ activates macrophage and vascular endothelial cells. These stimuli result in the activation and recruitment of other leukocytes from the circulation. Monocytes in particular are recruited; these differentiate to macrophages. The activated macrophages then kill the microorganism that initiated the reaction. With chronic stimulation macrophages can fuse to form multinucleate giant cells. Fibrin is also deposited causing induration. This response is termed *delayed type hypersensitivity* (DTH). Usually the immune response subsides without damage to the host tissue, but this is not necessarily the case. Cell-mediated immunity to intracellular organisms like *Mycobacterium tuberculosis* can cause significant tissue destruction and fibrosis.

Cytotoxic Lymphocytes and Viral Infections

Viral infections also induce CMI. The viral peptides are processed and expressed by MHC class I molecules. Viral infection induces IFNα/β secretion, which upregulates class I and inhibits viral replication and cell proliferation. Antigen-specific CD8+ T-cells recognize the viral peptides, become activated, and lyse the cells. Interferons also activate NK cells, which can kill virally infected cells.

DERANGEMENTS OF CELL-MEDIATED IMMUNITY

Cell-mediated immunity contributes to disease pathogenesis in a variety of ways. First, a normal immune response itself may cause considerable damage to the host in its attempt to contain a microorganism. Examples include TNF-mediated septic shock, which occurs in gram-negative septicemia; toxic shock syndrome, developing in response to staphylococcal exotoxins; and tissue damage at the site of *M. tuberculosis* infection or parasitic infestations. Likewise, granulomatous diseases like sarcoidosis and Wegener's granulomatosis may be due to CMI to an unknown organism. Arthritis following infection with a variety of organisms (reactive arthritis) is also well documented but the mechanisms underlying this response are less clear.

Immunodeficiency occurs when the key elements of the cell-mediated immune response do not function appropriately. The molecular basis of several forms of SCID have now been identified, including mutations of the γc subunit (XSCID), JAK3, and Zap-70. Other forms of immunodeficiency are discussed in Chapter 185.

Allergic responses are now recognized to be regulated by T-cells. The factors that govern the shift in the immune response from a cell-mediated response to an allergic response are now becoming better understood and should provide new avenues for the treatment of the most common form of immunologic disease, allergy. Moreover, understanding the principles that underlie Th1 versus Th2 development will have important implications in vaccine development and strategies for immunotherapy.

Finally, the advances in the understanding of the molecular basis of the cellular immune response have provided a variety of new therapies. Principal among these are cytokines or anticytokines that will be used clinically.

BIBLIOGRAPHY

Abbas AK, Lichtman AH, and Pober JS: *Cellular and molecular immunology,* ed 2, Philadelphia, 1994, Saunders.
Callard R, Gearing A: *The cytokine facts book,* London, 1994, Academic Press.
Fisher GH, Rosenberg FJ, Straus SE et al: Dominant interfering Fas gene mutations impair apoptosis in a human autoimmune lymphoproliferative syndrome, *Cell* 81:935-946, 1995.
Haas WP, Pereira, Tonegawa S: Gamma/delta cells, *Annu Rev Immunol* 11:637-686, 1993.
Johnston JA, Bacon C, Riedy MC, O'Shea JS: Signaling by the IL-2 and related receptors: JAKs, STATs and relationship to immunodeficiency, *J Leuk Biol* 60:441-452, 1996.
Kuhn R, Lohler J, Rennick D et al: Interleukin-10-deficient mice develop chronic enterocolitis, *Cell* 75:263-274, 1993.
Paul WE: Fundamental immunology, ed 2, New York, 1993, Raven Press.
Paul WE, Seder RA: Lymphocyte responses and cytokines, *Cell* 76:241-251, 1994.
Puck JM: Molecular and genetic basis of X-linked immunodeficiency disorders, *J Clin Immunol* 14:81-89, 1994.
Rosen FS, Cooper MD, Wedgwood RJ: The primary immunodeficiencies, *N Engl J Med* 333:431-440, 1995.
Samelson LE, Donovan JA, Isakov N et al: Signal transduction mediated by the T-cell antigen receptor, *Ann N Y Acad Sci* 766:157-172, 1995.
Schull MM, Ormsby I, Kier AB et al: Targeted disruption of the mouse transforming growth factor beta-1 gene results in multifocal inflammatory disease, *Nature* 359:693-699, 1992.
Yokoyama WM, Daniels BF, Seaman WE et al: A family of murine NK cell receptors specific for target cell MHC class I molecules, *Semin Immunol* 7:89-101, 1995.

CHAPTER

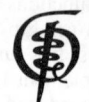

175 Complement System and Immune Complex Diseases

Robert H. Carter

The complement system is a group of soluble and cell-bound proteins (Tables 175-1 and 175-2). The system may be divided into components responsible for (1) initial recognition and labeling of targets, (2) attack functions, and (3) regulation of these processes. Potential targets include foreign molecules and organisms (viruses, bacteria, fungi), complexes of self and foreign molecules, and damaged self tissues. The basic mechanism of the system is a regulated cascade of a series of protein associations. When activated, some complement proteins acquire protease activity. Like the clotting system, the activation of a series of enzymes results in amplification of the number of molecules involved in a reaction; each protease catalyzes the cleavage of multiple molecules of the next protein in the cascade. However, the complement system has coevolved with cellular immunity, and the power of the complement system lies in its ability to recruit diverse cellular responses.

Most of the soluble complement components are synthesized in the liver and released into the circulation. Hepatic synthesis is increased in response to inflammatory cytokines, including IL-1, IL-6, and IFNγ, in the acute phase response to infection or tissue damage. Some complement proteins can be produced locally at sites of inflammation, including in the joints and brain.

Table 175-1   Complement serum (plasma) proteins

COMPONENT	MOLECULAR WEIGHT (DALTONS)	SERUM CONCENTRATION (MG/ML)
Classical		
C1q	410,000	150
C1r	90,000	100
C1s	85,000	50
C4	206,000	300
C2	117,000	15
Alternative		
Factor B	90,000	225
Factor D	25,000	3
Properdin	110,000-220,000	25
Both pathways		
C3	190,000	1200
Terminal components		
C5	185,000	85
C6	128,000	60
C7	120,000	55
C8	150,000	55
C9	79,000	60
Regulators		
C1 inhibitor	105,000	275
Factor I	88,000	35
Factor H	150,000	500
C4-binding protein	560,000	250
S protein	84,000	500
Anaphylatoxin inactivator	310,000	35
SP-40,40	80,000	50

Table 175-2   Complement membrane proteins

	MOLECULAR WEIGHT (DALTONS)	TISSUE DISTRIBUTION
Regulators		
DAF	70,000	All peripheral blood cells, epithelial and secretory cells, fibroblasts, endothelial cells
MCP	45,000-70,000	Same as DAF (but not on erythrocytes)
CD59	18,000	Same as DAF
Receptors		
CR1	190,000-280,000	Erythrocytes, monocytes/macrophages, neutrophils, B-cells, some T-cells, kidney podocytes
CR2	140,000	B-cells, some thymocytes, nasopharyngeal cells
CR3	160,000/95,000	Monocytes/macrophages, neutrophils, some lymphocytes
CR4	150,000/95,000	Monocytes/macrophages, neutrophils
C3aR	?	Mast cells, basophils
C5aR	42,000	Monocytes/macrophages, neutrophils

HISTORY AND NOMENCLATURE

More than a century ago the ability of serum to kill microorganisms was shown to require both heat-stable and heat-labile activities. The former, "antibody," was present only in the serum of individuals previously exposed to the specific pathogen. The heat-sensitive activity was present in all individuals, and was termed *complement* by Ehrlich. Over time, further physical and chemical means were used to demonstrate that this "classical" complement pathway consisted of multiple factors, which were numbered consecutively (C1, C2, etc.) as they were identified, rather than in the sequence in which they are activated in vivo. In parallel, lysis of microorganisms by serum through mechanisms that did not require antibody was also described. This activity was called *properdin,* and was also shown to involve a series of proteins, identified alphabetically as factors (factor A, factor B, etc.). Only later did students of the "classical" pathway accept that this "alternative" pathway was an intrinsic part of the complement system (factor A turned out to be C3). The initial focus on lysis of bacteria or foreign cells also resulted in underappreciation of the integration of complement with both innate and adoptive cellular immune systems.

As the enzymatic cascade proceeds, the complement factors are clipped into smaller fragments, which are identified by lower case letters (e.g., C3a, C3b, etc.). The same convention is used with the alternative factors (Ba, Bb). Activation is associated with formation of complexes of these proteins, which are written together (e.g., C3bBb) (the convention of Walport and Lachmann, using C2a to designate the smaller fragment of C2, will be used here).

COMPLEMENT ACTIVATION

The classical and alternative cascades are two mechanisms for activation of complement. They both consist of an initial recognition event, followed by formation of a multimolecular complex and a proteolytic cleavage reaction that generates a new enzyme. They both result in activation of C3, a crucial intermediate in complement activation (Fig. 175-1). The principal difference is in the mechanism of activation.

The Classical Pathway

The first step in the classical pathway is activation of C1. C1 is a complex molecule consisting of multimers of three subunits, C1q, C1r, and C1s. Each C1 molecule contains six C1q subunits. Each C1q has a globular head attached to a collagen-like stalk. In the presence of calcium the stalks come together to form a cohesive core. Within this core lie two C1r subunits and two C1s subunits. Binding of the globular heads of C1q initiates the reaction (Fig. 175-2). Although other means of binding C1q are known (e.g., C-reactive protein or certain viruses), IgM and IgG are ligands for C1q, and for this reason the classical pathway is activated following the prior interaction of antibody with foreign material. Single molecules of pentameric IgM, or multimeric arrays of IgG, but not IgA or IgE, are effective.

Mannose-binding protein (MBP) is similar to C1q in that it has multiple subunits and associates with C1r and C1s. MBP recognizes oligosaccharides present on the surface of bacteria. Binding of MBP to bacteria activates the associated C1r and C1s. This provides an antibody-independent means of activating the classical pathway. Deficiency of MBP increases susceptibility to infections during infancy when antibody levels are low. More recently MBP deficiency has been demonstrated to result in a life-long propensity to infection, demonstrating the importance of antibody-independent activation of the classical pathway.

C1r and C1s are both proteases. Binding of C1q leads to cleavage and activation of C1r and C1s, resulting in a catalytically active C1 molecule. C4 is the initial substrate for activated C1. One C1 cleaves multiple C4 molecules, producing an initial amplification of signal. C1 cleaves C4 into two fragments, C4a, which is smaller and diffuses away, and C4b. Buried within the C4b portion of the intact C4 molecule, protected from water, is a thioester between the side chains of a cysteine and a nearby glutamic acid. With cleavage of C4 and unfolding of the C4b portion, the thioester is exposed to create an unstable intermediate. This reacts with hydroxyl groups or amines in the vicinity of activation to form ester or amide linkages. The result is covalent deposition of multiple C4b molecules near the active C1 complex. C4b then acts as a scaffold and binds C2. C2 bound to C4b is also a substrate for activated C1. The larger fragment of C2, C2b, remains bound to C4b, forming a new complex, C4b2b, called a C3 convertase, that can cleave and activate multiple C3 molecules. The larger cleavage fragment of C3, C3b, also contains an internal thioester, similar to that in C4b, which becomes exposed and covalently links C3b to either the activating surface or to the C4b2b convertase itself (Fig. 175-3). The new complex, C4b2b3b, becomes active in proteolytic cleavage of a new substrate, C5.

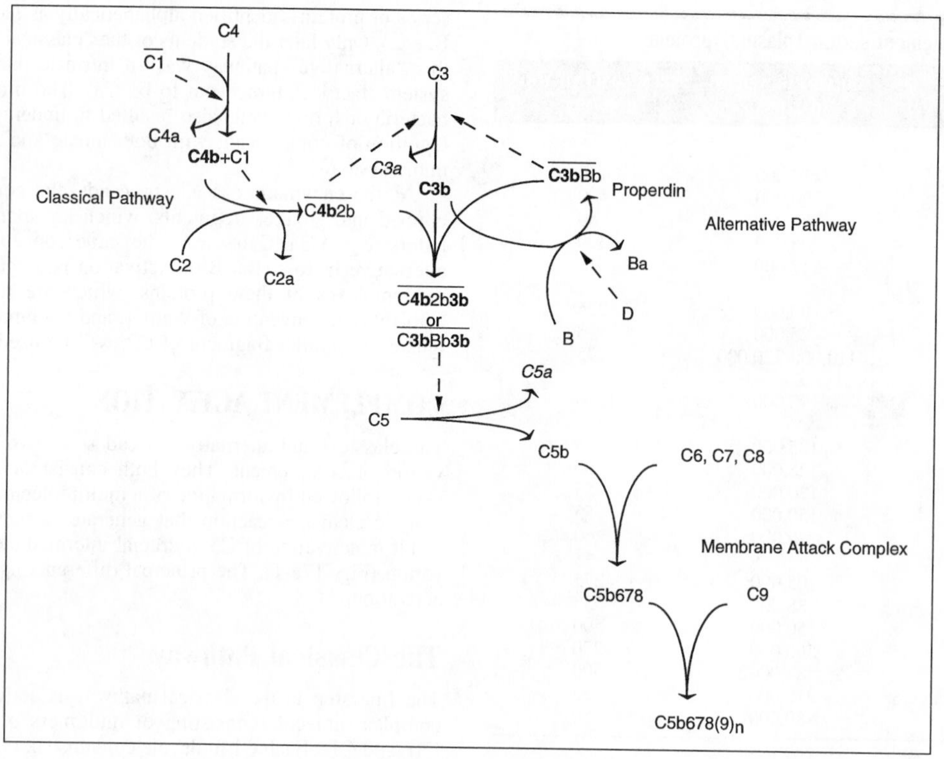

FIGURE 175-1   Summary of complement protein cascade, as described in the text. The cascade is initiated by either the classical or alternative pathway. In the classical, C1 is activated by specific binding proteins. The activated C1 cleaves C4 and C2, which form the active C4b2b complex. The alternative pathway is initiated by the spontaneous unfolding of C3 to generate a reactive intermediate that binds to local substrates. If the substrate is appropriate, factor B binds and is cleaved by factor D to generate the active C3bBb complex. Both C4b2b and C3bBb can cleave and bind additional C3 to form new complexes—C4b2b3b and C3bBb3b, respectively—both of which cleave C5 to initiate formation of the membrane attack complex. In this drawing, enzymatically active proteins or complexes are indicated by a bar above the molecule. The substrates on which these enzymes work are indicated by dashed lines. Molecules that become covalently bound to the activating surface or enzyme are indicated in bold. Soluble molecules released following enzymatic cleavage that are proinflammatory are shown in italics.

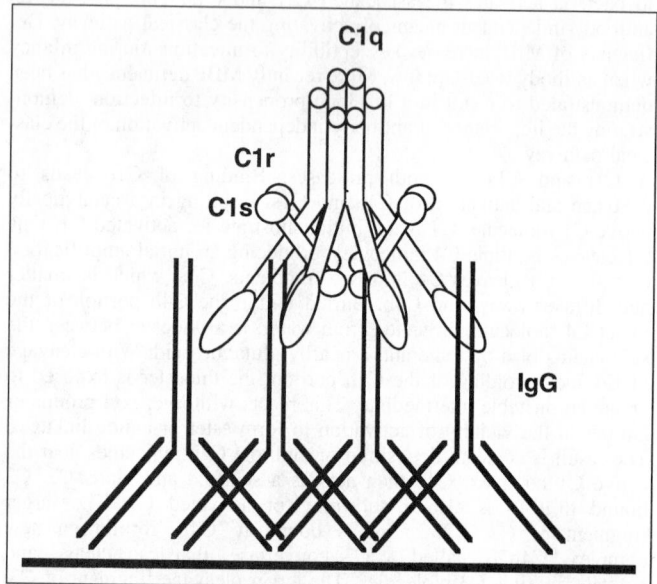

FIGURE 175-2   Model of C1 activation. The C1 consists of six C1q and two pairs each of C1r and C1s. The globular heads of C1q bind to multimeric arrays of IgG. This may induce a shift in the stalklike portions of the C1q that results in close contact between the catalytically active C1r molecules, which autoactivate and also cleave and activate C1s.

Modified from Columb M et al: *Philos Trans R Soc Lond Biol* 306:283, 1984.

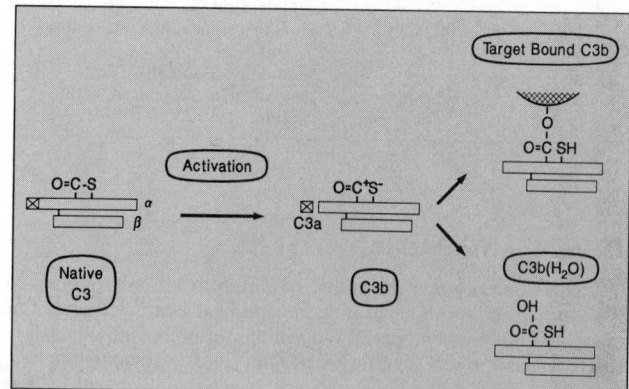

FIGURE 175-3   Activation of C3. Native C3 contains a highly reactive thioester bond (S − C = O) in its α chain. Activation of C3 by the C3 convertase liberates C3a and C3b. In this process the thioester bond within C3b is also broken, which allows metastable (a transiently reactive species) C3b to attach covalently to target surfaces or become inactive through an interaction with small molecules such as water.

Table 175-3   Regulatory proteins of complement

	MOLECULAR WEIGHT (DALTONS)	SERUM CONCENTRATION (MG/ML)	ACTION
Fluid phase			
Activation step			
C1 inhibitor	105,000	275	Inactivates C1r and C1s
Amplification step			
C4-binding protein	560,000	250	Binds C4b alone or in convertase and serves as cofactor for C4b degradation by factor I
Factor H	150,000	500	Binds C3b alone or in convertase and acts as cofactor for C3b proteolysis by factor I
Decay-accelerating factor (DAF)	70,000	Membrane	Accelerates decay of C3 convertases
Membrane cofactor protein (MCP)	45,000-70,000	Membrane	Cofactor for factor I–mediated proteolysis of C4b and C3b
Complement receptor one (CR1)	190,000-280,000	Membrane	Receptor, inhibitory profile similar to DAF and MCP
Factor I	88,000	35	Inactivates C4b or C3b
Membrane attack			
Vitronectin	84,000	500	Blocks fluid phase on MAC
CD59	18,000	Membrane	Blocks MAC on host cells
SP-40,40	80,000	50	Modulates MAC
Other			
Anaphylatoxin inactivator	305,000	35	Inactivates C4a, C3a, C5a

MAC, Membrane attack complex.

The Alternative Pathway

The alternative pathway is similar in that an initial reactive subunit binds to a surface, and then a multimolecular complex is assembled that can cleave C3. In contrast to the classical pathway, the alternative pathway is best viewed as a positive feedback loop—C3 is both the initial factor and the final substrate. C3 in serum unfolds spontaneously at a slow rate. This unfolding exposes the internal reactive thioester that binds covalently to an adjacent surface (see Fig. 175-3). The bound C3 acts as a scaffold and binds factor B. Like C2 when bound to C4, factor B bound to C3 is a substrate for a protease. The protease for factor B is factor D, which again clips off a small fragment to leave the larger fragment, Bb, bound to C3. The serum protein properdin stabilizes the C3Bb complex. The C3Bb complex, like the C4b2b complex, is a C3 convertase, and cleaves multiple additional C3 molecules. Again, C3b binds to either the convertase that produced it or to the adjacent surface. Amplification results from the association of additional factor B subunits with the C3b attached to the activating surface and cleavage of additional C3. Factor B can also associate with C3b produced by the C4b2b complex—the alternative pathway thus can amplify the C3 deposition initiated by either pathway. C3b that attaches to the C3bBb convertase creates a new convertase, C3bBb3b, which now cleaves the next protein in the complement cascade, C5. Thus either C4b2b3b or C3bBb3b can cleave C5, and both are called C5 convertases. C5 is cleaved to produce the soluble fragment C5a, and a larger fragment, C5b, which remains attached to the activating surface.

REGULATION

If unchecked, activation of complement would continue until all available C3 was consumed. To prevent this, each step is regulated (Table 175-3 and Fig. 175-4). In the classical pathway, activated C1 eventually activates and binds the inhibitor C1 INH, which blocks further C1 activity. The C4b2b complex can dissociate ("decay"), and C4b can be cleaved into inactive fragments. The further cleavage requires both a protease and a cofactor. A serum protein, C4 binding protein, displaces C2, thereby accelerating decay, and, when bound to C4b, serves as a cofactor for the cleavage of C4b by the protease factor I. These regulatory mechanisms effectively prevent fluid-phase activation of the classical pathway.

In the alternative pathway, the outcome of initial binding of auto-activated C3 is determined by a competition between binding of factor B, forming the convertase, and binding of another serum protein, factor H. Like C4 binding protein in the classical pathway, factor H not only physically disrupts the active alternative convertase complex, but also serves as a cofactor for cleavage of C3b by the protease factor I. The surface to which C3b is bound determines whether factor B or factor H can bind to the C3b. Surfaces rich in charged carbohydrates, such as sialic acid, favor binding of factor H to the C3b, blocking further amplification. Mammalian cells are rich in these types of carbohydrates, effectively blocking activation on an organism's own cells. Thus regulation of the initial activation steps of the classical and alternative pathways differs. The initial event in the classical pathway, the binding of C1q, is triggered by particular ligands, such as IgM or IgG. In contrast, the autoactivation of C3 occurs at a slow, steady rate, with attachment of C3b to whatever happens to be nearby. The outcome of this attachment depends on the competition between factor B and factor H for binding to the C3b. The carbohydrates on human cells favor factor H, resulting in cleavage and inactivation of the C3b by factor I. In contrast, most lower organisms do not possess sialic acid, favoring association of factor B with bound C3b, formation of the convertase, and further amplification. The alternative pathway represents, in contrast to antibody recognition, a nonadaptive but always present first line of defense for distinguishing foreign surfaces and labeling them as such by covalent deposition of C4b and C3b.

Cell surface proteins provide additional mechanisms for prevention of complement activation on self cells. Decay accelerating factor (CD55) promotes the dissociation of the C4bC2 and the C3bBb convertases. Membrane cofactor protein (CD46) acts as a cofactor for cleavage of C4b and C3b by factor I. These molecules are present on most cell types. Many hematogenous cells express complement receptor type 1 (CR1, CD35), which has both decay accelerating and cofactor activity. CR1 catalyzes the further degradation of C3 by factor I to produce a final fragment, C3dg, which remains attached to the activating surface.

Pathogenic organisms have adapted to evade complement attack. Some (herpes simplex, trypanosomes, *Leishmania*) express proteins that disrupt the convertases by mechanisms similar to the complement regulatory proteins. Others (human immunodeficiency virus) absorb regulatory proteins from host tissues. Measles virus uses binding to membrane cofactor protein to initiate fusion and entry into cells. Some bacteria strains have evolved sialic acid, thereby avoiding activation of the alternative pathway, and have increased virulence.

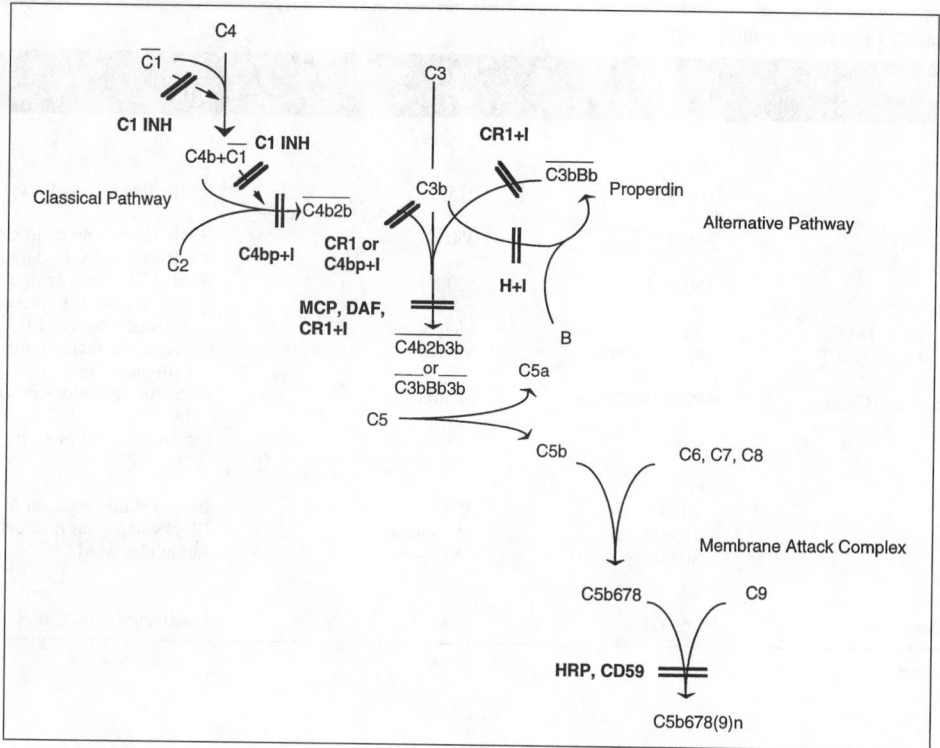

FIGURE 175-4   Regulation of complement activation. Regulatory molecules (shown in bold) and the steps they inhibit *(cross bars)* are shown on a simplified version of Figure 175-1. *C1 INH*, C1 Inhibitor; *C4bp*, C4 binding protein; *CR1*, complement receptor type 1; *MCP*, membrane cofactor protein; *DAF*, decay accelerating factor; *H*, factor H; *I*, factor I; *HRP*, homologous restriction protein.

EFFECTOR FUNCTIONS

The complement system promotes elimination of substrates by three mechanisms (Fig. 175-5). The core of the system is the covalent binding of C4b and C3b to surfaces, labeling them as targets for destruction. In this process, small soluble fragments are released that stimulate inflammation. The deposition of the terminal components of the complement system leads to formation of the "membrane attack complex" (see later discussion).

Coating for Recognition

Phagocytic cells express cell surface receptors, such as CR1 and complement receptor type 3, which bind the cleavage fragments of C3 and C4 covalently bound to activating substrates. The complement receptors promote the internalization of the material, such as bacteria, to which the C3b and C4b are bound, particularly in activated cells, as found at sites of inflammation. The process of deposition of proteins that enhance phagocytosis by binding to specific receptors on the phagocyte is termed "opsonization." Persons deficient in the complement proteins required to form the convertases or in the complement-binding proteins on phagocytes have severe problems with pyogenic infections. The contrast with the limited range of infections observed in patients with deficiencies of C5 or the later components illustrates the importance of the initial attachment of and opsonization by complement protein fragments (Chapter 186).

Complement is required for normal antibody responses when antigen is limited. Mice deficient in complement proteins show diminished antibody responses to protein antigens and fail to develop memory responses upon rechallenge. This is mediated by CR1 and complement receptor type 2 (CR2, CD21), which are found on B-lymphocytes and on cells in lymph nodes and the spleen called *follicular dendritic cells* (FDC), which serve to localize antigen for presentation to lymphocytes. While CR1 binds the larger fragments of C4 and C3, CR2 binds C3dg, the final fragment remaining bound at the site of activation. The complement proteins may serve two functions: trafficking and localization of antigen on the FDCs in the lymphoid centers, and enhancement of B-lymphocyte responses. These functions of complement also may play a role in the development of autoimmune diseases in persons with complement deficiencies.

Some pathogens have evolved surface proteins that engage complement receptors and use them to gain entry into cells. Epstein-Barr virus attaches to CR2, and measles virus attaches to membrane cofactor protein. These interactions enable the virion to fuse with the plasma membrane of the cell. In the case of Epstein-Barr virus, the expression of CR2 determines the tropism of the virus.

Release of Mediators

Multiple small fragments are generated during the proteolytic cascade of complement activation. The most potent of these is C5a, which is able to activate mast cells, basophils, and phagocytic cells, and is strongly proinflammatory. Mediators released from the mast cells and basophils result in vasospasm and increased vascular permeability, allowing cells and factors access to tissues. C5a acts both as a chemoattractant and to increase phagocytosis of opsonized material by neutrophils and macrophages. C5a also stimulates neutrophil respiratory burst and degranulation with release of mediators and enzymes that produce destruction of pathogens or tissues. In addition, C5a induces production of proinflammatory cytokines, including Il-1, IL-6, Il-8, and TNF. The C5a receptor is a seven membrane spanning protein typical of receptors associated with heterotrimeric GTP-binding proteins.

Membrane Attack Complex

In addition to release of small soluble fragments and covalent attachment of larger fragments, formation of the convertases also deposits C5b on activating surfaces. This molecule associates with lipid membranes through hydrophobic interactions. The additional complement

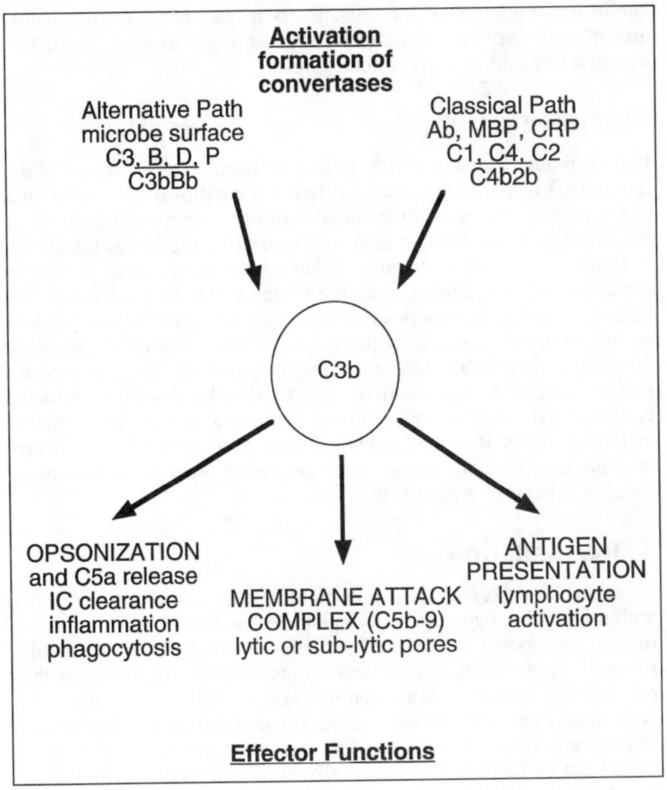

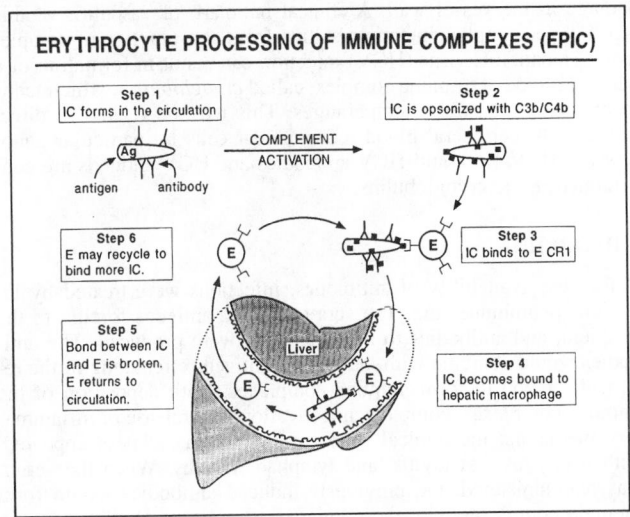

FIGURE 175-7 Schematic representation of erythrocyte *(E)* processing of immune complex *(IC)* mechanism.

Modified from Hebert LA, Cosio FG: *Kidney Int* 31:877, 1987.

IMMUNE COMPLEXES

Antibodies bind to foreign antigens through specific binding domains. As each antibody molecule is dimeric or, in the case of IgM, multimeric, one antibody molecule can bind to more than one molecule of antigen. As the response to a given antigen is polyclonal, different antibody molecules react to more than one site on an antigen. The result is a lattice of antibody and antigen molecules, particularly when there are approximately equivalent amounts of antigen and antibody, and this lattice is called an *immune complex*. Smaller complexes can be soluble within the blood. Larger complexes become insoluble, and precipitate either in tissues or along vessel walls. Other complexes may be formed around insoluble antigens already present in tissues, including those present on the surface of cells. Immune complexes activate complement, and C3b and C4b are covalently attached. Binding of C4 and C3 disrupts the lattice of large aggregates, promoting their solubilization and clearance. The C4b and C3b covalently bound to soluble complexes within the blood can bind to CR1, particularly on erythrocytes. The bound immune complexes are eliminated rapidly by reticuloendothelial cells on passage through the liver (Fig. 175-7). Insoluble complexes are targets for ingestion by phagocytic cells, attracted to the site by release of C5a. The phagocytic cells express CR1, CR3, and CR4 and receptors for the Fc portion of IgG. The complement receptors bind the fragments of C4 and C3 attached to the complexes, and Fc receptors bind the Fc regions of antibody molecules in the complex. If the phagocytic cells are properly activated, a local reaction ensues, with attempted ingestion of the opsonized material and/or degranulation and release of potentially damaging inflammatory mediators and enzymes. In infections, this promotes the isolation and destruction of the pathogen. However, in pathologic conditions complement activation can result in damage to host tissues.

PATHOLOGIC FORMATION
Infections

In most chronic infections the host mounts an immune response but is unable to eradicate the pathogen. Antibodies produced by the host combine with circulating antigens shed by the organism, forming immune complexes. Larger complexes may become insoluble and precipitate in blood vessels or be trapped in the kidney. A classic example is subacute bacterial endocarditis, which is often accompanied by glomerulonephritis and proteinuria. In chronic hepatitis B infections, immune complexes containing viral antigens deposit along blood vessel walls. Activation of complement and recruitment and activation of neutrophils results in vasculitis with inflammation and

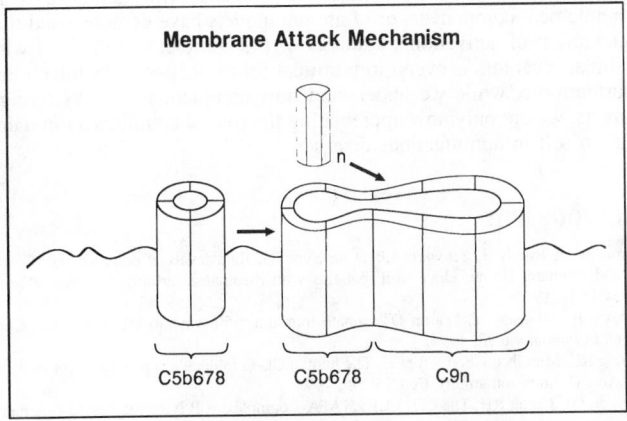

FIGURE 175-5 Overview of the activation and effector functions of complement. The classical (*Ab*, antibody; *MBP*, mannose binding protein; *CRP*, C-reactive protein) or alternative (*B*, factor B; *D*, factor D; *P*, properdin) pathways generate C3 convertases. These generate C3b. The C3b can function in opsonization and trafficking of immune complexes *(IC)* for activation of phagocytes and lymphocytes, respectively, and also forms the C5 convertase to induce formation of the membrane attack complex.

FIGURE 175-6 Mechanism of action of the membrane attack complex. When C8 joins C5b67, a small pore or channel is formed in the membrane. Binding of multiple C9 components accelerates lysis.

Modified from Frank MM. In Samter M, editor: *Immunological diseases*, vol I, Boston, 1988, Little, Brown.

components, C6, C7, and C8 form a complex with C5b partially within the membrane (Fig. 175-6). Multiple copies of the final protein, C9, associate with the C5b678 complex. If enough C9 attach, a pore through the membrane is formed, permitting leakage of salts and water and lysis of the cell. A cell surface protein, homologous restriction factor (CD59), prevents deposition of the membrane attack complex on our own tissues. In humans, the essential role of the terminal complement components is prevention of Neisserial infections.

damage in the vessel wall. A clinical hallmark of vasculitis of this type is hypocomplementemia resulting from consumption of complement. Hepatitis C virus (HCV) infection can result in formation of a particular type of immune complex, called *cryoglobulins,* which tends to precipitate at cooler temperatures. This may be related to direct infection of peripheral blood mononuclear cells by particular genotypes of HCV. Both anti-HCV antibodies and HCV antigens are concentrated in the cryoglobulins.

Iatrogenic

Before the availability of antibiotics, infections were treated by injections of immune sera. The sera contained antigens foreign to the recipient, and antibodies to these antigens were produced. The antibodies would combine with the foreign antigens circulating in the recipient's blood to form immune complexes. With deposition of the immune complexes, complement activation, and release of inflammatory mediators, the clinical syndrome of serum sickness appeared, with fever, rash, synovitis, and lymphadenopathy. When the serum was readministered, the previously induced antibodies would form immune complexes with the administered antigens locally either in the tissue at the site of injection or in the blood vessels adjacent to it. Complement activation would follow. Neutrophils would be recruited and bind to the complexes. A local inflammatory reaction would be induced ("Arthus's reaction"). Arthus's reaction was initially described as a complement-dependent result of local administration of foreign antigen to which the recipient had circulating antibodies. Interaction of Fc receptors on neutrophils with immunoglobulin in the deposited immune complexes is also required for this type of inflammatory reaction.

Injections of immune sera are now largely a thing of the past. However, antibodies may be produced against drugs, and continued administration can result in formation of immune complexes. With the development of new biologic therapeutic agents, Arthus's reactions and serum sickness may again become a problem.

Autoimmune

A similar inflammatory reaction resulting from activation of complement by locally formed or deposited immune complexes may be responsible for part of the tissue damage in many diseases, including most organs of the body. The autoantibodies with the most clinically apparent effects are those against blood cells, including red cells and platelets. Binding of these antibodies overcomes the regulatory mechanisms, and complement is activated. This results in destruction of these cells, by either phagocytosis or lysis, and anemia or thrombocytopenia ensues. Drugs may bind to these cells, and antibodies against the drugs may induce complement activation and elimination of the cells. Diseases are also caused by antibodies to noncirculating self-antigens in tissues. In Goodpasture's syndrome, antibodies are produced against basement membrane. Immune complexes form at sites where these antibodies bind, and these activate complement. The lung and the kidney are most dramatically affected, resulting in hemoptysis and glomerulonephritis.

Circulating immune complexes containing a variety of self antigens occur in systemic lupus erythematosus. Some of these become trapped in the kidney. Complexes of DNA and anti-DNA antibodies are characteristic of this disease and have increased propensity to become deposited, due in part to high amounts of charge on both the antibody and the antigen. Trapped complexes form "lumpy-bumpy" deposits seen on immunofluorescence staining of kidney sections, in contrast to the linear deposits seen when antibody reacts with tissue antigens. Immune complexes can also become trapped in other tissues that have high rates of blood flow, such as the choroid plexus in the brain. The immune complexes may also contribute to the abnormal antibodies produced in lupus through enhanced activation of B-lymphocytes by the bound complement fragments.

Rheumatoid factors are antibodies that bind to the Fc regions of other antibodies. Rheumatoid factors enhance lattice formation in immune complexes, increasing the likelihood of precipitation. Rheumatoid factors are increased in patients with rheumatoid arthritis, and likely contribute to the small vessel vasculitis that occurs in this disease. Rheumatoid factor production and complement activation occur in the synovium of inflamed joints in patients with rheumatoid arthritis and may contribute to pathogenesis and to joint destruction by attracting and activating neutrophils.

Physiologic

Injured tissue loses the ability to protect itself from complement activation. This marks the damaged tissue for removal and contributes to the process that leads to eventual healing. However, in some cases this leads to more damage than was caused by the initial insult. For example, reopening a recently stenosed coronary artery results in deposition of complement along the vessel wall in tissue that was previously ischemic but not dead. Neutrophils are recruited and produce an inflammatory reaction, with vessel occlusion and the eventual infarction of this tissue. Activation fragments of complement proteins induce increased expression of adhesion molecules on endothelial cells. Sublytic MAC complex formation may also provide a signal to endothelial cells. In animal models of ligation and reperfusion of coronary arteries, blocking complement activation reduces the area of infarction following reperfusion.

Transplantation

Liver or heart xenographs transplanted into humans are rejected within hours by a complement-dependent reaction *(hyperacute rejection)*. This process can be inhibited experimentally by either soluble molecules or by creating transgenic animal donors expressing on their cells human complement regulatory proteins that block complement activation. In animal models, xenografts under these conditions have relatively prolonged survival. Cell-mediated immune mechanisms would not be inhibited. Conceptually, such xenografts could be used as a bridge to allow patients undergoing acute organ failure a chance to survive long enough for recovery or transplantation with human organs.

SUMMARY

The initial thrust of the study of complement was to define the molecules that were responsible for lysis of foreign target cells. The complement components that make up the lytic pathway are now well characterized. However, studies of humans with deficiencies in complement components or of animal models have demonstrated that interaction of activation fragments of the complement proteins with cellular receptors is even more critical for protection from infections. Furthermore, while we understand how complement attacks foreign targets, we are only now appreciating the role of complement in damage to self in noninfectious diseases.

BIBLIOGRAPHY

Brodeur JP, Ruddy S, Schwartz LB et al: Synovial fluid levels of complement SC5b-9 and fragment Bb are elevated in patients with rheumatoid arthritis, *Arthritis Rheum* 34:1531, 1991.

Brown E, Atkinson JP, Fearon DT: Innate immunity: 50 ways to kill a microbe, *Curr Opin Immunol* 6:73, 1994.

Dorig RE, Marcil A, Chopra A et al: The human CD46 molecule is a receptor for measles virus (Edmonston strain), *Cell* 75:295, 1993.

Fearon DT, Carter RH: The CD19/CR2/TAPA-1 complex of B lymphocytes: linking natural to acquired immunity, *Ann Rev Immunol* 13:127, 1995.

Frank MM: Complement system. In Frank MM, Samter M, editors: *Samter's immunolgoic diseases,* Boston, 1995, Little, Brown.

Kinoshita T: Biology of complement: the overture, *Immunol Today* 12:291, 1991.

Lozada C, Levin RI, Huie M et al: Identification of C1q as the heat-labile serum cofactor required for immune complexes to stimulate endothelial expression of the adhesion molecules E-selectin and intercellular and vascular cell adhesion molecules 1, *Proc Nat Acad Sci* 92:8378, 1995.

Miletic VD, Frank MM: Complement-immunoglobulin interactions, *Curr Opin Immunol* 7:41, 1995.

Moore FD Jr. Therapeutic regulation of the complement system in acute injury states, *Adv Immunol* 56:267, 1994.

Thieblemont N, Delibrias C, Fischer E et al: Complement enhancement of HIV infection is mediated by complement receptors, *Immunopharmacol* 25:87, 1993.

Volanakis JE: Transcriptional regulation of complement genes, *Ann Rev Immunol* 13:277, 1995.

Walport MJ, Lachmann PJ: Complement. In Lachmann PJ, Peters K, Rosen FS et al, editors: *Clinical aspects of immunolgy,* Boston, 1993, Blackwell Scientific.

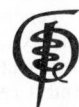

176   Immediate Hypersensitivity

Stephen I. Wasserman

In humans the term *immediate-type hypersensitivity reaction* refers to a collection of signs and symptoms comprising respiratory, cutaneous, cardiovascular, gastrointestinal, and systemic responses to a variety of pharmacologically active proinflammatory substances called *mediators*. These reactions require the concerted interaction of sensitizing antibody, specific target cells, and mediators. The most compelling evidence for their role in human pathobiology has been derived from observations in the skin and lung. Studies of patients with allergic asthma demonstrated that inhalation of a specific antigen induced both immediate and delayed (4 to 12 hours) airway dysfunction. Both early and late responses were independent of immunoglobulin G (IgG) antibody and could be abolished by pretreatment with disodium cromoglycate, a drug that can prevent mast cell–mediator release.

More elaborate experiments in the skin have demonstrated that intracutaneous administration of specific antigen to sensitized individuals or of antibody to human IgE can induce both early wheal-and-flare reactions and late inflammatory responses. Passive transfer of purified IgE antibody can prepare the skin of unsensitized hosts for antigen-induced early and late reactions. The early skin lesion is a classic pruritic wheal and flare, whereas the later response is inflammatory, manifested as a poorly demarcated erythematous swelling that persists for 4 to 24 hours. The early lesion reveals superficial edema formation with mast cell degranulation. The later inflammatory lesion consists of these elements and also a profound tissue infiltration comprising neutrophils, eosinophils, basophils, mononuclear leukocytes, and lymphocytes. In addition, vascular damage and even frank necrotizing vasculitis may ensue. In the lung, early responses are manifested by hyperemia, edema, and release of mucus. Later, infiltration by CD4-bearing T-lymphocytes and eosinophils is prominent. Any formulation of immediate-type hypersensitivity reactions therefore must also explain these late reactions.

Both the severity and the type of manifestations of either immediate or late reactions may reflect the concentration of the responsible reactants, the complex regulatory interactions involving target tissue sensitivities, or the availability and degradation of mediators. Although several mechanisms exist for generation of individual mediators, this does not diminish their importance in immediate hypersensitivity reactions but rather extends their potential contribution to non–IgE-mediated inflammatory disorders.

ANTIBODIES RESPONSIBLE FOR IMMEDIATE HYPERSENSITIVITY

Antibodies responsible for immediate hypersensitivity reactions (termed *reagins*) first were described by Prausnitz and Küstner in 1921, but protein purification was not accomplished until more than 40 years later. IgE is the reaginic antibody in humans. This unique antibody is composed of two light chains, κ or λ, and two ε heavy chains linked by disulfide bridges. IgE is a glycoprotein (190,000 daltons, 8 S sedimentation coefficient) digested by papain into two Fab′ fragments possessing the antigen-binding sites and an Fc fragment responsible for the special cell-binding characteristics of this immunoglobulin (Ig) class. As little as 4×10^{-5} ng antibody nitrogen/ml of human IgE can sensitize human tissues for a reversed passive anaphylactic reaction. This sensitization is caused by the ability of the Fc portion of IgE to bind tightly and persistently (half-life, 8 to 14 days) to specific high-affinity receptors (FcεRI). A second, lower-affinity receptor for the Fc portion of IgE, FcεRII, has been identified on lymphocytes (CD23).

The production of IgE antibody is under complex regulatory control. Genetic influences are important. Most humans have less than 100 units IgE/ml of serum, but IgE levels are higher in atopic indi-

viduals and their families. In animals, IgE synthesis requires both T- and B-lymphocytes. Removal of CD8 bearing T-cells by cytotoxic drugs or irradiation enhances IgE responses. Human T-lymphocytes secrete important regulatory factors for IgE synthesis. Interleukin 4 (IL-4) and 13 promote, and interferon γ (IFNγ) inhibits B-cell production of IgE. IgE-rich responses are thought to result from a specific helper T-cell population (Th2) that generates IL-4 but not IFNγ, whereas Th1 lymphocytes produce IFNγ but not IL-4 and inhibit IgE production. In the course of an immune response, CD4⁺ T-cells and B-cells bind via interaction of CD40 and CD40 ligand. In the presence of IL-4 (and probably IL-13) a switch from IgM to IgE synthesis occurs.

CELLS RESPONSIBLE FOR IMMEDIATE HYPERSENSITIVITY
Mast Cells and Basophils

The *mast cell* (Fig. 176-1) is a tissue cell derived from CD34⁺ bone marrow cells. They are present in humans at concentrations of 1 to 10×10^6 cells/g of tissue, prominently in submucosal loose connective tissue around blood vessels. Mast cells are also present in the mucosa of the upper and lower respiratory tract, in the gastrointestinal and genitourinary systems, and in skin; they also have been found free in the bronchial lumen. Production of mast cells in humans is driven by stem cell factor (SCF, kit-ligand). Their migration and life span are uncertain.

Two types of mast cells have been identified in humans. A *connective tissue* subset of mast cells predominates in skin and serosa, and a second, a *mucosal* subtype, is rich in the gastrointestinal mucosa and alveolar walls; its precursor matures under the influence of the T-lymphocytes. Factors produced by fibroblasts have been suggested to induce connective tissue mast cell differentiation. The connective tissue mast cell contains tryptic and chymotryptic proteases, a cathepsin G–like enzyme, and carboxypeptidase A. The mucosal mast cell lacks chymase. Individual mast cells contain several hundred metachromatically staining granules with a distinctive subgranular architecture. The mast cell plasma membrane is reduplicated, and within it reside 50,000 to 300,000 receptors for the Fc portion of IgE, functionally defined receptors for the anaphylatoxins (C3a, C5a), and SCF.

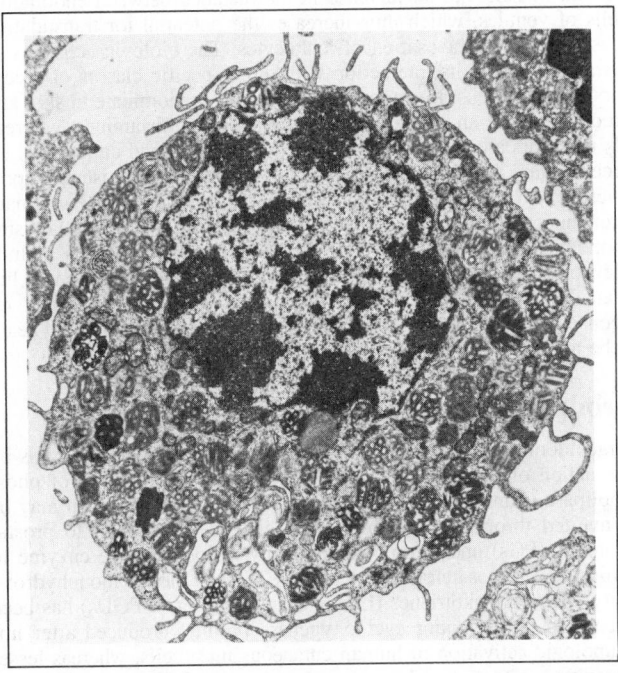

FIGURE 176-1   Electron micrograph of a human mast cell. Note the numerous membrane projections and presence of intragranular structures of mast cell. From Caulfield JP et al: *J Cell Biol* 84:299, 1980.

Basophils are bone marrow–derived polymorphonuclear leukocytes (PMNs) and are most closely related to eosinophils. Basophils and mast cells originate and develop independently. Basophils possess numerous metachromatically staining granules, but the granules are amorphous in appearance and lack tryptase and chymase. Receptors for the Fc portion of IgE, as well as for C3a and C5a, are present; SCF receptors are absent.

The antigen activation of mast cells and basophils requires cross-linking of two adjacent IgE molecules, which translates through the membrane receptor a signal that initiates degranulation. The sequence of noncytolytic secretory events that results in degranulation includes adenyl cyclase activation, tyrosine phosphorylation, phospholipase activation, arachidonic acid liberation, calcium influx, granule dissolution, granule-to-granule membrane fusion, granule-plasma membrane fusion, and finally, discharge of granule constituents to the external milieu. After antigen activation of sensitized mast cells, this entire sequence is completed in less than 5 minutes, but it requires 10 to 30 minutes in basophils. In addition to being degranulated by antigen and anaphylatoxin, connective tissue–type mast cells may be degranulated by such nonimmunologic stimuli as highly charged antibiotics, radiocontrast media, opiates, various neuropeptides, and adenosine triphosphate (ATP).

MEDIATORS

The activation and degranulation of mast cells and basophils cause the release of preformed, granule-associated *(primary)* mediators and the generation and release of unstored *(secondary)* mediators. Table 176-1 lists these mediators in terms of function. Such mediator functions include smooth muscle reactivity, chemotactic potential, enzymatic activity, and structural properties. Mediators also include a group of cytokines.

Smooth Muscle–Reactive Mediators

Histamine, the decarboxylation product of histidine, is ionically bound to the proteoglycan-protein backbones of mast cell and basophil granules. Histamine is displaced by sodium exchange in the extracellular fluid. Histamine is catabolized either by oxidative deamination (histaminase) or by combined demethylation and oxidative deamination (histamine *N*-methyltransferase plus monoamine oxidase). The effects of histamine are expressed as a constriction of smooth muscle and an increase in the distance between endothelial cells of venules, which thus increases the potential for transudation of serum and extravasation of leukocytes. The biologic activities of histamine follow its interaction with three specific classes of receptors on target cells. Receptors designated H_1 predominate in skin and smooth muscle and are inhibited by classic antihistamines, whereas H_2 receptors are selectively blocked by ranitidine and cimetidine. H_3 receptors are defined by selective agonists and regulate histamine production and release, particularly in the nervous system. Pulmonary bronchoconstriction, vasodilation, and increased cyclic guanosine monophosphate (cGMP) are H_1 effects, whereas H_2 effects include elevations in gastric acid secretion and cAMP and inhibition of human lymphocyte–mediated cytotoxicity. The wheal-and-flare response to histamine in the skin, adverse effects on the heart, and headache are caused by a combined effect of H_1 and H_2 receptors.

Products of Arachidonic Acid Oxidation

Arachidonic acid is mobilized from cell membrane phospholipids by the action of phospholipase A_2 or by the concerted action of phospholipase C and diacylglycerol lipase. Arachidonic acid then may be converted through a cyclooxygenase-dependent pathway to prostaglandins (PGs) and thromboxanes or by a lipoxygenase enzyme to hydroperoxyeicosatetraenoic acid (HPETE) and then to monohydroxy fatty acids or leukotrienes (LTs). *Prostaglandin D_2* (PGD_2) has been identified as the major cyclooxygenase product produced after immunologic activation of human cutaneous mast cells, whereas lesser amounts are generated by mucosal mast cells. PGD_2 constricts both animal and human smooth muscle, and it causes intense bronchoconstriction in asthmatic persons. PGD_2 is a potent inhibitor of platelet

activation and is thought to be responsible for flushing and hypotensive episodes in patients with mastocytosis. It can cause wheal-and-flare reactions in skin and potentiates chemotactic responses induced by other mediators (see later discussion).

The action of a 5-lipoxygenase enzyme found in mast cells, eosinophils, neutrophils, and mononuclear leukocytes generates 5-HPETE, which then is further metabolized to a monohydroxy fatty acid (5-HETE) or to leukotriene A_4 (LTA_4). LTA_4 is further metabolized to the chemoattractant dihydroxy fatty acid LTB_4 (mast cells, neutrophils), or by the addition of the tripeptide glutathione (cys-gly-glu), to LTC_4 (eosinophils, mast cells). Further metabolism of LTC_4 by γ-glutamyl transpeptidase to LTD_4 and by other peptidases, including a neutrophil dipeptidase to LTE_4, occurs. Three molecules (LTC_4, LTD_4, LTE_4) make up the *slow-reacting substance of anaphylaxis* (SRS-A).

These LTs are prominent products of human mast cells basophils and eosinophils. They interact with a specific receptor, and the sulfidopeptide and carbonyl domains appear most important to their function. LTs are degraded by oxidant reactions. The sulfidopeptide LTs are important constrictors of smooth muscle and induce bronchospasm, wheal-and-flare vasopermeability reactions, increased mucus release, and decreased cardiac performance, whereas LTB_4 depresses lymphocyte function. In most assays, LTD_4 is the most potent and LTE_4 the least active leukotriene. LTE_4 is thought to induce prolonged, nonspecific bronchial hyperreactivity.

Platelet-activating factor (PAF) is a unique phospholipid generated from mast cells by IgE-dependent mechanisms. Human macrophages, neutrophils, and eosinophils can also generate this molecule. Its structure is 1-*O*-acyl-2-acetyl-*sn*-glycerol-3-phosphorylcholine. The molecule is most active when the acyl group is C16 or C18; removal of the acetyl group or the choline moiety totally inactivates PAF. Thus PAF can be degraded by an acid-labile serum acetylhydrolase or by several phospholipases. PAF is capable of inducing aggregation of human platelets and secretion of their serotonin. In animals, PAF causes sequestration of platelets in the lung or skin and is a potent hypotensive agent. In humans, PAF is a strong bronchoconstrictor and can induce wheal-and-flare vasopermeability responses. Inhalation of PAF also induces long-lasting bronchial hyperreactivity to nonspecific irritants. In animals, PAF also produces neutrophil activation and aggregation, hypotension, and vascular collapse, as well as adverse effects on cardiac performance. Pulmonary mechanical changes depend on platelet activation, whereas the other effects of PAF do not.

The nucleoside *adenosine* is released from activated mast cells in vitro and is increased in the blood of humans after antigen-provoked bronchospasm. Adenosine is a potent inhibitor of platelet activation, enhances IgE-mediated mast cell responses, induces bronchospasm in asthmatic but not in normal individuals, is a potent coronary vasodilator, and can alter lymphocyte function. It is removed by its active uptake into cells or by destruction via adenosine deaminase. Adenosine interaction with receptors is prevented by xanthines, and its uptake is inhibited by dipyridamole.

Chemotactic Mediators

Eosinophil Chemotactic Factors. A low-molecular-weight peptide (300 to 500 daltons) has been identified in anaphylactic supernatants of challenged human lung, in isolated human lung mast cells, and in the circulations of patients with experimentally induced physical urticaria and antigen-induced bronchospasm. Also, human mast cells contain preformed, immunologically releasable, chemotactic factors (1500 to 3000 daltons) with specificity for eosinophilic PMNs. Factors of similar molecular weight and chemotactic specificity have been identified in the circulation of patients after experimental induction of physical urticaria or antigen-provoked bronchospasm.

High-Molecular-Weight Neutrophil Chemotactic Factor.

HMW-NCF has been described in human lung fragments, in leukemic basophils, and in the sera of patients with physical urticaria or asthma after physical or antigen challenge. HMW-NCF is a 660,000-dalton neutral protein that attracts and deactivates neutrophils.

Table 176-1   Vasoactive mediators

MEDIATOR	STRUCTURAL CHARACTERISTICS	FUNCTION	INHIBITION	INACTIVATION	DISEASE ASSOCIATION
Histamine (mast cells)	β-Imidazolyl-ethylamine (111 daltons)	Contracts smooth muscle Increases vascular permeability Stimulates suppressor T-lymphocytes (H_2) Generates prostaglandins Enhances (H_1) or inhibits (H_2) chemotaxis Elevates cAMP (H_2) and cGMP (H_1)	H_1 and H_2 antihistamines	Histamine (diamine oxidase) or histamine N-methyltransferase	Asthma Allergic rhinitis Urticaria Anaphylaxis Mastocytosis
Slow-reacting substance of anaphylaxis, or SRS-A (mast cells, monocytes, eosinophils)	Leukotrienes C = 5 (S)-OH-6(R)-S-glutathionyl-7,9-*trans*,11,14-*cis*-eicosatetraenoic acid D = 5(S)OH-6(R)-S-cysteinylglycyl-7,9-*trans*,11,14-*cis*-eicosatetraenoic acid E = 5(S)-OH-6(R)-S-cysteinyl-7,9-*trans*,11,14-*cis*-eicosatetraenoic acid	Increases mucus production Contracts smooth muscle Increases vascular permeability Synergistic with histamine Generates prostaglandins Vasodepressor Cutaneous Vasoconstriction (C) Vasodilation (D, E) Increases mucus production Depresses cardiac performance	FPL-55712	Peroxidases Lipoxygenase Peroxides Peptidases Hypochlorous acid	Anaphylaxis
Platelet-activating factor, or PAF (neutrophils, monocytes, mast cells, eosinophils)	1-*O*-acyl-2-acetyl-*sn*-glycerol-3-phosphorylcholine	Release of platelet amines Platelet and neutrophil aggregation Sequestration of platelets Decrease in blood pressure Bronchospasm Increased vasopermeability	Unknown	Phospholipases Acetylhydrolase	Anaphylaxis Physical urticaria
Prostaglandins D_2 (mast cells)	C_{20} fatty acids	Contracts smooth muscle Vasodepressor Elevates cAMP	Synthesis blocked by nonsteroidal antiinflammatory agents	Specific dehydrogenases	Asthma Allergic rhinitis Mastocytosis
E_2 (many cell types)		Relaxes smooth muscle, elevates cAMP			
$F_{2\alpha}$ (many cell types)		Lowers cAMP, contracts smooth muscle			
I_2 (many cell types)		Elevates cAMP, inhibits platelet aggregation, contracts smooth muscle			
Thromboxane A_2 (many cell types)		Contracts smooth muscle Stimulates platelet aggregation			
Endoperoxides (G_2, H_2) (many cell types)		Contract smooth muscle			
Prostaglandin-generating factor	Peptide (about 1400 daltons)	Induces prostaglandin production from surrounding cells			
Adenosine	Nuceloside	Inhibits platelet aggregation Enhances mast cell preformed-mediator release Constricts bronchial smooth muscle in asthmatic persons Coronary vasodilation	Xanthines	Adenosine deaminase	Asthma

cAMP, Cyclic adenosine monophosphate; *cGMP,* cyclic guanosine monophosphate.

Other Chemotactic Factors. Chemotactic factors with specificity for both neutrophilic and eosinophilic PMNs can be generated by the lipoxygenase-dependent pathway of arachidonic acid metabolism. PAF is also a potent leukoattractant, particularly for eosinophils. Less well characterized are factors chemotactic for T-lymphocytes, B-lymphocytes, monocytes, and basophils.

MAST CELL ENZYMES AND PROTEOGLYCANS
Tryptase

A preformed enzyme, *tryptase* is released subsequent to antigen challenge of IgE-sensitized human mast cells. This enzyme has a tryptic specificity and can cleave kininogen, C3, and other proteins susceptible to tryptic proteases. Tryptase is not inhibited by serum antitrypsins and is stabilized by its ionic binding to heparin. It is present in all human mast cells and may act as a smooth muscle mitogen. A captopril-insensitive, chymotryptic protease capable of generating angiotensin is present in connective tissue–type human mast cells. This enzyme stimulates mucus secretion. A cathepsin G–like protease and a carboxypeptidase are also present in connective tissue mast cells.

Lysosomal Enzymes

Myeloperoxidase, superoxide dismutase, arylsulfatases A and B, β-glucuronidase, hexosaminidases, and amino peptidase have been identified in isolated human or rat mast cells. These lysosomal enzymes can degrade ground substance proteoglycans.

Heparin

This sulfated, metachromatic mucopolysaccharide has been identified in the mast cells of human lung and skin. Human heparin interacts with human antithrombin to accelerate anticoagulation. Heparin may interfere with several complement function, liberates lipoprotein lipase, binds to platelet factor IV and to tryptase to prevent its inactivation, and is a potent endothelial growth factor.

Chondroitin 4-Sulfate and 6-Sulfate Proteoglycans

These proteoglycans predominate in human basophils. In mucosal mast cells, highly sulfated varieties of chondroitin sulfate also are present.

Cytokines

Human mast cells have been demonstrated to synthesize and release a variety of cytokines and growth factors, including tumor necrosis factor α (TNF-α); interleukins 3, 4, 5, and 6; and granulocyte-macrophage colony-stimulating factor (GM-CSF). Il-4 has also been identified in human basophils. A role for these cytokines has been postulated in mast cell growth and differentiation; in eosinophil growth, maintenance, recruitment, and activation; in IgE synthesis; and in fibrosis. The pattern of mast cell cytokine synthesis is similar to that of Th2 helper T-lymphocytes and may be an important contributor to allergic inflammation, such as that noted in asthma (see Chapter 188).

SUMMARY

The relevance of the preformed and newly generated mediators released by IgE-dependent and IgE-independent activation of mast cells and basophils to human immediate hypersensitivity reactions has been shown (1) by analysis of their varied and potent biologic effects using purified mediators, (2) by identification of mediators in blood or tissue in human allergic disorders, and (3) by the known pathophysiology of allergic disease.

Mediators have the ability to induce both immediate-onset short-lived, and delayed-onset prolonged inflammatory events. The former, presumably caused by the smooth muscle-reactive mediators, are exemplified by wheal-and-flare reactions, acute decrease in blood pressure, and smooth muscle contraction of the type noted in gastrointes-

tinal disturbances or airway dysfunction. The more persistent inflammatory reactions represent a response to the concerted effect of enhanced permeability, activation of other amplification mediators (complement, clotting, fibrinolytic, and kinin-generating systems), leukocyte infiltration resulting from chemotactic mediators, and cytokine release and tissue destruction by active enzymes. A good example is late-onset bronchospasm. The prolonged effect of antigen-induced inflammation may explain the chronic abnormalities seen in patients with asthma (bronchial hyperreactivity, mucus formation, smooth muscle hypertrophy, cellular infiltration, subepithelial fibrosis, epithelial damage) and also may explain the lack of immediate correlation between antigen exposure and asthmatic response noted in many patients.

BIBLIOGRAPHY

Costa JJ, Galli SJ: Mast cells and basophils. In Rich RR et al, editors: *Clinical immunology: principles and practice,* St Louis, 1995, Mosby.
Irani A, Schwartz LB: Mast cell heterogeneity, *Clin Exp Allergy* 19:143, 1989.
Ishizaka K: Control of IgE synthesis. In Middleton EE et al, editors: *Allergy: principles and practice,* ed 4, St Louis, 1992, Mosby.
Plaut M et al: Mast cell lines produce lymphokines in response to crosslinkage of FcERI or to calcium ionophore, *Nature* 339:64, 1989.
Valent P, Bettelheim P: The human basophil, *Crit Rev Oncol Hematol* 10:327, 1990.
Wasserman SI: Mediators of immediate hypersensitivity, *J Allergy Clin Immunol* 72:101, 1983.

CHAPTER

177 Tolerance and Autoimmunity

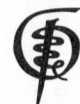

Alfred D. Steinberg

It has long been appreciated that autoimmune diseases involve some abnormality in normal self-tolerance. Advances in molecular immunology have provided some insights into the basic mechanisms by which tolerance is normally induced and maintained, as well as possible defects that predispose to impaired tolerance. The studies indicate that there are several partially overlapping mechanisms that play a role in tolerance induction and maintenance. An abnormality in one critical mechanism might predispose to the loss of tolerance, whereas an abnormality in another might not unless other factors stress the system. The following represents the present state of knowledge at the crossroads between descriptive phenomena and mechanistic explanation.

Since autoimmune diseases are characterized by immune responses against self antigens (autoantigens), the development of such anti-self responses must result from either a breakdown of regulatory processes that normally prevent autoimmunity or a bypass of those processes. Regulatory mechanisms that guard against autoimmune responses include "central tolerance," which operates largely through deletion of self-reactive lymphocytes in the organ in which the lymphocytes are generated (the thymus for T-cells), and peripheral tolerance, which involves a number of mechanisms including deletion and various forms of downregulation. These regulatory processes that prevent autoimmunity are collectively termed "self-tolerance." Numerous immune interactions relevant to tolerance are shown in Box 177-1.

Bypassing normal immune regulation can occur when, for example, the immune system is indifferent to a cryptic portion of a self antigen. If a cryptic part of the molecule induces an immune response, the body might, secondarily, react to additional portions of the self antigen. This spreading of the immune response may produce an autoimmune response to critical portions of the self antigen. A related bypass of immune regulation may occur when antiself B-cells are stimulated by nearby T-cells that are participating in another immune response (this has been termed a *bystander effect*).

One autoimmune disorder, systemic lupus erythematosus (SLE),

BOX 177-1
Factors that decrease or increase self-reactivity

I. Processes that tend to limit self-reactivity
Intrathymic deletion of thymocytes reactive with certain self-antigens
Deletion of peripheral T-cells reactive with certain self antigens
Downregulation of peripheral T-cells reactive with certain self antigens
Suppression of certain self-reactive T-cells by cells, factors
Deletion or downregulation of certain self-reactive B-cells by
  Interaction with antigen in a nonimmunogenic fashion
  T-cells, NK cells, dendritic cells
  Soluble factors
Clearance of self antigens and immune complexes by natural antibodies, complement, and the reticuloendothelial system

II. Factors that may augment self-reactivity
Defects in any of the processes listed in I.
  Impaired tolerance mechanisms
  Complement deficiencies
  Impaired deletion mechanisms (e.g., genetic inability to produce cell surface receptors necessary for apoptosis [Fas in *lpr/lpr* mice]—or the ligand to such a receptor [Fas-ligand in *gld/gld* mice] or other molecules involved in apoptosis)
Strong immune stimulation that overwhelms the processes in I.
  By cross-reactive foreign antigens
  By self antigens
    Encouraged by adjuvants (superantigens, other microbial stimulants, e.g., endotoxin)
    Encouraged by cytokine excesses or imbalances

ample, drug-induced tolerance, provides a simple framework for conceptualization. In this form of tolerance, an antigen is given. Lymphocytes able to recognize that antigen are stimulated. A cytotoxic drug is given to kill the stimulated lymphocytes. The result is preferential loss of lymphocytes able to recognize that antigen but not other antigens (with which the animal was not stimulated). For example, an animal is immunized with the antigen, tetanus toxoid. Tetanus toxoid stimulates many of the lymphocytes (T- and B-cells) reactive with the antigen. These cells are eliminated by administration of a cytotoxic drug, such as cyclophosphamide. The killing with cyclophosphamide (by itself not an antigen-specific agent) was rendered specific by the prior antigen administration. Since the cyclophosphamide selectively killed cells that were capable of responding to tetanus toxoid, subsequent immunization with tetanus toxoid leads to a blunted immune response. In this case, the tolerance to a potential infectious agent would be undesirable. On the other hand, if the antigen used could induce an autoimmune response, such tolerance might be desirable.

Several additional methods have been used to induce tolerance in animals: (1) giving an antigen to a very young animal; (2) deaggregating an antigen to make it less immunogenic and more toleragenic; (3) giving very small or very large doses of an antigen; (4) attaching an antigen or hapten to a molecule that tends to induce tolerance rather than immunity; (5) binding the antigen to an autologous cell, for example, thymocytes or dendritic cells; (6) placing the antigen directly in the thymus; (7) giving multiple injections of an antigen; and (8) feeding the antigen. Recent years have seen an emphasis on transgenic mice bearing the gene that encodes an antigen to which tolerance is to be induced, allowing expression of the protein from before birth. All these methods are designed to perturb the immune system so as to predispose to the induction of a hyporesponsive state with regard to the particular antigen.

Systemic Tolerance. Studies of superantigens (usually bacterial or viral products able to interact with T-cells bearing one or a limited number of TCR-v-beta receptors) have demonstrated that in vivo exposure can lead to tolerance by clonal deletion of T-cells reactive with the superantigen. In addition, clonal anergy may be induced in reactive T-cells that are not deleted—by downregulation of the TCR and CD8 on antigen-reactive T-cells and/or by impairment in their TCR-mediated signaling.

Since tolerance is maintained primarily by the T-cell population, it can be overcome by bypassing the T-cell tolerance so as to stimulate B-cells directly to produce antibody. Thus administration of bacterial lipopolysaccharide (endotoxin), 8-substituted guanosines, or other polyclonal B-cell activators may prevent or overcome tolerance. Thus a variety of specific and nonspecific factors could contribute to the impaired tolerance of patients with autoimmune diseases. In this regard, it has been noted that many patients have discrete autoimmune diseases, whereas others have features of more than one disease (e.g., lupus and polymyositis or autoimmune thyroiditis, type I diabetes, and pernicious anemia), suggesting an underlying generalized tolerance defect. A single population of cells retarding autoimmunity has been described in mice. These $CD4^+CD25^+$ T-cells appear capable of interfering, in an antigen nonspecific manner, with the development of autoimmunity, apparently by inhibiting T-cell activation. Related studies of postthymectomy-induced autoimmunity indicate that intrathymic tolerization to complexes of self peptides and MHC class II on adult antigen-presenting cells prevents several of the above autoimmune diseases. Thus although the mechanisms mediating suppression of these diseases are redundant, a great enough defect in one may be sufficient to allow autoimmune disease.

Oral Tolerance. Oral tolerance can be induced by active suppression and/or clonal anergy, depending upon the dose of antigen fed. In recent studies, antigen-specific T-cells were eliminated (apoptosis equals deletion; see later discussion) from intestinal Peyer's patches by oral antigen through mechanisms that depended upon the dose and frequency of antigen feeding. At lower doses of antigen, suppressor cells were induced, but not apoptosis. At higher doses, both Th1 and Th2 cells were activated, then eliminated. Thus orally administered antigen can induce active suppression, clonal anergy, and apoptosis (deletion).

is an organ-nonspecific syndrome characterized by the production of antibodies that are reactive with many different self antigens, including nuclear antigens. Polymyositis is a related disease characterized by a more limited autoantibody repertoire and by cell-mediated immunity against muscle cells. Certain autoimmune diseases are caused by antibodies that react with specific receptors, for example, Graves' disease (thyroid-stimulating hormone receptor) and myasthenia gravis (acetylcholine receptor). Other diseases involve cell-mediated immune reactions against a specific target organ or cell type. An apparent loss of self-tolerance occurs in all autoimmune diseases. In some disorders, measured autoreactivity may be critical to disease manifestations. In others, autoantibodies may not be pathogenic and may be merely markers of the disease.

Some autoimmunity originates from immune responses to foreign agents. For example, severe infection with particular strains of group-A β-hemolytic streptococci (especially strains characterized by thick capsules that make them highly virulent and immunogenic) may induce a vigorous immune response against streptococcal antigens; some of the antibodies induced also react with human heart antigens. Thus these group-A β-hemolytic streptococcal infections and resultant immune responses can cause acute rheumatic fever. Many individuals colonized by such potentially pathogenic streptococci do not develop autoimmunity—apparently because they do not mount a strong immune response. The magnitude of the immune response appears to be a critical factor in the development of rheumatic fever. In turn, many genetic and environmental factors influence the strength of the immune response. These principles should be kept in mind when dealing with other diseases in which the causes are less well understood: although autoimmunity might be induced by an exogenous agent, additional factors may be vital to the outcome. A schematic for such a process is given in Fig. 177-1.

EXPERIMENTAL TOLERANCE

Classically, experimental tolerance involved an initial treatment with a toleragenic form of an antigen so as to induce tolerance, and a later test with a standard immunogenic form of that antigen to determine whether tolerance had been induced by the initial treatment. Experimental tolerance may be induced in many different ways. One ex-

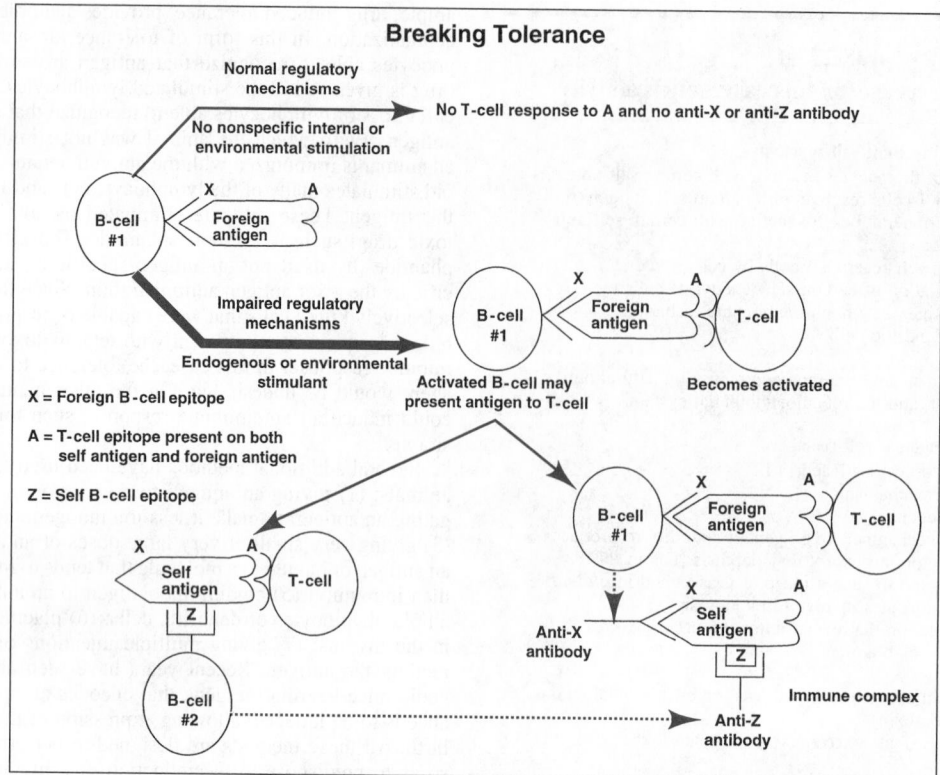

FIGURE 177-1   Among the many potential scenarios for breaking tolerance, this simplified figure provides an example. B-cell #1 interacts with a foreign antigen that is cross-reactive with a self antigen. In the presence of normal regulatory mechanisms and in the absence of unusual lymphocyte activation, there may well be no T-cell response to the common T-cell epitope (portion) of the antigen *(A)*. There also would be no antibody produced to the common B-cell epitope *(X)* or the self epitope Z. However, in the face of impaired regulatory mechanisms and/or the presence of endogenous or environmental stimulant(s), B-cell #1 may be sufficiently activated to present the foreign antigen to a T-cell such that the T-cell recognizes epitope A, receives additional stimulatory signals, and becomes activated. The activated T-cell then is capable of helping B-cells to produce anti-X antibodies. Anti-X antibodies are autoantibodies that recognize the X epitope present on both the foreign and self antigen. In addition, activated T-cells recognizing T-cell epitope A may help B-cell #2 to produce anti-Z antibodies that are antibodies recognizing the Z determinant present on the self antigen but not the foreign antigen. In such a manner, a foreign antigen cross-reactive with a self antigen, in the presence of immune regulatory abnormalities, may trigger an autoimmune response that could lead to disease.

Defective systemic and oral tolerance has been observed in lupus-prone NZB mice. Such an abnormality could result from either the lack of adequate suppressor function or some interference with such suppressor function. The data suggest that these mice have T-cells that prevent suppressor cells from functioning. If there is an expansion in lupus-prone mice of T-cells that produce factors able to drive B-cells to proliferate and differentiate, such T-cells would act in a manner analogous to exogenously administered lipopolysaccharide to bypass T-cell tolerance and directly stimulate B-cells to produce antibody. Such a mechanism may explain a defect in experimental tolerance in NZB mice. The same mechanism may contribute to a loss of self-tolerance in other disorders. On the other hand, NZB mice have excess antibody production and excess numbers of CD5$^+$ cells that are not very susceptible to tolerance induction. Thus a B-cell abnormality as well as T-cell abnormality may contribute to NZB disease. Indeed, evidence for defects in both populations comes from reconstitution experiments in NZB mice.

Apoptosis and Autoimmunity

An initial signal to a T-cell through its receptor for antigen (TCR) leads to activation, whereas a second signal occurring some time later leads to death (termed *activation-induced cell-death, programmed cell death,* or *apoptosis*). The induction of death by a second signal through the TCR serves to limit any particular immune response and to forestall the production of toxic cytokines (such as tumor necrosis factor [TNF]). Without this apoptosis, a toxic shock–like syndrome

might occur on stimulation with any strong and persisting antigen (it is currently observed only with certain bacterial toxins, superantigens able to stimulate large numbers of T-cells). Of special note, induction of cell death would limit any antiself immune responses because a second encounter with self antigen would lead to death of the reactive T-cell.

Certain self-reactive lymphocytes undergo apoptosis during selection in the thymus, a process regulated by several factors, including the tumor suppressor factor p53. In addition, peripheral apoptosis accounts for postthymic deletion of T-cells by a p53-independent mechanism that is influenced by the transcription factor IRF-1 (interferon regulatory factor 1). It now appears that several different pathways exist for induction of apoptosis in cells of the T-lineage.

Defects in apoptosis can play a critical role in certain murine autoimmune diseases. MRL-*lpr/lpr* mice develop a generalized autoimmune disorder with features of systemic lupus erythematosus (SLE), rheumatoid arthritis, and Sjögren's syndrome. The autoimmunity-associated *lpr* gene responsible for the lymphocyte proliferation observed in these mice encodes a defective *Fas* protein (CD95). Ordinarily, Fas is a receptor that mediates apoptosis in peripheral lymphocytes. In the absence of a normal Fas receptor, signals mediating apoptosis cannot function to cause the killing of self-reactive cells. As a result, self-reactive cells survive and therefore are poised to mediate autoimmune disease. The presence of a defective Fas protein in *lpr/lpr* mice leads to a receptor that cannot mediate signals provided by the Fas-ligand. This finding provides a mechanism for an association of widespread loss of tolerance and generalized autoimmunity.

The Fas (CD95) antigen affects not only T-cells but also B-cells. Ordinarily, antigen-specific CD4$^+$ T-cells trigger naive B-cells to proliferate and to produce specific antibody. B-cells that have been chronically exposed to the antigen express desensitized surface receptors for the antigen. When exposed to antigen-specific CD4$^+$ T-cells, those B-cells are eliminated. However, anergic B-cells from Fas deficient *lpr/lpr* mice are not eliminated. Instead, they are triggered to proliferate. Thus Fas deficiency can lead to retention of autoreactive B-cells both by failure of the B-cells to undergo apoptosis and failure of the T-cells to facilitate their elimination.

The defect of *lpr/lpr* mice is in fashioning a proper Fas receptor. In contrast, failure to produce a proper ligand for that receptor (Fas ligand) occurs in *gld/gld* mice that develop a similar autoimmune syndrome. Thus there is failure of apoptosis in these mice because the Fas receptor cannot be stimulated appropriately.

Lymphoproliferation and early death also occur in mice lacking the CTLA-4 antigen on T-cells. This antigen is expressed transiently after T-cell activation (for 2 to 3 days). It is a high-affinity receptor for the B7 family of antigens on antigen-presenting cells. Interaction with the CTLA-4 receptor serves to downregulate T-cell activation and proliferation. This downregulation is part of a balance that limits T-cell activation and proliferation after antigenic stimulation and diverts T-cells into a pathway toward memory cells that remain inactive until the antigen is presented again. Interference with the signal provided through the CTLA-4 receptor leads to uncontrolled T-cell activation and expansion and an autoimmune process. Activated T-cells are able to trigger self-reactive B-cells by a bystander effect and stimulate autoantibody production even when the triggering antigen was not a self antigen.

What is the relevance of these murine defects to human disease? For the moment, they point to mechanisms by which generalized cell-biologic abnormalities can lead to immune-mediated disorders. It is not likely that many patients with lupus will be found to have severe defects in either Fas or Fas-ligand. However, patients may be found with abnormalities in persistence of self-reactive lymphocytes for many different reasons. In view of the multiple other genes already known to influence apoptosis, including p53, Bcl2, Bax, Bcl-x$_L$, and Bcl-x$_S$, there undoubtedly are many possibilities for genetic contributions to autoimmune diseases.

It has long been suggested that patients with generalized autoimmune diseases manifest a bystander effect in which activated T-cells help bystander B-cells to produce antibody reactive with self antigens. Activated T-cells signal, via CD40-L (a membrane protein), the CD40 receptor of B-cells so as to block apoptosis of the B-cells. This apoptosis-blocking process is mediated by Bcl-x. Thus the presence of many activated T-cells could provide an environment for persistence of self-reactive B-cells and excess autoantibody production. Moreover, since B-cells are especially effective at presenting proteins to CD4$^+$ T-cells, the process represents a positive-feedback loop in which activated T-cells rescue B-cells from apoptosis and the B-cells activate the T-cells to further rescue B-cells from apoptosis—all the while the B-cells go on to produce autoantibodies.

Local Tolerance: Immunologically Privileged Sites and Tissues. The eye (anterior chamber) is an example of an immunologically privileged site in that transplants to the anterior chamber of the eye are protected from rejection. Privileged sites include the brain, testes, placenta, and pregnant uterus. A number of factors contribute to this privilege (only some of which are present in a given site) including blood-tissue barriers, absence of efferent lymphatics, an immunosuppressive microenvironment (due to production of such factors as transforming growth factor-β, vasoactive intestinal peptide, and α-melanocyte stimulating hormone), inhibitors of complement activation, and expression of the Fas-ligand. In the eye, several soluble factors serve to downregulate immunity, and the local production of Fas-ligand facilitates the induction of apoptosis in T-cells entering the eye.

In addition to privileged sites, certain tissues, when transplanted into nonprivileged sites, are less likely to be rejected. These privileged tissues include the cornea, testes, liver, and placenta. Mechanisms leading to such privilege include reduced expression of the major histocompatibility complex antigens, secretion of immunosuppressive factors, and expression of Fas-ligand.

The clinical relevance of immunologic privilege is immediately obvious when considering cornea transplants. These are the most successful of all transplants, in large measure because the organ being transplanted is an immunologically privileged tissue and the site to which it is transplanted is an immunologically privileged site. The pregnant uterus also is an immunologically privileged site and that property allows it to retain the embryo despite expression of paternal (foreign) antigens that would induce rejection if present at many other sites. Other possible advantages of privilege include maintenance of the integrity of critical organs that might be damaged by an excessive immune-mediated response to infectious agents. The brain, eye, and gonads are especially protected in this manner.

Studies of Transgenic Mice

Transgenic mice carry an introduced gene or genes that may be expressed from very early in development. Such mice allow studies of the interaction between gene expression and the immune system, a new approach to tolerance. Mice expressing the transgene for a protein and others carrying both an antibody transgene and a protein transgene have been studied. In the double-transgenic mice, tolerance occurs to the protein: antiprotein B-cells do not produce antibody. This tolerance is not caused by deletion of protein-reactive (self-reactive) B-cells, since transfer of those B-cells to nontransgenic mice allows them to produce antiprotein antibody when stimulated by protein and helper T-cells. In contrast, when the B-cells are transferred to protein single-transgenic mice, the continuous production of high concentrations of protein maintains tolerance. In vitro studies of B-cells from double-transgenic mice show that bacterial lipopolysaccharide is able to induce both proliferation and antibody production by previously tolerant B-cells. These studies suggest that certain forms of tolerance may involve downregulation (anergy) rather than deletion of self-reactive B-cells. Moreover, a loss of such tolerance may be induced by polyclonal immune activators such as bacterial lipopolysaccharide. Thus an endogenous immune stimulatory environment (equivalent in effect to exogenous lipopolysaccharide) or excessive sensitivity to environmental stimulators may contribute to loss of self tolerance.

In contrast to this transgenic tolerance model, relevant especially to humoral autoimmunity, other transgenic experiments point to deletion of self-reactive B-cells. Thus a mouse bearing the anti–major histocompatibility complex (MHC) class I Ig transgene demonstrates deletion of self-reactive B-cells. Such a mechanism may be especially important for avoiding organ-specific autoimmune diseases.

INDUCTION OF ORGAN-SPECIFIC AUTOIMMUNITY

Induction of organ-specific autoimmunity is somewhat more straightforward than that of organ-nonspecific autoimmunity. If transgenic mice are prepared so that they express the transgene product on cell surfaces after the neonatal period, a model for neoantigen expression is created. When such a neoantigen is expressed on an endocrine or exocrine gland, an immune response against that tissue takes place; if the response is sufficiently intense, destruction of the gland may occur. This same destructive process is induced by viral infection of a gland and expression of viral antigens on the cell surfaces. A similar destructive process may be brought about by induction of class II MHC gene products on glandular cell surfaces, so that self antigens are presented to the immune system in a manner analogous to foreign antigen presentation by Ia-bearing antigen-presenting cells. Destruction of the pancreatic islets in juvenile-onset diabetes may result from such a process.

Induction of MHC class II molecules on gland cell surfaces may occur through several different mechanisms; however, viral infection is likely to be one of the most important. If a viral infection causes an inflammatory response in a gland, local production of interferon (IFN) or tumor necrosis factor (TNF) induces MHC class II expression on cells in the gland. The Ia molecules could then serve to target adjacent self antigens to autoreactive T-cells, which would initiate an immune response against the gland. This process can lead to autoimmune thyroiditis. An unusual expression of MHC class II molecules has been demonstrated on the thyroid glands of patients with autoimmune thyroiditis.

A person's ability to mount an immune response against a self antigen by the mere induction of a class II MHC product on the cell surface indicates the fragile balance between health and disease. However, other factors appear necessary for disease. One important factor is the extent of the immune response. People with the genotype HLA-A1,B8,DR3 tend to be especially predisposed to autoimmune phenomena and make especially strong antibody responses to a variety of antigens. Such individuals probably manifest a shift in the immune thermostat toward increased immunity. Such a shift may have adaptive value in guarding against infections; however, the trade-off is increased predisposition to loss of self-tolerance and the development of autoimmune diseases.

Potential Role of Other Cells

Thus far, we have emphasized B- and T-cells, the prominent actors in the expression of immunity; however, other cells also participate and could be important in maintenance of self-tolerance or loss associated with autoimmunity. One such cell deserves special mention: the dendritic cell. Dendritic cells are found in many organs and appear to differ somewhat from one site to the next. These cells have extremely high expression of MHC class II molecules and are the most potent inducers of naive T-cells to help in antibody production. Such cells can induce a state of tolerance when covered with hapten and can induce neonatal tolerance. They also may normally present self antigen to the immune system. Diabetes in nonobese diabetic (NOD) mice can be prevented by the transfer of dendritic cells that had been exposed to islet cell antigens. Thus a defect in the function of dendritic cells would be expected to induce special susceptibility to autoimmunity.

CROSS-REACTIVITY AND MOLECULAR MIMICRY

A variety of antigens that cross-react with self antigens are potentially able to induce an immune response to self antigens. For example, bovine thrombin, used in surgery to promote hemostasis, cross-reacts with human thrombin. In rare patients, an immune response to bovine thrombin is sufficient to induce an antibody response to human thrombin that may subsequently lead to severe hemorrhage due to inadequate amounts of available, functional thrombin. Some individuals (without other autoimmune features) develop antibodies to their own thrombin without prior administration of bovine thrombin during surgery. Such antibodies could arise due to cross-immunization or due to loss of self-tolerance. Patients with systemic lupus or rheumatoid arthritis also may develop antithrombin antibodies.

By adaptive evolution, structure function–dictated coevolution, or purely random processes, many bacterial and viral products share striking structural homologies with mammalian proteins. The presence on viruses or bacteria of structures with strong homology to host self antigens leads to the possibility of antiself responses being commingled with normal defensive immunity. Moreover, the mimicry involved in such situations often is a critical adaptation to allow the foreign invader to enter cells or otherwise facilitate its life cycle. For example, a virus with a structure homologous to a hormone would be able to interact with the receptor for that hormone to facilitate entry into the cell. However, an immune response against such a virus might include an autoimmune component (see later discussion on idiotypy).

Cross-reactions due to molecular mimicry between foreign and human antigens have been demonstrated for B-cell epitopes and for T-cell epitopes. Cross-reactions with T-cell epitopes could be critical to both generalized and organ-specific autoimmunity. For example, it has been demonstrated that T-cells from patients with rheumatoid arthritis recognize and are stimulated by peptides from a mycobacterial heat-shock protein and that T-cells from patients with multiple sclerosis respond to viral peptides cross-reactive with myelin basic protein. Several investigators have also found spreading of mimicry with nuclear peptide antigens from T-cell epitopes to autoantibody production. Thus it is possible that some autoantibody production may represent a response to a T-cell epitope mimic such that the

source of the B-cell response is obscured. Such epitope spreading may occur in certain autoimmune diseases, with the antibody responses being either pathogenic or mere markers of the autoimmune process.

IDIOTYPY AS MECHANISM OF AUTOREACTIVITY

A process similar to molecular mimicry also may induce autoimmunity. This process involves not homology but a lock-and-key structural relationship. For example, some organisms have evolved so as to use receptors on mammalian cells for entry. An antibody response may be induced against the portion of the organism that serves as a ligand for the receptor. Such a response includes a population of antibodies (called *Ab 1*) having antibody with combining sites with structures *(idiotopes)* closely related structurally to portions of the original receptor. The structures or idiotopes are able to induce an antibody response: the resulting antibodies (*Ab 2*, or second antibody in the series) are called *antiidiotype antibodies* because they recognize the relatively unique structures (idiotopes) on a population of antibodies made by the body. However, the antiidiotype antibodies (Ab 2), by virtue of recognizing the idiotope, also recognize the closely related structure on the original receptor. Such antibodies may be observed as antireceptor antibodies.

Just as idiotypy may be found for antibody molecules, in an analogous fashion, idiotypy occurs for T-cell receptors for antigen critical for cell-mediated immunity. A variety of autoimmune diseases may result partly or completely from such a T-cell response. In addition, skewing of the T-cell repertoire toward T-cells that recognize Ia molecules might generally increase T-cell activation and lead to autoimmunity.

IMPLICATIONS FOR THERAPY

Understanding the mechanisms of tolerance induction and interference could lead to strategies for preventing or treating patients with autoimmune diseases. For many years, studies of experimental tolerance appeared to bear little relationship to human disease. A breakthrough came with the application of human immunology to Rh factor mismatches. An Rh (D)-negative woman fertilized by an Rh (D)-positive man is subject to being immunized by fetal Rh (D)-positive erythrocytes (Rh [D]-positive inherited from the father) that enter the maternal circulation at delivery. When such immunization occurs, maternal antibodies develop that, in subsequent pregnancies, enter the fetal circulation and react with fetal erythrocytes to produce erythroblastosis fetalis. Once it is produced, the maternal antibody cannot easily be inhibited. However, the antibody can be prevented by injecting the mother with antibodies to Rh (D) within 3 days of delivery. By extension, many possible manipulations of the immune system seem possible for dealing with a great variety of autoimmune diseases. Trials of oral tolerance with a self antigen have already been performed in patients with several autoimmune disorders. In animals, tolerance to a specific self antigen has been induced with a retroviral vector and autoimmune diabetes prevented. Further advances are eagerly awaited.

BIBLIOGRAPHY

Ally BA, Hawley TS, McKall-Faienza KJ et al: Prevention of autoimmune disease by retroviral-mediated gene therapy, *J Immunol* 155:5404-5408, 1995.

Bellgrau D et al: A role for CD95 ligand in preventing graft rejection, *Nature* 377:630, 1995.

Bonomo A, Kehn PJ, Payer E et al: Pathogensis of post-thymectomy autoimmunity, *J Immunol* 154:6602-6611, 1995.

Bottazzo GF, Pujol-Borrell R, Hanafusa T: Role of aberrant HLA-DR expression and antigen presentation in induction of endocrine autoimmunity, *Lancet* 2:1115, 1983.

Chen Y, Inobe J, Marks R et al: Peripheral deletion of antigen-reactive T-cells in oral tolerance, *Nature* 376:177-180, 1995.

Claman HN: Immunological tolerance. In Samter M, editor: *Immunological diseases*, Boston, 1988, Little, Brown.

Clare-Salzler MJ, Brooks J, Chai A et al: Prevention of diabetes in nonobese diabetic mice by dendritic cell transfer, *J Clin Invest* 90:741-748, 1992.

Fuchs EJ, Matzinger P: B-cells turn off virgin but not memory T cells, *Science* 258:1156, 1992.

Griffith TS, Brunner T, Fletcher SM et al: Fas ligand–induced apoptosis as a mechanism of immune privilege, *Science* 270:1189, 1995.

Karjalainen J et al: A bovine albumin peptide as a possible trigger of insulin-dependent diabetes mellitus, *N Engl J Med* 327:302, 1992.

LaSpada AR, Skalhegg BS, Henderson R et al: Fatal hemorrhage in a patient with an acquired inhibitor of human thrombin, *N Engl J Med* 333:494-497, 1995.

Lehmann PV et al: Spreading of T-cell autoimmunity to cryptic determinants of an autoantigen, *Nature* 358:155, 1992.

Marrack P, Kappler J: The staphylococcal enterotoxins and their relatives, *Science* 248:705, 1990.

Posselt AM et al: Prevention of autoimmune diabetes in the BB rat by intrathymic islet transplantation at birth, *Science* 256:1321, 1992.

Rathmell JC, Cooke MP, Ho WY et al: CD95 (Fas)-dependent elimination of self-reactive B cells upon interaction with CD4$^+$ T cells, *Nature* 376:181-184, 1995.

Sakaguchi S, Sakaguchi N, Asano M et al: Immunologic self-tolerance maintained by activated T cells expressing IL-2 receptor alpha-chains (CD25), *J Immunol* 155:1151-1164, 1995.

Schonrich G, Alferink J, Klevenz A et al: Tolerance induction as a multistep process, *Eur J Immunol* 24:285, 1994.

Segal BM, Klinman DM, Shevach EM: Microbial products induce autoimmune disease by an IL-12 dependent pathway, *J Immunol* 158:5087-5090, 1997.

Steinberg AD et al: Theoretical and experimental approaches to generalized autoimmunity, *Immunol Rev* 118:129, 1990.

Steinberg AD et al: Systemic lupus erythematosus, *Ann Intern Med* 115:548, 1991.

Tamura T, Ishihara M, Lamphier MS et al: An IRF-1-dependent pathway of DNA damage-induced apoptosis in mitogen-activated T lymphocytes, *Nature* 376:596-599, 1995.

Taylor AW, Streilein JW: Immunoreactive vasoactive intestinal peptide contributes to the immunosuppressive activity of normal aqueous humor, *J Immunol* 153:1080, 1994.

Tivoli EA et al: CTLA4Ig prevents lymphoproliferation, *J Immunol* 158: 5091-5094, 1997.

Watanabe-Fukunga R et al: Lymphoproliferation disorder in mice explained by defects in Fas antigen that mediates apoptosis, *Nature* 356:314, 1992.

Waternhouse P et al: Lymphoproliferative disorders with early lethality in mice deficient in CTLA-4, *Science* 270:985, 1995.

Webb SR, Hutchinson J, Hayden K et al: Expansion/deletion of mature T cells exposed to endogenous superantigens in vivo, *J Immunol* 152:586, 1994.

Weigle WO: The effect of lipopolysaccharide desensitization on the regulation of in vivo induction of immunologic tolerance and antibody production and in vitro release of IL-1, *J Immunol* 142:1107, 1989.

Wucherpfennig KW, Strominger JL: Molecular mimicry in T cell–mediated autoimmunity: viral peptides activate human T-cell clones specific for myelin basic protein, *Cell* 80:695, 1995.

II LABORATORY AND DIAGNOSTIC TESTS

CHAPTER

178 Complement Measurements

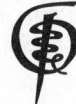

Robert H. Carter, M. Kathryn Liszewski, and John P. Atkinson

Serum concentrations of complement proteins reflect the balance between production and consumption. Failure of production most often reflects a genetic deficiency in a particular complement protein, which can be important diagnostically in autoimmune disorders and susceptibility to recurrent infections. Increased consumption can be an indicator of diseases associated with complement activation. Activation of the complement system leads to formation of complexes of the individual proteins that are proteolytically active, cleaving the next protein in the cascade. However, many complement proteins are acute phase reactants whose production is increased markedly in inflammatory conditions, including those associated with complement activation. To cause a decrease in serum levels, consumption must occur in the vasculature and must be enough to outstrip production. Thus although many diseases cause complement activation, hypocomplementemia on the basis of consumption is frequently associated with a chronic systemic illness with circulating high levels of immune complexes, such as systemic lupus erythematosus (SLE) or cryoglobulinemia.

METHODS OF MEASUREMENT

Complement can be assessed either by its hemolytic activity or by its reactivity in antigenic assays. The total hemolytic complement (THC, or CH$_{50}$) assay, which measures activation of the entire classical pathway, and immunoassays of individual components (e.g., C1, C4, C2, C3) are generally used in clinical practice. Antigenic assays for C4 and C3 are the most widely available. Radial immunodiffusion, which measures the size of a precipitin ring formed in an agarose gel containing specific antibody to an individual complement protein, has been largely replaced by nephelometric immunoassays, which detect changes in the intensity of light scatter as complement proteins interact with their specific antibodies. The detection of activation or cleavage products such as the anaphylatoxins (C3a, C5a), the cleavage peptides released from C4 (C4d), C3 (C3d), and factor B (Bb), or of neoantigens resulting from activation fragments is also becoming more available. Although these assays provide a measure of activation that is less dependent on synthesis, to date their role in clinical practice is limited.

INTERPRETATION OF TEST RESULTS

Several of the complement proteins (C1, C2, D) are heat labile. As a consequence, THC assays require careful collection, processing, and storage of specimens. A common cause of a depressed serum THC reading is improper specimen handling. The THC assay provides a functional assessment of the classical pathway based on the ability of the test serum to lyse sheep erythrocytes optimally sensitized with rabbit antibody. All nine components of the classical pathway (C1 to C9) are required to give a normal THC reading. A THC finding of 200 means that at a dilution of 1:200 the tested serum lysed 50% of the antibody-coated cells in the standard assay system.

The most common indication for ordering a THC assay is in the initial evaluation of a patient with a rheumatic disease or unexplained recurrent pyogenic (especially neisserial) infection. For an SLE patient, a THC value of 0 most likely indicates a severe depletion of the early components of the classical pathway or a deficiency of C2. However, for those with recurrent neisserial infections, a 0 value suggests a deficiency of C5, C6, C7, or C8 (Chapter 186).

The range of normal complement protein concentrations is quite broad, usually approximating plus or minus 50% of the normal population mean. Because complement proteins are acute phase reactants, levels tend to increase even with minor intercurrent illnesses, thereby increasing the scatter in the "normal" population. Thus the interpretation of an isolated static value from an individual may be difficult. Serial changes in levels for a given patient over time are generally more informative than is comparison with an absolute range of normal. Low values usually suggest ongoing disease, whereas normal or high values are less helpful.

ALTERATIONS IN DISEASE

Complement proteins are acute phase reactants and, as with several other proteins such as fibrinogen and C-reactive protein, tend to be elevated in many inflammatory conditions (Table 178-1). Such elevations are common and nonspecific and therefore of little clinical usefulness. In most infectious diseases, complement values are normal or elevated. Depressions associated with in vivo complement activation are more informative. Virtually any disease that gives rise to circulating immune complexes can cause hypocomplementemia, provided the complexes contain immunoglobulin G or M (IgG, IgM) antibodies capable of activating complement (Box 178-1).

In SLE, THC levels are depressed at some time in more than 50% of patients, whereas levels are generally normal in patients with discoid lupus. As a rule, complement depressions are associated with increased severity of disease, especially renal disease. Component analyses have demonstrated low levels of C1, C4, C2, and C3. Serial observations often reveal decreased levels preceding clinical exacerbations; reduction in C4 tends to occur before reduction in C3, THC, and other components. As attacks subside, levels return toward nor-

Table 178-1 Interpretation of complement tests

THC	C4	B	C3	INTERPRETATION	EXAMPLES
High	High	High	High	Acute phase response	Any inflammatory condition
Low	Low	Nl	Nl	Classical path activation or deficiency	SLE
					C1INH deficiency
					C4 deficiency
Low	Low	Nl	Low	Classical pathway activation	SLE or immune complex disease
Low	Nl	Nl	Low	Nephritic factor or deficiency	Membranous glomerulonephritis or C3 deficiency
Low	Nl	Low	Low	Alternative pathway activation or deficiency	Infection or deficiency of factor H or I
Nl	Nl	Low	Nl	Deficiency	Factor B deficiency
Low	Low	Low	Low	Alternative and classical path activation	Immune complex disease

Nl, Normal.

Table 178-2 Common tests for immune complexes

TEST	METHOD	ADVANTAGES	DISADVANTAGES
Physical	Centrifugation or precipitation	Gives measure of IC	Insensitive; IC can be contaminated with other proteins
C1q	Association of C1q with IC	Sensitive	Requires complement-activating IC, which depends on lattice and Ig subclass; other C1q-binding molecules can interfere
Rheumatoid factor	Competition of IC with aggregated IgG for binding of rheumatoid factor	Independent of complement activation by IC	Depends on lattice structure of IC; high concentrations of IgG can interfere
Raji	Binding of IC to Raji cells	Detects IC that have activated C3	Autolymphocyte autoantibodies can interfere
			Antilymphocyte autoantibodies

mal in reverse order, with C4 tending to remain depressed longest. However, certain considerations must be taken into account when interpreting the result of clinical assays. Normally, C4 and factor B are present in concentrations of one fourth to one sixth that of C3. For C3 to drop below normal, a substantial activation of either the classical or alternative pathway must be ongoing. In addition, the quoted normal levels represent plus or minus 2 standard deviations, and individual baseline (predisease) levels of C3 or C4 are usually not available. Since normal C4 levels are 16 to 48 mg/dl, it would require less classical pathway activation to depress C4 values from 20 mg/dl than from 40 mg/dl. Such considerations must be taken into account when interpreting the results of these clinical assays.

Serum levels of THC, C3, and C4 are usually normal or elevated in patients with rheumatoid arthritis. Depressed levels are associated with extraarticular manifestations of the disease, particularly vasculitis. Such patients usually also have high titers of rheumatoid factor and immune complexes in their serum. Synovial fluid complement levels are usually low in patients with rheumatoid arthritis when measured by activity determinations but may be normal when measured by immunoassay. The presence of antigenic fragments that are nonfunctional (which have not been cleared from the joint space and remain reactive in the immunoassay) may account for these findings. Because measurement of complement levels in joint, pleural, spinal, and pericardial fluids is complicated technically and difficult to interpret, such determinations are seldom helpful in clinical decision making.

Any cause of chronic antigenemia that is associated with an antibody response may lead to acquired hypocomplementemia, including subacute bacterial endocarditis; hepatitis B surface antigenemia; gram-negative sepsis; viremias, such as measles; or recurrent parasitemias, such as malaria. Essential mixed cryoglobulinemia, a disease characterized by arthritis or arthralgias, cutaneous vasculitis, and nephritis, is often accompanied by profound hypocomplementemia resulting from classical pathway activation by the cold-precipitating immune complexes that occur in this disease.

Most immune complex diseases show evidence of classical pathway activation, but type II membranoproliferative glomerulonephritis is associated with hypocomplementemia, a normal C4, and low C3; this combination of findings indicates activation of the alternative pathway. The responsible mechanism in some patients involves a circulating C3 nephritic factor, an autoantibody directed against the alternative pathway C3-cleaving enzyme. It combines with and stabilizes this enzyme, then promotes positive feedback through the amplification loop.

Certain inherited deficiencies of control proteins lead to uncontrolled cycling of the activation pathway to which they belong and to secondary consumption of complement protein with resulting hypocomplementemia. C1 inhibitor deficiency permits the unopposed cleavage of C4 and C2 by C1 and is associated with the clinical syndrome of hereditary angioedema. Deficiency of either of the control proteins, I or H, leads to uncontrolled cycling of the amplification loop with secondary depletion of C3 and other alternative pathway proteins. Clinically the deficiencies of H and I associated with recurrent pyogenic infections are presumably caused by impaired opsonization of the bacteria consequent to the low C3 levels (Chapter 186).

Paroxysmal nocturnal hemoglobinuria (PNH) is an acquired clonal disorder of hematopoietic stem cells. Such cells are deficient in an enzyme required for production of glycolipid tails that anchor certain proteins to the cell membrane. As a result, these cells lack these surface proteins. Decay-accelerating factor (DAF) and CD59 are glycolipid-anchored membrane proteins. Their deficiency produces PNH because of complement-mediated damage to the cell. THC, C3, and C4 levels, however, are normal because the amount of complement required for lysis is small.

MEASUREMENT OF IMMUNE COMPLEXES

Circulating immune complexes (ICs) play an immunopathologic role in a wide variety of diseases, including autoimmune disorders, vasculitic syndromes, infectious illnesses, and malignancies (see Box 178-1). As a consequence, the demonstration of ICs in tissues and biologic fluids can be of aid in elucidating the pathophysiology of certain conditions (Chapter 175).

Detection of Immune Complexes

In tissues, ICs are demonstrable by histologic, histochemical, and light and electron microscopic methods. Electron-dense accumulations of IC may be observed in subepithelial or subendothelial locations of kidney glomerular vessels. Scattered subepithelial deposits are characteristic of poststreptococcal glomerulonephritis, whereas extensive subepithelial deposits are the hallmark of membranous glomerulopathy. In lupus nephritis, electron-dense deposits are often observed in

BOX 178-1
Diseases associated with immune complexes

Autoimmune diseases
  Rheumatoid arthritis
  Felty's syndrome
  Systemic lupus erythematosus
  Sjögren's syndrome
  Mixed connective tissue disease
  Periarteritis nodosa
  Systemic sclerosis
Glomerulonephritis
  Exogenous and endogenous antigens
Neoplastic diseases
  Solid and lymphoid tumors
Infectious diseases
  Bacterial
    Infective endocarditis
    Meningococcal infections
    Disseminated gonorrheal infection
    Recurrent infections in children
    Infected ventriculoatrial shunt
    Streptococcal infections
    Leprosy
    Syphilis
  Viral
    Dengue hemorrhagic fever
    Cytomegalovirus infections
    Viral hepatitis
    Infectious mononucleosis
    Subacute sclerosing parencephalitis
  Parasitic
    Malaria
    Trypanosomiasis
    Schistosomiasis
    Filariasis
    Toxoplasmosis
Other conditions
  Dermatitis herpetiformis and celiac disease
  Ulcerative colitis and Crohn's disease
  Myocardial infarction
  Idiopathic interstitial pneumonia
  Cystic fibrosis
  Sarcoidosis
  Multiple sclerosis
  Amyotrophic lateral sclerosis
  Myasthenia gravis
  Uveitis
  Otitis media
  Atopic diseases
  Arthritis associated with intestinal bypass procedure for morbid
    obesity
  Sickle cell anemia
  Thrombotic thrombocytopenic purpura
  Primary biliary cirrhosis
  Kidney and bone marrow transplantation
  Pregnancy, preeclamptic and eclamptic syndrome
  Lyme arthritis
  Steroid-responsive nephrotic syndrome; xanthomatosis; vasectomy;
    oral ulceration and Behçet's syndrome
  Pemphigus and bullous pemphigoid
  IgA deficiency
  Thyroid disorders
  Ankylosing spondylitis
  Iatrogenic diseases

throughout the GBM and deposit evenly to produce a smooth, linear pattern, whereas ICs that randomly deposit from the circulation into the glomerular filter are detected as granular, interrupted deposits.

More than 30 different tests have been described for the measurement of IC in blood, yet no *one* test is particularly satisfactory for routine clinical use. Procedures for detecting ICs containing unknown antigens in biologic fluids are based on (1) physical properties of IC; (2) interactions of IC with certain serum factors, such as complement or rheumatoid factors (RFs); and (3) interactions with cells bearing Fc and C receptors, such as B-lymphocytes, macrophages, platelets, and erythrocytes (Table 178-2).

The Raji cell assay, a frequently used IC test, demonstrates some of the difficulties in this area. First, the assay is not only technically complex but also requires a tissue culture system to grow this human pre–B-lymphocyte tumor cell line. The Raji cell possesses complement receptor type II (CR2), which primarily binds the C3 breakdown product, C3dg, but does not contain CR1, which primarily binds C3b. Thus the assay detects only ICs with C3dg. Non–complement-fixing ICs either are not detected at all or are inefficiently measured by this assay. Finally, antilymphocyte antibodies are common in rheumatic diseases and give a false-positive test, since the Raji cell is a human B-cell tumor line.

Currently no universal and absolutely specific reagent is available for IC detection and quantitation. Most assays detect only complement-fixing, large-size complexes and do not differentiate between specific complexes and nonspecific aggregates. Moreover, the complement-dependent techniques may give false-positive results because of the presence of interfering substances in the serum sample, such as deoxyribonucleic acid (DNA) or endotoxin. The RF-based tests may be influenced by the presence of endogenous RF in the serum sample and high levels of serum IgG. Cellular techniques may give false-positive results because of the presence of anticellular antibodies frequently found in sera of patients with autoimmune disorders. Even in experienced hands, therefore, the screening for ICs in human sera may require the use of several tests, and considerable caution is essential in their interpretation.

Finally, it should be emphasized that detection of ICs in biologic fluids does not necessarily indicate that the pathology of the disease under study results from these complexes. The most direct test would be one that demonstrates IC in the affected tissue itself. However, experience over the past 10 years has pointed to the limited usefulness of IC measurements for decision making in clinical medicine. ICs are typically present in infectious diseases; malignancies; idiopathic chronic inflammatory conditions involving the lung, kidney, or liver; and most inflammatory rheumatic diseases.

On the more positive side, a correlation exists between levels of circulating IC and disease activity in patients with SLE with a relationship between IC levels, antibodies to DNA, low complement levels, and clinical manifestations. Also, in patients with bacterial endocarditis, a correlation has been found between circulating IC levels, duration of disease, and extravalvular manifestations.

Two clinical tests that are more frequently used than IC assays to provide useful information regarding the presence of ICs are those for complement and cryoglobulin.

1. *Complement assays.* The reduction in circulating components of the classical pathway of complement (i.e., C1, C4, C2, C3) is usually related to IC formation, since ICs activate this cascade (Chapter 175).
2. *Cryoglobulins.* Mixed cryoglobulins are special types of ICs: ones that precipitate from serum in the cold. Such complexes usually consist of IgG, a C3 fragment, RF (IgM), and antigen. This test provides a direct and quantitative measurement of an important IC (Chapter 202).

a subendothelial position. Of the immunohistochemical techniques available, the most widely used is immunofluorescence, which uses fluorochrome-labeled antibodies for detecting immunoglobulins (Ig) and complement (C) fragments within tissue specimens. The two major antibody-induced forms of glomerular injury (antiglomerular basement membrane, or anti-GBM glomerulonephritis; IC glomerulonephritis) display different patterns of Ig deposition under immunofluorescence. Anti-GBM antibodies react with antigen distributed

BIBLIOGRAPHY

Brouet JC et al: Biological and clinical significance of cryoglobulinemia: report of 86 cases, *Am J Med* 57:775, 1974.

Callegari PE, Williams WV: Laboratory tests for rheumatic diseases: when are they useful? *Postgrad Med* 97:65, 1995.

Frank MM: Detection of complement in relation to disease, *J Allergy Clin Immunol* 89:641, 1992.

Glovsky MM: Applications of complement determinations in human disease, *Ann Allergy* 72:477, 1994.

Hebert LA, Cosio FG, Neff JC: Diagnostic significance of hypocomplementemia, *Kidney Int* 39:811, 1991.

Schur PH: Complement studies of sera and other biologic fluids, *Hum Pathol* 14:338, 1983.

Scullion M, Balint G, Whaley K: Evaluation of the C1q solid-phase binding assay for immune complexes: a clinical and laboratory study, *J Clin Lab Immunol* 2:15, 1979.

Whaley K: *Methods in complement for clinical immunologists,* New York, 1985, Churchill Livingstone.

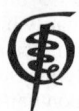

CHAPTER

179 Evaluation of Cellular Immune Function

John J. O'Shea

The initiation and regulation of the cellular immune response is dependent on the tightly orchestrated activities of a variety of specialized cells, principally involving lymphocytes and mononuclear phagocytes. The simplest screening test for integrity of cellular immunity remains in vivo skin testing. However, additional tests are available from clinical laboratories to analyze the presence and function of these cells. These tests include flow cytometry, immunofluorescence and immunohistochemistry, lymphocyte proliferation assays, and assays for lymphocyte cytotoxicity. As our understanding of the complexity of the immune response increases, new methodologies to assess various aspects of the interactions regulating the immune system have been developed. These new methodologies are identifying derangements of immune function characteristic of disease states. For example, advances in molecular biology have expanded our knowledge of the structure and function of the numerous soluble factors, termed *cytokines,* that regulate the immune response. The measurement of cytokines in body fluids and delineation of cytokine-producing cells in various diseases are areas of intense investigation. In addition, molecular techniques can define specific T-cell receptor usage in different diseases, and strategies may be devised to delete these pathogenic clones of cells. This chapter reviews the assays available to assess quantitative and functional aspects of the various lymphoid populations. Emphasis is on those most commonly used; more specialized techniques will be only briefly discussed. It should be stressed that immunologic tests are not in themselves diagnostic. The results from the laboratory need to be interpreted in the clinical context. A careful history and physical examination remain critical aspects of the evaluation of the patient with a suspected derangement in cellular immunity.

IN VIVO ASSESSMENT OF CELL-MEDIATED IMMUNITY: DELAYED-TYPE HYPERSENSITIVITY

Despite many recent technical advances in assessing the cellular immune response, the intradermal skin test remains the most straightforward initial screening procedure for evaluating cell-mediated immunity, although the test may be rendered negative by a variety of factors. A positive skin test requires a complex series of interactions involving most of the components of the cellular immune system and thus implies intact delayed-type hypersensitivity (DTH) and, with few exceptions, cell-mediated immunity. Failure to respond is termed *cutaneous anergy* and implies a defect in this process but does not localize this defect further. In addition to evaluating cellular immune function in the aggregate, skin testing can also be used to determine specific prior sensitization to various viral, bacterial, and fungal antigens, and this information can be useful diagnostically.

The skin test is performed by injecting a minute quantity of an antigenic preparation intradermally. At 24, 48, and 72 hours, the degree of skin induration is assessed clinically. Induration of more than 5 mm is commonly considered a positive result. When evaluating the tuberculin test, however, induration of 10 mm in diameter or greater

indicates probable exposure to *Mycobacterium tuberculosis,* whereas induration of 5 to 10 mm suggests that specific sensitization is questionable, and 0 to 4 mm is a negative test. Patients who develop 5 to 10 mm of induration may have had a previous bacillus Calmette-Guerin (BCG) vaccination or have been exposed to one of the atypical mycobacteria. Skin testing to assess established DTH is done with a battery of recall antigens including mumps, *Candida,* trichophytin, and tuberculin. When such a battery of antigens is used, it is unlikely that an individual will have failed to encounter at least one of them. More than 97% of normal persons develop at least one positive skin reaction when three or more antigens are used.

A variety of nonimmunologic and immunologic conditions are associated with cutaneous anergy (Box 179-1). Many of the nonimmunologic causes may have similar etiologies. For instance, zinc deficiency appears to play a role in the anergy seen in surgical patients, sickle cell anemia, and malnutrition. Immunologic causes include congenital T-cell immunodeficiencies like severe combined immunodeficiency (SCID), iatrogenic immunosuppression, and autoimmune disease. In addition, defects in macrophage antigen presentation func-

---

BOX 179-1
Causes of cutaneous anergy

I. Immunologic
   A. Acquired
      1. Acquired immunodeficiency syndrome (AIDS)
      2. Acute leukemia
      3. Carcinoma
      4. Chronic lymphocytic leukemia
      5. Hodgkin's disease
      6. Non-Hodgkin's lymphoma
   B. Congenital
      1. Ataxia telangiectasia
      2. Di George's syndrome
      3. Nezelof's syndrome
      4. Severe combined immunodeficiency
      5. Wiskott-Aldrich syndrome
II. Infections
   A. Bacterial
      1. Bacterial pneumonia
      2. Brucellosis
   B. Disseminated mycotic infections
   C. Mycobacterial
      1. Lepromatous leprosy
      2. Miliary and active tuberculosis
   D. Viral
      1. Varicella
      2. Hepatitis
      3. Influenza
      4. Infectious mononucleosis
      5. Measles
      6. Mumps
III. Immunosuppressive medications
   A. Cyclophosphamide
   B. Methotrexate
   C. Rifampin
   D. Systemic corticosteroids
IV. Other
   A. Alcoholic cirrhosis
   B. Anemia
   C. Biliary cirrhosis
   D. Burns
   E. Crohn's disease
   F. Diabetes
   G. Malnutrition
   H. Old age
   I. Pregnancy
   J. Pyridoxine deficiency
   K. Rheumatic diseases
   L. Sarcoidosis
   M. Sickle cell anemia
   N. Surgery
   O. Uremia

tion, such as deficiency of MHC class II, also result in anergy. Because a failure to respond properly to antigens in DTH skin testing is affected by so many factors, more specific tests need to be employed to make the correct diagnosis. Skin testing is useful, however, in that a positive response negates the need for more sophisticated testing, like measurement of in vitro lymphocyte proliferation, as this is rarely abnormal in the setting of normal skin testing.

FLOW CYTOMETRIC ANALYSIS OF PERIPHERAL BLOOD LEUKOCYTES

The initial evaluation of a suspected defect in cellular immunity is to determine if there is a sufficient number of the cells involved. A complete blood cell count (CBC) and differential will identify gross abnormalities in the number of circulating lymphocytes, as is found in chronic lymphocytic leukemia, systemic lupus erythematosus, or the acquired immunodeficiency syndrome (AIDS). However, this analysis is not sufficient to identify more subtle defects. Since the circulating lymphocyte pool is composed of several subpopulations, including B-lymphocytes, T-cells (including CD4$^+$ or helper T-cells and CD8$^+$ or cytolytic T-cells), and natural killer (NK) cells, a total lymphocyte count will not identify a deficiency in a specific population.

The most widely used technique to enumerate subsets of peripheral blood leukocytes is flow cytometry. This technique allows the examination of thousands of cells for size, shape, and membrane receptor expression. Using monoclonal antibodies, which recognize cell surface molecules and are specific for various leukocyte subsets, the proportion of the individual subset can be determined. In addition, as flow cytometric techniques have become increasingly sophisticated, techniques have been devised to measure characteristics other than surface receptor expression, including intracellular calcium levels, nucleic acid content, apoptosis, and synthesis of cytokines.

Peripheral blood leukocytes, separated by density gradient centrifugation or red blood cell depletion, are incubated with monoclonal antibodies labeled with a fluorescent dye. As an alternative, a primary antibody is bound to the cells followed by a labeled secondary antibody that binds to the primary antibody. A suspension of labeled cells is then aspirated into the cytometer, where the cells flow past a laser beam. Their size, granularity and fluorescence (a measure of the amount of fluorescently labeled antibody bound by the individual cell) can be simultaneously determined. Fluorescence intensity is then plotted as a function of cell number. Multiple antibodies with different specificities and distinct fluorescent emissions can be used. A list of the various surface molecules used to distinguish cell types is included in Table 179-1. The designation *CD* (cluster of differentiation) refers to surface molecules that are recognized by specific monoclonal antibodies. Because these structures are recognized by antibodies, they are also referred to as *antigens* or *markers*.

T-lymphocytes are enumerated on the basis of the expression of the T-cell receptor by antibodies reacting with the CD3 complex of proteins. T-cells are further divided into subpopulations that recognize MHC class I or MHC class II molecules by the coreceptors CD8 and CD4, respectively. Monocytes also express CD4, but they can be distinguished from T-cells by their lack of CD3 expression. Monoclonal antibodies can also be used to differentiate the γδ-subset of T-cells from the more numerous αβ T-cells. NK cells are determined by expression of CD56, an adhesion molecule specific for this leukocyte subset and CD16, an Fc receptor. Major antigens that are used to identify B-cells are: CD19, CD20, and CD22. B-cells also express IgM on their membranes.

Table 179-1   Cluster of differentiation (CD) nomenclature: selected cell surface molecules used to identify cell types

CD DESIGNATION	CHARACTERISTICS	CELL TYPE EXPRESSING
CD1a-c	43-49 kD	Thymocytes, B-cell
CD1d	43-49 kD associated with β2 microglobulin, functions in antigen presentation	Intestinal epithelium
CD2	50 kD, receptor for CD58, LFA-3	T-cells and NK cells
CD3	Complex of proteins including γ-, δ-, ε-, ζ-, and η-chains associated with TCR subunits	T-cells
CD4	59 kd, coreceptor for MHC class II, receptor for HIV, associated with Lck kinase	Class II restricted T-cells, monocytes
CD5	67 kD, receptor for CD72	T-cells and a subset of B-cells
CD6	100 kD	T-cells and a subset of B-cells
CD7	40 kD	T-cells
CD8	32 kd αα-homodimer and αβ-heterodimer, coreceptor for MHC, class I	Class I restricted T-cells
CD11a	170-180 kD, LFA-1 α-chain adhesion molecule, associated with CD18	T-cells
CD11b	iC3b receptor α-chain, associated with CD18	Monocyte/macrophages, neutrophils, NK cells
CD11c	p150/95, associated with CD18	Granulocytes, monocytes, and NK cells
CD14	55 kD receptor for complexes of LPS and LPS-binding protein	Monocytes
CD16	Low affinity IgG receptor (FcγRIII)	NK cells, activated monocytes, neutrophils
CD18	95 kD, associated with CD11a, b, c; mutated in leukocyte adhesion deficiency syndrome	Leukocytes
CD19	90 kDa	B-cells
CD20	35 and 37 kD, phosphoprotein	B-cells
CD22	135 kD	Mature B-cells, not plasma cells
CD25	55 kD, IL-2Rα subunit	Activated T-cells, B-cells, monocytes
CD28	44 kD monomers form homodimer. Key costimulatory molecule	T-cells
CD34	105-120 kD	Hematopoietic progenitor cells
CD40	45-50 kD	B-cells
CD40L	39 kD CD40 ligand, mutated in hyper IgM syndrome	T-cells
CD44	95 kD, deficient in Wiscott-Aldrich patients	T-cells, neutrophils, brain
CD45	220 kD transmembrane tyrosine phosphatase, differential splice variants	Leukocytes, naive T-cells (CD45RA), memory T-cells (CD45RO)
CD56	180-220 kD adhesion molecule	NK cells
CD69	55-65 kD, early activation marker	Activated T-cells, B-cells, NK cells, and macrophages
CD95	36-43 kD, Fas, mutated in autoimmune lymphoproliferative syndrome	Many cells
CD122	75 kD IL-2Rβ chain	NK, T-cells, and B-cells
CD127	65-75 kD IL-7R	T-cells, thymocytes, lymphocyte progenitors
CD130	130 kD, gp130, common β subunit of IL-6, IL-11, LIF, OSM, etc. receptors	—

Congenital immunodeficiencies can be distinguished based on cell populations analyzed by flow cytometry. For example, X-linked agammaglobulinemia, due to deficiency of the Bruton's tyrosine kinase (Btk), is characterized by the lack of B-cells and a normal number of T-cells. In contrast, some patients with severe combined immunodeficiency (SCID) lack T-cells and have variable numbers of B-cells. For instance, in X-linked SCID, (common γ-chain deficiency) and autosomal SCID due to JAK3 deficiency, T-cells are absent but B-cells are present (so-called T-B+ SCID). Moreover, in patients with SCID due to deficiency of Zap-70 (ζ-associated protein of 70 kD), there is absence of CD8+ T-cells with relative sparing of CD4+ T-cells. By comparison, in patients with SCID due to adenosine deaminase deficiency, there is progressive diminution of both T-cells and B-cells over time. Patients with Wiskott-Aldrich syndrome lack CD43 expression. In addition, a syndrome termed *leukocyte adhesion deficiency* is characterized by recurrent bacterial and fungal infections, progressive periodontitis, and/or delayed umbilical cord separation that is associated with a defect in the expression of CD18, which associates with three different subunits (CD11 a, b, and c) to form three receptors. CD11a/CD18 (LFA-1) is a surface molecule on T-cells involved in cellular adhesion. CD11b/CD18 is a receptor for a complement fragment, C3bi, and is expressed on monocytes and macrophages.

Similarly, flow cytometric analysis of lymphocyte subsets is invaluable in AIDS. Quantifying the number of CD4+ cells in patients with AIDS can be a useful indicator of prognosis, as those with fewer than 200 CD4+ cells per mm³ have a poor prognosis.

The clinical value of careful enumeration of mononuclear cell subsets is expanding. These tools have been used in characterizing various hematologic malignancies and have led to specific therapies based on the phenotype of the malignant cell. Flow cytometry can be used to establish clonality and assign lineage and level of cell differentiation. In addition, flow cytometry is used in assessing the response to therapy with agents like IL-2 that dramatically expand the number of NK cells in the peripheral blood, and experimental immunosuppressive drugs or monoclonal antibodies that target lymphocytes.

ANALYSIS OF IMMUNE CELLS IN TISSUES

Immunofluorescence and immunohistochemistry. Although it is useful to delineate the various subpopulations of lymphoid cells in the peripheral blood, the abnormalities observed may not be representative of events occurring in tissues affected by immunologic diseases. Histochemical and immunohistologic evaluation of tissue sections permits the direct examination of lymphoid subpopulations in the tissue. Lymph node morphology has been used for years to assess immunocompetence. Since the lymph node is divided into a paracortical area that contains T-cells and germinal centers and primary follicles that contain B-cells, routine histologic evaluation can identify various gross deficiencies. Isolated T-cell deficiencies result in either sparsely populated paracortical areas or paracortical areas in which T-cells are replaced by non–T cells, such as histiocytes or eosinophils. Isolated B-cell deficiencies are characterized by absence of germinal centers and plasma cells. Monoclonal antibodies that identify T-cells, B-cells, and monocytes have been used in analysis of inflammatory tissue lesions including skin test sites, various infectious processes, allograft rejection, sites of graft-versus-host disease, and malignancies. From these studies it has become clear that the predominant cell infiltrating sites of delayed-type hypersensitivity is the CD4+ T-cell. In contrast, CD8+ cells predominate during graft-versus-host disease, allograft rejection, and lepromatous leprosy.

FUNCTIONAL ASSESSMENT OF CELLULAR IMMUNITY IN VITRO

Although quantitation of lymphocyte subpopulations with flow cytometry is a powerful tool, in most cases it provides no information on the function of these cells. Moreover, delayed-type hypersensitivity skin tests measure activity of the entire system but cannot assess specific capabilities of the various cells involved in cell-mediated immunity. A number of in vitro assays are available to determine functional aspects of these cells, but if DTH responses are completely normal, there is little point in measuring lymphocyte proliferation in vitro.

Lymphocyte Proliferation. An in vitro correlate of cell-mediated immunity (CMI) is a determination of T-cell proliferation. This method evaluates the capacity of T-lymphocytes that have been primed in vivo to respond in vitro after culture with the appropriate antigen. The first step in this response is the interaction of antigen-specific T-cells with antigen-presenting cells. After recognition of the specific antigen, the T-cell undergoes a series of physiologic changes resulting in its transformation to a lymphoblast and culminating in cell division. Although a variety of changes can be measured, lymphocyte responsiveness is most commonly assessed by measuring DNA synthesis through the incorporation of radiolabeled thymidine. Measurements of T-cell DNA synthesis stimulated by specific antigens may suggest a specific defect in antigen responsiveness or a lack of antecedent sensitization, but a poor response to a single antigen does not necessarily imply a more global dysfunction of CMI.

Besides specific antigen, a variety of nonspecific stimuli can be used to activate T-cells in vitro. Mitogens, such as phytohemagglutinin or concanavalin A, are lectins that stimulate T-cells by nonspecifically aggregating membrane receptors. Since such mitogens activate cells irrespective of their antigen specificity, no previous sensitization is required. This activation, however, is dependent on an accessory cell such as the monocyte. Thus activation by mitogens can be used to test both the integrity of T cell–monocyte interaction and the ability of the T-cells to proliferate. T-cells can also be activated in the absence of accessory cells by crosslinking the TCR in conjunction with crosslinking a costimulatory molecule like CD28 with the appropriate monoclonal antibodies. As an alternative, pharmacologic stimuli can be used. These systems have the capacity to examine intrinsic T-cell function, independent of accessory cell function. Proliferation in response to IL-2 is also measured.

Altered lymphocyte function can result in abnormal responses to mitogens, manifested as either diminished peak responses or as shifts in either the dose-response curve or the kinetics of the response. Results from studies comparing delayed-type hypersensitivity skin testing and in vitro mitogen responses suggest there is a good correlation between the two. Anergic patients usually do not mount normal mitogen responses in vitro. However, since delayed-type hypersensitivity requires functions not tested by the in vitro analysis of mitogen responsiveness, such as chemotaxis of monocytes and lymphocytes, an occasional anergic patient responds to mitogens in vitro.

T-cells also respond vigorously to foreign (allogeneic) cells in a response that is known as the *mixed lymphocyte reaction* (MLR). The MLR does not require prior sensitization and is directed primarily at human leukocyte antigens, locus D (HLA-D)–region antigens, on the stimulator cells. This test is also used to determine the suitability of a donor in tissue transplantation.

Lymphocyte Cytotoxicity Assays. Cytolytic cells are heterogenous, and the ability to lyse cells can be accomplished by cytolytic T-cells, NK cells, and monocytes. The cytolytic activity is influenced by prior sensitization in the case of T-cells, but is also profoundly influenced by cytokines like IL-2, IL-12, INFα/β, and IFNγ. Cytotoxic T-cells are specifically committed effector T-cells that have the capacity to lyse target cells bearing antigens to which the cytotoxic cells have been primed. Cytotoxic T-cells primed to the major histocompatibility complex (MHC)-encoded antigens of the stimulator cells can be generated during the MLR. Cytotoxic T-cells directed at class I MHC antigens are usually of the CD8+ phenotype, whereas those directed at class II MHC antigens are usually CD4+ cells. Cytotoxic T-lymphocytes can be assayed by their capacity to lyse target cells labeled with radioactive chromium. The amount of released label is a measure of cytotoxicity. In general, T cell–mediated cytotoxicity plays a role in the host's defense against viral infection and perhaps in preventing neoplasia. Measurement of cytotoxic T-cells is used for pretransplantation screening, and antiviral cytolytic responses are also useful, particularly in the assessment of anti-HIV immunocompetence.

Natural killer (NK) cells recognize and kill targets without the need for antecedent sensitization; thus they play a role in the "natural resistance" of the host. They are thought to be important in resistance to malignancies and viral infections. NK function is assessed by culturing effector cells (from peripheral blood, spleen, or inflammatory exudates or tissue) with labeled targets. Target-cell lysis is quantified by measuring the release of the label. Thus the abilities of the effector cells both to bind and kill the target are evaluated. Target cells are usually malignant cell lines, such as the erythroleukemia cell line, K562. Since cytokines (administered in vivo or in vitro) enhance normal NK function, many studies examine NK cytolytic function following cytokine stimulation. NK cells can also kill immunoglobulin-coated targets via engagement of their Fc receptors, an assay termed *antibody-dependent cellular cytotoxicity* (ADCC).

NK cell dysfunction has been described in a variety of disease states including malignancy, infectious, and autoimmune disease, although the significance and pathogenetic basis of these alterations are unclear. Patients with Chediak-Higashi syndrome also have impaired NK function. Thus the clinical utility of measuring NK activity remains to be defined.

B-lymphocytes are genetically programmed with a surface receptor (immunoglobulin) specific for a particular antigen. Following antigen recognition and receptor engagement the B-cells proliferate and blasts transform and differentiate into plasma cells that produce large amounts of the receptor molecule in a soluble form, that is, antibody or immunoglobulin (Ig). B-cell Ig production is dependent upon T cell–B cell contact and appropriate T-cell cytokine stimulation. A crude but rapid assessment of the humoral (B-cell) immune system is provided by analysis of serum immunoglobulins (Chapter 173). Total Ig, Ig subclasses, and monoclonal Ig protein can be detected by available techniques. A number of assays can test the ability of T-cells to support B-cell Ig production. Most straightforward is to culture resting B-cells with activated T-cells and measure proliferation, and immunoglobulin in the culture supernatant. Mutations of CD4OL that occur in the disease Hyper IgM syndrome interfere with the ability to provide help to B cells. The requirement for T-cells can be bypassed by the use of a plant lectin–poke weed mitogen. In fixed tissues human plasma cells can be identified by their display of intracytoplasmic immunoglobulin as detected by fluoresceinated antibodies.

MEASUREMENT OF CYTOKINES AND CYTOKINE-PRODUCING CELLS

The importance of cytokines in cellular growth and differentiation, hematopoiesis, inflammation, and immunoregulation is now well established. In some cases, cytokine measurements in serum are routine and clinical utility has been established, for example, the measurement of erythropoietin levels. Other cytokines, like IL-6, TNFα, and IFNγ, are readily detected in the serum and increase with inflammation, but the clinical significance of measuring their levels has not been established. In addition, the serum concentration of a given cytokine may be a poor reflection of the amount produced in a specific tissue undergoing immunologic damage (e.g., synovial fluid).

A number of assays are available for measuring cytokines. Most are based on antibody recognition of epitopes on the cytokine as detected in an ELISA system. However, serum and tissues often contain large amounts of cytokine inhibitors, and soluble cytokine receptors that can interfere with the function of the particular cytokine being measured. Thus the balance between these factors must be appreciated when interpreting clinical significance of cytokine measurements. Cytokine mRNA can be demonstrated in whole tissues by the polymerase chain reaction (PCR) and in situ hybridization techniques have been developed to detect cytokine genes in individual cells. Combining these techniques with antibodies that identify cytokine protein and cell surface antigens allows a definition of the cells in a specific lesion responsible for the cytokine production. Intracellular cytokines can also be measured by flow cytometry. Although these techniques are primarily experimental at the present time, they likely will move from the research arena into the clinical laboratory in the not too distant future.

MONOCYTE-MACROPHAGE ASSAYS

Mononuclear phagocytes perform several important and necessary functions for immune responses. One function is antigen presentation, which is necessary to initiate cell-mediated immunity. Antigen presentation involves taking up native antigen, processing it, and presenting it to relevant T-cells. For activation, T-cells must see antigen in the context of class II products encoded by genes of the major histocompatibility (MHC) locus on the antigen-presenting monocyte. An inability to express MHC class II molecules has been described

in several patients with severe immunodeficiency. The integrity of antigen presentation is measured in lymphocyte proliferation assays.

Other functional tests of monocyte activity include assays of chemotaxis, bacterial killing, and cytotoxicity. Patients with lepromatous leprosy or neoplasia have been described with defects in chemotaxis and cytotoxicity, respectively. In addition, it has been suggested that patients with malacoplakia have a defect in monocyte killing of *Escherichia coli* organisms. The production of cytokines like IL-1, TNFα, GM-CSF, and IL-6 by monocytes can also be assessed. Another marker of monocyte activation is neopterin secretion. The only known cellular source of neopterin is macrophages, and increased levels in the blood and urine are found in rheumatoid arthritis, transplant rejection, tuberculosis and infections with other intracellular pathogens, and AIDS.

BIBLIOGRAPHY

Callard R, Gearing A: *The cytokine facts book,* London, 1994, Academic Press.
Coligan JE et al: *Current protocols in immunology,* New York, 1994, John Wiley & Sons.
Fleisher TA, Marti GE: Flow cytometry. In Rich RR, editor: *Clinical immunology: principles and practice,* St Louis, 1996, Mosby.
Howard MC, Miyajima A, Coffman R: T cell derived cytokines and their receptors. In Paul W, editor: *Fundamental immunology,* ed 3, New York, 1993, Raven Press.
Kurnick JT, Bhan AK, McCluskey RT: Analysis of cell mediated reactions. In Colvin RB, Bhan AK, McCluskey RT, editors: *Diagnostic immunopathology,* New York, 1995, Raven Press.
Rose NR, de Macario EC, Fahey JL et al: *Manual of clinical laboratory immunology,* ed 4, Washington, DC, 1992, American Society for Microbiology.
Rosen FS, Cooper MD, Wedgwood RJ: The primary immunodeficiencies, *N Engl J Med* 333:431-440, 1995.

CHAPTER

180   Laboratory Methods in Immediate Hypersensitivity

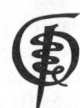

Stephen I. Wasserman

The clinical assessment of immediate hypersensitivity disease is based on the ability to reproduce in a controlled and localized fashion in vivo anaphylactic reactions to suspected antigenic substances. Precise and sensitive in vitro tests capable of measuring the amounts and antigenic specificity of individual immunoglobulins, particularly IgE, are also available.

IN VIVO TECHNIQUES
Skin Tests

Testing of antigens in the skin can be performed by intradermal and prick-puncture methods. The latter route is favored because of its reproducibility, lesser risk of systemic (anaphylactic) reactions, better specificity, and better patient acceptance. Skin-test sites (back or forearm) are cleansed, and a single drop of antigen solution is placed on the skin. A needle or commercial prick-puncture device is inserted into the skin through the antigen. Only superficial penetration is made, and no bleeding should occur. The antigen is removed by blotting 30 to 60 seconds after skin puncture, and the test site is measured for erythema (flare) and edema (wheal) 15 minutes later. Intradermal testing should be reserved for antigens that are of suspected clinical relevance but are nonreactive by prick-puncture techniques, recognizing that this technique is more sensitive but less specific than prick-puncture. Twenty to 50 microliters (0.02 to 0.05 ml) of antigen solution is injected intracutaneously, and the area of wheal and flare determined 15 minutes later. Various grading systems have been employed to describe the wheal-and-flare reaction and any associated pseudopodia. For both prick-puncture and intradermal techniques, appropriate controls are required to exclude unreported antihistamine ingestion, to verify skin reactivity, and to rule out dermographism. Use of diluent, histamine (0.01% intradermal, 1% prick-puncture),

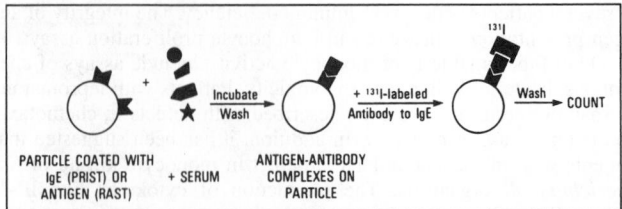

FIGURE 180-1 Principle of the radioimmunoassays (RAST and PRIST) used in the measurement of IgE or antigen-specific IgE.

and codeine (a nonspecific mast cell degranulator) provides negative and positive controls. Interpretation of skin tests, either prick-puncture or intradermal, requires that the response to diluent be absent or minimal (0 to 2 mm), and the response to histamine or codeine, or both, be present (8 to 10 mm intradermal, 5 to 6 mm prick-puncture). Because clinically irrelevant positive as well as false-negative reactions occur, it is essential that reactions be interpreted in light of the clinical history. In addition, the antigens employed must be fresh and must have antigenic reactivity, and the tests must have been properly administered. Since intradermal administration of concentrated antigens may cause wheal-and-flare reactions in a very high proportion of nonsensitive individuals, the more dilute the solution causing a positive response, the more likely the antigen is to be clinically relevant.

The skin also may be used for another form of testing—the P-K (Prausnitz-Küstner) reaction. Rarely performed because of the risk of introducing infection, this test employs sera from an individual in whom IgE antigenic sensitivity is suspected. A volunteer (nonallergic) is injected with 0.05 to 0.10 ml of the patient's serum intradermally, and this site and a control area are challenged with antigen (0.02 ml) 24 to 48 hours later. The test is read as for intradermal skin testing. This procedure was employed for research purposes and, occasionally, to evaluate food or drug sensitivity, but should be abandoned.

In rare cases, bronchial or nasal allergen challenge may be performed to assess allergic reactivity. These techniques, however, generally lack specificity and/or precision, more readily induce systemic reactions, are expensive, and may be confounded by nonspecific hyperirritability, which makes their interpretation more difficult. They should be reserved for unique situations. Since skin-test reactivity to an antigen is highly correlated with bronchial reactivity to the same antigen, such testing generally is redundant.

IN VITRO ASSAYS
IgE Measurement

Total serum IgE concentrations are too low to permit assessment by immunodiffusion techniques, therefore various radioimmunologic or enzymatic assays have been developed. The most commonly used test is the PRIST (paper disk radioimmunoassay technique, Fig. 180-1), in which the patient's serum is reacted with antibody to human IgE bound to a paper disk. After incubation, the disk is washed, and a radiolabeled antibody to human IgE is added; the disk is again washed. The amount of radioactivity bound to the paper disk correlates directly with the serum level of IgE. This technique is capable of measuring IgE in picogram quantities. IgE is reported as units or nanograms per milliliter. One unit is equivalent to 2.4 ng.

Antigen-specific IgE may be measured directly by the radioallergosorbent test (RAST, see Fig. 180-1) and by a number of other similar test systems or by measuring the antigen-induced release of histamine from basophil leukocytes. The RAST is similar in principle to the PRIST. In this test, specific antigens, rather than IgE molecules, are bound to a solid matrix and exposed to the patient's serum. The matrix is washed and reacted with radiolabeled antibody to human IgE. The amount of radiolabel bound to the solid phase is directly proportional to amounts of IgE in serum with specificity to the test antigen. The results are semiquantitative and are reported in comparison to a serum known to contain antigen-specific IgE. Modifications of this test employing fluorescence, luminescence, or color are available. This test also can be modified to assess antigen-specific IgG

BOX 180-1
Skin testing

Advantages	Disadvantages
Inexpensive	Requires discontinuation of antihistamines
Antigens are available	Can cause anaphylaxis
Rapid	Dermographism precludes testing
Precise	Extensive skin disease may preclude testing
Sensitive	Difficult to perform and/or interpret in some elderly patients

BOX 180-2
RAST testing

Advantages	Disadvantages
No risk of anaphylaxis	Expensive and slow
No risk of sensitization	Most tests use radioactivity
No need to interrupt antihistamines	Fewer antigens available
Dermographism or skin disease irrelevant	Lower sensitivity
	Lack of quantification
	Requires known positive serum
	High levels of antigen-specific IgG may interfere
	Does not directly measure clinical severity

antibodies. Such *in vitro* tests of specific IgE correlate well with other in vitro and in vivo tests of IgE reactivity, including skin testing, bronchial provocation, and leukocyte histamine release. Controversy exists over the relative utility of in vitro measurement of specific IgE compared with in vivo skin testing. The advantages and disadvantages (Boxes 180-1 and 180-2) must be weighed before either is utilized. At present, however, it appears that skin testing performed by a skilled individual with appropriate experience in interpretation is the cost-effective method of choice for assessing antigen-specific IgE in most clinical situations.

The release of histamine from peripheral blood basophils also can be used to define the presence and specificity of IgE in patients. Patient leukocytes, in whole blood or after washing to remove serum constituents, are interacted with various quantities of antigen, and the amount of histamine released is measured. This test requires fresh leukocytes in large numbers from patients not taking inhibitory drugs. Moreover, histamine measurements are laborious and expensive. Patient serum can be used to passively sensitize donor leukocytes, but this procedure suffers from the same difficulties as the direct test and is generally reserved for research purposes.

IMMUNOTHERAPY

Although not specifically a test or a diagnostic procedure, immunotherapy is directly linked to the proper interpretation of the demonstration of antigen-specific IgE. Allergen injection therapy, or immunotherapy, as it is generally known, has been utilized since the early 1900s, but at present is generally reserved for patients with IgE-dependent allergic diseases whose symptoms are not controlled by environmental manipulation or medications, or in whom such medications are contraindicated or not tolerated. Immunotherapy is efficacious in the treatment of allergic rhinitis, venom hypersensitivity, and asthma. Antigens that have been employed successfully include pollens, molds, danders, and insect and mite antigens. Foods are not used. Immunotherapy is complicated in patients receiving β-adrenergic blocking agents because of difficulty in treating anaphylaxis in this setting.

Immunotherapy is performed by the sequential (generally weekly) subcutaneous injections of gradually increasing amounts of antigen to which the patient has been shown to be sensitive by clinical and laboratory assessment. Initial dosage generally consists of 0.02 to 0.05 ml of a 1:100,000 concentration (weight:volume) or 100 protein nitrogen units (pnu) per milliliter of each antigen. Standardized allergens are increasingly available, and are preferable. Aqueous extracts of antigen generally are employed, but alum-precipitated antigen or polymerized antigens have been reported to be even more efficacious and/or safer. Weekly incremental doses of 0.05 to 0.10 ml are administered until, after 4 to 6 months, the patient is receiving 0.5 to 0.7 ml of a 1:100 w:v; 10,000 pnu or equivalent standardized allergen per milliliter of solution. Forms of immunotherapy that do not advance to high doses of antigen are ineffective. The skin site and patient should be observed 15 to 30 minutes after each injection, and any erythema, edema, tenderness, or allergic response noted. The rate of increase in concentrations of antigen may be slowed if large local reactions develop. Systemic reactions (wheezing, generalized pruritus, urticaria, hypotension) require a two-fold to ten-fold reduction in antigen dose and a slower schedule of advancement. A 2- to 3-year course of immunotherapy is associated with improvement in symptoms of allergic rhinitis in 60% to 75% of well-selected patients, and good results may be noted within the first year. The mechanism whereby immunotherapy provides relief remains elusive. Patients receiving immunotherapy initially experience a rise in serum antigen-specific IgE and IgG concentrations, but with time the IgE falls and IgG elevation persists. Postseasonal IgE rises are blunted or absent after immunotherapy and a diminished release of histamine from basophils, both to specific antigen and spontaneously, is observed. Finally, increases in antigen-specific CD8 lymphocyte reactivity, decreases in antigen-specific CD4 reactivity, an increase in antigen reactive Th1 and decrease in Th2 lymphocytes, and generation by macrophages of an inhibitor of histamine release have been reported to accompany clinically successful immunotherapy. Skin tests, which reflect mast cell sensitivity, generally do not change greatly with immunotherapy; however, successful immunotherapy with hymenoptera venom is associated in some patients with loss of skin reactivity. A more rapid procedure to initiate immunotherapy is used for hymenoptera venoms.

BIBLIOGRAPHY

Adkinson NF, Platts-Mills TAE: IgE and atopic disease. In Samter M et al, editors: *Immunologic disease,* ed 4, Boston, 1988, Little, Brown.

Bousquet J, Michel FB: In vivo methods for study of allergy: skin tests, techniques, and interpretation. In Middleton EE et al, editors: *Allergy: principles and practice,* ed 4, St Louis, 1993, Mosby.

Bryant DM, Burnes MW, Lazarus L: The correlation between skin tests, bronchial provocation tests, and the serum level of IgE specific for common allergies in patients with asthma, *Clin Allergy* 5:145, 1975.

Goodnow CC, Brink R, Adams E: Breakdown of self-tolerance in anergic B lymphocytes, *Nature* 352:532, 1991.

Hamburger HA, Katzaren JA: Methods in laboratory immunology: principles and interpretation of laboratory tests for allergy. In Middleton EE et al, editors: *Allergy: principles and practice,* ed 4, St Louis, 1993, Mosby.

Rocklin RE: Clinical and immunological aspects of allergen-specific immunotherapy in patients with seasonal allergic rhinitis and/or allergic asthma, *J Allergy Clin Immunol* 72:323, 1983.

Van Metre TE et al: A comparative study of the effectiveness of the Rinkel method and the current standard method of immunotherapy for ragweed pollen hay fever, *J Allergy Clin Immunol* 66:500, 1980.

181 Autoantibodies

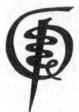

Liam Martin and Marvin J. Fritzler

Diseases associated with autoimmune phenomena tend to distribute themselves along a spectrum with organ-specific diseases at one end and non–organ-specific diseases at the other (Table 181-1). The organ-specific diseases, typified by Hashimoto's thyroiditis, are characterized by antibodies directed to, and inflammatory lesions within, a single organ. At the other end of the spectrum, typified by systemic lupus erythematosus (SLE), autoantibodies are directed against mul-

Table 181-1 Spectrum of autoimmune diseases and related autoantibodies

DISEASE	AUTOANTIBODY TARGET
Graves' disease	Thyroid peroxidase
Hashimoto's thyroiditis	Thyroglobulin
	Thyroid microsome
Myasthenia gravis	Acetylcholine receptors
	Striational skeletal and cardiac muscle
Insulin-dependent diabetes	Glutamic acid decarboxylase (GAD65)
	Carboxypeptidase
	Insulin
Insulin-resistant diabetes	Insulin receptor
Pernicious anemia	H^+, K^+ ATPase
	Vitamin B_{12} binding site on intrinsic factor
Addison's disease	Cytochrome p450 hydroxylase 21/17
Pemphigus vulgaris	Desmoglein3
Bullous pemphigoid	Basement membrane zone of skin and mucosa
Vitiligo	Melanocytes, tyrosinase
Idiopathic thrombocytopenic purpura	Platelet glycoprotein complex
Autoimmune hemolytic anemia	Erythrocytes
Primary biliary cirrhosis	Pyruvate dehydrogenase complex
	Primary biliary cirrhosis nuclear antigen
	PBC95/SP100
Chronic active hepatitis	Pyruvate dehydrogenase
	Nuclear lamin B
Goodpasture's syndrome	Type IV collagen (C-terminal domain)
Rheumatoid arthritis	γ-globulin
	Types II and III collagen
Sjögren's syndrome	SS-A/Ro, SS-B/la
	Nuclear mitotic apparatus (NuMA)
Scleroderma spectrum of diseases	Topoisomerase 1 (Scl-70)
	U3RNP (Fibrillarin)
	RNA polymerase
	PM/Scl
	Centromere proteins (CENPs)
Polymyositis	Jo-1 (histidyl tRNA synthetase)
	Other tRNA synthetases
	PM/Scl
Systemic lupus erythematosus	dsDNA
	snRNPs (U1-U6 ribonucleoproteins)
	Histones
	SS-A/Ro
Primary antiphospholipid antibody syndrome	Cardiolipin/B2-glycoprotein 1
Vasculitis	Proteinase 3
	Myeloperoxidase

tiple organs and the inflammatory lesions are widely disseminated. Common organs affected in organ-specific disease include thyroid, stomach, pancreas, and adrenal, whereas in non–organ-specific diseases, the kidneys, nervous tissue, skin, joints, and muscle are commonly involved. In organ-specific diseases, the lesions are relatively restricted, because the antigen in the organ serves as a target for the immune and inflammatory response. In non–organ-specific diseases, circulating immune complexes deposit systemically, giving rise to a widespread inflammatory response.

Interestingly, there are overlaps at each end of the spectrum. For example, thyroid antibodies are very prevalent in pernicious anemia patients, and these patients have a higher prevalence of autoimmune thyroid disease than is seen in the normal population. Similarly, patients with autoimmune thyroid disease have a high prevalence of parietal cell antibodies and, to a lesser extent, pernicious anemia. The systemic rheumatic diseases at the opposite end of the spectrum show considerable overlap. For example, features of scleroderma and polymyositis, or rheumatoid arthritis and SLE, are frequently seen in individual patients.

LABORATORY TESTS FOR SERUM ANTIBODIES IN AUTOIMMUNE DISEASE

The detection of autoantibodies in serum and other biologic fluids is carried out in the clinical laboratory primarily through (1) immunohistochemical techniques, such as immunofluorescence and enzyme-labeled antibody techniques; and (2) serologic techniques, such as latex particle aggregation, immunodiffusion, radioimmunoassay (RIA), enzyme-linked immunosorbent assay (ELISA), immunoprecipitation (IP), and Western immunoblotting (IB). The production of highly purified reagents in the form of monoclonal antibodies and recombinant antigens is now changing the laboratory approach to the investigation of autoimmune diseases.

Immunohistochemical techniques, RIA, and ELISA detect the presence of antibody through use of labeled molecules: for example, fluorescein-labeled molecules, enzyme-labeled (e.g., peroxidase) molecules, or radioisotope-labeled molecules. These techniques are highly sensitive for the identification of antibody binding to antigens. Tests involving secondary antigen-antibody reactions, such as agglutination (aggregation) or agar precipitation (immunodiffusion), are not as sensitive as the other techniques but are nevertheless quite suitable for the detection of certain antibodies.

The indirect immunofluorescence test is the most widely used immunohistochemical test to screen for serum autoantibodies (Fig. 181-1). Indirect immunofluorescence assays are performed by placing a test serum on antigen localized in tissue sections on a glass slide. The excess antibody is removed by washing and the bound antibody is detected by applying a "second" antibody—for example, a fluorescein-labeled antihuman immunoglobulin reagent—that has been raised in animals such as goats or rabbits. After the excess "second" antibody has been washed away, the slide is viewed in a microscope fitted with an ultraviolet light source. This procedure allows the technician to determine the antibody binding site in the cell and also, through grading the intensity of fluorescence, provides a semiquantitative measurement of the antibody concentration in the serum.

The technique of Western immunoblotting has proven useful in identifying target antigens in different substrates. IB is performed by reacting patients' sera with cellular or recombinant antigens that have been separated on polyacrylamide gels and electrophoretically transferred onto nitrocellulose sheets. Reactive antigens are visualized by applying conjugated second antibodies to the strip and reacting with an appropriate reagent to produce a color or photo signal. This technique is extremely sensitive and is useful in determining the specificity of antibodies.

The investigation of organ-specific autoimmune diseases dictates the use of slides that contain a variety of endocrine tissues, such as human thyroid, mouse stomach, or adrenal tissue. The detection of autoantibodies in non–organ-specific diseases relies on the use of tissue culture cells as a tissue substrate. The pattern of immunofluorescence (e.g., homogeneous, speckled, nucleolar, mitochondrial, or microsomal) can provide important information if it is interpreted in light of the antibody titer and the patient's clinical history.

INTERPRETATION OF TESTS FOR AUTOANTIBODIES

After a specific pattern of staining of the tissue substrate is detected, the titer of the antibody is the next most important component of the laboratory result. A high titer of autoantibody is significant, but a low, or even absent, autoantibody titer does not rule out a particular disorder. As examples of the latter, thyroid antibodies are present in low titer even in the presence of significant disease, and antibodies to some nuclear antigens in SLE (e.g., Ro antigen) may not be detected by standard autoantibody screening, such as the antinuclear antibody (ANA) test. In the case of low titers of thyroid antibodies, it is believed that the thyroid may serve as an immunosorbent of the anti-

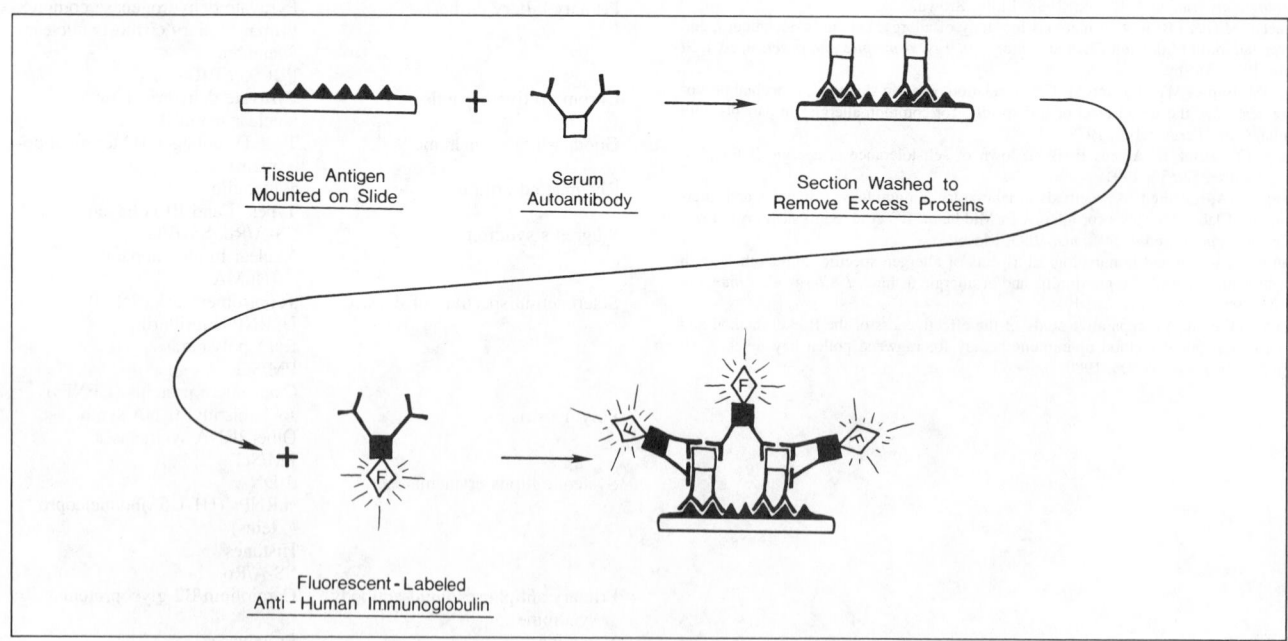

FIGURE 181-1   Indirect fluorescent-labeled antibody method for the detection of autoimmune antibody.

body. It is important to note that changing titers of some autoantibodies may relate to the severity, progression, or successful treatment of the disease, whereas other autoantibodies may not vary at all with disease course.

In addition to the false-negative results referred to earlier, the presence of autoantibodies in the patient's serum does not necessarily establish the diagnosis or the immunopathogenic origin of the disease. It should be remembered that many normal individuals have detectable titers of autoantibodies. Therefore when clinicians interpret the autoantibody test results they must recognize the potential for false-positive results, especially when autoantibody is present in low titer. In many of these individuals, the antibodies may persist through their lifetime with no apparent pathologic sequelae. False-positive results are particularly common in women, in patients on certain drugs (e.g., procainamide, hydralazine), in the first-degree relatives of patients with confirmed autoimmune disease, in acute viral or bacterial infections, in certain malignancies, and in the older (>60 years) population. The frequency and titer of antinuclear antibodies, for instance, rises in each decade after age 45.

SIGNIFICANCE OF COMMONLY ENCOUNTERED AUTOANTIBODIES
Thyroid Antibodies

Three types of thyroid autoantigens have been characterized that bind to antibodies in the sera of patients with Graves' disease or Hashimoto's throiditis: thyroglobulin, thyroid microsomal antigen, and the thyrotrophin receptor. Patients with Hashimoto's thyroiditis have autoantibodies to thyroglobulin and/or thyroid microsomal antigen in 95% of cases. A negative test with both antigens virtually rules out the diagnosis. Low to moderate titers of thyroglobulin antibody are present in myxedema, thyrotoxicosis, adenomatous hyperplasia, thyroid carcinoma, rheumatoid arthritis (RA), and SLE. Twenty percent of normal middle-aged women have antibodies to thyroglobulin. Two percent of healthy men and 6% of women have antibodies to thyroid microsomal antigen.

The thyroid microsomal antigen has been identified as thyroid peroxidase; the enzyme oxidizes iodine to a free radical form during the formation of thyroid hormones. Whether thyroid microsomal antibodies block in vivo production of thyroid hormones is unknown.

In Graves' disease, antibodies that react against the thyrotrophin receptor have been found. These antibodies are divided into stimulatory, thyroid-stimulating antibody (TSAb), and thyrotropin binding–inhibiting immunoglobulin (TBII). The TSAb includes the long-acting thyroid stimulator (LATS) and an antibody that prevents LATS binding, called *LATS protector.* Thyroid receptor–binding antibodies are measured by a radioreceptor assay.

Gastric Antibodies

Antibodies to gastric parietal cells are present in the sera of 90% of patients with pernicious anemia. These antibodies inhibit the activity of the proton pump in in vitro experiments, suggesting that they have a major role in the development of achylia in pernicious anemia. The antibody is detected in many patients with atrophic gastritis, is occasionally found in iron-deficient anemia, and is noted in thyroiditis and hyperthyroidism. Parietal cell antibodies, which increase with age, are present in Addison's disease (30%) and juvenile diabetes. Antibody to intrinsic factor is found in 50% to 70% of patients with pernicious anemia. Two types of intrinsic factor antibody exist: one prevents vitamin B_{12} binding to intrinsic factor, and the other binds to the intrinsic factor–B_{12} complex. Patients with smooth-muscle antibody also demonstrate gastric parietal cell–antibody activity; the cross-reacting antigen is related to F-actin.

Adrenocortical Antibodies

Up to 83% of patients with primary Addison's disease display antibodies to the cytoplasm of adrenocortical cells by indirect immunofluorescence assays. These antibodies react with a 54 kilodalton autoantigen that has been identified as the cytochrome p450 enzyme 21-hydroxylase. These antibodies are rarely seen in secondary adrenal insufficiency or other diseases of the adrenal gland.

Striated-Muscle Antibodies

These antibodies, detected by immunofluorescence, react with both skeletal and cardiac muscle. Fifty percent of patients with myasthenia gravis and 95% of myasthenia patients with a thymoma have antibodies that bind striated skeletal muscle. High titers of antibodies have been correlated with more severe disease, and generally, a titer of greater than 1:60 is specific for myasthenia. Some normal subjects also have the antibody, but the titers are usually less than 1:30. Patients with postpericardiotomy syndrome and occasional patients with dermatomyositis also display the antibody, but it is not found in patients with SLE or RA.

Cardiac muscle antibodies are found in one third of patients with rheumatic fever, as well as patients with recent streptococcal infections or acute glomerulonephritis. These antibodies are also observed in patients after cardiac surgery or trauma and in certain patients with ischemic heart disease.

Acetylcholine Receptor Antibody

Acetylcholine receptor (AChR) antibody is thought to be directly involved in producing the weakness in myasthenia gravis. Antibody may attach directly to the receptor or immediately adjacent to it, causing an increased turnover of the receptor. Patients with rheumatoid arthritis treated with penicillamine can develop AChR antibodies and myasthenia gravis. Antibodies to AChR are detected by radioimmunoassay.

Smooth-Muscle Antibodies

High titers of antibodies to smooth muscle are found in up to 70% of patients with chronic active hepatitis. These antibodies are also found in some patients with viral hepatitis, infectious mononucleosis, asthma, chronic bronchitis, chronic renal disease, and mycoplasmal pneumonia. Of normal individuals, 5% to 6% also have the antibody in their blood in low titer. The smooth-muscle antigen against which these antibodies react is F-actin. Moreover, smooth-muscle antibody titers in chronic active hepatitis may be higher (>1:80) and relatively more persistent than those seen in the other disorders. Primary biliary cirrhosis may be associated with smooth-muscle antibody titers of 1:10 to 1:40. There may be a decrease in titer of the antibodies during remission of chronic active hepatitis. Endomysial antibodies that are directed against the basement membrane of smooth muscle in the monkey esophagus are a reliable serologic marker for celiac disease.

Mitochondrial Antibodies

Ninety percent of patients with primary biliary cirrhosis (PBC) have antibodies to mitochondria. A high titer of mitochondrial antibodies (1:160 or greater) is consistent with PBC, although from 5% to 15% of patients may show low or trace amounts of the antibody. The titer of the antibody does not correlate with the severity or treatment of the disease. Several other diseases, including SLE, are accompanied by the presence of mitochondrial antibodies, but the titers are usually lower than those observed in PBC. Other conditions associated with mitochondrial antibodies include bile stasis, chronic active hepatitis, cryptogenic cirrhosis, and extrahepatic biliary obstruction. The reactive antigen is present on the inner mitochondrial membrane and has been characterized as a subunit of the pyruvate dehydrogenase complex (PDC), a major mitochondrial enzyme. Other related mitochondrial enzymes have also been identified as antigenic targets. In in vitro studies, mitchondrial antibodies can inactivate the catalytic activity of PDC and related enzymes.

Reticulin Antibodies

Antibodies to reticulin are present in up to 78% of patients with celiac disease. They tend to occur more frequently in pediatric than in adult patients and are usually of the IgA class. These antibodies are not specific for celiac disease and occur in adult patients with Crohn's disease, RA, and Sjögren's syndrome, and in normal individuals. The incidence of the antibody in dermatitis herpetiformis is between 12% and 68%. High titers of the antibody are suggestive of celiac disease. In patients treated with a gluten-free diet, the titer of reticulin antibodies falls. Reticulin antibodies are also useful predictors of disease relapse in patients who have undergone gluten challenge.

Myelin Antibodies

Myelin antibodies are found in a number of demyelinating disorders. In multiple sclerosis, antibodies to myelin basic proteins are described in the cerebrospinal fluid. Antibodies to myelin-associated glycoproteins (MAGs) are found in certain sensory-motor polyneuropathies, and antibodies to MAGs and myelin-associated glycolipids are described in Guillain-Barré syndrome.

Islet Cell Antibodies

Juvenile diabetics have pancreatic islet cell antibodies (ICA) in 80% of cases. The ICA gives a weak staining pattern, and a high concentration of antigen is required in the substrate. Four kinds of ICA have been described. The first two react with islet cell cytoplasm, and one of them fixes complement (CF-ICA); the third antibody is cytotoxic to islet cells; and the fourth one reacts with islet cell–surface antigens (ICSA). First-degree relatives of patients with juvenile diabetes, particularly those with CF-ICA in their serum, have an increased risk of developing diabetes. This risk is increased if they share one or two HLA-haplotypes with the affected sibling. Cytotoxic ICA and ICSA have also been recorded in the sera of patients for years prior to the development of diabetes. A subgroup of type II diabetics with no other endocrine disease who have ICA and an increased prevalence of HLA DR3 have been shown to become insulin-dependent.

Skin Antibodies

Antibodies to skin are found in some of the bullous diseases (Chapter 213). These antibodies are useful adjuncts to diagnosis, and the antibody titers are often related to disease activity. Antibodies to a keratinocyte cell surface glycoprotein have been identified in pemphigus vulgaris. This protein is a member of the cadherin family of cell adhesion molecules. In skin organ cultures these cadherin antibodies can cause loss of cell-cell adhesion. Antibodies to the basement membrane at the dermal-epidermal junction are seen in pemphigoid.

Cytoskeletal Antibodies

Antibodies to components of the cytoskeleton, particularly microfilaments, intermediate filaments, and microtubules, have been noted in many rheumatic and infectious diseases but they currently do not have any known disease specificity. There is also a high prevalence of these antibodies in low titer in the normal population.

Paraneoplastic Syndromes

Antibodies to neuronal specific proteins have been described in association with a number of paraneoplastic syndromes. Included amongst these are antibodies to Hu, a family of RNA binding proteins, which are found in paraneoplastic encephalomyelitis and paraneoplastic sensory neuropathy. Antibodies to Yo, a Purkinje cell antigen, are found in paraneoplastic cerebellar degeneration. Antibodies to different subtypes of calcium-channel blockers have been described in patients with the Eaton-Lambert syndrome.

Antinuclear Antibodies

Antinuclear antibodies (ANAs) react with a variety of nuclear antigens, including native, or double-stranded (ds) DNA; denatured, or single-stranded (ss) DNA; histones (basic nuclear proteins); nonhistone nuclear proteins; the nucleoli; nuclear lamins; and the nuclear matrix. ANAs occur in high frequency in systemic rheumatic diseases

Table 181-2 Autoantibody specificities and disease associations

ANTIBODY TO	DISEASE ASSOCIATION
1. Double-stranded (native) DNA	Highly specific for SLE (40%-60% incidence) when in moderate to high titer
2. Single-stranded (denatured) DNA	Present in SLE and other rheumatic and nonrheumatic diseases
3. Individual histones, H1, H2A, H2B, H3, H4	SLE (70%), drug-induced SLE (>95%), RA (15%)
4. Histone complexes H2A-H2B	Drug-induced SLE (>60%)
5. Sm (proteins complexed with U-RNAs)	SLE (30%), highly specific
6. U1-RNP (proteins complexed with U1-RNA)	MCTD (>95%), SLE (35%)
7. SS-A/Ro (proteins with small RNAs)	SS (70%), SLE (50%), other CTDs
8. SS-B/La (45K protein with RNA polymerase III transcripts)	SS (40%-50%), SLE (15%)
9. Proliferating cell nuclear antigen (PCNA)	SLE (<5%)
10. Ma antigen	SLE (20%)
11. Ki antigen	SLE (12%)
12. Scl-70 (topoisomerase I)	PSS (20%), highly specific
13. Centromere/kinetochore	CREST (70%-90%), diffuse scleroderma (10%-20%)
14. RANA (rheumatoid arthritis–associated nuclear antigen [EBV related])	RA (90%)
15. Mi-1	Dermatomyositis (10%)
16. Jo-1 (histidyl-tRNA synthetase)	Polymyositis (30%)
17. Ku	Polymyositis-scleroderma overlap (55%)
18. NuMa (nuclear mitotic apparatus) antigen	RA, Sjögren's syndrome
19. PM/Scl (PM-1)	Polymyositis-scleroderma overlap
20. Hu	Paraneoplastic encephalomyelitis and sensory neuropathy
21. Yo	Paraneoplastic cerebellar degeneration

EBV, Epstein-Barr virus; *SLE,* systemic lupus erythematosus; *MCTD,* mixed connective-tissue disease; *SS,* Sjögren's syndrome; *PSS,* progressive systemic sclerosis; *CREST,* calcinosis, Raynaud's phenomenon, esophageal hypomotility, sclerodactyly, and telangiectasis; *RA,* rheumatoid arthritis.

such as SLE, progressive systemic sclerosis (PSS), mixed connective-tissue disease (MCTD), and RA (Table 181-2). In situations in which the clinician is faced with a patient who has features of more than one autoimmune systemic disease, the diagnostic dilemma may be solved by knowing the specificity of the ANA.

Examples of commonly encountered ANA staining patterns observed by indirect immunofluorescence on tissue culture cells are shown in Fig. 181-2. The figure shows three staining patterns: (1) a homogeneous nuclear pattern, (2) a speckled nuclear pattern, and (3) a nucleolar pattern. Caution should be exercised in attempting to interpret immunologic specificities of ANA by pattern alone, as antibodies with different specificities may produce similar patterns. Further testing of sera by techniques such as immunodiffusion, ELISA, or immunoblotting is required to define the specificity of the antibodies.

Antibodies to DNA. High titers of dsDNA antibodies occur almost exclusively in patients with SLE, especially in patients with active nephritis or central nervous system disease. Low or absent titers are seen occasionally in other rheumatic diseases and in SLE in remission. Antibodies to ssDNA are seen in SLE, drug-induced SLE, and other rheumatic and nonrheumatic diseases. The antigenic determinants in dsDNA are felt to be present on the deoxyribosephosphate backbone. Antibodies to ssDNA probably react with purine and pyrimidine bases that are accessible in the single-stranded conformation. By immunofluorescence, antibodies to dsDNA produce a homoge-

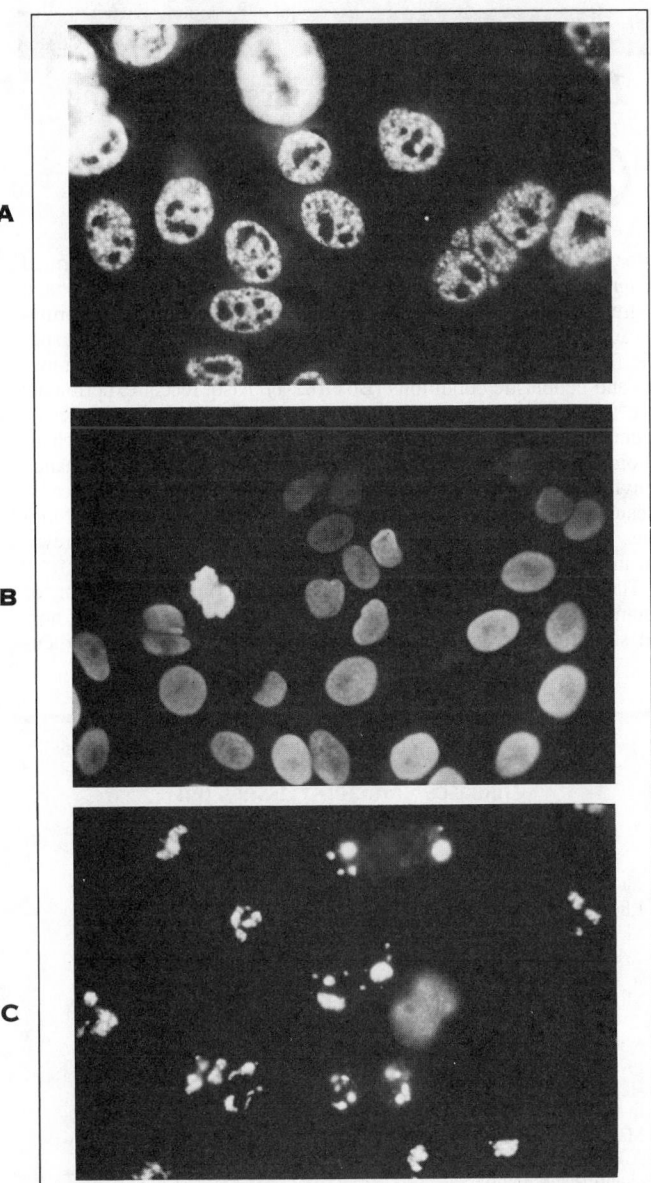

FIGURE 181-2   Composite showing different patterns of nuclear staining produced by antinuclear antibodies. **A,** Speckled nuclear staining with the absence of nucleolar staining. **B,** Homogeneous staining that includes the entire nucleus and nucleolus. **C,** Nucleolar staining. The substrate was HEp-2 cells grown on microscope slides. (×500.)

neous or rim pattern, but antibodies to ssDNA, when found in isolation, do not give a positive ANA. In certain patients the titer of antibodies to dsDNA may be used to monitor the patients' response to therapeutic measures.

Antibodies to Centromere/Kinetochore. Antibodies to the centromere/kinetochore region (ACA) of the chromosome display a characteristic speckled staining pattern on cultured cells by indirect immunofluorescence. These antibodies are most commonly associated with the scleroderma group of diseases, which includes systemic sclerosis, CREST syndrome, and Raynaud's phenomenon. The highest titer of ACA is found in the CREST syndrome, a less severe variant of systemic sclerosis.

Antibodies to Histone. Antibodies that bind to histone are present in up to 70% of SLE patients and 15% of RA patients when sera are screened by ELISA. In drug-induced SLE (DIL) 95% to 100% of patients have histone antibodies. These antibodies react with

all major classes of histone—H1, H2A, H2B, H3, and H4. Up to 75% of patients treated with procainamide or hydralazine develop histone antibodies. Of these patients, 15% develop overt clinical symptoms, including fever, malaise, myalgias, arthralgias, and pleural effusions. Other drugs associated with the development of histone antibodies include phenytoin and carbamazepine. Withdrawal of the offending drugs results in symptomatic relief and clearance of histone antibodies. By immunofluorescence on tissue culture cells, antibodies to histone produce a homogeneous staining pattern. The fact that antibodies to other nuclear proteins are absent in DIL may help to separate DIL from SLE, which is characterized by multiple autoantibody specificities.

Antibodies to Nonhistone Proteins. The other major class of ANAs in systemic autoimmune disease is characterized by reactivities with soluble nonhistone nuclear protein and protein-RNA complexes (see Table 181-2). Most of these proteins are easily extractable in physiologic buffers and are called *extractable nuclear antigens* (ENAs). Double immunodiffusion or related techniques are used to detect antibodies to these proteins. Antibodies to Smith (Sm) antigen are highly specific for SLE and are present in the sera of 15% to 30% of SLE patients. High titers of antibody to nuclear ribonucleoprotein (nRNP) are characteristic of MCTD, but low titers of this antibody may be found in SLE, PSS, and other connective tissue diseases. Sm antibodies bind to nuclear proteins that are complexed to uridine-rich RNA (U1, U2, U4, U5, U6), and these complexes of nuclear protein and RNA are called *small nuclear ribonuclear particles* (SnRNP). Antibodies to nRNP bind to proteins containing U1-RNA.

Antibodies against two other nuclear antigens, SS-A/Ro and SS-B/La, have been detected in high frequency in Sjögren's syndrome. Antibodies to SS-A/Ro antigen are present in 70% of patients with primary Sjögren's syndrome, in 15% of patients with secondary Sjögren's syndrome and RA, and in 40% of patients with SLE. Almost all newborns with the neonatal lupus syndrome have antibodies to SS-A/Ro. This syndrome consists of congenital heart block and/or a skin rash similar to that seen in subacute cutaneous lupus. Almost half of the mothers of these children have connective tissue disease. The remaining mothers are asymptomatic at delivery, but follow-up studies have shown that many of them eventually develop a systemic rheumatic disease such as SLE. Antibodies to SS-B/La antigen are present in approximately 50% of patients with Sjögren's syndrome and in 15% of SLE patients, but rarely are seen in any other connective tissue disease. Both antigens have been characterized at the macromolecular level.

An antibody that is reactive with a nuclear protein restricted to proliferating cells is present in SLE patients. The reactive antigen, termed *proliferating cell nuclear antigen* (PCNA), has been cloned and is known as elongation factor of DNA polymerase δ. Another ANA observed relatively frequently in sera from SLE patients is directed against the nuclear antigen named *Ma.*

Antibodies to the Jo-1 antigen have been noted in 30% to 50% of patients with polymyositis (PM), but they are uncommon in dermatomyositis and rare in other autoimmune disease. In PM the antibody to Jo-1 appears to be closely related to the development of pulmonary fibrosis. The Jo-1 antigen has been shown to be histidyl-tRNA synthetase. In patients with PM/PSS overlap and polymyositis, an antibody against the PM/Scl antigen has been observed in high frequency.

Current studies of ANA in progressive systemic sclerosis (PSS) patients using tissue culture cells, such as HEp-2 cells, have demonstrated ANA in almost all scleroderma patients. Various patterns of nuclear staining are seen in PSS sera, including speckled, nucleolar, and homogeneous. One such antibody is directed against a nuclear antigen Scl-70 and is highly specific for PSS, although it is of low sensitivity, being present in less than 30% of patients. The antibody has not been found in other connective tissue diseases.

Antibodies to nucleolar antigens are present in up to 50% of PSS patients, and antibody titers in PSS are higher than those found in other connective tissue diseases. Three distinct patterns of nucleolar staining can be seen by immunofluorescence: speckled, homogeneous, and clumpy patterns. Antibodies with a speckled pattern were shown to immunoprecipitate RNA polymerase 1 complex, the enzyme transcribing ribosomal genes in the nucleolus. This antibody is restricted to scleroderma and is associated with the diffuse form of the disease. Antibodies with a clumpy staining pattern are also restricted to PSS and recognize a protein that is part of the U3-RNP complex in the nucleolus. Antibodies to the PM/Scl antigen display a homogeneous pattern of nucleolar staining.

Antibodies to Phospholipids (anticardiolipin antibodies).

These antibodies are a hallmark of primary antiphospholipid syndrome (Chapter 212) but they are also found in up to 50% of patients with SLE and other systemic rheumatic diseases. They are correlated with the in vitro lupus anticoagulant test and the false-positive VDRL tests. Phospholipid antibodies are associated with a variety of clinical conditions, including recurrent fetal loss, recurrent venous and arterial thrombosis, thrombocytopenia, and labile hypertension. They are also associated with cerebrovascular accidents and early myocardial infarcts. Current opinion holds that IgG phospholipid antibodies are of greater pathologic significance than IgM antibodies.

Antineutrophil Cytoplasmic Antibodies

Antineutrophil cytoplasmic antibodies (ANCA) have been identified in a number of vasculitic disorders such as Wegener's granulomatosis, polyarteritis nodosa, and necrotizing and crescentric glomerulonephritis (Chapter 212). These antibodies have also been described in ulcerative colitis and sclerosing cholangitis, as well as in systemic rheumatic diseases. Three patterns of neutrophil staining are recognized by IIF: (1) granular cytoplasmic (cANCA); (2) perinuclear (pANCA); and (3) cytoplasmic and nuclear staining referred to as atypical (aANCA). The cANCA staining pattern is caused by reactivity with proteinase 3 (PR3), an enzyme component of the primary granules. Antibodies with the pANCA staining pattern are primarily directed against myeloperoxidase, but other target antigens include elastase, lactoferrin, and cathepsin G. The aANCA target antigens include myeloperoxidase and other antigens that remain to be identified. cANCA is a sensitive marker for Wegener's granulomatosis but antibody titers have not proven useful in determining the severity or activity of disease.

BIBLIOGRAPHY

Amagi M: Autoantibodies against cell adhesion molecules in pemphigus, *J Dermatol* 21:833-837, 1994.
Dalmau J, Posner JB: Neurologic paraneoplastic antibodies (anti-Yo, anti-Hu; anti-Ri): the case for a nomenclature based on antibody and antigen specificity, *Neurology* 44:2241-2246, 1994.
Harris E: The antiphospholipid syndrome: diagnosis, management, and pathogenesis, *Clin Rev Allergy Immunol* 13:3948, 1995.
Nickowitz RE, Wozniak RW, Schaffner F et al: Autoantibodies against integral membrane proteins of the nuclear envelope in patients with primary biliary cirrhosis, *Gastroenterology* 106:193-199, 1994.
Rao JK, Weinberger M, Oddone EZ et al: The role of cytoplasmic antibody testing in the diagnosis of Wegner's granulomatosis, *Ann Intern Med* 123:925-932, 1995.
Reichlin M: Autoantibodies to the RoRNP particles, *Clin Exp Immunol* 99:7-9, 1995.
Riley WJ: Enzymes as antigens in autoimmune endocrinopathies, *Clin Chem* 41:337-339, 1995.
Simmons-O'Brien E, Chen S, Watson R et al: One hundred anti-Ro (SS-A) antibody positive patients: a 10 year follow-up, *Medicine* 74:109-130, 1995.
von Muhlen CA, Tan EM: Autoantibodies in the diagnosis of systemic rheumatic disease, *Semin Arthritis Rheum* 24:323-358, 1995.

182 Rheumatoid Factors

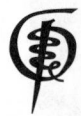

Dennis A. Carson

Autoantibodies against immunoglobulin G (IgG), commonly termed *rheumatoid factors,* are characteristic of rheumatoid arthritis and Sjögren's syndrome and may contribute to immune complex formation and tissue damage. However, IgM rheumatoid factors are not specific for rheumatic disease but are found in many chronic inflammatory and neoplastic conditions (Box 182-1). Also, recent experiments have shown that normal humans and animals regularly synthesize rheumatoid factors during anamnestic immune responses. The rheumatoid factors clear aggregated IgG from the circulation and enhance manyfold the presentation of antigens trapped in immune complexes. Because rheumatoid factors have these essential physiologic functions, immunoglobulin genes encoding rheumatoid factors are prevalent in all normal people.

The specificity of immunoglobulin M (IgM) rheumatoid factor for rheumatoid arthritis increases with serum titer. Compared with normal subjects, affected patients have more and higher-affinity rheu-

---

BOX 182-1
Diseases commonly associated with rheumatoid factor

Rheumatoid diseases
Rheumatoid arthritis
Sjögren's syndrome
Systemic lupus erythematosus
Scleroderma
Mixed connective tissue disease

Acute viral infections
Mononucleosis
Hepatitis
Influenza
Many others
After vaccination (may yield falsely elevated titers of antiviral or antibacterial antibodies)

Parasitic infections
Tryponasomiasis
Kala-azar
Malaria
Schistosomiasis
Filariasis
Others

Chronic inflammatory disease
Tuberculosis
Leprosy
Yaws
Syphilis
Brucellosis
Subacute bacterial endocarditis
Salmonellosis
Human immunodeficiency virus

Other hyperglobulinemic states
Hypergammaglobulinemic purpura
Cryoglobulinemia
Chronic liver disease
Sarcoid
Other chronic pulmonary disease

Modified from Kelley WN et al, editors: *Textbook of rheumatology,* ed 3, Philadelphia, 1996, WB Saunders.

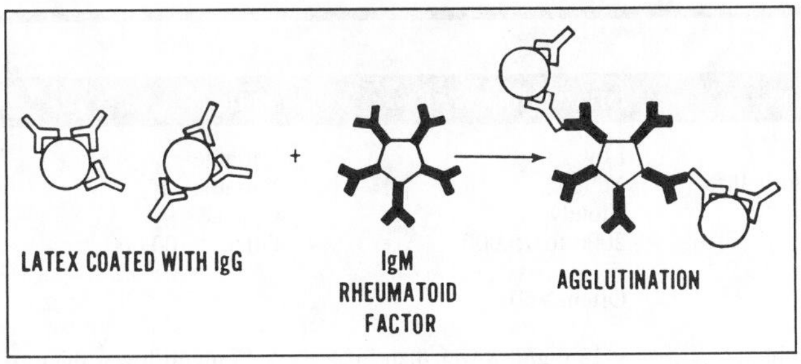

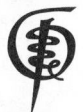

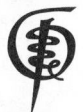

LATEX COATED WITH IgG + IgM RHEUMATOID FACTOR AGGLUTINATION

FIGURE 182-1 Latex fixation test for immunoglobulin M (IgM) rheumatoid factor.

matoid factor. Thus all patients suspected of the diagnosis should have a quantitative assay performed. IgM rheumatoid factors are multivalent and agglutinate IgG-coated latex particles to produce a visible flocculation (Fig. 182-1). IgM rheumatoid factor titers are expressed as the highest dilution of serum yielding detectable agglutination, as assessed visually or by nephelometry. Often, IgM rheumatoid factor titers are expressed as units, in comparison with a standard international serum preparation. At a serum dilution that excludes 95% of the normal human population, more than 70% of rheumatoid arthritis patients are seropositive. Individuals with borderline titers should be retested after several weeks. Only patients with IgM rheumatoid factor titers in the normal range on consecutive determinations should be considered seronegative.

Patients with very high IgM rheumatoid factor titers usually have more aggressive arthritis and more extraarticular rheumatoid disease than those with low titers. In some patients a remission in disease activity is heralded by a reduction in IgM rheumatoid factor titers. Small variations in IgM rheumatoid factor titers, however, are of little clinical significance in monitoring the response to therapy.

Rheumatoid factors of the IgG class, when compared with IgM rheumatoid factors, are inefficient agglutinators. Hence their measurement by agglutination is imprecise and requires the prior removal of IgM rheumatoid factors. IgG rheumatoid factors form part of the cryoprecipitating immune complexes that are quite common in rheumatoid synovial fluids. The appearance of cryoprecipitating rheumatoid factor in serum is a bad prognostic sign because it may be associated with vasculitis, Felty's syndrome, hyperglobulinemic purpura, or the hyperviscosity syndrome.

In the human infectious diseases associated with rheumatoid factor production the autoantibody disappears from the circulation after removal of the inciting antigen and the clearance of antigen-antibody complexes. The reasons for the persistence of rheumatoid factor in patients with rheumatoid arthritis are not known. Contributing factors probably include the localization of the rheumatoid factor–producing cells to the confined synovial membrane, where repeated trauma leads to cytokine and chemokine release, and the intermittent deposition of immune complexes containing normal environmental antigens.

Complement fixation by rheumatoid factor, as for other antibodies, depends on an exact stoichiometry between antigen and antibody. In the rheumatoid factor–synthesizing synovial membrane the concentration of normal IgG is low enough to permit extensive lattice formation and efficient complement consumption. Indeed, hemolytic complement levels characteristically are depressed in seropositive rheumatoid synovial fluids but are near normal in companion sera.

BIBLIOGRAPHY

Albani S, Carson DA: Etiopathogenesis of rheumatoid arthritis. In Koopman WJ, editor: *Arthritis and allied conditions*, ed 13, Baltimore, 1996, Williams & Wilkins.
Tighe H, Carson DA: Rheumatoid factor. In Kelley WN et al, editors: *Textbook of rheumatology*, ed 4, Philadelphia, 1996, WB Saunders.

183 Synovial Fluid Analysis

Nathan J. Zvaifler

Synovial fluid is readily obtained by aspiration from most joints, and its analysis is an essential evaluation of any patient with joint disease. Some disorders, such as gout, calcium pyrophosphate dihydrate (CPPD) deposition disease, and septic arthritis, can be diagnosed definitively by this procedure. Other diseases, including rheumatoid arthritis and systemic lupus erythematosus (SLE) may be considered or excluded. Indeed, synovial fluid analysis better reflects the events in the articular cavity than do abnormal blood tests, since antinuclear antibodies and increased erythrocyte sedimentation rate, elevated uric acid concentrations, or rheumatoid factors can be seen in normal individuals or in unrelated joint diseases.

NORMAL SYNOVIAL FLUID

Small quantities of a clear, pale-yellow or straw-colored, viscous, and slightly alkaline liquid are present in normal joints. The viscosity and mucinous characteristics of the synovial fluid depend on the integrity of hyaluronate, a large, highly polymerized mucopolysaccharide.

Synovial fluid is essentially a plasma dialysate, but because of the physical characteristics of the hyaluronate, certain molecules are preferentially excluded from the joint. Most electrolytes are present in amounts comparable to those in blood—including glucose, which approximates but is usually 10 mg/dl less than in blood. Proteins, particularly those with high molecular weight or asymmetric shape, are preferentially excluded. Because fibrinogen and many of the clotting factors are missing, normal synovial fluid does not clot. The total protein content is usually less than 2.0 g/dl, with the smaller molecules such as albumin disproportionately represented.

Normal synovial fluid is relatively acellular, with only a few hundred cells per cubic millimeter, predominantly mononuclear. Occasionally, large synoviocytes are seen. Red blood cells and platelets are absent. The cellular characteristics of the synovial fluid are independent of the peripheral blood cell count.

ARTHROCENTESIS

There are no absolute contraindications to synovial fluid aspiration, although patients with sepsis or taking anticoagulation therapy require special care, and the aspirating needle should not be placed through areas of tissue infection or cellulitis. The skin should be cleansed and aseptically prepared. A local anesthetic agent minimizes discomfort but should not be injected into the joint prior to fluid aspiration. The routes for arthrocentesis are varied, but sites of obvious bulging are most easily entered as long as vital anatomic structures are avoided. As much fluid as possible should be removed from the joint and allocated into containers appropriate for bacteriologic studies: a test tube with an anticoagulant (preferably heparin) for cell count and cytologic examination; a potassium oxylate–containing tube for glucose; and a clean, glass tube for special tests, such as complement or protein determination. When fluid is limited, the anticoagulant tube suffices for all studies. Simultaneous blood and serum samples for glucose, protein, and complement testing are advisable.

SYNOVIAL FLUID TESTS
Gross Examination

Observing the fluid obtained at the bedside helps plan subsequent studies, particularly if only small volumes are available. Generally, the cloudier the fluid, the more cells it contains. Occasionally an opacity results from crystalline materials, fibrin, or fragments of cartilage. As is seen in Table 183-1, fluids from degenerative, traumatic, or metabolic arthropathies and mechanical derangements of joints are

Table 183-1   Classification of synovial effusions

GROSS EXAMINATION	NORMAL	"NONINFLAMMATORY"	INFLAMMATORY	SEPTIC
Viscosity	High	High	Low	Variable
Color	Colorless to straw-colored	Straw-colored to yellow	Yellow	Variable
Clarity	Transparent	Transparent	Cloudy	Opaque
White blood cell count (per mm^3)	<200	200 to 2000	2000 to 75,000	Often >100,000
Polymorphonuclear leukocytes (%)	<25	<25	Often >50	>75
Glucose level (AM fasting)	Nearly equal to blood	Nearly equal to blood	<25 mg/dl lower than in blood	>25 mg/dl lower than in blood

usually colorless, in contrast to fluids from the inflammatory or septic rheumatic disorders. Streaks of blood can result from injury to small vessels during arthrocentesis, but grossly bloody fluids (hemarthrosis) are associated with a number of rheumatic disorders (Box 183-1).

Viscosity can be estimated by observing the rate at which synovial fluid extrudes from the syringe. Normally, because of high viscosity, a drop forms but leaves reluctantly; as it does, a long thread develops. Unusually viscous fluids are obtained from ganglia and in hypothyroid effusions. With increasing inflammation, viscosity is generally decreased, especially in chronic processes.

Cytology

Leukocyte counts are an essential part of synovial fluid analysis and form the basis for classification of joint effusions (Table 183-1). Those with leukocyte counts from 200 to 2000 cells/mm^3 are generally termed noninflammatory. Polymorphonuclear cells should constitute less than 25% of the total. As the count rises into the inflammatory and septic range, the proportion of polymorphonuclear leukocytes generally increases, not infrequently accounting for 90% of the total white blood cell population. Occasionally, however, in the early phases of rheumatoid arthritis or in certain infections such as tuberculosis, mononuclear cells may predominate. Leukocyte counts in excess of 100,000 cells/mm^3 are generally, but not exclusively, associated with joint infection; marked elevations are uncommonly seen in rheumatic fever, crystal-induced arthritides, rheumatoid arthritis, and Reiter's syndrome. Conversely, early in infectious processes or in those incompletely treated, counts of less than 100,000 cells/mm^3 are found. Gonococcal arthritis, tuberculosis, and certain fungal infections of joints regularly have lower counts (Fig. 183-1).

In general, the synovial fluid white blood cell count can be anticipated from the clinical examination. Joint redness and tenderness are usually paralleled by elevated leukocyte counts, with two significant exceptions. Systemic lupus erythematosus (SLE) and hypertrophic osteoarthropathy characteristically result in clinically inflamed joints but noninflammatory effusions. Both have elevated protein content, suggesting exudates; SLE fluids usually have very low hemolytic complement activity.

Wet Preparations

Examination of a drop of fresh synovial fluid by light microscopy is often the single most important test of synovial fluid. The slides and cover glasses must be scrupulously cleaned prior to use because dirt, minute pieces of glass, and fibers from lens paper can be confused with crystalline and fibrillar materials. Red and white blood cells are easy to distinguish and their numbers estimated.

Lipid droplets free in the synovial fluid usually signify fractures or trauma to the joint, but they can be seen in avascular necrosis, fat embolism, and, rarely, inflammatory effusions. Irregular strands of fibrin or fibrillar fragments of cartilage accompany degenerative arthritis. Both are faintly birefringent and should not be confused with crystalline materials.

All synovial fluids should be examined for crystals. Crystals of importance (as opposed to dust or debris) tend to have straight, parallel edges. Monosodium urate (MSU) appears as monotonously simi-

---

BOX 183-1
Conditions associated with hemarthrosis

Hereditary deficiency of clotting factors
Anticoagulation therapy
Sickle cell anemia
Thrombocytopenia
Pseudogout
Amyloidosis (xanthochromia only)
Pigmented villonodular synovitis
Synovial hemangioma
Rheumatoid arthritis
Infection
Trauma with or without fracture
Osteoarthritis
Neuropathic joints
Metallic joint prosthesis
Primary or metastatic neoplasm of joints
Myeloproliferative disease
Scurvy

---

lar 8- to 10-μ needle- or rod-shaped crystals. In contrast, calcium pyrophosphate dihydrate (CPPD) crystals assume multiple three-dimensional forms; rods, rhomboids, and parallelepipeds occur simultaneously. It is important to note whether the crystalline material is intra- or extracellular. During acute attacks of gout and "pseudogout," crystals are engulfed by leukocytes; in the intercritical periods, the crystals may lie free in the fluid. Crystal identification is greatly enhanced by compensated polarized light microscopy. Most rheumatologic textbooks discuss the theory of polarization microscopy; the principle is shown in Fig. 183-2.

Monosodium urate crystals appear as brightly birefringent rods or needles that have a yellow color when the crystal axis is parallel to the slow ray compensator. This is termed negative birefringence (see Color Plate VI-1). CPPD crystals are much less birefringent and, therefore, more difficult to identify. They have a positive birefringence; that is, their slow ray is in the long axis of the crystal, giving them a bluish appearance (see Color Plate VI-1). MSU crystals are virtually pathognomonic for gouty arthritis, and CPPD crystals are associated with CPPD deposition disease. However, two rheumatic diseases may coexist. This is particularly true for CPPD, which is present in the articular cartilages of 5% of the population. It is not surprising, therefore, that CPPD crystals have been identified in effusions from a number of inflammatory joint diseases. Acute infections and crystal-induced arthritis may also occur together and should be considered in any patient with unusually high joint fluid leukocyte counts or in whom articular inflammation fails to subside with appropriate therapy for the crystal-induced disorder.

Basic calcium phosphate (BCP) crystals, including apatite, octacalcium phosphate, and tricalcium phosphate, are associated with subcutaneous calcification and calcific periarthritis and tendinitis. Recently BCP crystals have been found in both acute and chronic synovitis (Chapter 208). Unfortunately, the size of BCP crystals is below

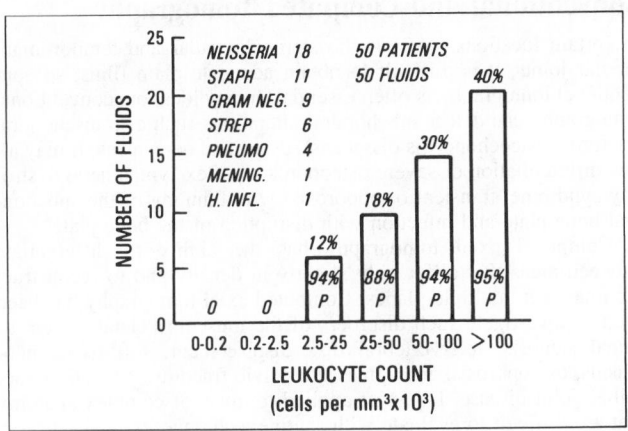

FIGURE 183-1 The leukocyte counts in 50 synovial fluids with various forms of septic arthritis. The percentage of the total sample that was present in each range of the white blood cell count appears above the bar; the percentage of polymorphonuclear (*P*) cells, within the bar.
From Krey PR, Bailen DA: *Am J Med* 67:436, 1979.

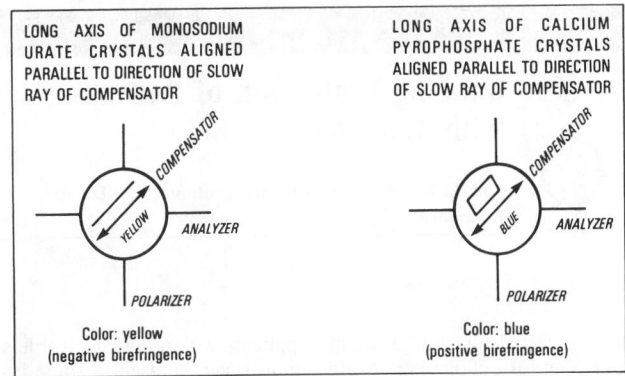

FIGURE 183-2 Use of the first-order red compensator (retardation plate), demonstrating the principles of polarized light microscopy as applied to the analysis of crystals in synovial fluid.
From Cohen AS: *Laboratory diagnostic procedures in the rheumatic diseases,* ed 3, New York, 1985, Grune & Stratton.

the limits of resolution of optical microscopy. However, these crystals do have a tendency to aggregate, giving them the appearance of shiny laminated printed "coins" by light microscopy. This appearance may suggest the need for further studies, of which transmission electron microscopy is the most readily available.

MSU or CPPD can be confused with other birefringent materials, including crystalline anticoagulants, such as calcium oxalate and ethylenediaminetetraacetic acid or repository forms of certain corticosteroid preparations (betamethasone and prednisolone *tert*-butylacetate are negatively and positively birefringent rods, respectively). Cholesterol crystals, usually found in chronic effusions of rheumatoid arthritis, are easily distinguished because of their large size and flat, platelike shape with notched corners.

Cytology

Wright's staining for cellular morphology provides accurate differential leukocyte counts. Typical LE cells may be found in centrifuged specimens from SLE effusions and, occasionally, in patients with Felty's syndrome. Large mononuclear cells are derived from the synovial lining (synoviocytes).

Gram's and Ziehl-Nielsen Stains

Smears, staining, and identification of organisms are performed in the usual manner on heparinized synovial fluid samples or specimens that have been concentrated by centrifugation. Interpretation is sometimes difficult because bacteria can be confused with precipitated hyaluronate (mucin).

Glucose

Generally, the intraarticular glucose concentration parallels the blood level, but the turnover in the joint differs; therefore, spurious results will be obtained if the sample is not obtained after prolonged fasting. Modest differences are not significant, particularly in the presence of large numbers (>50,000/mm³) of granulocytes, but a synovial fluid glucose reduction of more than 50 mg per deciliter, as compared with a companion blood sample, is most compatible with a joint infection.

Serum Proteins

Normally, most serum proteins are excluded from the articular cavity, but with increasing inflammation, large molecules gain access to the joint fluid. Thus, the protein content of fluids from acute and chronic inflammatory forms of arthritis exceeds the normal 1.5 to 2.0 g per deciliter and approach serum concentrations. In rheumatoid arthritis and certain other chronic inflammatory arthritides, there is also

a small contribution from local production of immunoglobulins or complement components. Pathologic fluids occasionally clot, owing to the presence of coagulation factors in the effusion that are normally absent from the joint. Antinuclear antibodies and rheumatoid factors produced in the chronically inflamed synovium are rarely detected when they are not demonstrable in the serum.

Complement

In general, the total hemolytic activity of synovial fluid is proportional to the white cell count or the concentration of total protein. For most inflammatory effusions, the complement activity is 50% or more of serum values. Effusions from patients with Reiter's disease have very high values, reflecting the fact that complement responds as an acute-phase reactant and is often markedly increased in the serum of these patients. In contrast, the joint fluids from patients with rheumatoid arthritis or SLE show low complement values as a result of intraarticular consumption. To avoid confusion caused by low serum levels of hemolytic activity (as might occur in SLE), the fluid complement value can be expressed as a percentage of the expected value based on comparison with serum concentrations of other proteins or individual complement components. Total hemolytic activity is usually less than 30% of the expected value in rheumatoid and SLE effusions. Similar low values may also be seen in certain immune complex forms of arthritis, such as acute hepatitis. Synovial fluid must be centrifuged and the supernatant frozen at $-70°$ C until tested to ensure correct total hemolytic complement determinations.

Measurements of complement components (e.g., C3, C4), although easier to perform, are less reliable because when activated they generate small-molecular-weight by-products (see Chapter 178) that are retained in the joint and are still detectable by the immunodiffusion techniques employed for their measurement.

BIBLIOGRAPHY

Freemoni AJ et al: Diagnostic value of synovial fluid microscopy: a reassessment and rationalisation, *Ann Rheum Dis* 50:101, 1991.

Gatter RA, Schumacher HR: *A practical handbook of joint fluid analysis,* ed 2, Philadelphia, 1991, Lea & Febiger.

Hasselbacher P: Arthrocentesis, synovial fluid analysis and synovial biopsy. In Schumacher HR (editor): *Primer on the rheumatic diseases,* ed 10, Atlanta, 1993, Arthritis Foundation.

McCarty DJ: Synovial fluid. In McCarty DJ, Koopman W (editors): *Arthritis and allied conditions,* ed 12, Philadelphia, 1993, Lea & Febiger.

Schumacher HR: Synovial fluid analysis and synovial biopsy. In Kelley WN et al (editors): *Textbook of rheumatology,* ed 5, Philadelphia, 1997, Saunders.

Wild JH, Zvaifler NJ: An office technique for identifying crystals in synovial fluid, *Am Fam Practitioner* 12:72, 1975.

Wild JH, Zvaifler NJ: Hemarthrosis associated with sodium warfarin therapy, *Arthritis Rheum* 19:98, 1976.

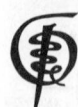

CHAPTER

184 Imaging Evaluation of Patients With Arthritis

Donald Resnick, David R. Marcantonio, and David J. Sartoris

The proper analysis and treatment of patients with articular disorders require careful radiographic examination. It can be used in some individuals whose clinical manifestations are confusing, allowing a specific diagnosis to be made. In other individuals in whom a clinical diagnosis is readily apparent, the radiographs document the extent and the severity of joint involvement. Furthermore, sequential radiographic examinations allow analysis of the efficacy of various therapeutic regimens.

Any summary of the radiographic evaluation of patients with arthritis must discuss the available imaging techniques and modalities, the cardinal roentgenographic signs of articular disease, and the peculiar predilection of certain disorders to affect specific "target areas" in the body.

IMAGING TECHNIQUES AND MODALITIES
Plain Film Examination

Initial plain film examination almost universally requires that more than one projection of a symptomatic joint be obtained. Reliance on a single projection frequently leads to misdiagnosis. For example, subtle osseous erosions in a hand or wrist of a patient with rheumatoid arthritis may not be detected on frontal or lateral views but are readily apparent on oblique projections.

In patients with polyarticular disease it is impractical to obtain a survey of all joints. The radiographic examination should emphasize articulations that are symptomatic and those that are common target sites of the disease in question. For example, the patient with rheumatoid arthritis requires careful roentgenographic analysis of the hands, wrists, feet, knees, shoulders, and cervical spine, and the patient with calcium pyrophosphate dihydrate (CPPD) crystal deposition disease requires careful analysis of the hands, wrists, knees, and pelvis.

Additional radiographs are required of certain sites in the evaluation of patients with ankylosing spondylitis (thoracic and lumbar spine, sacroiliac joints), diffuse idiopathic skeletal hyperostosis (thoracic and lumbar spine), and hemophilia (ankles, elbows).

Weight Bearing, Stress, and Traction Radiographs

In certain situations radiographs obtained during weight bearing, stress, or traction can supplement the plain film examination. In evaluating patients with osteoarthritis of the knee, radiographs obtained while the patient is standing on the affected leg can be extremely useful, allowing more precise documentation of the integrity of the articular cartilage. Furthermore, knee radiographs obtained during weight bearing allow analysis of the amount of displacement of the tibia on the femur and the degree of varus or valgus angulation. Slight flexion of the knees during the examination may be of added benefit. Weight-bearing radiography is less useful in the evaluation of other articulations.

Radiographs exposed during the application of stress across an articulation provide information regarding the integrity of surrounding ligaments and soft tissue structures. "Stress" radiographs are useful in the analysis of ligamentous injury of the knee, ankle, and first metacarpophalangeal joint. Analysis of the acromioclavicular joint after trauma may require the stress produced by tying a 5- or 10-pound weight to the wrist, whereas lateral radiographs of the lumbar spine obtained after prolonged standing with or without the application of additional weight may provide a more accurate assessment of any osseous defect in the neural arch (spondylolysis) and the presence of vertebral slippage (spondylolisthesis).

Conventional and Computed Tomography

In certain locations, such as the sternoclavicular and temporomandibular joints, it is difficult to obtain adequate plain films, so conventional tomography is often essential. In any location, conventional tomography can detect subchondral alterations such as transchondral fractures (osteochondritis dissecans), cysts, and neoplasms. It may allow differentiation of severe osteoporosis (reflex sympathetic dystrophy syndrome, transient osteoporosis) with thinning of the subchondral bone plate and infection with disruption of the bone plate.

Computed axial tomography has the ability to differentiate between areas that differ only slightly in density and to reconstruct the images in multiple planes. Computed axial tomography has been used to investigate such disorders of the musculoskeletal system as spinal stenosis, intervertebral disk displacement, soft tissue neoplasms, osteoporosis, and spinal and pelvic fractures, as well as sacroiliac joint disease. It is best applied to areas of complex anatomy that are difficult to evaluate with routine techniques.

Arthrography

Intraarticular injection of contrast media, air, or both has been used in investigating various articular problems. Knee arthrography, although now performed less frequently than in the past, can be employed in the analysis of meniscal injuries, as well as collateral and cruciate ligament tears, articular cartilage alterations, synovial processes, masses, and periarticular synovial cysts (popliteal cysts). In the hip, arthrography is most commonly employed to evaluate for the presence of prosthetic loosening or infection. Glenohumeral joint arthrography is helpful in the evaluation of rotator cuff tears, adhesive capsulitis, previous dislocations, synovial processes, infection, and bicipital tendon abnormalities. Indications for wrist arthrography include evaluation of synovial inflammation, ligamentous and capsular injuries, and soft tissue masses. Ankle arthrography may be used in the evaluation of ligamentous injuries, transchondral fractures, and intraarticular osteochondral bodies. It should be stressed, however, that the application of magnetic resonance imaging to analysis of the musculoskeletal system has lessened the need for arthrography.

Magnetic Resonance Imaging

Magnetic resonance imaging (MRI) has revolutionized musculoskeletal imaging over the past decade. Because of its excellent contrast sensitivity and satisfactory spatial resolution, it can be used to evaluate a variety of musculoskeletal processes. Important examples of such processes include intraspinal abnormalities, soft tissue infections and tumors, diseases leading to alterations in bone marrow, osteonecrosis, and intraarticular ligamentous and cartilage injuries. Magnetic resonance imaging has become the method of choice in evaluating internal derangements of the knee and shoulder, and it competes effectively with arthrography in assessing many wrist abnormalities. When combined with intravenous contrast enhancement, magnetic resonance imaging allows differentiation between inflamed synovial tissue and joint effusion. Special imaging sequences have also been developed for the analysis of articular cartilage abnormalities. Additional applications of magnetic resonance imaging include the evaluation of nerve entrapment syndromes, synovial cysts, and tendinitis.

CARDINAL ROENTGENOGRAPHIC SIGNS OF ARTICULAR DISEASE
Appendicular Skeleton

Soft Tissue Swelling. Soft tissue prominence may reflect an accumulation of intraarticular fluid, capsular distention, soft tissue edema, or periarticular or intraarticular masses. In rheumatoid arthritis, fusiform periarticular soft tissue swelling is characteristic (Fig. 184-1). A similar appearance may be identified in psoriatic arthritis, Reiter's syndrome (Fig. 184-2), juvenile chronic arthritis, and infection, as well as in hemophilia caused by the intraarticular accumulation of blood and the presence of synovial hypertrophy. In pigmented villonodular synovitis the soft tissue swelling may appear more nodular, creating a lobulated, radiopaque shadow. Magnetic resonance imaging in both hemophilia and pigmented villonodular synovitis may

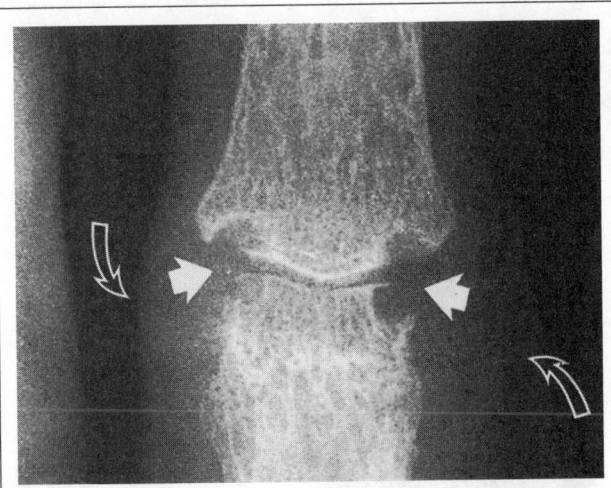

FIGURE 184-1   Rheumatoid arthritis. Findings include fusiform soft tissue swelling about the proximal interphalangeal joint *(curved arrows)*, diffuse joint space loss, periarticular osteoporosis, and marginal erosions *(arrowheads)*.

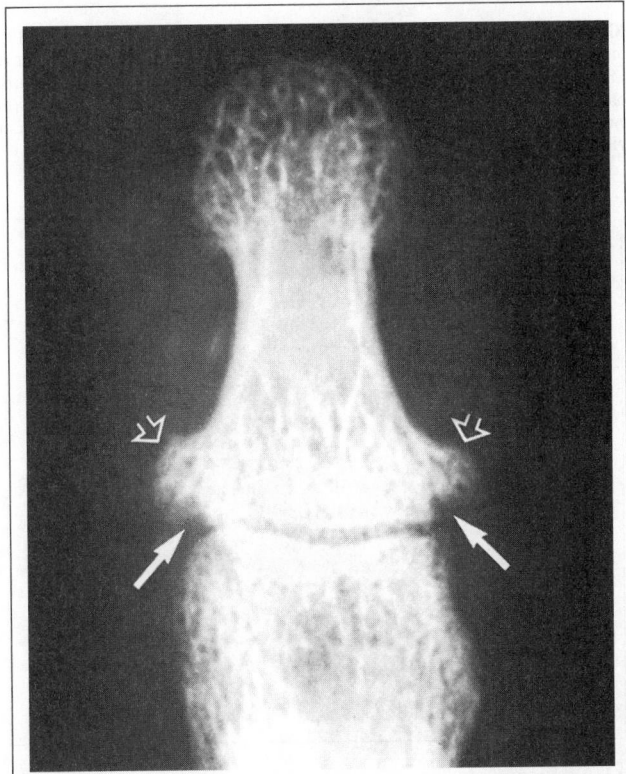

FIGURE 184-2   Reiter's syndrome. Observe the marginal erosions *(arrows)*, most evident along the base of the distal phalanx, and a characteristic proliferative component creating an ill-defined osseous surface *(arrowheads)*. The joint space is mildly narrowed, and there is no evidence of periarticular osteoporosis. Fusiform soft tissue swelling is evident. These changes occurring in a distal interphalangeal joint are more typical of psoriasis than Reiter's syndrome.

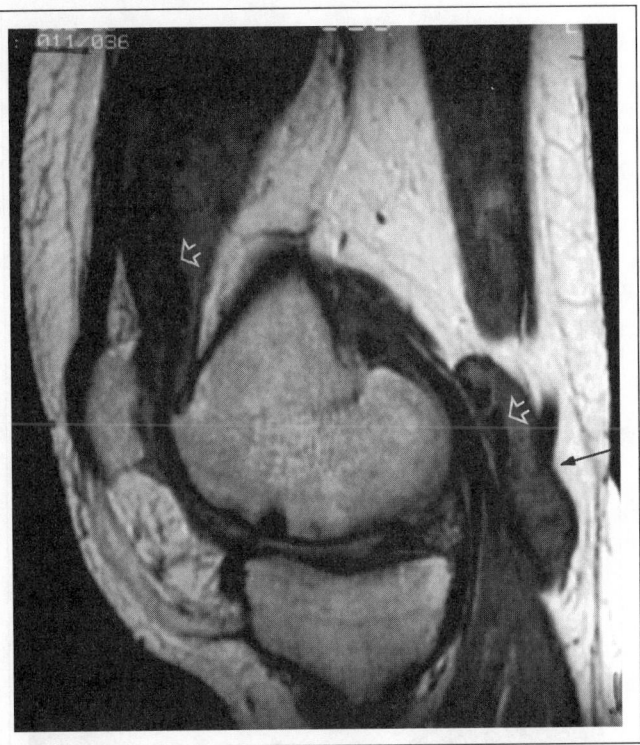

FIGURE 184-3   Pigmented villonodular synovitis. Sagittal proton density weighted (TR/TE, 2000/15) spin-echo magnetic resonance (MR) image shows a process involving both the joint space and posterior synovial cyst *(arrow)* with heterogeneous signal intensity. Areas of characteristic, very low signal intensity are also present in the joint space and synovial cyst, representing hemosiderin deposition in the synovium *(open arrows)*.

Courtesy V. Chandnani, MD, Honolulu.

"shoulder-pad" sign, is recognized in some cases of amyloidosis. Magnetic resonance imaging, with its superb soft tissue contrast, may be complimentary to routine radiographs in further assessment of nonspecific periarticular or intraarticular soft tissue swelling or prominence. Furthermore, contrast-enhanced magnetic resonance imaging may help in differentiation between inflamed and noninflamed soft tissues.

Reduction in Bone Density. Periarticular osteoporosis, an increased radiolucency of bone (osteopenia/porosis), is a well-recognized manifestation of certain articular disorders. In rheumatoid arthritis, synovitis with accompanying hyperemia leads to juxtaarticular osteopenia, especially in the hands, wrists, and feet (Fig. 184-1). In this disease similar osteopenia may occur about larger articulations such as the knee and the hip, although bony sclerosis or eburnation may be evident in these sites. During the acute inflammatory stage of certain of the seronegative spondyloarthropathies, periarticular osteopenia also may be evident, but it is more typical for these latter disorders to be unaccompanied by osteopenia, perhaps owing to the intermittent or episodic nature of the synovial inflammation (Fig. 184-2). Osteopenia is distinctly unusual in gouty arthritis and degenerative joint disease (osteoarthritis) and is infrequent in pigmented villonodular synovitis and idiopathic synovial osteochondromatosis. It may be apparent during acute episodes of pyogenic arthritis and during the course of tuberculosis and hemophilia.

Joint Space Narrowing. Cartilaginous destruction is accompanied by loss of the interosseous space *(joint space)*. In rheumatoid arthritis early cartilaginous destruction is typical and leads to diffuse loss of interosseous space (Fig. 184-1). This finding is especially prominent in the proximal interphalangeal and metacarpophalangeal joints of the hand; all the compartments of the wrist (Fig. 184-5); and the metatarsophalangeal joints of the foot, the knee, and the hip. Diffuse joint space loss is also common in ankylosing spondylitis, psoriatic arthritis, and Reiter's syndrome.

be diagnostic because of the specific imaging features of hemorrhage and hemosiderin deposition within the synovium (Fig. 184-3). Lobulated soft tissue swelling also is seen in gout (Fig. 184-4), xanthomatosis, and amyloidosis. In gouty arthritis the masses reflect the presence of tophi. Xanthomas are commonly encountered in tendinous structures such as the extensor tendons of the hand and the Achilles tendon. A peculiar prominence of the soft tissues of the shoulder, the

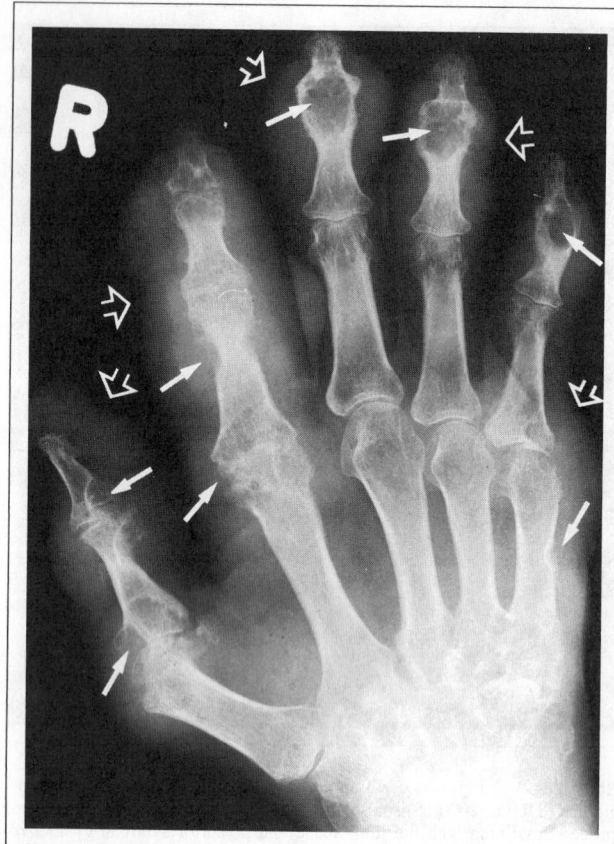

FIGURE 184-4 Gouty arthritis. Extensive involvement of the wrist and hand can be seen. All the compartments of the wrist, the metacarpophalangeal joints, and the proximal and distal interphalangeal joints are affected. Extensive intraarticular and periarticular erosions are evident *(arrows)*, without significant osteoporosis. Lobulated soft tissue swelling is apparent *(arrowheads)*.

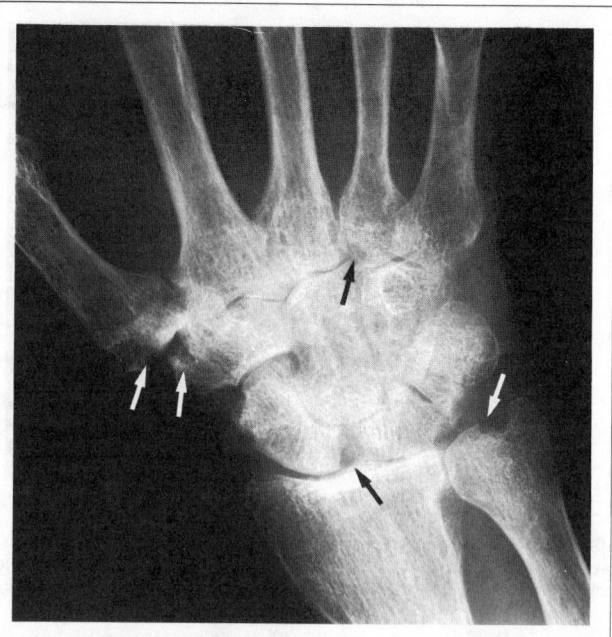

FIGURE 184-5 Rheumatoid arthritis. Note the diffuse involvement of all the compartments of the wrist, including the radiocarpal compartment, inferior radioulnar compartment, midcarpal compartment, common carpometacarpal compartment, and first carpometacarpal compartment. Marginal erosions *(arrows)*, soft tissue swelling, joint space narrowing, and mild osteoporosis are evident.

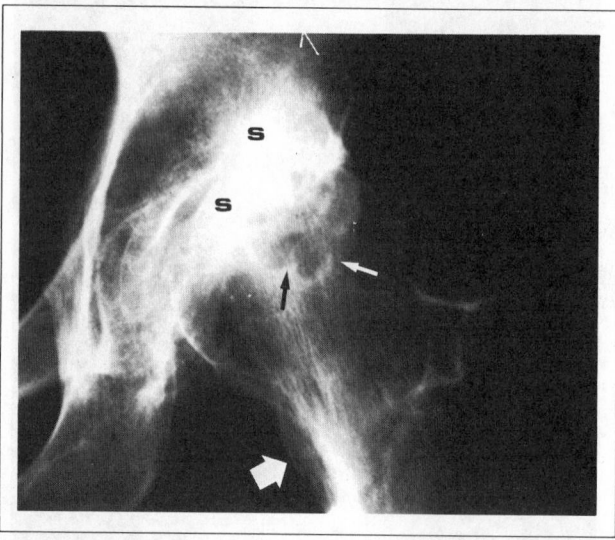

FIGURE 184-6 Osteoarthritis. The maximum area of joint space loss involves the superior aspect of the articulation. There is superior migration of the femoral head with respect to the acetabulum. Note the asymmetric nature of the joint space loss and the sclerosis *(S)* and cyst formation *(arrows)* on the superior aspect of the femoral head and adjacent acetabulum. There is thickening, or buttressing, along the medial aspect of the femoral neck related to new bone formation *(arrowhead)*. In this example, osteophytosis is not prominent.

In gouty arthritis joint space diminution is a less constant manifestation of the disease. In fact, the recognition of significant osseous erosion in the presence of a normal joint space is an important clue to the diagnosis of gout. The integrity of the articular space in gout is apparently related to the presence of relatively intact articular cartilage between areas of cartilaginous destruction.

Although joint space loss is also evident in degenerative joint disease (osteoarthritis), it involves limited areas of the articulation. The joint space narrows in the stressed area of the articulation. The hip joint space loss is usually maximum on the superolateral aspect of the joint (Fig. 184-6), whereas, in the knee it is the medial femorotibial space that is characteristically narrowed. Osteoarthritis of the interphalangeal and metacarpophalangeal joints of the hand and the first metatarsophalangeal joint of the foot may be accompanied by more diffuse loss of articular space (Fig. 184-7).

Pyogenic arthritis also is associated with early, diffuse loss of joint space. In tuberculosis and fungal disorders, such loss is a later radiographic manifestation.

Osteonecrosis of epiphyses of tubular bones, such as the femoral and humeral heads, is associated with considerable subchondral bony abnormality in the form of osteolysis, osteosclerosis, and cyst formation, in the absence of joint space narrowing. This combination of findings reflects the integrity of the articular cartilage, which derives most of its nutrition from the adjacent synovial fluid and therefore is unaffected by disruption of blood supply to the subchondral bone. Magnetic resonance imaging may show characteristic signal intensity changes of osteonecrosis (Fig. 184-8). In addition, magnetic resonance imaging may detect early osteonecrosis while plain films remain normal. Cartilage atrophy related to disuse or immobilization, in which the synovial fluid may not effectively nourish the cartilage, is accompanied by diffuse loss of interosseous space.

Preservation of interosseous space is common in patients with pigmented villonodular synovitis and idiopathic synovial osteochondromatosis.

Intraarticular Bone Ankylosis. Intraarticular bone ankylosis occurs in certain disorders. In rheumatoid arthritis this finding is usually limited to the carpal and tarsal areas. In psoriasis such ankylosis

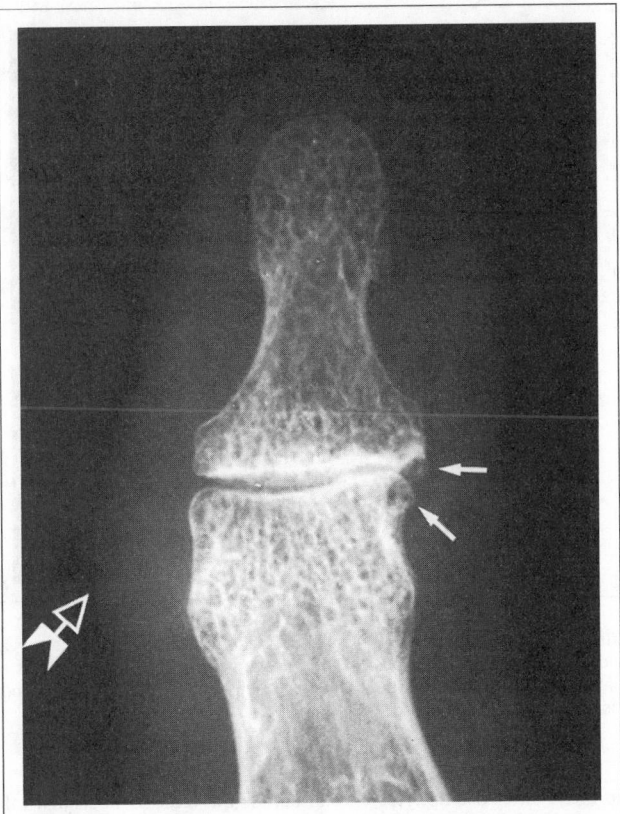

FIGURE 184-7   Osteoarthritis. Mild involvement of a distal interphalangeal joint is characterized by articular space diminution, and minimal eburnation of bone. Osteophytosis *(small arrows)* is not prominent. Soft tissue swelling is evident *(large arrows)*.

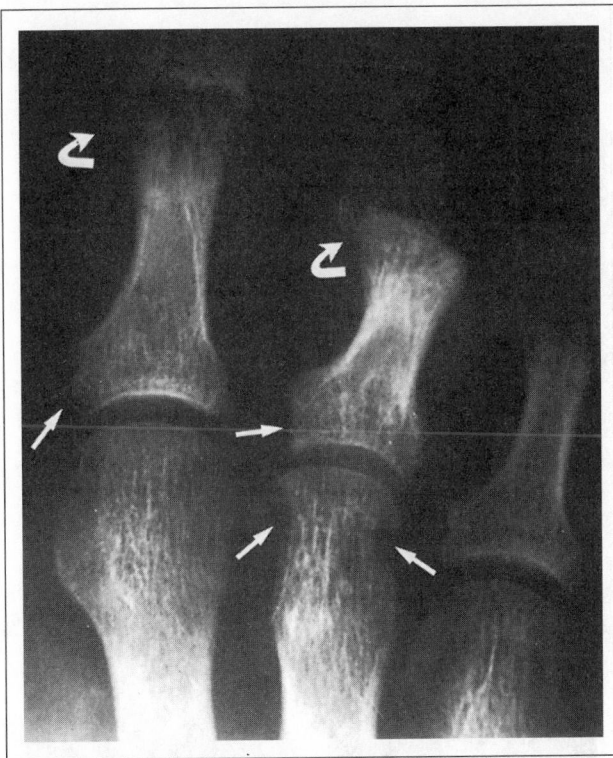

FIGURE 184-9   Psoriatic arthritis. Observe bony ankylosis involving interphalangeal joints of two toes *(curved arrows)*, accompanying soft tissue swelling, and marginal erosions of bone at the metatarsophalangeal joints *(straight arrows)*.

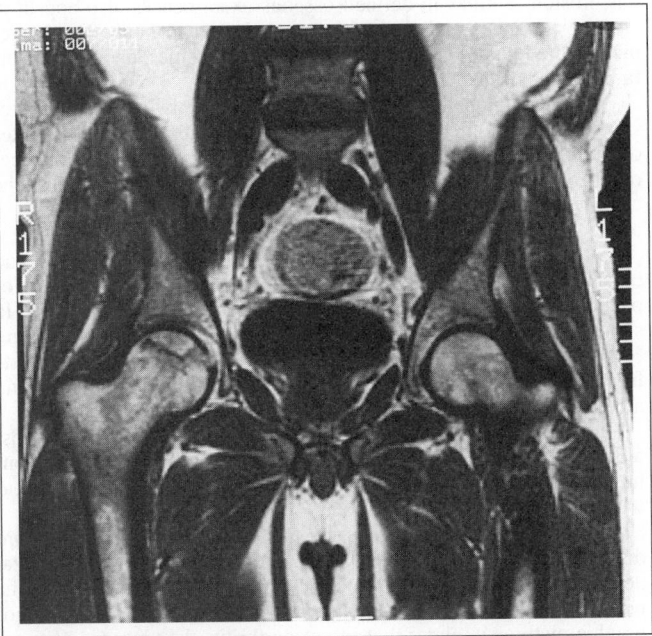

FIGURE 184-8   Osteonecrosis. Coronal T1-weighted (TR/TE, 600/20) spin-echo MR image demonstrates characteristic findings of osteonecrosis involving the right femoral head. A peripheral rim of low signal intensity representing sclerotic bone is seen surrounding an area of high signal intensity characteristic of preserved fatty marrow.

can be evident in interphalangeal joints of the hands and feet (Fig. 184-9) and in metacarpophalangeal and metatarsophalangeal articulations. In ankylosing spondylitis, large joints such as the hip may fuse.

Intraarticular bone ankylosis also is well recognized in the interphalangeal joints of patients with inflammatory or erosive forms of osteoarthritis. Bone ankylosis of joints in patients with gout, neuroarthropathy, tuberculosis, pigmented villonodular synovitis, and idiopathic synovial osteochondromatosis is uncommon, but it may be seen following pyogenic arthritis and in juvenile chronic arthritis.

Bone Erosion.   In some diseases osseous erosions are initially evident at marginal areas of the joint (marginal erosions), at sites where the synovium abuts bone that does not possess protective cartilage. Marginal erosions are early features of rheumatoid arthritis (Fig. 184-1) and other processes characterized by synovial inflammation such as psoriatic arthritis, Reiter's syndrome (Fig. 184-2), ankylosing spondylitis, and infection. With progression of disease, synovial inflammation leads to destruction of portions of subchondral bone as well. Transchondral extension of inflammatory synovial tissue or pannus also can create cystic lesions that may appear enclosed on radiographic examination.

In inflammatory forms of osteoarthritis central erosions may be identified within the interphalangeal joints of the hand. The distinctive central location of these osseous lesions may be related to the presence of bone collapse. Such erosions are accompanied by peripherally located osteophytes occurring at the attachment of the joint capsule, creating a "bird-wing" or "sea-gull" configuration.

Osseous erosions in gout occur in both intraarticular and extraarticular locations, frequently in relation to adjacent tophi (Fig. 184-4). Eccentric erosions arise at the margins of affected joints and progress slowly. They are well circumscribed and of variable size, and are commonly associated with a sclerotic margin and an elevated osseous spicule, the "overhanging-edge" sign. These erosions can occur in the absence of joint space narrowing and are usually accompanied by lobulated soft tissue swelling. Central osseous erosions also appear

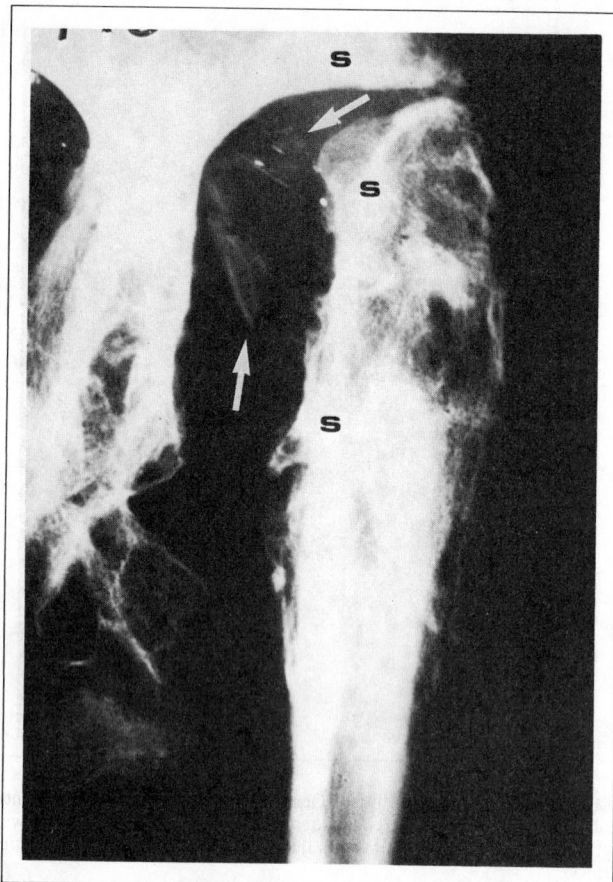

FIGURE 184-10 Neuroarthropathy (syphilis). Considerable sclerosis *(S)* and fragmentation *(arrows)* are seen. There is subluxation of the femoral head with respect to the acetabulum.

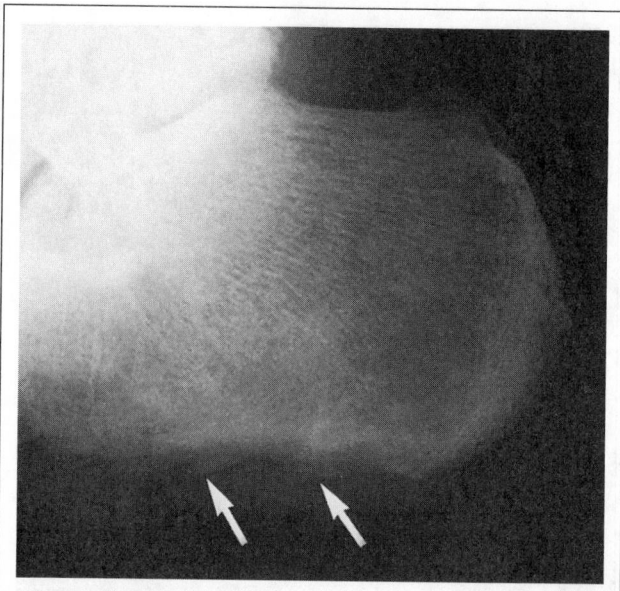

FIGURE 184-11 Psoriatic arthritis. Ill-defined proliferative bony changes are evident along the plantar aspect of the calcaneus *(arrows)*. These findings are compatible with psoriatic arthritis, Reiter's syndrome, or ankylosing spondylitis.

in gout, related to extension of cartilaginous deposits of urate into subchondral bone. Extraarticular erosions can appear anywhere in the skeleton beneath tophaceous deposits.

Intraarticular bone erosions may be evident in pigmented villonodular synovitis and idiopathic synovial osteochondromatosis, especially in the hip, elbow, and wrist. Single or multiple well-defined osseous defects appear in association with soft tissue prominence and, in the case of idiopathic synovial osteochondromatosis, intraarticular calcification and ossification.

Bone Sclerosis, Osteophytosis, and Proliferation. Sclerosis, or eburnation of subchondral bone, is a fundamental feature of osteoarthritis. It occurs in the stressed area of the affected articulation, in association with joint space narrowing and cyst formation. Sclerosis is especially prominent in osteoarthritis of the hip (Fig. 184-6) and knee.

Extreme sclerosis is characteristic of neuropathic disease of the skeleton, especially that occurring in syphilis and syringomyelia (Fig. 184-10). Other disorders associated with bone eburnation include CPPD crystal deposition disease, osteonecrosis, and pyogenic arthritis.

Osteophytosis also is a well-recognized feature of osteoarthritis. Typically the developing osteophyte is manifested as a ledge of bone at the margin of an articulation. Marginal osteophytes are especially characteristic along the medial aspect of the femoral head in association with osteoarthritis of the hip, and on the medial and lateral aspects of the distal femur and proximal tibia and posterior aspect of the patella in association with osteoarthritis of the knee. In the interphalangeal joints of the fingers, osteoarthritis is accompanied by capsular osteophytes related to outgrowths appearing at the osseous attachment of the joint capsule. One additional type of osteophyte that appears in osteoarthritis is related to bone irritation by the synovial membrane (the intraarticular counterpart of the periosteum). In the

hip these latter osteophytes extend across the femoral neck just inferior to the femoral head and are combined with proliferation along the medial aspect of the femoral neck, a phenomenon called *buttressing.*

Ill-defined osseous excrescences accompany bone erosions in the seronegative spondyloarthropathies, psoriatic arthritis, Reiter's syndrome, and ankylosing spondylitis. The affected bone appears "whiskered" because irregular outgrowths are seen about the sites of osseous erosion. Similar ill-defined osseous excrescences also appear at sites of tendinous and ligamentous attachment to bone. These sites include the femoral trochanters, humeral tuberosities, and plantar surface of the calcanei (Fig. 184-11).

In diffuse idiopathic skeletal hyperostosis (ankylosing hyperostosis of Forestier), well-defined bone outgrowths appear at osseous sites of tendinous and ligamentous attachment. These sites include the olecranon process of the ulna, the plantar and posterior surfaces of the calcaneus, and the anterior surface of the patella.

Subchondral Cyst Formation. In rheumatoid arthritis and other synovial inflammatory processes transchondral extension of pannus creates subchondral radiolucent lesions of variable size. In some instances the resulting cysts may lead to spontaneous fracture.

Cyst formation also is frequent in osteoarthritis. The cysts frequently are multiple, involving both sides of the articulation, and are accompanied by joint space loss and bone sclerosis.

In osteonecrosis, necrosis of bone and marrow is followed by osteoclastic resorption of dead trabeculae, with cyst formation. In contradistinction to the situation in osteoarthritis, these cysts may appear without loss of interosseous space.

Cyst formation is a recognized manifestation of the structural joint disease (pyrophosphate arthropathy) that accompanies CPPD crystal deposition disease. Additional structural changes include sclerosis, bone fragmentation, and osteophytosis. Although the resulting radiographic picture simulates that in osteoarthritis, the presence of cartilage calcification (chondrocalcinosis) and the involvement of unusual articular sites such as the wrist and elbow allow accurate diagnosis of CPPD crystal deposition disease in most instances.

Multiple subchondral cysts also can be seen in pigmented villonodular synovitis and hemophilia.

Bone Fragmentation and Collapse. Neuroarthropathy is the arthritic disorder that is associated with the most extensive fragmen-

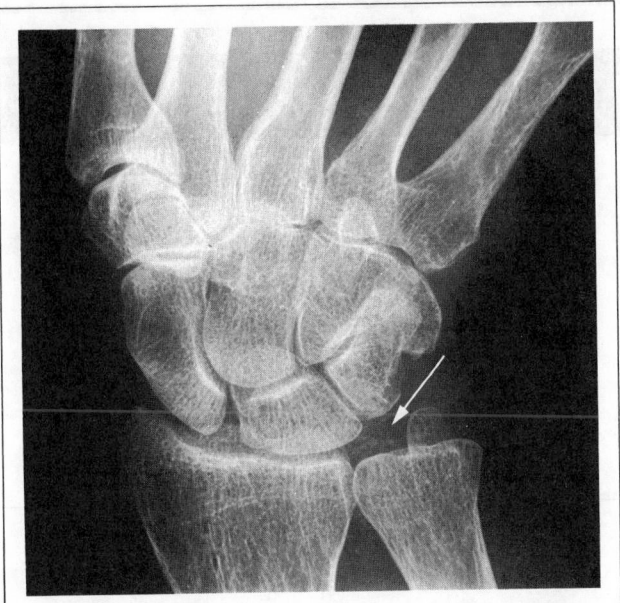

FIGURE 184-12 Calcium pyrophosphate dihydrate crystal deposition disease. The radiographic finding in this case is cartilage calcification (chondrocalcinosis) involving principally the triangular fibrocartilage of the wrist, creating a density adjacent to the distal ulna *(arrow)*.

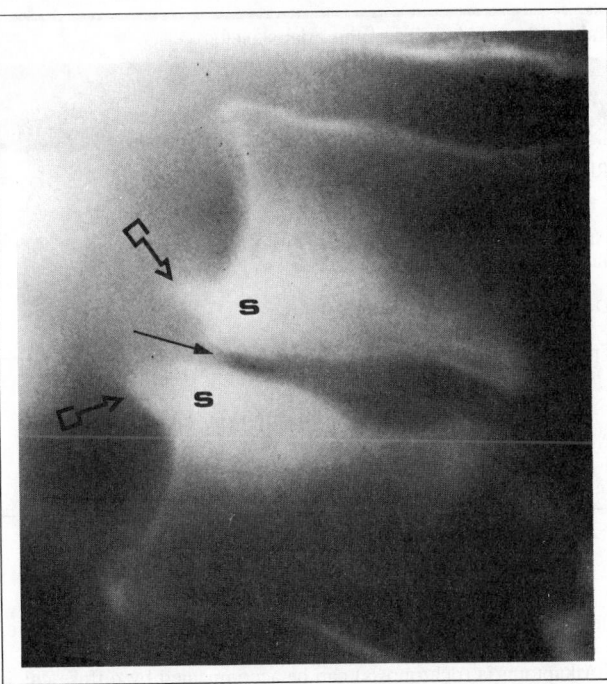

FIGURE 184-13 Degenerative disease of the nucleus pulposus. The radiographic abnormalities include considerable loss of intervertebral disk space height, a vacuum phenomenon creating a small radiolucency overlying the anterior aspect of the intervertebral disk *(solid arrow)*, and considerable reactive sclerosis *(S)* of the neighboring vertebral bodies. Triangular osteophytes are present along the anterior surface of the vertebrae *(open arrows)*.

tation and collapse of apposing articular surfaces (Fig. 184-10). Fragments of bone and cartilage may be displaced into the articular cavity, existing as "loose" bodies or becoming embedded in the synovial membrane at a distant site.

Pyrophosphate arthropathy can be associated with rapidly progressive fragmentation of bone. Other findings, such as chondrocalcinosis, provide helpful clues to the correct diagnosis. Fragmentation of subchondral bone is also evident in osteonecrosis and transchondral fractures (osteochondritis dissecans).

Intraarticular and Periarticular Calcification. Calcification of hyaline cartilage or fibrocartilage or both (chondrocalcinosis) is a fundamental radiographic sign of idiopathic CPPD crystal deposition disease (Fig. 184-12). The calcific deposits in fibrocartilage appear shaggy and are most commonly found in the menisci of the knee, triangular fibrocartilage of the wrist, and symphysis pubis. Hyaline cartilage calcification creates thin, curvilinear radiodensities that parallel the subchondral bone; any joint can be the site of such calcification. Synovial and capsular calcification also may be apparent.

Primary hyperparathyroidism and hemochromatosis can be associated with CPPD crystal deposition with chondrocalcinosis. Although cartilage calcification is occasionally observed in gout, the deposits are less extensive and usually are limited to one or two articulations.

Tendon calcification sometimes is evident in CPPD crystal deposition disease, but such calcification is much more frequent in hydroxyapatite crystal deposition disease, in which case it may lead to symptoms and signs of tendinitis. Calcific tendinitis is most common in the shoulder, although it may also be observed about other articulations such as the wrist, hip, and elbow. The radiograph outlines linear radiodensities within the substance of the tendon.

Cloudlike tumoral deposits of calcification about one or more articulations are observed in renal osteodystrophy with secondary hyperparathyroidism, collagen vascular disorders such as scleroderma and systemic lupus erythematosus, milk-alkali syndrome, hypervitaminosis D, and sarcoidosis. Tuftal calcification with or without resorption of the terminal phalanges is a well-recognized manifestation of scleroderma, and linear calcification in subcutaneous and muscular tissue can be evident in scleroderma, dermatomyositis, and systemic lupus erythematosus.

Axial Skeleton (Table 184-1)

Intervertebral Disk Space Narrowing. Degenerative disease of the nucleus pulposus of the intervertebral disk leads to progressive narrowing of the disk space associated with intradiskal collections of gas (vacuum phenomena) and sclerosis of the adjacent vertebral bodies (Fig. 184-13). The sclerotic vertebrae usually possess a well-defined margin bordering on the intervertebral disk. With magnetic resonance imaging of degenerative disk disease the intervertebral disk and adjacent marrow of the vertebral body undergo characteristic sequential changes in signal intensity.

Osteomyelitis of the spine frequently begins within the vertebral body and spreads to the neighboring intervertebral disk. The resulting radiographic findings include osteolysis and osteosclerosis of the vertebra and intervertebral disk space narrowing. Eventually, the adjacent vertebra also is involved. The margins of the affected vertebrae usually are ill defined, and the intervertebral disk lacks a vacuum phenomenon. These radiographic features usually allow differentiation of infection and degenerative disease of the nucleus pulposus. With increased sensitivity to subtle changes in bone marrow, magnetic resonance imaging can also play a role in the early detection of spinal osteomyelitis, often while plain films are normal. However, the signal intensity changes of early osteomyelitis must be distinguishable from the background normal marrow signal intensity, which is dependent on the distribution of red and yellow marrow at the anatomic site in question. Intravenous gadolinium administration may show areas of abnormal enhancement suggestive of infection, in the appropriate clinical setting. While magnetic resonance imaging of osteomyelitis is more sensitive than specific, when correlated with clinical information and routine radiographs, diagnostic accuracy is improved. Magnetic resonance imaging is also helpful in assessment of paraspinal and intraspinal involvement, such as epidural and paraspinal abscess.

Rheumatoid arthritis is associated with narrowing of the cervical intervertebral disks, with irregularity of the vertebral surface. Osteophytes are absent, but subluxation at one or more cervical levels (in-

Table 184-1   Arthritis of the axial skeleton

	INVERTEBRAL DISK SPACE NARROWING	VACUUM PHENOMENA	INVERTEBRAL DISK SPACE CALCIFICATION	BONE OUTGROWTHS	APOPHYSEAL JOINT EROSION	APOPHYSEAL JOINT ANKYLOSIS	ATLANTOAXIAL SUBLUXATION
Rheumatoid arthritis	+	−	−	−	+	±	+
Psoriatic arthritis, Reiter's syndrome	±	−	−	Paravertebral ossification	±	±	+
Ankylosing spondylitis	±	−	±	Syndesmophytes	+	+	+
Juvenile rheumatoid arthritis	+	−	±	−	+	+	+
Degenerative disease of the nucleus pulposus	+	+	−	−	−	−	−
Spondylosis deformans	−	−	−	Osteophytes	−	−	−
Diffuse idiopathic skeletal hyperostosis	−	−	±	Flowing anterolateral ossification	−	−	−
Alkaptonuria	+	+	+	Syndesmophytes (rare)	−	−	−
Infection	+	−	−	−	−	−	−

+, Common presentation; ±, uncommon; −, rare or absent.

cluding the atlantoaxial junction) and apophyseal joint erosions can be seen.

Alkaptonuria (ochronosis) can be accompanied by diffuse calcification of intervertebral disks and disk space narrowing. Multiple vacuum phenomena are common.

Other causes of intervertebral disk space narrowing and irregularity of adjacent vertebral bodies include neuroarthropathy, intraosseous diskal herniation (cartilaginous or Schmorl's node), trauma, and crystal deposition diseases. Such narrowing also occurs in dialysis spondyloarthropathy and may be related to amyloid deposition.

Osteophytosis and Other Bone Outgrowths. Degenerative changes in the anulus fibrosus of the intervertebral disk lead to spondylosis deformans, resulting in widespread spinal osteophytosis. The outgrowths are horizontally oriented and extend in an anterolateral direction.

Widespread spinal excrescences having a predilection for the lower thoracic and upper lumbar vertebrae are a fundamental feature of diffuse idiopathic skeletal hyperostosis (ankylosing hyperostosis) (Fig. 184-14). The radiographs reveal a flowing pattern of ossification along the anterolateral aspect of the spine, with a bumpy spinal contour and preservation of intervertebral disk height.

Ankylosing spondylitis is associated with thin vertical radiodense spicules (syndesmophytes) that extend from one vertebral body to its neighbor (Fig. 184-15). Syndesmophytes initially are evident at the thoracolumbar and lumbosacral junctions but soon extend to other portions of the spine. Additional findings include reactive sclerosis of the corners of the vertebral bodies (osteitis), straightening or squaring of the anterior vertebral margins, and apophyseal and costovertebral joint ankylosis. Eventually, widespread bone formation produces a "bamboo spine." Many of these findings in ankylosing spondylitis also are evident in the spondylitis accompanying inflammatory bowel diseases, such as ulcerative colitis and Crohn's disease.

Paravertebral ossification is seen in psoriatic arthritis and Reiter's syndrome. Such ossification creates initially ill-defined radiodense shadows separated from the edges of the vertebral bodies and intervertebral disks, particularly at the thoracolumbar junction, and eventually larger, better-defined excrescences that merge with the vertebrae and disks. It is their larger size and asymmetric distribution that distinguish these outgrowths from the syndesmophytes of ankylosing spondylitis and inflammatory bowel disorders.

Bone outgrowths of the spine also are seen in fluorosis, acromegaly, and hypoparathyroidism.

Intervertebral Disk Calcification. Extensive calcification of multiple intervertebral disks is virtually pathognomonic of alkaptonuria. Globular calcification of one or several intervertebral disks can occur on a dystrophic basis after injury or infection. In children calcification of one or more cervical intervertebral disks can be associated with significant clinical findings (diskitis) that disappear in

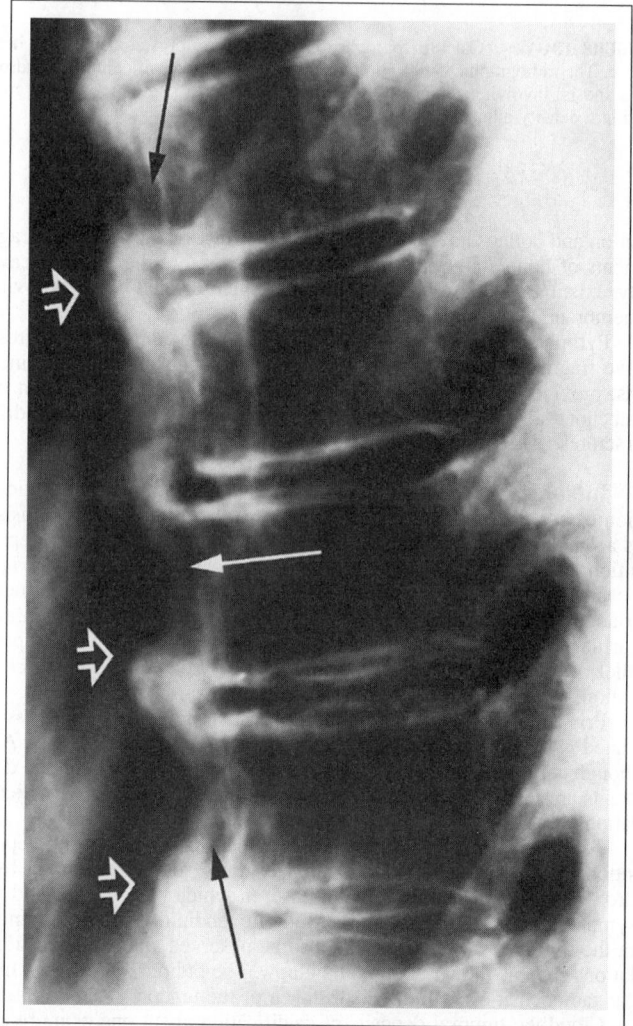

FIGURE 184-14   Diffuse idiopathic skeletal hyperostosis. In this disorder characteristic flowing ossification appears along the anterolateral aspect of the thoracolumbar spine. The bumpy spinal contour *(arrowheads)* and a radiolucency beneath the deposited bone, between it and the underlying vertebral body *(arrows)*, are evident.

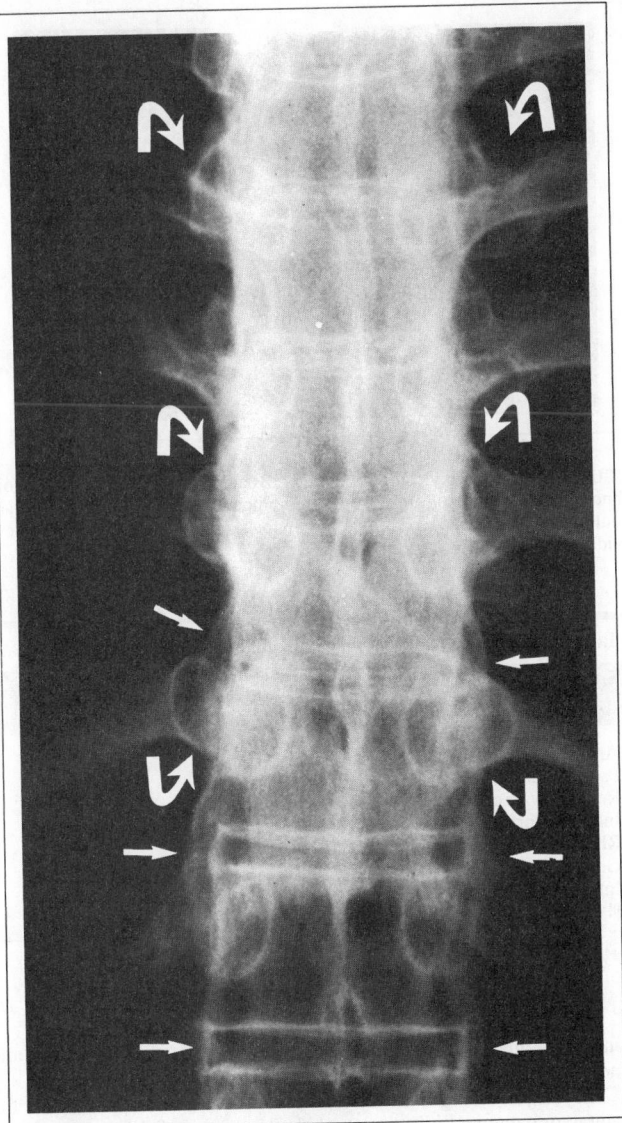

FIGURE 184-15 Ankylosing spondylitis. Syndesmophytes extend as vertical radiodensities between vertebral bodies *(straight arrows)*, producing bony ankylosis of the spine. Also evident is costovertebral joint ankylosis *(curved arrows)*.

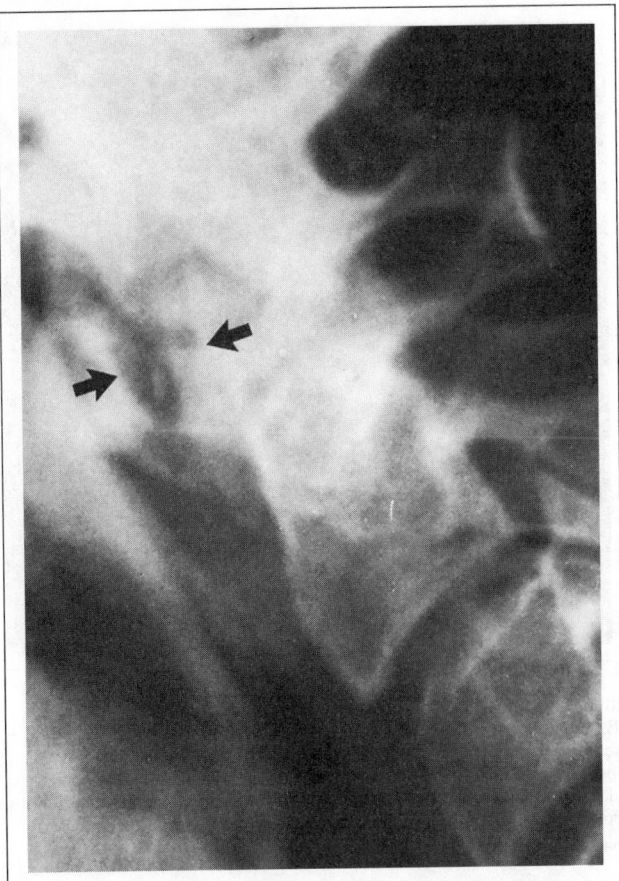

FIGURE 184-16 Rheumatoid arthritis. In this example prominent atlantoaxial subluxation is evident. This radiograph was exposed during flexion of the neck and demonstrates an increased distance between the anterior arch of the atlas and the odontoid process *(between arrows)*. Similar changes may be evident in other inflammatory synovial processes.

weeks or months. Calcification of the outer fibers of the anulus fibrosus may appear in CPPD crystal deposition disease. Diskal calcification also can occur in any disease that produces bone ankylosis between vertebral bodies or joint fusion in the corresponding apophyseal articulations.

Atlantoaxial Subluxation. Inflammation of the synovial sac between the transverse ligament of the atlas and the posterior surface of the odontoid process produces atlantoaxial subluxation, manifested as increased distance between the anterior arch of the atlas and the odontoid process of the axis on lateral films of the cervical spine, especially those exposed during neck flexion (Fig. 184-16). Rheumatoid arthritis, psoriatic arthritis, Reiter's syndrome, and ankylosing spondylitis show atlantoaxial subluxation, and each also may produce odontoid erosions on the anterior or posterior surfaces, or both. Magnetic resonance imaging can assist in evaluation of inflammation at the craniocervical junction and can also provide an assessment of secondary spinal cord complications (Fig. 184-17).

Paravertebral Swelling. Fusiform soft tissue masses about the spine can occur in association with a psoas abscess, seen in pyogenic infection of the spine as well as in tuberculosis. In the latter disease,

calcification of the psoas abscess may be identified. Paravertebral masses also can be evident with posttraumatic hemorrhage and with spinal neoplasms, indicating tumor extension.

CHARACTERISTIC TARGET AREAS OF ARTICULAR DISEASE

In addition to the morphologic features of articular lesions, the distribution of these lesions within the appendicular and axial skeleton provides clues to accurate diagnosis.

Hand

The articulations of the digits of the hand include the metacarpophalangeal, proximal interphalangeal, and distal interphalangeal joints and the interphalangeal joint of the thumb. Rheumatoid arthritis produces alterations that predominate in the metacarpophalangeal and proximal interphalangeal joints and in the interphalangeal joint of the thumb (Fig. 184-1). Although erosions may be apparent in distal interphalangeal joints, these are infrequent.

Osteoarthritis primarily involves the distal interphalangeal, proximal interphalangeal and, less commonly, the metacarpophalangeal joints (Fig. 184-7). Although changes may be isolated in distal interphalangeal or proximal interphalangeal joints, they are rarely isolated in the metacarpophalangeal joints. Extensive abnormalities in the last site should raise the possibility of CPPD crystal deposition disease.

Inflammatory or erosive osteoarthritis most frequently produces alterations in the distal interphalangeal and proximal interphalangeal joints. CPPD crystal deposition disease produces structural joint changes that predominate at the metacarpophalangeal joints. Gouty arthritis may affect any articulation of the digits (Fig. 184-4). Psori-

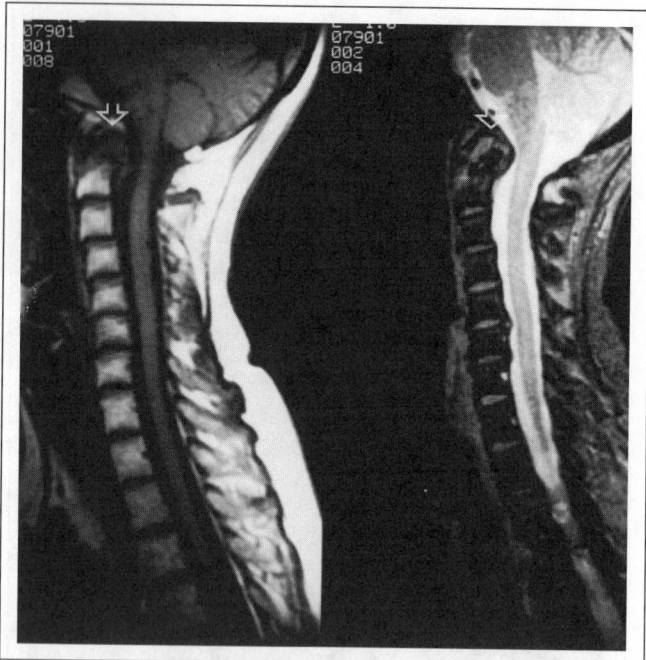

FIGURE 184-17 Rheumatoid arthritis. Sagittal T1-weighted spin-echo (TR/TE, 600/11) *(left)* and multiplanar gradient recalled (MPGR) *(right)* MR images of the upper cervical spine demonstrate an inflammatory mass causing erosive changes about the odontoid process *(open arrows)*, with secondary spinal cord distortion. High signal intensity inflammation can be seen about the odontoid process on the MPGR image *(open arrow)*.

Courtesy C. Gundry, MD, Minneapolis.

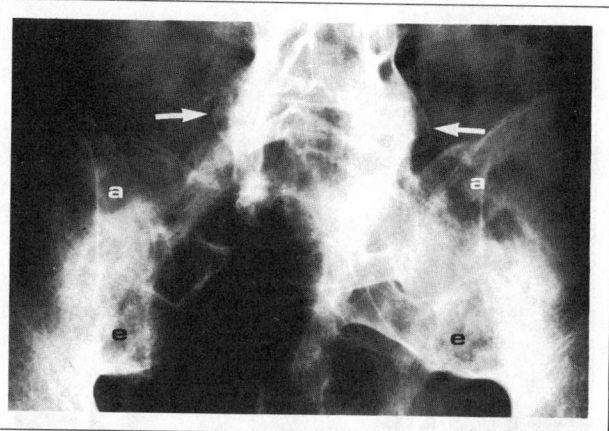

FIGURE 184-18 Ankylosing spondylitis. Bilateral symmetric sacroiliac joint abnormalities consist of erosion *(e)*, predominantly on the ilium, and intraarticular bony ankylosis *(a)*. Syndesmophytosis of the lower lumbar spine is evident *(arrows)*.

Table 184-2 Sacroiliac joint abnormalities

	BILATERAL SYMMETRIC	BILATERAL ASYMMETRIC	UNILATERAL
Ankylosing spondylitis	+		
Psoriatic arthritis	+	+	+
Reiter's syndrome	+	+	+
Inflammatory bowel disease	+		
Rheumatoid arthritis		+	+
Gout	+	+	+
Infection			+
Hyperparathyroidism	+		

+, Common presentation.

atic arthritis may be evident as a destructive arthritis of distal interphalangeal and proximal interphalangeal joints.

Wrist

The wrist is not a single joint; rather, it consists of a series of compartments: the radiocarpal compartment between the distal radius and proximal carpal row, the midcarpal compartment between the proximal and distal carpal rows, the common carpometacarpal compartment between the distal carpal row and metacarpals of the four ulnar digits, the first carpometacarpal joint between the trapezium and the first metacarpal, and the inferior radioulnar compartment between the distal radius and ulna. The radial aspect of the midcarpal compartment is conveniently termed the *trapezioscaphoid space*.

Rheumatoid arthritis initially involves the radiocarpal, midcarpal, inferior radioulnar, and pisiform-triquetral compartments, as well as the tendon sheaths and tendons of the wrists (Fig. 184-5). Eventually, all compartments of the wrist are altered.

Osteoarthritis produces alterations that are usually confined to the first carpometacarpal and trapezioscaphoid areas. Without a history of trauma, any process that appears degenerative but is not located within these typical compartments should not be designated as osteoarthritis until other possibilities, especially crystal deposition, are excluded.

Inflammatory osteoarthritis may result in abnormalities in the first carpometacarpal and trapezioscaphoid areas. Changes elsewhere in the wrist are unusual. Involvement in CPPD crystal deposition disease usually appears in the radiocarpal compartment. Gout can be associated with pancompartmental alterations, although the most severe involvement may be noted in the common carpometacarpal compartment. The findings in juvenile rheumatoid arthritis may be noted throughout the wrist, but the radiocarpal compartment often is spared.

Foot

The articulations of the foot are the distal interphalangeal, proximal interphalangeal, and metatarsophalangeal joints, the interphalangeal

joint of the great toe, and numerous articulations in the midfoot and hindfoot.

The major changes in rheumatoid arthritis are apparent in the metatarsophalangeal joints, interphalangeal joint of the great toe, and the articulations of the midfoot and hindfoot. The earliest changes in this disease may appear in the metatarsophalangeal articulations, especially in the fifth digit. Posterior calcaneal erosions and well-defined plantar calcaneal spurs are additional findings.

Gouty arthritis predominates in the first digit at both the metatarsophalangeal and interphalangeal joints, although any joint in the foot may be affected. Any articulation of the foot also may be altered in psoriasis and Reiter's syndrome, although sites of predilection include the metatarsophalangeal joints and interphalangeal joint of the great toe (Fig. 184-9). In both disorders proliferative erosions are noted on the plantar and posterior calcaneal surfaces (Fig. 184-11). Osteoarthritis may produce changes at the first metatarsophalangeal joint.

CPPD crystal deposition disease may be associated with selective involvement of the talonavicular area. The same articulation is also involved in neuroarthropathy accompanying diabetes mellitus.

Knee

Three spaces or compartments in the knee joint are the medial femorotibial, lateral femorotibial, and patellofemoral spaces. Rheumatoid arthritis and related synovial diseases such as ankylosing spondylitis produce symmetric loss of joint space in the medial and lateral femorotibial compartments. This involvement may be combined with alterations of the patellofemoral space.

Osteoarthritis produces asymmetric joint space narrowing. More frequently, it is the medial femorotibial space that is affected. In addition, the patellofemoral compartment may be altered in osteoarthritis, although abnormality in this area usually is combined with changes in the medial femorotibial space. Joint space narrowing con-

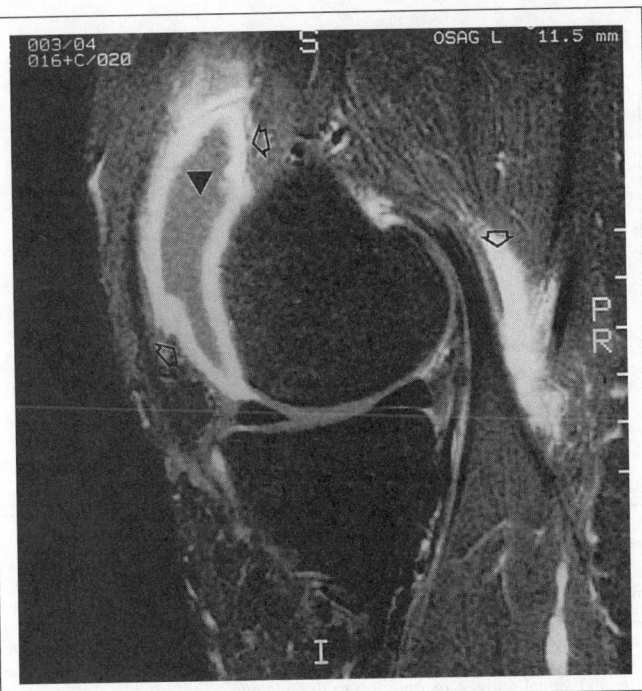

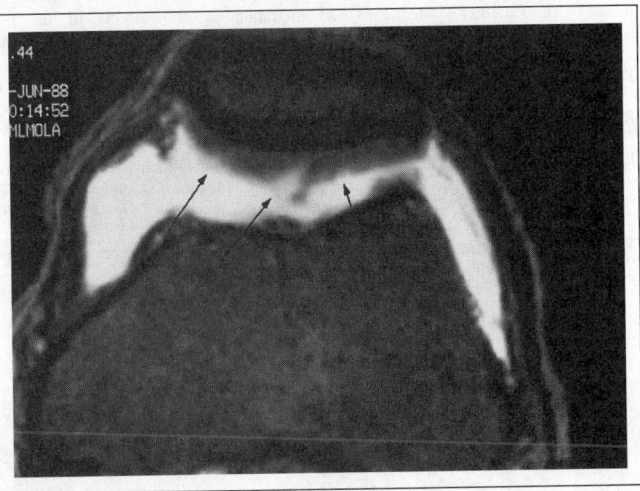

FIGURE 184-20 Articular cartilage abnormality. Transaxial three-dimensional MR image of the knee using fast imaging with steady-state precession (FISP) (TR/TE, 30/10; flip angle, 35 degrees) obtained following intraarticular injection of a gadolinium compound very clearly demonstrates irregularity of the articular cartilage of the patella *(arrows)*.
Courtesy J. Kramer, MD, Vienna, Austria.

FIGURE 184-19 Rheumatoid arthritis. Parasagittal fat-saturated, proton density–weighted spin-echo (TR/TE, 1600/30) MR image of the knee obtained immediately after intravenous injection of a gadolinium agent. A rim of high signal intensity representing enhancing pannus *(open arrows)* is evident surrounding an area of lower signal intensity representing joint effusion *(arrowhead)*. Differentiation was not possible without intravenous gadolinium. Enhancing inflamed synovium is also evident within a posterior synovial cyst *(open arrow)*.

fined to the patellofemoral compartment is more typical of CPPD crystal deposition disease. A similar predilection for patellofemoral compartmental alteration is seen in hyperparathyroidism.

Hip

The hip can be considered as a single articulation, but it is helpful to identify which area of the joint is predominantly affected.

In rheumatoid arthritis symmetric loss of joint space is the rule. This may eventually result in acetabular protrusion into the pelvis. A similar pattern may be noted in ankylosing spondylitis and in CPPD crystal deposition disease, although osteophytosis may accompany the loss of articular space in both disorders.

In osteoarthritis, joint space loss most characteristically occurs in the superior aspect of the joint (Fig. 184-6). Eventually, large osteophytes appear along the medial aspect of the femoral head, and the resulting radiographic picture may resemble symmetric loss of space.

Sacroiliac Joint

Many disorders are associated with erosion and sclerosis of the ilium and sacrum and widening or narrowing of the sacroiliac joint with or without intraarticular bone ankylosis; therefore it is the distribution of the changes that produces the most important clue to accurate diagnosis (Table 184-2). Changes may be bilateral and symmetric, as in ankylosing spondylitis (Fig. 184-18), or bilateral and asymmetric, as in Reiter's syndrome or psoriatic arthritis. Unilateral involvement always should suggest an infectious process, although this may be an early appearance in any of the spondyloarthropathies.

ADVANCED IMAGING METHODS

It is difficult in a short chapter to detail the many applications of current imaging methods with regard to the musculoskeletal system. Computed tomography and magnetic resonance imaging have the ad-

vantages of cross-sectional imaging capability and excellent contrast resolution. Although neither is used as a primary tool in the evaluation of arthritis, both have very definite roles in the approach to diagnosis and treatment.

Applications of computed tomography include evaluation of joints difficult to image with plain films, soft tissue extension of articular abnormalities, osseous destruction, communication of subchondral cysts with the joint space using intraarticular injection of air or iodinated contrast material, and computed arthrotomography for the detection of intraarticular osteochondral bodies.

Magnetic resonance imaging has revolutionized musculoskeletal imaging since its introduction just over 10 years ago. In addition to multiplanar imaging capability, magnetic resonance imaging has the further advantage of not utilizing ionizing radiation. With MRI there is excellent soft tissue contrast, allowing accurate evaluation of structures such as the menisci and cruciate and collateral ligaments of the knee, the rotator cuff of the shoulder, and the triangular fibrocartilage complex of the wrist. Signal intensity changes in bone marrow allow early detection of bone infarction (i.e., osteonecrosis) and infection (osteomyelitis). Magnetic resonance imaging has also improved spinal imaging and has nearly replaced myelography for most indications. Intravenous contrast-enhanced MRI can be used in the differentiation between inflamed synovium and joint effusion (Fig. 184-19). Magnetic resonance imaging performed with intraarticular injection of contrast material can be used in the evaluation of articular cartilage abnormalities (Fig. 184-20), transchondral fractures, and internal joint derangement and evaluation of possible communication between subchondral cysts and the joint space. Current areas under investigation include development of new imaging sequences for the evaluation of articular cartilage, as well as potential applications in the management of synovial inflammatory processes and other arthritidies.

BIBLIOGRAPHY

Aisen AM et al: Cervical spine involvement in rheumatoid arthritis: MR imaging, *Radiology* 165:159, 1987.

Berquist TH: *MRI of the musculoskeletal system*, ed 3, Philadelphia, 1996, Lippincott-Raven.

Kursunoglu-Brahme S et al: Rheumatoid knee: role of gadopentetate-enhanced MR imaging, *Radiology* 176:831, 1990.

Lawson TL et al: The sacroiliac joints: anatomic, plain roentgenographic, and computed tomographic analysis, *J Comput Assist Tomogr* 6:307, 1982.

Martel W: Erosive osteoarthritis and psoriatic arthritis: a radiologic comparison in the hand, wrist, and foot, *Am J Roentgenol* 134:125, 1980.

Martel W et al: Radiologic features of Reiter disease, *Radiology* 132:1, 1979.

Mitchel DG et al: Avascular necrosis of the femoral head: morphologic assessment by MR imaging with CT correlation, *Radiology* 161:739, 1986.

Resnick D: Patterns of femoral head migration in osteoarthritis of the hip: roentgenographic-pathologic correlation and comparison with rheumatoid arthritis, *Am J Roentgenol* 124:62, 1975.

Resnick D: Rheumatoid arthritis of the wrist: the compartmental approach, *Med Radiogr Photogr* 52:50, 1976.

Resnick D, Shaul S, Robins J: Diffuse idiopathic skeletal hyperostosis: extraspinal manifestations of Forestier's disease, *Radiology* 115:513, 1975.

Resnick D et al: Clinical, radiographic, and pathologic abnormalities in calcium pyrophosphate dihydrate deposition disease (CPPD): pseudogout, *Radiology* 122:1, 1977.

Sanchez RB, Quinn SF: MRI of inflammatory synovial processes, *Magn Reson Imaging* 7:529, 1989.

Thomas RH et al: Compartmental evaluation of osteoarthritis of the knee: a comparative study of available diagnostic modalities, *Radiology* 116:585, 1975.

III   CLINICAL IMMUNOLOGY

CHAPTER

185   The Primary Immunodeficiency Disorders

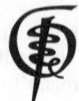

David L. Nelson

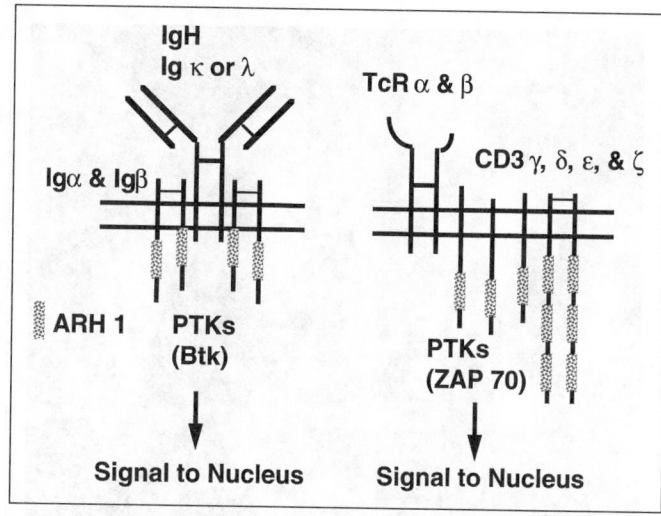

FIGURE 185-1   The components of the B-cell antigen receptor (BcR, *left*) and the T-cell antigen receptor *(TcR, right)*. In the BcR, antigen-binding immunoglobulin (Ig) heavy chains *(IgH)* and light chains (Ig κ or λ) are associated with a disulfide-linked heterodimer *(Igα and Igβ)* containing antigen receptor homology domains *(ARH1)*. The latter, which serve signal transduction purposes, associate with protein tyrosine kinases *(PTKs)*, in particular, *Btk,* and signal antigen recognition to the nucleus. Similarly, the TcR consists of the antigen binding TcRs α and β and the CD3 signal transduction proteins CD3 γ, δ, ε, and ζ. The latter complex of proteins associates with PTKs, including ZAP 70, for signal transduction to the nucleus.

Advances in the understanding of the human immune response over the past 20 years have brought our knowledge from the first morphologic definition of distinct lineages of lymphocytes to the current point at which the molecular cloning of the genes involved in the immune response has become commonplace. In part, these advances have been the result of the development of hybridoma-derived monoclonal antibody techniques, recent developments in molecular genetics and molecular biology technology, and the combination of these approaches. These techniques are currently being employed for the study of immunodeficiency diseases.

BASIC IMMUNOLOGY

Specific immunity is the result of two classes of lymphocytes termed B-cells and T-cells. Both are derived from progenitor cells in bone marrow: B-cells developing in the bone marrow and T-cells developing within the thymus gland. Both types of lymphocytes express receptors for foreign antigens on their surfaces: immunoglobulin or antibody molecules on B-cells and related T-cell antigen receptors on T-cells. B-cells differentiate into plasma cells, which secrete a great number of antibody molecules termed *immunoglobulins*. Immunoglobulins, which consist of one of five heavy chains (μ, δ, γ, α, and ε) paired with one of two light chains (κ or λ) to produce five forms or isotypes (immunoglobulins M, D, and G [IgM, IgD, and IgG; four subclasses], immunoglobulin A [IgA; two subclasses], and immunoglobulin E [IgE]) of antibody. T-cells are directly responsible for lysis of virally infected cells, the rejection of foreign tissue grafts, and the mediation of delayed-type hypersensitivity reactions. In addition to these direct effects, subsets of T-cells also perform regulatory functions amplifying and suppressing the immune response.

Of interest is the similarity of these antigen receptors at the genetic level and the commonality in the mechanisms responsible for generating mature receptors (Fig. 185-1). Indeed, the antigen receptors on T-cells and B-cells belong to a family of immunologically related molecules that has been termed the *immunoglobulin supergene family*. This similarity extends to the mechanism(s) by which transmembrane T-cell receptors (TcRs) and B-cell receptors (BcRs) signal within the cell that their cell surface receptors have encountered exogenous antigen.

The BcR consists of a single polymorphic immunoglobulin molecule (derived from the immunoglobulin heavy chain locus at 14q32 and either the κ light chain locus at 2p11 or the λ light chain locus at 22q11) that is noncovalently associated with a disulfide-linked heterodimer of two proteins termed Igα (CD 79α) and Igβ (CD 79β), which play no role in antigen recognition but rather serve as signal transduction molecules. Within their cytoplasmic tails, Igα and Igβ contain a sequence motif of approximately 26 amino acids variably termed the antigen-receptor homology motif 1 (ARH1), the antigen-recognition activation motif (ARAM), or the tyrosine-based activation motif (TAM). Phosphorylation of two tyrosine residues within the ARH1 are critical in signal transduction.

The TcR consists of a polymorphic disulfide-linked heterodimer consisting of an α chain derived from genes at 14q11 and a β chain derived from genes at 7q32. Rarely, an alternative TcR using a δ chain derived from 14q11 and a γ chain derived from 7p14 can be seen. This TcR complex is associated with a group of transmembrane proteins, termed the CD3 complex, consisting of γ, δ, ε, and ζ chains. The intracytoplasmic tail of each of the γ, δ, and ε chains contains a single ARH1 domain; the tail of the ζ chain contains three such domains.

T-cells recognize antigen in the context of major histocompatibility complex (MHC) antigens (which are also a part of the immunoglobulin supergene family). The antigens that T-cells recognize are small peptide fragments of larger antigens that are proteolytically degraded in endosomes. Exogenous antigens are taken up by antigen-presenting cells, such as monocytes, and by endocytosis and are largely loaded onto MHC class II antigens (HLAD, Dr), whereas endogenous antigens (such as viral proteins in virally infected cells) travel an endogenous pathway (Fig. 185-2) that includes being transported to the endoplasmic reticulum by a heterodimeric protein consisting of TAP1 and TAP2 (transporter of antigenic peptides 1 and 2). Within the endoplasmic reticulum these transported peptides are loaded onto MHC class I molecules (human leukocyte antigen [HLA] A, B, or C) before transport to the cell surface. T-cells of CD4 lineage generally recognize antigen in the context of MHC class II molecules, whereas T-cells of CD8 lineage recognize antigen in the context of MHC class I molecules.

Following antigen recognition, B-cells and T-cells become activated, express new novel protein molecules (particularly the CD40

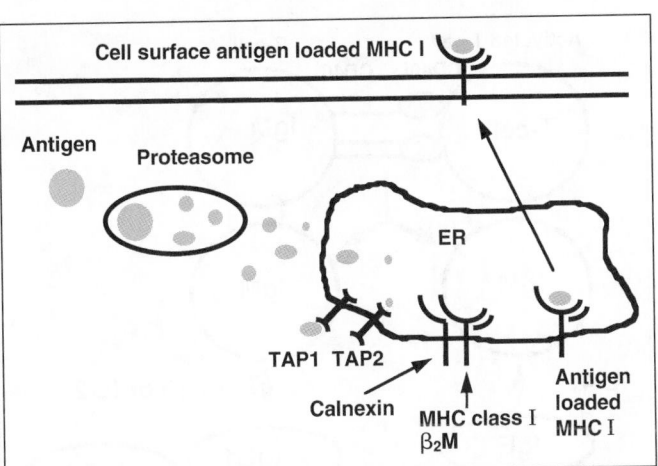

FIGURE 185-2 Endogenous pathway of antigen processing. Antigen enters proteasomes where it is degraded into small fragments. These small fragments are transported into the endoplasmic reticulum *(ER)* by the heterodimeric transporters of antigenic peptide *(TAP)* TAP1 and TAP2. Antigenic fragments displace calnexin from a complex of major histocompatibility complex (MHC) class I protein and associated β_2-microglobulin ($\beta_2 M$), and the latter complex is transported to the cell surface.

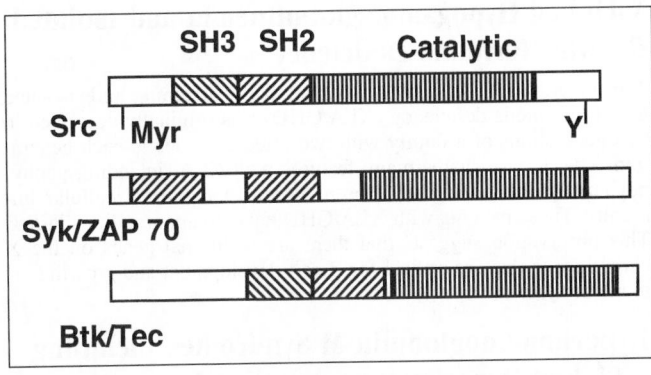

FIGURE 185-3 Families of protein tyrosine kinases (PTKs). The PTKs generally belong to one of three families of tyrosine kinases. The kinases contain an enzyme-active catalytic domain, SH3 domains, which bind to proline-rich domains of other proteins, and SH2 domains, which bind to phosphotyrosine residues on other proteins. The src family contains an amino-terminal myristilation site *(Myr)*, which governs localization within cells, and a carboxy-terminal tyrosine *(Y)*, which regulates src activity.

ligand on T-cells and the CD40 molecule on B-cells) on their surfaces, and secrete a series of low-molecular-weight soluble polypeptides called cytokines or interleukins such as interleukin-2 (IL-2). These activation events are the result of tyrosine phosphorylation of the ARH1 domains associated with the TcR and BcR. These phosphorylation events recruit additional enzymes termed protein tyrosine kinases (PTKs) to the ARH1s. The PTKs generally belong to one of three families—the *ras* family, the *syk/ZAP 70* family, or the *btk/tec* family (Fig. 185-3). These PTKs are responsible for downstream intracytoplasmic signaling to the nucleus that activation should occur, triggering the transcription of a number of immunologically important genes. In particular, *ZAP 70* has an association to the TcR, and *Btk* has an association with the BcR. These activated cells also express specific receptors for cytokines and interleukins. Following interaction of cytokines and/or interleukins such as IL-2 with their specific cell surface receptors, these activated cells undergo proliferative and differentiative events to mediate immunologic responsiveness.

EVALUATION OF THE IMMUNE SYSTEM

Patients with humoral immunodeficiencies usually come to medical attention with a history of recurrent pyogenic infections with high-grade encapsulated bacteria such as *Haemophilus influenzae* and *Diplococcus pneumoniae*. Recurrent sinopulmonary infections are the most common. Screening tests for a humoral immunodeficiency should include a determination of quantitative immunoglobulins of all classes and the measurement of "natural" antibodies such as antibodies to blood group substances or environmental antigens such as influenza. The ability of an individual to make an active humoral immune response can be discovered by collection of serum for determination of antibody titer before and after immunization with commonly available antigens such as Pneumovax, influenza vaccines, or diphtheria and tetanus toxoids. More advanced testing would usually be done in an immunology specialty laboratory.

Patients with cellular immunodeficiencies come to medical attention with recurrent opportunistic infections such as herpes and *Pneumocystis carinii* pneumonia. Evaluation of cellular immune responses should include a determination of the absolute lymphocyte count (complete blood cell count [CBC] and differential on three occasions) and the assessment of delayed-type hypersensitivity testing by the application of intradermal antigens that occur in the environment *(Candida)* or against which the individual has been immunized (diphtheria/tetanus).

Infection with human immunodeficiency virus (HIV) must always be given consideration in the evaluation of an immunodeficient pa-

tient. It must also be remembered that certain immunodeficiencies may interfere with the routine tests to diagnose certain infections such as humoral immunodeficiencies and HIV infection or cellular immunodeficiencies and tuberculosis.

IMMUNODEFICIENCY DISORDERS

The primary immunodeficiency disorders represent a set of inherited diseases that render affected individuals susceptible to recurrent infections and an increased incidence of cancer. The study of these diseases as "experiments of nature" has provided insight into the normal workings of the immune system and has contributed to our knowledge of abnormalities in immune function in both congenital and acquired deficiencies of immune function, including the acquired immunodeficiency syndrome. The World Health Organization (WHO) recognizes 18 primary specific immunodeficiency diseases, which can be separated into the following subgroups: (1) the predominantly antibody deficiency syndromes, (2) the combined immunodeficiency syndromes, and (3) other well-defined immunodeficiency syndromes. This classification provides a useful framework to consider the primary immunodeficiency disorders.

PREDOMINANTLY ANTIBODY DEFICIENCY SYNDROMES
X-Linked Agammaglobulinemia (Bruton's Agammaglobulinemia)

X-linked agammaglobulinemia (XLA) is an immunodeficiency state characterized by panhypogammaglobulinemia with absent peripheral B-cells and normal cell-mediated immunity. Patients often have recurrent infections at the time that maternally derived gammaglobulins disappear (3 to 6 months of age). Patients may acquire paralytic polio as the result of vaccination, and a dermatomyositis-like syndrome associated with meningoencephalitis and enteric cytopathic human orphan (ECHO) virus infection can develop. *Campylobacter jejuni* sepsis also occurs in these patients. In 20% to 40% of patients an arthritis (sterile effusion) develops. Gastrointestinal infections with *Giardia lamblia* and *Campylobacter* species occur, as does regional enteritis. Patients are unable to make specific antibody and have no B-cells. Recently this disorder has been shown to be the result of a deficiency in Bruton's tyrosine kinase *(Btk)*, a PTK intimately associated with the BcR on B-cells. In the bone marrow there is a block at the pre–B-cell stage (before the expression of the mature BcR on cell surfaces). Patients should be given treatment with intravenous immunoglobulin to maintain a "trough or nadir" level of at least 200 to 400 mg/dl. This usually requires an IgG dose of 350 to 500 mg/kg per month. Carrier testing of females in affected families is possible at specialized centers.

X-Linked Hypogammaglobulinemia and Isolated Growth Hormone Deficiency

The disorder of X-linked hypogammaglobulinemia and isolated growth hormone deficiency (XLA/GHD) was originally described in two generations of a family with two affected males in each generation. The disease shares many features with XLA, including panhypogammaglobulinemia with absent B-cells and normal cellular immunity. These patients with XLA/GHD have no abnormalities in *Btk*. This observation suggests that there are additional genes on the X chromosome that are critical for B-cell development and growth hormone production.

Hyperimmunoglobulin M Syndromes Including X-Linked Hyperimmunoglobulin M

Hyperimmunoglobulin M (hyper IgM) syndrome is a series of X-linked, autosomal recessive, and sporadic disorders characterized by normal or increased concentrations of serum IgM and IgD in some cases but decreased or absent IgG, IgA, and IgE. Patients have a high incidence of recurrent pyogenic infections, including otitis media, pneumonia, and septicemia. Patients have a high incidence of neutropenia, thrombocytopenia, and autoimmune disorders. Patients have normal numbers of IgM- and IgD-bearing B-cells in the periphery and may make IgM but not other isotypes of antibodies to some antigens. The X-linked form of the disorder is characterized by defective expression of the CD40 ligand on activated T-cells (Fig. 185-4). Failure of this ligand to bind to the CD40 molecule on activated B-cells leads to defective proliferation and differentiation of B-cells, including the capacity to make IgG, IgA, and IgE (isotype switching). Treatment of recurrent infections is with administration of intravenous immunoglobulins as for XLA. Other therapies (granulocyte colony-stimulating factor, antiinflammatories, and the like) may be directed at other parts of the disorder, if present.

Immunoglobulin Heavy Chain Deletions

Patients have been identified with multiple gene deletions within the heavy chain cluster at 14q32. Patients have been reported with only IgM, IgD, IgG3, IgE, and IgA2 in their serum. Immunoglobulin heavy chain deletions on one chromosome have been demonstrated in approximately 10% of all normal individuals. If symptomatic and lacking IgG antibodies and the ability to mount specific antibody responses, these patients may be given treatment with intravenous immunoglobulin.

Kappa Chain Deficiency

Patients have been reported with only λ-expressing immunoglobulins. There were point mutations in the constant regions of both κ alleles.

Selective Deficiency of Immunoglobulin G Subclasses

Selective deficiencies of IgG subclasses can occur with or without a deficiency of IgA. While any IgG subclass can be deficient, the most common pattern is that of IgG2 and IgG4 deficiency. If patients are having recurrent infections and fail to make antibody when challenged, particularly with polysaccharide antigens, intravenous immunoglobulin therapy should be instituted. In patients with concomitant IgA deficiency care must be taken to avoid production of anti-IgA antibodies, which have been associated with anaphylaxis.

Common Variable Immunodeficiency

Common variable immunodeficiency (CVID) is a term used to describe an aggregate of diseases of uncertain origin that share defective antibody production and for which other causes of immunodeficiency (e.g., XLA) have been excluded. B-cells may be present. Cell-mediated immunity is variable. Absence of eosinophils and/or pure red blood cell aplasia should suggest an associated spindle-cell thy-

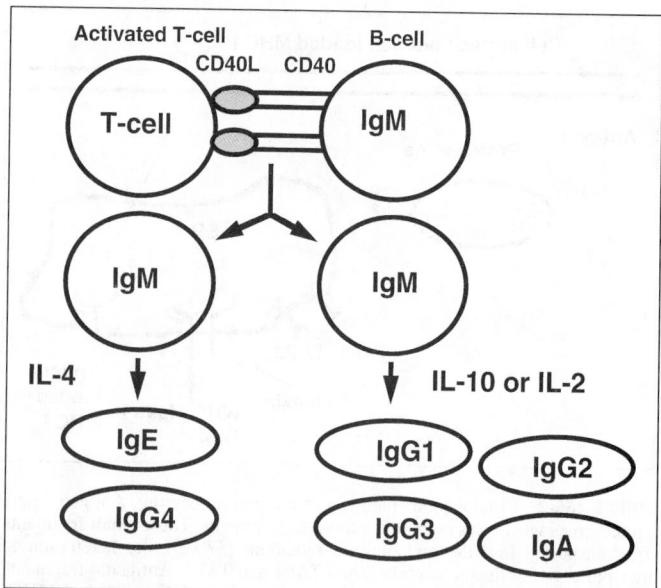

FIGURE 185-4   T-cells and B-cells cooperate to induce isotype switching. Activated T-cells express the CD40 ligand, which interacts with CD40 on the surface of B-cells. Ensuing B-cell proliferation and differentiation in the presence of lymphokines such as interleukins IL-4, IL-10, and IL-2 lead to the phenomenon of isotype switching and the generation of cells producing IgG1, IgG2, IgG3, IgG4, IgA, and IgE.

moma. Patients generally come to medical attention with recurrent sinopulmonary infections and/or gastrointestinal tract syndromes, including *G. lamblia* infection, which may be associated with nodular lymphoid hyperplasia of the gastrointestinal tract. Lymphoproliferative disorders, particularly carcinoma of the stomach, occur with some frequency. Some studies have indicated a candidate locus in the MHC class II and III gene locus on chromosome 6. Patients should receive intravenous gammaglobulin, and prompt attention should be paid to any infection. Some patients benefit from prophylaxis with a sulfonamide antibiotic or a rotation of several antibiotics.

Immunoglobulin A Deficiency

A selective deficiency of IgA occurs in about 1 in 500 to 1 in 700 normal white individuals. This contrasts with an incidence of 1 in 18,000 Japanese individuals. Most individuals with this disorder are asymptomatic; however, some have recurrent sinopulmonary infections and/or gastrointestinal tract disorders. Deficiency of IgA can occur in association with selective IgG subclass deficiencies and occurs more commonly in family members of CVID patients. Some studies have linked a candidate locus for the disease to the same general region as for CVID. Treatment is largely supportive. Anti-IgA antibodies may develop if patients are receiving blood products or gammaglobulins. Anaphylaxis can occur on reexposure to IgA.

Transient Hypogammaglobulinemia of Infancy

At birth infants have IgG levels comparable to their mother's, because of transplacental transfer of maternal IgG, whereas levels of IgM, IgG, IgA, and IgE are quite low. With time, this maternal IgG is catabolized, and at the same time, the infant's production of IgG is increasing as a result of exposure to antigens in the environment. As the IgG levels from two sources cross, there is a nadir in IgG levels, usually between 3 and 6 months of age. Occasionally there is a marked delay in the initiation of IgG synthesis, which leads to low IgG levels. These levels usually normalize by 2 years of age. Some of these individuals have relatives with other primary immunodeficiency disorders. Usually only careful observation and reassurances are needed.

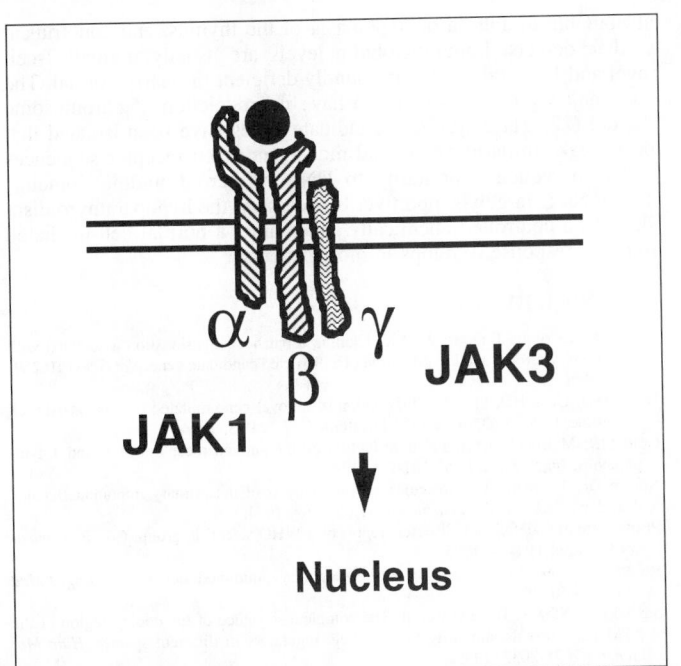

FIGURE 185-5   The high-affinity interleukin-2 (IL-2) receptor. The high-affinity IL-2 receptor (IL-2R) consists of at least three chains: IL-2Rα, IL-2Rβ, and IL-2Rγ. The β and γ chains are responsible for intracellular signaling and associate with the JAK1 and JAK3 kinases, respectively, which lead to downstream pathways signaling to the nucleus.

Severe Combined Immunodeficiency

Severe combined immunodeficiency (SCID) is a clinical syndrome encompassing several well-defined diseases, as well as some as yet undefined disorders. Patients come to medical attention with recurrent infections and failure to thrive that are often associated with diarrhea in the first few months of life. Skin rashes, including those resulting from *Candida* organisms, are common. Patients are generally hypogammaglobulinemic and lymphopenic; they have both pyogenic and opportunistic infections. Untreated, these diseases are often fatal in the first year of life. Although well recognized as pediatric disorders, these conditions are included because they are illustrative of critical defects in human immunity and some of them (adenosine deaminase [ADA] deficiency) have recently been described in adults. The well-characterized diseases within this syndrome follow.

X-Linked Severe Combined Immunodeficiency. Patients generally have normal numbers of B-cells associated with T-cell lymphopenia and hypogammaglobulinemia. This disorder is due to mutations in the γ chain of the interleukin-2 receptor (IL-2R). The high-affinity IL-2R consists of three chains: IL-2Rα, IL-2Rβ, and IL-2Rγ (Fig. 185-5). The β and γ chains are responsible for intracellular signaling in response to IL-2 binding to the receptor. The profundity of the deficiency of immune development in these patients may occur because the IL-2Rγ is also a component of the receptors for IL-4, IL-7, IL-9, and IL-15; therefore, deficient signaling by multiple lymphokines may be involved in the pathogenesis of this disorder. Treatment with intravenous immunoglobulin can be used as an interim therapy before bone marrow transplantation, which does not require immunosuppression.

Autosomal Recessive Severe Combined Immunodeficiency Resulting From JAK3 Deficiency. Some patients with autosomal SCID have hypogammaglobulinemia and a lymphocyte phenotype (T−, B+) similar to patients with X-linked SCID. The gamma chain of the IL-2 receptor, IL-2Rγ, is associated with a PTK termed JAK3. Patients with this form of autosomal SCID have de-

fective JAK3 activity as a result of point mutations in the JAK3 gene and thus a lack of signaling with all of the cytokines for which it is a part of their receptor (see earlier discussion). Treatment can include intravenous gammaglobulin until a bone marrow transplantation without immunosuppression can occur.

Adenosine Deaminase Deficiency. ADA deficiency is an autosomal recessive form of SCID. Patients lack ADA, an enzyme in the purine salvage pathway, as a result of point mutations in the ADA gene. Patients are born with a normal immune system, which undergoes atrophy in response to the accumulation of toxic products of the purine pathway (deoxy-adeonsine triphosphate [deoxy ATP]). Patients can be given treatment with bone marrow transplantation or polyethylene glycol–treated ADA. ADA deficiency was the first disease treated by an approved gene therapy protocol. Recently two adult women were reported with ADA deficiency. Both had received immunosuppressive therapy, which was followed by the onset of recurrent infections. The genetic defects in these women were typical of patients with early-onset disease.

Purine Nucleoside Phosphorylase Deficiency. Purine nucleoside phosphorylase (PNP) deficiency is a form of autosomal recessive SCID. Patients lack PNP, an enzyme in the purine salvage pathway. As with ADA deficiency, the accumulation of toxic metabolites (deoxy-GTP) leads to progressive lymphopenia and immunodeficiency. Transfusions with PNP containing packed red blood cells and bone marrow transplantation have been attempted.

Major Histocompatibility Complex Class II Deficiency. Patients with this form of autosomal recessive SCID have normal or decreased serum immunoglobulin levels associated with normal numbers of B-cells and T-cells. Diarrhea and failure to thrive are common. At least three different genetic lesions may account for this disorder. Two are due to defects in the genes for proteins (class II transcription activation [CIITA] and RFX5) that regulate transcription of the MHC class II genes on chromosome 6. In the absence of class II MHC genes the recognition of exogenous antigens by T-cells is impaired.

Severe Combined Immunodeficiency Resulting from TAP2 Deficiency. Two siblings with recurrent respiratory infections and no history of viral infections were found to express less than 1% of normal amounts of HLA class I molecules on the surface of their peripheral blood mononuclear cells. A defect in β2-microglobulin was ruled out, and both patients were shown to have defects in the TAP2 gene—one of the two TAP genes involved in loading MHC class I antigens in the endoplasmic reticulum with antigenic peptides, the displacement of calnexin, and the transport of MHC class I molecules to the cell surface.

Reticular Dysgenesis. Reticular dysgenesis is a rare autosomal recessive disorder that is often lethal shortly after birth. Many of the infants are "small for gestational age" or premature. Hematopathologic findings are characterized by near-normal numbers of lymphocytes or a profound lymphopenia (with a restricted TcR repertoire) and often a profound failure in the maturation of myeloid precursors (agranulocytosis). Erythrocytes and platelets are normal. Many have a rash that can appear like graft-versus-host disease, eczema, or epidermolysis bullosa. Hepatitis may be present. Some of these patients receive engraftment with maternal T cells. Treatment strategies have included bone marrow transplantation subsequent to immunosuppressive bone marrow ablation.

CD3γ or CD3ε Deficiency. This immunodeficiency is an autosomal recessive disorder with a variable T-cell phenotype, even within a family. Lymphocyte and serum immunoglobulin levels are normal. Deficient signaling through the TcR and variable expression of the TcR account for this rare immunodeficiency.

CD8 Deficiency. This autosomal recessive form of SCID results from mutations in the gene for ZAP 70 PTK that is involved in signaling through the TcR. Diagnosis is easy in these patients because they have normal immunoglobulin levels, normal numbers of CD4+ T-cells, and decreased or absent CD8+ cells in the peripheral blood. The CD4+ cells, however, do not respond to a variety of stimuli. Bone marrow transplantation has been successful in treating this disorder.

OTHER WELL-DEFINED IMMUNODEFICIENCY SYNDROMES
Wiskott-Aldrich Syndrome

The Wiskott-Aldrich syndrome (WAS) is an X-linked recessive disorder associated with thrombocytopenia, eczema, recurrent infections, and an increased incidence of cancer, particularly lymphoreticular neoplasia. The thrombocytopenia is associated with small platelets and is of a consumptive rather than a productive nature, since it responds to splenectomy. Patients have low levels of IgM and normal or elevated levels of IgG, IgA, and IgE. Cell-mediated immunity is variable. Patients are susceptible to all types of infection. Using a positional cloning approach, the gene responsible for WAS was cloned and the protein encoded by this gene was termed the WAS protein (WASP). A search of the available databases at the time did not reveal any homology to other known genes or proteins. The predicted protein contains 502 amino acids and a very proline-rich region. The WASP protein is present in platelets, the cytoplasmic but not the nuclear fraction of peripheral blood mononuclear cells (PMBCs), lymphocytes, monocytes, T-cells and non–T-cells, Epstein-Barr virus–transformed B-cell lines, but not fibroblast cell lines. Patients have been described who both make and fail to make WASP protein. X-linked thrombocytopenia and WAS have been shown to be allelic disorders at the WASP locus. The thrombocytopenia responds to splenectomy. Bone marrow transplantation is the definitive treatment and must be preceded by immunosuppressive bone marrow ablation. The long-term consequences of such therapy are unknown.

Ataxia-Telangiectasia

Ataxia-telangiectasia (AT) is an autosomal recessive immunodeficiency disorder associated with cerebellar ataxia, oculocutaneous telangiectasias, recurrent infections, and an increased incidence of malignancies. Patients have both humoral and cellular immunodeficiency. Most patients lack IgA and IgE. One third to half of patients produce low-molecular-weight IgM (monomeric versus pentameric). Cell-mediated immunity is variable, but immunity to viruses is particularly defective.

The gene encoding AT was mapped to 11q32 and has recently been isolated and termed *ATM,* using a positional cloning approach. The gene appears to encode a protein that may function in cell-cycle checkpoints and bears similarity to a family of signal transduction mediators involved in controlling the G1 phase of the eukaryotic cell cycle: the TOR1 and TOR2 proteins in yeast, as well as their mammalian homologs, designated mTOR or RAFT in the rat and FRAP in humans. The gene also shows strong similarity to two other yeast proteins— ESR1, an essential yeast protein required for DNA repair and meiotic recombination, and ESR1/MEC1. The carboxy-terminal 400 amino acids also show high similarity to the lipid kinase domain of the 100-kD catalytic subunit of the signal transduction mediator phosphatidylinositol-3' kinase (PI-3 kinase) of mammalian cells and the rad3 gene product in fission yeast required for the G2-M cell-cycle checkpoint where it monitors the completion of DNA damage repair and is essential for the correct coupling of mitosis and DNA synthesis. The gene is expressed in virtually every cell type of the body studied to date.

Treatment is largely supportive. Prompt attention to infections is warranted, and appropriate physical therapy techniques to maintain optimal function are essential.

DiGeorge Syndrome

The DiGeorge syndrome is a developmental field defect involving the third and fourth pharyngeal arches. Although often incomplete, the full syndrome becomes evident with neonatal hypocalcemic tetany resulting from parathyroid gland aplasia or hypoplasia, immune defects attributable to aplasia or hypoplasia of the thymus, and conotruncal cardiac defects. Immunoglobulin levels are usually normal; T-cell level and function can be profoundly deficient or nearly normal. The vast majority of cases (>85%) have microdeletion of chromosome 22, del (22)(q11.21q11.23). Candidate genes have been isolated that bear weak similarity to rat and mouse androgen receptor sequences and also sequence similarity to DNA or steroid-binding domains. Treatment is largely supportive. If necessary, the hypoparathyroidism should be controlled chemically. With time, a normal cell-mediated immune response develops in most patients.

BIBLIOGRAPHY

Budarf ML, Collins J, Gong W et al: Cloning a balanced translocation associated with DiGeorge syndrome and identification of a disrupted candidate gene, *Nat Genet* 10:269-278, 1995.

Derry JMJ, Ochs HD, Francke U: Isolation of a novel gene mutated in Wiskott-Aldrich syndrome, *Cell* 78:635-644, 1994 (erratum, *Cell* 79:923, 1994).

Gold MR, Matsuuchi L: Signal transduction by the antigen receptors of B and T lymphocytes, *Int Rev Cytol* 157:181-276, 1995.

Nelson DL, Kurman CC: Molecular genetic analysis of the primary immunodeficiency disorders, *Pediatric Clin North Am* 41:657-664, 1994.

Primary immunodeficiency diseases: report of a WHO scientific group, *Clin Exp Immunol* 99(suppl 1):1-24, 1995.

Rosen FS, Cooper MD, Wedgwood RJP: The primary immunodeficiencies, *N Engl J Med* 333:431-440, 1995.

Savitsky K, Sfez S, Tagle DA et al: The complete sequence of the coding region of the ATM gene reveals similarity to cell cycle regulators in different species, *Hum Mol Genet* 4:2025-2032, 1995.

Smith CIE, Notarangelo LD: Molecular basis for X-linked immunodeficiencies, *Adv Genet* 35:57-115, 1997.

Stewart DM, Notarangelo LD, Kurman CC et al: Molecular genetic analysis of X-linked hypogammaglobulinemia and isolated growth hormone deficiency, *J Immunol* 155:2770-2774, 1995.

Stewart DM, Trieber-Held S, Kurman CC et al: Studies of the expression of the Wiskott-Aldrich syndrome protein, *J Clin Invest* 92:2627-2634, 1996.

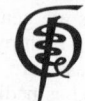

CHAPTER

186   Inherited Complement Deficiencies

Robert H. Carter, M. Kathryn Liszewski, and John P. Atkinson

Inherited deficiencies of complement components predispose an individual to bacterial infections and/or immune-complex excess syndromes such as systemic lupus erythematosus (SLE) (Table 186-1). Most complement deficiencies are inherited as autosomal codominant (recessive) traits except for C1 inhibitor deficiency (autosomal dominant) and properdin deficiency (sex linked). Complement deficiency states are associated with defects in complement-dependent functions. The activity of the individual protein is lost, as are the activities of

Table 186-1   Inherited complement deficiencies

COMPONENTS	ASSOCIATED ILLNESS
C1, C4, C2	Systemic lupus erythematosus, immune complex, infections
Mannose-binding protein	Infections
C3	Pyogenic infections, immune complex
C5 to C8	*Neisseria meningitidis* infection
Factor D	Pyogenic infections
Properdin	*N. meningitidis* infection
C1 inhibitor	Hereditary angioedema
Decay accelerating factor (DAF) and CD59	Paroxysmal nocturnal hemoglobinuria
Factors H and I	Infections, urticaria, hemolytic anemia

the proteins that follow in the cascade. However, the consequences of complement deficiencies in patients and in animal models are often unexpected. For example, the effects of C5 deficiency are much less severe than one might expect, whereas deficiencies of the components of the classical activation pathway are associated with difficulty with disposal of immune complexes. With some complement proteins many individuals who have deficiency appear entirely healthy, and population-based studies are required to detect increased susceptibility to infection or disease. The relative lack of severity of these deficiencies illustrates the development of multiple mechanisms for fighting infections.

CLASSICAL PATHWAY

Deficiencies of the early components of the classical pathway (C1, C4, and C2) are frequently associated with immune complex–mediated syndromes, especially SLE or a lupuslike illness. The latter is characterized by a low or negative antinuclear antibody (ANA) test result, although antibodies to ribonuclear proteins, especially anti-Ro (SS-A), are present in most of these patients. Except for an increased frequency of skin lesions, individuals with classical pathway deficiency show similar clinical manifestations to those in other SLE patients.

Normally the early complement components promote removal of immune complexes. The covalent attachment of C4 and C3 disrupts the lattice formed by antibody and antigen, enhancing solubility of the complex. Once solubilized, the complexes containing covalently attached C4b and C3b are bound by CR1 on erythrocytes and cleared in the liver by the reticuloendothelial system (see Chapter 175). Without such processing, immune complexes may accumulate in excessive quantities in plasma and deposit in inappropriate locations. Immune-complex deposition is a pathologic hallmark of SLE and is responsible for much of the tissue damage. In C2 or C4 deficiency, C3 may still bind to immune complexes via the alternative pathway. This attached C3 may be sufficient for trafficking of antigens contained in the complexes to lymphoid follicles. The impaired hematogenous solubilization and clearance of immune complexes results in increases in immune complexes that are available for promoting immune reactions. The attached C3 fragments may contribute to the abnormal antibody production characteristic of SLE.

Component C1

Deficiency in both the C1q subunit and the C1rC1s subunits has been described. Both deficiencies are associated with immune complex abnormalities and lupuslike disease in a high percentage of patients. The patients are also subject to an increase in pyogenic infections.

Mannose-Binding Protein

Binding of mannose-binding protein (MBP) to bacterial surfaces provides an antibody-independent mechanism for activation of the classical pathway. This is most important when antibody titers are low, particularly in infancy. Deficiency of MBP results in increased bacterial infections during this period, although a smaller increased risk persists throughout life.

Component C4

Component C4 is a pivotal protein of the classical pathway. On activation, it becomes covalently bound to a particle surface and can function as an opsonin or continue the cascade. A deficiency in C4 predisposes to SLE or autoimmune disorders. Approximately 90% of C4-deficient patients have SLE. In some patients with C4 deficiency there is an increased frequency of infection.

Plasma C4 is composed of two distinct but similar glycoproteins, termed *C4A* and *C4B*, coded for by two separate genes. C4A binds more efficiently to amino-containing (NH2) substrates, whereas C4B binds more effectively to hydroxyl (OH) groups. This genetic diversity thus allows C4 to react with a larger variety of pathologic substrates, a selective advantage for a host defense system.

A partial deficiency of C4 also predisposes to SLE or related disorders. Of white SLE patients, 10% to 15% are null (no protein produced) for C4A. In addition, C4A heterozygous deficiency (i.e., only one of the two C4A alleles is abnormal) is increased among SLE patients. C4A or C4B deficiency has been associated with scleroderma, immunoglobulin A (IgA) nephropathy, Henoch-Schönlein purpura, childhood diabetes mellitus, chronic forms of hepatitis, and subacute sclerosing panencephalitis. Whether the association is due to the deficiency of C4A itself or due to linkage of the C4A null gene with another locus, such as major histocompatibility complex (MHC) genes, remains controversial. However, the association is observed in multiple ethnic groups, arguing against linkage to the MHC as a causal mechanism.

Component C2

In C2 deficiency the classical pathway can proceed to covalently link C4b to antigens or immune complexes but could not assemble the C4b2b convertase for cleavage of C3. Thus clearance of immune complexes is only partially compromised. Perhaps for this reason, the risk of lupuslike disease is less in C2 than in C4 deficiency, although approximately 50% of individuals lacking C2 develop SLE or a related illness. These individuals also have a measurable but less severe propensity to infections. C2 deficiency is the most common of all the complement protein deficiencies.

ALTERNATIVE PATHWAY

Inherited defects of components of the factor D and properdin are exceedingly rare. Individuals with factor D deficiency have recurrent respiratory infections. Individuals with properdin deficiency usually have recurrent, severe infections, especially with *Neisseria meningitidis*. Their serum demonstrates impaired complement activation in the absence of specific antibody. Lupuslike illness is not a feature of these deficiencies, which is consistent with the idea that the classical pathway is primarily responsible for immune-complex clearance. Factor B deficiency has not been reported.

Component C3

Deficiency of C3, the component common to both the classical and alternative pathways, results in severe, recurrent infections with encapsulated bacteria that begin shortly after birth. The clinical course resembles that observed in congenital hypogammaglobulinemia. If they survive the infections, these patients also have problems associated with excess immune complexes, such as glomerulonephritis. These clinical problems relate directly to the critical role played by C3 in opsonization-phagocytosis and in immune-complex handling. However, in classic cases SLE does not develop, perhaps because of the inability of immune complexes lacking C3 fragments to stimulate lymphocyte activation.

Membrane Attack Complex

Deficiency of components of the membrane attack complex (MAC) (C5 to C8) is primarily associated with infection by *Neisseria* species. Otherwise, such affected individuals are surprisingly healthy. C9-Deficient individuals appear to be normal. The contrast between the pyogenic infections observed in C3 deficiency and the limitation to susceptibility to *Neisseria* infection in deficiencies of the components of the terminal pathway demonstrates the importance of the other functions of C3 and the early components.

Complement Receptors

Complete deficiencies of CR1 (C3b/C4b receptor) and CR2 (C3dg/Epstein-Barr virus receptor) have not been reported. An acquired reduction in the levels of CR1 occurs in immune complex–mediated syndromes, including SLE, presumably because of the mechanisms of clearance of CR1 with bound immune complexes in the liver.

Autoantibodies to CR1 may also be responsible for the reduced levels of CR1 in SLE. A deficiency of CR3 (CD11b/CD18) and CR4 (CD11c/CD18) occurs in association with deficiency of LFA-1

(CD11a/CD18), because of absence of the common CD18 chain. CR3 and CR4 are integrins that have an inactive fragment of C3b, iC3b, as one of their ligands. This condition, known as *leukocyte adhesion deficiency syndrome* (CD11-CD18 deficiency), causes recurrent, severe bacterial (*Staphylococcus aureus* or *Pseudomonas* species) infections. It may be suspected at birth if there is delayed separation of the umbilical cord and development of omphalitis. Most patients die in childhood of refractory infections involving soft tissue, mucosal surfaces, and the intestinal tract.

INHIBITOR DEFICIENCIES
C1 Inhibitor

The illness produced by functional deficiency of the C1 inhibitor (C1INH) is hereditary angioedema (HAE), a familial tendency toward recurrent episodes of nonpainful, nonpruritic, nonerythematous angioedema. Facial and extremity involvement are primarily a cosmetic problem, but severe abdominal pain may result when swelling involves the bowel wall, and edema of the larynx can be fatal. The attacks usually develop in adolescence and continue throughout life. Precipitating factors other than trauma are not known. Swelling resolves spontaneously within 48 to 72 hours, leaving no residua. Unlike genetic deficiencies of other complement components, heterozygotes are afflicted. The C1INH levels are decreased 5% to 20% from normal.

A deficiency of C1INH prevents the proper regulation of activated C1. As a consequence, plasma levels of C4 and C2, the substrates of C1, are chronically low. The C3 level is characteristically normal, demonstrating the ability of regulatory mechanisms to disrupt fluid-phase convertase activity. The diagnosis is suggested by the clinical history and the finding of low C4 levels. A normal C4 value, especially during an episode, excludes the diagnosis. The angioedema may be related to uncontrolled action of other serum proteins regulated by C1INH, including Hageman factor, clotting factor XIa, kallikrein, and plasmin. Treatment usually involves the administration of non-masculinizing androgens such as danazol to stimulate increased hepatic synthesis of the C1INH. Attacks subside as the C1 inhibitor level rises above 25% to 30% of normal. An adequate physiologic level of the C1INH is indicated by the normalization of C4.

Factors H and I

Recurrent infections, hemolytic anemia, and urticaria develop in individuals with deficiency of factor H or I. Since factors H and I regulate C3, a deficiency of either allows the alternative pathway to fire to exhaustion and thereby consume C3. Infusion of normal plasma as a source of factor H or I can temporarily alleviate clinical symptoms as C3 levels normalize.

Decay-Accelerating Factor and CD59

The membrane-anchored proteins decay-accelerating factor (DAF) and CD59 inhibit complement activation on host tissue. DAF inhibits the C3 convertases, and CD59 blocks binding of C8 and C9 to MAC as it assembles. A deficiency of DAF and CD59 on erythrocytes predisposes these cells to lysis and produces the illness paroxysmal nocturnal hemoglobinuria (PNH). DAF and CD59 are anchored to the membrane by a glycolipid scaffold. PNH represents an acquired somatic stem-cell defect in the attachment of this anchor to proteins. Mutations in the X chromosome gene PIG-A (the phosphatidylinositol glycan class A complementation group) result in defective biosynthesis of GlcNAc-PI, an intermediate in the synthesis of the glycosylphosphatidylinositol anchor.

NEPHRITIC FACTORS

A C3 deficiency state arises when an autoimmune antibody is made against the C3 convertase. The autoantibody against the alternative pathway convertase is called the *C3 nephritic factor.* The autoantibody stabilizes the convertase causing excessive C3 cleavage, which results in a secondary deficiency of C3. These patients, predominantly children, may come to medical attention with glomerulonephritis, partial lipodystrophy, or frequent infections with an encapsulated bacteria.

BIBLIOGRAPHY

Arnett FC, Reveille JD: Genetics of systemic lupus erythematosus, *Rheum Dis Clin North Am* 18:865, 1992.

Colten HR, Rosen FS: Complement deficiencies, *Annu Rev Immunol* 10:809, 1992.

Davies KA, Schifferli JA, Walport MJ: Complement deficiency and immune complex disease, *Semin Immunopathol* 15:397, 1994.

Figueroa JE, Densen P: Infectious diseases associated with complement deficiencies, *Clin Microbiol Rev* 4:359, 1991.

Frank MM: Complement and disease: inherited and acquired complement deficiencies. In Frank MM, Samter M, editors: *Samter's immunologic diseases,* Boston, 1995, Little, Brown.

Lachmann PJ: Complement deficiencies: genetic and acquired. In Lachmann PJ, Peters K, Rosen FS, Walport MJ, editors: *Clinical aspects of immunology,* Boston, 1993, Blackwell Scientific.

Mathieson PW, Peters DK: Deficiency and depletion of complement in the pathogenesis of nephritis and vasculitis, *Kidney Int Suppl* 42:S13, 1993.

Moulds JM, Krych M, Holers VM et al: Genetics of the complement system and rheumatic diseases, *Rheum Dis Clin North Am* 18:893, 1992.

Wurzner R, Orren A, Lachmann PJ: Inherited deficiences of the terminal components of human complement, *Immunodeficiency Rev* 3:123, 1992.

CHAPTER

187   Rhinitis

Robert S. Zeiger and Michael Schatz

The term *rhinitis* is used to describe disorders of the nasal mucosa. These diseases, with their associated symptoms of nasal discharge or obstruction, sneezing, rhinorrhea, pain, and anosmia, cause more than 28 million restricted days, 6 million bedridden days, and loss of 3 million work days and 2 million school days each year, at a medical cost of $500 million. Although not life threatening, rhinitis may substantially interfere with the quality and enjoyment of life. Simple diagnostic tests generally allow classification of the patient's problem and initiation of therapy programs that provide increased comfort and function.

APPLIED NASAL ANATOMY AND PHYSIOLOGY

The nose is composed of a 10- to 12-cm mucosal passage, extending from the nasal orifice to the nasopharynx and pharynx, that is occupied by three turbinates. The nasolacrimal duct opens beneath the inferior turbinate; the orifices of the frontal, anterior ethmoid, and maxillary sinuses extend from anterior to posterior in the order listed, beneath the middle turbinate, and together with the anterior ethmoid air cells make up the ostiomeatal complex. The openings of the posterior ethmoid and sphenoid sinuses empty into the superior meatus. Disruption, distortion, or swelling of the turbinates or meatal mucosal inflammation can occlude the orifices of the sinuses. In particular, disease of the ostiomeatal complex appears to predispose to chronic or recurrent maxillary, ethmoid, or frontal sinusitis. The vulnerable position of the eustachian tube orifice in the posterior nasopharynx is evidenced by the frequent auditory problems, serous otitis media, infection, or hearing loss associated with nasal mucosal and turbinate swelling.

On microscopic examination, the nasal mucosa is composed of stratified squamous epithelium in its anterior one third and of ciliated pseudostratified columnar epithelium interspersed with mucus-secreting goblet cells in the remainder. The lamina propria contains seromucous glands, blood vessels, nerves, and ground substance. This structure provides the substrate for the main nonolfactory functions of the nose: warming, humidification, and filtration of inspired air. Humidification is accomplished by the transudation of fluid from the fenestrated capillaries to the mucosal surface. Sinusoids situated over the turbinates provide accumulations of pooled blood, which transfer heat. Filtration occurs by a variety of mechanisms. The architecture of the nasal airway creates turbulent airflow that fosters deposition of large particles ($>$10 µm) on the anterior nasal surfaces, and local immune responses permit inactivation or neutralization of inspired foreign material. Beating cilia transport mucus and trapped particles posteriorly toward the nasopharynx at an average rate of 5 mm per minute, leading to clearance of particles in 10 to 15 minutes. Structural or functional ciliary abnormalities increase nasopharyngeal and/or sinus infection. The nose also acts as a "gas mask" by retaining 99% of inhaled water-soluble gases, including common pollutants (sulfur dioxide, formaldehyde, and ozone).

Nasal structures are controlled by autonomic reflexes generated from mucosal afferent fibers. The vasomotor fibers innervating the vasculature are parasympathetic efferents that dilate, and sympathetic (primarily α-adrenergic) efferents that constrict, vessels. The secretomotor fibers that innervate the glands are parasympathetic. Glandular secretion is indirectly affected by sympathetic activity through α-adrenergic innervation of its vasculature; however, cholinergic influence predominates.

A normal cycle of alternating constriction and dilation of the turbinate sinusoids every 2 to 4 hours leads to continual differences in patency between the nostrils. This turbinate cycle usually can be detected only by rhinometric flow-volume measurements. Patients with nasal disorders have an exaggerated turbinate cycle, which is described as alternating nasal congestion. Increased α-adrenergic activity, stimulated by normal homeostasis, exercise, or local or systemic sympathomimetics, leads to vasoconstriction and increased nasal patency, whereas its reduction because of drug administration (e.g., reserpine) or disease (hypothyroidism) results in vasodilation and decreased patency. Parasympathetic (cholinergic) stimulation (cold, odors, and irritants) causes vasodilation and hypersecretion.

Nasal vasomotor instability can be best understood as a local autonomic imbalance with hyperresponsive cholinergic reactivity leading to exaggerated nasal turbinate swelling and hypersecretion. This vasomotor instability is characterized clinically by alternating nostril congestion and symptoms in response to recumbency, alcohol intake, temperature and humidity changes, and other nonspecific irritants (inert dust, smoke, fumes, aerosols, powders, and strong odors). Any inflammatory, noninflammatory, or structural cause of chronic rhinitis may lead to vasomotor instability. Its presence is not diagnostic of a specific disorder but rather indicates a general nasal malfunction.

INCIDENCE

Chronic rhinitis is estimated to affect up to 20% of the population. Seasonal allergic rhinoconjunctivitis caused by pollen is most common in young adults and accounts for about half the cases; the various types of perennial rhinitis make up the remainder. Immunoglobulin E (IgE)–mediated reactivity against household dust mites, mold, and animal danders participates in the illnesses of about one third of patients with chronic perennial rhinitis; another one third of cases are caused by chronic infections, either nasopharyngitis or sinusitis. The remainder comprises perennial eosinophilic, nonallergic rhinitis (ENR) (15%), structurally related rhinitis (5% to 10%), rhinitis medicamentosa (less than 5%), and nasal mastocytosis (rare). ENR occurs later than allergic rhinitis (age at diagnosis, 38 versus 25 years), and nasal polyps occur in at least one third of patients with ENR. In an undefined proportion of patients, ENR is exacerbated by aspirin and other nonsteroidal antiinflammatory agents. The prevalence of nasal polyps in the population is about 1%; their occurrence increases with age and is associated with asthma (especially nonallergic) and aspirin idiosyncrasy.

PATHOPHYSIOLOGY
Allergic (Seasonal) Rhinitis

In the sensitized individual, inhaled allergen rapidly initiates release of chemical mediators from mast cells; these mediators cause variable degrees of vasodilation and edema (nasal congestion), increased mucus secretion and cellular recruitment (rhinorrhea), and increased capillary and mucosal permeability. The mediators probably also disturb the balanced nervous control of nasal function, leading to direct and reflex vascular dilation and hypersecretion. The sneezing threshold falls. After continued daily allergen exposure, lesser quantities of specific allergen cause severe nasal symptoms (priming). Similar mechanisms lead to the characteristic ocular symptoms of tearing and

itching associated with allergic rhinitis. Nonspecific nasal mucosal hyperreactivity (i.e., enhancement of symptoms by physical stimuli, irritants, or emotions) is characteristically coincident with allergic reactivity of the nasal mucosa.

Nonallergic (Perennial) Rhinitis

Our understanding of the pathophysiology of most types of nonallergic inflammatory rhinitis is limited. In ENR the specific stimulus for eosinophil attraction to nasal and sinus mucosa is unknown, but the presence of the eosinophils per se may lead to tenacious, viscid mucus, and release of eosinophil constituents such as major basic protein may produce mucosal damage. *Aspirin idiosyncrasy* refers to a clinical syndrome that, in its entirety, includes ENR, nasal polyps, hyperplastic and secondarily infected sinuses, and asthma. Respiratory and/or cutaneous manifestations, which are not immunologically mediated, follow ingestion of aspirin and nonsteroidal antiinflammatory agents. In nasal mastocytosis, presumably increased "spontaneous" or nonspecific triggered mediator release from increased numbers of mucosal mast cells leads to nasal symptoms. Although the pathophysiology of nasal or sinus infection may be straightforward, the factors that increase individual susceptibility to recurrent or chronic infectious rhinosinusitis (other than nasal or sinus obstruction) and the contributory role of noninfectious sinus mucosal inflammation are incompletely understood.

Noninflammatory (Vasomotor) Rhinitis

Vasomotor instability, which is present in patients with rhinitis medicamentosa, rhinitis associated with systemic autonomic states, high-output vascular conditions, endocrine disorders (typically hypothyroidism or hyperthyroidism), or pregnancy, and idiopathic vasomotor rhinitis are thought to result from a direct effect of medication or endocrine or neurologic factors on the nasal vasculature and/or the autonomic nervous system.

Structural Rhinitis

Anatomic disturbances such as nasal septal deviation, fractures, foreign bodies, tumors, or choanal atresia produce rhinitis by physical mechanisms specific to the abnormality. Secondary nasal mucosal hyperreactivity may also result from the structurally induced abnormalities of nasal air flow.

PATIENT EVALUATION: HISTORY, PHYSICAL EXAMINATION, AND LABORATORY EVALUATION

A proper evaluation of patients with chronic rhinitis requires a correlation of historical data, physical findings, and nasal cytologic findings. In many clinical circumstances the nose can be adequately examined physically by anterior rhinoscopy (using a nasal otoscope adapter or nasal speculum). Rhinopharyngeal endoscopy (flexible or rigid) in the hands of an experienced, skilled clinician allows better definition of mucosal edema, inflammation, pathologic drainage, or polyp formation in the entire nasal cavity, including accessible components of the ostiomeatal complex. Rigid endoscopy provides better image clarity than flexible endoscopy and allows sampling of purulent discharge from the middle meatus, the cultures of which have been shown to correlate with cultures of ipsilateral maxillary and ethmoid sinuses.

Nasal cytologic examination can be performed on expelled mucus but should preferably be performed on materials obtained by scraping the nasal turbinates and mucosal surfaces with a flexible nasal probe (Rhinoprobe).

Sinus radiographs are particularly revealing in patients with chronic, unremitting postnasal discharge in association with nasal neutrophilia, and such radiographs often demonstrate mucosal thickening, opacification, and/or air-fluid levels. Abnormal sinus radiographs also are observed in perennial nonallergic eosinophilic rhinitis and in aspirin hypersensitivity. More than 50% of children coming to allergy clinics with chronic rhinitis characterized by postnasal discharge and nasal neutrophilia demonstrate on sinus radiographs gross abnormalities that respond to antibiotics. For patients with clinical features of chronic or recurrent sinusitis, computed tomography scans of the sinuses in the coronal plane are the procedures of choice because they allow better definition of disease of the ostiomeatal complex.

Specific IgE should be determined by skin tests (preferable) or radioallergosorbent test (RAST) in patients who have a clear history of allergy and in those with nasal eosinophilia and/or basophilia. Skin tests are performed to confirm the diagnosis, to direct specific environmental measures, and to select immunotherapeutic extracts (see Chapter 180). An adequate battery of skin-test antigens includes household dust mites, clinically relevant danders, molds (of the genera *Alternaria*, *Hormodendrum*, *Penicillium*, *Aspergillus*, and *Helminthosporium*), and the prevalent local pollens.

Perennial allergens like danders and dust mites are of particular importance in the winter months, when the home is closed and forced air circulates. Atmospheric and indoor molds are also perennial problems in climates not affected by frost or snow. Pollen allergens generally follow a characteristic seasonal pattern in temperate climates (trees in early spring, grasses in late spring, and weeds in the fall). Grasses may become perennial allergens in subtropical climates, pollinating from February through December; nevertheless, a peak seasonal worsening can be elicited in the spring.

Rhinomanometry can provide objective, quantitative measurement of nasal airway resistance. However, for routine clinical evaluation rhinomanometry may not be particularly useful because of considerable overlap of nasal airway resistance in normal subjects and those with rhinitis. Rhinomanometry may be useful for serial measurements of changes in nasal patency after allergen or chemical challenges and drug therapy.

To evaluate for anosmia or hyposmia, the threshold for detecting inhaled pyridine or the University of Pennsylvania "sniff and scratch" test may be employed. A timed saccharin taste test is a useful screening procedure for mucociliary dysfunction.

TREATMENT
General Measures

Vigorous exercise induces sympathetic discharge and redistribution of blood flow and is the body's most efficient homeostatic control for reducing nasal obstruction. Increased patency develops rapidly and persists for at least 15 to 30 minutes. The maintenance of a regular exercise program provides an effective regimen for patients with chronic rhinitis and may counteract vasomotor instability. Increased nasal airway resistance characteristically occurs in recumbency but may be counteracted, in part, by the patient's lying supine with the head elevated.

The annoyance caused by profuse rhinorrhea can be reduced somewhat by occluding the anterior nares with absorbent, nonshredding facial tissue and replacing the tissue when saturated. Forceful blowing of the nose must be avoided to prevent epistaxis and unnecessary irritation.

Nasal tissue appears to benefit greatly from irrigation with warm saline. Its use should be considered for all patients with chronic rhinitis; benefit appears maximal for topical rhinitis medicamentosa, atrophic rhinitis, nasopharyngitis, and sinusitis. The most effective method of saline irrigation is provided by an adaptation of the Water-Pik device. Warm saline is delivered in a pulsating stream at 20 pulses per second through a special right-angled, rubber-tipped nasal adaptor placed loosely within one naris; the patient leans over a sink to perform the irrigation. As an alternative, a soft vinyl bulb syringe may be used for saline (8 ounces of water + ¼ teaspoon of salt) irrigation.

Specific Medications

Antihistamines and Decongestants. The antihistamines used to treat rhinitis are chemically diverse. These agents competitively antagonize histamine at its H_1-receptor site and exert varying degrees of anticholinergic, local anesthetic, central nervous system (CNS)–depressant, and ganglionic and adrenergic-blocking activities. In addition, a number of antihistamines, especially newer ones (e.g., ketotifen, azelastine), may inhibit mediator release from mast cells and basophils.

Antihistamines have been classified on the basis of their chemical structures. However, this classification appears to have limited value for predicting the efficacy or adverse effects of specific agents, and some of the newer agents do not fit readily into the traditional classification. Hydroxyzine appears to be the most potent of the first-generation antihistamines.

Use of first-generation antihistamines has been limited by their sedative and anticholinergic side effects. Approaches to minimize the sedative side effects have included bedtime dosing, gradually increasing daytime dosing, and combining antihistamines with sympathomimetic agents (which may also enhance their therapeutic efficacy). Recently, second-generation antihistamines that do not cross the blood-brain barrier and are devoid of anticholinergic or demonstrable sedative effects have become available (astemizole, cetirizine, fexofenadine, loratadine, and terfenadine). Neither sedation nor CNS impairment were found with the second-generation H_1-antihistamines compared with placebo when administered at manufacturers' recommended daily dosages (terfenadine and fexofenadine, each 60 mg twice a day, and astemizole, loratadine, and cetirizine each at 10 mg daily). Of these newer agents, only astemizole appears to be as effective as hydroxyzine and more effective than traditional agents such as chlorpheniramine, and these second-generation antihistamines are generally considerably more expensive than older antihistamines. Most of the second-generation H_1-antihistamines available today, with the exception of fexofenadine and cetirizine, are metabolized by oxidation and/or glucuronidation in the hepatic P_{450} system. Blood levels of these second-generation agents may increase markedly in hepatic dysfunction, in elderly individuals, and with concomitant use of macrolide antibiotics and the imidazole antifungal agents such as ketoconazole or other cytochrome P_{450} inhibitors. Prolongation of the QT_c interval associated with ventricular tachycardia, torsades de pointes, and cardiac arrest has been reported with overdosage of astemizole and terfenadine. As such, astemizole and terfenadine should be discontinued during macrolide antibiotic and imidazole antifungal treatment, reduced in elderly individuals, and probably avoided in patients with hepatic dysfunction and cardiac arrythmias. Fexofenadine, the active metabolite of terfenadine, has the advantage of being only 5% metabolized and therefore tolerated by patients with hepatic dysfunction. Moreover, unlike terfenadine and astemizole, fexofenadine has not been reported to cause changes in QT_c intervals when given concomitantly with erythromycin or ketoconazole.

In patients with daily symptoms, antihistamines should be taken regularly for best therapeutic results. Loss of clinical efficacy of a previously useful antihistamine may occasionally occur during continuous administration. Recent studies suggest that this is not generally caused by true tachyphylaxis but rather by the increased severity of the underlying disorder or secondary complications. When effective, antihistaminic agents may be used in rhinitis with coexisting asthma, except during status asthmaticus.

Oral sympathomimetic amines (decongestants) effectively reduce nasal congestion and are available singly or combined with antihistamines. Rebound rhinitis medicamentosa is rarely associated with chronic use of oral decongestants. These agents may cause insomnia and irritability and should be avoided in hypertensive patients and in those receiving monoamine oxidase inhibitors (MAOIs).

Intranasal Cromolyn. Disodium cromoglycate (cromolyn sodium as a 4% solution [Nasalcrom]) is an effective medication in the treatment of allergic rhinitis and reduces the need for antihistamine medication. The usual dosage for patients 6 years old and older is one (5.2 mg) spray in each nostril three to four times a day. If needed, the dose may be doubled. Treatment with nasal cromolyn is more effective if started before contact with the offending allergen. Adverse reactions are minimal and have included sneezing, nasal stinging, headache, and bad taste.

Corticosteroids. The usefulness of corticosteroids in the treatment of inflammatory disorders has been recognized for many years. Highly potent, surface-active, rapidly metabolized corticosteroids, such as beclomethasone dipropionate (Vancenase or Beconase), flunisolide (Nasalide), triamcinolone acetonide (Nasacort), budesonide (Rhinocort), and fluticasone proprionate (Flonase) have been introduced for intranasal use. Extensive clinical and toxicologic studies have documented their efficacy and safety in managing eosinophilic-associated rhinitis (seasonal or perennial allergic rhinitis, eosinophilic nonallergic rhinitis, and eosinophilic polyps). The usual recommended starting dosage is two sprays in each nostril one to two times per day. Higher doses may be necessary for more recalcitrant rhinitis. Clinical improvement should be achieved within 1 to 2 weeks, but may not be maximal for 4 to 6 weeks. After optimal improvement the dosage should be tapered by one spray in each nostril each week until the minimally effective dose is determined. Patients with allergic rhinitis without polyp disease may require therapeutic doses of topical corticosteroids during peak allergy triggering, followed by a tapering to low-dose maintenance therapy. Patients with perennial nonallergic rhinitis with eosinophilia usually require a moderate maintenance dose, and those with eosinophilic polyps a larger maintenance dose. Side effects of these agents have been minimal and include mild nasal bleeding (5%), irritation in the form of stinging or burning (40% of patients using flunisolide), and transient episodes of sneezing. Intranasal *Candida* infection and septal perforation are rare.

Antibiotics. Acute sinusitis generally is caused by *Streptococcus pneumoniae, Moraxella catarrhalis* (especially in children), or *Haemophilus influenzae,* whereas chronic sinusitis is more often caused by anaerobic organisms (especially in adults). Thus no antibiotic has a spectrum broad enough to cover all possibilities. Amoxicillin in doses of 500 mg three times daily in adults (40 to 50 mg/kg per 24 hours in children) is the drug of choice in non–penicillin-allergic persons, since approximately 80% of the usual organisms are susceptible, tissue penetration is good, and dosing intervals are convenient. Ampicillin is less expensive but requires more frequent administration and does not penetrate sinus tissues as well. β-Lactamase–producing *H. influenzae* and *M. catarrhalis,* however, are resistant. Amoxicillin-clavulanate or cefuroxime is usually adequate for β-lactamase–producing strains as well as the other usual organisms. In patients who are allergic to penicillin, the following may be alternates: doxycycline, trimethoprim and sulfamethoxazole, erythromycin and sulfisoxazole, or clindamycin. Coverage for anaerobes is generally provided by amoxicillin, clindamycin, erythromycin plus sulfonamides, cefuroxime, and metronidazole (which essentially only covers anaerobes).

Decreased postnasal discharge, pain, and clearing of nasal neutrophilia and bacteria usually occur within 3 to 4 days after starting therapy. Treatment should continue for at least 2 to 3 weeks, the exact duration depending on the chronicity of the condition. The use of prophylactic antibiotics, such as sulfisoxazole or tetracycline for 1 to 2 months, in a fashion analogous to that used in the treatment of frequent urinary tract infections, may be appropriate for patients with frequent relapses.

Other Medications. Mucoevacuants such as guaifenesin (600 to 1200 mg twice daily) or iodinated glycerol (two tablets four times a day) are being increasingly recommended for patients with chronic nasopharyngitis-sinusitis, although proof of their efficacy is lacking. Intranasal ipratropium (two sprays in each nostril twice daily) may be useful for patients with vasomotor rhinitis associated with watery rhinorrhea, the common cold, or to prevent reflux rhinorrhea in response to spicy foods (gustatory rhinitis) or cold air.

Immunotherapy

Immunotherapy, frequently termed *desensitization* or *hyposensitization,* is reserved for rhinitis caused by IgE-mediated hypersensitivity. Immunotherapy is beneficial in IgE-mediated allergic rhinitis in children and adults when (1) strict diagnostic criteria for clinically significant IgE reactivity are met and (2) administration of high doses of potent allergens is continued for a specified amount of time. The clinical benefit derived from immunotherapy can be measured in partial reduction in symptoms and/or medication usage, not in eradication or cure. Immunotherapy should be given a 12-month trial and, if effective, continued for 3 to 5 years and then evaluated for trial discontinuation. Because of potential life-threatening side effects, it should be carried out only by specialists trained in its use, and it should be reserved for patients whose disease is not adequately controlled by other means.

Allergic Rhinitis

Proper management begins with elimination or avoidance of the responsible allergen or allergens. Outdoor pollen exposure may be reduced by use of pollen masks and indoor pollen exposure by use of air-conditioners or air purifiers (containing high-efficiency particulate air [HEPA] filters). The most important aspects of mite environmental control are (1) encasing pillows and mattresses in plastic and (2) washing bed clothes in hot water every 7 to 10 days. Although maximal reduction of animal dander exposure entails elimination of pets from the home, recent studies suggest that regular bathing of the pet and use of air purifiers reduce animal dander antigen exposure. Mold control is facilitated by reducing indoor humidity and use of a fungicide in areas where mold is growing.

Symptoms can usually be controlled using as-needed or regular antihistamines or antihistamine-decongestant combinations, intranasal cromolyn, or (most effectively in moderate or severe disease) intranasal corticosteroids. Occasionally, oral corticosteroids are required for severe episodes. If these medications fail, a trial of immunotherapy is indicated in properly selected patients.

Eosinophilic Nonallergic Rhinitis

Regular use of antihistamines and decongestants may provide acceptable control, but intranasal steroids frequently are required. An occasional patient needs episodic or even long-term alternate-day oral corticosteroid therapy. Surveillance for secondary nasopharyngitis-sinusitis and the development of nasal polyps is particularly important.

Eosinophilic rhinosinusitis with or without complicating nasal polyps often is associated with sinus abnormalities. It is frequently difficult to know whether infection or eosinophilic infiltration remains responsible for the sinus abnormalities. Cytologic study of a postnasal mucus specimen may reveal infectious (neutrophilic) or noninfectious (eosinophilic) inflammation. Frequently a combination of appropriate antibiotic and short course of daily oral corticosteroid is necessary to ameliorate the condition. Radiologic as well as clinical improvement should be documented.

Nasopharyngitis-Sinusitis

Chronic or acute bacterial infection of the nasopharynx or paranasal sinuses may complicate other forms of rhinitis or may occur alone. Proper management requires control of the underlying rhinitis, regular saline lavage, and intermittent courses of appropriate antibiotics supplemented for 3 to 5 days with topical decongestants. Oral decongestant medications and mucoevacuants (guaifenesin, iodinated glycerol) are often recommended, although proof of their value is lacking. Corticosteroids, in addition to antibiotics, are occasionally useful for relief of severe noninfectious sinus or nasal inflammation complicating the infectious process. Long-term antibiotics and surgical sinus therapy must be considered for particularly recalcitrant cases.

Nasal Polyps

Long-term intranasal steroids are the mainstay of therapy. Intermittent courses of oral corticosteroids may be necessary to shrink the polyps to a size controllable by intranasal steroids. Some patients may require long-term alternate-day oral corticosteroid therapy. Appropriate treatment of secondary infection is essential. For patients requiring long-term corticosteroids or those who fail to respond, surgical therapy must be considered.

Rhinitis and Pregnancy

Chronic rhinitis may be the most frequently occurring medical illness during pregnancy. The physiologic increase in turbinate congestion associated with the normal hormonal changes of pregnancy and the frequency of allergic rhinitis in women of childbearing age contribute to this problem. Avoidance of allergens and nonspecific precipitants and the use of intranasal saline is the initial approach, supplemented by *intermittent* topical oxymetazoline. Nasal congestion not responding to short-term or intermittent topical therapy is usually effectively treated with oral decongestants (pseudoephedrine), whereas

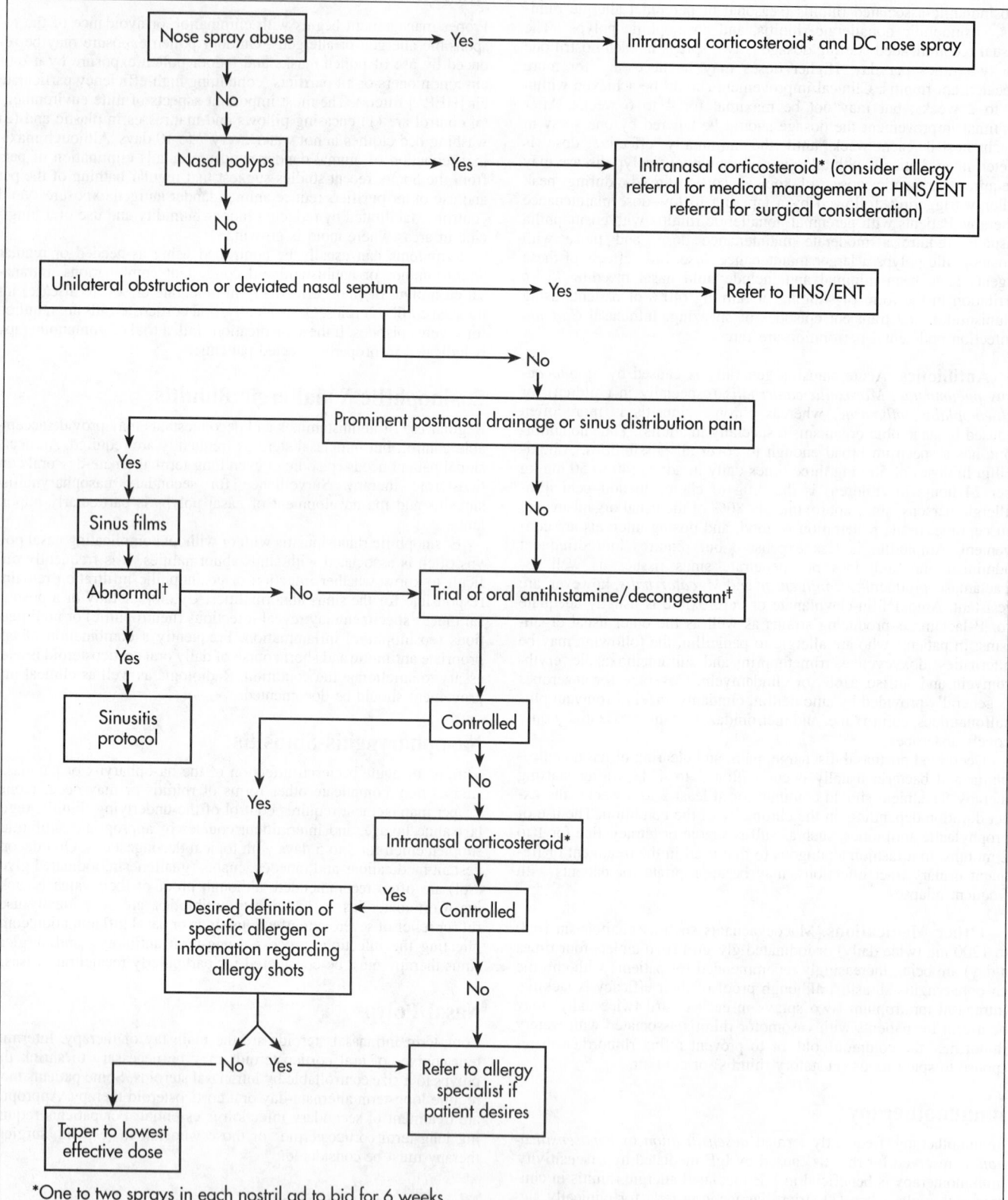

*One to two sprays in each nostril qd to bid for 6 weeks.
†Opacification, air fluid level, >8 mm mucosal thickening (asymptomatic solitary polyps or retention cysts do not need referral).
‡Generic Isochlor, Naldecon, Drixoral (chlorpheniramine for patients with high blood pressure).

FIGURE 187-1   Clinical practice guideline for the management of rhinitis (adult >12 years of age). *DC*, Decongestant; *HNS/ENT*, head and neck surgery or ear, nose, and throat.

✔ *WHEN TO REFER*

The frequency of rhinosinusitis demands that the generalist become competent in its recognition, treatment, and indications to refer to specialists. An algorithm to aid in this objective is presented in Fig. 187-1.

itching, sneezing, or rhinorrhea may require antihistamines (tripelennamine) or cromolyn. Intranasal steroids should be used for recalcitrant eosinophilic rhinitis or nasal polyps during pregnancy. Amoxicillin and erythromycin appear to be the drugs of choice for nasal or sinus infection during pregnancy; tetracycline is contraindicated. Cephalosporins are also generally considered safe during pregnancy, and sulfonamides may be considered in early or middle pregnancy.

BIBLIOGRAPHY

Bolger WE, Kennedy DW: Current perspectives on sinusitis in adults, *J Respir Dis* 13:421, 1992.
Incaudo GA: The diagnosis and treatment of rhinosinusitis during pregnancy and lactation. In Schatz M, Zeiger RS, editors: *Asthma and allergy in pregnancy and early infancy,* New York, 1993, Marcel Dekker.
Jalowayski A, Zeiger RS: Examination of nasal and conjunctival epithelial specimens. In Lawlor CJ, Fischer TJ, editors: *Manual of allergy and immunology: diagnosis and therapy,* ed 2, Boston, 1988, Little, Brown.
Juniper EF et al: Comparison of beclomethasone diproprionate aqueous spray, astemizole and the combination in the prophylactic treatment of ragweed pollen–induced rhinoconjunctivitis, *J Allergy Clin Immunol* 83:627, 1989.
Juniper EF et al: Comparison of the efficacy and side effects of aqueous steroid nasal spray (budesonide) and allergen-injection therapy (Pollinex R) in the treatment of seasonal allergic rhinoconjunctivitis, *J Allergy Clin Immunol* 85:606, 1990.
Meltzer ED, Schatz M, Zeiger RS: Evaluation and therapy of rhinitis. In Middleton E Jr et al, editors: *Allergy: principles and practice,* ed 3, St Louis, 1988, Mosby.
Mikaelian AJ: Vasomotor rhinitis, *Ear Nose Throat J* 68:251, 1989.
Mullarkey MF: Eosinophilic nonallergic rhinitis, *J Allergy Clin Immunol* 82:941, 1988.
Mygind N, Anggard A: Anatomy and physiology of the nose: pathophysiologic alternations in allergic rhinitis, *Clin Rev Allergy* 2:173, 1984.
Naclerio RM: Allergic rhinitis, *N Engl J Med* 325:860, 1991.
Settipane GA: Nasal polyps: epidemiology, pathology, immunology and treatment, *Am J Rhinol* 1:119, 1987.
Simons FER, Simons KJ: Antihistamines. In Middleton E Jr, et al, editors: *Allergy: principles and practice,* ed 4, St Louis, 1993, Mosby.
Slavin RG: Medical management of nasal polyps and sinusitis, *J Allergy Clin Immunol* 88:141, 1991.
Zeiger RS: Allergic and nonallergic rhinitis: classification and pathogenesis. I. Allergic rhinitis, *Am J Rhinol* 3:21, 1989.
Zeiger RS: Allergic and nonallergic rhinitis: classification and pathogenesis. II. Nonallergic rhinitis, *Am J Rhinol* 3:113, 1989.
Zeiger RS: Prospects for ancillary treatment of sinusitis in the 1990s, *J Allergy Clin Immunol* 90:478, 1992.

CHAPTER

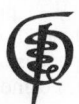

188 Asthma

Timothy D. Bigby and Stephen I. Wasserman

Asthma is a common disorder that is recognized on clinical examination as reversible airway obstruction with cough and/or wheeze. Recent advances in our understanding of the pathophysiology of asthma have expanded this definition to also include airway inflammation and hyperresponsiveness to a broad range of physical, chemical, and pharmacologic stimuli. An understanding of the pathogenesis and pathophysiology of this disorder provides the opportunity for improved therapeutic intervention. This chapter summarizes our basic understanding of asthma, places this understanding into a clinical context, and provides a framework for a modern approach to asthma management.

EPIDEMIOLOGY

Estimates indicate that asthma occurs in 4% to 6% of the population in the United States and is more common in urban than in rural populations and in African-Americans. Some estimates also suggest that asthma is more common in Hispanics, Southeast Asians, and Pacific Islanders. In childhood, the male-to-female ratio is 2:1, but this ratio equalizes in adulthood. The age at onset of disease is widely distributed. Asthma develops in half of the patients by the age of 10 years, but onset into the sixth and seventh decades is common. Less than 50% of childhood asthmatics continue to have asthma in adulthood; however, asthma that develops in adulthood rarely remits.

There is a trend in the United States and worldwide of increasing prevalence of asthma. The cause of this increase is unknown, but it may relate to increasingly urban living conditions with resulting greater exposure to environmental and occupational pollutants. There is also a strong association between passive exposure of children to tobacco smoke and the development of asthma and atopy.

PATHOLOGY

The lungs of patients dying of fatal exacerbations of asthma reveal evidence of hyperinflation with thick, tenacious mucus plugging of airways. These plugs may appear as spiral casts of the airways consisting of mucus and shed epithelial cells (Curschmann's spirals) or compact clusters of epithelial cells (Creola bodies), and may be composed of eosinophil lysophospholipase (Charcot-Leyden crystals). Microscopic examination of postmortem specimens of human airways reveals patchy denudation of the airway epithelium, airway edema, marked mucosal inflammatory cell infiltration, and evidence of smooth muscle hypertrophy. The most readily apparent and consistent features of the inflammatory cell infiltrate in asthma are the presence of eosinophils, lymphocytes, and, with special stains, mast cells. Neutrophils, monocytes, and macrophages are also present.

The pathologic features of asthma have also been investigated in patients by means of sputum examination, bronchoalveolar lavage, and endobronchial biopsy, all of which demonstrate increased numbers of inflammatory cells. Eosinophils in the sputum have been suggested as a marker of asthma, but this is neither sensitive nor specific. Bronchoalveolar lavage studies confirm these observations and also note a small increase in the number of mast cells. However, there is no specific profile of bronchoalveolar lavage cells in asthma, and lavage has no routine utility in its diagnosis or management. Endobronchial biopsy specimens reveal inflammatory cell influx similar to that found in postmortem specimens of airways, even when disease is relatively quiescent. Deposition of types III and V collagen below the basement membrane is also apparent.

ORIGINS, PATHOGENESIS, AND PATHOPHYSIOLOGY

Numerous hypotheses have been put forth to explain the clinical syndrome of asthma. An initial focus was on abnormalities in neural and humoral receptor control of airway smooth muscle. Although intriguing data regarding such a dysfunction have accumulated, these concepts have not provided a complete understanding of asthma. More recently, an appreciation of airway inflammation in asthma has led to a reexamination of the origins, pathogenesis, and pathophysiology of asthma. The terms "intrinsic" and "extrinsic" no longer adequately reflect our current understanding. We now appreciate that asthma is a heterogeneous disorder, with multiple triggers initiating the development of airway hyperresponsiveness and the clinical end-point of bronchoconstriction.

During the last decade attention has been focused on the relationship between the inflammatory response in the airway and the development of airway hyperresponsiveness and clinical asthma (Fig. 188-1). Experimental work indicates that viral respiratory tract infection, oxidant pollutants, some chemicals, and exposure to antigen are associated with inflammatory cell infiltration into the airway. These agents are also associated with the development of airway hyperresponsiveness. Most data suggest that airway inflammation precedes the development of hyperresponsiveness and therefore may be the prerequisite feature for the development of hyperresponsiveness and clinical bronchospasm. However, airway inflammation is not univer

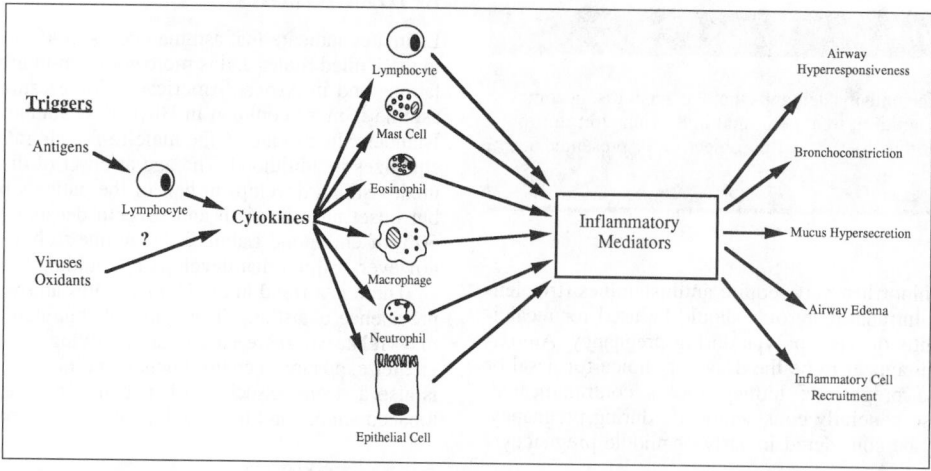

FIGURE 188-1   Proposed model of the pathogenesis of asthma. Antigen, oxidants, or viral respiratory tract infection triggers the release of cytokines that stimulate the recruitment of inflammatory cells to the airway and enhance their ability to release inflammatory mediators. These mediators in turn cause end-organ effects. Noninflammatory cells, such as epithelial cells, may participate in this process. In the case of antigens, lymphocytes seem to be the principal source of cytokines. With other triggers the source of cytokines is unknown.

sally associated with hyperresponsiveness. For example, purulent bronchitis or the purulent sputum of pneumonia can be present without the development of airway hyperresponsiveness or clinical bronchospasm. Thus airway inflammation may be a necessary but not a sufficient reason for the development of asthma, or as an alternative, there may be specific characteristics of the inflammatory response in this disorder.

The pathogenesis of allergic asthma has been studied extensively. Various in vivo and in vitro experiments suggest that, in susceptible hosts, a T-cell–mediated immune response to inhaled antigen occurs. Human T helper cells can be divided into subsets, TH_1 and TH_2, based on the profile of cytokines they produce (Chapter 174). In asthma the predominant CD4 helper cell in the lung produces an array of cytokines, including granulocyte-macrophage colony-stimulating factor (GM-CSF) and interleukins 3, 4, 5, and 10 (IL-3, IL-4, IL-5, and IL-10), characteristic of the TH_2 subset. The spectrum of cytokines contributed by activated TH_2 cells could explain features of allergic asthma including immunoglobulin E (IgE) synthesis (IL-4) and eosinophilia (GM-CSF and IL-5). In addition, IL-4 upregulates adhesion molecules on eosinophils, basophils, and vascular endothelium. Immunostaining shows these cytokines in the lung and skin of allergic individuals, and in situ hybridization demonstrates the expression of their genes. In addition, the same cytokines have been found in fluid lavaged from the airways of symptomatic asthmatics and are generated acutely during antigen-provoked bronchospasm. However, no available data permit the extrapolation of this scenario for allergic inflammation of the airway to the setting of inflammatory responses induced by other asthma triggers, such as oxidant pollutants and viral respiratory tract infection.

Controversy exists regarding the relative importance of different inflammatory cell types in asthma. Mast cells and eosinophils are prominent and easily discernible features of the inflammatory response in asthmatic airways. Mast cells are effector cells of an IgE-mediated allergic response. These cells are the source of vasoactive substances (Chapter 176) and a variety of cytokines including IL-4 and tumor necrosis factor alpha (TNF-α). Thus mast cells may complement the proinflammatory cascade of cytokines produced by TH_2 lymphocytes, which in turn contribute to the cellular and physiologic changes observed in asthma. The response to a specific antigen in the airway has been presumed to involve specific IgE on the surface of the mast cell; furthermore, responses that involve the mast cell have often been thought to be stimulated by specific antigen. However, we now understand that allergic responses and mast cell function are more complex. For example, IgE binds not only to mast cells but also to monocytes, macrophages, and platelets via specific receptors. Further, these cells can be stimulated by specific antigen.

On the other hand, mast cells are not stimulated exclusively by antigen. Other biochemical mediators and changes in osmolality may induce mast cell mediator release. Therefore some of the effects of antigen may not be mediated by mast cells, and some mast cell–mediated effects may not be stimulated by antigen.

There is substantial evidence that eosinophils play an important role in asthma. Increased numbers of eosinophils are found in the blood, sputum, and bronchoalveolar lavage of asthmatics. Eosinophil accumulation in the airway seems to be a prominent feature of the late asthmatic response to allergen challenge in allergic asthmatics as assessed by bronchoalveolar lavage and endobronchial biopsy. Eosinophils are attracted to the airway by the generation of IL-5 from TH_2 lymphocytes and by lipid or peptide chemoattractants. Eosinophils are prominent in the asthmatic airway in submucosal tissue, epithelium, and the airway lumen. They release a variety of mediators affecting the airway, including GM-CSF, transforming growth factor beta (TGF-β) and IL-5. These cytokines may have autoregulatory effects on eosinophils. Some of their other mediators include major basic protein, eosinophil cationic peptide, eosinophil peroxidase, and eosinophil-derived neurotoxin. These are highly basic molecules that are toxic to airway epithelial cells, causing desquamation of airway epithelium in vitro similar to that seen in clinical asthma. Eosinophils are also the source of a variety of other mediators with bronchoactive effects, including leukotriene C_4 and platelet-activating factor. The stimulus for eosinophil recruitment to the airway is uncertain, but eotaxin and platelet-activating factor potently stimulate eosinophil chemotaxis. The precise mechanism by which eosinophils are activated in asthma to generate lipid mediators or to degranulate remains uncertain, but immune complexes containing immunoglobulins G and A (IgG and IgA) are potent degranulation stimuli. In addition, GM-CSF, IL-5, and IL-3 prime the eosinophil to a more responsive state. When compared with peripheral blood eosinophils, those in the airway are hypodense and demonstrate granular dissolution, suggesting ongoing eosinophil activation in asthma.

Mast cells and eosinophils are not the only inflammatory cells in asthmatic airways. Neutrophils and macrophages are also present. These cells are capable of releasing mediators with effects on smooth muscle tone, mucus secretion, and airway edema. Transient airway hyperresponsiveness has been induced in the laboratory with agents that recruit neutrophils and macrophages into the lung. These and other data have been used to argue that neutrophils or macrophages may be responsible for the development of airway hyperresponsiveness. A substantial body of evidence obtained in animal models and human studies supports this hypothesis. Macrophages also participate in regulating the airway inflammatory response, in part through the

Table 188-1   Inflammatory mediators and asthma

MEDIATOR	EFFECTS
Histamine	Bronchoconstriction
Cyclooxygenase products: $PGF_{2\alpha}$, thromboxane, PGD_2	Bronchoconstriction
Leukotrienes	
LTB_4	Chemotaxis
LTC_4, LTD_4	Bronchoconstriction, mucus hypersecretion, edema
Platelet-activating factor	Eosinophil recruitment, bronchoconstriction, airway hyperresponsiveness
Neuropeptides: *Substance P*	Bronchoconstriction, airway edema, mucus hypersecretion
Oxygen radicals	Bronchoconstriction?
Peptide chemotactic factors: *IL-8*	Inflammatory cell chemotaxis
Proteases	Hyperresponsiveness
Cytokines: *GM-CSF, TNF-α, IL-3, IL-4, IL-5, Il-10*	Modulation of immune and inflammatory cell function

GM-CSF, Granulocyte-macrophage colony-stimulating factor; *IL,* interleukin; *TNF-α,* tumor necrosing factor alpha.

generation of specific cytokines, including IL-1, IL-6, IL-8, GM-CSF, TNF-α, and histamine-releasing factors.

The link between inflammation and airway hyperresponsiveness is thought to be provided by the ability of these inflammatory cells to synthesize and release a large number of potent chemical mediators (Table 188-1). A wide range of mediators, including histamine, prostaglandins, thromboxane A_2, leukotrienes, platelet-activating factor, proteases, neuropeptides, peptide chemotactic factors, and oxygen radicals, have been shown to have effects on airway function (Table 188-1). Hyperresponsiveness can be induced with leukotriene E_4 and platelet-activating factor. Mast cells and eosinophils are prominent sources of both of these compounds. Hyperresponsiveness has also been induced experimentally by mast cell tryptase. In addition, mast cells generate the vasoactive and spasmogenic compounds histamine, leukotriene C_4, prostaglandin D_2, and adenosine. A variety of chemoattractant molecules (some of which are specifically directed toward eosinophils), structural proteoglycans, heparin, tryptase, chymase, and cytokines are also products of mast cells, as previously noted. The concerted actions of these molecules can cause acute smooth muscle constriction, airway hyperemia, edema, and secretion of mucus. Some mediators released from inflammatory cells function primarily to amplify and extend the inflammatory response. The role of each mediator, however, has been difficult to determine without specific inhibitors. Although histamine has been shown to have significant effects on airway function, antihistamines have little effect in asthma. Likewise, platelet-activating factor has been shown to have significant effects on airway function and to recruit eosinophils to the lung, but initial clinical trials with antagonists have been disappointing. Additional studies also suggest that many of the effects of platelet-activating factor are mediated secondarily by the cysteinyl leukotrienes. The relative importance of proteases, neuropeptides, and oxygen radicals in human asthma is poorly defined at this time, and specific inhibitors do not exist for potential clinical use.

Slow-reacting substance of anaphylaxis (SRS-A) was demonstrated to induce sustained airway smooth muscle contraction more than 50 years ago. Since 1980, this mediator substance has been chemically characterized as the cysteinyl leukotrienes LTC_4, LTD_4, and LTE_4. These compounds are part of a larger family of mediators derived from arachidonic acid via the 5-lipoxygenase pathway. LTC_4 and LTD_4 induce not only sustained smooth muscle contraction in the airway, but also hypersecretion of mucus and airway edema. A related compound, leukotriene B_4 (LTB_4), is a potent chemotactic factor and is responsible in part for the recruitment of inflammatory cells to the airway and stimulation of inflammatory cell secretion. Clinical trials with 5-lipoxygenase inhibitors and LTD_4 receptor antagonists indicate efficacy in asthma, providing further evidence that leukotrienes are important mediators in asthma.

Specific triggers of asthma may also add to our fund of knowl-

edge about the cause of asthma. Exercise may be one of many triggers or the sole trigger of bronchospasm in asthmatic patients and is related to cooling and drying of the airway. The mechanism of hyperresponsiveness and bronchoconstriction in this case may be via neurogenic reflexes and leukotrienes, findings consistent with the knowledge that increased osmolarity, as occurs in drying of the airway, is known to stimulate mast cell–mediator release.

A unique form of asthma is associated with the use of nonsteroidal antiinflammatory drugs (NSAIDs). Aspirin and other NSAIDs may provoke manifestations of hypersensitivity that include rhinorrhea, flushing, eosinophilia, and nasal polyps in association with asthma. The reaction is not IgE mediated, but the molecular mechanism responsible for this syndrome is not known. Increased production of leukotrienes after aspirin ingestion has been demonstrated in these patients by the identification of increased amounts of leukotriene E_4 in the urine. The ability to induce this reaction is shared by all NSAIDs that inhibit cyclooxygenase activity, whereas salicylates that do not inhibit cyclooxygenase do not elicit this response. However, why this syndrome occurs in only a small fraction of patients taking NSAIDs remains unexplained.

The association of inflammation with asthma is clear. Virtually all data support a causal role for airway inflammation in the development of airway hyperresponsiveness and bronchoconstriction. Considering the substantial redundancy of the inflammatory cells and mediators involved in asthma, a single cell or a single mediator is inadequate to explain the syndrome. The pathogenetic trigger for this process is best worked out for allergic asthma. In this case the lymphocyte, specifically the TH_2 helper cell, seems to play a key role via release of cytokines that modulate cell function in the airway. In nonallergic asthma inflammation also plays a major pathogenetic role, but the relative importance of specific inflammatory cells is less well known. Both allergic and nonallergic airway hyperresponsiveness can be mimicked in the laboratory over the short term. However, in both allergic and nonallergic asthma the mechanism that sustains the inflammatory and hyperresponsive state of the airway over the long term, resulting in the chronic clinical disorder we call asthma, remains unknown.

Asthma is recognized as a complex genetic disorder that appears to involve multiple genes. These genes are not necessarily the same from individual to individual. Linkage in asthmatics has been demonstrated with the cytokine gene cluster on the long arm of chromosome 5 (5q31-33), the long arm of chromosome 11 (11q13) the high-affinity receptor for IgE, the long arm of chromosome 14, and the T-cell antigen receptor. Mutations in putative genes have been identified in the β_2 adrenergic receptor, the platelet-activating factor acetyl hydrolase, and the 5-lipoxygenase gene in asthmatics. The significance of these mutations is unknown at this time.

CLINICAL MANIFESTATIONS
History

In general the clinical hallmarks of asthma are episodic wheezing associated with dyspnea, cough, and sputum production. Between episodes of wheezing asthmatics have symptoms that improve and may completely remit. In describing the clinical manifestations of asthma, acute symptoms should be distinguished from chronic symptoms. However, the chronic symptoms of asthma are essentially the same as those observed acutely, but they usually lack severity and fluctuate over greater periods.

The symptoms of acute bronchospasm can range from subtle to dramatic. A vague sense of chest tightness can be the sole manifestation, but more often this is accompanied by wheezing, dyspnea, and cough. Most patients note wheezing as the development of a musical sound in their chest associated with respiration, and they may be able to discern differences in severity. However, some patients are unable to detect their wheezing. Dyspnea may develop gradually or suddenly and may become severe during acute bronchospasm. Occasionally cough can be the only symptom of asthma, and in the evaluation of chronic cough, asthma should be included in the differential diagnosis. The cough associated with asthma can be dry, but it often produces thick, tenacious sputum, which may contain mucus plugs. The patient may also note that the sputum becomes purulent as symptoms worsen. This may represent secondary infection but also can be caused by inflammatory cell infiltration in the lung without viral or bacterial suprainfection.

Related historical details are of benefit in the care of asthmatics. The age of onset, frequency of episodes, severity of disease, requirements for medications, hospitalizations, and prior need for mechanical ventilation are all key features. The patient should be questioned about a history of travel, gastrointestinal tract symptoms, and occupational or recreational exposure to dust, fumes, chemicals, and pets. A history of allergy, atopy, eczema, allergic rhinitis, or nasal polyps may be elicited. Medication allergies or symptoms associated with the use of NSAIDs may be associated with asthma. A seasonal component to symptoms or a temporal relationship associated with exposure to specific antigens is suggestive of allergy.

Physical Examination

The hallmark of acute bronchospasm is wheezing. This finding may change with the severity of obstruction. In general, less severe bronchospasm is associated with only expiratory wheezes. As severity increases, wheezing may be heard in inspiration and expiration. With profound bronchospasm, wheezing may be heard only on inspiration or may be absent with diminished air movement. However, the intensity and the phase of wheezing may not correlate well with the severity of obstruction. When wheezing is correlated with other physical examination findings, a more reliable assessment can be made of the severity of obstruction. For example, the expiratory phase of the respiratory cycle is prolonged by bronchospasm. Normally the inspiratory/expiratory ratio is less than 1:2, but this ratio increases in a graded fashion to 1:3 or 1:4 with increasing degrees of airway obstruction. When severe obstruction is present, the intensity of breath sounds also diminishes. During symptomatic episodes respirations may become labored, the patient may begin to use the accessory muscles of respiration, and intercostal or supraclavicular retractions may be present. With severely labored respirations the patient may become diaphoretic, anxious, and unable to speak in full sentences. A respiratory rate greater than 30 breaths per minute and a heart rate of 120 beats per minute suggest severe bronchospasm. A fall in systolic blood pressure of greater than 18 mm Hg with inspiration (pulsus paradoxus) also suggests a severe episode. Agitation, confusion, somnolence, and cyanosis are foreboding findings and suggest impending respiratory failure. Unilateral loss of breath sounds can be consistent with mucus plugging and secondary atelectasis, but these findings must raise the possibility that a pneumothorax has developed. Patients are at increased risk of barotrauma during a severe exacerbation of asthma. In addition to pneumothorax, pneumomediastinum may be a manifestation of barotrauma and is strongly suggested by the development of subcutaneous emphysema.

In the chronic setting findings associated with asthma are essentially the same but less severe. Furthermore, most patients have symptom-free intervals in which physical findings are essentially absent. The duration of these symptom-free intervals depends on the severity and the adequacy of control of the patient's disease. Exacerbating factors also play a role in the duration of these disease-free intervals. During symptom-free intervals wheezing can very often be elicited by forced expiration. However, this finding is not specific for asthma.

LABORATORY FINDINGS
Hematologic Findings

Blood cell counts may reveal evidence of eosinophilia, which is usually mild, representing 5% to 15% of the differential cell count. Profound eosinophilia (25% or greater, 3000 cells/μl or greater) should suggest another cause. In the setting of symptoms of asthma, transient pulmonary infiltrates, worldwide travel, and profound eosinophilia, tropical eosinophilia should be considered. Allergic bronchopulmonary aspergillosis and the hypereosinophilic syndrome are also causes of profound eosinophilia that may be confused with asthma.

Serologic Testing

Total IgE level is frequently elevated in serum in patients with asthma, but there is controversy regarding the frequency of this finding, the usefulness of these data in clinical practice, and the implications of elevated IgE levels in the pathogenesis of asthma. Large population surveys demonstrating high frequencies of asthma in groups with elevated serum IgE levels and relative absence of asthma in groups with low serum IgE levels have been interpreted as indicating an allergic basis for all asthma, but other studies have failed to show such an association. In general, total serum IgE level has little utility in the diagnosis and management of asthma. Antigen-specific IgE measurements may be of use in patients with a history compatible with specific allergy and asthmatic symptoms associated with that allergen. Very high elevations of IgE level should suggest a disorder such as allergic bronchopulmonary aspergillosis.

Sputum Examination

Wright's stains usually reveal inflammatory cells, including neutrophils and eosinophils, in the sputum of asthmatics, although this finding is of little diagnostic value. Sputum cultures during an acute exacerbation may occasionally reveal a specific predominant pathogen associated with bacterial bronchitis, but these cultures more often reveal normal oral flora. The presence of *Mycoplasma* organisms in the sputum may be significant. Examination of bronchoalveolar lavage fluid, a powerful research tool, has no current value in clinical diagnosis or management.

Pulmonary Function Studies

During acute bronchospasm, spirometry reveals evidence of obstruction with decreased forced expiratory volume in one second (FEV_1) and midexpiratory flows. The ratio of FEV_1 to forced vital capacity (FEV_1/FVC) is also reduced. In cases of more severe obstruction, hyperinflation is evident, with an increased residual volume and functional residual capacity. The flow-volume loop often reveals evidence of obstruction with diminished flows and coving inward of the expiratory limb. One of the hallmarks of asthma is partial or complete reversal of airway obstruction after the administration of a bronchodilator. This response can also be used to gauge the adequacy of treatment. However, the lack of response to a one-time dose of bronchodilator does not preclude a reversible component to the patient's obstruction. The diffusing capacity of the lung for carbon monoxide, also termed *transfer factor* in Great Britain, is often increased in asthmatics who do not smoke. The exact mechanism of this increase is unknown, but it is thought to represent an increase in pulmonary capillary blood volume associated with airway obstruction. Peak flow measurements are also reduced. Peak flow meters are inexpensive, simple devices that patients can use and interpret themselves. These provide patients with objective information about the severity of their airway obstruction.

Bronchial challenge testing can be used to establish the presence of airway hyperresponsiveness. Nonspecific bronchial hyperresponsiveness is demonstrated by exaggerated bronchoconstriction to inhaled histamine or methacholine. Most full-service pulmonary function laboratories can make these measurements, but they have been restricted by the availability of clinically approved challenge agents. These techniques have been partially supplanted by exercise or cold air challenge, but they are not as reliable as methacholine or histamine. Nonspecific bronchial challenge is most useful to assist in the evaluation of cough or to establish the diagnosis of asthma when the patient comes to medical attention with a compatible history but physical examination and pulmonary function evidence of obstruction are lacking. In addition, it has some utility during disability evaluations and medical-legal evaluations of pulmonary dysfunction. However, bronchial challenge can be a hazardous procedure and should not be performed when significant airway obstruction is present. A more reasonable diagnostic maneuver in the latter setting would be the administration of a bronchodilator to assess the degree of reversibility. Specific bronchial challenge has utility in selected cases. This can be performed to a broad range of provocative agents including exercise, cold air, specific antigen, dust, fumes, and oxidant pollutants. However, specific airway challenges should be performed only in specialized centers experienced with these procedures.

Arterial Blood Gas Studies

Assessment of arterial blood gases is usually not necessary in the management of asthma in either the acute or chronic setting. However, during moderately severe exacerbations pulse oximetry may be of value. During severe exacerbations or in the setting of a serious complicating condition, arterial blood gas studies are indicated. Hypoxemia is a frequent finding in this setting and is caused by a mismatch of ventilation and perfusion associated with bronchoconstriction, with a resultant increase in the alveolar-arterial oxygen pressure difference. Patients with mild to moderate obstruction hyperventilate, and thus the arterial carbon dioxide pressure (Pco_2) is decreased. However, during prolonged, severe episodes of airway obstruction respiratory muscle fatigue may develop and the Pco_2 may normalize or become elevated. A normal Pco_2 during a severe exacerbation of asthma is thought to be an ominous sign, suggesting impending respiratory failure. Some experts have recommended early intubation of such individuals to avoid profound respiratory muscle fatigue or respiratory arrest. However, clinical studies indicate that asthmatics with severe obstruction and normal or elevated Pco_2 do not necessarily require intubation and often improve with aggressive bronchodilator therapy, without mechanical ventilation.

Chest Radiography

In the setting of chronic asthma and in the absence of another underlying condition chest radiographs are normal. During an exacerbation chest radiographs are not required unless fever, sputum production, chest pain, leukocytosis, or physical evidence of barotrauma is present. Hyperinflation of the lung may be present during severe exacerbations, but the remainder of radiographic abnormalities in asthmatics are complications of their disease, such as pneumonia, pneumothorax, or pneumomediastinum. Infiltrates may be seen in allergic bronchopulmonary aspergillosis.

DIAGNOSIS AND DIFFERENTIAL DIAGNOSIS

The diagnosis of asthma is made principally on clinical grounds, and laboratory data are used in a supplementary or confirmatory fashion. A history of episodic wheezing in a nonsmoking patient with findings of wheezing on physical examination is strongly suggestive of asthma. Other causes of wheezing should be reasonably excluded. The diagnosis is confirmed with spirometry, which demonstrates obstruction (an FEV_1 of 80% of predicted value or less) that resolves or significantly improves with a bronchodilator. If pulmonary function is normal, spirometry should be repeated after a forced expiratory maneuver, which usually induces a fall in FEV_1 in asthmatics. If spirometry still remains normal, bronchial challenge testing should be considered. As an alternative, the patient can be followed over time with serial spirograms to demonstrate a variable obstructive ventilatory defect.

Not all patients who wheeze have asthma. Additional diagnoses should be considered in both the acute and chronic settings. Upper airway obstruction, tracheomalacia, and tracheal or bronchial masses can all masquerade as asthma. These disorders are usually distinguished by the presence of stridor on physical examination and flow limitation on a flow-volume loop. Laryngeal (vocal cord) dysfunction can be clinically indistinguishable from asthma. This disorder is caused by inappropriate apposition of the vocal cords during the inspiratory phase of the respiratory cycle and can be successfully treated by speech therapy. These patients with laryngeal dysfunction have often been misdiagnosed; when the dysfunction is severe, they have even been given treatment with systemic corticosteroids for presumed severe asthma. The clue to this diagnosis is inspiratory stridor on physical examination. Flow-volume loops demonstrate normal or near-normal expiratory flow with a flow-limited inspiratory limb. Vocal cord dysfunction is confirmed by direct laryngoscopy.

Patients with chronic fixed airway obstruction such as emphysema or chronic bronchitis may have acute wheezing episodes, which are most often associated with exacerbations of their disease. These patients often have airway hyperresponsiveness that is enhanced during their exacerbation. In the past these patients have been labeled as having asthmatic bronchitis. Whether they have a "reactive component" to their disease and actually represent an overlap between fixed and reversible airway obstruction is not clear. Such patients are usually older with a later onset of disease and a history of smoking. They are differentiated from asthmatics by a history of smoking, a component of their disease that responds poorly to aggressive bronchodilator therapy, and pulmonary function findings of an obstructive defect that does not reverse over time. However, acute bronchitis can be associated with the development of airway hyperresponsiveness. The most common clinical setting for this is the development of wheezing with viral respiratory tract infection. In children respiratory syncytial virus infection is frequently associated with the development of wheezing and an obstructive ventilatory defect. Most of them have transient symptoms that resolve spontaneously, but in a small subgroup sustained clinical asthma may develop. Similarly, other viral respiratory tract infections are associated with transient wheezing, with sustained asthma developing in some patients. The possibility that bacterial bronchitis might be associated with clinical wheezing in previously unaffected people has been suggested for *Mycoplasma* and *Chlamydia* organisms.

Other disorders are associated with wheezing. Patients with left ventricular failure can wheeze during episodes of fluid overload and show nonspecific bronchial hyperactivity. These patients are usually easily differentiated from asthmatics by clinical evidence of left ventricular dysfunction with an S_3 gallop, crackles, and jugular venous distention. However, the occasional patient may lack these clinical findings. The mechanism by which individuals with left-sided heart failure wheeze is unknown, but airway edema is suspected.

In 10% to 15% of patients with pulmonary embolus, wheezing develops. Although the wheezing associated with pulmonary embolus is short-lived, consideration of pulmonary embolus must be included in the differential diagnosis of patients who come to medical attention for the first time with dyspnea and wheezing. In the more chronic setting other diagnoses must also be considered. Patients with hypersensitivity pneumonitis, sarcoidosis, lymphangioleiomyomatosis, and pulmonary helminth infections can also have a component of wheezing and airway obstruction associated with their disease.

MANAGEMENT

The general goal for the treatment of asthma is maintenance of a normal or near-normal lifestyle without functional limitation. Other goals include the aggressive, early therapy of exacerbations to minimize or eliminate the need for emergency care. Nonpharmacologic interventions play a central role in optimal treatment. Most important among these interventions is patient education. Detailed understanding of asthma and its treatment allows patients to participate in their own care, to recognize potential problems, and to facilitate early treatment, thus avoiding severe exacerbations. Recognizing the stimuli that provoke bronchospasm, such as exercise, cold air, animal dander, dust, and perfumes, allows the patient to plan for these eventualities or to avoid them. Patients should also avoid medications such as NSAIDs and beta blockers. Pretreatment before exercise or cold exposure, as well as avoidance of antigens, contributes significantly to improved care. Although not a cause of asthma, anxiety or fatigue can contribute indirectly to symptoms. Knowledgeable patients can be instructed to initiate specific therapies such as increased inhaled β_2-agonist treatment or oral corticosteroids if specific symptoms develop. Written self-management protocols have been developed that can be individualized for appropriate patients. This approach prevents the delay associated with contacting the primary physician and may prevent worsening symptoms that dictate emergency care. Significant interventions by patients in their therapy must be followed by physician contact.

Aerosol Medications

Inhaled bronchodilators are central in the management of both acute and chronic asthma. These agents are inhaled as aerosols. The determinants of aerosol deposition in the lung are (1) size of the particle (1 to 5 μm), (2) the flow rate at which the particle is inhaled (i.e., higher flow rates favor impaction in the upper airway), (3) the duration for which the aerosol is in the lung, and (4) the device from which the aerosol is generated. Jet nebulizers and ultrasonic nebulizers have been suggested to have an advantage in patients with severe disease that is treated with inhaled bronchodilator. In contrast to this widely held belief, numerous studies show that metered-dose inhalers are at least as effective as nebulizers in both chronic and acute settings, provided the metered-dose inhaler is used correctly. However, proper use of a metered-dose inhaler is a major problem; as few as 20% of patients use this device correctly. The problem can be minimized by the use of spacing devices, which should be prescribed to all patients. Use of metered-dose inhalers in all clinical settings for the treatment of asthma would substantially reduce health care costs for these patients.

β_2-Adrenergic Agonists

One of the most important consequences of stimulation of β_2 receptors in the lung is direct relaxation of airway smooth muscle. Metaproterenol, albuterol, and terbutaline are intermediate-acting β_2-selective agonists commonly used in the United States. Recently a longer-acting agent, salmeterol, has been released in the United States. A current controversy surrounding β_2-agonist use focuses on the issues of drug tolerance, hyperresponsiveness, and mortality. Some experts suggest that tolerance to β_2 agonists in the lung may develop and that frequent, regular use of β_2 agonist may increase airway hyperresponsiveness. Some studies support this opinion. Recent studies have further suggested a link between the use of β_2 agonists and mortality from asthma. However, these observations do not distinguish between increased use of drug by patients with more severe disease, which may be fatal, and the possibility that β_2 agonists contribute to mortality by enhancing disease severity. The role of the longer-acting β_2 agonists such as salmeterol in the treatment of asthma is not yet clear. Thus far, salmeterol appears to be useful as a chronic maintenance medication with little evidence for the development of tolerance. However, because of its delayed onset of action, it should not be used as a rescue medication.

β_2 Agonists are also available for oral or parenteral administration. Oral preparations, especially long-acting forms, have been recommended for improved control of bronchospasm because they result in fewer fluctuations in drug levels throughout the day, but toxicity is greater with the oral route because of higher systemic levels of the drug. Furthermore, the maximal degree of bronchodilation achieved orally is less when compared with the inhaled route of administration. For these reasons the oral route is not recommended for β_2 agonists. In severe, acute exacerbations of asthma the parenteral administration of adrenergic agonists has been recommended for many years. Epinephrine and terbutaline have been given subcutaneously for this purpose. However, toxicity is greater via this route, and it does not offer any advantage in terms of bronchodilation. Thus in the emergency room setting the systemic administration of adrenergic agonists, especially epinephrine, should be discouraged. A selective β_2 agonist delivered via the inhaled route is preferred. If the clinical response is insufficient and if clinical signs of toxicity are absent, the drug may be readministered.

Theophylline

The mechanism of theophylline's action in asthma remains unclear. Theophylline is a phosphodiesterase inhibitor and therefore increases intracellular cyclic adenosine monophosphate levels, which in turn may relax smooth muscle. However, these effects occur at doses of theophylline that exceed the therapeutic range used in the treatment of asthma. Theophylline is also an adenosine-receptor antagonist, and this antagonism does occur in clinically relevant concentrations. Some related agents that are more potent adenosine-receptor antagonists, however, have no bronchodilating effects. Theophylline also may have modest antiinflammatory properties, but their relevance to clinical asthma is unknown.

Theophylline is an effective bronchodilator, about one fourth as potent as inhaled β_2 agonists. It enhances mucociliary clearance, increases diaphragmatic contractility, and can dilate pulmonary arteries and increase respiratory drive in the central nervous system. However, these additional effects are unlikely to be of great clinical importance in the treatment of asthma. Theophylline, given orally, is of proven benefit in the chronic management of asthma. The most convincing data pertain to asthmatics with relatively mild symptoms that occur primarily at night. With sustained-release preparations, these

patients have improved control and are thus better able to sleep than with the intermediate-acting inhaled β_2 agonists. When theophylline is added to a regimen of inhaled β_2 agonists, there is greater bronchodilation, but these effects are additive as opposed to synergistic.

In severe exacerbations the standard of care has been to administer intravenous theophylline (as aminophylline). There is not good evidence, however, that adding intravenous aminophylline to inhaled β_2 agonists in the emergency room setting is of clinical benefit. Moreover, intravenous aminophylline has a low therapeutic index and the consequences of theophylline toxicity can be profound. Therefore, if used intravenously to treat acute exacerbations of asthma, aminophylline should be employed judiciously and with monitoring of serum levels.

The resurgence in theophylline use with the development of long-acting preparations has been associated with a significant increase in serious theophylline toxicity. Risk factors for theophylline toxicity include advanced age, congestive heart failure, liver disease, profound hypoalbuminemia, and coadministration of drugs that interfere with theophylline's metabolism such as cimetidine, erythromycin, allopurinol, and some quinilone antibiotics.

Glucocorticosteroids

Corticosteroids have the potential to modify the severity of disease in asthma as well as to treat bronchospasm. The mechanism of action of corticosteroids is still controversial, but with the recognition that inflammation of the airway is associated with asthma the focus has been on their antiinflammatory and immunomodulatory properties. These agents are known to limit inflammatory cell recruitment and inflammatory cell stimulation. They also inhibit the arachidonic acid cascade, but the precise site and mechanism of this inhibition are currently controversial. The major effect of corticosteroids on arachidonic acid metabolism appears to be inhibition of the expression of the inducible form of cyclooxygenase. In the acute setting, however, corticosteroids may increase the number and affinity of β_2 receptors in the lung before affecting the inflammatory and immunologic cascades. Corticosteroids have been shown to modify disease severity by decreasing airway hyperresponsiveness in the long term.

Corticosteroids have been underused and misused in the treatment of asthma. For example, systemic steroids have been employed in settings where inhaled steroids would be adequate. Chronic systemic administration of corticosteroids may be necessary for patients with severe disease not controlled with other agents, but extended treatment is accompanied by profound side effects. The most important are bone mineral loss with secondary fracture, avascular bone necrosis, cataract formation, hyperglycemia, psychiatric disturbance, and opportunistic infection. For patients requiring continual systemic corticosteroids for control of severe disease, alternate-day treatment should be attempted to minimize long-term side effects. However, alternate-day therapy often fails in these patients. Short courses of systemic corticosteroids can be used with relative safety to gain control of acute exacerbations of chronic asthma. Most side effects associated with courses of less than 2 weeks are not life threatening and include sleep disturbance, increased appetite, and mood alterations, although avascular bone necrosis has been attributed to such use. Patients who receive treatment with corticosteroids for less than 2 weeks can have these drugs abruptly reduced or stopped. Tapering the corticosteroids in patients treated with high doses for long periods or with frequent short courses is more difficult. Although it seems logical to reduce the dose of corticosteroids rapidly, too aggressive a taper often precipitates a second exacerbation and ultimately results in the patient receiving systemic corticosteroids for a longer period. The maximal dose, the duration of therapy, and frequency of courses should all be considered in determining the rate of tapering systemic steroids. Patients who receive treatment with large doses of systemic steroids for 1 month or longer can demonstrate biochemical and/or clinical evidence of pituitary-adrenal insufficiency. The risk of adrenal insufficiency is directly correlated with dose, duration of therapy, and frequency of administration.

Inhaled corticosteroids provide a relatively safe and effective alternative to systemic steroids. Recent trends, supported by numerous clinical studies, favor earlier and more aggressive use of inhaled corticosteroids. Adrenal-suppressive effects of inhaled steroids are not seen with standard doses and have not been found with doses as high as four times the standard dose. Although most inhaled corticosteroids are recommended for three or four daily administrations, they are effective when used twice per day. Inhaled corticosteroids should, in general, be stopped and systemic corticosteroids substituted during acute exacerbations of asthma because of the tendency of many inhaled agents to stimulate cough or bronchospasm. However, they should be restarted as systemic corticosteroids are reduced. The known side effects of inhaled steroids are relatively few. Dysphonia and vocal cord atrophy are uncommon complications but do occur. Oral candidiasis develops in about 15% of patients but can be easily minimized by the use of a spacing device and rinsing the mouth after inhalations; treatment with antifungal drugs is occasionally necessary. The long-term consequences of inhaled corticosteroids, especially at high doses, have not been adequately examined with respect to effects on bone mineral metabolism, cataract formation, or other potential toxicities. Preliminary studies suggest that such long-term effects may be possible. Delayed long bone growth may result from the use of inhaled corticosteroids in children.

Cromolyn and Nedocromil

Cromolyn and nedocromil are agents that may modify the severity of asthma and decrease airway inflammation and hyperresponsiveness. Their mechanism of action is unknown, but they are thought to stabilize mast cells and prevent mediator release. They may also affect other cell types, including macrophages, neutrophils, and probably eosinophils by inhibiting secretion of mediators. The proper use of these agents in the treatment of asthma remains unclear. At clinical doses neither has direct bronchodilating effects, and they are used as disease-modifying and prophylactic agents. Predicting which patient will respond to these agents is difficult, but younger patients tend to respond more often than older patients. An allergic component to the patient's disease is not predictive of a clinical response. The significant advantage of cromolyn and nedocromil is their virtual lack of side effects, but their substantial expense and lack of a predictable clinical response limit their use. Cromolyn has been found effective and is recommended for use in exercise-induced asthma, but β_2 agonists are also effective and less expensive.

Anticholinergics

Anticholinergics block reflex bronchoconstriction, but they have no direct relaxing effect on airway smooth muscle. The introduction of ipratropium bromide has allowed the administration of inhaled anticholinergics without significant systemic toxicity. The onset of action of ipratropium is delayed up to 30 minutes after an inhalation, although it is then sustained for up to 6 hours. However, only a limited number of asthmatics have a significant response to ipratropium, and the responses are usually modest. Predictors of a response are lacking, although older patients are more likely to improve than younger patients. The effects of these medications should be determined with clinical or pulmonary function assessments.

Immunotherapy

Although specific immunotherapy has been advocated for patients with allergic asthma, allergen avoidance is the first line of treatment. The second line of therapy should be more conventional antiasthma drugs. If these fail or symptoms are severe, specific immunotherapy can be considered. Immunotherapy for allergic rhinitis has proven beneficial, but benefits in patients with asthma have proved to be more difficult to demonstrate. Data are available suggesting that specific immunotherapy is of benefit in some instances of dust mite, animal dander, and pollen-induced asthma. These benefits must be weighed, however, against the risk of a systemic reaction to allergen extract injections.

Antibiotics

Antibiotics are frequently used for treatment of purulent bronchitis in patients having an exacerbation of asthma, based on the assumption that purulent secretions are caused by a bacterial infection. However,

most respiratory tract infections in asthmatics are viral. Furthermore, in patients with asthma purulent secretions can develop during exacerbations as a result of inflammatory cell influx into the airway, rather than infection. Sputum cultures are difficult to interpret and are complicated by bacterial colonization of the respiratory tract in many patients or by oropharyngeal contamination of collected specimens. Specific changes in the rate of improvement have been difficult to demonstrate in exacerbations of asthma treated with oral antibiotics.

Leukotriene Receptor Antagonists and Synthesis Inhibitors

Antagonists of cysteinyl leukotrienes and inhibitors of the 5-lipoxygenase pathway inhibit acute bronchospasm induced by exercise and allergen. These agents are also effective for aspirin-induced bronchospasm. This class of drugs has both bronchodilator and antiinflammatory properties. Data on their efficacy in chronic stable asthma is limited. Studies suggest a 10% to 15% improvement in FEV_1 that is sustained, which is comparable to other bronchodilating drugs. One cysteinyl leukotriene receptor antagonist, zafirlukast, and one 5-lipoxygenase inhibitor, zileuton, have recently been released in the United States for use in mild to moderate asthma. They may be especially effective in the management of aspirin-sensitive asthma. Their precise role in the clinical management of asthma and their positioning relative to other drugs is currently not known.

Other Therapies

Other treatments of asthma are worthy of mention. Antihistamines have been evaluated through multiple studies as potential bronchodilators. The more sedating, less potent antihistamines such as chlorpheneramine have been shown to lack benefit in the treatment of asthma. More specific H_1 antagonists, including terfenadine, azelastine, and cetirizine, may blunt histamine or even antigen-induced acute bronchospasm in the short term, but they have little proven benefit in the treatment of chronic asthma. Ketotifen, an antihistamine with other antiinflammatory properties, is of questionable value in the treatment of asthma. Calcium channel blockers have been evaluated without convincing evidence of their efficacy. Intravenous or inhaled magnesium has been advocated in the treatment of acute bronchospasm in the emergency room setting based on limited clinical trials, demonstrating a modest short-term benefit.

A variety of other treatments are investigational or are potential therapies of the future. Troleandomycin (TAO) has been used in corticosteroid-dependent asthmatics as a steroid-sparing drug. TAO is known to prolong the half-life of corticosteroids by slowing their metabolism in the liver. Direct effects of TAO in asthma have also been suggested but never established. Clinical trials using TAO have reported conflicting results. Cytotoxic and immunosuppressive drugs have been tried in severe, steroid-dependent asthma. Methotrexate has been found by one group of investigators to have significant steroid-sparing effects in severe asthmatics, but substantial toxicity can be associated with its administration. Additional data are needed to evaluate the efficacy and long-term side effects of this drug before it can be recommended for treatment of severe asthma. Cyclosporin and gold are reported to be of value in the treatment of severe asthma, but further study is required.

Despite initial excitement about platelet-activating factor antagonists, the effect of these agents in clinical asthma has been disappointing.

MANAGEMENT STRATEGIES

The chronic management of asthma is changing (Table 188-2). Mild, intermittent symptoms may be controlled by inhaled β_2 agonists as needed. If symptoms are uncontrolled by this treatment, inhaled β_2 agonists can be increased to regular dosing intervals of every 4 to 6 hours. However, concerns about the effects of β_2 agonists on severity of disease have discouraged the regular use of these drugs and instead have favored the addition of an antiinflammatory agent such as inhaled corticosteroids, cromolyn, or nedocromil. Inhaled steroids have also been championed as first-line therapy. If symptoms are not controlled by inhaled β_2 agonists and inhaled corticosteroids, theoph-

Table 188-2   Guidelines for management

	THERAPY			
	FIRST LINE	SECOND LINE	THIRD LINE	ALTERNATIVES
Chronic asthma				
Mild	Inhaled β_2 agonists as needed	Inhaled corticosteroid two to four times a day		
Moderate	Inhaled β_2 agonists as needed	Inhaled corticosteroid two to four times a day (high dose)	Sustained-release theophylline (5 mg/kg twice daily)	Cromolyn, ipratropium
Severe	Inhaled β_2 agonists as needed	Corticosteroid (high dose inhaled or systemic)	Sustained release theophylline (5 mg/kg twice daily)	Consider above with or without systemic corticosteroids
Acute exacerbation				
Mild	Increased inhaled β_2 agonists			
Moderate	Increased inhaled β_2 agonists	0.5-1 mg/kg oral prednisone every day		
Severe	Increased inhaled β_2 agonists	1-2 mg/kg every 6 hours of oral prednisone or intravenous methylprednisolone		Oxygen, antibiotics, mechanical ventilation

ylline is a logical third choice. Theophylline should be started at a low dose and gradually increased with assessment of theophylline blood levels to guide adjustments in therapy and to evaluate symptoms that suggest toxicity. The therapeutic range is 5 to 15 µg/ml. The practice of increasing the theophylline level to the high therapeutic range adds little in terms of bronchodilation and should be discouraged because of the risk of toxicity. Cromolyn or nedocromil can be instituted early in this scheme, and efficacy evaluated after several weeks of therapy. Ipratropium bromide can also be tried if symptoms are uncontrolled. Patients may be considered for immunotherapy if demonstrable specific allergy plays a role in their disease and asthma symptoms are not controlled by medication. Chronic systemic administration of corticosteroids should be reserved for patients who have failed all other measures. Corticosteroid-sparing agents remain controversial at this time.

The management of acute exacerbations should rely heavily on inhaled β_2 agonists (Table 188-2). These should be delivered by metered-dose inhaler whenever possible. Systemic administration of these drugs should be avoided in the treatment of asthma. Furthermore, intravenous administration of aminophylline is controversial in the setting of an acute exacerbation and is not routinely recommended by the authors. Systemic corticosteroids are recommended if inhaled β_2 agonists do not rapidly result in clinical improvement. However, corticosteroids are relatively slow in their onset of action in the acute setting and may require 6 to 8 hours for beneficial effects to become evident. If the patient is well enough to return home but requires therapy in addition to inhaled β_2 agonists, 60 mg of prednisone by mouth followed by 60 mg daily for 7 days with a rapid taper is usually adequate. In severely ill patients corticosteroids are usually administered intravenously in the acute setting at doses of 60 to 120 mg of methylprednisolone every 6 hours. However, there is no evidence that intravenous corticosteroids are superior to oral. Ipratropium bromide can be tried if symptoms are uncontrolled with inhaled β_2 agonists, but this is not often of benefit. Overt respiratory failure necessitates intubation and mechanical ventilation. In patients whose lungs are difficult to ventilate because of high peak airway pressures and agitation, sedation and paralysis may be necessary to lower peak pressures and lessen the risk of barotrauma. Controlled hypoventilation is occasionally necessary for patients with profound respiratory failure.

PROGNOSIS

The long-term outlook for patients with asthma is age dependent. Whereas 25% or more of childhood asthmatics continue to have symptoms as adults, more than 90% of asthmatics with the onset of symptoms as adults continue to have symptoms throughout their lives. On the other hand, little is known about the evolution of severity of disease and whether severity increases or decreases with age.

✔ *WHEN TO REFER*

Most patients with asthma do not have severe disease and are effectively managed by their primary care provider using standard management strategies as outlined earlier. However, consultation with a specialist should be considered for any patient with poorly controlled symptoms that have not responded to aggressive conventional therapy. Pulmonary and allergy specialists are appropriate consultants and share expertise in this clinical area, but each have different strengths that may be advantageous in consultation regarding a particular patient. Patients who require regular systemic corticosteroids should also be referred for consultation. Any patient who has had a near-death episode or requires mechanical ventilation should be evaluated in the intensive care unit by a pulmonary specialist with expertise in critical care, and this patient should be followed up with outpatient consultation. Patients suspected of having a significant allergic component to their asthma benefit from referral for evaluation. Consultation with an allergist then allows development of avoidance strategies and consideration of desensitization to specific identified allergens.

Although mortality rates from asthma in the United States declined during the 1970s, they have steadily increased in the 1980s and are currently in excess of 1.7 deaths per 100,000 per year. Currently, estimates suggest that mortality exceeds 4500 deaths per year. Increases in asthma death rates have also been reported for New Zealand, Great Britain, Canada, France, Germany, and Denmark. A number of hypotheses have been put forward to explain these apparent increases. Some data suggest that the increase in the prevalence of asthma is associated with oxidant pollutants. Other possibilities include a perceived rather than real increase resulting from diagnostic coding trends, shifts in physician diagnostic patterns, an increase in the ability of the physician to detect asthma, and changes in health care access. Another possible explanation for the increase in asthma mortality is that specific therapies for asthma contribute to the severity of disease. Specific therapy could increase airway responsiveness, induce tolerance to that specific drug, or facilitate abuse of medications with resulting toxic side effects. One transient increase in asthma mortality in Great Britain in the 1960s was associated with the clinical use of a high-potency isoproterenol metered-dose inhaler. The role that medications may play in the current rise in asthma mortality is being examined and suggests an association between the long-acting inhaled β_2 agonist, fenoterol, and the rise in mortality in locations such as New Zealand, Great Britain, and Canada. Such a relationship between asthma mortality and beta agonists that are available in the United States has not been established.

Little is known about the long-term effects of asthma on the lung and lung function. Some studies suggest that fibrosis with narrowing of the airway and basement membrane thickening may be long-term consequences of asthma. The clinical correlate of these studies may be the development of fixed airway obstruction as a consequence of long-standing asthma. Recent data suggest that the normal age-related loss in FEV_1 is accelerated in asthmatic patients. These important issues warrant further investigation.

BIBLIOGRAPHY

Blake KV et al: Relative amount of albuterol delivered to lung receptors from a metered-dose inhaler and nebulizer solution, *Chest* 101:309, 1992.

Chan-Yeung M, Malo JL: Occupational asthma, *N Engl J Med* 333:107, 1995.

McFadden ER: Methylxanthines in the treatment of asthma: the rise, the fall, and the possible rise again, *Ann Intern Med* 115:323, 1991.

National Heart, Lung, and Blood Institute: *Guidelines for the diagnosis and management of asthma,* Bethesda, Md, 1997, U.S. Department of Health and Human Services.

Robinson DS et al: Predominant TH_2-like bronchoalveolar T-lymphocyte population in atopic asthma, *N Engl J Med* 326:298, 1992.

Sears MR et al: Regular inhaled beta-agonist treatment in bronchial asthma, *Lancet* 336:1391, 1990.

Sears MR et al: Relation between airway responsiveness and serum IgE in children with asthma and in apparently normal children, *N Engl J Med* 325:1067, 1991.

Sokol W: Vocal cord dysfunction presenting as asthma, *West J Med* 158:614, 1993.

Spitzer WO et al: The use of beta-agonists and the risk of death and near death from asthma, *N Engl J Med* 326:501, 1992.

Weiss KB, Gergen PJ, Hodgson TA: An economic evaluation of asthma in the United States, *N Engl J Med* 326:862, 1992.

Young S et al: The influence of a family history of asthma and parental smoking on airway responsiveness in early infancy, *N Engl J Med* 324:1168, 1991.

CHAPTER

189 Anaphylaxis

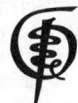

Diana L. Marquardt

Anaphylaxis is a sudden, untoward, often life-threatening event characterized by a constellation of signs and symptoms involving one or more organs or tissues. Classic anaphylaxis constitutes a systemic immediate hypersensitivity reaction induced by specific antigen cross-linking immunoglobulin E (IgE) molecules on the surface of tissue mast cells, resulting in the release of vasoactive, chemotactic, and enzymatic mediators, including measurable amounts of histamine and tryptase. In practical terms the precise mechanism of a particular anaphylactic reaction may not be understood, and the syndrome is better defined by clinical manifestations than by the involvement of a defined immunologic reaction. Thus the term *anaphylactoid,* used to describe non–IgE-mediated, systemic, life-threatening reactions or reactions of unknown immunologic basis, has become outmoded.

The clinical presentation of anaphylaxis may include respiratory, cardiovascular, cutaneous, or gastrointestinal tract manifestations (Box 189-1). Upper airway obstruction may be experienced as hoarseness, dysphonia, or a "lump in the throat" and may be evidenced as inspiratory stridor suggestive of laryngeal edema. The lower airway obstruction symptoms of chest tightness or wheezing may also ensue. In one large series of fatal anaphylaxis case reports, 70% of the deaths were attributed to respiratory causes, underscoring the importance of these findings. Primary cardiovascular events include hypotension, arrhythmias, and circulatory collapse; myocardial infarction may complicate anaphylaxis. Urticaria, angioedema, pruritus, and flushing are common dermatologic manifestations that are present in nearly 80% of anaphylaxis episodes and may precede more serious events. Abdominal cramping, nausea, vomiting, and diarrhea may occur as a result of gastrointestinal tract smooth-muscle spasm.

Although anaphylaxis caused by IgE-related mechanisms is perhaps best understood, immune complexes, agents that alter arachi-

---

BOX 189-1
Clinical manifestations of anaphylaxis

Respiratory
Bronchospasm
Laryngeal edema
Rhinorrhea

Cardiovascular
Hypotension, syncope
Dysrhythmias
Shock
Headache

Cutaneous
Urticaria
Angioedema
Flushing
Pruritus

Gastrointestinal
Nausea, vomiting
Diarrhea
Abdominal cramping

---

donic acid metabolism, direct mast cell–degranulating drugs, and idiopathic mechanisms have been implicated in anaphylaxis. In IgE-mediated anaphylaxis a previous, sensitizing exposure to antigen is required to induce synthesis of specific IgE antibodies to sensitize mast cells and basophils. Reexposure to a specific antigen, generally a large polypeptide or protein or a small molecule combining as a hapten with human protein, may elicit an anaphylactic response. Penicillin, hymenoptera venom, and allergenic extracts used in skin testing and desensitization are among the common causes of anaphylaxis today. Crustaceans and peanuts are the foods most commonly implicated. Anaphylaxis induced by latex antigen has become a major concern in spina bifida patients and health care workers. The risk of anaphylaxis is increased with the length and frequency of antigenic exposures, and a parenteral exposure is more dangerous than an oral one. Mucocutaneous exposures may induce anaphylaxis as well. The administration of whole blood, immunoglobulin, or serum products may be associated with immune-complex formation, complement activation, and anaphylaxis. This response is best illustrated by a patient lacking native immunoglobulin A (IgA) but possessing immunoglobulin G (IgG) or, less commonly, IgE antibodies to IgA by some prior exposure. Aspirin-induced anaphylaxis has been postulated to result from alterations in arachidonic acid metabolism because the nonsteroidal antiinflammatory drugs that similarly inhibit the cyclooxygenase enzyme also provoke the response. This is the most common medication group thought to cause anaphylaxis. It has been reported that platelets obtained from aspirin-sensitive individuals may be activated by aspirin to produce inflammatory mediators, whereas those of normal individuals lack this response. A group of agents apparently capable of directly inducing mast cell degranulation includes radiocontrast media, plasma expanders, and opiates. These agents require no previous host sensitization, although reexposure to radiocontrast media in an individual with a history of a previous adverse reaction carries a markedly increased risk of anaphylaxis. Idiopathic anaphylaxis implies an unknown mechanism underlying a documented anaphylactic episode. More than a third of cases of anaphylaxis fall into this category, and recurrent attacks are common. A small group of patients has been identified with exercise-induced anaphylaxis, and in others no precipitating factor can be determined. There is evidence of mast cell degranulation in this syndrome, but the mechanism underlying it is unknown.

Because the interval between antigenic exposure and life-threatening complications may be only a matter of minutes, the treatment of anaphylaxis is emergent. Subcutaneous epinephrine is the mainstay of therapy and is often sufficient to reverse the symptoms.

In more severe reactions airway patency is compromised and must be maintained, supplemental oxygen may be required, and intravenous fluids or pressors may be necessary to maintain blood pressure. Glucocorticoids may help to prevent a biphasic response or later recurrence of symptoms and should be administered early in all but mild cases. Antihistamines aid in symptomatic relief of pruritus or swelling and may assist in control of hypotension. With the possible exception of the perioperative period, both H_1 and H_2 blockers appear to be beneficial. Aminophylline may be useful for bronchospasm, and there are isolated reports of the benefit of naloxone and glucagon in particularly unrelenting cases. The symptoms of anaphylaxis usually respond to early appropriate therapeutic measures. However, patients receiving β-adrenergic blocking drugs may be resistant to the beneficial effects of beta agonists and are at greater risk for a severe, protracted course of symptoms. Patients undergoing chronic angiotensin-converting enzyme inhibitor or calcium channel–blocker therapy also may be more susceptible to severe manifestations of anaphylaxis.

> ✔ *WHEN TO REFER*
>
> Most patients who have anaphylactic reactions in which the antigen or inciting factor is unknown or unavoidable should be carefully counseled, provided with an injectable epinephrine supply, and evaluated by an allergy specialist.

STINGING INSECT HYPERSENSITIVITY

Stings from insects of the order Hymenoptera result in anaphylaxis in an estimated 0.5% of the population. Sensitivity to honey bee or vespid (yellow jacket, yellow hornet, and bald-faced hornet) venoms are mediated by IgE and may be confirmed by skin testing or radioallergosorbent test (RAST) with the specific venom extract. To develop IgE antibodies to insect venom, a patient must first be exposed to the venom. Therefore initial exposure stings should not result in an immediate hypersensitivity reaction. Adults who have had systemic allergic reactions to insect stings should have skin testing with hymenoptera venom. It is recommended that patients with positive skin test results should receive venom immunotherapy, which is effective in decreasing the likelihood and severity of future sting reactions. However, there is a developing controversy regarding this recommendation. Some recent reports using sting challenges of previous systemic reactors suggest that these patients are relatively unlikely to have subsequent severe reactions. Until more definitive data are available, the recommendation for immunotherapy still stands. Those who have had only large local sting reactions do not require venom immunotherapy, since the risk of subsequent systemic sting reactions is very small. Children less than 16 years of age with a history of strictly cutaneous sting reactions rarely have serious reactions on restinging and may not require immunotherapy.

Venom immunotherapy induces an increase in IgG-blocking antibodies to venom that correlates with clinical protection against serious sting reactions. However, the precise mechanism of desensitization with immunotherapy remains unclear, and no marker has been identified to document protection against stings. It requires several weeks to reach maintenance levels of immunotherapy, and after that point, regular venom immunotherapy should be administered at 4- to 6-week intervals. Current recommendations are for 5 years of immunotherapy, which can be discontinued after that time with little likelihood of severe adverse reactions to subsequent stings.

Patients with sting anaphylaxis but normal skin test results for IgE are not candidates for immunotherapy, and these and other patients with prior histories of systemic reactions to stings should be equipped with kits that allow self-administration of subcutaneous epinephrine. Preloaded syringes or spring-loaded, automatic-injection syringes containing measured doses of epinephrine have a shelf life of at least 18 months and should be immediately available. Patients given such syringes should be carefully instructed in their use and warned to seek medical treatment as soon as possible when symptoms require.

> ✔ *WHEN TO REFER*
>
> Adults with a history of generalized urticaria, angioedema, bronchospasm, hypotension, diffuse pruritus, or a combination of these symptoms that occur within minutes after an insect sting should be referred to an allergist for evaluation and consideration of immunotherapy. Skin testing may also be useful in differentiating an unwitnessed vasovagal response to an insect sting from an anaphylactic response.

Although much less common than Hymenoptera venom reactions, both fire ant venom and stings from insects of the genus *Triatoma* have been shown to induce anaphylaxis on an IgE-mediated basis in certain individuals. Immunotherapy has been effective in reducing the risk of serious reactions to these agents as well.

DRUG REACTIONS

In a general sense drug reactions are relatively frequent, varied, and often poorly understood. However, some types of drug reactions have a well-defined immunologic basis, and a subset of these can be predicted and/or prevented. IgE-mediated drug reactions result in signs and symptoms of the type described earlier for anaphylaxis. Penicillin and other beta-lactam antibiotics account for the largest group of IgE-mediated reactions, including more than 400 deaths yearly in the United States. Penicillin-sensitive individuals can be identified by skin testing with the major and minor haptenic determinants. Patients identified as penicillin allergic by skin testing who require penicillin therapy for a serious indication may be desensitized to penicillin under close supervision by a graded oral or parenteral regimen. Desensitization is effective but short-lived, and once a course of drug therapy has been discontinued, restarting therapy requires repeat skin testing and desensitization, if necessary. Penicillin allergy itself appears to be a dynamic process; patients receiving frequent, intermittent courses of antibiotic therapy develop a greater risk for reactions. Hypersensitivity often declines with time, and up to 80% of patients with documented penicillin allergy no longer exhibit positive skin test results 10 years after the last exposure. Therefore penicillin therapy should be avoided in patients with a history of penicillin reactions, but previously sensitive patients requiring penicillin for a life-threatening indication should have skin testing and be desensitized if necessary. The entire procedure must be repeated each time penicillin therapy is considered.

Other drugs that may cause IgE-mediated reactions that can be predicted by testing include cephalosporins (which cross-react to some extent with penicillins), insulin, streptokinase, egg-related vaccines, and some local anesthetics and muscle relaxants. Some studies to predict reactivity to sulfa drugs have indicated some potential utility for skin testing to these agents, but such tests are not yet in routine use. However, successful desensitization protocols have been developed to allow the short- or long-term administration of trimethoprim-sulphamethoxazole, sulfasalazine, and vancomycin.

Non–IgE-mediated drug reactions are generally unpredictable and often require symptomatic treatment rather than prophylaxis. An exception to this rule is the radiocontrast media reaction that may be prevented or limited by pretreatment of high-risk patients with antihistamines and glucocorticoids or by the use of nonionic low-osmolality agents. Reactions to iodinated radiocontrast media cannot be detected by skin testing, and an adverse reaction may occur on the first exposure to such agents. The strongest predictor for an adverse reaction is a previous adverse reaction, but greater risk for contrast media reactions has been reported for asthmatic individuals, patients receiving β-adrenergic blocking drugs, and those of female gender. Other types of immunologic drug reactions include cytotoxic reactions in which drug antigen interacts with cell membranes, inducing IgG and immunoglobulin M (IgM) cytotoxic antibodies. Hemolytic anemia, thrombocytopenia, and leukopenia are common clinical sequelae of these reactions, and penicillin and quinine are two drugs likely to produce them. Immune-complex drug reactions result from

BOX 189-2
Prevention of drug reactions

1. Take a thorough medical history.
2. Avoid agents known to have caused previous reactions, and educate the patient accordingly.
3. Require a clear indication for drug usage.
4. Observe the patient after injections and administer drugs orally when possible.
5. Test for drug allergy when feasible and desensitize or premedicate if necessary.
6. Maintain current immunizations.

deposition of antigen-IgG immune complexes within vessel walls or basement membranes and complement fixation. Serum sickness is based primarily on this immune mechanism. Cell-mediated or delayed hypersensitivity reactions are best exemplified by allergic contact dermatitis, characterized by topical sensitization and a subsequent eczematous outbreak up to 48 hours later.

Many drug reactions, including fixed drug eruptions, drug fevers, and some organ toxicities, have no defined immunologic basis and thus cannot be predicted or prevented. Any previous untoward drug reaction calls for a careful consideration of alternate therapeutic approaches. Other general methods of preventing severe drug reactions are noted in Box 189-2.

BIBLIOGRAPHY

Absar N et al: Desensitization to trimethoprim/sulfamethoxazole in HIV-infected patients, *J Allergy Clin Immunol* 93:1001, 1994.

Gold M et al: Intraoperative anaphylaxis: an association with latex sensitivity, *J Allergy Clin Immunol* 87:662, 1991.

Golden DBK, Schwartz HJ: Guidelines for venom immunotherapy, *J Allergy Clin Immunol* 77:727, 1986.

Golden DBK et al: Discontinuing venom immunotherapy: outcome after five years, *J Allergy Clin Immunol* 97:579, 1996.

Greenberger PA, Patterson R: The prevention of immediate generalized reactions to radiocontrast media in high-risk patients, *J Allergy Clin Immunol* 87:867, 1991.

Kemp SF et al: Anaphylaxis: a review of 266 cases, *Arch Intern Med* 155:1749, 1995.

Kivity S, Yarchovsky J: Relapsing anaphylaxis to bee sting in a patient treated with beta blocker and calcium blocker, *J Allergy Clin Immunol* 85:669, 1990.

Lang DM et al: Gender risk for anaphylactoid reaction to radiographic contrast media, *J Allergy Clin Immunol* 95:813, 1995.

Lieberman P: The use of antihistamines in the prevention and treatment of anaphylaxis and anaphylactoid reactions, *J Allergy Clin Immunol* 86:684, 1990.

Marquardt DL, Wasserman SI: Anaphylaxis. In Middleton EE et al, editors: *Allergy: principles and practice,* ed 4, St Louis, 1993, Mosby.

Reisman RE: Natural history of insect sting allergy: relationship of severity of symptoms of initial sting anaphylaxis to re-sting reactions, *J Allergy Clin Immunol* 90:335, 1992.

Schwartz H: Elevated serum tryptase in exercise-induced anaphylaxis, *J Allergy Clin Immunol* 95:917, 1995.

Schwartz LB et al: Tryptase levels as an indicator of mast cell activation in systemic anaphylaxis and mastocytosis, *N Engl J Med* 316:1622, 1987.

Sheffer AL, Austen KF: Exercise-induced anaphylaxis, *J Allergy Clin Immunol* 73:699, 1984.

Wong JT et al: Vancomycin hypersensitivity: synergism with narcotics and "desensitization" by a rapid continuous intravenous protocol, *J Allergy Clin Immunol* 94:189, 1994.

190 Periarticular Rheumatic Complaints

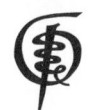

Harry G. Bluestein

Pain and stiffness of the soft tissues around joints commonly occurs after unaccustomed physical activities. Those acute symptoms are short-lived and generally resolve completely. Persistent subacute or chronic rheumatic complaints, however, require medical evaluation to differentiate symptoms caused by a variety of systemic illnesses from those caused by a primary rheumatic disorder. Recognition of the differences between arthritis, an intraarticular process, and periarthritis is essential (see Chapter 191). With periarticular involvement, physical examination shows that the pain is not localized to the articulation, and passive range of motion of the joint is usually minimally affected. Thus history and physical examination are generally sufficient to recognize most periarticular problem syndromes. Laboratory tests and radiographs contribute little, but they may play an important role in excluding alternative causes of the symptoms. Other imaging techniques such as magnetic resonance imaging (MRI), are more revealing but are usually not cost effective. An exception may be evaluation of the rotator cuff of the shoulder.

As a group, the periarticular musculoskeletal conditions entail complaints of pain and stiffness on motion, which are generally most severe in the morning. Each condition, however, has a relatively unique anatomic distribution. Most are regional, affecting a single joint or extremity. Primary diffuse rheumatic symptoms affecting periarticular tissues are also common and are problematic because they must be differentiated from symptoms resulting from other systemic illnesses and because they tend to be more chronically persistent. In evaluating diffuse symptoms, it is especially important to exclude malignancies, the myopathy of hypothyroidism, other endocrinopathies, and systemic rheumatic disorders. Among the last-mentioned, polymyalgia rheumatica is most important because it causes profound stiffness and pain, often in the absence of physical findings.

FIBROMYALGIA

Fibromyalgia, the currently preferred name for the most common diffuse periarticular rheumatic syndrome, is characterized by widespread musculoskeletal pain, chronic fatigue, and, often, disordered sleep. Typically the fibromyalgia patient is a middle-aged woman, although the disease can occur at any age and in both sexes. The etiopathogenesis is unknown, and the validity of fibromyalgia as a distinct nosologic entity remains controversial. To some authors, it is but one form of psychogenic rheumatism, the symptoms representing a somatization of psychologic stresses. In fact, many fibromyalgia patients do exhibit signs or symptoms of depressive anxiety. To others, the characteristic presentation of myofascial pain and stiffness with a bilateral distribution of tender-point sites that are reproducible from patient to patient marks a distinct entity. Those who believe it to be unique also point to the fact that many fibromyalgia patients are not depressed or anxious and that there is very little success in treating this condition with psychotherapy. Hypotheses to explain fibromyalgia pain have focused on abnormal sensitivities at afferent and efferent nerve endings causing heightened pain sensations and increased chronic regional muscle contractions. Pain appreciation is further modulated by central nervous system mechanisms related to emotional factors.

On clinical examination patients with fibromyalgia come to the physician with a history of chronic, widespread aching pain or burning, and stiffness with increased emphasis truncally. Most patients also have arthralgias involving the small joints of the hands and sometimes other joints. Examination reveals tenderness without other physical findings. Musculoskeletal trigger or tender points are multiple and localized to typical areas (Fig. 190-1). These are regularly

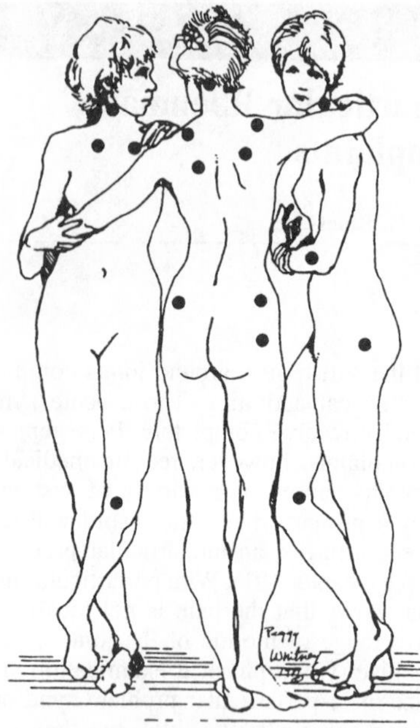

FIGURE 190-1 Tender-point locations for the 1990 American College of Rheumatology classification criteria for fibromyalgia (*The Three Graces,* after Baron Jean-Baptiste Regnault, 1793, Louvre Museum, Paris). See Box 190-1 for details of the tender-point locations.

From Wolfe F et al: *Arthritis Rheum* 33:160, 1990.

elicited by firm digital palpation. Often the rheumatic complaints are accompanied by profound fatigue, which is present throughout the day and indistinguishable from that described by patients with chronic fatigue syndrome. Also common are a variety of neurologic symptoms unmatched by abnormalities on neurophysiologic testing. Symptoms of carpal tunnel syndrome and varying paresthesias occur with normal nerve conduction. Subtle cognitive defects, dizziness, and clumsiness are frequent complaints. Tension headaches, irritable bowel syndrome, and symptoms of urethrocystitis in the absence of infection occur with a greater frequency in fibromyalgia patients than in controls.

The diagnosis of fibromyalgia can be made only on clinical grounds, since laboratory studies are normal, including the sedimentation rate and autoantibody profiles. Fibromyalgia must be considered in any patient with the characteristic complaints of musculoskeletal pains and stiffness plus the demonstration of typical tender points. Systemic illnesses that can produce diffuse musculoskeletal pain should be excluded. The diagnostic criteria of the American College of Rheumatology (Box 190-1) perform well, with a sensitivity of 88.4% and a specificity of 88.1%.

The natural history of fibromyalgia is not well defined, but it appears to be a chronic condition with fluctuating symptoms. Although tissue damage does not occur, many patients become disabled by their inability to function because of their pain. Treatment is generally unrewarding. Simple analgesics, muscle relaxants, and nonsteroidal antiinflammatory drugs are regularly employed but provide only minimal benefit. Small doses of tricyclic antidepressants help to reduce symptoms. Patients should also be instructed in an exercise regimen including daily stretching and every-other-day nonimpact exercises with the goal of an aerobic level of conditioning. Massage, acupuncture, and the injection of local anesthetics into tender points may provide temporary relief. Perhaps most important is the physician's support and constant reassurance that fibromyalgia is a benign condition and that physical damage to the body does not occur.

REGIONAL PERIARTICULAR SYNDROMES

Tendinitis, bursitis, and capsulitis are the major causes of pain around a single large or medium-sized joint. *Tendinitis* is usually caused by a mechanical stress to the involved tendon. Repeated injury to a ten-

---

BOX 190-1

The American College of Rheumatology 1990 criteria for the classification of fibromyalgia*

---

1. History of widespread pain.
Definition.
Pain is considered widespread when all of the following are present: pain in the left side of the body, pain in the right side of the body, pain above the waist, and pain below the waist. In addition, axial skeletal pain (cervical spine or anterior chest or thoracic spine or low back) must be present. In this definition, shoulder and buttock pain is considered as pain for each involved side. "Low back" pain is considered lower segment pain.

2. Pain in 11 of 18 tender point sites on digital palpation.
Definition.
Pain, on digital palpation, must be present in at least 11 of the following 18 tender point sites:
Occiput: Bilateral, at the suboccipital muscle insertions.
Low cervical: Bilateral, at the anterior aspects of the intertransverse spaces at C5-7.
Trapezius: Bilateral, at the midpoint of the upper border.
Supraspinatus: Bilateral, at origins, above the scapula spine near the medial border.
Second rib: Bilateral, at the second costochondral junctions, just lateral to the junctions on upper surfaces.
Lateral epicondyle: Bilateral, 2 cm distal to the epicondyles.
Gluteal: Bilateral, in upper outer quadrants of buttocks in anterior fold of muscle.
Greater trochanter: Bilateral, posterior to the trochanteric prominence.
Knee: Bilateral, at the medial fat pad proximal to the joint line.
Digital palpation should be performed with an approximate force of 4 kg.
For a tender point to be considered "positive" the subject must state that the palpation was painful. "Tender" is not to be considered "painful."

From Wolfe F et al: *Arthritis Rheum* 33:160, 1990.
*For classification purposes, patients will be said to have fibromyalgia if both criteria are satisfied. Widespread pain must have been present for at least 3 months. The presence of a second clinical disorder does not exclude the diagnosis of fibromyalgia.

don may result in calcium deposits, primarily in the form of calcium hydroxyapatite. *Calcific tendinitis,* as this condition is called, is hypothesized to result from the combination of diminished blood supply and recurrent trauma. *Bursitis* is an inflammation of a synovial-lined sac located at sites of maximum movement of tendons over bones. Like tendinitis, bursitis is often triggered by repetitive or excessive use. Often the process is indolent, but the bursa may become inflamed as part of a systemic inflammatory disorder. Gout and pseudogout, as well as bacterial infection, can produce a dramatic acute bursitis, whereas the chronic inflammatory arthritides may cause subacute bursitis. A swollen, inflamed bursa should always be aspirated and the fluid examined for monosodium urate or calcium pyrophosphate dihydrate crystals (see Chapter 183). Microbiologic studies are always advisable when large numbers of leukocytes are present.

The shoulder, because of its complex anatomy (Fig. 190-2), is particularly susceptible to multiple forms of periarthritis. *Bicipital tendinitis* is common and generally readily recognized. It is triggered by heavy lifting or repetitive movements affecting the long head of the biceps. Typically bicipital tendinitis becomes evident as pain or aching over the anterior shoulder and upper arm. Examination reveals tenderness along the tendon, particularly as it passes through the bicipital groove. The result of Speed's test, the sharp exacerbation of pain on anterior flexion of the shoulder against resistance with the arm outstretched in supination, is usually positive. *Rotator cuff tendinitis* is a more complex common cause of shoulder pain. It occurs after overuse of the shoulders, particularly with the arms over the head. The supraspinatus tendon, an essential part of the rotator cuff mechanism, is injured as a result of its impingement between the head

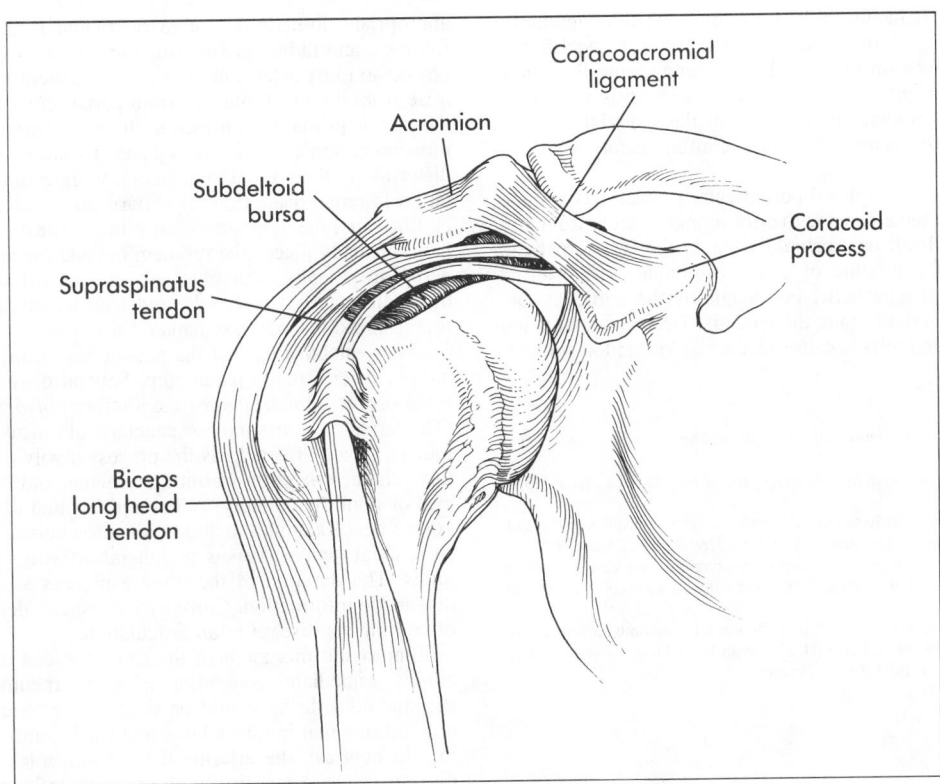

FIGURE 190-2   Anatomic relationships among periarticular structures of the shoulder. Note the susceptibility of the subdeltoid bursa and supraspinatus tendon to impingement between the humerus and the acromion and coracoacromial ligament when the arm is raised over the head.

of the humerus and the acromion, which occurs as the arm is abducted. With this form of tendinitis deep palpation elicits tenderness that is maximal on the lateral aspect of the shoulder over the greater tuberosity and below the acromion. Other physical findings may include Neer's sign—pain on forward flexion of a partially internally rotated humerus with forearm in pronation—and Hawkins' sign—abduction of the fully internally-rotated humerus. The supraspinatus tendon is the most frequent site of calcific tendinitis. Deposits of calcium hydroxyapatite accumulate in the region of the tendon where there is maximal stress from the shoulder impingement syndrome.

The shoulder is also the site of the most common examples of bursal inflammation, namely *subacromial* or *subdeltoid bursitis*. Physical findings often mimic those of rotator cuff tendinitis, and in fact bursitis and tendinitis tend to coexist. These subacute forms of inflammation in the periarticular tissues of the shoulder usually show no visible signs of inflammation. Indeed, if swelling, redness, and heat are detected, infection or crystal-induced disease is likely to be present. *Adhesive capsulitis* may be a sequela of unresolved tendinitis and bursitis at the shoulder. In this condition there is thickening of the capsule with adhesion to the underlying humerus, producing a markedly restricted range of motion often called a "frozen shoulder." Adhesive capsulitis can result from any condition that leads to prolonged immobilization of the shoulder. In addition to markedly restricted active and passive range of motion, there is diffuse tenderness around the shoulder. Arthrography documents a constricted capsule and reduced volume of the joint space. Once developed, stretching the capsule with intraarticular injections of a local anesthetic and nonabsorbable corticosteroids may hasten improvement and permit gradually advancing range-of-motion exercises.

At the elbow the olecranon bursa is susceptible to all of the potential pathogenic mechanisms that produce bursitis. In many cases a bland effusion is present, presumably attributable to trauma, although the injury may be unrecognized by the patient. An inflammatory effusion in the bursa may occur in rheumatoid arthritis (particularly in patients with rheumatoid nodules), acute gout, and infection. Tendi-

nitis at the elbow occurs directly at the site of attachment of tendons to the lateral or medial epicondyles. The extensor muscles to the hand insert laterally and the flexors medially. Tendinitis at the lateral epicondyle is more common. It is often called *tennis elbow* and results from repetitive, forceful extension at the wrist. The opposite motion, forceful flexion, leads to *golfer's elbow* or tendinitis at the medial epicondyle.

A common form of tendinitis occurring near the wrist is called *De Quervain's tenosynovitis*. It is an inflammation of the abductor pollicis longus and extensor pollicis brevis tendons of the thumb at the site where they pass over the medial end of the radius. Finkelstein's test, which triggers exquisite pain by ulnar deviation of the wrist while the flexed thumb is gripped by the fingers, is an important diagnostic finding.

The hip is the site of *trochanteric bursitis* localized to the bursa that underlies the insertion of the gluteal muscles into the lateral and posterior portions of the greater trochanter. Often there is no clear precipitating event, but it can occur with chronic irritation to the region as a result of leg-length discrepancy, persistent running across a slope, or repetitive use of the hip to push doors or other objects. Trochanteric bursitis becomes evident as pain on the lateral aspect of the hip, often radiating toward the knee. There is local tenderness at the edge of the greater trochanter, and the pain is aggravated by lying on the affected side.

Two common types of bursitis occur in the knee region. Prepatellar bursitis, commonly called *housemaid's knee*, produces pain in the front of the knee aggravated by bending the knee. A fluid collection is usually apparent directly over the patella. *Anserine bursitis* causes pain below the tibia-femoral articulation on the medial aspect of the knee. The anserine bursa underlies the insertion of the gracilis, sartorius, and semitendinosus muscles into the anteromedial condyle of the tibia. Pain from anserine bursitis is aggravated when climbing stairs. Palpation over the region of the bursa produces pain.

The most common periarticular problems about the ankle relate to the Achilles tendon. Achilles tendinitis occurs in long-distance runners or as part of a systemic inflammatory disorder, particularly the spondyloarthropathies (Chapter 200). Less often, Achilles tendinitis may be a symptom of gout or pseudogout. The retrocalcaneal bursa, which underlies the insertion of the Achilles's tendon into the calcaneus, can also become inflamed. Retrocalcaneal bursitis can occur from pressure from tight shoes or as a part of the synovial involvement of rheumatoid arthritis and other chronic inflammatory arthropathies.

Treatment for all of the regional periarticular problems is similar. It includes rest of the affected area with only enough exercise to maintain range of motion, local heat or cold as preferred by the patient, and local injection of a mixture of a nonabsorbable corticosteroid preparation and a local anesthetic. For tendinitis the corticosteroid should be injected around, not into, the tendons. This treatment is not advised for Achilles tendinitis because of the risk of tendon rupture.

BIBLIOGRAPHY

Bennett RM: Fibromyalgia: the commonest cause of widespread pain. *Compr Ther* 21:269, 1995.
Doherty M et al: *Rheumatology examination and injection techniques,* London, 1992, WB Saunders.
Frieman BG, Albert TJ, Fenlin JM: Rotation cuff disease: a review of diagnosis, pathophysiology, and current trends in treatment, *Arch Phys Med Rehabil* 75:604, 1994.
Wolfe F et al: The American College of Rheumatology criteria for the classification of fibromyalgia: report of the Multicenter Criteria Committee, *Arthritis Rheum* 33:160, 1990.
Yunus MB, Masi AT: Fibromyalgia, restless legs syndrome, periodic limb movement disorder, and psychogenic pain. In McCarty DJ, Koopman WJ, editors: *Arthritis and allied conditions,* Philadelphia, 1993, Lea & Febiger.

CHAPTER

191 Evaluation of Joint Complaints

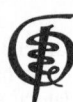

Nathan J. Zvaifler

Arthritis is a symptom. Indeed, patients may develop joint complaints during the course of more than 100 different illnesses. The relevance of this symptom and recognition of its cause usually can be ascertained in the course of a careful history and physical examination. The scheme shown in Fig. 191-1 is an approach that the author has found useful. It categorizes musculoskeletal complaints in a manner that leads to a proper diagnosis in most instances when combined with

appropriate observations of extraarticular manifestations, laboratory findings, and radiologic investigation. In the initial confrontation the physician must determine whether the patient's rheumatic symptoms arise from involved joints or from periarticular tissues. In the former, the pain is primarily confined to the articulation and is aggravated by movement or use of the affected part. Examination often demonstrates distortion of the normal joint anatomy, signs of inflammation, or limitation in range of motion. In periarthritis, such as tendinitis, bursitis, or fibrositis, the symptoms can mimic arthritis, but physical examination usually places the problem beyond the articulation. Moreover, periarthritis tends to involve only one, or a few, of the larger joints but spares the wrists, hands, and feet, which so often participate in true arthritic disorders, (Chapter 190).

After establishing that the patient has arthritis, recognition of the *pattern* of arthritis is paramount. Several distinctions are necessary: is the process *monarticular* (one joint) or *polyarticular* (many joints)? (The terms *oligoarticular* or pauciarticular usually imply that two to four joints are affected.) Is the process involving the joint inflammatory (characterized by warmth, erythema, and boggy synovial swelling) or noninflammatory? What is the actual distribution of joint involvement? Examples include symmetric versus asymmetric joint disease, axial (spinal) versus peripheral arthritis, or large versus small joints. The duration of the disease process also provides important diagnostic information. *Chronicity* is usually defined as 6 to 8 weeks of continuous disease in an articulation.

Employing this method, the examiner can develop a profile that allows immediate recognition of many rheumatic disorders. Thus rheumatoid arthritis would be described as a chronic inflammatory polyarthritis that involves large and small joints in a symmetric fashion. In contrast, the arthritis that accompanies inflammatory bowel disease is characteristically short-lived, inflammatory, and oligoarticular or polyarticular, but asymmetric and with a propensity to involve the large joints of the lower extremities.

The scheme outlined in Fig. 191-1, which places particular emphasis on recognition of inflammatory joint disease and the distribution of involvement, is similar to the approach presented in the examination of synovial fluid (Chapter 183) and in the radiologic evaluation of arthritis described in Chapter 184. The reader is encouraged to refer to these chapters.

MONARTICULAR DISEASE

Monarthritis can be acute or chronic. It is essential, however, that all monarticular arthritis be considered to be infectious arthritis until proved otherwise, because failure to recognize a pyogenic arthritis may result in permanent joint injury. Furthermore, and perhaps more important, most bacterial infections of joints are derived from the

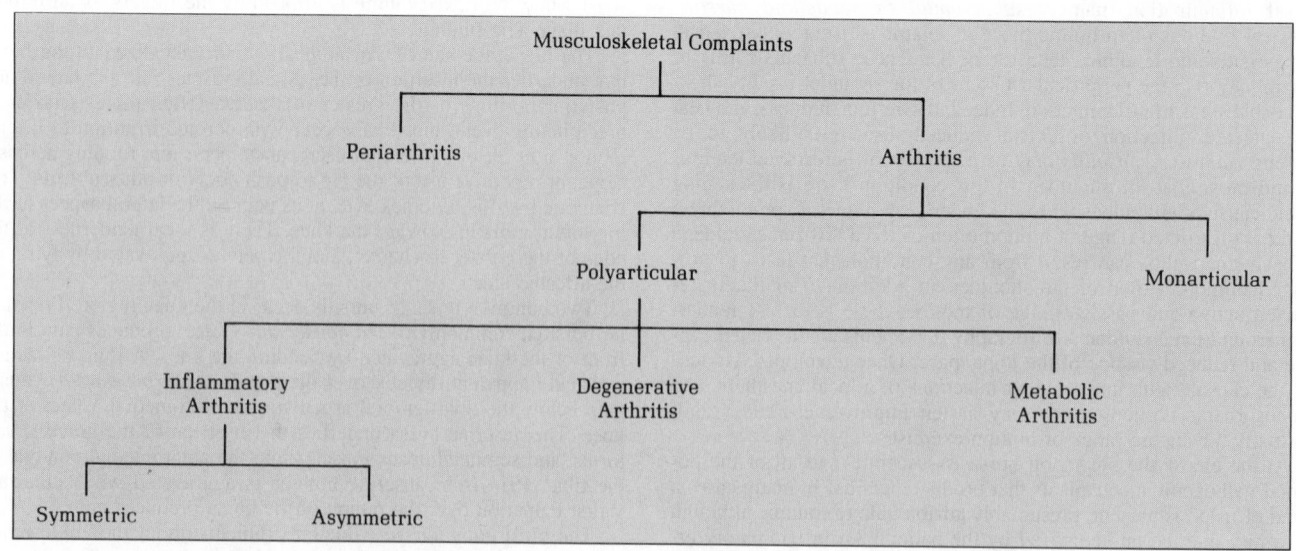

FIGURE 191-1   Systematic evaluation of musculoskeletal complaints.

BOX 191-1

Causes of monarthritis

Infection*, †, or ‡
Crystal-induced†
Trauma†
Hemarthrosis†,‡
Foreign body‡
Pigmented villonodular synovitis‡
Joint neoplasms‡
Aseptic necrosis‡
Osteochondritis dissecans‡
Mechanical internal derangement†,‡
Sarcoidosis‡
Neuropathic (Charcot's) joint†,‡
Onset of polyarthritis†,‡

*The most important diagnosis.
†Acute.
‡Chronic.

BOX 191-2

Causes of polyarthritis: Metabolic (deposition) joint diseases

Gouty tophi*
Calcium pyrophosphate dihydrate deposition disease*
Hydroxyapatite crystalline arthritis
Amyloidosis
Hyperlipidemia
Multicentric reticulohistiocytosis

*The most important diagnoses.

BOX191-3

Causes of polyarthritis: Degenerative joint diseases

Primary generalized (erosive) osteoarthritis*
Secondary osteoarthritis*
Calcium pyrophosphate dihydrate deposition disease
Neuropathic joint disease
Hyperparathyroidism
Acromegaly
Hemochromatosis
Wilson's disease
Ochronosis
Osteodystrophies
Heritable disorders of connective tissue

*The most important diagnoses.

---

bloodstream; therefore, coexistent foci of infection and septicemia are usually present. Any very painful joint may be septic. Once infectious arthritis is suspected, the diagnosis is suggested by the finding of an inflammatory joint fluid, often with more than 50,000 polymorphonuclear leukocytes per cubic millimeter, and confirmed by positive Gram's stain and/or culture. After infection the next most important condition to recognize is crystal-induced monarthritis. The diagnosis is easily made by microscopic examination of the synovial effusion and demonstration of the characteristic shape and birefringence of monosodium urate or calcium pyrophosphate dihydrate (CPPD) crystals. There are many other less common causes of acute and chronic monarthritis (Box 191-1). It is also important to recognize that disorders normally characterized by polyarthritis may begin in a monarticular form. This is particularly true of rheumatoid arthritis, and, occasionally, observation for many months may be required before the disease assumes its typical appearance.

POLYARTICULAR DISEASES

Polyarthritis can be divided into arthritides that are degenerative (generally noninflammatory), inflammatory, or metabolic in origin. The last-mentioned (Box 191-2) are most diverse. For example, chronic tophaceous gout may involve large or small joints in an asymmetric (usual) or symmetric (less common) fashion, whereas CPPD deposition disease may mimic a severe form of osteoarthritis, often in unusual locations such as the wrist, have a symmetric rheumatoid-like pattern, or appear as a degenerative process limited to one or a few weight-bearing joints. The joint symptoms of metabolic disease are usually caused by the deposition of materials in and around articulations; these deposits often give the joint an unusual configuration that is easily appreciated on physical examination. Thus deposits of monosodium urate (tophi) or lipid in capsular structures or tendons

tend to give the joint a lumpy, bumpy, asymmetric appearance, contrasting with the usually smooth contour produced by conventional inflammatory synovitis. Amyloid infiltration of the shoulders makes them seem unusually large and bulky (the shoulder-pad sign). In the rare destructive arthropathy known as *multicentric reticulohistiocytosis,* granulomas form about the nail beds or over the eyelids, where they may be confused with xanthelasma.

Degenerative Polyarthritis

The prototype of the degenerative form of polyarthritis is primary generalized osteoarthritis (Box 191-3). This disorder characteristically affects women around the time of menopause and involves the distal and proximal interphalangeal joints, the carpometacarpal articulation at the base of the thumb, and the hips, knees, lumbar spine, and first tarsometatarsal (bunion) joints. Symptoms are limited to individual joints and in the fingers may be accompanied by short episodes of redness and pain followed by the development of asymmetric, bony-hard swelling about the affected articulation. When present in the distal interphalangeal finger joints, these bony spurs are called *Heberden's nodes;* at the proximal articulation, *Bouchard's nodes.* Radiographs confirm the degenerative, osteosclerotic nature of the process, although erosions may be present, and synovial fluid examination discloses normal or only minimally cellular effusions.

Although the joints are affected one by one, the accumulation of irreversible changes may, in the end, produce a pattern that appears bilateral and symmetric. This is especially true in the hands, where the changes may be confused with rheumatoid arthritis unless careful attention is given to the additive, progressive manner in which the joint deformities develop. Similar deformities can develop in the absence of any inflammatory component. Secondary forms of osteoarthritis may be limited to a few joints when they are the result of trauma or may be widespread when they reflect metabolic abnormalities that influence the integrity of cartilage. The complicating joint injuries seen in athletes and industrial workers or the exaggerated degeneration that accompanies neurologic lesions are examples of the former; the arthropathy of acromegaly, hyperparathyroidism, hemochromatosis, and ochronosis are examples of the latter.

Inflammatory Polyarthritis

The causes of inflammatory polyarthritis are many (Table 191-1). In some, arthritis is the dominant feature, whereas in others it is merely one manifestation of a systemic disorder. The proper distinction of this group of diseases is facilitated by recognition of the duration of the inflammatory polyarthritis as well as the typical distribution of involved joints. For example, both rubella and acute infectious hepatitis can present with symmetric, inflammatory swellings of the proximal and metacarpophalangeal joints in a picture indistinguishable from that of rheumatoid arthritis. One reaches a correct diagnosis by recognizing that neither rubella arthritis nor the articular manifesta-

Table 191-1   Causes of polyarthritis: Inflammatory joint disease

	COURSE			DISTRIBUTION	
CAUSE	ACUTE	INTERMITTENT	CHRONIC	SYMMETRIC	ASYMMETRIC
Rheumatoid arthritis*		±	+	+	±
Systemic lupus erythematosus*		±	+	+	
Other connective tissue diseases		±	±	+	
Crystal deposition diseases		±	+	+	±
Neisserial infection	+			±	+
Hepatitis B	+		±	+	
Rubella	+			+	
Lyme arthritis	±	+	±		+
Bacterial endocarditis	+			+	±
Rheumatic fever	+			+	±
Erythema nodosum	+	±		+	±
Sarcoidosis	+	+	±	+	+
Hypersensitivity to serum or drugs	+	±		+	+
Henoch-Schönlein purpura	+			±	+
Relapsing polychondritis	±	+	±	+	+
Juvenile (rheumatoid) polyarthritis	±	±	+	+	+
Hypertrophic pulmonary osteoarthropathy	±		+	+	
Ankylosing spondylitis*		±	+	±	+
Reiter's disease*	±	±	±	±	+
Enteropathic arthropathy*	±	+	±	±	+
Psoriatic arthritis*		±	+	+	+
Reactive arthritis	+	±	±	±	+
Behçet's disease	±	+	±		+
Familial Mediterranean fever	±	+	±		+
Whipple's disease	±	+	±		+
Palindromic rheumatism		+		±	+

*The most important diagnosis.
+, Most common; ±, less common.

tions of acute infectious hepatitis persist more than a few weeks. Indeed, although rheumatoid arthritis may be difficult to diagnose correctly, especially early in its course, chronicity is a primary feature. Finally, however, it is the development of an inflammatory, bilateral, symmetric polyarthritis affecting both the large and small joints that distinguishes rheumatoid arthritis from the other important group of inflammatory polyarticular diseases, the spondyloarthropathies (Table 191-1).

A number of other disorders may mimic the pattern of rheumatoid arthritis. Most prominent among these are the connective tissue diseases, especially systemic lupus erythematosus (SLE). In general, their less-destructive nature and their accompanying systemic features allow them to be recognized. Thus the distinctive skin rashes, the polyserositis, and the hematologic, central nervous system, and renal abnormalities of SLE point the way to the correct diagnosis. So, too, do the thick skin, Raynaud's phenomenon, sclerodactylia, telangiectasia, calcinosis, and esophageal and gastrointestinal disturbances of scleroderma. Dermatomyositis is suggested by the typical edematous, dusky, violaceous, periorbital, and malar rash and by the symmetric weakness and occasional atrophy of the proximal muscles of the limb girdle, the neck, and the pharynx.

Other members of this group may have distinctive disease manifestations, such as the painful, necrotic pustules of gonococcemia, the palpable purpura of hypersensitivity angiitis or Henoch-Schönlein purpura, the tender pretibial erythematous nodules of erythema nodosum or erythema chronicum migrans, the hallmark of Lyme arthritis. The findings of clubbed fingers or floppy ears and saddlenose should alert the physician to hypertrophic osteoarthropathy and relapsing polychondritis, respectively.

The spondyloarthropathies, as the name implies, comprise a disparate group of diseases that share the features of an asymmetric, oligoarthritis or polyarthritis that favors the large joints of the lower extremities. They affect men predominantly. Periostitis, a characteristic radiologic feature often seen along the shafts of the digits, has its counterpart in the beefy, swollen toes (dactylitis, or "sausage toes") noted in patients with Reiter's disease and psoriatic arthritis and, less frequently, in the enteropathic or reactive joint diseases. Sacroiliitis and inflammatory disease of the apophyseal joints of the lumbar, tho-

racic, and cervical spine are regular features of ankylosing spondylitis; they affect many persons with Reiter's disease and a greater than expected (by chance alone) number of patients with psoriasis, reactive arthritis, and the various forms of inflammatory bowel disease. An association with the human leukocyte antigen haplotype B27 is seen in those who have spondylitis. Psoriatic arthritis may involve the distal joints of the fingers; almost invariably, however, the contiguous nail shows psoriatic changes, which facilitate the distinction from inflammatory (erosive) forms of generalized osteoarthritis.

BIBLIOGRAPHY

American College of Rheumatology Ad Hoc Committee on Clinical Guidelines: Guidelines for the initial evaluation of the adult patient with acute musculoskeletal symptoms, *Arthritis Rheum* 39:1, 1996.

Arnett FC et al: The American Rheumatism Association 1987 revised criteria for the classification of rheumatoid arthritis, *Arthritis Rheum* 31:315, 1988.

Gall EP: Evaluation of the patient: history and physical examination. In Schumacher HR Jr, editor: *Primer on the rheumatic diseases,* ed 10, Atlanta, 1993, Arthritis Foundation.

CHAPTER

192   Rheumatoid Arthritis

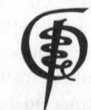

Nathan J. Zvaifler

Rheumatoid arthritis (RA) is a chronic systemic disorder with its primary manifestations in the joints. The causes and origins of RA remain obscure, although the pathogenesis is increasingly well understood. The disease is ubiquitous, occurs in both sexes (favoring women 3:1), and is seen in all parts of the world. Rural populations seem to be less affected than urban dwellers, and the disease may be more severe in developed countries. Variability is seen not only in populations but also in individuals. In epidemiologic studies, for instance, RA appears to be a modest and often remitting disease, whereas, when studied in the clinic, it is usually characterized by a relentless, progressive, destructive course. Patients who have a positive serologic test result for an antibody in the bloodstream known as rheumatoid factor (RF) and a particular genetic predisposition will display all the features of the prototype disease called RA. There is a significant concordance of disease in identical twins, but an analysis of families with more than one affected member suggests that RA is polygenic. Moreover, since genetic susceptibility accounts for only about 30% of the risk, there must be other important environmental factors, including an infectious origin. However, almost 80% of patients with seropositive (i.e., RF-positive) RA carry specific class II major histocompatibility complex (MHC) molecules, either human leukocyte antigen (HLA)-DR1 or HLA-DR4 (Dw4, Dw14, Dw15 haplotypes) (see Chapter 172). Genes for the HLA-DR subregion encode one alpha chain but several polymorphic HLA-DR beta chains. The beta chains contain regions of remarkable hypervariability, particularly in the amino acid sequences surrounding position 70 of the first domain of the HLA-DR β1 chain. Each of the haplotypes associated with susceptibility to RA have similar amino acids at positions 70 to 74.

In a susceptibility model these shared epitopes would be involved in disease induction, but evidence is accumulating that HLA-DR β1 genes represent severity markers and predict outcome in RA. The development of erosive and seropositive (RF) disease is almost an invariable accompaniment of these disease-associated gene sequences. Patients with extraarticular disease generally carry two disease-linked HLA-DR β1 alleles, whereas those with only moderate disease show one copy of the disease-linked sequence. An important reservation concerning the significance of the HLA-DR β1 alleles comes from studies of African-Americans who have similar disease severity, frequency and amount of RF, nodules, and radiographic evidence of cartilage and bone erosions to their white counterparts. Despite this similarity, African-Americans with RA have a low frequency of the rheumatoid epitope, and it is RF positivity, not the presence or the dose of the rheumatoid epitope, that explains disease severity.

The earliest events in RA are difficult to document, but the available evidence suggests that microvascular injury and mild synovial cell proliferation are the first lesions. The changes are probably nonspecific, since they are seen in other acute inflammatory joint diseases.

In established RA the tissues that line the joint (synovium) appear edematous and protrude into the joint cavity as slender villous projections. Light microscope examination discloses a characteristic, but not pathognomonic, constellation of histologic changes, including hyperplasia and hypertrophy of the synovial lining cells and focal or segmental vascular changes; in addition, the connective tissue stroma of the synovial villous, which normally has few cells, is packed with mononuclear cells, some collected into aggregates, particularly around small blood vessels (Fig. 192-1). Lymphocytes predominate in these follicles, with a mantle of plasma cells about their periphery. Multinucleated giant cells, when present, are usually in areas of synovial lining–cell hyperplasia. Abundant fibrinlike material is deposited on the synovial cell surface and in the intracellular matrix.

The rheumatoid synovium contains large amounts of immunoglobulin when examined by immunofluorescent technique. Deposits of immunoglobulin G (IgG) and immunoglobulin M (IgM), alone or in combination, are demonstrable in synovial lining cells, blood vessels, and the interstitial connective tissues. A significant number of the plasma cells in the rheumatoid synovium make an IgG RF that combines in the cytoplasm with similar IgG molecules ("self-associating IgG"), and de novo immunoglobulin synthesis can be demonstrated in rheumatoid synovial explants or continuous cultures of lymphocytes from synovium. Based on these findings, two pathogenetic mechanisms have been advanced to explain rheumatoid synovitis. The first—the "extravascular immune-complex hypothesis"—proposes an interaction of antigens and antibodies in synovial tissues and fluid. The antibodies are, in general, locally produced, especially the self-associating dimers and higher multiples of the IgG–anti-IgG complex. Other potentially important complexes are those in which the antigens are constituents of articular tissues or by-products of the inflammatory

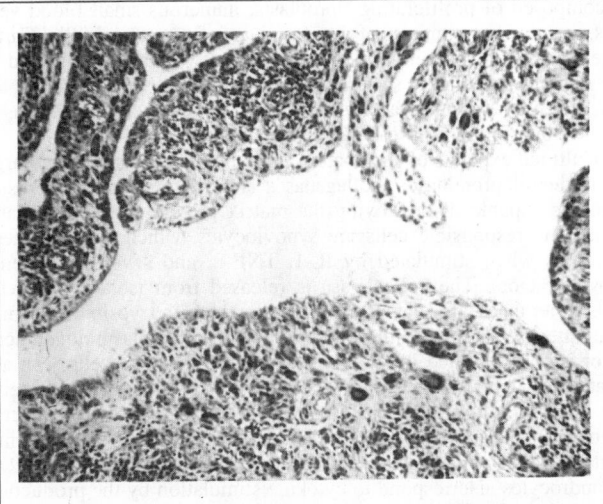

FIGURE 192-1 Active rheumatoid synovitis from a patient with seropositive rheumatoid arthritis. The redundant hypertrophic villous structures contain a dense infiltration of lymphocytes and occasional giant cells. The synovial lining cells are hyperplastic.

process—collagen, cartilage proteoglycans, fibrinogen or fibrin, partially digested IgG, and soluble nucleoproteins. Immune complexes that form in joint tissues activate the complement system, generating a number of biologically active products, which increase vascular permeability and allow an influx of serum proteins and cellular blood elements into the site where the complexes reside. In the articular cavity, polymorphonuclear leukocytes attracted by complement-derived chemotactic factors ingest the complexes, with subsequent release of large quantities of hydrolytic enzymes and production of toxic O_2 and OH radicals and arachidonic acid metabolites. Each may participate in the inflammation and tissue damage.

In the second scenario RA joint disease results from cell-mediated damage. Beneath the lining cells of the synovial membrane, CD4+ (helper/inducer) memory lymphocytes accumulate in perivascular areas. Dispersed among them are antigen-presenting cells, macrophages, and dendritic cells. An expected consequence of their interaction is the elaboration of soluble factors that cause T-cell proliferation, differentiation of B-cells into antibody producers, and the production of other cytokines. Despite the predominance of lymphocytes, the cytokines found in the RA synovium are mainly factors produced by fibroblast-like lining cells and macrophages, such as interleukin-1 (IL-1) tumor necrosis factor alpha (TNF-α), IL-6, and granulocyte-macrophage colony-stimulating factor (GM-CSF), with a paucity of interleukins made by activated T-cells. Thus, although T lymphocytes appear to be critical for the initiation of synovitis, as the inflammation becomes chronic they may be anergized or down-regulated by factors in the microenvironment. Macrophages and synoviocytes, however, remain unopposed and free to express their proinflammatory and destructive potential (see later discussion). The large number of memory lymphocytes in the synovium might reflect either the presence of autoantigens within the joint (type II collagen, articular proteoglycans, and heat shock proteins are favorite candidates) or an increased binding of T-cells to adhesion molecules induced on the endothelium of postcapillary venules by inflammatory cytokines. The ligands for such adhesion molecules are expressed on all T-cells, but in significantly greater amounts or with greater avidity on many CD4 cells. Thus they preferentially accumulate and are also retained in the inflamed synovium by virtue of their cell surface expression of other integrins, which are receptors for matrix proteins (see Chapter 174).

Chronic RA is characterized by destruction of articular cartilage, ligaments, tendons, and bone. The damage results from a dual attack—from without by inflammatory molecules derived from phagocytic leukocytes in the synovial fluid—and from above and below by granulation tissue (pannus). This vascular granulation tissue is composed of proliferating fibroblasts, numerous small blood vessels, and various numbers of mononuclear inflammatory cells. Cartilage matrix collagen and proteoglycans are enzymatically digested in the region immediately surrounding nests of these cells. In other areas a dense avascular, acellular, fibrous type of pannus acts as a mantle, interfering with cartilage nutrition.

Cultured explants of rheumatoid synovial fragments produce large quantities of proteinases (collagenases and stromelysin) and prostaglandins capable of destroying the matrix proteins in cartilage and bone. The responsible cells are synoviocytes, which produce these materials when stimulated by IL-1, TNF-α, and several mitogenic growth factors. The collagenase is released from isolated synovial cells in an inactive or latent form. Treatment with trypsin or plasmin (the latter is potentially important in vivo because plasminogen activator is demonstrated in cultured rheumatoid synovial cells) can activate the latent enzyme. Synoviocytes also produce metalloproteinase inhibitors, and inflammatory synovial fluid contains α_2 macroglobulins. These are potent inhibitors of collagenase, but these important regulatory mechanisms appear to be overwhelmed in RA. Chondrocytes also respond to cytokine stimulation by the production of proteinases and are probable participants in cartilage destruction. Some work suggests that chondrocytes can transform and become a fibrous type of pannus.

Using these observations the following scheme of joint destruction has been proposed. Inflammation of the synovium alters the display of adhesion molecules on the endothelium of small synovial blood vessels. These engage circulating blood cells, allowing them to accumulate in the joint. The lymphocytes and macrophage in the synovium, individually or in concert, release soluble products that cause tissue inflammation, further permeability of synovial blood vessels, and the production of proteinases and prostaglandins by synovial cells and chondrocytes. The proliferation and overgrowth of synoviocytes under the influence of these cytokines lead to irreversible damage of joint structures.

Extraarticular Manifestations of Rheumatoid Arthritis

The cause of the various vascular and parenchymal lesions of RA and their relation to one another have not been defined. A number of observations suggest that the lesions result from injury induced by circulating immune complexes. Anti–gamma globulins of the IgG and IgM classes, as well as IgG, are integral parts of these complexes. Their presence correlates somewhat with the severity of articular and extraarticular manifestations, but whether they are responsible for these changes or are merely markers for severe rheumatoid disease remains a question.

CLINICAL FEATURES

Rheumatoid arthritis is a highly variable disease, ranging from a mild pauciarticular illness of brief duration to a relentlessly progressive, destructive polyarthritis associated with a systemic vasculitis. The extent of articular involvement correlates poorly with constitutional symptoms and extraarticular manifestations, but both destructive arthritis and extraarticular features are more common in patients whose serum contains high titers of RFs (see Chapter 182).

Joint Disease

Rheumatoid arthritis often begins with prodromal symptoms such as fatigue, anorexia, weakness, and generalized aching and stiffness that is not clearly localized to articular structures. Joint symptoms usually appear gradually over weeks to months. Occasionally there are brief, remittent episodes of articular involvement before the development of more persistent arthritis, and approximately 20% of patients have an abrupt onset, with rapid development of polyarthritis that is often accompanied by severe constitutional symptoms.

Articular involvement is manifested on clinical examination by pain, stiffness, limitation of motion, and the signs of inflammation, that is, swelling, warmth, erythema, and tenderness. Difficulty in making a fist, poor grip strength, and morning stiffness lasting more than 30 minutes (and frequently several hours) are characteristic of RA. Joint

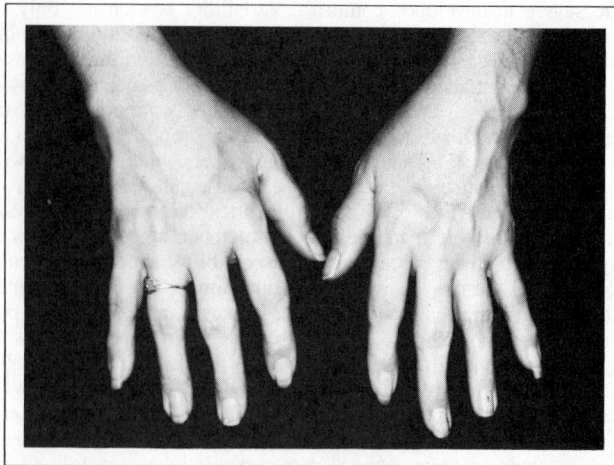

FIGURE 192-2 Early changes of rheumatoid arthritis in the hands, showing swelling, mainly limited to the proximal interphalangeal joints.

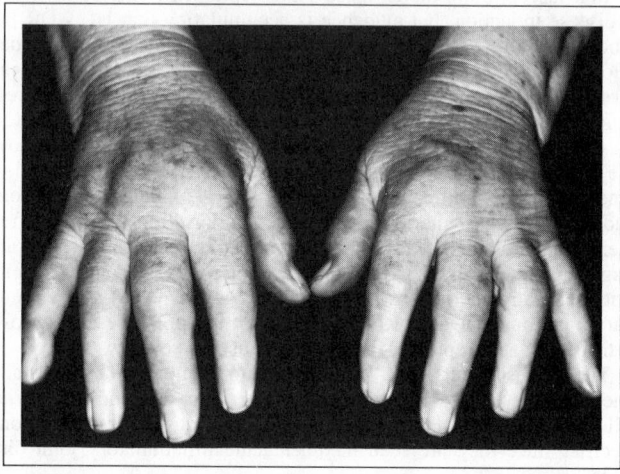

FIGURE 192-3 Advanced changes in the hand. Swelling and synovial hypertrophy are predominantly in the metacarpophalangeal articulations, especially the second and third; the early flexion contractures of the fingers are evident.

swelling results from synovial hypertrophy, thickening of the joint capsule, and frequently from an increase in the volume of synovial fluid. Initially pain limits motion, but later, capsular fibrosis, bony or fibrous ankylosis, and soft tissue contracture become responsible.

Rheumatoid arthritis can affect any diarthrodial joint; those most commonly involved initially are the small joints of the hands or feet, the wrists, and the knees. At the outset there may be any pattern of joint disease, although usually it is bilateral and polyarticular. In a small percentage of patients the disease remains unilateral or monarticular (commonly the knees) for periods of months to years. As the disease becomes established, the arthritis spreads to the elbows, shoulders, hips, ankles, and subtalar and sternoclavicular joints. Less often, the temporomandibular and cricoarytenoid joints are affected. Spinal involvement usually is limited to the upper cervical articulations.

Joint examination early in the disease reveals fusiform (spindle-shaped) swelling of the proximal interphalangeal (PIP) joints (Fig. 192-2). This swelling may diminish after a few years. Bilateral, symmetric swelling of the metacarpophalangeal (MCP) joints, particularly the second and third, is very common and remains long after PIP joint inflammation has subsided (Fig. 192-3). The distal interphalangeal (DIP) joints more often are spared. As the disease progresses, characteristic hand deformities develop, including ulnar deviation of the digits, hyperextension at the PIP joints with flexion at the DIP joints ("swan's neck" deformity), or a flexion deformity of the PIP joints, with extension of the DIP joints ("boutonniere" deformity). Rheumatoid involvement of the thumb causes hyperextension at the interphalangeal joints and flexion of the MCP joints with a resultant loss of pinch. Tenosynovitis is a cardinal feature of RA. A sudden loss of ability to extend the fingers—especially the third, fourth, and fifth digits—follows rupture of the extensor tendons or their dislocation into the intermetacarpal space.

Wrist disease is an almost invariable accompaniment of RA. Synovial hypertrophy and tenosynovitis on the volar aspect may compress the median nerve beneath the transverse carpal ligament, producing a "carpal tunnel syndrome," with paresthesia and dysesthesia of the thumb, the second and third digits, and the radial aspect of the fourth finger. Late in the disease, wrist immobility develops, and pronation and supination may be severely limited.

Flexion contractures of the elbow are frequent, even at an early stage of the disease. Shoulder involvement is not uncommon. Examination generally reveals limitation of motion together with tenderness just below and lateral to the coracoid process. Swelling is rarely seen.

Rheumatoid arthritis of the hip joints is less common, develops late in the illness, and is characterized by discomfort in the groin or buttocks. Hip disease may be recognized only because of gait abnormalities or limitation of joint motion. Aseptic necrosis of the femoral head, perhaps related to corticosteroid therapy, produces identical findings.

The knee joint is commonly affected, displaying synovial hypertrophy, chronic effusion, and, later, ligamentous laxity. A regular accompaniment of knee involvement is quadriceps atrophy, often of great severity. Pathologic enlargement of the normal gastrocnemius-semimembranosus bursa (Baker's cyst) may compress structures behind the knee, causing discomfort. Occasionally the bursa dissects or ruptures, giving rise to symptoms and signs mimicking acute thrombophlebitis. Arthrography usually confirms the diagnosis (Fig. 192-4) and should be performed in any patient with RA in whom acute unilateral tenderness, warmth, or edema of the lower leg (pseudophlebitis) develops.

Arthritis in the feet and ankles creates a number of vexing problems. Limited flexion and extension of the foot results from disease of the mortise joint, subtalar involvement impairs eversion and inversion, and pain on walking may result from bursitis beneath the insertion of the Achilles tendon into the calcaneus. In the foot proper, synovitis of the metatarsophalangeal (MTP) joints is particularly common, whereas interphalangeal joint involvement is less usual. Subluxation of the metatarsal heads, hallux valgus, and lateral deviation and clawing of the toes develop with progression of the disease.

In RA, intermittent cervical spine pain and stiffness are frequent, whereas neurologic complications are rare. Symptoms may result from spinal cord compression by anterior dislocation of the first cervical vertebra, by vertical subluxation of the odontoid process of the second vertebra, or by torsion and compression of the vertebral arteries, which causes vertebrobasilar insufficiency and syncope on downward gaze. Headache, a frequent complaint, is most commonly occipital but occasionally radiates over the top of the cranium. Neck examination discloses localized tenderness, muscle spasm, and limitation of rotary motion with retention of flexion and extension.

Extraarticular Manifestations

Systemic features of RA (Box 192-1) are frequent but usually occult and of limited clinical significance. Occasionally, however, they dominate the clinical picture.

Rheumatoid Nodules. At some time, subcutaneous nodules appear in 15% to 20% of patients as firm, nontender, rounded, or oval masses in the subcutaneous or deeper connective tissues, varying in size from less than 0.5 cm to several centimeters in diameter. Areas subjected to mechanical pressure are common sites, especially the olecranon and extensor surface of the forearms and the Achilles tendon. Unusual locations include the pleura, meninges, ears, and bridge of the nose. Subcutaneous nodules seldom cause symptoms, but they occasionally break down or become infected and may be overlooked

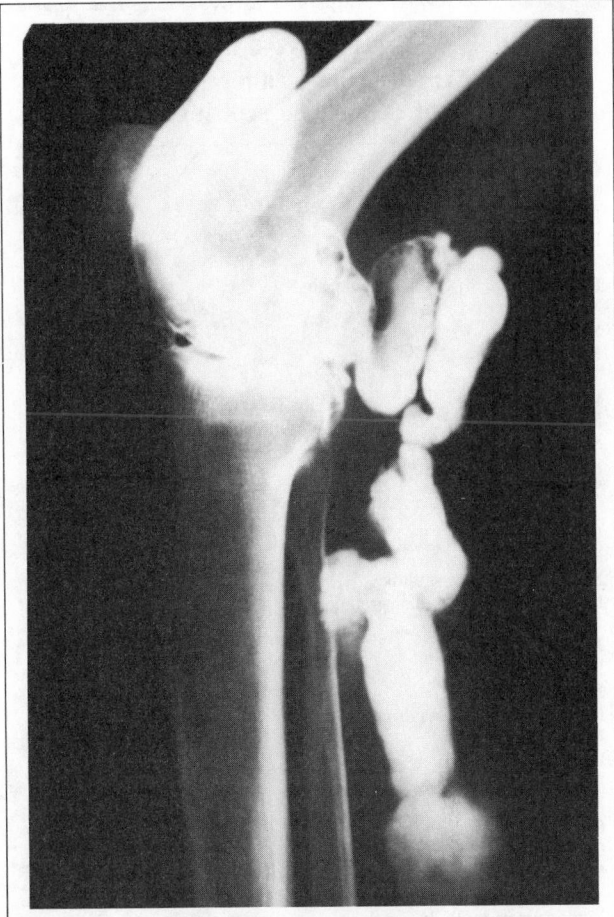

FIGURE 192-4   Dissecting popliteal (Baker's) cyst. Arthrogram of the knee in lateral projection demonstrating dissection of radiocontrast material into the lower leg.

as portals for bacteremia and septic arthritis. Typically they develop insidiously and persist, but regression is possible at any time. Because they are almost invariably found in patients with seropositive disease, rheumatoid nodules portend a more severe and destructive arthritis.

Vasculitis. Rheumatoid arthritis has a spectrum of vascular lesions: capillaritis and venulitis, which are thought to be important in the development of rheumatoid nodules and synovitis; a bland intimal proliferation commonly affecting digital and mesenteric vessels; subacute lesions of arterioles and venules in scattered locations; and an acute, widespread, necrotizing ateritis of small- and medium-sized arteries that may be indistinguishable from polyarteritis nodosum. This most severe form of rheumatoid vasculitis, designated *rheumatoid arteritis,* characteristically produces polyneuropathy, skin necrosis and ulceration, digital gangrene, ulceration or perforation of the nasal septum, and visceral infarction. When present, the neuropathy takes the form of an acute sensorimotor mononeuritis (mononeuritis multiplex) with dropped foot or wrist and a patchy sensory loss in one or more extremities. Ischemic skin lesions appear in crops as small, brown spots (not unlike splinter hemorrhages) in the nail beds, nail folds, and digital pulp. Large ischemic ulcerations can develop in the lower extremities, particularly over the malleoli. Fatal intestinal and myocardial infarction have been reported. Fever, polymorphonuclear leukocytosis, and thrombocytosis are common. Many patients have concomitant episcleritis, scleromalacia, pleuritis, myocarditis, and/or pericarditis. The prognosis in the untreated, fulminant form of vasculitis is exceedingly poor. The full-blown picture is rare, and individual features can exist independently, persist for long periods, and pose little threat to life.

BOX 192-1
Extraarticular manifestations
of rheumatoid arthritis

Constitutional
Weight loss
Fever, sweats
Fatigue

Lymphadenopathy and splenomegaly
Nodules
Subcutaneous
Parenchymatous

Ocular
Episcleritis
Scleritis
Scleromalacia
Sjögren's syndrome

Cardiac
Pericarditis
Myocarditis and vasculitis
Endocardial and valvular granulomata

Pulmonary
Pleuritis
Interstitial fibrosis
Nodules: Caplan's syndrome
Fibrosing alveolitis
Bronchiolitis obliterans

Neurologic
Cord compression
Cerebral vasculitis
Entrapment neuropathies
Distal sensory neuropathy
Mononeuritis multiplex

Vasculitis
Cutaneous necrotizing vasculitis
Dermal infarcts
Periunguinal infarcts
Digital gangrene
Leg ulcers
Polyarteritis

Hematologic
Anemia
Eosinophilia
Felty's syndrome

Miscellaneous
Myositis
Amyloid
Osteoporosis

Neuropathy. Rheumatoid arthritis tends to spare the central nervous system but causes a number of abnormalities in peripheral nerves, including the severe sensorimotor neuropathy (mononeuritis multiplex) accompanying vasculitis; entrapment neuropathies of the median, ulnar, or anterior tibial nerves; and a mild, generally benign, symmetric distal sensory or sensorimotor neuropathy.

Myopathy. Weakness and atrophy of skeletal muscle are commonly observed in the absence of neurologic abnormalities and are most pronounced in muscle groups that cross involved joints. The cause is unknown. Biopsy specimens show nodular infiltrates of lymphocytes, reduction in skeletal muscle fiber number and circumference, and condensation of sarcolemmal nuclei. Electromyograms (EMGs) may display myopathic changes. Neither biopsy nor EMG correlates well with clinical observations. Muscle enzymes are usually normal. In rheumatoid patients with proximal muscle weakness

the possibility of steroid myopathy or chloroquine neuromyopathy should be considered.

Cardiac Manifestations. The most common symptomatic lesion is acute pericarditis, which appears most often in males with seropositive disease. An associated pleural effusion is often detected. Characteristics of both pericardial and pleural fluids are a low glucose concentration, increased lactic dehydrogenase and gamma globulin levels, and low complement activity. The course of the pericarditis is variable, ranging from a mild, self-limited process to cardiac tamponade and death. A good response to steroid therapy can be expected, but chronic effusion or constriction may ensue and necessitate pericardiectomy. Recurrences are not uncommon. Less common are granulomatous lesions that are similar on histologic study to rheumatoid nodules and involve the epicardium, myocardium, and valves; also uncommon are focal interstitial myocarditis and arteritis of coronary vessels. Occasionally, valvular insufficiency or conduction abnormalities may be recognized during life, and, rarely, myocardial infarction occurs as a manifestation of coronary arteritis.

Pleuropulmonary Manifestations. The respiratory symptoms encountered in most rheumatoid patients can usually be ascribed to more common disorders, but some pulmonary abnormalities seem to be intimately related to the rheumatoid process. They include (1) pleurisy with or without effusion, (2) nonpneumoconiotic intrapulmonary rheumatoid nodules, (3) rheumatoid pneumoconiosis (Caplan's syndrome), (4) diffuse interstitial fibrosis and pneumonitis, and (5) an involvement of the intima of small pulmonary arteries and arterioles that leads to pulmonary hypertension. Considerable overlap exists among these syndromes. Upper airway obstruction with hoarseness and stridor may result from cricoarytenoid arthritis, and bronchiolitis obliterans is a recognized complication. The presence of numerous rheumatoid nodules in the lungs of patients with a history of pneumoconiotic exposure and in whom RA develops is referred to as *rheumatoid pneumoconiosis, or Caplan's syndrome.* First described in Welsh soft-coal miners, the same phenomenon occurs in asbestos and ceramic workers, gold and chalk miners, and others with arthritis and an appropriate industrial exposure. Radiographs reveal multiple, well-defined nodular opacities (0.5 to 5.0 cm in diameter) widely distributed throughout the lungs or large numbers of smaller nodules that present a "snowstorm" appearance. Occasionally nodules coalesce into large conglomerate masses, and cavitation has been observed. Typical lesions sometimes antedate the development of RA, occasionally by years. Although usually unexplained, diffuse pneumonitis may be caused by treatment with gold, penicillamine, or methotrexate.

Ocular Manifestations. Rheumatoid disease uncommonly but characteristically is associated with inflammatory lesions of the episclera and sclera. Episcleritis is a relatively benign, transient condition that causes mild discomfort in the eyes but does not interfere with vision. Scleritis is more serious, can cause blindness, and may proceed as an indolent, slowly progressing process or as recurrent subacute episodes of ocular inflammation. Lesions usually originate in the superior sclerae, surrounded by hyperemia of the deep scleral vessels. Inflammation may spread to other layers of the eye, ciliary body, and retina, resulting in secondary complications. The histologic finding is that of a rheumatoid nodule, and the lesions are most often found in patients with high titers of RF and subcutaneous nodules.

The most common ocular abnormalities of RA (approximately 15% to 20% of patients) are the corneal and conjunctival lesions associated with Sjögren's syndrome. This syndrome, which is more properly viewed as a concomitant of, rather than as a manifestation of, rheumatoid disease, is presented in detail in Chapter 193.

Renal Involvement. The kidneys are remarkably spared in RA, although unexplained, mild proteinuria and occasional red blood cells (RBCs) in the urine sediment may be found. More often, renal abnormalities are a consequence of drug therapy (i.e., interstitial nephritis from nonsteroidal antiinflammatory drugs [NSAIDs], gold nephropathy, or penicillamine glomerular nephritis). Complicating amyloidosis may produce a nephrotic syndrome.

Lymphadenopathy, Splenomegaly, and Felty's Syndrome. Lymph nodes may be enlarged proximal to inflamed joints or in areas remote from articular inflammation. Up to 10% of patients with RA have palpable splenomegaly. Felty's syndrome is a symptom complex of chronic RA associated with splenomegaly, leukopenia, skin hyperpigmentation, leg ulcers, lymphadenopathy, anemia, and thrombocytopenia. A rare finding is nodular regenerative hyperplasia of the liver. Commonly patients have high titers of RF and antinuclear antibodies, subcutaneous nodules, and manifestations of systemic rheumatoid disease. The leukopenia is in fact a selective neutropenia and may be profound; polymorphonuclear counts of less than 1000 cells/mm³ are frequent. Marrow examination usually reveals moderate hypercellularity with a paucity of mature neutrophils. Multiple explanations for neutropenia have been proposed, including hypersplenism, but splenectomy often fails to correct the abnormality. The incidence of gram-positive infections, however, can decline after splenectomy, even when the neutropenia remains unaltered. A portion of patients with Felty's syndrome have lymphocytosis caused by an expansion of an unusual (Tγ) large granular lymphocyte subpopulation. Splenectomy is contraindicated in these patients.

Complications

An increased frequency of infections is observed in RA patients, particularly those with systemic rheumatoid disease. Infections may be local (pyarthrosis) (see Chapter 203) or extraarticular. Herpes zoster is more common. Death from septicemia, pneumonia, lung abscess, empyema, or pyelonephritis is well recognized.

Clinically significant amyloidosis is infrequent and is rarely a cause of death. Amyloidosis should be considered in rheumatoid patients in whom renal insufficiency develops (especially with a nephrotic syndrome) and in those with unexplained gastrointestinal tract hemorrhage.

Osteoporosis, either generalized or involving thoracic or lumbar vertebrae, may complicate RA. The origin is probably multifactorial, with contributions from generalized malnutrition, the postmenopausal state, immobilization, steroid therapy, and perhaps the catabolic state imposed by chronic rheumatoid disease itself.

Rarely, a hyperviscosity syndrome occurs as a result of the intravascular interaction of large quantities of RF and circulating IgG. Symptoms may include a bleeding diathesis (with bruising, epistaxis, and gingival hemorrhage), confusion, vertigo, retinal hemorrhages, congestive heart failure, and intestinal ischemia.

LABORATORY FINDINGS

A normocytic, normochromic or hypochromic anemia, usually associated with a low serum iron level and a normal or low iron-binding capacity, is a common feature of RA. Large stores of unused iron are found in the bone marrow. The white blood cell count is usually normal, but a mild increase in polymorphonuclear leukocytes is not uncommon. Leukocytosis in general does not indicate enhanced disease activity, but eosinophilia, when present, is often associated with severe systemic rheumatoid disease. Thrombocytosis is common. The erythrocyte sedimentation rate (ESR) is elevated to a variable degree in most patients and roughly parallels disease activity.

Serum protein analysis may reveal elevation in the α_2 and gamma globulin fractions and a mild to moderate diminution in serum albumin. The gamma globulin increase is polyclonal. Liver and renal function test results are usually normal, as is the urinary sediment.

Conventional IgM RF is demonstrable in approximately 70% of adults with RA but is not specific for this disease. The presence and amount of the autoantibody have important prognostic and diagnostic significance (Chapter 182). Five percent to 10% of patients have false-positive test results for syphilis. At least 25% of seropositive rheumatoid patients have serum antinuclear antibodies, generally with a homogeneous pattern of nuclear immunofluorescence. Antibodies to native double-stranded DNA are very rare. Circulating immune complexes and cryoprecipitable proteins consisting of immunoglobulins, complement components, and RFs are demonstrable in the serum of some patients with RA, especially those with vasculitis or Felty's syndrome. Normal serum complement values are the rule, but depressed values are seen in patients with systemic complications.

Table 192-1   Factors that portend a poor outcome in rheumatoid arthritis

CLINICAL	LABORATORY
Number of inflammed joints (>14)	Persistently elevated acute-phase reactants (CRP, erythrocyte sedimentation rate)
Extraarticular manifestations	Immunoglobulin M rheumatoid factor
Rheumatoid nodules	RA "shared epitope" human leukocyte antigen (HLA)-DRβ1
Continuous diseases activity	Juxtaarticular bone erosions

Synovial fluid analysis can be of value in establishing the diagnosis of RA, although no one finding is specific (Chapter 183). Characteristically the fluid is exudative, with white blood cell counts ranging from 5000 to 20,000 cells/mm³; counts in excess of 50,000 cells/mm³ are occasionally encountered. Polymorphonuclear leukocytes make up at least two thirds of the cells, except very early in the disease. The synovial fluid is turbid in appearance, with reduced viscosity; it forms a loose, friable clot on addition of dilute acetic acid (the mucin clot test). The protein content, normally less than 2g/dl, often is elevated to levels exceeding 3.5 g/dl. Hemolytic complement is reduced to less than one third the serum values, especially in patients with seropositive disease; C4 and C2 levels are most profoundly depressed. Glucose concentrations may be low or normal, similar to rheumatoid effusions in other body fluids.

RADIOLOGIC FINDINGS

No roentgenographic features are pathognomonic of RA, but the diagnosis frequently is suggested by a characteristic pattern of joint erosions. The tendency toward symmetry in established disease and the predilection for certain anatomic sites—notably the MCP and PIP joints of the hands, wrists, and knees and the MTP joints of the feet—are important in differentiating RA from degenerative joint disease and from other inflammatory arthritides. So, too, is the relative lack of bone formation in the presence of advanced joint destruction, a feature that contrasts with the exuberant new bone formation often seen in ankylosing spondylitis, Reiter's syndrome, and psoriatic arthritis. Specific roentgenographic abnormalities are detailed in Chapter 184.

COURSE AND PROGNOSIS

It is impossible to reliably predict the course that RA will follow when the patient is seen at the inception of the disease. The "natural history" of RA (i.e., in the absence of therapy) is not completely understood, but there are several valid impressions. Of any 100 rheumatoid arthritis patients studied, approximately 15% have a short-lived joint disease that remits without significant residua. In another 15% to 25% the disease may persist for some time but then leaves with only mild to moderate damage to the joints. Fifty percent of patients have persistent activity of the arthritis punctuated by exacerbations and remissions but invariably leading to progressive deformity with a variable disability. The remaining 10% have a relentless disease that is unresponsive to therapy and eventuates in complete disability with the patient restricted to a bed or wheelchair existence (before the availability of joint replacement).

Features that portend either a favorable or a dismal outcome have been identified (Table 192-1). In general, remissions are most likely to occur during the first year of disease, especially after an acute onset with systemic manifestations. Men do better than women, and disease beginning before age 45 years seems to augur a better outcome. It is axiomatic that the longer an active progressive disease continues, the worse the outlook. The appearance of extraarticular disease is associated with a particularly poor prognosis, and patients in whom such features develop have twice the mortality rate of conventional rheumatoid patients. Factors that presage a less favorable course are an insidious onset of disease; persistence beyond 1 year without re-

BOX 192-2
Criteria for classification of rheumatoid arthritis

1. Morning stiffness in and around the joints lasting at least 1 hour before maximal improvement.
2. At least three joint areas with simultaneous soft-tissue swelling or fluid (not bony overgrowth alone) observed by a physician. The 14 possible joint areas are right or left PIP, MCP, wrist, elbow, knee, ankle, and MTP joints.
3. At least one joint area swollen as above in a wrist, MCP, or PIP.
4. Simultaneous involvement of the same joint areas (as in no. 2) on both sides of the body (bilateral involvement of PIP, MCP, or MTP is acceptable without absolute symmetry).
5. Subcutaneous nodules over bony prominences or extensor surfaces, or in juxtaarticular regions, observed by a physician.
6. Demonstration of abnormal amounts of serum "rheumatoid factor" by any method that has been positive in fewer than 5% of normal control subjects.
7. Radiographic changes typical of RA on posteroanterior wrist radiographs, including erosions or unequivocal bony decalcification localized to or most marked adjacent to the involved joints (osteoarthritic changes alone do not qualify).

Arnett FC et al: *Arthritis Rheum* 31:315, 1988.
MCP, Metacarpophalangeal; *MTP*, metatarsophalangeal; *PIP*, proximal interphalangeal.

mission; early appearance of bone erosions on radiologic examination of the joints; development of nodules; and, most important, the presence of serum RF, particularly in high titers. Patients with the HLA-DRβ1 shared epitope do worse, as do those with a low socioeconomic status or lack of education.

Patients rarely die of RA, although systemic vasculitis and atlantoaxial subluxation can be lethal. Rheumatoid patients may succumb to overwhelming sepsis or complications of drug or surgical therapy, but the majority die of the same diseases as age-matched cohorts, except 5 to 10 years sooner.

DIAGNOSIS

Like most diseases, RA can be diagnosed easily in its advanced and characteristic form, but early in the course the diagnosis is often obscured. Considerable diagnostic confusion results when the disease is manifested with only constitutional symptoms or when the initial joint disease is spotty or monarticular. The earliest features of the inflammatory synovitis usually appear in the wrists, PIP and MCP joints of the hands, and the MTP joints of the feet. The joints are painful, often appearing swollen and sometimes red. In time, the disease spreads, finally assuming its typical form as a bilateral, symmetric polyarthritis involving small and large joints in both the upper and lower extremities. The axial skeleton is usually spared, except for the cervical spine. The demonstration of subcutaneous nodules is especially helpful confirmatory evidence. Additional findings that substantiate the diagnosis are positive test results for RF, an exudative synovial fluid analysis showing polymorphonuclear leukocytosis and depressed complement values, and radiographic findings of bone demineralization and erosions about the affected joints. In the majority of patients the disease has assumed its more characteristic clinical features in 1 or 2 years.

The American College of Rheumatology criteria for the diagnosis of RA are outlined in Box 192-2. Any combination of four or more of this group of symptoms, signs, and laboratory findings in a patient whose disease has been continuous for at least 6 weeks is designated *rheumatoid arthritis*. It should be appreciated, however, that these criteria were not developed for the bedside diagnosis of rheumatoid arthritis, but rather to classify large groups of patients for inclusion in epidemiologic surveys, drug trials, and studies of the natural history of the disease. Therefore an individual's failure to meet an arbitrary set of criteria should not preclude the diagnosis of RA, especially in its early stages.

DIFFERENTIAL DIAGNOSIS

Joint symptoms are common and have a multiplicity of causes (detailed in Chapter 191). Some diseases, however, have chronic polyarticular inflammation as a major component, and it is these diseases that most often have to be distinguished from RA. Two groups are particularly important: the connective tissue diseases and the seronegative spondyloarthropathies. In the former, distinctive skin rashes, typical organ system involvement, and the availability in some instances of definitive serum antibodies help to make the correct diagnosis. The spondyloarthropathies, however, particularly when peripheral arthritis predominates, may prove more challenging. These disorders often have a chronic, destructive polyarthritis which, on examination, shows synovial hypertrophy and histologic features resembling those of RA. As a rule, the peripheral joint disease tends to be asymmetric, favoring the larger joints, and except for psoriatic arthritis, lower extremity involvement predominates. Psoriatic arthritis characteristically has a predilection for the distal interphalangeal joints of the hands, especially when there is disease of the associated fingernail. Reiter's disease, ankylosing spondylitis, and, less regularly, psoriatic and colitic arthritis produce remarkable erythema and swelling of individual proximal and distal joints of the toes, an uncommon location in RA. An important distinguishing feature is that sacroiliitis and spondylitis of the thoracic and lumbar articulations are common to the group, and iridocyclitis is a frequent accompaniment. The association with the HLA-B27 haplotype may be useful.

Rheumatoid arthritis can develop at any age and not uncommonly begins in the elderly. In patients with a positive test result for RF the disease course and prognosis appear to be similar to those in other age-groups. In a subset, however—those with symmetric inflammatory synovitis of the hands and feet, often associated with exaggerated peripheral edema—the process appears more benign. For some of these patients the articular manifestations may be an expression of underlying polymyalgia rheumatica (giant cell arteritis; see Chapter 195). Others may have the so-called benign synovitis of the elderly. In either instance the arthritis is remarkably sensitive to small doses of corticosteriods (5 to 10 mg of prednisone per day) and has a much better outcome than conventional RA.

For the various other joint diseases that occasionally may be confused with rheumatoid arthritis the reader is referred to the more extensive differential diagnosis of arthritis presented in Chapter 191.

MANAGEMENT

The natural course of RA is characterized by spontaneous remissions and exacerbations that make the evaluation of therapy difficult. Although there is a general agreement that certain treatment modalities are helpful in the short term, retrospective analysis of RA patients who receive treatment for more than 5 to 7 years shows that less than 25% are still taking their original medications. Since there is no known cure of RA, it follows that a variety of therapies have to be tried until an appropriate combination is found. An empathetic doctor-patient relationship, in which the physician devotes the time necessary to explain to the patient both the disease and the reasons for selecting one or another treatment, is an absolute prerequisite for success. A total management program requires the participation of a variety of medical and paramedical personnel: physiatrists, orthopedic surgeons, visiting nurses, and, when indicated, other medical specialists. No one physician's practice can encompass these many special areas; he or she must be willing to "orchestrate" this complex program.

Basic Program

Rest and Exercise. Rheumatoid arthritis has many of the manifestations of a constitutional disease. Fatigue is frequently a cause of considerable disability. Most patients recognize the need for rest but require specific directions as to when to rest and how much rest is necessary. There is disagreement about the importance of complete bed rest, but the unwillingness of insurers to fund prolonged hospitalization makes the issue moot. During periods of rest at home, individual inflamed joints should be supported with well-fitted splints or plastic shells. The mattress must be firm, and a bed board is useful. A bed cradle and a padded footrest to prevent deformities of the feet and ankles should be employed regularly. Positions that lead to contractures, such as pillows beneath the knees or lying on the side with the knees flexed, must be discouraged. Patients with hip disease ought to lie prone on a firm surface for 30 minutes twice daily to prevent hip flexion contractures.

As patients return to more regular activities, a rest period should be prescribed. For workers the most practical approach is to recline for 30 to 60 minutes during the lunch period. Homemakers should lie down for a similar period during the naptime of young children. Thirty minutes of rest before dinner is helpful. Weekend activities may have to be curtailed to provide additional rest, and others in the family should be recruited to perform the duties of the member with RA.

Exercises to maintain joint mobility and regain muscle strength are an integral part of the basic treatment program. It takes only 10 to 15 minutes to put all the joints through a complete range of motion, and this should be done twice daily. Isometric exercises prevent quadriceps atrophy, but resistance exercises should be avoided. Heating pads or hot packs applied to affected joints for 15 to 20 minutes three times daily give good relief of pain and allow greater range of motion; occasionally, cold applications are efficacious. Paraffin baths and whirlpool units are available for home use, but their use should be taught to the patient by a physical therapist before their introduction into a home program. Soaking the hands or a hot shower in the morning before starting the exercise program usually decreases muscle spasm and stiffness and allows more effective participation.

Drugs

An array of new drugs has been added to those already available for treating RA. No single drug is specific or universally successful, but for most patients some combination can be found that diminishes the articular disease. Several classes of such agents are recognized: analgesics; NSAIDs; glucocorticoids; remissive, slow-acting, or disease-modifying antirheumatic drugs (DMARDs); and immunomodulatory compounds. Early in the illness, RA is usually managed with NSAIDs only, but patients with poor prognostic signs or more aggressive or chronic disease have one of the DMARDs added. Various combinations are possible, all have been tried, and none appears appreciably better; failure with one combination does not preclude success with another. There are very few drug interactions between NSAIDs and DMARDs. Usually adrenocorticosteroids or immunosuppressive drugs are considered only after other modalities have been exhausted. A possible exception is methotrexate, which is increasingly used as the first drug in patients with features that portend a poor outcome (Table 192-1). The pharmacologic features, dosage schedules, and toxicity of the individual medications are considered in Chapter 205. Subsequent remarks in this chapter are limited to their use in RA.

Analgesics. Acetaminophen (Tylenol), 300 to 600 mg three or four times daily or propoxyphene hydrochloride (Darvon), 32 or 65 mg three or four times daily may be used for pain relief, although neither substitutes for the antiinflammatory effects of aspirin or NSAIDs. Severe pain is occasionally managed with oral codeine, but its potential for addiction when employed in a chronic disorder such as RA precludes its regular use.

Nonsteroidal Antiinflammatory Drugs. Aspirin remains an important drug for the treatment of RA. Its successful use depends on dosing at regular intervals and in large amounts, usually 3.6 to 5.4 g (12 to 18 tablets) per day. Administration immediately after meals or with food minimizes gastric irritation. The last dose is usually prescribed for bedtime. Some patients, particularly, elderly individuals cannot take these optimal amounts of aspirin. Tinnitus is a common side effect but is easily controlled by a slight reduction in dose. Gastric irritation is a frequent accompaniment of aspirin therapy. Buffered preparations, aspirin suspensions, or enteric-coated aspirin may be better tolerated. Other salicylate compounds may substitute for aspirin. Sodium salicylate, calcium salicylate, choline magnesium trisalicylate, benorylate, and diflunisal are all reported to produce significantly fewer gastrointestinal tract symptoms and blood loss. Chemical detection of small amounts of blood in the stool is not an indication to discontinue the medication. Other important toxicities include aspirin sensitivity and effects on platelet adhesiveness.

Despite the increased cost, most patients prefer NSAIDs because of the less frequent dosing (see complete list in Chapter 205). No one NSAID is significantly better than another, but most patients find one that provides relief. Therefore trials of each are indicated. Since their onset of action is rapid, trials need not exceed 2 to 3 weeks. There is no indication that combinations of NSAIDs and aspirin are better than either alone. Indomethacin is available in a slow-release form at a dose of 75 to 100 mg. Taken at bedtime, it is particularly effective in relieving night pain and the duration of morning stiffness.

Adrenocorticosteroids. Every attempt should be made to employ conservative measures and the disease-modifying agents listed later before instituting treatment with adrenocorticosteroids. Most rheumatologists, however, accept that in some patients this therapy is justified. Use of these drugs requires an intimate knowledge of their long-term toxicity (Chapter 205). Indications for the judicious use of corticosteroids for long periods are (1) as an aid in the rehabilitation of patients who otherwise might be invalided or remain housebound, (2) in treatment of disability resulting from acute systemic or febrile manifestations of the disease, and (3) in the presence of deterioration that has continued, despite all other conservative forms of treatment (not including cytotoxic agents).

There is relatively little advantage of one synthetic steroid over another. Cortisone and hydrocortisone have limited usefulness because of their salt-retaining effects. Prednisone and prednisolone are preferred because they are least expensive. If a decision to employ long-term corticosteroid therapy is made, the smallest possible daily total dose should be selected. The patient must be informed that this dose will not be exceeded, except under unusual circumstances. Generally the average daily prednisone dose for men should not be more than 7.5 mg and for women, 5.0 mg daily. Smaller doses should be prescribed for children and postmenopausal women, two groups that are particularly susceptible to side effects. Divided doses may be more effective than single morning or evening administration but result in more side effects. Alternate-day corticosteroids are usually not successful in the management of RA but may be worth a trial because of the lower frequency of undesirable side effects. Initiating therapy with large priming doses followed by a stepwise decrease is not recommended. "Pulse therapy" with intravenous methylprednisolone (Medrol) in 1 g doses may have short-term benefits.

Even with small maintenance doses of prednisone, suppression of adrenal gland function develops. Therefore the amount of corticosteroid must be sharply increased in situations of acute or overwhelming stress and before major surgery. Cortisone acetate or hydrocortisone sodium succinate (Solu-Cortef) (but not hydrocortisone acetate) should be administered intramuscularly in 50- to 100-mg doses 4 to 6 hours before operation and continued intravenously or intramuscularly at those intervals for 24 to 48 hours after surgery or until the patient begins oral feeding. Thereafter, a rapid reduction to the maintenance dose is permissible. Avascular necrosis of bones, particularly in the hip joints, can develop from prolonged or intermittent steroid therapy. Continued use of corticosteroids to treat the pain and limitation of motion attributable to osteonecrosis can compound an already difficult situation.

Intraarticular Corticosteroids. The intraarticular injection of microcrystalline suspensions of corticosteroids may be of use in patients with a limited number of involved joints or in whom a few joints are disproportionately inflamed. Joint aspiration to exclude infection is mandatory, and removing large effusions can decrease joint distention and reflex spasm of surrounding muscle groups. The dose employed depends on the size of the joint. In the knee, 20 to 40 mg of triamcinolone hexacetonide or a comparable, relatively nonabsorbable corticosteroid preparation is used. Lesser amounts are appropriate for smaller joints. Aside from pain and the potential for introducing infections, atrophy of the injection site is the only frequent complication. The response to intraarticular therapy is variable. Complete relief of inflammation and pain sometimes lasts many months. If it is short-lived, the risks outweigh the benefits, since joints that are repeatedly injected occasionally develop accelerated degenerative arthritis. Therefore it is wise to limit intraarticular therapy in a single joint to two or three times a year.

Disease-Modifying Antirheumatic Drugs.

This group of compounds includes gold, D-penicillamine, the 4-aminoquinolines, and sulfasalazine (Azulfidine). A description of the individual drugs is presented in Chapter 205. Each should be used separately and continued for 3 to 6 months before a decision is made about its effectiveness, unless toxicity supervenes. Improvement is always gradual, and a rebound in disease activity is not observed after discontinuation.

Gold compounds. Most rheumatologists advocate the use of gold. The disadvantages of weekly visits to the physician, injections, and additional laboratory tests to avoid toxic side effects are offset by the occasional dramatic responses obtained with this treatment. In general, one patient in five has an excellent result; an additional two patients receive significant benefits. Gold is recommended early in the disease, when there is active joint inflammation and before significant destructive changes have occurred, but control studies have shown benefits at every stage of rheumatoid arthritis.

Patients should be instructed to pay particular attention to pruritus, minor skin rashes, particularly in seborrheic areas, and a metallic taste in the mouth. These are all forerunners of more serious problems. There may be a long lag from the initiation of gold therapy until benefits are noted. Without this knowledge patients may become discouraged and discontinue treatment. Either gold sodium thiomalate (Myochrysine) or gold thioglucose (Solganal) is given intramuscularly at weekly intervals: 10 mg the first week, 25 mg the second week, and 50 mg weekly thereafter. Usually by the tenth to fourteenth injection, the patient notices signs of improvement. At this time, 50 mg of the drug can be given every other week for the next four to eight injections; and, with continued improvement, 50 mg can be given every third or fourth week, for a minimum of 2 years (and possibly indefinitely). Should symptoms return, weekly injections of 50 mg can be reinstituted, sometimes with good results. If the patient has not improved by the time 1 g of drug has been given, another form of treatment is indicated.

Undesirable side effects include proteinuria, thrombocytopenia, leukopenia, and, rarely, anemia and pancytopenia. A urinalysis and complete blood cell count must be checked before each injection for the first 4 weeks and biweekly or monthly thereafter. The drug should be discontinued if leukopenia or proteinuria develops. When the white blood cell count or urinalysis returns to normal, gold can be reinstituted at half the normal dose, and the effect observed. If there is no adverse reaction, the full treatment program can be continued. Similarly, when pruritus or dermatitis clears, therapy often can be reinstituted after a judicious trial at a smaller dose. Severe dermatologic complications may require antihistamines or steroids. Treatment with British anti-lewisite (BAL) should be reserved for patients with profound dermal, renal, or hematopoietic toxicity. Pneumonitis, hepatitis, peripheral neuritis, and enterocolitis are rare side effects of gold treatment.

An oral gold compound (auranofin) is now available. When prescribed at 3 mg twice a day, it is less effective than injectable gold but has less severe dermal, renal, and hematologic side effects. Diarrhea, however, can be a troublesome complication. Three months of treatment should be tried before abandoning this therapy.

D-Penicillamine. Although D-penicillamine is effective in patients with RA, its use is plagued with frequent and annoying, but generally reversible, side effects that limit its use. The percentages of good responses, type of toxicity, and delayed onset of improvement are similar to those with gold. Treatment is initiated at 250 mg daily and increased by that amount every 3 months until clinical improvement or toxicity intervenes or a dose of 1.0 g daily is reached. Skin rash, transient loss of taste, stomatitis, gastric upset, leukopenia, thrombocytopenia, and proteinuria are common and often can be controlled by reduction in dose. The frequency of dermatitis may be greater in patients who developed a rash from gold, but allergy to penicillin is not a contraindication. Rare complications include glomerulonephritis, Goodpasture's syndrome, and myasthenia gravis. Blood cell counts and urinalyses are required at least monthly. Treatment is continued indefinitely; after months or years tolerance sometimes develops.

Antimalarials (4-aminoquinolines). Chloroquine diphosphate is administered in a dose of 250 mg once daily, generally at bedtime; this tends to minimize complicating gastrointestinal tract or vasomotor symptoms. Hydroxychloroquine sulfate (Plaquenil) is taken in a dose of 200 mg twice daily. Patients in whom side effects of headache, nausea, abdominal cramping, diarrhea, or skin rash develop from one antimalarial may tolerate another. Improvement with these agents occurs slowly, seldom before 4 weeks; 3 to 6 months of drug administration is usually required before maximal benefits are achieved. If improvement occurs, the drug is continued, often at a reduced dose, but only if the patient has funduscopic examinations two or three times yearly by an ophthalmologist acquainted with the drug's rare but potentially severe ocular toxicity. Early detection of retinal abnormalities and immediate discontinuation of therapy may arrest or reverse the ocular damage.

Sulfasalazine. Sulfasalazine has some value in the treatment of RA with improvement occurring in 6 to 12 weeks. Enteric-coated tablets are given in an initial dosage of 500 mg twice a day and, if tolerated, the dosage is increased to 1000 mg two to three times daily. Nausea or dyspepsia are the major side effects of the drug. Rashes occur infrequently, and neutropenia is a rare serious complication. Hemolyses can occur in patients with underlying glucose-6-phosphate dehydrogenase (G6PD) deficiency (see Chapter 89).

Methotrexate. The folic acid analog methotrexate is currently the most widely used disease-modifying agent for the treatment of RA. Originally considered an antiproliferative, cytotoxic drug, its rapid onset of action and the recurrence of disease soon after its discontinuation suggest that its action in RA is antiinflammatory. An increase in local concentrations of adenosine at sites of injury probably accounts for the drug's antiinflammatory effects. Clinical improvement is seen in two thirds of patients, often within a few weeks of starting methotrexate, and almost half are still taking the medication 5 years later. This is a testimony to its efficacy, as well as the usually modest side effects, which most patients are willing to tolerate to retain the drug's benefits. Treatment is customarily initiated at 7.5 mg (three tablets) taken as a single dose once a week. Failure to respond in 4 to 6 weeks is reason to make upward adjustments to a total dose of 15 mg once a week. Larger doses, either by mouth or intramuscular injection, are occasionally efficacious but limited by side effects. Generally these reactions consist of nausea and a vague sense of feeling poorly that lasts a few days following administration. Stomatitis, vomiting, and diarrhea are less common complaints. Folic acid, 1 mg daily, tends to ameliorate gastrointestinal tract toxic effects without interfering with the therapeutic benefits of methotrexate. Radiologic evidence of bone erosion may be retarded by methotrexate treatment, but progression can be observed even in asymptomatic subjects. Withdrawal of methotrexate is almost invariably associated with prompt

---

✔ WHEN TO REFER

Referral to a rheumatologist is suggested when the patient is first seen if the diagnosis of RA is in question.

A rheumatologist should be consulted to outline early aggressive treatment for patients at high risk for developing severe, destructive RA.

Referral to a rheumatologist is indicated whenever conventional therapies have failed to control joint inflammation or destruction and treatment with cytotoxic agents, high doses of corticosteroids, combination drug therapy, or experimental modalities is being considered.

Rheumatologic consultation should be considered for those patients in whom "rheumatoid necrotizing vasculitis" (systemic rheumatoid disease) or Felty's syndrome develops.

Referral to an orthopedic surgeon is necessary for management of local complications (such as entrapment neuropathies or torn tendons), prophylactic synovectomies (especially wrists and finger joints), and reconstruction and replacement of seriously damaged joints.

Referral to a physiatrist is advisable for splinting or specialized exercises for specific joints.

return of disease activity. Although hematologic abnormalities are rare and hepatotoxicity is usually mild, it is advised that blood cell count and liver function studies be obtained monthly while patients take this medication. A threefold or greater increase in liver enzymes is an indication for discontinuation of treatment, but the drug can be restarted at a lower dose if the test results become normal. Many clinicians use methotrexate not only as the initial treatment in RA, but also in combination with other disease-modifying agents when patients are first seen with factors that predict a poor outcome (see Table 192-1). Although some reports on combination therapy have been encouraging, evidence that such treatment will change the long-term, natural history of RA is unproven. Additional information on this important subject is provided in Chapter 205.

Cytotoxic (Immunosuppressant) Drugs. Cytotoxic drug therapy should be limited to the small number of rheumatoid patients for whom all other therapeutic modalities have failed or who have life-threatening systemic complications or have had unacceptable corticosteroid side effects. The patient and the prescribing physician must have full knowledge of the serious immediate and potential long-term complications. Specific agents are described in Chapter 205. Immunomodulatory agents (e.g., levamisole), lymphoplasmapheresis, and total lymphoid irradiation are controversial therapies.

Surgical Management

Orthopedic surgery can be preventive or restorative. Synovectomy in joints unaffected by local or systemic therapy can improve function and eliminate swelling for a period of time. Soft tissue damage such as tendon rupture can be minimized or repaired. Excision of subluxated, painful metatarsal phalangeal joints aids ambulation, and realignment of finger joints improves hand function. For predictable relief of pain and restoration of function, however, the procedure of choice is total joint replacement.

The availability of prosthetic joints, especially hips and knees, has revolutionized the care of rheumatoid patients with multiple joint involvement. Early consultation with orthopedic surgeons to plan appropriate interventions is an essential part of the management program.

BIBLIOGRAPHY

Brooks PM, Day RO: Nonsteroidal antiinflammatory drugs: differences and similarities, *N Engl J Med* 324:1716, 1991.

Firestein G, Zvaifler NJ: Rheumatoid arthritis: a disease of disordered immunity. In Gallin JI, Goldstein IM, Snyderman R, editors: *Inflammation: basic principles and clinical correlates,* ed 2, New York, 1992, Raven.

Gordon DA, Stein JL, Broder I: The paradox of effective therapies but poor long-term outcomes in rheumatoid arthritis: a systemic analysis of 127 cases, *Am J Med* 54:445, 1973.

Harris ED Jr: Rheumatoid arthritis: pathophysiology and implications for therapy, *N Engl J Med* 322:1277, 1990.

Pincus T: The paradox of effective therapies but poor long-term outcomes in rheumatoid arthritis, *Semin Arthritis Rheum* 21(suppl 3):2, 1992.

Utsinger PD, Zvaifler NJ, Ehrlich GE: *Rheumatoid arthritis: etiology, diagnosis, management,* Philadelphia, 1985, Lippincott.

Van der Heijde DM et al: Prognostic factors for radiographic damage and physical disability in early rheumatoid arthritis: a prospective study of 147 patients, *Br J Rheumatol* 31:519, 1992.

Vollerstsen RS et al: Rheumatoid vasculitis: survival and associated risk factors, *Medicine* (Baltimore) 65:365, 1986.

Weyand CM et al: The influence of HLA-DRβ1 genes on disease severity in rheumatoid arthritis, *Ann Intern Med* 117:801, 1992.

193 Sjögren's Syndrome

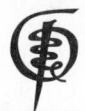

Robert I. Fox

Sjögren's syndrome (SS) is a chronic autoimmune disorder characterized by lymphocytic infiltration of the lacrimal and salivary glands, leading to severe dryness of eyes (keratoconjunctivitis sicca) and mouth (xerostomia). SS may exist as a primary disorder or in association with other autoimmune diseases (secondary SS), including rheumatoid arthritis (RA), systemic lupus erythematosus (SLE), or progressive systemic sclerosis (scleroderma, PSS). Patients with primary SS frequently have extraglandular manifestations including rash, arthritis, pneumonitis, nephritis, and nervous system involvement.

CLASSIFICATION CRITERIA AND EPIDEMIOLOGY

There has been considerable debate about the criteria for the diagnosis of SS, leading to confusion in clinical practice and in research studies. The specific criteria used for the diagnosis of SS at our institution are listed in Box 193-1. SS patients should have objective evidence of dry eyes, as measured by Schirmer's test (paper strips placed in the lower conjunctival sac) and installation of rose bengal or fluorescein to demonstrate keratoconjunctivitis sicca. Dryness of the mouth is documented by measurement of saliva flow using either a Lashley cup (a suction cup fitting over the opening of Stensen's duct), a sponge placed under the tongue, or simple observation of the decreased weight of a sugarless candy placed in the mouth for 3 minutes. When objective dryness of eyes and mouth is documented, the critical question is whether these problems result from an "autoimmune" attack on the glands. The presence of circulating autoantibodies and a minor salivary gland biopsy specimen with lymphocytic infiltration (described later) indicate SS as the cause of the sicca symptoms. Other disease processes can result in lacrimal and salivary gland swelling and chronic dysfunction (Box 193-2). These include sarcoid-

---

BOX 193-1
Criteria for diagnosis of primary and secondary Sjögren's syndrome

I. Primary Sjögren's syndrome
  A. Symptoms and objective signs of ocular dryness
    1. Schirmer's test less than 8 mm wetting per 5 minutes
    2. Positive rose bengal or fluorescein staining of cornea and conjunctiva to demonstrate keratoconjunctivitis sicca
  B. Symptoms and objective signs of dry mouth
    1. Decreased parotid flow rate using Lashley cups or other methods
    2. Abnormal biopsy of minor salivary gland (focus score of ≥2 based on average of four evaluable lobules)
  C. Evidence of a systemic autoimmune disorder
    1. Elevated titer of rheumatoid factor ≥1:320 or
    2. Elevated titer of antinuclear antibody ≥1:320 or
    3. Presence of anti-SS A [Ro] or anti-SS B [La] antibodies
II. Secondary Sjögren's syndrome
  Characteristic signs and symptoms of SS (described above) plus clinical features sufficient to allow a diagnosis of rheumatoid arthritis, systemic lupus erythematosus, polymyositis, or scleroderma
III. Exclusions include infectious diseases (hepatitis B, hepatitis C, human immunodeficiency virus, human T-leukemia viruses types 1 and 2), other causes of sicca symptoms including autonomic neuropathy, and other causes of infiltration of lacrimal or salivary glands including sarcoidosis, amyloidosis, and lipid storage disorders.

BOX 193-2
Causes of keratitis and salivary gland enlargement other than Sjögren's syndrome

Keratitis
1. Mucous membrane pemphigoid
2. Sarcoidosis
3. Infections: Virus (adenovirus, herpes, vaccinia), bacteria, or chlamydia (i.e., trachoma)
4. Trauma (i.e., after contact lens) and environmental irritants including chemical burns, exposure to ultraviolet lights or roentgen rays
5. Neuropathy including neutrotropic keratitis (i.e., damage to fifth cranial nerve) and familial dysautonomia (Riley-Day syndrome)
6. Hypovitaminosis A
7. Erythema multiforme (Stevens-Johnson syndrome)

Salivary gland enlargement
1. Sarcoidosis, amyloidosis
2. Bacterial (including gonococci and syphilis) and viral infections (i.e., infectious mononucleosis, mumps, human immunodeficiency virus)
3. Tuberculosis, actinomycosis, histoplasmosis, trachoma, leprosy
4. Iodide, lead, or copper hypersensitivity
5. Hyperlipoproteinemia, especially types IV and V
6. Tumors (usually unilateral) including cysts (Warthin's tumor), epithelial (adenoma, adenocarcinoma), lymphoma, and mixed salivary gland tumors
7. Excessive alcohol consumption

osis, lymphoma, tuberculosis, hepatitis C, and acquired immunodeficiency syndrome (AIDS). In comparison, the recently adopted European (EEC) classification criteria for SS do not require the presence of autoantibodies or an abnormal biopsy for diagnosis, nor do they exclude patients with infections such as hepatitis C, human T-leukemia virus, or human immunodeficiency virus (HIV). Also, other causes of sicca syndrome including autonomic neuropathy are not excluded. Since there are no uniform diagnostic criteria for SS, the incidence and prevalence vary widely in the literature. Using the stringent criteria listed in Box 193-1, the prevalence of primary SS is roughly 1/2500. The disease affects predominantly women, with a peak onset during the sixth decade of life and a less frequent onset during childhood or the third decade. Secondary SS is more common, since up to 20% of RA patients and up to 30% of SLE patients have significant sicca symptoms.

PATHOGENESIS

The initiating factors in SS remain unknown, but genetic and environmental factors are likely to play a role. Genetic factors include genes encoded by the major histocompatibility complex (MCH) (i.e., HLA-DR/DQ, HLA-DP, and associated genes on chromosome 6) and probably non-MHC genes related to the development and differentiation of the lacrimal and salivary glands. Among a small number of identical twins studied with primary SS the disease shows concordance in approximately 20%. The failure of the other identical twin to develop SS indicates the important role of extragenetic factors. No single environmental factor has been found as a trigger in SS, but indirect evidence has suggested Epstein-Barr virus (EBV) as a potential cofactor. A potential role for a retrovirus has been suggested in Japanese patients and in animal models of SS. Other candidate viruses include human herpes virus type 6 and hepatitis C, since each of these viruses may have a site of latency and reactivation within the salivary and/or lacrimal glands. It seems most likely that a variety of different environmental agents may play a role in intitiation or propagation of SS.

Salivary glands exhibit focal lymphoid infiltrates (Fig. 193-1, *A*) that are not detected in normal biopsy specimens (Fig. 193-1, *B*). Antibodies directed against salivary gland cells are not detected in most primary SS patients, and immune complexes are not detected at the basement membrane around the blood vessels or salivary gland epithelial cells. Taken together, these results suggest a cell-mediated immune mechanism rather than a humoral mechanism for glandular destruction. Cytokines, including interleukin-2 (IL-2), tumor necrosis factor alpha (TNF-α), and interferon-gamma (INF-γ) are made by T cells that infiltrate the gland, and IL-1 and IL-10 are produced by the grandular epithelial cells.

CLINICAL MANIFESTATIONS

The most common ocular symptom is a dry, gritty feeling caused by a decrease in the volume and alteration in the composition of the tear film. Dry mouth is another common complaint and often is accompanied by rampant periodontal problems. Many patients describe difficulty in swallowing food, problems in wearing dentures, change in their sense of taste, burning of the oral mucosa, intolerance of acidic or spicy foods, and inability to speak continuously for more than a few minutes because of dryness. Nutrition may be compromised and sleep disturbed by nocturia resulting from increased fluid intake.

Dryness of the skin has been attributed to a decrease in the secretory capacity of the sebaceous glands in some patients. Oral candidiasis, particularly angular cheilitis, is extremely common in these patients and an important contributing factor in their increased mouth pain and decreased sensation of taste.

Skin involvement in SS patients may become evident as leukocytoclastic vasculitis or as hypergammaglobulinemic purpura. Periungual telangiectasis may be detected in primary SS patients, but the presence of a large number of lesions suggests an increased chance of scleroderma.

Involvement of exocrine glands in the upper respiratory tract leads to dryness of the nasal passages in approximately 50% of the patients. Mucus plug inspissation associated with bronchospasm and dyspnea is a relatively common problem. This often occurs after upper respiratory tract infection when tenacious secretions cannot be adequately mobilized, especially in the postoperative setting. SS patients may develop pleurisy with and without effusion, and lymphoid interstitial pneumonitis. Clinically significant hypothyroidism develops in 10% to 15% of SS patients. Thus endocrine as well as exocrine glandular cells may be targets for immune attack in primary SS.

The most common functional renal abnormality noted in SS patients is the inability to acidify the urine in response to an administered acid load, such as ammonium chloride. In rare SS patients with clinically significant interstitial nephritis, hypokalemia may be severe enough to produce paralysis. Glomerulonephritis is uncommon in primary SS patients and generally suggests the development of SLE. However, glomerulonephritis may be associated with mixed cryoglobulemia or amyloidosis in the primary SS patient. SS patients can develop obstructive nephropathy resulting from enlarged lymph nodes or renovascular hypertension caused by vasculitis.

Hematologic disorders in the primary SS patient include an anemia of chronic disease, iron deficiency related to medications, and occasionally hemolytic anemia. Neutropenia in SS is frequent but rarely reaches a level of clinical significance. An increased frequency of non-Hodgkin's lymphoma, (up to 40-fold in comparison with controls) especially involving the salivary glands and cervical lymph nodes, occurs in SS patients. There is no evidence to suggest that other solid tumors are increased in these patients.

Central nervous system abnormalities, including vasculitis, transverse myelitis, and aseptic meningitis, may occur in primary SS patients in patterns similar to those seen in SLE patients. Demyelinating disorders of the central nervous system may appear; these present a diagnostic difficulty, since sicca complaints occur in patients with multiple sclerosis as a result of autonomic neuropathy. Peripheral sensory neuropathy affecting the lower extremities is relatively common, particularly in SS patients with hyperglobulinemic purpura. Mononeuritis multiplex caused by vasculitis occurs much less frequently.

LABORATORY FEATURES

SS patients generally have a positive antinuclear antibody (ANA) test because of the presence of anti-SS A and anti-SS B antibodies (see Chapter 181). The SS-A and SS-B antigens are identical to the "Ro" and "La" antigens, respectively. Although a sensitive indicator for SS,

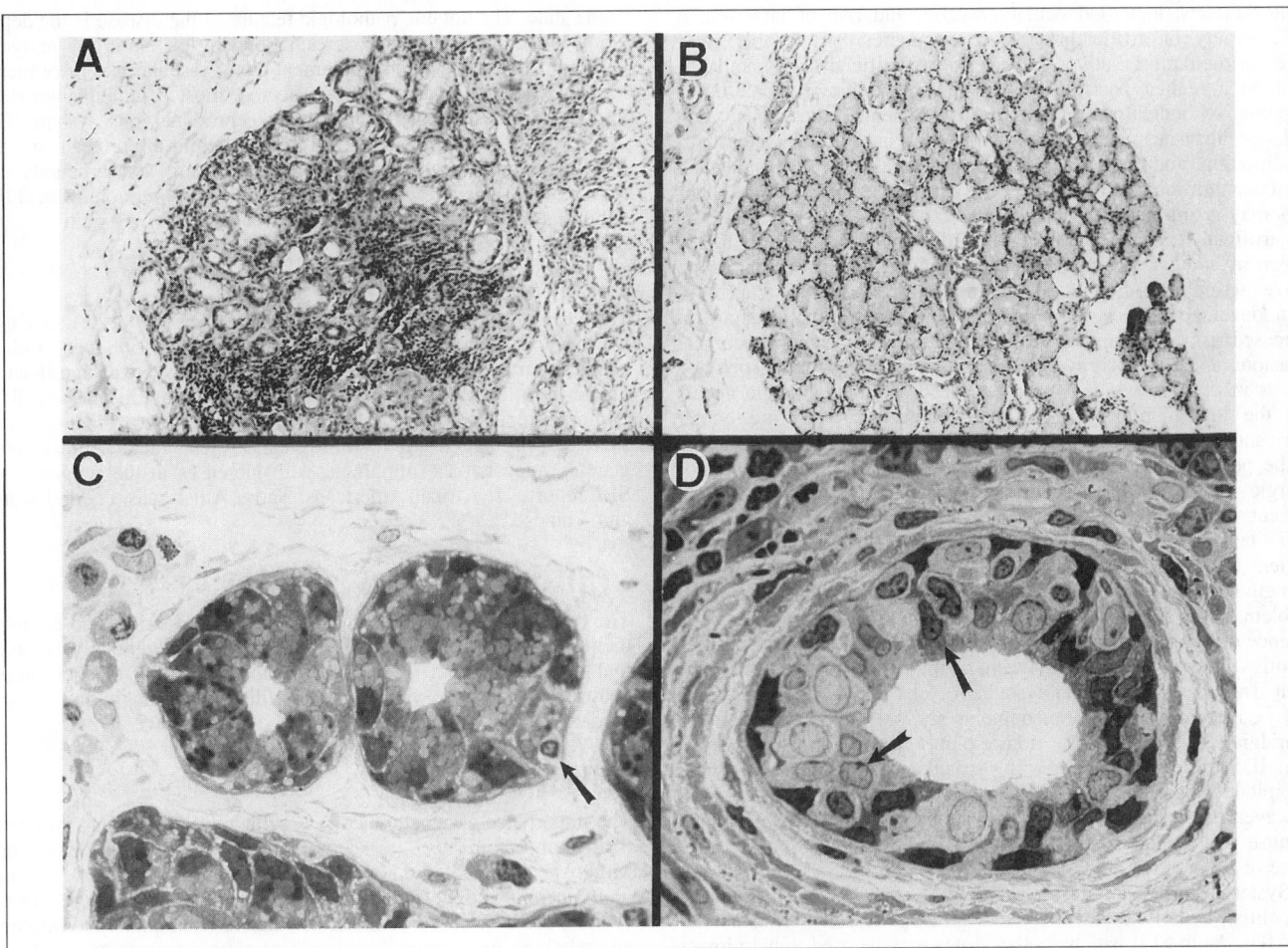

FIGURE 193-1   Salivary gland biopsy specimens, **A,** from a patient with Sjögren's syndrome and **B,** from a normal individual. **C** and **D,** Higher-magnification views of acini and ducts from the salivary gland in **A.** *Arrows,* lymphocytes (CD4 T cells) infiltrating glands.

anti-SS A antibodies are not specific for SS, since they also are present in SLE patients who lack SS symptoms. Anti-SS B antibodies are more consistently associated with sicca symptoms, but approximately half of the primary SS patients lack this autoantibody. These antibodies are associated with specific HLA-DR and DQ alleles and with specific T-cell antigen receptor polymorphisms.

Rheumatoid factor (RF) is an autoantibody directed against the Fc portion of immunoglobulin G (IgG). The titers of RF are relatively low (1:320 to 1:640) in most primary SS patients, so a very high titer (>1:10,000) in an SS patient suggests a superimposed problem such as rheumatoid arthritis or a monoclonal RF paraprotein.

Elevated liver function test results are uncommon and, when present, suggest viral hepatitis or toxic side effects of medications. In some patients SS coexists with biliary cirrhosis, which can be distinguished by antibodies against the mitochondrial enzyme 2-oxoacetic acid dehydrogenase. Elevated liver function test results in some SS patients may result from elevated levels of type II mixed cryoglobulins.

DIFFERENTIAL DIAGNOSIS

Sicca symptoms may accompany autonomic neuropathy associated with diabetes mellitus, multiple sclerosis, or SLE. Sicca complaints in patients with fibromyalgia are assumed to derive from central autonomic dysfunction, because of the relatively normal salivary gland biopsy specimens.

Dryness of the eyes and mouth can accompany aging; therefore dryness does not necessarily indicate a disease process. Often, the symptoms of dryness become clinically apparent in elderly individu-

als when they take medications with anticholinergic side effects such as tricyclic antidepressants, muscle relaxants, diuretics, cardiac medications, and over-the-counter cold remedies. Also, anxiety can lead to increased symptoms of dryness, since stimulation of the sympathetic nervous system leads to decreased glandular flow. Thus the vast majority of dry-eye patients do not have evidence of an autoimmune disorder, and it is important to reassure these individuals that they do not have a systemic disease.

Blepharitis results from the blockage and chronic low grade infection of the meibomian glands that line the eyelids. The release of exotoxin from these sites of infection can lead to symptoms of ocular discomfort as well as keratitis on examination.

In patients with significant dryness and salivary gland swelling, other processes such as retrovirus (HIV) infection, sarcoidosis, and lymphoma must be considered (Box 193-2). Less common causes of chronic bilateral salivary gland swelling include mycobacterial and fungal infections, amyloidosis, and salivary gland tumors. Suppurative (bacterial) parotitis should be suspected in any patient with a sudden increase in salivary gland size, particularly older patients in the postoperative setting.

TREATMENT

Dry eyes (keratoconjunctivitis sicca) can range in severity from a mildly annoying complaint to a significant clinical corneal abrasion that can lead to loss of employment and even blindness. The mainstay of therapy is topical treatment using artificial tears. Artificial tears containing corticosteroids are to be avoided when possible because of the significant complications, including subcapsular cataracts, increased ocular pressure, and risk of infection. A wide variety of artificial tears are commercially available; they differ in their preservatives and viscosity. Artificial tears should be used on a regular basis, and their frequency of use increased in response to increased local dry environmental conditions. This includes airplanes, department stores that use closed-system air-conditioning, and environments with dry winds. In some patients a particular artificial tear may cause a burning sensation in the eyes. This may result from topical irritation caused by the preservative in the artificial tear. The recognition of this problem can lead to the choice of another artificial tear preparation with a different preservative. Also, several types of preservative-free artificial tears have been developed. It is worth emphasizing that SS patients are at increased risk for complications during anesthesia, including corneal abrasions and postoperative pneumonitis resulting from inspissated mucus in the airways, because of the use of anticholinergic agents and the low humidity of the operating room. Therefore ocular lubricants are recommended for all SS patients during surgery and in the postoperative recovery room. Also, cautious use of anticholinergic agents, adequate hydration, and humidified oxygen help prevent these complications.

To help prevent progressive periodontal problems, intensive oral hygiene is required. Topical application of a neutral fluoride may help strengthen dental enamel and retard dental deterioration. A common problem in the SS patient is oral candidiasis, which may reflect the absence of naturally occurring antiyeast substances in saliva and frequently occurs in patients with recent antibiotic or corticosteroid treatment. Treatment with topical nystatin or clotrimazole for 4 to 6 weeks may be required to alleviate symptoms and prevent recurrences. For arthralgias and myalgias, nonsteroidal antiinflammatory drugs (NSAIDS) may be used, but with particular caution, since they may precipitate renal abnormalities in patients with interstitial nephritis. However, these agents can provoke esophageal injury in SS patients because they adhere to the drier walls of the esophagus in the absence of the normal salivary flow.

Systemic corticosteroids are generally reserved for life-threatening vasculitis, hemolytic anemia, and pleuropericarditis resistant to NSAIDs. As in SLE patients, other drugs may be used to help lower the dosage of corticosteroids, including hydroxychloroquine and azathioprine. When cyclophosphamide has been necessary for vasculitis, intravenous pulse therapy at 1 to 3-month intervals is preferred over daily therapy to decrease risk of lymphoma.

BIBLIOGRAPHY

Anderson LG, Talal N: The spectrum of benign to malignant lymphoproliferation in Sjögren's syndrome, *Clin Exp Immunol* 10:199-221, 1972.
Block KJ, Buchanan WW, Wohl MJ, Bunim JJ: Sjögren's syndrome: a clinical pathological and serological study of 62 cases, *Medicine (Baltimore)* 44:187-231, 1956.
Daniels TE, Whitcher JP: Association of patterns of labial salivary gland inflammation with keratoconjunctivitis sicca: analysis of 618 patients with suspected Sjögren's syndrome, *Arthritis Rheum* 37:869-877, 1994.
Fox R: Sjögren's syndrome: genetic, environmental, clinical and therapeutic aspects, *Curr Opin Rheumatol* 8:438-445, 1996.
Fox R, Saito I: Criteria for diagnosis of Sjögren's syndrome, *Rheum Dis Clin North Am* 20:391-401, 1993.

CHAPTER

194 Systemic Lupus Erythematosus

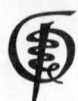

John H. Klippel

Systemic lupus erythematosus (SLE) is an immune-mediated, inflammatory disease with widespread organ involvement. Antibodies reactive with nucleoproteins ("antinuclear antibodies") are the hallmark of the disease. The etiology is unknown, although genetic, hormonal, and environmental factors are thought to contribute to the altered im-

mune state. The notable pathologic feature of the disease is the deposition of immunoglobulins, presumably in the form of antigen-antibody complexes, and complement along vascular basement membranes. Multiple organs may be affected, most commonly the skin, joints, serosal surfaces, kidneys, and central nervous system. The modes of presentation and clinical manifestations are protean, and the disease course is highly variable, with periods of exacerbations and remissions. Medical therapies are directed at suppression of local tissue inflammation, as well as suppression of immune function.

INCIDENCE AND PREVALENCE

The yearly incidence of SLE is estimated to be 50 to 70 new cases per million, with a prevalence of approximately 500 per million. Women, particularly during the reproductive years, are at significantly greater risk than are men with a female-to-male ratio of about 9:1. Although lupus may develop at any age, the highest incidence is observed in the age-group 20 to 40 years. Racial factors, presumably genetic, appear to be important, with increases in the frequency of SLE reported in African Americans, Native Americans, Puerto Ricans, and Chinese.

ETIOLOGIC FACTORS

The cause of SLE is unknown, but genetic, endocrine, and environmental factors are thought to be important. It is generally believed that these factors act synergistically, and depending on the relative contribution of these various factors, distinct serologic and clinical subsets may be produced.

Genetic Factors

The importance of genetic factors is evident by the finding of clinical SLE in approximately 1 of 10 first-degree relatives of SLE patients. Moreover, immunologic abnormalities such as diffuse hypergammaglobulinemia, antinuclear antibodies, and false-positive test results for syphilis are even more common in otherwise completely asymptomatic relatives. An intermediate degree of disease concordance is found in monozygotic, but not dizygotic, twin pairs. Studies of human leukocyte antigen (HLA) in SLE have found associations with class II antigens, in particular, HLA-DR3 and the linked specificities DR2 and DQw1. These confer a relative risk of approximately 3.

Inherited deficiencies of several complement components have been associated with lupuslike illnesses. The most common is a deficiency of the second component of complement (C2); deficiencies of other classic and alternate pathway components in patients with SLE have been noted (Chapter 186). Some are coded by autosomal recessive genes of the sixth chromosome, which are in linkage disequilibrium with HLA-DRw2. Whether the association of complement deficiencies with SLE is a consequence of linkage to HLA-D–region SLE disease genes or an inherent susceptibility induced by the complement deficiency itself is not known.

Environmental Factors

Environmental factors incriminated in SLE include ultraviolet light, bacterial and viral infections, and drugs (see Drug-Induced Lupus Syndromes later in this chapter). Presumably these factors share a common property of stimulating the immune system and altering its function. For instance, the exposure of cultured keratinocytes to ultraviolet light causes programmed cell death (apoptosis) with the formation of blebs on the cell membrane containing nucleoproteins to which antibodies are formed in SLE. Conceivably this might result in changes of the nucleoproteins such that they become antigenic, perhaps through the formation of thymidine dimers in DNA and RNA. Bacterial DNA and lipopolysaccharide fractions are potent polyclonal B-cell activators and, when administered to animals, induce the formation of circulating immune complexes and, subsequently, antibodies to both single- and double-stranded DNA. Viruses are postulated to play a major role in both murine and canine models of SLE. Theoretically the chronic infection of lymphocytes with a virus might account for immunologic abnormalities that are present in SLE. Indirect evidence for a persistent viral infection in SLE includes increases in antibodies to multiple DNA and RNA viruses; the presence of electron-dense paramyxovirus-like cytoplasmic inclusions, so-called tubuloreticular structures, along vascular endothelium and within circulating lymphocytes; and reports of type C oncornaviruses in involved renal and skin tissue. Recent studies have focused mainly on type C retroviruses. However, attempts to isolate retroviruses from SLE tissues by hybridization and cocultivation techniques have been largely unsuccessful. Thus the proposed viral origin of SLE remains an attractive, yet entirely unproved, hypothesis.

Endocrine Factors

The disproportionate number of women with SLE and the propensity for the disease to worsen during pregnancy and in the immediate postpartum period underscore a potentially important role for female sex hormones. Alterations in estrogen metabolism with increased hydroxylation of estrone that enhance estrogen activity have been described in SLE. Conversely, an increased frequency of SLE that occurs in patients with Klinefelter's syndrome suggests that androgens may have a protective function. Opposing effects of sex hormones on both humoral and cellular immunity have been described and may eventually explain these clinical observations.

PATHOGENESIS

The major immunologic defect in SLE is a state of spontaneous B-lymphocyte hyperactivity with the uncontrolled production of a wide variety of antibodies to both host and exogenous antigens. Whether this results from a primary failure of the B lymphocytes to respond to normal suppressor signals, from defects in T-regulatory lymphocytes, or from both is uncertain. For reasons that are unexplained, antibodies to nucleic acids and nucleic acid–protein complexes, such as the nucleosome made up of DNA and histones, predominate. These antibodies become deposited in the subendothelial layers of vascular basement membranes, either as antigen-antibody complexes directly from the circulation or as antibody reacting with antigens that are present in the basement membrane. The sites of deposition and pathologic consequences of complexes in the skin, kidney, choroid plexus, or serosal surfaces are dictated in part by physicochemical properties of the antigen or antibody, such as size, charge, molecular configuration, immunoglobulin class, and complement-fixing properties (Chapter 175). Once deposited, the immune complexes initiate a localized inflammatory response involving activation of complement, emigration of neutrophils, the release of kinins and prostaglandins, and, in all likelihood, antibody-dependent, cell-mediated tissue injury. Direct antibody-mediated injury may be associated with some manifestations of lupus, such as hemolytic anemia and thrombocytopenia.

PATHOLOGIC FEATURES

The earliest demonstrable pathologic event in SLE is an acute vasculopathy. The periarteriolar supporting tissue becomes edematous and infiltrated, first, with neutrophils and, later, with plasma cells and lymphocytes. The persistence of inflammation results in the local deposition of an acellular, homogenous eosinophilic material, similar on histologic study to fibrin and called *fibrinoid material*. In addition, nuclear debris from cellular necrosis within tissues reacts with antinuclear antibodies and coalesces to form intensely basophilic-staining material referred to as hematoxylin bodies.

When examined by indirect immunofluorescence, the vascular lesions can be shown to contain immunoglobulins, presumably complexed with antigen, complement components, and fibrin. These findings can be demonstrated along the basement membrane of skin, serosal surfaces, choroid plexus, pulmonary parenchyma, and renal glomeruli. Elution studies of the kidney have revealed the predominant antibodies to be of immunoglobulin G (IgG) and immunoglobulin M (IgM) classes, directed primarily against nucleoprotein antigens.

Involvement of the kidney results in several different forms of renal disease (Chapter 116). The most common type is characterized by an early infiltration of vascular tufts with neutrophils and lymphocytes, followed by swelling and proliferation of glomerular mesangial,

endothelial, or epithelial cells. A similar inflammatory reaction may be seen within the tubulointerstitium. By electron microscopy, dense deposits can be demonstrated in the mesangium and between endothelial cells and the glomerular basement membrane. Cellular proliferation that is confined to the mesangium is termed *mesangial nephritis*. Proliferative changes of the glomerular capillaries are classified as focal or diffuse nephritis depending on the extent and degree of the proliferative changes. Late in the process, sclerosis of the glomerulus or fibrosis of tubulointerstital tissues may be evident. In addition, adhesions may form between the vascular tufts and the parietal layer of Bowman's membrane, leading to epithelial crescents.

The other major form of SLE renal involvement is membranous nephropathy, which is indistinguishable on pathologic study from idiopathic membranous disease. When studied with light microscopy, the glomerular basement membrane is uniformly thickened by an eosinophilic material with no or minimal cellular proliferation. Thickening of the basement membrane may be accentuated in isolated glomerular tufts to produce a "wire-loop" appearance. On electron microscopy, dense deposits are seen in the subepithelial spaces with fusion of the glomerular foot processes (Chapter 116).

There is no good explanation for the different types of renal disease in SLE. It is speculated that physical properties of the deposited antibodies or immune complexes, dynamics of tissue deposition and clearance, or genetically determined differences in host reactivity may account for them.

CLINICAL FEATURES

The spectrum of clinical manifestations of SLE ranges from a mild systemic illness with a photosensitive facial rash and transient, diffuse arthritis to a fulminant presentation with life-threatening involvement of the heart, lungs, kidneys, or central nervous system. Episodes of disease exacerbations, or flares, are of varying severity and often quite individualized for any particular patient.

The disease course is remarkably unpredictable. Flares of the disease are often followed by periods of clinical remission. The duration of the cycles in this disease pattern are of various lengths, with transitions occurring abruptly, unexpectedly, and without obvious cause. The survival after diagnosis is currently estimated to be greater than 90% at 10 years. The highest mortality is in patients with progressive renal involvement or central nervous system disease. The most frequent causes of death are primary organ failure (renal or central nervous system), infections, and cardiovascular disease.

Constitutional signs and symptoms are extremely common and may be striking in severity. Most patients note fatigue, and malaise, anorexia, and weight loss are not infrequent. Fever, occasionally with rigors and night sweats, may suggest the presence of an underlying infection. The increased susceptibility of SLE patients to both common and opportunistic infections demands careful evaluation for occult infectious processes in all patients with febrile systemic presentations.

Mucocutaneous Features

The wide variety of mucocutaneous involvement can be seen in SLE. The acute erythematous, often maculopapular eruption on the malar region of the face ("butterfly rash") (Fig. 194-1, *A*) and the chronic scarring lesions of discoid lupus (Fig. 194-1, *B*) are most easily recognized. An interesting subset of generalized, nonscarring cutaneous lupus, termed *subacute cutaneous lupus,* is intermediate between these two common forms of lupus skin involvement (Chapter 212). Both papulosquamous (psoriasiform) and annular (polycyclic) variants have been described. A broad spectrum of other skin manifestations, including bullae, urticaria, verrucae, and angioedema, has been noted. Most lupus rashes are worsened by exposure to ultraviolet light.

Superficial vasculitis of dermal vessels produces erythematous, tender areas on the fingertips and palms, splinter hemorrhages of the nailbeds, and periungual infarctions. Livedo reticularis develops in patients with antiphospholipid antibodies, and dependent nonthrombocytopenic purpura develops in those with cryoglobulins. Peripheral vasomotor instability, often exacerbated by cold exposure or heightened emotions, leads to color changes of fingers and toes that are

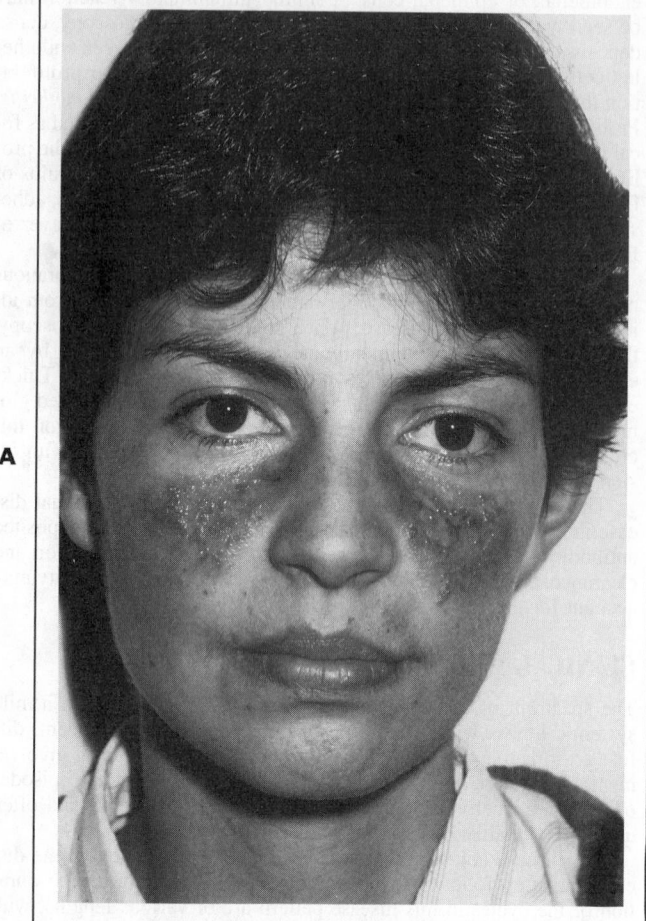

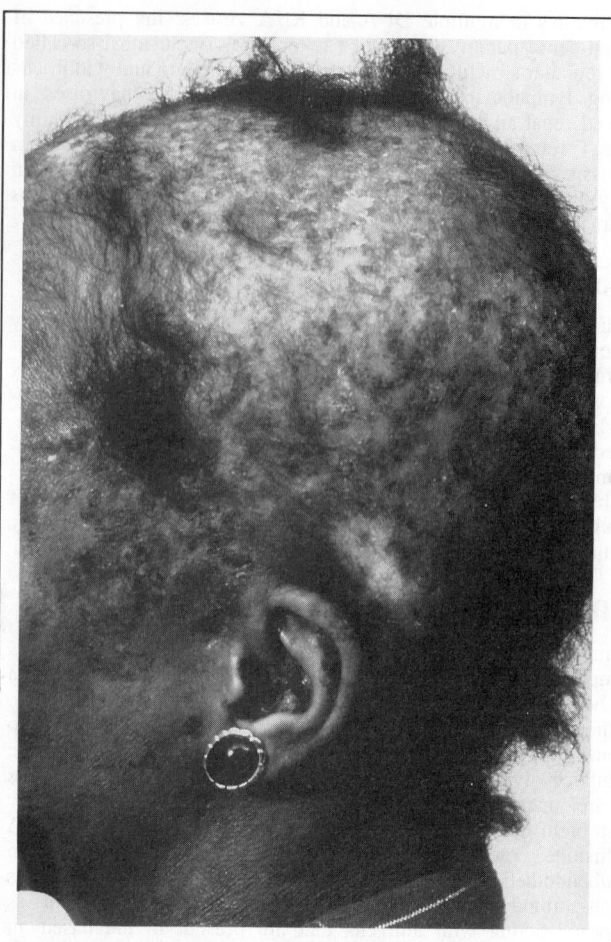

FIGURE 194-1   A, Erythematous malar ("butterfly") rash in patient with systemic lupus erythematosos (SLE). **B,** Scarring discoid rash of the scalp with extensive alopecia in patient with SLE.

From Dieppe PA et al, editors: *Atlas of clincial rheumatology,* London, 1986, Gower Medical.

characteristic of Raynaud's phenomenon. Inflammation in the subcutaneous fat (lupus profundus) can cause extensive skin ulceration with atrophy and calcifications on healing.

Superficial ulcerations of oral and genital mucous membranes are typically painless and often go undetected. Ulcerations of the nasal mucosa can lead to epistaxis and perforation of the nasal septum. Hair loss results in either diffuse or patchy alopecia. In the absence of scarring of the scalp by discoid lesions the alopecia generally is entirely reversible. The regrown hair in involved areas is often brittle, with a short, stubby appearance.

Musculoskeletal Features

The arthritis of SLE is typically a transient peripheral polyarthritis with symmetric involvement of both small and large joints. Despite complaints of joint pain, signs of joint inflammation with effusions and palpable synovial thickening are often absent. The joint complaints are rarely chronic and essentially are never associated with cartilage loss, subchondral cystic changes, or bony erosions. The development of persistent pain or synovitis in a single joint should suggest a superimposed complication such as osteonecrosis or septic arthritis. Periarticular structures, particularly tendon sheaths, may be involved, and involvement can lead to acute rupture of the Achilles or patellar tendons.

Reducible, rheumatoid-like hand deformities with ulnar deviation of the phalanges and flexion and extension abnormalities of the small joints of the fingers develop in about 10% of patients. In contrast to rheumatoid arthritis, however, bony erosions of the wrist, metacarpal heads, or interphalangeal joints are not present on radiographs. The

arthropathy is similar to the hand deformities described after rheumatic fever (Jaccoud's arthritis) and is thought to be caused by capsular and tendon laxity from recurrent chronic inflammation.

The major disabling chronic joint disease of SLE is the arthropathy of osteonecrosis (avascular necrosis), most commonly involving large weight-bearing joints such as the hips, knees, and ankles (Chapter 201). Nuclear magnetic resonance imaging studies are able to detect this complication before the development of classic late radiographic findings. Osteonecrosis is most frequently seen following the use of high-dose corticosteroids. Osteonecrosis may produce significant pain and disability, and orthopedic surgery with total joint replacement may be necessary.

Muscle pain and weakness may result from inflammatory myositis or occur as a complication of drug therapy, most commonly steroid myopathy or neuromyopathy from antimalarials. Similarly, symptoms of fibromylagia appear to be frequent in SLE patients.

Serositis

Inflammation of serosal surfaces may be associated with acute or chronic pleuritis, pericarditis, or peritonitis. The pain may be severe and may suggest myocardial infarction, pulmonary embolus, or acute abdominal crisis. Fluid accumulation is usually modest, although occasionally pericardial tamponade or massive ascites develops. In patients with fever or with chronic serositis, analysis of the fluid is necessary to exclude an underlying infection. Typically the fluid that accumulates with lupus serositis has a white blood cell count of less than 3000 cells/mm^3 (predominantly monocytes and lymphocytes), reduced levels of complement as compared with serum levels, and, often, the finding of LE cells formed in vivo.

Cardiac Features

Ischemic heart disease from coronary arteritis or, more commonly, atherosclerotic coronary disease with angina or myocardial infarction is an increasingly recognized complication in SLE. Patients with nephrotic syndrome or those who receive treatment with prolonged courses of corticosteroids are at increased risk. Noninfectious vegetations form on the ventricular surfaces of the mitral, aortic, and tricuspid valves (Libman-Sacks endocarditis), particularly in patients with antiphospholipid antibodies. The vegetations can easily be visualized by echocardiography. The endocardial lesions may produce valvular regurgitations that require valve replacement. In addition, the vegetations may break off to produce arterial emboli and are a potential nidus of superimposed bacterial infection.

An inflammatory process involving the myocardium can produce persistent tachycardia, ventricular arrhythmias, conduction abnormalities, and, occasionally, intractable congestive heart failure. It is often associated with a more generalized peripheral inflammatory myopathy. Chemistry studies reveal increased levels of muscle enzymes, particularly the MB isoenzyme of creatine phosphokinase.

Pulmonary Features

Although pulmonary function studies reveal minor diffusion and obstruction abnormalities in a high proportion of patients, clinical problems resulting from pulmonary involvement in SLE are distinctly unusual. Transient basilar pneumonic infiltrates ("lupus pneumonitis") with nonproductive cough, hypoxemia, and complaints of dyspnea must be distinguished from infection. Alveolar hemorrhage with massive hemoptysis and pulmonary hypertension are extremely rare but serious complications associated with a high mortality.

Gastrointestinal Tract Symptoms

Transient, nonspecific abdominal pain is common and generally considered to result from peritonitis. Acute or chronic pancreatitis is infrequent with active SLE and more commonly seen as complication of drug therapy, particularly with corticosteroids. Hepatic involvement is distinctly unusual. Hepatitis, when found, is typically attributable to the use of salicylates or nonsteroidal antiinflammatory drugs, fatty infiltration from corticosteroids, or other non–SLE-related causes. Primary biliary cirrhosis has been reported to be increased in SLE patients. Vasculitis of the mesentery and intraabdominal organs may lead to acute abdominal crises that require surgical exploration. Infarction and perforation of the bowel or viscera are associated with a high mortality.

Renal Features

Active renal involvement is first detected on urinalysis by the finding of proteinuria, red blood cells, white blood cells, or cellular or hyaline casts. Patients with massive proteinuria may occasionally come to medical attention with peripheral edema or the nephrotic syndrome. Hypertension is very common in patients with lupus nephropathy.

The role of renal biopsy in the clinical management of SLE is controversial. Biopsy is generally not needed for diagnostic purposes, except for rare instances in which drug toxicities or secondary complications such as amyloidosis are considerations. On the other hand, renal biopsy does provide valuable information as to the type of nephritis that is present—proliferative, membranous, or a combination—which is important in assessing prognosis and planning therapy (Chapter 116). Biopsy findings of mesangial nephritis are generally associated with a relatively benign disease course, whereas diffuse proliferative or membranoproliferative nephritis indicates a much less favorable renal outcome. Studies have shown that individual chronic biopsy features such as glomerular sclerosis, fibrous crescents, interstitial fibrosis, and tubular atrophy predict a poor outcome.

Aside from prognostic information derived from the renal biopsy,

the course of renal disease is highly unpredictable. Although progression is often associated with persistent clinical or serologic abnormalities, exceptions are sufficiently common to make these abnormalities unreliable monitors of renal inflammation. Loss of renal function may be acute, similar to that of rapidly progressive glomerulonephritis, or, more typically, chronic with a slowly progressive rise in serum creatinine level over the course of many years. End-stage renal failure can be successfully managed with dialysis or transplantation.

Neuropsychiatric Features

Neurologic and, in particular, psychiatric manifestations are frequent. Disturbances of mental function are most common and range from mild confusion, with memory deficits and impairments of orientation and perception, to frank psychiatric disturbances of hypomania, delirium, and schizophrenia. Seizures are usually of the grand mal type, although petit mal, focal, and temporal lobe epilepsy have been described. Severe headaches, often with scotomata typical of the fortification spectra of migraine, are increased in SLE patients. Strokes from hemorrhage or cerebral infarction occur, particularly in patients with antiphospholipid antibodies. Less common neurologic disturbances include cranial neuropathies, transverse myelopathy, aseptic meningitis, pseudotumor cerebri, chorea, hemiballismus, a parkinsonian picture, and both sensory and motor peripheral neuropathies.

Before signs and symptoms of central nervous system dysfunction are attributed to active SLE, other causes must be considered. Infections (meningitis, intracranial abscess), renal failure (azotemia, hypertension), drug effects (corticosteroids, antimalarials, anticonvulsants), mass lesions (tumors, subdural hematoma), structural defects (hydrocephalus, aneurysms), and arterial emboli from endocardial vegetations can all mimic central nervous system SLE.

Conventional studies performed to evaluate the central nervous system are of limited value in the assessment of these patients. The cerebrospinal fluid may show mild elevations of protein and IgG levels, oligoclonal bands on electrophoresis, and pleocytosis, usually lymphocytes. On the other hand, the fluid is often normal, even in the presence of major clinical dysfunction. The electroencephalogram may be normal or show local or diffuse changes. Arteriographic studies rarely demonstrate evidence of vasculitis of small or large vessels. Abnormalities of static pertechnetate brain scans, computed tomography, magnetic resonance imaging, and positron emission tomography (PET) scans have been reported.

Lymphadenopathy

Enlargement of peripheral and axial lymph nodes and splenomegaly occur but are usually transient. Biopsy specimens of lymph nodes demonstrate hyperplasia with preservation of the normal architecture. Chronic or massive lymphadenopathy should suggest either lymphoma, particularly in patients with secondary Sjögren's syndrome, or angioimmunoblastic lymphadenopathy.

LABORATORY FINDINGS

Patients with SLE display a host of laboratory abnormalities reflecting the multisystemic nature of the disease. Moderate anemia with normocytic, normochromic erythrocyte indices is a consistent feature. Although a positive Coombs' test result can occasionally be found in SLE patients, anemia resulting from actual hemolysis is extremely infrequent. Leukopenia, particularly lymphocytopenia, is common and often accurately reflects disease activity. Thrombocytopenia is usually of low grade; counts of 50,000 to 100,000 cells/mm³ are the rule. Lower platelet counts may be associated with bleeding and are an indication for aggressive treatment. Bone marrow aspirates in SLE are generally hypercellular. Cellular destruction within the marrow may lead to the phagocytosis of nuclear debris and the formation of in vivo LE cells.

Prolongation of the partial thromboplastin time results from antiphospholipid antibodies, which inhibit activation of prothrombin. False-positive serologic test results for syphilis are commonly seen in these patients as a result of cross-reactivity of the antibody with other phospholipids. Paradoxically, these patients with the

Table 194-1   Antibodies to nuclear antigens in systemic lupus erythematosus

ANTIBODY SPECIFICITY	SLE PATIENTS WITH ANTIBODY	CLINCIAL ASSOCIATION
1. DNA		
Double-stranded	60	Highly specific; titers parallel disease activity, particularly lupus nephritis
Single-stranded	60	Nonspecific, present in many other rheumatic diseases
2. Histones	70	Higher frequencies (90%) in patients with drug-induced forms of lupus
3. Ribonucleoproteins		
Sm	30	Found only in SLE (diagnostic)
U1 RNP	40	Common in lupus "overlap" syndromes
Ro (SS-A)	30	Common in lupus with Sjögren's syndrome or subacute cutaneous lupus; related to neonatal lupus and congenital heart block
La (SS-B)	15	Common in lupus with Sjögren's syndrome
Ribosomal P	5	Associated with lupus psychosis

so-called lupus anticoagulant have an increased incidence of venous and arterial thromboses rather than bleeding. Other antibodies against coagulation factors VIII, IX, XI, XII, and XIII have been described.

The most distinctive laboratory feature of SLE is the development of antibodies to host antigens, especially to nuclear antigens, including single- and double-stranded DNA, nuclear histones, and specific soluble ribonuclear protein antigens, notably the Smith (Sm) antigen. Routine screening studies to detect these antibodies use indirect immunofluorescent assays of cultured cell lines, fixed tissue sections, or the haemoflagellate *Crithidia luciliae*. Different specificities produce distinct patterns of immunofluorescence, commonly referred to as *homogeneous, speckled, nucleolar, or rim patterns* (Chapter 293). Sera from SLE patients are capable of producing all patterns, although the rim pattern, produced by antibodies to double-stranded DNA, is the most specific for the disease. Antinuclear antibodies may produce a false-positive beaded pattern in the fluorescent treponemal antibody (FTA) assay.

The antigen specificities of many of the antinuclear antibodies found in patients with SLE have been identified and assays developed to directly measure these antibodies (Table 194-1). Antibody to double-stranded DNA is commonly used to monitor the disease, particularly in patients with lupus nephritis. Antibodies to ribonuclear protein antigens are of interest; antibodies to the Sm antigen are essentially diagnostic of SLE; antibodies to U1-RNP, Ro (SS-A), and La (SS-B) are characteristically seen in SLE overlap syndromes.

Serum levels of complement proteins generally are reduced during states of clinically active SLE. Reductions result from a consumption of classic and alternate pathway components at the tissue sites of immune-complex deposition and as a result of impaired synthesis. Levels of total hemolytic complement (CH_{50}), C3, and C4 often are used as monitors of disease activity. Persistent, markedly reduced levels of CH_{50} should suggest the possible presence of an inherited complement deficiency, most commonly a deficiency of C2 (Chapter 228).

Nonspecific elevations in levels of immunoglobulins, particularly IgG and IgM, are frequent. A deficiency of IgA appears to be more common in SLE than in normal persons. Monoclonal gammopathies have been described occasionally. Marked increases in gamma globulins may result in a hyperviscosity syndrome or renal tubular acidosis. Serum cryoglobulins of the mixed IgG-IgM type are often found in patients with Raynaud's phenomenon, purpura, or renal involvement and hypocomplementemia.

DIAGNOSIS

The diagnosis of SLE poses little problem if the clinical and serologic features are classic and evolve over a brief time period. Frequently, however, clinical manifestations are atypical or occur so sporadically as to make diagnosis quite difficult. Moreover, serologic abnormalities, in particular antinuclear antibodies, can be found in a number of other conditions besides SLE (Table 194-2).

Classification criteria have been developed for SLE (Table 194-3). Any combination of four or more criteria over any time period has been found to be a sensitive, specific means of identifying patients with SLE. The high specificity of select laboratory studies such as antibodies to double-stranded DNA, antibodies to the ribonuclear pro-

Table 194-2   Conditions other than systemic lupus erythematosus with a positive antinuclear antibody

FINDING	CONDITION(S)
Normal	Usually in low titer; frequency increases with age, female sex, and family history of immunologic disease
Drug Induced	Hydralazine, procainamide, and others
Hematologic	Autoimmune hemolytic anemia; autoimmune thrombocytopenic purpura
Skin	Psoriasis, pemphigus vulgaris, lichen planus
Lung	Idiopathic pulmonary fibrosis, asbestosis, primary pulmonary hypertension
Hepatic	Autoimmune hepatitis, primary biliary cirrhosis, chronic viral hepatitis, alcoholic liver disease
Infectious	Chronic bacterial diseases (e.g. osteomyelitis, subacute bacterial endocarditis)
Endocrine	Diabetes mellitus, autoimmune thyroiditis, Graves' disease
Neurologic	Multiple sclerosis, subacute sensory neuropathy
Malignancies	Myelodysplastic syndromes, lymphoma, leukemia, melanoma, solid tumors (ovary, breast, lung, kidney, liver)

tein antigen Sm, or hypocomplementemia in the setting of multisystem disease makes these serologic studies valuable in diagnosis.

TREATMENT

The drug treatment of SLE is largely empiric and guided by the concept of SLE disease activity. Therapy is intensified during periods of acute flares, with the severity of the manifestation dictating drug selection, dose, and duration of treatment.

Nonsteroidal antiinflammatory drugs (NSAIDs) have a role in the treatment of fever, musculoskeletal symptoms, and mild pleurisy. Patients with SLE are particularly prone to the development of drug complications of NSAIDs, including hepatitis, impairments of renal function, skin rashes, and an aseptic meningitis syndrome that can easily be confused with active SLE. The complications are readily reversible on discontinuing the drug.

Adrenal corticosteroids should be reserved for patients who have failed to respond to NSAIDs or as first-line therapy in patients with acute, severe disease. The type of corticosteroid is less important than the dose. Oral prednisone is most commonly used and begun as a single, daily dose given in the morning; topical or intralesional corticosteroid preparations are used for cutaneous disease. Manifestations such as fever, fatigue, polyarthritis, or serositis typically respond promptly to treatment with low-dose prednisone (≤0.5 mg/kg). Severe or life-threatening manifestations such as pericarditis, myocarditis, hemolytic anemia, thrombocytopenia, acute glomerulonephritis, and central nervous system disease are indications for higher doses in the range of 1 mg/kg daily. Bolus intravenous methylprednisolone (1 g or 15 mg/kg) is a widely used alternative to conventional high-dose oral corticosteroids. In patients with severe disease who fail to

Table 194-3 American College of Rheumatology criteria for the classification of systemic lupus erythematosus (SLE)

CRITERION	FREQUENCY IN SLE (%)
1. Malar rash	57
2. Discoid rash	18
3. Photosensitivity	43
4. Oral or nasopharyngeal ulcers	27
5. Nonerosive arthritis	86
6. Pleuritis or	52
Pericarditis	18
7. Persistent proteinuria or	50
urinary casts	36
8. Seizures or	12
psychosis	13
9. Hemolytic anemia or	18
leukopenia ($<4000/mm^3$) or	46
lymphopenia ($<1500/mm^3$) or	—
thrombocytopenia ($<100,000/mm^3$)	21
10. LE cells or	73
DNA antibody or	67
Sm antibody or	31
false positive serologic test for syphilis	15
11. Antinuclear antibody	99

Tan E Et al: *Arthritis Rheum* 25:1271, 1982.

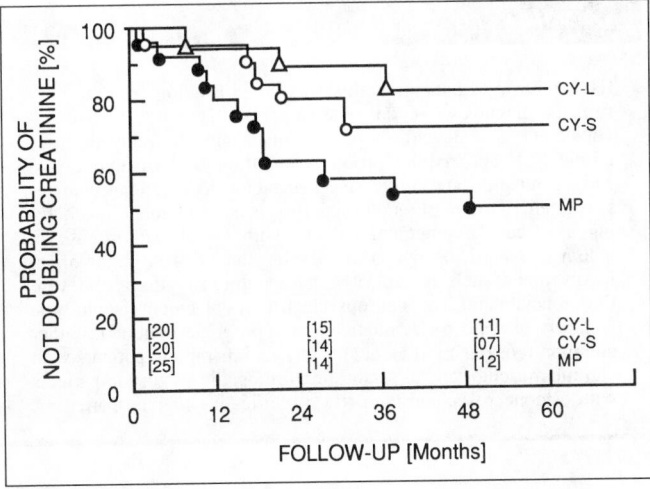

FIGURE 194-2 Cumulative probability of not doubling serum creatinine following treatment with intravenous methylprednisolone (MP) as compared with 6- (CY-S) and 30- (CY-L) month course of intravenous cyclophosphamide. From Boumpas DT et al: *Lancet* 340:741, 1992.

show substantial improvement within several days the prednisone should be given two or three times daily.

The prednisone dosage should be kept constant until symptoms and signs of SLE activity are well under control. However, complications of corticosteroids vary directly with dose and duration of administration. Thus a cautious reduction in dose, once inflammation has subsided, is critical in the prevention of corticosteroid toxicity. Patients who fail to respond to a 4-week course of high-dose corticosteroids (>1 mg/kg daily), relapse with dose reductions, or develop unacceptable toxicities are candidates for alternate forms of therapy.

The antimalarial drugs chloroquine, hydroxychloroquine, and quinacrine have an important role in the treatment of mild systemic features of SLE, especially mucocutaneous manifestations. Antimalarials should be used with caution in patients with glucose-6-phosphate dehydrogenase (G6PD) deficiency or in patients with liver disease. Hydroxychloroquine (200 to 400 mg daily) is the most commonly used antimalarial. Improvements are generally noted within the first several weeks of therapy; conversely, SLE flares may be seen in the immediate period following the discontinuation of antimalarials. The most serious potential toxic effect of antimalarials is retinal damage. The risks of retinal toxicity with the low doses used in SLE are exceedingly small; however, as a precaution, eye examinations for disturbances in color vision and retinal changes should be performed every 6 to 12 months during treatment. Additional complications of antimalarial drugs include rashes, photosensitivity, neuromyopathy, and pigmentary changes of skin, mucous membranes, and hair. Antimalarials have been associated with birth defects and are contraindicated during pregnancy and in patients wishing to become pregnant.

Immunosuppressive drugs are reserved for patients with life-threatening manifestations including severe lupus nephritis, central nervous system disease, cardiopulmonary events, or hematologic complications such as thrombocytopenia. Intravenous bolus cyclophosphamide, a nitrogen mustard alkylating agent, has been shown to prevent the loss of renal function and reduce the likelihood of end-stage renal failure (Fig. 194-2). Alternative immunosuppressive agents used in SLE include azathioprine, methotrexate, and cyclosporin A. Side effects of immunosuppressive drugs are potentially serious, and it is recommended that they be administered only by physicians experienced in their use.

Pregnant patients with SLE are at increased risk of disease flares during the pregnancy, as well as in the immediate postpartum period, and must be followed up closely. In general, it is recommended that pregnancy be avoided during periods of disease activity involving major organs, particularly nephritis. Premature delivery, fetal wastage, and spontaneous abortion are all increased in SLE. These complications are increased in mothers with high titers of anticardiolipin an-

---

BOX 194-1

Drugs capable of producing serologic and clinical features of systemic lupus erythenatosus

Antihypertensive

Hydralazine
Methyldopa

Aniarrhythmics

Procainamide
Practolol

Anticonvulsants

Phenytoin
Mephenytoin trimethadione
Ethosuximide
Primidone

Miscellaneous

Isoniazid
Penicillamine
Chlorpromazine
Propylthiouracil
Methylthiouracil
Chlorthalidone
Sulfonamides
Penicillin
Chlorprothixene

tibodies. The passive transfer of maternal antibodies across the placenta can produce transient abnormalities in the newborn (e.g., hepatosplenomegaly, cytopenias, and photosensitive rashes), which resolve as antibody titers decline.

Congenital heart block and other cardiac abnormalities are increased, particularly in infants born of mothers with antibodies to Ro(SS-A) (Chapter 293).

DRUG-INDUCED LUPUS SYNDROMES

A number of drugs (Box 194-1) are associated with the development of antinuclear antibodies and, less frequently, clinical syndromes resembling SLE. Two drugs in particular, procainamide and hydralazine, are extremely potent inducers of antinuclear, antierythrocyte, and antilymphocyte antibodies. In approximately 60% of patients re-

✔ *WHEN TO REFER*

Early referral of patients with suspected SLE is important to confirm the diagnosis, ascertain the extent and severity of organ involvement, and develop a plan of management. Many diseases mimic SLE and require prompt recognition and treatment, and early evaluation and aggressive management of major organ involvement, particularly lupus nephritis, is a key element in achieving a successful outcome. Patients with established disease in whom new signs or symptoms develop that suggest major organ involvement, such as nephritis, cardiopulmonary disease, severe thrombocytopenia, or neuropsychiatric involvement, should be similarly referred for evaluation and appropriate treatment. Other common referrals in SLE include physical therapy in patients with chronic musculoskeletal disabilities, orthopedic surgury in patients with osteonecrosis, and high-risk obstetrics in pregnant patients.

ceiving these drugs such antibodies develop. The antibodies themselves appear to be harmless and do not necessitate drug withdrawal. High antibody titers may persist for months without the development of any clinical symptom. Antibody titers may remain elevated for months and years, even after the drugs have been discontinued. However, in a small percentage of patients in whom the antibodies develop, a clinical syndrome with a predominance of musculoskeletal, pulmonary, and polyserositic symptoms that resembles SLE may develop. Renal and neurologic disease is distinctly uncommon. The clinical syndrome is generally reversible on discontinuing the suspected medication, although antiinflammatory drugs, including corticosteroids, may be required in the treatment of symptoms.

The mechanism whereby drugs induce autoantibodies is unknown. The rate of drug metabolism, host genetic factors, and drug influences on immune regulation are considered potentially important. The lupus-inducing drugs do not appear to exacerbate idiopathic SLE and thus can be used safely and as needed.

BIBLIOGRAPHY

Boumpas DT et al: Systemic lupus erythematosus: emerging concepts. I. Renal, neuropsychiatric, cardiovascular, pulmonary, and hematologic disease, *Ann Intern Med* 122:940, 1995.
Boumpas DT et al: Systemic lupus erythematosus: emerging concepts. II. Dermatologic and joint disease, the antiphospholipid antibody syndrome, pregnancy and hormonal therapy, morbidity and mortality, and pathogenesis. *Ann Intern Med* 123:42, 1995.
The Canadian Hydroxychloroquine Study Group: A randomized study of the effect of withdrawing hydroxychloroquine sulfate in systemic lupus erythematosus, *N Engl J Med* 324:150, 1991.
Lahita RG, editor: *Systemic lupus erythematosus,* New York, 1992, Churchill Livingstone.
McLaughlin JR et al: Kidney biopsy in systemic lupus erythematosus. III. Survival analysis controlling for clinical and laboratory results, *Arthritis Rheum* 37:559, 1994.
Mills JA: Systemic lupus erythematosus, *N Engl J Med* 330:1871, 1994.
Nossent HC et al: Systemic lupus erythematosus after renal transplantation: patient and graft survival and disease activity, *Ann Intern Med* 114:183, 1991.
Wallace DJ, Hahn BH, editors: *Dubois' lupus erythematosus,* Philadelphia, 1992, Lea & Febiger.
West SG: Neuropsychiatric lupus, *Rheum Dis Clin North Am* 20:129, 1994.

CHAPTER

195 Vasculitic Syndromes

Leonard H. Calabrese and George F. Duna

The vasculitides encompass a heterogeneous group of disorders, all sharing to varying degrees the pathologic features of vascular inflammation and vascular necrosis. Vasculitic syndromes may be conveniently classified as either primary or secondary. The primary vascu-

litides represent a diverse group of disorders with the vascular system as the primary target organ of disease pathogenesis and are believed to be immune mediated. Secondary vasculitis occurs when the vascular system is injured as a result of a wide variety of noxious stimuli, including infection or simple mechanical or chemical trauma.

PATHOGENESIS

Over the past 20 years there has been considerable progress in our understanding of the mechanisms of vascular inflammation. Immunologic factors are believed to be central in the pathogenesis of most vasculitic syndromes, although no uniform mechanism is likely to be operative in all cases. Although specific causes are rare, there is a growing body of clinical and experimental support for at least four mechanisms involved in vascular inflammation.

Immune Complexes

Evidence supporting the role of circulating immune complexes (ICs) in certain vasculitic conditions includes (1) animal models of immune-complex disease, (2) identification of immune complexes in tissues, (3) identification of immune complexes in the sera of patients with vasculitis, and (4) identification of discrete antigens responsible for certain vasculitic disorders. Among the primary vasculitides the strongest evidence in support of a pathogenic role for immune complexes is for the diseases within the hypersensitivity vasculitis group (see later discussion). True hypersensitivity vasculitis, which follows exposure to a discrete antigen (most commonly a drug), is often accompanied by evidence of complement activation and immunoglobulin and/or complement deposition in involved tissues. Additional evidence for a pathogenic role of immune complexes is found in Henoch-Schönlein purpura, cryoglobulinemia attributable to hepatitis C, urticarial vasculitis, and a fraction of patients with polyarteritis nodosa (PAN) attributable to hepatitis B virus infection.

Antibody-Associated Disease

Tissue-specific antibodies have been identified in a variety of vasculitic conditions and include antiendothelial cell antibodies and a variety of other tissue-specific and non–organ-specific antibodies. Most of these antibodies are not complement fixing, and it is unclear what role, if any, they have in pathogenesis.

Perhaps the greatest breakthrough in vasculitic research in the past decade has been the discovery of antineutrophil cytoplasmic antibodies (ANCAs). In 1982 ANCAs were identified by an immunofluorescent technique in a small number of patients with crescentic glomerulonephritis and vasculitis. This was followed in the mid-1980s by a series of observations identifying ANCA in association with Wegener's granulomatosis. Over the past few years the antigenic specificities of ANCA have been clarified, and laboratory techniques have been further defined. ANCAs are not specific for any particular form of vasculitis but are found in a family of vasculitic syndromes including Wegener's granulomatosis, microscopic polyarteritis nodosa, a subset of patients with PAN, and Churg-Strauss syndrome and in renal-limited forms of vasculitis.

ANCAs are divided on the basis of their immunofluorescent pattern and antigenic specificity. By immunofluorescence, ANCAs can be separated into those that produce cytoplasmic (C-ANCA) or perinuclear (P-ANCA) patterns. The antigen responsible for the C-ANCA pattern in most patients with vasculitis is a serine protease (29 kD in size) known as proteinase 3 (PR3). The antigen associated with the P-ANCA pattern in the setting of vasculitic disease is the enzyme myeloperoxidase (MPO). These substrates are found within the alpha or azurophilic granules of granulocytes and the cytosolic granules of monocytes. An important fact is that antibodies reacting with other antigens (i.e., non-PR3, non-MPO) can produce the C-ANCA or P-ANCA pattern, but these reactivities are currently of unknown clinical significance.

ANCAs are not associated with a single disease but are found in association with a family of diseases sharing certain pathologic features, including vasculitis with some granulocytic component (at least early in the course). In addition, these conditions share a similar renal pathologic picture described as "pauciimmune" glomerulonephritis, which implies little in the way of immune-complex and/or complement deposition, and frequent presence of cellular crescents. The sensitivity of ANCA in these diseases varies but may exceed 90% in patients with active multisystemic Wegener's granulomatosis. In general, antibodies to PR3 yielding the C-ANCA pattern are found in patients with Wegener's granulomatosis. Antibodies reacting in a P-ANCA pattern and directed at MPO are more likely to be found in patients with isolated renal disease (i.e., idiopathic, rapidly progressive glomerulonephritis). The specificity of ANCA depends on both technical factors and the nature of the control group. In laboratories performing both immunofluorescence and solid-phase assays directed against PR3 and MPO, specificity exceeds 95% for one of these families of specific vasculitic conditions.

Many other conditions have been reported to have ANCA positivity including Kawasaki's disease, certain infections including human immunodeficiency virus (HIV), inflammatory bowel disease, and sclerosing cholangitis. These reports have identified ANCA by immunofluorescence but have not confirmed reactivity to either PR3 or MPO. ANCAs are useful in the diagnosis of their associated vasculitic conditions and to some degree in monitoring disease activity.

It has been proposed that ANCAs may be directly pathogenic, but the evidence supporting this is incomplete. ANCAs under certain circumstances are capable of binding to neutrophils, causing release of their toxic products. Antibodies directed against either PR3 or MPO may bind to endothelial cells expressing these antigens on their surface.

Cell-Mediated or Endothelial Focus Disease

Certain vasculitic conditions are associated with neither circulating immune complexes nor specific autoantibodies. Giant cell arteritis and Takayasu's arteritis are such disorders and are notable for their pathologic appearance, which suggests a cell-mediated process. The ability of endothelial cells to become "activated" and to serve as antigen-presenting cells and sources of cytokine production forms a basis for their interaction with immune-competent cells. Endothelial cells also express multiple adhesion molecules that have the ability to interact with complementary ligands on immunocytes, leading to leukocyte binding and subsequent emigration. Evidence currently exists for endothelial cell activation and adhesion molecule expression in a variety of vasculitic conditions.

Immunoproliferative Disease

Several vascular inflammatory diseases (e.g., lymphomatoid granulomatosis) demonstrate strong evidence for a spectrum of lymphoproliferation ranging from benign to frankly malignant. These conditions are angiocentric and angioinvasive, predominantly involve T cells, and display little propensity for vessel necrosis. In the past these disorders have been included in the classification of the primary vasculitides, but in light of current immunohistochemical and immunogenetic data these probably represent lymphoproliferative disorders and are best treated as malignant lymphomas.

Although these immune-mediated mechanisms are discussed separately, it should be appreciated that most vasculitic syndromes probably represent admixtures of these proposed pathogenic mechanisms. For example, endothelium initially injured by immune complexes or antibody may subsequently become activated to secrete cytokines or display adhesion molecules, or both, to become the focus for further cell-mediated pathologic changes. A clearer understanding of the pathologic mechanisms involved in discrete syndromes will facilitate more specific therapies.

CLASSIFICATION

Numerous classifications have been proposed in an effort to better understand the vasculitides. Most of these schemes have been plagued by inherent inconsistencies and lack of clinical utility. In 1978, Fauci and others at the National Institutes of Health proposed a classification scheme that has been widely used. A modification of this scheme is presented in Box 195-1. This classification is based on clinical, pathologic, immunologic, and therapeutic variables that results in a system that is not only approachable in its clarity, but is also clinically useful.

> **BOX 195-1**
> **Current classification of necrotizing vasculitis**
>
> **Polyarteritis nodosa group**
> Classic polyarteritis
> Churg-Strauss syndrome (allergic granulomatosis)
> Microscopic polyarteritis
> Polyangiitis
>
> **Hypersensitivity vasculitis group**
> True hypersensitivity vasculitis
> Henoch-Schönlein purpura
> Cryoglobulinemic vasculitis
> Vasculitis associated with connective tissue disease
> Urticarial vasculitis
> Vasculitis associated with systemic diseases
>
> **Wegener's granulomatosis group**
> Wegener's granulomatosis
> Limited Wegener's granulomatosis
>
> **Giant cell group**
> Giant cell arteritis
> Takayasu's arteritis
>
> **Angiocentric lymphoproliferative disorders**
> Benign lymphocytic angiitis
> Lymphomatoid granulomatosis
> Angiocentric lymphoma
>
> **Miscellaneous vasculitides**

SYSTEMIC NECROTIZING VASCULITIS GROUP
Polyarteritis Nodosa

Polyarteritis nodosa is a vasculitic syndrome affecting primarily medium-sized muscular arteries. PAN is more common in males, with a sex ratio of approximately 2:1. All age-groups may be affected, but it is more common between the ages of 40 and 60 years.

Pathologic Findings. Necrotizing vasculitis with fibrinoid necrosis represents the characteristic active lesion. In some instances necrotizing lesions are eccentric and form a "blow-out" type of aneurysm. These aneurysms are clinically relevant, since they may be useful in diagnosis when identified on angiography and also serve as the focus of rupture and hemorrhage.

PAN has been reported in association with hepatitis B in approximately 15% to 30% of cases. In these instances ICs are believed to play an important role. Other underlying diseases that have been associated with a PAN-like syndrome include hairy cell leukemia, endocarditis, connective tissue diseases, and drug abuse.

Clinical Findings. Polyarteritis nodosa ranges from a mild, transient process to a fulminating and rapidly fatal disease. Virtually any organ may be affected at onset or during the course of the disease. There is no predominant presenting sign or symptom, making PAN a frequent diagnostic challenge. The most common signs of PAN relate to its multisystemic inflammatory nature. Constitutional symptoms including weakness and malaise, often accompanied by varying degrees of fever and weight loss, are common. Other clinical findings reflect the wide range of target organ involvement. Musculoskeletal symptoms are common, including an inflammatory polyarthritis that may mimic early-stage rheumatoid arthritis. Involvement of peripheral nerves is also common, manifesting as either a glove-and-stocking type of neuropathy or mononeuritis multiplex. Symptoms relating to the presence of gastrointestinal tract involvement ranging from vague abdominal pains to the picture of frank perforation may also be seen at any time.

The kidneys, involved in the vast majority of patients, display vasculitic involvement of the extraglomerular vasculature. True glomerulonephritis is uncommon in classic PAN. Microaneurysms identified by angiography, when present, are almost considered pathognomonic of PAN. Involvement of the renal vasculature frequently results in hypertension, which may at times be clinically severe or even malignant. Renal failure can occur and may be responsible for death in up to 50% of patients with PAN.

The neurologic system is involved in as many as 25% of patients with PAN and may include both the central and peripheral neurologic systems. Peripheral neuropathies are seen in nearly half the patients and may be a presenting sign. Central nervous system manifestations may become evident as strokes, altered mental status, cognitive impairment, seizures, or hemorrhage.

Muscle involvement may be manifested by simple myalgias or proximal myopathy mimicking polymyositis. Muscle enzyme levels may be normal or slightly elevated, and electromyograms may reveal patchy inflammatory myopathic changes.

Gastrointestinal tract problems are present in nearly half the patients. The clinical manifestations relate to ischemia, which may involve the mucosa, submucosa, or the entire thickness of the bowel. Other organs of the gastrointestinal system may be involved as well. The most severe complication of gastrointestinal tract involvement by PAN is visceral perforation. This complication is catastrophic in clinical practice when it occurs in the setting of uncontrolled disease and the patient is receiving immunosuppressive therapy.

Cardiac involvement occurs in up to 60% of patients with PAN and is second only to renal disease as a cause of death. Cardiac manifestations include myocardial infarction and congestive heart failure, which are often exacerbated by associated hypertension.

A variety of other target organs can be involved in PAN. Skin involvement is relatively infrequent compared with other categories of vasculitis, but skin may demonstrate inflammatory subcutaneous nodules or livedo reticularis. Testicular involvement has been considered a common pathologic finding, but active orchitis is relatively rare.

Differential Diagnosis. The differential diagnosis of PAN includes other forms of primary and systemic vasculitides, as well as any other condition capable of producing multisystem organ dysfunction. These conditions include disseminated infections and cancer.

The diagnosis of PAN can be problematic. There are no specific laboratory tests for PAN, and the most sensitive laboratory findings are elevation of the values of acute-phase reactants, including the erythrocyte sedimentation rate and C-reactive protein. ANCA has been reported in a small percentage of cases. The most important aspect of the diagnosis is a high index of suspicion. The diagnosis must be made based on either tissue evidence of necrotizing vasculitis or characteristic angiographic findings. The appropriate tissue for biopsy varies from patient to patient and, whenever possible, the clinically involved organ should be sampled first. Biopsy of symptomatic muscle or nerve may reveal the diagnosis, although even in the presence of documented disease these tissues may reveal false-negative results. Percutaneous renal biopsy specimens generally do not show glomerulonephritis. Biopsies of the skin are problematic because this organ can be involved as a result of so many other primary and secondary vasculitic syndromes and lacks specificity. When there is no obvious tissue to biopsy, visceral angiography may help by demonstrating multiple microaneurysms or vascular irregularities, or both (Fig. 195-1).

Management. Without treatment the 5-year survival rate for PAN is 10% to 15%. With the use of corticosteroids the 5-year survival rate is improved to 50%. In recent years the use of combination therapy with cyclophosphamide and high-dose corticosteroids has been reported to increase the 5-year survival rate to 80% or more. PAN in the presence of hepatitis B appears to have a more serious prognosis and may require specific therapies for the underlying infection, including the use of interferon-α.

CHURG-STRAUSS SYNDROME (ALLERGIC GRANULOMATOSIS)

Churg-Strauss syndrome is among the rarest forms of vasculitis and is characterized by necrotizing vasculitis, eosinophilia, and a history of adult-onset asthma or atopy, or both. In distinction to PAN, the lungs are nearly always involved, with x-ray changes being noted in

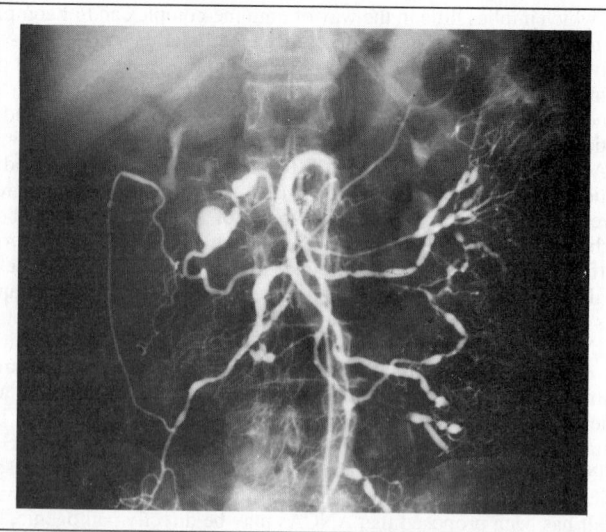

FIGURE 195-1   Mesenteric arteriogram in a patient with polyarteritis. Chacterisic multiple microaneurysms, as well as scattered luminal irregularities, are evident.

✔ WHEN TO REFER

Patients with PAN are challenging in clinical practice, from both a diagnostic and a therapeutic perspective. When the diagnosis is seriously entertained and strategies for biopsy of accessible tissues and/or angiography are being considered, consultation with a rheumatologist or immunologist with expertise in these disorders is appropriate. Long-term management in patients with PAN, which includes the use of alkylating agents and high-dose corticosteroids, is most appropriately carried out in conjunction with a clinician skilled in the use of such agents.

---

more than 90% of patients. Churg-Strauss syndrome has a strong predisposition for peripheral neurologic system involvement, which is seen in 60% to 70% of cases. Peripheral neuropathies, including symmetric glove-and-stocking sensory motor involvement as well as mononeuritis multiplex, may be the early or predominant manifestation of the disease. Cutaneous involvement is present in approximately two thirds of patients, which is far more frequent than in PAN. Gastrointestinal tract, cardiac, and renal involvement may also be observed. A history of adult-onset asthma, which may precede the vasculitic syndrome by 5 to 6 years or more, is characteristic. Churg-Strauss syndrome should be suspected in any patient with unexplained eosinophilia, particularly in the setting of adult-onset asthma. The diagnosis and management strategy for Churg-Strauss are similar to those for PAN. It is not clear whether Churg-Strauss has a better prognosis than PAN, but patients without renal disease can often be treated with corticosteroids alone.

MICROSCOPIC POLYARTERITIS NODOSA

Microscopic PAN may represent a variant of PAN with certain similarities to Wegener's granulomatosis. Patients with microscopic PAN generally demonstrate segmental necrotizing glomerulonephritis and varying degrees of small vessel involvement of other target organs including the lungs. In distinction to that with Wegener's granulomatosis, the inflammation is characteristically devoid of giant cells and granuloma formation. Diagnostic strategies for suspected microscopic PAN are similar to those outlined earlier for PAN, although angiography is generally not helpful because of the lack of microaneurysms. It is estimated that more than 50% of patients with microscopic PAN are ANCA positive, which may be useful in diagnosis. Treatment is similar to that for PAN with renal disease, including the long-term use of alkylating agent therapy such as cyclophosphamide and high-dose corticosteroids.

Treatment of the acute condition is generally instituted with prednisone at doses of 1 mg/kg per day and cyclophosphamide, 1 to 2 mg/kg per day. Milder cases without renal, pulmonary, or central nervous system involvement may at times be treated with corticosteroids alone. In fulminant cases or when there is a question of malabsorbtion, intravenous routes of administration are preferred and higher doses of corticosteroids may be needed. After the first several weeks of therapy and after the acute phase of the disease has subsided, the corticosteroids may be gradually consolidated to an every-other-day regimen. The treatment phase may be prolonged and is generally maintained for approximately 1 year after the disease has been deemed to be in clinical remission.

The combined use of high-dose corticosteroids and cyclophosphamide is associated with significant toxicity. Long-term studies of patients with Wegener's granulomatosis who were placed on a similar regimen reveal treatment-related toxic effects in more than 50%. Drug-induced granulocytopenia and infection are the greatest short-term toxic effects with this regimen, particularly during the acute phase of illness, when the patient is receiving both daily high-dose corticosteroids and cyclophosphamide. The use of a prophylaxis for *Pneumocystis carinii* pneumonia such as trimethoprim-sulfamethoxazole on an every-other-day basis is widely employed. Monitoring of complete blood cell counts and urinalysis is essential and should be done approximately every 2 weeks until the patient's condition is stabilized and every month thereafter. Long-term risks associated with the use of cyclophosphamide include permanent sterility, particularly in women, azoospermia in men, hemorrhagic cystitis, transitional cell carcinoma of the bladder, and an increased risk of lymphoreticular malignancy. Following gradual discontinuation of treatment, the risk of relapse is greatest in the first year after therapy.

POLYANGIITIS OR OVERLAP SYNDROME

In addition to PAN, Churg-Strauss syndrome, and microscopic PAN, the polyangiitis or overlap syndrome is included in the category of systemic necrotizing vasculitis. Polyangiitis may bear the features of each of these disorders and demonstrate clinical features of other vasculitic syndromes such as the hypersensitivity vasculitis group (HVG) or giant cell arteritis group (see later discussion). It is unclear whether polyangiitis represents a distinct nosologic entity, and the prognosis of this disorder is unclear. Patients fitting this description should be approached diagnostically and therapeutically as having PAN.

HYPERSENSITIVITY VASCULITIS GROUP

The concept that hypersensitivity mechanisms could result in vasculitis was first proposed by Zeek in 1948. The distinguishing features of the original condition included an apparent triggering by a drug or protein, prominence of skin involvement, and a vascular disease that tended to involve small vessels and display the feature of leukocytoclasis (nuclear fragmentation; Fig. 195-2). Since then, it has become well recognized that many patients with these features (i.e., cutaneous vasculitis and small vessel involvement with leukocytoclasis) have no history of exposure to drug or toxin. Other conditions associated with this clinical and pathologic picture include vasculitis attributable to a variety of connective tissue diseases; Henoch-Schönlein purpura; vasculitis associated with cryoglobulinemia, malignancy, and certain infections; and, occasionally, vasculitis as a manifestation of other forms of systemic vasculitis. At present we prefer the term hypersensitivity vasculitis group, which refers to a heterogeneous group of disorders all displaying the clinical and pathologic features previously described. The presence of these findings (i.e., vasculitic rash that on biopsy displays small vessel vasculitis with leukocytoclasia) should serve as a clinical starting point for the differential diagnosis of the disorders referred to in the classification scheme under this heading (Box 195-1).

Pathogenesis

The origins of these disorders are diverse, but within the hypersensitivity vasculitis group there is strong evidence for a shared mechanism of vascular inflammation mediated by immune complexes. Evi-

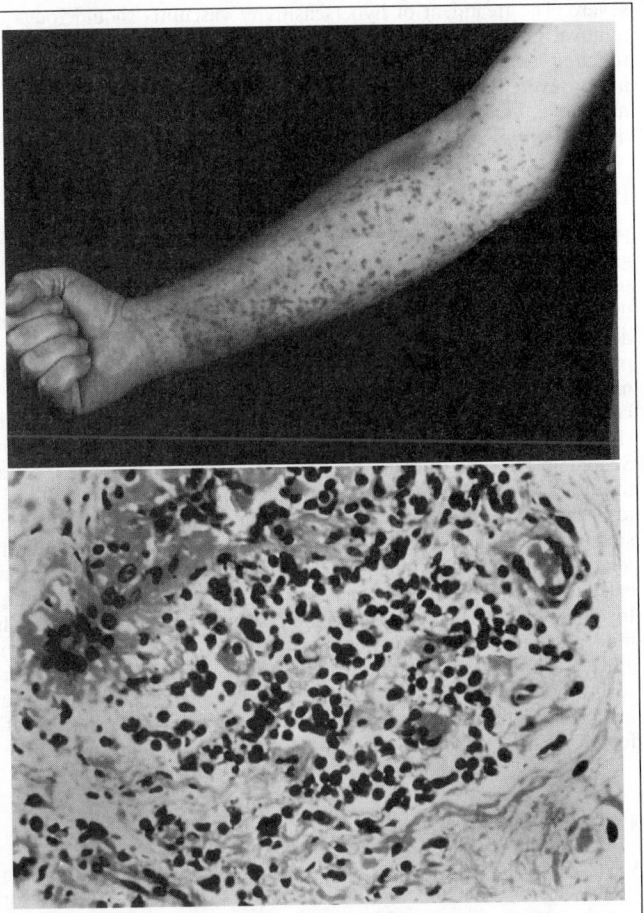

FIGURE 195-2 **A,** The arm of a patient with true hypersensitivity attributable to a drug reaction demonstrating palpable purpura. **B,** Hispathologic appearance of a biopsied lesion demonstrating acute leukocytoclastic vasculitis with extensive nuclear debris.

dence supporting an immune-complex pathogenesis includes the experimental model of serum sickness, which was elucidated more than 30 years ago. A large body of data supports the important role of immune complexes in humans including identification of soluble circulating immune complexes in peripheral blood and deposition in the target tissue. In a few diseases discrete antigens have been identified, such as hepatitis C, which has been found in the majority of patients with cryoglobulinemia.

The diseases within the hypersensitivity vasculitis group demonstrate a shared pathologic feature, namely, a small-vessel vasculitis predominantly involving the capillaries and postcapillary venules. The infiltrates may be either polymorphonuclear leukocyte or lymphocyte predominant and frequently display leukocytoclasia.

SPECIFIC SYNDROMES
Hypersensitivity Vasculitis

True hypersensitivity vasculitis resulting from exposure to exogenous antigen is the most common syndrome within the hypersensitivity vasculitis group. Incriminate antigens are diverse but include drugs, infections, chemicals, immunizations, and a wide variety of exposures including insect bites and foreign proteins. The clinical course of patients with hypersensitivity vasculitis is variable but is usually self-limited. Varying degrees of constitutional symptoms including fever, malaise, and weight loss may be observed. The skin is the most common target organ, and the most common rash is that of palpable purpura. Other cutaneous lesions may also be observed, including a maculopapular rash, ulcers, bullae, and even urticaria. Occasionally, with more serious target organ involvement (e.g., pulmonary, renal, central nervous system) the course may be more severe. The treatment of hypersensitivity vasculitis should focus on removal of the inciting antigen. For many patients no treatment is required, since the disease is self-limiting and mild. For others with more severe involvement it may be necessary to use adjunctive modalities including corticosteroids and for severe cases, cytotoxic drugs.

Henoch-Schönlein Purpura

Henoch-Schönlein purpura is a syndrome characterized by the presence of palpable purpura and varying degrees of gastrointestinal tract ischemia and glomerulonephritis. Other symptoms such as fever, arthritis, and constitutional symptoms are not uncommon. This disorder is most common in individuals younger than 18 years of age. On pathophysiologic study the condition appears to be mediated by immunoglobulin A (IgA)—containing immune complexes, which have been identified both in sera and within the target tissues including skin and kidney. Little is known about the origins of Henoch-Schönlein purpura, but the illness is preceded by an upper respiratory tract infection in 30% to 50% of the patients and has been linked to β-hemolytic streptococcal infections on etiologic grounds in some studies. The natural history of Henoch-Schönlein purpura is entirely related to the degree of renal involvement. In most cases that are clinically mild without clinical renal disease the disease is self-limiting. In those with renal involvement the disease may be progressive. In mild cases no treatment is necessary provided that renal function is adequately monitored, and outpatient care may be sufficient. For more severe cases with life-threatening disease the use of corticosteroids has been advocated. No specific therapy has been proven of benefit for progressive nephritis.

Cryoglobulinemia

Cryoglobulins are proteins that reversibly precipitate on cooling. Patients with cryoglobulinemia may display a systemic vasculitic disorder characterized by palpable purpura, arthralgias, fatigue, peripheral neuropathy, glomerulonephritis, and hepatosplenomegaly (Chapter 202). Cryoglobulins have been classified based on their composition and include type 1 cryoglobulins, which contain only monoclonal immunoglobulins, type 2 cryoglobulins, which contain a monoclonal immunoglobulin as well as a polyclonal component, and type 3 cryoglobulins, which contain only polyclonal immunoglobulin with or without complement. Patients with type 1 cryoglobulins generally have an underlying hematologic malignancy or a lymphoproliferative disorder. Type 2 cryoglobulinemia has long been considered idiopathic or essential in nature but in recent years has been associated with infection with hepatitis C. The natural history of cryoglobulinemic vasculitis depends on the distribution and severity of target organ involvement, particularly renal disease. Traditional therapy for type 2 cryoglobulinemia has been directed at decreasing the formation or deposition of cryoglobulins and has relied on the use of corticosteroids, cytotoxic drugs, and plasmapheresis. Recent studies have focused on the use of interferon-α therapy, which appears to be associated with some degree of success but is followed by frequent relapse when therapy is discontinued. Patients with cryoglobulinemia are at increased risk for lymphoproliferative disorders.

Differential Diagnosis

Various conditions are capable of mimicking the clinical picture of hypersensitivity vasculitis and include subacute bacterial endocarditis, inflammatory bowel disease, celiac disease, Behçet's syndrome, retroperitoneal fibrosis, and vasculitis associated with organ transplantation. Of particular importance is the recognition that some patients with systemic vasculitis traditionally associated with larger vessel involvement (e.g., PAN, Wegener's granulomatosis) may demonstrate similar cutaneous involvement.

Management

The management of patients with disorders within the hypersensitivity vasculitis group depends first on recognizing the underlying condition. As mentioned previously, for patients with true hypersensitiv-

---

✔ *WHEN TO REFER*

The patient who comes to medical attention with palpable purpura should not pose a diagnostic problem as to the nature of the underling skin lesion. The fact that the patient most likely has a small-vessel cutaneous vasculitis is certain, but the real question is, what is the nature of the underlying vasculitic condition? The basic evaluation should include a search for incriminate exogenous antigens such as drugs or infections, as well as serologic studies for connective tissue diseases and a careful assessment for underlying systemic diseases (i.e., malignancies, infections, inflammatory diseases, etc.). These investigations can be initiated by the primary care physician. For many patients no treatment may be required, but for patients with serious visceral disease such as renal, pulmonary, or neurologic involvement consultation with a specialist in vasculitis is advisable. As with all other forms of vasculitis in which patients require long-term, high-dose immunosuppressive therapy with corticosteroids and cytotoxic drugs, consultation with a clinician familiar with such therapies is advisable.

---

ity vasculitis, often no therapy is required other than removing the inciting precipitating factor. For patients with mild Henoch-Schönlein purpura no treatment may be required other than supportive care. The therapy of cryoglobulinemic vasculitis is still unclear, but suppression of immune-complex formation through the use of drugs or apheresis may still be required. The role of interferon-α therapy is not yet defined.

WEGENER'S GRANULOMATOSIS

Wegener's granulomatosis (WG) is a vasculitic syndrome with a striking predilection for the upper and lower respiratory tracts. WG affects both sexes equally and occurs in persons of any age (mean age, 40 years).

Pathologic Findings

Inflammatory lesions in WG are characterized by the presence of necrosis, vasculitis, and granuloma formation. Small vessels are primarily involved. Muscular arteries are infrequently affected, and microaneurysms are rare. Renal disease is characterized by a focal and segmental glomerulonephritis with varying degrees of fibrinoid necrosis and epithelial crescent formation. Immune-complex deposition is distinctly unusual.

Clinical Findings

Wegener's granulomatosis ranges from a mild, indolent process to a rapidly progressive disease. Although any organ may be affected, WG is characterized by involvement of the upper and lower respiratory tracts and in most cases the kidneys. Constitutional symptoms commonly occur and include fever, weight loss, and malaise.

Upper airway disease is the most common presenting feature of WG. Nasal disease is prominent and may lead to mucosal congestion, crusted ulcers, septal perforation, epistaxis, and external "saddle-nose" deformity (Fig. 195-3). Sinusitis occurs in most patients, often resulting in erosive, destructive bony changes. Otologic manifestations include serous otitis media and hearing loss. Subglottic stenosis may result in life-threatening upper airway obstruction.

Pulmonary disease is another cardinal feature of WG. Cough, hemoptysis, and pleuritis are the most common pulmonary symptoms. Many patients, however, are asymptomatic. The most common radiologic findings are fleeting pulmonary infiltrates and pulmonary nodules that frequently cavitate. Pulmonary function tests may reveal reduced lung volumes and carbon monoxide diffusion capacity. Bronchoscopy and broncheoalveolar lavage may demonstrate a neutrophilic alveolitis. Upper and lower respiratory tract disease may be complicated by infections.

Renal disease may range from mild to fulminant glomerulonephri-

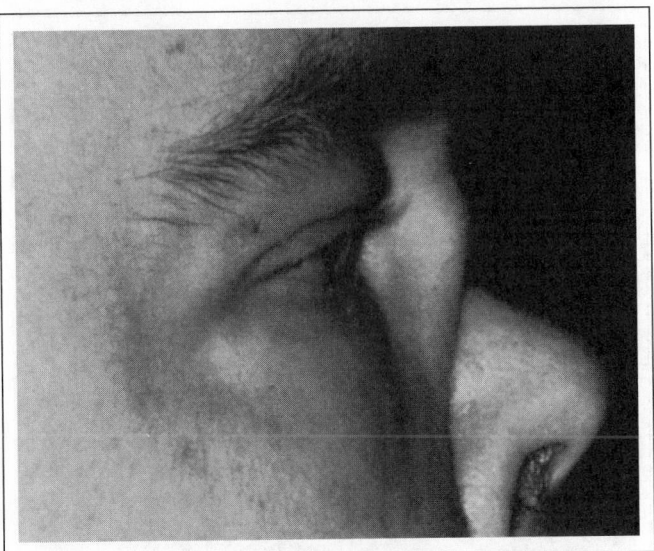

FIGURE 195-3 External nose deformity in a patient with Wegener's granulomatosis.

tis (rapidly progressing to end-stage renal failure). The presence of red blood cell casts in a freshly collected urine sediment allows early detection of kidney involvement, often before deterioration in renal function.

In addition, WG can target virtually any organ. Examples include ocular inflammatory disease, proptosis of the orbit, cutaneous ulcers, palpable purpura, arthralgias, myalgias, mononeuritis multiplex, cranial nerve palsies, cerebrovascular events, ischemic enterocolitis, pericarditis, and myocarditis.

Differential Diagnosis

The differential diagnosis of WG includes other systemic vasculitides (Churg-Strauss syndrome, microscopic PAN), lymphoproliferative disorders (angiocentric immunolymphoproliferative disorders, lymphoma), and various other pulmonary renal syndromes (systemic lupus erythematosus, Goodpasture's syndrome).

Cytoplasmic pattern ANCA (C-ANCA) or anti-PR3 antibodies may assist in the diagnosis of WG. The sensitivity of C-ANCA is about 90% in patients with active generalized (including renal) disease. On the other hand, only 50% of patients in remission or those with disease limited to the respiratory tracts have positive results. The specificity of C-ANCA or anti-PR3 antibodies in the diagnosis of WG exceeds 90%.

Pathologic evidence of disease represents the definitive proof of WG. A triad of necrosis, vasculitis, and granuloma formation is considered pathognomonic. Nonetheless, the diagnostic yield of a biopsy varies with the size of the pathologic specimen and how completely it is sectioned. Because of small sample size, a complete diagnostic triad is rarely described in sinus, nasal, cutaneous, or transbronchial pulmonary biopsies. On the other hand, open-lung biopsies reveal various combinations of the triad components in about 90% of cases. Kidney biopsy specimens reveal focal and segmental glomerulonephritis with varying degrees of necrosis and epithelial crescent formation. Although compatible with WG, such findings are not diagnostically specific.

Angiography is expected to be a low-yield diagnostic procedure in WG, since the involved vessels are small and microaneurysms are unusual.

Management

Without treatment the mean survival time of patients with WG used to be 5 months. The introduction of corticosteroids modestly increased mean survival time to 12 months. In recent years combination therapy with cyclophosphamide and high-dose corticosteroids has resulted in

✔ *WHEN TO REFER*

Management of the patient with WG requires a multidisciplinary team approach to achieve the best possible outcome. Early referral to a rheumatologist familiar with the disease is advised for prompt diagnosis and therapy, early detection of treatment-related complications, and their differentiation from active disease. Otolaryngologists play a particularly important role for patients with WG who may need drainage procedures for impacted sinuses, tympanostomies and drainage tubes for chronic otitis media, or tracheotomy and later reconstructive surgery for subglottic stenosis.

greater than 80% 5-year survival. In selected patients remission may be achieved with methotrexate in combination with corticosteroid therapy.

Traditional therapy for active Wegener's granulomatosis is similar to the treatment described in the discussion of management for patients with PAN. Combined high-dose corticosteroids and cyclophosphamide is the initial treatment of choice. The therapeutic regimen is similarly tapered, as for patients with PAN. As with PAN, the risk of relapse is greatest in the first year after discontinuation of therapy. Long-term sequelae such as late-onset hemorrhagic cystitis and transitional cell carcinoma of the bladder, as well as an increased incidence of lymphoreticular malignancy, must be kept in mind.

GIANT CELL GROUP
Giant Cell Arteritis

Also known as temporal arteritis, giant cell arteritis (GCA) is a large- and medium-sized vessel systemic vasculitis, generally affecting persons older than 50 years of age; the disease affects females slightly more often. It is the most common systemic vasculitis in adults.

Pathologic Findings. The diagnosis depends on a temporal artery biopsy. Granulomatous inflammation of the arterial wall, destruction of the internal elastic lamina, and giant cell formation represent the characteristic pathologic findings in GCA (Fig. 195-4). Active lesions tend to be patchy in distribution.

Clinical Findings. Although nonspecific constitutional symptoms such as fever, malaise, and weight loss are common, classic symptoms of GCA include persistent headache, visual impairment, scalp tenderness, and jaw claudication. On examination, the temporal artery may be tender or pulseless, or both. The clinical presentation is even more characteristic when associated with polymyalgia rheumatica, a syndrome of bilateral shoulder and hip girdle pain and stiffness occuring in about 50% of patients. Other symptoms of focal large and medium-sized vessel ischemia include transient ischemic attacks (TIAs), strokes, and extremity claudication. Involvement of the thoracic or abdominal aorta, or both, infrequently leads to aortic dilation and aneurysm formation.

Differential Diagnosis. When GCA becomes evident with nonspecific and predominantly constitutional symptoms, it may be confused with other systemic vasculitides, such as PAN, as well as a variety of infectious and neoplastic processes. In such instances the diagnosis depends primarily on consideration of GCA in the differential diagnosis. An elevated erythrocyte sedimentation rate is the most sensitive laboratory abnormality in GCA. Nonetheless, it lacks diagnostic specificity.

Temporal artery biopsy remains the gold standard for the diagnosis of GCA. Although a positive biopsy confirms the diagnosis with certainty, false-negative biopsies do occur. Failure to find characteristic histopathologic features may be due to inadequate sample size and the patchy nature of the vasculitic process. Careful sectioning of a substantial biopsy specimen (greater than 5 cm) optimizes the diagnostic yield of the procedure.

When GCA involves large vessels, angiography may suggest the diagnosis. Typical angiographic findings include smooth, linear

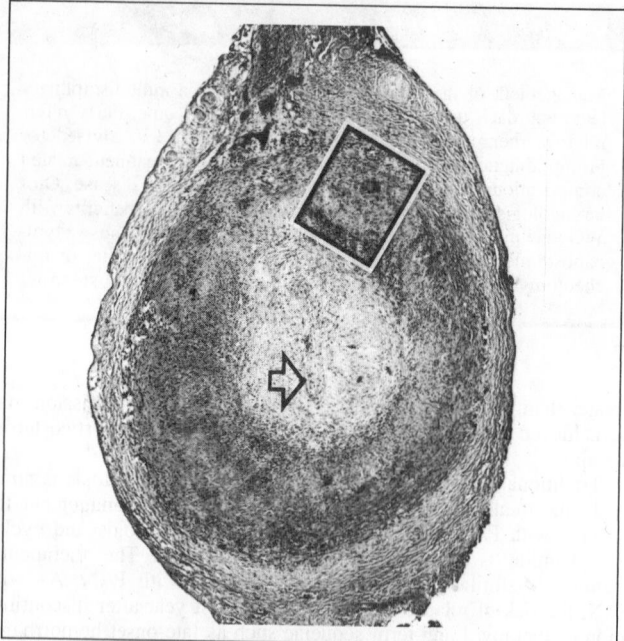

A

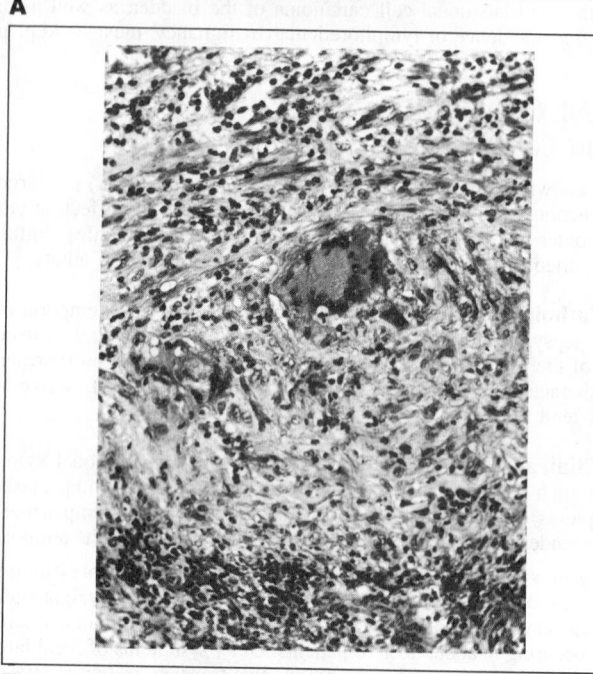

B

FIGURE 195-4   Temporal artery biopsy. **A,** Low-magnification view of cross-section of cordlike temporal artery showing granulomatous inflammation of the media and luminal occlusion caused by intimal proliferation. **B,** High-magnification view of boxed area in **A,** showing multinucleated giant cells in a predominantly lymphomononuclear inflammatory infiltrate (**A,** magnification ×40; **B,** magnification ×160).

narrowing or dilation of the thoracic or abdominal aorta and its branches.

Management. Once the diagnosis of GCA is strongly suspected, particularly in the presence of ocular symptoms, the condition is treated as a medical emergency. Treatment with high doses of glucocorticoids is initiated immediately to minimize the risks of ischemic complications such as blindness. Improvement in symptoms may be noted within 48 hours. Steroids are gradually tapered only after GCA is well under control, in about 6 weeks. The mean duration of disease is about 2 years.

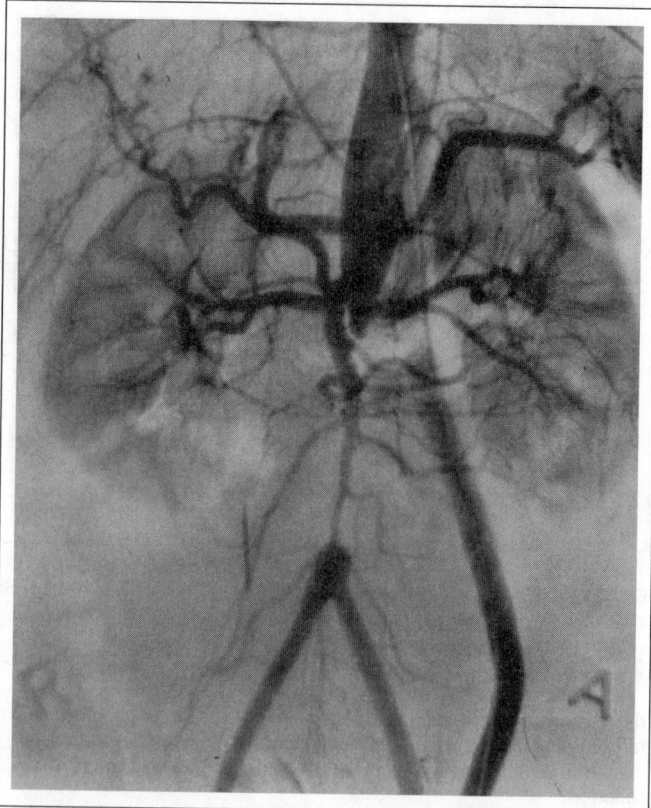

FIGURE 195-5   Takayasu's arteritis. Angiogram demonstrates complete occlusion of the lower aorta, perfusion of the lower aortic trunk via collaterals, and a functioning aortofemoral graft on the left.

✔ WHEN TO REFER

When the diagnosis of GCA is suspected, the evaluating physician should initiate treatment without delay. Patients are then referred for temporal artery biopsy as soon as possible. A complete ophthalmologic evaluation is also suggested. A rheumatology referral is indicated when doubt exists about the diagnosis (e.g., atypical symptoms or negative temporal artery biopsy), response to therapy is less than expected, or relapse of disease occurs, even with cautious tapering of glucocorticoids.

Takayasu's Arteritis

Takayasu's arteritis is a large-vessel vasculitis of the aorta and its major branches that occurs predominantly in young women. The manifestations of disease relate to progressive inflammatory stenoses and/or aneurysms of major branches of the aorta. The subclavian arteries are the most commonly involved vessels, followed by the aorta itself, common carotid, and renal arteries. In addition to constitutional symptoms and arthalgias, patients may complain of limb claudication and symptoms of cerebral, myocardial, or mesenteric ischemia. Vascular bruits and asymmetric pulses or blood pressure are the most common findings on examination. Involvement of the renal arteries may cause hypertension. The diagnosis is based on angiographic evidence of vascular stenoses and/or aneurysms in the appropriate distribution (Fig. 195-5). The treatment consists of glucocorticoids. Cytotoxic agents, including methotrexate, have been used in refractory cases. Surgical intervention may be needed to bypass a critically stenosed vessel.

KAWASAKI'S DISEASE

Kawasaki's disease (KD) is an acute systemic vasculitis primarily affecting young children. It is characterized on clinical examination by the presence of fever for 5 or more days, in addition to four of the following findings: bilateral nonpurulent conjunctivitis, fissured lips or oral mucous membrane erythema (strawberry tongue), truncal skin rash, erythema or desquamation of palms and soles, and cervical lymphadenopathy. Vasculitis of the coronary arteries is common and may result in aneurysm formation. The aorta, mesenteric, pulmonary, carotid, and subclavian arteries may also be involved. The illness is usually self-limiting within 4 to 8 weeks. Deaths occur in 1% to 2% of patients, usually as a result of acute thrombosis of coronary artery aneurysms. Intravenous immunoglobulins reduce the signs of systemic inflammation and, more important, prevent the occurrence of coronary artery aneurysms. High-dose salicylates provide symptomatic relief.

PRIMARY ANGIITIS OF THE CENTRAL NERVOUS SYSTEM

Primary angiitis of the central nervous system (PACNS) refers to vascular inflammatory disease that is isolated to the central nervous system and unassociated with other systemic diseases. Symptoms and signs are generally nonspecific, revealing either focal or diffuse neurologic deficits. The onset may range from insidious to fulminant, and the course can be self-limiting or chronic. The diagnosis generally relies on either pathologic evidence of central nervous system vasculitis or angiographic documentation of vascular stenosis or ectasia, or both, in multiple cerebral vessels. A variety of conditions can mimic PACNS and should be excluded by clinical evaluation and appropriate laboratory studies. Examples include infections, lymphoproliferative diseases, pharmacologic agents (sympathomimetics and drug abuse), connective tissue diseases, and systemic vasculitides. The treatment of PACNS is controversial and should be individualized. Glucocorticoids have been used successfully. In progressive cases the addition of cyclophosphamide may be beneficial. The role of calcium channel blockers remains to be defined.

ANGIOCENTRIC IMMUNOPROLIFERATIVE DISORDERS

Angiocentric immunoproliferative disorders represent part of a spectrum of lymphocytic vasculitis known as angiocentric immunoproliferative lesions (AILs). They share the common features of being angioinvasive and angiodestructive. Lymphomatoid granulomatosis is the best described of these conditions and tends to involve lung, skin, kidney, and the central and peripheral nervous systems. The vascular infiltrates in lymphomatoid granulomatosis demonstrate a high degree of cellular atypia and may be confused with malignant lymphoma. In 15% to 50% of cases of lymphomatoid granulomatosis, transformation into malignant lymphoma may be observed. These disorders are all characterized by T-cell infiltration of the vascular tissues. Originally, lymphomatoid granulomatosis was treated similarly to PAN and Wegener's granulomatosis. In view of the high rate of malignant transformation, such cases are probably best treated as a lymphoma from the outset.

CLINICAL APPROACH AND SUMMARY

The diagnostic approach to a patient with suspected vasculitis requires a working knowledge of the spectrum of vasculitic disorders, as well as a command of medicine in general. On diagnosis the signs and symptoms of vasculitis are nonspecific, merely reflecting vascular ischemia, regardless of cause. Certain vasculitic conditions are greater diagnostic challenges than others, such as PAN or Wegener's granulomatosis, since affected patients may come to medical attention with a nonspecific picture of fever, multisystem organ dysfunction, or arthritis, or a combination of these. Other presentations such as palpable purpura clearly delineate the likelihood of an underlying vasculitis, leaving the greater challenge in these patients of identifying the cause.

For most patients with vasculitis the origin remains unknown. In these instances the clinician should then attempt to define the basic

---

BOX 195-2

Warning signs and symptoms of vasculitis

1. Fever of unknown origin
2. Unexplained multisystem disease
3. Peripheral neuropathies
4. Unexplained inflammatory arthritis
5. Unexplained inflammatory myositis
6. Unexplained glomerulonephritis
7. Suspicious rash
8. Unexplained target organ ischemia

---

mechanism of vascular inflammation (e.g., immune complex, lymphoproliferative, or ANCA associated), the distribution and severity of target organ involvement, and the activity of the overall disease.

The most important principle underlying the diagnosis of vasculitis is a strong clinical suspicion. Box 195-2 enumerates a series of warning signs or symptoms that may be encountered in patients with systemic vasculitis. These findings should alert the clinician to the possibility of systemic vasculitis when a careful workup of other causes is not revealing. The warning signs and symptoms of vasculitis should be considered as follows:

1. Fever of unknown origin. Over the past several decades there have been changing patterns of diseases responsible for fever of unknown origin (FUO). Although certain diseases such as systemic lupus erythematosus are now infrequently responsible for FUO, the vasculitides remain prominently entrenched. Vasculitis should be suspected in any patient with an FUO, particularly in the presence of other warning signs or symptoms of systemic vasculitis.

2. Unexplained multisystem disease. In any patient who comes to medical attention with multisystem disease (e.g., pulmonary infiltrates, azotemia, central nervous system dysfunction, arthritis, myositis), a strong consideration should be given to the presence of a vasculitic syndrome. Clearly, disseminated infections, malignancies, and other inflammatory diseases must always be considered as well.

3. Peripheral neuropathies. The peripheral nervous system, by virtue of its vulnerable blood supply, is a frequent target organ of many of the vasculitic disorders. Different patterns of neuropathy can be seen, including glove-and-stocking pattern, mononeuritis multiplex, and even pure sensory neuropathy. Mononeuritis multiplex is perhaps the most specific peripheral neurologic manifestation of vasculitis, and in the absence of diabetes and demyelinating disease, vasculitis should be considered a leading etiologic factor.

4. Unexplained inflammatory arthritis. The arthritis associated with many forms of vasculitis is frequently symmetric, inflammatory, and painful but nonerosive. It may be confused with the early manifestations of rheumatoid arthritis or other forms of polyarthritis.

5. Unexplained inflammatory myositis. Muscle is a major target organ of many forms of vasculitis. Clinical manifestations may include myalgia or weakness, or both. Minor elevations of muscle enzyme levels and abnormal electromyograms may be seen.

6. Unexplained glomerulonephritis. The systemic vasculitides are always serious considerations in patients who come to medical attention with glomerulonephritis. This may be particularly true in patients with severe hypertension. There is no specific urinary sediment finding that can easily differentiate vasculitis from other forms of glomerulonephritis.

7. Suspicious rash. The skin is a prominent target organ of the systemic vasculitides, particularly the hypersensitivity vasculitis group. Certain rashes are highly specific for vasculitis, such as palpable purpura, whereas others such as urticaria are only rarely vasculitic. If the skin rash is unexplained in a patient with other signs or symptoms that raise suspicion of vasculitis, a biopsy should be performed.

8. Unexplained target organ ischemia. It should be kept in mind that virtually any target organ can be involved in patients with sys-

---

BOX 195-3
Conditions mimicking systemic vascultis

Cholesterol embolism
Atrial myxoma
Fibromuscular dysplasia
Anticardiolipin antibody syndrome
Sarcoidosis
Malignant angioendotheliomatosis
Ergotism
Human immunodeficiency virus infection

---

temic vasculitis. Findings such as unexplained myocardial infarction or stroke in a young person should, at least, raise the suspicion of a vasculitic cause.

From the perspective of diagnosis it should be kept in mind that a variety of conditions can mimic the presence of systemic vasculitis. These can lead to vascular occlusion resulting in end-organ ischemia and may closely mimic the primary vasculitides. These are listed in Box 195-3.

Proper treatment of vasculitis depends on prompt diagnosis; identification of the precise vasculitic syndrome, if possible, or, at least, the mechanism of inflammation involved; assessing the severity of the disease (i.e., the extent of target organ involvement); and the activity of the disease. Focal and transient cases may require little or no therapy; more severe, persistently active cases may require long-term treatment with immunosuppresive drugs. Careful monitoring in such cases is essential to avoid serious treatment-related complications.

BIBLIOGRAPHY

Bacon PA, Carruthers DM: Vasculitis associated with connective tissue disease, *Rheum Dis Clin North Am* 21:1077, 1995.

Calabrese LH, Clough JD: Hypersensitivity vasculitis group (HVG): a case-oriented review of a continuing clinical spectrum, *Cleve Clin Q* 46:17, 1982.

Fauci AS, Haynes BF, Katz P: The spectrum of vasculitis: clinical, pathologic immunologic and therapeutic considerations, *Ann Intern Med* 89:660, 1978.

Hoffman GS, Kerr GS: Recognition of vasculitis in the acutely ill patient. In Mandell BF, editor: *Acute rheumatric and immunologic disease,* New York, 1994, Marcel Dekker.

Hoffman GS et al: Wegener's granulomatosis: an analysis of 158 patients, *Ann Intern Med* 116:488, 1992.

Hunder GG: Giant cell (temporal) arteritis, *Rheum Dis Clin North Am* 16:399, 1990.

Kerr GS et al: Takayasu arteritis, *Ann Intern Med* 120:919, 1994.

Rosen S, Falk R, Jennette JC: Polyarteritis nododa: microscopic form and renal vasculitis. In Churg A, Churg J, editors: *Systemic vasculitis,* New York, 1991, Ikagu-Schion.

Sundy JS, Haynes BF: Pathogenic mechanisms of vessel damage in vasculitis syndromes, *Rheum Dis Clin North Am* 21:861, 1995.

CHAPTER

196 Raynaud's Phenomenon

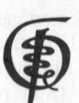

Richard M. Silver

Maurice Raynaud described the clinical syndrome of episodic digital ischemia provoked by cold or emotion. The classic attack of Raynaud's phenomenon (RP) is triphasic, that is, pallor followed by cyanosis, and then by hyperemia, often accompanied by numbness and discomfort. Actually, history of a tricolor response is not common, and RP will be underdiagnosed if all three phases, white, blue, and red, are required for diagnosis. Pallor is the most reliable sign of RP, and erythema is the least reliable sign in subjects with cold-sensitive digits.

BOX 196-1
Conditions associated with Raynaud's phenomenon

Occupational/environmental exposures
Vinyl chloride disease
Vibration injury
Cold injury
Posttraumatic injuries (e.g., hypothenar-hammer syndrome)

Drug exposures
Beta blockers
Ergotamines
Bleomycin

Occlusive vascular diseases
Arteriosclerosis obliterans
Thromboangiitis obliterans (Buerger's disease)
Thoracic outlet syndrome
Thromboembolism
Takayasu's disease
Other vasculitic syndromes

Connective tissue diseases
Systemic sclerosis (scleroderma)
Systemic lupus erythematosus
Polymyositis/dermatomyositis
Rheumatoid arthritis
Overlap syndromes or mixed connective tissue disease

Hematologic conditions
Polycythemia
Cryoglobulinemia
Cold agglutinin disease
Cryofibrinogenemia

Miscellaneous conditions
Primary pulmonary hypertension
Reflex sympathetic dystrophy
Myxedema
Carpal tunnel syndrome
Ovarian cancer

PREVALENCE

Reports of the prevalence of RP are variable and sometimes overestimated, depending upon the study population, the referral bias of the reporting center, and the method of assessment. In a carefully conducted population-based study, the prevalence of RP among adults living in the southern United States was estimated to be 4.6%. The prevalence may be higher in colder climates and in selected populations.

CLASSIFICATION

Raynaud's phenomenon may be a benign condition (Raynaud's disease, or primary RP), or it may be associated with an underlying disorder (secondary RP) (Box 196-1). It is important to evaluate patients having RP for the presence of an underlying condition, particularly connective tissue diseases such as systemic sclerosis in which RP may be the initial clinical manifestation (Box 196-2).

DIAGNOSIS

A history of a bicolor, cold-induced response, particularly if it includes white fingers, is sufficient for a diagnosis of RP. Provocative tests, for example, immersion of the hands in iced water, are unnecessary, painful, and may be dangerous. The following clinical features are seen in secondary but not in primary RP: late age of onset, digital ulcers, and asymmetric distribution. If present, an underlying condition should be sought. Prospective studies of individuals having RP have revealed two readily available tests that are highly predic-

BOX 196-2
Diagnostic evaluation of the patient
with Raynaud's phenomenon

History: including occupational and drug exposure, smoking, symptoms of connective tissue disease, frequency and duration of Raynaud's phenomenon attacks

Physical examination: including skin examination, palpation of peripheral pulses, auscultation for bruits

Laboratory studies: complete blood cell count, erythrocyte sedimentation rate, thyroid function tests, cryoglobulins, antinuclear antibodies (ANA), nailfold capillary microscopy

Ancillary tests: anticentromere, anti-Scl-70, and anti-DNA antibodies if screening ANA positive or connective tissue disease suspected; arteriography only if peripheral pulses asymmetric or diminished

Modified from Maricq HR et al: *Arthritis Rheum* 23:183, 1980.

tive of the presence or eventual development of a connective tissue disease: nailfold capillary microscopy and antinuclear antibodies (ANA).

The nailfold capillary bed at the edge of the cuticle can be visualized using in vivo microscopy or a handheld ophthalmoscope. Distinctively abnormal nailfold capillaries are present in the majority of patients with systemic sclerosis (Fig. 196-1), and many patients with dermatomyositis. The presence of abnormal nailfold capillaries in a patient with RP is highly predictive of the eventual development of clinically apparent connective tissue disease, especially a scleroderma-spectrum disorder.

A positive test result for ANA in a patient with RP may also be predictive of the presence of or evolution to a connective tissue disease. Certain types of ANA are specific and predictive of particular connective tissue diseases. For example, anticentromere antibodies are predictive of the CREST syndrome (limited cutaneous systemic sclerosis). Antibodies to topoisomerase I (anti-Scl-70) are specific for diffuse systemic sclerosis. All patients with RP should be screened with a complete history and physical examination searching for features of an underlying condition, and routine laboratory testing should include tests for ANA and nailfold capillary microscopy.

Other vascular processes that may mimic the cyanotic phase of RP include livedo reticularis, acrocyanosis, and chronic pernio. Each of these conditions lacks the episodic character of RP as well as the characteristic pallor. Livedo reticularis refers to a purplish appearance of the skin with a netlike pattern usually affecting the extremities. It is usually idiopathic and benign, but it may be associated with connective tissue diseases, vasculitis, cholesterol embolization, or blood dyscrasias. Acrocyanosis is a benign condition in which the hands and sometimes the feet are persistently cold and blue, regardless of ambient temperature. Pernio is a chronic vasospastic disorder in which hemorrhagic vesicles and ulcers occur on the toes, usually resolving in warm weather.

THERAPY

Treatment of RP per se depends on the severity (threshold, frequency, duration) and on the existence of any associated condition. Patients with mild primary or secondary RP may require no treatment other than modification of lifestyle to avoid undue exposure to cold or cigarette smoke. Biofeedback training is beneficial for some patients. Patients with more severe primary or secondary RP may require additional treatment. Calcium-channel blocking agents such as nifedipine are effective in many cases, more in primary than in secondary RP. Other vasodilator drugs that may be effective include prazosin, hydralazine, reserpine, and topical nitrates. The addition of antiplatelet agents may be beneficial for some patients.

Severe digital ischemia may progress to gangrene. Impending gangrene requires aggressive vasodilator therapy, and serial sympathetic ganglion blockade is sometimes beneficial. Surgical thoracic sympathectomy is not recommended because of the high rate of recurrence

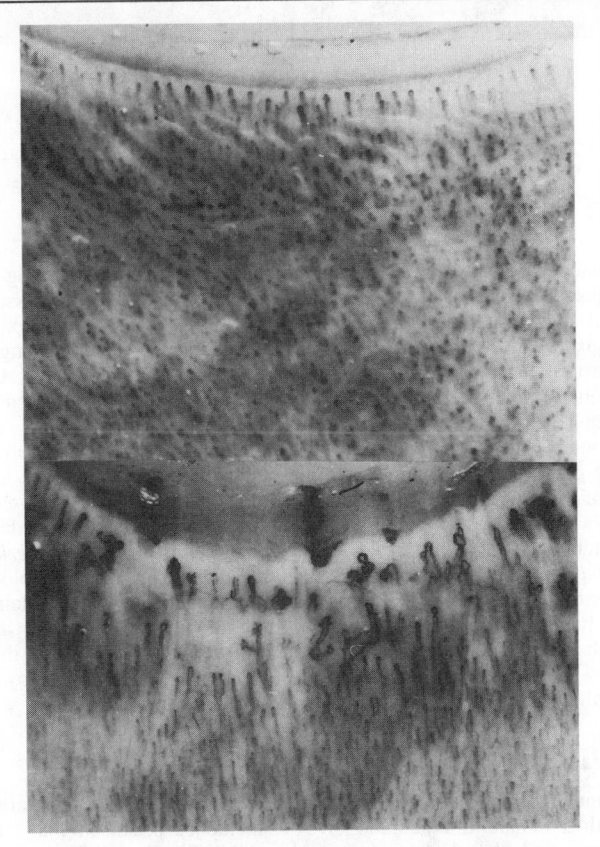

FIGURE 196-1   Nailfold capillary bed in a normal subject *(top)* and in a patient with systemic sclerosis *(bottom)*. Enlarged capillaries as well as areas of avascularity are present in the patient with systemic sclerosis, as are capillary hemorrhages in the cuticle.
From Maricq HR: *Dermatologica* 168:73, 1984.

of RP, but digital sympathectomy may provide long-lasting benefit in selected cases. Prostacyclin infusion may be effective and is warranted in severe cases. Dry, gangrenous digits should be allowed to autoamputate. Surgical amputation is reserved for patients with intractable pain or superinfection.

BIBLIOGRAPHY

Harper FE et al: A prospective study of Raynaud phenomenon and early connective tissue disease: a five-year report, *Am J Med* 72:883, 1982.

Kallenberg CGM, Wouda AA, The TE: Systemic involvement and immunological findings in patients presenting with Raynaud's phenomenon, *Am J Med* 69:675, 1980.

Luggen M et al: The evolution of Raynaud's phenomenon: a long-term prospective study, *J Rheumatol* 22:2226, 1995.

Maricq HR: Nailfold biopsy in scleroderma and related disorders, *Dermatologica* 168:73, 1984.

Maricq HR et al: Diagnostic potential of in vivo capillary microscopy in scleroderma and related disorders, *Arthritis Rheum* 23:183, 1980.

Maricq HR et al: Prevalence of Raynaud phenomenon in the general population, *J Chron Dis* 39:423, 1986.

Raynaud M: *On local asphyxia and symmetrical gangrene of the extremities.* Selected monographs, trans. Barlow T. London, 1888, New Sydenham Society.

Spencer-Green G: Raynaud phenomenon, *Bull Rheum Dis* 33:1, 1983.

CHAPTER

197 Systemic Sclerosis

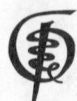

Thomas A. Medsger, Jr.

Systemic sclerosis is a chronic multisystem disorder resulting in thickening of the skin (scleroderma) and other connective tissues and involving other organ systems. A spectrum of disease exists (Box 197-1). With *limited cutaneous* involvement, skin thickening is most often restricted to the fingers and/or face. This variant has been termed the CREST (*c*alcinosis, *R*aynaud's phenomenon, *e*sophageal hypomotility, *s*clerodactyly, and *t*elangiectasia) syndrome. With *diffuse cutaneous* involvement, in contrast, the skin of the distal and proximal extremities (above the elbows), face, and trunk (chest, abdomen) is affected. Either of these forms of disease may coexist with features of other connective tissue disorders, notably polymyositis or systemic lupus erythematosus *(overlap syndrome)*. In both variants the dermis, internal organs, and blood vessels show increased deposition of connective tissue matrix (collagen, glycosaminoglycans), leading to organ dysfunction and ischemia. Distinctive serum autoantibodies are found in more than 90% of cases. The cause is unknown, and no specific therapy is available.

EPIDEMIOLOGY

Annual incidence is approximately 20 cases per million population with a female-to-male ratio of 3:1. Incidence peaks after age 60 years, and the disease is rare in childhood. Familial systemic sclerosis is uncommon. Although there is no obvious precipitating event or exposure, certain environmental "triggers" to scleroderma-like illnesses are recognized, including exposure to vinyl chloride, other organic hydrocarbons, silica dust, and the tumoricidal drug bleomycin.

PATHOGENESIS

Scleroderma skin fibroblasts synthesize excessive quantities of collagen precursors. The reason for this abnormality is unknown, but vascular and immunologic hypotheses have been proposed.

Clinical and pathologic evidence of vascular disease is abundant. Endothelial cell antigens and the products of platelet aggregation are found in increased amounts in peripheral blood. Ischemia is believed to play a role in fibroblast stimulation. Subintimal fibroplasia leads to narrowing of the lumens of small arteries (Fig. 197-1) and arterioles and to capillary obliteration.

The immunologic hypothesis is supported by the early appearance of mononuclear cell (T-cell) infiltration in the skin (Fig. 197- 2), lung, and other affected tissues. Cytokines produced by peripheral blood mononuclear cells can cause dermal fibroblast proliferation and increased collagen production in tissue culture. The presence of disease-specific serum autoantibodies also suggests participation of the immune system, but these antibodies are not themselves found in involved blood vessel walls or other affected tissues.

ORGAN INVOLVEMENT
Skin

In the early or edematous phase the fingers and hands are tight (puffy) and swollen (Fig. 197-3, *A*). This stage may last indefinitely or be replaced gradually after several weeks or months by skin thickening (indurative phase). At this time the most accurate method for establishing a diagnosis is careful palpation. In limited scleroderma (Box 197-1) skin thickening is generally restricted to the fingers, hands, and face, whereas diffuse scleroderma first affects the fingers and hands and then spreads at a variable rate to the forearms, upper arms, thighs, upper anterior chest, and abdomen. Hyperpigmentation with surrounding hypopigmentation leads to a "salt-and-pepper" appearance of the skin (Fig. 197-3, *B*). The patient's facial appearance may become pinched, immobile, and expressionless, with thin, tightly pursed lips and reduced oral aperture (Fig. 197-3, *B*). In limited cutaneous disease the most striking digital and facial finding is that of numerous telangiectasias (Fig. 197-4).

After several years the dermis tends to soften considerably or actually become thin (atrophic phase). Skin overlying bony prominences (extensor surfaces of the proximal interphalangeal joints, elbows) is extremely vulnerable to trauma and may break down, leaving painful, slow-healing ulcerations. Skin healing in other locations is normal.

Especially in limited scleroderma, there is a tendency to develop intracutaneous and subcutaneous calcification, chiefly in the digital

---

BOX 197-1
Classification of scleroderma

I. Systemic sclerosis (systemic scleroderma)
  A. With diffuse cutaneous involvement: symmetric, widespread skin changes affecting both distal and proximal extremities and often trunk and face; tendency to rapid progression of skin thickening and early appearance of visceral disease (pulmonary interstitial fibrosis, cardiomyopathy, renal involvement)
  B. With limited cutaneous involvement: symmetric, restricted skin thickening affecting distal extremities (often confined to fingers) and face; prolonged delay in appearance of distinctive internal manifestations (e.g., pulmonary arterial hypertension, biliary cirrhosis); prominence of calcinosis and telangiectasias
  C. With "overlap" syndrome: typical features of one or another connective tissue disease (e.g., polymyositis/dermatomyositis or systemic lupus erythematosus)
II. Localized forms of scleroderma
  A. Morphea: single or multiple (generalized) plaques
  B. Linear scleroderma: with or without melorheostosis; includes scleroderma *en coup de sabre,* with or without facial hemiatrophy
  C. Eosinophilic fasciitis
  D. Eosinophilia-myalgia syndrome
  E. Toxic oil syndrome

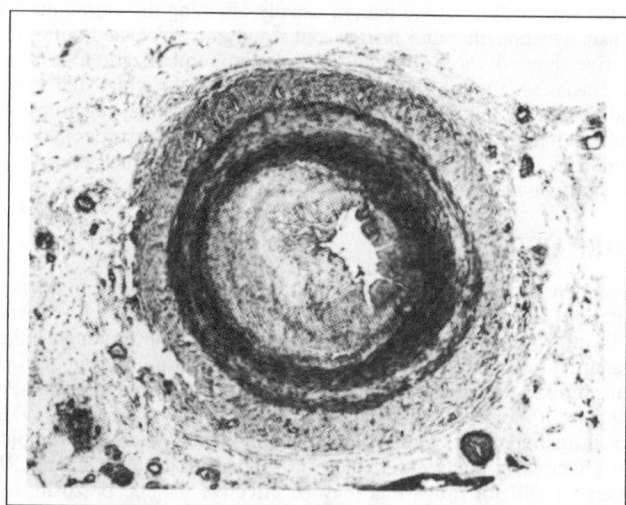

FIGURE 197-1 Photomicrograph of a digital artery obtained at autopsy from a 45-year-old woman with diffuse cutaneous systemic sclerosis who had Raynaud's phenomenon for more than 20 years before her death. There is near-occlusion of the lumen, owing to striking subintimal proliferation. Periadventitial fibrosis is also present.

pads and periarticular tissues, along forearm extensor surfaces, in the olecranon bursae, and in the prepatellar areas. Overlying skin may ulcerate, with extrusion of calcareous material and secondary bacterial infection.

Peripheral Vascular System

Raynaud's phenomenon is often the first symptom and occurs eventually in more than 95% of patients. Small areas of ischemic necrosis with ulceration of the fingertips heal, leaving pitted scars; rarely, terminal phalangeal gangrene may ensue. Angiographic studies disclose narrowing and obstruction of the digital arteries, which on histologic study show prominent subintimal connective tissue proliferation without inflammation, as well as adventitial fibrosis (Fig. 197-1). Concomitantly, nailfold capillary microscopy reveals that circulation is altered by the appearance of "giant loops" and in diffuse scleroderma a paucity of nailfold vessels ("dropout").

Joints, Tendons, and Bones

Symmetric polyarthralgias, joint stiffness, and carpal tunnel syndrome are frequent initial or early complaints, but palpable synovitis is unusual. Coarse, leathery crepitus (tendon friction rubs) may be felt during joint motion over the elbows, wrists, fingers, knees, and ankles. These rubs are relatively specific for diffuse scleroderma and often antedate an explosive increase in skin thickening. Flexion contractures of the fingers (Fig. 197-3, *A*) and other, larger joints usually become apparent within several months in the diffuse cutaneous variant, resulting in significant disability.

The most common bony radiographic abnormality is resorption of the tufts of the terminal phalanges of the digits. In a few patients severe, erosive changes of the finger joints develop. Other examples of bone resorption include "notching" of the posterior ribs and dissolution of the condyle and ramus of the mandible.

Skeletal Muscle

In most instances weakness and atrophy of skeletal muscle result from disuse caused by joint contractures or chronic disease. However, approximately 15% of patients have a primary myopathy. Of these, some have typical polymyositis, but the majority have a subtle, noninflammatory fibrous myopathy that tends to be nonprogressive.

Gastrointestinal Tract

Esophagus and Stomach. Esophageal dysfunction, the most common internal organ manifestation, occurs in nearly 90% of scleroderma patients. Dysphagia for solid foods and mild retrosternal burning pain, postprandial fullness, and regurgitation are frequent.

Radiographic and manometric abnormalities are found initially in 75% of patients, including some who have no esophageal symptoms, and consist of reduced peristalsis in the distal esophagus and gastroesophageal reflux. In limited scleroderma chronic peptic esophagitis is complicated by distal narrowing or stricture and, rarely, by serious bleeding from mucosal telangiectasias. Gastric atony is unusual. One recently recognized complication is "watermelon stomach," a striped appearance of the gastric antral mucosa on endoscopy attributable to bands of superficial ectatic blood vessels, which may be the source of recurrent major episodes of bleeding.

Small Intestine. In a few patients the illness is dominated by intestinal complaints, consisting of marked bloating, abdominal cramps, and episodic diarrhea. Severe bowel atony produces a functional ileus (pseudoobstruction), which may simulate mechanical obstruction. Hypomotility favors bacterial overgrowth in the proximal

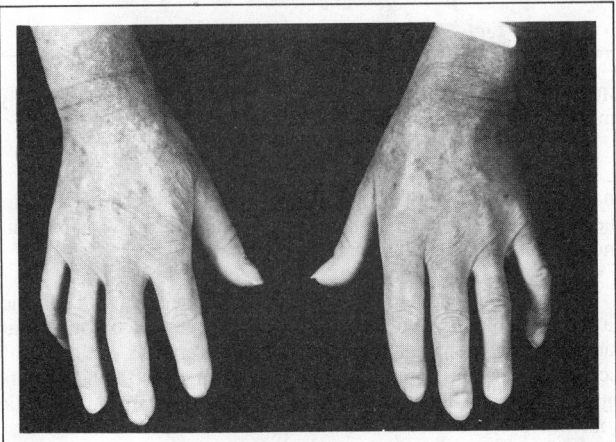

A

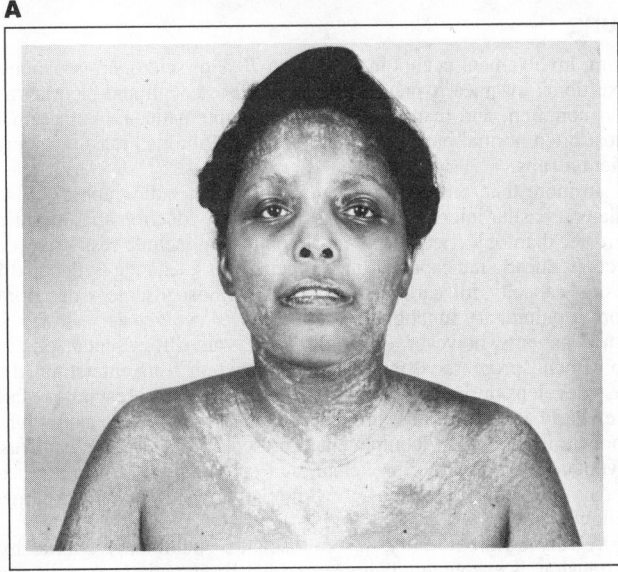

B

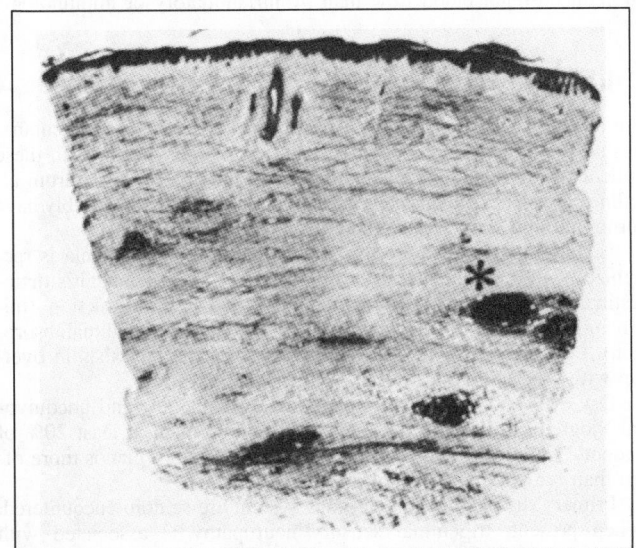

FIGURE 197-2   Photomicrograph of a skin-punch biopsy obtained from the dorsum of the forearm of a 53-year-old woman with diffuse cutaneous systemic sclerosis. Skin appendages are atrophic, and the dermis is markedly thickened by the deposition of dense collagenous connective tissue. Prominent collections of small round cells *(asterisk)* are present; they were identified as T lymphocytes.

FIGURE 197-3   The characteristic taut, thickened, shiny skin of scleroderma with pigmentary abnormalities. **A,** Hands showing typical skin changes with flexion contractures of the fingers. **B,** Typical facial features of a patient with scleroderma showing pursed mouth, prominent teeth, pinched nose, and loss of skin folds. Hyperpigmentation and hypopigmentation are evident on the anterior chest (diffuse cutaneous disease).

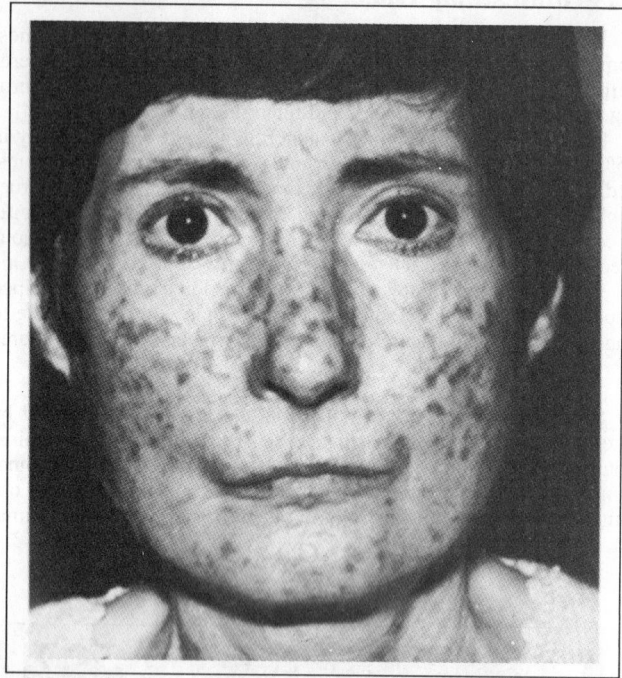

FGIURE 197-4   Face of a 45-year-old woman with limited cutaneous systemic sclerosis showing multiple telangiectasias.

small intestine and may lead to malabsorption with extreme wasting. These functional abnormalities are caused by atrophy of intestinal smooth muscle with collagenous replacement.

Colon. Constipation, either alone or alternating with diarrhea, may signal colonic involvement. Patchy atrophy of the muscularis leads to the development of wide-mouthed diverticula, which usually occur along the antimesenteric border of the transverse and descending colon. Rectal incontinence and prolapse are rare but disabling problems.

Lung

Lung involvement occurs in more than 70% of scleroderma patients. Exertional dyspnea is present in nearly 50%; cough and pleurisy are less common, and many patients are asymptomatic. Examination is most often normal but may reveal bibasilar "fibrotic" rales or pleural friction rubs.

In more than one third of patients the chest radiograph discloses bilateral basilar interstitial fibrosis. Pulmonary function abnormalities (greater than 65% frequency) most commonly include restrictive defects (reduced vital capacity) and impaired gas exchange (reduced diffusing capacity for carbon monoxide). In most instances deterioration of pulmonary function does not occur or evolves very slowly. In a few patients, however, especially those with diffuse cutaneous involvement, progressive pulmonary dysfunction from interstitial disease develops during the first several years, leading to respiratory failure. Early in disease a prominent alveolar macrophage and/or lymphocyte inflammatory component is present, but later there is diffuse alveolar, interstitial, peribronchial, and pleural fibrosis. Modest secondary pulmonary hypertension with relatively slow progression may follow.

A very different entity, severe "isolated" pulmonary arterial hypertension, is encountered almost exclusively in patients with limited cutaneous scleroderma, typically after 15 to 30 years of observation. Rapidly worsening dyspnea on exertion (over the course of several months) is a clue to this diagnosis. The chest radiograph is typically normal and restrictive physiology absent, but the diffusing capacity is extremely low. Diagnosis is confirmed by echocardiogram or by right-side heart catheterization. Right-sided cardiac failure ultimately develops. This complication is uniformly fatal, with a mean survival

of only 2 years. Pathologic findings include severe narrowing and/or occlusion of small pulmonary arteries caused by subintimal proliferative changes and medial smooth muscle hypertrophy without evidence of vasculitis.

Lung cancer, independent of smoking, occurs with increased frequency in late-stage systemic sclerosis, usually in the setting of longstanding pulmonary fibrosis.

Heart

Primary cardiac problems include pericarditis with or without effusion, left ventricular or biventricular failure, or serious supraventricular or ventricular arrhythmias without other origin or cause. Cardiac tamponade is rare in systemic sclerosis. Clinically apparent congestive failure caused by myocardial fibrosis occurs in less than 5% of patients, nearly all of whom have diffuse skin thickening. Radionuclide studies frequently reveal subtle resting-, exercise-, and cold-induced abnormalities of ventricular function in this patient subset. Cardiac arrhythmias, including complete heart block and other electrocardiographic abnormalities, are encountered. The typical pathologic finding in advanced cases is extensive replacement of myocardium and conducting system with fibrosis. Myocarditis has been reported in several patients with scleroderma in overlap with typical polymyositis.

Kidney

"Scleroderma renal crisis" is encountered in 20% of persons with diffuse scleroderma, especially those with rapidly advancing cutaneous involvement of less than 4 years' duration. This complication is characterized by the abrupt onset of malignant hyperreninemic arterial hypertension followed promptly by acute oliguric renal insufficiency. Accompanying findings include severe headache, visual symptoms from hypertensive retinopathy, seizures, sudden left ventricular failure, microscopic hematuria, and proteinuria. On occasion blood pressure remains normal, and azotemia and severe microangiopathic hemolytic anemia are the dominant features. The latter consists of anemia disproportionate to renal failure, schistocytes on the peripheral blood smear, increased lactate dehydrogenase and indirect bilirubin levels, reticulocytosis, and thrombocytopenia. Pathologic findings include subintimal proliferative changes of the intralobular arteries and fibrinoid necrosis of the walls of these vessels, afferent arterioles, and glomerular tufts. The pathogenesis of these renal circulatory abnormalities remains unclear, but they are more likely to be precipitated by reduced renal blood flow than by inflammatory or immunologic events.

Other Organs

Primary biliary cirrhosis occurs in some women with limited cutaneous scleroderma, often coexisting with Sjögren's syndrome. In these patients pruritus, jaundice, hepatomegaly, and elevation of serum alkaline phosphatase levels develop, and patients almost invariably have serum antimitochondrial antibodies.

Hematologic studies are usually normal, although anemia is recognized and may be caused by blood loss (peptic esophagitis or intestinal telangiectasias), excessive red blood cell destruction (microangiopathic hemolysis), or metabolic causes (intestinal malabsorption). Leukopenia is often present when scleroderma exists in overlap with other connective tissue diseases.

Dry eyes and dry mouth are frequent complaints, and unequivocal Sjögren's syndrome (Chapter 193) is present in at least 20% of patients. Lip biopsy shows fibrosis of minor salivary glands more often than lymphocytic infiltration.

Primary disorders of the nervous system are seldom encountered. When present, trigeminal sensory neuropathy is associated with serum anti-U1RNP antibodies. Vasculitis with sensory neuropathy and/or mononeuritis multiplex, impotence, and autonomic neuropathy all have been described. The most common association of these features and the likely cause of the neurologic findings is coexisting Sjögren's syndrome. Sjögren's syndrome–related vasculitis is characterized by palpable purpura, sensory and/or motor neuropathy, hypocomplementemia, and an increased frequency of anti-SSA

TABLE 197-1 Systemic sclerosis subsets according to serum autoantibodies

CLINICAL FEATURES	ACA	TH	U1RNP	PMSCL	U3RNP	RNA POL III	TOPO I
				AUTOANTIBODY SUBTYPE			
Antinuclear antibody staining pattern	Centromere	Nucleolar	Speckled	Nucleolar	Nucleolar	Speckled/nucleolar	Speckled/nucleolar
Proportion of patients	25%	<5%	10%	<5%	<5%	25%	20%
Skin classification	←———————Limited———————→					←———————Diffuse———————→	
Organ involvement	PHT	PHT Small bowel	Muscle	Muscle	Muscle PHT	Kidney	Lung (fibrosis) Kidney

PHT, Pulmonary hypertension.

antibody. Secondary nerve compression—for example, carpal tunnel syndrome attributable to fibrous tenosynovitis at the wrist—is frequent.

Hypothyroidism, often unrecognized on clinical examination, occurs in one fourth of patients and is frequently accompanied by serum antithyroid antibodies. As in the salivary glands, fibrosis is a prominent histologic finding, and lymphocytic infiltration typical of Hashimoto's thyroiditis is less common.

COURSE

The natural history of systemic sclerosis is extremely variable and certainly not always "progressive." With limited cutaneous disease, skin thickening tends to remain minimal over many years. The most reliable early signs predicting diffuse skin involvement are the appearance of cutaneous thickening before the onset of Raynaud's phenomenon, rapid proximal progression of scleroderma, and the presence of palpable tendon friction rubs and serum anti–topoisomerase I antibody. In limited cutaneous disease the more serious sequelae are infrequent and tend to occur late (e.g., after 10 to 25 years or more of disease). In contrast, patients with diffuse skin thickening are at greatest risk of internal involvement during the first 5 years after disease onset; thereafter the risk of new visceral disease is significantly lower.

The life span of patients with limited cutaneous disease is significantly longer than that of individuals with diffuse scleroderma. Persons with limited cutaneous disease may die of pulmonary hypertension or intestinal malabsorption, whereas those with diffuse disease are more likely to succumb to renal failure, cardiomyopathy, or interstitial lung disease, in part because in the former, myocardial or renal involvement rarely, if ever, develops. Cumulative survival 10 years after disease onset is approximately 80% in the limited cutaneous variant and 60% in the diffuse cutaneous subset.

LABORATORY TESTS

Routine laboratory test results are generally normal. The most consistent serologic abnormality is the presence of serum antinuclear antibodies, which are detected in nearly 95% of patients. During recent years several new autoantibodies have been identified that are relatively specific for systemic sclerosis (Chapter 181). Seven different autoantibodies now identify approximately 85% of patients (Table 197-1). Of the antibodies found in patients with limited cutaneous involvement, anticentromere accounts for 60% and anti-Th (nucleolar staining) for 10%. Anti-topoisomerase I (speckled and/or nucleolar staining) and anti-RNA polymerase III (speckled or nucleolar staining) together account for over 80% of patients with diffuse disease. Anti-U3RNP (nucleolar), U1RNP (speckled), or anti-Pm/Scl (nucleolar) antibodies are found in the majority of patients with systemic sclerosis who also have polymyositis or other overlap features.

Each of the previously mentioned autoantibodies has correlations with certain clinical and laboratory features (Table 197-1). Interestingly, it is rare to find two scleroderma-specific serum autoantibodies in a single patient. The production of several of these antibodies has been linked to genetic factors, for example, anti–topoisomerase I with human leukocyte antigen (HLA)-DR5 and anti-PM/Sclwith HLA-DR3.

DIFFERENTIAL DIAGNOSIS

The diagnosis of advanced systemic sclerosis is straightforward. Much more difficult is the identification of a specific connective tissue disease when only Raynaud's phenomenon is present. This symptom is relatively common in the general population (up to 6% of females and 3% of males), and in most instances no systemic disease origin or cause is found. However, in the majority of Raynaud's phenomenon patients in whom an underlying connective tissue disorder develops, the disorder develops within 2 years. Clues to such evolution include arthralgias or arthritis, tenosynovitis with tendon friction rubs, carpal tunnel syndrome, puffy or swollen digits, sclerodactyly, cutaneous hyperpigmentation, digital pitting scars, nailfold capillary changes, bibasilar rales, heartburn or distal esophageal dysphagia, and proximal muscle weakness. Unilateral and unidigital Raynaud's phenomenon is rarely found in connective tissue disease. Other causes for Raynaud's to be considered are extrinsic vascular compression (thoracic outlet syndrome), occupational trauma (vibratory tool use, such as chainsaw and jackhammer), and vasoconstricting drugs (ergot derivatives, beta blockers).

The several forms of localized scleroderma include morphea (patches of skin thickening), generalized morphea (widespread confluent patches), and linear scleroderma (bandlike involvement, often in a dermatomal distribution). Lesions of these several morphologic types may occur alone or in combination. Children and young women account for 80% of cases. In contrast to systemic sclerosis, localized scleroderma often involves the subcutaneous tissue, does not tend to symmetrically affect the digits, is often unilateral, and has no associated Raynaud's phenomenon or visceral disease. The individual active lesions are ivory-colored centrally with a surrounding erythematous border. They are usually located in the extremities, but truncal and facial involvement also may be seen. Histologic features include increased collagen deposition and perivascular and interstitial mononuclear cell infiltration without the vascular abnormalities typical of systemic sclerosis. Laboratory abnormalities include peripheral blood eosinophilia and anti–single-stranded DNA antibodies.

Eosinophilic fasciitis (Chapter 198) is distinguished from systemic sclerosis by a number of findings, including relative sparing of the digits; prominent involvement of the lower extremities (feet, lower legs); skin dimpling, signifying retraction of the subcutis; and absence of Raynaud's phenomenon, visceral involvement, and scleroderma-specific serum antinuclear antibodies. Two epidemic disorders, eosinophilia-myalgia syndrome caused by ingestion of contaminated L-tryptophan, and toxic oil syndrome attributed to ingestion of adulterated cooking oil, closely resemble eosinophilic fasciitis. However, they are more serious conditions that can result in pulmonary infiltration with hypoxia, pulmonary arterial hypertension, and severe ascending polyneuropathy, which may cause fatal respiratory muscle paralysis.

TREATMENT

The physician should take the time to discuss scleroderma with the patient and family, who are often unreasonably pessimistic. Such discussion helps to establish a strong patient-physician relationship, which is important in this chronic, demanding condition. When possible, classification as diffuse or limited cutaneous disease should be established since this distinction is helpful in predicting the future risk

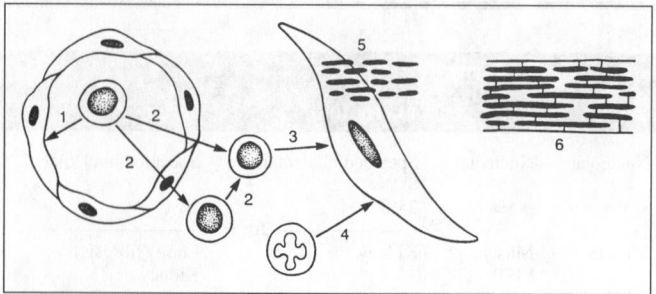

FIGURE 197-5 Schematic representation of pathophysiology of systemic sclerosis with possible sites for therapeutic intervention. Rational therapy would be designed (1) to prevent endothelial cell damage, (2) to alter communication between mononuclear cell subsets, (3) to prevent mononuclear cell stimulation of fibroblasts, (4) to prevent mast cell degranulation, (5) to block fibroblast production or extrusion of procollagen, or (6) to increase solubilization of preformed collagen.

From Koopman WJ, editor: *Arthritis and allied conditions: a textbook of rheumatology,* ed 13, Baltimore, 1996, Lea & Febiger.

of visceral complications. Evaluation of the effectiveness of treatment has proved difficult because of variability in disease severity and rate of progression, failure to classify patients into the previously mentioned recognized subsets, limitations in the availability and application of objective criteria for ascertaining improvement (or deterioration), and the influence of psychologic factors on symptoms.

At least six separate sites of intervention would appear to be useful in the treatment of systemic sclerosis, as illustrated in Fig. 197-5. Protecting vascular endothelium, modifying the immune response, down-regulating fibroblasts, and dissolution of collagenous deposits are worthy goals. The actions of present and future systemic therapies can be considered in this broad framework.

Drugs

No drug or combination of drugs is of proved value in systemic sclerosis. In general, antiinflammatory agents and corticosteroids have been disappointing, although relatively small doses of corticosteroids may be helpful in some patients with myositis, symptomatic serositis, and, on occasion, refractory arthritis or the "edematous" phase of skin involvement. High-dose corticosteroid therapy should be avoided, as it may precipitate renal crisis. Treatment with dipyridamole and aspirin, agents designed to protect injured endothelial cells, has resulted in laboratory but not clinical evidence of improvement.

In numerous uncontrolled studies D-penicillamine has been reported to reduce skin thickness and the frequency of new renal involvement and to improve pulmonary function and survival. Dosage recommended and toxicity encountered are similar to those in rheumatoid arthritis (Chapter 192). As many as 20% of patients cannot tolerate the drug. Other unproven remedies include colchicine, cytotoxic drugs (azathioprine, methotrexate, cyclophosphamide, cyclosporin A), interferon gamma, and pheresis (apheresis, photopheresis).

Supporting Measures
Raynaud's phenomenon. Avoidance of cold exposure, dressing warmly, and abstinence from tobacco are helpful. Various vasodilating drugs have been used, especially during the winter months, the most promising of which are the calcium-channel blockers, for example, nifedipine. When large vessels are involved, such as radial and/or ulnar arteries, microvascular reconstruction should be considered. Digital sympathectomies are recommended when ischemia is present and vasospasm is prominent. Digital tip amputation for gangrene may occasionally be required.

Calcinosis. Reliable treatment to eradicate calcinosis is not available. Surgical excision may be helpful in selected instances. Suppression of local inflammation surrounding calcinosis has been accomplished with colchicine.

Skin. Special lotions, soaps, and bath oils are used to relieve skin dryness. Excessive bathing and use of household detergents may ag-

gravate this symptom. Noninfected ulcers respond to occlusive dressings, such as Duoderm, that are also protective. Superficial bacterial infections (almost always caused by staphylococci) are treated with half-strength hydrogen peroxide soaks, gentle local debridement, and, sometimes, oral antibiotics. Deeper infections, especially septic arthritis or osteomyelitis, must be approached aggressively with intravenous antibiotics, excision of infected and devitalized tissue, joint fusion, and, rarely, amputation.

Joints and muscles. Articular complaints may be treated with salicylates and other nonsteroidal antiinflammatory drugs. Corticosteroids are seldom necessary, except in cases of active polymyositis. To minimize the progression of joint contractures sometimes common in the diffuse cutaneous subset, patients should be taught and encouraged to perform range-of-motion exercises for all joints and a program to maximize the oral aperture. Elective proximal interphalangeal joint replacement arthroplasties and fusions have been performed.

Gastrointestinal tract. Prokinetic drugs (metoclopramide, cisapride) improve esophageal motility in some patients, whereas nifedipine, a smooth-muscle relaxant, may reduce it. Reflux esophagitis can be minimized by sitting upright during and after eating, avoiding food before bedtime, raising the head of the bed on blocks, taking antacids, mucosal protective coating, histamine (H_2)–receptor blockade, and proton pump inhibition with omeprazole and related agents. Esophageal stricture may require periodic dilation or, rarely, surgical correction.

Bouts of intestinal pseudoobstruction should be treated by placing the intestine at rest; surgery should be avoided, since the problem is functional rather than structural, and extremely prolonged ileus may follow abdominal surgery in these patients.

Improvement in steatorrhea and other signs of malabsorption may follow the administration of tetracycline or other broad-spectrum antibiotics, but the underlying hypomotility is unaffected. Prokinetic drugs have not been successful in such advanced cases. Parenteral hyperalimentation may be necessary in this circumstance, but these malnourished patients all too often die of bacterial infection.

Lungs. In patients with pulmonary fibrosis, bacterial bronchitis or pneumonitis require prompt and vigorous antibiotic treatment. Prophylactic pneumococcal pneumonia vaccine and annual influenza vaccination should be given to these individuals. For inflammatory alveolitis caused by scleroderma and documented by high-resolution computerized tomography, bronchoalveolar lavage and/or open-lung biopsy, corticosteroids alone or in combination with an immunosuppressive drug (particularly cyclophosphamide) may be efficacious. D-penicillamine may limit progression in milder cases of interstitial fibrosis but apparently cannot alter the course of advanced involvement. When exercise results in hypoxia, supplemental oxygen is indicated. No effective vasodilator or other therapy is available for pulmonary arterial hypertension at present, although some promising data on intravenous prostaglandin analog administration by continuous pump have been reported. Only a handful of transplantations (heart-lung, single lung) have been performed.

Heart. Symptomatic pericarditis should be treated with nonsteroidal drugs or corticosteroids. Hemodynamically significant pericardial effusion may have to be managed with pericardiocentesis or, if recurrent, an open pericardial window. If myocarditis is suspected, glucocorticoids should be tried. The typical progressive left ventricular failure caused by myocardial fibrosis is unaffected by any therapy and is generally fatal. Because digitalis intoxication is common, greater reliance is placed on diuretics. Serious arrhythmias often complicate this situation and respond inconsistently to antiarrhythmic drugs.

Kidneys. The most important aspect of therapy of renal involvement is early detection; at highest risk are patients with rapidly progressive diffuse cutaneous disease. A recent significant elevation of blood pressure is likely to signal the onset of "renal crisis." The early, aggressive use of angiotensin-converting enzyme (ACE) inhibitors; other new, potent antihypertensive agents; and improved dialysis procedures and care have dramatically reduced mortality from this complication. Survival with adequate renal function is the rule today. Many patients receiving dialysis who continue a regimen of captopril or one of the other ACE inhibitors have slow reversal of renal

✔ *WHEN TO REFER*

Rheumatologists are the best-qualified physicians to confirm the diagnosis of systemic sclerosis and to determine the correct classification subset of the individual patient. Patients with uncomplicated, limited cutaneous involvement should be followed up by their primary care physician. For digital ischemia or infection, pulmonary fibrosis, pulmonary hypertension, esophageal stricture, and malabsorption problems an appropriate specialist's expertise should be sought. Individuals with diffuse, rapidly progressive skin thickening should be followed by a rheumatologist and by selected other specialists, depending on the visceral sequelae encountered. When skin thickening regresses in diffuse disease, the risk of new visceral involvement diminishes considerably, and more routine follow-up should be transferred to the primary care physician.

vascular damage and can be removed from dialysis after 3 to 24 months. Many instances of successful renal transplantation have been reported.

BIBLIOGRAPHY

Campbell PM, LeRoy EC: Raynaud's phenomenon, *Semin Arthritis Rheum* 16:92, 1986.

Cannon PJ et al: The relationship of hypertension and renal failure in scleroderma (progressive systemic sclerosis) to structural and functional abnormalities of the renal cortical circulation, *Medicine* 53:1, 1974.

Follansbee W: The cardiovascular manifestations of systemic sclerosis (scleroderma), *Curr Publ Cardiol* 11:242, 1986.

Jablonska S: Scleroderma-like conditions. In Jablonska S, editor: *Scleroderma and pseudoscleroderma*, Warsaw, 1975, Polish Medical Publishing.

Maricq HR: Widefield capillary microscopy: technique and rating scale for abnormalities seen in scleroderma-related disorders, *Arthritis Rheum* 29:1159, 1981.

Owens GR et al: Pulmonary function in progressive systemic sclerosis: comparison of CREST syndrome variant with diffuse scleroderma, *Chest* 84:546, 1983.

Steen VD, Medsger TA, Jr: Epidemiology and natural history of systemic sclerosis, *Rheum Dis Clin North Am* 16:1, 1990.

Steen VD, Medsger TA, Jr, Rodnan GP: D-Penicillamine therapy in progressive systemic sclerosis (scleroderma), *Ann Intern Med* 97:652, 1982.

Steen VD, Powell DL, Medsger TA, Jr: Clinical correlations and prognosis based on serum autoantibodies in patients with systemic sclerosis, *Arthritis Rheum* 31:196, 1988.

Steen VD et al: Outcome of renal crisis in systemic sclerosis: relation to availability of angiotensin-converting enzyme (ACE) inhibitors, *Ann Intern Med* 113:352, 1990.

Stupi A et al: Pulmonary hypertension (PHT) in the CREST syndrome variant of progressive systemic sclerosis (PSS), *Arthritis Rheum* 29:515, 1986.

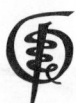

CHAPTER

198 Diffuse Fasciitis With Eosinophilia

Richard M. Silver

Eosinophilic fasciitis (EF) (diffuse fasciitis with eosinophilia or Shulman's syndrome) was first described in 1974. More than 200 cases have now been reported. It is a rare rheumatic disease that superficially may resemble systemic sclerosis (scleroderma), but whose treatment and course are quite different.

CLINICAL FEATURES

EF is characterized by the acute onset of aching stiffness in the extremities accompanied by cutaneous and subcutaneous edema and fibrosis. Increased numbers of eosinophils are present in the blood and usually in the affected tissues. In nearly half of all cases the onset occurs soon after strenuous exertion. Men and women are affected equally, usually between the third and seventh decades, although cases with childhood onset have been described.

Both upper and lower extremities may be affected by pain, swell-

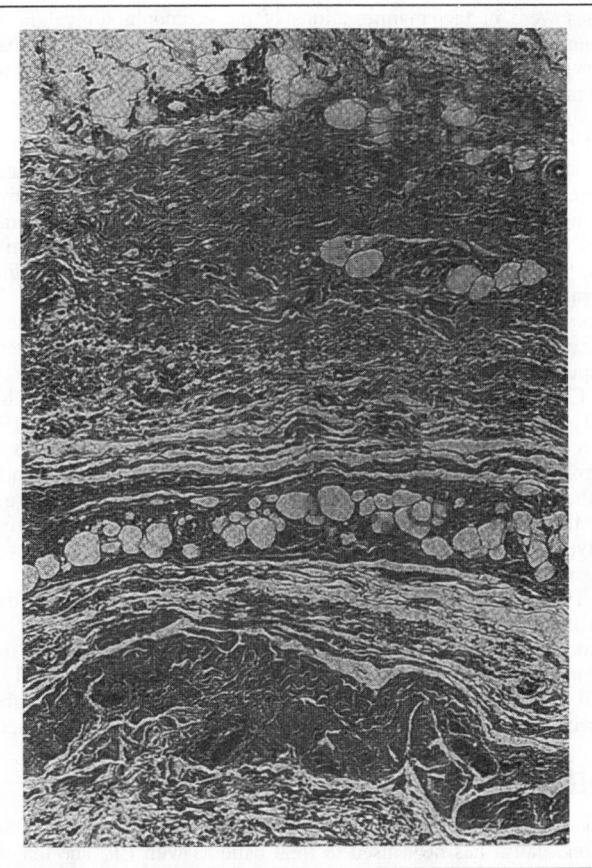

FIGURE 198-1   Subcutaneous inflammation in eosinophilic fasciitis *(EF)*. Inflammation tends to involve subcutaneous tissue and fascia. Plasma cells and eosinophils are often but not consistently present.

From Feldman SR, Silver RM, Maize JC: *J Am Acad Dermatol* 26:95, 1992.

ing, and extreme tenderness. Asymmetric involvement is not uncommon, and the trunk may also be affected. Facial involvement is rare and, although the distal extremities (forearms and calves) may be severely affected, the fingers and toes are spared. The absence of acrosclerosis, as well as the general absence of Raynaud's phenomenon, antinuclear antibodies, and abnormal nailfold capillaries, serves to distinguish EF from systemic sclerosis (scleroderma).

The skin is edematous in the acute phase, and the extremities often exhibit pitting edema. Carpal tunnel syndrome may result from the edema, and it may be the presenting manifestation. As the acute phase subsides, the skin develops a woody induration, which may evolve to a hidebound state. Joint flexion contractures may result. Some patients have a peau d'orange appearance to the skin; others may have plaques resembling localized scleroderma (morphea).

Arthralgia and inflammatory polyarthritis may be present in the early phase. Tests for rheumatoid factor are generally negative, and erosive arthritis is rare. Hypergammaglobulinemia is common, and the erythrocyte sedimentation rate (ESR) is often elevated. Hematologic abnormalities occur rarely, including thrombocytopenia, aplastic anemia, and leukemia.

PATHOLOGY AND ETIOLOGY

Histopathologic confirmation requires a full-thickness skin biopsy. The epidermis is normal or only mildly atrophic. The dermis may or may not be thickened because of edema, inflammation, and collagen deposition, but typically the most intense inflammation is present in the subcutis, including the fascia (Fig. 198-1). Eosinophils may be seen but are not always noticeable. The fascia is markedly thickened.

The origin of EF is unknown. Rare cases have been associated with hematologic or solid tissue malignancy. Many recently reported cases were in fact manifestations of the eosinophilia-myalgia syndrome (EMS) associated with the ingestion of contaminated L-tryptophan. This essential amino acid was frequently used to treat insomnia, depression, fibromyalgia, and premenstrual symptoms. The syndrome reached epidemic proportions in the United States in the fall of 1989. More than 1500 cases were reported to have fulfilled the strict criteria of the Centers for Disease Control and Prevention: (1) eosinophilia in excess of 1000 cells/mm^3, (2) myalgias severe enough to interfere with daily activities, and (3) exclusion of infection or malignancy that might also produce eosinophilia and myalgia. Common clinical manifestations of EMS that rarely occur in idiopathic EF include pneumonitis (eosinophilic) and neuropathy. The latter was sometimes severe, and many of the EMS-related deaths (2.5% of all reported EMS cases in the United States) were related to respiratory failure secondary to neuropathy.

EMS bears a striking resemblance clinically and histopathologically to the toxic oil syndrome (TOS) that occurred in Spain in 1981, affecting 20,000 individuals. In both syndromes, inflammation and fibrosis occurred in the subcutaneous fat and fascia, often extending to the perimyseal tissues. Serum aldolase levels were mildly elevated, but the creatine kinase was usually normal. Whereas EF tends to involve the subcutis alone, EMS and TOS tend to be pancutaneous and subcutaneous.

TOS was associated with the ingestion of adulterated rapeseed oil, but the precise etiologic agent was never identified. EMS has been associated with the ingestion of L-tryptophan containing trace amounts of a contaminant, 1′1-ethylidenebis[L-tryptophan] (EBT), as well as other trace contaminants. EBT can induce dermal and subcutaneous lesions in mice, similar to the skin lesions in EMS patients.

THERAPY

Moderate- to high-dose corticosteroid therapy (30 to 60 mg prednisone daily) has been used to treat patients with EF. The majority have a partial or complete response. Blood eosinophil levels and the erythrocyte sedimentation rate return promptly to normal. Early-phase edema usually resolves, but softening of the skin happens only gradually. Relapses occur rarely. Hydroxychloroquine has been useful in some patients, with or without concomitant corticosteroid therapy. Spontaneous remission of EF has been noted.

Patients with EMS also tended to respond to corticosteroid therapy if initiated in the acute phase, with prompt resolution of edema, dyspnea, and eosinophilia; myalgia improved but often recurred as corticosteroid doses were tapered. It is uncertain whether corticosteroid therapy affected other aspects of the syndrome, such as cutaneous sclerosis and neuropathy. The majority of EMS patients continue to have chronic symptoms.

BIBLIOGRAPHY

Blauvelt A, Falanga V: Idiopathic and L-tryptophan–associated eosinophilic fasciitis before and after L-tryptophan contamination, *Arch Dermatol* 127:1159, 1991.

Campbell DS, Morris PD, Silver RM: Eosinophilia-myalgia syndrome: a long-term follow-up study, *South Med J* 88:953, 1995.

Feldman SR, Silver RM, Maize JC: A histopathologic comparison of Shulman's syndrome (diffuse fasciitis with eosinophilia) and the fasciitis associated with the eosinophilia-myalgia syndrome, *J Am Acad Dermatol* 26:95, 1992.

Hertzman PA et al: The eosinophilia-myalgia syndrome: status of 205 patients and results of treatment 2 years after onset, *Ann Intern Med* 122:851, 1995.

Lakhanpal S et al: Eosinophilic fasciitis: clinical spectrum and therapeutic response in 52 cases, *Semin Arthritis Rheum* 17:221, 1988.

Mayeno AN et al: Characterization of "Peak E," a novel amino acid associated with eosinophilia-myalgia syndrome, *Science* 250:1707, 1990.

Shulman LE: Diffuse fasciitis with hypergammaglobulinemia and eosinophilia: a new syndrome? *J Rheumatol* 1(suppl):46, 1974.

Silver RM et al: Scleroderma, fasciitis, and eosinophilia associated with the ingestion of L-tryptophan, *N Engl J Med* 322:874, 1990.

Silver RM et al: A murine model of the eosinophilia-myalgia syndrome induced by 1,1′-ethylidenebis (L-tryptophan), *J Clin Invest* 93:1473, 1994.

Slutsker L et al: Eosinophilia-myalgia syndrome associated with exposure to L-tryptophan from a single manufacturer, *JAMA* 264:213, 1990.

199 Inflammatory Myopathies

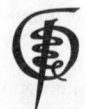

Paul H. Plotz

The inflammatory myopathies are a collection of uncommon diseases, primarily of skeletal muscle, that become evident most often as weakness (Box 199-1). The two best-known variants—polymyositis and dermatomyositis—occur alone, as a part of a related connective tissue disease, or accompanied by a malignancy. There are less common variants—inclusion body myositis, eosinophilic myositis, focal nodular myositis, and orbital myositis—and there is a childhood variant that most closely resembles dermatomyositis. These diseases are classified as autoimmune connective tissue diseases because they are chronic idiopathic inflammatory diseases characterized by lymphocytic infiltration of affected tissue and they are often accompanied by autoantibodies. Furthermore, the clinical manifestations overlap with those of other members of that disease family, and except for inclusion body myositis, they are more common in females. There are about 10 new cases per million per year in the United States.

ETIOLOGY AND PATHOGENESIS

It is certain that immune mechanisms are important in the pathogenesis of the idiopathic inflammatory myopathies. The major evidence that the humoral immune system is involved includes the presence of myositis-specific autoantibodies in many patients, the presence of other autoantibodies such as those found in systemic lupus erythematosus in some patients, and the deposition of complement components in the muscle, especially in patients with dermatomyositis. The major evidence for the involvement of the cellular immune system is the presence of an inflammatory infiltrate consisting largely of T cells in the muscle. The infiltrate may be perivascular, around the muscle fascicles, infiltrating the fascicles, and even within individual muscle cells. In polymyositis and inclusion body myositis, CD8+ (cytotoxic) cells predominate, while in dermatomyositis, there are more CD4+ (helper) cells.

Except for the few cases that can be ascribed to drugs or viruses (Box 199-2), the presumed etiologic agents in inflammatory myositis are unknown. Although viruses, especially picornaviruses, several of which can cause a myositis in humans and animals, are attractive candidates, there is little direct evidence that they play a role. A recent extensive search by sensitive molecular techniques in muscle biopsy specimens for all of the proposed candidate viruses was negative.

BOX 199-1
Classification of idiopathic inflammatory myopathies

Primary idiopathic polymyositis
Primary idiopathic dermatomyositis
Dermatomyositis or polymyositis associated with malignancy
Childhood dermatomyositis or polymyositis
Polymyositis or dermatomyositis associated with another connective tissue disease
Inclusion body myositis
Miscellaneous: eosinophilic myositis, localized nodular myositis, and others

---

From Schumacher HR: *Primer on the rheumatic diseases,* ed 10, Atlanta, 1993, Arthritis Foundation.

BOX 199-2
Differential diagnosis of idiopathic inflammatory myopathy

Neuromuscular disorders
Genetic muscular dystrophies
Spinal muscular atrophies
Neuropathies: Guillain-Barré and other autoimmune polyneuropathies, diabetes mellitus, porphyria
Myasthenia gravis and Eaton-Lambert syndrome
Amyotrophic lateral sclerosis
Myotonic dystrophy and other myotonias

Endocrine and electrolyte disorders
Hypokalemia, hypercalcemia or hypocalcemia, hypomagnesemia
Hypothyroidism, hyperthyroidism
Cushing's syndrome, Addison's disease

Metabolic myopathies
Familial periodic paralysis
Disorders of carbohydrate metabolism: McArdle's disease, phosphofructokinase deficiency, adult acid maltase deficiency, and others
Disorders of lipid metabolism: carnitine deficiency, carnitine palmitoyl transferase deficiency
Disorders of purine metabolism: myoadenylate deaminase deficiency
Mitochondrial myopathies

Toxic myopathies
Alcohol
Chloroquine and hydroxychloroquine
Cocaine
Colchicine
Corticosteroids
D-penicillamine
Ipecac
Lovastatin and other lipid-lowering agents
Zidovudine

Infections
Viral: influenza, Epstein-Barr virus, human immunodeficiency virus, coxsackievirus
Bacterial: staphylococcus, streptococcus, clostridia
Parasitic: toxoplasmosis, trichinosis, schistosomiasis, cysticercosis

Miscellaneous
Polymyalgia rheumatica
Vasculitis
Eosinophilia myalgia syndrome
Paraneoplastic syndromes

HISTORY, PHYSICAL EXAMINATION, AND LABORATORY FINDINGS

Patients complain of the progressive onset of weakness that affects actions requiring proximal arm and leg muscles (shoulder and pelvic girdles). They have difficulty lifting things above their heads or combing their hair, climbing stairs, getting into or out of a car, or lifting their head off a pillow. Less often, muscle pain or tenderness is the dominant complaint. Patients may have difficulty in swallowing—either food gets stuck in the throat, pharynx, or upper esophagus or liquids may regurgitate through the nose. Some patients notice a change in their voice. There is great variation in the rapidity of disease onset. Some patients, usually with severe disease, can name a day when the symptoms began, and disability can progress with frightening speed. Others may fail to notice a gradual decline in function or accept it as part of an aging process and not seek medical attention for years. Most often, a patient has symptoms for several months before first complaining to a physician, and several more months then elapse before the diagnosis is established.

When a rash accompanies the muscle complaints, the disease is called *dermatomyositis,* and occasionally a typical rash precedes the weakness by up to several months. The almost-diagnostic rashes of dermatomyositis are a purplish (heliotrope) discoloration of the eyelids (sometimes only along the edge of the upper lid, but sometimes involving all of both lids to give an owl's eye appearance); a raised, plaquelike, sometimes scaly eruption over the interphalangeal joints, or just erythema of those knuckles, called Gottron's sign; a related flat or scaly erythema of the interphalangeal joints of the toes, knees, elbows, or malleoli; a flat or slightly raised facial rash that may be sun sensitive, resembling the lupus erythematosus butterfly rash (but often distinguished from it because in dermatomyositis the nasolabial folds and forehead may be involved); a flat or slightly raised erythematous rash of the V region of the neck or over the upper back (shawl sign); and a flat or slightly raised erythematous rash of the scalp, which is often itchy.

Inflammatory myopathies rarely affect the facial or extraocular muscles, and muscle atrophy or contractures are not common early. The distal muscles are not usually much affected except in inclusion body myositis, where distal weakness and a mild accompanying peripheral neuropathy including foot drop may confuse the picture. Except in inclusion body myositis, involvement is generally symmetric.

Involvement outside the skeletal muscles may be very important in determining the outcome of the disease. Interstitial lung disease is the most common and threatening extraskeletal muscle manifestation, occurring mainly in patients with one of the myositis-specific autoantibodies, anti-Jo-1 (or the related autoantibodies anti–PL-7, anti–PL-12, anti-OJ, or anti-EJ). Cardiac involvement in the form of rhythm disturbances or, more rarely, frank myocarditis and cardiac failure is less frequent. Gastrointestinal tract involvement below the esophagus is uncommon but may cause diarrhea or even rectal incontinence.

The correct diagnosis of myositis depends on the typical findings by history and on examination and on several laboratory tests. The muscle-related enzymes, creatine kinase and aldolase, are most specific, but the levels of transaminases and lactase dehydrogenase (LDH) are usually elevated, too. The creatine kinase level is elevated in almost every patient with myositis, and if muscle disease is suspected, a serum creatine kinase level should be obtained, since an elevated level of the other enzymes alone may lead to an incorrect diagnosis of liver disease. The electromyogram helps rule out other neuromuscular diseases that may resemble myositis, such as myasthenia gravis or motor neuron disease. A muscle biopsy should be performed early in the course of disease in every patient in whom the diagnosis of an inflammatory myopathy is thought likely, to confirm the presence of the characteristic findings of degeneration and regeneration of muscle fibers and lymphocytic inflammation, to seek inclusion bodies (best seen on a snap-frozen specimen stained with trichrome), and to rule out the occasional surprise such as a dystrophy, sarcoidosis, amyloidosis, polyarteritis, or an unusual metabolic myopathy. A magnetic resonance image of muscles using the short inversion time inversion recovery (STIR) technique is a sensitive way to locate muscle inflammation and may be useful to help select a site for biopsy (Fig. 199-1).

DIFFERENTIAL DIAGNOSIS

The differential diagnosis of muscle weakness must take into account a broad range of conditions; the physician should consider diseases of the central and peripheral nervous system, genetic metabolic disorders of muscle, several endocrine diseases, electrolyte abnormalities, drug-induced myopathies, several infections, and a variety of other diseases such as polymyalgia rheumatica and the eosinophilia myalgia syndrome (see Box 199-2). A careful history and physical examination suffice to point to or away from inflammatory muscle disease. The following items point away from myositis: a family history of a similar muscle disease, symptoms in an adult that began in childhood, weakness that develops during or after exercise or after either eating or fasting, facial or extraocular muscle involvement, fasciculations or myotonia (difficulty relaxing a muscle after a prolonged contraction), involvement of only one muscle, and significant hypertrophy or atrophy. A search for drugs or toxins that cause myopathy is essential, especially for those that may be hidden or denied at first, such as alcohol, cocaine, ipecac, or zidovudine. Infections are not common as a cause of muscle weakness, but human immunodeficiency virus (HIV) infection—perhaps because it predisposes to other viruses or to bacterial pyomyositis—and Lyme disease and influenza may become evident as myositis. Of the endocrine diseases, myxedema can mimic polymyositis closely.

IMPORTANT VARIANTS

Several of the variants of inflammatory myopathy deserve special mention. *Inclusion body myositis* is a slowly progressive disease that closely resembles polymyositis and is found in older patients (rarely before age 40 years, except in a familial childhood type) in whom distal weakness, asymmetric involvement, isolated muscle atrophy, a history of unexpected falling, and the absence of rash, interstitial lung disease, and myositis-specific autoantibodies are distinguishing features. Occasionally, however, other autoantibodies or features of another connective tissue disease such as Sjögren's syndrome are present. Inclusion body myositis responds relatively poorly to standard treatment, although some investigators report that progression of weakness can be slowed or halted even if strength does not return. *Cancer-associated myositis* presents a difficult diagnostic problem. There is an increased incidence of cancer in the entire population of myositis patients. It is more likely to occur in older patients and those with dermatomyositis. A sensible approach to the patient with a recent diagnosis of myositis is to perform a meticulous history and physical examination, including pelvic and rectal examinations, and supplement it with a standard battery of laboratory tests, including stool specimens for occult blood and other tests such as a chest x-ray and mammography as dictated by good medical practice for a person of that age-group. Any abnormality not clearly related to myositis should then be followed up until a satisfactory explanation is obtained. *Connective tissue disease–associated myositis* is most often found in patients with lupus erythematosus, mixed connective tissue disease, or scleroderma, and it commonly responds very well to antiinflammatory therapy.

TESTS FOR AUTOANTIBODIES

Antinuclear or anti–extractable nuclear antigen (ENA) antibodies are often present in patients with myositis, but these autoantibodies are found in many other diseases. Of great interest is a series of recently described autoantibodies that occur almost exclusively in myositis.

Some patients have autoantibodies directed against a series of enzymes that join an amino acid to its proper transfer RNA—anti–Jo-1, anti–PL-7, anti–PL-12, anti-EJ, and anti-OJ. Some patients have autoantibodies to other intracellular proteins or particles such as the signal recognition particle (SRP) and Mi-2. Careful study of the clinical manifestations and the presence of serum autoantibodies has drawn attention to the fact that polymyositis and dermatomyositis may actually be a group of syndromes, some of which are characterized by a particular autoantibody. These differ from one another not only in their autoantibodies and clinical manifestations, but also in their extraskeletal muscle manifestations, racial predominance, human leukocyte antigen (HLA) type, rapidity or even season of onset, and re-

Table 199-1 Some syndromes associated with myositis-specific autoantibodies

AUTOANTIBODIES	GENDER HLA TYPE	CHARACTERISTIC CLINICAL FEATURES
Anti-Jo-1 Anti-PL-7 Anti-PL-12 Anti-OJ Anti-EJ	♀:♂ = 2.7 HLA DR3	Relatively acute onset; frequent interstitial lung disease, fever, Raynaud's phenomenon, arthritis, and "mechanic's hands." Moderate response to therapy, but persistent disease.
Anti–signal recognition particle (SRP)	♀:♂ > 6 HLA DR5	Very acute onset, often in fall, severe weakness, no rash, palpitations, ♀>♂, poor response to therapy.
Anti–Mi-2	♀:♂ = 12 HLA DR7	Relatively acute onset, classic dermatomyositis with V sign and shawl sign rashes, cuticular overgrowth, good response to therapy.

From Schumacher HR: *Primer on the rheumatic diseases,* ed 10, Atlanta, 1993, Arthritis Foundation.
HLA, Human leukocyte antigen.

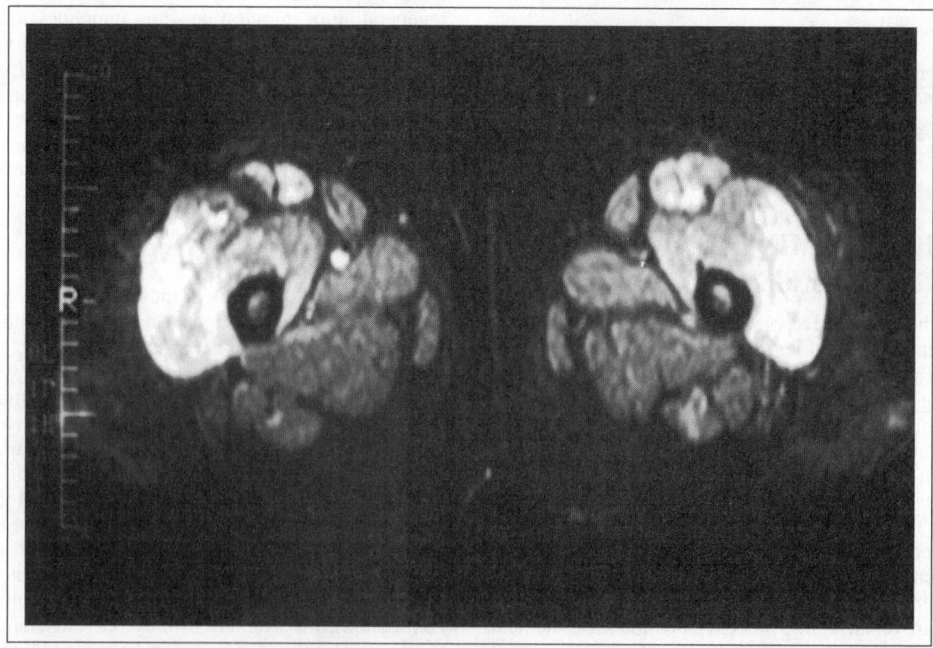

FIGURE 199-1 Magnetic resonance image obtained with the STIR technique demonstrates the appearance of inflammation as a bright signal, particularly in the anterior muscles of the thighs of this 31-year-old woman who came to medical attention with facial rash, pruritic chest rash myalgias, and an elevated serum creatine kinase level.

✔ *WHEN TO REFER*

If a patient's complaint of weakness appears to be due to muscle weakness as judged by history, physical examination, and abnormalities of muscle enzymes (creatine kinase or aldolase), early consultation is advisable because definitive diagnosis requires specialized testing. Almost always, a muscle biopsy is part of the workup, and electromyography, magnetic resonance imaging, and rheumatologic or neurologic evaluation may be required. It is important to establish a diagnosis of an inflammatory myopathy as early as possible, since the chances for recovery of strength are improved with early therapy. Likewise, ruling out an inflammatory myopathy by definitive testing is important to avoid inappropriate therapy with toxic medications.

---

sponse to therapy and prognosis. Table 199-1 presents features of several of these syndromes.

TREATMENT

When the diagnosis of polymyositis or dermatomyositis has been established, corticosteroids are the preferred first treatment, usually prednisone, 1 mg/kg per day in a single morning dose. This dosage is maintained until the creatine kinase reaches normal level and there is substantial symptomatic improvement, and it is then lowered slowly, by 10 mg per day each month. Few patients achieve a complete return to normal strength, and most require continuing low-dose corticosteroid therapy to maintain a remission. If a patient fails to respond to this regimen, if the disease recurs with tapering, or if steroid side effects are a major problem, a second agent should be considered—methotrexate at 7.5 to 25 mg once a week by mouth or up to 50 mg per week parenterally or azathioprine at dosages up to 2.5 mg/kg per day. Alternative therapies for which there is anecdotal evidence of efficacy include pulse corticosteroids, chlorambucil, cyclophosphamide, and cyclosporin A. Intravenous gamma globulin has been shown to be effective in severe dermatomyositis, but the disease often returns when the infusions are not continued. Plasmapheresis and lymphapheresis are ineffective. In unremitting cases of well-established disease, other vigorous regimens such as a combination of two cytotoxic agents may be justified, but a repeat muscle biopsy ought to be considered to hunt for inclusion body myositis. Steroid-related myopathy frequently complicates treatment and should always be considered in a weak patient who fails to respond to increasing therapy or whose weakness is not accompanied by elevated muscle enzyme levels. The rash of dermatomyositis may respond well to hydroxychloroquine (200 mg twice daily). If the diagnosis of inclusion body myositis has been established, the proper approach to therapy remains controversial. Unless there are contraindications to steroid and/or cytotoxic therapy, treatment should be undertaken, particularly if there is inflammation on muscle biopsy and the creatine kinase level is elevated. The goal is stabilization, not remission, and it may take a year or more of therapy and then a period off treatment to be sure that even this limited goal has been achieved.

Assessment of treatment should rest on the triad of history, strength testing, and creatine kinase levels. Sole reliance on only one, such as the creatine kinase level, may well lead to improper or unnecessarily erratic therapy. Attentive physical therapy, including active exercise after acute inflammation has subsided, is important to preserve or even restore strength and range of motion.

BIBLIOGRAPHY

Adams EM, Plotz PH: The treatment of myositis: how to approach resistant disease, *Rheum Dis Clin North Am* 21:179, 1995.

Adams EM et al: The idiopathic inflammatory myopathies: spectrum of MR imaging findings, *Radiographics* 15:563, 1995.

Dalakas MC et al: A controlled trial of high-dose intravenous immune globulin infusions as treatment for dermatomyositis, *N Engl J Med* 329:1993, 1993.

Engel AG, Arahata K: Mononuclear cells in myopathies: quantitation of functionally distinct subsets, recognition of antigen-specific cell-mediated cytotoxicity in some dis-

eases, and implications for the pathogenesis of the different inflammatory myopathies, *Hum Pathol* 17:704, 1986.

Leff RL et al: Viruses in idiopathic inflammatory myopathies: absence of candidate viral genomes in muscle, *Lancet* 339:1192, 1992.

Leff RL et al: The treatment of inclusion body myositis: a retrospective review and a randomized, prospective trial of immunosuppressive therapy, *Medicine* 72:225, 1993.

Love LA et al: A new approach to the classification of idiopathic inflammatory myopathy: myositis-specific autoantibodies define useful homogeneous patient groups, *Medicine (Baltimore)* 70:360, 1991.

Oddis CV et al: Incidence of polymyositis-dermatomyositis: a 20-year study of hospital-diagnosed cases in Allegheny County, PA—1963-1982, *J Rheumatol* 17:1329, 1990.

Plotz PH et al: Myositis: immunologic contributions to understanding cause, pathogenesis, and therapy, *Ann Intern Med* 122:715, 1995.

Sigurgeirsson B et al: Risk of cancer in patients with dermatomyositis or polymyositis: a population-based study, *N Engl J Med* 326:363, 1992.

Zuckner J: Drug-induced myopathies, *Semin Arthritis Rheum* 19:259, 1990.

CHAPTER

200 Spondyloarthropathies

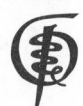 **Robert Inman**

The concept of the seronegative group of spondyloarthropathies (SpA group) had its origin in defining features that discriminated this family of arthritides from seropositive disease (i.e., rheumatoid arthritis [RA]). Over time, clinical and laboratory studies have added to a comprehensive body of data that has lent the SpA group increasing recognition by clinicians and increasing attraction for investigators. *Seronegative* refers to the absence of rheumatoid factor in blood or serum, and this feature has stood the test of time in differentiating SpA from RA. Although the differential diagnosis of seronegative polyarthritis is extensive, the finding of a positive rheumatoid factor is clearly of benefit for the clinician in orienting the diagnosis more toward RA than SpA. The *spondylo-* prefix refers to the predilection for involvement of the axial spine. As a generalization, this has some clinical value but is neither specific nor sensitive as a diagnostic marker in an individual case. RA can have significant axial involvement, particularly in the cervical spine. On the other hand, some patients with psoriatic arthritis may lack any axial involvement. This has led to a current discussion of revising the SpA nomenclature, but no consensus on new terminology has been achieved.

The SpA group generally refers to the following group of arthritides: ankylosing spondylitis (AS), reactive arthritis (ReA), Reiter's syndrome (RS), psoriatic arthritis (PsA), and enteropathic arthropathy or inflammatory bowel disease (IBD)–related arthropathy. Each of these has unique aspects that support its definition as a discrete disease entity, and these aspects are summarized separately in this chapter. There are several common features, however, that argue for regarding these entities as subcategories under the broader SpA title (Box 200-1). The male predominance of most of the SpA entities stands in contrast to RA and many autoimmune disorders in which there is a female predominance. If there is a hormonal basis to this

---

BOX 200-1
Features common to spondyloarthropathies

Male predominance
Human leukocyte antigen (HLA)-B27 association
Oligoarthritis (commonly asymmetric, lower extremity)
Enthesitis (Achilles tendonitis, plantar fasciitis)
Sacroiliitis
Acute anterior uveitis
Aortitis

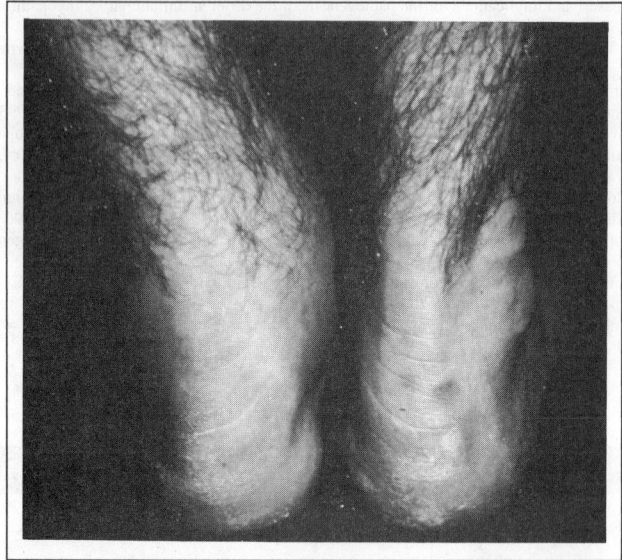

FIGURE 200-1   Swelling of the Achilles tendon of the left foot in a patient with reactive arthritis.

gender bias, it has not yet been characterized. The SpA group has an association with the class I human leukocyte antigen (HLA), B27 (strongest in AS). This contrasts with RA, which is associated with the class II antigen DR4. This B27 association has generated several hypotheses on the pathogenic role of HLA-B27 in SpA, including (1) presentation of an arthritogenic peptide to CD8+ cytotoxic T cells, (2) alteration of host-microbe interactions, and (3) molecular mimicry between B27 and microbial antigens. A striking experimental system on this issue is the B27-transgenic rat, which manifests a range of abnormalities in joints, nails, skin, bowel, and genitourinary tract that appear to encompass the whole range of clinical features in human SpA. In general the peripheral joint disease of the SpA group tends to be an oligoarthritis (four joints or fewer) with a tendency to involve lower extremities to a greater extent than upper extremities, commonly in an asymmetric joint distribution. Both of these features, when present, provide circumstantial evidence favoring SpA over RA in a differential diagnosis. Involvement of the sacroiliac joints is another characteristic articular manifestation of the SpA group that is not seen in seropositive disease. The pathophysiologic mechanism of sacroiliitis in SpA is unresolved. Lymphatic or venous drainage from the pelvis has been invoked as a conduit for microbial antigens of genitourinary or gastrointestinal tract origin, but this remains speculative. In addition to arthritis, inflammation in SpA commonly involves entheses (i.e., points of tendon insertion into bone). Enthesitis can occur at many sites but most characteristically becomes evident as heel pain, with either plantar fasciitis or Achilles tendonitis as the source of the pain (Fig. 200-1). This inflammation can lead to erosive changes in the calcaneus over time. Heel tenderness has proved to be a quite specific physical sign in the diagnosis of SpA and is an uncommon finding in other forms of polyarthritis. It is postulated that local neurogenic factors may play a role in the inflammation of the entheses, but the biologic basis for this localization has not been identified fully.

Of the extraarticular features shared by the SpA entities, the most common is acute anterior uveitis (AAU). This is typically a nongranulomatous, unilateral, relapsing iritis that generally responds to topical corticosteroid therapy. Studies conducted in ophthalmology clinics on patients who come to medical attention with AAU have documented that an underlying SpA (most often AS) is commonly found in such patients. The basis of this association appears to be a shared link with HLA-B27 as a marker of genetic predisposition, not only to SpA-associated AAU but to isolated, idiopathic AAU as well. The B27 link between the anterior uveal tract and the sacroiliac joint has intrigued researchers of the SpA group but awaits a definitive explanation. Just as a suggestion of low back pain in a patient with AAU

should raise the possibility of an underlying rheumatic disease to the ophthalmologist, so the onset of ocular redness, pain, or photophobia in a patient with SpA should suggest the onset of uveitis and should trigger a referral to an ophthalmologist for assessment. Less common extraarticular sites of inflammation in the SpA group are the ascending aorta and the aortic valve. The murmur of aortic insufficiency should alert the clinician to this manifestation when assessing a patient with SpA. There is a growing body of evidence that subclinical inflammation in the terminal small bowel is a common finding in SpA when systematic ileocolonoscopic studies have been performed. Effective control of the synovitis appears to coincide with resolution of the bowel inflammation, but which is the primary or secondary process remains unknown.

ANKYLOSING SPONDYLITIS
Pathophysiology

The pathogenesis of AS is not known, but both genetic susceptibility and an environmental trigger are probably involved. The strongest association for the former is HLA-B27, which is present in 90% of AS patients. Infection remains the speculative triggering event, albeit unproven and uncharacterized at present. For the internist the disease is likely to be declared on clinical examination in the late teens or early twenties, but for the pediatrician there is an important subset of juvenile RA that occurs with a pauciarticular onset, primarily in boys, and probably represents the clinical precursor of AS. The primary process represents inflammation at the sacroiliac joints and in the outer fibers of the anulus fibrosus. Reactive new bone formation and ankylosis are the hallmarks of this chronic inflammation, resulting in fusion of the sacroiliac joint for the former site and syndesmophyte formation for the latter. Enthesitis can occur at other sites as well, such as the superior iliac crest, the inferior rami of the pubis, and peripheral locations like the calcaneus. The lumbar spine zygoapophyseal joints are commonly involved, and involvement can lead to early restriction in spinal movement. Although HLA-B27 is implicated in the disease process, the mechanism whereby this class I HLA gene confers susceptibility to AS has not been fully resolved. The cellular basis of new bone formation also remains without an adequate explanation.

Diagnostic Approach

The patient's history is frequently the clue for the clinician that AS may be the origin of chronic or recurrent low back pain. Typically the setting is a man younger than 40 years of age, and the pain is insidious in onset and usually more than 3 months in duration by the time the patient seeks medical attention. Physical examination reveals decreased lumbosacral range of motion, which is quantified by the finger-to-floor distance on forward flexion or by the modified Schober's test. This test measures the increased increment in distance that occurs on forward flexion of two points sited at 10 cm above the posterior superior iliac spine and 5 cm below this line. The normal distraction is 5 cm. Direct pressure over the sacroiliac joints, lateral pressure on the pelvis, or flexion and abduction of the hip may reproduce the pain of sacroiliac inflammation. Chest wall expansion is reduced from the normal 5-cm difference from end expiration to full inspiration. Occiput-to-wall distance as a marker of cervical ankylosis serves as a simple, reproducible measure of cervical spine involvement. Laboratory examinations are of little value in assessing AS; the anemia of chronic disease and an elevation in the erythrocyte sedimentation rate (ESR) are characteristic of active disease but too lacking in specificity to be of diagnostic value. Although HLA-B27 may be of confirmatory value to support a clinical suspicion, the false-negative (10% of AS patients who are HLA-B27 negative) and false-positive (7% of North American whites are HLA-B27 positive) results are of sufficient frequency to limit the diagnostic value of the test.

Radiographic changes are often diagnostic (see Chapter 184), but if the clinical suspicion is strong, a bone scan may reveal abnormal uptake in the region of the sacroiliac joints before x-ray changes are evident. Characteristic radiologic features include blurring of the margins in the lower portion of the sacroiliac joint, followed by subchondral sclerosis, erosions, and bony ankylosis with obliteration of the joint space (Fig. 200-2). Early changes in the lumbar spine

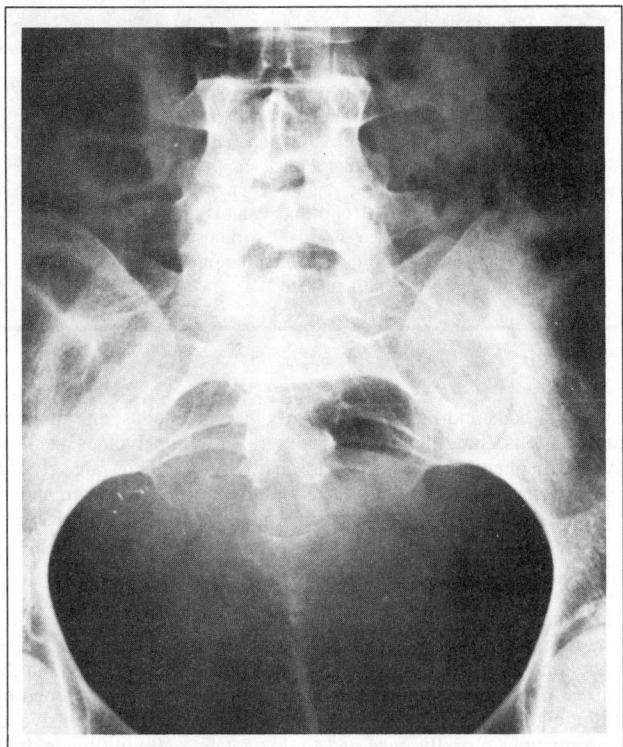

FIGURE 200-2 Ankylosing spondylitis. Total ankylosis of right sacroiliac joint and moderate change in left joint are visible. Juxtaarticular sclerosis, joint space narrowing, and irregularity with partial fusion are evident.

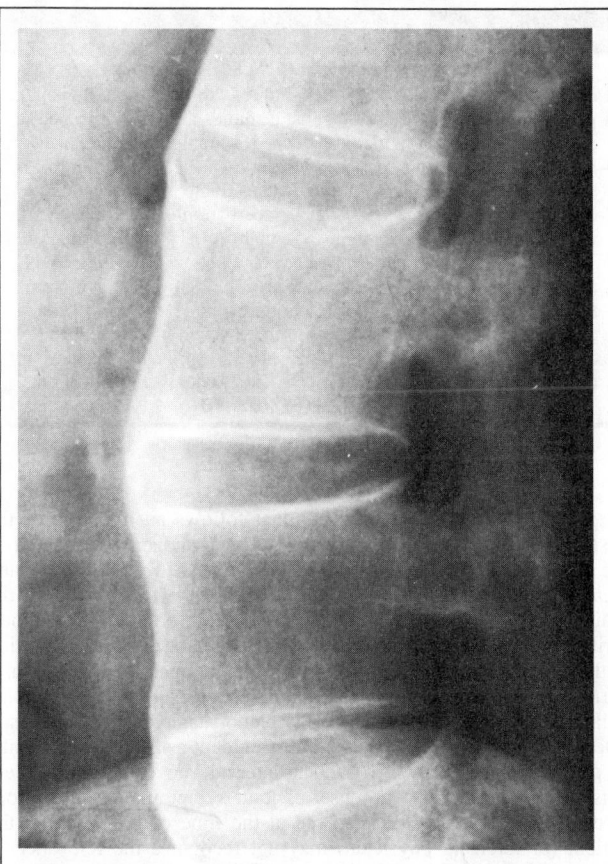

FIGURE 200-3 Same patient as shown in Fig. 200-2. Ossification in the anterior fibers of anulus fibrosus is evident between the lumbar vertebrae.

include squaring of the vertebral body (with loss of the anterior concavity of the vertebra) and "shiny corners" (local sclerosis at the anterior corner of the vertebra) (Fig. 200-3). The formation of the syndesmophyte (bridging the adjacent vertebral bodies) is a diagnostic change and may be seen anywhere in the spine (see Fig. 184-13). The end-stage disease is characterized by the bamboo spine appearance that is due to the syndesmophytes linking the vertebral bodies into a bony, immobile single unit. Other x-ray features may include sclerosis and whiskering in the symphysis pubis and iliac crests and new bone formation at sites of enthesitis, as in a calcaneal spur (see Fig. 184-9).

Differential Diagnosis

The usual differential diagnosis confronting the clinician is to exclude common noninflammatory back pain from the less common AS. The former usually represents degenerative disk disease or osteoarthritic change in the facet joints but often lacks a precise anatomic localization. In contrast to AS, back pain on this basis occurs in older individuals, is usually abrupt in onset, rarely is sustained over a 3-month period, and is generally improved with rest and worsened by exercise and mobilization. Morning stiffness is usually not a feature. Elevation in the ESR does not accompany isolated degenerative disk disease, nor should anemia. Radiographic studies show narrowing of the disk space with formation of osteophytes, which represent hypertrophic new bone formations extending in a horizontal plane (see Fig. 184-11), in contrast to the vertical orientation of the more delicate ossification of the syndesmophyte. Although less common, infection or malignancy can account for chronic back pain, particularly if the pain is unresponsive to conservative medical therapy. Constitutional symptoms such as fever or weight loss should alert the clinician to this possibility, and a bone scan may be indicated if plain radiographs leave the issue unresolved. Back pain that is steadily incremental in severity should always trigger a closer diagnostic investigation. More sensitive tests such as computed tomography (CT) scans or magnetic resonance imaging (MRI) may reveal structural abnormalities in the back that are unrelated to the symptoms, and the proper interpreta-

tion of those findings should recognize their common occurrence in normal asymptomatic adults.

Management

Education plays a key role in the management of AS. The patient should be well informed about the disease's natural history and about the importance of maintaining fitness and posture. An informed physiotherapist plays a key role in formulating a treatment plan. Exercises such as impact sports and repetitive loading of the back should be avoided; swimming is an ideal form of exercise. Satisfactory control of pain is usually achieved with regular dosages of nonsteroidal antiinflammatory drugs (NSAIDs), and these are generally well tolerated in the young adult population who make up most of the patients. Indomethacin 50 mg three times a day or diclofenac 50 mg three times a day has generally been found to be effective. The goal of treatment should be to decrease pain and stiffness to the point that an active exercise program can be sustained. For patients who are unresponsive to NSAID therapy, sulfasalazine, methotrexate, and short courses of oral prednisone (particularly for ocular inflammation) have been used (Chapter 205). Among these second-line agents, sulfasalazine alone has been subjected to prospective, randomized, controlled study, and its efficacy in improving axial symptoms is only marginal.

REACTIVE ARTHRITIS AND REITER'S SYNDROME
Pathophysiology

The current concept of both ReA and RS is that an extraarticular infection in an immunogenetically predisposed host triggers an aseptic arthritis that may (RS) or may not (ReA) be accompanied by characteristic extraarticular features. Although acute rheumatic fever would meet this minimal definition of ReA, the term is generally

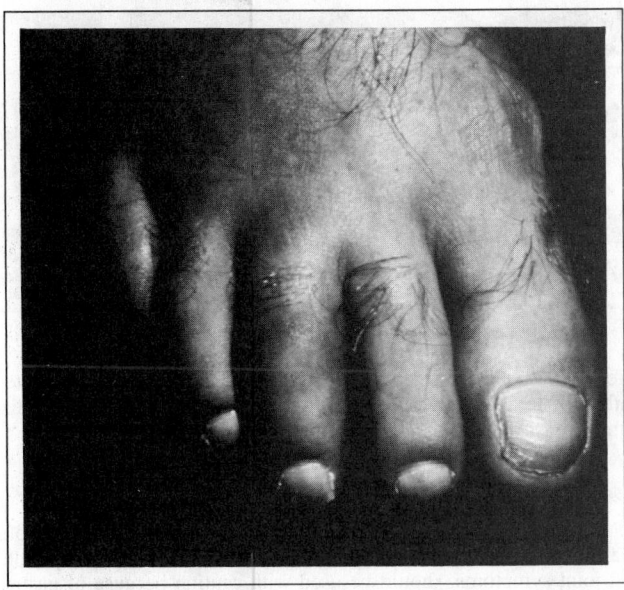

FIGURE 200-4   "Sausage digit," or dactylitis of the third toe.

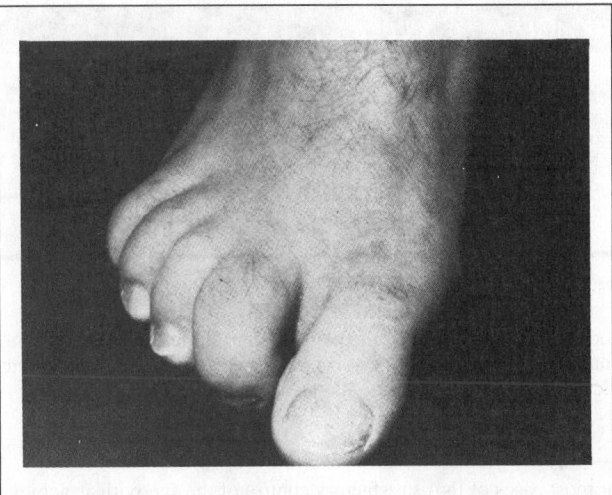

FIGURE 200-5   Appearance of the feet in psoriatic arthritis, showing the changes in the interphalangeal joints and the digits produced by periostitis.

Table 200-1   Forms of psoriatic arthritis

TYPE	APPEARANCE	APPROXIMATE FREQUENCY (%)
"Classic" psoriatic arthritis	Predominant involvement of distal interphalangeal joints and nail lesions	5-15
Symmetric "rheumatoid arthritis–like" arthritis	Bilateral symmetric large and small joint involvement	15-20
Oligoarticular arthritis	Asymmetric large or small joints; periostitis about the small joints leads to "sausage digits" and dactylitis	50-70
Ankylosing spondylitis	Sacroiliac or spinal joint disease; may be asymmetric; often associated with other types of peripheral joint involvement	5-20
Arthritis mutilans	Osteolysis of phalangeal and metacarpal joints; associated spondylitis	5

Diagnostic Approach

The physical examination is central to the diagnosis of PsA. A careful, comprehensive examination of the scalp and periumbilical and intertriginous regions of skin may reveal a psoriatic plaque unrecognized by the patient. Similarly, nail pitting or onycholysis may have been ignored or attributed erroneously to fungal infection. Five clinical categories of PsA have been described (Table 200-1). Distinctive but not pathognomonic features include dactylitis (diffuse swelling of a finger or toe) (Fig. 200-4), predilection for the distal interphalangeal joints, and an arthritis mutilans pattern accompanied by extensive deformities in the hand and telescoping of the digits (Figs. 200-5 and 200-6). There are no diagnostic laboratory tests for PsA. Elevation in ESR and a chronic anemia are common findings, but rheumatoid factor and ANA are absent. Synovial fluid analysis shows a nonspecific inflammatory effusion. Radiographs may show extensive erosive disease, most characteristically involving the distal interphalangeal joints. When radiographic sacroiliac involvement is observed, it is more frequently asymmetric than in AS.

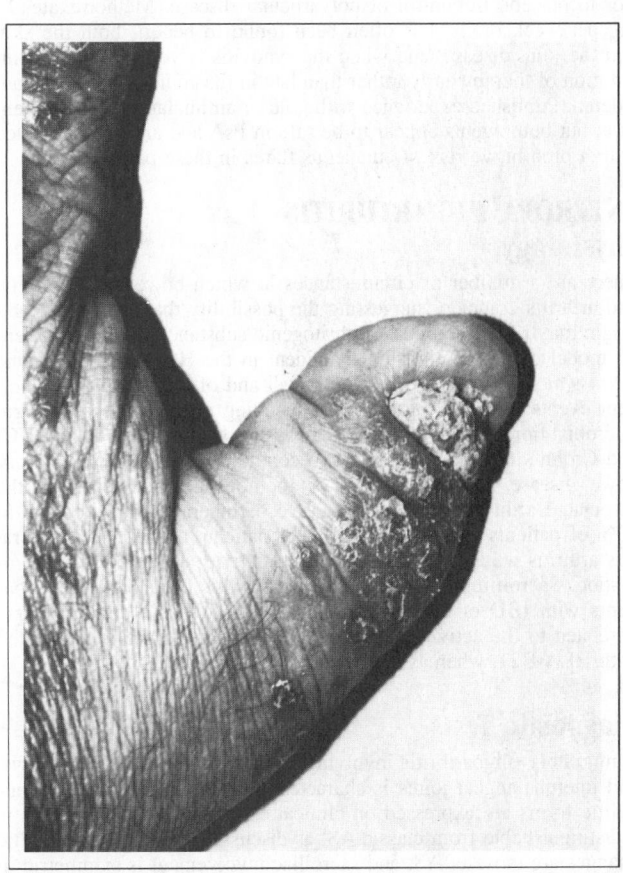

FIGURE 200-6   Severe psoriatic nail disease with arthritis in the distal interphalangeal joint. The thumb is short because of severe bony resorption (osteolysis) in the area of the affected joint.

Differential Diagnosis

Occasionally the skin and nail changes of RS can mimic psoriatic skin lesions, and the two entities may be confused. Ocular, genital, or mucosal inflammation points toward RS rather than PsA. Onychomycosis can mimic psoriatic nail dystrophy, and if there are adjacent osteoarthritic changes in the distal interphalangeal joints, the picture might resemble PsA. Although arthritis and a wide spectrum of skin

✔ *WHEN TO REFER*

With extensive skin involvement consultation with a dermatologist is warranted to outline a comprehensive strategy for control of the skin disease. If the arthritis has proved unresponsive to NSAID therapy, consultation with a rheumatologist is indicated to review and weigh the options for second-line agents in this disease.

✔ *WHEN TO REFER*

Diagnostic certainty is imperative before labeling a patient with IBD because of the chronicity and the need to exclude more reversible causes of diarrhea such as infection. A gastroenterologist should be consulted early in this regard, and usually a diagnostic colonoscopy is warranted. Peripheral or axial joint disease, particularly if unresponsive to NSAID therapy, should occasion a rheumatology consultation to outline a comprehensive treatment strategy.

lesions occur in lupus erythematosus, the clinical differentiation is usually not difficult if psoriatic plaques are present or if characteristic extraarticular features of lupus erythematosus are detected.

Management

For most cases of PsA satisfactory control of the synovitis is achieved with NSAID therapy. Diclofenac up to 200 mg per day in divided doses or indomethacin in similar dosage usually achieves a beneficial response. For patients who are not responsive to NSAID, sulfasalazine up to 3 g per day in divided doses has shown to be superior to placebo in control of polyarticular disease. Methotrexate, 15 mg per week orally, has often been found to benefit both the skin and the joint disease, and when the synovitis is very aggressive, institution of therapy early rather than late in the course should be considered. Published experience with gold or antimalarials is not extensive, but both agents appear to be safe in PsA and are not associated with a prohibitive risk of cutaneous flares in these patients.

ENTEROPATHIC ARTHRITIS
Physiology

There are a number of circumstances in which bowel inflammation and arthritis coincide, suggesting the possibility that antigens of gut origin may be the source of arthritogenic substances. An experimental model of the relationship is evident in the HLA-B27–transgenic rat in which inflammation of the bowel and of the joints are coincident events; both are modifiable depending on the state of the gut microbial flora. Just as the pathogenesis of both ulcerative colitis (UC) and Crohn's disease (CD), the two common forms of inflammatory bowel disease, remains unknown, so too does the pathogenesis of the associated arthropathy. A seronegative peripheral arthritis occurs in 10% of patients with UC and 20% of patients with CD. In general this arthritis waxes and wanes with the activity of the bowel inflammation. Sacroiliitis and ankylosing spondylitis occur in 15% of patients with IBD of either type and tend to follow a natural course unrelated to the activity of the IBD. The axial disease is associated with HLA-B27, whereas the peripheral arthritis is not.

Diagnostic Tests

A migratory oligoarthritis involving primarily knees, ankles, elbows, and interphalangeal joints is characteristic. The sacroiliac and spondylitic forms are expressed on clinical examination in a way that is indistinguishable from classic AS, as discussed earlier. Radiographic changes are those of AS, and sacroiliac involvement is symmetric in both cases. The critical diagnostic test is usually a bowel biopsy specimen obtained at the time of ileocolonoscopy.

Differential Diagnosis

The differential diagnosis of diarrhea and arthritis includes several entities besides enteropathic arthropathy. Perhaps the most common is postdysenteric ReA, and the key differentiating feature is a positive stool culture of the enteric pathogen. If cultures are nondiagnostic, it is sometimes only the clinical course of the bowel symptoms and the subsequent colonoscopic examination that settle the issue definitively. Whipple's disease may be evident in bowel and joint symptoms; again, a bowel biopsy may be necessary to make the diagnosis. Pseudomembranous enterocolitis caused by *Clostridium difficile*

infection, as well as gluten-sensitive enteropathy, has been associated with peripheral arthritis, but the clinical settings should easily be discriminated from IBD.

Management

Local steroid injections are usually sufficient for the peripheral oligoarthritis. NSAID therapy, although effective for axial and peripheral joint symptoms, should be used with caution because of gastrointestinal tract intolerance with underlying bowel inflammation. Sulfasalazine up to 3 g per day may have salutory effects on both the arthritis and the underlying IBD.

BIBLIOGRAPHY

Amor B, Dougados M, Khan MA: Management of refractory ankylosing spondylitis and related spondyloarthropathies, *Rheum Dis Clin North Am* 21:117, 1995.
Careless DJ, Inman RD: Etiopathogenesis of reactive arthritis and ankylosing spondylitis, *Curr Opin Rheumatol* 7:290, 1995.
Creemers MCW, van Riel PLCM, Franssen MJ, van de Putte LBA, Gribnau FWJ: Second-line treatment in seronegative spondyloarthropathies, *Semin Arthritis Rheum* 24:71, 1994.
Dougados M, van der Linden S, Leirisalo-Repo M et al: Sulfasalazine in the treatment of spondyloarthropathy, *Arthritis Rheum* 38:618, 1995.
Fan PT, Yu DTY: Reiter's syndrome. In Kelly WN , Harris ED, Ruddy S, Sledge CB, editors: *Textbook of rheumatology*, ed 4, Philadelphia, 1994, WB Saunders.
Inman RD: Seronegative spondyloarthropathies: treatment, In Klippel J, Wortmann R, Wyand C, editors: *Primer on the rheumatic diseases*, ed 11, 1997, The Arthritis Foundation.
Khan MA: Ankylosing spondylitis. In Klippel JH, Dieppe PA, editors: *Rheumatology*, St Louis, 1994, Mosby.
Michet CJ: Psoriatic arthritis. In Kelly WN, Harris ED, Ruddy S, Sledge CB, editors: *Textbook of rheumatology*, ed 4, Philadelphia, 1994, WB Saunders.
Mielants H, Veys EM: Enteropathic arthritis. In McCarty DJ, Koopman WJ, editors: *Arthritis and allied conditions*, ed 12, Philadelphia, 1993, Lea & Febiger.
Taurog JD, Richardson JA, Croft JT et al: The germ-free state prevents development of gut and joint inflammatory disease in HLA-B27 transgenic rats, *J Exp Med* 180:2359, 1994.
Thomson GTD, DeRubeis DA, Hodge MA, Rajanayagam C, Inman RD: Post *Salmonella* reactive arthritis: late clinical sequelae in a point source cohort, *Am J Med* 98:13, 1995.

CHAPTER

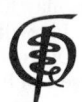

201 Uncommon Arthropathies

John H. Klippel and Nathan J. Zvaifler

INTERMITTENT ARTHROPATHIES
Familial Mediterranean Fever

Familial Mediterranean fever (FMF) is an inherited disorder of ethnic groups of eastern Mediterranean origin, especially Sephardic Jews and Armenians. The disease is transmitted by an autosomal recessive gene located on the short arm of chromosome 16; the function of the gene is unknown. The disease occurs more frequently in males, suggesting either incomplete penetrance in females or modulation by female sex hormones. Symptoms most commonly begin in the second decade of life, with recurrent paroxysms of fever, serositis, erysipelas-like rashes of the lower extremities, and arthritis. The acute attacks typically last several days. Leukocytosis, increased erythrocyte sedimentation rate, and elevations of acute-phase reactants such as C-reactive protein and fibrinogen may be evident during attacks. Joint pain or swelling, or both, most commonly involves the large joints, particularly the knees, ankles, and hips. Arthritis is often monarticular and may be associated with exquisite pain, synovial hypertrophy, and effusion. Occasionally, severe arthritis persists for several weeks or more after other clinical manifestations have resolved. Radiographs typically show only juxtaarticular osteoporosis, but after recurrent attacks joint space narrowing and osteophyte formation may be seen. Osteonecrosis may develop in the hip or knee, causing pain and disability. The most serious long-term consequence of FMF is amyloidosis, particularly nephropathy and renal failure. Attacks generally resolve spontaneously, and treatment is aimed at symptomatic relief. Colchicine (1.2 to 1.8 mg/day) has been shown to reduce the frequency of attacks and may prevent or retard amyloidosis.

Adult Still's Disease

Adult Still's disease is a rare disorder of young adults characterized by high-spiking fever, maculopapular rash, sore throat, hepatosplenomegaly, lymphadenopathy, and arthralgia or arthritis. Patients typically come to medical attention with fever of unknown cause; the pattern of the fever—daily or twice-daily fever spikes ($>39°$ C) that returns to below normal—is often a clue to the diagnosis. An evanescent salmon-pink rash on the trunk and proximal extremities may be evident with the fever spikes or may be elicited by rubbing the skin (Koebner's phenomenon) or by a hot bath. Complaints of severe joint and muscle pain are typical, and in the majority of patients a polyarthritis resembling rheumatoid arthritis eventually develops. In addition to elevation of the erythrocyte sedimentation rate, in most patients prominent leukocytosis and transaminase elevations may develop, particularly if treatment is with nonsteroidal antiinflammatory drugs (NSAIDs). Rheumatoid factor and antinuclear antibodies are absent, although antistreptolysin O titers may be elevated. Although bone erosions and subluxations of peripheral joints are uncommon, fusions of cervical apophyseal and carpometacarpal and intercarpal joints and progressive destruction of hip joints are relatively unique radiographic features that are evident in patients with chronic joint involvement. During the acute phases of the disease most patients respond readily to high-dose salicylate or aspirin (3.2 to 4.5 g/day) or other NSAIDs; corticosteroids are effective in patients who fail or develop toxicities from antiinflammatory drug therapy. Drug treatment for patients with chronic joint symptoms is similar to approaches used in rheumatoid arthritis and include drugs such as gold, hydroxychloroquine, and methotrexate.

Behçet's Disease

Behçet's disease is a systemic vasculitis with classic clinical features of recurrent oral and genital aphthous ulcerations, hypopyon uveitis, arthritis, thrombophlebitis, and neurologic manifestations. Pathologic findings of arteries and, in particular, veins are similar, with perivascular infiltration by lymphocytes and histiocytes, fibrinoid necrosis, and microthrombus formation. The disease occurs worldwide but with a particularly high frequency in countries of the eastern Mediterranean and in Japan.

Skin manifestations include erythema nodosum, a papulopustular eruption resembling acne vulgaris, and superficial thromobophlebitis. The development of a papular eruption 24 to 48 hours after a needle prick (pathergy reaction) is a characteristic and useful diagnostic sign in the majority of patients. Other important features include enterocolitis with mucosal ulcerations, occasionally perforating and sometimes complicated by the development of malabsorption; epididymitis and central nervous system involvement with dementia; and meningoencephalitis or a brain stem syndrome with forced laughter, spontaneous crying, and swallowing disturbances that may progress to fatal bulbar paralysis. Blindness occurs in up to 50% of patients in Japan. In most patients, self-limited recurrent episodes of a nonerosive, peripheral oligoarthritis of the knees, wrists, and ankles develop,

lasting 2 to 3 weeks. The synovial fluid is inflammatory with a predominance of neutrophils; synovial biopsy shows nonspecific findings of edema, hyperemia, and a paucity of infiltrating cells.

Diagnostic criteria established by an International Study Group require recurrent oral ulcerations (aphthous or herpetiform) at least three times in a 12-month period and two of the following: (1) recurrent genital ulceration, (2) anterior or posterior uveitis or retinal vasculitis, (3) skin lesions consistent with Behçet's disease, and (4) pathergy.

The mortality from the disease is low (3% to 4%); central nervous system involvement and major vessel disease account for most of the deaths. There is no specific therapy for Behçet's disease. Colchicine may reduce the orogenital ulcers and iritis, and corticosteroids and immunosuppressive therapy with azathioprine, chlorambucil, or cyclosporin A are indicated in patients with ocular or central nervous system disease.

Relapsing Polychondritis

Relapsing polychondritis is an episodic, inflammatory, and sometimes destructive disease of cartilaginous structures throughout the body. Classic clinical manifestations include inflammation of the cartilage of the ear, nose, and tracheobronchial tree. Fever, iritis, episcleritis, aortic insufficiency, and rapidly progressive glomerulonephritis are recognized complications. In about one third of patients the chondritis develops in association with an immunologic disorder such as systemic lupus erythematosus, rheumatoid arthritis, or systemic vasculitis. Arthritis is widespread, including both cartilaginous (symphysis pubis and manubriosternal) and synovial joints. The arthritis is typically asymmetric and affects peripheral joints, most commonly the ankles and wrists. Laboratory findings include an elevated erythrocyte sedimentation rate, an absent rheumatoid factor, hypergammaglobulinemia, and anemia. Joint radiographs are unrevealing. In the absence of typical clinical findings cartilage biopsy is generally required to establish the diagnosis. Corticosteroids are effective in controlling the cartilage inflammation and inflammatory eye disease. Dapsone, 50 to 200 mg per day, may be beneficial. Immunosuppressive drugs such as cyclophosphamide or cyclosporine are indicated in patients with serious, life-threatening manifestations that have failed to respond to high-dose corticosteroids.

Relapsing Seronegative Symmetric Synovitis With Pitting Edema

The relapsing seronegative symmetric synovitis with pitting edema (RS3PE) syndrome is associated with intermittent attacks of joint stiffness and symmetric polyarthritis, particularly involving small joints of the hands and feet. The onset is typically abrupt, and patients have profound pitting edema of the hands (often with carpal tunnel syndrome) and feet. The syndrome occurs almost exclusively in individuals over the age of 60 years and is more common in men. Rheumatoid factor is absent, and elevations of erythrocyte sedimentation rate may be seen. The synovitis and edema respond promptly with low doses of prednisone (5 to 15 mg daily), and complete remission after the corticosteroids are tapered is typical.

Palindromic Rheumatism

Palindromic rheumatism is characterized by recurrent attacks of painful swelling of joints with prominent periarticular inflammation. The onset is typically between the third and sixth decades of life. The attacks are abrupt in onset, without fever or other systemic findings, frequently lasting only hours and rarely more than a few days. The intervals between attacks vary from days to weeks to months. The knees, wrists, and shoulders are most commonly involved; however any joint can be affected. Periarticular attacks are marked by a swelling of the heels, finger pads, and palms that resembles angioedema; transient painful subcutaneous or tendon nodules may be found. The erythrocyte sedimentation rate is often elevated during the attack. The pattern of the disease is peculiar to individual patients and remains relatively unchanged for the duration of the illness, which may go on for decades. About one third of patients eventually progress into typical rheumatoid arthritis. Treat-

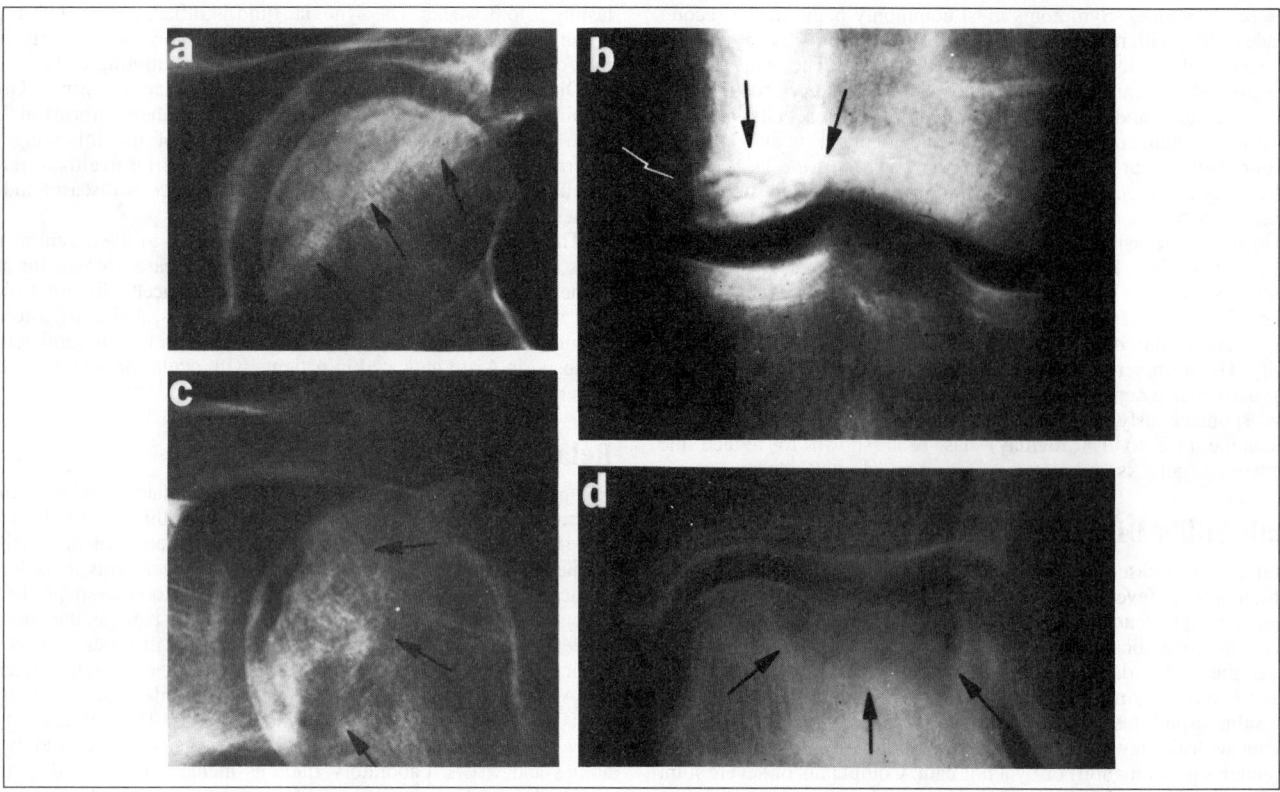

FIGURE 201-1   Osteonecrosis of femoral head *(a)*, medial femoral condyle *(b)*, humeral head *(c)*, and superior talus *(d)*. The margins of the necrotic segment undergo sclerotic change *(arrows)*.

ment with injectable gold, hydroxychloroquine, or sulfasalazine may be effective in chronic cases.

Intermittent Hydroarthrosis

Intermittent hydrarthrosis is a syndrome of episodic attacks of relatively painless effusions in large joints, most commonly the knees. The attacks occur with regular periodicity once or twice monthly; in women there is often a temporal association with the menses. The effusions accumulate rapidly and are resorbed over several days; joints are entirely normal in the interval between attacks. Laboratory studies during attacks are unremarkable, and joint fluids are noninflammatory. The condition is benign, with no long-term joint sequelae. No treatment has been shown to prevent or abort attacks, which remit spontaneously.

MONARTHROPATHIES
Osteonecrosis

Osteonecrosis is used to describe the joint disease resulting from death of trabecular bone beneath the articular surface. The two most common conditions responsible for osteonecrosis are trauma with disruption of the blood supply by fracture dislocation (femoral head osteonecrosis following hip fracture) and the use of high-dose corticosteroids. However, osteonecrosis occurs in a number of other settings including hemoglobinopathies (sickle cell disease and thalassemia minor), infiltrative marrow disorders (Gaucher's disease), air embolism (decompression sickness), alcoholism, pancreatitis, and systemic lupus erythematosus. Patients complain of severe pain, initially during weight bearing only but in late stages of the disease even at rest. The femoral and humeral heads, the femoral condyles, the navicular and lunate bones in the wrists, and the talus in the foot are all particularly susceptible.

Diagnosis rests on the recognition of symptoms of pain and limitation of motion in the affected joint and typical radiographic findings of subchondral rarefaction of bone, marginal sclerosis, and com-

pression fractures with disruption of articular surface (Fig. 201-1). Nuclear magnetic resonance imaging can detect necrotic bone even in the absence of radiographic changes and is the procedure of choice in the earliest stages of the disease. Bone decompression and grafting to enhance revascularization before the appearance of radiographic abnormalities may retard bone injury. Replacement arthroplasty is usually required in chronic stages of the disease.

Foreign Body Synovitis

Penetrating injuries of joints or periarticular tissues may induce acute or chronic inflammatory monarthritis, tenosynovitis, or dactylitis. The most common materials associated with synovitis are plant thorns (cactus needles, rose thorns, palm leaves), glass, metal, and sea urchin spines. The hands, feet, and knees are the most common joints affected. Fever is typically absent, except in instances when contaminating organisms or toxins are introduced, such as occurs with sea urchin spine injuries. Findings on radiographs are generally nonspecific, but radiopaque foreign bodies such as leaded glass, metal, or sea urchin spines may be detected. Ultrasonography, computerized tomography, and magnetic resonance imaging may be helpful in identifying the foreign material. Treatment requires wide excisional biopsy with synovectomy.

Pigmented Villonodular Synovitis

Pigmented villonodular synovitis is a benign tumor composed of matted masses of villae and synovial nodules. It generally becomes evident as a monarthritis in young adults. The knee is most commonly involved, but the hip, ankle, other joints, tendon sheaths, or bursae may be involved. Joint aspiration typically reveals a serosanguineous or xanthochromic fluid. Occasionally the process can be quite destructive of underlying bone, particularly in joints with a tight capsule, such as the hip. Radiographic examination shows soft tissue densities, diffuse rarefactions, and erosions. Magnetic resonance imaging is particularly useful in defining the synovial lesion and extent of bone erosion. The diagnosis is best made by arthroscopic biopsy. On histologic examination the synovium is infiltrated with lymphocytes, giant cells, and lipid-laden macrophages interspersed among areas of hemorrhage and synovial cell proliferation. Wide excision of the lesion is recommended, but recurrences are common. Recurrent lesions can be treated with intraarticular radiation synovectomy or by radiotherapy. Reconstructive surgery with total joint arthroplasty is indicated in patients with extensive joint destruction.

POLYARTHRITIS
Sarcoidosis

In patients with pulmonary sarcoidosis two distinct types of arthritis develop: (1) an acute transient polyarthritis associated with erythema nodosum and (2) a chronic, persistent polyarthropathy. The acute arthritis is migratory, involves large joints of the extremities, and typically appears at the onset of sarcoidosis, often in association with bilateral hilar adenopathy. Chronic arthritis is much less frequent and results from granulomatous inflammation of the synovium or juxtaarticular bone. It becomes evident as a chronic monarticular arthritis and, very rarely (almost exclusively in African Americans), as a destructive arthropathy. Diffuse swelling of the phalanges (dactylitis) is common. Radiographs may show the typical lacy cystic appearance of sarcoid bone disease. Synovial effusions are variably inflammatory with either mononuclear or polymorphonuclear predominance. Treatment is symptomatic and is usually limited to NSAIDs, but responses to chloroquine, colchicine, and corticosteroids have been reported.

Multicentric Reticulohistiocytosis

Multicentric reticulohistiocytosis (lipoid dermatoarthritis) is a rare and often very destructive polyarthritis affecting primarily adult women. The disorder is accompanied by firm, yellowish brown or red nodules appearing at the base of the fingernail or scattered throughout the upper extremities, face, and scalp. The skin lesions, which may be confused with xanthelasmas, tend to wax and wane, independent of the symmetric polyarthritis. The distal interphalangeal joints are invariably involved, although symmetric polyarthritis of large and small peripheral joints and the cervical spine may rarely be seen. Spontaneous remissions occur, but the arthritis often progresses to a mutilating, severely deforming condition. Radiographs of the joints confirm the extensive destructive changes and show loss of cartilage and striking resorption of subchondral bone. The skin and synovium are infiltrated by foamy histiocytic cells and by multinucleated giant cells that contain an undefined lipid or glycoprotein material. Nitrogen mustard alkylating agents appear to be an effective treatment.

Hyperlipoproteinemias

Individuals with type IIa hyperbetalipoproteinemia have tendinous and periosteal xanthomas, particularly over the extensor tendons of the fingers and over the Achilles tendons. Tendon involvement is usually asymptomatic, although it may rarely cause spontaneous tendon rupture. Acute monarthritis or oligoarthritis can be observed, most frequently in the knee or ankle. In children an acute migratory polyarthritis may develop that simulates rheumatic fever. Tendinous and intraosseous xanthomas develop in patients with type III dysbetalipoproteinemia. Intraosseous xanthomas appear as multiple, well-defined, small round or oval lucencies on radiographs and occasionally cause pathologic fractures. An association of arthralgia and transient synovitis has been described in type IV hyperlipoproteinemia. Lowering of serum cholesterol level can lead to reduction of the size of tendon xanthomas; surgical excision may be beneficial in selected cases but is associated with a high rate of recurrence.

PANNICULITIS

The subcutaneous fat is divided into lobules by fibrous septae through which course arteries and veins. Panniculitis may originate within the blood vessels or within fat lobules. Vasculitis, primarily of venules, is responsible for the panniculitis accompanying systemic illnesses and becomes evident on clinical examination as erythema nodosum or an immune-complex–induced arteriolitis such as lupus profundus or nodular vasculitis. Inflammation originating within the fat lobules results in relapsing nodular panniculitis (Weber-Christian syndrome). In pancreatic disease, vascular and primary fat-lobule inflammation have been implicated in nodular liquefying panniculitis. Bone and/or joint pain and inflammation may result from intramedullary and periarticular fat necrosis, respectively.

Erythema Nodosum

Erythema nodosum (EN) is characterized by the presence of raised, warm, painful, erythematous nodules of various sizes, occurring typically over both shins and less commonly on the thighs and forearms (Color Plate VII-1). Recognized causes include infections of the respiratory or gastrointestinal tracts; sensitivity to drugs such as sulfonamides, iodides, and birth control medications; inflammatory bowel disease; sarcoidosis; and neoplasms, including leukemias and Hodgkin's disease. In many patients, however, no cause is found. Biopsy of the lesion shows an early inflammatory infiltrate of lymphocytes and macrophages of the septum between fat lobules followed later by the formation of giant cells and granuloma. Vasculitis of the veins or arteries can be identified, together with occasional immunoglobulin and complement deposits. Two thirds of EN patients have joint pain, stiffness, or frank arthritis that often precedes the skin eruption. The arthritis primarily affects the knees, wrists, and ankles and usually resolves with the skin lesions but may persist for weeks or last several years, eventually clearing without deformity. Radiographs of the affected joints are normal; the erythrocyte sedimentation rate usually is elevated; and test results for rheumatoid factor are generally negative, except with underlying chronic infections, sarcoid, or leprosy. Joint symptoms usually respond to NSAIDs given in full doses; in the rare persistent case corticosteroids or potassium iodide may be required. Recurrences of both the erythema nodosum and joint symptoms are not uncommon.

Relapsing Febrile Nodular Panniculitis (Weber-Christian Syndrome)

The rare Weber-Christian syndrome probably represents several different forms of panniculitis that share similar clinical and pathologic manifestations. As its name indicates, it is characterized by recurrent attacks of tender, subcutaneous nodules with fever. The nodules may be mobile initially but generally become adherent to the dermis and leave an atrophic scar as the edema subsides. The nodules occur in crops on the trunk and proximal extremities. Liquefaction of the fat tissue may cause chronic sinus tracts with drainage of an oily, viscous material. Involvement of the pericardial fat, mesentery, and retroperitoneal tissues may accompany the subcutaneous lesions. A deficiency of α1-antitrypsin has been described in association with the syndrome. Corticosteroid therapy may be useful during acute phases, but there is no definitive therapy.

Pancreatic Diseases

In patients with acute and chronic pancreatitis or pancreatic neoplasms, a nodular, liquefying panniculitis may develop that is evident as tender, red subcutaneous nodules occurring primarily on the lower extremities. The nodules typically occur on the posterior aspect of the legs and, unlike EN, are generally movable when they first appear. On healing they leave a hyperpigmented, depressed scar. Polyarthritis, bone pain from osseous intramedullary fat necrosis, and serositis involving the pleura, mesentery, and pericardium can occur. Elevation of serum lipase level is a consistent finding, although the role of lipase in the pathogenesis of the fat necrosis is unclear.

ENTEROPATHIC ARTHROPATHIES
Inflammatory Bowel Disease

Similar inflammatory joint disorders occur with both ulcerative colitis and Crohn's disease. The characteristic peripheral arthritis becomes evident as an asymmetric, predominantly lower-extremity inflammation of knees, ankles, and, less commonly, small joints of the toes. It is often accompanied by periarticular inflammation and tendinitis, particularly involving the ankle and Achilles tendon. The arthritis generally appears after or concomitant with the onset of inflammatory bowel disease and tends to parallel the activity of the bowel disease. Peripheral arthritis is most closely correlated with EN, oral mucous membrane ulceration, and anterior uveitis, but not pyoderma gangrenosum.

In patients with inflammatory bowel disease an axial arthropathy (spondylitis) may also develop, with inflammatory low back and buttock pain and pain in the thoracic or cervical regions. Limitations of motion of the lumbar (Schober's test) and cervical (occiput to wall) regions are typically present, and chest wall expansion is reduced. Involvement of the hips or shoulders is common. The axial arthropathy often precedes bowel symptoms, and the course is typically independent of the intestinal disease. Radiographic changes are indistinguishable from ankylosing spondylitis with sacroiliitis, syndesmophyte formation, and eventual bony bridging of vertebral bodies.

Treatment of the peripheral and axial arthropathies of inflammatory bowel disease is similar. Primary emphasis should be placed on control of the underlying bowel disease, particularly in patients with peripheral arthritis. Physical therapy is important in patients with axial disease to relieve muscle spasm and maintain mobility of the spine. When necessary, joint symptoms may be treated with NSAIDs, although there is a risk of exacerbation of the bowel disease with these drugs. The peripheral arthritis is generally exquisitely sensitive to corticosteroid therapy when used for control of the bowel disease, but joint activity itself should generally not be considered an indication for the use of corticosteroids. Sulfasalazine may be effective in axial arthropathy.

Whipple's Disease

Articular complaints occur in the majority of patients with Whipple's disease, a rare disorder characterized by diarrhea, malabsorption with steatorrhea, fever, anemia, and hyperpigmentation (Chapter 245). In more than one third of the patients joint symptoms antedate apparent bowel involvement by 10 years or more. The joint involvement is generally episodic, inflammatory, and of abrupt onset; it involves predominantly the larger joints. It is often bilateral, however, and may involve the upper extremities as well, including the wrists and fingers. As the bowel disease progresses and steatorrhea becomes prominent, the arthritis often regresses.

Laboratory evaluation reveals negative rheumatoid factor studies and a mildly inflammatory joint fluid with a preponderance of mononuclear cells, but no findings are specific for this syndrome. Synovial biopsies have shown nonspecific mild inflammation and only infrequently show the period acid–Schiff stain (PAS)-positive inclusion bodies that characterize the small bowel histopathologic appearance in this disorder. A gram-positive actinomycete, *Troheryma whippelii,* has been isolated from duodenal tissues of patients with Whipple's disease, and a polymerase chain reaction provides a specific test for the disease. Treatment of the bowel disease with tetracycline generally leads to elimination of the arthritis within a few weeks.

HEMATOLOGIC DISORDERS
Coagulation Disorders

Hemophilia and related coagulation disorders are associated with recurrent hemorrhages into joints and adjacent soft tissues. Hemarthrosis occurs in 80% to 90% of hemophiliacs and causes exquisitely painful, warm, swollen joints. Recurrent episodes of bleeding may cause a chronic synovitis with the development of flexion deformities and a destructive arthropathy. In children repeated hemarthroses result in abnormalities of the epiphyseal plate and irregular bony overgrowth. Treatment requires infusion of plasma factors and immobilization of the joint in extension. Ice packs, analgesics, and NSAIDs may be helpful, and intraarticular corticosteroids are occasionally used. Patients are often made aware of impending hemarthrosis by a deep, burning pain in the joint and treat themselves with appropriate plasma factors at home. Hemarthrosis occasionally requires aspiration after appropriate replacement therapy, particularly if infection is suspected. The main long-term goal is to avoid muscle wasting, contracture, and joint deformity; performing physiotherapy to maintain joint motion and strengthen muscles is extremely important.

Sickle Cell Disease and Related Hemoglobinopathies

The crises of sickle cell disease are often associated with intense bone and joint pain, occasionally with an inflammatory arthritis resulting from small infarctions in the synovium and periarticular bone. In young children with sickle cell disease acute swelling of the hands and feet (dactylitis or "hand-foot syndrome") may occur in association with marked periosteal reaction along the phalanges, metacarpals, and metatarsals. Joint hemorrhages, a susceptibility to osteomyelitis, and in adults the development of hyperuricemia and gouty arthritis all produce complicating articular complaints. Osteonecrosis (presumably caused by thrombosis in epiphyseal vessels) is a recognized complication in individuals with sickle cell trait, sickle cell–hemoglobin C disease, and sickle cell thalassemia, as well as sickle cell anemia (SS) hemoglobinopathy.

ENDOCRINE DISEASES
Thyroid Disease

Hypothyroidism can be complicated by joint pain, stiffness, myopathy, pyrophosphate arthropathy, and symptoms of median nerve compression. Effusions, when present, are bland and hyperviscous. Muscle weakness may be associated with high levels of creatine kinase, causing confusion with polymyositis. Hyperthyroidism may cause muscular weakness, bone pain, and periarthritis of the shoulder. Thyroid acropachy (exophthalmos, pretibial myxedema, digital clubbing, and osteoarthropathy) is a rare syndrome that is seen in patients with treated hyperthyroidism. Musculoskeletal symptoms are common in patients with Hashimoto's thyroiditis, which is seen with increased frequency in patients with autoimmune connective tissue disorders and rheumatoid arthritis.

Diabetes Mellitus

A number of musculoskeletal disorders occur in patients with diabetes mellitus. Neuroarthropathy with osteolysis (Charcot's arthropathy) is seen in the forefoot and midfoot and in weight-bearing joints. Flexion contractures of the fingers with digital sclerosis resembling scleroderma (diabetic cheirarthropathy) and periarthritis of the shoulders with marked loss of movement (frozen shoulder) develop in patients with type I diabetes. Patients with type I and, in particular, type II diabetes are at increased risk for development of the diffuse idiopathic skeletal hyperostosis (DISH) syndrome. Calcifications and ossifications of the anterior longitudinal ligament of the spine and peripheral ligaments lead to back pain and an arthropathy of axial and peripheral joints. A diffuse scleroderma-like induration of the back and trunk (scleredema) also occurs in diabetes.

Parathyroid Disorders

Hyperparathyroidism has a recognized association with chondrocalcinosis and calcium pyrophosphate arthropathy. Articular manifestations also result from bone demineralization, subchondral trabecular fractures, collapse of cysts, and small-joint erosions, all related to the underlying metabolic bone disease. Spontaneous rupture of tendons is a recognized complication. Hyperparathyroidism resulting from renal failure has been associated with periarticular calcifications attributable to apatite crystal deposition, and a destructive, erosive spondyloarthropathy has been described. Hypocalcemic muscular cramps and subcutaneous nodular calcifications occur in patients with hypoparathyroidism, and an ankylosing spondylitis–like disorder with normal sacroiliac joints has been reported. In patients with pseudohypoparathyroidism shortened metacarpals and metatarsals develop.

Acromegaly

The increased levels of growth hormone in acromegaly produce an exaggerated growth of articular cartilage and bone. Hypertrophy of other structures, including the synovium, bursa, and tendon sheath, may cause effusions and symptoms of median nerve compression (carpal tunnel syndrome). Dorsal kyphosis of the spine and severe osteoarthritis of the hips may produce significant disability. Radiographs disclose thickening of the soft tissue and degenerative changes. Early in the process, particularly, there is a paradoxic widening of the cartilage space that is especially prominent in the small joints of the hands and feet. Mottling of the metacarpal and metatarsal heads and thickening of the trabecular bone occur. The vertebral bodies have a typical appearance produced by marked bony overgrowth on their anterior aspects.

Adrenal Disorders

In patients with cortisol excess (Cushing's syndrome), osteonecrosis, a proximal myopathy, and severe osteoporosis with compression fractures of the spine develop. Creatine kinase levels are normal in steroid myopathy. In cases of adrenal insufficiency severe muscle cramps and contractures of the legs are reversible with steroid replacement. Adrenal insufficiency is a recognized complication of the antiphospholipid syndrome. Pheochromocytoma has been associated with rhabdomyolisis caused by catecholamine-mediated vasoconstriction and muscle ischemia.

NEUROLOGIC DISORDERS
Neuropathic Joint Disease (Charcot's Joints)

The loss of sensation to a joint may result in a destructive arthropathy with joint instability, exaggerated degenerative and resorptive changes, and florid new bone formation. The prototype neuropathic arthropathy was described by Charcot in tabes dorsalis, and similar changes have been seen in a variety of neurologic disorders, including meningomyelocele, leprosy, paraplegia, diabetes mellitus, syringomyelia, and congenital indifference to pain. The affected joint is determined by the neural lesion: in tabes dorsalis the knees, hips, ankles, and vertebrae are affected; in diabetic neuropathy the forefoot and ankle; and in syringomyelia the shoulder or elbow. The joint disease is usually progressive, with insidious swelling and progressive instability. Occasionally, however, the onset is abrupt with associated inflammation of the surrounding soft tissues. Although generally painless, neuropathic joints may be painful but not in proportion to the joint destruction. Radiographs reveal only effusion initially, which is followed rapidly by cartilage loss, fragmentation, and resorption of subchondral bone and development of large, bulky, osteophytic bony overgrowths. Pathologic fractures are common. Management is limited to immobilization and restriction of weight bearing. Surgical arthrodeses are often unsuccessful, as are prosthetic joints.

Reflex Sympathetic Dystrophy Syndrome

Reflex sympathetic dystrophy (algodystrophy) is evident as severe pain, swelling, vasomotor dysfunction, and impaired mobility in an extremity. Involvement of the upper extremity produces edema and trophic skin changes of the hand and forearm, excessive perspiration and warmth of the hand, and pain and limitation of the ipsilateral shoulder (the so-called shoulder-hand syndrome). The symptom complex appears to be caused by an excessive or abnormal response of the sympathetic nervous system in an extremity to an injury or other insult. Common examples include neurologic disease (stroke with hemiplegia, spinal cord lesions, radiculopathies, and/or postherpetic neuralgia), atherosclerotic cardiovascular disease (myocardial infarction, severe angina pectoris, or coronary artery bypass surgery), endocrine disorders such as hyperthyroidism, and malignancies. Drugs such as isoniazid and barbiturates also have been implicated. A number of other trauma-related conditions such as causalgia, posttraumatic osteoporosis, traumatic vasospasm, and Sudeck's atrophy are included in this designation. After the initial inflammatory edematous stage, dystrophic changes begin to develop, with cool skin, cyanosis, and loss of motion. If spontaneous remission or response to treatment does not occur at this point, a superimposed atrophy of skin and soft tissue, contractures, osteopenia, and neuralgic pains with poor potential for reversibility occur. Bone scans show increased uptake, often in a periarticular distribution, before the detection of patchy osteoporosis

on radiographs, which occurs weeks to months later. There are no specific laboratory diagnostic findings. Treatment consists of pain management and early mobilization, application of local heat, and range-of-motion exercises to avoid joint contractures. Sympathetic nerve block and transcutaneous nerve stimulation have been used with some success. High-dose corticosteroids (60 mg prednisone daily for 1 to 2 weeks), or calcitonin (100-160 IU daily for 4 to 8 weeks) are used to reduce the high metabolic state, particularly in the acute stage.

MALIGNANCY
Hypertrophic Osteoarthropathy

Hypertrophic osteoarthropathy (HOA) produces prominent clubbing of the fingers in association with pain, swelling, tenderness, and stiffness of peripheral joints, especially the wrists and ankles. The adjacent long bones are often tender with edema and erythema of the overlying skin as a result of proliferation of the periosteum of tubular bones. Joint symptoms occasionally precede clubbing or radiologic evidence of periosteal change, although radionuclide bone scan identifies areas of increased uptake along the margins of the bone. The polyarthritis may be mistaken for rheumatoid arthritis, but the synovial fluid is characteristically noninflammatory.

Carcinoma of the lung is by far the most common cause of HOA, but numerous other malignant (mesothelioma, esophageal and gastric carcinoma, carcinoma of the liver) and nonmalignant (chronic infections, inflammatory bowel disease, pulmonary fibrosis) causes of the disease are recognized. A rare primary form (pachydermoperiostosis) produces clubbing, and bone changes occur in young boys with marked thickening of the skin of the face, forehead, and scalp and excessive sebaceous gland activity. NSAIDs or corticosteroids provide symptomatic relief. Resection of the primary neoplasm or eradication of other underlying causes occasionally produces dramatic relief of symptoms.

Paraneoplastic Syndromes

Malignancies may be associated with noninflammatory polyarthritis, including the occasional presentation of an occult malignancy as a seronegative peripheral polyarthritis. Carcinoma of the breast in women is the most common malignancy associated with the syndrome, although cases of pancreatic, lung, and cardiac tumors with arthritis have been described. In addition, dermatomyositis has been noted to be associated with a number of malignancies and ovarian carcinoma with an unusual palmar fasciitis. Most patients are found to have elevated sedimentation rates and noninflammatory joint effusions; serologic features such as rheumatoid factor and antinuclear antibody may be found in low titer. Musculosketetal symptoms resolve with effective treatment of the tumor and may reappear with tumor recurrence or as a sign of metastases.

Leukemia

In patients with leukemia, particularly children, an asymmetric polyarthritis may develop, involving the knees, ankles, and shoulders. Joint symptoms may precede recognition of the leukemia; nocturnal bone pain and unexplained fever are often clues to the diagnosis. The arthropathy may be due to direct infiltration of the synovium by leukemic cells or a response to periosteal reactions to the periarticular bone marrow. Polyarthritis and polyarteritis nodosa have been described in patients with hairy cell leukemia. The arthritis typically antedates the leukemia, whereas the vasculitis occurs late in the course, often after splenectomy has been performed for treatment. Gouty arthritis occasionally occurs in patients with leukemia, particularly following chemotherapy.

Angioimmunoblastic Lymphadenopathy

Angioimmunoblastic lymphadenopathy (AILD) is a lymphoproliferative disorder that shares many similarities with the connective tissue diseases, in particular, systemic lupus erythematosus and Sjögren's syndrome. Characteristic signs and symptoms include fever, weight loss, arthritis, hepatosplenomegaly, lymphadenopathy, and urticaria or maculopapular rash. Hemolytic anemia, thrombocytopenia, and hypergammaglobulinemia are commonly present, and antinuclear antibodies are found in most patients. Diagnosis is based on the classic appearance of the lymph node biopsy specimen with disruption of the normal architecture by proliferation of small blood vessels and infiltration by plasma cells and immunoblasts. The disease is self-limited in many patients, although treatment with corticosteroids and/or cytotoxic drugs may be required; in approximately one third of patients the disease progresses to malignant lymphoma.

BIBLIOGRAPHY

Bridges AJ, Hickman PL: RS3PE syndrome and polymyalgia rheumatica: distinguishing features, *J Rheumatol* 18:1764, 1991.

Dixey J: Erythema nodosum. In Klippel JH, Dieppe PA editors: *Rheumatology,* London, 1994, Mosby.

Garcia-Gonzalez A, Weisman MH: The arthritis of familial Mediterranean fever, *Semin Arthritis Rheum* 22:139, 1992.

Ginsburg WW et al: Multicentric reticulohistiocytosis: response to alkylating agents in six patients, *Ann Intern Med* 111:384, 1989.

Guerne PA, Weisman MH: Palindromic rheumatism: part of or apart from the spectrum of rheumatoid arthritis, *Am J Med* 93:451, 1992.

Hellmann DB: Sarcoidosis. In Schumacher HR, Klippel JH, Koopman WJ, editors: *Primer on the rheumatic diseases,* Atlanta, 1993, Arthritis Foundation.

International Study Group for Behçet's Disease: Criteria for diagnosis of Behçet's disease. *Lancet* 335:1078, 1990.

Klemp P et al: Musculoskeletal manifestations in hyperlipidaemia: a controlled study, *Ann Rheum Dis* 52:44, 1993.

Kozin F: The reflex sympathetic dystrophy syndrome, *Bull Rheum Dis* 36:1, 1986.

Leirisalo-Repo M: Enteropathic arthritis, Whipple's disease, juvenile spondyloarthropathy, uveitis, and SAPHO syndrome, *Curr Opin Rheumatol* 7:284-289, 1995.

Madhok R, York J, Sturrock RD: Haemophilic arthritis, *Ann Rheum Dis* 50:588, 1991.

Mankin HJ: Nontraumatic necrosis of bone (osteonecrosis), *N Engl J Med* 326:1473, 1992.

Michet CJ et al: Relapsing polychondritis: survival and predictive role of early disease manifestations, *Ann Intern Med* 104:74, 1986.

Myers BW, Masi AT, Feigenbaum SL: Pigmented villonodular synovitis and tenosynovitis: a clinical epidemiologic study of 166 cases and literature review, *Medicine* 59:223, 1980.

Panush RS et al: Weber-Christian disease: analysis of 15 cases and review of the literature, *Medicine* 64:181, 1985.

Pineda C et al: The spectrum of soft tissue and skeletal abnormalities of hypertrophic osteoarthropathy, *J Rheumatol* 17:773, 1990.

Pouchot J et al: Adult Still's disease: manifestations, disease course and outcome in 62 patients, *Medicine* 70:118, 1991.

Reginato AJ et al: Clinical and pathologic studies of 26 patients with penetrating foreign body injury to the joint, bursae, and tendon sheaths, *Arthritis Rheum* 33:1753, 1990.

Schwarzer AC, Schrieber L: Rheumatic manifestations of neoplasia, *Curr Opin Rheumatol* 3:145, 1991.

Slowman-Kovaks, Braunstein E, Brandt K: Rapidly progressive Charcot arthropathy following minor trauma in patients with diabetic neuropathy, *Arthritis Rheum* 33:412, 1990.

Steinberg AD et al: Angioimmunoblastic lymphadenopathy with dysproteinemia, *Ann Intern Med* 16:1379, 1988.

CHAPTER

202 Cryoglobulinemia

Peter D. Gorevic

Cryoglobulins are immunoglobulins that have the property of precipitating reversibly at low temperatures. Although cryoproteinemia associated with severe Raynaud's phenomenon was first described by Wintrobe and Buell in 1933 as a concomitant of multiple myeloma, it is now recognized that cryoglobulins may occur in a variety of infectious, neoplastic, and autoimmune diseases, the most common of which are listed in Table 202-1.

ETIOLOGY AND INCIDENCE

Monoclonal or single-component cryoglobulinemia is generally associated with multiple myeloma, macroglobulinemia, and other, rarer neoplastic proliferations of plasma cells and lymphocytes. These cryo-

Table 202-1 Types of cryoglobulins and their associated diseases

TYPE	FREQUENCY (%)
I. Monoclonal	25-40
A. Multiple myeloma (IgG, IgA)	
B. Macroglobulinemia (IgM)	
C. Chronic lymphocytic leukemia and other lymphoproliferative disorders	
D. Angioimmunoblastic lymphadenopathy	
E. Idiopathic	
II. Mixed (most often IgM-IgG*)	60-75
A. Infections	
1. Viral: hepatitis B, hepatitis C, infectious mononucleosis, cytomegalovirus	
2. Bacterial: subacute bacterial endocarditis, leprosy, poststreptococcal nephritis, intestinal bypass, syphilis	
3. Parasitic: schistosomiasis, toxoplasmosis, malaria, kala-azar, others	
B. "Autoimmune" diseases: systemic lupus erythematosus, rheumatoid arthritis, polyarteritis nodosa, Sjögren's syndrome; scleroderma, others	
C. Lymphoproliferative diseases: macroglobulinemia, various lymphomas, chronic lymphocytic leukemia, angioimmunoblastic lymphadenopathy, hairy cell leukemia	
D. Renal disease: proliferative glomerulonephritis	
E. Liver diseases: Laënnec's cirrhosis, biliary cirrhosis, chronic hepatitis	
F. Familial	
G. Essential	

*The division into groups with a "monoclonal" or "polyclonal" IgM is arbitrary and reflects the predominance of IgM components with kappa light chains, many of which bear specific idiotypic determinants.
IgA, IgG, IgM, Immunoglobulins A, G, and M.

globulins occur in large amounts (I to 5 g/dl) and are readily detected as monoclonal components on electrophoresis of whole serum or the isolated cryoprecipitate. In many instances production of these proteins does not cause clinical symptoms and they are detected accidentally during a routine laboratory analysis when a precipitate is noted in a serum that has been stored in a refrigerator. On occasion, however, they cause symptoms of cold intolerance marked by Raynaud's phenomenon, vascular ulcers, purpura, livedo reticularis, and in severe cases ischemia and gangrene of the extremities. In several large series of patients with cryoglobulins this type of cryoprotein constitutes approximately one third of those seen. As is the case with all immunoglobulin-producing tumors, immunoglobulin G (IgG) cryoglobulins are more common than immunoglobulin M (IgM) cryoglobulins, and these in turn are more common than immunoglobulin A (IgA) cryoglobulins. On occasion, Bence Jones proteins also are found to precipitate in the cold.

About two thirds of the cryoglobulins seen in most series are mixed cryoglobulins, so called because they consist of more than one class of immunoglobulin. In general, mixed cryoglobulins contain an IgM molecule together with IgG, although other combinations (such as IgA and IgG or IgM, IgG, and IgA) occasionally are present in these complexes. Mixed cryoglobulins may be difficult to detect, may precipitate slowly, and tend to be present in small amounts (50 to 500 mg/dl). Nevertheless, since they appear to be immune complexes, they very frequently give rise to systemic symptoms on clinical examination by causing vasculitis involving many different organ systems. Mixed cryoglobulins have been further subdivided into those in which one of the components, usually the IgM, appears to be monoclonal (since it contains only one type of light chain, most often of the kappa type) and those in which all components are polyclonal. These monoclonal IgMs share variable-region (i.e., idiotypic) antigenic determinants with similar molecules occurring in patients with known lymphoproliferative (e.g., chronic lymphocytic leukemia) or rheumatic (e.g., Sjögren's syndrome) diseases, reflecting in turn selective germ-line gene usage. However, although this subdivision is of obvious significance in individuals with malignancies of lymphocytes and plasma cells, it generally is of little importance in patients

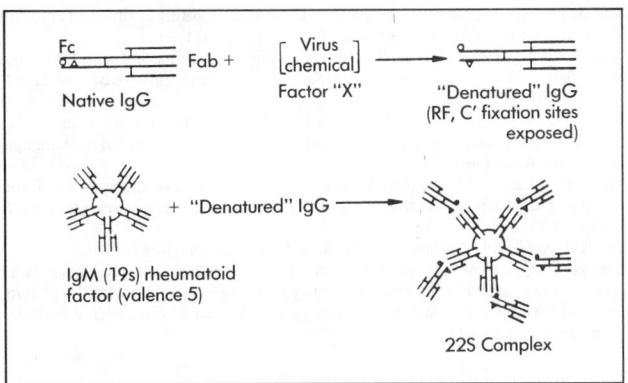

FIGURE 202-1   Possible mechanism for the formation of circulating immune complexes and their conversion to a mixed cryoglobulin (MC) through the formation of an immunoglobulin M (IgM)–anti-immunoglobulin G (IgG) with unusual solubility properties. Activation of complement then leads to vasculitis and/or nephritis with deposition of immune complexes. *RF,* Rheumatoid factor.

whose mixed cryoglobulins are associated with nonmalignant disorders such as hepatitis, systemic lupus erythematosus, rheumatoid arthritis, and other connective tissue diseases. In clinical and prognostic terms, too, there is little difference between the apparently monoclonal and the polyclonal mixed cryoglobulins in the nonneoplastic diseases.

PATHOPHYSIOLOGY

Monoclonal cryoproteins are usually products of a malignant clone of cells and are structurally indistinguishable from their noncryoprecipitable counterparts. Typical symptoms caused by these proteins are vascular occlusive phenomena, including acrocyanosis or bluing of the helices of the ears, probably resulting from their precipitation at the lower temperatures encountered in toes, fingers, and ears. In addition to the purely physical obstructive process, they may also initiate an inflammatory response via the activation of complement or through their direct interaction with various inflammatory cells.

Little is known about the cause or origin of the mixed cryoglobulins. However, their frequent association with chronic viral and bacterial infectious diseases (including hepatitis B and C viruses, infectious mononucleosis, and subacute bacterial endocarditis) and the discovery in some instances of specific antigens or antibodies in the cryoprecipitates suggest that perhaps a viral or bacterial infection results in the production, first, of antibodies to the infectious agent and then of antibodies directed against these antibodies (Fig. 202-1).

Mixed cryoglobulins are cold-precipitable immune complexes in which the major antibody activity is an IgM that has as its antigen IgG. Since this type of antibody activity was first described in the sera of patients with rheumatoid arthritis, it is commonly referred to as a rheumatoid factor (RF). In addition to IgM anti–gamma globulins and IgG (the latter of which may be oligoclonal or polyclonal), mixed cryoglobulins occurring in association with certain chronic viral infections (notably Epstein-Barr or hepatitis C virus) or autoimmune diseases (notably lupus erythematosus) may contain other antibody activities and occasionally have been found to contain viral or nuclear antigens to which these antibodies are directed. It appears quite likely that these and other unidentified substances represent the inciting antigens that lead to the production of the antibodies that ultimately give rise to the unusual cryoprecipitable IgM anti–gamma G globulins.

Patients with monoclonal mixed cryoglobulins tend to be markedly hypocomplementemic and most often have a severe depression of the C4 and C2 components of complement with less involvement of C3 or late-reacting components. These complement abnormalities may result from diverse mechanisms of in vivo or ex vivo activation and correlate only imprecisely with clinical evidence of disease activity. The presence in serum of cryoglobulins and other immune complexes associated with hypocomplementemia initiated a search for

each of these components in the vasculitic lesions, and in some instances it has proven possible to localize IgM, IgM RF, IgG, complement components, and at times, viral antigens in tissue lesions by immunohistochemical techniques. These observations suggest that many of the tissue lesions may be a consequence of the deposition of immune complexes in small vessels and/or glomeruli and the resultant inflammatory response, which initiates a systemic vasculitis and/or glomerulonephritis (Fig. 202-1). Why some patients with immune complexes have symptoms and others do not and the reason for differences in organ involvement in those with the disease remain to be elucidated. Determining factors may be related to the nature of the antigen, the type of antibody response, the size of the immune complexes, the function of the reticuloendothelial system, or the ability of the complex to activate complement or interact with specific complement or IgG (Fc) receptors. The lesions in patients with monoclonal cryoglobulins are most commonly a consequence of the fact that they are cold-insoluble proteins which occlude small vessels, initiating an inflammatory response and resulting in ischemia. Mixed cryoglobulins, on the other hand, resemble other types of immune complexes in that the vascular inflammation is a result of their deposition in the small vessels followed by activation of complement leading to an inflammatory response and vasculitis.

PATHOLOGIC FEATURES

Since cold insolubility may be rapid, especially if the protein is of high thermal amplitude and present in large amounts, care should be exercised in handling biopsy material to prevent ex vivo cryoprecipitation in tissue. The histologic hallmark of monoclonal cryoglobulinemia is the vascular occlusive lesion that stains for the specific immunoglobulin isotype. However, necrotizing vasculitis and immune-complex nephritis may also be seen. Conversely, patients with mixed cryoglobulins tend to have a vasculitic process involving small- and medium-size vessels in many organs, most often the skin and kidneys and less often the heart, adrenals, gastrointestinal tract, pancreas, muscles, lungs, and other organs. In the skin the typical lesion is a leukocytoclastic vasculitis, whereas in the kidneys the lesions resemble acute or subacute glomerulonephritis. Also characteristic in the kidney are hyaline inclusions in glomeruli that stain positively by indirect immunofluorescence for the components of the cryoglobulin.

CLINICAL AND LABORATORY FINDINGS

The most characteristic symptom complex associated with mixed cryoglobulinemia consists of arthralgias, dependent purpura, and one or more common manifestations such as Raynaud's phenomenon, cutaneous ulcers, cold urticaria, pericarditis, thyroiditis, Sjögren's syndrome, and other symptoms seen in many of the connective tissue diseases. The most severe manifestations of the presence of this type of cryoglobulin are the renal disease that develops as a consequence of an immune-complex type of nephritis and a peripheral neuropathy that may be due to a vasculitis of the peripheral nerves. The former can progress very rapidly, resulting in severe renal failure, or in about 25% of patients it can be arrested or halt spontaneously. Patients with mixed cryoglobulins often have hepatosplenomegaly, subclinical evidence of liver disease, and moderate lymphadenopathy.

Laboratory analysis reveals the cold-precipitable proteins and, often, an elevated erythrocyte sedimentation rate, moderate diffuse hypergammaglobulinemia, and the absence of a monoclonal spike on protein electrophoresis. A positive test for IgM RF is invariably found if sensitive assays are used.

The course of this disorder is variable and depends on the organs involved. In patients having only purpura and arthralgias, the course can be indolent and last for more than 25 years; in 40 patients, some of whom were followed over that long a period, the average length of follow-up among patients with no evidence of renal involvement was approximately 12 years, with only a small number of deaths in this group. Patients with renal disease, however, tend to have a poor prognosis with an average follow-up of approximately 6 years and a significantly higher mortality. At autopsy there are signs of systemic vasculitis involving the skin, kidneys, heart, adrenals, liver, pericardium, and many other organs. Overwhelming infections often contribute to death.

DIAGNOSIS

Serum that contains cryoglobulins becomes opalescent and forms a visible precipitate when incubated at 0° to 4° C. The quantity of cold-insoluble protein can be determined either as a cryocrit (percentage of total volume of serum separated at 37° C, stored 4 to 7 days at 40° C and spun down cold in a Wintrobe tube) or, better, by isolating the cryoglobulin and measuring the amount of protein precipitated. Further characterization of the type of protein in the precipitate is most readily carried out by immunoelectrophoresis or immunoglobulin quantitation. It should be remembered that symptoms are not related to the amount of cryoglobulins and that small amounts are often as significant as large ones.

Monoclonal cryoglobulins or myeloma proteins with the property of precipitating in the cold show no unique structural features that can readily explain this phenomenon. Cryoprecipitability may represent the tendency of certain molecules to interact with themselves or to change their conformation at low temperatures. Mixed cryoglobulins generally consist of several immunoglobulins, with the IgM component the most important. It was demonstrated in the 1960s that cryoprecipitability is not intrinsic in either of these components but requires the patient's IgM and the addition of IgG from almost any source. Thus mixed cryoglobulins appear to be antiimmunoglobulins with the IgM fraction behaving as a cold-insoluble RF. Since monoclonality, either in a single component or mixed cryoglobulin, raises the possibility of an underlying B-cell neoplastic condition, these patients should be further evaluated with a bone survey to look for lytic lesions (IgG or IgA), a computed tomography scan or comparable study of the abdomen to assess for retroperitoneal adenopathy and/or hepatosplenomegaly (IgM), and a bone marrow examination as indicated. Identification of low-grade lymphoproliferation in some instances may significantly guide the approach to treatment.

TREATMENT

Since the course of cryoglobulinemia may be quite variable, it is important to tailor therapy to the individual. In an asymptomatic or minimally symptomatic patient, no or only supportive (e.g., analgesic) therapy may be indicated. On the other hand, in the event that the cryoprotein results in severe cold intolerance or vascular insufficiency, plasmapheresis may be necessary to remove it until the disease can be brought under control by using other therapeutic agents. In some instances intravenous gamma globulin has also been used to ameliorate symptoms, particularly in IgG monoclonal cryoglobulinemia.

When underlying myeloma, macroglobulinemia, or other lymphoproliferative disease is identified or strongly suspected, treatment may be directed to these disorders. Management may be with cytotoxic agents such as melphalan, chlorambucil, azathioprine, or cyclophosphamide; in some instances alternative agents such as fludarabine have also been used.

The situation in patients with mixed cryoglobulins is somewhat different. Here again, treatment of the associated disease may be indicated. Recent studies have shown that the majority of patients with the idiopathic form of the disease, evident primarily as purpura and arthralgias, are infected by the hepatitis C virus. In these patients the presence of systemic symptoms such as renal disease, neuropathy, or severe debilitating ulcers often warrants more aggressive therapy. Several recent series have shown significant improvement in both the parameters of hepatitis C virus infection (e.g., liver function tests and viral copy number) and cryoglobulin level and symptoms in some patients who receive treatment with interferon-α. Similar to the general experience with chronic hepatitis C virus infection and hepatitis, however, some patients do not respond or only partially respond to interferon or relapse when the drug is discontinued.

Acknowledgements

This chapter is dedicated to my teacher, Dr. Edward Franklin, who made many seminal contributions to this field. Work was supported by the Arthritis Foundation.

BIBLIOGRAPHY

Brouet JC et al: Biological and clinical significance of cryoglobulins, *Am J Med* 57:775, 1974.

Galli M, Invernizzi F, Monteverde A, Monti G, editors: Hepatitis C virus and cryoglobulinemia, *Clin Exp Rheumatol* 13(suppl S-13):S-1–S-210, 1995.

Gorevic PD: Cryopathies: cryoglobulins and cryofibrinogenemia. In Frank MM, Austen KF, Claman HN, Unanue ER, editors: *Sampter's immunologic diseases,* ed 5, vol 2, Boston, 1995, Little, Brown.

Gorevic PD, Galanakis D, Finn AF, Jr.: In Rose NR, De Marcanio EC, Folds JD et al, editors: *Cryoglobulins: manual of clinical laboratory immunology,* ed 5, Washington, DC, 1997, ASM Press.

Gorevic PD, Frangione B: Mixed cryoglobulinemia cross-reactive idiotypes: implications for the relationship of MC to rheumatic and lymphoproliferative diseases, *Semin Hematol* 28:79, 1991.

Grey HM, Kohler PF: Cryoimmunoglobulins, *Semin Hematol* 10:87, 1973.

Wintrobe MM, Buell MV: Hyperproteinemia associated with multiple myeloma: with report of a case in which an extraordinary hyperproteinemia was associated with thrombosis of the retinal veins and symptoms suggesting Raynaud's disease, *Bull Johns Hopkins Hosp* 52:156, 1933.

CHAPTER

203 Infections of the Joints

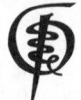

James S. Louie, Adolf W. Karchmer, and Michael H. Weisman

INFECTIOUS AGENT VERSUS HOST

The clinical presentations caused by different infectious agents affecting varied hosts challenge the skills of the clinician who must suspect and pursue the diagnosis, identify the offending microorganism, and initiate specific therapy to prevent the destruction of joint tissue. This continuing battle pits new and more virulent infectious agents with emerging patterns of antibiotic resistance against hosts beset with diseases and drugs that attenuate normal immune defenses. Because outcome depends on the rapidity of diagnosis and specific treatment, the initial efforts to identify the infectious agent by collecting and culturing infected fluids and tissue are critical before empiric antibiotic therapy is initiated. If these efforts are delayed, permanent damage and even death may occur. Antibiotic coverage is then reevaluated and changed when the infection is identified, the *in vitro* sensitivity to antibiotics is characterized, and the clinical response is reviewed. So the clinical paradigm is simple: when infectious arthritis is suspected, aspirate the joint, culture the fluid, initiate antibiotics, and monitor the response.

In infectious arthritis both bacterial products and the response of the host contribute to the joint damage. During acute experimental bacterial arthritis in rabbits the cytokines elaborated by host macrophages—interleukin-1 (IL-1) and tumor necrosis factor (TNF)—degrade cartilage by the induction of stromelysin and other metalloproteinases. When these factors are attenuated by monoclonal antibodies or steroids, cartilage degradation is minimized. In addition, bacterial products such as the staphylococcal toxic shock syndrome toxin 1 (TSST) may function as a superantigen to activate T lymphocytes and perpetuate synovial proliferation and cartilage degradation. Although these animal studies are preliminary, they emphasize the important interaction of bacteria and host in the initiation and perpetuation of infection and damage.

Clinical Features

Septic arthritis is monarticular in more than 80% of cases. Bacterial infections affect the knee, followed by the hip, shoulder, elbow, wrist, and ankle. The onset is abrupt, and pain and fever are common. The infected joint is usually tender, warm, erythematous, and swollen with effusion. Motion is limited by pain. In deeply situated joints such as the hip or sacroiliac joints inflammatory findings are less obvious. With infection of the hip, pain is referred to the anterior thigh or knee and is aggravated by range of motion, particularly internal rotation. With infection of the sacroiliac joint, pain is referred to the buttocks and low back and may be elicited by direct pressure.

Polyarticular septic arthritis is uncommon except in the syndrome

Table 203-1   Synovial fluid in untreated infectious arthritis

ORGANISM	LEUKOCYTE COUNT (CELLS/MM³)	POLYMORPHONUCLEAR LEUKOCYTES (%)	POSITIVE STAINED SMEAR (%)	CULTURE
Pyogenic bacteria	10,000->100,000	>90	65	Fluid
Mycobacteria	10,000-25,000	50-70	20	Tissue
Fungi	3000-25,000	<70	<20	Tissue

of disseminated gonococcal infection (DGI). Patients with DGI come to medical attention with fever, migratory polyarthralgias, tenosynovitis, and a characteristic rash with macules, papules, or pustules on an erythematous base in 20% of cases. Dissemination of gonococcal infection occurs in asymptomatic carriers with the onset of menstrual periods or in the latter half of pregnancy. Those with deficiencies of the late components of complement are prone to develop neisserial infections. In gonococcal infections a monarthritis may become the dominant clinical picture as the infection "settles" into a septic phase. In nongonococcal polyarticular septic arthritis, *Staphylococcus* is the causative organism in 50% to 80% of cases, affecting four joints on average. Patients in whom polyarticular septic arthritis develops include those with breaks in host defenses. In one series, half were patients with rheumatoid arthritis who displayed ulcerated callouses of the feet and were taking steroids and other immune-modulating drugs. The observation that septic arthritis tends to localize in one joint in normal individuals and in multiple joints in persons with attenuated immune defenses supports the role of host defenses in the control of disseminated infections.

The arthritis caused by fungi and mycobacteria has a more insidious onset and indolent course. The inflammatory features of pain, tenderness, warmth, erythema, swelling, and pain with movement are muted. Tenosynovitis and the carpal tunnel syndrome are common.

Etiologic Agents

The unique vulnerabilities of patients to bacterial invasion correlate with specific ages and the increased susceptibility to infection caused by immunosuppressive therapy and underlying diseases. Among children from 1 month to 2 years of age *Haemophilus influenzae* colonizes the upper respiratory tract and is the most frequent cause of septic arthritis, but this organism is a rare cause of arthritis after 5 years of age, and the incidence is likely to decrease with current immunization practices. *Neisseria gonorrhoeae* is the most common cause of acute bacterial arthritis among sexually active young adults, accounting for 65% of cases in this group. In contrast, among older adults gram-positive cocci account for 75% of acute joint infections. *Staphylococcus aureus* causes almost 60% of acute nongonococcal bacterial arthritis and an even larger proportion (80%) of joint infections superimposed on rheumatoid arthritis. In adults aerobic gram-negative bacilli are responsible for 10% to 20% of joint infections, especially in patients with coexisting extraarticular infection or significant underlying diseases. Septic arthritis associated with intravenous narcotic abuse may be caused by unusual organisms in unusual joints. Early studies reported gram-negative bacilli, including *Pseudomonas aeruginosa, Serratia marcescens, and Klebsiella* and *Enterobacter* species, in the sternoclavicular and sternochondral joints. More recently, *S. aureus,* in particular, strains resistant to methicillin, and groups A and G streptococci are described in the sacroiliac joints in these patients.

Chronic infectious arthritis is usually caused by *Mycobacterium tuberculosis;* atypical mycobacteria including *Mycobacterium kansasii* and *M. intracellulare,* and *Candida krusei* or fungi. Although rare causes of arthritis—any of the primary invasive fungi *(Sporothrix schenkii, Coccidioides immitis, and Blastomyces dermatitidis)*—may be responsible for joint infection. *Cryptococcus* and *Candida* species are more likely to be pathogens in immunocompromised hosts.

The indolent arthritis associated with prosthetic joints is usually caused by contamination of the joint at surgery with relatively avirulent organisms such as *Staphylococcus epidermidis,* α-hemolytic streptococci, and diphtheroids. In contrast, late-onset acute hematogenous infection involving prosthetic joints is caused by invasive bacteria including *S. aureus,* pneumococci, β-hemolytic streptococci, and gram-negative bacilli.

Although arthritis has been reported as an atypical feature of infection by viruses of many types, arthritis is an occasional event in mumps, parvovirus, rubella, alpha viruses, and hepatitis B virus (see later discussion, Viral Arthritis).

Laboratory Tests

Prompt diagnosis requires the recovery of synovial fluid or synovial tissue for the specific identification of the infectious agent by culture or other techniques. A *tentative* identification is derived from Gram's stain of bacteria within the cells recovered from the synovial fluid. Organisms should be visible in 60% of cases of nongonococcal bacterial arthritis, particularly if the cells are dispersed by a cytocentrifuge. *Specific* identification of the infectious bacteria traditionally depends on the culture and growth on supportive media. Some bacteria require special media and conditions to facilitate growth. When gonococcal arthritis is suspected, synovial fluid should be cultured on chocolate agar media and transported quickly to the laboratory for incubation in 5% to 7% carbon dioxide. For the identification of *Borrelia burgdorferi,* culture requires Barbour-Stroenner-Kelley media (Sigma B3528, Sigma Chemical Co., St. Louis) and incubation at 33° C. A new molecular technique to identify pathogens that are difficult to culture uses the polymerase chain reaction (PCR) to amplify minute quantities of specific bacterial DNA. Two different primers of oligonucleotides are selected to encompass a bacterial DNA sequence that codes for a characteristic bacterial protein. When these specific primers are added to synovial fluid samples with bacterial DNA together with sufficient nucleotides and a DNA polymerase within a thermocycler, a sequential process changes the temperature to dissociate the double strands of the bacterial DNA (approximately 96° C), anneal the primers to the single strands of bacterial DNA (approximately 56° C), and fill in the intervening nucleotides between the primers (approximately 72° C). This process constructs sufficient copies of the specific bacterial DNA fragments for identification by Southern blot testing. With this technique *N. gonorrhoeae, B. burgdorferi,* and other bacteria have been identified in synovial fluid even when cultures are negative. *M. tuberculosis* and the actinomycete *Trophyrema whippellii,* which produces Whipple's disease, have been identified in synovial tissue. Kits to assist in the PCR identification of elusive organisms are expected to be available in the United States soon.

When the synovial fluid leukocyte count is 50,000 cells/mm³ or more with 90% polymorphonuclear leukocytes, septic arthritis should be the working diagnosis (Table 203-1). Synovial fluid leukocyte counts less than 28,000 cells/mm³ occur in 50% of patients receiving immunosuppressive drugs, including those who are taking steroids, use intravenous recreational drugs, or have malignant neoplasms. Synovial fluid leukocytosis in this range overlaps with other inflammatory rheumatic diseases including rheumatoid arthritis, gout, and calcium pyrophosphate deposition disease (Chapter 183). Chemistry studies of synovial fluid, including glucose, protein, and lactate dehydrogenase testing, do not discriminate effectively between infectious and noninfectious inflammatory arthritis, but low synovial fluid–to-plasma ratios of glucose may be helpful in following the response to therapy. Clinical studies of cytokine profiles have not been validated for diagnostic use in humans.

The synovial fluid from joints with chronic infection caused by mycobacteria or fungi is less inflammatory (see Table 203-1). Synovial fluid leukocyte counts are low, and mononuclear cells predominate. Specifically stained smears of the joint fluid cells may reveal

Table 203-2 Suspected organisms causing septic arthritis based on Gram's stain of synovial fluid and age of the patient

| | SUSPECTED ORGANISMS | | | |
| | GRAM'S STAIN OF SYNOVIAL FLUID | | | |
AGE OF PATIENT	GRAM-POSITIVE COCCI	GRAM-NEGATIVE COCCI	GRAM-NEGATIVE BACILLI	NO ORGANISM SEEN[A]
Neonate	*Staphylococcus aureus*, group B or A streptococcus	*Neisseria gonorrhoeae*	Enterobacteriaceae	*S. aureus*, group B streptococcus, Enterobacteriaceae, *Candida* organism[b]
Child (2 months–5 years)	*S. aureus*, *Streptococcus pneumoniae*, group A streptococcus	*Haemophilus influenzae*[f]	Enterobacteriaceae, *H. influenzae*	*H. influenzae*, *S. aureus*, group A streptococcus, *S. pneumoniae*, Enterobacteriaceae
Child (5–15 years)	*S. aureus*, group A streptococcus, *S. pneumoniae*	*N. gonorrhoeae*,[c] *H. influenzae*	Enterobacteriaceae	*S. aureus*, group A streptococcus, *S. pneumoniae*, Enterobacteriaceae[b]
Adult (16–40 years)	*S. aureus*, group A streptococcus	*N. gonorrhoeae*[c]	Enterobacteriaceae, *Pseudomonas aeruginosa*[d]	*N. gonorrhoeae*,[c] *S. aureus*, group A streptococcus, Enterobacteriaceae,[b] *P. aeruginosa*[b,d]
Adult (>40 years)	*S. aureus*, group A streptococcus, *S. pneumoniae*, *Staphylococcus epidermidis*[e]	*N. gonorrhoeae*[c]	Enterobacteriaceae,[b] *P. aeruginosa*[b]	*S. aureus*, group A streptococcus, Enterobacteriaceae[b]

[a]Decreasing order of likelihood.
[b]Related to serious underlying disease or immunosuppressive conditions or hospital acquired.
[c]Sexual activity; possible exposure to *N. gonorrhoeae*. Will occasionally be *Neisseria meningitidis*.
[d]Related to parenteral drug abuse.
[e]Prosthetic joint.
[f]*H. influenzae* organisms are small rods or appear as coccobacilli; if true cocci, suspect gonococci (in setting of sexual abuse) or meningococci.

M. tuberculosis organisms by Ziehl-Neelsen–stained smears in 20% of cases and lepra organisms from patients with the heavy bacillary load of lepromatous leprosy. Synovial tissue retrieved by arthroscopic biopsy under direct vision increases the yield of mycobacterial and fungal identification by culture and histopathologic examination.

Indirect methods to identify specific infections test for specific antibodies in the host serum or synovial fluid. In Lyme disease enzyme-linked immunosorbent assay (ELISA) characterizes the quantity of antibodies attaching to *Borrelia* proteins coating the plastic microwells. Western blot gel assays then confirm the specificity of the antibodies to different molecular-weight proteins.

Other laboratory tests of systemic inflammation are occasionally helpful but are limited by nonspecificity. Elevations of the C-reactive protein and the Westergren erythrocyte sedimentation rate (ESR) are higher than recorded with idiopathic inflammatory diseases.

Radiographic procedures play a supportive role in the diagnosis of septic arthritis. Radiographs are important to rule out other mimicking or aggravating conditions such as an occult fracture or an adjacent focus of osteomyelitis. Occasionally, distention of the joint capsule and periarticular soft tissue swelling are evident, but narrowing of the joint space and subchondral erosions only reflect the delay in diagnosis and appropriate therapy. In long-standing arthritis destructive osteomyelitic lesions are often seen adjacent to joints infected by *C. immitis* or *B. dermatitidis*. Radionuclide scanning procedures identify foci of increased blood flow or collections of inflammatory cells. Technetium phosphate bone scans become abnormal within days, initially with an occasional "cold" photodeficient area attributable to intramedullary pressure causing restricted blood flow and subsequently a "hot" area of increased vascularity. Scans with gallium, which binds to transferrin, lactoferrin, and other leucocyte receptors, and indium-labeled peripheral white blood cells outline collections of white blood cells in bone, joints, and soft tissues. Computed tomography (CT scan) identifies early bony lesions when conventional radiographs may be difficult to interpret. Magnetic resonance imaging (MRI) affords the early detection of soft tissue changes including loculations of fluid. After administration gadolinium localizes within inflamed tissues and contrasts with the dark bone on T2-weighted images. Each of these procedures may identify inflammation and fluid in the hip, symphysis pubis, and sacroiliac joints when the pain and tenderness is nonlocalizing, but clinical correlation is required to support a diagnosis of infection.

Differential Diagnosis

An infectious cause should be strongly considered for any monarticular arthritis, even in the setting of a preexisting polyarticular disease.

When the presentation is accompanied by fever, an abrupt onset, or a synovial leucocytosis, or a combination of these, culture of the synovial fluid and other possible primary sites of infection and empiric antibiotics should be initiated.

Gout or calcium pyrophosphate dihydrate deposition disease can mimic the clinical and laboratory features of septic arthritis, but these diagnoses are established by identification of sodium urate or calcium pyrophosphate crystals, respectively, in synovial fluid cells examined by first-order, red-compensated microscopy (Chapter 183). Rarely, bacterial infection may coexist with crystal-induced arthritis in the setting of multiple myeloma or other immunologically compromised diseases.

The acute onset of rheumatoid arthritis, seronegative spondyloarthropathies, Reiter's syndrome, and acute rheumatic fever resembles an acute bacterial arthritis. The clinical presentation may highlight nonarticular signs, and the pattern of serologic tests may favor a rheumatic syndrome; occasionally, only the absence of organisms on Gram's stain and culture of the synovial fluid and the course of the illness, despite a wide spectrum of antibiotics, eliminate an infectious cause from consideration. In Reiter's syndrome that becomes evident with urethritis and arthritis, confusion with gonococcal arthritis might prompt antibiotic therapy until new features of the syndrome develop or the arthritis fails to respond to antibiotic treatment. As an alternative, PCR has identified gonococcal arthritis when the synovial fluid cultures did not support growth.

When chronic inflammatory monarthritis persists and rheumatoid arthritis, spondyloarthropathies, sarcoidosis, or Lyme disease is less likely on the basis of the clinical and laboratory test, synovial biopsy under the direct vision of the arthroscopist should yield tissues in which to identify mycobacterial or fungal organisms by appropriate culture and histologic techniques.

Treatment

Effective therapy of an infected joint requires prompt administration of an appropriate antimicrobial agent and adequate drainage of the joint space. Accordingly, antibiotics are selected to cover the pathogens most likely to be present and are initiated before the results of bacteriologic cultures are available. This choice is based on the age of the patient, clinical and epidemiologic information, and Gram's stain of the synovial fluid cells (Table 203-2). After identification of the bacterial pathogen and its pattern of in vitro sensitivity to antibiotics are reported, antibiotic therapy is revised (Table 203-3). With parenteral antibiotic therapy, therapeutic levels in synovial fluid and serum are achieved. Intraarticular injections of antibiotics are unnecessary and may irritate the synovium. With the exception of gono-

Table 203-3 Antibiotic therapy of acute septic arthritis in adults*

ORGANISM	DURATION (DAYS)	DRUG OF CHOICE	ALTERNATIVE DRUG/DOSAGE
Streptococci (nonenterococcal) or pneumococci	14	Penicillin G, 2 million U q4-6h IV	Cefazolin 1 g q8h IV
Enterococci	21-28	Penicillin G, 2 million U q4-6h IV, *plus* gentamicin,‡ 3-5 mg/kg/day IM or IV in q8h doses	Vancomycin, 1 g q12h,* *plus* gentamicin,‡ in doses noted
Staphylococcus aureus	21-28	Nafcillin or oxacillin, 2-3g IV in q6h	Vancomycin or cefazolin† in doses noted above
S. aureus or *Staphylococcus epidermidis* (methicillin-resistant)	21-28	Vancomycin, 1g q12h	—
Pseudomonas aeruginosa	21-28	Gentamicin, 3-5 mg/kg/day IV in q8h doses, *plus* piperacillin, 4-5 g q6h IV	An aminoglycoside‡ *plus* piperacillin, mezlocillin, or ceftazidine in full doses may be used in resistance encountered
Other facultative gram-negative bacilli (susceptibility permitting)	21-28	Gentamicin,‡ 5-6 mg/kg/day IM or IV in q8h doses, *plus* a broad-spectrum penicillin (mezlocillin or piperacillin) or a third-generation cephalosporin (cefotaxime, ceftizoxime, or ceftazidine) in doses for life-threatening infection	Tobramycin,‡ or amikacin,‡ *plus* either a third-generation cephalosporin, piperacillin, or mezlocillin, each in doses for life-threatening infection

*Recommended doses assume normal renal function. Many agents require dose adjustments if renal function is reduced.
†An equivalent cephalosporin antibiotic and doseage may be used.
‡Lean body weight used to calculate doses.
h, Hour; *IM,* intramuscularly; *IV,* intravenous; *q,* every.

coccal arthritis, oral antibiotics are not recommended as initial treatment for acute septic arthritis.

The in vivo efficacy of the antibiotic and drainage regimen is reflected by the clinical regression of systemic and local inflammation within the joint. The patient's chart should record the decrease in fever and joint fluid leucocytosis and volume within days to a week. If inflammation persists, even after adjustment of antibiotics according to the sensitivity profiles, radiologic and orthopedic procedures to rule out persisting infection in bone or loculated tissue are necessary.

Guidelines for empiric therapy in the setting of presumed septic arthritis will change as newer antibiotics and even newer antibiotic resistance patterns emerge. *Gram-positive cocci* suggest *Staphylococcus* or *Streptococcus* species. Since most *S. aureus* produce a beta lactamase, empiric therapy calls for β-lactamase–resistant penicillin with a bulky acyl side chain to prevent hydrolysis of the penicillin by the exoenzyme. Three parenteral antibiotic regimens are recommended; nafcillin or oxacillin four times a day; the less expensive cefazolin three times a day; or the more convenient ceftriaxone once a day. *Gram-negative bacilli* should be treated with a third-generation cephalosporin (ceftriaxone) or a quinolone (ciprofloxacin or levofloxacin). In an immunocompromised host, coverage for *Pseudomonas aeruginosa* includes a third-generation cephalosporin with antipseudomonas activity such as ceftazidime, a quinolone, or an extended-spectrum penicillin (piperacillin or mezlocillin) with an aminoglycoside. *Gram-negative cocci* reflect neisserial infections. Although gonococcal arthritis is usually caused by penicillin-susceptible strains, resistant strains including those that produce beta lactamase are being reported. Thus acute gonococcal arthritis should be treated with ceftriaxone 1 g intramuscularly (IM) or intravenously (IV) daily (or ceftizoxime or cefotaxime 1 g IV every 8 hours) for 7 to 10 days. If the patient has improved after 2 to 3 days of parenteral therapy, treatment may be completed with cefixime 400 mg, ciprofloxacin 500 mg, or ofloxacin 400 mg given orally twice daily. In patients who are highly allergic to penicillins or cephalosporins, spectinomycin 2 g IM twice daily, ciprofloxacin 400 mg IV twice daily, ofloxacin 400 mg IV twice daily, or levofloxacin, 500 mg once daily IV, is recommended. *Chlamydia trachomatis,* which often simultaneously infects the genital tract of patients with gonorrhea, is eradicated by the 7-day ofloxacin regimen; consideration should be given to treating this organism when therapy for gonococcal arthritis is provided (Chapter 265). When *no bacteria are identified on Gram's stain,* a first-generation cephalosporin is recommended unless the history suggests gonococcal or pseudomonal infection.

For patients with a nonimmediate type of penicillin hypersensitivity, cephalosporin antibiotics may be used to treat streptococcal (nonenterococcal), pneumococcal, and staphylococcal arthritis,

whereas in the setting of an immediate type of hypersensitivity, vancomycin should be used for these infections. Furthermore, vancomycin should be used in lieu of penicillin in all penicillin-allergic patients with enterococcal infection. Aminoglycoside and vancomycin dosages must be adjusted for patients with reduced renal function, as should doses of some penicillin and cephalosporin drugs if renal dysfunction is severe. Extraarticular infection, osteomyelitis, or preexisting structural joint disease may warrant more prolonged parenteral therapy in some patients. An alternative to vancomycin in the patient with penicillin allergy is clindamycin, which is particularly useful in beta hemolytic streptococcal infections.

Other important treatment interventions maintain the structural integrity of the infected joint. First, drainage of pyogenic joint infection to reduce intraarticular pressure, remove proteolytic enzymes, and facilitate antibiotic action is *essential* in protecting the articular cartilage. Most cases of pyogenic arthritis require repeated aspiration with a 20-gauge or larger needle at least once or twice daily. Arthrocentesis should continue for as long as effusions reaccumulate. Closed arthrocentesis is sufficient if the synovial fluid volume, white blood cell count, and percentage of polymorphonuclear leukocytes are decreasing and the cultures remain sterile. If synovial fluid analysis or radiologic procedures show persistent inflammation, arthroscopic or open drainage is indicated, particularly if the initial course of antibiotics was delayed beyond 72 hours.

An experimental staphylococcus arthritis in a goat was treated with cefuroxime and at 72 hours no differences were evident in the histochemical-histologic ratings, including the elaboration of IL-1, when the antibiotic coverage was combined with arthroscopy, arthroscopy with debridement, arthrotomy, or closed aspiration. However, open surgical decompression and drainage are recommended for septic processes in the hips in infants and small children, in whom a rapid increase in hip joint pressure can compromise the blood supply and destroy the femoral epiphysis. In addition, arthroscopic or open surgical drainage is preferred when antibiotic effectiveness or conditions for needle aspiration are compromised. These include delays in the diagnosis and treatment longer than 3 days, antibiotic-resistant organisms, and comorbid conditions that overwhelm or restrict host defenses, such as intravenous drug abuse, rheumatoid arthritis, malignancy, or patients taking steroids and immunosuppressive drugs. For example, the sternoclavicular arthritis associated with intravenous drug abuse is frequently associated with an adjacent osteomyelitis or posterior extension into the mediastinum and requires surgical excision for cure.

Infections of prosthetic joints represent a special kind of bacterial infection. If discovered early, particularly if the organism is gram-positive and sensitive to the antibiotic, a course of intravenous anti-

✔ *WHEN TO REFER*

Patients with a delayed diagnosis, particularly in the setting of diseases or drugs that compromise host responses, would benefit from referral to a rheumatologist or infectious disease specialist to assist in the recovery and processing of synovial fluid or synovial tissue for identification of the infectious organism, and for recommended antibiotic and closed-drainage therapies. Any delay in the response to initial therapies requires an orthopedic surgeon to facilitate open-drainage procedures. Pyogenic hip disease in a child is an absolute indication for orthopedic surgical intervention.

biotics may suffice. If the infection continues, despite antibiotics, the prosthesis has to be removed and the site sterilized with antibiotics for months before attempting a second prosthetic replacement. Various orthopedic innovations include custom-made implants to compensate for the deficient bone stock, antibiotic soaks for the implants, and antibiotic beads for the surgical site. Reports of eradication of infection in 95% and good to excellent clinical results in 65% of patients in a 4-year follow-up study, maintain some optimism, but occasionally in the fragile host the infected prosthesis is retained and infection is suppressed with continuous antibiotics.

Other important physical measures to rehabilitate the joint include immobilization of the painful joint until inflammation begins to subside. Passive range-of-motion exercises should be initiated as soon as possible, even as the inflammation is resolving, and active exercises begun as tolerated, to forestall venous thrombosis and emboli and contractures. Weight bearing is prohibited until all signs of active inflammation have cleared.

LYME DISEASE

First described in the area of Lyme, Connecticut, this tickborne illness caused by the spirochete *Borrelia burgdorferi* produces a multisystem disease of the skin, heart, nervous system, and joints (Chapter 274). Residence of the spirochete in different tick vectors may explain the different clinical presentations throughout the world. In the United States up to 60% of the *Ixodes dammini* nymphal and adult ticks may be infected with the spirochete, resulting in endemic Lyme disease in the Northeast and Midwest. The *Ixodes pacificus* ticks in the West infect lizards as an end vector, in addition to mammals, and are infected in less than 5%. In Europe, *Borrelia* organisms reside in the *Ixodes ricinus* and display a different spectrum of cell wall antigens, and infection becomes evident with more chronic skin manifestations and less arthritis.

Early clinical manifestations include a characteristic rash, erythema migrans (EM), which is noted in 75% of patients. Only 30% recall a tick bite at the site of the EM lesion within the previous month. The EM lesion begins as a red macule that expands with central clearing and develops into a large ring with a painless, warm, intense red border which contains the *Borrelia* organism. As the *Borrelia* organism disseminates from the skin, malaise, fatigue, headaches, fever, regional lymphadenopathy, and migratory musculoskeletal pain occur. Joint symptoms are usually limited to a few large joints in more than 50% of patients with untreated infection. The natural course of the arthritis is highly variable; the knee and other joints may be inflamed for weeks or months; then inflammation subsides. Recurrences are common but are unpredictable in frequency or duration. Joints are commonly more swollen than painful. Fatigue is often associated with arthritis, but fever and other systemic symptoms are rare. Synovial fluid contains from 500 to 75,000 cells/mm^3 with 80% polymorphonuclear leukocytes. In 10% of patients, particularly those with the human leukocyte antigen (HLA)-DR haplotypes DR2 or DR4, chronic arthritis with destruction of cartilage develops in large joints.

Although the relative roles of direct infection and of the immune reaction induced by the infecting spirochete in the pathogenesis of Lyme disease have not been clarified, most patients can be given effective treatment with antibiotics. Early treatment with doxycycline or amoxicillin reduces EM and associated symptoms and often prevents development of major late complications, including myocarditis, meningoencephalitis, and recurrent arthritis. Erythromycin is less effective. The treatment of choice for adults with early disease (EM or mild carditis) is doxycycline 100 mg orally twice daily or amoxicillin 500 mg orally three times daily for 10 to 21 days. In patients with neurologic manifestations, severe carditis, or arthritis, ceftriaxone 2 g IV or IM daily for 14 days is recommended. Although recovery proceeds slowly, 90% of patients with recurrent arthritis or neurologic symptoms respond to ceftriaxone. Doxycycline 100 mg twice daily or a combination of amoxicillin and probenecid, each 500 mg four times daily, has been used orally for 30 days to treat arthritis with response rates of 60% to 70%. Among patients with arthritis for whom these oral regimens fail, ceftriaxone cures 35% to 40%. Neither systemic nor intraarticular corticosteroids should be given because they may impair the response to antibiotics. Doxycycline should not be administered to women who are pregnant.

MYCOBACTERIAL AND FUNGAL ARTHRITIS

Tuberculosis and fungal infections are still commonly encountered, particularly in this era of acquired immunodeficiency syndrome (AIDS) and frequent use of steroids and immunosuppressive drugs. The articular features of these infections may dominate the clinical picture or be the presenting manifestation. Clinical suspicions are enhanced with any chronic monarticular arthritis, chronic tenosynovitis about the hands or wrists, or erythema nodosum skin lesions in individuals with significant immunodepressed states, even in the absence of other constitutional manifestations. Diagnosis requires the identification of the infected organism from synovial fluid or synovial tissue, although serologic and radiologic tests may be helpful.

Tuberculosis

The increase of pulmonary tuberculosis in the United States engendered by new immigration and immunocompromised diseases should increase the recognition of bone and joint disease that occurs in 5% of those infected with *M. tuberculosis*. The most common sites are the spine (called Pott's disease), hip, knee, ankle, and tendons of the hand and wrist. Sometimes a synovial mass occurs without osseous disease being evident on x-ray.

Although pulmonary findings may be absent in half of the cases, the result of the tuberculin skin test (purified protein derivative–standard [PPD-S]) is usually positive unless overwhelming disease or poor nutrition has induced an anergic state. The synovial fluid is variably inflammatory, and Ziehl-Neelsen stains identify organisms in only 20% of cases. Cultures of synovial fluid and, more reliably, synovial tissue are the standard for diagnosis but require 6 weeks of incubation for growth. As PCR tests become available, identification of various mycobacterial species should be available within a few days. Antituberculous chemotherapy is the cornerstone of management, and a combination of agents is recommended (Chapter 273).

Coccidioidomycosis

Coccidioidomycosis (see Chapter 276) occurs in the southwestern United States and Mexico and in similar climates in South America. Following inhalation of spores the benign, self-limited primary infection is characterized by fever, cough, and erythema nodosum with or without polyarthritis. The disease disseminates in 0.2% of cases, particularly in African Americans, Filipinos, and persons with AIDS. Bone infections occur in multiple sites, especially over bony prominences. Arthritis is usually monarticular, affecting the knee and the ankle. In 40% to 80% of reported cases bone or joint localization may be the *only* sign of disseminated disease. The diagnosis is made by identification of the organism in either synovial fluid or synovial tissues; the complement-fixation titer to *C. immitis* is usually positive in all forms of disseminated disease, including arthritis. Systemic administration of amphotericin B produces cure rates of 50% to 70%, but relapses are frequent. Amphotericin B is administered 0.6 mg/kg per day IV for a total of 1 to 2 g. The azoles, itraconazole and fluconazole, 400 mg per day by mouth, may become the drugs of choice.

Improved outcome for the patient with arthritis occurs when amphotericin or azoles are combined with synovectomy.

Other Fungal Infections

Blastomycosis (Chapter 276) is endemic in the Ohio and Mississippi river basins, the Middle Atlantic states, and the Southeast and may occur as a primary joint infection via hematogenous spread. The disease usually becomes evident as a monarticular arthritis of the lower extremities, often resembling an acutely septic joint. The diagnosis is made when the organism is grown from infected tissues. Because loculations are common, open drainage is often necessary. Treatment includes amphotericin B or itraconazole. Sporotrichosis occurs worldwide and is an occupational cutaneous and lymphatic infectious problem for people whose hands are commonly in soil. Systemic disseminated infection occurs in healthy hosts without prior skin or lung disease and may become evident as a unifocal infection of a bone or joint. In debilitated individuals the disease is more extensive and may be seen in multiple sites. Candidal septic arthritis virtually always occurs in a compromised host (e.g., transplantation patients, diabetics, immunosuppressed persons), frequently in the setting of widespread disseminated candidiasis that is obvious on clinical examination. Therapy is very difficult; amphotericin B and fluconazole may be useful, although the duration of therapy is not clear. Synovectomy is a useful adjunct.

Patients with AIDS are at risk for disseminated fungal and mycobacterial infection; these infections may involve joints and should be considered in the differential diagnosis of an AIDS patient with articular signs or symptoms. Therapy for tuberculosis follows standard guidelines, but atypical mycobacterial infection requires complex multidrug regimens (Chapter 273). Cryptococci may cause arthritis in patients with AIDS. In these patients cryptococcal capsular antigen is detectable in the synovial fluid and serum; infection may involve the meninges as well. Treatment similar to that given for cryptococcal meningitis should be considered, and lifelong suppressive therapy is warranted.

VIRAL ARTHRITIS

Acute, self-limited episodes of joint inflammation in small and large joints are observed in association with typical viral illnesses, including vaccinia, adenovirus, varicella, Epstein-Barr virus (infectious mononucleosis), herpes simplex, rubeola, influenza, echovirus, and lymphocytic choriomeningitis. During infection with other viruses arthritis may be a common aspect of the clinical illness: smallpox, mumps, alpha virus (chikungunya or O'nyong-nyong virus), rubella, parvovirus, and hepatitis B. An analysis of arthritis associated with viral illness has shown a heterogenous pattern of joint and periarticular inflammation, ranging from a symmetric polyarthritis of large and small joints to an oligoarthritis principally of the lower extremities. The inflammatory response in the synovium is also variable; cell counts ranging from 100 to 30,000 cells/mm^3 have been reported, with either polymorphonuclear leukocytes or mononuclear cells predominating. Different patterns may even be noted within patient groups infected by a single virus. There is evidence to suggest that immune-complex–mediated mechanisms account for hepatitis B–associated arthritis; comparable studies have not been performed in hepatitis C and other viral infections. Typically all of the virus-induced arthritides are of short duration and entirely reversible; however, some may be recurrent or persistent, and this leads to speculation that undiscovered viral infections may have an important role in the etiopathogenesis of chronic rheumatic diseases.

Hepatitis B virus infection gives rise to the most frequently diagnosed virus-associated arthritis (Chapter 355); besides being involved in a transient arthritis syndrome (see later discussion), this virus has been implicated in three other, more persistent systemic illnesses—a polyarteritis nodosa (PAN)-like necrotizing vasculitis, mixed cryoglobulinemia, and chronic glomerulonephritis. The arthritis begins abruptly, persists for 1 or 2 weeks, then disappears with the development of jaundice. Joint involvement is typically a symmetric polyarthritis of large and small joints, especially the metacarpophalangeal and interphalangeal joints. The hands often appear to have prominent periarticular swelling. Preceding the arthritis, 50% of the patients have a rash that is usually urticarial but may be macular or even frankly vasculitic (palpable purpura). Hepatitis B surface antigen and circulating immune complexes containing complement are detectable during the articular phase; as the arthritis resolves, the immune complexes containing complement disappear. Synovial fluid white blood cell counts are highly variable but usually show mild inflammation. Although the patients appear acutely ill and are febrile, the Westergren ESR is usually normal. The arthritis appears to be entirely self-limited.

Both the natural rubella infection and rubella vaccination may be associated with arthritis in a large number of individuals (estimated from 10% to 60%) (Chapter 251). Typically there is a sudden onset of a symmetric polyarthritis of large and small joints, which lasts less than 2 weeks. Postpubertal women appear more susceptible than men or children, perhaps because of the differential antibody responses. Vaccine-induced rubella arthritis is similar to the natural disease, but in some patients the arthritis is oligoarticular, confined to the knees. In addition, the vaccinated patients may have recurrent disease in the same joint for up to 3 years, especially those with knee involvement.

Arthralgias, polyarticular and migratory arthritis, and monarticular arthritis associated with mumps occur primarily in men. Large joints are involved most commonly. Symptoms may precede parotitis but usually occur 1 to 3 weeks after the onset of parotitis or systemic viral symptoms. Joint complaints resolve completely in several months and can be controlled by treatment with a nonsteroidal antiinflammatory agent. Visceral complications are seen with increased frequency in patients with mumps arthritis.

Parvovirus B19 has been associated with aplastic crisis of hemolytic anemias, erythema infectiosum (fifth disease) in school-age children, and arthritis-arthralgia in adults. Typically polyarthritis occurs abruptly in association with flulike symptoms. Women are affected more often than men. In the majority of cases the arthritis clears in 1 to 2 weeks; in a small number of cases it may persist for up to 2 years or recur later. The diagnosis is confirmed by demonstrating an immunoglobulin M antibody response to the B19 strain or by PCR.

In addition to causing AIDS, infection with the human immunodeficiency virus (HIV) has been associated with arthritis. Many HIV-infected patients come to medical attention with prominent skin changes and severe reactive arthritis that is not associated with HLA-B27 and is unresponsive to nonsteroidal antiinflammatory drugs. The synovial fluid contains 50 to 2600 white blood cells/mm^3, predominantly lymphocytes, and synovial biopsy specimens reveal mild chronic synovitis with mononuclear cell infiltration. Symptoms may abate with intraarticular corticosteroid treatment.

BIBLIOGRAPHY

Bayer AS et al: Gram-negative bacillary septic arthritis: clinical, radiographic, therapeutic, and prognostic features, *Semin Arthritis Rheum* 7:123, 1977.

Berney S, Goldstein M, Bishko F: Clinical and diagnostic features of tuberculous arthritis, *Am J Med* 53:3, 1972.

Chandrasekar PH, Narula AP: Bone and joint infections in intravenous drug abusers, *Rev Infect Dis* 8:904, 1986.

Dubost JJ et al: Polyarticular septic arthritis, *Medicine* 72:296, 1993.

Espinoza LR et al: Rheumatic manifestations associated with human immunodeficiency virus infection, *Arthritis Rheum* 32:1615, 1989.

Esterhai JL Jr, Gelb I: Adult septic arthritis, *Orthop Clin North Am* 22:503, 1991.

Fung MF, Louie JS: Infectious agent arthritis. In Weisman MH, Weinblatt ME: *Treatment of the rheumatic diseases*, Philadelphia, 1995, WB Saunders.

Gardner GC, Weisman MH: Pyarthrosis in patients with rheumatoid arthritis: a report of 13 cases and a review of the literature from the past 40 years, *Am J Med* 88:503, 1990.

Hansen BL, Anderson K: Fungal arthritis, *Scand J Rheumatol* 24:248, 1995.

Inman RD et al: Clinical and microbial features of prosthetic joint infection, *Am J Med* 77:47, 1984.

Jafari HS et al: Dexamethasone attenuation of cytokine-mediated articular cartilage degradation in experimental lapine *Haemophilus* arthritis, *J Infect Dis* 168:1186-1193, 1993.

Liebling MR et al: Nested polymerase chain reaction for the detection of *Borrelia burgdorferi* (Bb) in human body fluids, *Arthritis Rheum* 35:S183, 1992.

Liebling MR et al: Identification of *Neisseria gonorrhoeae* in synovial fluid using the polymerase chain reaction, *Arthritis Rheum* 37:702, 1994.

Masi AJ, Eisenstein BI: Disseminated gonococcal infection (DGI) and gonococcal arthri-

Acknowledgement:
I am grateful for the discussion and review by Dr. Milton Louie.

tis (GCA). II. Clinical manifestations, diagnosis, complications, treatment, and prevention, *Semin Arthritis Rheum* 10:173, 1981.

Nord KD et al: Evaluation of treatment modalities for septic arthritis with histological grading and analysis of uronic acid, neutral proteases, and interleukin 1, *J Bone Joint Surg* 77A:258-265, 1995.

Rynes RI et al: Acquired immunodeficiency syndrome–associated arthritis, *Am J Med* 84:810, 1988.

Shaw BA, Kasser JR: Acute septic arthritis in infancy and childhood, *Clin Orthop Relat Res* 257:212, 1990.

Small PM, Schecter GF, Goodman PC et al: Treatment of tuberculosis in patients with advanced human immunodeficiency virus infections, *N Engl J Med* 324:289, 1991.

Sutker WL, Lankford LL, Tompsett R: Granulomatous synovitis: the role of atypical mycobacteria, *Rev Infect Dis* 1:729, 1979.

Vincent GM, Amirault JD: Septic arthritis in the elderly, *Clin Orthoped* 251:241, 1990.

CHAPTER

204 **Rheumatic Fever**

Angelo Taranta

ETIOLOGY AND INCIDENCE

Rheumatic fever is an inflammatory syndrome that sometimes follows group A streptococcal infections of the throat (Chapter 261). Like the infections that lead to it, rheumatic fever affects mostly children 5 to 15 years of age but is seen also in young adults. Its incidence had been declining steadily in affluent countries, but recently a number of outbreaks have been recorded.

Sore throats have long been known to precede attacks of rheumatic fever. In modern times such "rheumatogenic" sore throats have been shown to be streptococcal, and rheumatic fever attacks not preceded by a sore throat have been shown to follow asymptomatic streptococcal infections by serologic techniques. Moreover, if streptococcal pharyngitis is treated so that streptococci are eradicated from the throat, rheumatic fever does not follow; if patients with previous attacks of rheumatic fever receive continual antibiotic prophylaxis, recurrences do not occur. In either case, the few failures of preventing rheumatic fever can be traced to failures to eradicate the streptococci from the throat or to prevent reinfection, respectively. These observations clinched the case for the streptococcal origin of rheumatic fever.

Although all attacks of rheumatic fever follow a streptococcal infection, only a few streptococcal infections are followed by rheumatic fever. Some streptococcal strains are more likely than others to cause rheumatic fever ("rheumatogenic streptococci"). Host factors may also be important, since the concordance rate for rheumatic fever is seven times higher in monozygotic twin pairs (18.7%) than in dizygotic twin pairs (2.5%).

PATHOPHYSIOLOGY

Although streptococci remain localized to the site of infection, their products diffuse out. Antibodies against these products (and T cells specifically sensitized to them) are demonstrable in the serum and in the skin (by tuberculin-type testing) or by in vitro lymphocyte responses. Several streptococcal antigens cross-react immunologically with mammalian tissue antigens, including several in the human heart. A circulating antibody response or a state of delayed hypersensitivity elicited by streptococcal membrane antigens may mediate tissue damage in rheumatic carditis.

PATHOLOGIC FEATURES

In patients dying of acute rheumatic fever a pancarditis is usually present, with exudative pericarditis, cardiac dilation, and verrucous lesions on heart valves. Fibrin and serosanguineous fluid may be present in the pericardium. With healing, fibrosis and adhesions develop, but constrictive pericarditis is rare.

A diffuse myocardial interstitial infiltrate, predominantly lympho-

cytic, is usually present, in addition to Aschoff bodies. Myocytolysis and complete loss of fibers occur in some areas.

Endocarditis resulting from acute rheumatic fever consists of verrucous lesions at the base and edges of one or more cardiac valves. Initially, there is a mass of eosinophilic material staining as fibrin. With progression, granulation tissue develops, and vascularization and progressive fibrosis occur. Pathologic changes involve the annulus as well as the valve cusps, and the chordae tendineae often are shortened as a result of scarring and thickening (see Chapter 25).

CLINICAL FINDINGS

The natural history of rheumatic fever begins with the streptococcal infection that precedes it. The infection need not be symptomatic but must be localized in the throat and must evoke an antibody response. After a 2- to 3-week latent period, the patient develops one or more of the "major" clinical manifestations of rheumatic fever described below.

Arthritis

The most common manifestation, arthritis, is benign, although acutely painful. Usually several joints are affected, those of the legs more than the arms, and the knees most of all. The joints of the axial skeleton and the temporomandibular joints are almost always spared, and the small joints of the hands and feet are usually not involved, especially by themselves alone. Each joint is affected for a week or so, but the process shifts from joint to joint with some overlap in time, one joint improving as another becomes inflamed. Thus the total duration of the arthritis may be 2 to 6 weeks if no treatment is given.

In any individual joint the arthritis reaches its acme quickly, usually within a day or two. There is tenderness, often exquisite, swelling, local warmth, and redness, accompanied by inability to move, but often not much effusion; the pain is sometimes more than one would expect from the physical findings. Characteristically, the arthritis of rheumatic fever heals completely even without treatment. Arthritis tends to be more common, more severe, less migratory, and longer lasting in adults than in children, but it still remains within the boundaries just described.

Carditis

Rheumatic carditis is the most important manifestation of acute rheumatic fever, and when severe, death may result from acute heart failure. More commonly, rheumatic carditis causes few or no symptoms and is diagnosed in the course of the examination of a patient who comes to medical attention because of arthritis or, less commonly, chorea. Patients with asymptomatic rheumatic carditis may later demonstrate rheumatic heart disease, despite the absence of a history of a recognized rheumatic attack.

Patients with acute rheumatic fever may have endocarditis, myocarditis, and pericarditis, often in combination. Important criteria for the diagnosis of carditis include organic heart murmur(s) not previously present, enlargement of the heart, congestive heart failure, and pericardial friction rubs or signs of effusion.

Organic murmurs are almost invariably present in patients with acute rheumatic carditis. The mitral valve is most commonly involved; a high-pitched, usually loud, apical systolic murmur is a common finding and indicates acute mitral regurgitation (Chapter 25). Valvulitis may be manifested by cusp thickening or verrucae, and depending on its extent, the murmur of mitral regurgitation may persist after the acute rheumatic attack or disappear. A middiastolic murmur, usually following a third heart sound, is commonly heard in patients with rheumatic fever and acute mitral regurgitation.

The second most common valvular lesion during acute rheumatic fever is aortic regurgitation. This lesion produces a soft, high-pitched decrescendo diastolic murmur that begins immediately after the second heart sound.

Congestive heart failure is the least common but most serious manifestation of rheumatic carditis. It usually develops in patients with combined severe valvular and myocardial inflammation. Congestive heart failure occurs in 5% to 10% of patients with first attacks of rheumatic carditis and is more common during recurrences.

Pericarditis occurs in up to 10% of patients with rheumatic fever, but always together with valvular involvement. Cardiac tamponade is rare.

Delayed atrioventricular (AV) conduction is a common finding during acute rheumatic fever, but it does not necessarily indicate clinical carditis. Various arrhythmias may occur, but atrial fibrillation is rare (in contrast to its frequency in patients with chronic mitral valve disease). In addition, the electrocardiogram (ECG) may show non-specific ST-T segment changes consistent with myocarditis, diffuse ST segment elevation or T-wave inversions caused by pericardial disease, or evidence of acute left atrial pressure elevation.

The chest radiograph is frequently normal but may indicate cardiac dilation and/or pulmonary venous hypertension. An echocardiogram is useful in patients with acute rheumatic fever for detecting the presence of pericardial effusion, chamber dilation, or valve abnormalities.

Chorea

Chorea is manifested by involuntary, abrupt, nonrepetitive limb movements and characteristic grimaces. The children so affected may cry or laugh inappropriately and may be extremely weak. Speech is often halting, jerky, or slurred. All of these symptoms disappear, without residua, in a few weeks or months.

Other Major Manifestations

Subcutaneous nodules are painless, roundish, firm lumps overlaid by normal skin. They range from a few millimeters to 1.5 cm in diameter, localize over bones and near joints, and rarely last longer than a month.

Erythema marginatum is a painless, evanescent, nonitching, macular, pink skin rash with the shape of smoke rings, but often festooned or circinate. It is limited to the skin of the trunk and proximal parts of the limbs, lasts for hours or days, and recurs.

Arthritis, carditis, and chorea may occur singly or in combination, but subcutaneous nodules and erythema marginatum are rarely, if ever, seen without carditis. Chorea typically occurs months, rather than weeks, after the provocative streptococcal infection.

In addition to these major clinical manifestations, patients with rheumatic fever have fever, malaise, and fatigue (especially when carditis and heart failure are present). The fever is usually moderate and without wide swings.

The long-term outlook depends on the presence and severity of carditis. Patients with no carditis during the acute attack have an excellent prognosis; those with carditis may lose all evidence of heart disease or may develop chronic, sometimes progressive, rheumatic heart disease. Whether the disease follows one course or the other depends primarily on the severity of the original carditis and on the effect of recurrences, if any.

LABORATORY FINDINGS

Antibody levels against one or more streptococcal extracellular products, such as streptolysin O, are regularly increased. Antistreptolysin O (ASO) is elevated in approximately 80% of cases; ASO levels of at least 250 units in adults and 333 units in children over 5 years of age are considered evidence of a recent streptococcal infection. In the remaining 20%, in whom ASO is low, elevations of levels of antihyaluronidase, antistreptokinase, or anti-DNase B are found almost invariably.

The erythrocyte sedimentation rate (ESR) is markedly elevated, the C-reactive protein (CRP) test result is positive, and the white blood cell count is moderately increased. None of these changes, of course, is specific for rheumatic fever.

DIAGNOSIS

Unlike pneumococcal pneumonia, which invariably affects the lungs, rheumatic fever has no obligate target organ. No single manifestation is diagnostic, but the greater the number of manifestations, the firmer the diagnosis. The most common presentation (also the least specific) is arthritis without carditis.

T. Duckett Jones proposed this empirical guide: the diagnosis is likely in the presence of two major manifestations or of one major and two minor manifestations (the minor being less specific than the major). Evidence of a preceding streptococcal infection was given a special status in the current revision (Box 204-1). In clinically questionable cases, exclusion of a previous streptococcal infection by repeated multiple streptococcal antibody determinations is helpful in ruling out rheumatic fever.

As noted earlier, not all streptococcal infections elicit an ASO response (only about 80% do); but all, by definition, elicit an antibody response to one or another streptococcal product.

TREATMENT

Aspirin is very effective in suppressing the arthritis of rheumatic fever, and a prompt response of the arthritis to aspirin strengthens the diagnosis. More vigorous antiinflammatory treatment, as with prednisone, is useful in controlling pericarditis and the congestive failure of acute carditis, but this treatment has no effect on the incidence of residual heart disease. Aspirin is administered to children in a dose of 80 mg/kg per day for the first 2 weeks, and 60 mg/kg per day for the following 6 weeks.

In patients with cardiomegaly, aspirin often is insufficient to control fever, discomfort, and tachycardia or does so only at toxic or near-toxic doses. These patients may then be treated with corticosteroids, as should all patients with definite evidence of heart failure. Prednisone may be started at a dose of 40 to 60 mg per day, to be increased if control of heart failure is not obtained. In extremely acute and severe cases, therapy may begin with intravenous administration of methylprednisolone (10 to 40 mg), followed by oral prednisone. After 2 or 3 weeks, prednisone should be slowly withdrawn, the daily dose being decreased at the rate of 5 mg every 2 to 3 days. When tapering is started, aspirin should be added at standard dose and continued for 3 or 4 weeks after prednisone is stopped. This "overlap" therapy reduces the incidence of posttherapeutic rebounds.

Patients who have had a definite attack of rheumatic fever should

---

BOX 204-1
Jones criteria (revised)* for guidance in the diagnosis of rheumatic fever

Major manifestations
Carditis
Polyarthritis
Chorea
Erythema marginatum
Subcutaneous nodules

Minor manifestations
Clinical
   Fever
   Arthralgia
   Previous rheumatic fever or rheumatic heart disease
Laboratory
   Markedly elevated erythrocyte sedimentation rate
   Positive C-reactive protein test
   Leukocytosis
   Prolonged PR interval

Plus
Supporting evidence of preceding streptococcal infection (increased antistreptolysin O [ASO] or other streptococcal antibodies; positive throat culture for group A streptococcus; recent scarlet fever)

---

*Courtesy of the American Heart Association.
NOTE: The presence of two major criteria, or of one major and two minor criteria, indicates a high probability of the presence of rheumatic fever if supported by evidence of a preceding streptococcal infection. The absence of the latter should make the diagnosis suspect, except in situations in which rheumatic fever is first discovered after a long latent period from the antecedent infection (e.g., Sydenham's chorea or low-grade carditis).

be protected from recurrences by the continual administration of antistreptococcal medication. Best results are obtained with the injection of 1.2 million units of benzathine penicillin G every 4 weeks. In developing countries where streptococcal exposure may be intense, an injection every 3 weeks is favored.

In patients intolerant of benzathine penicillin prophylaxis because of pain at the site of injection, continual oral medication is prescribed. Sulfadiazine (0.5 g once daily in children weighing less than 30 kg, 1 g in others) and oral penicillin (200,000 to 250,000 units twice a day) are about equally effective. Patients taking sulfadiazine should have a blood cell count after 2 weeks and also whenever they develop a rash in association with fever or sore throat. The drug should be stopped if the white blood cell count falls below 4000 cells/mm^3 or the neutrophils below 35%. For the exceptional patient sensitive to both penicillin and sulfa, erythromycin may be prescribed (100 to 250 mg twice daily).

The risk of recurrence is greatest during the first 3 to 5 years after an attack, and every effort should be made to maintain prophylaxis during this critical period. For patients with no evidence of cardiac involvement, prophylaxis is recommended until 20 years of age or at least for a minimum of 5 years. In patients with rheumatic heart disease, medication should be continued well into adult life, past the years when school-age children are in the home.

An attempt should be made to prevent first attacks of rheumatic fever by accurately diagnosing and effectively treating streptococcal infections. The most effective treatment is benzathine penicillin by injection (0.6 million units in children weighing less than 30 kg, and 1.2 million units in others). Penicillin by mouth (200 to 250,000 units three or four times a day for 10 days) is also effective, but compliance may be a problem.

BIBLIOGRAPHY

Bisno AL: Group A streptococcal infections and acute rheumatic fever, *N Engl J Med* 325:783, 1991.
Markowitz M, Kaplan EL: Reappearance of rheumatic fever, *Adv Pediatr* 36:39-65, 1989.
Stollerman GH: Rheumatic fever and streptococcal infection, New York, 1975, Grune & Stratton.
Taranta A, Markowitz M: *Rheumatic fever,* ed 2, Dordrecht, Boston, London, 1989, Kluwer Academic.
Taranta A: Rheumatic fever. In McCarty DJ, Koopman WJ, editors: *Arthritis,* ed 12, Philadelphia, 1993, Lea & Febiger.

CHAPTER

205 Antirheumatic Drugs

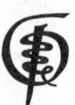

Joseph M. Cash

Rheumatic diseases are tremendously diverse, varying from regional myofascial pain syndromes (e.g., shoulder bursitis) and noninflammatory disorders (e.g., osteoarthritis) to immune-mediated diseases (rheumatoid arthritis, systemic lupus erythematosus, and others). As a consequence, antirheumatic drug approaches may be fundamentally analgesic (acetaminophen), antiinflammatory (nonsteroidal antiinflammatory drugs [NSAIDs] or glucocorticoids), or immunomodulatory (methotrexate or cyclophosphamide).

NONSTEROIDAL ANTIINFLAMMATORY DRUGS

Aspirin, nonacetylated salicylates, and NSAIDs reduce inflammation and pain and are thus useful in both inflammatory arthritis and noninflammatory pain syndromes.

Clinical Pharmacology

Aspirin and nonacetylated salicylates are rapidly absorbed from the upper gastrointestinal tract. Aspirin is metabolized by the liver to me-

tabolites, which are in turn excreted by the kidney. The half-life of aspirin may be as short as 15 minutes in low doses but as high as 12 hours at high doses, given the limited capacity of the liver to form metabolites. However, aspirin metabolism may accelerate with daily therapy, with steady states finally being reached in about 1 month. When giving treatment with antiinflammatory doses of aspirin, physicians should aim for a therapeutic level of 20 to 30 mg/dl.

NSAIDs are a diverse drug class: some members are active in ingested form and others are pro-drugs that require hepatic bioconversion to active metabolites. NSAID half-lives differ greatly, which may account for differences in therapeutic and toxic effects. Most NSAIDs are rapidly absorbed from the upper gastrointestinal tract and metabolized in the liver with subsequent renal elimination of metabolites. An effect of aging on the pharmacokinetics of NSAIDs has not been consistently demonstrated.

Mechanism of Action

NSAIDs and aspirin inhibit cyclooxygenase, leading to decreased enzymatic conversion of arachadonic acid to proinflammatory prostaglandins and thromboxanes. Cyclooxygenase has at least two forms—COX 1 and COX 2—and differential selectivity of NSAIDs for these isoenzymes may partially explain differences in efficacy and toxicity. However, the observation that nonacetylated salicylates produce similar analgesic and therapeutic effects without significant cyclooxygenase inhibition suggests that additional mechanisms of action may be important. These include inhibition of bradykinin release, effects on leukocyte function, and effects on vascular endothelial cell function. NSAIDs have myriad other effects, including analgesic effects, antipyretic effects, and antiplatelet effects, which are clearly important in certain clinical situations.

Efficacy

Aspirin, nonacetylated salicylates, and NSAIDs have all been shown in controlled studies to improve the symptoms of osteoarthritis and rheumatoid arthritis. In addition, several NSAIDs have demonstrated efficacy in acute gouty arthritis. In general, NSAIDs neither completely abolish pain nor completely abolish inflammation in patients with significant disease. Head-to-head studies have not demonstrated consistent efficacy advantages of any one NSAID over another. Moreover, modern nonsalicylate NSAIDs have never been demonstrated to be superior to aspirin alone. Therefore the choice of NSAID should be individualized and based on relative cost, convenience, and toxicity (Table 205-1).

TOXICITY OF NONSTEROIDAL ANTIINFLAMMATORY DRUGS
Gastrointestinal Tract

Gastrointestinal tract toxicity is a major concern with all NSAIDs except the nonacetylated salicylates. Dyspepsia is a common occurrence during NSAID therapy and does not necessarily indicate the presence of gastric erosions or ulcerations. NSAIDs produce a variety of gastrointestinal tract lesions, including erosions, ulcerations, and perforation. Gastrointestinal tract ulcerations may be asymptomatic (possibly as a result of the analgesic effect of NSAIDs) and may bleed profusely (as a result of antiplatelet effects). NSAID-associated ulcerations are usually found in the stomach, whereas idiopathic peptic ulcers typically occur in the duodenum. Risk factors for NSAID-associated gastric ulcer include preexisting peptic ulcer disease, old age, and multiple medical problems. In up to 4% of patients taking full-strength NSAIDs a symptomatic ulcer develops yearly. NSAIDs may produce ulcers either by direct gastric mucosal injury or via effects of circulating active drugs or active metabolites. Therefore the administration of parenteral preparations, rectal suppositories, or enteric-coated tablets may not completely protect patients from gastric ulceration. Cyclooxygenase inhibition (especially, COX 1) reduces the production of certain products (prostaglandins E_1, E_2 and I_2) that protect the gastric mucosa by maintaining mucosal blood flow and mucous production, as well as decreasing free-acid production. Nonacetylated salicylates that do not significantly inhibit cyclooxy-

Table 205-1   Commonly prescribed nonsteroidal antiinflammatory drugs

GENERIC	HALF-LIFE (HOURS)	DOSING INTERVAL*	COST*	GASTROINTESTINAL TRACT TOXICITY	COMMENTS
Salicylates					
Enteric-coated aspirin	4-15	6	$	+	Best-tolerated aspirin preparation
Choline + magnesium salicylate	4-15	8-12	$$$$	+	Tinnitus, large tablet size
Salsalate	4-15	8	$$	+	Tinnitus
Nonsteroidal antiinflammatory drugs (NSAIDs)					
Diclofenac	1	6-8	$$$$	+++	Hepatotoxicity
Tolmetin	1	6-8	$$$	++	Allergy
Ketoprofen	2	6-8	$$$	+++	—
Ibuprofen	2	4-8	$	++	Best-tolerated NSAID
Indomethacin	3-11	8-12	$$	+++	Headache, confusion in elderly
Ketorolac	4-6	4-6	$$$$	++++	Most toxic NSAID
Etodolac	6-7	6-12	$$$$	++	—
Naproxen	13	12	$$$	++	—
Sulindac	16	12	$$	++	Less renal toxicity than other NSAIDs
Oxaprozin	21	24	$$$$	+++	—
Nabumetone	23-30	12-24	$$$$	+	Rare gastrointestinal tract toxicity
Piroxicam	30-86	24	$$	+++	Frequently toxic in elderly patients

*Retail cost, northeastern Ohio, 1996.
$ to $$$$, Least expensive to most expensive; + to ++++, least toxic to most toxic.

genase and specific COX-2 inhibitors (nabumetone) are not associated with a substantial risk of peptic ulcer disease.

NSAIDs have several other important toxic effects. Most NSAIDs inhibit platelet function and thus prolong the bleeding time. Aspirin irreversibly acetylates platelet cyclooxygenase, thus prolonging the bleeding time for up to 2 weeks. Other NSAIDs prolong the bleeding time but via reversible mechanisms. Therefore the duration of bleeding time prolongation is a function of drug half-life. Elevated liver transaminase levels are common during NSAID therapy, although serious liver damage is rare with aspirin and NSAIDs. A variety of renal syndromes has been associated with NSAID therapy, including acute renal failure, nephrosis, and interstitial nephritis. For this reason NSAIDs should be used cautiously in patients with preexisting renal insufficiency or in patients with questionable renal blood flow. Allergic reactions (including bronchospasm and laryngeal edema) occur occasionally, especially with tolmetin and ketorolac. Aspirin allergy is associated with nasal polyps and asthma. Patients who have bonafide allergy to aspirin should not be prescribed NSAIDs unless under the supervision of an allergist. Central nervous system side effects including headache and disorientation occur occasionally with NSAID treatment, especially in elderly individuals. This side effect has been most closely associated with indomethacin therapy. Tinnitus is a dose-limiting side effect of salicylate and nonacetylated salicylate therapy.

Strategies for Safe Use

Clinicians considering use of NSAIDs must carefully weigh the potential benefit of treatment with the potential risks. For example, NSAIDs are an excellent choice for pain control in young patients with acute regional musculoskeletal syndromes. By contrast, NSAIDs are a much less attractive long-term treatment option in elderly patients with osteoarthritis. Aspirin or NSAID use is a reasonable first-line treatment in patients at low risk for gastrointestinal tract toxicity who have mild rheumatoid arthritis. However, because NSAIDs are not disease modifying, clinicians must carefully weigh the potential benefit (analgesia) with the potential risks when treating more serious cases of rheumatoid arthritis. NSAID toxicity can be limited when chronic therapy is indicated by using one or more of the following strategies:

1. Use the lowest effective dose. If patients receive significant analgesic benefit at less than the maximal prescribed dose, do not advance the dose further.
2. Use NSAIDs with shorter half-lives, which are in general safer than NSAIDs with longer half-lives. This may be especially important in elderly patients. Avoid prolonged NSAID treatment, es-

pecially with long half-life NSAIDs, in patients over the age of 65 years.
3. To minimize gastrointestinal tract toxicity, consider the following:
   a. Consider the use of nonacetylated salicylates. This drug class substantially reduces the probability of NSAID gastrointestinal tract toxicity, as well as effects of NSAIDs on platelet function. However, tinnitus may be a dose-limiting toxic effect.
   b. Consider the use of enteric-coated aspirin or NSAIDs. Enteric coating prevents aspirin and NSAIDs from being absorbed in the upper gastrointestinal tract, thus minimizing the local gastrotoxic effect. However, these preparations do not entirely protect the stomach because circulating active metabolites still inhibit mucosal cyclooxygenase.
   c. Consider coadministration of misoprostol. Misoprostol is a prostaglandin preparation that protects the stomach from NSAID-induced gastric injury.
   d. For primary analgesic effects consider the use of acetaminophen.

ANALGESICS

Simple analgesics (acetaminophen, tramadol, narcotics) may have a role as an adjunct to other antirheumatic drugs or as the sole therapeutic agent in noninflammatory pain syndromes. The goal of analgesic therapy is pain control, not reduction of inflammation or disease modification.

Acetaminophen

Acetaminophen, a derivative of *p*-aminophenol, is not structurally related to NSAIDs or narcotics. Although acetaminophen shares equivalent degrees of analgesic and antipyretic properties with NSAIDs and salicylates, it has no significant antiinflammatory activity. Acetaminophen is rapidly and nearly completely absorbed and has a relatively short plasma half-life (1 to 3 hours) necessitating dosing every 4 to 6 hours when used to treat chronic pain. A typical dosing regimen of acetaminophen in acute or chronic pain is 500 to 1000 mg four times per day. Acetaminophen should not be prescribed in doses exceeding 4 g/day in adults.

Acetaminophen is relatively safe at prescribed dosages. Gastrointestinal, hematologic, and dermatologic reactions are distinctly rare. Hepatic necrosis may be a fatal consequence of massive overdose, but liver abnormalities occur only rarely at standard dosages. However, alcoholics may be at increased risk of liver damage when concomitantly ingesting moderate dosages of acetaminophen. Analgesic nephropathy (chronic interstitial nephritis, renal papillary necrosis,

Table 205-2 Second-line antirheumatic drugs

DRUG	DOSING RANGE	ONSET OF ACTION (WEEKS)	RELATIVE EFFICACY*	MONITORING	MONITORING INTERVAL (WEEKS)
Auranofin	3-9 mg/day (PO)	8-16	+	CBC, UA	4-8
Azathioprine	75-150 mg/day (PO)	6-12	+++	CBC	4-12
Chlorambucil	2-6 mg/day (PO)	4-12	++++	CBC	2-8
Cyclophosphamide	50-150 mg/day (PO)	4-12	++++	CBC, UA	2-8
Cyclosporin A	2-5 mg/kg/day (PO)	6-16	+++	CBC, creatinine	2-8
D-Penicillamine	250-1000 mg/day (PO)	8-16	++	CBC, UA	4-12
Hydroxychloroquine	200-400 mg/day	12-24	++	Eye examination	26-52
Intramuscular gold	25-50 mg/week	12-20	+++	CBC, UA	2†
Methotrexate	5-30 mg/week (PO, IM, SQ)	3-8	++++	CBC, creatinine, SGOT, albumin	4-12
Minocycline	100-200 mg/day (PO)	8-24	++	CBC, creatinine, SGOT	26
Sulfasalazine	2000-4000 mg/day (PO)	4-12	+++	CBC	2-12

*+ to ++++, Minimal efficacy to strongest efficacy.
†Monitoring interval during loading phase. Complete blood cell count (CBC) and urinalysis (UA) should be checked monthly during maintenance phase.
IM, Intramuscular; *PO,* oral; *SGOT,* serum glutamate oxaloacetate transaminase (aspartate aminotransferase); *SQ,* subcutaneous.

and chronic renal failure) is the most important concern when acetaminophen is prescribed for long-term use. The relationship between acetaminophen and analgesic nephropathy remains controversial, although some reports suggest that increased long-term acetaminophen ingestion is more common in dialysis patients than in controls.

Acetaminophen is the drug of choice for initial treatment of symptomatic osteoarthritis. Acetaminophen is significantly less expensive than most prescription NSAIDs and is significantly safer. Acetaminophen provides degrees of pain relief to patients with symptomatic osteoarthritis of the knee similar to those provided by antiinflammatory dosages of ibuprofen. Acetaminophen may also be used as an adjunct to NSAID therapy in highly symptomatic patients, although this strategy is unproven.

Tramadol

Tramadol is a new, structurally unique analgesic that appears to work via opioid receptors. However, tramadol has less respiratory depression, constipation, and addictive potential than narcotics and is not a scheduled narcotic in the United States. Single doses of tramadol (50 to 100 mg) provide degrees of analgesia similar to those provided by moderate single dosages of codeine or propoxyphene. Tramadol has not been studied sufficiently in chronic pain models or in pain associated with rheumatic disease to fully define its relative efficacy and role. However, tramadol has a favorable side effect profile and may be a reasonable alternative in patients with chronic osteoarthritis if acetaminophen or NSAID therapy is either ineffective or contraindicated.

Narcotics

The decision to prescribe narcotics to any patient with chronic, nonmalignant pain is a difficult one. On the one hand, chronic narcotic use may lead to tolerance, addiction, excessive sedation, and other undesirable outcomes. On the other hand, NSAIDs and acetaminophen frequently provide inadequate pain relief. The experience with long-term narcotic therapy in cancer patients has largely been favorable with low rates of true addiction and tolerance. Therefore narcotics may be an appropriate option in selected patients with pain attributable to rheumatic conditions. Narcotics should be avoided in patients with a history of substance abuse, cognitive impairment, or severe character problems. In general, clinicians prescribing narcotics in this setting should become familiar with both the medical and legal ramifications of narcotic therapy. A trial of a short-acting narcotic (codeine, propoxyphene) in combination with acetaminophen is a reasonable first step, although many patients with chronic pain do best with longer-acting preparations.

DISEASE-MODIFYING ANTIRHEUMATIC AGENTS

Disease-modifying antirheumatic agents are chemically unrelated drugs that are primarily used for the treatment of rheumatoid arthritis

and other systemic rheumatic diseases (Table 205-2). All of these agents have a delayed onset of action and do not consistently induce disease remission. Each of these agents has a unique toxicity profile, which is frequently the most important issue guiding their use (Table 205-3).

Methotrexate

Methotrexate is an antimetabolite drug that is generally regarded as the most important disease-modifying antirheumatic agent for the treatment of rheumatoid arthritis. Methotrexate has a rapid onset of effect that is evident between 2 and 8 weeks, and a high percentage of patients with rheumatoid arthritis have sustained benefit over many years. Methotrexate also shows promise as a potential therapeutic agent in systemic lupus erythematosus, Wegener's granulomatosis, and other forms of systemic vasculitis.

Methotrexate inhibits the enzyme dihydrofolate reductase and ultimately the production of purines and DNA. Methotrexate has been shown to alter a variety of immunologic events including immunoglobulin M (IgM) rheumatoid factor synthesis, impairment of cytokine synthesis, impairment of leukotriene synthesis, interference of cell-to-cell adherence, and interference of leukocyte migration to the inflammatory site. The specific mechanism that leads to the therapeutic effect of methotrexate is unknown.

Oral methotrexate is well absorbed in most patients. Methotrexate may also be given by intravenous, intramuscular, or subcutaneous routes. Methotrexate is eliminated by the kidney; therefore its half-life and toxicity are enhanced in the presence of renal insufficiency. Treatment is usually started at a dosage of about 0.2 mg/kg per week (or 7.5 to 10 mg/week), which can be administered as a single dose. If this is not well tolerated, the dosage can be divided into two to three doses over a 24-hour period or the route of administration can be switched to subcutaneous or intramuscular injections. If patients do not improve in the ensuing 6 to 10 weeks, the dosage can be gradually escalated. Parental methotrexate may be better tolerated at higher doses than oral methotrexate. In addition, parental methotrexate may be preferable because of enhanced bioavailability compared with the variable absorption that may be associated with higher dosages of oral methotrexate. Weekly doses in excess of 30 mg are experimental and are not recommended outside formal study protocols.

The short-term efficacy of methotrexate has been established in a number of placebo-controlled and comparative trials. A high percentage of patients benefit from drug treatment with a sustained effect that may last for many years. Minor toxic reactions are common during methotrexate therapy and include stomatitis, elevated serum transaminase levels, transient fatigue, mild anemia, and macrocytosis. In rare cases nausea and stomatitis are a cause for discontinuation of medication. Folic acid 1 mg per day or leukovorin (folinic acid) 2.5 to 5 mg 24 hours after the methotrexate dose may be given to reduce the rate of minor methotrexate side effects.

The risk of severe hepatitis or cirrhosis of the liver from methotrexate has been substantially reduced in recent years as a result of

Table 205-3 Antirheumatic drug toxicity

TOXICITY	GLUE	NSAID	CPA	CHLOR	SSAL	AZA	MTX	CSA	D-PEN	MIN	IM GOLD	HCQ
Liver	−	+	−	−	+	+	+++	−	−	−	+	−
Gastrointestinal tract	++	+++	+++	+	++	+++	+++	−	+	++	++	−
Lung	−	−	+	−	+	+	+++	−	+	−	+	−
Mucocutaneous	−	−	++	++	++	+	+++	−	++	−	+++	−
Hematologic	−	+	+++	+++	++	+++	+	−	+	−	+++	−
Teratogenicity	−	+	+++	+++	−	+	+++	+	++	++	−	+
Malignancy	−	−	+++	+++	−	++	+	+	−	−	−	−
Infections	++	−	+++	+++	−	++	++	+++	−	−	−	−
Central nervous system	++	++	−	−	−	−	+	−	−	+++	−	−
Allergy	−	++	−	−	+++	−	−	−	−	−	+++	−
Autoimmunity	−	−	−	−	+	−	+	−	+++	−	−	−
Cystitis	−	−	+++	−	−	−	−	−	−	−	−	−
Hypertension	−	++	−	−	−	−	−	+++	−	−	−	−
Infertility	−	−	+++	+++	−	−	−	−	−	−	−	−
Renal	−	++	−	−	−	−	−	+++	−	−	+++	−

GLUC, Glucocorticoid; *NSAID*, nonsteroidal antiinflammatory drug; *CPA*, cyclophosphamide; *CHLOR*, chlorambucil; *SSAL*, sulfasalazine; *AZA*, azathioprine; *MTX*, methotrexate; *CSA*, cyclosporin A; *D-PEN*, D-penicillamine; *MIN*, minocycline; *HCQ*, hydroxychloroquine; *IM GOLD*, solgonol or myochrysine; + to +++, weak-to-strong association; −, little or no association.

careful prescreening of patients for chronic liver disease or alcohol use. Pretreatment liver biopsies are indicated if patients have risk factors for chronic liver disease (excessive alcohol ingestion, persistently elevated aspartate aminotransferase [AST], chronic hepatitis B or C). Patients receiving treatment with methotrexate should have a complete blood cell count, and serum glutamate oxaloacetate transaminase (SGOT), serum albumin, and serum creatinine levels should be checked every 4 to 12 weeks during therapy to monitor for toxic effects. If elevations of SGOT or reductions in albumin occur on a persistent basis, the dosage should be held or reduced. If concerns persist, a liver biopsy may be necessary.

Methotrexate should be avoided in patients with acute or chronic liver disease, alcoholics, and patients with morbid obesity associated with insulin-dependent diabetes because of the likelihood of serious liver toxicity. Methotrexate is teratogenic, and fertile women should be warned thoroughly regarding the necessity to practice adequate birth control during treatment. Methotrexate therapy should be avoided or used cautiously in patients with serum creatinine levels greater than 2.0 mg/dl.

Two large follow-up studies of psoriasis and germ-cell cancer patients who received treatment with methotrexate failed to show evidence of subsequent malignancy. In several patients who received treatment with methotrexate, lymphomas have been reported to develop, which subsequently resolved on removal of the drug. This occurrence appears to be rare, and a direct causative role of methotrexate in the development of lymphoma has not been established.

Gold Salts

Two intramuscular (Myochrysine and Solgonol) gold preparations and one oral (auranofin) gold preparation are available. Gold salts are used in the treatment of rheumatoid arthritis and, occasionally, psoriatic arthritis and cutaneous lupus erythematosus. The mechanism of action of gold is unknown, although the drug is not believed to be globally immunosuppressive.

Auranofin is an oral gold preparation given daily (3 to 9 mg). Intramuscular gold treatment typically begins with a 10- to 25-mg test dose followed by 50-mg weekly injections. Injections are continued weekly until a significant response is seen or a cumulative dose of 1 g is reached. The response to intramuscular gold is highly variable. A minority of patients have an excellent response, many patients have a partial response, and a significant minority of patients have no response whatsoever. In addition, many patients who have an excellent initial response to gold see the effect fade after 1 to 2 years.

Gold is among the most toxic of disease-modifying agents. Common toxicities include skin rash, oral ulcers, gastrointestinal tract upset, and most seriously, thrombocytopenia or proteinuria. As many as 40% of patients who receive treatment with intramuscular gold eventually discontinue the treatment because of side effects.

D-Penicillamine

D-penicillamine is used in rheumatoid arthritis and, in particular, as an important treatment of early systemic sclerosis. Common side effects include skin rash, gastrointestinal tract complaints, cytopenias, and proteinuria. In addition, D-penicillamine has the unique propensity to induce autoimmune syndromes including myasthenia gravis, Goodpasture's disease, inflammatory muscle disease, and systemic lupus erythematosus. D-penicillamine is an immune modulator and may also affect collagen structure—its presumed mechanism in systemic sclerosis.

Antimalarials

Three antimalarials (quinacrine, chloroquine, and hydroxychloroquine) are used to treat rheumatic disease, principally rheumatoid arthritis and systemic lupus erythematosus. Of these, hydroxychloroquine is by far the most important and most commonly used. Chloroquine has largely been discarded as an antirheumatic agent in the United States because of high rates of retinal toxicity. Antimalarial drugs are well absorbed and extensively distributed. The mechanism of action of these drugs in rheumatic disease is unknown, although a variety of immunomodulatory effects have been demonstrated.

Tolerability is the prime advantage of antimalarial treatment. Retinal toxicity is the most potentially serious side effect and can be minimized by using hydroxychloroquine at doses of 400 mg/day or less and obtaining screening ophthalmologic examinations every 6 to 12 months. Dermatitis, nausea, blood dyscrasias, and neuromyopathy are rare side effects.

Sulfasalazine

Sulfasalazine is a hybrid of a sulfa antibiotic (sulfapyridine) and a salicylate (5-aminosalicylic acid). Controlled trials have shown sulfasalazine to be an effective agent in the treatment of rheumatoid arthritis. Emerging evidence suggests that sulfasalazine may have a role in the management of ankylosing spondylitis and seronegative spondyloarthropathies, particularly if laboratory tests suggest serious inflammation and if these disorders are complicated by peripheral joint arthritis. There are limited data concerning the long-term efficacy of sulfasalazine in rheumatic diseases.

The initial dose is 500 to 1000 mg/day, which is later increased to 2000 to 4000 mg/day if tolerated. Several important toxicities may occur during sulfasalazine treatment. Skin rash, allergy, nausea, and vomiting are the most frequent causes of drug discontinuation. Neutropenia and thrombocytopenia are rare but serious problems, primarily in the first 3 months of therapy; thus lower initial dosages and close monitoring at the initiation of therapy is prudent.

Azathioprine

Azathioprine is used in rheumatoid arthritis, systemic lupus erythematosus, inflammatory muscle disease, and other rheumatic diseases. Minor gastrointestinal tract complaints such as nausea and vomiting are fairly common, as are minor reductions in the white blood cell count or platelet count. Rarely, severe cytopenias or hepatitis complicates therapy. In addition, patients receiving treatment with azathioprine have an increased susceptibility to herpes, cytomegalovirus, and human papillomavirus infections.

The major concern during long-term azathioprine therapy is hematologic malignancy, especially non-Hodgkin's lymphoma. This is especially important in renal transplantation patients. However, patients with rheumatoid arthritis and other autoimmune or inflammatory diseases may have an increased risk of non-Hodgkin's lymphoma independent of treatment. Limited data suggest that azathioprine exposure may mildly increase this risk. Because of these problems, azathioprine treatment should be restricted to patients who have either failed or not tolerated other disease-modifying antirheumatic drugs.

Alkylating Agents

Cyclophosphamide and chlorambucil are oral alkylating agents that are occasionally used in the treatment of refractory rheumatoid arthritis. In addition, intravenous pulse cyclophosphamide is commonly used in the treatment of nephritis associated with systemic lupus erythematosus, and intravenous pulse nitrogen mustard is an alkylating agent used at a few centers in the treatment of serious rheumatic diseases.

Both cyclophosphamide and chlorambucil are pro-drugs that are easily absorbed from the gastrointestinal tract. Both drugs undergo biliary conversion to active metabolites. Elimination is via both hepatic and renal routes. The most important difference between cyclophosphamide and chlorambucil is the production of the bladder-toxic metabolite acrolein following cyclophosphamide administration. Acrolein is not produced following hepatic metabolism of either chlorambucil or nitrogen mustard.

Alkylating agents are arguably the most effective agents for the treatment of severe rheumatoid arthritis and are the mainstay of treatment of life-threatening manifestations of vasculitis and systemic lupus erythematosus. The standard oral dosage of cylcophosphamide is 75 to 150 mg/day; the dosage range of chlorambucil is 2 to 6 mg/day. Intermittent "pulse" cyclophosphamide is infused in doses of 0.75 to 1.0 g/m^2 monthly in patients with normal renal function. The most reasonable way to give nitrogen mustard is via daily intravenous infusions of 3 to 5 mg with the total infused dose not to exceed 0.3 mg/kg. Alkylating agents reduce B- and T-cell numbers by direct cytotoxic effects. Function of both B cells and T cells is altered as well. Global immunosuppression results in and is responsible for both the favorable therapeutic effect, as well as increased susceptibility to infection—arguably the most important toxicity of alkylating agent therapy.

Toxicity concerns have severely restricted the use of alkylating agents in the treatment of rheumatic disorders that are not immediately life threatening. However, in the case of lupus nephritis or serious forms of vasculitis the potential therapeutic benefit may exceed the potential risk of toxicity. Cytopenias are dose related and common with all alkylating agents. Chlorambucil is particularly strongly associated with severe idiosyncratic granulocytopenia. All alkylating agents are associated with alopecia and nausea. Patients receiving treatment with alkylating agents have increased susceptibility to viral, bacterial, fungal, and atypical infections. This risk is particularly high during times of drug-induced neutropenia.

Gonadal toxicity is common during prolonged alkylating agent therapy, especially in women over the age of 30 years. All alkylating agents have been associated with the subsequent development of leukemia or lymphoma. In patients receiving treatment with oral cyclophosphamide a variety of bladder lesions may develop, ranging from hemorrhagic cystitis to bladder fibrosis to bladder cancer that appears to be dose related. This toxicity can be minimized by hydration and frequent voiding. Mesna is a compound that inactivates acrolein in the bladder. Mesna administration is practical only in patients receiving treatment with intravenous pulse cyclophosphamide and may reduce their risk of bladder-toxic effects.

Cyclosporine

Cyclosporine, a complex fungal-derived drug, is unique among antirheumatic drugs in that it specifically depresses T-cell function. As a consequence, it is a useful drug in T-cell–mediated diseases such as rheumatoid arthritis. Cyclosporine is noncytotoxic and inhibits the production of interleukin-2 (IL-2) and other T-cell–derived lymphokines.

Orally administered cyclosporine is variably and incompletely absorbed. It undergoes extensive first-pass hepatic metabolism with subsequent production of active and inactive metabolites. Elimination is primarily via biliary excretion. Metabolism is unaffected by renal failure but may be delayed in patients with liver disease.

The most important toxic effect of cyclosporine is renal insufficiency, which is generally reversible in patients who receive treatment for less than 1 year. However, patients who have sustained creatinine elevations during cyclosporine treatment or continue receiving the drug for more than 1 year may lose significant renal function. Hypertension is a common sequella of cyclosporine treatment and must be treated aggressively, since it may aggravate renal toxicity. NSAIDs, erythromycin, and ketoconazole may aggravate cyclosporine-induced renal insufficiency and should be avoided, if possible. Other toxic effects of cyclosporine include peripheral neuropathy, gingival hyperplasia, infection, and diabetes mellitus.

Toxicity can be minimized by initiating treatment at a dosage of 2 to 2.5 mg/kg per day. Renal function and blood pressure should be checked frequently at the initiation of treatment. If tolerated, the dosage can be slowly titrated upward. Dosages greater than 5 mg/kg per day are not recommended in patients with rheumatic diseases.

Minocycline

The tetracycline antibiotic minocycline has modest efficacy in rheumatoid arthritis. The mechanism of action of minocycline in rheumatoid arthritis is unknown; it remains unclear whether antibacterial effects or immunomodulatory effects are responsible for clinical improvement. Minocycline should be taken between meals, since food substantially reduces its absorption. Nausea and dizziness are common side effects and frequent causes of minocycline discontinuation. Minocycline has few serious adverse effects. The use of minocycline has not been established in other rheumatic diseases.

GLUCOCORTICOIDS

Synthetic glucocorticoids are widely used in the treatment of inflammatory rheumatic diseases. All glucocorticoids are 21-steroid molecules that are required for maintenance of blood pressure, muscle function, blood glucose and hepatic glycogen levels, as well as blood volume. Synthetic glucocorticoids are efficiently absorbed by the gastrointestinal tract and are highly protein bound in circulation. Glucocorticoids enter all cells, bind to intracellular glucocorticoid receptors, and then migrate to the nucleus where they enhance or inhibit gene expression. Glucocorticoid administration reduces the production of several mediators of inflammation, including prostaglandins, leukotrienes, thromboxanes, and nitric oxide. Glucocorticoids also decrease the synthesis of a variety of proinflammatory cytokines, including IL-1, IL-2, and tumor necrosis factor (TNF) and reduce transcription of the COX 2 gene. The net result of these effects is powerful down-regulation of inflammation.

Pharmacologic doses of glucocorticoids also have effects that extend beyond immunologic and inflammatory systems. Glucocorticoid therapy stimulates the appetite, leading to obesity and a cushingoid appearance in patients receiving treatment. Glucocorticoids promote hyperglycemia through increased hepatic glucose production and insulin resistance. Diabetes is a potential complication of glucocorticoid treatment, particularly in patients who were previously obese or have a tendency toward type II diabetes. All synthetic glucocorticoids have mineralocorticoid activity; thus patients receiving treatment may have problems with sodium retention, hypokalemia, and hypertension. Glucocorticoid therapy increases low-density lipoprotein (LDL) and total serum cholesterol levels. High-dose glucocorticoid treatment may damage muscle, leading to a myopathy characterized by proximal muscle weakness and, occasionally, myalgia. Glucocorticoids

Table 205-4 Common glucocorticoid treatment protocols for selected rheumatic diseases

RHEUMATIC DISEASE	HIGH-DOSE INDUCTION[A]	INTRAVENOUS PULSE[B]	INTRAMUSCULAR PULSE[C]	MID-DOSE ORAL[D]	LOW-DOSE ORAL[E]	INTRAARTICULAR[F]
Rheumatoid arthritis			X		X	X
Osteoarthritis						X
Lupus erythematosus with arthritis					X	X
Lupus erythematosus with nephritis	X	X				
Inflammatory muscle disease	X	X				
Polyarteritis nodosa	X	X				
Polymyalgia rheumatica				X		
Giant cell (temporal) arteritis	X					

[a]Prednisone 1 mg/kg daily for at least 1 month with gradual taper to 20 mg every other day if tolerated.
[b]One gram methylprednisolone intravenously (infused over 30 to 60 minutes); may be repeated daily for up to 3 days at onset of therapy or for flares.
[c]80 to 320 mg depo-methylprednisolone, intramuscular injection, for disease flares.
[d]10 to 20 mg prednisone per day initial dosage with subsequent taper as tolerated.
[e]1 to 7.5 mg prednisone per day, taper as tolerated.
[f]20 to 80 mg triamcinolone, intraarticular injection, for disease flares.

lead to thinning of the skin, thus predisposing patients to laceration with shear stress and extensive ecchymosis following minor trauma. Posterior subcapsular cataracts are seen occasionally during glucocorticoid treatment. Glucocorticoids also appear to increase the risk of complicated peptic ulcers associated with coexistent NSAID therapy.

Perhaps the most important consequence of sustained glucocorticoid therapy is osteoporosis. Glucocorticoids impair intestinal absorption of calcium and increase renal excretion of calcium, leading to a net negative calcium balance. Secondary hyperparathyroidism results and promotes bone resorption. In addition, glucocorticoids directly inhibit osteoblast differentiation, replication, and collagen matrix production. Taken together, osteoporosis is a near-universal consequence of sustained glucocorticoid therapy. Osteoporosis may be less serious in rheumatoid arthritis patients who receive treatment with low-dose prednisone (7 mg/day or less) as a result of the beneficial effect of increased mobility that is seen in patients with a therapeutic response. However, osteoporosis is a substantial cause of morbidity in patients receiving dosages greater than 10 mg/day.

Glucocorticoids may be administered by several different methods in highly variable dosing regimens, depending on the nature and severity of the condition being treated (Table 205-4). High-dose glucocorticoid therapy is strongly associated with the development of avascular necrosis (osteonecrosis), especially in renal transplantation patients and patients with systemic lupus erythematosus. The mechanism of this problem is probably a result of fat accumulation in the bone marrow and resultant increased venous pressure, venous stasis, and clot formation. As a result, bony areas with major weight-bearing function (hip or knee) are particularly prone to collapse attributable to bony necrosis. Patients taking more than 60 mg/day of prednisone or equivalent for more than 1 month are at highest risk.

Low-dose prednisone therapy is an effective and frequently necessary therapy in patients with moderate to severe rheumatoid arthritis. High-dose glucocorticoid therapy (1 mg/kg per day initially) is the mainstay of treatment of giant cell arteritis, other forms of systemic vasculitis, and serious manifestations of systemic lupus erythematosus. Although glucocorticoids are frequently necessary, clinicians should always prudently taper the dosage, searching for the lowest effective dose.

Several strategies may decrease glucocorticoid toxicity. Intraarticular glucocorticoids are particularly useful if inflammatory arthritis is limited to a single joint or two individual joints. Larger doses of glucocorticoids (250 to 1000 mg of methylprednisolone) may be infused over 1 hour ("pulse therapy") in patients who are critically ill, leading to an earlier onset of therapeutic effect and possibly reduced overall glucocorticoid exposure. Patients who require longer-term therapy for serious rheumatologic disease such as vasculitis, lupus erythematosus, or myositis frequently can be converted from every-day to every-other-day treatment. Every-other-day glucocorticoid treatment reduces the severity of cushingoid changes and weight gain but may not reduce the risk of osteoporosis.

BIBLIOGRAPHY

Adler RA, Rosen CJ: Glucocorticoids and osteoporosis, *Endocrinol Metabol Clin North Am* 23(3):641-654, 1994 (review).

Boumpas DT, Chrousos GP, Wilder RL et al: Glucocorticoid therapy for immune-mediated diseases: basic and clinical correlates, *Ann Intern Med* 119(12):1198-1208, 1993 (review).

Cash JM, Klippel JH: Second-line drug therapy for rheumatoid arthritis, *N Engl J Med* 330(19):1368-1375, 1994 (review).

Cash JM, Wilder RL: Refractory rheumatoid arthritis: therapeutic options, *Rheum Dis Clin North Am* 21(1):1-18, 1995.

Day RO: Aspirin and salicylates. In Kelley WN, Harris ED, Ruddy S, Sledge CB, editors: *Textbook of rheumatology,* Philadelphia, 1993, WB Saunders.

Felson DT, Anderson JJ, Meenan RF: Use of short-term efficacy/toxicity tradeoffs to select second-line drugs in rheumatoid arthritis: a metaanalysis of published clinical trials, *Arthritis Rheum* 35(10):1117-1125, 1992.

Furst DE: Clinical significance of long versus short serum half-life in NSAIDs: confounding and complicating factors. In Fancey JP, Paullus HE, editors: *Therapeutic applications of NSAIDs: subpopulations and new formulations,* New York, 1992, Marcel Dekker.

Garcia Rodriguez LA, Williams R, Derby LE et al: Acute liver injury associated with nonsteroidal antiinflammatory drugs and the role of risk factors, *Arch Intern Med* 154(3):311-316, 1994.

Graham DY, White RH, Moreland LW et al: Duodenal and gastric ulcer prevention with misoprostol in arthritis patients taking NSAIDs: Misoprostol Study Group, *Ann Intern Med* 119(4):257-262, 1993.

Griffin MR, Piper JM, Daugherty JR et al: Nonsteroidal antiinflammatory drug use and increased risk for peptic ulcer disease in elderly persons, *Ann Intern Med* 114(4):257-263, 1991.

Kirwan JR: The effect of glucocorticoids on joint destruction in rheumatoid arthritis: the Arthritis and Rheumatism Council Low-Dose Glucocorticoid Study Group, *N Engl J Med* 333(3):142-146, 1995.

Kremer JM, Alarcon GS, Lightfoot RW et al: Methotrexate for rheumatoid arthritis: suggested guidelines for monitoring liver toxicity—American College of Rheumatology, *Arthritis Rheum* 37:316-328, 1994.

Radis CD, Kahl LE, Baker GL et al: Effects of cyclophosphamide on the development of malignancy and on long-term survival of patients with rheumatoid arthritis: a 20-year follow-up study, *Arthritis Rheum* 38(8):1120-1127, 1995.

Singh G, Ramey DR, Morfeld D et al: Comparative toxicity of nonsteroidal antiinflammatory agents, *Pharmacol Ther* 62(1-2):175-191, 1994 (review).

Vane JR, Botting RM: A better understanding of antiinflammatory drugs based on isoforms of cyclooxygenase (COX-1 and COX-2), *Adv Prostaglandin, Thromboxane, Leukot Res* 23:41-48, 1995 (review).

IV JOINT DISEASES

CHAPTER

206 Osteoarthritis

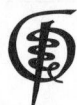

Kenneth D. Brandt

Osteoarthritis (OA), also called *osteoarthrosis* or *degenerative joint disease,* is the most common of all joint diseases to affect humans. Osteoarthritis is characterized by progressive loss of articular cartilage, thickening of subchondral bone, bony remodeling, and development of bony spurs (osteophytes). The clinical features include joint pain and stiffness, swelling, crepitus, low-grade synovitis, and loss of mobility. Osteoarthritis represents failure of the diarthrodial joint. In primary (idiopathic) OA no predisposing factor is recognizable. In secondary OA an underlying abnormality of the involved joint is apparent.

EPIDEMIOLOGY

Among the spectrum of specific joint diseases OA is the most frequent cause of rheumatic complaints. More than 80% of all people over the age of 55 years have radiographic evidence of OA; although not all of these individuals are symptomatic, as many as 30% of those affected have significant pain and disability. Osteoarthritis of the knee is the leading cause of chronic disability in the United States.

Aging

Age is the most powerful risk factor for OA. Only 21% of women under the age of 45 years, but 30% of those between 45 and 64 years of age and 68% of those age 65 or older, have radiographic evidence of OA. The same trend is seen in men. When all age-groups are considered, the prevalence of OA in men and women is comparable but women are more likely to be symptomatic.

Osteoarthritis is often considered to be a consequence of "aging," that is, of presumed senescence of the articular cartilage chondrocyte, with "running down" of its metabolic machinery. However, because joints accumulate mechanical insults throughout a lifetime, the distinction between aging and wear-and-tear is blurred. Furthermore, in normal human joint cartilage, only a modest reduction in cellularity occurs after maturity, and the cells remain metabolically active; indeed, the net rate of proteoglycan synthesis per cell is as high in normal cartilage from aged individuals as in that from younger adults. In OA, at least until the very late stages, the chondrocytes, rather than entering a hypometabolic state, synthesize increased quantities of proteoglycans, collagen, noncollagenous proteins, and DNA. Therefore, to call OA "degenerative joint disease" is patently incorrect. Although age-related changes occur in the chemical composition of normal articular cartilage, they are very different from those in OA cartilage and have not been clearly shown to predispose to OA.

Race and Genetics

Racial differences in the prevalence of OA are apparent. In the United States OA is more common in Native Americans than in the general population. Hip and interphalangeal joint OA are much less prevalent in South African blacks than in whites in the same population. Chinese in Hong Kong have a lower prevalence of hip OA than whites. Whether such variations are related to heredity or to cultural differences in joint usage is not known.

Other examples may be cited in which the etiologic role of ge-

netic factors is less ambiguous. In some instances the genetic defect results in a change in the gross structure of the joint, affecting congruity (e.g., acetabular dysplasia). In other cases it may lead to OA through systemic metabolic effects. Heberden's nodes (distal interphalangeal joint OA) clearly are inherited. Recently a point mutation in the cDNA coding for articular cartilage collagen was identified in several generations of a family with mild chondrodysplasia and secondary OA involving multiple joints. In ochronosis, a heritable disorder characterized by a deficiency of homogentisic acid oxidase, accumulation of homogentisic acid polymers leads to stiffening of articular cartilage and decreased ability of the tissue to transmit load (Chapter 209).

Joint Distribution and Relation of Osteoarthritis to Joint Overload and Trauma

Before age 55 years the pattern of joint involvement in men and women is similar. In older people OA of the interphalangeal joints and the thumb base is more common in women, whereas hip OA is more often seen in men.

In the normal joint some incongruity of the surfaces during loading is important for the "pumping" of nutrients from the synovial fluid into the cartilage and of catabolites from the cartilage into the fluid. Abnormalities in congruity caused by congenital or developmental defects have been considered to underlie most cases of idiopathic OA of the hip in humans. In such instances OA may be caused by mechanical "fatigue failure" of the matrix, increased contact stresses, or impaired nutrition of the chondrocyte.

Major joint trauma is an important risk factor for OA. Anterior cruciate ligament insufficiency, meniscus damage, and meniscectomy all lead to knee OA. Osteochondral fractures and fractures that heal with deformities which result in a concentration of the peak dynamic load (stress) within the joint also predispose to OA.

The site of involvement is strongly influenced by prior usage of the joint. For example, OA is common in ankles of ballet dancers, shoulders and elbows of professional tennis players, and metacarpophalangeal joints of boxers, although it is relatively unusual for OA to occur at these sites in the general population. Repeated overload of the joint by vocational or avocational use is an important—and potentially modifiable—cause of OA. Although jogging has been reported not to cause OA, selection bias (i.e., early cessation of the activity by those who incur joint damage) cannot be excluded in those studies.

Jobs requiring repeated knee bending and moderate physical demand appear to predispose to knee OA. The prevalence of hip OA is increased in farmers. Among groups of textile workers performing different repetitive manual tasks, OA was more prevalent in hand joints that were used repetitively for the task than in other hand joints.

Obesity

Obesity has long been associated with an increased prevalence of knee OA. Recent epidemiologic data indicate that obesity is not merely the result of decreased physical activity resulting from the painful knee, but may precede and represent an important risk factor for knee OA. In a strain of guinea pigs at risk for development of spontaneous knee OA, dietary restriction sufficient to decrease body weight by 28% decreased the severity of OA pathologic changes by 40%. Furthermore, in obese women weight loss reduced the risk of symptomatic knee OA. Whether metabolic factors as well as mechanical effects contribute to development of OA in obesity is unclear.

Risk Factors for Pain and Disability in Osteoarthritis

In general the association between the severity of pathologic changes of OA and joint pain is weak. Many subjects with advanced radiographic changes of OA are asymptomatic. The risk factors for pain and disability are poorly understood but are probably very different from the risk factors for cartilage damage. Psychosocial factors may be important determinants of who with OA becomes symptomatic and who does not; given comparable degrees of pathologic severity, women are more likely to be symptomatic than men, divorced individuals more likely than those who are married, and people on welfare more likely than those who are employed.

PATHOLOGIC FEATURES

Although loss of articular cartilage is the pathologic hallmark of OA, in the earlier stages of OA the cartilage is thicker than normal. Not only is the water content of the tissue increased, but increased synthesis of proteoglycans by the chondrocytes (see later discussion) results in an increase in the proteoglycan content of the extracellular matrix, which is readily apparent with histochemical staining. Localized softening of the cartilage (chondromalacia) develops in load-bearing areas. With progression of the disease the surface becomes disrupted and fissures develop (fibrillation). With joint motion the fibrillated cartilage is lost, exposing underlying bone that becomes thickened and eburnated. Microfractures of subchondral trabeculae may be seen. Bone cysts, reflecting localized osteonecrosis, form beneath the surface and weaken the osseous support for the overlying cartilage. New bone formation leads to osteophytes (spurs), which extend into the joint capsule and ligament attachments or into the joint space, where they may restrict joint movement. In addition, the subchondral plate thickens. On a radiograph of the OA joint subchondral "sclerosis" may be seen (Chapter 184).

Although mitosis of chondrocytes is never seen in normal adult articular cartilage, chondrocyte proliferation may be extensive in OA. Late in the disease, however, the cartilage is hypocellular. Capillaries from the underlying subchondral bone invade the tidemark and provide a basis for fibrocartilaginous outgrowths that may replace the defective hyaline cartilage. The repair cartilage, however, is inferior to the native cartilage in its ability to withstand mechanical stress. The synovium shows foci of inflammation, hyperplasia of the lining cells, and villus hypertrophy. The capsule thickens, further limiting joint motion. Periarticular muscle atrophy is common in OA and may contribute significantly to disability. In some cases, however, weakness may occur without atrophy as a result of neuronal reflex activity, with the afferent input from the diseased joint resulting in inhibition of efferent stimulation of periarticular muscles (arthrogenous muscle inhibition). Notably, synovial and cartilage disease may be as severe in those who are asymptomatic as in patients complaining of joint pain.

PATHOGENESIS

No single factor triggers the processes that result in cartilage destruction and new bone formation in OA. Most current theories of the pathogenesis of OA focus on the breakdown of the articular cartilage, which may be primary or attributable to abnormalities in subchondral bone, synovium, or extraarticular structures (ligaments, neuromuscular apparatus) (Box 206-1).

Articular cartilage is important because it fulfills two essential functions. First, it provides a remarkably smooth bearing surface so that one bone glides effortlessly over the other during movement of the joint. Second, cartilage is designed to prevent the concentration of stresses so that the bones do not shatter with loading of the joint.

OA develops in either of two settings: (1) the biomaterial properties of the articular cartilage and subchondral bone are normal but excessive loads applied to the joint cause the tissues to fail or (2) the applied load is physiologically reasonable but the material properties of the cartilage or bone are inferior.

Although mechanical "wear" is undoubtedly a factor in the loss of cartilage in OA, neutral matrix metalloproteinases (MMPs) and lysosomal proteases account for much of the loss of cartilage matrix. Whether their synthesis and secretion are stimulated by cytokines derived from the inflamed synovium (e.g., interleukin-1) or by other factors (e.g., mechanical stimuli), neutral metalloproteinases, plasmin, and cathepsins produced by the chondrocytes are central to the breakdown of articular cartilage in OA. Endogenous tissue inhibitors of these enzymes (e.g., tissue inhibitors of metalloproteinases [TIMP], plasminogen activator inhibitor) may stabilize the system, at least temporarily, and growth factors (e.g., insulin-like growth factor [IGF]-1 and transforming growth factor [TGF]-β) drive repair processes that may heal the lesion or at least stabilize the damage. In OA, stoichiometric imbalance exists between levels of matrix-degrading

---

BOX 206-1
Classification of osteoarthritis

I. Primary
 A. Idiopathic
 B. Generalized osteoarthritis
 C. Erosive osteoarthritis
II. Secondary
 A. Resulting from mechanical incongruity of joint
  1. Congenital or developmental defects, hip dysplasia, Legg-Calvé-Perthes disease, slipped femoral capital epiphysis, femoral neck abnormalities, protrusio acetabuli, multiple epiphyseal dysplasia, osteochondritis, Morquio's syndrome
  2. Posttraumatic
 B. Resulting from prior inflammatory joint disease (e.g., rheumatoid arthritis and variants, chronic gouty arthritis, pseudogout, infectious arthritis)
 C. Resulting from metabolic disorders (e.g., hemochromatosis, ochronosis, Wilson's disease, chondrocalcinosis, Paget's disease)
 D. Resulting from endocrinopathies (e.g., diabetes mellitus, acromegaly, sex hormone abnormalities, iatrogenic hyperadrenocorticism)
 E. Resulting from miscellaneous causes (e.g., osteonecrosis, hemarthrosis associated with blood dyscrasias)

---

enzymes—which may be several-fold higher than normal—and the level of TIMP, which is only modestly increased.

Which degradative enzyme (if any) is the key player in the breakdown of articular cartilage in OA is currently a subject of debate. Would a specific inhibitor of cartilage collagenase prevent development of OA or progression of cartilage damage? Of stromelysin? Or is an MMP inhibitor with broad specificity more likely to be effective? Are mechanisms for turnover of the cartilage matrix so redundant that none of the preceding therapeutic approaches would be effective? The answers are not known. Because analyses of cartilage and synovial fluid from patients with OA indicate a unique cleavage site in the core protein of aggrecan, the major proteoglycan of cartilage, which cannot be attributed to any of the known proteases, a major effort is under way to identify the putative "aggrecanase." There is some evidence that neutrophil collagenase (MMP-8) exhibits aggrecanase activity and that chondrocytes contain message for MMP-8, but it is not yet clear whether MMP-8 or any enzyme with aggrecanase activity is important in the pathogenesis of OA.

The chondrocytes in OA cartilage undergo cell division and are very active metabolically, producing increased quantities of collagen (which provides cartilage with tensile strength) and proteoglycans (which are responsible for the stiffness of the tissue and its ability to resist compression). Perhaps the earliest change in the cartilage in OA is a defect in the integrity of the collagen network, which normally constrains the proteoglycans within the tissue. This defect, which may be irreversible, leads to swelling of the cartilage and is accompanied by an increase in the synthesis of collagen, proteoglycans, and noncollagenous proteins which, however, are not integrated into the normal three-dimensional structure of the cartilage matrix. These homeostatic mechanisms may maintain the joint in a reasonable functional state for years. The repair tissue, however, does not hold up as well under mechanical stress as normal hyaline cartilage. Eventually, at least in some cases, the rate of proteoglycan synthesis declines and "end-stage" OA develops.

CLINICAL FEATURES

The joints most commonly involved in primary OA are the distal and proximal interphalangeal joints of the hands, the metacarpophalangeal joint of the thumb, the knees, hips, cervical and lumbar spine, and the metatarsophalangeal joint of the great toe. In primary OA most other joints are spared; if they are affected, secondary OA (Table 206-1) is probably present.

The predominant symptom of OA and the complaint that most of-

Table 206-1   Clinical features of primary osteoarthritis

Age	Usually elderly
Joint distribution	Monoarthritis or oligoarthritis
Most frequent sites	Distal and proximal interphalangeal joints of fingers, first carpometacarpal joint, first metatarsophalangeal joint, hips, knees, cervical spine, lumbar spine
Joints usually spared	Metacarpophalangeal joints, wrists, elbows, glenohumeral joints, ankles
Systemic manifestations	Absent
Characteristics of joint discomfort	Aggravated by use and relieved by rest (but pain also at rest with severe disease); gelling sensation; morning stiffness absent or less than 30 minutes in duration
Joint examination	Local tenderness, bony and/or soft tissue swelling, crepitus, effusion
Characteristics of synovial fluid	Normal viscosity, normal mucin test, mild leukocytosis ($<$2000 white blood cells/mm^3), predominantly mononuclear cells

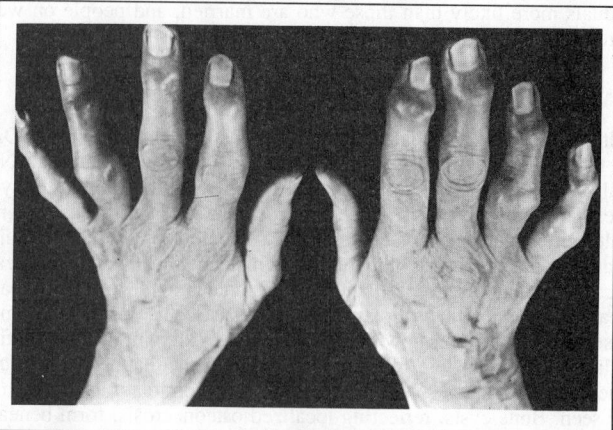

FIGURE 206-1   Osteoarthritis of the distal interphalangeal joints. Bony enlargement and deformity (Heberden's nodes) are evident. The node on the right index finger is inflamed, and the overlying skin is erythematous. Bony enlargement is present also at several proximal interphalangeal joints (Bouchard's nodes).

From Clinical slide collection on the rheumatic diseases, Copyright 1991, 1995; American College of Rheumatology.

ten leads the patient to seek medical attention is joint pain. Because the articular cartilage is not innervated, the pain cannot arise from that tissue. However, pain in OA may be caused by subchondral microfractures, irritation of periosteal nerve endings during remodeling or osteophyte formation, hemodynamic changes in subchondral bone resulting from distortion of the subchondral capillaries by thickened bony trabeculae, ligamentous strain, periarticular inflammation (bursitis, tendinitis), or low-grade synovitis.

The patient with OA complains of a deep ache, which is usually localized to the involved joint but occasionally is referred. Typically the pain occurs after joint usage and is relieved by rest, but in advanced OA it may be present also at rest. In severe hip OA night pain is common. Brief gelling of the joint after disuse is characteristic. Morning stiffness usually lasts less than 30 minutes. Constitutional features such as weight loss, anemia, fatigue, and fever, are not present in OA.

Physical findings include tenderness, bony crepitus, limitation of motion, and enlargement of the involved joint. Swelling may be caused by thickening of the synovium and capsule, effusion, or osteophytes. With progression of the disease gross deformity occurs with subluxation and marked bony enlargement.

When OA of the spine involves apophyseal joints, parasthesias, muscle weakness, and hyperreflexia may be caused by osteophytes, prolapse of a degenerated disk, or narrowing of neural foramina by apophyseal joint subluxation. In the cervical region osteophytes may compress the spinal cord, producing long tract signs. Osteophytes in the joints of Luschka may alter the course of the vertebral artery, producing vertigo, diplopia, scotomata, nystagmus, or ataxia. Symptoms of vertebral insufficiency in cervical OA may be related to the position of the neck.

PRIMARY OSTEOARTHRITIS
Heberden's Nodes

Heberden's nodes represent bony, cartilaginous, synovial, and capsular enlargements of the distal interphalangeal joints of the hands (Fig. 206-1). Similar changes may occur in the proximal interphalangeal joints (Bouchard's nodes). Nodal OA may be associated with flexion deformities and lateral deviation of the involved phalanges. Although the nodes are usually associated with little discomfort, they may become evident acutely with redness, swelling, and pain. Heberden's nodes are ten times more common in women than in men, and a strong hereditary tendency is apparent.

Erosive Osteoarthritis

Erosive osteoarthritis occurs particularly in postmenopausal women and affects distal and proximal interphalangeal joints and, occasionally, the metacarpophalangeal joints. Inflammation is much more

marked than in the typical patient with Heberden's nodes. Recurrent, acute, painful flare-ups are common. Radiographs show collapse of the subchondral plate and bony erosions, in addition to the typical features of OA (Chapter 184). Deformity may be severe, and ankylosis may develop. The synovium is infiltrated with lymphocytes and monocytes to a greater degree than usually seen in primary OA. Pannus, which is rare in other forms of OA, may develop. In 15% of patients with erosive OA rheumatoid arthritis may eventually develop, although test results for rheumatoid factor are negative.

Primary Generalized Osteoarthritis

Generalized OA is marked by involvement of three or more joints or groups of joints and, like erosive OA, occurs predominantly in middle-aged postmenopausal women. Interphalangeal joints of the hands and the first carpometacarpal joint are involved most often, but generalized OA also affects knees, hips, big toe, and spine. The course is typically episodic, with intermittent bouts of pain in the involved joint(s), often accompanied by warmth and effusion.

Chondromalacia Patellae

Chondromalacia patellae, a clinical syndrome of patellofemoral pain, occurs chiefly in young adults. Women are affected more than men. Softening of cartilage occurs where the patella comes in contact with the femur in midflexion of the knee. The changes are usually *not* progressive; in only a minority of cases does chondromalacia patellae seem to lead to OA.

Spondylosis Deformans

Spondylosis deformans refers to degenerative disease in the intervertebral disks rather than in the synovial joints of the spine. Progressive changes in the nucleus pulposus are similar to those in articular cartilage in OA. The vertebral endplates, which are composed of hyaline cartilage, fibrillate and disintegrate, leading to eburnation of subchondral bone. The nucleus pulposus may herniate into the vertebral body through the defective endplate (Schmorl's node). Vertebral osteophytes commonly develop.

SECONDARY OSTEOARTHRITIS

Osteoarthritis may occur as a sequel to a variety of diverse endocrine or metabolic disorders or to inflammatory joint disease (Box 206-1) when the capacity of the chondrocyte to maintain a normal matrix has been diminished, when joint congruity has been altered, or when the biomechanical properties of the cartilage or subchondral bone have been modified. For example, secondary OA commonly develops in the wake of rheumatoid arthritis or infectious arthritis. In such cases the cartilage is damaged initially by enzymes released from inflammatory cells in the synovium or joint space. Interleukin-1 and tumor necrosis factor, which are produced by mononuclear cells in the inflamed joint, suppress proteoglycan (PG) synthesis by the chondrocyte, on the one hand, and stimulate it to synthesize and release matrix-degrading proteases (e.g., stromelysin, collagenase, gelatinase) on the other. This "double hit" results in a matrix that is highly vulnerable to mechanical breakdown.

Hemochromatosis, Wilson's disease, ochronosis, gout, and calcium pyrophosphate dihydrate (CPPD) crystal deposition disease also may lead to secondary OA. In these instances deposits of hemosiderin, copper, homogentisic acid polymers, crystals of monosodium urate, or crystals of CPPD, respectively, may damage the chondrocyte. In some cases they may exert a direct mechanical effect, increasing cartilage stiffness and altering load forces.

LABORATORY STUDIES

No specific clinical laboratory abnormality is present in primary OA. The sedimentation rate is normal for the age of the patient. The synovial fluid shows only a slight increase in cell count (<2000 cells/mm^3) with normal viscosity and normal mucin. Fragments of cartilage and/or bone ("wear particles") or crystals of calcium hydroxyapatite or CPPD, or both, may be seen.

RADIOGRAPHIC EXAMINATION

The radiographic findings in OA are described in Chapter 184. A combination of joint space narrowing, sclerosis of subchondral bone, and bony outgrowths (osteophytosis) is typical. Subchondral cysts may be prominent, especially in the hip. Notably, in some patients with joint pain caused by OA, radiographs are normal even when arthroscopy reveals full-thickness ulceration of the articular cartilage. Osteophytes alone, without joint space narrowing, subchondral sclerosis or subchondral cysts, may be caused by aging and do not necessarily indicate underlying cartilage damage. Therefore they are not diagnostic of OA.

TREATMENT

The goals of treatment are to relieve pain, increase mobility, reduce disability, and prevent progression of the disease. Although many patients require only reassurance, a mild analgesic, and instruction about joint protection, cases of more severe OA warrant an aggressive, comprehensive approach using physical measures, drugs and surgery.

Reduction of Joint Loading

Osteoarthritis may be caused or aggravated by poor body mechanics. For example, genu varum or valgum or pronated feet may create excessive loading on the knee. This can be corrected with orthotics or osteotomy. Knee pain in individuals with patellofemoral OA can be significantly reduced by medial taping of the patella. The relief of pain may be maintained with an exercise program to strengthen the vastus medialis obliqus component of the quadriceps muscle to facilitate realignment of the patella. The taping procedure is simple, and most patients readily learn to apply the tape themselves after minimal instruction.

A wedged insole, which can be fabricated by a podiatrist, orthotist, or physical therapist, may reduce joint pain in patients with early-stage knee OA. Use of a running shoe with a well-cushioned sole as primary daily footwear may also be helpful.

Because the excessive load imposed by obesity may accelerate cartilage breakdown in lumbar spine and lower-extremity joints, the obese patient should be encouraged to lose weight. In such individuals loss of only a few kilograms may markedly reduce the risk of developing symptoms of knee OA; in patients who are already symptomatic, weight loss may decrease the severity of joint pain.

A cane (held in the contralateral hand) is helpful if hip or knee OA is unilateral; crutches or a walker are preferable if it is bilateral.

For symptomatic OA of the first carpometacarpal joint, splinting may be effective. For painful OA of the neck a cervical pillow may be useful. The patient should be instructed not to maintain prolonged neck flexion or extension (as when shampooing the hair, sitting in the front row of a theater, or viewing television while lying on a sofa). Repetitive cervical rotation (e.g., watching a tennis match from a midcourt seat) should also be discouraged.

Activities that cause excessive loading of the damaged joint should be avoided. For the patient with OA of the hip or knee the workplace may be modified to permit sitting instead of standing. Kneeling and squatting should be eliminated. Jogging and participation in racket sports should be discouraged; swimming and bicycling are good alternatives.

Physical and Occupational Therapy

Local application of heat or cold and an exercise program are useful adjuncts in management of OA. Patients with significant OA of the hip, knee, or lumbar spine are less active and tend to be less fit than normal individuals. Both musculoskeletal and cardiovascular fitness are impaired. Exercises should be designed to preserve or improve range of motion, strengthen involved muscles, and improve cardiovascular fitness. Aerobic exercises that may be recommended include swimming, dance or water exercises, bicycling, and walking. Pool exercises and swimming cause less stress on the joints than the other forms with regard to strengthening exercises. An effective aerobic conditioning program can be implemented in individuals with hip or knee OA without aggravating their joint disease or increasing their intake of nonsteroidal antiinflammatory drugs (NSAIDs) or analgesics.

Because the periarticular muscles play a major role in protecting the articular cartilage from stress and weakness of these muscles is common, attention should be paid to strengthening them. Strength training programs are effective even in very elderly persons and can be accomplished without increasing joint pain. Within weeks, quadriceps strengthening exercises may result in marked decrease in joint pain in the patient with knee OA, permitting reduction in the dose of NSAID or analgesic drug.

Psychosocial Issues

It is important to recognize that disability in patients with OA may be related to psychosocial problems. In a randomized controlled clinical trial in patients with moderately severe knee OA whose dose of NSAID or analgesic was held constant, periodic telephone calls by a trained lay person, presumably serving to enhance social support, led to significant improvement in joint pain and function.

Drug Therapy

Drug therapy for OA today is aimed at relief of pain; no pharmacologic agent has been shown to influence the natural progression of joint breakdown in humans. Although salicylates and other NSAIDs often produce symptomatic relief in patients with OA, in many cases this is a result of their analgesic properties rather than their antiinflammatory effects. Therefore an antiinflammatory dose of NSAID may be no more effective than a lower (essentially analgesic) dose or than a pure analgesic. Neither clinical evidence of joint inflammation (i.e., swelling, synovial tenderness) nor histologic evidence of synovitis predicts a better response to an NSAID than to an analgesic in OA. This is important because the major gastrointestinal tract side effects of NSAIDs (hemorrhage and perforation) are dose dependent. The annual rate of hospitalization for ulcer was found to increase from 4 per 1000 for non-users to more than 40 per 1000 for those using the highest NSAID doses. When NSAIDs are prescribed for patients with OA, treatment should be initiated with a lower (i.e., analgesic) dose rather than a higher (i.e., antiinflammatory) dose, and the dose should be increased on the basis of the symptomatic response. Subsequently, if the patient's clinical status permits, attempts should be made to reduce the dose of NSAID or to discontinue daily NSAID treatment in favor of intermittent use as needed (e.g., during flare-ups).

Until recently, palliation of OA pain essentially revolved around the selection of one or another NSAID. However, growing concern about the gastrointestinal tract side effects of NSAIDs, especially in elderly individuals, the segment of the population at greatest risk for OA; growing awareness that symptomatic relief of OA pain in many cases can be achieved as effectively with acetaminophen as with NSAIDs; and documentation of the efficacy of a variety of nonmedicinal measures have led to a change in the strategy for management of OA symptoms. The keystone of the treatment program today is a spectrum of nonpharmacologic measures with acetaminophen as the drug of choice for pain relief; if NSAIDs are required, they are used in the lowest doses possible and then, as *adjuncts* to the nonmedicinal measures rather than as monotherapy. This approach is consistent with recent guidelines for management of hip OA and knee OA published by the American College of Rheumatology.

Muscle relaxants may occasionally be useful when pain is due to spasm. A tricyclic antidepressant may be useful in patients with chronic neuropathic pain, even in the absence of clinical depression.

Systemic corticosteroids have no place in treatment of OA. However, intraarticular injection of a glucocorticoid may provide pain relief and improve motion. Because of concerns that too-frequent intraarticular steroid injections may lead to joint breakdown, the procedure is usually not repeated more often than every 4 to 6 months. Gold salts, antimalarials, penicillamine, and immunosuppressive drugs are not indicated in OA. Capsaicin cream, which depletes sensory nerve endings of substance P, a neuropeptide mediator of pain, can reduce joint pain when applied topically by patients with hand or knee OA, even when used as the sole therapy.

Considerable interest exists today in pharmacologic modification not merely of symptoms but of joint damage in OA. A wide variety of agents has been shown to prevent or retard progression of cartilage breakdown in animal models of OA. These agents, which are called *Disease Modifying OA Drugs (DMOADs)*, range from site-specific inhibitors of the catalytic site of a matrix metalloproteinase, to protease inhibitors with broad specificity, to agents that stimulate anabolic activity of the chondrocyte, to substances whose mechanism of action is obscure. To date, however, no agent has been shown convincingly to have a disease-modifying effect in humans.

Orthopedic Surgery

Total joint arthroplasty should be considered for patients with advanced OA who have unremitting pain or severely impaired function that is unresponsive to an aggressive approach encompassing the previously discussed measures. Surgery may be remarkably effective in such cases, especially in patients with hip or knee OA. In the earlier stages of OA, osteotomy, which redistributes compressive stresses, may relieve pain and prevent progression of the disease. Arthrodesis, which permanently eliminates joint motion, is used with some frequency for OA of the subtalar joint and first carpometacarpal joint.

Arthroscopic removal of loose cartilage fragments ("joint mice") may prevent locking, eliminate pain, and reduce abrasive wear of the joint surfaces. Saline lavage of the osteoarthritic knee—flushing out cartilage shards and other debris—may provide months of relief for

---

✔ WHEN TO REFER

Most of the nonmedicinal measures used for OA management can be implemented by the primary care physician, although referral to a physical therapist or an occupational therapist may be helpful in some cases. When intraarticular injection of steroid is indicated, if the primary physician is inexperienced with the procedure the patient should be referred to a rheumatologist or orthopedic surgeon. Referral to a rheumatologist is also appropriate for tidal irrigation of the knee. If a comprehensive approach employing the spectrum of medicinal and nonmedicinal measures described in this chapter does not result in sufficient symptomatic relief, referral to an orthopedic surgeon for consideration of arthroplasty (or osteotomy) is indicated.

---

patients whose joint pain has been refractory to pharmacologic measures, including intraarticular steroid injection. For individuals with knee OA the procedure may be equivalent to (and is much cheaper than) arthroscopy and can be performed in the office by primary care physicians experienced in knee arthrocentesis.

BIBLIOGRAPHY

Adams ME, Brandt KD: Hypertrophic repair of canine articular cartilage in osteoarthritis after anterior cruciate ligament transsection, *J Rheumatol* 18:428-435, 1991.

Bradley JD et al: Comparison of an antiinflammatory dose of ibuprofen, an analgesic dose of ibuprofen, and acetaminophen in the treatment of patients with osteoarthritis of the knee, *N Engl J Med* 325:87, 1991.

Brandt KD: Management of osteoarthritis. In Kelley WN et al, editors: *Textbook of rheumatology,* ed 5, Philadelphia, 1997, WB Saunders.

Brandt KD: Nonsurgical management of osteoarthritis: with an emphasis on nonpharmacologic measures, *Arch Fam Med* 4:1057-1064, 1995.

Brandt KD, Mankin HJ: Pathogenesis of osteoarthritis. In Kelley WN et al, editors: *Textbook of rheumatology,* ed 5, Philadelphia, 1997, WB Saunders.

Felson DT et al: Obesity and knee osteoarthritis: the Framingham study, *Ann Intern Med* 109:18-24, 1988.

Felson DT et al: Weight loss reduces the risk for symptomatic knee osteoarthritis in women, *Ann Intern Med* 117:535-539, 1991.

Griffin MR: Practical management of osteoarthritis: integration of pharmacologic and nonpharmacologic measures, *Arch Fam Med* 4:1049-1055, 1995.

Griffin MR et al: Nonsteroidal antiinflammatory drug use and death from peptic ulcer in elderly persons, *Ann Intern Med* 109:359-363, 1988.

Hochberg MC et al: Guidelines for the medical management of osteoarthritis. I. Osteoarthritis of the hip, *Arthritis Rheum* 38:1535-1540, 1995.

Hochberg MC et al: Guidelines for the medical management of osteoarthritis. II. Osteoarthritis of the knee, *Arthritis Rheum* 38:1541-1546, 1995.

Minor MA et al: Exercise tolerance and disease-related measures in patients with rheumatoid arthritis and osteoarthritis, *J Rheumatol* 15:905-911, 1988.

Rene J et al: Reduction of joint pain in patients with knee osteoarthritis who have received monthly telephone calls from lay personnel and whose medical treatment regimens have remained stable, 35:511-515, 1992.

Smalley WE et al: Nonsteroidal antiinflammatory drugs and the incidence of hospitalizations for peptic ulcer disease in elderly persons, *Am J Epidemiol* 141:539-545, 1995.

CHAPTER

207 Gout and Hyperuricemia

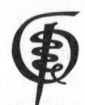

Robert A. Terkeltaub

The term *gout* denotes a heterogeneous group of disorders characterized by one or more of the following: (1) an increase in the serum concentration of uric acid (hyperuricemia); (2) recurrent attacks of a characteristic type of acute inflammatory arthritis in which microcrystals of the physiologic salt of uric acid, monosodium urate monohydrate, are demonstrable in synovial fluid leukocytes (acute gouty arthritis); (3) deposition of aggregates of monosodium urate monohydrate crystals (tophi) chiefly in and around joints and in soft tissues; (4) renal impairment associated with interstitial deposition of monosodium urate crystals (gouty nephropathy); and (5) uric acid urolithiasis. Hyperuricemia reflects a variety of metabolic or physiologic derangements that predispose to the clinical events just listed via the deposition of crystals of monosodium urate monohydrate or uric acid from supersaturated extracellular fluids. Although hyperuricemia is necessary, most often it is not sufficient for expression of gout. Therefore asymptomatic hyperuricemia is not a disease and should be distinguished in clinical practice from gout.

ETIOLOGY AND INCIDENCE

As a result of the evolutionary absence of the enzyme urate oxidase (uricase), humans are unable to oxidize uric acid to the soluble compound allantoin and must excrete the relatively insoluble compound uric acid as the end product of purine metabolism. In mice, which normally express the uricase gene, deletion of the uricase gene by homologous recombination induces hyperuricemia and renal deposition of uric acid crystals. Thus the lack of uricase predisposes the entire human species to the hazards of hyperuricemia and tissue deposition of crystalline uric acid. In addition, the sum of the complex array of renal mechanisms involved in uric acid excretion is net retention of more than 90% of urate filtered at the glomerulus, imposing a narrow margin of safety for serum urate concentrations. Specifically, the average serum urate concentrations in normal adult men and women are nearly 6 and 5 mg/dl, respectively, but the theoretic limit of solubility of monosodium urate in plasma is approximately 6.7 mg/dl.

Because many genetic and environmental influences govern and balance uric acid formation, transport, and disposal (discussed later), superimposition of one or more derangements in these processes can lead to hyperuricemia and gout. In fact, hyperuricemia (as defined by serum urate concentrations >7 mg/dl in men and >6 mg/dl in women) occurs in 5% to 10% of asymptomatic adult Americans. It appears that in less than 20% of this group clinically apparent urate crystal deposition develops, supporting conservative management for asymptomatic hyperuricemic individuals. The incidences of gouty arthritis and of uric acid urolithiasis among previously asymptomatic persons increase with the severity of hyperuricemia and become quite substantial when serum urate concentrations persistently exceed 9 mg/dl. However, recent data relevant to the long-term effects of hyperuricemia on renal function suggest that in most individuals higher degrees of hyperuricemia are tolerated with little apparent jeopardy to the kidney.

In 1986 the prevalence of self-reported gout in the United States was estimated at 13.6 per 1000 men and 6.4 per 1000 women. Gout is not only a common disease but also a significant public health problem because of its frequent association with short-term disability, occupational limitations, and the use of medical services. The prevalence of gout appears to have increased over the last few decades in the United States and in certain other countries with high standards of living. Gout is predominantly a disease of adult men and has a peak incidence in the fifth decade. In the United States, black men appear to have an incidence of gout higher than that of white men, possibly related to an increased prevalence of hypertension.

Gout rarely occurs in boys before adolescence or in women before menopause. These features correlate well with age-related patterns of serum urate concentration, which in men show a sharp increase during puberty with a subsequent plateau. In contrast, average serum urate concentrations during the reproductive period in women are nearly 1 mg/dl lower than those in age-matched men. The uricosuric effects of estrogens are believed to contribute to this phenomenon. Serum urate concentrations rise in women after menopause to levels comparable to those in men. The incidence of gout appears to be rising in elderly women and men in Western countries in association with lengthening of life expectancy and the frequent usage of diuretics in this group of individuals.

PATHOGENESIS
Purine Metabolism

Uric acid is the physiologic end-product of human purine metabolism (Fig. 207-1), and its remote sources are the ingestion of dietary purine-containing foods and the endogenous synthesis of purine nucleotides, which are building blocks in the synthesis of nucleic acids. Degradation of nucleic acids and free purine nucleotides to the purine bases xanthine and hypoxanthine and the sequential oxidation of these bases (mainly in the liver) to uric acid by the enzyme xanthine oxidase constitute the catabolic steps resulting in uric acid production. Urate circulates in the plasma predominantly in an unbound form. Renal excretion is the major route for uric acid disposal and accounts for about two thirds of the daily loss of this compound from the body. Extrarenal urate disposal is accomplished mainly by bacterial oxidation of urate secreted into the gut.

De Novo Synthesis. The synthesis of purine nucleotides involves a complex interplay of two alternative biochemical pathways. In the pathway of purine synthesis de novo, small-molecule precursors of uric acid are incorporated into a purine ring synthesized in 10 sequential steps on a ribose-phosphate backbone donated by 5-phosphoribosyl-1-pyrophosphate (PRPP) (Fig. 207-1). The first reaction committed to purine synthesis de novo is catalyzed by ami-

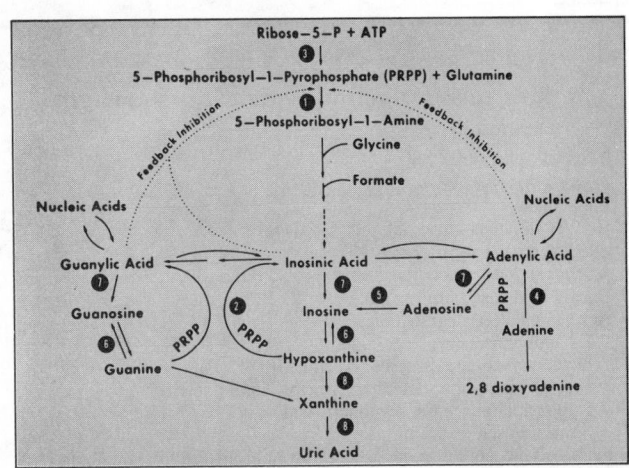

FIGURE 207-1   Outline of purine metabolism: *(1)* amidophosphoribosyltransferase, *(2)* hypoxanthine-guanine phosphoribosyltransferase, *(3)* PRPP synthetase, *(4)* adenine phosphoribosyltransferase, *(5)* adenosine deaminase, *(6)* purine nucleoside phosphorylase, *(7)* 5′-nucleotidase, *(8)* xanthine oxidase. From *Primer on the rheumatic diseases,* ed 11, Atlanta, 1997, Arthritis Foundation.

dophosphoribosyltransferase, which exerts a key rate-determining role in the pathway. Amidophosphoribosyltransferase activity is allosterically inhibited by purine nucleotide products of the pathway; feedback inhibition is reversed by PRPP, a substrate usually present in limiting concentration in the cell. The antagonistic interaction of purine nucleotides and PRPP at the level of activity of amidophosphoribosyltransferase appears to be of paramount importance in regulating the rate of purine synthesis de novo. Additional controls on the rate of purine nucleotide synthesis are exerted at the level of synthesis of PRPP and at the more distal branch point, which determine proportions of adenylate and guanylate nucleotides synthesized.

Base-Salvage Synthesis. The second pathway of purine nucleotide synthesis involves the two enzymes adenine phosphoribosyltransferase and hypoxanthine-guanine phosphoribosyltransferase (HGPRT), which catalyze single-step synthesis of purine nucleotides from the respective purine base substrates by reactions with PRPP (Fig. 207-1). The relationship between the rates of the base salvage and de novo pathways is likely to be governed in part by availability of the common substrate PRPP and by concentrations of the nucleotide products common to the pathways. Since the cell requires considerably less energy for purine base salvage than for purine synthesis de novo, preferential utilization of PRPP for purine base salvage is likely.

Production, Excretion, and Accumulation of Uric Acid

Measurements of uric acid synthesis and disposal have shown that the average readily miscible urate pool is about 1200 mg (range, 800 to 1600 mg) in normal men and is about half this value in normal women. Average uric acid production is about 750 mg per day in men; thus about two thirds to three fourths of the urate pool is turned over daily. Average urinary uric acid excretion in normal men receiving a purine-free diet, although somewhat variable, is 426 ±81 mg per day. The large discrepancy between daily urinary uric acid excretion and pool turnover is accounted for by extrarenal uric acid disposal. However, extrarenal urate disposal by the gut has only a limited capacity to be augmented in response to increases in serum uric acid.

From these considerations a number of potential mechanisms for excessive uric acid accumulation and thus hyperuricemia emerge. However, only diminished fractional uric acid excretion by the kidney, increased uric acid production, or both of these mechanisms acting in concert have been demonstrated to contribute substantially to the hyperuricemia of patients with the various forms of gout (Box 207-1).

The majority of patients with gout excrete normal total quantities

---

BOX 207-1
Working classification of hyperuricemia and gout

Uric acid overproduction
Primary hyperuricemia
Idiopathic
HGPRT deficiency (partial, and complete)
PRPP synthetase superactivity
Secondary hyperuricemia
Excessive dietary purine intake
Accelerated ATP degradation
    Ethanol abuse
    Glycogen storage diseases (types I, III, V, VII)
    Fructose ingestion, hereditary fructose intolerance
    Hypoxemia and tissue hypoperfusion
    Severe muscle exertion
Increased nucleotide turnover (e.g., myeloproliferative, lymphoproliferative disorders, hemolytic diseases, psoriasis, Paget's disease of bone)

Uric acid underexcretion
Primary hyperuricemia
Idiopathic
Secondary hyperuricemia
Diminished renal function
Inhibition of tubular urate secretion
    Competitive anions (e.g., ketoacidosis, lactic acidosis)
Enhanced tubular urate reabsorption
    Dehydration
    Diuretics
Mechanism complex or incompletely defined
    Lead nephropathy
    Hypertension
    Hyperparathyroidism
    Certain drugs (e.g., cyclosporine, pyrazinamide, ethambutol low-dose salicylates, dideoxyinosine)

---

of uric acid in urine. In the remaining individuals urinary uric acid excretion is excessive. The latter constitutes overexcretion, which has been defined by different laboratories as more than 600 to 700 mg per day in the presence of normal renal function in adult men with a purine-free diet or more than 800 to 1000 mg per day with a typical American diet. Increased rates of uric acid synthesis (overproduction) are almost invariably demonstrable by isotopic labeling studies in overexcreting individuals.

A working classification of hyperuricemia appears in Box 207-1. In this scheme patients in whom manifestations of urate deposition are prominent components of the overall clinical picture can be classified as having primary hyperuricemia, in contrast to patients in whom hyperuricemia and gout are generally minor clinical features resulting from any of a number of genetic or acquired processes.

Overproduction of uric acid can be associated with a primary derangement in the mechanisms regulating de novo purine nucleotide synthesis. Specific inherited enzyme aberrations can be identified in a small proportion of patients. In both the partial and virtually complete deficiencies of HGPRT, intracellular accumulation of PRPP resulting from diminished utilization of this regulatory substrate in purine base salvage drives purine synthesis de novo at an increased rate. In the case of variant forms of PRPP synthetase with excessive activity, increased PRPP availability for purine synthesis de novo results from increased synthesis of PRPP. Thus aberrations of these X-linked enzymes yield an increased uric acid synthesis by altering the balance of control of purine synthesis de novo toward increased production.

An increase in the net degradation of the adenine nucleotide adenosine triphosphate (ATP) has been proposed to be a factor in both the hyperuricemia of a subgroup of patients with primary gout and the hyperuricemia of a number of clinical disorders. First, the accelerated degradation of ATP to adenosine monophosphate (AMP) via the conversion of acetate to acetyl coenzyme A (CoA) in the metabolism of ethanol may be an important mechanism in hyperuricemia as-

sociated with alcohol ingestion. Furthermore, excessive alcohol consumption is a frequent feature in many individuals with gout. Second, hyperuricemia and gout are strongly associated with type I glycogen storage disease (glucose-6-phosphatase deficiency). There is evidence that hypoglycemia, a central feature of this disorder, stimulates uric acid synthesis via elevated levels of glucagon. Glucagon activates glycogen phosphorylase, and it is believed that an unopposed accumulation of phosphorylated sugars in the liver in the presence of glucose-6-phosphatase deficiency causes hepatic ATP depletion and the accumulation of AMP (adenylic acid), which is degraded to uric acid (Fig. 207-1). Third, fructose infusion and certain inborn errors of fructose metabolism have been reported to increase hepatic concentrations of phosphorylated sugars, consume hepatic ATP, and induce hyperuricemia. Fourth, in glycogen storage disease of types III, V, or VII, in which enzyme defects impair the resynthesis of ATP from adenosine diphosphate (ADP) in exercised muscle, moderate exercise provokes the enhanced release of uric acid precursors into the serum, resulting subsequently in hyperuricemia. In addition, the hyperuricemia known to occur with vigorous muscular exercise carried to exhaustion in normal individuals is associated with muscle ATP depletion and with marked elevations in levels of plasma hypoxanthine. Thus increased uric acid synthesis, not solely dehydration and hyperlacticacidemia, may contribute to the rise in serum urate and the occasional occurrence of uric acid nephropathy in this setting. Fifth, the marked hyperuricemia described in many acutely ill patients with disorders including hypotensive events or the adult respiratory distress syndrome is believed to partially reflect the systemic inhibition via hypoxia of ATP resynthesis from ADP in mitochondria, as well as the accelerated degradation of ADP to purine end-products. In these settings marked hyperuricemia (particularly a peak level >20 mg/dl), along with increases in plasma hypoxanthine, xanthine, and inosine, appears to indicate a poor prognosis. Sixth, overproduction of uric acid occurs with some frequency in a variety of acquired disorders in which there are excessive rates of cell turnover or tissue destruction. These conditions include several benign and malignant proliferative diseases.

In patients with gout and normal total uric acid excretion a relative deficit in the renal excretion of uric acid is the probable basis of hyperuricemia. That is, the excretion of normal amounts of uric acid is accomplished in these individuals only when serum urate concentrations are inappropriately high, a fact made apparent by the demonstration of decreased uric acid clearance in gouty normal excretors compared with normal individuals whose serum urate levels are experimentally made comparable by feeding of purine-rich diets. It is likely that virtually all plasma urate is filtered at the glomerulus, with more than 95% of the filtered load undergoing proximal tubular reabsorption. Subsequent tubular secretion contributes the major share to excreted uric acid, but the net urate excreted is modulated by substantial postsecretory tubular reabsorption.

There is no evidence that gouty "normal" excretors constitute a population with a single genetic or acquired renal defect. A diminished tubular secretory rate may contribute to hyperuricemia in some of these patients, and the possibility of increased tubular reabsorption in other patients with renal urate retention has not been dismissed. It is not certain whether such tubular abnormalities reflect primary defects in transport mechanisms or are caused by impairment of tubular processes by interfering metabolites (such as lactic acid) that accumulate in the course of one or more genetic metabolic disorders. Acquired, cryptic forms of renal impairment can be initially manifested by gouty arthritis alone. This is exemplified by the occurrence of gout in chronically lead-intoxicated users of unbonded ("moonshine") whiskey.

Gout patients as a group have a relatively high incidence of other diseases predisposing to diminished renal function, such as hypertension and diabetes mellitus. Another frequent factor in the occurrence of gout with normal total uric acid excretion is the administration of pharmacologic agents that alter renal tubular function either as a major action or as an unintended side effect. Among these agents are diuretics (including thiazides and furosemide), cyclosporine, pyrazinamide, ethambutol, and low-dose salicylates. The diverse actions of therapeutic agents on renal uric acid handling point out the many sites for potential alteration of uric acid metabolism that may result in the nonspecific end point of hyperuricemia.

Genetics and Gout

About 20% of gouty patients give family histories of the disease, and the incidence of hyperuricemia among close relatives of gouty individuals is 15% to 25%. However, pedigree analyses have not identified a unitary genetic aberration leading to hyperuricemia and gout in most individuals. Although inherited changes in the activities of a number of enzymes (Box 207-1) have been identified among patients with increased rates of purine synthesis and uric acid overproduction, alterations in the activities of the HGPRT and PRPP synthetase enzymes account for less than 10% of all patients with excessive purine nucleotide and uric acid production. The relative contributions of the other genetic defects underlying uric acid overproduction to clinical hyperuricemia and gout remain to be quantified.

Hereditary factors clearly influence renal urate handling in normal individuals, as demonstrated in twin studies. Furthermore, a number of kindreds with gout of relatively early onset and a markedly reduced fractional excretion of urate have been described. Genetic aberrations primarily affecting other metabolic pathways also are capable of altering renal urate handling, as exemplified by type I glycogen storage disease and maple syrup urine disease, in which lacticacidemia and ketonemia, respectively, can inhibit renal tubular urate secretion.

Hereditary influences appear to underlie the development of hyperuricemia in the majority of individuals with primary gout. In individual families this influence may be under polygenic or monogenic control and may be evident in disordered regulation of uric acid synthesis, inefficient uric acid excretion, or a combination of these mechanisms.

PATHOPHYSIOLOGIC AND PATHOLOGIC FEATURES OF URIC ACID CRYSTALLIZATION AND DEPOSITION

Although hyperuricemia has been associated on epidemiologic study with a number of abnormal processes (hypertension, obesity, glucose intolerance, and coronary occlusive disease), no pathogenetic relationships per se have been established. Similarly, a role for hyperuricemia per se as an isolated risk factor in the development of renal impairment is not proven. Rather, structural and functional kidney damage caused by uric acid excess from any cause is directly related to the physical deposition of crystals of monosodium urate at pH 7.4 or of crystals of undissociated uric acid in acidic urine (Chapter 349). In a minority of individuals with sustained hyperuricemia tophi and gouty arthropathy develop. Currently the factors that determine the predilection for urate crystal deposition are poorly understood. The diminished solubility of urate at the cooler temperatures of peripheral structures such as the toes and ears may help explain why urate crystals deposit in these areas. In addition, the propensity for marked urate crystal deposition in the first metatarsophalangeal joint may also relate to repetitive minor trauma there.

The observations that urate crystals often deposit in relatively avascular and proteoglycan-rich areas such as articular cartilage, that hemiplegia appears to have a sparing effect on the development of tophi and acute gout on the paretic side, and that tophi and acute gout occur within interphalangeal joints at the location of established osteoarthritic disease suggest the potential importance of both the structure and turnover of connective tissue matrix in urate crystal deposition. Although preliminary evidence has suggested that immunoglobulin may mediate the deposition of urate, the role of plasma proteins remains to be established. Interestingly, gout has been occasionally reported to occur in individuals without any past evidence of hyperuricemia, suggesting that decreased urate solubility alone may be sufficient for development of gout in a few individuals.

Macroscopic accumulations of urate can usually be visualized on arthroscopic examination in the synovial membrane by the time of the first gouty attack. Urate crystals found in joint fluid at the time of the acute attack may derive from rupture of these preformed synovial deposits or may have precipitated de novo, as exemplified in certain instances by the recognition of urate spherulites. In some individuals with gout, urate crystals can be found in asymptomatic metatarsophalangeal and knee joints that have never been involved in an acute attack of gout, confirming that gout can exist in an asymptomatic state.

Deposits of fine acicular monosodium urate crystals with a surrounding mononuclear cell inflammatory reaction and associated foreign body granuloma characterize the tophus, the pathognomonic lesion of chronic gout. Tophaceous deposits are common in cartilage (including articular cartilage), synovium, periarticular structures (including tendon sheaths and bursae), epiphyseal bone, and subcutaneous tissue; they can also occur in the renal interstitium. Tissue disruption and destruction proceed slowly, particularly as adjacent tophi coalesce, are joined by additional deposits, and provoke localized tissue responses such as pannus formation and osteoclasis in synovium and subchondral bone. The destructive effects of chronic tophaceous gout can progress even with antihyperuricemic therapy and are believed to be mediated by the ability of urate crystals to stimulate the release from mononuclear phagocytes and from synovial fibroblasts of inflammatory mediators implicated in bone and cartilage erosion and bone resorption. These mediators include interleukin-1 (IL-1), tumor necrosis factor–alpha (TNF-α), and prostaglandin E$_2$. Chronic multicentric urate deposition over a number of years can result in severe, deforming articular erosions, huge subcutaneous amorphous deposits, and localized tendon disruption or nerve entrapment. Tophi can appear rarely in visceral organs except for muscle, liver, spleen, and lung. They do not occur in the central nervous system because of the impermeability of the blood-brain barrier to uric acid and the inability of the central nervous system cells to generate uric acid as an end product of purine metabolism.

Interstitial deposition of monosodium urate in the kidney is associated with fibrotic and inflammatory changes in the renal medulla and pyramids resembling those of chronic pyelonephritis, with progressive damage in tubular epithelium of the loop of Henle and a peculiar form of glomerular sclerosis. The severity of gout correlates with vascular changes in the glomerular capillary bed and larger vessels.

At the usual acidic pH of urine the equilibrium between uric acid and urate is shifted in favor of the undissociated acid, the solubility of which is only 15 mg/dl. Even under physiologic conditions supersaturation of the urine with uric acid is required for excretion of the normal load of uric acid in a normal urine volume. With acutely increased loads uric acid crystal deposition in the collecting tubules can result in acute renal failure. More often, in hyperuricemic individuals in whom renal uric acid loads are chronically increased (overproducers), precipitation of uric acid crystals within a protein matrix in the renal pelvis, ureters, or bladder can lead to uric acid urolithiasis.

PATHOPHYSIOLOGY OF GOUTY ARTHRITIS

By far the most common clinical consequence of urate deposition is acute gouty arthritis, in which monosodium urate crystals liberated from deposits in and about the joint space or precipitated de novo appear to activate several humoral and cellular inflammatory mediator cascades, characteristically resulting in a severe bout of joint inflammation with extension of the process into periarticular tissues.

Crystal-induced activation of cells appears to be the central mechanism responsible for gouty inflammation. However, the precise roles of the individual inflammatory mediator systems in acute gout remain to be defined. Experimental evidence supports the belief that vasodilation, enhanced vascular permeability, and pain are promoted in part by the effects of urate crystal–induced prostaglandin release from cells within the joint space and the crystal-induced cleavage of biologically active complement peptides and kinins from inactive precursors. The release of a variety of cellular mediators (including IL-1, TNF, and interleukin-8 [IL-8]) from synovial mononuclear phagocytes and cartilage and humoral mediators (including C5a) probably triggers initial neutrophil adhesion to endothelium and neutrophil ingress into joints. Subsequent neutrophil phagocytosis of intraarticular urate crystals is believed to be associated with (1) the secretion of potent low-molecular-weight peptide chemoattractants for neutrophils (including IL-8) and arachadonic acid–derived chemotaxins (including leukotriene B$_4$ [LTB$_4$]) and (2) the release of lysosomal enzymes by secretion as well as by cell death. These events have been proposed to help establish a cycle of further neutrophil ingress, neutrophil activation by exposure to crystals and soluble mediators, and the amplification of inflammation. Furthermore, the systemic release from the gouty joint into the venous circulation of IL-1, TNF, interleukin-6 (IL-6), and IL-8 appears to be responsible for systemic manifestations (e.g., fever, leukocytosis, and hepatic acute phase protein response) in acute gouty arthritis and may help explain the capacity of the acute gouty attack to affect joints in more than one region.

The demonstration that experimental urate crystal–induced synovitis is markedly diminished when neutrophils are depleted by cytotoxic drugs or antineutrophil antiserum supports the critical role of polymorphonuclear leukocytes as the effector arm of acute gouty inflammation. Furthermore, the efficacy of colchicine in the prophylaxis of acute gout and in the treatment of early acute gout (discussed later) is believed to reflect its ability to suppress not only neutrophil adhesion to cytokine-stimulated endothelium but also the release of neutrophil chemoattractants from neutrophils exposed to urate crystals.

The mechanism whereby acute gouty paroxysms terminate (often without specific therapy) is probably multifactorial. Factors other than urate crystal dissolution or sequestration must play a role, since free urate crystals are often found in synovial fluid for weeks after subsidence of an acute gouty attack. Such factors are thought to include changes in the balance between proinflammatory and antiinflammatory factors, as well as modulation of crystal-leukocyte interaction via changes in the physical properties of the urate crystals. In addition, the limited functional life span (days) of normal neutrophils is believed to make continued ingress of neutrophils critical for the perpetuation of acute gouty inflammation.

CLINICAL FEATURES

Although it is presumed that patients with genetic gout possess from birth the underlying defects predisposing them to the disease, clinical expression is very infrequent in males before puberty and in women before menopause. However, uncommon exceptions to this observation exist and include type I glycogen storage disease in both sexes, in which severe derangements in the control of uric acid synthesis or disposal result in early and severe hyperuricemia. In addition, in the X-linked inherited states of partial deficiency of HGPRT and milder forms of superactivity of PRPP synthetase, early-adult-onset gout and a high incidence of uric acid urinary tract stones constitute the usual clinical phenotype in affected boys. Severe HGPRT deficiency is associated with spasticity, choreoathetosis, mental retardation, and compulsive self-mutilation (Lesch-Nyhan syndrome), in addition to clinical manifestations of hyperuricemia. Furthermore, in some individuals regulatory defects in PRPP synthetase are accompanied by sensorineural deafness and neurodevelopment defects. Women carriers of HGPRT deficiency and PRPP synthetase superactivity are predisposed to the development of symptomatic consequences of hyperuricemia in their postmenopausal years.

Clinical gout usually appears in men during middle life, a time in which the contributions of environmental factors and the attenuation of renal uric acid excretory function can combine with possible hereditary influences to produce hyperuricemia. In older individuals the propensity of urate crystals to deposit in osteoarthritic joints may make gouty arthritis more difficult to recognize.

Acute Gouty Arthritis

Acute gouty arthritis is characteristically (but not invariably) a disabling inflammatory process so dramatic in its onset and intensity as to have provoked numerous vivid literary descriptions. Often, the onset of exquisite pain and signs of inflammation occurs within minutes to hours, sometimes preceded by a few premonitory twinges in the affected area. Less frequently, the patient is warned of an impending attack by several days of slowly increasing discomfort, which eventuates in a full-blown episode. Typically the patient, well upon retiring, is awakened from sleep. The pain of acute gouty arthritis is usually so severe as to preclude weight bearing, and the patient may be unable to tolerate even the weight of a sheet on the inflamed area.

A precipitating event such as an injury, a surgical operation, a bout of excessive alcohol ingestion, an unusually heavy meal, an emotional stress, or a period of unaccustomed physical exertion may be related to the acute attack. Early in the course of treatment for hyperurice-

mia with uricosuric drugs or allopurinol, repeated acute gouty attacks are not uncommon. The precise manner in which these changes relate to urate deposition is unclear.

Certain characteristics of acute gouty arthritis are of value in establishing a specific diagnosis. These features include the pattern of joint involvement, the aforementioned qualities of typical gouty inflammation, and the course of the attack. Monarticular arthritis is the most common presentation, and a particular predilection is shown for the larger peripheral joints in the lower extremities. Podagra, acute gout of the metatarsophalangeal joint of the great toe, was described by Hippocrates, and the great toe remains the most common site of initial involvement in North Americans. Before the availability of effective treatment to reduce the frequency of gouty attacks, 90% of patients with gout had podagra at some point in the course of the disease. The ankle, midfoot (instep), and knee joints also are affected relatively frequently; upper-extremity involvement in the wrists, elbows, and metacarpophalangeal joints occurs occasionally. Bursal inflammation, particularly of the olecranon bursae, is common. The hips, shoulders, and spine very rarely are involved, especially early in the clinical course of gout.

Gouty inflammation involves not only the joint but also periarticular structures and skin, often yielding heat, redness, swelling, and tenderness in a wide area beyond the joint. The resulting appearance may suggest cellulitis, septic arthritis, osteomyelitis, or (especially in the foot) polyarticular arthritis. The tense, shiny skin overlying the area of inflammation may undergo desquamation as the attack subsides. Fever, leukocytosis, and elevated erythrocyte sedimentation rate may suggest an infectious process. If untreated, acute gouty arthritis usually resolves gradually but completely in 1 to 2 weeks. Occasionally, another attack in the same or another joint occurs during the recovery period.

After the initial attack about 10% of patients have no recurrence over many years, despite persistent hyperuricemia. More commonly, however, a symptom-free interval (intercritical gout) is terminated by a recurrent attack of arthritis, often during the first year after the initial episode. In the absence of treatment the ultimate course of gouty paroxysms is extremely variable; the majority of patients have an increase in the frequency of acute gouty attacks that may become more often polyarticular, more severe, and longer lasting. In other individuals the annual frequency of attacks may remain constant or even diminish, but in some the interval between episodes may decrease until gouty inflammation is virtually always present. A few patients do not exhibit the usual episodic course of early gouty arthritis, and their disease may proceed without obvious remission to joint destruction and disability in a relatively short time. In these patients gout occasionally may be confused with rheumatoid arthritis or other polyarticular inflammatory disorders.

Chronic Tophaceous Gout

In general, the interval between the initial attack of gout and the development of clinically visible tophi and crippling disease is prolonged, and tophi appear earlier and are more extensive in individuals with higher elevations in the serum urate concentration. However, great variability is evident in the development of structural changes in individuals at apparently comparable risk. Ten years after the initial attack more than half of the patients in one large series had either no tophi or minimal deposits. After 20 years, however, more than half of the patients had tophi and an appreciable proportion (24%) had deforming or disabling disease.

Clinically apparent tophi commonly appear as painless, firm deposits on the helix of the ear and less commonly on the antihelix. These tophi may be the sole urate deposits found or may be accompanied by irregular, occasionally large, deforming tophi on the fingers, hands, or feet. The olecranon bursae, the ulnar surface of the forearms, the tibial surfaces, and the Achilles tendons may harbor lumpy tophaceous deposits. The disruption of articular structures by tophi may potentiate the effects of repeated acute episodes of gouty arthritis and lead to chronic arthritis with irreversible erosion and deformity. Subcutaneous tophi may ulcerate through the skin and exude a white chalk or paste in which urate crystals are the major component. Such eroded tophi may drain for long periods and are susceptible to bacterial superinfection.

Uric Acid Urolithiasis

The incidence of uric acid urolithiasis in patients with primary gout is between 10% and 25% and appears to be related to the degree of hyperuricemia and hyperuricosuria. The mechanism of production, clinical symptoms, and management are discussed in Chapter 111.

Gouty Renal Disease

Urate crystal deposition and associated inflammation in the renal interstitium (urate nephropathy) and uric acid deposition in the collecting tubules (uric acid nephropathy) are relatively distinctive processes that can underlie the development of renal function abnormalities among gout patients. Nevertheless, the frequent concordance of gout and disorders such as hypertension and diabetes mellitus, both of which predispose to renal damage, and the association of lead poisoning with both nephropathy and hyperuricemia often render speculative the attribution of chronic renal impairment to gout. These issues are discussed in greater detail in Chapter 108.

LABORATORY AND OTHER DIAGNOSTIC TESTS

The interpretation of serum uric acid values and the definition of hyperuricemia are discussed earlier. When indicated, HGPRT and PRPP synthetase activity can be measured, but these assays currently are performed only by a limited number of specialized laboratories.

The diagnosis of acute or chronic gouty arthritis is unequivocally made by aspiration of the affected joint and visualization under compensated polarized light microscopy of strongly negatively birefringent, needle-shaped crystals (free and in leukocytes) in a smear of the synovial fluid, which typically demonstrates leukocytosis of 2000 to 50,000 cells/mm^3. The finding of urate crystals can be achieved in over 95% of joint aspirates in this disease (see Chapter 183), and a second joint aspirate is often positive for crystals in cases of gout when the initial aspirate was negative. The demonstration of typical crystals from tophaceous deposits is equally confirmatory, and studies have indicated some success and specificity in establishing a diagnosis of gout between acute attacks by demonstrating urate crystals in aspirates from asymptomatic first metatarsophalangeal joints.

Among typical radiographic features of gout are the presence of subcutaneous and periarticular masses adjacent to eroded bone, overall retention of bone density and joint spaces, asymmetric distribution of erosions (which may be periarticular or articular in location), and fine shelves of retained bone forming "overhanging edges" of erosions (Fig. 207-2).

Once a diagnosis of gout is established, it is important to ascertain whether the disease is primary or secondary (Box 207-1). A thorough history and physical examination, along with routine laboratory tests, including a hemogram and serum chemistry panel, can detect many diseases or environmental factors associated with hyperuricemia and gout, including (1) drug-induced hyperuricemia (e.g., diuretics, low-dose salicylates, cyclosporine, pyrazinamide, ethambutol, nicotinic acid), (2) chronic renal disease, (3) hematologic diseases (e.g., polycythemia vera, acute and chronic leukemias, sickle cell disease, hemolytic anemias) and other proliferative disorders (including psoriasis and Paget's disease of bone), (4) chronic lead intoxication, and (5) alcoholism.

In patients known to have intact renal function, it is advisable to establish whether hyperuricemia is accompanied by excessive or normal uric acid excretion, since the determination can be used in considering the options for hypouricemic therapy. If renal function is intact, this can be most readily ascertained by measuring the patient's urinary acid excretion during a 24-hour period (with excretion of greater than 1000 mg/day with a routine balanced diet generally defined as urate overproduction, as discussed earlier). Radiologic procedures employing contrast media and drugs that alter uric acid metabolism should be avoided in the midst of urine uric acid measurements.

DIFFERENTIAL DIAGNOSIS

The diagnosis of acute gouty arthritis is usually not difficult to establish, particularly in the setting of an attack of podagra or of acute

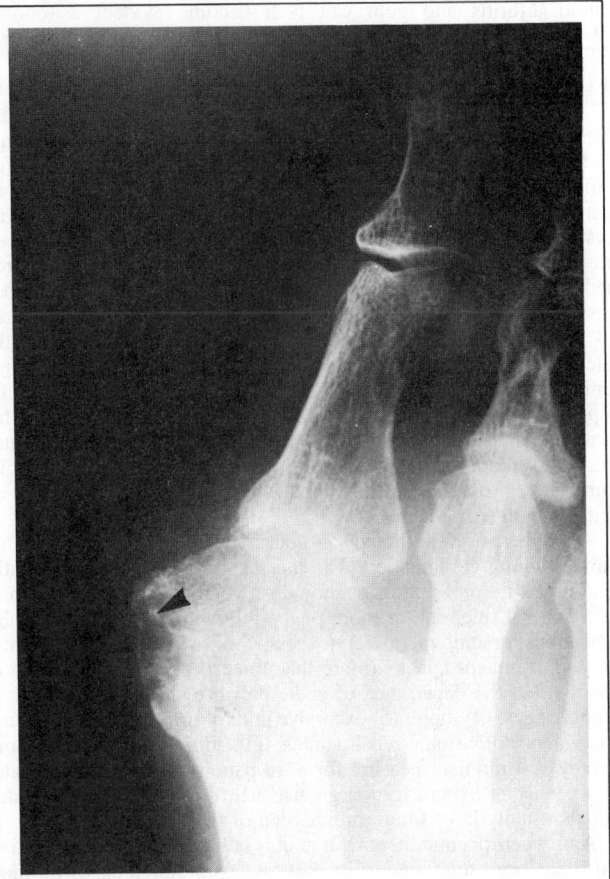

FIGURE 207-2   Chronic tophaceous gout involving the distal metatarsal and metatarsophalangeal joints of the great toe. The overlying soft tissue mass, the marginal and periarticular radiolucent bony defects (erosions) with a rim of cortical bone *(arrow)* forming an overhanging edge, and an area of stippled calcification within an erosion *(arrowhead)* are evident. In this oblique view, joint spaces and bone density are maintained.
Courtesy T. McDowell Anderson, MD.

monarticular peripheral arthritis in a hyperuricemic individual. Acute gout of the foot and ankle may mimic cellulitis, and cellulitis overlying a joint may mimic gout. Hyperuricemia is relatively frequent in the general population and is sometimes absent at the time of an acute gouty attack. Since other disorders (e.g., calcium pyrophosphate deposition disease, septic arthritis, Reiter's disease, and rheumatoid arthritis) can become evident as acute or subacute monarticular or oligoarticular arthritis, confirmation of the diagnosis should be sought by aspiration and examination of the synovial fluid from an affected joint, which must employ compensated polarized light microscopy. The possibility of infection coexisting with gout (or substituting for it) should be excluded by Gram's stain and culture of the fluid. Profound lowering of the synovial fluid glucose suggests septic arthritis or rheumatoid arthritis rather than gout. As discussed in Chapters 183 and 208, compensated polarized microscopy is required to distinguish calcium pyrophosphate dihydrate (CPPD) crystals, which are weakly, positively birefringent, from urate crystals.

A prompt, dramatic response to colchicine of attacks of acute gouty arthritis treated within 24 hours of onset is relatively but not absolutely specific, since responses in sarcoid arthritis, pseudogout, and rheumatoid arthritis are less complete and less frequent. Radiographs are of little diagnostic value early in the course of chronic gout but may show highly suggestive features once tophaceous deposits have developed, usually in areas of joints previously subjected to multiple acute attacks. Aspiration and examination of fluid from subcutaneous tophi or from a distended olecranon bursa are often indicated to confirm the diagnosis of chronic gout, in part because rheumatoid arthritis and gout can both become evident as chronic arthropathy with subcutaneous nodules.

MANAGEMENT

The aims of current therapeutic programs in gout and hyperuricemia are (1) to quickly resolve attacks of acute gouty arthritis with as few complications as possible; (2) to limit recurrences of acute gouty arthritis; (3) to prevent the disabling consequences of monosodium urate crystal deposition in articular, renal, and other tissues; (4) to prevent uric acid urolithiasis; and (5) to recognize and appropriately treat medical conditions commonly associated with gout, including hypertension, obesity, hyperlipidemia, chronic alcoholism, and chronic renal insufficiency. It is important to emphasize the distinctive rationale underlying use of antiinflammatory and antihyperuricemic drugs. Antiinflammatory drugs are used to treat or in the case of colchicine to prevent gouty inflammation, but they do not alter the state of hyperuricemia leading to the inflammation. Similarly, the uricosuric drugs and allopurinol reduce serum urate levels but have no antiinflammatory properties. In fact, their initiation during acute gouty arthritis is counterproductive.

Antihyperuricemic therapy in gout is potentially toxic, and it requires lifelong continuation. The therapeutic aims and the potential benefit-risk ratio of treatment should be weighed for each individual. As a general rule, one or more of the following serve as acceptable indications for antihyperuricemic therapy in patients with documented gout: (1) frequent attacks (more than three per year) of acute gouty arthritis, (2) the occurrence of acute polyarticular gout, (3) chronic joint changes, (4) tophi, (5) excessive urinary uric acid excretion, and (6) evidence of chronic renal damage. In addition, antihyperuricemic therapy is a rational measure for most patients with gout associated with persistent hyperuricemia greater than 8 mg/dl, since such individuals usually have future progression of the disease.

Antihyperuricemic therapy in gout is believed to be cost-effective, and it has been suggested to be cost-saving in individuals with more than one attack of acute gout per year. Allopurinol is believed to be more cost-effective than uricosuric drugs.

It is important to recognize that in some individuals the serum urate concentration can be successfully normalized without antihyperuricemic drugs by management of an associated condition or by removal of a specific etiologic factor (e.g., cessation of alcohol consumption, substitution of another class of antihypertensive agent for a thiazide in the treatment of hypertension, or improved treatment of Paget's disease of bone or psoriasis).

An important aspect of management relates to asymptomatic hyperuricemia. The great majority of individuals with this chemical aberration do not require drug treatment, although the adjunctive measures described later may be of value to the overall health of these people as well as patients with gout. The identification of individuals with asymptomatic hyperuricemia who are at highest risk and warrant specific therapeutic intervention, however, is an aim of management; conversely, avoidance of treatment in individuals in whom it is unnecessary is of equal importance.

Acute Gouty Arthritis

The severity of pain and disability associated with acute gouty arthritis demands prompt intervention, despite the usual spontaneous resolution of the process within 1 to 2 weeks. In general, the earlier treatment is initiated, the more rapid and complete the response to antiinflammatory agents. The involved joint should be placed at rest; on occasion, a narcotic analgesic may be required. Despite the impressive intensity of inflammation, gouty arthritis is usually quite successfully treated with any of a number of types of antiinflammatory drugs including the nonsteroidal antiinflammatory drugs (NSAIDs).

At present the NSAIDs are the preferred drugs in acute gouty arthritis. Indomethacin (50 mg three or four times daily for 2 to 3 days, with subsequent rapid tapering and discontinuation by 1 week) often leads to a prompt response, although headache and gastrointestinal tract side effects occasionally limit its use. Naproxen (initial dose, 375 to 500 mg twice daily) and sulindac (initial dose, 200 mg twice a day) also are generally effective. Many of the newer NSAIDs (see Chapter 205) are being used successfully in gouty arthritis. However,

salicylate-based drugs are not advocated for acute gout. Colchicine can also be used in low doses (0.6 mg by mouth twice daily if renal function is intact) as an adjunct to other agents for the therapy of severe acute attacks.

There are several primary treatment options for acute gouty arthritis in individuals who cannot take NSAIDs. First, oral colchicine is usually rapidly effective when administered in the first 24 hours after onset of symptoms (usual dose, 0.5 mg every hour until relief or side effects, most commonly diarrhea, occur or until a maximum total dose of about 5 to 6 mg [10 tablets] is reached). However, under most circumstances colchicine has the poorest therapeutic benefit-to-toxicity ratio of drugs used to treat acute gout. In particular, the diarrhea almost always provoked by oral colchicine may be severe. Thus colchicine use as the primary treatment for acute gout has been superseded by other modalities.

A valuable approach to the therapy of acute gout is the local intraarticular injection of a microcrystalline glucocorticosteroid ester. Such treatment is ideal and effective in a single large joint, regardless of the prior duration of the acute attack.

When the use of other agents is contraindicated, adrenocorticotrophic hormone (ACTH) has been employed successfully to manage acute gout (usual dose, 40 IU subcutaneously or intramuscularly with a repeat of this dose as often as every 12 hours for 1 to 3 days in incomplete responders). In severe, refractory cases of polyarticular gout intravenous administration of ACTH is often effective (usual dose, 40 IU units by slow intravenous infusion; this dose can be repeated the next day in incomplete responders). Systemic antiinflammatory corticosteroids are often useful when ACTH cannot be employed (e.g., in states of chronic severe adrenal suppression) or in refractory cases of acute polyarticular gout. Typical doses of prednisone are 30 to 60 mg prednisone per day, tapering to less than 20 mg per day by 1 week, followed by continuing therapy for 1 to 3 weeks. Intramuscular triamcinolone acetonide (60 mg as a single dose) or intravenous methylprednisolone (80 to 200 mg per day in divided doses) can be used in severe cases when the administration of oral drugs is contraindicated.

Acute gout can be observed in transplantation patients taking small maintenance doses of prednisone, illustrating the relatively low potency of systemic corticosteroids in acute gout. In addition, rebound attacks of acute gout can be observed after cessation of therapy with ACTH and systemic corticosteroids. Thus low-dose daily oral colchicine is particularly useful as adjunctive therapy in patients with acute gout who receive treatment with ACTH or systemic corticosteroids.

Intravenous colchicine is no longer advocated for general use in acute gout. The risk of serious drug-induced morbidity (and mortality) for intravenous use of this potent antimitotic cell toxin is significant, particularly in elderly individuals, persons with renal insufficiency, and individuals already receiving oral colchicine.

Improvement with the treatment of acute gouty arthritis usually begins within 6 to 12 hours and is often complete within 3 days. In a small proportion of patients, particularly those in whom treatment has been delayed, improvement is minimal and resolution slow. In some gouty patients attacks occur regularly after dietary excess, alcohol intake, or other identifiable precipitating events. Avoidance of these circumstances, when possible, can reduce the frequency of attacks. Patients should be encouraged to initiate preemptive therapy for recurrent attacks with an NSAID (or colchicine: typical dose, 0.6 mg/hour to a total of four tablets, not more than once every 3 days) at the first premonition or symptom of an impending episode.

Intercritical Therapy

Colchicine (0.6 mg once or twice daily with normal renal function; 0.6 mg every 2 to 3 days with renal insufficiency) is a highly effective agent in the prophylaxis of recurrent attacks of acute gouty arthritis. If regular NSAID treatment is required for chronic joint symptoms or for other reasons, colchicine may usually be omitted, since NSAIDs probably exert an adequate prophylactic effect. The propensity of gouty arthritis to occur repetitively in patients early in the course of antihyperuricemic therapy with either uricosuric agents or allopurinol is well established. Such attacks should not, however, prompt discontinuation of the antihyperuricemic drug, even during treatment for the acute episode. Thus colchicine (or an NSAID) is generally given on a prophylactic basis during the first 6 months of antihyperuricemic therapy. In patients who are still having recurrent gout attacks or in patients with chronic tophaceous gout more prolonged use of prophylactic colchicine is indicated. It should be recognized that in patients with diminished renal function who are taking "customary" prophylactic doses of colchicine (0.6 to 1.2 mg daily) over a prolonged period, bone marrow suppression or a proximal myopathy may develop accompanied by a mild axonal polyneuropathy and elevations of serum creatine kinase level. The myopathy is rapidly reversible on discontinuation of colchicine.

Tophaceous Gout

In gout with or without evident tophi the body pool of urate is expanded. Tophus formation represents crystal deposition from supersaturated extracellular fluids. Resolution of tophi, reduction of urate pool size to normal, and removal of the immediate source of further crystallization and clinical events are congruent aims that can be achieved by long-term reduction of serum urate concentration. In patients with normal renal function the desired therapeutic goal is a serum uric acid level below 6 mg/dl. In patients with renal insufficiency serum uric acid lowering to this extent is not attempted, since it is generally not possible without use of potentially toxic doses of antihyperuricemics.

Two classes of potent antihyperuricemic agents are available: uricosurics and xanthine oxidase inhibitors. Uricosuric drugs increase renal clearance of uric acid; allopurinol, the xanthine oxidase inhibitor, blocks uric acid production and is used more often by clinicians than are the uricosurics.

The uricosuric agents commonly used in the United States are probenecid and sulfinpyrazone. Both agents inhibit renal tubular uric acid reabsorption, thus increasing net uric acid excretion. It is essential to start uricosuric drug therapy at low doses to minimize the risk of uric acid urolithiasis. Adequate hydration via a daily fluid intake of 2 to 3 L and alkalinization of the urine with sodium bicarbonate are also important measures for this purpose. In addition, prophylactic colchicine should be administered during the introduction of uricosuric agents, for a period after serum urate concentration is normalized, and, in patients with tophi, until tophi are resolved.

The starting dose of probenecid is 0.25 g twice daily with a gradual increase over 3 to 4 weeks to a usual maintenance level of 0.5 g two or three times daily. If serum urate concentration remains greater than 6.0 mg/dl, an increase in the dose to 2.5 or 3.0 g daily should be tried. Sulfinpyrazone is given in a starting dose of 50 mg daily with a gradual increase to 100 mg three or four times a day.

Gastrointestinal tract symptoms and skin rash are the most common reactions to uricosuric agents; hepatic necrosis and bone marrow suppression occur very rarely. Aspirin and other salicylates are uricosuric at high blood levels; however, at lower levels the major effect of salicylates is uric acid retention resulting from inhibition of tubular urate secretion. They also interfere with the action of uricosuric agents and should not be used in the treatment of gout. Uricosuric agents are very effective as first-line drugs for many patients with gout and normal urinary uric acid excretion. Uricosuric agents are not first-line drugs in patients with excessive uric acid excretion, with previous histories of uric acid stones, or with renal insufficiency (as defined by a creatinine clearance <80 ml/minute). These patients and those in whom uricosuric drugs are ineffective should receive allopurinol. Although tophi may be dissolved with uricosuric treatment, the rate of dissolution is usually faster with allopurinol and most physicians consider the presence of tophi an indication for the latter drug.

Allopurinol is a hypoxanthine analog that undergoes oxidation to the metabolite oxypurinol, a potent competitive inhibitor of xanthine oxidase. In this way allopurinol reduces conversion of hypoxanthine to xanthine and xanthine to uric acid (Fig. 207-1). Hypoxanthine and xanthine are cleared efficiently by the kidney and do not accumulate in significant concentrations in the serum. Allopurinol also decreases the rate of purine synthesis de novo. Thus the reduced total purine load presented to the kidney, together with the redistribution of the purines into three compounds (hypoxanthine, xanthine, and uric acid) with independent solubilities, diminishes the likelihood of uric acid stone formation in patients with hyperuricemia and gout.

Allopurinol can be given in a single daily dose and initially should

generally be administered with prophylactic oral colchicine or an NSAID. A dose of allopurinol of 300 mg per day is usually appropriate for an average-size patient with normal renal function. The major active allopurinol metabolite, oxypurinol, is excreted by the kidneys, and its half-life is extended beyond 24 hours in patients with renal insufficiency. To avoid the accumulation of oxypurinol and minimize certain allopurinol toxicities that correlate with daily dosage (discussed later), progressively smaller doses of allopurinol are used in patients with renal insufficiency. Thus patients with a creatinine clearance rate of less than 30 ml per minute should receive 100 mg per day or less of allopurinol.

Although uncommon, adverse effects with allopurinol are more severe and occur more often than with uricosuric drugs. These reactions include fever, eosinophilia, dermatitis, elevation of hepatic enzyme levels, renal failure, headache, diarrhea, and occasional vasculitis. The allopurinol hypersensitivity syndrome, consisting of some or all of these features, has a high mortality (20% to 30% of reported cases), dramatizing the importance of reserving the use of this agent for patients in whom it is clearly indicated. The risk of allopurinol hypersensitivity is greatly augmented in patients receiving thiazide diuretic therapy and in patients with diminished renal function who have received standard doses of allopurinol. In patients receiving allopurinol, the dose of the chemotherapeutic agents azathioprine and 6-mercaptopurine should be much lower than usual to avoid excessive accumulation of the cytotoxic agent. Allopurinol may also enhance the toxicity of cyclophosphamide.

In patients with milder forms of allopurinol hypersensitivity (e.g., pruritis or isolated maculopapular rash) and severe gout, in whom uricosurics are contraindicated, oral and intravenous desensitization to allopurinol or oxypurinol (which at present is only available on a compassionate-use basis) has been employed with partial success.

Combined treatment with the two classes of antihyperuricemic drugs has been attempted. The greatest benefit of this combination may be to individuals with intact renal function whose serum urate levels are not satisfactorily controlled with either agent alone. In some patients with severe tophaceous gout allopurinol and a uricosuric agent may hasten dissolution of tophi.

Dietary restriction of purine-containing foods, although capable of diminishing serum urate slightly (on average, 1 mg/dl in hyperuricemic patients) is seldom necessary.

Asymptomatic Hyperuricemia

Epidemiologic associations between hyperuricemia and a variety of disorders, including atherosclerosis, have been made. However, there is no evidence that increased serum urate concentration is a causative factor in these disorders. There is also no evidence that treatment of hyperuricemia alleviates these conditions. Furthermore, neither hyperuricemia nor gout is clearly related to the development of clinically significant renal disease. The great majority of asymptomatic individuals with hyperuricemia are likely to live their lives without the development of clinical manifestations of gout. These considerations suggest that treatment of all individuals with asymptomatic hyperuricemia is unnecessary. Although the risk of gouty arthritis or uric acid urolithiasis appears to increase substantially with increases in serum urate concentrations above 9.0 mg/dl, these manifestations are readily treatable when they occur and should then present no long-term danger to the patient. Use of hypouricemic agents to reduce urate levels in individuals with asymptomatic hyperuricemia appears to be warranted only when (1) evidence of uric acid overproduction or overexcretion exists, that is, when daily urinary urate excretion in the presence of normal renal function exceeds about 1000 mg with a routine diet; or (2) there is a strong family history of gout, nephrolithiasis, or renal failure.

Adjuncts to Management

Although purine-restricted diets are infrequently advised in long-term management of gout, specific deletion of one or more purine-rich foods is sometimes advisable when identified as provocative agents in acute attacks. Weight reduction can contribute to lessening hyperuricemia and thus can lower the risk of gout through reduction in the rate of purine synthesis. Weight reduction to lean body mass, with special emphasis on reduced calorie and protein intake, is a general

Referral to a rheumatologist is appropriate to help establish a diagnosis of gouty arthritis when diagnoses other than gout (in particular, acute septic arthritis or CPPD deposition disease) are strong considerations and the expertise to aspirate an affected joint is limited or there is no access to a compensated polarized light microscope to properly examine the synovial fluid. Once established, the diagnosis of gout signifies that the patient has a well-understood and readily treatable medical condition. However, referral to a rheumatologist for further evaluation of established gout is appropriate in all patients with an age of onset of gout before 35 years, in all premenopausal women with gout, and in gout with demonstrable urate overproduction without an identifiable secondary origin or cause. Other appropriate indications for referral to a rheumatologist include frequent gouty attacks, despite therapy, or the presence of abundant or enlarging subcutaneous tophi. Large, draining subcutaneous tophi (e.g., of the olecranon bursae) may heal poorly with surgery, and referral to a rheumatologist for medical evaluation should generally be considered first. Erosive gouty polyarticular joint disease merits referral because it generally requires aggressive management to avoid further anatomic progression. Rheumatology referral is appropriate for patients with gout attributable to cyclosporine use, since gout is often rapidly progressive in this setting. Patients with advanced renal insufficiency from any cause, in whom management may be difficult because of adverse drug interactions, also may benefit from rheumatology referral. Referral is appropriate for patients with severe gout and allopurinol hypersensitivity when there are contraindications to the substitution of uricosuric drugs.

adjunctive measure that is especially likely to benefit the gouty population, in which obesity, hypertension, and hyperlipidemia are very common. Substitution of other antihypertensive therapies in the place of diuretics helps (and is sometimes sufficient) to reduce hyperuricemia. Reduction of alcohol consumption represents another approach applicable to the general population and is especially likely to benefit gouty patients whose hyperuricemia is potentiated by the effects of alcohol on both production and urinary excretion of uric acid.

BIBLIOGRAPHY

Cronstein BN et al: Colchicine alters the quantitative and qualitative display of selectins on endothelial cells and neutrophils, *J Clin Invest* 96:994, 1995.

Fam AG et al: Desensitization to allopurinol in patients with gout and cutaneous reactions, *Am J Med* 93:299, 1992.

Ferraz MB, O'Brien B: A cost-effectiveness analysis of urate-lowering drugs in nontophaceous recurrent gouty attacks, *J Rheumatol* 22:908, 1995.

Fox IH, Palella TD, Kelley WN: Hyperuricemia: a marker for cell energy crisis, *N Engl J Med* 317:111, 1987.

Hochberg MC et al: Racial differences in the incidence of gout: the role of hypertension, *Arthritis Rheum* 38:628, 1995.

Kuncl RW et al: Colchicine myopathy and neuropathy, *N Engl J Med* 316:1562, 1987.

Levinson D, Becker MA: Clinical gout and pathogenesis of hyperuricemia. In McCarty DJ, Koopman WJ, editors: *Arthritis and allied conditions,* ed 12, Philadelphia, 1993, Lea & Febiger.

Lin H et al: Cyclosporine-induced hyperuricemia and gout, *N Engl J Med* 321:287, 1989.

Roberts WN, Liang MH, Stern SH: Colchicine in acute gout: reassessment of risks and benefits, *JAMA* 257:1920, 1987.

Terkeltaub R: Pathogenesis and treatment of crystal-induced inflammation. In Koopman W, editor: *Arthritis and allied conditions,* ed 13, Baltimore, 1996, Williams & Wilkins.

208 Arthritis Associated With Calcium-Containing Crystals

Lawrence M. Ryan and Daniel J. McCarty

Various calcium-containing crystals cause or are associated with arthritis. The most commonly recognized, calcium pyrophosphate dihydrate ($Ca_2P_2O_7 2H_2O$ [CPPD]) crystals, were discovered in synovial fluid obtained from patients with acute goutlike attacks (pseudogout) when compensated polarized light microscopy was first applied as a diagnostic tool in 1960. Other forms of crystal arthritis may also cause acute goutlike attacks. Frequently the accumulation of CPPD crystals is sufficient to render cartilages radiodense. The radiologic appearance of calcified cartilage is called *chondrocalcinosis.* However, deposits of other types of radiodense crystals in cartilage, such as calcium oxalate, are indistinguishable on radiographs from CPPD deposits. Thus the terms pseudogout and chondrocalcinosis lack specificity. *Crystal deposition disease,* which embraces four specific, clinically polymorphic, metabolic arthropathies, was proposed. Thus gout is a clinical presentation of monosodium urate crystal deposition disease, and pseudogout is a clinical form of CPPD crystal deposition disease. Crystal aggregates composed of carbonate-substituted hydroxyapatite and octacalcium phosphate also occur in joint tissues and synovial fluid. Since these crystals are basic calcium phosphates (BCPs), the term *BCP crystal deposition disease* has been proposed. Calcium oxalate crystals deposit in cartilage, synovium, bone, skin, and other tissues in primary oxalosis and in azotemic patients receiving treatment with hemodialysis or peritoneal dialysis.

CPPD CRYSTAL DEPOSITION DISEASE
Etiology and Incidence

Chondrocytes in all hyaline articular cartilage and fibrocartilages secrete inorganic pyrophosphate (PPi). Whether overproduction or underdestruction of PPi or some peculiarity of the local cartilage is responsible for nucleation and growth of the calcium salt of PPi is uncertain. Cartilage is essentially a gel that contains cells. CPPD crystals have been grown in synthetic gels (e.g., gelatin) at an ambient physiologic pH. Since the smallest CPPD crystal clusters in human cartilage are perilacunar in the midzone of hyaline articular cartilage, it is likely that PPi secreted by chondrocytes or formed at their surface diffuses into the surrounding gel and under certain conditions precipitates as its calcium salt, which is sparingly soluble at neutral pH.

PPi levels in urine and plasma are normal in patients with CPPD crystal deposition disease. This is in contrast to the situation in gout in which extracellular anion (urate) is elevated systemically. However, joint fluid levels of PPi are predictably elevated in all patients with CPPD crystals. Thus local rather than systemic anion accumulation underlies CPPD crystal formation. The cause of PPi accumulation within joints is unclear and may be multifactorial. Potentially important elements include increased chondrocyte PPi elaboration by cells stimulated with transforming growth factor–β (TGF-β), increased expression of cell surface enzymes that generate extracellular PPi in the cartilage (nucleoside triphosphate pyrophosphohydrolase [NTPPPH]), and increased local concentration of substrate (synovial fluid adenosine triphosphate [ATP]) for the PPi-generating ectoenzymes. Formation of CPPD crystals would be further favored by matrix changes that promote crystal nucleation or growth, or both. NTPPPH activity is elevated in joint fluids containing CPPD crystals compared with fluids from patients with a variety of other forms of arthritis. Substrate levels (ATP) in joint fluid are also higher in patients with CPPD crystal deposits. Chondrocyte PPi elaboration in vitro is stimulated by certain growth factors such as TGF-β or by increased collagen synthesis. There appear to be multiple metabolic pathways of PPi elaboration by chondrocytes analogous to multiple pathways leading to hyperuricemia. In both gout and pseudogout, formation of a crystal is a final common etiologic pathway.

CPPD crystal deposits were found in the joints of about 5% of anatomic cadavers. Radiographic prevalence rates increase with age; nearly 30% of octogenarians are affected. The incidence of symptomatic disease is approximately equal to that of symptomatic monosodium urate (MSU) crystal deposition disease (gout).

Pathophysiologic Features

All CPPD crystals found in joint fluid are probably derived from articular cartilage. Tophuslike masses of crystals of varying size, possibly formed by coalescence of the smaller perilacunar deposits, may eventually become contiguous to the joint space or may be exposed to synovial fluid through cartilaginous fibrillation. These crystals are embedded in an organic matrix that stains differently than does the matrix of normal cartilage.

Since the CPPD crystals are in equilibrium with joint fluid Ca^{2+} and $P_2O_7^{4-}$, a fall in the concentration of either ion increases their solubility and loosens the crystals from their organic "mold," resulting in crystal "shedding" into the joint fluid. Major surgery, especially parathyroidectomy, lowers the level of serum calcium and consequently, joint fluid calcium level. Acute attacks of pseudogout occur typically after surgery on the second postoperative day, coincident with the nadir of the serum calcium level fall, and have been induced in knee joints lavaged with magnesium-containing buffers; magnesium chelates PPi and is a CPPD crystal solubilizer.

The PPi level in most arthritic joint fluids (2 to 20 μM) is higher than that of plasma (1 to 3 μM). The PPi levels in joint fluids in acute pseudogout are consistently lower than in chronically symptomatic joints. The intraarticular PPi pool turns over faster in inflamed joints; the lower PPi levels are caused by equilibration with plasma as a result of increased blood flow. Thus once crystal shedding begins, the resultant inflammatory response causes joint fluid PPi levels to fall, further increasing crystal solubility and accelerating the shedding process. The magnitude and duration of the inflammatory response may result from the number of crystals released and the rate of release. Experimental crystal-induced joint inflammation is related to the amount and nature of crystals injected. Other mechanisms that may cause CPPD crystal shedding are (1) joint trauma, particularly microfracture of subchondral bone and cartilage in weight-bearing joints; (2) digestion of the organic matrix holding the crystals in the cartilage by another cause of inflammation, such as sepsis or gout; and (3) metabolic perturbation of the composition of the organic matrix holding the crystals in cartilage. These mechanisms provide a conceptual framework for the finding of CPPD crystals in joint fluid after trauma, after joint inflammation resulting from other causes, and after treatment of myxedema with thyroid hormone.

CPPD crystals, like MSU, absorb various proteins, which are responsible for some of their biologic properties. Also like MSU, they are phagocytosed by neutrophils and cause release of a glycopeptide that is chemotactic for neutrophils.

Almost no dissolution of CPPD occurs in the synovial fluid, and the crystals are phagocytosed avidly by fixed synovial macrophage-like cells. Even crystals that have been "processed" by neutrophils probably enter these cells eventually, together with the remnants of the neutrophils. CPPD crystals are slowly solubilized in the acidic milieu of phagolysosomes within synovial cells with a half-life of about 1 to 3 months. Thus there appears to be a dynamic traffic of crystals in joints. The number of crystals in transit in joint fluid at a given time probably represents the net effect of release from cartilage and uptake by synovium.

Phagocytosis of CPPD crystals by synoviocytes in tissue culture stimulates the release of prostaglandin E_2 via stimulation of phospholipase A_2. These crystals also stimulate synthesis and secretion of metalloproteinases, including stromelysin, collagenase, and gelatinase, that may be related both to the destructive arthropathy seen in some patients and to the shedding of more crystals. CPPD and other calcium-containing crystals are potent mitogens for fibroblasts, synovial cells, and chondrocytes. After endocytosis they activate phospholipase C with resultant activation of the phosphoinositol pathways. They also activate the protooncogenes *C-fos, C-jun,* and *C-myc.* Their mitogenic activity might explain the synovial cell hyperplasia commonly evident on clinical examination in patients with such crystal deposits.

BOX 208-1

Conditions associated with calcium pyrophosphate dihydrate crystal deposition disease

Familial hypocalciuric hypercalcemia
Hyperparathyroidism
Hemochromatosis
Hemosiderosis
Hypophosphatasia
Hypomagnesemia
Hypothyroidism
Gout
Neuropathic joints
Aging
Osteochondritis dissecans
Amyloidosis
Trauma (including joint surgery)

Pathologic Features

CPPD crystals are deposited in hyaline articular cartilage but have a proclivity for deposition in fibrocartilages such as the menisci of the knee, the articular disk (triangular ligament) of the distal radioulnar joint, the glenoid and acetabular labra, the symphysis pubis, and the anulus fibrosus of the lumbar and dorsal intervertebral disks. In hyaline cartilage the smallest deposits are perilacunar in the midzone. Crystals are seen in normal-appearing cartilage, in the tophuslike masses already described, and lining clefts caused by fibrillation of degenerative cartilage. Less frequently, CPPD crystals occur in periarticular tissues other than cartilage such as synovial membrane. In these tissues they often appear to form in areas of chondroid metaplasia.

Clinical and Laboratory Findings

In our series of over 900 cases, men predominated in a 1.4:1.0 ratio. The mean age was 71.6 years (range, 36 to 98 years); the mean age at onset of symptoms of acute arthritis was 57 years (range, 30 to 90 years).

Cases of CPPD crystal deposition disease are classified as (1) familial; (2) associated with metabolic diseases or trauma, including joint surgery; or (3) sporadic. The absence of associated diseases (Box 208-1) in the familial cases is noteworthy. In two kindreds differing chromosomal assignment for the susceptibility gene has been reported.

In many joints CPPD crystal deposition appears innocuous; neither joint inflammation nor cartilage degeneration occurs. In others, for unknown reasons, recurrent acute attacks, subacute inflammation, or progressive joint degeneration—sometimes very severe—or a combination of these occurs.

Several patterns of arthritis can be distinguished on clinical examination. CPPD crystal deposition disease is a great mimic because it may resemble gout, rheumatoid arthritis, osteoarthritis, traumatic arthritis, or a neuropathic joint; rarely it even resembles ankylosing spondylitis, rheumatic fever, psychogenic arthritis, or generalized sepsis.

Radiographic Features

CPPD crystals in fibrocartilaginous structures, hyaline (articular) cartilage, ligaments, and joint capsules present a characteristic appearance that is helpful in diagnosis. Their typical location and appearance are shown in Fig. 208-1. Radiographic degenerative changes characteristic of CPPD crystal deposition are incorporated into the diagnostic criteria presented in Box 208-2 (see also Chapter 184).

An arthritic patient may be screened for CPPD with four suitably

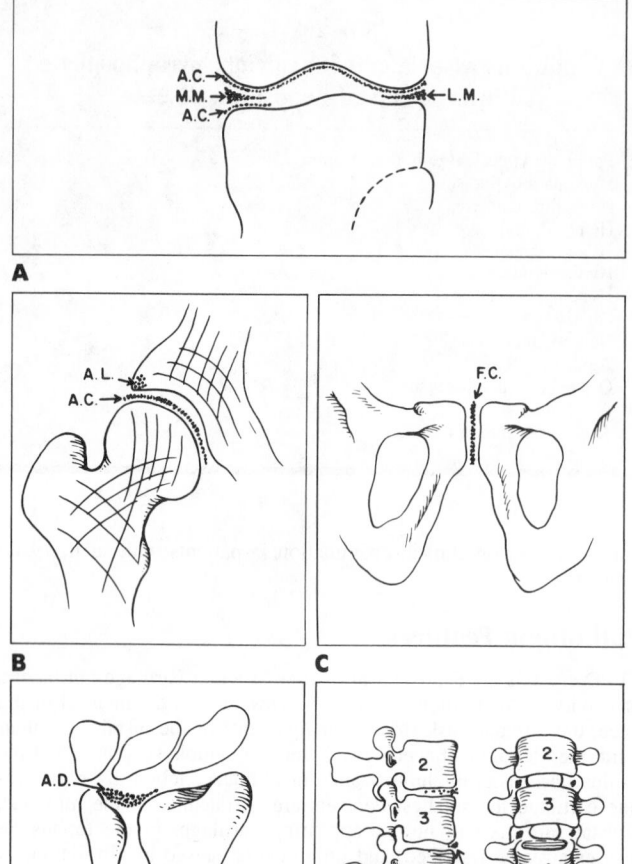

FIGURE 208-1   Typical location and appearance of calcium pyrophosphate dihydrate (CPPD) crystals. **A,** Anteroposterior view of knee; calcification of medial meniscus *(M.M.),* lateral meniscus *(L.M.),* and articular cartilage *(A.C.).* **B,** Anteroposterior view of hip; calcification of acetabular labrum *(A.L.)* and articular cartilage *(A.C.).* **C,** Anteroposterior view of pelvis; calcification appears as vertical line in the symphysis pubis (fibrocartilage *[F.C.]*). **D,** Anteroposterior view of wrist; calcification of articular disk *(A.D.)* of distal radioulnar joint. **E,** Lateral and anteroposterior views of lumbar spine; calcification in anulus fibrosus *(A.F).*

exposed radiographs: an anteroposterior view of each knee, an anteroposterior view of the pelvis, and a posteroanterior view of the wrists.

Diagnosis

Definite diagnosis rests on the specific identification of CPPD microcrystals (Chapter 183). The characteristic radiologic appearance of calcified cartilage and of certain degenerative changes is often helpful (Chapter 184). However, symptoms in such calcified joints can be caused by other types of arthritis, however, even if CPPD crystals are identified in joint fluid. The clinical picture is protean.

Therapy

Acute attacks may be treated with thorough aspiration of the joint, followed by injection of microcrystalline corticosteroid esters. Nonsteroidal antiinflammatory drugs in large doses are usually effective. Adrenocorticotropic hormone (ACTH) or corticosteroids are useful alternative treatments for pseudogout. The response to oral colchicine

---

BOX 208-2

Calcium pyrophosphate dihydrate crystal deposition disease: diagnostic criteria

Criteria

I. Demonstration of calcium pyrophosphate dihydrate (CPPD) crystals (obtained by biopsy, necropsy, or aspirated synovial fluid) by definitive means (e.g., characteristic "fingerprint" by radiographic diffraction powder pattern or by chemical analysis).
II. CPPD crystals on light microscopy or radiographs.
   A. Identification of crystals showing either no birefringence or weak birefringence on compensated polarized light microscopy.
   B. Presence of typical calcifications on radiographs.*
III. Characteristic clinical arthritis
   A. Acute arthritis, especially of knees or other large joints, with or without concomitant hyperuricemia.
   B. Chronic arthritis, especially of knees, hips, wrists, carpus, elbow, shoulder, and metacarpophalangeal (MCP) joints, especially if accompanied by acute exacerbations. The following features are helpful in the differentiation from primary osteoarthritis.
      1. Uncommon site (e.g., wrist, MCP joint, elbow, shoulder).
      2. Appearance of lesion radiologically (e.g., radiocarpal or patellofemoral joint space narrowing, especially if isolated).
      3. Subchondral cyst formation.
      4. Severity of degeneration: Progressive with subchondral bony collapse (microfractures), fragmentation, and formation of intraarticular radiodense bodies.
      5. Osteophyte formation: Variable and inconstant.
      6. Tendon calcifications, especially of Achilles, triceps, obturators.

Diagnostic categories

I. Definite: Criteria I or II A plus II B must be fulfilled.
II. Probable: Criteria II A or II B must be fulfilled.
III. Possible: Criteria III A or III B should alert the clinician to the possibility of underlying CPPD deposition.

*Heavy punctate and linear calcifications in fibrocartilages, articular (hyaline) cartilages, and joint capsules, especially if bilaterally symmetric. Faint or atypical calcifications may be caused by diacalcium phosphate dihydrate (CaHPO$_4$2H$_2$O) deposits or attributable to vascular calcifications. Both of these are also often bilaterally symmetric.

is unpredictable, but intravenous colchicine (1 mg) dramatically suppresses inflammatory symptoms. Prophylactic daily doses of colchicine reduced the number of acute attacks of pseudogout in controlled trials. Treatment of concomitant degenerative arthritis is the same as that for osteoarthritis (see Chapter 206). When the disease is associated with metabolic diseases, correction of the metabolic defect does not influence the course of the arthritis. For instance, removal of parathyroid adenomas, correction of iron overload in hemochromatosis, and correction of myxedema with thyroxine replacement do not result in resorption of the CPPD deposits.

Prognosis

Joint inflammation can be controlled in the great majority of patients with CPPD deposition disease, but joint degeneration, once established, often proceeds relentlessly and sometimes very rapidly to severe destructive arthropathy.

TYPES OF CPPD DISEASE
Type A: Pseudogout

The type A pattern is marked by inflammatory attacks of arthritis. Such episodes are self-limited and involve only one or a few joints. They can be severe, but less painful attacks occur and may outnumber full-blown attacks. About 25% of patients have this pattern.

Provocation of acute attacks by a surgical procedure or by medical illness is common in both gout and pseudogout. Trauma may provoke acute arthritis in either gout or pseudogout. Since both types of crystals are sometimes found in the same individual, joint aspiration and specific crystal identification are absolutely essential for precise diagnosis. Microbiologic examination has been useful in selected cases to exclude the possibility of septic arthritis.

The knee joint is to pseudogout what the bunion joint is to gout and is the site of more than half of all acute attacks. The patients are usually completely asymptomatic between attacks. Radiographic chondrocalcinosis is found in most patients who have this pattern.

Type B: Pseudorheumatoid Arthritis

Approximately 5% of patients have multiple joint involvement with subacute attacks lasting 4 weeks to several months. Nonspecific symptoms such as morning stiffness and systemic fatigue are common. Synovial thickening, limited joint motion caused by inflammation or attributable to flexion contractures, and elevated erythrocyte sedimentation rate are also found. About 10% of patients with CPPD-related arthritis have positive test results for rheumatoid factor, usually in low titer. CPPD deposits also have been described on both histologic and radiographic examination in patients with bona fide rheumatoid arthritis.

A variant of type B often causes confusion on clinical examination. The patient, usually elderly, has multiple acutely inflamed joints, marked leukocytosis, fever of 102° F to 104° F (39° C to 40° C), and disorientation. Systemic sepsis is suspected, and antibiotics are often prescribed, despite negative cultures. The entire picture reverses dramatically with antiinflammatory drug therapy.

Types C and D: Pseudoosteoarthritis

Approximately 50% of patients have had progressive degeneration of multiple joints. The knees are most commonly affected, followed by the wrists, MCP joints, hips, shoulders, elbows, and ankles. Involvement is generally symmetric, although the degenerative process is often further advanced on one side, especially in joints that have been subjected to trauma. CPPD crystal deposition should be suspected in patients with bilateral varus deformities or flexion contractures of the knees, or both, especially if accompanied by osteophytes and flexion contractures of other joints not ordinarily affected by primary osteoarthritis (wrists, elbows, shoulders, and MCP joints).

About half of patients with joint degeneration have episodic superimposed attacks of acute arthritis and have been classified as type C. Those without a clinically apparent inflammatory component have been classified as type D.

CPPD crystals often are found in joints without radiographically detectable cartilage calcifications, especially those with extensive degenerative change. Squaring of bone ends, subchondral cystic changes, and hooklike osteophytes, particularly in the MCP joints, are characteristic (see Chapter 184).

Heberden's nodes and other stigmata of primary osteoarthritis often coexist with the pattern of joint involvement peculiar to CPPD crystal deposition, probably a chance association of two common conditions affecting elderly persons.

Type E: Asymptomatic CPPD Crystal Deposition

Most joints with CPPD deposits plainly visible on radiographs are not symptomatic, even in patients with acute or chronic symptoms in other joints. Many patients with CPPD crystal deposits have neither acute attacks nor chronic joint symptoms.

Type F: Pseudoneurotrophic Joints

A destructive arthropathy resembling Charcot's joints may develop in some patients who have CPPD deposits and a normal neurologic examination.

Other Patterns

In some familial cases stiffening and straightening of the spine have been confused with ankylosing spondylitis. True bony ankylosis has

also been described in familial cases and is occasionally seen in the hips or knees of elderly patients. In some patients CPPD deposition and transient acute attacks are misdiagnosed as rheumatic fever or psychogenic arthritis. Hemarthrosis is not uncommon as a presenting feature. It is clear from the long-term observations of the natural history of CPPD joint deposition in familial cases that a given patient may show one pattern of arthritis early in the course of the disease and a different pattern later. Extensive crystal deposition with attendant tissue hypertrophy in the axial skeleton has been responsible for symptoms and signs of cord compression or radiculopathy, or both.

ASSOCIATED DISEASES

All putative disease associations are unproved; appropriately controlled comparisons either have not been made or, when made, have involved numbers so small as to make statistical application meaningless. The metabolic diseases listed in Box 208-1 affect connective tissue metabolism in some way. Since the prevalence of CPPD rises sharply with age, the question arises whether these metabolic conditions directly induce CPPD crystal deposition or cause a premature development of calcific deposits. CPPD crystal deposits associated with rare conditions such as hypophosphatasia and hypomagnesemia seem more likely to be "real" than do associations with glucose intolerance or hypertension. Although no causal relationships have been established, unsuspected metabolic abnormalities have been found repeatedly when appropriate laboratory studies have been performed. Measurements of serum calcium, phosphorus, alkaline phosphatase, magnesium, serum iron, transferrin, ferritin, and thyroid-stimulating hormone (TSH) levels are indicated in all new cases of CPPD crystal deposition occurring in individuals less than 60 years of age. Conversely, when arthritis supervenes in a patient with one of these metabolic conditions, the possibility of CPPD deposition disease should be considered. Screening for hypophosphatasia is unnecessary in elderly individuals, since CPPD deposition associated with this metabolic abnormality becomes evident at a young age.

Most series of patients with CPPD deposition show hyperparathyroidism in 5% to 15% of cases; about 20% of patients with hyperparathyroidism have radiologic evidence of chondrocalcinosis. Those with CPPD deposits are significantly older. The calcific deposits do not resorb after parathyroidectomy, and acute attacks often continue. Patients with radiographic chondrocalcinosis have an estimated 25% chance of having postoperative pseudogout following parathyroid adenoma removal.

Nearly half the patients with hemochromatosis have arthritis, and half of these have radiologic chondrocalcinosis (usually the older patients in a series). CPPD-related joint complaints may be present in patients with asymptomatic hemochromatosis. That iron may be directly related to the development of calcific deposits is suggested by reports of CPPD deposition in patients with transfusion hemosiderosis.

Hypothyroidism has been reported as being associated with asymptomatic CPPD deposits; joint inflammation is sometimes observed after treatment with thyroid hormone. Hyperuricemia, often accompanying mild azotemia, is common in elderly individuals. The coexistence of CPPD deposition disease and true gout with urate crystals has varied from 2% to 8% in most series.

BASIC CALCIUM PHOSPHATE CRYSTAL ARTHROPATHIES: MILWAUKEE SHOULDER/KNEE SYNDROME

The Milwaukee shoulder/knee syndrome is characterized by either stiff or hypermobile shoulders in elderly persons, mostly women. Glenohumeral degeneration and loss of the fibrous rotator cuff, often bilateral but most prominent on the dominant side, is accompanied by characteristic joint fluid findings including (1) BCP crystals (carbonate-substituted hydroxyapatite, octacalcium phosphate, and sometimes tricalcium phosphate) in microspheroid aggregates, (2) particulate collagens (types I, II, and III), (3) collagenase and other neutral protease activity, (4) low levels of α_1-antitrypsin and α_2 macroglobulin (two of the chief proteinase inhibitors found in serum or inflammatory joint fluid), and (5) leukocyte concentrations less than 500 cells/mm³. As many as 50% of joint fluids containing BCP crys-

✔ *WHEN TO REFER*

Patients with acute arthritis in whom pseudogout is suspected should be referred to rheumatologists experienced in joint aspiration techniques and analysis of synovial fluid. CPPD crystals are readily overlooked because of their small size and weak birefringence, and compensated polarized light microscopy is not available in many outpatient settings. Patients with recurrent attacks of pseudogout should be referred for consideration of prophylactic treatment. Those with refractory degenerative changes resulting from BCP or CPPD deposition may require orthopedic consultation and consideration of joint replacement.

tals also contain CPPD crystals. Symptoms occur late in the disease and are relatively mild. Pain after use and at night and decreased function of the affected arm are present most commonly, although the condition can be asymptomatic. Joint swelling is the rule, and hypermobility reflects dissolution of the rotator cuff.

Histologic examination shows focal synovial cell hyperplasia associated with intracellular BCP crystal aggregates. Extracellular crystal aggregates are present, scattered among collagen fibers. Endocytosis of BCP crystals by cultured synovial cells stimulates secretion of collagenase, gelatinase, and stromelysin. Incubation of tissues containing BCP crystals with collagenase in vitro results in release of the aggregates. If this process occurs in vivo, a cycle of crystal release, endocytosis, and protease release could account for the destruction of cartilage and rotator cuff that occurs in these patients. BCP, like other calcium-containing crystals, is mitogenic to cultured synovial cells, which could account for the synovial hyperplasia found in patients.

A similar destructive process associated with identical joint fluid findings occurs in the knees of patients with BCP crystal arthropathies, and the process is likely to involve the lateral tibiofemoral compartment associated with a valgus deformity, rather than the medial tibiofemoral compartment producing a varus deformity, as in primary "nodal" osteoarthritis. A role for mechanical trauma is suggested by the greater involvement of the shoulder of the dominant extremity. Osteochondromata are also often prominent radiographic features. It is likely that other large joints such as the elbow, hip, and ankle can also be involved by a similar process, but synovial fluid findings have not been presented to support this idea.

Treatment is symptomatic. Rest of the affected joint and nonsteroidal antiinflammatory drugs, analgesics, or a combination of these is probably helpful. Surgical replacement arthroplasty has been used with fair to good results.

CALCIUM OXALATE ARTHROPATHY

Interstitial fluid is supersaturated with calcium oxalate crystals when serum creatinine level exceeds about 8 mg/dl. These crystals have been associated with acute, subacute, or chronic joint symptoms in dialysis patients. They can also be deposited in the skin, blood vessel walls, and other tissues. These crystals, like MSU and CPPD, are phagocytosed by neutrophils during acute attacks.

BIBLIOGRAPHY

Halverson PB, McCarty DJ: Arthritis associated with apatite and other calcium phosphate crystals. In Koopman WJ et al., editors: *Arthritis and allied conditions*, ed 13, Baltimore, 1996, Williams & Wilkins.

Reginato AJ et al: Arthropathy and cutaneous calcinosis in hemodialysis oxalosis, *Arthritis Rheum* 29:1387, 1986.

Ryan LM, McCarty DJ: Calcium pyrophosphate dihydrate crystal deposition disease. In Koopman WJ et al., editors: *Arthritis and allied conditions*, ed 13, Baltimore, 1996, Williams & Wilkins.

Terkeltaub R: Pathogenesis and treatment of crystal-induced inflammation. In Koopman WJ et al., editors: *Arthritis and allied conditions*, ed 13, Baltimore, 1996, Williams & Wilkins.

CHAPTER

209　Ochronosis and Alkaptonuria

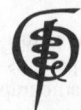

J. Edwin Seegmiller

ETIOLOGY AND INCIDENCE

Alkaptonuria results from a hereditary defect of tyrosine metabolism produced by a recessively inherited deficiency of the enzyme homogentisic acid oxidase. Consequently, instead of being oxidized in the tricarboxylic acid (TCA) cycle, homogentisic acid becomes the end product of both tyrosine and phenylalanine metabolism and is excreted in the urine throughout life (Fig. 209-1). Although this is a benign disorder during the first few decades of life, a black pigment derived from an oxidation product of homogentisic acid deposits progressively in the cartilage and connective tissue over the years, leading in the fifth or sixth decade of life to a severe degeneration of the cartilage of the spine and other major joints of the body. On microscopic examination of the black cartilage, Virchow in 1866 found a brownish, ocher-appearing pigment, which led to the pathologic designation of ochronotic arthritis.

The disease is generally regarded as a very rare disorder. In the former Czechoslovakia, however, a simple screening test applied to the urine of all newborns showed a frequency of alkaptonuria of 1 in 25,000 births, and the same test applied in the area of Cardiff, Wales, showed a frequency of 1 in 45,000 births (a far higher frequency than most geneticists would have expected in a British population).

Historically the disease has contributed substantially to the understanding of basic metabolic and genetic processes. The essential features of the one-gene, one-enzyme hypothesis were proposed in 1908 by Garrod as a result of studies of patients with alkaptonuria, 30 years before the more detailed development of this theory by microbiologists.

PATHOPHYSIOLOGIC FEATURES

Characteristically the urine turns dark on exposure to air, particularly if the urine is alkaline. Consequently, diapers of an affected child develop a brownish-black color if allowed to remain in contact with urine for any appreciable length of time. A similar darkening of clothing exposed to homogentisic acid in axillary perspiration and a darkening of axillary skin have been reported in some patients. In occasional affected children a lavender or even red appearance is found in diapers as a result of conjunction of homogentisic acid with certain amino acids but does not persist beyond the first year of life.

The amount of homogentisic acid excreted in the urine is directly related to the dietary intake of tyrosine and phenylalanine. The pathway of metabolism in which the block occurs normally serves to oxidize for energy production the surplus quantities of tyrosine in excess of those needed for protein synthesis and other metabolic functions.

Homogentisic acid has a renal clearance rate essentially equal to that of blood flow. Consequently, the concentration of homogentisic acid in plasma of affected patients remains extremely low. No difference has been found in ability of alkaptonuric and nonalkaptonuric individuals to excrete homogentisic acid rapidly after oral administration. A copper-containing enzyme, homogentisic acid polyphenoloxidase, may be involved in oxidation of homogentisic acid by a single electron transfer to a free radical hydroquinone, which then receives a second electron to become benzoquinone acetic acid before it can be deposited in connective tissue. The presence of the hydroquinone intermediate suggests the possibility of a free radical mechanism being involved in the damage produced in cartilage. Recent studies have shown that the portion excreted in the urine as benzoquinone acetic acid is substantially greater in adult patients than in infants. Benzoquinone acetic acid was reduced to undetectable amounts in adult patients receiving ascorbic acid, a known free radical scavenger, at a dose of 200 mg/kg per day for infants or 10 g per

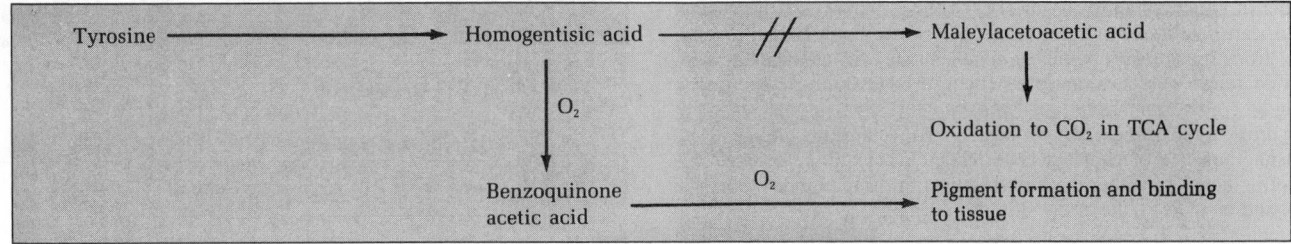

FIGURE 209-1   Metabolic block in alkaptonuria and possible mechanism of pigment formation and deposition leading to ochronotic arthritis. The tricarboxylic acid (TCA) cycle normally oxidizes the product of the missing enzyme to yield energy from surplus amounts of tyrosine and phenylalamine.

day for adults. The effect could also reflect the reducing action of ascorbic acid on preformed benzoquinone acetic acid. Also, an inhibition of proliferation of both rabbit and human cartilage cells in culture has been induced by concentrations of homogentisic acid quite comparable to those encountered in the serum of affected individuals. Benzoquinone acetic acid and its further oxidation products can readily react with sulfhydryl and amino groups, and the binding of this compound to connective tissues could well produce alterations in tissue components that lead to the cartilage degeneration that occurs in ochronotic arthritis.

PATHOLOGIC FEATURES

Despite minimal superficial pigmentary changes, deposition of pigment in cartilage and connective tissue is most dramatic. At postmortem examination dense pigmentation is found in cartilage of the larynx and in the costal cartilage in older alkaptonurics. Cartilage of the major joints of the body appears coal black. A similar pigmentation is also present throughout the body in fibrous tissue, tendons, ligaments, and fibrocartilage. Lesser degrees of pigment deposition are found in the intima of the large- and medium-size arteries and arterioles, arteriosclerotic plaques in the endocardium, stenotic aortic valves, various organs (kidney and lung), and the epidermis. Pigment can be both intracellular and extracellular and either granular or homogenous.

CLINICAL AND LABORATORY FINDINGS

The first clinical evidence of pigment deposition in cartilage appears in adults between 20 and 30 years of age and consists of a slight slate-blue or grayish color showing through the skin overlying the cartilage areas of the ears and occasionally of the nose. The ear cartilage feels thickened and irregular and is calcified in advanced cases. A dusky discoloration sometimes can be seen over the area of tendons in the hands. Another, more obvious site of pigment deposition is in the sclera of the eyes, where it is usually found about midway between the cornea and the outer and inner canthi in the general region of insertion of the rectus muscles. In some patients a more generalized pigmentation may also be detectable in the conjunctiva and cornea. With advanced disease the pigmentation may be noticed around the perifollicular areas of the skin of the hands or malar area of the face.

The earliest clinical symptoms are attributable to ochronotic spondylitis. Patients complain of stiffness and discomfort in the lower back, and in 10% to 15% of cases there is herniation of a nucleus pulposus. Stiffness of the lower back proceeds to rigidity with loss of the normal lordosis. Rigidity progresses to involve the dorsal and, later, the cervical spine. The first diagnostic radiologic evidence of the disease is a wafer of calcification of the lumbar intervertebral disks. Subsequently there is loss of joint space, and small osteophytes develop on the vertebral bodies (Fig. 209-2). In contrast to ankylosing spondylitis, the sacroiliac joints are not fused.

The peripheral joints are involved later, with some degree of limitation of motion in the knee joint or hip, or in some cases the shoulders. Most patients have periods of acute joint inflammation that may resemble rheumatoid arthritis on clinical examination. Later in the course of the disease the joints show marked limitation of motion.

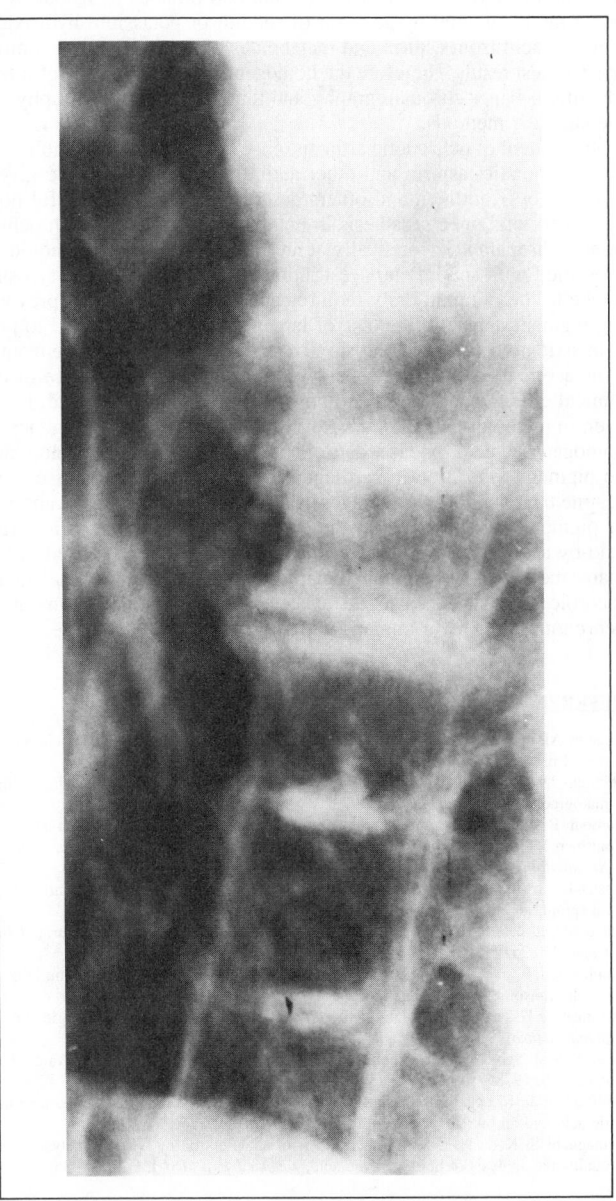

FIGURE 209-2   Alkaptonuric (ochronotic) spondylitis with widespread loss of disk space and waferlike calcification of multiple intervertebral disks.

Associated radiologic features include chondrocalcinosis and loose bodies in the joint space that may show calcification (see Chapter 184). Nuclear magnetic resonance imaging holds promise for detection of the pigment deposits in vivo. In many patients the pigmentation is so slight as to be scarcely noticeable, and the first diagnosis of the disease frequently is made with the discovery of the typical black cartilage at surgery for removal of loose bodies from a joint. The strong reducing properties of homogentisic acid can interfere with a wide range of colorimetric reactions used in clinical chemistry, including determinations of protein by the biuret reagent, 5-hydroxyindoleacetic acid by acidic ferric chloride, uric acid by phosphotungstate or cupric acetate reduction, creatinine by Jaffé reaction, glucose by either the copper reduction or the glucose oxidase test, and oxalate by the enzymatic determination.

DIAGNOSIS AND TREATMENT

Confirmation of the clinical or radiologic diagnosis is made by demonstrating the presence of homogentisic acid in the urine. A simple presumptive test consists of formation of a dark brown to black pigment on the surface layer of urine within 30 minutes to 1 hour of its being made alkaline by addition of sodium or potassium hydroxide. Gentisic acid from aspirin and metabolites of dopa can give a similar positive test result. Therefore the homogentisic acid must be definitely identified. Paper chromatography and thin-layer chromatography are the simplest methods.

Treatment of ochronotic arthritis, once the diagnosis is established, is symptomatic; aspirin and other antiinflammatory drugs are given. A report by Konttinen and others described the first successful noncemented total knee prosthesis in both knees of a patient with ochronotic arthropathy. Theoretically at an early stage the disease could be prevented with rigid dietary restriction of phenylalanine and tyrosine intake to the minimal daily requirements. The possibility of preventing pigment deposition by use of large doses of ascorbic acid to prevent oxidation of homogentisic acid to the more reactive benzoquinone acetic acid has been considered. No conclusive evidence of the clinical effectiveness of either approach has yet been obtained. However, in mice with alkaptonuria resulting from a genetic deficiency of homogentisic acid oxidase, ochronotic arthritis failed to develop, and no pigment deposition in cartilage was evident at 14 months of age, despite the excretion of homogentisic acid in their urine. This absence of pigment was attributed to the endogenous production of ascorbic acid by all mice in amounts comparable for size to those used in human studies. If so, lifelong dietary supplementation with adequate ascorbic acid should also be expected to prevent development of ochronotic arthritis in humans with alkaptonuria.

REFERENCES

Angeles AP et al: Chondrocyte growth inhibition induced by homogentisic acid and its partial prevention with ascorbic acid, *J Rheumatol* 16:512, 1989.

Feldman JM, Bowman J: Urinary homogentisic acid: determination by thin-layer chromatography, *Clin Chem* 19:459, 1973.

Kamoun P: Ascorbic acid and alkaptonuria, *Eur J Pediatr* 151:149, 1992 (letter).

Konttinen YT et al: Ochronosis: a report of a case and a review of literature, *Clin Exp Rheumatol* 7:435, 1989.

Koska L: Artifacts produced by homogentisic acid on the examination of urine from alkaptonurics, *Ann Clin Biochem* 23:354, 1986.

LaDu BN et al: The nature of the defect in tyrosine metabolism in alcaptonuria, *J Biol Chem* 230:251, 1958.

Montagutelli X et al: A mutation of the mouse homologous to human alkaptonuria maps on chromosome 16, *Genomics* 19:9, 1994.

Schumacher HR, Holdsworth DE: Ochronotic arthropathy. I. Clinical-pathologic studies, *Semin Arthritis Rheum* 6:207, 1977.

Srsen S et al: Screening for alkaptonuria in the newborn in Slovakia and in Wales, *Lancet* 2:576, 1978.

Wolff JA et al: Effects of ascorbic acid in alkaptonuria: alterations in benzoquinone acetic acid and an ontogenic effect in infancy, *Pediatr Res* 26:140, 1989.

Yamaguchi S, Koda N, Ohashi T: Diagnosis of alkaptonuria by NMR urinalysis: rapid qualitative analysis of homogentisic acid, *Tohoku J Exp Med* 150:227, 1986.

210   Amyloidoses

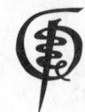

Merrill D. Benson

The amyloidoses are a heterogeneous group of protein deposition diseases characterized by specific chemical and physical properties of the tissue deposits (amyloid). Amyloid deposits are composed mainly of protein fibrils that are 7.5 to 10 nm in diameter when viewed by electron microscopy. They bind the histologic dye Congo red, and when Congo red–stained tissue sections are viewed through polarized light, the deposits show green birefringence, a characteristic considered specific for amyloid of all types. Other constituents of amyloid tissue deposits include proteoglycans, serum amyloid P component, and various lipoproteins, but all are considered secondary to the protein subunit of the fibril. There are a number of different types of amyloidosis, and each type is characterized by the specific protein that is found in fibrils of that type. In general, the proteins that make fibrils are plasma proteins, which are normally soluble but by means of various pathogenic mechanisms undergo a transition from solubility to insolubility and then aggregation to form fibrils. Common characteristics of amyloid deposits are that they are resistant to proteolysis and enlarge with time. It is generally assumed that disease expression is related to the disruption of normal tissue function, which is caused by the increasing size of the amyloid deposits. Of course, this process can lead to variable expression of the basic disease. For example, amyloid deposition in the heart leads to cardiomyopathy, amyloid deposition in the kidney leads to nephrotic syndrome or azotemia or both, and deposits in nerve lead to neuropathy. All these situations may occur alone or in combination to give a varied clinical presentation.

Since the different types of amyloidosis are characterized by specific precursor proteins, it is possible to classify these syndromes on a chemical basis (Table 210-1). It is important to remember that these are different diseases; although they may share some aspects of pathogenesis and they may have similar clinical features, as separate entities they have different prognoses and therapies.

IMMUNOGLOBULIN AMYLOIDOSIS

Immunoglobulin (AL) amyloidosis, also known as primary amyloidosis, is the most prevalent type of amyloidosis. It is the result of monoclonal plasma cell dyscrasia (either benign or malignant) in which the secreted immunoglobulin light chain (κ or λ) is incorporated into amyloid fibril structure. In the majority of cases of AL amyloidosis the monoclonal plasma cells retain normal features, although they may have increased amounts of cytoplasm indicating increased immunoglobulin synthesis. In a minority of cases malignant features are present and may allow a diagnosis of multiple myeloma or Waldenström's macroglobulinemia. In either case, organ dysfunction is related to fibril synthesis from the plasma cell light chain protein, not the benign or malignant character of the plasma cells.

The clinical manifestations of AL amyloidosis depend on the organ systems that are involved with amyloid deposits. The kidney, heart, and liver are the major vital organs that are often affected, resulting in nephrotic syndrome, cardiomyopathy, and hepatomegaly, respectively. Peripheral neuropathy (either sensory motor or carpal tunnel syndrome), gastrointestinal tract hemorrhage, purpura, macroglossia, and arthropathy (shoulder pad sign) may also be manifestations of AL amyloidosis. At initial medical evaluation these features may be present singularly, but more commonly features suggesting involvement of two or more organ systems are present. In particular, renal and cardiac amyloidoses often occur together, as may renal and hepatic amyloidoses. The nephrotic syndrome is an early manifestation of amyloidosis; the low serum albumin concentration from glo-

Table 210-1 Systemic amyloidoses

TYPE	CLINICAL NAMES	FIBRIL SUBUNIT PROTEIN (S)	DISTINGUISHING FEATURE
Immunoglobulin (AL)	Primary, myeloma associated	Immunoglobulin light chains (κ or λ)	Monoclonal immunoglobulin
Reactive (AA)	Secondary	Amyloid A	Inflammatory disease
Hereditary	Familial, heredofamilial, familial amyloid polyneuropathy	Transthyretin, apolipoprotein A-I, gelsolin, fibrinogen α-chain, lysozyme, cystatin C*	Autosomal dominant
β_2-Microglobulin (β_2M)	Dialysis	β_2M	Renal dialysis

*Usually restricted to intracranial blood vessels.

merular damage results in easily recognized clinical features. Cardiomyopathy may be fairly far advanced before angina syndrome or congestive heart failure is evident. Purpura, particularly periorbital, may be a presenting feature, but often major organ system involvement is also present.

Diagnostic Tests

Diagnostic testing usually reflects the organ system involved with amyloidosis. Nephrotic syndrome is frequently associated with proteinuria of 10 to 20 g per day, with the majority of this being albumin. The electrocardiogram in amyloid cardiomyopathy most frequently shows low voltage in the precordial leads and may also show conduction delays and either supraventricular or ventricular arrhythmia. The echocardiogram shows thickened intraventricular septum and left ventricular wall and usually enlargement of the left atrium, probably as a result of the restrictive nature of the left ventricle. None of these findings is specific for amyloid. There are, however, a few diagnostic tests that are very suggestive of AL amyloidosis. Since AL amyloid is the product of monoclonal light chain production, each patient with this disease has a monoclonal immunoglobulin dyscrasia. Eighty percent or more of individuals have an M component on immunoelectrophoresis of plasma or urine. Bone marrow aspirate usually has a slight increase in numbers of plasma cells (3% to 10%) but in the presence of multiple myeloma has more than 20% plasma cells with atypical features. These can be tested for monoclonality by histochemical analysis or fluorescence-activated cell sorter (FACS) analysis. AL amyloidosis is one of the few causes of clotting factor X deficiency, which leads to purpura. Partial thromboplastin time may be used to screen for this feature.

Treatment and Prognosis

AL amyloidosis has the worst prognosis of the different forms. Median survival varies among series but in most is 14 to 18 months from the time of tissue diagnosis. Median survival in patients who come to medical attention with heart failure and multiple myeloma is closer to 6 months. Five-year survival is approximately 20% in all series. The only specific treatment for AL amyloidosis has centered on cytotoxic therapy to reduce the population of monoclonal plasma cells. Combined melphalan and prednisone given orally in 6-week cycles has been used most extensively. Treatment with other alkylating agents such as chlorambucil and cyclophosphamide has also shown some success. Multidrug regimens in general tend to give less satisfactory results, since organ failure resulting from amyloidosis is a limiting factor. Recently, high-dose melphalan therapy with autologous bone marrow transplantation has been tried for a few patients, and results have been encouraging.

Nonspecific therapy for the different manifestations of AL amyloidosis is very important. Judicious use of diuretics, avoidance of negative inotropic cardiac drugs, and careful monitoring of nutritional and electrolyte status may be very important for the amyloid patient, especially during the early course of the disease after diagnosis, because the therapeutic effect of chemotherapy is usually delayed 4 to 6 months. Cardiac pacemakers may be indicated for conduction abnormalities, and kidney dialysis may be required for azotemia. Maintenance of normal sinus rhythm is important in preserving cardiac output in the presence of restrictive cardiomyopathy; however, calcium channel blockers and other potent negative inotropic drugs are generally contraindicated.

REACTIVE AMYLOIDOSIS

Reactive (amyloid A [AA]) or secondary amyloidosis is associated with chronic inflammatory diseases such as rheumatoid arthritis, ankylosing spondylitis, inflammatory bowel disease, osteomyelitis, and tuberculosis. The amyloid of familial Mediterranean fever (FMF) is in this group, since the primary disease is the periodic fever and the amyloidosis is a result of repeated episodes of inflammation. The fibril subunit protein, (AA) is a proteolytic product of serum apolipoprotein A (SAA), which is predominantly in the high-density lipoprotein (HDL) fraction of plasma. There are three functional genes coding for SAA—all located on the short arm of chromosome 11. Two gene products, SAA1 and SAA2, are acute-phase proteins synthesized by the liver. These two proteins participate in amyloid fibril formation. SAA4 is also synthesized by the liver, but in a constitutive fashion, and does not participate in amyloid fibril formation. An SAA3 gene that is expressed in some mammalian species is a pseudogene in humans. The function of acute-phase SAA (normally 1 to 3 μg/ml in plasma) is not known. During times of inflammation the plasma concentration may increase 500- to 1000-fold; therefore a function in removal of injured tissue or tissue repair has been hypothesized but not proven. The present incidence of reactive amyloidosis is low and probably reflects a lowered prevalence of chronic infectious diseases such as tuberculosis. Recent studies of subjects with chronic rheumatoid arthritis have shown an incidence of 6% to 8% for AA amyloidosis as demonstrated on gastric and duodenal biopsies. The incidence of clinically significant disease attributable to AA amyloidosis in rheumatoid arthritis patients is much lower.

Clinical Presentation

The most common clinical presentation of AA amyloidosis is the nephrotic syndrome, which may be present for several years before azotemia occurs. Liver and spleen amyloid deposits are also common but are of less concern until late in the course of the disease. Infiltration of gastrointestinal tract vessels, however, can lead to significant hemorrhage.

Treatment and Prognosis

Treatment of the chronic inflammatory process that is aimed at reducing the circulating levels of acute-phase SAA is recommended. In patients with rheumatoid arthritis who frequently have received prolonged treatment with antiinflammatory drugs the use of azathioprine or chlorambucil has been recommended. Colchicine is also given to patients with AA amyloidosis because it has a definite effect on the incidence of amyloidosis in FMF. Whether colchicine has a direct effect on other forms of AA amyloidosis is not known. Nonspecific forms of therapy are certainly indicated. These include renal dialysis for patients with azotemia. Reactive amyloidosis progresses more slowly than AL amyloidosis, does not result in peripheral neuropathy or macroglossia, and is less likely to be associated with purpura. It is less likely to result in cardiomyopathy. If life is prolonged with renal dialysis, hepatic decompensation resulting from amyloidosis is often the terminal event.

β₂-MICROGLOBULIN AMYLOIDOSIS

In a high percentage of individuals receiving long-term hemodialysis β₂-microglobulin (β₂M) amyloidosis develops. This type of amyloid deposition has a predilection for osseous and articular structures and often results in destructive lesions of the shoulder joints. Carpal tunnel syndrome is the most frequent initial manifestation and may occur in 50% to 70% of patients receiving dialysis for 10 years. Subsequently, diathroidal joints, particularly shoulders and hips, develop cystic lesions, and a painful articular syndrome ensues. Amyloid deposition in vertebral bodies also may occur and be life threatening. Pathogenesis is believed to be related to high levels of β₂M that cannot be cleared by hemodialysis. With the advent of long-term ambulatory peritoneal dialysis a similar pattern is emerging. β₂M, which is the light chain of the human leukocyte antigen (HLA) class I complex, is produced by all nucleated cells. Plasma levels may be as much as 60 times the normal level, and this presumably leads to the unaltered β₂M being deposited as amyloid fibrils. Structurally β₂M is similar to immunoglobulin molecules with extensive β-pleated sheet structure. The only specific treatment for β₂M amyloidosis is reestablishment of normal renal function. Renal transplantation has been effective in reversing this syndrome; however, many individuals with amyloidosis are not suitable candidates for renal transplantation. Therapy is often reduced to analgesics and surgical treatment of joint disease.

HEREDITARY AMYLOIDOSIS

Hereditary amyloidosis has become the most exciting area of study for amyloidosis, both in the basic research and clinical aspects. Many of the cases that were previously considered to be primary (AL) have now been shown to be hereditary, a finding of grave importance to both patient and physician. The majority of familial amyloidoses are associated with mutations of transthyretin, a normal plasma protein that transports thyroxine and retinol-binding protein–vitamin A (Table 210-2). However, a number of plasma proteins have mutated forms that are also associated with systemic amyloid syndromes (Table 210-3). In addition, a number of localized forms of amyloidosis may be associated with mutant proteins (e.g., familial Alzheimer's disease and the prion diseases including Gerstmann-Sträussler-Scheinker syndrome).

All the familial amyloidoses show autosomal dominant inheritance; however, they are of adult onset and sometimes come to medical attention very late in life, which tends to obscure the inheritance pattern. In addition, many of the transthyretin amyloidoses result in cardiomyopathy late in life, and this may be easily mistaken for the more common atherosclerotic cardiac disease.

The clinical manifestations of hereditary amyloidosis vary with the specific protein variant. Most of the transthyretin syndromes have some degree of generalized peripheral neuropathy or carpal tunnel syndrome, or both. Approximately one third of the transthyretin mutations are associated with amyloid deposits in the vitreous of the eye, and a very large number cause restrictive cardiomyopathy. Autonomic nervous system involvement results in orthostatic hypotension and gastrointestinal tract motility problems with resultant malnutrition. The sensory motor neuropathy typically starts with numbness and tingling in the lower extremities and progresses to involve more proximal areas. In some cases the neuropathy may be the most debilitating part of the disease; in others it may be mild. A few transthyretin mutations result in no neuropathy at all. Renal failure occurs in a minority of individuals; cardiomyopathy is more common. Of the amyloidosis associated with apolipoprotein A-I mutations, only the Arg26 mutation is associated with neuropathy (see Table 210-3). In general, the apo A-I syndromes result in renal and hepatic amyloid with death attributable to azotemia. Amyloidoses attributable to mutations in fibrinogen α-chain are all associated with renal amyloidosis and death as a result of azotemia, usually preceded by nephrosis and hypertension.

Clinical features that distinguish hereditary amyloidosis from AL amyloidosis include the absence of macroglossia and monoclonal protein in the plasma. Otherwise, the two diseases can be very similar on clinical examination, although hereditary amyloidosis usually progresses over a much longer time span. Very often patients

Table 210-2   Transthyretin amyloidoses

MUTATION	ORGAN INVOLVEMENT CLINICAL FEATURES	GEOGRAPHIC KINDREDS
Cys10Arg	Heart, eye, PN	US (Penn.)
Leu12Pro	LM, liver	United Kingdom
Asp18Glu	PN	South America
Asp18Gly	LM	Hungary
Val20Ile	Heart, CTS	Germany, US
Pro24Ser	Heart, CTS, PN	US
Val30Met	PN, AN, eye, LM	Portugal, Japan, Sweden, US
ValA30Ala	Heart, AN	US
Val30Leu	PN	Japan
Val30Gly	LM, eye	US
Phe33Ile	PN, eye	Israel
Phe33Leu	PN, heart	US
Phe33Val	PN	United Kingdom
Arg34Thr	PN, heart	Italy
Lys35Asn	PN, AN, heart	France
Ala36Pro	Eye, CTS	US
Glu42Gly	PN, AN, heart	Japan
Ala45Thr	Heart	US
Ala45Asp	Heart, PN	US
Gly47Arg	PN, AN	Japan
Gly47Ala	Heart, AN	Italy, Germany
Gly47Val	CTS, PN, AN, heart	Sri Lanka
Thr49Ala	Heart, CTS	France, Italy
Ser50Arg	AN, PN	Japan, French/Italian
Ser50Ile	Heart, PN, AN	Japan
Ser52Pro	PN, AN, heart, kidney	England
Glu54Gly	PN, AN, eye	England
Leu55Pro	Heart, AN, eye	US, Taiwan
Leu58His	CTS, heart	US (Md.)
Leu58Arg	CTS, AN, eye	Japan
Thr59Lys	Heart, PN, AN	Italy
Thr60Ala	Heart, CTS	US
Glu61Lys	PN	Japan
Phe64Leu	PN, CTS, heart	US, Italy
Ile68Leu	Heart	Germany
Tyr69His	Eye	US
Lys70Asn	Eye, CTS, PN	US
Val71Ala	PN, eye, CTS	France, Spain
Ser77Tyr	Kidney	US (Ill., Texas), France
Ile84Ser	Heart, CTS, eye, LM	US (Ind.) Hungary
Ile84Asn	Heart, eye	US
Glu89Gln	PN, heart	Italy
Ala97Gly	Heart, PN	Japan
Ile107Val	Heart, CTS, PN	US
Leu111Met	Heart	Denmark
Ser112Ile	PN, heart	Italy
Tyr114Cys	PN, AN, eye, LM	Japan
Tyr114His	CTS	Japan
Val122Ile	Heart	US
Δval122	Heart, PN	US, Ecuador

AN, Autonomic neuropathy; *CTS,* carpal tunnel syndrome; *eye,* vitreous deposits; *LM,* leptomeningeal; *PN,* peripheral neuropathy.

live 10 to 15 years after clinical presentation of the amyloid syndrome.

Treatment and Prognosis

Nonspecific therapy for hereditary amyloidosis is similar to treatment for the other systemic syndromes. Restrictive cardiomyopathy requires particular attention, since in the presence of autonomic neuropathy maintenance of blood pressure and cardiac output is difficult. In the last 5 years a number of liver transplantations have been performed as curative measures for the transthyretin amyloidoses. Transthyretin is synthesized predominantly in the liver, and liver transplantation results in rapid dissappearance of the variant protein from the plasma. Although liver transplantation halts the progression of the disease, no definite evidence of improvement in peripheral neuropathy has been documented. At present, one patient with fibrinogen α-chain amyloidosis has received liver as well as kidney trans-

Table 210-3 Mutant proteins (other than transthyretin) associated with hereditary systemic amyloidosis

PROTEIN	MUTATION	CLINICAL FEATURES	GEOGRAPHIC KINDREDS
Apolipoprotein A-I	Gly26Arg	PN, nephropathy	US
	Leu60Arg	Nephropathy	England
	Trp50Arg	Nephropathy	England
Gelsolin	Asp187Asn	PN, lattice corneal dystrophy	Finland, US, Japan Denmark,
	Asp187Tyr	PN	Czech countries
Cystatin C	Leu68Gln	Cerebral hemorrhage	Iceland
Fibrinogen	Arg554Leu	Nephropathy	Mexico
	Glu526Val	Nephropathy	US
	4904delG	Nephropathy	US
Lysozyme	Ile56Thr	Nephropathy, skin petechiae	England
	Asp67His	Nephropathy	England

PN, Peripheral neuropathy.

✔ *WHAT TO REFER*

Amyloidosis is a rare disease; therefore most physicians cannot expect to diagnose more than a few cases in their lifetimes. On the other hand, it is likely that several cases will come to medical attention at any major medical center during each year. One confounding aspect in the treatment of systemic amyloidosis is the multiorgan involvement. Individuals with amyloidosis may be referred to cardiologists, hematologists, gastroenterologists, nephrologists, or neurologists because of the presenting manifestation, but abnormalities may develop very quickly in other organ systems. For instance, azotemia in AL amyloidosis may be treated with dialysis; however, after only a few months of dialysis progression of the disease usually results in death attributable to cardiomyopathy or hepatic failure. A good suggestion is that after the diagnosis of amyloidosis is established the physician consult one of the major centers for the study of amyloidosis. Names and addresses of these referral centers can be obtained from the National Institutes of Health or the National Organization for Rare Disease.

plantation. Fibrinogen α-chain is synthesized predominently in the liver, and this measure may be curative. Gelsolin is synthesized by skeletal muscle, and lysozyme is synthesized by neutrophils. These syndromes are not amenable to organ transplantation. Apolipoprotein A-I, although predominently synthesized by the liver, is also synthesized by the intestine; therefore the effects of liver transplantation on the progression of this disease cannot be predicted.

LOCALIZED AMYLOIDOSIS

Alzheimer's disease is the most significant form of localized amyloidosis. The cerebral amyloid plaques contain a 42–amino acid residue degradation peptide of a large transmembrane protein called βPP. The function of this protein is not known, and the relationship between βPP or its degradation products and the dementia process is not known. Proteolytic processing of βPP protein leads to generation of β-peptide, the essential constituent of neuritic plaques. Amyloid β-peptide deposits also occur in leptomeningeal vessels and may lead to intracerebral hemorrhage, particularly in one hereditary form of βPP disease (hereditary cerebral hemorrhage with amyloidosis of the Dutch type) in which death results from cerebral hemorrhage rather than from dementia related to neuritic plaques. A similar cerebral hemorrhage syndrome occurs in Icelandic families with a mutation in the protease inhibitor, cystatin C. Although the high prevalence of Alzheimer's disease in individuals over 80 years of age is probably related to β-peptide deposits from normal βPP, a large percentage of cases of early-onset Alzheimer's disease (less than age 65 years) is related to mutations in either the βPP (chromosome 21), presenilin 1 (chromosome 14), or presenilin 2 (chromosome 1) genes.

Other forms of localized amyloidosis include type II diabetes melitis in which the islets of Langerhans in the pancreas are replaced with amyloid deposits from a locally produced protein, amyloid-associated polypeptide. Medullary carcinoma of the thyroid contains amyloid deposits synthesized from a fragment of calcitonin. Deposition of fibrils containing atrial naturetic factor (ANF) results in isolated cardiac atrial amyloidosis in many elderly individuals. Amyloidoses localized to the larynx, respiratory tract, and urinary tract are of the AL type and probably originate from local lymphocyte clones.

DIFFERENTIAL DIAGNOSIS

Diagnosis of systemic amyloidosis is a two-level process. First, it is necessary to recognize that the patient has amyloidosis. The clinical manifestations of systemic amyloidosis are protean; however, when there is multisystem disease, this diagnosis should be considered. Nephrotic syndrome in a patient with evidence of cardiomyopathy,

hepatomegaly, or peripheral neuropathy should immediately raise the possibility of amyloidosis in the differential diagnosis. Visual defects resulting from vitreous opacities should immediately suggest the diagnosis of hereditary transthyretin amyloidosis. Purpura, gastrointestinal tract hemorrhage, or macroglossia suggests the diagnosis of amyloidosis. The diagnosis of all forms of amyloidosis relies on biopsy of affected tissue and histologic demonstration of the typical amyloid deposits. Classically, rectal biopsy has been used for diagnosis of all forms of systemic amyloidosis. Sensitivity is 70% to 80%. Results of gastric and duodenal biopsies are similar. Abdominal fat pad aspirate has been reported to be as sensitive and have less morbidity. If these biopsy results are negative, biopsy of an affected organ such as kidney, liver, or heart may be necessary to establish the diagnosis.

Once the diagnosis of amyloidosis is established, it is crucial that the correct type of amyloidosis be ascertained. Counseling on prognosis and institution of therapy depends on proper classification of the amyloidosis. Cytotoxic drug therapy should be considered with AL amyloidosis but is definitely contraindicated in hereditary amyloidosis. Foremost in the minds of many patients is whether their disease is hereditary. Proper identification of familial forms of amyloidosis is important for genetic counseling.

BIBLIOGRAPHY

Benson MD: Treatment of AL amyloidosis with melphalan, prednisone and colchicine, *Arthritis Rheum* 29:683, 1986.

Benson MD: Amyloidosis. In Scriver CR, Beaudet AL, Sly WS, Valle D, editors: *The metabolic and molecular bases of inherited disease,* ed 7, vol 3, New York, 1995, McGraw Hill.

Benson MD: Amyloidosis. In Koopman W, editor: *Arthritis and allied conditions,* ed 13, Baltimore, 1996, Williams & Wilkins.

Holmgren G, Steen L, Ekstedt J et al: Biochemical effect of liver transplantation in two Swedish patients with familial amyloidotic polyneuropathy (FAP-met[30]), *Clin Genet* 40:242, 1991.

Husby G, Marhaug G, Dowton B et al: Serum amyloid A (SAA): biochemistry, genetics and the pathogenesis of AA amyloidosis, *Amyloid: Int J Exp Clin Invest* 1:119, 1994.

Kyle RA, Gertz MA: Systemic amyloidosis, *Crit Rev Oncol Hematol* 10:49, 1990.

211 Heritable and Developmental Disorders of Connective Tissue

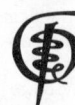

Stephen M. Krane

Skeletal dysplasias result from growth abnormalities in utero or in infancy and childhood. Disturbances in the proportions and length of the fetus may be caused by disorders of chromosomes or by genetically determined abnormalities of morphogenesis, skeletal growth, and maturation. Some become manifest only after birth as short stature or disproportionate body habitus. Hydrocephalus, cranial synostosis, cleft lip and palate, and change in facial appearance may be accompaniments. In addition to shortened limbs, there may be other abnormalities, such as polydactyly, syndactyly, clubbing of fingers and toes, joint dislocations, and multiple fractures. The skeletal dysplasias can be divided into two groups: those caused primarily by abnormal growth of cartilage and/or bone (osteochondrodysplasias) and those that involve malformations of individual bones or combination of bones (dysostoses). The osteochondrodysplasias have been considered in three categories:

1. Chondrodystrophies, which result from defects in growth of bones (e.g., achondroplasia)
2. Disordered development of cartilaginous and fibrous components of the skeleton (e.g., multiple exostoses)
3. Abnormal structure of metaphyseal and diaphyseal bone caused by disordered modeling and remodeling (e.g., some forms of osteogenesis imperfecta)

Although in most of these disorders the fundamental defect is unknown, some (e.g., certain of the chondrodystrophies and forms of osteogenesis imperfecta) may be considered among the heritable disorders of connective tissue. As defined by McKusick, these are generalized defects that involve primarily one component of connective tissue—for example, collagen, elastin, or proteoglycan—and are transmissible in mendelian patterns. Many appear to be distinctive, although the clinical phenotype may vary considerably. It is possible that some of these disorders will turn out to be mutations in genes that are homologous to the homeobox genes in *Drosophilia.*

Traditionally, this variability had been ascribed to differences in penetrance and expression of single genes. It is likely, however, that genetic heterogeneity plays a major role in the differences in clinical manifestations. Since the group of heritable disorders of connective tissue comprises over 100 distinct disease entities, it is not possible to describe any in detail here. Many of the disorders do share common clinical and pathologic features, depending on which component of the connective tissue is involved predominantly.

The term *connective tissue* is usually applied to cartilage, bone, tendons, fascia, ligaments, and the walls of blood vessels. Connective tissue is also considered the extracellular matrix of many other tissues. The character of any connective tissue is determined by the function of the specific cells that make up that tissue. Some components of the extracellular matrix are locally synthesized or modified by the component cells, whereas others are derived from the plasma.

The major fibrous proteins are collagen and elastin. The predominant nonfibrous (amorphous) components are the complex carbohydrates of the so-called ground substance, which include hyaluronic acid, the proteoglycans, and glycoproteins. Water and electrolytes derived from plasma are other important determinants of structure and function of many connective tissues. In bone, the presence of the calcium phosphate inorganic mineral phase contributes to its characteristics as a connective tissue. The particular organization of the cells and their extracellular matrices account for the mechanical properties of each tissue; included are such properties as ability to deform under load (articular cartilage), behavior as a rigid encasement to protect vital structures (bone of the skull), acting as levers for locomotion (long bones), or forming a flexible covering (dermis).

The heritable disorders of connective tissue may be considered ei-

Table 211-1 Major types of collagen and their tissue distributions*

TYPE	TISSUE
Fibrillar	
Type I	Bone, skin, tendons, ligaments, and dentin (all >80%)†; also other tissues
Type II	Articular cartilage, fibrocartilage, vitreous gel (all 50% to 90%); many tissues in early development
Type III	Large blood vessels (30%), and other tissues in association with type I (except bone)
Type V	Large blood vessels (5%), cornea, bone, and a few others
Type XI	Articular cartilage (5% to 20%)
Basement membrane–associated	
Type IV	All basement membranes (95%)
Type VII	Anchoring fibrils of epidermal-dermal junction
Fibril-associated	
Type IX	Cartilage (5% to 20%)
Type XII	Small amounts with type I
Type XIV	Skin, tendon
Short chain	
Type VI	Aorta, cornea, skin, placenta, ligaments, cartilage
Type VIII	Endothelial cells, Descemet's membrane
Type X	Hypertrophic cells of cartilage

*For more complete descriptions, see Prockop DJ, Williams CJ, Vandenberg P: Collagen in normal and diseased connective tissue. In McCarty DJ, Koopman WJ, editors: *Arthritis and allied conditions: a textbook of rheumatology,* ed 12, Philadelphia, 1993, Lea & Febiger.
†Numbers in parentheses indicate approximate percentages of total collagen in the tissues indicated.

ther from the point of view of each of the components of the extracellular matrix or by the characteristic pattern of clinical manifestations, which mainly involves skin, bones, joints, blood vessels, and eyes. We focus on the major components, about which there are considerable chemical data regarding structure and biosynthesis. These major components are collagens, elastin, and the proteoglycans.

COLLAGENS AND POSSIBLE DISORDERS OF COLLAGEN STRUCTURE AND METABOLISM

Collagens are a class of proteins, members of which have chemical and structural features in common, but each of which is a product of a different gene. One property of collagen molecules is the unique triple helix, a particular conformation of three component polypeptide (α) chains. Each of the mature α chains of the most abundant collagens that form banded fibrils (types I to III) contains approximately 1000 amino acids. The conformation of the chains is determined by the amino acid content, with glycine constituting a third of the total and occurring at every third position in the amino acid sequence. Two major classes of collagens are recognized: those that form banded fibrils and fibers and those that do not (Table 211-1). Type I collagen is the major type in most connective tissues, including skin, bone, and parenchymal tissues and blood vessel walls; type II is the major type in articular cartilage and nucleus pulposus; type III is particularly abundant in skin, blood vessel walls, and parenchymal organs but is not found in bone matrix. Other collagens—such as type IV, the predominant type in basement membranes—have unique structures distinct from those that form fibrils, mainly because of interruptions by noncollagenous sequences of the characteristic collagen helical sequences. In tissues the fibers contain characteristic mixtures of different collagens, for example, types I and III in skin or types II and IX in articular cartilage. The collagen also interacts with other components of the extracellular matrix—for example, proteoglycans—in specific ways. Each of the polypeptide (α) chains of the collagens is a product controlled by different genes. At least 18 different gene products have been characterized as among the subunits of at least 13 collagen molecules. The genes for these collagens are complex and huge, and may contain as many as 50 intervening (noncoding) sequences. The genes for several of the collagens have

Table 211-2   Osteogenesis imperfecta (OI)

TYPE	NAME	MODE OF INHERITANCE	MAJOR FEATURES
I (A and B)	OI: Mild long-bone disease; trias fragilitas ossium	Autosomal dominant	Mild to moderate severity; blue sclerae; deafness; little progression after puberty
II	Lethal perinatal OI; lethal OI congenita	Autosomal recessive	Severe; often stillborn or death soon after birth; multiple fractures; crumpled bones (broad bones); blue sclerae
III	Progressively deforming with normal sclerae	Autosomal recessive	Normal birthweight; fractures of long bones and spine at birth or onset of walking; progressive severe deformity; scoliosis; ligamentous laxity; white sclerae; dentinogenesis imperfecta common
IV	Dominant, with normal sclerae (blue in infancy)	Autosomal dominant	Variable severity at time of onset, with fractures of long bones and spine; hearing loss; some have dentinogenesis imperfecta (IVA)

been located on several different chromosomes. Even the genes coding for the two constituent chains of the most abundant collagen (type I) are present on separate chromosomes (α1 [I] on chromosome 17 and α2 [I] on chromosome 7). Biosynthesis of the collagen chains is a multistep process in which a precursor form (procollagen) is first synthesized, with peptide extensions at either end. During synthesis, several amino acids are uniquely modified posttranslationally (after incorporation into the polypeptide chains). These posttranslational modifications include hydroxylation of proline residues (hydroxyproline) and lysine residues (hydroxylysine) and addition of sugars (glucose and galactose) to the hydroxylysines, and formation of hydroxylysine and lysine aldehydes. Specific proteases act to cleave off the extensions of the procollagens to produce the processed collagen molecules, which can then polymerize to form fibrils and fibers.

Given the enormous complexities of structure and biosynthesis, it is not surprising that abnormalities of collagen have been frequently identified in a few uncommon human diseases and in a limited number of cases of common disorders that affect connective tissues.

Osteogenesis Imperfecta

Osteogenesis imperfecta (OI) is the term used to describe clinical phenotypes with hereditary bone fragility (tendency to fracture with minimal trauma). There is extreme variability in the manifestations, however, indicating clinical as well as genetic heterogeneity. Thus the OI syndrome has been subclassified using clinical and genetic criteria such as those shown in Table 211-2. Each of these types can be subclassified, and most are genetically and biochemically heterogeneous. Some individuals with OI cannot be placed in any of these categories. For example, there are patients with moderately severe bone disease, with or without blue sclerae, in whom the inheritance pattern does not fit that of autosomal dominant.

The dominant form with blue sclerae is the most widely recognized. Nearly 100% of persons with this syndrome have abnormally thin sclerae, which take on a slate or blue-black hue. Bones fracture with minimal trauma, beginning in infancy or early childhood. Osteopenia may be detected radiologically prior to fracturing. Perinatal fractures and severe deformities are unusual. Other manifestations include joint laxity, scoliosis, and easy bruising. Dentinogenesis imperfecta, common in the severe deforming (type III) OI, is uncommon in type I. A hearing defect indistinguishable from that of otosclerosis usually begins in the second and third decades and occurs in about one third of patients with OI type I. Since the skeletal manifestations tend to diminish after puberty, the results of therapy are difficult to evaluate. The use of sex hormones (androgens in males and estrogens in females) has been advocated to induce early puberty; short stature may result from such treatment, however, because of premature closure of epiphyses. Sodium fluoride therapy also has been used, but with limited success. Bones of patients with OI type III usually begin to fracture shortly after birth or even prenatally and frequently continue to fracture with the development of severe skeletal deformities that are seemingly independent of fracturing; kyphoscoliosis also develops. These patients do not have an increased incidence of deafness, and their sclerae are not blue. This form of OI is probably genetically heterogeneous, although recessive patterns have been documented. Therapy has been ineffective.

The findings of woven bone and abnormal patterns of deposition of collagen fibers in bone from patients with OI are difficult to interpret because clinical and histopathologic correlations are generally poor. Recently, techniques of protein chemistry and molecular biology have made it possible to demonstrate the nature of the defects in type I collagen structure because of specific mutations in most affected individuals. A decreased content of type I collagen and a relative increase in type III collagen have been found in the skin of patients with type I OI, particularly in those with the dominant form and blue sclerae. When compared with normal dermal fibroblasts, those cultured from such patients synthesize a higher ratio of type III to type I collagen. Since bone contains essentially only type I collagen, it is suggested that a decreased ability to synthesize this matrix component may be a basic defect.

Based on the results of recent studies, a considerable number of patients with OI have mutations in one or both structural genes of type I collagen. In some forms of OI—for example, the perinatal lethal form (type II)—most affected individuals have been shown to have such mutations. Many of the mutations are in different sites in the gene, yet produce apparently identical phenotypes. The consequences of the mutations are substitutions or deletions of single amino acids or deletion of whole exons (in phase) encoding multiple amino acids. Splicing mutations and others that produce frame-shifts have been described. In one example of the latter, a defect in the 3' portion of the pro-α_2(I) gene resulted in the absence of secreted α_2 chains and deposition of α_1(I)-chain trimers. Despite this extraordinary defect the mutation was not lethal. In some instances, an abnormal chain resulting from a mutation in one allele produces devastating effects (resulting from so-called protein suicide), whereas some nonfunctioning alleles that result in formation of no protein at all may have mild consequences. A particularly common mutation results in substitution of cysteine for glycine within the helix. This disrupts the helix, but depending on the location of the substitution within the chain, the defects vary from mild to lethal. Another common feature is "overmodification" of the lysine residues (formation of glycosylated hydroxylysine), because of delays in helix formation. Most of the mutations are dominant, and many are new mutations. In some kindreds the defect has not yet been identified, but linkage of the disorder with the collagen genes can be shown by analysis of restriction length polymorphisms.

Ehlers-Danlos Syndrome

A defect in collagen, particularly types I and III interstitial collagens, may be responsible for the Ehlers-Danlos syndrome (EDS). Clinical problems in this disorder include varying degrees (Table 211-3) of hyperextensible and soft, fragile skin, which may heal poorly when cut, leading to thin scars. Violaceous skin nodules (molluscoid pseudotumors), ecchymoses, and hyperpigmented skin may be found in areas subjected to repeated trauma. Calcified subcutaneous "spherules" may be palpated or detected radiologically. Some affected persons have hypermobile joints that display a tendency to dislocate recurrently. Other skeletal findings include intermittent joint pains, kyphoscoliosis, and deformities of the feet. Easy bruising is also common. In some people, sudden death results from rupture of a major blood vessel or viscera. Clinically and genetically, however, the Ehlers-Danlos syndrome is also heterogeneous, and it has been possible to subclassify the syndrome on these grounds.

Table 211-3   Types of Ehlers-Danlos Syndrome

TYPE	GENETICS	CLINICAL FEATURES	BIOCHEMICAL FEATURES
I, gravis	AD	Soft skin with scars, hypermobile joints, easy bruising	Unknown
II, mitis	AD	Less severe form of type I EDS	Unknown
III, familial, hypermobility	AD	Soft skin without scars, marked mobility of large and small joints	Unknown
IV, vascular	AD	Translucent skin; marked bruising; ruptured arteries, uterus, bowel; normal joint mobility	Defects in type III collagen synthesis or secretion
V, X-linked	XLR	Similar to Ehlers-Danlos syndrome type II	Unknown
VI, ocular	AR	Skin soft and extensible, scoliosis, ocular fragility, hypermobile joints	Deficiency of lysyl hydroxylase
VII, arthrochalasis multiplex congenita	AD	Congenital hip dislocation, hypermobile joints, skin soft without scars	Type I collagen defect: deletion of exon 6 in COL1A1 or COL1A2 encoding aminopeptidase cleavage site
VIII, periodontal	AD	Generalized periodontitis, skin soft and extensible, easy bruising, hypermobile joints	Unknown
IX	XLR	Soft, lax skin; bladder diverticula and rupture; bony occipital horns	Copper abnormality
X	AR	Mild joint hypermobility, easy bruising, abnormal platelet aggregation	Fibronectin defect

From Marini J: Heritable collagen disorders. In Klippel JH, Dieppe PA, editors: *Rheumatology,* London, 1998, Mosby.
AD, Autosomal dominant; *AR,* autosomal recessive; *XLR,* X-linked recessive.

Type I. In type I (gravis) EDS many of the clinical problems described previously may be present in the same affected person. Although a biochemical abnormality has not been identified, collagen fibers in skin and other tissues may be larger than normal and deposited in an irregular fashion.

Types II and III. In type II (mitis type) EDS all the manifestations are milder than in type I, and joint hypermobility is limited to the hands and feet. Cutaneous manifestations are mild or absent in type III EDS, whereas hypermobility of joints is generalized and severe.

Type IV. Individuals with type IV (arterial, ecchymotic, or Sack's variety) EDS have the poorest prognosis, with problems predominantly related to extensive bruising and fragility of arteries and veins. The skin, although not hyperextensible, is thin, particularly over acral parts, and the underlying venous network is prominent. There is a characteristic facies, with a pinched delicate nose, prominent eyes, and an appearance of premature aging. Vascular catastrophies or rupture of major viscera, such as the large intestine, occur in this group. Sudden death in EDS is a feature usually associated only with the types I and IV forms. The syndrome is also associated with mitral valve prolapse. Type IV EDS is biochemically, and probably genetically, heterogeneous; in several instances defective deposition of type III collagen has been demonstrated. Abnormalities in production of type III collagen have also been described in otherwise normal individuals with ruptured cerebral aneurysms. In some affected individuals, type III collagen could not be found on analysis of skin, parenchyma, or walls of blood vessels. Furthermore, their skin fibroblasts do not synthesize detectable type III procollagen. In other subjects, type III procollagen is synthesized but is not normally secreted. Still other individuals with an indistinguishable clinical phenotype have type III collagen present, presumably in normal and sufficient amounts.

Types V and IX. Type V EDS resembles type II; however, skin hyperextensibility may be striking, and the inheritance is X-linked. This syndrome may be related to cutis laxa, in that defective oxidation of lysine residues via the enzyme lysyl oxidase results in inadequate cross-linking of collagen molecules. Type IX EDS includes individuals with such manifestations as urinary bladder diverticuli and spontaneous bladder rupture, inguinal hernias, slight skin laxity, and a number of skeletal abnormalities—a peculiar feature being occipital hornlike exostoses. Lysyl oxidase activity is low in fibroblast cultures from these individuals and may result from impaired synthesis of enzyme protein. It is not yet clear whether these abnormalities are fundamentally different from those reported in type V EDS.

Type VI. A form of EDS (ocular-scoliotic type) has been described in individuals with severe kyphoscoliosis, joint laxity, and recurrent joint dislocations; microcorneas; and soft, hyperextensible skin with a "velvety" feel and slow wound-healing ability. Analysis of dermal collagen from individuals in different kindreds has revealed a marked decrease in hydroxylysine content, a defect at the level of posttranslational modification, with insufficient activity of lysyl hydroxylase. The mutation is probably in the gene that codes for this enzyme that catalyzes the hydroxylation of specific lysyl residues after their incorporation into the growing (nascent) polypeptide chain. This syndrome is also biochemically heterogeneous. Inheritance is probably autosomal recessive. Clinical abnormalities may be accounted for by defective collagen cross-linking, which critically requires hydroxylysine residues. All interstitial collagens are not equally affected (e.g., skin is much more deficient than bone), and this suggests that there may be multiple forms of lysyl hydroxylase, only one of which is affected by a mutation that leads to this syndrome.

Type VII. Type VII EDS is characterized by marked joint hypermobility and recurrent dislocations, moderate cutaneous hyperextensibility and bruisability, short stature, scoliosis, and a peculiar "scooped-out" facies with hypertelorism and epicanthal folds. Some have an abnormal type I collagen, the structure of which is consistent with partially processed procollagen. The incomplete processing of the procollagen is accounted for by abnormalities in the cleavage sites in the amino terminal portion of either procollagen chain caused by exon skipping and deletions of whole exons coding for 18 to 24 amino acids. A similar phenotype may also result from mutations in the enzyme responsible for the cleavage of the procollagen.

Type VIII. Type VIII EDS represents a distinct autosomal recessive entity characterized by moderate cutaneous fragility and severe generalized periodontitis, resulting in extensive alveolar bone resorption and premature loss of teeth. No biochemical defect has yet been identified.

Type X. A kindred has been described in which affected individuals had features of EDS with easy bruisability and a defect in platelet aggregation partially corrected by normal plasma or normal fibronectin. A defect in the structure of fibronectin might account for the bleeding abnormality as well as the connective tissue disorder, since fibronectin may function in adherence of cells to the extracellular, collagenous matrix.

Type XI. It has been suggested that the familial joint hypermobility syndrome be termed *type XI EDS,* although no specific biochemical defect has been identified.

Fibrillin and Marfan Syndrome

The Marfan syndrome includes a relatively common group of clinically heterogeneous heritable disorders of connective tissue. Initially believed to be a biochemical abnormality involving collagen, it has been shown that the defect resides in the fibrillin gene on human chromosome 15. Fibrillin, a (large 350-kD) connective tissue glycoprotein, is a component of microfibrils present in the connective tissue matrices of a variety of tissues, among which are the suspensory ligament of the lens, the wall of blood vessels, and the skin. Several point mutations in the gene segment 15q 15-21 plus abnormalities of fibrillin synthesis, extracellular transport, and incorporation into extracellular matrix have been reported in both familial and sporadic forms of Marfan syndrome.

The characteristic skeletal findings in the Marfan syndrome are dolichostenomelia (inappropriately long limbs compared with the trunk), arachnodactyly, pectus excavatum, and joint laxity. Scoliosis occurs at any level along the thoracolumbar spine; it is frequent and may worsen at the time of the pubertal growth spurt. Inguinal hernias are also common.

Over half of the Marfan cases have the classic ocular finding of ectopia lentis. The lens is usually displaced upward, but the zonules are intact and permit normal accommodation. In contrast, in homocystinuria, the lens is displaced downward; because the zonules are defective, accommodation is impaired. In addition, the globe is unusually long, and this contributes to a high frequency of myopia and an increased risk of retinal detachment.

Abnormalities of connective tissue may be found in the aortic wall and the heart. Histologic changes include disruption of elastic fibers in the blood vessel walls, increases in collagen deposition, and proliferation of smooth muscle cells. Such structural changes are manifested by enlargement of the aortic root, stretching of the aortic cusps, and progressive aortic regurgitation. The latter, if untreated, proceeds to left ventricular failure and death within a few years. Chest pain resembling angina pectoris may also develop. Aneurysms occur in the ascending and abdominal portions of the aorta. Aneurysms of the sinuses of Valsalva are common. Approximately a third of the patients have systolic clicks and murmurs, presumably of mitral origin. Echocardiographic abnormalities are detected in the majority of affected individuals. It would be unusual for a patient with strong clinical evidence of the Marfan syndrome not to have some cardiovascular finding that could be elicited either clinically or by echocardiography.

No therapy is available that can be directed against the fundamental defect or defects. Cardiovascular complications of the Marfan syndrome are managed like other forms of aortic and aortic valvular disease. Prophylactic repair of the ascending aorta prior to dilation is being investigated, as is the use of propranolol in patients who are unsuitable for surgery or in whom it is necessary to delay operation.

Cutis Laxa

Cutis laxa, or dermatolysis, is another clinically and genetically heterogeneous disease characterized by loose, hanging skin over all parts of the body. The condition is particularly noticeable over the face and around the eyes and produces a prematurely aged appearance. Although the skin is hyperextensible, it does not spring back into place. Easy bruisability is not apparent. Parenchymal involvement may occur in the lungs (emphysema) and in viscera with hernias, including diverticula of the gastrointestinal and genitourinary systems. The inheritance may be dominant, recessive, or X-linked. In one kindred in which the pattern has been X-linked, decreased activity of lysyl oxidase has been demonstrated.

Congenital Contractural Arachnodactyly

An autosomal dominant disorder called congenital contractural arachnodactyly (CCA) shares a number of musculoskeletal features with severe Marfan syndrome, but the patients have joint contractures rather than loose-jointedness. The eye and the aorta are not affected. CCA has been linked to a second fibrillin gene present on chromosome 5q 23-31.

ELASTIC TISSUE AND DISEASE

Elastic fibers interacting with collagens and other connective tissue components contribute to the distensible properties of structures such as arterial walls. The elastic fibers are comprised of two distinct proteins. The most abundant has an amorphous appearance by electron microscopy and the chemical composition of elastin. The other is a glycoprotein with a microfibrillar structure. Elastin consists of polypeptide chains rich in the amino acids glycine, alanine, and valine, but poor in polar amino acids. In mature elastin, these polypeptides are cross-linked through the side chains of lysines, some of which had been oxidized to aldehydes by the action of lysyl oxidase. In contrast, the microfibrillar component is rich in polar amino acids and does not contain these modified lysine residues and cross-links.

Pseudoxanthoma elasticum, a possible elastic tissue disease, is usually inherited in an autosomal recessive pattern, although a dominant pattern also has been described. Major manifestations occur in the skin and eye and the cardiovascular system. The skin shows thickened plaques and papules, most commonly localized to the face, neck, axillary and antecubital folds, lower abdomen, and thigh. The lesions may be 1 mm or less in diameter and barely visible, or they may be confluent yellowish plaques that tend to occur along skin creases. The typical ocular lesions are angioid streaks, which appear in the third or fourth decade, usually after the skin lesions. Angioid streaks result from cracks in Bruch's membrane, the structure located between the choroid and the retina. The vascular changes of pseudoxanthoma elasticum are usually confined to arteries, with occlusion of peripheral, coronary, and cerebral vessels. Bleeding may also occur, particularly into the gastrointestinal tract.

Histologically, in the skin, fibers accumulate that stain positively for elastic tissue, predominantly in the deeper dermis. The elastic fibers are swollen, irregularly clumped, and fragmented. These changes could result from a defect in elastin biosynthesis. The occurrence of calcium deposits and an increased content of proteoglycans are assumed to be secondary events.

COMPLEX CARBOHYDRATES OF THE GROUND SUBSTANCE AND THEIR DISEASES

The proteoglycans are composed of high-molecular-weight carbohydrates (glycosaminoglycans) attached covalently to a protein core. The glycosaminoglycans consist of repeating dimeric units of an amino sugar linked to a hexuronic acid or to galactose (as in keratan sulfate). The carbohydrate chains, in turn, are linked through xylose residues to the amino acids serine or threonine in the core protein. In articular cartilage, these proteoglycan subunits, containing many glycosaminoglycans, are attached, in association with a glycoprotein called *link protein,* to high-molecular-weight hyaluronic acid, the latter itself a glycosaminoglycan containing *N*-acetylglucosamine and glucuronic acid dimers.

The composition of the dimeric carbohydrate units of different glycosaminoglycans is unique; furthermore, the sugar residues may be sulfated at specific sites. For example, the dimeric unit of the chondroitin sulfate of cartilage consists of glucuronic acid and *N*-acetylgalactosamine, sulfated in the 4- or 6-position, whereas that of keratan sulfate consists of galactose and *N*-acetylglucosamine 6-sulfate. In dermatan sulfate, iduronic acid and acetylgalactosamine-6-sulfate make up the dimeric unit, whereas in heparan sulfate, glucuronic and iduronic acids are linked to either *N*-acetylglucosamine or glucosamine-*N*-sulfate.

In cartilage, the proteoglycans make up a significant portion of the extracellular matrix, although they are also found associated with the surfaces of cells in other tissues. Most diseases in which there has been a documented defect involving these substances, however, are due not to abnormal synthesis but to decreased degradation. The latter is ascribable to mutation in genes that code for the degradative enzymes or are responsible for some posttranslational modification. The secreted proteoglycans are taken up by cells through endocytosis, delivered to lysosomes, and then degraded by specific enzymes (endoglycosidases) that sequentially reduce the large carbohydrate chains to oligosaccharides. Thus, disorders of degradation are usually manifested by the intracellular accumulation of a polysaccharide modified no further than the site of defective enzymatic cleavage.

Clinical involvement is determined by the degree of enzymatic deficiency and tissue distribution relative to synthetic rates. The major organs most commonly involved are the skeleton, heart, nervous system, and eye. Although several of the disorders have their onset in infancy or early childhood with early death (e.g., Hurler's syndrome), others may not be recognized until the second decade of life and are compatible with relatively long survival (e.g., Scheie's syndrome). The consequences of lysosomal storage are enlargement and, occasionally, proliferation of cells, with secondary deposition of other connective tissue components (e.g., collagen), resulting in the alteration and compression of surrounding structures.

Although the prognosis often is grave, in some instances, these diseases run a relatively mild course. Attempts are being made to replace the missing enzyme directly or by cell, tissue, or even gene transplantation.

BIBLIOGRAPHY

Beighton P, editor: *McKusick's heritable disorders of connective tissue,* ed 5, St Louis, 1993, Mosby.

Byers PH et al: Perinatal lethal osteogenesis imperfecta (OI type II): a biochemically heterogeneous disorder usually due to new mutations in the genes for type I collagen, *Am J Hum Genet* 42:237, 1987.

Cole WG: Osteogenesis imperfecta. In Martin TJ, editor: *Bailliere's clinical endocrinology and metabolism,* London, Philadelphia, 1988, Bailliere Tindall, Saunders.

Dietz HC et al: Marfan syndrome caused by a recurrent de novo missense mutation in the fibrillin gene, *Nature* 352:337, 1991.

Kontusaari S et al: A mutation in the gene for type III procollagen (COL3 A1) in a family with aortic aneurysms, *J Clin Invest* 86:1465, 1990.

Krane SM: Genetic and acquired disorders of collagen deposition. In Piez KA, Reddi AH, editors: *Extracellular matrix biochemistry,* New York, 1984, Elsevier.

Kuivanieni H, Tromp G, Prockop DJ: Mutations in collagen genes: causes of rare and some common diseases in humans, *FASEB J* 5:2052, 1991.

Lee B et al: Linkage of Marfan syndrome and a phenotypically related disorder to two different fibrillin genes, *Nature* 352:330, 1991.

Maslen CL et al: Partial sequence of a candidate gene for Marfan syndrome, *Nature* 352:334, 1991.

Neufeld EF, Muenzer J: Mucopolysaccharidoses. In Scriver CR et al, editors: *The metabolic basis of inherited disease,* ed 6, New York, 1989, McGraw-Hill.

Prockop DJ, Williams CJ, Vandenberg P: Collagen in normal and diseased connective tissue. In McCarty DJ, Koopman WJ, editors: *Arthritis and allied conditions: a textbook of rheumatology,* ed 12, Philadelphia, 1993, Lea & Febiger.

Pyeritz RE: Heritable and developmental disorders of connective tissue and bone. In McCarty DJ, Koopman WS, editors: *Arthritis and allied conditions: a textbook of rheumatology,* ed 12, Philadelphia, 1993, Lea & Febiger.

Sakai LY, Keene DR, Engvall E: Fibrillin. A new 350-kD glycoprotein is a component of extracellular microfibrils, *J Cell Biol* 103:2499, 1986.

Spotila LD et al: Mutation in the gene for type I procollagen (COL1 A2) in a woman with postmenopausal osteoporosis; evidence for phenotypic and genotypic overlap with mild OI, *Proc Natl Acad Sci U S A* 88:6624, 1991.

Uitto J et al: Elastin in diseases, *J Invest Dermatol* 79(suppl):160S, 1982.

Uitto J et al: Biochemistry of collagen diseases, *Ann Intern Med* 105:740, 1986.

V DERMATOLOGY

CHAPTER

212   Cutaneous Manifestations of Connective Tissue Diseases

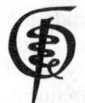

Thomas T. Provost, Wendy Lynch, and Eva Simmons-O'Brien

LUPUS ERYTHEMATOSUS

Cutaneous lesions are a common manifestation of lupus erythematosus, second only to arthritis. It has been estimated that approximately 15% to 20% of patients with classic systemic lupus erythematosus (SLE) possess coin-shaped scaring lupus lesions (discoid lupus erythematosus, [DLE]). In the past it was estimated that approximately 60% to 65% of SLE patients develop cutaneous manifestations during the course of their disease. However, this frequency is probably less today with the increased use of systemic steroids and hydroxychloroquine.

The cutaneous manifestations of lupus erythematosus are divided into specific and nonspecific lesions. The specific lesions include the coin-shaped scarring (discoid) lesions and the generally nonscarring annular and psoriasiform erythematous lesions of subacute cutaneous lupus erythematosus (SCLE) (Box 212-1).

Discoid Lupus

Discoid is a morphologic term meaning "coin- or disk-shaped," but unfortunately it has been employed incorrectly to differentiate cutaneous from systemic lupus erythematosus. Classic DLE lesions are round, annular, scarring lesions possessing an adherent scale and demonstrating telangiectasia. In addition, follicular plugging and hypopigmentation and hyperpigmentation may be prominent. Most DLE lesions are found on light-exposed areas. In black patients, DLE lesions are frequently associated with prominent pigment alterations and can be extremely disfiguring.

The relationship between DLE lesions and SLE has intrigued physicians for years. In general, DLE lesions occur in the absence of systemic features and serologic abnormalities (antinuclear antibodies, etc.). DLE lesions can be viewed as one end of a spectrum of a multisystem disease. The other end of the continuum are those lupus pa-

---

BOX 212-1

Clinical features associated with subacute cutaneous (SCLE) and discoid lupus (DLE) erythematosus lesions

SCLE

Nonscarring, minimal to moderate scale formation, no follicular plugging, very photosensitive.

30%-50% of SCLE patients satisfy diagnostic criteria for SLE.

DLE

Scarring lesion, prominent scale formation, follicular plugging, photosensitive but less than SCLE.

15%-20% of SLE patients have DLE lesions.

tients with significant systemic disease (i.e., renal disease, etc.) without evidence of cutaneous disease.

Approximately 5% to 10% of patients initially presenting with seronegative DLE lesions with time develop systemic disease. Therefore it is important to emphasize that it cannot be determined merely by examining the morphologic features of a discoid lupus lesion whether it occurs in the presence or absence of systemic disease. This can be determined only by a history and physical examamination and appropriate serologic testing.

Classic DLE lesions are seen in various forms. Discoid lupus lesions on the scalp produce a scarring, patchy alopecia. Over the malar eminences and the nose, they produce classic butterfly dermatitis. They may also occur as hyperkeratotic lesions, in which case the condition is termed *hypertrophic* or *hyperkeratotic lupus erythematosus*. Discoid lesions may also occur in association with a tender or nontender nodular induration of the dermis and subcutaneous tissue. This condition is referred to as *lupus profundus*. DLE can involve mucosal surfaces. These lesions are characterized by ulceration and erosions and, when biopsied, illustrate the same histopathologic features as classic discoid lupus lesions.

Discoid lupus lesions are characterized histologically by an inflammatory infiltrate composed predominantly of activated (HLA class II–positive) T-lymphocytes (both CD4 and CD8).

Subacute Cutaneous Lupus Erythematosus

The lesions of subacute cutaneous lupus erythematosus (SCLE) are annular, polycyclic, or psoriasiform with prominent scale formation. Unlike DLE lesions, those of SCLE generally do not scar and are not associated with follicular plugging or telangiectasia.

The serum of approximately 70% of SCLE patients contains anti-Ro (SSA) antibody. Photosensitivity is a dominant feature of these patients; and as many as 90% of patients with anti-Ro (SSA) antibody are photosensitive. In fact, in many of these patients, skin disease is activated by long-wave ultraviolet light, and their skin will burn when exposed to sunlight filtered through window glass.

Patients with distinctive SCLE cutaneous lesions have been described under a variety of headings, including antinuclear antibody–negative (ANA–negative) SLE; subacute cutaneous lupus erythematosus; late-onset lupus erythematosus; Sjögren's syndrome/lupus erythematosus overlap syndrome; and neonatal lupus infants' mothers (Table 212-1). Identical lesions of SCLE have been seen in patients with homozygous C_2 and C_4 complement deficiency and in neonatal lupus infants. In addition to extreme photosensitivity, approximately 30% to 50% of these SCLE patients satisfy the American College of Rheumatology criteria for the diagnosis of systemic lupus erythematosus. They lack, however, the increased frequency of severe renal disease associated with the presence of anti–double-stranded (native) DNA antibodies.

These annular polycyclic and psoriasiform lesions are most prominent in light-exposed areas and can involve widespread areas of the body. They may also involve the malar eminence and nose, producing classic butterfly dermatitis. Although SCLE lesions generally do not demonstrate the heavy lymphocytic infiltrate seen in the classic discoid lupus lesions, the inflammatory infiltrate is composed predominantly of CD4+ and CD8+ activated T-lymphocytes. Since these cutaneous lesions may be a prominent feature of neonatal lupus infants born of anti-Ro (SSA) mothers, it has been postulated that they arise, at least in part, by antibody-dependent cellular cytotoxicity mechanisms.

Prominent erythematous, edematous, "donutlike" lesions have been described in anti-Ro (SSA) antibody–positive Asian patients, especially Japanese lupus patients. Approximately 50% to 60% of Asian lupus patients are anti-Ro (SSA)–antibody positive (see Table 212-1). Furthermore, investigators have not found a striking increased frequency of photosensitivity associated with anti-Ro(SSA)–positive American patients. In a recent study of 100 anti-Ro(SSA) autoantibody–positive patients, a statistically significant earlier onset of disease and more aggressive organ involvement were found in black Americans compared to white Americans.

Photosensitivity

Photosensitivity is a major component of lupus erythematosus. Approximately 40% to 70% of SLE patients are photosensitive and most of their lupus lesions occur on light-exposed areas. Recent studies have demonstrated that both UVB (280 to 320 nm) and UVA (320 to 400 nm) are capable of inducing the formation of lupus lesions in some DLE, SCLE, and SLE patients.

Nonspecific Cutaneous Lesions in Systemic Lupus Erythematosus

In addition to the specific lesions listed earlier, lupus erythematosus patients frequently demonstrate a variety of nonspecific inflammatory and vascular lesions.

Alopecia is common in SLE (Color Plate VII-2). In addition to the scarring alopecia induced by DLE lesions, a diffuse alopecia may occur after flares of SLE. During these catabolic events, the normal growing hair bulbs (anagen) evolve prematurely into a resting phase (telogen). Approximately 3 months after induction of the telogen phase, the hair falls out (telogen effluvium), to be replaced by a normal (anagen) hair. This is a transient nonscarring diffuse alopecia.

In addition, the catabolic effect of an SLE flare may induce production of defective hair shafts that fracture a short distance above the scalp surface. This produces a characteristic thinning of the hair termed *lupus hair*. It is most prominent at the periphery of the scalp.

Inflammatory vascular disease in lupus erythematosus may manifest itself as short, linear telangiectasia in the cuticle nail folds; splinter hemorrhages; tender erythematous nodules on the tips of the fingers (Osler's nodes), and erythematous tender and nontender lesions on the thenar and hypothenar eminences (Janeway's spots). Urticaria-like lesions, livedo reticularis, and deep nodular lesions may also be manifestations of vasculitis. In addition, lupus patients may develop palpable and nonpalpable purpuric lesions over the lower extremities as manifestations of vasculitis; these lesions may or may not ulcerate. Histologically, most of these lesions demonstrate leukocytoclastic angiitis, but on occasion a mononuclear vasculopathy is seen.

Treatment. Cutaneous lesions of lupus erythematosus may be treated with a variety of preparations, including topical application and intralesional injection of corticosteroids and use of corticosteroid-impregnated tape. It must be stressed, however, that use of topical fluorinated corticosteroids, especially in the intertriginous areas of the groin, axillary regions, and the face, may produce atrophy and cosmetically objectionable telangiectasia.

Severe cutaneous lupus erythematosus may be successfully treated with a transient burst of parenteral corticosteroids (equivalent to 30 to 40 mg of prednisone daily and tapered over a period of 3 to 4 weeks). Pulse methylprednisolone therapy (1.0 g intravenously on 3 successive days) is an additional option. Hydroxychloroquine, either alone or together with a burst of methylprednisolone, may be used to control photosensitive lupus lesions. The patients are initially given

Table 212-1 Patient population associated with anti-Ro (SSA) antibodies

PATIENT POPULATION	FREQUENCY OF ANTI-RO (SSA) ANTIBODIES
Sjögren's syndrome	Variable; some cohorts by gel double diffusion ~ 30%-40% other cohorts by ELISA 80%-90%
Subacute cutaneous lupus erythematosus (SCLE)	~70%
Sjögren's syndrome/lupus erythematosus overlap syndrome (late-onset lupus erythematosus)	~80%-90%
Lupus-like disease associated with homozygous C_2 or C_4 complement deficiency	~50%-75%
Neonatal lupus infants' mothers	~95%
Japanese (all Asian?) lupus patients	~50%-60%

400 mg of hydroxychloroquine daily for 1 month and then 200 mg daily thereafter. Routine eye examinations are performed every 4 to 6 months to monitor for possible retinopathy. Quinacrine (Atabrine), 100 mg/day, has been effective in combination with hydroxychloroquine in controlling cutaneous lupus lesions. Quinacrine produces a characteristic yellow tint to the skin.

Recent studies have indicated that the skin lesions of some SCLE patients may respond to diaminodiphenylsulfone (Dapsone), 50 to 100 mg daily. This drug may be associated with a compensated hemolytic anemia, on unusual occasions with pancytopenia, and rarely with aplastic anemia. Glucose-6-phosphate dehydrogenase should be determined prior to initiating therapy, and at least monthly monitoring of a complete blood cell count is indicated in patients so treated.

In both Europe and the United States, thalidomide has been reported to be effective in treating refractory discoid lupus lesions. Also several reports indicate that retinoids (Etretinate) may be beneficial. In addition to these measures, lupus patients should be warned against excessive sun exposure. Protective clothing (i.e., long-sleeved shirts and blouses, wide-brim hats, etc.) should be encouraged. Sunscreens protective against long-wave (UV-A) and short-wave ultraviolet light (UV-B; sunburn spectrum) should be judiciously applied. Sunscreens with a sun-protective factor rating of 15 are advisable.

Antiphospholipid Syndrome (Anticardiolipin, Lupus Anticoagulant)

In recent years, many reports have documented the existence of a syndrome characterized by multiple venous and arterial thrombosis, fetal wastage, thrombocytopenia, pulmonary and systemic hypertension, and livedo reticularis with or without ulcerations. This syndrome was first recognized 40 years ago in systemic lupus erythematosus patients who had a suspected bleeding disorder and biologic false-positive serologic test for syphilis. Since then, a group of antiphospholipid antibodies, including anticardiolipin antibodies, lupus anticoagulant, and others, has been described. Current figures estimate the prevalence of anticardiolipin antibodies in SLE patients to range between 30% and 50%. Most of these patients have low titer anticardiolipin antibodies by ELISA (less than 5 standard deviations); only 5% to 10% of them have a history of a thrombotic episode.

The antiphospholipid antibodies (including lupus anticoagulant and the anticardiolipin antibody) are a group of related but distinct autoantibodies directed against negatively charged phospholipids (e.g., phosphotylcholine, phosphotylserine). Most recent experiments indicate that antiphospholipid antibodies require a cofactor present in normal sera. Several studies indicate that this cofactor is β_2-glycoprotein I. It appears that only negatively charged phospholipid combined with β_2-glycoprotein I is of pathologic significance (Chapter 181). The lupus anticoagulant interferes with the prothrombin activation complex (composed of activated factor X, factor V, platelet phospholipid, and calcium), prolonging the phospholipid-dependent coagulation tests, including the activated partial thromboplastin time, kaolin clotting time, Russell's viper venom time, and on occasion the prothrombin time. Mixing experiments with normal plasma fail to correct the prolonged coagulation times.

These autoantibodies produce in vivo thrombosis, and in vitro tests suggest a defect in coagulation. The exact pathogenesis is unknown but may involve inhibition of prostacyclin, fibrinolysis, or protein C activation.

The antiphospholipid (APL) syndrome can occur in the presence or absence of SLE. In the absence of SLE the condition is termed the *primary APL syndrome*. In general, there is a gross direct correlation with the presence of clinical features of the APL syndrome and the titer of anticardiolipin antibodies. However, abnormal quantities of anticardiolipin antibodies in the absence of disease are seen in association with some medications (chlorpromazine, hydralazine), infections, carcinoma, human immune deficiency syndrome, and endocrinopathies.

The most common dermatologic association with APL is livedo reticularis, characterized by a violaceous netlike pattern involving the lower extremities. Stellate leg ulcers, tiny digital ulcers, or large deep suprainfected ulcerations may be present. In unusual instances, gangrene of digits may occur. Less frequently, atrophie blanche (patches of ivory-white skin with telangiectasia surrounded by hyperpigmentation), thrombophlebitis, ecchymoses, subungual splinter hemorrhages, and purpura are observed. Prominent livedo reticularis of the lower extremities with central nervous system thrombosis (Sneddon's syndrome) is a manifestation of APL syndrome.

Treatment. At present, it is unclear what therapeutic modalities are effective in preventing this syndrome. Several therapeutic options exist. Anticoagulation with heparin and coumadin appears to inhibit the formation of new thrombi. However, complications arise, especially in patients with Sneddon's syndrome who have sustained strokes and are at risk for intracranial hemorrhage. Low-dose aspirin may also play a role in preventing the initiation of clot formation. Parenteral corticosteroids have been recommended (40 to 80 mg/day of prednisone). In fulminant cases, pulse intravenous methylprednisolone (1 g infused over 4 hours daily for 3 successive days) may be indicated. Plasmapheresis has been employed to remove the circulating autoantibody. Cytotoxic agents have also met with some success. A recent study indicates that coumadin is superior in preventing recurrent episodes.

DERMATOMYOSITIS

Dermatomyositis is an inflammatory disease characterized by inflammation most prominently of proximal muscles and the skin (Chapter 199). The amount or intensity of skin inflammation does not seem to be related to the degree of inflammation of the muscles. Rarely, the cutaneous manifestations of dermatomyositis can occur in the absence of muscle involvement (dermatomyositis sine myositis). In addition, it has been noted that despite successful treatment of the myositis with immunosuppressive agents and/or corticosteroids, the skin disease may fail to respond.

The cutaneous manifestations of dermatomyositis are characterized by erythematous, generally pruritic lesions that may involve the trunk, extremities, and face. Photosensitivity is frequent. Lesions may appear as patchy, violaceous erythematous blotches or linear streaks. At times the lesions may demonstrate atrophy, telangiectasia, and hypopigmentation, a condition termed *poikiloderma*. Facial lesions are characterized by periorbital edema and telangiectasia of the eyelids, giving a characteristic erythematous violaceous (heliotrope) appearance.

Involvement of the hands appears as erythematous, violaceous, slightly scaly papules over the extensor surfaces of the interphalangeal joints (Gottron's papules) (Color Plate VII-3). Similar violaceous erythematous papules can be found on the elbows and knees. Prominent cuticle nail fold telangiectasia is also frequently seen in dermatomyositis.

The pathologic features of the cutaneous lesions of dermatomyositis are quite similar to those of lupus erythematosus. The exact pathogenesis of these lesions is unknown, but there does not appear to be any relationship between cutaneous disease and the various autoantibodies associated with polymyositis and dermatomyositis (e.g., tRNA synthetase, [JO-1, PL-7, PL-12], and PM/Scl or Mi-2).

In patients with dermatomyositis, including those without myositis, there is an associated malignancy in 6% to 43% of the patients. This association is most striking in patients older than age 40 years. One recent study documented the difficulty in detecting ovarian carcinoma in associated female patients with the routine measures (physical examination, ultrasound, and computed tomography). Thus women with dermatomyositis should also undergo a transvaginal ultrasound and CA-125 if the previously mentioned studies are unremarkable (Chapter 222).

Corticosteroids (equivalent to 60 to 80 mg of prednisone per day) and immunosuppressive drugs (e.g., methotrexate 25 to 50 mg IM once weekly) are effective in treating most patients with dermatomyositis, but as noted earlier, the skin lesions may be resistant to this type of therapy. Chloroquine 250 mg daily or hydroxychloroquine 200 to 400 mg daily may control cutaneous manifestations. Antihistamines may also be needed to control the annoying pruritus so commonly associated with the cutaneous manifestations of dermatomyositis.

SCLERODERMA

There are three major forms of scleroderma: morphea, the limited form (CREST), and progressive systemic sclerosis (PSS).

Morphea is a form of scleroderma characterized by sharply demarcated porcelain-white plaques of indurated skin, with or without a surrounding halo of erythema, occurring on all areas of the body. Plaques of morphea may be multiple and involve large areas of the body *(generalized localized morphea).* Morphea may also present as atrophic hyperpigmented patches or as depressed sclerotic plaques in a linear configuration *(coup de sabre).* Typically morphea is not associated with any features that are seen with limited or progressive systemic forms of scleroderma.

The limited form of scleroderma is a chronic disease process characterized by sclerodactyly, cuticle nailfold injection, Raynaud's phenomenon, facial and oral involvement, esophageal dysmotility, and pulmonary diffusion abnormalities (Chapter 197). The sclerodactyly leads to resorption of the terminal tufts of the phalanges; painful recalcitrant "ice-picked" ulcerations frequently occur. Secondary infection is common and may eventually lead to surgical amputation of the digit.

Facial involvement is prominent, leading to effacement of the normal wrinkles and a sharpening of facial features. Inability to wrinkle the forehead with upward gazing, perioral tightening and contraction of the mouth are common.

The CREST syndrome, which is associated with anticentromere antibody, is a variant of the limited form of scleroderma. CREST is an acronym for *c*alcinosis, *R*aynaud's phenomenon, *e*sophageal dysmotility, *s*clerodactyly, and *t*elangiectasia. The telangiectasia in this syndrome can be very prominent over the face. Unlike the telangiectasia seen in hepatic disease or Osler-Weber-Rendu syndrome, the telangiectasia in scleroderma does not involve mucous membranes.

PSS, the third form of scleroderma, is characterized by a much more central onset with rapid, widespread dissemination and subsequent systemic involvement. Pulmonary, renal, cardiac, and gastrointestinal complications are common and often prove fatal. Antitopoisomerase 1 antibodies (anti-Scl-70) are frequently present in the sera from these patients.

The pathogenesis of the cutaneous lesions in scleroderma is unknown. A mononuclear inflammatory infiltrate occurs in the subcutaneous tissue beneath the dermis as the earliest change. Based upon in vitro studies that demonstrate that γ-interferon and interleukin 1 (IL-1) are capable of inducing resting fibroblasts to synthesize collagen, it has been proposed that the sclerosis may be the result of the action of lymphokines released by these inflammatory cells. Currently there is no explanation for the small-vessel vasculopathy characterized by thickening of the intima of small arterioles and the Raynaud's phenomenon.

The treatment of all forms of scleroderma is unsatisfactory. Topical and parenteral steroids, azathioprine, and cyclophosphamide have all been tried with little or no effect. Recent studies, both retrospective and prospective, have suggested that D-penicillamine may produce beneficial effects in some scleroderma patients.

BIBLIOGRAPHY

Cabiedes et al: Clinical manifestations of antiphospholipid syndrome in patients with SLE associated more strongly with anti-beta 2-glycoprotein-1 than antiphospholipid antibodies, *J Rheumatol* 22:1899, 1995.

Callen JP: Cutaneous lesions in connective tissue disorders, *Clin Rheum Dis* 7:325, 1982.

Grob JJ, Borderandi JJ: Thrombotic skin diseases as a marker of the cardiolipin syndrome, *J Am Acad Dermatol* 20:1063, 1989.

Laman SD, Provost TT: Cutaneous manifestations of lupus erythematosus, *Clin Rheum Dis* 20:195, 1994.

Provost TT et al: The relationship between anti-Ro(SSA) antibody in positive Sjögren's syndrome and anti-Ro(SSA) antibody positive lupus erythematosus, *Arch Dermatol* 124:63, 1988.

Simmons-O'Brien E et al: One hundred anti-Ro(SSA) positive patients: a 10 year follow-up, *Medicine* 74:109, 1995.

Sontheimer RD: The anticardiolipin syndrome, *Arch Dermatol* 123:590, 1987.

Sontheimer RD, Thomas JR, Gilliam JN: Subacute cutaneous lupus erythematosus: a cutaneous marker for a distinct lupus erythematosus subset, *Arch Dermatol* 115:1409, 1979.

Watson RM et al: Neonatal lupus erythematosus: a clinical serological and immunogenetic study with review of the literature, *Medicine* 63:362, 1984.

Whitmore SE et al: Ovarian cancer in patients with dermatomyositis, *Medicine* 73:153, 1994.

We would like to thank Michael D. Rader, MD for his contribution to the previous edition.

213 Bullous Diseases

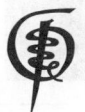

Hossein C. Nousari and Grant J. Anhalt

There are several skin diseases in which the primary lesion is a vesicle-bulla. Some etiologies of such diseases include infectious causes (bullous impetigo, herpes simplex, varicella). Others are caused by an inherited structural defect within the skin (epidermolysis bullosa), and some are caused by an allergic/hypersensitivity reaction to an antigen (allergic contact dermatitis, erythema multiforme). This chapter addresses a group of diseases referred to as *primary bullous diseases,* most of which are now proven to be caused by autoantibodies directed against cell adhesion molecules of the epidermis.

PEMPHIGUS

The term *pemphigus* refers to a group of bullous diseases that share two distinctive features: acantholysis (rounding and detachment of adjacent epidermal cells) and autoantibodies against specific epidermal antigens that are transmembrane cell adhesion molecules called *desmogleins.* The desmogleins are a subgroup of a superfamily of adhesion molecules called *cadherins* (calcium-dependent adhesion molecules). Epidermal desmogleins are unique cadherins that are expressed only in stratified squamous epithelium. This limited expression accounts for the localization of pemphigus lesions to skin and mucous membranes, and explains why lesions cannot occur in internal organs. The subsets of pemphigus vary according to the clinical appearance of lesions, the level of acantholysis within the epidermis, the epidemiology of cases, and ultimately, according to the specific cadherin to which autoantibodies are directed.

Pemphigus Vulgaris

This is a relatively rare disease but is the most common form of pemphigus—hence the term *vulgaris.* It affects both sexes, predominantly during the fourth and fifth decades of life and most often presents with painful oral erosions, which may last weeks or months prior to diagnosis. Most patients ultimately develop skin lesions, which appear as flaccid bullae that rupture rapidly, leaving persistent painful and crusted erosions. All mucous membranes with stratified squamous epithelium may become involved (mouth, pharynx, esophagus, nose, conjunctiva, glans, vagina, and anus). In extensive disease the scalp and upper trunk are consistently involved (Fig. 213-1, *A*). Pressure applied to an intact bulla leads to peripheral extension of the lesions, and shearing pressure applied to normal skin induces bulla formation (Nikolsky's sign). Data derived before the availability of oral corticosteroids showed the disease to be relentlessly progressive, with an approximately 50% mortality rate in the first 2 years and mortality approaching 100% by 5 years.

Histologic examination of early lesions reveals acantholysis in a suprabasilar location. Basal cells remain attached to the basement membrane (Fig. 213-1, *B*). The initial site of separation of epidermal cells from each other is within nondesmosomal areas. Ultimately desmosomes split, resulting in complete acantholysis of epidermal cells.

Direct immunofluorescence (IF) performed on skin adjacent to a lesion reveals deposition of IgG and to a lesser degree complement (C) components such as C3 on epidermal cell surfaces. All patients have serum anti–cell surface IgG antibodies as detected by indirect IF (Fig. 213-1, *C*). The autoantibodies are directed against desmoglein 3, a 130-kD desmosomal cadherin, also known as the *pemphigus vulgaris antigen.*

Pemphigus vulgaris (PV) is one of few autoimmune diseases in which the autoantibodies have been proven to be pathogenic. When patients' IgG is injected intraperitoneally into neonatal mice, the animals develop a disease that is identical to the human disease. The mechanism by which the IgG induces acantholysis is somewhat con-

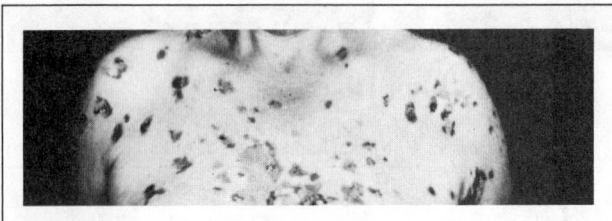

A

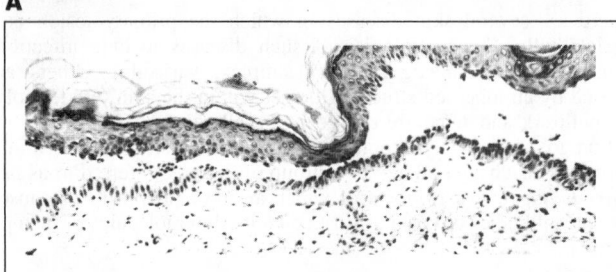

B

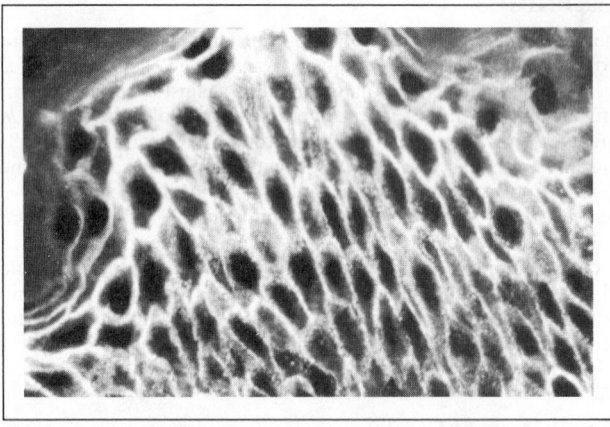

C

FIGURE 213-1   Pemphigus vulgaris. **A,** Clinical presentation with erosions over the chest wall; intact blisters are seen less commonly because they rupture easily. **B,** Hematoxylin and eosin examination of a blister reveals intraepidermal splitting due to suprabasilar acantholysis. **C,** Indirect immunofluorescence performed on cryosection of normal human skin using the serum of a patient with pemphigus and fluorescein-labeled antihuman IgG. Note binding of antibodies to the intercellular space between epidermal cells.

troversial. There is in vitro evidence that after IgG binds the epidermal cell surface, plasminogen activator is released from epidermal cells. This enzyme cleaves plasminogen into plasmin, which has proteolytic activity that may dissolve adhesion molecules of the cell surface and lead to acantholysis. On the contrary, there is also in vitro evidence in other cells that antibodies binding to cadherins can cause cell-cell detachment in the absence of any other inflammatory event. The mechanism of cell dysadhesion in the human disease is probably quite complex.

Despite the debate over mechanisms underlying acantholysis, it is clear that therapy must be aimed at clearing the pathogenic IgG autoantibodies. It is pointless to treat the target organ only (the skin), for the disease is a systemic autoimmune disease and disease activity is closely paralleled by increases and decreases of the serum autoantibody levels. Reduction of autoantibody synthesis is accomplished with long-term systemic corticosteroids such as prednisone in a 0.5 to 1.5 mg/kg/day dose. Pemphigus vulgaris has a chronic course, and long-term treatment with systemic steroids has potentially serious side effects. In addition, the disease may not be adequately controlled by corticosteroids alone, and immunosuppressives such as azathioprine, cyclophosphamide, methotrexate, or cyclophosphamide plus plasmapheresis are required for steroid-sparing effects in about one half of cases. Although patients with pemphigus vulgaris presently rarely die

of their disease, some (approximately 5%) ultimately succumb to the side effects of therapy.

Pemphigus Foliaceus

Also referred to as *superficial pemphigus,* this disease occurs as a sporadic form throughout the world or as an endemic form in South America (fogo selvagem).

The sporadic form most commonly affects the elderly. Lesions tend to appear and predominate over seborrheic areas such as the scalp, chest, and back. The primary lesion is a superficial vesicopustule, which may evolve into a scale-crust. The severity of the eruption can be trivial, with only several persistent lesions, or it may be life-threatening when a generalized exfoliative erythroderma develops. Unlike pemphigus vulgaris, mucosal lesions are extraordinarily rare and essentially "never" occur. This is a valuable clinical feature to differentiate pemphigus foliaceus from pemphigus vulgaris, in which mucosal lesions predominate.

Histologic examination reveals acantholysis within the granular cell layer with variable infiltration of neutrophils and/or eosinophils. Direct IF examination of skin reveals deposition of IgG (predominantly IgG4) and C3 on the epidermal cell surfaces. Indirect IF reveals circulating anti–cell surface IgG antibodies in the majority of patients, and the target antigen is a 160-kD desmosomal cadherin called desmoglein I.

Pemphigus foliaceus is also a tissue-specific autoimmune disease, and patients' IgG injected into neonatal mice induces characteristic cutaneous lesions. Remarkably, the epidermal lesions are superficial, as they are in affected humans. Again, it is thought that binding of IgG to the desmoglein I abolishes the protein's physiologic function of epidermal cell adhesion, thus leading to acantholysis.

Most patients with pemphigus foliaceus can be controlled using a lower corticosteroid dose than is needed with pemphigus vulgaris. A dose in the range of 0.50 to 1.0 mg/kg/day of prednisone is usually sufficient. Most treated patients respond rapidly, and the dose can be tapered over several months. The necessity to use steroid-sparing immunosuppressive agents in pemphigus foliaceus is uncommon.

Fogo Selvagem (Endemic Pemphigus Foliaceus)

This disease is similar to the sporadic variant of North American pemphigus foliaceous in every way, including causation by autoantibodies against desmoglein I. It differs, however, in its geographic distribution (occurring in developing areas near rivers in South America, especially central Brazil) as well as the typical age at onset (both children and adults are affected). An environmental agent, perhaps transmitted by an insect vector, is suspect in development of the disease in South America.

Pemphigus Erythematosus

This disease represents overlap of pemphigus foliaceus and lupus erythematosus. Patients exhibit a polymorphous eruption over the face and upper trunk that consists of vesicopustules and malar erythematous plaques that resemble lupus erythematosus. The histologic findings are similar to those of pemphigus foliaceus, but IF reveals both IgG on the epidermal cell surfaces and multiple immunoglobulins and C3 at the basement membrane zone (BMZ). Patients may have serologic abnormalities or clinical features suggestive of concurrent SLE. Some patients have an associated thymoma and occasionally myasthenia gravis. Therapy consists of corticosteroids and immunosuppressives.

Drug-Induced Pemphigus

Some patients using D-penicillamine, captopril, or rarely, other medications, develop a cutaneous disease that is indistinguishable from pemphigus foliaceus or, less commonly, pemphigus vulgaris. Such patients usually have autoantibodies against the cadherins that are recognized by sera from patients with idiopathic pemphigus foliaceus or vulgaris. These patients follow a course similar to that of those with the idiopathic disease.

IgA Pemphigus

This uncommon condition, also known as *intercellular IgA vesico-pustular dermatosis,* shares clinicohistologic features with idiopathic pemphigus foliaceus and subcorneal pustular dermatosis. Direct immunofluorescence shows IgA deposition on the superficial epidermal cell surfaces. An association with monoclonal gammopathies has been recently described. The inclusion of this entity within the pemphigus group remains controversial.

Paraneoplastic Pemphigus

There have been reports of cases of pemphigus associated with cancer, and these patients were presumed to have PV in association with malignancy. This association has recently been investigated further, and a new variant of pemphigus has been reported. Patients with paraneoplastic pemphigus (PNP) have a concurrent malignancy, and almost all cases are associated with one of a small number of neoplasms, including, in rank order of frequency: non-Hodgkin's lymphomas, chronic lymphocytic leukemia, Castleman's disease, thymomas, and poorly differentiated sarcomas. Lesions almost always begin within and around the oral and ocular mucosa as painful erythematous crusted erosions. At this stage the eruption is very similar to mucosal erythema multiforme/Stevens-Johnson syndrome. Later, generalized erythematous patches that undergo sloughing give the appearance of toxic epidermal necrolysis, or a more chronic, lichenoid eruption resembling a drug eruption can occur. Other mucosal epithelia can be affected. The course is rapidly progressive and often fatal within a few months when associated with a malignant neoplasm, but it usually resolves if a benign neoplasm (e.g., a thymoma or Castleman's tumor) is found and removed completely.

Histologic examination of early lesions reveals features of PV (suprabasilar acantholysis) as well as features of erythema multiforme (lymphocytic infiltrate and keratinocyte necrosis). IF studies of skin show deposition of IgG and C3 both on the cell surfaces and occasionally in the basement membrane. Indirect IF shows circulating antibodies reactive against the cell surfaces of stratified squamous epithelia (like other pemphigus variants) and transitional epithelia, simple epithelia, and other tissues where desmosomes are present (urinary bladder epithelium, hepatocytes, and intercalated disks of myocardium). These antibodies identify a complex of epidermal proteins including desmoplakins I and II (molecular weight 250 kD and 210 kD, respectively) that are components of desmosomes, the 230 kD bullous pemphigoid antigen, and two autoantigens (190 kD and 170 kD) whose identity remains unknown.

At present, the mechanism(s) by which these tumors induce this distinctive autoimmune disease remain speculative. When paraneoplastic pemphigus is associated with a malignant neoplasm such as non-Hodgkin's lymphoma, the prognosis is grave, although some patients have responded well to treatment with cyclosporine, 5 mg/kg/day and prednisone, 1 mg/kg/day. Aggressive therapy of the underlying neoplasm usually fails to halt progression of the disease and death. In cases associated with benign lesions (such as localized Castleman's tumor or thymoma), complete surgical excision results in a remission of the autoimmune disease.

PEMPHIGOID

The term *pemphigoid* is applied to bullous diseases characterized by blistering at the dermal-epidermal junction (DEJ) and anti–basement membrane zone (BMZ) antibodies that identify protein antigens of the hemidesmosome and lamina lucida. The different diseases are separated on the basis of their respective clinical presentations.

Bullous Pemphigoid

Bullous pemphigoid (BP), the most common of this group of diseases, predominantly affects the elderly. The onset can be abrupt or insidious and lesions predominate over flexural areas. Initially, urticarial plaques appear, which are later followed by tense, clear or hemorrhagic blisters (Fig. 213-2, *A*). Bullae rupture, leaving crusted erosions that, unlike those of PV, can heal within several days. Mucosal lesions occur only occasionally and are transient and trivial.

Histologic examination shows separation of the epidermis from

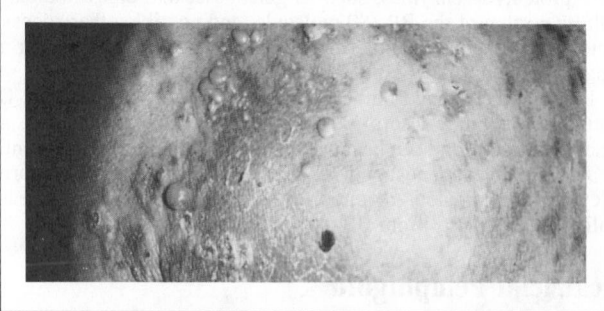

A

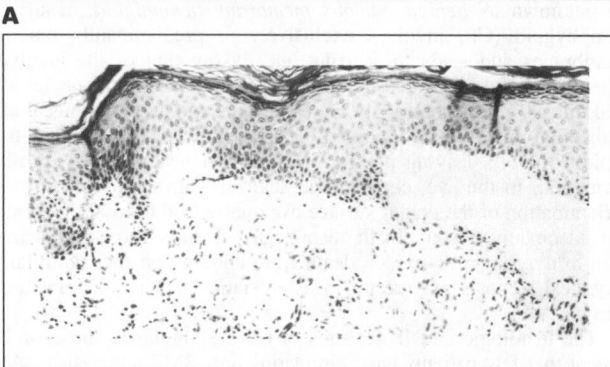

B

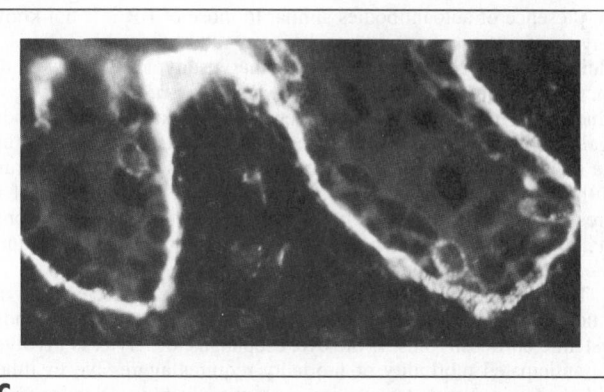

C

FIGURE 213-2   Bullous pemphigoid. **A,** Clinical presentation with intact bullae as well as healing lesions. **B,** Hematoxylin and eosin stain of a blister reveals dermal-epidermal separation and a dermal inflammatory cell infiltrate. **C,** Indirect immunofluorescence performed on cryosections of rat tongue using serum from a patient with bullous pemphigoid, and fluorescein-labeled antihuman IgG. Note the binding of antibodies to the basement membrane zone in a linear and continuous pattern.

the underlying dermis and a variable infiltrate of eosinophils and lymphocytes in the upper dermis (Fig. 213-2, *B*). The separation occurs through the lamina lucida between the basal cell membrane and the lamina densa (basal lamina). Direct IF of perilesional skin consistently reveals deposition of C3 and IgG (predominantly IgG4) at the DEJ. These IgG deposits are found within the lamina lucida in close proximity to the basal cell hemidesmosomes. Indirect IF reveals circulating anti-BMZ antibodies in 70% of patients (Fig. 213-2, *C*). These antibodies, like those of PV, bind only to stratified squamous epithelia, and they specifically identify proteins of the epidermal hemidesmosomes (molecular weight 230 kD and 180 kD).

It is now proven that circulating BP antibodies, specific for the 180-kD antigen (BP Ag 2), are directly responsible for blister formation. These antibodies bind the BP 180 antigen, and complement is activated. Complement components like C3a and C5a attract polymorphonuclear leukocytes to the BMZ either directly or by an anaphylatoxin action on mast cells with subsequent release of eosinophil chemotactic factors. The eosinophils then become activated and release proteolytic enzymes, such as gelatinase, that digest the extracellular portion of the BP 180 molecule (and possibly other adhesion molecules of the lamina lucida as well) and lead to dermal-epidermal separation.

It is relatively easy to induce remission in most patients with BP. Corticosteroids in a dose of 0.5 to 1.0 mg/kg/day of prednisone are usually sufficient and can be tapered over 6 to 8 months. Infrequently, the addition of immunosuppressive medications such as azathioprine or cyclophosphamide is required for adequate control of the disease. Unlike PV, mortality from BP is rare.

Cicatricial Pemphigoid

Also known as *benign mucous membrane pemphigoid,* cicatricial pemphygoid (CP) involves exclusively or predominantly mucous membranes and leads to scarring and dysfunction of the involved sites. The mucosal surfaces predominantly affected are the ocular and oral mucosae; less commonly the esophagus and nasopharyngeal and anogenital mucosae are involved. Lesions start as vesicles/bullae that rapidly rupture, leaving painful erosions that heal slowly with scar formation. In the eye, conjunctival scarring, entropion, and chronic inflammation of the ocular surface eventually lead to loss of vision if not adequately treated. In the esophagus, fibrosis and stenosis may lead to dysphagia or sudden death from choking on food. Similarly, laryngeal stenosis may result in asphyxiation and require tracheostomy.

The histologic and IF features of CP are similar to those of BP except that few patients have circulating anti-BMZ antibodies. Most patients with CP have antibodies that bind the BP 180 antigen. Given the presence of autoantibodies similar to those of BP, it is not known why these patients have mucosal lesions rather than skin lesions. In addition, a minority of patients with otherwise typical CP have a distinct form of the disease, called *antiepiligrin cicatricial pemphigoid,* which is characterized by the presence of circulating autoantibodies against epiligrin (now known as *laminin 5*). This protein constitutes the major component of the anchoring filaments, essential structures in the dermal-epidermal molecular interactions. Laminin 5 is of interest because it is the target of autoimmune antibodies in adult onset CP, but is congenitally deficient in a lethal variant of hereditary junctional epidermolysis bullosa.

Therapy of CP is determined by the tissues affected and the anticipated morbidity. Oral lesions can be treated with topical and/or systemic corticosteroids. If the eye, esophagus, or larynx is involved, the anticipated morbidity or mortality requires aggressive treatment with systemic corticosteroids and cyclophosphamide. Diaminodiphenylsulfone (dapsone) and azathioprine have been used with some success.

Pemphigoid Gestationis

More commonly known as *herpes gestationis* (HG), this is an uncommon disease that affects pregnant women and, rarely, women with ovarian tumors. The onset of the disease is during the late second or third trimester. Lesions appear first on the abdomen then spread to the rest of the trunk and proximal extremities and consist of urticarial papules and plaques followed by tense vesicles and bullae. The disease usually flares, but then resolves within several days to a few weeks after delivery. The disease often recurs in subsequent pregnancies and may also recur with menses and the intake of oral contraceptive hormones.

The histologic and direct IF findings are similar to those of BP. Sera of most patients have only trace amounts of IgG anti-BMZ antibody (formerly called the *HG factor*) that are undetectable by standard indirect IF testing. The HG factor is now known to be an IgG autoantibody, directed against the BP 180 antigen. The pathogenesis of HG is believed to be similar to that of BP, but the etiology remains uncertain and the importance of the underlying hormonal changes is unexplained.

Like BP, HG responds to moderate-dose systemic corticosteroid therapy. There may be a slightly increased risk of fetal morbidity and mortality in affected pregnancies, but this risk is very controversial.

EPIDERMOLYSIS BULLOSA ACQUISITA AND BULLOUS SYSTEMIC LUPUS ERYTHEMATOSUS

Epidermolysis bullosa acquisita (EBA) is an uncommon blistering disorder, with features that resemble congenital epidermolysis bullosa, porphyria cutanea tarda, inflammatory BP, or cicatricial pemphigoid. It affects predominantly the elderly but has been reported in children as well. Lesions predominate over the distal extremities and often are induced by trauma. Vesicles and bullae are usually followed by erosions that heal with scarring and milia formation.

Oral, ocular, and other mucosal surfaces may be involved, mimicking clinical features of CP. The disease tends to be chronic, with remissions and exacerbations. On histologic examination there is dermal-epidermal separation just beneath the lamina densa. There may be a dermal infiltrate of lymphocytes and neutrophils. Direct IF reveals IgG, IgM, IgA, and C3 at the BMZ of perilesional skin. Serum anti-BMZ antibodies are present in only 50% of patients. These antibodies react against a domain of the anchoring fibrils, which are composed of type VII collagen. There is a strong association with HLA-DR2 phenotype.

The pathogenesis is believed to involve antibody binding to type VII collagen with subsequent activation of complement, chemoattraction of polymorphonuclear leukocytes, and finally proteolytic destruction of the subbasal lamina/anchoring fibril area leading to blister formation.

Corticosteroids are of unpredictable benefit and many patients require the addition of azathioprine, cyclosporine, or other drugs for adequate control.

A condition known as bullous systemic lupus erythematosus (BSLE) is characterized by subepidermal blisters located preferentially in flexural areas. Those patients possess tissue-bound and circulating autoantibodies against type VII collagen. Thus EBA and BSLE share similar immunopathologic features, and BSLE may be caused by the development of anti–type VII collagen autoantibodies in the context of preexisting SLE. However, the relationship between these two anti–type VII collagen blistering disorders remains unclear.

LINEAR IGA BULLOUS DERMATOSIS AND CHRONIC BULLOUS DISEASE OF CHILDHOOD

These disorders are characterized by pruritic clusters of vesicles affecting the trunk and extremities, but mucosal involvement similar to CP is also seen. It is believed that these two conditions are part of the same spectrum. A transient drug-induced variant has been recently described, with vancomycin being the most commonly implicated drug.

Linear IgA, with or without a weaker IgG deposition, is characteristically seen along the BMZ. Autoantibodies against a 97-kd lamina lucida antigen and several other basement membrane components have been reported. Generally a relatively good response to dapsone, with or without concomitant oral prednisone, is achieved.

DERMATITIS HERPETIFORMIS

Dermatitis herpetiformis (DH) is an uncommon IgA-mediated bullous disease with a mean age at onset in the fourth decade. It is very rare in blacks and affects males more than females in a 3:2 proportion. Lesions classically involve the elbows, knees, buttocks, scalp, and face (Color Plate VII-4). The eruption is extremely pruritic, and primary lesions (grouped papulovesicles and papulopustules) are only rarely seen because they are very rapidly excoriated. The disease is lifelong and carries with it an increased incidence of intestinal lymphoma. Of DH patients, 80% have histologic evidence of gluten-sensitive enteropathy (GSE) similar to that seen in celiac disease, that is, small-bowel villous atrophy and lamina propria lymphocytic infiltration, but only 10% to 15% of patients have symptomatic GSE. There is no correlation between the severity of DH and that of the associated GSE.

Histologically there are neutrophilic microabscesses in dermal papillae that ultimately coalesce to form a subepidermal vesicopustule. Direct IF is diagnostic and reveals granular deposition of IgA in dermal papillae and along the BMZ, and the IgA is deposited on microfibrillar components around small elastic fibers in the upper dermis.

Indirect IF fails to reveal circulating antibodies against skin components.

DH has a strong immunogenetic background, and most patients have the HLA B8, DR3, DQW2 phenotype. However, the pathogenetic mechanisms responsible for IgA deposition in the skin are not clear.

DH responds dramatically to dapsone with cessation of pruritus within 24 to 48 hours, but patients require lifelong therapy. A gluten-free diet may lead to clearance of lesions in 6 to 36 months, and may decrease or eliminate the dapsone requirement for disease control, but only if the diet is strictly observed.

BIBLIOGRAPHY

Amagai M, Klaus-Kovtun V, Stanley JR: Autoantibodies against a novel epithelial cadherin in pemphigus vulgaris, a disease of cell adhesion, *Cell* 67:869, 1991.

Anhalt GJ et al: Induction of pemphigus in neonatal mice by passive transfer of IgG from patients with the disease, *N Engl J Med* 306:1189, 1982.

Anhalt GJ et al: Paraneoplastic pemphigus: an autoimmune mucocutaneous disease associated with neoplasia, *N Engl J Med* 323:1729, 1990.

Balding SD, Prost CP, Diaz LA et al: Cicatricial pemphigoid autoantibodies react with multiple sites on the BP180 extracellular domain, *J Invest Dermatol* 106:141, 1996.

Chan LS et al: Linear IgA bullous dermatosis: characterization of a subset of patients with concurrent IgA and IgG anti–basement membrane autoantibodies, *Arch Dermatol* 131:1432, 1995.

Domloge-Hultsch N et al: Antiepiligrin cicatricial pemphigoid: a subepithelial bullous disorder, *Arch Dermatol* 130:1521, 1994.

Gammon WR et al: Bullous SLE: a phenotypically distinctive but immunologically heterogeneous bullous disorder, *J Invest Dermatol* 100:28, 1993.

Katz SI, Strober W: The pathogenesis of dermatitis herpetiformis, *J Invest Dermatol* 70:63, 1978.

Liu Z, Giudice GJ, Swartz SJ et al: The role of complement in experimental bullous pemphigoid, *J Clin Invest* 95:1539-1544, 1995.

Mutasim DF, Diaz LA: The use of immunohistochemical techniques in the differentiation of subepidermal bullous diseases, *Am J Dermatopathol* 13:77, 1991.

Sigurgeirsson B, Agnarsson BA, Lindelof B: Risk of lymphoma in patients with dermatitis herpetiformis, *Br Med J* 308(6920):13, 1994.

Tanaka T, Furukawa F, Imamura S: Epitope mapping for epidermolysis bullosa acquisita autoantibody by molecularly cloned cDNA for type VII collagen, *J Invest Dermatol* 102:706, 1994.

Woodley DT et al: Identification of the skin basement membrane autoantigen in epidermolysis bullosa acquisita, *N Engl J Med* 310:1007, 1984

Zone JJ et al: Identification of the cutaneous basement membrane zone antigen and isolation of antibody in linear IgA disease, *J Clin Invest* 85:812, 1990.

214 Cutaneous Malignancies: Basal Cell Carcinoma and Squamous Cell Carcinoma

Margaret O'Neill and Stanley Miller

BASAL CELL CARCINOMA

Basal cell carcinoma (BCC) is the most common human malignancy, representing more than 25% of all cancers diagnosed in the United States each year. Incidence exceeds 600,000 cases annually. Predominantly a tumor of older individuals, BCC is increasing in frequency as the population ages. Nondermatologists need to be able to recognize this cancer because of its frequent occurrence.

The most common cause of BCC is chronic exposure to ultraviolet B waves in sunlight. Less often, BCCs may occur as the result of exposure to artificial light sources used in tanning salons, ionizing radiation, or arsenic. BCCs also develop within burn sites or other scars, and in association with underlying syndromes, such as xeroderma pigmentosum and basal cell nevus syndrome.

The typical BCC patient is a fair-skinned older man who has spent a significant amount of time outdoors. BCCs most commonly develop on sun-exposed areas of skin, especially on the head and neck region (85%), and particularly on the nose (25% to 30%). Several clinical

forms exist. More than half are noduloulcerative, appearing as erythematous-to-pearly, telangiectatic papules, often with central ulceration (Color Plate VII-5). A relatively rare form is the morphea-form BCC, which presents as an ill-defined, whitish, sclerotic or scar-like plaque, resembling a lesion of morphea (localized scleroderma). Pigmented BCCs are also uncommon and because of their coloration may be confused with a nevus or melanoma. Superficial BCCs often develop on less sun-exposed areas such as the trunk. Clinically they are atrophic, pink-to-red, scaly, well-demarcated plaques that may be mistaken for a persistent patch of eczema (Color Plate VII-5b).

If one lesion or especially multiple BCC lesions are noted in a patient in the first 2 or 3 decades of life, an underlying predisposing condition such as basal cell nevus syndrome, xeroderma pigmentosum, or chronic arsenic exposure should be considered. BCC is diagnosed by performing a skin biopsy. Because different modalities are used to treat the various histologic subtypes, a biopsy also helps to guide therapy.

Treatment modalities include curettage and electrodesiccation (C&E), excisional surgery, Mohs' micrographic surgery, cryotherapy, and radiation therapy. The method of treatment chosen depends on several factors, including the histologic subtype of the tumor (invasive or noninvasive features), the size of the lesion, cosmetic concerns in the area of treatment, and whether the tumor is primary or recurrent. Superficial and macronodular BCCs, especially on the trunk and extremities, are generally amenable to C&E, whereas this method is not appropriate for a morpheaform or an infiltrating BCC. For larger BCCs—especially in areas such as the face, where tissue conservation is vital—and for invasive subtypes or recurrent tumors, Mohs' micrographic surgery is the optimal form of therapy. Overall, recurrence rates are highest for morpheaform and basosquamous BCCs, lesions located on the nose or ear, larger BCCs (greater than 2-cm diameter), and tumors that are recurrent. The 5-year recurrence rate for treatment of a primary BCC is about 1% for Mohs' micrographic surgery, and averages 9% for C&E, surgical excision, radiation therapy, or cryotherapy.

With time, neglected BCCs can become locally destructive and erode into vital structures such as cartilage, bone, the orbit, and even the brain. Metastasis is extremely rare and is generally associated with larger tumor size, presence over a long period, and multiple recurrences. Once metastasis is diagnosed, survival is usually limited, averaging 8 months. Sites of metastasis, in order of frequency, are lymph nodes, lung, bone, skin, and liver. Therapies to date for metastatic BCC have been largely unsuccessful.

SQUAMOUS CELL CARCINOMA

Squamous cell carcinoma (SCC) is the second most common form of skin cancer. In most Caucasian populations, the SCC:BCC ratio is approximately 1:4. There is a linear correlation between lifetime exposure to ultraviolet light and rate of SCC occurrence. Factors favoring SCC development include poor ability to tan, tendency to sunburn, fair complexion, and blue eyes. Other high-risk conditions associated with SCC development include immunosuppressed states; a history of exposure to ionizing radiation, arsenic, polycyclic aromatic hydrocarbons or oncogenic human papillomaviruses (HPVs); chronic ulcers; burn scars; sinus tracts and scars; and chronic scarring dermatoses.

Ultraviolet-related SCC development involves a spectrum of disease. Histopathologically the earliest skin lesions reveal atypical cells confined to upper portions of the epidermis. Such lesions are termed *actinic keratoses* (AKs) and are considered precursors of SCC. Only a small percentage of AKs, however—probably less than 1%—evolve into fully developed SCCs. In situ SCC, also known as *Bowen's disease,* involves full-thickness atypia of the epidermis. Invasive SCC results when atypical cells break through the epidermal basement membrane, entering the dermal tissue. There is thus a spectrum of epidermal change in the process of SCC development, ranging from premalignant AKs to in situ carcinoma to invasive SCC. Individual lesions may remain static or progress to a more advanced stage within the disease spectrum.

The most common location for SCC is on the head and neck, followed by the extremities and trunk. AKs typically present as asymptomatic, flat, roughened, angular, scaly red papules that are often multiple. Lesions of in situ SCC can often be confused with a superficial BCC or a small plaque of eczema. Invasive SCC can variably present as a more substantive scaly red papule or plaque, a nodule, or even as a fungating mass or ulcer (Color Plate VII-6). Bleeding and crusting following minor trauma are common. Any chronic eczematous plaque or nonhealing wound, particularly arising in one of the high-risk settings described previously, should be considered as a possible SCC.

The diagnosis of SCC is made by skin biopsy. This allows for differentiation between in situ and invasive SCC, and permits identification of premalignant lesions that may be more hypertrophic and thus clinically confused with actual carcinoma.

The biologic behavior of SCC depends on multiple factors, including the degree of histologic differentiation of the tumor, its size, location, depth, status as a primary or recurrent tumor, associated etiologic factors, and the immune status of the host. The overall rate of local recurrence for SCCs of the skin is approximately 8%, and the rate of metastasis is about 5%. Cancers with a substantially higher rate of local recurrence and metastasis include tumors larger than 2 cm in diameter or deeper than 4 mm, lesions located on the ear and lip, tumors arising as a result of factors other than ultraviolet light exposure, those developing within radiation scars and chronic, non-healing wounds, poorly-differentiated, undifferentiated, and histologically infiltrative tumors, and those showing evidence of perineural invasion. Finally, organ transplantation patients and individuals receiving immunosuppressive agents for certain chronic illnesses have a markedly increased incidence of cutaneous SCCs, approximately 25-fold. The effect on the aggressiveness and metastatic potential of the individual lesions is less clear. Other immunosuppressive states probably predispose toward SCC in a similar fashion.

Treatment differs for the various forms of SCC. AKs are appropriately treated using cryotherapy or 5-fluorouracil cream, while in situ SCC generally requires curettage and electrodesiccation or surgical excision. Invasive SCCs should be surgically excised using conventional methods or Mohs' micrographic surgery, depending on the size, location, and potential for metastasis (see risk factors in earlier discussion). Radiation therapy has been employed for large, inoperable tumors, and recently success using oral retinoids in the treatment of advanced, inoperable local disease has been reported.

Cutaneous SCC most commonly (85%) metastasizes to regional lymph nodes. Lymph node dissection with or without adjuvant radiation therapy is the treatment of choice, and 5-year survival is approximately 50%. Distant metastatic disease is treated using chemotherapy protocols, and more recently, using biologic response modifiers such as retinoids and interferon.

BIBLIOGRAPHY

Edwards L et al: Treatment of cutaneous squamous cell carcinomas by intralesional interferon alfa-2b therapy, *Arch Dermatol* 128:1386, 1992.

Johnson SJ et al: Squamous cell carcinoma of the skin (excluding lip and oral mucosa), *J Am Acad Dermatol* 26:467, 1992.

Lippman SM, Meyskens FL: Treatment of advanced squamous cell carcinoma of the skin with isotretinoin, *Ann Intern Med* 107(4):499, 1987.

Miller SJ: Biology of basal cell carcinoma. I. *J Am Acad Dermatol* 24:1, 1991.

Miller SJ: Biology of basal cell carcinoma. II. *J Am Acad Dermatol* 24:161, 1991.

Rowe DE, Carroll RJ, Day CL: Prognostic factors for local recurrence, metastasis and survival rates in squamous cell carcinoma of the skin, ear, and lip, *J Am Acad Dermatol* 26:976, 1992.

Wingo PA, Tong T, Bolden S: Cancer statistics, 1995, *Cancer J Clin 45:8, 1995.*

215 Melanoma

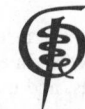

Susan E. Koch

EPIDEMIOLOGY AND ETIOLOGY

Malignant melanoma is the eighth most common cancer in the United States and is the cause of three quarters of deaths due to skin cancer. The incidence of melanoma in the United States has shown a progressive rise over the past several decades. In 1935, the lifetime risk of developing a melanoma was one in 1500. By the year 2000, one in 75 are estimated to develop melanoma during their lifetime. This trend has been associated with improved survival, largely due to earlier detection. The vast majority of melanomas occur in whites. In 1992, the U.S. death rate for melanoma was 0.4 per 100,000 in all other races compared with 2.5 per 100,000 in whites. Approximately one third of melanomas occur in those less than 45 years old.

There is considerable evidence that sun exposure is an important causal factor in whites. The rarity of melanoma among people of color is thought to be due to the protective influence of the darker skin types. Among whites, those who sunburn easily and tan poorly are at greatest risk. Those with even one sunburn early in life have an increased risk of melanoma in adulthood. Melanoma is most common on cutaneous surfaces subject to intermittent sun exposure, such as the legs in women and the back in men. Areas that are almost never exposed to the sun such as the bathing trunk area in males and the breasts in females are rarely affected.

Over the past two decades considerable attention has focused on the role of atypical (dysplastic) nevi and melanoma risk. Atypical melanocytic nevi are recognized clinically by ill-defined and irregular borders, color variegation, erythema, larger size (>5 mm or more), and mammillated surface. Histologically they demonstrate disordered architecture and may have cytologic atypia. Approximately 7% of the white population has at least one atypical nevus, and some individuals have dozens. The risk of melanoma for such individuals has been the subject of debate. Data from many centers suggest that having atypical nevi may place an individual at a higher risk. This risk is further increased if there is a family history of melanoma in a first-degree relative. Persons who have atypical nevi and one or more family members with melanoma are at great risk for melanoma. They should be identified and placed in a surveillance program to facilitate early detection and treatment. Individuals from these melanoma kindreds often have multiple primaries and develop melanoma at a younger age than do those with sporadic melanoma. Other risk factors for melanoma include immunosuppression and xeroderma pigmentosum. Large congenital nevi (>20 cm) may undergo malignant transformation in an estimated 6% of cases. The risk of melanoma in smaller congenital melanocytic nevi is disputed. Those individuals who have a history of melanoma are at an increased risk of developing another primary melanoma in the future (Color Plate VII-7).

CLINICAL FEATURES

Superficial spreading malignant melanoma, accounting for 70% of the tumors, is characterized by the following clinical features: asymmetry, border irregularity with notching, and variegation of color with shades of tan, brown, black, red, and white (Color Plate VII-8). The majority of the lesions are pigmented, but amelanotic melanoma also occurs as an erythematous plaque or nodule. Most melanomas are greater than 6 mm in diameter with a variable degree of surface elevation. Early tumors are flat and become more elevated as tumor thickness increases. Melanomas are often asymptomatic. Itching is the most common early symptom. Ulceration and bleeding may occur in advanced tumors. Early in situ melanoma may lack some of the previously mentioned classic features. A patient who notices any symptom or change in a preexisting nevus should be evaluated. In approximately 40% of superficial spreading melanomas, a preexisting melanocytic nevus is histologically identified. The remaining majority of cases occur *de novo*.

Nodular melanoma accounts for 15% of all melanomas and is characterized by its rapid grown and intense pigmentation. As with the superficial spreading variety, the most common sites of presentation are the legs in women and the trunk in men.

Acral lentiginous melanoma occurs on the skin of the palms, soles, and the subungual regions. This form of melanoma is one of the least common among whites but represents the majority of melanomas occurring in blacks, Asians, and Hispanics. The median age at the time of diagnosis is 65 years regardless of race. The most common location is the plantar surface of the foot, where the tumor presents as a flat or elevated irregularly shaped growth containing shades of brown, black, tan, red, and white—the latter indicative of regression. The average size of the tumor at presentation is 3 cm.

Subungual melanoma, which arises from the nail bed and matrix, is most commonly seen on the great toe and thumb. The pigmentation may be black or brown. *Hutchison's sign,* a brown discoloration of the proximal or lateral nail fold, is strongly suggestive of subungual melanoma. Amelanotic tumors present in as many as one fourth of cases of subungual melanoma and the erroneous diagnosis of pyogenic granuloma or paronychia is made.

Lentigo maligna represents an in situ melanoma occurring on actinically damaged skin of the face, neck, or upper extremities in older individuals. It is an asymptomatic, tan or brownish macule with an irregular border, which slowly enlarges. Initially it may resemble a solar lentigo. As it enlarges it becomes more cosmetically disturbing, and color variegation is common. In an estimated 5% to 30% of cases, the growth becomes invasive after a variable period of months to years. Invasion is generally suspected when nodular elevations develop within a preexisting macule.

DIAGNOSIS, LABORATORY EVALUATION, AND STAGING

The diagnosis of melanoma is confirmed by histologic examination of the tumor. The optimal procedure is an excisional biopsy, which enables the pathologist to confirm the diagnosis and accurately assess tumor thickness and level. Suspicious lesions occurring in cosmetically important areas may be best diagnosed with incisional biopsies before extensive therapeutic surgery is begun. Incisional biopsies should be taken from the most elevated portion of a tumor, and in flat lesions, through the darkest portion. The most important prognostic feature of the tumor is its Breslow thickness. This is a measurement from the top of the granular cell layer of the epidermis to the deepest portion of the tumor, reported in millimeters. Clark's level is used to describe the anatomic depth of invasion. Clark's level I melanoma is confined to the epidermis and is also referred to as *in situ melanoma*. Clark's II tumors invade the papillary dermis, and Clark's III tumors fill the papillary dermis but do not invade the reticular dermis. Clark's level IV melanomas extend into the reticular dermis, and Clark's level V tumors invade the subcutaneous fat. A patient's clinical stage is determined by clinical, histologic, and laboratory parameters. The formerly used three-stage system has largely been replaced with a four-stage system (Box 215-1).

The most common site of metastasis is to the regional lymph nodes. In-transit metastases occur between the primary site and the draining lymph node basin and appear as multiple dermal or subcutaneous nodules that may be darkly pigmented or nonpigmented. Metastasis also occurs to distant areas of the skin and subcutaneous tissues, and to the lungs, liver, brain, bones, and gastrointestinal tract. Any organ may be involved, and a laboratory evaluation takes into account the most common patterns of spread. At diagnosis and follow-up, every patient should have a complete cutaneous examination for distant cutaneous and subcutaneous metastases, in-transit metastases, second primary melanomas, and atypical nevi. Examination should include the regional and nonregional lymph node groups and the abdomen. A chest x-ray is indicated in all invasive melanomas to evaluate the presence or absence of pulmonary metastases. Liver function studies, particularly lactate dehydrogenase, are a sensitive but nonspecific indicator of occult liver metastasis. Possible gastrointestinal metastases may be evaluated by testing the stool for occult blood.

In situ melanoma is incapable of metastasis and therefore curable with appropriate surgical margins. The prognosis of invasive melanoma is dependent on its Breslow thickness. Other prognostic factors include ulceration, mitotic rate, regression, and presence or absence of lymphocytic infiltrate. Cases in older individuals and males, and those involving primary tumors of the head and neck and acral extremities have a poorer prognosis.

TREATMENT

The treatment of primary melanoma is surgical. The margins of excision around a biopsied tumor are based on its Breslow thickness. For in situ melanomas the recommended margin is 5 mm beyond the visible tumor. Invasive tumors that are less than 1 mm thick should be reexcised with 1 cm of surrounding skin through subcutaneous tissue to underlying fascia. Thicker tumors are subject to a excision of up to 3 cm of surrounding skin. Clinically suspicious lymph nodes should be biopsied. The role of elective lymph node dissection is controversial. More recently the use of *sentinel lymph node biopsy* shows promise in evaluating occult nodal disease while permitting selective lymph node dissection.

Therapy for metastatic melanoma is often ineffective, and the overall survival of patients with metastatic disease is 6 months. Treatment must be individualized based on the extent of the disease. Potential benefits of therapy must outweigh the morbidity of treatment. Surgical excision is a valuable treatment for isolated metastases of the lung, skin, and gastrointestinal tract. Radiation therapy is palliative and is used to treat intracranial metastases or bony involvement. A variety of chemotherapeutic regimens, immunotherapy with α-interferon, interleukin 2, and tumor vaccines are used in different centers with variable success.

FOLLOW-UP

All patients with a history of melanoma deserve careful periodic examination to detect recurrent disease, second primary tumors, lymphadenopathy, and hepatosplenomegaly. Physical examination should include the parameters mentioned earlier and careful review of systems to detect symptomatic recurrences. Patients who have had one melanoma are at increased risk of developing another primary tumor. This risk is particularly great in those individuals with atypical mole syndrome. In this selected population, careful surveillance—at least every 6 to 12 months—is warranted. The use of clinical photography to assess subtle changes in nevi may be of value. Family members should also be educated and examined periodically if they have atypical moles, for these individuals are at increased risk of developing melanoma as well. Follow-up examinations for patients with recently diagnosed melanoma should be scheduled every 3 to 6 months for the first few years following diagnosis, and at least yearly thereafter. Late recurrence, defined as a recurrence more than 10 years after treatment of the primary tumor, is well documented in melanoma; therefore, long-term follow-up of all patients is recommended.

BIBLIOGRAPHY

Balch CM et al: *Cutaneous melanoma,* ed 2, Philadelphia, 1992, Lippincott.
Barnhill RL, Mihm MC, Jr, Fitzpatrick TB et al: Neoplasms: malignant melanoma. In Fitzpatrick TB, Eisen AZ, Wolff K et al, editors: *Dermatology in general medicine,* ed 4, New York, 1993, McGraw-Hill.
Deaths from melanoma–United States, 1973-1992, *MMWR* 44:337, 1995.

BOX 215-1
Melanoma staging system

Stage I	Local disease; primary melanoma thickness 1.5 mm or less
Stage II	Local disease; primary melanoma thickness greater than 1.5 mm
Stage III	In-transit metastases or regional lymph node involvement
Stage IV	Distant metastases

Koh KH, Kligler BE, Lew RA: Sunlight and cutaneous malignant melanoma: evidence for and against causation, *Photochem Photobiol* 51:765, 1990.

Slade J et al: Atypical mole syndrome: risk factor for cutaneous malignant melanoma and implications for management, *J Am Acad Dermatol* 32:479, 1995.

CHAPTER

216 Psoriasis

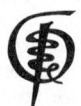

Frederick G. Wenzel and Warwick L. Morison

Psoriasis is a chronic inflammatory skin disorder that affects 1% to 2% of the world's population. It may be more common among Scandinavians and less common among Native Americans and black Africans. Both sexes are affected equally.

GENETICS

A family history can be found in 5% to 10% of patients with psoriasis. Recent evidence from HLA studies suggests a polygenic mode of inheritance. For example, certain class I MHC antigens (B13, B17, B37, B39, and Cw6) and class II MHC antigen DR7 occur with increased frequency in relatives of patients with psoriasis. A comparison of HLA haplotypes in 15 paired siblings with psoriasis revealed that 13 of the 15 pairs demonstrated identical HLA haplotypes, in contrast to the expected frequency of four identical HLA haplotypes. These results suggest that HLA-linked genes are in part responsible for the development of psoriasis. However, the fact that the concordance in homozygotic twins is only 66% suggests that environmental factors may also be important. A recent report provided evidence that, in some families, variation at a single non-HLA genetic locus on chromosome 17q is linked to psoriasis susceptibility.

The onset of psoriasis is usually bimodal, with the largest peak around the age of 16 to 20 years and a smaller peak from 50 to 60 years of age. Patients who develop psoriasis at an early age are more likely to have a positive family history, and approximately 85% are HLA-Cw6 positive. In contrast, patients with late-onset psoriasis usually do not have a family history and only 15% have the HLA-Cw6 haplotype. Patients with early onset often have more extensive disease and more nail involvement, and their course is often complicated by frequent relapses.

PATHOGENESIS

Although psoriasis may vary widely in its clinical appearance, the tendency of the epidermis to hyperproliferate is common to all patients. Keratinocyte turnover is ten times more rapid than usual, and maturation is abnormal. Transplantation studies of human skin to nude mice have demonstrated that keratinocytes from both lesional and nonlesional psoriatic skin are hyperproliferative. What stimulates the epidermis to become psoriasiform has been the major focus of investigation for the last 20 years. Increased production of leukotrienes in the epidermis has been shown in some studies. The 5-lipoxygenase inhibitor benoxaprofen (taken off the market because of hepatotoxicity) produced remissions of psoriasis. The pattern of cytokine production from both perivascular T-cells and keratinocytes, and the expression of adhesion molecules on endothelium have been the focus of more recent work. Tumor necrosis factor α (TNF-α) and interferon γ (IFN-γ) produced by mononuclear cells are probably responsible for stimulating keratinocytes to produce HLA-DR, intercellular adhesion molecule-1 (ICAM-1), interleukin-1 (IL-1), IL-6, IL-8, monocyte chemotactic activating factor (MCAF), and transforming growth factor α (TGF-α). Collectively these interactions result in keratinocyte activation and hyperproliferation, recruitment of inflammatory cells, and increased tortuosity of dermal papillary vessels, which are all characteristic of pso-

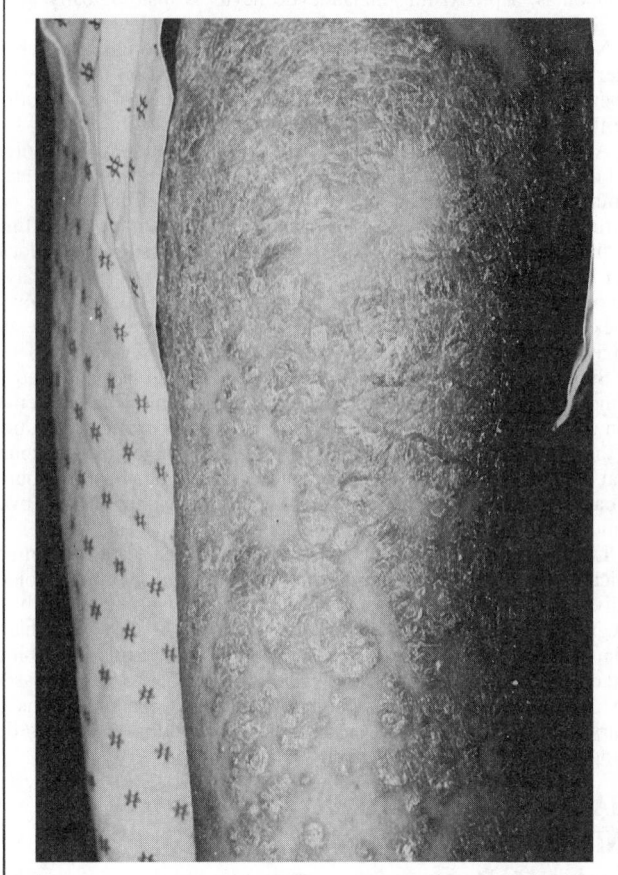

FIGURE 216-1   Plaque-type psoriasis.

riasis. It remains unclear whether the primary defect in psoriasis resides in the inflammatory infiltrate or within the epidermis itself.

CLINICAL PRESENTATION

The diagnosis of psoriasis is usually made on the basis of the clinical examination only. With the exception of certain unusual variants of psoriasis, the presentation is one of symmetric, well-demarcated, erythematous plaques with overlying silvery micaceous scales, often with accompanying pruritus (Fig. 216-1). Removal of the scale typically demonstrates pinpoint bleeding, which is called *Auspitz's sign.* Although psoriasis may affect any part of the body, it has a predilection for the knees, elbows, scalp, intergluteal cleft, palms, and soles. Nail involvement occurs in up to 50% of patients. The nail changes are often nonspecific, but pinhead-sized pits, onycholysis, and a red-brown discoloration resembling a drop of oil are some of the more characteristic findings (Fig. 216-2). Oral psoriasis may be demonstrated histologically in less than 2% of patients. Clinically it may mimic a geographic tongue. A seronegative inflammatory arthritis is seen in approximately 7% of patients. Patients with psoriatic arthritis are more likely to have nail abnormalities and scalp psoriasis. A complete description of the characteristics of psoriatic arthritis are given in Chapter 200.

A common feature of psoriasis is its tendency to develop at sites of minor trauma. This occurrence, known as *Koebner's phenomenon,* is not unique to psoriasis and can be seen in other papulosquamous dermatoses such as lichen planus. For example, scratches, tattoo applications, and surgical incisions have all been known to elicit psoriatic lesions. Indeed, chronic trauma may be why psoriasis typically affects the skin over the knees and elbows. Other factors that may exacerbate psoriasis include psychosocial stress, antecedent infection (especially streptococcal), HIV infection, childbirth, and specific drugs. Several drugs that exacerbate psoriasis are β-blockers, lithium,

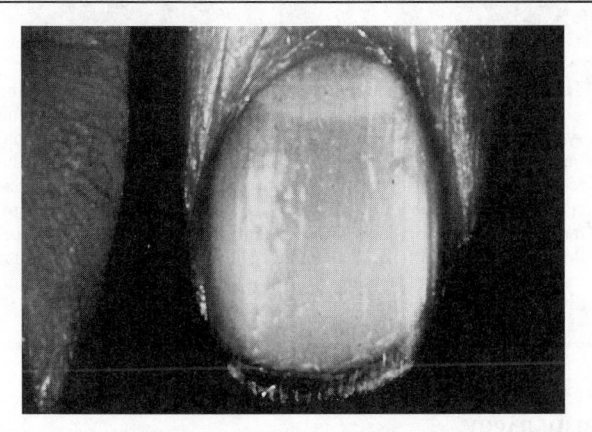

FIGURE 216-2   Nail pitting seen in psoriasis.

nonsteroidal antiinflammatory agents, interleukin-2, and, rarely, antimalarials. In addition, the use of systemic steroids, although helpful initially, may result in a dramatic flare, or the development of a pustular variant of psoriasis when the dose is reduced. Other dermatoses that might have a psoriasiform appearance include eczema, seborrheic dermatitis, tinea, cutaneous T-cell lymphoma, drug reactions, secondary syphilis, Reiter's syndrome, ichthyosis, and pityriasis rubra pilaris. When there is diagnostic confusion, a skin biopsy is often helpful. The histopathologic features of psoriasis are quite distinctive and are rarely confused with those of other dermatoses. Regular epidermal hyperplasia with focal parakeratosis, collection of neutrophils in the stratum corneum, and a mononuclear perivascular infiltrate are but a few of the characteristic changes.

There are five variants of psoriasis, which differ in their clinical appearance, severity, and response to treatment: plaque, guttate, inverse, pustular, and erythrodermic. *Plaque* type is the most frequently encountered variant. The lesions consist of indurated, sharply demarcated, oval to round plaques with the typical silvery scale (Color Plate VII-9). The lesions may be as small as a quarter or may expand to cover a large area. When lesions reach large sizes they may develop deep, painful fissures that make daily activities difficult. The *guttate* variety develops suddenly and often appears after a streptococcal infection. It consists of numerous small papules with slight scale. This variant may respond to oral antibiotics or remit spontaneously but may require traditional treatments to clear. *Inverse psoriasis* is often misdiagnosed as or coexists with a yeast or dermatophyte infection because of its location in the intertriginous areas. Psoriasis involving the axillary vault or inguinal region often lacks the characteristic scale because of the maceration that develops in such areas. *Pustular* psoriasis comes in three forms: plaques with a rim of pustules, palmoplantar pustules, and a rare generalized pustular eruption (Fig. 216-3). The latter form is the most severe with accompanying high fevers and leukocytosis. Aggressive treatment, often as an inpatient, including methotrexate or etretinate (Tegison), is often required. If psoriasis generalizes to involve the entire integument it is termed *erythroderma*. In this state, patients become hypermetabolic because of the water, protein, folic acid, and heat losses that develop as a consequence of a defective epidermal barrier. In patients with underlying coronary artery disease this hyperdynamic state may lead to high-output cardiac failure. A protein-losing enteropathy can also develop. Therefore an erythrodermic patient must be treated aggressively and may often require in-hospital management.

TREATMENT

Although there are no curative therapies for psoriasis, there are treatment options that adequately suppress the disease process and sometimes afford short periods of remission. The treatment is individualized based on the severity of a patient's disease, the patient's perception of his or her disease, accompanying medical problems, and the potential toxicities of each treatment. The treatments routinely offered

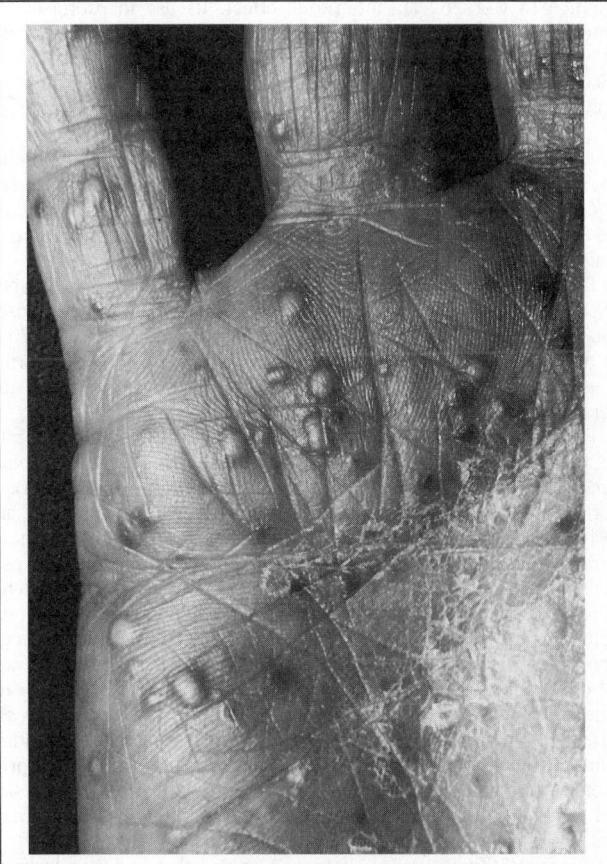

FIGURE 216-3   Pustular psoriasis.

fall in to five general categories: topical preparations, phototherapy, vitamin A analog, antimetabolites, and 5-lipoxygenase inhibitors.

Topical therapeutic agents include corticosteroids, vitamin D derivatives, anthralin, and tar preparations. Corticosteroids are the most commonly prescribed therapy for psoriasis in North America, but it should be noted that the incidence of side effects has increased with the advent of the superpotent fluorinated preparations. Only weak preparations, such as hydrocortisone, should be used on the face, perineum, and flexural areas. The major concerns with all corticosteroid preparations are dermal atrophy, skin fragility, fast relapse times, tachyphylaxis, and in rare cases, adrenal suppression resulting from systemic absorption. Calcipotriene, a derivative of vitamin D, has been recently approved for topical use on mild to moderate plaque psoriasis. Trials with this formulation have shown efficacy rates equal to a medium-potency steroid ointment, while avoiding the steroid-related side effects and tachyphylaxis. Potential risks include mild irritation and hypercalcemia, although this has not been observed with the recommended doses.

Anthralin, a synthetic derivative of tree bark extract, has been used since 1916. It is used widely in Europe as part of the inpatient Ingram's regimen. This regimen consists of a tar bath followed by exposure to ultraviolet B, which is followed in turn by an application of anthralin with salicylic acid. Repeating this sequence every 24 hours usually results in total clearing of extensive plaque-type psoriasis within 3 weeks. Anthralin can also be used as an Ingram's regimen in patients with limited, thick, plaque-type psoriasis. The anthralin is administered in strengths up to 1% and applied directly to the psoriatic plaque for 10 minutes to 1 hour daily. Commonly experienced side effects are irritation of surrounding skin, brownish discoloration of treated areas, and purple discoloration of bathtubs and clothing or linen. It is not suitable for the head and neck, genitalia, or flexural areas, where it is too irritating.

One of the oldest remedies for psoriasis is crude coal tar, which is assumed to work by an antimitotic effect. Its use in psoriasis was popularized by Goeckerman in the 1930s, and the regimen now bears his name. This treatment consists of the daily application of 2% to 5% crude coal tar combined with a tar bath and ultraviolet light. Many modifications of this program have been put forth, the Ingram's regimen being one of the more popular variants. Many psoriasis day care centers use a modification of Goeckerman's regimen for their patients. The criticisms of this treatment are the extended time commitments required of the patient and the associated mess. More recently, the use of liquor carbonis detergents (LCD) has replaced the use of crude coal tar.

Phototherapy refers to the use of sunburn-producing wavelengths (290 to 320 nm) of radiation (ultraviolet B) for treating dermatoses. This therapy is administered three to five times per week and 20 to 30 treatments are required for clearing. Patients with erythrodermic or generalized pustular psoriasis usually do not respond to this therapy.

Photochemotherapy or PUVA refers to the combination of orally administered 8-methoxypsoralen, a photosensitizing drug, and exposure 1 to 2 hours later to ultraviolet A radiation (320 to 400 nm). In North America treatments are usually given three times per week, and 20 to 30 treatments are required for clearing. This form of phototherapy is more effective than ultraviolet B for thick plaque-type psoriasis, pustular psoriasis, and generalized erythroderma, but it also has more side effects. The major concerns are premature photoaging, nonmelanoma skin cancers, and premature cataract formation. A recent report identified 30 genital tumors in 14 men receiving PUVA therapy out of a cohort of 892. These risks may be minimized by having the patient wear ultraviolet A screening sunglasses, protecting the patient's skin for 12 hours after ingestion of the psoralen, providing genital protection during PUVA therapy, avoiding patients with prior arsenic or ionizing radiation exposure, and conducting regular skin and ophthalmologic exams. This therapy, like most systemic therapies for psoriasis, is contraindicated in pregnancy.

Etretinate (Tegison) is a vitamin A analog that is particularly effective for acral or generalized pustular psoriasis. Etretinate is less effective in plaque-type psoriasis, in which other systemic therapies such as PUVA or methotrexate are preferred. Major side effects are mucocutaneous dryness, increased serum lipid concentration, and after prolonged treatment, skeletal changes. Etretinate is contraindicated in women capable of childbearing except in exceptional circumstances because it can persist in the body for 2 years or more.

Methotrexate, a methyl analog of folic acid, is the most commonly used antimetabolite for the treatment of psoriasis. Other antimitotic medications used less commonly include hydroxyurea and azathioprine. Methotrexate in doses of 2.5 to 25 mg per week is highly effective for extensive plaque-type psoriasis, pustular psoriasis, erythrodermic psoriasis, and psoriatic arthritis. It is thought to work by inhibiting DNA synthesis as well as neutrophil chemotaxis. Methotrexate is primarily used as a short-term treatment option to control psoriasis before switching to another therapy such as PUVA, UVB, or a topical regimen. Long-term methotrexate therapy is reserved for patients with severe psoriasis unresponsive to or intolerant of other less toxic treatments who have no contraindications to methotrexate as outlined by the American Academy of Dermatology in 1988. The major risks of long-term methotrexate treatment include hepatic fibrosis and cirrhosis, bone marrow suppression, and pulmonary toxicity. The most common side effects are nausea, loss of appetite, headaches, and alopecia. Conception must be avoided during treatment and for one menstrual cycle after completing treatment in women and 3 months after completing treatment in men.

Cyclosporine, currently not licensed for use in psoriasis, has been shown in many studies to quickly clear 90% of psoriasis in patients at a starting dose of 3 to 5 mg/kg a day orally. The risk of renal impairment and the consequences of immunosuppression have limited its use. Cyclosporine is most exciting because it may lead to a better understanding of the underlying immunologic mechanisms in psoriasis.

We would like to thank Lisa A. Beck, MD, for her contribution to this chapter in the previous edition.

✔ *WHEN TO REFER*

The treatment of each individual patient varies as dictated by the severity of the disease. Most patients experience both topical and systemic therapies during the course of their disease. For the patient with mild disease, topical treatments alone can yield adequate results. However, for the patient with moderate to severe psoriasis, consideration should be given to systemic and phototherapy treatments. It is not uncommon to combine therapies such as anthralin and PUVA, etretinate and PUVA, and methotrexate and PUVA to minimize the side effects of both treatment options and to shorten treatment times.

BIBLIOGRAPHY

Barker JNWN: The pathophysiology of psoriasis, *Lancet* 338:227, 1991.
Greaves MW, Weinstein GD: Treatment of psoriasis, *N Engl J Med* 332:581, 1995.
Henseler T, Christophers E: Psoriasis of early and late onset: characterization of two types of psoriasis vulgaris, *J Am Acad Dermatol* 13:450, 1985.
Morison W: *Phototherapy and photochemotherapy of skin disease,* ed 2, New York, 1991, Raven Press.
Roenigk HH et al: Methotrexate in psoriasis: revised guidelines, *J Am Acad Dermatol* 19:145, 1988.
Telfer NR et al: The role of streptococcal infections in the initiation of guttate psoriasis, *Arch Dermatol* 128:39, 1992.
Tomfohrde J et al: Gene for familial psoriasis susceptibility mapped to the distal end of human chromosome 17q, *Science* 264:1141, 1994.

CHAPTER

217 Dermatitis

S. Elizabeth Whitmore

Dermatitis and eczema are interchangeable terms used to describe inflammation of the skin inclusive of the more superficial epidermal compartment. The histologic changes, which include edema and a mononuclear cell infiltrate in the epidermis, surface serous exudation, and a perivascular mononuclear cell infiltrate in the upper dermis, lead to the visible surface changes of edematous papules, vesicles, crusting, scaling, erythema, and edema. When the process becomes more chronic, the epidermis reacts by thickening *(acanthosis)* with the clinical appearance of a washboard; this change is termed *lichenification.* Dermatitis is a very broad term and for this reason different types of dermatitis have been defined. These definitions are based on frequently associated disorders, as in atopic dermatitis; cause, as in contact dermatitis; morphology, as in nummular dermatitis; and location, as in hand dermatitis. The different types of dermatitis may be caused by purely endogenous factors, exogenous factors, or a combination of the two.

ATOPIC DERMATITIS

Atopic dermatitis is usually seen in association with other manifestations of atopy, including allergic asthma or rhinitis, or a family history of atopy. Although the etiology is not clear, it is considered an endogenous dermatitis. Various immunologic alterations have been described, including an elevated serum IgE antibody level, decreased delayed hypersensitivity responsiveness, decreased number or activity of T-suppressor and natural killer lymphocytes, and increased percentage of B-lymphocytes with surface-bound IgE1. Although these immunologic abnormalities may play a role in the pathogenesis of atopic dermatitis, they are not present in all patients.

Atopic dermatitis is classically divided into three types depending on the time of onset: infantile, childhood, and adult. Excluding infantile, in which extensor extremities and cheeks are usually affected, atopic dermatitis is generally considered a *flexural dermatitis* primarily involving the antecubital and popliteal fossae. Cutaneous changes include erythematous, edematous papules that frequently coalesce into plaques with secondary surface scale, erosions, crusts, and lichenification.

It is said that atopic dermatitis is the "itch that rashes," and therefore one of the fundamental goals of treatment is reduction of pruritus. This is accomplished with avoidance of low humidity and cold or very hot environments; the use of softened cotton clothing rather than wool or starched clothing, washing with mild moisturizing soaps (e.g., Dove, Aveeno Oilated, or Oilatum soaps), and frequent use of oil-based moisturizers (e.g., Eucerin lotion, Aquaphor ointment, or petrolatum). In addition, sedating antihistamines may be helpful purely because of their soporific effect. When dermatitis is present, the first line of treatment in adults includes moisturizers as listed previously and mid- (e.g., triamcinolone acetonide 0.1% and betamethasone valerate 0.1%) to high-potency (e.g., fluocinonide 0.05% and betamethasone dipropionate 0.05%) topical corticosteroid ointments. For facial, auricular, axillary, or genital dermatitis, only low-potency corticosteroids (e.g., hydrocortisone 1% over the counter and 2.5% by prescription) should be used. Not infrequently, patients also have recurrent infection or "dermatitis-aggravating" colonization with *Staphylococcus aureus* requiring oral antibiotics (e.g., cephalexin or dicloxacillin, 500 mg bid for 7 to 10 days).

While it is debated whether corticosteroids need to be applied once or twice daily, moisturizers clearly should be applied at least twice daily. Inappropriate or prolonged use of topical corticosteroids may cause permanent atrophy, striae, acne, bacterial or fungal infection, and even allergic contact dermatitis. Widespread application may also cause hypothalamic-pituitary-adrenal axis suppression. Patients should be warned to watch for skin thinning and striae, and therapy lasting longer than a few weeks should be monitored by the physician.

When the above treatments are ineffective, in-office phototherapy with ultraviolet B (UVB) radiation or photochemotherapy with ultraviolet A (UVA) in combination with the oral photosensitizer psoralen (PUVA), may be quite effective. Treatment is usually required three times weekly for 2 months, and then may be stopped or continued on a maintenance schedule, once every 1 to 3 weeks, as needed.

As atopic dermatitis is clearly aggravated by irritants contacting the skin, particularly the hands, the suggestion has been made that children with atopic dermatitis be dissuaded from choosing careers that involve a significant amount of wet work or frequent exposure to irritants.

NUMMULAR DERMATITIS

Nummular dermatitis is defined by its morphologic appearance of sharply circumscribed coin-shaped or discoid plaques of dermatitis.

Patients typically present with one or a few erythematous, nummular plaques formed by minute, coalescing papules or more inflammatory papulovesicles on the legs or arms. Early lesions usually have a moist surface due to serous exudate that quickly becomes crusted. With time, the lesions become dry, scaly, and flattened. Infrequently, generalized nummular dermatitis, often secondarily infected with *S. aureus*, may develop.

Similar to the therapy described earlier for atopic dermatitis, treatment includes avoidance of irritants and the use of moisturizers and mid- to high-potency topical corticosteroid ointments with oral antistaphylococcal antibiotics for secondary infection, as needed.

ASTEATOTIC DERMATITIS

Asteatotic dermatitis (eczema craquelé) occurs in individuals with dry (asteatotic, xerotic) skin and therefore is seen most frequently in the winter months in older persons exposed to environmental conditions that predispose to xerosis. These conditions include low ambient humidity and forced heat in the home, hot showers, and lack of emollient use. Once the skin becomes dry and develops microscopic cracks, it may sting, itch, and feel very tight. Patients present with chapped-appearing, erythematous areas with a surface netlike pattern of fine cracks, aptly also called *eczema craquelé*, typically affecting the legs, arms, and/or hands.

Treatment includes increasing the hydration of the skin and clearing the inflammation. Avoidance of irritants, warm instead of hot showers or baths followed by moisturizers, and low- to mid-potency topical corticosteroids, as described earlier for atopic dermatitis, are generally effective in treatment.

CONTACT DERMATITIS

Contact dermatitis may be divided into two types: irritant and allergic contact dermatitis. Unlike other forms of dermatitis in which estimates of incidence and prevalence are quite variable or unavailable, occupational contact dermatitis poses a major direct cost to industry; therefore reported epidemiologic statistics are believed to be fairly reliable. In this country, skin disease (90% of which is contact dermatitis) accounts for nearly 40% of all occupational illnesses, affecting approximately 0.1% of workers at an estimated cost of up to $1 billion per year.

Irritant contact dermatitis is a nonimmunologic reaction caused by a direct insult to the skin. Susceptibility to irritant contact dermatitis varies immensely among individuals. Patients with atopic dermatitis may develop irritant contact dermatitis from mild cleansers, while "resistant" individuals may experience no visible skin changes with exposure to harsh detergents. Irritant contact dermatitis is seen most commonly in persons who frequently wet and dry their skin, are exposed to cold outdoor winds or hot indoor forced heat, or any other factors that dry the skin and strip away the outermost cells of the skin or surface water-holding substances. The most commonly encountered irritants are alkaline solutions such as soaps and cleansers.

Exposure to a harsh chemical produces a localized scalded, erythematous, moist area with peeling back of the overlying epidermis, leaving a fine, lacy scale at the border. In contrast, a mild irritant only produces mild macular erythema. If exposure becomes chronic, secondary changes of scale and plaque formation develop. Treatment involves eliminating the contactant(s) and the use of moisturizers and mild soaps, as described earlier for atopic dermatitis.

Allergic contact dermatitis, a delayed hypersensitivity immune reaction, is less common than irritant contact dermatitis. It requires an initial sensitization phase in which a hapten applied to the skin binds a cutaneous protein, and is then processed by the antigen-presenting cell of the epidermis, the Langerhans' cell. The Langerhans' cell next moves into the dermis and travels through the lymphatics to the regional lymph nodes where it stimulates a clone of T-lymphocytes able to recognize the antigen. On subsequent exposure to the allergen, Langerhans' cells resident within the epidermis present the antigen to the circulating memory T-helper cells, which then release various cytokines including interleukin-2 and interferon γ. These mediators recruit and activate additional inflammatory cells, which also release various cytokines that act to enhance or dampen the inflammatory cascade. The resultant clinical reaction is that of an acute dermatitis.

The allergens that most commonly cause allergic contact dermatitis come from plants of the *Rhus* genus, including poison ivy, oak, and sumac. Exposure to the plant oleoresin containing urushiol in sensitized individuals usually leads to an acute, vesiculobullous eruption in the areas of contact. Other allergens tend to produce less dramatic reactions and sensitize a much smaller portion of the population. Such allergens include nickel, found in costume jewelry and various metal articles; neomycin, benzocaine, and merthiolate used as topical medicaments; and fragrances and preservatives found in most cosmetic and personal products, as well as dermatologic, ophthalmologic, and otic prescription and nonprescription formulations. Allergens encountered in various occupations include thiram, mercaptobenzothiazole, and carbamate rubber accelerators in all latex rubber products (including gloves); potassium dichromate in cement, dyes, or textiles; epoxy resin in adhesives, product finishes, and casings for electrical devices; rosin in adhesive materials; glyceryl monothioglycolate and paraphenylenediamine in permanent hair waves and dyes, respectively; and acrylates before fully cured (polymerized) in orthopedic "cement," dental bonding materials, and artificial nails.

Most often, persons with allergic contact dermatitis present with a chronic (as opposed to acute) dermatitis consisting of erythematous papules and lichenified plaques in the areas of contact. Patients with suspected allergic contact dermatitis should be referred to a dermatologist for patch testing. A meticulous history regarding both work and home exposures is required, followed by epicutaneous patch testing on the back with the application of various suspected chemical allergens for 48 hours. These sites are examined for localized reactions (erythema and edema, papules or vesicles) at 48 and 96 hours. Once the allergenic chemical(s) has been identified, avoidance of exposure is the cornerstone of treatment. In addition, mid- to high-potency corticosteroid ointments, as described for atopic dermatitis, are used for one to a few weeks to clear the chronic dermatitis, and ongoing use of moisturizers and avoidance of irritants is recommended to protect the altered skin from further damage.

CONTACT URTICARIA

An important type of contact reaction that is not dermatitis is contact urticaria, seen as a hive at the site of contact. When immunologically mediated, this reaction is caused by an IgE response to a protein in latex, bacitracin, neomycin, benzocaine, lindane, various metals, and other allergens, with latex allergy being most common. Studies in Europe and Canada have found the prevalence of latex contact urticaria in operating room personnel to be approximately 10%, with an over-representation among atopic individuals (30% affected). Also, patients with chronic parenteral exposure to latex, such as children with spina bifida or severe congenital urologic abnormalities requiring urinary catheterization and frequent surgical procedures are more likely to eventually develop latex contact urticaria; therefore prophylactic avoidance is recommended.

The presently rising incidence of sensitization to latex is thought to be due to the increased use of and declining quality of latex gloves, which leave more free protein antigen available to cause sensitization. Although the reaction in contact urticaria is usually localized to the site of contact, systemic signs of histamine release may occur, including generalized hives, mild wheezing to complete airway obstruction, and hypotension with tachycardia. Individuals who are allergic to latex are at greater risk for anaphylactic reactions when the antigen is encountered on mucosal surfaces such as the oral, vaginal, or rectal mucosa, or internally, as occurs with various invasive examinations and surgical procedures. Initial evaluation for this allergy includes a latex IgE RAST test; however, the sensitivity of this test is only approximately 70%, therefore patients with suspected allergy but negative RAST tests should be referred to an allergist or dermatologist specializing in this area for skin testing.

Recognition and diagnosis of this allergy with counseling on strict avoidance of latex exposures (latex gloves, balloons, condoms, etc.) and notification of these patients' physicians and dentists is absolutely essential, as both patients and physicians must recognize the potentially *life-threatening* nature of this lifelong disorder (patients require many specialized medical devices because face masks, catheters, tourniquets, dental dams, surgical gloves, and many other products all contain latex). Finally, patients should wear allergy-identifying Medic Alert bracelets and carry an epinephrine-containing pen for emergencies.

HAND DERMATITIS

Hand dermatitis is a term frequently applied to any dermatitic reaction on the hands; the actual primary disorder may be atopic dermatitis, irritant or allergic contact dermatitis predominantly affecting the hands, or "dyshidrotic hand dermatitis." This last-mentioned condition, unlike the former disorders, is always confined to the hands and has characteristic features. Patients usually present with a history of cyclic waves of pruritic, deep-seated, 1- to 2-mm vesicles on the sides of the fingers, and also often on the palms. As the lesions clear, there is subsequent overlying desquamation and drying of the skin. A "wave" generally lasts 1 to 3 weeks, and cycles may occur almost continuously or, at the other extreme, be a one-time occurrence. Despite the term *dyshidrotic,* the etiology is unknown, and there actually is no problem with hidrosis or sweating.

Treatment includes the avoidance of irritants and the application of hand cream (e.g., Cutemol or Neutrogena Hand Cream) and mid- to high-potency topical corticosteroid ointments as described earlier for atopic dermatitis, for flares of disease. Unresponsive disease may require in-office PUVA photochemotherapy, similar to that described earlier for atopic dermatitis, utilizing a smaller light box that exposes only the hands, rather than the entire body, to light. In addition, pa-

tients must be told that this is most often a chronic relapsing disorder for which there is no permanent cure.

INFECTIOUS ECZEMATOID DERMATITIS

Infectious excematoid dermatitis, or extensive secondary infection, may occur in any form of primary dermatitis. Marked serum crusting of the dermatitis is seen, with frequent extension of the dermatitis and infection to areas not previously affected. The mainstay of treatment for this disorder includes appropriate oral antibiotics (most often cephalexin or dicloxacillin, 1 to 2 g daily for 7 to 14 days, for treatment of *S. aureus,* the most common infectious agent), tap water or saline (2 teaspoons salt per quart of water) compresses or bathtub soaks, moisturizers, and topical corticosteroids as needed to control the primary dermatitis.

BIBLIOGRAPHY

Champion RH, Parish WE: Atopic dermatitis. In Rook A et al, editors: *Textbook of dermatology,* ed 5, Cambridge, Mass, 1992, Blackwell Scientific.
Domonkos AN, Arnold HL, Odom RB: *Andrews' diseases of the skin,* ed 8, Philadelphia, 1990, Saunders.
Rietschel RL, Fowler JR, Jr: *Fisher's contact dermatitis,* ed 4, Baltimore, 1995, Williams & Wilkins.

I would like to thank Dr. James Nethercott for his contribution.

CHAPTER

218 Acne Vulgaris

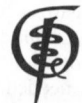

Charlotte E. Modly

Acne vulgaris currently affects 80% to 90% of young adults with sequelae that may persist indefinitely. Because of the physical and psychologic impact, an understanding of the pathophysiology, clinical manifestations, and treatment modalities of acne vulgaris is essential.

EPIDEMIOLOGY

Although acne vulgaris is traditionally associated with adolescence, it can occur in the neonatal period and into the fourth decade of life. Under the influence of maternal androgens, the neonate's sebaceous glands are stimulated; this may account for the prevalence of acneiform lesions during the first weeks of life. Sebaceous glands become quiescent again until puberty, and the peak incidence of acne is in the mid to late teens. It is slightly more common in males than in females, and the severe forms of acne are much more common in males. Hormonal factors are probably responsible for the higher incidence of acne in postadolescent women than men. Racial differences that have been reported include a higher prevalence in white American versus Japanese men, and a higher incidence of nodulocystic acne vulgaris in white versus black males.

PATHOGENESIS

The pathophysiologic events leading to the formation of an acne lesion occur within the microscopic structure known as the sebaceous follicle. Sebaceous follicles contain a small vellus hair and a large multilobulated sebaceous gland and are most concentrated on the face, back, chest, and shoulders. There are four principal components in the pathogenesis: (1) abnormal keratinization of follicular epithelium with the formation of the microcomedone (inspissated keratin, epithelial cells, sebum, and bacteria), (2) excess sebum production, (3) enzymatic activity of *Proprionobacterium acnes* and *Proprionobacterium granulosum,* and (4) chemotactic factors secreted by *P. acnes.*

Host factors such as heredity, environment, and emotional state also contribute to the development of acne lesions.

The formation of the microcomedone is universal to all acne lesions. Abnormal follicular keratinization prevents the loss of epithelial cells normally carried out of the follicle by the flow of sebum. The epithelial cells adhere and trap sebum and bacteria in the infrainfundibular portion of the follicle. The cohesiveness of follicular epithelial cells is thought to be related to a decrease in membrane coating granules; it is their lytic enzymes that allow normal differentiation to occur. The microcomedone is not clinically apparent but is the precursor of all other lesions.

Sebum is extremely important in the development of acne. Sebum production is regulated by androgens of gonadal and adrenal origins through the conversion of testosterone to 5-dihydroxytestosterone by the sebaceous follicle. Individuals with severe acne produce more sebum, and those with low levels of androgens, such as castrated or adrenalectomized patients, do not develop acne. Sebum alters the environment in the follicle via three mechanisms: it accumulates behind the microcomedone, causing follicular dilation; it provides a substrate for bacterial lipases that produce free fatty acids from the triglycerides in sebum; and it may contribute to abnormal follicular keratinization. The free fatty acids created are proinflammatory. In addition, the sebum from patients with severe acne is often relatively deficient in linoleic acid, an essential fatty acid required for normal epithelial differentiation.

The anaerobic diphtheroids, *P. acnes* and *P. granulosum,* are primarily responsible for the inflammation seen in acne. Bacterial lipases produce free fatty acids as mentioned earlier, but these are not as important as the recently identified low- and high-molecular-weight chemotactic peptides and proteolytic enzymes produced by the organisms. The peptides attract neutrophils, which in turn enter the follicle, phagocytize the bacteria, and release proteolytic enzymes. These enzymes disrupt the follicular epithelium. Higher molecular weight chemotactic factors are then released, and lymphocytes and macrophages are attracted. Recently it has been demonstrated that *P. acnes* is not the only source of chemotactic factors. Comedones may also secrete soluble factors that attract neutrophils into the follicle. Once the follicular contents contact serum in the dermis, complement is activated, and the inflammatory process continues.

CLINICAL MANIFESTATIONS

The lesions of acne vulgaris are heterogeneous. Localized primarily to the face and to a lesser degree to the back, chest, and shoulders, lesions can be inflamed or noninflamed. Erythematous papules, pustules, and large fluctuant nodules make up the inflammatory subset. Open comedones *(blackheads)* and closed comedones *(whiteheads)* are the noninflammatory lesions. In patients with the severe form of acne known as *acne conglobata,* inflammatory cysts with sinus tracts are present.

The differential diagnosis of acneiform lesions includes acneiform drug eruptions, acne rosacea, chloracne, and chronic sun damage. Drugs such as lithium carbonate, dilantin, actinomycin D, bromide- or iodide-containing medications, and systemic corticosteroids can produce acneiform lesions, but usually they are more homogeneous than those of acne vulgaris. Recently, acneiform lesions have been recognized as a manifestation of anabolic steroid abuse. Acne rosacea, which can present with papules and pustules, also demonstrates telangiectases and sebaceous gland hyperplasia. Chloracne represents a reaction to chlorinated hydrocarbons and manifests itself as open comedones. The facial lesions of tuberous sclerosis can also mimic acne but on close inspection are not follicular in distribution, are not heterogeneous or transient and are associated with the neurologic, ophthalmologic, and cutaneous stigmata of tuberous sclerosis.

TREATMENT

Treatment of acne vulgaris should be based on the pathogenic factors involved, that is, microcomedone formation, sebum production, and proliferation of *P. acnes.* Comedolytic agents include topical salicylic acid and topical tretinoin (transretinoic acid, Retin-A). Tretinoin is much more effective than salicylic acid, however, in preventing microcomedone formation and causing dissolution of mature comedones. Tretinoin normalizes epithelial differentiation and shedding, thereby preventing the cohesiveness that leads to microcomedone formation. It does not affect sebum production. Because the drug is now available in low-potency and less-irritating forms such as the 0.025% cream, tretinoin should be an essential part of the therapeutic regimen. Patients may experience some mild initial irritation and should be warned of enhanced photosensitivity while using tretinoin.

Sebaceous gland function can be altered through the use of hormonal therapy or isotretinoin. Estrogen and antiandrogen therapy is indicated in patients with evidence of ovarian androgen excess. Estrogens are usually prescribed in the form of oral contraceptives. Although it had been thought that at least 50 μg of estrogen per day are needed for a therapeutic response, recent evidence suggests that even 35 μg of estrogen, as is present in the newer triphasic contraceptives, may be sufficient to treat acne. Other antiandrogens, such as spironolactone, flutamide, and ciproterone acetate can be effective but usually require concomitant therapy with oral contraceptives to regulate menses. In patients with adrenal androgen excess, low-dose corticosteroids may be effective.

The most effective method of sebum suppression is through isotretinoin therapy. This systemically administered vitamin A derivative is reserved for severe cystic acne. It acts by markedly suppressing sebaceous gland function and abnormal keratinization and indirectly by decreasing bacterial growth. The impressive clinical performance of isotretinoin is tempered by the multitude of side effects, which range from universal drying of mucous membranes to hypertriglyceridemia and teratogenicity. Extreme caution should be used when prescribing isotretinoin to women of childbearing age. Concomitant contraceptive therapy is **mandatory.**

The antiinflammatory armamentarium includes the benzoyl peroxides, topical and systemic antibiotics, and intralesional corticosteroids. Recent evidence suggests that antimicrobial therapy may function to both kill *P. acnes* and decrease its inflammatory potential through nonlethal means. Low doses of antibiotics have been shown to decrease lipase and chemotactic factor production without altering bacterial viability. In addition, antibiotics can inhibit inflammatory cell migration. The benzoyl peroxides are lipophilic and antimicrobial without conferring resistance to the organisms. In addition, they may inhibit protein kinase C and be directly cytotoxic to leukocytes. No significant clinical difference has been detected between 5% and 10% benzoyl peroxides. Topical erythromycin and clindamycin phosphate are equally effective in reducing acne lesions and are easily applied as solutions, gels, or ointments. The benefit of adding zinc to topical erythromycin solutions is currently being evaluated. Combining a topical antimicrobial with tretinoin enhances penetration of the antibacterial agent.

Systemic antibiotics used in acne include tetracycline, doxycycline, minocycline, erythromycin, and trimethoprim-sulfamethoxazole. Although tetracycline (1 g/day) is used frequently and can be very effective, poor compliance can often interfere with therapeutic response. Doxycycline is also very effective but quite photosensitizing. Minocycline possesses better follicular penetrance and is very efficacious but expensive. Erythromycin (1 g/day) is a cost-effective form of acne therapy, but *P. acnes* develops resistance to it more rapidly than to the tetracyclines. Long-term antibiotic therapy can sometimes lead to a secondary gram-negative folliculitis that may require therapy with antibiotics such as trimethoprim-sulfamethoxazole or isotretinoin.

Acutely inflamed lesions of acne often respond well to intralesional administration of triamcinolone acetonide. Systemic steroids are used—rarely—in the acute setting to treat a severe flare of nodulocystic acne. Surgical therapy, such as chemical peels, dermabrasion, scar revision, and soft tissue augmentation, is directed toward treating the disfiguring sequelae of acne.

In summary, a rational first approach to treating acne vulgaris includes comedolytic therapy with tretinoin and antibacterial therapy with benzoyl peroxides and/or topical antibiotics. A response requires 2 to 3 months of therapy, and if the response is inadequate, systemic antibiotics are necessary. Isotretinoin and hormonal therapy should be reserved for the specific situations outlined earlier.

✔ *WHEN TO REFER*

Because of the prevalence of acne vulgaris, most practitioners will be confronted with a patient requesting treatment. Initiation of therapy with topical agents with proper patient education is appropriate. Should systemic and/or surgical therapy be necessary, consultation with a dermatologist should be considered.

BIBLIOGRAPHY

American Academy of Dermatology: Guidelines of care for acne vulgaris, *J Am Acad Dermatol* 22:676, 1990.

Pochi PE: Guidelines for prescribing isotretinoin (Accutane) in the treatment of female acne patients of childbearing potential, *J Am Acad Dermatol* 19:920, 1988.

Shalita AR: Acne revisited. *Arch Dermatol* 130:363, 1994.

Strauss JS: Biology of the sebaceous gland and the pathophysiology of acne vulgaris. In Soter NA, Baden HP, editors: *Pathophysiology of dermatologic disease,* New York, 1991, McGraw-Hill.

Strauss JS: Sebaceous glands. In Fitzpatrick TB, Eisen AZ et al, editors: *Dermatology in general medicine,* New York, 1993, McGraw-Hill.

Webster GF: Inflammation in acne vulgaris, *J Am Acad Dermatol* 33:247, 1995.

CHAPTER

219 Photodermatoses

Frederick G. Wenzel and Warwick L. Morison

Photodermatoses are disorders of the skin produced or exacerbated by exposure to sunlight or other sources of nonionizing radiation. Patients with these conditions are said to be photosensitive, and thus another name for these conditions is *photosensitivity disease*. Photodermatoses are common, and about 15% of people are photosensitive if exposed to a sufficient dose of sunlight. Fortunately, for most people the threshold of sensitivity is high. After one or two episodes these individuals usually appreciate their tolerance and subsequently avoid exposure of a duration sufficient to trigger the reaction. Thus they rarely consult a physician. There are many different and distinct photodermatoses, but, fortunately for the clinician, five conditions account for almost all cases of photosensitivity: polymorphous light eruption (PMLE), solar urticaria, lupus erythematosus (LE), drug and chemical photosensitivity, and porphyria. Other disorders are very rare.

Ultraviolet (UV) radiation in sunlight is arbitrarily divided into the shorter UVB wave band (295 to 320 nm) and the longer UVA wave band (320 to 400 nm). UVB radiation is mainly responsible for a sunburn, a suntan, and other normal responses to sunlight. However, photodermatoses are often triggered by UVA radiation. An important practical point is that window glass filters out UVB radiation, so if a patient describes a reaction caused by sunlight through window glass, such a reaction is almost certainly abnormal.

Everyone shows some response to sunlight, and therefore the first step in diagnosing a photodermatosis is to determine whether the response of the patient is greater than normal. Photodermatoses take two forms: exaggeration of the normal responses to sunlight and the development of a separate and distinct rash from a normal exposure to sunlight.

EXAGGERATED NORMAL REACTIONS TO SOLAR RADIATION

Sunburn can appear as an extremely severe response in several situations. Skin that lacks normal pigmentation is obviously prone to severe sunburning. Thus patients with albinism and vitiligo readily sunburn, and the underlying condition is usually quite evident. People

BOX 219-1
Common phototoxic agents

Psoralens (as medication and in plants and fruits)
Coal tar derivatives (in medications and cosmetics)
Vitamin A derivatives (Retin-A)
Para-aminobenzoic acid esters
Sulfonamides
Nalidixic acid
Doxycycline
Fluoroquinolones
Amiodarone

with so-called type I skin, who always sunburn and never tan because they lack normal-functioning melanocytes, are also prone to develop severe sunburns. Freckling of the skin is a common added problem in these patients.

A severe sunburn in an otherwise normal person—that is, a severity out of proportion with the duration of exposure—is usually caused by drug or chemical phototoxicity. Compounds that commonly produce this reaction are listed in Box 219-1. Systemic agents produce an exaggerated sunburn in all exposed areas, whereas topical agents produce a reaction limited to the area of contact exposed to sunlight. Phototoxic reactions may not follow the usual time course of a sunburn. They are often delayed in onset to 48 or 72 hours after exposure and may persist for a week or more. Dark pigmentation, often lasting for months, is a common sequela.

Several rare disorders should be considered in the diagnosis of a severe sunburn. In an infant or young child, repeated severe sunburns can be the first sign of xeroderma pigmentosum. Unfortunately this early warning is usually not appreciated until the patient begins to develop multiple skin tumors as a teenager or young adult. Widespread freckling of exposed skin is another sign of this disorder and usually precedes malignancies. Erythropoietic protoporphyria (EPP) is another rare disorder that can present as an exaggerated sunburn. More commonly, however, the child or young adult with this condition complains of pain and tingling in the skin within minutes of exposure to sunlight, and the early onset of an exaggerated sunburn is only a minor consideration.

ERYTHEMATOUS MACULOPAPULAR REACTIONS

Rashes that are erythematous and either elevated above the skin (papular) or not elevated (macular) are the most common type of photodermatoses. Three conditions are in this category: PMLE, solar urticaria, and LE. Several points are important in the diagnosis. First, these eruptions are discontinuous; individual lesions are separated by normal skin, a feature that clearly distinguishes them from sunburn. Second, the eruption is confined to exposed skin but usually does not affect *all* exposed skin; a maximally exposed site such as the face might be spared while the eruption is confined to the minimally exposed lower limbs. Finally, the eruption is related to a specific exposure to sunlight. The patient is normal, goes out into sunlight, develops a rash minutes to days later, and recovers in hours to a week or more. These reactions do not usually persist throughout summer.

PMLE affects about 10% of whites and is usually diagnosed as sun poisoning. The rash appears hours to a day or so after exposure to sunlight and persists for days or sometimes a week or more. Apart from macules and papules, vesicles may be present, plaques may form because of coalescence of lesions, and pruritus may change the lesions as a result of excoriations. LE can closely resemble PMLE, but the severity of the reaction, a history of burning through window glass, persistence beyond 1 week, scarring, and the presence of systemic symptoms help to warn that LE is the probable diagnosis (Chapter 194). Whenever in doubt, serologic tests, including an anti-Ro(SS-A) antibody determination to exclude a diagnosis of LE, are essential. Solar urticaria is a common skin condition in which hives appear after exposure to sunlight. This disorder is easily distinguished

BOX 219-2
Common photoallergens

Fragrances (musk ambrette and methyl coumarin)
Sunscreens
Halogenated salicylanilides (soaps and cosmetics)
Phenothiazines
Thiazides
Sulfonamides
Nonsteroidal antiinflammatory agents

✔ *WHEN TO REFER*

Any patient with persistent or recurrent photosensitivity should be referred to an experienced physician for further evaluation, including phototesting, photopatch testing, specialized laboratory evaluation, and photodesensitization, according to the clinical situation. Patients who are markedly incapacitated by their photosensitivity can be desensitized by deliberate exposure to selected wavelengths of radiation, but this should be done only in specialized centers.

from PMLE and LE because it begins within minutes of exposure and resolves within hours.

ECZEMATOUS REACTIONS

An eczematous reaction to sunlight may initially resemble a maculopapular reaction, but within a day the eruption becomes vesicular and continuous, with no intervening normal skin. The rash eventually becomes scaly and crusted. Pruritus is a prominent symptom, whereas it is usually mild or absent with a maculopapular reaction.

There are several types of sun-induced eczema. The most common variety is photoallergy, and some of the common photoallergens are listed in Box 219-2. A usual sequence includes an acute episode related to topical application of the photoallergen, followed by exposure to sunlight. Provided further contact does not occur, the reaction clears within a week or two. Systemic photoallergy is usually caused by ingested drugs, and if use of the agent is continued without awareness of the causal relationship, the reaction persists and ceases to be related to specific exposures to sunlight. Thiazides are the most common cause of systemic photoallergy. Often the rash persists throughout summer and then subsides to some extent during winter. It is important to identify photoallergens, because repeated exposure to these agents can lead to a persistent light reaction that continues in the absence of the photoallergen and may become a lifetime problem.

BULLOUS REACTIONS

The most common bullous reaction to sunlight is porphyria cutanea tarda, and in this condition the lesions are usually confined to or are more prominent on the dorsum of the hands and forearms (Color Plate VII-10). The onset of lesions is usually related to minor trauma of the skin rather than sunlight. Thus this is not a true photodermatosis, and the patient seldom complains of sunlight as a causal factor. Instead, the distribution of the rash suggests a photodermatosis.

Bullous pemphigoid and pemphigus can occasionally be triggered by exposure to sunlight, but this presentation is rare. More commonly, a bullous eruption caused by insect bites is confused with a photodermatosis because it occurs outdoors and is largely confined to exposed areas of skin.

DIAGNOSIS OF PHOTODERMATOSES

The process of establishing the correct diagnosis of a photosensitivity disease often differs from that in other disorders of the skin because patients tend to present after the event, with normal skin and only a history of the reaction. However, it is still essential to see the reaction, which may require provocative exposure to either sunlight or an artificial source of light. The first step is to establish that the patient does have a photodermatosis. The history of the relationship between exposure to sunlight and appearance of the reaction, plus the distribution of the response, are the key indicators. Photodermatoses are usually confined to exposed areas, exhibit sharp cutoffs at the margin of clothing, and spare relatively nonexposed areas such as behind the ears, under the chin, and the inner aspect of the arms.

Provocative testing is very useful when the patient has already recovered from a reaction or to determine if a reaction is normal. Sunlight is a convenient source of radiation. The patient should be asked to expose a forearm to sunlight for a time sufficient to produce the response. In the case of a rash, this permits its examination and also a biopsy of skin for histologic evaluation. Other special tests such as urine and red cell porphyrin levels, patch testing for photoallergens, and serologic testing for LE may be required for diagnosis of some patients.

TREATMENT OF PHOTODERMATOSES

Specific treatment is available for a few photodermatoses, including phlebotomy for porphyria cutanea tarda, β-carotene for EPP, and elimination of a phototoxin or photoallergen. The treatment of most photodermatoses, however, is nonspecific and consists of avoiding exposure to sunlight, using protective clothing and sunscreens, and taking measures to decrease photosensitivity. A sunscreen with a high sun-protective factor (SPF 15 or higher), broad-spectrum protection in both UVA and UVB ranges, and good substantivity (labeled "waterproof") should be applied before any significant exposure to sunlight. Sunscreens are very effective in blocking UVB radiation but provide less protection against UVA radiation. Therefore if a person is sensitive to these longer wavelengths, avoidance of exposure or physical protection with clothing is necessary.

BIBLIOGRAPHY

Epstein JH: Polymorphous light eruption, *J Am Acad Dermatol* 3:329, 1980.
Gould JW et al: Cutaneous photosensitivity diseases induced by exogenous agents, *J Am Acad Dermatol* 33:551, 1995.
Harber LC, Bickers DR, editors: *Photosensitivity disease,* ed 2, Toronto, Philadelphia, 1989, BC Decker.
Lim HW, Soter NA: *Clinical photomedicine,* New York, 1993, Marcel Dekker.
Morison WL: *Phototherapy and photochemotherapy of skin disease,* ed 2, New York, 1991, Raven Press.

CHAPTER

220 Superficial Fungal Infections

Constantino Costarangos and Bernard Cohen

Cutaneous fungal infections account for nearly 15% of all dermatologic complaints. Fungi are capable of infecting all keratinized tissues, including the skin, hair, and nails. Most superficial fungal infections are caused by dermatophytes, and yeasts including *Candida* and *Pityrosporum* species. Unlike *Candida* species, dermatophytes cannot survive on mucosal surfaces that do not contain keratin.

DERMATOPHYTE INFECTIONS

The dermatophytes belong to three genera, *Microsporum, Trichophyton,* and *Epidermophyton*. They all cause human infections and are acquired by contact with infected humans (anthropophilic fungi), animals (zoophilic fungi), or soil (geophilic fungi). The most common pathogenic dermatophyte cause of human infection in adults in the

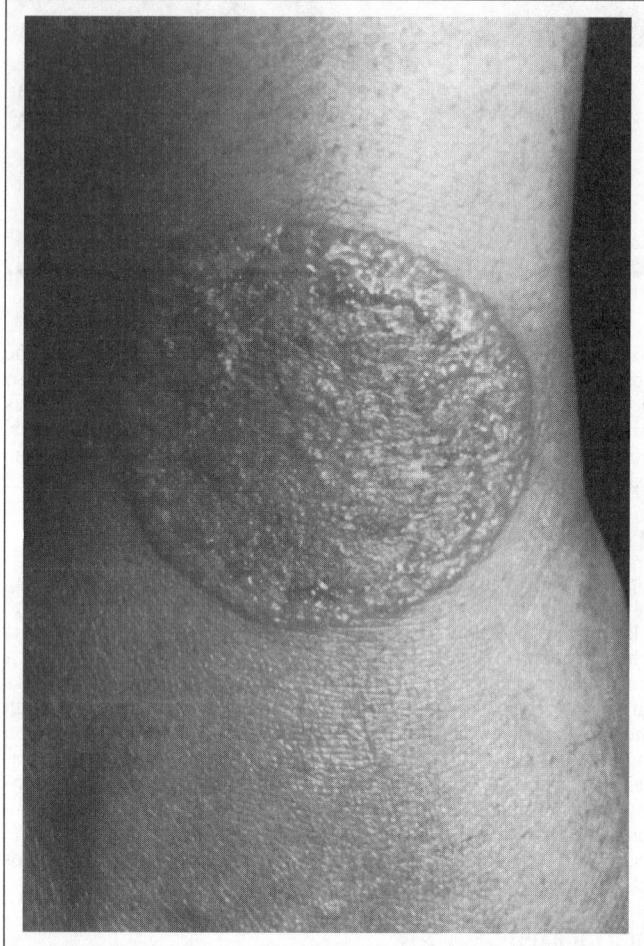

FIGURE 220-1   Tinea corporis—characteristic annular erythematous plaque with a raised border.

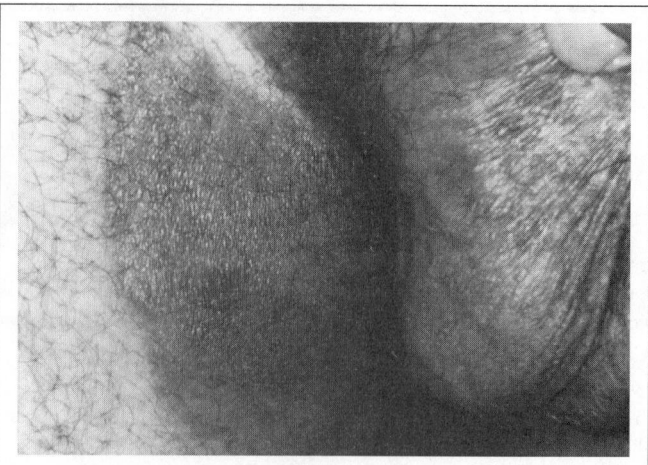

FIGURE 220-2   Tinea cruris—well-demarcated erythematous patch with fine wrinkling on the inner thigh.

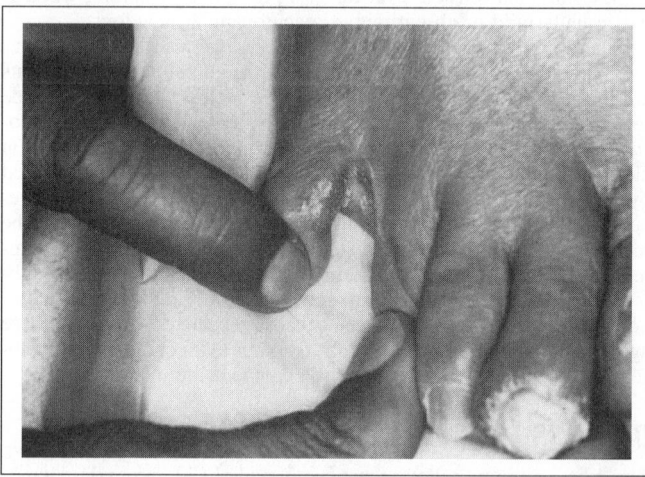

FIGURE 220-3   Tinea pedis—interdigital space with scaling and maceration.

United States is *Trichophyton rubrum* (anthropophilic fungus). *Trichophyton tonsurans* (anthropophilic fungus) is the second most commonly isolated organism from lesions in humans and is most common in children, followed by *Trichophyton mentagrophytes, Microsporum canis,* and *Trichophyton verrucosum* (zoophilic fungi, which are acquired by humans from infected animals such as cats, dogs, and cattle).

CLINICAL PRESENTATIONS

Tinea corporis (Fig. 220-1), a dermatophyte infection of the glabrous (nonhair) skin, usually presents with the classic "ringworm" appearance of an annular erythematous papulosquamous eruption with a raised scaly border and central clearing. The lesions begin as 2- to 3-mm red papules or pustules that expand peripherally. Pruritus is variable.

Tinea cruris (Fig. 220-2) also known as *jock itch* is a dermatophyte infection of the groin and sometimes the upper thighs, perianal, and perineal areas. It is usually associated with heat, humidity, excessive sweating, and occlusive undergarments, and it is more prevalent in teenage boys and men. The eruption presents as well-demarcated scaly patches with papulovesicular borders and partial central clearing, beginning in the inguinal creases. The scrotum is seldom involved and the penis is never involved, in contrast to candidal infections.

Tinea pedis (Fig. 220-3), commonly known as *athlete's foot,* is the most common symptomatic form of dermatophyte infection. It can generally be classified into three categories. Interdigital toe web infections usually present with scaling, peeling, maceration, and fissuring associated with variable itching and burning. Some patients de-

velop a scaly, hyperkeratotic "moccasinlike" appearance of the soles, which is usually caused by chronic *T. rubrum* infections. Infection may also involve the hands, *tinea manus* (Fig. 220-4), and nails, *tinea unguium.* "One hand, two feet" tinea is a peculiar but common presentation. Finally, an acute variant presents with an eruption of highly inflamed vesicles, bullae, and fissures of the feet. *Tinea pedis* is acquired in public health spas, showers, and swimming pools, and from contaminated carpets and floors.

Tinea capitis (Fig. 220-5) in the United States is caused almost universally by *T. tonsurans,* and is a disorder primarily affecting black school-age children. It is uncommon in adults. The majority of infections are associated with minimal inflammation and usually present as one or several annular scaly patches with minimal hair loss and may progress for months to widespread patches of alopecia. In classic "black-dot" ringworm, the weakened hairs break at the scalp. When more inflammation is present, chronic pustules mimicking bacterial folliculitis may develop and occasionally a tender, boggy, edematous, exudative plaque called a *kerion* (Fig. 220-6) appears in sensitized individuals. If left untreated, these kerions may heal spontaneously, with scarring and permanent hair loss.

Tinea unguium refers to onychomycosis caused by a dermatophyte. *T. rubrum* is the most common organism implicated in fungal infection of the fingernails and toenails. Three clinical forms of tinea unguium are recognized. The most common type is distal subungual disease. Superficial white onychomycosis, most com-

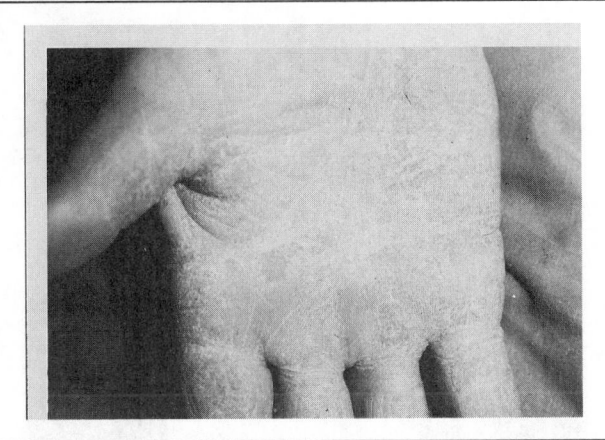

FIGURE 220-4 Thickened, hyperkeratotic palmar skin in a patient with tinea manus caused by *Trichophyton rubum.*

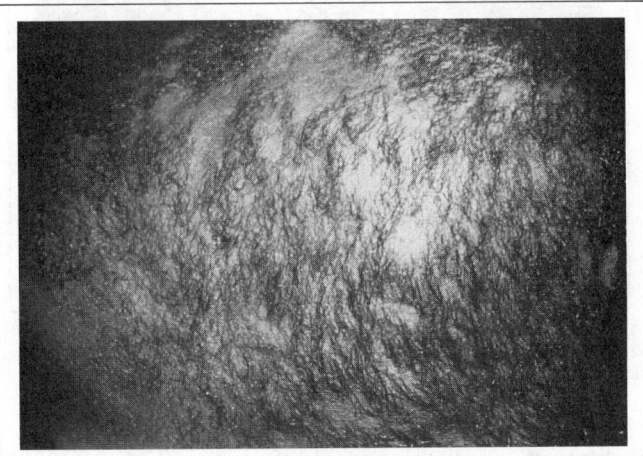

FIGURE 220-5 Tinea capitis—annular scaly patches of the scalp with hair loss.

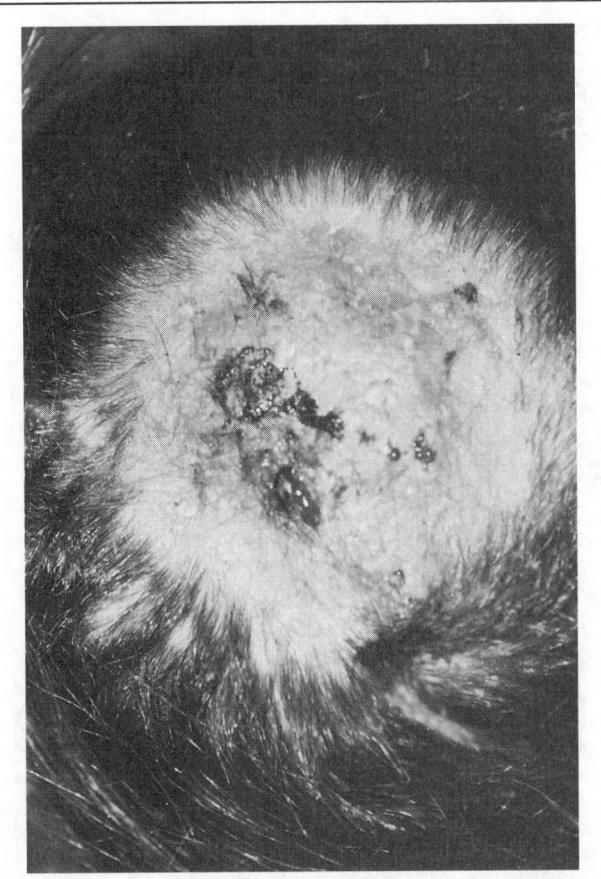

FIGURE 220-6 Typical kerion of the scalp manifested as a tender, crusted, boggy plaque with overlying alopecia.

monly caused by *T. mentagrophytes* is seen only on the toenails as one or several chalky, white spots on the surface of the nail. This is the only type of tinea unguium likely to respond to topical antifungal therapy. A third type is the proximal subungual disease, appearing as whitish yellow discoloration of the proximal nail plate and is the least common form of disease in the normal host but is more common in immunocompromised patients.

DIAGNOSTIC PROCEDURES

Clinical diagnosis is confirmed with a potassium hydroxide (KOH) or a fungal culture using appropriate media such as Sabouraud's agar or Dermatophyte Test Medium (DTM), particularly before committing a patient to long-term oral antifungal therapy. The presence of the characteristic fungal hyphae confirms the diagnosis by KOH culture (Fig. 220-7). In the case of tinea unguium, a KOH preparation of subungual debris should be performed and nail clippings may be cultured.

In tinea capitis, scrapings of scale and broken hairs from the involved scalp can be examined by KOH preparation and/or sent for fungal culture to confirm the clinical diagnosis.

THERAPY

Topical antifungal therapy may be used for localized dermatophyte infections of the skin, usually twice daily for 2 to 4 weeks. Imida-

zole agents, including ketoconazole (Nizoral), econazole (Spectazole), oxiconazole (Oxistat), clotrimazole, miconazole (Micatin, Monistat-Derm), and sulconazole (Exelderm) have become the mainstays of topical antifungal therapy (Table 220-1).

PITYROSPORUM INFECTIONS

Pityrosporum ovale is a lipophilic yeast, part of the normal skin flora, which is both a saprophyte and an opportunistic pathogen. It may be associated with pityriasis versicolor (more commonly known as tinea versicolor), *Pityrosporum* folliculitis, and seborrheic dermatitis (Fig. 220-8).

Pityriasis versicolor usually presents as asymptomatic or mildly pruritic hyperpigmented or hypopigmented, scaly patches that coalesce as they enlarge. Sites of predilection are the neck, sternal region, sides of the chest, abdomen, back, pubis, and intertriginous areas. Facial lesions are rare except in immunocompromised patients and infants. Some predisposing factors are warm climate, corticosteroids, and immunosuppressants. A KOH preparation of the scale shows blunt-ended hyphae and clusters of spores that form a "spaghetti and meatballs" pattern.

Pityrosporum folliculitis is characterized by pruritus, follicular papules, and pustules located primarily on the upper trunk, neck, and arms. It may be seen in healthy patients. Predisposing factors include immunosuppression, occlusion, antibiotic treatment, and diabetes mellitus.

Successful treatment of pityriasis versicolor has been reported with 2.5% selenium sulfide lotion applied to affected skin, left on for a period of 10 minutes to overnight as tolerated and then rinsed off. This can be repeated daily for 2 weeks and then weekly for several months. Prophylactic retreatment for 2 days of each month is recommended to prevent recurrence. Ketoconazole cream or shampoo, oral

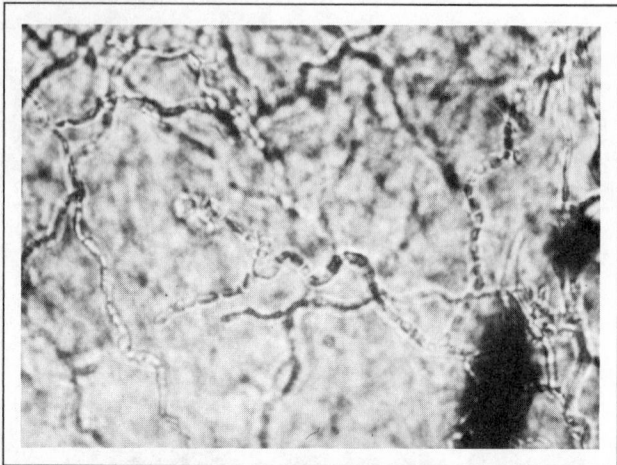

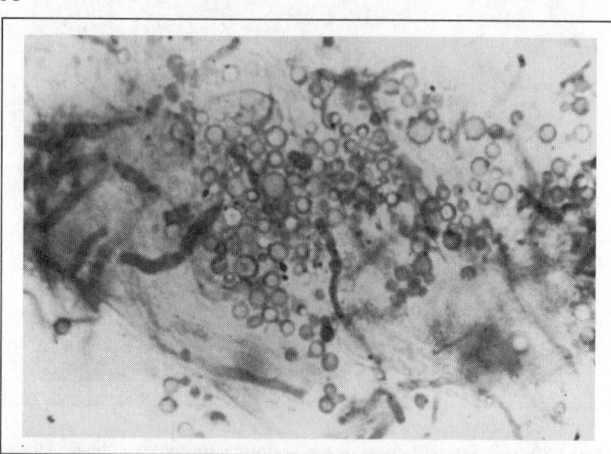

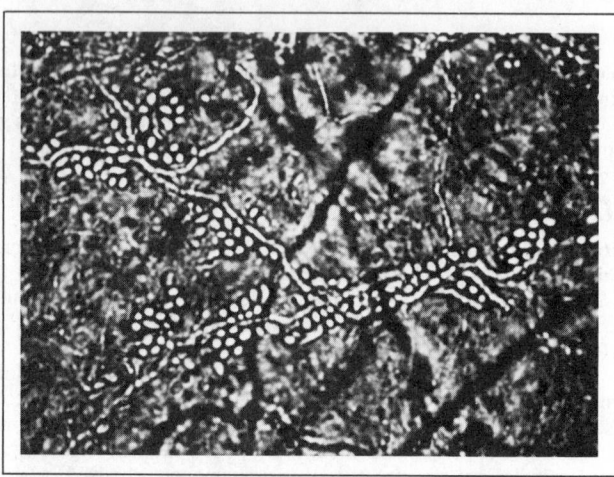

FIGURE 220-7   Fungal hyphae can be seen on a potassium hydroxide (KOH) preparation. **A,** Dermatophyte. **B,** KOH preparation, with blunt-ended hyphae and clusters of spores, characteristic of tinea versicolor. **C,** *Candida.*

ketoconazole, other imidazoles, and propylene glycol are also effective. A recommended regimen of oral ketoconazole is 200 mg daily for 5 days and repeated monthly for 2 months.

CANDIDIASIS

Candidiasis is an acute or chronic infection of the skin and mucous membranes caused most commonly by *Candida albicans*. Factors that

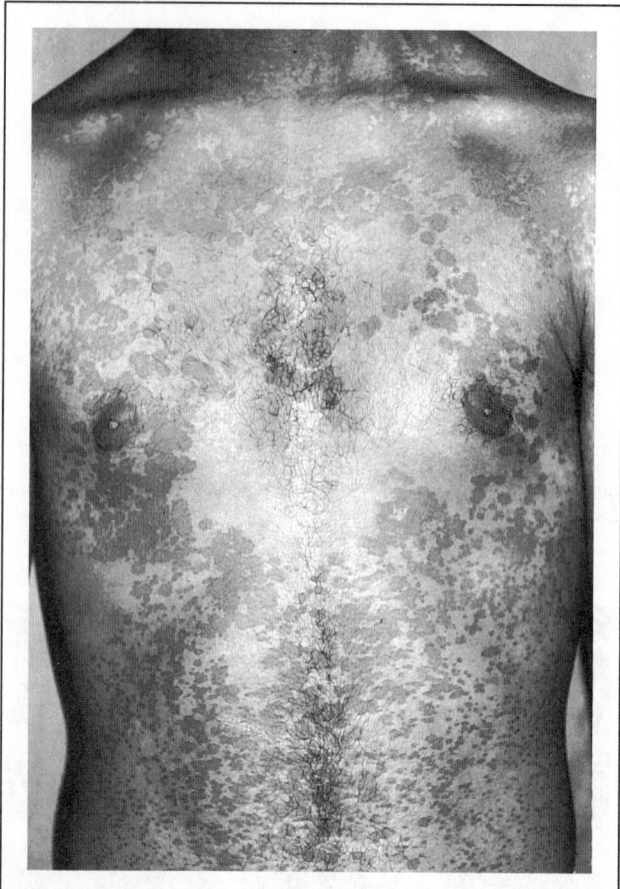

FIGURE 220-8   Typical scaly hyperpigmented macules on the trunk of a patient with tinea versicolor.

predispose to candidiasis include diabetes mellitus, birth control pills, pregnancy, antibiotics, systemic steroids, and immunosuppression. Warmth, moisture, and occlusion encourage the growth of *Candida.*

Mucosal Candidiasis

The clinical findings of oral candidiasis (thrush) include the typical creamy or cheeselike patches that adhere loosely to the underlying inflamed mucosa (Fig. 220-9). Predisposing factors include age extremes, intraoral prosthetic devices, malnourishment, antibiotics, and immunosuppression.

Vulvovaginal candidiasis most commonly presents with an acute vulvar pruritus and a thick "cottage-cheese" vaginal discharge. Other symptoms include vulvovaginal soreness, burning, dyspareunia, and dysuria. Balanitis due to *C. albicans* presents as small erythematous papules or fragile papulopustules in the coronal sulcus or on the glans. Predisposing factors to balanitis include an uncircumcised state, diabetes mellitus, and candidal vaginal infection in sexual partners.

Cutaneous Candidiasis

Candidal intertrigo is located commonly in the skin folds of the subaxillary, submammary, genitocrural, gluteal cleft, interdigital areas, and between the folds of skin of the abdominal wall. Clinically the affected skin consists of pruritic erythematous and macerated patches with satellite vesicopustules. The scrotum may be involved in candidiasis of the groin (Fig. 220-10).

Candida paronychia is characterized by swelling, redness, and tenderness of the paronychia area (Fig. 220-11). It tends to be chronic, and occasionally pus can be expressed from the base of the nail. Secondary nail changes, such as transverse nail ridging and onycholysis, can occur.

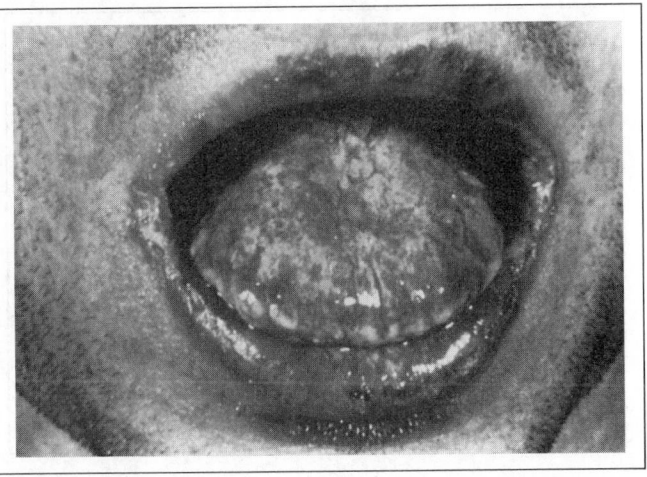

FIGURE 220-9 Thrush—characteristic creamy or cheeselike patches that adhere to the underlying inflamed mucosa. Angular cheilitis also present.

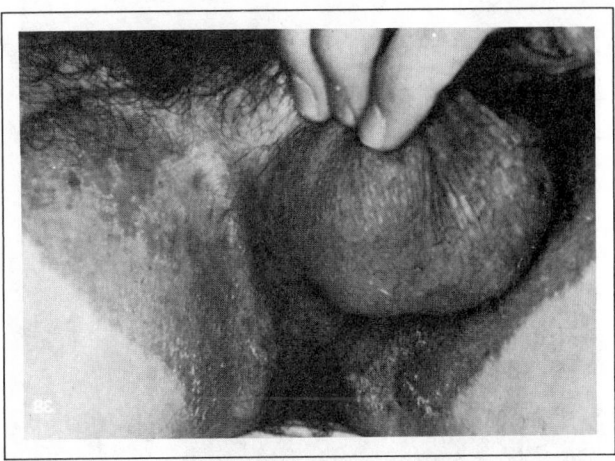

FIGURE 220-10 Candidal intertrigo with characteristic scrotal involvement.

Table 220-1 Treatment guidelines for common fungal infections

INFECTION	PHARMACOTHERAPY	COMMENTS
Tinea corporis	2-3 week therapy of antifungal cream (imidazoles, allylamines, ciclopirox, tolnaftate) 1-2 times a day; for multiple widespread or resistant lesions, oral griseofulvin, 15 mg qd up to a maximum of 500-1000 mg qd OR Oral ketoconazole 200 mg qd ± 4 weeks	Requires close monitoring of liver function in adults and children; perform periodic renal, hepatic, and hematopoietic function tests in adults. Photosensitivity is an occasional side effect; patients should be cautioned to wear sunscreen. Griseofulvin decreases activity of anticoagulants and efficacy of oral antibiotics; it may be antagonized by barbiturates and may potentiate alcohol.
Tinea cruris	Topical antifungal agents in a light cream-based vehicle	Loose fitting underwear, thorough drying after showering/bathing, and cool environment are adjunctive measures to promote healing.
Tinea pedis	Topical imidazoles In patients with severely symptomatic or widespread infection, oral griseofulvin for 2 weeks combined with a 3-4 week course of topical therapy Acute inflammatory lesions benefit from aluminum acetate, acetic acid, or cool tap water compresses	Allylamines, tolnaftate, and ciclopirox may be effective but have limited activity against secondary organisms. Cellulitis and lymphangitis should be treated with appropriate oral or parenteral antibiotics. Daily washing and thorough drying of the feet, lightweight shoes, cotton socks, and antifungal powder decrease the risk for recurrent infection.
Tinea unguium and onychomycosis	Oral itraconazole Oral griseofulvin Oral ketoconazole Oral terbinafine	FDA approved for onychomycosis; recommended dose is 200 mg qd for 12 consecutive weeks. May eradicate fungi in 6-18 months, recurrences exceed 50%. As with griseofulvin, this drug requires close clinical follow-up and monitoring. Drug levels remain high in nailbed for weeks; FDA approved for onychomycosis tablets; one 250-mg tablet once daily for 6 weeks for fingernail onychomycosis and for 12 weeks for toenail onychomycosis.
Tinea capitis	Twice weekly shampooing with selenium sulfide 2.5% shampoo Oral griseofulvin 15 mg/kg/day, 1-2 divided doses taken with food; increase dose until clinical response is evident or toxicity (nausea, vomiting, diarrhea) occurs OR Oral ketoconazole 4-6 mg/kg/day Oral itraconazole When kerion is present, therapy should include 2-week tapering course of oral prednisone to minimize scarring	Topical therapy is generally useless. Splitting the dose may relieve gastrointestinal upset. Patients should be warned to avoid sharing brushes, hats, combs, etc.; children may cover scalp to reduce spread in school.

Perlèche or angular cheilitis is analogous to intertrigo elsewhere and is usually caused by *C. albicans.*

Chronic Mucocutaneous Candidiasis

Chronic mucocutaneous candidiasis (CMC) is a term used to describe a collection of syndromes in which patients have recurrent or chronic infections of the oropharynx, mucous membranes, skin, and nails with

Candida. Although severe local infection may occur, there is little risk of disseminated disease. Associated disorders include thymoma, autoimmune disorders, polyendocrinopathies (such as hypoadrenalism, hypoparathyroidism, and hypothyroidism), and interstitial keratitis. CMC may begin in infancy or childhood and in many cases is seen in individuals with an underlying cell-mediated immune defect. Candidal infections in these patients usually do not respond to conventional topical therapy. By history, diaper dermatitis or oral lesions usually appear first, followed by lip fissures, angular cheilitis, paro-

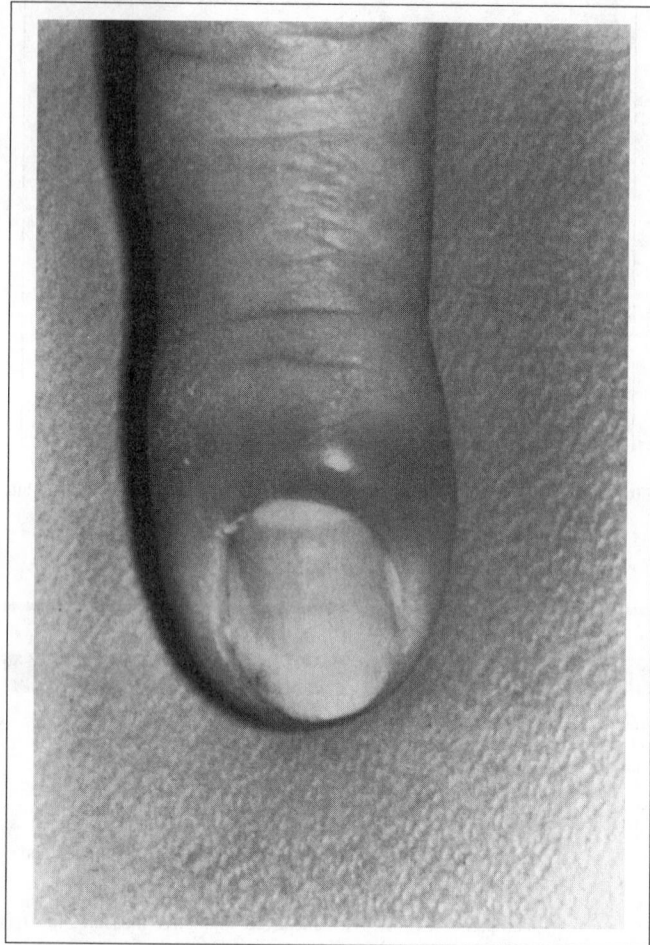

FIGURE 220-11   Candida paronychia—swelling and redness of paronychia area.

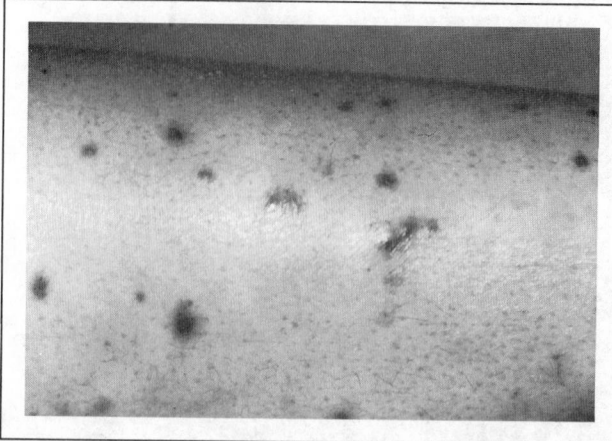

FIGURE 220-12   Hemorrhagic papules in an immunosuppressed patient with candidemia.

nychial and nail involvement, vulvovaginitis, and cutaneous involvement. Nail and skin lesions characteristically become crusted.

Cutaneous Manifestations of Systemic Candidiasis

Systemic candidiasis may manifest in the skin as nonspecific erythematous macules that become papular, pustular, and hemorrhagic and may progress to necrotic ulcers (Fig. 220-12). Those who are at risk include patients with malignancies, especially lymphomas and leukemias, and other immunosuppressed individuals. Other predisposing factors are intravenous lines, Foley catheters, intravenous drug abuse, and broad-spectrum antibiotics.

DIAGNOSTIC PROCEDURES

A KOH preparation and/or culture is used to confirm the diagnosis of cutaneous or mucosal candidiasis. To confirm the diagnosis of systemic candidiasis, a skin biopsy sent for culture or histopathology is necessary.

THERAPY

Successful topical treatment of oral candidiasis includes nystatin suspension "swish and swallow," and clotrimazole troches dissolved in the mouth several times daily. In the treatment of vulvovaginal candidiasis, topical agents should be considered the first line of therapy and they include nystatin, miconazole, clotrimazole, butoconazole, terconazole, and tioconazole vaginal tablet, suppository, or cream. The administration of oral fluconazole, itraconazole, and ketoconazole for

a period of 1 to 5 days in clinical trials has been shown to be effective in the treatment for acute vulvovaginal candidiasis in nonpregnant women. Treatment of candidal intertrigo should include the reduction of moisture in the area, correction of the predisposing factors, and the application of a topical antifungal cream.

The treatment for chronic mucocutaneous candidiasis depends on successful immunologic therapy, antifungal drugs, or a combination of both. Systemic therapy with oral ketoconazole, fluconazole, and low-dose amphotericin B is effective, but most patients relapse within a few weeks or months after antifungal treatment has been stopped; therefore long-term therapy is required. Good clinical results have been seen with the combination of systemic antifungals and *Candida*-specific transfer factors, which are small proteins that are extracted from the T-lymphocytes of immune donors and are administered to recipients who lack cell-mediating immunity.

The treatment for systemic candidiasis continues to be parenteral amphotericin B.

BIBLIOGRAPHY

Chapman SW, Daniel CR III: Cutaneous manifestations of fungal infection, *Infect Dis Clin North Am* 8:879-910, 1994.
Cohen B: Cutaneous fungal infections: diagnosis and management, *Cross Sect Dermatol* 1(4):1-7, 1995.
Faergemann J: *Pityrosporum* infections, *J Am Acad Dermatol* 31:518-520, 1994.
Hay RJ: Antifungal therapy of yeast infections, *J Am Acad Dermatol* 31:6-9, 1994.
Kirkpatrick CH: Chronic mucocutaneous candidiasis, *J Am Acad Dermatol* 31:14-17, 1994.
Martin AG, Kobayashi GS: Yeast infections: candidiasis, pityriasis (tinea) versicolor. In Fitzpatrick TB et al, editors: *Dermatology in general medicine*, ed 4, New York, 1993, McGraw-Hill.
Reef SE, Levine WC, McNeil MM et al: Treatment options for vulvovaginal candidiasis, *Clin Infect Dis* 20:80-90, 1995.

CHAPTER

221 Cutaneous Manifestations of Drug Reactions

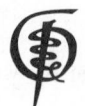

Antoinette F. Hood

Drugs are ubiquitous in our society, and adverse reactions to drugs are common. These may occur in any organ and often are accompanied by a wide spectrum of signs, symptoms, and laboratory abnormalities. The Boston Collaborative Drug Surveillance Program reported drug-induced skin reactions occurring in slightly more than 2% of all hospitalized patients. Although cutaneous drug reactions are only occasionally life threatening, they can produce significant morbidity, discomfort, and expense to the patient.

PATHOGENESIS

Drug eruptions can be produced by immunologic or nonimmunologic mechanisms. The basic pathogenic mechanisms involved in immunologic reactions are discussed in detail in Chapters 174 to 176 and are discussed only briefly here.

Immunoglobulin E (IgE)–mediated drug reactions (immediate type hypersensitivity), as typified by penicillin allergy, are characterized by pruritus, urticaria, laryngeal edema, bronchospasm, and, occasionally, by anaphylactic shock. Cytotoxic reactions induced by drugs are generally manifested in the skin by purpura. Immune complex–mediated drug reactions are characterized by fever, arthritis, nephritis, neuritis, edema, and a urticarial or papular eruption. Serum sickness is the classic example of an immune complex–dependent reaction. Delayed hypersensitivity, or *T cell–mediated reaction,* as typified by contact drug hypersensitivity, appears as a papulovesicular eruption. Factors involved in the production of immunologically mediated drug reactions include the molecular characteristics of the drug, immunogenic load, route of administration, and the patient's age and genetic ability to recognize antigenic determinants.

The pathogenesis of most cutaneous drug-induced reactions is not well understood. The terms *hypersensitivity* and *allergic* should be restricted to those reactions that are immunologically mediated or that can reasonably be presumed to be immunologically mediated. True allergic reactions affect a very small percentage of the population receiving a particular drug and require prior exposure or a latent period for development of an immune response.

Numerous nonimmunologic mechanisms can be implicated in the production of cutaneous drug reactions. Anagen alopecia and mucositis are examples of secondary side effects of antimitotic chemotherapeutic agents. These drugs are unable to distinguish between rapidly dividing tumor cells and rapidly dividing normal cells and therefore inadvertently produce these effects. Cumulative toxicity occurs when there is a prolonged exposure to certain drugs. The blue-gray skin discoloration (argyria) due to prolonged silver ingestion is a striking example of chemical accumulation. Certain drugs may produce exacerbation or precipitation of latent cutaneous disease in genetically susceptible individuals. The administration of iodides may provoke lesions of dermatitis herpetiformis; porphyria cutanea tarda may be induced by the administration of barbiturates, oral contraceptives, or busulfan. Alterations in normal flora by antibiotics, corticosteroids, and immunosuppressive agents may result in the overgrowth of yeast such as *Candida albicans* or may facilitate the growth of cutaneous dermatophytes. Finally, there may be nonimmunologic activation of effector pathways, which may stimulate an allergic reaction but are not antibody dependent. For example, certain drugs (e.g., codeine) can directly trigger the release of mast cell mediators and evoke a urticarial eruption.

The administration of drugs that produce alterations in the hematopoietic system, particularly agents used to treat malignancies, may result in a variety of cutaneous reactions resulting from modulation of the patient's immune system. An example of such a reaction is the eruption of lymphocyte recovery that occurs during the treatment of leukemia.

CLINICAL MANIFESTATIONS

In this chapter, drug reactions are categorized by the clinical appearance of the eruption. However, several points should be emphasized. First, the morphology of the cutaneous eruption does not usually identify the drug causing a particular reaction because similar skin eruptions may be caused by widely disparate drugs. Second, although repeated administration of a given drug usually provokes the same reaction in an individual patient, this is not entirely predictable, and occasionally different reactions may be produced. And last, the same drug may produce markedly different reactions in different individuals. Drugs commonly associated with various cutaneous reactions are listed in Box 221-1. In terms of frequency, the exanthematous reac-

tion occurs most commonly, followed by urticaria and/or angioedema, erythema multiforme, and Stevens-Johnson syndrome.

Acneiform Eruptions

Drug-induced acneiform eruptions are generally more papulopustular and less comedonal than typical acne vulgaris (Fig. 221-1). The pathogenetic mechanisms producing acneiform eruptions are quite varied. Some drugs, such as oral contraceptives, act on the sebaceous gland and exacerbate preexisting acne; other drugs, such as the halogens, lithium, and dactinomycin, induce pustular and inflammatory follicular lesions. Adrenocorticotropic hormone (ACTH) and corticosteroids produce comedonal lesions that are all in the same stage of development, presumably because of follicular occlusion.

Alopecia

Certain drugs, such as antimitotic agents, interfere with hair growth in the anagen or proliferative phase of the hair cycle, resulting in a so-called anagen effluvium. The mechanism of action for most of the other drugs that induce alopecia is not well understood, and therefore further classification is difficult. Diffuse alopecia may accompany administration of anticoagulants, antithyroid drugs, and vitamin A derivatives. Drug-induced alopecia is usually reversible on cessation of the offending agent.

Eczematous Eruptions

Many drugs are used both externally and internally. An eczematous type of drug eruption is similar in appearance to contact dermatitis and develops in patients who are already sensitized by topical exposure to a particular drug or to one chemically related to it. Subsequent systemic administration of the drug (by ingestion or injection) results in an acute papular and occasionally papulovesicular erythematous eruption. The reaction occurs within 2 days after the administration of the drug and is commonly localized to the site of previously existing allergic contact dermatitis. Patch testing may be used to demonstrate contact hypersensitivity to a suspected topical agent.

Agents present in topical preparations that frequently are associated with allergic contact dermatitis include neomycin, benzocaine, ethylenediamine diphenhydramine, and parabens.

Erythema Multiforme

Erythema multiforme is characterized by discrete erythematous macules, papules, or plaques. Bullae may develop in the center of some of the lesions. The pathognomonic iris or target lesion may not be present in drug-induced erythema multiforme. The lesions are characteristically found on the distal extremities and face. Severe erythema multiforme with fever and mucosal involvement is also known as the *Stevens-Johnson syndrome* (Color Plate VII-11). Although many drugs have been incriminated in the production of erythema multiforme, the most common agents are sulfonamides, penicillins, and anticonvulsant agents. Erythema multiforme may be precipitated by a wide variety of agents in addition to drugs. Without actually rechallenging the patient with the suspected drug to reproduce the reaction, it may be difficult to prove or disprove a causal relationship between a particular medication and erythema multiforme.

Erythema Nodosum

Regardless of its cause, erythema nodosum is manifested clinically by the sudden appearance of painful contusiform nodules on the legs (Color Plate VII-12). Drugs most commonly associated with erythema nodosum are halides, sulfonamides, gold, and oral contraceptives. No clinical signs or symptoms distinguish drug-induced erythema nodosum from that induced by infectious agents.

Exanthematous Eruption

This is the most commonly observed manifestation of a "drug rash." The pathogenesis of drug-induced exanthems is unknown (Color Plate

---

BOX 221-1
Drug-induced cutaneous eruptions

Acneiform eruptions
ACTH
Bromides
Corticosteroids
Cyanocobalamin (vitamin B_{12})
Dactinomycin
Iodides
Isoniazid (INH)
Lithium
Oral contraceptives
Phenytoin

Alopecia
Allopurinol
Amphetamines
Anticoagulants (coumarin, heparin)
Antithyroid drugs (carbimazole, thiouracil)
Chemotherapeutic agents
Heavy metals
Hypocholesterolemic drugs
Levodopa
Oral contraceptives
Propranolol
Retinoids

Eczematous eruptions (topical sensitizer/systemic medication)
Ampicillin
Chlorbutanol, chloral hydrate
Diphenhydramine (Caladryl, Benadryl)
Disulfiram (Antabuse)
Ethylenediamine, aminophylline, antihistamines
Iodine, iodides
Neomycin sulfate, streptomycin, kanamycin
Para-amino aromatic benzenes, para-aminobenzoic acid, sulfonamides, tolbutamide
Penicillin

Erythema multiforme
Allopurinol
Barbiturates
Chlorpropamide
Griseofulvin
Hydantoins
Nonsteroidal antiinflammatory agents
Penicillin
Phenothiazines
Sulfonamides
Thiazide diuretics

Erythema nodosum
Bromides
Codeine
Iodides
Oral contraceptives
Penicillin
Salicylates
Sulfonamides

Exanthematous eruptions
Allopurinol
Antibiotics
Anticonvulsants
Barbiturates
Benzodiazepines
Captopril
Chlorpropamide
Gold salts
Isoniazid
Nonsteroidal antiinflammatory agents
Para-aminosalicylic acid
Penicillamine
Phenothiazines
Quinidine
Thiazide diuretics

Exfoliative dermatitis
Allopurinol
Carbamazepine
Gold salts
Hydantoins
Isoniazid
Para-aminosalicylic acid
Phenylbutazone
Streptomycin
Sulfonamides

Fixed drug eruptions
Allopurinol
Barbiturates
Chlordiazepoxide
Nonsteroidal antiinflammatory agents
Phenolphthalein
Sulfonamides
Tetracycline

Leukocytoclastic vasculitis
Allopurinol
Cimetidine

Gold salts
Hydantoins
Nonsteroidal antiinflammatory agents
Phenothiazine
Sulfonamides
Thiazide diuretics
Thiouracils

Lichenoid and lichen planus–like eruptions
Antimalarials
Captopril
Chlordiazepoxide
Gold salts
Hydroxyurea
Para-aminosalicylic acid
Penicillamine
Quinidine
Thiazide diuretics

Photosensitivity eruptions
Griseofulvin
Nonsteroidal antiinflammatory agents
Phenothiazines
Sulfonamides
Sulfonylureas
Tetracyclines
Thiazide diuretics

Toxic epidermal necrolysis
Allopurinol
Aminopenicillins
Anticonvulsant agents
Imidazole antifungal agents
Nonsteroidal antiinflammatory agents (oxicam derivatives)
Sulfonamides
Tetracycline

Urticaria
Enzymes (L-asparaginase)
Indomethacin
Opiates
Penicillin and related antibiotics
Salicylates
Sulfonamides
X-ray contrast media

VII-13). Exanthematous or morbilliform eruptions are characterized by bright red, blanchable macules and/or papules that may coalesce to form large confluent patches or plaques. The lesions are widespread and typically involve the palms and soles. Fever is usually present. Manifestations of an exanthematous reaction typically occur 2 to 3 days after the offending agent is begun; however, some antibiotics and allopurinol may induce eruptions that do not appear until 2 weeks after initial administration of the medication. Many drugs have been associated with the production of exanthematous eruptions, but those most frequently implicated are antibiotics, nonsteroidal antiinflammatory drugs, thiazide diuretics, allopurinol, and gold salts. For reasons that are not known, exanthematous eruptions occur more commonly in certain populations: women have a higher incidence of this type of drug reaction than men, and patients with infectious mononucleosis taking ampicillin, and HIV-positive patients taking trimethoprim-sulfamethoxazole have unusually high reaction rates.

Exfoliative Dermatitis

Exfoliative dermatitis, or erythroderma, caused by drugs is indistinguishable from exfoliative dermatitis caused by primary underlying skin disorders. The eruption characteristically begins with erythema, which spreads gradually to involve the entire body. Extensive and prolonged vasodilation may result in abnormal temperature regulation, fluid imbalance, and right ventricular failure. The erythema is followed by diffuse desquamation. Gold salts and sulfonamides are frequently implicated offenders.

Fixed Drug Eruption

Fixed drug eruption is an uncommon reaction with a very characteristic clinical and histologic presentation. The skin lesions typically recur at the same sites with repetitive ingestion of the offending agent, hence the term *fixed eruption*. Initially there is an erythematous mac-

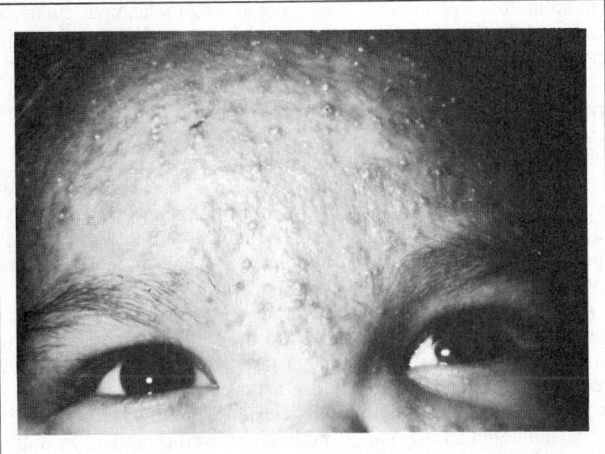

FIGURE 221-1 Acneiform eruption following the administration of adrenocorticotrophic hormone (ACTH). The individual lesions are papules and pustules and characteristically appear to be in the same stage of development.

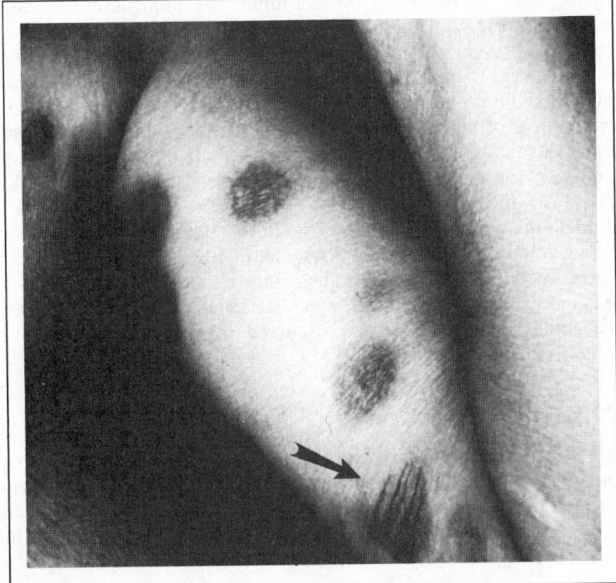

FIGURE 221-2 Fixed drug eruption characterized by bullous *(arrow)* and hyperpigmented lesions that recur with subsequent administration of the offending agent.

ule, which usually evolves to form a well-demarcated elevated lesion. Vesiculation and bullae formation may occur (Fig. 221-2). Resolution of the acute phase is usually accompanied by hyperpigmentation. The cause of fixed drug eruption is unknown. Drugs most frequently implicated in causing fixed drug reactions include phenolphthalein, tetracycline, and oxyphenbutazone.

Leukocytoclastic Vasculitis

Drug-induced leukocytoclastic vasculitis presents as palpable purpura that is clinically indistinguishable from idiopathic leukocytoclastic vasculitis or leukocytoclastic vasculitis precipitated by infection or systemic disease (Color Plate VII-14). The eruption clears when the drug is discontinued. The presumed mechanism for leukocytoclastic vasculitis is an immune complex–mediated reaction. Penicillins, sulfonamides, and allopurinol frequently are implicated in drug-induced leukocytoclastic vasculitis.

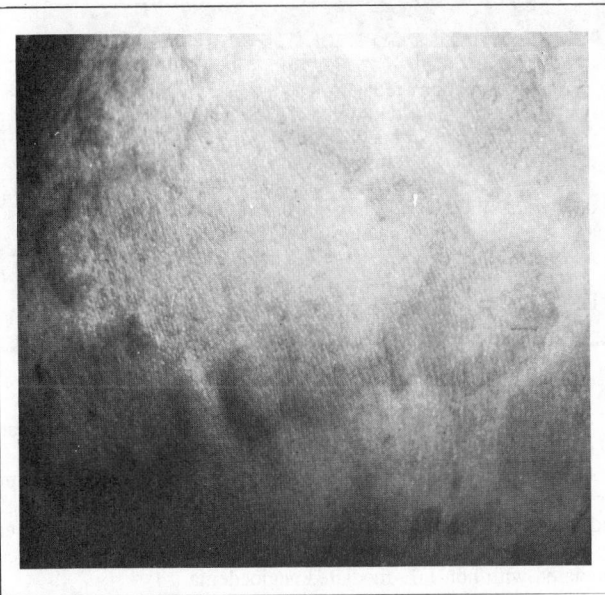

FIGURE 221-3 Urticarial lesion with serpiginous elevated erythematous blanchable borders.

Lichenoid and Lichen Planus–like Eruptions

Drug eruptions clinically indistinguishable from idiopathic lichen planus (purple polygonal papules) have been described; however, lichenoid drug eruptions in general tend to be more scaly and eczematous in appearance than lichen planus and may occur in a different distribution (i.e., sparing the mucous membranes and flexor surfaces). The accompanying pruritus is often intense. Irregular hyperpigmentation may be a disfiguring sequela.

Photosensitivity

Photosensitive drug-induced eruptions are discussed in Chapter 219, but some of the drugs associated with photosensitivity are listed in Box 221-1.

Toxic Epidermal Necrolysis

In toxic epidermal necrolysis, fever, and a diffuse, widespread macular erythema precede the formation of large flaccid bullae. Mucosal lesions such as stomatitis, pharyngitis, and conjunctivitis are common. Rupture of the blisters and loss of the overlying epidermis result in subsequent denudation of the skin (Color Plate VII-15). Fluid and electrolyte problems are similar to those occurring in a burn patient; secondary infection and sepsis are life-threatening complications. Mortality associated with toxic epidermal necrolysis is approximately 30%. Drugs most frequently implicated in this reaction include antibacterial sulfonamides, anticonvulsant agents, nonsteroidal antiinflammatory agents, and allopurinol. Survival of the acute episode is followed by healing, usually without scarring, in 2 to 4 weeks.

Urticaria and Angioedema

Urticarial lesions induced by drugs are second in frequency only to exanthematous eruptions. IgE-mediated urticarial reactions usually occur within minutes to hours of administration of the drug; urticarial lesions associated with serum sickness occur 7 to 10 days after administration of the drug. Some agents induce urticaria by nonimmunologic mechanisms such as local or systemic liberation of histamine from mast cells and basophils. Regardless of the pathogenic mechanism causing them, individual urticarial lesions should blanch, are usually pruritic, and should last less than 24 hours (Fig. 221-3). Agents most frequently implicated as a cause of urticaria are antibi-

✔ *WHEN TO REFER*

Most drug eruptions fall into reaction patterns that may be produced by more than one drug, may be induced by other agents (such as infection), or may be idiopathic. Experience with skin disease facilitates differentiation in pathogenesis, for example, distinguishing lichen planus from a lichenoid drug eruption. When a drug eruption is suspected, the presumed precipitating agent (usually the most recently administered) should be discontinued. If the reaction progresses or persists for more than a week, a skin biopsy and/or a consultation with a dermatologist may be beneficial to the patient and may avoid unnecessary changes in therapy.

otics, radiocontrast media, nonsteroidal antiinflammatory drugs, and opiates.

Angioedema is clinically characterized by circumscribed nonpitting edema typically involving the face, lips, and tongue. IgE-mediated angioedema is most frequently caused by penicillin and venoms (bee sting). Angiotensin-converting enzyme inhibitors have been associated with non-IgE–mediated angioedema.

EVALUATION AND MANAGEMENT OF A PATIENT WITH A DRUG ERUPTION

The evaluation of a patient presumed to have a drug eruption is most challenging when the patient is receiving multiple medications. When attempting to determine the offending agent, it is wise to remember that (1) most cutaneous drug reactions occur within 7 days of exposure to the medication, (2) certain drugs (e.g., antibiotics) have a higher incidence of cutaneous reactions than others, and (3) some drugs produce very characteristic reactions. A logical approach is to discontinue the most recently administered medication and/or drugs known to be frequent offenders.

Most drug eruptions are self-limiting and resolve promptly after the precipitating agent has been discontinued. Supportive treatment to control pruritus is often all that is required. Urticaria and angioedema may be life threatening and necessitate intervention with antihistamines, epinephrine, and/or corticosteroids. Toxic epidermal necrolysis requires hospitalization to manage areas of denuded skin, to prevent infection, and to monitor fluid and electrolyte balance.

BIBLIOGRAPHY

Bigby M et al: Drug-induced cutaneous reactions: a report from the Boston Collaborative Drug Surveillance Program on 15,438 consecutive inpatients, 1975-1982, *JAMA* 256:3358, 1986.
Bork K: *Cutaneous side effects of drugs,* ed 5, Philadelphia, 1988, WB Saunders.
Bruinsma W: *A guide to drug eruptions,* ed 5, Amsterdam, 1990, Excerpta Medica.
Horn TD, Redd JV, Karp JE et al: The cutaneous eruption of lymphocyte recovery, *Arch Dermatol* 125:1512, 1989.
Zürcher K, Krebs A: *Cutaneous drug reactions:* an integral synopsis of today's systemic drugs, ed 2, Basel, Switzerland, 1992, Karger.

CHAPTER

222   Cutaneous Manifestations of Internal Malignancy

Terri Dunn and Susan D. Laman

Cutaneous manifestations of internal malignancy include cutaneous metastases, paraneoplastic dermatoses, and some genodermatoses. This chapter reviews the cutaneous manifestations of the most common of these entities. The primary cutaneous malignancies—basal cell carcinoma, squamous cell carcinoma, and melanoma; cutaneous T-cell lymphoma; and the bullous diseases associated with malignancy are covered elsewhere.

CUTANEOUS METASTASES

Metastases to the skin from internal malignancy are uncommon; studies show frequencies ranging from 0.7% to 9.0%. In one retrospective study of 7316 patients with internal malignancy, skin involvement was the presenting sign of malignancy in only 0.8% of patients, but was present at the time of malignancy diagnosis in 1.3% of patients.

According to the current literature the most frequent primary sites of carcinoma that metastasizes to the skin are breast in women and lung in men. Cutaneous metastases invade the skin through direct extension and lymphatic, or hematogenous dissemination of neoplastic cells. Most commonly lesions present as nonhealing ulcers, indurated erythema, or nodules. A well-described nodule is the periumbilical Sister Mary Joseph's nodule associated with underlying gastric cancer. A skin biopsy of the lesion should be performed to establish the diagnosis, and patients must be referred for malignancy evaluation.

PARANEOPLASTIC DERMATOSES

Paraneoplastic dermatoses by definition are noncontiguous skin changes that show a causal relationship to an internal malignancy. The dermatoses may develop before, along with, or after the *clinical* diagnosis of the systemic malignancy. Practitioners should maintain a high index of suspicion for internal malignancy with development of any of these dermatoses. Most of the paraneoplastic dermatoses occur late in the course of a malignancy. Diagnostic modalities for the dermatoses include clinical recognition, a skin biopsy (in most cases), and possibly other laboratory work. A complete malignancy evaluation should be undertaken in any patient with development of one of these dermatoses. Most of the skin changes will at least partially clear with treatment or resolution of the tumor and may be treated symptomatically. The most common paraneoplastic dermatoses are discussed in the following sections (Table 222-1).

Acanthosis Nigricans

The lesions of acanthosis nigricans (AN) are symmetric, velvety plaques located in intertriginous areas and occasionally the oral mucosa. AN may be benign or associated with an endocrinopathy, medication, obesity, and/or a malignancy. Gastric adenocarcinoma is the most frequently associated cancer (see Color Plate VII-17).

Acquired Ichthyosis

Acquired ichthyosis usually has onset after age 20 years and is characterized by diamond-shaped hyperkeratotic scale, predominantly on the lower extremities. Hodgkin's lymphoma is the most frequently associated malignancy, but other solid malignancies have also been associated. Nonmalignant associations include sarcoidosis, leprosy, thyroid disease, AIDS, nutritional deficiencies, and cholesterol-lowering medications.

Primary Systemic Amyloidosis

The skin manifestations of primary systemic amyloidosis are pinch purpura, usually in the periorbital area; and waxy papules and plaques, which are most common on the face. Other less common skin findings include alopecia, bullous lesions, nail dystrophy, and pigment changes. Systemic manifestations include those associated with the deposition of amyloid in various organs and include macroglossia, peripheral neuropathy, carpal tunnel syndrome, cardiac decompensation, renal failure, hoarseness, and hepatomegaly. Approximately 25% of cases of primary systemic amyloidosis are associated with multiple myeloma, and many more are associated with a benign monoclonal gammopathy. Many researchers think that eventually all these patients with primary systemic amyloidosis will progress to multiple

Table 222-1 Paraneoplastic dermatoses

SYNDROMES	CUTANEOUS MANIFESTATIONS	OTHER ASSOCIATIONS	MOST COMMONLY ASSOCIATED INTERNAL MALIGNANCY
Acanthosis nigricans	Symmetric, intertriginous, hyperpigmented, velvety plaques	Obesity Diabetes	Gastric adenocarcinoma
Acquired ichthyosis	Diamond-shaped, hyperkeratotic scaling	AIDS Sarcoidosis Thyroid disease Medications Nutritional deficiencies	Lymphoma
Primary systemic amyloidosis	Pinch purpura on eyelids Waxy papules, nodules, plaques on face Alopecia Bullae Nail dystrophy Pigment changes	Macroglossia Peripheral neuropathy Cardiovascular failure Renal failure Hoarseness Hepatomegaly	Multiple myeloma
Bazex's syndrome	Psoriasiform, hyperkeratotic plaques on palms, soles, nasal bridge, ear helices		Carcinoma of the upper aerodigestive tract
Coagulopathies Trousseau's syndrome (superficial migratory thrombophlebitis)	Erythematous nodules coursing along superficial veins		Pancreatic carcinoma
Disseminated intravascular coagulopathy	Purpura Hemorrhagic bullae Gangrene	Infection Clotting factor abnormalities	Metastatic carcinoma
Deep venous thromboses	Tender cordlike lesion, with or without edema	Clotting factor abnormalities	Several malignancies
Dermatomyositis	Periorbital heliotrope discoloration Gottron's papules on dorsal hands Periungual telangiectasias Poikiloderma	Fatigue Proximal muscle weakness	Gastrointestinal malignancies
Erythema gyratum repens	Truncal polycyclic pattern with trailing scale		Bronchogenic carcinoma
Hypertrichosis lanuginosa acquisita	Fine, nonpigmented lanugo hair	Porphyria cutanea tarda Medications Thyrotoxicosis	Colon, lung, and breast carcinoma
Multicentric reticulohistiocytosis	Diffuse, erythematous papules and nodules on the face and upper trunk	Symmetric polyarteritis	Several malignancies
Necrobiotic xanthogranuloma	Yellow nodules or plaques	Paraproteinemia Cryoglobulinemia Anemia Leukopenia Increased ESR	Multiple myeloma
Necrolytic migratory erythema	Papulovesicular and eczematous eruptions—perineum, perioral, and flexural areas Glossitis Angular stomatitis	No malignancy Amino acid/zinc/essential fatty acid deficiency Glucose intolerance	Glucagonoma
Pruritus	Normal skin Excoriations Prurigo nodules Lichenification	Diabetes Renal impairment Hepatic impairment Anemia Polycythemia vera Thyroid disease Multiple sclerosis	Several malignancies
Sign of Leser Trélat	Sudden appearance or increased number of seborrheic keratoses		Gastric adenocarcinoma
Sweet's syndrome	Erythematous, pseudovesicular papules, nodules, and plaques		Acute myelogenous leukemia Lymphoma
Tripe palms	Accentuation of palmar dermatoglyphics	Acanthosis nigricans	Lung and gastrointestinal cancer

myeloma. Secondary amyloidosis rarely involves the skin and is rarely associated with malignancy.

Bazex's Syndrome

Bazex's syndrome (BS) (acrokeratosis paraneoplastica) is characterized by psoriasiform hyperkeratotic plaques most commonly located on the nasal bridge, helices of the ears, palms, and soles. BS is associated with malignancy of the oral cavity and upper respiratory or digestive tract in nearly 100% of cases (Fig. 222-1).

Coagulopathies

Coagulopathies that may be a marker for internal malignancy include superficial migratory thrombophlebitis (SMT), disseminated intravascular coagulation (DIC), and deep venous thrombosis (DVT). SMT is characterized by erythematous nodules coursing along superficial veins. It is most commonly associated with pancreatic carcinoma, but has been noted in association with several types of cancer. Approximately 50% of patients with SMT have a malignancy. Thrombotic complications of DIC may indicate metastatic malignancy and present as purpura, hemorrhagic bullae, or

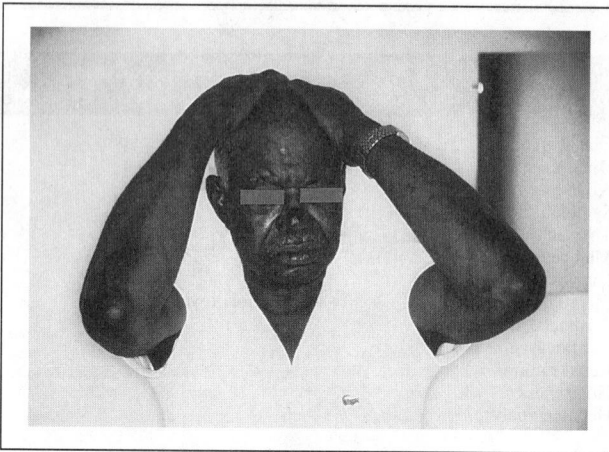

FIGURE 222-1   Bazex's syndrome with involvement of the skin of the nose, ear, and elbow.

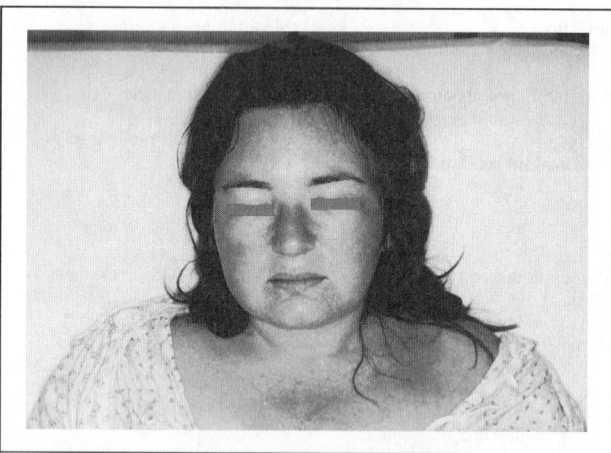

FIGURE 222-2   The heliotrope discoloration of dermatomyositis.

gangrene. A DVT occurring in an *unusual location* should arouse suspicion for an occult malignancy.

Dermatomyositis

The skin changes in dermatomyositis (DM) include a heliotrope discoloration involving the face and scalp (Fig. 222-2), Gottron's papules involving the dorsal hands (see Color Plate VII-3), periungual erythema and telangiectasias, and poikiloderma most frequently involving the flexor upper extremities. The muscle weakness associated with DM is proximal. DM sine myositis refers to the cutaneous changes without the muscle involvement and rarely occurs. As many as 40% of patients with DM have a malignancy. The malignancies occur most commonly in those older than 40 years of age and may precede or follow the diagnosis of DM. The most commonly associated malignancy is adenocarcinoma of the gastrointestinal tract. Several other malignancies are associated with DM and DM sine myositis. Ovarian carcinoma is noted to be particularly difficult to detect with routine measures (Chapter 171).

Erythema Gyratum Repens

Erythema gyratum repens (EGR) refers to the cutaneous changes of erythematous polycyclic bands with trailing scale, resembling grains of wood. The most common location is the trunk. Thus far all patients who have been reported have an associated malignancy, with bronchogenic carcinoma the most common.

Hypertrichosis Lanuginosa Acquisita

Hypertrichosis lanuginosa acquisita (Malignant Down) represents an acquired growth of fine, nonpigmented lanugo hair. It appears initially on the face, with the potential to spread diffusely. The most commonly associated malignancies include colon, lung, and breast carcinoma. Other associations include certain medications, porphyria cutanea tarda, and thyrotoxicosis. A congenital form of hypertrichosis lanugo, which is not associated with malignancy, has also been described.

Multicentric Reticulohistiocytosis

Multicentric reticulohistiocytosis (MRH) is characterized by infiltration of histiocytes in skin and internal organs. Cutaneous findings include periungual erythema and red-brown papules and nodules, which are most frequently located on the face and hands. The associated arthritis is symmetric and progresses to arthritis mutilans in approximately 50% of patients. As many as 28% of patients with MRH have one of several associated malignancies. Other systemic diseases associated with MRH include tuberculosis, diabetes mellitus, and thyroid disease.

Necrobiotic Xanthogranuloma

Necrobiotic xanthogranuloma is a destructive subcutaneous and dermal xanthogranuloma. The cutaneous lesions consist of red-yellow papules and nodules ranging in size up to 25 cm in diameter; they occasionally ulcerate. The most common location is the periorbital area, followed by the trunk, face, and extremities. Associated malignancies include multiple myeloma, lung carcinoma, and gastrointestinal carcinoma. Significant associated laboratory findings include benign monoclonal gammopathies, cryoglobulinemias, decreased complement levels, leukopenia, anemia, and increased erythrocyte sedimentation rates.

Necrolytic Migratory Erythema

Necrolytic migratory erythema (NME) is a papulovesicular skin eruption seen primarily in a perineal and perioral distribution. It is associated with glucagon-secreting α-cell tumors of the pancreas. Other associations include glossitis, angular stomatitis, glucose intolerance, and anemia. Necrolytic migratory erythema–like skin changes are seen in patients without a glucagonoma or other malignancy, and in those with zinc-essential fatty acid–amino acid deficiency states.

Pruritus

Pruritus may be a marker for malignancy, but it may also be associated with several primary dermatologic conditions and other non–cancer-related systemic diseases. The primary cutaneous associations include xerosis, scabies, bullous pemphigoid, dermatitis herpetiformis, and HIV-associated pruritus. The most common systemic associations include diabetes mellitus, anemia, polycythemia vera, paraproteinemias, renal failure, hepatic failure, thyroid disease, AIDS, and multiple sclerosis. Patients with persistent pruritus and none of the above associations should undergo a malignancy evaluation. Their skin may appear normal or xerotic, or it may be notable for lichenification or prurigo nodules.

Sign of Leser Trélat

The sudden appearance of multiple seborrheic keratoses in association with malignancy is defined as the sign of Leser Trélat. This occurs most frequently in the elderly. Gastrointestinal malignancies are the most frequently associated malignancy.

Sweet's Syndrome (Acute Febrile Neutrophilic Dermatosis)

Sweet's syndrome (SS) consists of fever, leukocytosis, and pseudovesicular erythematous papules, nodules, or plaques. The latter are most common on the upper body. SS is associated with

Table 222-2 Genetic disorders associated with cutaneous changes and malignancy

SYNDROME	INHERITANCE	CUTANEOUS ASSOCIATIONS	OTHER ASSOCIATIONS	ASSOCIATED INTERNAL MALIGNANCY
Ataxia telangiectasia (Louis-Bar Syndrome)	AR	Ocular and cutaneous telangiectasia Hypopigmented macules Café au lait macules Hirsutism	Cerebellar ataxia Mental retardation Immunologic defects Recurrent sinopulmonary infections	Lymphoreticular malignancies
Basal cell nevus syndrome (Gorlin's syndrome)	AD	Basal cell cancers Palmar and/or plantar pits	Skeletal abnormalities Odontogenic cysts Calcification of falx cerebri	Medulloblastoma
Cowden's syndrome	AD	Trichilemmomas Oral papillomatosis Acral keratoses	Fibrocystic breast disease Thyroid adenomas Ovarian cysts Hamartomatous GI polyps	Several carcinomas
Gardner's syndrome	AD	Osteomas Epidermoid inclusion cysts	Adenomatosis GI polyps Congenital retinal pigment	Colon carcinoma
Howell-Evans syndrome	AD	Palmoplantar hyperkeratosis		Esophageal carcinoma
Muir-Torre syndrome	AD	Sebaceous tumors Keratocanthomas	GI polyps	Colon and GU carcinoma
Peutz-Jeghers syndrome	AD	Mucocutaneous pigmented macules	Hamartomatous GI, GU, and respiratory polyps	Several malignancies

AD, autosomal dominant; *AR,* autosomal recessive; *GI,* gastrointestinal; *GU,* genitourinary.

cancer in approximately 20% to 30% of cases, most commonly acute myelogenous leukemia. Therapeutic options for SS include treatment of the underlying malignancy, if present, and immunosuppressive drugs.

Tripe Palms

Tripe palms (pachydermatoglyphy or acanthosis palmaris) are characterized by accentuation of the dermatoglyphic ridges. The most frequently associated malignancies include lung or gastric adenocarcinoma.

GENODERMATOSES WITH ASSOCIATED CUTANEOUS MANIFESTATIONS AND MALIGNANCY

Genodermatoses are skin changes associated with inherited syndromes, some of which are associated with malignancy. Thus recognition of the genodermatosis may allow early diagnosis of any associated internal malignancy. The most common genodermatoses associated with internal malignancies are summarized in Table 222-2.

Ataxia Telangiectasia

Ataxia telangiectasia (AT) (Louis-Bar Syndrome) is manifest in infancy with cerebellar ataxia. Patients may later develop oculocutaneous telangiectasias, mental retardation, and both cellular and humoral immune defects. The associated cutaneous findings include café au lait macules, mottled hypopigmentation and hyperpigmentation, hirsutism, and acanthosis nigricans. Patients with AT may develop lymphoreticular malignancies and, rarely, other malignancies.

Basal Cell Nevus Syndrome

The cutaneous manifestations of basal cell nevus syndrome (Gorlin's syndrome) include basal cell carcinomas (BCCs) and palmar and/or plantar pitting. The BCCs develop at an early age and become quite numerous. Other common features include odontogenic cysts, bifid ribs, kyphoscoliosis, frontal bossing, and calcification of the falx cerebri. The most commonly associated systemic malignancy is a medulloblastoma.

Cowden's Syndrome

The cutaneous features of Cowden's syndrome (Multiple hamartoma syndrome) are multiple facial papular warty growths (trichilemmomas), oral papillomatosis, acral keratoses, lipomas, and angiomas.

Breast carcinoma is the most frequently associated malignancy and has been described in up to 30% of affected women. Thyroid carcinoma is the second most commonly associated malignancy. Other associated tumors include thyroid adenomas, fibrocystic breast disease, and gastrointestinal polyps. The latter do not appear to be premalignant.

Gardner's Syndrome and Familial Adenomatous Polyposis

The cutaneous manifestations of Gardner's syndrome are epidermoid inclusion cysts, fibromas, and lipomas. Other findings include osteomas, desmoid tumors, congenital hypertrophic retinal pigmentation, and colonic polyps. There is nearly a 100% malignant transformation of polyps by the fifth decade. Siblings of Gardner's syndrome patients may have familial adenomatous polyposis (FAP). Further studies have demonstrated germline mutations in the adenomatous polyposis coli (APC) gene located on band 5q21 in more than two thirds of families affected by FAP and/or Gardner's syndrome. These observations indicate that FAP and Gardner's syndrome are variants of the same disease process.

Howell-Evans Syndrome

Howell-Evans syndrome (tylosis) is a rare syndrome of acquired palmar-plantar hyperkeratosis described in two English families. Esophageal squamous cell carcinoma was described in 30% of these patients. Nonfamilial palmar-plantar hyperkeratosis has been described in association with esophageal and lung carcinoma.

Muir-Torre Syndrome

Muir-Torre syndrome (MTS) describes patients with sebaceous neoplasms, visceral malignancies, and keratoacanthomas. The sebaceous neoplasms include sebaceous hyperplasia, adenomas, epitheliomas, carcinomas, and basal cell carcinomas with sebaceous differentiation. All are usually on the face. Adenocarcinomas of the gastrointestinal and genitourinary tracts are the most commonly associated malignancies.

Peutz-Jeghers Syndrome

The cutaneous manifestations of Peutz-Jeghers syndrome (PJS) include hyperpigmented macules on the lips, buccal mucosa, or in an acral location. The overall malignancy incidence in these patients ranges from 44% to 48%. The most commonly associated malignan-

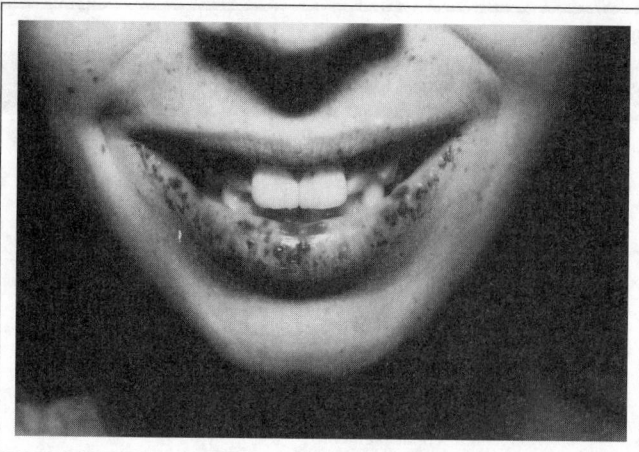

FIGURE 222-3   Peutz-Jeghers syndrome.
(Courtesy Dr. Bernard Cohen.)

cies include gastrointestinal, lung, breast, and gonadal tumors (Fig. 222-3).

SUMMARY

Certain dermatoses may reflect the presence of an internal malignancy. Any cutaneous finding that is known to be associated with malignancy should prompt a thorough systemic evaluation for that malignancy. It should be remembered that in any of these entities the dermatoses may precede, occur concurrently with, or parallel the *clinical* diagnosis of the tumor. For all dermatoses associated with an internal malignancy, early recognition of the cutaneous change may allow earlier recognition and treatment of the associated malignancy, thus enhancing patient survival.

BIBLIOGRAPHY

Callen JP: Skin signs of internal malignancy. In Callen JP, Jorizzo J, Piette W et al, editors: *Dermatologic signs of internal disease*, Philadelphia, 1995, WB Saunders.
Finan MC, Ray MK: Gastrointestinal polyposis syndromes, *Dermatol Clin* 7:419, 1989.
Kurzrock R, Cohen PR: Cutaneous paraneoplastic syndromes in solid tumors, *Am J Med* 99:207, 1995.
Kurzrock R, Cohen PR: Mucocutaneous paraneoplastic manifestations of hematologic malignancies, *Am J Med* 99:207, 1995.
Lookingbill DP, Spangler N: Skin involvement as the presenting sign of internal carcinoma, *J Am Acad Dermatol* 22:19, 1990.
Mehregan DA, Mehregan DR: Paraneoplastic syndromes, *Adv Dermatol* 9:25, 1994.
Mehregan DA, Winkelmann RK: Necrobiotic xanthogranuloma, *Arch Dermatol* 128:94, 1992.
Poole S, Fenske NA: Cutaneous markers of internal malignancy. I. Malignant involvement of the skin and the genodermatoses, *J Am Acad Dermatol* 28:1, 1993.
Poole S, Fenske NA: Cutaneous markers of internal malignancy. II. Paraneoplastic dermatoses and environmental carcinogens, *J Am Acad Dermatol* 28:147, 1993.
Skolnick M, Mainman ER: Erythema gyratum repens with metastatic adenocarcinoma, *Arch Dermatol* 111:227, 1975.
Whitmore SE et al: Ovarian cancer in patients with dermatomyositis, *Medicine* 73:153, 1994.

We would like to thank Ellen B. Rest, MD, for her contribution to this chapter in the fourth edition of this text.

223 Cutaneous Manifestations of Gastrointestinal Disease

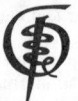

Van Ha and Susan D. Laman

Recognition of the cutaneous manifestations of gastrointestinal (GI) disease(s) is helpful, or in some cases pivotal, in establishing the diagnosis of the gastrointestinal disease(s). In this chapter, we address the cutaneous manifestations of various diseases associated with GI hemorrhage and inflammatory bowel disease. The skin manifestations of GI malignancy, the GI polyposis syndromes, the autoimmune blistering diseases, and the connective tissue diseases are covered in other chapters. Because of the limited scope of this text, the cutaneous manifestations of hepatic, pancreatic, and nutritional disorders are not addressed.

CUTANEOUS MANIFESTATIONS OF DISEASES ASSOCIATED WITH GASTROINTESTINAL HEMORRHAGE

Blue Rubber Bleb Nevus Syndrome

Blue rubber bleb nevus syndrome is a sporadic or autosomally dominant inherited disorder. Patients with this syndrome have cutaneous and GI tract hemangiomas. Histopathologically, the cutaneous lesions are cavernous hemangiomas. They vary from 1 mm to several centimeters in size and are occasionally painful. They do bleed, and although hemodynamically significant bleeding rarely occurs, patients often require iron supplementation and blood transfusions to treat their associated iron-deficiency anemia.

Cutis Laxa

Cutis laxa (CL) is a form of generalized elastolysis. In CL there are decreased, disorganized, and fragmented elastic fibers. Affected sites can include the skin, GI tract, and the cardiopulmonary systems. Dermatologic examination reveals loose, redundant skin folds around the eyelids, cheeks, and abdomen.

Degos Disease

Degos disease or malignant atrophic papulosis is a rare noninherited disorder of the skin, GI tract, central nervous system (CNS), and cardiopulmonary system. The cutaneous lesions develop slowly and are usually asymptomatic. The characteristic initial lesion is a pink or red dome-shaped papule less than 6 mm in diameter, which rapidly develops an area of central necrosis. The resultant lesion is a papule with an atrophic ivory center and an area of surrounding erythema. These lesions have a predilection for the proximal extremities and trunk. The GI, CNS, and cardiopulmonary manifestations usually develop after the skin changes (Table 223-1).

Ehlers-Danlos Syndrome

Ehlers-Danlos syndrome (EDS) is a group of disorders inherited in autosomal recessive, autosomal dominant, and x-linked fashion (Chapter 211). Type IV EDS can be inherited in both autosomal recessive and autosomal dominant forms and is the form of EDS associated most frequently with GI hemorrhage. The defect in type IV EDS lies in the synthesis and secretion of type III collagen. Patients have fragile skin and impaired wound healing, and they may suffer spontaneous rupture of the bowel.

Kaposi's Sarcoma

Kaposi's sarcoma is covered in detail in Chapter 227. The appearance of the cutaneous and mucosal lesions ranges from minute to very

Table 223-1 Diseases with cutaneous manifestations and GI hemorrhage

SYNDROME	INHERITANCE	CUTANEOUS MANIFESTATION	OTHER ASSOCIATED FINDINGS
Blue rubber bleb nevus syndrome	S/AD	Cutaneous cavernous hemangiomas	Iron deficiency anemia Hemangiomas in the liver, lungs, eyes, CNS
Cutis laxa	AD/AR/AC	Pendulous skin near eyelids, cheeks, abdomen	Tracheobronchomegaly Cardiomegaly Uterine prolapse Ruptured patellar tendon Aortic dilation
Degos disease		Papules with white atrophic centers	Episcleritis CNS infarcts Serositis
Ehlers-Danlos syndrome type IV	AD/AR	Impaired wound healing Skin fragility	Uterine hemorrhage Arterial aneurysms
Kaposi's sarcoma		Red-brown papules, nodules, plaques on skin and mucosal surfaces	Internal KS lesions
Osler-Weber-Rendu syndrome	AD	Macular and mat-like telangiectasia	Arterial venous malformations, aneurysms—GI, pulmonary, and CNS
Pseudoxanthoma elasticum	AD/AR	"Chicken skin" of the intertriginous areas	Angioid streaks of retina Arterial occlusion Hypertension

AD, autosomal dominant; *AR,* autosomal recessive; *AC,* acquired; *S,* sporadic.

large violaceous papules, plaques, and nodules. Hemorrhage can occur associated with the GI lesions.

Osler-Weber-Rendu (Hereditary Hemorrhagic Telangiectasia)

Osler-Weber-Rendu (OWR) syndrome or hereditary hemorrhagic telangiectasia (HHT) is a systemic disease with autosomal dominant inheritance. Patients have cutaneous, pulmonary, central nervous system (CNS), and gastrointestinal (GI) telangiectasia, arteriovenous malformations (AVMs), and aneurysms. The skin characteristically reveals sharply demarcated telangiectatic mats most commonly located on the face and hands, but they may be generalized. The initial symptom is recurrent epistaxis, which develops in most cases by puberty and eventually occurs in 80% of the cases. Patients are at risk for GI, pulmonary, and CNS hemorrhage (see Table 223-1). Patients with the CREST variant of scleroderma also have similar telangiectasia but no history of epistaxis. Therapeutic options for the cutaneous telangiectasia of OWR include electrocautery and laser treatment.

Pseudoxanthoma Elasticum

Pseudoxanthoma elasticum (PXE) is a rare disorder of connective tissue. Inheritance is in an autosomal dominant or autosomal recessive fashion. Histopathologic characteristics include calcification and degeneration of the elastic tissue. Patients' cutaneous lesions include soft, lax skin with overlying small yellow papules, fine wrinkling, and telangiectasia. This is most notable on the neck and flexural surfaces and is referred to as "plucked chicken skin." Other findings include arterial occlusion, hypertension, angioid streaks in the retina, and GI hemorrhage. The latter is more common in the upper GI versus lower GI tract.

CUTANEOUS FINDINGS IN INFLAMMATORY BOWEL DISEASE: CROHN'S DISEASE AND ULCERATIVE COLITIS

Crohn's disease (CD) and ulcerative colitis (UC) are both associated with several cutaneous manifestations (Table 223-2). The manifestations are similar in both diseases, although the frequency may differ. The presentation of some of these dermatologic manifestations may be the initial noted feature of inflammatory bowel disease (IBD), whereas other cutaneous changes may occur with or postdate the intestinal disease. The most common of all the dermatologic changes associated with IBD include pyoderma gangrenosum and erythema nodosum. Both will be discussed later in further detail.

Table 223-2 Cutaneous manifestations of inflammatory bowel disease

CUTANEOUS CHANGE	CROHN'S DISEASE	ULCERATIVE COLITIS
Erythema nodosum	++	++
Pyoderma gangrenosum	+	++
Oral apthae	++	++
Cutaneous polyarteritis nodosa	+	+
Leukocytoclastic vasculitis	+	+
Sweet's syndrome	+	+
Coagulation defects		+
Clubbing	++	++
Psoriasis	+	+
Nutritional deficiencies	+	
Metastatic Crohn's disease	+	

+, Infrequent; ++, common.

Erythema Nodosum

Erythema nodosum (EN) is more common in patients with CD than with UC. (Color Plate VII-12). EN is an inflammatory disorder of the subcutis, which is histologically defined as a septal panniculitis. Cutaneous examination reveals tender, erythematous, warm, nonsuppurative nodules typically located symmetrically overlying the pretibial surfaces. Other areas of potential involvement include the face, trunk, and upper extremities. EN may precede symptoms of IBD but is usually seen during IBD flares. In addition to the cutaneous changes, patients may also develop fever, arthralgias, and malaise. EN is not disease specific. It can be seen in other settings, including in association with certain medications, infections, sarcoidosis, pregnancy, and idiopathic inflammatory conditions. EN usually resolves over 3 to 6 weeks with bed rest; however, corticosteroids, dapsone, colchicine, and potassium iodide all have been tried with varied success for treatment.

Pyoderma Gangrenosum

Pyoderma gangrenosum (PG) is an idiopathic inflammatory disorder. It is characterized by the sudden onset of painful pustules, or nodules, that may quickly evolve to become large ulcers. The ulcers typically have liquefactive centers. The borders are violaceous, undermined, and frequently surrounded with hemorrhagic blisters. Healing occurs with cribiform scarring. PG is associated more with UC than

CD and is also linked to other disease processes including rheumatoid arthritis, leukemias, gammopathies, chronic active hepatitis, and sarcoidosis. PG manifests pathergy, which refers to development of new lesions at any site of trauma. Thus surgical treatment is almost never indicated. As with EN, PG can occur in IBD patients in remission but more often is seen during acute flares. Therapeutic options include oral corticosteroids, pulse corticosteroids, dapsone, azathioprine, cyclosporin A, clofazime, or rarely resection of the severely inflamed bowel.

BIBLIOGRAPHY

Apgar JT: Newer aspects of inflammatory bowel disease and its cutaneous manifestations: a selective review, *Semin Dermat* 10:138, 1991.

Burgdorf W: Cutaneous manifestations of Crohn's disease, *J Am Acad Dermatol* 5:689, 1981.

Danzi JT: Extraintestinal manifestations of idiopathic inflammatory bowel disease, *Arch Intern Med* 148:297, 1988.

Golitz LE: Heritable cutaneous disorders which affect the gastrointestinal tract, *Med Clin North Am* 64:829, 1980.

Greenstein AJ, Janowitz HD, Sachar DB: The extraintestinal complications of Crohn's disease and ulcerative colitis: a study of 700 patients, *Medicine* 55:401, 1976.

Gregory B, Ha VC: Cutaneous manifestations of gastrointestinal disorders, Part II, *J Am Acad Dermatol* 26:371, 1992.

Kafity AA, Pellegrini AE, Fromkes JJ: Metastatic Crohn's disease: a rare cutaneous complication, *J Clin Gastroenterol* 17:300, 1993.

Marks J: The relationship of gastrointestinal disease and the skin, *Clin Gastroenterol* 12:693, 1983.

Rankin GB: Extraintestinal and systemic manifestations of inflammatory bowel disease, *Med Clin North Am* 74:39, 1990.

Roberts N, Bunker C: The gut and the skin, *Brit J Hosp Med* 50:31, 1993.

We would like to thank Dr. Simmons-O'Brien and Dr. Lisa Beck for their contribution to the previous edition.

CHAPTER

224 Cutaneous Manifestations of Endocrine Disorders

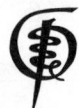

Diane Orlinsky and Susan E. Koch

Endocrine diseases frequently affect the skin, hair, nails, and mucous membranes. These changes often occur in association with signs and symptoms in other organ systems and may provide a clue to the underlying endocrine imbalance. The resolution of reversible changes may enable the clinician to monitor the effectiveness of therapy.

THYROID DISEASE

Although there are no pathognomonic cutaneous features of hypothyroidism, the integument is affected in the majority of individuals with deficient thyroid hormone (Table 224-1). The skin is pale, dry, and cool because of reduced sweating, vasoconstriction, and lower body temperature. Generalized myxedema, an accumulation of acid mucopolysaccharides in the dermis, imparts an edematous appearance to the face. Yellow discoloration most prominent on the palms, soles, and nasolabial folds occurs in longstanding hypothyroidism because of an accumulation of β-carotene resulting from reduced hepatic conversion of β-carotene to vitamin A. The hair is dull and coarse. Diffuse nonscarring alopecia of scalp hair is common and may be the presenting complaint. Loss of the lateral third of the eyebrows *(Hertough's sign)* occurs in one quarter of the patients but is not specific for hypothyroidism. Alopecia areata may be associated with the autoimmune forms of hypothyroidism. Nails are slow growing, brittle, and ridged. Other clinical manifestations are listed in Table 224-1. The majority of skin changes resolve with thyroid replacement therapy.

Table 224-1   Skin manifestations of thyroid disease

HYPOTHYROIDISM	HYPERTHYROIDISM
Pale, cool, dry skin	Warm, moist skin
Generalized myxedema	Easy flushing
Periorbital/acral nonpitting edema	Palmar erythema
Carotenemia	Hyperhidrosis
Malar blush	Hyperpigmentation
Decreased sweating	Vitiligo (autoimmune types)
Brittle, thin, ridged, slow-growing nails	Fine, soft scalp hair
Diffuse nonscarring alopecia	Diffuse nonscarring alopecia
Alopecia areata (Hashimoto's disease)	Alopecia areata
Eczema craquelé	
Loss of lateral third of eyebrow	Plummer's nails
	Pretibial myxedema (Graves' disease)
Keratoderma of palms/soles	Thyroid acropachy (Graves' disease)
Pruritus	Pruritus (rare)
Purpura, ecchymoses	Urticaria (rare)
Impaired wound healing	—

The cutaneous manifestations that result from excess thyroid hormone include warm, moist, erythematous skin resulting from peripheral vasodilation and hyperhidrosis. Flushing of the face and chest may occur and persistent erythema of the palms and elbows. Hyperpigmentation similar to that seen in Addison's disease is described. Vitiligo, found in as many as 7% of patients with Graves' disease, is not associated with other forms of hyperthyroidism and is not responsive to thyroid therapy. As with hypothyroidism diffuse nonscarring alopecia may occur. The hair loss correlates poorly with the degree of hyperthyroidism. Loss of the lateral third of the eyebrows may occur as with hypothyroidism. Alopecia areata is reported with Graves' disease. Nail changes include onycholysis with upward turning of the nails *(Plummer's nails),* which resolves with treatment. Thyroid acropachy refers to the painless clubbing of the fingers and toes associated with bony proliferation of the distal phalanges occurring in less than 1% of patients with Graves' disease.

Pretibial myxedema (thyroid dermopathy) occurs in 1% to 4% of patients with Graves' disease and rarely occurs in Hashimoto's thyroiditis and primary myxedema. It may be a presenting sign of Graves' disease, but more commonly it occurs months or years after the diagnosis. The vast majority of patients with pretibial myxedema have associated ophthalmopathy. The appearance of pretibial myxedema is one of bilateral, firm, erythematous to violaceous to yellowish brown thickened areas of skin with prominent follicular orifices imparting a *peau d'orange* appearance. The lesions occur on the pretibial areas and are asymptomatic but cosmetically undesirable. There are three major types: the nonpitting edema form (58%), the plaque form (21%), and the nodular form (20%). The less common elephantiasis form (1%) may cause significant functional problems. Pretibial myxedema is caused by the accumulation of acid mucopolysaccharides in the dermis and subcutaneous tissue.

ADRENAL DISEASE

The cutaneous changes in Addison's disease may result from a lack of glucocorticoid hormone or an excess of pituitary hormones, or as a result of autoimmune mechanisms. Cortisol insufficiency causes reduction of axillary hair; regrowth occurs after replacement therapy. Hyperpigmentation occurs with primary adrenal insufficiency due to elevated levels of anterior pituitary peptides that stimulate melanin production of the skin. It is not a feature of adrenal insufficiency due to pituitary failure. Hyperpigmentation may be generalized and appear as a persistent tan. It is accentuated in sun-exposed areas, palmar creases, newly acquired scars, and in areas of trauma such as the knees and elbows. Skin surfaces that are more heavily pigmented, such as the areola, nipples, and genitals, darken. Pigmented bands may occur on the fingernails, and the hair color may darken. Pigmentation of the buccal mucosa, tongue, and gums may occur. Gradual lightening of pigmentation occurs with replacement therapy. Vitiligo is also reported in a small percentage of patients. The

BOX 224-1
Cutaneous manifestations of Cushing's syndrome

Thin, fragile skin
Impaired wound healing
Petechiae/ecchymoses from trauma
Cutis marmorata of legs
Wide, violaceous striae
Moon facies/facial telangiectasia
Acne
Hyperpigmentation (Cushing's disease)
Acanthosis nigricans
Dermatophyte infection
Tinea versicolor

BOX 224-2
Cutaneous manifestations of diabetes mellitus

Infections
  Bacterial
  Fungal
Neurologic and vascular complications
  Autonomic dysfunction
  Mal perforans ulcers
  Ischemic ulcers
  Gangrene
Diabetic dermopathy
Necrobiosis lipoidica diabeticorum
Diabetic bullae
Lipid abnormalities
  Eruptive xanthomas
  Xanthelasma
Limited joint mobility and waxy skin syndrome
Pruritus
Other associations
  Acanthosis nigricans
  Granuloma annulare
  Vitiligo
  Hemochromatosis
  Glucagonoma
  Lichen planus
  Scleredema
  Perforating disorder of diabetes
  Werner's syndrome
  Lipodystrophy
  Kaposi's sarcoma
Reactions to insulin
  Allergic reactions
  Insulin edema
  Insulin-induced lipoatrophy or lipohypertrophy

cutaneous manifestations of glucocorticoid excess are listed in Box 224-1.

DIABETES MELLITUS

Almost all patients with diabetes mellitus develop cutaneous problems (Box 224-2). The skin findings in diabetes are varied and range in severity from mild to life-threatening. Diabetics are particularly susceptible to bacterial and fungal infections. Diabetic ketoacidosis can be triggered by infection or can predispose to infection; it is therefore important to look for infection in all patients who present with ketoacidosis. Volatile blood glucose levels and impaired function of neutrophils predispose patients to polymicrobial bacterial infections, which are difficult to treat. In addition, peripheral neuropathy and vascular disease also contribute to infections of the foot and lower extremities. These infections include paronychia, cellulitis, gas gangrene

(which may require amputation), and osteomyelitis. Diabetic patients have an increased incidence of superficial skin infections such as impetigo, erythrasma, erysipelas, folliculitis, carbuncles, and furuncles. Malignant external otitis, caused by *Pseudomonas aeruginosa,* is a rare but serious complication of diabetes with high morbidity and mortality rates. Candidal infections, including paronychia, angular stomatitis, thrush, balanitis, and vulvovaginitis, are also associated with poorly controlled diabetes. Candidiasis commonly occurs in known diabetics, and it may be the presenting sign of diabetes mellitus. Deep fungal infections, such as mucormycosis, are another complication of diabetes.

The neuropathy and angiopathy associated with diabetes can lead to other cutaneous complications. Autonomic dysfunction causes disturbances in sweating, including hypohidrosis or anhidrosis of the lower extremities and gustatory sweating. Chronic autonomic disturbances can culminate in erythema, edema, and atrophy of the affected area. Peripheral neuropathy contributes to the development of neuropathic perforating ulcers (mal perforans) of the soles, often further complicated by osteomyelitis of the underlying bone. The cutaneous manifestations of macroangiopathy of the lower extremities include mottled, atrophic skin, hair loss, dystrophic nails, and distal coldness and pallor.

The most common cutaneous sign of diabetes is diabetic dermopathy (shin spots). These asymptomatic lesions are small, atrophic, hyperpigmented scars located on the pretibial areas. They are variable in number and often bilateral. Although the origin of these lesions remains unclear, microangiopathy may be a contributing factor.

Necrobiosis lipoidica diabeticorum (NLD) is found in only 0.3% of diabetics, and is not unique to diabetes (Color Plate VII-16). At the onset of NLD, two thirds of patients are known to have diabetes. It has been shown that NLD may precede the diagnosis of diabetes mellitus by months to years. The presence of NLD, therefore, warrants an evaluation for diabetes as well as future monitoring. The initial lesions of NLD are characterized by small, red-brown plaques on the anterior and lateral lower legs. The lesions slowly evolve into larger yellow-brown plaques with erythematous borders, central atrophy, telangiectasias, and occasional ulceration. Involvement of the face, arms, and scalp occurs rarely.

Bullous lesions (bullous diabeticorum) are an uncommon finding in diabetes. They are found on the hands and feet, are asymptomatic, and usually resolve spontaneously. They must be distinguished from other bullous diseases, such as porphyria cutanea tarda, bullous impetigo, and bullous pemphigoid.

Although acanthosis nigricans is commonly thought of as a sign of internal malignancy, a benign variant of this skin condition occurs in conjunction with diabetes mellitus (Color Plate VII-17). It occurs as symmetric, velvety, thickened, hyperpigmented plaques typically located in the folds of the axillae, posterior neck, and the groin. This form of acanthosis nigricans has been linked to other endocrine disorders, such as acromegaly, Cushing's syndrome, hypothyroidism, insulin resistance, and polycystic ovary disease. It may also be seen in obese patients without endocrine disturbances.

HYPERLIPIDEMIA

Xanthomas are distinct skin lesions often associated with hyperlipidemia. Less commonly, they occur in patients who have paraproteinemia or normal lipid levels. Eruptive xanthomas are due to elevations in serum triglycerides. Conditions that cause hypertriglyceridemia, such as genetic disorders, diabetes mellitus, hypothyroidism, Cushing's syndrome, pancreatitis, and renal disease, can lead to eruptive xanthomas. These xanthomas appear suddenly as crops of small yellow papules most frequently on the buttocks and extensor aspects of the extremities (Color Plate VII-18). They resolve with normalization of serum triglyceride levels. Hypercholesterolemia is associated with tendinous, planar and tuberous xanthomas. Tendinous xanthomas are firm nodules typically located on the Achilles tendons and extensor tendons of the hands, elbows, and knees. Planar xanthomas are soft yellow macules or plaques that tend to occur on the trunk or eyelids (xanthelasma) (Color Plate VII-19). In approximately one half of cases, xanthelasma is seen in individuals with normal serum cholesterol levels. Tuberous xanthomas are soft yellow-orange plaques or nodules usually found on extensor surfaces, particularly over the elbows and knees. The presence of xanthomas warrants an evaluation for hyperlipidemia.

BIBLIOGRAPHY

Bijlmer-Iest JC, Vloten WA: Thyroid and the skin, *Curr Probl Dermatol* 20:34, 1991.
Fatourechi V, Pajouhi M, Fransway AF: Dermopathy of Graves' disease (pretibial myxedema): review of 150 cases, *Medicine* 73:1, 1994.
Feingold KR, Elias PM: Endocrine-skin interactions: cutaneous manifestations of adrenal disease, pheochromocytomas, carcinoid syndrome, sex hormone excess and deficiency, polyglandular autoimmune syndromes, multiple endocrine neoplasia syndromes, and other miscellaneous disorders, *J Am Acad Dermatol* 17:921, 1987.
Freinkel RK: Cutaneous manifestations of endocrine diseases. In Fitzpatrick TB et al, editors: *Dermatology in general medicine,* New York, 1993, McGraw-Hill.
Heymann WR: Cutaneous manifestations of thyroid disease, *J Am Acad Dermatol* 26:885, 1992.
Huntley AC: Cutaneous manifestations of diabetes mellitus, *Dermatol Clin* 7:531, 1989.
Jelinek JE: Cutaneous manifestations of diabetes mellitus, *Int J Dermatol* 33:605, 1994.
Kemmerly SA: Dermatologic manifestations of infections in diabetics, *Infect Dis Clin North Am* 8:523, 1994.
Parker F: Xanthomas and hyperlipidemias, *J Am Acad Dermatol* 13:1, 1985.

CHAPTER

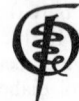

225 Cutaneous Manifestations of Sarcoidosis

Steven R. Feldman

The cutaneous manifestations of sarcoidosis are quite variable, sometimes isolated, but more often associated with pulmonary, ocular, and other systemic involvement (Chapter 53). Both specific and nonspecific lesions (Box 225-1) can be seen. Specific lesions are characterized by granulomatous inflammation; nonspecific lesions do not have a granulomatous basis. The importance of cutaneous sarcoidosis rests in its usefulness as a marker of systemic involvement, its ready access for histologic diagnosis, and its ability to cause disfigurement.

BOX 225-1
The cutaneous manifestations of sarcoidosis

Specific lesions
Papules and nodules
  Lesions in scars
  Annular patterns
  Lichenoid papules
Plaques
  Angiolupoid plaques
  Lupus pernio
Subcutaneous nodules
Hypopigmentation
Ichthyosis
Ulcerations
Generalized or photodistributed eruptions
Morpheaform lesions
Pruritic papulonodules
Scarring alopecia
Pterygium of the nail
Mucous membrane lesions

Nonspecific lesions
Erythema nodosum
Pruritus
Erythema multiforme
Digital clubbing
Calcinosis cutis

RELEVANT PHYSIOLOGY AND PATHOPHYSIOLOGY

The most common morphology of the specific lesions of cutaneous sarcoidosis is a papular eruption (Color Plate VII-20). The papules tend to be flesh-colored to hypopigmented in blacks and reddish-orange to violaceous in whites. The eruption is often symmetric and nonpruritic, and areas of predilection include the central face, posterior neck, and trunk. An annular arrangement of the papules may be seen, and it is not uncommon for the lesions to develop in scars. Plaques larger than 1 cm are common and may have a slightly scaly surface. The term *angiolupoid* is used to describe those plaques that have telangiectatic vessels on their surfaces. Chronic plaques present on the nose, ears, cheeks, and fingers are called *lupus pernio* (Color Plate VII-21).

Less common manifestations of sarcoidosis include subcutaneous nodules, hypopigmentation, ichthyosis, ulcerations, generalized or photodistributed eruptions, morpheaform lesions, pruritic papulonodules, scarring alopecia, and nail abnormalities. Mucous membranes also may be involved.

The nonspecific manifestations of sarcoidosis include erythema nodosum, calcinosis cutis, pruritus, and erythema multiforme. Of these, erythema nodosum is the most important. Clinically it consists of erythematous, warm, tender nodules that are usually located on the anterior legs. Biopsy discloses a septal panniculitis. When the onset of sarcoidosis is acute and manifested by erythema nodosum in association with arthralgias, elevated sedimentation rate, and hilar adenopathy, there is often a good prognosis with spontaneous regression.

LABORATORY AND OTHER DIAGNOSTIC TESTS

The histopathologic hallmark of sarcoidosis is granulomatous inflammation. In the skin, aggregates of epithelioid mononuclear cells are present in the superficial dermis, extending into the deep dermis and occasionally the subcutis. Multinucleated giant cells are often present, but in contrast to tuberculosis, there are few accompanying lymphocytes and no caseous necrosis. Asteroid bodies (stellate eosinophilic inclusions) and Schaumann bodies (lamellate round concretions) may be present in the giant cells but are also present in other granulomatous processes. Polarization microscopy should be performed to rule out foreign body reactions. Zirconium and beryllium can induce similar histologic patterns and should be excluded by history and special studies if needed.

Intradermal testing with heat-sterilized sarcoid tissue (the Kveim test) is of limited clinical utility but is a useful model for the immunopathologic study of sarcoidosis. Helper T-cells are present by 6 hours after injection; granulomas are found after 12 days. Studies from Europe report identifying mycobacterial DNA from some sarcoidal granulomas; this has not been confirmed in U.S. studies.

DIFFERENTIAL DIAGNOSIS

Most inflammatory dermatoses exhibit a characteristic lesion morphology. In contrast, patients with cutaneous sarcoidosis may have any one of a myriad of different morphologic patterns. Therefore sarcoidosis must be considered in the differential diagnosis of many eruptions, particularly in high-risk populations (e.g., African-Americans).

MANAGEMENT

The treatment of sarcoidosis must take into consideration its prognosis and severity. Acute involvement may resolve spontaneously and usually can be treated conservatively. At the other end of the spectrum, life-threatening internal organ involvement warrants aggressive attempts at management, including the use of systemic immunosuppressive agents. In general, cutaneous disease falls between these extremes, rarely justifying extreme measures except to prevent severe disfigurement. Because treatment for cutaneous involvement is based solely on the risk of disfigurement, serum angiotensin-converting enzyme levels and gallium scans are rarely helpful for managing cutaneous manifestations.

With only limited cutaneous involvement, in which potential scar-

✔ *WHEN TO REFER*

When a patient has cutaneous sarcoidosis, a careful search for systemic involvement must be initiated. Of special concern is possible retinal and pulmonary involvement. The presence of systemic involvement may dictate treatment with systemic corticosteroids. Otolaryngologic examination may be of value in patients with the *lupus pernio* pattern to detect involvement of the upper respiratory tract.

ring and disfigurement are minimal, potent topical corticosteroids may be used. Unfortunately, these agents have poor penetration to the granulomatous inflammation in the deep dermis, and their use is often complicated by the development of epidermal atrophy. Intralesional injection allows delivery of the corticosteroids through the full thickness of the dermis. This is particularly of value in the treatment of localized plaques and nodules.

Systemic corticosteroids are used only when there is widespread disfigurement, scarring alopecia, or systemic disease. For cutaneous disease, alternate-day regimens may be used, starting at 30 mg of prednisone and tapering to the minimal required dose. To avoid systemic corticosteroids or to reduce the dose, hydroxychloroquine therapy may be tried. For severe, treatment-resistant lesions, oral methotrexate may be used. Monitoring for side effects of methotrexate is essential; it may be difficult to distinguish the pulmonary effects of methotrexate from pulmonary sarcoidosis.

BIBLIOGRAPHY

Elgart ML: Cutaneous sarcoidosis: definitions and types of lesions. In Izumi T, editor: *Clinics in dermatology: sarcoidosis,* Philadelphia, 1986, Lippincott.
Fidler HM, Rook GA, Johnson NM et al: *Mycobacterium tuberculosis* DNA in tissue affected by sarcoidosis, *Br Med J* 306:546-549, 1993.
Ghossein RA, Ross DG, Salomon RN et al: A search for mycobacterial DNA in sarcoidosis using the polymerase chain reaction, *Am J Clin Pathol* 101:733-737, 1994.
Hanno R, Callen JP: Sarcoidosis. In Jordon RE, editor: *Immunologic diseases of the skin,* Norwalk, Conn, 1991, Appleton & Lange.
Jones E, Callen JP: Hydroxychloroquine is effective therapy for control of cutaneous sarcoidal granulomas, *J Am Acad Dermatol* 23:487, 1990.
Lower EE, Baughman RP: Prolonged use of methotrexate for sarcoidosis, *Arch Intern Med* 155:846-851, 1995.
White CR Jr: Predominantly mononuclear cell granulomas. In Farmer ER, Hood AF, editors: *Pathology of the skin,* Norwalk, Conn, 1990, Appleton & Lange.

CHAPTER

226 Cutaneous Manifestations of Human Immunodeficiency Virus Infection

Thomas D. Horn and Ciro R. Martins

Cutaneous signs of human immunodeficiency virus-1 (HIV-1) infection are divided into inflammatory, infectious, and neoplastic conditions (Box 226-1). Skin disease in the individual with HIV is frequently the presenting feature of the progressive immunologic failure of the acquired immunodeficiency syndrome (AIDS). The eruptions may be mild and usually represent conditions ordinarily encountered in healthy persons without HIV, such as seborrheic dermatitis, folliculitis, and molluscum contagiosum. As the peripheral CD4$^+$ lymphocyte number decreases, cutaneous disease tends to become more severe, more resistant to treatment, and more HIV restricted (e.g., cryptococcosis, Kaposi's sarcoma, *Mycobacterium haemophilum*). Thus clues that skin disease represent a manifestation of HIV infec-

---

BOX 226-1
Cutaneous signs of HIV-1 infection

Infectious
Viral
Oral hairy leukoplakia
Molluscum contagiosum
Epstein-Barr virus
Human papillomavirus
Cytomegalovirus
Herpesvirus infection (herpes simplex, herpes varicella-zoster)
Fungal
Oral candidiasis
Dermatophytosis
Pityrosporon ovale
Cutaneous manifestations of disseminated systemic infection
  Cryptococcus neoformans
  Histoplasma capsulatum
  Coccidioides immitis
  Sporothrix schenckii
Bacterial
Pyoderma, folliculitis, secondary impetiginization
Mycobacterium species
Syphilis
Rickettsial-bacillary angiomatosis
Protozoal
Acanthamoeba castellani

Inflammatory dermatoses
Xerosis, ichthyosis
Granuloma annular-like lesions
Exacerbation of preexisting skin disease, especially psoriasis
Drug eruptions
Papular (pruritic) eruption
Photosensitivity
Lichenoid dermatoses
Seborrheic dermatitis

Neoplasm
Lymphoma
Kaposi's sarcoma
Other vascular proliferations
  Angiomas
  Telangiectasia

---

tion include unusually wide distribution and large numbers of lesions, frequent recurrence, poor response to therapy, and identification of unusual infectious agents or neoplastic conditions (Table 226-1). Although cutaneous disease is rarely life-threatening, successful treatment greatly improves the quality of life and gives the patient a measure of control over the most visible aspects of the disease.

INFLAMMATORY CONDITIONS
Papular Eruption of HIV

Many individuals develop the rapid onset of skin-colored to erythematous papules on the trunk and extremities within several weeks to months of HIV infection. The eruption is asymptomatic or mildly pruritic and displays the nonspecific histologic findings of a predominantly lymphocytic perivascular inflammatory cell infiltrate with mild dermal edema and occasional eosinophils. This exanthem may be the first clinical manifestation of HIV infection. The cause is unknown. The treatment is symptomatic.

Psoriasis

Psoriasis affects approximately 1% of the population in the United States. In some patients with preexisting psoriasis, there is little change in disease severity with HIV infection, whereas in others, the erythematous, scaling plaques rapidly multiply and spread, often eventuating in erythroderma. Psoriasis may first appear during the course of HIV infection. Severely affected patients develop pustules

Table 226-1   Frequency of cutaneous features of HIV infection

	COMMON	LESS COMMON	RARE
Infections	Oral candidiasis Molluscum contagiosum Warts Herpes virus infections	Oral hairy leukoplakia *Pityrosporon* folliculitis Syphilis	Disseminated fungal infection Bacillary angiomatosis
Inflammatory dermatoses	Seborrheic dermatitis Drug eruption	Psoriasis Papular eruption	Granuloma annulare
Neoplasms	Kaposi's sarcoma	Basal cell carcinoma Melanoma	Lymphoma

and may experience fevers and arthralgias. Skin biopsy specimens of HIV-associated psoriasis are more likely to contain high numbers of plasma cells and fewer T-cells than tissue taken from patients without HIV. Mild disease may be treated with topical corticosteroid application, whereas more severe psoriasis requires therapy with ultraviolet B (UVB), psoralen plus ultraviolet A (PUVA), and/or systemic retinoid administration (etretinate). Methotrexate should be avoided. Remission of disease is rare; thus treatment is often lifelong.

Reiter's Syndrome

Reiter's syndrome may develop or worsen in association with HIV infection. The triad of arthritis, urethritis, and conjunctivitis is associated with lesions of psoriasis, discrete and confluent keratotic papules and pustules of the palms and soles (keratoderma blennorrhagica), and annular, scaling, erythematous patches on the penis (balanitis circinata). The individual manifestations of Reiter's syndrome in the patient with HIV are often more severe and recalcitrant than the usual case (Chapter 200).

Seborrheic Dermatitis

Seborrheic dermatitis is a common and early manifestation of HIV infection, occurring in up to 80% of patients. The primary lesion is an erythematous, scaling papule or plaque, with an oily or dry surface. The usual distribution is in the midfacial region, with extension to cover the entire face and scalp (Fig. 226-1). Heavy concentration in the eyebrows and nasolabial folds is characteristic. Erythema is often more intense in the person with HIV; this corresponds to the greater inflammatory cell infiltrate noted in biopsy specimens. The infiltrate is also deeper than usual, with scattered neutrophils and lymphocytoclasia. Therapy with topical corticosteroid and antifungal application is standard. The yeast *Pityrosporum ovale* is implicated in causing seborrheic dermatitis. The eruption often responds to topical or oral administration of ketoconazole.

Pruritus and Xerosis

Itching and dry skin are two very common manifestations of HIV infection. Pruritus may occur without any visible change in the skin and may become incapacitating. Antihistamine medication and skin lubrication may provide some relief, but severe cases require therapy with ultraviolet light. Psoralen plus ultraviolet A treatment generally results in improvement within 10 to 15 exposures. Xerosis may become progressively severe, leading to fish scale–like ichthyosis. Use of emollients such as petrolatum and decreased use of soap and exposure to hot water are usually beneficial.

Folliculitis and Prurigo of HIV

Folliculitis, characterized clinically by follicular inflammatory papules and pustules, is one of the most common cutaneous manifestations in late stages of HIV infection. The most commonly affected areas are the trunk, face, neck, and proximal extremities, but the eruption may be generalized, usually becoming a significant clinical prob-

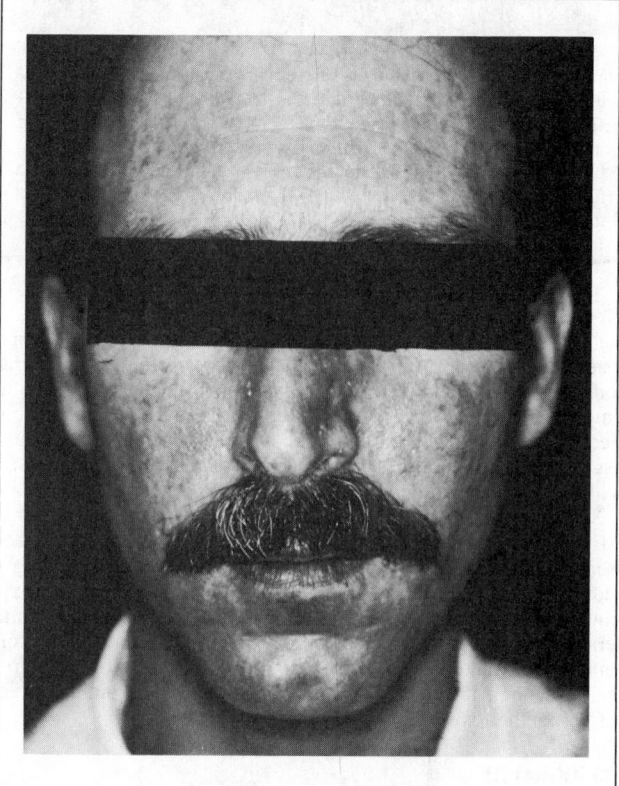

FIGURE 226-1   Seborrheic dermatitis in an individual with HIV.

lem when CD4 counts fall below 250 to 300 cells/mm^3. Possible infectious etiologies include bacterial *(Staphylococcus aureus),* fungal *(Pityrosporum ovale),* or parasitic *(Demodex folliculorum).* A fourth category of folliculitis, not associated with any known infectious agent, is the so-called eosinophilic folliculitis, histologically similar to the eosinophilic pustular folliculitis described by Ofuji. Specific diagnosis is aided by Gram stain and culture of a pustule, direct potassium hydroxide (KOH) examination of the follicular contents and, if necessary, by a biopsy specimen obtained from a follicular lesion. Whether treatment aimed at specific infectious agents is beneficial is unknown. In cases of eosinophilic folliculitis, phototherapy seems to be the only modality capable of inducing prolonged symptomatic relief.

Regardless of the etiology, folliculitis in HIV disease tends to be a chronic and recurring process. Pruritus is usually intense and results in picking, scratching, and rubbing. In response to these stimuli, lesions of prurigo nodularis may develop, characterized by hyperpigmented, hyperkeratotic papules with central erosion, ulceration, or crusting. Treatment of prurigo consists of decreasing the pruritus in order to break the "itching-picking" cycle and also decreasing the inflammatory reaction elicited by chronic trauma. Systemic antihistamines and topical corticosteroids are helpful in some cases. When recalcitrant disease ensues, phototherapy is often found to be effective.

Drug Reactions

Administration of trimethoprim-sulfamethoxazole is associated with a high incidence of cutaneous eruptions in individuals with HIV, consisting of widely distributed erythematous, often edematous macules and patches (Color Plate VII-13). The T-cells infiltrating the skin are often disproportionately CD8$^+$ compared with similar drug eruptions in persons without HIV. Itching may be severe. Certain individuals may develop stigmata of erythema multiforme (target lesions, ocular and oral erythema and erosion) and, rarely, toxic epidermal necrolysis (widespread, full-thickness epidermal necrosis with denudation).

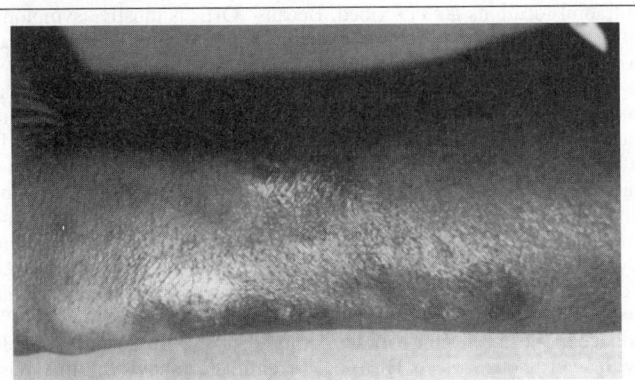

FIGURE 226-2   Lichenoid eruption on the extensor forearm of a man with late-stage HIV disease.

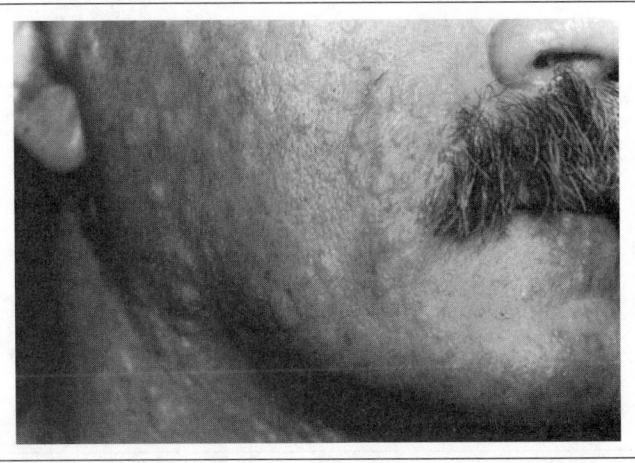

FIGURE 226-3   Widespread lesions of molluscum contagiosum. Notice the multiple flat-topped plaques and papules on the face, as well as the more typical dome-shaped lesions on the neck.

Such drug reactions may progress despite discontinuation of the offending agent. Supportive care, including scrupulous skin care, is the best treatment.

Azure blue lunulae of the nails may develop and extend distally because of azidothymidine (AZT) administration. This discoloration is especially notable in more darkly pigmented persons.

Photosensitivity Reactions

Some patients with HIV infection become highly sensitive to ultraviolet (UV) light. It is not clear whether HIV itself, other infectious agents, or medications predispose the patient to developing photosensitivity.

Examples of cutaneous diseases seen in HIV-infected persons that are triggered or exacerbated by UV light include porphyria cutanea tarda (PCT), chronic actinic dermatitis (an eczematous eruption), bullous photosensitivity (pseudo-PCT), photodistributed granuloma annulare, hyperpigmentation of sun-exposed areas, and lichenoid dermatitis.

Debate exists regarding the effect of UV light in promoting viral gene expression and possible activation of HIV. In vitro studies have demonstrated that sunlight, UVB, and PUVA (psoralen plus UVA) can activate HIV. Short-term in vivo studies, however, suggest that both PUVA and UVB do not cause any increase in viral load or clinical deterioration. UV light has been used for treatment of several skin diseases associated with HIV infection such as seborrheic dermatitis, pruritus, prurigo, and eosinophilic folliculitis. Further investigation is necessary.

Lichenoid Eruption of HIV

An inflammatory cutaneous eruption histologically characterized by lichenoid changes, on occasion affecting sun-exposed areas, occurs in association with HIV. The eruption is most commonly seen in African-American and other dark-skinned patients with advanced disease, when CD4 cell counts below 50 cells/mm^3. Clinically it is characterized by multiple violaceous, hyperpigmented, flat papules and plaques with a shiny surface (Fig. 226-2); scaling and eczematous changes may also be present. The frequent distribution of lesions in sun-exposed areas suggests photosensitivity as a causative factor. Affected patients may be receiving photosensitizing medications, including acyclovir, captopril, chloroquine, interferon, β-blockers, thiazide diuretics, ethambutol, and some nonsteroidal antiinflammatory drugs. The exact etiology of this eruption, however, remains to be determined.

Facial Flushing

Uncommonly, patients with HIV manifest a diffusely erythematous face with occasional telangiectasia and mild scale. The appearance is that of a deep flush. Its cause is uncertain. There are similarities to acne rosacea, but a definite association is not established. Treatment with systemic tetracycline or topical metronidazole may be of benefit.

Granuloma Annulare

Widespread papules and plaques with histologic features of granuloma annulare are reported in individuals with HIV. Biopsy specimens display the characteristic infiltrate of lymphocytes and histiocytes in a palisade around a subtly altered focus of collagen with increased mucin. The cause of granuloma annulare and the reason for an association with HIV infection are unknown.

INFECTIOUS CONDITIONS

In general, the microbes that infect the skin of individuals without HIV are also the most frequently encountered in the patient with HIV. Infections tend to be more severe, more resistant to treatment, and more often recurrent. Skin infections with *Staphylococcus aureus*, herpes simplex virus, varicella-zoster virus, molluscum contagiosum, *Candida* spp., and dermatophytes are most common, but vigilance must be maintained for unusual infectious agents in the skin. Cultures of the skin surface and skin biopsy specimens for histologic examination and tissue culture are very helpful in patient management. Cutaneous protozoal infections are reported in patients with HIV; however, this is exceedingly rare.

Viral Infections

Molluscum contagiosum is a pox virus that commonly infects homosexual patients with HIV. The typical lesion is a white, firm papule, often with a small central depression (Fig. 226-3). The papules frequently occur on the face and genitalia. Significantly larger lesions are referred to as *giant molluscum*. Progressive and recurrent disease is usual despite destruction with cryotherapy or curettage. Cutaneous cryptococcosis may mimic molluscum contagiosum; if in doubt, histologic confirmation is required (see later discussion).

The manifestations of herpes simplex virus infection are protean. The typical presentation of grouped vesicles on an erythematous patch may develop in any location, commonly perioral or perineal (Fig. 226-4). Severe ulcers may ensue, frequently perianally, where they may be coinfected with cytomegalovirus. Methods of documenting the presence of herpes simplex (and varicella-zoster) include Tzanck smear, viral culture, and histologic examination. A Tzanck smear is properly performed by firmly scraping the base of the vesicle or ulcer with a scalpel blade. The accumulated tissue is smeared on a glass slide, fixed, and stained with eosin and Wright's stain. Correctly executed, the Tzanck smear is a rapid and reliable test to establish the diagnosis of herpes simplex virus or varicella-zoster virus infection. A

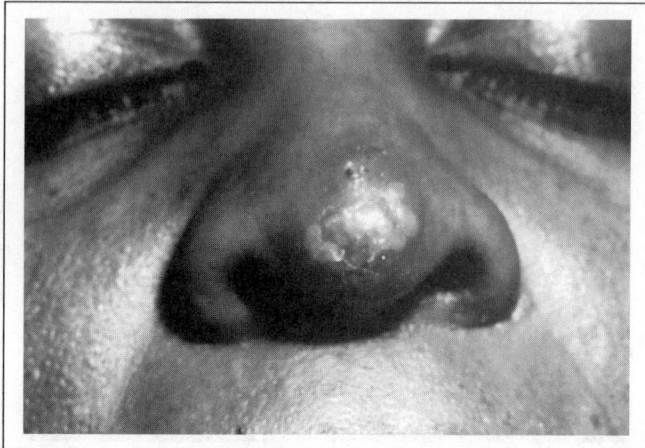

FIGURE 226-4   Herpes simplex infection on the tip of the nose of an otherwise asymptomatic woman with HIV.

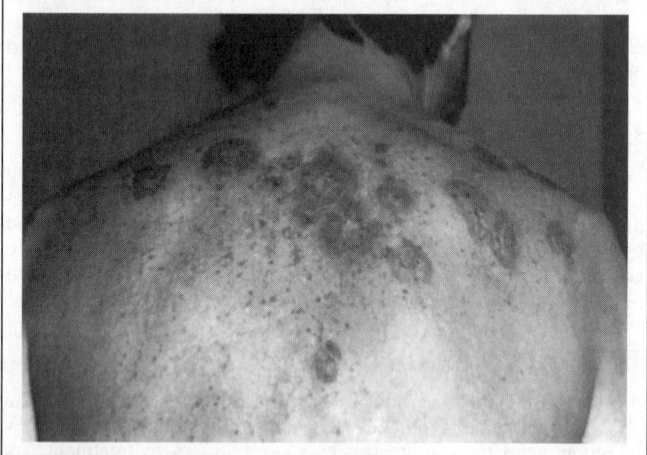

FIGURE 226-5   Disseminated lesions of herpes zoster not limited to a dermatomal distribution heralded the final stages of this patient's HIV disease.

positive smear contains multinucleated keratinocytes with molded nuclei and surrounding pale cytoplasm. Acyclovir, administered orally or intravenously, is the best treatment. Route of administration and dosage depend on the degree of immunosuppression and drug resistance. Resistant strains may respond to high doses or ganciclovir administration.

Shingles, caused by varicella-zoster virus reactivation, may be an early sign of immunosuppression in the person with HIV. As a rule, the eruption develops in the usual dermatomal patterns. Depending on the degree of immunosuppression, disseminated cutaneous disease (more than 10 lesions outside the dermatome of primary infection) may occur (Fig. 226-5). Disseminated secondary disease, as well as primary varicella infection, may eventuate in varicella pneumonia. As with herpes simplex virus, the typical primary lesions may be missed; the patient may have ulcers or disseminated lesions. Oral and intravenous acyclovir is the first-line treatment for these infections.

Perianal ulcers are the only cutaneous lesions repeatedly demonstrated to contain cytomegalovirus (CMV). Although the cytopathic effect of CMV may be identified histologically in skin biopsy specimens from a wide range of clinical lesions, cytomegalovirus is probably not the cause of the lesion examined through biopsy. Cutaneous lesions directly attributable to Epstein-Barr virus (EBV) infection do not exist, but EBV is implicated in the development of oral hairy leukoplakia (OHL). Oral hairy leukoplakia is a common manifestation of HIV infection and appears as white plaques with a warty surface, along the lateral margins of the tongue (Color Plate VIII-42). Other intraoral locations are described. Because OHL is mostly asymptomatic, treatment is not required. Human papillomavirus also may play a role in the cause of OHL.

Verruca vulgaris (wart) and condyloma are due to infection with the human papillomavirus (HPV). Warts proliferate with worsening immunosuppression. Usually the hands, feet, and perineum are most severely affected. Response to therapy is directly related to CD4 counts. In a large number of patients, treatment is palliative; the goal is to keep the size and distribution of lesions limited. Cryotherapy, podophyllum, and intralesional interferon injections are partially successful. Perianal condylomata are particularly recalcitrant; rectal lesions must be treated concomitantly if the goal is to clear the patient of lesions. Bowenoid papulosis may occur in individuals with HIV. This condition is HPV induced, and the lesion is a skin-colored or hyperpigmented papule with a verrucous surface. Histologic examination shows full-thickness epidermal dysplasia. Unlike the squamous cell carcinoma in situ of the genitalia, Bowenoid papulosis lacks metastatic potential.

Fungal Infections

Superficial infections with *Candida albicans* most often involve the oropharyngeal mucosa and intertriginous surfaces of the skin. Adherent, white plaques of variable extent and distribution can be found in the mouth. KOH examination readily shows pseudohyphae and spores. On the skin, candidiasis causes moist, eroded, erythematous plaques with peripheral pustules and erythematous papules. Potassium hydroxide examination and fungal culture confirm the diagnosis. More severe involvement is manifested by esophageal disease and by widely distributed cutaneous disease. Oral candidiasis responds to nystatin oral suspension given several times each day. Oral or cutaneous disease may require treatment with oral ketoconazole or fluconazole. As a sole agent, a topical antifungal preparation is of little benefit. Cutaneous septic emboli due to candidemia appear as violaceous, ulcerated nodules. This diagnosis is best established by skin biopsy and tissue culture.

Dermatophytosis is generally limited to the hands, feet, and inguinal region, but invasive dermatophyte infection may occur. Generally, the dermatophyte infection antedates HIV infection, but the condition worsens despite appropriate therapy. Nail involvement (onychomycosis) is largely resistant to all forms of therapy. The choice of treatment of dermatophytosis depends on the extent of involvement and the degree of immunosuppression. Localized diseases of the feet may respond to topical antifungal agents. More widespread infection is best treated with oral griseofulvin or ketoconazole.

Disseminated fungal infections occur uncommonly. The cutaneous eruptions caused by such infections are protean and often nonspecific. The new onset of any widely distributed or generalized cutaneous eruption is an indication for skin biopsy. Disseminated *Cryptococcus neoformans, Histoplasma capsulatum, Blastomyces dermatitidis,* and *Sporothrix schenckii,* among others, are reported in the population with HIV. Of these, cryptococcosis is perhaps most common, typically appearing as widely distributed white papules, mimicking molluscum contagiosum (Fig. 226-6). Identification of any disseminated fungal infection should prompt systemic evaluation. Examination of cerebrospinal fluid is important with the recognition of cutaneous cryptococcosis.

Pityrosporon ovale (Malassezia furfur) causes tinea versicolor in humans. *P. ovale* is implicated in the cause of a modestly inflammatory folliculitis seen commonly in persons with HIV. Follicular pustules with minimal or no erythema are present on the trunk and proximal extremities. Patients frequently complain of itching. Oral ketoconazole gradually lessens the eruption and improves the pruritus. Topical sodium thiosulfate lotion or selenium sulfide lotion helps reduce the growth of *P. ovale.*

Bacterial Infections

Folliculitis due to *Staphylococcus aureus* or *Streptococcus* spp. is the most common cutaneous bacterial infection associated with HIV infection. Deep-seated inflammation and abscess formation characterize the development of furuncles. Oral or intravenous antibiotics are generally helpful in conjunction with culture and determination of antibiotic sensitivities. In addition, furuncles may require incision and

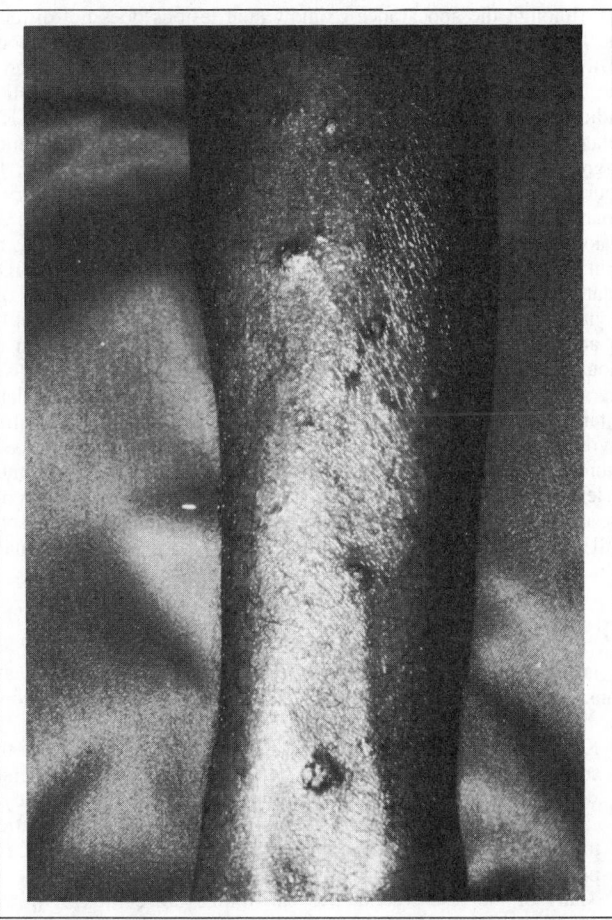

FIGURE 226-6 Disseminated cryptococcosis presenting with variable-sized cutaneous nodules resembling molluscum contagiosum.

drainage. Use of an antibacterial soap helps to decrease recurrent disease. Other cutaneous bacterial infections such as *Haemophilus influenzae* cellulitis and *Pseudomonas aeruginosa* ulcers are reported.

Any of the myriad cutaneous manifestations of syphilis may occur. The stigmata of secondary syphilis range from a few isolated papules to the classic generalized erythematous exanthem involving the palms and soles. Although serologic studies are less reliable than in individuals without HIV, confirmatory tests include the rapid plasma reagin (RPR), Venereal Disease Research Laboratory (VDRL), and fluorescent treponemal antibody absorption (FTA-ABS) tests; skin biopsy; and darkfield examination. Lesions of primary and secondary syphilis, especially condyloma lata, contain numerous spirochetes identifiable by correctly performed darkfield microscopy. The syphilitic chancre must be differentiated from chancroid and other causes of genital ulceration. Skin culture and biopsy are helpful when the diagnosis is uncertain. Appropriate therapy for syphilis is discussed in Chapter 274.

Mycobacterial infections primarily involving the skin are rare. Disseminated cutaneous tuberculosis and scrofuloderma are reported in individuals with HIV. Although systemic infection with *Mycobacterium avium-intracellulare* is fairly frequent, a specific skin lesion attributable to this "atypical" mycobacterium is not recognized. *Mycobacterium haemophilum* is reported to cause cutaneous ulceration in patients with HIV.

Bacillary angiomatosis (or epithelioid angiomatosis) is a rickettsial infection that causes a dermal lobular capillary proliferation. Clinically the lesions appear as erythematous to violaceous papules and nodules. The number and distribution of lesions are variable. The organisms involved, *Bartonella hanselae* and *Bartonella quintana*, are identified as clumps of pleomorphic bacilli staining with the Warthin-Starry silver stain.

NEOPLASIA
AIDS-associated Kaposi's Sarcoma

One of the most striking cutaneous manifestations of AIDS is Kaposi's sarcoma (Color Plates VII-22 and VIII-38). It is the most common malignancy associated with HIV disease in certain risk groups such as homosexual and bisexual men (Chapter 227).

Lymphoma

HIV infection predisposes patients to the development of lymphomas, and in some AIDS risk groups, particularly hemophiliacs, it is the most frequently associated neoplasm, with a higher relative risk compared to the other groups. In homosexual men with AIDS, lymphoma is the second most common malignant neoplasm, following Kaposi's sarcoma. The overall incidence of lymphoma in persons infected with HIV-1 is between 5% and 10%.

The overwhelming majority of tumors are non-Hodgkin's lymphoma (NHL) originating from B-cells, and since 1985, NHL has been recognized as an AIDS-defining illness. It is characterized by an aggressive nature, presentation at advanced stages, and very poor prognosis. Disease limited to lymph nodes is rare. An important feature of AIDS-NHL is the involvement of extranodal sites such as the central nervous system, gastrointestinal tract, bone marrow, and anorectal mucosa early in the disease course. Cutaneous involvement occurs with a frequency of 8.2%, approximately equal to that in non-HIV NHL. The majority of patients have one or a few skin-colored, erythematous, or violaceous nodules on the trunk. Multiple cutaneous nodules and plaques are uncommon.

Carcinoma

Although rare, squamous cell carcinoma arising in anal and perianal tissues is reported in homosexual men. An association is postulated between perianal squamous cell carcinoma and human papillomavirus infection. Basal cell carcinoma, squamous cell carcinoma in other sites, and melanoma are relatively common tumors in individuals without HIV. These cancers are reported in persons with HIV, but whether their incidences are higher than in the noninfected population is unknown.

BIBLIOGRAPHY

Berger T, Dhar A: Lichenoid photoeruptions in human immunodeficiency virus infection, *Arch Dermatol* 130:609-613, 1994.

Berger TG, Koehler JE: Bacillary angiomatosis, *AIDS Clin Rev* p. 43-60, 1993/1994.

Bruinsma W: A guide to drug eruptions—the file of side effects in dermatology, 29-31, E.F.S.E.D., Amsterdam, 1995, Free University.

Buchness MR, Sanchez M: HIV-associated pruritus, *Clin Dermatol* 9(1):111-114, 1991.

Goodman DS et al: Prevalence of cutaneous disease in patients with acquired immunodeficiency syndrome (AIDS) or AIDS-related complex, *J Am Acad Dermatol* 17:210, 1987.

Gregory N: Clinical manifestations of photosensitivity in patients with human immunodeficiency virus infection, *Arch Dermatol* 130:630-633, 1994.

Horn TD, Herzberg GZ, Hood AF: Characterization of the dermal infiltrate in HIV infected patients with psoriasis, *Arch Dermatol* 125:1462, 1990.

Horn TD, Hood AF: Cytomegalovirus is predictably present in perineal ulcers from immunosuppressed patients, *Arch Dermatol* 126:642, 1990.

Ofuji S et al: Eosinophilic pustular folliculitis, *Acta Derm Venereol (Stockh)* 50:195-203, 1970.

Rosenthal D et al: Human immunodeficiency virus–associated eosinophilic folliculitis, *Arch Dermatol* 127:206-209, 1991.

Ziegler JL, Dorfman RF: Overview of Kaposi's sarcoma history, epidemiology, and biomedical features. In *Kaposi's sarcoma: pathophysiology and clinical management*, New York, 1988, BC Decker.

227 Kaposi's Sarcoma

Kathryn A. O'Connell

PATHOPHYSIOLOGY

The AIDS epidemic in the United States was heralded in 1981 by the sudden appearance of Kaposi's sarcoma (KS) in young homosexual males. Before the AIDS epidemic, KS was a relatively rare neoplasm that occurred in three general groups of patients. Classic KS, initially described in 1872 by the Hungarian dermatopathologist Moritz Kohn Kaposi, is seen in elderly males, often of Mediterranean or Middle Eastern origin, and is sometimes associated with lymphoma. In the 1950s KS was recognized as a relatively common form of cancer in sub-Saharan Africa. This form of KS differs from the classic form in that it affects younger males and occasionally children. Like classic KS, an underlying immune deficit has not been identified. In the 1970s, however, a link with immune deficiency was strongly suggested by the greatly increased risk for this disease in iatrogenically immunosuppressed renal transplant recipients. The disease in immunosuppressed patients is far more aggressive, but it often resolves spontaneously if immune competence is restored. In iatrogenic KS, male predominance is minimal. The linkage to immunosuppression was, of course, greatly strengthened by the epidemic form of KS seen in AIDS. This form of KS provides many interesting epidemiologic clues because it is largely confined to homosexual males with AIDS. Indeed, KS in female AIDS patients is far more common in those who acquire HIV from a bisexual male than from an IV drug–abusing male. It is thought that this disease may in fact reflect infection of endothelial cells by an unknown sexually transmitted agent, superimposed on an immune deficit with aberrant cytokine networks.

In fact, however, the biologic basis for KS remains a mystery and there is no accepted model that provides a unifying conceptual framework for this fascinating disease in its four unique clinical presentations. Most recently, a great deal of interest has been generated by the discovery of a new human herpes virus, HHV8. The virion itself has been isolated, and genomic sequences have been identified in KS tissue from patients in all four groups. Subsequent work, however, has identified these sequences in body cavity–based lymphomas and in a variety of cutaneous tumors from organ transplant recipients without HIV; thus it is not yet clear what role this agent plays in the pathogenesis of KS. Research aimed at understanding this disease is of great practical importance since KS is a formidable clinical problem for a large cohort of AIDS patients in this country and patients both with and without HIV in Africa. KS arises multifocally, is not clonal, can regress spontaneously with immunocompetence, does not metastasize, and most likely has an infectious etiology. These unusual features provide important clues to understanding this fascinating biologic entity, an understanding that may alter the way we think about cancer and its management.

CLINICAL PRESENTATION AND DIFFERENTIAL DIAGNOSIS

Despite the clear-cut clinical presentations noted previously, the individual lesions of KS do not differ between these groups. In all patients with KS, the lesions usually begin as flat, violaceous patches or plaques that slowly enlarge, often developing a nodular component. As the lesions progress, there is often associated edema and ulceration, especially in dependent areas. It is critical to recognize, however, that KS lesions can occasionally mimic a multitude of unrelated skin lesions. These include simple ecchymoses, bacillary angiomatosis, malignant melanoma, nevi, hemangiomas, purpura, necrotizing vasculitis, erythema multiforme, granuloma annulare, prurigo nodularis, lichen planus, urticaria pigmentosum, pyogenic granuloma, cutaneous lymphoma, and even the great imitator itself, secondary syphilis (Color Plate VII-22).

Although the appearance of individual lesions does not differ in the four types of KS, the overall distribution, course, and response to therapy do. In classic KS the lesions usually remain confined to the lower extremities, follow an indolent course, respond well to radiotherapy, and rarely cause death. African endemic KS (non–HIV related) often presents like classic KS but tends to be more aggressive, sometimes invading bone. In the childhood form, the course resembles fulminant Burkitt's lymphoma and is refractory to treatment. Iatrogenic KS often arises abruptly with widespread lesions involving gastrointestinal and respiratory tracts as well as the skin; continued immunosuppression can lead to fatal KS. AIDS-related KS is unusual in that it most often involves the face, oral cavity, genitals, and trunk. Indeed, oral lesions should be sought out in any patient with a suggestive cutaneous lesion, since KS in the mouth can cause significant functional impairment, further aggravating AIDS-related weight loss. It is also clear that AIDS-related cutaneous KS is almost always accompanied by gastrointestinal involvement. Fortunately the gastrointestinal lesions tend to be submucosal and are usually asymptomatic. Pulmonary involvement is less common and has a grave prognosis. It is difficult to predict the course of AIDS-related KS for an individual patient since some will have widespread, rapidly progressing lesions and others maintain a more indolent course.

TESTING

It has been argued that histologic examination of lesions clinically consistent with KS is unnecessary. This author recommends biopsy for the following reasons:

1. KS is often the earliest clinical sign of HIV infection and in this setting, an AIDS-defining illness. The diagnosis of KS in a person with risk factors for HIV infection is grave news, and accuracy is essential. Definitive diagnosis of early-onset KS allows the patient to begin appropriate AIDS management before the occurrence of preventable opportunistic infections.
2. Many of the diseases that KS can mimic are curable if treated promptly and can be fatal if misdiagnosed, such as bacillary angiomatosis, malignant melanoma, and syphilis.

The workup for extracutaneous KS depends on the history and physical findings in each individual patient. Definitive diagnosis of pulmonary and intestinal KS generally involves bronchoscopic-endoscopic examination. KS involving the extremities is often accompanied by regional adenopathy, and biopsy and/or CT scan is often employed to establish fields for radiation therapy or to assess the need for systemic chemotherapy. All patients with a confirmed diagnosis of KS should be offered HIV testing regardless of whether they state risk factors for infection.

MANAGEMENT

There is no curative treatment for KS. The goals of treatment are to decrease functional impairment, pain, bleeding, infection, edema, and disfigurement with its attendant psychosocial and economic implications. As noted earlier, these goals are most easily achieved for patients with classic KS on the lower extremity who respond well to low-dose radiotherapy. African endemic KS is also responsive to radiotherapy and is often combined with α-interferon; too often, however, these modalities are unavailable, and the result is significant morbidity. Iatrogenic KS often resolves spontaneously if immunosuppressive drugs are discontinued. Patients with progressing iatrogenic KS are generally treated aggressively with systemic chemotherapy; the prognosis is usually poor.

AIDS-related KS presents formidable management problems because the lesions are often numerous and the underlying immunosuppression is irreversible. Options for cutaneous disease include radiotherapy, intralesional or systemic chemotherapy, and cryosurgery. The choice of treatment modality depends on the patient's underlying condition, the number, location, and size of the lesions, and the patient's wishes. Unfortunately, local injections and cryosurgery are very painful and must be repetitively administered, limiting their usefulness for patients with numerous lesions. Many patients with complications of AIDS are not candidates for systemic chemotherapy. In addition, patients with AIDS-related KS are often exquisitely sensitive to ra-

✔ *WHEN TO REFER*

In the early years of the epidemic, KS was rarely the cause of death in AIDS. This is changing because of advances in prophylaxis against opportunistic infections, and patients with KS are well-advised to seek care before the lesions become unmanageable. Patients with AIDS who are candidates for radiation therapy should be referred to radiation oncologists with specific experience in the treatment of AIDS-related KS, for the reason cited earlier. Intralesional chemotherapy and cryotherapy likewise require full knowledge of potential complications, such as ulceration and peripheral nerve injury. Physicians experienced in the treatment of cutaneous KS can also help patients formulate realistic expectations for aesthetic outcome, which is often less than ideal. Pulmonary involvement and/or widespread aggressive disease require systemic chemotherapy, and various combinations are in clinical trials. Again, these patients should be referred to oncologists experienced in management of Kaposi's sarcoma.

Other approaches being investigated include liposomal daunorubicin; various cytokines, especially the interferons; and experimental inhibitors of angiogenesis. Antiviral therapy has been suggested as a possible treatment, targeting the putative viral KS agent, but there is, as yet, no prospective study establishing efficacy. Although available treatments for widespread aggressive disease are inadequate and none have been shown to increase survival, significant improvement in quality of life is achievable for many patients and specialized referral is often helpful.

diation treatment and will develop debilitating ulceration, especially in the oral cavity.

BIBLIOGRAPHY

Friedman-Kien AE: Disseminated Kaposi's sarcoma syndrome in young homosexual men, *J Am Acad Dermatol* 5:468, 1981.
Moore PS, Chang Y: Detection of herpesvirus-like DNA sequences in Kaposi's sarcoma in patients with and without HIV infection, *N Engl J Med* 332:1181, 1995.
Orfanos CE, Husak R, Wolfer U et al: Kaposi's sarcoma: a reevaluation. *Recent Results Cancer Res* 139:275, 1995.

CHAPTER

228   Mycosis Fungoides and Sézary's Syndrome

Stanford I. Lamberg

RELEVANT PHYSIOLOGY AND PATHOPHYSIOLOGY

The term *mycosis fungoides* (MF) was an apt choice for the illness of a patient with mushroomlike, fungating tumors seen by Alibert in 1806. Sézary's syndrome (SS), now regarded as the leukemic phase of MF, was described in four persons with erythroderma and atypical circulating mononuclear cells in 1938. For the last 20 years, these and other lymphoreticular malignancies that originate in or predominantly involve the skin have been grouped under the name *cutaneous T-cell lymphoma* (CTCL). However, this term should not imply that these disorders are merely cancers of the skin, since evidence has accumulated that both MF and SS are systemic, low-grade, non-Hodgkin's lymphomas, either from the outset or early in their course. Although this review will deal only with MF and SS, classification has become more complex with the use of immunophenotyping and T-cell receptor gene rearrangement to assay tissue. Other T-cell lymphoma types recently defined include CD30-positive (Ki-1); HTLV-1

Table 228-1   Prognosis in mycosis fungoides and Sézary's syndrome

EXTENT OF DISEASE	SURVIVAL	
	3 YEAR	5 YEAR
Patches or plaques covering less than 10% of body surface AND with up to one clinically enlarged lymph node site	93%	83%
Patches or plaques covering less than 10% of the body surface AND more than one clinically enlarged lymph node OR patches or plaques covering 10% or more of the body surface AND up to one clinically enlarged lymph node site	80%	54%
Patches or plaques covering 10% or more of the body surface AND more than one clinically enlarged lymph node site OR presence of skin tumors	56%	50%
Generalized erythroderma (SS)	40%	35%
Visceral involvement (lymph nodes, bone marrow, peripheral blood, liver, spleen, lungs, etc.) in any skin or adenopathy stage	Further decrease	Further decrease

Modified from Lamberg SI et al: Clinical staging for cutaneous T-cell lymphoma, *Ann Intern Med* 100:187, 1984.

infection progressing to adult T-cell leukemia/lymphoma; angiocentric; subcutaneous; and primary and secondary large cell lymphoma. Nevertheless, 90% of T-cell lymphomas presenting in the skin are "typical" MF or SS, as described later.

CLINICAL FEATURES

MF typically begins with itchy patches, coin-sized to palm-sized, looking like "roses on wallpaper," most commonly in the bathing trunk area. SS most often begins with generalized redness, scale, and itching. Pathologic examination of skin biopsies may not be diagnostic of CTCL at this time. Early on the eruption may resemble a common benign disorder such as psoriasis or atopic eczema. It also may have the more distinctive patterns of poikiloderma atrophicans vasculare, which resembles radiation dermatitis; alopecia mucinosa, a patchy inflammatory scalp disorder with hair loss; or large plaque parapsoriasis, a patchy skin disorder that probably is an early form of MF. As MF advances, usually over many years, even decades, individual plaques first become thickened, reddish brown, flat, annular, or serpiginous, and later evolve to elevated tumors that may ulcerate. SS advances with worsening erythroderma, thickening of the facial features, enlarged lymph nodes, and large numbers of circulating atypical lymphocytes. Patients with MF may become generally exfoliative, however, and those with SS may develop tumors near the end of the disease course. In both cases, lymphadenopathy and other signs of visceral involvement also become more evident.

Survival is reduced with progression of skin and lymphadenopathy and with the appearance of abnormal pathologic findings in the viscera (Table 228-1). Although most patients survive for many years, many patients die of their disease or efforts to treat it, rather than an unrelated disorder. Death usually is from sepsis following tumor ulceration at a time when the patient is receiving chemotherapeutic agents.

LABORATORY AND OTHER DIAGNOSTIC TESTS

Workup of patients is directed at defining the extent of disease before initiating therapy. Although recent studies suggest that extracutaneous dissemination occurs early in the course of disease, it is unknown whether treatment aimed at systemic disease during this phase increases survival in this low-grade lymphoma. Since information about deeper tissue involvement, particularly in the early stages of the disease, has yet to be applied to the selection of therapy, patients continue to be treated with topical therapies in early clinical stages and systemic therapy in later clinical stages. Therefore the extent of laboratory and diagnostic evaluations can be limited to those items

Table 228-2 Workup of patients with mycosis fungoides and Sézary's syndrome

	ROUTINE*	INVESTIGATIONAL†
History and physical examination	x	
Skin mapping of lesions	x	
Chest x-ray	x	
Evaluation of signs or symptoms from history or physical examination	x	
Peripheral smear to count atypical lymphocytes	x	
Lymph node biopsy	x (Sometimes)	x
Bone marrow biopsy		x
Liver biopsy		x
Lymphangiogram, CT, MRI		x

*Obtained on all patients for the purpose of determining the type and extent of therapy needed.

†Items important to document if the patient is enrolled in a research protocol but would not likely alter treatment regimens at this time. It is assumed that pathologic diagnosis of cutaneous T-cell lymphoma already has been made based on appropriate biopsy material.

✔ **WHEN TO REFER**

A patient with persistent patches or plaques usually is referred to a dermatologist for evaluation. The diagnosis must be confirmed by skin biopsy, although several skin biopsies taken over time may be required to ensure the diagnosis. Routine care of patients with MF and SS may involve a primary care physician, a dermatologist, and specialists in radiation oncology and medical oncology. Ideally a medical center with a special interest in the disease also should participate if the patient is to be included in an ongoing protocol for these poorly understood disorders.

that alter treatment choices. Table 228-2 distinguishes between those tests needed to clinically stage patients for the purpose of choosing treatment and those more appropriate for patients in a research protocol.

DIFFERENTIAL DIAGNOSIS

The definitive diagnosis of MF and SS depends on confirmation by light microscopy. Electron microscopy, cell marker, and T-cell gene rearrangement analysis supplement light microscopy but need not be routine for most cases. Such studies may be needed to rule out various benign disorders in the earliest phase of MF and SS, and other lymphomas or leukemias in later or tumor phases. Distinguishing Sézary syndrome from other more benign causes of exfoliative erythroderma may be difficult by skin biopsy alone and may require examination of lymph nodes, blood, and bone marrow.

MANAGEMENT

The selection of either a conservative or aggressive management philosophy is controversial. In the conservative approach, one form of cutaneous therapy is given until the patient no longer responds, after which another form of cutaneous therapy is used. Various topical therapies continue to be given unless clinical signs of progression to visceral involvement appear or if the patient no longer responds to topical therapy, at which time systemic therapy is added. This approach seeks only palliation, although if the disease is purely cutaneous at the outset, intense topical therapy to the skin may effect a cure. In the aggressive approach, multimodal therapy, including total skin electrons and systemic chemotherapy, are combined in hopes of effecting a cure. A study from the National Cancer Institute (NCI) has shown that aggressive therapy in late-stage disease shortens survival, but no studies have been conducted with adequate numbers of patients with early-stage disease.

Topical therapies most often used for early-stage disease with limited numbers of thin patches or plaques include ultraviolet light combined with psoralen, topically applied nitrogen mustard (mechlorethamine) or nitrosourea BCNU (carmustine), topical corticosteroids, and radiotherapy with electrons. Treatment for later stage disease with visceral involvement includes radiation, interferon, systemic chemotherapy agents used for other lymphomas, and extracorporeal photopheresis.

BIBLIOGRAPHY

Bunn PA et al: Systemic therapy of cutaneous T-cell lymphomas (mycosis fungoides and the Sézary syndrome), *Ann Intern Med* 121:592, 1994.

Hoppe RT, Wood GS, Abel EA: Mycosis fungoides and the Sézary syndrome: pathology, staging and treatment, *Curr Prob Cancer* 14:295, 1990.

Kaye FJ et al: A randomized trial comparing combination electron-beam radiation and chemotherapy with topical therapy in the initial treatment of mycosis fungoides, *N Engl J Med* 321:1784, 1989.

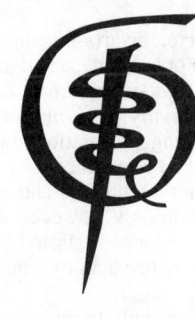

PART EIGHT

Infectious
Diseases

229 Basic Principles of Infectious Disease

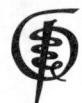

Peter Densen and Merle A. Sande

Infectious diseases, once thought to have been conquered, remain the most common cause of death worldwide, and, even in developed nations, a trend toward increasing mortality has occurred in recent years. Increasing attention is being focused on "emerging" infectious diseases, which in many instances reflect a reemergence of previously controlled infections or the recognition that previously described diseases (e.g., peptic ulcers and certain cancers) have an infectious origin.

In part, changing patterns of disease are a consequence of expanding and aging human populations, increased crowding, and a decline in governmental emphasis on public health standards. Modern transportation has brought with it the ability to rapidly carry pathogenic organisms from one corner of the world to another, from one relatively immune population to a more susceptible one, or to one with cultural or behavioral patterns that facilitate disease transmission.

An equally important aspect in this equation is that microbial agents have an inherent capacity for genetic change in response to environmental and other evolutionary pressures. This capacity, in conjunction with a short replication time, promotes the relatively rapid expression of new genetic information. The interaction of this genetic process with environmental, behavioral, and technologic changes within society provides a dynamic situation in which new agents emerge to cause new diseases (e.g., acquired immunodeficiency syndrome [AIDS]), old agents acquire resistance to standard therapy (e.g., plasmid-mediated antimicrobial resistance), and old agents are transmitted in new ways to cause typical disease in an atypical setting (e.g., corneal transplant–associated rabies).

Microorganisms surround us; they abound in our environment, on our skin, and on our mucosal membranes. Their acquisition from natural reservoirs in the environment, animals, or other humans requires an effective mode of transmission from and return to the reservoir. Transmission may occur by direct contact or through a common vehicle, or the microorganism may be airborne or vector-borne. For transmission to be successful, organisms must either adhere to body surfaces or gain access to subepithelial tissues directly. Acquisition may manifest itself as colonization (asymptomatic, little or no immune response), subclinical infection (asymptomatic, accompanied by an immune response), or active disease (symptomatic with or without an immune response). Delineation of the mode of transmission provides an opportunity for control of infection through the institution of primary preventive measures, such as hand washing or mosquito control. Identification of the biochemical determinants that account for adherence, invasiveness, and virulence, coupled with an understanding of the host immune response to these pathogenic features, provides the basis for primary prevention of infection through vaccination. The emergence of active clinical infectious disease heralds the need for therapeutic intervention (e.g., incision and drainage or specific antimicrobial therapy).

In the face of such varied and constant exposure, it is amazing that active disease is as uncommon as it is. Most microorganisms, however, are relatively avirulent, and these "nonpathogens" are restricted to their interface with the human host by an array of both nonspecific and specific host defense mechanisms (Table 229-1). Relatively few microorganisms are pathogenic for the normal host.

These organisms possess unique surface structures or secrete products that enhance their virulence. For a given organism, the risk of infection can be expressed by the following relationship:

$$\text{Risk of infection} \; \alpha \; \frac{\text{Dose (\# of organisms)} \times \text{Virulence}}{\text{Host resistance}}$$

or

$$\text{Infectious diseases} \; \alpha \; \frac{\text{Epidemiology} \times \text{Microbiology}}{\text{Anatomy} \times \text{Immunology}}$$

In some situations a single factor dwarfs the importance of the other variables in these equations. For example, a nationwide outbreak of sepsis caused by *Enterobacter cloacae* and *Enterobacter agglomerans* was associated with commercially available intravenous fluid that had become contaminated during preparation. In this situation ready access to the bloodstream by large numbers of relatively avirulent bacteria was a critical factor in the outbreak and overrode otherwise intact host defenses. More commonly, however, the balance between microbial factors and host resistance is shifted by disturbances in several variables simultaneously rather than by selective alteration of a single factor.

The principles just discussed also apply to patients with inherited or acquired immunodeficiency. These patients become infected at the same sites and with many of the same organisms as do normal individuals. Features that often characterize infection in these patients are increased frequency and severity, rapidity of onset, and slow resolution despite appropriate therapy. Relatively nonpathogenic organisms commonly cause infection in these patients and in individuals in whom local anatomic barriers to infection are breached by catheters, cytotoxic chemotherapy, or obstruction of a hollow viscus. The defect in host defenses permits these common "nonpathogens" to make their presence known.

Most organisms can be classified as either extracellular or intracellular pathogens. The former, typified by pyogenic cocci such as the pneumococcus, cause infection only while located extracellularly and are readily killed on ingestion by phagocytic cells. Intracellular pathogens like *Mycobacterium tuberculosis* possess virulence factors that inhibit the killing mechanisms of phagocytic cells. In their intracellular location they enjoy protection from humoral defense mechanisms as well as from many antibiotics. Such organisms generally cause chronic infection. Some organisms (e.g., *Staphylococcus aureus* and *Salmonella typhi*) are well adapted for an existence in either milieu.

An additional relationship exists between the site of infection, the microorganism, and the type of host defense primarily responsible for control of the infection (see Table 229-1). Most infections arise at the interface between the host and the environment. Thus knowledge of the organisms that colonize the skin and the various mucosal surfaces is valuable in predicting the range of likely causative organisms when infection arises from these sites. Conversely, identification of the infecting organism provides an important clue to the site of infection. Knowledge of these relationships is particularly useful when bacteremia is suspected as a complication of local infection or when it has been identified in the absence of an apparent site of infection.

The propensity of certain bacteria to cause infection affecting predominantly one organ system is known as tissue tropism. Examples of this phenomenon are the striking tendency of the meningococcus to cause meningitis, of viridans streptococci to cause subacute bacterial endocarditis, and of herpes simplex type 1 to cause encephalitis, while a close relative, herpes simplex type 2, causes primarily genital tract infection. Factors that contribute to tissue tropism include (1) specific biochemical moieties on the surface of the organism that are recognized by complementary structures on the surface of cells in the target organ, (2) the relative absence in the target organ of host defenses relevant for the organism in question, (3) the presence in the target organ of a specific nutrient critical for the growth of the organism, and (4) the local chemical environment as reflected by pH, tonicity, and redox potential. Sites in the human host that are partially immunocompromised include the relatively avascular heart valves; the cerebrospinal fluid, which contains few phagocytic cells

Table 229-1 Patterns of infection in patients with impaired host defense mechanisms

HOST DEFENSE MECHANISM IMPAIRED	CAUSE OF IMPAIRMENT	SITE OF INFECTION	COMMON INFECTING AGENTS
I. Anatomic and physiologic barriers to infection		Recurrent at site of abnormality	
A. Skin	Dermatitis Burns Intravenous catheters	Skin → blood	Staphylococci, streptococci, GNR
B. Skull	Skull fracture Cerebrospinal fluid leak	Meninges	Depends on site of leak: predominantly pneumococci but occasionally staphylococci or GNR if a dermal sinus is present
C. Mucociliary elevator	Alcohol Smoking Endotracheal tube Obstruction Immotile cilia (Kartagener's syndrome)	Bronchi, lungs	Colonizing flora
D. Gastric acid	Surgery, pernicious anemia, antacids	Intestine	*Salmonella* *Mycobacterium tuberculosis* Cholera
E. Intestinal motility or mucosal barrier	Blind loop syndrome, obstruction, tumor	Intestine → blood	Colonizing flora (*Streptococcus bovis*, clostridia, usually in the presence of a colonic neoplasm)
F. Urinary tract	Obstruction Catheterization Stones	Upper or lower urinary tract → blood	*Escherichia coli* "Urea splitters": *Proteus, Providencia*
G. Lymphatics	Obstruction	Lymphangitis	Group A streptococci
II. Immunologic barriers to infection			
A. Antibody IgG		Blood, meninges, broncopulmonary tree, sinuses, ears, intestine	Encapsulated bacteria* Enteroviruses *Giardia lamblia* *Pneumocystis carinii*
IgM	Acquired or inherited	Blood	Meningococci, GNR
IgA		Bronchopulmonary tree, sinuses	Colonizing flora
B. Complement	Acquired or inherited	Blood, meninges, bronchopulmonary tree, sinuses, ears	Encapsulated bacteria Disseminated gonococcal infection

C. Cell-mediated immunity	Acquired or inherited	Lungs, meninges, gastrointestinal tract	Bacteria
			  Listeria
			  M. tuberculosis
			  Atypical mycobacteria
			Viruses
			  Herpes simplex
			  Cytomegalovirus
			  Varicella zoster (shingles)
			Fungi
			  Candida
			  Cryptococcus
			Protozoa
			  P. carinii
			  Toxoplasma gondii
			  Cryptosporidium

D. Phagocytic function
  1. Neutrophils
    Deficient numbers
    (<500 cells/mm³)
	Neoplasia
	Cytotoxic chemotherapy
	Autoimmune neutropenia
		Skin, soft tissue, lung, blood	Staphylococci, GNR, *Candida, Aspergillus*

Defective function	Chronic granulomatous disease	Skin, soft tissue, lung, blood, bone, liver	Staphylococci, GNR, *Nocardia, Candida, Aspergillus*
	Job's (hyperimmunoglobulinemia E) syndrome	Skin, soft tissue	Staphylococci
	Chediak-Higashi syndrome	Skin, soft tissue	Staphylococci
	Myeloperoxidase deficiency	Lung	*Candida*
2. Reticuloendothelial function	Asplenia Hemoglobinopathies	Blood	Encapsulated bacteria*
	Cirrhosis	Blood	GNR

Streptococcus pneumoniae, Haemophilus influenzae, Neisseria meningitidis.
GNR, Gram-negative rods; *IgA, IgG,* and *IgM*, immunoglobulins A, G, and M.

and low levels of antibody and complement; bone; and the renal medulla. Treatment of infection in these sites generally necessitates prolonged administration of high-dose, parenteral, bactericidal antibiotics.

The host is not indiscriminately assailed by a multitude of organisms when anatomic abnormalities or genetic accidents create a specific rent in the host's armamentarium. Rather, infection usually is caused by a group of organisms with similar characteristics (see Table

229-1). Anatomic abnormalities frequently become evident as recurrent infection at exactly the same site. Defects in humoral immunity or in the complement cascade are associated with recurrent infection caused by encapsulated bacteria, and infections caused by *S. aureus* or gram-negative bacilli are common in patients with defective neutrophil function. Patients with defective cell-mediated immunity (e.g., as occurs in AIDS) become infected with intracellular pathogens such as the herpes type of viruses, toxoplasmosis, or *Pneumocystis cari-*

nii. When host defense is simultaneously impaired in different arms of the immune system, the pattern of infection reflects the sum of the defects. Thus patients with impaired humoral and cellular immunity (e.g., severe combined immunodeficiency) have recurrent infections caused by pyogenic cocci and intracellular pathogens. Combined patterns of infection are also observed when therapy for the underlying disorder has a toxic effect on other arms of the immune system, as may occur during treatment of hematologic malignancies. Patterns of infection also blur when concomitant broad-spectrum antibiotic therapy leads to the elimination of the critically important, protective nonpathogenic organisms, thereby providing for overgrowth of mucosal surfaces with resistant organisms. Nevertheless, the pattern of infections is an extremely valuable clue pointing to the site of immunologic or anatomic impairment and is important in directing the initial evaluation of patients efficiently and cost-effectively.

Redundancy and multiplicity are important characteristics of the immune system. Hence a single organism can be eliminated effectively by diverse but often overlapping mechanisms (see Table 229-1). The contribution of an individual mechanism to the defense against a given organism is determined by the specific location and the organism. For example, complement-dependent bactericidal activity is most important in protecting the bloodstream, whereas neutrophil phagocytic activity is more important in the soft tissues.

Infectious injury is produced in the host by means of a wide variety of mechanisms. Injury may occur systemically as well as locally and may be immediate or delayed. Local damage may be produced by cell-bound or secreted toxins that are cytotoxic or interfere with the normal function of a particular organ system in the absence of obvious anatomic disruption. The normal inflammatory response plays an important role in containing infection. The development of an exuberant response, however, contributes to tissue destruction through the unchecked action of cytokines, inflammatory proteases, and toxic metabolites released from phagocytic cells in response to microbial invasion. Damage is particularly likely to occur when infection occurs in a closed space (e.g., in a joint or in the brain) or when large numbers of different organisms are present (e.g., in the development of an anaerobic lung abscess). Resolution of the inflammatory response results in fibrosis or scarring and occasionally calcification. These healing processes may be responsible for delayed injury to the host (e.g., sterility in women recovering from pelvic inflammatory disease), the development of a new heart murmur during the healing phase of endocarditis, or the onset of seizures in patients with calcified intracerebral pork tape worm larvae (cerebral cysticercosis).

The expression of microbial antigens on the surface of epithelial and endothelial cells during intracellular replication of the pathogen can elicit the immune destruction of these cells. Other immunologic mechanisms of tissue injury include immune complex formation (endocarditis) and autoimmune hemolytic anemia, thrombocytopenia, or neutropenia that may occur during the polyclonal antibody response induced by infection of B lymphocytes with Epstein-Barr virus during infectious mononucleosis. Systemic injury may be initiated by ischemia and disseminated intravascular coagulopathy during septic shock.

It is clear from the foregoing discussion that the outcome of the encounter between the host and the microbe lies in dynamic balance. Infection with one organism (e.g., influenza virus) can alter this balance and set the stage for another infection (e.g., postviral bacterial pneumonia) caused by bacteria previously residing symbiotically in the host's oropharynx. It is also apparent that microorganisms owe their pathogenicity to virulence factors that enable the organism to colonize the host and elude host defense mechanisms. The value of specific immunity to the host is to negate the effect of microbial virulence factors by establishing an immune reaction on the organism itself or to its toxic products.

The remainder of Part Eight deals with the interaction between the human host and infectious agents. The chapters are grouped into four sections: Sections I and II provide a description of the specific host defenses, address the issue of the antibiotics used to aid these defenses, and describe methods used for identifying pathogens. Section III describes common clinical syndromes that result when infection occurs; the syndromes are enumerated and described according to how they are presented to the physician by the patient. In Section IV each agent that produces disease in humans—from the viruses to the helminths—is described in detail: its ecology, the host defenses it must overcome, how it produces infection, the specific disease it causes, and how the disease is diagnosed and most appropriately treated and prevented. The format of Part Eight should enable the clinician to quickly obtain necessary information derived either from the clinical setting (the patient) or from the microorganism (a positive culture). Cross-referencing has been used liberally to aid in the appropriate workup or therapy.

BIBLIOGRAPHY

Lorber B: Changing patterns of infectious diseases, *Am J Med* 84:569, 1988.

CHAPTER

230

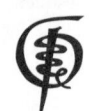

Host Defense Against Infection: The Roles of Antibody, Complement, and Phagocytic Cells

Peter Densen, David L. Weinbaum, and Gerald L. Mandell

HUMORAL IMMUNITY

Humoral immunity reflects protection from infection mediated by specific antibody. Protection depends on the highly specific capacity of a given antibody to recognize a given antigen and to trigger other aspects of host defense.

Properties and Distribution of Antibody

There are five classes of immunoglobulins: IgG, IgA, IgM, IgD, and IgE. Although IgE may play a role in limiting disease caused by some helminths, its function and that of IgD in host defense against infection have not been clearly delineated and will not be considered further here. IgG, which accounts for about 76% of the total plasma immunoglobulin, is distributed equally between the plasma and soft tissues and is the only immunoglobulin transported across the placenta to the fetus. There are four subclasses of IgG, numbered according to their decreasing concentration in plasma. Only IgG1 and IgG3 are efficient activators of complement and bind to neutrophils. The capacity of infants to synthesize different classes and subclasses of immunoglobulins matures at different rates. IgG2 and IgG4 synthesis matures more slowly than IgG1 and IgG3, and low levels of the former two are present for the first 18 to 24 months of life. Among the subclasses, IgG2 is particularly important in the response to polysaccharide antigens. These physiologic and functional attributes of IgG2 probably contribute to the high incidence of infection caused by encapsulated bacteria in young children and to the poor immunologic response of children under the age of 2 years to polysaccharide vaccines.

IgA, which accounts for 15% of the total plasma immunoglobulin, is distributed approximately equally between plasma and mucosal surfaces. Two subclasses are recognized: IgA1 predominates over IgA2 in serum (6:1), whereas the concentrations of the two subclasses are more nearly equal (2:1) on mucosal membranes. Secretory IgA (sIgA) functions primarily to prevent colonization of mucosal surfaces by microbial pathogens and to prevent absorption of inhaled or ingested potential allergens through a process known as *immune exclusion.* IgA is not transported transplacentally, but maternal sIgA present in breast milk helps protect newborn infants from infections caused by organisms in their shared environment during the maturation of the infant's ability to synthesize IgA.

IgM accounts for just 8% of the total plasma immunoglobulin and is confined principally (75%) to plasma. Much of the "natural" antibody present in serum against gram-negative organisms is found in the IgM class and presumably arises in response to unrecognized exposure to lipopolysaccharide antigens derived from gut flora. IgM is not transported transplacentally and IgM receptors are not present on phagocytic cells. Nevertheless, because of its pentameric structure, IgM is an efficient activator of complement.

The highly specific nature of the recognition of antigen by antibody imposes a requirement for antibody synthesis during the initial presentation of antigen. Consequently, a delay occurs before the beneficial effects of specific antibody are felt. The primary immune response is characterized by the synthesis of IgM followed by IgG. Subsequent exposure to the same antigen results in an anamnestic response with the rapid production of antibody, mainly IgG. This pattern is useful clinically in the serologic diagnosis of acute (elevated titer of specific IgM followed by an elevated titer of specific IgG) versus recurrent or chronic infection (elevated titer of specific IgG only). In addition, because IgM does not cross the placenta and because the capacity to synthesize IgM in response to a specific stimulus is acquired in utero, the presence in cord serum of IgM specific for a particular infectious agent, for example, *Toxoplasma gondii,* is indicative of in utero acquisition of infection.

Antibody Function in Infectious Diseases

Antibodies are bifunctional molecules, one end of which (Fab) recognizes and binds to antigen. The other end (Fc) triggers the biologic response of the host. Antibodies with differing antigenic specificities are produced by the host in response to the many antigens presented by an individual infectious agent. Thus more than one type of functional antibody may be produced during a single infection; conversely, a single antibody can mediate different functions, for example, opsonic and bactericidal. The triggering function of an antibody is determined in part by the chemical nature of the antigen—protein or polysaccharide; by the state of the antigen—soluble or particulate; by the properties of the antibody—class or subclass and complement or noncomplement fixing; and by its distribution.

IgA inhibits microbial attachment to the surface of mucosal cells by reacting with specific adhesion molecules on the microbial surface. *Neisseria gonorrhoeae, Neisseria meningitidis, Haemophilus influenzae,* and *Streptococcus sanguis* secrete a protease that specifically cleaves IgA1 into its component Fab and Fc fragments and probably contributes to the predilection of these organisms to cause mucosal infection or dental caries. Neutralizing antibodies are predominantly IgG molecules that neutralize microbial toxins, for example, tetanus or diphtheria toxins. They bind to the toxin and prevent its attachment or entry into the target cells of the host. Bactericidal antibodies (IgM and IgG) promote complement-dependent killing of susceptible gram-negative bacteria. Bactericidal activity requires recognition of specific (lytic) epitopes on the bacterial surface. For example, IgM specific for gonococcal lipopolysaccharide promotes killing of that organism, whereas IgM specific for outer membrane proteins does not. Opsonic antibodies promote ingestion of microorganisms by interacting with specific receptors on phagocytic cells. The interaction of antibody with its specific receptor also activates the microbicidal mechanisms of these cells. Only IgG1 and IgG3 function in this capacity by themselves. However, there are also neutrophil receptors for C3b and C3bi, opsonic molecules generated during complement activation. Thus both IgM and IgG also function as opsonins by virtue of their ability to activate complement. Opsonization requirements vary from organism to organism but in general, phagocytic uptake is most efficient when the organism is coated with both IgG and C3.

Immunoglobulin Deficiencies

Acquired immunoglobulin deficiencies result from decreased production, increased catabolism, or both. Decreased synthesis of immunoglobulin is most commonly observed in the setting of hematologic or lymphatic malignancy. Rarely, these deficiencies may arise as a postinfectious complication of certain viral infections (e.g., Epstein-Barr virus) in which the virus infects B-cells and appears to initiate an uncontrolled suppressor T-cell response. Increased catabolism of antibody is a well-described consequence of excessive protein loss

(e.g., the nephrotic syndrome, third-degree burns, or protein-losing enteropathies).

Inherited immunoglobulin deficiencies are relatively common, occurring in about 1 in 600 in the general population. Alone or in conjunction with an associated defect in cell-mediated immunity, these disorders constitute the majority (50% and 70%, respectively) of the primary immunodeficiency syndromes. The severity of these disorders is a function of whether all, several, or only one of the antibody classes or subclasses is affected and whether they are associated with defects in cell-mediated immunity. Patients with a global deficiency of IgG, IgA, and IgM experience recurrent pyogenic infections involving the sinopulmonary tract, ears, meninges, and bloodstream. These infections are caused predominantly by encapsulated organisms. Chronic or recurrent diarrhea occurs in many individuals with common variable hypogammaglobulinemia. An infectious etiology, primarily *Giardia lamblia,* is responsible for about 60% of these cases, whereas noninfectious causes, for example, gluten enteropathy, account for the remainder. Occasionally, plasma immunoglobulins will be normal in patients with this clinical history. In this situation, a selective deficiency of one of the IgG subclasses, in particular IgG2, should be sought. These patients may have a total plasma IgG within the normal range, as IgG1 accounts for an average of 70%, whereas IgG2 accounts for about 25%, of the total IgG.

Most patients with IgA deficiency are healthy, but some have atopic disease, gastrointestinal disorders, autoimmune disease, malignancy, or recurrent infection. When recurrent infection does occur, it usually involves the sinopulmonary tract, but an association with a specific group of organisms is reported infrequently. A high proportion of individuals with IgA deficiency and recurrent infection also has a selective deficiency of IgG2 or IgG4 or both.

Patients with a deficiency of IgM are at risk for bacteremia caused by gram-negative bacteria, in particular the meningococcus. This observation attests to the primary importance of IgM in host defense of the vascular space.

Therapy. Stable nonaggregating preparations of IgG that maintain their functional activity have recently been developed for intravenous infusion. Their use has been effective in decreasing the incidence of infection in patients with IgG deficiency. The increasing availability of preparations obtained from individuals with high titers of IgG against likely infectious agents, the ease of administration, and the low frequency of side effects have made these preparations the therapy of choice for deficient individuals. The dose of IV IG should be tailored to achieve postinfusion IgG concentrations in the 600 to 700 mg/dl range. IV IG infusions are generally necessary every 3 to 4 weeks to maintain a 25 to 40 day half-life for all four IgG subclasses. Infusions of fresh-frozen plasma or IgG should not be given to patients with complete selective deficiency of IgA because there is an increased risk of anaphylactic reactions because of the synthesis of antibodies to IgA.

The complications of chronic infection, pulmonary fibrosis, and bronchiectasis may progress despite immunoglobulin replacement therapy. Appropriate antibiotics should be used during periods of infection. Chronic antibiotic administration is not successful in preventing infection and may predispose to infection with resistant organisms. Close attention to good pulmonary drainage is important during periods of active infection and infection-free intervals.

HUMORAL IMMUNITY AND THE SPLEEN

Anatomically, the spleen is unique because it constitutes a quarter of the fixed lymphoid tissue and is located not in the lymphatic drainage, but in the systemic circulation. As a consequence of its content of macrophages, dendritic cells, and lymphocytes, the spleen plays a major role in filtration of the arterial circulation and is critical for the generation of a primary immune response to bloodborne antigens, especially when the antigen is a polysaccharide.

Absent splenic function occurs in cases of inherited or postsurgical asplenia. Decreased function has also been reported after infarction or irradiation, in systemic lupus erythematosus, inflammatory bowel disease, adult celiac disease, dermatitis herpetiformis, and in the hemoglobinopathies. The spleens of patients with sickle cell disease are nonfunctional by an average age of 13 months. The hyposplenic state can be readily established by examination of the peripheral blood smear for Howell-Jolly bodies.

Patients with splenic dysfunction are at increased risk of overwhelming sepsis caused by encapsulated bacteria. The overall risk of infection is increased 250-fold and is influenced by the underlying disease, ranging from 58 to 1000 times that in the general population for patients with splenectomies for trauma or thalassemia, respectively. The risk is greatest if splenectomy is performed during the first 3 years of life. The median time from splenectomy to infection is 5 years, but cases of overwhelming infection have been reported as many as 40 years after surgery. The pneumococcus is the most common pathogen and, together with *H. influenzae* and the meningococcus, accounts for 70% to 90% of cases. The bulk of the remaining cases are accounted for by *Staphylococcus aureus* and *Escherichia coli.*

As many as 70% of patients with postsplenectomy sepsis have no apparent primary site of infection. Gram stain of the buffy coat from peripheral blood demonstrates organisms in one third of patients. A positive smear indicates at least 10,000 organisms/ml of blood, approximately 100 times that in the blood of patients with intact spleens and bacteremia. Consequently, infection is fulminant, and disseminated intravascular coagulopathy occurs in 60% to 70% of patients. The overall mortality rate is about 50%, but ranges from 40% to 90% depending on the underlying disease.

Experiments in animals have shown that in the absence of specific anticapsular antibody, the spleen is essential for the removal of encapsulated pneumococci from the circulation and that this dependence increases with the degree of encapsulation. The effect of specific anticapsular antibody is to shift the major responsibility for bacterial clearance from the spleen to the liver.

These findings have led to the use of prophylactic antibiotics in children undergoing splenectomy before they are capable of responding to polysaccharide vaccines. In older children and adults, emphasis has been placed on vaccination with the multivalent pneumococcal and the tetravalent meningococcal vaccines. The response of splenectomy patients to polysaccharide vaccines is affected by the underlying disease and, in general, is not as good and does not persist as long as in normal individuals. Consequently, it may be advisable to periodically evaluate specific antibody titers and to consider repeating vaccination as necessary. Because of the possibility of intense local reactions, pneumococcal vaccination should not be repeated routinely.

THE COMPLEMENT SYSTEM IN INFECTIOUS DISEASES

The complement cascade functions chiefly as an amplification system. A recurrent theme is the cleavage of one component into two fragments, the smaller of which floats free whereas the larger is bound to the cell surface. The smaller fragments are potent mediators of the inflammatory response. These anaphylatoxins promote vascular dilation and enhance permeability (C3a, C5a) or act as a chemoattractant stimulus (C5a) for neutrophils, monocytes, and eosinophils. The larger cleavage products promote the continued sequential activation of the complement cascade, enhance phagocytosis (C3b, ic3b), and through the insertion of the membrane attack complex (C5b to C9) promote killing of susceptible organisms. Other actions include modulation of the immune response, promotion of neutrophil release from the bone marrow, and inhibition of precipitation and promotion of solubilization of immune complexes.

Complement activation proceeds by either the classical or alternative pathway. These pathways converge at the level of C3 and share a final activation sequence from C5 to C9. Because of positive feedback at the level of C3, activation of the classical pathway facilitates alternative pathway activation. A major feature of the classical pathway is its activation by antibody. As a consequence, activation occurs rapidly and efficiently, even at low concentrations of both antibody and complement. Antibody directs complement deposition to nearby structures and may itself serve as a site for complement binding. Proximity between antibody and complement on the microbial surface enhances the effector functions of these molecules.

Activation of the alternative pathway can occur in the absence of antibody. Hence the beneficial effects of complement as an amplification system can be expressed early in the course of microbial invasion before the synthesis of specific antibody. Although not required, antibody does facilitate alternative pathway activation. Activation is slow, taking two to three times as long as the classical pathway to achieve maximal activity and requiring a higher concentration of components for initiation.

Unlike the classical pathway, activation of the alternative pathway occurs continuously in the fluid phase, but its products are dissipated in a highly regulated manner by factors H and I, which interfere with the formation and function of C3bBb, the C3 convertase that is the critical product of alternative pathway activation. Properdin, another component, is a positive regulator of the alternative pathway and stabilizes C3bBb. Introduction of an appropriate cell surface shifts the balance from fluid phase control to complement activation and deposition. Thus the biochemical composition of the microbial surface is another determinant of activation. For example, the presence of sialic acid or sulfated acid mucopolysaccharides (heparin sulfate) on some cells enhances the binding of factor H to C3b, thereby promoting both the dissociation of Bb from C3bBb and the inactivation of C3b by factor I. Sialic acid is a prominent chemical constituent of the capsular polysaccharides of type III group B streptococci, K1 *E. coli,* and group B and C meningococci, whereas the capsule of K5 *E. coli* is composed of disulfoheparin. Thus the capsules of these organisms are nonactivators of the alternative pathway. It is noteworthy that these organisms are prominent causes of neonatal and infant sepsis. In these young individuals the absence of specific antibody to activate the classical pathway coupled with capsular polysaccharide-mediated inhibition of complement consumption via the alternative pathway may provide the ideal setting for infection with these organisms.

Recently a number of host cell membrane proteins have been identified that interact with specific activated complement components. These proteins fall into two general categories. The first group are complement receptors, which exhibit limited cellular distribution and subserve cell-specific functions. For example, CR-3 receptors are found primarily on phagocytic cells. Their genetic absence is associated with severe infections and death shortly after birth as a consequence of impaired neutrophil function. CR-2 receptors are present primarily on B-lymphocytes. Ligand interaction with this receptor augments antibody production. Epstein-Barr virus uses the CR-2 receptor to enter B-lymphocytes, thereby stimulating the polyclonal antibody response that characterizes the early phase of infectious mononucleosis. The second group of molecules are membrane proteins that inhibit complement activation. These proteins are widely distributed and prevent complement-mediated damage to host cells. They exert their influence by inhibiting either the cell-bound C3 convertases or assembly of the membrane attack complex. The deficiency of two of these membrane proteins, decay-accelerating factor and CD59, is the functional basis for the syndrome of paroxysmal nocturnal hemoglobinuria. Some microbial organisms (e.g., *Candida albicans* and herpes simplex type 1) express C3 binding proteins on their surface, which both protect the organism from complement activation and alter the ability of bound C3 to promote phagocytosis of the organism.

Complement Deficiency States

Complement deficiencies may be acquired or inherited. Acutely acquired deficiencies most commonly reflect consumption of complement components as occurs during overwhelming infection, severe burns, or hemodialysis. Total hemolytic complement is low and there is a global reduction of most of the individual components, which returns to normal after the acute event has subsided. Acquired chronic depression of complement activity is usually due to circulating immune complexes or, in rare situations, to antibody reacting with one of the components. These patients exhibit the same patterns of infection seen in individuals with inherited deficiencies of complement.

Homozygous complement deficiencies are found in approximately 1 in 10,000 persons, but the frequency is higher among patients with collagen vascular disease or certain infections. The pattern of infection varies with the deficiency and the nature of the accompanying defect in host defense effector mechanisms. For example, only 20% of patients with a classical pathway defect (C1, C2, or C4) experience infection, probably because their alternative pathway is intact.

Infection occurs early in life and is usually caused by encapsulated bacteria. On the other hand, immunologic diseases appear to be more common than infection, affecting 85% of these individuals.

Inherited defects of the alternative pathway are rare. The distinguishing feature of properdin deficiency is its X-linked mode of inheritance, which is reflected in a family history of meningococcal (often fulminant) infection occurring predominantly in teenage boys in skipped generations.

C3-deficient individuals experience both recurrent infection and immunologic disease. Opsonic, chemotactic, and serum bactericidal activity are defective in these patients. Infection typically occurs early in life, is recurrent, and is caused primarily by encapsulated bacteria. Patients with factor I or H deficiency are unable to inhibit the formation and activity of the alternative pathway C3 convertase, C3bBb. Hence their serum contains low levels of C3, and they exhibit a pattern of infection similar to that in patients with primary C3 deficiency.

Serum from patients with a deficiency of one of the terminal complement components (C5 to C9) lacks bactericidal activity but is capable of opsonizing organisms normally. Approximately half of these individuals never experience infection, and a minority develop immunologic disorders. The other half experience systemic meningococcal or gonococcal disease; of these, half suffer recurrent bouts of neisserial infection. Compared with the general population, meningococcal disease in these individuals is distinguished by (1) a 5- to 10,000-fold greater risk of infection, (2) a higher male/female ratio (3:1 vs. 1:1), (3) a higher median age of first infection (17 vs. 3 years), (4) a ten-fold greater relapse rate, (5) a higher recurrence rate (45% vs. <1%), (6) a higher rate of infection caused by group Y meningococci (44% vs. 10%), and (7) a paradoxically lower case fatality rate (2.9% vs. 19%) (Chapter 175).

Serum bactericidal activity plays a major role in protection against bloodborne infections. Both antibody and complement are critical for the expression of this activity and in their presence, bloodstream invasion is restricted to organisms that are naturally resistant to it. The physiologic nadir of antibody that occurs during the first year of life is reflected by absent serum bactericidal activity and the highest age-specific incidence of bacteremia and meningitis due to *H. influenzae* and *N. meningitidis*. These bacteria are readily killed by most adult sera. At the other end of the spectrum are patients with absent serum bactericidal activity because of a deficiency of one of the terminal complement components who experience an inordinate number of neisserial infections.

The frequency with which patients with hypogammaglobulinemia, hyposplenia, or complement deficiency experience infection caused by encapsulated bacteria, in particular *Streptococcus pneumoniae, H. influenzae,* and *N. meningitidis,* underscores the interplay between these host defense systems. In animal models of infection, elimination of these organisms from the bloodstream occurs in three phases: an early phase (0 to 1 hour) during which the bulk of the organisms are removed in an antibody-modulated manner by phagocytic cells within the spleen, liver, and lung; an intermediate phase during which further sterilization of the blood occurs as a consequence of complement-dependent killing of susceptible organisms; and a late phase, which is critically dependent on the contribution of the complement system to opsonization. In the absence of anticapsular antibody, complement fixation is less effective in promoting phagocytosis because C3b is deposited beneath the antiphagocytic polysaccharide capsule. Specific antibody promotes C3b fixation to the capsule itself. In this location, the cooperative opsonic function of C3b and antibody promotes ingestion and killing of these organisms. Patients with defective neutrophil function do not experience a higher frequency of these infections probably because of the large number of phagocytic cells and variety of mechanisms by which these cells can kill ingested organisms.

Diagnosis and Treatment of Complement Deficiency States

From the standpoint of infectious diseases, complement assays are used most commonly to evaluate the possibility of complement deficiency as an explanation for recurrent infection. In this setting, the most important screening test is the assay for total hemolytic complement (CH50). This assay measures the functional integrity of all nine

proteins in the classical pathway. It is important to realize that a normal result in the more commonly available antigenic assays for C3 or C4 does not exclude a defect elsewhere in the cascade.

Patients with complement deficiency states should receive the pneumococcal and meningococcal polysaccharide vaccines and the *H. influenzae* conjugate vaccine. Use of the classical pathway in patients with a defect in the alternative pathway is improved by vaccination. Conversely, the ability of specific antibody to facilitate alternative pathway activity independent of complement activation by the Fc portion of the immunoglobulin molecule provides a rationale for vaccinating patients with a defect in the classical pathway. Patients missing one of the terminal components benefit from vaccination as a consequence of improved opsonization and a shifting of the burden of host defense from complement-dependent bactericidal activity to phagocytosis. Fresh-frozen plasma can be used to restore complement component levels to normal but because of the short half-life of the components and development of antibody to the missing component, this approach should be reserved for life-threatening infections. Prophylactic antibiotics are necessary only rarely.

PHAGOCYTIC CELLS

Neutrophils, eosinophils, basophils, monocytes, and macrophages are all capable of ingesting invading pathogens and are classified as phagocytes. Neutrophils, eosinophils, and basophils are granulocytic phagocytes; monocytes and macrophages constitute the mononuclear phagocytic system. The cellular immune system (monocytes, macrophages, and lymphocytes) is discussed in detail in Chapter 174.

Neutrophils

Neutrophils are the most common phagocytes in the blood, constituting approximately 60% of the leukocytes on a blood smear. Development in the bone marrow consists of (1) a mitotic phase, in which myeloblasts divide and mature through promyelocytes and myelocytes, and (2) a nonmitotic phase of maturation, in which metamyelocytes mature to band cells and then to segmented neutrophils. The majority of mature neutrophils in the body are found in the nonmitotic compartment (i.e., the bone marrow reserve). It takes 9 to 11 days for the progeny of a myeloblast to leave the marrow, and in the adult, up to 10^{11} mature neutrophils enter the circulation per day. Once in the blood, neutrophils separate into two equal classes, actively circulating neutrophils and marginated neutrophils that adhere to blood vessel walls. The intravascular neutrophil half-life is 6 to 8 hours, after which neutrophils pass out of the bloodstream and migrate to mucosal surfaces or localize in areas of inflammation. Senescent neutrophils are themselves phagocytized by fixed tissue macrophages. Extravascular survival varies from hours to 4 days. Apoptosis (programmed cell death) promotes neutrophil death without releasing inflammatory substances. Granulocyte-monocyte colony-stimulating factor (GM-CSF) increases total neutrophil production by acting at the pluripotent stem cell. Granulocyte colony-stimulating factor (G-CSF) shortens periods of chemotherapy-induced neutropenia.

The mature neutrophil possesses at least two types of morphologically distinct cytoplasmic granules. The primary granule is a true lysosome, as it contains acid hydrolases in addition to myeloperoxidase, elastase, cationic proteins, lysozyme, and defensins. This granule appears to serve a microbicidal function. The specific granules outnumber the primary granules by 3:1 and contain lysozyme, lactoferrin, collagenase, and vitamin B_{12}–binding proteins. Specific granules discharge their contents into the extracellular fluid and may therefore function in part in the secretory regulation of the inflammatory response. The neutrophil membrane has surface receptors capable of binding the iC3b (CR3 receptor) and C5a components of complement, as well as the Fc end of immunoglobulin G.

The neutrophil's response in host defense against invading microbes may be divided into mobilization, adherence, locomotion, chemotaxis, phagocytosis, and intracellular killing. Although each of these events will be considered separately, they form a continuous process that may exist in all stages at once. Microbial invasion is followed by mobilization of both mature and band forms from the bone marrow, resulting in the leftward shift noted with many acute bacterial infections. These neutrophils become sticky and adhere to the vascular endothelium (margination). The cell then enters the tissues by locomoting between the endothelial cells (diapedesis). Once it is in the tissues, the neutrophil moves by chemotaxis (directed migration), in the direction of increasing concentrations of attractants (chemotactic factors). A large number of substances act as chemotactic factors for the neutrophil. The most important include (1) bacterial products, (2) complement components C3a and C5a obtained through either classical or alternative complement pathway activation, and (3) cellular products such as leukotrienes and cytokines derived from other neutrophils, lymphocytes, and macrophages. These factors include arachidonic acid metabolites, interleukin 1 (IL-1) (endogenous pyrogen), and tumor necrosis factor (cachectin). At the site of inflammation, the concentration of chemotactic factors is so strong that neutrophil chemotaxis is actually stopped and the cell becomes hyperadhesive.

Contact with the microorganisms initiates phagocytosis. Many virulent organisms resist ingestion by neutrophils. These organisms can be engulfed only by being trapped against a surface (surface phagocytosis) or by being opsonized. Once the microbe is bound to the neutrophil surface, the neutrophil membrane flows around it and encloses it in a vacuole called the *phagosome*.

Microbial attachment to the neutrophil initiates two events involved in intracellular killing, the "oxidative postphagocytic burst" and degranulation. The *oxidative burst* refers to a large increment in oxygen consumption and related metabolic changes by phagocytizing neutrophils. Most of this oxygen is converted to superoxide anion (O_2^-) and then hydrogen peroxide (H_2O_2). These oxygen metabolites are released into the phagosome, where they exert a microbicidal effect.

Degranulation, the other event in intracellular killing, begins before the phagosome is completely closed. The specific granules fuse with the developing phagosome and fire their contents. Because this fusion occurs before closure of the phagosome, specific granule contents are released into the extracellular fluid. The specific granule contains factors that generate chemoattractants for polymorphonuclear neutrophils (PMNs) and monocytes, have antimicrobial activity, and cause platelet activation. The primary granules fuse with the completed phagosome, and thus the contents of these granules usually stay in the phagosome. Inside the phagosome, granule contents and oxygen metabolites interact to kill microbes. Oxygen-dependent microbial substances include the active metabolites of oxygen (H_2O_2, O_2^-, the hydroxyl radical [$OH\cdot$], and singlet oxygen [$O\cdot$]) and myeloperoxidase from the primary granule. Hydrogen peroxide, a halide (iodide, bromide, or chloride), and myeloperoxidase act synergistically, increasing the microbicidal capabilities of H_2O_2 50-fold. Oxygen-independent microbicidal systems include the products of primary and specific granule fusion with the phagosome, namely, acidity, lactoferrin, lysozyme, cationic proteins, and defensins.

The multiple killing mechanisms of neutrophils are important, because microbes vary in their susceptibility to the different systems. Numerous defects of neutrophil function have now been identified (Box 230-1), and most lead to increased susceptibility to infection.

Mobilization. Problems in mobilizing sufficient numbers of neutrophils from the bone marrow to inflammatory sites usually result from insufficient bone marrow reserves. Neutropenia is the most common granulocyte abnormality seen in clinical practice. Cytotoxic drug–induced neutropenia accounts for the majority of cases, and infection remains the most important complication of the chemotherapy of malignant disease. The risk of infection increases with decreasing neutrophil counts, rising dramatically at peripheral blood neutrophil counts of less than 0.5×10^9/L (Chapter 236). Gram-negative rods, staphylococci, and fungal species account for the majority of infections in neutropenic patients. The lung, gut, skin, and urinary tract are common sites of local and disseminated infection, although bacteremia in which there is no demonstrable portal of entry is also common. Fever is usually present, but local signs of inflammation may be minimal because of the paucity of neutrophils.

Defects of Adherence and Locomotion. Abnormalities in adherence not only affect the neutrophil's ability to marginate and leave the bloodstream but also inhibit migration to infected tissue. Drug-induced defects are the most common and are often reversible when

---

BOX 230-1
Functional defects of neutrophils

Mobilization
Acquired neutropenia: drug-induced (i.e., by cytotoxic agents), autoimmune, leukemias
Congenital neutropenia: cyclic neutropenia, familial neutropenia, infantile genetic agranulocytosis

Adherence
Acquired: drug-induced (e.g., by corticosteroids), diabetes mellitus, leukemia
Congenital: leukocyte adhesion deficiency

Locomotion
Actin dysfunction
Bacteria-induced dysfunction
Leukocyte adhesion deficiency

Chemotaxis
Humoral defects: complement deficiency (C3 and C5), cell-derived agent deficiencies (e.g., lymphokines)
Inhibitors: Hodgkin's disease, sarcoidosis, lepromatous leprosy
Cellular defects: cells from neonates, Chédiak-Higashi syndrome, hyperimmunoglobulin E syndrome, thermal injury, hypophosphatemia

Phagocytosis (ingestion)
Opsonic defects: complement C3 deficiency, hypogammaglobulinemia, asplenia
Cellular defects: diabetes mellitus, systemic lupus erythematosus, hypophosphatemia, lazy leukocyte syndrome

Intracellular killing
Oxidative burst abnormalities: chronic granulomatous disease, glucose 6-phosphate dehydrogenase deficiency, glutathione peroxidase deficiency
Granule abnormalities: Chédiak-Higashi syndrome, myeloperoxidase deficiency, specific granule deficiency

---

the drug is discontinued. Corticosteroids and ethanol are prime offenders; their use may help explain the observed increases in their incidence. Rare congenital defects have been described in which the cells have abnormal surface glycoproteins. Leukocyte adhesion deficiency syndromes types 1 and 2 are examples.

Defects of Locomotion. Once it is adherent, the cell must be capable of moving out of the intravascular space. Defects of locomotion, such as the actin dysfunction syndrome, are separated from chemotactic defects by the inability of the neutrophil to move randomly as well as directionally (chemotaxis).

Chemotactic Defects. Inability of neutrophils to respond to chemotactic stimuli may be due to abnormal cells, absent or abnormal humoral factors, or humoral inhibitors of chemotaxis. Humoral defects include both congenital and acquired deficiency of the C3 and C5 complement components, as well as defective chemotactic lymphokines. Humoral inhibitors may be found in Hodgkin's disease, sarcoidosis, lepromatous leprosy, cirrhosis, uremia, and glomerulonephritis. Intrinsic cellular defects have been described in diabetes mellitus, the Chédiak-Higashi syndrome, thermal injury, neutrophil cytoskeletal defects, hypophosphatemia, and cells from neonates. Job's syndrome patients have defective neutrophil and monocyte chemotaxis and are characterized by markedly elevated levels of IgE, eczema, and recurrent "cold" staphylococcal skin infections (lacking signs of inflammation).

Although defective chemotaxis results in a delay in the establishment of an inflammatory focus, in most of these syndromes adequate numbers of neutrophils eventually reach the site of infection. Bacteremia, pneumonia, and deep visceral infections are uncommon. Abscesses of skin and soft tissue with regional adenopathy are the usual manifestations. Some patients suffer from otitis media and periodontal disease. *S. aureus* is the most common offending organism. Therapy consists of prolonged treatment with appropriate antimicrobials and surgical drainage of abscesses.

Defects of Phagocytosis. Decreased phagocytosis is most often related to opsonin defects, such as complement or immunoglobulin deficiencies. Rarely, a cellular defect is found. Anatomic or functional asplenia (i.e., sickle cell disease) may cause a deficiency of opsonic factors. Patients with these disorders have recurrent serious and, at times, life-threatening infections from encapsulated bacteria, primarily the pneumococcus and *H. influenzae*. Patients in this group should receive the pneumococcal and perhaps the *H. influenzae* vaccines, although the efficacy for these patients is unproved. Recently, diabetic hyperglycemia has been correlated with elevated neutrophil intracellular calcium levels and impaired phagocytosis. Correction of hyperglycemia reduced intracellular calcium and improved phagocytosis.

Defects of Intracellular Killing. Defects of intracellular killing involve abnormalities of either the oxidative burst or granule function. Chronic granulomatous disease (CGD) of childhood is a syndrome characterized by abnormal neutrophil oxidative metabolism. Affected persons suffer repeated severe infections involving the skin, lymph nodes, lungs, bones, liver, and spleen. Physical findings include an eczematoid dermatitis, lymphadenopathy, and hepatosplenomegaly. Laboratory abnormalities include leukocytosis, anemia, and hyperglobulinemia. Chest x-ray films often reveal pulmonary scarring from recurrent pneumonia. Noncaseating granulomas are a prominent histopathologic feature. *S. aureus* is the most common organism causing these lesions, followed by gram-negative rods (especially *Serratia marcescens*), *Nocardia,* and *Aspergillus* species. The usual course of the disease is one of recurrent infection leading to death in childhood, although some patients have milder forms of the disease. Chronic granulomatous disease occurs with a frequency of 1 in 1 million individuals. Classic CGD is an X-linked recessive disease with identifiable female carriers and accounts for two thirds of the cases. Autosomal recessive cases account for most of the remaining third.

The granulocytes and monocytes in this disease fail to exhibit a burst in oxygen uptake during phagocytosis, resulting in phagosomes that lack the microbicidal activity of superoxide anion and hydrogen peroxide. Neutrophils from X-linked CGD lack cytochrome b 558. Neutrophils from patients with autosomally inherited CGD lack a complete cytosol oxidase. Despite these genetic differences, the clinical presentation and biochemical "defects" in neutrophils from all CGD patients are similar. There is a failure of membrane-associated pyridine nucleotide oxidase to generate active oxygen metabolites during and after phagocytosis.

The diagnosis of CGD is made by demonstrating an abnormal oxidative burst during phagocytosis. A slide test that measures nitroblue tetrazolium reduction by neutrophils from a drop of patient blood is a sensitive screening test. Neutrophils from CGD patients cannot reduce the dye because they do not generate superoxide.

The granule abnormalities include myeloperoxidase deficiency and the Chédiak-Higashi syndrome. Myeloperoxidase deficiency may be the most common neutrophil functional defect occurring as either total (approximately 1 in 4000 persons) or partial (1 in 2000 persons) absence of myeloperoxidase in neutrophils and monocytes. The majority of patients with myeloperoxidase deficiency are free of infectious complications, although there is an association with systemic candidiasis and diabetes. In most patients, the disease is inherited in an autosomal recessive pattern. Specific granule deficiency is a rare disorder associated with defects in both chemotaxis and intracellular killing.

The Chédiak-Higashi syndrome is a rare autosomal recessive disease characterized by the presence of abnormal giant granules in all granule-containing cells. The clinical features include partial oculocutaneous albinism; rotatory nystagmus; peripheral neuropathy; recurrent skin, soft tissue, and respiratory tract infections; and an accelerated lymphoma-like phase characterized by widespread tissue infiltration by lymphoid cells. The diagnosis is made by the demonstration of giant granules in the neutrophils on the blood smear. They

---

BOX 230-2

**Noninfectious diseases
in which polymorphonuclear neutrophils
play a role in tissue damage**

Gout
Rheumatoid arthritis
Immune vasculitis
Neutrophil dermatoses
Glomerulonephritis
Inflammatory bowel disease
Myocardial infarction
ARDS
Asthma
Emphysema
Malignant neoplasms at area of chronic inflammation

Modified from Malech HL, Gallin JI: Neutrophils in human diseases, *N Engl J Med* 317:687, 1987.

Chemotaxis and intracellular killing are diminished, even though phagocytosis and the oxidative burst occur normally. Impaired killing is due to defective degranulation into the phagosome.

Neutrophil Mediation of Tissue Injury. The same microbicidal events used by PMNs to kill invading microbial pathogens can also act on host tissue to cause injury. Box 230-2 lists some noninfectious diseases in which neutrophils play a role. In the inflammatory arthritides, PMNs are attracted by nonmicrobial chemoattractants (complement components, leukotrienes, and cytokines). Escape from the neutrophil of both oxidative and nonoxidative factors causes destruction of adjacent tissue. This injury then attracts more PMNs. Similar events occur in autoimmune vasculitis. A role for the PMN has been proposed in potentiating tissue injury in inflammatory bowel disease and myocardial infarction as well.

The PMN appears to play a central role in pathogenesis of the acute respiratory distress syndrome (ARDS). Pulmonary vessels and parenchyma usually show large numbers of PMNs, suggesting that they are the major mediator of lung damage in this condition. ARDS can occur in the presence of severe neutropenia, however, and a unifying hypothesis suggests that a variety of stimuli (infection, trauma, toxic chemicals) trigger release of cytokines (IL-1, tumor necrosis factor, etc.), which activate PMNs and endothelial cells and cause ARDS.

Management. Appropriate antimicrobial therapy and surgical drainage of abscesses are standard treatment of infections resulting from abnormal neutrophil function. In *S. aureus* infections rifampin is often combined with other antistaphylococcal agents since it penetrates the neutrophil and promotes intracellular killing.

Trimethoprim-sulfamethoxazole is an effective prophylactic antibiotic in individuals with CGD. Interferon-γ improves phagocyte oxidative metabolism in some patients with CGD and has been shown to reduce infectious complications.

Granulocyte transfusions have been advocated for febrile neutropenic patients but are rarely used because of poor efficacy and frequent complications. Colony-stimulating factors (G-CSF and GM-CSF) have been administered to neutropenic patients with a resultant increase in neutrophil number and associated improvement in outcome with respect to both infection and underlying disease. Lastly, bone marrow transplantation has been attempted with mixed results in several patients with neutrophil defects.

Eosinophils

Eosinophils develop from a common granulocyte-monocyte stem cell in the bone marrow and function as tissue-based granulocytes. Their characteristic red-staining granules contain a myeloperoxidase distinct from that of the neutrophil and a crystalloid core. Their half-life in circulating blood is 2 hours, after which they migrate to tissues. Eosinophils are less efficient at phagocytosis than are neutrophils. They

✔ *WHEN TO REFER*

Most patients referred for evaluation because of "frequent infections" do not have identifiable defects of neutrophil function. However, a careful history, including a detailed family history, and physical examination will often identify patients who are most likely to have a significant defect. Clues include a positive family history, deep visceral infections requiring hospitalization, and multiple scars representing previous skin infections and drained abscesses. Determination of total white blood cell count with differential counts, total hemolytic complement, and immunoglobulin levels, and a nitroblue tetrazolium test will screen several of the more common previously mentioned defects. If suspicion is high and expertise is available, the more sophisticated studies to evaluate adherence, chemotaxis, phagocytosis, oxidative activity, and microbicidal activity can be performed.

are selectively attracted by an eosinophil chemotactic factor of anaphylaxis, histamine, and certain lymphokines. Eosinophils appear to be the most effective killer cells for helminths. Eosinophils are also involved in allergic responses.

The causes of eosinophilia ($>500/mm^3$ of blood) include drug reactions, helminthic infections, allergic disorders, collagen vascular diseases, malignancy, and idiopathic hypereosinophilic syndrome. Low-grade eosinophilia is often seen in Addison's disease. Charcot-Leyden crystals, a product of eosinophil degeneration, are seen in areas of eosinophil accumulation, such as respiratory secretions from patients with asthma.

Basophils

Basophils are also tissue-based granulocytes and are the least common blood granulocyte. They are related to mast cells and have IgE bound to their surface. Their granules are rich in histamine. Although basophils are capable of phagocytosis, they do not play a primary role in infection control but are involved in IgE-mediated allergic reactions.

Mononuclear Phagocytes

The mononuclear phagocyte system is composed of peripheral blood monocytes and their tissue counterparts, macrophages. Like neutrophils, monocytes and macrophages are capable of adherence, chemotaxis, phagocytosis, and intracellular killing. They function at a slower rate, as evidenced by their later arrival at infected areas and by their slower chemotaxis and phagocytosis in vitro.

The mononuclear phagocytes have three major functions: (1) they clear the body of damaged cells and cellular debris; (2) they are the first line of defense against intracellular pathogens that are not destroyed by neutrophils, such as *Mycobacterium tuberculosis* and *Histoplasma capsulatum;* and (3) they interact with lymphocytes to produce antibody and to form the cell-mediated immune system. The final stage of development of the mononuclear phagocyte is the giant cell. This cell characterizes inflammatory responses to organisms that require intact mononuclear phagocytes and cell-mediated immunity. Both monocytes and macrophages appear before giant cells, and it is felt that these cells fuse to form the multinucleated cells.

Cell-mediated Immunity. In 1891, Koch showed that inoculation of tubercle bacilli into guinea pigs led to rapidly disseminated and often fatal infection, yet when the survivors were rechallenged with the same bacilli, dissemination did not occur. In the 1940s this mechanism of resistance was further defined by showing that immunity to the tubercle bacillus could be transferred by lymphoid cells but not by serum (antibody) from immunized animals. This mechanism of host defense is now called the *cell-mediated immune system.* By complex interactions between T-cells and mononuclear phagocytes, this system kills organisms resistant to the usual humoral and phagocytic (neutrophil) microbicidal mechanisms. Some of the defects of the cell-mediated immune system are listed in Box 230-3.

BOX 230-3
Defects in the cell-mediated immune system

Monocytes
Chemotactic defects
  Chédiak-Higashi syndrome
  Chronic mucocutaneous candidiasis (thermal injury)
  Malignancy
  Viral infections

Microbicidal defects
HIV (AIDS)
Chédiak-Higashi syndrome
Malignancies
Viral infections

Lymphocytes
Primary
X-linked agammaglobulinemia
Hyper-IgM syndrome
Defects in expression of the major histocompatibility complex
  Thymic hypoplasia (DiGeorge's syndrome)
  Wiskott-Aldrich syndrome
  Chronic mucocutaneous candidiasis
  Purine nucleoside phosphorylase deficiency
  Severe combined immunodeficiency
  Common variable immunodeficiency
Secondary
Infections
  Viral: HIV (AIDS), measles, mumps, chicken pox, influenza, mononucleosis
  Bacterial: tuberculosis, leprosy, syphilis, typhoid fever
  Fungal: coccidioidomycosis, histoplasmosis, blastomycosis
  Parasitic: schiostosomiasis, toxoplasmosis
Malignancies
  Hodgkin's disease
  Melanoma
  Others
Drugs: cyclophosphamide, azathioprine, corticosteroids, antilymphocyte serum

BOX 230-4
Infections in patients with impaired cell-mediated immunity

Tuberculosis and atypical mycobacteria
Leprosy
Listeriosis
Herpes simplex and herpes zoster
Cytomegalovirus
Vaccinia
Aspergillosis
Cryptococcosis
Histoplasmosis
Coccidioidomycosis
Toxoplasmosis
Pneumocystis carinii
Salmonellosis
Cryptosporidiosis

Lymphocyte Defects

Primary Disorders of T-Cells. Thymic hypoplasia (DiGeorge's syndrome) is the prototype of disordered cell-mediated immunity. Patients with this disease are born lacking the thymus and parathyroid glands. The resultant defective cell-mediated immunity is associated with specific life-threatening infections (Box 230-4). The Wiskott-Aldrich syndrome is an X-linked disorder characterized by eczema, thrombocytopenia, and recurrent infections. There is progressive T-cell dysfunction with actual T-cell lymphopenia. Affected males rarely survive past the first decade. In other syndromes, such as chronic mucocutaneous candidiasis, ataxia-telangiectasia, and purine nucleoside phosphorylase deficiency, T-cell dysfunction with altered cell-mediated immunity is present.

Primary Disorders of B-Cells. X-linked agammaglobulinemia is a pure B-cell deficiency, which actually presents in boys during the first year of life. Recurrent pyogenic infections secondary to *H. influenza* and *S. pneumoniae* are the rule. Prophylaxis with intravenous immune globulin is now standard therapy.

Patients with hyper-IgM syndrome have elevated serum levels of IgM, no IgA, and very low levels of IgG. Both males and females are affected. These patients experience not only recurrent pyogenic infections, but also opportunistic infections, including pneumocystis, and autoimmune diseases affecting the cellular blood elements.

Primary Disorders of Both B-Cells and T-Cells. Severe combined immunodeficiency is an X-linked or autosomal recessive disorder. Because affected persons lack both T- and B-cells, both humoral and cell-mediated immune mechanisms are impaired. The disease is rapidly fatal, with few patients surviving beyond 2 years of age. Common variable immunodeficiency is an acquired disease of unknown cause that affects B-cells and sometimes T-cells. Antibody production, and sometimes T-cell function, is abnormal. A malabsorptive syndrome, often caused by *G. lamblia* infection of the small intestine, may be seen (Chapter 279).

Secondary Defects of T-Cell Function. T-cell function in secondary cell defects is suppressed by other conditions (Box 230-3). The most common cause of secondary T-cell defects is infection. Suppression of both delayed hypersensitivity skin test reactions and in vitro lymphocyte transformation has been associated with many viral, bacterial, and fungal infections. Cure of the underlying infection results in a return of normal cell-mediated immunity.

AIDS is a condition in which helper T-cells are selectively infected and destroyed by a retrovirus (the human immunodeficiency virus [HIV]), resulting in profound depression of the cell-mediated immune system (Chapters 248 and 256).

Various malignancies can also depress T-cell function and cell-mediated immunity. Hodgkin's disease is the best studied of these. The delayed hypersensitivity skin test reaction and lymphocyte transformation are often abnormal. The mechanism behind these defects is not known. Immunosuppressive drugs, including azathioprine, cyclophosphamide, corticosteroids, and antilymphocyte serum, make up the third group of causes. T-cell function and cell-mediated immunity usually return to normal when the drugs are stopped.

BIBLIOGRAPHY

Adams DH, Shaw S: Leukocyte-endothelial interactions and regulation of leukocyte migration, *Lancet* 343:831-836, 1994.

Alexiewicz JM et al: Polymorphonuclear leukocytes in non-insulin dependent diabetes mellitus: abnormalities in metabolism and function, *Ann Intern Med* 123:919-924, 1995.

Brown EJ, Joiner KA, Frank MM: The role of complement in host resistance to bacteria, *Springer Semin Immunopathol* 6:349-360, 1983.

Buckley RH: Immunodeficiency diseases, *JAMA* 258:2841-2850, 1987.

Crawford J et al: Reduction by granulocyte colony-stimulating factor of fever and neutropenia induced by chemotherapy in patients with small-cell lung cancer, *N Engl J Med* 325:164-170, 1991.

Densen P, Clark RA, Nauseef WM: Granulocytic phagocytes. In Mandell GL, Bennett JL, Dolin R, editors: *Principles and practice of infectious diseases,* ed 4, New York, 1995, Churchill Livingstone.

Densen P, Mandell GL: Phagocyte strategy vs. microbial tactics, *Rev Infect Dis* 2:817-838, 1980.

Densen P et al: Familial properdin deficiency and fatal meningococcemia, *N Engl J Med* 316:922-926, 1987.

Fearon DT: Complement, *J Allergy Clin Immunol* 71:520-529, 1983.

Figueroa JE, Densen P: Infectious diseases associated with complement deficiencies, *Clin Microbiol Rev* 4:359-395, 1991.

Gallin JI: Interferon-gamma in the management of infectious diseases, *Ann Intern Med* 123:216-224, 1995.

Henderson HR: The role of leukotrienes in inflammation, *Ann Intern Med* 121:684-697, 1994.

International Chronic Granulomatous Disease Cooperative Study Group: A controlled trial of interferon gamma to prevent infection in chronic granulomatous disease, *N Engl J Med* 324:510-516, 1991.

Johnston RB Jr: Current concepts: recurrent bacterial infections in children, *N Engl J Med* 310:1237-1242, 1984.

Johnston RB Jr: Monocytes and macrophages, *N Engl J Med* 318:747-752, 1988.

Locksley RM, Wilson CB: Cell mediated immunity and its role in host defense. In Mandell GL, Bennett JL, Dolin R, editors: *Principles and practice of infectious diseases,* ed. 4, New York, 1995, Churchill Livingstone.

Rosen FS, Cooper MD, Wedgewood RJP: The primary immunodeficiencies, *N Engl J Med* 333:431-440, 1995.

Sawyer DW, Donowitz GR, Mandell GL: Polymorphonuclear neutrophils: an effective antimicrobial force, *Rev Infect Dis* 2(7):S1532-S1544, 1989.

Schifferli JA, Ng YC, Peters DK: The role of complement and its receptors in the elimination of immune complexes, *N Engl J Med* 315:488-495, 1986.

Singer DG: Postsplenectomy sepsis, *Perspect Pediatr Pathol* 1:285-311, 1973.

Wara DW: Host defense against *Streptococcus pneumoniae:* the role of the spleen, *Rev Infect Dis* 3:299-309, 1983.

Weller PF: The immunobiology of eosinophils, *N Engl J Med* 324:1110-1118, 1991.

Yang KD, Hill HR: Neutrophil function disorders: pathophysiology, prevention, and therapy, *J Pediatr* 119:343-354, 1991.

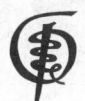

CHAPTER

231 Principles of Antiinfective Therapy

Robert C. Moellering, Jr., and George M. Eliopoulos

The introduction of sulfonamides into clinical use in the mid-1930s marked the beginning of the modern era of antimicrobial therapy. Few other advances in medicine have had such a striking impact on the morbidity and mortality of human disease. In the subsequent six decades, an impressive armamentarium of antimicrobial agents has become available; however, antibiotics have not been a panacea for clinical infections. The development of resistance to antimicrobial agents among pathogenic bacteria and the toxicity related to their use have remained significant problems, providing impetus for the development of new therapeutic agents. As a result, the annual cost of antibiotic use in this country has grown enormously, and antibiotic agents are now administered to more than a third of all hospitalized patients. The increased costs of antibiotics contribute significantly to the costs of caring for hospitalized patients. For these reasons the appropriate use of antimicrobial agents has been the subject of intense interest in recent years.

MECHANISMS OF ANTIMICROBIAL ACTION

An effective antimicrobial agent should be selectively toxic for the microbial pathogen, with little toxicity for the human host. Several structures or metabolic pathways within a bacterium are susceptible to such selective attack, either because they lack a counterpart in mammalian cells or because their sensitivity to antibiotic action greatly exceeds that of the mammalian cell. Categorization of antimicrobials by major site of action (Fig. 231-1) allows a useful overview of the ever-expanding number of available agents.

Cell Wall Synthesis

Bacteria are hyperosmolar with respect to mammalian tissue and interstitial fluid; thus they require a rigid cell wall to maintain their integrity when they colonize or infect humans. With no counterpart in the mammalian cell, this unique structure provides an ideal target for antibiotic action; inhibition of cell wall synthesis usually is bactericidal (i.e., results in bacterial cell death rather than simple inhibition of growth). The backbone of the cell wall, a polymer called *peptidoglycan,* is synthesized in three major steps, each inhibited by specific antimicrobial agents.

In the first step uridine diphosphate (UDP)-*N*-acetylmuramyl-pentapeptide is assembled in the bacterial cytoplasm. Cycloserine, a structural analog of alanine, inhibits the assembly of the pentapeptide chain. Next, UDP-*N*-acetylmuramyl-pentapeptide and *N*-acetylglucosamine are polymerized into linear peptidoglycan strands, which are then transferred across the plasma membrane and linked

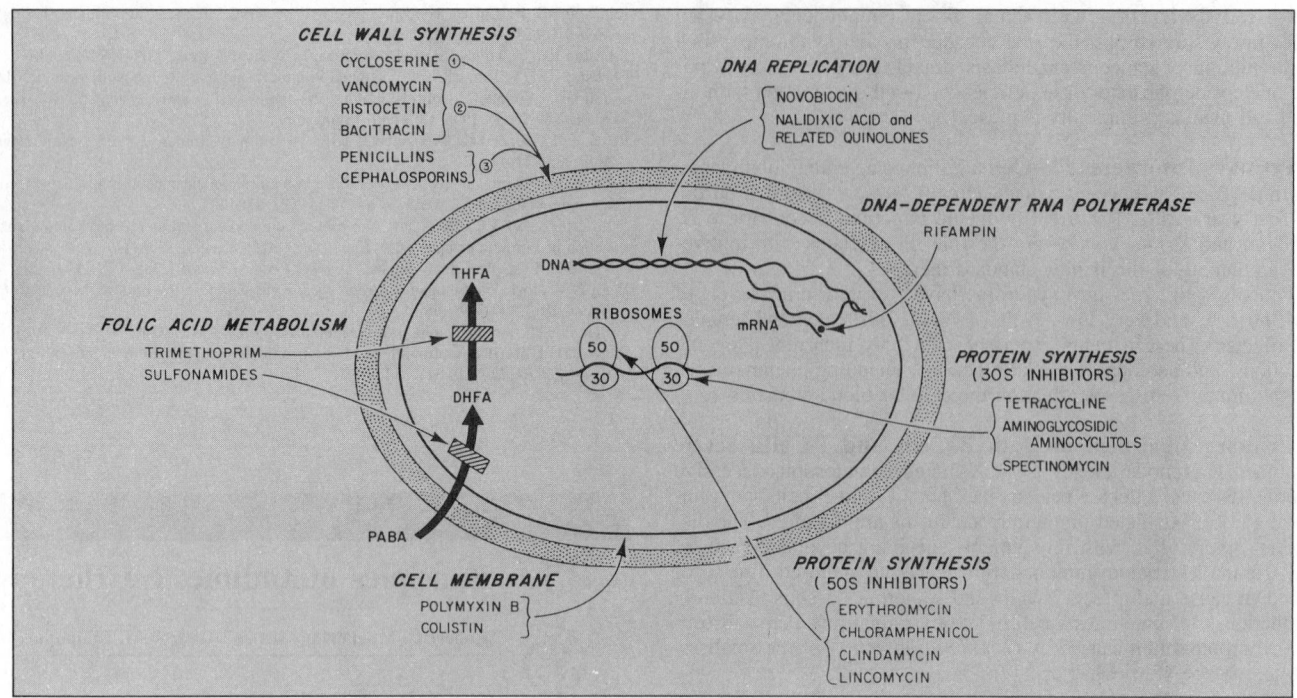

FIGURE 231-1 Mechanisms of action of antibacterial agents. *PABA,* Para-aminobenzoic acid; *DHFA,* dihydrofolic acid; *THFA,* tetrahydrofolic acid.

to the growing point of the bacterial cell wall. Several antibiotics, including vancomycin, teicoplanin, bacitracin, and ristocetin, inhibit this phase of cell wall synthesis. Outside the cell, the peptidoglycan strands are cross-linked via their pentapeptide side chains to create a three-dimensional polymer. Penicillins, cephalosporins, and other beta-lactam antibiotics inhibit this final polymerization step, called the *transpeptidation reaction.*

Penicillin binds to several distinct proteins in the bacterial cytoplasmic membrane. Each of these "penicillin-binding proteins" is believed to represent a distinct penicillin-sensitive enzyme involved in the final stage of peptidoglycan synthesis. One or more of these proteins would function as a transpeptidase that catalyzes the final cross-linking step, and others serve as carboxypeptidases or other enzymes that also act on cell wall precursors, but the function(s) of most penicillin-binding proteins in cell wall synthesis and remodeling is currently unknown.

The bactericidal effect of penicillin is an indirect process rather than a direct consequence of inhibition of wall synthesis. Penicillin-induced inhibition of peptidoglycan synthesis is followed by activation of an autolytic enzyme system within the bacterium. It is presumed that this system normally functions to break down the cell wall at points of growth or cell division; when triggered by penicillin, however, the autolytic system functions more extensively and is responsible for cell death and lysis. Mutants of bacteria that are defective in the autolytic system may demonstrate the phenomenon of tolerance; that is, their growth is inhibited by penicillin, but the cells are not killed.

Cell Membrane

The bacterial cytoplasmic membrane is an important regulator of the internal environment of the cell. The polymyxins are cationic detergents with specificity for polyphosphate-binding sites in bacterial membranes. Because disruption of the membrane is a lethal event, these antibiotics are bactericidal. However, mammalian cell membranes also bind the polymyxins, and as a result, these antibiotics are toxic.

DNA Synthesis and Replication

Novobiocin, nalidixic acid, and the fluoroquinolone antimicrobials inhibit the replication of bacterial deoxyribonucleic acid (DNA), prob-

ably through interaction with the complex formed by DNA and the enzyme DNA gyrase. Despite intensive investigation, the precise mechanism of action of these drugs is not completely understood. At low concentrations the fluoroquinolones are bactericidal, but at very high concentrations ribonucleic acid (RNA) and protein synthesis are also inhibited, and they become bacteriostatic.

DNA-Dependent RNA Polymerase

Rifampin selectively inhibits the enzyme DNA-dependent RNA polymerase, which catalyzes the transcription of genetic information onto messenger RNA (mRNA). Against most bacterial species this effect is bactericidal.

Protein Synthesis

A number of antibiotics inhibit bacterial protein synthesis by binding to ribosomes and blocking translation of mRNA. The bacterial ribosome is smaller than its mammalian counterpart and consists of two subunits, designated *50s* and *30s.* Four antibiotics bind to the *50s* subunit: erythromycins, clindamycin, lincomycin, and chloramphenicol. It appears that all four may share a similar binding site. Clindamycin, lincomycin, and chloramphenicol block the transfer of new amino acids onto the growing polypeptide chain, whereas erythromycin inhibits the translocation of the ribosomes on mRNA. These effects on protein synthesis are usually bacteriostatic.

Tetracycline and the aminoglycosidic aminocyclitols bind to the 30s ribosomal subunit. Tetracycline prevents attachment of the transfer RNA–amino acid complex and is bacteriostatic. The aminoglycosides bind irreversibly to the ribosome and cause cell death, although the exact mechanism of their bactericidal action is not entirely clear.

Folic Acid Metabolism

Most bacteria are unable to utilize preformed folic acid from their environment and rely on synthesis of tetrahydrofolate from para-aminobenzoic acid (PABA). The sulfonamides are structural analogs of PABA and competitively inhibit the first step in this process, that is, the conversion of PABA to dihydrofolic acid in the presence of dihydropteroate synthetase. Trimethoprim blocks a subsequent step (i.e., the reduction of dihydrofolate to tetrahydrofolate) by inhibiting the enzyme dihydrofolate reductase. Although these agents are bacteriostatic when given individually, in combination they are frequently synergistic and bactericidal.

Miscellaneous Mechanisms

Methenamine is a condensation product of formaldehyde and ammonia. It dissociates to release free ammonia and formaldehyde only at a pH of 5.5 or less. This characteristic restricts its antibacterial effect to the urinary tract and then only in an acid urine. Nitrofurantoin, another agent used in treatment of urinary tract infections, acts by a mechanism as yet incompletely defined.

MECHANISMS OF ANTIMICROBIAL RESISTANCE

Bacterial resistance to an antibiotic may be either an intrinsic property of a species or an acquired characteristic of an individual organism. Acquired resistance may result either from a chromosomal mutation or from the acquisition of exogenous DNA on a resistance plasmid, an extrachromosomal piece of DNA that codes for antibiotic-resistance genes, or on a transposon, a segment of DNA capable of insertion into either the bacterial chromosome or resident plasmids, or both. Most acquired resistance in clinical isolates is plasmid mediated. Mechanisms of antimicrobial resistance may be broadly viewed in four major classes.

Decreased Permeability

Decreased permeability to an antibiotic is a common cause of intrinsic resistance. Examples include the resistance of gram-negative bacilli by virtue of the relatively impermeable outer cell envelope to penicillin G, erythromycin, clindamycin, and vancomycin; the resistance of streptococci to the aminoglycosidic aminocyclitols; and the resistance of all gram-positive organisms to the polymyxins.

Acquired changes in permeability are usually the result of mutational events under selective antibiotic pressure. Examples include the small-colony variants of *Staphylococcus aureus* with decreased uptake of gentamicin, and the gram-negative bacilli with broad aminoglycoside resistance as a result of altered uptake of these agents.

Active Efflux

In the past, tetracycline resistance has been cited as an example of a plasmid-mediated alteration of antibiotic uptake. However, it is now known that the resistance determinant mediates an active efflux system for the antibiotic rather than affecting drug entry per se. Thus, although the net result of this resistance system is diminished intracellular levels of antibiotic, active removal rather than impaired entry accounts for this result. Efflux systems have now been shown to account for resistance to fluoroquinolones and other antimicrobials in some organisms.

Alteration or Inactivation of the Antibiotic

Alteration or inactivation of the antibiotic is the most common mechanism of acquired antimicrobial resistance and is frequently plasmid mediated. Several examples are found in both gram-positive and gram-negative organisms.

Beta-Lactamases. Acquired resistance to the beta-lactam antibiotics (the penicillins and cephalosporins) is largely determined by the production of enzymes (beta-lactamases) that hydrolyze the beta-lactam ring and inactivate the corresponding antibiotic. The genetic information for these enzymes may be carried either on the chromosome or on a plasmid, and their production may be either constitutive (produced at a constant rate) or inducible in the presence of an appropriate substrate.

The resistance of *S. aureus* to penicillin G was recognized in the 1940s, shortly after the introduction of penicillin into clinical use. Resistant strains were characterized by a plasmid-mediated inducible penicillinase that cleaved the beta-lactam ring of penicillin G. This staphylococcal beta-lactamase proved to have a narrow range of substrate specificity, and compounds such as the "penicillinase-resistant" penicillins (e.g., methicillin, nafcillin, oxacillin) and the cephalospo-

rins were resistant to inactivation; these compounds rapidly became the preferred agents for therapy of infections attributable to penicillinase-producing staphylococci. Although four physicochemically distinct beta-lactamases have been described in staphylococci, all appear to have similar substrate ranges and clinical significance.

The situation in gram-negative bacilli, however, is much more complicated, and many different types of beta-lactamases have been described. Unlike the gram-positive penicillinase, which has a narrow spectrum, these enzymes frequently have a broad substrate range and may be active against most of the available beta-lactam antibiotics. The development of beta-lactamase–resistant semisynthetic derivatives effective against gram-negative bacilli that produce these enzymes has been much more difficult than for *S. aureus*. The introduction of a new derivative has often been followed by prompt recognition of a beta-lactamase capable of inactivating it.

Important features of the gram-negative beta-lactamases are their broad dissemination and relative ease of transfer, both within and between species. The widespread emergence of high-level penicillin and ampicillin resistance in *Haemophilus influenzae* and *Neisseria gonorrhoeae* is the result of acquisition by these organisms of a beta-lactamase common in enteric gram-negative bacilli. Although rare, this enzyme has also been detected in penicillin-resistant clinical isolates of *Neisseria meningitidis*.

Chloramphenicol Acetyltransferase. Plasmid-mediated resistance to chloramphenicol is common in staphylococci, streptococci, and gram-negative bacilli. The mechanism of resistance involves inactivation of the antibiotic by plasmid-mediated acetylating enzymes.

Aminoglycoside-Modifying Enzymes. The aminoglycosides are important antibiotics in the treatment of gram-negative bacillary infections. Increasing resistance to the aminoglycosides, however, paralleled their increased use in clinical medicine. Resistance of clinical isolates to the aminoglycosides is largely determined by plasmid-mediated production of aminoglycoside-modifying enzymes. The following types of modification have been described:

1. Phosphorylation of hydroxyl (-OH) groups, with adenosine triphosphate as the phosphate donor
2. Adenylylation of hydroxyl groups, with adenosine triphosphate as the nucleotide donor
3. Acetylation of amino groups (-NH$_2$), with acetyl coenzyme A as the acetyl donor

Because the aminoglycosides contain many hydroxyl and amino groups potentially available for modification, a number of different aminoglycoside-modifying enzymes have been described. Bacterial strains are generally resistant to aminoglycosides against which their modifying enzymes are active. Semisynthetic aminoglycosides such as netilmicin and amikacin have been specifically tailored to resist modification by the more common enzymes, which enhances their spectrum against many plasmid-containing strains.

Alteration in the Target Site

Resistance to an antimicrobial may also result from a change in the target site at which it acts. This resistance may take one of three forms.

Increased Concentration of a Competing Substance. Sulfonamide inhibition of dihydropteroate synthetase may be overcome by increased concentrations of PABA, the natural substrate of the enzyme. A direct increase in PABA production is a mechanism of sulfonamide resistance in *S. aureus* and *N. gonorrhoeae*.

Synthesis of a Resistant Target. Bacteria may acquire a target resistant to antimicrobial action either by a mutation in the structural gene for that target or by plasmid-mediated modification of the target site. For example, rifampin resistance, is mediated by a chromosomal mutation in the structural gene for the RNA polymerase such that it no longer effectively binds rifampin. There are similar mechanisms for quinolone resistance in gram-positive and gram-negative bacteria, penicillin and sulfonamide resistance in pneumococci, and streptomycin resistance in enterococci.

Plasmid-mediated modification of a target site is exemplified by erythromycin and clindamycin resistance in *S. aureus*. In this situation the plasmid codes for an enzyme that methylates adenine residues in the ribosomal RNA of the *50s* ribosomal subunit. This alteration of the *50s* subunit blocks binding by erythromycin and clindamycin and confers resistance to these antibiotics.

Resistance to vancomycin in enterococci (which may be encoded by genes on plasmids or on the chromosome) is due in part to the production of a ligase with altered specificity that causes synthesis of cell wall precursors that do not have the D-ala-D-ala terminal pentapeptide sequence to which vancomycin normally binds.

Synthesis of an Alternative Target. Plasmid-mediated sulfonamide resistance in *Escherichia coli* results from the production of a second dihydropteroate synthetase enzyme, which is encoded by the plasmid and insensitive to sulfonamide inhibition. A similar mechanism of plasmid-mediated trimethoprim resistance (an altered dihydrofolate reductase) is also well established.

CHOICE OF APPROPRIATE ANTIMICROBIAL AGENTS

Armed with the basic information outlined here, the clinician can proceed to choose an appropriate antimicrobial agent for a given clinical setting. The following factors enter into the choice: (1) the identification of the infecting organism or a clinical estimate of the probability that a given organism is present, (2) knowledge of the antimicrobial susceptibilities of the organism(s), and (3) consideration of host factors that may affect the efficacy or toxicity of particular antimicrobial agents.

Identification of the Organism

In cases of suspected bacterial infection, cultures of appropriate sites should always be obtained before antibiotic therapy is begun. The results of these studies, however, are ordinarily not available for 24 to 48 hours. In situations in which immediate antimicrobial therapy is warranted, more rapid identification of the infecting organism is needed. Gram's stain smear of clinically infected material may provide useful preliminary information. Even if the appearance of Gram's stain is not diagnostic of a particular organism, it may limit the possibilities and guide initial choice of an antibiotic regimen. In fluids that are normally sterile, detection of bacterial antigens may be useful.

In certain situations no material will be available for either Gram's stain examination or attempts at bacterial antigen detection. In these cases the physician must use clinical experience in arriving at an estimate of the possible infecting organisms. For example, in a young child who comes to medical attention with acute otitis media the likely pathogens would be a virus, *H. influenzae,* the pneumococcus, or a group A streptococcus. Knowing these probabilities, the physician could choose appropriate initial antimicrobial therapy directed at this spectrum. Information presented in the later chapters on clinical infectious disease syndromes is of help in selecting appropriate initial antimicrobial therapy in patients in whom rapid presumptive identification of the pathogen cannot be made.

Antimicrobial Susceptibility Testing

Once an infecting organism has been either presumptively or definitely identified, knowledge of its antimicrobial susceptibilities is helpful. There is significant local variation in the pattern of antibiotic susceptibilities of most bacterial pathogens, and the physician should be aware of the latest information available in his or her particular area. Table 231-1 presents a listing of useful antimicrobials for infections caused by a variety of pathogens.

For certain organisms susceptibility to particular antibiotics can be reliably predicted, and specific testing is usually not necessary. For example, the group A streptococcus is uniformly sensitive to penicillins and cephalosporins at present. If erythromycin is used to treat a streptococcal infection, however, susceptibility to this drug should be determined because resistance is known to occur. In addition, some species that previously did not require susceptibility testing are now routinely checked because of the recent emergence of antibiotic resistance. The pneumococcus, for example, is checked for penicillin susceptibility when isolated from spinal fluid or blood, based on the worldwide appearance of strains that are resistant or relatively resis-

tant to penicillin. Similarly, *H. influenzae* is now routinely screened for ampicillin resistance because of the acquisition of a beta-lactamase, which has led to ampicillin resistance in as many as 40% of strains isolated in certain parts of the United States.

The organisms most frequently tested for antibiotic susceptibilities are the gram-negative bacilli and *S. aureus.* These organisms have a variety of antimicrobial resistance mechanisms, and susceptibility cannot be reliably predicted without specific testing. In addition, therapeutic choices may be limited or may involve the use of toxic agents. Susceptibility testing is mandatory to optimize these decisions.

A common method of susceptibility testing in the clinical laboratory is the disk-diffusion, or Bauer-Kirby, method. In this procedure a suspension of the bacterium to be tested is adjusted to a standard density and inoculated on the surface of a Mueller-Hinton agar plate. Filter paper disks impregnated with standard amounts of antibiotics are placed on the surface of the plate, which is then incubated overnight at 35° C. The diameter of the zone of inhibition around each antibiotic disk is measured and compared with a reference value. Organisms are scored as susceptible, intermediate, or resistant, based on the zone sizes of a large number of control organisms with known quantitative susceptibilities. A susceptible organism is one that is inhibited by a concentration of antibiotic achievable in serum (for most drugs) or urine (for drugs such as sulfonamides, nitrofurantoin, and nalidixic acid, the use of which is largely restricted to treatment of urinary tract infections). The disk-diffusion method is well suited for screening large numbers of organisms but provides only semiquantitative information and is not applicable to slowly growing or fastidious organisms.

Quantitative antibiotic susceptibilities may be determined by either the agar or broth dilution technique. The latter is now widely available for use in clinical laboratories with the advent of commercially prepared microdilution panels. Serial dilutions of antibiotic are made in either agar or broth medium, and a standard inoculum of bacteria is added. The lowest concentration of antibiotic preventing any visible growth after overnight incubation is termed the *minimum inhibitory concentration.* With the broth dilution method the inhibited tubes can then be subcultured for the determination of the minimum bactericidal concentration (i.e., the lowest concentration of antibiotic that achieves a specific level of killing, typically 99.9% of the original inoculum). Determination of quantitative susceptibilities may be important in infections that are difficult to eradicate, such as endocarditis (Chapter 24) and osteomyelitis (Chapter 243).

Host Factors

Despite precise identification of an infecting organism and determination of its antimicrobial susceptibility, several factors related to the host are of paramount importance in choosing an antimicrobial.

History of Allergy or Previous Reaction. Patients with a history of a major adverse reaction to an antibiotic should not ordinarily receive that agent again. Allergy to one member of an antibiotic class, such as the penicillin family, ordinarily implies allergy to all members of that group. Patients with a history of penicillin allergy may tolerate cephalosporins given cautiously if the past allergy was not immediate or life threatening. However, cross-allergenicity has been reported between these two groups of compounds.

Age. Even in patients without clinical evidence of renal disease, there is a progressive decrease in glomerular filtration (measured as creatinine clearance) with age. Because muscle mass also diminishes with age, the serum creatinine level often remains normal in this circumstance. For this reason, antimicrobials with a predominantly renal mechanism of excretion (see Impaired Renal Function) must often be administered to elderly patients in diminished dosage. In addition, the incidence of adverse effects associated with many antimicrobials increases with age. An example is isoniazid hepatitis, which is very unusual in patients younger than the age of 20 years but may occur in more than 2% of patients older than age 50 years.

Genetic and Metabolic Disorders. Deficiency of the enzyme glucose-6-phosphate dehydrogenase may be associated with hemo-

Table 231-1 Antimicrobial drugs of choice*

INFECTING ORGANISM	ANTIMICROBIAL OF CHOICE	ALTERNATIVE DRUGS
Gram-positive cocci		
Staphylococcus aureus or *Staphylococcus epidermidis*		
Nonpenicillinase-producing	Penicillin G or V	Cephalosporin,† vancomycin, clindamycin, erythromycin
Penicillinase-producing	Penicillinase-resistant penicillin‡	Cephalosporin,† vancomycin, clindamycin, erythromycin, imipenem
Methicillin-resistant	Vancomycin (±gentamicin and/or rifampin)	Trimethoprim-sulfamethoxazole, minocycline
Beta streptococci (groups A, B, C, G)	Penicillin G or V	Erythromycin, cephalosporin,† vancomycin
Streptococcus, viridans group	Penicillin G	Cephalosporin,† vancomycin, erythromycin
Streptococcus bovis	Penicillin G	Cephalosporin,† vancomycin, erythromycin
Enterococci		
Uncomplicated urinary tract infection	Ampicillin or amoxicillin	Nitrofurantoin, quinolone¶
Endocarditis or other serious infection	Penicillin G (or ampicillin) plus gentamicin or streptomycin	Vancomycin plus gentamicin or streptomycin
Pneumococci	Penicillin G or V	Erythromycin, cephalosporin,† chloramphenicol, vancomycin
Gram-negative cocci		
Neisseria gonorrhoeae	Ceftriaxone	Amoxicillin, penicillin G, spectinomycin, cefoxitin, cefixime, cefpodoxime, cefuroxime, cefotaxime, ceftizoxime, quinolone,¶ erythromycin
Neisseria meningitidis	Penicillin G	Chloramphenicol, cefuroxime, ceftriaxone, ceftizoxime, cefotaxime, sulfonamide, trimethoprim-sulfamethoxazole
Gram-positive bacilli		
Bacillus anthracis (anthrax)	Penicillin G	Erythromycin, tetracycline
Corynebacterium diphtheriae	Erythromycin	Penicillin G
Listeria monocytogenes	Ampicillin or penicillin G ±gentamicin)	Trimethoprim-sulfamethoxazole, chloramphenicol, tetracycline, erythromycin
Gram-negative bacilli		
Acinetobacter sp.	Imipenem, meropenem	Aminoglycoside,§ broad spectrum penicillin, trimethoprim-sulfamethoaxazole, doxycycline
Bordetella pertussis (whooping cough)	Erythromycin	Trimethoprim-sulfamethoxazole
Brucella sp. (brucellosis)	Doxycycline (±gentamicin)	Doxycycline (±streptomycin), doxycycline + rifampin, trimethoprim-sulfamethoxazole (±rifampin or aminoglycoside)
Campylobacter jejuni	Erythromycin	Tetracycline, gentamicin, quinolone¶
Enterobacter sp.	Aminoglycoside,§ imipenem broad spectrum penicillin,‖ trimethoprim-sulfamethoxazole, quinolone¶	Chloramphenicol, tetracycline
Escherichia coli		
Uncomplicated urinary tract infection	Trimethoprim-sulfamethoxazole or amoxicillin clavulante	Cephalosporin,† tetracycline, ampicillin, amoxicillin, trimethoprim, quinolone¶
Systemic infection	Aminoglycoside§ or cephalosporin†	Ampicillin,† broad-spectrum penicillin,‖ trimethoprim-sulfamethoxazole, chloramphenicol, ampicillin-sulbactam, ticarcillin-clavulanate, piperacillin-tazobactam, quinolone
Francisella tularensis (Tularemia)	Streptomycin	Tetracycline, chloramphenicol
Haemophilus influenzae		
Meningitis, epiglottis, bacteremia	Ceftriaxone, cefotaxime, or ceftizoxime	Trimethoprim-sulfamethoxazole, ampicillin + chloramphenicol initially (Chapter 266)
Other infections	Ampicillin or amoxicillin, ampicillin-sulbactam, amoxicillin-clavulanate	Trimethoprim-sulfamethoxazole, cefamandole, cefixime, cefprozil, cefpodoxime, loracarbef, cefuroxime, cefonicid, cefaclor, ceftriaxone, cefotaxime, ceftizoxime, sulfonamide, tetracycline, quinolone
Klebsiella pneumoniae	Aminoglycoside§ for serious infections, cefotaxime, ceftizoxime, ceftazidime, or ceftriaxone	Cephalosporin† (for serious infections, cefotaxime, ceftizoxime, ceftazidime, or ceftriaxone), ampicillin-sulbactam, trimethoprim-sulfamethoxazole, quinolone,¶ extended spectrum penicillin, chloramphenicol, tetracycline, ticarcillin-clavulanate, piperacillin-tazobactan, imipenem
Legionella pneumophila	Erythromycin	Add rifampin, quinolone
Pasteurella multocida	Penicillin G	Tetracycline, cephalosporin,† amoxicillin-clavulanate
Proteus mirabilis	Ampicillin	Cephalosporin,† aminoglycoside,§ broad spectrum penicillin,‖ trimethoprim-sulfamethoxazole, chloramphenicol, quinolone¶
Proteus, indole-positive	Aminoglycoside,§ cefotaxime, ceftizoxime, ceftriaxone, ceftazidime	Ticarcillin-clavulanate, broad-spectrum penicillin,‖ trimethoprim-sulfamethoxazole, chloramphenicol, tetracycline, quinolone,¶ imipenem, piperacillin-tazobactam

*Not all drugs listed are approved for that indication by the U.S. Food and Drug Administration. Antimicrobial susceptibility testing should be performed whenever possible. Not all drugs of a class can be used interchangeably, and some of the drugs listed may not be appropriate in specific settings.

†A first-generation cephalosporin is generally preferred for staphylococcal infections. Gram-negative bacilli may be more susceptible to second- or third-generation agents. Third-generation cephalosporins (cefotaxime and ceftriaxone) have been used for treating infections caused by penicillin-insensitive strains of pneumococci.

‡Methicillin, nafcillin, oxacillin, cloxacillin, dicloxacillin.

§Gentamicin, tobramycin, netilmicin, amikacin.

¶Ciprofloxacin, ofloxacin, levofloxacin, sparfloxacin, lomefloxacin (limited indications); norfloxacin, enoxacin (urinary tract infections only).

‖Mezlocillin, piperacillin.

Continued

Table 231-1   Antimicrobial drugs of choice*—cont'd

INFECTING ORGANISM	ANTIMICROBIAL OF CHOICE	ALTERNATIVE DRUGS
Pseudomonas aeruginosa		
Urinary infection	Broad-spectrum penicillin,‖ quinolone¶	Aminoglycoside,§ ceftazidime, imipenem
Other infection	Aminoglycoside§ ±broad-spectrum penicillin‖	Ceftazidime ±aminoglycoside, imipenem ±aminoglycoside, ciprofloxacin
Salmonella sp.	Quinolone¶ or ceftriaxone or cefotaxime	Ampicillin, amoxicillin, chloramphenicol, trimethoprim-sulfamethoxazole
Serratia marcescens	Aminoglycoside§ or cefotaxime, ceftazidime, ceftizoxime	Trimethoprim-sulfamethoxazole, broad-spectrum penicillin,‖ chloramphenicol, quinolone,† imipenem
Shigella sp.	Quinolone¶	Trimethoprime-sulfamethoxazole, ampicillin, chloramphenicol, tetracycline
Yersinia pestis (plague)	Streptomycin	Tetracycline, chloramphenicol
Anaerobes		
Anaerobic streptococci	Penicillin G	Clindamycin, chloramphenicol, cephalosporin,† erythromycin
Bacteroides sp.		
Oropharyngeal strains	Penicillin G	Clindamycin, cefoxitin, chloramphenicol, metronidazole, cefotetan, cefmetazole, imipenem, ampicillin-sulbactam, ticarcillin-clavulanate, piperacillin-tazobactam
Gastrointestinal strains	Clindamycin or metronidazole	Cefoxitin, chloramphenicol, cefotetan, cefmetazole, imipenem, ampicillin-sulbactam, ticarcillin-clavulanate, piperacillin-tazobactam
Clostridium perfringens	Penicillin G	Chloramphenicol, clindamycin, metronidazole

lytic episodes in response to oxidant stress. Antibiotics that may cause hemolysis in patients with this deficiency include the sulfonamides, nitrofurantoin, nalidixic acid, and chloramphenicol.

The rate of liver metabolism of certain drugs (e.g., isoniazid) is genetically determined. Persons who are "slow acetylators" of isoniazid have higher and more prolonged blood levels of the parent compound than others and an associated higher risk of isoniazid peripheral neuropathy. Persons who are "rapid acetylators," on the other hand, generate greater amounts of a toxic metabolite and may be more prone to the development of isoniazid hepatitis.

Patients with diabetes mellitus, especially those with associated vascular disease, may absorb intramuscular medications very poorly; if parenteral administration of a drug is required, the intravenous route is preferred in the diabetic patient. In addition, certain antibiotics (e.g., the sulfonamides, chloramphenicol) may potentiate the effect of oral hypoglycemic agents and should be used with caution in diabetic patients receiving these drugs.

Pregnancy and Lactation. Virtually all antibiotics cross the placenta and, as with other medications, should be avoided during pregnancy unless absolutely indicated. Moreover, certain antibiotics are associated with specific risks in this setting, and an alternative should be used if antimicrobial therapy is necessary. Trimethoprim and rifampin are teratogenic in rodents, and metronidazole is mutagenic in vitro; these agents should be avoided during gestation. The tetracyclines, including both minocycline and doxycycline, bind to growing bone and teeth. This effect may result in dysplastic changes of bone or enamel and discoloration of the teeth. In addition, pregnant women have an increased risk of tetracycline-induced hepatotoxicity. Because many alternatives are available, these agents should be avoided throughout pregnancy. The sulfonamides are probably safe in early pregnancy but should be discontinued before delivery. In fetal serum they compete with unconjugated bilirubin for albumin-binding sites and may increase the risk of kernicterus in the neonate. The aminoglycosides carry the theoretic risk of toxicity to the developing fetal ear. This risk has been documented only with streptomycin, however, and the ototoxicity was mild. Thus, if these agents are required for the treatment of severe infections, they probably are reasonably safe in the latter half of pregnancy.

When therapy with an antibiotic is required in the pregnant woman, certain agents are preferred for use. These agents include the penicillins, the cephalosporins, and erythromycin. It is recommended that clarithromycin not be used in pregnancy unless there is no alternative, because of adverse outcomes in various animal species. Data on other agents, such as clindamycin, chloramphenicol, vancomycin, and nitrofurantoin, are insufficient for an assessment of their safety during pregnancy.

The nursing mother also warrants special consideration in the selection of an antimicrobial agent. Many antibiotics appear in breast milk if administered to lactating women and may be associated with adverse effects in the infant; for example, because of the risk of kernicterus, sulfonamides should be avoided shortly after delivery if the mother is breast-feeding. Nitrofurantoin, nalidixic acid, and the sulfonamides may cause hemolysis in the infant with glucose-6-phosphate dehydrogenase deficiency. Chloramphenicol may reach relatively high levels in breast milk, which could result in the "gray syndrome" in a nursing infant. Perhaps the best approach is to discontinue breast-feeding temporarily during antibiotic administration while maintaining milk flow via a breast pump. When the antibiotic course is complete, breast-feeding may then be resumed.

Impaired Renal Function. The clinical use of drugs that are excreted primarily by the kidney may be affected in at least three ways by impairment of renal function. First, the dosage schedule for several of these antimicrobials must be changed. Table 231-2 presents dosage recommendations for the major antibiotics and suggested modifications in patients with various degrees of renal impairment. Second, the risk of toxicity associated with a drug may increase in patients with delayed excretion. Examples include impaired platelet function attributable to carbenicillin, tetracycline hepatotoxicity, and peripheral neuropathy caused by nitrofurantoin. Third, the efficacy of an agent in treating urinary tract infections may diminish as the rate of glomerular filtration of the drug falls. This is particularly important for the "urinary antiseptics" nitrofurantoin, nalidixic acid, and methenamine. Because of these considerations, an antimicrobial with a nonrenal route of excretion may be preferable for systemic infections in the patient with severe renal impairment.

Impaired Hepatic Function. Drugs that are predominantly metabolized in the liver should be used with caution in the patient with hepatic insufficiency. Included in this group are erythromycin, chloramphenicol, and clindamycin. In addition, the tetracyclines may exacerbate preexisting liver disease, and their use in this setting requires careful monitoring.

Site of Infection. To be effective, an antimicrobial agent must reach the site of an infection in a concentration adequate to inhibit the bacterial pathogen. For mild infections this goal can often be achieved with oral therapy. For more serious infections, however, the parenteral route is usually preferable. For infections in the pleural, pericardial, peritoneal, and synovial spaces, antibiotic penetration is relatively good, and parenteral administration of an effective drug is usually adequate for cure; direct, local instillation of the antibiotic is not necessary. For other sites of infection, however, antibiotic penetration is more marginal, and cure may require either the use of high-

Table 231-2   Dosage of antimicrobial agents

DRUG	NORMAL UNIT ADULT DOSE (ROUTE)	NORMAL DOSE INTERVAL (H)	ADJUSTED MAXIMUM DOSE IN RENAL FAILURE			REMOVAL BY DIALYSIS
			GFR >50 ML/MIN	GFR 10-50 ML/MIN	GFR <10 ML/MIN	
Aminoglycosides						
Gentamicin, tobramycin[a]	1.0-1.7 mg/kg (IM,IV)	8	1.0-1.7 mg/kg q(8 × creatinine)h or (1.0-1.7 mg/kg ÷ creatinine) q8h[b]			Yes(H,P)[c]
Netilmicin[a]	1.3-2.2 mg/kg (IM,IV)	8	1.3-2.2 mg/kg q(8 × creatinine)h or (1.3-2.2 mg/kg ÷ creatinine) q8h[b]			Yes(H,P)[d]
Kanamycin, amikacin[a]	5 mg/kg (IM,IV)	8	5 mg/kg q(8 × creatinine)h or (5 mg/kg ÷ creatinine) q8h[b]			Yes(H,P)[e]
Azithromycin	250-500 mg (PO)	24	Unknown	Unknown	Unknown	Unknown
Carbapenems, carbacephems						
Imipenem	0.5-1 g (IV)	6	0.5 g q6h[f]	0.5 g q8-12h	0.25-0.5 g q12h[g]	Yes(H)
Loracarbef	0.20-0.40 g (PO)	12	NC	0.20 g q12-24h	0.20 g q72-120h	Yes(H)
Cephalosporins						
Cefaclor	0.25-0.5 g (PO)	8	NC	NC	NC	Yes(H)
Cefadroxil	0.5-1.0 g (PO)	12	NC	0.5 g q12-24h	0.5 g q36h	Yes(H)
Cefamandole	1-2 g(IM,IV)	4	1-2 g q6h	1-2 g q6-8h	0.5-1.0 g q8-12h	Yes(H), No(P)
Cefazolin	0.5-1.5 g (IM,IV)	8	0.5-1.0 g q8h	0.5-1.0 g q12h	0.5-1.0 g q24-48h	Yes(H), No(P)
Cefixime	400 mg (PO)	24	NC[i]	300 mg q24h[j]	200 mg q24h[k]	No(H,P)
Cefmetazole	2 g (IV)	6-12	1-2 g q12h	1-2 g q16-24h	1-2 g q48h	Yes(H)
Cefonicid	1-2 g (IM,IV)	24	NC	1 g q24-48h	0.25-1.0 g q72-120h	No(H)
Cefoperazone	1-3 g (IM,IV)	8	NC	NC	NC	Yes(H)
Ceforanide	0.5-1.0 g (IM,IV)	12	NC	1 g q24-48h	1 g q48-72h	Yes(H), No(P)
Cefotaxime	1-2 g (IM,IV)	6	NC	1-2 g q6-12h	1-2 g q12-24h	Yes(H)
Cefotetan	2 g (IV,IM)	12	NC	1-2 g q12-24h	1-2 g q48h	Yes(H)
Cefoxitin	1-2 g (IM,IV)	4	1-2 g q6h	1-2 g q8-24h	0.5-1.0 g q12-48h[n]	Yes(H), No(P)
Cefpodoxime	0.10-0.40 g (PO)	12	NC	NC	125-250 mg q12-24h	Yes(H)
Cefprozil	250-500 mg (PO)	12-24	NC	125-250 mg q12-24h[h]	0.5-2.0 g q36-48h	Yes(H,P)
Ceftazidime	0.5-2.0 g (IM,IV)	8	0.5-2.0 g q8h	0.5-2.0 g q12-24h	0.5 g q12-24h	Yes(H,P)
Ceftizoxime	1-2 g (IM,IV)	6	NC	1-2 g q12h	NC[a]	No(H)
Ceftriaxone	1-2 g (IM,IV)	12-24	NC	NC	0.75 g q24h	Yes(H,P)
Cefuroxime	0.75-1.5 g (IM,IV)	6-8	NC	0.75-1.5 g q8-12h	NC	Yes(H,P)
Cephalexin	0.25-0.5 g (PO)	6	NC	NC	1 g q8-12h	Yes(H,P)
Cephalothin	1-2 g (IV)	4	1-2 g q6h	1-2 g q6h	1 g q8-12h	Yes(H,P)
Cephapirin	1-2 g (IV)	4	1-2 g q6h	1-2g q6h	1 g q12h	Yes(H,P)
Cephradine	1-2 g (IV)	4	1-2 g q6h	1 g q6h	NC	Yes(H,P)
Chloramphenicol	0.25-0.5 g (PO); 0.25-1.0 g (PO,IV)	6	NC	NC	NC	Yes(H), No(P)

GFR, Glomerular filtration rate; *H,* hemodialysis; *P,* peritoneal dialysis; *NC,* no change; *TMP,* trimethoprim.

[a]Serum level monitoring is recommended for therapy of the patient with renal impairment.
[b]When using the latter formula, a normal unit dose is necessary initially. Both formulas are valid estimates only if serum creatinine reflects GFR accurately.
[c]Following an initial loading dose, therapeutic levels can be maintained by administering a dose of 1 mg/kg after each hemodialysis or by adding 5 μg/ml to the peritoneal dialysis fluid.
[d]Following an initial loading dose, therapeutic levels can be maintained by administering a dose of 1.5 mg/kg after each hemodialysis or by adding 7.5 μg/ml to the peritoneal dialysis fluid.
[e]Following an initial loading dose, therapeutic levels can be maintained by administering a dose of 3.5 mg/kg after each hemodialysis or by adding 20 μg/ml to the peritoneal dialysis fluid.
[f]Dose adjustment generally required for creatinine clearance (C_{cr}) <70 ml/min/1.73 m².
[g]This range applies to C_{cr} 6-20 ml/min/1.73 m²; the upper range may be associated with increased risk of seizures. The drug should not be used when C_{cr} ≤ 5 ml/min/1.73 m² unless the patient is on hemodialysis.
[h]50% standard dose recommended for GFR ≤ 30 ml/min.
[i]If C_{cr} ≥ 60 ml/min.
[j]If C_{cr} 21-60 ml/min.
[k]If C_{cr} <20 ml/min.
[l]If C_{cr} 30-50 ml/min.
[m]If C_{cr} 5-29 ml/min.
[n]Administer dose q24h for C_{cr} < 30ml/min; for patients on hemodialysis, dose three times weekly after dialysis.
[o]Avoid if C_{cr} < 60 ml/min.

Table 231-2   Dosage of antimicrobial agents

DRUG	NORMAL UNIT ADULT DOSE (ROUTE)	NORMAL DOSE INTERVAL (H)	ADJUSTED MAXIMUM DOSE IN RENAL FAILURE			REMOVAL BY DIALYSIS
			GFR >50 ML/MIN	GFR 10-50 ML/MIN	GFR <10 ML/MIN	
Clarithromycin	250-500 mg (PO)	12	NC	250-500 mg q12-24h	250-500 mg q24h	Unknown
Clindamycin	0.6 g (IM,IV)	6-8	NC	NC	NC	No(H,P)
Erythromycin	0.15-0.3 g (PO)	6	NC	NC	NC	No(H,P)
	0.5-1.0 g (IV)	6	NC	NC	NC	
Metronidazole	0.25-0.5 g (PO)	6	NC	NC	NC	Yes(H), No(P)
	15 mg/kg load (IV), then 7.5 mg/kg (IV)	6				
Monobactams						
Aztreonam	1-2 g (IV)	8	NC	1 g q8h	0.5 g q6-12h	Yes(H,P)
Nitrofurantoin	50-100 mg (PO)	6	NC	Avoid[o]	Avoid[o]	Yes(H)
Penicillins						
Amoxicillin	0.25-0.5 g (PO)	8	NC	0.25-0.5 g q12h	0.25 g q12h	Yes(H), No(P)
Ampicillin	0.5-2.0 g (IM,IV)	4	NC	0.5-2.0 g q8h	0.5-2.0 g q12h	Yes(H), No(P)
	0.25-0.5 g (PO)	6	NC	0.25-0.5 g q8h	0.25-0.5 g q12h	
Azlocillin	2-3 g (IM,IV)	4	NC	3 g q6h	3 g q12h	Yes(H), No(P)
Carbenicillin	2-5 g (IM,IV)	4	NC	2-5 g q6h	2 g q8-12h	Yes (H,P)
Indanyl-carbenicillin	0.5-1.0 g (PO)	6	NC	NC	Avoid	No(H,P)
Cloxacillin	0.25-0.5 g (PO)	6	NC	NC	NC	No(H,P)
Dicloxacillin	0.25-0.5 g (PO)	6	NC	NC	NC	No(H,P)
Methicillin	1-2 g (IM,IV)	4	NC	NC	1-2 g q8-12h	Yes(H), No(P)
Mezlocillin	2-3 g (IM,IV)	6	NC	3 g q6-8h	2 g q6-8h	Yes(H), No(P)
Nafcillin	1-2 g (IM,IV)	4	NC	NC	NC	No(H,P)
Oxacillin	1-2 g (IM,IV)	4	NC	NC	NC	No(H,P)
Penicillin G	0.4-4.0 million units (IM,IV)	6	NC	NC	2 million units q4h	Yes(H), No(P)
Penicillin V	0.25-0.5 g (PO)	6	NC	NC	NC	Yes(H), No(P)
Piperacillin	2-3 g (IM,IV)	4	NC	3 g q6h	3 g q8h or 4 g q12h	Yes(H)
Ticarcillin	2-3 g (IM,IV)	4	NC	2-3 g q6h	2g q12h	Yes(H,P)
Polymyxins						
Polymyxin B	1.5-2.5 mg/kg/day (IV)	Continuous infusion	Avoid	Avoid	Avoid	No(H), Yes(P)
Colistin	0.8-1.7 mg/kg (IM)	8	Avoid	Avoid	Avoid	No(H), Yes(P)
Quinolones						
Nalidixic acid	0.5-1.0 g (PO)	6	NC	NC	Avoid	Unknown
Ciprofloxacin	250-750 mg (PO)	12	NC	250-500 mg q12h[l]	250-500 mg q18h[m]	No(<14%) (H,P)
	200-400 mg (IV)	12	NC	200-400 mg q18-24h[m]	200-400 mg q18-24h[m]	No(<14%) (H,P)
Lomefloxacin	400 mg (PO)	24	NC	200 q24h	Unknown	No(<14%) (H,P)
Norfloxacin	400 mg (PO)	12	NC	400 q24h	400 q24h	No (<14%) (H,P)
Ofloxacin	200-400 mg (PO,IV)	12	NC	200-400 mg q24h	100-200 mg q24h	Yes(H,P)
Sulfisoxazole	1 g (PO)	6	NC	1 g q8-12h	1 g q12-24h	Yes(H,P)
Tetracyclines						
Tetracycline	0.25-0.5 g (PO,IV)	6	0.25-0.5 g q8-12h	Avoid	Avoid	No(H,P)
Doxycycline	100 mg (PO,IV)	12-24	NC	NC	NC	No(H,P)
Trimethoprim-sulfamethoxazole	2-3 mg TMP/kg (IV)	6	NC	2-3 mg TMP/kg q12h	Avoid	Yes(H), No(P)
Trimethoprim	160/800 mg (PO)	12	NC	160/800 mg q24h	Avoid	Yes(H), No(P)
Vancomycin[a]	100 mg (PO)	12	NC	100 mg q24h	Avoid	No(H,P)
	1 g (IV)	12	1 g q24-72h[a]	[a]	[a]	

Table 231-3 Biliary concentration of antimicrobials*

CONCENTRATION	ANTIMICROBIAL
Exceeds serum levels	Penicillins (particularly nafcillin, ampicillin, azlocillin, mezlocillin, piperacillin), cephalosporins (particularly cefazolin, cefamandole, cefoxitin, cefoperazone, cefotaxime, moxalactam), tetracyclines (particularly doxycycline, minocycline), clindamycin, erythromycin, azithromycin, clarithromycin, metronidazole
Less than serum levels	Chloramphenicol, aminoglycosides, vancomycin, polymyxins, sulfonamides

*Assumes no obstruction is present.

dose, prolonged parenteral therapy or the direct, local instillation of the drug. Examples of these sites include the vegetations of bacterial endocarditis, areas of devitalized tissue, bone, the vitreous humor of the eye, and the cerebrospinal fluid (CSF). Knowledge of the achievable CSF concentrations of antimicrobials is an important factor in designing appropriate therapy for infections of the central nervous system (Chapters 239 and 240).

Concentration of antimicrobial agents in the bile may be an important factor in treating infections of the hepatobiliary system (Chapter 238). In Table 231-3, antibiotics are classified into two groups, based on whether biliary levels exceed those of serum in the unobstructed biliary tree. None of the antibiotics reliably achieves adequate biliary levels in the presence of obstruction, which usually requires drainage.

Almost all antimicrobial agents are concentrated in the urine (Chapter 246). The pH of the urine, however, may significantly affect the activity of particular drugs; methenamine, nitrofurantoin, and chlortetracycline are all more efficacious at an acid pH. In contrast, erythromycin, clindamycin, and the aminoglycosides are more active at an alkaline pH. In difficult therapeutic situations adjustment of the urine pH may increase the effectiveness of therapy. Antibiotic penetration of the prostate gland is not related to high urinary levels of drug. Erythromycin, trimethoprim, and various fluoroquinolones have produced satisfactory tissue levels at this site.

Host Defense Mechanisms. In the presence of normal host defense mechanisms there appears to be no difference in outcome whether patients are treated with a bactericidal or a bacteriostatic antibiotic. If host defenses are impaired, however, bacterial killing may largely depend on antibiotic action and simple bacteriostasis alone may be insufficient for cure. Such impairment of host defense may be either local, as in the vegetations of bacterial endocarditis or the open spaces of the CSF in meningitis, or global, as in the patient with neutropenia. In these situations the patient is best treated with bactericidal antibiotics.

SPECIFIC ANTIMICROBIAL AGENTS

Antimicrobial agents differ in their spectrum of activity, pharmacokinetic properties, and potential adverse effects. These considerations are important in selecting appropriate therapy.

Penicillins

Benzylpenicillin (penicillin G) was introduced into clinical use in the early 1940s. Since then, a number of derivatives of the basic penicillin nucleus have been developed in an attempt either to improve pharmacokinetic properties or to alter the spectrum of activity of the compounds. All these agents, however, share common toxic effects and cross-allergenicity.

Spectrum of Activity. Penicillin G is highly active against most gram-positive cocci, with the exceptions of penicillinase-producing *S. aureus,* the enterococci, and penicillin-resistant pneumococci. It is also effective against the following organisms: gram-positive bacilli, including *Corynebacterium diphtheriae,* variable numbers of other

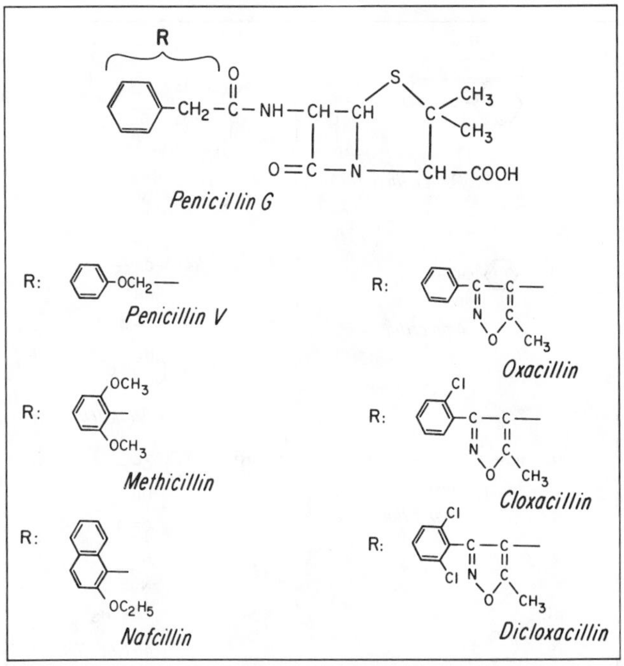

FIGURE 231-2 Structural formulas of penicillin and the penicillinase-resistant penicillins.

diphtheroids, *Listeria monocytogenes, Bacillus anthracis, and Erysipelothrix rhusiopathiae;* some gram-negative organisms, including many beta-lactamase–negative gonococci, meningococci, *Pasteurella multocida,* and *Streptobacillus moniliformis;* the spirochetes, including *Treponema pallidum,* leptospiras, and *Spirillum minus;* and most anaerobes except *Bacteroides* species. Penicillin V (phenoxymethylpenicillin) has a similar spectrum, although it is less active against some organisms (e.g., gonococci).

One of the important deficiencies in the spectrum of penicillin G is its ineffectiveness against penicillinase-producing *S. aureus.* Several derivatives of the penicillin nucleus have been developed to resist inactivation by the staphylococcal beta-lactamase; these include methicillin, nafcillin, oxacillin, cloxacillin, and dicloxacillin (Fig. 231-2). These agents are active against staphylococci, but methicillin-resistant strains, which are cross-resistant to the other penicillins and cephalosporins, have been recognized with increasing frequency in recent years. The mechanism of this resistance relates to an alteration in the penicillin-binding protein targets rather than to the production of penicillinase. The other organisms inhibited by penicillin G are generally less susceptible to the penicillinase-resistant derivatives. The high blood levels achievable with these derivatives, however, are usually sufficient to inhibit most strains. Enterococci, *Listeria,* and *Neisseria* species are exceptions; these organisms are not adequately treated with the antistaphylococcal penicillins.

Modifications have also been made in the penicillin nucleus to expand the spectrum of gram-negative coverage (Fig. 231-3); none of these broader-spectrum penicillins, however, is effective against penicillinase-producing *S. aureus.* Ampicillin and amoxicillin (as well as the closely related drugs bacampicillin and cyclacillin) provide excellent coverage for the same organisms as penicillin G. In addition, many strains of *H. influenzae, E. coli, Proteus mirabilis, and Salmonella,* and *Shigella* species are susceptible to these agents; however, resistance attributable to beta-lactamase production is now common except in *P. mirabilis,* and susceptibility testing is necessary. There is no significant difference between the spectrum of ampicillin and that of amoxicillin, except that the latter is less effective in clinical practice for shigellosis.

Carbenicillin, ticarcillin, azlocillin, mezlocillin, and piperacillin are other penicillins with enhanced spectra. Although often less active than ampicillin on a weight basis, they are effective against the same organisms. In addition, they are relatively resistant to certain

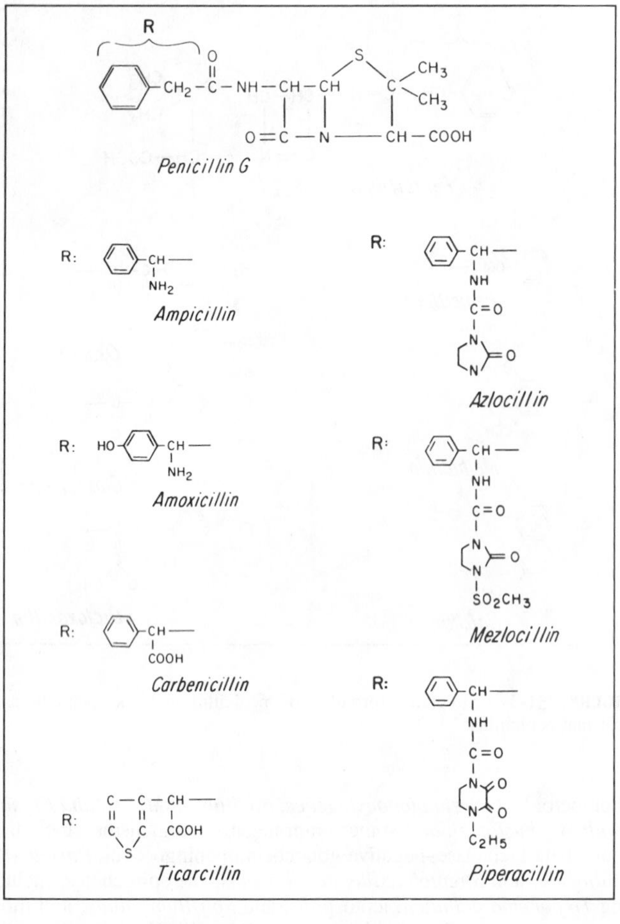

FIGURE 231-3   Structural formulas of the broader-spectrum penicillins.

gram-negative beta-lactamases and inhibit most strains of indole-positive *Proteus* species, *Enterobacter* species, and *Pseudomonas aeruginosa*. The minimum inhibitory concentrations of carbenicillin for *P. aeruginosa* are usually high (e.g., 75 to 100 µg/ml), but serum levels above this range can be achieved with high doses. Ticarcillin is twice as active by weight as carbenicillin against *P. aeruginosa* and therefore may be used in a lower dose; for other organisms the spectrum of activity of ticarcillin and carbenicillin is similar. Mezlocillin and piperacillin are more active against Enterobacteriaceae than the other two agents, particularly against strains of *Klebsiella pneumoniae*. Against strains of *P. aeruginosa,* the activity of mezlocillin parallels that of ticarcillin, whereas azlocillin and piperacillin are more active. In the treatment of serious gram-negative infections beyond the urinary tract these drugs are often combined with an aminoglycoside both to extend the antibacterial spectrum and in the hope of reducing the risk of the development of resistance.

Ampicillin has been combined with the beta-lactamase inhibitor sulbactam, both ticarcillin and amoxicillin are marketed with the beta-lactamase inhibitor potassium clavulanate, and piperacillin has been combined with tazobactam to extend the spectrum of each penicillin against some beta-lactamase–producing organisms. Such combinations typically demonstrate activity against *E. coli* and *K. pneumoniae*. These inhibitors are inactive against the chromosomal beta-lactamases of several gram-negative bacilli, which are troublesome nosocomial pathogens, such as *Enterobacter* species and *P. aeruginosa*.

Pharmacokinetics. Penicillin G is unstable in gastric acid and therefore unreliably absorbed by the oral route. Penicillin V is more acid stable and is preferred to penicillin G if oral therapy is appropriate. Methicillin and nafcillin are also poorly absorbed when taken orally, but oxacillin and, especially, cloxacillin and dicloxacillin are fairly well absorbed. One of the latter two agents is generally preferred for oral therapy of staphylococcal infections. Oral ampicillin

and amoxicillin are well absorbed, but the latter is more completely absorbed, with consequent higher and more prolonged blood levels. Amoxicillin may be given every 8 hours by mouth, compared with every 6 hours for ampicillin. Amoxicillin is also available in combination with potassium clavulanate for administration by mouth. Carbenicillin, ticarcillin, azlocillin, mezlocillin, and piperacillin are not absorbed orally, but the indanyl ester of carbenicillin is well absorbed and achieves adequate urine levels for the therapy of urinary tract infections attributable to susceptible organisms. It does not provide serum levels high enough for the treatment of systemic infections.

The penicillins are well absorbed intramuscularly, but intravenous infusion is generally preferred if large doses are required. Two repository forms of penicillin G are available for intramuscular use. Procaine penicillin G achieves therapeutic serum and tissue levels for up to 12 hours after intramuscular injection, and benzathine penicillin G achieves detectable serum levels for up to 30 days. The latter levels are low, however, and are useful only for exquisitely sensitive organisms.

All the penicillins except nafcillin are primarily cleared by the kidney. In general, active tubular secretion is more important than glomerular filtration. Most of these agents require dosage adjustment in the presence of severe renal disease (see Table 231-2). Nafcillin, on the other hand, is primarily metabolized by the liver and does not require a dosage change in cases of renal failure. Similarly, oxacillin can be given in full doses in renal failure, since in this setting it can be excreted by the liver.

Adverse Effects. The most common important adverse reactions to the penicillins involve systemic drug allergy; these reactions include anaphylaxis, various forms of skin rash, drug fever, and serum sickness. In addition, organ- and tissue-specific hypersensitivity may occur. Coombs' test–positive hemolytic anemia, immune thrombocytopenia, neutropenia, pulmonary infiltrates with eosinophilia, and drug-induced lupus may occasionally occur with any of the agents. Methicillin is the penicillin that has most commonly caused acute allergic interstitial nephritis, and oxacillin has been associated with hypersensitivity hepatitis. Like other antibiotics, the penicillins may cause pseudomembranous colitis as a result of colonic overgrowth of toxigenic *Clostridium difficile* (Chapter 263). Any of these drugs can cause milder forms of diarrhea or other gastrointestinal tract upset. Carbenicillin and ticarcillin in high doses may cause volume overload (sodium content, 5 mEq/g antibiotic), hypokalemic alkalosis (by acting as a nonresorbable anion in the distal renal tubule), and interference with platelet function with clinical bleeding. High CSF levels of any penicillin may cause neurotoxicity with coma, myoclonus, and seizures.

Cephalosporins

The first cephalosporin commercially available, cephalothin was released in the United States in 1964. Since then, many additional cephalosporins and related antibiotics have been approved for clinical use. All except cefoxitin, cefotetan, cefmetazole, and moxalactam are semisynthetic derivatives of the same basic nucleus, 7-amino cephalosporanic acid.

Spectrum of Activity. Seven available cephalosporins (cephalothin, cephapirin, cefazolin, cephradine, cephalexin, cefadroxil, and cefaclor) have very similar spectra of activity and have been termed *first-generation cephalosporins* (Fig. 231-4). In vitro susceptibility to these agents is routinely tested with a class antibiotic disk containing either cephalothin or cefazolin. Most gram-positive cocci are susceptible to these drugs, including penicillinase-producing *S. aureus*. However, enterococci, methicillin-resistant staphylococci, and *L. monocytogenes* are resistant. Penicillin-resistant strains of pneumococci also exhibit reduced susceptibility to these cephalosporins. Among gram-negative bacilli, most strains of *E. coli, P. mirabilis,* and *K. pneumoniae* are susceptible, as are most anaerobes, with the exception of *Bacteroides* species. Cefaclor has greater activity against *H. influenzae* than do the other oral derivatives in this class.

Several cephalosporins (cefamandole, cefonicid, ceforanide, cefmetazole, cefuroxime, cefoxitin, and cefotetan) have expanded spectra of activity against certain gram-negative bacteria and are termed *second-generation cephalosporins* (Fig. 231-5). These agents,

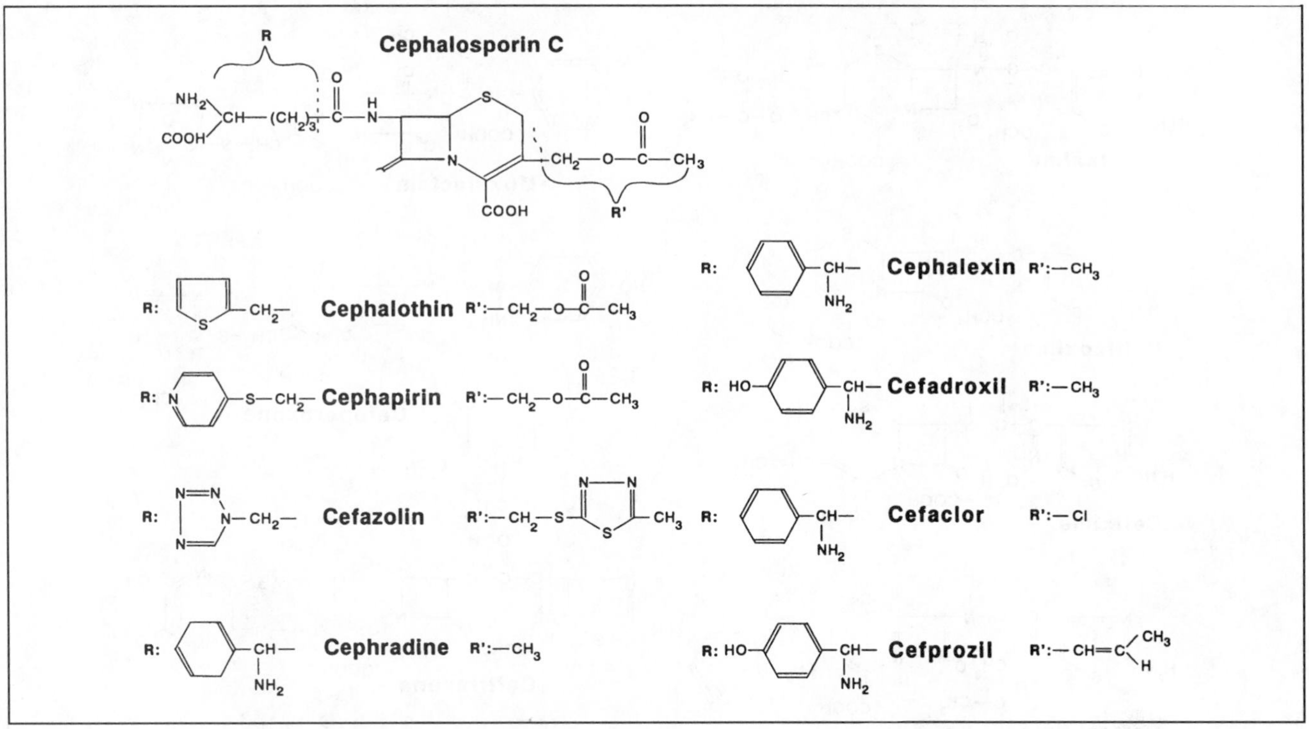

FIGURE 231-4   Structural formulas of the first-generation cephalosporins.

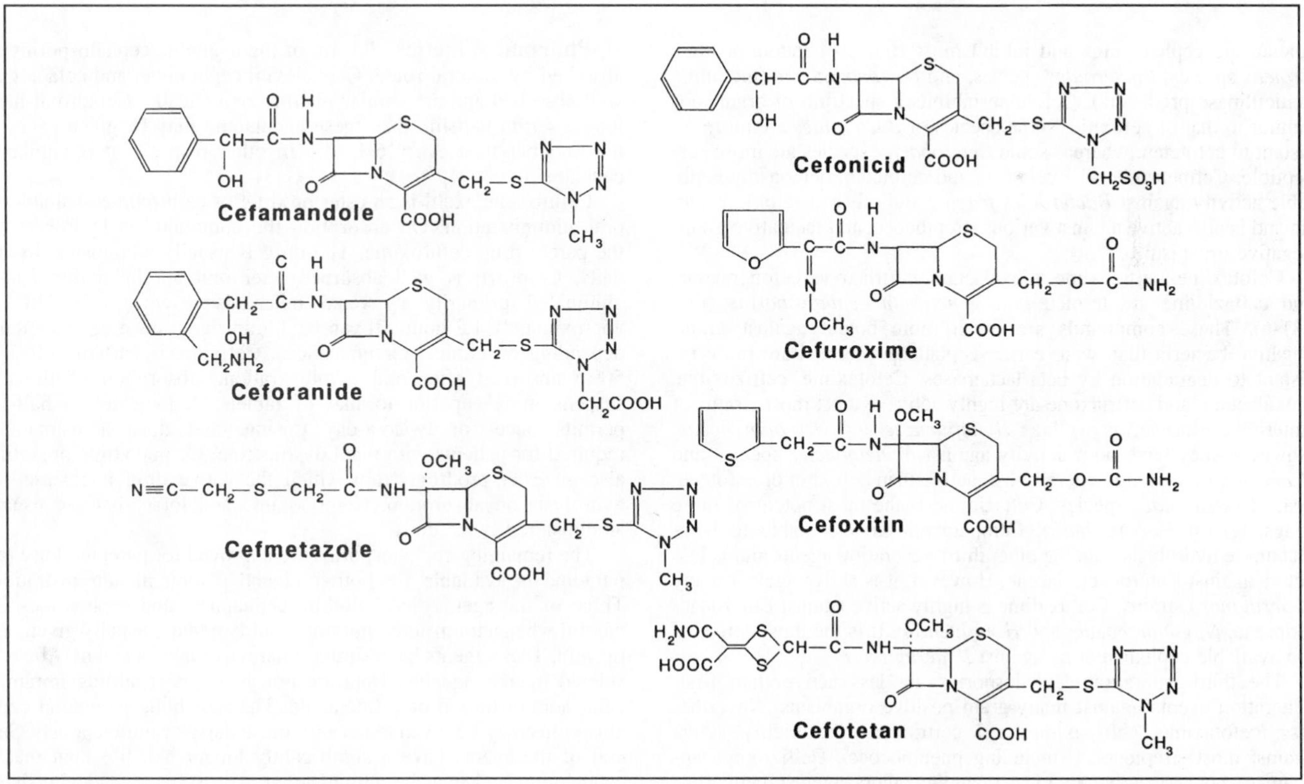

FIGURE 231-5   Structural formulas of the second-generation cephalosporins.

particularly cefotetan and cefoxitin, are often less active than first-generation cephalosporins against gram-positive organisms. All of these agents are active against *Klebsiella* species, *P. mirabilis,* and *E. coli*. Although these compounds (e.g., cefamandole) may appear to inhibit strains of *Enterobacter* species in vitro, derepression of the

inducible chromosomal beta-lactamases of these organisms renders them resistant to the cephalosporins. Cefuroxime is more active against *H. influenzae* than several of the other agents and has been approved for the treatment of meningitis attributable to selected pathogens, although other agents are now preferred. Cefoxitin and ce-

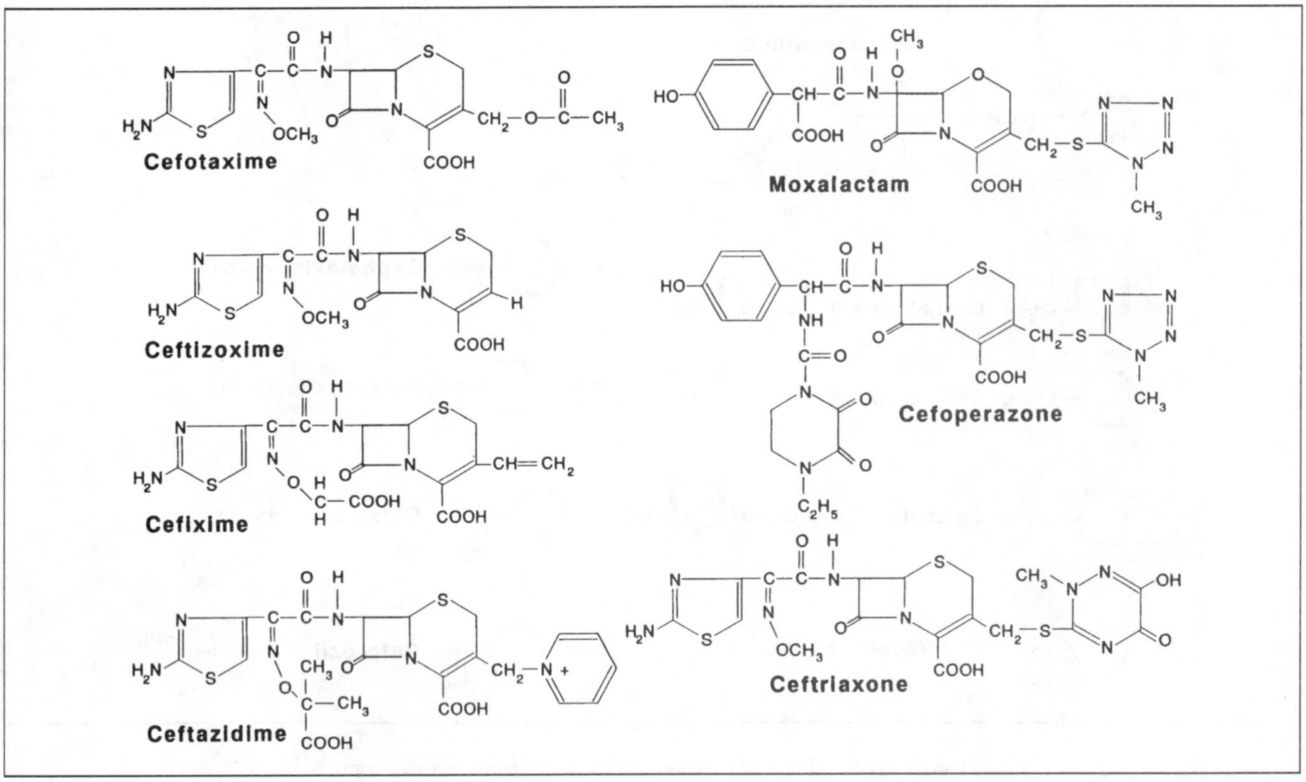

FIGURE 231-6   Structural formulas of the third-generation cephalosporins.

fotetan are cephamycins and inhibit most strains of indole-positive *Proteus* species, *Bacteroides* species, and *N. gonorrhoeae* (including penicillinase producers). Cefotetan inhibits a spectrum of organisms similar to that of cefoxitin; some species of *Bacteroides* are more resistant to cefotetan, whereas some *Enterobacter* species are more susceptible. Cefmetazole, like cefoxitin and cefotetan, demonstrates notable activity against *Bacteroides fragilis* and other anaerobic bacteria and is also active against various streptococci and faculative gram-negative organisms.

Cefotaxime, ceftizoxime, moxalactam, ceftriaxone, cefoperazone, and ceftazidime are termed *third-generation cephalosporins* (Fig. 231-6). These compounds are much more potent against gram-negative bacteria than were earlier cephalosporins and are more resistant to degradation by beta-lactamases. Cefotaxime, ceftizoxime, moxalactam, and ceftriaxone are highly active against most strains of Enterobacteriaceae, as well as *H. influenzae* and *N. gonorrhoeae*. However, they have poor activity against *Acinetobacter* species and *P. aeruginosa* and are generally less active than cefoxitin or cefotetan against *Bacteroides* species. Ceftazidime is the most potent of these drugs against *P. aeruginosa*. Cefoperazone is less stable to beta-lactamase hydrolysis than the other third-generation agents and is less active against Enterobacteriaceae. However, it is active against many *P. aeruginosa* strains. Ceftazidime is highly active against Enterobacteriaceae, *N. gonorrhoeae*, and *H. influenzae*. It is the most active of the available cephalosporins against *P. aeruginosa*.

The third-generation cephalosporins are less active than first-generation agents against many gram-positive organisms. Nevertheless, cefotaxime, ceftizoxime, and ceftriaxone are highly active against most streptococci, including pneumococci. Ceftizoxime appears to be less active in vitro than the others against penicillin-resistant pneumococci. Cefixime and cefpodoxime are oral agents classified as third-generation drugs based on activity against some gram-negative bacteria. Cefixime and ceftibuten exhibit poor activity against staphylococci, and ceftibuten is not as active as the other cephalosporins against pneumococci. Although technically a carbacephem antibiotic rather than a cephalosporin, loracarbef is an orally administered beta-lactam with an antimicrobial spectrum and clinical uses similar to those of the oral cephalosporins.

Pharmacokinetics. Several of the available cephalosporins are absorbed by the oral route. Cephalexin, cephradine, and cefaclor are well absorbed and are similar pharmacokinetically. Cefadroxil has a longer serum half-life than these agents and may be given every 12 hours rather than every 6 hours. In other respects, it is similar to cephalexin.

Cefuroxime axetil is an ester prodrug of cefuroxime available for oral administration. On absorption the compound is hydrolyzed to the parent drug cefuroxime. The drug is usually administered twice daily. Cefprozil is well absorbed after oral administration and is eliminated primarily by renal mechanisms with a half-life of approximately 1.2 hours. It can be administered once or twice daily, depending on clinical circumstances. Cefixime is partially (40% to 50%) absorbed after oral administration. Absorption of the oral suspension is superior to that of tablets. A long serum half-life permits once- or twice-a-day dosing, and dose adjustment is required for patients with renal dysfunction. Cefpodoxime proxetil is also an ester prodrug, from which the active drug is released by hydrolysis on absorption. Cefpodoxime and loracarbef are usually administered twice daily.

The remaining cephalosporins are approved for parenteral use (cephradine is available for both oral and parenteral administration). Three of the agents—cephalothin, cephapirin, and cephradine—are painful when administered intramuscularly and are usually given only by vein. These agents have similar pharmacokinetics and may be considered interchangeable. Data are not available regarding intramuscular administration of cefmetazole. The remaining parenteral cephalosporins may be given either intramuscularly or intravenously. Several of the agents have a significantly longer half-life than that of cephalothin and may be administered at less frequent dosing intervals (see Table 231-2). Ceftriaxone has a uniquely long half-life (6 to 8 hours) and can be administered intramuscularly or intravenously once or twice a day. The third-generation cephalosporins achieve excellent levels in CSF in the presence of meningeal irritation and (with the exception of cefoperazone, which is not approved for use in meningitis) have become the agents of choice for meningitis caused by the Enterobacteriaceae. Ceftriaxone, cefotaxime, and cefuroxime have also been used successfully in childhood meningitis.

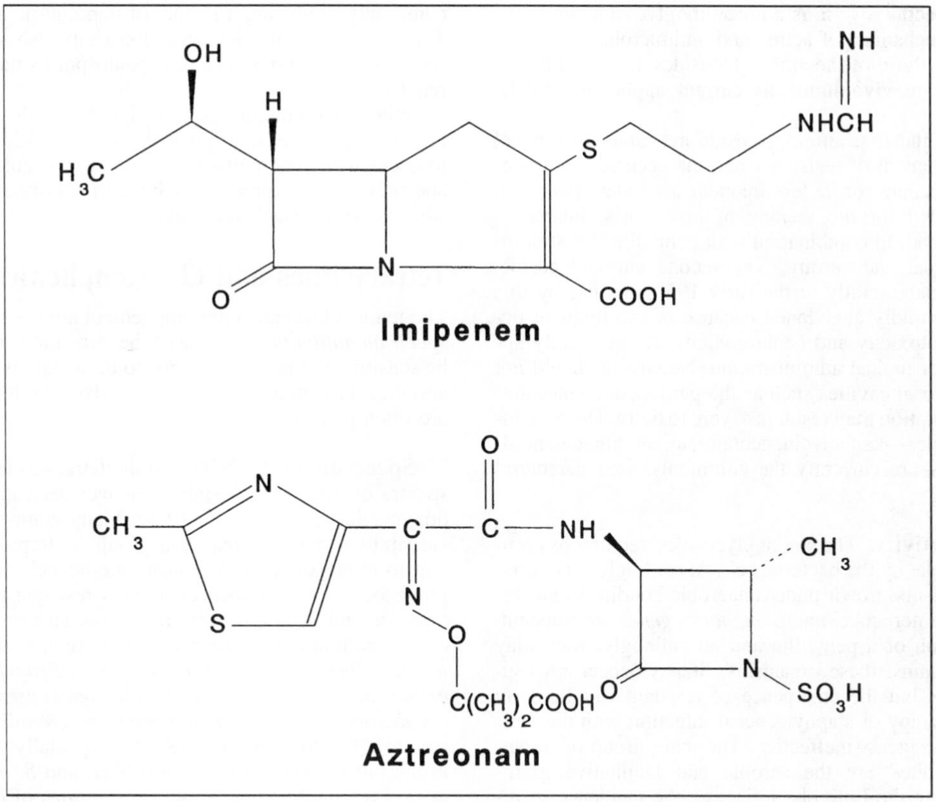

FIGURE 231-7 Structural formulas of imipenem and aztreonam.

Most of the cephalosporins are primarily excreted by the kidney, both by active tubular secretion and by glomerular filtration. Doses are modified in the presence of renal failure, as suggested in Table 231-2.

Adverse Effects. As with the penicillins, the most common major reactions to the cephalosporins involve systemic drug allergy. In addition, neutropenia and immune thrombocytopenia are occasionally seen. Cephalosporins rarely cause renal injury by themselves, but some appear to potentiate the nephrotoxicity of concurrently administered aminoglycosides.

Moxalactam, which is now infrequently used, was associated with a bleeding diathesis. This is believed to be related in part to the presence of a labile methylthiotetrazole side-chain. This moiety, which has also been associated with a disulfiram-like reaction after ingestion of alcoholic beverages, is also present with the use of cefoperazone, cefamandole, cefmetazole, and cefotetan. Bleeding diatheses have not been common with these other agents in standard clinical use.

Other Beta-Lactams

Two other beta-lactam antibiotics, which are neither penicillins nor cephalosporins, are also available for clinical use. Imipenem, the first carbapenem antibiotic approved for human use, is formulated in combination with the dehydropeptidase I enzyme inhibitor, cilastatin, which prevents renal metabolism of the drug. Aztreonam is the first available monobactam antibiotic. In contrast to penicillins, cephalosporins, and carbapenems, the nucleus of this agent contains only the single (beta-lactam) ring (Fig. 231-7).

Spectrum of Activity. Imipenem is active against a wide variety of gram-positive and gram-negative, aerobic and anaerobic pathogens. Notable exceptions include methicillin-resistant strains of *S. aureus,* some enterococci (especially *E. faecium*), and *Stenotrophomonas (Xanthomonas) maltophilia.* The latter produces a beta-lactamase, which inactivates the drug. Although most strains of *P. aeruginosa*

are susceptible to imipenem, resistance to the drug has emerged during therapy. The antimicrobial spectrum of aztreonam is limited to aerobic and facultative gram-negative bacteria. The drug is relatively resistant to hydrolysis by many common beta-lactamases, but enzymes capable of inactivating the drug do exist.

Pharmacokinetics. Imipenem is usually administered intravenously, which is appropriate for its use in severely ill patients. However, a formulation for intramuscular injection is available. The drug is eliminated primarily by the kidneys; doses are usually administered every 6 hours in adults with normal renal function. Adjustments in dosage are needed when renal function is decreased. Aztreonam can be given either intravenously or intramuscularly. Elimination is via the kidneys, with contributions of both glomerular filtration and tubular secretion. In healthy volunteers the serum elimination half-life is approximately 1.5 to 2 hours. Dose adjustment is necessary in patients with impaired renal function.

Adverse Effects. Adverse reactions to imipenem are similar to those seen with other β-lactam antibiotics. Nausea is a significant symptom in some patients. Adherence to dosing guidelines is recommended to minimize the risk of seizures or other adverse central nervous system effects, particularly when imipenem is used in patients with renal dysfunction. Although some penicillin-allergic patients prove to be allergic to aztreonam as well, it appears that the new drug can be given safely in most patients who are allergic to penicillin. In the authors' experience this feature has been a major factor in decisions to choose aztreonam from among alternative agents in selected beta-lactam–allergic patients.

Aminoglycosidic Aminocyclitols

Eight currently available antibiotics contain an aminocyclitol ring. They all share certain pharmacologic and antimicrobial properties. Seven of these antibiotics are aminoglycosidic aminocyclitols (usually referred to as *aminoglycosides*); that is, they have amino-containing sugars linked to an amino-cyclitol ring by glycosidic bonds. The eighth, spectinomycin, is a nonaminoglycoside aminocyclitol. Although its mechanism of action and antimicrobial spectrum are roughly similar to those of the aminoglycosides, the rapid development of resistance in vivo limits its current application to the therapy of gonorrhea.

Streptomycin was the first aminoglycoside available for clinical use. The rapid development of resistance and the occurrence of irreversible ototoxicity account for its less frequent use today. However, it is still recommended for the therapy of brucellosis, tularemia, plague, tuberculosis, and, in combination with penicillin, for streptococcal and enterococcal endocarditis. The second aminoglycoside, neomycin, was used parenterally in the early 1950s. Its use by this route, however, was rapidly abandoned because of the frequent occurrence of severe ototoxicity and nephrotoxicity. It is currently approved only for oral or topical administration. Neomycin should not be used to irrigate serosal cavities such as the peritoneum, since significant systemic absorption may result in severe toxicity. The remaining five aminoglycosides—kanamycin, gentamicin, tobramycin, netilmicin, and amikacin—are currently the commonly used parenteral agents.

Spectrum of Activity. The aminoglycosides require oxygen-dependent, active uptake by the bacterial cell. Accordingly, anaerobes and facultative organisms grown under anaerobic conditions are resistant. Streptococci, enterococci and *L. monocytogenes* are resistant, although a combination of a penicillin and an aminoglycoside may produce synergism against these organisms. Staphylococci are usually sensitive initially, but the emergence of resistant small-colony variants makes the therapy of staphylococcal infection with the aminoglycosides as single agents ineffective. The main group of organisms effectively inhibited are the aerobic and facultative gram-negative bacilli. Among the Enterobacteriaceae, the incidence of resistance to kanamycin is higher than that to the other four commonly used agents. In addition, *P. aeruginosa* is virtually always resistant to kanamycin. Gentamicin and tobramycin are similar in efficacy, and organisms resistant to one are usually cross-resistant to the other. Exceptions are *P. aeruginosa,* for which tobramycin is more active, and *Serratia marcescens,* for which gentamicin is more active. Netilmicin and amikacin are semisynthetic aminoglycosides designed to resist inactivation by many plasmid-mediated aminoglycoside-modifying enzymes. Amikacin has the broadest spectrum of activity of the currently available compounds.

Pharmacokinetics. None of the aminoglycosides is absorbed in clinically useful amounts by the oral route. Intramuscular and intravenous routes of administration produce similar blood levels. Intravenous infusion should be slow, given over 30 minutes. The four commonly used parenteral agents have nearly identical pharmacokinetics. Kanamycin and amikacin, however, are less active on a weight basis than are gentamicin, netilmicin, and tobramycin and consequently are given in higher doses. Therapeutic serum concentrations of kanamycin and amikacin are 20 to 25 μg/ml after a dose and less than 7 μg/ml before the next dose. For gentamicin, netilmicin, and tobramycin, therapeutic postdose levels are 4 to 8 μg/ml (6 to 10 μg/ml for netilmicin) and predose levels are less than 2 μg/ml. These levels pertain to the traditional use of these aminoglycosides in thrice-daily (or, for amikacin, thrice- or twice-daily) dosing. Recently there has been increasing interest in the use of these drugs on a once-daily basis, for which alternative monitoring methods must be used.

The aminoglycosides are excreted solely by glomerular filtration. Careful dosage adjustment is mandatory in the presence of renal impairment (see Table 231-2). Serum levels should be monitored to ensure appropriate therapy in this circumstance.

Adverse Effects. All the aminoglycosides are ototoxic. Streptomycin and gentamicin affect predominantly the vestibular system, whereas kanamycin, neomycin, and amikacin affect mainly auditory function. The effects of tobramycin and netilmicin are seen equally in the two systems. The risk of ototoxicity increases with age, longer duration of therapy, higher total dose, renal impairment, high serum levels of the drug, previous aminoglycoside therapy, and concurrent use of loop diuretics. Ototoxicity may be irreversible.

The aminoglycosides are also direct renal tubular toxins, most commonly producing a picture of nonoliguric acute tubular necrosis. The same factors that enhance ototoxicity also appear to worsen nephrotoxicity. Concurrent use of cephalosporins may increase the risk of renal injury.

When given rapidly in very high doses, the aminoglycosides may produce neuromuscular blockade. This blockade is much more likely to occur with concomitant use of neuromuscular blocking agents for anesthesia or with preexisting impairment of neuromuscular transmission, as with myasthenia gravis.

Tetracyclines and Chloramphenicol

The tetracyclines and chloramphenicol are often referred to as *broad-spectrum antibiotics* because of the wide range of organisms that may be sensitive to them. Resistance to these agents is common, however, and they may produce a number of adverse effects. Alternative agents are often preferred.

Spectrum of Activity. All the tetracycline analogs have similar spectra of activity, although the newer derivatives, minocycline and doxycycline, may be more active. Many gram-positive organisms are susceptible, but *S. aureus* and group A streptococci are often resistant to tetracycline, as are most enterococci. Significant numbers of pneumococci and gonococci are now resistant to tetracyclines. *H. influenzae* and meningococci are usually susceptible, as are a number of less common gram-negative organisms, such as *Pasteurella multocida, Vibrio cholerae, Yersinia pestis, Francisella tularensis, Brucella* species, *Burkholderia (Pseudomonas) pseudomallei, Haemophilus ducreyi,* and *Calymmatobacterium granulomatis.* Enteric gram-negative bacilli may be sensitive, especially to levels achieved in urine, but *P. aeruginosa, P. mirabilis,* and *S. marcescens* are nearly always resistant. On occasion, some strains of *P. aeruginosa* may respond to the concentrations of tetracycline that are achievable in the urine. Anaerobes may be susceptible, but other agents are usually preferred for the treatment of *B. fragilis* infections. Rickettsiae, chlamydiae, mycoplasmas, and spirochetes are generally inhibited by the tetracyclines.

Chloramphenicol is similarly active against a variety of organisms, including rickettsiae, chlamydiae, mycoplasmas, spirochetes, and most gram-positive and gram-negative bacteria, including anaerobes. Less toxic agents are usually preferred, however, and chloramphenicol is useful mainly for brain abscess, beta-lactamase–producing *H. influenzae* infections, meningococcal or pneumococcal meningitis in a penicillin-allergic patient, invasive salmonellosis, and infections involving *B. fragilis. P. aeruginosa* is uniformly resistant.

Pharmacokinetics. Based on differences in pharmacokinetics, the tetracyclines can be divided into the following groups: (1) the short-acting agents, chlortetracycline, oxytetracycline, and tetracycline, which are given every 6 hours; (2) the intermediate-acting group, methacycline and demeclocycline, which are given every 12 hours; and (3) the long-acting compounds, minocycline and doxycycline, which are administered at 12- to 24-hour intervals. All the compounds are well absorbed by mouth, although food, antacids, and iron therapy may interfere. Intramuscular injection is quite painful, but the short- and long-acting agents can be given intravenously in doses equivalent to those by mouth. The tetracyclines are excreted in the bile but reabsorbed from the intestine and eventually eliminated by the kidney. All the agents except doxycycline accumulate in the serum in the presence of renal failure and thus should be avoided in this setting.

Chloramphenicol is equally effective orally or intravenously. It is not approved for intramuscular administration. The drug is mainly metabolized in the liver, and dosage reduction may be necessary in hepatic insufficiency.

Adverse Effects. The tetracyclines may be associated with systemic drug allergy, photosensitization, aggravation of uremia, and dose-related hepatotoxicity, especially during pregnancy or in the presence of renal failure. Demeclocycline may cause nephrogenic diabetes insipidus. The potential for dysplasia and staining of teeth makes tetracyclines unsuitable for use in children and pregnant women.

Chloramphenicol produces two forms of bone marrow toxicity.

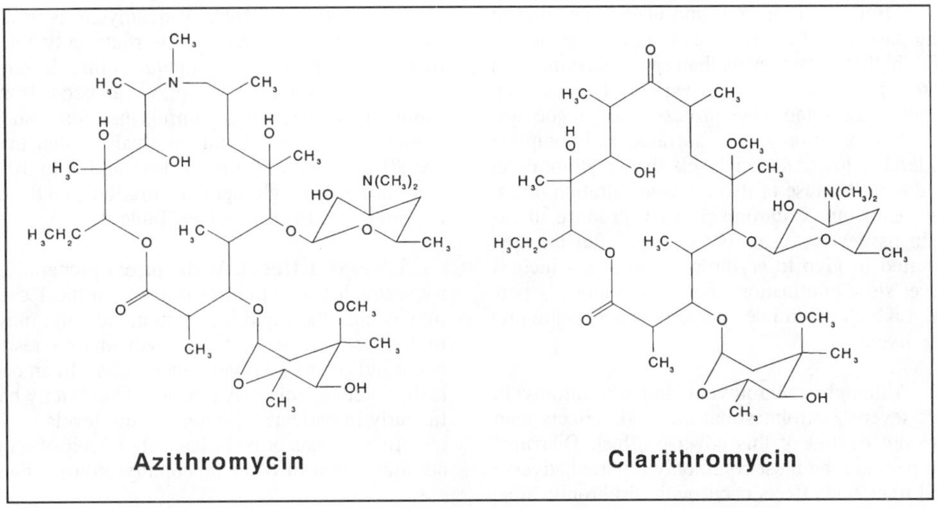

FIGURE 231-8   Structural formulas of azithromycin and clarithromycin.

One common form, reversible bone marrow suppression, is related to the dose and duration of therapy. The more serious toxicity, aplastic anemia, is rare (1 in 20,000 to 1 in 40,000) but usually fatal.

Erythromycin and Clindamycin

Although chemically unrelated, erythromycin and clindamycin have similar mechanisms of action and resistance, spectra of activity, and pharmacokinetics.

Spectrum of Activity. Erythromycin is active against most gram-positive cocci, but some strains are resistant, including 50% to 90% of enterococci. It is not recommended for the treatment of severe staphylococcal infections because of the potential development of resistance during therapy. In some parts of the world significant resistance to erythromycin has emerged among *S. pyogenes* and pneumococci as well. Erythromycin is also effective against the following organisms: many gram-positive bacilli, including *C. diphtheriae,* other diphtheroids, *L. monocytogenes, E. rhusiopathiae,* and *B. anthracis;* some gram-negative organisms, such as gonococci, meningococci, *Bordetella pertussis, Campylobacter jejuni,* and *Legionella pneumophila;* many anaerobes; treponemes; *Mycoplasma pneumoniae;* and some strains of *Chlamydia* and *Rickettsia* species. Enterobacteriaceae are resistant except as the pH approaches 8.5.

Clindamycin is a chemical derivative of the older antibiotic lincomycin, which it has now largely replaced because of better oral absorption and increased potency. It has activity against gram-positive cocci similar to that of erythromycin; enterococci, however, are nearly always resistant. In addition, erythromycin-resistant staphylococcal infections should not be treated with clindamycin, even if the organisms are initially sensitive, because of the risk of emergence of resistance during therapy. Clindamycin is more active than erythromycin against anaerobes and is an excellent drug for *B. fragilis* infections, although resistance does occur (Chapter 271). Some strains of peptococci and *Clostridium* species may be resistant, as are virtually all aerobic gram-negative bacilli. Clindamycin is not active against gonococci.

Pharmacokinetics. Both erythromycin and clindamycin are adequately absorbed when taken orally and are primarily metabolized by the liver. Clindamycin may also be given intramuscularly or intravenously, but parenteral erythromycin is only given intravenously because of pain on intramuscular injection. Neither drug is ordinarily given in altered dose in renal failure, but both may require adjustment of the dose with severe liver disease. Clindamycin achieves particularly high concentrations in bone and has been suggested as a useful alternative to the penicillins and cephalosporins in the treatment of osteomyelitis (Chapter 243).

Adverse Effects. Erythromycin is an exceptionally safe antibiotic. Apart from phlebitis with intravenous use, the only major adverse effect is hypersensitivity cholestatic hepatitis, which is seen primarily with erythromycin estolate. Drug fever and rash are rare complications of erythromycin use.

The major complication of clindamycin therapy is pseudomembranous colitis, a severe and sometimes fatal inflammatory colitis caused by *C. difficile* that may occur in 2% to 10% of patients taking the drug (Chapter 263). Rarely, clindamycin is associated with drug fever, rash, or leukopenia.

New Macrolides

The macrolide antibiotics are naturally occurring agents that have a large 14-, 15-, or 16-member lactone ring. Erythromycin is the best known macrolide and has a 14-member ring (Fig. 231-8). One of the major drawbacks of erythromycin is its lack of stability under acid conditions. The breakdown products on exposure to gastric acid are not only inactive, but are also responsible in large part for the gastrointestinal tract side effects seen in many patients who receive this drug. Chemical modification to prevent acid breakdown has resulted in the synthesis of a variety of new macrolides, including roxithromycin, dirithromycin, clarithromycin, and flurithromycin, which are more resistant to acid hydrolysis, better absorbed when given by the oral route, and produce fewer gastrointestinal tract side effects than erythromycin. A number of these agents are undergoing clinical trials. Clarithromycin, dirithromycin, and the 15-member azalide, azithromycin, have recently been approved for use in the United States. The 15-member macrolide has a nitrogen atom in the ring structure; as a result, it possesses unique characteristics.

Spectrum of Activity. The newer 14-member macrolides, including clarithromycin, are generally similar to erythromycin in spectrum of activity; thus the reader can refer to the section on erythromycin for more specifics. Because the 14-hydroxy metabolite of clarithromycin exhibits enhanced activity against *H. influenzae,* this drug appears more potent in vivo than erythromycin against *Haemophilus* species. In general, the spectrum of azithromycin against gram-positive organisms is similar to that of erythromycin as well, although on a weight basis it is slightly less active. It is approximately four times more active against *H. influenzae* than erythromycin and shows activity against a variety of Enterobacteriaceae and other gram-negative organisms. It is also quite active against *Chlamydia trachomatis* and other *Chlamydia* species (as is true for most of the macrolides). Both azithromycin and clarithromycin possess in vitro activity against *Mycobacterium* species, including *Mycobacterium avium-intracellulare* complex.

Pharmacokinetics. Both azithromycin and clarithromycin are well absorbed from the gastrointestinal tract, and clarithromycin, on a weight basis, produces higher serum levels than erythromycin. Both of these new agents are rapidly taken up by a variety of tissues and are concentrated in macrophages and other professional phagocytes. Indeed, the tissue uptake of azithromycin is so rapid and complete that it produces considerably lower serum levels than erythromycin when given in similar doses. Because of its high concentration in tissues and slow release therefrom, azithromycin may produce therapeutic concentrations in tissues for a number of days after therapy. Dirithromycin is converted in vivo to erythromycylamine, which is microbiologically active; slow elimination of these compounds permits once daily dosing. Like all macrolides, these new agents are primarily excreted via the liver.

Adverse Effects. Although azithromycin and clarithromycin produce fewer and less severe gastrointestinal tract side effects than erythromycin, they are not devoid of this adverse effect. Diarrhea, nausea, and abdominal pain are the most commonly reported adverse effects. Gastrointestinal tract side effects occur with dirithromycin as well. As noted earlier, clarithromycin use should be avoided in pregnancy.

Polymyxins

The polymyxins are cyclic polypeptide antibiotics; all derivatives except polymyxin B and E (colistin) are too toxic for human use.

Spectrum of Activity. Polymyxin B and colistin have identical spectra of activity. Gram-negative bacilli, particularly *P. aeruginosa,* are usually susceptible. *Proteus* species, *Providencia stuartii (Proteus inconstans),* and *S. marcescens* are nearly always resistant, as are gram-positive and anaerobic organisms. The availability of the aminoglycosides, newer beta-lactams, and fluoroquinolones for *P. aeruginosa* infections has relegated these toxic agents to rare use.

Pharmacokinetics. Neither agent is absorbed by mouth. Polymyxin B is usually given as a continuous intravenous infusion in a dose of 1.5 to 2.5 mg/kg per day. Colistin is given intramuscularly two or three times a day, in a total daily dose of 2.5 to 5.0 mg/kg. These drugs have poor tissue penetration and may not be effective in systemic infections; their main use now is for resistant urinary tract infections. In addition, polymyxin B can be given intrathecally in a daily dose of 5 to 10 mg for adults for the treatment of gram-negative meningitis. Both drugs are excreted by glomerular filtration and require major dosage change with renal insufficiency (see Table 231-2).

Adverse Effects. Nephrotoxicity in the form of acute tubular necrosis occurs in 20% of patients who received treatment with these drugs. In addition, neurotoxicity is common, ranging from circumoral paresthesias to neuromuscular blockade, apnea, and seizures.

Vancomycin

Vancomycin was introduced in the mid-1950s for therapy of infections attributable to penicillinase-producing *S. aureus.* With the development of the penicillinase-resistant penicillins, however, it was relegated to a secondary role because of its apparent toxicity. The emergence of methicillin-resistant staphylococci, which remain susceptible to vancomycin, and the availability of a purer compound with less toxicity have led to a resurgence of interest in this agent.

Spectrum of Activity. Most gram-positive organisms are susceptible, including penicillinase-producing *S. aureus,* methicillin-resistant *S. aureus,* enterococci, *S. epidermidis,* and penicillin-resistant pneumococci. Gram-negative bacilli and *Bacteroides* species are resistant. Strains of enterococci that are resistant to high concentrations of vancomycin have now emerged. Resistance is often plasmid mediated and transferable and appears to result from target-site modification. There is increasing awareness of rare pathogens that are intrinsically resistant to vancomycin, including *Leuconostoc, Pediococcus,* and *Lactobacillus* species.

Pharmacokinetics. Vancomycin is usually not absorbed by mouth, and it is given by this route only for bowel sterilization or treatment of pseudomembranous colitis. In rare patients with intense colitis some systemic absorption can occur from the enteral route. Intramuscular injection is painful; therefore vancomycin is given intravenously at 6- to 12-hour intervals. Usual therapeutic serum levels are 20 to 30 μg/ml after a dose and 5 to 10 μg/ml before a dose. Elimination is by glomerular filtration, and the dosage is changed with impaired renal function (see Table 231-2).

Adverse Effects. With current preparations of this drug, toxicity seems less common than it was in the 1950s and 1960s. Phlebitis may occur, and rapid intravenous infusion may produce a syndrome of hypotension and diffuse erythematous rash. Nephrotoxicity may occur but seems relatively uncommon. In an occasional patient fever, rash, or leukopenia may develop. Ototoxicity has been described, particularly in patients with high serum levels (>50 μg/ml), but the precise role of vancomycin has often been obscured by the concurrent administration of other potentially ototoxic compounds.

Sulfonamides and Trimethoprim

Spectrum of Activity. The sulfonamides have a broad spectrum of activity, including most gram-positive cocci (except enterococci), many gram-negative bacilli (except *P. aeruginosa* and *S. marcescens*), most *H. influenzae,* gonococci and meningococci, and *Chlamydia* and *Nocardia* species. Although sulfonamides are active in vitro against group A streptococcus, they do not eradicate this organism from the throat or prevent the nonsuppurative sequelae. Trimethoprim has a spectrum similar to that of the sulfonamides, and the combination is frequently synergistic, especially against the Enterobacteriaceae. The combination is also frequently used in the prophylaxis and therapy of *Pneumocystis carinii* pneumonia.

Pharmacokinetics. The sulfonamides are well absorbed by mouth and are distributed to most body tissues in high concentrations. Sulfadiazine has the lowest protein binding of this class and achieves the highest levels in spinal fluid. However, it is less soluble than the newer agents and may produce crystalluria. Sulfisoxazole, sulfamethoxazole, sulfamethizole, and sulfacytine are more soluble derivatives used for treatment of urinary tract infections. Sulfisoxazole is available for intravenous administration. The sulfonamides are metabolized by the liver, as well as filtered and secreted by the kidney; doses are changed in the presence of renal impairment (see Table 231-2). Trimethoprim is also well absorbed when taken by mouth and is available alone for oral use and in fixed combination with sulfamethoxazole for oral or intravenous administration.

Adverse Effects. The sulfonamides are associated with fairly frequent systemic drug allergy, including anaphylaxis, severe skin rash, vasculitis, and drug fever. In addition, they may occasionally cause aplastic anemia, agranulocytosis, immune hemolytic anemia, neutropenia or thrombocytopenia, pulmonary infiltrates with eosinophilia, and granulomatous hepatitis, sometimes with progression to chronic active hepatitis. Sulfadiazine may cause crystalluria and acute renal failure, but this is rare with the more soluble agents. Trimethoprim occasionally causes megaloblastic anemia or hyperkalemia.

Metronidazole

Spectrum of Activity. Metronidazole is highly active against the gram-negative anaerobic organisms (including *B. fragilis*), *Clostridium* species, and most strains of anaerobic gram-positive cocci. The anaerobic nonsporulating gram-positive bacilli and microaerophilic streptococci are often resistant, as are aerobic bacteria with the exception of *C. jejuni* and *Gardnerella vaginalis. Helicobacter pylori* is usually susceptible. Metronidazole may be ineffective as a single agent for mixed aerobic-anaerobic infections.

Pharmacokinetics. Oral metronidazole is well absorbed, giving serum levels similar to those after intravenous administration. The drug diffuses well into tissues and body fluids, including CSF and

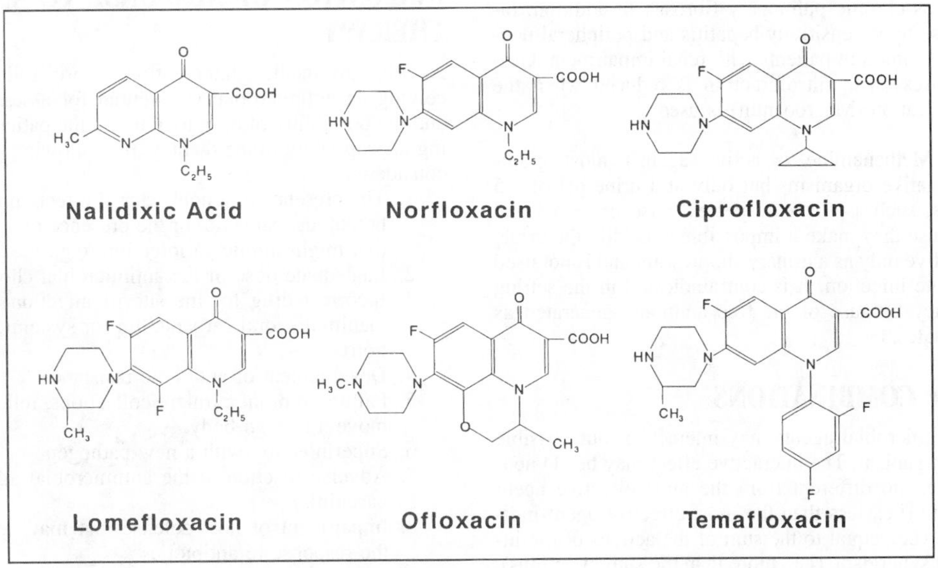

FIGURE 231-9 Structural formulas of nalidixic acid and the newer fluoroquinolone antimicrobial agents.

bile. The liver is the main site of metabolism, and no change in dose is necessary in the presence of renal failure. The presence of severe hepatic disease, however, may require a dosage reduction.

Adverse Effects. Frequent, minor side effects of metronidazole administration include nausea, dry mouth, an unpleasant metallic taste, and a disulfiram-like interaction with alcohol. Peripheral neuropathy may complicate high-dose therapy but is generally reversible if the drug is stopped promptly. Transient neutropenia has been observed with longer durations of therapy. Metronidazole is mutagenic in vitro and carcinogenic in rodents; the relevance of these observations to human use of the drug is unknown.

Quinolone Antibiotics

Nalidixic acid was synthesized in 1962 and is the prototypic drug of a class of antimicrobial agents referred to as the quinolones. The original representatives of this class lacked activity against gram-positive bacteria, anaerobes, *P. aeruginosa,* and *Serratia* species. Several important chemical modifications, including the addition of a fluorine atom at position 6 in the quinolone ring and key substitutions at positions 1 and 7, have resulted in a variety of new compounds with enhanced spectra of activity and decreased toxicity, against which bacteria are less likely to develop mutational resistance (Fig. 231-9). Norfloxacin, ciprofloxacin, ofloxacin, enoxacin, lomefloxacin, sparfloxacin, and levofloxacin have been approved for use in the United States. Other new quinolones such as pefloxacin and tosufloxacin are available in other countries, and a variety of additional compounds are currently undergoing clinical trials in the United States and elsewhere.

Spectrum of Activity. In general, the new fluoroquinolones all possess outstanding activity against Enterobacteriaceae and inhibit most other gram-negative bacilli, including *P. aeruginosa* and *Legionella* species. Of the currently available compounds, ciprofloxacin is most active against *P. aeruginosa.* They are also active against gram-positive organisms, but their activity against these bacteria, particularly that against streptococci, including *S. pneumoniae,* is not as impressive as their activity against gram-negative bacilli. Of the currently available compounds, ofloxacin appears to have the greatest activity against the pneumococci. Gram-negative diplococci such as gonococci and meningococci are generally susceptible to the new fluoroquinolones. Several of the fluoroquinolones demonstrate in vitro activity against various strains of *Chlamydia, Mycoplasma,* and *Rickettsia* species; however, at present only the use of ofloxacin in the treatment of *Chlamydia trachomatis* urethritis and cervicitis is ap-

proved. Although these antimicrobial agents possess excellent activity against methicillin-susceptible staphylococci, in many areas, the majority of methicillin-resistant staphylococci are now resistant to the new fluoroquinolones. The activity of these compounds against anaerobes is limited. Likewise, none has outstanding activity against enterococci.

Pharmacokinetics. As a rule, the new fluoroquinolones are all well absorbed when given orally. Indeed, the oral bioavailability exceeds 50% for all of these compounds, and in some cases (such as ofloxacin) it exceeds 95%. Although serum concentrations of most of these drugs are only modest, they penetrate well into a variety of tissues, including the prostate. Protein binding is low for all of the quinolones, and with the exception of enoxacin, none is more than 25% bound to serum proteins. Elimination of the ofloxacin is almost entirely by the renal route; both renal and nonrenal mechanisms are important for norfloxacin, ciprofloxacin, enoxacin, and lomefloxacin. All of the new fluoroquinolones are available for oral administration, and intravenous preparations of ciprofloxacin and ofloxacin are also available.

Adverse Effects. In general, the fluoroquinolones are relatively free of serious adverse effects. One member of this class, temafloxacin, was taken off the market because its use was occasionally associated with thrombocytopenia, hemolytic anemia, and renal failure. In many clinical trials the overall prevalence and severity of adverse effects to the quinolones have been lower than those to the comparative agents, including penicillins and sulfonamides. The majority of side effects are gastrointestinal (nausea, abdominal discomfort, vomiting, and diarrhea) followed by central nervous system symptoms (headache, dizziness, nervousness, and insomnia). Photosensitivity is occasionally seen in patients receiving fluoroquinolones. Although they cause cartilage erosions in the weight-bearing joints of certain experimental animals, these findings have not been documented in humans. These agents are *not* recommended for use in children or pregnant women.

Urinary Tract Antiseptics

Nitrofurantoin. Nitrofurantoin inhibits many enterococci and Enterobacteriaceae at concentrations achievable in the urinary tract. However, the majority of *Proteus* species and all *P. aeruginosa* strains are resistant. Achievable blood levels are low and are not effective for systemic therapy. Therefore the use of nitrofurantoin is limited to acute infections of the urinary tract and prophylaxis of recurrent infections. Toxic reactions include an acute pneumonic syndrome with eosinophilia, as well as chronic pulmonary fibrosis. In addition, nitrofurantoin may cause hypersensitivity hepatitis and peripheral neuropathy that is more common in patients with renal impairment. Gastrointestinal tract distress with nitrofurantoin is reduced when the macrocrystalline preparation (Macrodantin) is used.

Methenamine. Methenamine is active against most grampositive and gram-negative organisms but only at a urine pH of 5.5 or less. Urea splitters, such as *Proteus* species, raise urine pH and may be resistant because they make it impossible to acidify the urine. Methenamine is effective only as a urinary suppressant and is not used for the therapy of acute infection. It is contraindicated in the setting of hepatic insufficiency because of the free ammonia generated as the compound dissociates.

ANTIMICROBIAL COMBINATIONS

A combination of antimicrobial agents may interact in four possible ways against a microorganism. The interactive effect may be (1) neutral (or indifferent, i.e., no different from the most effective agent alone), (2) antagonistic (i.e., less than the most effective agent individually), (3) additive (i.e., equal to the sum of the actions of the individual drugs), or (4) synergistic (i.e., more than the sum of actions).

The use of synergistic antimicrobial combinations has been advocated for the treatment of endocarditis (Chapter 24) caused by drug-resistant organisms such as the enterococcus or *P. aeruginosa* and for the therapy of infections in settings in which bacterial killing by the host may be defective, as in the neutropenic patient (Chapter 236). Combinations of agents may produce synergy in several ways. They may inhibit serial or sequential steps in a biochemical pathway, as with trimethoprim-sulfamethoxazole. One of the drugs may block bacterial inactivation of the other, as exemplified by the combination of a beta-lactamase inhibitor, such as clavulanic acid, with a beta-lactam antibiotic. The best-studied mechanism involves enhancement of aminoglycoside uptake by a cell wall inhibitory agent such as penicillin. This is the mechanism that underlies penicillin-aminoglycoside therapy of serious enterococcal infections and probably accounts for beta-lactam aminoglycoside synergism against *P. aeruginosa* and other gram-negative bacteria.

The use of more than one antibiotic in therapy increases the risk of an adverse drug reaction and enhances the selective pressure for the emergence of resistant organisms. In addition, the possibility of antagonism between the agents, as previously mentioned, must be considered. The best-studied example of antibiotic antagonism involves the combination of a bacteriostatic agent, particularly tetracycline or chloramphenicol, with a beta-lactam, such as penicillin. The simultaneous in vitro use of these agents results in clear-cut antagonism against a variety of species. In a clinical study of patients with pneumococcal meningitis a group receiving both penicillin and chlortetracycline had nearly four times the mortality of a group receiving penicillin alone. In animal studies this effect is evident only if the static agent is given first. It is assumed that inhibition of bacterial growth by tetracycline or chloramphenicol may interfere with the mechanism of bacterial killing by the beta-lactam.

Other examples of potential antimicrobial antagonism include (1) the simultaneous use of more than one 50s ribosomal subunit inhibitor, which may produce competition for binding to the same site of action, and (2) the combination of the bacteriostatic agents tetracycline or chloramphenicol with the bactericidal aminoglycosides. In the second example the bacteriostatic agent may interfere with active aminoglycoside transport into the cell and inhibit bacterial killing. The phenomenon of antimicrobial antagonism is probably of clinical significance only in situations of impaired host defense, in which bacterial killing is most dependent on antibiotic action. Examples include local impairment of host defense (e.g., endocarditis and meningitis) and systemic impairment, as with neutropenia.

Whenever possible, a single antimicrobial agent is preferred for therapy of infectious diseases. Use of combination therapy has been advocated only in the following specialized situations: (1) prevention of emergence of resistant organisms, when this is common with a single agent; (2) polymicrobial infections; (3) initial therapy of sepsis of unknown cause, pending identification of the pathogen; and (4) infections in which synergistic killing has been shown to be of benefit.

EVALUATION OF RESPONSE TO ANTIMICROBIAL THERAPY

As with any medical intervention, careful follow-up of a patient receiving an antimicrobial is essential for assessing clinical response and the possibility of drug toxicity. In the patient who is not responding appropriately to the therapy, the following possibilities should be considered:

1. The presence of a nonbacterial infection (e.g., viral, fungal, tuberculous, parasitic) or the presence of a noninfectious process that might mimic an infection (e.g., vasculitis, lymphoma)
2. Inadequate dose of the antimicrobial chosen
3. Incorrect drug for the site of infection (e.g., cephalothin for meningitis, oral carbenicillin for systemic *P. aeruginosa* infection)
4. Development of antibiotic resistance
5. Failure to drain purulent collections, relieve obstruction, or remove a foreign body
6. Superinfection with a new pathogen
7. Adverse reaction to the antimicrobial agent (e.g., drug fever, vasculitis)
8. Impairment of host defense that may delay or interfere with the response to antibiotics

The choice of appropriate antimicrobial therapy is best made with a detailed knowledge of the anatomic and pathophysiologic correlates of the specific infectious disease processes. This material is reviewed in subsequent chapters on specific infectious diseases.

BIBLIOGRAPHY

Abramowicz M, editor: *Handbook of antimicrobial therapy,* New Rochelle, NY, 1992, Medical Letter.

Anonymous: Clarithromycin and azithromycin, *Med Lett Drugs Ther* 34:47, 1992.

Bennett WM et al: Drug prescribing in renal failure: dosing guidelines for adults, *Am J Kidney Dis* 3:155, 1983.

Beutler E: Glucose-6-phosphate dehydrogenase deficiency, *N Engl J Med* 324:169-174, 1991.

Calderwood SB, Moellering RC Jr: Common adverse effects of antibacterial agents on major organ systems, *Surg Clin North Am* 60:65, 1980.

Donowitz GR, Mandell GL: Beta-lactam antibiotics, *N Engl J Med* 318:419-426, 490-500, 1988.

Eliopoulos GM: Antibiotic resistance in *Enterococcus* species: an update. In Remington, JS, Swartz, MN, editors: *Current clinical topics in infectious diseases,* vol 16, Cambridge, MA, 1996, Blackwell Scientific, pp. 21-51.

Fass RJ et al: Platelet-mediated bleeding caused by broad-spectrum penicillins, *J Infect Dis* 155:1242-1248, 1987.

Geddes AM, Stille W: Imipenem: the first thienamycin antibiotic, *Rev Infect Dis* 7:(suppl 3), 1985.

Goldman P: Metronidazole, *N Engl J Med* 303:1212, 1980.

Hooper DC, Wolfson JS: The fluoroquinolones: pharmacology, clinical uses, and toxicities in humans, *Antimicrob Agents Chemother* 28:716, 1985.

Hooper DC, Wolfson, JS, editors: *Quinolone antimicrobial agents,* ed 2, Washington, DC, 1993, American Society for Microbiology.

Kirst H, Sides GD: New directions for macrolide antibiotics, *Antimicrob Agents Chemother* 33:1413, 1989.

Kitzis MD et al: Dissemination of the novel plasmid-mediated β-lactamase CTX-1, which confers resistance to broad-spectrum cephalosporins, and its inhibition by β-lactamase inhibitors, *Antimicrob Agents Chemother* 32:9-14, 1988.

Mandell GL, Sande MA: Antimicrobial agents: drugs used in the chemotherapy of tuberculosis and leprosy. In Gilman AG et al, editors: *The pharmacological basis of therapeutics,* ed 8, New York, 1990, Macmillan.

Mandell GL, Sande MA: Antimicrobial agents: penicillins, cephalosporins, and other beta-lactam antibiotics. In Gilman AG et al, editors: *The pharmacological basis of therapeutics,* ed 8, New York, 1990, Macmillan.

Mandell GL, Sande MA: Antimicrobial agents: sulfonamides, trimethoprim-sulfamethoxazole, and agents for urinary tract infections. In Gilman AG et al, editors: *The pharmacological basis of therapeutics,* ed 8, New York, 1990, Macmillan.

Mazzei T et al: Chemistry and mode of action of macrolides, *J Antimicrob Chemother* 31(suppl C):1-9, 1993.

McOsker CC, Fitzpatrick PM: Nitrofurantoin: mechanism of action and implications for resistance development in common pathogens, *J Antimicrob Chemother* 33(suppl A):23-30, 1994.

Moellering RC Jr: Principles of antiinfective therapy. In Mandell GL et al, editors: *Principles and practice of infectious diseases,* ed 4, New York, 1995, Churchill-Livingstone.

Moellering RC Jr, editor: Tissue-directed antibiotic therapy, *Am J Med* 91(suppl 3A):1S-45S, 1991.

Moellering RC Jr, Elopoulos GM, Sentochnik DE: The carbapenems: new broad-spectrum beta-lactam antibiotic, *J Antimicrob Chemother* 24(suppl A):1-8, 1989.

Moellering RC Jr, Krogstad DJ, Greenblatt DJ: Vancomycin therapy in patients with impaired renal function: a nomogram for dosage, *Ann Intern Med* 94:343, 1981.

Neu HC, editor: Aztreonam: a monocyclic beta-lactam antibiotic, *Am J Med* 78(2A):1-80, 1985.

Ristuccia AM, Cunha BA: The aminoglycosides, *Med Clin North Am* 66:303, 1982.

Sande MA, Mandell GL: Antimicrobial agents: the aminoglycosides. In Gilman AG et al, editors: *The pharmacological basis of therapeutics,* ed 7, New York, 1985, Macmillan.

Sande MA, Mandell, GL: Antimicrobial agents. In Gilman AG et al, editors: *The pharmacological basis of therapeutics,* ed 8, New York, 1990, Macmillan.

Sanford JP, Gilbert DN, Sande M, editors: *The Sanford guide to antimicrobial therapy–1995,* Dallas, 1995, Antimicrobial Therapy, Inc.

Smith LG, Sensakovic J: Trimethoprim-sulfamethoxazole, *Med Clin North Am* 66:143, 1982.

Tartaglione TA, Polk RE: Review of the second-generation cephalosporins: cefonicid, ceforanide, and cefuroxime, *Drug Intell Clin Pharm* 19:188-198, 1985.

Ward A, Richards DM: Cefotetan: a review of its antibacterial activity, pharmacokinetic properties, and therapeutic use, *Drugs* 30:382-426, 1985.

Weber DJ, Tolkoff-Rubin NE, Rubin RH: Amoxicillin and potassium clavulanate: an antibiotic combination, *Pharmacotherapy* 4:122-133, 1984.

Wolfson JS, Hooper DC: The fluoroquinolones: structures, mechanisms of action and resistance, and spectra of activity in vitro, *Antimicrob Agents Chemother* 28:581, 1985.

Yost RL, Ramphal R: Ceftazidime review, *Drug Intell Clin Pharm* 19:509-513, 1985.

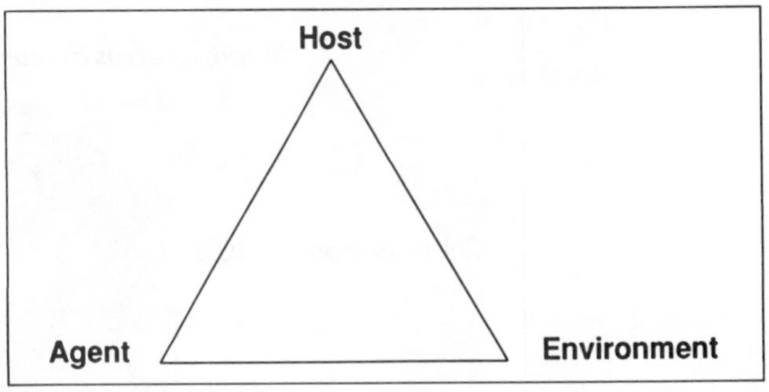

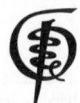

FIGURE 232-1 Triangular model of disease showing that the interplay of host, agent, and environment is important in understanding the causation of disease and its control.

CHAPTER

232 Hospital Infection Control

R. Michael Massanari and Richard P. Wenzel

Modern health care has been acclaimed for accomplishments in preserving life and sustaining dysfunctional organ systems; however, these advances are not achieved without a price. Intervention in the natural history of disease, whether with highly technical surgical procedures or with toxic chemicals, is often accompanied by adverse events with serious sequelae for the patient. In general, the risk of adverse events and the impact of adverse outcomes are poorly understood. Nosocomial infections are an exception to this generalization; this subset of adverse outcomes of medical care has been the subject of intense investigation for several decades.

Nosocomial infections are infections that occur in the course of health care delivery. Because these infections often occur during hospitalization, they have also been designated hospital-acquired infections. The term *nosocomial infections* is preferable to *iatrogenic infections* because the latter inappropriately implicates the physician in the causation of infection. Estimates of the frequency of nosocomial infections suggest that 5% of patients admitted to acute care institutions in the United States will acquire an infection; this translates to approximately 2 million patients per year. The impact of hospital-acquired infections on the patient and on society is significant. Estimates are that 20,000 to 70,000 patients die as a direct result of nosocomial infections. For those who recover, 4 days will be added to the hospital stay on average, with an overall cost to society of $2 billion. With the shift of health care delivery to ambulatory settings, the risk of nosocomial infections is probably decreased. For some populations of patients, rates of nosocomial infections for those entering modern hospitals may be increased because of their greater severity of illness compared with those admitted to hospitals a decade ago. However, there have been no systematic studies of the risks of nosocomial infections in this environment.

Nosocomial infections are not an inevitable consequence of health care. With proper attention to prevention and proactive medical care, up to 33% of nosocomial infections can be prevented. Before considering prevention, the complexity of the problem and the factors that contribute to the risk of nosocomial infections must be understood. A conceptual model of disease may be helpful in analyzing hospital-acquired infections. The "triangular" model of disease (Fig. 232-1) comprises the following components: the host or infected patient, the agent or nosocomial pathogen, and the environment or context in which the disease occurs. To understand causation of nosocomial infections, one must recognize the interplay of these components.

HOST

Hospitalized patients are a unique subset of the population in terms of risk for infection. Conditions that predispose the host to infection can be categorized into those that are intrinsic to the patient and those that are imposed by the health care system.

Intrinsic Conditions

Age is generally considered an important determinant of risk for nosocomial infections. Neonates, particularly low-birth-weight infants, are at considerably increased risk for infection. Immature mechanisms of host defense are important determinants of host susceptibility. Whether age is an independent risk factor for patients in the eighth and ninth decades is still a matter of debate.

The nutritional status of the patient has been considered an important risk factor for infection. Undernutrition results in significant alterations in immunologic responses, and cellular immunity is particularly impaired among patients with severe malnutrition; however, the importance of malnutrition as an independent risk factor for hospitalized patients has not been well documented. Overnutrition or obesity also contributes to infection, particularly to postoperative wound infections.

The most significant risk factors for infection in hospitalized patients are the underlying diseases. In patients with severe burns the skin is denuded, depriving the host of a vital mechanical barrier that prevents invasion by environmental microorganisms. Nosocomial infections constitute a major threat to survival for burn patients. Patients with leukemia and aplastic anemia are at risk for nosocomial infections because the underlying disease interferes with the production of phagocytic cells, which are essential in the defense against infection. Patients with the acquired immunodeficiency syndrome (AIDS) are at increased risk for nosocomial infection by virtue of impairment of cellular immune responses. Thus any disease that interferes with or impairs normal mechanical or physiologic host defense mechanisms increases susceptibility to nosocomial infections.

Conditions Imposed by the Health Care System

Every diagnostic and treatment modality used by the physician, however simple and seemingly harmless, is accompanied by a risk of adverse reaction(s). Pertinent to nosocomial infections, medications used to treat malignant diseases or to modulate immunologic responses alter the capacity of the patient to control infection. Some medications augment the risk of infection as a direct consequence of the pharmacologic effects. Antacids and β_2-blockers, routinely administered to patients in intensive care units to reduce the risk of gastrointestinal tract bleeding, may increase the risk of gram-negative lower respiratory tract infections by interfering with the secretion of gastric acid.

An assortment of paraphernalia, usually plastic or metal cannulas and tubes, is introduced through normal protective barriers such as skin and mucous membranes or into a hollow viscus. These foreign bodies interfere with normal physical barriers and protective mecha-

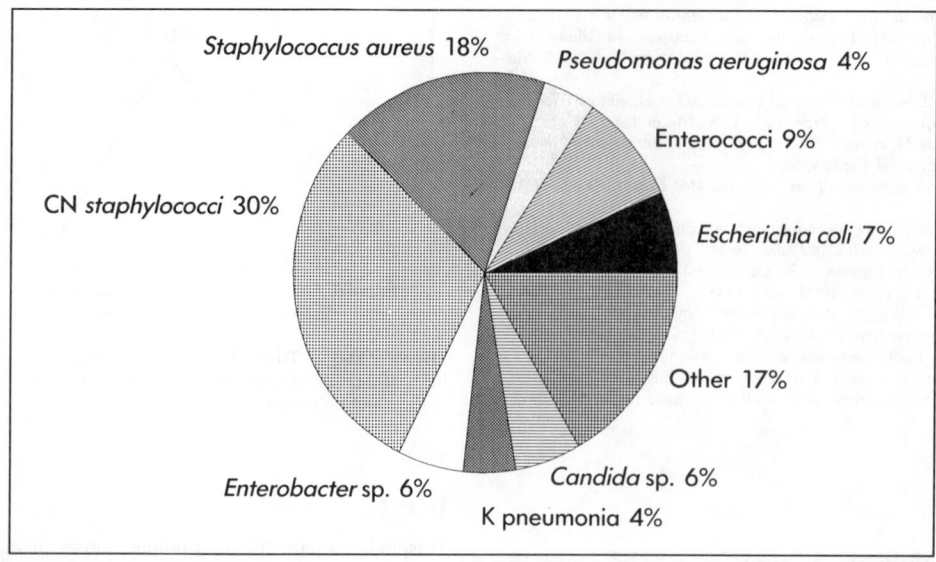

FIGURE 232-2   Distribution by species of more than 10,000 bloodstream isolates from the National Nosocomial Infection Surveillance System, 1986 to 1989.

nisms. Intravenous cannulas, urinary catheters, pressure monitoring devices, dialysis catheters, and intubation tubes predispose to severe and sometimes fatal nosocomial infections.

It is routine during surgical interventions to enter the sterile internal milieu of the host. Despite the most sophisticated techniques to maintain a sterile environment, inoculation of even small numbers of organisms into the operative site may be sufficient to establish a nidus of infection.

AGENTS

The biologic agents capable of producing nosocomial infections are myriad. Viruses, bacteria, fungi, protozoa, and arachnids have all been implicated. Nosocomial bacterial and fungal infections are most significant in terms of frequency, morbidity, and mortality. Although many species of bacteria and fungi have been associated with nosocomial infections, a few common pathogens account for most of the infections. The Centers for Disease Control and Prevention (CDC) maintains the only national database on nosocomial infections in the United States. More than 100 hospitals voluntarily report summary information on nosocomial infections to the National Nosocomial Infection Surveillance (NNIS) System. The distribution of nosocomial pathogens isolated from the bloodstream and reported by NNIS between 1986 and 1989 are summarized in Fig. 232-2. The four most frequent pathogens isolated from blood cultures account for more than 50% of bacteremias: coagulase-negative staphylococci, *Staphylococcus aureus,* enterococci, and *Escherichia coli.* The relative frequency with which specific strains of pathogens have been associated with nosocomial infections has changed over time. Group A β-hemolytic streptococci, presently a rare cause of nosocomial infections, were a frequent source of serious infections in the early twentieth century. In 1995 the first nongovernmental national surveillance system for antibiotic resistance among nosocomial bloodstream isolates was begun. The program—SCOPE—is directed by investigators at the Medical College of Virginia and the University of Iowa and surveys 50 hospitals in the United States. From the 1940s through the 1960s *S. aureus* was the predominant pathogen. During the next two decades gram-negative bacilli such as *E. coli, Enterobacter* species, *Klebsiella* species, and *Pseudomonas* species emerged as predominant pathogens. During the past decade coagulase-negative staphylococci and *Candida* species, commensal flora once regarded as contaminants, have emerged as increasingly important pathogens.

The changing ecology of nosocomial pathogens during the latter half of the twentieth century reflects changing technologies and the ability to care for and preserve patients with severe chronic diseases. Use of antibiotics, in particular, has changed the distribution of noso-

comial pathogens. Commensurate with changes in species of nosocomial pathogens has been the emergence of expanding patterns of multiple antimicrobial resistance. The emergence of multiple-drug-resistant (including vancomycin-resistant) *Enterococcus faecium* as an important nosocomial pathogen illustrates this alarming trend. Paradoxically, the emerging pathogens are sometimes less virulent as measured by their capacity to produce disease in healthy hosts. The major concern of clinicians and epidemiologists alike today is the threat that the gene for vancomycin resistance will be transferred from enterococci to *S. aureus.* Several traits render these organisms virulent in the hospital environment.

Adherence

The first step in the infectious process is adherence of the microbe to host tissue. Intrinsic properties of the agent that facilitate adherence enhance the capacity of an organism to produce disease. *E. coli, Proteus mirabilis,* and other gram-negative bacteria contain fimbriae (pili), which are tiny projections on the surface of the bacterium. Specific chemicals located on the tips of pili enable organisms to attach to selected sites in tissues of the host (e.g., *E. coli* to urinary tract endothelium). Similarly, the cell walls of *S. aureus* contain teichoic acids that adhere to host epithelial cells (Chapter 260). *Staphylococcus epidermidis* produces a layer of "slime," a biofilm consisting of glycocalyx that surrounds the organism. A potentially important property of the biofilm is attachment to foreign material such as intravascular cannulas, prosthetic valves, and prosthetic joints. This intrinsic property of *S. epidermidis* may explain in part why this organism has emerged as one of the most frequent nosocomial pathogens.

Toxin Production

Microbes produce toxic substances that may be important in the pathogenesis of nosocomial infections. *S. aureus* produces several exotoxins such as leukocidin, which is cytotoxic for neutrophils. *S. aureus* also produces enterotoxin F, a toxin responsible for toxic shock syndrome, and exfoliatin, a toxin responsible for the "scalded skin syndrome." Exotoxin A is an enzyme released by *P. aeruginosa* that produces diphtheria toxin–like effects on cells. The toxin is lethal for mammalian cells and may be important in the pathogenesis of disease in humans. A virulence factor common to all gram-negative bacteria is endotoxin (Chapter 245). The active component of endotoxin is lipid A, a structural component of the cell walls of gram-negative bacteria. Endotoxin plays a pivotal role in gram-negative septicemia and shock by triggering the release of endogenous mediators of inflammation, such as tumor necrosis factor and leukotrienes, and by activating several host protein "cascades" including complement, co-agulation, kallikrein-kinin, and other pathways. Despite the role of toxic substances in the pathogenesis of nosocomial infections, "viru-lence" factors are not imperative for inducing disease. Bacteria such as enterococci and coagulase-negative staphylococci produce little in the way of toxic substances. Despite this apparent impotence, these organisms are among the most frequent pathogens responsible for nosocomial infections and may be associated with significant mor-bidity and mortality.

Antimicrobial Resistance

To ensure survival in "hostile" environments, bacteria have acquired several mechanisms for combating the toxic effects of antimicrobial agents. In an environment where antibiotics are used frequently, this intrinsic property is important to ensure survival of nosocomial patho-gens. Antibiotic resistance, coupled with the capacity to transmit this genetic information rapidly to other bacteria by conjugation and trans-duction, accounts for the emergence of endemic strains of multiply resistant bacteria in the hospital environment.

Environmental Adaptability

Several nosocomial pathogens are able to adapt to a variety of envi-ronmental temperatures. *Legionella pneumophila* survives in water if the temperature varies between 5° C (41° F) and 45° C (113° F). The capacity to withstand changes in ambient temperatures enhances the opportunity for transmission from one environmental niche to another. Both *Pseudomonas* and *Legionella* species are capable of surviving in water reservoirs with minimal energy requirements. Thus organ-isms are able to establish a niche in a variety of sites within a hospi-tal.

ENVIRONMENT

The third component of the model that determines susceptibility to nosocomial infections is the biologic and physical environment in which the patient receives care.

Biologic Environment

A reservoir is that site in the environment where microbes reside. The reservoir provides a source of nutrients and a niche conducive to sur-vival and replication of the organism. Microbes are found in humans, animals, plants, and inert material in the environment. Reservoirs may be categorized with reference to the patient as exogenous or endog-enous.

Exogenous reservoirs include air, water, food, equipment, medi-cations, and animate sources (e.g., the health care worker). Epidem-ics associated with *Aspergillus* species in air, *L. pneumophila* in wa-ter, and *Salmonella* species in food have been reported in hospitals. Past experience and attention to hospital design have eliminated many exogenous reservoirs; however, sometimes elusive reservoirs continue to create problems for the immunocompromised patient. Once iden-tified, these reservoirs can usually be controlled, but often at consid-erable cost to the hospital. Medical equipment, particularly that which uses water reservoirs or nebulizers, provides potential reservoirs for aquaphilic nosocomial pathogens. Medical personnel constitute a critically important reservoir and contribute to infections by carrying and shedding organisms or by serving as vectors who carry organ-isms from reservoirs to the uninfected patient. For example, 15% to 30% of the population carry *S. aureus* in the nasal antrum. A sub-group of carriers are prone to shed organisms into the environment, thereby creating a risk for patients. Health care workers also transmit disease during acute infections with communicable agents (e.g., in-fluenza, rotavirus, and respiratory syncytial virus).

The most important reservoir for nosocomial pathogens is endog-enous flora found in or on the patient. Humans are colonized with myriad gram-positive and gram-negative bacteria. This symbiotic re-lationship between host and commensal is easily disturbed during hos-pitalization. The severity of the underlying disease and frequent use of antibiotics alter the normal flora that reside on the skin and in the upper airway and bowel. When antibiotic-susceptible flora are eradi-cated during the course of antibiotic therapy, patients become colo-

nized with large numbers of intrinsically resistant flora such as en-terococci, *S. epidermidis,* and *Candida* species, or with resistant En-terobacteriaceae and *Pseudomonas* species. In the compromised host these "new" flora invade and establish a nidus of infection. Unlike exogenous reservoirs that can be disinfected or eradicated, little can be done to eradicate nosocomial pathogens from endogenous reser-voirs.

Transmission of microorganisms from exogenous reservoirs to the patient occurs via several mechanisms. Some organisms (e.g., *Myco-bacterium tuberculosis*) remain viable when suspended in air and are spread by aerosols. Aerosolized particles may be as small as 1 to 5 µm in diameter; when inhaled the organism is carried to and depos-ited in the alveoli of the lung. The recent emergence of multiple-drug–resistant *M. tuberculosis* and the threat to both patients and health care workers have generated renewed attention to this mode of trans-mission. Organisms are also spread by direct contact between per-sons. The most frequent person-to-person contact in hospitals occurs between health care worker and patient. Without vigorous hand wash-ing, staphylococci and a variety of gram-negative bacilli may be car-ried as superficial flora on the hands and spread from one patient to another.

Physical Environment

Recognizing the importance of reservoirs and modes of transmission in nosocomial infections makes the role of the structural environment in determining risks of nosocomial infections apparent. Improper ven-tilation may disseminate airborne organisms from patient to patient or patient to employee. Potable water, which harbors *Legionella* or-ganisms, can aerosolize bacteria from shower heads and water spig-ots. Inadequate space allocation or inadequate attention to traffic pat-terns in the hospital may contribute to spread of organisms from res-ervoir to patient.

Medical equipment, particularly that which requires direct patient contact such as respirators, dialyzers, and endoscopes, may predis-pose to infections when improperly cleaned and disinfected. This situ-ation is a particular problem when a new technology is introduced. Sophisticated new technologies often limit alternatives for disinfec-tion and simultaneously introduce unsuspected reservoirs and new modes of transmission.

INFECTION SITES

Nosocomial infections may occur at any conceivable anatomic site. Most (80%) occur in one of four sites: urinary tract, surgical wound, lower respiratory tract, or bloodstream. Lower respiratory tract infec-tions are discussed elsewhere in the text (Chapter 237).

Urinary Tract Infections

The urinary tract is the most frequent site of infection, accounting for 40% of nosocomial infections. Most infections are associated with some form of instrumentation of the urinary tract. Four factors have been identified as independent risk factors for infection with indwell-ing urinary catheters: duration of catheterization, breaches in proper care of catheters, absence of systemic antibiotics, and female gender. Nosocomial urinary tract infections are associated with increased risk of septicemia and mortality. Because of the morbidity and mortality associated with urinary tract infections, the physician must be sure that the benefits of catheterization outweigh the risks of the interven-tion (Chapter 246).

Postoperative Wound Infections

Wound infections after surgical procedures have a significant impact on morbidity by prolonging hospitalization and convalescence. Con-tamination of the wound by the inciting pathogen may occur from endogenous or exogenous reservoirs. Endogenous reservoirs include the skin and, when mucous membranes are transected during surgi-cal procedures, the bowel or airways. Exogenous sources include op-erating room personnel and surgical equipment. Contamination often occurs during a breakdown in surgical technique.

Several factors or conditions have been associated with increased risk of wound infections. Some of these conditions are summarized

---

BOX 232-1

Conditions that increase the risk of postoperative wound infections

Preoperative

Age
Underlying disease (e.g., obesity, remote infection)
Duration of preoperative hospital stay
No preoperative shower
Shaving the operative site

Intraoperative

Duration of the procedure
Use of electrocautery
Use of surgical drains
Technical care of the wound

From Mayhall CG. In Wenzel RP, editor: *Prevention and control of nosocomial infections*, ed 2, Baltimore, 1993, Williams & Wilkins.

in Box 232-1. The most consistent predictors of risk of postoperative wound infections include (1) severity of illness of the patient as reflected in the American Society of Anesthesiologists' preoperative assessment score, (2) duration of the operative procedure (a reflection of the complexity of the operative procedure and skill of the surgeon), and (3) level of contamination as classified by a contaminated or dirty wound (e.g., perforated bowel, compound fracture).

Several of the factors that predispose to wound infections can be controlled or managed. Results from the Study for Efficacy of Nosocomial Infection Control (SENIC) conducted by the CDC suggested that at least 33% of wound infections are preventable by careful attention to techniques. Furthermore, prophylactic antibiotics reduce the incidence of wound infections. Optimal chemoprophylaxis requires that the antibiotic inhibit the growth of potential nosocomial pathogens, that it penetrate the site of infection, and that administration precede the operative procedure. Prophylactic antibiotics should be initiated within 2 hours before the incision is made and continued for no longer than 24 hours after the procedure is completed.

Bacteremia

Hospital-acquired bloodstream infections occur less frequently than infections at other sites, accounting for approximately 10% of nosocomial infections. The incidence of bacteremia among hospitalized patients has been increasing. This trend may reflect a selection bias created by national efforts to reduce hospital use by limiting admission to only the sickest patients. Nosocomial bacteremias are serious infections resulting in 7 to 14 additional days of hospitalization and an attributable mortality rate of 25%. Bacteremias may occur without an apparent source (primary) or secondary to infections at another site. The distinction between primary and secondary bacteremia is important for epidemiologic as well as clinical reasons. Secondary bloodstream infections occur as a complication of 1% to 5% of urinary tract infections, 3% of postoperative wound and pulmonary infections, and 5% of cutaneous infections. The usual pathogens are *E. coli, S. aureus, Klebsiella pneumoniae,* and *P. aeruginosa.* Identification of the source allows treatment of both the underlying condition and the complicating bacteremia. For example, bacteremia developing in patients with a urinary tract infection should always suggest the possibility of obstruction, which may require surgery as well as antibiotics.

Primary bacteremias are often associated with intravascular cannulas. In large referral hospitals, 90% of patients receive intravenous infusions. When primary bacteremias occur, cannulas should lead the list of suspected sources of infection. Increasing reliance on technologies such as hyperalimentation, arterial monitors, and Swan-Ganz and tunneled catheters has added to the risk of nosocomial bacteremia. Prevention of this hazardous infectious complication requires discretion in deciding when patients will benefit from the technology and

careful attention to asepsis when inserting and maintaining intravascular cannulas.

PREVENTION

As knowledge regarding risk factors and causation in nosocomial infections increased, a discipline emerged that is dedicated to the study and prevention of these untoward events. Infection control programs have become the standard of care in acute care hospitals. The components of these programs are summarized here.

Infection Control Committee

The committee provides the authority for control programs. It is usually appointed by the hospital administration and includes representatives from the physician staff, nursing, administration, engineering-maintenance, central sterilizing, pharmacy, and other departments deemed appropriate by the administrator. The charge to the committee is to formulate and execute policies related to the control of hospital-acquired infections.

Infection Control Staff

The committee retains a staff who is responsible for implementing committee policies. In most small hospitals the staff includes the committee chairperson, usually a physician with interest in infectious diseases, who serves as "hospital epidemiologist." In larger institutions hospital epidemiologists are specially trained for this task and commit a significant portion of professional time to this effort. In most hospitals the principal staff person is the infection control practitioner, usually a nurse or microbiologist who has received specific training for this task and who commits most of his or her professional time to this effort. For larger hospitals it has been recommended that optimal staffing should include one practitioner for every 250 beds. The tasks of the infection control staff are described in the next sections.

Surveillance

Surveillance is a method for identifying, counting, and monitoring nosocomial infections. It is used to establish endemic rates of nosocomial infections and to identify epidemics. The success of surveillance programs depends on establishing explicit definitions for infections and adhering to the definitions over time. Surveillance data are most useful when converted to rates, for example, the number of events per patients at risk (number of infections per 100 admissions) or number of events per time at risk (number of events per 1000 patient-days). The data are usually reported monthly (when), by service or by physician (who), by patient care area (where), by pathogen (what), and by procedure (how). The information is used by the infection control committee to analyze problems, establish program priorities, and design interventions. The information may also be disseminated to health care providers in the institution to increase awareness regarding methods for preventing nosocomial infections.

Control Programs

A second important component of the infection control program is the implementation of effective interventions to control the spread of infection in hospitals. In most circumstances this effort entails implementation of guidelines set forth by the CDC or the American Hospital Association. These guidelines for the control of nosocomial infections are usually based on scientific studies that have passed the scrutiny of experts in the field. Some controls emerge from local efforts to control institution-specific problems. These measures can be equally important, as long as they have been demonstrated to be effective. Controls are generally designed to disinfect, to contain known reservoirs, or to interfere with known modes of transmission. Methods for containing hospital biohazards may be categorized into engineering or administrative controls.

Engineering Controls. Engineering controls are incorporated into the design and structure of the hospital. They include everything

---
BOX 232-2

Guidelines for intravenous line use

---

1. Use only when indicated
2. Choose a low-risk site (upper extremity)
3. Use good technique
   a. Wash hands
   b. Use aseptic preparation
   c. Date and label the site
4. Maintain appropriately
   a. Discontinue emergency sites within 24 hours
   b. Observe daily
   c. Remove in 48 hours
5. Discontinue as early as possible
6. With unexplained sepsis, suspect the intravenous site

BOX 232-3

Universal precautions to reduce risk of infection

---

1. All health care workers should use barrier precautions* when contact with infectious body fluids is anticipated.
2. Wash hands if contaminated and immediately after removing gloves.
3. Avoid sharp injuries.
4. Use mouthpieces, resuscitation bags, or other ventilation devices for emergency resuscitation.
5. Health care workers who have exudative lesions or weeping dermatitis should refrain from direct patient care.
6. Pregnant health care workers should be especially familiar with and strictly adhere to precautions to minimize risk of exposure to blood-borne agents.

---

*Gloves (routine); goggles, masks, and gowns (when indicated). From Centers for Disease Control and Prevention: *MMWR* 36(suppl 2S):2, 1987.

from the proper design of ventilation systems to the simple placement of hand-washing sinks in convenient locations. Protection of the environment in high-risk areas such as operating suites includes the proper exchange of fresh air (20 L/hour) through high-efficiency filters to remove potential airborne pathogens. For hospitals in which outbreaks of legionellosis have been documented, special engineering controls may be required to eradicate and control *Legionella* organisms in the potable water system. Currently available options include infusion of heavy metal ions, hyperchlorination, raising the hot water temperature, and ultraviolet light. Infection control staff must be cognizant of these important aspects of control programs and review all new construction plans to ensure that these measures have been addressed.

Administrative Controls. Administrative controls must be implemented at the volition of the health care worker. Because the success and efficacy of administrative controls depend on the knowledge and initiative of health care workers, education and reinforcement are important elements in a successful prevention program. Examples of administrative controls include the following:

Guidelines for procedures. The insertion of an intravenous line (e.g., intravenous cannula) is accompanied by a measurable risk of infection. The risk of infection may be reduced by adhering to certain guidelines regarding insertion, maintenance, and removal. Guidelines for proper insertion of an intravenous line are summarized in Box 232-2. Similarly, infection control programs must ensure adherence to proper guidelines for all procedures that impose a risk of infection for patients.

Isolation and universal precautions. Isolation or segregation precautions are procedures that have been traditionally used in hospitals to contain transmissible pathogens and protect employees and other patients. These administrative controls are implemented after establishing a presumptive diagnosis of a transmissible disease.

The AIDS epidemic has heightened concern for the risk of transmission of disease from patients to health care workers and from health care workers to patients. Blood-borne nosocomial pathogens such as hepatitis B, human immunodeficiency virus (HIV), and the agent of Creutzfeldt-Jakob disease pose a particular risk to health care workers because of their exposure to body fluids and secretions. These exposures often occur when health care workers encounter patients with undiagnosed, asymptomatic disease. To reduce the risk of infection, it has been recommended that health care workers avoid direct contact with body fluids by exercising universal precautions with all patients. These precautions, summarized in Box 232-3, include the routine use of gloves when exposure to potentially infectious fluids is anticipated and use of goggles and masks when there is risk of droplet contact with mucous membranes. Special attention must be given to reducing accidental needle sticks (e.g., no recapping of used needles and using puncture-resistant containers for disposal of used needles). It is assumed that when universal precautions are used as part of routine patient care practices, an added level of protection against transmission of blood-borne pathogens is afforded both health care workers and patients.

Hand washing. Hand washing is a simple hygienic measure that interrupts the transmission of nosocomial pathogens from a patient reservoir to an otherwise uninfected, uncolonized patient. Despite repeated reports that confirm Semmelweis's original observation on the efficacy of hand washing in 1847, clusters of preventable nosocomial infections continue to occur because of careless inattention to hand washing by health care personnel.

Employee health. Two important objectives of an employee health program include protection of patients from transmissible diseases carried by health care workers and protection of the employee against communicable diseases in patients. These objectives may be accomplished by screening employees for disease (e.g., tuberculosis) at the time of job entry and periodically during the term of employment. The latter is especially important in the current era of multiple-antibiotic–resistant strains of tuberculosis (Chapter 273). Employee health programs also screen employees to ensure that they are protected by vaccination against a variety of communicable diseases. When previous exposure or vaccination cannot be documented, many institutions provide vaccination against hepatitis B and rubella for employees. The employee health program should also include counseling, volunteer testing, and follow-up for health care workers parenterally exposed to HIV or other blood-borne pathogens. The programs should have provisions for evaluation of acute illnesses to ensure that employees with acute transmissible infections are excused from work. Because of the threat of HIV and multiple-drug–resistant tuberculosis for health care workers, Occupational Health and Safety Administration (OSHA) has devised and mandated complex work rules for ensuring employee safety. Implementation of these rules usually resides with employee health programs working in concert with infection control programs.

Efficacy of Infection Control Programs. It has been estimated that the cost of an effective infection control program in a 250-bed hospital ranges between approximately $78,000 (1989 dollars) and $200,000 (1994 dollars). Because infection control programs do not generate revenue, one may query whether prevention programs can be justified. In a large national study (SENIC) conducted by the CDC in the mid-1970s, it was observed that hospitals incorporating all elements of an infection control program had a 33% reduction in the rates of nosocomial infections. Based on estimates of cost for increased lengths of stay following nosocomial infections, the program should "break even" when the infection rate is reduced by as little as 10%. A recent comparison of the cost to save a life and extend life-years of hospitalized patients and similar costs for other public health programs suggests the relative benefits of an excellent infection control program. Thus effective infection control programs are not only effective in reducing rates of nosocomial infection but also are cost effective. This observation is all the more compelling under prospective reimbursement, in which the financial risk of unnecessary hospitalization because of nosocomial infections is assumed by the health care provider.

BIBLIOGRAPHY

Beck-Sague C, Jarvis WR: Secular trends in the epidemiology of nosocomial fungal infections in the United States, 1980-1990, *J Infect Dis* 167:1247-1251, 1993.

Bennett JV, Brachman PS, editors: *Hospital infections,* ed 3, Boston, 1992, Little, Brown.

Centers for Disease Control and Prevention: Recommendations for prevention of HIV transmission in health-care settings, *MMWR* 40:1-9, 1991.

Centers for Disease Control and Prevention: Nosocomial enterococci resistant to vancomycin: United States, 1989-1993, *MMWR* 42:597-599, 1993.

Centers for Disease Control and Prevention: Guidelines for preventing the transmission of *Mycobacterium tuberculosis* in health-care facilities, *MMWR* 43:RR-13, 1994.

Classen DC et al: The timing of prophylactic administration of antibiotics and the risk of surgical wound infection, *N Engl J Med* 26:281-286, 1992.

Cruse PJE, Foord R: The epidemiology of wound infection: a 10-year prospective study of 62,939 wounds, *Surg Clin North Am* 60:27-40, 1980.

Doebbeling BN, Stanley GL, Sheetz CT et al: Comparative efficacy of alternative handwashing agents in reducing nosocomial infections in intensive care units, *N Engl J Med* 327:88-93, 1992.

Driks MR et al: Nosocomial pneumonia in intubated patients given sucralfate as compared with antacids or histamine type 2 blockers: the role of gastric colonization, *N Engl J Med* 317:1376-1382, 1987.

Edmond MB, Wenzel RP, Pasculle AW: Vancomycin-resistant *Staphylococcus aureus:* perspectives on measures needed for control, *Ann Intern Med* 24:329-334, 1996.

Federal Register: Standard for bloodborne pathogens, *Fed Reg* 56 (235):64175-64182, 1991.

Haley RW et al: The nationwide nosocomial infection rate: a new need for vital statistics, *Am J Epidemiol* 121:159-167, 1985.

Haley RW et al: The efficacy of infection surveillance and control programs in preventing nosocomial infections in U.S. hospitals, *Am J Epidemiol* 121:182-205, 1985.

Helms CM et al: Legionnaires' disease associated with a hospital water system: a 5-year progress report on continuous hyperchlorination, *JAMA* 259(16):2423-2427, 1988.

Ishak MA et al: Association of slime with pathogenicity of coagulase-negative staphylococci causing nosocomial septicemia, *J Clin Microbiol* 22:1025-1029, 1985.

Kunin CM: *Detection, prevention, and management of urinary tract infections,* ed 4, Philadelphia, 1987, Lea & Febiger.

Maki DG: Nosocomial bacteremia: an epidemiologic overview, *Am J Med* 70:719-732, 1981.

Martone WJ, Garner JS, editors: Proceedings of the Third Decennial International Conference on Nosocomial Infections, *Am J Med* 91(3B):1-333, 1991.

Massanari RM et al: Reliability of reporting nosocomial infection in the discharge abstract and implications for receipt of revenues under prospective reimbursement, *Am J Public Health* 77:1-3, 1986.

Miller PJ, Wenzel RP: Etiologic organisms as independent predictors of death and morbidity associated with bloodstream infections (BSI), *J Infect Dis* 156:471-477, 1987.

Pittet D, Wenzel RP: Nosocomial bloodstream infections: secular trends in rates, mortality, and contibution to total hospital deaths, *Arch Intern Med* 155:1177-1184, 1995.

Selden R, Lee S, Wang WL: Nosocomial *Klebsiella* infections: intestinal colonization as a reservoir, *Ann Intern Med* 74:657-664, 1971.

Sheth NK, Franson TR, Sohnle PC: Influence of bacterial adherence to intravascular catheters on in vitro antibiotic susceptibility, *Lancet* 2:1266-1268, 1985.

Stamm WE: Catheter-associated urinary tract infections: epidemiology, pathogenesis, and prevention, *Am J Med* (suppl 3B)91:65S-71S, 1991.

Voelker R: Disease detectives are turning to molecular techniques to uncover emerging microbes, *JAMA* 275:176-178, 1996.

Wadowsky RM et al: Effect of temperature, pH, and oxygen level on multiplication of naturally occurring *Legionella pneumophila* in potable water, *Appl Environ Microbiol* 49:1197-1205, 1985.

Wenzel RP: The economics of nosocomial infection: Lowbury Lecture for 1994, *J Hosp Infect* 31:79-87, 1995.

Wenzel RP, editor: *Assessing quality health care: perspective for clinicians,* Baltimore, 1992, Williams & Wilkins.

Wenzel RP, editor: *Prevention and control of nosocomial infections,* ed 2, Baltimore, 1993, Williams & Wilkins.

II LABORATORY TESTS

CHAPTER

233 Use of Laboratory Tests in Infectious Diseases

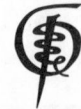

Thomas A. Drake

Identification of an etiologic agent is essential for the diagnosis of and choice of therapy for most infectious diseases. Laboratory techniques to identify etiologic agents can be grouped into three categories: isolation of the organism in culture, demonstration of the organism or its specific components at sites of infection, and measurement of specific immune response.

Isolation of pathogenic organisms in culture, except when culture is not feasible, has long been the mainstay of diagnostic methods, with other techniques providing supportive information. A major drawback with culture and serologic techniques, however, is the length of time normally required to establish a diagnosis. The need for more immediately available information, coupled with recent technologic developments, has dramatically increased interest in direct detection techniques, techniques encompassing a variety of tests ranging from simple morphologic stains on direct specimens to the newly developed tests of antigen detection by monoclonal antibodies and pathogen-specific DNA detection. Although relatively few of these procedures have replaced culture as the standard diagnostic technique, they will be used more and more as methodologies are improved to provide timely results.

TEST INTERPRETATION

The usefulness of any laboratory technique varies with the nature of the infection and must be evaluated clinically in terms of predictive value, timeliness, and cost. The *predictive value* of a test is the frequency with which a disease is accurately predicted to be present or absent by a particular positive or negative test result, respectively. (A positive predictive value of 60% means that of 100 patients with positive tests, 60 will actually have the disease and 40 will not.) To assess predictive value, test sensitivity (frequency of positive test result among patients with the disease), test specificity (frequency of negative test results among persons without the disease), and disease prevalence (probability of the presence of disease in the population being evaluated) must be known or reasonably approximated. The details of predictive value theory are available elsewhere and are not presented here (see Bibliography). The concepts involved, however, are directly applicable to testing in clinical microbiology.

For tests in which the ranges of values obtained from reference and patient populations overlap, test sensitivity and specificity are determined by the cutoff value chosen to separate positive and negative results; a gain in one will result in a loss in the other. One can illustrate this relationship by reference to coliform urinary tract infections (the presence of coliform bacteria in urine obtained by suprapubic aspiration or catheterization) in symptomatic women. The traditional diagnostic criterion of 10^5 bacteria per milliliter of midstream urine yields 99% specificity but only 51% sensitivity (Chapter 246) for this group of patients (in which the prevalence of infection is 50%). In this setting predictive values of positive and negative results are 98% and 67%, respectively. If the criterion for a positive test result in this group is revised to 10^2 bacteria per milliliter, specificity is 85%, sensitivity is 95%, and predictive values of positive and negative results are 86% and 94%, respectively. Thus use of the lower cutoff value produces more clinically acceptable predictive values of positive and negative results. Other tests for which established cutoff values are of comparable import include purified protein derivative (PPD) skin testing (diameter of induration), some enzyme and radioimmunoassays (degree of enzymatic activity or radioactivity measured), and many titrated serologic tests.

A second important aspect of laboratory testing, which is often not appreciated intuitively, is the significant influence that the probability of disease has on a test's predictive value. To continue the preceding example, although the cutoff of 10^2 bacteria per milliliter was clinically useful in a high-prevalence (50%) population, application of this criterion in a low-prevalence setting (e.g., 6% in certain asymptomatic patients) would result in an unacceptably low predictive value of a positive result (29%). The predictive value of a negative result, however, would be high (>99%). In low-prevalence settings test specificity becomes a critical determinant of positive predictive value. With 1% prevalence, the latter drops from 91% to 50%, to 17% when test specificity changes from 99.9% to 99%, to 95%, respectively. Because many tests do not have 99.9% sensitivity or are used in even lower disease-prevalence populations, positive results may need to be confirmed by independent means, as is accepted practice for the serologic diagnosis of syphilis and human immunodeficiency virus (HIV) infection. In general, in low-prevalence settings positive results should be questioned, whereas in high-prevalence settings negative findings should prompt further investigation.

CULTURE OF PATHOGENIC MICROORGANISMS IN CLINICAL MEDICINE
Bacteria

Specimen Collection and Handling. Avoidance of contamination, adequacy of sampling, and preservation of viability are critical factors in proper specimen collection and handling. Effort must always be made to obtain appropriate specimens before the institution of antibiotic therapy. Details regarding specimen collection from specific body sites are presented in other chapters; general guidelines are presented in Box 233-1. Submission of inappropriate, contaminated, or mishandled specimens creates potentially confusing and dangerous clinical situations. The patient is placed at risk if effective therapy is withheld or if unnecessary therapy is administered, and the cost of care is increased.

The human body harbors abundant flora of commensal bacteria on the skin and mucous membranes and in the intestinal tract (Table 233-1). Skin should be disinfected with tincture of iodine, iodophor, chlorhexidine, or alcohol before being traversed to obtain specimens. Alcohol is the least rapidly acting, requiring 1 to 2 minutes of contact to afford maximum antibacterial effect. The practice of replacing needles on syringes before inoculating blood culture bottles should be abandoned, since it does not reduce contamination and increases the risk of needle-stick injury. When sites of infection are in continuity with the skin (e.g., via sinus tracts or open wounds), superficial

or sinus tract material should be considered contaminated, and acceptable samples are those taken only at deep sites.

Specimens may be collected directly into sterile containers (cerebrospinal fluid [CSF], urine, stool, tissue), via syringe (blood, body fluid, and tissue aspirates), or with a swab (mucous membranes). Cotton swabs are adequate for most purposes but Dacron- or calcium alginate–tipped swabs should be used when *Neisseria gonorrhoeae, Bordetella pertussis,* or *Corynebacterium diphtheriae* are sought. The volume of a specimen submitted is important in situations where pathogenic bacteria may be present in low numbers. Maximal recovery of organisms from blood is obtained by culturing a total of 30 ml of blood in two or three draws. At least 5 ml of CSF should be obtained for routine bacterial culture, and 10 ml for mycobacterial culture. In addition, bulk stool samples more frequently yield pathogens than do rectal swabs.

Procedures for specimen transport must ensure viability of pathogens, as well as limitation of contaminant growth. The best means to accomplish these goals are through use of appropriate transport systems and prompt delivery to the laboratory. Transport media such as Stuart and Amies media are formulated to maintain organism viability but restrict rapid growth and should be used for swabs and tissue samples. Urine and stool should be transported in sealed sterile containers and refrigerated if not processed within 1 hour of collection. In contrast, blood and CSF should be incubated at 37° C if processing is delayed. All other specimens, including sputum, should be kept at room temperature. Certain pathogens such as *Neisseria* and *Haemophilus* species are killed when exposed to the cold, whereas others such as group A streptococci are quite hardy.

Blood specimens are inoculated immediately into culture bottles to optimize organism recovery. Adequate dilution (1:5 to 1:10) in medium is important to minimize natural antibacterial properties of blood. This is also facilitated by having sodium polyethylene sulfonate (SPS) as a component of blood culture medium, which also serves as an anticoagulant. *Neisseria* species and *Peptostreptococcus anaerobius* are inhibited by SPS, however, and SPS-free media should be used when presence of these organisms is suspected. Sucrose-supplemented media designed for recovery of cell wall–deficient organisms have not proved useful for routine use. Media containing resins to absorb and inactivate antibiotics are of limited benefit; these methods appear to be most advantageous when used with small-volume systems like the BACTEC (Becton-Dickinson Diagnostic Instrument Systems, Towson, Md.). One novel blood culture system, the lysis centrifugation method (Isolator, DuPont Co., Wilmington, Del.) avoids the use of liquid culture media. Blood is drawn directly into an evacuated tube containing a blood cell lysing solution. Tubes are centrifuged to sediment bacteria, and the bottom layer is plated directly to agar media.

The recognized spectrum of disease associated with anaerobic bacteria has broadened as improved techniques for recovery, isolation, and identification have been developed. Although some anaerobes can survive extended exposure to oxygen, others are oxygen sensitive; thus specimens that may harbor such anaerobes should not be exposed to air. Fluids should be collected in a syringe, the air immediately expressed, and the contents injected into an anaerobic transport tube. Swabs should not be used because air remains trapped among the fibers. Tissue specimens should be placed in anaerobic transport containers. A variety of these systems is currently commercially available; the simplest of them is the carbon dioxide–filled, stoppered tube. When the tube is held upright during opening and insertion of the specimen, the carbon dioxide does not flow out of the bottle, and the atmosphere remains anaerobic if the container is recapped quickly. Preservation of *N. gonorrhoeae* requires that carbon dioxide be added to the incubation atmosphere, as is provided by the traditional candle jars or various commercially available systems.

Isolation and Identification. Inoculation of agar plates, properly streaked, allows isolation of separate colonies. This separation is essential for identification of bacteria and may also provide a crude estimate of relative numbers of bacteria. The concentration of organisms in a liquid sample (such as urine) can be determined by plating a defined amount of dilution of the sample uniformly over the surface of an agar plate. Inoculation of broth medium precludes quantitation but permits culture of a larger sample volume and may be more

---

BOX 233-1
Do's and don'ts of specimen collection and handling

1. Collect specimen from site of infection.
2. Use appropriate collection technique to avoid contamination by indigenous flora.
3. Do not use swabs for anaerobic cultures.
4. Avoid contaminating specimen for culture when Gram's stain or other stain is prepared at the time of collection.
5. Use proper technique when culture medium is directly inoculated.
6. Label specimen and provide a specific description of the source and the testing desired.
7. Use appropriate transport medium to preserve organism viability.
8. Avoid delays in specimen transport.
9. Never freeze specimen or expose to heat; refrigerate only stool and urine; incubate only blood and cerebrospinal fluid.

Table 233-1 Normal human microbial flora*

ORGANISM	GRAM'S STAIN/MORPHOLOGY†	SKIN	NOSE/NASOPHARYNX	MOUTH/OROPHARYNX	CONJUNCTIVA	COLON	VAGINA	EXTERNAL GENITALIA	ANTERIOR URETHRA
Aerobic and facultative anaerobic bacteria									
Staphylococcus									
Coagulase-negative	+/c	++	++	++	++	±	++	++	++
S. aureus	+/c	+	+	+	+		±	+	
Streptococcus									
β-Hemolytic	+/c	±	±	±	±	+	+	+	+
S. pneumoniae	+/c		±	+	±	+	±		
Enterococci	+/c	±		±		±	±	±	
Viridans	+/c	+	++	++	±	+	+	±	+
Corynebacterium	+/cb	++	±	±	±	±	±	±	±
Branhamella	–/c	±	+	+	±				
Neisseria	–/c	±	±	+	±	+	±		+
Haemophilus	–/cb	±	±	+	±		±		
Gardnerella	–/cb						+		
Enterobacteriaceae	–/b	±	±	±		++	±	+	±
Acinetobacter	–/b					+			±
Moraxella	–/b		±	±					
Pseudomonas	–/b					+	+		+
Treponema	/s			±		±	±		+
Mycobacterium	af/b	±					±	+	+
Mycoplasma, ureaplasma							±	++	±
Anaerobic bacteria									
Peptococcus, Peptostreptococcus	+/c	+	+	+		+	+		
Actinomyces	+/b			++		±	±		±
Bifidobacterium	+/b			+		+	+		
Clostridium	+/b	±		±		++	±		
Eubacterium	+/b			+		++	±		
Lactobacillus	+/b	±		±		+	++		±
Bacteroides	–/b			±		++	±		
Fusobacterium	–/b			+		++	±		
Propionibacterium	–/b	++	+	+	+	+	±	++	+
Veillonella	–/b			+		+	±		±
Fungi									
Candida		±		±	+	±	±		
Torulopsis		±		±	+	±	±		
Rhodotorula		±		±	++	±			
Cryptococcus		±		±					
Aspergillus		±		±					
Penicillium		±		±					
Pityrosporon		+		+					

*Relative presence at each body site is indicated: ++, prominent; +, common; ±, irregular.
†Gram's stain/morphology: +, gram-positive; –, gram-negative; af, acid-fast; c, coccus; cb, coccobacillus; b, bacillus; s, spirochete.

conducive to growth. Specimens from normally sterile body sites should be inoculated to a medium that will support the growth of suspected pathogens. Usually this medium includes blood and chocolate (laked blood) agar plates and a nutrient broth. When specimens are obtained from areas of the body normally harboring bacteria, selective culture media and environments are often necessary. In selective media the nutrient, chemical, and inhibiting composition is varied to allow growth of only certain organisms. These media are necessary for isolation of certain enteric pathogens and are commonly used to improve recovery of group A streptococci from throat cultures.

The time needed to grow, isolate, and identify different organisms varies considerably. The more common aerobic pathogens grow rapidly, and preliminary reports based on morphologic and growth characteristics can be expected from the laboratory within 24 hours. Use of automated or rapid identification techniques applied to isolated colonies yields definitive identification within several hours to a day in most cases. Anaerobes generally grow more slowly, and plates are not usually examined for 48 hours. Most pathogenic mycobacteria require at least several weeks of incubation before identifiable colonies form. However, application of immunologic or nucleic acid–based direct detection techniques on early cultures can substantially reduce the time needed for identification. Several species of pathogenic bacteria (e.g., *Treponema pallidum, Borrelia* species, and *Mycobacterium leprae*) cannot be isolated on artificial media. Assessments of mixed organism growth as "normal (e.g., fecal, oral) flora" in specimens from contaminated sites are made simply by inspection of culture plates, without specific organism identification.

Blood cultures are incubated in the collection bottle and monitored regularly, with Gram's stain and subcultures performed if there is evidence of bacterial growth. Several automated systems (BACTEC; BacT/Alert, Organaon Technika Corp., Durham, N.C.; ESP, Difco Laboratories, Detroit, Mich.) have automated monitoring based on carbon dioxide or other gas production by growing organisms, which reduces the time needed for a culture to be recognized as positive. The Septi-chek system (Roche Diagnostics Systems, Nutley, N.J.) consists of a device with an enclosed agar paddle that is attached to the top of the blood culture bottles after inoculation. When the bottles are inverted, the paddle is flooded; hence one is effectively performing a subculture without entering the system. This technique reduces the time needed to make bacterial colonies available for identification and susceptibility testing. Blood cultures are held for at least 7 days before being reported as negative and discarded. The laboratory should be notified if a longer incubation is indicated, as for suspected brucellosis.

Laboratory personnel should always be notified if plague (*Yersinia pestis*) or tularemia (*Francisella tularensis*) is suspected. These agents are highly infectious in culture, and isolation should be attempted only in laboratories using adequate safety precautions. Usual laboratory precautions are also insufficient for safe handling of specimens that contain *Coccidioides immitis* or hemorrhagic fever viruses (Box 233-2).

Management of Specimens From Specific Body Sites. Principal discussions of aspects of management of specimens are found in the following chapters presenting the major clinical syndromes associated with each: blood, Chapters 245, 275, and 279; CSF, Chapter 239; upper and lower respiratory tract specimens, Chapter 237; gastrointestinal tract specimens, Chapter 242; urine, Chapter 246; genital tract specimens, Chapter 244; and skin and soft tissue specimens, Chapter 241.

Clinicians should familiarize themselves with specimen handling and culture protocols of the clinical microbiology laboratory they use to ensure that they will obtain the clinical information needed without excessive testing (and its attendant cost). For example, throat cultures may routinely include only a search for group A streptococci or, conversely, might entail identification and susceptibility testing of all possible pathogens. Another example is urine cultures, where a screening procedure may or may not be used and policies for detection and susceptibility testing of fewer than 10^4 or 10^5 organisms per milliliter can vary.

Viruses

It is possible to culture viruses through the use of tissue culture systems. Viruses causing human disease that can be routinely cultured are listed in Table 233-2, and those primarily detected by nonculture techniques are listed in Table 233-3. With time, it is expected that use of direct detection techniques, particularly nucleic acid amplification methods, will replace culture as the diagnostic method of choice for most viruses. Viral diagnostic services are available in most hospital and commercial laboratories. A discussion with laboratory personnel facilitates proper and expeditious treatment of specimens.

Specimen Collection and Handling. Maximum recovery of virus depends on obtaining samples as early as possible in the course of the patient's illness and minimizing the time from specimen procurement to laboratory processing. In contrast to most bacterial infections, sampling of sites other than the focus of infection may yield the causative virus (see Table 233-2).

Swabs are convenient for obtaining specimens from the throat, nasopharynx, rectum, external urogenital tract, conjunctiva, and skin lesions. Because viruses multiply intracellularly, recovery depends on obtaining a sufficient number of infected cells when sampling. Swabs should be placed in appropriate transport media, preferably a specific viral transport medium (usually buffered saline with added protein

Table 233-2 Appropriate agents and specimens for diagnostic viral culture

AGENT	SPECIMENS
Enteroviruses	Feces, throat swab; CSF if indicated
Influenza viruses	Throat swab
Parainfluenza virus	Throat swab
Respiratory syncytial virus	Nasopharyngeal wash (preferable to throat swab)
Mumps virus	Throat swab, urine; CSF if indicated
Measles virus (rubeola)	Throat swab
Rubella virus	Throat swab, urine
Herpes simplex virus	Skin or mucosal lesion (swab from base); involved tissue (e.g., brain)
Varicella-zoster virus	Vesicle fluid or swab
Cytomegalovirus	Throat, urine, blood leukocytes
Adenovirus	Throat swab, feces

CSF, Cerebrospinal fluid.

Table 233-3 Human viruses detected primarily by nonculture techniques

DIRECT DETECTION	SEROLOGIC DIAGNOSIS
Hepatitis B	Hepatitis A, B, C
Human immunodeficiency virus	Human immunodeficiency virus
Papillomavirus	Epstein-Barr virus
Polyomavirus	Arboviruses
Rotavirus	Human T lymphotrophic virus I, II
Norwalk virus	
Rabies virus	

BOX 233-2

Organisms hazardous to laboratory personnel if handled without special precautions

Francisella tularensis (tularemia)
Yersinia pestis (plague)
Coccidioides immitis (coccidioidomycosis)
Hemorrhagic fever viruses (Lassa fever and others)

and antibiotics). If samples are to be processed within 4 hours, a routine transport medium (e.g., Stuart or Amies medium or the Culturette system [Marion Scientific Corp., Rockford, Ill.]) is acceptable. Cerebrospinal fluid, urine, feces, and tissues can be placed directly into sterile containers, as for bacterial culture. Vesicular skin lesions can be aspirated and the fluid injected into a small volume of liquid viral transport medium (and the syringe flushed with same) before the base of the lesion is swabbed. Blood for viral culture should be collected in heparinized tubes to allow recovery of leukocyte fractions.

Delays in transport before processing should be minimized; in some instances it may be desirable to inoculate tissue culture tubes at the bedside. Respiratory syncytial virus, varicella-zoster virus, and cytomegalovirus are particularly labile. Otherwise, specimens should be kept at 4° C until processed; blood should be held at room temperature. Freezing is detrimental to most viruses and should be avoided unless samples must be held for more than several days.

Isolation and Identification. Viruses are cultured in living mammalian cells. Because no single type of cultured cell supports the growth of all viruses, specimens are inoculated to two or more types of cells (usually including primary monkey kidney cells and human fetal diploid fibroblast cells). Culture medium is biochemically complex to maintain cell viability and contains antibiotics to prevent growth of bacteria or fungi. Highly contaminated specimens such as stool are pretreated with antibiotics, and a filtrate of centrifuged supernatant is used to inoculate cell cultures.

Characteristics used to identify specific viruses include the cell lines that support replication, the morphologic appearance of the cytopathic effect, and the results of a variety of tests (e.g., hemadsorption to infected cells, hemagglutination inhibition, and direct immunofluorescence). Providing a brief statement of the clinical situation assists laboratory personnel in choosing appropriate cell lines for inoculation and tests to perform to identify likely pathogens. The time required to isolate and identify viruses by traditional methods varies considerably, depending on the type of virus and the infecting inoculum (Table 233-4). However, these times may be shortened to 24 to 72 hours by centrifuging inoculum onto cell monolayers to enhance infectivity and using direct immunofluorescence to detect viral replication before the cytopathic effect is observed (the "shell vial" technique).

Fungi

Nearly all pathogenic fungi are readily cultured when appropriate media are used. Methods of procurement and transport of most specimens are similar to those for bacteria. Skin lesions should be sampled by obtaining scrapings, preferably from the margins of the lesion. As with mycobacteria, recovery of fungal material is greater with larger volumes of fluids (CSF, urine, effusions) than are normally obtained for culture of the usual bacteria. If fungemia is suspected, blood should be inoculated in special culture bottles containing a biphasic medium (broth plus agar slant) or collected using the Isolator system (DuPont Company, Wilmington, Del.), which may provide optimum recovery. Specimens should never be frozen. The time required for

growth and identification varies considerably among species, ranging from only several days (or less) for some, such as *Candida* species, to several weeks for others, such as *Histoplasma capsulatum*. Characteristics used for identification include growth rate, colony and microscopic morphologic features, and, for yeasts, biochemical reactions such as carbohydrate assimilation and fermentation.

Penicillium species are a frequently encountered contaminant. Although *Candida* and *Aspergillus* species are potentially pathogenic, isolation of these fungi from normally nonsterile sites commonly represents only colonization and should prompt further attempts to document true infection.

Chlamydiae, Rickettsiae, and Mycoplasmas

Laboratories providing viral diagnostic services usually also isolate *Chlamydia trachomatis*, since these organisms grow intracellularly and are cultured in cell monolayers. However, direct antigen or nucleic acid detection methods are more commonly used, and *Chlamydia psittaci* and *Chlamydia pneumoniae* are best diagnosed by serologic means (Chapter 257). Rickettsiae are also obligate intracellular parasites that can be cultured only in animals, embryonated eggs, or tissue culture. Diagnosis rests on serologic testing or direct detection in infected tissue (Chapter 259). *Mycoplasma* species can be isolated on artificial agar-based media, but the availability of services for their culture remains limited (Chapter 258). Swabs may be used to collect specimens and are best transported in a protein-containing medium formulated specifically for *Mycoplasma* species.

DIRECT DETECTION TECHNIQUES

These techniques, of widely varying complexity and cost, are capable of rapid, direct detection of microorganisms in body samples and in some instances supplant culture as the diagnostic method of choice. They often complement culture techniques, however, particularly in cases in which culture is the more sensitive technique or when isolation of the organism is necessary for further characterization (e.g., antibiotic susceptibility testing). These techniques are also used to more rapidly identify organisms isolated in culture.

Microscopy

Wet mounts. The wet mount is the simplest of microscopic methods and allows for observation of the motility and morphologic features of the living organism (Color Plate VIII-1). A drop of fresh specimen is placed on a slide, and a cover glass is added (with margins petrolatum-sealed to prevent desiccation, if desired). Samples may be examined with bright-field (this is the usual way; lowering the condenser provides the necessary contrast) or phase-contrast microscopy. Stool and vaginal pool specimens are commonly examined by this method. Use of the dark-field condenser provides a clearer outline of organisms—although internal detail is lacking—and is most commonly used in examining exudates for *T. pallidum* to diagnose syphilis (Color Plate VIII-2). Contrast can also be provided by the addition of India ink (traditionally used for demonstration of *Cryptococcus neoformans* in CSF [see Chapter 278]) or methylene blue (Box 233-3). Potassium hydroxide solution dissolves host cells and keratinous debris and facilitates visualization of fungi in skin scrapings and vaginal secretions (Box 233-4). Iodine solution, although it renders trophozoites immotile, is also useful, especially for identification of ova and parasites in stool samples. For Neufeld's reaction, or quellung reaction, a highly sensitive and specific test for identifying pneumococci in clinical specimens, the specimen is prepared as a wet mount to which antibody to the capsular polysaccharide is added, making the capsule refractile and thereby visible (Color Plate VIII-3).

Stains for Smears and Imprints. Various stains are available for use on air-dried or alcohol-fixed smears or touch preparations (Box 233-4). Gram's stain, the most widely used, should be performed on specimens submitted for bacterial or fungal culture (Color Plates VIII-4 to VIII-9). Organisms are grouped as gram-positive or gram-negative based on their ability to retain crystal violet dye after exposure to an acetone-alcohol solution. Reactivity depends on cell wall

Table 233-4   Time to detection for viruses in tissue culture

AGENT	USUAL TIME (DAYS)	RANGE (DAYS)
Enteroviruses	2-5	1-14
Influenza viruses	5-7	3-14
Parainfluenza virus	5-10	3-14
Respiratory syncytial virus	5-7	2-10
Mumps virus	5-10	3-14
Measles virus (rubeola)	5-10	3-14
Rubella virus	10-14	10-21
Herpes simplex virus	1-4 (1)*	1-10
Varicella-zoster virus	7-10	5-21
Cytomegalovirus†	5-28 (3)*	3-42
Adenovirus	5-10	3-28

*Using direct immunofluorescence on inoculated cell monolayers.
†Time varies considerably depending on patient population.

BOX 233-3
Wet-mount microscopic procedures

India ink preparation
1. Place a drop of specimen on a clean glass slide.
2. Cover with coverslip, preferably a larger size.
3. Place a small drop of India ink on the slide, touching the coverslip; it will be drawn under the coverslip and provide a gradient suspension of the ink particles.
4. Examine using bright-field microscopy; scan the slide to find the point at which suspension is optimal for observing capsules or organisms.

Potassium hydroxide preparation
1. Place a small portion of specimen on a clean glass slide.
2. Add a drop of 10% potassium hydroxide solution; if necessary, mix with specimen using an applicator stick.
3. Cover with a coverslip, then heat gently by passing through a flame (do not heat excessively; several minutes or more of setting may be necessary to dissolve material composed of keratin).
4. Examine using bright-field microscopy; adjust substage condenser to optimize contrast.

Methylene blue stain for fecal leukocytes
1. Place a small portion of liquid stool on a clean glass slide.
2. Add a drop of methylene blue stain and mix with the specimen; place coverslip.
3. Let stand several minutes, then examine with bright-field microscopy.

BOX 233-4
Staining procedures for smears and imprints

Gram's stain procedure
1. Air dry the smear, and fix by heating.
2. Flood with crystal violet solution, let stand 1 minute, and then rinse briefly with tap water.
3. Flood with iodine solution, let stand 1 minute, and then wash with tap water as before.
4. Flush the slide with decolorizer solution until the stain no longer elutes from the thinner areas of the smear, and then rinse with tap water.
5. Apply safranine counterstain, let stand 10 seconds, and then flush with tap water and blot dry.

Kinyoun acid-fast stain procedure
1. Air dry the smear, and fix well by heating.
2. Flood with Kinyoun carbolfuchsin, let stand 2 minutes (no heating), and then wash briefly with tap water.
3. Flush with acid alcohol decolorizer for 1 minute, and then wash with tap water.
4. Apply methylene blue counterstain for 20 to 30 seconds, flush with tap water, and blot dry.

Wright's stain
1. Make a thin peripheral blood smear on a clean glass slide and allow to air dry.
2. Flood horizontally placed slide with undiluted stain solution and let sit for 5 minutes.
3. Without removing stain, add an equal volume of buffer and mix by blowing gently on the liquid surface; let sit 10 to 20 minutes.
4. Wash off stain thoroughly with water and air dry.

Tzanck preparation
1. Obtain cells from the base of a lesion or mucosal surface by gentle scraping or with a swab moistened in saline.
2. Apply to a limited area of a clean glass slide (do not smear); if using a swab, roll it across the surface.
3. Allow specimen to air dry (fix in methyl alcohol for 1 minute or more if using Giemsa stain).
4. Stain as described for Wright's stain.

---

characteristics. Bacteria stain positively or negatively (with a few exceptions such as *Legionella* species in clinical specimens and mycobacteria, which do not stain at all). Fungi are uniformly gram-positive. Carbolfuchsin stain (1% solution) can be substituted for safranine as a counterstain to provide more intense staining of gram-negative organisms that may otherwise be difficult to see. Although the stain is easy to accomplish and its interpretation is often straightforward, it must be examined critically. Whether the material is representative of the site of infection (e.g., sputum versus saliva) and whether the staining was properly performed should be determined. Overdecolorization is often feared but is easily evaluated by examining the degree of staining of neutrophils or other cells (nuclei should stain purple, cytoplasm pink). Morphologic appearance is as important as the staining because both aging and exposure to antibiotics may alter an organism's reactivity to stain; antibiotics may also distort the organism's usual morphology. Gram's stain aids in determining whether an infection is present and, if so, what organisms are present. The findings should also be used to interpret the culture results: anaerobes, other fastidious organisms, or organisms exposed to antibiotics may be seen with Gram's stain but fail to grow in culture.

Mycobacteria stain with the Ziehl-Neelsen and Kinyoun methods (Box 233-4), as well as with auramine-rhodamine fluorescent stain. The latter stain requires the use of a fluorescence microscope but is more sensitive than the former methods and permits rapid screening of slides. *Nocardia* species and some nontuberculous mycobacteria may be less acid-fast, requiring a modified staining procedure. Acridine orange is a fluorescent stain that stains all bacteria. Methenamine silver and toluidine blue stain fungi and *Pneumocystis carinii* cysts (Color Plate VIII-10). Giemsa stain (Color Plates VIII-11 and VIII-12) provides excellent cellular detail and demonstrates fungi, many parasites including *Toxoplasma* species and *P. carinii* trophozoites, and viral inclusions (Tzanck cell test) (Color Plate VIII-13). Wright's stain (Box 233-4) can also be used for Tzanck preparations and is generally more available to the clinician. Iron hematoxylin and trichrome stains are useful in screening for intestinal parasites. Wright's and Giemsa stains demonstrate parasites in blood (Color Plates VIII-14 to VIII-17), with the exception of leptospiras. Antibody staining for direct fluorescence microscopy (discussed next) is applicable to smears, imprints, and many histologic sections.

Immunologic Tests

Direct Immunofluorescence and Related Methods. These methods identify microorganisms or viral-infected cells on slide preparations of specimens and thus are similar to routinely stained smears, except that selectivity and visualization of staining are achieved by using labeled, specific antibody. Slides are prepared by rolling a swab over a limited area of the surface or applying a drop of sediment from centrifuged fluid specimens; they are then air dried and fixed. Specific antibody labeled with fluorescent compound is layered over the slide, which is then incubated and washed. Specifically bound antibody remains attached, and the organisms or cells carrying the antigen appear brightly stained against a dark background when viewed through a fluorescence microscope. The alternative use of enzyme-conjugated antibody eliminates the need for a fluorescence microscope but requires the additional step of incubating with enzyme substrate, which is deposited as a colored precipitate. The technique is also applicable to frozen or paraffin-embedded histologic sections of tissue.

Direct immunofluorescence and immunoenzyme techniques are used to detect *C. trachomatis* in genital and conjunctival specimens, *Legionella* species, *B. pertussis, P. carinii,* and various viruses (respiratory syncytial virus, influenza, parainfluenza, cytomegalovirus, and adenovirus) in respiratory samples, *Cryptosporidium* species in stool, and herpes simplex virus in skin and mucous membrane samples and tissue biopsy specimens.

Agglutination Tests. Antigen-antibody interactions in agglutination tests are observed as visible clumping of microscopic particles

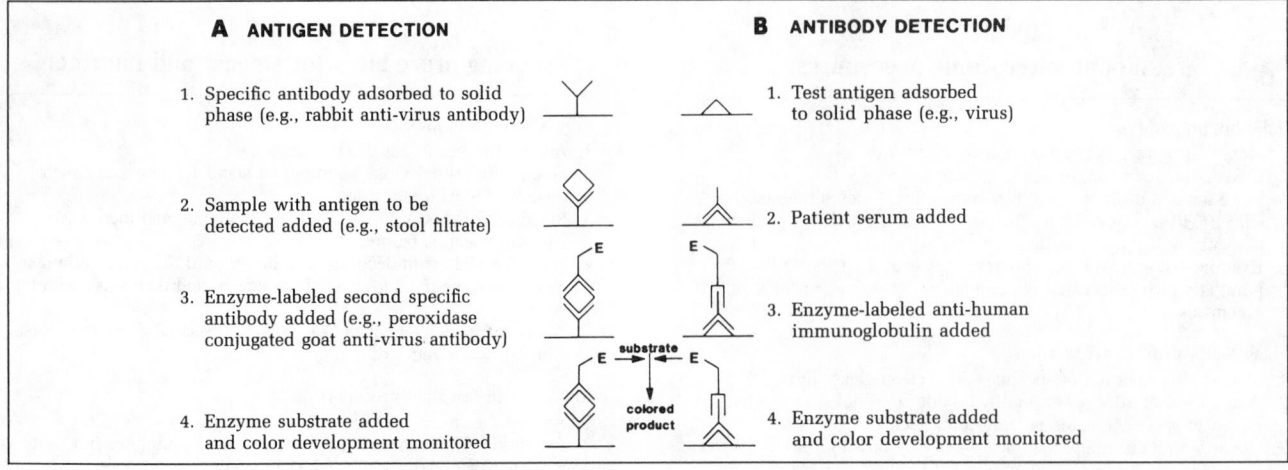

FIGURE 233-1   Technique of solid-phase, enzyme-linked immunosorbent assay (ELISA) for, **A,** antigen or, **B,** antibody. Washes are performed after steps 2 and 3 to remove unbound reactants.

in suspension. A particulate-phase suspension is mixed with a soluble-phase solution in test tubes or on flat surfaces, and visible clumping is assessed in minutes to hours. Direct agglutination tests are those in which a particulate antigen (e.g., bacteria in suspension) reacts directly with specific antibody in solutions. Indirect (or passive) agglutination tests have antibody in the particulate phase (e.g., coating latex beads) reacting with antigen in solution or suspension. Semiquantitative results can be obtained by titrating samples. In both the direct and indirect tests, interacting antigen and antibody bridge adjacent particles, causing visible agglutination.

These methods are rapid and sensitive and have been applied to direct detection of microorganisms and their soluble antigens in various clinical specimens, having replaced counterimmunoelectrophoresis (CIE) methods. Applications include detection of group A streptococci in throat swabs, capsular polysaccharide antigens of *Streptococcus pneumoniae, Haemophilus influenzae, Neisseria meningitidis,* group B streptococci, and *C. neoformans* in CSF, serum, and urine, and *Clostridium difficile* toxin in stool. False-positive reactions may occur (often as a result of rheumatoid factor in serum samples) but should be detected in most cases by the use of proper controls.

Radioimmunoassays and Enzyme Immunoassays. Radioimmunoassay (RIA) and enzyme immunoassay (EIA) procedures are extremely sensitive techniques, analogous in principle and differing only in the "label" that is measured. Fluorescent compounds are less commonly used alternative labels. Enzyme immunoassays can be as sensitive as RIAs and are often preferred. Enzymes and substrates are chosen to yield a colored product, thus permitting quantitation using spectrophotometry or qualitative results by visual inspection. The numerous exact RIA and EIA methodologies are variants of two basic methods, competitive binding and immunosorbent assays.

The enzyme-linked immunosorbent assay (ELISA) is the most widely used immunosorbent, or "sandwich," technique (Fig. 233-1). Specific antibody is bound to a solid substrate of the reaction system, which may be the wall of the chamber itself (tubes or microtiter plate wells) or a removable component (e.g., beads, a stick, or a disk). The test sample is incubated in the chamber; the antigen, if present, binds to the fixed antibody. Radio-labeled or enzyme-labeled antibody directed against the antigen is then added, and unbound antibody is removed by washing. The amount of specifically bound labeled antibody is proportional to the amount of antigen present in the test sample. Quantitation is made by comparison with a standard curve that is prepared by assaying known quantities of antigen.

In competitive binding assays, antigen in test samples competes with an added known amount of purified labeled antigen for binding to specific antibody. After separation of antigen-antibody complexes from free antigen, the amount of antibody-bound, labeled antigen

(which is inversely proportional to the concentration of antigen in the test sample) is measured.

Although these techniques have enjoyed widespread application in the research setting, their use in the routine clinical microbiology laboratory for direct detection of antigen is just now increasing. RIAs and EIAs are established methods for detecting hepatitis B surface and core antigens in serum and rotavirus in stool. Other commercially produced assays that have become available will detect chlamydia, gonococci, and herpes simplex virus in genital specimens, group A streptococci in throat specimens, respiratory syncytial virus in nasal secretions, *Legionella pneumophila* antigen in urine, enteric adenoviruses in stool, and HIV antigens in serum.

Nucleic Acid–Based Tests

Advances in molecular biology, particularly the development of the polymerase chain reaction (PCR), have made it feasible to use nucleic acid–based tests for direct detection of microorganisms in clinical specimens, as well as for identification of microorganisms isolated by culture techniques. These techniques have the potential to be highly specific, sensitive, and relatively rapid. The specificity of these tests derives from the fact that each specific organism has unique sequences in its genetic code, which can be detected through the use of synthesized or cloned complementary nucleic acid sequences, referred to as probes or, in the case of amplification assays, primers. Under certain conditions native double-stranded DNA in samples can be released from cells and separated into single strands. On reversal, complementary DNA (native DNA or the exogenously added probe or primer) anneals (hybridizes) by reforming hydrogen bonds between matched base pairs. Consecutive sequences of matched base pairs must be present for the stable reassociation of DNA strands, accounting for its exquisite molecular specificity.

By using labeled probes and separating complexed DNA from the residual single-stranded probe, target DNA can be directly detected. For example, in southern blot analysis the target DNA is bound to a solid membrane. Other test configurations use alternative forms of solid supports or are performed entirely in solution. In general, however, these methods are insufficiently sensitive for direct detection of microorganisms in clinical samples because of insufficient target DNA. An exception is the use of probes specific for ribosomal RNA, as there are generally at least 1000-fold more copies of ribosomal RNA than chromosomal DNA in organisms. Currently available tests using this technique include those for direct detection of *Legionella* species, *N. gonorrhoeae,* and *C. trachomatis.*

Amplification assays, of which the PCR technique is the most widely used, overcome the problem of low numbers of target DNA sequences in samples by enzymatically amplifying the target sequence more than 100,000-fold in a matter of hours. The amplified target sequence is then sufficiently abundant to be detected by a variety of methods. In the PCR technique specificity is largely determined by the choice of primers, which are synthetic oligonucleotides complementary to either end of a much longer (usually 200 to 1000 bases) target DNA sequence. Sequential and repetitive activity of nucleic acid replicating enzymes, which depend on stable hybridization of the primers to the target, replicate exponentially the intervening sequence between the primers. Multiple targets can be amplified simultaneously; such a test format is referred to as multiplexing. RNA viral sequences can be detected by first transcribing the RNA strand to a complementary DNA strand ("reverse transcribed" PCR [rt-PCR]). Further discussion and an illustration of PCR is presented in Chapter 10 (see Fig. 10-6). A variety of alternative methods for nucleic acid amplification are under development for commercial use, such as the self-sustained sequence reaction (3SR), transcription-mediated amplification, strand displacement amplification, and nucleic acid sequence–based amplification.

The recent introduction of commercial automated or semiautomated systems will facilitate widespread use of these techniques, which include direct detection of mycobacteria, common sexually transmitted disease organisms, and some viruses, such as cytomegalovirus, HIV, and hepatitis viruses; this list will undoubtedly expand over time. Research applications have been extensive, often targeting fastidious or noncultivatable organisms. Although the tests as generally used are qualitative, quantitative detection is feasible and is useful in certain settings such as determining HIV load in blood.

Sample collection and transport conditions employed for culture or antigen detection are generally sufficient for these tests, since DNA is relatively stable. For blood, ethylenediamine tetraacetic acid (EDTA) is the preferred anticoagulant, and freezing should be avoided before component separation. Use of swabs with aluminum shafts should be avoided because of potential inhibition of the amplification reaction by the metal. Interference has also been described for hemoglobin, mucus, urine, and phosphates; most of these can be dealt with during the processing stage in the laboratory. Some commercial systems provide special collection devices for optimal performance, which facilitate release of nucleic acid from cells and prevent its degradation during transport and storage.

In practice, PCR and other nucleic acid amplification techniques may be less sensitive than is possible in theory, and test performance may vary according to specimen source. Nevertheless, studies have generally found nucleic acid–based techniques to be comparable to or exceed the performance of culture for detecting microorganisms in clinical samples. Assay specificity should approach the ideal when appropriate methods are used to detect amplified product and avoid sample contamination. As PCR and related nucleic acid amplification tests are introduced, it will be important to define the clinical significance of positive and negative results, as well as appropriate test usage in a cost-conscious environment. This will vary by microorganism, body site, and clinical situation and is addressed where appropriate in the relevant chapters.

SEROLOGY

The primary humoral immune response to an antigenic stimulus is an initial production within 1 to 2 weeks of immunoglobulin M (IgM) antibodies, followed by a more prolonged production of immunoglobulin G (IgG) and a gradual fall in specific IgM levels. The secondary response occurs several days after reexposure to an antigen and consists predominantly of IgG production. The nature of the primary and secondary responses has important implications for the use of serologic testing as a diagnostic tool. Given the time necessary to mount a response to a primary infection, antibody may not be demonstrable until several weeks after the onset of the illness, often too late to be of practical diagnostic use. For certain agents with a significant latent period, such as hepatitis A, the appearance of antibody precedes or coincides with the clinical syndrome (Chapter 355).

Persistence of IgG antibody may preclude the association between detectable antibody and the current illness in patients in whom previous infection has occurred with the same or an antigenically related organism. In these instances detection of IgM-specific antibody may distinguish between recent and remote infections, as is possible for hepatitis A and toxoplasmosis. Otherwise, one relies on demonstration of a fourfold increase in titer between acute and convalescent sera (2 to 3 weeks or more apart) or a standing titer that is significantly higher than that found in the general population. Specific titers obtained for the same sample may vary among laboratories or even in one laboratory if the sample is assayed at different times. Therefore, when serial titered serologic tests are used to document or follow an infection, samples should be tested in parallel in the same laboratory.

All microorganisms are antigenically complex, and the onset, nature, and duration of the antibody response can vary for each antigenic component. In some cases advantage can be taken of this spectrum of response by varying either the antigen or the method used (e.g., precipitin vs. complement-fixation procedures), as in serologic tests for rubella.

Precipitin Reactions

Precipitin reactions are based on direct visualization of a precipitated antigen-antibody complex. The reaction can occur in either liquid medium (tube precipitin tests) or, more commonly, in gel medium (radial and Ochterlony immunodiffusion tests). Except for radial immunodiffusion, reactions are qualitative, and serial dilutions of the test sample must be run to obtain a semiquantitative result ("antibody titer"). Precipitin and immunodiffusion assays are commonly used in the serologic diagnosis of systemic mycoses and various parasitic infections.

Agglutination Reactions

The principle and performance of agglutination assays are similar to those for direct detection of antigens. When designed for detection of specific antibody, however, the solid phase carries the appropriate antigen, which may be intact organisms (e.g., formalinized bacteria) or soluble antigen bound to carrier particles such as erythrocytes or latex beads. Common uses of these techniques are the nontreponemal tests for syphilis (Chapter 244) and the detection of heterophilic antibodies in infectious mononucleosis (Chapter 255). A related technique, hemagglutination inhibition, is used to detect antibodies to rubella (Chapter 251).

Neutralization Tests

Neutralization tests are used to detect protective antibody to viruses, including rubella, polio, and rabies. Dilutions of serum are incubated with given amounts of virus, and ability to block infection in cell culture is determined. Neutralization of hemolytic or enzymatic activity is also the basis for detecting antistreptolysin O, antideoxyribonuclease B, and antihyaluronidase antibodies in group A streptococcal infection (Chapter 261).

Complement-Fixation Assays

Although technically complicated, complement-fixation assays are used extensively in serologic testing, particularly in reference laboratories. The assays are performed in two phases. The first phase is based on the ability of certain immunoglobulins to bind, or fix, complement when they form antigen-antibody complexes; the second is based on the ability of unbound complement to lyse red blood cells. Results are reported as the maximum dilution of serum causing a given degree of complement inhibition. Assays require several days to complete and are not usually performed in routine clinical microbiology laboratories.

The technique has been widely applied but for many pathogens has been supplanted by other, more rapid-acting and easily performed assays. However, complement-fixation assays are still commonly used for detecting antibody to *C. immitis, H. capsulatum* (Chapter 277), and various viruses.

Indirect Immunofluorescence Assays

Indirect immunofluorescence assays are designed to detect specific antibody and are similar in performance to the direct immunofluorescence assays described for detection of antigen. For indirect assays the antigen in question, usually intact organisms or virus-infected cells, is fixed to microscope slides. Dilutions of test serum are incubated over the surface, and unbound antibody is removed by washing. Bound antibody is detected by a second incubation with a fluorescence or enzyme-labeled antihuman immunoglobulin. The latter may be selected or prepared to detect bound IgG or IgM, or both. Results are reported as the maximum dilution of serum producing a given degree of specific fluorescence. These assays are sensitive and relatively simple to perform and are used for detection of antibody to *Legionella* species, *T. pallidum,* chlamydiae, rickettsiae, Epstein-Barr virus, HIV, toxoplasma, and *Entamoeba histolytica.*

Radioimmunoassays and Enzyme Immunoassays

Radioimmunoassays and enzyme immunoassays for antibody detection are usually immunosorbent types of assays. Their design and execution is similar to that described for direct detection of antigen, but the sequence of steps is altered, being analogous to those of indirect immunofluorescence assays (Fig. 233-1). First, antigen is bound to a solid phase of the system. A dilution of test serum is then incubated with the solid phase; a second incubation using labeled antihuman immunoglobulin follows, with washes after each. Labeled staphylococcal protein A, which binds to the Fc portion of IgG, may also be used to detect bound antibody.

Results are reported as positive or negative by comparing the amount of label activity from a given test serum dilution with the range of activities found in negative control sera at the same dilution. The sensitivity and specificity of these assays depend on the cutoff level chosen to separate positive from negative samples. In some cases this necessitates establishing an indeterminate range if the separation is not clear-cut. Quantitative results, if reported, may be expressed as absolute activity units (counts per minute for RIAs, or optical density or absorbance for EIAs) or as a ratio of sample activity to that of a strongly positive reference serum.

The preceding techniques have broad application, but in the clinical serologic laboratory they have generally not replaced assays that were well established before EIA development. Radioimmunoassay and EIA are the primary methods for detecting antibody to hepatitis A, B, and C and HIV (Chapter 248) and are alternative techniques for detecting many other agents, including toxoplasma, rubella, cytomegalovirus, herpes simplex virus, and the Lyme disease spirochete (Chapter 274).

Western Blot Assay

The technique of Western blot assay, common in research laboratories, has become a diagnostic test for confirmation of HIV antibody in serum. In the procedure proteins in a mixture extracted from cultured virus are separated electrophoretically according to molecular weight then replica transferred ("blotted") to nitrocellulose paper. After incubation with the patient's serum, bound antibody is detected, which allows determination of the specific proteins against which antibodies are directed. Because some proteins are more specifically associated with infection than others, test specificity is better than that of EIAs, which use whole-virus homogenates as the substrate antigen. Simpler procedures such as EIAs that use purified proteins or protein fragments are likely to supplant this test for diagnostic purposes in the future.

SKIN TESTING

In contrast to the many in vitro methods available to measure the antibody response to infection, the in vivo delayed hypersensitivity skin test is still the only routinely used method for evaluating the cellular immune response to infection. The test is performed by placing 0.1 ml of antigen solution intradermally using a 25- or 27-gauge needle. The site of inoculation is marked and is examined 24, 48, and sometimes 96 hours later, and the diameter of the area of induration is measured. Erythema often occurs but is generally not of significance in interpreting the test, except in the case of mumps antigen (Chapter 251). Other methods, such as multiple puncture devices, are less well standardized; therefore the results are less reliable. By convention,

induration of 5 mm or more in diameter is considered a positive reaction, although 10 mm is the accepted cutoff value for tuberculin testing in normal populations (Chapter 273). It should be realized that in a truly positive population (i.e., those infected with or exposed to the organism) the measured values form a continuum, including those of persons with no response. Interpretation in any given case should be flexible, depending on the question being asked, because sensitivity varies inversely with specificity, depending on the cutoff set.

The optimal concentration of each antigen for testing has been standardized, and for some antigens, such as tuberculin, lower and higher concentrations are available. In patients in whom a severe reaction may be anticipated, the lower dose may be used initially; if the reaction is negative, the test is repeated with a standard dose. When no reaction occurs with the standard concentration, a negative response to a higher ($\times 10$) dose is more definitive evidence of anergy or lack of primary exposure. However, interpretation of a measurable response to the higher concentration must be made with caution. Negative responses in the presence of current or past infection may be a result of local skin abnormalities, anergy, or technical faults in test administration. Antigen should not be injected into areas of skin with dermatologic lesions such as atopic dermatitis.

Anergy is associated with numerous conditions, including congenital and acquired immune deficiencies and a variety of infections, especially extensive tuberculous and fungal infections. If anergy is suspected, a battery of skin tests is used to determine its presence. This should include at least three antigens to which most persons have been exposed and to which they will react. Those currently available for use include *Candida* and *Trichophyton,* streptokinase-streptodornase, mixed respiratory vaccine, and staph-phage lysate. A kit is available that simultaneously applies seven antigens with a negative control (Multitest CMI, Pasteur Merieux, Lyon, France).

Administration of skin tests generally does not immunize the patient, although serologic responses may occur after histoplasmin, *Brucella* species, mumps, and lymphogranuloma venereum testing; these antigens should be avoided in situations in which serologic testing has greater diagnostic value. The Frei test for lymphogranuloma venereum is now obsolete.

BIBLIOGRAPHY

American Society for Microbiology: Cumulative techniques and procedures in clinical microbiology, Washington, DC, The Society.

Baselski VS: The role of molecular diagnostics in the clinical microbiology laboratory, *Clin Lab Med* 16:49, 1996.

Murray PR et al, editors: *Manual of clinical microbiology,* ed 6, Washington, DC, 1995, American Society for Microbiology.

Needham CA: Rapid detection methods in microbiology: are they right for your office? *Med Clin North Am* 71:591, 1987.

Rose NR et al, editors: *Manual of clinical laboratory immunology,* ed 4, Washington, DC, 1992, American Society for Microbiology.

Smith TF et al: New developments in the diagnosis of viral diseases, *Infect Dis Clin North Am* 7:183, 1993.

Sox HC Jr: Probability theory in the use of diagnostic tests, *Ann Intern Med* 104:60, 1986.

III CLINICAL SYNDROMES

CHAPTER

234 Fever of Unknown Origin

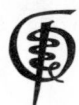

Martin G. Täuber

Body temperature is one of the most frequently monitored physical signs in modern medicine. The normal upper limit of orally measured temperature is generally considered to be 98.6° F (37.0° C). Normal temperature varies among healthy individuals, however, so that many persons, particularly younger adults and women in the second half of their menstrual cycle, may have temperature readings as much as 1.5° F (0.8° C) higher. Physical exercise and heavy meals also increase body temperature. In addition, body temperature physiologically shows diurnal changes of up to 1.8° F (1° C). The lowest temperatures are in the early morning hours, and the highest are in the late afternoon. Axillary temperature is usually about 1° F (0.6° C) lower, and rectal temperature is approximately the same amount higher than oral temperature.

FEVER

Fever is defined as an elevation of body temperature above normal limits induced by regulatory processes of the nervous system that originate in the hypothalamus. The rise of body temperature to a higher level is achieved by a combination of increased internal heat production and reduced external heat loss. Shivering in skeletal muscles is the major source of increased heat production; peripheral vasoconstriction results in conservation of body heat.

The key pathophysiologic factor in the patient with fever is the adjustment of the hypothalamic temperature set point to a higher than normal level by a disease process usually distant to the hypothalamus. The release of prostaglandins, primarily of the E class, from endothelial cells of the cerebral microvasculature in the vicinity of the thermoregulatory area appears to be instrumental in increasing the temperature set point. This release can be stimulated by two classes of substances circulating in the bloodstream of febrile patients: endogenous and exogenous pyrogens. Several members of the family of cytokines function as endogenous pyrogens, including interleukin-1 and -6, cachectin/tumor necrosis factor, and interferons. Prototype exogenous pyrogens are the lipopolysaccharides (endotoxin) that are released from gram-negative bacteria during infection, but gram-positive organisms also release potent pyrogens.

In the great majority of illnesses associated with fever, the underlying disease process stimulates the release of pyrogenic cytokines which then act on the hypothalamus. The primary sources of cytokines are phagocytic monocytes/macrophages, although other leukocytes and other types of cells have also been shown to release endogenous pyrogens. Furthermore, some evidence suggests that pyrogenic cytokines may be released locally in the hypothalamus under the influence of other pyrogens. A large variety of disease processes, such as infections, tumors, and immunologic reactions, can precipitate the secretion of pyrogenic cytokines from macrophages and other sources. Exogenous pyrogens both act directly on the thermoregulatory center and stimulate the release of cytokines from macrophages. Consequently, it is evident that the pathogenesis of fever follows the same final pathway in many different, unrelated diseases. This makes fever a highly nonspecific sign, a fact that should be kept in mind when considering fever of unknown origin.

Pathologic states other than fever may also result in an elevation of body temperature. In hyperthermia, for instance, impairment of pe-

ripheral heat-dissipating mechanisms or unusual internal heat production results in a body temperature above that set by the central regulation. Hyperthermia due to disturbed heat dissipation is found in heat stroke or in states of prolonged peripheral vasoconstriction caused by pheochromocytoma, Addison's disease, or anticholinergic drugs. Malignant hyperthermia, a rare disorder characterized by excessive muscular heat production induced by some anesthetics, is a typical example of hyperthermia due to excessive heat production. Primary or metastatic tumors, trauma, and inflammatory processes that directly involve the thermoregulatory center in the hypothalamus may also alter body temperature. In these patients hypothermia is usually observed, whereas hyperthermia is extremely rare.

FEVER OF UNKNOWN ORIGIN

The wide variety of diseases that can cause fever makes the medical evaluation of a febrile patient a constant challenge. A thorough medical history and a physical examination, supplemented by routine laboratory tests, enable identification of the cause of fever in most patients. In a few febrile patients, however, the underlying disease eludes diagnosis even after a prolonged period of illness and despite careful medical evaluation. These patients are then given the tentative diagnosis of having a fever of unknown origin (FUO).

Diagnostic criteria for FUO have been strictly defined for study purposes. Although details of these definitions may need adjustments to account for changing practices in medicine, the three principles defining the concept of FUO have retained their validity. Febrile patients should be given this diagnosis only if the illness has persisted long enough to make the presence of a common, self-limiting viral disease unlikely (usually at least 3 weeks); the patient must have been carefully examined and had routine laboratory tests and chest radiographs, in order for all readily detected causes of fever to have been ruled out. In addition, the fever has to be significant on several occasions (usually above 101° F [38.3° C]). This latter point is particularly important, as many patients may have slightly elevated body temperatures for many months or years without evidence of serious underlying diseases. In some cases, exaggerated diurnal temperature variations are interpreted as fever ("habitual hyperthermia"). Patients with the *chronic fatigue syndrome,* a syndrome of undetermined etiology, also often complain of low-grade fever, although the predominant symptom is disabling fatigue. It is important in these instances to avoid the extensive and invasive evaluations that have to be considered in patients with FUO.

The large majority of cases of FUO are caused by infections, neoplasias, and collagen vascular diseases. A fourth group includes diseases categorized as granulomatous disorders. Numerous miscellaneous diseases are responsible for the rest of the patients in whom a cause for FUO can be identified (Table 234-1).

The spectrum of diseases found in several series examining FUO shows some variation according to the population studied and the study period (Table 234-1). In children, infections tend to be the most frequent cause of FUO, whereas neoplasms and connective tissue disorders are more frequent in the elderly. In patients with FUO lasting more than 1 year, infections and neoplasias decrease in frequency, whereas granulomatous diseases are the single most important category. Diagnostic advances may continuously change the spectrum of causes of FUO. For example, serologic tests have reduced the importance of systemic lupus erythematosus as a cause of FUO, and modern imaging techniques facilitate early detection of abscesses and solid tumors.

In all studies, a substantial number of patients evaluated for FUO remained without a definite diagnosis (Table 234-1). A follow-up of these patients usually shows a benign long-term course, especially in those patients whose fever is not accompanied by a substantial weight loss or by other signs of a serious underlying disease. This pattern suggests that intensive diagnostic evaluation of patients with FUO results in identification of most serious diseases that initially manifested themselves with a FUO.

Causes

Factitious Fever. The possibility of factitious fever should be considered in every patient with prolonged fever before engaging in

Table 234-1   Causes of fever of unknown origin

DISEASE CATEGORY	PETERSDORF AND BEESON (100 PATIENTS, 1952-1957)	HOWARD et al. (100 PATIENTS, 1969-1976)	LARSON et al. (105 PATIENTS, 1970-1980)	KNOCKAERT et al. (199 PATIENTS, 1980-1989)
Infections	**36 (36%)**	**37 (37%)**	**32 (30.5%)**	**45 (22.6%)**
Tuberculosis	11	3	5	10
Abdominal abscess	4	9	8	4
Hepatobiliary	7	7	4	1
Endocarditis	5	9	0	3
Urinary tract	3	4	3	1
Cytomegalovirus	0	0	4	8
Others	6	5	8	18
Malignancies	**19 (19%)**	**31 (31%)**	**33 (31.4%)**	**14 (7.0%)**
Lymphoma	6	20	11	2
Leukemia	2	3	5	4
Solid tumors	9	8	6	7
Others	2	0	11	1
Collagen vascular and autoimmune disorders	**13 (13%)**	**13 (13%)**	**8 (7.6%)**	**21 (10.6%)**
Juvenile rheumatoid arthritis	2	1	4	6
Systemic vasculitis	0	5	1	6
Lupus erythematosus	5	3	0	1
Rheumatic fever	6	0	1	0
Others	0	4	2	8
Granulomatous disorders	**6 (6%)**	**7 (7%)**	**9 (8.6%)**	**28 (14.1%)**
Granulomatous hepatitis	2	0	4	3
Crohn's disease	0	4	2	4
Sarcoidosis	2	0	2	4
Giant cell arteritis	2	3	1	17
Miscellaneous	**19 (19%)**	**7 (7%)**	**10 (9.5%)**	**43 (21.6%)**
Factitious fever	3	0	3	7
Periodic fever	5	0	0	2
Pulmonary emboli	3	0	1	5
Drug fever	0	2	0	6
Others	8	5	6	23
Undiagnosed	**7 (7%)**	**5 (5%)**	**13 (12.4%)**	**48 (24.1%)**

From Petersdorf RG, Beeson PG: *Medicine (Baltimore)* 40:1, 1961; Howard P et al: *Tex Med* 73:56, 1977; Larson EB, Featherstone HJ, Petersdorf RB: *Medicine (Baltimore)* 61:269, 1982; Knockaert DC et al: *Arch Intern Med* 152:51, 1992.

extensive and invasive procedures. Factitious fever is responsible for up to 10% of the cases of FUO and is most commonly encountered among young adults within the health professions. Frequently, there is evidence of psychiatric problems or a history of multiple hospitalizations in different institutions. Rapid changes of body temperature without associated shivering or sweating, large differences between rectal and oral temperature, and discrepancies between fever and pulse rate or general appearance are typically seen in patients who manipulate or exchange their thermometers, the most common cause of factitious fever. Alternatively, fever may be caused by injection of nonsterile material, such as feces or milk, resulting in atypically localized abscesses or polymicrobial infections.

Infections
Bacterial diseases
Abscesses. Abscesses are most frequently located intraabdominally and must be considered in patients with FUO even in the absence of localizing symptoms (Chapter 238). Previous abdominal operations, trauma, or a history of diverticulosis, peritonitis, endoscopy, or gynecologic procedures all increase the likelihood of an occult intraabdominal abscess. The most common abscess locations are the subphrenic space, the liver, the right lower quadrant, the retroperitoneal space, and in women, the pelvis.

Tuberculosis. Tuberculosis continues to be an important cause of FUO (Chapter 273). Several factors may prevent its prompt diagnosis. Dissemination, which typically occurs in patients with reduced immunocompetence, may initially be present with constitutional symptoms lacking localized signs, and with normal chest radiographs. Patients with disseminated tuberculosis or with early tuberculosis may have negative purified protein derivative (PPD) tests, and cultures

take 4 to 6 weeks to become positive. Tuberculous infections of the kidney, female genitalia, or mesenteric lymph nodes tend to manifest themselves as FUO because of a lack of characteristic, localized manifestations. Disseminated, visceral infections with atypical mycobacteria have also been implicated as a cause of FUO. Most of these patients have some underlying hematologic malignancy or are infected with the human immunodeficiency virus (HIV) (see later discussion).

Hepatobiliary infections. Cholangitis sometimes occurs without local signs and with only mildly elevated or normal liver function tests (Chapter 364). Similarly, acute cholecystitis or gallbladder empyema (Chapter 364) has been responsible for cases of FUO because of the lack of right upper quadrant pain or jaundice, especially in elderly patients. A rare cause of FUO is bacterial hepatitis, caused by α-hemolytic streptococci, *Propionibacterium acnes,* or *Actinomyces israelii.* The only abnormal finding in these patients may be an elevated alkaline phosphatase level.

Urinary tract infections. These infections are rare causes of FUO because urinalysis is an easily performed routine test that detects most cases of urinary tract infections. In young children, however, the collection of clean-catch urine specimens may be difficult. Furthermore, perinephritic abscesses sometimes fail to communicate with the urinary system and can thus yield a normal urine analysis (Chapter 246). Anatomic abnormalities of the urinary tract in a patient with FUO should raise the possibility of an occult urinary tract infection.

Endocarditis. Endocarditis (Chapter 24) has become a rare cause of FUO. Failure to diagnose endocarditis may be due to the absence of a murmur, or the failure of blood cultures to yield the organism. Culture-negative endocarditis is reported in 5% to 10% of endocarditis cases in the literature. Prior antibiotic therapy is the most frequent reason for negative blood cultures.

Other causes of culture-negative endocarditis include organisms that are difficult to culture (nutritionally variant streptococci, *Brucella* spp., anaerobes, members of the HACEK group [*Haemophilus* spp., *Actinobacillus actinomycetocomitans, Cardiobacterium hominis, Eikenella corrodens, Kingella* spp.]), obligate intracellular organisms (*Coxiella burnetii,* chlamydiae), uremia, and very late stages of untreated endocarditis. Manifestations of endocarditis (such as cerebrovascular stroke, nephritis, or musculoskeletal symptoms) involving organs other than the heart may detract from the correct diagnosis in febrile patients with sterile blood cultures.

Osteomyelitis. Osteomyelitis almost always causes localized pain or discomfort at least intermittently (Chapter 243). The most frequent reason that this diagnosis is missed is the failure to consider osteomyelitis in a febrile patient with musculoskeletal symptoms. A typical example is the elderly patient with back pain, in whom degenerative changes are thought to be responsible. Low-grade fever or a history of urinary tract infection should raise the possibility of vertebral osteomyelitis in these patients. Radiographs fail to show changes suggestive of osteomyelitis sometimes for weeks after the development of symptoms. Radionucleotide studies (technetium 99m bone scanning) are more sensitive than conventional radiology but lack specificity.

Other bacterial diseases. Some systemic bacterial illnesses may occasionally manifest themselves as FUO. Among these, brucellosis, which is still prevalent in Latin America and the Mediterranean, is the most important (Chapter 270). It should be considered in patients with persisting fever and a history of contact with cattle, swine, goats, and sheep, or consumption of raw milk products. Systemic infections due to *Salmonella* (Chapter 269), *Neisseria meningitidis* (Chapter 264), or *Neisseria gonorrhoeae* (Chapter 265) have been described as causes of FUO. Cutaneous changes may be the only sign other than fever in neisserial infections. Cultures and serologic tests are necessary to establish the diagnosis of these infections. Spirochetes also occasionally cause FUO. The most important among these is *Borrelia recurrentis,* which is transmitted by ticks and is responsible for causing sporadic cases of relapsing fever (Chapter 274). Febrile episodes lasting 3 days with intervals of approximately 7 days occur in these patients. Ratbite fever, caused by *Spirillum minor,* has also been described as a cause of FUO (Chapter 274). *Borrelia burgdorferi* (responsible for Lyme disease) (Chapter 274) and *Treponema pallidum* (causing syphilis) (Chapter 274) are other spirochetes that rarely can cause FUO.

Viral diseases
Herpes viruses. Two members of the herpesvirus family, the cytomegalovirus and the Epstein-Barr virus, can cause prolonged febrile illnesses with constitutional symptoms and no prominent organ manifestations, particularly in the elderly (Chapter 255). Infections by each of these viruses typically cause enlarged lymph nodes, but these may be missed on physical examination when they are small. Lymphocytosis with atypical lymphocytes should direct attention to the correct diagnosis, which can be confirmed by appropriate serologic tests. These tests may initially be negative and should be repeated in suspected cases 2 to 3 weeks after the onset of illness.

Human immunodeficiency virus. Prolonged febrile episodes are frequent in patients with advanced HIV infection (Chapter 248). In these patients, fever may be caused by a large variety of opportunistic infections, by lymphomas, or by the HIV itself. Typical and atypical mycobacteria and cytomegalovirus are opportunistic infections that frequently cause prominent constitutional symptoms, including fever, with few localizing or specific signs. Rarely, other opportunistic infections, such as salmonellosis, histoplasmosis, or toxoplasmosis, can also elude rapid diagnosis in febrile acquired immunodeficiency syndrome (AIDS) patients and thus present as FUO. Lymphomas involve extranodal sites, including the brain, in over 80% of AIDS patients and can at times be difficult to diagnose promptly. Extensive diagnostic workup, including imaging studies, are necessary to exclude these opportunistic diseases in HIV-infected patients with prolonged fever, before the fever can be attributed to the HIV infection itself (Centers for Disease Control and Prevention stage IVA).

Other infectious causes
Fungi. Immunosuppression, the use of broad-spectrum antibiotics, and intravascular devices all predispose to disseminated infections with opportunistic fungi, such as *Candida albicans* (Chapter

277). Systemic infection can remain undiscovered in these patients because blood cultures are negative in approximately 50% of cases. *Malassezia furfur* has caused FUO and line infections in patients on total parenteral nutrition receiving intravenous lipid preparations. Fever can sometimes be the most prominent symptom in patients who have reticuloendothelial involvement by histoplasmosis without clinical manifestations in other organs (Chapter 277).

Parasites. Toxoplasmosis should be considered in febrile patients with lymph node enlargement, but because the lymph nodes may be small, diagnosis is sometimes difficult (Chapter 279). Rising antibody titers and immunoglobulin M (IgM) antibodies confirm the diagnosis. Malaria can be missed as a cause of fever if the physician is unaware of a history of recent travel to an endemic area and if the fever pattern is nonsynchronized. Other parasites (Chapter 279) that can rarely cause FUO include *Trypanosoma* and *Leishmania* organisms and amebae.

Chlamydia. Chlamydia psittaci, the cause of psittacosis, should be considered in a patient with FUO who has a history of contact with birds (Chapter 257). Lymphogranuloma venereum may on rare occasions also manifest itself as FUO. Serologic study is essential for the diagnosis of these chlamydial infections.

Rickettsia. Chronic infections with *C. burnetii,* chronic Q fever, or Q fever endocarditis have been identified in patients with FUO (Chapter 259). Signs of hepatic involvement are frequent. The infection is transmitted from cattle and sheep, and serologic tests should be performed in suspected cases.

Neoplastic Diseases
Lymphomas. Both Hodgkin's disease (Chapter 93) and non-Hodgkin's lymphoma (Chapter 93) frequently cause fever, night sweats, and weight loss. The correct diagnosis can be delayed if the tumor is difficult to detect, as is the case when the disease is confined to the retroperitoneal lymph nodes. Anemia may be the most prominent laboratory abnormality in patients with lymphomas.

Malignant histiocytosis. This rare, rapidly progressive malignant disease that manifests itself with high fevers; weight loss; and enlargement of lymph nodes, liver, and spleen is occasionally found in patients with FUO (Chapter 91).

Leukemias. Acute leukemias are another important neoplastic cause of FUO. In aleukemic or preleukemic states, the peripheral blood smear and bone marrow aspirate may not reveal the correct diagnosis, and a bone marrow biopsy is necessary (Chapter 92).

Solid tumors. Among the solid tumors, hypernephromas are most commonly associated with FUO, with fever as the only presenting symptom in 10% of the cases (Chapter 126). Hematuria may be absent in about 40% of cases, whereas anemia and a highly elevated sedimentation rate are frequent. Other solid tumors that may cause fever as the presenting symptom include primary liver carcinomas; adenocarcinomas of the breast, colon, or pancreas with metastases to the liver; and sarcomas of the retroperitoneum. If bronchogenic carcinomas cause fever, it is usually because of bronchial obstruction with subsequent pneumonia. Benign leiomyomas can sometimes cause fever and may be difficult to detect when they originate in the gastrointestinal tract.

Myxomas are rare tumors of the heart that are well recognized as a cause of FUO (Chapter 33). They frequently cause fever along with a high sedimentation rate and anemia, whereas a cardiac murmur may be absent or intermittent. Myxomas are easily detected by echocardiography.

Collagen Vascular and Autoimmune Diseases. A variety of different diseases of uncertain etiology are summarized as collagen vascular and autoimmune diseases. These diseases can present as FUO if fever precedes other, more specific manifestations, such as arthritis, pneumonitis, or renal involvement. Systemic lupus erythematosus (Chapter 194) was a relatively common cause of FUO 20 years ago. Today, it is readily diagnosed in most cases by demonstration of antinuclear antibodies. Systemic-onset juvenile rheumatoid arthritis is a difficult to diagnose cause of fever (Chapter 192). High-spiking fevers, nonpruritic rashes, arthralgias and myalgias, pharyngitis, and lymphadenopathy are typically present. Laboratory abnormalities include pronounced leukocytosis, elevated sedimentation rate, anemia, and abnormal liver function tests. All these findings prompt the search for an infectious cause and thus delay the correct diagnosis.

Other collagen vascular diseases that need to be considered because of their potential for nonspecific presentations are periarteritis nodosa, rheumatoid arthritis, and mixed connective tissue disease. Rheumatic fever can be difficult to diagnose because it has become rare in the developed world, despite an apparent recent increase in some areas in the United States, and because some of the classic criteria may be absent (Chapter 204).

Granulomatous Diseases

Giant cell arteritis. This disease occurs almost exclusively in persons over 60 years of age. In this age-group giant cell arteritis is the single most common diagnosis leading to FUO (Chapter 195). The diagnosis may be obscured when typical symptoms such as headache, tender temporal arteries, and polymyalgia rheumatica are absent. Anemia, a high sedimentation rate, and elevation of α_2 serum proteins are typical laboratory findings. The diagnosis can usually be confirmed by biopsy of an involved artery. Because of the frequency of giant cell arteritis in causing FUO in elderly patients, some experts recommend a temporal artery biopsy in all patients over 60 years of age with FUO. When no diagnostic biopsy is performed, therapy with corticosteroids should be instituted in all suspected cases, since the untreated disease may rapidly lead to blindness and other serious central nervous system sequelae.

Regional enteritis. Crohn's disease is the most common gastrointestinal cause of FUO. Diarrhea and other abdominal complaints may be absent in a few patients, particularly in young adults (Chapter 341). The diagnosis is made in these patients by endoscopy and biopsy.

Sarcoidosis. Very rarely, sarcoidosis manifests itself with fever and malaise in the absence of evidence of lymph node and pulmonary involvement (Chapter 53). Erythema nodosum is sometimes present. The diagnosis should be suspected if noncaseous granulomas are found in the liver.

Granulomatous hepatitis. In some patients with hepatic granulomas, none of the diseases usually associated with this nonspecific reaction, such as tuberculosis, syphilis, brucellosis, sarcoidosis, Crohn's disease, or Hodgkin's disease, can be found. These patients often have fever that may be accompanied by slight hepatomegaly, asthenia, and sometimes arthralgias and myalgias for many months or years (Chapter 358). Elevated alkaline phosphatase level is the most consistent laboratory abnormality. The long-term prognosis is excellent, with about half of the patients recovering spontaneously. The other half respond to corticosteroid treatment ranging from a few weeks to several years.

Idiopathic granulomatosis. Noncaseating granulomas involving multiple organs are associated with fever and other nonspecific signs and symptoms in patients with this recently described disease. The etiology is unclear and the disease runs a prolonged course with a fairly good prognosis. Many patients have been treated with corticosteroids or other immunosuppressive agents.

Miscellaneous Causes

Inherited diseases. Familial Mediterranean fever is most often, but not exclusively, found in patients of Mediterranean descent (Chapter 201). Recurrent febrile episodes at varying intervals are associated with pleural, abdominal, or joint pain due to polyserositis. The diagnosis can be made only after exclusion of other causes of fever and polyserositis. Other inherited diseases that cause febrile episodes and have been reported as causing FUO include Fabry's disease and hypertriglyceridemia.

Drug fever. Although a wide variety of drugs can cause drug fever, those more frequently involved include alpha-methyldopa, quinidine, diphenylhydantoin, β-lactam antibiotics, procainamide, and isoniazid. A history of allergy, skin rashes, or eosinophilia is often absent in cases of drug fever; neither the fever pattern nor the duration of previous therapy is a helpful parameter in establishing the diagnosis. Whenever drug fever is suspected, the incriminated drug should be discontinued. This cessation leads to defeverescence within 2 days in the vast majority of cases if the drug was in fact responsible for the fever.

Others. Peripheral pulmonary emboli as well as occult thrombo-

phlebitis can cause FUO. These diagnoses should be considered in patients with predisposing conditions, particularly previous surgery, traumas, or prolonged bed rest. Another possible cause of fever in a patient after surgery or trauma is an undiscovered hematoma, usually intraabdominal.

A self-limiting necrotizing lymphadenitis (Kikuchi's disease) has recently been described as a cause of FUO. It causes prolonged fever, constitutional symptoms, laboratory evidence of chronic inflammation, and sometimes liver function abnormalities. The etiology of the disease is not known.

Fever can occur in patients with Laennec's cirrhosis (Chapter 357). If there is lack of evidence for a hepatic disease, it may be classified as FUO. Whipple's disease should be considered in a patient with abdominal complaints and central nervous system symptoms (Chapter 340). Other diseases that on rare occasions may cause FUO include idiopathic pericarditis, thyroiditis, renal angiomyolipoma, and complex partial status epilepticus.

Diagnostic Approach to Adults

The numerous possible causes of FUO in an individual patient combined with the availability of a broad armamentarium of diagnostic tests make the rational evaluation of a patient with FUO a demanding task. Experiences of many investigators document the best strategy for the initial approach to such patients as being a careful clinical examination combined with a limited set of diagnostic "routine" tests (see Box 234-1). Based on a detailed knowledge of the possible causes of FUO, these basic evaluations usually provide the clinician with clues to the nature of the underlying disease. The subsequent evaluations should then attempt to confirm or refute the diagnostic possibilities raised by the initial evaluation. Nonselective application of numerous tests within a short time is likely to result in high costs, a heavy burden to the patient, and findings that may be difficult to interpret.

History. The history of a patient with FUO is best structured to cover three areas.

1. Inquiries regarding symptoms from all major organ systems should be made, including a detailed history of general complaints such as fever, weight loss, night sweats, headaches, and rashes. All complaints should be recorded, even if they have disappeared before the examination.
2. Previous health history is important including surgery, dental history, and psychiatric illnesses.
3. A detailed evaluation should include the family history; immunization status; the workplace situation; travel; nutrition, including consumption of dairy products; drugs; a sexual history; recreational habits; and animal contacts, including possible exposure to ticks and other vectors.

Physical Examination. The unambiguous documentation of fever and the exclusion of factitious fever are obvious early steps in the physical examination of a patient with FUO. Over 25% of the patients evaluated for FUO at the National Institutes of Health were ultimately found to have no fever, whereas another 9% had factitious fever. Fever should be measured more than once in the presence of a nurse to exclude manipulation of thermometers. Electronic thermometers facilitate the rapid and unequivocal documentation of fever.

The pattern of fever (continuous, remittent, or intermittent) is usually of little help in the evaluation of a patient with FUO, as, in general, there is a weak correlation between fever patterns and specific diseases. Exceptions are tertian and quartan malaria (Chapter 279), but these should not present as FUO because of their suggestive fever pattern. Other diseases, such as brucellosis, borreliosis, or Hodgkin's disease, tend to cause recurrent episodes of fever, but the fact that these diseases are typical causes of FUO underscores the limited diagnostic value of fever patterns.

A regular physical examination should be repeated daily while the patient is hospitalized for the evaluation of FUO. Special attention should be directed to rashes, new or changing cardiac murmurs, signs of arthritis, abdominal tenderness or resistances, lymph node enlargement, and funduscopic changes. The latter may be the only localized

BOX 234-1
Stage-specific diagnostic approach to fever of unknown origin

Stage 1: Screening (in all adult patients with fever of unknown origin)

History: Specific symptoms, review of systems, immunization, travel, animal exposure, medications and drugs, sex, work, recreation

Physical examination: Fever documentation; general examination with special attention to skin, lymph nodes, fundi, heart and lungs, abdomen, joints

Hematology: Complete blood cell count and differential, ESR

Chemistry: Liver function tests, protein electrophoresis

Urine analysis: Cells; chemistry

Cultures: Blood (aerobe and anaerobe, mycobacteria, fungi, viruses); urine; cerebrospinal fluid and other body fluids, if obtained

Serologies: Brucellosis, syphilis, Lyme, HIV, CMV, EBV, amebiasis, toxoplasmosis, chlamydia; antinuclear antibodies, rheumatoid factors, antistreptolysin-O

Imaging: Regular chest radiogram; abdominal ultrasound

Others: Skin tests (purified protein derivative and control); electrocardiogram; bone marrow aspirate (?)

Stage 2: Noninvasive approach to suspected diagnoses

Computed tomography scan: Abdomen (intraabdominal tumors or abscesses; liver abscesses); chest (lung tumors); head (lymphoma, toxoplasmosis, abscess)

Radiograms: Intravenous pyelogram (urinary tract abnormalities); bone films (osteomyelitis); retrograde cholangiography (cholangitis)

Endoscopies: Gastrointestinal tract (Crohn's disease); bronchial tree (bronchus tumors)

Radionucleotide studies: Bone (osteomyelitis); thyroid gland (thyroiditis); pulmonary perfusion/ventilation (emboli)

Echocardiogram (cardiac tumors, endocarditis)

Stage 3: Invasive approach to suspected diagnosis

Biopsies: Lymph nodes, tumors, skin lesions, liver, bone marrow

Laparoscopy (if evidence of intraabdominal abscess obtained during stage 1 or 2)

Stage 4: Failure to establish a diagnosis

Reevaluate patient at regular intervals (if clinical status not rapidly deteriorating)

Empiric therapy: Nonsteroidal antiinflammatory drugs; corticosteroids; antituberculous drugs; antibiotics

CMV, Cytomegalovirus; *EBV,* Epstein-Barr virus; *ESR,* erythrocyte sedimentation rate; *HIV,* human immunodeficiency virus.

physical finding in patients with disseminated mycobacterial or fungal infections.

Basic Laboratory Tests and Procedures. Despite the rationale for a carefully selected approach to the patient with FUO, it is reasonable to routinely perform a set of basic laboratory tests and procedures (Box 234-1). These tests and procedures are discussed later.

Blood cell count and microscopic examination. Anemia is an important sign and suggests a serious underlying disease in a patient with FUO. Leukemias can be missed in aleukemic cases. Lymphocytosis with atypical cells should raise the suspicion of a herpesvirus infection. A leukocytosis with a "left shift" (increase in band forms) suggests an occult bacterial infection. Malaria and spirochetal diseases can be diagnosed by direct examination of the peripheral blood smear, but repeated examinations are often necessary.

Urinalyses. It is important to exclude urinary tract infections and malignant tumors of the urinary tract. Not all urinary tract infections or tumors are consistently associated with pathologic findings in the urine, however, and a single normal urinalysis is insufficient to exclude a urinary tract infection.

Serum chemistry. At least one liver function test is usually abnormal in patients with FUO, in whom the underlying disease originates in the liver or causes nonspecific alterations of the liver, such as granulomatous hepatitis. Most other chemistry tests rarely contribute to the diagnosis in patients with FUO, although they are frequently ordered. Protein electrophoresis is almost routinely performed and can sometimes suggest a specific diagnosis, such as giant cell arteritis.

Cultures. Blood cultures for aerobic and anaerobic pathogens are essential in the evaluation of all patients with FUO (Chapter 233). However, more than a total of approximately six blood cultures are not required. Urine should also be cultured routinely; cultures of sputum and stool (Chapter 233) may be helpful in the presence of signs or symptoms suggestive of pulmonary or gastrointestinal tract disease. All normally sterile tissues and liquids that are sampled during the further workup of patients with FUO need to be cultured for bacteria, mycobacteria, and fungi. These tissues and liquids include cerebrospinal fluid, pleural or peritoneal fluid, liver, bone marrow, and lymph nodes (Chapter 233).

Serologic tests. Serologic tests are most helpful if paired samples show a significant, usually fourfold increase of antibodies specific to an infectious microorganism (Chapter 233). Causes of FUO that can be diagnosed by serologic testing include brucellosis, lues, cytomegalovirus, infectious mononucleosis, HIV infection, amebiasis, toxoplasmosis, and chlamydial diseases. In the majority of patients with FUO, however, serologic tests are of limited diagnostic value.

Antibodies directed against host-specific tissue components, rheumatologic tests, and the detection of circulating immune complexes are frequently performed tests in patients with FUO. These tests are helpful in diagnosing a few diseases such as systemic lupus erythematosus or thyroiditis, but their diagnostic accuracy is limited in other autoimmune and collagen vascular diseases.

Imaging. Chest radiographs are routinely performed in all patients with FUO. Routine abdominal ultrasound examinations may also be justified, even in the absence of signs of an intraabdominal process. However, in a patient with signs or symptoms suggestive of an intraabdominal process, a negative ultrasound examination should not give rise to the exclusion of such a process.

Additional Noninvasive Procedures. The use of additional noninvasive procedures in patients with FUO should be guided by clinical or laboratory findings. The relative diagnostic value of these noninvasive procedures in the evaluation of a patient with FUO has been studied only to a limited degree. In general, adding a second or even third test to the evaluation of the same organ or body region increases the likelihood of detecting a disease process. The possibility that at least one of the test results will be false-positive, however, also increases. Thus the choice of these procedures should be carefully considered.

Computed tomography scans. If ultrasound studies fail to reveal the diagnosis, computed tomography (CT) scans of the abdomen are indicated in all patients with symptoms suggestive of an intraabdominal process, in patients with suspected retroperitoneal tumors or infections, or in those with abnormal liver function tests. Intravenous pyelography may be more sensitive than the CT scan in detecting processes involving the descending urinary tract, but for most other processes of the retroperitoneal space, the CT scan is the preferred method today. The few data comparing CT scanning and magnetic resonance imaging (MRI) currently provide no evidence for the superiority of MRI in patients with FUO. There is no reason to routinely perform both examinations in these patients.

Endoscopy. Endoscopic examination of the upper and lower gastrointestinal tract, including retrograde cholangiography where indicated, must be performed when searching for Crohn's disease, Whipple's disease, biliary tract diseases, and gastrointestinal tract tumors. Sometimes, it may be necessary to complement these endoscopic studies with barium enemas or upper gastrointestinal tract series.

Radionucleotide studies. Ventilation and perfusion radionucleotide studies are necessary to document pulmonary emboli. If suspicion of pulmonary emboli persists despite negative scanning studies, pulmonary angiography is indicated. If osteomyelitis is suspected in a patient without compatible changes in conventional radiography, technetium bone scan may be a more sensitive method for documenting skeletal involvement. Radionucleotide studies using gallium citrate or indium-111-labeled granulocytes are recommended by some authors for the diagnosis of occult abscesses. Although these tech-

✔ *WHEN TO REFER*

Evaluation of a patient with FUO is a multidisciplinary task performed by primary care physicians or internists in close collaboration with subspecialists (e.g., infectious diseases, rheumatology, hematology, and gastroenterology). Often, multiple diagnostic tests including CT scans, MRIs, or invasive procedures are necessary to establish a diagnosis. Efficient evaluation of a patient with FUO is best performed at a medical center where all the necessary specialties and diagnostic tools are readily available. Typically, patients are hospitalized initially so that they may be examined daily, and to assess the patient's condition and need for supportive therapy and quickly search for the common causes of FUO. If a diagnosis cannot be readily established, further workup can be performed on an outpatient basis if the clinical condition is sufficiently stable.

niques have been successful in some studies, other authors have found a high number of false-positive and false-negative results with both of these techniques.

Echocardiography. This technique is highly sensitive in diagnosing cardiac tumors, such as myxomas. In addition, the diagnosis of endocarditis is frequently possible by echocardiography, particularly when transesophageal echocardiography is available (Chapter 24).

Invasive Procedures and Biopsies. In many instances of FUO, the final diagnosis is based on direct examination of involved tissue. Therefore any indication of organ involvement should raise the question of a biopsy. Biopsies are readily performed in enlarged, accessible lymph nodes, other peripheral tissues, and the bone marrow. For the latter, there may be some justification for routine examination in all patients with FUO, independent of signs of bone marrow involvement. The decision to perform biopsy is more difficult if it necessitates an exploratory surgical procedure, such as laparotomy. Experiences with modern imaging techniques suggest that laparotomy should be performed only in those patients in whom noninvasive testing has revealed an indication of an intraabdominal process. If all noninvasive examinations are negative, it is unlikely that the laparotomy will reveal a diagnosis. The same holds true for liver biopsy. Liver biopsy rarely results in important information in patients without abnormal liver findings, although it is a valuable tool in patients with abnormal liver function tests or morphologic alterations of the liver.

Empiric Treatment

If all efforts to establish a cause of FUO fail, empiric treatment may be considered. The decision to treat should depend on the general condition of the patient, on symptoms associated with fever, and on clinical considerations about the underlying illness. In general, empiric therapy with antibiotics or antituberculous drugs rarely produces favorable results. Most often, corticosteroids are used as initial empiric therapy. As an alternative, nonsteroidal antiinflammatory drugs may be used. It appears, however, that in the patient lacking symptoms making an empiric therapy mandatory, repeated clinical evaluation is more prudent than empiric therapy.

BIBLIOGRAPHY

Aduan RP et al: Factitious fever and self-induced infection: a report of 32 cases and review of the literature, *Ann Intern Med* 90:230, 1979.
Davis SG, Gravie NW: The role of indium-labelled leukocyte imaging in pyrexia of unknown origin, *Br J Radiol* 63:850, 1990.
Dinarello CA, Cannon JG, Wolff SM: New concepts on the pathogenesis of fever, *Rev Infect Dis* 10:168, 1988.
Durack DT, Street AC: Fever of unknown origin: reexamined and redefined, *Curr Clin Topics Infect Dis* 11:35, 1991.
Gelfand JA, Wolff SM: Fever of unknown origin. In Mandell GL, Bennett JE, Dolin R, editors: *Principles and practice of infectious diseases*, ed 4, New York, 1995, Churchill Livingstone.
Howard P et al: Fever of unknown origin: a prospective study of 100 patients, *Tex Med* 73:56, 1977.

Knockaert DC, Vanneste LJ, Bobbaers HJ: Fever of unknown origin in elderly patients, *J Am Geriatr Soc* 41:1187, 1993.
Knockaert DC et al: Fever of unknown origin in the 1980s: an update of the diagnostic spectrum, *Arch Intern Med* 152:51, 1992.
Knockaert DC et al: Clinical value of gallium-67 scintigraphy in evaluation of fever of unknown origin, *Clin Infect Dis* 18:601, 1993.
Larson EB, Featherstone HJ, Petersdorf RG: Fever of undetermined origin: diagnosis and follow-up of 105 cases—1970-1980, *Medicine (Baltimore)* 61:269, 1982.
Liu GT et al: Visual morbidity in giant cell arteritis: clinical characteristics and prognosis for vision, *Ophthalmology* 101:1779, 1994.
Mackowiak PA, LeMaistre CF: Drug fever: a critical appraisal of conventional concepts, *Ann Intern Med* 106:728, 1987.
McNeil BJ et al: A prospective study of computed tomography, ultrasound, and gallium imaging in patients with fever, *Radiology* 139:647, 1981.
Miralles P et al: Fever of uncertain origin in patients infected with the human immunodeficiency virus, *Clin Infect Dis* 20:872, 1995.
Petersdorf RG, Beeson PB: Fever of unexplained origin: report of 100 cases, *Medicine (Baltimore)* 40:1, 1961.
Telenti A, Hermans PE: Idiopathic granulomatosis manifesting as fever of unknown origin, *Mayo Clin Proc* 64:44, 1989.
Zoutman DE, Ralph ED, Frei JV: Granulomatous hepatitis and fever of unknown origin: an 11-year experience of 23 cases with three years' follow-up, *J Clin Gastroenterol* 13:69, 1991.

CHAPTER

235 Fever and Rash

Peter K. Lindenauer and Merle A. Sande

The patient in whom fever and rash develop poses a challenging and often urgent diagnostic problem. To provide optimal care, the clinician must be familiar with the wide variety of disease processes that become evident in this manner, especially those that may be acutely life-threatening. A successful evaluation begins with an initial assessment of the degree of illness and follows with a detailed history, close observation of the rash itself, recognition of relevant physical findings, and judicious use of laboratory testing. Therapy may be specific, as in the case of recognized bacterial infection; supportive, as in most viral infections; or presumptive, for the "toxic-appearing" patient with petechial skin lesions.

PATHOGENESIS

Exanthems may be caused by the direct effects of a pathogen or by the immunologic response of the body toward an antigen. Bloodstream spread of an infecting organism can lead to multiplication in the skin itself or to invasion of the cutaneous vessels. The vesicular rash of the herpesviruses is an example of direct cutaneous invasion with a cellular response characterized by multinucleated giant cells and inclusion bodies. In Rocky Mountain spotted fever (RMSF) the rickettsiae invade the vasculature of the integument and internal organs via endothelial cells (Color Plate VIII-18) and can be demonstrated in vessel walls by immunofluorescence. Recent investigation has demonstrated that tumor necrosis factor (TNF), a product of lipopolysaccharide (LPS)-activated macrophages, is the major mediator of the Shwartzman reaction. This interaction of LPS and TNF leads to the adherence of leukocytes and eventually fibrin within the capillary endothelium and is thought to be the mechanism through which meningococcal and other bacillary gram-negative infections cause their characteristic hemorrhagic and necrotic skin lesions. The recognition of direct invasion of the skin or cutaneous vessels is important because a direct aspirate or biopsy specimen may lead to an immediate definitive diagnosis (Chapter 259) (Color Plate VIII-19). Bacterial toxin production is another mechanism of cutaneous injury, and is seen in both staphylococcal scalded-skin syndrome and toxic shock syndrome (TSS).

Infectious organisms or other antigens may invoke an immune response that leads to the development of a rash. This rash can represent an antigen-antibody reaction, delayed hypersensitivity, or, less commonly, an immediate hypersensitivity reaction. The erythematous rashes of drug reactions, measles, mononucleosis, hepatitis B infection, leptospirosis, typhoid fever, and rheumatic fever are examples of exanthems mediated largely by antigen-antibody reactions. The rash of a drug reaction may also be initiated by a nonimmunologic mechanism. Delayed hypersensitivity has been shown to be essential to vesicle formation in vaccinia infection and may be important in other vesicular eruptions. Urticarial rashes, such as those seen with serum sickness or drug ingestion, are probably mediated by an allergic reaction, although this mechanism is not common in exanthems caused by infectious agents. Skin rash is a common manifestation of many of the rheumatologic disorders (systemic lupus erythematosus, dermatomyositis, Behçet's disease, and Reiter's syndrome) and is a by-product of a diverse group of autoimmune mechanisms.

APPROACH TO THE PATIENT AND DIFFERENTIAL DIAGNOSIS

The differential diagnosis of fever and a rash includes a wide variety of disease processes, some of which are potentially life threatening (Tables 235-1 and 235-2). In approaching the patient, one must first consider the severity of illness because many such patients are unable to provide a history and some may require urgent intensive care. When an infectious origin is likely, the clinician must judge whether the patient requires immediate, often empiric, antibiotics. During this initial evaluation thought should also be given to the role of patient isolation when airborne spread of pathogens is of concern.

Obtaining a complete medical history and performing a thorough physical examination are crucial for both diagnostic success and for drug selection when empiric therapy is required. The history should focus on travel outside the local area, including contact with rural or natural environments, wild animals or insects, occupational exposures, and contacts with ill individuals. A thorough exploration of prescription and nonprescription drug use, including over-the-counter drugs, herbal and folk remedies and injection drug use, is required. A review of dietary habits and a detailed sexual history often provide valuable clues toward diagnosis. Important items in the medical history include prior illnesses and immunizations, immunologic status including known human immunodeficiency virus (HIV) infection or HIV risk factors, recent chemotherapy, use of immunosuppressive agents or steroid use, the presence of valvular heart disease, and prior adverse drug reactions. The clinician should inquire about the onset of the rash in relation to other signs of illness and the rash's geographic distribution and progression over time. The examination should allow time for dermatologic classification of the rash and for noting the presence of physical findings such as generalized adenopathy, mucosal involvement, neurologic abnormalities including meningismus, and arthritis or tenosynovitis.

An appreciation of the influence of season and geographic setting is essential. RMSF is almost exclusively a disease of late spring to early fall, coinciding with increased exposure to the tick vectors *Dermacentor variabilis* or *Dermacentor andersoni*. Lyme disease, another arthropod-borne illness, arises following exposure to the infected tick nymph *Ixodes dammini* or *Ixodes pacificus* and, like RMSF, occurs most commonly in the late spring and summer months. Outbreaks of exanthems caused by enteroviruses (Chapter 250) also occur in the warmer months, whereas meningococcal and streptococcal diseases usually occur in late winter and early spring. The eastern and southern plains regions have the majority of cases of RMSF, but the disease has been reported in every state, with the exception of Vermont and Hawaii. Lyme disease cases cluster in three distinct geographic zones: the Northeast, the Upper Midwest, and the Far West. Although the human erhlichioses, a newly described group of tick-borne diseases, are now recognized causes of acute febrile illness, the rarity of rash as a manifestation of disease has given rise to the nickname "Rocky Mountain spotless fever." A history of travel to endemic areas is usually found in cases of coccidioidomycosis (southwestern United States), and in viral hemorrhagic fever and scrub typhus (Southeast Asia).

A history of exposure to an infected contact can often be obtained in cases of viral, streptococcal, gonococcal, meningococcal, and chlamydial infections. Contact with livestock or contaminated water should raise the possibility of leptospirosis, whereas exposure to rodents might suggest rat-bite fever. A history of tick exposure is obtainable in approximately 60% of patients with RMSF but in only 30% of patients with Lyme disease. *Erysipelothrix* infection is seen primarily in patients having occupational or recreational contact with fish, swine, or cattle. Ingestion of undercooked pork or bear meat may result in trichinosis, whereas raw seafood is associated with *Vibrio vulnificus* infection in patients with preexisting liver disease. Sporotrichosis is usually seen in farmers, gardeners, or florists who have extensive contact with soil or vegetation.

Almost any drug may produce fever and cutaneous eruption. The diagnosis of drug eruption, however, is usually one of exclusion. A medication history should be taken. Hospitalized patients receiving multiple medications are a particularly susceptible group. Drug reactions produce myriad cutaneous manifestations that may be maculopapular (morbilliform), urticarial, vesiculobullous, petechial, purpuric, nodular, acneiform, or desquamating. The same drug may cause different findings in different patients. Frequently implicated medications include penicillins, phenytoin, sulfonamides, sulfones, and barbiturates. The presence of fever and rash in an injection drug user should suggest hepatitis B infection or infective endocarditis.

Although tampon use during menses was initially described in the vast majority of patients with toxic shock syndrome, this now accounts for little more than half of the 300 cases reported annually. The remaining cases of toxic shock are due primarily to staphylococcal infections such as abscesses and other cutaneous infections, postoperative and postpartum infections, and infections associated with burns.

The hospitalized patient in whom fever and rash develop presents a special situation. Neutropenic or immunosuppressed patients are at particular risk of bacterial infection with *Pseudomonas aeruginosa*, *Clostridium* spp., and α-hemolytic streptococci, all of which are commonly associated with rash. Disseminated candidiasis, aspergillus, and herpesvirus infections are common complications of neutropenia, and occasionally rash is one of the signs of infection. The development of fever and rash during broad-spectrum antibiotic therapy or parenteral hyperalimentation in any patient should suggest the possibility of systemic candidiasis. Indwelling intravascular catheters, pacemakers, prosthetic heart valves, and dialysis shunts pose a significant risk of bacteremia or endocarditis.

Patients with HIV infection frequently come to medical attention with fever and a rash. An exanthem associated with a "viral syndrome" (fever, headache, aseptic meningitis, pharyngitis, and myalgias) may be associated with acute HIV seroconversion (Chapter 248). Common dermatologic disorders in HIV-infected individuals include seborrheic dermatitis, eosinophilic folliculitis, papular dermatitis, and psoriasis. Common bacterial infections such as pyoderma furunculosis and folliculitis may complicate HIV disease. Cutaneous manifestations of systemic infections may occur, and cutaneous infections may occur in severe forms. Varicella-zoster and herpes simplex lesions are common and sometimes severe in HIV-infected patients. Cryptococcal, histoplasmal, candidal, and coccidioidal fungal infections may involve the skin; mycobacterial infections may rarely involve the skin. Neoplasms that affect the skin include Kaposi's sarcoma and, occasionally, malignant lymphomas. Bacillary angiomatosis, which has been increasingly recognized in HIV-infected patients, is caused by a rickettsia, *Bartonella henselae* or *Bartonella quintana*. The clinical syndrome can be varied and may include skin lesions (usually friable red papules or nodules) with or without systemic involvement such as fever, malaise, hepatosplenomegaly, lymphadenopathy, and lytic bone lesions. Infection caused by *B. quintana* or *B. henselae* can also cause fever, bacteremia, and hepatosplenomegaly with blood-filled cysts (peliosis hepatis and peliosis splenis) in the absence of cutaneous findings.

Drug reactions are common in HIV-infected patients and often become evident as fever with a rash. Trimethoprim-sulfamethoxazole is a common offender; some studies have reported that rash developed in more than 50% of patients taking this drug, and up to 30% of patients need to change therapy because of severe skin toxicity. Rash with or without fever has also been reported to accompany treatment with dapsone, pentamidine, clindamycin, fluconazole, foscarnet, sulfadiazine, didanosine (DDI), zalcitabine (DDC), and zidovudine (AZT).

Associated symptoms may provide important clues in considering

Table 235-1   Identification of life-threatening diseases associated with fever and rash

DISEASE	HISTORY	CHARACTERISTICS OF RASH	DISTRIBUTION OF RASH	ASSOCIATED CLINICAL FINDINGS	DIAGNOSTIC AIDS
Rocky Mountain spotted fever	Tick exposure (60%) May-September occurrence in temperate-zone states Heaviest endemic area middle Atlantic states and Southeast	Initial maculopapular petechiae appearing on 2nd to 6th febrile day and usually painless (Plates VIII-18 and VIII-19)	Begins on wrists, ankles, forearms, spreading within 6-8 hours to palms, soles, trunk	Prodrome of fever, headache, myalgias Hyponatremia, normal to slightly increased white blood cells, thrombocytopenia, hypoalbuminemia	Biopsy of involved skin with immunofluorescence and other serologic tests Serology: Complement-fixation more sensitive and more specific than Weil-Felix agglutination
Meningococcemia*	Tends to occur in late winter, early spring Outbreaks in military recruits, crowded living conditions	*Acute:* May be maculopapular initially. Small petechiae with irregular borders ("smudging"), at times with vesicular or grayish ulcer. May coalesce. Painful (Plate VIII-21) *Chronic:* Maculopapules, petechial vesicles, or pustules; tender nodules	*Acute:* Extremities and trunk in random fashion *Chronic:* Extremities, particularly over joints	*Acute:* Meningitis, disseminated intravascular coagulation, shock, acidosis *Chronic:* Rash appears with recurrent cycles of fever over 2-3 months	*Acute:* Aspiration of center of skin lesions for Gram's stain, culture (up to 70% positive). Blood cultures. Cerebrospinal fluid culture and Gram's stain *Chronic:* Blood culture usually positive during febrile episode. Biopsy findings resemble leukocytoclastic angiitis
Disseminated gonococcal infection	Incidence higher in women than in men Young, sexually active Onset often related to menstruation	Pustules on erythematous base most characteristic. Also, macules, papules, pustules, and bullae less commonly (Plate VIII-22)	Over extremities, with relative sparing of face and trunk. Usually few (5-40) lesions	Migratory polyarthralgia, tenosynovitis, septic arthritis	Gram's stain of lesion Blood, joint fluid culture (50%) prove diagnosis Cervical, rectal, throat cultures support diagnosis
Staphylococcal septicemia	Nosocomial: Indwelling catheters, pacemakers, dialysis shunts, wound infections Drug abuse	Pustules, purulent purpura, subcutaneous nodules, infarcts	Widespread, with infarcts having predilection for distal extremities	Endocarditis, with valvular incompetence, meningitis, multiple-organ involvement	Aspiration of lesions for Gram's stain culture Blood, cerebrospinal fluid (where indicated) cultures Teichoic acid antibody suggestive of deep-seated infection
Pseudomonas septicemia	Hospitalized patients, especially with neutropenia or burns	*Vesicles:* Isolated or in small clusters rapidly becoming hemorrhagic *Ecthyma gangrenosum:* Round, indurated, ulcerated painless lesions with central gray eschar (Plate VIII-23) *Maculopapular lesion:* Small erythematous lesion resembling "rose spots" Gangrenous cellulitis	Random Axillary or anogenital area, thigh Trunk Localized	Generally extremely toxic with fever; septic picture	Aspiration of lesion for Gram's stain, culture Cultures of blood, urine, sputum, etc.

Disease					
Candida septicemia	Broad-spectrum antibiotics, leukemia, immunosuppression, hyperalimentation, cardiac surgery	Multiple discrete pink maculopapular lesions 2-5 mm in diameter	Trunk and extremities	Toxic state; associated ophthalmitis, esophagitis, cystitis	Punch biopsy of lesion with stains for fungus Buffy coat of blood Blood cultures (definitive diagnosis) Examination and culture of stool, urine, sputum (supportive of diagnosis with multiple-site involvement) Barium or endoscopic examination of esophagus
Infective endocarditis	Indwelling catheters, pacemakers, dialysis shunts, valvular heart disease, prosthetic valves, intravenous drug abuse, preceding dental or surgical manipulations	*Petechiae:* Often in small groups *Osler's nodes:* Pea-sized, tender, erythematous nodules *Janeway lesions:* Small erythematous or hemorrhagic macules	Conjunctivae, palate, upper chest, distal extremities Pads of fingers and toes Palms and soles	Heart murmur, valvular incompetence, metastatic abscesses, infarcts, Roth's spots, splenomegaly, hematuria, glomerulonephritis, etc.	Serology not yet reliable Blood cultures (3-5 sets) Echocardiogram Circulating immune complexes
Toxic shock syndrome	Young female predominance 1-4 days prodrome of fever, myalgias, arthralgias, and diarrhea Onset during or soon after menses (has also been reported in men and unassociated with menses in women)	*Erythroderma:* Seen at presentation. Diffuse, blanching, macular (deep-red "sunburned" appearance). Resolves within 3 days, followed 5-12 days later by desquamation, most commonly of hands and feet (Plate VIII-20) *Mucosal hyperemia:* Pharynx, conjunctivae, vagina	Diffuse, hands and feet predominantly	Fever, severe hypotension, multisystem involvement (gastrointestinal, muscular, renal, hepatic, hematologic, central nervous system)	Clinical criteria (see text) Negative serologic results for Rocky Mountain spotted fever, leptospirosis, measles Identification of toxin-producing strain of *Staphylococcus aureus*
Lyme disease	Tick exposure 30% from endemic areas—Northeast, Midwest (Minnesota/Wisconsin), and West (California/Oregon) Usually begins in summer	*Erythema chronicum migrans:* Expanding annular erythema (median diameter, 15 cm) from central macule or papule. Secondary annular lesions seen	Commonly thigh, groin, axilla. Any site can be involved	Fever, chills, malaise, myalgias, lymphadenopathy Late (weeks to months) central nervous system, cardiac, and joint involvement	Primarily history and clinical criteria Organism can be cultured (difficult; special media) Serologic testing

*Acute syndrome may occasionally be caused by *Haemophilus influenzae* and *Streptococcus pneumoniae*, especially in splenectomized patients.

Table 235-2 Differential diagnosis of fever and rash based on appearance of rash

Macules or macules and papules	*Bacterial:* Scarlet fever, erysipelas, meningococcemia, *Pseudomonas* septicemia, secondary syphilis, infective endocarditis (Osler's nodes), leptospirosis, toxic shock syndrome, Lyme disease, chlamydia *Viral:* Rubeola, rubella, enteroviruses, erythema infectiosum, mononucleosis, cytomegalovirus, hepatitis B, roseola, adenovirus, atypical measles, human immunodeficiency virus, coxsackie virus *Rickettsial:* Rocky Mountain spotted fever (early), murine and scrub typhus *Fungal:* Disseminated candidiasis, coccidiodomycosis, sporotrichosis, cryptococcosis, histoplasmosis, blastomycosis *Other:* Drug reactions, mycoplasmal pneumonia, toxoplasmosis, trichinosis, erythema multiforme, erythema marginatum, erythema nodosum, systemic lupus erythematosus, dermatomyositis, serum sickness, sarcoidosis, Behçet's syndrome, Reiter's syndrome, inflammatory bowel disease, familial Mediterranean fever
Vesicles	*Bacterial:* Staphylococcal scalded-skin syndrome, bullous impetigo, *Pseudomonas* septicemia *Viral:* Herpes simplex, varicella-zoster, hand-foot-and-mouth disease, eczema herpeticum, disseminated vaccinia *Rickettsial:* Rickettsialpox *Other:* Drugs, mycoplasmal pneumonia, Stevens-Johnson syndrome, inflammatory bowel disease, porphyria, pemphigus, pemphigoid
Petechiae, purpura, or purpuric macules, papules or pustules	*Bacterial:* Meningococcemia, sepsis with disseminated intravascular coagulation, gonococcemia, *Pseudomonas* sepsis, staphylococcal sepsis, infective endocarditis, listeriosis *Viral:* Atypical measles, viral hemorrhagic fevers, enterovirus (occasional) *Rickettsial:* Rocky Mountain spotted fever, epidemic typhus *Other:* Drug, trichinosis, Henoch-Schönlein purpura, thrombotic thrombocytopenic purpura

many of the disease processes included in the differential diagnosis of fever and rash. Usually, RMSF begins after a 3- to 12-day incubation period with fever, headache, and myalgias, with the rash appearing on or about the fourth febrile day (range, 2 to 6 days). Disseminated gonococcal infection is more common in women than in men, and the onset is often related to menstruation. Low-grade fever, migratory polyarthralgia, and tenosynovitis often accompany the rash (Chapter 265). Prominent articular symptoms accompanying a rash should also suggest a primary immunologic process, such as collagen vascular disease, serum sickness, or inflammatory bowel disease. Meningococcemia may become evident as a mild febrile illness, with headache, weakness, and general malaise but can very rapidly accelerate to fulminant sepsis. In patients with enteric fever from *Salmonella* organisms, diarrhea often develops after a period of constipation that appears in conjunction with the rash. Staphylococcal bacteremia may be associated with symptoms of cardiac, central nervous system, or pulmonary involvement.

DIFFERENTIAL DIAGNOSTIC VALUE OF RASH

The skin responds to infection or immunologic challenge in limited ways. Exanthems can be generally divided into the following groups: (1) macular and maculopapular lesions, (2) vesicular or bullous lesions, and (3) pustular, petechial, or purpuric lesions (Table 235-2). It should be realized, however, that although these divisions are helpful in the initial appraisal of the patient, they do not represent absolute distinctions. Not only do many processes become evident with a similar rash, but also one agent may produce more than one type of rash. Exanthems may also change with time; for example, RMSF progresses from an erythematous maculopapular eruption to a petechial rash.

A macular or maculopapular rash is the most common exanthem elicited by nonherpetic viruses, but such a rash does not always signify a benign process. Examples of more serious infections that may become evident with a maculopapular rash include RMSF, meningococcemia, gonococcemia, *Pseudomonas* septicemia, typhoid fever, and disseminated candidiasis.

Lyme disease becomes evident with with the characteristic erythema migrans (EM) rash in more than 60% of patients 1 to 36 days after a tick bite (mean, 7 to 10 days). This rash begins as a small red papule that gradually expands to a ring of erythema at the site of innoculation, often with central clearing. The axilla, thigh, and groin are most commonly involved, but any site may be affected. In a significant percentage of individuals, similar-appearing, although smaller, secondary lesions develop within several days at sites distant from the primary EM lesion.

Toxic shock syndrome (Chapter 260) is characterized by a "sunburned-appearing," deep red, macular erythroderma in association with fever, hypotension (systolic blood pressure less than 90 mm Hg) and diffuse myalgias or arthralgias. The so-called streptococcal

toxic shock–like syndrome shares many of the clinical features of TSS but is caused by exotoxin-producing strains of group A streptococci. Although the skin or mucous membranes are the suspected pathways of entry for this infection, a definitive entry site can be identified in only a minority of cases. Moreover, when identified, local trauma at these sites often appears minor. Unlike in TSS, the majority of patients with toxic streptococcal infections have soft tissue involvement as a component of the illness. This often takes the form of severe myositis or necrotizing fasciitis, and many patients require extensive debridement and, at times, amputation. This virulence is reflected in the case fatality rates for toxic streptococcal syndrome, which are five times those for TSS.

Drugs typically produce maculopapular exanthems that are frequently cherry-red. The "slapped-face" rash of erythema infectiosum, the "target" lesion of erythema multiforme, and the rapidly spreading macule around a pale center of erythema marginatum are examples of maculopapular lesions distinctive enough to suggest a specific diagnosis. Desquamation is common with scarlet fever, Kawasaki disease, TSS (Color Plate VIII-20), and severe erythroderma caused by drug reactions.

Vesicular lesions are caused by a number of viruses including herpes simplex, varicella-zoster, vaccinia, and some enteroviruses. Similar lesions may also be seen with mycoplasmal infections, usually in association with ulcerative stomatitis. The staphylococcal scalded-skin syndrome is characterized by large bullae that rupture, leaving areas of bright red, denuded skin resembling a burn. *Pseudomonas* septicemia may be associated with single or clustered vesicles that rapidly become hemorrhagic or with the centrally necrotic lesions of ecthyma gangrenosum. Vesicular lesions of the Stevens-Johnson syndrome prominently involve the oral mucosa as well as the skin. Ulcerative colitis or regional enteritis may be associated with vesicular lesions that progress to chronic ulceration and may also have prominent mucosal involvement in the form of aphthous stomatitis.

Petechial, purpuric, or pustular skin lesions frequently indicate life-threatening disease. The identification of such a rash should immediately direct the clinician's attention to treatable bacterial or rickettsial infections, such as meningococcemia (Color Plate VIII-21), gonococcemia (Color Plate VIII-22), RMSF (Color Plate VIII-18), infectious endocarditis, and disseminated intravascular coagulation associated with septicemia. The petechial rash of atypical measles, which may also have vesicular and urticarial components, may mimic RMSF. It is seen in patients previously vaccinated with killed measles vaccine after an exposure to live virus. Rarely, enterovirus infections produce petechial lesions. In travelers returning from an endemic area it is important to consider the syndrome of severe *Plasmodium falciparum* infection that can become evident with hemolysis, thrombocytopenia, and renal failure accompanied by petechiae. Other causes include various collagen vascular diseases, notably the vasculitides, Henoch-Schönlein purpura, and thrombotic thrombocytopenic purpura.

The distribution of an exanthem is of diagnostic significance. A nonvesicular rash involving the palms and soles should suggest RMSF, meningococcemia, infective endocarditis, mycoplasmal infection, scarlet fever, or bacteremia. The copper-colored, scaly macules and papules of secondary syphilis, as well as drug exanthems, atypical measles, and Kawasaki's disease, may also affect these sites. Kawasaki's disease, or mucocutaneous lymph node syndrome, has recently been described in adults. Skin involvement is characterized by an indurative, erythematous, desquamative rash of the palms and soles and a polymorphous, nonvesicular rash. Maculopapular rashes attributable to viruses usually spare the palms and soles, whereas these sites may be involved in vesicular exanthems caused by the herpesviruses and certain coxsackievirus strains (e.g., hand-foot-and-mouth disease). Exanthems that have a predilection for the extremities include gonococcemia, Henoch-Schönlein purpura, dermatomyositis, ecthyma gangrenosum (Color Plate VIII-23), and sporotrichosis (Color Plate VIII-24). The rash of scarlet fever begins on the face and neck and spreads to the trunk and extremities within 36 hours to localize in body folds and antecubital areas and on the palms and soles. Rubeola usually begins behind the ears, spreads first to the forehead, then involves the entire body within 1 day without confluence. The "rose spots" of typhoid fever and the maculopapular lesion associated with *Pseudomonas* septicemia are generally confined to the trunk.

ASSOCIATED PHYSICAL FINDINGS

Associated physical findings are often of diagnostic value. Many processes that involve the skin also involve the mucous membranes. Thus a careful search for enanthems should be undertaken. Koplick's spots, which are diagnostic of rubeola, are bluish-gray specks on a red base, resembling a grain of sand on the buccal mucosa opposite the second molar. A "strawberry tongue" suggests Kawasaki disease, TSS, or scarlet fever and in the latter may be associated with purpuric macules on the soft palate. Palatal petechiae are seen in up to 50% of patients with infectious mononucleosis, usually at the junction of the hard and soft palate; they are also seen in patients with infective endocarditis. Vesicular or ulcerative mucosal lesions may be seen in hand-foot-and-mouth disease, Behçet's syndrome, Reiter's syndrome, inflammatory bowel disease, and the Stevens-Johnson syndrome.

Meningitis or neurologic changes may be seen with meningococcemia, RMSF, staphylococcal bacteremia, leptospirosis, Kawasaki disease, TSS, the "aseptic meningitis" caused by enterovirus infection, and as a late finding in Lyme disease. Generalized adenopathy may be prominent in mononucleosis, toxoplasmosis, syphilis, sarcoidosis, systemic lupus erythematosus, and drug hypersensitivity. Cervical adenopathy is common in scarlet fever with streptococcal pharyngitis, rubella, and mucocutaneous lymph node syndrome. Hilar adenopathy may be prominent in sarcoidosis and atypical measles. The presence of a heart murmur should raise the possibility of infective endocarditis even in the absence of the "classic" but unusual findings of splinter hemorrhages, Janeway lesions, or Osler's nodes. Prominent joint involvement is suggestive of disseminated gonococcal infection or immunologic disorders (e.g., collagen vascular diseases, drug reactions, the prodrome of hepatitis B, or inflammatory bowel disease). The rash of the inflammatory bowel disease generally accompanies exacerbations of gastrointestinal tract symptoms. Rash, fever, and pneumonia should suggest mycoplasmal infection, atypical measles, RMSF, mononucleosis, coccidioidomycosis, or septicemia associated with staphylococcal or *Pseudomonas* pneumonia. Multisystem involvement is frequently seen in systemic lupus erythematosus and TSS.

LABORATORY DIAGNOSIS

Diagnostic attempts should be directed initially toward procedures that may give immediate results (Table 235-3). Pustular, petechial, and purpuric lesions should be aspirated or scraped, and any obtainable fluid cultured and examined microscopically. Gram-negative, biscuit-shaped cocci can be found in the skin lesions of up to 70% of patients with meningococcemia and petechial lesions, although some authors suggest that this may be overly optimistic. Vesicular lesions should be unroofed with a scalpel blade and the contents examined

Table 235-3   Diagnostic tests useful in fever and rash

TEST	APPLICATION
Aspirate of lesion for Gram's stain and culture	Most helpful in pustular or petechial lesions. Positive in up to 70% of meningococcemias
Wright's or Giemsa stain of vesicular fluid	Up to 70% of herpesvirus infections show multinucleated giant cells or cytoplasmic inclusion bodies
Biopsy	Fungal infections, vasculitis, granulomatous disease
	Immunofluorescence: Rocky Mountain spotted fever, systemic lupus erythematosus
Cultures of distant sites Blood	All cases of possible bacteremia, fungemia
Throat, rectal swab	Viral infections
Throat, rectum, urethra, cervix, joint	Disseminated gonococcal infection
Serologic testing	Streptococcal and rickettsial infections, syphilis, typhoid fever, leptospirosis, Lyme disease (*Borrelia burgdorferi* spirochete), *Mycoplasma* species, coccidioidomycosis, hepatitis B, Epstein-Barr virus, cytomegalovirus, measles, atypical measles, systemic lupus erythematosus, trichinosis, enterovirus and adenovirus infections

✔ WHEN TO REFER

The many disease processes that become evident with fever and rash cross the boundaries of conventional medical subspecialties. In so doing, they call upon the full complement of skills possessed by the general internist, in particular, the ability to take a careful history and synthesize data pertaining to a number of organ systems simultaneously. Nevertheless, patients with many of the conditions discussed in this chapter are ill enough to warrant early consultation with an infectious disease specialist or dermatologist. As a general rule, if the initial history, physical examination, and laboratory analysis leave the attending physician with little confidence in a diagnosis and the patient is extremely ill, or if after a conservative trial of empiric antibiotics the patient has failed to respond, a consultation with an infectious disease specialist is in order. Because a punch biopsy is frequently used as part of the overall diagnostic approach and because the experience of a dermatologist in evaluating complex rashes is often valuable, it is reasonable to consider consulting these specialists early in the course of illness.

with Wright's or Giemsa stain for multinucleated giant cells or inclusion bodies characteristic of herpesvirus infection. In the immunocompromised patient aspiration of maculopapular lesions may reveal gram-negative *Pseudomonas aeruginosa* bacilli, and strong consideration should also be given to performing a punch biopsy with fungal staining for *Candida* organisms. Needle aspiration and punch biopsy appear to be effective methods to rapidly diagnose group A streptococcal infections in patients with necrotizing fasciitis or myositis, often providing a firm diagnosis before blood cultures have had sufficient time to yield an organism. Biopsy may also be helpful in identifying vasculitis or granulomatous disease. Immunofluorescence of skin biopsy specimens in RMSF may be positive as early as the fourth day of illness and should be considered an early diagnostic aid. Immunofluorescence is also valuable in the diagnosis of systemic lupus erythematosus, pemphigus vulgaris, and pemphigoid. Serologic testing in early Lyme disease is hampered by an unacceptably high false-negative rate, and diagnosis of Lyme disease is largely a clinical one.

Examination and culture of cerebrospinal fluid, joint fluid, or urethral or cervical discharge may yield a bacteriologic diagnosis, especially in meningococcal or gonococcal infection. Blood cultures should be performed in all cases in which bacteremia is considered. Throat, rectal, and cerebrospinal fluid cultures for viruses are becoming increasingly useful and available. Throat, rectal, urethral, and cervical cultures should be performed in patients suspected of having disseminated gonococcal infection. Serologic tests may be useful in selected cases. A list of diseases in which they may be helpful is given in Table 235-3.

BIBLIOGRAPHY

Berger T, Perkocha LA: Bacillary angiomatosis, *AIDS Clin Rev* 81-95, 1991.

Bohach GA et al: Staphylococcal and streptococcal pyrogenic toxins involved in toxic shock syndrome and related illnesses, *Crit Rev Microbiol* 17(4):251, 1990.

Dumler JS, Bakken JS: Ehrlichial diseases of humans: emerging tick-borne infections, *Clin Infect Dis* 20:1102–1110, 1995.

Heymann WR: Noninfectious causes of fever and a rash, *Int J Dermatol* 28(3):145, 1989.

Kingston ME, Mackey D: Skin clues in the diagnosis of life-threatening infections, *Rev Infect Dis* 8(1):1, 1986.

LeBoit P: Dermatopathologic findings in patients infected with HIV, *Dermatol Clin* 10(1):59, 1992.

Lee BL: Drug interactions and toxicities in patients with AIDS. In Sande MA, Volberding PA editors: *The medical management of AIDS*, ed 4, Philadelphia, 1992, WB Saunders.

Mastin DB et al: Atypical measles in adolescents and young adults, *Ann Intern Med* 90:877, 1979.

Medina I et al: Oral therapy for *Pneumocystis carinii* pneumonia in the acquired immunodeficiency syndrome, *N Engl J Med* 323(12):776, 1990.

Meyers SA, Sexton DJ: Dermatologic manifestations of arthropod-borne diseases, *Infect Dis Clin North Am* 8(3):689-712, 1994.

Milgrom H et al: Kawasaki disease in a healthy young adult, *Ann Intern Med* 92:467, 1980.

Nadelman RB, Wormser GP: Erythema migrans and early lyme disease, *Am J Med* 98(suppl 4A):15S-24S, 1995.

Spencer LV, Callen JP: Cutaneous manifestations of bacterial infections, *Dermatol Clin* 7(3):579, 1989.

Tyring SK: Natural history of varicella zoster virus, *Semin Dermatol* 11(3):211-217, 1992.

van Deuren M et al: Rapid diagnosis of acute meningococcal infections by needle aspiration or biopsy of skin lesions, *Br Med J* 306:1229-1232, 1993.

Walker DH: Rocky Mountain spotted fever: a seasonal alert, *Clin Infect Dis* 20:1111-1117, 1995.

Weber DJ, Cohen MS: The acutely ill patient with fever and rash. In Mandell GL, Douglas RG, Bennett JE, editors: *Principles and practice of infectious disease*, ed 4, New York, 1995, Churchill Livingstone.

Wolf JE, Rabinowitz LG: Streptococcal toxic shock–like syndrome, *Arch Dermatol* 131:73–77, 1995.

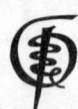

CHAPTER

236 Fever in the Compromised Host

Lowell S. Young

Many patients who are immunologically compromised are at risk for development of serious infection. The initial clinical manifestation of this infectious process is usually fever. For the purposes of definition, fever represents an elevation in core body temperature in excess of 38° C or 100.2° F. Such definitions are arbitrary, however, and some individuals may have a normal body temperature within 1° above or below 37° C. Fever is the hallmark of infection but is not diagnostic of it. Indeed, the opposite of fever—hypothermia—can occasionally be an important clinical finding that suggests infection in markedly debilitated patients. Perhaps most important, a change in body temperature in a compromised patient—particularly if measured at a rectal source, which approximates core body temperature—should alert the clinician to the possibility of an incipient infectious process, prompt an immediate and comprehensive clinical evaluation, and lead to the consideration of empiric antimicrobial therapy.

More difficult to define than an actual elevation in body temperature is the term *compromised* or *immunocompromised*. The term implies an impaired ability to resist infection. Susceptibility to infection can result from purely mechanical factors such as major trauma or damage to the integument. However, the term *compromised* usually refers to patients who have impaired ability to resist infection that results from an immunologic defect. The prime examples of compromised hosts are individuals with hematologic malignancies (e.g., acute leukemia), recipients of organ transplants, and patients treated with corticosteroids or ionizing radiation. Some individuals are born with congenital immunodeficiencies and obviously qualify for the classification.

The nature of the immunologic defects predisposing to infection has been covered in other chapters but may be categorized according to the following concepts. First, the number of the phagocytic cells belonging to the neutrophil or polymorphonuclear leukocyte series may be reduced or their function impaired. These cells respond to acute infection, and severe impairment in the function of such cells either qualitatively (as in chronic granulomatous disease of childhood) or quantitatively (as in the case of acute leukemia in which blast cells exceed the production of normal, functioning neutrophils in the bone marrow) results in markedly increased susceptibility to bacterial infection. Second, a relatively slower-acting population of phagocytic cells includes circulating monocytes and tissue macrophages, and the fixed mononuclear phagocytes of the reticuloendothelial system may be functionally impaired. These cells collaborate with T helper cells in defense against intracellular pathogens, particularly slow-growing bacteria such as *Mycobacterium tuberculosis*. This component of immunity, often referred to as cell-mediated immunity, seems critical in the defense against a variety of viral, parasitic, and fungal pathogens. Third, there may be quantitative defects in humoral factors that are important in host defense. These include circulating antibodies of the immunoglobulins A, G, and M class (IgA, IgG, and IgM), as well as an enzymatic system such as the complement cascade, which results in direct lysis of some bacteria and viruses. Clearly, however, this segregation of the components of host defense is artificial. To optimize host defense, antibodies bind to bacteria or other microbes (a process known as *opsonization*) and prepare them for ingestion by phagocytic cells. The great majority of patients who are immunologically compromised have defects of one or more of these components in host defense. Not to be overlooked, however, is the fact that therapeutic intervention with cytotoxic anticancer drugs or the use of immunosuppressing medications such as corticosteroids can have profound effects on humoral antibody production and can reduce the number or impair function of phagocytic cells and lymphocytes. Quite often, combinations of defects are present. Therapy with cytotoxic or immunosuppressive medications superimposed on a preexisting immunologic defect results in markedly enhanced infection risk.

PATHOGENESIS OF FEVER

The mechanisms of inflammation leading to fever are much better understood now than when earlier investigators identified a crude substance elaborated by phagocytic cells that, different from endotoxin, triggered fever in experimental animals. Initially termed *endogenous pyrogen*, it was hypothesized that phagocytosis led to the elaboration of a humoral factor that then acted centrally on brain centers that regulate body temperature. Elaboration of endogenous pyrogen would then be the signal to hypothalamic temperature control centers for the triggering of muscular activity (e.g., shivering) that results in elevation of core temperatures. It is now recognized that *endogenous pyrogen* describes the effects of several cytokines elaborated by mononuclear phagocytes. The best known is interleukin-1 (IL-1), a chemically sequenced protein that triggers fever in experimental animals and in humans. Endotoxin administration, as well as other stimuli, causes release of IL-1. Other pyrogenic substances, however, are elaborated by mononuclear phagocytes after exposure to infectious stimuli such as bacteria, viruses, and parasites. These inflammatory mediators include tumor necrosis factor (also known as cachetin) and the interferons. It seems probable that antigen-antibody complexes, as may occur in collagen vascular diseases, can trigger the elaboration of endogenous pyrogens such as IL-1. Furthermore, various neoplastic processes seem also to result in the release of pyrogens from the reticuloendothelial system. Thus a variety of mechanisms from the progression of underlying disease to a hypersensitivity reaction can provoke fever in both normal and compromised patients.

CLINICAL APPROACH TO THE PATIENT

The clinician must be alert to the fact that the development of fever in a patient with impaired immunity may be due to multiple causes and that multiple infectious processes may be present simultaneously. The cardinal principle with regard to clinical management is that infection should clearly be suspected as the most likely cause of fever, and, depending on the immune status of the host, measures to diagnose and treat infection should be rapidly initiated.

The onset of fever should prompt a meticulous yet expeditious bedside evaluation of the patient that should be completed in a matter of minutes. Particular areas of concern during the physical examination should be the head and neck for evidence of central nervous system infection, the oropharynx for evidence of bacterial pharyngitis, the lungs for evidence of any infectious process therein, the abdomen, the urinary tract, the perirectal area, and the integument. If a patient has a foreign body in place, such as an intravenous or intraarterial catheter, it should be carefully examined and cultures drawn through the catheter channel(s). Immunosuppressed patients are likely to have a limited or impaired inflammatory response. A frank purulent reaction (abscess or sputum production) is rare in severely neutropenic patients. Laboratory studies should focus on studies that give prompt results (e.g., Gram's stains of body fluids and aspirates). Some processes involving the lung or brain are notoriously difficult to diagnose without a biopsy, and empiric therapy may have to be initiated before invasive diagnostic measures. Cultures for suspected aerobic and anaerobic organisms and for fungi should be taken immediately. Blood cultures should be obtained before the initiation of any antimicrobial therapy and before appropriate serologic tests are obtained. One cannot criticize the latter measures, but serologic results will not be forthcoming for days, so such studies are largely for confirmatory purposes. If the patient has any central nervous system finding, a chest x-ray film of the lung, routine urinalysis, and lumbar puncture should be obtained as quickly as possible, depending on the underlying clinical urgency. In a hypotensive patient, treatment should be initiated within a matter of minutes.

Epidemiology

The source of infectious fever may be categorized as either endogenous or exogenous. Normal hosts are colonized by myriad microorganisms that generally are harmless. Given the presence of impaired immunity, staphylococci colonizing the skin (coagulase negative) or nares *(Staphylococcus aureus)* can invade and cause life-threatening diseases. This process may be abetted by foreign bodies such as vascular or urinary catheters. Perhaps more than the majority of documented infections in compromised individuals are endogenous, with the natural reservoir being the skin or gastrointestinal tract. Gram-negative bacilli, the most common cause of life-threatening bloodstream invasion, are usually regarded as endogenous pathogens, and the same concept applies to *Candida* species. The great majority of normal individuals, however, are not carriers of *Pseudomonas aeruginosa* or *Klebsiella* species. Careful studies have shown that compromised individuals acquire these organisms from food or environment, and the organisms are often colonized in the gut before systemic invasion. In a hospital setting the potential for transmission of infection from person to person or from an environmental source to a high-risk patient is increased when the host is immunocompromised. Additional examples of exogenous infections are *Aspergillus* pneumonia or transfusion-associated infection. The setting of a critical care unit presents many opportunities for transmission of infection from patient to patient or from the inanimate environment to patient.

DIFFERENTIAL DIAGNOSIS OF INFECTIOUS DISEASE SYNDROMES IN THE COMPROMISED HOST

Table 236-1 summarizes some of the major clinical syndromes and the causative agents that the clinician should seek to identify in febrile, immunocompromised patients. These syndromes and agents can be conveniently categorized in terms of anatomic localization of symptoms: central nervous system, respiratory tract, gastrointestinal tract, and skin and soft tissues. Some febrile patients, however, may not demonstrate any localizing signs of infections, and these patients may be among those who are most seriously ill.

Central Nervous System Infection

In the immunocompromised host both gram-positive and gram-negative bacillary pathogens cause brain abscess or meningitis, but one organism should always be considered: *Listeria monocytogenes.* In many series this organism is the most common cause of bacterial meningitis. However, encapsulated bacteria such as pneumococci and staphylococci (usually from a bacteremic source) may cause metastatic central nervous system disease. Patients with compromised cell-mediated immunity (Hodgkin's disease or acquired immunodeficiency syndrome [AIDS]) are at particular risk for development of cryptococcal or even *Listeria* meningitis. The cryptococci are probably the most important fungal pathogens, but occasionally *Candida* and *Aspergillus* species can cause central nervous system disease. The herpesviruses, including cytomegalovirus (CMV), Epstein-Barr, and herpes simplex, may cause central nervous system disease, although the exact proportion of attributable causes is a matter of controversy. The human immunodeficiency virus type I (HIV-I) can cause central nervous system reactive pleocytosis. Reactivated or quiescent central nervous system syphilis should also be considered in patients with severe immunologic impairment. Parasites rarely cause central nervous system disease in immunocompromised patients.

Respiratory Tract

The lungs offer a particular challenge for the evaluation of fever in the compromised patient. Often, it is clear that the patients have respiratory tract symptoms manifested by cough, hypoxia, and shortness of breath. Despite the ready detection of pulmonary abnormalities, diagnosis is difficult because of problems in accurately obtaining pulmonary secretions or in obtaining an adequate sampling of lung parenchyma. Community-acquired pathogens such as pneumococcus and *Haemophilus influenzae* can cause lobar and sometimes even diffuse pneumonia. Gram-negative bacilli are often associated with opportunistic pneumonia in patients with intubated tracheas; these lung infections are associated with extraordinarily high mortality rates. Depending on epidemiologic circumstances, *Legionella* species may cause life-threatening infections in patients who are debilitated, receiving organ transplants, or receiving immunosuppressive therapy associated with transplantation or cancer treatment. The primary parasitic cause of diffuse pneumonia in immunocompromised patients has clearly been *Pneumocystis carinii.* However, *Toxoplasma* and *Strongyloides* species can cause pulmonary infiltrates.

The most common opportunistic fungi causing lung infection include the *Aspergillus* species and cryptococci. Even *Candida* organisms, however, may involve the lung on a fungemic basis. One should not overlook the possibility of mycobacterial disease, particularly in patients with impaired cell-mediated immunity. The pulmonary involvement is usually primary for tuberculosis but can be secondary for the atypical mycobacteria (e.g., *Mycobacterium avium-intracellulare* complex).

Viral infections are often difficult to diagnose in immunocompromised patients. Respiratory tract pathogens such as adenovirus, measles, and respiratory syncytial virus have long been known to complicate immunosuppression. However, the predominant pathogen in patients after organ transplantation is CMV. This agent can cause diffuse interstitial pneumonitis that is indistinguishable from *Pneumocystis* infection; indeed, CMV may coexist with pneumocystosis. Other viral causes of lung disease in compromised patients include varicella-zoster virus. Interestingly, *Mycoplasma* and *Chlamydia* spe-

Table 236-1   Origins of infectious disease syndromes in the compromised host

| | PATHOGENS TO CONSIDER | | | |
PATTERN OF INVOLVEMENT	BACTERIA	FUNGI	VIRUSES	PARASITES
Disseminated disease with skin lesions (vasculitis or abscesses, or both)	*Staphylococcus aureus* *Pseudomonas aeruginosa* *Aeromonas hydrophila* Other gram-negative bacteria *Nocardia* sp. *Noncholera vibrios* Mycobacteria	*Candida* sp. *Aspergillus* Phycomycetes *Trichosporon* sp.	Herpes simplex Varicella-zoster	
Diffuse interstitial pneumonia*	Any gram-negative or gram-positive organism, including *Nocardia* sp. and mycobacteria	*Aspergillus* sp. *Candida* sp. Mucor sp. Cryptococci	Herpes simplex Varicella-zoster Cytomegalovirus Measles	*Pneumocystis carinii*† *Toxoplasma gondii* *Strongyloides stercoralis* *T. gondii*
Central nervous system infection, meningoencephalitis, possibly brain abscess	*Listeria monocytogenes* *Nocardia* sp. S. aureus P. aeruginosa Mycobacterium tuberculosis	*Cryptococcus neoformans* *Aspergillus fumigatus* *Phycomycetes* sp. *Candida* sp.	Varicella-zoster	*T. gondii*
Oroesophageal syndromes	Anaerobes Aerobes: Streptococci and gram-negative rods, particularly *P. aeruginosa*	*Candida* sp. *Aspergillus* sp.	Herpes simplex Cytomegalovirus	
Diarrhea	*Clostridium difficile* *Campylobacter* sp. *Salmonella* sp. *Shigella* sp.		Adenovirus Coxsackievirus Rotavirus	*Giardia lambla* *Cryptosporidium* sp. *Microsporida* sp. *Isospora belli*

*Consider also underlying disease, radiation therapy, and drug reactions.
†May be reclassified as a fungus.

cies, despite their major role as a cause of pneumonia in young adults, are not common pathogens in immunosuppressed patients.

Gastrointestinal Tract

The multiple causes of diarrhea in immunosuppressed patients are listed in Table 236-1. Conventional enteric pathogens such as *Salmonella, Shigella,* and *Campylobacter* should be considered, bearing in mind that diarrhea can stem from the toxins of *Clostridium difficile,* whose overgrowth is a result of selection by antimicrobial therapy; *Isospora belli* and *Cryptosporidium* organisms are two acid-fast–staining parasites associated with impaired cell-mediated immunity, especially AIDS. Their role as a cause of diarrhea has been recognized in other immunosuppressed patients. Pain on swallowing has commonly been linked to *Candida* mucosal overgrowth (thrush and esophagitis). Herpes simplex and CMV, however, may cause identical symptoms as well as a similar radiologic appearance on esophagram. Occasionally, severe cellulitis of the posterior pharynx can be caused by streptococci and even *P. aeruginosa* in the markedly neutropenic host.

Cutaneous Syndromes

Occasionally the sudden onset of bacteremia such as is due to streptococci or staphylococci, may be manifested by cutaneous involvement. Ascending cellulitis of an extremity that is due to streptococci can occur in immunosuppressed as well as normal patients. Metastatic abscesses are common with *S. aureus* bacteremia. In systemic gram-negative infections, necrotizing vasculitis such as the ecthyma gangrenosum of *P. aeruginosa* infection is considered to be virtually diagnostic of this particular pathogenic disease (Color Plate V-23). Fungal pathogens such as *Aspergillus* or *Candida,* however, have been associated with metastatic lesions, and their appearance may be in-

distinguishable from gram-negative vasculitis. The obvious approach in this situation is not to rely on morphologic interpretation of the findings but to carry out aspirations and biopsies of suspected lesions. The information gained therefrom may be more valuable than a blood culture, and the results may be returned sooner than the results of blood cultures.

EMPIRIC ANTIMICROBIAL THERAPY

One of the major important decisions that the clinician must make at the bedside is whether to initiate empiric therapy for the patient who has fever. In some patients it is not possible to discern, on clinical grounds alone, the difference between infectious fever and fever resulting from a neoplasm, drug reaction or hypersensitivity reaction (including reactions to blood products). Whereas the recent administration of blood products might lead the clinician to temporize in the administration of empiric antimicrobial therapy, the basic tenet that underlies all major initial therapeutic choices should be the clinical status of the host. If the patient's immunologic status is severely impaired, as evident in a circulating normal neutrophil count of less than 500 cells/μl, and the patient's overall clinical condition appears to be deteriorating, it is prudent to obtain diagnostic studies mentioned previously and begin broad-spectrum antimicrobial treatment. If a reasonable likelihood exists that the fever is due to a hypersensitivity reaction or underlying disease, diagnostic measures including cultures should be obtained and the patient very carefully observed over the ensuing hours. For the patient who is markedly neutropenic (white blood cell count less than 100 cells/μg) or severely neutropenic (white blood cell count less than 500 cells/μg), a broad-spectrum regimen is preferred as initial therapy unless specific clues identify a likely causative microorganism. Examples of the latter might be transtracheal aspirates, urine Gram's stains, or the aspiration of infected material from an abscess.

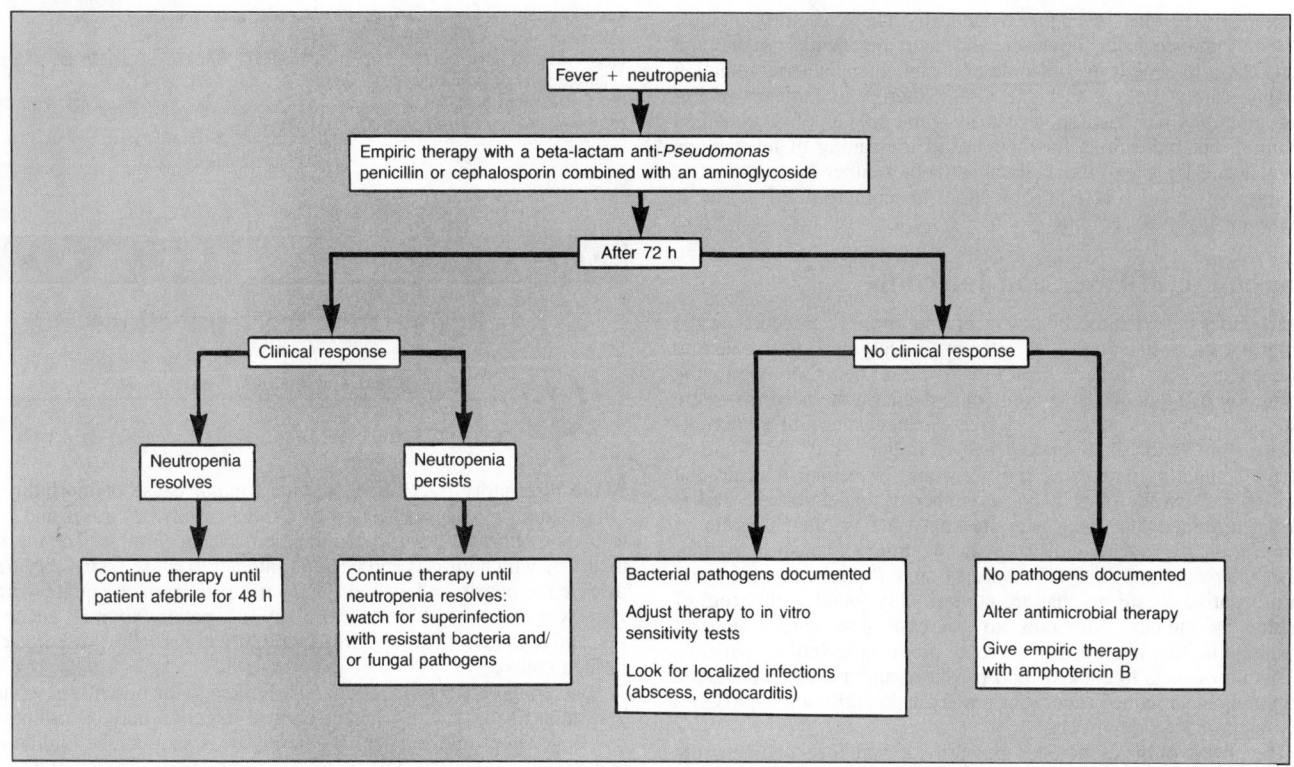

FIGURE 236-1   Empiric approach in febrile neutropenic patients.

Choice of Empiric Therapy

Despite many advances in laboratory diagnosis, there is no clear-cut way to distinguish between gram-negative sepsis and gram-positive infection. Therefore an initial choice of antimicrobial agents should provide broad-spectrum coverage (Fig. 236-1) (Chapter 231). Traditional choices have included an aminoglycoside such as gentamicin, tobramycin, or amikacin for gram-negative activity paired with another broad-spectrum agent of another class that covers *P. aeruginosa*. That broad-spectrum agent may be a β-lactam compound such as carbenicillin, ticarcillin, azlocillin, or mezlocillin, or one of the cephalosporins with reliable anti-pseudomonal activity (cefoperazone or ceftazidime). Alternative choices would include imipenem, aztreonam or one of the intravenous quinolones. The gram-positive activity of the aforementioned compounds is variable, and some clinicians would consider the additional use of vancomycin as initial therapy if the likelihood of gram-positive infection is significant.

Many therapeutic trials have been carried out to evaluate the efficacy of one, two, or three antimicrobial agents as empiric therapy. No convincing evidence suggests that three or more antimicrobial compounds are more effective than double-agent therapy. Several studies performed over the last decade suggest that dual-agent combination therapy may provide synergistic antibacterial activity and minimize the emergence of resistance. Some recent reports, however, suggest that monotherapy with an agent such as ceftazidime or imipenem may be adequate to sustain a neutropenic immunocompromised patient for the first 48 hours until the results of cultures may identify the target of specific antimicrobial therapy. Such a decision should be based on the predictability that most disease-causing bacteria in an institution is susceptible in vitro. For relatively susceptible organisms such as *Escherichia coli* or *Klebsiella* species, a potent β-lactam compound may be sufficient as monotherapy. For *P. aeruginosa* infections the weight of evidence favors the continued use of combinations. For *S. aureus* bacteremia the evidence points toward the continuing efficacy of monotherapy, provided that the organism is susceptible in vitro. For deep-seated staphylococcal infections, however, the combination of a penicillinase-stable β-lactam plus ri-

fampin or an aminoglycoside, may lead to more rapid clinical improvement.

The identification of a specific infecting agent may permit more targeted treatment. A therapeutic dilemma, however, relates to patients who have persistent neutropenia, yet no organism is identified as the cause of pyrexia (Fig. 236-1). Indeed, between 50% and 80% of febrile neutropenic patients may have no identified cause of fever, yet they respond to broad-spectrum therapy. It has been suggested that such patients have incipient nonbacteremic infection (e.g., from a gastrointestinal tract source) and that early treatment arrests further spread of infection. Some clinicians prefer to continue antibiotics until the neutrophil count rises above 500 cells/μL. Usually, however, antibiotics may be discontinued after 3 to 5 afebrile days, and patients are very carefully followed. If this regimen is followed, patients must be monitored to avoid the development of a catastrophic "rebound" septicemia. A greater challenge, however, is what to do for the persistently febrile patient who has undocumented infection. Some controlled studies suggest that in the face of persistent immunosuppression and fever the most prudent choice after the initiation of antibacterial treatment is to initiate empiric antifungal therapy with amphotericin B (Fig. 236-1). The agents that are active against the opportunistic fungi (such as amphotericin B with or without flucytosine) are toxic, and the decision to initiate empiric antifungal therapy should not be made lightly. On the other hand, controlled clinical studies suggest the benefits of such empiric treatment with amphotericin alone in the febrile neutropenic patient who has not responded to 5 to 7 days of empiric antibacterial therapy and in whom no apparent cause of the fever is identified. The role of the new azoles, including fluconazole and itraconazole, for empiric therapy in place of amphotericin B, requires further evaluation.

Augmentation of host defenses in compromised patients is a highly desirable goal. In practice, however, routine use of granulocyte transfusions has not been more efficacious than optimal antibacterial therapy, and significant side effects have been associated with granulocyte transfusions. Granulocyte and granulocyte-macrophage colony-stimulating factors (G-CSF and GM-CSF) accelerate recovery of leukocytes in neutropenic patients and are reported to reduce parenteral antibiotic usage when given prophylactically. These recombinant moieties may induce fever, however, and their therapeutic use has not been shown to benefit the outcome of documented bacterial infection or significantly prolong survival. Use of therapeutic antisera or immunoglobulins has been supported by some studies of documented infection, but indications for their use in the setting of fever alone are unclear. The role of monoclonal antibodies either for treatment or for prevention of bacterial infection in compromised hosts is unproven.

Prevention of Fever and Infection

Clearly, measures for the treatment of opportunistic infection in the compromised host represent an attempt to deal with life-threatening emergencies, but from a cost-effectiveness point of view, the prevention of fever and infection would decrease the need for costly systemic antibiotics as well as decrease patient morbidity. Microorganisms are part of humans' native milieu, and to eliminate potential infecting pathogens entirely would be neither realistic and nor feasible. On the other hand, a number of epidemiologic studies have determined that the gastrointestinal tract is often the site of colonization by potential disease-causing microorganisms, particularly *P. aeruginosa, Klebsiella* species, and *Proteus, Serratia,* and gram-negative organisms that are not normally found in the stool of healthy individuals. Measures to decrease gastrointestinal tract carriage via the monitoring of food products given to patients, restriction of diets to cooked food products, and use of prophylactic antibiotics have gained favor, but prophylactic antibiotic approaches have significant side effects.

The advent of the quinolones may provide both local and systemic prophylaxis against the majority of gram-negative and many of the important gram-positive opportunistic bacterial pathogens. More extensive use of prophylactic agents to "decontaminate" the gastrointestinal tract with nonabsorbable antibiotics has not met with uniform success. Anticandidal prophylaxis may be accomplished with agents such as clotrimazole (topically) or fluconazole (systemically). Acyclovir provides prophylaxis against viral opportunistic infections caused by herpesviruses. Agents such as trimethoprim-sulfamethoxazole prevent *P. carinii* pneumonia in patients with leukemia or impaired cell-mediated immunity. Attempts to minimize the environmental acquisition of potential pathogens have met with limited success. Nonetheless, meticulous infection control measures (hand washing, reverse isolation, avoidance of unnecessary procedures) appear to have some effect in reducing the opportunistic infection.

Immunoprophylaxis has clear-cut appeal, and use of killed or recombinant vaccines such as those directed against pneumococci or hepatitis B is justified. However, humoral antibody responses in immunosuppressed patients are often poor. An alternative approach is passive immunization with exogenous antibodies. Prophylactic use of immunoglobulins in hypogammaglobulinemic individuals can prevent fever and documented infection.

There is still some debate about suppressing fever. If an infectious organism is readily identified and patients are elderly and have extreme discomfort and tachycardia with possible cardiovascular complications, suppression of fever with salicylates or acetaminophen may minimize patients' symptoms. If the cause of the fever is unknown, however, it seems prudent to delay suppression of body temperature elevation because this physical finding may represent one of the earliest clues to an initial or ongoing infection.

BIBLIOGRAPHY

EORTC International Antimicrobial Therapy Cooperative Group: Ceftazidime combined with a short or long course of amikacin for empirical therapy of gram-negative bacteremia in cancer patients with granulocytopenia, *N Engl J Med* 317:1692, 1987.

Gastinne H et al: A controlled trial in intensive care units of selective decontamination of the digestive tract with nonabsorbable antibiotics, *N Engl J Med* 326:594-599, 1992.

Ginema Infection Program: Prevention of bacterial infection in neutropenic patients with hematologic malignancies: a randomized, multicenter trial comparing norfloxacin with ciprofloxacin, *Ann Intern Med* 115:7-12, 1991.

Infectious Diseases Society of America: Guidelines for the use of antimicrobial agents in neutropenic patients with unexplained fever, *J Infect Dis* 1997, in press.

Lieschke GJ, Burgess AW: Drug therapy: granulocyte colony-stimulating factor and granulocyte-macrophage colony-stimulating factor, *N Engl J Med* 327:28-35, 99-106, 1992.

Mackowiak PA, editor: *Fever: basic mechanisms and management,* New York, 1991, Raven.

Pizzo PA et al: Empiric antibiotic and antifungal therapy for cancer patients with prolonged fever or granulocytopenia, *Am J Med* 72:101-111, 1982.

Rubin RH, Young LS: *Clinical approach to infection in the compromised host,* ed 3, New York, 1994, Plenum.

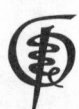

CHAPTER

237 Respiratory Tract Infections

Birgit Winther and Jack M. Gwaltney, Jr.

Acute respiratory tract infections are a major cause of morbidity in all age-groups. They are caused by a large variety of viruses and bacteria that, either alone or in combination, produce illness. The mechanisms by which viruses and bacteria interact to cause respiratory tract disease are poorly understood. The major pathogenic respiratory tract viruses include the rhinovirus, myxovirus, paramyxovirus, adenovirus, and coronavirus groups. Most viral infections follow a short, self-limited course.

Bacterial colonization is generally limited to the nostrils, nasopharynx, mouth, and throat, whereas clinical infection may occur both in colonized areas and in normally sterile areas such as the middle ear and paranasal sinuses. *Streptococcus pneumoniae, Haemophilus influenzae,* and group A β-hemolytic streptococci are the most common bacterial pathogens in upper respiratory tract infection. Other important, although less common, bacterial pathogens include *Moraxella catarrhalis, Staphylococcus aureus,* other streptococcal species, and anaerobic species, including *Fusobacterium* and *Bacteroides.*

THE COMMON COLD

Despite its mild and self-limited nature, the common cold is the leading cause of acute morbidity in the United States. As such, it is the most frequent reason for nonelective physician visits, as well as for industrial and school absenteeism. The most important common cold viruses are the rhinoviruses (Chapter 250) and coronaviruses (Chapter 251), although other respiratory tract viruses may also cause the syndrome (Table 237-1). The cause of approximately one third of colds in adults remains unknown: presumably, they are caused by undiscovered viruses.

One reason colds occur frequently is because of the large number of pathogenic viruses. Currently 100 antigenically different types of rhinovirus produce specific immunity. In some studies more than three fourths of persons with coronavirus colds had neutralizing antibody, indicating a previous infection.

Epidemiology

Observation of families in the home has provided important information on the frequency and epidemiology of colds. Overall, children have an average of six to eight colds per year; however, young chil-

Table 237-1 Viruses associated with the common cold

VIRUS GROUP	PERCENTAGE OF CASES
Rhinovirus	30-35
Coronavirus	≥10
Parainfluenza virus	
Respiratory syncytial virus	10-15
Influenza virus	
Adenovirus	
Other known viruses	5
Presumed undiscovered viruses	30-35

dren in nursery school can have up to 10 to 12 colds per year. Adults have an average of only two to three per year. Boys have a slightly higher incidence of colds through adolescence. Most frequently, school children introduce respiratory tract viruses into the home. After a cold is introduced, the spread among family members depends on both the age of the person with the index case and the age and immune status of the exposed person. Adults without children in the home have fewer colds than do persons with this exposure.

Different respiratory tract viruses tend to predominate during specific times of the year (Table 237-2). Rhinovirus colds are most common in the early fall and late spring; parainfluenza virus infections peak in late fall; and coronavirus colds are most often seen in midwinter. Other viruses, such as influenza and respiratory syncytial virus, usually produce a distinct annual outbreak, which generally occurs during the winter or early spring.

The mechanism(s) for the spread of respiratory tract viruses has not been well established. Transmission may occur by large or small aerosol spread or by direct contact with infectious secretions on skin and environmental surfaces. Rhinovirus is produced primarily in the nose and nasopharynx and is shed in highest concentration in nasal secretions (Chapter 250). Peak viral titers in nasal mucus usually occur on the third day of experimental infection and coincide with the period of maximum symptoms. Many persons with natural or experimental rhinovirus colds have recoverable virus on the hands. From there, virus can be transmitted experimentally to the hands of other susceptible persons, in whom colds can be initiated by self-inoculation of the nasal or conjunctival mucosa. These findings suggest that direct contact may be an important mode of rhinovirus transmission. Other respiratory viruses, such as rubeola and coxsackievirus A21, are believed to spread by droplet nuclei as true airborne infections. Influenza and adenovirus are also thought to be transmitted by the airborne route in some cases. More experimental studies are required to establish with certainty the natural mechanism of transmission of each of the common respiratory viruses.

Pathogenesis

The pathogenesis of rhinovirus colds has become better understood in recent years, but much remains to be learned. Indeed, little research has focused on the pathogenesis of other cold viruses. Viral deposition into the nose is the first step in rhinovirus pathogenesis. Virus may reach the nose directly or by way of the eye and lacrimal duct. A very small amount of virus is sufficient to initiate infection. After deposition into the nose, virus is carried posteriorly by the mucociliary escalator to the adenoid, where M cells and nonciliated cells with high expression of the ICAM-1 rhinovirus receptor may transport rhinovirus to immunocompetent cells. Viral cytopathic effect on the nasal epithelium is minimal in rhinovirus infection but is believed to be important as the stimulus for triggering various inflammatory events in the airway. These inflammatory reactions, which are associated with both soluble mediators and neurogenic reflexes, result in vasodilation, vascular transudation, mucous gland secretion, pain, cough, and sneezing. Symptoms begin approximately 16 hours after viral inoculation. Over the second and third days of infection the virus ap-

pears to spread anteriorly from the nasopharynx to ciliated epithelial cells in the nasal passages. The amount of viral excretion from the nose is reduced after several days, but viral shedding persists on average for 3 weeks and then ceases. Inflammatory mechanisms activated in rhinovirus colds include α-adrenergic and parasympathetic nervous pathways, as well as interleukin-1, 6, and 8, prostaglandin, and kinin systems.

Clinical Features

The incubation period of rhinovirus colds is generally 16 to 20 hours. The most prominent symptoms include nasal discharge, nasal congestion, sore throat, sneezing, and cough. Malaise and myalgias may be present, but constitutional symptoms are not prominent in rhinovirus and coronavirus infections. A temperature elevation of more than a degree is distinctly uncommon in adults; infants and young children may have more marked febrile responses. The nasal and pharyngeal symptoms reach their peak on the second and third days of illness and rapidly decline thereafter. Cough and laryngeal symptoms, when present, subside more slowly. One fourth of rhinovirus colds last longer than 1 week.

The clinical manifestations of the common cold are so typical that the diagnosis is usually made by the patient. The only conditions that frequently mimic these symptoms are allergic and vasomotor rhinitis, which may be recognized by their recurrent or chronic clinical history. Findings on physical examination may be minimal, despite the patient's subjective discomfort, but the patient may look congested, with oral respiration, and may have the characteristic nasal voice (rhinolalia clausa). Anterior rhinoscopy may show secretions in the nasal cavity, but the mucous membrane often appears normal. Mild pharyngeal and tonsillar injection without exudate are considered typical but may not be prominent. Pulmonary abnormalities are limited to rhonchi without rales or other evidence of pulmonary alveolar consolidation. No clinical features have been found that distinguish between infections caused by different rhinovirus types or between rhinovirus colds and those caused by other viruses. Diagnosis of the specific viral causative agent is usually not possible on the basis of clinical findings. In certain epidemiologic settings some acute respiratory infections such as influenza and pharyngoconjunctival fever can be recognized without viral culture or serologic tests. Knowledge of the characteristic seasonal patterns for the different viruses may aid in the identification of a particular infection (Table 237-2).

Diagnosis

The main challenge to the physician is to distinguish the uncomplicated cold from the 10% of cases of streptococcal pharyngitis and the estimated 5% to 10% of cases of secondary acute bacterial sinusitis or otitis media. Streptococcal antigen detection tests and throat cultures are useful for diagnosing streptococcal pharyngitis, but recognizing bacterial infection of the sinus and ear is difficult because of the lack of simple, noninvasive diagnostic tests for these complications.

Table 237-2   Seasonal incidence of colds caused by different respiratory viruses

MONTH	RHINOVIRUS	CORONAVIRUS	RESPIRATORY SYNCYTIAL VIRUS	PARAINFLUENZA VIRUS	ADENOVIRUS	INFLUENZA VIRUS
September	++++			+	++	
October	++			++	+	
November	+	++	+	++	+	+
December	+	+++	++	+	++	+++
January	+	+++	+++	+	++	+++
February	+	+++	+++	+	++	+++
March	++	+	++	+	++	+++
April	+++			+	+	++
May	++			+	+	
June	++				++	
July	++				++	
August	+++				++	

Relative frequency: ++++, most common; +, least common.

Table 237-3　Microbial causes of acute pharyngitis

TYPE OF MICROORGANISM	SYNDROME OR DISEASE	ESTIMATED INCIDENCE (%)
Viral		
Rhinovirus	Common cold	20
Coronavirus	Common cold	5
Adenovirus	Pharyngoconjunctival fever	5
Herpes simplex virus	Gingivitis, stomatitis, pharyngitis	4
Parainfluenza virus	Common cold, croup	2
Influenza virus	Influenza	2
Coxsackievirus A	Herpangina	<1
Epstein-Barr virus	Infectious mononucleosis	<1
Cytomegalovirus	Infectious mononucleosis	<1
Human immunodeficiency virus (HIV)	Primary HIV infection	<1
Bacterial		
Streptococcus pyogenes	Pharyngitis, tonsillitis	15-30
Mixed anaerobic infection	Gingivitis, stomatitis (Vincent's angina), peritonsillitis, peritonsillar abscess (quinsy)	<1
Neisseria gonorrhoeae	Pharyngitis	<1
Corynebacterium diphtheriae	Diphtheria	<1
Mycoplasmal		
Mycoplasma pneumoniae	Pneumonia, bronchitis, pharyngitis	<1
Unknown		40

The pharynx, nasal cavity, ears, and sinuses should be thoroughly examined. Pharyngeal or tonsillar exudate should raise suspicion of streptococcal or adenovirus infection, mononucleosis, Vincent's angina, or diphtheria. A vesicular eruption on the soft palate is characteristic of herpes simplex and coxsackievirus A infection. Radiologic examination of the maxillary and frontal sinuses is a valuable procedure in the diagnosis of acute sinusitis; however, a "fresh common cold" can also produce abnormalities in the paranasal sinus as early as days 3 to 5 after the onset of symptoms. Examination of the ears is directed at pathologic features of the tympanic membrane during acute otitis media. Pneumatic otoscopy is helpful in differentiating chronic middle ear effusion (secretory otitis media) from acute otitis.

Most respiratory viruses can be grown in cell culture, but this is currently not possible in most laboratories. Rapid techniques of viral identification using nucleic acid probes, fluorescent antibody, and other immunodiagnostic procedures on respiratory tract secretions are being developed and will be useful if antiviral chemotherapy becomes available. The serologic diagnosis of influenza, parainfluenza, respiratory syncytial virus, and adenovirus infection may be made retrospectively with paired sera obtained in the acute phase of illness and approximately 3 weeks later. A fourfold or greater rise in antibody titer is indicative of infection. Serologic diagnosis of rhinovirus infection is not practical because of the numerous antigenic types.

Treatment

Treatment of patients with an uncomplicated common cold is symptomatic. Rest during the initial day or so of illness is advisable, not only for the comfort of the patient, but also to reduce the exposure of others during the period of maximum virus shedding. Regular hand washing and care to avoid contamination of the environment with nasal secretions may help to prevent spread. The topical intranasal administration of interferon α-2b made by the recombinant technique is effective when given prophylactically in experimental rhinovirus colds. In addition, contract prophylaxis with interferon α-2b prevented natural rhinovirus colds in the family setting. Antiviral chemotherapy with a low dose of topical interferon α-2b and symptomatic therapy with two antimediators (oral naproxen and topical ipratropium) has been shown in a blind, placebo-controlled study to significantly diminish the overall morbidity of the cold (total symptom score, rhinorrhea, cough, and malaise). The optimal concentration of interferon and other antimediators are currently being tested. Nonsedating antihistamines have been shown to provide minimum benefit in the symptomatic management of sneezing and rhinorrhea. Antibiotics have no place in the treatment of uncomplicated colds. Evalua-

tion of published studies suggests that vitamin C is not effective in either prophylaxis or treatment of colds. Attempts to develop vaccines have been thwarted by the great number of causative viruses.

ACUTE PHARYNGITIS

A variety of respiratory viruses and a number of bacteria cause acute pharyngitis. The majority of cases are of viral origin and are self-limited in their clinical course. Accurate diagnosis of these infections is important for two reasons: first, to recognize infections that are amenable to treatment, specifically group A β-hemolytic streptococcal infection and its major postinfectious complication; and second, to detect the causes of pharyngitis that may be associated with serious systemic illness, such as infectious mononucleosis and diphtheria.

Etiologic Factors

The results of epidemiologic investigations are influenced by the season, the age of the population, the severity of the illness, and the diagnostic methods employed. In most studies common cold viruses cause about 25% of all cases of pharyngitis, and other recognized respiratory viruses account for an additional 10% to 15% (Table 237-3). Pharyngitis caused by rhinovirus and coronavirus infections is generally mild, whereas pharyngitis produced by adenoviruses and herpes simplex virus may be severe.

Streptococcus pyogenes (group A β-hemolytic streptococci) is the leading bacterial pathogen, accounting for 15% to 30% of all cases of acute pharyngitis (Chapter 261). The importance of non–group A β-hemolytic streptococci as a cause of pharyngitis remains uncertain. Infection with these strains does not carry the risk of acute rheumatic fever or poststreptococcal glomerulonephritis. Other causes of bacterial pharyngitis include mixed anaerobic infection (Vincent's angina), *Corynebacterium diphtheriae*, *Mycoplasma pneumoniae*, and *Neisseria gonorrhoeae*. The role of *Chlamydia pneumoniae* as a cause of pharyngitis is not defined but has been suggested in some studies.

Clinical Features of the Various Types

The common cold frequently produces mild or moderate pharyngeal discomfort. Additional respiratory symptoms, especially nasal complaints and coughs, usually accompany the sore throat. Posterior pharyngeal erythema and edema, if present, are mild. Pharyngeal and tonsillar exudate and painful regional adenopathy are not present. Temperature elevation is not usually seen in adults and adolescents.

Influenza virus infection may produce moderate to severe pharyngeal discomfort in addition to systemic complaints of myalgia, headache, and cough. Fever is common in adults as well as children and may reach 38.5° C (101.3° F) or higher. Pharyngeal exudate and painful adenopathy are not present. Defervescence occurs in 3 to 4 days, but fever may last for more than a week.

Adenovirus generally produces more severe pharyngeal and systemic symptoms than do the common cold viruses. In addition to the prominent sore throat accompanied by malaise, myalgia, headache, dizziness, and chills, conjunctivitis occurs in up to half of the patients. Such cases of so-called pharyngoconjunctival fever may occur as summertime water-borne epidemics, as well as during the respiratory tract disease season. Tonsillar or pharyngeal exudate may be present. The average duration of fever and symptoms is 5 to 7 days.

Mild cases of herpes simplex pharyngitis cannot be distinguished from other viral causes of pharyngitis (Chapter 255). Severe disease is marked by a prominent ulcerative and exudative pharyngitis. Coxsackievirus pharyngitis, also known as herpangina, may be recognized by a relatively sparse vesicular eruption on the soft palate, uvula, and anterior tonsillar pillars, primarily in children with prominent fever and dysphagia (Chapter 250).

Infectious mononucleosis resulting from Epstein-Barr virus is associated with an exudative pharyngitis or tonsillitis in half the patients, in addition to the characteristic systemic symptoms and signs of persistent anorexia, malaise, fatigue, generalized adenopathy, and splenomegaly (Chapter 255). The mononucleosis syndrome is also associated with cytomegalovirus infection, but exudative pharyngitis is typically absent.

Acute streptococcal pharyngitis varies greatly in severity. It may be mild and indistinguishable from the pharyngitis associated with the common cold. In contrast, the severe disease is characterized by marked pharyngeal pain, dysphagia, fever, and the physical findings of exudative posterior pharyngitis and tonsillitis with tender cervical lymphadenitis. Strains of *S. pyogenes* that produce erythrogenic toxin also cause the characteristic rash of scarlet fever.

Another bacterial pharyngitis that may have distinguishing clinical features is Vincent's angina, which is caused by mixed anaerobes and spirochetes. It produces necrotic tonsillar ulceration with a gray membrane and foul breath. Peritonsillar abscess (quinsy) is also a mixed anaerobic infection that occurs most commonly in young adults. Pharyngeal discomfort is severe, with associated dysphagia. The characteristic physical findings include peritonsillar swelling with medial displacement of the tonsil on the involved side. Bilateral involvement may occur.

In unimmunized persons, diphtheritic pharyngitis continues to occur (Chapter 263). The onset of symptoms tends to be insidious, and pharyngeal discomfort is mild. The characteristic tonsillar membrane is gray and firmly adherent to the mucosa.

Diagnosis

Diagnosis of streptococcal pharyngitis by the clinical features of the illness, even with the aid of explicit scales and prediction rules, is often difficult. The diagnosis can be made in cases with pharyngeal exudate, fever, and tender adenopathy, although a similar presentation may occur with adenoviral and herpetic pharyngitis. In cases without exudate it is difficult to distinguish streptococcal pharyngitis from that caused by common cold viruses and influenza. Therefore laboratory confirmation of the diagnosis is often necessary. Rapid diagnosis by streptococcal antigen detection is highly specific but only moderately sensitive compared with throat culture. Specimens with only sparse growth on culture are likely to have a false-negative antigen detection test result. In a substantial proportion of patients with false-negative antigen detection test results, serologic responses to group A streptococci develop, indicating an invasive infection. For this reason, throat culture should be performed in patients with pharyngitis who have negative streptococcal antigen test results.

A crystal violet–stained smear of pharyngeal exudate demonstrates the presence of numerous *Fusobacterium* organisms and spirochetes in Vincent's angina. Throat culture on Löffler's medium should be obtained in all suspected cases of diphtheria. Cultures and serologic tests for influenza viruses, adenovirus, herpes simplex virus, cytomeg-

alovirus, and *M. pneumoniae* are available in some large laboratories.

Treatment

Although streptococcal pharyngitis is ordinarily self-limited, antibiotic therapy has been shown to shorten the duration of clinical illnesses. Antimicrobial therapy prevents suppurative complications and reduces the risk of subsequent development of acute rheumatic fever. Because initiation of antimicrobial therapy within a week of the onset of streptococcal pharyngitis prevents the subsequent development of acute rheumatic fever, therapy may be withheld until the result of the throat culture is known. For patients who are not allergic to penicillin, oral therapy should include penicillin V, 250,000 units every 6 to 8 hours in adults, and 200,000 units for children <5 years old and 400,000 units for children >5 years old, divided into two doses each day for 10 days. A single dose of long-acting benzathine penicillin (1.2 million units intramuscularly in adults) is also effective. Penicillin-allergic patients should be given treatment with a 10-day course of erythromycin.

Oral penicillin in the preceding dosages is the treatment of choice for peritonsillitis and Vincent's angina. Peritonsillar abscess also generally requires surgical drainage. The treatment of viral pharyngitis remains symptomatic, but amantadine is beneficial when given early in the course of illness in patients with presumed influenzal pharyngitis occurring during known influenza A epidemics. Chronic oropharyngeal herpetic infection in an immunosuppressed patient should be treated with acyclovir, but acyclovir is not recommended in otherwise healthy persons with acute herpetic pharyngitis.

The standard supportive measures of bed rest, saline gargles, minor analgesics, and adequate hydration are sufficient in most cases of viral and streptococcal pharyngitis.

Active immunization is available for types A and B influenza and diphtheria. Attenuated adenovirus vaccines have been successful in certain high-risk populations such as military recruits but are not available for general use.

ACUTE LARYNGITIS, CROUP, AND EPIGLOTTITIS

Acute laryngitis usually occurs as part of more generalized upper respiratory tract illnesses. Hoarseness may be a major complaint during infection with any of the respiratory tract viruses. It is not known whether secondary bacterial infection plays a role in cases of acute laryngitis. *M. catarrhalis* has been isolated from the nasopharynx of a majority of a group of adults with acute laryngitis. The significance of this finding remains to be determined. The diagnosis of acute laryngitis is usually evident from the clinical history and is confirmed when mirror examination of the larynx reveals hyperemia and edema. There is no evidence that antimicrobial agents are of value in the treatment of acute laryngitis. Supportive care includes humidification of inhaled air and resting the voice.

Croup is a clinical syndrome in children that is characterized by inspiratory stridor and a barking cough. Viral laryngotracheobronchitis is most commonly responsible, and parainfluenza viruses are the most frequently identified pathogens. The diagnosis depends on recognition of the clinical syndrome and exclusion of acute bacterial epiglottitis or the presence of a laryngeal foreign body.

Acute epiglottitis caused by group B *H. influenzae* is primarily a disease of childhood and may be mistaken for croup or laryngitis. Clinical differentiation is not always possible, although in acute epiglottitis the patient appears toxic and the clinical course is more rapidly progressive (Chapter 266). Visualization of the inflamed epiglottis with either a tongue blade or a laryngoscope must be undertaken with extreme care to avoid precipitating acute airway obstruction. Blood cultures are frequently positive for *H. influenzae*. Hospitalization, nasotracheal intubation, and intravenous chloramphenicol (50 to 75 mg/kg per day in four divided doses) has been the standard treatment. Intravenous cefuroxime (100 to 200 mg/kg per day in three divided doses) or a third-generation cephalosporin such as cefotaxime (100 to 150 mg/kg per day in four doses) is also an acceptable treatment for acute epiglottitis. The incidence of acute

Table 237-4   Causative organisms in acute maxillary sinusitis and acute otitis media

ORGANISM	ACUTE MAXILLARY SINUSITIS (%)	ACUTE OTITIS MEDIA (%)
Streptococcus pneumoniae	30	50-60
Haemophilus influenzae	25	20
Anaerobic bacteria	6	
Staphylococcus aureus	4	2
Streptococcus pyogenes	2	5-10
Moraxella catarrhalis	2	5-10
Gram-negative bacteria	9	10

epiglottitis has declined markedly since the use of the *H. influenzae* vaccine.

ACUTE SINUSITIS

The majority of cases of acute sinusitis occur as a complication of viral upper respiratory tract infection. A smaller proportion of cases are associated with dental infection, allergic rhinitis, or nasal anatomic abnormalities. An important new concept in understanding the pathogenesis of sinusitis is the recognition of the importance of the osteomeatal area of the nasal cavity. Obstruction of this narrow passageway—into which drain the frontal, maxillary, and ethmoid sinuses—is recognized as a major risk factor for inflammatory sinus disease. The sinuses normally remain sterile as a result of continuous mucociliary clearance of particulate matter entering the sinus cavity. Colds, influenza, and other acute respiratory tract infections cause inflammation in the nasal passages, which leads to narrowing or obstruction of the osteomeatal area in up to 80% of patients as judged by computed tomography (CT) imaging studies. In addition, respiratory tract viruses have been recovered from sinus aspirates of patients with acute sinusitis and may infect the ciliated epithelial cells lining the sinus cavities. Both of these processes could disrupt the normal cleansing mechanism and increase the susceptibility of the sinus to secondary bacterial invasion. The resulting exudative effusion usually contains more than 5000 polymorphonuclear leukocytes/ml^3, with bacterial titers usually exceeding 10^5 colony-forming units (CFU)/ml. The maxillary sinus may also be infected by direct extension of dental root abscesses of the upper molars.

Etiologic Factors

The infectious agents responsible for acute maxillary sinusitis in adults have been identified by direct sinus puncture and culture of the aspirated fluid (Table 237-4). This approach avoids contamination of the culture specimen by nasopharyngeal flora. *S. pneumoniae* and unencapsulated strains of *H. influenzae* account for approximately half the cases; smaller numbers of cases are due to *S. aureus, S. pyogenes, M. catarrhalis,* and gram-negative bacteria. Mixed anaerobic infection is usually associated with contiguous dental disease. Respiratory tract viruses, including rhinovirus, influenza virus, and parainfluenza virus, have been recovered alone or in combination with bacteria in about 20% of patients. A small proportion of cases of sinus disease result from fungal infections, particularly aspergillosis, phaeohyphomycosis, zygomycosis (mucormycosis), pseudallescheriasis, and hyalohyphomycosis (penicillosis). Presumably the causes of infections of the frontal, ethmoid, and sphenoid sinuses are similar to those of the maxillary antra.

Diagnosis

The clinical features of acute sinusitis may be difficult to distinguish from those of a prolonged cold. Uncomplicated colds last, on average, about a week; thus illnesses lasting longer probably have sinus involvement. Facial discomfort, purulent nasal discharge or postnasal discharge, and tonal changes in the voice are common features of sinusitis, and these symptoms may be accompanied by moderate headache. The findings on physical examination are variable. Tempera-

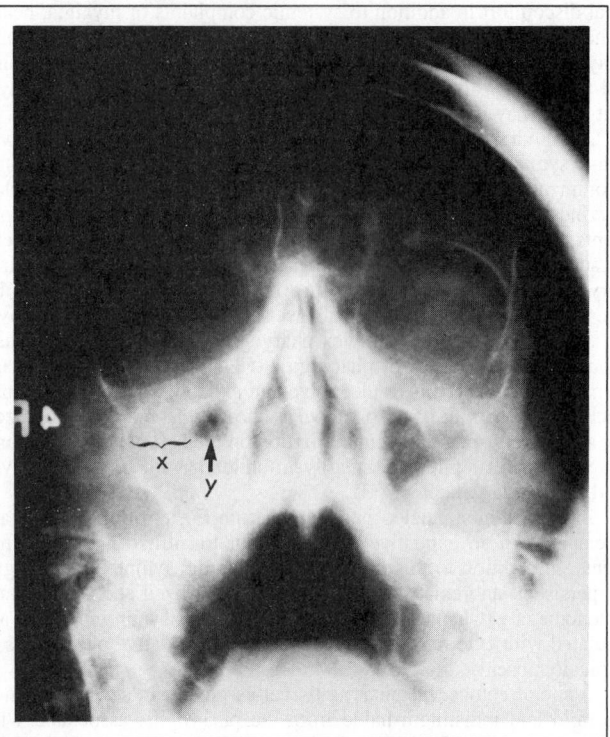

FIGURE 237-1   Waters' projection x-ray of a patient with acute maxillary sinusitis. The right-side maxillary sinus shows evidence of significant mucosal thickening *(x)* and an abnormal air-fluid level *(y)*.

ture elevation occurs in less than half of adults with acute maxillary sinusitis documented by sinus aspiration. Erythema, swelling, and tenderness may be found over the involved sinus but are not present in most patients, and their absence does not exclude the diagnosis. Periorbital edema and increased lacrimation are characteristic findings in ethmoid sinusitis.

Transillumination of the maxillary and frontal sinuses is useful in a patient with previously normal sinuses. The procedure should be undertaken in a completely darkened room using a sinus transilluminator. For examination of the maxillary sinuses the tip of the instrument is placed on the infraorbital ridge and is directed downward toward the hard palate. The finding of complete opacity is strong evidence for the presence of active infection. The presence of "dullness" (diminished but not complete absence of light transmission) is also suggestive of infection. The finding of normal transillumination is good evidence that no infection is present. Transillumination is less helpful in patients with chronic sinusitis, in whom reduced light transmission may be a persistent finding. Normal variations in bone thickness may cause different intensity of transillumination among different individuals.

X-ray examination of the sinuses has traditionally been used for diagnosis. The finding of complete opacification, an abnormal air-fluid level, or mucosal thickening is strong evidence for the presence of active infection (Fig. 237-1). It is now recognized that, although standard radiographs are satisfactory for detecting disease of the frontal, antral, and sphenoid sinuses, they are insensitive for diagnosing ethmoid sinusitis. For this reason, limited CT examination of the sinuses is now being offered by some radiology departments at costs comparable to those of a standard sinus x-ray series. CT examination also allows evaluation of the osteomeatal complex for evidence of narrowing and anatomic obstruction. In patients with chronic sinusitis the presence of persistent radiographic abnormalities limits the usefulness of imaging techniques in the diagnosis of active infection.

Culture of nasal secretions or sinus washings obtained through the natural ostium are not useful for diagnosis because of contamination with the resident nasopharyngeal flora. Specimens for culture that are

Table 237-5   Antimicrobials for treating acute community-acquired sinusitis

ANTIMICROBIAL	ADULT DOSE
Trimethoprim-sulfamethoxazole, double strength	160 mg/800 mg bid
Cefuroxime axetil	250 mg bid
Amoxicillin/clavulanate	500/125 mg tid
Loracarbef	400 mg bid

bid, Twice daily; *tid,* three times a day.

collected from the mouth of the sinus ostium under direct vision by endoscopy have not been compared with those obtained by sinus puncture and cannot be considered free from extraneous microbial contamination. Direct sinus puncture is the accepted way to collect specimens for culture but is not practical in the usual case of sinusitis. Sinus puncture is generally reserved for patients with unusually severe infection, those not responding to therapy, or those in whom intracranial spread of infection is suspected. Because routine bacteriologic diagnosis is not possible, it is necessary to base antimicrobial treatment on the known causes of sinusitis (Table 237-4).

Treatment

Treatment of acute community-acquired sinusitis is a course of antimicrobial therapy that covers the major known causes of infection. The ampicillins recommended previously are no longer considered adequate because of the increasing importance of β-lactamase–producing strains of *H. influenzae* and *M. catarrhalis.* Studies of sinus puncture before and after treatment have shown several antimicrobials to be effective for treating the usual bacterial causes of acute sinusitis, including the β-lactamase–producing strains (Table 237-5). In selecting from among these agents, cost and the potential for side effects are the major considerations, since all appear equally effective, with bacteriologic cure rates of greater than 90%. A 10-day course of treatment is recommended in the usual case. Supportive therapy generally includes nasal decongestants and analgesics if required.

Management of therapeutic failures can be difficult. If the response to the initial course of treatment is not satisfactory, a sinus puncture is recommended to provide a specimen for bacterial culture and antimicrobial sensitivity testing, and to obtain the therapeutic benefits of sinus lavage. An additional, more prolonged course of antimicrobial treatment based on culture results, if available, is then recommended. Topical corticosteroids are also used in the hope of reducing swelling and promoting sinus drainage, although their effectiveness is unproven. If the condition still does not clear, allergy and immunology evaluations may be helpful. Most important, CT imaging of the osteomeatal complex and sinuses should be performed to determine whether there are anatomic abnormalities that require surgical correction.

Repetitive bacterial infections, particularly when untreated or inadequately treated, may produce irreversible changes in the sinus mucosa. In chronic sinus disease squamous cells may replace the normal ciliated epithelium, and sinus sterility cannot be maintained by the normal clearance mechanisms. Although the sinus becomes colonized with bacteria, antimicrobial therapy is usually not helpful for controlling the symptoms of chronic sinus disease. Exacerbations of acute infection can occur, however, and should be treated in the same way as an acute infection in persons with normal sinuses. Surgical correction of obstructive lesions is most important in the treatment of chronic sinus disease.

OTITIS MEDIA

Acute otitis media is an inflammation of the middle ear mucosa and may be classified as suppurative or nonsuppurative based on the characteristics of the fluid present in the middle ear. The most important predisposing factor in the development of this disease is an acute infection, usually viral, involving the eustachian tube in the posterior nasopharynx. Eustachian tube dysfunction and abnormal middle ear pressures have recently been observed in young adults with experi-

mental rhinovirus infection. If local host defense mechanisms are inadequate, microbial proliferation results in infection.

Etiologic Factors

Several viruses have been isolated from middle ear fluid, either alone or in combination with bacteria. These include rhinovirus, adenovirus, respiratory syncytial virus, parainfluenza virus, and coxsackievirus. Bacterial pathogens identified by diagnostic tympanocentesis include many common inhabitants of the nasopharynx. *S. pneumoniae* is the most important, accounting for more than half of the cases. Next in importance are *H. influenzae, M. catarrhalis,* and *S. pyogenes* (Table 237-4). Nose and throat cultures obtained at the time of tympanocentesis have yielded a variety of potential pathogens but are not useful in determining the bacterial cause of acute otitis media. In infants younger than 6 weeks of age, a considerable fraction of cases are due to coliform organisms and *S. aureus,* in addition to the more common pathogens such as *S. pneumoniae* and *H. influenzae.*

Clinical Features and Diagnosis

Acute otitis media is often preceded by an upper respiratory tract illness. In the typical history an earache develops in a patient with a cold that has been improving. Fever is often present, and hearing is slightly impaired. The diagnosis of acute otitis media is based on otoscopic examination of the tympanic membrane that typically in the early phase shows a bright-red bulging of the posterosuperior part of the drum. Later, the redness extends to most of the tympanic membrane and the landmarks disappear. Within hours to days a spontaneous perforation may occur with normalization of the temperature and relief of pain. The characteristics of the fluid in the middle ear vary from clear to mucopurulent, and it may be blood tinged at the time of perforation. Closure of the perforation usually occurs within hours, and normalization of the hearing usually occurs within 1 to 2 weeks. Small children younger than 1 year of age may have more prolonged illness. Tympanocentesis is required for an etiologic diagnosis but is not routinely performed in clinical practice. Its use is generally limited to neonates, older children, or adults with complications that require identification of the pathogen to guide antimicrobial therapy.

Treatment

Antimicrobial therapy in the uncomplicated case of acute otitis media should be directed against *S. pneumoniae, H. influenzae,* and *M. catarrhalis.* Augmentin, cefuroxime axetil, and trimethoprim-sulfamethoxazole provide such coverage, or other agents may be chosen on the basis of examination of the middle ear fluid. Myringotomy may be beneficial in patients with severe earache caused by a bulging tympanic membrane. The usefulness of therapy for symptoms, including oral antihistamines and decongestants, is controversial.

Complications following acute otitis media are rare but include acute mastoiditis, labyrinthitis, and meningitis. Chronic middle ear effusion (secretory otitis media) may persist for several months and may be caused by eustachian tube dysfunction, probably resulting from recurrent viral infections. Chronic effusions may produce a degree of conductive hearing loss that requires treatment by the placement of pneumatic equalization tubes. However, surgery should be withheld for 3 or more months to permit the highest rate of spontaneous resolution.

Prophylactic antibiotics have been shown to be of value in the prevention of recurrent infections in selected patients. Corticosteroid treatment in addition to antibiotics has not been beneficial.

In children with recurrent acute otitis media and chronic middle ear effusion (secretory otitis media) locally produced secretory immunoglobulin A antibody is usually present in the nasopharynx. However, patients who have repeated bacterial infections of the middle ears or sinuses, or both, should be evaluated for immunoglobulin deficiency.

BIBLIOGRAPHY

de Arruda E et al: Localization of rhinovirus replication in vitro with in situ hybridization, *J Med Virol* 34:38, 1991.

Gwaltney JM Jr: Viral vaccines in the control of otitis media: Workshop on Vaccines for Otitis Media, Children's Hospital of Pittsburgh, *Pediatr Infect Dis J* 8:578, 1989.

Gwaltney JM Jr: Combined antiviral and antimediator treatment of rhinovirus colds, *J Infect Dis* 166:776-782, 1991.

Gwaltney JM Jr: Computed tomographic study of the common cold, *N Eng J Med* 330:25-30, 1994.

Gwaltney JM Jr et al: The microbial etiology and antimicrobial therapy of adults with acute community acquired sinusitis: a 15-year experience at the University of Virginia and review of other selected studies, *J Allergy Clin Immunol* 90:457, 1992.

Hayden FG et al: Prevention of natural colds by contact prophylaxis with intranasal alpha 2-interferon, *N Engl J Med* 312:71, 1986.

McBride TP et al: Alterations of eustachian tube, middle ear and nose in rhinovirus infection, *Arch Otolaryngol Head Neck Surg* 115:1054, 1989.

Naclerio RM et al: Kinins are generated during experimental rhinovirus colds, *J Infect Dis* 157:133, 1988.

Schlager TA et al: Optical immunoassay for rapid detection of group A β-hemolytic streptococci, *Arch Pediatr Adolesc Med* 150:245-248, 1996.

Sperber SJ et al: Effects of naproxen in experimental rhinovirus colds, *Ann Intern Med* 117:37, 1992.

Turner BW et al: Physiologic abnormalities in the paranasal sinuses during experimental rhinovirus colds, *J Allergy Clin Immunol* 90:474, 1992.

Winther B et al: Sites of rhinovirus recovery after point inoculation of the upper airway, *JAMA* 256:1763, 1986.

Winther B et al: Distribution of the human rhinovirus receptor, ICAM-1, on epithelia of the upper airways, (unpublished).

CHAPTER

238 Intraabdominal Infections

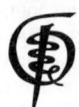

Matthew E. Levison

Intraabdominal infection attributable to bacteria and fungi may take several forms. Infection may be in the retroperitoneal space or within the peritoneal cavity. Intraperitoneal infection may be diffuse or localized in one or more abscesses. Intraperitoneal abscesses may form in dependent recesses, such as the pelvic space or pouch of Morison, in the various perihepatic spaces, within the lesser sac, and along the major routes of communication between intraperitoneal recesses, such as the right paracolic gutter. Abscesses also often form about diseased viscera—pericholecystic, periappendiceal, pericolic, and tuboovarian—and between adjacent loops of bowel (i.e., interloop abscesses). In addition, infection may be contained within the intraabdominal viscera, such as in hepatic, pancreatic, splenic, or renal abscesses.

Intraperitoneal infection has been divided into two categories: primary, in which an intraabdominal source is not clinically evident, and secondary, in which an intraabdominal source is evident. Secondary intraperitoneal infection is far more common than the primary variety. Tertiary peritonitis has been conceived recently as a later stage in the disease, when clinical peritonitis and systemic signs of sepsis (e.g., fever, tachycardia, tachypnea, hypotension, elevated cardiac index, low systemic vascular resistance, leukopenia or leukocytosis, and multiorgan failure) persist after treatment for secondary peritonitis and either no organisms or low-virulence pathogens, such as enterococci and fungi, are isolated from the peritoneal exudate.

PRIMARY INTRAPERITONEAL INFECTION
Pathogenesis

Primary peritonitis usually is seen in children with nephrosis or adults with cirrhosis. The presence of ascites appears to be the common feature among the various underlying conditions associated with primary peritonitis. The route of infection in primary peritonitis is presumed to be hematogenous, lymphogenous, or transmural migration through an intact gut wall from the intestinal lumen or the lumen of the fallopian tubes from the vagina. The hematogenous route is most likely in patients with cirrhosis, as the reticuloendothelial system of the liver is known to be normally a major site for removal and destruction of bacteria from blood. The transmural migration of bacteria is the probable route of infection in the majority of patients with anaerobic primary peritonitis.

A single species of bacteria is usually isolated. The organisms that most commonly cause primary peritonitis in children are *Streptococcus pneumoniae* and group A streptococci, followed in frequency by gram-negative enteric bacilli. In cirrhotic patients, enteric organisms, especially *Escherichia coli,* account for up to 69% of the pathogens, followed by streptococci (e.g., *S. pneumoniae* and group A streptococci) and anaerobes.

Other causes of primary peritonitis include *Neisseria gonorrhoeae, Chlamydia trachomatis,* and *Mycobacterium tuberculosis.* Gonococcal or chlamydial perihepatitis (Fitz-Hugh–Curtis syndrome) may develop in women, presumably from asymptomatic infection of the fallopian tubes that spreads from the pelvic space along the right paracolic gutter to the perihepatic space. Tuberculous peritonitis may result from the direct entry into the peritoneal cavity of tubercle bacilli from the lymph nodes, intestines, or genital tract or via hematogenous dissemination from remote foci.

Clinical Manifestations

Primary peritonitis occurs at all ages. In the preantibiotic era it accounted for about 10% of all pediatric abdominal emergencies but now is responsible for less than 1% to 2%. Primary peritonitis in children usually accompanies postnecrotic cirrhosis or the nephrotic syndrome. It may precede other manifestations of nephrosis, and repeated episodes may occur. Primary peritonitis may present as an acute febrile illness that is often confused with appendicitis. In adults, primary peritonitis occurs in about 10% of those presenting with cirrhosis and ascites. The onset may be insidious, and findings of peritoneal irritation may be absent in an abdomen distended with ascites. Indeed, ascitic fluid with a positive culture, but few leukocytes, has been noted in patients without clinical findings of peritonitis (so-called bacterascites) and may represent early infection of the peritoneum, before a host response. Primary peritonitis in cirrhotic patients is generally associated with other features of end-stage liver disease (hepatorenal syndrome, progressive encephalopathy, variceal bleeding).

Gonococcal or chlamydial perihepatitis most often occurs in women and simulates acute cholecystitis. It presents with the sudden onset of pain in the right upper quadrant of the abdomen; at times, the pain is referred to the right shoulder. There may be low-grade fever, right upper quadrant tenderness, guarding, and a friction rub over the liver. In patients with primary gonococcal or chlamydial peritonitis, the source would not be clinically evident, but in other patients the peritonitis may be secondary to clinically apparent uterine cervicitis and/or salpingitis.

Primary tuberculous peritonitis usually is gradual in onset, with fever, weight loss, malaise, night sweats, and abdominal distention. The abdomen may not be rigid and is often characterized as being "doughy" on palpation.

SECONDARY INTRAPERITONEAL INFECTION
Pathogenesis

Secondary intraperitoneal infection may occur as a result of any one of a variety of primary intraabdominal processes (Box 238-1). Most have in common contamination of the peritoneal cavity with organisms that normally reside on the mucosal surfaces of the gastrointestinal tract or vagina. The resultant infection is usually polymicrobial, and the composition reflects the predominantly anaerobic mucosal microflora at these sites.

The surface microflora of the digestive tract varies quantitatively and qualitatively from region to region along its length and is different again from that of the vagina. For example, the gingival crevice in the oral cavity has an enormous microflora, with over 100 different species in total numbers of 10^{11} to 10^{12} organisms/g. (By way of comparison, a colony of solid-packed bacteria on the surface of an agar plate has a density of 10^{12} organisms/g.) Obligate anaerobes outnumber the aerobes in the gingival crevice.

The stomach, because of its acidity, normally has a sparse flora (less than 10^3 organisms/ml), which consists of the more acid-tolerant species of mouth organisms such as lactobacilli and yeast. In the presence of achlorhydria or gastric obstruction, however, an abundant flora that is derived from the oral cavity or from contaminated food or water may be in the stomach.

BOX 238-1

Primary intraabdominal processes leading to peritonitis

Perforation of peptic ulcer
Traumatic perforation of uterus, urinary bladder, stomach, bowel
Spontaneous bowel perforation (typhoid, tuberculosis, amebic or *Strongyloides* ulcers)
Appendicitis, diverticulitis
Intestinal neoplasms
Gangrene of bowel (strangulation, obstruction, vascular insufficiency)
Suppurative cholecystitis
Bile peritonitis
Pancreatitis
Operative contamination or disruption of surgical anastomosis
Female genital abnormalities (e.g., septic abortion, puerperal sepsis, postoperative uterine infection, endometritis from intrauterine device, nongonococcal salpingitis)
Suppurative prostatitis
Rupture of any intraperitoneal abscesses
Chronic ambulatory peritoneal dialysis
Peritoneovenous and ventriculoperitoneal shunts

Similarly, few organisms normally inhabit the upper small bowel, but in the presence of slowing of small bowel motility (as occurs in scleroderma), small bowel obstruction (as may occur in Crohn's disease), blind loops, diverticula, and gastric achlorhydria or gastric obstruction, an abundant flora may be present in the small bowel. Patients with cirrhosis, intestinal pseudoobstruction, gastrocolic or jejunocolic fistula, immunoglobulin deficiencies, or malnutrition, and some elderly patients with malabsorption also may have more than normal numbers of bacteria in the small bowel.

Members of the large bowel flora may be found in the terminal ileum in counts of 10^6 to 10^7 organisms/ml, but only in the relatively stagnant large bowel is an enormous, predominantly anaerobic microflora normally present. The colonic microflora is similar in density (10^{11} to 10^{12} organisms/g) and complexity (over 200 different species) to that of the gingival crevice; however, the species differ at the two sites. For example, bile-sensitive, anaerobic gram-negative bacilli (e.g., *Prevotella melaninogenica*, *Prevotella intermedia*, and *Porphyromonas gingivalis*) are found in the oral microflora, whereas the bile-resistant species, members of the *Bacteroides* group, are the major constituents of the normal colonic microflora and are uncommon in the oral microflora. *Clostridium perfringens*, another important pathogen, is not normally isolated from the mouth, stomach, or small bowel but is usually found in the fecal flora. The predominant aerobes in colonic flora include *E. coli* and enterococci, which are usually not found in the oral microflora. The large bowel flora is relatively stable but may be altered by antibiotic therapy.

The vaginal microflora is much less dense (10^7 to 10^8 organisms/ml) and less complex than the oral or colonic flora. It consists predominantly of anaerobic lactobacilli and to a lesser extent of non-*fragilis* species of *Bacteroides*. As with the gingival crevice flora, the vaginal flora is normally characterized by the absence of *B. fragilis*, *E. coli*, and enterococci in large numbers. However, the vaginal microflora may resemble that of the colon in certain circumstances, such as soon after gynecologic surgery.

Not all members of the microflora are found in an established intraabdominal infection. The extremely oxygen-sensitive components of the anaerobic flora do not seem to be as pathogenic as the relatively aerotolerant anaerobes (e.g., *B. fragilis* and *P. melaninogenica*), which are encapsulated by a surface polysaccharide, their presumed virulence factor. These two species, together with *Fusobacterium nucleatum*, various anaerobic gram-positive cocci (including the microaerophilic *Streptococcus intermedius*), and *C. perfringens*, account for over 80% of anaerobic isolates. As part of the polymicrobial flora characteristic of established infection, the facultative anaerobic copathogens include *E. coli* and enterococci, especially when the intra-

abdominal infection is of colonic origin. Together with highly antibiotic-resistant strains of enteric gram-negative bacilli, *Pseudomonas aeruginosa* is more frequently isolated from patients who develop their intraabdominal infection while in the hospital, after having received broad-spectrum parenteral antimicrobials. However, recent studies have noted *P. aeruginosa* to compose a more significant portion of the aerobic isolates in community-acquired intraabdominal infection than had been noted previously. Anaerobic gram-positive cocci, *P. melaninogenica*, *Prevotella disiens*, and *Prevotella bivia*, are found more frequently than *B. fragilis*, *E. coli*, and enterococci in intraabdominal infections of gynecologic origin, as would be predicted from the composition of normal vaginal flora. These anaerobes may be found with or without *N. gonorrhoeae*. However, *B. fragilis* may be a more common pathogen when a tuboovarian abscess is present.

Peritonitis that occurs in patients receiving chronic ambulatory peritoneal dialysis is usually due to contamination of the catheter with skin microflora, since gram-positive organisms (most commonly *Staphylococcus epidermidis*, followed by *Staphylococcus aureus*, *Streptococcus* species, and diphtheroids) constitute 60% to 80% of isolates. Gram-negative organisms account for 15% to 30% of isolates, in which case, enteric bacteria presumably gained access to the peritoneal cavity by transmural migration through an intact intestinal wall after the introduction of dialysis solutions into the peritoneum.

Candida peritonitis has also been observed as a complication of peritoneal dialysis, gastrointestinal surgery, or perforation of a viscus, and its occurrence in the latter two instances is related to numerous factors that increase the rate of *Candida* colonization in the gastrointestinal tract. These include immunosuppression, prolonged hospitalization, and antimicrobial therapy.

Endogenous infections depend primarily on defects of local host defense mechanisms that otherwise limit the invasive activities of indigenous bacteria. Disruption of the mucosal surface would allow escape of indigenous bacteria. Once in tissues beneath the epithelium, pathogenic anaerobes require low oxidation-reduction potential, low oxygen concentration, and abundant nutrients to support optimum growth. These requirements are usually met by tissue devitalized by ischemia, trauma, neoplastic growth, or previous infection with facultative organisms. In this environment, anaerobic organisms can attain growth rates similar to those seen with aerobic enteric bacilli. The rapidly expanding bacterial and inflammatory cell mass, frequently accompanied by gas production, can then interrupt blood supply to the surrounding tissue and cause further tissue necrosis. The organisms themselves possess several virulence factors, such as polysaccharide capsules, endotoxin, and the production of proteolytic enzymes and heparinase, which promote additional tissue necrosis, local spread, and hematogenous dissemination.

Each component of the pathogenic mixture of organisms may contribute in different ways to produce the clinical picture. For example, after implantation of fecal contents in rats, *E. coli* is responsible for bacteremia and early mortality, whereas *B. fragilis* is responsible for late abscess formation.

Infectious material can be spread over much of the peritoneal cavity within a short time by gravity, movement of the diaphragm, and peristaltic movement of the gastrointestinal tract. The extent and rate of intraperitoneal spread of contamination depend on the volume and nature of the exudate, the course of the primary disease process, and the effectiveness of the localizing processes. If peritoneal defenses, aided by appropriate supportive measures, control the inflammatory process, the disease may end by resolution; abscesses may develop only about diseased organs, such as the appendix or gallbladder; or an abscess may be confined in the peritoneal space, usually in the pelvis, perihepatic spaces, or right paracolic gutter. When the peritoneal and systemic defense mechanisms cannot localize the inflammation, diffuse peritonitis results.

Clinical Manifestations

Peritonitis. Primary and secondary peritonitis may present clinically in an identical way, but on occasion the clinical presentation is masked either by the underlying disease in patients with primary peritonitis (e.g., hepatic encephalopathy in patients with ascites and end-stage cirrhosis) or by the primary disease process in patients with secondary peritonitis. Moderately severe abdominal pain is almost always the predominant symptom. The pain is aggravated by any motion, including respiration. The progression of abdominal pain is a function of the rate of dissemination of the material producing the pain stimulus. Rupture of a peptic ulcer, with massive spillage of gastric contents, produces catastrophic epigastric pain, which, within minutes, may spread to involve the entire abdomen. The spread of pain from a lesion such as a ruptured appendix is much more gradual. Decreased intensity and extent of pain with time usually suggests localization of the inflammatory process.

Anorexia, nausea, and vomiting commonly accompany abdominal pain. Patients may also complain of feverishness, sometimes with a chill, thirst, scanty urination, inability to pass feces or flatus, and abdominal distention.

Body temperatures may reach 41° C (106° F). Subnormal temperature in the range of 35° C (95° F) is often seen in the early stages of chemical peritonitis (e.g., bile peritonitis) and late in the course of continuing intraabdominal sepsis or septic shock and is a grave sign.

Initially in peritonitis, there is hypermotility, which is followed by paralysis of the bowel and accumulation of fluid and electrolytes in the lumen of the adynamic bowel. Marked abdominal tenderness to palpation is present and is usually maximum over the organ in which the process originated. Rebound tenderness, both direct and referred, signifies parietal peritoneal irritation. This finding is sometimes more accurate than direct palpation in locating the point of maximum tenderness, as well as in delineating the extent of peritoneal irritation.

Muscular rigidity of the abdominal wall is produced both by voluntary guarding and by reflex muscle spasm. Hyperresonance due to gaseous intestinal distention can usually be demonstrated by percussion. Pneumoperitoneum from a ruptured hollow viscus may produce decreased liver dullness to percussion. Rectal and vaginal examination may reveal tenderness and the presence of a pelvic abscess and may indicate a primary focus in the female pelvic organs.

Abdominal muscle spasm may be deceptively absent in some patients. Those with lax abdominal musculature (e.g., patients in the postpartum period, with ascites due to cirrhosis, or with marked cachexia) may not have abdominal rigidity. Similarly, patients in shock or receiving glucocorticosteroid therapy, or in whom loculated intraabdominal abscesses are not in contact with the anterior abdominal wall (e.g., subphrenic, lesser sac, and pelvic abscesses) may not exhibit marked abdominal wall spasm. Absent bowel sounds may be the only manifestation of peritonitis; a high index of suspicion is necessary to make a diagnosis in such patients.

Shifts of isotonic, protein-rich fluid into the peritoneal cavity as a consequence of inflammation, combined with fluid shifts into the bowel lumen, can produce a profound fall in circulating blood volume and elevation of the hematocrit. Fluid and electrolyte losses are further exaggerated by coexisting fever, vomiting, occasional diarrhea, and loss of gastrointestinal tract fluid via intestinal intubation. As the process continues, the decreased venous return to the right side of the heart results in a drop in cardiac output, causing hypotension. In addition, endotoxic or bacteremic shock may develop (Chapter 245).

The intraperitoneal inflammation results in a relatively high and fixed diaphragm and considerable pain on respiration, leading to basilar atelectasis with intrapulmonary shunting of blood. In some patients, pulmonary edema develops due either to increased pulmonary capillary leakage as a consequence of hypoalbuminemia or to the direct effects of bacterial toxins (adult respiratory distress syndrome). In these patients, progressive hypoxemia develops with decreasing pulmonary compliance and requires volume-cycled ventilatory assistance with increasingly higher concentrations of inspired oxygen.

INTRAPERITONEAL ABSCESS

The clinical picture associated with the formation and progression of an intraperitoneal abscess may be acute but is often gradual: the patient who seemed to be recovering from peritonitis or an abdominal operation stops improving; fever returns, and localizing symptoms may develop. Local symptoms and signs vary widely with the location and source of the abscess. Subphrenic abscesses are usually accompanied by pleural or pulmonary involvement, whereas subhepatic abscesses have more dominant signs in the upper abdominal or subcostal area and fewer pulmonary changes.

RETROPERITONEAL ABSCESSES

Abscesses in the retroperitoneal spaces have been associated with prolonged morbidity and high mortality because of their insidious course and frequently vague clinical manifestations, which have resulted in delayed diagnosis and delayed or inadequate treatment. These infections arise most commonly from disease in organs that lie within or adjacent to one of the spaces in the retroperitoneum. Less commonly, retroperitoneal abscesses result from hematogenous dissemination of infection at a distant site.

The retroperitoneum extends from the diaphragm to the brim of the true pelvis. The lateral borders of the quadratus lumborum muscles correspond to its lateral margins. It is divided into anterior and posterior spaces by the anterior layer of the renal fascia. The anterior space contains the pancreas and retroperitoneal portions of the duodenum and colon. Abscesses in the anterior retroperitoneal space may originate, for example, from perforation of the duodenum as a result of peptic ulceration or trauma, from trauma or inflammation of the pancreas, from appendicitis, or from colonic perforation due to diverticulitis, inflammatory bowel disease, or carcinoma. The posterior retroperitoneal space contains on each side a kidney and ureter surrounded by renal fascia, and in the midline the abdominal aorta, inferior vena cava, lymphatics, and lymph nodes surrounded by renal fascia.

Infections of the abdominal aorta or suppurative lymphadenitis may be the cause of abscess in the medial portion of the posterior retroperitoneum. Pyelonephritis is the usual cause of abscesses in the perinephric space (Chapter 246).

Most retroperitoneal space infections lateralize to one side or the other, but extension across the midline can cause bilateral abscesses. Lack of an anatomic barrier inferiorly favors spread of infection downward into the pelvis.

Posterior to the retroperitoneum are the retrofascial spaces, which are occupied by the quadratus lumborum and psoas muscles. Abscesses in the retrofascial spaces arise from infection in the disk spaces or vertebral bodies or from infection in the retroperitoneum. Osteomyelitis of the lumbar spine can be associated with contiguous infection of the abdominal aorta.

The clinical course of retroperitoneal and retrofascial infection is frequently chronic. In over 50% of patients symptoms are present for more than 3 weeks before diagnosis and consist of fever, sweats, generalized malaise, cachexia, and back, flank, or hip pain, which may radiate into the legs. A tender mass may be palpable in the flank or back. Scoliosis and abdominal disturbance are less common. The thigh may be held in a flexed position and pain elicited by extension and internal rotation of the thigh, which indicates involvement of the psoas space (psoas sign). Retrofascial infection points into the groin, either above Poupart's ligament or in the inguinal region of the thigh. Infection may also extend into the pleural space, mediastinum, or peritoneal cavity. Periureteral inflammation may result in sterile pyuria.

Polymicrobial infection involving obligate and facultative anaerobes would be expected in abscesses arising from disease in the duodenum or colon, whereas single species, either *E. coli* or *S. aureus,* would be expected in abscesses secondary to either ascending or hematogenous pyelonephritis, respectively, or to vertebral osteomyelitis.

VISCERAL ABSCESSES
Liver Abscess

For a discussion of liver abscess, see Chapter 361.

Splenic Abscess

Pathogenesis. Splenic abscesses are uncommon lesions and are usually multiple. The multiple small abscesses usually develop as a complication of hematogenous dissemination. Splenic abscesses that develop during the course of bacterial endocarditis are usually due to *S. aureus* or streptococci. Enterobacteriaceae (e.g., *Salmonella*) and anaerobic microorganisms have also been recovered. Some are related to infection in contiguous organs and others result from infected traumatic hematomas or infarcts of the spleen (e.g., in patients with sickle cell hemoglobinopathies). Positive blood cultures have been reported in 70% of patients with multiple splenic abscesses but in only 14%

with solitary abscesses. Fungal splenic abscesses, often occurring as part of the syndrome of hepatosplenic candidiasis, have been noted in patients predisposed to candidial infections (e.g., patients receiving high-dose corticosteroids or cancer chemotherapy).

Clinical Manifestations. Left upper quadrant abdominal pain and fever are the usual manifestations of splenic abscesses. Irritation of the adjacent diaphragm may result in pain referred to the left shoulder. Splenic enlargement and tenderness are usually present, with high, spiking temperatures; occasionally a splenic rub is heard. Clinical findings may be absent in some patients with multiple small splenic abscesses.

Pancreatic Abscess

For a discussion of pancreatic abscess, see Chapter 366.

Pathogenesis. Pancreatic abscesses develop in about 1% to 9% of patients following acute pancreatitis, which may be either biliary, alcoholic, postsurgical, or posttraumatic in origin. A pancreatic abscess occasionally follows penetration by a peptic ulcer or occurs as a complication of endoscopic retrograde cholangiopancreatography.

About one third to half of pancreatic abscesses have been reported to be polymicrobial, involving mainly facultative microorganisms, such as *E. coli* and other Enterobacteriaceae, enterococci, *viridans* streptococci, and occasionally *S. aureus*. Modern anaerobic bacteriologic techniques have also documented the presence of anaerobes. The mixed enteric bacterial origin of many pancreatic abscesses suggests that bacteria may reach the pancreas by reflux of contaminated bile. The hematogenous route probably accounts for infections caused by *S. aureus*.

Clinical Manifestations. The clinical presentation of pancreatic abscesses varies. The patient may fail to respond to therapy for pancreatitis, or 1 to 3 weeks after the onset of pancreatitis the patient's condition may deteriorate after an initial response. Nausea, vomiting, and abdominal pain that frequently radiates to the back are present in more than 80% to 90% of patients. A body temperature of more than 38.3° C (101° F) and abdominal tenderness are usually present. Less frequently, jaundice, abdominal distention, or an abdominal mass or signs of generalized peritonitis may be present. The serum amylase level is elevated in 20% to 70% of patients and may remain elevated.

ACUTE CHOLECYSTITIS AND CHOLANGITIS

For a discussion of cholecystitis and cholangitis, see Chapter 364.

DIAGNOSIS OF INTRAABDOMINAL INFECTION

The diagnosis of primary peritonitis is one of exclusion of a primary intraabdominal source of infection (Chapter 342) and can be made with certainty only after a thorough laparotomy. Under certain circumstances, however, laparotomy may be avoided on the basis of an appropriate clinical setting, such as cirrhosis or nephrosis, and findings in peritoneal fluid obtained by paracentesis (e.g., if gram-positive organisms are found, a diagnosis of primary peritonitis can usually be made and exploratory laparotomy deferred). In children, if gram-negative organisms, a mixed flora, or no organisms are obtained, full exploratory laparotomy is indicated to rule out possible intraabdominal sources of peritoneal contamination. In patients with end-stage cirrhosis, exploratory laparotomy may be very life threatening, and the likelihood of finding a primary intraabdominal focus may be small. It is best to defer operation in these patients while awaiting a response to antimicrobial therapy. Patients with primary peritonitis usually respond to appropriate antimicrobial therapy within 48 hours. Paracentesis for smear and culture is indicated in all cirrhotic patients with ascites and in children with marked proteinuria and abdominal pain, whether or not the diagnosis of nephrotic syndrome has been previously established.

Paracentesis is not without hazard, especially in patients with hemorrhagic tendencies or bowel distention. Rarely, major complications can occur, including perforation of the bowel followed by general-

ized peritonitis, abdominal wall abscess, and serious hemorrhage. If no fluid can be aspirated, peritoneal lavage with Ringer's lactate solution can provide fluid for examination. Taps should not be attempted in the region of abdominal scars, where bowel may be adherent to the underside of the scar. The aspirate should be examined for blood, pus, bile, digested fat, and amylase; the sediment should be Gram-stained, and the fluid should be cultured aerobically and anaerobically (Chapter 233).

In patients with primary peritonitis, the leukocyte count in peritoneal fluid usually is greater than 300 cells/mm^3, with granulocytes predominating unless *M. tuberculosis* is the pathogen. Gram's stain of the sediment is frequently diagnostic but may be negative in up to 60% or more of patients with cirrhosis and ascites.

The diagnosis of tuberculous peritonitis often requires operation or laparoscopy and is confirmed by histologic study of the peritoneal biopsy and bacteriologic examination of the peritoneal biopsy specimen and fluid. Multiple nodules scattered over the peritoneal surface and omentum are observed. Adhesions and a variable amount of peritoneal fluid are usually present. Ascitic fluid may have an elevated protein concentration (>3 g/dl) and a lymphocytic pleocytosis, but neither may be present. *Coccidioides immitis* can cause a similar granulomatous peritonitis with a variable clinical presentation. The diagnosis of *C. immitis* peritonitis can be made from a wet mount of ascitic fluid, on finding *C. immitis* by culture, and by histologic examination.

A peripheral leukocytosis of 17,000 to 25,000 cells/mm^3 is usual in acute intraabdominal infections, the differential count showing polymorphonuclear predominance and a moderate to marked shift to the left. Although there may be fewer than 5000 white cells/mm^3 in the circulating blood, the differential smear usually shows an extreme shift to immature polymorphonuclear forms. Hematuria and pyuria without bacteriuria may reflect intraabdominal inflammatory disease (e.g., appendicitis, adjacent to the urinary tract). Elevated serum amylase levels may be seen in peritonitis due to almost any cause, but very high levels are seen only in acute pancreatitis. Hyponatremia may be seen in patients given water to replace isotonic fluid losses, but it is also characteristic of porphyria. Acidosis is present in severe and late peritonitis.

Supine, upright, and lateral decubitus radiographs of the abdomen may reveal distention of both small intestine and colon, with adynamic loops of bowel or features of mechanical intestinal obstruction, volvulus, intussusception, or vascular occlusion. Inflammatory exudate and edema of the intestinal wall produce a widening of the space between adjacent loops. Peritoneal fat lines and psoas shadows may be obliterated. Free air may be visible if a viscus is ruptured. Chest radiographs should always be taken to rule out a pulmonary or thoracic problem as the cause of the abdominal distress and best determine the presence of air beneath the diaphragm.

Gas with a fluid level, or mottling due to gas, may also be visible in intraperitoneal or visceral abscesses. Calcification in the gallbladder or other organs may also be observed on x-ray film.

The search for intraperitoneal or visceral abscesses may be aided by routine and contrast radiography, radionuclide scanning, ultrasonography, angiography, and especially by computed tomography (CT). Some radiographic findings of a right-sided subphrenic or liver abscess include right-sided pleural effusion, basilar atelectasis, elevation of the diaphragm, and loss of diaphragmatic movement on fluoroscopy. Left subphrenic, splenic, or pancreatic abscess may be accompanied by left-sided pleuropulmonary findings. Radiography may also reveal displacement of viscera by an abscess; for example, the stomach may be outlined with barium or air to reveal displacement due to a left perihepatic, lesser sac, or pancreatic abscess. Intravenous cholangiography has been replaced by sensitive and specific hepatobiliary scanning with one of the technetium 99m–labeled acetanilid iminodiacetic acid (IDA) derivatives for the diagnosis of acute cholecystitis, even in the presence of moderately severe liver dysfunction. In acute cholecystitis, the common duct and small bowel are visualized, but because the cystic duct is occluded, the gallbladder is not visualized. Obstruction of the common bile duct also can be diagnosed by hepatobiliary scanning. In this case, no component of the biliary system or small bowel is visualized, despite adequate hepatic uptake. In obstructive cholangitis, however, ultrasonography is preferred due to decreased dependability of IDA scintigraphy in the pres-

Table 238-1 Susceptibility of clinically important pathogens to antimicrobial agents used in empiric regimens*

	AMPICILLIN	CEFAZOLIN	CEFAMANDOLE	CEFOXITIN	THIRD-GENERATION CEPHALOSPORIN	CEFTAZIDIME
Escherichia coli	R	R	S	S	S	S
Proteus mirabillis	S	S	S	S	S	S
Klebsiella sp.	R	S	S	S	S	S
Enterobacter sp.	R	R	S	R	R†	R†
Serratia sp.	R	R	R	R	R†	R†
Pseudomonas aeruginosa	R	R	R	R	R†	R†
Bacteroides fragilis	R	R	R	R	R	R

*Antimicrobial susceptibility may vary locally. The local institutional clinical microbiology laboratory should be consulted for the prevailing patterns of antimicrobial susceptibility.
†These species produce routinely inducible, chromosome-encoded β-lactamase and also mutate at a high frequency for constitutive β-lactamase production.
R, Clinically significant resistance (>10% of isolates); *S*, sensitivity.

ence of severe jaundice. Percutaneous transhepatic cholangiography and endoscopic retrograde cholangiography are extremely valuable in evaluating bile duct obstruction. However, it is seldom feasible to use these techniques in the acutely ill patient with cholangitis.

Technetium 99m sulfur colloid liver-spleen scan visualizes the entire organ and delineates abnormal areas as "cold spots" due to decreased uptake of the isotope. Two other radionuclide scans that are at times helpful in detecting intraabdominal abscesses are scans of leukocytes tagged with gallium 67 (Ga 67) and indium 111 (In 111). Unlike ^{99m}Tc, Ga 67 and In 111 accumulate in areas of inflammation and appear as areas of increased radioactivity or "hot spots." Gallium is excreted into the intestinal tract and Ga 67 and In 111 can accumulate in any inflammatory process. For these reasons, false-positive scans may result from misinterpretation of radioactivity within the lumen of the bowel, within the wall of an inflamed bowel, or within a noninfected operative site in the process of healing.

Ultrasound is helpful in determining the size, shape, consistency, and anatomic relationships of an intraabdominal abscess or collection of peritoneal fluid. Ultrasound can be used to determine gallbladder size and the presence of stones and bile duct dilation; however, common duct obstruction can be present without bile duct dilation. CT has proved to be especially well suited for the diagnosis of intraabdominal abscess. Definition is unimpeded by intraluminal gas and postoperative changes, except in the presence of metallic surgical clips or residual barium, which may disrupt the image. Observed findings consistent with abscess include a low-density tissue mass and a definable capsule. CT can detect extraluminal gas, a finding highly suggestive of abscess. Contrast material is commonly administered orally, rectally, and intravenously when an attempt is being made to diagnose intraabdominal abscess. The intraluminal contrast helps to distinguish loops of bowel from abscess cavities, and the parenteral contrast may enhance a surrounding capsule, thus allowing for easier identification.

Magnetic resonance imaging (MRI) requires no administration of contrast material and eliminates exposure to radiation but is costly, and its usefulness in relation to CT and ultrasound remains to be demonstrated.

Under favorable circumstances, percutaneously placed catheters, guided by CT and ultrasonography, can be used to drain intraabdominal abscesses and thus confirm the presence and position of the abscess with certainty. Gram's stain and culture of the purulent material obtained allow specific antibiotic therapy to be initiated earlier in the course of illness.

With these new methods of determining the location and extent of intraabdominal infection, subsequent operative treatment can be more direct. In some cases percutaneous catheter drainage and antibiotic therapy may avert the need for surgery. Overreliance on any single technique is dangerous, and the diagnosis should be confirmed by other methods and by clinical findings.

TREATMENT OF INTRAABDOMINAL INFECTION

Antimicrobial therapy should be initiated immediately after appropriate specimens (e.g., blood and peritoneal fluid) are obtained for Gram's stain and culture. Initial antimicrobial therapy is therefore em-

piric, based on the predicted sensitivities of the most likely pathogens. In vitro sensitivity reports allow subsequent adjustment of the initial regimen to more specific therapy.

Primary bacterial peritonitis due to either *S. pneumoniae* or group A streptococci is best treated with penicillin G. Suspected *S. aureus* peritonitis should be treated with a penicillinase-resistant penicillin or a first-generation cephalosporin (e.g., cefazolin), unless a methicillin-resistant strain is identified, when vancomycin is appropriate. Suspected Enterobacteriaceae or *P. aeruginosa* infection should be treated initially with an appropriate β-lactam antibiotic, such as ampicillin, ticarcillin, a ureidopenicillin, aztreonam, imipenem, or a cephalosporin with or without gentamicin or tobramycin.

If the infection is community-acquired, Enterobacteriaceae, such as *E. coli, Proteus mirabilis,* or *Klebsiella pneumoniae,* are likely to be involved, and if hospital-acquired, more antibiotic-resistant Enterobacteriaceae such as *Enterobacter* or *Serratia* species, or *P. aeruginosa* may be involved. The antimicrobial activity that can be expected from agents used in empiric regimens against commonly encountered facultative gram-negative bacillary pathogens is shown in Table 238-1. As many as 30% to 40% of both community-acquired and nosocomial infections caused by *E. coli* are resistant to ampicillin on the basis of β-lactamase production, and even over 10% may be resistant to first-generation cephalosporins. *P. mirabilis* is likely to be sensitive to ampicillin, the broad-spectrum penicillins (e.g., ticarcillin or piperacillin), first-, second-, and third-generation cephalosporins, imipenem, and aztreonam. *K. pneumoniae* is sensitive to all of the forementioned, except ampicillin and the broad-spectrum penicillins (e.g., ticarcillin or piperacillin), to which it is resistant on the basis of β-lactamase production.

β-lactamases produced by *E. coli* and *K. pneumoniae* and the β-lactamases produced by *B. fragilis* and *S. aureus*, are inhibited by clavulanic acid, tazobactam, and sulbactam. When these β-lactamase inhibitors are combined in formulations with ticarcillin (Timentin), piperacillin (Zosyn), amoxicillin (Augmentin), and ampicillin (Unasyn), the antibiotics become active against these β-lactamase-producing organisms. These inhibitors, however, do not inhibit the inducible, chromosome-encoded β-lactamases produced by commonly encountered nosocomial pathogens, such as *Enterobacter cloacae, Serratia marcescens, Citrobacter freundii, Morganella morganii,* and *P. aeruginosa.* Addition of clavulanic acid therefore does not improve the activity of ticarcillin against these β-lactamase producers. These organisms are resistant to ampicillin or amoxicillin, first-generation cephalosporins, and, frequently, second-generation cephalosporins on the basis of mechanisms other than β-lactamase, so addition of β-lactamase inhibitors does not improve the activity of ampicillin or amoxicillin against these organisms.

These nosocomial pathogens, which produce inducible, chromosome-encoded β-lactamases, have an additional mechanism for resistance to β-lactam antibiotics: they have a sufficiently high rate of mutational loss of the variable expression of β-lactamase production that about 1 in 10^7 colony-forming units (CFU) are "stable-derepressed" mutants. These mutants constitutively produce large amounts of β-lactamase. In infected tissue that usually contains 10^{8-10} CFU/g, there are large numbers of these stable-derepressed mu-

AZTREONAM	AMOXICILLIN/CLAVULANATE, AMPICILLIN-SULBACTAM	BROAD-SPECTRUM PENICILLINS	PIPERACILLIN-TAZOBACTAM, TICARCILLIN-CLAVULANATE	IMIPENEM MEROPENEM	CEFIXIME AMINOGLYCOSIDE QUINOLONES
S	S	S	S	S	S
S	S	S	S	S	S
S	S	R	S	S	S
R†	R	R†	R†	S	S
R†	R	R†	R†	S	S
R†	R	R†	R†	S	S
R	S	R	S	S	R

tants even before initiation of antimicrobial therapy. These mutants may become predominant and cause persistent infection during therapy with most β-lactam antibiotics, especially third-generation cephalosporins, including ceftazidime, and are highly resistant to all β-lactam antibiotics, except imipenem, meropenem, and cefixime. There is no cross-resistance among these strains to quinolones, aminoglycosides, or trimethoprim-sulfamethoxazole. If anaerobic bacteria are suspected, antibiotics active against *B. fragilis* (see later discussion) should also be used initially.

The role of antimicrobial therapy in the outcome of localized infection due to anaerobes or a mixture of anaerobes and facultative microorganisms is extremely difficult to assess, as there is usually a dramatic response to surgical drainage and debridement alone. Antimicrobial therapy significantly reduces mortality among patients with bacteremic infections due to Bacteroidaceae or Enterobacteriaceae. Antimicrobial drugs also control early metastatic foci of infection, reduce suppurative complications if given early, and prevent local spread of existing infection. Once a sufficiently large abscess has formed, antimicrobial drugs alone, without drainage, will not eliminate the infection, but they may mask some of the clinical manifestations of abscess formation.

Because anaerobic infections are commonly polymicrobial, a broad spectrum of antimicrobial activity is required. Drugs active against anaerobic bacteria may be inactive against the accompanying aerobic or facultative pathogens in mixed infections, and vice versa. For this reason, combinations of two or three drugs are used. However, some drugs, such as imipenem, ticarcillin plus clavulanic acid, piperacillin plus tazobactam, or ampicillin plus sulbactam, are active against both aerobes and *B. fragilis* and can be used alone. Drugs are selected for their activity against most of the more virulent pathogens in the infective mixture, for example, the Enterobacteriaceae and *B. fragilis,* which frequently cause bacteremia and abscesses in these patients. However, the antibiotics need not be active against every pathogen isolated. It is apparent that if most of the organisms are eliminated, their synergistic effect is removed, and the patient's defenses may be able to eradicate the remaining organisms. Although enterococci were not considered significant pathogens in polymicrobial infection in the past, this organism may be the sole intraabdominal pathogen, at times associated with enterococcal bacteremia, especially in patients with polymicrobial intraabdominal infection that was treated with an antimicrobial agent that lacked activity against the enterococcus.

If present, enterococcal infection may be treated with ampicillin, penicillin G, imipenem, or a ureidopenicillin. Enterococci are less susceptible to other β-lactam antibiotics such as carbenicillin or ticarcillin and are least susceptible to the antistaphylococcal penicillins and cephalosporins. Recently, enterococci have been identified with increasing frequency in monomicrobial and polymicrobial infections and nosocomial outbreaks. These organisms frequently are (1) highly resistant to ampicillin, either because of β-lactamase production in *E. faecalis* or because of loss of affinity of penicillin-binding bacterial cell membrane proteins in *E. faecium;* (2) resistant to glycopeptides (i.e., vancomycin or teicoplanin) due to plasmid-encoded synthesis of a membrane protein in both *E. faecalis* and *E. faecium;* or (3) resistant to aminoglycosides due to the presence of plasmid-encoded aminoglycoside inactivating enzymes.

Some strains of enterococci are resistant to all penicillins, glyco-

peptides, and aminoglycosides. Emergence of clinically significant infection due to strains that are resistant to traditional antibiotic therapy requires routine antimicrobial susceptibility testing of enterococci, which may have been abandoned in the recent past. Either combinations of β-lactamase inhibitors with a β-lactam antibiotic, such as sulbactam-ampicillin (Unasyn), clavulanic acid–amoxicillin (Augmentin), or tazobactam-piperacillin (Zosyn), or glycopeptides are effective for treatment of infection due to β-lactamase–producing *E. faecalis.* Glycopeptides are effective for treatment of infections due to *E. faecium* that is highly resistant to ampicillin but still sensitive to glycopeptides. Teicoplanin, an investigational antibiotic, is no longer available in the United States for compassionate use, for treatment of infections due to vancomycin-resistant, teicoplanin-sensitive strains (van B phenotype glycopeptide resistance). Some strains are both vancomycin and teicoplanin resistant (van A phenotype resistance), highly resistant to ampicillin (especially if *E. faecium*), and aminoglycoside resistant. Treatment of infections due to multiresistant strains should be based on results of susceptibility tests; potential antimicrobial agents include chloramphenicol or doxycycline. Synercid, an investigational antibiotic that can be obtained from Rhone-Poulenc Rorer Pharmaceuticals Inc. for compassionate use, is usually active against vancomycin-resistant strains of *E. faecium,* but not *E. faecalis.*

Nearly 100 percent of strains of *B. fragilis* are sensitive to imipenem (0.5 to 1.0 g IV q6h), chloramphenicol (50 to 100 mg/kg/day), ticarcillin plus clavulanic acid (3 g ticarcillin IV q4-6h), ampicillin plus sulbactam (2 g ampicillin intravenously every 6 hours), piperacillin-tazobactam (3 g piperacillin intravenously every 6 hours), or metronidazole (loading dose of 15 mg/kg intravenously and then 7.5 mg/kg every 6 hours intravenously or by mouth.) However, chloramphenicol may be active against these organisms only at concentrations that are close to serum levels (i.e., 20 to 25 μg/ml), above which predictable bone marrow suppression occurs if therapy is longer than 1 week. Clindamycin (300 to 600 mg intravenously every 6 to 8 hours) and cefoxitin (1 to 2 g every 4 hours) are active against anaerobic gram-negative bacilli, although resistance has been reported at some medical centers.

Only about 85% of *B. fragilis* strains are sensitive to cefoxitin; 90% are sensitive to ticarcillin or ureidopenicillins, that are not combined with a β-lactamase inhibitor. At present, in most clinical microbiology laboratories, no standardized in vitro method is commonly used to determine the antibiotic sensitivity of anaerobes. Thus in seriously ill patients with *B. fragilis* infection, the use of imipenem, ticarcillin-clavulanic acid, piperacillin-tazobactam, ampicillin-sulbactam, or metronidazole, which has almost 100% predictable activity against *B. fragilis,* is advised.

The other anaerobic pathogens in polymicrobial infections are usually sensitive to β-lactam antibiotics, clindamycin, or chloramphenicol. However, anaerobic and microaerophilic gram-positive cocci may not be sensitive to metronidazole. If this agent is used for its *B. fragilis* activity, an additional antibiotic (e.g., ampicillin) should be given for the treatment of these gram-positive cocci. The facultative or aerobic components (e.g., *E. coli* or *P. mirabilis*) may not be sensitive to some of the antibiotics active against *B. fragilis,* and initial therapy should include an aminoglycoside (e.g., 1.7 mg gentamicin or tobramycin/kg every 8 hours intravenously or intramuscularly in patients with normal renal function). A β-lactam antibiotic (ampicillin or cephalosporin) should be substituted for the potentially nephrotoxic and ototoxic aminoglycoside if sensitivity testing indicates appropriate activity.

The newer cephalosporins (e.g., cefotaxime, ceftizoxime, ceftazidime, and ceftriaxone) and other, similar β-lactam antibiotics (e.g., imipenem) have demonstrated significantly better activity against the Enterobacteriaceae than the older cephalosporins, but, except for imipenem, they have poor activity against *B. fragilis.* Thus the newer cephalosporins can be used to replace aminoglycosides in empiric regimens, combined with either metronidazole or clindamycin, and avoid the risk of aminoglycoside toxicity.

Ampicillin-sulbactam or piperacillin-tazobactam can be used as a single empiric agent in community-acquired infections, because of its activity against both aerobic and anaerobic pathogens, including susceptible enterococci. Imipenem, because of its broad-spectrum activity, which encompasses many organisms resistant to other antimicrobial agents, can be used as a single empiric agent in nosocomial infections (e.g., postoperative peritonitis occurring in hospitalized patients or those who have recently received broad-spectrum antibiotics). Optimally, initial empiric treatment should be modified to reflect the specific antimicrobial susceptibilities of the pathogens isolated from cultures of blood and intraabdominal specimens. However, empiric treatment for anaerobic bacteria should be continued when anaerobic infection is suspected (i.e., multiple morphotypes seen on Gram-stained specimens, or putrid odor to the specimens, gastrointestinal tract perforation), even when no anaerobes are isolated from clinical specimens, because of the well-known problems of isolating these fastidious pathogens in the routine clinical microbiology laboratory.

The duration of therapy is usually prolonged to prevent relapse, since host defenses may not eradicate the pathogens from sequestered areas of extensive tissue necrosis and abscess formation. Not all these areas are accessible to adequate surgical drainage.

Operation for peritonitis is performed to stop continuing contamination, to remove foreign material and devitalized tissue from the peritoneal cavity, and to provide drainage of purulent collections. Operation is generally not indicated in the following situations:

1. Primary peritonitis
2. Moribund patients whose condition continues to deteriorate, despite vigorous supportive therapy
3. Patients in whom the disease process subsides and localizes while they are being prepared for surgery
4. Patients with peritonitis resulting from pelvic inflammatory disease (which usually responds to nonsurgical therapy)

In localized pyogenic infection such as intraperitoneal or visceral abscess surgical drainage is usually required. Immediate operation is indicated for the suppurative complications of acute cholecystitis and for severe forms of cholangitis.

Percutaneous catheter drainage guided by ultrasonography or CT has been used successfully as an alternative to surgery and appears most effective with unilocular abscess cavities when a safe route of approach is present. Surgery may be required for more complete drainage of multiloculated or highly viscous abscesses, for abscesses not in contact with the abdominal wall (e.g., interloop or mesenteric abscesses), or for correction of instigating factors (e.g., biliary tract obstruction or perforated bowel). Complications or percutaneous catheter drainage may occur in up to 15% of patients and include septicemia, hemorrhage, peritoneal spillage, and fistula formation. However, the morbidity and mortality associated with percutaneous drainage may be less than that associated with surgery.

Drainage of the general peritoneal cavity is physically impossible, since exudate and adhesions rapidly isolate and occlude the drains and may increase the risk of secondary infections. However, drains are often placed in a dependent point to which fluid can be expected to gravitate or in an area of devitalized tissue that cannot be removed.

REFERENCES

Bohnen JMA: Operative management of intraabdominal infections, *Infect Dis Clin North Am* 6:511, 1992.

Bohnen JMA, Solomkin JS, Dellinger EP et al: Guidelines for clinical care: antiinfective agents for intraabdominal infections, *Arch Surg* 127:83, 1992.

Dellinger EP et al: Surgical infections stratification system for intraabdominal infection, *Arch Surg* 120:21, 1985.

Do H, Lambiase RE, Deyoe L et al: Percutaneous drainage of hepatic abscesses: comparison of results in abscesses with and without intrahepatic biliary communication, *Am J Roentgenol* 157:1209, 1991.

Dunn DL, Simmons RL: The role of anaerobic bacteria in intraabdominal infections, *Rev Infect Dis* 6(suppl 1):S139, 1984.

Finegold SM, Lance WL, editors: Anaerobic infections in humans, San Diego, 1989, Academic.

Finegold SM, Wexler JM: Therapeutic implications of bacteriologic findings in mixed aerobic-anaerobic infections, *Antimicrob Agents Chemother* 32:611, 1988.

Joiner KA, Gorbach SL: Acute septic complications in gastrointestinal emergencies, *Clin Gastroenterol* 10:93, 106, 1981.

Levinson MA: Percutaneous versus open drainage of intraabdominal abscesses, *Infect Dis Clin North Am* 6:525, 1992.

Mosdell DM, Morris DM, Voltura A et al: Antibiotic treatment for surgical peritonitis, *Ann Surg* 214:543, 1991.

Mueller PR, Simeone JF: Intraabdominal abscess: diagnosis by sonography and computed tomography, *Radiol Clin North Am* 21:425, 1983.

Nelken N, Isnatius J, Skinner M et al: Changing clinical spectrum of splenic abscess: a multicenter study and review of the literature, *Am J Surg* 154:27, 1987.

Nichols RL: Intra-abdominal infections: an overview, *Rev Infect Dis* 7(suppl 4):S709, 1985.

Root RK, Trunkey DD, Sande MA, editors: *Contemporary issues in infectious diseases,* vol 6, Focus on infection: new surgical and medical approaches, New York, 1986, Churchill Livingstone.

Saklayen MG: CAPD peritonitis: incidence, diagnosis and management, *Med Clin North Am* 74:997, 1990.

Sawyer MD, Dunn DL: Antimicrobial therapy of intraabdominal sepsis, *Infect Dis Clin North Am* 6:545, 1992.

Stantan R, Frey CF: Comprehensive management of acute necrotizing pancreatitis and pancreatic abscess, *Arch Surg* 125:1269, 1990.

Wilcox CM, Dismukes WE: Spontaneous bacterial peritonitis: a review of pathogenesis, diagnosis and treatment, *Medicine (Baltimore)* 66:447, 1987.

Wilson SE, Finegold SM, Williams RA, editors: *Intraabdominal infection,* New York, 1982, McGraw-Hill.

CHAPTER

239 Acute Meningitis

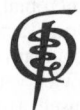

Allan R. Tunkel and W. Michael Scheld

Acute inflammation of the central nervous system (CNS) may be caused by a wide variety of etiologic agents. Because of their overall frequency, this chapter focuses on meningitis due to the most important pathogens: bacteria, viruses, and fungi.

EPIDEMIOLOGY AND ETIOLOGY
Bacterial Meningitis

Although the exact incidence of bacterial meningitis in the United States is not known, in a surveillance study of 27 states from 1978 through 1981, the overall annual attack rate was 3.0 cases per 100,000 population. Attack rates have been reported to vary by age, sex, and geographic area with the highest rates in the Pacific region (Washington and Oregon) and lowest rates in the mid-Atlantic region (Arkansas and Louisiana). The disease is more common worldwide, especially in certain regions, such as the sub-Saharan "meningitis belt" of Africa. In addition, a review of all cases (~4100) of bacterial meningitis admitted to an isolation-fever hospital in Salvador, Brazil, between 1973 and 1982 revealed an average annual incidence of 45.8 cases per 100,000 population, illustrating the global importance of the meningitis problem.

Bacterial meningitis is a significant problem in hospitalized patients. In a recent review of 493 episodes of bacterial meningitis in adults aged 16 years and older at the Massachusetts General Hospital from 1962 through 1988, 40% of episodes were nosocomial in origin, and these episodes carried a high mortality rate (35% for single episodes of nosocomial meningitis).

Over 80% of all cases of bacterial meningitis are due to one of three major organisms: *Haemophilus influenzae, Neisseria meningitidis,* and *Streptococcus pneumoniae.* All are more common in the winter months except *H. influenzae,* which demonstrates a biphasic

Table 239-1 Causes of bacterial meningitis: age-related incidence (%)*

ORGANISM	UNDER 2 MONTHS OF AGE	2 MONTHS TO 6 YEARS OF AGE	OVER 6 YEARS OF AGE
Haemophilus influenzae	0-2	5-10	5
Neisseria meningitidis	0-1	20-50	25-45
Streptococcus pneumoniae	1-8	10-30	40-70
Escherichia coli (and other gram-negative bacilli)	30-40	1-4	5
Streptococcus agalactiae	30-60	2-5	1-3
Staphylococci	2-5	1-2	5
Listeria monocytogenes	2-15	1-2	5-15
Others (including unidentified organisms)	5-10	5-10	5-10

*Numbers are approximate

pattern in the northern states with peak incidences in spring and fall, although in southern states the peak incidence is also in the winter months. The attack rate is higher in members of the lower socioeconomic groups. The frequency of bacterial meningitis is age-related (Table 239-1). Nearly 75% of cases occur in children under 6 years of age, and males are affected more commonly than females in all age-groups (1.5 to 2:1). In infants 2 months old or younger, the most common etiologic agents are *Escherichia coli,* other gram-negative bacilli, and group B streptococci *(S. agalactiae).* Between the ages of 2 months and 6 years, *H. influenzae* is the predominant pathogen. Beyond age 6, meningococci and pneumococci cause the majority of cases, with a second peak after age 50 years for pneumococci and gram-negative bacilli.

H. influenzae (Chapter 266) until recently was the most common cause of meningitis in the United States (40% to 50% of cases), and capsular type b strains accounted for over 90% of serious *H. influenzae* infections. Over 50% of patients with *H. influenzae* meningitis have concurrent pharyngitis or otitis media on presentation. Disease due to this organism after age 6 is rare and suggests an underlying host defect, for example, chronic parameningeal foci of infection (sinus or mastoids), sickle cell disease, splenectomy, diabetes mellitus, hypogammaglobulinemia, CNS trauma with a cerebrospinal fluid (CSF) leak, or alcoholism. Unencapsulated *H. influenzae* strains may also cause meningitis. Recently the incidence of invasive infections, specifically in young children, caused by *H. influenzae* type b in the United States has been profoundly reduced (by 76% to 90%) in part because of the recent widespread use of conjugate vaccines against *H. influenzae* type b that have been licensed for routine use in all children beginning at 2 months of age.

Meningococcal meningitis (Chapter 264) is primarily an illness of children and young adults; less than 10% of cases occur after age 45. It differs from other types of bacterial meningitis in that it may occur in epidemics (usually due to serogroups A and C), now primarily outside the United States. Deficiency of the terminal complement components (C5, C6, C7, C8, and perhaps C9) predisposes to disseminated *Neisseria* infections, including gonococcemia and meningococcemia. The distribution of meningococcal serogroups in a surveillance study of 27 states from 1978 through 1981 was as follows: A, 4.7% (especially in the indigent populations of Seattle and Anchorage); B, 51.1%; C, 22.3%; Y, 5.8% (higher incidence in military personnel with a predilection for pneumonia); others (especially W135), 6.4%; and unclassifiable, 9.7%. Recently, however, there has been an increase in the incidence of serogroup C disease in North America equaling or surpassing that caused by serogroup B; emergence of this clonal group of virulent serogroup C meningococcal strains has led to an increase in the rate of meningococcal disease in some regions, an increased number of outbreaks, and a higher case fatality rate.

Pneumococcal meningitis is the most common form in adults and is frequently associated with other suppurative foci: pneumonia (25%), otitis media or mastoiditis (30%), sinusitis (10% to 15%), and endocarditis (<5%) (Chapter 24). Previous head trauma (with or without a CSF leak) is found in approximately 10% of patients with pneumococcal meningitis, and the pneumococcus causes the overwhelm-

ing majority of recurrent meningitis cases. Other conditions (sickle cell disease, splenectomy, hypogammaglobulinemia, multiple myeloma, alcoholism) also predispose to systemic pneumococcal infection, including meningitis. Among the 84 known serotypes of pneumococci, 18 cause the majority (82%) of cases of bacteremic pneumococcal pneumonia, and there is a close correlation between bacteremic serotypes and those responsible for meningitis.

Gram-negative bacillary meningitis is encountered only in specific clinical settings: in neonates, in head trauma, after neurosurgical procedures, during gram-negative septicemia, in underlying defects in host defenses, and in association with strongyloidiasis (Chapter 281) in the hyperinfection syndrome, in which meningitis caused by enteric bacteria occurs secondary to seeding of the meninges during persistent or recurrent bacteremias associated with the migration of infective larvae; alternatively, the larvae may carry enteric organisms on their surfaces or within their own gastrointestinal tracts as they exit the intestine and subsequently invade the meninges. The most common etiologic agents, in approximate order of frequency are *Klebsiella* species, *E. coli,* and *Pseudomonas aeruginosa,* although a wide variety of other organisms may be responsible. Nosocomial meningitis is increasing in frequency, as is the proportion of cases that are due to aerobic gram-negative bacilli.

Group B streptococcal disease (Chapter 262) in neonates has been divided into two types: early-onset septicemia associated with premature rupture of the membranes and low-birth-weight infants, and late-onset (>7 days after birth) meningitis. In early-onset disease, the organism is acquired from the maternal genital tract; the risk of transmission from the mother to her infant is increased when the inoculum of organisms and number of sites of maternal colonization are high. Intrapartum chemoprophylaxis with penicillin or ampicillin directed at parturient women with high-risk factors (colonized with group B streptococci, prolonged rupture of amniotic membranes [>18 hours], fever, and low-birth-weight infant [<2.5 kg]) could effectively reduce the incidence of early-onset disease. The source of the organism (nearly always serotype III) in late-onset disease remains unknown, as 40% of affected infants are born to culture-negative mothers. Nosocomial transmission from other colonized infants or nursery personnel is possible. This organism is the most common cause of serious neonatal infection in many large centers. Although the incidence of group B streptococcal infection varies in different geographic areas, the overall incidence has remained the same ($\cong$ 1 to 3 cases per 1000 live births) in recent years. An estimated 12,000 cases occurred in the United States in 1979. The group B streptococcus can also cause meningitis in adults. Risk factors include age beyond 60 years, diabetes mellitus, being a parturient woman, cardiac disease, collagen vascular diseases, malignancy, alcoholism, hepatic failure, renal failure, and corticosteroid therapy; no underlying illnesses were found in 43% of patients in one study.

The other bacterial etiologic agents of meningitis are relatively uncommon. *Listeria monocytogenes* causes disease in neonates and immunosuppressed adults (especially renal transplant recipients) but should also be considered in the elderly, alcoholic, or cancer patient (Chapter 263). *Listeria* meningitis is found infrequently in patients with human immunodeficiency virus (HIV) infection, despite its increased incidence in patients with deficiencies in cell-mediated immunity. Thirty percent of all cases occur in presumably normal persons. Outbreaks have been associated with the consumption of contaminated food, especially dairy products. More than 300 patients with listeriosis were reported in two separate outbreaks in California and Switzerland in the late 1980s resulting from contaminated cheese. Encephalitis, especially involving multiple cranial nerves, is relatively common with *Listeria* meningitis. *Staphylococcus aureus* may initiate meningitis after open head trauma or a neurosurgical procedure, or in association with endocarditis. *Staphylococcus epidermidis* is the most common cause of an infected CSF shunt, followed in frequency by *S. aureus,* gram-negative bacilli, and diphtheroids.

Viral Meningitis

The exact incidence of viral meningitis is unknown. It peaks in incidence in late summer and early autumn (for the enteroviruses), and nearly all patients are under 40 years of age. A wide variety of etiologic agents is responsible, but the enteroviruses (Chapter 250) are most commonly implicated in the United States. Frequently encountered enteroviral isolates are ECHO virus 9,4,6,11,18,33 and coxsackievirus A9 or B4. Mumps is particularly common in Scandinavian series, but the incidence in the United States has declined dramatically since the introduction of mumps vaccine in 1967. A wide variety of other viruses may be responsible: herpes simplex types 1 and 2, poliovirus, adenoviruses, measles virus, cytomegalovirus, herpes zoster virus, lymphocytic choriomeningitis virus (LCM), hepatitis viruses, Epstein-Barr virus, human herpesvirus 6, and various arboviruses. The arboviruses produce an encephalitic clinical picture (Chapter 253). In addition, the human immunodeficiency virus type 1 (HIV-1) may cause aseptic meningitis, more commonly in the otherwise asymptomatic seropositive patient. Specific clues may aid in determining the causative organism: parotitis, pancreatitis, orchitis, or oophoritis with mumps; contact with mice or hamsters (winter peak) with LCM; a coexisting typical skin rash with varicella-zoster and measles; and genital lesions with herpes simplex type 2. Despite vigorous virologic culturing techniques, the cause of aseptic meningitis remains unknown in up to 70% of cases.

Fungal Meningitis

Numerous fungal species may infect the nervous system and produce meningitis, encephalitis, or brain abscess (Chapter 276). Some are encountered nearly exclusively in immunocompromised hosts or diabetic patients (e.g., *Aspergillus* species, *Mucor* species) (Chapter 276). Two species cause most fungal meningitis in the United States. Meningitis due to *Cryptococcus neoformans* (Chapter 276) is encountered in patients with lymphoma, the acquired immunodeficiency syndrome (AIDS), sarcoidosis, organ transplantation, collagen vascular diseases, diabetes mellitus, chronic hepatic failure, chronic renal failure, and patients receiving corticosteroid therapy; up to 50% of patients have no underlying disease. Currently patients with AIDS are in the highest risk group; clinical studies suggest that 6% to 13% of AIDS patients develop cryptococcal meningitis. *Candida albicans* meningitis is rare but may develop in debilitated patients receiving hyperalimentation or broad-spectrum antibiotics, including recent therapy for bacterial meningitis, and is also associated with prematurity, malignancy, chronic granulomatous disease, diabetes mellitus, thermal injuries, and insertion of central venous catheters. Disseminated coccidioidomycosis, histoplasmosis, or blastomycosis may involve the nervous system and become evident as subacute or chronic meningitis (Chapter 276).

PATHOGENESIS AND PATHOPHYSIOLOGY

Several factors affect the pathogenesis of bacterial meningitis: (1) host defense mechanisms; (2) microbial virulence factors; (3) microbial route of invasion of the CNS; and (4) pathophysiologic alterations as a result of CNS infection.

Mucosal Colonization and Systemic Invasion

Multiple defects in host defense (splenectomy, hypogammaglobulinemia, complement-deficiency states, defects in cell-mediated responses) may predispose the patient to the development of bacterial meningitis. The most important predisposing factors, however, are recent colonization of the nasopharynx by an appropriate pathogen and the absence of specific antibody. Many of the major meningeal pathogens possess surface characteristics that enhance mucosal colonization. The fimbriae of *N. meningitidis* mediate adhesion of the organism to nasopharyngeal epithelial cells. After attachment via a specific cell-surface receptor, meningococci are then transported across nonciliated nasopharyngeal columnar epithelial cells within a phagocytic vacuole. This series of events appears to be essential for development of invasive meningococcal disease. Fimbriae have also been implicated in the adhesion of *H. influenzae* to upper respiratory tract epithelial cells, although fimbriae have not been found on CSF or blood isolates of *H. influenzae* type b in patients with invasive disease.

Bacterial meningitis is more likely to occur if the nasopharynx has been recently colonized by *H. influenzae,* pneumococci, or meningococci when circulating bactericidal or opsonizing antibody

against the appropriate serotype is absent. The common occurrence of *E. coli* sepsis and meningitis in the premature infant may be related to delayed passage of opsonizing immunoglobulin G2 (IgG2) antibody to K1, which crosses the placenta only in the late stages of gestation.

Bacteremia

Once bacteria gain access to the bloodstream, they must overcome additional host defense mechanisms for survival. An important virulence factor in this regard is bacterial capsule, which through its ability to resist classic complement pathway bactericidal activity and inhibit neutrophil phagocytosis, facilitates development of a high-grade bacteremia. The host possesses several defense mechanisms to counteract the antiphagocytic activity of bacterial capsule. One is the alternative complement pathway, which is activated by the capsular polysaccharides of pneumococci, resulting in cleavage of C3 with attachment of C3b to the bacterial surface, thereby facilitating opsonization, phagocytosis, and intravascular clearance of the organism. Activation of the complement system is also an essential defense mechanism in protection from invasive disease caused by *N. meningitidis*. However, a recent study has shown that a qualitative relationship exists among the level of circulating meningococcal lipopolysaccharide (LPS), a fatal outcome, and the degree of complement activation, indicating that the prognosis is worse in patients with an intact complement system.

Meningeal Invasion

There are three potential bacterial routes of entry into the CSF: hematogenous, via a contiguous structure, and direct implantation. The hematogenous route is the most common; the primary foci of infection may be the nasopharynx, skin, lung, heart, gastrointestinal or genitourinary tract, umbilical stump, or elsewhere. Bacteria may enter the CSF through the dural sinuses or the choroid plexus—the precise mode of penetration is unknown. There is evidence that preexisting sterile inflammation (as in the cribriform plate area after nasopharyngeal colonization) may selectively localize organisms in these areas if bacteremia occurs.

Recent studies have shown that cells in the choroid plexus and/or cerebral capillaries possess receptors capable of mediating adherence of some meningeal pathogens, with subsequent transport into the subarachnoid space. For example, *E. coli* strains expressing S fimbriae bind to the luminal surface of the vascular endothelium and to the epithelium lining the choroid plexus and brain ventricles. Another pathogenic mechanism that may promote CNS invasion by meningeal pathogens is the association of the organism with circulating monocytes, with bacteria gaining access to the CSF in association with monocytes migrating along normal pathways.

When bacteria reach the CSF from contiguous structures (sinusitis, otitis media, mastoiditis, dental infection, petrositis, facial or scalp infections), three routes are possible: septic thrombosis of emissary veins with intracranial spread; association with secondary osteomyelitis; or via paraspinal lymphatics (not applicable to intracranial infection when lymphatics are absent). Bacteria may also be directly implanted within the CSF by a skull fracture (recent or remote, with CSF leak), lumbar puncture, neurosurgical procedure, or skin communication (meningomyelocele, dermal sinus, decubitus ulcer).

Alterations of the Blood-Brain Barrier

A major host defense against the development of meningitis is the integrity of the blood-brain barrier. The barrier separates the brain from the intravascular compartment and functions as a regulatory interface. An experimental rat model has been used to investigate the blood-brain barrier alterations that occur during bacterial meningitis. After the intracisternal inoculation of meningeal pathogens, there was a uniform host response at the level of the cerebral capillary endothelial cell characterized morphologically by an early and sustained increase in pinocytotic vesicle formation and a progressive increase in separation of intercellular tight junctions. These morphologic changes correlated functionally with increased penetration of albumin across the blood-brain barrier. Increased permeability occurred in the near absence of CSF leukocytes, although the presence of leukocytes augmented changes in permeability late in the disease course. The major bacterial virulence factor responsible for this increased permeability after challenge with gram-negative organisms is LPS, probably through LPS-induced release of various inflammatory cytokines (e.g., interleukin-1, tumor necrosis factor) within the CNS. The site of the blood-brain barrier injury during bacterial meningitis has recently been localized to the meningeal venules.

Bacterial Survival Within the Subarachnoid Space

Once bacteria enter the subarachnoid space, host defense mechanisms are inadequate to control the infection. Concentrations of antibody and complement are extremely low in normal CSF and in infected CSF early in the disease course; functional opsonic and bactericidal activity are often absent in CSF. These properties are necessary for adequate phagocytosis and killing of encapsulated organisms, including the most common etiologic agents of bacterial meningitis. It has been suggested that during bacterial meningitis, leukocyte proteases degrade complement components crossing the blood-brain barrier, further resulting in inefficient phagocytic activity at the site of infection.

Bacterial meningitis produces an inflammatory exudate within the subarachnoid space that may exert both beneficial and detrimental effects. A high bacterial concentration with a low leukocyte concentration in purulent CSF is associated with a poor prognosis in meningitis. However, a study of experimental pneumococcal meningitis in leukopenic animals found no differences in bacterial growth rates in normal as compared with leukopenic animals, suggesting that bacterial eradication from the CSF during the early phase of bacterial meningitis is not leukocyte dependent.

The pathway of neutrophil traversal into the CSF is unknown. Adherence of neutrophils to vascular endothelium may be a necessary prerequisite. Pretreatment of endothelial cells with various inflammatory cytokines has induced formation of specific adhesion molecules such as intercellular adhesion molecule 1 and endothelial leukocyte adhesion molecule 1, although these adhesion molecules have not yet been demonstrated conclusively in cerebral endothelium. Recent studies in an experimental rabbit model have suggested that the intravenous inoculation of a monoclonal antibody (IB4) against the CD18 family of integrin receptors on leukocytes blocks accumulation of leukocytes in CSF, despite intracisternal challenge with meningeal pathogens or their potential virulence factors. Although the site of leukocyte traversal into CSF is unknown, most evidence supports entry through postcapillary venules. Purulent CSF is chemotactic for leukocytes in vitro. One putative substance has been identified as C5a, and the intracisternal inoculation of C5a into rabbits causes a rapid, early influx of leukocytes into CSF.

Induction of Subarachnoid Space Inflammation

The induction of a subarachnoid space inflammatory response is a critical event leading to many of the pathophysiologic consequences of bacterial meningitis. Although bacterial capsule is crucial for intravascular and subarachnoid space survival of meningeal pathogens, capsular polysaccharides are remarkably noninflammatory. Recent studies have investigated the surface-exposed virulence factors of meningeal pathogens responsible for induction of this inflammatory response. For *S. pneumoniae* it is predominantly the cell wall, and for *H. influenzae* type b it is LPS. Release of these virulence factors after bacteriolytic therapy may further augment the subarachnoid space inflammatory response. In addition, these virulence factors elicit inflammation through the CSF release of inflammatory cytokines such as interleukin-1 and tumor necrosis factor. In fact, increased CSF concentrations of tumor necrosis factor may be specific for bacterial meningitis, as tumor necrosis factor concentrations, measured in mice and humans with either bacterial or viral meningitis, were elevated in CSF only during bacterial meningitis. Other inflammatory cytokines, such as interleukin-6, interleukin-8, and interleukin-10, have also been detected in the CSF of patients with bacterial meningitis, although additional studies are needed to precisely define their contributions to disease. Elevated CSF concentra-

tions of platelet-activating factor have been observed in children with *H. influenzae* meningitis, correlating with bacterial density, and CSF LPS and tumor necrosis factor (TNF) concentrations; these elevated concentrations of TNF and platelet-activating factor were associated with severity of disease.

Increased Intracranial Pressure

A major pathophysiologic consequence of bacterial meningitis is the development of increased intracranial pressure, primarily due to the development of cerebral edema; the edema may be vasogenic, cytotoxic, and/or interstitial in origin. Vasogenic cerebral edema is primarily a consequence of increased blood-brain barrier permeability (see earlier discussion). Cytotoxic cerebral edema results from swelling of the cellular elements of the brain, most likely due to release of toxic factors from neutrophils and/or bacteria. Interstitial edema occurs secondary to obstruction of normal CSF pathways as in hydrocephalus. CSF outflow resistance (defined as factors that inhibit the flow of CSF from the subarachnoid space to the major dural sinuses) has been shown to be markedly elevated in experimental animal models of bacterial meningitis, suggesting that attenuation of the normal CSF absorptive mechanisms during meningitis may decrease the ability of the brain to compensate in situations of increased intracranial pressure. These concepts have been solidified in greater detail by measuring brain water content (indicative of cerebral edema if elevated), CSF lactate, and CSF pressure in animals with pneumococcal meningitis. All three parameters were elevated in infected animals, and early, specific antibiotic therapy normalized CSF pressure and brain edema.

Alterations in Cerebral Blood Flow

Cerebral blood flow may also be altered in patients with bacterial meningitis. Intracranial vessels passing through the inflammatory exudate are often involved with secondary parenchymal changes (e.g., infarction, hemorrhage, abscess). In an infant rhesus monkey model of *H. influenzae* meningitis, certain areas of the cerebral cortex (postcentral, temporal, and occipital) were hypoperfused relative to the hypothalamus and midbrain, whereas the brainstem may be hyperperfused, suggesting that one of the initial physiologic changes in *H. influenzae* meningitis is cerebral cortical hypoperfusion with resultant cerebral anoxia. Recent studies in an experimental model of pneumococcal meningitis have demonstrated disturbances in cerebral autoregulation, in which even minor fluctuations of mean arterial blood pressure are likely to have adverse consequences for patients with meningitis, with risk of brain injury from either transient hypotension or hypertension. Blood flow alterations may lead to regional hypoxia, increased brain lactate concentration secondary to utilization of glucose by anaerobic glycolysis, and CSF acidosis, which may be precursors to encephalopathy.

The transport capacity of the barrier is also disturbed, and this, in concert with an increased utilization by intracranial tissues, is the major cause of the depressed CSF glucose content (hypoglycorrhachia) seen in bacterial meningitis. Glucose utilization by microorganisms or leukocytes within the CSF appears to play only a minor role in this process.

Neuronal Injury

Recent data have accumulated suggesting that reactive oxygen species may contribute to the cerebral edema, increased intracranial pressure, changes in regional blood flow, and neuronal injury during bacterial meningitis. In experimental animal models of pneumococcal meningitis, therapy with conjugated superoxide dismutase, deferoxamine, or catalase attenuated the increase in regional cerebral blood flow, brain water content, and intracranial pressure. Nitric oxide may also be important; it has been shown to account for regional cerebral blood flow changes and pial arteriolar dilation in the early phase of meningitis and is involved as a mediator of brain edema and meningeal inflammation.

A potential role of excitatory amino acids in the pathogenesis of brain injury in bacterial meningitis has also been proposed. In an experimental animal model of pneumococcal meningitis, elevated CSF concentrations of glutamate, aspartate, glycine, taurine, and alanine, as well as elevated glutamate concentrations in the brain extracellular space, were detected, suggesting that excitotoxic neuronal injury may play an important role in bacterial meningitis.

CLINICAL MANIFESTATIONS

The classic findings in adults with meningitis (Table 239-2) include fever, headache, nuchal rigidity, and signs of cerebral dysfunction. Shaking chills, profuse sweats, weakness, anorexia, nausea, vomiting, myalgias of the lower extremities or back (especially with meningococcal disease), and photophobia are common. Patients able to speak usually describe the headache as generalized and extremely severe. Neck stiffness may be subtle or marked and accompanied by Brudzinski's and Kernig's signs. Cerebral dysfunction is manifested as confusion, delirium, or a declining level of consciousness, from lethargy to coma. Cranial nerve palsies (principally involving cranial nerves III, IV, VI, and VII) occur in approximately 10% of patients, whereas seizures (due to the underlying disease, fever in infants, or penicillin neurotoxicity) are somewhat more frequent. Focal cerebral signs are unusual (10% to 20%) and include hemiparesis, visual field defects, and dysphasia. These may be transitory (e.g., Todd's paralysis) or may appear late in the disease course as a result of the development of intracranial venous thrombophlebitis, subdural empyema, brain abscess, hemorrhage, or infarction. Signs of increased intracranial pressure (coma, hypertension, bradycardia, third nerve palsy) appear late in the disease course and are ominous prognostic signs. Papilledema is rare and should suggest an alternate diagnosis (e.g., intracranial mass lesion).

A rash develops in approximately 50% of meningococcal infections. An erythematous maculopapular eruption, chiefly centrifugal in location (e.g., volar aspect of the forearms, wrists, ankles, and occasionally the palms and soles), is present early and is easily confused with numerous other entities, including enteroviral aseptic meningitis syndromes. A petechial, purpuric, or ecchymotic rash is suggestive of meningococcal infection but may be seen in other types of meningitis due to ECHO virus type 9, *Acinetobacter* species, *S. aureus,* and, rarely, *H. influenzae* or *S. pneumoniae.* An indistinguishable skin rash may be present in Rocky Mountain spotted fever, *S. aureus* endocarditis, and rapidly overwhelming *S. pneumoniae* or *H. influenzae* bacteremia in patients who have undergone splenectomy. In patients who have suffered basilar skull fractures in which a dural fistula is produced between the subarachnoid space and the nasal cavity, paranasal sinuses, or middle ear, meningitis is usually caused by *S. pneumoniae.* These patients commonly come to medical attention with rhinorrhea or otorrhea due to a CSF leak, and a persistent defect is a common explanation for recurrent bacterial meningitis. Patients with *L. monocytogenes* meningitis have an increased tendency to have seizures and focal deficits early in the course of infection, and some patients may come to medical attention with ataxia, cranial nerve palsies, or nystagmus caused by rhomboencephalitis, although there may be no evidence of parenchymal brain involvement.

The classic findings may be less apparent in several clinical settings. Neonates usually do not demonstrate nuchal rigidity and may have normal temperatures. The only clues may be listlessness, high-pitched crying, fretfulness, refusal to feed, irritability, and other nonspecific abnormalities. Full or tense fontanels are a late sign of disease and are often absent. Similarly, elderly patients with various underlying conditions (e.g., diabetes mellitus, cardiopulmonary disease) may become lethargic or obtunded; thus other clues to the meningitis, including fever, may not be revealed. Signs of meningeal irritation are variable, and the onset may be insidious. The postneurosurgical patient or the patient who has undergone head trauma also presents a unique clinical situation, as these patients already have many of the symptoms and signs from their underlying disease process that are similar to those seen in patients with meningitis. When doubt arises, lumbar puncture is indicated. Meningitis is more common in the febrile alcoholic patient, and an altered mental state should not be ascribed to delirium tremens or other causes unless meningitis has been excluded by CSF examination.

Nearly all the preceding findings may be present with viral meningitis (Chapter 250), although the illness is usually milder, with less derangement of higher integrative functions and fewer cranial nerve palsies, focal neurologic deficits, and seizures. Extracranial manifes-

Table 239-2   Symptoms and signs in bacterial meningitis

FINDINGS	RELATIVE FREQUENCY (%)
Headache	≥90
Fever	≥90
Meningismus	≥85
Brudzinski's sign	≥50
Kernig's sign	≥50
Altered sensorium	>80
Vomiting	~35
Seizures	~30
Petechiae	~50
Focal findings	10-20
Cranial nerves	~10
Hemiparesis	<5
Papilledema	<1
Myalgia	30-60
Other suppurative foci (pneumonia, otitis, sinusitis, etc.)	0-30

tations such as herpangina, exanthems, parotitis, or pleurodynia may suggest a viral cause.

The mode of onset has important diagnostic and prognostic implications. Approximately 20% of all patients come to medical attention with acute disease of less than 24 hours' duration and rapidly progressive signs. In almost all these patients, the disease is due to pyogenic bacteria and requires rapid therapeutic intervention (see Treatment). Despite such intervention, however, mortality remains high (≥50%). In the subacute form, signs and symptoms have been present for 1 to 7 or more days, the differential diagnosis is extensive, and mortality, even when a bacterial cause is established, is lower (≤25%). The disease in these patients is commonly preceded by an upper respiratory tract infection (e.g., pharyngitis), which may have resolved by the time meningitis becomes evident. The symptoms and signs of another infectious focus (e.g., otitis, sinusitis, mastoiditis, pneumonia, endocarditis) may be evident on admission.

A variety of epidemiologic and clinical features may be useful in predicting the etiologic agent in meningitis (Table 239-3).

LABORATORY INVESTIGATION
Blood Studies

Certain serum chemistry studies and blood tests are helpful in the diagnosis and management of meningitis. Hyponatremia is common and may indicate the presence of the syndrome of inappropriate antidiuretic hormone secretion. Severe renal failure necessitates an alteration in dosage of many antibiotics. A leukocytosis with a shift to the left suggests a bacterial origin, but there is a large overlap. In patients with petechiae, purpura, hypotension, or shock, clotting variables may reflect disseminated intravascular coagulation. Blood cultures should be obtained in all patients; they are positive in 40% to 80% of cases of bacterial meningitis and are occasionally positive when CSF cultures are negative. If a petechial rash is present, aspiration of the lesion may demonstrate the pathogen when examined by Gram's stain. Wright's stain of the buffy coat (or even a peripheral blood smear) may reveal intraphagocytic meningococci (or pneumococci) in fulminant cases, even when the CSF stains are negative.

Radiographic Studies

If pyogenic meningitis is suspected or established, radiographic studies of the sinuses, mastoids, and chest should be obtained to exclude suppurative foci in these locations. When papilledema or focal neurologic signs are present, a computed tomography (CT) scan is necessary in the initial evaluation to exclude a space-occupying intracranial lesion (e.g., brain abscess, subdural empyema) before attempting lumbar puncture. CT or magnetic resonance imaging (MRI) may also be useful in patients with prolonged fever several days after initiation of antimicrobial therapy, or in those with prolonged obtundation or coma, new or recurrent seizure activity, signs of increased intracranial pressure, or focal neurologic deficits. MRI is better than CT

Table 239-3   Epidemiologic and clinical clues to the etiologic agent in acute meningitis

FEATURE	MICROORGANISM(S) SUSPECTED
Age	See Table 239-1
Seasonal incidence	
Winter, spring	Meningococci, pneumococci, mumps, LCM
Late summer, fall	Enteroviruses, arboviruses, leptospires
Sibling with meningitis	Meningococci, *Haemophilus influenzae*
Military recruit	Meningococci, *Mycoplasma* sp., adenovirus
Epidemic	Meningococci, enteroviruses, arboviruses
Swimming, freshwater lake	Amebas (*Naegleria* sp.)
Contact with water, rats, domestic animals	Leptospires
Contact with mice, hamsters	LCM virus
Contact with tuberculosis	*Mycobacterium tuberculosis*
Contact with pigeon excreta	*Cryptococcus neoformans*
Recurrent meningitis	Pneumococci
During, after treatment of bacterial meningitis	*Candida* sp.
Geographic area	*Coccidioides immitis*
Homosexuality, intravenous drug abuse	HIV
Associated condition	
Alcoholism	Pneumococci, *Listeria monocytogenes*, *H. influenzae*
Diabetes mellitus	Pneumococci, Enterobacteriaceae, *Staphylococcus aureus*, *Cryptococcus neoformans*, rhinocerebral mucormycosis (with acidosis)
Cancer	Enterobacteriaceae, pneumococci, *Listeria monocytogenes*, *Cryptococcus neoformans*, *S. aureus*, carcinomatous abscess (*Aspergillus* + *Nocardia* sp.)
Steroids, immunosuppressives	*Listeria, Cryptococcus neoformans; M. tuberculosis*
AIDS	*Cryptococcus neoformans*, toxoplasmosis, PMLE, and others
Sickle cell anemia	Pneumococci
Splenectomy	Pneumococci, *H. influenzae*
Hypogammaglobulinemia	Pneumococci, *H. influenzae*
Skull fracture (closed)	Pneumococci, *H. influenzae*, Enterobacteriaceae
Skull fracture (open) or craniotomy	Enterobacteriaceae, *S. aureus*, pneumococci, clostridia (rare)
CSF otorrhea or rhinorrhea	Pneumococci, *H. influenzae*, Enterobacteriaceae, *S. aureus*
CSF shunt	*Staphylococcus epidermidis*, *S. aureus*, Enterobacteriaceae, diphtheroids
Strongyloidiasis	Enterobacteriaceae
Associated infections and physical findings	
Pharyngitis	Viruses, *H. influenzae*, meningococci, pneumococci
Otitis media	*H. influenzae*, pneumococci, mixed anaerobes
Malignant otitis externa	*Pseudomonas aeruginosa*
Sinusitis	Pneumococci, *H. influenzae*, anaerobes
Pneumonia	Pneumococci, meningococci
Endocarditis	Pneumococci, *S. aureus*
Cellulitis	Streptococci, *S. aureus*
Arthritis	Meningococci, pneumococci, *S. aureus*, *H. influenzae* (rare)
Brain abscess, subdural empyema	Anaerobes, *S. aureus*, Enterobacteriaceae
Petechiae, purpura	Meningococci, ECHO virus 9, Rocky Mountain spotted fever, *S. aureus* endocarditis, pneumococci or *H. influenzae* (splenectomy)
"Typical" skin rash	Measles, varicella
Herpes progenitalis	Herpesvirus type 2
Conjunctival suffusion	Leptospires
Parotitis	Mumps
Choroid tubercles	*M. tuberculosis*

AIDS, Acquired immunodeficiency syndrome; *CSF,* cerebrospinal fluid; *HIV,* human immunodeficiency virus; *LCM,* lymphocytic choriomeningitis virus; *PMLE,* progressive multifocal leukoencephalopathy.

for evaluation of subdural effusions, cortical infarctions, and cerebritis, although it is more difficult to obtain an MRI scan in a critically ill patient, limiting its usefulness in many patients with bacterial meningitis.

Cerebrospinal Fluid Examination

The diagnosis of meningitis rests on careful examination of the CSF. The opening pressure is elevated (e.g., 200 to 300 mm H$_2$O) in virtually all cases of meningitis. Values over 600 mm H$_2$O suggest extensive cerebral edema, intracranial suppurative foci, or communicating hydrocephalus due to the exudate in the subarachnoid space.

In acute, untreated, bacterial meningitis, the CSF white blood cell count usually ranges from 100 to 10,000 cells/mm^3, with a median count of approximately 2000 and polymorphonuclear leukocyte predominance. Very high white blood cell counts ($\geq$50,000 cells/mm^3) are unusual and suggest intraventricular rupture of a brain abscess. Occasionally, the white blood cell count may be very low (0 to 20 cells/mm^3) while the CSF is turbid because of a high bacterial concentration; the prognosis is poor in such cases. Therefore, Gram's

stain and culture should be performed on the CSF from all patients with suspected meningitis even if the cell count is zero. A lymphocytic predominance is found in the majority of cases with the aseptic meningitis syndrome (Table 239-4), and this may be helpful in differential diagnosis. The CSF protein concentration is elevated in virtually all types of meningitis (Table 239-4) and often exceeds 100 mg/dl. Huge elevations (>1000 mg/dl) suggest subarachnoid block or inadvertent insertion of the spinal needle into an epidural or subdural abscess instead of the subarachnoid space. Similar elevations are also commonly seen in gram-negative bacillary ventriculitis in infants. A CSF glucose value of 40 mg/dl or less, or a CSF blood sugar ratio of less than 0.5, is found in approximately 60% of bacterial meningitis patients and suggests this diagnosis. However, a wide variety of other conditions can produce hypoglycorrhachia of this magnitude (Table 239-4) and must be considered: fungal or tuberculous meningitis and rare cases of viral meningitis, sarcoidosis, meningeal carcinomatosis, hypoglycemia, and subarachnoid hemorrhage. A recent analysis found that a CSF glucose value less than 34 mg/dl, a CSF blood glucose ratio less than 0.23, a CSF protein concentration greater than 220 mg/dl, more than 2000 CSF leukocytes/mm^3, or more than

1180 CSF neutrophils/mm^3 was an individual predictor of bacterial, as opposed to viral, meningitis with 99% certainty or better.

Bacterial concentration is usually very high (generally, $\geq 10^5$ colony-forming units (CFU)/ml and often $\geq 10^7$ CFU/ml) and correlates directly with the antigen titer in the CSF. Higher values are associated with a more prolonged and severe illness and perhaps a worse prognosis. Gram's stain permits identification of the causative agent in about 80% of patients with untreated bacterial meningitis (Plates VIII-8 and VIII-9). The probability of detecting the organism through staining techniques correlates with bacterial concentrations in CSF; CSF bacterial concentrations less than or equal to 10^3 CFU/ml are associated with poor microscopic results (organisms seen 25% of the time), whereas microscopy is positive in 97% of cases when CSF bacterial concentrations are greater than or equal to 10^5 CFU/ml. The recent administration of antibiotics reduces this frequency to approximately 60% and may result in diagnostic confusion. If sufficient numbers of organisms are present, a positive quellung reaction with specific antisera establishes a pneumococcal origin. Cultures are positive in 70% to 85% of cases of bacterial meningitis but are often negative in tuberculous or fungal meningitis (Table 239-4).

Many CSF enzymes (e.g., lactate dehydrogenase, glutamic-oxaloacetic transaminase, creatine kinase) are increased in bacterial meningitis, but the precise tissue(s) of origin remains unknown. Because these elevations may also accompany other conditions, none of these enzymatic assays is used in routine diagnosis. Lysozyme is present in increased concentrations in the CSF in a wide variety of CNS infections and is not diagnostically useful. The CSF lactic acid concentration is increased in bacterial meningitis, whereas it is usually normal in "aseptic" meningitis due to viruses. This test may be helpful (measured by gas-liquid chromatography or various simpler chemical methods) in differentiating partially treated bacterial meningitis (or others with a negative Gram's stain) from a viral syndrome.

Several specific diagnostic tests have been developed. The lysate of the amebocytes of the horseshoe crab *(Limulus)* gels on exposure to small quantities of bacterial endotoxin (≤ 10 ng/ml). A positive *Limulus* lysate test result indicates that a gram-negative organism is the cause of the meningitis (e.g., meningococci, *H. influenzae,* gram-negative bacilli), but speciation is not possible.

Counterimmunoelectrophoresis (CIE) is available for the detection of specific antigens in the CSF due to meningococci (serogroups A or C), *H. influenzae* type b, pneumococci (omniserum representing 83 serotypes), type III group B streptococci, and *E. coli* K1. These tests are variably sensitive (positive in 62% to 95%) but highly specific. Cross-reactions may occur. The tests may be useful in the rapid diagnosis (results generally available in 1 hour) of suspected bacterial meningitis when Gram's stains are negative.

Recently, several new tests using staphylococcal coagglutination or latex agglutination have been described for detection of bacterial capsular polysaccharide antigen in the CSF of patients with meningitis attributable to one of the three major pathogens. These newer tests are both more rapid and more sensitive (they detect $\cong 1$ ng/ml) than CIE and are commercially available (e.g., Directigen, Bactigen, Wellcogen). They are less expensive than CIE, require less technical sophistication for performance in the laboratory, and can be applied in outpatient (and even field) settings. Currently available latex agglutination tests detect the antigens of *H. influenzae* type b, *S. pneumoniae, N. meningitidis, E. coli* K1, and group B streptococci. However, many of the kits do not include tests for group B meningococcus, and others probably are poor detectors of this antigen because of the limited immunogenicity of group B meningococcal polysaccharide. These procedures should be performed on compatible CSF specimens with a negative Gram's stain. Polymerase chain reaction (PCR) has also been used to amplify DNA from patients with meningitis caused by *N. meningitidis* and *L. monocytogenes.* In one small study of CSF samples from patients with meningococcal meningitis the sensitivity and specificity of PCR were both 91%. Further refinements in PCR may demonstrate its usefulness in the diagnosis of bacterial meningitis when the CSF Gram's stain, bacterial antigen test results, and cultures are negative.

Because culture and India ink preparations are positive in only $\cong 50\%$ of cases of cryptococcal meningitis, detection of cryptococcal polysaccharide antigen in CSF, serum, or urine is very helpful in the diagnosis of this infection (Chapter 233).

DIFFERENTIAL DIAGNOSIS

As noted, multiple infectious and noninfectious processes may be responsible for the acute meningitis syndrome. Bacterial meningitis must be recognized rapidly and separated from the aseptic meningitis syndrome by the epidemiologic, clinical, and laboratory clues that have been enumerated. This differentiation often depends on a thorough examination of the CSF (see Table 239-4). Because many other causes of the aseptic meningitis syndrome also require aggressive therapy, up to 50% of patients with a presumptive diagnosis of bacterial meningitis will have received antibiotics before the initial lumbar puncture. Although this practice may obscure Gram's stain or culture results (usually, 60% or more positive), usually a granulocytic

Table 239-4   Typical cerebrospinal fluid findings in acute meningitis

TEST	BACTERIAL MENINGITIS	ASEPTIC MENINGITIS SYNDROME
Cell count	<100 to >10,000, usually 1000 to 5000	<10 to >1000, usually 100 to 500
Percentage of granulocytes	≥ 80	$\leq 50^*$
Protein	100 to 500, occasionally >1000	100 to 500
Glucose	≤ 40	Normal†
Gram's stain	Positive 75% to 80%	Negative‡
Culture	Positive 70% to 85%	Negative§
Acid-fast stain	Negative	Positive in tuberculosis ($\leq 25\%$)
India ink	Negative	Positive in cryptococcal disease (50% to 75%)
Cytology	Negative	Positive in cryptococcal or neoplastic ($\geq 70\%$) disease
Wet mount	Usually negative	Positive in amebic meningitis
Counterimmunoelectrophoresis	Positive‖	Negative
Lactate	Positive (≥ 35 mg/dl)	Negative
Limulus lysate	Positive¶	Negative
Cryptococcal antigen	Negative	Positive in cryptococcal ($\geq 95\%$) disease
Enzymes (e.g., lactate dehydrogenase)	Often elevated	Often elevated
C-reactive protein	Positive	Negative

*May be $\geq 50\%$ in early tuberculous, fungal, amebic, spirochetal, or viral meningitis; in tuberculous meningitis an initially lymphocytic predominance may become neutrophilic with therapy.
†Commonly, cerebrospinal fluid glucose level is low in meningitis due to *Mycobacterium tuberculosis, Cryptococcus neoformans,* and other fungi; neoplasia; chemicals; sarcoidosis ($\sim 10\%$); syphilis (50% to 55%); and subarachnoid hemorrhage. It is under 40 mg/dl in less than 5% of viral cases (especially mumps and lymphocytic choriomeningitis virus).
‡May be positive in fungal meningitis (e.g., 40% with *Candida* sp.).
§Positive in tuberculous ($\geq 80\%$) and cryptococcal (50%) meningitis, and, rarely, in viral syndromes.
‖Positive response rates on CIE, staphylococcal coagglutination, and latex agglutination vary with infecting organisms (see text).
¶The *Limulus* lysate test is positive only in gram-negative meningitis ($\geq 90\%$).

pleocytosis, high protein, and hypoglycorrhachia persist in the CSF and suggest this diagnosis. Other procedures (e.g., CIE, staphylococcal coagglutination, and latex agglutination; *Limulus* lysate test; CSF lactate concentration) may be very helpful in differentiating this entity from viral, tuberculous, or fungal meningitis.

Tuberculous meningitis (Chapter 273) usually becomes evident in a subacute or chronic aseptic form, but an acute presentation with a granulocytic predominance in the CSF may occur in immunosuppressed hosts or during the course of miliary tuberculosis. Cranial nerve palsies (presumably due to the predominantly basilar exudate) are common. The CSF protein may be high, and hypoglycorrhachia is usual. Smears of the CSF for acid-fast bacilli are usually negative (≥75%), and cultures, although eventually positive in more than 80% of cases, are not helpful in the acute situation. Other procedures may be necessary to secure this diagnosis (e.g., a tuberculin skin test, a chest x-ray, or bone marrow or liver biopsies). The occurrence of meningitis with hyponatremia and a negative CSF Gram's stain is suggestive of tuberculous meningitis. Several rapid diagnostic tests are under development, the most promising of which are the presence of tuberculostearic acid in CSF and use of PCR to detect fragments of mycobacterial DNA in CSF.

Meningitis due to fungi is also usually chronic and progressive, but acute presentations do occur. Epidemiologic features, such as treatment for bacterial meningitis, hyperalimentation (*Candida* sp.) geographic locale (*Coccidioides* sp., and rarely, *Histoplasma* sp.), lymphoma, or immunosuppression (cryptococci), may suggest the diagnosis. In the acute presentation, the CSF findings may be indistinguishable from those of bacterial or tuberculous meningitis, but a lymphocytic pleocytosis or an aseptic picture is usually evident. Cryptococci may be seen on India ink or cytologic preparations; they are cultured in the majority of cases. The yield is enhanced if large volumes of CSF (e.g., >10 ml) are cultured. Cultures of blood, urine, sputum, or stool may also be positive. Cryptococcal polysaccharide antigen can be detected in the CSF by latex fixation in approximately 95% of cases; serum cryptococcal polysaccharide antigen may also be detected, particularly in severely immunocompromised patients (e.g., those with AIDS), although the value of the serum polysaccharide antigen for screening patients suspected of having meningeal disease has not been established. Yeast cells are present on CSF smear in 40% of cases of *Candida* meningitis, and most cases are confirmed rapidly by culture. Coccidioidal meningitis is rarely acute, and the CSF usually demonstrates a lymphocytic predominance. The skin test is usually negative, but the presence of complement-fixing antibody to the causative organism in the CSF is confirmatory in approximately 95% of cases; CSF complement-fixing antibodies are present in at least 70% of patients with early meningitis and are obtained from virtually all patients as disease progresses.

Parameningeal foci of infection, such as epidural abscess, subdural empyema, or brain abscess, are often suggested by the clinical setting (Chapter 240), but they may also produce the CSF findings typical of aseptic meningitis. Other procedures (e.g., CT or MRI, myelograms) are necessary for diagnosis. A combined surgical and medical (antibiotic) approach is usually required.

CNS syphilis (Chapter 274) may be manifested in many different ways; acute meningitis may be the first clue to this disease in 25% of patients. The CSF reflects the typical abnormalities of the aseptic meningitis syndrome, although hypoglycorrhachia is present in 55% of patients. The presentation is usually subacute, and cranial nerve palsies or seizures are common. Serologic tests for syphilis must be performed on the serum and CSF in all cases of the aseptic meningitis syndrome. Although the specificity of the CSF VDRL for the diagnosis of neurosyphilis is high, the sensitivity is low (reactive tests in only 30% to 70% of patients), so a nonreactive result does not exclude the diagnosis. Based on difficulties in the diagnosis of neurosyphilis, elevation of CSF concentrations of white blood cells or protein in the appropriate clinical and serologic setting should lead to initiation of appropriate antimicrobial therapy. A transient deterioration in neurologic function on initiation of penicillin therapy (Jarisch-Herxheimer reaction) also suggests this diagnosis.

Lyme disease, due to *Borrelia burgdorferi*, may produce meningitis during its second stage (weeks to months after the initial infection) in which patients have symptoms of headache, stiff neck, nausea, vomiting, malaise, and fever of several weeks' duration that may alternate with periods of milder symptoms. Serum test results for antibodies to *B. burgdorferi* are usually positive in the majority of cases during this stage.

Free-living amebas (*Naegleria* sp.) may produce a fulminant, acute purulent meningitis with a high fatality rate (Chapter 279). The diagnosis is suggested by a history of swimming in warm freshwater lakes or swimming pools and is confirmed by noting freely motile amebas on fresh preparations of unrefrigerated, unspun CSF. Despite therapy with amphotericin B and miconazole, mortality remains high.

Herpes simplex type 1 infection of the CNS usually produces progressive, often fatal encephalitis, whereas herpes simplex type 2 infection may become evident as a progressive meningoencephalitis in neonates or immunosuppressed patients or as a benign aseptic meningitis in normal adults (Chapter 255). The definitive diagnosis of type 1 infections usually requires a brain biopsy, although CT, MRI, or electroencephalogram findings localizable to the temporal lobe are suggestive. Since herpes simplex type 1 remains the only viral CNS infection for which antiviral therapy (i.e., acyclovir) has been proven to be beneficial in controlled clinical trials, an empiric course should be administered for patients with presumed viral encephalitis; a brain biopsy is only indicated in unusual cases. PCR for the detection of herpes simplex virus in CSF is promising as an aid to early diagnosis. Adenine arabinoside and acyclovir have reduced mortality in these infections; acyclovir is recommended based on its ease of administration and good safety profile.

Neurologic disease associated with HIV may take the form of encephalitis, meningitis, ataxia, or myelopathy. Aseptic meningitis usually occurs in the asymptomatic seropositive patient, although it may manifest before seroconversion or in patients with full-blown AIDS. The CSF typically shows a mononuclear pleocytosis with normal glucose level and slightly elevated protein concentration. Direct HIV infection of the meninges is the presumed cause of the meningitis, as the virus is readily isolated from the CSF.

The neurologic complications of bacterial endocarditis (Chapter 24) are myriad and may overshadow other stigmata of the disease. An acute meningitis syndrome with a purulent CSF (often negative on culture) may represent the "cerebritis" that is particularly common in acute staphylococcal endocarditis. Careful attention to other peripheral manifestations of this disease, heart murmurs, or splenomegaly usually suggests this disorder.

Multiple causes of the aseptic meningitis syndrome do not require antimicrobial or surgical therapy; the most important of these are viral (Chapter 250) and leptospiral (Chapter 275) meningitis. The epidemiologic clues to these infections are outlined in Table 239-3; the CSF findings are usually typical of the aseptic meningitis syndrome (Table 239-4), with a lymphocytic CSF pleocytosis, mildly elevated protein concentration, and normal glucose level. Occasionally, the CSF white blood cell count is high (e.g., ≥1000 cells/mm^3 with LCM virus), and glucose level is depressed in up to 5% of cases (mumps, LCM, occasionally ECHO viruses). Viral isolation should be attempted by throat, stool, and CSF cultures, although the CSF culture is rarely positive. If an agent is isolated, diagnosis is confirmed by a fourfold difference in antibody between acute and convalescent sera. Although leptospires can occasionally be cultured on special media or seen by dark-field examination (e.g., of urine), the diagnosis usually rests on specific serologic procedures.

A wide variety of other, presumably noninfectious processes may produce the aseptic meningitis syndrome, including neoplasia, cerebritis in systemic lupus erythematosus, granulomatous angiitis, sarcoidosis, lymphomatoid granulomatosis, cyst-related meningitis, chemically induced meningitis (e.g., radiographic dyes or anesthetics), and various poorly understood chronic or recurrent syndromes (Mollaret, Behçet's, Vogt-Koyanagi-Harada). These are rarely confused with acute bacterial meningitis.

TREATMENT

The successful management of the acute meningitis syndrome is based on the following principles: (1) recognition that meningitis is present (through an appreciation of the clinical setting, physical findings, and presumed etiologic agents) (Table 239-4); (2) rapid identification of the pathogen (through rapid techniques of CSF examination, for example, Gram's stain, CIE and agglutination tests, *Limulus*

Table 239-5　Antibiotics of choice for bacterial meningitis

ORGANISM	ANTIBIOTIC(S) OF CHOICE	ALTERNATIVES
Neisseria meningitidis	Penicillin G	Ampicillin, chloramphenicol, third-generation cephalosporin‡
Streptococcus pneumoniae		
PCN MIC <0.1 µg/ml	Penicillin	Third-generation cephalosporin‡
PCN MIC 0.1-1 µg/ml	Third-generation cephalosporin‡	Vancomycin, meropenem
PCN MIC ≥2 µg/ml	Vancomycin plus a third-generation cephalosporin‡	Meropenem
Haemophilus influenzae (β-lactamase–negative)	Ampicillin	Chloramphenicol, third-generation cephalosporin‡
H. influenzae (β-lactamase–positive)	Cefotaxime or ceftriaxone	Chloramphenicol
Enterobacteriaceae	Third-generation cephalosporin‡	Aminoglycosides, extended-spectrum penicillins, aztreonam, quinolones, trimethoprim-sulfamethoxazole
Pseudomonas aeruginosa	Ceftazidime (? plus an aminoglycoside*)	Extended-spectrum penicillin plus an aminoglycoside, aztreonam, quinolones
S. agalactiae	Penicillin G or ampicillin (? plus an aminoglycoside*)	Third-generation cephalosporin, chloramphenicol
Listeria monocytogenes	Ampicillin (? plus an aminoglycoside*)	Trimethoprim-sulfamethoxazole
Staphylococcus aureus (methicillin-sensitive)	Nafcillin or oxacillin	Vancomycin (? plus rifampin)
S. aureus (methicillin-resistant)	Vancomycin	Trimethoprim-sulfamethoxazole
Staphylococcus epidermidis	Vancomycin (? plus rifampin)	Penicillin G
Mycobacterium tuberculosis	Isoniazid plus rifampin plus pyrazinamide (? plus ethambutol)	Quinolones, ethionamide, imipenem, amoxicillin–clavulanic acid
Candida sp.	Amphotericin B	Fluconazole
Cryptococcus neoformans	Amphotericin B (? plus 5-fluorocytosine)	Fluconazole
Coccidioides immitis	Amphotericin B†	Fluconazole

PCN MIC, Penicillin minimum inhibitory concentration.
*Value of aminoglycoside addition unproved.
†Intraventricular administration is usually required in addition to systemic route.
‡Cefotaxime or ceftriaxone.

lysate test, lactate level); (3) rapid initiation of therapy; and (4) observation and treatment of complications (e.g., shock, disseminated intravascular coagulation) and sequelae.

Initial Approach

Once meningitis is recognized, the initial approach is designed to optimize early therapy. If the mode of onset is acute, pyogenic meningitis is likely, and the prognosis is less favorable than if the onset had been more prolonged. The first consideration is the rapid (within 30 minutes of encountering the patient) initiation of therapy. The same procedure should be followed if the patient is comatose.

If focal neurologic signs are absent, the next step is rapid evaluation of the CSF through a lumbar puncture and appropriate diagnostic tests. If focal neurologic signs are present, a CT scan should be obtained immediately to exclude a brain abscess or other intracranial mass lesion, as lumbar puncture is relatively contraindicated in this setting. If there is any delay in obtaining a CT scan, empiric antibiotics should be started immediately, with the choice based on age and the underlying disease status of the patient (see later discussion).

The diagnosis of bacterial meningitis rests on the initial battery of tests (e.g., CSF Gram's stain, lactate level, CIE or agglutination tests, *Limulus* lysate, examination of peripheral blood or skin lesions for organisms, purulent CSF without a positive Gram's stain) and clinical judgment. Antimicrobial therapy should be started on the basis of the most likely etiologic agent. If pyogenic meningitis is unlikely and the diagnosis is consistent with the aseptic meningitis syndrome (e.g., CSF pleocytosis with a lymphocytic predominance, normal glucose), treatable causes must be ruled out (e.g., partially treated bacterial meningitis, parameningeal foci, fungal or tuberculous meningitis, herpes simplex encephalitis, as previously outlined). If one of these treatable conditions is likely, specific therapy (antibiotics with or without surgery) should be started; if they are not, careful observation, often with a follow-up lumbar puncture in 6 to 8 hours, is a reasonable approach.

Complications may be present and adjunctive measures may be required. If the patient is comatose and/or signs of increased intracranial pressure are present, the intracranial pressure should be monitored and kept in the normal range (see Adjunctive Therapy). If shock, disseminated intravascular coagulation, or suppurative complications are present, the patient should be placed in an intensive care environment, monitored, and aggressively treated.

Antimicrobial Therapy

Because host defenses are relatively inadequate at the site of infection in bacterial meningitis, only parenteral bactericidal antibiotics should be used. The choice of a particular agent is influenced by its ability to penetrate the blood-brain barrier (Chapter 231). In addition, bacterial meningitis is the only infection in which definite in vivo antibiotic antagonism has been demonstrated. Thus potentially antagonistic combinations of a bactericidal and a bacteriostatic agent, such as chloramphenicol-gentamicin for gram-negative bacilli, or penicillin-tetracycline for pneumococci, should be avoided in the treatment of this disease. The current antimicrobial agents of choice (with alternative agents) for the treatment of meningitis are listed in Table 239-5, with recommended dosages for adults in Table 239-6. In the patient with presumed bacterial meningitis and a negative CSF Gram's stain, treatment is directed at the most likely etiologic agent, depending on age, as shown in Table 239-7.

Penicillin (20 to 24 million units/day intravenously) and ampicillin (12 g/day intravenously) are equally effective against sensitive pneumococci. However, antimicrobial resistance patterns have modified recommendations for the therapy of pneumococcal meningitis, with the emergence of strains that are relatively (minimal inhibitory concentration [MIC] range of 0.1 to 1.0 µg/ml) and highly (MIC ≥2.0 µg/ml) resistant to penicillin; the frequency of penicillin resistance has exceeded 20% to 25% in many areas of the United States and is even higher in many locations throughout the world. The third-generation cephalosporins (i.e., cefotaxime or ceftriaxone) have been considered the treatment of choice for pneumococcal meningitis caused by relatively penicillin-resistant strains, and vancomycin is recommended for highly resistant isolates. However, there are reports of treatment failure and emergence of pneumococcal strains that are resistant to the third-generation cephalosporins (MIC range of 4 to >32 µg/ml).

In addition, a recent report documented therapeutic failure of vancomycin in 4 of 11 patients with CSF-culture–proven pneumococcal

Table 239-6 Dosages of antimicrobials in meningitis (adults with normal renal function)

DRUG	DAILY DOSE	DOSING INTERVAL
Penicillin G	20-24 million U	Continuous infusion or 4 million U q4h
Ampicillin	12-16 g	2 g q4h
Chloramphenicol	4-6 g*	1.0-1.5 g q6h
Nafcillin, oxacillin	12 g	2 g q4h
Cefotaxime	12 g	2 g q4h
Ceftriaxone	4 g	2 g q12h
Ceftazidime	6 g	2 g q8h
Vancomycin	2-3 g	1 g q8-12h
Gentamicin, tobramycin	3-5 mg/kg	1.7 mg/kg q8h
Amikacin	15 mg/kg	5 mg/kg q8h
Trimethoprim-sulfamethoxazole	10 mg/kg	5 mg/kg q12h
Isoniazid	300-600 mg	Daily (oral)
Rifampin	600 mg	Daily (oral)
Amphotericin B	0.5-0.7 mg/kg	Daily
5-Fluorocytosine	100-150 mg/kg	q6h
Fluconazole	400 mg	Daily

*Higher dose recommended if used for pneumococcal meningitis.

Table 239-7 Empiric therapy of purulent meningitis*

AGE	STANDARD THERAPIES	ALTERNATIVE THERAPIES
0-3 weeks	Ampicillin plus cefotaxime	Ampicillin plus an aminoglycoside
4-12 weeks	Cefotaxime or ceftriaxone plus ampicillin	
3 months to 18 years	Cefotaxime or ceftriaxone	Ampicillin, chloramphenicol, ampicillin plus chloramphenicol
18-50 years	Cefotaxime or ceftriaxone	Chloramphenicol
>50 years	Third-generation cephalosporin plus ampicillin	Ampicillin plus an aminoglycoside, trimethoprim-sulfamethoxazole

*Vancomycin should be added to empiric therapeutic regimens when highly penicillin- or cephalosporin-resistant *S. pneumoniae* is suspected.

meningitis, indicating the need for careful monitoring of patients receiving vancomycin therapy for pneumococcal meningitis. Based on these data, penicillin can never be recommended as empiric therapy in suspected pneumococcal meningitis. We recommend the combination of vancomycin plus a third-generation cephalosporin (cefotaxime or ceftriaxone) pending susceptibility testing. However, if a highly resistant strain is isolated, therapy with vancomycin plus the third-generation cephalosporin should be continued; this recommendation is based on experimental animal studies that suggest that this combination is synergistic in the killing of highly resistant pneumococci. The addition of rifampin has also been recommended by some authorities. Intrathecal or intraventricular vancomycin may be a reasonable option in patients who are not responding to therapy otherwise.

N. meningitidis meningitis can also be treated with either penicillin G or ampicillin. However, the frequency of meningococci that are relatively resistant to penicillin has been increasing in Spain; the mechanism of this resistance is due to decreased affinity of penicillin to penicillin-binding protein 3. The clinical significance of these isolates is unclear because patients have recovered uneventfully with standard penicillin therapy. In the United States the prevalence has remained low and has not changed significantly over the past decade. In addition, β-lactamase–producing isolates have been reported in Africa. Although they have not yet been reported in the United States, it would seem prudent to analyze the MICs for all meningococcal isolates.

Therapy of meningitis due to *H. influenzae* type b has been markedly altered as a result of the emergence of β-lactamase–producing

strains, accounting for approximately 24% and 32% of CSF isolates overall in the United States in 1981 and 1986, respectively. Resistance to chloramphenicol has also been described, although it occurs more commonly in Spain (>50% of isolates) than in the United States (<1% of isolates). Currently third-generation cephalosporins (cefotaxime or ceftriaxone) are recommended as therapy when β-lactamase–producing strains of *H. influenzae* type b are suspected or isolated. Despite initial studies suggesting its efficacy, cefuroxime should not be used for the treatment of bacterial meningitis based on findings in a recent prospective, randomized study in which ceftriaxone was found superior to cefuroxime in rapidity of CSF sterilization in children with bacterial meningitis. In addition, ceftriaxone was associated with a reduction of hearing impairment when compared with cefuroxime.

Ampicillin is generally recommended for the therapy of meningitis due to group B streptococci or *L. monocytogenes*. However, the combination of ampicillin and gentamicin is synergistic in vitro and in vivo, and such treatment appears reasonable for these infections. As an alternative, trimethoprim-sulfamethoxazole can be used for the treatment of *L. monocytogenes* meningitis.

In patients with a CSF shunt, meningitis is most commonly caused by coagulase-negative staphylococci. Initial therapy should consist of vancomycin with close monitoring of CSF levels during treatment. If the patient fails to improve, the addition of rifampin may be warranted. Removal of the shunt is important adjunctive therapy. *S. aureus* meningitis should be treated with nafcillin or oxacillin, with vancomycin reserved for patients allergic to penicillin or when methicillin-resistant organisms are isolated or suspected.

The therapy of gram-negative bacillary meningitis remains problematic. Most strains are resistant to ampicillin, and chloramphenicol is bacteriostatic. Until recently, the aminoglycosides were considered the drugs of choice. However, these agents penetrate poorly into the CSF during parenteral therapy alone, and intrathecal administration (via lumbar puncture) fails to produce reliable antibiotic concentrations at a site where infection (ventriculitis) is usually present.

The introduction of the third-generation cephalosporins has changed the approach to therapy of gram-negative bacillary meningitis in many patients. These agents have excellent in vitro activity against the major gram-negative meningeal pathogens and enter purulent CSF in bactericidal concentrations. Therapy with cefotaxime for gram-negative bacillary meningitis (due to susceptible strains) in adults results in cure rates of 74% to 94% in contrast to the mortality rates of 40% to 90% or more achieved with older regimens (e.g., aminoglycosides and/or chloramphenicol). These agents must be considered the drugs of choice for this disease. One particular agent, ceftazidime, has been shown to be efficacious for the treatment of *P. aeruginosa* meningitis, resulting in cure in 19 of 24 patients in one study when administered either alone or in combination with an aminoglycoside. Intrathecal or intraventricular aminoglycoside therapy should be considered only if there is no response to systemic therapy. This mode of administration is rarely needed at present. The fluoroquinolones (e.g., ciprofloxacin or pefloxacin) have been used successfully in some patients with gram-negative bacillary meningitis, but at present should only be used in adult patients with gram-negative bacterial meningitis who are failing conventional therapy or when the causative organism is resistant to standard drugs. Due to the poor activity of third-generation cephalosporins against some major meningeal pathogens (all agents of this class against *L. monocytogenes*), none of these agents should be used alone for purulent meningitis of unclear origin.

Treatment for acute bacterial meningitis is usually continued for 10 to 14 days for the more common forms of meningitis and often longer (e.g., 3 weeks) for gram-negative bacillary meningitis. Several studies have demonstrated the efficacy and safety of short-course therapy (7 days) in infants and children with *H. influenzae* meningitis, but despite successes, the duration of therapy should be individualized.

Tuberculous meningitis is best treated with two tuberculocidal agents: isoniazid (300 to 600 mg by mouth daily) and rifampin (600 mg by mouth daily) (Chapter 273). Both attain excellent CSF concentrations. More recently, regimens have taken advantage of the newly appreciated merits of pyrazinamide and its intracellular microbicidal activity. For tuberculous meningitis in nonimmunocompromised patients, a 6-month treatment regimen is recommended consisting of isoniazid, rifampin, and pyrazinamide for the first 2 months, followed by 4 months of isoniazid and rifampin. Some authors, however, recommend 9 months of treatment for CNS tuberculosis. In addition, HIV-1 infected patients may require longer courses of treatment. Ethambutol should be added in cases of suspected drug resistance. Of great concern are the recent reports of outbreaks of multidrug-resistant tuberculosis, especially in HIV-infected patients. In patients who have tuberculous meningitis caused by multidrug-resistant organisms, therapy should be guided by CSF penetration. Ethionamide, the fluoroquinolones (e.g., ciprofloxacin, ofloxacin), imipenem, and amoxicillin-clavulanic acid are agents that may be considered. Steroids appear to exert a beneficial effect in this disease and should be administered in selected cases with extreme neurologic compromise, elevated intracranial pressure, impending herniation, or impending or established spinal block. Some authors also recommend corticosteroids in patients with CT or MRI evidence of either hydrocephalus or basilar meningitis. Prednisone, 1 mg/kg per day, tapered over 1 month, is often recommended, although varying doses of dexamethasone or hydrocortisone have also been used.

Amphotericin B is the mainstay of therapy for fungal meningitis (Chapter 277). Intravenous therapy alone (0.5 to 0.7 mg/kg per day intravenously) is indicated for *Candida* meningitis (Chapter 277). The addition of 5-fluorocytosine allows a reduction in dosage of amphotericin B to 0.3 mg/kg per day for the treatment of cryptococcal meningitis. This combination of fluorocytosine and amphotericin B for 6 weeks is as efficacious (with more rapid sterilization of the CSF) as 0.4 mg/kg per day of amphotericin B alone for 10 weeks. Fluorocytosine alone cannot be recommended because of the development of resistance and a low cure rate. Leukopenia, thrombocytopenia, and diarrhea may occur with peak fluorocytosine serum levels of 100 µg/ml or more. It is advisable to monitor complete blood cell counts biweekly and reduce the fluorocytosine dose if azotemia occurs. In a recent study a shorter course of combined amphotericin B and fluorocytosine therapy for 4 weeks was recommended for patients with the following characteristics: no underlying disease or immunosuppressive therapy; meningitis that is recognized early and not complicated by neurologic abnormalities; a CSF white blood cell count before treatment of greater than or equal to 20 cells/mm^3; a pretreatment serum cryptococcal antigen titer less than 1:32; a negative CSF India ink preparation after 4 weeks of therapy; and serum and CSF cryptococcal antigen titers less than 1:8 at 4 weeks (Chapter 279).

Fluconazole, a new triazole antifungal agent, has been evaluated in the treatment of cryptococcal meningitis in patients with AIDS. In one trial the failure rate with fluconazole (8 of 14 patients) was much greater than in patients receiving combination therapy with amphotericin B plus 5-fluorocytosine (0 of 6 patients). A subsequent study by the Mycoses Study Group found no significant differences in the number of patients who were cured, improved, or died whether they received treatment with amphotericin B (at least 0.3 mg/kg per day) or fluconazole (200 mg/day). However, there was a trend toward early mortality in patients who were initially randomly selected to receive therapy with fluconazole. Based on these findings, we recommend that AIDS patients with cryptococcal meningitis receive initial therapy with amphotericin B (0.5 to 0.7 mg/kg per day) with or without 5-fluorocytosine for a period of about 2 weeks. This regimen is then followed by fluconazole (400 mg/day) to complete a 10-week course (Chapter 248). Due to the high rate of relapse in AIDS patients with cryptococcal meningitis, maintenance antifungal therapy should then be instituted for life; the maintenance therapy of choice is fluconazole, 200 mg/day.

Intraventricular administration of amphotericin B is usually necessary for meningitis due to *Coccidioides immitis* but is rarely required for cryptococcal disease. The benefit of adding agents other than 5-fluorocytosine (e.g., rifampin, tetracyclines) to amphotericin B remains unproved, despite in vitro susceptibility studies with strains of *Histoplasma* or *Aspergillus*. In patients who fail to respond to amphotericin B, the newer antifungal agents (e.g., fluconazole) in maximum tolerated doses may be considered (Chapter 276).

Adjunctive Therapy

Some patients with bacterial meningitis should receive treatment with adjunctive dexamethasone therapy to attenuate the subarachnoid

space inflammatory response associated with antibiotic-induced bacterial lysis and reduce many of the pathophysiologic consequences of bacterial meningitis, such as cerebral edema and increased intracranial pressure. The value of corticosteroid therapy in bacterial meningitis has recently been examined in several controlled clinical trials. In one double-blind, placebo-controlled trial, infants and children with predominantly *H. influenzae* type b meningitis were randomly selected to receive antibiotics (cefuroxime or ceftriaxone) with either dexamethasone or placebo. The patients who received antibiotics plus dexamethasone became afebrile sooner, had more rapid normalization of CSF parameters, and were significantly less likely to acquire moderate to severe sensorineural hearing loss. The benefits in terms of morbidity, however, were statistically significant only in the patients receiving antibiotic therapy with cefuroxime, not in those receiving ceftriaxone.

In a second study from Egypt performed in children and adults with bacterial meningitis, there was a significant reduction in mortality rate and overall neurologic sequelae in patients with pneumococcal meningitis who received adjunctive dexamethasone concomitant with antibiotics (ampicillin plus chloramphenicol). However, no significant differences were observed in time to afebrility or improvement in CSF parameters. The antibiotics were given intramuscularly, an extraordinarily high percentage of patients came to medical attention in a comatose state, and there were no significant differences in outcome for meningitis caused by *N. meningitidis* or *H. influenzae* type b.

In a third recently published trial from Costa Rica, infants and children with bacterial meningitis were given treatment with cefotaxime with or without adjunctive dexamethasone administered 15 to 20 minutes before the first antibiotic dose. At 24 hours the clinical condition and mean prognostic scores were significantly better among the patients who received adjunctive dexamethasone therapy. When the patients were followed up for a mean of 15 months, those who received adjunctive dexamethasone had a significantly decreased incidence of one or more neurologic sequelae, although there was only a trend in reduction of audiologic impairment.

A fourth published, prospective, placebo-controlled, double-blind study from Switzerland of adjunctive dexamethasone in 115 children with acute bacterial meningitis revealed that neurologic sequelae (at 3, 9, and 15 months of therapy) were fewer in the dexamethasone group.

Several recent multicenter, randomized, placebo-controlled trials conducted in the United States and Canada in infants and children with bacterial meningitis have questioned the use of adjunctive dexamethasone therapy. These trials demonstrated no significant differences in neurologic or audiologic sequelae with adjunctive dexamethasone, although the dexamethasone was given after initiation of antimicrobial therapy (>4 hours in many patients) and some patients had incomplete follow-up.

Based on the preceding data, the use of adjunctive dexamethasone therapy (0.15 mg/kg every 6 hours for 2 to 4 days) is recommended for infants and children with *H. influenzae* type b meningitis. Dexamethasone should be administered concomitant with or just before the first dose of an antimicrobial agent for optimal attenuation of the subarachnoid space inflammatory response. Patients should be carefully monitored for the possibility of gastrointestinal tract hemorrhage. In adults or in patients with bacterial meningitis caused by other organisms the routine use of adjunctive dexamethasone is not recommended, pending results of ongoing studies. Although some authorities recommend its use in all cases of bacterial meningitis with a likely bacterial origin or cause (i.e., demonstrable bacteria on CSF Gram's stain, which may predict the patients at greatest risk of bacteriolysis-induced exacerbation of inflammation), there are no clinical data to support this recommendation. The use of dexamethasone is of particular concern in patients with pneumococcal meningitis who are given treatment with vancomycin, since a diminished CSF inflammatory response may significantly reduce CSF vancomycin penetration; steroid therapy may prove harmful in this circumstance.

When cerebral edema and raised intracranial pressure appear likely (e.g., by CT scan or neurologic examination) and the patients are comatose or have markedly abnormal neurologic examinations, making the detection of further deterioration difficult, a pressure-monitoring device should be placed intracranially. The patient should be monitored regularly in an intensive care environment and measures instituted to maintain the intracranial pressure in the normal range. These measures may include forced hyperventilation with respiratory muscle paralysis, hypothermia, osmotic agents such as mannitol or glycerol, and dexamethasone. However, some authorities believe that hyperventilation should not be used to reduce intracranial pressure in patients with bacterial meningitis who have evidence of cerebral edema on CT scan because intracranial pressure would be decreased at the expense of a reduction in cerebral blood flow, possibly approaching ischemic thresholds. Glycerol, which can be administered orally, has been evaluated in a trial of infants and children with bacterial meningitis in which patients were randomly selected to receive adjunctive intravenous dexamethasone, oral glycerol, dexamethasone plus glycerol, or none of these; 7% of glycerol-treated patients and 19% of those not given glycerol had neurologic or audiologic sequelae.

If shock complicates acute bacterial meningitis, vigorous supportive measures are necessary. The septic arthritis that occasionally develops usually responds to systemic antibiotics and repeated needle aspiration, but open surgical drainage is indicated in a minority of patients. Seizures can be managed acutely with anticonvulsant therapy, and the presence of focal seizures should raise the question of brain abscess or subdural empyema.

PROGNOSIS

With appropriate therapy, mortality for the various forms of meningitis in the United States is as follows: *H. influenzae*, 3% to 6%; *N. meningitidis*, 5% to 10%; *S. pneumoniae*, 20% to 35%; *E. coli*, 30%; *L. monocytogenes*, 15% to 40%; group B streptococci, 10% to 30%; viruses, less than 1%; and fungi, 10% to 50% or more, depending on the organism. The rates are higher in neonates and in adults over 50 years of age. Coma and selected CSF abnormalities (high bacterial concentrations, low leukocyte counts, glucose levels ≤13 mg/dl, lactate values >10 mEq/L) all adversely influence the prognosis. Sequelae such as mental retardation, deafness and other cranial nerve abnormalities, and seizures are present in up to half the survivors of neonatal or childhood meningitis. The development of hydrocephalus may necessitate CSF shunt insertion.

BIBLIOGRAPHY

Ashwal S et al: Bacterial meningitis in children: pathophysiology and treatment, *Neurology* 42:739-748, 1992.
Bonadio WA: The cerebrospinal fluid: physiologic aspects and alterations associated with bacterial meningitis, *Pediatr Infect Dis J* 11:423-432, 1992.
Bozzette SA et al: A placebo-controlled trial of maintenance therapy with fluconazole after treatment of cryptococcal meningitis in the acquired immunodeficiency syndrome, *N Engl J Med* 324:580-584, 1991.
Bryan JP et al: Etiology and mortality of bacterial meningitis in Northeastern Brazil, *Rev Infect Dis* 12:128-135, 1990.
Dismukes WE et al: Treatment of cryptococcal meningitis with combination amphotericin B and flucytosine for four as compared with six weeks, *N Engl J Med* 317:334-341, 1987.
Dunne DW, Quagliarello V: Group B streptococcal meningitis in adults, *Medicine* 72:1-10, 1993.
Durand ML et al: Acute bacterial meningitis in adults: a review of 493 episodes, *N Engl J Med* 328:21-28, 1993.
Feigin RD et al: Diagnosis and management of meningitis, *Pediatr Infect Dis J* 11:785-814, 1992.
Friedland IR, McCracken GH Jr: Management of infections caused by antibiotic-resistant *Streptococcus pneumoniae*, *N Engl J Med* 331:377-382, 1994.
Geisler PJ et al: Community-acquired purulent meningitis: a review of 1,316 cases during the antibiotic era, 1959-1976, *Rev Infect Dis* 2:725-745, 1980.
Gray LD, Fedorko DP: Laboratory diagnosis of bacterial meningitis, *Clin Microbiol Rev* 5:130-145, 1992.
Hollander H, Stringari S: Human immunodeficiency virus–associated meningitis: clinical course and correlations, *Am J Med* 83:813-816, 1987.
Jackson LA et al: Prevalence of *Neisseria meningitidis* relatively resistant to penicillin in the United States: 1991, *J Infect Dis* 169:438-441, 1994.
Kilpi T et al: Oral glycerol and intravenous dexamethasone in preventing neurologic and audiologic sequelae of childhood bacterial meningitis, *Pediatr Infect Dis J* 14:270-278, 1995.
Larsen RA et al: Fluconazole compared with amphotericin B plus flucytosine for cryptococcal meningitis in AIDS: a randomized trial, *Ann Intern Med* 113:183-187, 1990.
Paris MM et al: Effect of dexamethasone on therapy of experimental penicillin- and cephalosporin-resistant pneumococcal meningitis, *Antimicrob Agents Chemother* 38:1320-1324, 1994.
Paris MM et al: Management of meningitis caused by penicillin-resistant *Streptococcus pneumoniae*, *Antimicrob Agents Chemother* 39:2171-2175, 1995.
Pfister HW et al: Mechanisms of brain injury in bacterial meningitis: workshop summary, *Clin Infect Dis* 19:463-479, 1994.

Powderly WG et al: A controlled trial of fluconazole or amphotericin B to prevent relapse of cryptococcal meningitis in patients with the acquired immunodeficiency syndrome, *N Engl J Med* 326:793-798, 1992.
Prober CG: The role of steroids in the management of children with bacterial meningitis, *Pediatrics* 95:29-31, 1995.
Quagliarello VJ, Scheld WM: Treatment of bacterial meningitis, *N Engl J Med* 336:708-716, 1997.
Quagliarello V, Scheld WM: Bacterial meningitis: pathogenesis, pathophysiology, and progress, *N Engl J Med* 327:864-872, 1992.
Radetsky M: Duration of treatment in bacterial meningitis: a historical inquiry, *Pediatr Infect Dis J* 9:2-9, 1990.
Saag MS et al: Comparison of amphotericin B with fluconazole in the treatment of acute AIDS-associated cryptococcal meningitis, *N Engl J Med* 326:83-89, 1992.
Schaad UB et al: A comparison of ceftriaxone and cefuroxime for the treatment of bacterial meningitis in children, *N Engl J Med* 322:141-147, 1990.
Scheld WM, Wispelwey B, editors: Meningitis, *Infect Dis Clin North Am* 4:555-854, 1990.
Schlech WF et al: Bacterial meningitis in the United States, 1978 through 1981: the national bacterial meningitis surveillance study, *JAMA* 253:1749-1754, 1985.
Schmutzhard E et al: A randomized comparison of meropenem with cefotaxime or ceftriaxone for the treatment of bacterial meningitis in adults, *J Antimicrob Chemother* 36(A):85-97, 1995.
Spanos A et al: Differential diagnosis of acute meningitis: an analysis of the predictive value of initial observation, *JAMA* 262:2700-2707, 1989.
Tunkel AR, Scheld WM: Pathogenesis and pathophysiology of bacterial meningitis, *Clin Microbiol Rev* 6:118-136, 1993.
Tunkel AR, Scheld WM: Acute bacterial meningitis, *Lancet* 346:1675-1680, 1995.
Tunkel AR et al: Bacterial meningitis: recent advances in pathophysiology and treatment, *Ann Intern Med* 112:610-623, 1990.
Viladrich PF et al: Evaluation of vancomycin for therapy of adult pneumococcal meningitis, *Antimicrob Agents Chemother* 35:2467-2472, 1991.
Wenger JD et al: Bacterial meningitis in the United States, 1986: report of a multistate surveillance study, *J Infect Dis* 162:1316-1323, 1990.

CHAPTER

240 Brain Abscess and Perimeningeal Infections

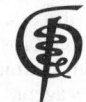

Michael R. Chicoine and Ralph G. Dacey, Jr.

Localized intracranial and intraspinal infections present formidable difficulties in diagnosis and treatment. Recent improvements have been made in microbiologic techniques of bacterial isolation, antimicrobial chemotherapy, neuroimaging, and neurosurgical techniques; nevertheless, brain abscess and perimeningeal infections are potentially fatal diseases. Optimal management of the patient with these conditions demands timely cooperation between the primary physician and neurosurgeon.

BRAIN ABSCESS
Pathophysiology and Etiology

In 80% of patients brain abscess is associated with known extracerebral sources of infection. The most common primary sites of infection are found either in close proximity to the central nervous system (CNS) (e.g., in the paranasal sinuses) or in distant locations, usually within the chest (Table 240-1). In addition to gram-positive cocci and Enterobacteriaceae, microaerophilic and anaerobic organisms form brain abscesses up to 40% of the time; therefore anaerobic cultures should be obtained in all patients. Multiple organisms have been reported in up to 50% of patients harboring a brain abscess. The causative organism can often be predicted from the site of the abscess—an important fact when choosing initial antibiotic therapy. Additional factors that aid in prediction of the causative organism are the patient's age, geographic region of residence, and travel history.

Bacteria may gain access to the brain from contiguous sites of infection by direct spread or presumably via infected thrombi in the emissary veins that penetrate the cranial vault. Cerebral abscesses formed by spread from a contiguous site are generally solitary. Otitis media and complicating mastoiditis may cause abscesses in the adjacent temporal lobe or cerebellar hemisphere. Common bacterial iso-

Table 240-1 Brain abscess: predisposing conditions, locations, and microbiology

PREDISPOSING CONDITION*	SITE OF ABSCESS	USUAL ISOLATE(S) FROM ABSCESS
Contiguous site of primary infection		
Otitis media and mastoiditis	Temporal lobe or cerebellar hemisphere	Streptococci (anaerobic or aerobic), *Bacteroides fragilis*, Enterobacteriaceae
Frontoethmoidal sinusitis	Frontal lobe	Predominantly streptococci: *Bacteroides* species, Enterobacteriaceae, *Staphylococcus aureus*, and *Haemophilus* species
Sphenoidal sinusitis	Frontal or temporal lobe	Same as in frontoethmoidal sinusitis
Dental sepsis	Frontal lobe most common	Mixed *Fusobacterium, Bacteroides,* and *Streptococcus* species
Penetrating cranial trauma or postsurgical infection	Related to wound	*S. aureus,* streptococci, Enterobacteriaceae, *Clostridium* species
Distant site of primary infection		
Congenital heart disease	Multiple abscess cavities; middle cerebral artery distribution common, but may occur at any site	Streptococci (*viridans*, anaerobic, and microaerophilic), *Haemophilus* species
Lung abscess, empyema, bronchiectasis	Same as in congenital heart disease	*Fusobacterium, Actinomyces, Bacteroides* species; streptococci; *Nocardia asteroides*
Bacterial endocarditis	Same as in congenital heart disease	*S. aureus,* streptococci
Compromised hosts (immunosuppressive therapy or malignancy)	Same as in congenital heart disease	*Toxoplasma* species, fungi, Enterobacteriaceae
Acquired immunodeficiency syndrome	Any location	*Toxoplasma* species; less likely are *Cryptococcus* species, tuberculosis, cytomegalovirus encephalitis (consider PML and primary lymphoma)

*Predisposing conditions identified in approximately 80% of cases.
PML, Progressive multifocal leukoencephalopathy.

lates from otogenic abscesses are aerobic and anaerobic streptococci, *Bacteroides fragilis,* and Enterobacteriaceae, often in mixed culture. Frontal lobe abscess is usually associated with frontal, ethmoid, or sphenoid sinusitis. The most common bacterial isolates in frontal lobe abscesses are aerobic and anaerobic streptococci (especially the *Streptococcus milleri* group), although Enterobacteriaceae, *Bacteroides* species, and other organisms are also reported. In brain abscess resulting from penetrating craniocerebral trauma, traumatic cerebrospinal fluid (CSF) drainage from skull fractures, or neurosurgical wound infection, *Staphylococcus aureus* is usually the causative agent, although Enterobacteriaceae and *Clostridium* species are also found.

Brain abscess in association with a distant primary source of infections is the result of hematogenous dissemination of the infecting organism. Such abscesses are often multiple. These metastatic abscesses may occur at any location within the brain, although there appears to be a predisposition for sites in the distribution of the middle cerebral artery, particularly at the corticomedullary junction. Most metastatic brain abscesses occur as a result of suppurative pulmonary disease such as lung abscess, empyema, or bronchiectasis. Isolates from this group of patients include *Fusobacterium* and *Actinomyces* species, *Nocardia asteroides,* and *Bacteroides* and *Streptococcus* species. Brain abscess occurs in patients with right-to-left shunting caused by congenital heart disease or, less commonly, resulting from pulmonary arteriovenous malformations as in the Rendu-Osler-Weber syndrome (hereditary hemorrhagic telangiectasia). Streptococci (aerobic, microaerophilic, and anaerobic) are isolated from most brain abscesses in patients with congenital heart disease. Brain abscess is a rare complication of bacterial endocarditis.

Immunosuppressive therapy, underlying malignancy, acquired immunodeficiency syndrome (AIDS), and other causes of impaired immunity also increase the risk of development of brain abscess. Fungi (*Candida, Aspergillus, Cryptococcus, Blastomyces,* and *Histoplasma* organisms and the Zygomycetes [*Mucor* and *Rhizopus* species]) and parasites (*Toxoplasma* species) are important diagnostic considerations in this group of patients. Ten percent to 20% of AIDS patients initially have neurologic symptoms. In 40% to 60% of patients with AIDS neurologic impairments develop, and up to 75% have postmortem findings of CNS involvement. Many of these patients have focal mass lesions identified by computed tomography (CT) or magnetic resonance imaging (MRI) caused by *Toxoplasma gondii,* primary CNS lymphoma, progressive multifocal leukoencephalopathy (PML), or fungal sources (Chapter 279). Biopsy of these lesions may be in-

dicated, since appropriate therapy varies drastically depending on histologic and culture data, but current recommendations (as discussed later) generally begin with an empiric trial of antitoxoplasmal chemotherapy followed by serial CT scanning (every 2 to 3 weeks) (Chapter 248).

Patient age and travel history also lend important clues to the origin of brain abscesses. Meningitis is a more common predisposing condition in neonates and infants, and gram-negative organisms (especially *Proteus* and *Citrobacter* species) are the most frequent causative agents. Patients who have lived in or traveled to Mexico or Central or South America and who have enhancing lesions on CT or MRI must be considered at risk for cysticercosis (Chapter 281).

Clinical Manifestations and Differential Diagnosis

Brain abscesses are most common in males in the first three decades of life. Diagnosis is often delayed because patients with brain abscess may have little evidence of neurologic deficit and few signs of an infectious process, but modern imaging techniques have led to more rapid diagnosis of cerebral abscesses. Any neurologic illness in a patient with one of the predisposing conditions (Table 240-1) should suggest the diagnosis of brain abscess at an early point in the course of the disease. The classic triad of fever, headache, and focal neurologic deficit is present in less than 50% of patients. The most common symptom is headache, which is seen in approximately 70% of patients. Fever occurs in 50% to 60% of adults but is more common in children. The focal nature of brain involvement by the abscess is demonstrated in approximately 80% of patients by either a localizable neurologic deficit or seizures. Other indicators of increased intracranial pressure, such as nausea, vomiting, and lethargy, are less common but are important, since they may point to incipient decompensation and require urgent surgical management. Papilledema and cranial nerve deficits are seen in a minority of patients. Brain abscess may sometimes mimic bacterial meningitis in its presentation, with signs of meningeal inflammation that may indicate close proximity of the abscess to the ventricles or subarachnoid space.

Brain abscess must be differentiated from other intracranial infections such as meningitis, subdural empyema, mycotic aneurysm, and epidural abscess. CT or MRI or both are essential for accomplishing this differentiation. Other conditions to be distinguished from brain abscess include primary or metastatic brain tumors, cerebral infarc-

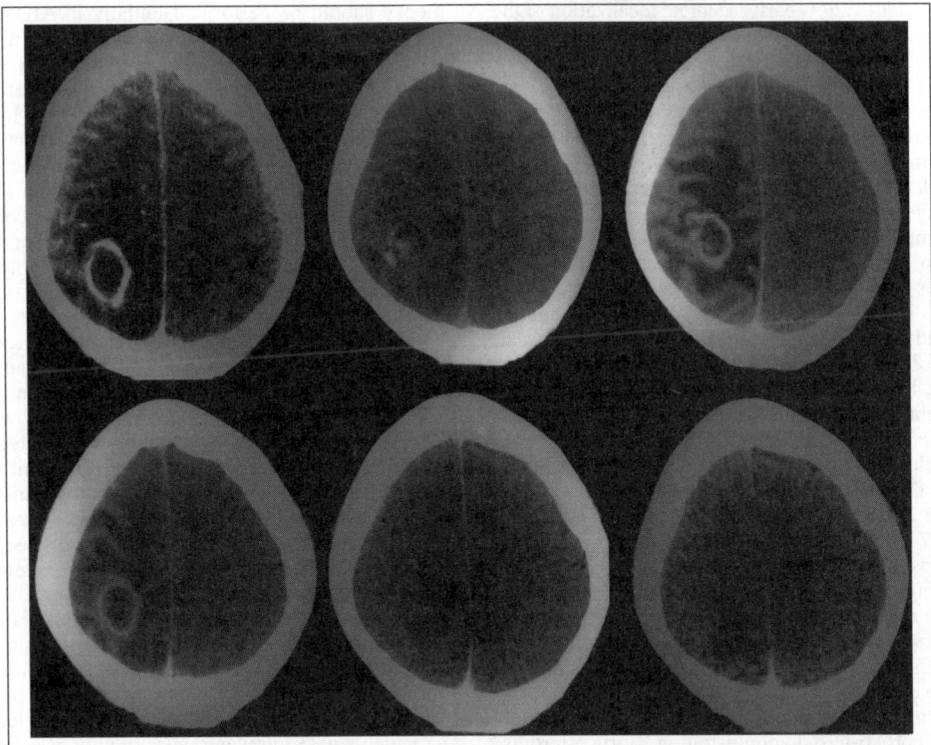

FIGURE 240-1   Serial computed tomography (CT) scans of head (with intravenous contrast) in 30-year-old man who sought medical advice with headache and mild left-side hemiparesis without fever 2 days after tooth extraction for abscess. **A,** Initial scan demonstrated right-side parietal ring-enhancing lesion with surrounding edema. **B,** Two days later, after stereotactic needle biopsy and aspiration, CT demonstrated punctate area of air along needle tract and decompression of the abscess. Cultures grew *Streptococcus viridans*. Serial scans at, **C,** 1 week; **D,** 1 month; **E,** 3 months; and **F,** 6.5 months after aspiration demonstrated evolution and resolution of abscess.

tion, viral encephalitis (predominantly herpes simplex), and chronic subdural hematoma.

Laboratory Diagnosis and Radiologic Evaluation

Periperal leukocyte counts are elevated in less than 50% of patients with brain abscesses. The erythrocyte sedimentation rate (ESR) is moderately elevated in up to 90% of patients with cerebral abscesses. Elevated serum C-reactive protein level may be even more sensitive in differentiating between infectious and neoplastic origins but, like peripheral leukocyte counts and ESR, it is also nonspecific. Blood cultures infrequently recover the offending organism.

Lumbar puncture should not be performed in patients with known or suspected intracranial abscess for two reasons. First, the analysis of the CSF is not diagnostic. Findings include elevated CSF protein level, variable pleocytosis, and a normal glucose level. Second, lumbar puncture may precipitate brain herniation if a mass lesion is present. As a consequence, the diagnosis of intracranial abscess rests with the patient's history and the imaging studies, either CT or MRI. In a patient with an apparent intracranial infection and a focal neurologic deficit or a history of a predisposing condition (Table 240-1), a CT or an MRI scan should be obtained to exclude an abscess before lumbar puncture.

CT is more quickly obtained and more safely performed than MRI in the acutely ill patient. Its sensitivity is comparable to MRI; however, CT may miss early inflammatory changes. This fact is rarely clinically significant because few patients come to medical attention in the early cerebritis stage of abscess formation. Noncontrasted images usually show white matter edema and mass effect. Depending on the location, hydrocephalus may also be present. With the infusion of intravenous contrast material, ring enhancement is observed in the mature abscess (Fig. 240-1). This pattern of edema and en-

hancement, however, is similar to that observed in some tumors. One potential distinguishing factor is that the wall of the abscess capsule is often thinned along its medial aspect. Nonetheless, the diagnosis most often must be made by aspiration or biopsy.

CT is particularly helpful in defining paranasal sinus disease. The standard transaxial examination may detect the underlying frontal, ethmoid, sphenoid, or mastoid sinus infection that is responsible for the intracranial abscess. Coronal images of the sinuses provide an even more detailed examination for underlying sinus disease (Fig. 240-2, *D*). This examination is more expensive but more sensitive than plain films.

MRI provides greater definition of the intracranial anatomy and better sensitivity for edema and early inflammatory changes such as those seen in cerebritis. In addition, it is not limited by bone artifact in the posterior fossa. The pattern and timing of enhancement with gadopentate dimeglumine (gadolinium–diethylenetriamine penta-acetic acid [DPTA]) is similar to iodinated contrast medium in CT; therefore a mature abscess shows ring enhancement (Fig. 240-2, *A-C*). This appearance, however, is not specific, and a neoplasm must still be ruled out.

Both MRI and CT may be used for stereotactic biopsies or aspirations of suspected lesions. Follow-up scans are invaluable for verification of the resolution of the abscess and for assessment for disease recurrence. One must bear in mind that complete resolution of the abscess on imaging studies may lag behind a clinical cure by 3 to 6 months.

Treatment

Most patients with brain abscess require a combination of surgical and antibiotic therapy. Despite adequate treatment, as high as 25% to 30% mortality from brain abscess has been reported, with permanent neurologic sequelae occurring in 30% to 55% of cases. However, contemporary imaging techniques allow early, accurate localization of the lesion, and mortality and morbidity have each been reduced to less than 10% in recent large clinical series.

The initial choice of antibiotic therapy should be based on the location of the abscess and the site of the underlying primary infection (if one can be identified) because these features can be used to predict the probable bacteriologic isolate. Specific therapy should be prescribed when culture data from the abscess cavity become available. Before surgical drainage, therapy should be initiated with penicillin G, 20 to 24 million units per day, and metronidazole, 500 mg intravenously (IV) every 6 hours. Metronidazole may be preferable to chloramphenicol in this setting because it achieves a higher concentration in the abscess cavity and is bactericidal against *Bacteroides* species. This combined treatment is effective against streptococcal, *Bacteroides,* and *Fusobacterium* species and many Enterobacteriaceae, although recent increases in these organisms and in *Pseudomonas aeruginosa* (chronic ear infections) may suggest adding stronger gram-negative coverage such as an aminoglycoside or a third-generation cephalosporin such as ceftazidime. Methicillin or nafcillin (8 to 12 g/day IV) should be substituted for penicillin G when *Staphylococcus aureus* is the likely causative organism (Table 240-1). Vancomycin (1 g IV every 12 hours) may be used if the patient is penicillin allergic. Consultation with an otolaryngologist is recommended for patients with concomitant sinus infection.

Dexamethasone, 20 to 30 mg/day, or methylprednisolone, 100 to 150 mg/day, appears to be beneficial in reducing periabscess edema and hence intracranial pressure, although the use of these drugs in brain abscess is controversial because they may slow the macrophage and glial response. Formation of an abscess capsule may also be deleteriously inhibited by corticosteroid administration. Corticosteroids, however, do not appear to decrease antibiotic delivery to the abscess.

Pyrimethamine and sulfadiazine are effective therapy for toxoplasmosis of the CNS in patients with AIDS, but prolonged suppressive therapy may be necessary to prevent relapse. In AIDS patients with acute intracranial lesion(s) suggesting toxoplasmosis, empiric coverage with these two agents should be initiated. A clinical and radiologic response should be noted by 10 and 14 days, respectively; otherwise, a biopsy should be performed to rule out other diagnoses. A

biopsy should be performed initially in AIDS patients if the CT or MRI scan is atypical for toxoplasmosis or if impending herniation precludes waiting for a response to antibiotic therapy.

Prophylactic antiepileptic therapy is generally recommended for patients with supratentorial brain abscess(es). The optimal duration for prophylactic anticonvulsants is not well defined, but some authors recommend 1 to 2 years before withdrawal of anticonvulsant medications. Male patients with frontal, temporal, or multiple abscesses have the highest risk for development of epilepsy.

There are two accepted methods for the surgical treatment of brain abscess—complete excision and stereotactic needle aspiration. Complete excision of the well-encapsulated abscess in an accessible location may be superior to stereotactic aspiration, but results with either excision or aspiration appear equivalent. Surgical excision is preferred for posterior fossa lesions, as well as for brain abscesses caused by fungi, since available antifungal therapy is unsatisfactory. The use of CT or MRI for serial evaluation of patients with brain abscess and for facilitation of stereotactic biopsy in selected patients has lowered mortality rates for this disease. Several recent series document a diagnostic yield of 94% to 96% with a low transient morbidity (4% to 6%) associated with stereotactic biopsy. Repeated aspiration is occasionally necessary. Recent reports have discussed the addition of endoscopy as a further improvement on the stereotactic technique for aspiration of cerebral abscesses. Endoscopy may be particularly useful in drainage of multiloculated or multifocal abscess and may enhance intraoperative assessment of the adequacy of abscess aspiration. Regardless of the method, surgical drainage should be accomplished immediately in patients who demonstrate a progressive neurologic deficit or a decreasing level of consciousness.

Patients with intraventricular rupture of a cerebral abscess and resultant ventriculitis have a much worse prognosis. Such patients may require intrathecal antibiotics, in addition to surgical drainage and an extended course of intravenous antibiotics. Other patients with poor prognosis include those with early, rapid progression and those with profound neurologic deficits on presentation.

Some reports have suggested that management for selected patients with brain abscess may be with antibiotic therapy alone. Patients with early abscess or cerebritis, patients with small abscesses (i.e., diameter less than 2 cm), and alert patients without neurologic deficits may be candidates for nonsurgical therapy. Radiographic or clinical evidence of deterioration indicates the need for surgical drainage. The nonsurgical approach to treating brain abscesses poses several potential problems. Because the causative agent is not identified, the choice of antibiotic may be incorrect. Moreover, the proper treatment of brain tumors and vascular lesions mistakenly diagnosed as brain abscess may be critically delayed. In addition, research has indicated that antibiotic efficacy is impaired by the acidic environment of the abscess cavity and that alkalization can be accomplished only by aspiration of the abscess contents. Nonetheless, if such a treatment course is chosen, the physician must exercise extraordinary care in monitoring the patient's neurologic status to detect subtle changes that may herald sudden deterioration. Antibiotic therapy should be continued for 4 to 6 weeks parenterally, followed by oral treatment for 2 to 6 months, although this regimen is empiric and probably excessive for some organisms. Therefore the decision to treat the condition by medical means alone should be made jointly with the neurosurgeon. All patients should undergo serial imaging studies to document resolution of the abscess in the months after completion of treatment. Five percent to 10% of patients have been reported to have recurrent cerebral abscesses. Abscess most frequently recurs at the original site within 6 weeks after treatment ends.

INTRACRANIAL SUBDURAL EMPYEMA
Pathogenesis and Etiology

Infection within the subdural space has many etiologic similarities to brain abscess. Most cases (35% to 60%) of subdural empyema are related to paranasal sinusitis, most often frontoethmoid. Infections in the middle ear and temporal bone account for around 15% of cases, and the remainder are metastatic infections from distant sources or related to surgery or traumatic injuries. Most of the metastatic cases arise from purulent bronchopulmonary disease.

The most common site for subdural empyema is in the anterior

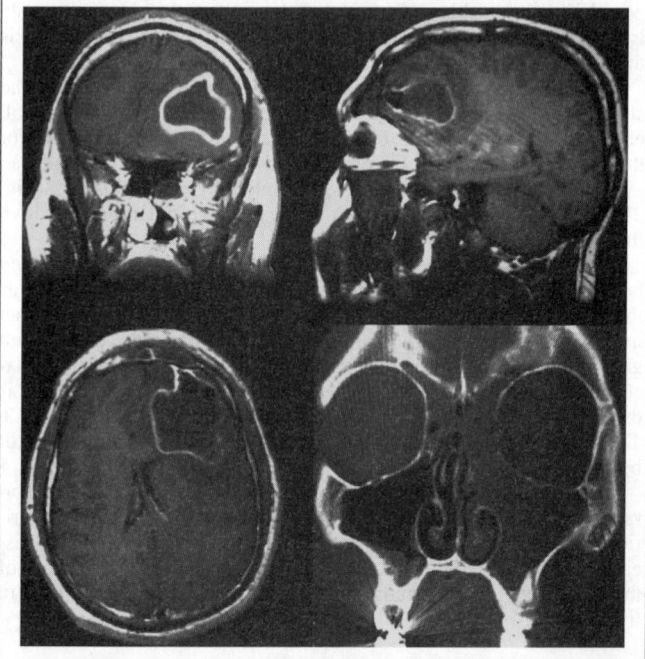

FIGURE 240-2   Magnetic resonance imaging (MRI) of the head in coronal **(A),** sagittal **(B),** and axial **(C)** planes after intravenous administration of gadolinium and noncontrast coronal CT scan **(D)** demonstrated infection in maxillary, ethmoid, and frontal sinuses and large, left-side frontal ring-enhancing lesion in a 21-year-old man.

cranial fossa as a result of paranasal sinusitis. Otogenic subdural empyema occurs over the temporal and occipital lobes or in the posterior fossa. Frontal subdural empyema may be bilateral or situated between the two hemispheres, or both. Infection in the subdural space is often associated with septic venous thrombosis and subsequent hemorrhagic cortical infarction. This pathologic finding may be responsible for the high incidence of focal seizures in this condition.

Aerobic, microaerophilic, and anaerobic streptococci, Enterobacteriaceae, and *B. fragilis* are the most common bacterial isolates. Subdural empyema in infants is almost always associated with meningitis caused by *Haemophilus influenzae* or gram-negative bacteria, but the incidence of *H. influenzae* infections has declined significantly since the introduction of the *H. influenzae* vaccine in 1987.

Clinical Manifestations

Most patients with subdural empyema are males with paranasal sinusitis (the male-female ratio is 3:1). There is a peak incidence in the second and third decades. The presence of localized severe headache (75%) and fever (85%), later becoming associated with lethargy and focal seizures (50%), should suggest the diagnosis of subdural empyema. Meningismus is frequent as well. Papilledema is noted in fewer than half of the patients, but other indicators of increased intracranial pressure (e.g., lethargy, nausea, and vomiting) are common.

Laboratory Diagnosis and Radiologic Evaluation

Peripheral leukocyte count and ESR are more consistently elevated in patients with subdural empyema than in patients with abscess, but these are nonspecific findings. CSF findings in subdural empyema are also nonspecific and rarely permit culture of the causative organism. Lumbar puncture is generally contraindicated, since it is nondiagnostic and may precipitate cerebral herniation.

MRI is superior to CT in detecting extracerebral infections such as subdural or epidural empyema. Small amounts of extracerebral fluid or pus may be difficult to detect with CT but are visible with MRI because of the lack of bone artifact, the better separation of CSF and brain, and the capability of multiplanar imaging. The signal char-

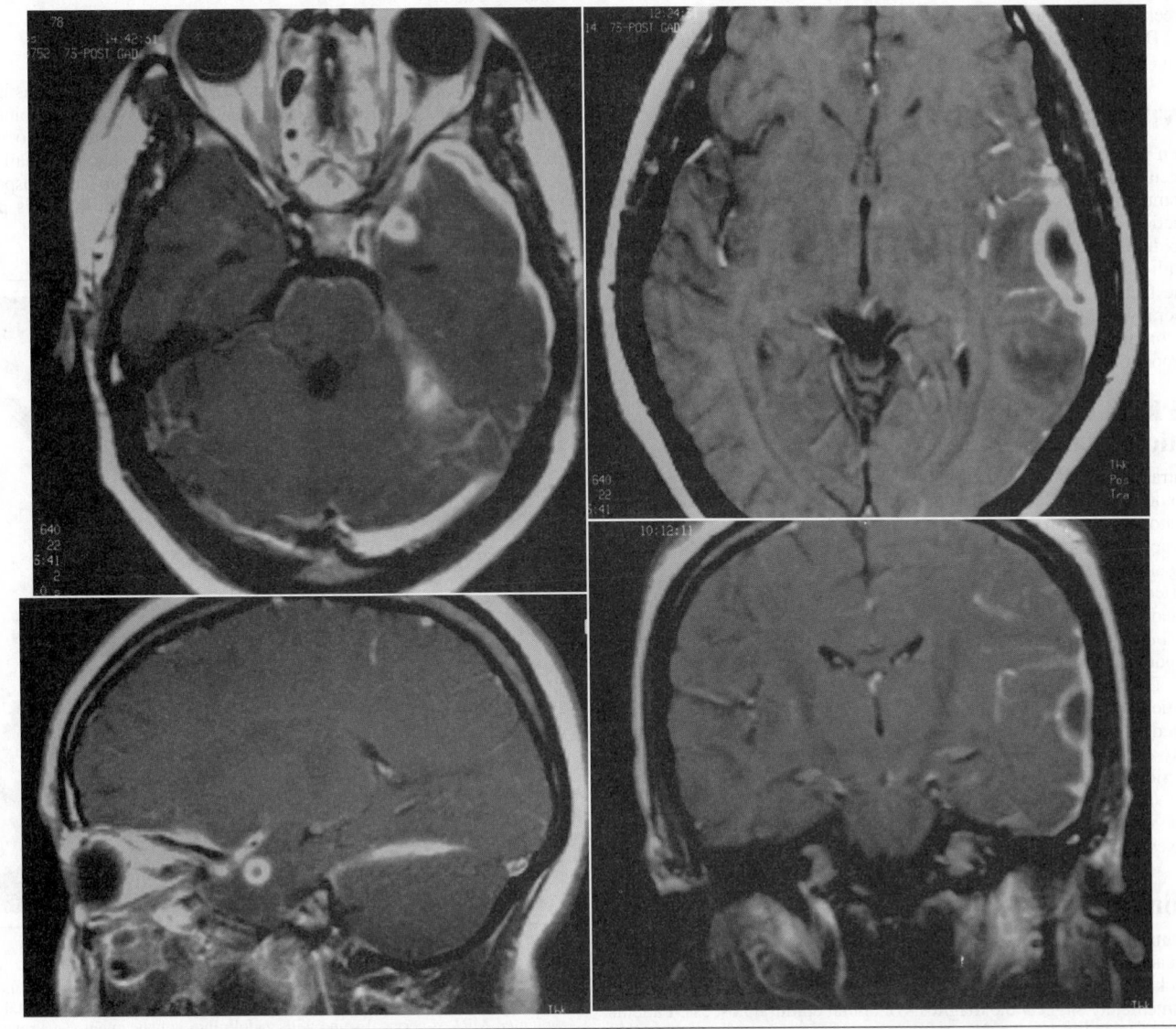

FIGURE 240-3 MRI scan of head (T1-weighted, after intravenous administration of gadolinium) of a 14-year-old girl with multiple foci of intracranial infection, both brain abscesses and subdural empyemas secondary to spread of sinus infection. Views in, **A** and **B,** axial; **C,** sagittal; and, **D,** coronal planes demonstrate left-side temporal brain abscess and subdural empyema.

acteristics of the fluid collection can also be used to differentiate a benign effusion from a more complex purulent collection.

The CT scan typically demonstrates an extracerebral fluid collection with surrounding low attenuation and enhancement. MRI detects even more subtle amounts of parenchymal edema as high signal on T2-weighted images. The T1-weighted images delineate the margins of the extracerebral collection. Gadolinium enhancement is similar to that seen on CT (Fig. 240-3).

Treatment

The clinical suspicion or radiologic diagnosis of subdural empyema requires the immediate use of antibiotic therapy. Either penicillin G, nafcillin, or vancomycin and metronidazole and a third-generation cephalosporin should be initiated after appropriate cultures are made. β-Lactamase–resistant antibiotics should be used in traumatic or post-surgical cases in which the presence of *S. aureus* is likely. Corticosteroids may be useful in patients with increased intracranial pressure. As for cerebral abscess, antiepileptic therapy is usually instituted for supratentorial subdural empyema.

Burr holes and irrigation accomplish adequate drainage in some patients, but craniotomy is usually necessary for thorough evacuation of pus. Fluid for aerobic and anaerobic cultures must be obtained intraoperatively. Parenteral antibiotic therapy is continued for 4 to 6 weeks after surgical drainage.

Despite medical and surgical therapy, mortality in subdural empyema is 15% to 30%, primarily because the diagnosis is often delayed.

INTRACRANIAL EPIDURAL ABSCESS

Ten percent of epidural abscesses occur intracranially; the remainder occur in the spine. These abscesses share with subdural empyema the common causes of sinusitis, mastoiditis, and postoperative wound infection. Subdural empyema and osteomyelitis commonly coexist with epidural abscesses. Epidural abscess should be suspected in patients with sinusitis or otitis who come to medical attention with cellulitis of the face or scalp. Treatment should consist of appropriate antibiotic therapy and drainage of pus by means of burr holes or craniectomy. If a communication between the epidural space and a sinus cavity exists, proper closure should be accomplished to prevent recurrent infection.

SPINAL EPIDURAL ABSCESS
Etiology and Pathogenesis

Intraspinal bacterial infections occur most often within the posterior epidural space. Bacteria may gain access to the epidural space by hematogenous spread from distant infections, usually in the skin or pelvic structures, or by contiguous spread from an adjacent vertebral osteomyelitis. Penetrating injuries may also implant bacteria in the epidural space. *S. aureus* is the most common causative organism, being isolated in 60% to 90% of cases. *Escherichia coli, P. aeruginosa, Streptococcus pneumoniae,* and *Klebsiella* and *Proteus* species have been reported. Tuberculosis of the spine may also involve the epidural space.

The thoracic spine is the site of the abscess in 50% to 80% of patients, followed in frequency by the cervical and lumbar spine. Isolated epidural abscesses resulting from hematogenous spread generally occur dorsal to the thecal sac, whereas contiguous spread of infection from an underlying osteomyelitis collects anterior to the thecal sac. Spinal epidural abscess may extend over many spinal levels. The epidural mass may consist of pus and granulation tissue in acute cases or of fibrous granulation tissue in chronic cases.

Clinical Manifestations

Spinal epidural abscess occurs most commonly in the fifth to seventh decades of life with a slight male preponderance. The triad of fever, back pain, and neurologic symptoms of spinal cord dysfunction should immediately suggest the diagnosis of spinal epidural abscess. Patients often notice localized back pain that subsequently becomes associated with a radicular component. Weakness, dysesthesia, and urinary or fecal incontinence or retention may subsequently be followed by complete paralysis. Physical examination demonstrates spinal tenderness on percussion (unless the infection is predominantly subdural) in

nearly all patients with spinal epidural abscesses, and signs of root or cord compression are common. Diabetes mellitus, intravenous drug abuse, and other causes of immunocompromise are predisposing factors for the development of spinal epidural abscess.

Laboratory Diagnosis and Radiologic Evaluation

Peripheral leukocyte counts are elevated in the majority of patients with spinal epidural abscess, and virtually all patients have an elevated ESR. In addition, serial ESR evaluation is important to assess the adequacy of treatment. Cerebrospinal fluid findings are nonspecific, and because of the risk of introduction of infection into the subdural space, lumbar puncture is contraindicated.

MRI has replaced CT myelography as the radiologic procedure of choice for the detection of epidural abscess. Although both techniques are equally sensitive, MRI is superior to CT myelography in specificity. MRI better defines the rostral and caudal extent of the abscess, as well as the degree of cord compression (Fig. 240-4). In addition, MRI is equal to combined bone and gallium scans in sensitivity (96%) and specificity (92%) for underlying vertebral osteomyelitis. MRI offers the additional advantage of not requiring a lumbar puncture. Plain radiographs continue to serve as the screening examination for suspected disk space infection, paravertebral soft tissue mass, or spinal malalignment.

Treatment

As with other perimeningeal infections, treatment should be instituted as soon as the diagnosis is made and should consist of a combination of antibiotic therapy and surgical drainage. Antistaphylococcal therapy (methicillin, nafcillin, or vancomycin) should initially be combined with aminoglycosides or third-generation cephalosporins until intraoperative culture data are available. Corticosteroids prob-

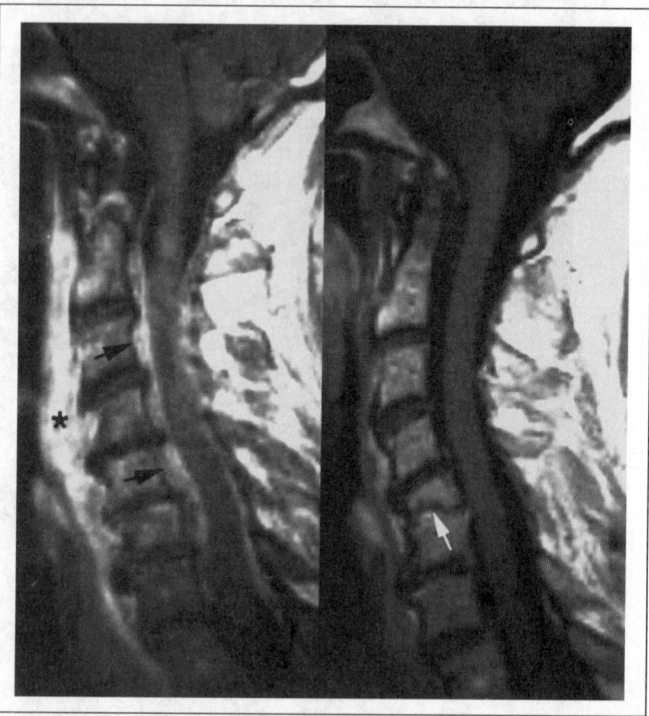

FIGURE 240-4 This fifty-seven-year-old man sought medical advice with epidural abscess and discitis in the cervical spine resulting from cutaneous infection with *Staphylococcus aureus*. At the time of presentation sagittal T1-weighted MRI of cervical spine with gadolinium enhancement *(left)* revealed epidural abscess primarily anterior to cervical cord *(black arrows)*, and enhancement in the prevertebral space *(asterisk)*. Five months after anterior surgical drainage of abscess and 6-week course of intravenous oxacillin, MRI with gadolinium demonstrated resolution of infection, as well as postoperative changes *(white arrow)*.

ably should be given perioperatively to patients with spinal epidural abscess to reduce edema, but this remains controversial.

Surgical drainage should be performed as an emergency procedure consisting of laminectomy and irrigation of the epidural space. Lesions with associated bony destruction and spinal instability resulting from osteomyelitis may require more extensive debridement, stabilization, and fusion. The subdural space should not be violated. Despite combined therapy, mortality rates remain as high as 10% to 20%, and morbidity can be catastrophic (e.g., paraplegia). Early diagnosis and rapid treatment offer the best chance for reducing mortality and morbidity.

BIBLIOGRAPHY

Baker AS et al: Spinal epidural abscess, *N Engl J Med* 293:463, 1975.

Bok APL, Peter JC: Subdural empyema: burr holes or craniotomy? A retrospective computerized tomography–era analysis of treatment in 90 cases, *J Neurosurg* 78:574, 1993.

Brock DG, Bleck TP: Extraaxial suppurations of the central nervous system, *Semin Neurol* 12:263, 1992.

Ciricillo SF, Rosenblum ML: Imaging of solitary lesions in AIDS, *J Neurosurg* 74:1029, 1991 (letter).

Ciricillo SF, Rosenblum ML: Use of CT and MR imaging to distinguish intracranial lesions and to define the need for biopsy in AIDS patients, *J Neurosurg* 73:720, 1990.

Cowie R, Williams B: Late seizures and morbidity after subdural empyema, *J Neurosurg* 58:569, 1983.

Dacey RG Jr: Central nervous system infections: brain abscesses and shunt infection. In Root RK, Trunkey DD, Sande MA, editors: *Contemporary issues in infectious diseases*, vol 6, Focus on infection: new surgical and medical approaches, New York, 1986, Churchill Livingstone.

Duma CM, Kondziolka D, Lundsford LD: Image-guided stereotactic management of non–AIDS-related cerebral infection, *Neurosurg Clin North Am* 3:291, 1993.

Hasemir MG, Ebeling U: CT-guided stereotactic aspiration and treatment of brain abscesses: an experience with 24 cases, *Acta Neurochir* 125:58, 1993.

Hellwig D, Bauer BL, Dauch WA: Endoscopic stereotactic treatment of brain abscesses, *Acta Neurochir* 61:102, 1994.

Hlavin ML et al: Spinal epidural abscess: a ten-year perspective, *Neurosurgery* 27:177, 1990.

Itakurg T et al: Stereotactic operation for brain abscess, *Surg Neurol* 28:114, 1987.

Kagawa M et al: Brain abscess in congenital cyanotic heart disease, *J Neurosurg* 58:913, 1983.

Kondziolka D, Duma CM, Lundsford LD: Factors that enhance the likelihood of successful treatment of brain abscesses, *Acta Neurochir* 127:85, 1994.

Koszewski W: Epilepsy following brain abscess: the evaluation of possible risk factors with emphasis on new concept of epileptic focus formation, *Acta Neurochir* 113:110, 1991.

Latchaw RE, Hirsch WL, Yock DH: Imaging of intracranial infection, *Neurosurg Clin North Am* 3:303, 1992.

Levy RM: Brain abscess and subdural empyema, *Curr Opin Neurol* 7:223, 1994.

Levy RM, Berger JR: HIV and HTLV infections of the nervous system. In Tyler KL, Martin JB, editors: *Infectious diseases of the nervous system*, Philadelphia, 1993, FA Davis.

Luft BJ, Remington JS: Toxoplasmic encephalitis, *J Infect Dis* 157:106, 1988.

Lunsford LD: Stereotactic drainage of brain abscesses, *Neurol Res* 9:270, 1987.

Mampalam TJ, Rosenblum ML: Trends in the management of bacterial brain abscess: a review of 102 cases over 17 years, *Neurosurg* 23:451, 1988.

McAlister WH, Lusk R, Muntz HR: Comparison of plain radiographs and coronal CT scans in infants and children with recurrent sinusitis, *Am J Roentgenol* 153:1259, 1989.

Modic MT, Feiglin DH, Piraino DW: Vertebral osteomyelitis: assessment using MR, *Radiology* 157:157, 1985.

Nussbaum ES, Rigamonti D, Stadiford H et al: Spinal epidural abscess: a report of 40 cases and review, *Surg Neurol* 38:225, 1992.

Obana WG, Rosenblum ML: Nonoperative treatment of neurosurgical infections, *Neurosurg Clin North Am* 3:359, 1992.

Osenbach RK, Loftus CM: Diagnosis and management of brain abscess, *Neurosurg Clin North Am* 3:403, 1992.

Rea GL, McGregor JM, Miller CA, Miner ME: Surgical treatment of the spontaneous spinal epidural abscess, *Surg Neurol* 37:274, 1992.

Redekop GJ, Del Maestro R: Diagnosis and management of spinal epidural abscess, *Can J Neurol Sci* 19:180, 1992.

Rodesch G et al: Nervous system manifestations and neuroradiologic findings in acquired immunodeficiency syndrome (AIDS), *Neuroradiology* 31:33, 1989.

Salzman C, Tuazon CU: Value of the ring-enhancing sign in differentiating intracerebral hematomas and brain abscesses, *Arch Intern Med* 147:951, 1987.

Schoendorf KC, Adams WG, Kiely JL, Wegner JD: National trends in *Haemophilus influenzae* meningitis mortality and hospitalization among children: 1980 through 1991, *Pediatrics* 93:663, 1994.

Schroth G et al: Advantage of magnetic resonance imaging in the diagnosis of cerebral infections, *Neuroradiology* 29:120, 1987.

Smith AS, Blaser SI: Infectious and inflammatory processes of the spine, *Radiol Clin North Am* 29:809, 1991.

Stapleton SR, Bell BA, Uttley D: Stereotactic aspiration of brain abscess: is this the treatment of choice? *Acta Neurochir* 121:15, 1993.

Sze G, Zimmerman RD: The magnetic resonance imaging of infections and inflammatory diseases, *Radiol Clin North Am* 26:839, 1988.

Tyler KL, Martin JB, Scheld WM: Focal suppurative infections of the central nervous system. In Tyler KL, Martin JB, editors: *Infectious diseases of the nervous system*, Philadelphia, 1993, FA Davis.

Walder LA, Anastasia LF, Spodick DH: Pulmonary arteriovenous malformation and brain abscess, *Am Heart J* 127:27, 1994.

Wingarten K et al: Subdural and epidural empyemas: MR imaging, *Am J Neuroradiol* 10:81, 1989.

Wispelwey B, Scheld WM: Brain abscess, *Semin Neurol* 12:273, 1992.

Yildizhan A, Pasoglu A, Kandemir B: Effect of dexamethasone on various stages of experimental brain abscess, *Acta Neurochir* 96:141-148, 1989.

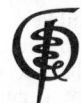

CHAPTER

241 Skin and Subcutaneous Infections

Richard E. Bryant

PRIMARY INFECTIONS OF SKIN
Impetigo

Impetigo is a superficial pyoderma that is usually caused by *Staphylococcus aureus*, mixtures of *S. aureus* and *Streptococcus pyogenes*, or less often by *S. pyogenes* alone. Impetigo is rarely caused by group C or G streptococci. In neonates it may be caused by group B streptococci. Impetigo is highly contagious in families or institutions where crowding, poor hygiene, and recurrent abrasions enhance the likelihood of infection, especially in preschool children.

Bacteria colonize the skin several weeks before disease occurs after minor trauma (Chapter 261). Lesions start as small vesicles beneath the stratum corneum and quickly become pustules and rupture to produce the characteristic honey-colored "stuck-on" crusts. Lesions on exposed surfaces often coalesce to form large crusts. Autoinoculation frequently produces separate lesions. Lymphadenopathy occurs often, but constitutional symptoms are mild or absent.

Diagnosis is usually suspected based on clinical appearance and confirmed by Gram's stain and culture. Serologic confirmation of *S. pyogenes* skin infection is obtained by a rising titer of antibody to antideoxyribonuclease B or antihyaluronidase. Antistreptolysin O titers do not rise predictably after impetigo. The differential diagnosis of impetigo includes secondary infection of primary skin lesions such as insect bites, eczema, or dermatophytosis. Early lesions of varicella or herpes simplex are usually larger and persist longer than do vesicles associated with impetigo. Viral diagnosis can be confirmed by Tzanck test, fluorescent antibody test, or viral culture. Cost-effective treatment options include oral erythromycin, topical mupirocin, or oral cephalosporins given twice daily.

Bullous Impetigo

Bullous impetigo is caused by *S. aureus* strains that produce an exfoliative exotoxin. The staphylococci are in phage group II, usually type 71. Nasal colonization is usually the reservoir from which bacteria spread to the skin, where invasion occurs after minor trauma. Bullous impetigo occurs primarily in neonates and young children and is less common than nonbullous impetigo.

Lesions begin as small vesicles and progress to large, flaccid blisters containing clear yellow fluid. Bullae rupture to form a thin, light-brown crust. Lymphadenopathy is rare, and systemic symptoms are usually mild. Diagnosis is made from Gram's stain showing clusters of gram-positive cocci and cultures growing *S. aureus*. Staphylococcal impetigo is easily differentiated from primary bullous diseases such as pemphigus because in patients with impetigo, cultures and smears are positive and Nikolsky's sign is negative. A penicillinase-resistant penicillin given orally is the treatment of choice. Erythromycin or mupirocin may be used for penicillin-allergic patients.

Ecthyma

Ecthyma is an ulcerative crusting infection caused by group A streptococci that occurs on exposed skin areas, especially the legs of children after abrasions, cuts, or insect bites. It may affect all sites and age-groups but in adults usually is associated with poor hygiene. Lesions caused by *Pseudomonas aeruginosa* or *S. aureus* can have a similar appearance.

Lesions begin as vesicles that become pustular and rupture to form dried, grayish, "punched-out," crusted lesions on a red, indurated base. Lesions extend below the epidermis and therefore heal more slowly than do those of impetigo and often leave scars. Patients with acquired immunodeficiency syndrome (AIDS) may have severe infection and bacteremia. Penicillin is the treatment of choice.

Erysipelas

Erysipelas is a distinctive superficial cellulitis of the skin that is usually caused by group A streptococci (rarely by group B, C, G, or D streptococci), *S. aureus,* or *Haemophilus influenzae.* Infection may occur at any age but is more common in infants, young children, and elderly individuals. Abdominal erysipelas may develop from umbilical infection in infants, whereas in children and adults the face and lower extremities are more often involved. Infection may occur at sites of minor trauma or surgery. Pelvic erysipelas may occur after surgery or radiotherapy. Erysipelas of the vulva may be caused by group B streptococci. Erysipelas often represents a complication of lymphatic obstruction that may be congenital (Milroy's disease) or iatrogenic (e.g., saphenous vein donor graft sites, cancer surgery, irradiation).

Illness usually begins as a localized, tender, red lesion that rapidly becomes bright-red, hot, painful, and indurated and develops a raised, advancing border reflecting the dermal involvement (Color Plate VIII-25). Malaise, headaches, and fever are common, and chills may occur. Lymphatic obstruction during infection produces the *peau d'orange* appearance of the skin. Lymphatic obstruction may persist after infection and predispose to recurrent erysipelas at the same site.

Erysipelas is diagnosed by its distinctive clinical appearance, blood and throat cultures, or serologic confirmation of a group A streptococcal infection.

Early stages of herpes zoster may mimic erysipelas but are distinguished by pain and hyperesthesia, which precede development of vesicular lesions. Angioedema and severe contact dermatitis may mimic erysipelas.

Early in its course erysipelas can usually be managed with oral antibiotics. Penicillin is the drug of choice, and erythromycin, newer macrolide analogs, or cephalosporins are alternatives. Patients with extensive disease and systemic symptoms should be hospitalized and receive parenteral antibiotics. Bacteremia occurs in 20% of patients. Superficial desquamation may be seen at the site of infection.

Cellulitis

Cellulitis is an acute infection of the skin with prominent involvement of subcutaneous tissue. *S. aureus* and group A streptococci are the most common infecting organisms. In young children *H. influenzae* causes a distinctive violaceous cellulitis of the face, neck, or upper body (Color Plate VIII-26). The origin of cellulitis is suggested by circumstances, bacterial features, and host-specific features of clinical presentation. Intravenous drug addicts have a high frequency of infection caused by *S. aureus, S. pyogenes,* and, more rarely, gram-negative bacilli or anaerobes. Diabetic patients have recurrent cellulitis and polymicrobial anaerobic infection of their insensate, traumatized feet. Deep-seated polymicrobial infections of the oropharynx or perirectal areas may become evident as cellulitis. Leukemic patients with neutropenia may have cellulitis caused by gram-negative bacilli, anaerobes, or fungi. Cellulitis after surgery is usually staphylococcal or streptococcal but may be polymicrobial and anaerobic if associated with gastrointestinal tract procedures or fecal soilage. Cellulitis after animal bites is usually caused by streptococci, staphylococci, or *Pasteurella multocida* and less often by anaerobic or polymicrobial infections. Human bites are often polymicrobial and have a higher frequency of anaerobic pathogens. Cellulitis after trauma in aqueous environments may be caused by *Erysipelothrix rhusiopathiae, Aeromonas hydrophila,* or *Vibrio* species. Cellulitis may be a presenting sign of bacteremia caused by *Vibrio vulnificus* in the chronic alcoholic or immunocompromised patient after ingestion of raw seafood.

Cellulitis usually originates at sites of previous injury of the skin or more rarely by hematogenous spread (*H. influenzae*). Initial local tenderness and erythema are followed by rapid intensification of heat, swelling, and pain. Involved skin is red and hot but, unlike with erysipelas, has indistinct borders because of the depth of infection. Central areas may become necrotic or blister. Regional lymphadenopathy, chills, and fever often occur, and lymphangitis may be present.

Information gained by microscopic examination of smears and Gram's stains can direct initial antibiotic therapy and should be modified by results of cultures and sensitivity studies. Representative material is usually obtained from the more central, purulent areas of infection rather than from the advancing borders of cellulitis. Skin biopsies are especially helpful for diagnosing fungal infection in immunocompromised patients.

The type and route of antibiotic administration are determined by the infecting organism and the extent and severity of infection. More extensive disease may require surgical debridement. Patients with cellulitis complicating dermatophytosis should have treatment for the underlying fungal infection.

Patients with recurrent cellulitis associated with lymphatic obstruction often benefit from prolonged therapy with oral penicillin.

Lymphangitis

Lymphangitis is an infection of the lymphatic vessels, usually involving an extremity. Group A streptococci and *S. aureus* are the most common causative organisms. The site of entry is often less conspicuous than the red, tender streaking of the skin overlying the inflamed lymphatic channels. Proximal lymph nodes are enlarged and usually tender. Fever and leukocytosis typically occur. Diagnosis is made by clinical appearance and confirmed by Gram's stains of the primary lesion or by blood cultures. Antibiotic therapy is directed toward suspected bacterial pathogens. Since lymphangitic streaking can also occur with herpetic infection, it is important to exclude that entity by careful history and follow-up examination.

Elephantiasis nostras is a chronic cellulitis caused by recurrent lymphangitis and lymphadenitis. The progressively worsening lymphedema leads to thickening of the skin and nodulation, ulceration, and hypertrophy that mimics elephant skin (Color Plate VIII-27).

Folliculitis

Folliculitis is an infection of hair follicles usually caused by *S. aureus,* but it may be caused by streptococci, Enterobacteriaceae, Pseudomonadaceae, fungi, or viruses, or it may be sterile. Involvement of the follicle may be superficial or deep and may follow mechanical occlusion of follicles after superficial irritation. Sycosis barbae is deeper folliculitis of the bearded area caused by *S. aureus. P. aeruginosa* is a common cause of folliculitis on the buttocks, hips, or axillae that may be acquired from "hot tubs" or from heavily contaminated water (Color Plate VIII-28). This lesion may be preceded by pruritic and papular lesions. Folliculitis adjacent to intertriginous yeast infection may be caused by *Candida* organisms. Patients with bone marrow transplants can have lesions mimicking folliculitis caused by *Pityrosporum* organisms. Severely immunocompromised patients may have folliculitis caused by *Malassezia furfur.*

Superficial folliculitis usually responds to local measures such as cleansing and topical antibiotics, but oral antibiotics may be required for management of deep or recurrent folliculitis. Some patients may require ciprofloxacin therapy for *Pseudomonas* folliculitis.

Patients with AIDS may have a widespread acneiform eruption, recurrence of adolescent acne, necrotizing folliculitis, or eosinophilic pustular folliculitis.

Noninfectious folliculitis may be seen with pustular psoriasis, acne, occupational acne, corticosteroid or lithium therapy, acne rosacea, and a variety of disorders of uncertain origin.

Furuncles and Carbuncles

These lesions are abscesses (boils) of deeper skin structures caused by *S. aureus*. Lesions usually begin as folliculitis and are found in hairy areas of the face, neck, buttocks, extremities, or axillae that are sites of heavy perspiration and frequent irritation. Furuncles begin as painful, red nodules that expand and liquefy centrally in the characteristic stages of development of a "boil." Deeper lesions with multiple interconnecting subcutaneous furuncles are termed *carbuncles*. These lesions usually drain to overlying skin at several sites. Carbuncles are most common on the back of the neck, the back, and the thighs.

Furuncles appear to be more common in obese and diabetic patients and are recognized as complications of corticosteroid therapy or underlying immunologic disease, immunoglobulin deficiency, or neutrophil dysfunction. Linkage between iron deficiency and recurrent furunculosis remains unproved. Leukocytosis, fever, and constitutional symptoms usually reflect more extensive cellulitis and tissue involvement.

Recurrent furunculosis may be caused by the predisposing conditions already cited but more often reflects persistent colonization or reinfection of a normal host, or both. Nasal colonization is usually the site of primary carriage. Less often, colonization may be in perineal or other skin sites as well. Recurrent furunculosis may be perpetuated in some patients by recolonization through cross-contamination from family members.

Topical application of moist heat that promotes localization and drainage is often adequate treatment for simple furuncles. Antistaphylococcal antibiotics are recommended for extensive involvement or lesions located on the midface or for patients thought to have bacteremia or those at risk of colonization of previously damaged heart valves or prosthetic devices.

Patients with boils and compromised host defenses from diabetes mellitus, rheumatoid arthritis, organ transplantation, or leukemia should receive antistaphylococcal antibiotics. Patients requiring parenteral therapy for infection with methicillin-resistant staphylococci (MRSA) should receive vancomycin. Surgical drainage is an integral part of managing large furuncles or carbuncles. Furunculosis is usually a self-limited process. Patients with recurrent furunculosis are best treated with regimens containing rifampin to eradicate staphylococcal carriage (Chapter 260). Topical application of antibiotics to the nose or use of various staphylococcal vaccines are not of proven value. However, topical mupirocin is an effective means of eradicating staphylococcal colonization of the nose and is active against MRSA. Prolonged therapy with oral clindamycin or ciprofloxacin eradicates carriage in some patients.

Staphylococcal Scalded-Skin Syndrome

In this syndrome extensive bullae formation and exfoliation of the skin (Chapter 260) are caused by phage group II *S. aureus* organisms that produce an exfoliative exotoxin. Toxin-producing staphylococci may primarily involve the conjunctivae, pharynx, umbilicus, abscesses, or the blood stream, but in contrast to bullous impetigo, the lesions of the scalded-skin syndrome are sterile. Lesions are characterized on histologic examination by a cleavage plane high in the epidermis. This feature aids in differentiating this disease from toxic epidermal necrolysis, which involves subepidermal layers that can be distinguished on histologic study (Color Plate VIII-29).

Staphylococcal scalded-skin syndrome is seen almost exclusively in young children and has caused epidemics in neonatal nurseries. The disease appears rapidly but may follow a recognized staphylococcal infection by several days. Pain, fever, and generalized erythema and edema of the skin are followed by development of large, flaccid bullae that are easily ruptured and demonstrate a positive Nikolsky's sign. Skin sloughs off with light lateral pressure. Extensive denudation of skin may cause problems with fluid and electrolyte balance. There is little difficulty differentiating this disease from toxic epidermal necrolysis. The latter is usually caused by drug allergy, may involve mucous membranes, occurs most often in adults, and involves the subepidermis.

Treatment of the staphylococcal scalded-skin syndrome includes penicillinase-resistant penicillins (nafcillin) and supportive therapy. Corticosteroids are not recommended.

Scarlet Fever

Scarlet fever is a classic exanthematous disease of childhood associated with acute group A streptococcal pharyngitis. The erythrogenic toxin responsible for the rash is coded for by a bacteriophage infecting the streptococcus. Immunity to the toxin precludes recurrence of this syndrome (Chapter 261).

Symptoms of pharyngitis usually develop 1 to 2 days before appearance of the rash. Headache, fever, malaise, and submandibular adenopathy are often present. The pharynx is erythematous, with enlarged tonsils and a purulent exudate. The tongue has prominent papillae that protrude through a whitish coating. Over several days this coating clears, leaving a bright-red tongue with accentuated papillae, giving rise to the term *strawberry tongue*. The exanthem begins on the upper chest, with subsequent spread to the neck and extremities. It is a confluent erythema composed of small puncta that impart a rough feel to the skin. The rash is accentuated in the flexural creases, where it may assume a linear petechial appearance (Pastia's lines). The exanthem persists for 5 to 10 days and desquamates on clearing. Desquamation begins on the face, where it produces a fine scale, and subsequently progresses to the trunk and limbs. Desquamation is often most marked on the hands and the feet, where large areas of skin may slough. Scarlet fever is often accompanied by an elevated white blood cell count. Throat cultures grow group A streptococci, and serologic evidence of infection is provided by rising titers to antistreptolysin O. Penicillin is the drug of choice.

Staphylococcal scarlet fever may mimic many of the features of streptococcal scarlet fever. The syndrome is presumed to represent an incomplete form of the staphylococcal scalded-skin syndrome caused by exfoliative exotoxin. The rash can be identical, but staphylococcal scarlet fever does not produce an enanthem and is not associated with pharyngitis but may arise from a surgical wound infection. The treatment of choice is a penicillinase-resistant penicillin.

Streptococcal Toxic Shock

Streptococcal toxic shock is a term applied to fulminant streptococcal infection associated with progressive multiorgan failure and a mortality rate of 30% to 60% (Chapter 261). One study found positive tissue cultures in 95% and bacteremia in 65% of patients. None of the patients had a classic rash of scarlet fever. Patients had a brief, nonspecific prodrome that was quickly followed by hypotension, renal failure, adult respiratory distress syndrome, mental status changes, and disseminated intravascular coagulation. The primary site of infection may be inapparent or may become evident with local pain, swelling, and erythema.

Streptococcal toxic shock syndrome has occurred with pharyngitis, cellulitis, otitis, osteomyelitis, necrotizing fasciitis, myositis, postpartum myometritis, endocarditis, and peritonitis. Women may have this syndrome as a complication of pregnancy, gynecologic surgery, or pelvic inflammatory disease. Patients with fulminant pneumonia may have rapidly progressive pleural effusions and empyema.

Staphylococcal Toxic Shock Syndrome

The multisystem toxic shock syndrome is caused by a pyrogenic enterotoxin producing staphylococci and occurs in conjunction with menstrual and nonmenstrual illness (Chapter 260). Criteria for diagnosis include a temperature of 38.9° C (102° F) or greater, diffuse erythroderma, hypotension, involvement of three or more organ systems, and desquamation of the skin on the palms and/or soles late in the course of illness (Chapters 235 and 260). The rash is scarlatiniform, may be evanescent, and may resemble a sunburn. There is often prominent mucous membrane involvement with conjunctivitis, pharyngitis, and vaginal hyperemia or erythema. Changes in cognitive function may be severe. Leukocytosis, thrombocytopenia, and microscopic hematuria are often present. Elevation of creatinine values and liver function test abnormalities are common. Myoglobinuria and increased serum creatine kinase levels occur in patients with muscle injury. By definition, patients with bacteremia are excluded from this syndrome complex, but identical symptoms may occur in patients with deep-seated staphylococcal infection or postoperative staphylococcal infection. Infected wounds causing toxic shock usually appear minimally inflamed and must be explored to confirm the diagnosis by Gram's stain and culture.

Toxic shock syndrome usually occurs within 2 days but may occur more than a week after surgery. Virtually all wounds, lesions, or bites are at risk of this complication. Toxic shock associated with nasal packing for epistaxis appears analogous to tampon-related disease but has occurred in the absence of absorbent materials. Approximately 50% to 70% of toxic shock syndrome cases occur in association with menstruation and tampon use. Most patients are young white women. In black and Hispanic women toxic shock syndrome rarely develops unless it complicates surgery or deep-seated infection. The syndrome may occur in conjunction with influenza, sinusitis, pharyngitis, tracheitis, infected burns, or abscesses.

Appropriate management includes removal of tampons and vaginal irrigation or drainage of infected sites in patients with associated deep-seated infection. Patients should be monitored carefully and should receive aggressive fluid volume replacement and treatment for shock and ventilatory insufficiency. Corticosteroids are probably helpful early in the course of shock. Antistaphylococcal therapy is helpful in eradicating toxin-producing organisms and reduces the likelihood of recurrent disease.

Erythrasma

Erythrasma is a chronic superficial infection of the skin caused by *Corynebacterium minutissimum.* It generally affects the intertriginous zones such as the groin, axillae, toe clefts, and inframammary folds but occasionally may be widespread. The clinical lesion appears as a well-demarcated brownish-red patch with a fine scale. Patients are usually asymptomatic or mildly pruritic. Erythrasma is a common condition that occurs more often in men than in women and is seen more frequently in a humid climate.

Tinea cruris may resemble erythrasma, although tinea may appear more inflammatory. The distinction between the two is made by a positive potassium hydroxide examination in tinea and by Wood's light examination, which shows a characteristic coral-red fluorescence in erythrasma. Erythromycin, 250 mg qid for 7 to 14 days, produces excellent therapeutic results.

Trichomycosis Axillaris

Trichomycosis axillaris is a superficial infection of the axillary and pubic hairs caused by diphtheroids. Although the etiologic agent has been said to be *Corynebacterium tenuis,* multiple types of organisms appear to be responsible, sometimes in the same patient. This asymptomatic condition becomes evident with the formation of yellow, red, or black nodules on the hair shaft. The sweat may be similarly colored. Treatment consists in shaving the affected area and applying a topical erythromycin ointment.

NECROTIZING SOFT TISSUE INFECTIONS

Many infections may lead to necrosis of skin and soft tissues. These diseases should be classified primarily on the basis of their anatomic involvement and secondarily on their microbial origin or cause. They may be divided into superficial cellulitis, fascial-level infection, or myonecrosis and are best characterized at surgery. Deep infections may dissect along fascial planes and involve muscles and fat to a greater extent than is suspected on clinical examination. Prompt, aggressive surgical intervention, deep biopsy, and adequate debridement are the keys to reduced mortality. Broad-spectrum antibiotics are selected empirically and changed on the basis of smears and culture results. These infections have been linked with group A streptococcal infection but may occur with staphylococci, gram-negative bacilli, *Vibrio vulnificus,* mucormycosis, or *Aspergillus* organisms. Polymicrobial infection with anaerobic and aerobic organisms is probably the most common cause of this entity.

Necrotizing Fasciitis

Necrotizing fasciitis is a life-threatening infection of subcutaneous tissue and fascial planes. It may occur in normal persons after minor trauma or may occur in surgical wounds. Such infections occur more frequently in the elderly, debilitated diabetic patients, indigent alcoholic or homeless patients, or drug abusers. Tissue necrosis follows hemorrhage and dissection of infection along fascial planes with secondary vascular thrombosis and gangrene. Lesions begin as tender, red, swollen areas that may spread over 24 to 48 hours to become indurated and cyanotic, with blisters containing reddish-black fluid. Lesions are tender but may become anesthetic in gangrenous areas. Black eschar formation may resemble a deep burn (Color Plate VIII-30). Surrounding skin is often undermined and can be easily separated from deep fascia by manipulation with a probe. Patients have chills, fever, and prostration. Persistent fever and clinical deterioration typically occur, despite apparently adequate antibiotic therapy, because tissue-space fluid collections are overlooked and undrained.

Cultures of blood and involved tissue are usually positive, and diagnosis can be confirmed by Gram's stain, biopsy of involved skin, or computed tomography–guided or ultrasound-guided aspiration of tissue fluid collections. Leukocytosis is marked, and anemia requiring transfusion may be present.

Necrotizing fasciitis must be distinguished from other acute cutaneous infections. The necrotic areas of skin separate it from simple erysipelas or cellulitis. Clostridial cellulitis and nonclostridial crepitant cellulitis usually have more crepitus and few cutaneous changes. Gas gangrene characteristically affects underlying muscle, whereas necrotizing fasciitis does not. Radiographic evidence of gas suggests a diagnosis other than necrotizing fasciitis. Since both gangrene and necrotizing fasciitis require surgery, the differential diagnosis is often best made at surgery. Needle aspiration of fluid after demonstration of fluid collections by imaging techniques may be especially useful in streptococcal gangrene but is not adequate for management of other forms of fasciitis. Surgery should be performed promptly.

One must remember that aggressive surgical debridement is the key to effective therapy of necrotizing fasciitis and that appropriate parenteral antibiotic therapy plays a vital but ancillary role. Although diabetes and atherosclerosis may adversely affect survival, the worst prognostic factors include delayed recognition or incomplete surgical debridement.

Clostridial Cellulitis

Clostridial cellulitis (Chapter 263) is a superficial infection that does not extend to involve muscles. It is characterized by a longer incubation period, but less pain, edema, and systemic toxicity than gas gangrene. A thin discharge is present, and crepitus and gas formation are often prominent.

Gram's stain and culture of the exudate establish the clostridial nature of the process. Radiographs show the presence of gas without involvement of muscle. Diagnosis is confirmed at surgery. Therapy consists of simple wound debridement and administration of penicillin, cefoxitin, or a β-lactamase inhibitor combination.

Nonclostridial Crepitant Cellulitis

Nonclostridial crepitant cellulitis, a gas-forming infection, probably occurs more often than gas gangrene. It frequently mimics clostridial cellulitis. The infection is usually polymicrobial and may contain coliforms, streptococci, and bacteroides. Diabetic patients are predisposed to this syndrome and often have a more aggressive course than do nondiabetic patients. There may be abundant gas dissecting along tissue planes, but there is characteristically little systemic toxicity and no muscle involvement (Chapter 271).

Local surgical debridement and drainage are indicated. Antibiotics are eventually dictated by culture results, but broad-spectrum coverage should be instituted initially because of the variety of potential pathogens.

Gas Gangrene

Gas gangrene is a fulminant, life-threatening infection of subcutaneous tissue and muscle caused by *Clostridium* species (usually *C. perfringens*) (Chapter 263). It follows trauma complicated by wound contamination and may be associated with cholecystectomy or other surgical procedures, compound fractures, or vascular insufficiency. Contamination may originate from soil containing spores of *C.*

perfringens or may arise from normal skin flora that contain this organism in large numbers. Invasiveness of this pathogen is enhanced by its production of more than a dozen exotoxins, of which the alpha toxin is the most important. Infectivity is increased a millionfold when organisms lodge in injured muscle tissue with a compromised vascular supply. Thus both contamination and a properly anaerobic environment are necessary for development of overt disease.

Onset of infection may occur within a few hours to a few days after the inciting event. Pain may increase dramatically after an initial improvement and appear disproportionate to early changes in the wound appearance. Marked edema soon follows; muscle may herniate through wounds, and surrounding skin may form dark blisters and

undergo necrosis. Crepitus is rarely prominent early, and gas may be obscured by extensive edema. The wound has a foul-smelling, thin discharge. Gram's stain of this material shows many large, grampositive bacilli but very few neutrophils. Delirium, tachycardia, and shock may follow rapidly, but fever may be mild. In overwhelming infection this process may evolve and lead to death in several hours.

The diagnosis of gas gangrene is made on clinical grounds, substantiated by Gram's stain smears and by radiographs showing gas spreading linearly along muscle and fascial planes, and proved at surgery by demonstration of gas in tissues and myonecrosis. Bacteremia is rare.

Prompt, aggressive surgical debridement with removal of all in-

Table 241-1   Distinctive skin signs and risk factors associated with specific infections

DISEASE (INFECTIOUS AGENT)	RISK FACTORS	SKIN SIGNS AND PRESENTATION
Ecthyma gangrenosum (*Pseudomonas aeruginosa*) (Chapter 236)	Immunocompromised patients, especially those with neutropenia and leukemia or lymphoma; prognosis significantly better if not bacteremic	Single or multiple lesions evolving from vesicles to round indurated necrotic ulcers or eschars, often involving skin folds (Color Plate VIII-23)
Toxic shock syndrome (TSS) (*Staphylococcus aureus*) (Chapter 261)	Menstruating women (usually young whites); may occur postpartum	Sunburnlike rash, conjunctivitis, "strawberry tongue," pharyngitis with fever, hypotension, and prostration; desquamation of palms and soles several days to 1 to 2 weeks later (Color Plate VIII-20)
	TSS related to wound, medical procedure, or injury (any sex or race)	Wound usually only slightly red, indurated, and not purulent
Vibrio vulnificus–related *Vibrio* species cellulitis (Chapter 268)	Immunocompromised patients: alcoholism, cirrhosis, diabetes, leukemia, renal failure, or steroid recipient having contact with sea water, brackish water, or shellfish	May begin as pustules, cellulitis, or lymphangitis, progressing to large hemorrhagic bullous lesions that ulcerate
Anthrax (*Bacillus anthracis*) (Chapter 263)	Contact with infected animals or animal products (wool, hides, ivory, hair) imported from countries with endemic disease (e.g., Africa, India, Pakistan, Haiti)	Malignant pustule usually on exposed skin of face, neck, hands, or arms; bullae develop in 1 to 5 days with edema and erythema; signs of sepsis possibly severe
Plague (*Yersinia pestis*) (Chapter 270)	Fleaborne disease from infected animals (rabbits, bobcats, prairie dogs) in Southwest United States to sightseers, hunters, or vacationers or to pets, from which owners are secondarily infected	Rarely prominent flea bite with papule or vesicopustule; may have associated tender lymphadenopathy (buboes) and serious systemic illness
Tularemia (*Francisella tularensis*) (Chapter 270)	Avocational, vocational, or domestic exposure to ticks or infected animals	Ulcerative lesion with raised margins at site of injury; may have marked regional adenopathy and systemic illness; may have oculoglandular syndrome
Cutaneous diphtheria (*Corynebacterium diphtheriae*) (Chapter 263)	Poor hygiene; more common in "skid row" population of South and Northwest United States	Lesions may be primarily or secondarily infected; often a persistent punched-out ulcer with a pustule or gray shaggy membrane
Lyme disease (*Borrelia burgdorferi*) (Chapter 274)	Tick bite that usually goes undetected in endemic area	Quite variable: Characteristic lesion of erythema chronicum migrans begins as red macule or papule, developing bright-red outer margins with central clearing
"Hot tub" folliculitis	Recent use of hot tubs, whirlpools, or spa pools (usually within 1 to 4 days); diagnosed by culture of lesion	Folliculitis with papules, vesicles, or pustules over exposed areas; spares face and neck; may have fever, adenopathy, and mastitis; usually self-limited (Color Plate VIII-28)
Elephantiasis nostras	Chronic cellulitis and edema of extremity caused by lymphangitis and lymphadenitis	Progressively worsening lymphedema with recurrent infection; thickening and hardening of skin with nodulation, ulceration, and hypertrophy of skin to form pachydermatosus appearance (Color Plate VIII-27)
Clostridium septicum sepsis	Gas gangrene caused by hematogenous spread, usually from underlying malignancy that may be inapparent	"Spontaneous" gas gangrene with rapid development of edema, blisters, bulla formation, and subcutaneous air
Erysipeloid (*Erysipelothrix rhusiopathiae*)	Usually secondary infection of cut or abrasion by contact with fish, crustaceans, or meat products	Violaceous, warm, tender lesion with raised margins; lesion may clear centrally with brownish discoloration; few constitutional symptoms
Epithelioid (bacillary) angiomatosis	Disseminated cutaneous and multiorgan bacillary infection of patients with acquired immunodeficiency syndrome	Vascular lesion with 2- to 6-mm papules resembling Kaposi's sarcoma or pyogenic granuloma; silver-staining bacilli seen in areas of necrosis
Sporotrichosis (*Sporothrix schenckii*) (Chapter 276)	Secondary infection of abrasion or cut of skin from thorns, splinters, sphagnum moss, or mine timbers colonized with fungus	Papules, pustules, or nodules that become indurated and ulcerate, producing multiple lesions by lymphangitic spread (Color Plate VIII-24)
Mycobacterium marinum (Chapter 273)	Exposure to fish, aquariums, or swimming pools	Violaceous papule, ulcer, or scaling lesion at site of injury; lesions may resemble sporotrichosis (Color Plate VIII-31)

volved tissue is required for successful therapy. Although high-dose penicillin is the drug of choice for gas gangrene, empiric therapy is usually broadened to cover polymicrobial infection, including gram-negative bacilli and anaerobes. Clindamycin may reduce toxin elaboration by clostridia and enhance efficacy of alternative regimens, including cefoxitin, imipenem, or β-lactamase inhibitor combinations. Hyperbaric oxygen therapy, when available, may be a valuable adjunctive therapy but is not a substitute for surgery.

Synergistic Nonclostridial Anaerobic Myonecrosis

Synergistic nonclostridial anaerobic myonecrosis may involve subcutaneous tissue, fascia, and muscle. It is caused by combinations of aerobic gram-negative bacilli (e.g., *Escherichia coli* or *Klebsiella, Enterobacter,* or *Proteus* species) and anaerobes (*Bacteroides* species and/or anaerobic streptococci).

Synergistic necrotizing cellulitis occurs most frequently in the perineal region or lower extremities of patients with diabetes and/or renal disease and vascular disease. A variant, Fournier's gangrene, which can be caused by staphylococci and streptococci in addition to the organisms just cited, involves prominent necrotizing fasciitis of male genitalia. The distinction is artificial because Fournier's gangrene may be predominantly cellulitis or may extend to involve muscles of the abdominal walls and extremities.

The infection may begin as vesicles that form tender skin ulcers which drain thick, foul-smelling, "dishwater" pus. Necrotic skin is quite tender and is surrounded by florid erythema and edema. Crepitus may be present. Patients appear toxic, and many are bacteremic.

Radical surgical debridement is the cornerstone of successful therapy. Amputation may be necessary, but tissue recovery is often better than expected. Broad-spectrum antimicrobial therapy is started empirically and is modified by the results of smears and cultures. Mortality is high even with adequate management.

Table 241-2   Antimicrobial therapy of dermal infection

INFECTION	USUAL ORGANISMS	ANTIBIOTIC TREATMENT
Impetigo		
Nonbullous	*Staphylococcus aureus* more than *Streptococcus pyogenes*	Oral macrolide, mupirocin, antistaphylococcal β-lactam (ASB)
Bullous	*S. aureus*	As above
Ecthyma	*S. pyogenes*	Oral Pen-G or Pen-V (parenteral Pen for sepsis)
Erysipelas	*S. pyogenes*	Oral Pen (parenteral for sepsis)
	S. aureus	Antistaphylococcal β-lactam (parenteral for sepsis or associated vascular insufficiency)
Cellulitis		
Usual	*S. aureus, S. pyogenes*	ASB (parenteral for sepsis, associated vascular insufficiency, or compromised host, followed by specific oral therapy)
Water injury	*Vibrio vulnificus*	Tetracycline + Imi, Cipro, or chloramphenicol
	Aeromonas hydrophila	Cipro, SMX/TMP, Imi, or expanded-spectrum cephalosporin (ESC)
	Erysipelothrix rhusiopathiae	Pen-G, Amp, Erythro, oral cephalosporin
Diabetic foot		
Early	Aerobic gram-positive cocci	Pen-G, Pen-V, Clind
Late	Anaerobes, aerobic gram-negative bacilli, streptococci	Ticar/Clav, Pip/TAZO, Imi, Amp/Sul ± Aztreo (parenteral for severe disease and sepsis)
		Oral Amox/Clav, Clind + Cipro, Metro + Cipro or ASB
Bite wound	*S. pyogenes, S. aureus, Pasteurella multocida, Eikenella corrodens, Capnocytophaga canimorsus*	Amox/Clav, Amp/Sul, ESC, tetracycline
Necrotizing dermatitis	—	*Aggressive surgery for diagnosis and therapy*
Necrotizing fasciitis	*S. pyogenes*	Parenteral Pen-G
	Polymicrobial anaerobic and aerobic gram-negative bacilli	Imi, Ticar/Clav, Pip/TAZO, Amp/Sul + Aztreo, or Amp + Clind + Gent
Clostridial	Clostridial cellulitis	Pen-G, Cefox, Ticar/Clav, Amp/Sul, Pip/TAZO
	Gas gangrene	Imi + Clind, Pen-G + Clind
Synergistic nonclostridial anaerobic myonecrosis	Anaerobes, aerobic gram-negative bacilli and streptococci	Imi, Ticar/Clav, PIP/TAZO, Amp/Sul + Aztreo, Amp + Clind + Gent
Meleney's ulcer	Combined infection: *S. aureus,* microaerophilic streptococci (±*Entaemoeba histolytica*)	ASB (Metro if *E. histolytica* present)

DRUG GROUPING	COMMENTARY AND ABBREVIATIONS
β-Lactams	Penicillins, cephalosporins, carbopenems, or monobactam
Macrolides	Erythromycin (Erythro): cheapest to use, less well tolerated
	Clarithromycin, azithromycin: active versus *Haemophilus influenzae,* broader spectrum but not active versus Erythro-resistant *S. aureus* or *S. pyogenes*
	Clindamycin (Clind): good anaerobic spectrum, poor versus *H. influenzae*
Antistaphylococcal β-lactams	
Oral penicillins	Dicloxacillin, amoxicillin/clavulanate (Amox/Clav)
Oral cephalosporins	Cephradine, cefadroxil, cefuroxime, axetil, cefaclor
Parenteral penicillins	Nafcillin, ampicillin/sulbactam (Amp/Sul), ticarcillin/clavulanate (Ticar/Clav), imipenem (Imi)
Parenteral cephalosporins	Cephalothin, cephapirin, cefazolin, cefuroxime
Penicillin	Penicillin G (Pen-G): oral or parenteral
	Penicillin V (Pen-V): oral
Expanded-spectrum cephalosporins	Cefmenoxime, cefotaxime, ceftizoxime, ceftriaxone, ceftazidime
Miscellaneous	Sulfamethoxazole/trimethoprim (SMX/TMP), ciprofloxacin (Cipro), cefoxitin (Cefox), aztreonam (Aztreo), gentamicin (Gent), metronidazole (Metro), Piperacillin taxobactam (Pip/TAZO)

Progressive Bacterial Synergistic Gangrene

Progressive bacterial synergistic gangrene was first described by Meleney, who was thought to have produced similar lesions in animals by combined infection with staphylococci and streptococci but not by either alone. The synergistic infection induced in animals was a more fulminant infection than the disease described by Meleney and led some observers to suggest that Meleney's synergistic gangrene was actually cutaneous amebiasis. The disease is a rare complication of surgical or traumatic wounds caused by microaerophilic or anaerobic streptococci along with *S. aureus* or, rarely, a gram-negative bacillus.

The lesion begins as a painful ulcer that classically enlarges to contain three discrete parts. The central necrotic ulcer and gangrenous skin are surrounded by a zone of intense purplish discoloration, which is surrounded by an erythematous zone of cellulitis. Untreated lesions expand to involve contiguous areas, and subsequent systemic complications occur. Cultures show that the outer edge of the infection contains streptococci, whereas central ulcerated lesions contain staphylococci. Lesions should be carefully examined for amebae, and amebic serologic studies should be obtained.

Radical surgical debridement and intensive antibiotic therapy are needed for optimal management of patients with affected wounds.

Table 241-1 lists the skin signs and risk factors for specific infections. Table 241-2 lists antimicrobial therapy for various dermal infections.

BIBLIOGRAPHY

Ahrenholz DH: Necrotizing soft tissue infections, *Surg Clin North Am* 68:199, 1988.

Allen TA et al: Toxic shock syndrome associated with use of latex nasal packing, *Arch Intern Med* 150:2587, 1990.

Bufill JA et al: *Pityrosporum* folliculitis after bone marrow transplantation, *Ann Intern Med* 108:560-563, 1988.

Caplan ES, Kluge RM: Gas gangrene: review of 34 cases, *Arch Intern Med* 136:778, 1976.

Chartier C, Grosshans E: Erysipelas, *Int J Dermatol* 29:458, 1990.

Davson J, Jones DM, Turner L: Diagnosis of Meleney's synergistic gangrene, *Br J Surg* 75:267, 1988.

Demidovich CW et al: Impetigo: current etiology and comparison of penicillin, erythromycin, and cephalexin therapies, *Am J Dis Child* 144:1313, 1990.

Farmlett EJ et al: Computed tomography in the assessment of myonecrosis, *J Am Assoc Radiol* 38:278, 1987.

Feingold DS: Gangrenous and crepitant cellulitis, *J Am Acad Dermatol* 6:289, 1982.

Harawi SJ et al: Cutaneous diseases associated with HIV infection, *Pathol Annu* 26:265, 1991.

Herman LE et al: Folliculitis: a clinicopathologic review, *Pathol Annu* 26:201, 1991.

Hewitt WD, Farrar WE: Care report: bacteremia and ecthyma caused by *Streptococcus pyogenes* in a patient with acquired immunodeficiency syndrome, *Am J Med Sci* 295:52, 1988.

Kingston D, Seal DV: Current hypotheses on synergistic microbial gangrene, *Br J Surg* 77:260, 1987.

Koehler JE, Tappero JW: Bacillary angiomatosis and bacillary peliosis in patients infected with human immunodeficiency virus, *Clin Infect Dis* 17:612, 1993.

Mertz PM, Maishall DA, Eaglstein WH et al: Topical mupirocin treatment of impetigo is equal to oral erythromycin therapy, *Arch Dermatol* 125:1069, 1989.

Neefe LI et al: Staphylococcal scalded-skin syndrome in adults: case report and review of the literature, *Am J Med Sci* 277:99, 1979.

Riseman JA et al: Hyperbaric oxygen therapy for necrotizing fasciitis reduces mortality and the need for debridements, *Surgery* 108:847, 1990.

Sanders LJ, Slomsky JM, Berger-Caplan C: Elephantiasis nostras: an eight-year observation of progressive nonfilarial elephantiasis of the lower extremity, *Cutis* 2:406, 1988.

Sarkany I, Taplin D, Blank H: The etiology and treatment of erythrasma, *J Invest Dermatol* 37:283, 1961.

Stamenkovic I, Lew PD: Early recognition of potentially fatal necrotizing fasciitis: the use of frozen-section biopsy, *N Engl J Med* 310:1689, 1984.

Stevens DL: Streptococcal toxic-shock syndrome: spectrum of disease, pathogenesis, and new concepts in treatment, *Emerging Infect Dis* 1:69, 1995.

Stevens DL et al: Spontaneous, nontraumatic gangrene due to *Clostridium septicum*, *Rev Infect Dis* 12:286, 1990.

Sudarsky LA et al: Improved results form a standardized approach in treating patients with necrotizing fasciitis, *Ann Surg* 206:661, 1987.

CHAPTER

242 Gastrointestinal Tract Infections

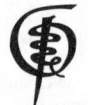

Herbert L. DuPont

Although diarrheal illness is a major cause of absenteeism from work and school in industrialized regions, it is of greater importance in developing nations, where it is often the major cause of infant mortality and serious morbidity in travelers from areas of lower disease endemicity. Laboratory procedures available during the past two decades have provided convincing evidence that most of the acute diarrhea occurring throughout the world is of infectious origin. Thus with these laboratory techniques the disease is now subject to study with the aim of defining etiologic factors, describing specific epidemiologic modes of spread and patterns of susceptibility, and developing effective means of treating, controlling, and even preventing the disease. This chapter focuses on the responsible etiologic agents in gastrointestinal tract infection; discusses their mechanisms of disease production; and offers a perspective on diagnosis, therapy, and prevention. Acute diarrhea is the primary focus. The other important clinical presentation of intestinal infection, enteric (typhoidlike) fever, also is discussed briefly.

PATHOPHYSIOLOGY

Most forms of enteric infection lead to the occurrence of diarrhea with variable associated symptoms. Diarrhea is generally defined as the passing of a greater number of stools of decreased form than is customary. A more rigid definition is not practical. Three factors acting together or separately lead to the passage of unformed stools: intestinal secretion, nonabsorption of intraintestinal constituents (often disaccharides), and altered intestinal motility. In acute infectious diarrhea, available evidence suggests that the first two mechanisms are important, and the third, which is largely unstudied in acute states of diarrhea, is of particular importance in chronic diarrhea of noninfectious origin (i.e., irritable bowel syndrome and idiopathic ulcerative colitis). The ways infectious microorganisms produce increased luminal fluid are reviewed briefly when the specific etiologic agents are described.

ETIOLOGIC AGENTS AND THEIR VIRULENCE PROPERTIES

The various microbial agents capable of producing active infection of the intestinal tract make up a formidable list, which will not be reviewed in its entirety in this chapter. Rather, the focus will be on the more important agents that are recognized as producing a measurable amount of illness or on newly described organisms that might soon be shown to play important roles in disease occurrence.

Bacterial Agents

Bacterial enteropathogens probably account for between 30% and 80% of acute diarrhea, depending on the setting. The bacterial agents appear to be particularly important in tropical areas and are responsible for most of the morbidity among persons traveling from low- to high-risk areas ("traveler's diarrhea"). Table 242-1 lists important bacterial causes of acute diarrhea. Additional bacterial enteropathogens are discussed later in the chapter.

Vibrio cholerae. Cholera characteristically is a severe, dehydrating illness caused by *V. cholerae* O1 and *V. cholerae* 0139 and occurs in certain endemic areas of Asia, Africa, the Middle East, and Latin America. Within the past 25 years, cholera has been endemic along the U.S. Gulf Coast (Chapter 268). The *V. cholerae* found in the United States has been hemolytic, biotype El Tor, serotype Inaba. An important widespread epidemic of cholera is currently occurring in South and Central America. Cases have been imported into the

Table 242-1   Important bacterial enteropathogens, their virulence properties, and world occurrence

ETIOLOGIC AGENT	VIRULENCE PROPERTIES	OCCURRENCE
Vibrio cholerae	Heat-labile enterotoxin	Endemic areas primarily in Asia, Africa, and Latin America
Enteropathogenic and enteroadherent *Escherichia coli*	HEp-2 cell adherence	Infantile diarrhea, worldwide
Enterotoxigenic *E. coli*	Colonization factor antigen, heat-stable and heat-labile enterotoxins	Developing regions, tropical countries, infants, and travelers
Invasive *E. coli*	*Shigella*-like invasiveness	Rare epidemics, endemic in South America and eastern Europe
Hemorrhagic colitis *E. coli*	Shigalike toxin	Beef source in industrialized areas
Shigella spp.	Shigalike toxin, invasiveness	Worldwide
Salmonella spp.	Cholera-like toxin production, invasiveness	Worldwide
Campylobacter jejuni	Cholera-like toxin production, invasiveness	Worldwide
Aeromonas spp.	Hemolysin, cytotoxin, enterotoxin	Worldwide, especially Thailand, Australia, and Canada
Yersinia enterocolitica	Heat-stable enterotoxins, invasiveness	Worldwide, primarily Scandinavia, Canada, and South Africa

United States primarily through contaminated foods obtained in outbreak areas. Diarrhea caused by non-*cholerae Vibrios* may be severe, and in many cases these strains produce septicemia, particularly in immunocompromised patients. The source of non-*cholerae Vibrios* infection in this country has generally been uncooked oysters, although infection has also been acquired by world travelers. To isolate *Vibrio* spp. the laboratory must use a *Vibrio*-selective medium (e.g., thiosulfate citrate bile salts sucrose [TCBS]).

Escherichia coli. Discussing *E. coli* as a cause of diarrhea is a complex task and is getting more so daily. A growing body of evidence suggests that the rubric *E. coli* encompasses a variety of agents showing biochemical similarities but strikingly different virulence properties, epidemiologic features, and clinical features. The organisms collectively might be referred to as diarrheagenic *E. coli*.

E. coli was first described as a cause of diarrhea in the 1940s and 1950s, when a limited number of serotype-identified organisms were shown to produce diarrhea outbreaks in hospital newborn nurseries. Serologic schemes were developed in the 1950s to type the *E. coli* by the somatic and flagellar antigens, and the serotypes epidemiologically implicated in nursery outbreaks were collectively called enteropathogenic *E. coli* (EPEC). Although it is currently thought that these strains are important causes of infantile diarrhea, their rate of occurrence and general epidemiology need additional study. A factor limiting such study has been the lack of reliable reagents for serotype identification. Recently, EPEC strains have been shown to focally adhere to HEp-2 tissue culture cells; this property may serve as a screening procedure (Fig. 242-1). The property of adherence has also been shown for EPEC in infants with diarrhea, where the organism has been shown to adhere to the epithelial surface and produce damage to microvilli, terminal web, and glycocalix without invasion. *E. coli* strains showing various patterns of attachment to tissue culture cells (local, diffuse, or aggregative types) not belonging to EPEC serotypes have been associated with diarrhea. The biologic significance of these strains and their relationships are currently being studied.

In the early 1970s, strains of *E. coli* were identified as causes of diarrhea in persons from the United Kingdom or the United States during military stationing in the Middle East and Southeast Asia. These strains, shown to variably produce heat-labile choleralike toxin (LT) or heat-stable enterotoxins (ST), have been called enterotoxigenic *E. coli* (ETEC). Both LTs and STs produce transudation of fluid and electrolytes and thus lead to dilation of the bowel (Fig. 242-2). Strains of ETEC are now known to be a major cause if not the most important cause of diarrhea among infants living in tropical areas and are also responsible for just under half the cases of traveler's diarrhea. The ETEC organisms possess colonization fimbriae, which render them adherent to the upper gut of the infected host. Host specificity of the various colonization fimbriae or pili may prevent transmission of ETEC between animals and humans.

When ETEC were first studied, a large outbreak of diarrhea occurred in the United States due to *E. coli,* which possessed the property of *Shigella*-like invasiveness. The organism had contaminated Camembert and Brie cheese imported from France. The clinical disease resembled shigellosis; persons affected commonly complained of fever, severe abdominal pain, and bloody diarrhea. These invasive *E. coli* have not been shown to be important causes of endemic diarrhea, although they seem to be regularly found in urban Brazil and some areas in eastern Europe. The property of invasiveness of these strains of *E. coli,* like strains of *Shigella,* is associated with a mixture of soluble bacterial proteins encoded by a 140-megadalton plasmid. In some strains, a portion of the chromosome also controls the property of invasiveness.

The most recent addition to the growing list of diarrheagenic *E. coli* has been associated with diarrhea outbreaks traced to contaminated beef. The illness is distinctive: patients are afebrile or have low-grade fever yet commonly pass grossly bloody stools. An intense colitis is characteristically found on endoscopy. The clinical syndrome (bloody diarrhea without fever) has been called hemorrhagic colitis. The implicated etiologic agents, an O157:H7 and less commonly other *E. coli,* have been shown to produce a cytotoxin immunologically related to if not the same as that produced by the Shiga bacillus (*Shigella dysenteriae* type 1). This organism, including others that produce Shigalike toxin, may produce the hemolytic uremic syndrome during the course of infection.

***Shigella* Species.** For *Shigella* strains, with worldwide distribution, the human is the only important reservoir (Chapter 269). The most important virulence property of this organism is invasiveness, although a Shigalike toxin is also produced and may play a role in the early, watery, small-bowel phase of the illness. Later in the disease the colon is the target organ, and here extensive mucosal invasion occurs, leading to the passage of many small-volume stools containing blood and polymorphonuclear leukocytes and patient complaints of abdominal pain, cramps, fecal urgency, and tenesmus. Because of the low dose of *Shigella* organisms required to transmit the illness, secondary spread from an index case characteristically occurs.

***Salmonella* Species.** *Salmonella* organisms occur throughout the world in both humans and animals (Chapter 269). The strains are invasive to the intestinal mucosa but are less destructive locally than *Shigella* species. In *Salmonella* gastroenteritis, an intestinal polymorphonuclear leukocyte reaction occurs after invasion by the organisms, and the organisms are contained locally. In typhoid or enteric fever, the organisms stimulate an intestinal mononuclear leukocyte reaction, which may facilitate the dissemination of the infecting strain into the regional and then systemic circulation.

Campylobacter jejuni. This microaerophilic *Vibrio*-like organism is a major cause of diarrhea in all regions of the world (Chapter 267). The reservoir most closely resembles that of *Salmonella;* animals, particularly poultry, and unpasteurized milk are important vehicles of transmission. The organism is invasive to intestinal mucosa,

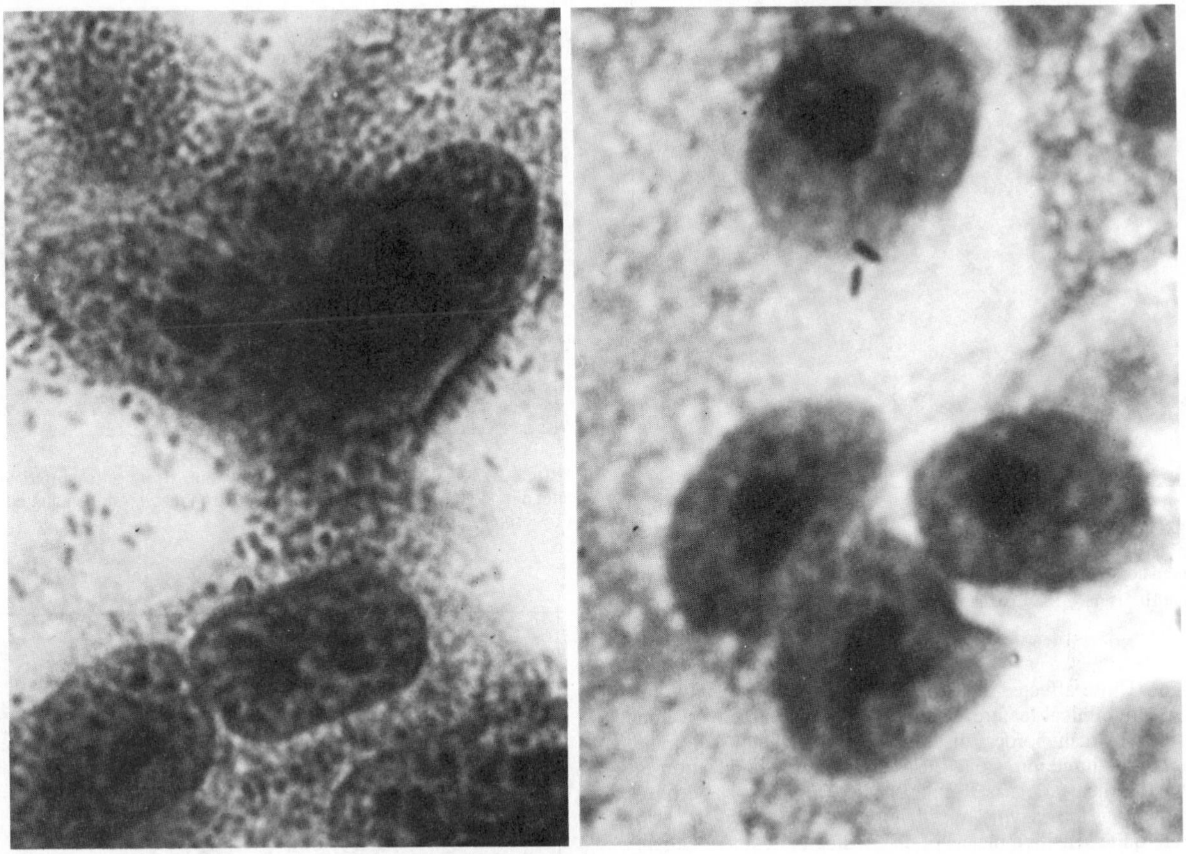

A   B

FIGURE 242-1   HEp-2 cell adherence assay. **A,** An enteropathogenic. *Escherichia coli* (serogroup O119) is shown to be adherent to the tissue culture cells while a nonpathogenic strain of *E. coli* remains nonadherent. **B,** Wright-Giemsa stain, magnification ×1000.

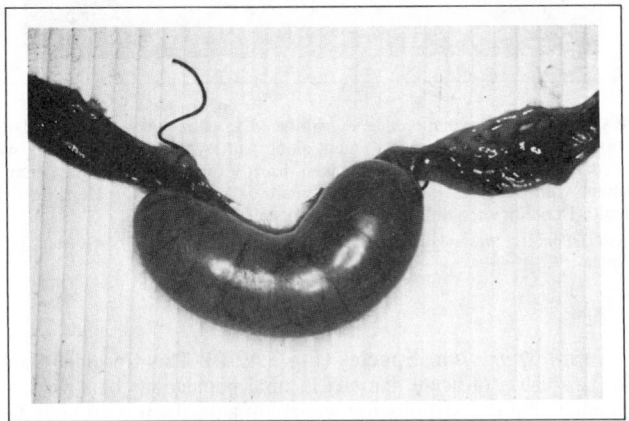

FIGURE 242-2   Rabbit ileal intestinal loop test for *E. coli* enterotoxin. Dilation has occurred 18 hours after injection of a filtrate containing heat-labile enterotoxin.
From DuPont HL: *Med Clin North Am* 62:945, 1978.

which explains the occurrence of bloody stools and an inflammatory intestinal exudate. The importance of the cholera-like toxin produced by *C. jejuni* strains is not known.

Aeromonas* Species and *Plesiomonas shigelloides. *Aeromonas* species (especially *A. hydrophila* and *A. sobria*) have been associated with diarrhea in all regions. A high frequency of occurrence has

been seen only for certain areas, however, including Thailand, western Australia, and Canada. The organisms produce a number of impressive virulence properties as demonstrated in the research laboratory—hemolysins, a cytotoxin in adrenal cells, and an enterotoxin in the suckling mouse model—and invasiveness in rabbit ileal loops has been shown for one strain. Yet *Aeromonas* organisms are often found in stools of asymptomatic persons living in endemic areas, and several strains possessing the virulence characteristics in laboratory studies failed to produce illness when ingested by adult volunteers in high doses. *P. shigelloides* is an occasional cause of diarrhea. Infection by this organism is particularly common among travelers and those ingesting seafood.

Yersinia enterocolitica. *Y. enterocolitica* clearly shows geographic preferences (Chapter 270). It likes colder regions of the world, such as Canada and Scandinavia, although it is characteristically a summer pathogen in these areas. The organism produces heat-stable enterotoxins differing in methanol solubility, and it can be invasive to intestinal mucosa.

Viral Agents

Viruses play important roles in producing diarrheal diseases. Two unrelated viruses or groups of viruses, rotavirus and the small, round viruses such as Norwalk virus, are particularly noteworthy. Enteric adenoviruses, astroviruses, and caliciviruses cause diarrhea, but their frequency and epidemiology are largely unstudied.

Rotavirus. No agent can rival rotaviruses as important causes of gastroenteritis in industrialized areas (Chapter 254). Rotaviruses probably produce more deaths associated with diarrhea than any other

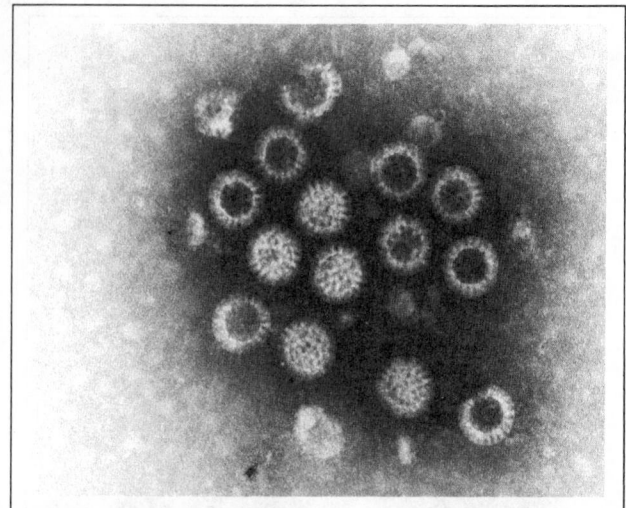

FIGURE 242-3   Representative electron micrograph of rotavirus in diarrheal stool from a 10-month-old infant from rural Central America. (Phosphotungstic acid hematoxylin, magnification ×259,000.)

From DuPont HL, Portnoy BL, Conklin RH: *Annu Rev Med* 28:167, 1977.

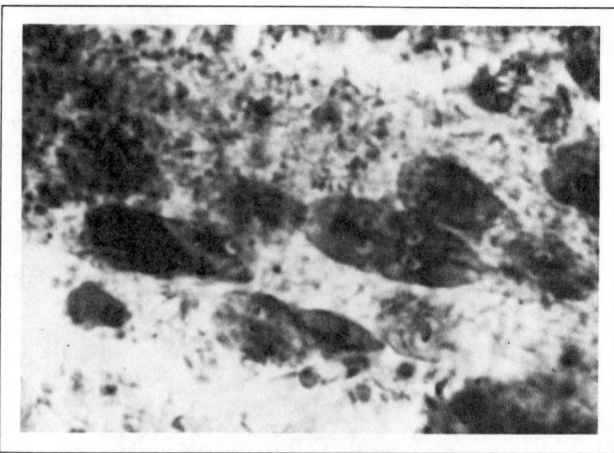

FIGURE 242-4   *Giardia lamblia* trophozoites from an asymptomatic infant attending a Houston day-care center. The trophozoites are entangled in debris. (Trichrome, magnification ×1000.)

single agent. Those affected are less than 3 years of age, and vomiting is the major clinical feature. Because of the frequent involvement of small-bowel brush border, disaccharidase deficiency commonly follows rotavirus infection. Rotaviruses are detected by electron microscopy in diarrheal stools as 70-nm particles (Fig. 242-3). Serologic procedures such as the enzyme-linked immunosorbent assay are available and are quite sensitive means of diagnosing the etiologic agents.

Norwalk Virus. The Norwalk virus and related viruses, 26- to 27-nm particles seen by immune electron microscopy, probably explain a majority of the water-borne outbreaks of gastroenteritis in the world (Chapter 254). All age-groups appear to be susceptible. In developing tropical countries Norwalk virus infects a majority of persons by the time they reach 3 years of age (like rotavirus). Vomiting is common, as is secondary disaccharidase deficiency. Two U.S. laboratories have cloned the Norwalk virus, which will be important in producing the reagents needed for organism detection.

Parasitic Agents

Although numerous parasites are capable of producing diarrhea, and their ubiquity, particularly in the developing regions of the world, makes them all potentially important, only four agents will be considered briefly here, since their importance is established as enteric pathogens in healthy persons: *Giardia lamblia, Entamoeba histolytica,* and *Cryptosporidium* and *Cyclospora* species. It appears likely that occasionally patients will have symptomatic infection due to *Blastocystis hominis, Trichomonas hominis,* or *Dientamoeba fragilis.*

Giardia lamblia (Fig. 242-4). In the developing world this protozoan is so commonly encountered that it is impossible to implicate it as a common cause of acute diarrhea (Chapter 279). It does cause acute diarrhea in industrial areas, particularly in persons exposed to water in mountainous areas or in infants attending day-care centers. The reservoir includes infected persons, although animals may play an important role as sources of infection in certain areas. The relationship between animal and human strains of *G. lamblia* needs additional study.

Entamoeba histolytica (Fig. 242-5). *E. histolytica* is a cause of morbidity primarily in less developed areas. All age-groups are affected in these regions, and chronic or recurrent symptoms occur. The potential for development of liver abscess is a fact about which all students of medicine need to be aware (Chapter 279).

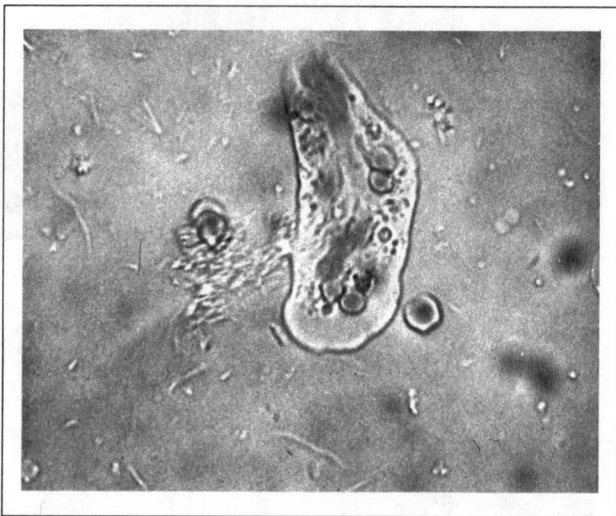

FIGURE 242-5   Live *Entamoeba histolytica* trophozoite with ingested red blood cells. Unidirectional movement along with cytoplasmic streaming was noted. This photomicrograph was taken directly from stool specimen from a patient with diarrhea. Prepared by Bernard J. Marino of the Houston City Health Department; saline preparation, magnification ×1000.

From DuPont HL, Pickering LK: *Infections of the gastrointestinal tract,* New York, 1980, Plenum.

Cryptosporidium Species (Fig. 242-6). This Coccidia organism is a cause of acute diarrhea in rural populations of developing nations living in proximity to a variety of animals. It is an important cause of severe, cholera-like diarrhea in patients with acquired immunodeficiency syndrome (AIDS) (Chapter 248) (Color Plates VIII-32 and VIII-33) and in infants attending day-care centers. The important reservoir of *Cryptosporidium* species is probably drinking water.

Cyclospora Species. *Cyclospora* organism is an emerging coccidial pathogen of humans. It causes prolonged watery diarrhea in immunocompromised hosts (especially those with AIDS) and in travelers to certain international settings including Nepal, Haiti, and Mexico. There is growing evidence that the organism may be seen in sporadic cases of diarrhea and occasionally in water-borne or berry-associated outbreaks of illness in previously healthy persons in industrialized regions of the world. The organism is seen as 8- to

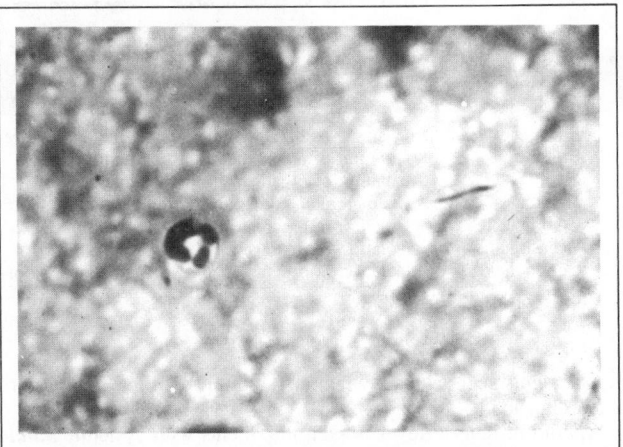

FIGURE 242-6   *Cryptosporidium* oocyst in diarrheal stool obtained from a patient with acquired immunodeficiency syndrome. (Permanent modified Kinyoun acid-fast stain.)

Table 242-2   Relative importance of enteropathogens in endemically acquired diarrhea

AGENT Δ	INDUSTRIALIZED REGIONS: CHILDREN (%)	DEVELOPING AREAS*: CHILDREN (%)	TRAVELER'S DIARRHEA† (%)
Rotavirus	20-30	15-30	<10
Enterotoxigenic *Escherichia coli*	<4	20-30	10-40
Enteropathogenic *E. coli*	4	4	<1
Shigella spp.	3-15	3-12	3-15
Salmonella spp.	4	4	7
Campylobacter jejuni	3-12	3-12	3-15
Giardia lamblia	4	4	<3
Unknown	40	<40	20

*Non–cholera-endemic areas.
†U.S. adults traveling to Mexico.

10-μm spheric bodies on standard microscopy examination of stool specimens.

FREQUENCY OF OCCURRENCE OF ETIOLOGIC AGENTS
Endemic Diarrhea

The relative importance of the various enteropathogens in endemic settings differs according to patient age, time of year, and geographic location. Table 242-2 summarizes the results of a number of studies that attempted to characterize the occurrence of the different pathogens as causes of endemically acquired diarrhea. Three groups or settings are identified in Table 242-2: diarrhea in children in industrialized regions such as the United States; diarrhea occurring in children in developing areas where cholera is not endemic; and diarrhea that occurs among U.S. adults traveling to tropical regions (traveler's diarrhea). Rotavirus is an important cause of diarrhea in infants and children under 3 years of age in all areas. It shows an impressive wintertime predisposition in temperate areas; this seasonal peak is blunted in more tropical regions. The less developed the region, the more important ETEC becomes, again primarily in infants and children. These strains usually are the most important causes of diarrhea in infants and children in the less developed areas, which explains their presence and importance as causes of traveler's diarrhea. Immunity occurs secondary to rotavirus and ETEC infections. Travelers from the United States are susceptible to ETEC because of the rarity

of these strains in the United States; they are less susceptible to rotavirus, which is endemic to both areas. *Shigella* and *Campylobacter* species are important in all settings. In semitropical Mexico and Morocco, ETEC is the major summertime cause of traveler's diarrhea. In fall and winter, ETEC rates fall and *C. jejuni* infection rates rise in travelers.

Food-Borne Diarrhea

Food is an excellent culture medium for enteric pathogens and represents an extremely important vehicle of disease transmission, particularly in tropical areas. Development of clinical symptoms when a contaminated food is ingested by a healthy person depends on one of two factors: (1) the number of organisms in the food and (2) the presence of a highly virulent organism in the vehicle. Nearly any bacterial species is capable of producing at least mild diarrhea and other intestinal complaints if swallowed in sufficient numbers. A far smaller inoculum is necessary to produce symptoms if the agent is a high-grade (virulent) pathogen, such as *Shigella, Salmonella, Campylobacter,* or *Cryptosporidium* species. Table 242-3 summarizes the clinical features of the most common forms of food-borne diarrhea, which are useful in separating the various etiologic agents. Determining the presence of associated cases, constructing the incubation period, and assessing the degree of vomiting and fever can suggest the etiologic diagnosis of food-borne illness before laboratory confirmation is received. In the United States the most common forms of food-borne diarrhea outbreaks unassociated with fever in the affected are *Staphylococcus aureus* (a true food poisoning) and *Clostridium perfringens;* the incubation period usually allows differentiation. *Bacillus cereus* produces two forms of food-borne illness, which resemble either *S. aureus* food poisoning or *C. perfringens* disease. Isolation of the organism is necessary to determine the presence of *B. cereus.* Finding fever in a percentage of cases suggests strongly that an invasive agent is responsible (i.e., *Salmonella, Shigella,* or *Campylobacter* species). *Vibrio parahaemolyticus* is a possible agent in diarrhea outbreaks (which may be extensive) secondary to ingestion of contaminated seafood. Laboratory identification of one of the invasive pathogens from stool and/or less commonly from food is required to make a definitive diagnosis.

Gay Bowel Syndrome

Certain male homosexual patients have diarrhea with a high frequency. Diarrhea in male homosexual persons should be approached in a special way. Because of sexual practices of many of these patients, they more frequently have fecal-oral contamination and therefore show accelerated transmission of all the agents spread by this route (*Shigella, Salmonella, Campylobacter, G. lamblia, E. histolytica,* etc.). Also, they may have unique enteric infections. Perhaps through direct rectal inoculation, proctitis occurs, which may be due to *Neisseria gonorrhoeae, Chlamydia trachomatis,* herpes simplex, or *Treponema pallidum.* Male homosexual patients with AIDS may have diarrhea due to intestinal infection secondary to *Cryptosporidium, Isospora,* and *Cyclospora* species; Microsporidia; *Salmonella;* herpes viruses (herpes simplex and cytomegalovirus); human immunodeficiency virus (HIV) itself; and *Mycobacterium* of the *avium-intracellulare* complex.

Persistent Diarrhea

Most patients with enteric infection have diarrhea for no more than a week. When diarrhea lasts 2 weeks, certain agents or processes should be considered (Box 242-1). Although *G. lamblia* is the cause of diarrhea in no more than 4% of unselected cases of acute illness, this protozoan can be found in one third or more cases of persistent illness, as defined here. The agents that infect the small bowel (rotavirus, Norwalk agent, and *G. lamblia*) may lead to a disruption of disaccharidase production by cells of the intestinal brush border. Failure to split disaccharides, most particularly milk lactose, may lead to an osmotic and fermentative diarrhea. Alteration of diet with restriction of milk consumption may be all that is necessary to control symptoms. In selected cases of acute diarrhea, small-bowel motility patterns are disturbed, leading to stasis in the upper gut and overgrowth

Table 242-3   Major forms of food-borne diarrhea

AGENT	INCUBATION PERIOD (HOURS)	FEVER	VOMITING	DIAGNOSIS
Staphylococcus aureus	1-5	Absent	Profuse	Characteristic epidemiologic and clinical picture
Bacillus cereus	2-5	Absent	Profuse	Isolation of organism from food and/or stool
	8-22	Absent	Yes	Isolation of organism from food and/or stool
Clostridium perfringens	8-22	Absent or low-grade	Minimal	Characteristic epidemiologic and clinical picture
Salmonella sp.	8-24	Common	Common	Isolation of organism from food and/or stool
Shigella sp.	7-120	Common	Occasional	Isolation of organism from food and/or stool
Vibrio parahaemolyticus	12-24	Occasional	Occasional	Isolation of organism from seafood and/or stool

---

BOX 242-1

Causes of diarrhea lasting more than 1 to 2 weeks (persistent illness)

Parasitic infection (*Giardia, Isospora, Cyclospora,* or *Microsporidium* species)
Disaccharidase deficiency
Bacterial overgrowth syndrome
Bacterial enterocolitis (due to *Shigella, Salmonella, Campylobacter,* or *Yersinia* species or diarrheagenic *E. coli*)
Less defined agents (Brainerd agent)
Host deficiencies (immunodeficiency, micronutrient deficiency)

---

of colonic bacteria. Bacterial species in high numbers in the small bowel interfere with absorption of dietary constituents at least partially through deconjugation of bile salts. Small bowel intubation will reveal heavy growth ($>10^5$ colonies/cc) of normally nonpathogenic bacteria in these cases. A favorable response of the subacute illness to empiric anti-*Giardia* therapy with metronidazole may represent treatment of giardiasis or an anaerobic bacterial overgrowth syndrome. Other parasitic agents may cause persistent diarrhea, including *Isospora, Cyclospora,* and *Microsporidium.* The conventional bacterial enteropathogens (*Shigella, Salmonella, Campylobacter,* and *Yersinia* species and EPEC) may occasionally produce more protracted diarrhea, as has been seen most clearly for EPEC and other adherent *E. coli* in young infants. Stool culture should reveal one of these agents.

ETIOLOGIC DIAGNOSIS OF ENTERIC INFECTION
Clinical Aspects

Certain enteric pathogens tend to produce characteristic clinical symptoms. In general, invasive bacterial enteropathogens (*Shigella, Salmonella, Campylobacter*) produce more intense diarrhea when compared with the viral or parasitic agents and infections. *Shigella* and *Campylobacter* strains characteristically lead to the passage of bloody stools (occurring in about 30% to 50% of cases). Bloody stools are passed in about 8% of patients with salmonellosis. Other less common causes of dysentery (bloody stools) are *E. histolytica, V. parahaemolyticus, A. hydrophila,* and *Y. enterocolitica.* Viral agents (rotaviruses and Norwalk-like agents) produce vomiting in most cases. In classic giardiasis, the patient describes intermittent diarrhea associated with abdominal pain and cramping, bloating, and flatulence. Despite these clinical characteristics of enteric infection when in the classic presentation, it is extremely difficult to diagnose most cases of diarrhea clinically. For this reason laboratory diagnosis is necessary.

In most patients with persistent diarrhea, an etiologic agent cannot be identified. Further research will identify new agents. An interesting syndrome known as "Brainerd diarrhea," first described during an outbreak in Brainerd, Minnesota, is associated with consumption of unpasteurized milk or untreated surface water. The illness characteristically lasts longer than 1 year and is unresponsive to antimicrobial agents. The cause of the syndrome remains undefined. In developing regions where malnutrition is common, deficiency in

micronutrients such as zinc, vitamin A, or folic acid may lead to protracted diarrhea.

Typhoid or enteric fever is seen in patients with systemic *Salmonella* infection (Chapter 269). In Latin America, Asia, and Africa, it usually corresponds to bacteremic infection by *Salmonella typhi,* or less commonly *Salmonella paratyphi.* In the United States, bacteremia and typhoidlike disease are more frequently caused by nontyphoid strains of *Salmonella.* Symptoms and signs include fever, which may be impressive, headache, and abdominal symptoms. The abdominal findings are variable and may consist of constipation, diarrhea, pain and cramps, distention, and ileus. On physical examination patients may have small, delicate erythematous macules that blanch on pressure, clustered in small numbers usually around the abdomen (rose spots). In addition, steady deep palpation of the abdomen often reveals segmental ileus, felt as air and fluid being displaced by the pressure. Patients typically have leukopenia and a pulse-temperature deficit. Other infections resembling typhoid fever are rickettsial infection, brucellosis, tularemia, yersiniosis, babesiosis, leptospirosis, and *Campylobacter fetus* infection.

Use of the Laboratory

For most cases of mild to moderately severe diarrheal disease (≤ 5 unformed stools without fever and/or without bothersome cramps, pain, nausea, and vomiting), an etiologic assessment is unnecessary and treatment can be given empirically. For more severe diarrhea (≥ 6 unformed stools or the other clinical findings are of concern or are disabling to the patient), the laboratory can offer invaluable help in determining how best to manage the patient. Table 242-4 summarizes the tests described below (Chapter 233).

Fecal Leukocyte Test. In patients to be further evaluated, the fecal leukocyte test can give rapid useful information. By mixing stool (if present, mucus is preferred) with dilute methylene blue and looking at the wet-mount preparation under a coverslip, or after heat-fixing the specimen, adding the same stain, and allowing it to dry, one can determine microscopically the presence of leukocytes and a rough quantitation of their number. The finding of numerous leukocytes (Fig. 242-7) indicates diffuse colonic inflammation rather than a specific etiology. Thus the test is useful in defining the pathology of the infection. Not all patients with invasive bacterial diarrhea will have numerous leukocytes on fecal smears. Early in a *Shigella* infection the small bowel is the site of infection, and late in the disease the inflammatory character of the colitis is reduced. In both situations stools are positive for *Shigella,* but the stool examination for leukocytes may be negative. The infectious process also may be focal (e.g., in selected cases of antibiotic-associated colitis), and leukocytes will be sparse due to dilution by the luminal contents. Understanding these limitations of the test, one can consider the agents that are likely to produce diffuse colonic inflammation and therefore characteristically produce a fecal leukocyte exudate. The three most common causes of leukocyte-positive stools are *Shigella, Salmonella,* and *Campylobacter* organisms. Other recognized causes of numerous stool leukocytes are *Clostridium difficile* (antibiotic-associated colitis), *Y. enterocolitica, A. hydrophila, V. parahaemolyticus,* and invasive *E. coli.* Patients with idiopathic ulcerative colitis and certain patients with other serious forms of allergic colitis will also be found to have fecal leukocytes. Finding stools with many leukocytes in the presence of

Table 242-4   Use of the laboratory in determining origins or causes of sporadic cases of diarrhea

LABORATORY TEST	INDICATIONS	PROBABLE DIAGNOSIS IF RESULT IS POSITIVE
Fecal leukocytes	All moderately to severely ill cases	Diffuse colonic inflammation (see text)
Stool culture	Moderately to severely ill cases; those with fever or positive fecal leukocytes; male homosexuals	*Shigella; Campylobacter; Salmonella* spp.
Blood culture	Enteric fever and all clinically septic patients	*Salmonella* bacteremia; less likely, sepsis associated with *Campylobacter* or *Yersinia* spp.
Parasite examination (stool or small-bowel fluid)	Diarrhea of >2 week's duration; travel to special areas (see text); day-care center–associated case; male homosexuals	*Giardia lamblia; Entamoeba histolytica; Cryptosporidium* sp.; *Cyclospora*
Rotavirus antigen	Hospitalized infants <3 years of age	Rotavirus

moderate to severe diarrheal illness generally is an indication for either performing a stool culture, *C. difficile* toxin assay, or treating the patient empirically with an antimicrobial agent.

Stool Culture. It should be realized that the routine laboratory should be able to recover *Shigella, Salmonella,* and *Campylobacter* organisms from culture of stool. The indications for performing a stool culture include moderate to severe illness (particularly those with fever or requiring hospitalization) and cases positive for fecal leukocytes. In hamburger-associated diarrhea cases, stools should be cultured for *E. coli* O157:H7. In selected cases, the laboratory can be instructed to culture stool for *V. cholerae, V. parahaemolyticus* (on TCBS agar), *Y. enterocolitica,* or *C. difficile.*

Blood Culture. In patients with clinical typhoid or enteric fever or in any ill, hospitalized patient who has intestinal symptoms, blood cultures should be performed. The diagnosis of typhoid fever is generally made in the proper clinical setting by a positive blood culture for the causative agent. If the patient has received antimicrobial therapy preceding the evaluation, culturing bone marrow aspirate material will give a higher yield. Other systemic enteric infections are diagnosed etiologically by blood culture. Nontyphoid salmonellae, *C. fetus,* and *Y. enterocolitica* are included in this category.

Parasite Examination (Figs. 242-4 to 242-6). Indications for parasite examination include (1) all patients with diarrhea lasting more than 2 weeks, (2) illness originating during travel to the Rocky Mountains, Russia, or developing regions of the world, (3) diarrhea in a person exposed to day-care centers, or (4) a male homosexual patient. Evidence suggests that in *G. lamblia* and *Cryptosporidium* sp. infection, stools are negative for the protozoan in half the cases. When *Giardia* infection is strongly suspected and stools are negative, it is advisable to collect small-bowel fluid or mucus, perform a small-bowel biopsy to look for the agent, or treat the patient empirically without establishing a diagnosis. The nylon string test (Entero-

Test) can be tried to sample small-bowel mucus but will be helpful in a limited number of patients.

Special Tests. Commercial kits for rotavirus detection (e.g., Rotazyme) are readily available. Because there is no specific treatment for viral gastroenteritis, the test has limited applicability. The major indication for the serologic study for rotavirus is hospitalization of an infant under 3 years of age with gastroenteritis. A positive rotavirus antigen test result in such a patient should lead to fluid, but not antimicrobial therapy. The best laboratory test for diagnosing antibiotic-associated colitis is to assay for *C. difficile* toxin by tissue culture or serologic procedure (Chapters 233 and 263). This is a reliable indicator of antibiotic-associated colitis in the older child and adult. Young infants and children may have toxin in stool without evidence of a pathologic process. In the patient with typhoid or enteric fever, serologic studies are of limited value in making a diagnosis. Serologic diagnosis of typhoid fever (Widal's reaction) is useful in parts of the world where the illness is endemic, because of the relative importance of *S. typhi.* In areas where typhoid fever is unusual (e.g., the United States), serologic changes suggesting typhoid fever are more likely to be due to exposure to other cross-reacting gram-negative rods than to the typhoid bacillus.

TREATMENT OF DIARRHEA

For all patients with diarrhea, fluid and electrolyte replacement is advisable. Although this treatment is not usually critical to well-nourished adults with mild to moderate diarrhea, it can be lifesaving to the very young or the elderly patient with dehydrating illness. All patients with active diarrhea should be encouraged to drink Gatorade, Pedialyte, Lytren, or soft drinks augmented with saltine crackers. In dehydrating illness, oral rehydration salts or intravenous fluids should be given. Packets of salts containing NaCl 3.5 g, NaHCO$_3$ 2.5 g, NaHCO 2.5 g, KCl 2.5 g, and glucose 20 g are available to add to 1 liter of fluid, giving the following chemical composition: Na$^+$ 90 mmol, Cl$^-$ 80 mmol, K$^+$ 20 mmol, HCO$_3$$^-$ 30 mmol, and glucose 111 mmol. Diet should be altered during diarrhea. Calories must be provided to facilitate enterocyte renewal. For infants, breast milk or lactose-free formula is given. For all patients boiled starches or cereals with some salt should be given. Crackers, bananas, yogurt, soup, and boiled vegetables also should be provided. When stools are formed, diet may return to normal. Milk products should be withheld for the first day or two for older children and adults.

Empiric Therapy

In mild to moderate diarrhea or when illness develops in a person away from home, it is often not practical to use the laboratory to help establish an etiologic diagnosis. In this instance, therapy can be given empirically based on clinical features of illness (Table 242-5). Although mild symptoms need not be treated with anything other than fluids, moderate illness in an older child or an adult may be optimally managed with a drug to nonspecifically improve the illness, such as bismuth subsalicylate (Pepto-Bismol) or loperamide (Imodium). Bismuth subsalicylate will reduce the diarrhea by 50% and is most effective in treating a secretory type of illness. The dose is 30 ml every 30 minutes for eight doses (one 8-ounce bottle over 3½ hours). This therapy can be repeated on the second day. Loperamide

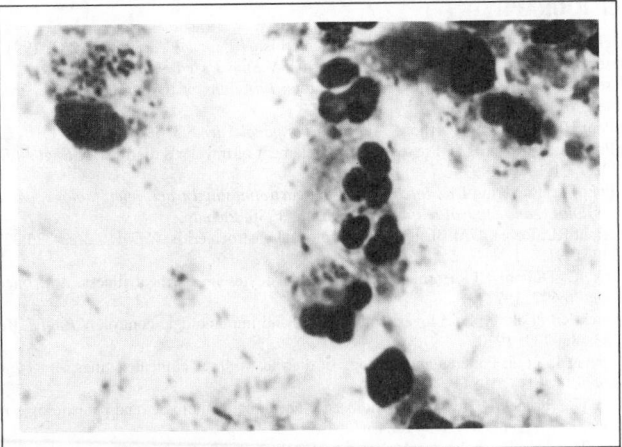

FIGURE 242-7   Fecal leukocytes in a patient with diffuse colitis of unknown origin. (Methylene blue permanent, magnification ×1000.)

Table 242-5   Therapy of acute diarrhea according to clinical and laboratory findings (see text for details)

LABORATORY RESULTS	CLINICAL ASPECTS	THERAPY
None performed	Mild diarrhea (illness does not require change in activities)	Fluids only
	Moderate diarrhea (illness requires change in activities, but the patient is able to adequately function)	Loperamide or bismuth subsalicylate (Pepto-Bismol)
	Severe diarrhea (patient is disabled by the illness)	Antimicrobial therapy
Culture positive for *Campylobacter* sp.	Any situation	Erythromycin or quinolones
Culture positive for *Shigella* sp.	Any situation	Trimethoprim-sulfamethoxazole (TMP-SMX) or quinolone
Culture positive for *Salmonella* sp.	Asymptomatic or mild to moderate gastroenteritis*	Fluids only
	Severe gastroenteritis, septic or hospitalized patient	Quinolone or TMP-SMX

*If high-risk condition exists (immunocompromised, hemodialysis patient or elderly individual) treat as severe gastroenteritis.

even more impressively reduces symptoms and is given in a dose of two capsules (4 mg) initially followed by one capsule after each unformed stool not to exceed eight capsules in 24 hours; prescription dosing is 16 mg/day maximum dose or 4 mg initially followed by 2 mg (liquid or caplet) after each unformed stool not to exceed 8 mg (over-the-counter dosage not requiring a prescription). Patients with fever or dysentery (bloody stools), or those worsening on therapy, should not receive loperamide-like drugs.

Antimicrobial agents are given to patients with severe diarrhea or those with fever and perhaps to those found to have fecal leukocytes on microscopic examination. For adults with traveler's diarrhea acquired in the interior of Mexico during rainy summer months, trimethoprim-sulfamethoxazole (TMP-SMX) is the optimal empiric therapy. The dose is one double-strength tablet (160 mg TMP/800 mg SMX) twice daily for 3 days. Drugs effective for most forms of moderate to severe traveler's diarrhea during all seasons and in nearly all international settings are norfloxacin 400 mg twice a day by mouth or ciprofloxacin 500 mg twice a day by mouth or ofloxacin 300 mg twice a day by mouth for 3 days for adults. Milder illness may be treated with a single dose of one of the antimicrobials listed.

Specific Therapy

Ideally, the laboratory can be used to make a presumptive or definitive diagnosis. Culture-positive cases of campylobacteriosis are best treated with erythromycin. When stool cultures are positive for *Shigella,* TMP-SMX is given unless TMP-resistant *Shigellae* are common in the area. For patients with *Salmonella* gastroenteritis, no antimicrobial therapy is given for mild to moderate or asymptomatic cases. If, on the other hand, the patient is clinically septic, has a severe bout of illness due to *Salmonella,* is ill enough to justify admission to the hospital, or is immunocompromised, undergoing hemodialysis, or elderly, antimicrobial agents should be given to treat bacteremic illness. For typhoid (enteric) fever, a fluoroquinolone such as ciprofloxacin or ofloxacin is given twice a day for 10 days. Relapses occur in typhoid fever and should be treated with a second short course of therapy. For nontyphoid bacteremic salmonellosis, one of the quinolones or TMP-SMX is preferred because ampicillin resistance among these strains is common. Many persons feel that 10 days of fluoroquinolone represents optimal therapy for bacteremia *Salmonella* (typhoid or nontyphoid).

PROPHYLAXIS FOR TRAVELER'S DIARRHEA

Diarrhea occurs in approximately 40% of persons traveling from low-risk (United States, Canada, northwestern Europe) to high-risk areas (Latin America, Asia, and Africa). The problem can be reduced by exercising care about where and what one eats. Heat kills microbes, and steaming hot foods should be sought. Other usually safe items include bread and other dry goods, citrus fruit, and bottled (particularly carbonated) liquids.

For certain travelers, drug prophylaxis (antimicrobial drugs or bis-

muth subsalicylate) can be given. Because of side effects of the conventional antimicrobials (intestinal reactions, skin rashes, acquisition of resistance by intestinal flora, etc.), we currently advise that they be used only for a minority of persons making critical trips and for persons at risk of developing a more serious illness or suffering greater consequence if they acquire an illness. Persons with achlorhydria, or those who have had gastric resection or regularly take maximum doses of omeprazole might be considered in the latter category. A traveler should use this form of prophylaxis only after receiving approval from a physician and after the risks and benefits are clearly understood. Three agents are currently recognized as useful in preventing the illness: TMP-SMX, a quinolone, and bismuth subsalicylate. The antimicrobial agents are 80% to 90% effective and are given in the dose of one double-strength tablet of TMP-SMX (160 mg TMP/800 mg SMX) during summertime travel to the interior of Mexico and other areas where TMP resistance among bacterial enteropathogens is unusual, and norfloxacin 400 mg, ciprofloxacin 500 mg, or ofloxacin 300 mg once daily beginning the day of travel and continuing for 1 to 2 days after returning home. Studies to determine the optimum dose of the tablet form of bismuth subsalicylate for use in treatment and prophylaxis indicate that bismuth subsalicylate is between 60% and 65% effective in preventing the illness and should be administered in a dosage of two tablets just before meals and at bedtime four times a day. Prophylactic agents are most practical for short-term use (less than a week) and probably should be restricted to trips of 3 weeks or less. For many international travelers, cautious food selection and early treatment of illness (fluids, nonspecific drugs, or antimicrobials, depending on severity of symptoms) are the optimal ways to prevent or treat diarrhea.

BIBLIOGRAPHY

Blacklow NR, Greenberg HB: Viral gastroenteritis, *N Engl J Med* 325:252-263, 1991.
Blaser MJ, Reller LB: *Campylobacter* enteritis, *N Engl J Med* 305:1444, 1981.
Blaser MJ, Smith PD, Ravdin JI et al, editors: *Infections of the gastrointestinal tract,* New York, 1995, Raven.
DuPont HL: Infectious diarrhoea, *Ailment Pharmacol Ther* 8:3, 1994.
DuPont HL, Ericsson CD: Prevention and treatment of traveler's diarrhea, *N Engl J Med* 320:1021-1027, 1993.
DuPont HL, Pickering LK: *Infections of the gastrointestinal tract: microbiology, pathophysiology, and clinical features,* New York, 1980, Plenum.
Guerrant RL, Bobak DA: Bacterial and protozoal gastroenteritis, *N Engl J Med* 325:327-339, 1991.
Harris JC, DuPont HL, Hornick RB: Fecal leukocytes in diarrheal illness, *Ann Intern Med* 76:697, 1972.
Hornick RB et al: Typhoid fever: pathogenesis and immunologic control, *N Engl J Med* 283:686, 739, 1970.
Koopman JS et al: Patterns and etiology of diarrhea in three clinical settings, *Am J Epidemiol* 119:114, 1984.
Navin TR, Juranek DD: Cryptosporidiosis: clinical, epidemiologic, and parasitologic review, *Rev Infect Dis* 6:313, 1984.
Quinn TC et al: The polymicrobial origin of intestinal infections in homosexual men, *N Engl J Med* 309:576, 1983.

243 Osteomyelitis

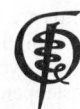

Jon T. Mader

Osteomyelitis describes infection in bone. The root words *osteon* (bone) and *myelo* (marrow) are combined with *-itis* to define the clinical state in which bone is infected with microorganisms. Based on etiologic and clinical considerations, bone infections have traditionally been classified as either hematogenous osteomyelitis or osteomyelitis resulting from a contiguous focus of infection. Contiguous focus osteomyelitis has been further subdivided into osteomyelitis in patients who have relatively normal vascularity and osteomyelitis in patients with generalized vascular insufficiency.

PHYSIOLOGY AND PATHOPHYSIOLOGY

Osteomyelitis may be acute or chronic. The acute disease is characterized by a suppurative infection accompanied by edema, vascular congestion, and small-vessel thrombosis. The vascular supply to the bone is compromised as the infection extends into the surrounding soft tissue. Large areas of dead bone (sequestra) may be formed when both the medullary and periosteal blood supplies are compromised. Viable colonies of bacteria may be harbored within the necrotic and ischemic tissues even after an intense host response, surgery, and therapeutic antibiotics. Once the antibiotics are discontinued or the host response declines, the organisms may again proliferate and lead to a recurrence of the infection. The hallmarks of chronic osteomyelitis are a nidus of infected dead bone or scar tissue, an ischemic soft tissue envelope, and a refractory clinical course.

Hematogenous Osteomyelitis

Long bone hematogenous osteomyelitis occurs mainly in infants and children. The metaphyses of the long bones (tibia, femur) are most frequently involved. The anatomy in the metaphyseal region seems to explain this clinical localization. Nonanastomosing capillary ends of the nutrient artery make sharp loops under the growth plate and enter a system of large venous sinusoids where the blood flow becomes slow and turbulent. The metaphyseal capillaries lack phagocytic lining cells, and the sinusoidal veins contain functionally inactive phagocytic cells. These capillary loops are essentially end-artery branches of the nutrient artery. Any end-capillary obstruction could lead to an area of avascular necrosis. Minor trauma probably predisposes the infant or child to infection by producing a small hematoma, vascular obstruction, and subsequent bone necrosis that is susceptible to inoculation from transient bacteremia. The acute infection initially produces a local cellulitis, which results in a breakdown of leukocytes, increased bone pressure, decreased pH, and decreased oxygen tension. The cumulative effects of these physiologic factors further compromise the medullary circulation and enhance the spread of infection.

The infection may proceed laterally through the haversian and Volkmann's canal systems, perforate the bony cortex, and separate the periosteum from the surface of the bone. When this process is coupled with the presence of medullary extension, both the periosteal and endosteal circulations are lost and large segments of dead cortical and cancellous bone are formed. In the infant the medullary infection may spread to the epiphysis and joint surfaces through capillaries that cross the growth plate. In the child over 1 year of age the growth plate is avascular, and the infection is confined to the metaphysis and diaphysis. The joint is usually spared unless the metaphysis is intracapsular. Thus cortical perforation at the proximal radius, humerus, or femur infects the elbow, shoulder, or hip joint, respectively, regardless of the age of the patient.

A single pathogenic organism is almost always recovered from the bone in hematogenous osteomyelitis. Polymicrobic hematogenous os-

teomyelitis is rare. In the infant, *Staphylococcus aureus*, *Streptococcus agalactiae*, and *Escherichia coli* are the most frequently recovered bone isolates; in children over 1 year of age, *S. aureus*, *Streptococcus pyogenes*, and *Haemophilus influenzae* are the most commonly isolated organisms. After age 4, however, the incidence of *H. influenzae* osteomyelitis decreases.

Infants and children have different presentations of osteomyelitis or clinical examination. Neonatal osteomyelitis is characterized by a paucity of systemic and local findings. Local findings that may be present include edema and decreased motion of a limb. A joint effusion or septic joint adjacent to the bone infection is present in 60% to 70% of cases. Classically, children with hematogenous osteomyelitis come to medical attention with abrupt fever, irritability, lethargy, and local signs of inflammation 3 weeks or less in duration. However, 50% of children now come to medical attention with vague complaints including pain in the involved limb 1 to 3 months in duration and minimal temperature elevation.

Because infants and children with hematogenous osteomyelitis usually have normal soft tissue enveloping the infected bone and are capable of a very efficient metabolic response to infection, they have the potential to resorb large sequestra and generate a significant periosteal response to the infection. The latter feature leads to substantial formation of bone (called an involucrum) at the margin of the infection. The involucrum affords skeletal continuity and a maintenance of function during the healing phase. If antimicrobial therapy directed at the responsible pathogen is begun before extensive bone necrosis, the infection has an excellent probability for arrest.

Hematogenous osteomyelitis is also found in adults. The infection usually begins in the diaphysis but may spread to involve the entire medullary canal. Extension into the joint may occur because the growth plate has matured and once again shares vessels with the metaphysis. Cortical penetration usually leads to a soft tissue abscess, since the periosteum is firmly adherent to the bone. In time, sinus tracts form, connecting the sequestered nidus of infection to the skin by way of the soft tissue extension(s). In the adult *S. aureus*, *Staphylococcus epidermidis*, and aerobic gram-negative organisms account for the majority of the bone or blood isolates.

Adults usually seek medical advice with vague complaints of nonspecific pain and few constitutional symptoms of 1 to 3 months' duration. However, acute clinical presentations with fever, chills, swelling, and erythema over the involved bone(s) are sometimes seen. The clinical signs resulting from soft tissue extension often dominate the findings at presentation and can lead to inappropriate diagnostic and therapeutic measures unless the possibility of an osseous origin is considered.

Vertebral Osteomyelitis

Vertebral osteomyelitis in adult patients is usually hematogenous in origin but may be a result of trauma. A preceding history of urinary tract infection or intravenous drug abuse often is present. An early involvement of the anteroinferior edge of the vertebral body suggests spread from the bony entrance of the anterior spinal artery; however, retrograde infection via Batson's plexus of veins is also postulated. The lumbar vertebral bodies are most often involved, followed in frequency by the thoracic and cervical vertebrae. Spread to adjacent vertebral bodies may occur rapidly through the rich venous networks in the spine. Posterior extension may lead to epidural and subdural abscesses or even meningitis. Anterior or lateral extension may lead to paravertebral, retropharyngeal, mediastinal, subphrenic, retroperitoneal, or psoas abscesses.

On clinical examination the patient usually has vague symptoms and signs consisting of dull, constant back pain and spasm of the paravertebral muscles. More specific complaints may be localized to a soft tissue abscess. The presence of point tenderness over the involved vertebral body is a characteristic finding. Fever may be low grade or absent.

The infection is usually monomicrobic when hematogenous in origin. The most commonly isolated organism is *S. aureus*. However, aerobic gram-negative rods are found in 30% of the cases. *Pseudomonas aeruginosa* and *Serratia marcescens* have a high incidence of isolation among intravenous drug abusers.

Contiguous Focus Osteomyelitis With No Generalized Vascular Insufficiency

In contiguous focus osteomyelitis the organism may be directly inoculated into the bone at the time of trauma or may extend from adjacent soft tissue infections. Common predisposing conditions include open fractures, surgical reduction and internal fixation of fractures, and chronic soft tissue infections. In contrast to hematogenous osteomyelitis, multiple bacterial organisms are usually isolated from the infected bone. The bacteriology is diverse, but *S. aureus* remains the most commonly isolated pathogen. In addition, aerobic gram-negative bacilli and anaerobic organisms are frequently isolated. Bone necrosis, soft tissue damage, and loss of bone stability occur regularly, which makes this form of osteomyelitis difficult to manage.

Contiguous Focus Osteomyelitis With Generalized Vascular Insufficiency

The small bones of the feet are commonly involved in this category of osteomyelitis. Inadequate tissue perfusion predisposes the patient to the infection by blunting the local inflammatory response. The infection commonly develops after minor trauma to the feet, infected nail beds, cellulitis, or trophic skin ulceration. Multiple bacteria are usually isolated from the infected bone. The most common organisms are *S. aureus, S. epidermidis, Enterococcus* species, gram-negative rods, and anaerobes. Although cure is desirable, a more attainable goal of therapy is to suppress the infection and maintain the functional integrity of the involved limb. Even after successful treatment, recurrent or new bone infection occurs in the majority of patients. In time, resection of the infected bone is almost always necessary.

Chronic Osteomyelitis

Both hematogenous and contiguous focus osteomyelitis can progress to a chronic bone infection. No exact criteria separate acute from chronic osteomyelitis. In clinical practice newly recognized bone infections are considered acute, whereas a relapse of a treated infection represents a chronic process; however, this simplistic classification is clearly inadequate. As mentioned, the hallmark of chronic osteomyelitis is the simultaneous presence of organisms, necrotic bone, and a compromised soft tissue envelope. The infection will not regress until the nidus for the persistent contamination is removed. Persistent drainage and/or sinus tract(s) are common. Antibiotic therapy alone is usually unsuccessful in the treatment of chronic osteomyelitis.

Multiple species of bacteria are usually isolated from biopsies of infected granulations from deep within the wound, except in chronic hematogenous infection, in which a single organism is often recovered from patients even after years of intermittent drainage. The prospects of arresting the infection are reduced when the integrity of the soft tissue surrounding the infection is poor or the bone itself is unstable as a result of an infected nonunion or an adjacent septic joint.

LABORATORY AND OTHER DIAGNOSTIC TESTS

The bacteriologic diagnosis of long bone bacterial osteomyelitis rests on the isolation of the causative bacteria from bone or blood. In hematogenous osteomyelitis, positive blood cultures can often obviate the need for a bone biopsy when there is associated radiographic or radionuclide scan evidence of osteomyelitis. Chronic osteomyelitis is rarely associated with a bacteremia unless there is an acute extension of the infection into the soft tissues. Sinus tract cultures are not reliable for predicting which organisms will be isolated from the infected bone. Antibiotic treatment of osteomyelitis should be based on deep-bone biopsy specimen cultures and specific antimicrobial susceptibilities.

Sedimentation rates, C-reactive protein level, and leukocyte counts are frequently elevated before therapy in the acute disease. The white blood cell count rarely exceeds 15,000 cells/mm³. The leukocyte count is usually normal in patients with chronic osteomyelitis. The sedimentation rates, C-reactive protein level, and leukocyte counts may fall with appropriate therapy; however, these values may elevate contemporaneously around each debridement surgery. A sedimenta-

tion rate and C-reactive protein level that return to normal during the course of therapy are favorable prognostic signs. These laboratory determinations, however, are not reliable in the compromised host, since these patients are constantly challenged by minor illnesses and peripheral lesions that may elevate these indices.

Radiographic changes in acute hematogenous osteomyelitis are often difficult to interpret and lag at least 2 weeks behind the evolution of infection. The earliest radiographic changes are soft tissue swelling, periosteal thickening and/or elevation, and focal osteopenia. These findings are subtle and may be missed. The more diagnostic lytic changes are delayed and often associated with an indolent infection of several months' duration. Later, when the patient is receiving appropriate antimicrobial therapy, radiographic improvement may lag behind clinical recovery. In contiguous focus and chronic osteomyelitis the radiographic changes are even more subtle, are often found in association with other nonspecific radiographic findings, and require a careful clinical correlation to achieve diagnostic significance.

An earlier diagnosis of osteomyelitis may be achieved with radionuclide imaging. However, the actual mechanism of labeling bone with radiopharmaceuticals is still unclear. The technetium 99m polyphosphate (^{99m}Tc) scan demonstrates increased isotope accumulation in areas of increased blood flow and reactive new bone formation. The result is usually positive in biopsy-confirmed cases of hematogenous osteomyelitis as early as 48 hours after the initiation of the bone infection. Negative results of ^{99m}Tc scans that have been reported in documented osteomyelitis may be related to impaired blood supply in the infected area.

A second class of radiopharmaceuticals used for the evaluation of osteomyelitis includes gallium citrate and indium chloride. Gallium or indium attaches to transferrin, which leaks from the bloodstream into areas of inflammation. Gallium or indium scans also show increased isotope uptake in areas concentrating polymorphonuclear leukocytes, macrophages, and malignant tumors. Because these scans do not show bone detail well, it is often difficult to distinguish between bone and soft tissue inflammation; a comparison with a ^{99m}Tc scan helps resolve this problem. In contrast to gallium citrate, indium chloride is more heavily concentrated by hematopoietic tissue. When first evaluating a suspected case of osteomyelitis, x-ray studies, technetium bone scans, and gallium or indium scans are selectively ordered to assist in the diagnosis, assess the extent of involvement, and guide the site selection for the bone biopsy. In most cases of osteomyelitis clinical and radiographic evaluation are all that is needed.

Indium-labeled leukocyte scans are less useful in the evaluation of osteomyelitis. Results of indium leukocyte scans are positive in about 40% of patients with acute osteomyelitis and 60% of patients with septic arthritis. Patients who had chronic osteomyelitis, bony metastases, and degenerative arthritis often have negative scan results.

Computed tomography (CT) may have a role to play in the diagnosis of osteomyelitis. Increased marrow density occurs early in the infection, and intramedullary gas has been reported in patients with hematogenous osteomyelitis. The CT scan is also useful to help identify areas of necrotic bone and to assess the involvement of the surrounding soft tissues. In a recalcitrant infection the CT scan may identify the surgical approach and augment a thorough debridement. One disadvantage of this study is the scatter phenomenon that occurs when metal is present in or near the area of bone infection. The scatter results in a significant loss of image resolution.

Magnetic resonance imaging (MRI) is a useful modality for differentiating between bone and soft tissue infection. Initial MRI screening usually consists of a T1-weighted and a T2-weighted spin-echo pulse sequence. In a T1-weighted study tissue edema is dark and fat is bright. In a T2-weighted study the reverse is true. The typical appearance of osteomyelitis is a localized area of abnormal marrow with decreased signal intensity on T1-weighted images and increased signal intensity on T2-weighted images. On occasion there may be decreased signal intensity on T2-weighted images. Post-traumatic and surgical scarring of the bone marrow shows a region of decreased signal intensity on T1-weighted images with no change on the T2-weighted image. Sinus tracts are seen as areas of high signal intensity on the T2-weighted image extending from the marrow and bone through the soft tissues and skin. Differentiation of infection from neoplasm on the basis of the MRI may be difficult; therefore clinical and radiographic correlation is mandatory. Metallic implants in the region of interest may produce focal artifacts, decreasing the utility of the image.

The diagnosis of vertebral osteomyelitis relies on the isolation of a causative organism from the infected vertebral body, disk space, paravertebral abscess, or blood. A closed biopsy for culture and histologic study may be performed under fluoroscopy or CT guidance. An open biopsy is indicated when a closed biopsy carries a high risk of possible complications. Tissue must be sent both for cultures and for histologic confirmation, since the differential diagnosis includes metastatic or primary tumors, mycoses, and tuberculosis. The earliest radiographic change is a subtle rarefaction of the vertebral end plate. Narrowing of the adjacent joint and involvement of the vertebral body occur later in the course of the disease.

The technetium scan is useful in vertebral infection, and the result is usually positive in biopsy-confirmed cases of axial osteomyelitis. The gallium or indium scan is difficult to interpret because of the high concentrations of hematopoietic tissue in the vertebral bodies. CT and MRI are used to assess the extent of vertebral, paravertebral, and soft tissue involvement.

DIFFERENTIAL DIAGNOSIS

A number of conditions may become evident similarly to osteomyelitis. Malignant and benign tumors including Ewing's sarcomas, osteosarcomas, fibrous histiocytomas, fibrosarcomas, lymphomas, and benign giant cell bone cysts may be confused with osteomyelitis. Patients with leukemias may have bony infiltrates that may resemble osteomyelitis. Bone infarcts resulting from sickle cell anemia or other hemoglobinopathies and noninfected nonunions and old trauma may mimic osteomyelitis. In the preceding conditions radiographs and scans may be consistent with osteomyelitis, but the patients generally lack symptoms and signs of infection including fever, erythema, and drainage. The correct diagnosis is usually based on histologic studies and culture results.

MANAGEMENT
Acute Hematogenous Osteomyelitis

Acute long bone hematogenous osteomyelitis is primarily a medical disease in children. In the adult debridement surgery, incision with drainage of soft tissue abscesses, or both are often required. Identification of the causative pathogen is essential. The infection is usually susceptible to specific antimicrobial therapy (Chapter 231). Mismanagement with inappropriate antibiotic(s) encourages disease extension, sequestra formation, and the development of a refractory infection. Surgical intervention is indicated if the patient has not responded to specific antimicrobial therapy within 48 hours or has evidence of a persistent soft tissue abscess, or if joint sepsis is diagnosed or suspected. The first step is to obtain appropriate culture material. A bone biopsy is necessary unless the patient has positive blood cultures along with radiographic studies or bone scan findings consistent with osteomyelitis. After cultures are obtained, a parenteral antimicrobial regimen is initiated to cover the clinically suspected pathogens. Once the organism is obtained, the antibacterial activity of different antibiotic classes can be determined by appropriate sensitivity methods. The disk diffusion method is often a sufficient guideline for antibiotic therapy. However, quantitative antibiotic sensitivity testing by the macrodilution or microdilution techniques on all aerobic bone isolates is a prerequisite to determine the minimum concentration of the antibiotic required to inhibit (minimum inhibitory concentration [MIC]) and kill (minimum bactericidal concentration [MBC]) the pathogenic organism(s). It is best to choose an antibiotic or antibiotic combination that has a low MIC/MBC ratio relative to its expected serum concentration. The antibiotic regimen may be continued or changed on the basis of sensitivity results. The patient is treated for 4 to 6 weeks with appropriate parenteral antimicrobial therapy dated from the initiation of therapy or after the last major debridement surgery. The goal of the therapy is to prevent a refractory infection. If the initial medical management fails and the patient is clinically compromised by a recurrent infection, medullary and/or soft tissue debridement is necessary in conjunction with another course of antibiotics.

Oral antibiotic therapy can be used for treatment of childhood osteomyelitis. However, it is recommended that the patient first receive 2 weeks of parenteral antibiotic therapy before changing to an oral regimen. In addition, the patient must be compliant and agree to close outpatient follow-up. Absorption and activity of the orally administered antibiotic should be monitored by the measurement of the serum bactericidal activity against the causative pathogen. A peak bactericidal dilution of at least 1:8 or greater should be present and maintained. Pediatric patients cannot be given oral antimicrobial therapy with the quinolone class of antibiotics.

Vertebral Osteomyelitis

The therapy for vertebral osteomyelitis requires parenteral antibiotics and may include early surgery and stabilization. The choice of an antibiotic is guided by the biopsy or debridement culture results. The antibiotic is given for 4 to 6 weeks, usually dated from the initiation of therapy or from the last major debridement surgery. The indications for surgery are the same as for all other hematogenous infections of bone: failure of medical management, soft tissue abscess formation, and an impending instability. The neurologic status of the patient must be closely monitored at frequent intervals. Fusion of adjacent infected vertebral bodies is a major goal of therapy. The decision to advise an orthosis as opposed to internal fixation or bed rest is best individualized. The failure rate with bed rest alone is not statistically different from that for stabilization with a cast, corset, or brace.

The therapy for vertebral osteomyelitis has improved over the years. The current mortality rate is approximately 5%. Nearly 90% of patients who receive treatment for vertebral osteomyelitis have uneventful recoveries. About 6% have permanent neurologic defects.

Osteomyelitis Resulting From Contiguous Focus Infection or Chronic Osteomyelitis

The types of osteomyelitis discussed in this section share the common denominators of infected necrotic bone and poorly perfused soft tissue enveloping the bone. Adequate drainage, thorough debridement, obliteration of dead space, wound protection, and specific antimicrobial coverage are the mainstays of therapy. After the diagnostic evaluation a bone biopsy is performed. Aerobic and anaerobic cultures are taken from these bone samples. The patient receives antibiotics only after the results of the cultures and their sensitivities are known. If immediate debridement surgery is required, however, the patient may receive antibiotics to cover the clinically suspected pathogens before the bacteriologic data are reported. These antibiotics may be modified, if necessary, when results of the debridement cultures and sensitivities are determined.

When possible, debridement surgery is performed after specific antibiotic therapy has been initiated. Antimicrobial therapy initiated before surgery decreases the risk of bacteremia at surgery, helps marginate the wound, and produces more supple soft tissues at the time of surgery. Surgical exposure is direct and atraumatic and is designed to avoid unnecessary devitalization of bone and soft tissue. If necessary, the wound is debrided every 48 to 72 hours until all nonviable tissue and superfluous hardware have been removed. The cortical and cancellous bone remaining in the wound after debridement surgery must bleed uniformly to ensure antibiotic perfusion and avert continued sequestration.

Appropriate management of the dead space created by debridement surgery is mandatory to arrest the disease and maintain the integrity of the skeletal part involved. The goal of dead space management is to replace dead bone and scar tissue with durable vascularized tissue. For this reason, secondary infection healing is discouraged because the scar tissue that fills the defect may later become avascular. Suction irrigation systems are now rarely used because of the high incidence of associated nosocomial infections and the unreliability of these setups. Complete wound closure should be attained whenever possible. Local tissue flaps or free flaps may be used to fill dead space. Cancellous bone grafts may be placed beneath local or transferred tissues when structural augmentation is necessary. Careful preoperative planning is crucial to make efficient use of the patient's limited cancellous bone reserves. Open cancellous grafts without soft tissue coverage are useful when a free tissue transfer is not a treatment option and local tissue flaps are inadequate. If motion is present at the site of infection, measures must be taken to achieve permanent stability of the skeletal unit. Antibiotic-impregnated acrylic beads are occasionally used to sterilize and temporarily maintain a dead space. The beads are usually removed within 2 to 4 weeks and replaced with a cancellous bone graft. The evolution of local antibiotic therapy is rapidly taking place.

Bone reconstruction of segmental defects and difficult infected nonunions has been accomplished using the Ilizarov external fixation method. This method uses distraction or compression histogenesis, a process of bone regeneration to fill bone defects or to compress nonunions and correct malunions. In one clinical series, 92% of patients had chronic osteomyelitis with segmental defects (ranging from simple nonunions to 8-cm gaps) that were successfully reconstructed. The technique is labor intensive, and a long period of treatment (average, 8.5 months in the device) is required.

Antibiotics are used to treat live infected bone and to protect bone undergoing revascularization, since it takes bone 3 to 4 weeks to revascularize after debridement surgery. The patient is given 4 to 6 weeks of antimicrobial therapy, usually dated from the last major debridement surgery; however, the duration of antibiotic administration for osteomyelitis remains controversial. Outpatient intravenous therapy is now possible and feasible. The long-term intravenous access catheters make outpatient intravenous treatment possible and decrease hospitalization time. A responsible patient or visiting nurse can be taught to administer the antibiotic at home using the implanted catheter. Outpatient intramuscular antibiotic administration is also feasible.

Oral therapy with the quinolone class of antibiotics is currently being used in adult patients with gram-negative osteomyelitis. The currently available quinolones have relatively poor activity against *Streptococcus* and *Enterococcus* species and anaerobes. The quinolones have modest activity against *S. aureus* and *S. epidermidis,* but resistance is increasing. Coverage of aerobic, gram-positive organisms should be obtained with other antibiotics such as clindamycin or ampicillin-sulbactam. Before changing to an oral regimen, it is recommended that the patient initially receive 2 weeks of parenteral antibiotic therapy. Then the patient must receive 4 to 6 weeks of oral therapy, be compliant, and agree to close outpatient follow-up.

Osteomyelitis Resulting From Contiguous Focus Infection With Vascular Disease

Osteomyelitis associated with vascular insufficiency is difficult to treat because of the relative inability of the host to participate in the eradication of the infection process. Since these infections are insidious, they are often beyond simple salvage by the time the patient seeks medical therapy. The determination of the vascular status of the tissue at the infection site is crucial in the evaluation of these patients. Several methods are used to determine the vascular status. The measurement of cutaneous oxygen tensions and pulse pressures, however, is most commonly used. Cutaneous oxygen tensions are obtained by a modified Clark electrode, which is applied to the skin surface. Cutaneous oxygen tensions provide guidelines for determining the location of adequate tissue perfusion. The values also aid in the assessment of whether local debridement surgery can be performed and in selecting surgical margins where wound healing can be expected to occur. Hyperbaric oxygen therapy may allow healing in areas where marginal tensions are present.

Management may be by suppressive antibiotic therapy, local debridement surgery, or ablative surgery. Judgment regarding which type of treatment to offer the patient depends on tissue oxygen perfusion at the infection site, the extent of the osteomyelitis, and the preference of the patient.

The patient may be given long-term suppressive therapy when a definitive surgical procedure would lead to unacceptable patient morbidity or disability or when the patient refuses local debridement or ablative surgery. Even with suppressive antibiotic therapy, in time, most of these patients require ablative surgery.

Local debridement surgery and a 4-week course of antibiotics may be used in the patient who has localized osteomyelitis and good tissue oxygen perfusion. If these criteria are not present, the wound fails to heal and ultimately an ablative procedure becomes necessary.

BOX 243-1
Cierny and Mader classification of osteomyelitis

Anatomic type

Stage 1	Medullary osteomyelitis
Stage 2	Superficial osteomyelitis
Stage 3	Localized osteomyelitis
Stage 4	Diffuse osteomyelitis

Physiologic class

A Host	Normal host
B Host	Systemic compromise (Bs)
	Local compromise (B1)
C Host	Treatment worse than the disease

Systemic or local factors that affect immune surveillance, metabolism, and local vascularity

Systemic (Bs)	Local (B1)
Malnutrition	Chronic lymphedema
Renal, liver failure	Venous stasis
Diabetes mellitus	Major vessel compromise
Chronic hypoxia	Arteritis
Immune disease	Extensive scarring
Malignancy	Radiation fibrosis
Extremes of age	Small vessel disease
Immunosuppression or immune deficiency	Complete loss of local sensation
Tobacco abuse	

The patient with extensive osteomyelitis and poor tissue oxygen perfusion usually requires some type of ablative surgery. Digital and ray resections, transmetatarsal amputations, midfoot disarticulations, and Syme's amputations allow the patient to ambulate without a prosthesis. The amputation level is determined by the vascular status of the tissues proximal to the site of infection and the requirements of a thorough debridement. The patient is given 4 weeks of antibiotics when infected bone is surgically transected. Antibiotics are given for 2 weeks when the infected bone is completely removed but some residual soft tissue infection remains. When the amputation is performed proximal to the bone and soft tissue infection, the patient is given standard prophylaxis.

STAGING

The following major factors influence the treatment and prognosis of osteomyelitis: (1) the degree of necrosis, (2) the condition of the host, (3) the site and extent of involvement, and (4) the disabling effects of the disease itself. These factors must be considered when assessing treatment results and efficacy of treatment alternatives.

The current classification of hematogenous and contiguous focus osteomyelitis with or without generalized vascular insufficiency is vague and does not adequately define the anatomic nature of the disease, take into account the quality of the host, determine treatment, or identify prognostic factors. Cierny and Mader have developed an alternate classification, which includes these factors (Box 243-1). In this approach the infection and host are staged using four anatomic types and three physiologic classes. The paradigm is determined by the status of the disease process, regardless of its origin or regionality. The anatomic types of osteomyelitis are medullary, superficial, localized, and diffuse. *Medullary osteomyelitis* denotes infection confined to the intramedullary surfaces of the bone. Hematogenous osteomyelitis and infected intramedullary rods are examples of this anatomic type. Superficial osteomyelitis, a true contiguous focus infection of bone, occurs when an exposed, infected necrotic surface of bone lies at the base of a soft tissue wound. Localized osteomyelitis is usually characterized by a full-thickness, cortical sequestration, which can be removed surgically without compromising bony stability, whereas diffuse osteomyelitis is a through-and-through process

✔ *WHEN TO REFER*

The management of osteomyelitis is a team approach usually involving the primary care physician, an infectious diseases physician, and an orthopedic surgeon. The primary care physician is responsible for optimizing the clinical condition of the patient, especially when the patient is a compromised host. If the defect(s) of the compromised host can be minimized, the patient will have a better response to therapy. The infectious diseases physician is responsible for initiating a regimen of optimal antibiotics and for monitoring their use. The orthopedic surgeon performs appropriate debridement surgery, dead space management, and if necessary, bony stabilization. On occasion, a plastic surgeon is necessary to place a local or microvascular flap to cover a soft tissue defect. Also, a vascular surgeon may perform a bypass of diseased vessels in the patient with peripheral vascular disease or vascular disease accompanying diabetes mellitus.

that usually requires an intercalary resection of the bone for cure. Diffuse osteomyelitis includes infections with a loss of bony stability either before or after debridement surgery.

The patient is classified as an A, B, or C host. An A host represents a patient with normal physiologic, metabolic, and immunologic capabilities. The B host (Box 243-1) is either systemically or locally compromised, or both. When the morbidity of treatment is worse than that imposed by the disease itself, the patient is given the C host classification. The terms *acute* and *chronic osteomyelitis* are not used in this staging system, since areas of macronecrosis must be removed, regardless of the acuity or chronicity of the infection. The stages are dynamic and interact according to the pathophysiologic features of the disease; the stages may be altered by successful therapy, host alteration, or treatment. This staging system provides a framework for describing and developing experimental models of osteomyelitis, planning medical and surgical treatments, and comparing the results of therapy among institutions.

SKELETAL TUBERCULOSIS

Skeletal tuberculosis is the result of hematogenous spread of *Mycobacterium tuberculosis* early in the course of a primary infection (Chapter 273). In rare instances skeletal tuberculosis may result from the contiguous spread of infection from a caseating lymph node or direct inoculation. A primary or recurrent bone infection initially elicits an acute inflammatory reaction that gradually matures to an indolent, granulomatous process. Bony sequestration is not uncommon. Cartilage and bone are destroyed slowly by granulation tissue. Thus articular cartilages are retained and recognizable on both clinical and radiographic examination late in the disease process. The symptoms are usually related to biomechanical alterations in articular function, fractures, or the sequela of extraosseous extension of the infection.

Any bone may be involved in skeletal tuberculosis; however, the infection is usually monostotic. In children and adolescents the metaphyses of the long bones are the most frequently infected sites, as in any pyogenic infection. In the adult, axial skeleton involvement is most common, followed in frequency by the proximal femur, knee, and small bones of the hands and feet. A vertebral infection usually begins in the anterior portion of a vertebral body adjacent to an intervertebral disk in a thoracic vertebral body. The lumbar and cervical vertebrae are less commonly involved. Adjacent vertebral bodies may become infected, and a soft tissue abscess may develop. Fifty percent of the patients with skeletal tuberculosis have evidence of extraosseous infection.

Tissue for culture and histologic study is almost always required for the diagnosis of skeletal tuberculosis. Cultures for tuberculosis are positive in approximately 80% of the cases, but 6 weeks may be required for growth and identification of the organism. Histologic findings of granulomatous tissue compatible with tuberculosis and a positive tuberculin skin test result are sufficient evidence to begin tuberculosis therapy. However, a negative skin test result does not rule out

skeletal tuberculosis. Therapy involves prolonged chemotherapy and in some cases surgical debridement surgery or stabilization, or both.

FUNGAL OSTEOMYELITIS

Bone infections may be caused by a variety of fungal organisms, including coccidioidomycosis, blastomycosis, cryptococci, histoplasmosis, and sporotrichosis (Chapters 276 and 278). The most common presentation is a cold abscess overlying an osteolytic lesion. Joint extension occurs most frequently in coccidioidomycosis and blastomycosis. Therapy for fungal osteomyelitis involves surgical debridement and antifungal chemotherapy.

BIBLIOGRAPHY

Calhoun JH, Anger DM, Mader JT: The Ilizarov technique in the treatment of osteomyelitis, *Tex Med* 87:56, 1991.

Calhoun JH, Mader JT: Osteomyelitis of the diabetic foot. In Fryberg RG, editor: *The high-risk foot in diabetes mellitus*, New York, 1991, Churchill Livingstone.

Cierny G, Mader JT: Adult chronic osteomyelitis, *Orthopedics* 7:1557, 1984.

Cierny G, Mader JT, Penninck JJ: A clinical staging system of adult osteomyelitis, *Contemp Orthopedics* 10:17, 1985.

Davidson PT, Horowitz I: Skeletal tuberculosis: a review with patient presentations and discussion, *Am J Med* 48:77, 1970.

Sapico FL, Montgomerie JZ: Pyogenic vertebral osteomyelitis: report of nine cases and review of the literature, *Rev Infect Dis* 1:754, 1979.

Waldvogel FA, Medoff G, Swartz MM: Osteomyelitis: a review of clinical features, therapeutic considerations, and unusual aspects, *N Engl J Med* 282:198, 260, 316, 1970.

CHAPTER

244 Sexually Transmitted Diseases (Urethritis, Vaginitis, Cervicitis, Proctitis, Genital Lesions)

Michael F. Rein

EPIDEMIOLOGY

A variety of microorganisms can be transmitted during sexual contact (Box 244-1). They differ markedly in taxonomy, virulence factors, growth requirements, and response to therapy. They are grouped together because sexual transmission plays an important role in their overall epidemiology. None of the sexually transmitted diseases (STDs) is acquired solely via coitus. In some cases (e.g., shigellosis and candidiasis) sexual transmission plays a relatively minor role, although for other conditions, such as infection with *Chlamydia trachomatis*, sexual transmission is the major route of acquisition in the United States.

Recognizing a disease as sexually transmitted has several practical consequences for the clinician. It allows one to identify a population at very high risk for the same infection, specifically the sexual partners of the infected patient. Rough estimates of the prevalence of infection among sexual partners of patients with STDs are listed in Table 244-1. The estimates are averages and do not reflect the risk of acquiring an STD from a single exposure to an infected sexual partner. Some sexual partners will have been exposed but once, and these people are at considerably lower risk of infection than are those who have had frequent contact with the infected patient. In most cases the rates of infection among sexual partners are so high that, when identified as such, they are immediately given treatment for the infection, even before the diagnosis has been confirmed. The rationale for such "epidemiologic treatment" is that complications may develop in these patients, or they may further transmit the infection while awaiting the results of confirmatory laboratory tests. In this setting the risks of antibiotic administration are outweighed by the risks of waiting to confirm the diagnosis. Epidemiologic treatment is a cornerstone of control of many STDs (see Box 244-1).

Failure to treat sexual partners simultaneously for many of these

BOX 244-1
Sexually transmitted microbial pathogens

Viruses

Herpes simplex virus
Cytomegalovirus
Molluscum contagiosum (poxvirus)
Human papillomavirus (HPV)
Epstein-Barr virus
Hepatitis A, B*, C
Human immunodeficiency virus (HIV)

Mycoplasmas

Mycoplasma hominis
*Ureaplasma urealyticum**
Mycoplasma genitalium

Bacteria

*Neisseria gonorrhoeae**
Neisseria meningitidis
*Treponema pallidum**
*Haemophilus ducreyi**
Shigellae
Group B streptococci†
Gardnerella vaginalis
Salmonellae†
Listeria monocytogenes†
*Calymmatobacterium granulomatis**
Campylobacter fetus

Chlamydiae: *Chlamydia trachomatis**
Fungi: *Candida* species
Endoparasites

*Entamoeba histolytica**
*Trichomonas vaginalis**
*Giardia lamblia**

Ectoparasites

*Phthirus pubis**
*Sarcoptes scabiei**

*Epidemiologic treatment is appropriate.
†Role of sexual transmission is less well defined.

Table 244-1 Prevalence of infection among sexual partners of heterosexual patients with sexually transmitted diseases

TYPE OF INFECTION IN INDEX PATIENT	PERCENTAGE OF CONSORTS INFECTED	
	MALE	FEMALE
Gonorrhea	60 (40-90)	60 (37-92)
Syphilis	30-50	30-50
Chlamydia trachomatis	30	60-75
Trichomoniasis	30-70	90
Herpes genitalis	75	75
Venereal warts	60	60
Donovanosis	0.4-60.0	0.4-60.0

infections may permit them to reinfect each other sequentially, resulting in so-called Ping-Pong infection. Apparent relapse or treatment failure often results from one sexual partner's remaining untreated. Sympathetic, nonjudgmental questioning about sexual partners and practices may yield information about an untreated sexual partner that is essential to eradicating the disease in a patient.

The STDs are largely diseases of lifestyle, and their incidence is higher among patients with multiple sexual partners. Patients whose activities place them at high risk for STDs should be screened regularly. Routine screening of high-risk women for chlamydial infection can reduce the incidence of complications such as pelvic inflammatory disease (PID). As a second consequence, the coexistence of many

STDs is prevalent in groups with high levels of sexual activity. Patients whose patterns of sexual behavior predispose them to one STD predispose them to others. Thus multiple venereal infections are common. Faced with the diagnosis of a single sexually transmitted infection in a patient, the clinician should carefully rule out others. Patients with any STD should be considered at increased risk for infection with human immunodeficiency virus (HIV) and should be offered antibody testing (Chapters 248 and 256). Patients with an STD should be counseled regarding high-risk sexual behavior and should be educated regarding means to reduce their risk (e.g., safer sexual practices and barrier contraceptives). Management of STDs always involves consideration of more than one patient. The clinician should make efforts to ensure that the source of the patient's infection and sexual contacts following infection are adequately managed. Cases of gonorrhea, syphilis, lymphogranuloma venereum, chancroid, donovanosis, acquired immunodeficiency syndrome (AIDS), and in some states, asymptomatic HIV infection, must be reported to local health departments.

Infections dependent on sexual contact for their transmission occupy their epidemiologic niche for a number of reasons. In general, the organisms do not survive well in the environment, and transmission by fomites is rare. In addition, the organisms tend to have somewhat restricted anatomic ranges. For example, cornified squamous epithelium is resistant to primary infection with *Neisseria gonorrhoeae* or *C. trachomatis,* organisms that can infect the epithelium of the urethra, endocervix, pharynx, rectum, and conjunctiva. *Trichomonas vaginalis* can infect only the urogenital tract. Organisms must be inoculated into these sites to produce disease. The lesions or discharges that characterize most STDs and that contain the highest concentration of organisms tend to occur on the genitalia. Therefore transmission of these infections requires intimate contact of susceptible epithelia with anatomic sites containing relatively large numbers of fresh organisms.

Sexually transmitted diseases generally enter into the differential diagnosis of signs and symptoms affecting the genitalia. However, the primary lesions of STDs may also affect the mouth, eye, and rectum, and disseminated infection may involve distant sites.

DIAGNOSIS
History

The patient should be asked about the onset and progression of symptoms, with specific emphasis on skin lesions, discharges, and discomfort. Association of symptoms with the menstrual period and sexual activity should be investigated, and specific details of the methods of contraception and recent antibiotic use should be obtained. It is helpful to ask whether the patient has a specific reason to suspect an STD. An estimate of the incubation period may be obtained by determining the patient's last sexual contact or last contact with a new partner. It is important not to assume that patients are heterosexual. The history should be taken referring to sexual partners in gender-neutral terms until the sexual preference of the patient has been established. Sympathetic questioning with regard to the gender of partners and the orifices used for sexual contact is essential to the management of patients with STD.

Physical Examination

Male genitalia are best examined with the patient standing in front of the seated examiner. The entire genital area should be evaluated, and inguinal adenopathy and skin lesions involving the pubis, thighs, and buttocks should be noted. The penis should be examined for skin lesions, and one should note the presence of perimeatal erythema, which can suggest urethritis, and the quantity and character of urethral discharge. The patient's underwear may reveal staining and give an indication of the amount of discharge, if he has urinated shortly before examination; recent micturition can eliminate much inflammatory discharge. If no urethral discharge is spontaneously present, the urethra should be gently stripped. This is best accomplished by grasping the penis firmly between the thumb and forefinger with the thumb pressing on the ventral surface. The examiner's hand is then moved distally, compressing the urethra. This maneuver expresses small amounts of discharge. The urethral meatus can be gently spread, and the degree of erythema of the urethra can be estimated. If no urethral discharge is expressed, a calcium-alginate urethral (or nasopharyngeal) swab should be inserted at least 2 cm into the urethra. The use of cotton-tipped swabs is contraindicated because their large size makes insertion extremely uncomfortable and the cotton fibers may inhibit the growth of certain fastidious organisms. Scrotal contents should be palpated for masses or tenderness. In men practicing receptive anal intercourse, the anus and perianal skin should be carefully examined. Anoscopy is a helpful addition to the diagnostic workup in selected patients.

The female genitalia are best examined with the patient in the lithotomy position. Lesions around the labia are sought, and labial edema, erythema, or excoriation is noted. The labia minora are spread and the urethral orifice examined. Periurethral erythema suggests urethritis. Urethral discharge can be expressed by gently stripping the urethra with the forefinger inserted into the vagina. The examiner should attempt to palpate Bartholin's glands in the labia minora; they should be neither palpable nor tender. Any discharge expressible from the orifices of these glands should be carefully examined.

A vaginal speculum is inserted using warm water as the only lubricant, since jelly contains antibacterial substances that can interfere with the recovery of fastidious pathogens. The cervix should be visualized, and cervicitis or cervical discharge noted. The vaginal walls are also examined for erythema, punctate hemorrhages, or tiny ulcerations. The character (e.g., color, adherence, frothiness) and amount of vaginal discharge should be noted. Endocervical specimens are obtained by inserting a swab into the endocervix. Vaginal specimens are obtained by sweeping a swab through the anterior and posterior vaginal fornices. After all suitable specimens for cultures and microscopic examination are obtained the speculum is removed, and discharge collected in the blade is examined as described in the next section. A bimanual examination is conducted. Specific attention should be directed to tenderness in the adnexae or discomfort on cervical traction. The vaginally contaminated finger should not be inserted into the rectum; the examiner should change gloves between the vaginal and rectal examinations. Rectal mucosa is susceptible to infection with a variety of sexually transmitted pathogens, and it is possible that these organisms could be transmitted from the vagina to the rectum on the examiner's glove. Inguinal adenopathy and lesions of the pubic area, thighs, and buttocks should be sought in patients of either sex.

Laboratory Examinations

Urethral discharge should be applied to a microscope slide by rolling the swab across the slide. This material should be prepared with Gram's stain and examined with the oil immersion objective. Squamous epithelial cells from the distal portion of the urethra will be seen, and cuboid epithelial cells will be observed if the specimen has been obtained by inserting a swab into the urethra. The distal portion of the urethra has a normal flora consisting primarily of gram-positive cocci and rods, but these have no specific diagnostic significance. The presence of polymorphonuclear neutrophils (PMNs) is abnormal. Although a strong association between the presence of five PMNs per oil immersion field and acute urethritis has been suggested, many patients with urethritis may display fewer PMNs, particularly if they have urinated shortly before the examination. The slide should be carefully scanned for gram-negative, cell-associated diplococci, which confirm a diagnosis of gonorrhea in 95% of infected, symptomatic men (Chapter 265).

Endocervical discharge collected on a cotton swab should be examined against a white background. A yellow or green tinge suggests mucopurulent cervicitis. The swab is then rolled over an area of 2 cm² on a microscope slide, and Gram's staining is performed. PMNs are normally found in the endocervical mucus, but they should arouse suspicion of mucopurulent cervicitis if present in sheets. Vaginal flora always contaminate the endocervical specimen, and rigid criteria must be applied to the diagnosis of gonorrhea on the basis of an endocervical smear. The smear is positive in only 50% of infected women.

The pH of vaginal discharge should be assessed by inserting a piece of indicator paper in the discharge that has pooled in the speculum. We have found nitrazine paper useful because it has a pH range of 4.5 to 7.0. The normal vaginal pH is 4.5, and this pH is preserved in vulvovaginal candidiasis. On the other hand, an elevated vaginal pH is associated with trichomoniasis or bacterial vaginosis. The apparent pH can be artifactually elevated by contamination with cervical discharge or semen.

After testing the pH, one should add one or two drops of 10% potassium hydroxide (KOH) to the discharge. The preparation is then examined for the presence of a pungent, fishy, aminelike odor. This odor constitutes a positive "whiff test" result and suggests trichomoniasis or bacterial vaginosis. The whiff test result is negative in candidiasis.

Vaginal discharge should be examined by means of a wet-mount slide, which may be prepared by agitating the swab carrying vaginal discharge in a test tube containing a small amount of normal saline. A drop of this material is then transferred to the microscope slide, a coverslip is applied, and the preparation is examined at 100× and 400× magnifications with the substage condenser racked down to increase contrast; vaginal squamous epithelial cells are transparent, and their edges are sharp and easily discerned. The presence of large numbers of coccobacilli adhering to the surface of these cells (clue cells) and obscuring their edges suggests bacterial vaginosis. The presence of approximately one polymorphonuclear leukocyte per epithelial cell is normal; increased numbers are distinctly unusual in bacterial vaginosis but are seen with some other forms of vaginitis and with cervicitis. The appearance of an excessive number of PMNs in a specimen containing clue cells should suggest a second process.

The normal flora consist of large rods. In bacterial vaginosis the flora consist primarily of sheets and clumps of coccobacilli. Motile trichomonads are approximately the size of a PMN, are most easily recognized by their characteristic twitching motility, and are seen in about 70% of infected women. Spermatozoa may be seen up to 10 days after the last sexual contact; motile spermatozoa suggest coitus within 24 hours. *Candida* organisms are recognized as budding, ovoid yeasts or as elongated pseudohyphae.

A KOH preparation is made by combining a drop of the wet-mount suspension with a drop of 10% KOH, applying a coverslip, and gently warming the slide before microscopic examination. All cellular elements except bacteria and fungi are destroyed. The KOH preparation is more sensitive and more specific than the wet mount for the diagnosis of candidiasis but obviously cannot be used for diagnosis of other genital infections. Vaginal discharge can be examined with Gram's stain, and bacterial vaginosis can be diagnosed therefrom, but *Candida* organisms and trichomonads are best recognized on the wet-mount preparation.

Gram's stain of the rectal mucosa reveals large numbers of bacteria; gonococci can be identified in about 50% of rectal infections. The sensitivity can be increased by taking the specimen through an anoscope, recovering flecks of mucus or mucopus for microscopic examination.

Material from lesions can be examined with the Tzanck preparation for multinucleated giant cells, which is diagnostic of herpesvirus infection (Chapter 255) or by dark-field microscopy for the spirochete of syphilis (Chapter 274).

Cultures for *N. gonorrhoeae* should be taken from the urethra in men, from the endocervix and possibly from the rectum in women, and from any mucosal surface used for sexual contact. Thus the throat and rectum should be cultured in homosexual men who have participated in receptive oral or anal intercourse. Vaginal discharge can be cultured on appropriate media for *Candida* and *Trichomonas* organisms and *Gardnerella vaginalis*.

In the past, tissue culture techniques were required for identification of herpes simplex virus and *C. trachomatis* (Chapter 257). Newer, culture-independent techniques such as antigen detection (e.g., direct fluorescent antibody, enzyme-linked immunosorbent assay [ELISA]), DNA probes, and genomic amplification techniques (e.g., polymerase chain reaction) have significantly increased the sensitivity and decreased the cost of identifying these sexually transmitted organisms as well as *Haemophilus ducreyi*, *Trichomonas vaginalis*, and *N. gonorrhoeae*.

C. trachomatis can be recovered from the urethra, endocervix, or other sites by tissue culture (Chapter 257). Direct fluorescence microscopy with monoclonal antibodies, ELISA, and DNA probes have been used to identify *C. trachomatis* in genital smears with high accuracy, rapid turnaround time, and low cost compared with culture (Chapter 257).

SPECIFIC CLINICAL SYNDROMES

Sexually transmitted diseases often enter into the differential diagnosis of specific syndromes associated with genital infections.

Urethritis

Patients with urethritis (Chapter 246) generally come to medical attention with some combination of urethral discharge and dysuria (Table 244-2).

Gonococcal and Nongonococcal Urethritis. Gonorrhea accounts for approximately half of the cases of urethritis seen in STD clinics but for as few as 10% of the cases of acute urethritis seen in private practice and student health care settings. Acute urethritis of any other origin is referred to as nongonococcal urethritis (NGU). The clinical spectrum of gonorrhea differs from that of NGU (Table 244-2); however, there is sufficient clinical overlap that accurate differential diagnosis must be based on microscopic examination of the urethral specimen.

Shorter incubation periods tend to be associated with gonorrhea; longer incubation periods are more suggestive of NGU. The onset of symptoms in gonorrhea is often abrupt, whereas the symptoms of NGU are generally subacute. They may increase gradually over several days or may fluctuate, sometimes almost completely disappearing, only to reappear 2 to 3 days later. These stuttering symptoms often greatly prolong the time until patients seek medical care. Most men with gonorrhea seek attention within 2 to 3 days of the development of symptoms, whereas delays of more than a week are common with NGU. The symptoms of gonorrhea tend to be more severe than those of NGU, with almost three fourths of the patients complaining of discharge and dysuria. Patients with NGU tend to complain of discharge or dysuria rather than both. Most commonly, patients seek medical advice with dysuria and do not notice the discharge, which is revealed on examination.

The discharge of acute gonococcal urethritis is usually purulent; a purulent discharge visible at the meatus on initial examination strongly suggests gonorrhea. The discharge of NGU may be equally purulent but is more likely to be mucoid or mucopurulent, that is, clear with purulent flecks. The discharge of NGU is usually not obvious until it is expressed from the urethra.

Even if untreated, the symptoms of urethritis gradually subside over months. Untreated gonorrhea may progress to *gleet,* a chronic inflammatory condition characterized by very little dysuria and a mucoid discharge reminiscent of NGU.

The definitive diagnosis is made on the basis of Gram's stain of the urethral discharge. Gram-negative, cell-associated diplococci are seen in 95% of patients whose discharge subsequently grows gonococci. Since the sensitivity of the culture is less than 100%, discrepancies between Gram's stain and the culture may indicate a failing of the culture rather than of Gram's stain. A patient with acute urethritis and Gram's stain suggestive of gonorrhea should be given treatment for that disease, whereas a patient with Gram's stain revealing PMNs but no gram-negative, cell-associated diplococci should be given treatment for NGU. An important shortcoming of the urethral Gram's stain is its inability to detect coincident NGU in the presence of gonorrhea. Miscellaneous bacteria often observed on Gram's stain represent the normal flora of the anterior urethra and are of no diagnostic significance.

Nongonococcal urethritis includes several different infections. *C.*

trachomatis causes fewer than half of cases of NGU, and its relative role as a cause of this syndrome appears to be decreasing. *Ureaplasma urealyticum* is responsible for some fraction of the remainder. From the practical standpoint, these two organisms probably account for more than 70% of cases of NGU and the syndrome can be effectively treated with regimens consisting of tetracycline or macrolide antibiotics. Thus when Gram's stain of urethral discharge does not display gram-negative, cell-associated diplococci, the disease is probably caused by a tetracycline-sensitive infection. *T. vaginalis* is usually carried asymptomatically by men but may be responsible for 5% of cases of NGU. Syphilis, lymphogranuloma venereum, and occasionally infection with either herpes simplex virus or Enterobacteriaceae can cause urethral discharge, but these conditions are rare.

Postgonococcal Urethritis. *C. trachomatis* is not eradicated by the single doses of antimicrobials usually used to treat gonococcal urethritis. Because these agents are extremely prevalent in sexually active populations, men may acquire gonococci and chlamydiae from the same sexual exposure. Such patients initially respond to appropriate single-dose therapy, but a reexacerbation of symptoms occurs in the absence of reexposure. Treatment with a tetracycline eradicates the chlamydiae and cures the patient. Patients who have a recurrence of urethral symptoms after treatment for gonorrhea, however, may be reinfected or may be true treatment failures. Thus a workup with a urethral Gram's stain and culture is necessary in a patient who comes to medical attention with a recrudescence of symptoms.

Asymptomatic Urethral Infections. The gonococcus and the agents of NGU can be carried asymptomatically. In about 3% of men acquiring gonococcal infection of the urethra, symptoms never develop. Because these men do not seek treatment, their number tends to grow. They are usually identified because of the development of the complications of gonorrhea or because the diagnosis is made in a sexual partner. Women whose gonorrhea is diagnosed because complications have developed or because a routine screening culture was positive are likely to have acquired the infection from an asymptomatic man. Up to 40% of the asymptomatic male sexual partners of such women are infected, and all the sexual partners of a patient with gonorrhea should receive medical attention. It has been shown that 5% of asymptomatic men in venereal disease clinics carry *C. trachomatis.* The asymptomatic male sexual partners of women known to have chlamydial infection should receive epidemiologic treatment. Asymptomatic carriers of *N. gonorrhoeae* or *C. trachomatis* may have small numbers of PMNs on Gram-stained smears of material recovered from urethral swabs. Trichomonal infestation of the urethra is usually asymptomatic.

Urethritis in Women and the Urethral Syndrome. Dysuria in women may be a symptom of classic upper or lower urinary tract infection (UTI) (Chapter 246). Among sexually active women, however, it is a relatively nonspecific complaint and is more likely to result from vulvovaginitis than from UTI. It is helpful to question women regarding whether the dysuria is perceived to occur inside or outside the body. The former suggests urethritis or UTI, whereas the latter suggests vulvovaginitis. Fifty percent of women with symptomatic UTI have levels of bacteriuria far lower than the traditional 10^5 organisms/mm^3. Women with dysuria who do not have vaginitis or routine UTI have been said to have the urethral syndrome. Some of these women also have pyuria, as defined by placing some uncentrifuged midstream urine in a hemacytometer and finding more than 8 white blood cells/mm^3. It is now clear that many of these symptomatic women with pyuria have sexually transmitted urethritis caused by *N. gonorrhoeae* or *C. trachomatis.* Women are generally unaware of urethral discharge, although it can sometimes be identified on physical examination. These same organisms are likely to cause coincident cervical infection, and detection of mucopurulent cervicitis on physical examination lends support to the diagnosis. However, some women with chlamydial infection appear to be infected only at the urethra, and a negative test result for chlamydia from the cervix does not rule out urethritis. Unless the sexually transmitted nature of these infections is recognized, asymptomatic male sexual partners of these women will not be treated, and frequent, frustrating recurrence of symptoms from reinfection will result. Since chlamydial and gono-

Table 244-2   Clinical features of acute gonococcal and nongonococcal urethritis

CLINICAL FEATURE	GONOCOCCAL	NONGONOCOCCAL
Incubation period	Shorter: ≤4 days, 70% ≤2 weeks, 90%	Longer: ≤4 days, 40% 2-3 weeks, ~30%
Onset of symptoms	Abrupt	Gradual, fluctuating
Discharge and dysuria	70%	40%
Discharge	Purulent	Mucoid or mucopurulent

coccal infection may well respond, at least initially, to regimens prescribed for UTI (e.g., quinolones, trimethoprim-sulfamethoxazole [TMP-SMX], amoxicillin), the clinician should consider STD in the patient with recurrent "culture-negative" UTI. Even if the initial infection were, in fact, cured by the urinary tract regimen, recurrence could result from reinfection by an untreated sexual partner (Chapter 246).

Treatment of Acute Urethritis. Nongonococcal urethritis, which is most likely the result of a tetracycline- or macrolide-sensitive organism, may be treated orally with azithromycin, 1 g as a single oral dose. Single-dose therapy has the obvious advantage of independence from concerns regarding patient compliance. Azithromycin remains relatively expensive, although the powder form, which is administered mixed in water, is less expensive than the same dose comprising four capsules. Doxycycline, 100 mg twice a day, or erythromycin, 500 mg four a day, either for 7 days, is considerably cheaper. Minocycline, long avoided because of its tendency to induce middle ear disturbances, can in fact be used as a 100-mg dose administered at bedtime for 7 nights. Urethritis or cervicitis can also be treated with ofloxacin, 300 mg orally twice a day for 7 days, a regimen that is also expensive but may have a role in special circumstances in which the etiologic differential diagnosis includes *N. gonorrhoeae* or the Enterobacteriaceae (e.g., salpingitis, epididymitis). The treatment of gonorrhea is discussed in Chapter 265. The tetracycline regimens, once highly effective in the treatment of gonorrhea, are now associated with high failure rates in certain areas. Treatment for urethritis of unknown origin should include a single dose that is effective for gonorrhea and a regimen that is active against the agents of NGU.

The patterns of recurrent NGU can be helpful in deciding on future therapy. Some patients have a prompt resolution of symptoms but note recurrence after sexual exposure. Such cases probably represent reinfection, and the patient can be retreated with the initial regimen. Of course, it is important to ensure that all sexual partners receive appropriate treatment. Other patients note an initial symptomatic response, but their symptoms return after discontinuation of therapy even though they have not been reexposed. Such cases are often successfully treated with longer courses of doxycycline (e.g., 100 mg twice a day for 4 weeks). As an alternative, erythromycin in doses of 500 mg four times daily can be used for the same interval. A few patients note no response of symptoms to doxycycline. These patients are likely to be infected with a tetracycline-resistant organism, principally *T. vaginalis* or tetracycline-resistant *U. urealyticum*. Trichomoniasis is diagnosed only with great difficulty in men, usually depending on the culture results rather than on direct microscopic examination. Trichomoniasis responds to metronidazole, 2 g as a single, oral dose, and ureaplasmal infection to azithromycin or erythromycin in the doses mentioned earlier. Persistent relapses or treatment failures should prompt referral to a urologist.

Because up to 40% of men with acute gonococcal urethritis are also infected with *C. trachomatis,* gonorrhea might best be treated with a single dose of an appropriate drug (see Chapter 265) followed by a regimen of doxycycline, erythromycin, or azithromycin that is effective against chlamydia. Ofloxacin in a regimen of 300 mg orally twice a day for 7 days or azithromycin as a single 2 g dose cures both chlamydial and gonococcal infection, but the cost is higher than those two drug regimens using doxycycline or erythromycin.

Other Urethritides. Nongonococcal urethritis can accompany Stevens-Johnson syndrome and is a part of Reiter's syndrome. In both cases the diagnosis is made on the basis of extragenital manifestations. Many cases of Reiter's syndrome seem to follow urethral infection with *C. trachomatis* and probably represent a disordered immune response to the pathogen. Because of this association, patients with Reiter's syndrome should initially receive a course of doxycycline.

Cervicitis

Under the influence of estrogens the vaginal epithelium cornifies and becomes resistant to several important sexually transmitted pathogens. Thus a number of venereal diseases involve the cervix while sparing the vagina. Acute cervicitis usually becomes evident with an increased cervical discharge, mucoid or purulent, and inflammation around the cervical os.

Increased cervical discharge is seen in pregnancy, during the use of oral contraceptives, and in some patients wearing an intrauterine contraceptive device. The discharge is generally mucoid rather than purulent and does not contain abnormally large numbers of PMNs. The appearance of cervical erythema can result from the outgrowth of columnar epithelium onto the cervix. Such ectropion is usually symmetric around the os, is more common in younger women and those taking oral contraceptives, and may increase the risk of acquiring chlamydial infection.

Purulent or mucopurulent cervical discharge usually accompanies cervicitis of gonococcal or chlamydial origin. Gram's stain of the discharge reveals large numbers of PMNs, as well as gram-negative, cell-associated diplococci in about 50% of women with gonorrhea; a negative Gram's stain does not rule out gonococcal infection. The smear may be misleading because of the presence of other gram-negative diplococci in normal vaginal secretions.

Gonococci or chlamydiae are isolated from 60% to 90% of the sexual partners of men with gonococcal or chlamydial urethritis. Chlamydiae have been isolated from 50% to 90% of sexually active patients with a specific form of cervicitis characterized by erosion, congestion, edema, and hypertrophy about the cervical os. The lesion is generally intensely red, asymmetric about the os, and often friable, bleeding when it is abraded during the examination. A purulent cervical discharge usually accompanies this type of cervicitis. Women who come to medical attention with the syndrome of hypertrophic cervicitis (and their sexual partners) should receive treatment for chlamydial infection. After adequate treatment the hypertrophic cer-

Table 244-3   Vulvovaginitis

CLINICAL AND LABORATORY FINDING	TRICHOMONIASIS	CANDIDIASIS	BACTERIAL VAGINOSIS
Symptoms			
Pruritus	+++	+++	+
Discharge	+++	+	++
Odor	+	+	+++
Menses	Increased after	Increased before	Not related
Discharge	Thin, purulent	Thick, adherent	Thin, adherent
Froth	++		+
Color	White, yellow, green	White	Grayish white
pH	Elevated	4.5	Elevated
Whiff test	++		+++
Microscopy			
Flora	Rods or coccobacilli	Rods, yeasts, pseudohyphae	Coccobacilli
Polymorphonuclear neutrophils	+++	May be present	
Epithelial cells	Normal	Normal	Clue cells

+, Minimal if present; ++, often described; +++, prevalent and pronounced.

Table 244-4   Differential diagnosis of genital lesions

MORPHOLOGIC FEATURE	NUMBER	DISTRIBUTION	SURFACE	BASE
Ulcers	?Single (55%) or multiple	Penis, labia, cervix	Clean	Indolent
	Single	Penis	Purulent	Inflamed
	Single	Penis, labia	Beefy red, granulation tissue	Friable
	Single	Penis, labia	Eroded papule	Benign
	Multiple	Penis, vulva, thigh, cervix, grouped	Clean	Clean, all same size
	Multiple (30%) or single (70%)	Penis, vulva, thigh	Necrotic	Variable size, ragged
Papules	Single	Penis, labia	Clean or small erosion	Benign
	Multiple	One or more rows behind corona	Clean	Benign
	Multiple	Penis, labia, vagina, often grouped	Verrucous	Benign
	Multiple	Penis, labia, pubic hair, thighs, buttocks	Umbilicated, with tiny plug	Benign
	Multiple	Disseminated, palms, soles	Coppery	Benign
	Multiple	Penis, labia, thighs, buttocks, wrists, and ankles	Crusted	
Vesicles	Multiple	Penis, labia, thighs, cervix, grouped	Umbilicated	Erythema
Crusts	Multiple	Grouped		Erythema
	Multiple	Disseminated		Erythema may be present
Erythema	Patches	Glans, shaft of penis, labia, vulva	Intense erythema	

vicitis usually resolves to a simple cervicitis. About 50% of women with gonorrhea also have chlamydial infection, and women with gonococcal cervicitis should receive treatment with a double regimen as described for gonococcal urethritis.

Herpes simplex virus is recovered from the cervix of 80% of women with primary herpes genitalis and can cause an acute cervicitis that may not be associated with lesions of the external genitalia. The cervix may show discrete, grouped, or coalescent ulcerations, and there may be frank cervical necrosis. This type of cervicitis is often accompanied by a mucoid discharge.

Vulvovaginitis

Vulvovaginitis is a common clinical syndrome and is the most frequent cause of genital symptoms in women. Treatment should be based on a specific etiologic diagnosis, which can usually be made at the time of initial evaluation. Although the infectious vaginitides have different manifestations (Table 244-3), there is so much clinical overlap that initial evaluation must include bedside laboratory evaluation.

Candidiasis. More than 80% of vulvovaginal yeast infections are caused by *Candida albicans* (Chapter 277); 3% to 15% are due to *Candida (Torulopsis) glabrata*. Other species of *Candida* are rarely implicated. Although a matter of chronic concern, there is very little evidence to suggest that the percentage of cases caused by species other than *C. albicans* has increased in response to current therapeutic practices. The problem of diagnosing this common infection is compounded by the fact that *Candida* organisms can be isolated from the vaginas of many healthy, asymptomatic women. Thus screening asymptomatic women for the presence of yeasts is not indicated. Broad-spectrum antibiotics predispose to the development of vulvovaginal candidiasis by reducing the normal bacterial content of the vagina and allowing the yeasts to overgrow. *Candida* organisms are carried more frequently by women receiving oral contraceptives, and these women have a higher incidence of candidal vulvovaginitis. The disease is also more common in diabetic patients and during pregnancy, and many women describe a recrudescence or exacerbation of symptoms in the immediate premenstrual period. Severe, recalcitrant vulvovaginal candidiasis can be a manifestation of AIDS.

Patients with candidal vulvovaginitis generally complain of perivaginal pruritus and relatively little discharge. External dysuria is frequently described. On examination the labia minora may be pallid or erythematous. The vulva is often intensely red, and excoriation attests to the marked pruritus. Satellite lesions, tiny papulopustules located beyond the main erythematous border, may be observed. The discharge is characteristically thick and adherent to the vaginal walls. On speculum examination it is often evident as curds resembling cottage cheese. Sometimes, however, a thin discharge will be seen. Vaginal pH is normal, and the whiff test result is negative. Wet-mount slides and KOH examinations often, but by no means always, reveal budding yeasts and variable, often normal numbers of PMNs. The diagnosis of candidal vulvovaginitis is best based on a combination of clinical and microscopic findings, since up to 50% of infected, symptomatic women have negative results of microscopic examinations for yeasts. Culture may be useful in these cases.

The infection is usually treated by the local application of an antifungal drug. Commercial preparations of imidazole antifungals (miconazole, clotrimazole, butoconazole, terconazole, or econazole) are effective agents. Seven-day, 3-day, and single-dose regimens have been shown to be reasonably efficacious, and there is no evidence that any specific drug or formulation is superior. Treatment with a single oral dose of the triazole fluconazole, 150 mg, is also highly effective and convenient. Other drugs such as nystatin, boric acid, or gentian violet are less effective but may be useful in cases of imidazole or triazole resistance. Recurrence is a major problem and should cause a search for risk factors that can be eliminated. Unnecessary use of antibiotics should be avoided, and switching to a lower-dosage oral contraceptive may be useful. There is no good evidence that simultaneous treatment of a rectal focus with oral nystatin reduces the frequency of relapse. Some patients with frequently recurring disease have prolonged remission following 6 months of treatment with an oral agent.

Sexual transmission seems to contribute relatively little to the overall epidemiology of vulvovaginal candidiasis. In up to 10% of the sexual partners of infected women, however, a candidal balanitis may develop that is characterized by intense erythema and pruritus of the glans. This condition appears to be sexually transmitted and responds to topical anticandidal medication.

Trichomoniasis. The incidence of trichomoniasis in the United States appears to be decreasing, possibly in response to the widespread use of metronidazole for bacterial vaginosis (see later discussion). This infection is almost always sexually transmitted, although trichomonads can survive for several hours on wet surfaces,

EDGE	PAIN	ADENPATHY	INCUBATION PERIOD	SUGGESTED DIAGNOSIS
Indurated	Mild (30%)	Moderate	<21 days (up to 90 days)	Syphilis
Ragged	Mild to severe	Mild or absent	<24 hours	Human bite, other trauma
Serpiginous		Inguinal granulomas	1-12 weeks	Donovanosis
Benign	Lesion often goes entirely unnoticed	Moderate, but usually appears after lesion resolves	2 weeks	Lymphogranuloma venereum
Erythema	Severe: prodome of paresthesia	Moderate, tender	3-7 days, recurrent	Herpes genitalis
Undermined erythema	Moderate	Moderate, tender	2-5 days	Chancroid
Benign			2 weeks	Early lymphogranuloma venereum
Benign				Pearly penile papules
Benign			3-30 weeks	Venereal warts
Benign			2-26 weeks	Molluscum contagiosum
Benign	Occasional, mild	Prominent	6-12 weeks	Secondary syphilis
Linear tracks may be seen	Intense pruritus	Rare superinfected excoriation	4 weeks	Scabies
	Mild	Moderate, tender	2-5 days	Herpes genitalis
	Mild	Mild	2-5 days	Healing herpes genitalis
	Pruritus	Mild or absent	4 weeks	Scabies
Satellite lesions	Pruritus		Undefined	Candidiasis

and nonvenereal transmission probably occurs in certain rare instances. Affected women usually complain of pruritus and discharge, which may begin or be exacerbated during or immediately after the menstrual period.

On examination the labia are often erythematous, and a discharge may be present on the perineum. Through the speculum the vaginal walls are seen to be erythematous, sometimes with punctate hemorrhages, which give a granular appearance to the mucosa. The discharge is loose and collects in the posterior fornix. It is frothy in about 40% of cases. The diagnosis may be made by wet-mount examination of the discharge, which contains numerous PMNs and reveals motile trichomonads in about 70% of cases. Of women coming to venereal disease clinics, 25% of those in whom trichomonads are isolated from the vagina are asymptomatic. These women should receive treatment, however, because symptoms will develop in about half of them within the next 6 months and they constitute an important reservoir of infection.

Treatment of trichomoniasis is with metronidazole, which can be administered as a single, 2-g dose or in doses of 250 mg orally three times daily or 500 mg twice daily for 7 days. Metronidazole, like disulfiram, causes nausea, vomiting, and flushing if consumed with alcohol, and patients should be suitably cautioned. The drug is contraindicated in early pregnancy, and treatment of trichomoniasis in this setting is less than ideal. Clotrimazole, 100 mg intravaginally each night, may relieve symptoms and occasionally produces a cure. Just before delivery, infected women should receive definitive treatment with metronidazole to prevent possible spread of infection to the infant during the birth process. Trichomonads resistant to metronidazole are being recognized with increasing frequency. Infections with these organisms are very difficult to cure but are sometimes eradicated by a 2-week course of metronidazole, 2 g orally per day, along with 500 mg (broken tablet) intravaginally each night.

Trichomonads can be isolated in 30% to 70% of the male sexual partners of infected women. Most of these men are asymptomatic, but they should receive treatment as a public health measure and because the long-term effects of chronic trichomonal carriage are unknown.

Bacterial Vaginosis. Bacterial vaginosis has become the most common vaginal infection in the United States. Affected women are usually sexually active and complain of a vaginal discharge that may be relatively scanty and, unlike that of trichomoniasis, is usually non-irritating. More so than with the other vaginitides, affected women complain of a vaginal odor that they may describe as "fishy." Symptoms bear little relation to the stage of the menstrual cycle, and there is very little vulvar inflammation. The discharge is thin but often adheres to the vaginal walls. There may be enough to pool in the posterior fornix, and it is often seen to contain small bubbles. If present in smaller amounts, it appears as increased moistness of the vaginal walls, often yielding a light reflex during examination. The vaginal pH is elevated, usually to 5.0 or higher, and the whiff test result is positive. Microscopic examination of the discharge reveals clue cells, vaginal epithelial cells studded with tiny coccobacilli. These organisms often obscure the nucleus or the edges of the cells. Among the epithelial cells there are relatively few PMNs; the presence of large numbers of PMNs suggests a coincidental inflammatory process. The bacterial flora consist of sheets or clumps of gram-negative coccobacilli. The diagnosis can, indeed, be made when Gram's stain of vaginal discharge reveals that the normal flora of gram-positive rods (lactobacilli) have been replaced by these organisms.

The coccobacilli that are present in large numbers are *Gardnerella vaginalis* and are one component of a synergistic infection with vaginal anaerobes that produce the amines responsible for the characteristic odor. Carriage of *G. vaginalis* alone does not produce clinical disease, but these organisms may replace the normal flora of hydrogen peroxide–producing lactobacilli, which normally keep anaerobic bacteria in check. The anaerobic bacilli elaborate amines responsible for the characteristic odor. Curved anaerobic rods, such as *Mobiluncus curtisii,* and mycoplasmas are often present and may play a role in the infection. Although initially thought to be a benign condition, bacterial vaginosis and its associated organisms have been significantly associated with PID, amnionitis, postpartum fever and endometritis, and low-birth-weight infants.

Treatment of bacterial vaginosis consists of metronidazole, which is active against vaginal anaerobes, in doses of 500 mg orally twice a day for 7 days. A single, 2-g dose appears less effective. Pregnant women may be given treatment with clindamycin, 300 mg orally twice a day for 7 days. Topical clindamycin and topical metronidazole are now available and are also effective. Somewhat surprisingly, initial management of infected women need not involve treatment of male sexual partners. Some women with recurrent disease, however, can be cured only by simultaneous treatment of sexual partners.

Skin and Mucous Membrane Lesions

The skin of the genital area is involved in many generalized dermatoses, but STDs are a frequent cause of genital lesions among adults. One can occasionally estimate the incubation period of STDs by obtaining a history of a single recent sexual contact or a recent contact with a new sexual partner. When available, an estimate of the incubation period can be helpful in the differential diagnosis of genital lesions (Table 244-4).

Recently there has been an increase in the incidence of chancroid in the United States, but chancroid and lymphogranuloma venereum are still considerably more common in the Far East and Africa than in the United States. Donovanosis is endemic in India, New Guinea, the West Indies, and some parts of Africa and South America. It is now extremely rare in the United States. In these days of rapid intercontinental travel, recent sexual exposure in an endemic area can increase the probability of these otherwise rare diseases.

Medications occasionally produce a fixed drug eruption involving the genitalia, and broad-spectrum antibiotics may predispose to the development of candidiasis and may alter or completely eliminate the lesions of syphilis.

Although the typical syphilitic chancre (Color Plate VIII-34) is described as nontender, up to 30% of patients with primary syphilis describe either pain or tenderness of the lesions. Significant pain usually accompanies the lesions of chancroid, herpes genitalis, and tularemia.

Because lesions often change over time, a history of the initial manifestation may be crucial to making the diagnosis. Genital ulcerations that began as vesicles point to a diagnosis of herpes genitalis.

Morphologic Characteristics of Genital Lesions. In many cases the appearance of genital lesions is sufficiently distinctive to permit accurate differential diagnosis without resorting to laboratory tests (Table 244-4). Herpes genitalis and chancroid both produce painful genital ulcerations. Grouped clusters of vesicles or small ulcerations are characteristic of herpes genitalis. These lesions tend to be of approximately the same size and appear relatively clean; the ulcers of chancroid tend to vary in size and look ragged and necrotic. Herpes characteristically begins as vesicles, although by the time the patient comes to the physician, all of these may have ruptured to form shallow ulcers. Recurrence is characteristic of herpes genitalis but not of chancroid. Patients with the former sometimes note a prodrome of local paresthesias preceding the eruption of vesicles by about 12 hours. Vesicles are not a manifestation of chancroid, and a history of vesicles can simplify the differential diagnosis. If the differential diagnosis is in doubt, material from an ulcer can be subjected to one of the newer culture-independent techniques for identification. Particularly in the developing world, multiple infections are simultaneously present.

Pruritic patches in the groin may represent candidiasis or dermatophytosis. Candidiasis is usually intensely red rather than the brown to violet discoloration that accompanies *Tinea* species infection. Dermatophytes usually spare the scrotum, whereas *Candida* organisms involve it. Satellite lesions, tiny papulopustules beyond the main area of erythema, strongly suggest candidiasis. A potassium hydroxide preparation of skin scrapings establishes the diagnosis.

Healing herpes genitalis and scabies both result in crusted lesions in the genital area. Intense itching, often worse at night or immediately after bathing, is characteristic of scabies. Herpetic lesions are usually restricted to the genitalia, whereas itching around the belt line, ankles, wrists, or in the interdigital webs strongly suggests a diagnosis of scabies.

The lesions of STDs may be found in the perianal region in patients practicing receptive anal intercourse and in the perioral or oral area in patients engaging in orogenital contact.

Other conditions should be considered in the differential diagnosis of genital lesions, including Behçet's syndrome, in which recurrent genital ulcerations are associated with recurrent lesions in the mouth and systemic symptoms. Malignancy is part of the differential diagnosis of subacute or chronic lesions, particularly in older patients. In endemic areas tick-borne tularemia can produce a painful genital ulcer that is usually associated with regional adenopathy and systemic toxicity.

Inguinal Adenopathy

Inguinal adenopathy accompanies a variety of genital lesions in STDs (Table 244-4). Tender adenopathy is more common with gonococcal than with nongonococcal urethritis but is not a common finding with either disease. Adenopathy, usually bilateral, is seen in about 80% of patients with primary herpes genitalis and usually begins during the second week of illness. Tender adenopathy usually accompanies lesions of chancroid as well. Occasionally, patients with infectious mononucleosis come to medical attention with isolated inguinal adenopathy, although generalized lymphadenopathy is more common. Relatively painless inguinal adenopathy accompanies primary syphilis, and the involved nodes are discrete, firm, and freely movable. Suppuration is rare.

The inguinal adenopathy of lymphogranuloma venereum usually appears weeks after resolution of the primary lesion. Indeed, the primary lesion is so subtle that it is described by only about 30% of infected men and by virtually no infected women. The adenopathy of lymphogranuloma venereum may be extensive and may involve nodes above and below the inguinal (Poupart's) ligament. This adenopathy gives the appearance of a single mass of nodes bisected by a groove, a sign highly suggestive of lymphogranuloma venereum. The nodes in lymphogranuloma venereum may eventually suppurate and drain, and they are sometimes described as giving a bluish discoloration to the overlying skin. The complement-fixation test for lymphogranuloma venereum is sensitive by the time nodes have appeared, and a negative test result goes far to ruling out the disease. The test result is positive, however, in patients who have had other chlamydial exposure, and because NGU is relatively common in sexually active populations, a positive test result is not by itself diagnostic of lymphogranuloma venereum. Serologic tests may be of assistance in diagnosing plague and tularemia. The diagnosis of syphilitic adenopathy is often confirmed on serologic study.

Patients with inguinal adenopathy should be carefully examined for associated findings suggesting STD, as well as for evidence of infection of the lower extremities. The diagnosis may be assisted by needle aspiration of nodes. Material recovered should be examined by dark-field microscopy for *Treponema pallidum* and Gram's stain and cultured for bacteria and chlamydiae (Color Plate VIII-2).

In endemic areas plague and tularemia must be considered in the differential diagnosis of acute inguinal adenopathy in a young person. Affected patients are usually systemically ill, and their diseases represent medical emergencies. In appropriate areas the diagnosis should be pursued vigorously. In young children staphylococci and streptococci spreading from infections of the lower extremities are the most common cause of inguinal adenopathy.

Miscellaneous Syndromes

Acute epididymitis has been associated with gonococcal and chlamydial infection. Patients with chlamydial epididymitis usually have an accompanying nongonococcal urethritis (Chapter 246). Older men with epididymitis may be infected with gram-negative rods. These men usually do not have a urethral discharge but may notice scrotal swelling and erythema. Various viruses can also cause acute orchiepididymitis.

Bartholinitis has been associated with gonorrhea, as well as with various aerobic and anaerobic bacteria. Material expressed from Bartholin's glands should be cultured on a medium selective for gonococci as well as on routine media. Gram's stain of expressed discharge may be extremely helpful in determining the cause.

Acute proctitis can be caused by *N. gonorrhoeae* and is usually evident as a mild change in bowel habits and the appearance of mucus or pus in the stool. Most rectal gonococcal carriers are completely asymptomatic, and gonococci can be isolated from the rectums of 40% of women with gonorrhea. At the other end of the spectrum is a rare colitis syndrome with bloody diarrhea. *C. trachomatis* has also been isolated from the rectums of asymptomatic men and men with acute colitis. Lymphogranuloma venereum may involve the rectum years after genital symptoms have subsided, with the development of rectal strictures that sometimes require operation. Herpetic proctitis has been described in homosexual men. Amebic proctocolitis is associated with homosexual practices and should enter into the differential diagnosis of homosexual men who come to medical attention with large-bowel symptoms. *Shigella* dysentery has also been acquired by homosexual practices. Recently infection with *Campylobacter* species and so-called *Campylobacter*-like organisms has been associated with diarrheal disease in homosexual men (Chapter 267). Giardiasis is a common cause of small-bowel symptoms in this same population. All these infections are components of what has been termed the *gay bowel syndrome*.

BIBLIOGRAPHY

Centers for Disease Control and Prevention: 1993: sexually transmitted diseases treatment guidelines, *MMWR* 42(No RR-14):1, 1993.

Corey L et al: Genital herpes simplex infection: clinical manifestations, course, and complications, *Ann Intern Med* 98:958, 1983.

Fox KK et al: Vaginal discharge: how to pinpoint the cause, *Postgrad Med* 98:87, 1995.

Goode MA et al: Infectious vaginitis: selecting therapy and preventing recurrence, *Postgrad Med* 96:91, 1994.

Joesoef MR et al: Bacterial vaginosis: review of treatment options and potential clinical indications for therapy, *Clin Infect Dis* 20:S72, 1995.

McCoy MC et al: Bacterial vaginosis in pregnancy: an approach for the 1990s, *Obstet Gyncol Survey* 50:482, 1995.

Nickel P et al: Nongonococcal urethritis, *Curr Prob Dermatol* 24:97, 1996.

Quinn TC: Recent advances in diagnosis of sexually transmitted diseases, *Sex Transm Dis* 21:S19, 1994.

Rein MF, editor: Sexually transmitted diseases, vol 5. In Mandell GL, editor: *Atlas of infectious diseases,* Philadelphia, 1996, Current Science.

Schmid GP et al: Evolving strategies for management of the nongonococcal urethitis syndrome, *JAMA* 274:577, 1995.

Sobel JD: Epidemiology and pathogenesis of recurrent vulvovaginal candidiasis, *Am J Obstet Gynecol* 152:924, 1985.

CHAPTER

245 Gram-Negative Bacteremia and the Sepsis Syndrome

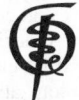

Lisa Istorico Sanders and C. Glenn Cobbs

The purpose of this chapter is to describe an approach to the patient with suspected or proven gram-negative bacteremia. In addition, we consider the so-called sepsis syndrome, a disorder that frequently accompanies gram-negative bacteremia, but one that may also accompany invasive disease caused by gram-positive bacteria, fungi, protozoa, and viruses as well as noninfectious illnesses.

Because of the imprecise nature of the terms *sepsis* and *sepsis syndrome,* a consensus conference of critical care physicians was held in 1991 and the following definitions were proposed. The term *systemic inflammatory response syndrome* (SIRS) was defined as an inflammatory reaction to any one of a number of insults including infection, burns, and trauma. It was evident with at least two of the following: (1) temperature greater than 38° C or less than 36° C; (2) heart rate greater than 90 beats per minute; (3) tachypnea, defined as respiratory rate greater than 20 breaths per minute or hyperventilation with an arterial carbon dioxide pressure ($Paco_2$) less than 32 mm Hg; and (4) alteration of white blood cell count to greater than 12,000 cells/mm^3, less than 4000 cells/mm^3, or greater than 10% immature neutrophils. Furthermore, *sepsis* was defined as SIRS caused by infection, and *severe sepsis* as illness complicated by organ dysfunction, hypoperfusion abnormality (lactic acidosis, oliguria, or mental status changes), or hypotension (systolic blood pressure <90 mm Hg or reduction of 40 mm Hg or more from baseline that is not due to other causes). The term *septic shock* was reserved for an illness associated with hypotension that is not responsive to fluid resuscitation. These definitions have since proved useful in describing common clinical presentations and for classifying patients for clinical trials. They are less useful in predicting outcome for an individual patient and are not defined by the origins or causes of the illness. Nonetheless, the terminology is increasingly being encountered in

medical literature. It will probably continue to be used until we have more precise diagnostic means to rapidly differentiate the various causes. The use of the term *sepsis syndrome* was not encouraged at the consensus conference, but it has most often been used to refer to sepsis with altered organ perfusion manifested by hypoxemia, increased serum lactate level, oliguria, or altered mentation.

Sepsis is the leading cause of death in noncoronary intensive care units and results in as much as $10 billion in annual health care expenditures. Death rates from sepsis increased 83% from 1980 to 1992. These increases are likely to continue because of the invasive nature of medicine today and the increasing number of immunocompromised patients surviving with multiple medical problems.

Enterobacteriaceae (including *Escherichia coli, Klebsiella* and *Proteus* species, and others) and *Pseudomonas* species are the microorganisms most commonly responsible for gram-negative bacteremia. When these organisms invade the blood stream, it appears that endotoxin, a component of gram-negative bacterial cell walls, triggers a cascade of host inflammatory responses leading to the major detrimental effects. Although other organisms can trigger a similar response, it is useful to consider gram-negative bacteremia as a distinct entity because of its characteristic epidemiology, pathogenesis, pathophysiology, and treatment.

EPIDEMIOLOGY

The true incidence of gram-negative bacteremia can only be estimated. The best estimates of incidence come from certain medical centers that have tracked bloodstream infections over a number of years and from data collected nationwide from sentinel hospitals by the Centers for Disease Control and Prevention (CDC). Both sources indicate that the incidence of gram-negative bacteremia has increased. At Boston City Hospital, the incidence of gram-negative bacteremia between 1935 and 1972 rose from less than 1 to 10 cases/1000 medical or surgical admissions. The CDC has estimated that annual cases of septicemia in the United States more than doubled from 1979 to 1987, increasing from 164,000 cases to 425,000. The proportion of these cases attributable to gram-negative bacteria was not stated, but current estimates indicate that about 200,000 cases of gram-negative bacteremia occur yearly in the United States.

Numerous factors may account for this increase. Invasive devices such as central venous catheters are being used more frequently in both inpatient and outpatient settings. Large numbers of patients are now being treated with immunosuppressive and cytotoxic therapies. The proportion of elderly patients and patients with serious underlying diseases in our society is steadily increasing.

Bacteremia may be classified as either community acquired or hospital acquired (nosocomial). The incidence of community-acquired gram-negative bacteremia has increased slightly in the past few years. Most cases still occur as a complication of urinary tract infection in otherwise healthy individuals. In contrast, hospital-acquired gram-negative bacteremia has increased steadily over the past 25 years. More episodes of polymicrobial bacteremia and multiple bacteremic episodes in the same patient have also been noted. Although gram-negative bacteria still account for a significant proportion of nosocomial infections, coagulase-negative staphylococci, enterococci, and yeast have emerged as important bloodstream pathogens as well.

The incidence of gram-negative bacteremia varies in different hospital settings. Tertiary care institutions generally have twofold to fourfold higher rates of bacteremia than do smaller community hospitals. Moreover, the percentage of bacteremia episodes that are nosocomially acquired is much higher for tertiary care centers (up to 75% vs. 40% to 50% for community hospitals). These differences presumably reflect the relative severity of patient illness as well as the average length of stay at the two types of institutions.

The overall in-hospital mortality rate for patients with gram-negative bacteremia is approximately 30%. Mortality rates for patients with septic shock exceed 60%. The most important factor predicting mortality is the presence of severe underlying disease. In their study of outcome in patients with gram-negative bacteremia, McCabe and Jackson classified patients into risk categories: rapidly fatal disease (e.g., terminal malignancy), ultimately fatal disease (death anticipated within 4 years), and nonfatal disease. Mortality in these three groups was 91%, 66%, and 11%, respectively. Additional predictors of poor prognosis identified in more recent studies include the presence of shock, organ system failure, nosocomial infection source, granulocytopenia, hypothermia, inappropriate antimicrobial therapy, and elevated circulating levels of certain cytokines.

MICROBIOLOGY

The genitourinary tract is the site of disease responsible for gram-negative bacteremia in approximately 35% of patients. In otherwise healthy individuals, urinary tract infections are most often caused by *E. coli*. In contrast, individuals with urinary tract obstruction or those who develop infection after instrumentation frequently become infected with bacteria such as *Enterobacter, Klebsiella, Proteus, Serratia,* and *Acinetobacter.* Prior antimicrobial therapy, especially in the presence of foreign bodies in the urinary tract, predisposes to uropathogens with multiple antimicrobial resistance patterns. The presence of the sepsis syndrome associated with a urinary tract infection should raise suspicion for urinary tract obstruction.

Pulmonary infections are responsible for 10% to 15% of episodes of gram-negative bacteremia. *E. coli, Klebsiella* species, and resistant microorganisms such as *Pseudomonas, Serratia,* and *Acinetobacter* are frequently encountered. The upper respiratory tract may be colonized by gram-negative bacteria in patients with chronic illnesses, recent hospitalizations, or recent antibiotic therapy, and the majority of nosocomial gram-negative bacillary pneumonias result from aspiration of colonizing strains. When gram-negative bacillary pneumonia occurs, bacteremia complicates the disease in approximately 15% of patients. It occurs most often when there is associated lung abscess and/or endobronchial obstruction.

An intraabdominal source (including perforated appendix, perforated diverticulum, ischemic bowel, peritonitis, liver abscess, and biliary tract disease) is found in approximately 15% of patients with gram-negative bacteremia. In such cases, the microorganism isolated from the blood presumably reflects the preexisting bowel flora. Anaerobic species, especially *Bacteroides,* may cause bacteremia in this setting, and polymicrobial bacteremia is also encountered with serious intraabdominal disease (Chapters 242 and 271).

Patients with burns are at particular risk for microbial invasion of skin, both because of the loss of this natural barrier to infection and because of compromise of immune defenses as a consequence of the injury. Care in the burn center is directed at prevention of skin colonization by topical application of creams with broad activity against many species of bacteria, rigorous debridement of necrotic tissue, and use of parenteral antibiotics. The microorganisms that colonize a particular burn unit are usually responsible when invasion occurs.

Gram-negative bacilli are also important etiologic agents of nosocomial intravascular catheter infections, accounting for approximately half of bacteremic episodes. The genera encountered reflect the particular hospital's ecology and include *Klebsiella, Enterobacter, Acinetobacter, Pseudomonas,* and *Escherichia.*

Patients with profound granulocytopenia are susceptible to bacteremia as a result of invasion of mucosal surfaces by resident flora. The oropharynx and gut appear to serve as sites of bacterial invasion in the granulocytopenic patient with occult gram-negative bacteremia (Chapter 236).

Despite thorough evaluation, a primary source cannot be determined in up to 30% of patients with gram-negative bacteremia.

Patients with human immunodeficiency virus (HIV) infection appear to be at increased risk of gram-negative bacteremia. "Spontaneous" *Pseudomonas aeruginosa* bacteremia is particularly common in patients with advanced HIV infection. These infections carry a high mortality, and relapse is common.

PATHOGENESIS
Host-Parasite Interactions

The pathogenesis of bacterial infection is a dynamic process in which colonizing microorganisms interact with host defenses. The virulence of the particular bacterial species and the status of the host's immune system are the variables that determine the likelihood of subsequent disease. Our present understanding of host defense against microbial invasion is discussed in detail in Chapter 229; specific factors related to gram-negative infection are discussed here.

Host Defense Factors

Anatomic barriers are an important first line of defense against bacterial infection. Disruption of the skin barrier as a result of trauma, burns, or intravascular catheterization may allow entry of gram-negative bacteria, as does urinary tract catheterization. The integrity of the intestinal mucosa may be compromised by ischemia or malnutrition, making bacterial translocation more likely.

Both the humoral and cell-mediated arms of the immune system play a role in preventing gram-negative disease, and patients with defective function of either of these arms may be at increased risk.

Burn patients have numerous defects in their immune defenses, which further predispose them to infection. These patients have low levels of immunoglobulins, increased suppressor T-cell activity, decreased helper T-cell activity, and perhaps, most important, defects in neutrophil function.

Polymorphonuclear leukocytes are the host's primary defense against pyogenic bacteria that have penetrated external mechanical barriers. Patients with profound granulocytopenia are especially susceptible to invasive bacterial disease.

Occasionally, therapy directed at preventing other nosocomial complications may predispose to infection. Gastric alkalization used to prevent stress ulceration in ill patients may allow bacterial overgrowth in the upper gastrointestinal tract, leading to an increased risk of nosocomial pneumonia should aspiration occur.

Microbial Virulence Factors

For a potential pathogen to cause bacteremia, it must (1) attach to host epithelial surfaces, (2) evade local defenses, (3) multiply, and (4) disseminate from the site of primary infection.

Attachment of invading microorganisms frequently involves specific interactions between receptors on the bacterial surface and carbohydrate moieties or other ligands on the host cell membrane. Fimbriae are cellular appendages that bacteria use to attach to epithelial or environmental surfaces. P fimbriae of *E. coli* allow attachment to susceptible uroepithelial cells, and it is likely that *Vibrio cholerae* attach to intestinal epithelial cells via fimbriae before delivery of toxin. Fibronectin normally coats mucosal cells in the oropharynx and covers cell surface receptors for gram-negative bacilli, thereby blocking their adherence. In ill patients, fibronectin may be digested by elastase released by inflammatory cells and gram-negative colonization may occur.

Bacterial proliferation and invasion at local sites are facilitated by the production of a variety of extracellular bacterial enzymes and toxins. Many species of gram-negative bacilli produce hemolysins, proteases, and elastases, which break down tissue barriers, degrade immunoglobulins, and damage phagocytic cell membranes. A pseudomonal toxin, exotoxin A, inhibits host cell protein synthesis by inactivating elongation factor 2, a necessary cofactor for ribosome function.

Some gram-negative bacteria possess extracellular capsules composed of long-chain acidic polysaccharides.

In the absence of specific antibody, these capsules act as virulence factors by protecting the microorganism from the opsonic effects of alternative complement pathway components. Moreover, capsular polysaccharide is often poorly immunogenic, leading to an inadequate host antibody response. For example, *E. coli* K5 capsule is structurally quite similar to an intermediate molecule in the biosynthesis of heparin and the capsule apparently is perceived as a "self" antigen by the host immune system (Table 245-1).

Cell wall components of gram-negative bacilli clearly contribute to their virulence. Endotoxin is a lipopolysaccharide (LPS) component of gram-negative bacterial outer membranes. It is composed of three segments (Fig. 245-1), an outermost series of oligosaccharides that are antigenically diverse and determine the O serotype of the bacteria; a connecting series of core oligosaccharides, which are relatively conserved among gram-negative bacteria; and an innermost lipid segment, lipid A. Lipid A is the toxic portion of the molecule and directly or indirectly appears to trigger many of the systemic effects associated with gram-negative bacteremia (see later discussion). The O-polysaccharide side chains also contribute to the microorganism's virulence. Strains that lack these polysaccharide antigens have a characteristic rough colony appearance and may be more suscep-

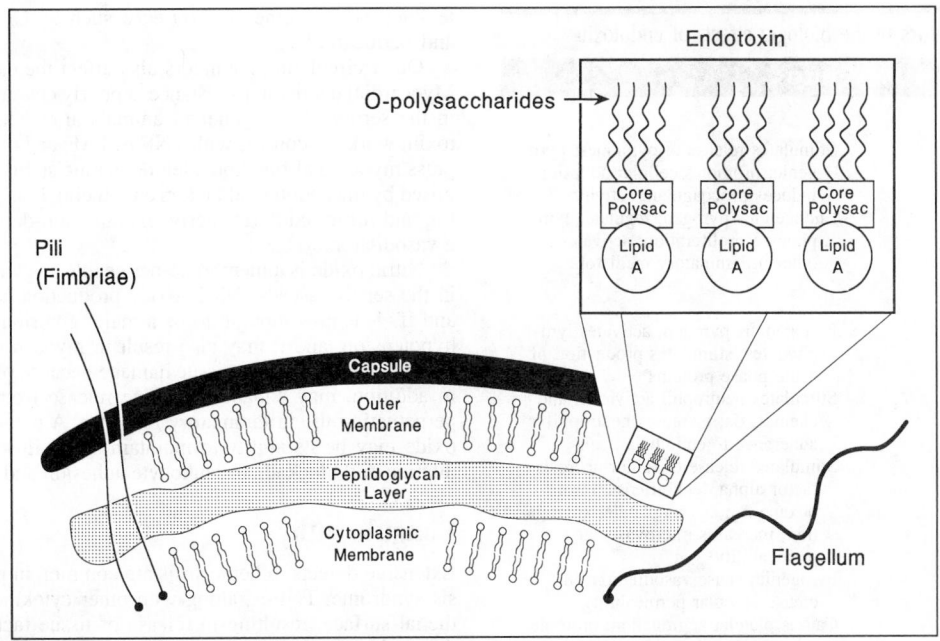

FIGURE 245-1   Cell wall structure of a typical gram-negative microorganism.

Table 245-1   Virulence factors of gram-negative bacteria

VIRULENCE FACTOR	ACTIVITY	EXAMPLE
Fimbriae	Promote adherence	P fimbriae of *Escherichia coli*
Enzymes, exotoxins	Degrade immunoglobulins, damage phagocytes	Pseudomonas exotoxin A, Shiga toxin
Capsules	Inhibit opsonization and phagocytosis	*Haemophilus influenzae,* type B
		Klebsiella species
		K1 capsule of *E. coli*
O polysaccharides	Impair antibody-mediated complement killing	Virulent gram-negative bacilli
Endotoxin: Lipid A	Triggers sepsis cascade	Most gram-negative bacilli

tible to the lytic action of complement and other products that attack the bacterial cell wall.

PATHOPHYSIOLOGY

The complex pathophysiologic events that lead from localized bacterial disease to sepsis and multiple organ dysfunction remain incompletely understood. It is clear, however, that host inflammatory response plays a major role in the development of severe sepsis. In the host, bacterial products trigger defense mechanisms mediated by the release of cytokines and other circulating substances, the activation of plasma factors such as the complement and coagulation cascades, and the recruitment of cellular components. These responses may abrogate microbial invasion and disease but may cause significant damage to host tissues as well. Pathophysiologic events surrounding gram-negative organism infection are most thoroughly studied, but similar events may also be triggered by other microorganisms.

In the case of gram-negative organism infection, LPS appears to be the most important activator of host defenses. When injected into experimental animals, purified LPS can produce many of the signs of septic shock, including fever, chills, hypotension, coagulopathy, and death. Studies have shown that LPS in the circulation binds via its lipid A moiety with high affinity to a host protein, LPS-binding protein (LBP). The LPS-LBP complex then attaches to monocytes and macrophages via a specific cell surface receptor, CD14, inducing release of tumor necrosis factor alpha (TNF-α) and interleukin-1 (IL-1) from these mononuclear cells. In addition to inducing release of cytokines and other inflammatory mediators, LPS also contributes to

the activation of the complement and coagulation cascades that occur with sepsis (Table 245-2).

Role of Tumor Necrosis Factor Alpha and Interleukin-1

Evidence implicating TNF-α in the pathogenesis of the sepsis syndrome includes increases in TNF-α levels in animals and human volunteers given endotoxin, the duplication of signs and symptoms of sepsis by TNF-α infusion, and the finding of elevated TNF-α levels in patients with the sepsis syndrome. TNF-α stimulates macrophages to release IL-1, and there appear to be at least two important results of the interaction of TNF-α and host endothelial cells: induction of procoagulant activity, which may trigger the coagulation cascade (see discussion later), and increased expression of adhesion molecules promoting white blood cell adherence. In some instances, TNF-α may not be uniquely responsible for the sepsis syndrome, since TNF-α levels may be elevated in patients with a variety of conditions unrelated to sepsis, including rheumatoid arthritis, leprosy, and acquired immunodeficiency syndrome (AIDS). Furthermore, TNF-α is not detectable in some patients with the sepsis syndrome.

IL-1 shares many biologic activities with TNF-α, including pyrogenic effects and induction of procoagulant activity and adhesions on endothelial cells. IL-1 also results in release of platelet-activating factor (PAF) and an inhibitor of tissue plasminogen activator. This latter effect results in increased platelet aggregation and coagulation. IL-1 plays a role in the host immune response by initiating activation of T lymphocytes, aiding in B-cell replication and antibody production, and activating polymorphonuclear leukocytes.

Table 245-2   Mediators of the biologic effects of endotoxin

MEDIATOR	EFFECTS
Primary mediators	
Tumor necrosis factor	Stimulates release of cytokines; pyrogenic; promotes cellular adhesion; induces procoagulant activity
Interleukin-1	Endogenous pyrogen; regulates lymphocyte proliferation; activates other inflammatory mediators
Additional mediators	
Interleukin-6	Endogenous pyrogen; activates lymphocytes; stimulates production of acute-phase proteins
Interleukin-8	Stimulates neutrophil activation and chemotaxis; increases neutrophil adherence to endothelial cells
Platelet-activating factor	Stimulates release of tumor necrosis factor alpha, leukotrienes, thromboxane A_2; causes platelet aggregation; increases microvascular permeability
Prostaglandins	Pyrogenic; cause vasodilation; increase vascular permeability
Thromboxane A_2	Causes platelet aggregation; promotes release of nitric oxide; causes vasoconstriction
Leukotrienes	Promote neutrophil chemotaxis; increase vascular permeability
Myocardial depressant substance	Causes reversible ventricular dilation; decreases myocardial contractility
Endothelin-1	Causes intense vasoconstriction
Nitric oxide	Causes vasodilation; inhibits platelet aggregation

Additional Inflammatory Mediators

Multiple other cytokines are involved in the perpetuation and regulation of the inflammatory response. In addition to TNF-α and IL-1, other proinflammatory cytokines include interleukins 6 and 8 (IL-6 and IL-8) and interferon gamma (IFN-γ), whereas interleukins 4, 10, and 13 (IL-4, IL-10, and IL-13) and transforming growth factor beta seem to downregulate the immune response. In addition, antagonists of and soluble receptors for some of the cytokines discussed earlier are found in the serum of patients with sepsis. These factors also serve to blunt immune responsiveness.

A variety of important inflammatory mediators and regulatory hormones (PAF, arachidonic acid metabolites [prostaglandins, leukotrienes], and related molecules) are derived from the phospholipid component of cell membranes. Endotoxin, directly or indirectly through the effects of TNF-α and IL-1, leads to generation of a number of these molecules.

PAF is released from cell membranes of many cell types including monocytes, macrophages, platelets, neutrophils, and endothelial cells in response to endotoxin. PAF causes platelet aggregation and thrombosis as well as a marked increase in microvascular permeability. It also has a negative ionotropic effect on the heart and causes hypotension. It leads to increased production of arachidonic acid metabolites in a similar manner to TNF-α and IL-1.

Arachidonic acid, generated from cell membrane phospholipids, may be metabolized to produce prostaglandins and thromboxane via the cyclooxygenase pathway or leukotrienes via the lipoxygenase pathway. These substances appear to mediate many of the systemic effects of TNF-α and IL-1. Specific inhibitors of cyclooxygenase blunt the effects of experimentally administered endotoxin in humans, and lipoxygenase inhibitors have similar effects in animals. Prostaglandin I_2 is a potent vasodilator that at least contributes to the hypotension seen during gram-negative sepsis. Prostaglandin E_2 contributes to the fever seen in gram-negative sepsis through its effects on the hypothalamus. Leukotriene B_4 is a powerful chemotactic and activating factor for polymorphonuclear leukocytes, and other leukotrienes such as C_4 affect vascular tone and permeability.

Other circulating mediators also affect the cardiovascular system. Myocardial depressant substance, a poorly characterized moiety found in the serum of experimental animals after administration of endotoxin, works in concert with TNF-α, PAF, and other cytokines to suppress myocardial function. Hemodynamic stability is further compromised by the endothelial factors endothelin-1, an intense vasoconstrictor, and nitric oxide (formerly, endothelium-derived relaxing factor), a vasodilator.

Nitric oxide is a membrane-permeable gas with multiple functions in the sepsis cascade. Nitric oxide production, stimulated by TNF-α and IL-1, is now thought to be a major contributor to sepsis-induced hypotension, and it may also result in myocardial depression. Nitric oxide may contribute to tissue damage because of its cytotoxicity and, in addition, may enhance cytokine release from other cells, further perpetuating the inflammatory response. A potential benefit of nitric oxide may be its ability to maintain blood flow to tissues via vasodilation and blockade of leukocyte adhesion and platelet aggregation.

Coagulopathy

Extensive defects in hemostasis are common in patients with the sepsis syndrome. TNF-α, along with other cytokines, attacks the endothelial surface, resulting in release of tissue factor and activation of the extrinsic pathway of coagulation. Endotoxin directly activates factor XII (Hageman factor), which triggers the intrinsic coagulation pathway through activation of factor XI. Evidence suggests that the activation of the extrinsic pathway plays a more significant role in LPS-mediated coagulation than intrinsic pathway activation; nonetheless, the net result is excess thrombin generation, the formation of platelet-fibrin microthrombi, and disseminated intravascular coagulation (DIC). Factor XII also stimulates the conversion of prekallikrein to kallikrein, which converts kininogen to circulating bradykinin. Kinins then play a role in the hypotension and increased vascular permeability encountered during bacteremia.

Complement Activation

Complement components are an important group of humoral mediators activated during the sepsis syndrome. Complement may be activated during bacteremia by the classic pathway (interaction of microbial antigens and specific antibodies) or the alternative pathway (nonspecific activation by bacterial cell wall components). Complement may also be activated through interaction with the coagulation or fibrinolytic pathways. C3a and C5a function as anaphylatoxins causing vasodilation, increased vascular permeability, and histamine release from mast cells. C5a is a potent chemotactant for neutrophils and has been further implicated as a stimulus for producing prostaglandins and other bioactive arachidonic acid products.

Role of Neutrophils

Many of the events discussed earlier contribute to the activation of neutrophils. Although these cells are crucial in defense against bacterial infections, it is now recognized that they also are major contributors to the tissue injury seen in sepsis. Neutrophils are activated by LPS, TNF-α, and IL-1. Other substances such as complement component C5a and IL-8 are potent chemotactic agents that induce neutrophil migration and degranulation. During sepsis, neutrophil adherence to the endothelial surface is enhanced by increased expression of various adhesion molecules. Once stimulated, neutrophils produce active oxygen species, proteases, hydrolases, cytokines, and other substances necessary to combat bacterial invasion and perpetuate the immune response. In the process these substances may cause widespread endothelial damage leading to multiple organ dysfunction and the adult respiratory distress syndrome.

The net result of the complex interactions described earlier are fever, hypotension, myocardial depression, DIC, and altered organ system function, the clinical manifestations of the sepsis syndrome. Figure 245-2 is an attempt to illustrate the proposed interaction of LPS and cellular and humoral factors.

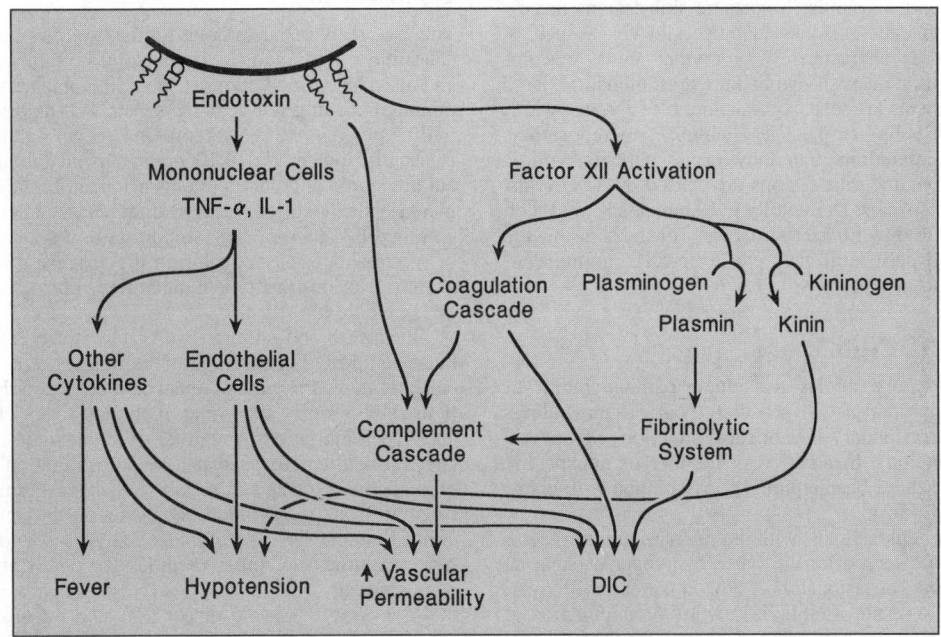

FIGURE 245-2   Diagram of the interaction of host inflammatory mediators during gram-negative sepsis. *TNF-α,* Tumor necrosis factor alpha; *IL-1,* interleukin 1; *DIC,* disseminated intravascular coagulation.

CLINICAL MANIFESTATIONS

Fever, often accompanied by shaking chills, is the most common clinical manifestation of bacteremia (Table 245-3). In a series of 612 patients with gram-negative bacteremia reported by Kreger and others fever (temperature 37.6° C [>99.6° F]) was seen in 82% of patients. Thirty patients did not mount a febrile response within the first 24 hours after the onset of bacteremia. These patients had a higher incidence of shock and death than did those with fever. Hypothermia (temperature <36.4° C [<97.6° F]) was seen in 83 bacteremic patients (13%). These patients had outcomes similar to those patients who presented with fever. Although the majority of bacteremic patients have fever, a significant percentage of patients who present with hypothermia are also found to be bacteremic. Of 85 consecutive patients with hypothermia admitted to San Francisco General Hospital, 33 were bacteremic, 19 with gram-negative microorganisms. In patients with unexplained hypothermia, blood cultures should be obtained and consideration given to beginning empiric antibiotics. Age, renal insufficiency, corticosteroid or antipyretic administration, and malignancy all increase the likelihood that a bacteremic patient will not mount a febrile response.

Respiratory manifestations frequently accompany gram-negative bacteremia, and acute onset of tachypnea with respiratory alkalosis is among the earliest and most consistent finding. The adult respiratory distress syndrome (ARDS) occurs in as many as 20% of patients with gram-negative sepsis, and the mortality rate approaches 90% in this subgroup.

Mental status changes may occur in patients with gram-negative bacteremia. Changes may range from mild anxiety or restlessness to profound confusional states. Change in mentation is a particularly important diagnostic clue in elderly patients who may exhibit few other early signs of disease.

Shock develops in up to 40% of patients with gram-negative bacteremia, and its presence is a predictor of increased mortality risk. The characteristic hemodynamic findings early in septic shock are an increased cardiac index and decreased systemic vascular resistance. Studies have also shown a decreased left ventricular ejection fraction and acute left ventricular dilation, perhaps due to circulating myocardial depressant factor. These abnormalities usually revert to normal by 7 to 10 days. Of course, prolonged hypotension may lead to de-

Table 245-3   Clinical and laboratory manifestations of gram-negative bacteremia

FINDING	COMMENT
Physical examination	
Fever	Hypothermia also occurs
Tachypnea	Occurs early via direct stimulation of central respiratory center by endotoxin
Altered mental status	Multifactorial, important early sign
Hypotension	Related to decreased systemic vascular resistance, decreased myocardial contractility
Cyanosis	Low cardiac output syndrome
Petechiae, purpura	Manifestation of disseminated intravascular coagulation
Muscle tenderness	Associated with bacteremic localization in muscle
Laboratory studies	
Leukopenia	May occur transiently early or later with overwhelming infection
Leukocytosis	Common
Thrombocytopenia	Present to some degree in 50% of patients
Hyperglycemia, hypoglycemia	Impaired glucose regulation
Abnormal renal or liver function	Secondary to poor perfusion
Respiratory alkalosis	Direct stimulation of central respiratory center
Hypoxemia	Multifactorial; right-to-left shunt, noncardiogenic pulmonary edema
Metabolic acidosis	Due to lactate accumulation

velopment of end-organ failure, including acute myocardial infarction, acute renal tubular damage, and respiratory failure.

A number of dermatologic manifestations have been described in patients with gram-negative bacteremia. Skin may be the primary site of disease leading to bacteremia (especially in the presence of percutaneous intravascular devices), or skin manifestations may develop secondary to hematogenous seeding. Metastatic skin lesions are especially prominent with infections caused by certain *Vibrio* species. Ecthyma gangrenosum is characterized by erythematous, maculopapular lesions with central necrosis. On histologic examination, large numbers of microorganisms are seen, some within blood vessel walls, and few inflammatory cells are present. Ecthyma gangrenosum is most commonly encountered in granulocytopenic patients with *P. aeruginosa* bacteremia, but similar lesions are caused by *Aeromonas* or other gram-negative species. Dermatologic lesions associated with sepsis that are not due to direct bacterial invasion of the skin include petechiae, purpura, and peripheral gangrene from DIC, immune injury, or vasoconstriction, respectively.

LABORATORY FINDINGS

Results of routine laboratory studies are seldom pathognomonic of bloodstream invasion by gram-negative bacteria, but certain findings may suggest primary or secondary sites of focal infection (e.g., pyuria with urinary tract infection). In addition, a number of nonspecific laboratory abnormalities have been reported in association with gram-negative sepsis (Table 245-3).

Polymorphonuclear leukocytosis with an increase in immature forms typically develops soon after the onset of pyogenic bacterial infection. Leukopenia may occasionally develop in patients with overwhelming infections as a result of rapid destruction or aggregation of granulocytes or possibly suppression of bone marrow function by bacterial toxins or host inflammatory mediators. Leukopenia is more commonly seen in infants, the elderly, alcoholics, and others with decreased bone marrow reserve. Morphologic changes in polymorphonuclear cells may occur with sepsis, including the nonspecific findings of toxic granulations and Döhle's bodies and the more specific finding of vacuolization.

Abnormalities of coagulation are common during bacteremia. In one series, 126 of 222 bacteremic patients had laboratory evidence of thrombocytopenia. DIC with increased fibrin split products and depressed levels of clotting factors was noted in 25 (11%) patients in the same report. Clinically, however, significant bleeding was uncommon (3%). If very sensitive tests for detection of thrombin and plasmin activation are used, evidence of DIC can be found in almost all patients with bacteremia and less than 50,000 platelets/μL.

A number of metabolic derangements have been described during gram-negative bacteremia. Insulin resistance may be an early clinical sign of bacteremia in diabetic patients, but hypoglycemia has also been reported. Serum amino acid levels rise as a result of muscle proteolysis, and serum triglycerides are characteristically elevated due to increased fat breakdown and alterations in use. Increases in blood urea nitrogen and creatinine coincide with renal hypoperfusion and acute tubular damage. Immunologically mediated renal injury with abnormalities of urinary sediment may also occur. A recent series reported depressed serum levels of ionized calcium in 12 of 40 patients with gram-negative bacteremia versus none of 20 patients with gram-positive bacteremia.

Elevation of serum bilirubin levels disproportionate to other liver function tests has been described during bacteremia, even among patients with nonabdominal primary sites. Hemolysis and increased tissue breakdown as well as toxic or metabolically mediated hepatocellular dysfunction may be responsible. Serum transaminase levels may also be elevated from long-standing hypotension and ischemic hepatic injury.

Varying degrees of hypoxemia may develop during sepsis as a result of pneumonia, ARDS, or other causes of intrapulmonary arteriovenous shunting. At the same time, the arterial/venous oxygen difference is often decreased. This apparent inefficiency in blood oxygen extraction by the tissues may be caused by derangement of microvascular blood flow regulation and/or a poorly characterized primary defect in cellular oxidative metabolism. Unless cardiac output is maintained or increased, tissue oxygen delivery may become impaired at a time when fever and stress of infection greatly raise cellular energy requirements. Lactic acidosis is often a manifestation of bacteremic shock, reflecting both an increase in anaerobic glycolysis and impairment of hepatic lactate clearance.

DIAGNOSIS

The diagnosis of bacteremia ultimately rests on the isolation of the causative microorganism from blood cultures. At least two aerobic and anaerobic blood cultures should be obtained before antibiotic administration. In gram-negative sepsis, the majority of such specimens will be positive, but bacteremia may occasionally be intermittent and is usually low grade (<10 organisms/ml blood). Hypertonic blood culture media or culture systems using antibiotic removal devices may increase the yield of positive cultures in patients already receiving antimicrobial therapy. It is important to note that the entire spectrum of septic shock may develop in the absence of demonstrable bloodstream invasion if sufficient quantities of bacterial cell wall fragments or toxins are absorbed.

Because blood culture results may not be available for 24 to 48 hours, empiric diagnosis and therapy must often be based on a clinical judgment. Physicians must be alert for early clinical manifestations of the sepsis syndrome, including fever, changes in mentation, and hyperventilation. A number of large studies of patients with suspected gram-negative sepsis have shown that only about 30% to 40% of patients suspected clinically will have gram-negative organisms isolated from their blood. Because of the imprecise nature of a clinical diagnosis of gram-negative sepsis and delay in obtaining blood culture data, other methods for confirming a diagnosis have been studied.

Assays now exist to detect LPS and many of the cytokines that contribute to the development of gram-negative sepsis. The chromogenic limulus amebocyte lysate assay is the best test currently available for LPS detection. Using this test, LPS can be detected in 60% to 80% of patients with gram-negative bacteremia. Sensitivity declines if patients with sepsis have gram-negative infection without bacteremia. Some studies have found a correlation between LPS levels and subsequent mortality, whereas others have not. TNF-α is detectable more frequently than IL-1, and high levels of TNF-α generally correlate with increased mortality. IL-6, IL-8, IL-10, endogenous LPS antibodies, and cytokine antagonists are also demonstrable in the circulation of a varying percentage of patients with sepsis. For the present, measurement of LPS and other sepsis mediators remains a research tool and is not useful for diagnosis or prognosis.

The evaluation of any patient with suspected bacteremia should include a diligent search for evidence of a primary focus of infection. Examination should include the skin surface, including the perirectal area. In addition to blood cultures, a chemistry profile, urinalysis, and complete blood cell count with differential should also be obtained. Arterial blood gas determination may reveal respiratory alkalosis, evidence of hypoxia, or metabolic acidosis. Radiographic evaluation should include chest x-ray film and possibly abdominal films. For patients with a suspected abdominal (including renal) source, sonography, or computed tomography may also be indicated.

Hemodynamic monitoring with a pulmonary artery catheter may be diagnostically and therapeutically useful in selected patients presenting with hypotension. The characteristic finding of sepsis, namely, increased cardiac output with very low systemic vascular resistance, is seen in only a small number of other conditions (e.g., hypotension caused by drugs such as nitroprusside, narcotics, and psychotropic drugs). The finding may also occur in patients with anaphylaxis, addisonian crisis (see later discussion), or shock resulting from neurogenic injury.

Differential Diagnosis

Infections with gram-positive bacteria, viruses, fungi, protozoa, and metazoa can mimic gram-negative sepsis. Toxic shock syndrome resulting from either staphylococcal vaginal colonization, staphylococcal cellulitis, or staphylococcal pneumonia (Thucidides syndrome) or from group A streptococcal disease may produce the signs and symptoms of sepsis (Chapters 260 and 261). A characteristic "sunburn" rash, mucosal erythema, and multiorgan failure should suggest this diagnosis. Pneumococcal bacteremia in the asplenic host, overwhelming staphylococcal disease without rash, and meningococcal bacteremia syndrome without meningitis may closely resemble gram-negative bacteremia and shock. Rickettsial disease, particularly Rocky

Mountain spotted fever and epidemic typhus, may mimic gram-negative bacteremia early in its course. History of tick bite, headache, and rash developing several days after fever support the diagnosis of Rocky Mountain spotted fever. Other infectious diagnoses to be considered include disseminated fungal infection (e.g., *Candida* or related species in leukopenic patients or *Histoplasma capsulatum* in HIV-infected patients), disseminated tuberculosis, falciparum malaria, and disseminated viral infection (e.g., cytomegalovirus in transplant recipients).

Several important noninfectious conditions must be differentiated from gram-negative bacteremia. Myocardial infarction may become evident with hypotension and occasionally fever. In this setting cardiac output is initially low, with elevated systemic vascular resistance.

Pulmonary embolus may be especially difficult to differentiate from bacteremia; fever, hypoxia, tachypnea, and hypotension may all be present. Usually, fever is low grade, and pulmonary and systemic vascular resistance are both increased. Leukocytosis with left shift is usually absent.

Patients with acute pancreatitis come to medical attention with fever, tachypnea, tachycardia, and altered blood pressure. In hemorrhagic pancreatitis the patient may be in shock. A history of abdominal pain, abdominal tenderness on physical examination, and elevated levels of amylase and lipase should confirm the diagnosis.

Several endocrine disorders, including adrenal insufficiency and thyroid storm, may mimic the findings of bacteremia. Acute adrenal insufficiency, in particular, may become evident with hypotension, mental status changes, and fever.

Some collagen vascular diseases may be confused with the sepsis syndrome. Vasculitis may become evident with fever, skin lesions, and end-organ damage. Hypotension and decreased vascular resistance, however, are not typical features of systemic vasculitis.

Two unusual reactions to medications can simulate many of the features of the sepsis syndrome. An uncommon syndrome of severe lactic acidosis associated with the use of nucleoside analog (azidothymidine [AZT], dideoxyinosine [ddI], and dideoxycytidine [ddC]) therapy in HIV-infected patients has been reported. Patients may come to medical attention in shock with rapidly progressive liver failure. Mortality rates are over 50% even with discontinuation of the offending medication. The absence of a source of infection and laboratory test results reflecting worsening liver function can help differentiate this syndrome.

Chronic salicylate intoxication can result in a "pseudosepsis" syndrome characterized by fever, leukocytosis, hypotension, increased cardiac output, decreased systemic vascular resistance, and multiple system organ failure. This syndrome should be considered in older adults who are taking aspirin regularly for chronic pain or inflammatory conditions and in whom a source of infection cannot be identified.

THERAPY

The treatment of gram-negative bacteremia has traditionally involved three basic principles: (1) identification and management of the primary focus of infection, (2) ongoing assessment of physiologic parameters with intervention to support vital organ perfusion, and (3) specific antimicrobial therapy (Box 245-1). Recently, attention has focused on a fourth method, modulation of the host inflammatory response through use of genetically engineered molecules. Figure 245-3 details points in the progression of gram-negative infection at which various therapies may be successful.

General Measures

The physician should always attempt to identify primary sites of infection, as the resolution of bacteremia may depend on successful management of such a focus. Rapid identification of the microorganism responsible for bacteremia may also be possible based on Gram's stain of clinical specimens (sputum, urine, cerebrospinal fluid, synovial fluid, etc.). Specific therapeutic goals should include drainage of abscesses, relief of obstruction (e.g., an obstructed ureter in pyelonephritis), excision of dead tissue (e.g., infarcted bowel), and removal of infected prosthetic devices.

All patients with suspected gram-negative bacteremia should be

---

BOX 245-1
Management of gram-negative bacteremia

Seek to identify a primary site of gram-negative disease
  Gram's stain and culture of inflammatory material, sputum, urine, etc.
Monitor physiologic parameters
  Vital signs, mental status, urine output, arterial blood gas values, electrolyte and creatinine levels, coagulation studies
Maintain tissue perfusion if hypotensive
  Expand intravascular volume
  Sympathomimetic amines if volume expansion fails
  Dopamine: Begin at 2 to 5 μg/kg per minute
  Dobutamine: Begin at 2 μg/kg per minute
  Isoproterenol: Begin at 2 μg per minute
  Norepinephrine: 0.05 μg/kg per minute if other agents are ineffective; causes intense vasoconstriction
  Consider physiologic monitoring with Swan-Ganz catheter
Administer antibiotics
  See text and Table 245-4
Consider modulation of host inflammatory response
  See text and Table 245-5
Support if organ system failure develops
  Mechanical ventilation, hemodialysis, etc.

---

hospitalized. Although some patients with gram-negative bacteremia have relatively mild symptoms, many require aggressive supportive care in an intensive care unit. Vital signs, including temperature, pulse, blood pressure, and respiratory rate, should be monitored continuously or determined at frequent intervals. Intravenous and oral fluid intake and urinary, stool, and gastric outputs should also be recorded. Invasive monitoring of pulmonary artery pressure may be required for optimal management of patients with severe hypotension or ARDS.

For the patient with septic shock, aggressive repletion of circulatory volume may be lifesaving. Vascular pooling and increased vascular permeability during sepsis lead to decreased effective blood volume. An isotonic fluid challenge should be administered promptly. Normal saline is appropriate, although some authorities believe that colloid solutions such as albumin or hetastarch are more effective volume expanders. Packed red blood cells provide effective volume replacement for patients with significant anemia.

Because of pulmonary artery constriction during sepsis, simple central venous pressure determinations cannot be relied on to accurately reflect volume status. Monitoring pulmonary capillary wedge pressure (PCWP) with a Swan-Ganz catheter may be useful in guiding the volume expansion of severely hypotensive patients, patients with underlying cardiac dysfunction, and ventilatory-dependent patients requiring positive end-expiratory pressure. Cardiac output is usually optimal at a PCWP of approximately 12 cm H_2O. Critics of "routine" use of a pulmonary artery catheter point out that adequate controlled trials have not been performed to demonstrate that patient survival is improved by the use of these devices. Furthermore, complications of pulmonary artery catheterization include bleeding, pneumothorax, catheter-related infection, and arrhythmias. Clearly, the pulmonary artery catheter is a potentially valuable tool but should be used judiciously and only by a physician adequately trained in its proper use. Retrospective studies have shown that patients managed in intensive care units by trained critical care physicians have improved survival rates over those who are not managed in this way.

Vasopressors may be beneficial for patients who remain hypotensive despite fluid replacement. Dopamine at a starting dose of 2 to 5 μg/kg per minute is the agent preferred by most authorities; the final dose must be titrated for each patient. Other agents such as dobutamine or isoproterenol may also be used instead of or in addition to dopamine. As with dopamine, these must be titrated to desired effect. Occasional patients may require the use of more potent agents, such as norepinephrine, but excessive vasoconstriction may further impair tissue perfusion and lead to gangrene.

Renal function may be severely impaired during sepsis due to poor

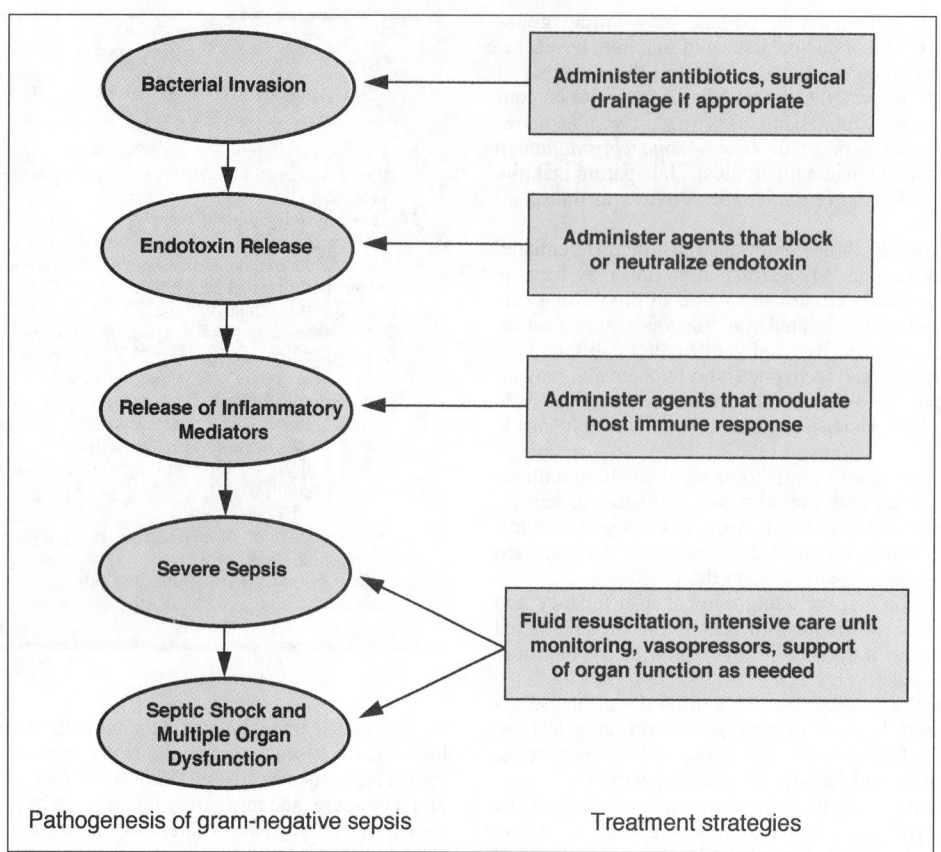

Pathogenesis of gram-negative sepsis   Treatment strategies

FIGURE 245-3   Potential therapeutic strategies for the treatment of gram-negative sepsis.

renal perfusion pressure. Dopamine augments renal blood flow when used in a dose up to about 10 μg/kg per minute, but higher doses lead to renal vasoconstriction. Patients who remain oliguric after fluid challenge and correction of hypotension should be monitored closely for signs of acute renal failure. Hemodialysis may be required to correct fluid and electrolyte imbalances in some patients.

Many patients with pneumonia or ARDS require intubation and mechanical ventilatory support. Maintenance of adequate blood oxygenation is critical, as tissue oxygen delivery in sepsis is highly dependent on oxygen delivery. Positive end-expiratory pressure may be necessary for patients with severe ARDS, but must be used with caution in patients with depressed cardiac outputs.

Lactic acidosis often complicates tissue hypoperfusion during sepsis. Although the administration of bicarbonate solutions should be considered for patients with arterial pH of less than 7.0, management is primarily directed toward restoring tissue oxygen delivery. Bicarbonate infusion may correct acidemia, but a controlled trial has shown that it does not improve hemodynamics.

Antimicrobial Therapy

In patients with suspected gram-negative bacteremia, antimicrobial therapy is almost always initiated before the precise bacterial pathogen and its antimicrobial susceptibilities are known. Furthermore, it may be difficult at times to determine whether an infectious disorder is caused by a gram-negative bacteria, a gram-positive one, or even a yeast or mold. For example, in certain clinical settings (patients with advanced HIV disease, organ transplant recipients, and profoundly granulocytopenic patients) it may be appropriate to include initial coverage for a variety of microbial pathogens.

In the case of suspected gram-negative bacterial disease, combination antimicrobial therapy is used to provide coverage against a broad spectrum of pathogens, to help prevent the emergence of resistant strains during therapy, and to provide possible synergistic bactericidal activity against specific microorganisms. An example of this

synergism is that produced by the combination of an aminoglycoside and an antipseudomonal penicillin for treatment of *P. aeruginosa* infection.

Table 245-4 indicates examples of initial antimicrobial therapy in patients with suspected gram-negative bacteremia in a variety of clinical settings. In most situations, an aminoglycoside is recommended in combination with a β-lactam agent with activity against gram-negative bacilli (penicillin, cephalosporin, carbapenem, or monobactam) (Chapter 231). Among patients at high risk for nephrotoxicity or ototoxicity, a broad-spectrum β-lactam, such as a third-generation cephalosporin or imipenem, may be used alone initially. For the penicillin-allergic patient, aztreonam, which appears to have a low incidence of cross-reactivity with other β-lactam drugs, or a parenteral quinolone may be used with or without an aminoglycoside.

An educated guess as to the origin or cause of suspected gram-negative bacterial disease may be possible on the basis of clinical setting, ancillary culture data such as a urinary tract pathogen, skin or other surveillance cultures, or examination of inflammatory material. After isolation and identification of the etiologic microorganism and determination of its sensitivities, the physician should reevaluate antimicrobial therapy to select the safest and most effective therapeutic regimen.

Bacteremia may persist or recur in up to 10% of patients despite appropriate therapy and may be a clue to the presence of an occult abscess or intravascular site of infection. In addition, persistent bacteremia may indicate inadequate serum antimicrobial concentrations and prompt the assessment of serum bactericidal activity.

Therapies Directed Toward Modulation of Host Immune Response

Despite the availability of broad-spectrum antimicrobial agents, the mortality associated with gram-negative bacteremia has remained at about 30% for the past three decades. Further advances in the treatment of gram-negative bacteremia may depend on interrupting the

Table 245-4   Suggested initial drug therapy based on clinical setting

CLINICAL SETTING	ANTIBIOTICS	COMMENT
Urinary tract	Ampicillin* plus aminoglycoside†	Combination also covers enterococci
Respiratory tract:		
Community-acquired	Erythromycin* and third-generation cephalosporin‡ OR First- or second-generation cephalosporin§ plus aminoglycoside	Gram-negative bacteria cause 10% to 20% of community-acquired pneumonias requiring hospitalization; *Haemophilus influenzae, Klebsiella pneumoniae,* and others implicated; consider *Legionella* species if patient is elderly or immunosuppressed
Hospital-acquired	Antipseudomonal β-lactam‖ plus aminoglycoside	Must treat for more resistant organisms including *Pseudomonas aeruginosa*
Intraabdominal and biliary tract	β-Lactam inhibitor¶ plus aminoglycoside OR Imipenem plus aminoglycoside	Use regimen active against enteric gram-negative bacteria and anaerobes
Unknown source	Imipenem or β-lactam inhibitor plus aminoglycoside	Add vancomycin if gram-positive infection is a consideration
Burns	Antipseudomonal β-lactam plus aminoglycoside	Choose agent with greatest antipseudomonal activity at particular hospital
Catheter infection	Vancomycin* plus ceftazidime OR Vancomycin plus aminoglycoside	Include vancomycin for methicillin-resistant staphylococci
Granulocytopenia	Antipseudomonal β-lactam plus aminoglycoside	Add vancomycin for *Staphylococcus* species if intravascular catheter is present
Human immunodeficiency virus infection	Antipseudomonal β-lactam plus aminoglycoside	Rule out *Pneumocystis* pneumonia, disseminated histoplasmosis, disseminated *Mycobacterium avium,* or provide coverage; stop nucleoside analogs if lactic acidosis is present

*Others: Ampicillin 1-2 g every 4-6 hr; erythromycin 0.5-1 g every 6 hr; ticarcillin-clavulanate 3.1 g every 4-8 hr; vancomycin 1 g every 12 hr.
†Gentamicin, tobramycin 3-5 mg/kg/day divided every 8 hr; amikacin 15 mg/kg/day divided every 8 hr. Must adjust for renal dysfunction.
‡Cefotaxime 1-2 g every 6-8 hr; ceftriaxone 1-2 g every 24 hr; ceftazidime 1-2 g every 8 hr.
§Cefazolin 1 g every 8 hr; cephalothin 1-2 g every 4-6 hr; cefuroxime 1 g every 8 hr.
‖Pipracillin, mezlocillin, ticarcillin 3 g every 4 hr; ceftazidime 1-2 g every 8 hr; imipenem 500 mg every 6 hr.
¶Ticarcillin clavulanate 3.1 g every 4-6 hr; piperacillin/tazobactam 3 g every 4-6 hr.

underlying pathophysiologic mechanisms responsible for tissue damage. The initial enthusiasm for this approach has waned as multiple attempts to affect outcomes with immune-modulating agents have failed. Although many agents have shown promise in animal models, duplicating these results in humans has proved difficult. What has become clear is that the pathophysiology of the sepsis syndrome is extraordinarily complex and that intervention with a single agent at a single point in the process is unlikely to be effective. In addition, many of the patients who are susceptible to serious gram-negative organism infections have many other medical problems that may affect their immune responsiveness and contribute to mortality. It may be that a certain combination of adjunctive therapies is appropriate in a neutropenic patient with *P. aeruginosa* bacteremia and that a different combination is effective for an elderly patient with a perforated diverticulum. Important studies with immune-modulating agents are discussed in this section. These and additional agents that have been tested or are in development are described in Table 245-5.

Corticosteroids have been studied extensively in gram-negative sepsis because of their ability to attenuate the inflammatory response. In animal studies pretreatment with corticosteroids prevented lethal effects of injected endotoxin. Among more than 600 bacteremic patients evaluated in several large human trials, however, mortality rates for patients receiving corticosteroids and those receiving placebo were similar.

Opiate receptor blockers such as naloxone have also received considerable attention. As with corticosteroids, animal models suggest improved survival when naloxone is administered early in the course of septic shock. However, at least one small prospective human trial failed to show any significant difference in outcome among patients receiving naloxone versus those receiving placebo.

Neutralization of endotoxin is an attractive theoretic approach to the treatment of gram-negative sepsis. Initial studies in humans using antibodies to endotoxin involved the administration of human polyclonal antisera raised against the core polysaccharide and lipid regions of endotoxin. This antiserum was produced in human volunteers who were immunized with mutant rough bacterial strains (such as *E. coli* J5) that lack the antigenically diverse external O polysaccharides. In

a human study of more than 200 bacteremic patients, mortality was significantly reduced among patients receiving adjunctive treatment with antisera directed against *E. coli* J5 as compared with controls. Problems with production of antisera and the potential for transmission of infection prevented the widespread use of this product. Hybridoma technology has made possible the production of specific monoclonal antibodies directed against lipid A, which have overcome the feasibility problems of human antisera.

Two monoclonal antibodies, HA-1A and E5, have undergone extensive clinical testing. Initial studies suggested that certain subgroups of patients with sepsis, identified retrospectively, benefited from monoclonal antibody therapy. When these subgroups were studied prospectively in additional trials, benefit was not confirmed and mortality was no different than with no treatment.

Other approaches to blocking the effects of LPS include administration of nontoxic lipid A precursors, which have enhanced survival of animals with gram-negative bacteremia, and infusion of proteins such as bactericidal or permeability-increasing protein, which bind to and neutralize the effects of LPS.

Multiple compounds that block cytokines involved in the pathogenesis of gram-negative sepsis have been developed. Large, randomized trials of a monoclonal antibody to TNF-α and of a receptor antagonist of IL-1 have not shown survival benefits over placebo. Other therapeutic strategies involve blocking secondary mediators of the sepsis syndrome, inhibiting activation of the complement and coagulation cascades, and blunting the responsiveness of neutrophils. Although theoretically these approaches may be attractive, no data from human trials as yet have confirmed any significant benefit. An additional concern is the cost of many of these new technologies. In addition to showing clinical benefit, trials are also being designed to explore the cost-benefit ratio of widespread use of these agents.

PREVENTION

Because gram-negative bacteremia is a potentially lethal disorder, even with appropriate therapy, prevention is crucial. Simple procedures, such as strict adherence to approved hand-washing techniques

Table 245-5   Agents that may modify host response to gram-negative infection

TARGET	AGENT(S)	TRIAL RESULTS	COMMENT
Endotoxin (lipopolysaccharide [LPS])	Monoclonal antibodies (MAbs) to LPS	Large trials of HA-1A, E5 showed no benefit	Retrospective analysis showing benefit in subgroups not confirmed when prospectively studied
	LPS-neutralizing proteins	Benefit in animal models; human trials planned	Bactericidal or permeability-increasing protein most promising of these
	Lipid A analogues	Animal studies show protection against LPS challenge; increased survival if given with antibiotics	Difficult to use in humans because of large infusion of lipid required; more potent agents being developed
Tumor necrosis factor alpha (TNF-α)	MAbs to TNF-α	No benefit in randomized, placebo-controlled trial with 994 patients	Trend toward decreased mortality in patients in shock
	Soluble TNF-α receptors	Benefit in animal models	Possible increase in mortality of treated patients in one study
	Phosphodiesterase inhibitors	Benefit in animal models; decreased fever, TNF-α after LPS infusion in volunteers	Decreases TNF-α mRNA production; pentoxifylline is best-studied agent
Interleukin-1 (IL-1)	IL-1 receptor antagonist	No benefit in randomized, placebo-controlled trial with 893 patients	Retrospective analysis showing benefit in subgroups not confirmed when prospectively studied
IL-6	MAbs to IL-6	Conflicting data in animal studies	
IL-8	MAbs to IL-8	Benefit in animal models	
Platelet activating factor (PAF)	PAF receptor antagonists	In 262 septic patients, benefit only in those with proven gram-negative infections	Additional human studies ongoing
Arachidonic acid metabolites	Inhibitors of cyclooxygenase, lipoxygenase	Protective in animal models of septic shock, minimal human data	Agents include ibuprofen, ketoconazole
Nitric oxide	Nitric oxide synthase inhibitors	Variable results in animal trials; increased blood pressure but decreased cardiac output in septic patients	N-monomethyl-L-arginine (L-NMMA) is best-studied agent
Coagulation cascade	Antithrombin III (AT III)	Decreased mortality in animal studies not confirmed in human studies	AT III inactivates thrombin, other clotting factors; reduction of severity of disseminated intravascular coagulation seen in most human studies
	Protein C	Benefit in animals; preliminary human study promising	Inhibits factors Va and VIIa
Complement activation	C1-esterase inhibitor	Decreased complement activation, clinical improvement in small number of patients	
	MAbs to C5a	Protective in primate model, no human data	Also inhibits neutrophil chemotaxis
Neutrophils	MAbs to IL-8, C5a	Discussed above	
	MAbs to adhesion molecules	Protection from tissue damage in animals	Concern for use in active infection

✔ *WHEN TO REFER*

In general, most general internists and family practitioners are capable of the management of gram-negative bacteremia. It is likely that patients with severe sepsis and septic shock will require care in an intensive care unit (ICU), so patients should be hospitalized in a facility that has available ICU beds. If transportation to another facility is necessary, blood and other appropriate cultures should be obtained and antibiotics begun before transport. When ICU care is required, the collaboration of a critical care specialist may be desired, particularly if invasive monitoring devices are necessary. For gram-negative infections relating to a specific clinical condition (e.g., cancer chemotherapy–induced neutropenia or urinary tract obstruction) consultation with an expert in that particular field may be required.

and meticulous care of intravascular catheters, are important in decreasing the incidence of nosocomial infection. Moreover, both intravascular and urinary tract (Foley) catheters should be used only when needed and removed as soon as possible. Surgical correction of anatomic defects may be useful in preventing bacteremia in selected patients with recurrent urinary tract infections.

Colonizing oropharyngeal and gastrointestinal tract bacteria are often implicated in gram-negative infections; hence, strategies to reduce colonization have been attempted. Aerosolized polymyxin B sulfate and endotracheal gentamicin have been shown to decrease colonization; however, resistant organisms may emerge. Other studies have assessed selective decontamination of the digestive tract with topical nonabsorbable antibiotics. Results of these studies are conflicting, but a recent study of 445 intubated patients in Europe demonstrated no difference in the incidence of pneumonia or in mortality rates. Prophylactic oral antibiotics are occasionally used to prevent gram-negative infections. Trimethoprim-sulfamethoxazole has been shown to prevent urinary tract infections in renal transplant patients and in patients with recurrent urinary tract infections. This agent and, more recently, quinolones have been used to prevent infections in neutropenic cancer patients. Also in neutropenic patients, colony-stimulating factors that increase neutrophil counts have been shown to reduce fevers and decrease antibiotic use.

BIBLIOGRAPHY

Abraham E et al: Efficacy and safety of monoclonal antibody to human tumor necrosis factor α in patients with sepsis syndrome: a randomized, controlled, double-blind, multicenter clinical trial, *JAMA* 272:934, 1995.

Banerjee SN et al: Secular trends in nosocomial primary bloodstream infections in the United States, 1980-1989, *Am J Med* 91:S86, 1991.

Bone RC: The pathogenesis of sepsis, *Ann Intern Med* 115:457, 1991.

Bone RC et al: A controlled clinical trial of high-dose methylprednisolone in the treatment of severe sepsis and septic shock, *N Engl J Med* 317:653, 1987.

Bone RC et al: ACCP/SCCM Consensus Conference: definitions for sepsis and organ failure and guidelines for the use of innovative therapies in sepsis, *Chest* 101:1644, 1992.

Centers for Disease Control and Prevention: Increase in national hospital discharge survey rates for septicemia—United States, 1979-1987, *MMWR* 39:31, 1990.

Eykyn SJ, Gransden WR, Phillips I: The causative organisms of septicaemia and their epidemiology, *J Antimicrob Chemother* 25:S41, 1990.

Fisher CJ et al: Recombinant human interleukin-1 receptor antagonist in the treatment of patients with sepsis syndrome: results from a randomized, double-blind, placebo-controlled trial, *JAMA* 271:1836, 1994.

Glauser MP et al: Septic shock: pathogenesis, *Lancet* 338:732, 1991.

Goldie AS et al: Natural cytokine antagonists and endogenous antiendotoxin core antibodies in sepsis syndrome, *JAMA* 274:172, 1995.

Harris RL et al: Manifestations of sepsis, *Arch Intern Med* 147:1895, 1987.

Kreger BE, Craven DE, McCabe WR: Gram-negative bacteremia. IV. Re-evaluation of clinical features and treatment in 612 patients, *Am J Med* 68:344, 1980.

Lynn WA, Cohen J: Adjunctive therapy for septic shock: a review of experimental approaches, *Clin Infect Dis* 20:143, 1995.

McCabe WR, Jackson GG: Gram-negative bacteremia, *Arch Intern Med* 110:83, 1962.

McCloskey RV et al: Treatment of septic shock with human monoclonal antibody HA-1A: a randomized, double-blind, placebo-controlled trial, *Ann Intern Med* 121:1, 1994.

McGowan JE: Changing etiology of nosocomial bacteremia and fungemia and other hospital-acquired infections, *Rev Infect Dis* 7:S357, 1985.

Michie HR et al: Detection of circulating tumor necrosis factor after endotoxin administration, *N Engl J Med* 318:1481, 1988.

Moncada S, Higgs A: The L-arginine-nitric oxide pathway, *N Engl J Med* 329:2002, 1993.

Morris DL et al: Hemodynamic characteristics of patients with hypothermia due to occult infection and other causes, *Ann Intern Med* 102:153, 1985.

Morrison DC, Ryan JL: Endotoxins and disease mechanisms, *Ann Rev Med* 38:417, 1987.

National Institutes of Health Conference: Selected treatment strategies for septic shock based on proposed mechanisms of pathogenesis, *Ann Intern Med* 120:771, 1994.

Parrillo JE: Pathogenetic mechanisms of septic shock, *N Engl J Med* 328:1471, 1993.

Rackow EC, Astiz ME: Pathophysiology and treatment of septic shock, *JAMA* 266:548, 1991.

Scheckler WE, Scheibel W, Kresge D: Temporal trends in septicemia in a community hospital, *Am J Med* 91:S90, 1991.

Schumann RR et al: Structure and function of lipopolysaccharide binding protein, *Science* 249:1429, 1990.

Veterans Administration Systemic Sepsis Cooperative Study Group: Effect of high-dose glucocorticoid therapy on mortality in patients with clinical signs of systemic sepsis, *N Engl J Med* 317:659, 1987.

Zeigler EJ et al: Treatment of gram-negative bacteremia and shock with human antiserum to a mutant *Escherichia coli*, *N Engl J Med* 307:1225, 1982.

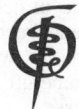

CHAPTER

246 Urinary Tract Infections

**Donald Kaye, Allan R. Tunkel, and
George R. Fournier, Jr.**

Infection of the urinary tract indicates the presence of microorganisms (almost always bacteria) within the urinary system. The definitive diagnosis depends on the isolation of these organisms from the urine. Under normal circumstances urine within the bladder is sterile. On voiding, however, it becomes contaminated by the bacterial flora that normally colonize the mucosal surface of the anterior urethra. Other sources of contamination are the vagina and surrounding skin. Therefore in culturing voided urine, it is necessary to make a decision about what numbers of bacteria in the urine indicate probable infection of the urinary tract and which are likely to be due to contamination from the urethra. Although specimens collected by urethral catheterization or suprapubic aspiration more accurately reflect the microbiologic status of the urine, such procedures are invasive and uncomfortable; thus it is usually necessary to rely on cultures of voided urine for diagnosis of urinary tract infection. In the majority of patients with urinary tract infection, voided urine contains at least 10^5 organisms/ml of urine. In contrast, urine from healthy subjects usually contains less than 10^4 organisms/ml of urine. Significant bacteriuria therefore means 10^5 or more organisms/ml of urine. Its presence defines a high probability of the existence of a urinary tract infection. Other studies suggest that a threshold of 10^2 coliform bacteria/ml of urine may be a more sensitive indicator of infection in acutely symptomatic women and yields only slightly more false-positives than a value of 10^5 organisms/ml. Thresholds of 10^3 and 10^2 organisms/ml have been suggested as significant bacteriuria in symptomatic men and catheterized patients, respectively.

Urinary tract infection includes the clinical entities of *cystitis,* reflecting symptoms related to the bladder and urethra (lower tract), and *pyelonephritis,* reflecting symptoms related to the kidneys (upper tract). Cystitis is associated with the presence of dysuria (Chapter 106), frequency, urgency, and occasionally suprapubic tenderness. Acute pyelonephritis describes the clinical syndrome characterized by flank pain, fever, and flank tenderness and is often associated with dysuria, frequency, and urgency.

It is important to recognize, however, that the correlation between symptoms and the presence of infection can be very poor. Urinary tract infections (upper or lower tract) may be asymptomatic (asymptomatic bacteriuria), and patients with upper tract infection may have only lower tract symptoms. Lower urinary tract symptoms commonly occur in patients (usually females) with less than 10^5 bacteria/ml of urine. The term *urethral syndrome* has been used to describe this entity. Of patients with urethral syndrome (after excluding vaginitis and herpes as causes of the frequency, urgency, and/or dysuria), some—about one third of sexually active women—are found to have bacteria in bladder urine and therefore have urinary tract infection (presumably lower tract infection); the remaining patients with urethral syndrome have *Chlamydia trachomatis* (Chapter 257) or less commonly *Neisseria gonorrhoeae* urethritis or symptoms of unknown etiology. *Ureaplasma urealyticum* and noninfectious etiologies of urethritis (trauma, psychologic, allergic, and chemical) have been postulated as possible causes. Bacterial urinary tract infection and *C. trachomatis* or *N. gonorrhoeae* urethritis are associated with pyuria (greater than or equal to eight leukocytes/mm³ uncentrifuged urine), whereas the other causes of the urethral syndrome are not associated with pyuria. Upper tract symptoms may also occur in the absence of infection and may be associated with renal infarction or renal calculi.

A urinary tract infection may occur as a single event or as part of a pattern of recurrent infections. Recurrences may be either relapses or reinfections. The term *relapse* means that the same infecting organism is causing recurrent infection in spite of appropriate therapy and implies that the organism is being harbored somewhere within the urinary tract. Relapses occur within 1 to 2 weeks after stopping antimicrobial therapy and are often associated with renal infection, underlying structural abnormalities of the urinary tract (e.g., stones), or the presence of chronic bacterial prostatitis. In *reinfection,* different organisms cause the recurrence each time; therefore reinfection is a new infection. Occasionally, a reinfection with the same microorganism, which may have persisted in the vagina or feces, may occur within 2 weeks and may be mistaken for a relapse.

The terms *chronic urinary tract infection* and *chronic pyelonephritis* are confusing, meaning different things to different authors. Chronic urinary tract infection literally means a continuing infection, and this definition fits the patient with persistent urinary tract infection who relapses. However, multiple reinfections should not be categorized as "chronic." Chronic pyelonephritis has come to refer to a morphologic appearance of the kidney that may be caused by bacterial infection but is also seen in other disease entities, such as chronic urinary tract obstruction, analgesic nephropathy, and uric acid nephropathy. The situation would be clearer if these morphologic findings, which are really nonspecific, were termed *chronic interstitial nephritis,* with the term *chronic pyelonephritis* reserved for cases with a proven bacteriologic cause.

PATHOGENESIS

Bacteria can presumably gain access to the urinary tract and cause infection through three pathways: through the bloodstream to the kidneys, by lymphatic channels to the kidneys from a possible source in the bowel or pelvis, or by ascending from the urethra into the bladder and then up to the kidneys through the ureters. There is variable clinical and experimental evidence to support each of these pathways. The kidney is frequently a site of abscesses in patients with staphylococcal bacteremia or endocarditis. Experimental pyelonephritis can be induced by intravenous inoculation of large numbers of *Candida, Staphylococcus aureus,* or enterococci. It is difficult, however, to produce pyelonephritis in animals by the intravenous injection of gram-negative bacilli (the organisms that usually cause infection in humans) unless the kidney is manipulated in some way to produce either extrarenal or intrarenal obstruction (e.g., by ureteral ligation or renal cautery). Extrapolating this evidence to humans, together with clinical observations, suggests that pyelonephritis caused by gram-negative organisms rarely occurs by the hematogenous route.

The role of lymphatic spread of bacteria in the pathogenesis of pyelonephritis is based on indirect (and tenuous) evidence consisting of the demonstration in animals of lymphatic connections between the upper and lower urinary tracts and the possible existence of lymphatic channels between the colon and right kidney.

Most clinical and experimental evidence clearly supports the ascending pathway in the vast majority of urinary tract infections. Organisms that cause urinary tract infection in women usually colonize the vaginal introitus and periurethral area from a fecal reservoir before urinary tract infection occurs. The female urethra, by virtue of its anatomic location in proximity to the warm, moist vulvar and perirectal areas, is very prone to contamination; and its short length provides easy access to the bladder. Men appear to be relatively protected from ascending infection because of the male urethra's different anatomic location and also perhaps because of prostatic secretions that exhibit antibacterial activity. These facts may help explain the much higher incidence of urinary tract infections in females as compared with males. Further clinical evidence for the importance of the ascending route is provided by the fact that urethral catheters with open drainage systems result in urinary tract infections in essentially all patients within 96 hours. Presumably, bacteria enter the bladder by moving up through the lumen of the catheter from the collecting bag or along the exudative material between the urethral mucosa and catheter.

Colonization of the periurethral areas and subsequent urinary tract infection depend on an interplay between the infecting organism and the host defense mechanisms. Inoculum size certainly is important, having a positive correlation with the risk of infection. Certain virulence factors have been identified in bacteria. The presence of fimbriae has been demonstrated to be important for attachment of *Proteus mirabilis* and *Escherichia coli* to urinary tract epithelium. These hairlike structures project outward from the organism and contain highly specific polysaccharides that attach to specialized receptors on the uroepithelium. The adhesins most commonly and specifically expressed by pyelonephritic strains of *E. coli* are P and S fimbriae, whereas type 1 fimbriae appear to play a more important role in colonization of the vagina, perineum, and bladder. Changes in just one simple sugar render the organism unable to attach and avirulent in producing urinary tract infections. Bacterial lipopolysaccharide likely plays an important role in inducing the local inflammatory response and in producing constitutional symptoms and signs during both cystitis and pyelonephritis. In addition, both interleukin-1 and interleukin-6 are measurable in the urine more frequently in bacteriuric than nonbacteriuric elderly patients. *E. coli* possessing high quantities of certain K antigens (K1, K2, K5, and K13 or K51) appear to be more virulent pathogens than other *E. coli* strains, as they are more likely to infect the kidney. Resistance to serum bactericidal activity, presence of aerobactin, and hemolysin production are other potentially important virulence factors. Bacterial production of urease has also been shown to increase the risk of pyelonephritis in experimental animals. Urease production, together with the presence of bacterial motility and fimbriae, may favor the production of upper tract infection by organisms such as *Proteus*.

The host in turn possesses mechanisms that defend against bacterial invasion. The urine is a good but variable culture medium. Anaerobic bacteria and other fastidious organisms that make up most of the normal urethral flora do not generally multiply well in urine. Extremes in urine osmolality, a low pH, and a high urea concentration inhibit growth of many bacteria. The bladder mucosa appears to have its own intrinsic antibacterial defense mechanisms. Uromucoid or urinary slime (Tamm-Horsfall protein) rich in mannose residues avidly binds *E. coli* and may prevent attachment of *E. coli* to uroepithelial cells; the increased risk of urinary infection in the elderly has been attributed, in part, to the lower urinary excretion rates of Tamm-Horsfall protein found in the elderly. Natural antiadherence mechanisms have also been identified in the bladders of several animal species (dogs, rabbits, rats, and mice). These mechanisms can be reversed after brief treatment of the bladder with dilute hydrochloric acid, supporting the concept of a superficial acid-sensitive natural antiadher-

ence mechanism. Further information is needed, however, to precisely define the importance of antiadherence mechanisms as defense mechanisms against urinary tract infections. In addition, the flushing mechanism of the bladder is an important defense mechanism. Urine flow first dilutes the bacterial inoculum, and then voiding flushes it from the bladder. Any interference with normal voiding, such as obstruction, the presence of a foreign body, or incomplete bladder emptying, can compromise these bladder defense mechanisms and lead to bacterial retention and multiplication.

Lactobacilli in the vagina also probably serve as a defense mechanism against colonization with Enterobacteriaceae. Lactobacilli lower vaginal pH, produce lactic acid from glycogen, and may compete for receptor sites used by Enterobacteriaceae for adherence. All of these factors may be important in protecting against vaginal colonization by Enterobacteriaceae. Elimination of lactobacilli by the antibacterial effects of spermicides or by the postmenopausal state predisposes to colonization and urinary tract infection with Enterobacteriaceae. Estrogen replacement (with either a topically applied vaginal cream or an orally administered agent) in postmenopausal women results in replacement of lactobacilli and may lead to a decrease in colonization and urinary tract infection caused by Enterobacteriaceae.

The different regions of the kidney have different susceptibilities to infection. Animal studies have shown that the medulla is generally much more susceptible to bacterial infection than the cortex. This same susceptibility correlates with human kidney disease in which the earliest lesions occur in the renal pelvis, with an area of inflammation and exudate extending from the pelvis and medulla to the cortex in a triangular wedge. This particular vulnerability of the medulla has been attributed to the high concentration of ammonia, which may inactivate the fourth component of complement, and to high osmolality, low pH, and low blood flow, which inhibit leukocyte mobilization to the area.

PATHOLOGY

Morphologically, the acutely infected kidney may be enlarged, with small abscesses scattered throughout the parenchyma. Abscesses that occur beneath the capsule give the surface a studded, nodular appearance. They may coalesce, producing a renal carbuncle that can perforate through the capsule and result in a perinephric abscess. The pelvis appears hemorrhagic and ulcerated. An intense neutrophilic infiltrate surrounds the tubules and eventually produces areas of necrosis. White cell casts may be found within the tubules and become hallmarks for the laboratory diagnosis of acute pyelonephritis when they are detected in the voided urine. Generally, the glomeruli and blood vessels are spared in the acute inflammatory process.

The circulation to the most distal part of the medulla and papilla is easily compromised. In certain populations—specifically patients with diabetes mellitus, sickle cell disease, or chronic obstruction, or analgesic abusers—vascular disease is present and can lead to ischemia and infarction of the papilla. In these patients, papillary necrosis can become a serious complication of acute pyelonephritis (and can also occur in the absence of infection). The papilla may slough, with the remnant being voided in the urine. The papilla can also obstruct, producing renal colic, oliguria, and suppurative hydronephrosis. Death may follow from rapidly progressive renal insufficiency or bacteremia.

Chronic pyelonephritis is characterized morphologically by caliceal dilation and cortical scarring. Involvement of the kidney is focal and unequal, and kidney size may be variable, ranging from large (early) to small shrunken kidneys (late). Microscopically, lymphocytes, plasma cells, and macrophages are present in the interstitium. The tubules are atrophied and dilated and may be filled with casts, giving the appearance of thyroid tissue. The glomeruli and blood vessels are spared until late in the disease course, when the glomeruli exhibit sclerosis, and fibrotic thickening of the intima of the small arteries develops. As mentioned previously, these morphologic changes are nonspecific and have multiple causes. In a strict sense, the term *chronic pyelonephritis* should be applied only to patients in whom past or present infection can be documented.

Most patients in whom urinary tract infections develop have anatomically and functionally normal urinary tracts, but many predisposing factors increase the risk that infection will develop. Obstruction to urine flow with impairment of normal bladder function and stasis within the urinary system is the most important factor. It markedly increases the risk of urinary tract infection from the hematogenous and the ascending routes. Obstruction can be caused by any number of factors. Extrarenal obstruction may be the result of (1) congenital anomalies of the ureters or urethra (valves, bands); (2) calculi (which also harbor bacteria, making eradication of infection extremely difficult); (3) extrinsic ureteral compression; and (4) an enlarged prostate gland. Obstruction may also be intrarenal in conditions such as nephrocalcinosis, uric acid nephropathy, polycystic kidney disease, and scars. Males of any age appear to be much more prone to obstructive lesions of the urinary tract than are women.

The importance of vesicoureteral reflux in the pathogenesis of urinary tract infection and the development of subsequent renal damage has become apparent in recent years. Reflux of contaminated urine from the bladder provides a direct route to the pelvicaliceal system and obviously predisposes to ascent of infection. Reflux also tends to perpetuate infection by maintaining a residual pool of infected urine in the bladder after voiding. Reflux, most common in young children, can be due to a congenital abnormality or to bladder overdistention, such as occurs in bladder outlet obstruction. It can be caused by bladder infection alone, the inflammation and edema inhibiting the competency of a marginally competent vesicoureteral junction. Reflux in the presence of infection in a child is associated with development of renal scarring and lack of growth of the kidney. Infants and preschool-aged children are at the highest risk for developing renal damage. These children may have severe degrees of reflux, which may eventually cause enough scarring to lead to end-stage renal disease. The progression of scars or the development of new ones becomes less common after the age of 5 years and is rare after full growth of the kidney. There is thus a population of patients (infant or preschool-aged) in whom bacteriuria and reflux can produce significant renal damage. On the other hand, it is clear that sterile reflux per se can result in renal scarring. Reflux tends to decrease with the treatment of bacteriuria, and mild to moderate degrees disappear over time, even with persistent infection, probably because of the maturation of the vesicoureteral junction. Progressive renal disease rarely develops in adults in association with urinary tract infections, except in the presence of obstruction or other significant renal disease that in itself can cause renal damage.

MICROBIOLOGY

Enterobacteriaceae are the most common pathogens involved in urinary tract infection. *E. coli* is responsible for the vast majority (85%) of the cases of acute urinary tract infection. Patients with recurrent infections, those with structural abnormalities of the urinary tract, those who have had urethral instrumentation, and those whose infections were acquired in the hospital have an increased frequency of infection caused by *Proteus, Klebsiella-Enterobacter* species, *Pseudomonas*, enterococci, and staphylococci. *E. coli* accounts for about 50% of urinary tract infections in hospitalized patients. Generally, gram-positive organisms are much less important as causes of urinary tract infection than are gram-negative bacilli. When *S. aureus* causes infection, the illness may be acute, and renal infection may be secondary to bacteremia. Coagulase-negative staphylococci (usually *Staphylococcus saprophyticus*) account for up to 10% to 15% of urinary tract infections, mainly in young, sexually active females. Infections caused by urease-producing organisms (e.g., *Proteus, Providencia, Morganella*, strains of *Pseudomonas* and *Klebsiella, S. saprophyticus*) tend to alkalinize the urine by converting urea into ammonia, leading to formation and precipitation of struvite crystals, a predominant component of urinary calculi and encrustations on urinary catheters. Anaerobic organisms rarely cause urinary tract infection.

Candida albicans is the most common fungus isolated from the urinary tract, accounting for 48% to 59% of positive fungal cultures; *Torulopsis glabrata* is the second most common fungus isolated (5% to 21% of cultures). Particularly in women, vaginal or perineal fungal colonization may contaminate urine cultures. Low growth of candidal colonies in urine (10^3 to 10^4 organisms/ml) probably should be used as a diagnostic threshold for fungal urinary tract infection.

EPIDEMIOLOGY

As previously stated, urinary tract infection is much more common in females than in males. It is interesting to note, however, that infant males have a higher prevalence of infection than do infant females. This higher frequency is presumably secondary to the higher incidence of anomalies of the urinary tract in male infants. In addition, studies have suggested that uncircumcised male infants are more likely than circumcised infants to have urinary tract infections during the first year of life. After infancy, the prevalence of urinary tract infection in males drops to less than 0.1% until the ages when prostatic disease occurs. In these later years, the prevalence of urinary tract infection in men increases to 4% to 10%.

Urinary tract infection in males is frequently associated with urologic abnormalities. However, a small number of men between 20 and 50 years of age suffer acute, uncomplicated urinary tract infections. The exact reason for such infections is unclear; one possible explanation is homosexual intercourse.

In males with infection, it is usually important to evaluate for structural abnormalities of the urinary tract. Ultrasonography should be performed to rule out nephrolithiasis and obstructive uropathy. Further evaluation, including intravenous pyelography with postvoiding views of the bladder, cystoscopy, and radionuclide evaluation may also be necessary. When infection is eradicated in a man, he tends not to become infected again unless there is catheterization or instrumentation of the urethra.

At least 10% to 20% of the female population have a symptomatic urinary tract infection sometime during their lives, and up to one third of elderly women have asymptomatic urinary tract infections when populations are screened. During the preschool years, the period prevalence (i.e., percentage with infection sometime during the pre-school years) of significant bacteriuria has been reported to be 4.5% for girls and 0.5% for boys. Infection during this period is often symptomatic, and it is believed that much of the renal damage that occurs from infection in both males and females occurs at this time.

Bacteriuria is common in females of school age, is often asymptomatic, and frequently recurs. The prevalence of bacteriuria is about 1%, and about 5% of schoolgirls have significant bacteriuria at least once before leaving high school. Each year on resurvey, about 25% of those reported as infected in the previous year's survey are cured either spontaneously or with antibiotics but are replaced by an equal number in whom bacteriuria has developed. The same girls tend to have multiple reinfections. Thus the prevalence remains the same from year to year. Within 3 months after marriage, over 50% of the women who had childhood bacteriuria have bacteriuria again. From these data it appears that in women, bacteriuria in childhood defines a population at increased risk for the development of bacteriuria in later life.

Once adulthood is reached, the prevalence of bacteriuria increases in the female population, the increase being positively correlated with increasing age and parity. Sexual activity is associated with an increased risk of urinary tract infection and probably plays a permissive role in facilitating inoculation of bladder urine with urethral flora. It has been demonstrated that use of the diaphragm with spermicidal jelly or use of spermicidal foam with a condom markedly alters normal vaginal flora and strongly predisposes to vaginal colonization and bacteriuria with Enterobacteriaceae.

The prevalence of bacteriuria in young nonpregnant women is about 1% to 3%, rising to 33% in elderly women. On yearly resurveys of populations, bacteriuria has cleared in about 25% of bacteriuric women, and they are replaced by an equal number who have become infected. The same women tend to become infected repeatedly. Therefore, it is apparent that "cure" of urinary tract infection in a female applies only to the episode being treated. It is likely that it will be followed by future infections.

The prevalence of asymptomatic bacteriuria during pregnancy ranges from 4% to 7%, with much of the bacteriuria already present during the first trimester. Symptomatic pyelonephritis develops during pregnancy in about 20% to 40% of bacteriuric patients. Most cases of acute pyelonephritis can be prevented by treating and eliminating asymptomatic bacteriuria in the early stages of pregnancy. This fact is very significant, not only because of the decrease in maternal morbidity but also because of the apparent association between acute pyelonephritis of pregnancy and an increased frequency of premature delivery and infant morbidity and mortality. Asymptomatic bacteriuria per se may also increase the frequency of prematurity and fetal wastage. Therefore it seems justified to screen for urinary tract infection in pregnancy and to treat bacteriuria in pregnant women.

The incidence of funguria in hospitalized patients has been increasing. Predisposing conditions include presence of an indwelling catheter, antimicrobial therapy, diabetes mellitus, and immunocompromised states.

CLINICAL SYMPTOMS AND DIAGNOSIS

The manifestations of urinary tract infections in adults are usually easy to recognize. Lower tract symptoms result from inflammation and irritation of the urethral and bladder mucosa, causing frequent and painful urination of small amounts of turbid urine. Patients sometimes complain of suprapubic heaviness or pain. Occasionally, the urine is blood tinged or grossly bloody, reflecting damage to superficial blood vessels in the bladder mucosa. Fever tends to be absent in infection limited to the lower tract. The classic clinical manifestations of upper tract involvement include fever, sometimes accompanied by chills, flank pain, flank tenderness, and often lower tract symptoms of frequency, urgency, and dysuria. The lower tract symptoms may antedate the appearance of fever and upper tract symptoms by 1 or 2 days. Localization studies indicate that as many as 30% of patients who have only clinical lower urinary tract symptoms may have subclinical upper urinary tract involvement. Pain from the kidney can occasionally be localized near the epigastrium and can radiate to one of the lower quadrants.

As previously mentioned, there can be a poor correlation between symptoms and the presence of infection. About 40% of sexually active females who have lower tract symptoms have the urethral syndrome with sterile urine or insignificant bacteriuria. Only about one third of these patients have urinary tract infection; the rest have urethritis caused by *Chlamydia* (Chapter 257) or other infectious or noninfectious etiologies. There is also a poor correlation between symptoms and signs and the site of infection. About one third of patients with no symptoms or with only symptoms of cystitis have renal bacteriuria.

The definitive diagnosis of a urinary tract infection depends on the isolation of bacteria from the urine in significant numbers. Microscopic examination of the urine can be helpful. The presence of at least one bacterium per high power field in properly collected midstream clean-catch, Gram-stained, uncentrifuged urine correlates with 10^5 or more bacteria/ml of urine (i.e., significant bacteriuria). The absence of bacteria in several fields of a stained sedimented specimen indicates the probability of less than 10^4 bacteria/ml and is evidence against significant bacteriuria.

The major reason for obtaining a urine culture before therapy in a woman with apparent lower urinary tract infection is to detect those with the urethral syndrome (who will have $<10^5$ bacteria/ml urine). In this group are patients with chlamydial urethritis, which often has more serious implications than urinary tract infection (Chapter 257). Therefore if significant bacteriuria is present by microscopic examination, it is reasonable in the nonpregnant woman with lower tract symptoms to take a culture only if symptoms do not respond to therapy or recur after therapy is discontinued. Isolates can then be submitted for antimicrobial susceptibility testing.

The presence or absence of pyuria, as defined by more than 5 to 10 leukocytes per high power field in sedimented urine, correlates poorly with bacteriuria. About 20% of urine samples with pyuria have less than 10^5 bacteria/ml. Conversely, about 30% of the specimens with at least 10^5 bacteria/ml do not have increased numbers of white cells. However, the vast majority of patients with symptomatic infection have pyuria. According to a stricter definition of pyuria (at least 10 leukocytes/mm^3 of midstream urine), the vast majority of patients with either symptomatic or asymptomatic bacteriuria will have pyuria; however, pyuria without infection remains common, especially in elderly women.

The measurement of pyuria has been simplified by the use of a rapid assay to determine the presence in the urine of leukocyte esterase, an enzyme found in primary neutrophil granules. The assay is a reasonable method to quickly determine the presence of significant pyuria (sensitivity of 75% to 96%), and it is used most appropriately as a screening test to determine the need for urine cultures in symptomatic patients for whom routine microscopy is either unavailable or impractical.

White cell casts in the presence of urinary tract infection are strong evidence for pyelonephritis. Although mild proteinuria is common in urinary tract infections, excretion of 3 g or more of protein in 24 hours suggests the presence of glomerular disease and should not be attributed to infection alone. Occasionally, microscopic or gross hematuria is seen in the urine of patients with infection, reflecting hemorrhagic cystitis. Red cells, however, may indicate other disorders, such as the presence of calculi, vasculitis, glomerulonephritis, or renal tuberculosis.

Interpretation of a culture depends on both the clinical setting and the manner in which the specimen was obtained. The standard urine culture in most laboratories is performed on midstream, clean-catch specimens collected in sterile containers. In women, the external genitalia are washed two to three times with a cleaning agent to reduce urethral contamination. This cleaning procedure is of questionable value in men, although it is widely practiced. After collection, specimens should be processed expeditiously. A urine specimen that is allowed to sit at room temperature for several hours may yield falsely elevated bacterial colony counts. Counts of bacteria are relatively stable for up to 24 hours when urine is stored at 4° C.

In general, there are two separate but overlapping populations. One has bacterial counts between 0 and 10^4 bacteria/ml of urine, which usually represents contamination. The second, which represents true bacteriuria, has counts of more than 10^5 bacteria/ml. The two populations overlap mainly between 10^4 and 10^5 bacteria/ml. If there are more than 10^5 bacteria/ml in a clean-catch urine specimen from an asymptomatic female, there is an 80% probability that this represents true bacteriuria. If two different specimens demonstrate at least 10^5 of the same bacterium per milliliter, the probability increases to 95%. Thus two clean-catch specimens should be obtained in an asymptomatic female to confirm the diagnosis. In a symptomatic patient, one titer of 10^5/ml or more is sufficient to establish the diagnosis. When the number of bacteria per milliliter is between 10^4 and 10^5 in an asymptomatic female, a confirmatory second specimen (preferably a first-voided morning specimen) will contain 10^5 bacteria/ml in only 5% of instances. Thus 95% of the time, titers between 10^4 and 10^5 bacteria/ml represent contamination. However, in males, in whom contamination is less likely, a titer of 10^4 organisms/ml is more suggestive of infection. These criteria apply only to the Enterobacteriaceae. Gram-positive organisms, fungi, and bacteria with fastidious growth requirements may not reach titers of 10^5/ml in patients with infection and may be in the range of 10^4 to 10^5/ml. Isolation of Enterobacteriaceae in low-titer counts (e.g., 10 to 10^4/ml) in patients with frequency, urgency, and dysuria (i.e., the urethral syndrome) usually indicates lower tract infection caused by these organisms.

Localization of Infection

Several methods have been used to localize the site of infection in the urinary system. One method involves inserting an indwelling catheter and sterilizing the bladder by washing it with antibiotic solutions. Serial quantitative urine cultures are then taken at frequent intervals through the catheter. Because all bacteria previously in the bladder have theoretically been killed, organisms found in the early serial specimens will have collected in the bladder from the ureters, thus localizing infection to the upper tract. Another method involves direct catheterization of the ureters for quantitative cultures. These two methods, though reliable, are invasive techniques and not routinely recommended.

A noninvasive technique has been developed based on the fact that bacteria in urine of renal origin are coated with antibody. Fluorescein-conjugated antihuman globulin is added to the bacteriuric urine, and the urine is examined under a fluorescence microscope. Fluorescence indicates antibody-coated bacteria and usually correlates with upper tract infection. The predictive value of associating a positive test for fluorescence with upper tract infection is 88% as established by several studies. The predictive value of associating a negative test with bladder infection is 76%. The relatively high false-positive and false-negative rates render this test useful mainly for clinical studies and not for management of individual patients. False-positive results may be observed in children, in men with a prostatic focus of infection, in women whose urine becomes contaminated with vaginal contents, in men and women with proteinuria, and with hemorrhagic cystitis, bladder tumors, bladder stones, indwelling catheters, and organisms that fluoresce even if not coated (e.g., yeasts and pseudomonads). False-negative results may be observed in children, in early acute pyelonephritis, and with inability of antibody to combine with certain bacteria (e.g., mucoid-coated pseudomonads).

MANAGEMENT

All antimicrobial agents have side effects, and the associated possible morbidity must be weighed against the anticipated benefit to the patient. Infections in nonpregnant adult (especially elderly) women are characterized by their frequency and propensity to reinfect and/or relapse. The prognosis in this population is good in that progressive renal impairment and damage are rare after recurrent infections except when there is obstruction or other underlying abnormality that by itself can cause damage. Furthermore, no study has demonstrated decreased morbidity or mortality resulting from treatment of these patients with asymptomatic bacteriuria. With present information, considering that the cost and toxicity of antimicrobial therapy may be more significant than the infection itself, therapy is not warranted in the nonpregnant woman who has asymptomatic bacteriuria. It is necessary, however, to treat symptomatic patients to relieve their symptoms even though infection may recur.

In contrast to the benign course in nonpregnant women, bacteriuria in preschool-aged children of either sex (and to a lesser degree in older children) can result in significant morbidity, with impaired kidney growth, scar formation, and even renal insufficiency. Similarly, in pregnant women, bacteriuria has significant consequences for the health of the newborn and mother; these include low birth weight, premature labor, hypertension-preeclampsia, maternal anemia, and amnionitis. However, some studies have shown no increased delivery rate of low–birth weight infants to women with urinary tract infection. Therapy in children and pregnant women is beneficial and should be aggressively undertaken.

Bacteriuria in males is uncommon except in the elderly, as previously described, and its presence implies the possibility of a structural abnormality of the urinary system (e.g., obstruction). These patients therefore must have a diagnostic workup for structural abnormalities. Children and males of any age experiencing their first episode of urinary tract infection, and women who have a relapse after appropriate therapy, are at risk of urologic abnormalities and should have imaging studies of the urinary tract (ultrasonography in adults and children and intravenous urography in selected children and adults to delineate renal architecture). However, recent data have suggested that radionuclide cystography (to detect vesicoureteral reflux) and renal cortical scintigraphy (to detect pyelonephritis and renal scarring) have become the mainstays for evaluation of pediatric urinary tract infection. Renal cortical scintigraphy with dimercaptosuccinic acid (DMSA) Tc 99m has been shown to be more sensitive than intravenous urography in detection of renal scars (probably because functional alterations of the renal cortex appear earlier than anatomic lesions), although intravenous urography provides more precise information on the severity and extent of any permanent renal damage. These studies are unnecessary in women with their first episode of urinary tract infection, but after three or four reinfections, evaluation may be indicated.

Management of urinary tract infection (Fig. 246-1) includes nonspecific modalities and specific antimicrobial therapy. Forcing fluids has been advocated as a part of therapy. Theoretically, hydration results in a rapid reduction of bacterial counts and flushes bacteria from the bladder. It also decreases renal medullary hypertonicity, thus enhancing leukocyte migration to the area. It may, however, hinder therapy by producing increased urine output, thereby lowering urinary concentrations of antimicrobial agents. Because there is no evidence that hydration improves the results of appropriate antimicrobial therapy, its routine use is not recommended.

Changing the urinary pH has also been recommended as an adjunct to therapy. Lowering urinary pH enhances the antibacterial activity of urine by increasing the concentration of undissociated molecules of organic acids normally found in urine. The undissociated molecules probably penetrate better into the bacterial cell than do those in the ionized form present at a high pH. Urinary pH also affects the activity of many chemotherapeutic agents. The activity of methenamine mandelate, methenamine hippurate, and nitrofurantoin is increased at low urinary pH, whereas the aminoglycoside antibiotics are more effective at an alkaline pH. However, pH change is not necessary or even desirable except when methenamine mandelate or methenamine hippurate is used. For these agents to be effective, the urinary pH must be maintained at 5.5 or less. Acidification can be achieved by the use of ascorbic acid or methionine; by a modification of diet; and by restricting milk, sodium bicarbonate, and fruit juices except for cranberry juice; cranberry juice increases the urinary concentration of hippuric acid, which has antibacterial activity at low urine pH. Urinary acidification can be difficult to achieve and can cause precipitation of urate stones. Urinary analgesics, for example, phenazopyridine hydrochloride (Pyridium), have little place in the routine management of symptomatic infections. The dysuria usually responds rapidly to antibacterial therapy.

Selection of an appropriate antibiotic has become complex because of the increasing number of compounds available. Ideally, the agent chosen should not affect anaerobic bacteria (to avoid *Candida* vaginitis and *C. difficile* colitis) and should have low toxicity. There is no evidence to support any superiority of bactericidal over bacteriostatic drugs. It is also important to note that the correlation between the response of bacteriuria and inhibitory blood levels of antimicrobial agents is poor. In contrast, inhibitory urine levels are essential. Many oral antimicrobial agents in the dosages commonly used for urinary tract infection do not achieve serum levels above the minimum inhibitory concentration for most urinary pathogens. Yet these agents are effective because concentration in the urine results in high antibacterial urinary levels. Achieving blood levels therefore does not seem to be important in treating most urinary tract infections, although adequate blood levels are necessary in bacteremia. In patients with renal insufficiency, dosage modifications are necessary for agents that are excreted primarily by the kidneys and cannot be cleared by any other mechanism. In renal failure, there is also an inability of the kidney to concentrate antibiotics in the urine, making it difficult to eradicate bacteriuria. This fact may be a particularly important factor when using aminoglycosides, but with the penicillins and cephalosporins, adequate urine concentrations are generally attained in spite of impaired renal function.

Symptomatic Urinary Tract Infection

Most patients with symptomatic urinary tract infection are women of childbearing age. The onset of symptoms is frequently related to sexual intercourse. No one antimicrobial agent is unequivocally the drug of choice in these patients. Some useful agents are ampicillin, amoxicillin, cephalexin, tetracycline, trimethoprim-sulfamethoxazole, trimethoprim alone, norfloxacin, ciprofloxacin, ofloxacin, and nitrofurantoin. Effective therapy results in a marked decrease in bacterial titers within 48 hours after the onset of treatment. However, many of the organisms that commonly cause community-acquired urinary tract infections (including *E. coli*) are now resistant to amoxicillin and sulfonamides. Amoxicillin-clavulanic acid, trimethoprim-sulfamethoxazole, and the newer fluoroquinolones are active against the great majority of these organisms. Trimethoprim-sulfamethoxazole and the fluoroquinolones have the added advantage of having poor activity against the anaerobic flora of the vagina and gut.

A symptomatic response can be an unreliable index of efficacy, as symptoms can abate spontaneously without antimicrobial therapy, although bacteriuria persists. In patients with pyelonephritis severe enough for hospitalization and when gram-negative bacillary bacteremia is suspected by the presence of high fever, shaking chills, and/or hypotension, antibiotic therapy should be parenteral and must have activity against all potential pathogens (Chapter 245).

Evidence has accumulated that upper urinary tract infection requires more prolonged therapy than lower tract infection. A number of investigators have demonstrated that with infections limited to the lower urinary tract, single doses of antibacterial therapy have been sufficient to eradicate bacteriuria in women. To date, a number of agents (i.e., various sulfonamides, kanamycin, amoxicillin, trimethoprim-sulfamethoxazole, trimethoprim alone, and a fluoro-

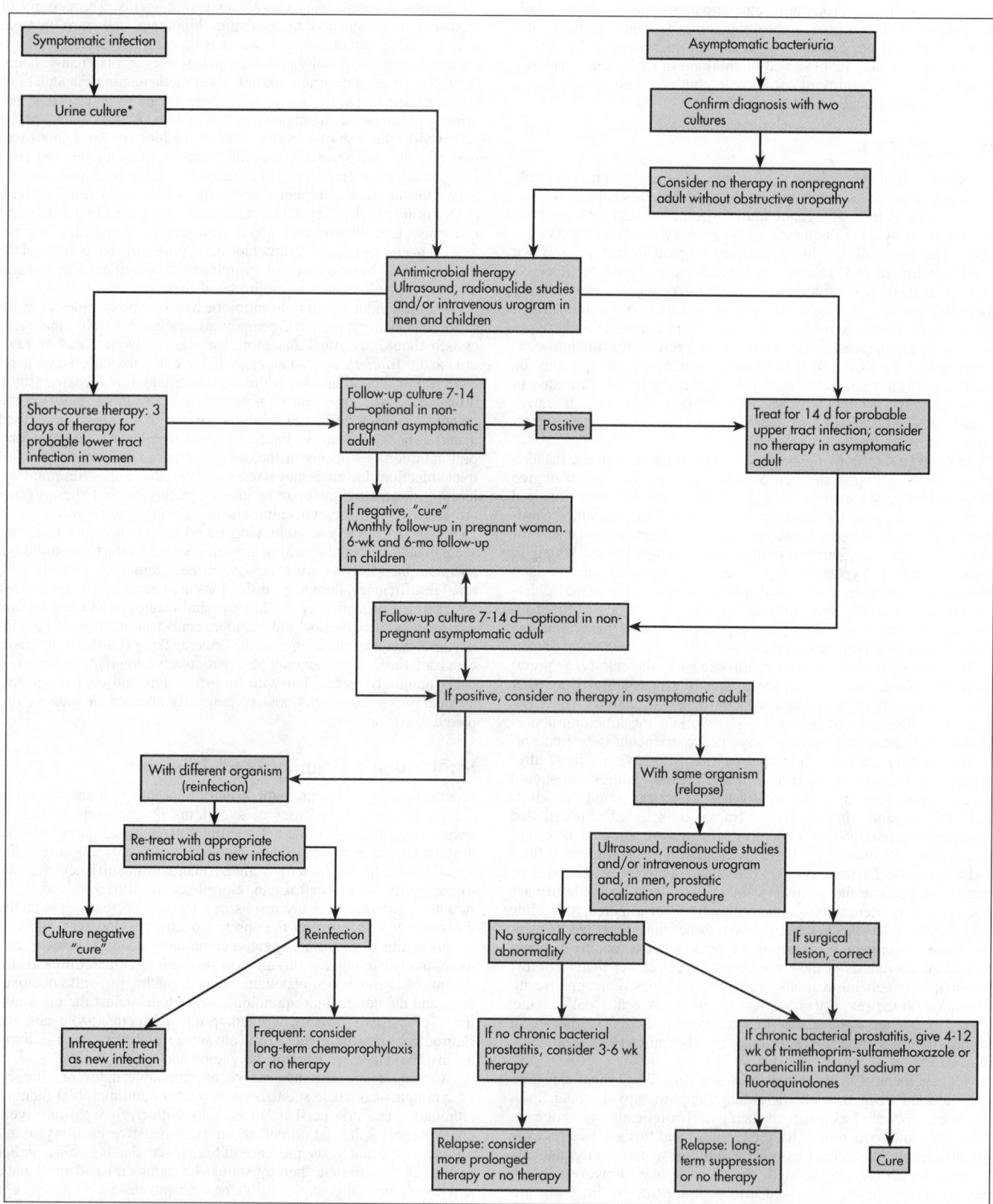

FIGURE 246-1 Management of urinary tract infections. *Not mandatory in women with only lower tract symptoms.

quinolone) have been shown to be effective in single-dose regimens. However, single-dose therapy with a fluoroquinolone is particularly prone to failure in patients infected with *S. saprophyticus*. Although it is likely that short courses (1 to 3 days) of any antimicrobial agent active against the infecting organism will be effective in lower urinary tract infection, 3 days of therapy are much more likely than single dose or 1 day of therapy to eliminate the organism from the gut and vagina, decreasing the risk of reinfection. Furthermore, 3 days of therapy may cure some unsuspected upper tract infections.

As an additional observation, it has become clear that therapy with trimethoprim-sulfamethoxazole, trimethoprim, or a fluoroquinolone is more likely to result in eradication of Enterobacteriaceae from the vagina and colon than therapy with β-lactam antibiotics. This results in lower reinfection rates. It seems reasonable, therefore, to treat women who have only lower tract symptoms (i.e., no fever, flank pain, or flank tenderness) with 3 days of one of these drugs.

In contrast to lower tract infection, patients with upper tract infection require at least 2 weeks of treatment. In the absence of nausea and vomiting and if the patient's overall degree of illness is mild, therapy can safely be given orally in the outpatient setting. Patients with nausea, vomiting, or moderate-to-severe illness and those who are pregnant often require hospitalization for initial parenteral therapy.

Urine cultures should be obtained in all children, all men, and women with upper tract symptoms or fever, before initiating therapy. Cultures are not mandatory in women with lower tract symptoms.

A patient who relapses after short-course therapy may have upper tract infection, and in symptomatic patients a 2-week course of antimicrobial therapy is indicated. In children and pregnant women, follow-up cultures should be obtained again at 6 weeks and 6 months (children) or monthly (pregnant women) to detect reinfections. In the nonpregnant adult who remains asymptomatic after therapy, a follow-up culture is probably not cost effective.

Asymptomatic Bacteriuria

Most patients with asymptomatic bacteriuria are women, usually in the older age group, with reinfection (and occasionally relapse) occurring very commonly after therapy. As previously discussed, potentially toxic and expensive therapy in this type of patient must be weighed against the apparently benign nature of the infection. In general, asymptomatic bacteriuria in the elderly should not be treated, particularly in view of the high rate of reinfection or relapse, and the high rate of adverse drug reactions in this population. If there are pressing reasons to treat asymptomatic bacteriuria, (i.e., before undergoing an invasive genitourinary tract procedure), 3 days of therapy should be the first approach.

Asymptomatic infection in children, pregnant women, and adults with evidence of obstruction should not be ignored because of the associated morbidity. These patients should be managed as described for symptomatic infection, with initial therapy directed at lower tract infection (i.e., short-course therapy).

Relapsing Urinary Tract Infection

If there is a relapse after appropriate antimicrobial therapy, renal infection (the usual cause of relapse in women), a structural abnormality of the urinary tract such as stone or obstruction, or chronic bacterial prostatitis must be considered. The ultimate success of therapy in the presence of a significant abnormality depends on its correction. Many recurrent infections in men are relapses, presumably because of a persistent focus in the prostate (i.e., chronic bacterial prostatitis). These patients usually have no prostatic signs or symptoms but have recurrent urinary tract infections, always with the same organism. Recurrences of urinary tract infection may be frequent or as infrequent as every several months.

In all patients who have a relapse, an investigation for structural abnormalities should be considered with radiographic evaluation and, in males, an attempt to diagnose chronic bacterial prostatitis should be made using a quantitative bacterial localization technique (see Chronic Bacterial Prostatis later in this chapter).

Women without structural abnormalities who have a relapse (pre-sumably from a renal focus) have a higher cure rate with long courses of therapy. In a woman who has a relapse after a 14-day course and who has no structural abnormalities, a more prolonged course (e.g., 3 to 6 weeks) should be considered. Even longer-term therapy (e.g., 6 weeks to 6 months) may be given but only in selected patients, such as adults with continuous symptoms or those who are at high risk for the development of renal damage, such as children. Asymptomatic adults without obstruction probably should not receive these longer courses. If bacteriuria persists or relapses during antimicrobial therapy, indicating the development of resistance, the antimicrobial agent should be changed. All patients should be followed with urine cultures every 1 to 2 months while on therapy. The antimicrobial agents that can be used for long-term therapy include amoxicillin, sulfisoxazole, trimethoprim-sulfamethoxazole, trimethoprim alone, nitrofurantoin, carbenicillin indanyl sodium, oral cephalosporins, and fluoroquinolones.

Trimethoprim-sulfamethoxazole is effective therapy for chronic bacterial prostatitis because of its superior penetration into the noninflamed prostate. Oral carbenicillin indanyl sodium may also be useful. Nevertheless, only about a third of patients with chronic bacterial prostatitis can be cured with these agents, even with 12-week courses. The fluoroquinolones are also concentrated in the noninflamed prostate and are useful in chronic bacterial prostatitis. Patients with chronic bacterial prostatitis or relapsing urinary tract infection who are not cured can be managed by treating each flare-up of urinary tract infection or by daily low-dose suppressive therapy with an agent that is active against the infecting organism.

Reinfection of Urinary Tract

Patients with reinfections can be divided into two groups: those who have relatively infrequent reinfections, perhaps every 2 to 3 years or up to several times each year, and those in whom frequent reinfections develop. Of recurrent urinary tract infections in women, 80% are reinfections. Reinfections are uncommon in young and middle-aged males. Women with infrequent reinfections can be treated with a 3-day course of therapy for each recurrence as a new episode of infection.

Many patients with frequent reinfections are middle-aged or elderly women with infection limited to the lower urinary tract. Most asymptomatic reinfections in this group need not be treated. If, however, the episodes are very frequent and symptomatic, or if there is the likelihood of renal damage (i.e., the presence of uncorrectable obstruction), these patients can be treated on a long-term basis. Long-term therapy should also be instituted in children because of the risk of the development of renal parenchymal damage. This approach is actually prophylactic and is aimed at decreasing the number of reinfections. Trimethoprim-sulfamethoxazole and nitrofurantoin are particularly useful agents for long-term prophylaxis, because, with prolonged use, they are unlikely to allow the emergence of antimicrobial-resistant bacteria in the periurethral area. Trimethoprim-sulfamethoxazole also has the ability to penetrate into vaginal secretions, helping prevent colonization of the periurethral area with bacteria from a fecal source. As little as 40 mg of trimethoprim and 200 mg of sulfamethoxazole (half of a regular-strength tablet) three times a week at bedtime is effective in preventing recurrent infection. Patients receiving long-term prophylaxis should have urine cultures every 1 to 2 months. Therapy is continued with the same agent as long as the patient remains abacteriuric. If bacteriuria persists or recurs, the therapy should be altered, using the response of the bacteriuria as the criterion of efficacy.

If this approach is used, a 6-month trial of prophylaxis can be tried, after which the regimen is discontinued and the patient observed for further infection. Another approach for women who have documented recurrent symptomatic infection is self-administration of a 3-day antimicrobial regimen at the onset of symptoms of urinary tract infection.

In some women, symptomatic reinfections are associated with sexual activity. These episodes may be prevented by voiding within 15 minutes after intercourse and/or by the administration of a single dose of an antimicrobial agent immediately before or after coitus.

Fungal Urinary Tract Infection

In patients with suspected funguria, therapy should be directed toward predisposing factors. Unnecessary indwelling catheters should be removed, nutritional status should be optimized, and antimicrobial therapy should be discontinued, if possible, to reduce fungal colonization. If these measures fail to clear the infection and systemic fungal infection is not present, antifungal therapy can be initiated with amphotericin B bladder irrigation. Various oral therapies (e.g., flucytosine, azoles) have also been examined, with variable response rates. More recently, studies utilizing oral fluconazole therapy have demonstrated significant efficacy in the treatment of funguria, with success rates greater than 75% to 80%. Further evaluation of fluconazole is needed, however, to define the optimal dosage and duration of therapy.

In patients with upper urinary tract fungal infection, the presence of a fungus ball and accompanying obstruction should be assessed; these patients are especially prone to development of fungemia. Placement of a percutaneous nephrostomy tube to relieve the obstruction is often required; this tube may also be used to instill an antifungal agent or remove the fungus ball.

PREVENTION

Catheterization of the urinary bladder should be avoided if possible (Chapter 232). The risk of infection after a single catheterization in an ambulatory patient is about 1% but is higher in elderly or debilitated patients, patients with urologic abnormalities, and pregnant women. Patients with indwelling catheters have a much greater risk of infection. Infection develops within 4 days in essentially all patients with an open drainage system. The use of a triple-lumen catheter with a continuous rinse of neomycin plus polymyxin B or use of a closed sterile drainage system delays the development of bacteriuria for up to 10 days in most patients. One of these systems should be used when an indwelling catheter cannot be avoided. Other alternatives include intermittent catheterization by insertion of a sterile or clean catheter every 3 to 6 hours for periodic bladder emptying, and suprapubic catheterization, which yields lower rates of bacteriuria because of the lower density of bacteria on the anterior abdominal skin than in the urethra. Although use of prophylactic antimicrobial therapy has been suggested as one means to reduce bacteriuria and symptomatic urinary tract infection in persons practicing intermittent bladder catheterization, adverse drug reactions and breakthrough bacteriuria with resistant organisms limit the usefulness of this practice.

Catheters coated or impregnated with silver ions, which are bactericidal, have shown reduced incidence of catheter-associated urinary tract infections in some studies but not in others.

Although it is possible to eradicate urinary tract infection with antimicrobial therapy in the presence of a sterile drainage system, reinfection is the rule. The patient in whom symptoms of infection develop in the presence of an indwelling catheter must be treated. In the absence of symptoms, however, it is better to avoid treatment until removal of the catheter, at which time eradication of infection becomes easier.

PROSTATITIS

The term *prostatitis* means prostatic inflammation and should be interpreted as a generic term having four major subcategories: acute bacterial prostatitis, chronic bacterial prostatitis, nonbacterial prostatitis, and prostatodynia. Acute bacterial prostatitis is an acute, usually gram-negative, bacterial infection of the prostate gland that coexists in the majority of cases with acute bacterial cystitis. Chronic bacterial prostatitis is a subclinical or indolent chronic infection of the prostatic acini by bacteria that can be localized to the prostatic secretions. Nonbacterial prostatitis is a chronic inflammatory condition of the prostatic acini for which there is no identifiable etiologic organism; associated symptoms can be indolent or totally subclinical. Prostatodynia refers to a clinical condition in which irritative voiding symptoms and pelvic pain suggest an acute inflammatory process but with minimum or no evidence of inflammatory cells in the prostatic secretions. In all forms of prostatitis except prostatodynia there are usually more than 10 white blood cells per high power field on examination of the expressed prostatic secretions.

Acute and chronic bacterial prostatitis constitute the two conditions of greatest general medical interest. Both conditions can result from ascent of bacteria in the urethra, reflux of infected urine into the posterior urethral prostatic ducts, lymphatogenous spread of bacteria from the rectum, or hematogenous spread. The first two routes of infection are thought to be the most common. In acute bacterial prostatitis, marked inflammation is present in part or all of the gland, with diffuse stromal hyperemia and edema, polymorphonuclear leukocyte infiltration within and around the acini, varying degrees of lymphocyte and macrophage invasion, intraductal glandular cell desquamation, and microabscess formation. Large abscesses are a late complication.

In chronic bacterial prostatitis, the inflammatory reaction is less pronounced, more focal, and characterized by lymphocyte, plasma cell, and macrophage infiltration within and around the acini and stroma. Because such changes have also been observed to lesser and greater degrees in 98% of prostatectomy specimens from patients with prostatic hypertrophy, the diagnosis of this form of prostatitis rests on the demonstration of bacteria in the prostatic secretions and not merely on the presence of inflammatory changes in the tissue.

The bacteriology of both forms is similar, with *E. coli, Pseudomonas* species, and enterococci being the most common pathogens. Cases resulting from nosocomial infections following instrumentation may be due to highly resistant gram-negative organisms.

Acute Bacterial Prostatitis

Clinical Manifestations. In acute bacterial prostatitis the symptoms are usually of short duration before presentation and typically consist of perineal pain, dysuria, frequency, urgency, and nocturia, all of which may at times be complicated by urinary retention. The perineal pain may radiate to the sacral region of the back, down the penis and suprapubic area, or to the rectal area. Less severe obstructive symptoms (e.g., urinary hesitancy and a decreased force and caliber of the stream) may occur. Gross or microscopic hematuria may be present, as may a purulent urethral discharge. Fever with or without chills and malaise are almost always present. In the more severe form of infection, the patient appears ill and may be frankly septic, with positive blood cultures. The prostate is typically painful to palpation, but in subacute cases the pain may be minimal. Complications of acute bacterial prostatitis include formation of abscesses (which may rupture into the urethra, perineum, or rectum), pyelonephritis, acute epididymitis and orchitis, and septic shock. Although uncommon, progression to chronic bacterial prostatitis can occur if the acute phase is not adequately treated.

Diagnosis. Vigorous prostatic massage may produce serious complications, such as spread of infection to the epididymis or kidney, or bacteremia. However, a careful rectal examination of the prostate to ascertain degree of tenderness, determine consistency of the gland, and rule out the presence of a perirectal abscess, tumor, or foreign body is indicated. It is not necessary to express prostatic secretions to make the diagnosis of acute bacterial prostatitis because the urine is almost always infected and culture of a voided specimen will identify the offending organism. Likewise, instrumentation of the urethra should be avoided in cases complicated by urinary retention. In such situations urologic consultation should be obtained for suprapubic urinary diversion.

Chronic Bacterial Prostatitis

Clinical Manifestations. Chronic bacterial prostatitis is usually asymptomatic when the infection is confined to the prostate proper, but should be suspected when relapsing urinary tract infection secondary to bacteria of the same serotype is documented. Eradication of the bladder bacteria leads to disappearance of symptoms, despite the fact that bacteria can still be cultured from the prostatic secretions.

Diagnosis. The diagnosis is established by performing the bacterial localization studies described by Meares and Stamey, which demonstrate a higher bacterial count in the expressed prostatic secretions, or preferably an ejaculate, as compared to that in the urine (quantitative methods that detect small numbers of bacteria must be used). In brief, the localization test, performed after eradicating bladder bacteria with an antibiotic that does not diffuse into the prostatic secretions (e.g., nitrofurantoin, amoxicillin, or cephalexin), consists of three sets of cultures: (1) an initial 10-ml aliquot and an additional 10-ml aliquot of urine (voided bladder urines, or VB_1 and VB_2, respectively), which are cultured separately; (2) the expressed prostatic fluid following prostatic massage; and (3) a 10-ml aliquot of urine that is subsequently collected (VB_3). The infection is localized to the prostatic secretions if the bacterial count in the secretions is ten-fold greater than the count in the VB_2 urine culture. If the bacterial count in VB_2 exceeds 10^3 bacteria/ml, the infection cannot be localized and the localization procedure must be repeated after additional antimicrobial administration. Because chronic inflammation and fibrosis are present in the gland, the prostate may be firm and irregular and thus suggestive of cancer; the demonstration of infected prostatic secretions does not rule out this possibility. If the consistency of the gland does not return to normal after adequate antibiotic therapy or if a nodule persists, a transrectal ultrasound examination with guided biopsies is indicated to rule out cancer.

Chronic granulomatous prostatitis is a rare inflammatory condition (0.8% of all benign inflammatory diseases) frequently associated with a recent urinary tract infection. This condition is notable in that it mimics prostate cancer on digital rectal examination and is rarely due to specific granulomatous disease. Irritative voiding symptoms are the most common symptoms and in most patients tend to resolve within a few months.

Therapy of Acute and Chronic Bacterial Prostatitis.

As a general rule, treatment should be guided by the results of bacterial cultures and the overall clinical situation. Therapy of serious acute bacterial prostatitis may require parenteral antibiotics until the acute phase of the infection has been overcome, followed by a 1-month course of oral antibiotic therapy. Therapy of less serious bouts of acute prostatitis consists of a 3- to 4-week course of oral antibiotics. Because penetration by most antibiotics is good in the acute phase of infection, any antibiotic demonstrated to be effective on sensitivity studies can be used.

Therapy of chronic bacterial prostatitis is less clear-cut, because this form of prostatitis is notoriously refractory to treatment. Most urologists would treat for a minimum of 4 weeks with trimethoprim-sulfamethoxazole, a fluoroquinolone, or carbenicillin indanyl sodium, agents that penetrate well into the nonacutely inflamed prostate, and then repeat cultures.

Longer periods of therapy are justified if initial therapy fails. If the infection persists after 12 weeks despite appropriate antibiotic therapy, switching to another of the aforementioned drugs is reasonable. Unfortunately, some patients with this form of prostatitis are not cured with antimicrobial therapy alone and at the same time do not have clear indications for surgery, such as secondarily infected prostatic calculi or significant benign prostatic hypertrophy. In these patients, consideration should be given to treating symptomatic infection when it occurs or to instituting a regimen of chronic suppressive therapy (e.g., low daily doses of trimethoprim-sulfamethoxazole or nitrofurantoin) to avoid episodes of symptomatic urinary tract infection.

Chronic Nonbacterial Prostatitis and Prostatodynia

In general the symptoms of chronic nonbacterial prostatitis and prostatodynia are the same and include chronic irritative symptoms along with varying degrees of perineal pain and discomfort in the absence of any conventionally demonstrable infection. Chronic nonbacterial prostatitis is often associated with symptoms that can be indolent or totally subclinical, although in symptomatic cases irritative voiding symptoms are present. Symptoms associated with prostatodynia tend to be more severe (irritative voiding symptoms, pelvic pain) and in unusual cases incapacitating. In both conditions various urodynamic derangements of voiding are observed, leading to hyperirritability of the bladder and incoordination of the urethral sphincteric mechanism. Symptoms associated with nonbacterial prostatitis probably result from the chronic inflammatory process within glandular acini; the ob-

served urodynamic abnormalities associated with prostatodynia may result from a primary neurologic (sensory or motor) disorder. The major difference between these two forms of prostatitis is that the white blood cell count in prostatic secretions is by convention higher in chronic nonbacterial prostatitis (more than 10 white blood cells per high power field) than in prostatodynia. Thus the distinction between the two entities can be rather vague and arbitrary. Because symptoms of transitional carcinoma of the prostatic urethra can mimic symptoms of chronic prostatic irritation (i.e., frequency, urgency, and nocturia), a urologic consultation should be obtained and urinary cytologies performed. From a practical standpoint, as long as serious disorders (such as adenocarcinoma of the prostate or transitional cell carcinoma of the prostate, bladder, or urethra) and surgically correctable anatomic abnormalities (such as urethral strictures) are ruled out, then in the vast majority of cases the long-term morbidity to the patient is minimal. Antibiotic therapy is of no value in the management of these forms of prostatitis. Antiinflammatory agents, such as ibuprofen, may be helpful in patients with severe symptoms. Those with a congested prostate may be relieved by regular prostatic massage. Some patients may respond to zinc sulfate because the prostatitis is mainly due to a low zinc concentration in the prostate. Tuberculosis of the prostate can masquerade as nonbacterial prostatitis, but in this condition it would be expected that other upper tract stigmata indicating a more generalized genitourinary tubercular infection would also be present.

Prostatic Infections in Patients With HIV Infection

Prostatic infections in men with HIV infection are caused not only by the typical bacteria seen in immunocompetent men, but also by atypical bacteria, fungi, and viruses. Acute and chronic prostatitis and prostatic abscess have been reported, and the symptoms of each type of prostatitis are not significantly different from those in patients who are seronegative for HIV. However, patients with HIV infection frequently receive antibiotic prophylaxis, and routine urine cultures are often negative despite the presence of pyuria and symptoms. For this reason the evaluation should include urine cultures for acid-fast bacilli, viruses, and fungi as well as imaging of the prostate using transrectal ultrasound to rule out an abscess. If an abscess is found, it should be drained transurethrally. If no abscess is seen and if routine urine cultures are negative, then consideration should be given to a transrectal biopsy of the prostate, and tissue samples sent for special stains and cultures looking for acid-fast bacilli, fungi, and viruses. Biopsy should be avoided in patients with diarrhea, but transrectal ultrasound should be done to rule out an abscess.

BIBLIOGRAPHY

Abrutyn E, Mossey J, Berlin JA et al: Does asymptomatic bacteriuria predict mortality and does antimicrobial treatment reduce mortality in elderly ambulatory women? *Ann Intern Med* 120:827-833, 1994.

Eggli DF, Tulchinsky M: Scintigraphic evaluation of pediatric urinary tract infection, *Semin Nuclear Med* 23:199-218, 1993.

Hooton TM et al: A prospective study of the risk factors for symptomatic urinary tract infection in young women, *N Engl J Med* 335:468-474, 1996.

Kaye D, editor: Urinary tract infections, *Med Clin North Am* 75:241-520, 1991.

Kim ED, Schaeffer AJ: Antimicrobial therapy for urinary tract infection, *Semin Nephrol* 14:551-569, 1994.

Kunin CM: Urinary tract infections in females, *Clin Infect Dis* 18:1-12, 1994.

Leigh DA: Prostatitis-an increasing clinical problem for diagnosis and management, *J Antimicrob Chemother* 32(A):1-9, 1993.

Nicolle LE: Urinary tract infection in the elderly, *J Antimicrob Chemother* 33(A):99-109, 1994.

Raz R, Stamm WE: A controlled trial of intravaginal estriol in postmenopausal women with recurrent urinary tract infection, *N Engl J Med* 329:753-756, 1993.

Ronald A: Sex and urinary tract infection, *N Engl J Med* 335:511-512, 1996.

Rosenfeld DL, Fleischer M, Yudd A et al: Current recommendations for children with urinary tract infection, *Clin Pediatr* 34:261-264, 1995.

Smellie JM: The intravenous urogram in the detection and evaluation of renal damage following urinary tract infection, *Pediatr Nephrol* 9:213-220, 1995.

Sobel JD, Kaye D: Urinary tract infections. In Mandell GL, Bennett JE, Dolin R, editors: *Principles and practice of infectious diseases*, ed 4, New York, 1995, Churchill Livingstone, pp. 662-690.

Spach DH, Stapleton AE, Stamm WE: Lack of circumcision increases the risk of urinary tract infection in young men, *JAMA* 267:679-681, 1992.

Stamm WE: Catheter-associated urinary tract infections: epidemiology, pathogenesis, and prevention, *Am J Med* 91(3B):65S-71S, 1991.

Stamm WE, Hooton TM: Management of urinary tract infections in adults, *N Engl J Med* 329:1328-1334, 1993.

Stapleton A et al: Postcoital antimicrobial prophylaxis for recurrent urinary tract infection: a randomized, double-blind, placebo-controlled trial, *JAMA* 264:703-706, 1990.

Voss A, Meis JFGM, Hoogkamp-Korstanje JAA: Fluconazole in the management of fungal urinary tract infection, *Infection* 22:247-251, 1994.

CHAPTER

247 Infections in Travelers

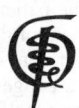 **Philip J. Rosenthal**

Travel to developing countries puts individuals at risk for many infectious diseases that are rarely contracted in developed areas. Clinicians managing patients who travel should be familiar with the features of common travel-related infections, should provide appropriate pretravel advice, and should understand the reasonable management of individuals who return from travel with an illness.

COMMON INFECTIONS OF TRAVELERS
Traveler's Diarrhea

Diarrhea is by far the most common infectious problem of travelers, occurring in up to 50% of travelers to some areas. Infection results from the ingestion of contaminated food or water. Such contamination is common in underdeveloped countries where water purification may be inadequate and where food is often contaminated with enteric pathogens.

More than 80% of diarrhea in travelers is likely bacterial (Box 247-1). The most common pathogen is enterotoxigenic *Escherichia coli*. Other important bacterial pathogens include *Shigella* species, *Campylobacter jejuni*, *Salmonella* species, *Aeromonas*, *Plesiomonas shigelloides*, and *Vibrio* species. Less common causes of traveler's diarrhea are viruses, including rotavirus and Norwalk virus, and protozoan parasites, including *Giardia*, *Entamoeba histolytica*, and *Cryptosporidium*. Cholera is endemic in many areas and now epidemic in much of Latin America, but it appears to be a minor risk to travelers.

Traveler's diarrhea typically presents as a watery diarrhea, often beginning within a week of the onset of travel. The illness includes the passage of 3 to 10 unformed stools per day, usually for 3 to 5 days. Abdominal pain and cramps commonly accompany the diarrhea. In about 10% to 20% of individuals, generally those infected with invasive organisms (Box 247-1), fever, vomiting, or the passage of bloody stools may occur.

Simple traveler's diarrhea responds well to treatment. Management begins with fluid and electrolyte replacement. Specific effective therapies include bismuth subsalicylate, antimotility agents, and antibiotics. Recent studies have shown the most effective regimens to be combinations of an antibiotic and an antimotility agent such as loperamide. Considering antibiotic resistance patterns, the most appropriate regimen for most areas is a short (1 to 3-day) course of a fluoroquinolone and loperamide. Beginning this regimen shortly after the onset of diarrhea has been shown to rapidly limit the illness. For those wishing to avoid antibiotic therapy, either bismuth subsalicylate or loperamide alone are fairly effective at relieving the symptoms of traveler's diarrhea. When the illness includes fever or bloody diarrhea, an antimotility agent should not be used; stool cultures should be obtained for a microbiologic diagnosis, and empiric antibiotic therapy with a fluoroquinolone should be instituted.

Malaria

Malaria is the most common potentially life-threatening infection to confront travelers. In the United States, about 1000 cases are reported each year in returning travelers and immigrants (Table 247-1), and many additional cases are unreported or occur in Americans while traveling. Malaria in travelers is about equally divided between *Plasmodium falciparum*, which can progress rapidly to critical illness and death, and *Plasmodium vivax*, which rarely causes dangerous complications. Much less common are infections with *Plasmodium malariae* and *Plasmodium ovale*. Malaria is transmitted by anopheline mosquitoes, which bite only in the evening and at night.

The specific risk of malaria for a traveler depends on the area visited. In Subsaharan Africa, the risk is high, even in many urban areas. Malaria can also be transmitted in cities on the Indian subcontinent but is generally not transmitted in urban areas of other parts of Asia or in South America or Oceania. Overnight stays in rural areas remain a risk in most countries in these regions. *P. falciparum*, the most dangerous malaria parasite, is commonly resistant to antimalarial drugs. The risk of acquiring falciparum malaria is greatest in Subsaharan Africa. The risk of acquiring multiply drug resistant parasites is greatest in Southeast Asia, although drug resistance is increasing through nearly all regions endemic for malaria.

Malaria presents as a febrile illness, usually without the classically described regular fever pattern but often with additional nonspecific symptoms such as cough or diarrhea. With falciparum malaria, this presentation can progress rapidly to dangerous multiorgan system involvement including cerebral malaria with coma, profound anemia, noncardiogenic pulmonary edema, and renal failure. Clinical malaria can present within 1 to 2 weeks of an infecting mosquito bite, but the incubation period can also be much longer. In the United States, falciparum malaria almost always presents within 1 to 2 months of the patient's return from travel, whereas the other malarial

---

BOX 247-1

Causes of traveler's diarrhea (listed in approximate order of importance)

Secretory diarrhea
Enterotoxigenic *E. coli*
Norwalk agent
Rotavirus
Giardia lamblia
Cryptosporidium
Vibrio species
Aeromonas species
Plesiomonas species
Vibrio cholerae

Invasive diarrhea
Shigella species
Salmonella species
Invasive *E. coli*
Campylobacter jejuni
Entamoeba histolytica
Yersinia enterocolitica

Table 247-1   Imported malaria in the United States, 1986 to 1992

AREA OF ACQUISITION	TOTAL CASES	PERCENTAGE OF ALL CASES	PERCENTAGE OF *P. FALCIPARUM* FROM THIS AREA
Africa	2985	43.3	73.4
Asia	2126	30.9	13.2
Central America*	1342	19.5	8.4
South America	120	1.7	23.8
Oceania	227	3.3	18.9
Unknown	88	1.3	23.4
TOTAL	6888	100	39.5

Data from Centers for Disease Control and Prevention.
*Includes Mexico and the Caribbean.

species may commonly present many months, and occasionally more than a year, after the return.

The diagnosis of malaria continues to rely on a Giemsa-stained blood smear. Thin smears are generally adequate for diagnosis. Thick smears increase sensitivity, but can be difficult to interpret by inexperienced personnel. The four malarial species that infect humans can usually be readily distinguished based on morphologic criteria. In addition, geographic and temporal factors, as discussed earlier, can be helpful in distinguishing falciparum malaria from the other species, which is the only discrimination necessary in the initial management of an ill patient.

The therapy of malaria is complex because of the increasing resistance of malaria parasites to available drugs. *P. falciparum* parasites are now often resistant to chloroquine in all areas endemic for this parasite except for Central America above the Panama Canal, Haiti, and the Middle East. Resistance to other drugs, including folate antagonists (pyrimethamine-sulfadoxine [Fansidar], proguanil), mefloquine, and halofantrine, is also increasing in many areas, and quinine resistance has appeared in Southeast Asia. Recently, *P. vivax* resistant to chloroquine has been reported from South Asia and Oceania, although this is not yet a significant problem. Sensitive falciparum parasites and other species can be treated with chloroquine. *P. vivax* and *P. ovale* infections also require the subsequent administration of primaquine to eradicate chronic liver forms that are not killed by chloroquine. Falciparum malaria from areas with known chloroquine resistance should usually be treated with quinine. A second slow-acting drug (e.g., doxycycline) can be given concurrently to shorten the needed course of quinine, which is often poorly tolerated. Seriously ill patients (parasitemia >2% to 3%, any signs of organ-system dysfunction) should initially be treated with intravenous quinidine in an intensive care unit. Other drugs that are generally effective for treatment, that are better tolerated than quinine but entail some risk of resistance and toxicity, include Fansidar, mefloquine (not approved for therapy in the United States), and halofantrine.

Typhoid

Approximately 500 cases of typhoid are reported per year in the United States, mostly in travelers and immigrants. Travelers with extended stays or those who have difficulty complying with standard dietary precautions are at particular risk. Typhoid is caused by *Salmonella typhi*, which is acquired from contaminated food or water, but some other *Salmonella* species may cause similar systemic illnesses. After a variable incubation period, usually 1 to 2 weeks, fever is the presenting symptom, often accompanied by headache and abdominal pain. Without therapy, the illness can progress to involve serious complications, including intestinal hemorrhage and perforation; the mortality rate is 10% to 15%.

The diagnosis of typhoid is made by the isolation of *Salmonella typhi* from blood, stool, or urine. An early diagnostic workup is important, as blood cultures are positive in 90% of patients in the first week of illness but are positive in only 50% after 3 to 4 weeks. Stool cultures may typically be negative early in the illness, but they are more likely to be positive after a number of weeks. With increasing worldwide antibiotic resistance, trimethoprim-sulfamethoxazole or a fluoroquinolone should generally be used empirically for suspected typhoid, and the sensitivity pattern of the infecting organism should guide definitive therapy. With appropriate early therapy, typhoid uncommonly progresses to severe complications or death.

Arboviral and Animal-Transmitted Viral Infections

Dengue fever is a fairly common infection in travelers and has been increasing in many areas, including Mexico, the Caribbean, and Central and South America, in recent years. Four dengue serotypes are distributed in tropical areas worldwide and are principally transmitted by *Aedes aegypti* mosquitoes, which are common in urban areas. Dengue fever has an incubation period of 2 to 7 days, followed by an illness characterized by fever, malaise, severe frontal headache, and joint and muscle pain. Gastrointestinal and respiratory symptoms may develop. A maculopapular rash typically appears 3 to 5 days after the onset of fever and spreads from the trunk to the face and extremities. Diagnosis can be made based on serologic examination. No treatment is available, but dengue fever is generally self-limited, with resolution of the acute illness after about 1 week. Dengue hemorrhagic fever, a severe illness that often includes shock and hemorrhage, usually occurs in individuals with prior immunity to a serotype other than that causing the acute infection. Because travelers are unlikely to have a prior history of dengue infection, presentation with hemorrhagic fever is rare in this group.

Other arboviral infections are rare in travelers but should be considered in immunization strategies and in differential diagnoses of returning travelers with unusual illnesses. Yellow fever is a severe, often fatal febrile illness transmitted by *Aedes* and other mosquitoes in South America and Africa. Japanese encephalitis virus, which is transmitted by *Culex* mosquitoes, causes many asymptomatic infections, but it also causes fatal encephalitis in East Asia from Japan to India, primarily in rural, rice-growing areas. Between 1978 and 1992, 24 cases of Japanese encephalitis, many of which were fatal, occurred in expatriates residing in Asia. Rift Valley fever virus is transmitted by mosquitoes in eastern and southern Africa and causes a febrile illness that is usually benign but can be complicated by blinding ophthalmologic complications, fulminant hepatitis, and fatal encephalitis. Numerous other uncommon hemmorhagic fever viruses are transmitted by mosquitoes and ticks. Other systemic febrile syndromes can be transmitted directly by infected animals. Hemorrhagic fever with renal syndrome is caused by a number of hantaviruses transmitted by the excreta of rodents, most commonly in Asia.

Viral Hepatitis

Hepatitis A is the most common serious illness in travelers that is nearly fully preventable by immunization. In developing countries nearly all of the population is infected by the hepatitis A virus in childhood, usually as an asymptomatic infection. In developed countries, most adults have not been infected with hepatitis A virus and therefore remain at high risk of infection when they travel in areas of high prevalence. Although the risk of infection is greatest for those with protracted stays in rural areas and those not following standard enteric precautions, infection of travelers taking appropriate precautions in major tourist areas is not uncommon. Transmission may occur by person-to-person contact or from contaminated water or food.

Hepatitis B, C, and D viruses are all transmitted by the parenteral route and thus do not generally pose very high risks for travelers. However, rates of hepatitis B antigenemia are very high in some developing areas, where more than 50% of adults may have been infected with the virus. Individuals participating in health care activities and those who are sexually active with new partners while traveling should be vaccinated. Hepatitis C, though less contagious, is transmitted by the same routes as hepatitis B. Hepatitis D, caused by an incomplete virus that requires hepatitis B infection for its propagation, is a risk in individuals with acute or chronic hepatitis B virus infection.

Hepatitis E is a newly described enterically transmitted viral hepatitis with an incubation period of 4 to 8 weeks. As with hepatitis A infection, the disease is usually self-limited and there is no progression to chronic hepatitis. Progression to fulminant hepatitis may be more common with hepatitis E than with other viral hepatitides (reportedly 1% to 2% of patients), and this risk is particularly high in pregnant women. Outbreaks of hepatitis E have been described in many developing countries, including India, the Middle East, Subsaharan Africa, South Asia, and Mexico. Diagnosis is made based on serologic examination; an IgM antibody signifies acute infection.

All of the viral hepatitides can present similarly, with malaise, fatigue, anorexia, and fever, progressing to abdominal symptoms and often jaundice. Diagnosis in a classic case is not difficult, but early stages of hepatitis may resemble other nonspecific febrile illnesses commonly presenting in travelers.

Other Protozoan Infections

A febrile illness including bloody diarrhea or abdominal pain should lead to the consideration of amebiasis, which is transmitted by contaminated food or water, and which can cause severe colitis and extraintestinal abscesses, particularly in the liver. Diagnosis is made by identifiying ova of *Entamoeba histolytica* in stool or, for nonintestinal infections, by serologic testing. Treatment is with metronidazole, which eliminates tissue trophozoites, and iodoquinol or paromomycin to eliminate intestinal cysts. Free-living amoebae *(Naegleria, Acanthamoeba),* which are usually acquired from contact with warm fresh water, can rarely cause severe neurologic infections, which are usually fatal.

Leishmaniasis, transmitted by sand flies, presents either with a chronic skin ulcer (cutaneous leishmaniasis) or a febrile wasting syndrome with hepatosplenomegaly and anemia (visceral leishmaniasis or kala-azar). Both syndromes, which are caused by different leishmanial species, occur in many regions of the developing world and may present many months after the initial infection. Cutaneous leishmaniasis from the New World can also be complicated in some areas by destructive mucosal infections that often appear long after the initial skin ulcer. A new syndrome, viscerotropic leishmaniasis, was recently identified in American soldiers who, after stays in the Persian Gulf region, had relatively mild signs and symptoms of visceral leishmaniasis caused by species that usually cause only cutaneous disease. Travelers to the Middle East may be at risk for this syndrome. Treatment for leishmaniasis is usually with sodium stibogluconate, a fairly toxic drug requiring a 20-day course of parenteral therapy.

Trypanosomal infections are uncommon in travelers but can occur in those traveling to rural areas. African trypanosomiasis, transmitted by the tsetse fly, presents with a painful bite wound and a febrile illness lasting approximately a week. This illness is followed by a severe acute (West African trypanosomiasis) or chronic (East African trypanosomiasis) illness that often includes neurologic and myocardial dysfunction. American trypanosomiasis (Chagas' disease), transmitted by reduviid bugs, presents with a painful bite wound and usually no systemic symptoms. Chronic asymptomatic infection then ensues for years to decades, followed by the signs of severe myocardial or smooth muscle dysfunction. Unfortunately, the available drugs for African (suramin, melarsoprol) and American (nitrofurtimox) trypanosomiasis are highly toxic and of quite low efficacy.

Helminth Infections

Infections with a number of helminths, although considered exotic when encountered in the United States, are extremely common in developing countries. The finding of eosinophilia in a returned traveler is suggestive of infection with a tissue-invasive helminth. A number of roundworms, including *Ascaris, Trichuris,* and hookworms may be isolated from the stool of returning travelers, but they uncommonly cause disease at the low parasite densities generally present in these individuals. *Strongyloides stercoralis* differs from the other helminths in that it can complete its life cycle in the human host and thus multiply to high numbers through autoinfection. *Strongyloides* may cause diarrhea or perirectal itching years after a traveler has returned from the tropics. It can cause much more severe disease, with multiorgan involvement and gram-negative bacteremia, if an individual is in an immunocompromised state because of steroid use, AIDS, or other factors either at the time of infection or at some later time. *Trichinella spiralis* causes trichinosis, which is acquired by ingesting larvae in undercooked meat, and presents with intestinal symptoms followed by fever, periorbital edema, petechiae, and occasionally severe multiorgan involvement. Roundworms are treated with mebendazole except for strongyloidiasis and trichinosis, which are treated with thiabendazole.

Acute tapeworm infections, acquired though the ingestion of undercooked meat or fish containing larvae, are usually not medically serious. However, two syndromes can present long after the ingestion of ova of the pork tapeworm *Taenia solium* (cysticercosis) or echinococcal animal tapeworms (hydatid disease). Cysticercosis presents most commonly with neurologic sequelae, including seizures; cysts can be visualized on CT scans. Echinococcosis presents with symptoms related to the presence of massive cysts in the liver or other organs. Intestinal tapeworm infections and cysticercosis are treated with praziquantel. Echinococcosis is treated with albendazole and, when possible, surgical removal of the cyst.

Disease from a number of trematodes can occur in travelers. Schistosomiasis is contracted when swimming or wading in fresh water in tropical areas. Manifestations in travelers include swimmer's itch, a pruritic rash that occurs when cercariae invade the skin, and acute schistosomiasis (Katayama fever), a febrile syndrome coinciding with larval migration (2 to 10 weeks after infection), which occasionally causes severe manifestations, including neurologic abnormalities, in travelers. The inflammatory changes of the mesenteric or bladder vasculature and their sequellae caused by chronic schistosomal infection are rare in travelers. Other trematodes that may occasionally present in travelers are the liver flukes *Clonorchis sinensis* and *Opisthorchis,* which are transmitted by raw fish principally in East Asia; the liver fluke *Fasciola hepatica,* which is transmitted worldwide by raw watercress contaminated by sheep or cattle excreta; the lung fluke *Paragonimus westermani,* which is transmitted by raw crab in Asia and Africa; and a number of intestinal flukes that are transmitted by raw water vegetables or fish, mostly in Asia. Trematode infections are generally treated with praziquantel.

Filarial infections may be a common cause of eosinophilia in travelers, but they rarely progress to severe disease, probably because of the limited organism load in most infected travelers. Lymphatic filariasis, caused by *Wucheria bancrofti* and *Brugia* species in many tropical areas, is transmitted by night-biting mosquitoes. Patients seek health care, usually after an extended stay in the tropics, with lymphangitis progressing to lymphatic obstruction and its sequellae. *Onchocerca volvulus* causes river blindness in Africa and Central and South America. This infection is tranmitted by *Simulium* blackflies, which breed in fast-flowing water. Infected individuals have a pruritic rash or conjunctivitis, and chronic infection can progress to blindness. Loa loa, which is transmitted by deerflies and horseflies in Africa, presents most commonly with pruritic skin nodules. Diagnosis of filarial infections, which can be difficult, involves identifying microfilariae in blood or infected tissues. Treatment is also difficult because the agents used (diethylcarbamazine, ivermectin) may not kill all forms of infecting parasites but may cause significant host toxicity from dying organisms.

Sexually Transmitted Diseases

Sexually transmitted diseases are a problem worldwide, but travelers may be at increased risk due to changes in personal behavior that may occur during travel and to differences in risk groups for certain infections in different countries. The human immunodeficiency virus is very common in young adults in much of Africa and parts of Latin America and Asia. The prevalence of infection continues to rise at an alarming rate in many developing countries. Individuals in the well-known American risk groups (injection drug users, homosexual men) but also all heterosexually active young adults, are at high risk of contracting HIV infection while traveling. Acute HIV infection typically presents with fever, malaise, headache, lymphadenopathy, pharyngitis, and rash beginning some weeks after the initial infection and lasting for 2 to 4 weeks.

Well-known sexually transmitted diseases such as gonorrhea, chlamydia, herpes simplex virus infection, and syphilis are common in most developing countries. In addition, diseases that are little seen in the United States, including chancroid, lymphogranuloma venereum, and granuloma inguinale are common in many areas. Chancroid, which is caused by *Haemophilus ducreyi* and is more common than syphilis in some regions, presents with painful genital ulcers and is treated with erythromycin. Lymphogranuloma venereum, caused by specific strains of *Chlamydia trachomatis,* is endemic in many developing countries. It presents as marked inguinal lymphadenopathy following a minor genital lesion and is treated with tetracyclines or erythromycin. Granuloma inguinale, caused by *Calymmatobacterium granulomatis,* has a sporadic endemicity in the tropics; it presents with painless, nodular genital lesions and is treated with tetracyclines.

PRETRAVEL ADVICE

Because individuals traveling to developing countries will be at risk of numerous bothersome and dangerous infectious problems, appropriate counseling before travel is very important. Such counseling should go beyond the simple provision of required vaccines and should include a detailed discussion of risks and the means by which these risks can be minimized. Up-to-date information regarding appropriate malaria prophylaxis, immunizations, and other precautions for all travel destinations is available from the Centers for Disease Control and Prevention in an annually published book (*Health Information for International Travel*), through a telephone hotline ([404] 332-4559) and via the World Wide Web (http://www.cdc.gov).

Prevention of Enteric Infections

Where the safety of tap water is questionable, as is the case in most of the tropics, it should be avoided. Canned or bottled carbonated beverages, beer and wine, and coffee and tea made from boiling water are generally safe. Uncarbonated bottled water may not be safe. Ice should be avoided, as it is usually made from tap water. Water can be treated by a number of methods. Vigorous boiling provides the greatest safety, but it is often impractical. Disinfection with iodine (tincture of iodine or tetraglycine hydroperiodide) will eliminate most pathogens, but *Cryptosporidium* cysts will not be destroyed. Commercial portable filters are convenient and probably very effective in removing bacteria and parasites but not viruses, although their effectiveness has not been well studied.

Precautions to avoid enteric infections from food include the avoidance of salads and uncooked, unpeeled fruit and vegetables; the avoidance of unpasteurized dairy products, including cheese; and the assurance that cooked meals are served very hot. Undercooked or raw meat, fish, and shellfish should be avoided. Food from street vendors is also at higher risk of containing enteric pathogens than is that served in restaurants or private homes.

Bismuth subsalicylate offers moderate (approximately 65%) protection against traveler's diarrhea when taken with meals four times a day. A number of antibiotics have been shown to prevent 80% to 90% of cases of traveler's diarrhea. The use of these agents for the prophylaxis of traveler's diarrrhea is not generally recommended, however, because of the potential toxicity of drug therapy and possible effects of widespread antibiotic use on bacterial resistance patterns. For short-term travel (less than 3 weeks) when diarrhea would be intolerable, however, the use of bismuth subsalicylate or an antibiotic (usually a fluoroquinolone at once-daily dosing) for the prophylaxis of traveler's diarrhea may be appropriate. Individuals taking prophylactic medications should understand that they remain at risk for diarrhea, and so should follow all of the precautions listed earlier.

Prevention of Malaria and Other Vector-Borne Diseases

Because drug resistance has limited the utility of all available antimalarial drugs, and because numerous other infections are transmitted by arthropods, it is essential that patients be counselled about the avoidance of insect bites. Malaria is transmitted by anopheline mosquitoes, which bite in the evening and at night, and, with the exception of Africa and parts of India, are primarily a problem in rural areas. Other important vectors, including nonanopheline mosquitoes (dengue, yellow fever, lymphatic filariasis), sand flies (leishmaniasis), tsetse flies (African trypanosomiasis), reduviid bugs (American trypanosomiasis), blackflies (onchocerciasis), and deerflies and horseflies (Loa loa) may bite day or night. Measures to prevent insect bites include wearing long-sleeved clothing, using insect repellants and insecticides, and sleeping under mosquito netting when window screens are not available. Permethrin insect repellants can be used on clothing and bedding. Permethrin-treated bednets have been shown to significantly limit malaria transmission in Africa. Topically administered repellants should contain diethylmethylbenzamide (DEET), though concentrations above 30% are not recommended because of potential toxicity to humans.

Chemoprophylaxis for malaria is no longer simple, because resistance of malaria parasites to chloroquine and other drugs is now widespread (Table 247-2). For areas without reported drug resistance (Central America above the Panama Canal, Haiti, the Middle East) chloroquine remains safe and effective. For areas with chloroquine-resistant falciparum malaria, mefloquine is recommended by the Centers for Disease Control and Prevention. This drug is generally effective, but its use can be complicated by central nervous system toxicity, including seizures and personality changes, and it may also fail because of the presence of resistant parasites in some areas. In

Table 247-2 Chemoprophylaxis of malaria*

DRUG	REGIMEN	NOTE
Areas without chloroquine resistance		
Chloroquine	500 mg weekly	Safe in pregnancy
Areas with chloroquine resistance		
Mefloquine	250 mg weekly	First-line regimen recommended by CDC; occasional neurologic toxicities
Chloroquine and Proguanil†	500 mg weekly 200 mg daily	A reasonable alternative to mefloquine in many areas, though resistance is common, especially in Southeast Asia
Doxycycline	200 mg daily	Especially for regions of Southeast Asia with multidrug resistance; photosensitivity and GI toxicity common

*Recommendations may change, because resistance to all available drugs is increasing. Travelers to remote areas should consider carrying effective therapy (quinine, Fansidar, or mefloquine) for use if they develop a febrile illness and cannot reach medical attention quickly. For all of these drugs, begin 1 to 2 weeks before and continue for 4 weeks after travel.
†Not available in the United States but widely available in other countries.

Southeast Asia, where resistance is greatest, doxycycline appears to be effective in preventing malaria. Doxycycline requires daily administration and may be limited by gastrointestinal toxicity and photosensitivity. In those who cannot tolerate mefloquine, another regimen that is advocated for many areas (but not Southeast Asia) is the combination of chloroquine and proguanil, which is not available in the United States but is widely available and used in other countries. For travelers to remote areas, it may be prudent to carry an effective treatment for resistant malaria (quinine, Fansidar, or mefloquine) for use when a serious febrile illness develops and medical attention is not available.

Other General Precautions

Travelers should be counseled to avoid swimming or wading in fresh water; most bodies of fresh water in the tropics are contaminated with schistosomes, and risks of leptospirosis and primary amebic meningoencephalitis are present in some areas. Swimming in seawater does not entail these risks, but some areas may be contaminated with fecal material. Travelers should not walk barefoot in any area potentially contaminated by animal or human feces; this will reduce the risk for the transmission of cutaneous larva migrans, hookworm infections, or strongyloidiasis by the invasion of bare skin by infecting larvae. Rabies remains a common infection in many developing countries. Close contact with wild and unvaccinated domestic animals should be avoided.

Immunizations

The specific travel plans, activities, and health status of a traveler must be considered in making specific vaccine recommendations (Table 247-3). Those without a history of tetanus immunization should be fully immunized, and all individuals should have received a booster within 10 years. For individuals traveling to remote areas, giving a tetanus booster every 5 years may be considered, because with this schedule even a dirty wound does not require a booster, which may be difficult to obtain while traveling. Primary polio vaccination in adults is with the inactivated vaccine. For previously vaccinated individuals, a single booster with either the inactivated or oral vaccine should be given once. For individuals born after 1956 and previously vaccinated for measles, mumps, and rubella, single measles and rubella boosters are indicated.

The most important new immunization for travelers is the hepatitis A vaccine, which became available in the United States in 1995, and which replaces immune globulin for almost all travelers. A single

Table 247-3   Immunizations for international travelers

VACCINE	INDICATION	DOSE
Recommended for nearly all travelers to developing countries		
Tetanus/diphtheria		
Primary series	Unimmunized adults	Doses at 0, 1, 6 months
Booster	All adults	One dose every 10 years
Measles/mumps/rubella	Susceptible individuals born after 1956	Two doses 1 month apart
Polio		
Inactivated polio vaccine (IPV)		
Primary series	Unimmunized adults	Doses at 0, 1, 6 months
Booster	Travelers	One dose (needed only once)
Oral polio vaccine (OPV)		
Primary series	Not recommended in adults	
Booster	Travelers	One dose (needed only once)
Hepatitis A	All travelers	Two doses 6 months apart
Recommended for certain travelers		
Typhoid	Extensive travel to rural areas; poor compliance with enteric guidelines	
Attenuated live (Ty 21a)		
Primary series		Four doses over 8 days
Booster		Repeat regimen every 5 years
Polysaccharide (Vi)		
Primary series		One dose
Booster		One dose every 2 years
Yellow fever	High-risk travel or requirement of vaccination	
Primary series		One dose
Booster		One dose every 10 years
Meningococcal	Travel to high-risk areas	One dose
Rabies	Significant exposure risk	
Primary series		Doses on days 0, 7, 28
Booster		One dose every 2 years
Japanese encephalitis	Extended travel to rural South Asia	Doses on days 0, 7, 30
Plague	Significant exposure risk	Doses at 0, 1, 3 to 6 months
Hepatitis B	Health care workers; sexually active adults	Doses at 0, 1, 6 months

dose of the vaccine provides fairly high levels of protection within 2 weeks and strong immunity within a month. A second dose 6 months later appears to provide long-term immunity; it is not yet clear whether additional booster doses of the vaccine will be needed. The only remaining indication for immune globulin in travelers is for those needing immunity to hepatitis A within less than 2 to 4 weeks of the time of vaccination.

Two new immunizations for typhoid have replaced an older, poorly tolerated whole cell vaccine. An oral attenuated *Salmonella typhi* (Ty 21a) vaccine has been available since 1990. A polysaccharide vaccine (Vi) that is administered parenterally became available in 1995. Both vaccines offer 50% to 80% efficacy in preventing typhoid and are well tolerated. Typhoid vaccination is not necessary for most travelers, but those who may not be able to follow enteric precautions and those with extended stays in developing countries should be vaccinated with either of the available new vaccines.

Travelers with protracted stays in high-risk areas should be considered for immunization against meningococcus (restricted areas of Subsaharan Africa and the Indian subcontinent), plague (primarily desert regions), and Japanese encephalitis (rural, rice-growing areas of South Asia). Health care workers and those who may be unable to follow appropriate recommendations regarding the avoidance of sexually transmitted diseases should be immunized against hepatitis B. Travelers working with animals should be vaccinated against rabies.

Yellow fever vaccination is required in a small number of countries for travelers entering directly from the United States, but a number of other countries require vaccination if an entering traveler first passes through an endemic area. Thus the traveler's full itinerary must be examined in making recommendations. Meningococcal vaccination is required only for those individuals traveling to Mecca, Saudi Arabia for the annual Hajj.

Smallpox has been eradicated, and vaccination is no longer required or available in any area. Cholera remains an important problem, but the poor efficacy and toxicity profile of the whole cell vaccine, which was previously heavily used, has led to its abandonment. Cholera vaccination is no longer required by any country. Careful en-

teric precautions, rather than immunization, should be relied on for the prevention of cholera in high-risk areas.

Advice for Pregnant and Immunocompromised Individuals

All immunizations are best completed before pregnancy. During pregnancy, live vaccines should be avoided, but immunizations that do not include live components are probably safe and can be used when indicated. When yellow fever vaccination is required, unless a pregnant patient's travel plans entail a considerable risk, she should obtain written documentation that this live vaccine is medically contraindicated.

Pregnant women should take particular care to follow enteric precautions while traveling. Extensive use of iodides to treat water should be avoided because of a theoretic risk of causing a fetal goiter. Chemoprophylaxis and treatment of diarrhea with bismuth subsalicylate or antibiotics should be avoided when possible, because the most effective drugs are generally not safe to use during pregnancy. Fluid and electrolyte replacement for diarrhea is of utmost importance.

Malaria is a particular concern in pregnant women because chemoprophylaxis is difficult, and falciparum malaria in pregnant women is often severe. Women should seriously consider whether travel during pregnancy to an area with chloroquine-resistant malaria is necessary. Assiduous measures to prevent nocturnal mosquito bites are very important. Chemoprophylaxis with both chloroquine and proguanil appears to be safe in pregnancy; a regimen combining these two drugs will be effective in many areas with chloroquine-resistant malaria but may commonly fail in Southeast Asia. Mefloquine is not recommended for chemoprophylaxis in pregnant women, although it is not known to be teratogenic, and is probably safe after the first trimester of pregnancy. For the treatment of malaria during pregnancy, the significant risk of malaria to mother and fetus far outweighs any potential risk of standard therapies.

Live-organism vaccines should be avoided in immunocompromised individuals. Certain infections are a much greater risk in indi-

---

BOX 247-2
Common infections in returning travelers
(listed by presentation)

Fever
Malaria
Typhoid
Dengue
Viral hepatitis
Acute HIV infection
Amebiasis
Tuberculosis
Brucellosis
Leptospirosis
Rickettsial illnesses
Other protozoans

Diarrhea
Enterotoxigenic *E. coli*
Shigella
Salmonella
Campylobacter
Aeromonas
Plesiomonas
Rotavirus
Norwalk agent
Giardia
Entamoeba histolytica
Cryptosporidium

Eosinophilia
Acute schistosomiasis
Strongyloidiasis
Filariasis
Ascariasis
Hookworms
Other helminths

BOX 247-3
Initial evaluation of illnesses in returned travelers

Fever
Blood smears
Blood cultures

Diarrhea
Stool culture
Stool ova and parasites

Eosinophilia
Stool ova and parasites
Serology or specific tests for helminths

---

viduals with AIDS, transplants, and other immunodeficiencies. These include cryptosporidiosis, which commonly causes severe unremitting diarrhea; leishmaniasis, which often presents as severe disseminated disease; tuberculosis, which more commonly progresses rapidly after infection to active disease; salmonellosis, which can cause chronic bacteremias; strongyloidiasis, which can cause hyperinfection with multiorgan failure and bacteremia; and endemic fungal infections (histoplasmosis and paracoccidioidomycosis in Latin America, *Penicillium* in Thailand), which very commonly disseminate.

EVALUATION OF HEALTH PROBLEMS AFTER INTERNATIONAL TRAVEL
Fever

Any febrile presentation may represent dangerous illnesses, and so the exact pattern or characteristics of the fever are generally not helpful. Most important is to rule out dangerous and treatable causes of fever, in particular malaria and typhoid (Box 247-2). Other common problems, such as dengue and viral hepatitis, are not specifically treatable, but a prompt diagnosis is helpful. The evaluation of a febrile returning traveler should include a careful physical examination and appropriate studies to rule out common causes of fever. Unless a straightforward explanation is found, it is necessary to rule out malaria with blood smears and typhoid with cultures of blood and stool (Box 247-3). Amebiasis, when not affecting the intestinal tract or liver, and early viral hepatitis may not present with typical localizing findings, and can be diagnosed serologically. Other illnesses presenting primarily with fever in travelers include dengue, acute schistosomiasis, acute HIV infection, primary tuberculosis, and, less commonly, numerous protozoan, helminthic, and viral infections discussed earlier. Additional bacterial infections to be considered in travelers with specific risks include melioidosis (Southeast Asia),

leptospirosis, brucellosis, rickettsial infections, bartonellosis (South America), plague, and relapsing fever.

Enteric Infections

Traveler's diarrhea lasts for more than a week in 10% of individuals, and so it quite commonly presents in returned travelers. Uncomplicated diarrhea without evidence of inflammatory changes (i.e., no fecal blood or leukocytes) can be treated with an antibiotic and an antimotility agent as discussed earlier. If fever or significant systemic symptoms are reported or if fecal blood or leukocytes are noted, stools should be evaluated with cultures and examination for parasites (Box 247-2). Presumptive treatment for bacterial enteritis with a fluoroquinolone is appropriate in most cases of inflammatory diarrhea; antimotility agents should be avoided. Evaluation for parasites is usually negative in these cases but may reveal *Entamoeba histolytica,* which can be treated with metronidazole, or *Cryptosporidium,* which unfortunately lacks an effective therapy.

Chronic diarrhea is common following travel. Evaluation for parasites is usually negative but may reveal giardiasis, which can be treated fairly successfully with metronidazole or paromomycin. If no cause of the diarrhea is identified or only parasites that are generally considered nonpathogens are identified, a therapeutic trial of metronidazole may be helpful. Chronic diarrhea with malabsorption and/or abdominal pain developing after a long stay in the tropics may represent tropical sprue, a disease of unknown etiology that responds to treatment with folate and tetracycline, or gastrointestinal tuberculosis. Imaging procedures and/or endoscopy are required for diagnosis. Many returned travelers express great concern regarding risks of intestinal parasitic infections. Stool evaluation for enteric parasites is often helpful to rule out these infections and thus reassure patients.

Eosinophilia

Unexplained eosinophilia in returned travelers is often due to infection with tissue-invasive helminths (Box 247-2). Other possible causes include tuberculosis, fungal infections, allergic diseases, malignancy, and collagen vascular diseases.

Helminths likely to cause eosinophilia include organisms that transiently migrate through tissue (*Ascaris,* hookworms, *Strongyloides,* visceral and cutaneous larva migrans), and those that live within tissue (schistosomes and other flukes, filariae, *Trichinella,* cysticercosis, echinococcosis). Unusual helminths that should be considered in travelers eating raw seafood, primarily in East Asia, include *Gnathostoma, Anisakis,* and *Angiostrongylus.* The specific symptoms that led to the evaluation for eosinophilia, the patient's specific travel history, and any physical findings should guide the initial evaluation (Box 247-3). Gastrointestinal symptoms suggest an intestinal parasite, which can usually be diagnosed by stool evaluation. Cutaneous pruritis or swellings suggest filariasis, which can be diagnosed by identifying microfilariae in blood or infected tissues. Serology can be helpful in early presentations of intestinal parasites that may not yet be excreting ova in the stool (e.g., acute schistosomiasis) and in unusual helminthic diseases.

✔ WHEN TO REFER

Specific advice for travelers regarding immunizations and malaria chemoprophylaxis can be obtained from the CDC (*Health Information for International Travel,* published annually; travelers' hotline: [404] 332-4559; World Wide Web site [http://www.cdc.gov]) or local health departments. Clinics specializing in travel medicine are also available in some areas. Patients presenting after travel with severe manifestations of malaria or other infections discussed in this chapter should be seen by an infectious diseases specialist. Patients with a persistent gastrointestinal illness and negative stool studies for bacteria and parasites should be evaluated by a gastroenterologist; endoscopic studies will often be helpful in diagnosing some difficult-to-diagnose infections (e.g., giardiasis, intestinal tuberculosis) and other conditions (e.g., tropical sprue, inflammatory bowel disease). Persistent febrile illnesses and symptomatic eosinophilia following travel warrant consultation with a specialist in infectious diseases.

BIBLIOGRAPHY

American College of Physicians Task Force on Adult Immunization and Infectious Diseases Society of America: *Guide for adult immunization,* Philadelphia, 1994, American College of Physicians.

Barry M, Bia F: Pregnancy and travel, *JAMA* 261:728-736, 1989.

Bradley DJ, Warhurst DC: Malaria prophylaxis: guidelines for travellers from Britain, *BMJ* 310:709-714, 1995.

Centers for Disease Control and Prevention: *Health information for international travel,* Washington, DC, US Government Printing Office, published annually.

Dupont HL, Ericsson CD: Prevention and treatment of traveler's diarrhea, *N Engl J Med* 328:1821-1827, 1993.

Gardner P et al: Adult immunizations, *Ann Intern Med* 12:35-40, 1996.

Wolfe M, editor: Travel medicine, *Med Clin North Am* 76:1261-1535, 1992.

Wyler DJ: Malaria chemoprophylaxis for the traveler, *N Engl J Med* 329:31-37, 1993.

CHAPTER

248 Acquired Immunodeficiency Syndrome

Julie Louise Gerberding and Merle A. Sande

In 1981 a group of homosexual men with an unusual presentation of Kaposi's sarcoma and *Pneumocystis carinii* pneumonia were identified in the United States. This cluster of cases proved to be the beginning of what has become an enormous pandemic. The term *AIDS* (acquired immunodeficiency syndrome) was defined by the Centers for Disease Control (CDC) to describe patients who lacked other causes for impaired immunity and who developed unusual malignancies, such as Kaposi's sarcoma, or opportunistic infections. It is now obvious that human immunodeficiency virus (HIV) is responsible for AIDS and a myriad of earlier and less severe manifestations of progressive immunodeficiency. This chapter describes the spectrum of disease associated with HIV infection.

ETIOLOGY AND PATHOPHYSIOLOGY

HIV (type 1) infection and the human diseases it causes appear to be new, although some studies have demonstrated antibodies to this retrovirus in sera obtained in Africa as early as the mid-1950s. HIV is found in many body fluids including blood, semen, saliva, vaginal secretions, and breast milk, either as free or cell-associated virus, and is transmissible by direct inoculation of any of these fluids. It is trophic for T-cell lymphocytes and other cells that possess CD4 surface receptors, including macrophages, promyelocytes, intestinal immuno-

cytes, astrocytes, oligodendrocytes, epidermal Langerhans' cells, and certain fibroblasts (Chapter 256).

The CD4 or helper T-cell is the critical target for HIV, and its destruction over time leads to the manifestations of immunodeficiency and the clinical disease known as AIDS. The CD4 cell is infected with HIV when activated (e.g., by cytokines), which results in expression of the CD4 receptor on its surface. The virus attaches to this receptor and is internalized, and its RNA is reverse-transcribed onto host DNA by an enzyme, reverse transcriptase (a target for antiretroviral drugs). The altered DNA is then transported to the nucleus, where it is integrated into the cell's genes by another enzyme (integrase). The virus may lie dormant in this integrated state, but when the cell is activated by external signals (e.g., foreign antigens, cytokines), the virus is activated by the host's normal activation processes. With the help of other viral enzymes, especially protease (another target for antiretroviral drugs), this results in the development of mature viral particles. It is thought that when these viruses are then released, the T-cell dies.

After initial inoculation, the virus most likely infects one of the local resident cells (usually dendritic cells), leading to release of cytokines and attraction and stimulation of lymphocytes, which in turn allows for expression of CD4 receptors and infection of these T-cells. It is likely that in some instances the infection is contained and aborted at this stage; lymphocytes from several groups of individuals exposed to infected secretions (via needlestick or vaginal intercourse) have been shown to have immunologic memory to HIV antigens, but these individuals did not develop progressive infection or antibody. In cases in which infection is established, the cells are apparently drained by regional lymph nodes, where an amplification of the cycle of immune stimulation, virus replication, and cell destruction with further infection of new T-cells occurs at increasing rates. During this phase of HIV infection, high titers of virus are released into the circulation, CD4 cells may drop transiently, and the patient may develop symptoms of a nonspecific viral infection like mononucleosis.

Within several weeks, the virus is cleared from the circulation in association with an immune response (antibodies as detected by enzyme-linked immunosorbent assay [ELISA] and Western Blot begin to appear) and the patient becomes asymptomatic. This symptom-free period may last for several years (average is 10.5 years, depending on the population); some so-called long-term persisters have been infected for 20 years and show no signs of symptoms or decline in numbers of CD4 cells. During this period of clinical latency the virus remains surprisingly active in the various lymph nodes throughout the body. It has been estimated that between a billion and a trillion viruses are generated each day, which is countered by the production of as many as a billion CD4 cells. The only clinical signs may be the presence of enlarged lymph nodes, so-called generalized lymphadenopathy. In time the virus wins the war: CD4 cell numbers begin to decline; the germinal centers in the enlarged lymph nodes are emptied, with resulting disappearance of the "adenopathy;" viral titers begin to increase in the bloodstream; and the patient becomes symptomatic (see later discussion). There are likely many unknown factors that determine the rate of disease progression, but several have been identified: the height of viral load during the initial infection with HIV correlates directly with disease progression, and the ability of the infecting strain to produce syncytial formation (fusion of infected and noninfected CD4 cells into giant cells) is associated with more rapid progression, as is the presence of various coinfections such as tuberculosis (perhaps by heightening the degree of T-cell activation).

The major manifestations of HIV infection (opportunistic infections and malignancies) are a consequence of the immune defects that result from destruction of helper T-cells (CD4 lymphocyte counts of less than 200/mm^3 are usually but not always associated with symptoms) and other target cells. Infection is also associated with a release of various lymphokines (likely resulting in many of the nonspecific symptoms of progressive HIV, including wasting) and nonspecific stimulation of B-cells (resulting in hypergammaglobulinemia).

EPIDEMIOLOGY

HIV infection is a global disease, and the pandemic is expected to spread to more than 50 million persons by the year 2000. Infection is transmitted by three main mechanisms: (1) sexually, through unprotected heterosexual or homosexual contact with an infected partner; (2) parenterally, by direct inoculation of infected blood (transfusion of blood products, sharing contaminated injection drug equipment, occupational injury among health care workers); and (3) perinatally, from infected mothers to their offspring. Early in the epidemic, infection appeared to be confined to individuals populating "high-risk groups." It is now clear, however, that activities leading to infection do not necessarily correlate with membership in just these risk groups, and it is more appropriate to assess HIV risk in terms of high-risk behaviors.

The importance of these risk behaviors in perpetuating the epidemic varies throughout the world. Three main epidemiologic patterns have been described by the World Health Organization. The first pattern predominates in developed countries, including the United States, and is primarily related to sexual transmission among homosexual men and contact with contaminated blood among injection drug users. The second pattern is evident in Africa, Latin America, and the Caribbean, where heterosexual and perinatal transmission predominate. In these areas, HIV has penetrated into the general population to such an extent that more than 20% of the adult population in some locales is seropositive, and the number of cases among women equals or exceeds that among men. The third pattern of transmission is seen in Asia, India, Eastern Europe, and the Pacific rim, where the epidemic became apparent in the late 1980s and has spread rapidly among sexually active heterosexual and homosexual adults and injection drug users. There is some evidence that genetic differences in viral strains isolated from these various geographic areas may be responsible in part for these unique epidemiologic characteristics.

A distinct but genetically related virus, HIV type 2 (HIV 2), is found in western Africa and has not yet spread extensively outside of this region. Although the clinical presentation and natural history of infection with HIV 2 are not as clearly defined as for HIV 1, HIV 2 does appear to be less transmissible from mother to fetus and less rapidly progressive than HIV 1. Otherwise the pathophysiology and outcome of infection with these two retroviruses appear to be similar. To date, the cases of HIV 2 infection in the United States have occurred predominantly in persons previously residing in HIV 2 endemic areas. Nevertheless, the blood supply is now screened with tests that detect infection with both agents.

It is difficult to determine factors that influence transmissibility, but some helpful information has accumulated. Among homosexual men, rectal receptive intercourse without condom protection, traumatic intercourse, and multiple sexual partners are factors highly correlated with transmission. Among intravenous drug users, exposure to contaminated blood via shared needles and contaminated drug paraphernalia increases transmission risk. Sexual transmission is also important in this population, especially when prostitution is practiced to finance drug use. With the advent of donor screening protocols recommended by the blood bank community, the current risk of acquiring HIV from blood transfusion in the United States is estimated to be less than 1/50,000 units transfused. Infected blood products such as clotting factor preparations were an important source of infection among hemophiliacs and other blood product recipients early in the epidemic, but these products are treated with a process proven to reliably inactivate HIV and other bloodborne pathogens. Unfortunately, transfusions continue to transmit HIV in the developing world where donor screening is not always available.

Children acquire HIV perinatally or from infected blood products. The exact mode(s) of perinatal transmission have not been clearly delineated, but treatment of the infected mother with an antiretroviral drug (zidovudine) during the third trimester and at delivery, and of the infant during the first 6 weeks of life reduces infection rates in affected infants from 25% to 8.3%. Breastfeeding is also a proven route of HIV transmission. Current recommendations in the United States argue against breastfeeding when maternal infection is documented, but this approach has not been advocated in developing countries where it is believed that the benefits of breastfeeding may outweigh the risks of HIV transmission.

Heterosexual partners of individuals in all risk categories have acquired HIV, but transmission appears to be more efficient from man to woman. About 40% of steady male sexual partners of infected women have HIV infection, whereas about 60% of female partners of infected men acquire the disease. The efficiency of sexual transmission is believed to increase in the presence of concomitant genital lesions such as chancroid, syphilitic chancres, and perhaps herpesvirus infections that disrupt the integrity of the mucosal barrier. In Africa, aggressive sexually transmitted disease (STD) intervention (early diagnosis and treatment) resulted in nearly a 50% reduction in HIV transmission. Treatment of certain STDs has been shown to markedly reduce HIV viral RNA in semen. Lack of circumcision in Africa is also associated with an increased risk of infection, but this is not established with certainty in the United States.

There is no evidence to suggest that HIV is spread by casual contact, by the airborne route, by insects, by direct exposure to tears or saliva, or by environmental contamination. People having nonsexual household contact with infected individuals do not acquire HIV.

Occupational transmission to health care workers is now well documented and poses a challenge to those responsible for providing care to the increasing number of infected patients. Prospective studies of providers who sustained exposure to HIV through needlesticks or similar percutaneous injuries demonstrate that the magnitude of overall risk is 0.2% to 0.3%. However, certain factors markedly increase transmission risk, such as exposure to large volumes of blood (injections, large-bore hollow needles, deep penetration) or exposure to blood containing high titers of HIV (e.g., source patients with advanced stages of HIV infection). The risk may be less when the exposure involves minimal amounts of blood (superficial injuries, suture needlesticks, needles passing through gloves before contacting the skin) or when the source patient has early stages of HIV infection and is not highly viremic. It has now been shown that postexposure administration of an antiretroviral agent (zidovudine) to the health-care worker reduces the risk of acquiring HIV infection by 80%. The risk from contamination of mucous membranes or nonintact skin is too low to be reliably quantified in the studies that have been performed to date, but most authorities agree that these exposures are less risky than percutaneous exposures unless prolonged contact with relatively large volumes of blood occurs via a break in the integument or some other portal of entry.

CLINICAL STAGES OF HIV INFECTION
Acute Viral Syndrome

A majority of patients (but not all) infected with HIV develop an acute mononucleosis-like illness characterized by fever, headache, lymphadenopathy, pharyngitis, macular rash, and malaise within one to several weeks of exposure. Aseptic meningitis, hepatosplenomegaly, extreme fatigue, weakness, arthralgias, and myalgias are also frequently associated with this syndrome. Heterophile and monospot tests are negative, but atypical lymphocytes may be present on peripheral blood smear. Symptoms usually resolve within 2 to 4 weeks, but rapid progression with early development of an AIDS-defining condition has been described. The acute illness is temporally associated with seroconversion and high titer viremia. Some authorities have speculated that this illness could also be caused by lymphokines released during nonspecific activation of multiple clones of lymphocytes by HIV antigens that behave as superantigens.

HIV infection should be suspected in any person at risk who has an unexplained febrile viral-like illness. Initially, HIV screening tests may not demonstrate antibody. However, tests for viral RNA (branched DNA or quantitative pcr assays) or viral antigens (p24 antigen) will invariably demonstrate evidence of HIV. Data now exist that suggest that the height of this viral load correlates with the eventual rate of progression of disease, and some authorities suggest that treatment of the acute disease with antiretroviral agents might "reset the thermostat" by reducing viral burden and thus slow overall progression to AIDS.

Persistent Generalized Lymphadenopathy

Lymphadenopathy, defined in this setting as enlargement of the lymph nodes in at least two extrainguinal sites for a minimum of 3 months in the absence of any illness or drug known to cause lymphadenopathy, is usually present and, as noted earlier, results from the massive viral replication and immunologic response (lymphocyte recruitment and proliferation). Biopsy reveals reactive hyperplasia and expansion of germinal centers. The presence of persistent lymphadenopathy does not influence prognosis; however, a decrease in the size of the involved nodes correlates with the onset of AIDS and portends a poor prognosis.

Symptomatic Infection

Nonspecific complaints of fever, weight loss, diarrhea, and malaise; lymphadenopathy; and oral thrush are frequently noted in patients who have been infected with HIV for more than 5 years and whose CD4 counts are generally dropping toward 200/mm^3 or below. In the past, these symptoms and signs defined a condition known as AIDS-related complex (ARC), but now once the CD4 count reaches 200/mm^3, patients are classified as having AIDS.

A distinct subgroup of patients with CD4 counts at any level develop immune thrombocytopenic purpura (ITP), which is clinically similar to ITP in other patients. Although platelet counts less than 50,000 are common, bleeding is rare unless drugs adversely affecting platelet function are administered. Optimal treatment for AIDS-related ITP remains controversial. Platelet counts improve after antiretroviral therapy with zidovudine is instituted in some patients; others seem to benefit from corticosteroids. Splenectomy is rarely necessary.

Diseases suggestive of modest immune deficiency, such as dermatomal varicella zoster infection, chronic herpes simplex lesions, cutaneous fungal infections, and oral leukoplakia portend progression to AIDS-defining infections. Recurrent infection with encapsulated bacteria and nontyphoid *Salmonella* species also occurs in these patients. The risk of reactivating tuberculosis is increased to >30% (Chapter 273). Tuberculosis may present as upper lobe pulmonary disease in HIV-infected patients with high CD4 counts, but with increasing immunosuppression, disseminated diseases with adenopathy, soft, diffuse, small, nodular pulmonary infiltrates, and bacillemia are more likely.

The diagnosis of AIDS is readily established when the patient has obvious manifestations such as Kaposi's sarcoma or *P. carinii* pneumonia. In many patients, however, the initial symptoms and signs are subtle and necessitate careful evaluation to establish a definitive diagnosis. The CDC surveillance definition of the syndrome was initially based solely on clinical manifestations; it was later expanded to incorporate HIV antibody positivity as a requirement in certain instances, and now it includes CD4 lymphocyte counts as criteria for diagnosis.

Onset of AIDS may be gradual or abrupt. In most patients a history of prodromal symptoms is elicited for variable periods before diagnosis. Some patients present with isolated Kaposi's sarcoma lesions and no evidence of prodrome or opportunistic infection; overall they have a better short-term prognosis than those who have opportunistic infections or neurologic disease.

A rational approach to evaluating individuals with suspected HIV disease has several objectives: (1) to diagnose HIV infection at an early point at which medical intervention is effective, (2) to establish the presence and severity of immune deficiency, (3) to exclude other causes of the clinical findings, (4) to identify preventable and/or treatable components of the illness, and (5) to diagnose life-threatening complications expediently. No single protocol can be provided to accomplish these objectives in all patients, but the following general approach can be individualized.

DIAGNOSING HIV INFECTION

In the AIDS era, it is essential to incorporate a careful history to elicit information about risk behaviors for acquiring HIV infection into the routine medical history for all adult patients. Sufficient information should be sought to accurately assess risk from sexual practices, recreational drug use, and blood product transfusions. All patients for whom HIV infection cannot be excluded with reasonable certainty on the basis of history should be offered HIV testing, or at the very least, should be referred to appropriate community resources for such testing. History alone is an unreliable method for excluding HIV infection; many patients are reluctant to disclose risk behaviors, and

many (especially women) may not realize that their sexual partners are at risk for infection.

Pretest counseling should assess individual risk, provide risk reduction education, and explain the importance of testing and the meaning of a positive and a negative test. Third-party risks should also be addressed. The procedures for recording test results and protecting the patient's confidentiality are also important components of this process.

Licensed tests for HIV use three general techniques for detection of the antibody: ELISA, IFA (immunofluorescent assay), and Western Blot. The commercially available ELISA tests are extremely sensitive but relatively nonspecific, whereas the IFA and Western Blot are more specific but are more labor intensive and expensive to perform. The ELISA tests are useful screening tests; the Western Blot or IFA is then used as a confirmatory test for repeatedly reactive ELISA-positive serum. Using this protocol, HIV testing is one of the most accurate laboratory procedures currently available. Rapid tests for HIV antibody are not yet in widespread use, but they may prove useful in settings where delays in obtaining test results are problematic. These rapid tests are very sensitive but lack specificity. Thus they are most useful in excluding the diagnosis of HIV infection, but positive results should be confirmed with conventional tests.

Although a negative antibody test does not exclude the diagnosis of HIV, it makes it extremely unlikely unless the individual has been exposed in the previous 6 months. If the patient believes exposure has occurred, a repeat test should be offered 3 to 6 months later. Although documented cases of delayed seroconversion (after 1 year) have appeared, this phenomenon is rare, and the vast majority of patients will have antibody within 6 months of initial infection. Antibody to HIV may disappear in the preterminal phases of the disease in some patients.

Two serum tests for quantitation of viral activity are currently available that will be useful for establishing diagnosis of infection before antibody is detectable (during acute infection) and have changed the way that patients are managed after diagnosis. The branched DNA assay detects viral RNA that is released into the bloodstream (probably from the lymph nodes), which correlates with total body viral replication. It is highly sensitive (down to 500 copies of RNA/ml) and employs a method of magnifying the signal used to detect the RNA. The quantitative polymerase chain reaction (PCR) is similarly sensitive and employs the PCR method of multiplying the RNA itself to detectable levels. Both tests give quantitative measures of viral replication and are remarkably consistent from day to day. The measure of viral RNA in serum has been shown to correlate remarkably well with rate of progression of disease, especially in patients with >300 CD4 cells/mm^3, and is being touted as a more useful measure than CD4 count for determining when to start antiretroviral therapy and for monitoring therapeutic effect.

Posttest counseling should include an assessment of mental status (especially if a positive test result was obtained), an explanation of the meaning of the result, a review of third-party risks and confidentiality procedures, appropriate referral for psychologic support and drug rehabilitation if needed, and a follow-up appointment. If a positive result is returned from a patient at low risk, testing should be repeated. Those at increased risk but not already infected should be referred for relevant programs to reduce behavioral risks.

INITIAL EVALUATION AND MANAGEMENT OF THE INFECTED PATIENT

A comprehensive medical evaluation should be performed for all newly diagnosed patients with HIV infection. The history should include assessment of general health status; immunizations, drug, and medication history; sexual history (including obstetric and gynecologic information in women); and assessment of travel, geographic, and occupational exposures that increase the risks of specific opportunistic infections. The physical examination should document initial height and weight and include a careful funduscopic, oral, lymphatic, cutaneous, and genital examination (including pelvic examination with Pap smear).

Laboratory studies are helpful in establishing the presence of immune dysfunction and overall health status. The CD4 lymphocyte count provides essential prognostic information and is necessary to guide medical interventions. However, significant diurnal variation in CD4 count is well documented, and results can vary among laboratories. Many clinicians recommend repeating CD4 counts when they are used as the sole criterion for clinical decisions. In some cases, measuring the CD4 cell count as a percentage of total lymphocyte count is a more useful index of immunosuppression. A measure of viral RNA (see earlier discussion) is of value in determining viral activity and making decisions about therapy. Nonspecific markers of disease progression include elevated erythrocyte sedimentation rate and β-2-microglobulin, but these tests have largely been rendered obsolete by more specific CD4 count and viral RNA quantitation.

Hematologic abnormalities are common in HIV infection and may be multifactorial. A decreased white blood cell count ($<3000/mm^3$) is often seen, usually with concomitant absolute lymphopenia ($<1500/mm^3$). Lymphopenia may correlate with the immune suppression. Thrombocytopenia may be induced by antiplatelet antibodies as in ITP (see earlier discussion). In addition, many of the chemotherapeutic and other therapeutic agents administered to patients are toxic to the bone marrow. The bone marrow should be examined if the etiology is in doubt since disseminated fungal, *Mycobacterium tuberculosis*, and *Mycobacterium avium-intracellulare* infection and lymphoma can be associated with pancytopenias and can be detected in the bone marrow.

Minor abnormalities in liver function tests are not uncommon. Alkaline phosphatase elevation is the most common and correlates with cytomegalovirus infection but is also increased in AIDS cholangiopathy and various infiltrative diseases of the liver (MAI, mTb, fungal infections, peliosis hepatis caused by *Bartonella* infection, and lymphoma). Serum lactate dehydrogenase enzyme may be increased, and many clinicians obtain this test at the time of initial evaluation so that the baseline value can be compared to that obtained when pneumocystic pneumonia is later suspected. A polyclonal gammopathy is typically present. A serologic test for syphilis, antitoxoplasma IgG titer, and a chest radiograph are also advisable.

Most but not all AIDS patients are anergic when a battery of at least four intradermal skin tests for delayed hypersensitivity is applied. A smaller proportion of those with earlier stages of infection are anergic, and purified protein derivative (PPD) testing is routine for all patients. Those with a PPD response greater than 5 mm and those exposed to active cases of tuberculosis are at high risk for active disease and should be given isoniazid prophylaxis, regardless of age.

Initial health care maintenance is directed toward improving overall health status. Nutrition, smoking cessation, drug rehabilitation, safer sex, and psychosocial issues should be explored. Reproductive counseling is extremely important and all too often is overlooked. Pneumococcal vaccine, influenza vaccine (annually), hepatitis B vaccine (especially if the patient is sexually active or sharing needles), and hemophilus B vaccine are recommended. Although the response to these vaccines declines as immunodeficiency develops, a proportion of patients will achieve protective titers and immunization is strongly encouraged. There is evidence that immunization may transiently increase viral RNA levels, but currently no information exists that this significantly accelerates disease progression.

Antiretroviral Therapy

The indications for antiretroviral therapy have undergone dramatic changes in recent years, and recommendations for their use remain in flux. Numerous new therapies have been introduced since 1996; their dosages, side effects, toxicities, and drug interactions are listed in Table 248-1. In addition, the development of sensitive quantitative assays of viral load have now made it possible to measure directly the influence of the therapies on the virus itself. Updated references should be consulted for current treatment recommendations, but the following treatment principles are accepted by most experts:

1. Serum viral RNA levels are predictive of disease progression and are more valuable than CD4 counts for determining when to initiate therapy and for monitoring antiviral effectiveness.
2. The goal of antiviral treatment is to reduce viral RNA levels to below the level of detection (or at least as low as possible) for as long as possible.

3. Combination therapy (use of two or more antiviral drugs) is now recommended to obtain maximal antiviral treatment effect and to reduce the emergence of drug-resistant HIV isolates; monotherapy (single drug regimens) should be avoided.
4. Drug combinations that include two reverse transcriptase inhibitors and a protease inhibitor are the most likely to produce a sustained antiviral effect and lower viral levels below the level of detection.
5. Strict adherence to the antiviral treatment regimen is essential to obtain the desired benefit and to avoid the emergence of drug resistance and clinical failure.
6. None of the HIV antiviral drugs has been proved to be safe for use in pregnant women (FDA Category A). However, treatment to prevent perinatal HIV transmission is recommended. Updated guidelines are expected when data from recent clinical trials become available.

The optimal time to initiate therapy has not been firmly established for all stages of HIV disease. For now, the following approach is recommended.

1. The optimal time to initiate treatment is when the patient is willing to adhere to the treatment regimen.
2. The initial regimen should include three drugs (two reverse transcriptase inhibitors and a protease inhibitor).
3. Treatment is definitely recommended for patients with AIDS, CD4 counts >500, rapidly declining CD4 counts, or viral load greater than 10,000. Some experts recommend treating patients with any detectable serum viral RNA.
4. Treatment of initial infection to lower the total body viral load and improve long-term outcomes is recommended by many experts, but data to prove the long-term clinical benefit of this approach are not available.

The quantitative viral RNA level should be measured 3 to 8 weeks after initiating therapy. If the viral RNA has not decreased by at least a log or become nondetectable, then the treatment is failing and another regimen should be employed. When changing regimens, at least two new drugs should be used.

If the patient responds to treatment, tolerates the regimen, and remains asymptomatic with stable CD4 counts, then it is reasonable to monitor viral RNA every 3 to 6 months. If titers increase, evaluate adherence to the current regimen and consider changing regimens. If drug toxicities dominate the clinical picture, or if viral RNA titers increase despite treatment, it may be prudent to stop therapy, especially if the CD4 count is approaching 0.

Prophylaxis for Opportunistic Infections (Table 248-1)

When the CD4 count is less than 200, patients are at high risk for the development of pneumocystic pneumonia (PCP). Prophylaxis with trimethoprim-sulfamethoxazole (TXS) (1 double-strength tablet every day or three times a week) is advised. Dapsone (50 to 100 mg every day) may also be effective, but methemoglobinemia must be monitored and G-6PD deficiency contraindicates treatment. Several other regimens have also been tested and appear promising (Chapter 280). These oral regimens are now believed to be superior in efficacy to aerosolized pentamidine, which has been relegated to second-line drug status. The decline in incidence of pneumocystic pneumonia as the index diagnosis for AIDS attests to the benefit of routine primary prophylaxis.

The value of prophylaxis of some of the other common opportunistic infections has now been established:

1. Toxoplasmosis (usually as toxoplasmic encephalitis) develops in up to 40% of patients with a positive serum antibody test for *Toxoplasma gondii* during the course of AIDS and prophylaxis is warranted. TXS administered as previously described for PCP prevention is effective. If not tolerated, pyrimethamine (50 mg/wk) plus dapsone (50 to 100 mg/day) is also effective.
2. Disseminated tuberculosis develops in up to 40% of patients with a positive PPD (5 mm induration) during the course of AIDS and isoniazid (300 mg/day) for 1 year is effective in preventing activation.
3. *Mycobacterium avium-intracellulare* infection occurs in up to

Table 248-1   Prevention and treatment of common opportunistic infections in AIDS patients

INFECTION	PREVENTION AND TREATMENT
Bacterial infections	
Bacillary angiomatosis	*Treatment:* Erythromycin 500 mg PO or IV qid × 2-4 months *OR* Doxycycline 100 mg PO bid *Suppression:* Erythromycin 250-500 mg PO qid
Mycobacterium tuberculosis	*Primary prophylaxis:* Indicated for patients with positive purified protein derivative or high-risk behaviors; isoniazid 5 mg/kg/day (max 300 mg/day) PO qid, *plus* pyridoxine 25-50 mg PO × 12 months *Treatment* (isoniazid resistance rate <4%): Isoniazid 5 mg/kg (max 300 mg/day) PO × 6 months, *plus* rifampin 10 mg/kg (max 600 mg/day) PO × 6 months, *plus* pyrazinamide 15-30 mg/kg (max 2 g/day) PO × 2 months *Treatment* (isoniazid resistance rate not known or ≥4%): Add ethambutol 15-25 mg/kg (max 2.5 g) PO daily
Mycobacterium avium-intracellulare complex	*Primary prophylaxis:* Indicated when CD4 count <50/mm³. Clarithromycin 500 mg PO bid *OR* azithromycin 1200 mg PO weekly *Treatment:* Clarithromycin 500 mg PO bid *OR* azithromycin 500 mg PO qd, *plus* ethambutol 15-25 mg/kg/day ± rifabutin 300 mg PO qd *Suppression:* Always necessary (clarithromycin or azithromycin) ± ethambutol (lower dose to 15 mg/kg/day)
Fungal infections	
Esophagitis (fluconazole sensitive)	Fluconazole 200 mg PO × 1, then 100 mg qd × ≥3 weeks (or 2 weeks after symptoms resolve) *OR* itraconazole oral solution 100-200 mg PO qd × ≥3 weeks
Coccidioidomycosis	*Primary prophylaxis:* Not recommended for most patients *Pulmonary and extrapulmonary (not meningitis) treatment:* Fluconazole 400-800 mg PO qd for ≥9 months *OR* itraconazole 200 mg bid PO with food or acidic cola *OR* amphotericin B 0.5-1.0 mg/kg/day IV × 7 days then 0.8 mg/kg IV qod. Total dose ≥2.5 g
Cryptococcal meningitis	*Treatment:* Amphotericin B (initial Rx) with fluconazole completion Rx. Amphotericin B: 0.7-1.0 mg/kg/day IV until afebrile and headache, nausea, and vomiting cease. Then discontinue amphotericin B and start fluconazole 400 mg PO qd to complete 8-10 week course. Then maintain on fluconazole 200 mg PO qd indefinitely. If using amphotericin B only, total dose approximately 2.5 g *Suppression:* Fluconazole 200 mg/day PO indefinitely (lifetime)
Histoplasmosis	*Treatment:* Amphotericin B 0.5-1.0 mg/kg/day IV × 7 days, then 0.8 mg/kg qod or (3 ×/week) IV to total dose of 10-15 mg/kg and then suppressive Rx *OR* itraconazole 300 mg PO bid × 3 days, then 200 mg PO bid for 12 weeks or 400 mg qd × 12 weeks (85% to 90% response) and then chronic suppression *Suppression:* Itraconazole 200 mg capsules PO bid indefinitely
Parasitic infections	
Cryptosporidium parvum	*Treatment:* No therapy proven efficacious but paromomycin 500-750 mg PO tid or qid for 10 days to several months or 1.0 g PO bid may be beneficial
Isospora belli	*Treatment:* Trimethoprim-sulfamethoxazole 1 double-strength tablet (trimethoprim 160 mg, sulfamethoxazole 800 mg) PO qid × 10 days then bid × 3 weeks *Suppression* (maintenance Rx): Trimethoprim-sulfamethoxazole 1 double-strength tablet 3 ×/week
Enterocytozoon bieneusi and septata intestinalis	*Treatment:* Albendazole 400 mg PO bid and then chronic suppression
Pneumocystis carinii	*Primary prophylaxis* (initiate when CD4 count <200/mm³ or in patients with rapidly decreasing CD4 count or constitutional symptoms or oral thrush): Trimethoprim-sulfamethoxazole 1 double-strength tablet (trimethoprim 160 mg, sulfamethoxazole 800 mg) PO qd or 3 ×/week *Treatment* (if patient **NOT** acutely ill, able to take oral drugs, PaO_2 >70 mm Hg): Dapsone 100 mg PO qd, *plus* trimethoprim 5 mg/kg PO tid × 21 days *OR* trimethoprim-sulfamethoxazole 2 double-strength tablets PO q8h × 21 days and then chronic suppression *Treatment* (if patient acutely ill, PaO_2 <70 mm Hg): Prednisone 15-30 min before first dose of trimethoprim-sulfamethoxazole: 40 mg PO bid × 5 days, then 40 mg PO qd × 5 days, then 20 mg PO qd × 11 days, *plus* trimethoprim-sulfamethoxazole (15 mg trimethoprim/kg/day) IV divided q6h or q8h × 21 days. Start chronic suppression posttreatment *Suppression:* Same as primary prophylaxis (see above)
Toxoplasma gondii	*Primary prophylaxis* (when CD4 ≤100/µl and IgG antibody positive for *Toxoplasma*): Trimethoprim-sulfamethoxazole 1 double-strength (160 mg trimethoprim) tablet PO qd. NOTE: For HIV-infected pregnant women who are seropositive for *T. gondii* antibodies and have CD4 count <200/mm³: spiramycin 1.0 gm PO tid throughout pregnancy *Treatment:* Pyrimethamine 200 mg PO (loading dose), then 50-100 mg PO qd, *plus* folinic acid (leucovorin) 10-20 mg PO (or IV) qd, *plus* either sulfadiazine 1.0-1.5 g PO q6h *OR* clindamycin 600 mg PO *OR* 600-1200 mg IV q6h × 3-6 weeks *Suppression:* Sulfadiazine 1.0 g PO qid, *plus* pyrimethamine 50 mg PO qd, *plus* folic acid 10 mg PO qd
Viral infections	
Retinitis	*Treatment:* Ganciclovir 5.0 mg/kg IV (at constant rate over 1 hour) q12h × 14-21 days *OR* foscarnet 60 mg/kg (adjusted for renal function) IV at constant rate (requires infusion pump) over minimum of 1 hour q8h (or 90 mg/kg q12h) × 14-21 days *OR* combination of intraocular ganciclovir implant (delivers 1-2 µg/hr × 6-7 months), *plus* either concomitant IV ganciclovir as above *OR* oral ganciclovir 1.0 g tid *Suppression* (may be indefinite): Ganciclovir 5 mg/kg IV qd or 6 mg/kg IV qd 5 days/week *OR* foscarnet 90-120 mg/kg/day IV with hydration and dose adjusted for renal function

30% of patients during the course of AIDS. Clarithromycin (500 mg/day), azithromycin (250 mg/day), or rifabutin (300 mg/day) have all been shown to reduce disseminated infection by >50% and prolong survival. It is reasonable to initiate prophylaxis with one of these drugs once the CD4 count has reached the 50 to 75 cells/mm³ range.

A reduction in frequency of fungal infections including cryptococcal meningitis, candida esophagitis, and oral thrush, but not histoplasmosis, resulted when fluconazole (200 mg/day) was given to patients with <200 CD4 cells/mm³ but because of potential emergence of resistant fungi and other drug interactions, most authorities use the drug to treat established infection and do not routinely use it

for prophylaxis. Patients who respond to antiretroviral treatment may demonstrate improvements in CD4 counts. Preliminary data suggest that this increase reflects clonal expansion of residual lymphocytes, not reconstitution of all previously destroyed clones. Thus once started, opportunistic infection prophylaxis should be continued even when CD4 count rises above the threshold level (often 200/mm³) for initiation.

CLINICAL SYNDROMES ASSOCIATED WITH HIV

Improving the quality of life and increasing the survival time of patients infected with HIV through appropriate antiretroviral therapy,

Table 248-2   New AIDS therapies

DRUG	DOSE	MAJOR TOXICITIES	DRUG-DRUG INTERACTIONS	CROSS-RESISTANCE PATTERNS
Reverse transcriptase inhibitors				
Didanosine (DDI, Videx)	200 mg bid; (<60 kg, 125 mg bid)	Neuropathy, pancreatitis, diarrhea	Pentamidine, ganciclovir, zalcitabine	Unknown
Lamivudine (3TC, Epivir)	150 mg bid	In combination with AZT, same as AZT alone	—	DDI, DDC
Stavudine (D4T, Zerit)	40 mg q12h (<60 kg, 30 mg bid)	Neuropathy	Avoid use with agents that may cause peripheral neuropathy	AZT, DDI, DDC
Zalcitabine (DDC, Hivid)	0.75 mg q8h	Neuropathy, stomatitis, pancreatitis, LFT increases	Didanosine, pentamidine	DDI, 3TC, D4T
Zidovudine (AZT, ZDV, Retrovir)	200 mg tid or 300 mg bid	Cytopenia, GI intolerance, LFT increase/hepatitis, asthenia, myopathy	Ribavirin	
Delavirdine (DEL, Rescriptor)	400 mg tid	Rash, headache, LFT increase	Increased concentration of terfenadine, astemizole, ergot derivatives, alprazolam, midazolam, triazolam, dihydropyridines (e.g., nifedipine), cisapride, decreased delavirdine concentrations; carbamazepine, phenobarbital, phenytoin, rifabutin, rifampin	NVP
Nevirapine (NVP, Viramune)	200 mg qd × 2 wk then 200 mg bid	Rash, fever, LFT increase	Reduced concentrations of oral contraceptives, saquinavir	DEL
Protease Inhibitors				
Indinavir (IND, Crixivan) Inhibits CYP 3A	800 mg tid on empty stomach	Nephrolithiasis, indirect hyperbilirubinemia, hyperglycemia	Midazolam (Versed), triazolam (Halcion), carbamazepine (Tegretol), astemizole (Hismanal), terfenadine (Seldane), rifampin (Rifadin, Rimactane), cisapride (Propulsid)	RIT, NEL, SAQ
Ritonavir (RIT, Norvir) Inhibits CYP 2D6, 2C9, 2C19, 3A; Induces CYP 1A2, 3A	300 mg bid with food, then dose escalation over 2 wk to 600 mg bid	GI intolerance, circumoral paresthesias, increased cholesterol/lipids, hyperglycemia/diabetes, LFT increases	Meperidine (Demerol), prioxicam (Feldene), propoxyphene (Darvon, Darvocet), alprazolam (Xanax), clorazepate (Tranxene), diazepam (Valium), estazolam (ProSom), flurazepam (Dalmane), zolpidem (Ambien), midazolam (Versed), triazolam (Halcion), amiodarone (Cordarone), encainide (Enkaid), flecainide (Tambocor), propafenone (Rythmol), quinidine (Quinidex, Quinaglute), bupropion (Wellbutrin), carbamazepine (Tegretol), astemizole (Hismanal), terfenadine (Seldane), beta blockers, rifabutin (Mycobutinin), clozapine (Clozaril), pimozide (Orap), cisapride (Propulsid), various ergotamines	IND, NEL, SAQ
Saquinavir (SAQ, Invirase) Inhibits CYP 3A	600 mg tid with fatty meals	GI intolerance, hyperglycemia/diabetes, LFT increases	Midazolam (Versed), triazolam (Halcion), carbamazepine (Tegretol), phenobarbital (Luminal, Barbita), phenytoin (Dilantin), itraconazole (Sporanox), astemizole (Hismanal), terfenadine (Seldane), rifampin (Rifadin, Rimactane), rifabutin (Mycobutin), cisapride (Propulsid)	Unknown
Nelfinavir (NEL, Viracept) Inhibits CYP 3A	750 mg tid	Mild diarrhea	Midazolam (Versed), triazolam (Halcion), astemizole (Hismanal), terfenadine (Seldane), oral contraceptives	Unknown

prophylaxis for common infectious complications, and prompt treatment of complicating illnesses is a realistic goal. Recognition of the wide variability in presentation and the more common manifestations of involvement of the various organ systems is necessary for appropriate diagnosis and management. See Table 248-2 for new AIDS therapies.

Fever

Fever is not uncommon in patients infected with HIV who have CD4 cell counts of <500/mm³, and night sweats are frequently associated. When fever accompanies an accelerated catabolic state with weight loss and anorexia, the presence of opportunistic infection or malignancy signifying the onset of AIDS should be suspected.

In sexually active adults, sexually transmitted diseases and anorectal infections often go unrecognized as sources of fever. Serologic tests for syphilis and proctologic examination with cultures for *Neisseria gonorrhoeae, Chlamydia trachomatis,* and herpes simplex virus should be performed. Blood cultures should be obtained and processed for isolation of bacteria, mycobacteria, and fungi. In the absence of other symptoms, infection with disseminated *M. tuberculosis* (Chapter 273), *M. avium-intracellulare, Histoplasma capsulatum, Coccidioides immitis* (Chapter 276), and *Cryptococcus neoformans* (Chapter 278) should be excluded. Nontyphoid salmonella bacteremia can also present with fever alone and is often recurrent despite appropriate treatment.

Cytomegalovirus (CMV) infection is a cause of fever, and CMV may be cultured from the blood and urine (Chapter 255). Because this organism is prevalent in persons infected with HIV, a causal relationship with fever can be implied only when no other pathogen is detected.

Hypotension suggests hypoadrenalism, especially if electrolyte disturbances are noted. Adrenal insufficiency is very common in AIDS patients and has been attributed to HIV-induced abnormalities in steroid synthesis, adrenalitis from CMV infection, and ketoconazole therapy. Disseminated histoplasmosis may present with a septic shock syndrome with hypotension, fever, DIC, and adult respiratory distress syndrome (ARDS). The fungus may be found within macrophages by examining the peripheral blood smear or bone marrow and can be cultured from the blood or marrow.

Lymphadenopathy

In patients with HIV, lymph node biopsy typically reveals reactive hyperplasia (Color Plate VIII-35), and biopsy of nodes in patients with persistent generalized lymphadenopathy is not routinely required. Biopsy should be performed to exclude disseminated tuberculosis, *M. avium-intracellulare* infection (Color Plate VIII-36), histoplasmosis, toxoplasmosis, bacillary angiomatosis (Chapter 270), lymphoma, and Kaposi's sarcoma, when asymmetric, regional, or painful lymphadenopathy occurs. Increasing numbers of patients with aggressive B-cell lymphomas have been recognized in the past several years (as many as 30% of patients on retroviral therapy followed for more than 3 years in one study).

Enlargement of the hilar or mediastinal nodes is unusual and should suggest lymphoma, mycobacterial or fungal infection, or Kaposi's sarcoma. If no other tissue is available for examination, these nodes can also be studied on biopsy.

Although hepatosplenomegaly in combination with lymphadenopathy and fever may be a manifestation of HIV, it may also be a sign of disseminated fungal or mycobacterial infection or lymphoma. Liver biopsy may be of value if blood cultures are negative, accessible peripheral lymph nodes are not enlarged, and no contraindications are present.

Dysphagia

Complaints of dysphagia or odynophagia usually signify mucosal infection with *Candida albicans* (Chapter 277) or herpes simplex virus. Infection may extend from the oral mucosa into the esophagus or upper respiratory tract and often results in anorexia and weight loss from decreased caloric intake. Candida infection may be diagnosed by scraping the typical patchy white mucosal lesions and identifying hyphae after wet-mount preparation in 10% potassium hydroxide. Virus cultures should be performed if wet-mount preparations are negative. Cytomegalovirus may be cultured in both symptomatic and asymptomatic patients and should be considered pathogenic only when other causes have been excluded and histologic findings are consistent. The presence of painful superficial ulcers in the mouth or esophagus may represent aphthous ulcers, which, if resistant to steroids, may respond to thalidomide.

Oral candidiasis can be treated topically with nystatin in oral suspension or clotrimazole troches. Systemic therapy with fluconazole should be considered for more extensive mucosal involvement. Acyclovir should be administered intravenously to patients with documented herpes simplex esophagitis (Chapter 255).

Diarrhea

Diarrhea is a frequent complaint. Symptoms range from frequent loose stools to fulminant diarrhea producing profound weight loss and malabsorption. A thorough evaluation is warranted because virtually any gastrointestinal pathogen may be found (Box 248-1) (Chapter 242). Stool for bacterial cultures; testing for ova and parasites, including microsporidia and cryptosporidia (Chapters 339, 346, and 279); and proctosigmoidoscopy should be included in the initial diagnostic workup.

Common bacterial pathogens cultured include *Campylobacter* species (Chapter 267), *Salmonella* species, *Shigella* species (Chapter 269), and *Yersinia* species. If any of these organisms is isolated, specific antibiotic treatment is indicated.

Although parasites are frequently identified in stool specimens from asymptomatic homosexual men, they may produce diarrhea and treatment is indicated. In addition to *Giardia lamblia* and *Entamoeba histolytica* (Chapter 279), unusual parasites such as *Isospora belli, Blastocystis hominis,* microsporidium, and *Cryptosporidium parvum* may produce symptoms. Cryptosporidia are readily demonstrated by direct examination of the stool with a modified Kinyoun stain (Color Plate VIII-32). Therapy with trimethoprim-sulfamethoxazole is usually effective in eradicating *Isospora* organisms. To date, treatment for cryptosporidiosis has been disappointing, and diarrhea in these patients may persist or may wax and wane indefinitely. Limited success with paramomycin (500 mg tid), a nonabsorable aminoglycoside, has been reported.

BOX 248-1
Gastrointestinal infections commonly associated with AIDS and the pathogens frequently causing these infections

Proctitis
Herpes simplex virus
Neisseria gonorrhoeae
Treponema pallidum
Chlamydia trachomatis

Colitis
Salmonella species
Campylobacter species
Shigella species
Entamoeba histolytica
Cytomegalovirus

Enteritis
Cryptosporidium species
Isospora belli
Giardia lamblia
Strongyloides stercoralis
Mycobacterium avium-intracellulare
Cytomegalovirus
Microsporidia

When stool examination and culture fail to reveal a pathogen, more invasive diagnostic tests are indicated. Sigmoidoscopy and colonoscopy with mucosal biopsy are necessary to thoroughly evaluate the lower intestinal tract. A duodenal aspirate may be necessary to definitively diagnose *G. lamblia* and *I. belli* infection. Small bowel biopsy may reveal evidence of parasitic infection, Kaposi's sarcoma, *M. avium-intracellulare* infection, Whipple's disease, or intestinal lymphoma. Cytomegalovirus has been implicated as a cause of diarrhea when mucosal biopsy reveals histologic evidence of intracellular inclusions in areas of active inflammation and hemorrhage and no other cause is found (Color Plate VIII-37).

A history of recent antibiotic use should suggest *Clostridium difficile* toxin. Evidence of pseudomembrane formation and mucosal inflammation are usually seen on lower endoscopy (Chapter 263).

A specific cause for the diarrhea in many AIDS patients (20% to 40%) will not be found despite extensive evaluation. Treatment of symptoms with antimotility drugs may afford some relief to some patients, but the diarrhea may persist relentlessly, resulting in profound weight loss and debilitation.

Perirectal Pain

Anorectal pain with purulent discharge usually signifies localized infection. Anoscopic examination with cultures for herpes simplex virus and *N. gonorrhoeae* may be diagnostic. The presence of mucosal ulcerations suggests herpes simplex virus, *Treponema pallidum,* or *C. trachomatis* infection. Perirectal abscesses are occasionally seen, particularly in the homosexual population (Chapter 31). Rectal malignancies such as squamous cell carcinoma and cloacagenic carcinoma are increasingly found in individuals with AIDS, and these patients may have proctologic symptoms. Kaposi's sarcoma lesions can also be etiologic.

Acute Abdominal Pain

Patients with AIDS occasionally develop symptoms of intraabdominal catastrophe or peritonitis. Bowel perforation secondary to gastrointestinal lymphoma may occur, and prognosis is poor. Symptoms of peritoneal irritation as an isolated finding may also occur. Gastrointestinal tuberculosis, CMV infection, and disseminated fungal infections have been reported in this setting.

Cutaneous Lesions

The lesions of Kaposi's sarcoma are often the first sign of AIDS to appear, particularly in homosexual men. These nontender, raised, violescent tumors may occur on any part of the body (Color Plate VIII-38), and a scrupulous search for lesions should be undertaken during the initial evaluation of any patient in whom AIDS is suspected. Kaposi's sarcoma may initially present in the oral cavity, on the soles of the feet, and in the rectal mucosa and other inconspicuous sites, as well as in the gastrointestinal tract (Color Plate VIII-39). Biopsy of any suspicious lesion will be diagnostic if Kaposi's sarcoma is present.

Bacillary angiomatosis should be considered in patients with raised, tender, nonblanching but friable angiomatous lesions on the skin (Color Plate VIII-40). These patients usually have fever and may also have hepatomegaly (peliosis hepatitis). The condition results from infection with *Bartonella henslei* or *Bartonella quintana,* which induces proliferation of vascular endothelial cells. These bacteria can now be cultured from the skin or blood in some laboratories. The Warthin-Starry silver stain will also reveal the bacilli in biopsied tissue. Treatment with erythromycin is effective (Chapters 270 and 346).

Herpesvirus infection can be diagnosed by viral culture of the typical cutaneous vesicles and mucosal ulcerations. Herpes simplex (types I and II) produces localized or disseminated lesions, which are not always distinguishable from varicella zoster infection without culture. Therapy with acyclovir may be useful in severe local infections or disseminated disease (Chapter 255).

Cutaneous bacterial infections including impetigo, folliculitis, and ecthyma caused by *Staphylococcus aureus* occur in many patients. These conditions usually respond to oral systemic therapy but tend to recur. Psoriasis, maculopapular rashes, and basal cell carcinomas also appear with increased incidence in patients infected with HIV. *C. neoformans* and, rarely, other fungi can produce molluscum contagiosum–like lesions or chronic cutaneous infections of the skin, nail beds, and genitalia. Fungal cultures should be obtained any time such an infection does not respond promptly to antibacterial therapy.

Dyspnea

Shortness of breath with exertion in a patient with risk factors for acquiring AIDS usually signifies the onset of *Pneumocystis carinii* pneumonia (Chapter 280). A dry hacking cough, fever, and tachypnea are common presenting complaints; but any symptom suggestive of respiratory involvement warrants a diagnostic evaluation aimed at identifying this opportunistic pathogen. Symptomatic patients should be evaluated with a chest radiograph and arterial blood gas determination. The chest radiograph usually reveals bilateral, diffuse, fine reticulonodular infiltrates, but infiltrates may also be alveolar or well localized. Occasionally the chest radiograph is entirely normal. Pleural effusion is atypical for pneumocystis infection and suggests pleural involvement with Kaposi's sarcoma or other opportunistic pathogens. Pleuritic chest pain suggests pneumothorax, a complication of recurrent pneumocystic pneumonia, which may also be more common in patients who received aerosolized pentamidine prophylaxis. Arterial blood gas analysis usually demonstrates a mild respiratory alkalosis and hypoxemia (Po$_2$ 50 to 60 mm Hg). Pulmonary function tests and gallium scanning may be of value in symptomatic patients with normal chest radiographs. A restrictive pattern with abnormal diffusing capacity to carbon monoxide is almost always demonstrated.

The organism can be identified on direct examination of induced sputum (induced with saline nebulization) with Giemsa staining (Chapter 233) (Color Plate VIII-10) in more than half of patients. Bronchoscopy performed with transbronchial lavage followed by immediate examination of specimens with Giemsa, silver methionine, or fluorescent antipneumocystis antibody tests reveals the diagnosis in more than 90% of patients. Bronchoscopic biopsy may increase the yield of this approach but is not usually required. Open lung biopsy is rarely indicated.

P. carinii pneumonia still contributes to the morbidity and mortality of HIV infection despite effective prophylactic therapy. Treatment with trimethoprim-sulfamethoxazole or pentamidine is effective in the majority of patients, but the infection is fatal in as many as 15% of

initial episodes. Relapse occurs in at least 20%, and mortality increases with recurrent infection.

In addition to *P. carinii,* a multitude of other organisms may invade the respiratory tract in AIDS patients and cause disease. *M. tuberculosis, H. capsulatum, C. immitis* and *C. neoformans* are not uncommonly detected; infection with *Legionella* species has also been reported. These organisms can usually be identified by careful culturing of specimens obtained at bronchoscopy and by histologic examination with special stains (acid-fast, PAS, Giemsa, and silver methionine). Procedures for processing specimens should be carefully coordinated with the microbiology and pathology services to facilitate diagnosis. Isolation of CMV and MAI is common, but they rarely cause symptomatic pulmonary disease. Infection with *Streptococcus pneumoniae* or other common respiratory bacterial pathogens should be considered when the chest radiograph reveals lobar consolidation, because this radiographic pattern is not common in pneumocystic or fungal pneumonias.

Not all pulmonary disease in AIDS patients is directly related to the immune deficiency. Pulmonary embolism should be considered, particularly after prolonged bed rest. Diagnosis usually requires arteriography because many patients have other pulmonary abnormalities, making ventilation-perfusion scanning nondiagnostic.

Headache

The symptoms and signs of central nervous system (CNS) involvement in AIDS patients are often subtle, and opportunistic infections of the CNS therefore may go unrecognized unless careful history and neurologic examinations are performed. Chronic or progressive headache is the most prevalent symptom suggesting CNS involvement.

Toxoplasma gondii has emerged as the most frequent cause of encephalitis in AIDS patients (Chapter 279). Headache and focal neurologic signs and seizures are typical, although patients may have no localizing findings. The absence of antitoxoplasma antibody as assayed by the Sabin-Feldman dye test or other equally sensitive test for IgG makes the diagnosis much less likely, but false-negative antibody tests have been reported. Computed tomography (CT) usually demonstrates multiple ring-enhancing lesions, but other findings such as focal edema and large lesions with mass effect have also been described (Fig. 248-1). Delayed scanning after double-dose contrast infusion improves the yield of the procedure. CT scans may be completely normal in some patients in whom toxoplasmosis is documented at autopsy. Magnetic resonance imaging (MRI) is more sensitive and may reveal lesions not evident on CT (Fig. 248-2).

In patients with HIV infection and <200 CD4 cells/mm^3, a trial of treatment for toxoplasmosis with pyramethamine and sulfadiazine is justifiable without obtaining a tissue diagnosis, providing the clinical and radiographic findings are consistent with the diagnosis. However, brain biopsy is recommended if the CT scan or MR image is atypical, or if the patient deteriorates or does not improve on clinical or radiographic examination after 7 to 10 days of therapy. In patients who have a high probability of toxoplasmosis based on clinical findings and in whom scans reveal large lesions with mass effect, dexamethasone for 5 to 7 days is useful. If deterioration is noted after dexamethasone is discontinued, biopsy is recommended.

Other pathophysiologic processes that have been identified in patients with headache or other CNS symptoms and abnormal CT scans include infection with *M. tuberculosis, H. capsulatum,* herpes simplex virus, CMV, HIV itself, and progressive multifocal leukoencephalopathy (see later discussion). The most likely cause is primary CNS lymphoma, which may present with exactly the same symptoms as toxoplasmic encephalitis but is more likely to demonstrate a single lesion on scan and a negative toxoplasmosis serology. It is important to establish this diagnosis by biopsy, because most patients will respond at least transiently to radiation therapy.

Headache is also the most frequent complaint of AIDS patients with meningitis. Evidence of meningeal irritation is present in only 25% of affected patients. *C. neoformans* is by far the most common cause of meningitis in AIDS patients (Chapter 278). India ink preparation of the spinal fluid demonstrates the typical encapsulated fungus in about 75% of cases, but the cryptococcal antigen test of serum and cerebrospinal fluid is more sensitive (>95%). The serum cryp-

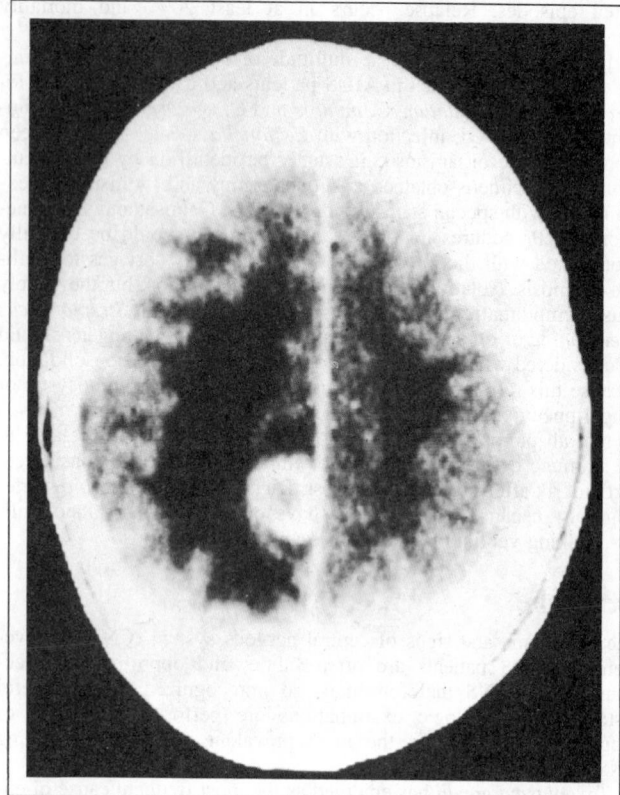

FIGURE 248-1   Computed tomography brain scan of patient with biopsy-proved *Toxoplasma* infection.

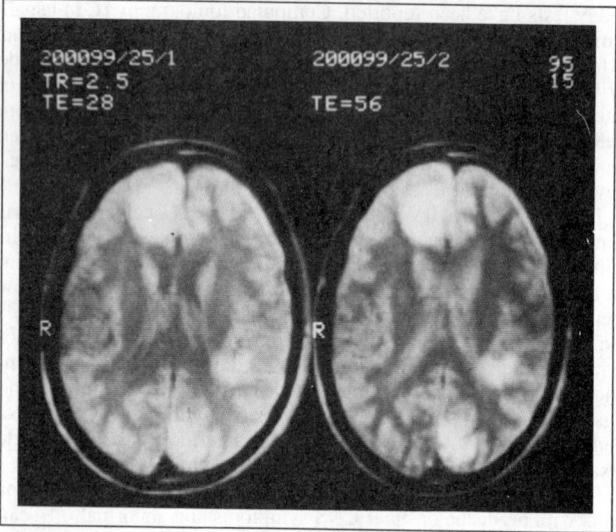

FIGURE 248-2   Magnetic resonance image of patient with multiple *Toxoplasma* lesions in the central nervous system.

tococcal antigen titer (CrAg) is a good screening test in this clinical setting.

Once the diagnosis is established, therapy with amphotericin (0.5 to 0.7 mg/kg/day IV) in the sicker patient or fluconazole (400 mg/day po) in the stable patient is recommended. Most patients respond to therapy: the organism disappears from the cerebrospinal fluid and antigen titers decrease. Definitive cure, however, is rare, and relapse occurs within 4 to 6 months. Maintenance therapy with fluconazole (200 mg/day) is recommended to reduce the likelihood of relapse.

Other opportunistic fungi, *M. tuberculosis,* lymphoma, and, rarely, *Listeria monocytogenes* also produce meningitis in AIDS patients. HIV can be cultured from the spinal fluid, but pleiocytosis is unusual, and isolated elevation of protein is the only clue to diagnosis. Bacterial meningitis caused by *Pneumococcus, Haemophilus, Listeria,* or *Meningococcus* organisms also occurs and usually presents in typical fashion.

Seizures

CNS involvement in AIDS patients may first be manifested by seizures. By far the most common cause of seizures is toxoplasma encephalitis, although CNS lymphoma and herpesvirus infection may also produce seizures. CT should be performed before lumbar puncture to avoid precipitating herniation. Therapy is aimed at treating the underlying disorder and preventing seizure activity with anticonvulsants.

Dementia

More than half of all AIDS patients will have evidence of neurologic abnormalities on initial presentation when careful mental status and neurologic examinations are performed. Mild to moderate dementia is not uncommon, but the true incidence may have been overestimated in early reports. However, as immunosuppression progresses, the frequency of AIDS dementia complex (ADC) (a condition that most likely results from HIV infection of CNS macrophages and release of cytokines) increases. The preservation of alertness is important in differentiating ADC from structural lesions that usually present with coexisting lethargy, obtundation, or coma. Patients typically demonstrate memory loss, poor judgment, and, later in the course of their disease, apathy and withdrawal. CT scans usually reveal only atrophy. Psychiatric disturbances secondary to the stress inherent in coping with this debilitating and ultimately fatal disease or unmasking of underlying psychiatric problems certainly contribute to the high incidence of neurologic abnormalities in these patients, but opportunistic infection and neoplasm must also be excluded.

Histopathologic studies of brain tissues from biopsy specimens or autopsy have provided convincing evidence to support a role for viral infection in many of these patients. As noted, HIV has been identified in patients with progressive encephalopathy and may also produce sensory neuropathy and vacuolating myelopathy. Likewise, CMV inclusions have been associated with a more acute syndrome characterized by psychosis and rapid death. Papova viruses, particularly SV-40 and JC viruses, have been implicated in progressive multifocal leukencephalopathy in several patients.

Blindness

Visual disturbances, a serious complication of HIV infection, are usually the result of CMV infection (Chapter 255). CMV produces a progressive retinochoroiditis, which may rapidly progress to visual field defects and ultimately blindness (Color Plate VIII-41). Ophthalmologic examination reveals white plaques and focal hemorrhages. Early lesions are commonly asymptomatic. The use of intravenous ganciclovir (5 mg/kg q12h for 14 to 21 days followed by 6 mg/kg qd 5 days/wk for life) is effective in controlling infection and reducing symptoms, but bone marrow suppression is a common complication. Foscarnet (60 mg/kg IV q8h ×14 days followed by 90 to 120 mg/kg qd for life) is also effective but extremely expensive, and it is associated with renal and electrolyte abnormalities. *Candida* species and *T. gondii* also produce patchy retinal exudates that may interfere with vision. Treatment is indicated but requires close ophthalmologic follow-up.

Miscellaneous Conditions

Pericardial effusions have been seen in AIDS patients and are most often secondary to Kaposi's sarcoma invading the pericardial surfaces. Hemodynamic compromise is uncommon, and the diagnosis is often apparent only on postmortem examination. Murantic endocarditis without clinical manifestations has also been described as an incidental finding at autopsy.

Primary renal disease is not common in AIDS patients, but a picture of nephrosclerosis with proteinuria progressing to renal failure appears to result from HIV infection itself. Impaired kidney function secondary to nephrotoxic drugs is also common.

A peculiar oral lesion termed *hairy cell leukoplakia* has been identified in patients with HIV. This condition produces whitish plaques on the lateral borders of the tongue, which may be confused with thrush (Color Plate VIII-42). Epstein-Barr and papilloma viruses are both present within the lesion. The condition temporarily responds to high doses of acyclovir, but relapse is expected and treatment is not indicated unless symptoms are present.

Infection of the paranasal sinuses may produce symptoms of acute sinusitis in AIDS patients. Although common bacterial pathogens are often isolated, antral aspirates from these patients have demonstrated a high incidence of *Candida* species and *Pseudallescheria boydii* (a normally saprophytic fungus, which has only rarely been associated with sinusitis in immunocompromised hosts). Otolaryngology consultation should be obtained therefore if symptoms do not respond to antibacterial therapy.

PROGNOSIS AND TREATMENT GOALS

The course of AIDS is dictated by the severity of the immune deficiency and the resulting clinical manifestations. The long-range impact of the newer antiretroviral therapy on slowing progression of HIV infection is yet to be determined. Patients who have Kaposi's sarcoma tend to have a longer median survival period than do those who have opportunistic infections. Although individual infections can be treated with varying degrees of success, the course is usually relentless in its progression. Typically the patient eventually becomes infected with multiple pathogens, including *P. carinii, M. avium-intracellulare, T. gondii,* and aggressive CMV, which themselves accelerate HIV infection. Death is most often the result of progressive wasting, respiratory insufficiency, or CNS involvement.

Medical care should focus on providing comfort, preventing the opportunistic infections, and managing the new complexities of antiretroviral therapy. Treatment of the infections and malignancies associated with the disease is largely palliative and should be instituted only after careful consideration of the potential complications of therapy. A thorough discussion of these facts with the patient will facilitate realistic treatment expectations. The use of life-support measures, including cardiopulmonary resuscitation and artificial ventilation, should also be addressed as early as possible. The survival rate for AIDS patients with respiratory failure has actually improved in the last few years, and intensive care is certainly not contraindicated; but the expected benefit from aggressive measures must be balanced against the overall quality of life in the face of a progressive disease.

An organized team approach, with involvement of counselors, nurses, and physicians, can offer valuable contributions to the medical and psychosocial care of the patient with AIDS. Home health aides and hospice care can maximize the number of days that patients remain outside of the hospital and in their own environment. Involvement of family members and loved ones can also contribute dramatically to the patient's ability to cope with the disease.

PREVENTION

Vaccine against the AIDS retrovirus is not yet available, and prevention of infection depends on preventing transmission of the virus. Family members and household contacts should be reassured that the disease is not transmitted by casual contact and must be instructed in the use of good hygienic practices. Patients and their sexual partners should be counseled about the potential for sexual transmission of the virus. Women with HIV infection should be treated with antiretroviral drugs when pregnant to reduce transplacental transmission.

BIBLIOGRAPHY

Carpenter CC et al: Antiretroviral therapy for HIV infection in 1997, *JAMA* 277:1962, 1997.
International AIDS Society: Guidelines for using antiretroviral agents.
Saag M, Holodniy M, Kuritzkes D et al: HIV viral load markers in clinical practice, *Nature Med* 2:625-629, 1996.
Sande MA, Volberding PA, editors: *The medical management of AIDS*, ed 5, Philadelphia, 1997, WB Saunders.
Sanford JP, Gilbert DN, Sande MA, editors: *The Sanford guide to HIV/AIDS therapy*, Dallas, 1997, Antimicrobial Therapy Inc.
USPHS/IDSA Prevention of Opportunistic Infections Working Group: USPHS/IDSA guidelines for the prevention of opportunistic infections in persons infected with human immunodeficiency virus: disease-specific recommendations, *Clin Infect Dis* Aug 21 (suppl 1):532-543, 1995.

CHAPTER

249 Fever in the Hospitalized Patient

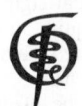 **Rafael Jurado and John E. McGowan, Jr.**

Many patients have fever while hospitalized; a study in a county hospital in Atlanta, Georgia, found that 29% of hospitalized patients had oral temperatures ≥38° C during the course of their hospital stay, with the highest frequencies of occurrence in patients on medicine and surgical services. Although many published studies focus on the problem of prolonged fever or fever of unknown origin (Chapter 234), management of fever of short duration represents the problem for the majority of patients who experience hospital-acquired (nosocomial) fever. The likely sources of such fevers differ from those of fevers acquired before hospitalization and those of extended duration.

On occasion the source of fever is readily apparent, such as in surgical wound infection with copious exudate. More often, the source of the fever is at first obscure. Careful history and physical examination of the febrile patient must be combined with consideration of the procedures and instrumentations that the patient has experienced and the medications initiated during the hospitalization to make an effective plan for diagnosis. In many cases the fever is alleviated by removing one or more of these elements of the patient's care (e.g., an intravenous catheter or a drug) rather than by adding new therapies.

DIFFERENTIAL DIAGNOSIS OF HOSPITAL-ACQUIRED FEVER

This chapter focuses on the causes most often associated with patients admitted to an internal medical service. Both infectious and noninfectious processes have been associated with nosocomial fever in these patients. The relative proportion of each can vary dramatically from center to center (Table 249-1). Such distribution depends largely on the patient population served, the types of services offered at the facility, and the availability and use of diagnostic procedures to determine cause. More recent studies show similar results.

Table 249-1 Sources of hospital-acquired* fever episodes in medical service patients

	GRADY MEMORIAL HOSPITAL, ATLANTA	VA HOSPITAL, MINNEAPOLIS
Total fever episodes	184	123
Proportion caused by		
Infection	50%	66%
Inflammatory diseases	4%	12%
Malignancy	16%	10%
Vascular diseases	10%	6%
Procedure complications	6%	2%
Drug reactions	3%	3%
Miscellaneous and unknown sources	11%	1%

Grady Memorial Hospital data from McGowan et al: *Am J Med* 82:580, 1987; VA Hospital data from Filice et al: *Arch Intern Med* 149:319, 1989.
*Episodes with onset after first 24 hours of hospitalization.

For example, a prospective study of patients with fever beginning at least 48 hours after admission to Presbyterian University Hospital in Pittsburgh, published by Arbo and others in 1993, showed 56% of fevers were due to infection, 25% to noninfectious sources, and the remainder were of unknown cause. Relevant diagnostic possibilities are discussed in the following sections.

Infections Commonly Leading to Nosocomial Fever

1. *Sepsis associated with intravascular therapy:* infection at the cannula, in the subcutaneous tunnel, or in the fluid delivery system is frequently a source of febrile episodes in patients who have received intravascular therapy for 48 hours or more. Fever caused by septic thrombophlebitis is particularly difficult to identify, because development of the typical signs of abscess formation in the underlying vein may require an extended period. Incision and drainage of the loculated exudate inside the vessel often are required for management.

2. *Catheter-associated bacteriuria:* colonization of the bladder with microorganisms is the most frequent nosocomial infection today and is closely associated with catheterization of the bladder, whether indwelling or periodic. Many patients with newly acquired bacteriuria remain asymptomatic, but in some infection manifested by fever develops (Chapter 246).

3. *Lower respiratory tract infection:* lower respiratory tract infection is the third most frequent site of nosocomial infection today. It is especially likely in patients who have been on ventilator therapy. Especially susceptible are postoperative patients who received general anesthesia, patients with respiratory insufficiency, and elderly patients (all of whom are likely to aspirate). Use of H2-blockers and enteral nutrition appear to be associated with a higher risk of gram-negative rod pneumonia than is sucralfate. This is probably due to the permissive effect of decreased gastric acidity on bacterial growth. Increased gastric flora then become the source of colonization of the pharynx, from which organisms may be aspirated into the lower airways. Fever usually accompanies these pneumonias or other pulmonary infections.

4. *Surgical wound infection:* infection of surgical wounds afflicts those who have undergone surgical procedures; overall it occurs in about 1 of 200 hospitalized patients. Superficial wound infections (stitch abscess, etc.) often have few associated systemic signs such as fever, but abscess or infection deeper in the wound is often accompanied by fever.

5. *Cardiac bypass:* cardiac bypass procedures subject patients to postperfusion syndrome, caused by cytomegalovirus or Epstein-Barr (EB) virus (Chapter 255).

6. *Upper respiratory infection:* upper respiratory infection may be manifested as a general malaise with fever, especially before localizing signs or symptoms appear. For example, sinusitis can be relatively hard to identify as a fever source. Paranasal sinusitis is especially prominent in patients hospitalized in an intensive care unit and is associated with obstruction created by the devices inserted through the patient's nose, such as a gastric tube or nasotracheal tube. Viral infections transmitted within the institution can appear after several days of hospitalization; these can be as serious as influenza or as trivial as a common cold (Chapter 237).

7. *Pacemaker and prosthesis infections:* infection caused by pacemakers and other prosthetic devices may be manifest only by onset of fever. Data pointing to the source may not be obtained until the infection has continued for an extended period.

8. *Skin or soft tissue infection:* skin or soft tissue infection, especially at points where pressure is applied during a hospital stay, is likely to worsen during the stay. Sometimes these sites produce fever as their presenting manifestation (Chapter 241).

9. *Incubating infections:* infections that are incubating at the time of admission may be responsible for fever during hospital stay, especially when the incubation period is prolonged. For example, development of illness associated with varicella or hepatitis infection acquired in the community may occur only

after a patient has been admitted. In addition, fevers associated with some infections tend to be intermittent or low-grade and may be absent or unremarkable at the time of hospital admission. Increased activity of these processes may lead to the conclusion that the fever and the process have begun after hospitalization.

10. *Bacteremia:* bacteremia without an apparent underlying source may have fever as its only indicator. Peduzzi and colleagues have documented that detecting such cases is difficult, and the only defense against overlooking such a potentially severe source is routinely obtaining blood cultures of patients whose fever with hospital onset is not readily explained. Endocarditis, especially on the tricuspid valve, may account for this clinical manifestation but remain unapparent until specific search is made for this possibility (Chapter 24).

Likely Noninfectious Causes

Reactions to therapeutic agents (medications, contrast dyes, etc.) frequently are manifested by development of fever. Approximately 15% of hospitalized patients experience some drug-related side effect. Usually this cause is recognized because other signs of drug toxicity, such as rash or eosinophilia, are present concurrently. Of special interest are those begun recently and those for which fever is a frequent adverse effect (e.g., β-lactams, isoniazid, phenytoin). Some drugs are more likely than others to produce inflammation at the site of administration when given parenterally. For example, erythromycin compounds for parenteral administration, which have low pH, often cause phlebitis at the intravascular cannula site, and this possibility should be considered if a patient has fever after parenteral erythromycin therapy is begun. Therapeutic immunoglobulins or immunologic products such as interferon also may lead to fever. Many affected patients have no history of prior drug reactions, and some will manifest no other symptoms or signs that suggest the diagnosis of drug-induced fever.

Surgical procedures commonly are followed by fever. Fevers that develop more than 48 hours after the procedure usually are due to infection. Of those fevers occurring in the first 48 hours, most resolve without specific antimicrobial or other therapy. Postcardiotomy syndrome is a special case of postoperative fever that should be considered in patients who have undergone this type of procedure. Pleural or pericardial rub may help indicate the source.

Intravascular-catheter-induced inflammation without concurrent infection can serve as a source of fever in patients who have received intravascular therapy. Only about half of patients with positive intravenous catheter tip culture findings have phlebitis at the site of catheter insertion at the time the catheter is removed.

Fever after blood transfusion has diverse causes. The most common is the so-called pyrogenic reaction, due to immune destruction of leukocytes and/or platelets. A rare but more severe form is transfusion-associated acute lung injury (TRALI), in which the recipient's leukocytes are activated by donor leukocyte antibodies, leading to a self-limited form of adult respiratory distress syndrome (ARDS). Hemolytic transfusion reactions are characterized by fever, flushing, pain at the infusion site, and hemoglobinuria, and have the potential to lead to acute renal failure. Bacteria such as *Yersinia enterocolitica* can contaminate the blood product, causing severe sepsis, but this occurs extremely rarely.

Thrombophlebitis is a potential threat to any hospitalized patient, because enforced bed rest and inactivity increase the risk of venous stasis. Local inflammation of veins in the legs or pelvis is a particular concern in patients who have diseases that increase pressure on vessels, have undergone extensive abdominal or pelvic surgery, or have experienced other procedures that make phlebitis more likely (Chapters 31 and 85). Infection may be present, but inflammation in the absence of infection is common. Abdominal or pelvic tenderness may provide the clue to this process.

Pulmonary embolus can be associated with fever in the absence of readily apparent signs of phlebitis, endocarditis, or other predisposing factors. Because the pulmonary signs and symptoms associated with embolus and the accompanying infarction of lung tissue are often mild or absent, only a high index of suspicion will lead to the testing that documents this reason for hospital onset of fever in some cases. The fever often lasts 2 to 3 days after the acute event, but recurrent emboli can prolong the period.

Instrumentation other than that described previously can lead to fever in hospitalized patients. Inflammation may develop at the site of hemodialysis catheters, in the presence or absence of active infection. Angiography, colonoscopy, duodenoscopy, fiberoptic bronchoscopy, endoscopic retrograde cholangiopancreatography, and so on, all have been associated with fever episodes after being used.

Therapeutic devices and procedures can cause fever in the hospital setting. For example, fever can be associated with nasotracheal intubation even if no infection develops in the area of physical trauma to the upper airways. This is especially likely when the devices are used improperly. Fever arising later in the hospital course also can be caused by sterile abscesses or other inflammation associated with repeated intramuscular injections.

Noninfectious illnesses can have their onset during hospitalization, and fever may result. Similarly, diseases producing fever only intermittently may demonstrate this manifestation only after the patient has been hospitalized for an extended period. Immune-mediated diseases such as arthritis and neurologic events such as subarachnoid or subdural hemorrhage, intracerebral bleeding, or seizure must be considered. Hepatitis, cholangitis, appendicitis, pancreatitis, myocardial infarction, vascular ischemia of an extremity, perforation of a gastrointestinal ulcer, acute gout or pseudogout, and similar events unrelated to hospital care also can produce episodic fever that sometimes appears during the hospital stay. The relationship between malignancy and fever is considered in Chapter 234; nonhematologic malignancies were associated with fever as often as leukemia and lymphoma in the investigation of Filice et al. Fever associated with ethanol withdrawal may be delayed for a day or two after admission, depending on circumstances leading to the patient's hospitalization and details of recent alcohol consumption.

Fraudulent (self-induced) fever may be produced at any time, and on occasion appears to be nosocomial in onset. Contamination of intravascular delivery lines with mouth or other endogenous flora, alteration of thermometry, self-injection of skin and joint spaces, and use of nonprescribed drugs all may be sources of fever in hospitalized patients. *Factitious* fever is produced by alterations of thermometry and often is seen in individuals with paramedical or medical backgrounds and borderline personality disorders.

Hospital-Acquired Fever in Selected Populations of Patients

In certain well-defined groups of patients, causes of fever are rather stereotyped. Such "conditional" profiles of likely causes of fever are quite useful in the diagnostic evaluation, as long as it is remembered that patients in these specific risk categories are not immune to other, more mundane causes of fever. Among such groups are patients in the intensive care unit, those with HIV infection, and those who have received organ transplants. The interested reader is referred to the Bibliography for articles that consider these and other special groups in detail.

DIAGNOSTIC APPROACH

When a patient becomes febrile in the hospital, the following steps should be included in the evaluation:

1. Quickly evaluate the patient for a localizing sign or symptom that indicates the fever source. Signs and symptoms such as a new cough productive of purulent sputum or a hot, swollen joint obviate extensive investigations of other possible causes. Bornstein stresses that the nature of the patient's underlying illness often provides clues. For example, concomitant esophageal stricture or altered mental status may make the possibility of mixed aerobic/anaerobic aspiration pneumonia more likely.

2. The next most important step is detailed review of the patient's clinical course since hospitalization, with particular attention to procedures, instrumentation, medications, and other interventions that have been part of clinical care. Because many sources of nosocomial fever are linked to procedures or instruments, this can be an efficient way to determine the source.

3. If the patient is receiving intravascular therapy, inspect the site of cannula insertion for phlebitis. Determine whether the cannula has been in place longer than the recommended period (Chapter 232). If so, or if no other steps define the likely fever sources, remove the entire intravascular therapy system and, if such therapy is still required, insert a new system at a different location. Send the cannula tip for semiquantitative bacterial culture evaluation. Examine the site of cannulation carefully for signs of venous thrombophlebitis that might require incision and drainage or ligation of the infected vein. Milk the vein backward to the point of catheter insertion to see whether pus can be expressed. If it can, septic thrombophlebitis is possible. Fluid-associated sepsis is more rare, so culture of the fluid being administered is less frequently requested or found to be the source. Examine the fluid container for cracks, cloudy fluid, blood, or other signs of contamination, and send the fluid for culture evaluation if any of these findings is present.

4. If the patient currently has an indwelling urinary catheter or was subjected to bladder catheterization earlier in the hospitalization, examine a urine specimen for presence of white blood cells, bacteria, and yeast. If any of these is present, obtain a culture specimen of the urine for evaluation for bacteria and yeast. Evaluate the urine sediment for presence of casts or other evidence of inflammatory diseases of the urinary tract. Presence of periurethral abscess or epididymitis can be detected by careful examination.

5. Patients currently or previously on ventilator therapy should be evaluated for the presence of pneumonia by physical and radiologic examination. Respiratory secretions obtained through the endotracheal tube (or any sputum being produced, if the patient is not intubated) should be examined for amount, purulence, and Gram-stain appearance. If findings warrant, cultures then are evaluated for bacteria and yeast. Consider the possibility of pulmonary embolus in any patient with hospital-acquired fever, as only high suspicion allows diagnosis of this potentially lethal process to be made in patients when other manifestations are relatively weak or absent.

6. Operative or traumatic wounds should be inspected for signs of inflammation, and any drainage present should have culture evaluation for bacteria and fungi. Signs and symptoms suggestive of deep abscess in the trauma or operative region should be sought, and imaging or other tests undertaken if this possibility remains likely (Chapter 238). In particular, perirectal or prostatic abscess can be overlooked if meticulous attention is not given to physical examination. Fever early (within the first 48 hours) after surgical procedures may be due to atelectasis or release of pyrogens after intraoperative tissue trauma, but these should be considered only after other potentially serious possibilities have been eliminated. Sensitization resulting from exposure to halothane or other anesthetic agents that produce severe pyrexia may be recognized as such, but less dramatic increases still may be produced by general anesthetic agents and should be considered.

7. Special aspects of the patient's care should be evaluated if surgery has been performed. For example, use of certain anesthetic agents can produce sensitization manifested in part by fever (e.g., halothane reaction). Likewise, thyroid storm can be precipitated by surgery on this gland. Malignant hyperthermia is a dramatic event manifested by acute hyperpyrexia and muscle rigidity after exposure to certain anesthetics.

8. The patient's list of medications should be surveyed for drugs known to be associated with fever production. All nonessential medications should be discontinued, especially those that have recently been prescribed. Parenteral drugs likely to produce inflammation at the site of administration (e.g., erythromycin) should be discontinued or replaced, if possible. Because fever will not necessarily remit within 24 to 48 hours of the time that the drug is discontinued, patience in observing the patient's response may be needed.

9. Review the patient's record and laboratory testing summaries to determine whether blood or blood product transfusion has

---

BOX 249-1

Work flow approach to history and physical examination in diagnosis of hospital-acquired fever

---

History

What procedures, instrumentations, or other interventions have been performed since this patient was hospitalized? Has anesthesia been administered?

What new medications, immunoglobulins, or transfusion products has the patient received since hospitalization?

Has the patient been treated with antipyretics or other drugs that affect fever?

Have contrast dyes or other diagnostic products been administered as part of imaging or other diagnostic procedures?

What underlying diseases does the patient have that may be manifested by intermittent fever, which may have created the false appearance of fever as nosocomial?

Has the patient manifested new symptoms that may signal acquisition of a likely nosocomial pathogen (e.g., nosocomial diarrhea as a manifestation of *Clostridium difficile* infection, sputum production as a manifestation of nosocomial pneumonia)?

Physical examination

Head

Nasogastric or gastric tube in place? Evaluate for sinusitis.

Chest

On ventilator now or recently? Operative procedure with general anesthesia since admission?

New onset or change in character of sputum production or of respiratory function? Careful chest examination for infection or inflammation, follow-up diagnostic studies (radiograph, scanning, etc.) as warranted.

Murmur or other sign of cardiac dysfunction? If operative or invasive diagnostic procedure performed, evaluate possibility of endocarditis, especially if prophylaxis for the procedure was suboptimum. Blood culture evaluation should be made if there is any suspicion that the fever represents bloodstream invasion.

Are the patient's prior course and care consistent with a focus for pulmonary emboli?

Gastrointestinal

Onset of diarrhea in the hospital? Evaluate for *Clostridium difficile* infection, especially if the patient has recently been treated with antimicrobial agents. Perhaps more likely, which new medication could be causing local irritation of the gut?

Genital

Urinary catheter in place now or recently? Obtain urine specimen for microscopic examination (pyuria, hematuria, bacteriuria); if appropriate, follow with Gram's stain and culture.

Operative site or site of trauma

Signs of superficial or deep infection? Possibility of loculated areas requiring imaging techniques for evaluation?

Extremities

Are signs of thrombophlebitis or manifestations of extremity ischemia present?

Skin

Skin rashes are probably the most common and easily noted manifestations of febrile drug reaction, transfusion reaction, and viral or other infections.

Intravascular therapy administered now or recently? Examine closely for phlebitis or exudate at the site of cannulation. Attempt to milk fluid back from vein, and palpate for possible septic thrombophlebitis. Examine fluid container for cracks or cloudy fluid.

Signs of decubitus or other ulcer, especially one that has broken down since hospital stay began?

---

taken place. Febrile reactions associated with this procedure usually occur during or just after transfusion, but fever with onset months afterward may be associated with infection produced by hepatitis viruses, especially hepatitis C virus, acquired at the time of transfusion.

10. Of hospital-acquired fevers 10% to 20% may remain undiagnosed. Some resolve spontaneously. With long-term follow-up evaluation, causes of others eventually become clear as new symptoms or findings appear. Collagen diseases, factitious fever, lymphoma, chronic granulomatous disease of the liver, and chronic viral infections such as those produced by Epstein-Barr virus (EBV) or cytomegalovirus (CMV) often become more obvious as time progresses.

These 10 general approaches to evaluation of nosocomial fever are related to aspects of the history and physical examination listed in Box 249-1.

MANAGEMENT

Therapy and preventive measures depend on the findings of the diagnostic evaluation. Use of antipyretics often is discouraged until the source of the fever has become clear, although Styrt and Sugarman note that in some patients the comfort produced by antipyretics outweighs the relative benefit of observing fever pattern, and in some patients the drugs are needed to reduce the risk of adverse effects associated with underlying cardiac disease.

Because hospital-acquired fever frequently has noninfectious causes, routine use of antimicrobial agents when fever begins is not recommended. Of course, if a patient has hypotension or other manifestations of suspected bacterial infection, empiric antimicrobial therapy may be wise. Organisms causing nosocomial infections frequently are resistant to many commonly used antimicrobial agents, so the choice of empiric therapy depends on patterns of resistance in the specific institution. The most important step in many cases is re-

---

✔ *WHEN TO REFER*

Management of several of the potential sources of hospital-acquired fever may require skills and services of other professionals, ranging from the surgeon to the radiologist. Although these consultants may be needed to provide specific procedures, decisions about the need for such services and the further care of the patient after completion of such actions usually are best made by the patient's personal physician.

---

moval of the predisposing catheters and other devices that have been listed.

BIBLIOGRAPHY

Arbo MJ et al: Fever of nosocomial origin: etiology, risk factors, and outcomes, *Am J Med* 95:505, 1993.

Cunha BA, Shea KW: Fever in the intensive care unit, *Infect Dis Clin North Am* 10:185, 1996.

Donowitz GR: Fever in the compromised host, *Infect Dis Clin North Am* 10:129, 1996.

Filice GA et al: Nosocomial febrile illnesses in patients on an internal medicine service, *Arch Intern Med* 149:319, 1989.

Fischer SA, Trenholme GM, Levin S: Fever in the solid organ transplant patient, *Infect Dis Clin North Am* 10:167, 1996.

McGowan JE Jr et al: Fever in hospitalized patients, with special reference to the medical service, *Am J Med* 82:580, 1987.

Peduzzi P et al: Predictors of bacteremia and gram-negative bacteremia in patients with sepsis, *Arch Intern Med* 152:529, 1992.

Styrt B, Sugarman B: Antipyresis and fever, *Arch Intern Med* 150:1589, 1990.

IV ORGANISMS INFECTIVE TO HUMANS

VIRAL DISEASES

250 Common Viral Infections, Picornavirus, and Orthomyxovirus Infections (Rhinovirus, Enterovirus, and Influenza)

R. Gordon Douglas, Jr.

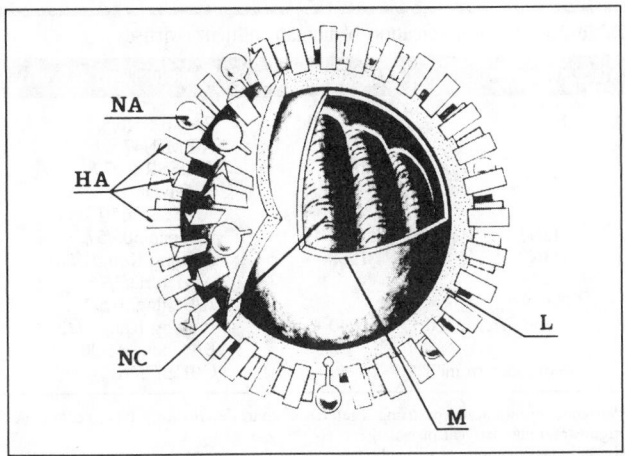

FIGURE 250-1   Diagrammatic representation of influenza virus. *HA* and *NA*, Hemagglutinin and neuraminidase subunits, respectively; *NC*, nucleocapsid that consists of nucleoprotein and viral RNA; *M*, matrix protein; *L*, lipid bilayer.

From Stuart-Harris CH, Schild GC: *Influenza: the viruses and the diseases*, Littleton, Mass, 1976, Publishing Sciences Group.

The picornavirus family consists of a large number of serologically distinct viruses that are similar in structure and physical and chemical properties. They are responsible for many asymptomatic infections and for a spectrum of illnesses ranging from common colds to pneumonia, myopericarditis, aseptic meningitis, paralytic poliomyelitis, and hepatitis.

The orthomyxoviridae contain only one genus, *Influenza*, and three types (species): A, B, and C. Types A and B cause a variety of acute respiratory disease syndromes in humans, the most notable being influenza, an acute respiratory disease with fever and prominent systemic symptoms. Both types A and B spawn recurring epidemics of varying severity in human populations. Type C virus appears to be endemic and primarily causes minor respiratory illness in young children.

Table 250-1   Human picornaviruses

GENUS AND SPECIES	NUMBER OF IMMUNOTYPES
Enteroviruses	
Poliovirus	3
Coxsackievirus A	23
Coxsackievirus B	6
Echovirus	30
Enterovirus	5
Rhinovirus	>100
Hepatitis A virus	1

CHARACTERISTICS

Picornaviruses are small, icosahedral, nonenveloped, ether-resistant viruses. The capsid, which is 20 to 30 nm in diameter, is composed of 60 subunits (capsomers) that are synthesized from four structural polypeptides (VP1 through VP4); VP1 is the dominant antigen. The capsid encloses a linear, single-stranded ribonucleic acid (RNA) genome with a molecular weight of 2.6×10^6. The RNA functions as a monocistronic messenger, yielding a polyprotein of molecular weight 2.5×10^5 that subsequently undergoes specific cleavages to form the structural polypeptides of the capsomers. In addition, a virus-coded RNA polymerase and other polypeptides required for viral replication are produced.

Influenza virus particles are spherical, with a diameter of 80 to 120 nm; however, filamentous particles of varying lengths may also be seen. The helical viral nucleocapsid is composed of nucleoprotein and RNA (Fig. 250-1). The RNA genome is single stranded and divided into separate segments. There are eight segments for types A and B and seven for type C. Structural stability is provided by matrix protein, and the viral core is surrounded by an outer lipid bilayer into which the surface subunits are inserted. Two different surface subunits, hemagglutinin and neuraminidase glycoproteins, are present on types A and B particles, whereas a single glycoprotein, a hemagglutinin-esterase glycoprotein, is present on type C particles.

Attachment of the virus to susceptible cells is mediated by the hemagglutinin subunit. The red blood cell receptor is a neuraminic acid–containing glycoprotein; probably a similar receptor is involved in initiation of infection of eukaryotic cells. Penetration is by pinocytosis, and uncoating results from fusion with the endosomal membrane. New viral RNA is replicated through a complementary RNA

messenger, and this takes place in the cell nucleus. Viral proteins are synthesized in the cytoplasm. Nucleocapsid assembly takes place in the cell nucleus, and virion assembly takes place at the cell surface. Virion surface subunits orient on the cell plasma membrane, and virus is released by budding through the membrane. During the latter process the lipid bilayer is acquired.

Newly synthesized virus contains neuraminic acid residues that promote aggregation at the cell surface. Neuraminidase activity disrupts or prevents occurrence of these aggregates, a phenomenon that results in an increase in free infectious particles. From initiation to completion, replication takes 6 hours. Infected cells produce new virus over a period of several hours, then cell death ensues.

CLASSIFICATION

Picornaviruses are very small, nonenveloped RNA viruses. Three genera infect humans: rhinovirus, hepatitis A virus, and enterovirus. More than 100 immunotypes of rhinovirus have been described (Table 250-1). Hepatitis A virus was originally classified as enterovirus type 72 but now is thought to represent a new genus (Chapter 355).

Originally, the enteroviruses were subdivided into three groups—polioviruses, coxsackieviruses, and echoviruses—on the basis of antigenic relationships and differences in host range. In recent years, as new enteroviruses have been isolated, it has become clear that basing their classification on host range is not the best approach. Thus newly discovered enteroviruses have been given the designation of enterovirus types 68 to 72, whereas the enterovirus immunotypes previously classified as poliovirus, coxsackievirus group A, coxsackievirus group B, and echoviruses have retained the original designation.

The human influenza viruses are classified as shown in Table 250-2. All three types are similar in biochemical and biophysical properties. However, distinctive differences in antigenic determinants of

Table 250-2   Classification of human influenza viruses

TYPE	SUBTYPE	YEARS OF PREVALENCE	REPRESENTATIVE VARIANTS*
A	H1N1†	1918-1957‡	Puerto Rico/8/34
			A/FM/1/47
		1977-	A/USSR/92/77
			A/Taiwan/1/86
			A/Texas/36/91
	H2N2	1957-1967	A/Japan/305/57
	H3N2	1968-	A/Hong Kong/1/68
			A/Victoria/3/75
			A/Beijing/32/92
B	None determined	1940-§	B/Hong Kong/5/72
			B/Panama/45/90
C	None determined	1949-‖	C/JHB/2/66

*Variants are monitored by using a reference strain described by type, geographic origin/strain number/year of isolation.
†Earlier classifications of this subtype included the separate designations $H_{Sw}1N1$, HON1, and H1N1. All are now designated as the H1N1 subtype.
‡An influenza virus was first isolated from swine in 1931 and from humans in 1933; retrospective serologic studies indicated that a virus resembling swine/31 became prevalent in humans in 1918.
§First isolated from humans in 1940.
‖First isolated from humans in 1949.

major structural subunits provide a basis for a classification that reflects biologic and epidemiologic behavior.

Types A, B, and C viruses contain different but antigenically stable nucleoprotein antigens. Type A viruses may exhibit major and minor antigenic variation of their surface hemagglutinin and neuraminidase subunits. When new type A viruses that lack serologic cross-reactivity with one of the surface subunits of earlier viruses (major change) appear, a subtype designation is assigned. This phenomenon has been called *antigenic shift,* and usually such an occurrence has led to widespread epidemic or pandemic influenza. Three distinct human subtypes have been described: H1N1, H2N2, and H3N2.

Separate and distinct subtypes of type A virus have also been described for equine and avian species. Because of antigenic relatedness, type A viruses of swine (formerly $H_{Sw}1N1$) are designated as H1N1 viruses. Virus types B and C have not exhibited antigenic shift, and no indigenous occurrence in animals has been described.

The most likely explanation for antigenic shift among type A viruses is that new surface antigens are acquired from an animal virus by genetic reassortment, and this is followed by subsequent spread among humans. The existence of a segmented genome facilitates reassortment of genes (recombination) in a mixed infection.

Both virus types A and B exhibit minor antigenic change of the hemagglutinin and neuraminidase subunits; in these instances, serologic cross-reactivity between subunits is demonstrable. This type of change has been called *antigenic drift* and is presumed to result from mutability of the virus genome and selective pressure of population immunity. Such changes may lead to epidemic influenza. A prototype strain representative of each of these variants is designated by geographic origin, strain number, and year of isolation (see Table 250-2).

Antigenic differences among type C viruses are minimal.

EPIDEMIOLOGY
Enteroviruses

The epidemiology of most enteroviruses is similar. Enteroviruses are distributed worldwide, but their epidemiologic behavior is affected by climate, season, age, and socioeconomic and other factors. In temperate climates, enteroviruses are strikingly more prevalent in the summer and autumn months, predominantly August through October, but often beginning earlier and extending well into winter months. This seasonal periodicity has never been satisfactorily explained, but it is not observed in the tropics, where enteroviruses are endemic year-round. Age is another important epidemiologic factor. Outbreaks of enteroviral infections are highest in children less than 1 year of age, and children invariably have higher attack rates than adults. Antibody incidence is at least three to six times higher in the lower socioeco-

nomic classes, and multiple infections are common in these situations, where such conditions as poor hygiene and overcrowding may be present.

In urban areas of the United States, several immunotypes of enteroviruses usually dominate each season, but the types may vary from city to city or region to region and, further, from year to year. Occasional epidemics with a single immunotype (e.g., echovirus type 9) have occurred nationwide or even worldwide. The most frequent nonpolio isolates reported to the World Health Organization and the Centers for Disease Control and Prevention in recent years include echovirus types 11, 9, 4, 6, 3, and 7; coxsackievirus types B5, B2, B4, and B3; and coxsackievirus type A9. These types accounted for two thirds of all isolates.

Enteroviruses are spread predominantly via the fecal-oral route, principally from person to person directly, although enteroviruses have been isolated from flies, cockroaches, food naturally exposed to flies, dog feces, and a number of other vehicles. Direct person-to-person, fecal-oral transmission is consistent with the higher antibody incidence in children and in the lower socioeconomic groups. Enterovirus infections often cluster in families, and the home may be the setting where most transmission takes place. The period of maximum contagiousness corresponds to the period of maximum virus excretion. Once virus has been introduced into a household, secondary attack rates are close to 100% for wild polioviruses, about 75% for coxsackieviruses, and 50% for echoviruses. Presumably, the lower rate for echoviruses is due to their being shed for shorter periods and in lower quantities than polioviruses or coxsackieviruses. There are exceptions (e.g., coxsackievirus A21 behaves like a respiratory virus). Respiratory spread of other enteroviruses may occasionally be important. Enterovirus type 70, the agent of acute hemorrhagic conjunctivitis, appears to be spread by fomites, fingers, and ophthalmologic instruments contaminated with virus.

The last case of endemic poliomyelitis in the United States occurred in 1979. All of the 5 to 10 cases that occur annually are associated with the use of live oral polio vaccine. Approximately 40% occur in vaccine recipients and 60% in contacts of recipients.

Rhinoviruses

The epidemiology of rhinovirus infections differs considerably from that of enteroviruses. The seasonal pattern is not so abrupt. Rhinovirus infections tend to occur year-round, with fall and spring peaks of infection. In the United States, an early fall peak occurs shortly after the opening of school and a second peak occurs in the early spring. However, continuing rhinovirus infections are observed each month of the year.

Like enteroviruses, rhinoviruses have a worldwide distribution. In a given geographic area, one or several immunotypes may be prevalent at any time, only to be replaced during the next peak by one or several other immunotypes. Studies of the incidence of antibody show rapid acquisition of antibody during childhood and adolescence, with a peak incidence in young adults. There is little evidence that any of the more than 100 immunotypes predominates. Rhinovirus infections are among the most common human virus infections. Studies indicate infection rates of at least 1.2 per person per year in children under the age of 1 year and 0.7 in young adults.

Recent studies have elucidated the mechanisms of transmission. Most rhinovirus infections appear to be transmitted in the home after introduction of infection by a child of school age. The incubation period is 2 to 6 days, and secondary attack rates in family members range from 25% to 70%. Infection is initiated via the respiratory tract. Virus spreads from person to person by transfer of contaminated secretions from an infected donor to a susceptible recipient. Such transfer may occur from hand to hand or from hand to fomite to hand, followed by autoinoculation of nasal or conjunctival mucosa by the susceptible subject. Infection also may be transmitted by large- or small-particle aerosols.

Influenza

Influenza viruses were probably a cause of disease in ancient times; retrospective tracing has dated the occurrence of influenza epidemics at least to 1173. Thereafter there is a nearly continuous record of epidemics, which are periodically interspersed with extensive pandemics (worldwide epidemics). During the past century, serologic tests of sera from elderly persons have permitted an assessment of epidemic disease. In 1889 a pandemic occurred with a type A virus containing an H3-like hemagglutinin and an equine 2 (now N8)–like neuraminidase. Little is recorded of influenza in the intervening years preceding the devastating pandemic of 1918, which was caused by an H1N1 (formerly called swine) virus. That pandemic caused about 500,000 deaths in the United States and about 20 million fatalities worldwide.

The modern history of influenza began with isolation of influenza virus from humans in 1933. Since that time two shifts causing pandemics have occurred, one in 1957, caused by H2N2 (Asian) virus, and a less extensive one in 1968, caused by H3N2 virus. In the intervening years antigenic drift and epidemics of varying severity occurred.

The pattern exhibited by a typical type A epidemic in an urban community is shown in Fig. 250-2. In the initial phases of an epidemic, infection and illness appear predominantly in school children, and this is reflected by a sharp rise in school absenteeism, physician visits, and pediatric hospital admissions. These children carry the virus into the home, where preschool children and adults acquire the infection. Infection and illness among adults are then reflected in industrial absenteeism, adult hospital admissions, and mortality associated with influenza or pneumonia.

The duration of an epidemic is generally 3 to 6 weeks, although virus is present in the community for a variable number of weeks before and after the epidemic period. During the epidemic period the duration of an outbreak in subsegments of the population may be brief (e.g., the complete course of epidemic influenza may occur in an institutionalized population in a period of 2 weeks).

Influenza type B presents a similar pattern of epidemic occurrence, except that excess mortality may not be apparent. Influenza type C has not been shown to produce epidemic disease.

Epidemics in temperate climates typically occur in winter, although fall and spring epidemics may also be seen. Both virus types A and B (and probably C) cause infections and illness every winter; however, an epidemic does not occur unless the constellation of factors required for epidemic spread occurs. The relative significance of crowding, environmental conditions, and other factors for development of an epidemic is uncertain, but the most important factor is population susceptibility, an occurrence primarily attributable to antigenic variation.

Antigenic shift occurs at a point location, and the new virus then spreads throughout the world along transportation routes; the source and spread of antigenic drift viruses are less certain. Community "seeding" with a new virus may occur during the "off season," and as much as 2 years may precede the occurrence of epidemic disease. Such a pattern of infection would imply a summer survival mechanism or repeated community introductions of new viruses; evidence favors the latter.

Influenza virus is transmitted primarily by the airborne route, but direct contact is probably also important. The incubation period varies between 1 and 5 days. Attack rates of illness during epidemics vary between 10% and 50%. The highest attack rates during epidemics of types A and B are in the 5- to 19-year-old age-group; however, high frequencies occur in preschool children and adults of all ages. Attack rates are usually lower for type B in preschool children and adults.

Mortality attributable to influenza has proved to be a reliable index of epidemic influenza, but it tends to minimize the magnitude of a type B epidemic because there may be no excessive mortality. The severity and frequency of influenza epidemics are variable. Only in a general way can the magnitude be related to the occurrence of antigenic shift. Thus the consequences of antigenic drift must be considered to be of equal significance.

PATHOGENESIS
Enteroviruses

Most enteroviruses initially produce infection of the mucosal and lymphoid tissue of the pharynx and gut. In some instances, viremia occurs, with subsequent involvement of other target organs, such as the heart, brain, meninges, and skin. In contrast, rhinoviruses exclusively

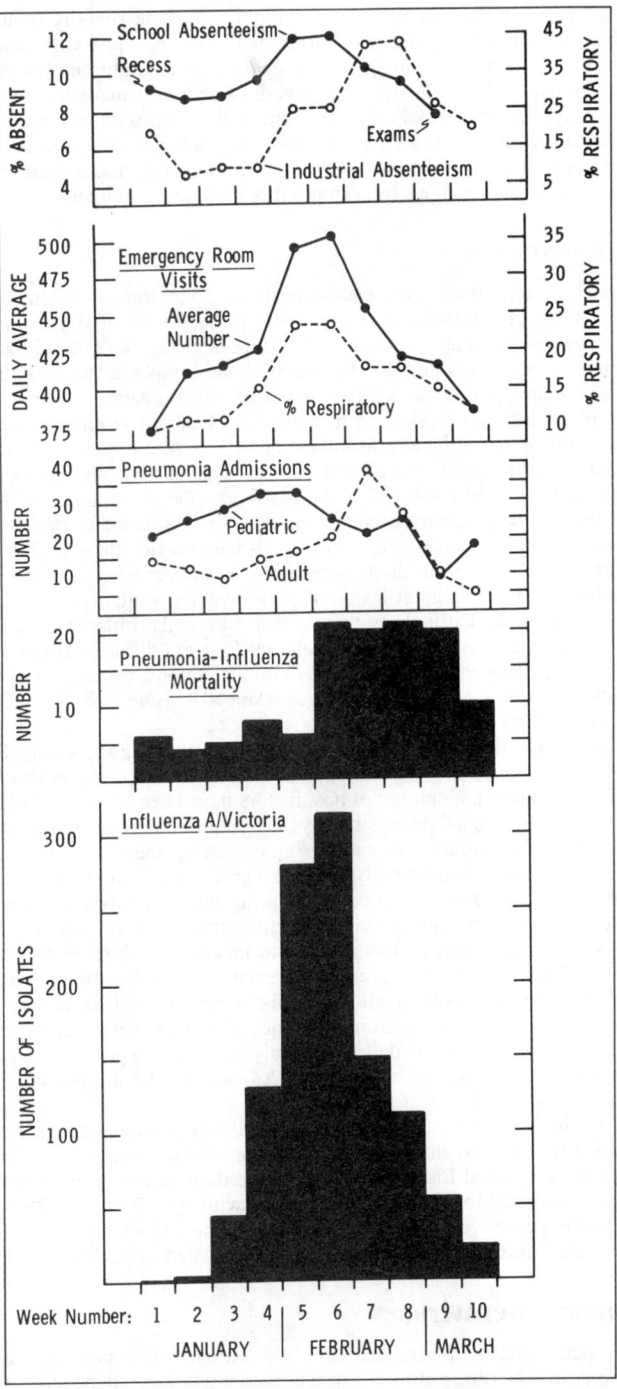

FIGURE 250-2   Correlation of the nonvirologic indices of epidemic influenza with the number of isolates of influenza A/Victoria virus according to week, Houston, 1976.

From Glezen WP, Couch RB: Interpandemic influenza in the Houston area, 1974-76, *N Engl J Med* 298:587, 1978.

infect the upper respiratory tract; they have not been demonstrated to disseminate to distant sites in the body (Table 250-3).

Rhinovirus

The pathologic findings of rhinovirus infection include hyperemia and edema of the mucous membranes, with exudation of serous and mucinous fluid and engorgement of the turbinates. On histologic examination, subepithelial edema with sparse cellular infiltrates is seen. Virus is recovered from the nose, throat, and saliva, but the nose appears to be the predominant site of replication. The severity of the illness parallels the quantity of virus shed in the nasopharyngeal secretions. Direct viral damage to the epithelium is slight, and symptoms most likely result from the release of chemical mediators such as bradykinin and lysylbradykinin. The pathogeneses of enterovirus and rhinovirus infections are contrasted in Table 250-3. There is no apparent effect of exposure to cold on the frequency and severity of common colds resulting from rhinovirus infection in humans.

Poliovirus

Among enteroviruses, the pathogenesis of poliovirus infection has been most clearly worked out, and the pathogenesis of most other enteroviruses probably resembles that of poliovirus. The initial infection with poliovirus involves the mucosal and lymphoid tissue of the pharynx and gut. Virus shortly thereafter disseminates to regional lymph nodes, and replication in these sites leads to viremia, which may correspond clinically to mild illness. Viremia may or may not result in infection of the central nervous system and other susceptible sites. In only 1% to 2% of the cases does the virus penetrate the central nervous system. Although it is most likely that the central nervous system is invaded across the blood-brain barrier, the possibility of transmission of virus along nerve fibers has never been completely excluded. The prominent lesion of poliomyelitis results from infection of neurons, particularly the anterior horn cells. Inflammation is secondary and consists of perivascular cuffing and diffuse infiltration of mononuclear cells. In other enterovirus infections, the target organ of the viremia may be the meninges, skeletal muscle, testicle, skin, heart, or other sites.

It is clear that there are differences in virulence among strains of poliovirus, which may in part explain differences in paralysis attack rates. In addition, a number of host factors have been associated with an increased risk of paralysis. Boys are more commonly paralyzed than girls. Fatigue and strenuous exercise during the first 3 days of the major illness substantially increase the incidence and severity of paralysis. Conversely, strict bed rest during this period has a sparing effect on paralysis. Intramuscular injection, trauma, or surgery within 2 weeks of the onset of illness tends to localize paralysis to the involved limb. Tonsillectomy, even in the remote past, increases the incidence of bulbar poliomyelitis. The incidence, but not the severity, of poliomyelitis is increased in pregnancy. Finally, genetic factors appear to increase the incidence of paralysis; histocompatibility antigens human leukocyte antigen 3 (HLA3) and HLA7 are associated with an increased risk of paralysis.

In the last decade, children with hereditary immunodeficiencies who were exposed through vaccination or contact with vaccine recipients accounted for 14% of cases of paralytic poliomyelitis in the United States. Most cases have occurred with type 2 or type 3 oral poliovirus vaccine. Both isolated B-cell immunodeficiency and severe combined immunodeficiency syndrome have been implicated.

Other Enteroviruses

The pathogenesis of coxsackievirus and echovirus infections may be similar to either the poliovirus or the rhinovirus model, depending on the strain and other factors. In the case of viruses that produce primarily upper respiratory infections, the pathogenesis is presumed to be similar to that described for rhinovirus infection. In the case of enterovirus infections that result in aseptic meningitis with or without exanthema, the pathogenesis may be similar to that for poliovirus, except that the target tissues in the final phase are the meninges and skin instead of the spinal cord gray matter.

Host risk factors, such as those identified with poliovirus infections, have not been observed in other human enterovirus infections. However, in experimental coxsackievirus myopericarditis in mice, adrenal corticoids, exercise, exposure to cold, alcohol, male sex, genetic factors, and chronic undernutrition have been associated with increased virulence of infection. It is not known whether these factors play a role in coxsackievirus infection in humans.

In both poliovirus and rhinovirus infection, the mechanism of cellular injury is believed to be the cytolysis that results from virus replication. Immunologic mechanisms may also be involved in some enterovirus infections. Patients with isolated agammaglobulinemia have persistent enterovirus infections. In patients with myopericarditis, coxsackievirus can be detected in the myocardium or pericardium, and cytolysis may result directly from viral replication early in the illness. Later in the illness, an immunologic basis for continuing lesions is suggested by the absence of infectious virus and the presence of immunoglobulins and complement on immunofluorescent staining in the heart of patients with myopericarditis. An immunologic pathogenesis is consistent with the findings in experimental coxsackievirus myocarditis in mice: an early "infectious phase" and a later "immunologic phase."

Influenza

The initial deposition site of inhaled aerosol particles is the tracheobronchial mucosa. The covering mucous blanket includes mucoproteins that contain the neuraminic acid receptor. Binding undoubtedly occurs, but the action of viral neuraminidase could induce release and liquefaction of mucus, thereby further promoting access of virus to the mucosal surface. The primary site of infection is the superficial columnar epithelium. Completion of the viral replicative cycle in these cells results in cellular death and desquamation. Edema and mononuclear cell infiltration of involved areas result, and these changes are accompanied by a prominent cough. A similar sequence occurs in the nasopharynx, where virus may also be deposited. Changes at these sites lead to nasal and pharyngeal symptoms.

During the incubation period the extent of involvement of the cellular mucosa increases, and this change is reflected in an increase in the quantity of virus detected in secretions. There is a direct relationship between the quantity of virus detected and the severity of the illness in uncomplicated cases. After a 2- to 3-day period, a fall in the quantity of virus in secretions occurs; this fall is accompanied by an improvement in symptoms, but virus shedding and symptoms may last for 5 to 8 days. Although severe myalgias are a feature of acute influenza, viremia has rarely been detected.

Recovery from acute influenza generally ensues before antibody is detectable in either serum or secretions. A role for interferon in recovery is suggested by its appearance in secretions just as the progressive reduction in the quantity of virus begins. Cell-mediated cytotoxicity for virus-infected cells has been demonstrated; T-cells, natural killer cells, and cells mediating antibody-dependent cellular cytotoxicity may contribute to clearance of the localized infection. When antibody appears in secretions, virus is no longer detectable, suggesting a role for local antibody in the final clearance of virus.

On occasion, particularly in persons with underlying heart or lung disease, viral involvement of alveolar tissues of the lung may occur and produce an interstitial pneumonia. Virus titers in secretions from these patients may be very high (10^{7-9}TCID$_{50}$/ml) and the duration of viral shedding prolonged. Sometimes, marked accumulation of lung edema, with hemorrhage, hyaline membrane formation, extensive mononuclear infiltration, and pulmonary fibrosis, is seen.

Pneumonia in association with influenza is most commonly caused by bacteria. In these cases, viral infection has presumably impaired the normal lung defense mechanisms so that invasion by pneumococci, staphylococci, and gram-negative bacteria is promoted. Such cases exhibit the histologic features of bacterial pneumonia, although, if the pneumonia occurs early in the course of influenza, the histologic features of both viral and bacterial pneumonia may be exhibited.

Table 250-3 Comparative pathogenesis of enterovirus (poliovirus) and rhinovirus infections

PATHOGENESIS	POLIOVIRUS	RHINOVIRUS
Method of transmission	Fecal-oral	Respiratory
Site of viral deposition	Gastrointestinal mucosa	Upper respiratory mucosa
Virus isolation	Throat and feces	Nose and throat
Viremic	Yes	No
Central nervous system involvement	Yes	No

Antibody is the primary defense mechanism against acquisition of infection. Locally synthesized immunoglobulin A (IgA) antibody is the primary mediator of protection for the upper respiratory passages, whereas serum-derived IgG antibody mediates protection of the lower respiratory passages. The latter measure is used to assess immunity, because a direct correlation exists between serum antibody titer and resistance to infection. In general, a hemagglutination-inhibition titer of 1:32 against the epidemic virus is associated with substantial resistance. Antibody directed toward the hemagglutinin is required to prevent infection, whereas antibody directed toward either the hemagglutinin or the neuraminidase reduces the level of infection, the likelihood of occurrence of illness, and the severity of illness.

The risk of febrile illness in persons lacking either hemagglutinin or neuraminidase antibody is about 80%, whereas in most circumstances some antibody is present, and the febrile illness risk is about 50%.

DISEASES IN HUMANS

All the picornaviruses produce subclinical infection in humans (Table 250-4). In the case of the enteroviruses, the majority of infections are asymptomatic, whereas for rhinoviruses the proportion of asymptomatic infections is probably around 30% to 40%. Picornaviruses contribute to a broad clinical spectrum of illnesses.

Common Colds and Other Respiratory Illnesses

The predominant illness resulting from rhinovirus infection is a typical common cold, which is indistinguishable from that produced by other respiratory viruses (Chapter 237). Rhinoviruses are the single most important cause of common colds in older children and adults. Although all picornaviruses presumably contribute to the total causes of common colds, the relative proportion of colds attributable to enteroviruses is small.

Acute Febrile Undifferentiated Illness

Undifferentiated febrile illnesses caused by most enterovirus immunotypes may be accompanied by upper respiratory symptoms, such as sore throat and occasionally cough and coryza. These illnesses are clinically indistinguishable from the "flulike" syndromes caused by rhinoviruses, parainfluenza viruses, adenoviruses, and influenza viruses, except that they commonly occur in the summer months, when influenza, for example, is almost entirely absent in the northern hemi-

sphere. These illnesses may be unaccompanied by any respiratory signs or symptoms. Their occurrence in the summer months is suggestive of enterovirus infection, especially when other evidence of enterovirus infection (e.g., aseptic meningitis, exanthem) is present in the community.

Enteroviruses occasionally also produce the syndromes attributable to other respiratory viruses, such as pharyngitis, laryngitis, tracheobronchitis, and pneumonia. During outbreaks of other types of enteroviral disease (e.g., aseptic meningitis, pleurodynia), cases of viral respiratory illness such as viral pneumonia are encountered.

Paralytic Poliomyelitis

Clinical Findings. The incubation period of paralytic poliomyelitis is 9 to 12 days. The manifestations are extremely variable, ranging from inapparent infection to severe paralysis and death. Approximately 95% of poliovirus infections are subclinical. In 4% to 8% of infections, an illness known as abortive poliomyelitis occurs, causing fever, headache, sore throat, listlessness, anorexia, vomiting, and pain in the muscles or abdomen. The physical findings are normal, and the illness lasts only a few hours to days. Nonparalytic poliomyelitis occurs in 1% to 2% of all infections and differs from abortive poliomyelitis in that aseptic meningitis is present. In addition to stiffness of the neck and back, the patient generally has more headache and higher fever and appears more toxic than in abortive poliomyelitis. Frank paralysis occurs in roughly 0.1% of all poliovirus infections in children. There is a biphasic course in a third of affected children, beginning with a "minor" illness, resembling abortive poliomyelitis, which coincides with viremia and lasts 1 to 3 days. The patient then appears to be recovering and remains symptom-free for 2 to 5 days before the abrupt onset of meningitic symptoms and signs of "major" illness: headache, fever, malaise, vomiting, and neck stiffness. The temperature is generally 98.6° to 102.2° F (37° to 39° C) and is often accompanied by chilliness and, rarely, by rigors. In older children and in most adults, the illness consists of a single phase, with a more prolonged prodrome and a more gradual onset of paralysis.

The occurrence of spontaneous muscle pain is the most important characteristic of the major illness. Most commonly involved are muscles of the neck and lumbar region, but muscles of the flank, abdomen, or limbs also may be involved. The pain is relieved by motion, and the patient may pace nervously to work it off.

The meningitic phase of the major illness, accompanied by muscle pain, is generally present for 1 to 2 days before the characteristic asymmetric paralysis ensues. The proximal muscles of the extremities tend to be more involved than the distal muscles. The legs are

Table 250-4   Diseases associated with picornaviruses*

SYNDROME	POLIOVIRUSES	COXSACKIEVIRUSES GROUP A	COXSACKIEVIRUSES GROUP B	ECHOVIRUSES	ENTEROVIRUSES	RHINOVIRUSES
Asymptomatic infection	1-3	All types	All types	All types	All types	All types
Common cold	1-3	All types	All types	All types	All types	All types
Acute febrile, undifferentiated illness	1-3	All types	All types	All types	All types	
Paralysis	1-3	4,6,7,9,11,14,21	1-6	1-4,6,7,9,11,14,16,18,19,30	70,71	
Aseptic meningitis	1-3	1-11,14,16-18,22,24	1-6	All except 24,26,29,32	70,71	
Encephalitis		2,5-7,9	1-5	2-4,6,7,9,11,14,17-19,25	70,71	
Herpangina		2-6,8,10,22				
Hand-foot-mouth syndrome		5,7,9,10,16			71	
Lymphonodular pharyngitis		10				
Exanthem		2,4,5,9,16	1,3-5	1-9,11,14,18,19,25,30,32,33	71	
Pleurodynia			1-5			
Myopericarditis			1-5			
Generalized disease of the newborn			1-5			
Orchitis			1-5			
Neonatal diarrhea				11,14,18		
Chronic meningoencephalitis in agammaglobulinemics				2,3,5,9,11,19,24,25,30,33		
Acute hemorrhagic conjunctivitis	24				70	

*Numbers indicate the immunotype associated with indicated syndrome. Hepatitis produced by hepatitis A virus (formerly enterovirus 72) is excluded.

more commonly involved than the arms, and large muscle groups of the hand are at greater risk than small ones. Any combination of limbs may be paralyzed; the most common pattern is involvement of one leg, followed by involvement of one arm or both legs and both arms. Both the extent and rapidity of paralysis are highly variable. Most commonly, paralysis progresses over 2 to 3 days and almost invariably halts when the patient becomes afebrile. Sensory loss does not occur in poliomyelitis, and its presence should strongly suggest other diagnoses, such as Guillain-Barré syndrome.

In bulbar poliomyelitis, there is paralysis of muscle groups innervated by cranial nerves, especially the muscles of the soft palate, pharynx, and larynx. Other cranial nerve nuclei are frequently involved but rarely pose a threat to life. The frequency of the bulbar form of the disease varies between 5% and 35%.

Encephalitis, manifested primarily by confusion, disturbances of consciousness, and seizures, is an uncommon form of poliomyelitis occurring principally in infants.

Coxsackievirus A7 and enterovirus 71 are neuropathogenic in monkeys and have been recognized as the cause of small outbreaks of poliomyelitis. Other enterovirus immunotypes have also been associated with sporadic cases of paralytic disease that is usually milder than poliomyelitis. Frank paralysis, which is less common than muscle weakness, is usually not permanent. Poliomyelitis caused by administration of oral poliomyelitis vaccines to children with hereditary immunodeficiencies occurs after an incubation period of 7 to 21 days. In contacts, usually young adults, the incubation period is 20 to 29 days. In immunocompromised children, the illness is protracted, and paralysis may progress over several weeks. Mortality is high (40%) and prolonged fecal excretion of virus is characteristic.

Complications. The complications of poliomyelitis include respiratory failure caused by paralysis of the respiratory muscles, and airway obstruction from involvement of cranial nuclei or lesions in the respiratory center. Other complications include aspiration pneumonia, pulmonary edema, pulmonary embolism, viral myocarditis, gastrointestinal hemorrhage, paralytic ileus and gastric dilation, and development of urinary calculi.

Differential Diagnosis. Poliomyelitis usually presents a clear-cut clinical picture that differs from that of Guillain-Barré syndrome. In Guillain-Barré syndrome, paralysis is symmetric and is accompanied by sensory loss; facial diplegia is common, and paralysis may progress over a period of up to 2 weeks. Hysteria, diphtheria, botulism, tick paralysis, pseudoparalysis, and encephalitis may mimic poliomyelitis in some instances.

Laboratory Findings. The peripheral white cell count may be normal or elevated. Cerebrospinal fluid findings are similar to those of aseptic meningitis, with pleocytosis and a minimally elevated protein concentration. The cell count usually returns to normal within 2 to 3 weeks, but minor protein abnormalities may last longer. Polioviruses can be isolated from throat secretions in the first week of the illness and may often be isolated from feces for several weeks. They are rarely isolated from cerebrospinal fluid.

Prognosis. The overall mortality of paralytic poliomyelitis in epidemics in the past was 5% to 10%. In bulbar poliomyelitis mortality is high, and most patients with poliovirus encephalitis die. Some degree of permanent damage is observed in about a third of poliomyelitis victims. Full return of function is less likely in severely paralyzed muscles than in mildly paralyzed ones. Patients requiring mechanical ventilation because of spinal respiratory paralysis rarely recover without some sequelae. Although bulbar poliomyelitis causes the greatest threat to life in the first week of illness, it is rarely responsible for permanent damage in surviving patients. Some estimate of the eventual outcome can be made at 1 month. No additional return of function can be expected beyond 9 months. New onset of weakness in the previously affected muscle groups has been reported years later and apparently is due to gradual deterioration of motor neurons, not to infections or immunologic mechanisms.

Treatment. There is no specific antiviral treatment. Therapy for symptoms includes hospitalization, bed rest, a bed board and foot-board, moist heat packs, and management of problems threatening the respiratory tract, including the use of mechanical ventilators.

Aseptic Meningitis

Clinical Findings. Acute aseptic meningitis (acute viral meningitis) is a syndrome characterized by signs and symptoms of meningeal irritation with mononuclear pleocytosis of the cerebrospinal fluid (Chapter 239). The attack rates for aseptic meningitis are highest in children younger than 1 year of age. The disease is also seen in older children and young adults, but enteroviral aseptic meningitis after the age of 40 is rare.

The onset may be gradual or abrupt. Typically, the patient feels chilly and has fever and headache for only a few hours before frank signs of meningitis are present. Nausea and vomiting are common, especially in children. Some patients also complain of sore throat. The illness may be biphasic, as in poliomyelitis, and fever and myalgia are present for a few days, followed by defervescence and absence of symptoms for 2 to 10 days before the sudden reappearance of fever, headache, and stiff neck. Signs of meningeal irritation may be absent in neonates, and even in older children and adults these signs are usually mild. Stiffness of the neck and back, sometimes with muscle spasms, is the only neurologic sign in most cases. Kernig's and Brudzinski's signs are present in about a third of patients.

Laboratory Findings. The peripheral white blood cell count is usually normal. The cerebrospinal fluid is clear but may be under mildly increased pressure. The total white blood cell count is usually 30 to 300/mm^3 but may on occasion exceed 1000/mm^3. Cell counts of less than 10/mm^3 or even normal are not rare, especially in neonates. Typically, the white cells are predominantly lymphocytes, but in the first 24 hours of illness, polymorphonuclear leukocytes may outnumber lymphocytes. The cerebrospinal fluid glucose and protein concentrations are usually normal.

Echoviruses and coxsackieviruses can be isolated from the cerebrospinal fluid in the first few days after the onset of meningitis but rarely after the first week. More frequently, and for longer periods, such viruses may often be isolated from throat or anal swab specimens. Because of the multiplicity of immunotypes, serologic diagnosis is not practical in most hospital viral diagnostic laboratories.

Treatment. The patient with aseptic meningitis is treated for symptoms. Fever and signs of meningeal irritation subside in a few days to 1 week. Cerebrospinal fluid pleocytosis may persist for some time after the fever and signs of meningeal irritation are resolved.

Encephalitis

Some patients with enteroviral infection and meningitis develop confusion and changes in the highest integrative functions. These are indicative of encephalitis. In neonates, disseminated disease, including encephalitis with lethargy, convulsions, bulging fontanelles, and cerebrospinal fluid pleocytosis, may develop.

Herpangina

Herpangina is a specific infectious disease characterized by a vesicular enanthem of the fauces of the soft palate, accompanied by fever, sore throat, and pain on swallowing. It is caused predominantly by group A coxsackieviruses but has also infrequently been associated with other enterovirus infections. It primarily affects children between the ages of 3 and 10 years but is occasionally seen in older children and adults. The illness begins suddenly with a fever of 99.8° F (37.7° C) to 104.9° F (40.5° C). Vomiting, myalgia, and headache are common at onset but generally do not persist. Sore throat and pain on swallowing are the most prominent symptoms and precede the appearance of the enanthem by several hours to a day. Inspection of the throat reveals erythema, a mild exudate on the tonsils, and the characteristic enanthem, which must be carefully sought to avoid missing it. The lesions, usually 2 to 6 in number (rarely, 12) are painful. They are located on the soft palate, on the free-hanging margin between the tonsils and the uvula; less commonly, they are on the surface of the tonsils or the posterior pharyngeal wall. They begin as punctate macules that evolve over a 24-hour period to 2 to 4 mm papules that vesiculate centrally and eventually ulcerate. The usual clinical laboratory diagnostic tests are not helpful. Symptoms can be treated.

Lymphonodular Pharyngitis

Lymphonodular pharyngitis is a variant of herpangina. It consists of tiny nodules of packed lymphocytes, which eventually recede without undergoing vesiculation or ulceration.

Hand-Foot-Mouth Syndrome

Hand-foot-mouth syndrome is a distinctive vesicular eruption most commonly caused by coxsackievirus A16 but also by enterovirus 71 and less commonly by other enteroviruses. The illness is mild and lasts for 1 week or less. It occurs predominantly in children and consists of sore throat or mouth, refusal to eat, fever of 100.4° to 102.2° F (38° to 39° C), which lasts for 1 to 2 days, and vesicles in the oral cavity, chiefly on the buccal mucosa and tongue. Several lesions may coalesce to form bullae that frequently ulcerate by the time they are seen by a physician. Lesions of the skin are less constant, occurring in 75% of patients. They are most commonly seen on the hands and feet, where either the extensor surfaces or the palms or soles may be involved. Less commonly, lesions occur more proximally in the extremities or buttocks and, rarely, on the genitalia.

The cutaneous lesions of hand-foot-mouth disease are tender and consist of mixed papules and clear vesicles with a surrounding zone of erythema. They are located subepidermally and are accompanied by mixed lymphocytic and polymorphonuclear inflammation and extensive acantholysis of the overlying epidermis. The lesions may resemble those caused by herpes simplex or varicella-zoster viruses, but they usually can be distinguished clinically by the number and distribution of lesions.

Exanthems

One of the most interesting features of enteroviral infections is the occurrence of exanthems. Once recognized, they are important as indicators of the prevalence of enterovirus infections in the community. On the other hand, they may be confused with other infective exanthems of greater medical significance. Fine, maculopapular rashes resembling rubella but occurring during summer epidemics have been reported with echovirus type 9, although a number of other enteroviruses may produce this syndrome. The rash characteristically occurs simultaneously with fever and begins on the face, then spreads to the neck, chest, and extremities. It consists of innumerable faint, pink macules that do not itch or desquamate. The rash is transient, but it may last 5 days or more on the face. Lesions may coalesce, giving the cheeks a violaceous hue. Helpful features in distinguishing enteroviral rash from rubella are the summertime occurrence and absence of lymphadenopathy in the posterior cervical and postauricular regions. Rash associated with echovirus type 9 and coxsackievirus A9 may have a petechial component. Petechial enteroviral exanthem associated with signs of meningeal irritation can be confused with meningococcemia.

A number of enterovirus infections may produce roseoliform exanthems. As in roseola, the rash does not appear until defervescence. The prototype is the Boston exanthem, first of the known enterovirus exanthems to be recognized and now known to be caused by echovirus type 16. Multiple cases often occur sequentially in families, and the mean age of those affected is 3 years. Before the rash, the temperature is 100.4° to 102.2° F (38° to 39° C), and there may be pharyngitis without cough or coryza.

Epidemic Pleurodynia

Epidemic pleurodynia (Bornholm disease) is an acute infectious disease characterized by fever and sharp spasmodic chest or abdominal pain. It is a disease of muscle, not of the pleura or peritoneum. Group B coxsackieviruses are the most important cause of epidemic pleurodynia. The illness occurs mainly in children 5 to 15 years of age and their parents.

There is no prodrome. The illness begins with the abrupt onset of spasmodic pain, typically over the lower rib cage or upper abdomen. Fever of 100.4° to 103.1° F (38° to 39.5° C) reaches its peak within 1 hour after the onset of each paroxysm and subsides as the pain recedes. In some outbreaks, sore throat and headache have been prominent, but cough and nasopharyngeal symptoms are usually notably absent. The intensity of the discomfort varies from a mild ache to severe pain. It is most often described as stabbing or constricting pain, occurring along the costal margin or occasionally the subxyphoid region. Half of the patients, especially adults, have pain primarily in the thorax. In the other half, pain occurs primarily in the upper abdomen. Periumbilical pain or pain in the lower abdominal quadrants is more common in children. In an individual patient, only one site or at most two are usually involved.

The spasmodic and paroxysmal character of the pain is characteristic of this disease. Each paroxysm typically lasts 2 to 10 hours. The first paroxysm is the most severe; subsequent paroxysms are shorter and are accompanied by less severe fever. During a paroxysm, if the pain is mild and the patient is ambulatory, he or she stoops forward or leans to the side, splinting the chest. With more severe pain, the patient lies in bed, resists being turned, and appears acutely ill and apprehensive. Chest pain limits deep inspiration; consequently, respirations are rapid and shallow. In most patients, tenderness mimicking the spontaneously occurring pain is elicited by pressing on the affected muscles, and palpable, often visible muscle swelling may be observed. Auscultation of the chest reveals nothing abnormal. Pleural friction rubs are rare. As the pain subsides and the temperature drops to normal, profuse sweating may occur. Although dull aching of muscles often persists, the patient may look and feel entirely healthy between paroxysms. About a fourth of patients experience multiple recurrences, often after they have been free of pain for a day or more and have felt well enough to return to work or school. Most patients are ill for 6 days or less. In keeping with the multiple disease manifestations of enteroviruses, during any given outbreak of pleurodynia caused by a particular enterovirus, a number of patients may appear with aseptic meningitis, pericarditis, and mildly symptomatic disease caused by the same immunotype.

Pleurodynia may be confused with many other illnesses because of the variable location of the disease. The usual clinical laboratory findings are normal. Therefore during the enterovirus season, pleurodynia should be considered in adults or children who have acute onset of fever and pain in the chest or abdomen.

Myopericarditis

Coxsackieviruses rarely attack the myocardium without attacking the pericardium; however, signs of either myocarditis or pericarditis may be dominant. In infants, myocarditis tends to be predominant and the disease fulminant. In contrast, the disease is usually much milder in adults and consists clinically of signs and symptoms of pericarditis or a mixed picture of myocarditis and pericarditis. Most cases are due to group B coxsackievirus types 1 to 5, although other enteroviruses may produce this syndrome.

In the newborn, the illness typically begins abruptly at about 1 week of age with listlessness, anorexia, and fever. These symptoms persist for about 2 days before clinical evidence of heart disease becomes apparent. In a third of patients the illness is biphasic, with a hiatus of 1 to 7 days of apparent well-being between the initial febrile illness and the appearance of frank myocarditis. With the onset of heart failure, respiratory distress, marked tachycardia, cardiomegaly, a systolic murmur, and electrocardiographic evidence of myocardial injury are seen. Clinical or electrocardiographic evidence of pericarditis is usually absent. In severely affected infants, cyanosis and circulatory collapse develop rapidly. In fatal cases, disseminated viral infection involving the central nervous system, liver, pancreas, and adrenal glands is often seen.

In older children and adults, the disease occurs at least twice as frequently in males as in females. An upper respiratory tract illness usually precedes the onset of cardiac manifestations by about 2 weeks. Symptoms include dyspnea, chest pain, fever, and malaise. Pain in the precordial area is usually dull, but it may resemble angina pectoris or be sharp and pleuritic; pain may be aggravated by lying down and relieved by sitting up and leaning forward. There is a pericardial friction rub in 35% to 85% of patients. Enlargement of the cardiac silhouette on chest radiographs may be due to either effusion or dilation. Signs of frank congestive heart failure are observed in 20% of cases. Electrocardiographic abnormalities, consisting of ST segment elevation or nonspecific ST and T wave abnormalities, are invariably present. More severe myocardial disease may lead to the development of Q waves, arrhythmias, and heart block. Serum levels of myocardial enzymes and white blood cell counts are frequently elevated.

Neonatal coxsackievirus myocarditis has a mortality rate of about 50%, and death usually occurs within 1 week of onset. Most older children and adults recover uneventfully. However, one fifth of patients experience one or more recurrences of myopericarditis several weeks to more than 1 year after the initial illness. Persistent electrocardiographic abnormalities, cardiomegaly, and chronic congestive heart failure indicate that permanent myocardial injury sometimes occurs. Chronic constrictive pericarditis has occurred following coxsackievirus myopericarditis after intervals of 5 weeks to 1 year.

Virus has been isolated rarely from myocardium or pericardial fluid in adults and only occasionally from other sites. The diagnosis can be established only by demonstrating a four-fold rise in antibody titer. The presumptive diagnosis is based on high levels of antibody in convalescent sera specimens.

Specific antiviral agents are not available, and therapy must be for symptoms only. Corticosteroids are of no proven benefit.

Chronic Meningoencephalitis in Agammaglobulinemias

Echoviruses have been responsible for persistent, sometimes fatal infection of the central nervous system in patients with agammaglobulinemia. The illness is commonly associated with a syndrome resembling dermatomyositis.

Acute Hemorrhagic Conjunctivitis

Acute hemorrhagic conjunctivitis is a recently recognized ocular infection caused by enterovirus type 70 and coxsackievirus A24. Unlike most enteroviral infections, it is probably transmitted primarily from fingers or fomites directly to the eye.

Acute hemorrhagic conjunctivitis emerged simultaneously in Ghana and Indonesia as a newly recognized disease in 1969. Since then, its spread has been explosive and pandemic. It has reached all parts of the world including North America, but the Western Hemisphere has not experienced the same widespread epidemics as have Asia and Africa. The disease apparently spreads more rapidly in crowded and unsanitary conditions.

Acute hemorrhagic conjunctivitis begins abruptly, and the illness reaches its peak on the first day. Symptoms appear first in one eye and then a few hours later in the other. The major symptoms are a burning sensation, ocular pain, photophobia, swelling of the eyelids, and a watery discharge. Constitutional symptoms, such as fever, malaise, and headache, are observed in a fifth of patients. The most distinctive sign is subconjunctival hemorrhage, which is present in 70% to 90% of patients with enterovirus type 70 infection, but it is seen much less frequently in disease caused by coxsackievirus A24. The hemorrhages may be pinpoint or may occupy the entire bulbar conjunctiva and are precipitated by everting the upper lid or rubbing the eye. Small follicles appear on the tarsal conjunctiva after 3 to 5 days in 90% of the patients. Corneal erosions or a fine punctate epithelial keratitis is also present in most patients. The ocular discharge is serous or seromucous. The preauricular lymph nodes are often enlarged and tender. Recovery usually begins by the second or third day and is complete by 10 days.

Fortunately, serious complications are very rare. Some cases of motor paralysis (poliomyelitis) have occurred in association with the disease. Symptoms can be treated. Antimicrobial agents are not indicated, and antiviral agents are not available. Attention to aseptic technique should decrease transmission.

Hepatitis

Hepatitis A is caused by hepatitis A virus, a picornavirus belonging to a separate genus (Chapter 355).

Other Illnesses

Enteroviral infections have been associated with a number of other illnesses. In most instances, there is no evidence that such associations are causal. For example, many reports indicate recovery of enteroviruses from stool specimens of patients with nonbacterial gastroenteritis. In most controlled studies, however, the rate of isolation of enteroviruses from control subjects is about the same as that from ill subjects. There is stronger evidence that echovirus types 11, 14, and 18 are associated with epidemic diarrhea of the newborn. Overall, it appears that the role of enteroviruses in diarrheal diseases is minor.

Hepatitis has occurred in disseminated enteroviral infections, generally those produced by group B coxsackieviruses, but there is no known relationship between enteroviral infections (other than hepatitis A virus) and hepatitis occurring in the absence of other manifestations. Pancreatitis and orchitis have occurred in patients with group B coxsackievirus infections. A role for coxsackievirus B4 in the pathogenesis of juvenile diabetes mellitus has been suggested.

Uncomplicated Influenza

The influenzal syndrome is a febrile illness of sudden onset, with tracheitis and marked myalgias. The case of a typical patient treated with amantadine appears in Fig. 250-3. After an incubation period of 1 to 5 days, patients have a sudden onset of headache, chilly sensations, fever, malaise, myalgias, anorexia, and sore throat. Shaking chills may occur, but rarely recur after the onset of fever. Fever rapidly ascends to a level of 101° to 104° F (38.3° to 40.0° C), and respiratory symptoms ensue. A nonproductive cough is characteristic; sneezing, rhinorrhea, and nasal obstruction are common. The nonproductive cough frequently occurs in paroxysms and is accompanied by substernal soreness; these findings indicate the presence of tracheitis. Patients may also report photophobia, hoarseness, nausea, vomiting, diarrhea, and abdominal pain. Gastrointestinal symptoms are more prominent in children than in adults and are noted more frequently with type B than with type A infection.

Physical examination reveals an acutely ill patient who is usually coughing. Lid slits may be narrowed as a result of eye pain, and minimum to moderate nasal obstruction or discharge may be present. Despite complaints of sore throat, minimum inflammation is seen on examination, but tender anterior cervical nodes are commonly present. The trachea may be tender on lateral motion, and cough that is precipitated by deep breathing with the mouth open confirms the presence of tracheitis. Examination of the chest reveals nothing abnormal or an occasional dry crackle. Muscles may be tender on palpation, but the remainder of the physical findings are unremarkable.

Most adults ill with influenza virus infection do not exhibit the exact syndrome that has been described. Moreover, the influenzal syn-

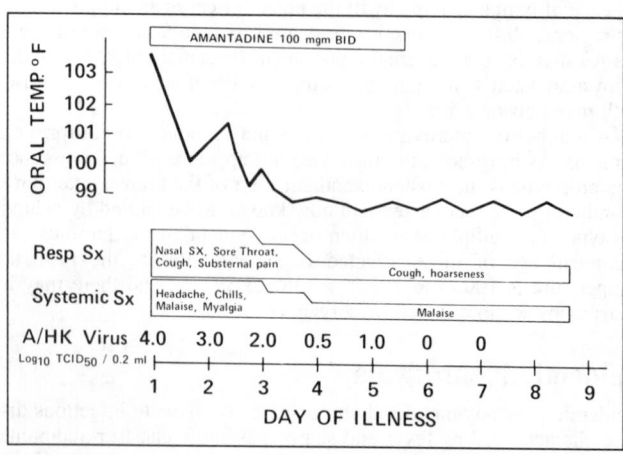

FIGURE 250-3   Case of uncomplicated acute influenza in a healthy 24-year-old man.

Courtesy of Dr. V. Knight.

drome is uncommon in children and is not seen in infants. Predominant symptoms in a particular patient may be sneezing, nasal obstruction, and discharge (common cold); nasal obstruction, discharge, and sore throat (upper respiratory illness); sore throat with erythema (pharyngitis); hoarseness (laryngitis); or cough (tracheobronchitis). Fever may or may not be present.

The duration of prominent respiratory and systemic symptoms is 1 to 5 days. Thereafter a progressive improvement ensues, although the nasal symptoms, malaise, and cough may continue for several days. The total duration of overt illness rarely exceeds 10 days, although many patients complain of lassitude for an additional 1 to 2 weeks.

Pulmonary Complications of Influenza

Lung involvement represents more extensive disease or influenza in a patient with preexisting chest disease. Some patients with influenza exhibit moist or dry crackles over a localized area of the lung on physical examination, and some exhibit diffuse inspiratory and expiratory wheezes. The moist or dry crackles are usually over a lower lobe and represent a segmental pneumonia that may or may not be apparent on the chest radiograph; the wheezes represent bronchiolitis. Such patients initially appear very ill, but apart from a tendency to remain febrile and acutely ill for a longer period than usual, the course of their illness is similar to that of patients without chest findings. Fewer than 5% of healthy adults exhibit one of these disease patterns, but they are common in infants and small children (Box 250-1).

As a consequence of influenza infection, exacerbations of acute respiratory insufficiency may occur in patients with chronic obstructive pulmonary disease. Such patients may have increased coughing and sputum production and new chest findings, or they may simply exhibit fever and respiratory insufficiency. Some permanent deterioration in lung function may result from the infection.

Extensive influenzal pneumonia was a prominent disease during the pandemics of 1918 and 1957. The disease is most likely to occur in persons with underlying heart or lung disease, but about half of the cases in recent years have occurred in persons thought to be otherwise healthy. A case in an otherwise healthy person is shown in Fig. 250-4. The disease at onset is similar to other cases of influenza, but instead of improving by the third to fifth day of illness, patients continue to be febrile, and progressive air hunger and cyanosis develop. Chest examination initially reveals bilateral moist crackles and wheezes without signs of consolidation; chest radiographs reveal bilateral interstitial disease, sometimes accompanied by areas of local consolidation. Sputum is often scanty but may be copious, frothy, and pink-tinged if the patient has underlying heart disease. Bacteriologic tests reveal normal flora, and such patients do not respond to antibiotics. Blood gas studies reveal marked hypoxia, and ventilatory assistance may be required. The mortality rate is very high.

Mixed viral and bacterial pneumonia may also occur. The clinical appearance is of typical influenza at onset, but after 2 to 5 days, a cough productive of purulent or bloody sputum and chest pain that is sometimes pleuritic develops. These findings usually indicate the onset of a superimposed bacterial pneumonia. Chest examination reveals an area of consolidation, and examination of sputum reveals predominance of a lung pathogen. The most likely cause of the bacterial pneumonia is the pneumococcus, but staphylococci and *Haemophilus influenzae* also are commonly found. If the patient was receiving antibiotics or was hospitalized before the onset of bacterial superinfection, a gram-negative organism may be responsible. Mortality is variable, depending on the presence of an underlying disease and the bacterium responsible for the pneumonia.

The most common pattern of pneumonia with influenza is postinfluenzal bacterial pneumonia. This disease occurs most commonly in persons with an underlying chronic disease, particularly cardiovascular or lung disease. Patients have influenza, and remission of fever and symptoms ensues. Then during or just after recovery they experience the reappearance of fever and the onset of chest pain, which may be pleuritic, and a cough productive of purulent or bloody sputum. The physical examination, chest radiograph, sputum studies, and leukocyte counts reveal findings typical of a bacterial pneumonia. These patients respond to appropriate antibiotics, and the mortality rate is low.

Neurologic Complications

The occurrence of encephalitis and encephalopathy in association with acute influenza, particularly in children, is well documented, although rare. Virus is not isolated from the cerebrospinal fluid, and the pathogenesis is uncertain.

Reye's syndrome may be seen after both type A and type B influenza. It is most prominent after influenza in older children but occurs in young adults as well.

Guillain-Barré syndrome and transverse myelitis have also been reported after influenza, but the absence of a relationship between epidemic influenza and the incidence of Guillain-Barré syndrome suggests that influenza infection is rarely associated with this disease.

BOX 250-1
Clinical presentations of influenza

Uncomplicated influenza
  Common cold
  Upper respiratory illness
  Pharyngitis
  Laryngitis
  Tracheobronchitis
  Influenzal syndrome
Complications of influenza
  Pneumonia
    Segmental influenzal
    Extensive influenzal
    Mixed viral bacterial
    Postinfluenzal bacterial
    Exacerbation of acute respiratory insufficiency
  Neurologic
    Encephalitis, encephalopathy
    Reye's syndrome
    Guillain-Barré syndrome
    Transverse myelitis
  Other
    Sinusitis, otitis

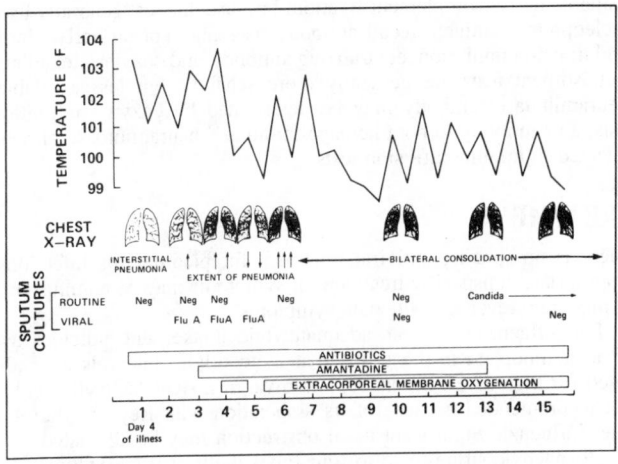

FIGURE 250-4   Case of fulminant influenzal pneumonia leading to death in an otherwise healthy 48-year-old man. Day 1 of hospitalization was day 4 of the illness.

Data from Lefrak et al: Extracorporeal membrane oxygenation for fulminant influenza pneumonia, *Chest* 66:385, 1974.

Other Complications

Sinusitis and otitis media may occur as a consequence of upper respiratory illness (Chapter 230). Although otitis is reported to be caused by influenza virus directly, in most cases the ear and sinus symptoms are probably caused by pressure changes secondary to obstruction of the eustachian tube or sinus foramina. Frank secondary bacterial sinusitis and otitis media may, however, occur.

Myositis may be seen in children, particularly with influenza type B infection.

Myocarditis, pericarditis, disseminated intravascular coagulation, and myositis with myoglobinuria have accompanied acute influenza but are rare.

DIAGNOSIS

Specific tests for isolation of picornavirus or to measure antibody responses may be available from local laboratories, state health laboratories, or the CDC for severe cases, such as paralytic poliomyelitis or encephalitis. Presumptive diagnoses can often be made from the characteristic clinical picture.

A presumptive diagnosis of influenza may be made if a patient has an acute respiratory disease with fever and without pneumonia during a community epidemic of influenza. Supporting information is provided by a throat culture finding negative for group A streptococci in patients with prominent pharyngitis and by the absence of significant peripheral blood leukocytosis and neutrophilia.

A definite diagnosis of influenza requires demonstration of influenza virus in a patient's respiratory secretions or a rise in titer of specific antibody. The optimum specimen for virus detection is a combined nasal wash and throat swab specimen, but a nose and throat swab specimen will do. Such tests are often available. Methods for rapid detection of virus are being increasingly used, and some methods are commercially available. Specificity for types A and B viruses is high; sensitivity is also high for acutely ill hospitalized children, but data for outpatients and adults are limited.

For virus isolation a protein stabilizer must be added to nasal wash specimens with saline, but a swab specimen may be directly inserted into a protein-containing medium. Storage at 4° C for up to 5 days does not alter isolation rates from febrile patients, but testing should be done as early as possible.

Both tissue cultures and embryonated chicken eggs are suitable for isolation, with the optimal system varying for the different influenza viruses. Virus is detected after a 3-day period of incubation in 85% to 90% of cases, although 7 to 10 days may be required. Methods for rapid detection of virus in respiratory epithelial cells or respiratory fluids can provide a specific diagnosis on the day of collection.

A rise in titer of antibody between acute and convalescent sera may be detected with several serologic procedures. The most readily available test is complement fixation; because this test generally uses nucleoprotein antigen, recall antibody rises may appear early. Hemagglutination inhibition, neutralizing antibody, and enzyme-linked immunosorbent tests are generally more sensitive but less available. Neuraminidase antibody may be determined by enzyme inhibition tests, and antibody to both hemagglutinin and neuraminidase may be detected in immunodiffusion tests.

TREATMENT

There is no specific antiviral treatment for picornavirus infections. Appropriate nonspecific treatment of symptoms may be administered to moderate fever and alleviate symptoms.

For influenza, bed rest, adequate fluid intake, and judicious use of acetaminophen in 0.6 g doses at 3- to 6-hour intervals are indicated for high fever, headache, and myalgias. Acetylsalicylic acid is not recommended because of its association with Reye's syndrome after influenza. Significant nasal obstruction may be alleviated with 0.25% phenylephrine three to four times daily or 0.1% xylometazoline twice daily by nasal spray or drops. Significant cough may be relieved by guaifenesin syrup with dextromethorphan in doses of 5 to 10 ml every 3 to 4 hours.

Specific treatment is available for type A influenza. Amantadine hydrochloride in doses of 100 mg twice daily or rimantadine in doses of 100 mg twice daily hastens the disappearance of fever and symptoms, but, to be effective in uncomplicated influenza, they must be started within the first 48 hours of illness. When type A influenza is known to be the cause of disease in a community, amantadine or rimantadine is recommended for all persons with a chronic underlying disease who have acute influenza and for healthy persons with clinically severe influenza. Central nervous system side-effects, such as drowsiness, dizziness, nervousness, and insomnia occur in 5% to 7% of healthy persons taking amantadine, but they are less frequent with rimantadine. Such symptoms are not generally apparent in acutely ill persons. Because of renal excretion of amantadine, caution must be used in persons with compromised renal function, and reductions in dosage are indicated. Schedules for dosages based on level of renal function are available. Because of the general reduction in renal function among elderly persons, therapy with only 100 mg per day is recommended for patients 65 years and older. Caution must be exercised in medicating persons with central nervous system disease and in those receiving drugs with central nervous system activity. Rimantadine is not primarily excreted by the kidneys.

Persons presumed to have primary influenzal pneumonia or mixed influenza and bacterial pneumonia should also receive amantadine or rimantadine, in the doses indicated, although the benefit is uncertain. Patients with mixed viral-bacterial pneumonia and bacterial pneumonia after influenza should receive appropriate antibiotics (Chapter 231).

Emergence of viral isolates resistant to amantadine and rimantadine among treated patients has created concern about use of these drugs for treatment. This is of practical importance only if an unhealthy or elderly person in the same household contracts influenza from a person treated with amantadine or rimantadine, since acquisition of a drug-resistant virus severely limits treatment options.

Ribavirin, a nucleoside analog, is approved for small-particle aerosol treatment of severe respiratory syncytial virus infections in infants. It also has been shown to be effective for treatment of uncomplicated type A and B influenza in healthy adults, and results of treatment of severe disease are encouraging. It is not approved for treatment of acute influenza.

PREVENTION
Vaccines

No vaccines exist for rhinovirus, coxsackievirus, echovirus, or the more recently discovered enterovirus infections. However, one of the most dramatic demonstrations of vaccine efficacy has been the eradication of paralytic poliomyelitis in much of the world by use of oral (OPV) and inactivated (IPV) poliovirus vaccines. Both vaccines have excellent records of safety and efficacy.

Leading Polio Vaccines. Wild poliovirus infection has been eliminated from the Western Hemisphere and other large geographic regions. The World Health Organization predicts global eradication by the year 2000.

OPV elicits both circulatory and secretory antibodies and induces immunity that may be lifelong. One advantage of this vaccine is that nonvaccinated persons may become immunized by contact with vaccinated persons, and the circulation of wild viruses is prevented by alimentary immunity. However, 8 to 10 cases of paralytic poliomyelitis associated with the use of OPV occur each year in the United States. The benefits of OPV have diminished with the elimination of wild virus–associated poliomyelitis in the Western Hemisphere and the reduced threat of poliovirus importation into the United States. Furthermore, the risk of vaccine-associated poliomyelitis with OPV is less acceptable.

Recently a more potent inactivated poliovirus vaccine was licensed. It confers humoral but not secretory immunity, provided three initial doses and subsequent boosters are given. Its advantages are that it cannot undergo mutation or reversion to virulence, and it is safe to administer to immunodeficient or immunosuppressed persons. It is the preferred vaccine for previously unvaccinated adults and immunodeficient persons.

At present in the United States, the preferred regimen is two doses of IPV at 2 and 4 months of age, followed by two doses of OPV at 12 to 18 months and 4 to 6 years of age. This regimen combines the inherent safety of IPV with the broader immunologic response of OPV. As an alternative, four doses of OPV at 2, 4, and 6 to 18 months and at 4 to 6 years of age is acceptable in certain situations (e.g., to reduce the number of injections), but this regimen should not be used for immunocompromised persons or as primary immunization of persons older than 18 years of age. For these two groups exclusively, and as an acceptable alternative in infants, four doses of IPV may be given.

Hepatitis A Vaccines. Inactivated hepatitis A vaccines have recently been approved in the United States and some other countries. They are indicated for active prophylaxis in persons 2 years of age or older. They are recommended for persons at high risk, including travelers to areas of high endemicity, including Africa, Asia, Eastern Europe, Mexico, Central and South America, the Mediterranean basin, and parts of the Caribbean; military persons; persons living in areas of high endemicity; persons engaging in high-risk sexual activity; and users of illegal drugs. Two doses of vaccine, optimally 6 months apart, are given. For persons requiring postexposure prophylaxis, immune globulin is given. Vaccine may be given simultaneously at a separate site.

Influenza Vaccines. Inactivated influenza virus vaccines are prepared as follows: virus is grown in embryonated chicken eggs, inactivated by formalin, and partially purified to remove adventitial egg material. The resulting virus is either left intact (whole virus vaccine) or disrupted and sometimes further purified (split product and subunit vaccines). The formulation is determined by immunization advisory committees of the World Health Organization and the Centers for Disease Control and Prevention in Atlanta. Currently circulating types A and B viruses are included annually, with selection of particular variants based on antigenic novelty and recent epidemiologic experience. Because of the persistence of H3N2 viruses since the appearance of H1N1 virus in 1977, recent vaccines have contained H3N2, H1N1, and B variants. The dosage is standardized for hemagglutinin content.

Protection against influenza among persons given influenza virus vaccine generally varies between 50% and 90%. The degree of protection has varied with the potency of the vaccine, the extent of influenza activity, and the degree of antigenic relationship of the vaccine virus to the challenge virus. For most years, the vaccine may be assumed to convey about 70% protection against illness caused by influenza virus infection.

Annual vaccination is recommended for persons with a chronic underlying disease that increases the likelihood that they will have pneumonia and die of influenza. These diseases include cardiovascular and pulmonary disease, renal disease, metabolic disease, severe anemia, and diseases that compromise immune function.

Vaccine is given by intramuscular injection, and any of the different types may be used in adults, but only split product is recommended for those 6 months to 12 years of age. Persons with previous exposure to the vaccine components need be given only one dose, whereas those without previous exposure to one of the components should be given two doses of that component 1 month apart. Two doses of vaccine are recommended for persons less than 9 years of age who are receiving influenza vaccine for the first time.

Current vaccines have minimal side-effects. Persons with allergy to eggs or egg products should not be given vaccine. In the past, some pain, redness, or swelling at the vaccination site was reported by about 10% of adults in the 48 hours after vaccination, and systemic symptoms were reported in about 2%. Such reactions were usually mild, but moderately severe local and systemic reactions occurred. More recent reports of U.S. vaccines indicate still fewer reactions; among elderly populations there is little to no detectable reactogenicity. During the 1976 national immunization program for swine influenza in the United States, an increase in the incidence of the Guillain-Barré syndrome was noted in the 8-week period after vaccination. The risk that the syndrome would develop was about 1 in 100,000 vaccinations, and risk increased with increasing age. However, 3 subsequent years of vaccine monitoring did not reveal a similar increased risk, and no increased risk was noted in the military vaccine program. Thus the basis of the association of Guillain-Barré syndrome with swine influenza immunization is uncertain, but it does not appear to be a complication attributable to all influenza vaccines.

✔ WHEN TO REFER

Rhinovirus, enterovirus, and influenza infections are among the most common human afflictions. Many patients do not seek medical attention, and the vast majority of those who can be treated by the generalist. Patients with more severe illnesses may require the attention of an infectious diseases specialist, pulmonologist, or neurologist as appropriate. Examples of severe illnesses include influenza, viral or bacterial pneumonia, picornavirus aseptic meningitis, encephalitis, paralysis, myopericarditis, or rhinovirus infection complicated by sinusitis that requires drainage.

Chemoprophylaxis

Amantadine or rimantadine, given before exposure, prevents about 50% of type A influenza virus infections and about 70% of illnesses. They are not effective for type B influenza. They are recommended for the same persons for whom vaccine is recommended if they are unvaccinated or were vaccinated with a variant unrelated to the epidemic virus. The drug should be given in a dosage of 100 mg twice daily, starting administration at the beginning of a type A epidemic and continuing until the epidemic ceases, generally for 4 to 6 weeks. Persons 65 years and older should be given 100 mg daily; side-effects should be less of a problem among elderly persons at this lower dosage, yet effectiveness should remain high.

An alternative use is to provide prophylaxis against epidemic type A disease during the early phase of an epidemic while an antibody response to vaccine given at the beginning of the epidemic develops. For this purpose, a 14-day course is recommended.

Amantadine and rimantadine may also be used for influenza A outbreak control in nursing homes. When used in this way, drug therapy should be administered to all residents, regardless of whether they have received vaccine, for the duration of the community epidemic. Dosage for either drug is 200 mg daily for young persons and 100 mg daily for elderly persons; reductions in these dosages may be needed for amantadine depending on renal function.

Nausea, headache, and central nervous system side-effects (see the section on Treatment), which may occur with amantadine therapy, are usually mild and begin within the first 48 hours of drug use. They may disappear with continued drug usage and cease on withdrawal of the drug. Severe central nervous system side-effects, including seizures and hallucinations, may occur with high blood levels in patients with reduced renal function. Side effects with rimantadine are less frequent.

BIBLIOGRAPHY

Barker W et al: Case control study of influenza vaccine effectiveness in preventing pneumonia hospitalization among older persons, Monroe County, New York, 1989-1992. In Hannoun C et al, editors: *Options for the control of influenza II,* Amsterdam, 1993, Elsevier.

Barker WH, Mullooly JP: Pneumonia and influenza deaths during epidemics: implications for prevention, *Arch Intern Med* 142:85, 1982.

Centers for Disease Control and Prevention: Certification of poliomyelitis elimination—the Americas, 1994, *MMWR* 43:720-722, 1994.

Couch RB et al: Influenza: its control in persons and populations, *J Infect Dis* 153:431, 1986.

Dalakas MC et al: A long-term follow-up study of patients with post-poliomyelitis neuromuscular symptoms, *N Engl J Med* 314:959, 1986.

Degelau J et al: Amantadine resistant influenza A in a nursing facility, *Arch Intern Med* 152:390-392, 1992.

Doyle WJ et al: A double-blind placebo-controlled clinical trial of the effect of chlorpheniramine on the response of the nasal airway, middle ear and eustachian tube to provocative rhinovirus challenge, *Pediatr Infect Dis* 7:222, 1988.

Gwaltney JM Jr: Combined antiviral and antimediator treatment of rhinovirus colds, *J Infect Dis* 166:776-782, 1992.

Hayden FC, Couch RB: Clinical and epidemiological importance of influenza A viruses resistant to amantadine and rimantadine, *Rev Med Virol* 2:89, 1992.

Hendley JO, Gwaltney JM Jr: Mechanisms of transmission of rhinovirus infections, *Epidemiol Rev* 10:242, 1988.

Hull HF et al: Paralytic poliomyelitis: seasoned strategies, disappearing disease, *Lancet* 343:1331-1337, 1994.

Johnston SL, Bloy H: Evaluation of rapid enzyme immunoassay for detection of influenza A virus, *J Clin Microbiol* 31:142-143, 1993.

McBean AM et al: The serologic response to oral polio vaccine and enhanced potency inactivated polio vaccines, *Am J Epidemiol* 128:615, 1988.

McKinney RE Jr, Katz SL, Wilfert CM: Chronic enteroviral meningoencephalitis in agammaglobulinemic patients, *Rev Infect Dis* 9:334, 1987.

Monto AS, Arden NH: Implications of viral resistance to amantadine for control of influenza A, *Clin Infect Dis* 15:363-367, 1992.

Naclerio RM et al: Kinins are generated during experimental rhinovirus colds, *J Infect Dis* 157:133, 1988.

Newman RW et al: Immune response of human volunteers and animals to vaccination with egg grown influenza A (H1N1) virus is influenced by three amino acid substitutions in the haemagglutinen molecule, *Vaccine* 11:400-406, 1993.

Nichol KL et al: Achieving the national health objective for influenza immunization: success of an institution-wide vaccination program, *Am J Med* 89:156, 1990.

O'Neil KM et al: Chronic group A coxsackievirus infection in agammaglobulinemia: demonstration of genomic variation of serotypically identical isolates persistently excreted by the same patient, *J Infect Dis* 157:183, 1988.

Prevots DR et al: Completeness of reporting for paralytic poliomyelitis, United States, 1980 through 1991, *Arch Pediatr Adolesc Med* 148:479-485, 1994.

Rorabaugh ML et al: Aseptic meningitis among infants less than two years of age: acute illness and neurologic complications, *Pediatrics* 92:206-211, 1993.

Rose NR et al: Post-infectious autoimmunity: two distinct phases of coxsackievirus B3-induced myocarditis, *Ann NY Acad Sci* 475:146, 1986.

Shaw MW, Arden NH, Maassab HF: New aspects of influenza viruses, *Clin Microbiol Rev* 5:74, 1992.

Strebel PM et al: Epidemiology of poliomyelitis in the United States one decade after the last reported case of indigenous wild virus–associated disease, *Clin Infect Dis* 14:568-579, 1992.

Strikas RA, Anderson LJ, Parker RA: Temporal and geographic patterns of isolates of nonpolio enteroviruses in the United States, *J Infect Dis* 153:346, 1986.

Wright PF: Strategies for the global eradication of poliomyelitis by the year 2000, *N Engl J Med* 325:1774, 1991.

251 Paramyxovirus (Parainfluenza, Mumps, Measles, and Respiratory Syncytial Virus), Rubella Virus, Coronavirus, and Adenovirus Infections

Eurico Arruda and Frederick G. Hayden

PARAMYXOVIRUS INFECTIONS
Classification

The paramyxoviridae family is a group of medium-sized (150 to 300 nm) pleomorphic ribonucleic acid (RNA) viruses that includes several important human (Table 251-1) and veterinary pathogens. Their common characteristics include a helical nucleocapsid that contains a linear, single-stranded RNA; a lipid-containing envelope; cytoplasmic replication; and, unlike influenza viruses, antigenic stability without recognized genetic recombination. One glycoprotein (HN) on the surface of paramyxoviruses has hemagglutinin and sometimes neuraminidase activity and is responsible for adsorption of virus to host cell receptors. Another protein (F), which has hemolyzing and membrane-fusing activity, is responsible for viral penetration into cells and the formation of multinucleated giant cells, a major cytopathic effect of paramyxoviruses.

The family is subdivided into three genera: (1) The paramyxovirus genus includes parainfluenza viruses types 1 to 4, mumps virus, and Newcastle disease virus, which causes respiratory tract disease in chickens and may accidentally infect humans. These viruses have both hemagglutinin and neuraminidase activities. (2) Measles virus has a hemagglutinin but no neuraminidase and is grouped in the morbillivirus genus. (3) Respiratory syncytial virus has neither hemagglutinin nor neuraminidase and is classified in the pneumovirus genus. There is no antigen common to all paramyxoviruses, but considerable cross reactivity in complement fixation or neutralization tests is present in members of the paramyxovirus genus. An unusual form of severe hepatitis characterized histologically by giant multinucle-

ated syncytial hepatocytes has been linked to a paramyxoviral infection of undefined type. In addition, cases of fatal pneumonia and central nervous system disease have been linked to zoonotic infection by a novel equine morbillivirus in Australia.

PARAINFLUENZA VIRUSES
Characteristics

The human parainfluenza viruses are separated into types 1 to 4 and type 4 into subtypes A and B on the basis of antigenicity. This group of viruses is relatively homogeneous, with a slow rate of evolution. They share common antigens, and heterotypic antibodies are detected during infection.

Epidemiology

Parainfluenza viruses have a worldwide distribution and infect most persons initially during childhood. They are the most commonly identified cause of acute laryngotracheobronchitis (croup) in children and are second only to respiratory syncytial virus as a cause of lower respiratory tract disease causing hospitalization of infants. Parainfluenza virus infection is documented in 31% to 42% of croup, 7% to 17% of pneumonia, and 7% to 18% of bronchiolitis cases in children. The incidence of croup and other lower respiratory tract disease produced by parainfluenza virus type 1 or 2 infection is highest between 4 months and 4 to 6 years of age. Parainfluenza virus type 3 can cause bronchiolitis or pneumonia in very young infants despite the presence of maternal antibody. Reinfections with parainfluenza viruses are common, are rarely severe, and account for nearly all the parainfluenza viral illness of adults. In children, reinfections with the same serotype have occurred within months.

Parainfluenza types 1 and 2 typically cause epidemics lasting up to several months during alternate years in the fall. Overlapping outbreaks involving both types 1 and 2 may occur. Parainfluenza type 3 causes sporadic infection throughout the year but also epidemics in spring and summer months. Transmission of parainfluenza viruses occurs within families, and outbreaks with high attack rates have occurred in closed populations, such as nurseries, day care centers, and hospitals. It is estimated that parainfluenza virus types 1 and 2 cause approximately 250,000 visits to emergency rooms and 70,000 hospitalizations in the United States during an epidemic year. Up to 10% of acute upper respiratory diseases in adults is caused by parainfluenza viruses.

The virus is transmitted from person to person in infected respiratory secretions by direct contact or by large droplets. The incubation period ranges from 2 to 8 days. The duration of viral shedding is 3 to 10 days, although persistent shedding of parainfluenza types 1 and 3 for months has been reported.

Pathogenesis

Although dissemination of infection has been reported rarely, the principal features of parainfluenza virus infection are replication and cytolytic change in the respiratory tract mucosa. The virus can be localized to ciliated columnar epithelial cells. Viral shedding tends to reflect the severity of illness and may be prolonged in immunocompromised hosts. Severe giant cell pneumonia has developed in patients who have deficits in cell-mediated immune function.

Levels of serum neutralizing antibody correlate partially with protection against infection and illness, but immunity is more closely associated with neutralizing antibody levels in the respiratory tract secretions. The nasopharyngeal secretion concentrations of parainfluenza virus–specific IgE and of histamine are higher in patients with croup or wheezing than in those with upper respiratory illness alone.

Clinical Features

Initial infections with parainfluenza virus types 1 to 3 commonly cause febrile rhinitis, pharyngitis, laryngitis, and/or bronchitis. Up to 30% of children with primary infections have evidence of lower respiratory disease. The principal severe form of illness in type 1 and 2 infection is croup, manifested by inspiratory stridor, barking cough,

Table 251-1   Human paramyxoviridae

VIRUS	TYPES	CLINICAL SYNDROMES	VIRUS DETECTION		SEROLOGIC TESTS†	VACCINE
			SPECIMEN	METHOD*		
Parainfluenza	1-4	Colds Pharyngitis Croup Bronchitis Bronchiolitis Pneumonia	Nasal aspirate/wash, throat/NP swabs, sputum	VI, IF, EIA, RT-PCR	NT, CF, HAI, ELISA	Investigational
Mumps	1	Parotitis Orchitis Oophoritis Pancreatitis Aseptic meningitis Encephalitis Arthritis	Saliva, urine, CSF	VI	CF, NT, HAI, IF, ELISA	Live virus
Measles	1	Typical measles Modified measles Atypical measles Pneumonia Encephalitis	Throat/NP swabs, urine, blood	VI, IF, RT-PCR	CF, HAI, NT, ELISA	Live virus
Respiratory syncytial	1 (2 subgroups)	Colds Bronchitis Bronchiolitis Pneumonia	Nasal aspirate/wash, sputum, NP/throat swabs	VI, IF, EIA, RT-PCR	CF, NT, ELISA	Investigational

*VI, Viral isolation; IF, immunofluorescence; EIA, enzyme immunoassay; RT-PCR, reverse transcription-polymerase chain reaction.
†NT, Neutralization; CF, complement fixation; HAI, hemagglutination inhibition; ELISA, enzyme-linked immuno-sorbent assay; IF, immunofluorescence.

and hoarseness caused by subglottic edema. Bacterial suprainfections are rare in croup but may complicate other respiratory tract infections produced by parainfluenza viruses. Type 3 infection causes croup, bronchiolitis, or pneumonia. Type 4 infections are mild and are infrequently recognized. However, they may also cause significant lower respiratory tract illness in some patients. All four types of parainfluenza virus can also cause severe lower respiratory tract infection in adults and children who have undergone bone marrow or solid organ transplantation.

Reinfection with parainfluenza virus is frequently asymptomatic, but it may be associated with lower respiratory disease in children. Symptomatic infections in adults are manifested as common colds, usually without fever, pharyngitis, tracheobronchitis, influenza-like illness, exacerbations of chronic bronchitis, and, rarely, pneumonia. Parainfluenza virus has been associated with parotitis and has been isolated from patients with Guillain-Barré syndrome, aseptic meningitis, and acute renal transplant rejection.

Diagnosis

Throat and nasopharyngeal swabs or nasal washings contain the virus at the onset of symptoms. The duration of viral shedding averages 8 days, but it decreases significantly in reinfections. Parainfluenza virus types 1 to 3 can often be isolated within 3 days and usually within 10 days after inoculation from specimens from infants and children. Isolation of type 4 virus or virus from specimens during reinfections may require 2 to 3 weeks. Virus detection is accomplished in monkey kidney cells by hemadsorption of guinea pig erythrocytes, and confirmation is by immunofluorescence. Immunofluorescent staining of shell vial cultures provides a means of more rapid diagnosis. Immunofluorescence of respiratory tract cells has been used for rapid diagnosis.

Antibodies to parainfluenza viruses can be measured by a variety of serologic techniques (Table 251-1). A four-fold or greater titer rise constitutes evidence of infection, but a serotype-specific diagnosis cannot be reliably made because of the common occurrence of heterotypic antibody responses. Complement fixation or hemagglutination inhibition antibodies increase in only one half of adults infected with type 1 or type 3 virus.

Treatment and Prevention

Supportive care and close monitoring are indicated in patients with severe lower respiratory involvement. Management of croup typically consists of mist therapy and supplemental oxygen. Racemic epinephrine nebulization is commonly used in hospitalized patients under close observation. Short-term, high-dose corticosteroids appear beneficial and may reduce the duration of hospitalization. Inhaled steroids are effective in mild to moderately severe croup. Aerosolized ribavirin has been used in immunodeficient children with severe parainfluenza virus infection. A parainfluenza virus type 3 vaccine is currently under development.

MUMPS VIRUS
Characteristics

Only one serotype of mumps virus is known to exist, although antigenic differences between strains have been detected by monoclonal antibodies. The soluble (S) antigen derived from the nucleocapsid and the viral (V) antigen associated with the envelope elicit complement-fixing antibodies detectable early and late after infection, respectively. Mumps virus can be propagated in embryonated eggs and a variety of cell cultures, including monkey kidney, human embryonic kidney, or HeLa cells, and can be detected by cytopathic effects and hemadsorption of guinea pig red blood cells.

Epidemiology

Mumps virus is endemic worldwide and humans are the only known natural host. Before wide-scale immunization, mumps was primarily a disease of childhood, with 90% of the cases occurring in those less than 14 years of age. Since the introduction of the live attenuated vaccine, the annual reported incidence of mumps has decreased 99% in the United States. Outbreaks, some involving highly immunized populations, have occurred among groups of high school and college students, in work settings including hospitals, and in other closed populations such as those in military barracks or prisons in the early 1990s. These outbreaks have been related to vaccine failure and failure to vaccinate. However, the overall incidence of mumps in all age-groups has continued to decrease in the United States, and fewer than two cases per 100,000 population are reported per year. The disease occurs throughout the year, with a peak incidence in late winter to early spring in temperate climates.

Mumps virus is transmitted in infected saliva or respiratory secretions by direct contact or droplets that enter the upper respiratory tract. More intimate contact is needed than for transmission of measles or varicella. The infection rates in outbreaks involving susceptible, closed populations have been as high as 80%. The period of peak communicability extends from several days before to several days after the onset of parotitis, but virus has been isolated as many as 7 days before and 9 days after the appearance of parotitis. Virus can be present in saliva in cases of inapparent infection or in those without parotitis, and these persons may be contagious. The incubation period averages 14 to 18 days, with a range of 7 to 25 days. Natural mumps infection is thought to confer lifelong immunity. The frequency and manifestations of reinfection are uncertain.

Pathophysiology

After primary infection, the virus replicates in the upper respiratory tract epithelium and regional lymph nodes during the incubation period. Viremic dissemination then leads to secondary localization in glandular and neural tissue and to subsequent clinical disease. Infection has been produced experimentally by direct instillation of the virus into the parotid (Stensen's) duct.

The infected salivary glands show a diffuse interstitial edema, with a serofibrinous exudate containing mononuclear cells. The ductal epithelium shows degenerative changes, but the glandular cells are relatively spared. Involved pancreas or testes show similar changes with more hemorrhage and polymorphonuclear cell infiltration. Local areas of infarction may develop because of vascular compromise, and atrophy of the germinal epithelium with hyalinization and fibrosis can ensue.

In mumps encephalitis the brain may show widespread neurolysis typical of a primary viral encephalitis or changes consistent with a postinfectious encephalitis (i.e., perivenous demyelination, perivascular mononuclear cuffing, and an increase in microglial cells, with relative sparing of neurons). Virus-specific cytotoxic T-lymphocytes have been demonstrated in peripheral blood and cerebrospinal fluid of children recovering from mumps meningitis. Unlike in other paramyxovirus infections, severe illness is not recognized in immunosuppressed patients.

Clinical Features

Mumps virus causes an acute, generalized infection in susceptible hosts, with characteristic involvement of the salivary glands and other organ systems. Approximately a third of infections are asymptomatic. The prodromal symptoms are nonspecific and include fever, anorexia, malaise, and headache. The higher frequency of complications in postpubertal persons is important with respect to the recent increase in mumps cases in older age-groups.

Sialitis. Most patients with clinical mumps have parotitis. Other salivary glands can be affected in 10% of cases, but they are rarely affected alone. Parotid involvement usually begins with complaints of earache or jaw tenderness on mastication. Pain worsens over a 2- to 3-day period, as the gland reaches maximum size, and is exacerbated by sour stimuli, such as citrus fruit.

Parotid involvement is bilateral in three fourths of patients. Swelling in one gland usually precedes that in the other by 1 to 5 days. It occurs at the angle of the jaw, with eventual obliteration of the angle. The lower portion of the ear is lifted up and out, increasing the angle between the earlobe and the side of the neck. Neck asymmetry is particularly obvious when viewed from behind, and a bull-neck appearance may be seen. The gland feels doughy and edematous, with indistinct borders. The orifices of Stensen's ducts may be red and swollen, but without expressible pus. This characteristic helps to distinguish this disease from bacterial sialitis. In the presence of submandibular gland involvement, the distinction between mumps and cervical adenitis may be difficult. Although uncommon, sublingual gland involvement is usually bilateral and causes submental

swelling, which also can involve the floor of the mouth and the tongue. Presternal edema has been described, possibly secondary to obstruction of cervical lymphatic drainage. During the first 3 days of illness, the temperature may range from normal to 104° F (40° C). Defervescence and resolution of parotid tenderness and swelling occur within 1 week. Late complications of parotitis (sialectasia and recurrent sialadenitis) are rare.

Orchitis-Epididymitis and Oophoritis. Mumps orchitis is rare before adolescence but occurs in 20% to 30% of postpubertal males and is bilateral in a fourth of the patients. Epididymitis precedes or accompanies orchitis in 85% of cases. Orchitis usually occurs 1 to 2 weeks after the onset of parotitis, but it may precede or occur without parotitis. Symptoms begin abruptly, with fever, nausea, vomiting, and headache, followed by testicular swelling and tenderness. The testicle may enlarge to three or four times normal size. Pain and swelling diminish in conjunction with defervescence, usually by 7 to 10 days. Some degree of atrophy develops in approximately 50% of affected testicles. Although abnormalities in sperm count follow mumps orchitis, sterility is a rare sequela, and impotence is not a recognized complication. An increased risk of testicular neoplasia after mumps orchitis has been debated.

Oophoritis is reported to occur in 5% of postpubertal females. Involvement of the right ovary can mimic appendicitis. Infertility or premature menopause after mumps oophoritis has been reported rarely.

Central Nervous System. Asymptomatic cerebrospinal fluid (CSF) pleocytosis can be found in up to a half of patients with mumps. Clinical meningitis accompanies mumps parotitis in up to 15% of patients, more frequently in males than in females. Meningeal symptoms develop between 1 week before and 2 weeks after parotitis, but up to half of the cases occur in the absence of parotitis.

The clinical manifestations are typical of viral meningitis (Chapter 239). Lymphocytic pleocytosis, with less than 500 cells/mm^3, is usual, but CSF white counts may increase to over 2000/mm^3. Up to a fourth of patients have an initial polymorphonuclear predominance. Glucose level is usually normal, but hypoglycorrhachia occurs in 6% to 30% of patients. Protein concentration is normal to slightly elevated. Clinical and laboratory abnormalities usually return to normal in 7 to 10 days. Sequelae of mumps meningitis are rare.

Encephalitis is estimated to occur in 1 in 400 to 6000 cases. Manifestations usually develop 7 to 10 days after parotitis and include high fever, alterations in the sensorium, seizures, focal neurologic signs, ataxia, movement disorders, and rarely cortical blindness. Although recovery is usually complete, death occurs in approximately 1% of patients and is more likely in adults. Sequelae of psychomotor retardation, seizures, and aqueductal stenosis with hydrocephalus have been reported. Other neurologic syndromes associated with mumps include cerebellar ataxia, facial palsy, polyradiculitis, transverse myelitis, and cranial neuropathies.

Other Complications. Acute pancreatitis, manifested by nausea, vomiting, deep epigastric pain, fever, and chills, occurs in approximately 5% of patients. Recovery usually occurs over 5 to 7 days but in severe cases may take several weeks (Chapter 366).

Electrocardiographic abnormalities, including altered atrioventricular conduction, depressed ST segment, and inverted T waves, occur in 4% to 15% of adults with mumps, but symptomatic myocarditis is rare. Sudden infant death and fatalities caused by heart failure have occurred.

Arthritis following mumps occurs in less than 1% of patients. Adult males are most commonly affected, and in about three fourths of the cases arthritis follows parotitis by 1 to 3 weeks. It can occur before or in the absence of parotitis. Although it is usually a nondeforming, migratory polyarthritis involving large joints, monoarticular arthritis has also been described. Arthritis is commonly accompanied by fever, leukocytosis, and elevated erythrocyte sedimentation rate, as well as by other, visceral complications (orchitis, pancreatitis). Resolution usually occurs within 1 month.

Transient high-frequency hearing loss occurs in less than 5% of patients. Complete, permanent hearing loss occurs in approximately

1 in 20,000 patients with mumps and is occasionally associated with vestibular dysfunction. The hearing loss is unilateral in three fourths of patients. Onset is usually sudden, with vertigo, tinnitus, nausea, and vomiting, followed by permanent deafness. The cause is likely either acoustic neuritis or an endolymphatic labyrinthitis.

Mumps in pregnant women is generally no more severe than in nonpregnant females. Transplacental infection can occur, but teratogenic effects are unproven. An increase in fetal mortality rate and possibly an increased frequency of low birth weight may follow maternal mumps infection during the first trimester.

Mumps virus has been implicated as a cause of juvenile-onset diabetes mellitus. Many reports document the onset of diabetes from 10 days to 5 weeks after clinical mumps. A similar 7-year periodicity of mumps and diabetes with a period of 3 to 4 years between peaks has been found in epidemiologic studies. Other reported complications of mumps virus infection include ocular disease (conjunctivitis, iritis, retinitis, uveitis, optic neuritis), hemolysis, thrombocytopenia, thyroiditis, prostatitis, nephritis, splenic rupture, and neonatal pneumonia.

Diagnosis

The differential diagnosis of mumps parotitis includes other infectious, as well as noninfectious, etiologies of acute parotitis. Viral causes of parotitis include coxsackievirus, Epstein-Barr virus, influenza A, lymphocytic-choriomeningitis virus, parainfluenza, herpes simplex, cytomegalovirus, and echovirus.

The peripheral white blood cell count is variable, but relative lymphocytosis is common. In the presence of orchitis or meningitis, the white count may exceed 20,000/mm³ with a polymorphonuclear predominance. The level of serum amylase, principally the salivary isoenzyme, is elevated in 90% of patients with parotitis. A normal serum lipase level may be helpful in differentiating the high amylase level from that seen in pancreatitis. The levels of salivary and pancreatic amylase isoenzymes may not correlate well with the clinical diagnosis of mumps pancreatitis. Transient hematuria and decreased urine concentrating ability and creatinine clearance are common during the course of mumps.

Saliva, urine, and, in the cases of central nervous system disease, CSF all contain virus. Virus is usually present in saliva for 4 to 5 days after the onset of parotitis. It is usually present in urine during the first 5 days and occasionally up to 2 weeks. Cerebrospinal fluid culture results may be positive during the first 6 days of illness.

Serologic tests are useful in diagnosis and determination of immune status. S antigen complement-fixation antibody titer levels rise in the first week of illness and disappear over several months. V antigen complement-fixation antibody titer levels rise 1 to 2 weeks later and persist at low levels for years. A four-fold rise in convalescent titer level is diagnostic. An acute phase serum that contains an elevated anti-S titer level and a low anti-V titer level is presumptive evidence of acute mumps infection. Detection of mumps-specific IgM by ELISA or immunofluorescence assay is a sensitive and specific means of establishing the diagnosis with a single serum specimen. Measurement of virus-specific IgG by ELISA has been found to be more sensitive than conventional assays for assessment of immune status. Skin testing is not reliable for the diagnosis or assessment of immune status and may provoke an antibody rise that can obscure the serologic diagnosis.

Treatment

Specific therapy is not available for mumps virus infection. Treatment of mumps orchitis has included scrotal elevation or support, ice packs, and antiinflammatory agents. Glucocorticoids, diethylstilbestrol, anesthetic block of the spermatic cord, and incision of the tunica albuginea have not been proved beneficial.

Prevention

A live attenuated mumps vaccine prepared in chick embryo cell culture has been available in the United States since 1968 and is 75% to 95% effective in preventing mumps. Immunization can be given any time after 1 year of age and is usually given at 15 months in combination with measles and rubella vaccination. Mumps vaccine should be given to all susceptible persons, unless contraindicated by documented anaphylactic reaction to egg proteins or to neomycin, immunodeficiency states, or pregnancy. In particular, susceptible adults should be immunized because of the increased risk of mumps-associated complications. Immunization may be ineffective if given within 3 months of blood transfusions or treatment with immunoglobulin for any reason.

Complications following vaccination are rare. Parotitis, rash, pruritus, febrile seizures, unilateral deafness, and meningoencephalitis with virus recovery from CSF have been reported in the 30 days following vaccination.

Postexposure administration of mumps immune globulin is of doubtful value in preventing mumps, although its use has been reported to decrease the risk of orchitis in men with mumps. The globulin is not licensed or available in the United States. Immune serum globulin is not recommended for postexposure prophylaxis. Postexposure administration of mumps vaccine may not be protective, but there is no contraindication.

Patients with mumps should be considered to be infectious until parotid swelling has subsided.

MEASLES VIRUS
Characteristics

Wild measles virus is pathogenic only for humans and certain old world primates. Only one strain of wild measles virus is recognized. Infection confers lifelong protection, although asymptomatic reinfections can occur and may contribute to the persistence of antibody.

Epidemiology

In the prevaccine era, measles caused epidemics of 3 to 4 months' duration every 2 to 5 years, especially in populous areas. In the United States, 90% of reported cases occurred in those less than 10 years old. Vaccine use has been associated with an over 95% decrease in the incidence of measles and a marked change in the age distribution of cases. Despite the existence of an effective vaccine, measles is one of the leading causes of childhood mortality in the world, with an estimated over 1 million deaths annually, virtually all among underprivileged, nonimmunized populations. An upsurge in measles incidence in the United States in the late 1980s, related primarily to outbreaks in unimmunized preschool children, prompted the recommendation for a second vaccine dose at school entrance age. In the last 3 years the reported cases of measles in the United States have been fewer than 1000/year. The majority of the remaining cases are due to outbreaks among unvaccinated children and young adults.

Measles is among the most contagious infections of humans and can spread despite high levels of herd immunity. Measles transmission occurs primarily in schools or households, although up to 4% of measles cases are nosocomially acquired. While immunization rates above 80% have been associated with protection against outbreaks in urban populations, rates over 95% have not prevented outbreaks in closed populations, such as schools. Airborne transmission without face-to-face contact has been implicated in outbreaks linked to physicians' waiting rooms and other medical settings.

Measles virus is transmitted to the respiratory tract or conjunctiva by airborne droplets or by direct contact with infectious secretions. The virus remains infectious in small-particle aerosols for several hours. Patients are most infectious during the late prodrome, when sneezing and coughing contribute to dissemination of infected respiratory secretions, but virus may be shed for several days after the onset of rash. Although virus is present in blood and urine, transmission by these sources is believed to be uncommon. The incubation period is usually 10 to 14 days but may last up to 3 weeks in adults.

Pathogenesis

Measles virus initially infects the respiratory epithelium. A number of isoforms of the human cofactor protein CD46 act as cellular receptors for the measles virus. Viremia then leads to infection of reticuloendothelial cells. A secondary viremia corresponding to the prodromal stage of illness results in virus dissemination to the skin, respiratory tract, and other sites. Giant cells may be present in the tonsils, appendix, other lymphoid organs, and multiple sites in the respiratory tract. Leukopenia, particularly lymphocytopenia, may be secondary to direct destruction of leukocytes. Measles infection is associated with immune suppression, in part manifested by suppression of delayed hypersensitivity reactions and depressed natural killer cell activity for at least 3 weeks after rash onset. This seems to stem from a relative impairment of IL-12 production caused by the infection of monocytes/macrophages, which favors the development of a CD4$^+$ Th2 immune response. Skin and mucous membrane lesions contain multinucleated giant cells and other markers of viral replication. The onset of the exanthem corresponds temporally to the appearance of specific immune responses. The ensuing virus-specific polyclonal immune activation mediates recovery from the disease and establishment of long-term immunity. In addition, it has an important role in the pathogenesis of some of the disease manifestations. Cellular immunity plays a major role in viral clearance. Skin rash develops in agammaglobulinemic patients with measles, whereas in patients with deficient cell-mediated immunity, progressive giant-cell pneumonia without rash may occur.

The histopathologic changes in involved organs include lymphoid hyperplasia, mononuclear cell exudates, and multinucleated giant cells with eosinophilic intranuclear and intracytoplasmic inclusions. Severe lower respiratory tract involvement is marked by destruction of ciliated respiratory epithelium, interstitial pneumonia, epithelial cell hyperplasia, and giant-cell formation.

Clinical Features

Typical Measles. The prodrome of measles lasts 2 to 4 days (range up to 8 days) and is characterized by fever up to 105° F (40.5° C), malaise, anorexia, cough, coryza, and conjunctivitis with photophobia and excess lacrimation. Koplik's spots, red-based lesions with central bluish gray specks, appear on the buccal or labial mucosa, typically opposite the second molars, toward the end of the prodromal period and last for several days. The enanthem may involve the soft or hard palate or may become hemorrhagic in more extensive cases. The skin eruption begins about the face and neck behind the ears as discrete erythematous macules, which proceed downward to cover the trunk and extremities, including the palms and soles. Lesions enlarge, become maculopapular, and often coalesce on the face, shoulders, and upper trunk. In adults, gastrointestinal (abdominal pain, vomiting, diarrhea) and musculoskeletal complaints are common. The eruption clears after 5 to 6 days in its order of appearance, often with brownish discoloration and fine desquamation. Defervescence and improvement of symptoms usually occur several days after the appearance of the rash, but cough may persist.

Modified Measles. The administration of immune serum globulin after measles exposure may alter the course by prolonging the incubation period, shortening the prodrome, and ameliorating the clinical manifestations, including conjunctivitis, Koplik's spots, and rash.

Atypical Measles. In adults who received the inactivated measles vaccine between 1963 and 1968, an unusual, often severe constellation of clinical manifestations may develop 1 to 2 weeks after exposure to wild virus. This syndrome has also occurred after sequential killed live virus immunizations or, rarely, after live vaccine alone. The illness begins abruptly with fever, headache, myalgia, vomiting, abdominal pain, and nonproductive cough. Dyspnea, coryza, sore throat, and pleuritic pain are common. After 3 to 4 days, an erythematous maculopapular rash begins on the distal extremities and spreads proximally for 3 to 5 days. Vesicles singly or in crops, petechiae, purpura, and/or urticarial lesions can develop, along with peripheral edema. Because of the polymorphous nature of the eruption, atypical measles may be mistaken for varicella, scarlet fever, meningococcemia, or Rocky Mountain spotted fever. The face is often spared, Koplik's spots are absent, but conjunctivitis and glossitis with strawberry tongue may occur. Pneumonia occurs in most cases, and chest radiograph changes include patchy,

diffuse, or dense lobar infiltrates; pleural effusion; and hilar adenopathy. Leukocyte counts are low to normal, but left shift, eosinophilia, increased transaminase levels, coagulopathy, and elevated erythrocyte sedimentation rate are common. The fever and other symptoms resolve in 1 to 3 weeks. The course is self-limited, although acute respiratory failure has been described. Residual nodular pulmonary infiltrates may persist for years.

Serologic studies show low or absent initial measles antibody titers, with high titers in samples from convalescent patients. Measles virus has been isolated rarely from these patients. This syndrome is probably the result of an altered immune response to wild measles virus exposure in a previously sensitized host. Recurrences have not been documented.

Measles in Immunosuppressed Patients. Measles is associated with high frequency of complications, most frequently pneumonitis and encephalitis, and with higher mortality, in patients with deficient cell-mediated immunity, including patients infected with HIV, patients with malignancies, and malnourished children from underprivileged populations. Rash may be inapparent in up to 40% of these patients. Measles giant-cell pneumonitis occurs in up to 80% of the patients with advanced HIV infection and in up to 60% of those with malignancies. The case fatality rate is estimated to be 40% in patients infected with HIV, 70% in patients with malignancies, and up to 20% in malnourished children. An inclusion-body encephalitis resulting from persistent measles virus infection may develop in up to 20% of patients with malignancies in 1 to 12 months after initial exposure. Its manifestations include focal myoclonic seizures, personality changes, and a rapid-course coma with case fatality rate of greater than 80%. The CSF, computed tomography (CT), and magnetic resonance imaging (MRI) may be normal, and serologic studies may be nondiagnostic.

Complications

Immunologic status, nutrition, age, race, and availability of medical services influence the outcome of infection. The mortality rate of measles in developed areas with good medical services is usually 0.03% to 0.1%, but is 10- to 100-fold higher in the developing world. The morbidity rate is highest in the very young, adults, one third of whom are hospitalized, and those with underlying immunodeficiency or malnutrition. Most deaths follow respiratory tract and/or neurologic complications.

Respiratory Tract. Lower respiratory tract complications develop in 4% to 50% of patients. Direct viral infection of the respiratory tract is manifested as bronchitis, pneumonia, and, in children, croup or bronchiolitis. In young adults, a multilobar reticulonodular infiltrate is the most common radiographic finding, and pleural effusion or lobar consolidation is uncommon. Giant cell pneumonia develops rarely in apparently normal persons. Secondary bacterial pneumonia is commonly associated with measles pneumonia, and acute sinusitis and serous or suppurative otitis media often follow measles.

Central Nervous System. Electroencephalograph abnormalities with slowing occur transiently in over half of patients with uncomplicated measles. Lymphocyte pleocytosis occurs in about one third of ordinary measles cases. Acute encephalitis, manifested by fever, headache, seizures, altered sensorium, and sometimes focal signs, occurs in 1 in 1000 to 2000 patients. Onset is usually 4 to 7 days after the appearance of the exanthem, but it may precede the rash by 10 days. Cerebrospinal fluid findings include mild elevations in protein level and lymphocytic pleocytosis. Although virus has been demonstrated rarely in the brains of patients who died, in most cases the pathologic changes of demyelination, gliosis, and mononuclear cell infiltrate suggest an immune-mediated, postinfectious encephalomyelitis. Cell-mediated immune responses to myelin basic protein are present in about one half of patients. Death occurs in about 10% of affected persons. The sequelae include behavioral and intellectual changes, seizures, and motor deficits. Subacute sclerosing panencephalitis is a rare, late complication of measles infection.

Other Clinical Presentations. Viral mesenteric adenitis or appendicitis can cause abdominal pain and signs of peritonitis. Such an occurrence during the prodromal stage may present a particularly confusing differential diagnostic problem. Mild viral keratitis occurs commonly and may progress to corneal ulceration in a small portion of cases. Blindness has been reported in 1% of those with ocular involvement. Icteric hepatitis occurs in up to 8% of adult cases, and two- to three-fold elevations of serum AST, LDH, and/or CPK values are common in adults with measles. Transient electrocardiographic changes occur in about 20% of patients, but clinical signs of cardiac disease are rare. Although not a recognized cause of congenital anomalies, measles infection during pregnancy has been associated with spontaneous abortion, premature delivery, and perinatal mortality. Tuberculin reactivity may be depressed for up to 4 weeks after infection. Measles may activate tuberculosis.

Laboratory Diagnosis

Classic measles is easily diagnosed clinically, but laboratory diagnosis may be helpful when the physician is unfamiliar with the infection in areas of decreasing measles prevalence, or in cases of atypical measles.

Leukopenia is common during the prodrome and early eruptive stage of measles, and if it is pronounced (<2000 cells/mm^3), is associated with a poor prognosis. The development of leukocytosis suggests bacterial superinfection or other complications. Measles virus may be isolated from the blood, urine, and throat or conjunctival secretions during the prodrome and up to several days after the exanthem appears. Virus isolation from clinical specimens can be performed in different types of cells, such as human embryonic kidney and primary monkey kidney cells. The characteristic cytopathic effect of multinucleated giant-cell formation usually develops in 5 to 10 days. Immunofluorescence of spin-amplified shell vial cultures of A549 cells can reduce the detection time to 1 to 2 days. Cytologic studies of respiratory and conjunctival secretions or urinary sediment may reveal multinucleated giant cells with characteristic intranuclear inclusions. Immunofluorescence staining of cells from these sites may demonstrate measles virus antigens. Detection of measles virus RNA in respiratory secretions by RT-PCR has been developed and is potentially more practical than cell culture.

Serologic studies of paired specimens constitute the most practical method of laboratory diagnosis of acute and atypical measles. Antibody appears rapidly, so that specimens collected within several days in the first week of rash may demonstrate seroconversion. Because of its technical simplicity and greater sensitivity than the complement-fixation test, the hemagglutination-inhibition method is commonly used for antibody measurement. Among the available assays (Table 251-1), ELISA is the most sensitive and simple to perform. Detection of measles-specific immunoglobulin M (IgM) by ELISA is a sensitive indicator of recent infection and can yield positive findings within 1 week of rash onset. Detection of antibodies in saliva is a satisfactory practical alternative to serum for seroprevalence studies. For the diagnosis of subacute sclerosing panencephalitis, CSF antibody measurements should also be obtained.

Prevention

The live attenuated measles virus vaccine currently used in the United States is prepared in chick embryo cell culture. This vaccine provides durable immunity in at least 95% of recipients vaccinated at 15 months or older. Antibody titers elicited by immunization tend to decrease with time, and secondary vaccine failures occur. All school-aged children, including college and high school students, and health care workers should have documented immunity to measles (i.e., birth before 1957, physician-diagnosed measles, prior immunization with two doses of vaccine, or seropositivity). Combined measles-mumps-rubella (MMR) vaccine is preferred because mumps can also occur in highly vaccinated populations. A two-dose schedule is now advocated for all children, with the first dose at age 15 months and the second at entrance to school. The first dose should be given at 12 months of age for children in some areas with recurrent measles transmission. Immunization is indicated for asymptomatic children infected with human immunodeficiency virus (HIV) and should be con-

sidered in symptomatic ones, especially those in populations with active measles transmission. However, in light of a reported case of measles pneumonitis after MMR vaccine, it may be prudent to withhold measles-containing vaccines from persons infected with HIV who are severely immunosuppressed (<750 CD4$^+$ T-lymphocytes for children <12 months of age, <500 for children 1 to 5 years of age, <200 for persons 6 years of age or older). Among underprivileged populations of developing countries, where earlier loss of maternal antibodies occurs, the World Health Organization's (WHO) Expanded Program on Immunizations (EPI) recommends that a dose of monovalent measles vaccine be given at 9 months of age, followed by the routine vaccination schedule. Persons whose initial vaccine may have been ineffective are also candidates for revaccination. This includes those who received inactivated measles vaccine (available 1963 to 1968), a close sequence of inactivated and live virus vaccines (3 months between injections), concurrent administration of immune serum globulin, vaccine before 12 months of age when maternal antibody may suppress an active response, and in general those whose immunization status cannot be documented. Most persons born before 1957 are likely to have been naturally infected.

The most common side-effects associated with measles vaccination are fever, rash, or both, occurring in 5% to 15% of recipients between 5 and 12 days after inoculation. Febrile convulsions, and, rarely, meningoencephalitis have also been described. Contraindications to live measles vaccine include pregnancy; primary or acquired immunodeficiency states; recent immunoglobulin therapy; anaphylactic reaction to egg ingestion or neomycin; and intercurrent febrile illness, which may increase the rate of primary vaccine failure. Revaccination of those who previously received inactivated vaccine is sometimes accompanied by fever, rash, and localized induration, erythema, and vesiculation at the injection site.

Postexposure prophylaxis of measles with passive immunization is indicated for susceptible persons who are at increased risk of complications, including pregnant women and immunocompromised patients. Immunoglobulin may prevent or modify measles if given within 6 days of exposure. The recommended dose of immunoglobulin is 0.25 ml/kg (0.5 ml/kg for immunocompromised individuals) to a maximum of 15 ml. Exposed symptomatic patients infected with HIV should receive immunoglobulin regardless of vaccine status. In normal hosts, postexposure administration of vaccine usually prevents disease if administered within 3 days after exposure to natural measles. Hospitalized patients require respiratory isolation.

Treatment

Short-term administration of vitamin A (200,000 IU/day for 2 days) reduces morbidity and mortality in severe measles in children. Parenteral and/or aerosolized ribavirin and immunoglobulin have been used in immunocompromised patients with measles pneumonia.

RESPIRATORY SYNCYTIAL VIRUS
Characteristics

Two major subgroups (A and B) are distinguished principally by antigenic differences in the G surface glycoprotein, which mediates attachment to host cells. The importance of strain variation in clinical or immunologic responses is unresolved, but infections by subgroup A strains may be more severe. Natural infection occurs only in humans and chimpanzees.

Epidemiology

Respiratory syncytial virus (RSV) has worldwide distribution. In temperate climates, it causes annual outbreaks for up to 6 months in the late fall, winter, and spring months. Most children have specific serum antibody by 2 years of age, and reinfections in children and adults are common. Strains of both subgroups of RSV appear to cocirculate during epidemic periods but in varying proportions.

Respiratory syncytial virus is the major cause of lower respiratory tract illness in infants and young children. It accounts for 60% to 90% of bronchiolitis and up to 40% of pneumonia cases in this age group. RSV is associated each year with an estimated 90,000 hospitalizations and 4500 deaths from lower respiratory tract disease in the United States. Most severe infections occur in infants less than 6 months old, although high levels of maternal RSV antibody may be associated with protection against lower respiratory tract disease. Other risk factors for lower respiratory tract disease include male gender, lack of breastfeeding, crowding, lower socioeconomic status, day care attendance, and parental smoking. RSV activity correlates with winter peaks in respiratory deaths of infants less than 1 year of age. Secondary infection in family contacts of an index case are common. RSV is a major nosocomial pathogen, and high attack rates occur in patients and staff during outbreaks in hospitals, day care centers, and geriatric units. Nosocomial outbreaks of RSV infection have involved up to one half of hospital staff and patients. The average incubation period is 5 days, with a range of 2 to 8 days. RSV transmission requires close contact, with spread either by large-particle aerosols or by contamination of hands with infectious secretions and inoculation into the eye or nose.

Pathogenesis

Respiratory syncytial virus primarily infects the respiratory tract, and cell-to-cell spread of the virus may lead to involvement of the entire length of the respiratory mucosa. Lymphocytic peribronchiolar inflammation, later necrolysis and proliferation of the bronchiolar epithelium, and inflammatory exudate contribute to small airway obstruction in RSV bronchiolitis. Air trapping with hyperinflation and atelectatic collapse results. Eosinophilic cytoplasmic inclusions in epithelial cells and multinucleated giant cells, severe fibrosis, and hyaline membrane formation may occur in fatal RSV pneumonia. Increased respiratory secretion titers of RSV-specific IgE, histamine, eosinophil cationic protein, and leukotriene LTC4 play a role in airway bronchospasm and inflammation and correlate with the occurrence of wheezing in children.

Naturally acquired immunity to RSV is incomplete and of short duration, but the severity of the illness decreases with reinfections. Local antibody concentration correlates better with protection from illness than does serum antibody level. The role of cell-mediated immunity in recovery from infection is unresolved, but severe infections may occur in immunocompromised children and adults.

Clinical Features

The majority of infections in both children and adults are symptomatic. In infants and young children, upper respiratory illness accompanied by fever and otitis media is common. Lower respiratory tract involvement is manifested as pneumonia, bronchiolitis, tracheobronchitis, or, less often, croup. Bronchiolitis in infancy has been associated with an increased risk of subsequent recurrent wheezing, and lower respiratory RSV disease early in life may be followed by chronic alterations in pulmonary function. Infants with congenital heart disease or prematurity-associated lung disease and immunocompromised hosts of any age are at risk for severe infection. RSV infection has been associated with apneic spells, particularly in premature infants, and with sudden infant death syndrome.

The most common syndrome observed in adults is upper respiratory illness with coryza and cough, often accompanied by low-grade fever. The illness tends to be more severe and prolonged than rhinovirus colds. Bronchitis, influenza-like symptoms, pneumonia, sinusitis and otitis, and exacerbations of asthma and chronic bronchitis have also been associated with RSV infection in adults. Bronchial hyperreactivity measured by pulmonary function testing may last for several months after infection. RSV causes illness indistinguishable from influenza virus infections in the elderly. Bronchopneumonia or secondary bacterial pneumonia complicates a high proportion of infections in the elderly. Rarely, RSV infections may be associated with diffuse, life-threatening pneumonia in previously healthy adults. Immunocompromised hosts, particularly bone marrow transplant recipients in the early transplant period, have an increased risk of severe RSV infection with high mortality rate. Uncommon manifestations of RSV infection include meningitis, myelitis, exanthems, and myocarditis.

Diagnosis

Nasal secretions obtained by nasopharyngeal aspiration or washing, as well as sputum or lower respiratory samples, are appropriate specimens for virus isolation. Because the virus is heat-labile, freezing and delays in processing of clinical specimens should be avoided. Human heteroploid HEp-2 cells are most frequently used for virus isolation. RSV causes characteristic syncytia formation in HEp-2 cells after an average of 3 to 5 days. An increasing number of techniques for detection of viral antigens in clinical specimens are available. Immunofluorescence staining of exfoliated respiratory cells is a sensitive method for the rapid (less than 2 hours) direct detection of RSV in clinical samples and for the confirmation and typing of isolates in cell culture. Rapid detection of RSV antigens by several commercially available membrane-based EIA assays is also sensitive and specific and, combined with isolation in cell cultures, provides the best RSV detection rates. RT-PCR assays have shown sensitivity and specificity equivalent to other RSV detection methods in clinical samples, including middle ear effusion fluids.

Treatment

Management of lower respiratory disease includes correction of hypoxemia and close monitoring of respiratory status. Corticosteroids and bronchodilators have not been found to be beneficial. The only currently approved antiviral drug for lower respiratory tract RSV infections of infants is ribavirin, delivered by small-particle aerosol. Several studies reported that ribavirin reduced illness severity, blood gas abnormalities, and number of days on mechanical ventilation in previously healthy and high-risk infants hospitalized with RSV bronchiolitis or pneumonia. More recent studies, however, have not confirmed its efficacy. It may be considered in infants and young children with underlying conditions such as congenital heart disease, bronchopulmonary dysplasia, cystic fibrosis, immunosuppressive diseases or therapies, severe illness, or younger than 6 weeks of age. Aerosolized ribavirin is generally well tolerated, but is expensive and its administration requires prolonged periods of exposure. Aerosol ribavirin combined with intravenous immunoglobulin containing high titers of anti-RSV antibody may benefit bone marrow transplant patients with RSV pneumonia.

Prevention

No vaccine against RSV is currently available. Several investigational vaccines are under study, and one of these, a purified fusion (F) protein vaccine, has been shown to reduce RSV lower respiratory illness in children with cystic fibrosis. In addition, passive immunization of high-risk infants with underlying cardiac and pulmonary diseases with immunoglobulin containing high titers of anti-RSV neutralizing antibody during the RSV season reduces infection rates and hospitalizations. One polyclonal product is commercially available. Attenuated and glycoprotein subunit RSV vaccines are currently under development. Thorough hand washing and regular use of eye-nose goggles may be effective in preventing nosocomial RSV spread. Use of gowns and gloves, decontamination of surfaces and fomites, cohorting of infected cases, and perhaps protective isolation of high-risk contacts are additional control measures.

RUBELLA VIRUS
Classification

Rubella is a spherical, enveloped, single-stranded RNA-containing virus. Although its clinical and epidemiologic behavior is similar to that of the paramyxoviruses, rubella is classified in the togavirus family. Only one serologic type is recognized.

Epidemiology

During the prevaccine era in the United States, epidemics of rubella occurred every 6 to 9 years, and most reported cases occurred in children under 10 years of age. A major epidemic in 1964 resulted in the birth of approximately 20,000 infants with congenital rubella defects, and, on the basis of the periodicity of reported rubella, another significant epidemic was forecast for the early 1970s. When live attenuated rubella virus vaccine became available in 1969, mass vaccination of children 1 year of age and older was recommended to reduce transmission of rubella from children to susceptible pregnant women. The incidence of rubella has declined over 99% compared to the pre-vaccine era. Approximately 200 cases have occurred annually in the United States in recent years.

Unfortunately, disease activity during the 1970s remained relatively constant among adolescents and young adults, and outbreaks of rubella were described among high school and college students, military trainees, prison inmates, hospital employees, and even discotheque clientele. Several outbreaks occurred among populations with rates of immunity greater than 90%; moderate levels of herd immunity have not reliably prevented transmission. Increased emphasis was therefore placed on the identification and vaccination of susceptible adolescents and adults, especially women, and levels of reported rubella in these older age groups dropped markedly in the 1980s.

Pathogenesis

Transmission of rubella is primarily via respiratory droplets or direct contact with an infected patient. The period of communicability is from approximately 7 days before to 5 days after rash onset. Patients differ markedly in their ability to spread infection, perhaps related to the presence of respiratory symptoms, such as sneezing and coughing, that facilitate dissemination. Persons with subclinical rubella can transmit infection. Infants with congenital rubella often shed large amounts of virus for prolonged periods (in some cases, over 1 year) and pose an important infection hazard to nonimmune caretakers.

After infection of the upper respiratory tract, the virus multiplies locally, and eventually viremia results. The incubation period averages 18 days (range 14 to 21 days). The rash is believed to be immunologically mediated. Rubella virus can be isolated from rash lesions and also from adjacent areas of normal skin. Virus has also been isolated from joint effusions in persons with rubella arthritis.

Naturally acquired immunity against rubella is usually life long, but reinfections, mostly subclinical, have been reported. Such reinfections are more common in persons with vaccine-induced immunity, especially those with low antibody titer levels. Viremia is probably extremely rare in such persons, and gestational reinfection appears to pose minimum risk to the fetus.

Clinical Features

Rubella is commonly inapparent. When clinical illness occurs, it is generally mild and is manifested by rash and lymphadenopathy, with mild constitutional symptoms. Discrete, pink maculopapules appear first on the face and then spread to the chest, abdomen, and extremities. The lesions may coalesce, especially on the face, and may desquamate during convalescence. An enanthem of punctate or larger red macules (Forchheimer spots) may appear on the soft palate before or coincident with the rash onset. The usual duration of rash is 2 to 5 days. Rash may be totally absent. The postauricular, posterior cervical, and suboccipital lymph nodes are often tender and swollen; the discomfort is usually short-lived, but palpable nodal enlargement may persist for weeks. Splenomegaly may be observed. In children, rash is usually the first sign of the illness, but many adults experience a prodrome consisting of low-grade fever, malaise, anorexia, headache, sore throat, and, in severe cases, cough, coryza, and conjunctivitis, as seen in rubeola. Arthralgia and arthritis are infrequent in children, but are more common among adult women. Joint symptoms usually appear 2 to 3 days after the onset of rash and persist only a few days. Thrombocytopenic purpura and encephalitis are infrequent complications. Testalgia may indicate orchitis.

Congenital Infection. In marked contrast to the usually mild nature of postnatal rubella, gestational rubella can be potentially devastating to the developing fetus and may produce the congenital rubella syndrome. Defects of virtually every organ system have been described, but the most notable involvement is of the eyes (e.g., cataract, glaucoma), heart (especially patent ductus arteriosus and pulmonary stenosis), and central nervous system (e.g., sensorineural

deafness, psychomotor retardation). A fulminant neonatal presentation, with hepatosplenomegaly, jaundice, thrombocytopenic purpura, and radiolucent bone lesions, may also occur. More subtle changes, such as learning disabilities and behavioral disturbances, may not be recognized until years after birth. Endocrinopathies, especially diabetes mellitus, and a late-onset, progressive encephalitis may be other late manifestations. The risk of major anomalies is greatest for infection during the first trimester.

Diagnosis

Because of the nonspecific nature of the signs and symptoms, clinical diagnosis of postnatal rubella is difficult in a nonepidemic setting. The virus can often be detected in throat, blood, or urine specimens, but viral isolation is difficult and requires special techniques, since the virus does not produce cytopathic effect in cell cultures. Recently developed RT-PCR assays provide an alternative to cell culture.

Diagnosis is best accomplished by demonstration of a four-fold rise in antibody titer in paired sera. The hemagglutination inhibition (HI) technique has been the standard method for many years, but has been supplanted by alternative methods, such as EIA, radioimmunoassay, latex agglutination, radial hemolysis, and immunofluorescence. Using these methods, the criteria for a significant rise in antibody level vary by type of assay and by laboratory. The presence of rubella-specific IgM antibodies in a single specimen obtained during the subacute stage strongly suggests recent primary infection. Single antibody determination in serum or saliva is useful for epidemiologic surveys.

In screening for rubella susceptibility using the time-honored hemagglutination-inhibition technique, the presence of any level of rubella antibody has generally been considered to indicate previous infection (or immunization) and presumed immunity; the absence of such antibody indicates probable susceptibility. Clinical experience with the newer serologic methods is less extensive, but any antibody level above the standard positive cut-off value for that particular assay is likewise generally considered presumptive evidence of immunity. An undocumented history of rubella illness is unreliable and should not be accepted as evidence of immunity.

The diagnosis of congenital rubella infection may be strongly suggested in some instances by the history and physical examination. In other instances, however, the clinical presentation does not allow easy differentiation of rubella from other types of congenital infection, including toxoplasmosis, cytomegalovirus, herpes simplex, and syphilis.

The diagnosis of congenital rubella infection in an infant can be confirmed by the presence of rubella-specific IgM antibodies or by a significant titer level of rubella antibody between 6 and 11 months of age (by which time levels of passively acquired maternal antibody should be negligible). Viral isolation is also diagnostic and can be helpful even after the immediate neonatal period, because viral persistence and shedding may be prolonged for 6 months or longer after birth.

Prevention and Treatment

There is no specific therapy for rubella, but treatment of symptoms may be helpful for patients with significant fever, malaise, or arthritis.

Since the time of its licensure in 1969, over 180 million doses of live attenuated rubella virus vaccine have been distributed in the United States. The vaccine strain currently available in this country (RA 27/3) is grown in a human diploid cell line and, though more immunogenic than the previously used strains, has no increase in side-effects. Rubella vaccine is available as a monovalent antigen or in combination with live measles and/or mumps vaccines.

Vaccine reactions are uncommon in children but may include fever, rash, lymphadenopathy, arthralgia, arthritis, and peripheral neuritis. Joint symptoms are more common in adult women than in children and begin 1 to 10 weeks after immunization. These symptoms are usually short-lived and do not result in permanent disability or deformity. Recurrent joint symptoms and frank arthritis are very unusual but have been reported. All joint reactions are less frequent and less severe with rubella vaccine than with rubella illness.

The durability of vaccine-induced immunity is of crucial importance, because it was hoped that vaccination during childhood might protect a woman through her childbearing years. Since antibody titers are lower after vaccination than after natural disease, continued surveillance is necessary to determine the possible need for booster vaccinations. At this time, however, booster of rubella vaccination is not routinely indicated.

Rubella vaccine virus can cross the placenta and infect the fetus of a susceptible vaccinee. However, more than 800 susceptible women have been vaccinated inadvertently during early pregnancy, and, despite serologic evidence of infection in some exposed infants, none had defects compatible with congenital rubella syndrome. The theoretic risk of malformation is less than 2%. However, rubella vaccination remains contraindicated during pregnancy, and women of childbearing age should not become pregnant for 3 months after vaccination. Vaccine may be given to children whose mothers are pregnant, because the vaccine virus is nontransmissible.

Rubella vaccination is currently recommended for all children, many adolescents, and some adults, particularly women, unless it is otherwise contraindicated. Routine vaccination of infants and enforcement of state laws requiring immunization of schoolchildren should ensure continuously high levels of immunity among young children. Many persons who receive the currently recommended second dose of measles vaccine are given the combined measles-mumps-rubella vaccine. This second dose of rubella vaccine serves to increase the overall level of rubella immunity. Identification and vaccination of susceptible adolescent and adult women are also essential for optimum rubella control. Situations that lend themselves well to serologic screening for rubella susceptibility include the premarital examination, entrance into educational or training institutions (such as colleges or military bases), and visits to family-planning clinics and employee health services. Serologic documentation of susceptibility in potential vaccinees of childbearing age is sometimes desirable but should not be considered mandatory, especially in outbreaks. No known ill effects result from vaccination of persons with preexisting immunity. Screening at prenatal visits allows vaccination of susceptible persons immediately after delivery. Breast-feeding and previous administration of $Rh_o(D)$ immune globulin or blood products are not contraindications to postpartum vaccination. In this latter instance, however, serologic testing is recommended 6 to 8 weeks later to ascertain whether seroconversion has occurred.

The traditional concern with nosocomial rubella has been that a pregnant hospital employee would contract rubella from an infected patient. Female hospital employees of childbearing age who are in contact with patients should be required to prove rubella immunity for their own protection. In several recent outbreaks, hospital employees with rubella have exposed large numbers of susceptible pregnant patients. It is therefore advisable for all hospital employees, male or female, who are in contact with pregnant patients to undergo similar screening for patient protection.

There is no evidence that rubella vaccine is either helpful or harmful in the management of patients recently exposed to rubella, but it is often given to provide future protection if the recognized exposure has not resulted in incubating infection. Immune serum globulin given after exposure may suppress or modify symptoms but does not reliably prevent infection or viremia. Limited experience with high-titer-level human rubella immunoglobulin has been favorable, but this material is not generally available. Prophylactic use of immune serum globulin after exposures during early pregnancy is not of proven benefit and should be considered only among women who would not contemplate therapeutic abortion under any circumstances. Serologic testing done promptly after such exposures often establishes preexisting immunity and reassures the involved persons.

CORONAVIRUS INFECTIONS
Classification and Characteristics

Coronaviruses are medium-sized, pleomorphic, lipid-enveloped viruses that contain a single-stranded RNA genome. The term *coronavirus* refers to the widely spaced, club-shaped spikes that radiate from the virus surface in electron microscopic preparations and impart a crownlike appearance. The surface projections, or peplomers, contain glycoproteins that have cell receptor binding, membrane fusing, and in some strains, hemagglutinating activities. They replicate in the cytoplasm of infected cells and cause a cytocidal effect.

The two best characterized strains of human coronavirus, 229E and OC43, are in separate antigenic groups. Most isolates from the respiratory tract are antigenically similar to one of these two strains. Human enteric coronaviruses have been recovered from cases of acute gastrointestinal infection, and coronavirus-like particles (CVLPs) detected by electron microscopy in the stool of both symptomatic and asymptomatic persons.

Epidemiology

Coronaviruses are the second most frequently recognized cause of the common cold and account for approximately 15% of all colds. Coronaviruses have been found throughout the world. In temperate climates, infection occurs principally in the winter and spring months, although outbreaks have been described during summer. The proportion of colds caused by coronaviruses is as high as 35% during periods of peak activity. Strain 229E causes outbreaks at 2- to 4-year intervals. The prevalence of antibody rises rapidly during the first 5 years of life, and most adults have antibody to OC43 and 229E. Reinfection with the same serotype appears to be common, and the level of circulating antibody correlates to a limited extent with protection from infection.

Coronaviruses are transmitted by the respiratory route, whereas enteric coronaviruses are presumably spread by the fecal-oral route. The seasonal (fall-winter) and age (2 years old) patterns of diarrhea associated with fecal shedding of CVLPs are similar to those with rotaviruses. There are no recognized animal reservoirs or vectors of human coronaviruses.

Clinical Features

The full spectrum of human coronavirus infections has not been determined. One third to one half of respiratory coronavirus infections are asymptomatic. The usual manifestations of infection are typical common colds (Chapter 237). In experimentally induced infections, the incubation period (2 to 5 days) is longer than in rhinovirus colds, and the average duration of illness is 6 to 7 days. Low-grade fever occurs in about one fifth of infected persons. In addition to nasal symptoms, cough and sore throat occur frequently. Virus excretion is detectable at the time symptoms begin and lasts for 1 to 4 days. Coronavirus infections have been associated with exacerbations of asthma and chronic bronchitis, recurrent wheezy bronchitis in children, and, uncommonly, lower respiratory tract disease or pneumonia in selected groups, including infants, young children, and military recruits.

Coronaviruses have been implicated as causes of acute gastroenteritis in young children and rarely of outbreaks of necrotizing enterocolitis in neonates. In addition to diarrhea, fever, and vomiting, more severely affected infants may show abdominal distention, blood in the stool, and radiologic evidence of pneumatosis intestinalis. CVLPs have been detected in adults with diarrhea, including some patients with acquired immunodeficiency syndrome (AIDS), but also in a high proportion of asymptomatic persons, particularly in tropical climates. Excretion of these agents may be prolonged and has been associated with poor hygiene. A reported association between coronavirus infection and multiple sclerosis remains to be proven.

Diagnosis

Laboratory diagnosis of coronavirus infections is technically difficult, because human coronaviruses have fastidious growth requirements. HCV-OC43 usually requires human organ culture for primary isolation. HCV-229E is more easily grown in cell culture. Immunoassays and nucleic acid hybridization assays have been described for detection of coronavirus in nasopharyngeal secretions. RT-PCR–based assays for human coronavirus have been developed and are a promising alternative to other methods of detection. Serologic diagnosis of 229E and OC43 infections by EIA is sensitive and specific and is useful in epidemiologic surveys.

Treatment and Prevention

Intranasal interferon protects against experimental coronavirus infection, but no specific antiviral therapy or vaccine is currently available. Treatment is for symptoms only.

ADENOVIRUS INFECTIONS
Classification and Characteristics

Adenoviruses are nonenveloped, icosahedral viruses that contain double-stranded deoxyribonucleic acid (DNA). The surface of the virus is relatively complex and consists of three types of capsomers (subunits): hexons, pentons, and rodlike structures that project from the penton base, known as fibers (Fig. 251-1). The capsomer types differ from each other morphologically, antigenically, and functionally. The hexon and penton bases contain group antigens that are common to all human adenovirus types, whereas the fibers have primarily type-specific antigens. Adenoviruses are distinguished antigenically on the basis of these group-specific (A to F) and type-specific (1 to 49) antigens. The adenoviruses most important for human disease are the lower serotypes (types 1 to 8, 11, 14, and 21). Many adenovirus serotypes can persist in latent state in tonsillar tissues of asymptomatic children and may be shed in stools for prolonged periods. With the exception of the enteric adenoviruses, types 40 and 41, other serotypes usually are associated with asymptomatic colonization.

Some adenoviruses are oncogenic for tissue culture and newborn animals, but the highly oncogenic types (12, 18, and 31) are isolated infrequently from humans. There is no definitive evidence that adenoviruses are a cause of human cancer.

Adenoviruses are regularly accompanied by a small single-stranded DNA parvovirus known as *adeno-associated virus* (AAV). These viruses cannot undergo productive replication in tissue culture or in animals without the association of adenoviruses (cytomegalovirus also can provide this helper function), although latent infection may occur. Adenovirus infection in humans is commonly accompanied by infection with adeno-associated virus, although the latter does not produce any unique disease syndrome. Most persons have antibodies to at least one of the four adeno-associated virus serotypes by 10 years of age.

Epidemiology

Adenoviruses, like the enteroviruses and many other nonenveloped viruses, are hardy agents and capable of transmission by a number of routes. Transmission within families and among children seems to be primarily via fecal–oral spread. Asymptomatic fecal excretion of adenoviruses may continue for years after initial infection, especially in children. Respiratory transmission by aerosols has been found in military populations and may also occur in civilian adults. Transmission by fomites or direct contact has been associated with swimming pools and physicians' offices in which sterilization or hand washing has been inadequate. Asymptomatic infection and a chronic carrier state are common with adenoviruses.

Infection with the lower serotypes tends to occur very early in life. Infection in children results in disease approximately half the time and is associated almost exclusively with isolation of the virus from the upper respiratory tract. Adenovirus infections appear to account for between 5% and 20% of cases of respiratory disease in children and for approximately 5% of cases of pneumonia and bronchitis. Adenovirus infections in adults tend to be sporadic, involve primarily the upper respiratory tract, and are strongly associated with contact with children. Adenovirus rarely produces pneumonia in civilian adults.

Pathogenesis

Adenoviruses may infect the respiratory tract, ocular mucosa, intestinal tract, and genitourinary tract. In the case of respiratory tract disease, adenovirus infection is associated with cytopathology and necrosis of cells of the respiratory tract. Presumably this is a direct effect of the virus, because complete virus as well as isolated virus components, primarily the penton base, may cause identical cytopathologic changes in tissue culture. Tissue invasion with viremia may occur and may result in disseminated infection in immunocompromised hosts. Most infections result in a brisk serum antibody response. Immunity to adenovirus infection is due to the presence of type-specific neutralizing antibody. Protection is afforded against both illness and infection. Heterotypic immunity does not occur. The degree of illness may be inversely proportional to the amount of specific secretory immunoglobulin A (IgA) present in nasal secretions, suggesting a moderating role for local antibody. Ocular infections may occur even in the presence of significant levels of serum antibody, and a role for local antibody in protection against these infections is presumed. Efforts at adenovirus vector-mediated transfer of the cystic fibrosis transmembrane conductance regulator (CFTR) gene to the respiratory epithelium have been hampered by local inflammatory and specific immune responses in cystic fibrosis patients.

Latent infection is common with these agents but appears to occur by a mechanism of low-level replication on mucosal surfaces or in lymphoid tissue rather than by integration of the viral genome into the host cell DNA. Latent infections lasting months to years have been described in the respiratory tract (human tonsils) and in the gastrointestinal tract. Latent infections are probably important in maintenance of the virus in populations, but there is no evidence that ill health results from the chronic carrier state.

Clinical Syndromes

Respiratory disease produced by adenovirus may involve all parts of the respiratory tract and is most frequently caused by adenoviruses types 1 to 7, 14, and 21. Pharyngitis is a common manifestation of adenovirus infection and may be associated with fever, pharyngeal exudate, and anterior cervical adenopathy, thus closely mimicking streptococcal pharyngitis. Although adenovirus has been detected in the middle ear of patients with chronic otitis media with effusion, its role in the etiology of this syndrome remains to be conclusively established. Pneumonia occurs commonly in infants and in military recruits and has also been reported in immunocompromised patients. Adenovirus infection also has been associated with a whooping cough syndrome, which may result occasionally from isolated adenovirus infection but is more frequent during dual adenovirus–*Bordetella pertussis* infection. A severe form of destructive airway disease called *bronchiolitis obliterans* may follow adenoviral infections. Adenoviruses appear to be a major cause of postinfectious bronchiectasis of childhood.

Pharyngoconjunctival fever, probably the best-characterized syndrome attributed to adenoviral infections, is an illness characterized by fever, pharyngitis that is often exudative, and conjunctivitis or keratoconjunctivitis. It is commonly due to adenoviruses types 3 and 7, may be epidemic or endemic, and is primarily seen in young children during the summer months. Epidemics have been associated with swimming pool water contaminated with adenoviruses, usually occurring because of inadequate chlorination or failure of the filtration

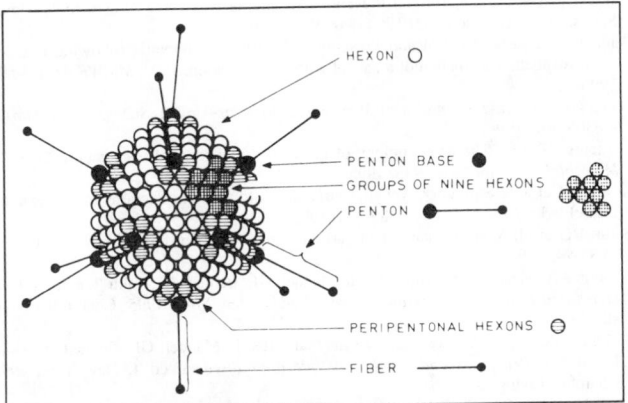

FIGURE 251-1 Structure of adenovirus virion.

From Phillipson L et al: *Molecular biology of adenoviruses: virology monographs 14,* New York, 1975, Springer-Verlag.

system. Adenovirus conjunctivitis without pharyngitis also has been seen in this setting. Nosocomial epidemics of pharyngoconjunctival fever also have occurred.

Epidemics of pneumonia and febrile lower respiratory tract infections in military recruits have been ascribed to adenoviruses, particularly type 4 and, to a lesser extent, types 7 and 21.

Epidemic keratoconjunctivitis, also known as *shipyard eye,* is also due to adenovirus infection. This disease is usually caused by adenovirus type 8 and has been spread by ocular tonometers that were inadequately sterilized between uses and by physicians' unwashed hands. Keratoconjunctivitis may cause lasting impairment of vision.

Conjunctivitis is usually caused by adenovirus type 3, 7, or 8, is usually relatively mild, and may be associated with pharyngitis. Adenovirus conjunctivitis is usually self-limited.

Hemorrhagic cystitis may occur with infection of the bladder; adenovirus 11 is the type most commonly involved. This illness occurs primarily in children and may be either epidemic or endemic. In contrast to bacterial cystitis, adenovirus cystitis tends to affect males three times as often as females. The symptoms are similar to those seen in patients with bacterial cystitis. The illness is self-limited, with the hematuria clearing within 1 or 2 days and the other manifestations clearing within a week. Asymptomatic urinary shedding of adenoviruses is common in patients with AIDS.

Adenovirus has been isolated infrequently from the cerebrospinal fluid in patients with meningoencephalitis. The infection is mild and self-limited, with primarily meningeal manifestations. Occasionally CNS involvement is part of multisystem disease. Chronic meningoencephalitis caused by serotypes 7, 12, and 32 has been documented in hypogammaglobulinemic patients.

Gastrointestinal infection with adenoviruses is usually asymptomatic in adults. However, enteric adenoviruses types 40 and 41 can cause up to 20% of infantile diarrhea, which is usually manifested by watery stools and fever, and lasts 1 to 2 weeks. Adenovirus infection of the gastrointestinal tract has been associated with intussusception in infants and children, but pathogenetic relationship is unproven.

Disseminated infections with adenoviruses have been described in infants and very young children and in patients with immunodeficiencies. All organ systems may be affected, but pneumonia, hepatitis, myocarditis, encephalitis, colitis, and nephritis are clinically prominent.

Adenovirus infections are common in patients with late-stage HIV disease. More than one third of these patients may have an adenoviral infection, most frequently gastrointestinal, but over 50% of them remain asymptomatic. Bone marrow and solid organ transplant recipients are also at increased risk of adenovirus shedding and invasive disease.

Diagnosis

Adenoviruses can be identified in clinical specimens by culture, detection of viral antigens (e.g., by immunofluorescence or enzyme-linked immunoassay), or detection of viral DNA. Depending on the site of infection, adenoviruses can be isolated from pharynx, sputum, stools, conjunctival scrapings or swabs, and fresh urine. Culture is satisfactory for many clinical situations except enteric infections (because of the less easily cultured adenovirus types 40 and 41), where antigen detection by EIA is the preferred method. Sensitive and specific detection of adenovirus DNA by PCR in clinical samples with group-specific or type-specific primers is an attractive alternative to viral isolation.

Both group-specific and type-specific antibodies are induced by adenovirus infection. Complement-fixing antibodies are group-specific, whereas neutralizing and hemagglutination-inhibition antibodies are type-specific. Paired acute and convalescent serum specimens may be screened for adenovirus infection using group-specific antigens and then tested for type-specific antibodies if necessary. Serologic testing for group-specific antibody alone detects 80% to 90% of symptomatic adenovirus infections, particularly in adults.

In patients with respiratory or ocular disease, culture of an adenovirus, especially one of the lower serotypes (types 1 to 15), strongly suggests an etiologic relationship to the illness. However, asymptomatic infections with prolonged virus shedding are common, particularly with higher serotypes (types 22 to 39) and in the gastrointesti-

nal tract; if there is doubt, the relationship between the virus isolated and the clinical findings can be reinforced by showing a rise in antibody titer between acute and convalescent serum specimens.

Treatment and Prevention

At the present time, there are no chemotherapeutic agents of proven effectiveness for adenovirus infection. Antivirals active in vitro include ciclofovir, ganciclovir, and possibly ribavirin. In immunocompromised patients, successful therapy of severe adenoviral infections has been reported with intravenous ribavirin.

Oral, live vaccines have been developed by the novel technique of packaging wild-type (nonattenuated) live adenovirus in enteric-coated capsules. Enteric-coated adenovirus vaccines types 4 and 7 that have been used in military recruits ensure enteric infection without infection of the respiratory tree and appear safe and effective. The enteric infection in adults is asymptomatic but results in the production of protective serum antibody. Transmission of these viruses occurs within families by the fecal-oral route.

Environmental manipulation also may be important for the control of adenovirus infections. Disease in military recruit populations may be minimized by not mixing incoming recruits with recruits who have already been in training for several weeks or by reducing the size of the recruit training groups. Adenovirus infections may spread through improperly sterilized tonometers, through contact with physicians' hands, and through swimming pool water; proper environmental controls must be applied in these areas. Swimming pool chlorination and filtration should be carefully monitored, particularly during periods of heavy use. Ophthalmologists and other physicians who examine patients with infective conjunctivitis should either wear gloves or scrupulously wash their hands between patients. Materials placed in patients' eyes, particularly tonometers, should be sterilized between examinations by a method known to be effective against adenoviruses.

BIBLIOGRAPHY

American Academy of Pediatrics Committee on Infectious Diseases: Reassessment of the indications for ribavirin therapy in respiratory virus infections, *Pediatrics* 97:137-140, 1996.

Baum SG: Adenovirus. In Mandell GL, Bennett JE, Dolin R, editors: *Principles and practice of infectious diseases,* ed 4, New York, 1995, Churchill Livingstone.

Baum SG, Litman N: Mumps virus. In Mandell GL, Bennett JE, Dolin R, editors: *Principles and practice of infectious diseases,* ed 4, New York, 1995, Churchill Livingstone.

Best JM: Rubella vaccines: past, present and future, *Epidemiol Infect* 107:17, 1991.

Briss PA et al: Sustained transmission of mumps in a highly vaccinated population: assessment of primary vaccine failure and waning vaccine-induced immunity, *J Infect Dis* 169:77-82, 1994.

Centers for Disease Control: Measles prevention: recommendations of the Immunization Practices Advisory Committee, *MMWR* 38:1, 1989.

Centers for Disease Control: Rubella prevention: recommendations of the Immunization Practices Advisory Committee (ACIP), *MMWR* 39:1, 1990.

Centers for Disease Control and Prevention: Update: childhood vaccine-preventable diseases–United States, 1994, *MMWR* 43:718-720, 1994.

Centers for Disease Control and Prevention: respiratory syncytial virus activity–United States, 1995-96 season, *MMWR* 44:900-902, 1995.

Centers for Disease Control and Prevention: Measles pneumonitis following measles-mumps-rubella vaccination of a patient with HIV infection, 1993, *MMWR* 45:603-606, 1996.

Centers for Disease Control and Prevention: Measles–United States, 1995, *MMWR* 45:305-307, 1996.

Clements CJ et al: The epidemiology of measles: thirty years of vaccination, *Curr Top Microbiol Immunol* 191:13-33, 1995.

Falsey AR et al: Respiratory syncytial virus and influenza A infections in the hospitalized elderly, *J Infect Dis* 172:389-394, 1995.

Gellin BG et al: Measles: state of the art and future directions, *J Infect Dis* 170(suppl 1):S3-14, 1994.

Gershon AA: Measles virus (rubeola). In Mandell GL, Bennett JE, Dolin R, editors: *Principles and practice of infectious diseases,* ed 4, New York, 1995, Churchill Livingstone.

Hall CB, McCarthy CA: Respiratory syncytial virus. In Mandell GL, Bennett JE, Dolin R, editors: *Principles and practice of infectious diseases,* ed 4, New York, 1995, Churchill Livingstone.

Henrickson KJ, Ray R, Belshe R: Parainfluenza viruses. In Mandell GL, Bennett JE, Dolin R, editors: *Principles and practice of infectious diseases,* ed 4, New York, 1995, Churchill Livingstone.

Kaplan LJ et al: Severe measles in immunocompromised patients, *JAMA* 267:1237-1241, 1992.

Khoo SH et al: Adenovirus infections in human immunodeficiency virus–positive patients: clinical features and molecular epidemiology, *J Infect Dis* 172:629-637, 1995.

Knott AM et al: Parainfluenza viral infections in pediatric outpatients: seasonal patterns and clinical characteristics, *Pediatr Infect Dis J* 13:269-273, 1994.

Knowles MR et al: A controlled study of adenoviral-vector-mediated gene transfer in the nasal epithelium of patients with cystic fibrosis, *N Engl J Med* 333:823-831, 1995.

McCarthy AJ et al: Intravenous ribavirin therapy for disseminated adenovirus infection, *Ped J Infect Dis* 14:1003-1004, 1995.

McIntosh K: Coronavirus. In Mandell GL, Bennett JE, Dolin R, editors: *Principles and practice of infectious diseases,* ed 4, New York, 1995, Churchill Livingstone.

Morris DJ et al: Polymerase chain reaction for rapid detection of ocular adenovirus infection, *J Med Virol* 46:126-132, 1995.

Murray K et al: A morbillivirus that caused fatal disease in horses and humans, *Science* 268:94-97, 1995.

Myint SH: Human coronaviruses: a brief review, *Rev Med Virol* 4:35-46, 1994.

Olsen MA et al: Isolation of seven respiratory viruses in shell vials: a practical and highly sensitive method, *J Clin Microbiol* 31:422-425, 1993.

Piedra PA et al: Purified fusion protein vaccine protects against lower respiratory tract illness during respiratory syncytial virus season in children with cystic fibrosis, *Pediatr Infect Dis J* 15:23-31, 1996.

Rubin EE et al: Infections due to parainfluenza virus type 4 in children, *J Infect Dis* 17:998-1002, 1993.

Shimizu H et al: Polymerase chain reaction for detection of measles virus in clinical samples, *J Clin Microbiol* 31:1034-1039, 1993.

Van Loon FPL et al: Mumps surveillance–United States, 1988-1993, *MMWR* 44(suppl 3):1-14, 1995.

Werdt CH et al: Parainfluenza virus respiratory infection after bone marrow transplantation, *N Engl J Med* 326:921, 1992.

Whimbey E et al: Combination therapy with aerosolized ribavirin and intravenous immunoglobulin for respiratory syncytial virus disease in adult bone marrow transplant recipients, *Bone Marrow Transplant* 16:393-399, 1995.

Wong RD et al: Clinical and laboratory features of measles in hospitalized adults, *Am J Med* 95:377-383, 1993.

Wood DL, Brunell PA: Measles control in the United States: problems of the past and challenges for the future, *Clin Microbiol Rev* 8:260-267, 1995.

CHAPTER

252 Rabies

Steven L. Chuck

VIROLOGY

Classic rabies virus is one of at least five rhabdoviruses known to cause the disease rabies in humans. Mokola virus, Duvenhage virus, and two serotypes of European bat Lyssaviruses are more restricted geographically and have been reported as rare causes of rabies in humans. These viruses have a bullet shape that suggests the name of the group (*rhabdos,* Greek for "rod").

Classic rabies virus contains a single nonsegmented negative strand of genomic RNA with five nonoverlapping genes, each of which encodes a single, distinct protein. The order of the genes is similar to that in other rhabdoviruses: from the 3' end, nucleocapsid protein, phosphoprotein, matrix protein, glycoprotein, and polymerase. The nucleocapsid protein, phosphoprotein, and polymerase, together with the genomic RNA, form the helical core of ribonucleocapsid. Antibody directed against the nucleocapsid protein is useful for detecting intracytoplasmic inclusions of rabies virus (Negri bodies). The nucleocapsid acts as an exogenous superantigen in humans, and monoclonal antibodies to epitopes in the nucleocapsid protein protect against experimental infection. An envelope of lipid bilayer derived from host cells covers this core. The matrix protein appears to be anchored on the inner aspect of the lipid membrane, and the glycoprotein coats the outer surface of the virus. This glycoprotein plays a large role in the virulence of the virus. Point mutations leading to a single amino acid substitution at one critical location in the glycoprotein can render the virus nonlethal in a mouse model, and neutralizing antibodies directed against the glycoprotein spikes confer immunity.

The virus is susceptible to inactivation by drying, heating, or exposure to sunlight, ultraviolet light, ethanol, formalin, and quaternary ammonium compounds. Importantly, the virus can also be inactivated by 20% soap solutions.

EPIDEMIOLOGY

Rabies virus exists in an enzootic cycle of warm-blooded animals transferred by bite from one animal to another. Worldwide, domestic dogs and cats account for the majority of cases. In areas where vaccination programs have been successfully implemented, the principal reservoir of rabies is in wild animals. In the United States the infected animals reported most commonly are skunks, raccoons, bats, foxes, and dogs. Although skunks are the most common carrier of rabies, bats are more widely distributed, being found in 48 states. Along the Mexican–United States border, stray dogs are a major carrier of rabies virus. Among domestic animals in the United States, cattle, cats, and dogs are most commonly infected. In Europe and Canada, foxes are the principal vector. Vampire bats, mongooses, jackals, and wolves are prominent sources of rabies elsewhere in the world. Rabies has rarely been reported in rodents, and no cases of human rabies have resulted from a rodent bite. Control of rabies in wild or domestic animal populations can be achieved with vaccination.

Human rabies usually results from the bite of an infected animal. Contamination of an open wound or mucous membranes with virus, however, can lead to rabies; a few cases have been reported in spelunkers investigating bat-infested caves and in laboratory workers preparing homogenates of infected brain. Human-to-human transmission has been documented only in recipients of corneal transplants from donors who died of undiagnosed rabies.

PATHOPHYSIOLOGY

The saliva of diseased animals contains infective rabies virus for several days before outward manifestations of illness, so bites from seemingly normal animals may lead to rabies. Most animals die of rabies, although some recover and then no longer secrete the virus in their saliva. Some bats have been found with virus in their fat; they apparently secrete the virus in their saliva during periods of stress.

After a bite by a rabid animal, the virus may replicate in nearby striated muscle cells or directly enter exposed nerve endings. After replication and amplification in muscle cells, the virus enters unmyelinated peripheral nerves. Immune responses appear to be protective only if induced before this step. Rabies virus moves through peripheral neurons via axoplasmic flow toward the central nervous system. Upon reaching the cell body, such as in the dorsal root ganglia, the virus replicates, infects adjacent cells, and continues to move proximally. In the brain, the virus involves the neurons of the limbic system early on but replicates and spreads rapidly, causing widespread neural dysfunction. Rabies virus then disseminates centrifugally from the central nervous system through nerves to many tissues. Subsequently the virus may be demonstrated in saliva, urine, cerebrospinal fluid, corneal cells, and skin.

Infected brains typically are edematous and infiltrated in either a focal or diffuse manner with lymphocytes, particularly around small blood vessels. Diffuse degenerative changes are seen in the neurons of the brain and spinal cord. Pathognomonic Negri bodies are seen in three fourths of cases. These eosinophilic, oval cytoplasmic inclusions may be stained with fluorescent antibodies for nucleocapsid material (Color Plate VIII-43). Negri bodies are most often seen in the ganglion cells of Ammon's horn in the hippocampus but may also be seen in neurons of the cerebellum, cortex, and spinal cord.

CLINICAL MANIFESTATIONS

After an incubation period, human rabies occurs in three stages: a prodrome, acute neurologic phase, and coma followed by death. Incubation usually occurs over 20 to 90 days, but periods of 10 days to several years have been reported. The incubation period tends to be shorter in children, when the bite is on the head or neck, and after a severe, deep bite. Symptoms are related only to the wound during the incubation period.

Nonspecific prodromal symptoms consist of apathy, malaise, anorexia, fatigue, fever, chills, and headache. Anxiety, irritability, and depression may occur. At the wound, hyperesthesia, pruritus, or pain radiating proximally may all occur. Other less common symptoms include cough, sore throat, abdominal pain, nausea, vomiting, diarrhea, and dysuria; an upper respiratory tract infection or gastroenteritis may be diagnosed initially. The prodrome may last from 1 to 10 days.

In three fourths of patients, the disease progresses to "furious" rabies, so named because of the neurologic hyperactivity. Agitation, excitement, and marked motor activity interspersed with calmness are soon followed by dysphagia and hydrophobia. Occuring in over half the cases of rabies, hydrophobia is virtually pathognomonic of rabies and results from fear of pain and choking produced by laryngeal and pharyngeal muscle spasms. Drooling may result from increased salivation and avoidance of swallowing. Hypersensitivity of the skin may lead to avoidance of stimulation even by air (aerophobia). Cortical hyperactivity is manifested in bursts of aggressiveness marked by thrashing, biting, hallucinations, and disorientation lasting several minutes separated by periods of full orientation and calmness. Seizures may also occur. Autonomic hyperactivity is common and may consist of supraventricular arrhythmias, deregulation of blood pressure, and tachypnea. Typically 2 to 7 days after the onset of symptoms, death or coma supervenes.

In about one quarter of patients, however, hyperactivity is not prominent, and the prodrome is followed instead by predominantly "paralytic" or "dumb" rabies. Paresis or paralysis accompanied by pain may develop either predominantly in the bitten extremity, diffusely, or in an ascending fashion similar to the Guillain-Barré syndrome. Hydrophobia occurs late if at all. The mental status declines, leading to disorientation, obtundation, and then coma.

Neurologic, cardiac, and pulmonary complications occur most commonly when the patient is comatose. Cerebral edema, increased intracranial pressure, seizures, inappropriate secretion of antidiuretic hormone or diabetes insipidus, and autonomic dysfunction resulting in alterations in blood pressure, heart rate and rhythm, or temperature regulation are the most frequent neurologic complications. Cardiac arrhythmias include atrial premature contractions, sinus bradycardia, and sinus arrest. Hypotension may develop from myocarditis, bradyarrhythmias, autonomic dysfunction, fluid depletion, or congestive heart failure. Hyperventilation with respiratory alkalosis is common. Hypoxia, hypoventilation, and abnormalities in the pattern of breathing may culminate in respiratory arrest. Aspiration, superinfection, or pulmonary edema from congestive heart failure or the adult respiratory distress syndrome may develop. Death occurs an average of 12 days after the onset of symptoms.

Once symptoms have begun, survival is unusual. Three cases of nonfatal rabies developing after preexposure or postexposure prophylaxis have been reported. Two persons developed rabies after postexposure prophylaxis had been given, and in both persons, recovery was reportedly complete. A third person, who had been immunized prior to exposure, recovered with some permanent loss of speech and motor function.

DIAGNOSTIC TESTS

Unfortunately, tests to diagnose infection with rabies virus before the onset of clinical manifestations are not available. The diagnosis may be confirmed antemortem by isolation of the virus, antibody testing, immunofluorescent staining of viral antigens in tissues, and detection of viral RNA in brain by polymerase chain reaction (PCR). During the first 2 weeks of illness, the virus may be found in saliva, cerebrospinal fluid, or urine. Isolation of the virus, however, is not a very sensitive test and requires an incubation period in the laboratory of up to 3 weeks. Rabies antibody can be detected in serum 6 to 15 days after the onset of illness in both vaccinated and unvaccinated patients. Such neutralizing antibodies are first found around day 10 in unvaccinated patients and then sharply increase to levels significantly higher than those seen in vaccinated patients. Vaccinated patients develop measurable titers of antibody in their serum about 8 days after vaccination. The presence of rabies antibody in the cerebrospinal fluid is diagnostic. These antibodies appear a few days after the rise in serum antibodies. Many patients, however, die before developing appreciable titers of neutralizing antibody. Viral antigens may be detected in half of patients during the first week of the disease by immunofluorescent staining. A full-thickness punch biopsy

of the skin overlying the back of the neck above the hairline is optimal because it is close to the central nervous system, it is readily accessible, and hair follicles are densely innervated. Corneal impressions are no longer recommended. Immunofluorescent staining of neck skin is perhaps the most reliable diagnostic test early in the disease. Recently the enormous sensitivity of PCR has been used to detect viral RNA in brains of dogs and humans. It may be possible to use PCR to detect the viral genome in bites from animals before the development of clinical rabies.

DIFFERENTIAL DIAGNOSIS

Antemortem diagnosis can be difficult if a clear history of exposure is absent and symptoms are atypical. The differential diagnosis encompasses all forms of encephalitis including infections from arboviruses, enteroviruses, and herpesviruses. Encephalomyelitis occurring 2 weeks after vaccination with phenol-inactivated neural tissue vaccines can be difficult to distinguish from rabies (see later discussion). Delirium tremens and toxic ingestions should also be considered. A person exposed to an animal at risk for rabies may develop "rabies hysteria," in which his or her extreme fear of the lethal infection is accompanied by marked agitation, anxiety, abnormal behavior, and movements that can be mistaken for seizures. Such a patient may be uncooperative, in contrast to the cooperation during periods of calmness exhibited by a patient with rabies. Paralytic rabies may be confused with poliomyelitis, Guillain-Barré syndrome, or transverse myelitis.

MANAGEMENT

Because specific therapy does not improve outcome once clinical signs are noted, treatment of human rabies, except for postexposure prophylaxis, consists of supportive care. A variety of antiviral agents have been tried, including human leukocyte interferon, but none has been beneficial when given after the onset of illness. Because the virus may be present in the saliva, urine, and cerebrospinal fluid of an infected patient, these fluids should be handled and disposed of properly. Although virus has not been isolated from blood of infected humans, precautions are warranted. Exposed personnel should be given the standard postexposure prophylaxis.

PREVENTION

Prevention of rabies involves vaccination of domestic animals and administration of immunoprophylaxis to exposed persons. Since the institution of legal requirements for vaccination of dogs, the incidence of human rabies has dropped markedly in the United States. Domestic cats, however, are less often required to be vaccinated and remain a potential transmitter of rabies.

Vaccination of humans dates to 1881, when Louis Pasteur developed the first successful vaccine for a human infection from dried spinal cords of rabid animals. Modified phenol- inactivated neural tissue vaccines are still used in some countries in Africa and Asia because of their low cost and ease of preparation. However, encephalomyelitis develops after 1 out of every 200 to 1600 vaccinations with neural tissue vaccine and is fatal in 15% of cases. Postvaccinial disease usually occurs 2 weeks after vaccination. Other vaccines, such as those derived from suckling mouse brain (SMB) and duck embryos (DEV), were developed because of the high rate of neurologic side-effects associated with nerve tissue vaccines. Because of the neurologic side-effects of SMB and low potency of DEV, however, these vaccines are no longer distributed, and human diploid cell vaccine (HDCV), composed of inactivated whole virions, has been the main vaccine used in the United States for over 15 years. A new cell culture–derived, adsorbed vaccine (rabies vaccine, adsorbed or RVA) was approved in 1988; several other inactivated virus vaccines are also under development. In addition, viral proteins expressed from cloned cDNA elicit protective antibody responses in mice, and ribonucleocapsid has been demonstrated to be an oral immunogen.

Immunoprophylaxis against rabies in humans may occur before or after exposure to the virus. The effectiveness of these regimens has been well demonstrated in animals and humans. Successful preexposure vaccination protects the host against subsequent infection with rabies virus. Postexposure protection consists of both early passive immunity conferred via injection of immunoglobulins and long-lasting immunity induced simultaneously with HDCV. Without postexposure prophylaxis, the risk of developing human rabies after an animal bite has been estimated at 15% to 40%; with the proper administration of serum and vaccine, no cases of rabies have occurred.

Preexposure Prophylaxis

Preexposure prophylaxis with HDCV is indicated for persons at high risk of subsequent exposure to rabies, such as veterinarians, animal handlers or trainers, some laboratory workers, spelunkers, travelers, or any other persons likely to contact rabid animals. Three 1-ml injections of HDCV given intramuscularly into the deltoid on days 0, 7, and 21 or 28 have led to adequate antibody responses in all persons vaccinated.

Preexposure prophylaxis has also been administered intradermally in the lateral upper arm with three 0.1-ml doses on days 0, 7, and 21 or 28. The intradermal route should not be used if the patient is concomitantly receiving chloroquine phosphate for malaria prophylaxis or if all three intradermal doses of vaccine cannot be given 30 days before travel to an area with endemic rabies.

Serologic testing for adequate antibody after preexposure prophylaxis is not recommended for routine cases, but antibody titers can be checked if the patient is immunosuppressed or an atypical regimen is used. In addition, persons with ongoing exposure to rabies should have measurements of antibody every 2 years. If the titer is inadequate, they should receive a booster dose of either 1 ml intramuscularly or 0.1 ml intradermally. Booster injections should be given only when clearly indicated because they have been associated with serum sickness reactions in approximately 6% of patients.

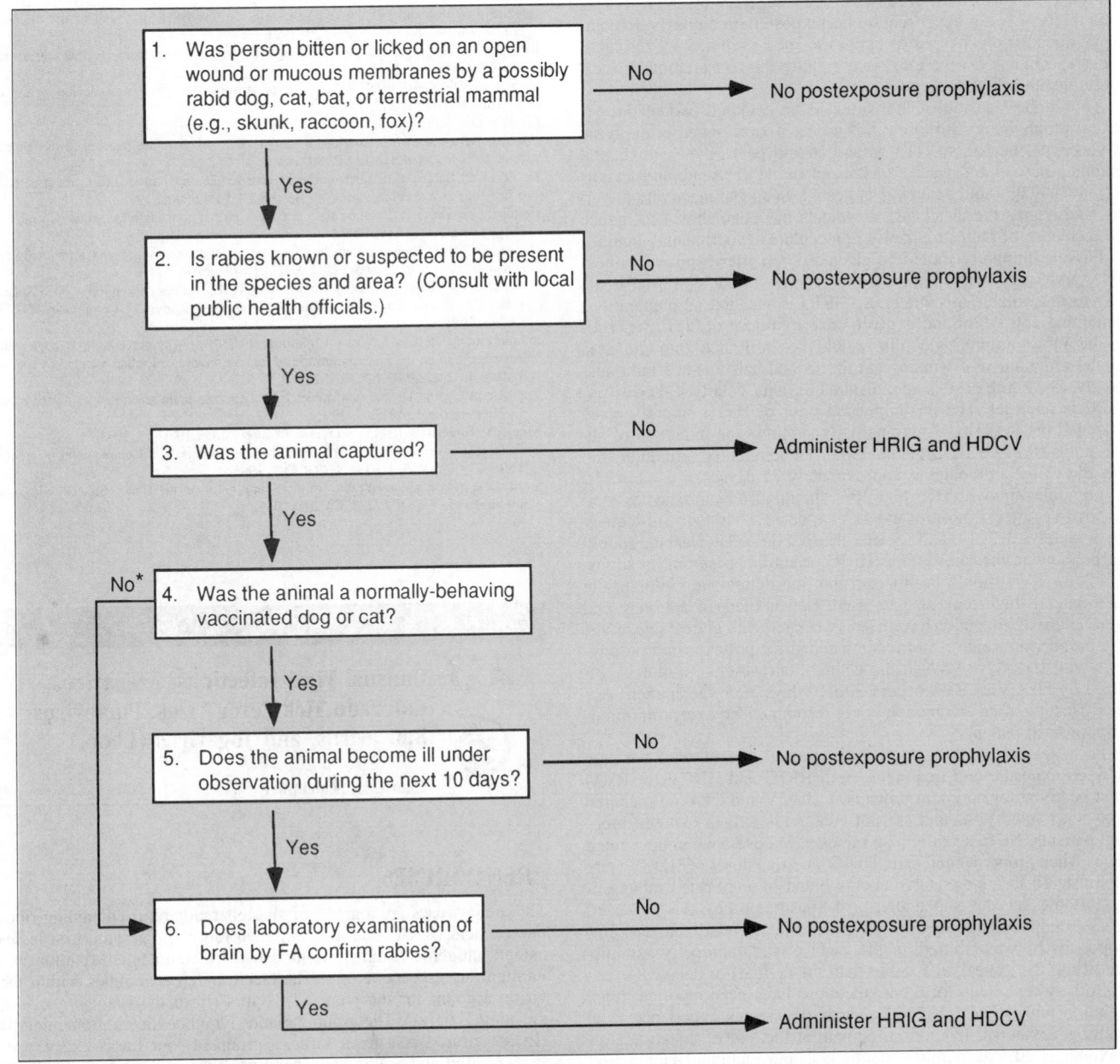

FIGURE 252-1   Algorithm for postexposure prophylaxis of rabies. *If the captured animal is not a normally behaving vaccinated dog or cat, postexposure prophylaxis may be initiated pending quarantine or examination of the brain.

Postexposure Prophylaxis

Postexposure prophylaxis (Fig. 252-1) includes thorough cleaning of the wound, passive immunization with human rabies immunoglobulin (HRIG), and active immunization with HDCV or RVA. Persons with a known immune response to preexposure prophylaxis should receive HDCV on day 0 and again on day 3 in addition to meticulous wound care. All other persons, including those with an unknown antibody response to preexposure prophylaxis, should receive the full postexposure regimen.

Initiation of postexposure prophylaxis should begin after consideration of the type of exposure (bite or nonbite), the species of the animal involved, the vaccination status of the animal, the local epidemiology of rabies, the appearance of the animal, and whether the attack was provoked. Postexposure prophylaxis is recommended after any bite by a known or suspected rabid dog, cat, skunk, bat, raccoon, fox, or other carnivore unless the animal is shown to be nonrabid by fluorescent-antibody staining of the brain. Healthy dogs or cats should be confined if possible for 10 days; rabies prophylaxis should be given only if the animal develops rabies in that time. If the dog or cat has escaped, local public health officials can be consulted regarding the occurrence of rabies in the area. Bites by small rodents and rabbits virtually never require postexposure prophylaxis. Recommendations for other types of exposure, such as to aerosolized laboratory specimens or livestock, may require the consultation of local public health officials.

Thorough cleansing of the wound is an essential part of postexposure prophylaxis. Too often, this aspect is overlooked in the haste to vaccinate the patient. The wound should be washed with liberal amounts of soap and water, devitalized tissue debrided, and tetanus vaccine and antibiotics given if indicated. Soap can inactivate the virus, and aggressive cleansing of wounds has been shown to reduce the incidence of rabies markedly in inoculated experimental animals.

Passive immunity should be given as soon after exposure as possible, preferably with HRIG although equine antirabies serum is the only form available in some areas. HRIG is available in preparations containing 150 IU/ml and is given once in a dose of 20 IU/kg. Half of the rabies immunoglobulin should be infiltrated into the area around a nonmucosal wound, and the second half injected intramuscularly. The entire dose is administered intramuscularly if the site exposed is mucosal. The recommended dose of HRIG should not be exceeded because HRIG may partially suppress the induction of active antibodies. HRIG provides rapid but temporary immunity; the half-life of the antibodies is approximately 21 days.

Immunization with HDCV or RVA should also be initiated as soon as possible after exposure and is completed with four subsequent doses on days 3, 7, 14, and 28 after the first dose. The vaccine should not be given at the same site as HRIG or antirabies serum. In adults, HDCV or RVA should be injected into the deltoid; in children, the anterolateral thigh may also be used. Lower titers of antibody and even failure of protection have been associated with gluteal injections. The intradermal route is not recommended for postexposure prophylaxis with HDCV or RVA in the United States. Active immunity induced by HDCV or RVA occurs 7 to 10 days after vaccination. Antibody testing after vaccination is not recommended except in immunosuppressed patients.

Postexposure prophylaxis is recommended regardless of the time between exposure and treatment. Both HRIG and HDCV (or RVA) must be given for optimum protection. HDCV and RVA are prepared from inactivated virus and are not contraindicated in exposed pregnant patients. No cases of human rabies have developed in the United States when proper wound care, HRIG, and five doses of HDCV were administered to hundreds of patients bitten by confirmed rabid animals. Rabies has developed after postexposure prophylaxis, however, in 13 patients outside the United States when wound care was improper, HRIG was omitted, or the vaccine was improperly administered (into the gluteal area rather than the deltoid) or delayed.

Both systemic and local complications have been reported in association with HDCV. Up to one half of patients experience local swelling, erythema, induration, or pain at the site of injection. Approximately 20% have mild systemic reactions including nausea, myalgias, malaise, fever, headache, adenopathy, or nonspecific abdominal pain. Three cases of Guillain-Barré syndrome have occurred, and both recovered without sequelae within 2 weeks. Anaphylaxis is rare;

fatal anaphylaxis has not been reported. Booster injections of HDCV have been associated with serum sickness. False-positive ELISA tests for human immunodeficiency virus have been reported after vaccinations for rabies.

✔ *WHEN TO REFER*

Known or suspected cases of rabies should always be referred to public health officials for investigation of other contacts of the afflicted animal. In addition, specialists in critical care and infectious diseases should be consulted for the management and prophylaxis of rabies.

BIBLIOGRAPHY

Baer GM, Fishbein DB: Rabies post-exposure prophylaxis, *N Engl J Med* 316:1270, 1987 (editorial).

Bernard KW, Fishbein DB: Pre-exposure rabies prophylaxis for travellers: are the benefits worth the cost? *Vaccine* 9:833, 1991.

Brochier B et al: Large-scale eradication of rabies using recombinant vaccinia-rabies vaccine, *Nature* 354:520, 1991.

Centers for Disease Control: Rabies vaccine, adsorbed: a new rabies vaccine for use in humans, *MMWR* 37:217, 1988.

Fishbein DB: Rabies, *Infect Dis Clin North Am* 5:53, 1991.

Fishbein DB et al: Administration of human diploid-cell rabies vaccine in the gluteal area, *N Engl J Med* 318:124, 1988 (letter).

Fu ZF et al: Rabies virus nucleoprotein expressed in and purified from insect cells is efficacious as a vaccine, *Proc Natl Acad Sci USA* 88:2001, 1991.

Helmick CG, Tauxe RV, Vernon AA: Is there a risk to contacts of patients with rabies? *Rev Infect Dis* 9(3):511, 1987.

Hooper DC et al: Rabies ribonucleocapsid as an oral immunogen and immunological enhancer, *Proc Natl Acad Sci USA* 91(23):10908, 1994.

Immunization Practices Advisory Committee (ACIP): Rabies prevention–United States, 1984: recommendation of the Immunization Practices Advisory Committee, *MMWR* 33:393, 1984.

Immunization Practices Advisory Committee (ACIP): Rabies prevention: a supplementary statement on the preexposure use of human diploid cell rabies vaccine by the intradermal route, *MMWR* 35:767, 1986.

Kamolvarin N et al: Diagnosis of rabies by polymerase chain reaction with nested primers, *J Infect Dis* 167(1):207, 1993.

King AA, Turner GS: Rabies: a review, *J Comp Pathol* 108(1):1, 1993.

National Association of State Public Health Veterinarians, Inc: Compendium of animal rabies control, 1995, *MMWR* 44(RR-2):1, 1995.

Smith JS et al: Unexplained rabies in three immigrants in the United States: a virologic investigation, *N Engl J Med* 324:205, 1991.

CHAPTER

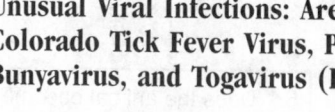

253 Unusual Viral Infections: Arenavirus, Colorado Tick Fever Virus, Parvovirus, Bunyavirus, and Togavirus (Ebola)

Charles J. Schleupner

ARENAVIRUSES

The arenaviruses are a group of single-stranded viri containing ribonucleic acid (RNA) that are similar in morphologic and, to a lesser extent, antigenic features, as indicated by complement-fixation and immunofluorescence assays. The electron-dense granules within the virion account for the name arenavirus (from the Latin *arenaceus,* meaning "sandy"). The group includes lymphocytic choriomeningitis (LCM) virus, Lassa fever virus, a group of four Lassa-like viruses from Central and South Africa, and the Tacaribe group of eleven viruses. Only LCM virus, Lassa virus, and four members of the Tacaribe group—Junin, Machupo, Sabia, and Guanarito viruses—are pathogenic for humans under natural circumstances. Junin virus in-

Table 253-1   Frequency of signs and symptoms during lymphocytic choriomeningitis virus infection

CHARACTERISTICS	FREQUENCY (%)
Fever with rigors	90-100
Malaise	100
Myalgias	80-93
Headache	85
Anorexia, nausea	50-80
Photophobia	25-80
Sore throat	25-70
Arthralgias	60
Vomiting	35-40
Scalp hair loss	≤47

fection results in Argentinian hemorrhagic fever, infection with Machupo virus produces Bolivian hemorrhagic fever, and Guanarito virus is associated with Venezuelan hemorrhagic fever. Sabia virus was isolated in Brazil in 1990; three cases of infection with this virus have been recognized; one was naturally acquired and two were in laboratory workers. Lymphocytic choriomeningitis virus, first isolated in 1933, is the prototype of the arenavirus group.

Epidemiology

Rodents are the natural reservoirs for most of the arenaviruses, in which there is an enzootic viral cycle of replication. Human infection represents accidental transmission through rodent bites or through contact with or aerosol exposure to their excreta. Exceptions to these routes of exposure may include Lassa fever and, rarely, Argentinian or Bolivian hemorrhagic fever, for which human-to-human transmission is also believed to occur via similar mechanisms.

Lymphocytic Choriomeningitis

Lymphocytic choriomeningitis virus infection occurs worldwide. Latent inapparent infection of wild and laboratory mice is the primary natural reservoir for sporadic LCM. Estimates of the virus carrier rate in mice have ranged from 4% in New York City to 27% in Washington, D.C. Isolated cases have also been related to infected dogs and guinea pigs. Syrian golden hamsters, found both in the laboratory setting and as household pets, have been epidemic sources. Lymphocytic choriomeningitis has been noted to occur less frequently in the summer months than in the other seasons of the year. This may be related to entry of field mice into homes during the colder months.

Although both acute illness, followed by recovery or death, and chronic infection are observed in rodents, persistent infection with LCM virus is not seen in humans. Furthermore, few acute cases have been studied in sufficient detail to define the pathogenesis of LCM. Because an influenza-like illness predominates, at least early in the course of disease in most patients, the route of acquisition of LCM virus is assumed to be most often pulmonary, with subsequent viral replication in the respiratory epithelium. A secondary viremia is then presumed to lead to multisystem involvement, including the central nervous system, when meningitis develops. Intact cell-mediated immunity is believed to be most important for host defense and recovery, as defined in the murine model of this infection. The correlation of interferon levels with the severity of illness and limitation of viral replication, and the correlation of the cytotoxic lymphocyte response with recovery in the mouse have not yet been established in humans.

Subclinical disease appears to be common. When symptomatic, LCM becomes evident initially as an influenza-like illness of varying severity with an incubation period of 5 to 12 days. The initial phase of the illness lasts 3 to 7 days. In the 25% to 50% of patients with a biphasic illness, a period of remission for 3 to 5 days ensues and is followed by a less severe recrudescence of illness lasting another 3 to 5 days, during which clinically evident meningitis or meningoencephalitis develops in 5% to 15% of patients.

The initial influenza-like illness and the second phase of illness are typified by the signs and symptoms presented in Table 253-1. In the initial phase myalgias are usually severe; headache, often retrobulbar, is associated with pain on eye motion. Less common complaints include testicular and parotid pain, dysesthesias, chest pain, and nonproductive cough. Physical findings are limited to a relative bradycardia, apathy (90%), and pharyngeal injection without exudate (65%).

The second phase of the illness, although generally milder, is typified by more severe headache; other findings include varied types of skin eruptions (10% to 20%), arthritis (10% to 20%), orchitis, parotitis, alopecia, and meningeal or encephalitic signs (5% to 15%), including confusion and nuchal stiffness. Convalescence takes 2 to 4 weeks and is characterized by easily becoming fatigued, excessive need for sleep, and myasthenia. Recovery is usually complete, and death is rare. Encephalitis may leave neurologic residua, including hydrocephalus, in 25% of cases. During pregnancy, LCM may lead to spontaneous abortion or congenital infection with anomalies and psychomotor retardation.

Laboratory abnormalities include leukopenia (<4000 white blood cells/mm^3 in 90% of cases), thrombocytopenia (<150,000 platelets/mm^3 in most cases), and modest elevations of serum levels of enzymes (aspartate aminotransferase [AST] and lactic dehydrogenase). Abnormalities of spinal fluid include pleocytosis (100 to 1500 cells/mm^3, predominantly mononuclear), an elevated protein level (50 to 300 mg/dl), and hypoglycorrhachia (25% to 50% of cases).

The diagnosis of LCM is suggested in a patient who has leukopenia and thrombocytopenia with a nonspecific, biphasic, febrile illness associated with severe myalgias. Meningeal symptoms associated with hypoglycorrhachia and a history of contact with mice or hamsters further support the diagnosis. The definitive diagnosis is established by LCM virus isolation from blood or cerebrospinal fluid until early in the second week of illness. Because viral isolation (in experimental animals) is impractical, the indirect immunofluorescent antibody test is the optimal serologic procedure for the diagnosis of acute LCM because of the rapid appearance of these antibodies and the sensitivity and specificity of this test. The complement-fixation antibody test is too insensitive, and the test for neutralizing antibody is impractical for other than epidemiologic investigations.

There is no specific therapy for LCM virus infection. Symptomatic management is usually adequate. Referral to a neurologist is indicated when signs of encephalitis develop (confusion and/or focal neurologic findings). An infectious diseases consultant could assist with rapid diagnostic considerations and with the more serious differential diagnostic considerations. Prevention of this disease relies on public education about the risks associated with pet hamsters. No vaccine is available.

Lassa Fever

Since its first description in 1969, Lassa fever has been seen in many countries of West Africa, and the prevalence of seropositivity extends into Central Africa. The reservoir, a multimammate rat, is widespread throughout the African continent. This rodent remains infected for life and excretes large quantities of virus in the urine. In addition to primary human infection transmitted through direct contact and contamination of food with rodent excreta, nosocomial and community human-to-human transmission are believed to occur through close unprotected contact. In Sierra Leone, where 8% to 52% of the population is seropositive, Lassa fever has been well studied. The ratio of clinical to subclinical disease in Sierra Leone is believed to be as low as 1:4 to 1:10; this ratio may be much higher in other settings. Up to 25% of populations studied undergo seroconversion each year; however, some of these seroconversions are suspected to be reinfections because 6% of some populations revert to seronegativity each year. Laboratory-acquired infection has also been reported. Clusters of Lassa fever cases have occurred throughout the year; illness occurs more frequently between February and May in Sierra Leone. Individuals of all ages are affected, but pregnant women seem prone to severe disease, especially during the third trimester. Furthermore, Lassa fever is a common cause of septic abortion.

The pathogenesis of Lassa fever is incompletely understood. Viremia has been documented for up to 16 days after the onset of clinical disease, and its magnitude has been directly associated with fatality rates. On pathologic study the most marked findings include eosinophilic necrosis of hepatocytes without an inflammatory response; Lassa virions are found within hepatocytes. Despite these findings, the degree of hepatic necrosis is insufficient to account for death in fatal cases. Similar necrosis occurs in the spleen surrounding depleted lymphoid follicles and in the adrenal gland. Involvement of other organs is reflected by edema and variably by hemorrhage and perivascular cuffing with round cells, as well as by parenchymal inflammation.

Disseminated intravascular coagulation (DIC) is not observed commonly in cases of Lassa fever and does not contribute to death. An inhibitor of platelet aggregation in the plasma of patients with Lassa fever has been defined between days 1 and 10 of illness; the amount of platelet inhibition is proportional to disease severity. In addition, deficient in vitro prostacyclin production by endothelial cells from infected moribund primates has been demonstrated. These reversible platelet and endothelial defects are believed to account for microcirculatory dysfunction leading to the fluid and solute loss from the intravascular compartment seen during severe Lassa fever. Plasma from patients with Lassa fever has been shown to inhibit neutrophil function during the same period of illness when platelet aggregation is also abnormal. Therefore a role for global disarray of cellular function accounting for illness severity has been suggested during Lassa fever.

The severity of Lassa fever ranges from subclinical disease to a severe, progressively fatal illness. After an incubation period of 7 to 18 days the onset of Lassa fever is insidious, with fever (peak of 39° to 41° C) and malaise present universally; these complaints are often accompanied by headache, which is predominantly frontal but persistent; and myalgias, which are frequently worse in the lumbar area. The frequency and timing of these and other signs and symptoms that develop as the disease worsens are shown in Table 253-2. Sore throat may be severe enough to cause dysphagia. Physical findings may include hypotension (80%); pharyngitis (70%) with a white, patchy exudate (40%); facial and neck swelling (30%); abdominal tenderness (45%); crackles; conjunctival edema and injection; a macular rash; and, less commonly, abnormal bleeding with petechiae. In mild and moderately severe cases recovery occurs during the second and third weeks; in more severe cases associated with fatalities the disease progresses to the development of an altered sensorium; pulmonary and peripheral edema; the accumulation of pleural, pericardial, and ascitic fluid; and hypovolemia and shock, probably as a result of diffuse capillary breakdown. During a case-control study of Lassa fever in Sierra Leone, the best clinical predictor of fatality was bleeding, usually from mucosal surfaces and from the respiratory, gastrointestinal, and genitourinary tracts. Symptoms and signs may be similar in children, but in endemic areas the disease is usually mild in this age-group; the most common manifestations are fever, hepatosplenomegaly, malaise, cough, and abdominal complaints. Lassa virus infection has been associated with hearing deficits of sudden onset in approximately one third of acutely ill hospitalized patients; the presence of residua after Lassa infection has been suggested by the 18% prevalence of sensorineural hearing deficits among seropositive residents of West Africa.

Laboratory findings include early leukopenia (40%), elevated he-

matocrit level (attributable to dehydration), proteinuria (67%, often massive), azotemia, and elevated serum enzyme levels (AST, creatinine kinase). Chest radiographs have revealed patchy infiltrates or pleural effusions. Electrocardiograph findings may be consistent with myocarditis.

Recovery from Lassa fever is usually complete, although unilateral or bilateral deafness may be permanent. Oculogyric crisis is an occasional distinctive feature of convalescence. Many patients have alopecia during convalescence. Although the mortality rate was first reported to be 40% to 50%, more recent estimates among hospitalized patients range from 9% to 38%, suggesting a geographic variation of virulence of Lassa virus strains; the exceptions to these mortality rates are individuals who have nosocomial infections and pregnant women, who seem to be at high risk and have had fatality rates of 52% and 67%, respectively. The overall mortality rate among all infected patients is estimated at 1% to 2%. A useful predictor of mortality is an AST value greater than 150 IU/L (55%); viremia levels greater than $10^{3.6}$ tissue culture infectious doses/ml have also been associated with a fatal outcome (76%).

The diagnosis of Lassa fever is suggested in a patient who has high fever, prostration, erosions or a membranous exudate in the pharynx, marked myalgias of the limbs or back, retrosternal pain, proteinuria, and a history of recent travel to West Africa; these findings in a person caring for a similarly ill patient with a history of such travel would also suggest this diagnosis.

Definitive diagnosis is accomplished by isolation of Lassa virus from serum or throat washings; isolation can be attempted up to 15 days after onset of illness, but throat washings are insensitive for diagnosis. Viruria is detectable in only 3% of patients. However, attempts to isolate the virus should be made only in maximum-containment laboratories because of the high risk of working with this agent. The polymerase chain reaction (PCR) has been applied successfully to both serum and urine to detect Lassa viral RNA during acute infection. The PCR on a serum specimen may be up to 79% sensitive on the day of admission. Lassa antigen detection in serum by enzyme-linked immunosorbent assay (ELISA) is a rapid method for early diagnosis during acute disease. Serologic diagnosis is best performed with immunoglobulin M (IgM) and immunoglobulin G (IgG) specific indirect immunofluorescent or ELISA antibody testing as early as 1 to 2 weeks into the illness. The presence of IgM antibody at more than 1:4 dilution of serum or a fourfold to eightfold rise in IgG antibody titer comparing acute and convalescent serum specimens would be diagnostic.

The therapy of Lassa fever is largely supportive; attention should be directed to careful fluid and electrolyte management. Critical intensive care may be necessary, along with appropriate strict isolation. Referral to a tertiary care setting is usually necessary. Physicians with expertise in hematology, critical care, and infectious diseases can often be helpful in the management of these cases. For patients with moderate or severe Lassa fever, intravenous (IV) (or oral, although less effective) ribavirin should be given for 10 days. When IV ribavirin is given within 6 days of fever onset, the mortality rate is reduced from between 61% and 75% to between 5% and 9%. The treatment regimen is given in Box 253-1. Adverse effects are limited to reversible anemia. Lassa immune globulin or plasma has been shown

Table 253-2 Approximate day of onset and frequency of signs and symptoms during acute Lassa fever

SIGN OR SYMPTOM	DAY OF ONSET	FREQUENCY (%)
Arthralgia (large joints)	3-4	50
Myalgia	3-4	35-65
Cough (nonproductive)	3-4	65
Headache	4-5	75
Sore throat	4-5	70
Chest pain (retrosternal, sharp)	3-4	70
Abdominal pain (crampy)	4-5	65
Vomiting	4-5	75
Diarrhea	4-5	75
Dizziness	7-21	75
Dysuria	—	35
Hearing loss	10-15	5-18

BOX 253-1
Ribavirin treatment and prophylaxis for Lassa fever*

Treatment regimen (total of 10 days)
  30 mg/kg IV as a loading dose, followed by
  16 mg/kg IV every 6 hours for 4 days and
  8 mg/kg IV every 8 hours for 6 days
Prophylaxis
  500 mg orally every 6 hours for 7 days

*Centers for Disease Control and Prevention telephone numbers for managing Lassa fever: (404) 639-1344 or (404) 639-3308.

to have minimal or no effect on mortality and is not recommended. In severe Lassa fever, exchange transfusion has anecdotally been reported to reverse platelet dysfunction (apparently by removing platelet inhibitors in plasma) and to result in clinical improvement. Maintenance of strict patient isolation and scrupulous specimen-handling procedures are vital to the prevention of secondary nosocomial cases of Lassa fever. Patients should be kept in strict isolation for 3 weeks, and known contacts should be observed for a similar period.

Persons with percutaneous or mucosal exposure to materials likely to contain Lassa virus should be considered for prophylactic oral ribavirin (see Box 253-1). Recombinant vaccinia virus vaccines containing the Lassa virus glycoprotein genome are being tested, but the persistence of Lassa viremia during clinical illness, despite the presence of antibody, raises concern about the potential efficacy of traditional vaccine approaches against this infection. Rodent control in dwellings is most important for prevention of Lassa fever in Africa.

Hemorrhagic Fevers

Argentinian hemorrhagic fever (AHF) occurs in a progressively expanding area radiating from Buenos Aires and now covering 120,000 km². This enzootic infection is continuing to spread northward, involving previously unimplicated rodent species. Infection occurs primarily in male farm workers between February and August when a wound is contaminated with urine from a chronically infected field mouse. Mucosal contamination with virus-contaminated airborne dust is another potential mechanism for acquisition. Transmission via contaminated foods also seems likely. Approximately 12% of the population in the endemic area is seropositive; one of three infections is subclinical. Thus almost 90% of the population remains susceptible. A mean of 360 cases per year has been seen for the last 5 years. Although Bolivian hemorrhagic fever (BHF) had been less common recently because of improved rodent control, an epidemic within a family occurred in 1994 without an obvious mechanism of transmission. The likely routes of transmission of BHF have been presumed to be similar to those of AHF.

In September 1989 an epidemic of a severe hemorrhagic illness occurred in the Portuguesa state of Venezuela and was initially thought to be caused by dengue virus. This epidemic of Venezuelan hemorrhagic fever (VHF) is now known to be caused by a new member of the Tacaribe complex of arenaviruses, Guanarito virus. The mechanism for transmission from the reservoir, the cotton rat, to humans is believed to be similar to that of the other arenaviruses.

The pathogenesis of AHF, BHF, and VHF is poorly understood. Initial viral replication in tissue phagocyte organs, especially in monocytes (macrophages), with a secondary viremia and ensuing capillary lesions, is believed to be important in AHF. Complement activation is involved in the early stages of AHF, but consistent evidence for involvement of immune complexes in its pathogenesis has been lacking. Other documented abnormalities include thrombocytopenia, presence of a concomitant plasma inhibitor of platelet aggregation (possibly interrelating with observed perturbations of the membrane calcium and sodium/potassium adenosine triphosphate [ATP]–dependent pumps), prolonged partial thromboplastin time, and low factor VIII:C activity with low levels of persistent ongoing coagulation and fibrinolysis. Endogenous alpha-interferon levels have been directly associated with fever, chills, and backache during AHF and VHF and inversely correlated with recovery. Generalized vasocongestion with hemorrhage is noted as a pathologic finding with bone marrow depletion in severe cases.

The clinical features of AHF, VHF, and BHF are similar. After an incubation period of 5 to 19 days, illness appears with gradual onset of fever, chills, malaise, severe myalgia, headache, dizziness, retroocular pain, anorexia, nausea and vomiting, and cutaneous hypoesthesia. The physical findings include toxicity, conjunctival injection, cutaneous and mucosal rashes, adenopathy, and mucosal petechiae. In BHF, nosebleed and gastrointestinal tract bleeding occur early in the disease. Pharyngitis is more common during VHF. Toward the end of the first week of the illness clinical findings worsen with the development of hypotension, relative bradycardia, and oliguria. In severe cases shock, neurologic abnormalities, hypothermia, a bleeding diathesis, and in fatal cases a capillary leak syndrome supervene. In individual cases the findings are primarily either hemorrhagic or neu-

rologic. Convalescence in either disease begins at 10 to 15 days of illness and is often marked by alopecia. Mortality rates vary from 5% to 34%; average rates are 16% to 18% in AHF and BHF. Highest mortality rates occur with VHF (34%).

Laboratory findings include leukopenia (neutropenia with AHF), thrombocytopenia, proteinuria, and depressed levels of selected complement components and some clotting factors. Diminished plasminogen activity has been detected during AHF. Absolute numbers of B and T lymphocytes, as well as T-helper and T-suppressor cells, are decreased; mononuclear leukocyte mitogen responses are also depressed during acute illness. Humoral antibody is not detected until as late as 3 to 4 weeks after onset. Possibly related to these immunologic changes and neutropenia are secondary bacterial pulmonary infections, which have been noted during AHF. There is no evidence of immune complex disease during either illness. Electrocardiographic findings are consistent with myocarditis.

The diagnosis of AHF, BHF, or VHF is suggested by the epidemiologic and clinical history. Viral isolation from blood, throat washings, or urine during the acute illness establishes the diagnosis. In up to 96% of patients with AHF, Junin virus has been isolated from peripheral blood mononuclear cells by cocultivation with vero cells. A fourfold rise in the neutralizing, indirect immunofluorescent, or complement-fixation antibody titer against the etiologic virus also supports the diagnosis, as does the presence of IgM antibodies. PCR has also been successfully used for the diagnosis of AHF with 98% sensitivity.

The therapy of the hemorrhagic fevers is supportive. Referral to a tertiary care setting with appropriate critical care and hematologic and infectious diseases support is usually helpful in the management of these cases. The mortality rate is reduced to 2% or less when immune plasma is given within 8 days of onset of AHF; the dose of immune plasma should provide more than 3000 therapeutic units of neutralizing antibody per kilogram. However, although these reports of therapeutic benefit are promising, in an alarming 10% of treated patients cerebellar dysfunction developed 4 to 6 weeks after recovery. Preliminary results of ribavirin therapy for late-stage, severe AHF are encouraging.

Prevention of AHF, BHF, and VHF is presently limited to improved rodent control. However, the high rates of seronegativity to these hemorrhagic fever viruses among the affected population underscore the need for effective vaccines. Optimism can be derived from the success of a candidate glycoprotein subunit vaccine for AHF in guinea pigs. A live, attenuated Junin virus vaccine (Candid 1) is currently undergoing clinical tests. Tacaribe virus, a nonpathogen for humans, has also been proposed as a human vaccine candidate agent because of its broad cross-reactivity with Junin virus.

COLORADO TICK FEVER

Colorado tick fever (CTF) is a benign viral infection transmitted by ticks that occurs primarily in the western mountainous regions of the United States and Canada. Because the early clinical syndromes of CTF and the rickettsial disease Rocky Mountain spotted fever (North American tick typhus) are similar, the two diseases are often confused (Chapter 259).

Classification and Characteristics

Colorado tick fever virus, a double-stranded RNA virus, is a member of the family Reoviridae and the Coltivirus genus because of its biochemical, serologic, and electron microscopic properties. Its taxonomic status has recently been changed to a Coltivirus because of the number of segments (12) in its RNA genome. The virus is stable at 4° C for up to 16 months in clotted blood. It is usually isolated from human plasma or erythrocytes by subinoculation into suckling mice.

Epidemiology

The geographic occurrence of CTF is determined by the presence of its primary vector, the hardshelled wood tick *Dermacentor andersoni,* and its definitive hosts and reservoirs, including the golden-mantled ground squirrel, the chipmunk, and other mammals. The virus has been identified in Colorado, Idaho, Nevada, Utah, Wyoming, and Montana; in the eastern sections of Washington, Oregon, and California; in the northern portions of Arizona and New Mexico; and in Alberta and British Columbia, Canada. Reports of CTF virus isolation from ticks on Long Island remain unconfirmed. Antibody to CTF virus (or a CTF-like virus) has recently been demonstrated in mammals from western California, where a viral isolate similar or identical to CTF virus has also been recovered from a rabbit. This area is outside the known distribution of *D. andersoni* and the common mammalian hosts of CTF virus. Therefore CTF may be a more widespread zoonosis than was previously suspected. Furthermore, because a few documented human infections from western California have occurred, additional possible vectors and/or mechanisms of transmission of CTF to humans are now being considered.

During the spring and summer months viral replication results from transmission between larval or nymphal ticks and small rodents during the life cycle of the virus. These rodents also serve as reservoirs because of their protracted viremia, which lasts up to several months. In this way they may contribute to overwintering of the virus. After molting to the adult stage, ticks feed on large mammals, including humans, who become incidental "dead-end" hosts. The virus is carried transstadially (not transovarially), and after hibernation infected nymphs reinitiate the cycle during the following spring.

Most cases of CTF occur between April and August, with the peak incidence in May and June. The several hundred cases reported annually probably represent a significant underestimate of true disease incidence. Although up to 90% of patients relate tick exposure, only 50% may report a tick bite. Because of occupational exposure outdoors, most cases occur in men younger than 60 years of age.

Physiology and Pathophysiology

After human inoculation via tick bite, CTF virus causes no local cutaneous reaction, and the mechanism and site(s) of early replication are unknown. Virus can be detected free in serum or plasma, usually during the first week of illness and occasionally during the second week. Intraerythrocytic viremia appears, and peak titers are reached during the second and third weeks of illness. The virus has been isolated occasionally from erythrocytes for up to 101 days after the onset of clinical illness, and viral antigen has been shown to persist in circulating erythrocytes for up to 135 days. Prolonged viremia is believed to be related to viral replication within infected erythropoietic precursors as they differentiate, resulting in protection of intraerythrocytic virus from humoral antibody. Transfusion-associated CTF has been documented.

Symptoms of central nervous system, pulmonary, pericardial, testicular, dermal, and ocular involvement during CTF suggest the potential for pantropism (ability to infect any tissue) of this virus in humans. Some of these manifestations may be immunologically mediated. Recent work does document a relationship of serum interferon levels to body temperature elevation. Despite evidence for murine teratogenicity, CTF has not been clearly related to human fetal abnormalities.

Clinical Disease

Asymptomatic illness is infrequent. Within 3 to 6 days after a tick bite most patients have a sudden onset of fever with chills, lethargy, headache (usually retrobulbar), and myalgias, which primarily affect the extremities and back. Although these complaints are nonspecific, other complaints are less common and more variable: vomiting, abdominal pain, diarrhea, stiff neck, vertigo, and sore throat. The acute illness often lasts 7 to 10 days. After 2 to 3 days fever often remits, leaving the patient very weak, only to recur within another 2 to 3 days. This biphasic, "saddleback" fever pattern occurs in 50% of patients and is virtually diagnostic of CTF in the correct epidemiologic setting. Rash, when present, is commonly macular or maculopapular and is usually located on the trunk. When the rash is petechial, it is often peripherally located. Conjunctival injection may accompany fever. Palpable splenomegaly may occur. Unusual but potentially severe complications in children include encephalitis, meningitis, and meningoencephalitis. Pericarditis, pleuritis, myocarditis, orchitis, and bleeding diathesis are rare.

Leukopenia (<4500 white blood cells/mm^3 and often 2000 to 3000 white blood cells/mm^3) is the most consistent and diagnostically helpful laboratory finding, occurring in two thirds of patients with confirmed disease early in the course. Lymphocytes and granulocytes are usually equally affected. Mild to marked thrombocytopenia may be seen. Neurologic involvement is often associated with cerebrospinal fluid lymphocytosis (fewer than 500 white blood cells/mm^3).

Recovery from CTF is eventually complete, with resultant lifelong immunity. Fifty percent or more of the patients, especially adults more than 30 years old, have a prolonged convalescence with asthenia that is unrelated to persistent viremia. Occasional residua have been reported after CTF accompanied by neurologic syndromes. Infection during pregnancy is usually benign.

Diagnosis and Differential Diagnoses

The differential diagnostic considerations include dengue fever, Rocky Mountain spotted fever, ehrlichiosis, and, when neurologic involvement is evident, viral meningitides, arboviral encephalitides, and tick paralysis. Because of the nonspecificity of the clinical manifestations of CTF, a specific diagnosis requires isolation of the virus from serum (or plasma), blood clot, or cerebrospinal fluid. In addition to viral isolation, viral antigen may be demonstrated in erythrocytes with a direct fluorescent antibody test for prolonged periods into convalescence. The direct fluorescent antibody test result is not usually positive before the sixth day of illness. The indirect fluorescent antibody method for detecting antibodies to CTF virus becomes positive earliest and is the most sensitive serologic test for the diagnosis of this disease. Neutralizing antibodies are delayed in appearance. Complement-fixing antibodies also appear slowly and are present in only 75% of patients.

Management and Prevention

The therapy for CTF is symptomatic and can usually be managed by the primary care physician once the diagnosis is likely. Prevention relies on public education concerning avoidance of tick-infested areas and use of protective clothing and insect repellents. The use of experimental inactivated and live attenuated vaccines is limited because of the small number of persons routinely exposed. Patients should be restricted from serving as blood donors for 5 to 6 months after the illness. Avoidance of aspirin for symptomatic therapy in children seems advisable because of the bleeding tendencies seen among patients with CTF in this age-group.

PARVOVIRUS INFECTIONS

The parvoviruses are one of three genera in the family Parvoviridae, which includes the dependoviruses (including human adeno-associated virus) and densoviruses (of insects). The parvoviruses were thought to be pathogens of a broad range of nonhuman vertebrate hosts until 1975, when Cossart identified a parvovirus-like structure in the sera of persons being screened for hepatitis B antigen. One of these sera was identified as B19, a designation that remains for this virus, which was subsequently identified by French, British, and Japanese investigators. B19 was first associated with symptomatic human infection in 1980. Subsequently it was linked with aplastic crises in patients with sickle cell disease in 1981, with erythema infectiosum and stillbirths in 1984, and with arthritis in 1985. Its clinical relevance is now well established.

Parvovirus B19 is a small, nonenveloped, single-stranded deoxyribonucleic acid (DNA) virus with a host range limited to humans. The virus has been grouped into six genome types by PCR and nucleotide sequencing (I, II, IIIa and IIIb, IV, and V). It is difficult to propagate in culture, requiring human erythroid bone marrow cells and exogenous erythroprotein. B19 binds to the erythrocyte P antigen, which is also present on cardiac myocytes. The major source of viral antigen for antibody assays is the serum of infected patients with hemolytic disorders or immunocompromise. B19 inhibits erythroid colony formation by infecting progenitor cells of the erythroid series. The virus probably also replicates in other tissues, including fetal myocardial cells and possibly peripheral blood leukocytes.

Table 253-3 Age distribution of cases of erythema infectiosum during an outbreak

AGE-GROUP (YEARS)	PERCENTAGE OF CASES
<5	10
5 to <15	70
≥15	20

Modified from Lauer BA et al: *Am J Dis Child* 130:252, 1976.

The most common clinical forms of B19 infection, erythema infectiosum (EI) and aplastic crisis (AC), occur in school-age children. The age distribution of cases in one outbreak is depicted in Table 253-3. Although there is no gender bias among primary cases, previously uninfected mothers within households more frequently acquire secondary cases of EI than do fathers, presumably as a result of closer contact with an infected child. The risk of secondary case acquisition within households ranges from 15% to 50%; the inverse relationship of risk for secondary cases to their age suggests a protective role for antibody, because 40% to 60% of adults older than 20 years of age are seropositive. When arthritis is part of the clinical presentation, adult women are most often affected.

Additional epidemiologic settings for B19 transmission, other than child-to-child contact in schools and play settings, include pediatric wards, day-care centers, and classrooms, where several adults and children may be exposed in the same setting. In each of these circumstances susceptible adults (up to 50%) may be exposed, leading to the potential for more consequential infection, especially in the pregnant female. B19 transmission and infection have also been documented by transfusion of pooled coagulation factor concentrates but rarely after single donor transfusion.

Parvovirus B19 is believed to be spread by respiratory droplets. During volunteer studies B19 DNA has been detected in respiratory secretions 7 to 11 days after intranasal inoculation, with concomitant viremia, fever, malaise, and pruritis.

During the second week of experimental infection, IgM antibody appears when no peripheral reticulocytes are detected and mild neutropenia, lymphopenia, and thrombocytopenia are found. The subsequent rash develops on day 17 or 18, after secretions have become negative for viral DNA. Hematologic abnormalities resolve by the third week after infection. Therefore it is presumed that B19 infection after respiratory exposure results in the rash of EI at a time when the patient is briefly or no longer infectious by the respiratory route. If arthritis develops, it often accompanies the rash during the third week after infection, as the IgG antibody response appears, suggesting an immune complex mechanism for the arthropathy.

Erythema infectiosum (or fifth disease) was recognized as a distinct entity in 1896 among a group of pediatric exanthems that had been numbered, including rubeola, scarlet fever, rubella, and roseola; its cause remained unrecognized until 1983 to 1984. EI usually occurs in outbreaks during late winter and spring. After exposure the incubation period for EI is 4 to 14 days, followed by the sudden onset of a "slapped-cheek" appearance (50% to 100% of cases of EI during outbreaks) with evolution to a lacy, generalized maculopapular rash on extremities and trunk. A prodrome of fever, coryza, malaise, cervical or generalized adenopathy, and sore throat may precede the rash in 20% to 60% of cases. The generalized rash typically waxes and wanes with varied stimuli, including irritation, bathing, stress, sunlight, and temperature change. This rash persists or recurs over less than 10 days in 55% of patients, for more than 20 days in 15%, and for more than 80 days in 1% or less of patients. The truncal rash may be varied in appearance: morbilliform, circinate, confluent, papular, vesicular, or purpuric. Despite the rash, most children with EI feel well and have only a low-grade fever; pruritis may complicate the course.

Results of most laboratory studies during acute EI are normal, with the exception of the previously mentioned hematologic abnormalities. In up to 80% of adults with EI, arthralgias or arthritis develops, more commonly in women, usually after the rash; the peripheral joints, especially the small joints of the hands, the knees, wrists, ankles, feet, and elbows, are primarily affected symmetrically. The pain is moder-

---

BOX 253-2

Clinical and hematologic sequelae of parvovirus B19 infection

Acute infection

Erythema infectiosum (with reticulocytopenia, lymphopenia, neutropenia, and/or thrombocytopenia)
Aplastic crisis (in patients with an abnormality of erythrocytes resulting in increased turnover)
Fetal infection and anemia leading to hydrops fetalis and spontaneous abortion (low risk)

Postinfectious complications

Arthritis or arthralgia
Purpura
Kawasaki's syndrome
Vasculitis
Lupuslike syndrome
Hemophagocytic syndrome

Chronic syndrome

Chronic bone marrow suppression in immunocompromised hosts
Fibromyalgia

---

ately severe but typically resolves in 2 to 4 weeks, occasionally lasting several months or years. The predominant manifestations and sequelae of B19 infection may vary in any outbreak among those which are hematologic, dermatologic, or rheumatic (Box 253-2). B19 infection may mimic acute seronegative rheumatoid arthritis or Lyme disease. The spectrum of disease associations for B19 is ever broadening. B19 infection during childhood has been linked with Kawasaki's syndrome and immune-mediated inner ear disease; during both childhood and adult years B19 infection has also been associated with a necrotizing vasculitis, a systemic lupus-like syndrome, a hemophagocytic syndrome, and an acute carpal tunnel syndrome. B19 continues to be a small risk after transfusion of pooled blood products because of the rare potential for prolonged viremia in the blood donor. B19 infection may cause some cases of fibromyalgia.

By using IgG antibody seroconversion or development of an acute IgM antibody to define infection, studies have demonstrated that in more than half of infected individuals rash does not develop; 17% to 25% are asymptomatic; and the remainder of those without rash have systemic, gastrointestinal, or respiratory tract symptoms.

After the initial descriptions of the association of B19 with AC, a number of subsequent studies have concluded that B19 is the cause of 90% or more of AC in patients with increased red blood cell turnover (Chapter 89). These settings include hemolytic anemias caused by hemoglobinopathies, pyruvate kinase deficiency, hereditary spherocytosis and stomatocytosis, and various acquired hemolytic disorders. Chronic bone marrow suppression may also occur in B19-infected patients with acquired immunodeficient states produced by hematologic malignancy, connective tissue disorders, and human immunodeficiency virus type 1 (HIV-1), as well as in apparently normal individuals. Most of these patients relate a viral prodrome followed by development of weakness and pallor. The severity of the anemia parallels the hemolytic process; the mechanism is presumed to involve B19 infection and inhibition of erythroid precursors. The course may be complicated by an acute glomerulonephritis with proteinuria. Children and presumably adults with AC may be particularly infectious because of the absence of rash during viral excretion at, before, or for 1 week or more after onset of disease. Virus appears to be present in large quantities in both blood and respiratory secretions.

B19 infection of pregnant women has become a concern since reports appeared of fetal hydrops and death after maternal infection. The virus causes fetal anemia, resulting in heart failure in the fetus. However, no fetal anomalies after maternal B19 infection have been documented. Overall, B19 is an infrequent cause of fetal infection or spontaneous abortion. The risk of B19-related fetal hydrops has been

Table 253-4 IgM and IgG antibody responses to parvovirus B19 infection detected by enzyme immunoassay according to day after onset of illness

DAY AFTER ONSET	PERCENTAGE OF POSITIVE RESULTS	
	IGM	IGG
0-2	78	42
3-7	93	90
8-28	93	100
29-56	74	94
57-112	74	91
>112	67	100

Modified from Anderson RD et al: *Pediatr Infect Dis* 2:243, 1983.
IgG, Immunoglobulin G; *IgM*, immunoglobulin M.

estimated at 1.6% to 5% after acute maternal infection within the first 18 weeks of gestation. Fetal myocarditis and hepatitis have also been described.

There is no risk estimate for women exposed after 20 weeks of gestation. The American Academy of Pediatrics has recommended that a pregnant (seronegative) woman not care for a patient with AC because such patients may be very infectious.

The differential diagnoses of acute B19 infection include rubella, hepatitis B, adenovirus, echovirus, coxsackievirus, and Epstein-Barr virus infection; Lyme disease; and serum sickness. For more subacute syndromes when B19 produces pharyngitis, fever, arthritis and rash, acute rheumatic fever, juvenile rheumatoid arthritis, and Still's disease must be considered differentially. The diagnosis of parvovirus B19 infection is complicated by the lack of a ready source of viral antigen. However, an enzyme immunoassay (EIA), a radioimmunoassay (RIA), immunofluorescence, and hemadherence assays have been adapted using antibody capture techniques with amplification to detect both IgM and IgG antibodies and viral antigen. The EIA has been shown to be both sensitive and specific (Table 253-4). The IgM assay is the most sensitive for detection of recent infection, but IgM antibody may persist for up to 6 months. Newer EIAs have used synthetic viral peptides as antigens with promising results.

Successful use of very sensitive hybridization and nested PCR assays for viral DNA has been reported. Viral DNA may persist for up to 2 months after the onset of clinical illness. B19 may be identified in tissues by detection of intranuclear inclusions in formalin-fixed tissues, which are not evident in routinely processed, air-dried preparations. Electron microscopic examination of infected tissues may reveal parvovirus-like particles for diagnostic purposes.

There is no treatment for acute EI, other than symptomatic management. In the adult with arthralgias or arthritis, nonsteroidal antiinflammatory agents are of value. Referral to a tertiary care center is appropriate for patients with AC, chronic B19 infection, and the pregnant, acutely infected woman. For patients with AC or chronic B19 infection, immune serum globulin has been of value in some cases. Intrauterine transfusion for fetal hydrops holds promise.

Currently there is no vaccine to prevent B19 infection. Because most patients with acute B19 infection are no longer infectious when clinical symptoms occur, prevention of transmission is not feasible. Patients with AC or chronic B19 infection may be infectious and should be managed in the hospital setting with respiratory isolation (in addition to universal blood and body fluid precautions). Pregnant women should be educated about the potential risks of caring for such patients and about preventive measures; they can be given the option of not providing care for such patients. Immunoglobulin prophylaxis after exposure of a pregnant woman to a patient with EI or AC has been suggested as a possible course of action, although efficacy data are not available.

ARTHROPOD-BORNE VIRUSES

The classic arthropod-borne animal viruses (arboviruses) are now taxonomically classified into several families. The majority belong to either the Togaviridae or Bunyaviridae families and cause such clinical disease syndromes as viral encephalitis, yellow fever, dengue fever, and hemorrhagic fevers.

The arboviruses are a heterogeneous group of more than 500 viruses, of which approximately 150 cause human disease. Ten genus-level taxa are required for classification, although most arboviruses belong to three genera, in either the Togaviridae (alphavirus), Flaviviridae or Bunyaviridae families. The major viruses responsible for human disease, which are discussed in this chapter, are classified in Table 253-5. The California serogroup of encephalitis viruses are the most frequently reported arbovirus infections in the United States.

Characteristics

The alphaviruses, flaviviruses, and bunyaviruses are spheric particles bound by a host-derived lipoprotein envelope with virus-specified glycoprotein projections from their surfaces and hemagglutinins. The Alphavirus and Flavivirus genera and the Bunyavirus family contain at least 92 and 258 member viri, respectively. Most possess hemagglutinins and are destroyed by lipid solvents such as ether. The members of both families are unstable in the environment. RNA comprises the genome of these three families of viruses, but the genome of the alphaviruses and flaviviruses consists of a continuous single strand (42S) that is infectious when extracted from the virion. The bunyaviruses, however, have a segmented genome composed of three single strands of RNA (32S, 26S, and 16S) that are not infectious after extraction. The single-stranded genome of these families allows for frequent single nucleotide base substitutions, thereby accounting for the antigenic and phenotypic variation observed.

The morphogenesis of the arboviruses is not uniform even within genera, but all mature in the cytoplasm. For example, in the Togaviridae family, the alphaviruses form nucleocapsids intracellularly and usually acquire a peripheral coat by budding through the cell membrane. Release of flaviviruses and bunyaviruses from the cell is believed to occur by either exocytosis or cell lysis.

Epidemiology

Mosquitoes are the predominant arthropod vector for most arbovirus infections, with the exception of Powassan and Russian spring-summer encephalitides, which are caused by ticks. Table 253-6 lists the common vectors, hosts, and geographic areas of classic arbovirus infections. The mosquito acquires the infection by ingesting the blood of a viremic host. The virus rapidly infects most tissues of the mosquito, eventually multiplying in the salivary glands. The mosquito's bite remains infectious for the lifetime of the insect. The time from the initial blood meal until virus is produced in the salivary glands is usually a few days, after which the mosquito can transmit infection. After the mosquito bites another vertebrate, another cycle of infection is established. In some cases the vertebrate hosts appear healthy and unaffected (e.g., birds with western equine encephalitis [WEE]), whereas in others, illness and death result (e.g., simian species with sylvan yellow fever; horses with Venezuelan equine encephalitis [VEE]). Except for dengue and urban yellow fever, most of these viruses cause zoonoses among wild animals, and humans are incidental rather than primary hosts.

The epidemiology of yellow fever was elucidated by the Yellow Fever Commission headed by Walter Reed in Cuba. Commission members, initially using themselves as subjects, discovered that the *Aëdes aegypti* mosquito was necessary for transmission. By use of mosquito control, yellow fever was eliminated from Havana shortly thereafter and later from many other parts of the world. However, *A. aegypti* mosquitoes have subsequently repopulated many of these areas, and the specter of the return of yellow fever to urban centers by reintroduction from the enzootic jungle cycle is ever present.

Yellow fever has two epidemiologic patterns: (1) the sylvan (endemic or enzootic) cycle, in which several mosquito species spread the disease among forest-dwelling primates, with humans being only incidental hosts; and (2) the urban (epidemic) cycle, in which spread occurs from human to human via an infected *A. aegypti* mosquito. Dengue is transmitted exclusively from human to human by *Aëdes* mosquitoes.

Within the family Bunyaviridae there are five genera, including the Bunyavirus genus (California and LaCrosse encephalitis viruses)

Table 253-5   Classification of selected alphaviruses, flaviviruses, and bunyaviruses causing human disease

FAMILY	GENUS	VIRUS SPECIES	MEAN NUMBER OF CASES PER YEAR IN UNITED STATES
Togaviridae	Alphavirus	Eastern equine encephalitis	5
		Western equine encephalitis	34
		Venezuelan equine encephalitis	—
		Chikungunya	—
		O'Nyong-nyong	—
		Sindbis	—
Flaviviridae	Flavivirus	Dengue fever types 1 to 4	0-5 (imported)
		St. Louis encephalitis	86
		Yellow fever	—
		Powassan encephalitis	1-2
		Russian spring-summer encephalitis	—
		West Nile encephalitis	—
		Japanese B encephalitis	—
Bunyaviridae	Bunyavirus	California encephalitis viruses	
		LaCrosse	71
		Tahyna	—
	Phlebovirus	Rift Valley fever	—
	Hantavirus	Hantaan virus (Korean hemorrhagic fever with renal syndrome)	—
		Muerto Canyon virus (*Hantavirus* pulmonary syndrome)	Unknown

Table 253-6   Epidemiology of selected alphaviruses, flaviviruses, and bunyaviruses

VIRUS GENUS	VECTOR*	NORMAL HOST	GEOGRAPHIC RANGE	VECTOR HABITAT
Alphavirus				
Eastern equine encephalitis	*Culiseta melanura* and various *Aëdes* species	Birds, mammals	Eastern United States; rarely Caribbean	Coastal freshwater hardwood swamps
Western equine encephalitis	*Culex tarsalis* (western United States)	Birds, mammals	Predominantly United States; also South America and Canada	Agriculture irrigation projects, among others
Venezuelan equine encephalitis	*Culex* species	Water birds, rodents, equines	Southern United States (Everglades), Central America, South America	Freshwater swamps and slow-moving bodies of water
Flavivirus				
Dengue	*Aëdes aegypti*	Humans	Caribbean and Central America, Mexico, South Pacific, Australia, Southeast Asia, Hawaii	Tropical-subtropical urban areas
Japanese B encephalitis	*Culex tritaeniorhyncus*	Birds (pigs)	Eastern Asia, Japan, Korea, Siberia, Taiwan	
Murray Valley encephalitis	*Culex annulirostris* and others	Birds	Australia	
Powassan encephalitis	*Ixodes cookei*	Rodents	Northern United States, Canada	
Russian spring-summer encephalitis	*Ixodes ricinus* and *Ixodes persulcatus*	Forest mammals (occasionally birds)	Northern Europe, Russia	Forest regions
St. Louis encephalitis	*Culex tarsalis, Culex pipiens, Culex nigripalps,* and others	Birds	Western Hemisphere	
Yellow fever				
Urban	*Aëdes aegypti*	Humans	South America, Caribbean islands, Africa	Urban areas predominantly, although *A. aegypti* in Africa can be both domestic and wild
Sylvan	*Aëdes* species	Simian species	South America, Africa	Jungle canopy, ground-level clearings, and jungle residence
Bunyavirus				
California encephalitis	*Aëdes melanimon*	Ground squirrels	United States	
LaCrosse subtype	*Aëdes triseriatus*	Chipmunks, squirrels	North central and northeastern United States	Tree holes or breeding sites
Hantaan	Aerosolized excreta	Fieldmouse	Eastern Asia, eastern Europe	Fields frequented by farmers and military troops
Muerto Canyon virus	Aerosolized excreta	Deermouse	Western and midwestern United States	Peridomestic areas with alternating drought and rains
Phlebotomus fever viruses	Phlebotomus sandfly species	Not identified	Mediterranean, Middle East, India, Pakistan	Sandy areas near ground level

Modified from Downs WG. In Evans AS, editor: *Viral infections of humans,* New York, 1979, Plenum.
*All are mosquito vectors except tick *Ixodes.*

and the viruses within the Hantavirus genus, including defined agents of hemorrhagic fever with renal syndrome (Hantaan, Seoul, Puumala, Dobrava, and Prospect Hill viruses). Disease caused by these agents had been previously recognized largely outside the United States, with the exception of the Prospect Hill virus, which was first isolated in Frederick, Maryland, and Seoul virus. In May 1993 the epidemiology of a new agent, a Hantavirus called Muerto Canyon virus (or Sin Nombre virus), emerged as an epidemic of hemorrhagic fever with pulmonary syndrome developed. This agent is maintained in nature in the deermouse and deposited in the environment via this rodent's excreta. Periods of drought followed by heavy rains potentiate the rodent population and allow for aerosolization of excreta containing this virus. When inhaled by humans, the disease process ensues. In addition to Muerto Canyon virus, there are two other new Hantavirus agents recently isolated in the United States. These include two similar but antigenically distinct agents, one isolated in Louisiana and another in Florida. Their epidemiology awaits further definition.

Summer is the major season for transmission of arboviruses in temperate regions. The incidence of all reported cases of encephalitis and the incidence of arthropod-borne encephalitis are both highest in the summer months, although no etiologic diagnosis is made for many cases of encephalitis. The higher incidence in the summer corresponds to the increased mosquito population. Elimination of the mosquito vector by either insect control or cold weather terminates the epidemic season. In tropical zones endemic disease may occur perennially with increased activity in the rainy season, when mosquito numbers increase.

The demographic distribution of disease caused by these viruses is shown in Table 253-6. Several indigenous cases of dengue fever have been reported in Texas. In addition, a newly introduced *Aëdes albopictus* mosquito vector has established itself in northern as well as southern states; thus the potential for more indigenous transmission of dengue fever by both the *A. aegypti* and *A. albopictus* vectors exists.

Pathophysiology

Encephalitis Viruses. The lesions produced by St. Louis encephalitis, WEE, eastern equine encephalitis (EEE), and VEE are sufficiently similar so that morphologic examination cannot be used to differentiate etiologic agents. The murine VEE model is cited to generalize about the events that occur after infection with the arboviruses that cause encephalitis.

Within 24 hours, virus is detected in the blood and peripheral tissues, such as lymph nodes, bone marrow, spleen, lung, liver, and other organs. Disease in these organs becomes evident on histologic study by infiltration with tissue monocytes-macrophages, which initiate cell-mediated immunity and the basis for recovery from viral infections. After 2 days marked lymphocyte destruction and lymph node necrosis are observed. On the fourth day the lymph nodes are extensively destroyed and replaced by macrophages, the bone marrow is depleted, and megakaryocytes are degenerating; yet minimum encephalitis is seen. As the virus titer in peripheral tissues decreases, the titer in the brain increases, eventually surpassing levels in other tissues. At 6 days the brain (predominantly the gray matter), spinal cord, and meninges are extensively involved, with severe lymphocytic perivascular cuffing, marked gliosis, and neuronal necrosis.

Primary Dengue Fever. After an incubation period of 5 to 8 days after mosquito bite, fever and viremia develop, with as many as 10^6 human infectious doses per milliliter of blood. A maculopapular rash appears 3 to 4 days later. Skin biopsy shows endothelial cell swelling, perivascular edema, and mononuclear cell infiltrates. Type-specific antibody to the infecting dengue virus develops, conferring long-term homologous protection; reinfection with another serotype can occur.

Dengue Hemorrhagic Fever and Dengue Shock Syndrome. Dengue hemorrhagic fever and dengue shock syndrome are primarily seen in southern and southeastern Asia in children, most of whom are between 3 and 6 years of age and have been infected a second time with dengue virus. These diseases are also seen in children 7 to 8 months of age who are born to mothers who have preex-

isting dengue antibodies. Most geographic areas where these syndromes are seen have endemic disease with two or more serotypes of dengue. These data suggest, but do not prove, that dengue hemorrhagic fever and dengue shock syndrome may be due to an immune complex disease that occurs after a second infection with a different dengue serotype. Various complement components, fibrinogen, and platelets are depressed, suggesting consumptive coagulopathy. Petechial hemorrhages in many tissues are seen in fatal cases, along with vasodilation, congestion, and edema. Gastrointestinal tract hemorrhages may produce hematemesis and melena.

Yellow Fever Virus. With yellow fever, disease is primarily confined to the liver, kidney, heart, and gastrointestinal tract. The liver demonstrates a characteristic lack of inflammatory cells, even in severe cases, in which there may be acute coagulative necrosis of the midzonal portion of the liver lobule with formation of intracellular hyaline deposits called Councilman's bodies. Serum enzyme and serum bilirubin values (reflecting hepatic function) and prothrombin time are abnormal. The proximal renal tubules exhibit cloudy swelling and fatty degeneration and are filled with granular debris. The renal failure observed during yellow fever has been attributed to hemoglobinuric nephrosis. The heart, when involved, is dilated and pale with scattered pericardial petechial hemorrhages. Myocardial fiber degeneration is seen on microscopic examination. These findings are associated with vascular collapse on clinical examination. Gastrointestinal tract hemorrhage is a frequent event during yellow fever. Hemorrhages may also be found in the mucous membranes and skin.

Hemorrhagic Fever With Pulmonary Syndrome. The pathophysiology of hemorrhagic fever with pulmonary syndrome is presumed to involve (after aerosol entry) viral replication in the lungs and spread via the vascular tree to the endothelium of the heart, kidneys, adrenal glands, pancreas, and skeletal muscle. A systemic inflammatory response syndrome ensues and is associated with the adult respiratory distress syndrome, myocardial depression, and coagulation abnormalities.

Clinical Manifestations

The patterns of clinical syndromes occurring during Alphavirus, Flavivirus and Bunyavirus infections are shown in Tables 253-7 and 253-8. These infections in many cases are asymptomatic; seroconversion may be the only evidence of infection (see Table 253-8).

Encephalitis Viruses. Few distinguishing characteristics allow an etiologic diagnosis of an Alphavirus or Flavivirus infection on clinical grounds alone. Clinical presentations may include a mild, undifferentiated febrile illness or a syndrome indistinguishable from influenza. The common clinical signs and symptoms of encephalitis include fever, headache, vomiting, nuchal rigidity, alteration in consciousness, lethargy, and convulsions. Physical findings include neck stiffness with a positive Kernig's sign. Pathologic reflexes, generalized muscular weakness, and paralysis may be variably present. Lumbar puncture usually reveals a pleocytosis with less than 500 cells/mm^3 and rarely more than 1000 cells/mm^3. Mononuclear cells predominate, but polymorphonuclear leukocytes may be seen in the early phases (days 1 and 2) during any of these infections. The protein level may be mildly elevated, but the glucose level is normal.

Clinical recovery, when it occurs, lasts 5 to 14 days with a potentially protracted convalescence. The mortality rate in symptomatic cases varies according to the etiologic agent (Table 253-8). The incidence of EEE in the general population is low because of the swamp-breeding characteristic of its vector, but the mortality rate is high. In contrast, the incidence of the family Bunyavirus infections (LaCrosse and California viruses) is very high in exposed populations, although the sequelae are few and the mortality rate is low. The incidence of sequelae attributable to infection with the alphaviruses and flaviviruses is predominantly age dependent. For example, with EEE and WEE most sequelae are found among the young, whereas after St. Louis encephalitis, severe disease occurs more frequently in the elderly. The reported sequelae range from such nonspecific complaints as persistent headaches, tremors, and nervousness to severe impairments in speech, sight, and gait; paralysis of extremities; and convulsions.

Dengue Fever. There are two clinical patterns in dengue fever: primary classic dengue fever and secondary dengue hemorrhagic fever, often associated with a shock syndrome.

Classic dengue fever starts after a 5- to 8-day incubation period with nonspecific flulike symptoms of headache, backache, stiffness, general malaise, and flushed skin. The onset is sudden, with a rapid rise in temperature to 102.2° to 104° F (39° to 40° C). The fever may last for 5 to 6 days or be associated with a temporary remission after the third day; hence the name "saddleback fever." The fever is accompanied by retroorbital pain on eye movement, photophobia, backache, and joint pain so severe that the disease is often called "breakbone fever." During the later days of the fever, a maculopapular morbilliform or scarlatiniform rash may develop over the thorax, spreading to the extremities and face. Scattered petechiae may be present during resolution of the illness. Lymphadenopathy, a relative bradycardia, and leukopenia are common during the second febrile phase.

Dengue Hemorrhagic Fever. The incidence of dengue hemorrhagic fever has been increasing in the Americas since 1984. Dengue hemorrhagic fever is characterized by a worsening of clinical illness 2 or more days after the onset of dengue fever and associated with hypoproteinemia and one or more bleeding abnormalities (thrombocytopenia of <100,000 cells/mm^3, prolonged bleeding time, or an elevated prothrombin time). *Dengue shock syndrome* refers to a subgroup of patients with dengue hemorrhagic fever in whom hypotension, hypoalbuminemia, a capillary leak syndrome, and hemoconcentration develop, usually with elevated serum transaminase levels and pleural or abdominal fluid accumulation. Patients may have melena or hematemesis, or both. Physical findings include petechiae, purpura, ecchymosis, epistaxis, and a positive tourniquet sign. Laboratory values may also show a reduction in serum complement. The mortality rate in some epidemics has been 10% (30.5% in patients with the shock syndrome); death usually occurs on the fourth or fifth day of illness. Acetaminophen is preferred to aspirin as an antipyretic, along with other supportive therapy.

Yellow Fever. The classic syndrome of yellow fever starts after a 3- to 6-day incubation period with the sudden onset of fever and chills. Headache, backache, generalized pain, nausea and vomiting, flushed face, conjunctival injection, and leukopenia are common. After 3 days of symptoms the fever typically remits. In the classic syndrome, the fever reappears after several days, along with jaundice, punctate soft-palate hemorrhages, epistaxis, gingival bleeding, and hematemesis. In up to 50% of patients, Faget's sign develops, which is a relative bradycardia inappropriate for the fever, possibly as a result of direct cardiac involvement. Shock may occur if cardiac damage is extensive. Coma and death occur in 10% to 60% of patients within 6 to 8 days of illness onset.

Yellow fever may appear as a mild illness of less than 1 week's duration, simulating dengue fever, influenza, malaria, or typhoid. The classic syndrome may mimic viral hepatitis, leptospirosis, or carbon tetrachloride poisoning.

Muerto Canyon Fever. The clinical characteristics of the Hantavirus pulmonary syndrome include a prodromal phase of 3 to 6 days, associated with fevers and myalgia. Gastrointestinal tract complaints, including nausea, vomiting, and abdominal pain, may be prominent. Headache and dizziness may also be associated complaints. Although the physical examination and laboratory results remain normal dur-

Table 253-7   Patterns of host response to *Alphavirus, Flavivirus,* and *Bunyavirus* infections in humans

RESPONSE	EXAMPLES
Asymptomatic infection	WEE, SLE, bunyaviruses
Mild febrile illness	WEE, SLE, bunyaviruses, yellow fever
Influenza-like illness with aching and joint pains	Dengue, chikungunya, Hantaan, phlebotomus fever
Encephalitis, mild	Bunyaviruses, WEE, SLE
Encephalitis, severe	SLE, EEE, WEE, tick-borne encephalitis
Jaundice, proteinuria	Yellow fever
Hemorrhagic fever with renal syndrome	Dengue (chikungunya?), Hantaan and other hantaviruses
Hemorrhagic fever with pulmonary syndrome	Muerto Canyon virus
Shock syndrome	Dengue (after secondary infection with a different dengue serotype)

WEE, Western equine encephalitis; *SLE,* St. Louis encephalitis; *CE,* California encephalitis; *EEE,* eastern equine encephalitis.

Table 253-8   Prognosis and sequelae in *Alphavirus, Flavivirus,* and *Bunyavirus* infections

VIRUS	INAPPARENT/APPARENT CASE RATIO	SEROLOGIC INCIDENCE IN ENDEMIC AREA	APPROXIMATE MORTALITY RATE IN SYMPTOMATIC PATIENTS (%)	AGE OF AFFECTED POPULATION AND SEQUELAE
Alphavirus				
Eastern equine encephalitis	23:1	Rare	50-80	Children: severe disease with sequelae; adults: few sequelae if recovery occurs
Western equine encephalitis	—	—	3-4	Sequelae occur in children
Venezuelan equine encephalitis	—	Frequent in areas of epidemic equine disease	1	Most deaths in children
Flavivirus				
St. Louis encephalitis	64:1	10%-70% in epidemic area	5-20	Greater severity in elderly
Dengue	—	High in endemic area	Rare	All ages
Dengue hemorrhagic fever and dengue shock syndrome	—	—	30-50	Children almost exclusively
Yellow fever	9:1	Rare	Up to 50 in severe cases	All ages
Bunyavirus				
California encephalitis	≥1,000:1	11%-60%	0.3	Sequelae uncommon; disease mostly in children <15 years of age
LaCrosse encephalitis	Commonly asymptomatic	—	≤1	Children; ≤10% with emotional lability, seizures
Muerto Canyon	—	—	55	Adults

Table 253-9   Diagnosis, prevention, and vaccination for *Alphavirus, Flavivirus,* and *Bunyavirus* Infections

VIRUS	ISOLATION OF VIRUS	PREVENTION	VACCINE
Alphaviruses			
Eastern equine encephalitis	Brain, Blood and CSF (poor yield)	Equine vaccine and mosquito control in epizootic disease	Equine and human use through U.S. Army
Western equine encephalitis	Brain, Blood and CSF (difficult)	Mosquito control for epizootic disease or epidemics	Equine and human use through U.S. Army
Venezuelan equine encephalitis	Blood and throat swab (high yield)	Equine vaccine	TC-83 live attenuated vaccine, predominantly for horses (occasionally used for laboratory personnel)
Flaviviruses			
Dengue fever	Blood	Mosquito control	Experimental
St. Louis encephalitis	Brain, Blood and CSF	Mosquito control in epidemics	None
Yellow fever	Blood Liver (biopsy not recommended because of bleeding)	Vaccine, mosquito control	Chick embryo live attenuated vaccine (17D) Revaccinate every 10 years
Bunyaviruses			
California and LaCrosse encephalitis	None reported	Protective clothing, mosquito repellent	None

CSF, Cerebrospinal fluid.

ing this prodromal phase, the cardiopulmonary phase ensues with progressive complaints of cough and shortness of breath. Physical findings include tachypnea, fever, and hypotension, as well as tachycardia. Associated findings during the course of illness also include hemoconcentration, thrombocytopenia, a prolonged partial thromboplastin time and an increasing shift toward immature granulocytes in the peripheral blood. Serum enzymes become elevated, along with leukocytosis. The only abnormality on urinalysis is proteinuria. Renal function usually remains intact. Up to 90% of patients require intubation and mechanical ventilation. Hemodynamic findings include a normal or elevated level of systemic vascular resistance but a depressed cardiac output. Intractable hypotension leads to renal failure and a terminal cardiac arrhythmia 2 to 16 days after the disease onset. In patients who recover, a rapid progression to improved oxygenation and hemodynamic function may ensue. Recovery has been complete for survivors. At postmortem examination increased pulmonary vascular permeability is noted, with interstitial and alveolar edema associated with interstitial lymphocytosis.

Diagnosis

The differential diagnoses of the encephalitides include noninfections (cerebrovascular events, tumors, toxins, and connective tissue disorders) and other infectious causes; the latter include herpes simplex virus, mumps, influenza, lymphocytic choriomeningitis, Lyme disease, acquired immunodeficiency syndrome (AIDS), and Reye's syndrome, among others. The patient's age, the seasonal setting, and whether there are ill patients in the community must be considered in formulating the differential diagnoses.

The diagnosis of most *Alphavirus, Flavivirus,* and *Bunyavirus* infections is most often established by examining acute and convalescent sera for neutralization (the most specific), hemagglutination inhibition, or complement-fixing antibodies, or for IgM by ELISA. This last technique is frequently used for rapid serodiagnosis. There is a high degree of cross-reactivity of hemagglutination inhibition and complement-fixing antibodies within genera. Virus may be detected in tissues by immunofluorescence or EIA. Nucleic acid hybridization and PCR have been used to detect viral RNA; these latter two techniques are commonly used today in lieu of antibody detection for acute diagnosis.

In some instances the diagnosis may be established by isolation of the virus from blood, cerebrospinal fluid, throat swabs, or

necropsy specimens of brain (encephalitis) or liver (yellow fever) (Table 253-9).

Liver biopsy for the antemortem diagnosis of yellow fever is not recommended because of the high complication rate. The histologic changes in the liver are pathognomonic (see earlier discussion). Routine postmortem liver biopsies have been used to monitor the incidence of disease in South America. The lesions of encephalitis caused by alphaviruses, flaviviruses, and bunyaviruses are not specific enough to allow identification of the various agents. The diagnosis of the Hantavirus pulmonary syndrome may be difficult because of the nonspecificity of signs and symptoms. Initial differential diagnoses often include pneumococcal bacteremia, severe atypical pneumonia or other less common pulmonary infections. At present, the only reliable method for diagnosis is serologic. Hantavirus IgM and IgG antibodies may be detected in serum by use of EIA. Hantavirus antigen may be detected in tissue by immunohistochemistry or by the use of PCR to detect RNA.

Treatment and Prevention

The treatment of patients with any of the encephalitides, dengue fever, or yellow fever is symptomatic. Patients with dengue hemorrhagic fever and yellow fever must be carefully observed for signs of shock and DIC and must be given appropriate treatment. No antiviral therapy is available.

Treatment of Hantavirus pulmonary syndrome is largely supportive. Therapeutic trials using ribavirin have been attempted, but results were disappointing. Oxygenation, mechanical ventilation, and the use of inotropic and vasopressor agents serve as the mainstay for management.

Prevention of infection by the arthropod-borne virusues is achieved primarily by mosquito control; vaccination is useful in some cases (Table 253-9). The live yellow fever vaccine is the only vaccine regularly used for humans. Although two vaccines for yellow fever have been developed, the 17D chick embryo vaccine developed by Theiler in 1937 is used exclusively because it produces less postvaccination encephalitis than does the French neurotropic vaccine.

Vaccines for equine and human use have been developed for EEE, WEE, and VEE. Vaccination of horses against VEE may help to terminate an epidemic in humans. Human epidemics of VEE often follow the first observation of equine disease by several weeks. The horse-mosquito transmission cycle is important because the high equine levels of viremia that develop are capable of reinfecting more mosquitoes. Interruption of the equine-mosquito cycle by horse vaccination generally leads to a gradual decrease in human disease. In contrast, in equines (or humans) the levels of viremia in WEE and EEE do not become sufficiently high to infect mosquitoes. Thus immunization of equines has little effect on interrupting the natural transmission cycle in WEE or EEE.

Mosquito control and prevention of mosquito bites are valuable preventive measures in all the arthropod-borne infections. Various means have been used, including removal of mosquito breeding areas in urban areas, irrigation management, use of persistent organophosphorus larvicides, and spraying of organophosphorus insecticides in ultra-low volumes from aircraft. Some mosquitoes, such as *A. aegypti* in the Americas, exist primarily as domestic species, and eradication stops the epidemic. On the other hand, other mosquitoes exist as both domestic and wild species (e.g., *A. aegypti* in Africa) or live in vast territories in the wild; therefore eradication is impractical. The surveillance program to detect infected mosquitoes has been successful in monitoring disease prevalence to help decide when to practice mosquito control. Mosquito repellents, netting, and protective clothing are useful individual measures for decreasing the chances of being bitten by an infected mosquito.

Prevention of the Hantavirus pulmonary syndrome necessitates education of the population groups who will be exposed in various areas throughout the United States; they must be cautioned to avoid inhalation of rodent excreta when feasible. Knowledge about the potential presentation of such a syndrome among potentially infected populations is vital to early recognition and prompt management. Recommendations for risk reduction have been published by the Centers for Disease Control and Prevention.

BIBLIOGRAPHY

Anderson LJ: Human parvoviruses, *J Infect Dis* 161:603, 1990.

Anderson LJ et al: Detection of antibodies and antigens of human parvovirus B19 by enzyme-linked immunosorbent assay, *J Clin Microbiol* 24:522, 1986.

Ater JL et al: Circulating interferon and clinical symptoms in Colorado tick fever, *J Infect Dis* 151(5):966, 1985.

Barry M et al: Brief report: treatment of a laboratory-acquired sabiá virus infection, *N Engl J Med* 333:294-296, 1995.

Brown KE et al: Erythrocyte P antigen: cellular receptor for B19 parvovirus, *Science* 262:114-117, 1993.

Butler JC, Peters CJ: Hantaviruses and Hantavirus pulmonary syndrome, *Clin Infect Dis* 19:387-395, 1994.

Calisher CH: Medically important arboviruses of the United States and Canada, *Clin Microbiol Rev* 7:89-116, 1994.

Cartter ML et al: Occupational risk factors for infection with parvovirus B19 among pregnant women, *J Infect Dis* 163:282, 1991.

Centers for Disease Control and Prevention: Bolivian hemorrhagic fever: El Beni department, Bolivia—1994, *MMWR* 43:943-946, 1994.

Centers for Disease Control and Prevention: Management of patients with suspected viral hemorrhagic fever, *MMWR* 37(suppl S3):1, 1988.

Centers for Disease Control and Prevention: Outbreak of acute illness: southwestern United States—1993, *MMWR* 42:421-424, 1993.

Centers for Disease Control and Prevention: Hantavirus infection: southwestern United States: interim recommendations for risk reduction, *MMWR* 42(RR-11):1-13, 1993.

Centers for Disease Control and Prevention: Imported dengue: United States—1993 to 1994, *MMWR* 44:353-356, 1995.

Centers for Disease Control and Prevention: Arboviral disease: United States—1994, *MMWR* 44:641-644, 1995.

Cohen B: Parvovirus B19: an expanding spectrum of disease, *Br Med J* 311:1549-1552, 1995.

Cummins D: Acute sensorineural deafness in Lassa fever, *JAMA* 264:2093, 1990.

Duchin JS et al: Hantavirus pulmonary syndrome: a clinical description of 17 patients with a newly recognized disease, *N Engl J Med* 330:949-955, 1994.

Emmons RW: Ecology of Colorado tick fever, *Annu Rev Microbiol* 42:49, 1988.

Enria DA et al: Importance of dose of neutralizing antibodies in treatment of Argentine hemorrhagic fever with immune plasma, *Lancet* 2:255, 1984.

Erdman DD et al: Human parvovirus B19–specific IgG, IgA, and IgM antibodies and DNA in serum specimens from persons with erythema infectiosum, *J Med Virol* 35:110, 1991.

Frame JD: Clinical features of Lassa fever in Liberia, *Rev Infect Dis* 11(suppl 4):S783, 1989.

Frickhofen N et al: Persistent B19 parvovirus infection in patients infected with human immunodeficiency virus type I (HIV-1): a treatable cause of anemia in AIDS, *Ann Intern Med* 113:926, 1990.

Garcia-Tapia AM et al: Spectrum of parovirus B19 infection: analysis of an outbreak of 43 cases in Cadiz, Spain, *Clin Infect Dis* 21:1424-1430, 1995.

Gillespie SM et al: Occupational risk of human parvovirus B19 infection for school and day-care personnel during an outbreak of erythema infectiosum, *JAMA* 263:2061, 1990.

Goodpasture HC et al: Colorado tick fever: clinical, epidemiologic, and laboratory aspects of 228 cases in Colorado in 1973, *Ann Intern Med* 88:303, 1978.

Gratacós E et al: The incidence of human parvovirus B19 infection during pregnancy and its impact on perinatal outcome, *J Infect Dis* 171:1360-1363, 1995.

Guerina NG: Management strategies for infectious diseases in pregnancy, *Semin Perinatol* 18:305-320, 1994.

Halstead SB: Selective primary health care: strategies for control of disease in the developing world. XI. Dengue, *Rev Infect Dis* 6(2):251-264, 1984.

Hammon WM, Ho M: Viral encephalitis, *Dis Mon, 1-47*, February 1973.

Huggins JW: Prospects for treatment of viral hemorrhagic fevers with ribavirin, a broad-spectrum antiviral drug, *Rev Infect Dis* 11(suppl 4):S750, 1989.

Jundt JW, Creager AH: STAR complexes: febrile illnesses associated with sore throat, arthritis, and rash, *South Med J* 86:521-528, 1993.

Khan AS et al: Hantavirus pulmonary syndrome: the first 100 U.S. cases, *J Infect Dis* 173:1297-1303, 1996.

Koch WC et al: Manifestations and treatment of human parvovirus B19 infection in immunocompromised patients, *J Pediatr* 116:355, 1990.

Kurtzman G et al: Pure red-cell aplasia of 10 years' duration due to persistent parvovirus B19 infection and its cure with immunoglobulin therapy, *N Engl J Med* 321:519, 1989.

Levis SC et al: Endogenous interferon in Argentine hemorrhagic fever, *J Infect Dis* 149(3):428, 1984.

Luban NLC: Human parvoviruses: implications for transfusion medicine, *Tranfusion* 34:821-827, 1994.

Markoff L: Alphavirus. In Mandell GL, Bennett JE, Dolin R, editors: *Principles and practice of infectious diseases,* ed 4, New York, 1995, Churchill Livingstone.

McCormick JB et al: Lassa fever: effective therapy with ribavirin, *N Engl J Med* 134(1):20, 1986.

McCormick JB et al: A case-control study of the clinical diagnosis and course of Lassa fever, *J Infect Dis* 155:455, 1987.

McCormick JB et al: A prospective study of the epidemiology and ecology of Lassa fever, *J Infect Dis* 155:437, 1987.

Molinas FC et al: Hemostasis and the complement system in Argentine hemorrhagic fever, *Rev Infect Dis* 11(suppl 4):S762, 1989.

Monath TP: Flaviviruses (yellow fever, dengue, dengue hemorrhagic fever, Japanese encephalitis, St. Louis encephalitis, tick-borne encephalitis). In Mandell GL, Bennett JE, Dolin R, editors: *Principles and practice of infections diseases,* ed 4, New York, 1995, Churchill Livingstone.

Naides SJ et al: Rheumatologic manifestations of human parvovirus B19 infection in adults, *Arthritis Rheum* 33:1297, 1990.

Peters CJ, Johnson KM: Lymphocytic choriomeningitis virus, Lassa virus, and other Arenaviruses. In Mandell GL, Bennett JE, Dolin R, editors: *Principles and practice of infectious diseases,* ed 4, New York, 1995, Churchill Livingstone.

Peters CJ et al: Pathogenesis of viral hemorrhagic fevers: Rift Valley fever and Lassa fever contrasted, *Rev Infect Dis* 11(suppl 4):S743, 1989.

Plotkin SA et al: Parvovirus, erythema infectiosum and pregnancy, *Pediatrics* 85:131, 1990.

Spruance SL, Bailey A: Colorado tick fever: a review of 115 laboratory-confirmed cases, *Arch Intern Med* 131:288, 1973.

Tesh RB: The emerging epidemiology of Venezuelan hemorrhagic fever and Oropouche fever in tropical South America, *Ann N Y Acad Sci* 740:129-137, 1994.

Tsai TF: Arboviruses. In Murray PR, Baron EJ, Pfaller MA, Tenover FC, Yolken RA, editors: *Manual of clinical microbiology,* ed 6, Washington, D.C., 1995, ASM Press.

Umene K, Nunoue T: A new genome type of human parvovirus B19 present in sera of patients with encephalopathy, *J Gen Virol* 76:2645-2651, 1995.

Vainrub B, Salas R: Latin American hemorrhagic fever, *Infect Dis Clin North Am* 8:47-59, 1994.

Vanzee BE et al: Lymphocytic choriomeningitis in university hospital personnel: clinical features, *Am J Med* 58:803, 1975.

Weissenbacher MC et al: Argentine hemorrhagic fever, *Curr Top Microbiol Immunol* 134:79, 1987.

Zeitz PS et al: A case-control study of Hantavirus pulmonary syndrome during an outbreak in the southwestern United States, *J Infect Dis* 171:864-870, 1995.

CHAPTER

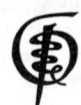

254 Rotavirus and Norwalk-Like Virus Infections

Suzanne M. Matsui

Acute infectious gastroenteritis is an extremely common disease worldwide and has a significant public health impact. Its most devastating effects are seen in developing countries in Asia, Africa, and Latin America, where 3 to 5 billion cases of diarrhea occur each year and lead to death in 5 to 10 million individuals. Approximately 40%

of these deaths are linked to rotavirus infections that primarily affect children younger than the age of 2 years. In developed nations the effect of infectious gastroenteritis on morbidity and mortality rates is less pronounced but still not trivial. For example, acute gastroenteritis is the second most common illness encountered in American families, with an incidence in the range of 10% to 15%. In American children, epidemiologic studies indicate that gastroenteritis is responsible for approximately 800,000 to 1 million hospital admissions and approximately 250 deaths per year. Elderly patients (>74 years old), particularly those residing in long-term care facilities, are also at higher risk of dying of diarrhea or its associated complications. In younger adults, acute gastroenteritis tends to run a self-limited course, but its economic impact, as measured in days lost from work, may be substantial (Chapter 242).

It is currently estimated that viruses account for 30% to 40% of the cases of infectious gastroenteritis in the United States. This exceeds the number of cases that can be attributed to bacterial and parasitic pathogens. These estimates are sure to require adjustment in the future because the cause of gastroenteritis cannot be determined with concurrent diagnostic tests in approximately 40% of cases.

Five major groups of viruses have been identified in association with acute gastroenteritis. This chapter focuses on the two groups that are the most important from a medical and public health standpoint: the human rotaviruses and Norwalk-like viruses. Detailed discussion of enteric adenovirus, astroviruses, and classic caliciviruses is beyond the scope of this chapter, and the reader is referred to recent reviews for more information.

ROTAVIRUS INFECTIONS
Characteristics

Rotaviruses are members of the family Reoviridae. The viral genome is composed of 11 segments of double-stranded ribonucleic acid (RNA) and is enclosed in a triple-layered, icosahedral capsid that measures approximately 75 nm in diameter. With one exception, each of the gene segments encodes a single viral protein. Classification of rotaviruses has depended on the serologic characteristics of three structural proteins. Viral protein 6 (VP6) the most abundant structural protein, is a determinant of group (A to G) and subgroup (I or II for group A rotaviruses) specificity. Commercial immunoassays are based on reactivity with antigenic regions of VP6. The two proteins that the outer capsid comprises, VP4 and VP7, are the primary targets to which neutralizing antibodies are directed. Viral serotype is determined by VP7, the viral surface glycoprotein. At least 10 serotypes of human rotavirus have been identified. Most infections, however, appear to be caused by only four of these (types 1 through 4).

The genome of rotavirus, like that of influenza virus, is segmented. This means that during mixed infection with two parental strains of rotavirus, each gene segment of the progeny viruses is contributed by one parent or the other. Thus gene reassortment has the potential to produce a wide array of progeny viruses with different combinations of parental genes. Although this feature has been useful in the laboratory setting to determine the gene(s) responsible for a specific viral phenotype and for vaccine development, it has not been shown conclusively that new or more virulent strains of rotavirus have evolved in nature by this mechanism.

Epidemiology

Group A rotaviruses are the most important cause of severe, dehydrating diarrhea in infants throughout the world. (Unless otherwise specified, the term *rotavirus[es]* is used to indicate group A rotavirus[es]). Recently, two antigenically distinct groups of rotaviruses (groups B and C) have been linked with human disease. Group B rotaviruses have caused large outbreaks of waterborne diarrhea among adults in China; group C rotaviruses have been found in association with sporadic cases of childhood diarrhea in various parts of the world. Rotaviruses of groups D and E appear to be strictly animal pathogens.

Group A rotavirus is primarily a pathogen of childhood. By age 3 years, nearly every child throughout the world will have had at least one rotavirus infection and will have developed antibodies to rotavirus. Symptomatic infections appear to occur most frequently in young

children between the ages of 6 and 24 months. Of hospitalizations for childhood diarrhea, 30% to 50% are due to group A rotavirus. In adults, group A rotavirus infection is generally milder or asymptomatic, but severe or prolonged infections have been reported among elderly, institutionalized patients and immunocompromised individuals. Rotavirus is also a minor cause of traveler's diarrhea.

Rotavirus infection tends to occur in the cooler winter months in temperate climates. For example, in the United States the rotavirus "season" begins in November in the Southwest and gradually moves eastward, peaking on the East Coast in February and March. In warmer, tropical climates infection occurs year-round, but some increase in incidence is observed during the cooler, rainy season.

Infected patients shed large numbers of viral particles in the feces (10^7 to 10^{10} or more virions/g), and the infectious dose is low. Rotavirus is most likely transmitted by the fecal-oral route. There is little evidence to suggest that aerosols or fomites are important vehicles of transmission. Rotaviruses are heat stable and acid stable and can remain infectious on environmental surfaces for hours to days. They are resistant to a variety of antiseptic agents, although 95% ethanol is an effective disinfectant. Therefore improved hygienic and socioeconomic conditions may not be sufficient to reduce the incidence of rotavirus diarrhea but may result in a more favorable outcome for infected individuals.

Pathophysiology

Rotavirus infects and replicates in the mature, columnar, epithelial cells of small intestinal villous tips. Infection begins in the proximal small bowel and may spread to involve the entire small bowel. Diarrhea and dehydration are presumed to result from the loss of these mature absorptive cells during infection. Abnormalities in D-xylose absorption, disaccharidase levels, and lactose tolerance have been observed but may not be clinically significant in all cases. Adenylate cyclase stimulation, a feature of enterotoxin-induced diarrheas, is not seen with rotavirus-induced illness. However, recent studies of mice indicate that a rotavirus nonstructural protein, NSP4, may function as an enterotoxin similar to *Escherichia coli* heat-stable toxin B. Pathologic features indicated by light microscopy include shortening and blunting of the villi, infiltration of the lamina propria by mononuclear cells, and elongation of the villous crypts. Electron microscopic analysis shows swelling of mitochondria, dilation of the endoplasmic reticulum, and destruction of microvilli. Rotavirus particles have been visualized in the dilated endoplasmic reticulum and lysosomes of columnar epithelial cells.

Rotavirus-induced diarrhea in immunocompetent individuals is usually self-limited. Pathologic features and their functional correlates return to normal as virus is cleared from the intestinal tract and diarrhea ceases. Prolonged or chronic symptomatic infection may be seen in immunocompromised individuals.

In most children serum antibodies develop by 2 to 3 years of age. The level of one's preexisting serum antibody does not accurately predict susceptibility or resistance to disease. Local immunity, measured by the level of immunoglobulin A (IgA) antibodies in intestinal fluids, appears to correlate more reliably with protection. IgA in human colostrum and breast milk may be responsible for the observation that rotavirus-infected infants who are breast-fed appear to shed smaller quantities of rotavirus in feces. In recent studies IgA antibodies, directed to VP6 and secreted from a backpack tumor in a mouse model of rotavirus infection, protected these animals from rotavirus infection. Anti-VP6 IgA antibodies did not have neutralization activity in vitro and did not protect mice from rotavirus infection when administered in the intestinal lumen. It is hypothesized that virus is inactivated intracellularly during the process of transcytosis of the IgA through the intestinal epithelial cell.

Clinical Disease

Rotavirus infection can result in a wide range of manifestations from no symptoms to mild diarrhea, to severe diarrhea with dehydration and occasional fatalities. As mentioned previously, children in the 6- to 24-month age-group appear to be most susceptible to symptomatic infection and may require hospitalization or aggressive fluid resuscitation. In natural infections the average incubation period is 1 to 3 days. Fever, vomiting, and in some cases respiratory symptoms may precede the onset of diarrhea. Vomiting usually resolves in 2 to 3 days with proper fluid replacement. Diarrhea is watery and nonbloody and lacks fecal leukocytes. Diarrhea generally begins later than the other symptoms and lasts 5 to 6 days. Viral shedding may persist for up to 10 days. Full clinical recovery is seen in most patients. Laboratory abnormalities such as elevated urine specific gravity, elevated blood urea nitrogen level, and hyperchloremic metabolic acidosis indicate the level of dehydration in the patient.

Adult volunteers given a rotavirus inoculum had an incubation period of 1 to 4 days. Vomiting and fever began as early as 1 day after inoculation; the diarrhea phase generally began 2 to 4 days after inoculation and lasted up to 7 days. Associated symptoms included anorexia and abdominal discomfort. In general, illness in adults tended to be milder than in symptomatic childhood infection.

Immunocompromised individuals are at risk for prolonged or chronic infections. Rotaviruses with genome rearrangements and other abnormalities have been identified in rotavirus-infected, immunocompromised patients.

Diagnosis

Although the clinical presentation combined with the epidemiologic pattern frequently suggests the diagnosis, it may be necessary to confirm the diagnosis by detection of virus or viral antigens and/or demonstration of a serologic response. Because rotaviruses are shed in large quantity in infected stools and the viral particles have characteristic surface features, they can be easily and accurately identified by electron microscopy of an unconcentrated, negatively stained specimen. Electron microscopy has the added advantage of recognizing not only group A rotaviruses but other rotavirus groups as well. Rotavirus antigen can also be detected by a number of commercially available enzyme immunoassays (EIAs) or latex agglutination tests that recognize VP6, the inner capsid protein that is a determinant of group specificity. These tests are sensitive, specific, relatively inexpensive, and rapid. In addition, the presence of rotavirus in fecal samples may be determined by extraction of viral RNA from these specimens and subsequent analysis by polyacrylamide gel electrophoresis. Molecular techniques, such as dot-blot hybridization and polymerase chain reaction, also appear to be sensitive and specific. Serologic response can be evaluated in several ways, including EIA, neutralization, inhibition of hemagglutination, immune electron microscopy, and complement fixation.

Management

The primary goal of therapy is to prevent or reverse dehydration and to correct electrolyte abnormalities. In most cases this can be accomplished with a glucose-based oral rehydration solution (ORS) tailored to the severity of fluid or electrolyte imbalance. According to recommendations from the American Academy of Pediatrics, solutions used for rehydration should contain 75 to 90 mEq/L of sodium (as found in the World Health Organization ORS). For patients in whom maintenance of hydration status or prevention of dehydration is the goal, solutions lower in sodium (40 to 60 mEq/L, as found in Pedialyte or Ricelyte) may be used. Administration of these glucose-based ORSs does not decrease the duration of diarrheal illness. Thus early feeding and adequate caloric intake are important adjuncts to ORS in promoting recovery in these patients. Intravenous fluid resuscitation is rarely needed and is reserved for advanced cases of dehydration or hypovolemic shock.

Antiviral chemotherapy is not likely to help much in the treatment of rotavirus diarrhea because viral replication and intestinal damage precede the onset of diarrhea. In immunocompromised children passive immunotherapy with human milk containing rotavirus antibodies has been shown to shorten the course of rotavirus infection.

Prevention and control of rotavirus infection can occur if fecal-oral transmission is interrupted. While improved hygienic and socioeconomic conditions alone may not affect the incidence of rotavirus diarrhea but may decrease the numbers of severe and fatal cases. Parents, hospital/institutional workers, and child care providers must be educated in proper disinfection techniques, isolation strategies, and appropriate use of gloves and hand washing. Another approach to prevention of rotavirus infection is immunoprophylaxis. The efficacy of immunoprophylaxis with live, attenuated vaccines is currently being tested. Oral tetravalent reassortant vaccines that target the four predominant human rotavirus serotypes have been developed. In field studies these live, attenuated vaccines have protected more than 80% of recipients from developing severe rotavirus diarrhea, a rate similar to that seen with natural infection. Although these vaccines may be licensed for use in the near future, alternative vaccine strategies that incorporate the recent discoveries of rotavirus virulence and immunity are also being investigated.

NORWALK-LIKE VIRUS INFECTIONS
Characteristics

Norwalk virus is the prototype strain of a group of small (27 to 40 nm), round, icosahedral viruses with relatively amorphous surface features revealed by electron microscopy. Viruses in this group are best known as causes of outbreaks of gastroenteritis in older children and adults but may also cause illness in younger children. Because these viruses have not been fully characterized, most of them bear the names of the outbreak locations such as Norwalk (Ohio), Hawaii, Snow Mountain (Colorado), Montgomery County (Maryland), and Taunton (United Kingdom). The Marin County (California) virus was originally thought to be yet another Norwalk-like virus but has now been classified as an astrovirus.

The Norwalk virus was identified by immune electron microscopy in 1972, but progress in characterizing the Norwalk-like viruses has been hampered by the inability to cultivate these viruses in vitro, the inability to cause productive infection in animal models, and the small amount of virus ($<10^6$ virions/g of feces) that is shed for brief periods during infection. Much of the currently available information has been derived from human volunteers who were administered a safety-tested viral inoculum from the original Norwalk outbreak. More recently, molecular cloning and expression have yielded a vast amount of new information. Norwalk and related viruses are now classified in the family Caliciviridae. These viruses have a genome composed of about 7.5 kb of single-stranded RNA of positive polarity.

Epidemiology

Norwalk and Norwalk-like viruses are a major cause of epidemic gastroenteritis. At least 30% to 40% of the outbreaks examined in two separate studies were due to Norwalk and serologically related viruses, as determined by the presence of viral antigen in clinical samples or serum immune responses. It has been estimated that serologically distinct viruses with similar electron micrographic features may be the etiologic agents of an additional 20% to 25% of such outbreaks.

In the United States serum antibodies to Norwalk virus are rarely detected in childhood, increase in incidence during the teenage years and early adulthood, and are found in approximately 60% of 40- to 60-year-old adults. In contrast, antibodies to Norwalk virus are acquired early in childhood in developing nations. These observations support the hypothesis that transmission of Norwalk virus occurs by the fecal-oral route. The association of serum antibody levels and protection from illness is less well understood. A paradoxic relationship between serum antibody response and long-term (>2 years) protection from illness has been observed in adult volunteers in the United States. This suggests that immune response is not the only determinant of susceptibility to infection.

Exposure to Norwalk virus can occur year-round in a variety of settings. Outbreaks of gastroenteritis have been reported aboard cruise ships, at family gatherings, and in nursing homes, summer camps, and schools. Contaminated food and/or water has been responsible for many of these outbreaks. Transmission through infected food handlers and from person to person has also been reported. Some of the largest epidemics of Norwalk gastroenteritis have involved the ingestions of contaminated clams and oysters. Standards for shellfish safety are typically based on fecal coliform counts. It has been shown, however, that the absence of fecal coliforms in shellfish may not accurately reflect the level of viral contamination in the shellfish.

Norwalk virus is also a minor cause of traveler's diarrhea, as evidenced by the outbreak of gastroenteritis in a military unit in Operation Desert Shield in which serum immune responses to Norwalk virus were demonstrated. In immunocompromised patients the importance of Norwalk-like viruses has not been clearly established. Two independent studies failed to agree on the incidence of Norwalk virus–induced diarrhea in acquired immunodeficiency syndrome (AIDS) patients. A recent prospective study found Norwalk-like infection in 6% of human immunodeficiency virus (HIV)-infected patients with diarrhea.

Pathophysiology

Experimental infection of adult volunteers with Norwalk or Hawaii viruses resulted in histologic changes in the small intestine. More specifically, during the symptomatic phase of infection intestinal villi were broadened and flattened and epithelial lining cells appeared vacuolated and disorganized. Mononuclear and polymorphonuclear cell infiltrates in the lamina propria and crypt cell hyperplasia were also observed. Effects of viral infection indicated by electron micrographs included dilation of the endoplasmic reticulum, multivesiculate bodies, widened intercellular space, and shortened microvilli. No viral particles were identified within these cells. Some of the asymptomatic, infected patients also demonstrated a few of these histologic changes on biopsy. In general, however, more severe biopsy lesions were seen in the more symptomatic volunteers. Repeat biopsy during recovery (a few weeks after the acute phase of infection) indicated complete resolution of these abnormalities.

Functional abnormalities observed during symptomatic infection included transient malabsorption of fat, D-xylose, and lactose and decrease in brush border enzyme levels compared with individual baseline values. Although histologic abnormalities were not found in the stomach or colon, gastric motility was decreased during infection. This may account for the nausea and vomiting that are prominent features of this illness. Altered adenylate cyclase levels were not observed.

Clinical Features

The clinical features of Norwalk virus–induced illness have been investigated in a controlled manner in adult volunteers. In a typical study volunteers were given a safety-tested oral inoculum derived from a secondary case of the original Norwalk epidemic. In approximately 50% of the infected volunteers clinical disease developed after an average incubation period of approximately 24 hours. Nausea was reported by nearly all of the ill volunteers, and vomiting occurred in more than 90%. Diarrhea was reported by more than 50% of the volunteers. Some volunteers also complained of fever, headache, myalgias, and abdominal cramps. Mild leukocytosis was occasionally detected. Symptoms generally resolved within 72 hours of onset. Experimental infection with Snow Mountain and Hawaii viruses caused illness that was indistinguishable on clinical examination from Norwalk virus illness.

Gastroenteritis associated with Norwalk-like viruses in the field is characterized by the sudden onset of nausea and vomiting with or without diarrhea. The clinical course resembles that of the ill volunteers. The illness is generally self-limited, lasting 12 to 60 hours. Although vomiting is a frequently reported symptom, severe dehydration is only occasionally seen, and the patient rarely requires hospitalization or aggressive fluid resuscitation. Elderly, debilitated patients may be more susceptible to severe dehydration, and occasional deaths related to complications of Norwalk gastroenteritis have been reported in this group.

Diagnosis

Recent advances in understanding the molecular biology of Norwalk-like viruses have led to the development of sensitive and specific PCR assays. In addition, expression of large quantities of recombinant viral particles in an insect cell system have facilitated the development of new antigen and antibody EIAs. The antigen EIA is highly strain-specific, whereas the antibody EIA is more broadly reactive. All of these assays are currently available only in research laboratories.

✔ *WHEN TO REFER*

Stool samples from patients suspected to be involved in an outbreak of viral gastroenteritis may be referred to state health department laboratories for further evaluation.

Management

Because illness with Norwalk and related viruses is generally self-limited, specific treatment is usually not necessary. If significant dehydration develops, oral or intravenous fluid resuscitation should be administered. No antiviral chemotherapy is available.

Large epidemics have been associated with the consumption of raw or undercooked shellfish. Until adequate seafood safety standards regarding virus contamination are established, it is prudent to advise the public of the risks of eating raw shellfish and the proper way to ensure that shellfish is fully cooked. For example, clams open after 1 minute of steaming, but 4 to 6 minutes of steaming is necessary to ensure that the internal temperature of the clam reaches that required to inactivate viruses (100° C).

The role for immunoprophylaxis is not clear, given the paradoxical association between the level of immune response and protection from disease. Further research in this area is needed before vaccine development can begin.

BIBLIOGRAPHY

Ball JM et al: Age-dependent diarrhea induced by a rotaviral nonstructural glycoprotein, *Science* 272:101, 1996.
Bernstein DI et al: Evaluation of rhesus rotavirus monovalent and tetravalent reassortant vaccines in U.S. children: US Rotavirus Vaccine Efficacy Group, *JAMA* 273:1191, 1995.
Burns JW et al: Protective effect of rotavirus VP6–specific IgA monoclonal antibodies that lack neutralizing activity, *Science* 272:104, 1996.
Blacklow NR, Greenberg HB: Viral gastroenteritis, *N Engl J Med* 325:252, 1991.
Duggan C et al: The management of acute diarrhea in children: oral rehydration, maintenance, and nutritional therapy, *MMWR* 41(RR-16):1, 1992.
Greenberg HB, Matsui SM: Astroviruses and caliciviruses: emerging enteric pathogens, *Infect Agents Dis* 1:71, 1992.
Grohmann GS et al: Enteric viruses and diarrhea in HIV-infected patients, *N Engl J Med* 329:14, 1993.
Hyams KC et al: Diarrheal disease during Operation Desert Shield, *N Engl J Med* 325:1423, 1991.
Jiang X et al: Sequence and genomic organization of Norwalk virus, *Virology* 195:51, 1993.
Kapikian AZ, Chanock RM: Norwalk group of viruses. In Fields BN, Knipe DM, Howley PM et al, editors: *Fields virology*, Philadelphia, 1996, Lippincott-Raven.
Kapikian AZ, Estes MK, Chanock RM: Norwalk group of viruses. In Fields BN, Knipe DM, Howley PM et al, editors: *Fields virology*, Philadelphia, 1996, Lippincott-Raven.

CHAPTER

255 Herpesvirus Infections (Herpes Simplex Virus, Varicella-Zoster Virus, Cytomegalovirus, and Epstein-Barr Virus)

David A. Katzenstein and M. Colin Jordan

CHARACTERISTICS

The eight herpesviruses that infect humans are herpes simplex virus (HSV-1 and HSV-2), varicella-zoster virus (VZV), cytomegalovirus (CMV), Epstein-Barr virus (EBV), human B cell lymphotropic virus (HBLV) or human herpesvirus 6 (HHV-6), and Kaposi's sarcoma–associated herpesvirus (KSHV or HHV-8). Human herpesvirus 7 (HHV-7) has been isolated from blood leukocytes but is not associated with a disease at present. All are symmetric, icosahedral enveloped viruses containing a DNA genomic core that is 30 to 45 nm in diameter. An electron-dense capsid consisting of 162 capsomers surrounds the deoxyribonucleic acid (DNA) core. The entire virion, including the envelope, ranges from 120 to 250 nm in diameter; the nucleic acid has a molecular weight of approximately 150×10^6. Although the clinical manifestations produced by each virus are diverse, there are several common features. The herpesviruses are among the most ubiquitous human pathogens. In general, infection is more frequent and occurs in younger age-groups in populations of lower socioeconomic status. With the exception of VZV, most infections are asymptomatic. Once infection is established in the host, the virus persists indefinitely in a nonreplicating, dormant state in specific cells and tissues. Under certain conditions the virus may be induced to replicate, producing either secondary disease or asymptomatic viral shedding. In the severely immunocompromised host, life-threatening disease may result from local viral invasion or widespread dissemination.

HERPES SIMPLEX VIRUS

The two strains of HSV that cause human disease, HSV-1 and HSV-2, are closely related antigenically and share nearly 50% DNA homology. HSV-1 is the more common cause of orolabial lesions (cold sores or fever blisters), whereas the majority of genital infections are caused by HSV-2. With certain exceptions, notably, herpetic encephalitis, which is nearly always the result of HSV-1 infection, and meningitis, which is usually caused by HSV-2, the two HSVs may cause identical lesions and disease.

Epidemiology

HSV-1 infection is frequently acquired in the first decade of life. By adulthood as many as 85% of the population have been infected as determined by serologic surveys. Nevertheless, only 15% to 25% of individuals have recurrent orolabial herpetic infection. Between symptomatic episodes HSV may be present in oral secretions in as many as 5% of healthy adults with a history of cold sores. Such asymptomatic shedding of HSV presumably plays an important role in the spread of viral infection in the normal population. HSV-2 infection is more closely linked to sexual activity in that the prevalence of antibody rises rapidly after puberty and is related to the age of first intercourse and the number of sexual partners. In women, asymptomatic shedding of HSV-2 in cervicovaginal secretions can be detected between episodes of clinically apparent genital infection. Asymptomatic HSV shedding from the urethra may occur in men. These states of asymptomatic shedding presumably account for cases of genital infection that occur in individuals with no known exposure to an index case.

Pathogenesis

The pathogenesis of infections with herpesviruses is summarized in Table 255-1. Vesicular lesions caused by HSV are the result of lytic infection of epithelial cells of the skin and mucous membranes. Typically lesions begin in crops of painful, small, fluid-filled vesicles. On the mucous membranes of the mouth, vagina, or rectum the vesicular stage may not be evident, and shallow circular ulcers develop. On the epidermis vesicles may contain clear fluid or appear pustular; they ulcerate, forming crusting lesions after 3 to 5 days; they usually heal without scarring. In the course of primary infection HSV enters the sensory nerve endings in the skin or mucous membrane and then migrates to the sensory nerve ganglia that innervate the affected area. In the neuron the virus establishes a nonreplicating latent infection. An "antisense" messenger RNA transcribed from a region of the viral genome encoding a regulatory protein (ICP-O) has been detected in latently infected neurons; no later gene products have been found, suggesting that HSV replication is restricted at a very early phase. Virus within neurons is capable of repeated reactivation, causing recurrent lesions or asymptomatic viral shedding. Frequently, prodromal dysesthesias or paresthesias are produced by migration of the virus down the nerve axon to the skin or mucous membrane. At the level of the vesicular lesion, cell-mediated immunity appears to play a crucial role in containment of the lytic infection. There is some experimental evidence to suggest that specific antiviral antibody is important in modulation of the latent HSV infection of neurons. During primary infection or in immunosuppressed patients, bloodborne virus may be carried to visceral organs.

Clinical Features

Orolabial Infection. Orolabial HSV-1 infection is usually acquired during childhood when infectious virus comes in contact with skin or mucous membranes. Primary infection is most often asymptomatic or results in only a few scattered vesicular lesions on the lips. In a small number of children and adults primary oral infection results in severe gingivostomatitis characterized by confluent vesicles or ulcers on the tongue, buccal and sublingual mucosa, and pharynx and by submandibular lymphadenopathy with fever.

Recurrent orolabial lesions (fever blisters or cold sores) are usually limited to the vermillion border of the lip and do not involve the oral mucosa. In a given individual, vesicles tend to recur in the same location, and often the appearance of lesions is preceded by hyperesthesia in the affected area and local lymphadenopathy. Recurrences are associated with exposure to intense sunlight, fever, stress, or injury to the trigeminal ganglion. In severely stressed patients the rate of shedding of oral virus may be as high as 20%.

Genital Infection. Genital herpes is more commonly caused by HSV-2 and is acquired through contact with oral or genital secretions that contain infectious virus (Chapter 244). Rarely, genital infection results from autoinoculation in patients with oral or digital lesions. The incubation period after sexual contact ranges from 2 to 7 days. In most patients the primary acquisition of genital herpes is asymptomatic, and the infection is manifested only by recurrent disease months or years later. In women, herpes lesions occur on the labia, vaginal mucosa, or cervix, or on the skin of the perineum. Occasionally crops of lesions may appear on the buttocks or thighs. In men, lesions most frequently involve the shaft of the penis, the foreskin, and, less often, the scrotum, thighs, and buttocks. Lesions on the glans penis frequently appear macular and fail to vesiculate. Male homosexuals often have perianal or rectal lesions.

Morbidity associated with primary and recurrent genital infection is widely variable. The initial primary genital infection may result in widespread lesions and a systemic illness with fever and malaise persisting for weeks. In some individuals frequent recurrences may oc-

Table 255-1 Pathogenetic sequence of uncomplicated infection with herpesviruses

VIRUS	PRIMARY INFECTION	CHRONIC INFECTION	LATENT INFECTION	REACTIVATION
HSV	Often asymptomatic Mucocutaneous lesions	Intermittent shedding in saliva, vagina, and tears	Neurons in sensory ganglia	Shedding; mucocutaneous lesions; neuropathy
VZV	Varicella in 95%	Hyperkeratotic lesions in AIDS	Sensory ganglia	Zoster
CMV	Usually asymptomatic; mononucleosis	Shedding in urine, saliva, vagina, semen, breast milk	Peripheral leukocytes ?Other tissues	Shedding dissemination
EBV	Usually asymptomatic; mononucleosis	Shedding in pharynx	B lymphocytes	Shedding; B-cell lymphoma

AIDS, Acquired immunodeficiency syndrome; *CMV*, cytomegalovirus; *EBV*, Epstein-Barr virus; *HSV*, herpes simplex virus; *VZV*, varicella-zoster virus.

cur for years; in others there are no further episodes. Recurrent lesions are preceded by prodromal hyperesthesia and frequently occur in association with menstruation or after vigorous sexual activity. In some women, recurrent cervical HSV infection may be evident only as a watery vaginal discharge. In general, recurrent episodes of genital herpes become less frequent and less severe over months to years. However, genital infection tends to recur more frequently than does orolabial disease; this greater relative frequency appears to be due to HSV-2 per se, because HSV-1 genital infection recurs much less often. Shedding of HSV in cervical secretions has been demonstrated during symptom-free periods in a small percentage of women. Complications of genital infection include urinary retention and cystitis, proctocolitis, and aseptic meningitis. Any of these may become a recurrent process. Transverse myelitis with irreversible neurologic deficits has also been reported.

Herpes Encephalitis. HSV-1 is an important cause of sporadic necrotizing encephalitis in all age-groups. It may occur in patients with or without a clinical history or serologic evidence of previous infection. The predominant clinical manifestations relate to the focal nature of the disease in most cases, characteristically involving the temporoparietal or frontotemporal region of one cerebral hemisphere. Thus differential diagnosis includes focal suppurative lesions such as brain abscess or subdural empyema, mycotic aneurysm, brain tumors, vascular lesions, cysts, and granulomas. Initial symptoms of HSV-1 encephalitis are usually fever, headache, olfactory hallucinations, personality changes, and alterations of consciousness. These are frequently followed rapidly by the onset of focal hemispheric signs such as hemiparesis, focal or major motor seizures, and unilateral cranial nerve palsies. Profound coma may develop and is a grave prognostic sign. In addition, the intensity of the necrotizing inflammation and cerebral edema may lead to increased intracranial pressure, producing papilledema and in some instances cerebral herniation. Spinal fluid examination usually demonstrates mononuclear pleocytosis with an elevated protein concentration, a normal glucose level, and the presence of red blood cells. However, initial lumbar puncture findings are normal in about 10% of cases. Because HSV-1 cannot be recovered from the spinal fluid, definitive diagnosis depends on isolation of virus from brain tissue after surgical biopsy or at autopsy. Fluorescence staining for HSV antigens in brain tissue yields a positive result in 70% of cases. More recent studies indicate that HSV DNA can be detected in the spinal fluid of 93% to 96% of cases of HSV-1 encephalitis by the polymerase chain reaction (PCR). Electroencephalography, technetium brain scans, and computed tomography usually demonstrate focal cerebral abnormalities with surrounding edema. Because approximately 50% of cases of suspected herpes encephalitis are found to have a variety of other infectious, malignant, or vascular lesions at brain biopsy, the procedure is recommended for definitive diagnosis if the PCR assay is negative.

Herpetic Whitlow. Periungual inoculation of HSV results in recurrent infection of the pulp of the finger, or herpetic whitlow. This disease occurs most often in medical and dental personnel after direct contact with herpes lesions or secretions containing HSV. Occasionally, whitlow results from autoinoculation in patients with oral or genital HSV infection. The appearance of vesicles or pustules is preceded by pain, redness, and swelling of the affected finger, and lesions may be accompanied by lymphangitis and regional lymphadenopathy. Some individuals have repeated bouts of herpetic whitlow. The primary value in diagnosis is the prevention of repeated attempts at incision and drainage and needless antibiotic therapy.

Herpes Keratitis. Corneal epithelium can be a site of primary as well as recurrent HSV infection. Herpes keratitis begins with small punctate vacuoles in the cornea that coalesce to form dendritic lesions. In advanced disease after frequent recurrences corneal ulcers and scarring may result. The signs of infection include a foreign body sensation followed by follicular conjunctivitis and preauricular lymphadenopathy. It is important to avoid the use of corticosteroid-containing ophthalmic solutions in patients with suspected ocular herpes infection.

Infection in Compromised Hosts. Oral and genital HSV infection may cause life-threatening disease in severely immunosuppressed patients. Reactivation of endogenous virus frequently occurs in patients with hematologic malignancies, bone marrow and organ transplants, and acquired immunodeficiency syndrome (AIDS). In these patients, herpetic lesions involve extensive areas of epidermis, the oropharynx, and the esophagus. Occasionally, hematogenous dissemination of HSV in compromised hosts produces extensive skin lesions resembling varicella. In patients with extensive skin damage from burns, pemphigus, Sézary syndrome, and eczema, HSV infection can involve large areas of denuded and intact epithelium and can be disseminated to visceral organs. In compromised patients receiving endotracheal intubation, tracheobronchitis and pneumonitis caused by HSV may develop. Rarely, systemic dissemination of HSV with lethal, fulminant hepatitis in pregnant women and transplant recipients has been observed (Table 255-2).

Congenital and Neonatal Infection. Transmission of virus to the fetus in utero is a rare complication of HSV infection in pregnancy. The clinical manifestations are similar to those of other congenital infections in which microcephaly, jaundice, hepatosplenomegaly, chorioretinitis, and thrombocytopenia are present at birth. Acquisition of HSV by the infant during passage through an infected birth canal is much more common, especially after recent primary infection of the mother. Clinical manifestations develop within 2 to 10 days after birth and include fever, cranial nerve palsies, seizures, and lethargy progressing to coma. Because characteristic herpetic skin lesions occur in only 60% of infected infants, the disease is frequently mistaken for neonatal sepsis. When it is untreated, the mortality rate is 50% to 60%, usually as a result of necrotizing encephalitis and hepatic necrosis (Table 255-2).

Diagnosis

In most cases of HSV infection the diagnosis is apparent on clinical examination. Examination of stained cells from the base of an ulcer (Tzanck preparation) often demonstrates characteristic multinucleate giant cells and intranuclear inclusions (Color Plate VIII-13). The clinical diagnosis can be confirmed by culture of vesicle fluid or cells scraped from the base of an ulcer. HSV produces distinct cytopathic effects in a variety of cell cultures within 24 to 96 hours, and culture remains the most sensitive and specific means of diagnosis (Chapter 233). Because most neonatal HSV infections occur in children born of mothers with no history of symptomatic genital lesions, routine screening cultures of pregnant women with a history of genital herpes are of no value. New diagnostic reagents, biotin, and fluorescein-labeled monoclonal antibodies have been developed that may provide rapid diagnosis based on antibody binding to infected cells. Currently the ability of these tests to exclude HSV infection is not resolved. In the case of brain biopsy for suspected herpes encephalitis, fluorescein-labeled antibody staining appears to be a useful adjunct to histopathologic evaluation and culture of biopsy specimens. Serologic detection of neutralizing or complement-fixing antibodies against HSV has little role in clinical diagnosis. However, it has been useful as a means of distinguishing "true primary" HSV infection from "recurrent primary" infection. In the former case, serum antibody is absent at the time of the first clinical episode of HSV, and antibody titers are present 2 to 4 weeks later. In "recurrent primary" infection, antibody is present, indicating antecedent infection before the initial clinical presentation. Diagnosis of HSV infection by serologic testing is further complicated by cross-reactivity between HSV-1 and HSV-2 antibodies and fluctuations in titers caused by other diseases.

Treatment

The recent development of antiviral compounds that specifically inhibit the replication of HSV has greatly altered the outcome of primary infection in both immunocompetent and immunocompromised hosts.

The approach to management is reviewed in Table 255-3. Topical use of such drugs is effective in herpetic keratitis, in which application of idoxuridine, adenine arabinoside (vidarabine [ara-A]), trifluridine, and acycloguanosine (acyclovir [ACV]) has been shown to speed resolution and prevent corneal ulceration and visual impairment. In genital herpetic infection, topical ACV has modest efficacy for primary episodes but none for recurrent bouts. Treatment does not

Table 255-2   Complications of herpesvirus infection

VIRUS	CONGENITAL INFECTION	PERIPARTUM INFECTION	PRIMARY INFECTION	RECURRENT INFECTION	ASSOCIATED NEOPLASMA
HSV	Microcephaly Hepatosplenomegaly Thrombocytopenia	Disseminated visceral and cutaneous disease	Encephalitis Keratitis Stomatitis Proctitis Whitlow Hepatic necrosis Aseptic meningitis Tracheobronchitis	Erythema multiforme Aseptic meningitis Whitlow Sensory and autonomic neu- ralgia	Cervical carcinoma
VZV	Limb atrophy Skin lesions Eye lesions Nervous system abnormali- ties	Varicella	Pneumonitis Meningoenocephalitis Hepatitis Reye's syndrome	Disseminated zoster	None
CMV	Cytomegalic inclusion disease Asymptomatic infection	Interstitial pneumonitis	Hepatitis Guillian-Barré syndrome Interstitial pneumonitis Encephalitis Pancreatitis Chorioretinitis Colitis	Same as primary	Kaposi's sarcoma
EBV	None known	None known	Polyclonal B-cell prolifera- tion Complications of mono- nucleosis	Poorly defined	Nasopharyngeal carcinoma Burkitt's lymphoma B-cell lymphoma

CMV, Cytomegalovirus; *EBV,* Epstein-Barr virus; *HSV,* herpes simplex virus; *VZV,* varicella-zoster virus.

appear to alter the frequency of subsequent recurrent episodes. Recent studies indicate that oral ACV is effective for treatment of primary herpes genitalis and prevention of recurrent episodes and is indicated for treatment of severe orolabial HSV-1 disease in immunocompromised patients. Again, however, the frequency of recurrence of lesions is not altered by therapy once treatment is stopped. HSV mutants resistant to ACV have been recovered, particularly from AIDS patients undergoing multiple courses of therapy. In HSV-1 encephalitis, intravenous therapy with ACV or ara-A significantly reduces mortality rate, particularly if treatment is begun before coma supervenes. However, many survivors of herpetic encephalitis have moderate to severe neurologic impairment. Acyclovir has fewer side effects and greater efficacy than ara-A. In disseminated herpetic infection of the newborn, intravenous treatment with ACV or ara-A substantially reduces mortality rate. HSV infections resistant to ACV can be effectively treated with foscarnet, but it must be given intravenously.

VARICELLA-ZOSTER VIRUS
Epidemiology

Varicella (chickenpox) is a very common childhood disease with a peak incidence in late winter and early spring. Approximately two thirds of the cases occur in the 5- to 9-year-old age-group. Despite the fact that chickenpox is a highly communicable disease, demonstration of infectious VZV in respiratory secretions is difficult. Nevertheless, airborne droplet spread is presumed to be the mode of transmission. In contrast to other herpesvirus infections, in the vast majority of cases VZV infections are clinically apparent and only 5% occur silently. The incubation period of chickenpox ranges from 10 to 21 days. Shingles or zoster is a nonseasonal reactivation of VZV that occurs most often in older age-groups and in immunosuppressed patients. In nonimmune individuals chickenpox may develop after contact with individuals who have zoster (shingles).

Pathogenesis

Varicella-zoster virus causes varicella as a primary infection, generally in childhood, and then may cause recurrent disease later in life in the form of zoster. A relationship between the two diseases was recognized nearly a century ago when it was observed that children could acquire chickenpox after exposure to adults with zoster. More recently, characterization of the viruses has provided convincing evi-

dence that the same agent causes both diseases. In the case of varicella, the virus is probably introduced into the host via the respiratory tract or oropharyngeal mucosa. After local virus replication a viremia ensues, during which VZV is carried to mucosal and cutaneous sites elsewhere in the body. The viremia is most likely cyclic, because cutaneous vesicles tend to develop in crops. Within a few days specific humoral and cell-mediated immune responses appear, and interferon concentrations in the vesicle fluids rise. Virus eventually disappears from the lesions as the cellular inflammatory infiltrate heightens. The mechanism by which the sensory ganglia are infected with VZV is not clear (i.e., whether virus seeds the ganglia hematogenously or is carried to the ganglia via sensory nerves). Shingles, which may occur decades after varicella, results when dormant virus in the sensory ganglia begins to replicate and migrates down the sensory nerve axon to the skin. In most cases, cutaneous lesions are distributed in the area of a single dermatome. Although the precise immune deficit allowing activation of virus in the ganglia has not been identified, waning cell-mediated immunity associated with advancing age is probably an important factor. Dissemination of VZV via the bloodstream may occur in some patients, particularly those with impaired immune mechanisms caused by underlying lymphoma, leukemia, AIDS, or chemotherapy.

Clinical Features

Varicella. Chickenpox results from primary infection with VZV in an immunologically naive host and characteristically becomes evident as widely disseminated cutaneous disease. Varicella is communicated by close, but not necessarily intimate, contact, probably by shedding of infectious virus in oropharyngeal secretions for 2 to 4 days before the clinical illness. Direct contact with vesicle fluid of either varicella or zoster may also result in acquisition of the virus. The first symptom of varicella in children is usually the characteristic exanthem. Small, irregular erythematous macules appear in a centripetal distribution, with lesions more prominent on the trunk, head, and proximal extremities. Within individual lesions tiny vesicles (1 to 4 mm) containing clear fluid appear. These either rupture or, if left undisturbed, become cloudy. Within hours to days the vesicles burst to form dry, crusted lesions on an erythematous base. New crops of lesions appear for 2 to 4 days, and characteristically, all three stages of lesions—macular, vesicular, and crusted—are present simultaneously.

Clinical evidence of disease in varicella varies from mild illness

Table 255-3   Chemotherapy of herpesvirus infections*

Virus	Host	Disease	Drug	Route	Treatment vs. Prophylaxis	Virus Shedding	Healing	New Lesion Formation	Documentation of Efficacy by Clinical Trials; Comments
Herpes simplex	Normal or immunocompromised	Initial genital, orofacial, or other mucocutaneous infection	Acyclovir	Topical	Treatment	++	+	0	Excellent documentation for genital infection; poor for other sites of infection. Oral or intravenous therapy should be employed in every case of initial infection
			Acyclovir	IV	Treatment	++++	+++	+++	
			Acyclovir	Oral	Treatment	+++	++	+++	
		Recurrent genital, orofacial or other	Acyclovir	Topical	Treatment	+/0	0	0	Excellent documentation for genital infection; fair for recurrences at other sites
			Acyclovir	Oral	Treatment	++	+	N/A	
			Acyclovir	Oral	Prophylaxis	N/A	N/A	++++	
			Famciclovir	Oral	Treatment	++	++	++++	
			Valacyclovir	Oral	Treatment	++	++	++++	
		Encephalitis	Vidarabine	IV	Treatment	N/A	++	+++	Acyclovir has been shown to be superior to vidarabine in two comparative clinical trials
			Acyclovir	IV	Treatment	N/A	+++	+++	
		Disseminated infection in the neonate	Vidarabine	IV	Treatment	+++	++	+++	Acyclovir and vidarabine are comparable
			Acyclovir	IV	Treatment	+++	+++	+++	
		Keratitis	Idoxuridine, Vidarabine, Trifluorothymidine	Topical	Treatment	+++	+++	+++	Activity of these drugs topically is approximately equivalent
Varicella zoster	Normal	Chickenpox (initial infection)	Acyclovir	Oral	Treatment	++++	++	++	Controversial because of benign nature of varicella
		Zoster	Acyclovir	IV	Treatment	+++	++	+++	No effect of acyclovir on postherpetic neuralgia
			Acyclovir	Oral	Treatment	+++	++	+++	Famciclovir and valacyclovir may reduce rate of postherpetic neuralgia
			Famciclovir	Oral	Treatment	+++	+++	++++	
			Valacyclovir	Oral	Treatment	+++	+++	++++	
	Immunocompromised	Chickenpox	Vidarabine	IV	Treatment	+++	++	+++	Acyclovir is more effective
			Acyclovir	IV	Treatment	++++	+++	++++	
		Zoster	Vidarabine	IV	Treatment	+++	++	+++	No comparative studies; most authorities prefer acyclovir (less toxic; possibly more effective)
			Acyclovir	IV	Treatment	+++	+++	++++	
Epstein-Barr virus	Immunocompromised	Lymphoma or progressive infection	Acyclovir	IV	Treatment	+/0	+/0	N/A	Documentation of clinical efficacy is poor
Cytomegalovirus	Immunocompromised	Various (retinitis, colitis, esophagitis, etc.)	Vidarabine	IV	Treatment	0	0	0	Foscarnet and ganciclovir equivalent for retinitis in AIDS. Pneumonitis in bone marrow transplant patients has generally responded less well than disease at other sites
			Acyclovir	IV	Treatment	0	0	0	
			Ganciclovir	IV	Treatment	+++	+++	+++	
			Foscarnet	IV	Treatment	+++	+++	+++	
			Ganciclovir	Oral	Prophylaxis	++	++	N/A	
			Cidofovir	IV	Treatment	+++	+++	++	

*Table prepared by Dr. John Mills.
†0, No effect; +++, maximum effect.

in which only a few vesicles are present to widespread infection covering the entire body with lesions. Fever may occur for 1 to 2 days before the onset of skin lesions and during the first 2 to 3 days of illness in children. In adults varicella is a more severe illness with prolonged fever, malaise, arthralgias, and frequently pulmonary involvement (varicella pneumonia). The pneumonia may be micronodular, interstitial, or even lobar in distribution and has a high mortality rate in pregnant women. After convalescence, pulmonary diffusion capacity may remain abnormal for several months. Less common complications include cerebritis, encephalitis, Guillain-Barré syndrome, and myocarditis. Especially in patients with poor hygiene, the skin lesions of varicella may become superinfected by bacteria (usually group A β-hemolytic streptococci or staphylococci).

Congenital and Neonatal Varicella. On rare occasions, in utero infection of the fetus occurs when the varicella develops in the mother in the first or second trimester. Afflicted children may have atrophy of a limb, cicatricial skin lesions, various ocular disorders, cortical atrophy, and seizure disorders (Table 255-2). Maternal varicella near the end of pregnancy may result in chickenpox in the newborn. If the maternal illness occurs within 2 weeks before delivery, the risk of varicella in the infant is approximately 25%. Mortality rate approaches 30% when the onset of varicella in the newborn is between 5 and 10 days after delivery. Overall, the mortality rate is approximately 10%.

Zoster. Herpes zoster (shingles) is the result of the reactivation of dormant VZV in the sensory ganglia in an individual who has had varicella previously. The incidence of zoster increases with age from less than 0.1% per year in the first decade of life to more than 1.0% per year after the age of 80. Most patients who have shingles do not have underlying malignancy. However, drugs and diseases that impair cell-mediated immunity may trigger the development of zoster, leading to the conclusion that cellular mechanisms are more important than humoral in the suppression of latent VZV infection. Herpes zoster characteristically causes pain and paresthesias that precede the development of a vesicular eruption in a single dermatomal distribution. Thoracic dermatomes are most commonly involved, followed by disease in the distribution of a single cervical, facial, lumbar, or sacral ganglion. The prodromal neuralgic symptoms may include pruritis, tingling, exquisite tenderness, and deep pain in an affected area for 1 to 2 days before skin lesions develop. The rash begins as maculopapules, which rapidly develop into crops of vesicles on an erythematous base. New lesions continue to appear for 3 to 5 days as the older ones ulcerate and crust. However, crusting lesions and pain in the affected area may persist for several weeks. In the absence of bacterial superinfection there is complete healing without scarring.

The most prominent complication (Table 255-2) of herpes zoster is the occurrence of persistent or intermittent pain in the affected area for months to years after resolution of acute zoster infection (postherpetic neuralgia). Postherpetic neuralgia is common in patients older than age 60 years and is rare in children. Involvement of motor and sympathetic nerves adjacent to the involved sensory ganglion also may complicate zoster. Sacral lesions may be accompanied by bowel or bladder dysfunction. Zoster in the distribution of the second or third cervical dermatome can cause facial muscle paralysis with or without involvement of cranial nerve VIII (Ramsay Hunt syndrome). Involvement of the ophthalmic branch of the trigeminal ganglion may result in conjunctivitis and, rarely, keratitis and iritis. Disseminated zoster can develop in both normal and immunocompromised patients, although this is much more common in patients with impaired immunity.

Zoster in Immunocompromised Patients. The increased incidence of zoster in the setting of certain diseases (AIDS, lymphoma, Hodgkin's disease, lupus erythematosus) and in association with immunosuppressive therapy (steroids and antineoplastic drugs) has served to demonstrate the importance of the immune system in maintenance of VZV in a latent state. Of patients with various malignancies, approximately 13% to 15% eventually have shingles. In addition, immunosuppressed patients and transplant recipients may have a risk of dissemination of virus approaching 25% to 30% if zoster develops. Generalization of the vesicular exanthem usually occurs 7

to 10 days after onset of the localized eruption. Virus may also invade the lungs, central nervous system, pancreas, or liver.

Treatment and Prevention

Ordinarily, varicella and zoster do not require specific therapy. In older patients with shingles, data are conflicting as to whether a short course of corticosteroids given early in the illness may reduce the risk of postherpetic neuralgia. No deleterious effects have been described in the normal host. However, corticosteroids should not be given to immunocompromised patients with zoster because of the risk of dissemination. Famciclovir, a newer agent similar to acyclovir but with a much longer intracellular half-life (in the form of penciclovir) may reduce the rate of development of postherpetic neuralgia in individuals over 50 years of age. Studies of valacyclovir are in progress. Adenine arabinoside at an intravenous dose of 10 mg/kg per day or ACV at 20 mg/kg per day appears to accelerate healing of lesions and to diminish the rate of dissemination if given early in immunocompromised patients (Table 255-3). It is ineffective, however, once dissemination has begun. In one study, early administration of acyclovir appeared to halt further progression even after dissemination had begun. Vidarabine, acyclovir, and interferon have all been shown to have a modestly beneficial effect in chickenpox occurring in immunocompromised children if therapy is started early. In patients with AIDS who have received multiple courses of ACV, a new syndrome of chronic zoster has been described. Painful hyperkeratotic papules or ulcers continue to yield VZV on culture, despite high-dose oral or intravenous ACV. The VZV strains recovered are highly resistant to ACV but susceptible to foscarnet.

A live, attenuated vaccine against VZV has recently been licensed in the United States to prevent chickenpox in children. Passive immunization with VZV immune globulin (VZIG) is available for certain high-risk patients who are exposed to cases of chickenpox or shingles. It should be administered within 72 hours of exposure to patients with leukemia, lymphoma, or congenital or acquired immunodeficiency, to patients receiving immunosuppressive drugs or high-dose steroids, and to newborn infants whose mothers had varicella within 5 days before delivery.

CYTOMEGALOVIRUS INFECTION
Epidemiology

CMV infections, most of which are subclinical, are extremely common throughout the world. The prevalence of CMV infection in a given population is directly related to lower socioeconomic status, crowded living conditions, and poor hygiene. Although little is known about the means of virus spread among individuals, the risk of acquisition of CMV infection is partially understood for certain age-groups. In the newborn infant infection may be acquired during passage through the birth canal, where cervicovaginal secretions may contain infectious virus. CMV may also be transmitted during the neonatal period by breast milk. Subsequently, shedding of CMV in urine or saliva is common in healthy young children, particularly in day-care centers, where as many as 60% have viruria. It is likely that widespread infection among asymptomatic children plays an important role in the spread of virus to other children and adults. Although the risk of infection appears to be low from any given encounter with an asymptomatic virus shedder, the virus is so ubiquitous that repeated opportunities for exposure undoubtedly occur. There is evidence that suggests that in adolescence and adulthood, infectious CMV in vaginal secretions, semen, and saliva may also be spread by sexual activity. In any age-group virus may be transferred from donor to recipient by blood transfusion and organ transplantation (kidney, heart, lung, and liver).

In the United States approximately 2% of all newborn infants are infected with CMV in utero as evidenced by the detection of virus in urine at birth. Most of these children appear normal and do not have obvious cytomegalic inclusion disease. Two studies, however, have indicated that in a small percentage psychomotor retardation, sensorineural hearing loss, and/or deficiency of intelligence quotient subsequently develops. Overt cytomegalic inclusion disease is present at birth in approximately 10% of infants infected in utero.

Pathogenesis

The following different types of virus-host interaction are recognized with respect to CMV (Tables 255-1 and 255-2):

1. Primary infection in which initial acquisition of virus occurs. The vast majority of these infections are asymptomatic in the normal host, although transplacental passage of the virus during pregnancy may produce cytomegalic inclusion disease of the fetus. Mononucleosis is the most common clinical manifestation of CMV infection in previously healthy adults. In immunocompromised individuals, primary infection may result in widespread CMV disease, particularly interstitial pneumonitis, hepatitis, colitis, and central nervous system involvement.

2. Chronic or persistent infection in which asymptomatic viral shedding occurs in various sites (urine, saliva, semen, cervicovaginal secretions) for months or years, despite a specific humoral and cell-mediated host immune response. This type of infection probably has special significance in the spread of CMV in the normal population.

3. Latent infection or persistence of CMV in a nonreplicating form in host cells or tissues. Although the cellular repository of the dormant virus has not yet been identified definitively, CMV in this state can be transmitted by blood transfusion or organ transplantation. The clinical consequences of virus transfer are more severe when the recipient has not previously been infected with CMV.

4. Reactivation or recurrent infection in which CMV reappears in a replicating form. Reactivation may result in asymptomatic viral shedding or in severe disseminated disease, particularly in the immunocompromised host (e.g., the patient with AIDS). In addition to reactivation by immunosuppression, latent CMV may be activated in pregnancy or during lactation.

In congenital infection, recent studies indicate that reactivation of endogenous CMV in the mother is the most common mechanism of fetal infection. However, symptomatic cytomegalic inclusion disease in the infant results predominantly, if not exclusively, when the mother acquires the virus as an exogenous primary infection. The vast majority of maternal infections in this setting are not associated with symptomatic maternal disease, although a few cases of CMV mononucleosis with transplacental passage of the virus have been described. Primary maternal CMV infection in the first trimester of pregnancy may be more likely to result in congenital disease.

In virtually all cases of congenital or acquired CMV disease, viremia can be detected by recovery of virus from peripheral blood leukocytes in tissue culture. Frequently the viremia antedates the development of tissue injury, particularly interstitial pneumonitis and retinitis. CMV can be recovered primarily with the polymorphonuclear leukocyte population of blood cells during viremic infection.

Clinical Features

Congenital Infection. As noted, 85% to 90% of infants infected with CMV in utero appear normal at birth, whereas cytomegalic inclusion disease is apparent in 10% to 15%. Manifestations include jaundice, hepatosplenomegaly, thrombocytopenia, petechiae, and various neurologic conditions. Microcephaly, motor disability, chorioretinitis, cerebral calcifications, and seizure disorders have also been described. Mental retardation and hearing loss may subsequently become apparent in children who survive. In general, neurologic manifestations persist or worsen, whereas hepatosplenomegaly, jaundice, and hemorrhagic phenomena may subside eventually.

Cytomegalovirus Mononucleosis

CMV is responsible for approximately two thirds of the cases of heterophil-negative infectious mononucleosis that meet conventional hematologic and clinical criteria. The disease may occur spontaneously in previously healthy individuals or within 3 to 8 weeks after blood transfusion. In spontaneous illness the age of the individuals afflicted (18 to 30 years) is somewhat higher than in EBV infectious mononucleosis. On clinical examination, CMV mononucleosis is characterized by less impressive tonsillopharyngitis and lymphadenopathy than EBV disease, although considerable overlap has been reported. Exudative pharyngitis is particularly rare in CMV mononucleosis. Although the heterophil test result is always negative, other evidence of disordered immunoregulation seen in CMV disease includes positive rheumatoid factor tests findings, cryoglobulinemia, high-titered cold agglutinins, positive results for antinuclear antibody, and false-positive syphilis serologic findings. As in EBV mononucleosis, complications such as Bell's palsy, Guillain-Barré syndrome, and a maculopapular rash after administration of ampicillin may be seen. Rare complications include thrombocytopenia, hemolytic anemia, myopericarditis, pneumonitis, and meningoencephalitis.

Infection in the Compromised Host

CMV infection is most likely to be life threatening when it occurs in the host whose defense mechanisms are impaired by underlying disease or superimposed immunosuppressive therapy. Patients with hematologic malignancies, recipients of organ transplants, and individuals with AIDS are particularly susceptible to disseminated CMV infection. In this setting the virus may involve the liver, pancreas, colon, adrenals, ocular structures, and the central nervous system. However, the major threat to life results from interstitial pneumonitis with progressive hypoxemia, which is now the most common cause of death in recipients of marrow transplants. In the latter, CMV infection is closely associated with graft-versus-host disease. In the case of CMV-seronegative renal and cardiac transplant recipients, the highest risk of CMV disease is in patients who receive an organ from a CMV-seropositive donor. On the other hand, marrow transplant recipients appear to have CMV disease primarily after reactivation of endogenous latent virus. CMV infection of homosexual men and patients with AIDS is extremely common. Symptomatic CMV disease usually occurs late in the progression of AIDS. Chorioretinitis is the most common initial manifestation. CMV esophagitis and colitis also occur frequently. Polyradiculitis appears to be increasing in frequency. At autopsy, CMV involvement of the central and peripheral nervous system, pneumonitis, hepatitis, and necrotizing adrenalitis are common findings in patients who died of AIDS.

Diagnosis

CMV infection can be diagnosed by recovery of the virus in human diploid cell cultures. Specimens appropriate for virus culture include urine, saliva, breast milk, semen, cervicovaginal secretions, peripheral blood leukocytes, intraocular fluids, and tissues obtained for biopsy or at autopsy. Depending on the amount of infectious virus present in the sample, 7 to 30 days is usually required for recovery of CMV. Although culture is specific for CMV infection, it does not distinguish between asymptomatic shedding and invasive disease in a given patient. As previously noted, however, recovery of virus from peripheral blood leukocytes is a valuable correlate of active or impending CMV disease. Positive "buffy coat" culture results have been reported in patients with congenital disease or CMV mononucleosis and in immunocompromised patients with disseminating infection. More rapid methods for detection of CMV in clinical specimens using centrifugal "shell vial" assays and monoclonal antibodies are now available. Newer assays include detection of CMV antigens in blood leukocytes ("antigenemia") and detection of viral DNA in cells or plasma by PCR. For diagnosis of CMV interstitial pneumonitis, open lung biopsy may be necessary to provide tissue for histologic examination and virus culture. Occasionally, characteristic inclusion-bearing cells indicating CMV infection can be detected in bronchial washings or lavage.

A variety of serologic tests are now available for detection of CMV antibody in serum, including complement fixation, immunofluorescence, anticomplementary immunofluorescence, indirect hemagglutination, and enzyme-linked immunosorbent assay (ELISA) (Chapter 233). In these tests a seroconversion from negative to positive or a fourfold or greater rise in titer in paired sera is necessary to confirm the presence of active CMV infection. CMV-specific immunoglobulin M (IgM) antibody can be demonstrated by either immunofluorescence or ELISA. Its detection suggests recent or active infection as opposed to more remote CMV infection. CMV-specific IgM antibody can be detected in approximately 75% of cord blood specimens from infants infected in utero; however, rheumatoid factor may cause a false-positive result.

Prevention and Treatment

Field trials of an attenuated CMV vaccine are in progress. The risk of serious CMV disease can be reduced in transplant recipients by use of CMV-seronegative donors and blood transfusions and by administration of prophylactic acyclovir, CMV-specific immunoglobulin, or ganciclovir (the latter in marrow recipients). In marrow recipients, administration of ganciclovir when CMV is detected in routinely obtained blood leukocyte cultures ("preemptive therapy") substantially reduces the risk of subsequent CMV disease. Ganciclovir (5 mg/kg twice daily intravenously) has proven efficacy for treatment of CMV retinitis in AIDS and probably in other forms of CMV disease. However, indefinite maintenance therapy with single daily infusions of 5 to 6 mg/kg of ganciclovir is virtually always necessary to prevent symptomatic relapse. CMV may become resistant to ganciclovir after multiple courses. Efficacy of ganciclovir for treatment of interstitial pneumonitis in marrow recipients is enhanced when it is combined with immunoglobulin. The main side effect of ganciclovir therapy is neutropenia. Foscarnet is available for use in treatment of CMV retinitis in AIDS and is active against ganciclovir-resistant strains of CMV. Its main side effects are nephrotoxicity, hypocalcemia, and seizures. Cidofovir has the advantage over the older agents in that it can be given once weekly for 2 weeks ("induction therapy") and then every other week during maintenance therapy.

EPSTEIN-BARR VIRUS
Epidemiology

Infections with EBV as measured by the presence of serum viral capsid antibody are extremely common throughout the world. In general, infection occurs early in life among individuals in lower socioeconomic groups and in developing countries. In some parts of the world virtually 100% of the population has had EBV infection by the age of 10 years. The vast majority of these infections are asymptomatic or perhaps associated with mild, nonspecific respiratory symptoms. Infectious mononucleosis occurs most often in older children or in young adults from the upper socioeconomic groups. The incidence is highest among university students and military cadets, where the rate of EBV infection among susceptible persons ranges from 12% to 30% per year. Infectious mononucleosis develops in approximately half of infected individuals. Presently the exact means of transmission of EBV is not well defined. On the basis of protracted shedding of virus in the oropharyngeal secretions of individuals recently infected, it appears likely that EBV is spread via the respiratory route. Relatively intimate contact (e.g., kissing) appears to be necessary. The incubation period of infectious mononucleosis appears to be 4 to 7 weeks. EBV may also be transmitted by blood transfusion, although transfusion-associated infections are much less common with EBV than with CMV.

Pathogenesis

Among the herpesviruses, EBV is unique in several respects. The virus cannot be propagated in conventional tissue culture cells. It does replicate in vitro in human B lymphocytes, although most of these cells are abortively infected (i.e., progeny virus is not produced and the cells are not lysed by EBV). The infected B cells are "immortalized" by the viral infection and proliferate indefinitely in vitro. In general, EBV infection of lymphocytes is a prerequisite for the immortalization response. Several new antigens appear on the membranes of EBV-infected B cells, including the nuclear antigen, the viral capsid antigen, and the lymphocyte-determined membrane antigen. EBV genetic material persists indefinitely in the form of an extrachromosomal plasmid, many copies of which are present in infected B lymphocytes.

The pathogenesis of infectious mononucleosis induced by infection with EBV is now understood to an extent, although several aspects remain to be defined. The virus is introduced into the susceptible host as a result of close contact (e.g., kissing) with another individual who is shedding EBV in the oropharynx. Initial virus replication occurs in the epithelial cells of the oropharynx and the salivary glands. A localized inflammatory response produces the pharyngeal exudate. Subsequently virus is carried via the lymphatics to local lymph nodes, and a viremia ensues. Local and generalized lymphad-

enopathy as well as splenomegaly then develop. Whether proliferation of lymphoid cells in these sites involves EBV-infected B cells themselves or is caused indirectly by "reactive" T cells is not yet clear. In the peripheral blood, EBV infection can be demonstrated in only a very small percentage of B cells. The vast majority of atypical lymphocytes, which are the hallmark of infectious mononucleosis, are T cells. These cells are apparently produced in response to infected B lymphocytes that express novel viral antigens on their surfaces. Initially, suppressor or cytotoxic T cells predominate in association with cutaneous anergy. Later, helper or inducer T cells are produced and correlate with eventual recovery. Production of the heterophil agglutinin, which is a macroglobulin, and several other aberrant antibodies results from polyclonal activation of infected B cells. Characteristically, EBV is shed in the oropharynx for many months after recovery from the clinical illness.

After initial subclinical infection or after infectious mononucleosis, EBV is permanently established in its latent form in B lymphocytes. In contrast to the other herpesviruses, in EBV infection no disease syndromes are clearly associated with reactivation of the dormant virus. However, EBV infection is strongly associated with several malignant disorders, including Burkitt's African lymphoma and nasopharyngeal carcinoma. High titers of EBV antibody are found in individuals with these diseases, and large quantities of viral DNA have been detected in the tumor cells. Non-Hodgkin's lymphomas in recipients of kidney, bone marrow, and heart transplants who receive immunosuppressive drugs on a long-term basis appear to be induced by EBV. A diffuse polyclonal lymphoma of the B-cell type has been described repeatedly in immunodeficient hosts, including recipients of organ transplants (particularly those receiving cyclosporin A), patients with severe combined immunodeficiency and ataxia-telangiectasia, and patients with AIDS. An X-linked lymphoproliferative syndrome has also been reported in males.

Clinical Features

Infectious Mononucleosis. The hallmark symptoms of infectious mononucleosis (IM) caused by EBV (EBV mononucleosis) include fever, fatigue, cervical adenopathy, and sore throat. The onset is often insidious, with the gradual development of increasing malaise, fever, and chills for less than a week, followed by the onset of pharyngitis. The pharyngitis may be mistaken for streptococcal infection. However, administration of ampicillin (and to a lesser extent other penicillins) results in the rapid appearance of a generalized maculopapular rash in the majority of patients with IM. Findings on physical examination often include periorbital edema; palatal petechiae; cervical, axillary, and epitrochlear lymphadenopathy; splenomegaly and hepatomegaly; and a variety of skin rashes. Rarely, IM caused by EBV may become evident as an aseptic meningitis or meningoencephalitis with a normal cerebrospinal fluid glucose level and a mononuclear pleocytosis. Neurologic manifestations of EBV infection, which occur in approximately 1% of patients, include Guillain-Barré syndrome, transverse myelitis, Bell's and other cranial nerve palsies, and mononeuritis multiplex. Hematologic complications include hemolytic anemia confirmed on Coombs' test and profound thrombocytopenia in less than 4% of cases. The acute splenic congestion and subcapsular hemorrhages in IM place patients at risk for splenic rupture caused by relatively minor trauma or exertion. The acute symptoms of EBV mononucleosis usually last from 2 to 4 weeks, although malaise, fatigue, and depression can be protracted and may be exacerbated by injudicious exercise. Splenomegaly and enlarged lymph nodes may persist for several months after the abatement of symptoms. In older adults EBV infection is more likely to be evident as a typhoidal illness with fever and malaise without splenomegaly or lymphadenopathy.

Laboratory features. The hallmark laboratory features of IM produced by EBV are the presence of heterophil antibodies, atypical lymphocytosis, and mildly elevated hepatic enzymes serum glutamate oxaloacetate transaminase [SGOT] and serum glutamate pyruvate transaminase [SGPT] levels. Heterophil antibodies are IgM antibodies, which selectively agglutinate erythrocytes of other species, including sheep red blood cells (the Paul Bunnell test) and horse red blood cells (the basis for the rapid agglutination or "monospot" test). Although these antibodies are usually detected at the time of presentation in more than 85% of patients with EBV infection, in a small number of patients the heterophil antibody test result may not be positive until 3 to 4 weeks after the onset of the illness. IM caused by EBV usually is characterized by leukocytosis ($>10^9$ cells/L) and relative and absolute lymphocytosis, and at least 10% of the lymphocytes have the characteristics of activated lymphocytes. The atypical lymphocytes characteristic of IM—"Downey cells"—are T lymphocytes with surface marker phenotypes of suppressor/cytotoxic T cells.

Diagnosis

Although the diagnosis presents little difficulty in most instances, there are several diagnostic pitfalls of which to be aware.

1. A diagnosis of streptococcal pharyngitis may be made if the systemic nature of the illness is not appreciated.
2. The heterophil agglutinin may take 3 to 4 weeks to appear.
3. Polymorphonuclear leukocytosis may be present initially, although many of the lymphocytes present are atypical.
4. Tonsillopharyngeal involvement, lymphadenopathy, and splenomegaly may be minimal or absent ("typhoidal" presentation).
5. The characteristic findings may be overshadowed by complicating features (neurologic manifestations, jaundice, thrombocytopenia with hemorrhage, hemolytic anemia, or splenic rupture).

In most cases the diagnosis of EBV mononucleosis is confirmed by the presence of heterophil antibody and atypical lymphocytosis. However, in heterophil-negative mononucleosis or in the absence of atypical lymphocytosis, EBV-specific serologic evaluation may be helpful. In these cases the presence of IgM antibodies against EBV is virtually diagnostic of acute infection, as is the development of antibody against the EBV nuclear antigen in paired sera. The absence of antibody against the viral capsid antigen of EBV after 2 weeks of illness excludes EBV infection.

CMV mononucleosis may closely mimic EBV-induced disease in terms of the hematologic manifestations, neurologic complications, production of aberrant antibodies, and ampicillin-induced rash. However, the heterophil test result is always negative. On clinical examination, CMV mononucleosis is characterized by less intense tonsillopharyngeal involvement (exudate is extremely uncommon) and lymphadenopathy. Other disorders that may have features similar to those of IM include toxoplasmosis, hepatitis A, adenovirus or herpes simplex, pharyngitis, enteroviral infections, Hodgkin's disease, angioimmunoblastic lymphadenopathy, and drug reactions (allopurinol, diphenylhydantoin, paraaminosalicylic acid, hydralazine, and methyldopa). In these entities, however, the atypical lymphocytosis is less intense and of much shorter duration.

Prevention and Treatment

There is currently no effective means of preventing EBV infection. EBV mononucleosis is usually a benign, self-limited illness in which treatment is confined to the relief of symptoms. Headache, fever, and painful pharyngitis should be treated with acetaminophen; aspirin should be avoided in EBV mononucleosis because of the risk of subcapsular splenic hemorrhage. Patients with EBV mononucleosis who have skin rashes after inadvertent administration of ampicillin should be reassured that the reaction is not a specific drug allergy and will not occur on rechallenge.

Treatment with oral corticosteroids (prednisone, 40 mg/day for 5 to 7 days) is indicated for patients with severe tonsillar enlargement that may result in upper airway obstruction. Parenteral administration of prednisone may be necessary if swallowing is difficult. Other indications for a brief course of corticosteroids are severe hemolytic anemia or thrombocytopenia and possibly aseptic meningitis or encephalitis. Corticosteroids do not benefit patients with protracted fatigue and malaise caused by EBV mononucleosis. Patients should be cautioned to avoid exertion during the acute illness and during convalescence. Relapses of fever and malaise commonly occur in patients who prematurely return to their customary level of activity.

HUMAN HERPESVIRUS 6

Human herpesvirus 6 (HHV-6) has been isolated from lymphocytes of patients with lymphoproliferative disorders and human immunodeficiency virus infection. Infection with HHV-6 appears to be relatively common among the normal population, where antibody prevalences of 20% to 40% have been detected. The virus has also been recovered from saliva of normal individuals. At present, no diseases have been definitively associated with the infection, except exanthem subitum (roseola infantum).

HUMAN HERPESVIRUS 8

Human herpesvirus 8 (HHV-8) has been detected by PCR amplification of viral DNA in essentially all forms of Kaposi's sarcoma (AIDS-related and more classic forms). DNA sequence analyses place HHV-8 in the β-herpesvirus subfamily, along with EBV and *Herpesvirus saimiri*, which cause lymphomas in humans and monkeys, respectively. Whether HHV-8 is the cause of Kaposi's sarcoma is not yet known. Peripheral blood mononuclear cells of patients with AIDS contain HHV-8 DNA, which is associated with an increased risk of development of Kaposi's sarcoma. Unusual serosal B-cell lymphomas that arise in the body cavities (chest and abdomen) of AIDS patients also contain HHV-8 DNA.

BIBLIOGRAPHY

Balfour H et al: Acyclovir halts progression of herpes zoster in immunocompromised patients, *N Engl J Med* 308:1448, 1983.

Brown ZA et al: Effects on infants of a first episode of genital herpes during pregnancy, *N Engl J Med* 317:1246, 1987.

Cesarman E et al: Kaposi's sarcoma–associated herpesvirus-like DNA sequences in AIDS-related body-cavity-based lymphomas, *N Engl J Med* 332:1186, 1995.

Corey L, Spear PG: Infections with herpes simplex viruses, *N Engl J Med* 314:686, 749, 1986.

Erice A et al: Progressive cytomegalovirus disease due to ganciclovir-resistant virus in immunocompromised patients, *N Engl J Med* 320:289, 1989.

Evans AS, Niederman JC, McCollum RW: Seroepidemiological studies of infectious mononucleosis with EB virus, *N Engl J Med* 279:1121, 1968.

Ho M: *Cytomegalovirus: biology and infection*, ed 2, New York, 1991, Plenum.

Holland GN et al: Cytomegalovirus diseases. In *Ocular immunity and infection*, ed 2, St Louis, 1996, Mosby.

Jacobson MA et al: Acyclovir-resistant varicella-zoster virus infection after chronic oral acyclovir therapy in patients with the acquired immunodeficiency syndrome, *Ann Intern Med* 112:187, 1990.

Jacobson MA, Mills J: Serious cytomegalovirus disease in the acquired immunodeficiency syndrome (AIDS), *Ann Intern Med* 108:585, 1988.

Jones JF et al: T-cell lymphomas containing Epstein-Barr virus DNA in patients with chronic Epstein-Barr virus infections, *N Engl J Med* 318:733, 1988.

Meyers JD, Fluornoy N, Thomas ED: Nonbacterial pneumonia after allogenic marrow transplantation: a review of 10 years' experience, *Rev Infect Dis* 4:1119, 1982.

Moore PS, Chang Y: Detection of herpesvirus-like DNA sequences in Kaposi's sarcoma in patients with and those without HIV infection, *N Engl J Med* 332:1181, 1995.

Prober CG et al: Use of routine viral cultures at delivery to identify neonates exposed to herpes simplex virus, *N Engl J Med* 318:887, 1988.

Stagno S et al: Congenital cytomegalovirus infection: the relative importance of primary and recurrent maternal infection, *N Engl J Med* 306:945, 1982.

Straus SE et al: Suppression of frequently recurring genital herpes: a placebo-controlled double-blind trial of oral acyclovir, *N Engl J Med* 310:1545, 1984.

Tyring S et al: Famciclovir for the treatment of acute herpes zoster: effects on acute disease and postherpetic neuralgia, *Ann Intern Med* 123:89, 1995.

Weller TH: Varicella and herpes zoster: changing concepts of the natural history, control, and importance of a not-so-benign virus, *N Engl J Med* 309:1362, 1434, 1983.

Whitley RJ et al: Vidarabine versus acyclovir therapy in herpes simplex encephalitis, *N Engl J Med* 314:144, 1986.

CHAPTER

256 **Human Retrovirus Infections**

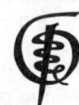

Jay A. Levy

Retroviruses have been found in association with three different pathologic conditions in humans: adult T-cell leukemia (ATL), tropical spastic paraparesis (TSP), and acquired immunodeficiency syndrome (AIDS). A retrovirus of an oncovirus type has been recovered from ATL patients, who are found primarily in southwestern Japan, the Caribbean basin, and certain areas of the southwestern United States. A similar agent isolated from patients with TSP has been frequently found in the Caribbean islands and Japan. A retrovirus with the biologic, morphologic, and molecular features of a lentivirus has been isolated from AIDS patients. Both of these human viruses preferentially replicate in human T cells. The virus associated with ATL induces the cells to divide continuously; the virus associated with AIDS causes cytopathic changes leading to cell death.

CHARACTERISTICS

A retrovirus is a 100-nm, lipid-enveloped, single-stranded ribonucleic acid (RNA) virus. Its genome consists of regions responsible for its assembly, including the gag (core region), pol (polymerase), env (envelope), and other portions coding for proteins that may be involved in replication and transformation. For example, with the AIDS virus,

certain accessory gene products have been identified (e.g., Vif, Nef, Tat, Rev) that can up-regulate or down-modulate virus replication. Likewise, certain regions of a retrovirus (oncogene or *onc*) may be responsible for the induction of cell transformation. Retroviruses derive their name from the presence of an enzyme (RNA-dependent deoxyribonucleic acid [DNA] polymerase or reverse transcriptase) that enables these viruses to make a copy DNA (cDNA) of their genomic RNA. This cDNA duplicates itself, circularizes, and subsequently integrates into the host cell chromosome. The virus then exists as a provirus in the cell and can be passed with the host genome to future cell generations.

By morphologic, biologic, and genetic properties the retrovirus family has been divided into seven genera, which include the oncoviruses, the spumaviruses, and the lentiviruses. The human retroviruses consist of the oncovirus associated with ATL, the retroviruses resembling a lentivirus found in AIDS, and the human foamy virus, a spumavirus. The latter, the first human retrovirus identified (in 1971), has not been associated with any disease in humans. Thus each of the three previously designated subfamilies of animal retroviruses has a human counterpart.

The ATL-associated retrovirus is characterized by its morphologic features when budding from the cell surface. An incomplete core is formed at the cell membrane, and the full virion develops by budding into immature and mature forms containing a nucleoid of about 92 nm (Fig. 256-1, *A* and *B*). The AIDS-associated lentivirus is characterized by a similar budding process, but the core can be complete before budding and the nucleoid in the mature form is cone-shaped (Fig. 256-1, *C* and *D*). Thus on cross section by electron microscopy, a lentivirus has a 42-nm core, but on tangential section it has a cone-shaped nucleoid (Fig. 256-1, *D*). Because of their lipid envelope, retroviruses are sensitive to polar solvents and heating in liquid form.

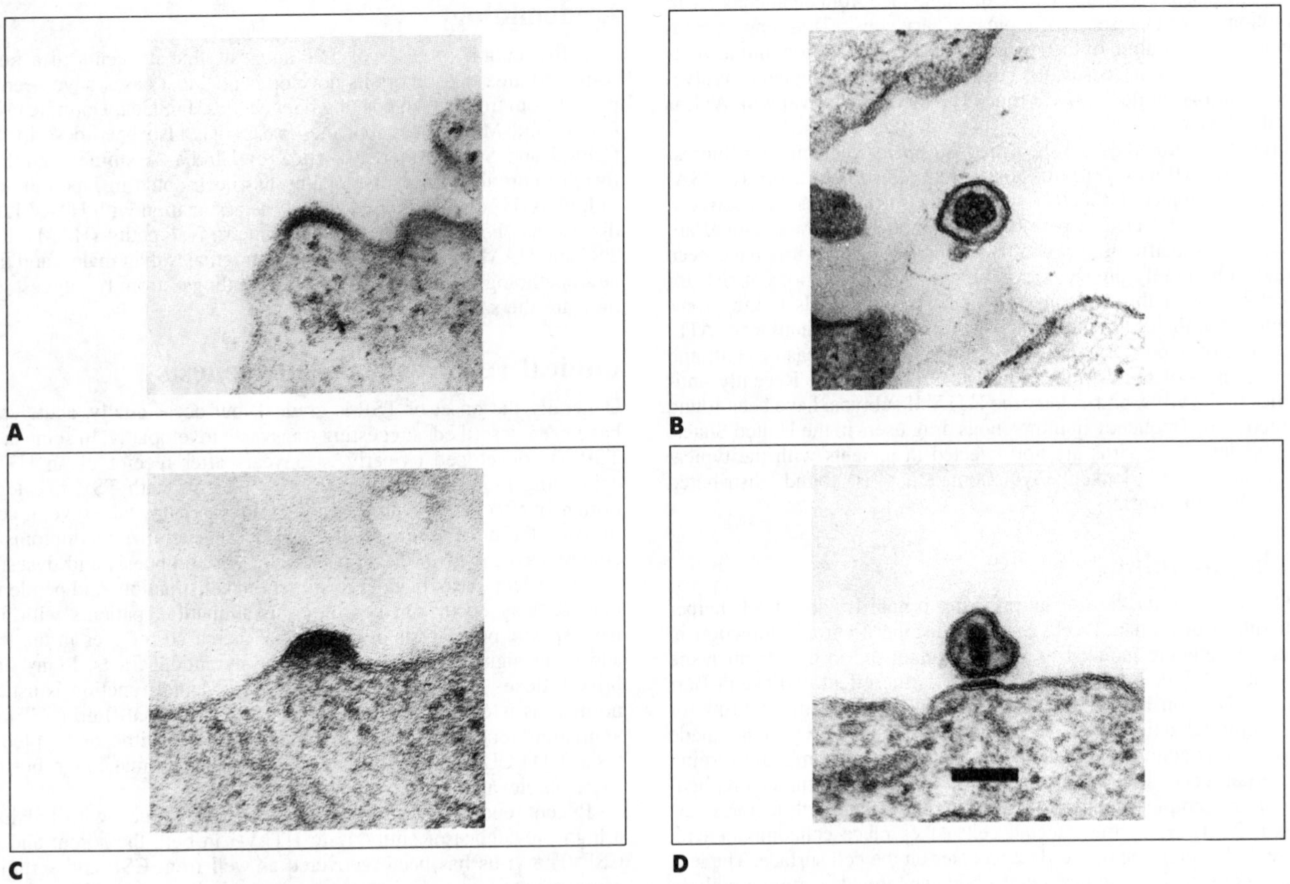

A

B

C

D

FIGURE 256-1   Electron micrographic examination of the human T-cell leukemia virus type I (HTLV-I) and the human immunodeficiency virus (HIV). **A,** Budding HTLV-I. **B,** Mature HTLV-I. **C,** Budding HIV type 1 (HIV-1). **D,** Mature HIV-1. Cone-shaped core is evident. Marker, 100 nm.

Photographs provided by Dr. Lyndon S. Oshiro, California State Public Health Laboratory, Berkeley.

However, when dried in the presence of proteins, they can withstand heating up to 68° C for several hours.

The retroviruses associated with human disease preferentially infect helper T cells but can infect other cells of the immune system. The AIDS retroviruses can also infect cells of the neurologic and gastrointestinal systems.

The human type C retrovirus associated with ATL has been called human T-cell leukemia virus type I (HTLV-I). It is also known as adult T-cell leukemia virus (ATLV) for the original isolate found in Japan. HTLV-II, which resembles HTLV-I, was recovered from a cell line established from a patient with hairy cell leukemia. HTLV-II appears to preferentially infect CD8+ T cells. This virus has not been consistently found associated with any disease.

The retrovirus recovered from AIDS patients is known as the human immunodeficiency virus (HIV) and is a lentivirus with morphologic, virologic, and molecular features distinct from the viruses responsible for ATL.

ADULT T-CELL LEUKEMIA
Epidemiology and Clinical Features

Adult T-cell leukemia has been a recognized disease entity since 1977. It occurs primarily in clusters in southern Japan, namely, the islands of Kyushu, Shikoku, and Okinawa (Chapter 92). The disease also is present with some frequency in blacks in the Caribbean basin and in individuals in the southeastern United States. By clinical and pathologic criteria, ATL encompasses human T-cell leukemias characterized by (1) onset in adulthood, (2) usually acute but somewhat chronic course, (3) leukemic cells with T-cell properties and pleiomorphic features (indented and lobulated nuclei are also frequently found), (4) lymphadenopathy and hepatosplenomegaly, (5) absence of mediastinal lymph node involvement, (6) frequent lytic changes in bone with hypercalcemia, and (7) in some cases leukemic cell infiltration of the skin. The disease generally can be distinguished from cutaneous T-cell lymphoma by (1) absence of typical Sézary cells, (2) absence of leukemic cell infiltration of the epidermis despite infiltration into the dermis or subcutaneous tissue, (3) bone marrow and pulmonary involvement, and (4) shorter survival time. The median survival with ATL is usually 1 year or less.

HTLV-I antibodies are measured by an indirect immunofluorescence assay (IFA) or enzyme-linked immunosorbent assay (ELISA) using virus-infected T cells or purified viral antigens, respectively. Virus can be detected in peripheral lymphocytes by monoclonal antibodies to specific viral proteins. Antibodies to the virus have been found to be highly prevalent in ATL patients; populations at risk for development of this leukemia, particularly individuals living in endemic areas in Japan; and family members of individuals with ATL. Evidence of exposure to the virus is also found in areas of Haiti and other islands of the Caribbean and in Central Africa. Recently antibodies to the virus, particularly the HTLV II subtype, have been found in increasing frequency in intravenous drug users in the United States. Antibodies to the virus are not detected in patients with the typical cutaneous T-cell leukemia/lymphoma that is found distributed throughout the world.

Pathophysiology

HTLV-I causes its disease by infecting primarily the CD4+ helper cell subset of human T cells and establishing a chronic infection in which T cells are induced to grow continuously. In this manner, the infection of T cells by HTLV-I resembles the effect of Epstein-Barr virus (EBV) on human B cells (Chapter 255). The mechanism for this immortalization is not yet known. It may involve proteins made by the virus acting at a distance from the viral genome and turning on certain genes in the virus or the cell to induce continuous replication. For example, production of the lymphocyte growth factor, interleukin 2 (IL-2), by the infected cells takes place concomitant with increased expression of the IL-2 recepter on the cell surface. The leukemic cells then spread through the body and invade certain lymphoid areas. The bone lesions in this disease may result from circulating humoral substances that induce osteoclastic activity rather than from invasion by malignant cells. Only very few HTLV-infected people de-

velop ATL. The reason for this difference in susceptibility to malignant changes in lymphocytes is not known.

HTLV-I also causes fusion of cells in tissue culture. It may use this mechanism for entering and spreading among lymphocytes and other cells in the body. The virus appears to be passed in the infected individual by cell-to-cell contact because cell-free transmission is a rare event in the laboratory. The T cells infected by the virus generally do not show evidence of this infection by expression of viral proteins in vivo. Virus is detected only after the cells are placed in culture. From experimental studies it is evident that many different T cells are initially infected, but eventually one autonomous clone grows out into the leukemic line. The route of transmission of the virus between individuals is unknown, but it may be passed via blood and body secretions (seminal and vaginal fluids) containing infected T cells. It can also be passed by milk from mother to child. The virus has been reported in mothers and their children and in spouses. It appears that many individuals are infected with the virus, and antibodies to it develop without causing leukemia. These antibodies can be of the virus-neutralizing type. In some individuals, antibodies to the virus have appeared 10 to 30 years before the development of leukemia. Because other types of T-cell leukemias are not associated with HTLV-I infection, the virus may act not as an initiator but as a cofactor in promoting the emergence of autonomous clones of malignant T cells.

Treatment

No specific therapy is available. Standard chemotherapy can lead to a prompt reduction in tumor cell mass, but long-term survival of patients is rare. Hypercalcemia can be managed with oral phosphates, calcitonin, or mithramycin.

TROPICAL SPASTIC PARAPARESIS
Epidemiology

The distribution of cases of TSP suggests that it occurs in a rather restricted area that favors its development. Most cases have been reported from tropical islands (e.g., Seychelles, Jamaica, Dominican Republic, and Martinique), but the disease has also been described in Central and South America, Africa, and India. A similar or related form of chronic spastic myelopathy has been noted in Japan in areas of high ATL prevalence. Because of the association with HTLV-I, this disease has been called HTLV-associated myelopathy (HAM). Both TSP and HAM occur more frequently in females than males, and their neuropathologic picture and clinical findings strongly suggest that they are the same syndrome.

Clinical Features and Pathogenesis

Generally the onset of TSP is gradual, but occasionally, acute cases have been described, suggesting transverse myelopathy. In some cases TSP has developed as early as 3 years after receipt of an HTLV-containing blood transfusion. In most patients with TSP, one leg is primarily affected. The progression is slow and may take several years to reach the most severe level of disease. Generalized symptoms include weakness of the legs, back pain, leg numbness, and dysesthesia of the feet. Also, bladder dysfunction, constipation, and penile impotence may occur. On neurologic examination, patients with TSP have spastic paraparesis or paraplegia, increased reflexes in the legs, and other signs of involvement of the pyramidal tracts. Many have brisk reflexes in the upper limbs as well. Mental function is usually normal, as is cranial nerve function. Cerebral spinal fluid (CSF) examination generally yields normal findings with little or no pleocytosis. CD4/CD8 cell ratios are usually in the normal range but can show an elevated CD4 lymphocyte value.

Recent reports have now confirmed that individuals with TSP have a high prevalence of antibody to HTLV-I in both the serum and the CSF. The virus has been recovered as well from CSF and serum of some patients, and the isolates are very similar to the HTLV-I associated with ATL. All this information emphasizes the potential neuropathic effects of HTLV-I. The pathogenesis involved in the disease is not known. Perivascular cuffing of some small vessels by lymphocytes penetrating the central nervous system has been reported, as well as demyelination of the spinal cord and brain. The disease may result from direct infection of nerve cells by the virus, secondary effects of autoimmune responses, or inflammation caused by infiltrating HTLV-I–containing cells present in the spinal cord. Because high levels of antibodies to HTLV are associated with TSP, a hypothesized autoimmune or immunologic mechanism has been favored. Neurologic cases with antibodies to HTLV-I are being classified as a separate group to follow their prognosis and potentially specific clinical features.

Treatment

Some patients with TSP have shown improvement with prednisone, but whether corticosteroids or other immunosuppressive agents can be helpful is not clear. Other drugs being considered are antiretroviral agents, such as 3-azidothymidine (Zidovudine, AZT).

ACQUIRED IMMUNODEFICIENCY SYNDROME
Epidemiology

Acquired immunodeficiency syndrome was first recognized in the United States in 1981, when *Pneumocystis carinii* pneumonia and/or Kaposi's sarcoma was identified in an unusually large number of homosexual men (Chapter 248). Subsequently these conditions, as well as B-cell lymphomas, in some patients were found to be associated with an acquired immunodeficiency state that on epidemiologic study appeared to be spread by a virus. Retrospective studies identified AIDS cases initially in New York, Haiti, and Africa as early as 1978. Initially the individuals primarily at risk in Western countries were homosexual and bisexual men (73%) and intravenous drug abusers (17%). The disease was also found in recipients of blood transfusions and blood products (hemophilia A and B patients), in heterosexual contacts of infected individuals, and in infants born of mothers who were in one of the risk groups (Chapter 248). These findings supported the conclusion that transmission occurred by intimate sexual activity, blood, and intrauterine exposure. In Africa, heterosexual activity is the major source of virus transmission, most likely because of the concomitant presence of venereal diseases. At present, heterosexual transmission has increased substantially in developed countries, but blood-derived cases (e.g., transfusion and hemophilia) have been essentially prevented by screening of blood donors and donations and the heat treatment of blood products.

Pathophysiology

The human immunodeficiency virus has a host range that involves preferential infection and replication in human T cells with the helper-cell phenotype. However, the virus can also infect other immune cells such as macrophages, and B lymphocytes, particularly if they carry the helper cell (OKT4A, Leu 3) marker. This CD4 protein may be a major receptor for attachment of the virus to cells. Other cellular receptors for HIV are probably present because CD4-negative cells (e.g., fibroblasts, bowel, and glial cells) can be infected by the virus. One alternative receptor in brain- and bowel-derived cells has been identified as galactosyl ceramide. Most recently, co-receptors for HIV infection have been identified. They include the chemokine receptors, CCR5 and CXCR4. The co-receptors are utilized by different HIV strains to enter a cell after virus attachment to CD4. The virus causes a cytopathic effect in lymphocytes, leading to fusion and formation of mononucleated cells, which eventually die. This preferential infection of certain helper T cells contributes to a gradual reduction in the helper T-cell number and a reversal of helper/suppressor T-cell ratios (normally 2:1) to less than 1.0, as observed in AIDS patients. Autoantibodies to helper T cells may also have a role in this disorder. This deficit in immune function leads to the opportunistic infections and cancers (B-cell lymphomas, Kaposi's sarcoma) characteristic of AIDS. Cofactors such as infection with EBV and cytomegalovirus (CMV) also appear important in depressing the helper/suppressor T-cell ratios in AIDS. These viruses alone can cause these changes in T-cell ratios (Chapter 248). The AIDS retrovirus can also infect the central nervous system, where it gives rise to neurologic syndromes, including headaches, dementia, global encephalopathy,

and sensory neuropathy. Cerebrospinal fluids contain the AIDS virus and show generally elevated protein levels without pleocytosis. Vacuolating myelopathy in the spinal cord of some patients has been described and appears to be caused directly by the virus.

Chronic diarrhea is a common symptom in individuals infected with HIV. In Africa it has been termed "slim disease." Some studies indicate direct infection of crypt cells of the bowel (including enterochromaffin cells) by the virus. This finding may explain the malabsorption and fluid loss observed in some infected individuals.

Transmission of HIV occurs via blood and body secretions, particularly seminal fluid. Unlike HTLV-I, the AIDS retrovirus can be transferred in a cell-free state, but the virus-infected cell appears to be the major source of transmission. The virus has been isolated in very small amounts from saliva, but epidemiologic evidence does not suggest this route as a mechanism for its spread. Studies in Africa strongly suggest that a major cofactor for heterosexual transmission is venereal disease, particularly genital ulcers caused by herpes virus or by *Haemophilus ducreyi* (chancroid), as well as the increased number of virus-infected cells in genital fluids associated with the inflammation.

Antibodies to HIV develop days to weeks after the infection, and, rarely, individuals without anti-HIV antibodies who are healthy on clinical examination can be found with virus in their lymphocytes and plasma. Most individuals experience seroconversion within 1 to 3 months after infection, and it is generally agreed that by 6 months all infected individuals show antibodies to the virus. Asymptomatic individuals probably handle HIV infection by the following different mechanisms: (1) On very rare occasions, they ward off the infection and eliminate the virus. (2) They keep the virus latent in the system, as with EBV infection of B lymphocytes. (3) They are "carriers" of the virus and can pass it to others through seminal (and vaginal) fluid and blood. (4) They are healthy except for a persistent lymphadenopathy, which reflects infection with the virus and perhaps a host response to the agent. The lymphadenopathy syndrome may represent an immunologic reaction of the individual against the virus because individuals who have shown no lymphadenopathy and develop AIDS often have a much more contracted course.

Neutralizing antibodies are produced against the virus in some individuals, but the virus envelope may change rapidly, enough to escape their protective effect. Antibodies to other HIV proteins are present in nearly all individuals with AIDS and can be detected by IFA, ELISA, Western blot, and radioimmune precipitation tests using virus-infected cells or purified viral antigens. Antibody levels decrease with severity of disease and may be extremely low at death, when most of the antibody-producing cells have been reduced by the overwhelming virus and opportunistic infections. Like HTLV-I, the AIDS retrovirus can remain with minimal expression in clinically healthy individuals but then gradually (or suddenly) replicate to high levels associated with the immune abnormalities and clinical findings characteristic of AIDS. The CD8+ lymphocyte may be an important cell involved in suppressing this virus replication and preventing the subsequent induction of disease. Thus variations in the virus (e.g., its pathogenic potential) and the host (e.g., immunologic response) determine progression to disease.

Kaposi's sarcoma could result from the release by normal cells of immune-modulating factors with angiogenesis-promoting activity. These factors may induce endothelial cell proliferation leading to Kaposi's sarcoma. Similarly, the B-cell lymphomas may be caused by hyperresponsive immune cells with cytokine production which results from the compromise of the T-cell function that generally controls B-cell growth. In Kaposi's sarcoma a new human herpesvirus (HHV-8) has recently been discovered that may play a role as an initiator or a promoter of the disease. EBV may have a similar function in B-cell lymphomas (Chapter 255).

Clinical Features

AIDS is characterized by a deficit in the cellular immune system, including T cells, B cells, and macrophages. The T cells involved are primarily those of the helper subset. The pathologic features of AIDS (as outlined previously) involve a destruction of immune mechanisms, which permits the superinfection of individuals with a variety of organisms normally not pathogenic to humans, including *P. carinii*, CMV mycobacteria, toxoplasma, and certain intestinal parasites. Malignancies, as noted, also can appear in infected individuals. In some people neurologic symptoms such as encephalopathy and dementia can appear without major abnormalities in the immune system. Moreover, some patients have primarily gastrointestinal tract problems caused in some cases by direct infection of the bowel by HIV. Most recent studies suggest that it takes at least 10 years for AIDS to develop in 50% of infected individuals; 25% will have symptoms, and the rest will still be healthy on clinical examination. In the latter group a number of long-term survivors have been identified who have been clinically healthy for more than 10 years and have normal CD4+ cell counts without antiviral therapy. These people, also called long-term nonprogressors, have low virus levels in their blood and strong cellular anti-HIV immune responses. The latter activity seems to be responsible for their long-term survival.

Diagnosis

Epidemiologic, clinical, pathologic, and sociologic factors are important in making the diagnosis of AIDS. AIDS, as defined by the Centers for Disease Control and Prevention, includes a very low CD4+ cell count and/or the presence of specific opportunistic infections and cancer (Chapter 248). Definitive proof of retrovirus infection can be obtained through the study of antibodies to HIV or isolation of the virus from blood. However, as with HTLV-I, antibodies to the agent in clinically healthy individuals cannot yet be interpreted conclusively in terms of the chance of developing AIDS.

Treatment and Prevention

There is no curative treatment yet for AIDS. Several attempts with antiretrovirus compounds have met with some success in reducing symptoms and prolonging life. New drugs and approaches against the opportunistic infections have been particularly helpful. The anti–reverse transcriptase drug AZT was the first drug to show promise in prolonging a healthy state in individuals with HIV infection. In some cases it extends life, but usually viral resistance to AZT develops. Thus recent therapeutic approaches include the use of two or three drugs in treatment. Other anti–reverse transcriptase inhibitors and drugs against the viral protease are now being evaluated. Immune-modulating factors (e.g., interferon and IL-2) have not been universally helpful but are receiving further consideration. Prevention has been achieved through selection of blood and blood products that are free of the virus and emphasized by recommended avoidance of contact with body fluids from virus-infected individuals. Studies have shown that heating (68° C) lyophilized factor VIII and factor IX products for several hours eliminates infectious virus. No vaccine is yet available.

BIBLIOGRAPHY

Barre-Sinoussi F et al: Isolation of a T-lymphotropic retrovirus from a patient at risk for acquired immune deficiency syndrome (AIDS), *Science* 220:868, 1983.

Franchini G: Molecular mechanisms of human T-cell leukemia/lymphotropic virus type I infection, *Blood* 88:5619, 1995.

Gallo et al: Frequent detection and isolation of cytopathic retrovirus (HTLV-III) from patients with AIDS and at risk for AIDS, *Science* 224:500, 1984.

Levy JA et al: Isolation of lymphocytopathic retroviruses from San Francisco patients with AIDS, *Science* 225:840, 1984.

Levy JA: Infection by human immunodeficiency virus—CD4 is not enough, *N Engl J Med* 335:1528, 1996.

Levy JA: *HIV and the pathogenesis of AIDS*, Washington, DC, 1997; ASM Press.

Lochelt M, Flugel RM: The molecular biology of human and primate spuma retroviruses. In Levy JA, editor: *The retroviridae*, vol 4, New York, 1995, Plenum.

Poiesz BJ et al: Detection and isolation of type C retrovirus particles from fresh and cultured lymphocytes of a patient with cutaneous T cell lymphoma, *Proc Natl Acad Sci U S A* 7:7415, 1980.

Roman GC: The neuroepidemiology of tropical spastic paraparesis, *Ann Neurol* 23:S113, 1988.

Sugamura K, Hinuma Y: Human retroviruses: HTLV-I and HTLV-II. In Levy JA, editor: *The retroviridae*, vol 2, New York, 1993, Plenum.

Yoshida M et al: Viruses detected in HTLV-1–associated myelopathy and adult T-cell leukaemia are identical on DNA blotting assay, *Lancet* 1:1085, 1987.

CHLAMYDIAL AND MYCOPLASMAL DISEASES

CHLAMYDIAL DISEASES

CHAPTER

257 Chlamydial Infections

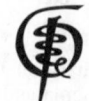

Julius Schachter

CLASSIFICATION

The chlamydiae are members of a genus of obligate, intracellular, gram-negative bacteria that are distinguished from all other bacteria by a unique growth cycle. They are placed in their own order, Chlamydiales, in the family Chlamydiaceae, with a single genus, *Chlamydia*, having four species, *C. psittaci, C. trachomatis, C. pneumoniae,* and *C. pecorum.* Only the first three are recognized as human pathogens. *C. trachomatis* is sensitive to sulfonamides, produces inclusions that stain with iodine because they contain a glycogen-like material, and causes trachoma, conjunctivitis, and pneumonia in infants and several sexually transmitted diseases in adults. *C. psittaci,* on the other hand, is resistant to sulfonamides; its inclusions do not contain enough glycogen to stain with iodine, and it causes psittacosis in humans. What were called the TWAR strains of *C. psittaci* have been classified as a new species, *C. pneumoniae,* based on morphologic features and lack of DNA relatedness.

CHARACTERISTICS

The chlamydial infectious particle is a coccal elementary body that is approximately 250 to 400 nm in diameter. *C. pneumoniae* elementary bodies are pear shaped. It attaches to the host cells in a process that may involve specific receptor sites. The coccal elementary body is then ingested by the susceptible host cell. This uptake process is selective and is induced by the chlamydiae. The chlamydiae remain within an endosome throughout their developmental cycle. Chlamydiae suppress phagolysosomal fusion. The entire growth cycle of the *Chlamydia* organism takes approximately 48 hours. During the first 8 hours the infecting particle changes into a larger (approximately 1 μm in diameter), ribonucleic acid (RNA)–rich reticulate particle that is metabolically active and divides by binary fission. The reticulate particles are noninfectious. Metabolic processes of the chlamydiae peak between 8 and 24 hours. At approximately 24 hours the reticulate bodies (also called initial bodies) begin to condense into infectious elementary bodies. At approximately 48 hours the inclusion bursts and releases the infectious coccal elementary body progeny.

C. psittaci contains many serologic types and biovars. There are no convenient laboratory methods for identifying these types; thus their relevance in different diseases and conditions in humans or animals cannot be determined. Only one *C. pneumoniae* serovar has been identified. With *C. trachomatis,* however, serovars have been identified by two tests: a mouse toxicity prevention test and a microimmunofluorescence test. It has been found that four of the *C. trachomatis* serovars (A, B, Ba, and C) are associated with endemic trachoma. Three of the serovars (L1, L2, and L3) are the causative agents of lymphogranuloma venereum (LGV) and represent a separate biovar (in terms of pathogenicity and receptor sites) within *C. trachomatis.* The other serovars of *C. trachomatis* (D to K) are usually transmitted sexually. Monoclonal antibodies to most of the serovars are available.

ECOLOGIC NICHE: EPIDEMIOLOGY
Chlamydia psittaci

C. psittaci is a common pathogen of domestic and feral mammals, in which it causes a wide variety of diseases. Most chlamydiae are transmitted by a fecal-oral or respiratory route. In their infectious cycles they often colonize the gastrointestinal tract. These mammalian chlamydiae, although economically significant because of the morbidity they produce in domestic mammals, are of little significance in terms of human health.

C. psittaci is virtually ubiquitous among avian species: more than 130 different avian species have been identified as hosts. Although the respiratory tract of birds may be infected, the infections are usually gastrointestinal. Inapparent or latent infections are common in birds or mammals. Stress (e.g., caused by crowding, aging, nutritional deficits, or breeding) may activate the inapparent infection, resulting in clinical evidence of disease. Healthy carriers or diseased birds may shed *C. psittaci* in feces. Because *C. psittaci* is highly stable, this shedding may result in environmental contamination.

C. psittaci strains of avian origin are highly infectious for humans, in whom they produce the disease psittacosis. Human respiratory tract infection usually results from exposure to aerosols of infective feces. The term *psittacosis* has been used historically to refer to *C. psittaci* infection in human or psittacine species, whereas the term *ornithosis* has been used to designate this infection in extrapsittacine birds. Exotic pet birds are often the reservoir for human infections. Poultry, particularly turkeys in the United States and ducks in eastern Europe, have also been important sources of human infection with *C. psittaci*. This infection may be considered an occupational hazard and is particularly important to those working in poultry processing plants.

Chlamydia pneumoniae

C. pneumoniae appears to have no animal reservoir. Apparently it is exclusively a human pathogen, although similar strains have been reported in horses and koalas. Seroepidemiologic studies indicate that infections are acquired relatively early in childhood. Seroprevalence rates reach 30% to 45% in many communities, indicating that exposure to this organism is common in most parts of the world.

Chlamydia trachomatis

C. trachomatis is considered exclusively a human pathogen, but similar strains have been isolated from swine and rodents. The agent is spread by close personal contact. In trachoma-endemic areas *C. trachomatis* is spread from child to child or within families in households. Moisture-seeking flies that feed on ocular discharges may act as mechanical vectors. In adults (particularly in industrialized societies) *C. trachomatis* is largely transmitted by sexual activity and is one of the most common of the sexually transmitted pathogens. In the United States the current estimate is that 4.5 million infections occur each year.

Vertical transmission of *C. trachomatis* also occurs. An infant born through an infected birth canal may acquire the infection. In the infant the eye, upper and lower respiratory tracts, gastrointestinal tract, and vagina may be infected.

Although chlamydial infections may cause severe disease, clinically inapparent infections are common. In adults, inapparent infection occurs in both the male urethra and the female cervix. In infants, clinically inapparent nasopharyngeal infections appear to be common, as do, to a lesser extent, gastrointestinal tract infections.

PATHOPHYSIOLOGY

Although some virulence factors are associated with the chlamydiae (i.e., surface antigens that appear to induce phagocytosis and prevent phagolysosomal fusion), there is no clear understanding of the pathogenesis of human chlamydial disease. *C. psittaci* strains appear to have a broad host-cell spectrum in vivo and are often found replicating within mononuclear phagocytic cells. *C. trachomatis* (with the exception of LGV strains) appears to be restricted to columnar epithelial cells for replication. All chlamydial species are cytocidal in that they kill cells as part of their growth cycle. It is probable that much of the disease associated with *C. trachomatis* represents the host's inflammatory reaction to this lethal effect of chlamydial infection on some of its cells. LGV strains cause far more damage and are far more invasive than the other *C. trachomatis* strains. *C. psittaci* strains are more destructive than *C. trachomatis* strains.

There is an abundant immune response to chlamydial infection, although immunity to these infections is poor and highly specific. Challenge infection with heterologous serovars may result in more severe disease (as may homologous reinfection when immunity wanes). Animal experiments suggest that the hypersensitivity or hyperreactivity seen in second infections is a response to a genus-specific antigen. A heat shock protein related to the groEL antigens has been identified as a sensitizing antigen candidate.

DISEASES PRODUCED IN HUMANS
Chlamydia psittaci

Human infection with *C. psittaci* (psittacosis) has two clinical forms. The one most commonly recognized is a form of atypical pneumonia, which is often termed *flu-like* and is characterized by fever, severe headache, nonproductive cough, and a protracted course. The second form of human psittacosis is often referred to as a typhoidal or toxic disease. It lacks the respiratory component and is characterized by severe headache, a protracted course, fever, and chills. In either instance the pulse rate may be slow relative to the fever. Hepatosplenomegaly is common. Hepatitis, myocarditis, endocarditis, and meningitis are among the many complications known to occur.

Chlamydia pneumoniae

C. pneumoniae appears to cause a respiratory disease in young adults that is indistinguishable on clinical examination from atypical pneumonia caused by *Mycoplasma pneumoniae* (Chapter 258). The symptoms may include severe pharyngitis. Severe, even fatal, pneumonias may occur in older individuals with underlying disease. The potential role of *C. pneumoniae* in inducing asthma is being actively investigated. Because the organism is such a common pathogen, many studies have suggested a broader clinical spectrum, including coronary disease and pneumonia in acquired immunodeficiency syndrome (AIDS) cases. Further studies are needed to define a chlamydial role in these conditions.

Chlamydia trachomatis

Lymphogranuloma Venereum. Lymphogranuloma venereum is a systemic, sexually transmitted infection (Chapter 244). In males, the disease usually becomes evident as inguinal lymphadenopathy. The male:female ratio for inguinal buboes is often as high as 20:1. Systemic signs, such as fever, shaking chills, and severe headache, are often associated with the inguinal lymphadenopathy. The disease is often described in stages. A primary lesion (a shallow ulcer or vesicle on the penis) is the first sign of the infection. The appearance of a bubo is the secondary stage, and the late sequelae, such as proctitis, rectal strictures, and proctocolitis, represent the tertiary stage. In the female, the vaginal tract's lymphoid drainage is retroperitoneal, so inguinal lymphadenopathy does not usually develop in women. Women are seen with late complications of LGV, such as perirectal strictures or the anogenital syndrome, which may involve stricture, proctitis, or rectovaginal fistula. These conditions result from a combination of inflammation, tissue destruction, and fibrosis. Although proctocolitis is generally considered one of the later lesions, a relatively severe form (often associated with weight loss and fever) may be seen as an early form of LGV in homosexual males.

Such complications as hepatitis and joint and central nervous system involvement are known. Lymphadenopathy may occur at many sites. For example, ocular infection may result in a diagnosis of Parinaud's oculoglandular syndrome. Respiratory tract infection has been a common result of exposure produced by laboratory accident.

Trachoma. Trachoma is a chronic follicular conjunctivitis that may afflict all members of a community or household in hyperendemic areas. Active disease is seen in young children, and virtually all of them will be infected before they are 2 years old. (This pattern changes; as living conditions improve, the age of onset of disease increases.) The infection is chronic, and reinfections may follow spontaneous clearance. The natural tendency of chlamydial infections to decrease in severity is interfered with by the secondary bacterial infections (pneumococci, *Haemophilus influenzae, Haemophilus aegyptius,* and *Moraxella* species) that are often common and may be seasonal in trachoma-endemic regions. As a result of severe trachoma, there may be necrosis that produces conjunctival scarring. Although the active disease occurs in young children, blindness occurs in adults. It takes many years for the shrinkage of scars to turn the upper lid inward so that the eyelashes abrade the cornea. These lesions, trichiasis and entropion, are the blinding lesions of trachoma.

***Chlamydia trachomatis* in the Male Genital Tract.** The most common disease resulting from *C. trachomatis* infection in men is nongonococcal urethritis (Chapter 244). This condition may be clinically indistinguishable from gonorrhea, although there is a tendency for the discharge to be scanty and mucoid rather than frankly purulent. *C. trachomatis* is the major cause of acute epididymitis in young men. Rectal infection may result in proctitis.

Many men with gonorrhea have concomitant chlamydial infection. If these men are given treatment with penicillin, which is not active against chlamydiae, postgonococcal urethritis, a specific subset of nongonococcal urethritis, usually develops.

***Chlamydia trachomatis* in the Female Genital Tract.** The cervix is the most common site of chlamydial infection in women. There are no pathognomonic findings to indicate the presence of the infection, and inapparent infections occur. When disease develops, it is an endocervicitis, and *C. trachomatis* may be significantly associated with a mucopurulent endocervical discharge and hypertrophic cervical erosions. Many women with chlamydial infections have involvement of the urethra, and dysuria is a common symptom. Chlamydia may cause bartholinitis. *C. trachomatis* is also a cause of infection in the upper female genital tract. The organism clearly causes endometritis, although data concerning the frequency of this condition are not available. *C. trachomatis,* however, is a major cause of acute salpingitis and appears to be the leading cause of perihepatitis (Fitz-Hugh–Curtis syndrome). Chlamydial salpingitis is usually milder than salpingitis caused by gonococci or anaerobes, but the risk of infertility appears to be approximately the same for chlamydial salpingitis as for other forms. Chlamydial salpingitis can be clinically inapparent. Many women who have tubal factor infertility or ectopic pregnancy have no history of acute salpingitis but show serologic evidence of previous chlamydial infection. Because of the inability to make an early diagnosis and because the condition is of polymicrobial origin, therapy for salpingitis should include antibiotics that are active against chlamydiae as well as the other causative agents.

Inclusion Conjunctivitis. Inclusion conjunctivitis occurs in infants or adults who are exposed to infected genital tract discharges. An acute mucopurulent conjunctivitis develops in the infant approximately 5 to 14 days after birth. If the infection is untreated, it tends to be self-limited, usually resolving within 2 months. In some infants, however, chronic infections that may threaten sight develop. In infants who do not receive treatment early, some scarring of the conjunctiva and a micropannus may develop, although there is usually no deleterious effect on vision.

Acute follicular conjunctivitis develops in adults (infants usually do not have follicular conjunctivitis until they are 1 to 2 months of age) and persists for months. Keratitis and micropannus are common. In severe cases the disease is clinically indistinguishable from acute trachoma.

Extraocular Infection in Infants. The most severe chlamydial disease in infants is a characteristic pneumonia syndrome, which can develop between the ages of 2 weeks and 4 months. The infants are afebrile, have a protracted course, and have tachypnea (occasionally apnea) and a dry, hacking cough. Many of the infants have conjunctivitis that is indicated either by history or by examination. Some of these pneumonias are associated with an acute serous otitis media. Radiographs show a diffuse interstitial pneumonia with hyperinflation. Elevated levels of immunoglobulins are usually found (particu-

larly immunoglobulin M [IgM]), and a relative eosinophilia is common. Although chlamydial pneumonia is not a life-threatening disease, affected infants may have permanent lung damage. Rhinitis and bronchiolitis are part of the spectrum of chlamydial infections of the respiratory tract in infants, but the incidence of these conditions is not known. Rectal and vaginal infections occur but have not been clearly associated with disease at these sites.

Respiratory Tract Infections in Adults

Serologic studies have implicated *C. trachomatis* as a cause of acute pharyngitis or pneumonia in adults. It is probable that most of these studies were actually detecting cross-reacting, genus-specific antibodies to *C. pneumoniae,* which is now recognized as a common respiratory tract pathogen. Occasionally, *C. trachomatis* has been isolated from lungs of patients with pneumonia and AIDS.

PERTINENT DIAGNOSTIC TESTS

Methods of diagnosing chlamydial infection are essentially the same as those used for diagnosing other bacterial diseases. The agent may be demonstrated directly in tissue samples. This does not apply to human psittacosis, but some of the infections with *C. trachomatis* may be diagnosed by appropriate staining of epithelial cell scrapings (Plate VIII-11). It is imperative that an adequate sample of epithelial cells be obtained to demonstrate the characteristic intracytoplasmic inclusions. Giemsa stain can be of particular use in identifying inclusion conjunctivitis in infants and in adults. Acute trachoma may also be diagnosed on cytologic study. Cytologic procedures are not routinely useful for diagnosing genital tract infections; isolation is much more sensitive. A number of nonculture diagnostic tests are available. The most commonly used tests are based on antigen detection and include enzyme immunoassay for genus-specific lipopolysaccharide (LPS) and use of fluorescein-conjugated monoclonal antibodies against a *Chlamydia* species–specific antigen to detect elementary bodies in clinical specimens. These tests have a sensitivity of 80% to 90% and specificity of about 97%, as compared with culture for diagnosis of genital tract infections. They offer the possibility of placing chlamydial diagnosis in laboratories that currently cannot perform tissue culture. Antigen detection methods seem best suited for use in high-risk populations. Because of potential false-positive results, these antigen detection methods should not be used in low-prevalence settings, where the results may have medicolegal implications. In moderate-risk and low-risk populations the positive nonculture test results should be considered presumptive and should be confirmed by either a confirmatory assay or another test based on a different principle. In high-prevalence settings such as sexually transmitted disease clinics the results of the initial test may be accepted.

Direct DNA probes are commercially available but are about as sensitive as antigen detection methods. Recently introduced DNA amplification procedures, polymerase chain reaction (PCR) and ligase chain reaction (LCR), are more sensitive than isolation. Both tests are highly specific. First-catch urine specimens have been found to be useful for screening asymptomatic men and women with these highly sensitive tests. Because the tests are expensive, research is being conducted to determine how to best use them.

Serologic tests are usually useful in diagnosing psittacosis, *C. pneumoniae* infection, and LGV in which exuberant antibody responses are seen. Paired acute and convalescent sera usually show a fourfold rise in complement-fixing antibodies when the patient has psittacosis. With LGV, very high titer levels are seen, but it is difficult to demonstrate rising titer levels because patients are usually examined well into the course of the disease. Genital tract infections with *C. trachomatis* are seldom diagnosed on serologic study because of the high prevalence of antibodies in sexually active populations and the chronic nature of the disease. This makes it difficult to time the collection of paired serum specimens appropriately. In patients having their first bouts of the disease, seroconversion is usually demonstrated, but microimmunofluorescence techniques must be used because the complement-fixation procedure is too insensitive. Serodiagnosis may be more useful for the systemic complications of *C. trachomatis* infections (epididymitis in men, salpingitis in women, pneumonia in infants) than for the more common superficial mucous

Table 257-1 Treatment of chlamydial infection

ORGANISM AND CONDITION	FIRST CHOICE		SECOND CHOICE	
	DRUG	DOSAGE	DRUG	DOSAGE
C. psittaci; Psittacosis	Tetracycline	500 mg qid × 3 weeks	Erythromycin	250 mg qid × 3 weeks
C. trachomatis				
LGV strains	Tetracycline	500 mg qid × 3 weeks	Sulfamethoxazole	1 g bid × 3 weeks
Non-LGV strains				
Genital tract infections	Doxycycline	100 mg bid × 1 week	Azithromycin	1 g orally
Pregnant women	Erythromycin	500 mg qid × 1 week	Amoxicillin	500 mg tid × 1 week
Infant pneumonia	Erythromycin	10 mg/kg qid × 2 weeks	Sulfisoxazole	37.5 mg/kg qid × 2 weeks
Inclusion conjunctivitis (infants)	Erythromycin	10 mg/kg qid × 2 weeks	Sulfisoxazole	37.5 mg/kg qid × 2 weeks
Inclusion conjunctivitis (adults)	Tetracycline	250 mg qid × 3 weeks	Erythromycin	250 mg qid × 3 weeks

LGV, Lymphogranuloma venereum; *bid,* twice a day; *qid,* four times a day; *tid,* three times a day.

membrane infections. The systemic infections result in higher levels of immunoglobulin G (IgG) or IgM antibodies, and in infants IgM antibody titers are particularly useful. Infants with *Chlamydia* pneumonia may show relative eosinophilia, and they virtually always have elevated serum globulin levels, particularly those of the IgM class.

Isolation of the infectious agent is seldom accomplished with *C. psittaci. C. pneumoniae* is particularly difficult to isolate, although use of HL or Hep-2 cells improves recovery. Because of superficial localization, *C. trachomatis* agents may be readily isolated. Inoculation of the collected specimens into McCoy cells treated with cycloheximide enhances chlamydial replication. Specimens containing epithelial cells must be collected directly from the involved site. Culture of discharges is less than optimal. Sensitivity of cultures probably varies by the site and the disease involved. It is probably as high as 95% for inclusion conjunctivitis of newborns but, more likely, between 70% and 80% for uncomplicated genital tract infections; because of sampling problems, it certainly would be less than that for some of the systemic complications of *C. trachomatis* infections.

TREATMENT

The treatment of choice for any chlamydial infection of adults is considered to be tetracycline (Table 257-1). The regimen may vary with the disease. Thus human psittacosis should be treated for 3 weeks with 1 g of tetracycline per day (250 mg four times a day). Shorter courses may result in relapse. No controlled treatment trials for *C. pneumoniae* infection exist. Published experience indicates that erythromycin at 1 g/day for 3 weeks is effective. Tetracyclines at equivalent dosage would also be expected to be active. *C. trachomatis* infections are usually more responsive to chemotherapy; LGV, however, does not respond rapidly to the antibiotic. In treating LGV, it is common to obtain a rapid response in terms of constitutional signs; thus the fever and chills may disappear quickly, but the buboes may take months to resolve. Adults with genital tract disease caused by non-LGV *C. trachomatis* respond to treatment with tetracycline (1 g/day for 14 days or 2 g/day for 7 days). Erythromycin at equivalent doses is considered to be the alternative drug of choice and is the drug that should be used in treating infants. Erythromycin succinate (40 mg/kg in four divided doses daily) for 2 weeks should be given to infants with chlamydial pneumonia or inclusion conjunctivitis of the newborn. Topical treatment is inadequate for this conjunctivitis. Failure rates as high as 50% have been observed for infants receiving topical therapy with sulfonamides or tetracycline. It is clear that most of these children have nasopharyngeal infections and often reinfect themselves after topical treatment.

Topical treatment is the standard for mass therapy of trachoma in developing countries. By analogy with chlamydial infection in infants in industrialized societies, it is easy to see that this regimen would fail if the children in trachoma-endemic areas also had extraocular infections. This is known to occur, and it is likely that some form of systemic treatment will be required to ensure a cure.

Sulfonamides (sulfisoxazole, 4 g/day for 7 to 14 days) are effective in treating most *C. trachomatis* infections. This is not considered a treatment of choice for the chlamydial infections of the genital tract because many of these infections are not specifically diagnosed as a result of lack of laboratory facilities and thus must be treated empirically. For example, with nongonococcal urethritis the standard procedure would be to determine the presence of urethritis, rule out gonorrhea, and treat with tetracyclines because they are effective against both *C. trachomatis* and a putative cause of this disease, *Ureaplasma urealyticum* (which is resistant to sulfonamides).

Treatment of gonorrhea with tetracycline for a week (as recommended for nongonococcal urethritis) after immediate treatment with amoxicillin or ampicillin plus probenecid (Benemid) reduces the incidence of postgonococcal urethritis in men and postgonococcal cervicitis and salpingitis in women.

In 1993, azithromycin was recommended for treatment of uncomplicated lower genital tract infections with *C. trachomatis.* The standard treatment regimen is 1 g given as a single dose. Thus this antibiotic presents the promise of minimizing the compliance problems inherent in the longer terms of therapy that have been previously required. In clinical trials, a single 1 g dose of azithromycin was found to be equal in effect to a 1-week course of doxycycline in treating uncomplicated lower genital tract infections with *C. trachomatis.*

PREVENTION

There are no effective vaccines available for human chlamydial infection. Control of sexually transmitted diseases also requires identification and treatment of contacts. A chlamydial infection in an infant, such as conjunctivitis or pneumonia, is an indicator of genital tract infection in the mother, and she and her sexual contact(s) should receive treatment. Adults with inclusion conjunctivitis require systemic treatment because they invariably have genital tract infections. Their sex partners should also be given treatment. Neonatal ocular prophylaxis is not effective. In high-prevalence settings pregnant women should be screened for chlamydial infection and receive treatment as needed.

Prevention of the serious consequences of sexually transmitted *C. trachomatis* infection requires more than simple treatment of the symptoms. Because of the high prevalence of asymptomatic infections in both sexes, screening of high-risk male and female populations is needed to identify infected individuals and reduce the reservoir.

BIBLIOGRAPHY

Beem MO, and Saxon EM: Respiratory tract colonization and a distinctive pneumonia syndrome in infants with *Chlamydia trachomatis, N Engl J Med* 296:306, 1977.

Grayston JT: *Chlamydia pneumoniae,* strain TWAR pneumonia, *Annu Rev Med* 43:317, 1992.

Grayston JT et al: A new *Chlamydia psittaci* strain, TWAR, isolated in acute respiratory tract infections, *N Engl J Med* 315(3):161, 1986.

Holmes KK et al, editors: *Sexually transmitted diseases,* ed 2, New York, 1990, McGraw-Hill.

Jascheck G et al: Direct detection of *Chlamydia trachomatis* in urine specimens from symptomatic and asymptomatic men by using a rapid polymerase chain reaction assay, *J Clin Microbiol* 31(5):1209-1217, 1993.

Lee HH et al: Diagnosis of *Chlamydia trachomatis* genitourinary infection in women by ligase chain reaction assay of urine, *Lancet* 345(8944):213-216, 1995.

Mardh PA et al: *Chlamydia trachomatis* infection in patients with acute salpingitis, *N Engl J Med* 296:1377, 1977.

Martin D et al: A controlled trial of a single dose of azithromycin for the treatment of chlamydial urethritis and cervicitis, *N Engl J Med* 327(13):921-925, 1992.

Moulder JW: Looking at chlamydiae without looking at their hosts, *ASM News* 50(8):353, 1984.

Oriel JD, Ridgway GL: *Genital infection by* Chlamydia trachomatis. London, 1982, Edward Arnold.

Saikku P: *Chlamydia pneumoniae* infection as a risk factor in acute myocardial infarction, *Eur Heart J Suppl* K:62-65, 1993.

Schachter J: Chlamydial infections, *N Engl J Med* 298:428, 490, 540, 1978.

Schachter J, Dawson CR: *Human chlamydial infections,* Littleton, Mass, 1978, Publishing Sciences Group.

Schachter J, Grossman M: Chlamydial infections, *Annu Rev Med* 32:45, 1981.

Sweet RL et al: Failure of beta-lactam antibiotics to eradicate *Chlamydia trachomatis* in the endometrium despite apparent clinical cure of acute salpingitis, *JAMA* 250(19):2641, 1983.

Westrom L et al: Pelvic inflammatory disease and fertility: a cohort study of 1,844 women with laparoscopically verified disease and 657 control women with normal laparoscopic results, *Sex Transm Dis* 19(4):185-192, 1992.

CHAPTER

258 Mycoplasmal Infections

John Mills

The first mycoplasmal bacterium was discovered by Nocard and Roux in 1898. This organism, now known as *Mycoplasma mycoides,* caused bovine pleuropneumonia and thus was originally termed *pleuropneumonia-like organism* (PPLO). The clinical syndrome of cold agglutinin–positive primary atypical pneumonia (distinct from bacterial pneumonias) was delineated between 1938 and 1943. In 1944, Eaton cultured a filterable agent from patients with atypical pneumonia in chick embryos which caused pneumonia when inoculated into in cotton rats; convalescent sera from these patients neutralized the organism. Between 1960 and 1962, Chanock, Marmion, Clyde, and co-workers showed that the Eaton agent was a *Mycoplasma* organism, later named *Mycoplasma pneumoniae.* Koch's postulates were satisfied when *M. pneumoniae* cultured from patients caused pneumonia when inoculated into volunteers.

MICROBIOLOGY

Mycoplasma and *Ureaplasma* species belong to the family Mycoplasmataceae, class Mollicutes. They are considered to be related to bacteria on the basis of nucleic acid homology and their intracellular organization and metabolism. However, unlike bacteria, mycoplasmas lack a cell wall, and unlike bacterial spheroplasts (which also lack a cell wall), they cannot synthesize cell wall precursors. The mycoplasmas are the smallest free-living organisms known, varying between 125 and 150 nm in diameter. The organisms are pleomorphic and are bound by a triple-layer cell membrane containing sterols.

More than 10 species of *Mycoplasma* and one *Ureaplasma* species have been recovered from humans. Many other species pathogenic for other animals and plants are known. The only species that are known to cause disease in humans are *M. pneumoniae, M. hominis,* and *U. urealyticum,* the latter two often referred to together as the genital mycoplasmas. Only 1 serotype of *M. pneumoniae* is known, whereas there are at least 7 serotypes of *M. hominis* and 14 of *U. urealyticum.* Growth of wild-type strains of *Mycoplasma* and *Ureaplasma* is slow (this is particularly true of *M. pneumoniae*), and 1 to 3 weeks may elapse before colonies are detected. Only *M. pneumoniae* can hemolyze sheep and guinea pig erythrocytes. *Ureaplasma* is regarded as a separate genus based on its size and biochemistry.

As shown in Table 258-1, mycoplasmas other than *M. pneumoniae* are commonly recovered from the oropharynx or urogenital tract but, with the exception of the genital mycoplasmas (*M. hominis* and *U.*

Table 258-1   Common Mycoplasmataceae recovered from humans

SPECIES	USUAL LOCATION
Mycoplasma pneumoniae	Oropharynx, lung
Mycoplasma salivarium	Oropharynx
Mycoplasma orale types 1-3	Oropharynx
Mycoplasma fermentans	Urogenital tract
Mycoplasma hominis	Oropharynx, urogenital tract
Ureaplasma urealyticum	Urogenital tract

urealyticum), have not been associated with any disease processes. On the other hand, recovery of *M. pneumoniae* from patients is almost invariably associated with disease.

EPIDEMIOLOGY

Mycoplasma pneumoniae is transmitted most commonly by means of aerosols, although occasional contact transmission may occur. Since the incubation period is 2 to 3 weeks, spread of disease is slow even among family members; however, the ultimate risk of infection to susceptible persons within a family is greater than 90%. Mini-epidemics are occasionally reported, especially in closed or crowded populations such as military camps and long-term care facilities. Two well-documented point-source outbreaks have also been described among persons attending a college fraternity pledge initiation ceremony that "degenerated into a gross bachanal" and among employees of a dental prosthodontics laboratory constructing and altering dental prostheses with drills and grinding wheels. Presumably *M. pneumoniae* was transmitted in both instances via heavily infective aerosols from a single individual.

Mycoplasma pneumoniae infection occurs throughout the year, although the incidence of disease is usually increased during the fall. Infection rates vary widely from year to year. Mycoplasma infection appears to be a common cause of pneumonia in all parts of the world, accounting for up to 10% to 20% of all pneumonic illnesses. People of all age-groups except neonates may be affected, although the disease is most commonly seen from age 5 years through the third decade. Prolonged carriage in the pharynx of infected individuals may occur even after antibiotic therapy and may account for persistence of the infection in large populations.

PATHOGENESIS AND PATHOPHYSIOLOGY

Mycoplasma pneumoniae is predominantly a pulmonary pathogen. Information on the pulmonary lesions caused by this organism is sparse because the disease is rarely fatal. Interstitial pneumonia and acute bronchiolitis with peribronchial lymphocytic infiltrates and edema of the bronchiolar wall have been described in the few patients on autopsy. Transbronchial clearance of small particles is impaired, presumably as a result of alterations in the respiratory epithelium and ciliostasis. Bacterial superinfection, however, is rare, although an increased risk of meningococcal meningitis was noted in one study in Africa.

Virulence factors of *M. pneumoniae* have not been well characterized. The organism attaches to specific glycoprotein receptors on the cell membrane of respiratory epithelium by means of a specialized surface protein. After attachment there is interruption of host-cell RNA and protein synthesis, leading to ciliostasis and cell death. Because *M. pneumoniae* is not an alveolar pathogen, the pulmonary infiltrates in mycoplasmal pneumonia may partly result from the host's immune response. Infection early in life (<3 years of age) is rarely associated with pneumonia, whereas infection occurring after 4 or 5 years of age, by which time the vast majority of the population has sensitized lymphocytes, is often associated with pulmonary infiltrates. The pathogenesis of the extrapulmonary disease caused by *M. pneumoniae* is unclear. Both direct cytopathic effects and immunologic injury have been postulated as disease mechanisms.

Persons with high antibody titers from previous exposure to the organism are relatively protected from illness, although such expo-

Table 258-2 Symptoms and findings in patients with documented *Mycoplasma pneumoniae* pneumonia

SYMPTOM	PERCENTAGE OF PATIENTS
Cough	99
Fever ≥100° F (37.8° C)	94
Fever ≥ 102° F (38.9° C)	77
Family size of four or more persons	91
Malaise	89
Headache	66
Chills	58
Sore throat	54
Sputum production	45
Hoarseness	37
Earache (subjective)	31
Ear infection (objective)	21
Nausea and/or vomiting	29
Coryza	29
White blood cell count ≥10,000/mm^3	27
White blood cell count ≥15,000/mm^3	5
Recurrent pneumonia	22
Skin rash	17
Diarrhea	15
Preexisting disease	14
Pleuritis	2
Hospitalization	2

From Foy HM et al: *JAMA* 214:1666, 1970.

sure may still result in infection and shedding of organisms from the oropharynx. Immunity acquired after natural infection apparently lasts 1 to 5 years, although reinfection with production of illness (i.e., second attacks) has been documented as early as 1 year after the previous exposure.

CLINICAL SYNDROMES

Disease is usually localized to the respiratory tract. Pneumonia, the best known clinical manifestation of infection, occurs in only 10% to 30% of infected individuals during endemic disease. Most *M. pneumoniae* infections cause rhinitis, pharyngitis, and tracheobronchitis that are indistinguishable on clinical examination from acute respiratory tract infection produced by other agents.

After an average incubation period of 2 to 3 weeks, mycoplasma pneumonia becomes evident with the gradual onset of fever, cough, malaise, and headache (Table 258-2). Cough is usually distressing but nonproductive; pleurisy and hemoptysis are rare. Upper respiratory tract symptoms often accompany or precede the pneumonic manifestations. Frequently, other family members have had recent respiratory illness. The patient usually appears to be only mildly ill, and hospitalization is seldom required. Cyanosis, dyspnea, and tachypnea are rare. Fever, which is proportional to the severity of the pneumonia, seldom exceeds 104° F (40° C). Physical examination reveals tympanic membrane inflammation in no more than 20% of patients. The incidence of true bullous myringitis is less. This condition may not develop until late in the course of mycoplasmal pneumonia and may occur without pneumonia. Conjunctivitis and pharyngitis, occasionally with a tonsillar exudate, and cervical adenopathy may be present. The chest findings may be normal in the presence of radiographically defined pulmonary infiltrates, but localized rales and rhonchi without signs of consolidation or effusion are usually present.

The importance of mycoplasma pneumonia in patients with impaired immune responses has not been established. The disease in patients with sickle cell anemia may be unusually severe, with prolonged fever, respiratory distress, severe pleuritic chest pain, large pleural effusions, and pneumonia involving more than one lobe occurring frequently. In patients with impaired humoral immunity the disease may result in moderate weight loss, prolonged fever, and cough, in some cases without pulmonary infiltrates.

The white blood cell count may be slightly elevated but is usually less than 15,000 cells/mm^3. The differential blood cell count is often normal but may show polymorphonuclear predominance. The erythrocyte sedimentation rate is frequently elevated. Occasional positive

---

BOX 258-1
Nonrespiratory manifestations of *Mycoplasma pneumoniae* infection

Dermatologic
  Maculopapular rashes
  Vesicular rashes
  Urticaria
  Erythema multiforme minor
  Erythema multiforme major (Stevens-Johnson syndrome)
  Erythema nodosum
Neurologic
  Meningoencephalitis
  Toxic psychosis
  Peripheral neuropathy
  Guillain-Barré syndrome
  Cerebellar ataxia
Cardiovascular
  Myocarditis
  Pericarditis
  Raynaud's phenomenon
  Arterial occlusions
Gastrointestinal
  Hepatitis
  Pancreatitis
  Gastroenteritis
Hematologic
  Hemolytic anemia
  Thrombocytopenic purpura
Musculoskeletal
  Polyarthritis

Coombs' test results and false-positive serologic test results for syphilis have been noted. Gram-stained sputum reveals inflammatory cells and alveolar macrophages without significant bacteria; routine bacterial cultures show no growth or scant normal oral flora.

The radiographic appearance of mycoplasma pneumonia is variable and cannot be distinguished reliably from that of other causes of pneumonia. Reticular and interstitial infiltrates are usually unilateral and involve one of the lower lobe segments. Bilateral disease has been reported in 10% to 40% of cases. Upper-lobe disease, multiple segmental infiltrates, lobar infiltrates, consolidation, pneumatoceles, abscesses, coin lesions, hilar adenopathy, and significant pleural effusions are unusual.

Untreated patients with mycoplasmal pneumonia gradually recover over a period of 2 to 6 weeks. Headache and fever resolve in 10 to 14 days, but the cough and pulmonary infiltrates resolve more slowly, lasting, on average, 3 to 4 weeks and sometimes longer. Rarely, fulminant mycoplasmal pneumonia may develop, which may cause rapidly progressive pulmonary insufficiency that may be fatal. This complication is invariably unexpected, since it tends to occur in healthy young men.

Mycoplasma pneumoniae may affect organ systems other than the respiratory tract (Box 258-1). When this occurs, it most frequently occurs concomitant with respiratory disease, although primary nonpulmonary involvement has been described. The pathogenetic relationship between *M. pneumoniae* infection and bullous myringitis, skin rashes, and hemolytic anemia is well established. Polyarthritis is very rare, and *M. pneumoniae* has been isolated from the joint fluid in a few cases. Likewise, the organism has been recovered from cerebrospinal fluid in some cases of meningoencephalitis and one case of pericarditis, suggesting a pathogenetic relationship. The other extrarespiratory complications have not been firmly established as related to mycoplasmal infection.

The hemolytic anemia found with mycoplasmal pneumonia is uncommon but may be severe, with up to 70% reduction in hemoglobin levels. Hemolysis usually occurs during the second or third week of illness, when titers of cold agglutinins are highest (≥1:512). The cold agglutinins in these patients exhibit a high thermal maximum (>25° C). Hemolysis may follow cooling in these patients, as during bathing or alcohol sponging. The hemolysis is usually transient and is followed in a few days by recovery, manifested as a reticulocytosis with gradual restoration of normal hemoglobin levels. Occasional patients may have severe hemolysis or vascular complications such as Raynaud's phenomenon or arterial thrombosis. Mild hemolysis without reductions in hemoglobin may be common in patients with *M. pneumoniae* infection because 83% in one series had a positive direct Coombs' test result and 64% had reticulocytosis above 2%.

DIAGNOSIS

Because *M. pneumoniae* is difficult to culture, diagnosis of *M. pneumoniae* infection has traditionally relied on detection of antibodies. *M. pneumoniae* infection results in the production of autoantibodies that agglutinate erythrocytes at 4° C but not at 37° C. These cold agglutinins are oligoclonal immunoglobulin M (IgM) antibodies that bind the erythrocyte I antigen. Erythrocyte agglutination occurs at 4° C and reverses at 37° C. The presence of cold agglutinins, especially in low titer, is nonspecific and can be found in other conditions, including infections by adenovirus, Epstein-Barr virus, and cytomegalovirus. Cold agglutinin titers of 1:64 or greater are present in 40% to 70% of cases of *M. pneumoniae* pneumonia and are rare in other infections. In general, the height of the cold agglutinin response is directly proportional to the severity of the disease.

A simple bedside test for cold agglutinins can be performed by adding about 0.4 ml of blood to a tube containing 0.2 ml of 3.8% sodium citrate solution (e.g., the tubes used for prothrombin time determinations) and then placing the tube in ice water for 30 seconds. Floccular agglutination of red blood cells can be observed by tilting the tube on its side; the agglutination must reverse on rewarming to 37° C. This positive result corresponds to a cold agglutinin titer of 1:64 or greater, highly suggestive of *M. pneumoniae* infection.

Specific antibodies to *M. pneumoniae* have been measured by a variety of techniques. The IgM response to *M. pneumoniae* (measured by enzyme-linked immunosorbent assay [ELISA]) is a sensitive and specific test for acute infection but only becomes positive 1 to 2 weeks into infection. The presence of fourfold or greater rises in immunoglobulin G (IgG) antibodies is also a sensitive test for infection but, obviously, requires comparing acute and convalescent specimens. A fourfold rise in antibodies using the older complement fixation test has a sensitivity of about 75%, and these antibodies rise somewhat earlier than IgG antibodies measured by ELISA. A single, high titer level (≥1:32) of complement-fixing antibody is also highly suggestive of recent infection because complement-fixing antibodies are usually short-lived.

The leading edge of mycoplasma pneumonia diagnosis is direct detection of *M. pneumoniae* antigens or nucleic acids in respiratory secretions. Mycoplasmal antigens in respiratory secretions have been detected by immunofluorescence or ELISA, and these tests appear to be sensitive and specific. Mycoplasmal DNA or RNA also can be detected in respiratory secretions, either directly or after polymerase chain reaction amplification; these tests also had good sensitivity and specificity. One commercially available kit uses a radioiodinated DNA probe to detect multicopy ribosomal RNA sequences in *M. pneumoniae*, and is reported to have a sensitivity and specificity above 90%. Given the rapid progress in this area of diagnosis, consultation with the clinical laboratory is warranted.

DIFFERENTIAL DIAGNOSIS

Without specific laboratory testing, the pneumonitis caused by *M. pneumoniae* cannot be differentiated from other "atypical" pneumonias caused by chlamydiae, rickettsiae, or viruses and often cannot be differentiated from bacterial pneumonia. The presence of bullous myringitis, skin rashes, and other unusual extrarespiratory tract manifestations increases the likelihood of *M. pneumoniae* disease, but laboratory confirmation is still recommended.

TREATMENT AND PREVENTION

Only patients with lower respiratory tract or extrarespiratory tract manifestations of *M. pneumoniae* infection warrant treatment. *M. pneumoniae* is susceptible in vitro to macrolide and tetracycline an-

---

> ✔ **WHEN TO REFER**
>
> Like patients with other types of pneumonia, patients with mycoplasma pneumonia who are seriously ill based on clinical (e.g., extreme dyspnea) or laboratory findings (arterial oxygen pressure <80 torr) should be hospitalized for treatment. Consultation should be sought if respiratory failure, Stevens-Johnson syndrome, or neurologic disease is present. Symptomatic hemolytic anemia generally warrants consultation as well.

tibiotics. Because the organisms lack a cell wall, they are resistant to β-lactam antibiotics. Erythromycin shows greater in vitro activity against *M. pneumoniae* than tetracycline, but on clinical study these two antibiotics are equally effective in shortening the duration of symptoms. Treatment should be with 1.5 to 2.0 g/day for 10 to 14 days or up to 3 weeks in cases of severe disease. Doxycycline, 100 mg twice a day, has in vitro activity and a cost equivalent to tetracycline and appears to be better tolerated than either tetracycline or erythromycin, and its absorption is unaffected by food.

The new macrolides such as azithromycin and clarithromycin are more active toward *M. pneumoniae* in vitro than erythromycin or tetracycline, and clinical trials have suggested that they may offer a slight benefit over conventional therapy. However, this slight clinical benefit must be balanced by the 20- to 40-fold increase in cost of therapy. Fluoroquinolones (e.g., ciprofloxacin and lomefloxacin) are also active against *M. pneumoniae,* but likewise are 20 to 30 times more expensive than either tetracycline or doxycycline.

Antimicrobial treatment of mycoplasma pneumonia reduces the duration of fever by an average of 4 days and the duration of cough and pulmonary infiltrates by about 6 days. *M. pneumoniae* can still be recovered from many patients during therapy and for up to 3 months after treatment. Rare instances of tetracycline-resistant *M. pneumoniae* have been reported.

Patients with fulminant mycoplasma pneumonia and respiratory insufficiency should receive oxygen or mechanical ventilation as required, in addition to specific chemotherapy. Anecdotal reports suggest that high-dose glucocorticoids may be beneficial.

Patients with *M. pneumoniae* infection should be instructed to cough into a handkerchief to limit spread of infectious droplets. Respiratory isolation of the rare patient requiring hospitalization is not necessary because transmission requires prolonged close contact. Ten days of tetracycline prophylaxis for family members of an index case was effective in prevention of illness, although colonization still occurred. Vaccines are not available.

GENITAL MYCOPLASMAS

Mycoplasma hominis and *U. urealyticum* are referred to as the genital mycoplasmas. Both organisms are found commonly in the urogenital tract of healthy adults, and this high incidence of colonization in persons without evidence of disease has been the cause of considerable difficulty in assigning genital mycoplasmas a pathogenic role (Chapter 244). *Mycoplasma hominis* and *U. urealyticum* can be isolated from one third and one half, respectively, of sexually active adults. Colonization occurs during birth (vertical transmission) and by sexual contact; thus the prevalence of colonization increases with greater promiscuity. Women are more readily colonized with genital mycoplasmas than men are. The relative virulence of different serotypes of genital mycoplasmas is not known.

Ureaplasma urealyticum is one cause of nongonococcal urethritis in men, although its role in this syndrome is still questioned by some authors (Chapter 244). Evidence of the pathogenicity of *U. urealyticum* in nongonococcal urethritis comes from studies in which men given treatment with antibiotics active only against *Chlamydia* species were not cured if both *Ureaplasma* and *Chlamydia* organisms were initially present. More compelling, of three investigators inoculated intraurethrally with a pure culture of *U. urealyticum,* urethritis developed in two. *Mycoplasma hominis,* on the other hand, is not a cause of urethritis.

Mycoplasma hominis has been isolated from the fallopian tubes of women with salpingitis, and these patients usually exhibit a rise in serum antibody titers to the organism. The overall importance of *M. hominis* as an etiologic agent in pelvic inflammatory disease is unclear, although it is probably insignificant in comparison with that of the gonococci, anaerobic and aerobic enteric bacteria, and *Chlamydia* organisms. *Ureaplasma urealyticum* probably plays even less of a role. *Mycoplasma hominis* is also the cause of some cases of postpartum and postabortal fever or sepsis and a rare cause of pyelonephritis, septic arthritis, and peritonitis.

Both *M. hominis* and *U. urealyticum* are susceptible to macrolides, tetracyclines, and quinolones; a tetracycline (preferably doxycycline, 100 mg twice daily for 7 days) is the drug of choice for treatment of both. Some strains of *M. hominis* and *U. urealyticum* are resistant to tetracycline; in this instance a macrolide or fluoroquinolone is recommended.

Several mycoplasmas, including *M. fermentans* (formerly, *M. incognitus*), *M. penetrans,* and the newly discovered species *M. pirum,* have been shown to infect patients with human immunodeficiency virus (HIV) infection, and it has been suggested that such infection may accelerate or worsen HIV-related disease. However, the exact relationship between infection by these mycoplasmas and HIV-induced disease remains unclear.

BIBLIOGRAPHY

Baum SG: Mycoplasma disease: introduction. In Mandell GL, Douglas RG Jr, Bennett JE, editors: *Principles and practice of infectious diseases,* ed 4, New York, 1995, Churchill Livingstone.

Baum SG: *Mycoplasma pneumoniae* and atypical pneumonia. In Mandell GL, Douglas RG Jr, Bennett JE, editors: *Principles and practice of infectious diseases,* ed 4, New York, 1995, Churchill Livingstone.

Blanchard A, Montagnier L: AIDS-associated mycoplasmas, *Ann Rev Microbiol* 48:687, 1994.

Chan ED, Welsh CH: Fulminant *Mycoplasma pneumoniae* pneumonia, *West J Med* 162:133, 1995.

Lo S-C et al: Newly discovered mycoplasma from patients infected with HIV, *Lancet* 2:1415, 1991.

Luttrell LM et al: Septic arthritis due to *M. hominis, Clin Infect Dis* 19:1067, 1994.

Razin S: DNA probes and PCR in diagnosis of mycoplasma infections, *Mol Cell Probes* 8:497, 1994.

Taylor-Robinson D: *Ureaplasma urealyticum* (T-strain mycoplasma) and *Mycoplasma hominis*. In Mandell GL, Douglas RG Jr, Bennett JE, editors: *Principles and practice of infectious diseases,* ed 4, New York, 1995, Churchill Livingstone.

RICKETTSIAL DISEASES

CHAPTER

259   Rickettsial Infections

David T. Durack and David H. Walker

The genus *Rickettsia* comprises a heterogeneous group of microorganisms whose definitive hosts are arthropods or small mammals. Some 10 species in this genus can cause disease in humans (Table 259-1), but this number is likely to increase because new strains are being identified. Current comparisons of genetic sequences are elucidating the relationships between species and will lead to future revisions of the taxonomy of the Rickettsiaceae.

Electron microscopic study reveals that rickettsiae are typical bacteria with a structure very similar to that of gram-negative bacilli. They are obligate intracellular parasites and therefore cannot be cultured on standard laboratory media. Typically these organisms cause disease by proliferating inside the endothelial cells of small blood vessels, producing vascular injury. In this chapter Rocky Mountain spotted fever (RMSF) is described in detail as a paradigm of rickettsial infection and the most important rickettsiosis in the United States. Other rickettsial diseases are summarized.

HISTORICAL NOTE

Louse-borne epidemic typhus fever has been important throughout human history. The disease, which was endemic in Europe, Africa, South and Central America, and Asia, flared periodically into major epidemics during periods of war, poverty, and social upheaval. For example, notable epidemics occurred during the Thirty-Years War, the Napoleonic wars, and World War I. During these conflicts, deaths related to illness, especially typhus fever, often outnumbered deaths in battle. Many thousands of cases occurred in Germany, Poland, and Egypt during World War II.

The historic studies done by Ricketts in western Montana from 1906 to 1909, which led to his discovery of the etiologic agent and vector for RMSF, constitute the scientific basis for our understanding of this disease. No specific treatment was then available; later, treatment with various antisera and *para*-aminobenzoic acid benefited some patients. The introduction of chloramphenicol in 1947 provided the first reliable cure for rickettsial diseases.

EPIDEMIOLOGY

Within the United States RMSF is the most prevalent rickettsial disease. The number of reported cases appears to show cyclic variations. A 10-year decline began in 1950, followed by a 20-year resurgence; from 1977 to 1983 more than 1000 cases were reported in the United States each year. This peak has been succeeded by another downward cycle, with approximately 600 cases reported annually after 1988. North Carolina and Oklahoma usually report more cases than any other state. Paradoxically, the disease has become distinctly uncommon in the Rocky Mountain states, probably as a result of declining populations of infected ticks in that area.

Of the other rickettsial diseases that occur in the United States, the ehrlichioses are most common. Imported boutonneuse fever, murine typhus, and Q fever are uncommon; typhus, recrudescent typhus (Brill-Zinsser disease), and rickettsialpox are rare. Basic facts regarding the geographic distribution of rickettsial diseases are given in Table 259-1. Seroepidemiologic studies show that various rickettsial diseases are highly prevalent in different regions. For example, infection with *Rickettsia conorii* (and a related strain for which the name *Rickettsia africae* has been proposed) is endemic in parts of Africa; *Rickettsia sibirica* in Asiatic Russia, northern China, and Mongolia; and *Rickettsia japonica* in Japan. A detailed discussion of the complex worldwide epidemiology of the Rickettsiaceae is beyond the scope of this chapter.

All the rickettsioses are zoonoses. They may be accidentally transmitted to humans by arthropod vectors (Table 259-1), but humans do not play an important role in the natural life cycle of these organisms, except in the case of epidemic typhus. It is possible that mammalian hosts serve as a reservoir or as a mechanism for amplification of the infected tick population, but transovarial transmission of rickettsiae from one generation of female ticks to the next appears to be the most important mechanism for maintenance of *Rickettsia rickettsii* in nature. In any case, the infected tick is the primary means by which *R. rickettsii* is introduced into humans. Activities that bring humans into contact with infected arthropods favor the development of disease. These relationships are clearly illustrated by the epidemiology of RMSF. When adult ticks of the species *Dermacentor variabilis* (the common dog tick), *Dermacentor andersoni* (the wood tick), or *Rhipicephalus sanguineus* (the brown dog tick found in Mexico) that are infected with *R. rickettsii* feed on a human for several hours, inoculation of organisms from the ticks' salivary glands into the dermal blood vessels can occur. Persons who spend time outdoors in areas where active, infected ticks abound are most likely to contract RMSF. In the United States RMSF occurs most frequently in boys in South Atlantic and South Central states, between April and September.

PATHOPHYSIOLOGY

The hallmark of infections by members of the genera *Rickettsia* and *Orientia* is vascular damage. Rickettsiae are first introduced into der-

Table 259-1   Some characteristics of the major human rickettsioses

DISEASE	ORGANISMS (RICKETTSIA AND OTHERS)	VECTOR	VERTEBRATE HOST	MEANS OF TRANSMISSION TO HUMANS	GEOGRAPHIC DISTRIBUTION	MORTALITY RATE (%) UNTREATED	TREATED
Spotted fever group							
Rocky Mountain spotted fever	R. rickettsii	Ticks (e.g., Dermacentor variabilis, Dermacentor andersoni)	Rodents	Tick bite	North, Central, and South America	20-25	3
Boutonneuse fever	R. conorii	Ticks	Rodents	Tick bite	Africa, Asia, and Mediterranean basin	?	1-3†
North Asian tick typhus	R. sibirica	Ticks	Rodents	Tick bite	Asia	0	0
Queensland tick typus	R. australis	Ticks	Rodents, marsupials	Tick bite	Eastern Australia	2	0
Rickettsial pox	R. akari	Mites	Mice	Mouse to mite to human	United States, Russia, possibly worldwide	0	0
Flinders Island spotted fever	R. honei	Unknown	Unknown	Presumed tick bite	Australia	0	0
Oriental spotted fever	R. japonica	Ticks	Unknown	Presumed tick bite	Japan	0	0
Typhus group							
Epidemic typhus	R. prowazekii	Body louse	Humans	Human to louse to human	Worldwide	15-30*	5*
Murine typhus	R. typhi (R. mooseri)	Rat fleas	Rats	Rat to rat flea to human	Worldwide	1	0-1†
Cat flea typhus	R. felis	Cat fleas	Opossums	Cat flea to human	Texas and California	0	0
Scrub typhus group							
Scrub typhus	Orientia tsutsugamushi	Larvae of mites (chiggers)	Rats, other rodents, birds	Mite to human	Asia, Pacific islands, and Australia	5	1
Other genera							
Q fever	Coxiella burnetii	Ticks (but usually by aerosol)	Cattle, goats, sheep, other mammals	Livestock to human, by aerosol	Worldwide	5	0‡
Human monocytic ehrlichiosis (HME)	Ehrlichia chaffeensis	Ticks (e.g., Amblyomma americanum)	Deer	Tick bite	North America and Europe, possibly worldwide	2-5	02
Human granulocytic ehrlichiosis (HGE)	HGE agent	Ticks (e.g., Ixodes dammini)	Rodents, deer	Tick bite	North America, possibly worldwide	2-5	0-2

*Mortality can be high in debilitated, malnourished patients; otherwise, it is lower than that for Rocky Mountain spotted fever.
†In hospitalized patients
‡Excluding Q fever endocarditis, which causes significant mortality.

mal tissue by feeding ticks (RMSF, boutonneuse fever, and other spotted fevers), by mites (scrub typhus, rickettsialpox), or by scratching when the skin is contaminated with infected feces of the human body louse (epidemic typhus) or fleas (murine typhus and cat flea typhus). Then rickettsiae spread via the bloodstream to infect vascular endothelial cells. *Rickettsia rickettsii* infects vascular smooth muscle cells as well.

Initial attachment to endothelial cells may be mediated by surface binding proteins, after which the attached organisms can be internalized by endothelial cells and macrophages. When specific antibodies are present, the rickettsiae remain within macrophage phagolysosomes and are killed, but in nonimmune hosts virulent rickettsiae can escape into the cytoplasm and multiply. Acute intracellular infection stimulates endothelial cells to produce cytokines such as interleukin-1 (IL-1), prostaglandins, and tissue factor, which presumably play an important role in pathogenesis of the acute-phase response, increased vascular permeability, and hemostasis. The spotted fever group of rickettsiae spread from cell to cell, whereas typhus-group rickettsiae remain inside until they achieve large numbers and burst the host cell.

Foci of vascular damage develop at sites where virulent rickettsiae injure or kill host cells (Plates VIII-44 and VIII-45). The inflammatory infiltrate consists primarily of mononuclear cells with a few polymorphonuclear leukocytes. These foci are the direct cause of the rash, encephalitis, interstitial pneumonitis, portal triaditis, interstitial nephritis, myocarditis, and, presumably, the vasculopathic consumption coagulopathy that may occur.

Disseminated infection of the cells lining the blood vessels has two important pathophysiologic consequences: increased vascular permeability and multifocal vasculitis at sites where injury induced by rickettsiae is most intense. Altered vascular permeability is manifested by edema and focal hemorrhages, not only in the skin and subcutaneous tissues (Plate VIII-45) but also in the viscera. Noncardiogenic pulmonary edema, hypovolemia, and acute renal failure can result. Focal vasculitis is more common than frank thrombosis of involved vessels. Intravascular thrombi are usually eccentric and nonocclusive (Plate VIII-44), and seldom result in infarction, although peripheral gangrene attributable to small-vessel involvement occurs in 4% of cases. The combined effects of increased vascular permeability, multifocal vasculitis, and associated coagulopathy account for the clinical features of these diseases. Any organ may be affected, but involvement of the skin (Plate VIII-45), lung, and brain usually is most important.

Specific cell-mediated immune responses have been documented in humans, and experimental studies in animals indicate that these are important for providing immunity to rickettsial diseases. T-lymphocytes are the major effector cells; interferon gamma (INF-γ) and tumor necrosis factor–alpha (TNF-α) activate intracellular killing of rickettsiae. The interaction of cellular and humoral responses achieves clearance of rickettsiae and provides long-term immunity in the great majority of patients who recover.

Vasculitis is not a typical manifestation of *Coxiella burnetii* infection, called Q fever. This species of *Rickettsia* can cause mild or severe, acute, subacute, or chronic systemic infection with fever, pneumonia, granulomatous hepatitis, and, occasionally, infective endocarditis, osteomyelitis, or central nervous system (CNS) involvement. Q fever may be transmitted by tick bite but is most often acquired by aerosols of *C. burnetii* shed into the air by infected livestock or animal products. After entering macrophages, coxiellae multiply following acid-activation in phagolysosomes. *C. burnetii* possesses an analogue to the macrophage infectivity potentiator (Mip) protein of *Legionella organisms*.

CLINICAL MANIFESTATIONS

The cardinal features of RMSF are fever, headache, and rash in a patient with a history of tick bite or exposure. However, only a small minority of RMSF patients have the full syndrome at presentation. This explains why the correct diagnosis is made in only about half of RMSF cases at first contact with a physician, the time when treatment is most likely to be effective.

The incubation period of RMSF after inoculation by an infected tick ranges from 2 to 12 days, with a median of 7 days. The onset of illness is often abrupt, with severe headaches and moderately high,

continuous fever. Myalgias and muscle tenderness are common, as are mild or moderate conjunctival redness and photophobia. Chills occur, but true rigors are uncommon.

The rash usually develops after the patient has already been ill for 3 to 5 days, but it may appear earlier or much later. It is absent entirely in up to 10% of patients; in such cases it is sometimes referred to as Rocky Mountain "spotless" fever. The rash may easily be overlooked in dark-skinned persons. The mortality rate is higher in patients without a rash because the diagnosis is often delayed in these cases. The rash itself consists of maculopapular pink or purplish spots 1 to 5 mm in diameter. These usually appear first on the extremities, especially around the ankles and wrists, on day 3 to 5 of illness. Over the next 1 to 2 days the rash spreads centripetally, sometimes involving the entire body. The rash typically extends to the palms and soles, often later in the course, but spares the face in most patients. In about 50% of cases the lesions become petechial or ecchymotic (Plates VIII-18 and VIII-45), but usually only after the fifth day of illness. Frank purpura may develop, especially in patients with thrombocytopenia (Plate VIII-19). Necrosis of the skin and peripheral gangrene occur in about 5% of hospitalized patients with RMSF. These are due to extensive small-vessel thrombosis in response to vasculitis, rather than to occlusion of large arteries or to fully developed disseminated intravascular coagulation, which is uncommon in RMSF.

Gastrointestinal tract symptoms are common. Nausea, vomiting, diarrhea, or abdominal pain, or a combination of these, occur in about two thirds of patients, often early in the illness. Therefore the initial diagnosis is often "gastroenteritis."

Involvement of vessels in the lung is evidenced by cough, interstitial and alveolar infiltrates, and development of noncardiogenic pulmonary edema in some severe cases.

Central nervous system manifestations are frequent and important. Most patients have headache, which often is severe. This symptom is useful in evaluation of adults and older children but not in very young children, who cannot describe headache in words. Signs of CNS involvement range from lethargy, confusion, and delirium to focal deficits, papilledema, seizures, and coma. About one fourth of patients have a stiff neck, which can be due to myalgia or to meningismus. Cranial and peripheral nerve lesions are rare.

As the disease progresses, diffuse edema develops in many patients because of leakage of plasma from damaged vessels. Attempts to correct hypotension with infusion of saline or colloid solutions may lead to worsening of the edema, which persists until the vasculitis resolves. Acute renal failure, which occurs in 10% to 15% of patients, is a result of hypovolemia produced by damaged, leaking vessels rather than rickettsial vasculitis in the kidney itself.

Most clinical reports of RMSF have described hospitalized patients, who are more likely to have severe disease and complications than outpatients. However, some patients with RMSF have mild disease and may be managed safely as outpatients. Because some patients undoubtedly recover spontaneously, remaining undiagnosed and untreated, the true incidence of mild or subclinical forms of RMSF is not yet known. Serologic surveys suggest that subclinical infection with a spotted fever group *Rickettsia* species which shares antigens with *R. rickettsii* is common in endemic areas.

DIFFERENTIAL DIAGNOSIS

The diagnosis of RMSF poses a serious problem for the physician of first contact because symptoms and signs are nonspecific, early treatment is needed to reduce mortality, and no laboratory test is available to confirm the diagnosis immediately except direct demonstration of *R. rickettsii* in skin lesions by immunofluorescence or immunoperoxidase. Rickettsemia can be detected by the polymerase chain reaction, but this technique is not sufficiently sensitive to be useful.

In the United States, meningococcemia (Chapter 264), enteroviral infections (Chapter 250), and ehrlichioses are the most common alternative diagnoses in patients who have a syndrome compatible with RMSF, and vice versa. Other initial diagnoses sometimes made in patients with RMSF include pneumonia, scarlet fever, Henoch-Schönlein purpura, various vasculitides and viral encephalitides, rubella, mononucleosis, typhoid fever, and hepatitis. Atypical measles in a partially immune host also should be considered (Chapter 251).

In developing countries measles, malaria, dengue, hemorrhagic fevers, other rickettsial infections, and many other locally endemic, acute febrile syndromes may be included in the extensive differential diagnosis.

The detection of purulent meningitis in a patient with fever, headache, and petechial or purpuric rash strongly suggests meningococcal infection, even in a region where RMSF is endemic. However, in patients whose spinal fluid is normal or shows only mild pleocytosis or a slightly elevated protein concentration, or both, it may be impossible to decide on clinical grounds whether the patient has RMSF or meningococcal infection. Such patients should be treated with chloramphenicol, the only antimicrobial agent that is fully effective against both diseases.

LABORATORY DIAGNOSIS AND IMMUNE RESPONSE

Only one fourth of patients with RMSF have leukocytosis, despite their toxic clinical appearance. The majority have normal or low white blood cell counts in peripheral blood. However, about three fourths show an increased proportion of band forms, often with toxic granulation of neutrophils. Sometimes band forms outnumber segmented neutrophils. The combination of a low or low-normal white blood cell count with a striking left shift in a febrile patient in an endemic area should raise the possibility of rickettsial infection. The platelet count is often low, less than 150,000 cells/μL in about half the patients, and less than 100,000 cells/μl in 10% to 20%.

Significant hyponatremia occurs in about half the patients. The serum albumin concentration falls below 3 g/dl in severe cases. Elevations of levels of serum transaminases, alkaline phosphatase, and/or bilirubin occur in 10% to 40%. Striking elevations of creatine phosphokinase serum concentrations have been reported, confirming the presence of myositis.

Thus when a patient from an endemic area has fever and headache in spring or summer, the combination of a low or low-normal total leukocyte count in peripheral blood with a striking left shift indicated on smear, hyponatremia, and thrombocytopenia strongly suggests the diagnosis of RMSF. However, these abnormal laboratory findings are nonspecific and not present in all patients; their absence does not exclude RMSF.

Cerebrospinal fluid (CSF), which usually is obtained to help differentiate RMSF from meningococcal meningitis, is abnormal in approximately half of RMSF patients. In these cases, the CSF profile is consistent with mild aseptic meningitis; from 5 to 200 leukocytes/μL may be present, with a predominance of either mononuclear or polymorphonuclear cells. The protein concentration may be slightly or moderately elevated. The glucose concentration usually is normal but occasionally is mildly reduced. The finding of more extreme abnormalities in the CSF during RMSF is unusual.

The etiologic diagnosis of any infectious disease is best achieved by isolation of the causative organism. Rickettsiae are highly biohazardous agents that have caused laboratory-acquired infections and deaths, especially in the preantibiotic era. Isolation of rickettsiae still requires complex systems such as inoculation of embryonated hens' eggs, cell cultures, or laboratory animals. These cumbersome, prolonged, and somewhat hazardous procedures are rarely useful in the care of an individual patient, but isolation and identification in research laboratories are necessary if we are to learn whether the numerous other species of rickettsiae found in ticks, insects, and animals in the United States (e.g., *R. montana, R. canada, R. amblyommi, R. parkeri, R. rhipicephali, R. bellii*) cause human disease. Recently the shell vial centrifugation-enhanced cell culture technique, which has proved useful in isolating some viruses from blood, has been adapted to isolate *R. conorii* efficiently.

The diagnosis of rickettsial disease usually can be confirmed by measurement of an immune response in survivors. The inherent delay in the appearance of a detectable serologic response to infection means that most patients require evaluation and treatment before a positive result is available. Eventual serologic confirmation is important, not only for epidemiologic and public health reasons but also for the individual patient, who can expect to be immune to RMSF after one confirmed attack, and for the treating physicians, who need to know whether their clinical diagnoses are accurate.

The Weil-Felix test, using agglutination of cross-reacting *Proteus* species OX-19, OX-2, and OX-K antigens, has been the main diagnostic test for rickettsial infection for many years. A fourfold rise in titer after an illness compatible with RMSF or murine typhus is confirmatory. Lack of specificity and sensitivity are major drawbacks to the Weil-Felix test. Diverse other conditions, including *Proteus* species urinary tract infections, leptospirosis, and various liver diseases, can cause false-positive test results. Single titers in the range of 1:160 are equivocal. More recently developed methods that yield both sensitive and specific results include indirect fluorescent antibody, passive hemagglutination, latex agglutination, and enzyme-linked immunosorbent assay (ELISA) tests. For routine diagnostic purposes the Weil-Felix test should now be replaced by indirect fluorescent antibody or latex agglutination tests.

Rapid, specific diagnosis of RMSF has been achieved by use of immunofluorescence or immunoperoxidase to demonstrate *R. rickettsii* in biopsy specimens from skin lesions. Although success of those techniques requires the presence of a rash and selection of an appropriate biopsy site, the procedure is moderately sensitive and highly specific. Positive results can be expected in about 70% of cases; the sensitivity falls if the patient has received treatment for 1 day or more with an antibiotic that is active against rickettsiae. A positive test result indicates the need for specific treatment, alerts the physician to possible complications, and eliminates the need for isolation and treatment for possible meningococcemia.

In nonimmune hosts, virulent rickettsiae taken up by macrophages can escape from phagosomes into the cytoplasm, where multiplication proceeds unhindered until the host cell lyses. When specific antibody is present, the rickettsiae remain within macrophage phagolysosomes and are killed. However, these same antibodies do not prevent rickettsiae from multiplying inside their endothelial target cells. Thus effective in vivo immunity requires the interaction of both cellular and humoral responses.

Specific cell-mediated immune responses have been documented in humans, and experimental studies in animal models indicate that such responses are of major importance in providing immunity to rickettsial diseases. T lymphocytes, INF-γ, and TNF appear to be important components of the normal host immune response, which achieves clearance of rickettsiae and provides long-term immunity in most patients who have recovered from rickettsial infection.

OTHER RICKETTSIAL DISEASES
Louse-Borne Epidemic Typhus

Louse-borne epidemic typhus fever ranks with RMSF as the most virulent of the rickettsioses. The human body louse, which is responsible for transferring typhus from human to human, is itself infected and eventually killed by *Rickettsia prowazekii*. Humans are considered to be the principal reservoir; if true, this feature would be unique among the rickettsioses. However, in the eastern United States, natural infection occurs among flying squirrels and can be the source of human infection. These squirrels may constitute reservoirs other than humans for *R. prowazekii*. Stupor and inanition are even more marked in typhus than in RMSF, and the typhus rash usually spares the palms and soles; otherwise, the clinical manifestations of these diseases share many similarities.

Late recrudescences many years after the original infection result in a milder form of typhus known as Brill-Zinsser disease. Fully virulent *R. prowazekii* can be recovered from the blood of such patients, perhaps explaining how typhus can reemerge in epidemic form after long periods of quiescence if social conditions favor proliferation of lice.

Murine Typhus

Murine typhus (caused by *Rickettsia typhi*) is transmitted from rats to humans by the rat flea. Sporadic cases occur in the United States, particularly in Texas and California, where the diseases can be transmitted by cat fleas in a cycle involving opossums. *Rickettsia typhi* can cause serious illness, but usually the disease is much milder than epidemic typhus, with approximately 1% mortality.

Rickettsialpox

Rickettsialpox begins with a localized papule that develops 7 to 10 days after inoculation via the bite of an infected mite carrying *R. akari.* This papule grows into a fluid-filled vesicle on an inflamed base, forms a black eschar, and finally heals with scarring. Systemic symptoms, including fever, headache, myalgia, and generalized maculopapular rash, appear a few days after the primary lesion. Rickettsialpox is not a fatal disease, but it should be treated because its symptoms respond well to tetracycline. The Weil-Felix reaction remains negative in this disease, but serologic diagnosis can be provided by an indirect immunofluorescence complement-fixation test.

Scrub Typhus

Scrub typhus, caused by *Orientia* (formerly *Rickettsia*) *tsutsugamushi,* is common in Asia, the western Pacific region, and northern Australia. Recent molecular studies have indicated that the genome of this pathogen is sufficiently different from the other rickettsiae to justify reclassification into a new genus, *Orientia.* The disease afflicts both local populations and transients, such as U.S. soldiers who served in Vietnam. An eschar forms at the site of a chigger bite during a 7- to 14-day incubation period, with associated lymphadenopathy. Systemic disease follows, with fever, rash, and splenomegaly. Central nervous system involvement or pneumonitis, or both, is frequently prominent. The eschar may be absent in many patients with scrub typhus. The death rate in untreated cases is about 5%, but treatment with tetracycline or doxycycline is usually effective. Doxycycline-resistant strains have been identified; based on recent animal studies, azithromycin may provide an effective alternate treatment.

Boutonneuse Fever

The important and widespread infection boutonneuse fever, caused by *R. conorii,* occurs in the Mediterranean basin, the Middle East, and many countries in Africa. In the United States, occasional imported cases occur in tourists returning from Europe and Africa. The disease has many local names such as Mediterranean spotted fever, South African tick bite fever and Kenyan tick typhus. A local eschar (called a "tache noire") develops at the site of inoculation of *R. conorii* by *Rhipicephalus sanguineus* or another tick species, according to region. However, the eschar occurs in only about half the cases. Associated lymphadenopathy is noted in approximately half of patients with an eschar. Development of an eschar is followed a few days later by fever and a generalized rash. The disease is generally much less severe than RMSF or typhus, but some patients require hospitalization and occasional fatalities occur.

Q Fever

Q fever is unique among rickettsial diseases in several ways: it is usually transmitted by inhalation rather than by an arthropod vector, it is not associated with a rash, and it may cause infective endocarditis.

Q fever occurs worldwide and is strongly associated with exposure to animals, especially farm livestock. Farmers, veterinarians, laborers who handle animal products, and laboratory workers are at particular risk. Epidemics have arisen from exposure to infected parturient cats and wild rabbits.

The disease can consist of an acute, self-limited fever with or without atypical pneumonia or can linger in subacute or chronic forms. It has been reported to be a common cause of atypical pneumonia in France, and most cases in North America probably remain undiagnosed. Q fever endocarditis has a high mortality rate, but sometimes patients can be cured by valve replacement and long-term antibiotic therapy. Late relapses, even after years, can occur in this form of the infection.

The antibody response to natural infection is complex, involving the immunoglobulin M (IgM), immunoglobulin G (IgG), and immunoglobulin A (IgA) titers to phase 1 and phase 2 antigens of *C. burnettii.* High IgG and IgA titers to phase 1 antigen suggest chronic Q fever infection with endocarditis.

Ehrlichiosis

The term "ehrlichiosis" refers to several diseases of humans and animals caused by obligate intracellular bacteria of the genus *Ehrlichia.* *E. canis* causes pancytopenia in dogs, *E. equi* causes equine granulocytic ehrlichiosis, *E. risticii* causes Potomac horse fever, and *E. phagocytophila* causes granulocytotropic infections in cattle, sheep, and deer. The first-recognized human disease caused by this genus was sennetsu fever, an infectious mononucleosis-like disease caused by *E. sennetsu* that occurs in Japan and Malaysia. Recently other important human infections have been identified.

At least two forms of ehrlichiosis occur in the United States: human monocytic ehrlichiosis (HME) and human granulocytic ehrlichiosis (HGE).

HME is an infection of mononuclear leukocytes caused by *Ehrlichia chaffeensis,* which is transmitted by ticks, particularly *Amblyomma americanum.* The disease is most common in the southern and southeastern United States, where it is associated with outdoor activities such as hunting, military training, and searching for golf balls near a wildlife reserve. Seven to 21 days after a tick bite, fever, chills and rigors, headache, myalgias, and anorexia develop. Only one third of patients have a rash. Leukopenia, thrombocytopenia, and elevated liver enzyme levels in serum are typical. The disease can be severe: more than 1500 cases have been tallied, and a majority of those analyzed by the Centers for Disease Control and Prevention required hospitalization. The fatality rate among hospitalized patients is 2% to 4%. Treatment with tetracycline or doxycycline effectively reverses the disease process. Serologic confirmation of *E. chaffeensis* infection is provided by fourfold or greater rise in immunofluorescent antibody titers. Serologic studies indicate that either many infections are asymptomatic or many persons are exposed to an antigenically related organism. Ten percent to 15% of patients with an RMSF-like illness but negative serologic results for RMSF have actually had ehrlichiosis. The organism can be grown in vitro in several cell lines.

HGE is an infection of polymorphonuclear leukocytes caused by an *Ehrlichia* species that is extremely closely related to the veterinary pathogens *E. equi* and *E. phagocytophila.* Near-identity by DNA homology results in shared antigens, so human infection with the HGE agent induces antibodies to both these species. Most cases described so far have been in the upper Midwest and Northeast regions of the United States, in Minnesota, Wisconsin, New York, and New England. The recognized range of this infection is likely to expand to other areas of the United States and Europe because of better case ascertainment and the geographic spread of infected tick populations. After inoculation of ehrlichiae into the skin by ticks such as *Ixodes scapularis* (which also carries Lyme disease) high fever and chills develop in patients, with prominent headache and myalgias. At this stage the illness cannot be distinguished on a clinical basis from other rickettsial and viral infections. Blood cell counts frequently reveal leukopenia, low platelet counts, and sometimes anemia, with increased liver enzymes in serum. In some cases the organisms can be seen as morulae within granulocytes in blood films.

HGE can be severe; death occurs in 2% to 5% of hospitalized patients, but most patients respond rapidly to treatment with a tetracycline. Some untreated illnesses persist for more than 1 month. The organism can be cultured in vitro in a leukemia cell line, but diagnosis is normally confirmed by serology. In the future, tests based on nucleic acid amplification are likely to become the standard methods for diagnosis of ehrlichiosis.

TREATMENT

Rickettsiae are generally susceptible to chloramphenicol and the tetracyclines. Treatment of RMSF and typhus fever with these drugs is usually effective, reducing the mortality rate by fivefold to tenfold (Table 259-1). The morbidity of rickettsial infections that seldom cause death, such as rickettsialpox or murine typhus, can also be reduced by antibiotic treatment. Rocky Mountain spotted fever should be treated with tetracycline 25 to 50 mg/kg per day orally; chloramphenicol 30 to 50 mg/kg per day orally in four divided doses; or doxycycline 200 mg/day in two oral doses, continuing for 2 to 3 days after resolution of fever. In severely ill patients the initial doses should be given parenterally. Although chloramphenicol has been used successfully for many years, doxycycline appears to be moderately more effective. For ehrlichiosis the efficacy of chloramphenicol is not established to the same degree as for other rickettsioses. Based on the results of in vitro studies, rifampin may be the best second-line drug.

Most cases of louse-borne typhus and scrub typhus can be cured with a single 200-mg dose of doxycycline. Occasional relapses occur, requiring retreatment. Boutonneuse fever responds to treatment with fluoroquinolones such as ciprofloxacin and ofloxacin, which would probably also be effective against other rickettsioses.

Corticosteroids probably do not affect the primary infectious process but can provide symptomatic improvement in patients with typhus fever. Their value in RMSF is unproved. Likewise, no proof exists that heparin is useful in severe cases, even in the few individuals in whom true disseminated intravascular coagulation develops.

The child living in an area where RMSF is endemic who has a febrile illness during the summer presents a special problem. Most have minor or self-limited infections requiring no specific treatment. However, it is evident that the few children who have RMSF must receive treatment early to reduce morbidity and mortality rates. In practice, it is reasonable to give treatment in potentially exposed children who have persistent fever for more than 2 days with doxycycline 4 mg/kg per day orally in two divided doses for 5 days. This is especially appropriate for those with prominent headache (after consideration of the possibility of bacterial meningitis and the indications for a spinal tap), while remembering that young children do not describe headache in the same way as older children and adults. The danger of inducing tooth discoloration in children with such a short course of tetracycline is low and is even lower if doxycycline is used; it is negligible in children older than 6 years of age. Because most of these children have self-limited diseases other than RMSF, it is undesirable to expose them to even a small risk of drug-induced marrow aplasia by using chloramphenicol too freely.

Intensive medical and nursing care is needed for severe cases of rickettsial disease. Hypovolemic shock, respiratory failure, or renal failure (which often coexist in patients with severe disease) requires management in an intensive care unit. Surgery is occasionally needed in the patients who have extensive cutaneous necrosis or gangrene of the extremities. In severe cases of RMSF, long-term neurologic sequelae including pareses, incoordination, incontinence, and language disorders may occur.

PREVENTION

Louse-borne epidemic typhus disappeared from the United States more than 50 years ago as a result of improving social and economic conditions. However, effective prevention of other rickettsial diseases in the United States has not yet been achieved. Prophylactic antibiotic treatment of patients after tick bite, even in areas where RMSF is endemic, is not indicated because less than 1% of the ticks carry virulent *R. rickettsii*. Moreover, chloramphenicol and tetracycline are rickettsiostatic, not rickettsiocidal drugs. Therefore attempted prophylaxis with antibiotics after exposure to ticks, mites, or fleas might merely prolong the incubation period until the rickettsiostatic drug is discontinued; it is not recommended.

The use of environmental acaricides, tick repellents, and protective clothing has had no decisive impact on the incidence of RMSF. Eradication of the infected tick population is probably not feasible. Thus the single effective preventive measure presently available is to avoid tick exposure and, if exposed, to search the body and remove ticks several times daily when ticks are active, with special attention to the scalp, axillae, and pubic regions. Attached ticks should be removed with care, to minimize the chance of inoculating rickettsiae by crushing them during removal.

Scrub typhus can be prevented by taking doxycycline once weekly while in endemic areas.

No licensed RMSF vaccine is available. Previously available vaccines made from whole, killed rickettsiae were only marginally effective; they have been withdrawn from use. A vaccine based on recombinant *R. rickettsii* outer membrane protein A expressed in baculovirus is effective in guinea pigs but has not been tried in humans. A typhus vaccine is not needed in the United States because the disease is so rare.

BIBLIOGRAPHY

Anderson BE, Dawson JE, Jones DC, Wilson KH: *Ehrlichia chaffeensis:* a new species associated with human ehrlichiosis, *J Clin Microbiol* 29:2838, 1991.

Bakken JS, Dumler S, Chen S-M et al: Human granulocytic ehrlichiosis in the upper midwest United States: a new species emerging? *JAMA* 272:212, 1994.

Bakken JS, Krueth J, Wilson-Nordskog C et al: Clinical and laboratory characteristics of human granulocytic ehrlichiosis, *JAMA* 275:199, 1996.

Chen S-M, Popov VL, Feng H-M et al: Cultivation of *Ehrlichia chaffeensis* in mouse embryo, Vero, BGM, and L929 cells and study of *Ehrlichia*-induced cytopathic effect and plaque formation, *Infect Immun* 63:647, 1995.

Everett ED, Evans KA, Henry RB, McDonald G: Human ehrlichiosis in adults after tick exposure, *Ann Intern Med* 120:730, 1994.

Fishbein DB, Dawson JE, Robinson LE: Human ehrlichiosis in the United States: 1985 to 1990, *Ann Intern Med* 120:736, 1994.

Goodman JE, Nelson C, Vitale B et al: Direct cultivation of the causative agent of human granulocytic ehrlichiosis, *N Engl J Med* 334:209, 1996.

Helmick CG, Bernard KW, D'Angelo LJ: Rocky Mountain spotted fever: clinical, laboratory, and epidemiologic features of 262 cases, *J Infect Dis* 150:480, 1984.

Higgins JA, Radulovic S, Schriefer ME, Azad AF: *Rickettsia felis:* a new species of pathogenic rickettsia isolated from cat fleas, *J Clin Microbiol* 34:671,1996.

McDade JE, Newhouse VF: Natural history of *Rickettsia rickettsii, Am Rev Microbiol* 40:287, 1986.

Radulovic S, Higgins JA, Jaworski DC, et al: Isolation, cultivation, and partial characterization of the ELB agent associated with cat fleas, *Infect Immun* 63:4826, 1995.

Raoult D, Weiller PJ, Chagnon A et al: Mediterrean spotted fever: clinical, laboratory and epidemiological features of 199 cases, *J Trop Med Hyg* 35:851, 1986.

Raoult D, Zuchelli P, Weiller PJ et al: Incidence, clinical observations and risk factors in the severe form of Mediterranean spotted fever among patients admitted to hospital in Marseilles: 1983 to 1984, *J Infect* 12:111, 1986.

Sawyer LA, Fishbein DB, McDade JE: Q fever: current concepts, *Rev Infect Dis* 9:935, 1987.

Schriefer ME, Sacci JB, Jr, Dumler JS et al: Identification of a novel rickettsial infection in a patient diagnosed with murine typhus, *J Clin Microbiol* 32:949, 1994.

Sexton DJ, Kanj SS, Wilson K et al: The use of a polymerase chain reaction as a diagnostic test for Rocky Mountain spotted fever, *Am J Trop Med Hyg* 50:59, 1994.

Telford SR, Lepore TJ, Snow P et al: Human granulocytic ehrlichiosis in Massachusetts, *Ann Intern Med* 123:277, 1995.

Walker DH, editor: *Biology of rickettsial diseases,* Boca Raton, Fla, 1988, CRC.

Walker DH: Rocky Mountain spotted fever: a seasonal alert, *Clin Infect Dis* 20:1111, 1995.

Walker DH, Barbour AG, Oliver JH et al: Emerging bacterial zoonotic and vector-borne diseases: ecological and epidemiological factors, *JAMA* 275:463, 1996.

Walker DH, Dumler JS: Emergence of the ehrlichioses as human health problems, *Emerg Infect Dis* 2:18, 1996.

Winkler HH: Rickettsia species (as organisms), *Ann Rev Microbiol* 44:131, 1990.

Yevich SJ, Sanchez JL, DeFraites RF et al: Seroepidemiology of infections due to spotted fever group rickettsiae and *Ehrlichia* in military personnel exposed in areas of the United States where such infections are endemic, *J Infect Dis* 171:1266, 1995.

BACTERIAL DISEASES

CHAPTER

260 Staphylococcal Infections

John N. Sheagren

ORGANISMS

Staphylococcus aureus is now acknowledged to be the most important bacterial pathogen of humans; it is the single most frequent isolate from *truly positive* blood cultures in hospitalized patients. Paradoxically, *Staphylococcus epidermidis* is in fact the single most frequent blood culture isolate, most of which are contaminants. *S. aureus* usually produces localized disease but can be rapidly invasive, spreading through the tissues, invading bone, and seeding the bloodstream to produce a fulminant picture of septic shock, disseminated intravascular coagulation, and rapid demise. It can persist deep within tissues, being carried for years without causing symptoms or disease. The balance between host and parasite that results in these kinds of

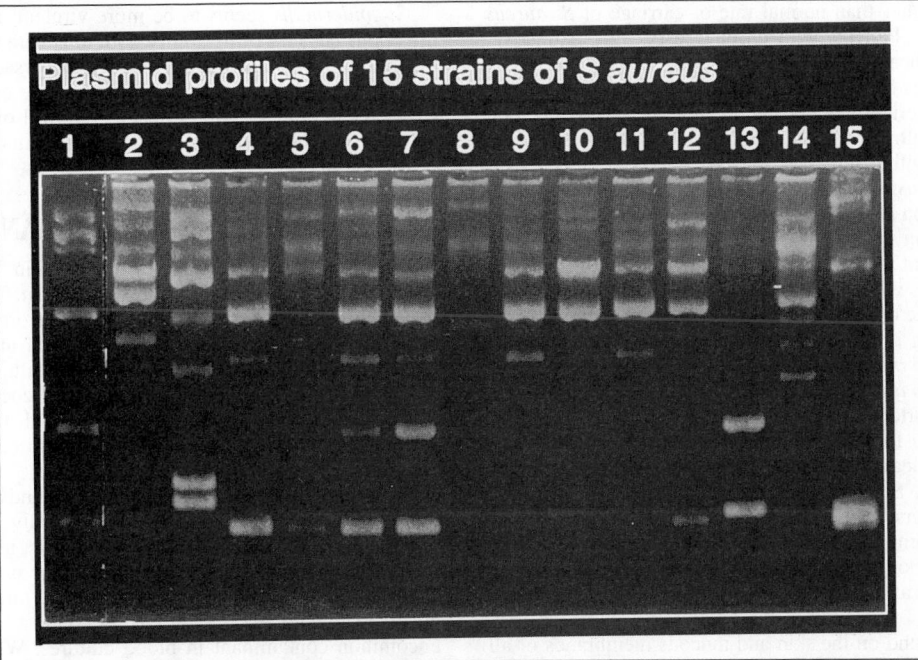

FIGURE 260-1   Plasmid profiles of 15 strains of coagulase-negative staphylococci showing the differences and similarities of plasmid DNA fragments from the various strains. Plasmids are isolated and treated with restriction endonucleases, and the resulting DNA fragments are separated by electrophoresis to reveal the profile.

From Herwaldt LA. In Doebbeling BN et al: *Current concepts: hospital-acquired infections: new challenges,* Kalamazoo, Mich, 1991, Upjohn.

relationships is only partially understood. There are only a few other clinically important species of the family Micrococcaceae, of which *S. epidermidis* and *Staphylococcus saprophyticus* are notable; for example, *S. saprophyticus* is the second leading cause of urinary tract infections in otherwise healthy young women.

Characteristics

Staphylococci are gram-positive cocci (0.5 to 1.5 μm in diameter) of the family Micrococcaceae. The two genera of clinical significance in this family are the *Micrococcus* and the *Staphylococcus*. Both produce catalase, but micrococci are differentiated from staphylococci by their inability to produce acid anaerobically from glucose. The differentiation of *S. aureus* from other staphylococci is accomplished in the clinical laboratory by two tests: *S. aureus* coagulates rabbit plasma and produces acid anaerobically from mannitol, whereas other staphylococci do not. There are now several methods of rapidly detecting *S. aureus*. Coagulase-negative staphylococci found on human skin have been divided into more than 20 species by DNA-DNA homology studies and biochemical testing. However, the majority of coagulase-negative staphylococci isolated from clinical specimens are *S. epidermidis*. The other clinically important coagulase-negative staphylococcus is *S. saprophyticus*.

S. aureus (the species designation *aureus* meaning "gold") is a gram-positive coccus that grows in clusters in liquid or semisolid media or within tissues when causing infection (Color Plate VIII-19). It grows well on blood agar plates, producing small, shiny, ultimately golden-yellow colonies that usually are surrounded by a clear zone of beta hemolysis. Although the colonies may initially look dull gray or even white, they rapidly turn a golden-yellow when the plates are exposed to air. The organisms grow well anaerobically or aerobically; in blood culture media both bottles of a single set are usually positive.

There are no reproducible serologic typing schemes available to classify subtypes of *S. aureus*; however, bacteriophage typing has been useful in identifying strain characteristics and providing epidemiologic data on organism spread. Bacteriophages are viruses that at-

tach to the mucopeptide–teichoic acid complex of the cell wall. Five major groups of organisms that have generally similar characteristics (phage groups I to V) have been designated. For example, some phage groups of staphylococci are more likely to produce certain toxins than are others. Recently, plasmid profiles and immunoblotting techniques have produced staphylococcal "fingerprints," which have been useful in epidemiologic study. As increasing percentages of strains of *S. aureus* have not been phage-typeable, plasmid-profile typing has increased in usefulness. Plasmid-profile analysis is carried out by separating plasmid contents from other *S. aureus* cell components and characterizing the isolated plasmids with restriction endonucleases. The resultant DNA fragments can be separated by electrophoretic techniques, and the pattern produced by a given strain of *S. aureus* can be compared with others (Fig. 260-1). Plasmid-profile typing seems most reliable during focused outbreaks of infection, since the plasmid content of a given *S. aureus* strain may not be stable over a prolonged period.

The identification of epidemiologically related strains of *S. epidermidis* has been facilitated in recent years by using plasmid-profile typing. This technique can be used to associate epidemiologically linked isolates or to separate infecting from contaminating organisms, a major problem with coagulase-negative staphylococci recovered from clinical specimens.

Epidemiology

Staphylococci may colonize almost all animal species. However, certain strains of *S. aureus* are limited to humans, whereas others are found in cattle, swine, and other animals. Humans carry *S. aureus* primarily in the nasopharynx, and heavily colonized individuals may become a source of recurrent infections both to themselves and to others. Most humans probably carry a few *S. aureus* organisms among the normal flora of every body site but in such low numbers that routine cultures rarely reveal the organism. Individuals regularly or intermittently using needles to inject substances either intravenously (such as drug addicts or patients receiving hemodialysis) or subcutaneously (such as insulin-dependent diabetics or patients receiving allergy shots) have a higher than normal rate of carriage of *S. aureus* in the nose and throat. Patients with chronic, especially exudative, skin diseases also are heavily colonized.

In newborn nurseries the rate of colonization increases rapidly after birth. In most nurseries it is not uncommon to see colonization rates of about 25%, with most infants remaining asymptomatic. Yet outbreaks of disease within nurseries may be traced to more "virulent" strains of *S. aureus,* sometimes traceable to a common personnel carrier. Colonization of hospitalized adults increases throughout hospitalization. Once an individual is a carrier, spread may occur to other areas of the patient's own body, as well as to clothing and other items and to individuals with whom the patient comes in contact. The most effective technique of stopping transmission from person to person in a hospital setting is simple: *meticulously washing one's hands immediately before and immediately after examining a patient essentially halts transmission and acquisition of staphylococci.* Hand washing is particularly important when one is examining patients with obvious staphylococcal lesions or chronic exudative dermatoses, since such patients may be heavily colonized, resulting in larger numbers of acquired organisms. Some strains of staphylococci not only are more virulent than others but also seem to spread more aggressively in a hospital environment. Outbreaks may occur, during which 20% to 30% of hospital personnel and patients entering the hospital may acquire the epidemic strain; subsequent multiple individual infections may occur.

S. epidermidis is found on the skin and mucous membranes of all warm-blooded mammals and is the most numerous aerobic component of normal skin flora. It rarely is responsible for infection in normal hosts outside the hospital. In the hospital it is the most common organism cultured from air and wounds during surgery, but it rarely causes disease. Infections have resulted from direct operative contamination but are usually associated with the insertion of indwelling foreign devices. Hospital-associated *S. epidermidis* infections are caused by organisms usually resistant to multiple antibiotics, including penicillin, semisynthetic penicillinase-resistant penicillins, cephalosporins, and aminoglycosides; infections acquired outside the hospital are usually due to antibiotic-susceptible organisms. Hospital personnel and patients appear to be reservoirs for these resistant organisms.

Pathophysiology

S. aureus is a ubiquitous and highly pathogenic organism. It produces a large number of enzymes that, together with its surface and cell wall components, contribute to its pathogenicity. Any strain of *S. aureus* from either an environmental or a personal culture is almost inevitably more virulent in an animal model than non–coagulase-producing staphylococci; however, there is substantial strain-to-strain variation in pathogenicity, even among strains of *S. aureus.* Virulence is probably related to the sum of enzyme production that permits the organism to resist degradation by environmental substances, resist phagocytosis by polymorphonuclear leukocytes (PMNs), produce specific exotoxins that may directly cause damage to tissues or cells, or possess surface receptors that permit it to adhere to inflamed or traumatized tissues. Most strains of *S. aureus* release a multitude of such toxins, including hemolysins, toxins that cause hemolysis and injure leukocytes and other tissues. Another enzyme, leukocidin, is particularly toxic to white blood cells.

In contrast to *S. aureus,* coagulase-negative staphylococci are relatively avirulent for humans and laboratory animals. The failure of *S. epidermidis* to produce coagulase and lethal toxins, the absence of protein A in the cell wall to inhibit opsonization, and the absence of surface ligands that bind human proteins such as fibronectin and fibrinogen may all contribute to the lesser virulence of this organism as compared with *S. aureus.* This lack of virulence probably contributes to the indolent nature of *S. epidermidis* infections and the capacity of the organism to lie dormant in tissue for long periods of time after surgical contamination before causing symptomatic disease. *S. epidermidis* commonly persists only in areas where host defense mechanisms are locally impaired, such as in endocarditic vegetations and tissues surrounding prosthetic devices, shunts, catheters, and sternal surgical incisions. Antibiotic therapy is often ineffective until all foreign material is removed from the area of infection.

S. epidermidis seems to be more virulent in foreign body–related infections because of its ability both to adhere to foreign material and to produce abundant quantities of exopolysaccharide or "slime," a characteristic that seems to be unique to the coagulase-negative species *S. epidermidis.* Slime impedes removal of the organism by host defense systems and allows organisms to remain fixed to the surfaces of foreign bodies.

DISEASES PRODUCED IN HUMANS

Because *S. epidermidis* is part of normal skin flora, it frequently contaminates cultures obtained by crossing skin. Therefore it can be implicated as a cause of disease only when the organism is cultured from a site at which there is clinical evidence of infection, when it is the only organism recovered, or when it is cultured on more than one occasion. Ideally, clusters of gram-positive cocci should also be identified in stained smears of infected material. In contrast, any culture growing *S. aureus* should be considered to be infected until proved otherwise.

S. aureus readily grows in both aerobic and anaerobic cultural conditions. Microbiology laboratories are usually readily able to identify the organism in culture media. The clinician usually is first informed that gram-positive cocci are growing in a patient's blood cultures. Over the next 24 to 48 hours, when these turn out to be coagulase-positive staphylococci, *S. aureus,* in contrast to *S. epidermidis,* is an uncommon contaminant in blood cultures. When present, *S. aureus* usually grows in several blood culture bottles; however, even a single positive blood culture for *S. aureus* is usually significant. Presence of *S. aureus* in the urine is difficult to interpret: although it may be a contaminant, it usually indicates a significant infection of the upper or lower urinary tract and may have resulted from a previously unrecognized bacteremic episode. Diagnosis of the organism as the cause of a variety of deep infections depends on how aggressively material is obtained for Gram's stain and culture. For example, patients with chronic bone or joint infections should promptly undergo deep aspiration or operative culture of the involved area.

Diseases Produced by *S. aureus* (Box 260-1)

Diseases Related to Toxin Production. The syndrome of gastroenteritis is produced by enterotoxin ingestion (Chapter 242). The ingestion of the preformed enterotoxin in foodstuffs causes acute gastroenteritis without requiring the presence of living organisms. Another gastroenteric syndrome that was thought in the past to have been caused by *S. aureus* was called "acute staphylococcal enterocolitis." This disease occurred in patients receiving broad-spectrum antibiotics and was characterized by fever, tachycardia, abdominal cramps, diarrhea (not infrequently with blood), and in some cases nausea and vomiting. A pseudomembrane was often demonstrable on sigmoidos-

---

BOX 260-1
Diseases produced by *Staphylococcus aureus*

Toxin production
Gastroenteritis
Staphylococcal scalded skin syndrome (SSSS)
Toxic shock syndrome (TSS)

Direct invasion
Cutaneous infections (paronychiae, cellulitis, boils, furuncles, carbuncles, surgical wound)
Pyomyositis
Osteomyelitis and septic arthritis (hematogenous or contiguous spread)
Pneumonia
Meningitis, cerebritis

Primary staphylococcal bacteremia
Transient
Complicated (associated with metastatic abscess formation)

copy. Gram's stain of stool predominantly showed clusters of *S. aureus*. Undoubtedly, many cases diagnosed as staphylococcal enteritis in the past were actually cases of antibiotic-associated colitis, now known to be caused by *Clostridium difficile*.

The staphylococcal scalded skin syndrome (SSSS) is also produced by the systemic effect of a toxin called the "exfoliative toxin." This syndrome occurs mainly in infants and young children but may be seen in adults, especially those who are immunosuppressed (patients with chronic renal failure who are receiving dialysis, patients who have had kidney transplantation, or patients who have been receiving cytotoxic or steroid therapy). The patient usually has a primary focus of infection, which may not be readily apparent; infection of the umbilicus in the neonate, conjunctivitis, or an earlier staphylococcal infection may have been minor, completely localized, and unnoticed. Patients first have tender skin and a bright red rash, either diffuse (as in scarlet fever) or macular. Blisters and bullae form as the upper epidermis splits off in large sheets (positive Nikolsky's sign). This phenomenon results directly from the action of exfoliative toxin, which attacks the skin in the middle layers of the epidermis. The finding of intraepidermal separation on skin biopsy differentiates this condition from the more severe, drug-related disease called toxic epidermal necrolysis, a variant of erythema multiforme or the Stevens-Johnson syndrome. Staphylococci producing the exfoliative toxin are usually classified by phage typing as phage group II organisms.

Toxic shock syndrome (TSS) has emerged because various strains of *S. aureus* have acquired the genetic capability to produce a new protein toxin. It is now known that the genetic material to produce the toxin is acquired by lysogeny (genetic material carried into the staphylococcus by a temperate bacteriophage). Two groups of investigators originally described an immunologically identical toxin called either staphylococcal pyrogenic exotoxin C or enterotoxin F. That toxin is now named toxic shock syndrome toxin-1 (TSST-1). Its mechanism is still unclear, but it appears (either directly or indirectly) to be a very powerful cytotoxin that injures cell surfaces. Two theories have attempted to explain how TSST-1 produces the septic shock/multiple organ system failure syndrome. First, TSST-1 may enhance the effect of subtoxic amounts of bacterial endotoxin. Second, TSST-1 may (at least in part because of its ability to be a superantigen) stimulate the production of one or more cell-damaging mediators, the most important of which seem to be tumor necrosis factor (cachetin) and/or interleukin-1 (IL-1), now known to play central roles in bacteremic shock.

Individuals colonized with one of the toxin-producing strains may have a low-grade, localized infection such as vaginitis during menstruation, especially if a superabsorbent tampon is used, or a small, peripheral abscess or wound infection. The toxin is produced at the site of the low-grade infection and, when absorbed systemically, causes a dramatic, multisystem disease characterized by all or most of the following: high fever, headache, confusion, myalgias, scarlatiniform rash followed by desquamation, conjunctival suffusion, subcutaneous edema, vomiting, profuse watery diarrhea, oliguria, a propensity to acute renal failure, hypocalcemia, liver function abnormalities, disseminated intravascular coagulation, and often severe, prolonged shock. In contrast to the group of patients with bacteremic (endotoxin-like) shock, these patients are rarely bacteremic with the causative organism. Yet, as noted, the substances mediating this variety of septic shock may be the same as those mediating bacteremic shock syndromes. Therapy is directed at drainage and eradication of the peripheral focus of infection using antistaphylococcal antibiotics as well as surgery; however, meticulous supportive care of the patient in shock plays the major role. Approximately 10% of patients who are severely ill with TSS who are promptly recognized and receive adequate supportive care will die. Patients with menstruation-associated TSS should not use tampons during subsequent menstrual cycles. Despite debate, antibiotic therapy *is* important: the recurrence rate is 70% without antibiotic therapy and only 20% if antibiotics are used during the initial episode and tampon use is subsequently discontinued. Nonmenstrual cases of TSS, however, now account for about one third of all patients.

Diseases Related to Direct Invasion

Dermal infections. Most minor skin infections are due to either *S. aureus* or group A, β-hemolytic streptococci. Infections around nails (paronychiae) occur with great frequency, as do furuncles and boils. Cellulitis may develop around sites of a minor abrasion or cut and progress rapidly to lymphangitis. On clinical examination, however, there is no way to differentiate between group A β-hemolytic streptococcal infections and those caused by *S. aureus,* a point of therapeutic importance. *S. aureus,* together with group A β-hemolytic streptococci, may cause classic impetigo in children, although the bullae are said to be larger ("bullous impetigo") when caused by *S. aureus.* Larger, localized skin infections are called furuncles and carbuncles. When a patient with a localized *S. aureus* skin infection has fever and chills, bacteremia must be considered and prompt diagnostic and therapeutic intervention must be initiated (see Primary Staphylococcal Bacteremia).

Bone and Joint Infections. *S. aureus* has a predilection for seeding to bones or joints (see Chapters 243 and 203). This seeding can result from direct inoculation, as in trauma or penetrating wounds, or from a transient bacteremic episode, the latter event often stemming from cutaneous infections. As noted, because of the presence of surface receptors for disrupted tissues and/or products of coagulation or inflammation, the circulating bacteria tend to lodge in recently traumatized or chronically inflamed tissues or around a foreign body. Thus the syndrome of acute osteomyelitis tends to occur in children with a bruised extremity and is particularly common in teenage athletes (e.g., wrestlers and football players). The traumatized area, usually the ankle, knee, or shin, becomes acutely red, warm, and swollen and may at first appear simply to be a primary cellulitis. Fever, shaking chills, and positive blood cultures are common.

Hematogenous osteomyelitis or arthritis in adults is usually less acute. The syndrome of vertebral osteomyelitis often occurs in elderly patients, many of whom are diabetic. This syndrome manifests itself as chronic back pain and low-grade fever; *S. aureus* may be cultured either from the blood or from an aspirate of the bone. Patients receiving hemodialysis may have osteomyelitis related to bacteremia, often asymptomatic, from infected shunts. Drug addicts may have primary osteomyelitis almost anywhere, related to the parenteral injection of their nasally carried strain of *S. aureus* along with the narcotics. Isolated staphylococcal septic arthritis often occurs as a complication of chronic underlying arthritis (such as rheumatoid arthritis or osteoarthritis) and also results from asymptomatic bacteremia seeding to one of the previously inflamed joints. Symptoms usually increase in one joint and are accompanied by fever; joint aspiration then reveals a purulent effusion containing the organism. *S. aureus* also commonly infects implanted joint prostheses.

Pneumonia. Many cases of staphylococcal pneumonia follow viral infections of the lower respiratory tract and are most common in children, especially infants. *S. aureus* pneumonia should be considered whenever such a patient has a high fever in the course of a lower respiratory tract infection. The chest radiograph usually reveals patchy infiltrates, which may rapidly excavate to produce pneumatoceles. Rapid development of pleural effusions, empyemata, or pneumothoraces, or a combination of these, may occur. Such children are usually bacteremic. Recurrent *S. aureus* bronchitis and pneumonia also are seen in children with cystic fibrosis.

Adult patients with influenza have an increased incidence of *S. aureus* pneumonia. The patient usually has typical symptoms of influenza, begins to improve, but then rapidly develops fever and chills with chest pain. Gram's stain of the sputum reveals clumps of gram-positive cocci. Mortality rate in this syndrome is high and is related to serious, localized, rapidly progressive pulmonary disease and the accompanying bacteremia.

Meningitis-cerebritis. Staphylococcal meningitis unassociated with endocarditis usually develops as a complication of a diagnostic or surgical procedure on the central nervous system (Chapter 239). Occasionally, *S. aureus* meningitis occurs in patients with endocarditis. Thus the features of this syndrome are similar to those in patients bacteremic with *Streptococcus pneumoniae* in whom meningitis develops. Interestingly, in some patients purpura and vascular collapse develop, and differentiation from meningococcal meningitis is difficult. The cerebrospinal fluid from patients with cerebritis (multiple, patchy, poorly defined brain abscesses) is also typically purulent, with pleocytosis, an elevated protein level, and low to normal glucose level; Gram's stain, however, usually reveals no organisms, and culture results are usually negative.

Endocarditis. *S. aureus* causes the majority of cases of the syndrome of acute bacterial endocarditis but may also produce the syndrome of subacute bacterial endocarditis (SBE; Chapter 24). Endocarditis may be present in any bacteremic patient, but most cases (as with SBE) occur in individuals with previously damaged valves. Typically an individual with a history of heart murmur develops a high fever, chills, and systemic toxicity; *S. aureus* grows in almost all blood cultures. Over the next several days the murmur may change, and multiple embolic phenomena (e.g., Janeway lesions, cutaneous infarcts, and petechiae) occur, substantiating the diagnosis of the valvular infection. Parenteral drug users exhibit a somewhat different syndrome: they have a high incidence of tricuspid valve endocarditis, often do not have a history of previous valvular lesions, and may not have a murmur audible on admission to the hospital (Chapter 247). Septic pulmonary emboli are common.

The syndrome of "spontaneous staphylococcal bacteremia" occurs when a young, otherwise healthy person without a portal of entry spontaneously develops high fever and chills and *S. aureus* grows from all blood cultures. The majority of these patients have endocarditis, and a changing murmur, usually aortic insufficiency, may develop. A recent review by Bayer et al. of patients with *S. aureus* bacteremia with and without endocarditis identified the following parameters that predicted endocarditis: (1) absence of an obvious primary site of infection, (2) community-acquired infection, (3) metastatic sequelae, and (4) echocardiographically demonstrable vegetations. The *absence* of an obvious primary focus of infection in a patient bacteremic with *S. aureus* is very strong evidence favoring the presence of endocarditis. The mortality rate in endocarditis produced by *S. aureus* is still very high and is approximately related to age and underlying physical condition. In chronically ill, elderly patients with left-sided endocarditis, the mortality rate, even with therapy, exceeds 50%; in the young drug user, however, it is less than 10%.

Primary Staphylococcal Bacteremia.

Occasionally, as noted earlier, staphylococcal bacteremia may develop in young persons in the absence of a peripheral site of infection. It is presumed that the organism disseminates from a minor skin infection (acne or a follicular lesion) or from the nose or pharynx in carriers who have a mild viral upper respiratory tract infection. Hospital-associated staphylococcal bacteremias are common in patients who have long, complicated medical and surgical illnesses; often, the source is a peripheral intravenous site that becomes infected. Organisms may then seed to a variety of peripheral sites, including the aortic or mitral heart valves, causing endocarditis. *S. aureus* is now known to be the most common organism isolated from hospital-acquired bacteremic episodes. Hospitalized patients are more likely to have impaired host-defense mechanisms, either from underlying disease or from therapy; therefore, bacteremia may have disastrous results. In otherwise healthy persons without underlying organic valvular lesions, endocarditis or metastatic infection of any other organ is unusual; thus the majority of relatively healthy patients who have staphylococcal bacteremia in the hospital require only brief treatment (2 weeks of parenteral antibiotics). The standard approach to such patients should be the following:

1. Over the 10- to 14-day period after the bacteremic episode the patient should be examined daily for a new or changing heart murmur, evidence of embolic phenomena, and signs of metastatic infection in bones, joints, kidneys (positive urine culture finding), meninges, lungs, or other organs.

2. If metastatic abscess formation is discovered, appropriate local drainage and more prolonged course of antibiotic therapy (e.g., at least 4 weeks) are required. In this subgroup of patients an echocardiographic study may make the diagnosis of endocarditis.

3. If no clinical evidence of metastatic seeding is found at the end of 14 days, the decision regarding the need for further therapy can be helped by the antibody titer to *S. aureus* teichoic acids (discussed later). If the titer of antibodies has increased fourfold, the infection is very likely to have seeded to some organ, and more prolonged therapy, either intravenous or oral, should be given. Also, deep foci of infection should be sought with computed tomography or radionuclide scans, or both. If, as occurs in the vast

majority of patients, the titer of teichoic acid antibodies does not rise, the infection probably has not seeded and antibiotics can be discontinued. The negative predictive value of the test for teichoic acid antibodies is probably of most value.

Infections in Immunocompromised Patients. Although *S. aureus* regularly causes both superficial and deep infections in normal hosts, it produces more serious infections with increased frequency in patients with impaired immune systems. Patients with reduced function or numbers of polymorphonuclear leukocytes (PMNs) are most susceptible (e.g., neutropenic patients and patients with functional defects in PMN killing functions such as those with chronic granulomatous disease or Chédiak-Higashi syndrome). Patients with isolated B-cell (antibody) or T-cell (cell-mediated) immunodeficiencies are not, in particular, more susceptible to *S. aureus* infections. Patients with acquired immunodeficiency syndrome (AIDS), however, considered primarily as having a T-cell deficit, in fact have multifactorial immunodeficiency with PMN problems as well as a B-cell impairment. Overall, AIDS patients have a substantial increase in staphylococcal infections, especially those attributable to *S. aureus*.

Diseases Produced by Coagulase-Negative Staphylococci

As stated earlier, coagulase-negative staphylococci are the most common organisms grown from blood cultures in the hospital. Approximately 75% of such cultures are contaminants; thus care should be taken in interpreting blood cultures growing these organisms. The source of the bacteremias caused by these microbes is usually a chronic, indwelling intravenous catheter; the highest incidence is in neonatal intensive care units and on hematology-oncology wards.

Endocarditis

Native valve endocarditis. Coagulase-negative staphylococci cause approximately 5% of cases of endocarditis on native cardiac valves. Coagulase-negative species other than *S. epidermidis* account for 50% of this group. In contrast to the increase in the number of cases of coagulase-negative staphylococcal prosthetic valve endocarditis in recent years, the incidence of native valve endocarditis has remained constant in the antibiotic era. Native valve endocarditis caused by coagulase-negative staphylococci becomes evident as a classic syndrome of SBE with nonspecific symptoms of fever, weight loss, and anorexia that may continue for many months (Chapter 24). There is little to distinguish its presentation, clinical findings, and laboratory values from those of viridans streptococcal endocarditis. The vegetations virtually always occur on rheumatic or previously abnormal valves.

Prosthetic valve endocarditis. One of the major changes in the epidemiology of endocarditis in the antibiotic era has been the emergence of *S. epidermidis* as one of the most common organisms infecting prosthetic heart valves. In contrast to native valve endocarditis, this species accounts for more than 95% of infecting coagulase-negative staphylococci. *S. epidermidis* and non–group A streptococci are responsible for 60% to 70% of the cases of prosthetic valve endocarditis (PVE). Streptococcal PVE generally occurs more than 1 year after surgery, can usually be treated with antibiotics alone, and has a low mortality rate; however, *S. epidermidis* PVE usually occurs within the first year after valve surgery, is often caused by an antibiotic-resistant organism, and has a mortality rate of up to 60%. *S. epidermidis* is probably inoculated into the area of the rigid sewing ring of the prosthesis at the time of surgery; the causative organisms are hospital associated (and thus antibiotic resistant) and are in an avascular area protected from antibiotics. The high mortality rate is largely due to hemodynamic factors caused by valve dehiscence, obstruction of the valve orifice by large vegetations that grow over the valve orifice from the valve ring, or conduction disturbances resulting from spread of infection outward to the conduction system.

Although *S. epidermidis* is acquired at the time of surgery, PVE may not appear for months to more than a year. This slow incubation period probably reflects the lack of virulence of the organism and its propensity for causing indolent infections associated with minimal symptoms. Half of the cases of *S. epidermidis* PVE have classic symptoms of endocarditis, whereas the other half have few signs or symptoms and no peripheral embolic phenomena. The latter patients simply come to medical attention with acute hemodynamic decompensation caused by valve dysfunction or with conduction abnormalities.

Diagnosis depends on detecting bacteremia; all patients with prosthetic cardiac valves who have fever, new murmurs, or any new valve dysfunction, regardless of the absence of signs or symptoms of classic endocarditis, should have blood cultures obtained. It is essential to obtain several blood specimens that are drawn at different times through separate venipunctures to eliminate contamination. Once positive blood cultures establish the diagnosis of *S. epidermidis* PVE, prognosis depends on the degree of valve dysfunction assessed by echocardiography, serial electrocardiograms, and cineangiography. Also important are what additional corrective procedures are feasible.

Cerebrospinal Fluid Shunt Infections. *S. epidermidis* causes 60% or more of the infections of ventriculoatrial and ventriculoperitoneal shunts used in the treatment of hydrocephalus. Meningitis and bacteremia are associated with infections of ventriculoatrial shunts, whereas meningitis and peritonitis are seen with ventriculoperitoneal shunt infections. One third of these infections begin as wound infections in the early postoperative period, whereas the remaining two thirds are seen from 1 month to more than 1 year after surgery. Fever and evidence of shunt malfunction are the most common manifestations of infection. Organisms occasionally can be repeatedly cultured from shunt tubing when there is little evidence of infection and only minimum cerebrospinal fluid pleocytosis. It is not clear whether this represents colonization or early infection. Organisms probably also gain access to the central nervous system by contamination at the time of surgery, as with PVE. The majority of organisms are resistant to multiple antibiotics and resemble strains isolated from patients with PVE. Mortality rate directly related to infection varies from 6% to 35%, depending on the series being reviewed. Related devices, such as reservoirs used for instillation of chemotherapy and ventriculostomy catheters used to decompress acutely increased intracerebral pressure, also commonly become infected with *S. epidermidis*.

Prosthetic Joint Infections. Infections of total hip and knee arthroplasties are uncommon, occurring in only 1% of implanted prostheses (Chapter 203); however, such infections usually require surgical replacement and often result in loss of ambulation. *S. epidermidis* accounts for approximately 40% of these infections and is second only to *S. aureus* in this regard. As with infections of other prosthetic devices, in prosthetic joint infection *S. epidermidis* is implanted into the wound at the time of surgery, may not produce symptoms of fever and pain for years, and is usually antibiotic resistant. Diagnosis is often difficult, since radiographs do not show changes of osteomyelitis until late in the infection. Bacteremia is uncommon.

Infections of Indwelling Catheters, Vascular Shunts, and Vascular Grafts. Chronic indwelling plastic catheters such as these used for hyperalimentation, chemotherapy, or peritoneal dialysis; vascular shunts used as access for hemodialysis; and vascular grafts all can become infected with *S. epidermidis*. Infections of vascular catheters and shunts become evident as fever with positive blood cultures (discussed earlier); infections of peritoneal dialysis catheters, as fever and abdominal pain with positive cultures of dialysis fluid; and infections of vascular grafts, as fever, local wound purulence, and graft malfunction.

Sternal Osteomyelitis After Cardiac Surgery. *S. epidermidis* causes approximately 30% to 50% of cases of sternal osteomyelitis and costochondritis that occur in the median sternotomy wound after cardiac surgery (Chapter 243). Together, *S. aureus* and *S. epidermidis* cause 50% to 60% of these infections, which occur in 1% to 2% of patients who have cardiac surgery. Outbreaks have taken place, however, in which *S. epidermidis* sternal wound infections occurred in a much higher percentage of patients. Such factors as improper placement of wire suture, hemodynamic instability during bypass, overuse of bone wax, and faulty skin antisepsis have all been thought to be important in the pathogenesis of these infections. Diagnosis is often difficult in the immediate postoperative period because fever and chest pain can be due to many other factors. Organ-

isms are antibiotic resistant, and medical therapy alone is rarely successful. Surgical debridement is essential to cure.

Urinary Tract Infections. Although urinary tract infections with *S. epidermidis* are very uncommon, another species of coagulase-negative staphylococcus, *S. saprophyticus,* is the second most common cause (next to *E. coli*) of urinary tract infections in otherwise healthy young women. Symptoms are indistinguishable from those experienced during *E. coli* urinary tract infections. *S. saprophyticus* is differentiated from *S. epidermidis* in the laboratory by its resistance to the antibiotic novobiocin. Infections respond readily to usual urinary tract antimicrobials, and relapse is uncommon. Because *S. saprophyticus* grows slowly, there may be fewer of these organisms in infected urine than the number ($>10^5$ colony-forming units/ml) with gram-negative bacteria. *S. epidermidis* occasionally causes infections in urinary tracts of elderly individuals, in patients with indwelling catheters, and in patients undergoing genitourinary surgery.

Infections in Immunosuppressed Patients. Coagulase-negative staphylococci are becoming important causes of bacteremia in immunosuppressed, neutropenic patients undergoing therapy for malignancy. The pathogenesis of bacteremia has been variously attributed to gut colonization with *S. epidermidis* after the use of oral antibiotics for gut sterilization or infection of long-term, indwelling plastic catheters used for administration of chemotherapy.

TREATMENT

The vast majority (more than 90%) of both community-acquired and hospital-acquired staphylococcal strains are resistant to penicillin. Thus patients suspected of having a staphylococcal infection require a penicillinase-resistant antibiotic. In the patient who is not allergic to penicillin, dicloxacillin (orally) or nafcillin or oxacillin (parenterally) are the drugs of choice (Chapter 231). Localized dermal and soft tissue infections can be treated orally for 10 to 14 days after drainage has been completed. Systemic infections require parenteral therapy. Four weeks of therapy should suffice in the uncomplicated case of endocarditis. In adult patients with osteomyelitis, 4 to 6 weeks of therapy usually should be combined with wide surgical debridement and drainage. After discharge, oral therapy for 3 to 6 months may prevent late relapses.

A rise in methicillin-resistant (better termed β-lactam antibiotic–resistant) staphylococcal organisms is becoming a significant problem. All staphylococci that show in vitro resistance to methicillin should be considered resistant to all β-lactam antibiotics (i.e., both penicillins and cephalosporins and probably even the newer β-lactam–like agents such as imipenem). Over the last 5 to 10 years, large university and community hospitals across the country have been reporting an increasing number of infections with these organisms. Thus far, essentially all β-lactam antibiotic–resistant organisms have remained sensitive to vancomycin, and many are sensitive to trimethoprim-sulfamethoxazole. The quinolone group of antibiotics may also be effective. Ciprofloxacin is the most commonly used quinolone. It is orally well absorbed, making it an option for outpatient therapy of a variety of deep staphylococcal infections, even some of those produced by β-lactam antibiotic–resistant strains; increasing resistance, however, of staphylococcal strains to the quinolones is now being reported more often.

The first patient with a documented infection to a *Staphylococcus aureus* strain with reduced susceptibility to vancomycin (MIC, 8 μg/ml) was described in Japan in May 1996. Previous infections with coagulase-negative staphylococci with reduced susceptibility to vancomycin have occasionally been reported. No patients with vancomycin-resistant *S. aureus* have yet been reported in the United States; however, the CDC has issued interim guidelines (CDC, 1997). These infections are anticipated to be very difficult to treat, probably requiring access to investigational antimicrobial agents.

Most infections with coagulase-negative staphylococci are hospital acquired; therefore these isolates should be considered resistant to the usual antistaphylococcal antibiotics. Many clinical laboratories report *S. epidermidis* isolates to be susceptible to semisynthetic penicillinase-resistant penicillins (particularly nafcillin) and cephalosporins when these isolates are actually resistant. Susceptibility test-

Table 260-1   Therapy for coagulase-negative staphylococcal infections

| | ANTIMICROBIAL AGENT* | | |
SITE OF INFECTION	METHICILLIN-SUSCEPTIBLE	METHICILLIN-RESISTANT	DURATION
Infected prosthetic cardiac valve, joint, or vascular graft; osteomyelitis	Nafcillin or oxacillin; ±gentamicin for 2 weeks (vancomycin or cefazolin if penicillin allergic)	Vancomycin ±rifampin; ±gentamicin for 2 weeks †	6 Weeks
Native valve endocarditis	Same	Vancomycin; ±gentamicin for 2 weeks	4 Weeks
Catheter infection	Nafcillin or oxacillin	Vancomycin	2 Weeks
Urinary tract infection	Amoxicillin or trimethoprim-sulfamethoxasole (*S. saprophyticus*)	Vancomycin	3 Days (lower UTI) or 2 weeks (upper UTI)
CSF shunt	Systemic nafcillin or oxacillin and intraventricular methicillin and/or gentamicin	Systemic rifampin and intraventricular vancomycin and/or gentamicin	2 Weeks

*See text for exact dosage.
†It may be possible to use a quinolone or trimethoprim/sulfamethoxazole in place of gentamicin-resistant organisms, but there are scant data in human infections to support this regimen.
CSF, Cerebrospinal fluid; *UTI,* urinary tract infection.

ing using modified methods has revealed that this heteroresistant (methicillin-resistant) phenotype can be detected in more than 80% of *S. epidermidis* from such hospital-acquired infections as intravenous catheter–associated bacteremia, PVE, and infections of cerebrospinal fluid shunts.

Heteroresistant strains of *S. epidermidis* are still uniformly susceptible to vancomycin, but *Streptococcus hemolyticus,* a coagulase-negative staphylococcus occasionally isolated from patients with nosocomial infections, may be resistant. Both rifampin and gentamicin are extremely active in vitro against most isolates; however, the emergence of rifampin-resistant mutants after brief drug exposure, the rapid increase in plasmid-mediated gentamicin resistance among staphylococci in some hospitals, and the nephrotoxicity of gentamicin have somewhat limited the utility of these two antibiotics in the treatment of coagulase-negative staphylococcal infections. Although both methicillin-resistant and methicillin-susceptible coagulase-negative staphylococci appear to be moderately susceptible to quinolones (ciprofloxacin, ofloxacin, and temofloxacin) in vitro, there are few data on the role of these antimicrobial agents in treating documented infections caused by coagulase-negative staphylococci. However, on the basis of data showing rapid emergence of ciprofloxacin-resistant coagulase-negative staphylococci in areas where use of the drug is high and of the poor record of ciprofloxacin in therapy of methicillin-resistant *S. aureus* infections, quinolones should probably not be used to treat coagulase-negative staphylococcal foreign-body infections until more studies documenting their efficacy become available. Likewise, up to half of nosocomial coagulase-negative staphylococci are susceptible to trimethoprim-sulfamethoxazole, but the role of this antimicrobial in foreign-body infections is unknown. The high rate of resistance of nosocomial isolates to clindamycin (more than 60% are resistant) generally limits its use.

All patients who have infections caused by hospital-acquired *S. epidermidis* or other coagulase-negative staphylococci should be treated with vancomycin, 1 g intravenously every 12 hours or 500 mg every 6 hours, until appropriate laboratory tests accurately define the susceptibility. Rifampin 300 mg orally every 8 hours or 600 mg every 12 hours and/or gentamicin, 1 mg/kg intravenously or intramuscularly every 8 hours may be added to vancomycin to increase serum bactericidal activity. Rifampin-resistant mutants have been recovered from patients with PVE receiving only vancomycin and rifampin. The addition of gentamicin as a third drug for the first 2 weeks of treatment prevented the emergence of rifampin resistance but led to increased nephrotoxicity. In most cases it is impossible to eradicate infections of indwelling foreign devices with antibiotics alone, without surgical removal of the devices. This is particularly true of prosthetic cardiac valves and prosthetic joints. In some cases, however, apparent cure of long-term indwelling intravenous catheter and peritoneal dialysis catheter infections has been achieved by the vancomycin-rifampin combination without catheter removal. Similarly, occasional cerebrospinal fluid shunt infections have responded

to intraventricular vancomycin (10 to 20 mg/day for adults) and/or gentamicin (5 to 8 mg/day for adults) administration and rifampin without shunt removal. The rare, truly methicillin-susceptible organism can be treated with systemic nafcillin or oxacillin (discussed later) and intraventricular methicillin (1 to 2 mg/kg twice a day). Some authorities consider methicillin (rarely used at present) to be less epileptogenic than other β-lactams for intraventricular administration.

An important issue in the treatment of staphylococcal infections is whether vancomycin is as effective as the semisynthetic penicillins for the treatment of infections caused by β-lactam antibiotic–*sensitive* strains. Vancomycin is certainly the drug of choice for β-lactam–resistant strains, since few alternatives are available. Several studies evaluating efficacy of vancomycin versus that of semisynthetic penicillin (usually nafcillin) suggest that *S. aureus* bacteremia is terminated less rapidly with vancomycin. Thus a consensus is emerging that therapy of β-lactam–sensitive staphylococci should employ nafcillin or oxacillin rather than vancomycin.

Coagulase-negative staphylococcal infections that routinely respond to conventional antistaphylococcal antibiotics are native valve endocarditis and outpatient (*S. saprophyticus*) urinary tract infections. Isolates from patients with native valve endocarditis who did not acquire their infections in the hospital are virtually always susceptible to semisynthetic penicillinase-resistant penicillins, but most produce penicillinase and are resistant to penicillin G. Nafcillin or oxacillin should be given in dosages of 8 to 12 g/day for 4 weeks. Cephalosporins may be given to penicillin-allergic patients who do not have a history of anaphylactic shock, and vancomycin may be given to those who do. A compilation of therapeutic recommendations is shown in Table 260-1.

With chronic infections when prosthetic devices are present, the standard approach to the treatment is to initiate antibiotic therapy and *remove* the prosthesis. If the involved prosthesis is critical to life function (e.g., a prosthetic heart valve), suppressive therapy may be tried. In such instances, if the patient is otherwise doing well, prolonged (possibly permanent) suppressive therapy should be administered, first parenterally, then orally.

In an *S. aureus* infection of a prosthetic heart valve, early operative intervention is mandatory, especially if the patient is showing any sign of valvular malfunction. Approximately half of such patients do well even if the operation has been carried out in the presence of active infection. As noted earlier, in the patient who is severely allergic to penicillin, vancomycin is the drug of choice; cephalosporins may be used in less severe allergies. Clindamycin is acceptable for bone and soft tissue infections but should not be used in bacteremic patients or in those with endocarditis because of high relapse rates.

A particularly difficult problem for the internist is the patient who has recurrent skin and soft tissue infections with *S. aureus.* Such patients initially may respond to antibiotics plus incision and drainage; however, relapse is common. Most of these patients are found to be carrying the infecting organism in the nose. In such instances, cultures of all family members should be made to ensure that the organism is not being passed back and forth. *S. aureus* carriers can then be treated with a combination of intensive cleansing (hand washing, nasal disinfectant soaps, and antibiotic creams) and a 5-day course of mupirocin calcium ointment intranasally twice a day. Intranasal mupirocin has been shown to eradicate nasal *S. aureus* carriage, subsequently reducing hand and skin colonization and, in several studies, decreasing the incidence of *S. aureus* bacteremias in hemodialysis patients. Other approaches to decreasing nasal carriage include the use of combined oral rifampin and dicloxacillin. By suppressing the nasal *S. aureus* carrier state, the episodes of recurrent superficial skin infections usually are terminated. Recently, *S. aureus* sternotomy infections after cardiac surgery have been linked to the nasal carriage of the organism; thus it may be prudent in high-risk patients (e.g., insulin-requiring diabetics and patients receiving hemodialysis) to eradicate the carried state in advance of cardiac surgery.

In the hospital setting, physicians, nurses, and others involved in patient care *must* wash their hands before and after examination of every patient to reduce the likelihood of both patient-to-patient and physician- or nurse-to-patient transfer of carried organisms. Hospital personnel who are recalcitrant nasal carriers respond to brief courses of mupirocin therapy; this will decrease nasal carriage and subsequent hand contamination.

PREVENTION

Measures for the prevention of staphylococcal infections should focus primarily on the hospital environment and should be based on meticulous infection control techniques (Chapter 232). Hospital personnel must be educated as to how these organisms are transmitted among individuals, and hand washing must be emphasized for all patient care team members. Meticulous attention must be paid to the use of medical devices that breach mucosal or dermal barriers. The placement of both routine and long-term intravenous lines (e.g., for hyperalimentation) should be performed according to specific protocols developed by the hospital's infection control committee. Increasingly, as data are further produced documenting the association between a patient's being a nasal carrier of *S. aureus* and his or her risk of nosocomial and postoperative infections, identification and treatment of nasal carriers will probably play an important role in prevention.

Prophylactic antibiotics have been shown to reduce postoperative staphylococcal infections, especially those complicating implantation of prosthetic devices and orthopedic and neurosurgical procedures. Such regimens usually use a cephalosporin or vancomycin (to cover *S. epidermidis* as well as *S. aureus*), and the drug should be given 30 to 60 minutes before the procedure to produce an adequate blood or tissue level, or both, during the operation. Prophylactic antibiotics should *not* be continued for more than 48 hours. Antibiotic prophylaxis, however, has the following deleterious effects: coagulase-negative staphylococci that are resistant to the antibiotics used as prophylaxis cause most of the infections of implanted devices, and prophylactic antibiotics select antibiotic-resistant skin flora, especially antibiotic-resistant coagulase-negative staphylococci, which may be spread from patients to hospital staff and thus increase the hospital reservoir of these organisms. Minimizing the duration of prophylaxis may ease some of the selective pressure for colonization with resistant organisms and decrease this reservoir. With the recent dramatic increase in vancomycin-resistant enterococci, extra effort will have to be made to reduce or restrict both prophylactic and therapeutic vancomycin usage.

Although clean-air systems (e.g., laminar air flow) reduce the number of airborne bacteria during surgery, there has been no clear demonstration that these systems are important in reducing the number of postoperative infections of implanted foreign devices. Meticulous surgical technique and appropriate barrier precautions during surgery remain the most important factors in the prevention of postsurgical infections.

BIBLIOGRAPHY

Archer GL: Antibiotic resistance in coagulase-negative staphylococci. In Mårdh P-A, Schleifer KH, editors: *Coagulase-negative staphylococci*, Stockholm, 1986, Almquist and Wiksell.

Bayer AS et al: *Staphylococcus aureus* bacteremia: clinical, serological, and echocardio-

graphic findings in patients with and without endocarditis, *Arch Intern Med* 147:457, 1987.

Caputo GM et al: Native valve endocarditis due to coagulase-negative staphylococci: clinical and microbiologic features, *Am J Med* 83:619, 1987.

Centers for Disease Control: Interim guidelines for prevention and control of staphylococcal infection associated with reduced susceptibility to vancomycin, *MMWR* 46:626-635, 1997.

Christensen GD et al: Nosocomial septicemia due to multiple antibiotic-resistant *Staphylococcus epidermidis*, *Ann Intern Med* 96:1, 1982.

Easmon CSF, Adlam C, editors: *Staphylococci and staphylococcal infections: clinical and epidemiological aspects*, vol 1, London, 1983, Academic.

Easmon CSF, Adlam C, editors: *Staphylococci and staphylococcal infections: The organism in vivo and in vitro*, vol 2, London, 1983, Academic.

Haley RW: Methicillin-resistant *Staphylococcus aureus*: do we just have to live with it? *Ann Intern Med* 114:162, 1991.

Jordan PA et al: Urinary tract infection caused by *Staphylococcus saprophyticus*, *J Infect Dis* 142:510, 1980.

Karchmer AW, Archer GL, Dismukes WE: Staphylococcus epidermidis prosthetic valve endocarditis: microbiologic and clinical observations as guides to therapy, *Ann Intern Med* 98:447, 1983.

Kloos WE, Bannerman TL: Update on clinical significance of coagulase-negative staphylococci, *Clin Microbiol Rev* 7:17, 1994.

Lowy FD, Hammer SM: *Staphylococcus epidermidis* infections, *Ann Intern Med* 99:834, 1983.

Marrack P, Kappler J: The Staphylococcal enterotoxins and their relatives, *Science* 248:705, 1990.

Musher DM, Lamm N, Darouche RO et al: The current spectrum of *Staphylococcus aureus* infection in a tertiary care hospital, *Medicine* 73:186, 1994.

Quie PG, Belani KK: Coagulase-negative staphylococcal adherence and persistence, *J Infect Dis* 156:543, 1987.

Schaberg DR, Culver DH, Gaymes RP: Major trends in the microbial etiology of nosocomial infection, *Am J Med* 91(3B):72, 1991.

Schoenbaum SC, Gardner P, Shillito J: Infections of cerebrospinal fluid shunts: epidemiology, clinical manifestations, and therapy, *J Infect Dis* 131:543, 1975.

Scully BE et al: Mupirocin treatment of nasal staphylococcal colonization, *Arch Intern Med* 152:353, 1992.

Sheagren JN: Inflammation induced by *Staphylococcus aureus*. In Gallin JI, Goldstein IM, Snyderman R, editors: *Inflammation: basic principles and clinical correlates*, New York, 1988, Raven.

Sheagren JN: *Staphylococcus aureus*: the persistent pathogen, *N Engl J Med* 310:1368, 1437, 1984.

Sheagren JN: Staphylococcal infections in immunocompromised patients. In Crossley K, Archer GL, editors: *Staphylococci and staphylococcal diseases*, New York, 1997, Churchill Livingstone.

Sheagren JN, Schaberg DR: Staphylococcal infections: a current concepts monograph, Kalamazoo Mich, 1992, Upjohn.

Smith IM, Vickers AB: Natural history of 338 treated and untreated patients with staphylococcal septicaemia (1936-1955), *Lancet* 1:1318, 1960.

Wade JC et al: *Staphylococcus epidermidis*: an increasing cause of infections in patients with granulocytopenia, *Ann Intern Med* 97:503, 1982.

Winston DJ et al: Coagulase-negative staphylococcal bacteremia in patients receiving immunosuppressive therapy, *Arch Intern Med* 143:32, 1983.

CHAPTER

261 *Streptococcus pyogenes* Infections

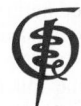

Dennis L. Stevens

Streptococcus pyogenes (group A streptococcus), perhaps more than any other pathogen, has developed an intimate relationship with the human host. In some acute infections and certainly in the well-known postinfectious sequelae, it is the host response elicited by this unique relationship that accounts for the morbidity and mortality. This chapter emphasizes these host-microbe relationships to explain the unique epidemiologic and pathogenic features of *S. pyogenes*.

EPIDEMIOLOGY

The declining prevalence of both rheumatic fever and serious infection caused by group A streptococci (GAS) throughout the 20th century in much of the Western world has been attributed to improved socioeconomic conditions, timely antibiotic treatment of streptococcal pharyngitis, and secondary prophylaxis for rheumatic fever. Some have argued that this decline is due to cyclic virulence changes in the

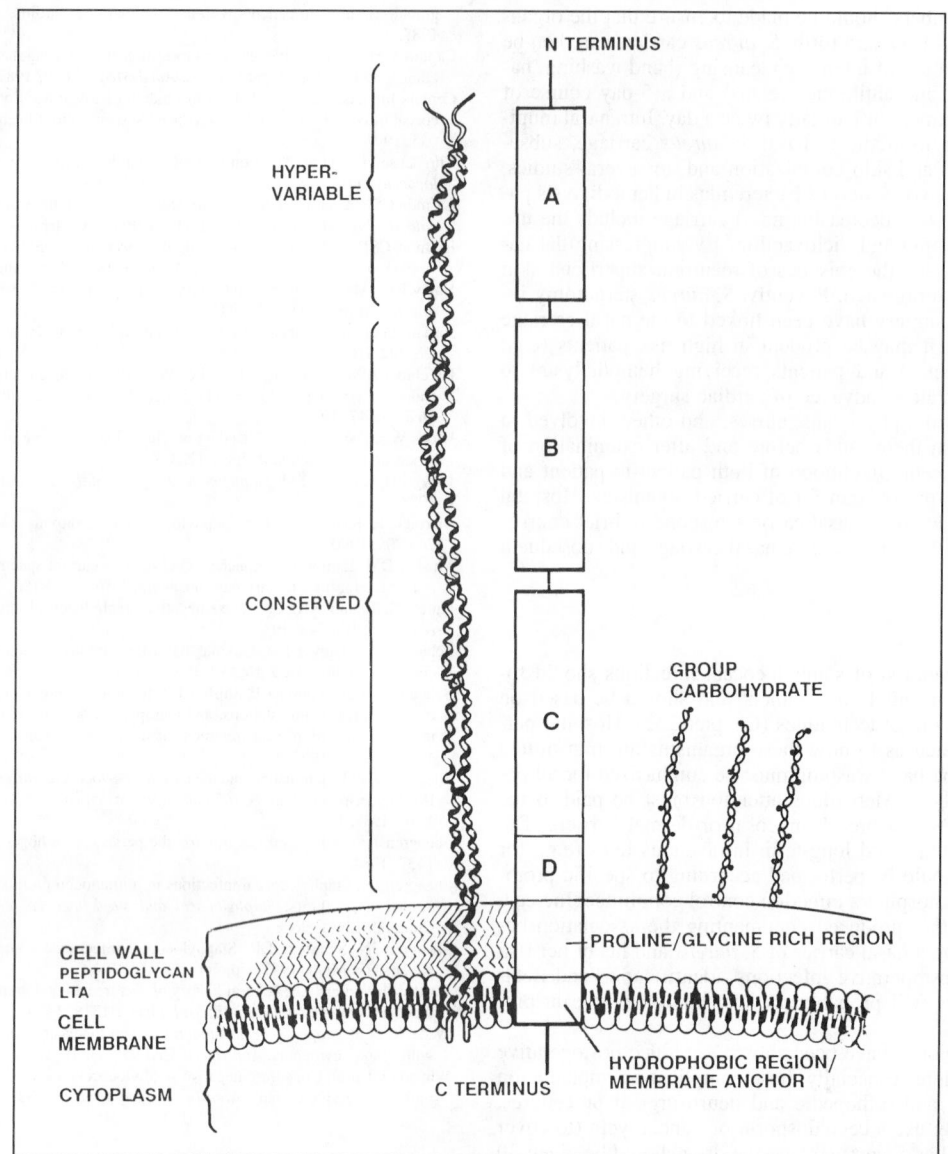

FIGURE 261-1 Structural components of M protein. M protein is a coiled coil consisting of four regions of repeating amino acids (*A* to *D*), a proline/glycine-rich region that serves to intercalate the protein into the bacterial cell wall, and a hydrophobic region that acts as a membrane anchor.

From Fischetti VA: *Sci Am* 264:58, 1991.

organism. The recent outbreaks of pharyngitis, acute rheumatic fever, and the newly recognized streptococcal toxic shock syndrome (strep TSS) support this concept.

The greatest reservoirs of *S. pyogenes* are the skin and mucous membranes of humans, and nearly 5% of all people, regardless of age, carry the organism in their throats.

BACTERIAL CELL STRUCTURE AND EXTRACELLULAR PRODUCTS
Capsule

Some strains of GAS possess luxuriant capsules of hyaluronic acid resulting in large mucoid colonies on blood agar. M protein, especially M type 18, may also impart a mucoid phenotype.

M Proteins

More than 80 different serotypes of GAS based on the M protein expressed are currently recognized. The protein is a coiled coil consist-ing of four regions of repeating amino acids (A to D), a proline/glycine-rich region that serves to intercalate the protein into the bacterial cell wall, and a hydrophobic region that acts as a membrane anchor (Fig. 261-1). Region A near the N terminus is highly variable, and antibodies to this region confer type-specific protection. Within the more conserved B to D regions lies an area that binds one of the complement regulatory proteins (factor H), stearically inhibiting antibody binding and complement-derived opsonin deposition and effectively camouflaging the organism against immune surveillance. M protein inhibits the phagocytosis of *S. pyogenes* by polymorphonuclear leukocytes (PMNLs), although this property can be overcome by type-specific antisera. Fragments of M protein can also act as superantigens. The regulation of M-protein synthesis is not firmly established but may be controlled by genetic elements of a vir gene composed of an upstream control sequence coupled to gene segments coding for M protein, immunoglobulin binding proteins, and C5a peptidase. Observations by Lancefield suggested that the quantity of M protein produced decreases with passage on artificial media and, conversely, increases rapidly with passage through mice. During untreated pharyngitis the

Table 261-1 The interplay between *Streptococcus pyogenes* and the human immune system

HOST FACTOR	COMPONENT	PATHOGENIC MECHANISM
Fibronectin	Fimbriae	Adherence to epithelium
Complement (C3)	Streptokinase	Inactivation of C3
Complement (C5a)	C5 peptidase	Destruction of chemotactic factor
Plasminogen	Streptokinase	Production of unregulatable form of plasmin
IgG	M-like protein	Binding or inactivation of IgG
Fibrin	Streptokinase	Dissolution of clot
PMNL	M protein	Prevention of phagocytosis
	SLO	Degranulation Increased expression of adherence glycoprotein Cytolysis Generation of oxygen radicals
Monocytes	SPEA SPEB SLO	Induction of TNF, IL-1,* IL-6
	Cell wall LTA Peptidoglycan	Induction of TNF
Lymphocytes	SPEA	Action as a superantigen Induction of lymphocyte production of TNF
NK cells	SPEA	Introduction of natural killer activity

*SLO and SPEA interact synergistically to induce IL-1-beta.
IgG, Immunoglobulin G; *PMNL*, polymorphonuclear leukocyte; *SLO*, streptolysin O; *SPEA*, pyrogenic exotoxin A; *SPEB*, pyrogenic exotoxin B; *LTA*, lipoteichoic acid; *TNF*, tumor necrosis factor; *IL-1*, interleukin-1; *NK*, natural killer.

quantity of M protein produced by an infecting strain progressively decreases during convalescence.

Cell Wall

The cell wall comprises a peptidoglycan backbone with integral lipoteicoic acid (LTA) components. The function of LTA is not well known; however, both peptidoglycan and LTA have important interactions with the host (Table 261-1).

Cytoplasmic Membrane

Little is known about the function and composition of the cytoplasmic membrane, although it is clear that the membrane does serve as a site of cell wall synthesis. This process is orchestrated by five different penicillin binding proteins (PBPs) found within membrane fragments. The regulation of autolysis and cell wall synthesis during chain elongation is a dynamic process whose control is a reflection of the metabolic activity of the cell, which becomes dysregulated in the presence of cell wall active antibiotics. All PBPs are expressed during log-phase growth of GAS, and it is at this stage that penicillin's effects are greatest.

Group Carbohydrate

Rebecca Lancefield is credited with providing a classification scheme for streptococci based on carbohydrate antigen obtained by acid extraction of cell wall material. Currently, groups of streptococci from A to O have been defined by such typing. The role of carbohydrate antigen in pathogenesis is vague and probably not as important as other factors. Streptococcal typing has been simplified with the development of commercially available rapid latex agglutination schemes. Although the bacitracin susceptibility test has proved very reliable as a presumptive marker for group A, both false-negative and false-positive results are problematic.

Streptolysin O

Streptolysin O belongs to a family of oxygen-labile, thiol-activated cytolysins (TACs) and causes the broad zone of beta hemolysis surrounding colonies of GAS on blood agar plates. TAC toxins bind to cholesterol moieties on eucaryotic cell membranes, creating toxin-cholesterol aggregates that contribute to cell lysis via a colloid-osmotic mechanism. Exogenous cholesterol inhibits hemolysis both in vitro and in situations where serum cholesterol is high (e.g., nephrotic syndrome); thus elevated antistreptolysin O (ASO) titers occur because either cholesterol or anti-ASO antibody neutralizes streptolysin O. Several TAC toxins including SLO have been cloned and sequenced, and there exists striking homology among SLO, perfringolysin O, and pneumolysin in a 13– to 15–amino acid sequence upstream from the cysteine residue. The significance of SLO in pathogenesis is discussed later in this chapter.

Deoxyribonucleases A, B, C, and D

Expression of deoxyribonucleases (DNases) in vivo elicits production of anti-DNase antibody during and after infection. Antibodies to DNase A and DNase B have proved useful in the serologic diagnosis of pharyngeal and skin infections. The importance of these enzymes in the pathogenesis of GAS infections has not been proved.

Hyaluronidase

The extracellular enzyme hyaluronidase hydrolyzes the hyaluronic acid in deeper tissues and may facilitate the spread of GAS infections along fascial planes. Its clinical importance is unknown; however, a rise in antihyaluronidase titers follows GAS infections in general, especially those involving the skin.

Pyrogenic Exotoxins A, B, C, MF, and SSA

The pyrogenic exotoxins A, B, C, MF, and SSA (also called scarlatina toxins and erythrogenic toxins) function to induce lymphocyte blastogenesis, potentiate endotoxin-induced shock, induce fever, suppress antibody synthesis, and act as superantigens.

The gene for pyrogenic exotoxin A (speA) is transmitted by bacteriophage, and stable toxin production depends on lysogenic conversion in a manner analogous to diphtheria toxin production by *Corynebacterium diphtheria*. Control of pyrogenic exotoxin A (SPEA) production is not yet understood, although the quantity of SPEA produced can vary dramatically from decade to decade. Historically, SPEA-producing strains have been associated with severe cases of scarlet fever and, more recently, with strep TSS.

Although all strains of GAS are endowed with genes for pyrogenic exotoxin B (SPEB [speB]), like SPEA, the quantity of toxin produced varies greatly. SPEB is related to the proteinase precursor, and the role of each in pathogenesis has only recently been investigated.

Pyrogenic exotoxin C (SPEC), like SPEA, is bacteriophage mediated, and its expression is likewise highly variable. Mild cases of scarlet fever in England have been associated with strains of GAS producing SPEC.

Streptococcal superantigen (SSA) has recently been described in an M type 3 GAS strain isolated from a patient with strep TSS. This toxin has similar characteristics to other pyrogenic toxins and also functions as a superantigen. Its distribution among strains of GAS and its role in pathogenesis has not been defined.

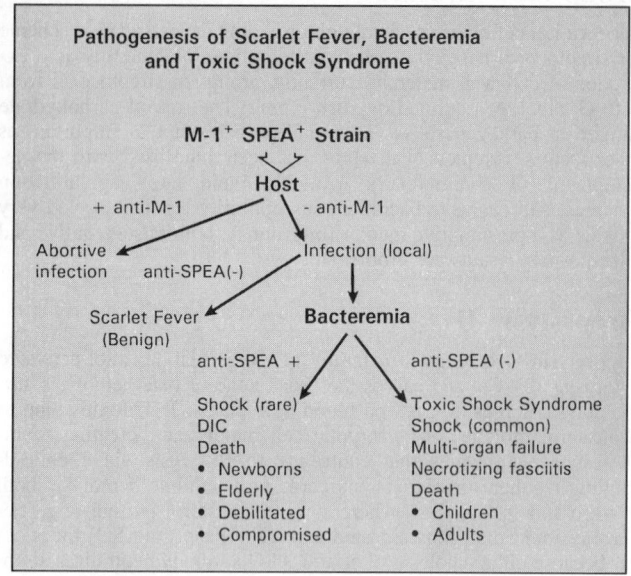

FIGURE 261-2   Pathogenesis of scarlet fever, bacteremia, and streptococcal toxic shock syndrome.
M-1⁺ SPEA⁺, A GAS strain that contains M protein type 1 and pyrogenic exotoxin A (SPEA); + *anti-M-1*, presence of antibody of M protein type 1; − *anti-M-1*, absence of antibody to M protein type 1; *anti-SPEA +*, antibody to SPEA; *DIC*, disseminated intravascular coagulation; *GAS*, group A streptococci.
From Stevens DL: *Clin Infect Dis* 14:2, 1992.

Mitogenic factor (MF), the latest superantigen to be discovered, has all the features of other pyrogenic exotoxins, is a potent inducer of cytokines and lymphokines, and has been found in most strains of GAS that have been examined.

Protein F is a fibronectin binding protein that, in conjuction with peptidoglycan, lipoteichoic acid, and M protein, plays an important role in adherence of GAS to epithelial surfaces.

CLINICAL FEATURES OF INFECTIONS
Pharyngitis and the Asymptomatic Carrier

Streptococcus carriage rate may rise from 5% to 15% to above 50% in school-age children during epidemics of GAS pharyngitis. Transmission occurs via aerosolized droplets from the upper airway of one host to another. Patients with GAS pharyngitis (most frequently children 5 to 15 years of age) have sore throat, submandibular adenopathy, fever, and pharyngeal erythema with exudates. Acute pharyngitis is sufficient to induce antibody against M protein, SLO, DNase and hyaluronidase, and, if present, pyrogenic exotoxins. GAS pharyngitis may proceed to scarlet fever, bacteremia, suppurative head and neck infections, streptococcal toxic shock syndrome, carrier state, rheumatic fever, or poststreptococcal glomerulonephritis. Thus the outcomes depend on the interaction between streptococcal virulence factors and the host (Fig. 261-2).

During GAS epidemics, particularly where rheumatic fever or a poststreptococcal glomerulonephritis are prevalent, treatment of asymptomatic carriers may be necessary, and at times, programs that use monthly injection of benzathine penicillin have greatly reduced the incidence of GAS pharyngitis as well as rheumatic fever.

Scarlet Fever

In the last decade, outbreaks of scarlet fever in the United States have often been associated with strains of GAS producing pyrogenic exotoxin C. The cases have been notably mild and the illness has been referred to as "pharyngitis with rash." Historically this form was known as benign scarlet fever, although scarlet fever has not always

been a mild disease: around the turn of the century mortality rates of 25% were common.

Scarlet fever has been divided into the following groups: mild, moderate, toxic, and septic (Table 261-2). Thus benign scarlet fever may be either mild or moderate, and the fatal or malignant form may be either septic or toxic. The toxic cases invariably began with a severe sore throat, marked fever, delirium, skin rash, and painful cervical lymph nodes. In severe toxic cases, fulminating fevers of 107° F, pulse rates of 130 to 160 beats per minute, severe headache, delirium, convulsions, little if any skin rash, and death within 24 hours were the usual findings. These cases occurred before the advent of antibiotics, antipyretics, and anticonvulsants, and deaths were the result of uncontrolled seizures and hyperpyrexia. The term *septic scarlet fever* refers to the form characterized by local invasion of the soft tissues of the neck and complications such as upper airway obstruction, otitis media with perforation, profuse mucopurulent drainage from the nose, bronchopneumonia, and death. Necrotizing fasciitis and myositis were not observed in association with scarlet fever; the only exception was locally invasive infection of the soft tissues of the neck as a complication of pharyngitis.

Soft-Tissue Infection (also see Chapter 241)

Erysipelas. Erysipelas is caused exclusively by *S. pyogenes* and is characterized by an abrupt onset of fiery red swelling of the face or extremities. Distinctive features are well-defined margins, particularly along the nasolabial fold; scarlet or salmon-red color; rapid progression; and intense pain. Flaccid bullae may develop during the second to third day of illness, yet extension to deeper soft tissues is rare. Surgical debridement is not necessary, and treatment with penicillin is very effective. Swelling may progress despite treatment, although fever, pain, and intense redness diminish. Desquamation of the involved skin occurs 5 to 10 days into the illness. Infants and elderly adults are most commonly afflicted, and erysipelas was more severe before the turn of the century.

Streptococcal Pyoderma (Impetigo Contagiosa). The thick, crusted skin lesions of streptococcal pyoderma frequently have a golden-brown color resembling that of dried serum. Children between 2 and 5 years of age are most commonly infected. Epidemics occur throughout the year in tropical areas or during the summer months in more temperate climates and are usually associated with poor hygiene. Initially colonization of the unbroken skin occurs either exogenously from infected persons or endogenously by oropharyngeal organisms. Development of impetiginous lesions requires 10 to 14 days and probably is initiated by minor abrasions, insect bites, and the like, all of which serve as a means of intradermal inoculation. Patients should receive penicillin, although, unlike treatment of rheumatic fever, penicillin may not prevent poststreptococcal glomerulonephritis. About 50% of cases of impetigo are caused by *Staphylococcus aureus*.

Cellulitis. GAS may invade the epidermis and subcutaneous tissues, resulting in local swelling, erythema, and pain. The skin becomes indurated and, unlike erysipelas, is a pinkish color. Patients with lymphedema attributable to lymphoma, filariasis, or surgical node dissection (e.g., mastectomy or carcinoma of the prostate) are predisposed to development of GAS cellulitis, as are those with chronic venous stasis. Saphenous donor site cellulitis may be due to group A, C, or G streptococci. In such patients there may not be a site of inoculation. Cellulitis associated with a primary focus (e.g., an abscess or a boil) is more likely caused by *S. aureus*. Aspiration of the leading edge and punch biopsy yield a causative organism in 15% and 40% of cases, respectively. Patients respond quickly to penicillin, although in some cases, when staphylococcus is of concern, nafcillin or oxacillin may be a better choice. If bluish or violet discoloration develops or if bullae become apparent, a deeper infection such as necrotizing fasciitis or myositis should be considered (see Necrotizing Fasciitis). In such cases, systemic toxicity is usually present. A serum creatine phosphokinase (CPK) level should be obtained and if elevated, prompt surgical inspection and debridement should be performed.

Table 261-2   Comparison of the clinical characteristics of types of scarlet fever

	OTHER NAMES	CLINICAL PRESENTATION	COMPLICATIONS	AGE (YEARS)	PREDISPOSING FACTORS
Scarlet fever	Benign scarlet fever Moderate scarlet fever Scarlet fever simplex	Fever Pharyngitis Scarlatina rash Desquamation	Late ARF or AGN Death rare	<10 (90%)	None
Septic scarlet fever	Scarlatina anginosa Malignant sore throat Garrotillo Morbus strangulatoris Ulcerative angina	Scarlet fever with local suppuration and invasion of deeper structures	Otitis Sinusitis Meningitis Airway obstruction Bacteremia Cavernous vein thrombosis	<10 (90%)	Before antibiotic era
Toxic scarlet fever	Malignant scarlet fever Atactic scarlet fever	Scarlet fever with hyperpyrexia and either neurologic complications or cardiovascular collapse; rash evanescent or absent	Convulsions Coma Sudden death	<10 (90%)	Before antibiotics, anticonvulsants, intravenous fluids

ARF, Acute rheumatic fever; *AGN,* acute glomerulonephritis.

Lymphangitis. Cutaneous infection with bright red streaks ascending proximally is invariably due to GAS. Prompt antibiotic treatment is mandatory because bacteremia and systemic toxicity develop rapidly.

Necrotizing Fasciitis. Necrotizing fasciitis, originally called streptococcal gangrene, is a deep-seated infection of the subcutaneous tissue that results in progressive destruction of fascia and fat but may spare the skin itself. *Necrotizing fasciitis* is now the preferred term for the entity because *Clostridium perfringens, Clostridium septicum,* and *S. aureus* can produce a similar pathologic process (Chapters 263 and 260). Infection may begin at the site of trivial or inapparent trauma. Within the first 24 hours, swelling, heat, erythema, and tenderness develop and rapidly spread proximally and distally from the original focus. During the next 24 to 48 hours the erythema darkens, changing from red to purple and then to blue, and blisters and bullae that contain clear yellow fluid form. On the fourth or fifth day the purple areas become frankly gangrenous. From the seventh to the tenth day the line of demarcation becomes sharply defined, and the dead skin begins to reveal extensive necrosis of the subcutaneous tissue. Patients become increasingly prostrated and emaciated and may become unresponsive, mentally cloudy, or even delirious. Use of aggressive fasciotomy, debridement, and Dakan's solution irrigation achieved mortality rates as low as 20% even before antibiotics were available. The increased severity of necrotizing fasciitis that has occurred among recent cases of strep TSS relative to shock, multiorgan failure, and mortality could be due to the emergence of increased virulence of GAS themselves.

Myositis. Historically, streptococcal myositis has been an extremely uncommon GAS infection, and only 21 cases were documented from 1900 to 1985. Recently an increased prevalence of GAS myositis has been reported in the United States, Norway, and Sweden. Translocation of GAS from the pharynx to the muscle site must occur hematogenously because penetrating trauma is usually not sustained. Further, most patients have not reported symptomatic pharyngitis or tonsillitis. Severe pain may be the only presenting symptom, swelling and erythema may be the only signs of infection, and muscle compartment syndromes may develop rapidly. In most cases a single muscle group is involved; however, because patients frequently have bacteremia, there may be several sites of myositis or abscess. Distinguishing streptococcal myositis from spontaneous gas gangrene caused by *C. perfringens* or *C. septicum* may be difficult, although the presence of crepitus or gas in the tissue would favor a diagnosis of clostridial infection. Myositis is easily distinguished from necrotizing fasciitis anatomically by means of surgical exploration or incisional biopsy, although clinical features of both conditions overlap. In published reports the case-fatality rate of necrotizing fasciitis is between 20% and 50%, whereas that of GAS myositis is between 80% and 100%. Aggressive surgical debridement is of extreme importance because of the poor efficacy of penicillin described in human cases as well as in experimental streptococcal models of myositis (see Antibiotic Efficacy).

STREPTOCOCCAL TOXIC SHOCK SYNDROME

In the late 1980s, reports of invasive GAS infections associated with bacteremia, deep soft-tissue infection, shock, and multiorgan failure began to appear in North America and Europe. Previously healthy individuals between the ages of 20 and 50 years have been most commonly afflicted; overall, 30% of patients die, despite aggressive modern treatment.

Acquisition of Group A Streptococci and Predisposing Factors

The portal of entry of streptococci could not be ascertained in 45% of cases, and preceding symptomatic pharyngitis was rare. Most infections occurred sporadically, although minor epidemics have been reported. Most commonly, the streptococcal infection occurred at a site of minor local trauma that frequently did not result in a break in the skin. Surgical procedures and viral infections such as varicella and influenza provided portals of entry in other cases.

A virus like prodrome suggestive of influenza preceded the onset of TSS by several days in adults. The use of nonsteroidal antiinflammatory agents to treat pain may mask the presenting symptoms or predispose the patient to more severe complications such as shock.

Symptoms

Pain is a common initial symptom of strep TSS; it is severe and abrupt in onset and may not be associated with tenderness or physical findings. The pain most commonly involves an extremity but may also mimic peritonitis, pelvic inflammatory disease, acute myocardial infarction, or pericarditis.

Physical Findings

Fever is the most common presenting sign, although on admission to the hospital, 10% of patients in one report had profound hypothermia attributable to shock. Confusion may be present in more than half of the patients, and in some it progresses to coma or combativeness. In our 1989 report, on admission 80% of patients had tachycardia and 55% had systolic blood pressure of less than 110 mm Hg. Although 45% of patients had normal blood pressure (systolic pressure, >110 mm Hg) on admission, in all of these patients hypotension developed within the subsequent 4 hours. Soft tissue infection evolved to necrotizing fasciitis or myositis in 70% of cases, and in these cases surgical debridement, fasciotomy, or amputation was required. An ominous sign was the progression of soft tissue swelling to formation of

Table 261-3   Antibiotic therapy of group A streptococcal disease

	ROUTE	DOSAGE
Pharyngitis and impetigo		
Benzathine penicillin	IM	1.2 million units (>27 kg)
Penicillin G (or V)	PO	200,000 units qid for 10 days
Erythromycin	PO	40 mg/kg/day (up to 1 g/day)
Rheumatic fever prophylaxis		
Benzathine penicillin	IM	1.2 million units every 28 days
Penicillin G	PO	200,000 units bid
Sulfadiazine	PO	1 g/day (>27 kg) 500 mg/day (<27 kg)
Erythromycin*	PO	250 mg bid

Modified from Kaplan EL et al: *Circulation* 55:S1, 1977.
*For use only in patients with sensitivity to both penicillin and sulfonamides.

vesicles and then bullae, which took on a violaceous or bluish coloration. Among patients with no soft tissue infection on admission a variety of clinical presentations were observed; these included endophthalmitis, myositis, perihepatitis, peritonitis, myocarditis, and overwhelming sepsis. Patients who have shock and multiorgan failure without clinical evidence of local infection have a worse prognosis because definitive diagnosis and surgical debridement may be delayed.

Laboratory Test Results

Evidence of renal involvement was apparent at the time of admission by the presence of hemoglobinuria and elevated serum creatinine level. The serum albumin level was moderately low (3.3 g/dl) on admission and dropped further (2.3 g/dl) by 48 hours. Hypocalcemia, including ionized hypocalemia, was detectable early in the hospital course. The serum creatine kinase level is a useful test to detect deeper soft-tissue infections, such as necrotizing fasciitis or myositis.

The initial laboratory studies demonstrated only mild leukocytosis but a dramatic left shift (43% of white blood cells were band forms, metamyelocytes, and myelocytes) (Table 261-3). The mean platelet count was normal on admission but dropped to approximately 120,000 cells/mm³ within 48 hours, frequently in the absence of criteria for disseminated intravascular coagulopathy.

Bacteriologic Cultures

GAS was isolated from blood in 60% of cases and from deep tissue specimens in 95%.

Clinical Course

Shock was apparent early in the course, and management was complicated by profound capillary leak. Adult respiratory distress syndrome (ARDS) occurred frequently (55%) and complicated fluid resuscitation. Renal dysfunction preceded hypotension in many patients and progressed or persisted for 48 to 72 hours, despite treatment. In all patients who survived, serum creatinine levels returned to normal within 4 to 6 weeks. Overall, 30% to 70% of patients have died, despite aggressive treatment, including administration of intravenous fluids, colloid, pressors, and mechanical ventilation and surgical intervention including fasciotomy and debridement, exploratory laparotomy, intraocular aspiration, amputation, and hysterectomy.

Characteristics of Clinical Isolates

M types 1, 3, 12, and 28 of GAS have been the most common isolates from patients with shock and multiorgan failure in studies made worldwide. Pyrogenic exotoxin A or B, or both, has been found in isolates from the majority of patients with severe infection. Infections

in Norway, Sweden, and Great Britain have been primarily due to M type 1 strains of GAS that produce pyrogenic exotoxin B.

POSTINFECTIOUS SEQUELAE
Rheumatic Fever

The prevalence of acute rheumatic fever (ARF) in the Western world decreased dramatically after World War II (0.5 to 1.88 cases/100,000 school-age children/year). In contrast, in India and Sri Lanka the prevalence of ARF has remained 140/100,000 for children between 5 and 19 years of age. Socioeconomic factors seem to be important because the highest rates in all countries have been among the impoverished in large cities. Although improved living conditions and the development of penicillin have had important roles in reducing the prevalence of ARF in the United States, the decreases had begun before antibiotics were available. In addition, a resurgence of ARF has occurred among U.S. military recruits and predominantly among white middle-class civilians. A particularly frightening aspect of these recent civilian cases was the low incidence of symptomatic pharyngitis (24% to 78%). Thus our modern primary prevention strategy (diagnosis of acute GAS pharyngitis with penicillin treatment within 10 days) would not have prevented ARF in these cases.

Variations in the expression of virulence factors of "rheumatogenic strains" of *S. pyogenes* may best explain these fluctuations in ARF. M types isolated from rheumatic fever patients (i.e., M-1, 3, 5, 6, 14, 18, 19, and 24) have a common antigenic domain, which is immunologically cross-reactive with human heart tissue. Understanding this molecular mimicry holds great promise in the elucidation of the immune mechanisms resulting in clinical ARF. One other marker for rheumatogenicity is the mucoid appearance of fresh pharyngeal isolates from patients with ARF. In recent times in the United States, such strains have been of M type 18.

Although certain M types are strongly associated with ARF, such strains may cause other GAS infections as well. For example, M types 1 and 3 have also been associated with poststreptococcal glomerulonephritis and TSS. Further, epidemics of pharyngitis caused by M-1 are not invariably associated with epidemics of rheumatic fever. That host factors determine the clinical outcome of GAS is suggested by the observation that individuals with certain human leukocyte antigen (HLA) class II antigens are predisposed to development of ARF. Further, Stollerman suggested that a gradual acquisition of susceptibility to ARF by schoolchildren occurs after repeated infections. This is supported by the observations that ARF is uncommon in children younger than 2 years old and that antibody response to streptococcal antigens is exaggerated in children with ARF compared with those with GAS pharyngitis alone. In addition, patients with ARF demonstrate increased expression of the B cell alloantigen D8/17 in comparison to unaffected family members, including identical twins. That some strains of GAS can cause ARF in any individual is suggested by the observation that the attack rate of ARF can vary from 388 cases/100,000 soldiers in World War II to 1/100,000 in the general population today. Such fluctuations among relatively homogenous populations separated in time suggest changes in relative rheumatogenicity of GAS and not unique host factors.

The clinical manifestations of ARF are multiple and, because each is not specific for ARF, several criteria must be met to establish a definitive diagnosis. Simply put, two major manifestations or one major and two minor manifestations plus, in either case, evidence of an antecedent GAS infection are required for definitive diagnosis. The major manifestations and the frequency with which they occur during first attacks of ARF are as follows: arthritis (75%), carditis (40% to 50%), chorea (15%), and subcutaneous nodules (<10%). The minor manifestations are fever, arthralgia, heart block, presence of acute-phase reactants in the blood (C-reactive protein, leukocytosis, and elevated erythrocyte sedimentation rate), and history of ARF or rheumatic heart disease. Carditis, when present, occurs during the first 3 weeks of illness and may involve pericardium, myocardium, and endocardium. Patients with pericarditis may have chest pain or pericardial effusion, whereas those with myocarditis may have intractable heart failure. Manifestations of acute endocarditis involve the development of new murmurs of mitral regurgitation or aortic regurgitation, the latter being sometimes associated with a low-pitched apical middiastolic flow murmur (Carey Coombs murmur). Murmurs of mitral stenosis and aortic stenosis are not detected during first attacks of ARF but are chronic manifestations of rheumatic heart disease. Migratory arthritis involves several joints, most frequently the knees, ankles, elbows, and wrists, in more than 50% of patients. Each involved joint has evidence of inflammation that characteristically resolves within 2 to 3 weeks with no progression to chronic arthritis or articular damage. Subcutaneous nodules occur several weeks into the course of ARF and are found over bony surfaces or tendons. They last only 1 to 2 weeks and have in some cases been associated with severe carditis. Erythema marginatum is an evanescent, nonpainful erythematous eruption occurring on the trunk or proximl extremities. Individual lesions can develop and disappear within minutes, but the process may wax and wane over several weeks or months. Sydenham's chorea often occurs later in the course than other manifestations of ARF and is characterized by rapid, nonpurposeful choreiform movements of the face, hands, and feet. Attacks usually disappear during sleep but may persist for 2 to 4 months.

Poststreptococcal Glomerulonephritis

Acute glomerulonephritis (AGN) can follow either pharyngeal infection or skin infection and is associated with GAS strains possessing M types 12 or 49, respectively. During epidemics of skin or pharyngeal infection produced by a nephritogenic strain, attack rates of 10% to 15% have been documented with latent periods of 10 days after pharyngitis and 3 weeks after pyoderma. Nonspecific symptoms include lethargy, malaise, headache, anorexia, and dull back pain. The classic signs of AGN are all related to fluid overload and are evident initially in edema, both dependent and periorbital. Hypertension develops in most patients and is usually mild. Severe cases may be characterized by ascites, pleural effusion, encephalopathy, and pulmonary edema, although evidence of heart failure per se is lacking. Evidence of glomerular damage by renal biopsy has been documented in nearly 50% of contacts of siblings with AGN, suggesting that, as in ARF, subclinical disease is not uncommon after infection with certain strains of GAS. Unlike rheumatic fever, but similar to scarlet fever, glomerulonephritis occurs most commonly in children between 2 and 6 years of age. Like ARF and scarlet fever, AGN may affect several members of the same family. Recurrences or secondary attacks occur only rarely, and there is little to suggest that AGN progresses to chronic renal failure.

The differential diagnosis of poststreptococcal AGN must include Henoch-Schönlein disease, polyarteritis nodosa, idiopathic nephrotic syndrome, leptospirosis, hemolytic uremic syndrome (*Escherichia coli* 0157:H7), and malignant hypertension. The diagnosis is simpler if there is a recent history of symptomatic GAS pharyngitis, impetigo, or scarlet fever. Elevated or rising antibody titers to streptococcal antigens such as ASO, anti-DNase A or B, and/or antihyaluronidase are helpful, although ASO concentration may be low in patients with pyoderma. A careful urinalysis to document proteinuria and hematuria should be performed, but it is mandatory to demonstrate red blood cell casts because the latter is the hallmark of glomerular injury. The blood urea nitrogen and creatinine values are elevated and, if nephrotic syndrome is present, the serum cholesterol level is elevated and serum albumin concentration is low. Twenty-four hour excretion of protein is usually less than 3 g, and total hemolytic complement and C3 levels are markedly reduced.

Pathogenesis

Streptococcus pyogenes has great adaptive capacity for survival in the human host. Table 261-1 depicts some streptococcal components that interact with human host factors to facilitate invasion and contribute to pathogenesis.

Adherence of cocci to the mucosal epithelium occurs via the complex interaction of fibronectin binding protien, lipoteichoic acid, peptidoglycan, and M protein with cell surface structures including fibronectin. How GAS penetrates cells or cell junctions to reach the deeper tissue is not understood. Recent studies suggested that carbon dioxide and oxygen may alter expression of M protein and fibronectin-binding protein. Once within the tissues, the organism evades the host's inflammatory defenses by destroying or inactivating complement-derived chemoattractants and opsonins and by binding or inactivation of immunoglobulin. Expression of M protein, in the absence of type-specific antibody, protects the GAS from phagocytosis by PMNLs and monocytes, and secretion of SLO in high concentration destroys approaching phagocytes. Distal to the focus of infection, lower concentrations of SLO stimulate PMNL adhesion to endothelial cells, effectively preventing continued granulocyte migration. A unique feature of the pyrogenic exotoxins and some M protein fragments is their ability to interact with certain V_{beta} regions of the T-cell receptor in the absence of classic antigen processing by antigen-presenting cells. In the nonimmune host, SLO, SPEA, and other streptococcal components stimulate host cells to produce tumor necrosis factor (TNF) and interleukin-1 (IL-1). In addition, the superantigens associated with GAS not only induce IL-1 and TNF-α from monocytes but also induce clonal proliferation of T lymphocytes with massive production of the lymphokines, gamma interferon, IL-2 and TNF-β. These monokines and lymphokines together then mediate hypotension and stimulate leukostasis, resulting in shock, microvascular injury, multiorgan failure, and death.

TREATMENT
Emergence of Erythromycin Resistance

The first erythromycin-resistant strain of *Streptococcus pyogenes* (GAS) was isolated in Great Britain in 1959, and by 1975, resistant strains had also been isolated in the United States, Canada, and Japan. Although the prevalence of erythromycin resistance among GAS has remained low (3.6% to 4.0%) in most Western countries, in Japan resistance increased from 8.5% to 72% between 1971 and 1974. Similarly, erythromycin resistance had been a rare finding in Sweden; however, in 1984 an epidemic of pharyngitis (294 cases) caused by erythromycin-resistant GAS was reported. Erythromycin resistance has also been documented in Finland, Australia, and Spain.

Sulfonamide Resistance

Sulfonamide resistance currently is reported in less than 1% of GAS isolates.

Therapeutic Failure of Penicillin

The recommended antibiotic therapies for GAS diseases are shown in Table 261-3. The major problem in the treatment of GAS infections with penicillin is a lack of in vivo efficacy, despite in vitro susceptibility to penicillin. Penicillin failure in pharyngitis, tonsillitis, or mixed infections has been attributed to inactivation of penicillin in situ by β-lactamases produced by colonizing organisms such as *Bacteroides fragilis* or *S. aureus*. Further, active selection of these β-lactamase–producing organisms following treatment with penicillin is well documented and leads to a higher percentage of treatment failures. For example, the failure rate of penicillin treatment of GAS pharyngitis may approach 10% to 25% and, with a second treatment with penicillin, increase to 40% to 80%. In contrast, cures of 90% of such failures are possible if the second treatment consisted of amoxicillin plus clavulanate compared with only 29% cure with a second regimen of penicillin. In addition, antibiotics that are unaffected by β-lactamase activity (e.g., amoxicillin, clavulanate, or clindamycin) have a greater efficacy than penicillin in patients with recurrent GAS tonsillitis.

Genotypic penicillin tolerance could also explain penicillin's lack of efficacy in tonsillitis or pharyngitis. Tolerant strains demonstrate a slower rate of growth, a slower rate of bacterial killing by penicillin, and an absence of β-lactam–induced cell lysis. Penicillin-tolerant GAS strains have been isolated from 11 of 18 cases of penicillin treatment failure in acute tonsillitis compared with isolation in 0 of 15 cases that were successfully treated. Penicillin-tolerant strains have also caused epidemics of pharyngitis.

Recently, reports that describe penicillin's reduced efficacy in the treatment of severe streptococcal infections in humans (i.e., streptococcal bacteremia, pneumonia, myositis, and strep TSS) have surfaced. Studies made in animals demonstrated that penicillin was effective if given early or if small numbers of GAS were used to initiate infection. With larger inocula or if treatment was delayed, penicillin was no more effective than placebo. Thus penicillin's efficacy was lost as the in-

✔ *WHEN TO REFER*

When encountering a patient with unexplained severe pain and fever, the physician should refer the patient to an infectious disease consultant. Soft tissue radiographs, complete blood cell count with differerential count, platelet count, serum creatinine and creatinine phosphokinase (CPK) concentrations, and albumin and calcium levels are also useful in the early diagnosis of strep TSS. If the patient has the symptoms and signs just described, together with hypotension or tachycardia out of proportion to the fever, the patient should be referred to the hospital for admission and resuscitation. General surgery or orthopedics consultation should be obtained when there is evidence of soft tissue infection with severe systemic signs of sepsis, since necrotizing fasciitis or myonecrosis is likely. Although radiographs do not show gas or localized abscess, systemic toxicity and soft tissue infection should prompt surgical exploration. The presence of violaceous bullae suggests necrotizing soft tissue infection and should also prompt surgical consultation. Children with chickenpox who have fever after day four of the illness may have a secondary bacterial infection with GAS and should be referred to the emergency room and or an infectious disease consultant. Women with postpartum fever should be referred to an infectious disease or obstetrics-gynecology consultant, since puerperal sepsis that is due to GAS has been described with increasing frequency in the United States.

fection became more severe. In contrast, clindamycin had excellent efficacy even if treatment was delayed up to 16 hours. Recently it was demonstrated that GAS in log-phase cultures produce five PBPs, whereas in stationary phase they do not. Thus in fulminant infections GAS have reached a stationary phase of growth, and subsequent treatment with penicillin fails because of an abscence of its high-affinity targets, the PBPs. Clindamycin's greater efficacy could be due to its ability to suppress M-protein synthesis, its longer postantibiotic effect, its indifference to in vivo inoculum or stage of growth, and its ability to attenuate TNF synthesis by human monocytes.

BIBLIOGRAPHY

Bisno AL: Group A streptococcal infections and acute rheumatic fever, *N Engl J Med* 325(11):783-93, 1991.

Bisno AL, Stevens DL: Current concepts: streptococcal infections of skin and soft tissues, *N Engl J Med* 334(4):240-245,1996.

Cleary R et al: A virulence regulon in *Streptococcus pyogenes*. Third International ASM conference on Streptococcal Genetics, Minneapolis, MN, 1990, (abstract 19), American Society for Microbiology (ASM).

Fischetti VA: Streptococcal M protein, *Sci Am* 264(6):58-65, 1991.

Harris RW, Sims PJ, Tweten RK: Evidence that *Clostridium perfringens* theta-toxin induces colloid-osmotic lysis of erythrocytes, *Infect Immunol* 59(7):2499, 1991.

Johnson LP, Tomai MA, Schlievert PM: Bacteriophage involvement in group A streptococcal pyrogenic exotoxin A production, *J Bacteriol* 166:623, 1986.

Kehoe MA et al: Nucleotide sequence of the streptolysin O (SLO) gene: structural homologies between SLO and other membrane-damaging, thiol-activated toxins, *Infect Immunol* 55:3228, 1987.

Kohler W, Gerlach D, Knoll HL: Streptococcal outbreaks and erythrogenic toxin type A, *Zentralbl Bakteriol Hyg* 266:104, 1987.

Lancefield RC: Current knowledge of type specific M antigens of group A streptococci, *J Immunol* 89:307, 1962.

Nida SK, Ferretti JJ: Phage influence on the synthesis of extracellular toxins in group A streptococci, *Infect Immunol* 36(2):745, 1982.

Smith TD et al: Efficacy of β-lactamase–resistant penicillin and influence of penicillin tolerance in eradicating streptococci from pharynx after failure of penicillin therapy for group A streptococcal pharyngitis, *J Pediatr* 6:601, 1987.

Stevens DL: Invasive group A streptococcus infections, *Clin Infect Dis* 14:2, 1992.

Stevens DL et al: Reappearance of scarlet fever toxin A among streptococci in the Rocky Mountain West: severe group A streptococcal infections associated with a toxic shock–like syndrome, *N Engl J Med* 321(1):1, 1989.

Stollerman GH: *Rheumatic fever and streptococcal infection,* New York, 1975, Grune & Stratton.

Wannamaker LW et al: Prophylaxis of acute rheumatic fever by treatment of the preceding streptococcal infection with various amounts of depot penicillin, *Am J Med* 10:673, 1951.

Watson DW, Kim YB: Erythrogenic toxins. In Montie TC, Kadis S, Ajl SJ, editors: *Microbial toxins,* vol 3, Orlando, Fla, 1970, Academic.

ENTEROCOCCI

262 Enterococcal and Other Non–Group A Streptococcal Infections

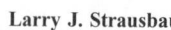

Larry J. Strausbaugh

CHARACTERISTICS AND CLASSIFICATION

Enterococci are gram-positive, facultatively anaerobic bacteria that are ovoid and appear on smears as short chains, pairs, or single cells. Their colonies are 1 to 2 mm in size and appear somewhat "buttery" in consistency. On blood agar plates they exhibit no hemolysis most frequently, alpha hemolysis occasionally, and beta hemolysis rarely. Enterococci usually possess the Lancefield group D antigen, an intracellular glycerol teichoic acid associated with the cytoplasmic membrane. Other distinguishing features include the ability to hydrolyze esculin, to grow in media containing 40% bile, to grow in 6.5% sodium chloride, to hydrolyze L-pyrrolidonyl-beta-naphthylamide (PYR), and to grow at both 10° C and 45° C.

For many years enterococci were classified in the genus *Streptococcus,* but on the basis of nucleic acid hybridization studies they were reassigned to a new genus designated *Enterococcus.* From a medical viewpoint the most important species are *E. faecalis* and *E. faecium.* The 17 other proposed enterococcal species are rarely isolated from human specimens.

EPIDEMIOLOGY

Enterococci can be recovered from water, soil, food, and a variety of animals. They also reside in the gastrointestinal tract of most normal adults. They are present in small numbers in the upper gastrointestinal tract but may achieve concentrations of 10^5 to 10^7 colony-forming units/g in feces. As a rule, *E. faecalis* is recovered more frequently and in greater numbers than *E. faecium,* but age, diet, underlying disease, prior antimicrobial therapy, and geography affect this finding. Enterococci, especially *E. faecalis,* have also been isolated from the oropharynx, the hepatobiliary tract, the vagina, anterior urethra, and skin of 5% to 35% of healthy individuals. Enterococci are also frequently isolated from the soft tissue wounds and cutaneous ulcers of hospitalized patients, and they can be recovered from environmental surfaces within the hospital as well.

Enterococci are common causes of human disease (Table 262-1). Their role in community-acquired infections such as endocarditis has long been recognized. In the last 15 years they have also been recognized as nosocomial pathogens. Data from the Centers for Disease Control and Prevention's (CDC's) National Nosocomial Infection Surveillance (NNIS) system indicate that enterococci are the third most frequently isolated pathogen. Moreover, data from several medical centers have indicated that the incidence of nosocomial enterococcal urinary tract infections and bacteremias has increased steadily during the last 20 years. *E. faecalis* is responsible for 80% to 85% of all enterococcal infections, and *E. faecium* for the majority of the remainder.

Until the last decade most enterococcal infections were thought to arise from the patient's own indigenous flora, and this is probably true for patients with community-acquired infections. Nosocomial infections, especially those caused by antimicrobial-resistant strains, arise most frequently from exogenous strains acquired in hospital as a result of person-to-person spread. Transient carriage of enterococci on the hands of medical personnel has been an important mode of transmission in several hospital outbreaks and one interhospital outbreak, suggesting that enterococci behave like methicillin-resistant staphylococci and gram-negative bacilli in this regard.

Table 262-1   Principal human diseases associated with enterococci

TYPE OF INFECTION	FREQUENCY OF ENTEROCOCCAL ISOLATION (%)
Community-acquired	
Endocarditis	5-15
Intraabdominal and pelvic*	25
Urinary tract	<5
Hospital-acquired	
Urinary tract	15
Surgical wound	12
Other cutaneous*	9
Bacteremia*	7

*Enterococci often isolated with other bacterial pathogens.

BOX 262-1
Intrinsic antimicrobial resistance of enterococci

Resistance to:
   Antistaphylococcal penicillins
   Cephalosporins
   Clindamycin
   Aminoglycosides
   Polymyxin
   Aztreonam
   Trimethoprim-sulfamethoxazole*

Higher minimum inhibitory concentrations of penicillin G, ampicillin, mezlocillin, and piperacillin than those of other streptococci.
Tolerance to bactericidal effect of virtually all antimicrobial agents.
Low-level production of aminoglycoside 6′-acetyltransferase by strains of *Enterococcus faecium* renders them more resistant to tobramycin, netilmicin, and sisomicin.

*May appear active against enterococci in vitro, but clinical treatment failures and lack of efficacy in animal models have been reported.

Vancomycin-resistant enterococci (VRE), which appeared in Europe a decade ago, have been spreading rapidly throughout the United States since 1988. In 1989 only 0.3% of nosocomial enterococcal isolates (submitted to the CDC's NNIS system) were VRE, but by 1993 this percentage had risen to 7.9%. Of the isolates recovered from patients in intensive care units, 0.4% were VRE in 1989, whereas 13.6% were VRE in 1993. VRE are present in at least 33 states, and outbreaks have occurred in a variety of urban hospitals across the country. As a rule, colonization and infection with VRE occur in hospitalized patients with severe underlying disease and prolonged lengths of stay who have been subjected to surgery, the use of invasive devices such as urinary catheters, and broad-spectrum antimicrobial therapy. Colonization is 5 to 10 times more common than infection. Both colonized and infected patients constitute an important reservoir for additional cases.

PATHOGENESIS

The pathogenicity of enterococci has traditionally been ascribed to their place of residence. When disease or injury breaches the integrity of the bowel or the lower urogenital tract, enterococci find their opportunity to invade. Even so, they have often been viewed as reluctant pathogens, and their pathogenic potential in the abdomen and pelvis has been debated. Nevertheless, the rising incidence of enterococcal bloodstream infections and their attendant 30% to 65% case fatality rates have generated a new respect and a renewed search for specific virulence factors. Recent studies have focused on aggregation substance, an adhesin that may promote colonization of mucosal surfaces, and extracellular products such as cytolysin and coccolysin, which may damage host cells and tissues.

Antimicrobial resistance also contributes to the pathogenic potential of enterococci. This property provides a selective advantage in the hospital environment and almost certainly explains the enterococcus's expanding role as a nosocomial pathogen. Its resistance is of two types: intrinsic and acquired. Intrinsic resistance, an inherent property of the bacterium that is universally present, has a number of important therapeutic consequences (Box 262-1). It limits therapeutic options; it necessitates the use of high dosages of penicillin G or other penicillin derivatives for the treatment of serious infections; it necessitates the use of synergistic combinations (e.g., ampicillin and gentamicin) for the treatment of endocarditis when bactericidal activity is required; and it limits the number of aminoglycoside combinations available for *E. faecium* infections—ampicillin or vancomycin combinations with tobramycin, netilmicin, and sisomicin do not demonstrate a synergistic bactericidal effect against this species.

Enterococci readily exchange genetic material among themselves and with other genera. This property has enabled them to acquire resistance to a number of antimicrobial agents, including penicillin G, ampicillin, other penicillins, imipenem, vancomycin, and fluoroquinolones (Table 262-2). Most acquired resistance depends on either the production of enzymes that inactivate the antimicrobial agent or changes in the molecular target of the antimicrobial agent.

The prevalence of acquired resistance varies considerably. Resis-

---

Table 262-2   Acquired antimicrobial resistance of enterococci

ANTIMICROBIAL AGENT	MECHANISM OF RESISTANCE
Aminoglycoside (high level)	
Streptomycin	Induction of ribosomal resistance, production of adenyltransferase
Kanamycin	Production of phosphotransferase
Gentamicin, kanamycin, tobramycin, amikacin, netilmicin	Production of fusion protein with phosphotransferase and acetyltransferase activity
Beta lactams	
Penicillin G, ampicillin, piperacillin, mezlocillin	Production of β-lactamase
Penicillin, ampicillin, imipenem	Altered penicillin binding protein (PBP) 5 or overproduction of PBP 5 in *E. faecium*
Glycopeptides	
Vancomycin, teicoplanin, and others	Production of ligase with altered specificity that results in synthesis of cell wall precursors that fail to bind glycopeptides
Vancomycin alone	Possibly same mechanism but different regulation
Miscellaneous	
Chloramphenicol	Production of chloramphenicol acetyltransferase
Erythromycin	Methylation of ribosomal RNA (also confers high-level clindamycin resistance)
Tetracyclines	Protection of ribosome from tetracycline inhibition
	Induction of active transport system to remove tetracycline from cell
Fluoroquinolones	
Ciprofloxacin	Unknown

---

tance to chloramphenicol, erythromycin, tetracycline, and streptomycin has been common for several decades. High-level resistance to gentamicin and all other aminoglycosides appeared in *E. faecalis* during the early 1980s and has disseminated widely since then. It has subsequently been recognized in *E. faecium*. Penicillinase-producing strains of *E. faecalis* have appeared in various parts of the world during the last few years but remain uncommon. Resistance of *E. faecium* to penicillin G, ampicillin, piperacillin, mezlocillin, and imipenem, which is not mediated by β-lactamases, also has increased. In some centers more than 50% of clinical isolates exhibit this type of resistance.

Most clinical isolates of enterococci possess several different forms of resistance, and this phenomenon complicates the therapy of enterococcal infections. This problem has reached its zenith in the appearance of the VRE strains of *E. faecium,* which are frequently resistant to all commercially available antimicrobial agents. They exhibit resistance to all β-lactam, glycopeptide, and fluoroquinolone antibiotics and express high-level resistance to all aminoglycoside antibiotics. Not surprisingly, these strains of *E. faecium* have been dubbed the "nosocomial pathogen of the 1990s." Another troublesome form of multiple resistance is high-level resistance to all commercially available aminoglycoside antibiotics in strains from patients with endocarditis. These strains are not killed by β-lactam–aminoglycoside or vancomycin-aminoglycoside combinations; hence, these combinations do not provide the bactericidal therapy necessary for the cure of endocarditis.

CLINICAL MANIFESTATIONS
Endocarditis

Enterococcal endocarditis almost always occurs on previously damaged aortic or mitral valves, even in intravenous drug addicts. It usually becomes evident in a subacute manner, although acute presentations are not unknown. In most case series men outnumber women 2 to 1. Male patients are generally in their fifth or sixth decade of life and often describe antecedent genitourinary tract procedures or infections. Women patients are generally in their childbearing years and often relate histories of gynecologic or obstetric events that may have induced bacteremia. Other features of this illness are described in Chapter 24.

Bacteremia Without Endocarditis

Overall, enterococci are isolated from 5% of all positive blood cultures. Approximately 25% to 35% of bacteremias occur in patients with community-acquired infections, principally endocarditis, biliary tract or other intra abdominal infections, and urinary tract infections.

Sixty-five percent to 75% of enterococcal bacteremias are nosocomial. As a rule, these occur in men and women over 50 years of age with serious underlying diseases (e.g., malignancies, traumatic injuries, or complicated surgeries). The bacteremias often occur more than 3 weeks after admission to the hospital and after prolonged antimicrobial therapy, especially broad-spectrum cephalosporin therapy. Bacteremias caused by VRE have been especially frequent in liver transplant recipients. Common sources for nosocomial enterococcal bacteremias include biliary tract and other intraabdominal or surgical wound infections (15% to 40% of cases), urinary tract infections (15% to 40%), burn wounds and other cutaneous infections (15% to 30%), and intravenous catheter infections (5% to 20%). The source of the bacteremia remains obscure in 15% to 20% of patients.

Twenty-five percent to 45% of enterococcal bacteremias are polymicrobial; gram-negative bacilli and staphylococci are isolated most frequently in association with enterococci. Patients with polymicrobial enterococcemia generally have more severe signs and symptoms of infection, including hypotension and disseminated intravascular coagulation. In contrast, patients with only enterococci in the blood tend to have more indolent disease characterized mainly by fever and signs referable to the primary site of infection.

Urinary Tract Infections

Enterococci account for approximately 2% of urinary tract infections in young, healthy women. They play a larger role in elderly men with prostatic disease and achieve prominence as a cause of nosocomial urinary tract infections, especially in patients undergoing urologic procedures and in patients with genitourinary tract structural abnor-

malities or indwelling urinary catheters. The clinical manifestations of enterococcal infections are similar to those caused by other bacteria (Chapter 246).

Intraabdominal and Pelvic Infections

Enterococci are frequently isolated from patients with secondary peritonitis, intraabdominal or pelvic abscesses, biliary tract disease, and other infections that derive from bowel or vaginal flora. The organisms are usually isolated in association with other members of the normal flora from these sites, but in patients who have received broad-spectrum antimicrobial therapy, the organism may be the sole isolate. The clinical significance of enterococci in these mixed infections is not always clear, but bacteremia can arise from such infections, especially in immunocompromised patients. Clinical features are discussed in Chapters 238 and 361.

Skin and Soft Tissue Infections

Enterococci are commonly isolated in mixed cultures from burns, decubitus ulcers, diabetic foot infections and wounds associated with abdominal surgery. The organisms are clearly opportunists in this setting, affecting only previously damaged tissue. Here again, it is difficult to assess the enterococcus' contribution in these conditions, but the frequency of bacteremia arising from these sources suggests that its involvement is not always benign. Clinical features are discussed in Chapter 241.

Miscellaneous Infections

Enterococci are rare causes of meningitis, pneumonia, and empyema. They are occasionally isolated from patients with infected medical devices such as orthopedic prostheses, central nervous system shunts, and peritoneal dialysis catheters.

DIAGNOSIS

Although finding chains of gram-positive cocci on Gram's stain of unspun urine or pus from intraabdominal abscesses strongly suggests enterococcal involvement, a definitive diagnosis is established by culture. Since enterococci rarely contaminate specimens from normally sterile body fluids, their isolation from blood, cerebrospinal fluid (CSF), synovial fluid, and the like indicates infection. Their isolation from mucosal surface exudates, however, is more difficult to interpret.

Once enterococci are isolated from clinical specimens, speciated, and subjected to standard susceptibility tests, special susceptibility tests may also be needed. Isolates from patients with endocarditis require tests for high-level resistance (minimum inhibitory concentration [MIC] >2000 mg/L) to streptomycin and gentamicin. Nitrocefin testing of blood and CSF isolates appears warranted to detect penicillinase-producing strains of *E. faecalis* because routine susceptibility tests do not detect this property. All isolates of enterococci require testing against vancomycin in either agar diffusion or conventional dilution assays using incubation periods of 24 hours. Fully automated methods of testing enterococci for resistance to vancomycin may be unreliable. Enterococci from infections that persist or recur, despite appropriate therapy, also merit special susceptibility tests to determine occult resistance.

TREATMENT

Enterococcal endocarditis and probably both meningitis and severe infections in patients with compromised host defenses require bactericidal therapy with synergistic combinations of antimicrobial agents (Chapter 24). Ampicillin or vancomycin therapy alone suffices for other serious enterococcal infections (Table 262-3). Before the identity and susceptibility pattern of the infecting organism are known, three considerations influence the choice of antibiotics: the likelihood of encountering an ampicillin- or vancomycin-resistant strain; the patient's drug allergy history; and the concurrent need to treat other bacteria involved in a polymicrobial infection (e.g., the necessity for cov-

Table 262-3 Therapy for noncardiac enterococcal infections*

TYPE OF INFECTION	FIRST CHOICES	ALTERNATIVES
Severe: with sepsis syndrome (e.g., bacteremia or cholecystitis)†	Ampicillin 2 g IV q4h or Vancomycin 1.0 g IV q 12h	Mezlocillin 5 g IV q6h or Piperacillin 3 g IV q4h or Imipenem 0.5-1.0 g IV q6h or Ampicillin 2 g and sulbactam 1g IV q6h or Piperacillin 3 g and tazobactam 375 mg IV q6h or Ciprofloxacin 0.4 g IV q12h or Ofloxacin 0.4 g IV q 12h
Mild: little systemic toxicity (e.g., uncomplicated urinary tract infection)	Amoxicillin 500 mg po tid or Ampicillin 500 mg po qid or Ciprofloxacin 250-500 mg po bid or Ofloxacin 200-400 mg po bid	Nitrofurantoin‡ 100 mg po q6h or Norfloxacin‡ 400 mg po bid

*See text for therapy of highly resistant strains of *E. faecalis* and *E. faecium.*
†Meningitis and serious infections in immunocompromised patients should be treated similarly to endocarditis with synergistic antimicrobial combinations.
‡Urinary tract infection only.

ering gram-negative bacilli and anaerobes in a patient with a diverticular abscess).

Ampicillin and sulbactam, piperacillin and tazobactam, and imipenem provide alternatives to vancomycin for treating penicillinase-producing strains of *E. faecalis* but offer no help for treating ampicillin-resistant strains of *E. faecium.* Vancomycin or a fluoroquinolone may be useful against such strains, but clinical experience with fluoroquinolones is limited, and certain strains of enterococci are clearly resistant.

Endocarditis caused by enterococci with high-level resistance to all aminoglycosides poses a special problem. Therapeutic considerations include 8 to 12 weeks of parenteral therapy with ampicillin or vancomycin, administration of ampicillin by continuous infusion, and surgical excision of the infected valve. Therapy of infections caused by multidrug-resistant strains of *E. faecium* (VRE) are even more problematic. Nitrofurantoin may be useful for uncomplicated urinary tract infections. Although some VRE strains may appear susceptible to tetracyclines and chloramphenicol in vitro, resistance to these agents can emerge rapidly during therapy. Investigational agents such as teicoplanin, a glycopeptide antibiotic under development by Merrill Dow, and the combination of quinupristin/dalfopristin (Synercid), a streptogrammin antibiotic under development by Rhone-Poulenc-Rorer, are the only choices for serious infections caused by multidrug-resistant *E. faecium.*

✔ WHEN TO REFER

Patients with enterococcal endocarditis caused by strains with high-level resistance to aminoglycoside antibiotics warrant consultation with an experienced specialist in infectious diseases who is knowledgeable about therapeutic options. All patients with enterococcal endocarditis in whom signs and symptoms of congestive heart failure, life-threatening arrhythmias, recurrent embolic phenomena, or other complications develop require the attention of a cardiologist or cardiovascular surgeon for consideration of valve replacement. Similarly, patients with intraabdominal or pelvic abscesses may also require the services of a surgeon or an interventional radiologist for drainage of a visceral abscess. Patients with invasive infections caused by multiply resistant strains of *E. faecium* often need the services of an infectious diseases specialist to obtain investigational antimicrobial agents from their manufacturers.

OTHER NON–GROUP A STREPTOCOCCI

Table 262-4 delineates the principal characteristics of four groups of medically important streptococci. Diagnosis rests on culture results from appropriate specimens. When isolated from blood, CSF, or other normally sterile body fluid, the diagnosis is definitive. When recovered from other specimens (e.g., swabs of wound exudates), it may be difficult to assign an etiologic role to these streptococci with precision. Nonetheless, the availability of commercial reagents for Lancefield typing has facilitated detection of these organisms. During the last 20 years their role in human disease has been more clearly defined and recognized with increasing frequency.

Most of these streptococci are normal flora or pathogens of various mammals; all are, to greater or lesser extents, colonizers of humans. Some infections result from animal contact. Most, however, derive from colonizing organisms that become invasive when trauma or disease provides opportunities to evade host defenses of the skin or the respiratory, gastrointestinal, or genitourinary tract. Infection may be localized to the site of invasion or disseminated via blood or lymph to distant sites.

Penicillin G is the drug of choice for virtually all of the nonenterococcal streptococci. Dosages as high as 20 to 30 million units/

Table 262-4　Characteristics and ecology of nonenterococcal, non–group A streptococcal pathogens

CATEGORY AND SPECIES	MICROBIOLOGIC PROPERTIES	ANIMAL SOURCES	HUMAN COLONIZATION*
Nonenteroccal group D 　S. bovis	Usually alpha hemolysis; hydrolyze esculin; grow in 40% bile; do *not* grow in 6.5% NaCl	Commonly isolated from feces of cattle, swine, and sheep	Oropharynx rare Colon 5% to 15%
Group B S. agalactiae	Narrow-zone beta hemolysis; eight serotypes on basis of polysaccharide capsular and protein antigens	Pathogen of cattle	Oropharynx <1% to 20% Vagina 5% to 40% Rectal up to 40%
Group C and G *Streptococcus pyogenes*–like 　S. equi 　S. equisimilis 　S. canis	Large colonies with a broad band of beta hemolysis	S. equi pathogen of horses; S. canis pathogen of dogs; some group members isolated from cattle, swine, sheep, and other mammals	Skin transient but probably frequent Oropharynx <1% to 20% Vagina <1% to 5% Colon <1% to 13%
S. intermedius group or S. milleri group 　S. anginosus 　S. intermedius 　S. constellatus	Minute, slow-growing colonies; microaerophilic or carboxyphilic; variable types of hemolysis; variable Lancefield groups: none, G, or F common, A and C uncommon; caramel-like odor associated with agar cultures	Not established	Skin—probably rare Oropharynx 1% to 11% Vagina 3% to 18% Colon 16% to 67%

*Site of colonization in humans and estimates or ranges of recovery from healthy adults.

day are employed for severe infections. An aminoglycoside antibiotic is often added for its synergistic bactericidal effect in the treatment of patients with endocarditis. Various cephalosporin antibiotics, erythromycin, vancomycin, and clindamycin are used for the nonenterococcal infections in patients who are allergic to penicillin.

NONENTEROCOCCAL GROUP D STREPTOCOCCI

Streptococcus bovis, the principal member of this group, accounts for approximately 5% of infective endocarditis cases and occasional cases of bacteremia in older adults. Both endocarditis and bacteremia commonly arise from a colonic source; in fact, the association of either condition with unrecognized colonic neoplasms is sufficiently strong to justify a thorough examination of the colon whenever *S. bovis* is isolated from blood. Unlike enterococci, *S. bovis* is highly susceptible to penicillin G, and therapy for endocarditis conforms to that recommended for the viridans streptococci (Chapter 24).

GROUP B STREPTOCOCCI

Streptococcus agalactiae, the only species of Group B streptococci, was initially recognized as a cause of meningitis and other serious infections in the newborn. More recently, it has been recognized as a cause of gynecologic, opportunistic, and nosocomial infections in adults. A CDC report in 1991 estimated the annual incidence of group B streptococcal infections in adults to be 2.4 infections per 100,000 population in metropolitan Atlanta. These organisms account for 8% of nonneonatal streptococcal bacteremias. Endomyometritis and, occasionally, urinary tract infections occur in women postpartum, whereas wound infections and pelvic cellulitis occur following gynecologic surgery. These infections are often polymicrobial and may give rise to bacteremia in up to one third of cases; in fact, *S. agalactiae* accounts for 10% to 20% of positive blood cultures in obstetric services.

In older adults with major underlying diseases, especially malignancies, diabetes mellitus, and neurologic impairments, *S. agalactiae* infections are more diverse and involve a number of different organ systems. Skin and soft tissue infections such as cellulitis, infected decubitus ulcers, and postoperative wound infections predominate in most case series. Urinary tract infections, pneumonias, endocarditis, and primary bacteremias also occur. In some series a substantial number of infections involve intravenous or intraarterial access devices. Bacteremia has been common in published cases, and secondary infections at distant sites have not been unusual. Case fatality rates in older adults usually exceed 40%.

GROUPS C AND G *pyogenes*–LIKE STREPTOCOCCI

These bacteria, which closely resemble *Streptococcus pyogenes* (Chapter 261), cause a wide variety of suppurative infections: pharyngitis, pneumonia, cellulitis, and other skin and wound infections. Bacteremia may ensue and lead to endocarditis, meningitis, arthritis, osteomyelitis, and other infections at sites far removed from the portal of entry. Group G streptococci account for approximately 10% and group C for approximately 1% of all β-hemolytic streptococcal bacteremias. Food-borne outbreaks of pharyngitis caused by groups C and G streptococci have been reported, and poststreptococcal glomerulonephritis has been observed to follow a few cases of group C streptococcal pharyngitis.

Serious groups C and G streptococcal infections often occur in older adults with significant underlying disease such as cancer, diabetes mellitus, and alcoholism. They may produce substantial mortality and morbidity in this population: endocarditis has a case fatality rate greater than 30%, and many survivors require valve replacement. Pneumonia frequently leads to empyema; approximately half of the reported patients with meningitis have died.

Streptococcus intermedius GROUP

Despite confusing and unresolved taxonomy issues, the diverse *Streptococcus intermedius* group of streptococci have increasingly been recognized to cause a variety of serious human infections. They are most frequently associated with abscesses, especially hepatic, dental, appendiceal, and brain abscesses (Chapters 238 and 240). In some case series *S. intermedius* group organisms have been isolated from as many as 80% of patients with liver abscesses, more than 50% of patients with appendiceal abscesses, and more than 50% of patients with brain abscesses. The organisms are recovered less frequently from patients with pneumonia, empyema, primary bacteremia, endocarditis, arthritis, wound infections, and the like. In approximately half of the cases, *S. intermedius* group organisms are recovered in association with other bacterial pathogens.

BIBLIOGRAPHY

Bradley SF, Gordon JJ, Baumgartner DD et al: Group C streptococcal bacteremia: analysis of 88 Cases, *Rev Infect Dis* 13:270-280, 1991.
Chenoweth C, Schaberg D: The epidemiology of enterococci, *Eur J Clin Microbiol Infect Dis* 9:80-89, 1990.

Colford JM Jr, Mohle-Boetani J, Vosti, KL: Group B streptococcal bacteremia in adults: five year's experience and a review of the literature, *Medicine* 74:176-190, 1995.

Edmond MB, Ober JF, Weinbaum DL et al: Vancomycin-resistant *Eneterococcus faecium* bacteremia: risk factors for infection, *Clin Infect Dis* 20:1126-1133, 1995.

Eliopoulos GM, Eliopoulos CT: Therapy of enterococcal infections, *Eur J Clin Microbiol Infect Dis 9:118-126, 1990.*

Gossling J: Occurrence and pathogenicity of the *Streptococcus milleri* group, *Rev Infect Dis* 10:257-284, 1988.

Herman DJ, Gerding DN: Antimicrobial resistance among enterococci, *Antimicrob Agents Chemother* 35:1-4, 1991.

Herman DJ, and Gerding DN: Screening and treatment of infections caused by resistant enterococci, *Antimicrob Agents Chemother* 35:215-219, 1991.

Hoge CW, et al: Enterococcal bacteremia: to treat or not to treat: a reappraisal, *Rev Infect Dis* 13:600-605, 1991.

Jett BD, Huycke MM, Gilmore MS: Virulence of enterococci, *Clin Microbiol Rev* 7:462-478, 1994.

Lewis CM, Zervos MJ: Clinical manifestations of enterococcal infection, *Eur J Clin Microbiol Infect Dis* 9:111-117, 1990.

Morris JG Jr, Shay DK, Hebden JN et al: Enterococci resistant to multiple antimicrobial agents, including vancomycin: establishment of endemicity in a university medical center, *Ann Intern Med* 123:250-259, 1995.

Murray BE: The life and times of the enterococcus, *Clin Microbiol Rev* 3:46-65, 1990.

Schwartz B et al: Invasive group B streptococcal disease in adults, *JAMA* 266:1112-1114, 1991.

Spera RV, Farber BF: Multidrug-resistant *Enterococcus faecium*: an untreatable nosocomial pathogen, *Drugs* 48:678-688, 1994.

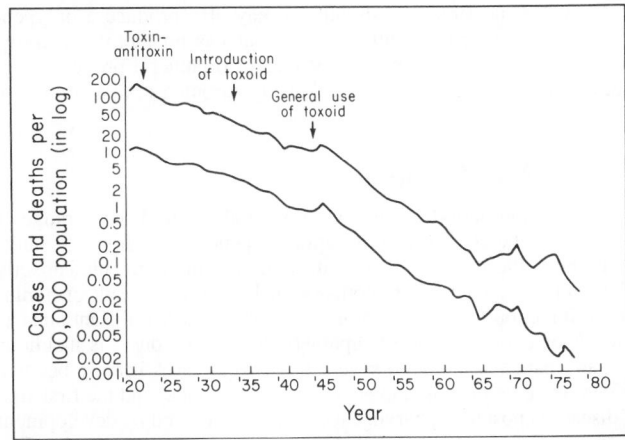

FIGURE 263-1   Diphtheria cases and death rates in the United States–1920 to 1978.

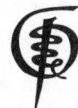

263 Gram-Positive Bacillary Infections and Clostridial Infections

Ronald Dworkin and James Leggett

CORYNEBACTERIUM AND OTHER CORYNEFORM ORGANISMS
Classification and Characteristics

There are two major taxonomic branches of gram-positive organisms. The actinomycete group, characterized by high guanine-plus-cytosine (G+C) base content of the DNA and an irregular cell shape, includes the genera *Corynebacterium, Actinomyces, Arcanobacterium, Mycobacterium,* and more than 15 others. The term *coryneform* (club-shaped) is actually a misnomer for many of these organisms. The second group, characterized by a lower G+C content and a more regular morphologic appearance, contains the clinically important genera *Streptococcus, Staphylococcus, Bacillus, Clostridium, Erysipelothrix, Listeria,* and others.

Corynebacteria are gram-positive, aerobic, nonmotile, catalase-positive, pleomorphic rods. Cells are arranged singly, in palisades of parallel cells or in groups that may take on the appearance of Chinese letters. *Corynebacterium diphtheriae* is the type species of its genus and causes the disease diphtheria. Other coryneform bacteria, often referred to as diphtheroids, have traditionally been considered to be nonpathogenic for humans, although they may occasionally cause severe infections *(C. diphtheriticum, C. minutissimum, C. striatum, C. xerosis, C. urealyticum,* and *C. jeikeium).* They are part of the normal flora of skin, mucous membranes, and intestine. In stained smears, *C. diphtheriae* organisms exhibit a club-shaped appearance and are arranged in palisades. Four distinct subspecies of *C. diphtheriae (gravis, mitis, intermedius,* and *belfani)* can be identified from their appearance on tellurite agar and their ability to ferment glycogen and starch. All four are capable of producing diphtheria toxin and clinical disease.

Epidemiology

Humans are the only known reservoir of *C. diphtheriae.* Transmission between persons is usually via aerosolized droplets. In some tropical areas where skin infections with *C. diphtheriae* are common, the organisms may be spread by direct contact. Fomites, dust, and milk rarely have been implicated as disease vectors. Conditions that favor crowding are associated with increased transmission, which explains the higher prevalence of disease in cold weather.

The Centers for Disease Control and Prevention (CDC) has been charting the cumulative incidence of diphtheria, a disease in which reporting is mandated. The improvement of health conditions and the introduction of diphtheria toxoid immunization in the 1920s have significantly reduced the number of cases in the United States (Fig. 263-1). The number of reported cases has decreased from more than 200,000 in 1921 to only a few per year at present. Because 77% of the recent diphtheria cases occurred in persons above the age of 15 years, as compared with the period between 1971 to 1981, when the rate in children younger than 15 years of age was four times that of adults, a loss of immunity may account for this shift to an older age-group. Many older adults (25% to 50%) are susceptible to diphtheria. Attack rates of diphtheria in Native Americans, Mexican Americans, and blacks are 10 times higher than in the rest of the population. Seventy-five percent of these cases occur in nonimmunized persons. Diphtheria remains a worldwide problem, particularly in developing countries. Outbreaks of diphtheria in developed countries have been reported in lower social economic groups as a result of crowding and increased opportunities for aerosol transmission. Diphtheria in immunized persons is usually mild and without either membrane formation or toxemia. Although a serum antitoxin level above 0.01 IU/ml is protective against disease acquisition, such individuals may serve as asymptomatic carriers of the organism.

Pathogenesis

Corynebacterium diphtheriae colonizes and multiplies on mucosal and epithelial surfaces. It can survive for up to 6 months in dust and fomites around patients with nasopharyngeal and cutaneous diphtheria. Other *Corynebacterium* species are found on the skin and in the gastrointestinal tracts of humans and animals. *C. diphtheriae* most commonly invades the upper respiratory tract. The serious manifestations of diphtheria are due to a potent toxin elaborated by the bacilli; however, the probability for disease acquisition may be influenced by genetic factors controlling virulence.

Diphtheria toxin is a heat-labile polypeptide exotoxin with a molecular weight of about 62,000 daltons. It is produced only by strains of *C. diphtheriae* infected with a lysogenic bacteriophage. The toxin contains two fragments, A and B, which carry out different functions. Fragment B is responsible for the transport of the toxin into cells. Fragment A inhibits polypeptide chain elongation by inactivating elongation factor 2 within cells. Protein synthesis is halted, leading to other metabolic alterations. One molecule of fragment A can produce cell death. The toxin affects all cells in the body, especially the heart (myocarditis) and nerves (demyelination).

Nontoxigenic strains of diphtheria may also produce a polypeptide that is similar to diphtheria toxin but has no biologic activity. Both toxigenic and nontoxigenic strains of diphtheria produce other biologically active substances, such as hyaluronidase, that contribute to the mild local inflammatory reaction.

Clinical Manifestations

The incubation period of diphtheria is usually 2 to 4 days (range, 1 to 7 days). The clinical manifestations depend on the immune status of the host, the location of the infection, and the toxigenic capacity of the microorganism. Symptoms occur locally as a result of noninvasive infection of the respiratory tract or skin and at distant sites as a result of dissemination of diphtheria toxin. The onset is insidious in many patients, although severe pharyngeal cases usually become evident in acute fashion. Fever is usually low grade, and the first sign of disease is posterior pharyngeal erythema, followed by development of an asymmetric membrane that evolves into a dirty-gray color. The extent of the membrane correlates with the severity of symptoms. As the toxin gains access to the circulation, symptoms related to myocarditis and neuritis develop. The frequency of symptoms and the severity of disease are inversely proportional to the patient's immunization history. Mortality rates of 3% to 12% have not changed in the last 50 years.

Types of Diphtheria

Faucial Diphtheria. Diphtheria involving the posterior structures of the mouth and proximal pharynx is the most common clinical entity. The onset of tonsillar diphtheria is usually sudden. A thin, patchy, readily removable exudate forms over one or both tonsils but is replaced within hours by a greenish-gray, firmly adherent, thick membrane. A sore throat is present in almost all cases. Cough, hoarseness, and dysphagia are present in 25% of patients. The membrane may extend to adjacent structures such as the faucial pillars, uvula, soft palate, and pharyngeal wall. Cervical lymphadenopathy and soft tissue swelling may give the appearance of a "bull neck," and cause respiratory stridor.

Extension of the diphtheria lesion into the larynx occurs in about 25% of patients. The membrane usually involves the epiglottis and, less commonly, the glottis and supraglottic structures. Hoarseness is common. Dyspnea, tachycardia, fever, and leukocytosis are poor prognostic signs.

Cutaneous and Anterior Nasal Diphtheria. Cutaneous diphtheria is most common in tropical areas. Lesions appear as chronic, nonhealing ulcers over the extremities. The presence of β-hemolytic streptococcal and staphylococcal infection may influence the clinical expression of cutaneous diphtheria. Constitutional symptoms and cardiac and neurologic complications are rare. Diphtheria involving the nasal area manifests itself in a purulent or serosanguinous nasal discharge, which may become crusted around the external nares and upper lip. Diphtheria conjunctivitis, corneal ulcers, and otitis media may develop.

Complications

Respiratory failure may result from severe pharyngeal or laryngeal involvement accompanied by airway obstruction. Myocarditis and polyneuritis are the major complications that result from the absorption of diphtheria toxin. Bacteremia is a rare event.

Clinical evidence of myocarditis develops in 10% to 25% of cases and accounts for half of diphtheria deaths. The incidence of myocarditis is highest in pharyngeal and laryngeal diphtheria, and circulatory failure results in up to 9% of patients. The onset of myocarditis is usually insidious. Electrocardiographic abnormalities develop during the first or second week of illness, as the oropharyngeal disease is improving. They are characterized by ST-T wave changes and atrial and ventricular arrhythmias. Elevations of serum aspartate aminotransferase (AST) levels, which correlate with the intensity of myocarditis, may be used to follow its course.

Nervous system involvement is a late complication that may occur up to a month or longer after the onset of illness in as many as 10% of patients. Local paralysis of cranial nerves IX and X occurs in 50% of patients with neurologic involvement, resulting in aspiration and nasal regurgitation of liquids. Paralysis of the oculomotor and ciliary nerves is common. Rarely, multiple cranial nerves may be involved. One third of the patients with neurologic complications have peripheral neuritis, which develops later and is principally a motor defect. In a large number of cases there is both cranial and peripheral nerve involvement. Almost all neuropathies resolve without sequelae within 2 weeks of onset of neurologic symptoms.

Infections Caused By Other Coryneform Bacteria (Diphtheroids)

Diphtheroids have traditionally been considered nonpathogenic for humans. These ubiquitous organisms colonize the skin and frequently contaminate blood cultures but may also produce significant disease. Their clinical significance is highly dependent on the clinical context in which they are isolated. Septicemia, endocarditis, and other serious infections are being encountered more frequently as immunocompromised patients and those with prosthetic devices increase in number. Endocarditis and infections of prostheses are the most commonly reported diseases. *C. jeikeium* has been associated with septicemia, endocarditis, meningitis, peritonitis, pneumonia, and other infections, particularly in immunocompromised hosts or patients with prosthetic devices. *C. urealyticum* (CDC group D2) has been isolated in the urine of patients with struvite stones or cystitis. *Arcanobacterium haemolyticum* causes pharyngitis among older children and young adults, often accompanied by a rash, suggestive of a scarlet fever syndrome that is due to *Streptococcus pyogenes*. Although "*C. ulcerans*" is now considered part of the *C. diphtheriae* group, some strains that do not cause a diphtheria-like illness have also caused pharyngitis. *C. minutissimum* may cause erythrasma, a pruritic intertriginous skin infection in which its macular lesions fluoresce coral-red under Wood's lamp. *C. xerosis, C. striatum,* and *C. pseudodiphthericum* are normal skin and oropharyngeal flora that have also been associated with pneumonia. *C. aquaticum,* Oerskovia species, and *Rothia dentocariosa* have all been reported to cause endocarditis or septicemia. *Rhodococcus equi* is emerging as a potentially important pathogen in immunocompromised patients. Treatment of coryneform bacteria depends on susceptibility testing. Although some species are susceptible to penicillins, many, including *C. jeikeium* and *C. urealyticum,* are resistant to common antibiotics except vancomycin. Initial therapy with vancomycin is encouraged for serious systemic infection.

Diagnostic Tests

The differential diagnosis of faucial diphtheria includes streptococcal or viral pharyngitis or tonsillitis, mononucleosis, Vincent's angina, and acute epiglottitis. A definitive diagnosis of diphtheria requires culture of the organism and the demonstration of toxin production. In patients with oropharyngeal diphtheria, however, it is often necessary to initiate therapy on the basis of the clinical diagnosis. In the past, when the disease was more common, presumptive diagnosis was often made by the presence of metachromatic granules (granules that stain deeply with methylene blue). However, methylene blue stains of exudate material may be confused with other organisms (diphtheroids, actinomyces) that have similar morphologic characteristics. Material from the lesion or, preferably, a piece of membrane should be cultured on Loeffler's or tellurite-selective media and a blood agar plate before antibiotics are given. The recovery of β-hemolytic streptococci should not rule out the diagnosis of diphtheria because these organisms are recovered from the pharynx in 20% to 30% of cases of confirmed diphtheria. Final identification requires biochemical tests.

Diphtheria-like organisms must be studied further for a determination of toxin production. Guinea pig inoculation or the more popular gel diffusion test (Elek plate method) is used to determine toxigenicity. The latter technique consists in placing a filter paper soaked in antitoxin on an agar plate and streaking a heavy inoculum of the organism at a right angle to the filter paper. If diphtheria toxin is elaborated, a precipitin line is formed by the toxin and the antitoxin. The test, fraught with several potential sources of error, should be performed only by an experienced reference laboratory.

Table 263-1 Summary of disease patterns, etiologic organisms, toxin production, and toxin target for major illnesses due to clostridial species

DISEASE PATTERN	CLOSTRIDIA	TOXIN	TOXIN TARGET
Gastrointestinal illness			
Food poisoning	*C. perfringens*, type A	Enterotoxin	Mucosal cells of the ileum
Enteritis necroticans	*C. perfringens*, type C	Beta toxin	Mucosal cells of the small bowel
Antibiotic-associated diarrhea/colitis	*C. difficile*	Toxin A–enterotoxin	Mucosal cells of the colon
		Toxin B–cytotoxin	
Neurologic syndromes			
Botulism	*C. botulinum*	Botulinal toxins, A, B, E, and F	Peripheral cholinergic synapses
Tetanus	*C. tetanus*	Tetanospasmin	Inhibitory neurotransmitters
Skin/soft tissue			
Necrotizing fasciitis	*C. perfringens*	Multiple toxins especially alpha toxin	Multiple cell membranes (e.g., capillary
	C. ramosum	(lecithinase) of *C. perfringens*	endothelial cells, erythrocytes, plate-
Myonecrosis	*C. bifermentans*		lets)
	C. septicum		
	C. novi		
	C. histolyticum		
	C. fallax		

Treatment

In suspected cases, diphtheria antitoxin should be administered promptly after cultures are obtained. Antitoxin is active only against free toxin before its entry into cells, so antitoxin must be given as soon as a presumptive diagnosis is made. The minimum effective dose of antitoxin has not been determined. Empiric intravenous or intramuscular dosing recommendations are based on the duration of illness and extent of membrane formation: 20,000 to 40,000 units of antitoxin for pharyngeal or laryngeal disease of 48 hours' duration, 40,000 to 60,000 units for nasopharyngeal lesions, and 80,000 to 100,000 units for extensive disease of 72 hours' duration or longer and for anyone with brawny swelling of the neck. Because up to 10% of the population may have allergic reactions to horse serum, a skin or conjunctival test should be performed by using 0.1 ml of a 1:20 saline dilution of the antitoxin. A positive reaction requires desensitization with increasing doses of the antiserum.

Antibiotics should be administered to prevent multiplication of the organism at the site of infection and to eliminate the carrier state. Both penicillin and erythromycin are effective agents and should be given for 7 days in diphtheria carriers and 12 to 14 days if clinical evidence of disease is present. Diphtheria patients should be isolated until antibiotic treatment is completed and three negative culture results from the lesion are obtained.

Bed rest and care to prevent aspiration pneumonia are important in the management of diphtheria. Patients with suspected myocarditis should have cardiac monitoring. Indirect laryngoscopy is recommended by some authorities because laryngeal involvement may not be suspected on clinical examination. Tracheostomy should be considered whenever laryngeal disease is present because progression of the infection may be rapid and lead to airway obstruction.

The prognosis in diphtheria varies with the age of the patient, the severity of the disease, and the promptness with which antitoxin is administered. Laryngeal edema has a grave prognosis. The case/fatality ratio in one series was 0.27% when antitoxin was injected on the first day of illness, and it increased to 1.67%, 2.77%, and 11.39% when antitoxin was administered on the second, third, and fourth days of illness, respectively; however, in recent reports the case/fatality ratio of clinical diphtheria was less than 5%. Reversible paralysis was observed in as many as 35% of the cases.

Prevention

The decline of diphtheria in industrialized countries is due largely to effective immunization programs. Children should receive five doses of diphtheria toxoid as part of the combined diphtheria-pertussis-tetanus (DPT) vaccine at 2, 4, 6, and 18 months, with a booster at the time of school entry. For continued protection, tetanus-diphtheria toxoid (Td) booster immunizations are recommended every 10 years. In a recent randomized, stratified sample of urban adults, the overall protective level of antitoxin (greater than or equal to 0.01 IU/ml) was demonstrated in 26% of men and 21% of women. Other serosurveys have confirmed that 25% to 50% of adults are susceptible to diphtheria. Particular attention should be also be directed at revaccinating adults, especially travelers to countries with higher endemic disease. For continued protection, booster immunizations are recommended at 25 years of age and every 10 years thereafter. For children 6 to 12 years of age, primary immunization consists of two doses of pediatric diphtheria-tetanus (DT) toxoid vaccine 6 weeks apart, with a booster 6 to 12 months later. For persons older than 12 years of age, a smaller dose of diphtheria-tetanus toxoid should be used with the same schedule. The larger doses of diphtheria toxoid in DPT and DT may cause systemic reactions in older persons who have become sensitized by previous exposure to products of *C. diphtheriae*. Patients should receive toxoid immunization in the convalescent stage of their disease, since infection does not always induce protective antitoxin levels.

CLOSTRIDIAL INFECTIONS
Bacteriology

Clostridia are gram-positive, spore-forming anaerobic bacteria found in soil and as part of the normal flora of the intestinal tract of humans and animals. More than 80 species have been recognized, and approximately 30 species have been associated with human infections. All species grow better under anaerobic conditions, but some, such as *Clostridium perfringens*, can survive exposure to oxygen for as long as 72 hours. Spore formation is characteristic but not universal with standard laboratory culture conditions.

Clostridia have been found in the intestinal tract of virtually all animals studied. In 70% of humans, clostridia are found in concentrations of 10^8 to 10^9 organisms/g of stool. Less often, clostridia can be isolated from the normal flora of the female genital tract, the oral cavity, and the skin. *C. perfringens* is the most common clinical isolate and the most frequent clostridial constituent of human fecal flora.

The major virulence factor of clostridia is toxin production. Often, the target of toxin activity explains the clinical pattern of illness (Table 263-1). The neurotoxins of *Clostridium botulinum* and *Clostridium tetani* are the most potent microbial poisons known: the lethal dose for humans is estimated at 10^{-9} mg/kg body weight.

Gastrointestinal Tract Illness

Clostridia cause three distinctly different gastrointestinal tract illnesses: food poisoning (*C. perfringens,* type A), *C. difficile* toxin–induced antibiotic-associated diarrhea, and enteritis necroticans (*C. perfringens,* type C). The same clostridia that cause gastrointestinal tract illness may cause extraintestinal disease (e.g., *C. perfringens* is the most common cause of gas gangrene [myonecrosis]). Other clostridia may use the gastrointestinal tract as a portal of entry, but the manifestations of their toxin activity are extraintestinal (e.g., the neurotoxicity of *C. botulinum* in patients with foodborne botulism).

Food-borne Disease Caused by Clostridial Species

Clostridium perfringens Food Poisoning

Incidence, etiology, and epidemiology. *C. perfringens* is the second or third most common cause of food poisoning in the United States. Because symptoms are mild and the illness self-limited, many outbreaks, especially those resulting from home food preparation, are probably not reported.

Disease results from the production of an extracellular 35-kD enterotoxin by type A *C. perfringens.*

Meat, meat products, and poultry are the suspected foods in most outbreaks. Identified epidemics are usually associated with commercial food production, in which it is often necessary to prepare food well in advance of serving.

Pathogenesis. *C. perfringens* is found in 30% to 80% of the carcasses of chicken and cattle in slaughterhouses. Contaminating organisms survive cooking by forming spores if the maximum temperature or duration of cooking is inadequate. Ingestion of 10^8 to 10^9 viable bacteria is necessary to cause disease. This can occur either by prolonged warming of initially cooked foods at 43° C to 47° C, or, more often, by rewarming of leftover foods. The organism is ingested in the vegetative state, and the toxin is then elaborated in the intestinal tract rather than being ingested preformed.

The enterotoxin is a protein with molecular weight of about 35 kD. The toxin binds to receptors on the mucosal cells of the ileum, inhibits glucose transport, causes protein loss, and promotes sodium secretion. Further, cellular macromolecular synthesis is inhibited, there is an influx of calcium into the cell, the cell's cytoskeleton collapses, and cell death ensues.

Clinical features and therapy. After an incubation period of 8 to 24 hours the patient has diarrhea (90% of cases) and moderate to severe cramping with midepigastric pain (80%); additional findings include nausea (25%) and infrequently vomiting (9%) and fever (24%). The illness is self-limiting and resolves in less than 24 hours.

Therapy is supportive with adequate fluid replacement as the major objective. There is no indication for use of an antimicrobial agent. In theory, drugs that inhibit peristaltic activity may prolong illness.

Laboratory diagnosis. The laboratory diagnosis requires demonstration of more than 10^5 *C. perfringens* organisms/g of suspect infected food, presence of more than 10^6 *C. perfringens* spores/g of stool of ill person(s), and isolation of the same serotype of *C. perfringens* from the stool of infected person(s) and from the suspect contaminated food. The latter criterion is difficult. More than 90 serotypes of type A *C. perfringens* are recognized; of all strains isolated from patients, only 40% are typeable. Hence, serotyping is best employed in epidemic situations only. Alternative methods of detecting the enterotoxin have been described (e.g., an enzyme-linked immunosorbent assay [ELISA] and a reverse passive latex agglutination test).

Prevention. To prevent *C. perfringens* food poisoning, cooked foods must be maintained above 60° C or cooled to below 10° C within 2 to 3 hours. Previously cooked and then refrigerated foods should be reheated to a minimum internal temperature of 75° C immediately before serving to ensure destruction of vegetative bacteria.

Enteritis Necroticans. Enteritis necroticans, a serious disease of the small intestine, is caused by the beta toxin of *C. perfringens,* type C. Epidemics of disease, called *darmbrand,* occurred in malnourished individuals from Norway and Germany at the end of World War II. The same disease is endemic in the highlands of New Guinea, where it is called *pigbel* because of the association with pig feasts.

The target of the toxin is the mucosal cell of the small bowel. Patients have acute abdominal pain, bloody diarrhea, vomiting, shock, and peritonitis. The mortality rate is 15% to 40%. Pathologic examination demonstrates an acute segmental ulcerative process of the small bowel mucosa. The mucosa lifts off the submucosa, leaving a large denuded area; the partially sloughed epithelium may form pseudomembranes.

Table 263-2   Historical evolution of the recognition of *Clostridium difficile* toxin as a cause of antibiotic-associated diarrhea/colitis

YEAR	EVENT
1893	Pathologic description of idiopathic pseudomembranous colitis (PMC)
1950	Increased incidence of PMC attributed to *Staphylococcus aureus*
1970	Recognition and investigation of "clindamycin" colitis
1974	Description of pathogenetic role of *C. difficile* toxin
1979	Report of cytotoxicity assay for *C. difficile* toxin
1992	*C. difficile* toxin recognized as usual cause of PMC and of 15% to 30% of cases of antibiotic-associated diarrhea

It is believed that the disease results from a deficiency of proteolytic enzymes (trypsin) which normally break down type C toxin. This may result from a combination of the following factors: (1) a low-protein diet; (2) the simultaneous consumption of food containing trypsin inhibitors such as sweet potatoes; and (3) the parasitization of some individuals by *Ascaris* worms that secrete trypsin inhibitors. Antitoxin titers are demonstrable in patients who survive the disease; hence the apparent predilection for children may reflect absence of protective antibody.

Medical therapy includes nasogastric suction, support with intravenous fluids, and use, if available, of antitoxin against the beta toxin. Resectional surgery is necessary in about half the patients. The role of antibiotics directed against the organism as opposed to broad-spectrum antibiotic therapy for intestinal perforation is unknown. In the endemic area, a beta-toxoid vaccine is recommended for prevention in children.

Clostridium difficile Toxin–Mediated Diarrhea and Colitis

History. Pseudomembranous colitis (PMC), although rare, was a recognized pathologic entity many years before the availability of antibiotics, although this pathologic lesion is now strongly associated with use of antibiotics. In retrospect, it is likely that many of the patients with an entity known as "staphylococcal pseudomembranous colitis" had *C. difficile* toxin–mediated enterocolitis. By the 1970s the pathogenetic role of *C. difficile* toxin (CDT) was recognized, and a specific sensitive biologic assay to detect the toxin became available (Table 263-2).

Pathophysiology. *C. difficile* toxin–mediated diarrhea and colitis (PMC) are caused by elaboration of two cytotoxins, A and B, by *C. difficile.* Mucosal invasion by the *C. difficile* organism does not occur.

Toxins. Toxins A and B are large proteins synthesized during rapid bacterial growth. Toxin B is a more potent cytotoxin in vitro in tissue culture, but toxin A is an enterotoxin and is believed to be responsible for clinical and pathologic findings. The mechanism of toxicity is incompletely understood. Most strains of *C. difficile* produce both toxins.

Toxin production. The factors that stimulate toxin production in patients are unclear. On experimentation, some strains increase toxin production in the presence of clindamycin. Constituents of the culture medium in vitro can influence toxin production. Sporulation and presence or absence of plasmids do not correlate with toxin production. In the hamster animal model and in human patients, administration of antimicrobial agents directly or indirectly stimulates an increase in the number of intestinal *C. difficile* and CDT production.

Epidemiology. The vast majority of patients with *C. difficile* toxin–mediated diarrhea or colitis have received antibiotic therapy in some form. Virtually all agents with antibacterial activity have been associated with the disease, especially those having the greatest activity against colonic flora. Clindamycin, ampicillin or amoxicillin, and cephalosporins are most often implicated on a case per treatment course basis. Other penicillins, quinolones, erythromycin, and trimethoprim-sulfamethoxazole are involved less often; aminoglycosides, sulfonamides, and tetracycline are seldom implicated. Both metronidazole and, rarely, vancomycin have been implicated, despite

Table 263-3   Results of tissue culture assays for *Clostridium difficile* toxin and stool cultures for *C. difficile*

PATIENT/DISEASE CATEGORY	PERCENTAGE OF PATIENTS WITH POSITIVE RESULTS	
	TISSUE CULTURE ASSAY FOR *C. DIFFICILE* TOXIN	STOOL CULTURE FOR *C. DIFFICILE*
Antibiotic-associated pseudomembranous colitis (PMC)	95-100	95-100
Antibiotic-associated diarrhea without confirmed PMC	15-25	25-50
Antibiotic exposure without diarrhea	2-8	10-25
Gastrointestinal tract disease unrelated to antimicrobial exposure	0-0.5	3-5
Healthy adults	0	3
Healthy neonates	5-63	5-70

From Bartlett JG: *Clin Infect Dis* 15:576, 1992.

their use as treatment for the condition. In addition, antimetabolite cancer chemotherapeutic agents have been implicated as causes of this disease, as have intestinal surgical procedures.

C. difficile is found as colonic flora in 2% to 3% of the general population but may be acquired nosocomially. Ten percent to 30% of hospitalized patients receiving antibiotics may be found to harbor the organism. Outbreaks have been reported in hospitals and nursing homes, spread on the hands of health care providers or by rectal thermometers, commode equipment, or the hospital environment when cleansing measures have been inadequate.

C. difficile *acquisition.* *C. difficile* has been isolated from sand, soil, mud, and feces of domestic animals. The organism is found as part of the fecal flora of 2% to 3% of asymptomatic adults. Carriage rate is higher in the elderly, infants, and patients with cystic fibrosis.

Clinical manifestations. The most common symptom is diarrhea, consisting of watery or loose stools without visible blood. This may begin at any time during a course of antibiotics or for up to 6 weeks after discontinuation, but usually within 2 weeks. Severity of illness is variable ranging from only mild, watery diarrhea to severe diarrhea with fever and prostration. Rarely, patients may come to medical attention with abdominal pain and fever, and postoperative patients may have ileus with fever and abdominal pain. Rarely, patients have come to medical attention with toxic megacolon or colonic perforation that has been ascribed to *C. difficile* but no history of diarrhea.

Diagnosis. Since 75% to 85% of cases of diarrhea occurring while patients are taking antibiotics are not due to *C. difficile,* making a specific diagnosis of *C. difficile*–associated diarrhea is important.

Pseudomembranous colitis is one end of the spectrum of disease caused by *C. difficile.* This diagnosis requires demonstration of typical pseudomembranes endoscopically on colonic examination. Up to one third of cases involve the right-side colon only; hence sigmoidoscopy may be inadequate to exclude the diagnosis.

Pseudomembranes are raised, punctate, yellow-white plaques 2 to 10 mm wide. Lesions may become confluent in severe cases. On histologic examination the colonic epithelium shows necrosis and infiltration of the lamina propria with polymorphonuclear leukocytes (PMNs) and eosinophilic exudate. The pseudomembrane is attached to the underlying epithelium by a stalk and is itself composed of fibrin, mucin, and PMNs.

Colonic appearance in patients with diarrhea associated with antibiotic use ranges from normal to erythema or edema, friability, ulceration or hemorrhage, to pseudomembrane formation. Pseudomembranous colitis is the anatomic diagnosis that is most clearly associated with *C. difficile,* since the toxin can be demonstrated in 95% to 100% of cases (Table 263-3).

Definitive diagnosis requires demonstration of CDT in the stool. Mere demonstration of the presence of the organism is inadequate. The gold standard assay for CDT is the tissue culture assay in which a stool filtrate applied to a tissue culture monolayer causes toxic dis-

ruption, which is neutralized by antisera to *C. difficile* or *Clostridium sordellii.* This assay generally takes 48 hours to complete.

More rapid results may be obtained by the use of either enzyme immunoassays for toxins A and B or a latex agglutination test. However, the sensitivity and specificity of these tests are not as good as the tissue culture assay, and many laboratories perform the tissue culture assay as a backup, despite offering the more rapid assays.

Treatment (Table 263-4). When possible, discontinuation of the offending antibiotic is the treatment of choice; this often results in resolution of symptoms in patients with mild disease. Antiperistaltics should be avoided. Patients with persistent or moderate to severe illness require drug therapy. Intravenous hydration and, often, hyperalimentation are required in patients with severe illness. Discussion of the major drugs used to treat CDT-mediated diarrhea follows.

Metronidazole. Metronidazole is the drug of choice for patients who are mildly to moderately ill, because of its low cost and good response rates (95% to 100%). Metronidazole is absorbed rapidly from normal bowel; the drug is less well absorbed in the presence of colitis. Mean fecal concentrations of 10 μg/ml were reported in patients with PMC given 500 mg orally four times a day. Similar fecal concentrations are reported after the intravenous administration of metronidazole. No reported clinical trials compare the efficacy of different dosage regimens. Response rates are similar with 500 mg three or four times a day.

Of interest, the in vitro activity of metronidazole is bactericidal and dose dependent. At concentrations similar to those found in feces, a 99.99% reduction of *C. difficile* occurs in vitro. The reported relapse rate with metronidazole varies from 5% to 32%. The mechanism of relapse with metronidazole may relate to improved drug absorption as the CDT-mediated colitis resolves with less drug delivered to the colon. Lower fecal levels of metronidazole are reported in patients with CDT-mediated diarrhea as opposed to the levels found in patients with PMC. Hence, during or after a course of metronidazole therapy, colonic levels may fall sufficiently to allow germination of spores, toxin production, and relapse of diarrhea. Generic oral metronidazole is relatively inexpensive. With the regimen of 500 mg three times a day for 10 days the approximate cost to the pharmacist is $2.

Vancomycin. Vancomycin taken orally is not absorbed to any substantial degree even from an inflamed gastrointestinal tract. Conversely, intravenous vancomycin does not achieve measurable levels in the lumen of the colon. Initially, a dose of 500 mg four times a day was employed; subsequently, the dose was reduced to 125 mg four times a day, with a response rate of nearly 100%. Even with the reduced dosage, fecal concentrations approximate 1000 μg/ml. Despite the high concentrations, spores of *C. difficile* survive vancomycin therapy and are recoverable from feces during and after therapy; the posttreatment strains remain vancomycin susceptible in vitro. When *C. difficile* is incubated in vitro with the concentrations of vancomycin found in feces, vancomycin is bacteriostatic. Resolution of diarrhea and colitis may result from the combination of vancomycin inhibition of *C. difficile,* peristalsis-induced washout of colonic content, and perhaps some reconstitution of the inhibitory influence of "normal flora."

Disadvantages of oral vancomycin are (1) its expense (appropriate cost to pharmacist, $160 for 10-day course) and (2) the risk of inducing vancomycin resistance in the resident gastrointestinal tract flora (especially enterococci). Despite these disadvantages, some authorities prefer vancomycin to metronidazole for seriously ill patients.

Other therapy. Alternative therapies employ bacitracin and cholestyramine. These drugs are used less often, and data on fecal concentrations are not available.

Oral bacitracin is given as 25,000 units (approximately 500 mg) four times per day for 7 to 10 days. The drug is bitter and must be specially prepared in capsule form to prevent nausea. Systemic absorption across inflamed mucosa and frequency of relapse need study.

Cholestyramine is an anion exchange resin that was used to treat PMC before the cause of the disease was known. It is now known that cholestyramine binds CDT A and B; the resin also binds vancomycin, precluding combination therapy. The oral adult dose is 4 g three to four times daily. Reported response rates vary from as low as 50% to as high as 95%.

Table 263-4   Alternative therapies for *Clostridium difficile* toxin–mediated antibiotic-associated diarrhea or pseudomembranous colitis*

DRUG	MECHANISM OF ACTION	TREATMENT REGIMEN (po)	FECAL CONCENTRATION (μg/ml)	RESPONSE RATE (%)	RELAPSE RATE (5%)	EXPENSE FOR 10 DAYS†
Vancomycin	Inhibits *C. difficile*	125 mg qid × 7-10 days	1000	97	5-55	$110-160
Metronidazole	Cidal for *C. difficile*	500 mg tid × 7-10 days	10	95-100	5-32	$1
Bacitracin	Anti–*C. difficile*	25,000 U qid × 7-10 days	NA‡	80-100	33-344	$44
Cholestyramine	Binds *C. difficile* toxin A and B, and vancomycin	4 g qid × 7-10 days	NA	50-95	?	$29-40

*For all patients: (1) if possible, discontinue all antimicrobial therapy; (2) avoid drugs with antiperistaltic actions (e.g., diphenoxylate with atropine [Lomotil]).
†Cost to pharmacist as of March, 1993.
‡*NA*, not available.

Treatment of pseudomembranous colitis in patients with adynamic ileus. Drug delivery to the lumen of the colon is difficult in patients with ileus. The absence of peristalsis may promote more toxin-induced injury with an increased risk of complications (e.g., bowel perforation and toxic megacolon).

There is no standardized treatment regimen because individual circumstances vary. One regimen reported to be effective used intracolonic vancomycin, 2 g, followed by 100 mg every 6 hours plus 100 mg after each stool via "pigtail" catheter into the cecum.

Treatment of relapse. The reported frequency of relapse varies from 5% to 55% of patients who receive treatment. The accumulated data indicate that relapses are due to CDT production by the original strain of *C. difficile;* the organisms do not display in vitro resistance to the commonly prescribed drugs.

With relapses, typically, all symptoms of diarrhea or PMC subside during therapy, only to recur 3 to 10 days after completion of metronidazole or vancomycin administration. There is no uniform recommendation for relapse management. Patients and physicians frequently become frustrated because 10% of patients may have two or more relapses and 5% may have three or more relapses. Conceptually, without availability of a drug to eradicate fecal vegetative or spore forms of *C. difficile,* giving repeated courses of therapy is an attempt to control toxin production until "normal" fecal flora are reestablished, with concomitant cessation of toxin production.

Relapses are initially managed by repeated 7- to 10-day courses of vancomycin or metronidazole in the same regimen employed for the initial episode. If a second course of therapy fails, repeat therapy with the combination of vancomycin in the initial dosage and rifampin, 600 mg, twice a day for 7 to 10 days may be tried.

Prevention. There is increasing consensus that *C. difficile* is acquired in the hospital environment. Numerous hospital outbreaks and case clusters have been described. The prevalence of asymptomatic fecal carriage of *C. difficile* is high in patient populations, whereas the carriage rate is low in the general adult population.

Mode of transmission in the hospital is unclear. *C. difficile* spores survive on inanimate objects in the immediate environment of the patient, but the significance is not known. Spread by the hands of hospital personnel is postulated. Reduction in incidence of *C. difficile* diarrhea was accomplished by mandated glove use by hospital personnel in one report. More aggressive control measures, such as treatment of all carriers with vancomycin or metronidazole, are expensive but might be considered in a true epidemic. Mainstays of prevention are judicious use of antimicrobial agents and implementation of universal precautions, especially use of gloves and hand washing, in patient care.

Neurologic Syndromes

Botulism
Definition. Botulism is a life-threatening neuroparalytic disease caused by toxins produced by *C. botulinum* and, rarely, other clostridial species. The disease is categorized by the circumstances under which it occurs: (1) food-borne botulism, (2) infant botulism, (3) wound botulism, and (4) unclassified cases.

History. The name of the disease is derived from the Latin word for sausage, *botulus.* Outbreaks of "sausage poisoning" were common in the nineteenth century. In 1895, Van Ermengem isolated an anaerobic, spore-forming bacillus from a ham suspected to have caused illness; subsequently he demonstrated that both the ham and a toxin from the organism could cause a paralytic illness in cats. Shortly after World War I the rapid increase in both commercial and home canning resulted in many epidemics of botulism. Most of the recent cases of food-borne botulism are the result of improper home-canning procedures. Infant botulism was not recognized until 1976.

Etiology and pathogenesis. *C. botulinum* is an anaerobic, spore-forming rod with subterminal spores that synthesizes and releases a potent exotoxin during growth and autolysis. In young cultures the organism stains gram-positive; after 18 hours of incubation the organism may stain gram-negative. Each strain produces one of eight antigenically distinct toxins, which are designated by letters. Types A, B, E, and, rarely, F cause human disease. Over the last 20 years type A has been the most frequent cause of food-borne outbreaks.

On a weight basis, botulinus toxins are the most potent poisons known. They are polypeptides with a molecular weight of approximately 150,000 daltons. The toxins are hematogenously disseminated and block neuromuscular transmission in cholinergic nerve fibers by preventing acetylcholine release. The motor–end-plate remains responsive to acetylcholine. In humans, central nervous system cholinergic pathways and adrenergic fibers are not affected. The result is hypotonia with a descending, symmetric flaccid paralysis. Recovery occurs by sprouting of new axons.

Spores of organisms producing type A or B toxins are widely distributed in soil throughout the world. Strains that produce type A toxin are most common in the western United States, whereas type B toxin producers are most common in the eastern United States and in Europe. Type E toxin is found in organisms from water samples from northern latitudes, possibly accounting for the high incidence of type E strains in fish-borne botulism.

Spores of *C. botulinum* can withstand temperatures of 100° C for hours; however, the toxins are relatively heat-labile: boiling for 10 minutes or heating at 80° C for 30 minutes inactivates the toxins. Hence, terminal heating of toxin-containing food can prevent illness. Strict anaerobic conditions are not always necessary for toxin production. Toxin synthesis is optimal at 30° C but can occur at refrigerator temperatures. With some exceptions, home-canned acidic foods such as tomatoes are safer than alkaline foods because a low pH retards spore germination and toxin production.

Toxins are absorbed from the stomach and small intestine. Digestive enzymes do not denature toxin, and pancreatic trypsin may enhance the toxicity of type E toxin. Slow toxin absorption may occur from the colon. If *C. botulinum* organisms or spores are ingested and reach the colon, toxin production can occur in the human gastrointestinal tract. The latter may explain the presence of toxin in the bloodstream days after the ingestion of contaminated food.

Food-borne Botulism
Epidemiology. Food-borne botulism results from the ingestion of preformed toxin in inadequately prepared food. On average, 15 "outbreaks" occur each year in the United States, but usually only a single case is involved per outbreak. Home-canned foods with a putrid odor are the most frequently implicated vehicle. However, some contaminated food may look and taste normal.

Botulism can occur when the following conditions are met: (1) a food product contains viable *C. botulinum* bacilli or spores; (2) conditions allow spore germination; (3) time and conditions permit production of toxin before ingestion; (4) food is heated insufficiently to destroy toxin; and (5) the toxin-containing food is ingested by a susceptible host.

High-risk foods include home-canned or home-processed low-acid fruits and vegetables, fish and fish products, and condiments such as relish and chili peppers. Commercially processed foods and improperly handled fresh foods have been implicated in outbreaks of botulism. In addition, some native traditional food preparation practices may perpetuate the problem.

Clinical manifestations. The hallmark of the disease is descending paralysis. Fever is absent unless there is an intercurrent infection. Incubation period averages 18 to 36 hours after ingestion of contaminated food but may be shorter or longer. Ptosis and weakness of the extraocular muscles are frequent findings; failure of accommodation occurs in some patients. Neuromuscular blockade results in symmetric weakness of the facial muscles, tongue, palate, larynx, diaphragm and intercostal muscles, and the extremities. Mild degrees of asymmetric muscle weakness may be encountered. Ileus of the intestinal tract and distention of the bladder may be present. Deep tendon reflexes vary with the severity of the illness; Babinski's sign is absent. The sensory examination finding is always normal. Gait disturbances and incoordination are due to generalized weakness. Impaired function of cholinergic autonomic pathways may result in reduced salivation and lacrimation, constipation, and urinary retention. Nausea and vomiting may occur.

From the onset of symptoms the disease progresses quickly over several days. The magnitude of neuromuscular impairment can progress hourly. Stabilization then occurs, with subsequent recovery over weeks to months. As in tetanus, recovery from botulism does not confirm long-term immunity. Rare examples of a second episode in the same patient are described.

Laboratory diagnosis and neurologic tests. Routine laboratory tests are not helpful in the diagnosis. The most sensitive test remains injection of patient serum and stool and extracts of suspected food intraperitoneally into mice, with some mice given polyvalent and type-specific monovalent botulinum antitoxins. In a positive test result, all mice die within 24 to 48 hours, except those protected by the polyvalent and type-specific antisera. The isolation of *C. botulinum* from the stool of an ill person is considered confirmatory, since the organism is rarely encountered in the intestinal flora of normal individuals. These tests are generally conducted in the laboratories of health departments or the CDC. Mouse bioassay and culture isolation have an overall case recognition rate of approximately 85%.

Except for occasional mild elevations in protein concentration, the spinal fluid is normal. Mild nonspecific electrocardiogram abnormalities may occur. Results of nerve conduction studies are normal; however, electromyographic examination of involved muscle groups frequently reveals decreased amplitude of the muscle action potential and facilitation during rapid repetitive or posttetanic stimulation. These results are similar to the abnormalities found in patients with the Eaton-Lambert syndrome.

Differential diagnosis. The diseases most frequently confused with botulism are those which produce generalized weakness. Patients with the Guillain-Barré syndrome almost always have mild sensory abnormalities and an increase in the spinal fluid protein concentration. The Miller-Fisher variant of Guillain-Barré is characterized by ophthalmoplegia, ataxia, and/or areflexia; again, elevation of the spinal fluid protein concentration assists in diagnosis. The course of myasthenia gravis is more insidious, and the deep tendon reflexes and pupils are normal. An edrophonium chloride (Tensilon) test may help exclude myasthenia gravis; however, patients with botulism may have transient partial test responses. In tick paralysis the weakness has an ascending pattern, paresthesias may be present, and a tick is found. Patients with diphtheria frequently have a history of pharyngitis, with subsequent weakness of the palate. Patients with poliomyelitis have asymmetric weakness, sparing of the ocular muscles, and cerebrospinal fluid pleocytosis. Cerebrovascular disease of the brain stem causes associated cerebellar or corticospinal tract abnormalities. Atropine or scopolamine poisoning produces toxic delirium and marked pupil dilation. In contrast, organophosphate insecticide poisoning causes cho-

linergic excess with miotic pupils. Other entities to consider include shellfish poisoning, familial periodic paralysis, and aminoglycoside antibiotic-induced neuromuscular blockade.

Treatment. Respiratory failure is the most important threat to the survival of patients with botulism. For this reason, patients with symptoms or known exposure should be hospitalized and observed closely. Sequential determinations of vital capacity should be made with consideration given to intubation if vital capacity is less than 12 ml/kg, or if hypoxemia or CO_2 retention is present. Many patients require intubation and ventilatory support for days to months. Tracheostomy may prove necessary to manage secretions.

If bowel sounds are present, cathartics and enemas are given to remove unabsorbed botulinum toxin from the intestine. Magnesium salts (citrate or sulfate) should not be given, since the magnesium can potentiate the toxin-induced neuromuscular blockade.

Other supportive care includes nasogastric suction and intravenous hyperalimentation if a severe ileus is present, use of a Foley catheter for bladder atonia, meticulous skin care, physical therapy, and close observation for hospital-acquired pneumonia or urinary tract infection.

As soon as the diagnosis is suspected, public health authorities* should be contacted, the case reported, and arrangements made to acquire trivalent botulinum type ABE antitoxin (Connaught Laboratories, Swiftwater, Penn). Retrospective data suggest that type-specific antitoxin is beneficial in patients with type E intoxication. The value in type A and B disease is less certain, especially if paralysis has already occurred. Because the toxin binds irreversibly to nerve endings and only circulating toxin is neutralized, antitoxin should be given as early in the course of the illness as possible. The antitoxin is of equine origin, and patients should be tested for hypersensitivity to horse serum. One can test for immediate hypersensitivity with either a skin test or instillation into the conjunctival sac; the latter method is preferred. Nonfatal hypersensitivity reactions occur in 15% to 20% of patients who receive the antitoxin. Patients who react to a test dose must be desensitized (regimen included in the package). The dose is two vials of antitoxin, one given intravenously and one intramuscularly. These may be repeated in 2 to 4 hours.

In the absence of infectious complications, antibiotic therapy has no role in food-borne botulism. Antibiotics in other forms of botulism are discussed later.

Guanidine hydrochloride may produce some improvement in cranial nerve palsies or extremity muscle strength. However, improvement in vital capacity rarely occurs; hence the use of guanidine is not recommended.

Prognosis. In the United States the mortality rate of food-borne botulism is approximately 10%, with higher mortality rates with type A than with type B or E. The time for recovery ranges from 30 to 100 days. Full neurologic recovery is usual.

Prevention. Promptly notifying public health authorities of a suspected case may prevent further consumption of a contaminated home-canned or commercial food product. The disease is best prevented by adherence to recommended home-canning techniques. High-temperature pressure cooking is necessary to ensure spore elimination from low-acid fruits and vegetables. The toxin itself is heat labile and is destroyed by boiling food. Laboratory-acquired botulism has been reported from other countries. Laboratory workers who routinely work with *C. botulinum*, or its toxin should receive the pentavalent botulinum toxoid vaccine.

Wound Botulism. First recognized in 1943, more than 30 cases of wound botulism have been reported in the United States. The typical patient is a young, previously healthy adult male who sustained severe trauma, with open fractures contaminated by soil. Fewer than 10 cases have occurred in individuals who abuse parenteral drugs. Disease caused by toxins A and B has been documented.

The disease is similar to food-borne botulism, except that nausea, vomiting, and diarrhea usually do not occur; fever generated by wound infection may be present; and the incubation period is longer,

---

*Centers for Disease Control and Prevention 24-hour phone numbers are (404) 639-2206 (weekdays) and (404) 639-2888 (nights and weekends).

with a median of 7 days (range, 4 to 18 days). The case fatality rate is approximately 17%.

After serum is obtained for bioassay for toxin, botulinum antitoxin is administered as for food-borne botulism, and the wound is debrided, even if it appears normal on gross examination. Anaerobic cultures of the wound should be performed to attempt to isolate *C. botulinum.* High-dose penicillin therapy (10 to 20 million units intravenously per day if renal function is normal) is usually administered, although its efficacy is not proved. The disease is best prevented by prompt, thorough debridement of contaminated wounds. Prophylactic use of antimicrobial agents after trauma cannot be relied on to prevent the disease.

Infant Botulism. Infant botulism was not recognized until 1976. It is now the most common form of botulism in the United States, with 30 to 80 cases documented annually.

Age appears to be an important factor in pathogenesis; 90% of recognized cases have occurred in children less than 6 months of age. In animals the illness can be reproduced only during a few days of early life. In distinction to food-borne botulism, it is believed that the intestinal tract of infants first becomes colonized with *C. botulinum;* then toxin is produced and absorbed, producing a slowly progressive disease. Quantitative studies demonstrated 10^3 to 10^8 *C. botulinum* organisms/g of feces. Studies that compare the fecal flora of infants with botulism to those of infants without the syndrome suggest three possible factors in colonization of the intestine with *C. botulinum:* delay in establishment of a normal fecal flora, presence of other bacterial flora that inhibit or promote colonization, or altered intestinal function that promotes germination and growth of ingested spores.

Diet plays a role in the pathogenesis of infant botulism. Spores of *C. botulinum,* but not the toxin, are found in approximately 10% of honey samples, and honey exposure is associated with approximately one third of cases. As a result, it is recommended that children less than 12 months old not ingest honey. Honey does not contain botulinum toxin; hence it is safe for older children and adults. In the majority of cases no definite source of the *C. botulinum* spores is identified. Breast-feeding may be relatively protective, but iron supplementation may increase susceptibility to the disease.

The earliest sign is constipation, which often appears 1 to 3 weeks before neurologic signs. Lethargy, listlessness, and anorexia then appear, accompanied by a weak cry, a decreased gag reflex, decreased sucking, and drooling. The child may have difficulty holding his or her head erect, ptosis may develop, and the child may become floppy. This dramatic picture is typical of hospitalized patients. The full disease spectrum runs from mild constipation to sudden death. Complete recovery requires several weeks to months.

Meticulous supportive care is the mainstay of therapy. Because toxin is rarely detected in serum and because of risk of hypersensitivity reactions, botulinum antitoxin is usually not given. Oral or parenteral penicillin therapy has no role. In contrast to adults with respiratory failure who often require a tracheostomy, the disease in many infants is managed successfully with endotracheal intubation. No evidence shows that cathartics or enemas influence the course of the disease; however, this approach may be tried cautiously if no ileus is present. The mortality rate for hospitalized patients is 2%.

Unclassified Botulism. Some patients above the age of 12 months have typical symptoms and signs of botulism, but no clear exposure is identified. It is possible that some cases result from production of toxin in vivo in a fashion analogous to that described for infant botulism.

Tetanus

Definition. Tetanus is an acute neurologic syndrome, often fatal, caused by a neuroexotoxin produced by *Clostridium tetani.* Tetanus is characterized by increased rigidity and convulsive spasms of the patient's skeletal musculature.

Etiology. *Clostridium tetani* is an anaerobic, gram-positive, motile bacillus. The vegetative form of the organism forms a single, spheric, terminal endospore that swells the end of the organism with a resulting drumstick or tennis racket shape. The vegetative forms of the organism are very susceptible to heat, disinfectants, and other adverse conditions, whereas the spores can survive in soil for months to years, are highly resistant to antiseptics, and are moderately resistant to heat. Killing of spores requires boiling for a minimum of 4 hours or exposure to an autoclave for 12 minutes at 121° C.

It is possible to separate *C. tetani* into 10 types, based on their flagellar antigens. All 10 types produce the major toxin, tetanospasmin. Because the tetanospasmins produced are nearly identical antigenically, only one antitoxin is needed to neutralize the tetanus toxins produced by all strains. Tetanospasmin has a molecular weight of approximately 150,000 daltons and is composed after cleavage of a heavy (100,000 mw) and light (50,000 mw) chain joined by a disulfide bond. Along with botulism toxin, tetanospasmin is one of the most potent microbial toxins. One milligram of tetanospasmin can kill 50 to 70 million mice.

Epidemiology. The tetanus bacillus can be found in 20% to 65% of soil samples and as part of the normal flora of the intestinal tract of certain animals and humans. The highest yields of the organism are found in cultivated land; in hot, damp climates; in densely populated regions; and in soil rich in organic matter. The organism has also been found in house dust, operating rooms, and contaminated heroin.

The incidence of tetanus in the United States decreased from 560 reported cases in 1947 to 53 reported cases in 1988. Tetanus in the United States is a disease of older adults. Of the 109 tetanus patients reported to the CDC in 1989 and 1990, 59% were older than 50 years of age and 6% were younger than 20 years of age. There was one case of neonatal tetanus.

The age distribution suggests inadequate immunity of older adults. Serologic surveys since 1977 indicate inadequate circulating tetanus antitoxin levels in 6% to 11% of adults 18 to 39 years of age and 49% to 66% of adults older than 60 years. Clinical evidence of tetanus occurs virtually exclusively among unvaccinated or inadequately vaccinated persons or in individuals whose vaccination histories are unknown or uncertain.

Tetanus has occurred after surgery and seemingly harmless procedures such as skin testing or intramuscular injections of medication. Drug addicts represent another risk group. "Skin poppers" who inject drugs subcutaneously appear to be at particularly high risk. Of interest, heroin is often diluted with quinine, which lowers oxygen tensions at the site of injection and hence favors the growth of *C. tetani.*

A large problem exists in underdeveloped countries as a result of poor immunization standards and low levels of hygiene. One example is the practice of applying local dried clay to the umbilical stump of babies born to unimmunized mothers. The global incidence of tetanus is estimated to be 1 million cases per year with 800,000 neonatal deaths.

Pathogenesis. Because *C. tetani* is noninvasive, clinical tetanus can occur only when local tissue conditions allow toxin production and the host has no circulating antitoxin. Portals of entry of the organism include puncture wounds and lacerations, surgical wounds, subcutaneous injection sites, chronic skin ulcers, burns, infected umbilical cords, otitis media with tympanic membrane perforation, abortion, and the postpartum female genital tract. Neonatal tetanus usually follows infection of the umbilical stump. In the United States most cases result from cut or puncture wounds incurred while working, gardening, or handling animals. The injuries are often trivial. In 10% to 20% of cases, no history of injury or portal of entry is identified. Because the spores are ubiquitous in the environment, most cases result from contamination from an exogenous source. Endogenous infection is possible in rare cases that follow surgery on the intestinal tract.

Spores of *C. tetani* undoubtedly contaminate wounds frequently, but tetanus develops rarely because sporulation to the vegetative state requires an oxygen tension below that normally encountered in tissue. Occasionally, spores survive in a wound for months to years and ultimately produce disease after subsequent trauma that alters local conditions. Wound toxin production occurs under those conditions that reduce the local oxidation-reduction potential. Examples include the presence of suppuration, foreign body, necrotic tissue, and calcium salts. After conversion to the vegetative form, the tetanus bacillus stays localized, but the tetanospasmin enters peripheral nerve terminals and is carried within axons in membrane-bound vesicles toward the spinal cord at a rate of 250 mm per day. In the central nervous system the toxin reaches presynaptic terminals, where it blocks release of neurotransmitter used by inhibitory afferent motor neurons (gamma-aminobutyric acid [GABA]). Loss of inhibition results in unrestrained action potentials and sustained muscle contraction. The result is muscle rigidity from uninhibited afferent stimuli entering the central nervous system from the periphery. Spasms result from more vigorous stimuli; even emotional and visual stimuli can result in muscle spasm. Tetanus toxin can also produce neuromuscular blockade similar to that of the toxin of botulism. Tetanus toxin can act directly on muscles to produce contraction. Some of the clinical manifestations suggest that the toxin has an excitatory effect on the sympathetic nervous system, probably also via GABA inhibition.

Toxin binding is irreversible, and recovery requires sprouting of new axon terminals. A histopathologic change in the brain stem of patients who die of tetanus has been reported, and a toxic myocarditis has been described.

Clinical Manifestations. The incubation period is 7 to 21 days, but cases can appear as early as 2 days or as late as 56 days after time of injury. The short incubation period indicates severe disease, usually after trauma. In general, the length of the incubation period reflects the distance of the site of injury from the central nervous system.

Regardless of severity, the patient usually has nonspecific symptoms such as restlessness, headache, and irritability. The most common presenting complaints are pain and stiffness in the jaw, abdomen, or back with associated difficulty swallowing; as the disease evolves, muscle stiffness becomes muscle rigidity and patients often complain of difficulty opening the mouth (trismus). Trismus is the most common sign of tetanus and is given the familiar descriptive name "lockjaw." As more muscles become involved, rigidity becomes generalized and the sustained contractions of the facial musculature result in a characteristic expression called *risus sardonicus*. Reflex muscle spasms develop within 24 to 72 hours of the first symptoms; the interval between first symptoms and reflex spasm is referred to as the onset time. A short onset time is associated with a poor prognosis. Any sudden increase in intensity of afferent stimuli arising in the periphery can cause painful, dangerous spasms. The spasms can interfere with respiration either by tonic contraction of the respiratory muscles or by production of laryngospasm. The resulting hypoxia can lead to irreversible central nervous system damage and death.

Clinical evidence of tetanus can be generalized (including neonatal tetanus) or localized (to include cephalic tetanus). Patients with local tetanus complain of pain and stiffness in the area of the wound. Localized increases in muscle tone are often present. Cephalic tetanus is a rare form of local tetanus that results from contamination of wounds of the head or neck and may complicate otitis media or a head injury. Cephalic tetanus is manifested by ocular muscle palsies and evidence of facial nerve dysfunction. Generalized tetanus is manifested initially by abdominal and back pain, stiffness of the neck and jaw, and dysphagia. Spontaneous muscle contractions (spasms) may occur. Physical examination reveals an alert, restless patient with trismus, rigid abdominal wall, and increased deep tendon reflexes. Low-grade fever is often present. Spasm of the facial muscles may result in risus sardonicus. Generalized tetanus may be mild, moderate, or severe. Mild cases have an incubation period of 10 days or longer, and symptoms and signs develop over 4 to 7 days. Paroxysmal spasms are few. Patients with moderate tetanus have an incubation period of less than 10 days, and symptoms and signs develop over 3 to 6 days. In addition to generalized muscle rigidity, these patients have dysphagia. Spasms occur but do not result in respiratory impairment. Patients with severe tetanus have incubation periods of less than 7 days, and symptoms evolve over 3 days or less. Frequent, severe spasms result in respiratory impairment and opisthotonos. Patients with severe tetanus may have autonomic instability, paroxysmal hypertension and hypotension, tachycardia, arrhythmias, high fever, and profuse sweating. The usual duration of disease, regardless of severity, is 3 to 4 weeks.

Tetanus neonatorum is generalized tetanus that results from infection in neonates within 10 days of birth. The child demonstrates irritability, facial grimacing, difficulty sucking, excessive crying, flexion of the arms, clenched fists, extension of the legs, plantar flexion of the toes, and intense rigidity, which may produce opisthotonos. The mortality rate usually is greater than 70%.

In the United States the overall mortality for mild to moderate tetanus is approximately 6%, whereas it may reach 60% or more for severe tetanus. Neonatal tetanus mortality is 90% or greater. Recovery from moderate to severe tetanus requires 3 to 6 weeks but is generally complete.

Complications of tetanus include hypoxia from inadequate ventilation and the ever-present threat of aspiration of oropharyngeal contents as a consequence of difficulty in swallowing. Involvement of the sympathetic nervous system can result in severe vasoconstriction, hypertension, tachycardia, and arrhythmias. Myocarditis can produce pulmonary edema and hypotension. Patients generally do not have a high fever; high fever usually indicates the presence of a secondary infection. Common secondary infections include pneumonia, infection of the original wound, infected decubiti, and infections of the urinary tract in patients with indwelling bladder catheters. Midthoracic vertebral fractures can occur as a result of severe muscle spasms and occur more often among children and adolescents. Gastrointestinal tract complications include paralytic ileus, constipation, and acute peptic ulceration.

Laboratory Findings and Diagnosis. The laboratory findings in patients with tetanus are nonspecific. One third of patients demonstrate leukocytosis. Results of blood chemistry panels are almost always normal initially. Electrocardiogram shows nonspecific changes only. The spinal fluid examination is normal.

The diagnosis of tetanus is made on the basis of clinical criteria. Culture for *C. tetani* has low sensitivity and specificity, but attempt is warranted in suspected cases. The organism is identified in the laboratory with standard anaerobic culture and morphologic characteristics plus the demonstration of toxin production in mice.

No other disease is easily confused with full-blown tetanus. In the early stages the differential diagnosis includes dystonic reaction caused by phenothiazine toxicity, subarachnoid hemorrhage, severe hypocalcemia or alkalosis with tetani, meningitis, and strychnine poisoning. Strychnine poisoning produces symptoms similar to those of tetanus, but in contrast, patients with strychnine poisoning recover after 24 to 48 hours, once exposure to the drug has ceased. The possibility of meningitis can be excluded by lumbar puncture.

Treatment

General measures. All patients should be admitted to an intensive care unit after initial evaluation. Any recognized wound should be debrided. Abscesses require drainage. Stimulation should be minimized.

Airway protection, cardiopulmonary monitoring, prevention of aspiration and decubiti, and nutrition are the focus of routine care.

Antitoxin. Therapy is directed toward removing the source of the toxin and neutralizing circulating toxin. Circulating tetanospasmin is neutralized by the intramuscular administration of human tetanus immunoglobulin (TIg). No evidence shows that local infiltration at the site of the suspected wound or injury is of value. TIg has a half-life of 25 days, which results in substantial antitoxin levels for up to 16 weeks. One study indicated that 500 units is as effective as higher doses.

If human antitoxin is not available, equine tetanus immunoglobulin in the dosage of 50,000 to 100,000 units intramuscularly is equally effective. Because of the equine source of the antisera, the rate of reactions is high. Aqueous epinephrine in 1:1000 dilution should be readily available. Equine immunoglobulin is less expensive than TIg, and hence is used extensively in underdeveloped countries.

Subsequent to recovery, patients require active immunization. The disease does not confer natural immunity.

Muscle spasms. Benzodiazepines are first-line therapy for the muscle spasms of tetanus. Since they are GABA agonists, they indirectly antagonize the central nervous system effects of tetanospasmin. They are not oversedating and thereby do not exacerbate the hypoventilation associated with the disease. Diazepam or lorazepam are commonly used, and large doses may be required. Intravenous formulations of these contain propyleneglycol, which may produce lactic acidosis. Intravenous midazolam does not, but it must be given by continuous infusion because of the short half-life. Propofol may also be used. Barbiturates cause respiratory depression and are no longer indicated in routine management of tetanus.

When muscle spasms are severe or interfere with ventilation, neuromuscular blocking agents such as pancuronium or vecuronium are used. Great care must be used to ensure that paralyzed patients are provided controlled mechanical ventilation and close observation. Paralysis is best reserved for the treatment of severe tetanus not adequately controlled by other measures.

Tracheostomy. Tracheostomy must be considered in the management of patients with tetanus. Tracheostomy prevents hypoxemia caused by laryngospasm, reduces the risk of aspiration of oropharyngeal secretions, and facilitates the use of mechanical ventilators. If tracheal secretions are copious, tracheostomy should be performed early in the course of the disease. Tracheostomy should be performed electively rather than as an emergency.

Antibiotics. The role of antibiotics in tetanus management remains controversial. Parenteral penicillin, 10 to 12 million units daily for 10 days, is administered to eradicate vegetative cells. Clindamycin, metronidazole, tetracycline, and erythromycin are active against the organism. A clear benefit to antimicrobial therapy has not been shown. In one study, oral metronidazole was compared with intramuscular penicillin and showed better survival in the metronidazole group. This may reflect a negative effect of penicillin, which itself is a GABA antagonist.

Prevention. Nearly all cases of tetanus occur in nonimmunized or inadequately immunized individuals. Immunization of children should begin at 6 to 8 weeks of age. The alum-adsorbed toxoid is preferred. Diphtheria-pertussis-tetanus (DPT) vaccine is the preferred preparation for administration to infants and children less than 7 years of age, unless contraindications exist, whereas the diphtheria-tetanus toxoid is used in older children and adults.

DPT is given to children at 2, 4, 6, and 15 months and at 4 to 6 years of age. Protective levels of serum antitoxin persist for at least 10 years in individuals who complete the primary injection series. Tetanus and diphtheria (Td) toxoids adsorbed for adult use are recommended every 10 years at approximately ages 15 years, 25 years, and so on. The primary immunization schedule for nonimmunized individuals older than 7 years of age is Td initially, after 4 to 8 weeks, at 6 to 12 months after the second dose, and then every 10 years. A recent proposal by the American College of Physicians to forego the 10-year booster for a single booster at age 55 years has been controversial. Approximately 95% of the cases in the United States occur in persons who have not received the primary series of tetanus toxoid. Immunized mothers confer protection to their infants via transplacental maternal antibodies.

Of all individuals who receive emergency medical care for injuries known to predispose to tetanus, 1% to 6% receive less than the recommended prophylaxis. In 1987 and 1988, 58% of tetanus patients reported did not seek medical care for their injuries; of those who sought care, 81% did not receive the prophylaxis recommended by the CDC.

Postinjury tetanus prophylaxis requires good wound management, insistence on adequate immunity, and, perhaps, antibiotic prophylaxis. Surgical debridement removes purulent collections, foreign bodies, and necrotic tissues and hence reduces the risk of environmental conditions that promote spore germination. The need for tetanus toxoid (active immunization) with or without tetanus immune globulin as passive immunization depends on the nature of the wound and the tetanus immunization history of the patient (Table 263-5).

For passive immunization, human TIg is recommended strongly; protection is longer than that provided with antitoxin of animal origin and produces fewer adverse reactions. The dose of TIg is 250 units intramuscularly; if it is given with tetanus toxoid, the two should be prepared in separate syringes and administered at separate sites.

MYONECROSIS AND OTHER CLOSTRIDIAL INFECTIONS

The isolation of *Clostridium* species from a clinical specimen must be taken in context and is not necessarily diagnostic of tissue invasion and infection. An outline of infections other than intestinal disorders, botulism, and tetanus wherein the clostridia play a role is presented in Box 263-1.

Table 263-5 Guide to tetanus prophylaxis in routine wound management

HISTORY OF ABSORBED TETANUS TOXOID (DOSES)	CLEAN, MINOR WOUNDS		ALL OTHER WOUNDS*	
	Td†	TIg	Td†	TIg
Unknown or <3 doses	Yes	No	Yes	Yes
Three or more doses‡	No§	No	No‖	No

Modified from *MMWR* 40(RR-10):1991.
*Wounds contaminated with dirt, feces, soil, and saliva; puncture wounds; avulsions; and wounds resulting from missiles, crushing, burns, and frostbite.
†For children <7 years old; DTP (DT, if pertussis vaccine is contraindicated) is preferred to tetanus toxoid alone. For persons ≥7 years of age, Td is preferred to tetanus toxoid alone. *DPT,* Diphtheria-pertussis-tetanus vaccine; *Td,* combined tetanus-diphtheria toxoid; *DT,* diphtheria and tetanus vaccine.
‡If only three doses of fluid toxoid have been received, then a fourth dose of toxoid, preferably an absorbed toxoid, should be given.
§Yes, if >10 years since last dose.
‖Yes, if >5 years since last dose. (More frequent boosters are not needed and can accentuate side effects.)

BOX 263-1
***Clostridium* spp. infections other than intestinal disorders, botulism, and tetanus**

Simple contamination
Focal suppurative infection
Intraabdominal
Cholangitis
Tuboovarian and pelvic abscess
Empyema

Skin and subcutaneous tissue
Localized infection
Anaerobic "cellulitis"
Perirectal abscess
Foot ulcers in diabetics
Amputation stump infections in diabetics and patients with severe peripheral vascular atherosclerotic disease
Suppurative myositis in heroin addicts

Diffuse spreading "cellulitis" and fasciitis
Myonecrosis (gas gangrene)
Extremities
Uterus
Spontaneous

Bacteremia

Clostridia are part of the intestinal flora of 70% of humans and many animal species, with fecal concentrations as high as 10^8 to 10^9 organisms/g of stool. Thirty or more species are present in the intestine; *C. ramosum* and *C. perfringens* are the most frequent clinical isolates. Clostridia can be isolated from the skin of the perineum and occasionally from other skin sites. Often, clothing harbors large numbers of clostridial spores. Soil samples consistently contain *Clostridium* species in concentrations up to 10^4 bacteria/g.

The organism most often incriminated in producing tissue damage is *C. perfringens*. *C. perfringens* is relatively aerotolerant, causes "stormy fermentation" in milk, and is known to produce 12 toxins, as well as an enterotoxin. *C. perfringens* is divided into five types (A through E), based on the production of four major toxins: alpha, beta, epsilon, and iota. The alpha toxin is incriminated as causing the most tissue damage. Alpha toxin is a phospholipase C that hydrolyzes lecithin into phosphorylcholine and diglyceride. Alpha toxin is hemolytic, lyses platelets, and causes widespread capillary damage. When given intravenously, the toxin causes massive intravascular hemolysis and damages hepatic mitochondria. In experimental animals, the higher the concentration of alpha toxin in culture supernatant fluid, the smaller the inoculum necessary to cause tissue damage. The protective value of antiserum to the toxins of *C. perfringens* is proportional to the antiserum content of alpha antitoxin. Although beta, epsilon, and iota toxins can cause increases in capillary permeability, they do not have the histotoxic potential of alpha toxin.

Simple Contamination

Most culture isolations of clostridial species represent simple contamination. In the preantibiotic era, clostridia were cultured from 10% to 30% of the posttraumatic wounds in civilians and from 80% of combat injuries. In the Korean conflict 27% of the war wounds were contaminated by clostridia without evidence of suppuration. In posttraumatic wounds there is no difference in the frequency of culture isolation of clostridia from well-healing open wounds versus suppurative wounds. Because of the ubiquitous nature of clostridia, the diagnosis of a clostridial infection cannot be made solely on bacteriologic grounds.

Focal Suppurative Infections

Clostridia are most often part of a polymicrobic infection. In one study of soft tissue infection harboring clostridia, 84% of the cultures contained other pathogenic bacteria. As stated earlier, *C. perfringens* is the most common clostridial species isolated, although *C. ramosum* is nearly as frequent. Clostridia species can be isolated from severe localized suppurative processes without any clinical evidence of local or systemic damage caused by clostridial toxins.

Intraabdominal Infections. Infections complicating bowel perforation have a high likelihood of harboring clostridia. Gas gangrene is generally absent, and the flora are mixed aerobic/anaerobic organisms; hence it is not possible to distinguish on clinical grounds which infections will be culture-positive for clostridia. A clostridial intraabdominal infection, especially *C. septicum* infection, has been associated with underlying carcinoma (e.g., silent perforation of a colon carcinoma, occult carcinoma of the pancreas, and leukemia or lymphoma).

Cholangitis. *C. perfringens* is found in 10% to 20% of diseased gallbladders cultured at surgery. *Emphysematous cholecystitis* refers to severe cholangitis with gas formation in the biliary tract radicals and in the wall of the gallbladder; clostridial species are isolated in 50% of cases. There is a clinical association with diabetes mellitus. There is no evidence of muscle invasion or of systemic signs of clostridial toxin.

Tuboovarian and Pelvic Abscess. Among 200 patients with pelvic infections, clostridia were isolated in 6%. Clostridia were encountered most frequently in patients with pelvic or tuboovarian abscess. Before the availability of antibiotics, *C. perfringens* was isolated so frequently from patients with mild endometritis after septic abortion that one author referred to the organism as a "harmless saprophyte." Rarely, uterine gas gangrene can occur even in an uncomplicated delivery (discussed later).

Empyema. Clostridia have been isolated from a variety of pulmonary infections; however, clostridia have been noted most often in patients with empyema as a complication of chest trauma or, less often, in association with underlying aspiration pneumonia. Usually there is no sign of local or systemic toxin production; thus the clinical presentation is indistinguishable from that of other microbial causes of empyema or aspiration pneumonia.

Skin and Subcutaneous Tissue

Localized Infection. *Cellulitis* connotes inflammation of skin and subcutaneous tissue with sparing of underlying fascia and muscle. Perirectal abscesses, foot ulcers in diabetic patients, and infections of inadequately perfused amputation stumps are examples of localized clostridial infections. If inadequately treated, any of these infections can extend to fascial planes and muscles with concomitant severe systemic disease and signs of toxemia.

Clostridial infections of the skin and subcutaneous tissue may be indolent, with slow spread to contiguous areas. Clostridia may be present in pure or mixed culture. No systemic signs of toxicity are evident. Minimal pain and edema occur; perhaps because of the lack of edema, tissue gas may be more evident than in patients with myonecrosis. By definition, there is no necrosis of, or gas in, muscle tissue.

A localized form of suppurative myositis may develop in heroin addicts. Local pain and tenderness develop in discrete areas, often on the thigh or forearm, with the subsequent evolution of crepitance and fluctuation that requires surgical drainage. The process is unusual in that the local suppuration does not necessarily develop at sites of trauma or heroin injection, and the abscesses remain localized without systemic signs of toxicity. Histologic examination demonstrates the presence of subcutaneous abscesses and purulent myositis-fasciitis from which clostridia can be recovered in pure culture.

Diffuse Spreading "Cellulitis" and Fasciitis. In contrast to the focal processes, spreading cellulitis and fasciitis are associated with systemic signs of clostridial toxemia and death within 48 to 72 hours of onset. The disease may appear suddenly and spread through fascial planes, producing suppuration and diffuse crepitance. On examination, the involved area is only slightly painful, presumably because of necrosis of the dermal nerves, and diffuse subcutaneous crepitance is present. The crepitance is often palpable and can be detected with the diaphragm of a stethoscope. The extent of crepitance may be documented with soft tissue radiographs. Shock, renal failure, and intravascular hemolysis develop. Microscopic examination demonstrates intense inflammation of subcutaneous tissue and fascial planes with only minimal muscle inflammation. None of the muscle necrosis that typifies gas gangrene is evident; surgical debridement may not be beneficial, since there is no gangrenous muscle to be removed. Bedside surgical incision may be useful for diagnostic purposes.

Myonecrosis (Gas Gangrene). Clostridial myonecrosis results from bacterial invasion of healthy muscle from adjacent traumatized muscle or soft tissue that has been contaminated with clostridia. This disease is uncommon after through-and-through bullet wounds but develops after penetration of shrapnel fragments, which cause necrosis of deep muscles. Any trauma with muscle necrosis and absent exposure to atmospheric oxygen favors germination of clostridial spores.

The incubation period is short. Symptoms can begin less than 24 hours after the initiating trauma or surgery. The average incubation period is 4 days, with a range of 8 hours to 20 days. The patient suffers the sudden onset of pain in the wound, and over a few hours, the pain spreads beyond the wound margins. On examination the skin is edematous with a color that is initially pale and then evolves into a reddish-blue hue. Large hemorrhagic bullae often develop. At this early stage, crepitance may be detected. The wound develops a thin, sweet-smelling, watery discharge that on microscopic examination demonstrates the presence of few inflammatory cells and many large, gram-positive bacilli. Approximately 15% of patients have associated clostridial bacteremia.

A tachycardia develops that is disproportionate to the minimal elevations in temperature. Subsequently, shock and renal failure develop. Despite the gravity of the illness, the patient remains alert and oriented. Often, patients verbalize their sense of doom in a fashion unnerving to the physician. Just before death, toxic delirium and then coma ensue.

Definitive diagnosis and treatment require surgical intervention. In the early stages the muscle is pale, edematous, and does not contract when probed with instruments. In later stages the muscle turns beefy red and ultimately appears black and friable. If the stage of the disease is in doubt, a frozen section may help.

The differential diagnosis includes at least two other entities that become evident with rapidly spreading soft tissue infection. Group A streptococci can cause the clinical picture of necrotizing fasciitis (streptococcal gangrene of the skin) with or without myonecrosis. Similarly, mixtures of aerobic and anaerobic bacteria can produce synergistic infections, sometimes with gas formation that mimic clostridial fasciitis and myonecrosis.

The pathophysiologic mechanism of gas gangrene postulates initial necrosis of muscle in the presence of impairment of blood supply as a consequence of either the initial injury or associated peripheral vascular disease. The milieu for toxin production requires a low redox potential, anoxia, and the availability of amino acids, peptides, and calcium. The toxins synthesized then produce necrosis of adjacent tissue, and the process becomes self-perpetuating.

In 80% of myonecrosis cases, *C. perfringens* is isolated. Most of the other 20% of cases are caused by *C. novyi, C. septicum,* or *C. bifermentans.* The initial trauma wounds are often contaminated with other miscellaneous aerobic and anaerobic bacteria. The mortality rate of gas gangrene is 40% to 60%. The highest mortality rate is in cases involving the abdominal wall; the lowest rate is in cases involving a single extremity.

Spontaneous clostridial myonecrosis. An interesting variant is the patient in whom the classic picture of clostridial myonecrosis, usually on an extremity, develops without preceding trauma and without an apparent source. *C. septicum* has been implicated in the majority of reported cases. Most patients have an underlying intestinal abnormality, such as silent colon carcinoma, bowel wall infiltration by leukemia or lymphoma, or mucosal damage produced by cancer chemotherapy. The underlying bowel processes allow clostridial bacteremia. However, it is unclear how the anoxic conditions necessary for bacterial replication and toxin production are provided in nontraumatized muscle. This variant often follows a fulminant course, with hemolysis, hypotension, and renal failure eventuating in death within the first 24 to 48 hours of illness.

Uterine myonecrosis. Clostridial destruction of the myometrium starts 2 to 3 days after a septic abortion or, rarely, after an uncomplicated normal delivery. Jaundice caused by massive alpha toxin–induced hemolysis develops rapidly. Renal failure occurs as a consequence of hemoglobinuria. Findings on pelvic examination may be minimal, but radiographs demonstrate gas in the wall of the uterus and adjacent tissues. Hypotension is usually present.

Milder forms of the disease result from toxin generation by organisms in small foci of residual placental tissue; this process is often successfully addressed with simple curettage. In severe cases, invasion and necrosis of uterine muscles occur, with spread into adjacent pelvic structures. Even with total hysterectomy and debridement, the prognosis is grave.

CLOSTRIDIAL BACTEREMIA

Up to 3% of positive blood cultures in some medical centers yield clostridial species. *C. perfringens* accounts for 50% to 60% of the isolates. A positive blood culture finding for clostridia does not correlate with a predictably stormy clinical course. In patients with septic abortion, positive blood culture results occurred in up to 27% of cases; yet the syndrome of uterine gas gangrene was rare. Most patients with clostridial bacteremia have a variety of associated conditions, and the significance of the clostridia is enigmatic. Occasionally, the patient has an associated mixed flora infection (e.g., aspiration pneumonia, decubitus ulcer, or intraabdominal abscess), which represents the presumed portal of entry. Associated gas gangrene is rare. *C. perfringens* accounts for approximately 60% of positive blood isolate findings. Isolation of *C. septicum* from blood cultures suggests an underlying hematologic malignancy, neutropenia, or colonic carcinoma.

Diagnosis

The diagnosis of clostridial disease is made primarily on clinical grounds. Clostridia are present in many wounds, and their presence at any site, including blood, does not necessarily indicate the presence of severe disease. Gram's stains of exudates at sites of clostridial invasion demonstrate many large gram-positive bacilli as well as other organisms. Samples for culture require an appropriate anaerobic transport mechanism. Specimens are cultured in an anaerobic environment in selective media.

Patients with severe clostridial disease have protein and casts in their urine. The presence of hemolytic anemia results in hemoglobinemia and hemoglobinuria; muscle necrosis causes myoglobinuria. Renal failure often results. In severe disease, disseminated intravascular coagulation may occur. The clostridia may be visible on stains of peripheral blood or buffy coat.

Radiographic demonstration of gas in muscles, subcutaneous tissue, or the wall of the uterus or gallbladder is consistent with the diagnosis. However, atmospheric gas may enter traumatized wounds. Also, other bacteria, especially other anaerobic bacteria, mixed with aerobic organisms, may produce gas.

Treatment

Surgical Debridement. The combination of surgical debridement and antibiotic therapy is the mainstay of therapy. The use of polyvalent gas gangrene antitoxin and hyperbaric oxygen is controversial. Simple wound contamination requires only mechanical cleansing. Localized infection of the skin and soft tissue, without evidence of extension to adjacent tissue or associated fever, can be managed primarily with debridement without systemic antibiotics. Fasciitis and myonecrosis require extensive debridement with excision or amputation of all necrotic tissue. In severe cases amputation, hysterectomy, or excision of the entire anterior abdominal wall may prove necessary. Because the extent of tissue necrosis is difficult to judge at surgery, it is reasonable to return the patient to the operating room within a few hours for repeat debridement to ensure excision of all necrotic tissue.

Antimicrobial Therapy. The use of antibiotics depends on the clinical situation. No antibiotic therapy is necessary for simple contamination or even for clostridial bacteremia if there are no concomitant signs or symptoms consistent with active infection. Localized skin and soft tissue infection may require administration of antibiotics in addition to surgical debridement.

For fasciitis or myonecrosis, intravenous penicillin G is the drug of choice. With normal renal function the recommended dose is in the range of 20 million units per day. In the penicillin-allergic patient, alternative agents include chloramphenicol, clindamycin, and cefoxitin.

In severe clostridial disease, thought should be given to patterns of antibiotic resistance. Virtually all *C. perfringens* and 95% of other clostridia are susceptible to penicillin G in vitro. In contrast, 15% to 20% of clostridial strains may be resistant to clindamycin. This is unfortunate because animal experiments indicate greater efficacy of clindamycin than of penicillin when the infecting organism is susceptible to both drugs. *C. ramosum, C. tertium, C. sporogenes,* and some strains of *C. perfringens* may demonstrate in vitro resistance to clindamycin and even to penicillin G. Up to 25% of *C. perfringens* strains are resistant in vitro to metronidazole. Combination therapy is necessary for mixed aerobic/anaerobic infections.

Hyperbaric Oxygen. Controlled experiments in animals indicate an increase in survival of approximately 10% in animals who had debridement, treatment with penicillin, and exposure to hyperbaric oxygen, as compared with animals managed with combined penicillin therapy and surgical debridement. No controlled human studies have been conducted. At present, the use of hyperbaric oxygen should be considered adjunctive only and should not be a reason to delay surgical debridement or antibiotic therapy.

Antitoxin. Some authorities still recommend polyvalent gas gangrene antitoxin. However, the antitoxin is not produced in the United States, and available products are prepared in horses. Because of questionable efficacy and risk of hypersensitivity to horse serum, most centers have discontinued the use of antitoxin.

LISTERIA INFECTIONS
Classification and Characteristics

Listeria organisms are small, nonsporulating, nonencapsulated gram-positive aerobic bacilli within the *Clostridium* subbranch, together with the genera *Staphylococcus, Streptococcus,* and *Lactobacillus. Listeria monocytogenes* was first recognized as a cause of disease in humans in 1929. It is the only important human pathogen of this genus.

Because of its coccoid appearance and uneven staining, *L. monocytogenes* may be confused with pneumococci, *Haemophilus influenzae,* and diphtheroids in stained smears of clinical specimens. *Lis-*

teria organisms are distinguished by their motility, catalase reaction, and ability to hydrolyze esculin and to produce beta hemolysis. *Listeria* species may be serotyped by their somatic (O) and flagellar (H) antigens.

Epidemiology

L. monocytogenes is worldwide in distribution. Although its primary habitats are soil and decaying vegetable matter, the organism has been isolated from a great variety of domestic and wild animals. Human fecal excretion of *Listeria* organisms occurs in about 1% of the normal population, in 4.8% of abattoir workers, and in 26% of contacts of patients with listeriosis. Transplacental and vaginal transmission of *Listeria* organisms is responsible for fetal and neonatal infection. Because of its widespread occurrence, *L. monocytogenes* frequently contaminates food production and processing environments. There have been documented instances of listeriosis after the ingestion of contaminated cabbage, milk, cheese, mushrooms, and poultry (turkey franks). In California in 1985, 142 cases with 45 deaths were attributed to a single source of contaminated cheese. It is likely that *Listeria* organisms are enterically acquired in most cases, and invasive systemic listeriosis occurs in a small percentage of these individuals.

In the United States the incidence of listeriosis is not known because limited surveillance was started only in 1988. On the basis of active surveillance of 19 million persons in four states in the United States, the aggregate incidence was 7.4 per million (1850 cases/year). In pregnant women the incidence of listeriosis is 223 per million. Listeriosis is manifested as a wide spectrum of diseases in risk groups, such as pregnant women, infants, elderly adults, and immunocompromised hosts. It is rarely seen in persons with intact immunity. Pregnancy-related infection accounts for approximately one fourth of the sporadic cases of listeriosis.

Pathogenesis

The pathogenesis of listeriosis is not well understood. *Listeria* has the ability to invade and propel itself through intestinal epithelial cells, allowing entry into the circulation. The association of human listeriosis and compromised host-defense mechanisms, as well as experimental animal studies, indicates that intact cellular and humoral immunity is important in the prevention of clinical disease. Gastric neutralization predisposes to acquisition of listerial enteritis and bacteremia. Immunosuppression by corticosteroids may increase the risk of meningitis.

Clinical Manifestations

The spectrum of disease caused by *L. monocytogenes* ranges from a transient asymptomatic carrier state to an acute fulminant septicemia. The different syndromes of human listeriosis are pregnancy infections, granulomatosis infantisepticum (disseminated microabscesses), sepsis, meningoencephalitis, and localized infections.

Listeriosis of pregnancy may be asymptomatic or may become evident as an acute febrile illness. Most commonly, women develop a flulike illness of fever and myalgias, sometimes with symptoms suggesting a respiratory, gastrointestinal, or urinary tract infection. The diagnosis is established only by obtaining a positive blood culture because there are no characteristic clinical findings. The infection most commonly occurs during the last trimester of pregnancy and may seriously affect the fetus, causing amnionitis, premature labor, premature rupture of membranes, and stillbirth. There are documented cases of bacteremic infections without fetal damage.

Granulomatosis infantisepticum results from transplacental infection and is characterized by disseminated visceral abscesses and granulomas. Infants should receive prompt treatment if the diagnosis is suspected. Cultures of blood, spinal fluid, and meconium should be obtained, as well as cultures of the maternal vagina and lochia.

Listeria sepsis may occur in infants infected during vaginal delivery or in immunosuppressed adults. There are no characteristic clinical findings, and the diagnosis must be established by blood culture. The presentation may be similar to that of gram-negative sepsis but is more likely to be meningitis.

Nonperinatal meningoencephalitis is usually a disease of immunosuppressed patients (Chapter 239). The infection also occurs in patients with cirrhosis of the liver and, occasionally, in normal individuals. The clinical illness may be insidious in onset, with anorexia, lethargy, behavioral changes, and low-grade fever; or it may be acute and fulminant. Pharyngitis, otitis media, and cranial nerve palsies may be present, together with signs of meningitis and encephalitis. The cerebrospinal fluid (CSF) is abnormal, but a wide range of values for CSF white blood cell count and protein and glucose levels exists. Despite its name, listeriosis is not commonly associated with monocytosis in either the CSF or blood. The CSF findings alone do not distinguish *Listeria* infection from other forms of pyogenic or aseptic (viral) meningitis.

Recent clinical reports suggest that septicemia without an identified focus is the most common clinical manifestation of listeriosis. *Listeria* sepsis cannot be distinguished on clinical grounds from that caused by other organisms. Localized *Listeria* infection may follow direct contact with the organism (skin, conjunctiva) or may result from a bacteremia (arthritis, osteomyelitis, endocarditis, peritonitis, pleurisy). Skin and eye infections may be associated with granulomatosis infantisepticum. Culture of the organism is necessary to establish an etiologic diagnosis because there are no characteristic clinical findings.

Diagnostic Tests

The protean manifestations of listeriosis and the lack of pathognomonic findings preclude diagnosis on clinical features alone. Isolation of the organism from either blood or infected tissues and secretions is required. Although *Listeria* organisms grow readily in routine media, isolation from nonsterile sites may be enhanced by selective media and the use of polymerase chain reaction technology. The differential diagnosis of prematurity, spontaneous abortion, or stillbirth includes Group B streptococcal or *Escherichia coli* infection, toxoplasmosis, and syphilis. The presence of colonies showing subdued β-hemolysis on blood agar from normally sterile sites should suggest the possibility of *Listeria* organisms. *Listeria* organisms in CSF specimens may closely resemble streptococci on Gram's stain and have caused up to 10% of adult meningitis cases in recent studies. If the clinical setting suggests listeriosis, the laboratory should be alerted to its possibility and should carefully evaluate all diphtheroid-like isolates.

Treatment

The optimal antibiotic therapy of *L. monocytogenes* has not been well defined by controlled clinical trials. In vitro the organism is susceptible to penicillin, ampicillin, erythromycin, gentamicin, rifampin, and chloramphenicol, but many of these drugs are only bacteriostatic and/or do not penetrate intracellularly. Penicillin or ampicillin with or without an aminoglycoside is most commonly recommended. Trimethoprim/sulfamethoxazole has been used successfully. Treatment failures are common with cephalosporins, which should not be used.

The optimal duration of antimicrobial therapy is not established and varies with the type and severity of the infection and with the patient's underlying disease. Two weeks of therapy may be adequate in uncomplicated listeriosis in most patients. Granulomatosis infantisepticum, endocarditis, and infections in severely immunosuppressed patients probably should be treated for 3 to 6 weeks.

Prevention

Although the current understanding of the epidemiology and pathogenesis of listeriosis is incomplete, it is prudent to advise persons at high risk for listeriosis that they eat only thoroughly cooked foods, wash raw vegetables thoroughly before eating, and avoid unpasteurized dairy products. Prevention of exposure to the organism is not practical, because *L. monocytogenes* has been isolated from virtually every animal species cultured, as well as from soil, water, sewage, and dust. Prompt recognition of disease, particularly in high-risk persons, and early therapy reduce morbidity and mortality rates.

BIBLIOGRAPHY

Bartlett JG: Antibiotic-associated diarrhea, *Clin Infect Dis* 15:573, 1992.

Berry PR: Evaluation of ELISA, RTPLA, and Vero cell assays for detecting *Clostridium perfringens* enterotoxin in faecal specimens, *J Clin Pathol* 41:458, 1988.

Bretzke ML et al: Diffuse spreading *Clostridium septicum* infection, malignant disease and immune suppression, *Surg Gynecol Obstet* 166:197, 1988.

Burke GW: Absence of diarrhea in toxic megacolon complicating *Clostridium difficile* pseudomembranous colitis, *Am J Gastroenterol* 83:304, 1988.

Carthier G et al: Protection against experimental pseudomembranous colitis in gnotobiotic mice by use of monoclonal antibodies against *Clostridium difficile* toxin A, *Infect Immunol* 59:1192, 1991.

Centers for Disease Control and Prevention: Tetanus surveillance: United States–1989-1990, *MMWR* 41:1, 1992.

Centers for Disease Control and Prevention: Diphtheria, tetanus, and pertussis: recommendations for vaccine use and other preventive measures: recommendations of the Immunization Practices Advisory Committee, *MMWR* 40(RR-10):1, 1991.

Centers for Disease Control and Prevention: Summary of notifiable diseases: United States–1991, *MMWR* 40(53):57, 1992.

Coyle MB, Lipsky BA: Coryneform bacteria in infectious diseases: clinical and laboratory aspects, *Clin Microbiol Rev* 3:227, 1990.

Durand ML et al: Acute bacerial meningitis in adults: a review of 493 episodes, *N Engl J Med* 328:21, 1993.

Farber JM, Peterkin PI: *Listeria monocytogenes:* a food-borne pathogen, *Microbiol Rev* 55:476, 1991.

Fekety R: Antibiotic-associated colitis. In Mandell GL et al, editors: *Principles and practice of infectious diseases,* ed 3, New York, 1989, Churchill Livingstone.

Gellin BG, Broome CV: Listeriosis, *JAMA* 261:1313, 1989.

Gorbach SL: Other *Clostridium* species (including gas gangrene). In Mandell GL et al, editors: *Principles and practice of infectious diseases,* ed 3, New York, 1989, Churchill Livingstone.

Halpern JL et al: Sequence homology between tetanus and botulinum toxins detected by an antipeptide antibody, *Infect Immunol* 57:18, 1989.

Harnish JP et al: Diphtheria among alcoholic urban adults, *Ann Intern Med* 111:71, 1989.

Harvey RL, Sunstrum JC: *Rhodococcus equi* infection in patients with and without human immunodeficiency virus infection, *Rev Infect Dis* 13:139, 1991.

Johnson S et al: Nosocomial *Clostridium difficile* colonization and disease, *Lancet* 336:97, 1990.

Johnson S et al: Prospective controlled study of vinyl glove use to interrupt *Clostridium difficile* nosocomial transmission, *Am J Med* 88:137, 1990.

Kain KC et al: *Arcanobacterium hemolyticum* infection: confused with scarlet fever and diphtheria, *J Emerg Med* 9:33, 1991.

Karzon DT, Edwards KM: Diphtheria outbreaks in immunized populations, *N Engl J Med* 318:41, 1988.

Kato N et al: Identification of toxigenic *Clostridium difficile* by the polymerase chain reaction, *J Clin Microbiol* 29:33, 1991.

Lawrence JD et al: Impact of active immunization against enteritis necroticans in Papua, New Guinea, *Lancet* 336:1165, 1990.

Lecour H et al: Food-borne botulism, *Arch Intern Med* 148:578, 1988.

Levett PN: Time-dependent killing of *Clostridium difficile* by metronidazole and vancomycin, *J Antimicrob Chemother* 27:55, 1991.

Linnan MJ et al: Epidemic listeriosis associated with Mexican-style cheese, *N Engl J Med* 319:823, 1988.

Lund BM: Food-borne disease due to *Bacillus* and *Clostridium, Lancet* 336:982, 1990.

Lyerly DM et al: *Clostridium difficile:* its disease and toxins, *Clin Microbiol Rev* 1:1, 1988.

Martin RR: *Clostridium tetani* (tetanus). In Mandell GL et al, editors: *Principles and practice of infectious diseases,* ed 3, New York, 1989, Churchill Livingstone.

McCarthy JD et al: Fever, dyspnea, and slurred speech following lower extremity trauma, *Rev Infect Dis* 13:172, 1991.

McFarland LV et al: Risk factors for *Clostridium difficile* carriage and *C. difficile*–associated diarrhea in a cohort of hospitalized patients, *J Infect Dis* 162:678, 1990.

Moore R et al: *C. difficile* toxin A increases intestinal permeability and induces Cl-secretion, *Am J Physiol* 259:G165, 1990.

National Heart, Lung, and Blood Institute Workshop Summary: hyperbaric oxygen therapy, *Am Rev Respir Dis* 144:1414, 1991.

Rappuoli R et al: Molecular epidemiology of the 1984-1986 outbreak of diphtheria in Sweden, *N Engl J Med* 318:12, 1988.

Schaffner W: *Clostridium botulinum* (botulism). In Mandell et al, editors: *Principles and practice of infectious diseases,* ed 3, New York, 1989, Churchill Livingstone.

Schreiner MS et al: Infant botulism: a review of 12 years' experience at the Children's Hospital of Philadelphia, *Pediatrics* 87:159, 1991.

Schuchat A et al: Epidemiology of human listeriosis, *Clin Microbiol Rev* 4:169, 1991.

Shaffer N et al: Botulism among Alaska natives: the role of changing food preparation and consumption practices, *West J Med* 153:390, 1990.

Soriano F et al: Skin colonization by *Corynebacterium* groups D2 and JK in hospitalized patients, *J Clin Microbiol* 26:1878, 1988.

Soriano F et al: Urinary tract infection caused by *Corynebacterium* group D2: report of 82 cases and review, *Rev Infect Dis* 12:1019, 1990.

Stevens DL: Lethal effects and cardiovascular effects of purified alpha and theta toxins from *Clostridium perfringens, J Infect Dis* 157:272, 1988.

Stevens DL et al: Spontaneous, nontraumatic gangrene due to *Clostridium septicum, Rev Infect Dis* 12:286, 1990.

Wren BW: Identification of toxigenic *Clostridium difficile* strains by using a toxin A gene-specific probe, *J Clin Microbiol* 28:1808, 1990.

264 *Neisseria meningitidis* Infections

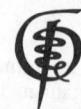

James A. Reinarz

THE ORGANISM
Characteristics

Neisseria meningitidis (meningococcus) is a gram-negative, nonmotile, non–spore-forming, oxidase-positive, encapsulated coccus. The organism is fastidious and usually requires chocolate blood agar or other enriched media (e.g., Mueller-Hinton) for primary isolation. It is aerobic and grows best on surface plates or in agitated liquid media under 5% to 10% supplemental carbon dioxide at 37° C. Differentiation from *Neisseria gonorrhoeae* and other members of the family Neisseriaceae is based on glucose and maltose metabolism; *N. gonorrhoeae* does not use maltose. Separation of *N. meningitidis* from "nonpathogenic" *Neisseria* spp. requires immunologic (serologic) testing.

Meningococci are divided into subgroups on the basis of their capsular polysaccharide immunogenicity. Most human diseases are caused by *N. meningitidis* groups A, B, and C, although groups X, Y, Z, 29E, and W135 may cause severe and fatal illness.

Virulence factors for meningococci are incompletely understood. The capsular polysaccharide inhibits phagocytosis by polymorphonuclear leukocytes and may be important to intravascular replication. The meningococcal cell wall contains a lipopolysaccharide complex (endotoxin) considered to be one of the primary mediators of tissue injury.

Epidemiology

Serious outbreaks of spinal meningitis have been reported since the 1800s. Epidemic meningococcal disease has been documented in the United States at 7- to 10-year intervals during this century. Major epidemics occurred during World War I, World War II, the Korean War, and the Vietnam conflict. Meningococcal disease remains a worldwide problem, and major outbreaks are reported regularly in Africa and South America. These epidemics involve thousands of individuals and have high morbidity and mortality rates. Group A *N. meningitidis* remains the primary cause in these areas. Most meningococcal disease in the United States occurs in young infants, children, and military recruits. Sporadic cases occur in any age-group without regard to social status or geographic location.

Until the 1960s most epidemic disease in the United States was caused by group A *N. meningitidis.* In the early 1960s group B emerged as the predominant serogroup. In 1967 to 1968, group C succeeded as the predominant cause of both sporadic and epidemic disease in closed populations, especially military training centers. In the 1980s and early 1990s groups B and C remained predominant, although groups Y and W135 recently have been reported with increasing frequency in Western Europe and the United States. Group Y is commonly associated with pneumonia.

Meningococci are confined entirely to human beings. No animal vectors have been detected. Spread presumably occurs from person to person by aerosol droplets, with subsequent colonization of the nasopharynx. In nonepidemic periods, nasopharyngeal carriage is approximately 5% to 15%, but it may approach 60% to 80% in closed populations with or without coexistent meningococcal disease. Nasopharyngeal carriage is almost always asymptomatic. Carriage usually persists for several weeks, although chronic carriers are not uncommon. Nasopharyngeal acquisition is followed in 7 to 10 days by a highly specific serologic response (usually immunoglobulin M [IgM]) to the group-specific polysaccharide of the colonizing strain. Evidence strongly suggests that invasive meningococcal disease is most likely to occur within days of acquisition of a new strain of *N. meningitidis,* that is, before the development of a specific antibody.

Virtually all strains of *N. meningitidis* were once extremely sensitive to commonly used antimicrobials, including sulfa drugs (sulfadiazine). However, within an extremely short interval during the early 1960s, most group B and group C *N. meningitidis* strains became resistant to sulfa. Unlike in the gonococcus, β-lactamase production by *N. meningitidis* has been rare, and penicillin-resistant strains are not a clinical problem. However, relatively resistant strains are being documented in Europe and may be a harbinger of future problems. At present, penicillin remains the antibiotic of choice.

Pathophysiology

Although acquisition of the organism is an essential antecedent to invasive meningococcal disease, host factors appear to be extremely important also. Invasive or disseminated meningococcal disease occurs almost exclusively in persons who have no measurable specific antimeningococcal bactericidal antibody to the colonizing group of *N. meningitidis*. The importance of this specific antibody-complement bactericidal system is further supported by the occurrence of multiple episodes of group-identical meningococcal disease in persons congenitally lacking terminal complement components C5 to C9, whose serum is thus incapable of complement-mediated bacteriolysis (Chapter 230). Recently an inordinate frequency of meningococcal disease has been described in several kindred with congenital deficiencies in the alternative complement pathway. In addition, susceptible individuals frequently experience a viral or mycoplasmal respiratory illness in the several days preceding bloodstream invasion. In some manner, perhaps secondarily to virus-induced defects in polymorphonuclear leukocyte function, antecedent viral illnesses may predispose to invasive meningococcal disease.

Once bloodstream invasion has occurred, the organism may replicate at an astonishing rate. The resulting disease varies from a transient, benign, almost asymptomatic bacteremia to a devastating, rapidly fatal illness. Few clinical diseases rival the fulminance of meningococcemia; within hours, a patient may deteriorate from good health to irreversible shock, obtundation, marked hemorrhagic diathesis, and death. *N. meningitidis* exhibits marked tropism for the central nervous system, especially the meninges, and skin. Tropism is also apparent for synovial joints, serosal surfaces, and adrenal glands. The most common clinical presentation is a composite of septicemic and meningitic features. Rarely, a relatively benign chronic meningococcemia may result.

Factors determining the clinical expression are poorly understood. Endotoxin is thought to play a role in more fulminant forms. Although endotoxin is difficult to detect and quantitate in vivo, the severity of clinical disease correlates with concentrations of circulating capsular polysaccharide, which is closely bound to the cell wall lipopolysaccharide (endotoxin). Endotoxin activates the clotting and complement cascades and produces extensive endothelial damage, both directly and indirectly (Chapter 239). Circulating tumor necrosis factor has been demonstrated in meningococcemia and may be a major factor in mortality.

Although adrenal involvement occurs frequently with meningococcemia, adrenal insufficiency does not explain the clinical syndromes, the profound shock, or the Waterhouse-Friderichsen syndrome. In fact, serum cortisol concentrations are usually markedly elevated during the illness, and adrenal function remains normal in most patients who recover. Additionally, in some patients who die of the Waterhouse-Friderichsen syndrome, the adrenal glands have been normal morphologically.

CLINICAL SYNDROMES
Nasopharyngeal Involvement

Primary meningococcal infections, almost always in the nasopharynx, are usually asymptomatic or indistinguishable from viral coryzal syndromes. Diagnosis is rarely made unless frequent nasopharyngeal cultures are made of individuals at risk during epidemic periods. In most cases, nasopharyngeal colonization is entirely benign and is beneficial because it results in the production of protective bactericidal antibodies. Recently urethritis that is easily confused with *N. gonorrhoeae* urethritis has been reported.

Meningococcemia

Meningococcemia (alone or in association with meningitis) is the most frequently encountered clinical presentation. Early clinical features are protean, nonspecific, and difficult to distinguish from those of a viral respiratory disease or influenza syndrome. However, fever (usually in excess of 102° F), chilliness, shaking chills, myalgias, and other systemic symptoms of toxicity appear rapidly.

Skin manifestations are the hallmark of meningococcal disease. A migratory evanescent macular rash, especially over the trunk, is indistinguishable from the "rose spots" associated with typhoid fever. Skin eruptions also may be papular or maculopapular. The macular eruption is subtle and is frequently overlooked by the inexperienced observer. Petechiae, almost universally present, can occur over the entire skin surface but are particularly prominent on the lower extremities, trunk, wrists, and palpebral and bulbar conjunctivae (Color Plate VIII-21). Petechiae may rapidly increase in number and may coalesce to form ecchymoses. Subungual petechiae are unusual, but palmar and plantar petechiae and pustules are common. Unfortunately, the diagnostic value of petechiae is diminished by their frequency in active persons, such as military recruits, and in many other diseases. Furthermore, skin manifestations may be absent or inapparent during the initial physical examination, making repeated assessments essential, an almost impossible task in outpatients except in high-risk populations or during epidemic disease.

Headache, neck soreness, nuchal rigidity, confusion, lethargy, obtundation, and other features of meningeal involvement may be presenting symptoms or may not be manifested for hours or days, if at all (Chapter 239). Alternatively, meningitis may be the predominant clinical expression, with few or subtle suggestions of meningococcemia. In adolescents and adults, purulent meningitis and a petechial rash must be considered to be caused by *N. meningitidis,* although *Haemophilus influenzae* may produce similar clinical features in young children (Chapter 266).

An extensive or progressive petechial or ecchymotic eruption, hypotension, peripheral cyanosis, tachypnea, confusion, and obtundation, especially if present on initial evaluation or developing rapidly, strongly suggest fulminant meningococcemia (Waterhouse-Friderichsen syndrome). Disseminated intravascular coagulation with resultant consumptive coagulopathy produces a marked bleeding diathesis from mucosal surfaces and skin puncture sites. The illness, progressing with astonishing rapidity, may end in death within hours.

Septic Arthritis

Migratory arthralgias are common during meningococcemia. Occasionally an isolated septic arthritis may be manifested during or after meningococcemia (Chapter 203). The joint (usually a large joint) becomes erythematous, painful, and tender and develops an effusion. Tenosynovitis, commonly associated with gonococcemia, is unusual.

Myocarditis

Myocardial involvement is frequent in meningococcal disease. A majority of persons who die of meningococcal disease have extensive focal myocarditis. Decreased cardiac output, cardiac dilation, and electrocardiographic changes occur with sufficient frequency to suggest that myocarditis is common among those destined to survive. Pericardial friction rubs and pericardial effusions may occur during active disease or convalescence; during the latter period these serous membranes probably represent immunologic reactions. Purulent pericarditis also may occur.

Pneumonia

Pulmonary infiltrates are common in meningococcemia produced by the major serogroups, although clinical pneumonia is infrequent. However, with increasing frequency, meningococcal pneumonia is being recognized as a distinct syndrome. The clinical syndrome is similar to other bacterial pneumonias, with fever, chills, cough, pleuritic chest pain, tachypnea, bloody sputum, and occasionally, pleural effusion (Chapter 237). No features are pathognomonic. Group Y *N. meningitidis* is the most frequently implicated serogroup.

Chronic Meningococcemia

Chronic meningococcemia is a rare condition of recurrent febrile episodes with petechiae. This entity is often confused with immunologically induced purpuric vasculitides. Blood culture findings are positive during bacteremic episodes, and the disease is promptly eradicated by treatment. On occasion, chronic meningococcemia may suddenly deteriorate into a syndrome similar to acute meningococcemia.

DIAGNOSIS

Definitive diagnosis of meningococcal diseases is made by recovery of *N. meningitidis* from a normally sterile site, such as blood, cerebrospinal fluid (CSF), joint fluid, petechial aspirate, or transtracheal aspirate. A presumptive diagnosis may be made by demonstrating group-specific polysaccharide in serum, CSF, or joint fluid or by demonstrating gram-negative diplococci in CSF or petechial or buffy-coat smears. Antisera are available commercially for groups A, C, D, and Y. Reliable antiserum is not available for group B, which is responsible for a great percentage of cases in the United States. A positive CIE finding is supportive of the diagnosis; a negative CIE finding has little value. A specific antibody response may be diagnostic during convalescence.

In most cases, treatment must be based on a presumptive clinical diagnosis; to await confirmatory cultures is hazardous. A highly probable diagnosis is usually apparent in a febrile patient with fulminant meningococcemia or with extensive petechial eruption, nuchal rigidity, and purulent CSF. With more subtle clinical presentations, however, the diagnosis may be extremely difficult. The principal clue is a skin rash, especially if petechiae are prominent. If there is any doubt, the individual should be hospitalized and evaluated further. A progressive petechial eruption is very suggestive. It must be emphasized, however, that not all individuals manifest cutaneous lesions, even with rapidly progressive illness. In these circumstances, the clinician is laboring under a great disadvantage. If meningococcal disease is suspected, cultures should be obtained and therapy started. The polymerase chain reaction (PCR) may permit retrospective diagnosis.

Gram-stained smears of petechial aspirates may be very helpful. These smears are obtained by slightly puncturing or excoriating a fresh petechia with the point of a sterile scalpel blade or a large-bore needle. Care must be taken not to incise deeply into the dermis and produce overt bleeding. The transudate of clear or slightly bloody fluid should be smeared on a glass slide and also applied onto a warmed plate containing chocolate blood agar for culture (Chapter 233). Numerous leukocytes and intracellular and extracellular gram-negative diplococci may be seen. Such a finding is strong presumptive evidence of meningococcemia. Negative smear results should be interpreted with caution.

Two or three blood cultures should be obtained at short intervals before treatment. To minimize temperature shock, which might kill the organism, the medium optimally should be warmed to body temperature before culturing. Air should be added to the culture bottle, because *N. meningitidis* is aerobic. Recovery of the organism may be enhanced if the bottle is agitated during incubation and the contents are subcultured to solid media within 12 to 24 hours.

Lumbar puncture is indicated in most, if not all, suspected cases of meningococcemia and all suspected cases of meningitis. If the diagnosis seems highly probable on clinical grounds, however, therapy should not be delayed for results of CSF analysis or lengthy study of petechial or buffy-coat smears. Indeed, in some patients with fulminant disease, institution of therapy should take precedence even over performance of the lumbar puncture.

Other laboratory data offer little support in diagnosis. A leukocytosis with a left shift is common, but normal hemogram findings are not unusual. Neutropenia may occur during fulminant disease. Thrombocytopenia is common and suggests disseminated intravascular coagulation. Decreased P_{CO_2} and metabolic acidosis secondary to tissue hypoperfusion are frequent. Prolonged prothrombin and partial thromboplastin times and decreased serum fibrinogen level are noted only in severe disease and suggest a poor prognosis.

Differential diagnosis requires discrimination among a wide array of viral, bacterial, and rickettsial infections. The more commonly confused entities include the viral exanthemata (rubeola, rubella, echoviruses), arthropod-borne encephalitides, Rocky Mountain spotted fever (Chapter 259), endemic typhus, and other forms of pyogenic meningitis.

TREATMENT

Penicillin G administration is the treatment of choice for all forms of meningococcal disease. For adults, 10 to 20 million units should be administered intravenously daily; high doses are required to ensure adequate CSF and joint fluid concentrations. For children the dosage of penicillin is 100,000 to 250,000 units/kg/day. For clinical purposes, strains of all serogroups are almost universally sensitive to very low concentrations of penicillin. Therapy should be continued for 7 to 10 days or until the patient has been afebrile for 5 days. For individuals with a known serious allergic reaction to penicillin, chloramphenicol in a dosage of 50 mg/kg/dl (1 gm q6h) is a reasonable alternative. Meningococci are sensitive to first-generation cephalosporins. However, these agents cannot be relied on to yield adequate CSF concentrations. Cefuroxime and several third-generation cephalosporins are effective and achieve high CSF concentrations. Clinical experience with these antimicrobials is very limited. No data are available to support the use of penicillin and a third-generation cephalosporin, and use of this combination should be discouraged. Because of unpredictable sensitivity, sulfonamides should not be considered for treatment. There is no advantage to using combined regimens, and some data suggest that chloramphenicol and penicillin together are less effective than either alone.

Supportive treatment is extremely important (Chapter 245). Adequate replacement of intravascular volume deficits and correction of acidosis and hypoxemia are essential.

Data are contradictory regarding the efficacy of heparin used either prophylactically or in treatment of documented disseminated intravascular coagulation (DIC). Glucocorticoids have no proven value.

Generally, replacement of clotting factors and platelets or the administration of ε-aminocaproic acid (EACA) is contraindicated. However, a serious consumptive coagulopathy should be managed in consultation with a hematologist.

Clinical studies to assess the value of high-titer immunoglobulins with antibody to core antigen and to tumor necrosis factor have shown no therapeutic benefit. Commercially available intravenous immunoglobulin has no documented value in clinical disease. At present, immunotherapy has no documented value. Monoclonal antiendotoxin has been reported to be effective in uncontrolled studies.

PROPHYLAXIS

Family contacts of patients with active meningococcal disease probably are at significant risk of nasopharyngeal colonization and development of meningococcemia. These individuals should receive prophylactic antimicrobial agents that achieve effective concentrations in the nasopharynx. Rifampin is the drug of choice, and 600 mg should be administered every 12 hours for 2 days (for children, 10 mg/kg every 12 hours for 2 days). For pregnant women, ceftriaxone, 125 mg administered as a single intramuscular dose, should be used rather than rifampin. Minocycline is effective, but a high incidence of vertigo is associated with its use. Even large doses of penicillin, erythromycin, and the various tetracyclines are incapable of eradicating the organism from the nasopharynx and are useless for prophylaxis. Sulfonamides are very effective if the isolate is sensitive; however, sensitivity data may be unavailable when most needed. Several quinolones produce good mucosal concentrations and may emerge as useful prophylactic antibiotics in adults. The value of chemoprophylaxis for persons other than family contacts (e.g., co-workers) is much less certain. Population prophylaxis (e.g., of military personnel) with rifampin rapidly induces rifampin-resistant strains of *N. meningitidis* and cannot be recommended. Prophylaxis of hospital personnel is not indicated unless extensive contact (e.g., through mouth-to-mouth resuscitation) has occurred. The data regarding prophylaxis of school, classroom, and dormitory contacts and co-workers are equivocal. In general, such prophylaxis should be discouraged.

Immunoprophylaxis is a very valuable adjunct in high-risk populations. Purified tetravalent polysaccharide vaccines are available for groups A, C, Y, and W-135. A single injection of 50 μg rapidly induces protective antibody. Until very recently, the vaccine has produced only limited immunogenicity in infants; however, recent modifications offer hope of active immunization of infants who are at highest risk naturally. At present no passive prophylaxis is available, and intramuscular γ-globulin is ineffective. Vaccine should be offered to individuals with splenectomy.

Adult meningococcal disease warrants a careful history for meningococcal infection or other fulminating infections in family members. A positive family history or repeated episodes of meningococcal disease mandates an evaluation of both the classic and alternative complement pathways. The hemolytic complement assay (CH_{50}) detects most complement deficiencies and is recommended for screening adults with sporadic infections. Immunization is strongly recommended for those with complement deficiencies. Frequency for booster immunizations has not been determined.

BIBLIOGRAPHY

Apicella MA: *Neisseria meningitidis.* In Mandell GL, Douglas RG Jr, Bennett JE, editors: *Principles and practice of infectious diseases,* New York, 1995, Wiley.

Densen P et al: Familial properdin deficiency and fatal meningococcemia: correction of the bactericidal defect by vaccination, *N Engl J Med* 316(15):922, 1987.

Ellison RT et al: Meningococcemia and acquired complement deficiency: association in patients with hepatic failure, *Arch Intern Med* 146(8):1539, 1986.

Gaebler J et al: Prophylaxis of contacts of patients with meningococcal infection, *J Indiana State Med Assoc* 76(12):828, 1983.

Gardlund B: Prognostic evaluation in meningococcal disease: a retrospective study of 115 cases, *Intensive Care Med* 12(4):302, 1986.

Giraud T et al: Adult overwhelming meningococcal purpura: a study of 35 cases, 1977-1989, *Arch Intern Med* 151:310, 1991.

Goldschneider I, Gotschlich EC, Artenstein MS: Human immunity to the meningococcus. I. The role of humoral antibiotics, *J Exp Med* 129(6):1307, 1969.

Goldschneider I, Gotschlich EC, Artenstein MS: Human immunity to the meningococcus. II. Development of natural immunity, *J Exp Med* 129(6):1327, 1969.

Greenwood BM: Selective primary health care: strategies for control of disease in the developing world. XIII. Acute bacterial meningitis, *Rev Infect Dis* 6(3):374, 1984.

Halstensen A et al: Antimicrobial therapy and case fatality in meningococcal disease, *Scand J Infect Dis* 19:403, 1987.

Koppes GM, Ellenbogen C, Gebhart RJ: Group Y meningococcal disease in United States Air Force recruits, *Am J Med* 62(5):661, 1977.

Kristiansen BE et al: Rapid diagnosis of meningococcal meningitis by polymerase chain reaction, *Lancet* 337:1568, 1991.

Lepow ML, Gold R: Editorial retrospective: meningococcal A and other polysaccharide vaccines: a five-year progress report, *N Engl J Med* 308(19):1158, 1983.

Mellado MC et al: Endotoxin liberation by strains of *N. meningitidis* isolated from patients and healthy carriers, *Epidemiol Infect* 106:289, 1991.

Moore PS et al: Respiratory viruses and *Mycoplasma* as cofactors for epidemic group A meningococcal meningitis, *JAMA* 264:1271, 1990.

Pinner RW et al: Meningococcal disease in the United States–1986, *J Infect Dis* 164:368, 1991.

Shulman ST, Pharr JP et al: *The biological and clinical basis of infectious diseases,* ed 5, Philadelphia, 1997, WB Saunders.

Waage A, Halstensen A, Espevik T: Association between tumour necrosis factor in serum and fatal outcome in patients with meningococcal disease, *Lancet* 1(8529):355, 1987.

265 *Neisseria gonorrhoeae* Infections

Edward W. Hook III

THE ORGANISM
Characteristics

Neisseria gonorrhoeae is a gram-negative, oxidase-positive, non–spore-forming coccus; it usually is seen in pairs exclusively and causes infection of human mucosal surfaces. The organism is aerobic; grows best at 35° to 37° C, and its growth is facilitated in 5% carbon dioxide. It may be differentiated from *Neisseria meningitidis* and other *Neisseria* species on the basis of its ability to utilize glucose but not maltose, lactose, or sucrose for growth or by using monoclonal antibody reagents specific for the organism's major outer membrane protein, protein I. Gonococci grow well on supplemented

chocolate agar. For isolation from mucosal surfaces colonized by mixed bacterial flora, Thayer-Martin or an alternative selective medium containing antimicrobials to inhibit growth of other microorganisms is preferred.

On artificial media, gonococcal colonies may take one of three morphologic forms, designated P^+, P^{++}, or P^- (formerly designated T_1 and T_2, T_3, or T_4, respectively). Forms P^+ and P^{++} are small colonies obtained from patients on primary isolation and contain gonococcal cells covered by surface pili, which enhance attachment to epithelial cells and block phagocytosis by polymorphonuclear leukocytes. The P^- colonial forms are larger and contain less virulent, nonpiliated organisms. P^+ or P^{++} gonococci may give P^- progeny during serial culture.

Gonococcal colonies of each type (P^+, P^{++}, or P^-) may also differ in opacity. Organisms in opaque colonies contain outer membrane proteins, termed *Opa (opacity) proteins,* whereas transparent colonies do not. Opa proteins promote aggregation of gonococci and mediate adherence of organisms to mammalian cells. Although opaque and transparent colonies are usually present in the same culture, opaque colonies predominate in men with gonococcal urethritis and in women midway through the menstrual cycle (day 15). Transparent colonies predominate in isolates from women at times other than midcycle and in isolates from blood, synovial fluid, and fallopian tubes in patients with complicated gonococcal infection. Transparent colonies are more resistant than organisms from opaque colonies to killing by normal human serum.

Several methods of distinguishing different strains of gonococci have been developed. An auxotyping system that differentiates organisms according to their ability to grow on media lacking nutrients (e.g., certain amino acids and pyrimidines) is widely used and differentiates more than 30 different gonococcal strains. There are correlations between auxotypes and differences in cell-surface antigens and susceptibility to the bactericidal activity of human serum and the propensity to cause disseminated or asymptomatic disease. More recently, typing systems have been based on antigenic variability of protein I, the major outer membrane of the gonococcus. Early protein I typing systems based on the specificity of absorbed polyvalent antisera have been supplanted by monoclonal antibody–based typing systems, which facilitate use of gonococcal typing for epidemiologic and pathophysiologic studies. Other methods that differentiate gonococci by using pilus and lipopolysaccharide antigens or by pulse–gel electrophoresis have been developed but are not yet as widely used as the auxotyping and protein I–based systems for epidemiologic studies.

Epidemiology

The true incidence of gonorrhea is unknown because of incomplete reporting, treatment of the disease by nonmedical personnel, and presence of undetected carriers. The figures reported by the Centers for Disease Control and Prevention (CDC), however, may represent as little as one half the true incidence of gonorrhea infections. In addition, because reporting is more complete from publicly funded clinics that disproportionately serve people in lower socioeconomic classes and minority clients, gonorrhea reporting may be more complete for blacks and other racial minorities than for whites. Despite these limitations, reporting of gonorrhea in the United States is probably better than in most countries.

In the United States, gonorrhea rates peaked in the mid-1970s when more than one million cases per year were reported. Since then, gonorrhea incidence reached a plateau and subsequently has declined. Infection rates initially fell as a result of factors such as changes in the proportion of the population aged 16 to 24 (the ages at which risk for gonorrhea acquisition is greatest) and the success of national gonorrhea control efforts by the U.S. Public Health Service. Nationwide changes in contraceptive practices away from the oral contraceptive pill (which may slightly increase risk for gonorrhea acquisition) in favor of barrier methods such as diaphragms, spermicidal preparations, and condoms (which reduce risk for gonorrhea) may likewise have contributed to falling rates. More recently, behavioral changes among both heterosexuals and homosexually active men in response to the threat of human immunodeficiency virus (HIV) infection have probably also contributed to declining gonorrhea rates.

From 1984 to 1994 the number of cases of gonorrhea reported fell more than 52%, from 878,556 to 418,068. The impressive decline in gonorrhea incidence has not occurred uniformly throughout the population. For instance, gonorrhea rates among adolescents ages 15 to 19 years declined only 29%, from 1077.8 to 763.4/100,000 population. Similarly, while rates in whites declined more than 77%, from 104.7 to 30.1 per 100,000 population, rates for non-Hispanic blacks fell only 33.4%, from 1830.9 to 1219.3 per 100,000 population.

The disease is almost exclusively transmitted by sexual contact, although perinatal transmission to infants occurs, and transmission by fomites has been described in children under conditions of crowding and poor hygiene. In the United States the highest incidence is in the 16- to 25-year-old age-group, with 78% of patients younger than 30 years of age. Military personnel, urban dwellers, members of lower socioeconomic classes, homosexual males, and prostitutes all tend to have higher frequencies of gonococcal infections.

The spread of gonococcal disease occurs largely through contact with individuals with asymptomatic or ignored symptomatic infection. It is estimated that one fifth of infected men acquire infection after a single sexual exposure to a female with gonococcal cervicitis. The risk of transmission from infected male to female has not been well studied, but it is probably higher. The proportion of new infections that are asymptomatic probably varies, depending on regional differences in virulence of prevalent strains of gonococci.

Pathophysiology

Primary gonococcal infection in adults occurs almost entirely at sites lined with columnar or transitional epithelium: the mucous membranes of the urethra, cervix, rectum, and pharynx. Although the mode of transmission dictates these areas as primary sites of infection, the gonococcus has a number of characteristics that may facilitate initiation of infection.

Attachment of gonococci to cell surfaces is important in the pathogenesis of infection. The presence of extracellular pili appears to be a virulence factor for initiation of gonococcal infections. Pili present on the surface of P^+ and P^{++} colonial variants facilitate attachment to human mucosal cells. Piliated gonococci have a much higher affinity for attachment to mucosal cells than to other human cells (e.g., leukocytes, erythrocytes, or fibroblasts). At least one other class of surface proteins (the Opa proteins) also mediates attachment to mucosal cells. In addition, gonococci produce an extracellular immunoglobulin A1 (IgA1) protease that cleaves secretory IgA1. Secretory IgA has been demonstrated to inhibit adherence of the organism to human mucosal cells. The pathogenetic significance of IgA1 protease production by the gonococcus, however, remains unclear because other types of secretory IgA are produced by patients with gonococcal infection, and the duration of local antibody production is relatively short.

Local gonococcal infection elicits an inflammatory response, which, if untreated, leads to formation of fibrous deposits and adhesions. This fibrous scarring is subsequently responsible for many complications, such as urethral stricture or fallopian tubal abnormalities, which, in turn, lead to ectopic pregnancy and infertility.

Most gonococci that cause disseminated infection display resistance to complement-mediated bactericidal activity of human serum; this differentiates these organisms from the majority of gonococcal strains. Approximately 90% of serum-resistant strains isolated from patients with disseminated infection share the same major outer membrane protein (termed *protein I*) serotype and auxotype. Thus certain strains, through their resistance to serum bactericidal effects, are more likely to cause disseminated disease.

Under the selective pressure of therapy for gonococcal infections, the organisms have developed two distinct types of antimicrobial resistance. Since the mid-1950s most gonococci causing local disease have demonstrated a stepwise increase in resistance to penicillin. In 1954, 300,000 units of procaine penicillin G reliably cured gonococcal urethritis. Gradually increasing resistance necessitated stepwise increments in dosage up to 4.8 million units of procaine penicillin G plus 1 g of probenecid. In 1989, continued increases in resistance resulted in the decision that penicillin could not be recommended for routine therapy of gonorrhea for the first time since its introduction. This gradually increasing, low-level resistance (most gonococcal isolates in the United States continue to have minimal inhibitory concentrations for penicillin of less than 1 μg/ml) is the result of at least five separate chromosomal mutations resulting in altered susceptibility of the gonococcus to penicillin G. *N. gonorrhoeae* with clinically significant chromosomally mediated resistance to penicillin G are usually also less susceptible to other antimicrobials, including tetracycline, erythromycin, and occasionally even spectinomycin.

The second form of gonococcal antimicrobial resistance is plasmid mediated. Gonococci have now been recognized with plasmids mediating high-level resistance to either penicillin or tetracycline. Organisms with plasmids for penicillin resistance produce a β-lactamase that inactivates penicillin. A number of different β-lactamase plasmids have been described that vary in molecular weight. Several different β-lactamase plasmids may be found in a single community at the same time. The prevalence of penicillinase-producing gonococci varies from one area of the globe to another. In parts of Southeast Asia, 30% to 60% of gonococcal isolates produce β-lactamase. In the United States, the incidence of infection with β-lactamase–producing gonococci now accounts for about 8% of all reported gonorrhea and shows substantial regional variation.

In 1985 gonococci were recognized with minimal inhibitory concentrations of tetracycline ≥ 16 μg/ml, which contained a conjugative plasmid carrying the tet M gene first described in streptococci. These organisms are essentially impervious to clinically attainable serum levels of tetracycline. An increased number of gonococcal isolates throughout the United States have plasmids for resistance of both penicillin and tetracycline.

In 1987, to monitor national trends and geographic patterns of antimicrobial resistance in *N. gonorrhoeae,* the CDC initiated nationwide sentinel surveillance of gonococcal susceptibility. This surveillance program now provides data that allow anticipatory adjustment of gonorrhea treatment recommendations based on laboratory results rather than on observed treatment failures, as was previously the case.

CLINICAL SYNDROMES (Chapter 244)
Asymptomatic Carrier

Although the prevalence of asymptomatic infection varies, asymptomatic carriers are a major source of new gonococcal infections. The belief, however, that gonococcal infection is usually asymptomatic in females and rarely asymptomatic in males is probably incorrect. The symptoms of genital gonococcal infection in women—dysuria, urinary frequency, increased vaginal discharge, and abnormal menses—are often transient and attributed to other causes such as "cystitis" and treated without confirmation. Both *N. gonorrhoeae* and *Chlamydia trachomatis* have been established as important causes of urethritis in young women. Tracing and treating asymptomatic contacts of men or women who have symptomatic, recently acquired gonorrhea is an important element of public health control efforts. Routine screening cultures also are recommended during pregnancy and in certain high-risk populations. However, awareness of the symptoms of gonococcal genital infections in women and proper use of diagnostic testing when clinically indicated in patients who are at risk or who have characteristic symptoms are equally important.

Gonococcal Urethritis in Males (Chapter 244)

In males, the rarity of other urinary tract infections before age 40 justifies the assumption that dysuria in young, sexually active men usually represents sexually transmitted infection. Nongonococcal urethritis is two to three times as common as gonococcal urethritis in men in the United States. Gonococcal urethritis represents the bulk of gonococcal disease seen in male patients. Clinical disease usually is manifested after a 2- to 7-day incubation period as urethritis with urethral discharge. The discharge is usually purulent but may be clear. Discharge and/or dysuria usually prompt males to seek evaluation and therapy. Untreated, discharge may persist an average of 8 weeks before remitting. Complications such as epididymitis (previously occurring in 5% to 10% of untreated males), prostatitis, and urethral stricture are now uncommon as the result of increased awareness and availability of appropriate therapy.

Gonococcal Proctitis in Homosexual Men

Although many homosexually active men have modified their behavior in response to the epidemic of HIV, homosexual men with multiple sex partners remain at a significant risk for development of gonorrhea, including proctitis. Gonococcal anorectal infection results from receptive anal intercourse with men who have urethral infection. Anorectal gonorrhea may be asymptomatic or may cause symptomatic proctitis with tenesmus, anorectal pain, bloody rectal discharge, and constipation. Homosexually active men with symptomatic proctitis should be evaluated for other sexually transmitted organisms, including syphilis, amebiasis, and *Chlamydia, Campylobacter, Shigella,* and herpes simplex virus infections, as well as for gonorrhea. About 40% of homosexual males with proctitis have anorectal gonorrhea, but it is not unusual to discover several pathogens in patients with symptomatic proctitis. Men who have had receptive rectal intercourse with sex partners who have urethral gonococcal infection should be treated and have cultures for gonorrhea, irrespective of the presence of symptoms.

Gonococcal Infection in Females

The usual primary site of gonococcal infection in the female is the endocervix, although organisms also are recovered frequently from the vagina, the urethra, and the rectum. Endocervical infection with *N. gonorrhoeae* or *C. trachomatis* either may be associated with no signs or symptoms or may cause mucopurulent cervicitis, which is manifested by purulent cervical secretions and easily induced cervical bleeding. Symptoms in females are often nonspecific and mild; most women with uncomplicated infection probably do note dysuria, frequency, abnormal menstruation, or change in vaginal discharge. As many as 40% of women with cervical gonorrhea have coexistent *C. trachomatis* infection; concomitant infection with *Trichomonas vaginalis* occurs in about 20% of women with gonorrhea.

Gonococcal Salpingitis

The major complication of gonorrhea in women is contiguous spread of infection, which gives rise to salpingitis. This complication occurs in 10% to 15% of untreated women and may result in infertility caused by bilateral tubal obstruction or an increased likelihood of tubal pregnancy. Gonococcal pelvic inflammatory disease (PID) often manifests during menses or a few days after the onset of menstruation; clinically, it tends to be more acute than nongonococcal PID. In the United States, 40% or more of cases of PID are associated with gonococcal infection. Other pathogens implicated as causes of PID include *C. trachomatis, Mycoplasma hominis,* and mixed aerobic-anaerobic infections. The most common presenting symptom of gonococcal salpingitis is relatively acute onset of lower abdominal pain, which is usually bilateral. Other findings may be history of recent dysuria, abnormal vaginal discharge, or abnormal menstruation. Physical examination may show bilateral adnexal tenderness that is worsened by movement of the cervix, and cervicitis, with increased leukocytes in cervical and vaginal secretions. Fever, localized rebound, guarding, and lower abdominal tenderness are also frequently present. The clinical diagnosis of PID is imprecise at best; however, given its sequelae (e.g., sterility, ectopic pregnancy), it is an important consideration in evaluating lower abdominal pain and pelvic tenderness in young women. Fever, leukocytosis, and elevated erythrocyte sedimentation rate, when present with adnexal tenderness and cervicitis, increase the likelihood of PID but need not be present. Infrequently, PID may cause the so-called Fitz-Hugh–Curtis syndrome, a perihepatitis that manifests with fever and subacute, pleuritic right upper quadrant pain and tenderness. Chronic right upper quadrant pain may result from "violin-string" adhesions between the liver and the abdominal wall. Both *N. gonorrhoeae* and *C. trachomatis* have been implicated as causes of perihepatitis complicating PID.

Acute gonococcal infection may lead to other local complications as well, the most common of which are acute Bartholin's gland inflammation or abscess. These are manifested as pain and swelling along the posterior third of the labia minora. Chronic Bartholin's gland cysts rarely involve active gonococcal infection. Similar, albeit less frequent, infections may involve the Skene's gland.

Gonococcal Pharyngeal Infection

Pharyngeal infection occurs in about 20% of persons engaging in fellatio with males with urethral gonococcal infection. Although pharyngeal infection is usually asymptomatic, it may be associated with exudative pharyngitis and cervical adenitis. Pharyngeal gonococcal infection is less common after cunnilingus with infected females.

Disseminated Gonococcal Infection

Only a very small percentage of gonococcal infections become hematogenously disseminated. Nonetheless, gonococcal arthritis is the most common cause of septic arthritis seen in young persons in the United States. Individuals with disseminated gonococcal infection (DGI) are often unaware of primary genital, oral, or rectal infection and discover their illness with the onset of polyarthritis or skin rash. Unlike many patients with other bacteremic illnesses, patients with DGI rarely have high fever, dramatic leukocytosis, or other signs of clinical toxicity; most patients with DGI have temperatures of less than 38° C by mouth and peripheral leukocyte counts of less than 10,800/mm^3. The arthritic component of the syndrome, present in greater than 75% of DGI, includes tenosynovitis, arthralgia, or purulent arthritis. Joints most commonly involved are knees, ankles, and wrists, but any joint may be involved. Skin rash is frequently seen with gonococcemia as well (Chapter 235). The rash is characteristically described as between 5 and 30 pustules on erythematous bases and located primarily on extremities (Color Plate VIII-22). The rash may present as petechiae, papules, hemorrhagic bullae, or necrotic papules, as well as pustules. Disseminated gonococcal infection may follow an acute or subacute course. The onset in women often occurs with the initiation of menses. Gonococcal endocarditis and meningitis are rare, albeit devastating, complications of gonococcemia.

It is of interest that a single auxotype (requiring arginine, hypoxanthine, and uracil for growth) is associated with both the majority of disseminated gonococcal infections in whites and a disproportionate percentage of asymptomatic infections of males. This strain of gonococcus is usually resistant to the complement-mediated bactericidal activity of human serum and is significantly more susceptible to penicillin and tetracycline than are strains isolated from patients with symptomatic uncomplicated genital infection. Recently a number of cases of DGI caused by β-lactamase–producing gonococci (PPNG) or gonococci with chromosomally mediated antibiotic resistance have been reported.

Individuals with inherited deficiency of C5, C6, C7, or C8 components of complement are uniquely predisposed to dissemination of gonococcal and other neisserial infections (Chapter 229). These patients' sera lack bactericidal activity against gonococci, even against those normally sensitive to serum. Although less than 5% of patients with DGI have complement deficiency syndromes, individuals who have multiple systemic gonococcal or meningococcal infections should have serum hemolytic complement activity (CH$_{50}$) tested to screen for complement deficiency.

GONORRHEA IN PREGNANCY

Retrospective studies show that pregnant women with gonorrhea detected at term are more likely to have premature delivery, a low–birth weight infant, delayed delivery after rupture of membranes, and chorioamnionitis. Thus screening for gonorrhea in pregnancy, even for individuals believed to be at low risk for infection, is recommended.

Gonorrhea in Children

During childbirth, infants passing through the birth canal may be infected with gonorrhea. The chief sites of infection in neonates are conjunctiva, pharynx, and anal canal. Gonococcal ophthalmia neonatorum is now largely prevented by routine screening for gonorrhea during pregnancy, by treatment of infected women, and by silver nitrate instillation in eyes of infants at birth. *C. trachomatis* has replaced the gonococcus as the leading cause of neonatal conjunctival infection and is not prevented by silver nitrate prophylaxis.

Between 1 year of age and puberty, gonococcal infection is unusual; most cases in this age-group are vulvovaginitis in females sexually molested by a household member. For medicolegal and diagnostic purposes, complete bacteriologic evaluation is important.

DIAGNOSIS

In males, the diagnosis of gonococcal urethritis often can be made on the basis of Gram stain alone. Gram-negative intracellular diplococci in urethral exudate are virtually diagnostic. The diagnosis of symptomatic gonococcal urethritis by Gram stain can provide 95% sensitivity and 98% specificity. Urethral culture is confirmatory in Gram stain–positive patients and significantly increases diagnostic yield in patients without demonstrable discharge.

In homosexual males, rectal culture should be part of screening procedures. In homosexual males with proctitis, Gram stain is useful for detection of leukocytes (indicative of proctitis or colitis) and may show gonococci or *Campylobacter.* However, anorectal Gram stain smears often are hard to interpret, are not highly sensitive for detection of gonococci, and always should be supplemented by culture for *N. gonorrhoeae.* Patients with symptomatic proctitis should always undergo anoscopy, a simple office procedure. Those without gonorrhea should be investigated for *Chlamydia, Salmonella, Shigella,* and *Campylobacter* species; herpes simplex virus; and amebae, any of which may be present (Chapters 255, 257, 267, 269, and 279).

Pharyngeal cultures for *N. gonorrhoeae* are most useful in patients with DGI or symptomatic pharyngitis incurred as a result of practicing fellatio. The need for routine pharyngeal cultures in other settings is debatable, because most asymptomatic gonococcal infections of the pharynx subside spontaneously without therapy and without complication or further spread.

In testing women patients for gonococcal infection, one cervical culture provides the diagnosis in 80% to 90% of cases. Culture of the rectum and urethra increase yield by less than 5% each. Gram stain of cervical specimens showing gram-negative intracellular diplococci provides 60% diagnostic sensitivity, with greater than 90% specificity in high-risk populations, but staining alone cannot be relied on in diagnosing genital gonorrhea in women.

Although PID is often a clinical diagnosis, microbiologic studies may support the diagnosis. In women with lower abdominal pain and adnexal tenderness, isolation of *N. gonorrhoeae* and/or *C. trachomatis* from the cervix supports the diagnosis of salpingitis. The clinical value and cost-effectiveness of routine hospitalization or laparoscopy for the diagnosis of salpingitis are debated. Certainly hospitalization and laparoscopy should be strongly considered in women with suspected PID who have atypical presentation, early pregnancy, or poor response to therapy.

Disseminated gonococcal infection is often a clinical diagnosis as well, with only 50% of patients with suspected DGI having positive blood, joint fluid, skin, or cerebrospinal fluid cultures. A presumptive diagnosis can be made on the basis of appropriate clinical presentation, positive culture for *N. gonorrhoeae* from genital sites, pharynx, or rectum, and significant clinical improvement within 48 hours of beginning therapy. The probability of isolating the organism from blood is highest during the first 48 hours after onset of symptoms. Synovial fluid cultures are more often positive later in the course or when synovial fluid leukocyte counts are in excess of $20,000/mm^3$.

Careful culture techniques significantly increase the likelihood of positive culture findings. Small urethrogenital calcium alginate or dacron swabs on wire shafts are preferred for intraurethral culture in males. Specimens should be inoculated directly onto culture media at the time of collection. Commercially available modified Thayer-Martin medium packaged in small plastic bags to retain carbon dioxide generated after inoculation are cheap and efficient. Biplates containing Thayer-Martin medium and chocolate agar medium without antibiotics are increasingly popular because a variable percentage of gonococci are inhibited by the vancomycin in Thayer-Martin medium (vancomycin concentration should not exceed 3 μg/ml). Blood, synovial fluid, or cerebrospinal fluid should be inoculated into broth medium, but many gonococcal isolates are inhibited by the sodium polyanethol sulfonate (SPS) present in standard blood culture media. This inhibitory effect may be counteracted by the addition of 1% gelatin to this medium.

In many settings testing for *N. gonorrhoeae* is currently performed using nonamplified nucleic acid probe tests, which permit a single swab specimen to be used for both gonorrhea and *C. trachomatis* testing. While these tests are less sensitive than optimally performed culture for either organism, their low cost, ease of transport, and the ability to test for both pathogens using a single swab have contributed to their increasing use. Testing practices for *N. gonorrhoeae* will likely continue to change. An amplified nucleic acid test for gonorrhea diagnosis (a ligase chain reaction [LCR] test), which permitted diagnosis of infections using swabs or voided urine was approved and marketed in 1996. The LCR tests appear to be as sensitive as well-performed culture and offer increased ease of transport and specimen collection. At present, however, they are more costly than culture or nonamplified nucleic acid detection tests.

Serologic tests currently being marketed for gonococcal screening have not been useful because of the inability to determine whether antibodies present represent previous or current infection, because of cross-reaction with meningococcal infection, and because of low sensitivity. The predictive value of a positive test result with the serologic tests marketed in the United States up to 1982 was only 5% to 10%. Thus 90% to 95% of patients with "reactive" serologic findings indicated by these tests did not have gonorrhea.

In areas where β-lactamase–producing gonococci or gonococci with high-level, chromosomally mediated antimicrobial resistance are prevalent, culture diagnosis (rather than Gram-stain diagnosis) should be encouraged, and gonococcal isolates should be tested for antimicrobial resistance and for β-lactamase production.

TREATMENT

Although many gonococci remain sensitive to a variety of antibiotics, including penicillin G, ampicillin, spectinomycin, cefoxitin, trimethoprim-sulfamethoxazole, and several third-generation cephalosporins, the continued development of antimicrobial resistance has resulted in deletion of penicillins from the list of drugs recommended for gonorrhea therapy. Treatment of gonococcal infection should be approached with consideration of efficacy, ease of administration, potential side-effects, and cost. Single-dose therapy is preferable for patients in whom compliance with several days of therapy may be a problem.

In 1989 the CDC issued new guidelines for gonorrhea therapy; these guidelines recommended ceftriaxone 125 to 250 mg for uncomplicated gonorrhea. These regimens have the advantages of proven efficacy for infections caused by gonococci with all currently recognized forms of antibiotic resistance at genital, rectal, and pharyngeal sites. Alternative single-dose regimens recommended for treatment of uncomplicated gonorrhea include ciprofloxacin, 500 mg by mouth (PO); ofloxacin, 400 mg PO; or cefixime, 400 mg PO, each given as a single dose.

Although high-level spectinomycin resistance in gonococci has reduced the utility of this drug for gonorrhea treatment in the Far East, only a few infections caused by spectinomycin-resistant gonococci have been reported across the United States to date. Neither spectinomycin nor the quinolones (ciprofloxacin or ofloxacin) are active against *Treponema pallidum,* and experience with each of the cephalosporin regimens currently recommended is limited. Therefore repeat serologic testing for syphilis 1 month after treatment is recommended for all patients with gonorrhea. Similarly, none of the currently recommended regimens is effective for coexistent *C. trachomatis* infections. Concomitant treatment for chlamydia of all gonorrhea patients using a single 1 g dose of azithromycin or 7 days of doxycycline, tetracycline, or erythromycin is recommended. As a result of increasing numbers of treatment failures and antibiotic resistance, doxycycline, 100 mg, or tetracycline, 0.5 g, four times daily for 7 days, can no longer be considered effective for treatment of genital gonococcal infection. However, these drugs are effective in eradicating concomitant *C. trachomatis* infection, which is present in up to 20% of men and 40% of women with gonorrhea. Treatment of heterosexual patients with uncomplicated gonorrhea using single-dose therapy plus 7 days of doxycycline, tetracycline, or erythromycin for possible *C. trachomatis* coinfection reduces the risk of complications due to chlamydia and is preferred to single-dose therapy alone. For patients with penicillin allergy, single-dose therapy alone may be preferred.

Follow-up ("test of cure") culture for patients with gonorrhea is

Table 265-1 Therapy of gonococcal infections in hospitalized patients

DISEASE	THERAPY
Acute salpingitis* (pelvic inflammatory disease)	Optimal therapy for acute salpingitis has not been established. Initial therapy should ideally include agents active against gonococci, chlamydiae, genital anaerobes, *Mycoplasma hominis,* and facultative gram-negative rods
Disseminated gonococcal infection	Ceftriaxone, 1 g IM or IV every 24 hr daily until improvement occurs, followed by oral cefuroxime axetil, 500 mg twice daily, or amoxicillin, 500 mg with clavulanic acid three times a day, to complete 7 days of therapy or Ceftizoxime, 1 g IV every 8 hr daily until improvement occurs, followed by oral cefuroxime axetil, 500 mg twice daily, or amoxicillin, 500 mg with clavulanic acid three times a day, to complete 7 days of therapy or Ceftizoxime, 1 g IV every 8 hr daily until improvement occurs, followed by oral cefuroxime axetil, 500 mg twice daily, or amoxicillin, 500 mg with clavulanic acid three times a day, to complete 7 days of therapy or Spectinomycin, 2.0 g IM twice daily for 3 days (treatment of choice for disseminated infections caused by penicillinase-producing *N. gonorrhoeae,* or PPNG)

*Certain third-generation cephalosporins (e.g., ceftriaxone, cefotaxime, and cefuroxime) and cefoxitin, which are highly active in vitro against PPNG, are probably effective for complicated gonococcal infections caused by PPNG, as well as for penicillin-allergic patients with complicated gonococcal infections.

no longer advised because of the high efficacy of currently recommended treatment regimens. At the same time, however, individuals with recently diagnosed gonorrhea are at increased risk for reinfection, thus rescreening at 3 to 6 months is suggested. Although the most common cause of recurrent infection is reinfection resulting from failure to locate and treat contacts of the initial case, any gonococci isolated on reculture should be tested for β-lactamase production.

The therapy of acute gonococcal PID should be directed against gonococci, chlamydiae, facultative gram-negative bacilli, and the anaerobic bacteria associated with the illness, unless differentiation of etiologic agents has been carried out. Although efficacy is unproved, removal of intrauterine devices from women with acute PID is recommended. Patients in whom the diagnosis is unclear, who are unable to comply with outpatient therapy, who are suspected to have pelvic abscess, or who are not responding to outpatient management should be reevaluated and hospitalized. Hospitalization of all women with PID is desirable to confirm the diagnosis, initiate parenteral therapy, ensure compliance, and monitor the clinical response. Although firm therapy guidelines for PID are not warranted on the basis of available data, the use of antibiotic combinations active against the major pathogens seems reasonable (e.g., cefoxitin plus doxycycline for initial parenteral therapy, until clear-cut clinical improvement occurs, followed by doxycycline 100 mg PO twice daily to complete a 10- to 14-day total duration of therapy). Sex partners of all patients with PID should be screened and treated for sexually transmitted diseases.

In general, the organisms causing disseminated gonococcal infection are significantly more sensitive to penicillin and tetracycline than most strains causing symptomatic urethritis. However, DGI caused by gonococci with both chromosomally and plasmid-mediated antimicrobial resistance has been reported. In addition, because of the risk of meningitis, endocarditis, and septic arthritis, patients with disseminated infection should initially be hospitalized and observed. Initial therapy should be ceftriaxone 1.0 g IV or IM daily (Table 265-1). Significant clinical response should occur within 48 hours of ini-

tiation of therapy. After clinical improvement, the patient may be followed as an outpatient while he or she is completing a 7- to 10-day course of oral therapy using cefixime 400 mg or ciprofloxacin 500 mg twice daily. Patients with high synovial fluid white blood cell counts may require repeated joint aspiration and irrigation to reduce inflammation. Painful joints may be ameliorated in some cases by a brief period of immobilization. As with all gonococcal infections, examination and treatment of the patient's contacts are of great epidemiologic importance.

PREVENTION

At present, useful preventive measures for reducing spread of gonococcal disease are treatment of acute infection, patient education, and careful tracing and treatment of contacts of patients with gonococcal disease. Use of condoms can prevent passage of infection between partners. Vaccines are not available. Prophylactic antibiotics, although effective, are expensive and carry the risk of increasing resistance of gonococci to antibiotics presently in use.

BIBLIOGRAPHY

Centers for Disease Control and Prevention: Sexually transmitted diseases treatment guidelines, *MMWR* (No RR-14):47-66, 1993.

Centers for Disease Control and Prevention, Division of STD Prevention: Sexually Transmitted Disease Surveillance–1994, Sept 1995, U.S. Department of Health and Human Services, Public Health Service.

Cohen MS, Sparling PF: Mucosal infection with *Neisseria gonorrhoeae:* bacterial adaptation and mucosal defenses, *J Clin Invest* 89:1699, 1992.

Dallabetta G, Hook EW III: Gonococcal infections, *Infect Dis Clin North Am* 1:25, 1987.

Eschenbach DA et al: Polymicrobial etiology of acute pelvic inflammatory disease, *N Engl J Med* 293:166, 1975.

Faruki H et al: A community-based outbreak of infection with penicillin-resistant *Neisseria gonorrhoeae* not producing penicillinase (chromosomally mediated resistance), *N Engl J Med* 313:607, 1985.

Gorden SM et al: The emergence of *Neisseria gonorrhoeae* with decreased susceptibility to ciprofloxacin in Cleveland, Ohio: epidemiology and risk factors, *Ann Intern Med* 125:465, 1996.

Handsfield HH et al: Treatment of the gonococcal arthritis dermatitis syndrome, *Ann Intern Med* 84:661, 1976.

Handsfield HH et al: Epidemiology of penicillinase-producing *Neisseria gonorrhoeae* infections: analysis by auxotyping and serogrouping, *N Engl J Med* 306:950, 1982.

Handsfield HH et al: A comparison of single dose cefixime with ceftriaxone as treatment for uncomplicated gonorrhea, *N Engl J Med* 325:1337, 1991.

McGee ZA, Johnson AP, Taylor-Robinson D: Pathogenic mechanisms of *Neisseria gonorrhoeae:* observations on damage to human fallopian tubes in organ culture by gonococci of colony type 1 or type 4, *J Infect Dis* 143:413, 1981.

Quinn TC et al: The polymicrobial origin of intestinal infections in homosexual men, *N Engl J Med* 309:576, 1983.

Upchurch DM et al: Behavioral contributions to acquisition of gonorrhea in patients attending an inner city sexually transmitted disease clinic, *J Infect Dis* 161:938, 1990.

CHAPTER

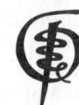

266 Infections Caused by *Haemophilus* Species

David T. Durack and John R. Perfect

THE ORGANISMS
Classification

Haemophilus is a genus of small, pleomorphic, nonmotile, facultatively anaerobic coccobacillary gram-negative bacteria, several species of which are commonly present in the normal flora of humans. Encapsulated strains are important human pathogens, especially for young children and some immunocompromised adults.

The major pathogen in this group of organisms is *Haemophilus influenzae* type b, which causes a wide range of infections including pneumonia, bacteremia, meningitis, and cellulitis. This pathogen was isolated and described in 1892 by Richard Pfeiffer, who found it in

Table 266-1 Relationship between age and the frequency* of major infections caused by *Haemophilus influenzae*

INFECTION	3 TO 24 MONTHS	2 TO 5 YEARS	5 YEARS AND OLDER
Otitis, sinusitis mastoiditis	+++	+++	++
Meningitis	+++	++	+
Bacteremia	+++	++	+
Pneumonia	++	+++	+
Cellulitis	+++	+	Rare
Epiglottitis	+	+++	Rare
Pyarthrosis	++	+	Rare
Endocarditis	Rare	Rare	Rare

*+++, most common; ++, less common; +, occasional.

the upper respiratory secretions of many patients with influenza, hence the name of the species. This led to the erroneous belief that this bacterium caused influenza, which persisted until influenza A virus was identified in the 1930s.

Characteristics

Haemophilus species require accessory growth factors, including heat-stable factor X (derived from hemoglobin) and heat-labile factor V (nicotinamide-adenine dinucleotide [NAD]), for successful cultivation in vitro. These requirements are supplied by special media, such as rabbit blood, Levinthal medium, Fildes enrichment, or chocolate agar. Some species have an absolute or relative requirement for carbon dioxide. Recovery of *Haemophilus ducreyi* has been improved with enriched chocolate agar containing Isovitalex, supplemented GC agar, or supplemented Mueller-Hinton agar with vancomycin. These special nutritional requirements, together with the ability of some species to hemolyze blood, are used routinely to identify and speciate *Haemophilus* in the laboratory. Strains can be further subdivided into five biotypes by biochemical tests for indole production, urease, and ornithine decarboxylase. Proper collection of specimens, prompt inoculation into suitable media, and correct decolorization of Gram stains are necessary for isolation and identification of these relatively fastidious organisms. Standard antisera are used to determine whether strains of *H. influenzae* recovered from clinical specimens are type b (see later discussion).

Epidemiology

Haemophilus influenzae. Members of the species *H. influenzae* reside only on living hosts, are not found free in the environment, and cause disease only in humans. Strains of *H. influenzae* are present in the normal flora of the nasopharynx of a majority of healthy children and adults. Most of these strains are unencapsulated, and therefore untypeable; because of *H. influenzae* type b vaccine they may become relatively even more common. Of the encapsulated strains, about half are type b. The colonization rate with this type is very low in neonates, rising to approximately 5% in 5-year-old children. Nasopharyngeal colonization itself usually does not cause symptoms, but it provides the source for most cases of invasive disease.

Strains of *H. influenzae* can be found in the vaginal flora of normal women. From this site invasive infection can arise, sometimes as a complication during pregnancy and delivery.

The relative frequency of the various kinds of infection at different ages is summarized in Table 266-1. *H. influenzae* has a special predilection for children less than 5 years old, in whom type b strains caused more than 95% of systemic *Haemophilus* infections before the development of conjugate vaccines. Before the introduction of the first of four currently licensed polysaccharide protein conjugate vaccines in 1987, approximately 1 in every 1000 children in the United States less than 5 years of age had systemic *Haemophilus* infection each year. Rates are higher among blacks, Native Americans, Native Alaskans, and children of low socioeconomic status groups. Factors that increase exposure include crowding, presence of young siblings, and attendance at day care centers. Other factors that influence sus-

ceptibility of individual children are duration of breast-feeding, parental smoking, and history of recurrent respiratory infections. Since introduction of the conjugate vaccines in the United States, there has been a reported 95% decrease in cases of *Haemophilus* type b infection.

In older children and adults, a variety of conditions, including sickle cell anemia, asplenia, agammaglobulinemia, alcoholism, Hodgkin's disease, and acquired immunodeficiency syndrome (AIDS), predispose to *H. influenzae* infection. The incidence of systemic disease caused by *H. influenzae* in adults in the United States seems to have increased during the past 2 decades. In one study, nearly one quarter of isolates from patients with invasive *Haemophilus* infection were from patients older than 18 years of age, and the percentage is likely to increase with childhood immunizations. Whether the overall incidence of systemic infections in certain age-groups has increased significantly remains controversial because apparent increases may be due more to variable reporting patterns and geographic differences than to real changes. However, it is clear that with the introduction of conjugate vaccines, the number of invasive infections in young children has dramatically fallen. Definitive assessment of the long-term impact of these vaccines will have to await the results of prospective studies but the immediate results are impressive.

Other Species of *Haemophilus*

Renewed interest in isolation and identification of the other species of the genus *Haemophilus* has expanded our knowledge of their ecology and pathogenicity for humans. Many of these species reside in the upper respiratory tract, forming part of the normal flora. *H. parainfluenzae* can be recovered from 10% to 25% of normal children. *H. haemolyticus* and *H. parahaemolyticus* are also commonly present in the upper respiratory tract. *H. aphrophilus* has been recovered from one third of healthy persons, and *H. paraphrophilus* also has been found in the mouths and throats of healthy individuals. These species can be recovered from a wide variety of clinical specimens and sites, and all occasionally may cause invasive infection (Table 266-2). For example, *H. parainfluenzae* can be found in the flora of the throat, vagina, and urethra of adults (2% to 13%) and can be sexually transmitted, as can the known sexually transmitted pathogen *Haemophilus ducreyi*. When *Haemophilus* species are isolated from infections in soft tissue or bone, or infections related to the genitourinary or gastrointestinal tracts, polymicrobial infection with other bacteria is common.

CLINICAL DISEASES
Pathophysiology and Immune Responses

The pathogenicity of *H. influenzae* and the host's immune responses to infection with this important pathogen have been studied for nearly a century, but our understanding is not yet complete. The most important determinant of pathogenicity is the outer capsule of these organisms, which is composed of complex carbohydrate polymers. There are six antigenically distinct capsular types (designated *a* to *f*), each containing different sugars. Strains possessing the type b capsule, which contains polymers of ribose and ribitol phosphate (PRP), are strikingly more virulent than strains with other capsular types or nonencapsulated (untypeable) strains. Nonencapsulated strains often are associated with sinusitis, otitis media, and bronchitis, but they seldom produce invasive, systemic disease such as bacteremia or meningitis except in neonates. Why the great majority of systemic infections are caused by strains with the type b capsule is not fully understood. The proven ability of the polysaccharide capsule to impede phagocytosis by leukocytes presumably is a key factor. Possession of the PRP capsule also favors intravascular survival of this organism.

It can be shown experimentally that the genes that control production of the type b capsule confer greater invasive potential than genes for other capsular types. For example, the gene for PRP, which is located within two 17-kilobase direct repeats in the chromosome of *H. influenzae* type b, can be inserted into a nonvirulent, capsule-deficient type d strain. The transformed type d strain produces capsule, survives better in the bloodstream, and becomes virulent. Genetic studies have also suggested that the lipopolysaccharide is important in enhancing the efficiency of *H. influenzae* translocation from the nasopharynx into the bloodstream. The precise mechanisms gov-

Table 266-2   Relative frequency* with which *Haemophilus* species are isolated from various sites and clinical specimens

ORGANISM	BLOOD AND/OR CSF	THROAT†, SINUSES, EARS	SPUTUM	PUS‡	ENDOCARDITIS	CONJUNCTIVITIS	CHANCROID
H. influenzae (encapsulated)	+++	+	++	++	Rare	−	−
H. influenzae (untypeable)	Rare	+++	+++	+	−	−	−
H. parainfluenzae	+	+	+	+	+	−	−
H. haemolyticus and *para-haemolyticus*	+	++	++	Rare	Rare	−	−
H. aphrophilus	Rare	+	+	+	+	−	−
H. paraphrophilus	Rare	+	+	+	+	−	−
H. aegyptius	+§	−	−	−	−	+	−
H. ducreyi	−	−	−	−	−	−	+

*+++, most common; ++, less common; +, occasional; −, does not occur.
†Including epiglottis.
‡Empyema, septic arthritis, pericarditis, osteomyelitis.
§Brazilian purpuric fever.

erning virulence currently are being studied by molecular techniques. Recently *H. influenzae* became the first microorganism to have its entire genome sequenced. With this genetic information, *H. influenzae* has become a model pathogen for study of bacterial virulence mechanisms. Molecular techniques such as DNA fingerprinting for epidemiology studies and PCR-based detection systems of *H. influenzae* from clinical specimens are available but presently remain primarily research procedures.

Infection with *H. influenzae* can result in production of specific bactericidal and anticapsular antibodies. Concentrations of 0.15 µg/ml are considered to be protective, whereas 1.0 µg/ml indicates long-term protection. Unfortunately, most children younger than 2 years of age and a few apparently normal older children fail to produce protective quantities of antibody even after recovering from a major, invasive *Haemophilus* infection such as meningitis. Infants possess some maternal immunoglobulin G (IgG) antibody before 3 months of age and usually develop adult levels of bactericidal and anticapsular antibodies by 3 to 5 years of age. These antibodies are low or absent in the serum of most normal children between 3 months and 3 years of age, the period of greatest susceptibility to invasive *Haemophilus* disease. These observations indicate that bactericidal and anticapsular antibodies play a crucial role in normal host resistance to *H. influenzae*. However, susceptibility cannot always be predicted solely on the basis of presence or absence of these antibodies; it is presently believed that other antibodies to nonencapsulated protein antigens, termed *antisomatic antibodies,* also may contribute to immunity. The significance of mucosal immunity, including secretory IgA antibodies and influence of bacterial IgA1 proteases for colonization and infection, remains an important area of study. Another important defense mechanism that matures during the first few years of life is the ability of fixed macrophages of the reticuloendothelial system to clear circulating microorganisms. Notably, patients with anatomic or functional asplenia are several times more susceptible to *Haemophilus* infection, as are patients with human immunodeficiency virus (HIV) infection. The relative importance of cellular immunity and of genetic predispositions (such as IgG subclass II deficiency, complement deficiencies, or G2m(n) allotype) to *Haemophilus* infections remains to be further defined.

Clinical Syndromes

The spectrum of *H. influenzae* infections is wide and characteristically different at various ages (see Table 266-1). Localized lumenal infections of the ears, paranasal sinuses, and bronchi occur in patients of all ages, but invasive infection is overwhelmingly more common in young children than in adults. The median age of children with pneumonia or epiglottitis is between 2 and 5 years, which is older than the median age for meningitis and bacteremia.

Meningitis. *H. influenzae* type b used to be the most common cause of bacterial meningitis in young children, but in a vaccinated population, it has probably been reduced in incidence below pneumococcal meningitis (Chapter 239). The organisms originate in the nasopharynx, usually reaching the meninges by way of the blood-

stream through the choroid plexus. In some cases, they invade locally, directly from colonized or infected paranasal sinuses or mastoids to the meninges. Cranial trauma with resulting cerebrospinal fluid leak can lead to *Haemophilus* meningitis, although pneumococcal meningitis is still more common in this setting. Very young children manifest nonspecific symptoms including fever, vomiting, irritability, lethargy, and anorexia. Signs include somnolence, convulsions, coma, pain on handling or movement, hyperreflexia, cranial nerve pareses, and bulging fontanelles. In older patients, headache and meningismus are more prominent. These manifestations are indistinguishable from those of meningitis caused by *Neisseria meningitidis* or *Streptococcus pneumoniae.*

With modern antibiotic and supportive therapy, overall mortality can be reduced to about 1%. Mortality rate is higher in infants and in those in whom treatment is delayed until coma and/or cardiovascular collapse supervenes. Most patients who survive the first 2 days in the hospital recover, but up to one third suffer permanent sequelae, including deafness or reduced intelligence of varying degree. These defects may not be recognized until long after the acute illness has resolved. In some children, long-term sequelae improve slowly with the passage of time. Children are commonly treated with dexamethasone in addition to antibiotic during the first 2 or 3 days; this appears to reduce the frequency and severity of sequelae in children by mitigating inflammation, edema, and damage mediated by bacteria and cytokines, and has been shown to reduce hearing loss. The value of dexamethasone for treatment of meningitis in adults is less certain.

H. influenzae meningitis is much less common in adults than in children. In contrast to the high frequency of hematogenous seeding in children, in adults the bacteria often reach the meninges by spread from a contiguous focus of infection or site of trauma involving the paranasal sinuses or mastoids. The clinical picture is similar to that found in other common forms of bacterial meningitis.

Bacteremia. In children, bacteremia occurs most often in association with invasive localized disease, such as pneumonia, meningitis, or cellulitis. However, children less than 2 years of age who have fever and leukocytosis may have positive blood culture results for *H. influenzae* despite the lack of any sign of localized infection. These children must be treated and watched closely for later-developing signs of a focus of infection. Although presence of a rash is unusual, in a few children with *H. influenzae* bacteremia a syndrome indistinguishable from acute meningococcemia, including a petechial or purpuric rash, develops.

In adults, *H. influenzae* bacteremia occurs most commonly in association with pneumonia, in patients who are compromised by alcoholism, hypogammaglobulinemia, bronchiectasis, chronic obstructive pulmonary disease, or HIV infection. In asplenic patients, *H. influenzae* can cause fulminant septicemia. Although pneumococci are the most common cause of this syndrome in both children and adults, patients known to be asplenic who have signs of fulminant septicemia should be treated initially for *H. influenzae* as well as *S. pneumoniae* infection until the cause is known (Chapter 262).

Otitis, Sinusitis, Mastoiditis. Otitis media in children is commonly caused by *H. influenzae.* The causal organisms usually are untypeable strains that may be isolated in mixed culture together with pneumococci (3% of cases) and/or other potential bacterial pathogens, including *Staphylococcus aureus* and anaerobes. In adults, acute maxillary sinusitis and mastoiditis often are caused by nonencapsulated strains of *H. influenzae* together with pneumococci (Chapter 237).

Lower Respiratory Tract Infection. *H. influenzae* type b causes 20% to 30% of bacterial pneumonias in children, and 3% to 8% of those in adults. *Haemophilus* pneumonia cannot be distinguished clinically or radiologically from other bacterial lobar or bronchopneumonias. Bacteremia occurs in about 20% of patients with *H. influenzae* pneumonia. The prognosis is good for treated cases, except when the patient has serious underlying disease such as chronic obstructive airway disease, or when a complication, for example, empyema, develops. Resolution is usually complete, without abscess formation or parenchymal scarring. The sputum of patients with chronic bronchitis usually contains *H. influenzae, Moraxella,* and pneumococci, but because these potential pathogens colonize the nasopharynx, as well as abnormal bronchi, their potential role in pathogenesis or persistence of chronic bronchitis is difficult to confirm. Certainly antibiotics given for treatment of chronic bronchitis or prevention of recurrences should be active against *Haemophilus* species (Chapter 237).

Cellulitis. Cellulitis of the head or neck in young children is commonly caused by *H. influenzae* (Chapter 241). Buccal, orbital, or periorbital cellulitis may represent a primary infection or may be associated with underlying ear or sinus disease. A characteristic bluish purple color may be present when the cheek is involved. *H. influenzae* type b cellulitis is an invasive infection that may progress to form an abscess or may spread to the meninges. *H. influenzae* rarely causes cellulitis in adults but should be considered in the differential diagnosis of cellulitis of the head, neck, and chest.

Epiglottitis. Epiglottitis is a serious illness that generally has an abrupt onset. Fever, sore throat, and dysphagia with drooling develop, usually in a child 2 to 5 years of age. Stridor with respiratory distress may soon follow, so this condition must be treated as an emergency (Chapter 237). When acute epiglottitis is suspected, the child should be taken quickly to an operating room. There a lateral radiograph of the neck to demonstrate swelling of the epiglottis may be performed to confirm the diagnosis, followed by direct visualization under conditions in which intubation or tracheotomy to secure the airway can be performed at once if necessary. If examination confirms the diagnosis of acute epiglottitis, immediate elective intubation is preferable to observation. Tracheotomy is not needed in most cases because the endotracheal tube can be left in place for several days until the soft tissue swelling resolves during antibiotic treatment. Epiglottitis may occur in adults but is much less common than in children and usually less severe.

Pyarthrosis. Although septic arthritis is less common than the other forms of invasive infection discussed, *H. influenzae* was the leading cause of pyarthrosis in children from 6 months to 2 years of age, before the recent introduction of the conjugate vaccine (Chapter 203). Involvement of a single large, weight-bearing joint is typical. Associated osteomyelitis is rare.

Infection at Other Sites. Pyogenic local infections (e.g., cholecystitis and osteomyelitis) occasionally are caused by *H. influenzae.* Such infections are clinically indistinguishable from those caused by more common bacterial pathogens. *H. influenzae* is found occasionally in the vaginal flora, giving rise to cases of endometritis, salpingitis, postpartum bacteremia, or neonatal infection that can mimic streptococcal group B sepsis. Despite the high frequency of bacteremias caused by this organism, *H. influenzae* endocarditis is rare.

Diagnosis

Recovery of the organism by culture from the blood or cerebrospinal fluid, or from a normally sterile body site such as the pleural cavity or a joint, provides definitive evidence of infection. The possible significance of respiratory isolates must be evaluated in light of clinical findings. When *H. influenzae* is isolated from purulent sputum, it should be regarded as a potential rather than a proven pathogen; the natural history of the disease and the response to antibiotic treatment may indicate its significance in individual patients.

Gram stain of the cerebrospinal fluid (Color Plate VIII-8) correlates with culture results in about 70% of meningitis cases; the other 30% consist of false-negative and false-positive results in roughly equal numbers. Soluble type b capsular antigen can be detected in body fluids by latex agglutination or staphylococcal coagglutination tests. Detection of *H. influenzae* type b by one of these means may be diagnostically useful in cases of meningitis in which the Gram stain result is inconclusive or in which antibiotics were started before cultures were taken. However, even these modern tests yield approximately 25% false-negative results and occasional false-positive findings.

Treatment

H. influenzae is likely to be sensitive in vitro to a variety of antimicrobial agents, including β-lactams, chloramphenicol, tetracyclines, rifampin, sulfonamides, and trimethoprim-sulfamethoxazole (Chapter 231). Ampicillin was reliably effective until 1974, when plasmid-mediated resistance appeared. Since then, these β-lactamase–producing strains have proliferated worldwide. Although wide local variations exist, the overall incidence of ampicillin resistance in the United States has risen to about one third, with a range from 20% to 40%. Type b strains are about twice as likely to be resistant as non–type b isolates. Chloramphenicol, cefamandole, cefuroxime, cefotaxime, ceftriaxone, tetracycline, rifampin, and trimethoprim-sulfamethoxazole usually remain effective, but up to 2% of clinical isolates show resistance to one or more of these first-line drugs. Erythromycin, cephalexin, and sulfisoxazole are less active.

These findings have important implications for treatment. The rate of resistance is high enough in all areas that ampicillin alone should not be used for treatment of serious *Haemophilus* infections. Current practice favors use of a third-generation cephalosporin such as cefotaxime, 200 mg/kg/day divided into doses every 6 hours, or ceftriaxone, 75 to 100 mg/kg/day once daily or divided into doses every 12 hours for meningitis (dose not to exceed 4 g/day) as first-line treatment for invasive *Haemophilus* infections in the United States (Chapter 239). The combination of ampicillin, 200 to 400 mg/kg/day, plus chloramphenicol, 100 mg/kg/day, remains appropriate as an alternative, but clinicians and microbiologists must be alert for possible multidrug-resistant strains that could cause treatment failure.

For localized infections such as otitis, sinusitis, or mastoiditis, the β-lactam agents ampicillin, amoxicillin, or amoxicillin plus clavulanic acid usually provide safe and effective treatment. For patients allergic to penicillins or not responding to treatment, alternatives are available in trimethoprim-sulfamethoxazole, a series of new oral cephalosporins, erythromycin plus sulfonamide, and macrolides such as azithromycin and clarithromycin. These drugs are usually effective against both β-lactamase–negative and β-lactamase–positive strains. Some failures must be expected with any antibiotic regimen.

Patients with meningitis who remain febrile or suffer a recurrence of fever during treatment may have a complication such as a subdural effusion, drug fever, or nosocomial infection. Provided the organism does not possess primary resistance to the antibiotic used, persistent fever is usually due to causes other than antibiotic failure.

Prevention

Vaccination. Because *H. influenzae* infection is very common in infants and young children, much effort had been expended to develop an effective vaccine. Unfortunately, various earlier PRP vaccines failed to induce protective antibody levels reliably in children less than 18 months of age, the very group that most needs protection. The strategy of conjugating PRP to a protein such as tetanus or diphtheria toxoid has been more successful, conferring 80% to 90% protection against invasive *H. influenzae* disease. It also reduces acquisition of *H. influenzae* type b colonization but will not rapidly terminate carriage of organisms by colonized individuals. Four conjugate vaccines (PRP-T, HbOC, PRP-OMPC, PRP-D) have been licensed. The Public Health Service Immunization Practices Advisory Committee presently recommends that all children receive conjugate vaccine at 2, 4, and 6 months of age, with a booster dose at 12 to 15 months. Conjugate vaccines should not be considered to double as an immunization against either tetanus or diphtheria, even though they contain toxoids; the normal schedule for diphtheria and tetanus immunization should be followed (see Appendix—Adult Immunization in the United States).

Although the vaccines are very effective, cases of infection do occur in vaccinated children. The vaccine immunity may be less effective when used in the neonatal period, with low–birth-weight infants, and in some individuals with HIV infection. Although the *H. influenzae* type b polysaccharide has stimulated replication of HIV in vitro and the vaccine may be less effective in some patients infected with HIV, it should still be considered for this population.

The new polysaccharide-protein conjugate vaccines are immunogenic for patients with Hodgkin's disease, patients undergoing splenectomy, and some adults with HIV infection. Therefore vaccination of adults known to be at higher than normal risk of infection may be considered.

Chemoprophylaxis. Secondary prevention after an index case is much less of an issue in the era of vaccine use. It will probably be used only in outbreaks where vaccination status is unknown, in unvaccinated populations, and in children in an immunocompromised condition. It has been known that children less than 5 years of age who live in the same house or attend the same day care center as an individual who has an index case of invasive *H. influenzae* type b infection are at somewhat increased risk of developing this disease during the next few days (coprimary cases) or weeks (secondary cases). The attack rate in this age-group was as high as 5% before the advent of effective vaccines, which is actually higher than the known risk for development of meningococcal infection in contacts of a patient with meningococcal disease. A short course of rifampin may protect these children and may eradicate the carrier state. Prophylaxis with rifampin, 600 mg orally twice daily for 2 days, is nonetheless recommended for both child and adult family members if there are any unvaccinated or immunocompromised children less than 4 years of age living in the same household, or children younger than 2 years old attending day care, in the exposed group. This form of attempted prophylaxis may also be given to children exposed to actual cases (not carriers) in day care centers where children have not received vaccinations.

INFECTIONS CAUSED BY OTHER *HAEMOPHILUS* SPECIES

Little is known about specific host defense mechanisms against *Haemophilus* species other than *H. influenzae*. Under most circumstances these species appear to be much less virulent, yet paradoxically they cause infective endocarditis more commonly than either typeable or untypeable *H. influenzae*. They are sometimes involved in polymicrobial infections arising from oral, respiratory, gut, or genitourinary flora and can act as opportunistic pathogens in compromised hosts.

Haemophilus parainfluenzae

Bacteremia with the *H. parainfluenzae* organism has been associated with endocarditis, pneumonia, epiglottitis, meningitis, pharyngitis, and arthritis. The organism has been recovered from dental and brain abscesses. *H. parainfluenzae* causes the subacute form of endocarditis; patients may have no history of underlying heart disease. A significant feature of these cases is development of large vegetations, giving rise to a fairly high frequency of major arterial embolization.

Haemophilus aphrophilus and Haemophilus paraphrophilus

The species *H. aphrophilus* and *H. paraphrophilus* have been recovered in a variety of infections, including endocarditis, otitis media, sinusitis, laryngoepiglottitis, arthritis, peritonitis, meningitis, pneumonia, empyema, bacteremia, and osteomyelitis. They also have been isolated from brain abscesses and wound infections. An association with malignancy has been noted in approximately one fourth of the reported cases of *H. aphrophilus* infection.

Haemophilus aegyptius

The name *H. aegyptius* is applied to strains of *H. influenzae* isolated from the conjunctival sac, where they may cause an acute contagious conjunctivitis. They are indistinguishable from *H. influenzae* by routine microbiologic tests; special biochemical tests show that they belong in biotype III.

The syndrome of epidemic purpura fulminans in Brazilian children, associated with antecedent purulent conjunctivitis, has been named *Brazilian purpuric fever*. *H. aegyptius* was isolated from the blood of a high proportion of cases; these strains carried a plasmid not found in isolates from the conjunctivae of children who did not have the septicemia syndrome. A Brazilian study group has concluded that *H. aegyptius* probably causes this syndrome. The onset of *Haemophilus* septicemia follows 3 to 15 days after onset of conjunctivitis, by which time the ocular finding may have resolved. The disease carries a very high fatality rate.

Haemophilus ducreyi

Chancroid is a sexually transmitted disease characterized by painful, sharply demarcated, nonindurated genital ulceration (Chapters 244 and 265). Clinical disease usually appears 2 to 5 days after exposure. Initially, a tender papule forms; this lesion then becomes pustular and ulcerates. A single ulcer is most common, but several lesions may occur. Regional lymphadenitis that is usually unilateral and painful and sometimes involves the overlying skin is common. Chancroid can easily be confused with primary syphilis, herpes genitalis, or lymphogranuloma venereum. The diagnosis is confirmed by demonstration of *H. ducreyi* on smear and culture from the primary lesion or the secondary bubo. Gram-stained preparations should show gram-negative coccobacilli in chains or in a "school of fish" pattern. Culture of material taken from the ulcer or aspirated from the bubo should be placed on supplemented agars, incubated for 14 to 21 days, and subcultured at intervals. Because patients may contract syphilis simultaneously with chancroid, serologic characteristics should be checked after treatment. Genital ulcers promote transmission of HIV; thus chancroid may play a significant role in the epidemiology of AIDS in high-prevalence areas.

Treatment

Ampicillin has been used more than any other antibiotic for treatment of these infections, usually with good results despite the fact that ampicillin-resistant strains of *H. aphrophilus* and *H. paraphrophilus* are common. For endocarditis caused by one of these species, treatment with high-dose ampicillin for 3 to 4 weeks is usually effective, but some cases can be cured only by longer courses and/or valve replacement. However, ceftriaxone has become the drug of choice for serious infections, particularly endocarditis. Overall mortality rate for endocarditis caused by these organisms is presently about 15%. Addition of an aminoglycoside could result in synergistic antibacterial action, but the potential benefit of combined therapy has not been validated in clinical practice. Unfortunately, it is technically difficult to perform antibiotic sensitivity tests and bactericidal assays on these fastidious, slow-growing organisms. Chancroid is effectively treated with ceftriaxone, 250 mg IM in a single dose, or erythromycin, 500 mg qid PO for 7 days, or ciprofloxacin, 500 mg bid PO for 3 days. Alternatives are trimethoprim-sulfamethoxazole or amoxicillin and clavulanic acid. Aspiration of a bubo may be therapeutically useful in that it prevents spontaneous rupture and drainage.

Prevention

Most *Haemophilus* species other than *H. influenzae* cause human infection too infrequently to require any specific preventive measures. Identification and treatment of infections with potentially invasive strains may help to limit their spread. Use of a condom should prevent transmission of *H. ducreyi*.

BIBLIOGRAPHY

Barbour ML, Mayon-White RT, Coles C et al: The impact of conjugate vaccine on carriage of *Haemophilus influenzae. J Infect Dis* 171:93-98, 1995.

Bieger RC, Brewer NS, Washington JA II: *Haemophilus aphrophilus:* a microbiologic and clinical review and report of 42 cases, *Medicine* 57:345, 1978.

Brazilian Purpuric Fever Study Group: *Haemophilus aegyptius* bacteremia in Brazilian purpuric fever, *Lancet* 2:757, 1987.

Casadevall A et al: *Haemophilus influenzae* type b bacteremia in adults with AIDS and at risk for AIDS, *Am J Med* 92:587, 1992.

Chunn CJ et al: *Haemophilus parainfluenzae* infective endocarditis, *Medicine* 56:99, 1977.

Coll-Vincent B, Suris K, Lopez-Soto A et al: *Haemophilus paraphrophilus* endocarditis: case report and review, *Clin Infect Dis* 20:1381-1383, 1995.

Dajani AS, Asmar BI, Thirumoorthi MC: Systemic *Haemophilus influenzae* disease: an overview, *J Pediatr* 94:355, 1979.

Daum RS et al: Epidemiology, pathogenesis, and prevention of *Haemophilus influenzae* disease, *J Infect Dis* 165(suppl 1):1, 1992.

Doern GV: National collaborative study of the prevalence of antimicrobial resistance among clinical isolates of *Haemophilus influenzae, Antimicrob Agents Chemother* 32:180, 1988.

Farley MM et al: Invasive *Haemophilus influenzae* disease in adults: a prospective, population-based surveillance, *Ann Intern* Med 116:806, 1992.

Granoff DM: *Haemophilus influenzae* type b in a day care center: relationship of nasopharyngeal carriage to development of anticapsular antibody, *Pediatrics* 65:65, 1980.

Hand WL: *Haemophilus* species. In Mandell GL, Douglas RG Jr, Bennett JE, editors: *Principles and practice of infectious diseases,* ed 4, New York, 1995, Wiley.

Immunization Practices Advisory Committee: Recommendations of the Immunization Practices Advisory Committee (ACIP), *MMWR* (40:No. RR-1 and No. RR-12), 1991.

Kniskern PF, Marburg S, Ellis RW: *Haemophilus influenzae* type b conjugate vaccines, *Pharm Biotechnol* 6:673-694, 1995.

Moxon ER: *Haemophilus influenzae.* In Mandell GL, Douglas RG Jr, Bennett JE, editors: *Principles and practice of infectious diseases,* ed 4, New York, 1995, Wiley.

Moxon ER, Kroll JS: Type b capsular polysaccharide as a virulence factor of *Haemophilus influenzae, Vaccine* 6:113, 1988.

Schlamm HT, Yancovitz SR: *Haemophilus influenzae* pneumonia in young adults with AIDS, ARC, or risk of AIDS, *Am J Med* 86:11, 1989.

Spagnuolo PJ: *Haemophilus influenzae* meningitis: the spectrum of diseases in adults, *Medicine* 61:74, 1982.

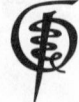

CHAPTER

267 Infections Caused by *Campylobacter* and *Helicobacter* Species

Jean-Paul Butzler

In the last decade certain members of the genus *Campylobacter* have emerged as a cause of human disease. Frequent in animals, particularly in ovines and bovines, campylobacteriosis has been known for more than 40 years as a veterinary disease. The first cases in humans, in a milk-borne outbreak, were described in 1946 by Levy, and organisms resembling *Campylobacter jejuni* were seen in blood cultures from several of the victims. *Campylobacter fetus* ssp. *fetus* was first found in humans by Vinzent, who isolated it from the blood of three pregnant women hospitalized because of fever of unknown origin. In 1957, King was the first to link *C. jejuni* with enteritis in humans, but her observations were based on only a few cases. The reason for this paucity of reports was that the selective culturing techniques necessary for the isolation of *Campylobacter* were not known at that time. It was not until 1972 that the first successful fecal isolations were reported in Belgium. This was the breakthrough that led to the discovery that *C. jejuni* enteritis is a common disease. The pathology caused by *C. fetus* ssp. *fetus* differs from that caused by *C. jejuni. C. fetus* ssp. *fetus* nearly always attacks debilitated individuals; *C. jejuni* is the most common cause of bacterial diarrhea.

Eight *Campylobacter* species of clinical importance have now been described (Table 267-1). *C. jejuni* and *Campylobacter coli* are by far the species most frequently isolated from humans, mostly with enteric disease. These species will therefore be discussed in this review. Since they are almost identical in behavior and epidemiology,

Table 267-1 *Campylobacter* species of clinical importance

APPROVED NAME	SITE ISOLATED	PATHOGENICITY
Campylobacter fetus ssp. *fetus*	Blood, various other body fluids	Systemic campylobacteriosis in immunocompromised patients
Campylobacter jejuni	Feces	Acute enterocolitis
Campylobacter coli	Feces	Acute enterocolitis
Campylobacter lari	Feces	Acute enterocolitis
Campylobacter upsaliensis	Feces	Acute enterocolitis
Campylobacter hyointestinalis	Feces	Acute enterocolitis
Campylobacter jejuni ssp. *doylei*	Feces	Acute enterocolitis
*Campylobacter butzleri**	Feces	Acute enterocolitis

*This species has been shown to belong to the genus *Arcobacter.*

wherever the name *C. jejuni* is used in this review the enteric *Campylobacter* species are implicated as well.

PATHOPHYSIOLOGY

All *Campylobacter* organisms, including *C. jejuni,* have a flagellum at one or both ends and are able to reach and attach to the mucosal surface. The spiral shape of *Campylobacter* organisms enables them to "corkscrew" their way through thick mucus. Specific outer membrane proteins have been found in *C. jejuni* that bind to epithelial cells, but intact functioning flagella appear to be necessary for cell invasion. *Campylobacter* organisms, like other gram-negative bacteria, possess lipopolysaccharides in their cell wall, so tissues are exposed to damage from endotoxin. Cholera-like toxins are produced by many strains but in small amounts. Toxins with cytopathic activity have also been detected in supernatant fluids of *C. jejuni* cultures. The significance of these various toxins is in doubt, because strains producing no detectable enterotoxin and minimal cytotoxic activity are fully virulent in human volunteers, and patients do not develop neutralizing antibodies to the toxins. The frequent finding of dysenteric stools suggests that mucosal damage due to an invasive process analogous to that seen in shigellosis is important in the pathogenesis. Indeed, the fact that many patients have erythrocytes and leukocytes in their stools suggests colonic involvement. In cases of *Campylobacter* colitis, sigmoidoscopy has shown an inflamed, friable, edematous mucosa, and rectal biopsies show decreased numbers of epithelial cells with irregular spacing and reduced mucus production, crypt abscesses, and infiltration of the lamina propria with neutrophils, plasma cells, and lymphocytes. In some cases the appearance is indistinguishable from that of an acute ulcerative colitis or Crohn's disease. *C. jejuni* bacteremia occasionally occurs, and in such cases the organism is usually isolated both from blood and feces.

There are several reasons for the scarcity of reports on *C. jejuni* septicemia: the unlikelihood of growing *Campylobacter* by routine blood culture techniques; the rarity with which blood from patients with enteritis, even when patients are febrile, is sent in for culture; and the bactericidal activity on *C. jejuni* of normal human serum. Persons with hypogammaglobulinemia are unusually susceptible to *C. jejuni,* just as they are to infection with *Giardia lamblia* and *Salmonella.* The tendency seems to be greater for *C. fetus* ssp. *fetus* than *C. jejuni* to cause bacteremia. One explanation is that *C. fetus* ssp. *fetus* is resistant to the bactericidal activity of normal human serum. The experimental oral or intragastric inoculation of *C. jejuni*–susceptible animals occasionally results in systemic spread, but the bacteremia is transient. The prodromal febrile illness, often with rigors, suffered by many patients with *Campylobacter* enteritis is in keeping with the concept of early bacteremia.

The brisk antibody response shown by infected patients also indicates an invasive process. Specific IgG, IgM, and IgA antibodies appear in the serum, and IgA antibodies appear locally in intestinal secretions in response to infection. Those specific for flagellar and surface proteins confer protection from reinfection with homologous strains and presumptively a range of other strains, because children in developing countries develop general immunity after only a few infections. This immunity is reflected by a progressive rise of specific serum IgA antibody during early childhood. This may explain why in developing countries where *C. jejuni* is hyperendemic, rates of infection and illness due to this organism decline with age. Studies with volunteers have demonstrated short specific immunity to *C. jejuni*.

With regard to the minimum infective dose of *C. jejuni*, several factors tend to suggest that it is about 10^5. First, only 500 organisms (in milk) are needed to initiate illness. Second, below a dose of 10^4 organisms, illness is infrequent in volunteers. Third, outbreaks did result from contaminated food vehicles at ambient temperatures and atmosphere. Probably the infectivity of *C. jejuni* lies somewhere between that of *Shigella* (about 10^2) and *Salmonella* (about 10^8), but it must be emphasized that in addition to possible strain variation, such variables as the type of food or drink containing the organisms and host factors such as the contents of the stomach may greatly influence the size of the infective dose.

CAMPYLOBACTER JEJUNI INFECTIONS
Clinical Presentations and Differential Diagnosis

Acute enterocolitis, the most common presentation of *C. jejuni* infection, can affect persons of all ages (Chapter 242). *C. jejuni* has been found in virtually every country where it has been sought. Not all *Campylobacter* infections produce symptoms. Asymptomatic excreters commonly occur among the close contacts of infected patients, although their incidence in the total population is less than 1%. The signs and symptoms of a *C. jejuni* infection are not distinct, and it is not possible to differentiate infection by this pathogen from illnesses caused by other pathogens. Symptoms may last for only 24 hours and may be indistinguishable from those associated with viral gastroenteritis. The incubation period is commonly 2 to 5 days, but estimates have extended up to 10 days. In about half of the patients, diarrhea is preceded by a febrile period with malaise, headache, myalgias, and abdominal pain; fever of 104° F (40° C) associated with confusion or delirium may be present. The stools rapidly become liquid and foul-smelling, then watery; fresh blood may appear by the third day. Fecal samples examined microscopically show an inflammatory exudate with leukocytes, and it is usually possible to see numerous campylobacters, owing to their characteristic morphology. Vomiting is rare. The diarrhea persists about 2 or 3 days, but abdominal pain and discomfort may persist after the diarrhea has stopped. The abdominal pain is typically periumbilical or epigastric, intermittent, and colicky, and it may radiate to the right iliac fossa or the lower abdomen. Therefore differential diagnosis with appendicitis can sometimes be difficult, and a number of patients are admitted to a surgical ward because of suspected appendicitis. Indeed, *C. jejuni* may cause pseudoappendicitis. In most cases, the removed appendix is normal. Enlarged mesenteric nodes (mesenteric adenitis) and terminal ileitis may be responsible for these symptoms.

In a significant proportion of patients, the stools contain fresh blood, pus, or mucus, and this suggests that colorectal inflammation is not uncommon in *Campylobacter* infection. Laparotomy, sigmoidoscopy, colonoscopy, and postmortem examinations—carried out on patients who have succumbed from the disease—have shown that mucosal damage may occur during the course of this infection. The pathologic features may vary from no gross changes of the mucosal bowel to inflammation and edema of the full thickness of the bowel, hemorrhagic lesions, or even frank necrosis, gangrene, and perforation.

Thus the pathologic findings on rectal biopsy are nonspecific, and the clinical presentation and radiographic findings are also nondiagnostic. This clinical picture and the propensity of *Campylobacter* infection in young adults make differential diagnosis with ulcerative colitis sometimes difficult. Since treatment with steroids can have serious consequences, it is imperative that the correct diagnosis be established. Crohn's disease may also be difficult to distinguish from *C. jejuni* colitis, in which the segmental mucosal edema, loss of vascular pattern with ulceration, and cobblestone appearance found may be identical to the lesions observed in Crohn's disease. Histologic ex-

amination of mucosal biopsy specimens from infected patients has shown depletion of goblet cells, infiltration of polymorphonuclear leukocytes in the crypt walls with crypt abscesses, and mixed inflammatory infiltrate in the lamina propria comprising polymorphs and plasma cells.

Surgeons can be confronted with *Campylobacter* colitis for several reasons.

1. It may mimic an intraabdominal emergency such as intestinal intussusception, appendicitis, or cholecystitis; some of these patients are operated on unnecessarily, because the abdominal pain is followed only later by diarrhea, or the diarrhea may be totally absent.
2. It may mimic Crohn's disease or ulcerative colitis; therefore *Campylobacter* should be excluded as a cause in "relapses" of inflammatory bowel disease.
3. It can be associated with a "real and true" surgical emergency such as acute appendicitis, acute cholecystitis, or mesenteric lymphadenitis.

C. jejuni colitis may induce toxic megacolon; it may be the cause of massive lower gastrointestinal hemorrhage; or *Campylobacter* colitis may be complicated by bowel necrosis. Finally, *Campylobacter* colitis may mimic colon cancer during barium enema examination; colonoscopy of these patients may reveal a bleeding, ulcerated, mass-like lesion in the transverse colon attributable to *Campylobacter*, but mimicking carcinoma of the transverse colon. *C. jejuni* may cause infectious proctitis in homosexual men.

The incidence of *C. jejuni* bacteremia has increased; it is no longer a "bacteriologic curiosity." *C. jejuni* bacteremia is probably more frequent than is clinically suspected, since extension to the blood is part of the pathogenesis in the early stages of the disease. There are a number of reasons for the scarcity of reports on septicemia, as discussed earlier. *C. jejuni* is isolated more frequently from the blood of enteric patients if the sample is taken in the early stages of the disease and if the cultures are incubated under the right conditions. Strains of *C. fetus*, which are intrinsically resistant to killing by serum, are more likely to be isolated from the blood and other extraintestinal sites. The most common form of *C. fetus* infection is a pure septicemia without dissemination and splenomegaly. *C. fetus* chiefly attacks debilitated patients with impaired defenses against infection. The pathology caused by *C. fetus* is extremely varied and includes pyogenic meningitis and meningoencephalitis, abortion, endocarditis, thrombophlebitis, septic arthritis, and icterus associated with hepatosplenomegaly. Other systemic manifestations of *C. jejuni* infection include meningitis and septic arthritis. In pregnant women, *C. jejuni* bacteremia has potentially severe consequences to the fetus and should therefore be treated with antimicrobial drugs. Some patients develop erythema nodosum or reactive arthritis after *Campylobacter* enteritis, regardless of whether they possess HLA-B27. Infection with *C. jejuni* often precedes the Guillain-Barré syndrome and is associated with axonal degeneration, slow recovery, and severe residual disability. Although the pathogenesis of this association is not understood, it is suggested that antibodies directed against *Campylobacter* may cross-react with human peripheral nerve myelin proteins. Furthermore, Chinese paralytic syndrome, an acute neurologic disease similar to Guillain-Barré syndrome in northern China, is also associated with *Campylobacter* infection based on serologic studies. Hypogammaglobulinemic and AIDS patients develop severe, persistent, and relapsing infections due to *C. jejuni*. Therefore early antimicrobial therapy is needed in these patients. Although infection with *Campylobacter* occurs frequently with HIV disease, relapse, systemic toxicity, and septicemia are less common than with salmonellosis.

Diagnosis

Campylobacter enteritis can be readily diagnosed by direct microscopic examination of fresh feces. With either a dark-field examination or phase-contrast optical system, campylobacters can be seen and distinguished from other organisms by virtue of their extremely rapid darting and spinning motions. The introduction of selective media has made the diagnosis of campylobacter enteritis a simple procedure for a clinical microbiologist. It is essential to incubate the cultures under conditions of reduced oxygen tension, ideally 5%. The thermophilic nature of *C. jejuni* means that cultures can be incubated to best advantage at 42° C. Although they may also grow well at 37° C, incubation at the higher temperature provides increased selection and quicker results. *Campylobacter* plates should be examined at 24 to 48 hours for small or mucoid, gray, nonhemolytic colonies. If a suspicious colony is seen, identification begins with a Gram stain. *C. jejuni* is a gram-negative bacillus, which can appear as short curves, S shapes, gull-wing shapes, and long spirals. When the Gram stain appears to be *Campylobacter*-positive, oxidase and catalase tests should be used to confirm the diagnosis; biotyping and serotyping complete further identification.

The disease can also be diagnosed serologically. The great majority of patients develop antibody to *Campylobacter* during the first few days of illness; the antibody level quickly reaches a maximum titer and then declines during the ensuing few months. In culture-negative cases of *C. jejuni* infection, for example in reactive arthritis and erythema nodosum, serologic diagnosis is useful. A complement-fixation test is commercially available.

Management

In general, *Campylobacter* enteritis carries a good prognosis, and the isolation of campylobacters from stools does not warrant chemotherapy. By the time a bacteriologic diagnosis is made, the patient is usually recovering. In the absence of chemotherapy the feces of patients remain positive for about 2 to 7 weeks after the illness. Patients with mild cases excrete the organism for only a few days; occasionally, patients may excrete the organism for longer periods. Antimicrobial treatment is indicated in patients with prolonged disease with severe symptoms, high fevers, or bloody stools; in relapses during pregnancy; and in immunocompromised persons. The clinical course of *C. jejuni* diarrhea in AIDS patients very often requires long-term treatment.

Erythromycin has been advocated as the agent of choice for the treatment of *Campylobacter* enteritis. It has excellent in vitro activity, low toxicity, a fairly narrow antibacterial spectrum, and relatively low cost. Resistant strains are on the whole rare and almost confined to *C. coli*. It probably matters little what preparation of erythromycin is given (other than enteric-coated pills). There are theoretical reasons for favoring the stearate, at least for adults. Apart from being acid-resistant and stable, it is incompletely absorbed, so there is the chance of a contact action in the bowel lumen, as well as a systemic action in the blood. A dosage of 500 mg twice daily for 5 days has proved satisfactory in practice; higher doses of the stearate are liable to cause acute abdominal pain. Erythromycin ethylsuccinate at 40 mg/kg/day in divided doses is recommended for children. The newer macrolides (roxithromycin, rokitamycin, and clarithromycin) may have a future because of their pharmacologic advantages. Until now there has not been sufficient evidence to prove that these drugs are superior to erythromycin and they may be better tolerated. Several clinical trials have shown that ciprofloxacin (and other fluoroquinolones) is an efficient treatment for *Campylobacter* enteritis. These drugs are also active against other causes of dysentery and constitute a sensible treatment for enteritis of unknown etiology, as well as for cases in which cultural confirmation of the causative agent is pending. Unfortunately, as the use of fluoroquinolones has expanded (especially in veterinary practice), the rate of resistance of *Campylobacter* organisms to these agents has increased. Sensitivity tests should be conducted because erythromycin and tetracycline resistance have been described. In the industrialized countries, dehydration caused by *C. jejuni* is infrequent, but fluid and electrolyte replacement are sometimes necessary in infected infants. The best treatment for *C. jejuni* infections in developing countries could well prove to be different.

Factors such as low socioeconomic status and malnutrition may determine the severity of a *C. jejuni* infection and its great prevalence in very young children. Vomiting and watery diarrhea are frequent, and sometimes oral rehydration is required in children. Antibiotics should be reserved for very severe cases. It is certain that education and better hygiene have far greater roles in reducing infections than do antibiotics.

HELICOBACTER PYLORI INFECTION

Today there is overwhelming evidence that *Helicobacter pylori* is the major etiologic agent of chronic active (type B) gastritis and that it may further predispose to peptic ulceration. This evidence includes histologic observations, the effect of therapeutic eradication of the organism on the underlying inflammation, challenge studies in human volunteers, experimental models, and possible pathogenetic mechanisms. Recent developments in *H. pylori* research indicate progress in the detection of subtypes of *H. pylori* that may be responsible for the wide variability in clinical outcome; the most severe clinical outcome is maltoma (mucosa-associated lymphoid tissue lymphoma) and gastric cancer.

Pathophysiology

Studies from Australia, Canada, the United States, and Europe have shown a close correlation between *H. pylori* colonization of the gastric mucosa and clinical histologic gastritis. Evidence exists that *H. pylori* causes the gastritis and is not simply an opportunist harmlessly occupying a favorable ecologic niche. In infected patients the bacteria colonize the surface gastric epithelium (protected by gastric mucus) in enormous numbers. Colonization is associated with thinning of the epithelium and the presence of polymorphonuclear leukocytes. Sections of gastric biopsy material show that the organisms lie in the mucus layers covering the epithelium and on the epithelial surface at the intracellular junctions of the mucus-secreting cells. This observation has led to the hypothesis that *H. pylori* has a spiral morphology that enables it to move efficiently in a viscous environment and that the bacteria are attracted to the epithelial surface by the chemotactic influence of preferred metabolites diffusing from the tissue. *H. pylori* is susceptible to acid, but bacterial cells are protected from gastric acid by the mucus layer in which they reside; they are also protected physiologically by a powerful urease that splits transudated plasma urea into ammonia and carbon dioxide. The inflammation produced probably benefits the bacteria by increasing the transudation of nutrients, but how the bacteria cause the inflammation is unknown. They are not invasive, so their action must be mediated indirectly through soluble substances. Some strains produce a vacuolating cytotoxin, and there is evidence that the urease is toxic. The vacuolating cytotoxin has been genetically characterized and is now widely accepted as a major factor involved in ulcerogenicity. The role of *H. pylori* in peptic ulceration is well established by a large number of clinical trials that show the cure of ulcer disease after the cure of infection. On the other hand, the pathogenesis of ulcer formation is still incompletely understood.

Laboratory and Other Diagnostic Tests

The diagnosis of *H. pylori*–associated gastritis can be made either by histologic or microbiologic examination of gastric biopsy specimens. Several staining methods (Warthin-starry silver stain, hematoxylin-eosin, Gram stain, Giemsa, or fluorescent labeling with acridine orange) have been investigated and found effective for identifying campylobacter organisms. Isolation and identification of *H. pylori* by culture methods are easily achieved, providing that appropriate transport and incubation conditions are respected. Sufficient decontamination of the endoscopes and the biopsy channels must be performed to avoid bacterial outgrowth by contaminants. Three to 6 days are necessary for culture because of the slow growth rate of this bacterium. *H. pylori* is a gram-negative, oxidase- and catalase-positive curved or spiral rod that requires a microaerophilic environment for growth. The most peculiar characteristic of this organism is its ability to produce a large amount of urease. This property can be exploited as a rapid presumptive test for diagnosis and may be proposed as a reliable alternative test to culture and direct examination when laboratory facilities are not available. Because endoscopies consume considerable resources, noninvasive tests could provide an alternative, or at least a confirmatory, means of diagnosis. These tests are available in the form of serologic tests and the urease breath test. In the latter, urea-incorporating isotopic carbon is given to the patient and the output of the isotope in CO_2 is measured in the breath; the urease activity of *H. pylori* causes high output. Current enzyme-linked immunosorbent assay (ELISA) techniques are sufficiently sensitive and specific to monitor patients who come to gastroenterology clinics and to eliminate antibody-negative patients from endoscopic investigation, unless they are receiving nonsteroidal antiinflammatory drug therapy or have symptoms of reflux. In follow-up of antimicrobial chemotherapy, repeated endoscopies are rarely indicated. A carefully performed and well-validated noninvasive test can be relied on in these two groups of patients.

Management

In vitro antimicrobial work continues to be essential in the search for the most appropriate treatment. In vitro *H. pylori* is susceptible to a wide range of antimicrobial agents, including β-lactams, quinolones, erythromycin, and tetracycline. Vancomycin, sulfamethoxazole, and trimethoprim are not inhibitory. *H. pylori* is susceptible to bismuth but not to cimetidine, sucralfate, or carbenoxolone. Obviously, antagonists of the histamine H$_2$ receptor are effective in promoting ulcer healing. However, this therapy does not promote healing of the antral gastritis or eradication of *H. pylori*. Residual organisms and the associated gastritis or duodenitis are thought to be responsible for recurrence of the ulcer. Several studies have shown that *H. pylori* was cleared by bismuth salts in 50% to 70% of patients; however, relapse was extremely common, and long-term clearance was achieved in only 30% of patients. Relapse usually occurred within 3 months. Because of side-effects and poor compliance, therapies using a proton-pump inhibitor with an antibiotic were evaluated. The regimens used were a 2-week course of omeprazole 20 to 40 mg twice daily plus amoxicillin 1 g twice daily or 500 mg four times daily; and a 2-week course of omeprazole 40 mg once in the morning and clarithromycin 500 mg three times daily. The eradication rates did not surpass 75% and were considered insufficient. Encouraging results of several pilot studies showed that 1-week low-dose therapies comprising omeprazole, clarithromycin, and a nitroimidazole or amoxicillin allow a cure of the infection in more than 90% of patients. These short-term triple therapies may be the treatment of the future, but monitoring the resistance of *H. pylori* to the agents used is necessary.

BIBLIOGRAPHY

Bazzoli F et al: Short-term low-dose triple therapy for the eradication of *Helicobacter pylori, Eur J Gastroenterol Hepatol* 6:773, 1994.

Butzler JP et al: *Campylobacter* and *Helicobacter* infections, *Curr Opin Infect Dis* 5:80, 1992.

Butzler JP et al: Macrolides in *Campylobacter* enteritis. In Bryskier A et al, editors: *Macrolides: chemistry, pharmacology and clinical uses,* Paris, 1993, Arnette Blackwell.

Glupczynski Y et al: Surveillance of *Helicobacter pylori* resistance to antimicrobial agents in Belgium from 1989 to 1994, *Gut Suppl* 37:A56, 1995 (abstract 223).

Griffiths PL, Park RWA: Campylobacters associated with human diarrhoeal disease, *J Appl Bact* 69:281, 1990.

Kosunen TU, Mégreaud F: Diagnosis of *Helicobacter pylori, Curr Opin Gastroenterol Suppl* 11:5, 1995.

Labenz J, O'Morain C: Eradication, *Curr Opin Gastroenterol Suppl* 11:47, 1995.

Mishu Allos B, Blaser M: *Campylobacter jejuni* and the expanding spectrum of related infections, *Clin Infect Dis* 20:1092, 1995.

Sanchez R et al: Evolution of susceptibilities of *Campylobacter* spp. to quinolones and macrolides, *Antimicrob Agents Chemother* 38(9):1879, 1994.

Skirrow MB: Diseases due to *Campylobacter, Helicobacter* and related bacteria, *J Comp Path* 111(2):113, 1994.

Suerbaum S, Wadström T: Bacterial pathogenic factors, *Curr Opin Gastroenterol Suppl* 11:11, 1995.

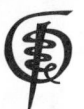

CHAPTER

268 Infections Caused by *Vibrio* Species

Mary E. Wilson, Aldo A.M. Lima, and Richard L. Guerrant

With the reemergence of cholera in the Americas for the first time in nearly 100 years and the emergence of the new, non-O1 (O139 Bengal) strain causing epidemic cholera since 1993, this most-feared epidemic disease of the nineteenth century has awakened new concerns about diagnosis, epidemiology, and control of "infections caused by vibrios." After its abrupt appearance in Peru in January 1991, 391,000 cases and nearly 4000 deaths were reported in 1991 to the Pan American Health Organization—more than the total number reported worldwide over the previous 5 years. Cholera has since become a concern throughout the Americas, with cases occurring in almost every country in North and South America (including Mexico and the United States). In addition to epidemic cholera, there are other potentially life-threatening *Vibrio* infections associated with seafood or seacoast exposure. The astute physician and knowledgeable microbiologist must sustain a high index of suspicion to promptly treat *Vibrio* infections, as is treatment often required before the microbiologic diagnosis is available (Chapter 242).

THE ORGANISMS
Classification and Characteristics

Members of the genus *Vibrio* are short, curved, gram-negative bacilli found commonly in seawater and in salt-water shellfish, fish, and crustaceans in many parts of the world. Historically, *Vibrio cholerae* O1, the organism that causes cholera, has been of primary interest to clinicians and epidemiologists, and other members of the genus were referred to as "noncholera vibrios" (NCV) or "nonagglutinable vibrios" (NAG). Subsequently, many of the NCV group were found also to be pathogenic for humans. Other members of the family Vibrionaceae include *Aeromonas* and *Plesiomonas,* which are also associated with human enteric disease.

Of the 35 recognized *Vibrio* species, at least 13 have been associated with disease in humans. In the laboratory, *Vibrio* species grow on usual media such as blood, chocolate, and Mueller-Hinton agars. They can be differentiated from Enterobacteriaceae, *Aeromonas,* and *Plesiomonas* because pathogenic *Vibrio* species are oxidase-positive and all tolerate relatively high salt concentrations and can therefore grow on thiosulfate citrate bile salts sucrose (TCBS) agar. Culture on TCBS agar is recommended whenever *Vibrio* infection is suspected. The potential human pathogens listed in Table 268-1 can be further differentiated by the ability of some species (*V. cholerae* and *Vibrio mimicus*) to grow in only trace concentrations of salt (nonhalophilic), whereas the remaining (halophilic) organisms require at least 0.5% sodium chloride to support their growth.

As would be predicted from their growth requirements in vitro, *Vibrio* species are most often isolated from environmental sources in coastal waters, although they have been found in nearly all geographic locations in the United States. Inland the organisms can survive in brackish waters. Infections caused by *Vibrio* species are more common in the warmer months of the year, when aquatic bacterial counts are highest and when people increase their exposure to seawater through recreational habits. The organisms adhere to plankton, and since mollusks and crustaceans filter seawater and retain plankton along with their associated vibrios, *Vibrio*-induced gastroenteritis is commonly associated with a history of ingestion of raw or undercooked shellfish. The seafood most commonly associated with *Vibrio* infection in the United States is raw oysters. Similarly, wound infections caused by vibrios are often associated with a history of exposure of wounds to seawater or of handling sea fish or shellfish. An increased awareness of these infections by physicians, improved iso-

Table 268-1   Clinical syndromes seen with *Vibrio* infections

	WATERY DIARRHEA	DYSENTERY	SEPTICEMIA	WOUND INFECTION	OTITIS
Nonhalophilic					
V. cholerae (O1)	++				
V. cholerae (non-O1)[a]	+	+	±	+	±
V. mimicus[a]	+	+			±
V. albensis[b]				(±)	
Halophilic					
V. parahaemolyticus	+	+	(±)	+	+
V. vulnificus (L+)[a]			++	++	±
V. alginolyticus				+	+
V. fluvialis (EF6)	+	+			
V. furnisii[c]	+				
V. damsela				+	
V. hollisae[a]	+	(±)			
V. metschnikovii			(±)		
V. cincinnatiensis[d]			(±)		
V. carchariae[e]				(±)	

++, Commonly causes life-threatening disease; +, causes disease that is usually nonfatal; ±, rarely reported; (±), one reported case.
[a]Disease is associated with the consumption of raw oysters.
[b]A single case of postoperative endophthalmitis caused by this organism is reported.
[c]Isolated from human stool specimens but not proven to be a pathogen.
[d]Associated meningitis is reported.
[e]Isolated from an infected shark bite wound.

lation techniques, and an increase in exposure to these aquatic organisms through foreign travel, consumption of raw shellfish, and water-based recreational activities have resulted in an increase in reported *Vibrio* infections over recent years. In addition, the enlarging population of immunocompromised patients, either undergoing treatment for malignancies or infected with the human immunodeficiency virus, has increased the population of individuals at risk.

Clinical manifestations of *Vibrio* infections fall into one of five categories. *V. cholerae* serogroup O1 is the cause of cholera, the profuse watery diarrheal disease that can rapidly lead to severe dehydration, shock, and death if not promptly treated with adequate rehydration (Chapter 242). The stool characteristically has few or no polymorphonuclear leukocytes and no erythrocytes. Other vibrios may also cause diarrhea, which may mimic the watery diarrhea of cholera or may present as dysentery with bloody diarrhea and fecal leukocytes on microscopic examination. Extraintestinal syndromes caused by vibrios include primary septicemia (often bacteremia), wound infections, and otitis (media or externa). As outlined in Table 268-1, infections with the different *Vibrio* species tend to manifest characteristic disease patterns. In some cases, pathogenic factors that may account for these differences in clinical manifestations have been identified. For instance, *V. cholerae* O1 is able to adhere to small intestine luminal cells and elaborate a potent secretion-inducing enterotoxin, whereas some strains of *V. parahaemolyticus* are more likely to adhere to the colonic mucosa, produce a cytotoxin, and cause local cell destruction and dysentery. The peculiar ability of *V. vulnificus* to cause septicemia may be related to its ability to survive in human serum, in contrast to other *Vibrio* species. The aggressive nature of *V. vulnificus* wound infections may relate to its potent extracellular toxins and enzymes, which cause profuse local cellular destruction. Recognition of characteristic clinical syndromes in the appropriate setting may result in earlier diagnosis and more effective treatment of the various types of *Vibrio* infections.

CHOLERA
Epidemiology

Cholera has been recognized as the cause of epidemic and endemic disease for several centuries, and as the cause of seven multinational pandemics. In the 1850s John Snow linked the development of cholera to the consumption of fecally contaminated water. The etiologic agent *(V. cholerae)* was discovered by Robert Koch in 1884 in Calcutta. Since then *V. cholerae* has been recognized as the cause of endemic disease in Bengal and of several near-global pandemics. Like other vibrios, *V. cholerae* displays flagellar (H) and somatic (O) antigens; *V. cholerae* O group 1 is the cause of cholera. This group can

exist as two biotypes, classical and El Tor, both of which can be further divided into three serotypes reflecting differences in O antigens: Ogawa (which expresses the O antigens A and B), Inaba (A and C), and Hikojima (A, B, and C). The Hikojima serotype is rare, but the other two are frequently isolated from infected humans. The two biotypes, El Tor and classical (each of which may include all three serotypes), correspond historically and clinically to human disease syndromes.

The first recognized cholera pandemic began in 1817 in India and Russia. Subsequently there were six major pandemics in the eighteenth and early nineteenth centuries. From 1883 through 1960 the classic biotype of *V. cholerae* (presumably) dominated both endemic and epidemic disease. After its discovery in 1905, the El Tor biotype caused four outbreaks between 1937 and 1958, which were confined to Indonesia. In 1961 the current outbreak of El Tor cholera began in the Celebes Islands and subsequently spread across Asia, the Middle East, Africa, and parts of Europe, constituting the seventh cholera pandemic. The El Tor biotype actually displaced the classic biotype from the endemic regions of cholera along the Ganges River and in Bangladesh. Factors favoring the spread of the El Tor biotype were a lower ratio of cases to carriers and longer viability of the organism in the environment. The classic biotype returned to Bangladesh in 1982 and has replaced El Tor as the predominant endemic strain in that area. However, the El Tor biotype continues to spread with the current pandemic. In 1991, epidemic cholera was reported in Peru, the first occurrence of the disease in South America in nearly 100 years. Since then, cholera has become endemic throughout Latin America with more than 1.3 billion cases and more than 11,000 deaths in the first 5 years. Involved countries include Ecuador, Columbia, Brazil, Bolivia, Chile, Venezuela, Mexico, Guatemala, El Salvador, Panama, Honduras, and the United States, among others. Vehicles responsible for spread of the disease have included public water supplies and sewage systems, water used for irrigation with resultant contamination of vegetables, seawater used for bathing, and fresh water crustaceans and shellfish. The nonhemolytic El Tor, Inaba *V. cholerae*, is closely related to the seventh pandemic isolates from Asia and Africa, and is quite different from the *V. cholerae* O1 isolates from the U.S. Gulf Coast noted in later discussion.

During the nineteenth century approximately 250,000 Americans died during three cholera epidemics. This was followed by a long disease-free period beginning in 1911 during which cholera was thought to be eradicated from the United States. In 1973, a sporadic case occurred in Texas from an unknown source. Between 1974 and 1985 there were three sporadic cases and 27 outbreak-related cases, including a 1978 outbreak of 11 cases in Louisiana that was attributed to the ingestion of locally harvested crabs. In 1981 there was an outbreak in Texas caused by the ingestion of contaminated rice. This was followed in 1986 by the largest recent outbreak in Louisiana, involving 18 persons and resulting in one fatality. Many of the infected individuals had recently consumed either crabs, raw oysters, or cooked shrimp.

Since 1973, the *V. cholerae* strain implicated in U.S. cholera cases has been a hemolytic toxigenic *V. cholerae* O1 serotype Inaba strain, which contains the phage VcA-3. This strain is identical to *V. cholerae* O1 strains isolated from the Gulf Coast waters; thus it is designated as the Gulf Coast strain. In 1991, however, U.S. Food and Drug Administration researchers isolated from the coastal waters in Mobile Bay, Alabama, a *V. cholerae* O1 serotype Inaba, biotype El Tor that does not contain VcA-3. This strain is identical to the seventh pandemic strain by phage type, enzyme electrophoresis, and pulse field gel electrophoresis. Although the strain has not been implicated as a cause of autochthonous cholera in the United States, the isolation from the environment indicates that the potential for spread of cholera within the United States exists. To date, cases of cholera caused by the pandemic strain have been imported by travelers or in seafood either served on airplanes or imported into the United States from countries affected by the pandemic.

The question of a reservoir for cholera between outbreaks is obscure, since no animal reservoir is known. Chronic human carriers of the disease have been documented but are rare. *V. cholerae* may actually be able to survive and multiply in the environment and may not require human transmission. Nontoxigenic O1 *V. cholerae* has been isolated from seawater and shellfish, and it may be that *V. cholerae* survives in association with marine life or in sea-water sludge. *V. cholerae* O1 produces a chitinase that may facilitate its attachment to the exoskeletons of crabs and shrimp, which contain chitin. Similar to other *Vibrio* infections, cholera is manifested primarily in the summer and early fall months, when environmental water is at its warmest. During outbreaks, water-borne fecal-oral spread is the dominant mode of transmission.

In October 1992, the eighth cholera pandemic began in the Indian subcontinent with the emergence of a novel toxigenic strain of *V. cholerae,* which does not agglutinate with the O1 antiserum but possesses the potential to cause severe disease and spread swiftly, both traits that were formerly the prerogative of the O1 serogroup of classical or El Tor cholera. This strain has been assigned a new serogroup, O139 Bengal, to indicate its initial isolation from areas along the coast of the Bay of Bengal. Studies on virulence-associated genes and proteins expressed by *V. cholerae* O139 show that this strain is likely an O antigen mutant of an El Tor strain with an array of virulence determinants typical of El Tor biotype O1, and not a non-O1 strain that acquired virulence genes by genetic transfer.

Pathophysiology

Establishment of cholera involves the ability of *V. cholerae* to pass beyond the acid environment of the stomach, to colonize the small intestine, and to produce its characteristic toxin. A pH of less than 2.4 is vibriocidal, and raising the gastric pH increases an individual's susceptibility to cholera. Thus the ingestion of *V. cholerae* with food, the use of antacids or H_2 blockers, achlorhydria for any reason, or partial gastrectomy decreases the required infective inoculum from 10^8 to 10^3 organisms.

Once past the stomach, *V. cholerae* penetrates the intestinal mucus and actively moves to the small intestinal mucosa, where it adheres and multiplies. On the brush border, the organism produces cholera toxin, which binds via its B subunit to the ganglioside GM_1 present on intestinal cells. The A subunit is then translocated into the cell, where, by ADP-ribosylating the stimulating G_s-protein, it stimulates the cellular adenylate cyclase to produce cyclic adenosine monophosphate. Cyclic adenosine monophosphate stimulates the net secretion of chloride and decreases absorption of sodium chloride by the mucosal epithelium. Prostaglandin and platelet activating factor synthesis is also stimulated by cholera toxin and likely also contributes to fluid and electrolyte secretion. The result is the loss of massive amounts of electrolytes and water into the gut lumen, leading to hypovolemic shock, metabolic acidosis, and total body potassium depletion. Hypoglycemia may occur, particularly in children, despite the fact that the mechanism for glucose absorption in the gut remains in-

tact. Manifestations of the disease are attributable to severe dehydration, metabolic acidosis, and electrolyte imbalance. Stool is isotonic, with sodium and chloride levels slightly lower and potassium concentrations slightly higher than those of serum.

The virulence of *V. cholerae* depends on both its ability to bind to intestinal mucosa and its ability to produce the enterotoxin. Antigens expressed by *V. cholerae* thought to be important for its virulence include cholera toxin, a secreted hemolysin, and the pilus TcpA, among others. TcpA has been found to facilitate attachment of the organism to intestinal mucosa, an important component of colonization. Furthermore, the ability of strains to produce cholera toxin A subunit, encoded by the gene *ctxA,* and the pilus encoded by *tcpA* are coregulated by the same protein, ToxR. Thus *toxR* expression is probably critical for the expression of virulence.

Natural infection with *V. cholerae* induces some immunity to the disease, as evidenced by the fact that in endemic regions, cholera is most common in children under 5 years of age, whereas epidemics affect all age-groups. Patients who have had cholera develop circulating antibodies to H and O antigens and to cholera toxin, although the presence of antitoxin antibodies is not well correlated with clinical immune status. The development of local immunity in the gut, with the production of *Vibrio*-specific secretory IgA by Peyer's patch lymphocytes, is more likely to be associated with protective immunity than are systemic antibodies. Indeed, the importance of local gut immunity provides the basis for recent attempts to develop an oral vaccine that protects humans against challenge with the organism.

Clinical Manifestations

Symptoms of cholera may range from an asymptomatic infection or mild diarrhea to a severe dehydrating illness, with death often occurring within hours to several days after the onset of diarrhea. Death resulting from massive fluid loss into the bowel has occurred even before the first watery stool. The syndrome usually begins as painless watery diarrhea, which soon becomes clear and odorless, with a typical "rice water" appearance (Chapter 242). Vomiting may be present, but typically there is little abdominal pain. Symptoms progress quickly because of rapid fluid losses and dehydration. Patients experience thirst and muscle cramps, and their mental status is detached or otherwise depressed. They may progress to shock within hours of the onset of symptoms. Laboratory data often reveal hyperchloremic acidosis and hemoconcentration. Hypoglycemia may occur, especially in children, and may lead to coma or seizures. Finally, either hypokalemia or hyperkalemia may be present; the former may lead to ileus or arrhythmias, and the latter is usually associated with severe acidosis and dehydration. Serious complications of cholera include renal failure secondary to hypoperfusion with acute tubular necrosis, or aspiration of vomitus.

The diagnosis of cholera can often be made on the basis of examination of the stool. Generally, few or no fecal leukocytes or erythrocytes are present, and *V. cholerae* can be detected by dark-field examination in 80% of cases. The organism has a characteristic "shooting star" motility, and it can be immobilized by specific *V. cholerae* antiserum. The sensitivity of the dark-field examination can be enhanced by first incubating stool in bile peptone broth for 8 to 18 hours at 37° C, increasing the yield to 95% of cases. Culture of the stool on selective TCBS media usually yields results within 48 hours. Rapid diagnosis has also been achieved with fluorescent antibody-labeling techniques. Serology is reserved for epidemiologic studies, since a rise in titer occurs too late for practical use in any individual case. Vibriocidal antibodies usually show a four-fold rise by the fourteenth day after the onset of illness, and they may remain elevated for up to 2 to 3 months after symptoms subside.

Prevention

The mode of transmission of *V. cholerae* O1 has been shown to be fecal-oral, usually in contaminated water or through the consumption of inadequately cooked or contaminated seafoods. The organism survives in food held at 55° to 60° C, indicating that great care must be taken in preparation to avoid contamination of foods after cooking. Thus the mainstay of prevention of cholera involves adequate sanitation. In regions where cholera is endemic and municipal water supplies are not adequately chlorinated, avoidance of contaminated water, ice, fruits, and raw vegetables or seafood greatly decreases the risk of disease.

Treatment

Prompt replacement of fluid and electrolytes is essential for the management of patients with cholera. In many instances this can be accomplished orally. The World Health Organization recommends an oral solution containing 3.5 g sodium chloride, 2.5 g sodium bicarbonate, 1.5 g potassium, and 20 g glucose (or 40 g sucrose) per liter of water. If these reagents are unavailable, a solution containing 5 g of sodium chloride and 20 g of glucose (or 40 g of sucrose, or 30 to 80 g of rice powder) per liter has also been shown to be effective. For patients with severe diarrhea (more than 100 ml/kg/day), abnormal mental status, or vomiting, intravenous (IV) replacement is advisable. Correction of hypoglycemia may be necessary, and glucose should be administered as an emergency measure if seizures or abnormal mental status are observed.

A historical perspective underscores the effectiveness of adequate oral replacement of fluids in the treatment of cholera. Mortality rates during the six major cholera pandemics of the nineteenth century exceeded 50% in major cities. In regions where recommended treatment with catharsis and blood-letting was practiced, mortality rates rose to greater than 90%. However, when IV fluids were utilized the mortality decreased to 33%, and the inclusion of bicarbonate in IV fluids decreased this mortality rate to 15%. The discovery that glucose and sodium transport are coupled in the small intestine, so that glucose accelerates the absorption of salt and water, led to the development of oral rehydration solution by researchers working in Dhaka and Calcutta in the 1960s. Widespread distribution of instructions for oral rehydration and packets of salts and sugar reduced the mortality rate to less than 4% when more than 4000 patients were treated for cholera during the Bangladesh War of Independence. Finally, the exemplary response of Peruvian physicians largely averted a potentially disastrous outcome of the current epidemic of cholera in that country. Through the widespread use of oral and IV rehydration and appropriate use of antibiotics, the mortality rate during the epidemic has been less than 0.5% in Lima, the epicenter of the epidemic. Mortality rates of less than 5% have been achieved even in remote regions of the jungle in Peru.

Antibiotics have been shown to shorten the duration of diarrhea and to decrease stool output in patients with cholera. A combination of antibiotic therapy with IV or oral hydration greatly decreases the duration of disease, and thus the expense of treatment. *V. cholerae* is often resistant to β-lactam antibiotics, and either tetracycline (250 mg orally every 6 hours for 3 days) or doxycycline (300 mg once or 100 mg bid for 3 days) is considered the drug of choice in older children and adults. Other agents are also effective, including trimethoprim-sulfamethoxazole and chloramphenicol. Outbreaks of cholera caused by strains resistant to doxycycline, chloramphenicol, gentamicin, and trimethoprim-sulfamethoxazole have been identified in Bangladesh, Africa, and South America, sometimes by a plasmid-borne resistance factor. For this reason, antibiotic susceptibility should be tested when possible. The quinolone antibiotics (e.g., ciprofloxacin) may be useful in treatment of resistant strains in older children and adults.

Vaccine Development

A vaccine of killed *V. cholerae* in suspension is currently available for intramuscular, subcutaneous, or intradermal administration, but it affords protective immunity in only approximately 50% to 70% of cases and requires a booster every 3 to 6 months. It was previously administered to meet international immunization requirements, but there are no longer any countries that require the administration of this vaccine. Because natural disease confers protection, researchers are concentrating on the development of a vaccine that can be administered orally and stimulate an immune response similar to that in natural infection. Several oral vaccines have been tested. One consists of a whole-cell vaccine of killed *V. cholerae* of both biotypes, along with the cholera toxin B subunit. A trial of this vaccine in Bangladesh revealed 85% efficacy in preventing cholera, but this declined to 50% after 36 months. More recently, genetically engineered live

cholera vaccines containing deletions to render them nonpathogenic have also been tested. The *Salmonella typhi* Ty21a vaccine strain expressing *V. cholerae* O antigens was only 25% protective against cholera. In contrast, immunization studies with a *V. cholerae* O1 strain with the toxin subunit deleted resulted in higher levels of protection. However, the latter resulted in an unacceptable rate of side-effects with mild diarrhea and cramps, and therefore was abandoned. Finally, a vaccine strain in which both the enterotoxin and accessory toxins are deleted (CVD 103) is well tolerated, immunogenic, and protective in preliminary trials. Further studies of this strain for vaccination of populations at risk, including young children, are under way.

As the pandemic of cholera spreads to new areas in the Caribbean and South America, the need to educate peoples in diverse regions regarding treatment with oral rehydration therapy and antibiotics increases, as does the need to develop an effective vaccine. History teaches us that the pandemic is likely to continue because of contamination of environmental sources such as seawater, seafood, human water supplies, and sewage. An organized and unified approach to the treatment of this disease, such as was effected in Peru, will have tremendous impact in preventing mortality from this disease. In addition, we can hope that cholera will now drive the sanitary revolution in Latin America, Africa, and South Asia as it did in the United States and Europe a century ago.

OTHER PATHOGENIC VIBRIOS
Non-O1 *V. cholerae*

Much more common than cholera as a cause of gastroenteritis in the United States is a group of organisms that are genetically identical to *V. cholerae* but do not agglutinate in O group 1 antisera. Called *non-O1 V. cholerae,* these bacteria were previously referred to as *non-cholera vibrios* or as *nonagglutinable vibrios,* a misnomer because they do agglutinate in their own specific antisera. A typical disease syndrome is difficult to describe because of a marked variability in the pattern of illness. More than one half of the cases in the literature involve a diarrheal illness, although extraintestinal manifestations also occur. Several outbreaks and many sporadic cases have been reported. The spectrum of illness ranges from severe watery cholera-like diarrhea to a dysentery-like syndrome with fever, abdominal pain, bloody diarrhea, and fecal leukocytes (Chapter 242). The severity of the clinical presentation is probably determined by whether an isolate possesses one of a number of virulence factors. Some non-O1 *V. cholerae* produce a cholera toxin–like enterotoxin. Other putative virulence factors include an El Tor–like hemolysin, Kanagawa hemolysin, shigalike toxin, hemagglutinin, and heat-stable enterotoxins. Furthermore the non-O1 *V. cholerae* produce two colony types on agar plates: opaque and translucent. The opaque morphology has been found to be correlated with increased virulence, an increased polysaccharide coat, and resistance to serum bactericidal activity. Some non-O1 *V. cholerae* have been noted to have invasive properties, unlike O1 *V. cholerae.* Treatment of non-O1 *V. cholerae* gastroenteritis consists primarily of fluid replacement. Whether antibiotics are of benefit is unclear. However, invasive disease with bacteremia definitely warrants antibiotic therapy.

Non-O1 *V. cholerae* organisms have been isolated from several extraintestinal sites, including bile, gallbladder, blood, wounds, ear drainage, sputum, and cerebrospinal fluid. Patients infected at these sites frequently are afflicted with an underlying disease such as cirrhosis, malignancy, diabetes, peripheral vascular disease, or conditions resulting in achlorhydria. These organisms are widely distributed in the environment in seawater, sewage, and brackish surface waters, with an increase in environmental isolates and disease prevalence during the warmer months. Non-O1 *V. cholerae* enteritis has been noted in association with the ingestion of undercooked shellfish or untreated surface water. In addition, the organism has been implicated as a cause of diarrhea in travelers to coastal areas throughout many tropical countries.

Vibrio parahaemolyticus

Vibrio parahaemolyticus has been recognized since the 1950s as the agent causing 70% of gastroenteritis cases in Japan, and is probably related to the common practice of consuming raw fish. It has also been noted since the 1950s as the cause of numerous outbreaks and sporadic cases of diarrhea and extraintestinal disease along the Pacific, Gulf, and Atlantic coasts in the United States and elsewhere. The organism has been isolated from seawaters during the warmer months and from sediment out of Chesapeake Bay during the winter. Its reservoir is believed to be saltwater fish and shellfish. It has been isolated from environmental samples associated with salt water or sewage in the Pacific Northwest, particularly when the ambient temperature exceeds 20° C. Because of this temperature variation, disease caused by *V. parahaemolyticus* tends to occur in the summer months in temperate climates and the dry season in equatorial regions. Outbreaks are often noted in association with consumption of raw seafood (e.g., raw oysters) or undercooked or poorly handled shellfish, in which the organism is able to multiply as rapidly as every 9 minutes. In addition, *V. parahaemolyticus* has been implicated as a cause of travelers' diarrhea.

Although both severe cholera-like illness and severe dysentery have been reported, *V. parahaemolyticus* gastroenteritis is more often mild and self-limited. Diarrhea, abdominal cramps, nausea, vomiting, headache, and fever are the most common manifestations, with temperatures rarely exceeding 102.5° F (38.9° C). Extraintestinal isolates have most often come from infected wounds, although one case each from blood, ear, and synovial fluid has been reported. Pathogenicity in strains of *V. parahaemolyticus* has been associated with the Kanagawa phenomenon, the ability to produce a hemolysin that can lyse blood in high salt–mannitol agar containing human erythrocytes (Wagatsuma agar). The majority of clinical isolates (96.5%) but very few environmental isolates (1%) exhibit the Kanagawa phenomenon. Virulence depends not only on the production of toxins, but also on the ability to colonize human intestine. There is evidence that *V. parahaemolyticus* pili facilitate binding of the bacteria to human intestinal mucosa. Up to 70% of clinical *V. parahaemolyticus* isolates have recently been found to possess a urease, which may prove to be yet another disease-associated biotype marker.

Vibrio vulnificus

V. vulnificus, also referred to as *lactose-positive (L+) Vibrio,* is associated with a higher mortality rate than other *Vibrio* species. In contrast to *V. cholerae* and *V. parahaemolyticus, V. vulnificus* infections are usually extraintestinal. Two distinct clinical syndromes have been noted: primary sepsis and wound infection. The latter may or may not be associated with bacteremia. Primary sepsis occurs almost exclusively in patients with underlying disease, especially hepatic disease (present in 75% in one series), or disorders associated with increased serum iron such as hemochromatosis, hepatitis, or thalassemia major. Less often the syndrome occurs in patients with malignancy or after gastrectomy. The route of acquisition of the organism is usually through ingestion of contaminated food, often raw oysters or raw fish (sushi). These patients are bacteremic with *V. vulnificus,* and in a large portion hypotension is either found on presentation or develops subsequently. Early in the illness metastatic cutaneous lesions are common (75% of cases). Typically, the lesions develop bullae or vesicles and sometimes necrosis; microscopic examination reveals a necrotizing vasculitis. Osteomyelitis, peritonitis with associated sepsis, and secondary massive rhabdomyolysis caused by *V. vulnificus* have been reported. Surgery may be required to eradicate localized peripheral lesions. However, primary *V. vulnificus* sepsis is associated with a mortality of approximately 50% in published series.

In contrast to patients with primary sepsis, wound infections with *V. vulnificus* most often occur in patients without underlying disease. These usually arise in conjunction with a history of exposure of a wound to seawater, or in an injury occurring in the sea. Wounds often progress to vesicles, bullae, and necrosis, and may extend to adjacent areas or cause secondary bacteremia. Surgical debridement is often required to arrest the progressive infection. Many *V. vulnificus* isolates are susceptible to the penicillins, cephalosporins, chloramphenicol, gentamicin, tetracycline, rifampin, and sulfisoxazole. Animal and human studies suggest that tetracycline and an aminoglycoside may be the drug combination of choice, although there are many examples of successful therapy with other agents. Mortality from *V.*

vulnificus wound infections is approximately 16% and is closely correlated with the presence or absence of underlying disease.

Although the evidence for gastroenteritis from *V. vulnificus* is limited, the organism has also been isolated from patients with gastrointestinal illness, and many patients with primary septicemia develop diarrhea, nausea, and vomiting before their bacteremic disease. There are also cases that suggest that asymptomatic gastrointestinal *V. vulnificus* infection may serve as the route of entry for primary septicemia. As further evidence for this, almost all patients with primary septicemia have a history of consumption of raw oysters within 24 hours of admission. Alcohol abuse and the consumption of antacids or H_2- blockers may predispose to the development of *V. vulnificus* gastrointestinal infection.

In some studies, more than 50% of oyster lots sampled during selected months have been culture-positive for *V. vulnificus*. However, not all individuals ingesting these oysters become infected, illustrating that both bacterial virulence factors and host immune defenses must contribute to the development of symptomatic *V. vulnificus* disease. The extreme pathogenicity of *V. vulnificus* is related to a number of bacterial virulence factors. The organism produces a cytotoxin-hemolysin, an elastolytic protease, a collagenase, and various phospholipases, all of which have been hypothesized to aid in the invasion of this organism into a host. Virulent strains of *V. vulnificus* are surrounded by a capsule that is associated with the production of opaque colonies on culture plates, as opposed to nonvirulent translucent colonies. The capsular antigen in opaque variants enables the organism to resist phagocytosis by neutrophils and to evade the bactericidal activity of human serum, both of which predispose to the development of bacteremia. Finally, the propensity of some patients with liver disease or hemochromatosis to develop primary sepsis probably relates to the ability of encapsulated isolates to use transferrin-bound iron for growth if the transferrin is 100% saturated. The bacteria require high concentrations of iron, and the increased iron load in patients with cirrhosis or hemochromatosis facilitates the growth of the organism in their serum.

Vibrio alginolyticus

The pathogenicity of this organism in humans was not recognized until 1973. Since that time there have been a number of case reports of extraintestinal infections with *V. alginolyticus*. Most commonly reported are wound infections, infected cutaneous ulcers, or otitis. Rare cases of *V. alginolyticus* conjunctivitis and bacteremia in compromised hosts have been reported as well. The majority of wound infections occur after exposure to seawater, and cases of otitis media have been reported in patients with perforated tympanic membranes. In most cases, the infected individuals do not have underlying diseases and are not seriously ill. As with other vibrios, the organism can be cultured from seawater during the warm summer and early fall months.

Vibrio mimicus

Vibrio mimicus is a nonhalophilic species previously classified as biochemically atypical non-O1 *V. cholerae*. It was subsequently found by DNA analysis to constitute a separate species. *V. mimicus* has been isolated primarily from patients with diarrhea, but 13% of clinical isolates are derived from patients with internal or external otitis. The diarrhea is often associated with abdominal cramps, vomiting, and fever. Inflammatory diarrhea occurs in fewer than half of cases. On epidemiologic study, *V. mimicus* gastroenteritis has been linked to consumption of raw oysters, and otitis usually occurs after exposure to seawater.

Investigators have found a toxin immunologically and biologically similar to cholera toxin elaborated by *V. mimicus,* but this is rare (10% of clinical, 1% of environmental isolates). Examination of *V. mimicus* strains from Bangladesh revealed that 75% of whole-cell cultures of patient isolates were cytotoxic according to two assays, but this was not caused by an elaborated enterotoxin. In the same study, 25% of environmental isolates exhibited cytotoxicity as well. Finally, the production of a metalloprotease by *V. mimicus* has been associated with fluid secretion into rabbit intestines. The clinical significance of these cytotoxic and proteolytic activities is unclear.

Vibrio fluvialis and Other Species

Between 1976 and 1977, 4.9% of patients with diarrhea in Bangladesh (constituting more than 500 cases) were found to harbor *V. fluvialis*. These patients often had a severe watery diarrhea with dehydration mimicking cholera, but some were observed to have bloody diarrhea. Seventy-five percent of the patients were proved to have fecal leukocytes, demonstrating the organism's ability to invade the intestinal mucosa. Consistent with this finding, *V. fluvialis* isolates have been found to elaborate enterotoxins. The organism is widely distributed in marine environments in Great Britain as well, and it has been reported in association with wound infections in addition to gastroenteritis. Other *Vibrio* species (*V. furnisii, V. damsela, V. hollisae, V. metschnikovii, V. cincinnatiensis, V. carchariae,* and *V. albensis*) have also been associated with human disease (see Table 268-1).

Treatment

Most cases of gastroenteritis caused by vibrios other than *V. cholerae* O1 are self-limited, and treatment other than fluid and electrolyte replacement is not usually required. Extraintestinal disease such as otitis, conjunctivitis, cellulitis, and bacteremia, however, often requires specific antibacterial therapy. Antibiotics effective against most *Vibrio* organisms include tetracycline, doxycycline, chloramphenicol, and the β-lactams may or may not be effective, as indicated by in vitro drug susceptibilities. The quinolones such as ciprofloxacin and norfloxacin are very active in vitro against *Vibrio* organisms, and trials have shown that ciprofloxacin or ofloxacin have equivalent or better efficacy against *v. cholerae* than doxycycline does. Whether antibiotics are administered enterally or parenterally should be determined by the severity of the disease. Finally, some cases of wound infection in normal hosts (e.g., caused by *V. damsela*) can be effectively treated with surgical debridement alone and do not require specific antibiotic therapy.

BIBLIOGRAPHY

General

Janda JM et al: Current perspectives on the epidemiology and pathogenesis of clinically significant *Vibrio* spp., *Clin Microbiol Rev* 1:245, 1988.

Cholera

Almeida RM et al: Vibriophage VcA-3 as an epidemic strain marker for the U.S. Gulf Coast *Vibrio cholerae* O1 clone, *J Clin Microbiol* 30:300, 1992.
Attridge S: Oral immunization with *Salmonella typhi* Ty21a-based clones expressing *Vibrio cholerae* O-antigen: serum bactericidal antibody responses in man in relation to preimmunization antibody levels, *Vaccine* 9:877, 1991.
Carpenter CCJ: The treatment of cholera: clinical science at the bedside, *J Infect Dis* 166:2, 1992.
Clemens JD et al: Field trial of oral cholera vaccines in Bangladesh: results from three-year follow-up, *Lancet* 335:270, 1990.
DePaolo A et al: Isolation of Latin American epidemic strain of *Vibrio cholerae* O1 from U.S. Gulf Coast.
Finch MJ et al: Epidemiology of antimicrobial resistant cholera in Kenya and East Africa, *Am J Trop Med Hyg* 39:484, 1988.
Galen JE et al: Role of *Vibrio cholerae* neuraminidase in the function of cholera toxin, *Infect Immun* 60:406, 1992.
Glass RI, Libel M, Brandling-Bennett AD: Epidemic cholera in the Americas, *Science* 256:1524, 1992.
Guerrant RL, Fang GD, Thielman NM et al: Role of platelet activating factor in the intestinal epithelial secretory and Chinese hamster ovary cell cytoskeletal responses to cholera toxin, *Proc Natl Acad Sci USA* 91:9655-9658, 1994.
Herrington DA et al: Toxin, toxin-coregulated pili, and the *toxR* regulon are essential for *Vibrio cholerae* pathogenesis in humans, *J Exp Med* 168:1487, 1988.
Khan WA et al: Randomised controlled comparison of single-dose ciprofloxacin and doxycycline for cholera caused by *Vibrio cholerae* O1 or O139, *Lancet* 348:296-300, 1996.
Khin-Maung U, Greenough WB III: Cereal-based oral rehydration therapy. I. Clinical studies, *J Pediatr* 118:S72, 1991.
Levine MM: Modern vaccines: enteric infections, *Lancet* 335:958, 1990.
Lima AAM: Cholera: molecular epidemiology, pathogenesis, immunology, treatment, and prevention, *Curr Opin Infect Dis* 7:592-601, 1994.
Lowry PW et al: Cholera in Louisiana, *Arch Intern Med* 149:2079, 1989.
Migasena S et al: Preliminary assessment of the safety and immunogenicity of live oral cholera vaccine strain CVD 103-HgR in healthy Thai adults, *Infect Immun* 57:3261, 1989.
Ramamurthy T et al: Emergence of a novel strain of *V. cholerae* with epidemic potential in southern and eastern India, *Lancet* 341:703, 1993.
Waldor MK, Mekalanos JJ: Tox R regulates virulence gene expression in non-O1 strains of *V. cholerae* that cause epidemic cholera, *Infect Immun* 62:72, 1994.
Winner L III et al: New model for analysis of mucosyl immunity: intestinal secretion of specific monoclonal immunoglobulin A from hybridoma tumors protects against *Vibrio cholerae* infection, *Infect Immun* 59:977, 1991.

Other Pathogenic Vibrios

Abbott SL, Jamda JM: Severe gastroenteritis associated with *Vibrio hollisae* infection: report of two cases and review, *Clin Infect Dis* 18:310-312, 1994.
Arita M et al: Purification and characterization of a new heat-stable enterotoxin produced by *Vibrio cholerae* non-O1 serogroup Hakata, *Infect Immun* 59:2186, 1991.
Bode RB et al: A new *Vibrio* species, *Vibrio cincinnatiensis,* causing meningitis: successful treatment in an adult, *Ann Intern Med* 104:55, 1986.
Brennt CE et al: Growth of *Vibrio vulnificus* in serum from alcoholics: association with high transferrin iron saturation, *J Infect Dis* 164:1030, 1991.
Chowdhury MAR, Miyoshi S-I, Shinoda S: Role of *Vibrio mimicus* protease in enterotoxigenicity, *J Diarrhoeal Dis Res* 9:332, 1991.
Johnson JA, Panigrahi P, Morris JG Jr: Non-O1 *Vibrio cholerae* NRT36S produces a polysaccharide capsule that determines colony morphology, serum resistance, and virulence in mice, *Infect Immun* 60:864, 1992.
Kelly MT, Stroh EMD: Temporal relationship of *Vibrio parahaemolyticus* in patients and the environment, *J Clin Microbiol* 26:1754, 1988.
Morris JG: *Vibrio vulnificus*—a new monster of the deep? *Ann Intern Med* 109:261, 1988.
Nakasone N, Iwanaga M: Pili of a *Vibrio parahaemolyticus* strain as a possible colonization factor, *Infect Immun* 58:61, 1990.
Pavia AT et al: *Vibrio carchariae* infection after a shark bite, *Ann Intern Med* 111:85, 1989.
Penman AD et al: *Vibrio vulnificus* wound infections from the Mississippi Gulf coastal waters, *South Med J* 88:531-533, 1995.
Tendolkar UM, Deodhar LP: *Vibrio albensis* as a cause of post-operative endophthalmitis, *J Infect* 20:261, 1990.
Wachsmuth IK et al: Difference between toxigenic *Vibrio cholerae* O1 from South America and U.S. Gulf Coast, *Lancet* 337:1097, 1991.

---

269 Infections Caused by *Salmonella* and *Shigella* Species

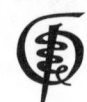

David Bangsberg and Merle A. Sande

SALMONELLA
Classification and Characteristics

Salmonellae are gram-negative, non–spore-forming bacilli that belong to the family Enterobacteriaceae. They have undergone several taxonomic reclassifications. The Kauffmann-White schema classified salmonellae according to their serologic reactions against polyvalent antisera against their somatic (O) and flagellar (H) antigens. The O-antigens determined their serogroup, which was divided into serogroups A through I. The strains that cause human disease were predominantly in serogroups A through E. These serogroups were divided into more than 2000 serotypes, according to their H antigens. The most recent classification divides salmonellae by their DNA-DNA hybridization patterns into six groups, with most strains that cause human disease in subgroup 1. In this classification, the group Arizona is included in the *Salmonella* genus. Another classification schema divided the genus *Salmonella* into three primary species, *Salmonella typhi, Salmonella cholerasuis,* and *Salmonella enteritidis; S. enteritidis* was divided into more than 2000 serotypes. Under this schema, a serotype may be formally designated as *S. enteritidis* serotype *heidelberg,* but by convention and convenience, the strain is named *S. heidelberg.* This latter classification system is still widely used for epidemiologic and clinical purposes.

NONTYPHOIDAL SALMONELLA
Epidemiology

The *Salmonella* infection incidence data in the United States are derived from a national surveillance program. From 1976 to 1991 the population-based isolation rate of *S. enteritidis* increased from 56,000 to 306,000. There were 43,323 cases of nontyphoidal *Salmonella* reported in 1994, which is a low estimate of total cases because of underreporting. *Salmonella typhimurium* and *S. enteritidis* are the most

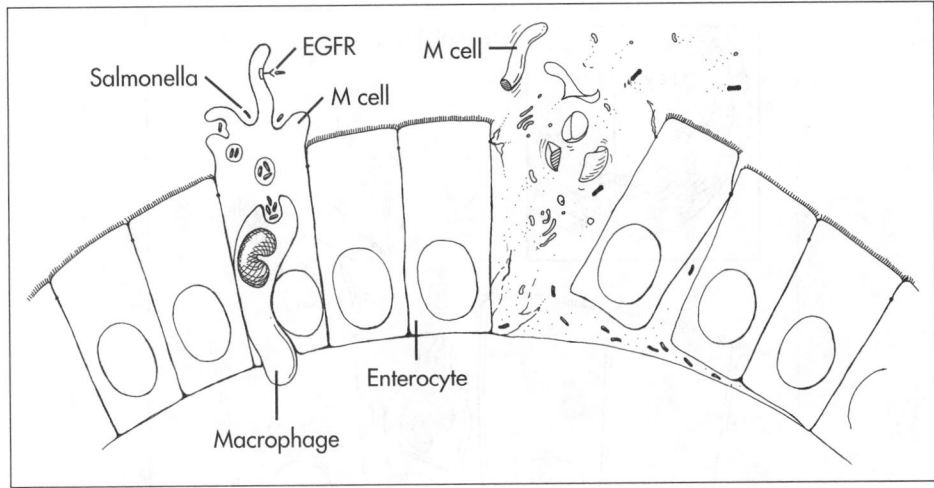

FIGURE 269-1   Nontyphoidal *Salmonella* invade M cells through membrane ruffling and EGF receptor–dependent pathways. M cells are destroyed with bacterial replication, which disrupts epithelial tight junctions and exposes the basolateral surfaces to infection.

common isolates in the United States. The majority of outbreak-associated *Salmonella* infections are associated with food service establishments, but hospital and nursing home outbreaks have the highest case fatality rate (3% vs. 0.043% for the general public). The most common source of *S. enteritidis* in both outbreak and sporadic infections is undercooked chicken eggs. Although fresh eggs contain 10 or fewer organisms, storage or preparation in inappropriate temperature conditions allows multiplication of the organism and an increase in the infectious dose. Other reservoirs of *Salmonella* include turkeys, ducks, cattle, swine, sheep, dogs, turtles, lizards, snakes, and insects. Salmonellae can be transmitted person to person, by fomites, from pets (turtles), and, rarely, by blood products or medical instruments (endoscopy).

Pathophysiology

The consequences of ingesting viable *Salmonella* organisms are determined by host and microbial factors. The determinants of symptomatic infection include the serotype or strain of *Salmonella*, type of vehicle, route of transmission, inoculum, and health status of the host. A large inoculum is usually required to produce disease in healthy subjects.

Intestinal motility and normal flora are intrinsic defenses of the small intestine. The administration of antimicrobial agents may reduce the inoculum required to produce disease because changes in the normal flora favor multiplication of Salmonellae within the intestine. A decrease in intestinal motility and a reduced transit time may prolong the period of illness and the convalescent carrier state.

Salmonellae produce a wide spectrum of disease. Most strains cause either an asymptomatic infection or self-limited diarrheal illness.

Salmonellae are invasive intracellular pathogens. Intracellular invasion is facilitated by decreased oxygen tension in the small intestine. Salmonellae infect M cells in the terminal ileum. They may enter cells either by binding to the epidermal growth factor (EGF) receptor or though EGF-independent membrane ruffling. Internalization in membrane-bound vesicles leads to calcium mobilization and phospholipase A2 and 5-lipoxygenase activation, resulting in leukotriene production and cytoskeletal reorganization. In this process, the M cells are destroyed and tight junctions are disrupted, which allows Salmonellae to invade adjacent enterocytes. Cytokine activation leads to lymphoid cell proliferation and migration from adjacent Peyer's patches and, in combination with enterocyte disruption, contributes to clinical diarrhea. Enterocyte infection and disruption is the primary pathophysiologic process in nontyphoidal gastroenteritis, whereas Peyer's patch invasion, proliferation, and necrosis constitute the primary pathophysiologic process of typhoidal enteric fever (Figs. 269-1 and 269-2).

Salmonella bacteremia is frequent in patients with impairments in cellular and humoral immunity. The specific mechanisms have not been determined, but patients with *Salmonella* bacteremia have an increased incidence of underlying diseases, including AIDS, lymphoma, leukemia, and sickle cell disease. There is also an increased incidence of *Salmonella* infection and bacteremia in patients with hemolysis caused by bartonellosis and malaria.

Clinical Disease

The clinical manifestations of nontyphoidal *Salmonella* infection are quite varied. Asymptomatic infection is the most common sequela of ingesting salmonellae. When clinical disease develops, it usually takes the form of one of the following syndromes: enterocolitis, bacteremia, localized infection, or a chronic carrier state.

Enterocolitis.   Gastrointestinal symptoms predominate in two thirds of symptomatic *Salmonella* infections. The usual incubation period is 12 to 72 hours, but it varies with the size of the inoculum. Incubation periods of up to 2 weeks have been reported. Nausea, vomiting, and chills are common initial symptoms. They are rapidly followed by colicky abdominal pain, diarrhea, and fever. The severity of the diarrhea ranges from a few loose stools to up to 30 bowel movements daily. The stools are characteristically watery and green, with an offensive odor, and they have variable amounts of mucus. Depending on the degree of colonic involvement, there may be a dysenteric presentation, with high fever and blood-tinged or frankly bloody mucoid stools. Symptoms usually subside within 5 days but may persist for as long as 2 weeks.

Enterocolitis is a self-limited illness that should be treated only with symptomatic therapy (fluid, electrolytes), unless there is evidence or suspicion of either an associated bacteremia or a localized infection. Antimicrobial therapy should be given to patients with impaired host-defense mechanisms (lymphoma, sickle cell disease, AIDS), because such patients have an increased risk of bacteremia. Uncomplicated enterocolitis should not be treated with antibiotics. Antibiotics may prolong the period of convalescent excretion of the organism. The median duration of *Salmonella* fecal excretion is about 5 weeks in adults; children less than 5 years old have a prolonged excretion period. The fecal excretion of nontyphoidal *Salmonella* organism for periods of days, or even months, after infection is not uncommon. Positive stool cultures are obtained in 10% to 15% of enterocolitis patients for 1 to 2 months after the illness. These patients have been termed *convalescent carriers*. The need to eradicate the organism in convalescent carriers who are health care workers is often raised, but nosocomial outbreaks of salmonellosis are rare in the United States, despite the high frequency of prolonged convalescent

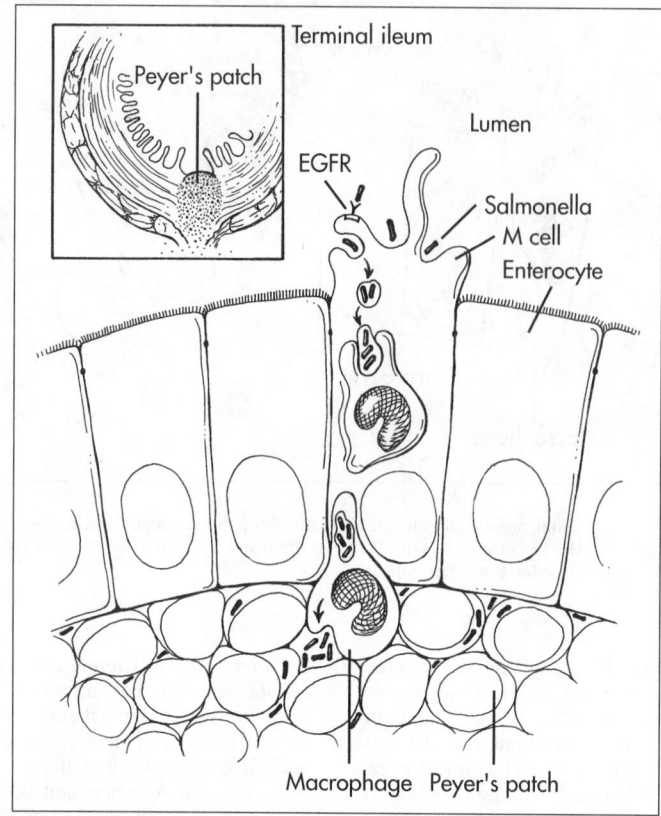

FIGURE 269-2 *Salmonella typhi* invade M cells through membrane ruffling and EGF receptor–dependent pathways. Macrophages originating from Peyer's patch take up *S. typhi* in close association with M cells. *S. typhi* replicate in Peyer's patches and then enter the lymphatic system, leading to bacteremia. Replication in Peyer's patches causes hypertrophy followed by necrosis, which can cause intestinal perforation.

carriage. Hence, attempts to eradicate the organism in such persons are not justified and may not be effective.

Bacteremia. Bacteremia occurs in less than 5% of nontyphoidal infections. It occurs in patients with underlying chronic diseases such as diabetes, malignancy, end-stage renal disease, systemic lupus erythematosus, cirrhosis, or AIDS. Mortality is high among bacteremic adults but infrequent in children. *S. cholerasuis* infections are associated with bacteremia in 50% of cases, and bacteremia is also common in serogroup type B. *Salmonella* infection in these patients may be manifested only by fever and positive blood cultures, and not by the usual gastrointestinal symptoms. Bacteremia and localized infections usually are treated with either chloramphenicol, ampicillin, a third-generation cephalosporin, or a fluoroquinolone. If the organism is susceptible, ampicillin is preferred for localized disease.

Uncomplicated bacteremia without localized infection may be treated with either chloramphenicol, ampicillin, a third-generation cephalosporin, or a fluoroquinolone for 10 to 14 days. Extraintestinal salmonellosis resistant to ampicillin and chloramphenicol is usually treated with trimethoprim-sulfamethoxazole, which may be particularly useful for prostatic and urinary tract infections.

Localized Infection. During *Salmonella*-associated bacteremia, localized infection may develop. In some patients, the infection develops in sites of preexisting disease such as vascular aneurysms, bone infarcts, congenital cysts, injection sites, and calculous gallbladders. Infection of an abdominal aorta aneurysm may present as prolonged fever, back pain, or recurrent bacteremia after gastroenteritis and has a high mortality without surgical therapy. *Salmonella* is the most common cause of osteomyelitis in patients with sickle cell anemia. The infection localizes in previously infarcted or ischemic bone. Meningitis occurs primarily in neonates, whereas pneumonia and empyema are most common in elderly persons and in patients with underlying

disease. Abscesses of the spleen, liver, and soft tissue rarely are encountered. Endocarditis may develop on natural or prosthetic valves. Osteomyelitis and intravascular infections require 6 or more weeks of therapy.

TYPHOIDAL SALMONELLA
Epidemiology

There are about 33 million cases of typhoid fever worldwide each year. Most cases occur in the developing world, specifically South and East Asia, Africa, Latin America, and India. Transmission of typhoid fever has become rare in the United States because of improved water treatment, although food-associated outbreaks are occasionally reported. There were 441 cases in the United States in 1994. Mortality in the United States is less than 1% but can approach 30% in developing countries. Humans are the only natural reservoir for *S. typhi,* the etiologic agent of typhoid fever.

Pathophysiology

Ingestion of 10^7 *S. typhi* organisms caused typhoid fever in 50% of exposed persons. Volunteer studies have shown that an inoculum of 10^5 organisms produced disease in 28% of subjects, whereas 10^9 organisms produced disease in 95%. However, a smaller inoculum can cause disease if the organism is ingested with foods that buffer the gastric acid (e.g., milk) or if the host has had a gastrectomy or is achlorhydric. The initial events after ingestion of *S. typhi* are similar to those related to nontyphoidal *Salmonella*. In severe infections, necrosis of Peyer's patches can occur, leading to bowel perforation and/or bacterial invasion of the lymphatic system, resulting in systemic bloodstream infection. Bacteria are cleared from the blood by mononuclear phagocytes, principally in the liver and spleen. Replication of *S. typhi* occurs primarily in Peyer's patches, resulting in a bacteremic, febrile illness with abdominal tenderness, whereas replication in nontyphoidal gastroenteritis occurs primarily in the epithelial cells of the intestinal lumen, resulting in a diarrheal illness (see Figs. 269-1 and 269-2). The organism possesses a surface antigen that impedes phagocytosis and killing by serum factors. This antigen has been termed *Vi antigen* (virulence), and it contributes to the ability of *S. typhi* to survive normal host-defense mechanisms.

Clinical Presentation

Enteric fever is a clinical syndrome characterized by fever, headache, prostration, cough, splenomegaly, and leukopenia. Without therapy, the illness is prolonged and associated with serious complications. The classic syndrome is produced by *S. typhi;* however, a less severe syndrome can be infrequently produced by *Salmonella paratyphi* A, B, and *S. typhi* C. The term *typhoid fever* has been applied when the causative organism is *S. typhi*, and the term *paratyphoid fever* is used when *S. paratyphi* is implicated.

The incubation period of typhoid is usually 7 to 14 days. There is an inverse relationship between the inoculum size and the incubation period, with the latter ranging from 3 to 60 days. The onset of illness is usually insidious. Fever is the earliest indication of disease. The temperature usually remains elevated, but a remittent pattern may occur. A dull headache often accompanies the fever. Right lower quadrant or diffuse lower abdominal pain occurs in 20% to 40% of cases. Abdominal tenderness is characteristic. Relative bradycardia, although classically described, is uncommon. Erythematous maculopapular lesions 2 to 4 mm in diameter that blanch on pressure and are referred to as *rose spots* may appear on the upper abdomen and lower thorax during the first or second week of illness. Rose spots usually appear in crops of 10 or fewer lesions and resolve in hours or days. They are present in a minority of patients and may not be visible in dark-skinned individuals. Hepatomegaly and splenomegaly are detectable after the third week of illness in one third and one half of patients, respectively. Cough is present in one third of patients, and nausea, vomiting, and diarrhea occur in up to one half of patients. Some patients may have constipation as their most prominent gastrointestinal complaint. Anemia and leukopenia can occur, and elevated transaminases, creatinine phosphokinase, lactate dehydrogenase, and alkaline phosphatase are common. Diagnosis is made from isolation of *S. typhi* or *S. paratyphi* from blood, stool, urine, rose spots, or bone marrow. The organism is recovered from blood cultures in 50% to 70% of cases but can be recovered in up to 90% of cases when bone marrow is cultured. Stool examination reveals mononuclear cells.

In the preantibiotic era, patients either slowly recovered or developed serious complications during the third and fourth weeks of illness. Mortality rates were 10% to 15%; intestinal hemorrhage (5% to 20%) or perforation (2% to 5%) were the most serious complications. The mortality rate for typhoid fever is now less than 1% and symptoms resolve within 3 to 5 days with appropriate antimicrobial therapy and supportive care.

Typhoid and enteric fever should be treated with antimicrobial agents. They have been successfully treated with chloramphenicol IV or PO (50 mg/kg/day), ampicillin IV or PO (100 mg/kg/day), amoxicillin PO (4 g/day), trimethoprim-sulfamethoxazole (320 to 640 mg; 1600 to 3200 mg, respectively) daily, ciprofloxacin (1000 to 1500 mg), and ceftriaxone IM (1000 mg) daily. Ciprofloxacin and ceftriaxone have excellent activity against *S. typhi* (MIC = 0.01 to 0.1 mg/ml). They are active against intracellular organisms and are concentrated in the biliary tract. Chloramphenicol, ampicillin, and amoxicillin are given in four divided doses, and trimethoprim-sulfamethoxazole and ciprofloxacin in two divided doses. The recommended duration of therapy is 2 weeks. The clinical response of typhoid fever patients is slow, regardless of the antibiotic used. Most patients require 3 to 5 days of therapy to become afebrile. Because ciprofloxacin and ceftriaxone are expensive and ciprofloxacin is not approved for use in children, chloramphenicol remains the drug of choice in most parts of the world. Although it has good in vitro activity, aztreonam has been associated with poor clinical response rates.

Relapse occurs in 5% to 10% of untreated patients and in 10% to 20% of patients receiving chloramphenicol. The symptoms in relapse are usually milder than those of the initial illness and begin about 2 weeks after discontinuation of the antimicrobial therapy.

Drug resistance is a growing problem worldwide. Ampicillin-resistant *S. typhi* has been reported from Mexico, France, South Asia, and Southeast Asia. Chloramphenicol-resistant *S. typhi* has been reported from these areas and West Africa, the Middle East, and India. Initial therapy with both chloramphenicol and ampicillin has been recommended in areas where resistance to these agents has been reported. If the organism is sensitive to both drugs, chloramphenicol is continued, if it is resistant to one antibiotic, the other antibiotic is continued alone. Fortunately, it is quite rare for *S. typhi* to acquire resistance to both ampicillin and chloramphenicol. In that situation, trimethoprim-sulfamethoxazole, ceftriaxone, or a fluoroquinolone would be indicated. Drug resistance is also a growing problem in the United States. Fourteen percent of *Salmonella* isolates reported to the Centers for Disease Control and Prevention (CDC) demonstrated resistance to ampicillin in 1989-1990. Five percent were resistant to gentamicin, and 1% were resistant to trimethoprim-sulfamethoxazole. Resistance to quinolones and third-generation cephalosporins is rare thus far. Factors associated with drug resistance include prior hospitalization, age less than 1 year, black race, and recent antimicrobial therapy. The choice of antimicrobial agent should be influenced by knowledge of the local epidemiology of drug-resistant isolates and results of in vitro sensitivity testing.

Corticosteroid therapy is recommended for all patients with confirmed typhoid fever who are delirious, obtunded, stuporous, comatose, or in shock. In one study, dexamethasone, 3 mg/kg body weight as an initial dose, followed by eight doses of 1 mg/kg every 6 hours, significantly reduced the case-fatality rate. Before corticosteroids are administered, malaria, in which corticosteroids are contraindicated, should be considered in the differential diagnosis.

Intestinal hemorrhage can be managed with antibiotic therapy and transfusion, whereas intestinal perforation requires surgery.

Chronic Carrier State

A chronic intestinal carrier state, defined as documented fecal excretion of *S. typhi* for a minimum period of 1 year, is observed in 1% to 3% of typhoid fever patients. The gallbladder is the site of persistent intestinal infection. *S. typhi* is excreted in the bile, and stool contains 10^6 to 10^9 organisms per gram of feces. They are asymptomatic but serve as the natural reservoir for *S. typhi*. The chronic carrier state may persist for the lifetime of an individual if antibiotic therapy and/or biliary tract surgery are not undertaken.

Chronic carriers are usually treated with oral ampicillin, 4 to 6 g daily, and probenicid, 2 g daily, each in four divided doses for 6 weeks. Relapses occur in 30% to 50% of these patients. Relapsing patients usually have biliary tract disease, and cure often requires cholecystectomy. However, case reports in chronic relapsing carriers with gallbladder involvement describe clearing of organisms with ciprofloxacin, 750 mg twice daily for 3 weeks.

Diagnostic Tests

The diagnosis of *Salmonella* infection is established by isolating the organism from stool, urine, blood, or other infected secretions and tissues. Serologic tests are of no value in establishing a diagnosis early in the illness but may be useful retrospectively. Their greatest value is in epidemiologic investigations.

Salmonella in HIV Infection

There are increased rates of both typhoidal and nontyphoidal *Salmonella* infection in people with HIV infection in high prevalence areas. Typhoidal *Salmonella* infection may include fulminant diarrhea and/or colitis. In nontyphoidal *Salmonella* infection, there is an increased rate of bacteremia with persistent fever, and the gastrointestinal symptoms may be absent. Initial response to therapy is good in both typhoidal and nontyphoidal disease, but relapses occur frequently that may require chronic suppressive therapy. This can be accomplished with a prophylactic dose of trimethoprim-sulfamethoxazole or a quinolone. Recommended initial therapy

---

✔ *WHEN TO REFER*

Infectious disease referral should be considered when infections occur in immunocompromised hosts or in patients with multiply drug-resistant organisms. Immunocompromised individuals who plan to travel to *Salmonella*-endemic areas should also seek infectious disease consultation regarding the need for vaccination. Failure to eradicate the chronic carrier state may require either infectious disease consultation for further antibiotic treatment or surgical consultation for cholecystectomy.

---

includes either a quinolone or third-generation cephalosporin, depending on sensitivity results. Zidovudine also has antimicrobial activity against *Salmonella*.

Prevention

Adequate protection of water supplies, vaccination of persons at risk, pasteurization of milk products, sanitary disposal of human excreta, and identification, isolation, and treatment of chronic typhoid carriers are the primary measures for control of typhoid fever. Since humans are the only natural reservoir for *S. typhi,* these measures have been very successful in developed countries. Typhoid fever can also be prevented by vaccines. Killed whole parenteral vaccines are associated with unacceptably high rates of systemic and local reactions. An orally administered vaccine made from an attenuated, nonpathogenic strain of *S. typhi* using 10^9 organisms (Ty21a) is administered in four doses every other day for a 5-day period. The oral vaccine has yielded 43% to 96% efficacy in field trials. The parenteral vaccine made from the Vi antigen capsular polysaccharide can be administered in one dose. Local or systemic reactions are uncommon, and field efficacy is 75%. Although these vaccines have demonstrated reasonable efficacy in endemic areas, vaccination of the traveler is controversial. The incidence of traveler-associated typhoid in U.S. travelers was 6.1 per million travelers between 1982 and 1984. It is highest in travelers to the Indian subcontinent and Peru. Protection in travelers originating from nonendemic areas is reduced because of the lack of naturally acquired immunity. Protection by these vaccines may be adequate only for water exposures and not for higher inoculums associated with food-borne exposures. Travelers should follow the administration protocol of the oral vaccine carefully, including avoidance of antibiotics such as mefloquine for malarial prophylaxis, which will kill the attenuated live bacteria.

Control of nontyphoidal *Salmonella* requires proper food handling, storage, and preparation, in conjunction with outbreak surveillance and control.

World Wide Web Information

Recent developments in *Salmonella* outbreaks, pathophysiology, therapy, and vaccine development can be accessed on the "Microbial Underground's *Salmonella* Page" at this World Wide Web address: http://www.qmw.ac.uk/~rhbm001/salmopage.html.

SHIGELLA
Classification and Characteristics

Shigellae are gram-negative, non–spore-forming bacilli that belong to the family Enterobacteriaceae. Shigellae are classified according to their somatic (O) antigens. The genus is divided into four species, *Shigella dysenteriae, Shigella flexneri, Shigella boydii,* and *Shigella sonnei,* which include more than 40 serotypes. These species frequently are referred to as subgroups A, B, C, and D, respectively.

Epidemiology

Shigellosis occurs throughout the world and is responsible for more than 576,000 deaths each year among children less than 5 years of age. There were 29,769 isolations of Shigellae reported to the CDC

in 1994. During the 5-year period between 1986 and 1990, there was an increase of nearly 20% in the average annual reported incidence compared to the 5-year period a decade earlier. *S. sonnei* is the most common species in the United States and Western Europe, whereas *S. flexneri* predominates in most developing countries. *S. dysenteriae,* the cause of dysentery pandemics, was the most common species isolated during the early 1900s. It virtually disappeared, only to emerge as the cause of pandemics in Central America (1969-1973), Bangladesh (1972-1977), southern India (1972-1978), central Africa (1979-1986), eastern India (1984), and Thailand and Myanmar (1984-1986).

Shigellosis is most common in late summer and is primarily a disease of children less than 4 years of age. Humans are the only known reservoir of the organism. Transmission is predominantly from direct person-to-person contact, rather than from ingestion of contaminated food or water. However, food-borne outbreaks have been reported after ingestion of tofu salad at a Michigan commissary, iceberg lettuce from Spain, and German potato salad on a cruise ship. Day care settings have been the source of community-wide epidemics. A day care center outbreak in Kentucky led to 219 infections, which accounted for 47% of the *Shigella* infections reported in the community. Transmission was associated with staff who both changed diapers and prepared food and with a high toddler-to-toilet ratio. The secondary attack rate in family members was 33% but has been reported to be as high as 60% in other outbreaks. Although traditional outbreak control measures failed to control the Kentucky outbreak, community-wide emphasis and monitoring of hand washing brought a rapid end to transmission.

Fecal excretion of Shigellae may continue for up to 6 weeks in untreated patients. Long-term carriage is rare. When it occurs, there is persistence of organisms in the colon, rather than in the biliary tract as in cholera and salmonellosis.

Pathophysiology

The inoculum of *Shigella* organisms required to produce disease is the lowest of any of the enteric bacterial pathogens. Ten *S. dysenteriae* bacilli produce illness in 10% to 20% of healthy adults, and 200 *S. flexneri* or *S. sonnei* bacilli cause disease in 40% of subjects. Shigellae are more resistant to acid than are salmonellae or *Vibrio cholerae* organisms. *S. dysenteriae* and certain strains of *S. flexneri* and *S. sonnei* elaborate an enterotoxin, which may be responsible for the early phase of the diarrhea.

Although *Salmonella* infection is limited to the small intestine, *Shigella* organisms invade intestinal epithelial cells in both the small and large intestine and are unable to directly infect the apical surface of epithelial cells. Shigellae obtain entry to the submucosa through infecting M cells. They then enter the submucosa through actin-mediated transcytosis into macrophages that originate from lymphoid follicles. Shigellae replicate in macrophages, which subsequently undergo apoptosis, or programmed cell death. Intracellular replication and macrophage apoptosis require the presence of a 22-kilodalton plasmid. Absence of the 22-kilodalton plasmid renders Shigellae nonpathogenic. Macrophage apoptosis leads to the release of preformed interleukin-1, which initiates the inflammatory response. Polymorphonuclear migration through epithelial tight junctions in response to IL-1 exposes the basolateral surface of epithelial cells to bacterial invasion. After epithelial invasion, Shigellae can infect adjacent cells through transcytosis at epithelial intermediate junctions, which is driven by an actin-based intracellular motor (Fig. 269-3). As a result, Shigellae disseminate through the epithelium and lamina propria to form microabscesses and diffuse ulceration. Since involvement below the submucosa is rare, bacteremia is uncommon. Production of Shiga toxin contributes to local mucosal destruction and large-volume watery diarrhea seen in the early course of the disease. The strong inflammatory response explains the presence of polymorphonuclear leukocytes on microscopic stool examination.

Clinical Disease

Shigellosis is usually abrupt in onset, with an incubation period of 1 to 3 days. Watery diarrhea, crampy abdominal pain, and fever up to 104° F (40° C) are the most common early symptoms and coincide

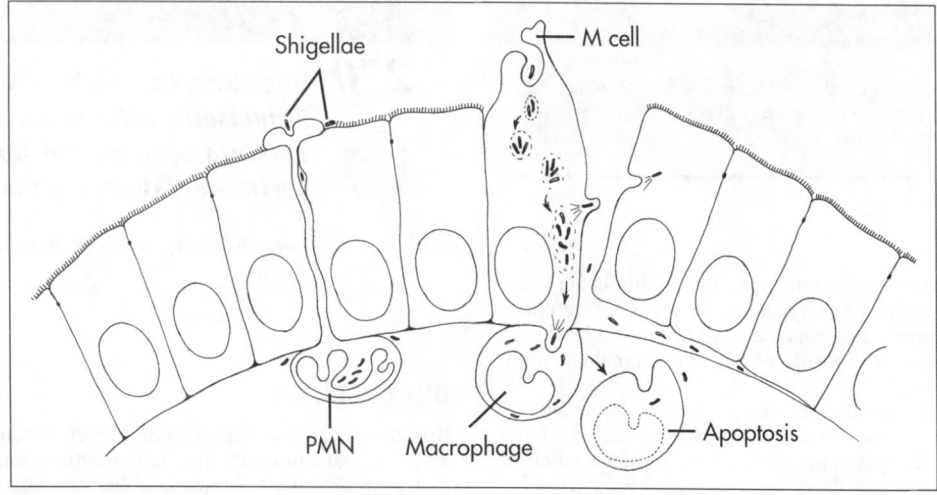

FIGURE 269-3   Shigellae infect M cells, followed by uptake in macrophages. After infection, macrophages undergo apoptosis, which releases Shigellae to infect the basolateral surfaces of intestinal epithelium. Shigellae also gain entry to basolateral surfaces by polymorphonuclear (PMN) intrusion through tight junctions in response to chemotactic signals. An intracellular actin motor drives transcytosis between cells.

with infection of the small intestine. This phase of the illness lasts for several days in most patients. With infection of the colon, tenesmus, fecal urgency, and the passage of bloody, mucoid stools occur. Fever becomes less prominent, and the volume of the stools is decreased. This second phase of illness may last for 2 to 3 weeks without antimicrobial therapy.

Shigella bacteremia is a rare event. It most often occurs in patients younger than 5 years of age, the elderly, and immunocompromised individuals.

The severity of shigellosis is related to the infecting organism. *S. sonnei* produces the mildest illness, *S. flexneri* is intermediate, and *S. dysenteriae* type 1 causes the most serious illness. Many patients infected with *S. sonnei* are asymptomatic or have only a brief episode of watery diarrhea. In contrast, gross blood and mucus are present in the stool of a majority of patients infected with *S. dysenteriae*. Strain differences also are reflected in mortality rates. Shigellosis caused by *S. sonnei* is fatal in less than 1% of patients in most areas, whereas *S. dysenteriae* outbreaks have a mortality as high as 20% to 30%. Geographic differences also influence mortality figures. In Bangladesh, the case-fatality rates among hospitalized children were highest (10%) in those infected with *S. sonnei* in 1974-1988.

Convulsions are common in children less than 4 years of age. In one series, seizures developed in 25% of children with a temperature exceeding 103° F (39.4° C). The incidence of seizures in children with a temperature of less than 103° F was about 6%. Hyperpyrexia may not be an independent variable, since dehydration and electrolyte abnormalities may be more severe in infants with higher temperatures. Complications of shigellosis that can lead to death have been identified in a 15-year study in Bangladesh and include intestinal perforation, toxic megacolon, dehydration, sepsis, hyponatremia, hypoglycemia, seizures, hemolytic-uremic syndrome, and pneumonia. Sepsis and hypoglycemia were found to be the most common causes of death.

Shigella in AIDS

Shigella is an uncommon cause of gastroenteritis in patients with HIV, and the incidence in homosexual men with and without HIV does not appear to differ. Once infected, there is an increased incidence of bacteremia in patients with HIV. Although individuals with intact immune systems recover spontaneously, individuals infected with HIV should be treated with antimicrobial therapy. Response to therapy is usually rapid and, unlike with *Salmonella* infections, relapses are uncommon, which makes chronic suppressive therapy unnecessary in most cases.

Diagnostic Tests

A definitive diagnosis of shigellosis is established by isolation of Shigellae from stool or a swab of colonic lesions. Shigellae survive for only a short time in stool so fresh specimens should be inoculated promptly on appropriate culture media. In severe dysenteric cases, it is very important to test a suspected *Shigella* colony on a plate with a panel of group antisera to rapidly rule out *S. dysenteriae* type 1 because of this organism's tendency to cause widespread epidemics. Serology is unhelpful in diagnosis because antibodies do not develop until after clinical resolution and are helpful only as an aid in tracking epidemics.

Microscopic examination of methylene blue–stained stool preparations is useful in distinguishing shigellosis from toxigenic or viral diarrheal syndromes. Numerous fecal polymorphonuclear leukocytes are usually found in shigellosis, whereas fecal leukocytes are absent in toxin-induced or viral diarrhea. Fecal leukocytes also occur in salmonellosis, *Campylobacter* enteritis, and ulcerative colitis. Sigmoidoscopy reveals diffuse mucosal inflammation, often with multiple shallow ulcers 3 to 7 mm in diameter.

Treatment

The correction of fluid, electrolyte, and glucose abnormalities is the mainstay of therapy and is particularly important in elderly and very young patients. Although the use of antibiotics in adults with shigellosis is controversial, therapy shortens the period of symptomatic illness and decreases the duration of fecal excretion of Shigellae. Fever and diarrhea usually respond within 1 to 2 days of initiating effective therapy, and mortality is reduced to less than 0.1%. Organisms resistant to multiple antibiotics are common, especially in Africa, Asia, and South America. In a study by the CDC, 32% and 7% of United States *Shigella* isolates were resistant to ampicillin and to trimethoprim-sulfamethoxazole, respectively. Isolates associated with foreign travel were resistant to trimethoprim-sulfamethoxazole in 20% of cases; no quinolone resistance was encountered.

Trimethoprim-sulfamethoxazole (160 mg and 800 mg, respectively) every 12 hours for 5 days is the treatment of choice for shigellosis not associated with foreign travel. Children may be given trimethoprim-sulfamethoxazole (10 mg/kg/day and 50 mg/kg/day, respectively) in two divided doses for 5 days. Ampicillin (500 mg PO qid for 5 days) is effective for sensitive organisms, as is a single oral dose of tetracycline (2.5 g). Fluoroquinolones such as norfloxacin and ciprofloxacin are effective drugs, especially for foreign travel–related shigellosis, but these drugs are not approved for pediatric use. Preferred treatment is 500 mg PO bid for 5-7 days for acute infection,

✔ *WHEN TO REFER*

Infectious disease consultation should be considered either in immune-compromised patients or severely ill patients infected with a multiply drug-resistant organism.

and perhaps 750 mg for recurrent infection. Amoxicillin is not effective because of low intraluminal antibiotic levels. Oral cefixime, cephalexin, and intravenous cefamandole have been associated with high failure rates, presumably because of low intraluminal and intracellular concentrations.

Antiperistaltic agents such as diphenoxylate hydrochloride with atropine sulfate (Lomotil) should be avoided because of the possibility that they will exacerbate symptoms and prolong fecal excretion of organisms.

Prevention

The most important control measure is to institute proper sanitary and hygienic measures. Hand washing is extremely important in decreasing direct transmission of organisms. Asymptomatic and convalescent carriers should also be excluded from involvement in food preparation and handling. A live attenuated oral vaccine is under development.

BIBLIOGRAPHY

Bennish ML: Potentially lethal complications of shigellosis, *Rev Infect Dis* 13(suppl 4):S319, 1991.

Galan JE et al: Involvement of the epidermal growth factor receptor in the invasion of cultured mammalian cells by *Salmonella typhimurium, Nature* 357:588, 1992.

Gotuzzo E: Association between the acquired immunodeficiency syndrome and infection with *Salmonella typhi* or *Salmonella paratyphi* in an endemic typhoid area, *Arch Intern Med* 151:381, 1991.

Hedberg CW et al: Role of egg consumption in sporadic *Salmonella enteritidis* and *Salmonella typhimurium* infections in Minnesota, *J Infect Dis* 167:107, 1993.

Jones BD, Ghori N, Jones BD: *Salmonella typhimurium* initiates murine infection by penetrating and destroying the specialized epithelial M cell of the Peyer's patches, *J Exp Med* 180:15, 1994.

Jones BD et al: *Salmonella typhimurium* induces membrane ruffling by a growth factor–receptor-independent mechanism, *Proc Nat Acad Sci* 90:10390, 1993.

Lee LA et al: Increase in antimicrobial-resistant *Salmonella* infections in the United States, 1989-1990, *J Infect Dis* 170:128, 1994.

Levine WC et al: Epidemiology of non-typhoidal *Salmonella* bacteremia during the human immunodeficiency virus epidemic, *J Infect Dis* 164:81, 1991.

Li A et al: Safety and immunogenicity of the live oral auxotrophic *Shigella flexneri* SFL124 in adult Vietnamese volunteers, *Vaccine* 11:180, 1993.

Mishu B et al: Outbreaks of *Salmonella enteritidis* infections in the United States, 1985-1991, *J Infect Dis* 169:547, 1994.

Mohle-Boetani JC et al: Community shigellosis: control of an outbreak and risk factors in child day-care centers, *Am J Public Health* 85:812, 1995.

Neill MA et al: Failure of ciprofloxacin to eradicate convalescent fecal excretion after acute salmonellosis: experience during an outbreak in health care workers, *Ann Int Med* 114:195, 1991.

Pace J, Hayman MJ, Galan JE: Signal transduction and invasion of epithelial cells by *S. typhimurium, Cell* 72:505, 1993.

Perdomo JJ, Gounon P, Sansonetti PJ: Polymorphonuclear leukocyte transmigration promotes invasion of colonic epithelial monolayer by *Shigella flexneri, J Clin Invest* 93:633, 1994.

Perdomo OJ et al: Acute inflammation causes epithelial invasion and mucosal destruction in experimental shigellosis, *J Exp Med* 180:1307, 1994.

Sai-Cheong L et al: Bacteremia to non-typhi *Salmonella:* analysis of 64 cases and review, *Clin Infect Dis* 19:693, 1994.

Salam MA, Bennish ML: Antimicrobial therapy for shigellosis, *Rev Infect Dis* 13(suppl 4):S332, 1991.

Woodruff BA, Pavia AT, Blake PA: A new look at typhoid vaccination: information for the practicing physician, *JAMA* 265:756, 1991.

Zychlinsky A et al: Interleukin 1 is released by murine macrophages during apoptosis induced by *Shigella flexneri, J Clin Invest* 94:1328, 1994.

CHAPTER

270 Infections Caused by *Brucella, Francisella tularensis, Pasteurella, Yersinia* Species, and *Bordetella pertussis* (Whooping Cough)

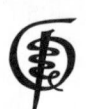

Nancy K. Henry, Walter R. Wilson, and J. Owen Hendley

BRUCELLOSIS

Brucellosis (undulant fever, Malta fever, Mediterranean fever) is an infection that causes abortion in domestic animals and may be transmitted incidentally to humans. In humans, the acute form is characterized by fever without localized findings. Chronic infection causes fever, weakness, and vague symptoms that may persist for months to years.

Classification and Characteristics

Marston, in 1863, provided the first description of the clinical presentation in humans; the etiologic agent was isolated by Bruce in 1886. In 1897, Bang reported that *Brucella abortus* was the cause of contagious abortion in cattle. There are at least six species of the genus *Brucella*. Three of these, *Brucella melitensis* (goats), *Brucella abortus* (cattle), and *Brucella suis* (pigs), are responsible for the majority of infections in humans. Rarely, a fourth species, *Brucella canis* (dogs, especially beagles), has been isolated from infected humans.

The Brucellae are small, non–spore-forming, nonencapsulated, gram-negative coccobacilli. Growth is best at 37° C in trypticase soy broth or tryptose phosphate broth at a pH of 6.7 in an atmosphere containing 10% carbon dioxide. Brucellae do not ferment carbohydrates, and the species may be distinguished from each other by their requirements for carbon dioxide atmosphere for growth, growth in the presence of dyes, production of hydrogen sulfide and urease, and specific agglutination in antisera. On solid media, the colonies are usually slow growing; small; smooth; translucent; and blue, white, or amber; they require at least 2 days to demonstrate growth.

Epidemiology

The natural reservoir of brucellosis in the United States is domestic animals, especially cattle, sheep, goats, and swine. Recently, brucellosis has been identified in wild bison herds in the western portion of the United States. The disease is transmitted to humans primarily by contact with infected animals. The organisms may invade through the conjunctivae, nasopharynx, gastrointestinal tract, or genitourinary tract, or through abraded skin or inadvertent subcutaneous inoculation. Human-to-human transmission probably does not occur.

Brucellosis is primarily an occupational disease involving meat-packing plant employees, veterinarians, laboratory personnel, farmers, and ranchers. Less commonly, brucellosis may be acquired by ingestion of unpasteurized dairy products. The enactment of local and state ordinances for animal surveillance and for pasteurization of dairy products has resulted in a steady decline in the reported number of cases of human brucellosis from the 1940s to the 1980s. The increased mobility of populations resulting from international air travel has resulted in more frequent diagnosis of brucellosis in the United States among travelers who live in areas of the world such as the Middle East, where brucellosis is endemic. In the Middle East, camels harbor *Brucella* and infection is transmitted to humans by direct contact with infected animals or by ingestion of unpasteurized camel's milk or milk products.

The usual male/female ratio is 6:1, with the peak incidence in 20- to 50-year-old males.

Currently, *B. abortus* and *B. suis* are the species most frequently

Table 270-1   Syndromes and treatment of disorders caused by *Brucella*, *Francisella*, *Pasteurella*, and *Yersinia*

ORGANISM	SYNDROMES	ANTIMICROBIAL THERAPY
Brucella *B. abortus* *B. melitensis* *B. suis* *B. canis*	Acute	Doxycycline 200 mg/day plus rifampin 600-900 mg/day for 6 weeks *or* tetracycline 2 g/day for 6 weeks plus streptomycin* 1 g/day *or* gentamicin 5 mg/kg/day for 2 weeks
	Endocarditis	Antibiotics as above plus cardiac valve replacement
	Central nervous system	Third-generation cephalosporin plus rifampin for 6 weeks
Francisella tularensis	Ulcerglandular Oculoglandular Pulmonary Typhoidal	Streptomycin 15-20 mg/kg/day *or* gentamicin 3-5 mg/kg/day for 7-14 days *or* doxycycline 200 mg/day *or* tetracycline 2 g/day *or* chloramphenicol 2 g/day for 14 days
Pasteurella multocida	Soft tissue Respiratory Endocarditis Osteomyelitis Bacteremia	Penicillin V 2 g/day *or* doxycycline 200 mg/day *or* TMP/SMX 1 DS tablet for 7-10 days Aqueous penicillin G 10-20 × 10⁶ units/day *or* parenteral cephalosporin for 2-4 weeks
Yersinia pestis	Bubonic Pneumonic Septicemic	Streptomycin* 2 g/day *or* gentamicin 5-7 mg/kg/day *or* tetracycline 2 g/day for 10 days
	Meningitis	Chloramphenicol 2 g/day for 10 days
Y. enterocolitica	Diarrhea Mesenteric adenitis	TMP/SMX 1 DS tablet twice daily *or* ciprofloxacin 500 mg-1 g/day *or* doxycycline 200 mg/day for 7-10 days
	Bacteremia	Gentamicin 5 mg/kg/day *or* parenteral TMP/SMX, ciprofloxacin, *or* doxycycline as above
Y. pseudotuberculosis	Mesenteric adenitis	Drug therapy controversial and includes aminoglycoside, chloramphenicol, tetracycline, or TMP/SMX

*Streptomycin is no longer manufactured by U. S. pharmaceutical companies. It may be difficult to obtain. Gentamicin therapy may be substituted for streptomycin if streptomycin is unavailable.
DS, double strength.

isolated from human infections in the United States. On a worldwide basis, *B. melitensis* is the most common cause of brucellosis.

Pathophysiology

After invasion of the human host, the Brucellae localize intracellularly in such tissues of the reticuloendothelial system as lymph nodes, bone marrow, liver, spleen, and kidneys. The bacilli are engulfed by macrophages, in which they may be killed rapidly, or the organisms may replicate and destroy the phagocytic cells, releasing more bacteria into the environment. This results in proliferation in the reticuloendothelial system and a characteristic but nonspecific reaction of these tissues. Granuloma formation occurs with the appearance of epithelioid cells, giant cells of the foreign body or Langhans' types, lymphocytes, and plasma cells. Although the granulomas typically are noncaseating, caseous necrosis may occur, especially with *B. suis* infections. Brucellae may reside intracellularly in phagocytes, in which they are relatively protected from antibody and from antimicrobial agents. In most instances, the granulomas undergo a process of healing, with fibrosis, death of the organisms, and frequently, calcification. Uncommonly, suppuration and caseation of the granulomas may occur, and Brucellae may survive for months to years, with periodic episodes of fever and nonspecific symptoms; or abscesses may develop in the reticuloendothelial system, testes, epididymides, ovaries, kidneys, brain, and other organs.

In animals, brucellae proliferate in the cytoplasm of the chorionic epithelial cells of the placenta as a consequence of the presence of high concentrations of erythritol, a carbohydrate that stimulates growth of brucellae. Erythritol is plentiful in the placentas of cattle, swine, goats, and sheep, but not humans. Possibly for this reason, brucellosis is a common cause of abortion in animals, but human abortion occurs no more frequently with this disease than with bacteremias caused by other microorganisms.

Clinical Manifestations

The four species of *Brucella* that affect humans differ in their virulence for humans. *B. abortus* infection is mild and usually self-limited; severe complications are uncommon. *B. suis* infection is characterized by a destructive, suppurative disease often associated with

a prolonged chronic localized infection. *B. melitensis* is the most virulent species and is associated with severe acute infection and the highest mortality rate. *B. canis* infection is similar to that caused by *B. abortus*.

Asymptomatic Brucellosis. Asymptomatic infections may be the most common form of brucellosis. Approximately 50% of meat-packing plant employees and 33% of veterinarians who had positive serologic titers for brucellosis were unaware of a previous acute infection. Infection in children is also frequently asymptomatic (Table 270-1).

Acute Brucellosis. The incubation period is usually from 5 to 14 days, although many months may elapse between the time of infection and the first appearance of symptoms. Bacteremia occurs without specific localizing signs. Most patients complain of malaise, fever, lethargy, weakness, weight loss, and anorexia. Fever from 38° C to 40° C is characteristically prominent in the afternoon or evening and is frequently associated with shaking chills and profuse sweats. Myalgias, headache, and backache occur frequently and are often severe. Approximately 20% of patients develop a monoarticular arthralgia affecting the large joints, especially the knee, shoulder, ankle, or elbow.

Abnormal physical findings, aside from tachycardia and fever, are often few or absent. Diffuse nontender lymphadenopathy and splenomegaly occur in 10% to 20% of patients, and hepatomegaly in 5% to 10%. On occasion, patients develop tender testicles and, infrequently, acute epididymitis.

Localized Brucellosis. Localized brucellosis occurs uncommonly, and less than 33% of these patients have fever, chills, malaise, and weight loss. Because the serologic titers in these patients may be low or absent, diagnosis is usually made by biopsy and isolation of the organism from culture. The most common sites of involvement of localized brucellosis (roughly in decreasing order of frequency) are bone and joint, spleen, endocardium, lung, genitourinary tract, and nervous system.

Bone and joint. Arthralgias and myalgias occur frequently in acute brucellosis, but these symptoms usually are self-limited or disappear with antimicrobial therapy. When localized disease occurs, the most frequent sites involved are the spine and knee. Sacroiliitis is the most commonly reported site of involvement. Spondylitis involves the intervertebral disk and adjacent structures. Localized pain and nerve root irritation are prominent complaints. Osteoporosis, periosteal thickening, or paravertebral abscess may occur. With healing, dense sclerosis results in the formation of a characteristic x-ray appearance of "parrot-beak" osteophytes. Differential diagnosis includes tuberculosis and *Staphylococcus aureus* osteomyelitis (Chapter 243).

Gastrointestinal. Brucellosis may present as an enteric fever with anorexia, abdominal pain, nausea, vomiting, diarrhea, or constipation. Gastrointestinal complaints occur in up to 80% of patients with brucellosis. Multiple or single splenic abscesses of various sizes may occur. The characteristic x-ray appearance of splenic brucellosis is one of splenomegaly with multiple calcific lesions or concentric "bull's-eye" calcifications. Splenic brucellosis may be associated with sporadic febrile episodes of irregular periodicity. The episodes may occur frequently or may recur after 20 or more years of quiescence. In approximately 30% to 50% of patients with brucellosis, liver function tests become abnormal. Granulomatous hepatitis may occur, especially with *B. abortus* infection.

Infective endocarditis. Infective endocarditis occurs in less than 2% of patients. Brucellar endocarditis is an acute ulcerative process usually involving the aortic valve. Because most available antibiotics are bacteriostatic against brucellae, relapse rates have been reported to be high. Cardiac valve replacement is usually necessary to eradicate the infection.

Respiratory tract. Hilar adenopathy, often bilateral, and peribronchial and perihilar pulmonary infiltrates characterize the pulmonary form of brucellosis. Pleural effusion or empyema also may occur. Pulmonary nodules may be indistinguishable from carcinoma. Healed pulmonary brucellosis may be associated with multiple calcified granulomas that resemble histoplasmosis on chest x-ray.

Genitourinary tract. *B. suis* is the most common cause of renal brucellosis. Perinephric abscess or chronic granulomatous pyelonephritis may occur. Brucellae may be isolated from urine culture in these patients. Brucellosis and renal tuberculosis should be considered in the differential diagnosis of pyuria with negative routine microbiologic urine cultures. Testicular swelling and tenderness occur in at least 5% of cases, and *B. suis* is more commonly associated with testicular abnormalities than are other species. Sterility in the male occurs rarely. In women, tuboovarian and pelvic abscess with chronic endometritis and cervicitis have been described.

Nervous system. Rarely, brucellosis may cause meningoencephalitis, peripheral neuropathy, myelitis, or myelopathy. In chronic meningitis, pleocytosis is present, but cerebrospinal fluid cultures for Brucellae are rarely positive.

Strain 19 Vaccine Disease. Strain 19 vaccine is a live brucella vaccine used by veterinarians to immunize cattle against *B. abortus.* Inadvertent self-inoculation of veterinarians, either through the skin or by conjunctival spray or ingestion, is relatively common. Vaccine-associated disease is usually milder than the naturally acquired form and is manifested by fever, chills, headache, fatigue, and myalgia. Multiple episodes of inadvertent self-inoculations are not uncommon. The condition is self-limited.

Chronic Brucellosis. Chronic brucellosis is a poorly understood condition in which a small percentage of patients with acute brucellosis develop a chronic state of ill health that may persist for months or years. These patients complain of weakness, fatigue, mental depression, vague pains, and intermittent fever; they usually have no abnormal physical findings referable to brucellosis, except splenomegaly. These patients should be evaluated for possible sites of chronic suppuration, especially in the spleen, liver, or kidneys. Blood cultures are negative, and serologic tests are of little value in the diagnosis of chronic brucellosis.

Diagnosis

Brucellosis should be suspected in patients who have been febrile for a week or more and who have a history of occupational or other exposure to animals, travel to endemic areas, or ingestion of unpasteurized dairy products. Although the physical examination is usually normal, generalized lymphadenopathy or hepatosplenomegaly may be present. Routine laboratory tests are of minimal value in the diagnosis. Leukopenia or a normal white blood cell count occurs more commonly than does leukocytosis. The organism may be isolated from blood, urine, bone marrow, or tissue cultures. Bone marrow cultures are positive more often than blood cultures are. It is important to notify the microbiology laboratory that brucellosis is suspected. Cultures must be kept for at least 3 to 4 weeks, and the use of biphasic trypticase soy broth and agar (Casteneda's medium) with a carbon dioxide atmosphere facilitates the isolation of brucellae from culture.

Serum antibody titer measured by the standard agglutination test primarily measures circulating IgM antibody. Within the first few weeks of acute infection, the standard agglutination titer increases four-fold to eight-fold. A titer equal to or greater than 1:160 is considered significant. Despite appropriate antimicrobial therapy, the standard agglutination titer may remain persistently elevated for a prolonged period (up to 2 years) in 5% to 7% of patients. As a consequence, the standard agglutination titer may not be useful in differentiating acute infection or acute relapse of a chronic infection from other causes of fever in patients with chronic brucellosis. A false-positive standard agglutination titer may occur as a result of immunologic cross-reactivity in patients with tularemia, *Yersinia* infection, or cholera, or with vaccination against these infections.

The 2-mercaptoethanol agglutination test destroys IgM antibody and measures IgG antibody. Although this test is not as sensitive as the standard agglutination test, a significantly elevated titer ($\geq$1:60) correlates better with activation of infection in patients with chronic brucellosis. Moreover, the 2-mercaptoethanol test is more often useful in predicting recovery from *brucella* infection. Titers usually disappear within 6 months after appropriate antimicrobial therapy. Radioimmunoassay or enzyme-linked immunosorbent assay detects IgM and IgG antibody and may be useful in distinguishing acute from chronic infection, as well as acute exacerbation of chronic infection. The brucella skin-test antigen is of little diagnostic use and is probably best avoided. The use of polymerase chain reaction or enzyme-linked immunosorbent assay (ELISA) is reportedly useful for the diagnosis of brucellosis. These tests have not yet been standardized but likely will be in the relatively near future.

Treatment

Many patients with brucellosis recover spontaneously, and patients should be reassured that with appropriate therapy, recovery from infection is anticipated. Adequate rest, nutrition, hydration, and other supportive measures are important in managing patients with active infections.

Antimicrobial therapy shortens the duration and reduces the frequency of complications of acute brucellosis (Table 270-1). The use of a single antimicrobial agent for the treatment of patients with brucellosis is associated with a higher relapse rate than the use of combination therapy. Previously the World Health Organization (WHO) recommended the use of tetracycline for 6 weeks together with streptomycin for the first 3 weeks of therapy. Streptomycin must be administered intramuscularly, a factor that complicates therapy. Presumably, gentamicin may be substituted for streptomycin but limited clinical data are published on the use of gentamicin therapy for brucellosis. Currently the World Health Organization recommends the use of doxycycline together with rifampin for 6 weeks (Table 270-1), and this regimen is probably the treatment of choice for patients with brucellosis. Patients unable to tolerate doxycycline, such as pregnant women or children, may be treated with a combination of trimethoprim-sulfamethoxazole and rifampin. More seriously ill patients should be treated with tetracycline for 4 to 6 weeks, together with streptomycin for 2 to 3 weeks, or co-trimoxazole together with streptomycin. Therapy with rifampin may be added to either regimen for 4 to 6 weeks. Patients with infective endocarditis or central nervous system infection should be treated with a combination of antimicrobial agents as listed previously, but the duration of therapy should be at least 3 to 6 months. Most patients with *Brucella* endocarditis require cardiac valve replacement in addition to antimicrobial therapy. Although some fluoroquinolones are active in vitro against *Brucella,* the relapse rate following therapy with a fluoroquinolone is unacceptably high.

Relapse occurs frequently after completion of treatment and may be treated with another course of antimicrobial agents. Relapse occurs less frequently after combined tetracycline-streptomycin therapy than with tetracycline therapy alone. Approximately 5% of patients receiving antimicrobial therapy experience a Jarisch-Herxheimer reaction. Severe reactions may be treated with prednisone, 20 mg/day for 3 to 4 days.

The therapy of localized brucellosis depends on the site involved and the nature of the infection. All patients should receive appropriate antimicrobial therapy. Abscesses should be excised and drained; spondylitis may be treated with antimicrobials and immobilization. Splenectomy may be necessary in patients with splenic brucellosis associated with multiple relapses, splenomegaly, or large, calcific splenic granulomata.

The treatment of chronic relapsing brucellosis is frustrating. Localized areas of suppuration should be treated surgically. Antimicrobial therapy in these patients is usually ineffective, and psychotherapy, good nutrition, and reassurance are often more important than the use of antibiotics. Occasionally, the use of short-term (3 to 4 days) corticosteroid therapy is necessary for control of debilitating, episodic symptoms.

The mortality rate for untreated cases of brucellosis is low (3% to 5%). Deaths are most often associated with infective endocarditis. With appropriate antimicrobial therapy, the mortality rate is less than 1%. Complications occur in approximately 1% to 2% of patients. With adequate therapy, patients are able to return to work in 6 weeks or less.

Reinfection may occur. Immunity induced by one attack is only relative, and multiple reinfections may occur in individuals at high risk of exposure. Some individuals who have recovered from one or more infections acquire hypersensitivity to Brucella antigen. Veterinarians are especially susceptible to this problem, and accidental exposure to strain 19 may result in brief, violent, local and systemic reactions.

Prevention

The only practical means of eliminating brucellosis is to eliminate the animal reservoir of the disease. A federally funded eradication program in the United States has drastically reduced the number of bovine cases. Porcine brucellosis remains a serious problem for individuals working in pork-processing plants. There is no entirely sure means of eliminating exposure to brucellosis for meat-packing plant workers, veterinarians, laboratory workers, or livestock workers. Employees should use protective gloves, eyeglasses, and clothing. Cuts or other skin abrasions should be dressed carefully. Ingestion of unpasteurized dairy products should be avoided. An active educational program should be instituted for high-risk individuals. No satisfactory vaccine for human use is available.

FRANCISELLA TULARENSIS
Classification and Characteristics

Francisella tularensis causes tularemia (rabbit fever, deerfly fever), an infectious disease of animals that may be transmitted to humans by direct contact or by insect vector. In humans, infections are characterized by the presence of a cutaneous or mucocutaneous lesion, lymphadenopathy, high fever, and severe constitutional symptoms, which, if untreated, may persist for weeks to several months.

F. (Pasteurella) tularensis is a small, gram-negative, nonmotile, aerobic, pleomorphic coccobacillus. Special culture media (e.g., glucose-cysteine blood agar, thioglycolate broth, or other cysteine-supplemented media) are required for growth. Growth is optimal at 37° C, and small, smooth, opaque colonies appear after 24 to 48 hours of incubation. The organism may be identified on the basis of its morphology, growth requirements, fluorescent staining, and agglutinins with specific antisera.

Cross-reactions with serum agglutinins of brucellosis and plague may occur because *F. tularensis* is related antigenically to their causative organisms.

Epidemiology

F. tularensis has been isolated from more than 100 wild mammals; from amphibians, fish, birds, ticks, deerflies, and mosquitoes; and from water samples. In the United States, the most important reservoirs are rabbits and ticks.

Humans are highly susceptible to tularemia. Infection is most com-monly acquired through the bite of an infected arthropod, through dermal or mucosal contact, or through inhalation of aerosolized organisms from tissue or body fluids of an infected animal. The gastrointestinal tract is relatively resistant to *F. tularensis* and, uncommonly, the infection may be acquired by ingestion of contaminated water or undercooked meat. The organism is highly infectious for laboratory personnel, and microbiologic cultures and infected animals should be handled with caution. Laboratory personnel who process these specimens should always be warned when tularemia is suspected. Culture plates should be handled in vented hoods to avoid inhalation of aerosolized organisms. Tularemia occasionally is transmitted by occupational exposure; veterinarians, trappers, meat-packing plant employees, and livestock workers are at risk.

Cases usually occur sporadically, but clusters and small epidemics have been reported. An epidemic in Vermont was attributed to infected muskrats. Human-to-human transmission probably does not occur.

The incidence of human tularemia in the United States reached a peak in the late 1930s and has declined steadily to levels of 0.6 to 0.7 per million population. The disease is most common in Texas, Arkansas, Illinois, Tennessee, Missouri, and Virginia. Most cases occur during the spring and summer months in areas where tick-borne cases predominate. During winter months, rabbit-associated cases are more common. Infection rates are highest among adult men.

Pathophysiology

In humans, as few as 50 organisms can cause infection if injected intradermally or inhaled, whereas at least 10^8 organisms are required when ingested orally. The most common portals of entry in humans are the skin and mucous membranes. *F. tularensis* is capable of penetrating intact skin, but more often the organisms are inoculated by insect bite or enter inapparent abrasions or anatomic openings such as hair follicles. Approximately 48 hours after the bacilli gain entry into the skin, a macular erythematous lesion develops and becomes papular. The papule is pruritic; it enlarges, and ulceration occurs, usually within 4 to 7 days after initial contact. The evolution of the cutaneous lesions is associated with fever, chills, regional lymphadenopathy, and bacteremia. The organisms are engulfed by cells of the reticuloendothelial system, in which they may survive intracellularly for long periods.

Evisceration of animals infected with tularemia may cause aerosolization of organisms, and in humans, inhalation results in the pneumonic form of tularemia. Bacteremia after cutaneous infection may also cause tularemic pneumonia. Ingestion of a large number of *F. tularemia* organisms may cause pharyngitis and cervical lymphadenopathy or a nonspecific febrile illness with no localized findings. The gastrointestinal form of tularemia occurs uncommonly, and a greater hazard associated with the ingestion of contaminated food may be aerosolization and inhalation of organisms during mastication.

Early lesions are characterized on histopathologic examination by focal necrosis occurring especially in organs of the reticuloendothelial system. Subsequently, the necrotic areas may undergo granulomatous reactions with multinucleated giant cells and, occasionally, with caseation. Healing is associated with fibrosis and calcification of the granulomata.

Clinical Manifestations

After an incubation period of 2 to 7 days, the large majority of patients with tularemia have an abrupt onset of fever and chills. Fever of 39° to 40.6° C is continuous or mildly intermittent. Severe generalized headache and myalgias occur commonly. In untreated cases, fever may persist for a month or longer. Hepatosplenomegaly is common, especially in untreated cases. A generalized maculopapular rash occurs in approximately 25% of cases.

Patients with tularemia have one of the following clinical syndromes.

Ulceroglandular. The ulceroglandular form of tularemia (75% to 85% of cases) is characterized by the development of an indurated skin lesion at the portal of entry and by regional lymphadenopathy. The involved lymph nodes are exquisitely tender, warm, erythematous, and fluctuant. Drainage may occur spontaneously. Regional lymphadenopathy in patients with tularemia is usually more prominent and painful than that accompanying infections caused by other organisms. Generalized adenopathy may occur, but the regional lymph nodes are involved most prominently. In 10% of cases, the skin lesion may be inapparent (glandular form). In rabbit-associated cases, the skin lesion is located on the finger or hand in more than 90% of cases; in tick-borne cases, the ulcer is usually located on the lower extremity, perineum, or trunk. The location of the skin lesion accounts for the higher frequency of axillary or epitrochlear lymphadenopathy in rabbit-associated cases and for inguinal and femoral adenopathy characteristic of infections transmitted by tick bite.

Typhoidal. The typhoidal form (5% to 15% of cases) may occur after intradermal, respiratory, or gastrointestinal tract entry. Fever, chills, weight loss, and hepatosplenomegaly without localized findings occur. Skin lesions and regional lymphadenopathy are absent, and the only clue to the diagnosis may be a history of possible exposure.

The mortality among patients with typhoidal tularemia is higher than in patients with ulceroglandular disease. Factors associated with a higher mortality are delayed diagnosis and antimicrobial therapy, pneumonia, and abnormal renal function.

Oculoglandular. The conjunctiva is the portal of entry for oculoglandular tularemia (1% to 2% of cases), and patients have unilateral painful purulent conjunctivitis together with preauricular or cervical lymphadenopathy. Small nodular lesions or ulcerations of the conjunctiva may be present in some patients.

Oropharyngeal. Rarely, after gastrointestinal challenge, an acute exudative or membranous pharyngitis with cervical lymphadenopathy may occur (in less than 1% of cases).

Pulmonary. Pleuropulmonary complications occur in approximately 10% to 15% of ulceroglandular, and in as many as 80% of typhoidal, cases of tularemia. The pneumonic form of tularemia may occur as a result of direct inhalation of aerosolized organisms or as a result of bacteremia. Cough is usually nonproductive. Physical examination of the chest frequently reveals no abnormalities. Bilateral patchy infiltrates or, occasionally, lobar pneumonia is visible on x-ray (Fig. 270-1). Pleural effusion may occur.

Complications. Meningitis, osteomyelitis, endocarditis, pericarditis, and peritonitis are rare complications of tularemia.

Diagnosis

Ulceroglandular tularemia must be distinguished from other conditions and infections associated with the clinical syndrome of fever, a cutaneous ulcer, and regional lymphadenopathy.

A thorough history is important in the diagnosis of tularemia. Contact with wild animals, ticks, or deerflies, or exposure in the case of veterinarians or laboratory personnel, should suggest the diagnosis of tularemia in a patient with an acute febrile illness, especially if such factors are associated with a cutaneous lesion and lymphadenopathy. The typical features of ulceroglandular infection are often so characteristic of tularemia that this diagnosis is self-evident. Tularemia may be unsuspected in atypical cases or in the typhoidal form. As many as 80% of patients with the typhoidal form reportedly do not have a history of vector contact. Often, a high index of suspicion for tularemia in endemic areas is necessary to establish a diagnosis.

Gram-stained smears of sputum or exudate from ulcers or lymph nodes only rarely demonstrate *F. tularensis;* special culture media are necessary to isolate the microorganism. Because of the high risk to laboratory personnel, most laboratories are reluctant to attempt isolation of *F. tularensis* from clinical specimens or animals. Preferably, only those laboratories with experienced personnel and adequate facilities for processing specimens and cultures should attempt microbiologic studies of *F. tularensis*. The agglutination test is a reliable, standard, and safe method for diagnosing tularemia. A four-fold increase in titer is diagnostic of infection; a single convalescent titer of 1:160 or greater is highly suggestive of recent or current infection. Agglutination titers are usually negative during the first week of ill-

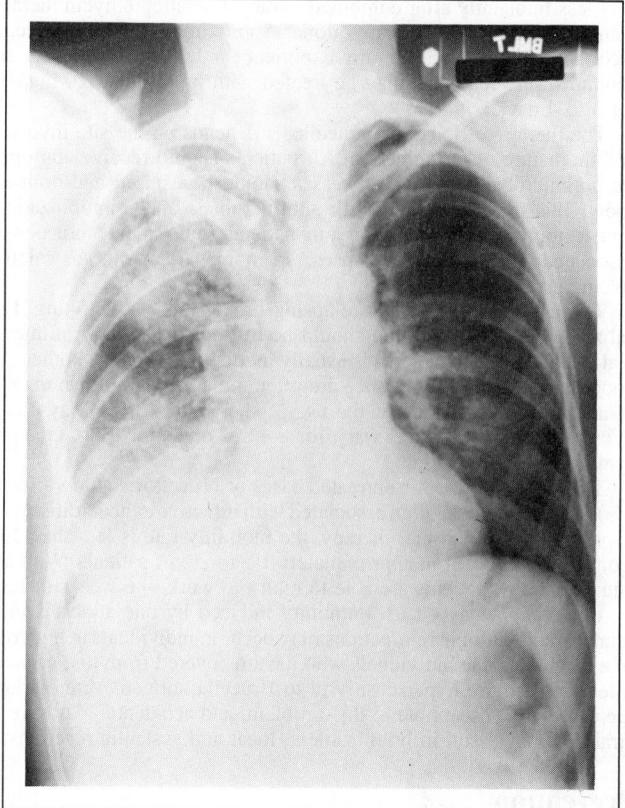

FIGURE 270-1   *Tularemia* pneumonia.

ness and become positive in 50% of patients during the second week. Titers reach a maximum after 4 to 8 weeks and may remain elevated for months to years after an acute infection. Agglutinins for brucellosis may appear and increase during tularemia infection, but the antibody is present in low titer.

Treatment

Streptomycin or gentamicin administered alone is the drug of choice for treating all forms of tularemia. Streptomycin therapy for 7 to 14 days is highly effective. Gentamicin therapy may be preferable in patients with preexisting vestibular dysfunction or in patients over 65 years of age. Adjustments of streptomycin or gentamicin dosage must be made in patients with abnormal renal function (Chapter 231). For patients unable to tolerate streptomycin or gentamicin, tetracycline or chloramphenicol may be administered for 14 days. Relapse is not caused by resistant microorganisms and should be treated with another course of the same antimicrobial drug. A variety of other antimicrobial agents are active in vitro against *F. tularensis,* including some fluoroquinolones, erythromycin, rifampin, cefotaxime, and ceftriaxone, but clinical experience with these agents is limited. For the treatment of meningitis caused by *F. tularensis,* a combination of gentamicin and chloramphenicol should be used.

The mortality rate among untreated patients is 5% to 15%; the typhoidal form is associated with the higher figure. With appropriate antimicrobial therapy, mortality is less than 1%. Immunity after acute infection with *F. tularensis* is lifelong.

Prevention

Avoidance of contact with possible sources of infection is the most effective means of prevention. A live attenuated tularemia vaccine is available for high-risk individuals from the Centers for Disease Control and Prevention (CDC) in Atlanta, Georgia. The vaccine is administered intradermally by multiple-puncture techniques like those for vaccinia; it is effective but does not provide complete protection.

The attack rate and severity of the infection are markedly reduced in vaccinated individuals.

Antimicrobial prophylaxis following tick or other insect bites is not recommended. Antibiotic prophylaxis with streptomycin or gentamicin after known exposure to *F. tularensis,* for example, among laboratory workers, protects against infection. The prophylactic use of tetracycline or chloramphenicol, however, does not protect against infection and simply prolongs the incubation period.

PASTEURELLA SPECIES
Classification and Characteristics

Pasteurellae are primarily animal pathogens, but they occasionally produce infection in humans; these infections range from small, localized cutaneous abscesses to septicemia, osteomyelitis, and endocarditis. *Pasteurella multocida* is the species most often associated with disease in humans. Very rarely, human infections have been caused by other pasteurellae *(Pasteurella haemolytica, Pasteurella pneumotropica, Pasteurella ureae).*

Pasteurellae are small, non–spore-forming, nonmotile, bipolar, gram-negative coccobacilli. Growth occurs in aerobic or facultatively anaerobic conditions at 37° C on ordinary culture media and is enhanced by blood- or serum-enriched agar under carbon dioxide atmosphere. The different species of *Pasteurella* may be distinguished by their ability to cause hemolysis on blood agar and pathogenicity in laboratory animals. Four serotypes of *P. multocida* have been identified.

Epidemiology

P. multocida has been isolated from a great number of wild and domestic animals. The highest carriage occurs in cats (50% to 90%), dogs or swine (50%), and rats (15%). The majority of human infections are associated with animal bites or scratches, especially those of cats and dogs. Human infection may also occur in association with animal exposure other than bites. These infections occur in persons who have frequent contact with animals and usually involve the upper respiratory tract, extremities, or intraabdominal organs. Some patients with *P. multocida* infection (approximately 15%) have no known animal contact. Infection in these patients usually involves the upper respiratory tract or occurs intraabdominally. *P. multocida* has been isolated from the nasopharynx of apparently normal individuals exposed to animals.

Pathophysiology

After cutaneous or subcutaneous inoculation, a local inflammatory reaction occurs; this is followed by necrosis and, in some cases, by abscess formation. Cellulitis and, infrequently, lymphangitis may occur. The oropharyngeal form is characterized by exudative pharyngitis, occasionally with the formation of tonsillar or peritonsillar abscess. Rarely, bacteremia occurs, and microabscesses may develop in multiple organs such as bone, brain, lung, or endocardium. The virulence of *P. multocida* is related to the degree of encapsulation; strains with large capsules are more resistant to phagocytosis and are more aggressive than those with small or absent capsules.

Clinical Manifestations

The most common manifestation in humans is a localized soft tissue infection (usually on an extremity) that develops after direct animal contact, especially dog or cat bite. Within hours to several days after exposure, patients complain of pain of acute onset, erythema, and swelling at the site of inoculation. Serosanguineous drainage of the cutaneous lesion often occurs 1 to 2 days after onset of symptoms. A low-grade fever and regional lymphadenopathy occur commonly. Abscesses may form, and, rarely, osteomyelitis complicates local infection of the extremity.

P. multocida has been isolated, alone or in combination with other microorganisms, from the nasopharynx or sputum of patients with chronic obstructive pulmonary disease or with no apparent underlying condition. Many of these patients have no history of recent animal exposure. Rarely, *P. multocida* has been isolated from patients with sinusitis, pharyngitis, pharyngeal abscess, otitis, bronchiectasis, empyema, peritonitis, or pyelonephritis. *P. multocida* is a rare cause of infective endocarditis.

Diagnosis

P. multocida infection should be suspected in patients with a history of animal exposure and a cutaneous infection, especially that following a cat or dog bite. Gram-negative bipolar bacilli may be visualized on gram-stained smears of pus, exudate, or other specimens. Confirmation of this diagnosis requires isolation of *P. multocida* from culture.

Treatment

Penicillin is the drug of choice for the treatment of *P. multocida* and other *Pasteurella* species infections. Localized cutaneous infection without osteomyelitis may be treated successfully with penicillin V or amoxicillin/clavulanate potassium (Augmentin) administered orally for 7 to 10 days. Severe infections, for example, bacteremia, endocarditis, or meningitis, should be treated with intravenous penicillin for 2 to 4 weeks or longer, depending on the nature of the infection. Patients unable to tolerate the penicillins may be treated with parenteral second- or third-generation cephalosporins, tetracycline, co-trimoxazole, or chloramphenicol. Orally administered cephalosporins such as cephalexin, cefaclor, and cefadroxil are less active than penicillin in vitro and should not be administered to patients with *P. multocida* infection. Ciprofloxacin is quite active in vitro against *P. multocida,* but few data are published concerning the efficacy of ciprofloxacin therapy in humans. Appropriate surgical drainage or debridement is important in treating abscess, osteomyelitis, and other deep-seated infections. Death occurs very rarely in patients with *P. multocida* infections and is usually associated with endocarditis or meningitis.

Prevention

Avoidance of contact with wild and domestic animals is probably the only means of preventing human *P. multocida* infections. Animal bites, scratches, or other wounds should be cleaned, debrided, and dressed adequately.

YERSINIA SPECIES

The genus *Yersinia* includes *Yersinia pestis, Yersinia enterocolitica,* and *Yersinia pseudotuberculosis.* These organisms cause disease primarily in animals; humans most often acquire infection as a result of direct contact with infected animals or animal products. In humans, *Y. pestis* causes plague; mesenteric lymphadenitis and enterocolitis are caused by *Y. enterocolitis* or *Y. pseudotuberculosis.*

Yersinia pestis

Classification and Characteristics. Throughout history, plague has been a source of dread and fascination. Pandemics of plague have caused human suffering and death unequaled by those of any other infectious disease. At least three great pandemics of plague have occurred in the last 1500 years. The first authentic pandemic was recorded in the sixth century AD. The second pandemic, known as the "black death," swept through Europe, Asia, and Africa during the fourteenth century, killing an estimated one fourth of the world's population (60 million deaths). The last major pandemic originated in China in 1894 and reached the United States in 1900.

Y. pestis is a gram-negative, nonmotile, non–spore-forming, bipolar-staining, pleomorphic bacillus. The organism is an aerobe or facultative anaerobe that grows well at 37° C on many routine culture media. Growth is somewhat slow, and cultures should be held a minimum of 48 to 72 hours before being discarded as negative. The colonies are small and transparent and have the appearance of beaten copper.

Virulence is related to the production of endotoxin, exotoxin, and a substance called *fraction 1.* Fraction 1 is a soluble protein that makes the organism relatively resistant to phagocytosis. A lipopolysaccharide endotoxin is responsible for most of the clinical manifestations of plague.

Epidemiology. Plague occurs worldwide as an enzootic disease affecting more than 200 species of mammals, notably rodents. Disease in wild rodents (sylvatic plague) serves as a reservoir for infection for domestic rats (murine or rat plague), which, along with their ectoparasites (fleas), often live in close association with humans. The principal murine hosts, which have worldwide distribution, are the domestic rat *(Rattus rattus)* and the ectoparasite vector, the oriental rat flea *Xenopsylla cheopis.* Infection of the flea occurs by ingestion of blood from a bacteremic animal. The organisms multiply in the gastrointestinal tract of the flea and are regurgitated when the flea ingests another blood meal. Rat fleas will attack humans, especially during periods when the population of rats declines because of plague-associated deaths. Humans acquire the disease as a direct result of the flea bite or by scratching the regurgitated gastrointestinal contents of the flea into the bite.

Infection may also be acquired by direct contact with infected animals during evisceration, skinning, or, rarely, by animal bite. Human-to-human transmission may occur by inhalation of droplet nuclei from patients with the pneumonic form of plague. Airborne infection is highly contagious to individuals caring for patients with pneumonic plague, and such patients should be placed in strict isolation.

In the United States, the majority of cases occur in the southwestern states, especially New Mexico and Arizona. Male patients predominate, and two thirds of patients are less than 20 years of age. In New Mexico, the majority of cases occur among native Americans living in rural areas.

Pathophysiology. After the flea-borne *Y. pestis* organisms gain access to a human host, the bacilli are phagocytized quickly by polymorphonuclear leukocytes and macrophages. The flea-borne bacilli are relatively resistant to intracellular killing and replicate rapidly, with the production of capsular antigen (factor 1) and other toxins. Lysis of phagocytes releases a large number of virulent microorganisms that are resistant to phagocytosis. A marked inflammatory response usually occurs in regional lymph nodes. Bacteremia results in metastatic foci of infection in the lungs, other lymph nodes, and viscera. A marked hemorrhagic diathesis develops as a result of a direct effect of plague toxin on blood vessels or as a consequence of disseminated intravascular coagulation. Profound toxemia ensues, and even patients treated with appropriate antimicrobial therapy may die of fulminant toxemia despite eradication of the microorganism. The precise mechanisms of the severe tissue damage and toxemia caused by *Y. pestis* are not understood fully.

Clinical Manifestations. Human plague usually presents in three clinical forms: bubonic, pneumonic, or septicemic. These forms may appear singly or in combination.

Bubonic plague. Bubonic plague is the most common form of plague (90% to 95% of cases). After an incubation period of 1 to 12 days (usually 2 to 4 days), patients develop an acute, often fulminant illness. Symptoms begin abruptly with fever (39° to 41° C), shaking chills, nausea, vomiting, headache, delirium, and marked prostration. The flea bite portal of entry is rarely visible. If present, it is a vesiculopapular lesion that becomes pustular. More than two thirds of patients develop painful regional lymphadenopathy in the first 2 days of illness. Lymphadenopathy occurs most commonly in the inguinal area and (in decreasing order of frequency) in the axillary, cervical, and epitrochlear areas. Generalized lymphadenopathy occurs in approximately 15% of cases. Lymph nodes (buboes) are matted, tender, 2 to 5 cm in diameter, and surrounded by a zone of boggy hemorrhagic edema. Suppuration and drainage occur after 1 to 2 weeks of illness. Petechiae and large ecchymotic skin lesions occur, and hemorrhage into a serous cavity or viscus or into the gastrointestinal tract, respiratory tract, nasopharynx, or genitourinary tract is common. Occasionally, patients with disseminated intravascular coagulation develop gangrene of the fingers, toes, nose, or penis. The term *black death,* used to describe cases of plague during the Middle Ages, is derived from the appearance of the hemorrhagic complications.

The course of bubonic plague is characterized by an irregular fever that often declines with the appearance of buboes and then in-

creases again. In favorable outcomes, the fever decreases gradually, concomitantly with generalized improvement. In fatal cases, a precipitous increase or decrease in fever, often to a subnormal level, occurs just before death. Most fatalities occur during the first week of illness.

Pneumonic plague. Approximately 5% of patients with bubonic plague develop bacteremic pneumonia. Primary pneumonic plague occurs as a result of inhalation of droplet nuclei from a patient with pneumonic plague or as a result of laboratory-acquired infection. A large amount of blood-streaked, mucoid sputum is produced, which contains an enormous number of *Y. pestis* bacilli. Pneumonic plague is a fulminant illness accompanied by marked prostration, dyspnea, cyanosis, and death within 1 to 5 days in virtually 100% of untreated patients.

Septicemic plague. In approximately 5% to 10% of patients, an acute, prostrating febrile illness occurs without detectable lymphadenopathy. Manifestations are otherwise identical to those of bubonic plague. Untreated patients die as a result of endotoxemic shock and disseminated intravascular coagulation, usually within 3 to 5 days from onset of symptoms (Chapter 245).

Diagnosis. The diagnosis of plague should be suspected in individuals with fever and painful lymphadenopathy who reside in or travel to endemic areas. Bubonic plague mimics many diseases, including tularemia, severe staphylococcal or streptococcal infection, lymphogranuloma venereum, and cat-scratch fever. The septicemic form, or the early stage of infection before the appearance of localized signs, resembles typhoid fever, rickettsial infection, or malaria. *Y. pestis* may be isolated from blood culture or aspirate of buboes in at least 80% of patients with bubonic plague. Virtually all patients with the septicemic form have positive blood cultures, and the bacteremia often reaches very high levels (10^4 to 10^6/ml). Gram-stained smears of bubo aspirates, or sputum from patients with pneumonic plague, demonstrate gram-negative bacilli. The classic bipolar staining is best demonstrated by Wright-Giemsa stains of aspirates or peripheral blood. Serologic diagnosis is helpful for retrospective confirmation.

Treatment. Strict hospital isolation of patients with plague is mandatory until the completion of several days of antimicrobial therapy. High-dose streptomycin administered for 2 to 3 days followed by lower dosages to complete a total of 10 days of treatment is effective therapy. Although streptomycin remains the drug of choice for the treatment of plague, gentamicin may be substituted. Tetracycline administered orally or intravenously in divided doses for 10 days is also effective. Patients with plague meningitis should be treated with chloramphenicol for 10 days.

The mortality rate for untreated bubonic plague is estimated to be 50% to 90%. Virtually all untreated patients with septicemic or pneumonic plague die. With appropriate treatment, mortality in cases acquired in the United States has been reduced to 10% to 15%.

Prevention

Individuals in endemic areas should avoid contact with wild animals, particularly rodents. A formalin-killed plague vaccine is available for persons at high risk of exposure in plague-endemic areas and for laboratory personnel who work with *Y. pestis.*

Chemoprophylaxis should be administered to individuals who have had close contact with patients with suspected or confirmed plague pneumonia and for household contacts of flea-borne plague cases. Tetracycline 30 mg/kg/day or sulfonamide 30 to 60 mg/kg/day administered orally in divided doses for 7 days is an effective chemoprophylactic agent.

Yersinia Species

Classification and Characteristics. *Y. enterocolitica* and *Y. pseudotuberculosis* are microorganisms that primarily inhabit a large variety of wild and domestic animals. *Y. enterocolitica* is a relatively common cause of enterocolitis and mesenteric lymphadenitis in Scandinavia. *Y. pseudotuberculosis* has been isolated from cases of mesenteric adenitis and septicemia.

Y. enterocolitica and *Y. pseudotuberculosis* are gram-negative, pleomorphic bacilli that do not ferment lactose, are urease-positive, and can be distinguished from each other and from *Y. pestis* by serologic and biochemical tests, pathogenicity in animals, and bacteriophage sensitivity patterns. *Y. enterocolitica* and *Y. pseudotuberculosis* grow well on conventional culture media at 37° C and in buffered saline at 4° C. Both are motile at 22° to 25° C but nonmotile at 37° C. At least 34 serotypes of *Y. enterocolitica* and 5 serotypes of *Y. pseudotuberculosis* have been identified. *Y. enterocolitica* produces a heat-stable enterotoxin and lipopolysaccharide endotoxin similar to that produced by other gram-negative bacilli. The virulence of *Y. pseudotuberculosis* appears to be related to the production of lipopolysaccharide endotoxin and to its ability to survive intracellularly.

Epidemiology. The incidence of *Y. enterocolitica* infections is highest in Scandinavia; sporadic cases have been reported in the United States. The means of transmission is unclear. The organism has been isolated from a large variety of wild and domestic animals, from fresh water, and from a number of foods, including meat, shellfish, tofu, and dairy products. Presumably, transmission from animals to humans occurs. Food-borne transmission to humans has been documented among school children. Infections occur most frequently in children and adolescents during the winter months.

Y. pseudotuberculosis has been isolated from many species of wild and domestic animals and from food, water, and environmental sources. Humans probably acquire infection as a result of contact with animals or through ingestion of contaminated food or water. The highest incidence occurs among Scandinavian children and adolescents during the winter months. Sporadic cases have been reported in the United States.

Pathophysiology. The presumed portal of entry for human cases of *Y. enterocolitica* and *Y. pseudotuberculosis* infections is the gastrointestinal tract. Human pathogenic strains of *Y. enterocolitica* cause mucosal ulcerations in the terminal ileum, necrosis of Peyer's patches, and mesenteric adenitis. Bacteremia occurs rarely and may be associated with metastatic abscess formation. Polyarthritis has been reported in association with *Y. enterocolitica* infection, especially among persons with histocompatibility antigen HLA-B27.

Y. pseudotuberculosis causes ulcerative lesions in the terminal ileum; it also causes mesenteric adenitis. Bacteremia may occur rarely. On histopathologic examination, suppurative granulomatous lesions occur, and in bacteremic cases, the liver, spleen, and other organs may be involved.

Clinical Manifestations. Enterocolitis is the most common clinical manifestation of *Y. enterocolitica* infection (Chapter 242). Most patients are less than 5 years of age and exhibit fever, abdominal pain, and diarrhea usually lasting 1 to 3 weeks. Fecal leukocytes are present on stool examination, and, occasionally, patients have bloody diarrhea. Mesenteric adenitis or terminal ileitis occurs in older children and adolescents and presents a syndrome that is clinically indistinguishable from acute appendicitis.

Polyarthritis involving the knees, ankles, wrists, fingers, and toes occurs in 10% to 30% of Scandinavian adults with *Y. enterocolitica* infection. Typically, arthritis begins a few days to a month after the onset of diarrhea. Symptoms often persist from 1 to 4 months. Erythema nodosum occurs in approximately 20% to 30% of cases. The presence of HLA-B27 in patients with *Y. enterocolitica* infection has been related to Reiter's syndrome and in Scandinavia to arthritis and sacroiliitis.

Diagnosis. *Yersinia* organisms may be isolated from specimens of stool, mesenteric lymph nodes, blood, or abscess material. Inoculation of duplicate sets of cultures for incubation at 37° C and 25° C, respectively, enhances isolation of the microorganism. Serologic tests are helpful in the retrospective diagnosis of *Yersinia* infection.

Therapy. Patients hospitalized with *Yersinia* infection should be placed in enteric isolation. Cases of mesenteric lymphadenitis and terminal ileitis are usually self-limited, and the efficacy of antimicrobial therapy in these patients is unclear. The mortality associated with bacteremia caused by *Y. enterocolitica* or *Y. pseudotuberculosis* is high—50% to 75%—and these patients require prompt antimicrobial therapy. *Y. enterocolitica* is usually susceptible in vitro to aminogly-

cosides, chloramphenicol, tetracycline, co-trimoxazole, cefuroxime, fluoroquinolones, and third-generation cephalosporins. These microorganisms are usually resistant in vitro to penicillin, ampicillin, and first- and second-generation cephalosporins (other than cefuroxime). *Y. pseudotuberculosis* is usually susceptible in vitro to ampicillin, co-trimoxazole, tetracycline, chloramphenicol, cephalosporins, and aminoglycosides. The optimal antimicrobial therapy for patients with bacteremia caused by *Y. enterocolitica* or *Y. pseudotuberculosis* is not yet established. Empiric therapy with a parenterally administered aminoglycoside in combination with co-trimoxazole, a third-generation cephalosporin, or chloramphenicol is suggested. Antimicrobial therapy may be adjusted once the results of in vitro susceptibility tests are known.

Prevention. No specific preventive measures are known. General measures include those aimed at preventing ingestion of food or water contaminated with animal excreta.

BORDETELLA PERTUSSIS INFECTION (WHOOPING COUGH)

Pertussis (whooping cough) is an acute contagious disease of all age-groups and is caused by *Bordetella pertussis,* a strictly human pathogen. In children, infection of the ciliated epithelium of the respiratory tract with *B. pertussis* results in the pathognomonic symptom complex of paroxysmal cough followed by an inspiratory "whoop." In contrast, infection in adults characteristically causes a mild illness that mimics prolonged bronchitis.

Classification

B. pertussis is a nonmotile, gram-negative coccobacillus approximately 0.5×1.0 μm in size; it produces β-hemolysis on Bordet-Gengou (B-G) agar. The genus *Bordetella* can be distinguished from *Haemophilus,* with which it was formerly classified, by the lack of growth requirements for factors X and V and lack of production of nitrate or indole. In addition to *B. pertussis,* the genus *Bordetella* includes *Bordetella parapertussis* and the enzootic *Bordetella bronchiseptica. B. parapertussis* infrequently produces mild disease in humans, in spite of the fact that immunity to *B. pertussis* does not protect against infection with *B. parapertussis.*

B. pertussis, like other gram-negative bacteria, has a wide array of antigens. Several are of interest because of the effort to produce an effective acellular vaccine to replace the vaccine containing whole organisms. Antigens elaborated by the organisms include filamentous hemagglutinin (FHA) and lymphocytosis promoting factor (LPF), also called *pertussis toxin.* Absorbed LPF may cause systemic effects such as the lymphocytosis in patients with pertussis. Serotyping of *B. pertussis,* begun in the 1950s, was based on demonstrating agglutinogens on the bacteria. Serotyping was simplified during the 1980s as workers in England established that *B. pertussis* has fimbriae of two antigenically distinct types, which correspond to agglutinogens 2 and 3 under the old scheme.

Epidemiology

Pertussis occurs worldwide with little seasonal variation. After widespread pertussis vaccination of infants in the late 1940s, the incidence of pertussis in children decreased by more than 50%. In North America, the age-specific attack rate of pertussis has shifted from a peak in preschool and school-age children to higher attack rates in infants and adolescents. The shift to the older age-group is consistent with the loss of vaccine-induced immunity after 10 to 12 years.

Pertussis is most severe in infants younger than 6 months of age, and mortality is greatest in this age-group. The occurrence of disease in young infants emphasizes the unusual lack of immunity in the newborn. Low levels of antibody in women of childbearing age may contribute to an absence of transplacentally acquired protective antibody.

Humans are the only known source of *B. pertussis* in nature. In spite of this, asymptomatic carriage is extremely uncommon; this distinguishes *Bordetella* from the majority of bacterial respiratory pathogens. Transmission occurs from case to case, usually within families. Unimmunized household contacts of patients with pertussis may have an attack rate of up to 100%. Adults with undiagnosed disease are an important source of infection for children and other adults within a household.

Pathophysiology

B. pertussis is found exclusively in association with ciliated respiratory epithelial cells (Fig. 270-2), which emphasizes the unique capability of the organism to attach to cilia. *B. pertussis* does not invade the respiratory epithelium. The characteristic lymphocytosis of pertussis can be attributed to absorption of pertussis toxin from the respiratory tract, but the pathophysiology of the prolonged paroxysmal cough remains unknown.

Adenoviruses have been associated with pertussis by seroconversion and viral isolation from the nasopharynx. An independent role for adenovirus in causing this disease is unlikely, however.

Clinical Disease

The clinical picture of pertussis varies with the age of the affected patient. In children, the hallmark of pertussis is the paroxysmal cough. After an incubation period of 7 to 10 days, the typical illness progresses through three stages, each of about 2 weeks' duration (Fig. 270-3). The catarrhal phase is initiated by rhinorrhea and low-grade fever. The disease is most contagious during this stage, yet it is difficult to recognize clinically because symptoms resemble those of the

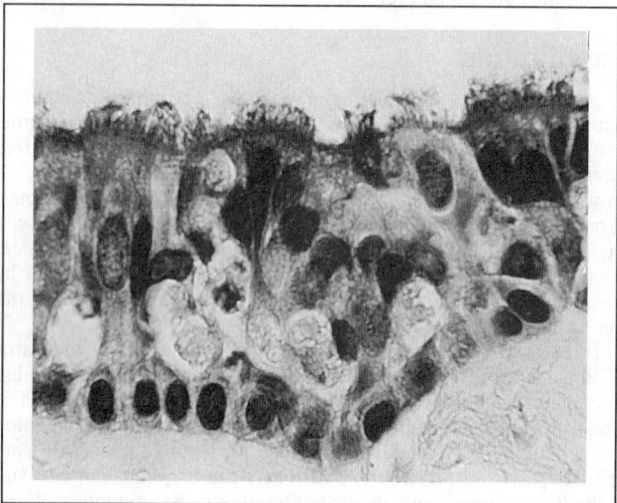

FIGURE 270-2   *Bordetella pertussis* enmeshed in the cilia of respiratory epithelium (human nose).
Courtesy Dr. Per Larsen, Gentofte Hospital, Copenhagen, Denmark.

"common cold." Late in the catarrhal stage, a cough appears that becomes paroxysmal. During the paroxysmal stage, exhausting paroxysms of coughing may occur two to three times per hour. The relentless, repetitive cough leads to facial plethora and expectoration of viscid, tenacious mucus. Long paroxysms may terminate with cyanosis, apnea, vomiting, or a gasping inspiratory whoop. Pertussis is commonly called *whooping cough,* but the inspiratory whoop is by no means a constant feature of the disease. During the convalescent phase, the frequency and severity of paroxysms gradually diminish. Convalescence, however, may be punctuated by relapses of paroxysmal coughing.

Peripheral lymphocytosis, often exceeding 30,000 cells/mm^3, develops late in the catarrhal phase and continues into the paroxysmal phase. This characteristic finding is often the only laboratory datum supporting the clinical impression of pertussis. Perihilar infiltrates may be seen on chest radiographs.

Clinical manifestations in adults may be similar to those in infants. More commonly, however, adults suffer only a nonspecific prolonged "bronchitis" and do not develop the characteristic paroxysmal cough. Lymphocytosis rarely accompanies adult disease.

The complications of pertussis have diminished significantly since the advent of antibiotics and improved supportive care. Secondary bacterial infection, such as otitis media or bacterial pneumonitis, may occur. Bacterial pneumonia, which is uncommon but may contribute to mortality, may be heralded by consolidation on chest x-ray and a shift from lymphocytosis to leukocytosis. Atelectasis and pneumothorax are infrequent, and long-term pulmonary sequelae are now rare. Convulsions and central nervous system damage (pertussis encephalopathy) may result from hypoxia and increased venous pressure accompanying cough paroxysms or perhaps from an undefined neurotoxin produced by the organisms.

Diagnosis

Recovery of *B. pertussis* from respiratory secretions provides a definitive diagnosis of pertussis. Obstacles to isolation of the organisms include culturing too late in the illness for organisms to be present, nonviable organisms resulting from antibiotic therapy before culture, and laboratory inexperience in growing the organisms. B-G agar, which was developed in 1900 with the use of secretions from Bordet's son who had pertussis, is the standard medium for isolation of *B. pertussis.* Nasopharyngeal (not oropharyngeal) secretions should be obtained with a calcium alginate swab during the first 3 weeks of infection (see Fig. 270-3) and inoculated directly onto agar. Tiny white colonies surrounded by a small zone of β-hemolysis appear after 3 to 5 days of incubation at 36° C. Fluorescent antibody staining of respiratory secretions by experienced laboratories correlates well with positive cultures.

Serologic diagnosis of infection has not been reliable in the past, but an enzyme-linked immunosorbent assay (ELISA) for IgG, IgM, and IgA antibodies to *B. pertussis* developed in Finland is now used for accurate serologic diagnosis. Specific antigens such as FHA, LPF,

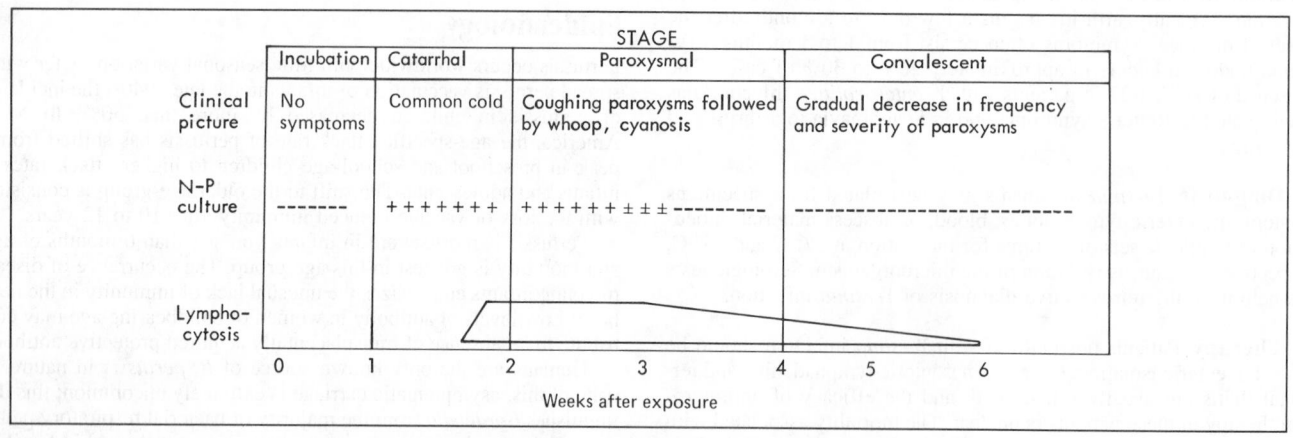

FIGURE 270-3   Clinical course of pertussis. *N-P,* Nasopharyngeal.

and pertactin (a 69-kilodalton outer membrane protein) are used as the antigen in ELISA testing of sera obtained from patients in the acute and convalescent stages of infection. Interpretation of serologic findings is complicated by the fact that both IgG and IgM antibodies are generated after vaccination as well as with infection. The IgG antibodies persist for years. On the other hand, IgA antibodies are produced only by infection (not vaccination), and IgM antibodies have a short half-life. Serologic evidence of infection is provided by either a four-fold rise in IgG antibody titer to *B. pertussis* antigen(s) or elevated IgM and/or IgA titers during or after illness. Studies utilizing ELISA serology in addition to culture have demonstrated that culture is positive in fewer than half of the cases of pertussis infection diagnosed with serology.

The use of the polymerase chain reaction (PCR) with appropriate primers is a promising new tool for accurate detection of *B. pertussis* in nasopharyngeal secretions. It has the advantage over serology of early diagnosis, whereas infection is ongoing. In addition, PCR appears to be much more sensitive than culture in detecting infection.

Therapy

The therapy of pertussis is largely supportive, although erythromycin rapidly eliminates viable organisms. Nursing care and adequate nutrition are essential. In the acute paroxysmal stage, unnecessary manipulation of the child should be discouraged, since stimulation, particularly suctioning of the upper respiratory tract, may precipitate additional paroxysms of coughing.

Antibiotic therapy renders the patient noncontagious and may abort disease if administered during the incubation period or the catarrhal stage. However, once the paroxysmal stage is reached, antibiotics are not thought to alter the course of pertussis disease. *B. pertussis* is sensitive in vitro to ampicillin, erythromycin, chloramphenicol, tetracycline, and trimethoprim-sulfamethoxazole. Ampicillin does not reliably eradicate the organism from the nasopharynx. Nasopharyngeal shedding of the organism can be eradicated within 3 days with oral erythromycin (40 to 50 mg/kg/day in four divided doses; 1 g/day in adults). Therapy should be continued for 14 days to prevent the reappearance of shedding that can occur after shorter antibiotic courses.

Pertussis immune globulin is of no benefit in treatment of pertussis. Corticosteroids in conjunction with erythromycin reduced the frequency of paroxysms of coughing in one controlled trial. Since complicating infections might be potentiated by this therapeutic regimen, however, additional study is needed before it can be recommended for routine use in pertussis. Albuterol (salbutamol) in a dose of 0.1/ mg/kg tid. by mouth is commonly employed as adjunctive therapy in Europe.

Prevention

Erythromycin prophylaxis (40 to 50 mg/kg/day for 14 days) of household contacts of a case of pertussis has been advocated as a means of preventing or attenuating disease in the contacts. Although its efficacy is unproven, prophylaxis should be provided to infants and small children in view of the severity of disease in this age-group.

Active immunization with pertussis vaccine is the only effective method of disease control. Use of the whole-cell vaccine was based on efficacy trials conducted in the late 1940s. Pertussis vaccine is not given to persons over 6 years of age, despite evidence that individuals vaccinated more than 12 years before exposure are again susceptible to disease. The side effects of the whole-cell pertussis vaccine have been a source of great controversy, although the established protective efficacy is 70% to 90%.

The antigens of *B. pertussis* in the whole-cell vaccine that are responsible for stimulating vaccine-induced immunity have not been defined. This has posed problems for rational design and testing of acellular vaccines. Proposed protective antigens include LPF (pertussis toxin), FHA, fimbrial agglutinogens 2 and 3, and pertactin, a 69-kilodalton outer membrane protein. Recent trials in Europe of a variety of acellular vaccines have documented acceptable efficacy (≥80%) of several products in infants. All contained LPF and FHA; some also contained pertactin and/or fimbrial antigen. All of the acellular vaccines were significantly less reactogenic than whole-cell vaccine. Acellular vaccines containing two or more components of the

organism are now licensed in the United States for prevention of this serious disease in infants.

BIBLIOGRAPHY

Ad Hoc Group for the Study of Pertussis Vaccines: Placebo-controlled trial of two acellular pertussis vaccines in Sweden—protective efficacy and adverse events, *Lancet* 1:955, 1988.

Ariza J et al: Treatment of human brucellosis with doxycycline plus rifampin or doxycycline plus streptomycin, *Ann Intern Med* 17:25, 1992.

Committee on Infectious Diseases-AAP: Acellular pertussis vaccine: recommendations for use as the initial series in infants and children, *Pediatrics* 99:282, 1997.

Deen JL et al: Household contact study of *Bordetella pertussis* infections, *Clin Infect Dis* 21:1211, 1995.

Edelman K et al: Detection of *Bordetella pertussis* by polymerase chain reaction and culture in the nasopharynx of erythromycin-treated infants with pertussis, *Pediatr Infect Dis J* 15:54, 1996.

Halperin SA, Marrie TJ: Pertussis encephalopathy in an adult: case report and review, *Rev Infect Dis* 13:1043, 1991.

He Q et al: Comparison of polymerase chain reaction with culture and enzyme immunoassay for diagnosis of pertussis, *J Clin Micro* 31:642, 1993.

Long SS et al: Widespread silent transmission of pertussis in families: antibody correlates of infection and symptomatology, *J Infect Dis* 161:480, 1990.

Mousa AR et al: The nature of human brucellosis in Kuwait: study of 379 cases, *Rev Infect Dis* 10:211, 1988.

CHAPTER

271 Infections Caused by *Bacteroides* and Other Mixed Nonsporulating Anaerobes

Anthony W. Chow

THE ORGANISMS
Classification and Characteristics

Obligate anaerobes are a heterogeneous group of bacteria that require reduced oxygen tension for growth. By convention, they are defined as microorganisms that are unable to survive on the surface of solid media in air (18% oxygen). In contrast, facultative bacteria can grow either in the presence or the absence of air, whereas microaerophilic or capnophilic bacteria grow poorly or not at all in air but grow better in the presence of 10% carbon dioxide in air or anaerobically. Within this broad definition, obligate anaerobes vary greatly in their sensitivity to oxygen. Extremely oxygen-sensitive anaerobes, for example, spirochetes and certain strains of *Clostridium,* cannot tolerate even 5 minutes of exposure to low concentrations of oxygen. As a general rule, obligate anaerobes commonly associated with infective processes are relatively aerotolerant and can survive for as long as 72 hours (but cannot replicate) in low concentrations of oxygen.

Obligate anaerobes are part of the indigenous microflora on mucocutaneous surfaces, especially the oropharynx, skin, gastrointestinal tract, and genital tract. Infections involving these microbes, therefore, are primarily acquired endogenously. Such infections characteristically entail multiple organisms (polymicrobial), both anaerobic and facultative (mixed), reflecting the combined influence of the complex commensal flora and the unique microbiota of the underlying conditions. Clostridia (sporulating anaerobes) and actinomycetes are considered elsewhere (Chapters 263 and 277, respectively).

Taxonomic Considerations. The generic classification of currently recognized, clinically important anaerobic bacteria, with their prevalence as normal flora or in infection, is presented in simplified form in Table 271-1. In the past, confusion over the nomenclature and taxonomy of obligate anaerobes was a major deterrent to recognition of the clinical significance of these microorganisms. More recently, aided by gas-liquid chromatographic analysis of acid endproducts, carbohydrate fermentation patterns, and other biochemical

Table 271-1 Generic classification and prevalence of major anaerobic bacteria in normal flora and infection

ANAEROBIC BACTERIA	GENERA	NORMAL FLORA				COMMON CLINICAL ISOLATES
		SKIN	OROPHARYNX	INTESTINE	GENITALIA	
Sporulating bacilli	*Clostridium*	0	±	2	±	*C. perfringens, C. difficile, C. ramosum, C. septicum, C. novyi*
Nonsporulating bacilli						
Gram-negative	*Bacteroides*	0	2	2	1	*B. fragilis, B. vulgatus, B. thetaiotaomicron, B. distasonis,*
	Prevotella	0	2	1	1	*P. melaninogenica, P. intermedia, P. bivia, P. disiens*
	Porphyromonas	0	2	1	1	*P. asaccharolytica, P. gingivalis*
	Fusobacterium	0	2	±	1	*F. nucleatum, F. necrophorum, F. varium, F. mortiferum*
Gram-positive	*Actinomyces*	0	1	±	0	*A. israelii, A. naeslundii, A. viscosus*
	Bifidobacterium	0	±	2	±	*B. eriksonii, B. breve*
	Eubacterium	±	1	2	±	*E. lentum, E. limosum*
	Lactobacillus	0	±	1	2	*L. casei, L. plantarum, L. acidophillus*
	Propionibacterium and *Arachnia*	2	±	±	1	*P. acnes, P. granulosum, A. propionica*
Cocci						
Gram-negative	*Veillonella* and *Acidaminococcus*	0	2	1	1	*V. parvula, A. fermentans*
Gram-positive	*Peptostreptococcus*	1	2	2	1	*P. asaccharolyticus, P. prevotii, P. magnus, P. variabilis, P. anaerobius, P. micros, P. parvulus, P. productus*
Spirochetes	*Treponema*	0	1	±	±	*T. vincentii, T. denticola*

0, Absent or rare; ±, irregularly present; 1, usually present; 2, predominant.

tests, clinically important anaerobes can be readily identified to species. The routine adoption of vastly improved culture techniques to achieve anaerobiosis; the introduction of prereduced, anaerobically sterilized media; and careful attention to specimen collection and transport have greatly enhanced the recovery of even very fastidious anaerobes from clinical material. This improved recovery has resulted in greater appreciation for the significance of these microorganisms. In addition, the unique association of specific nonsporulating anaerobes with certain clinical syndromes (e.g., *Prevotella intermedia* and *Porphyromonas gingivalis* in periodontal infections, and *Prevotella bivia* and *Prevotella disiens* in female genital infections) is being increasingly recognized. Such taxonomic differentiation clearly has important implications, not only in diagnostic and therapeutic considerations, but also in studies of the pathogenesis of these infections. In this regard, the not infrequent practice of referring to any gram-negative obligately anaerobic bacillus as a *"Bacteroides"* and to those resistant to ampicillin and penicillin as *"Bacteroides fragilis"* without further bacterial speciation is not to be condoned.

Ecologic and Host-Parasite Considerations

Indigenous microflora. Quantitatively, obligate anaerobes are the predominant bacteria present as normal microflora on mucocutaneous surfaces. They outnumber facultative bacteria by a factor of 10 to 1000 at several body sites, particularly the oropharynx, colon, and vagina (Table 271-2). Despite the complexity of the microbial composition, it is important to recognize the unique ecologic niches associated with these indigenous bacteria. For example, in the oral cavity, *Streptococcus sanguis, Streptococcus mutans, Streptococcus mitis,* and *Actinomyces viscosus* preferentially colonize the tooth surface; in contrast, *Streptococcus salivarius* and *Veillonella parvula* have a predilection for the tongue and buccal mucosa. *Bacteroides vulgatus, Bacteroides thetaiotaomicron, B. fragilis,* and *Bacteroides distasonis* are primarily indigenous in the colon; *P. bivia* and *P. disiens* are primarily resident in the female genital tract.

The precise role of the indigenous microflora remains controversial. A prevailing view is that the presence of the indigenous flora provides a mucosal defense against colonization and subsequent invasion by organisms more traditionally associated with disease ("colonization resistance"). To accomplish this, these microbes must overcome many adverse host conditions to successfully colonize selective human mucosal surfaces. Some of these host conditions are mechanical, such as the flow of fluids over the epithelium, mucociliary clearance, and epithelial cell turnover. Some pertain to local environmental conditions, such as supply of essential nutrients, pH, oxidation-reduction potential (Eh), and oxygen tension. Still others relate to local immune factors that involve both specific and nonspecific antimicrobial systems. Thus the mere introduction of an organism to a site does not ensure its establishment in the stable resident flora. It is likely that a highly specific microbe-host interaction ("adherence") is necessary for the indigenous flora to gain a selective advantage to be retained at a particular site, where the rate of microbial proliferation exceeds the rate of removal. Although the normal flora play an important role in the mucosal host defenses, these same organisms have the potential to cause invasive disease under certain clinical conditions.

Although the microbial composition of the indigenous microflora at a given site in a specific individual appears to be relatively constant, this ecosystem is readily influenced by a variety of host and environmental factors. Thus physiologic conditions such as pregnancy, menses, and age; underlying processes such as malignancy; and host factors such as diet, hospitalization, antimicrobial therapy, and recent surgery may all affect the indigenous microflora (Table 271-3). Knowledge of the anatomic location of the primary source of infection and the underlying condition of the host, therefore, is essential in predicting the probable organisms implicated in anaerobic and mixed infections associated with the indigenous microflora.

Pathophysiology

Obligate anaerobes implicated in mixed infections are generally of poor pathogenicity. However, under special circumstances that lead to either structural alterations in the normal mucosal barrier or tissue ischemia and lowered oxidation-reduction potential, these opportunistic organisms can proliferate and invade surrounding healthy tissues. Therefore, conditions that predispose to anaerobic infections are those that cause local ischemia or tissue necrosis, such as trauma, bite, foreign body, surgical manipulation, irradiation, or neoplasm.

Apart from impairment of local host defenses, certain microbial

Table 271-2   Concentrations and distribution of major normal microflora at various body sites

SITES	ANAEROBES		AEROBES	
	BACTERIAL CONCENTRATION	PREDOMINANT GENERA	BACTERIAL CONCENTRATION	PREDOMINANT GENERA
Skin	10^4-10^5/cm^2	*Propionibacterium*	10^2-10^3/cm^2	*Staphylococcus* *Micrococcus* "Diphtheroids"
Oropharynx	10^6-10^{11}/ml	*Peptostreptococcus* *Veillonella* *Actinomyces* *Bacteroides* *Fusobacterium*	10^4-10^6/ml	*Streptococcus*
Intestine				
Stomach and upper small bowel	10^1-10^4/ml	*Peptostreptococcus* *Veillonella*	10^1-10^4/ml	*Streptococcus* *Lactobacillus*
Lower small bowel	10^4-10^7/ml	*Bacteroides* *Bifidobacterium*	10^4-10^7/ml	"Coliforms"
Colon	10^{11}-10^{12}/ml	*Bacteroides* *Bifidobacterium* *Eubacterium* *Clostridium* *Peptostreptococcus* *Veillonella*	10^8-10^9/ml	*Escherichia* "Enterococci" *Lactobacillus*
Genitalia				
Vagina and endocervix	10^8-10^{10}/g	*Peptostreptococcus* *Lactobacillus* *Bacteroides*	10^7-10^9/g	*Lactobacillus* *Streptococcus* *Staphylococcus*

Table 271-3   Effect of host conditions on the indigenous microflora at various body sites

SITE	HOST FACTOR	CHANGE OF FLORA
Gingiva	Dental caries and periodontal disease	Increased motile anaerobic gram-negative bacilli and spirochetes
Oropharynx	Hospitalization, antibiotics, or serious illness	Increased facultative gram-negative bacilli
Upper small bowel	Achlorhydria, vagotomy, and pyloroplasty	Increased *Escherichia coli, B. fragilis,* and *Bifidobacterium*
Small bowel	Regional enteritis, decreased motility, or stasis secondary to blind loop, obstruction, diverticula, irradiation, etc.	Colonic flora
	Disrupted anatomic continuity after bowel resection or bypass	Colonic flora
Large bowel	Colonic resection with ileostomy	Decreased anaerobes and some facultative bacteria
Vagina	Parturition, hysterectomy, or irradiation	Increased *E. coli* and *B. fragilis*

virulence factors may be particularly important for disease potential among some obligate anaerobes. This concept is supported by the observation that the anaerobic pathogens commonly isolated in clinical infection often are not the organisms that are numerically dominant in the indigenous microflora. For example, in intraabdominal infection after colonic perforation, *B. fragilis* is almost always present, whereas *B. distasonis* and *B. vulgatus* are not, even though the latter organisms are more predominant in the normal colonic flora. It is now known that only *B. fragilis* is encapsulated, which accounts for its enhanced virulence, whereas the other members of the group are not.

Microbial factors considered important in the pathogenesis of anaerobic infections are summarized in Table 271-4. Obligate anaerobes are known to possess a number of extracellular or membrane-bound enzymes that may promote tissue destruction, provide nutrients, or allow microbial survival in a hostile environment. These enzymes include lipases, proteases, nucleases, and heparinases. Membrane-bound enzymes (e.g., superoxide dismutase and β-lactamases) may be important for protecting virulent organisms from the toxic effects of oxygen and β-lactam antibiotics, respectively. Catalase may serve a function similar to that of superoxide dismutase. Organisms lacking these enzymes are susceptible to killing by toxic oxygen radicals and common antibiotics in the environment and thus are less effective as pathogens.

B. fragilis and other anaerobes produce various short-chain fatty acids in vitro and in vivo. These fatty acids have been shown in several model systems to be deleterious to mammalian and bacterial cell function. Infections associated with *B. fragilis* are associated with production of high concentrations of succinic acid, which impairs the

Table 271-4   Microbial virulence factors important in mixed anaerobic infections

MICROBIAL FACTORS	PATHOGENIC EFFECT
Histolytic enzymes (e.g., collagenase, fibrinolysin, hyaluronidase, protease, lipase, ribonuclease, deoxyribonuclease, etc.)	Tissue destruction
Oxygen-scavenging enzymes (e.g., superoxide dismutase, catalase, peroxidase)	Survival in aerobic environment
Endotoxin	Direct toxicity
	Hageman factor and complement activation
Capsular polysaccharide	Inhibition of phagocytosis
	Abscess formation
Surface ligands and charge	Adherence and bacterial interaggregation
IgA protease	Impairment of secretory and mucosal immunity
Heparinase	Promotion of coagulation and tissue ischemia
β-lactamase	Resistance to β-lactam antibiotics
Bacteriocin and metabolites (e.g., fatty acids, H$_2$S, NH$_3$, etc.)	Inhibition of normal flora

generation of the respiratory burst and profoundly reduces phagocytic killing and chemotactic responses of neutrophils. This effect is most evident at low pH and low Eh, conditions present in abscesses and mixed infections. It has been suggested that succinic acid production may represent an important virulence mechanism by *Bacteroides* species in the pathogenesis of synergistic mixed infections.

B. fragilis, Prevotella melaninogenica, and a number of anaerobic gram-positive cocci are encapsulated. Possession of a capsule by these organisms is associated with increased virulence, as evidenced by their enhanced ability for abscess formation and systemic invasion. Interestingly, although nonencapsulated organisms by themselves may be unable to induce abscesses during experimental infection, many such strains become heavily encapsulated after a mixed infection with other facultative and anaerobic bacteria. These heavily encapsulated strains are able to induce abscesses thereafter when inoculated alone. The selection of encapsulated anaerobes occurs in the presence of other encapsulated, or unencapsulated, but abscess-forming facultative or anaerobic organisms. This phenomenon may help to explain how nonpathogenic organisms that are part of the normal host flora can become pathogens. It should be noted that although encapsulated anaerobes are more virulent than their nonencapsulated variants during experimental infection, and that encapsulated strains are more prevalent than nonencapsulated organisms at clinically infected sites, encapsulation is clearly not the only virulence factor important in the pathogenicity of polymicrobial infections containing obligate anaerobes. The capsular materials of *B. fragilis* and *P. melaninogenica* have been extracted and purified. These large–molecular weight polysaccharides have been demonstrated to inhibit phagocytosis in vitro and promote abscess formation in several animal models in vivo. In addition, several oral anaerobes, for example, *P. melaninogenica, Porphyromonas gingivalis,* and *Prevotella intermedia,* are found to secrete IgA proteases that may impair secretory and local mucosal immunity.

Anaerobic gram-negative bacteria also possess lipopolysaccharides (LPS) in their outer cell membrane similar to their aerobic counterparts. However, the structure and biologic activity of LPSs from several anaerobic bacteria are distinctly different from those of the classic LPS of Enterobacteriaceae. For example, LPSs of *B. fragilis* and *P. intermedia* lack 2-keto-3-deoxyoctanoic acid and L-glycero-D-mannoheptose, and they have little endotoxic potency. The LPSs of *Fusobacterium nucleatum* and *V. parvula,* on the other hand, have biochemical and biologic properties similar to those of classic endotoxin.

Microbial Synergy. Two thirds of infections in which obligate anaerobes can be isolated are mixed infections involving both anaer-

obes and facultative bacteria. The infectivity of obligate anaerobes in these instances is often facilitated by the coexistence of facultative organisms. Such examples of bacterial synergy are well demonstrated in periodontal infection, in progressive synergistic gangrene of Meleney, and in various animal models of intraabdominal and subcutaneous abscesses. A synergistic potential has been demonstrated between *Bacteroides* species and several facultative bacteria, between *Bacteroides* species and most anaerobic gram-positive cocci, and between most anaerobic gram-positive cocci and *Pseudomonas aeruginosa* or *Staphylococcus aureus.* Participation by symbiotic facultative bacteria may be essential for the anaerobes by providing necessary growth factors, by lowering the oxidation-reduction potential of the environment, or by impairing local host defenses. Conversely, the presence of obligate anaerobes may benefit coexisting facultative bacteria either by growth enhancement, by protection from phagocytosis (e.g., succinic acid production by *Bacteroides* spp.), or by protection from β-lactam antibiotics (e.g., β-lactamase production). Microbial synergy for infection between an anaerobe and a facultative bacterium is best demonstrated within tissues where bacterial clearance is normally slow (e.g., subcutaneous abscesses, or fibrin clot in intraperitoneal infection) or is hampered by underlying disease. An understanding of the dynamic interactions between different components of a complex flora in mixed infections has important therapeutic implications. Microorganisms in mixed infections may handle antimicrobial agents differently from those in monomicrobial infections, and it may not be necessary to eradicate every bacterial species in mixed culture to achieve a cure.

CLINICAL PRESENTATIONS OF ANAEROBIC INFECTIONS

Anaerobic infections may involve any tissue or organ. Prospective studies utilizing modern anaerobic culture techniques indicate that anaerobic bacteria are particularly prevalent in infections of the head and neck, lung and pleural space, intraabdominal organs, female genital tract, and necrotic skin and soft tissues (Table 271-5). Salient clinical features of these infections are highlighted in the following discussions.

Head and Neck Infections

Anaerobic infections of the head and neck most commonly involve the oral cavity and are odontogenic in origin (Chapter 237). These include dentoalveolar and periodontal infections and orofacial space abscesses. Anaerobes are also commonly present in chronic otitis me-

Table 271-5   Infections commonly or rarely associated with anaerobes

SITE	INFECTIONS LIKELY TO INVOLVE ANAEROBES	PERCENTAGE WITH ANAEROBES	INFECTIONS UNLIKELY TO INVOLVE ANAEROBES
Head and neck	Periodontal and apical abscess	100	Acute infections of
	Fascial space infections	85	Sinuses
	Chronic sinusitis	50	Nasopharynx
	Chronic otitis media	50	Middle ear
Central nervous system	Brain abscess (not traumatic)	85	Meningitis
	Subdural empyema	($\cong$50)*	
Pleuropulmonary	Aspiration pneumonia	85	Bronchitis
	Necrotizing pneumonitis	85	Lobar pneumonia
	Abscess	90	
	Empyema	75	
Intraabdominal	Peritonitis and abscess	95	Primary and "spontaneous" peritonitis
	Hepatic abscess	50	Cholecystitis or ascending cholangitis
			Pancreatitis
Female genital tract	Vulvovaginal abscess	75	Cystourethritis
	Salpingitis and pelvic peritonitis	50	Pyelonephritis
	Tuboovarian abscess	90	
	Posthysterectomy wound infection	70	
	Septic abortion and postpartum endometritis	75	
Skin, soft tissue, and bone	Crepitant cellulitis	(High)*	Septic arthritis
	Myonecrosis	100	Osteomyelitis of long bones
	Necrotizing fasciitis	(High)*	
	Synergistic cellulitis	(High)*	

*Percentages unavailable.

dia and mastoiditis and in tonsillar and peritonsillar abscesses. Acute sinusitis is seldom caused by anaerobic organisms unless it is associated with a dental infection. The clinical manifestations of these infections are largely dictated by the anatomic location and the extent and predetermined routes of spread (Fig. 271-1). Mandibular osteomyelitis may also result from infection complicating tooth extraction, from open fractures, or in association with debilitation, diabetes mellitus, radiation therapy, and malnutrition. Such infections not only may produce significant local symptoms but on rare occasions may also result in life-threatening complications, for example, mediastinal or intracranial extension, retropharyngeal spread with airway obstruction, pleuropulmonary suppuration, and hematogenous dissemination.

The concept of microbial specificity in odontogenic and other head and neck infections has been appreciated only recently. In the healthy periodontium, the microflora is sparse, consisting mainly of gram-positive organisms such as *S. sanguis* and *Actinomyces* species. In the presence of gingivitis, the subgingival flora shifts to a predominantly anaerobic gram-negative flora with *P. intermedia* as the most common isolate. In advanced periodontitis, the flora further increases in complexity, with a preponderance of anaerobic gram-negative motile bacilli and spirochetes; *P. gingivalis* is then most commonly isolated. Overall, some pigmented anaerobic bacilli (particularly *Porphyromonas asaccharolytica, P. gingivalis, P. intermedia,* and *P. melaninogenica), F. nucleatum, Peptostreptococcus* species, *Actinomyces* species, and streptococci are the most prevalent isolates in pyogenic orofacial infections arising from odontogenic sources. *Fusobacterium* and anaerobic gram-positive cocci are also commonly isolated in chronic or recurrent maxillary sinusitis. *Fusobacterium necrophorum* and *P. melaninogenica* are most frequently recovered from tonsillar and peritonsillar abscesses. Although the anaerobes associated with orofacial and upper respiratory infections were considered to be universally susceptible to penicillin in the past, recent data indicate that β-lactamase–producing strains, particularly the pigmented anaerobic gram-negative bacilli, have become increasingly prevalent. Furthermore, rapid emergence of β-lactamase–producing anaerobes, as well as facultative bacteria, has been documented after a single course of penicillin therapy for acute tonsillitis. Such organisms not only can survive penicillin therapy, they may also protect other penicillin-susceptible bacteria by the release of β-lactamase in infected tissue. The selection of β-lactamase–producing bacteria during therapy may account for suboptimal responses to penicillin in some cases of head and neck infections. Except in selected patients with serious underlying illness, facultative gram-negative bacilli and staphylococci are not commonly involved in head and neck infections.

Central Nervous System Infections

Anaerobic bacteria are frequent pathogens in intracranial infections, particularly those caused by contiguous spread from chronic otitis media, mastoiditis, or sinusitis (Chapter 240). Intracranial extension may result in brain abscess, subdural empyema, epidural abscess, or suppurative thrombophlebitis of cortical vessels or venous sinuses. Anaerobic intracranial infections may also occur by hematogenous dissemination, particularly from chronic and suppurative pulmonary foci, or in the presence of cyanotic congenital heart disease. Purulent meningitis, except in the newborn, seldom involves anaerobic bacteria. Cerebral abscesses of sinus or dental origin are more probably caused by *Streptococcus milleri,* either alone or in mixed culture with other oropharyngeal anaerobes and facultative bacteria. Otogenic cerebral abscesses, on the other hand, frequently involve *B. fragilis, Proteus* spp. and streptococci.

Pleuropulmonary Infections

Anaerobic bacteria are important pulmonary pathogens, particularly after aspiration of oropharyngeal secretions (Chapter 237). Anaerobic pleuropulmonary infections include aspiration pneumonitis, putrid lung abscess, necrotizing pneumonia, and empyema. Pneumonitis is usually the initial lesion, and related symptoms in the early phases may be indistinguishable from other causes of acute bacterial pneumonia. However, if untreated, pulmonary abscess may occur after 8 to 14 days. Approximately one half of patients with lung abscess develop putrid-smelling expectorations. The subsequent clinical course depends largely on the nature of the underlying pulmonary pathologic condition. About 10% of patients with anaerobic infections of the lung parenchyma develop empyema. Necrotizing pneumonia is characterized by multiple small cavities within a pulmonary segment or lobe. The course is often fulminant, with rapid extension into adjacent segments.

Anaerobic pleuropulmonary infections are typically polymicrobial in nature. Predominant anaerobic isolates include *Peptostreptococcus* species, *F. nucleatum,* and the saccharolytic black-pigmented anaerobic gram-negative bacilli *(P. melaninogenica* and *P. intermedia).* Aerobic and microaerophilic streptococci (e.g., *Streptococcus intermedius)* are also frequently isolated. Hospital-acquired infections have a higher coisolation rate of facultative bacteria such as *S. aureus, Escherichia coli, Klebsiella pneumoniae,* and *P. aeruginosa* than does community-acquired aspiration pneumonia.

Intraabdominal Infections

Intraabdominal sepsis most commonly results from bacterial contamination of intraperitoneal or retroperitoneal spaces after intestinal perforation (Chapter 238). The initial event is peritonitis, either generalized or localized, with subsequent abscess formation. Common predisposing conditions include penetrating trauma, perforated appendicitis or diverticulitis, inflammatory bowel disease, intestinal malignancy with strangulation or obstruction, and anastomotic leak following intestinal surgery. Although a multiplicity of anaerobic and facultative bacteria may be isolated in intraabdominal infections—particularly *B. fragilis, Peptostreptococcus* spp., *Clostridium* spp., Enterobacteriaceae, and *Enterococcus faecalis*—it is not always clear which components are the primary pathogens and which are merely symbionts or commensals. Animal studies of experimental peritonitis simulating intestinal perforation have further elucidated the pathogenesis of such infections and suggest a biphasic process. Early peritonitis and bacteremia are related to facultative coliform bacteria, whereas late abscesses are caused by anaerobes, often in synergy with facultative bacteria. Apart from the causative agents in abscess formation, other intestinal bacteria not involved initially may subsequently translocate into the abscess. The most common translocating intestinal bacteria include enterococci and *E. coli.* The exact mechanism for this translocation, whether by hematogenous or lymphatic channels, by transmural migration from the intestinal lumen, or by phagocytic transport, is presently unknown. The presence of fibrin in the peritoneal cavity during peritonitis also appears to predispose to abscess formation. Fibrin appears to inhibit phagocytic function by entrapment of bacteria and neutrophils, impairing phagocytosis. The therapeutic implications of these studies are clear: both microbial components of intraabdominal sepsis should receive appropriate an-

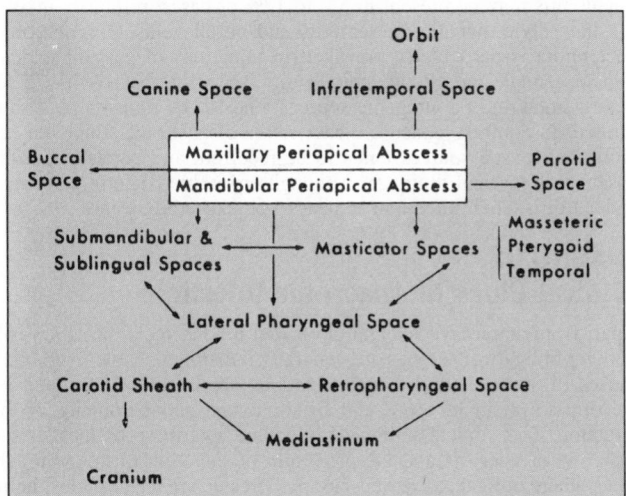

FIGURE 271-1   Potential routes of spread of deep fascial space infections.

From Chow AW: Infections of the oral cavity, neck, and head. In Mandell GL, Bennett JE, Dolin R, editors: *Principles and practice of infectious diseases,* ed 4, New York, 1995, Churchill Livingstone.

Table 271-6 Predominant microorganisms in female genital tract infections

	MAJOR PATHOGENS IMPLICATED		
TYPE OF INFECTION	EXOGENOUS STD AGENTS	ENDOGENOUS MIXED AEROBES AND ANAEROBES	GENITAL MYCOPLASMAS
Periurethral and labial pyrogenic infections	+	++	±
Vulvovaginitis	±	++	±
Cervicitis, endometritis, and salpingitis	++	++	+
Tuboovarian abscess	±	++	
Posthysterectomy and other pelvic infections		++	
Postpartum and postcesarean section infections		++	+

STD, Sexually transmitted disease; +, less common; ++, most common; ±, not present.

timicrobial attention. Early surgical debridement of fibrinous exudate and necrotic debris is critical. Use of fibrinolytic agents (e.g., trypsin) may be a useful adjunct in preventing abscess formation postoperatively.

Obstetric and Gynecologic Infections

Most female genital tract infections, including the classic sexually transmitted diseases (STDs), are polymicrobial and frequently involve both facultative and anaerobic bacteria. In general, three major classes of microorganisms have been implicated: (1) those considered to be exogenous STD pathogens (e.g., *Neisseria gonorrhoeae, Chlamydia trachomatis,* herpes simplex, *Trichomonas vaginalis*), (2) mixed facultatives and anaerobes indigenous to the cervicovaginal normal flora, and (3) genital mycoplasmas (e.g., *Mycoplasma hominis* and *Ureaplasma urealyticum*) (Table 271-6). Mixed facultatives and anaerobes are particularly important in closed-space infections such as vulvovaginal, adnexal, or tuboovarian abscesses, and in postsurgical and postpartum infections. Other common gynecologic and obstetric infections involving a mixed facultative and anaerobic flora include acute and chronic salpingitis, infections associated with contraceptive intrauterine devices, postpartum or postcesarean section wound infections, endometritis, and amnionitis. The most common anaerobes found include *Prevotella* spp. (especially *P. bivia, P. disiens,* and *P. melaninogenica*), *Peptostreptococcus* spp., and *Actinomyces* spp. The most common facultative pathogens are Enterobacteriaceae (especially *E. coli*), and aerobic or microaerophilic streptococci. *B. fragilis* is not a common organism in the normal vagina, but its prevalence is increased in posthysterectomy and postcesarean section infections, and in pelvic infections associated with malignancy and immunosuppressive therapy. The entity of "nonspecific vaginitis" or bacterial vaginosis also appears to be a polymicrobial infection involving both facultatives and anaerobes. Apart from *Gardnerella vaginalis,* high concentrations of *Prevotella* spp., *Peptostreptococcus* spp., and *Mobiluncus* spp. (a motile anaerobic curved gram-negative bacillus) can be regularly isolated from vaginal secretions compared with uninfected control specimens.

Necrotic Skin and Soft Tissue Infections

Necrotic wound and soft tissue infections are particularly prone to develop in areas that have been injured by trauma, ischemia, or surgery (Chapter 241). Anatomic sites regularly exposed to fecal or oral contamination are particularly at risk, such as wounds associated with intestinal surgery, decubitus and diabetic ulcers, human bites, and infected pilonidal cysts. Clinical manifestations include crepitant cellulitis, synergistic necrotizing cellulitis or gangrene, myonecrosis, and necrotizing fasciitis. The range of bacterial isolates in such infections is enormous. Anaerobes, including *Bacteroides* spp., anaerobic cocci, and clostridia, are almost universally present in mixed culture.

Anaerobic Bacteremia and Endocarditis

Obligate anaerobes account for 9% to 14% of all significant positive blood cultures from a general hospital population (Table 271-7). *Bacteroides* spp. are the predominant isolates, followed by *Peptostreptococcus* and *Clostridium* spp. *B. fragilis* has been reported as the third

Table 271-7 Prevalence of anaerobes in bacteremia

	HARBOR–UCLA MEDICAL CENTER	VANCOUVER GENERAL HOSPITAL
Total number of patients with bacteremia	1348	686
Number with anaerobes (%)*	185 (14)	62 (9)
Number polymicrobial (%)*	42 (23)	12 (19)
Major isolates (%)*		
Bacteroides	46	61
Peptostreptococcus	16	13
Clostridium	10	22
Fusobacterium	4	2

*Percentage of cases with anaerobic bacteremia.

most common cause of gram-negative bacillary bacteremia, surpassed only by *E. coli* and *K. pneumoniae.* The clinical manifestations of anaerobic bacteremia and the specific organisms involved depend to a large extent on the portal of entry and the nature of the underlying disease. For example, *B. fragilis* is most common in bacteremia of gastrointestinal and necrotic soft tissue origin. Bacteroidaceae bacteremia of the female genital tract and odontogenic origin rarely involves *B. fragilis;* more commonly, a *Peptostreptococcus* sp. is isolated. The latter is also associated with bacteremia related to necrotic soft tissue infections, and occasionally in necrotizing pneumonia and empyema. *Fusobacterium* spp., when isolated, are usually oropulmonary or pelvic in origin. Several clinical features are particularly distinctive in anaerobic bacteremia. Excessive jaundice with hyperbilirubinemia has been noted in 10% to 40% of cases. Suppurative thrombophlebitis may be present in 5% to 12% of cases, primarily involving the pelvic, hepatic, mesenteric, and portal veins. Polymicrobial bacteremia is particularly prevalent in infections of gastrointestinal, female genital, and odontogenic origin. Anaerobic bacteremia of female genital and odontogenic sources tends to be transient and self-limited. In contrast, anaerobic bacteremia of gastrointestinal and necrotic soft tissue sources tends to be recurrent and persistent in the absence of surgical drainage. Although anaerobic bacteria can cause endocarditis, such infections appear to be exceedingly rare.

DIAGNOSIS
Clinical Clues to Anaerobic Infections

Apart from actinomycosis and clostridial myonecrosis, infections involving obligate anaerobes are generally indistinguishable from other causes of sepsis. Clinical manifestations are largely determined by the organ system involved and by the extent and chronicity of the infection. The clinical setting of infection suggestive of local tissue ischemia or necrosis and the proximity of infection to mucosal surfaces where obligate anaerobes normally reside are the two most helpful clues. The presence of putrid, foul-smelling discharge is virtually diagnostic of infection involving anaerobes, although the absence of foul odor does not rule out this possibility. Similarly, the finding of crepitus or black discoloration of affected tissue is only suggestive

Table 271-8 Recommended procedure for specimen collection for anaerobic culture

SOURCE	PROCEDURE
Pulmonary	Percutaneous transtracheal aspiration or bronchoscopic aspiration with protected catheter or brush
Pleural	Thoracentesis
Odontogenic space infections	Extraoral aspiration of abscess
Female genital	Laparoscopic aspiration, culdocentesis, or dilation and curettage per cervical os
Sinus tract or draining wounds	Needle and syringe aspiration of wound edge through intact skin; specimen obtained by tissue biopsy or curettage, or at surgery from depths of wound

evidence. A well-performed Gram stain of appropriately collected clinical material is a very useful diagnostic tool. Anaerobic infections are typically polymicrobial, and the characteristic cellular morphology of certain anaerobic pathogens may be recognized by an accomplished microscopist. The finding of "sterile" pus by conventional culture methods in the face of a positive Gram stain should be considered presumptive evidence of an anaerobic infection. In the final analysis, however, the accurate diagnosis of anaerobic infection depends on the ability of the laboratory to isolate these fastidious organisms from clinical material likely to yield meaningful bacteriologic data.

Specimen Collection and Transport

One of the major handicaps in the recovery of anaerobic bacteria is improper specimen collection and transport (Chapter 233). Care must be taken to avoid specimens that may be potentially contaminated by commensal flora of mucocutaneous surfaces where anaerobes normally reside (e.g., throat swabs, expectorated sputum, voided urine, bronchoscopic and nasotracheal aspirates, vaginal secretions, feces, colostomy effluent, or superficial wound swabs). Blood and other body fluids that are normally sterile and aseptically obtained should be routinely cultured for anaerobic bacteria. Other clinical materials and special procedures likely to yield meaningful bacteriologic data for anaerobic infections are summarized in Table 271-8.

Apart from judicious selection of appropriate specimens for culture, proper specimen transport to preclude aeration and adequate anaerobic culture techniques are equally important for documentation of an anaerobic infection. Many fastidious organisms are extremely oxygen-sensitive and cannot withstand even a brief moment of exposure to air. Fluid transport media such as thioglycolate broth or Stuart's medium support growth of facultatives as well as anaerobes. In the presence of a mixed infection, facultative organisms, which grow faster than anaerobes, frequently preclude recovery of the latter. An ideal transport system, therefore, should be nonselective and nonbactericidal, and have sufficiently low oxidation-reduction potential and minimum susceptibility to oxidation. Such an ideal system is costly and not readily available commercially. The closest substitute consists of gas-filled containers, usually flushed with carbon dioxide. Specimens are collected with a sterile needle and syringe, and care is taken to expel the air in the syringe before instillation of the specimen into the transport vial. If commercial anaerobic transport vials are not available, specimens should be retained within the needle and syringe, capped to minimize aeration, and delivered immediately to the clinical laboratory. If swabs are to be used, it is recommended that they be prepared, stored, and transported in gas-filled containers under anaerobic conditions. Immediate processing of specimens by the laboratory also improves recovery, but in practice, this is often not feasible.

Radiologic and Imaging Studies

Noninvasive tests such as computed tomography, magnetic resonance imaging, ultrasonography, and gallium or indium scanning are most useful for localization of suppurative infections in the central nervous system, and in intraabdominal and pelvic organs. The sensitivity and specificity of these tests in detection of abscess and differentiation from tumor, hematoma, and other noninflammatory space-occupying lesions in various sites remain to be determined by careful prospective study. In general, it may be said that a positive scan is highly suggestive, particularly when supported by the clinical picture; however, a negative scan is much less useful in ruling out infection.

THERAPY
Antimicrobial Susceptibility and Empiric Therapy

Successful treatment of anaerobic infections requires rational antibiotic selection in conjunction with judicial surgical resection and drainage. Choice of appropriate antibiotics should be guided by culture results and antibiotic susceptibility data on the specific organisms involved (Chapter 231). Unfortunately, there is considerable method-related variability in susceptibility results, and as yet there is no general agreement as to the "gold standard" method that should be followed in the clinical laboratory. For these reasons, and because certain drugs are essentially always active against certain anaerobes, it has been accepted that not all clinical anaerobic isolates require in vitro susceptibility testing. Susceptibility testing is important, however, particularly in clinical settings where there has been persistence of infection or suboptimal response to empiric antibiotic regimens. Which specific anaerobic isolate to test when several are present and which drugs to be included remain somewhat controversial issues. Certainly organisms that are recognized as virulent and are frequently resistant and antibiotics that are frequently used as empiric therapy should be considered for testing. The former includes some members of the *B. fragilis* group, pigmented anaerobic gram-negative bacilli, *P. bivia, P. disiens,* certain *Fusobacterium* species, and *Clostridium* species. The latter includes penicillin G, certain broad-spectrum ureidopenicillins (e.g., ticarcillin, piperacillin, mezlocillin) and carbapenems (e.g., imipenem-cilastatin, meropenem), clindamycin, and certain cephalosporins (e.g., cefoxitin, ceftriaxone, cefotetan, cefotaxime, ceftizoxime, ceftazidime).

In the absence of specific culture or susceptibility data, initial antibiotic therapy requires empiric choices based on knowledge of the pathogens most likely to be present in a particular clinical setting, predicted in vitro susceptibility patterns (Table 271-9), and the toxicologic and pharmacokinetic characteristics of the agents being considered.

Although penicillin G has been considered the agent of choice for a number of mixed aerobic-anaerobic infections at various sites above the diaphragm (particularly in oropulmonary and head and neck infections), recent experience suggests that this general recommendation may no longer be tenable. This concern has arisen based on the following findings: (1) β-lactamase production has been observed with increasing frequency among clinical isolates of anaerobic bacteria besides *B. fragilis* (particularly *P. bivia, P. disiens,* and some pigmented anaerobic gram-negative bacilli); (2) β-lactamase production is increasingly found among aerobic isolates, which may protect coisolated penicillin-sensitive anaerobes (e.g., *Branhamella catarrhalis, Haemophilus influenzae, Staphylococcus* species); (3) β-lactamase activity can be detected directly in clinical specimens; and (4) failure of penicillin therapy has been well documented. These data highlight the need to reassess the role of β-lactamase production both as a virulence mechanism and as a cause for therapeutic failure in mixed infections. It remains to be seen whether routine use of a β-lactamase inhibitor (such as clavulanic acid or sulbactam) in combination with penicillin will resolve these current concerns. Among the β-lactams, susceptibility of obligate anaerobes to ampicillin is comparable to that of penicillin G, whereas penicillin V and semisynthetic penicillins (e.g., methicillin and cloxacillin) are distinctly less active. Among the cephalosporins, only cefoxitin, cefotetan, and ceftizoxime have enhanced antianaerobic spectrum. These agents appear to have comparable activity against *B. fragilis,* with resistance rates ranging from 3% to 17%, and none is as active as clindamycin or metronidazole. Other cephalosporins (e.g., cefazolin, cephalexin, cefamandole, cefuroxime, ceftriaxone, cefoperazone, ceftazidime, etc.) are much less active.

Table 271-9   Comparative in vitro antibiotic activity against major anaerobes

	ABOVE DIAPHRAGM		ABOVE/BELOW DIAPHRAGM		BELOW DIAPHRAGM	
ANTIBIOTIC	FUSOBACTERIUM	BACTEROIDES MELANINOGENICUS GROUP	PEPTOSTREPTOCOCCUS	ACTINOMYCES	BACTEROIDES FRAGILIS GROUP	CLOSTRIDIUM
Penicillin	S	S-R	S	S	R	S*
Ampicillin-sulbactam†	S	S	S	S	S	S
Piperacillin, ticarcillin, mezlocillin	S	S	S	S	S-R	S
Piperacillin-tazobactam	S	S	S	S	S	S
Imipenem	S	S	S	S	S	S
Cefazolin	S	S-R	S	S	R	S
Cefoxitin	S	S-R	S	S	S	S-R
Cefotetan	S	S	S	S	S-R	S
Ceftizoxime	S	S	S	S	S	S-R
Cefotaxime	S	S	S	S	S-R	S
Ceftriaxone	S	S-R	S	S	S-R	S
Cefoperazone	S	S	S	S	S-R	S
Ceftazidime	S	S-R	S	S	S-R	S
Clindamycin	S*	S	S*	S	S	S-R
Chloramphenicol	S	S	S	S	S*	S
Metronidazole	S	S	S-R	R	S	S
Tetracycline	S	S-R	S-R	S	S-R	S-R

S, >80% strains sensitive; S-R, 30%-80% strains sensitive; R, <30% strains sensitive.
*Emerging resistance noted.
†Similar combinations currently available are amoxicillin-clavulanic acid and ticarcillin-clavulanic acid; they have comparable activities against anaerobes.

Table 271-10   Empiric antimicrobial regimens for suspected anaerobic or mixed infections

SITE	TREATMENT OF CHOICE	ALTERNATE REGIMENS
Pleuropulmonary, odontogenic, or human bite infections	Penicillin G IV, 1-4 MU q4h or ampicillin-sulbactam IV, 1-2 g q6h	Clindamycin IV, 600 mg q6h Cefoxitin IV, 1-2 g q6h Cefotaxime IV, 2 g q6h
Brain abscess or subdural empyema	Penicillin G IV, 4 MU q4h + metronidazole IV, 500 mg q6h	Penicillin G IV, 4 MU q4h + chloramphenicol 500 mg q6h
Intraabdominal, pelvic, or necrotic soft tissue infections	Clindamycin IV, 600 mg q6h or metronidazole IV, 500 mg q6h; each + tobramycin 1.5 mg/kg IV, q8h or ciprofloxacin IV, 200 mg q12h	Cefoxitin IV, 2 g q6h; cefotetan IV, 2 g q12h; ceftizoxime IV, 3 g q8h; piperacillin IV, 3 g q4h; imipenem IV, 500 mg q6h; or piperacillin-tazobactam IV, 2-4 g q4-6h; each + tobramycin IV, 1.5 mg/kg q8h or ciprofloxacin IV, 400 mg q12h

Among the penems, imipenem-cilastatin and meropenem are the most broadly active. They have the added advantage of excellent antipseudomonal and antistaphylococcal spectrum. The monobactam aztreonam is inactive against both anaerobes and gram-positive aerobes.

Clindamycin remains highly active against *B. fragilis* and other anaerobes, although emerging resistance has been noted in some centers. Erythromycin is not considered useful for anaerobic infections because of relative resistance by *B. fragilis* and some strains of *Fusobacterium*. It is difficult to administer parenterally, and only low blood levels are achieved by the oral route. The role of newer macrolides (e.g., roxithromycin, azithromycin, clarithromycin) remains to be determined.

Metronidazole has excellent activity, particularly against *B. fragilis*, *Fusobacterium* spp., and *Clostridium perfringens*. However, *Peptostreptococcus* and *Bacteroides* species other than *B. fragilis* are only moderately sensitive, whereas nonsporulating gram-positive bacilli are relatively resistant to therapeutic levels of metronidazole. Metronidazole lacks activity against facultative bacteria and should not be used as a single agent during empiric therapy, since most infections involving anaerobic bacteria are in fact mixed infections. It is important to note that metronidazole is the only agent with consistent bactericidal activity against *B. fragilis*, and it crosses the blood-brain barrier well. For these reasons, it is particularly useful for treating anaerobic brain abscess or endocarditis.

Chloramphenicol is active against a wide range of anaerobic bacteria, including *B. fragilis*, and like metronidazole, no resistance to it by these strains has been noted. Because of its myelotoxic proper-

ties, it should be reserved for treating selected patients with anaerobic infections involving the central nervous system.

Tetracycline and its analogs can no longer be recommended as empiric treatment of anaerobic infections because of the substantial resistance acquired by *B. fragilis* and virtually all classes of other anaerobic bacteria. Tetracycline, however, remains useful in the treatment of actinomycosis.

Trimethoprim-sulfamethoxazole, vancomycin, and the fluoroquinolones have only limited activity against anaerobic bacteria. Vancomycin is effective against some gram-positive anaerobes (particularly *Clostridium difficile*) but has no activity against gram-negative anaerobes. Similarly, among the quinolones, ciprofloxacin is more active than enoxacin, ofloxacin, or norfloxacin, but none are reliable as single-agent therapy for anaerobic or mixed infections.

Aminoglycoside antibiotics are uniformly inactive against obligate anaerobes. These drugs are often included in antimicrobial regimens directed at facultative gram-negative bacilli for the therapy of mixed infections.

The recommended regimens for empiric therapy of various anaerobic or mixed infections at different sites are summarized in Table 271-10. In general, therapy should be directed at both the facultative and anaerobic components of the suspected microflora. Although a broad-spectrum single agent (e.g., cefoxitin, ceftizoxime, cefotetan, ampicillin-sulbactam, piperacillin-tazobactam, ticarcillin-clavulanic acid, imipenem-cilastatin, or meropenem) may be used to minimize toxicity and reduce cost, combination therapy is sometimes preferred to achieve synergistic activity (e.g., penicillin, clindamycin, metronidazole, or enhanced cephalosporins, each plus an aminoglycoside). A parenteral route for administration, relatively high dosages, and prolonged duration of treatment (3 to 6 weeks) are usually required because of the extent of tissue necrosis and tendency for relapse with these infections.

Surgical Drainage of Abscesses

Although surgical resection and drainage may be the decisive therapeutic modality for most suppurative anaerobic infections, several exceptions are noteworthy. In lung abscess, nonsurgical treatment alone is often effective, perhaps because of spontaneous drainage and expectoration of abscess contents through the tracheobronchial tree. Recent experience indicates, however, that certain cerebral abscesses may also respond to antibiotics alone even when well encapsulated. A similar experience has been noted with hepatic and tuboovarian abscesses. These data indicate that abscesses do not always require drainage, although it is not clear what factors are reliable predictors of a favorable response to antibiotics alone.

Adjunctive Measures

Apart from surgical and antimicrobial therapy, adjunctive measures such as topical wound irrigations with hydrogen peroxide solution and hyperbaric oxygen treatment may further hasten eradication of infection and promote healing. Although data from well-controlled studies are lacking, hyperbaric oxygen therapy has been recommended for selected cases of necrotic soft tissue infections, and for recalcitrant anaerobic osteomyelitis involving the maxilla or mandible.

PREVENTION

Anaerobic infections can be prevented by avoiding conditions that predispose to invasion by surface microflora. In traumatic wounds, the most effective prophylaxis is thorough debridement and cleansing of the wound, elimination of foreign bodies and dead space, and reestablishment of good circulation. The complex gastrointestinal or vaginal flora can be numerically reduced before surgery. Mechanical cleansing of the bowel with a low-residue or liquid diet followed by cathartics, enemas, and luminal antibiotics effectively reduces the bacterial concentration in the colon preoperatively. Parenteral perioperative antibiotics also have been used prophylactically in gastrointestinal and gynecologic surgery when there is a possibility of contamination with normal microflora at the operative site. Those operations that may benefit from prophylactic antibiotics include elective colorectal surgery, gastroduodenal surgery when intraluminal bacterial overgrowth is anticipated, cesarean section after rupture of the membranes and labor, vaginal hysterectomy in the premenopausal woman, and radical pelvic or head and neck surgery for malignancy. Several studies have shown significant reduction in the frequency of postoperative infections from about 20% to 30% to 4% to 8% after prophylactic administration of antibiotics in clean, uncontaminated surgery. Cephalosporins have been particularly useful in prophylactic regimens for head and neck, pelvic, and gastrointestinal surgery. Comparative studies have indicated that for surgical prophylaxis involving colorectal or pelvic procedures, a first-generation cephalosporin, such as cefazolin, may be as effective as some second- or third-generation cephalosporins, including cefonicid, cefoxitin, cefotetan, ceftizoxime, or cefotaxime. In contaminated or "dirty" surgery, early *treatment* rather than prophylaxis is essential for reduction of postoperative morbidity.

BIBLIOGRAPHY

Aldridge KE et al: Discordant results between the broth disk elution and broth microdilution susceptibility tests with *Bacteroides fragilis* group isolates, *J Clin Microbiol* 28:375, 1990.
Appleman MD, Heseltine PNR, Cherubin CE: Epidemiology, antimicrobial susceptibility, pathogenicity, and significance of *Bacteroides fragilis* group organisms isolated at Los Angeles County–University of Southern California Medical Center, *Rev Infect Dis* 13:12, 1991.
Bartlett JG: Anaerobic bacterial infections of the lung and pleural space, *Clin Infect Dis* 16(suppl 4):S248-S255, 1993.
Brook I: Diagnosis and management of anaerobic infections of the head and neck, *Ann Otol Rhinol Laryngol Suppl* 155:9-15, 1992.

✔ **WHEN TO REFER**

Anaerobic and necrotizing infections of the central nervous system, pleuropulmonary spaces, intraabdominal and pelvic organs, and skin and soft tissue infections are often life threatening and require a multidisciplinary approach (including various medical and surgical subspecialties, as well as critical care) for optimal management. The services of an infectious disease specialist, medical microbiologist, and a clinical pharmacist may be invaluable to assist in the diagnosis and management of these complicated and serious infections.

Brook I: The role of encapsulated anaerobic bacteria in synergistic infections, *FEMS Microbiol Rev* 13:65-74, 1994.
Chow AW: Life-threatening infections of the head and neck, *Clin Infect Dis* 14:991-1004, 1992.
Finegold SM: Overview of clinically important anaerobes, *Clin Infect Dis* 20(suppl 2):S205-S207, 1995.
Gorbach SL: Antibiotic treatment of anaerobic infections, *Clin Infect Dis* 18(suppl 4):S305-S310, 1994.
Hentges DJ: The anaerobic microflora of the human body, *Clin Infect Dis* 16(suppl 4):S175-S180, 1993.
Hillier SL, Krohn MA, Cassen E et al: The role of bacterial vaginosis and vaginal bacteria in amniotic fluid infection in women in preterm labor with intact fetal membranes, *Clin Infect Dis* 20(suppl 2):S276-S278, 1995.
Jousimies-Somer HR: Update on the taxonomy and the clinical and laboaortry characteristics of pigmented anaerobic gram-negative rods, *Clin Infect Dis* 20(suppl 2):S187-S191, 1995.
Kurtesz D, Chow AW: Infected pressure and diabetic ulcers, *Clin Geriat Med* 8:835-852, 1992.
McClean KL, Sheehan GJ, Harding GKM: Intraabdominal infection: a review, *Clin Infect Dis* 19:100-106, 1994.
Rosenblatt JE, Brook I: Clinical relevance of susceptibility testing of anaerobic bacteria, *Clin Infect Dis* 16(suppl 4):S446-S448, 1993.
Summanen P: Recent taxonomic changes for anaerobic gram-positive and selected gram-negative organisms, *Clin Infect Dis* 16(suppl 4):S168-S174, 1993.
Tanner A, Stillman N: Oral and dental infections with anaerobic bacteria: clinical features, predominant pathogens, and treatment, *Clin Infect Dis* 16(suppl 4):S304-S309, 1993.

CHAPTER

272 Infections Caused by Legionellae

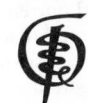

Washington C. Winn, Jr. and Christopher J. Grace

THE ORGANISM
Classification and Characteristics

Legionella pneumophila, the most important member of the family Legionellaceae, is an aerobic, gram-negative bacillus that produces sporadic and epidemic respiratory illness ranging from a self-limited flulike syndrome to severe pneumonia and occasionally disseminated disease. Although this bacterium was identified first as an important human pathogen after an outbreak of respiratory disease at an American Legion convention in 1976, it was isolated from the blood of a patient with pneumonia in 1947. On the basis of cell wall composition, physiology, and DNA hybridization studies, the bacillus is unrelated to any previously recognized human pathogen.

In subsequent years a group of related bacteria that are distinct from *L. pneumophila* has been identified. The classification of the Legionellaceae is detailed in Box 272-1. *Legionella micdadei,* originally designated *Pittsburgh pneumonia agent,* was the first member of the genus to be isolated; it was recovered in 1943 from the blood of a soldier who had a nonfatal illness that was included in the designation "Fort Bragg fever." Approximately 90% of reported *Legionella* infections have been caused by *L. pneumophila* and *L. micdadei.*

BOX 272-1
Classification of legionellaceae

Species isolated from humans	Species isolated from environment only
L. pneumophila (14 sero-groups)	*L. cherrii*
ssp. *pneumophila*	*L. erythra* (2 serogroups)
ssp. *fraseri*	*L. jamestownensis*
ssp. *pascullei*	*L. parisiensis*
L. micdadei	*L. shakespearei*
L. bozemanii (2 serogroups)	*L. santicrucis*
L. dumoffii	*L. steigerwaltii*
L. feeleii (2 serogroups)	*L. adelaidensis*
L. gormanii	*L. fairfieldensis*
L. hackeliae (2 serogroups)	*L. brunensis*
L. israelensis	*L. moravica*
L. jordanis	*L. quinlivianii* (2 serogroups)
L. sainthelensi (2 sero-groups)	*L. gratiana*
L. longbeachae (2 sero-groups)	*L. quateirensis*
	L. nautarum
	L. worsleiensis
L. maceachernii	*L. londiniensis*
L. oakridgensis	*L. geestiana*
L. wadsworthii	*L. rubrilucens*
L. birminghamensis	*L. spiritensis*
L. cincinnatiensis	*L. waltersii*
L. anisa	unnamed genomospecies
L. tucsonensis	
L. lansingensis	

L. pneumophila is a short, gram-negative bacillus, measuring 0.5 to 0.7 μm by 2 to 4 μm, with occasional filamentous forms up to 20 μm in length. Slightly tapered ends and central constrictions are present frequently. Gram stain detects the bacterium if large numbers of organisms are present, as in lung biopsy specimens. Prolonged staining with safranin or addition of carbolfuchsin to the counterstain improves the sensitivity of the Gram stain. Crystal violet (the "half Gram stain"), the Gimenez stain, and the Giemsa stain also demonstrate the bacilli. In tissue, one of the silver impregnation stains, for example, the Dieterle stain, is useful. None of these stains is specific for Legionellae. They are, however, useful for screening specimens in which bacteria have not been demonstrated by conventional means or in which Legionellae have not been detected by available fluorescent conjugates.

Fourteen serogroups of *L. pneumophila* are recognized currently. Antigens that are serogroup-specific and others that are more broadly cross-reactive have been described. The majority of clinical isolates of *L. pneumophila* (at least 60%) have been serogroup 1 strains.

L. pneumophila is non–spore-forming and non–acid-fast, and it requires the addition of cysteine to media for growth. Biochemical characterization is not useful for identification. Definitive identification may require genetic analysis. For practical purposes, serologic characterization of an isolate that requires cysteine for growth and resembles *Legionella* morphologically is sufficient. If such an isolate does not react with available sera, it should be sent to a reference laboratory.

Epidemiology

Infection with *L. pneumophila* is widespread in the United States and elsewhere. Although infection with these organisms is clearly not restricted in its geographic distribution, serosurveys indicate that exposure to the organism varies widely from one location to another. In some populations, up to one third of individuals have serologic evidence of previous infection with *L. pneumophila* or related organisms. In other areas, only 1% of sample groups are seropositive. Studies from several centers have shown that as many as 5% of pneumonias are caused by these organisms. Thus *L. pneumophila* appears to be a common respiratory pathogen with a wide distribution.

Legionella pneumonia has been described principally as an epi-

demic infection, with many cases related to a common source of exposure. Sporadic cases also occur, even in areas that have not experienced epidemic disease. *L. pneumophila* has been isolated from a variety of fresh-water sources, including drinking water. A cloud of droplets generated by cooling towers and evaporative condensers has produced *L. pneumophila* infection. Other types of equipment that generate aqueous aerosols, for example, contaminated shower heads, humidifiers, and nebulizers, also have been implicated as sources of infection. Home heating systems may be a source for sporadic cases. Application of contaminated tap water to healing surgical wounds has caused nosocomial *Legionella dumoffii* infection. It is important to realize, however, that recovery of *L. pneumophila* from environmental sources has usually not been associated with disease. *L. pneumophila* infection occurs most commonly in the summer and early fall. Both epidemic and sporadic cases follow the same seasonal pattern. Nevertheless, infections have been seen year-round.

L. pneumophila pneumonia has been reported in all age-groups, although most patients are over 50 years of age. A striking male predominance is seen. Patients with underlying chronic diseases and immune suppression are at increased risk for severe *Legionella* infection. A high index of suspicion is warranted for patients with chronic heart, lung, or renal disease; diabetes mellitus; solid organ or bone marrow transplantation; or chronic alcoholism. Patients who smoke cigarettes, recipients of antineoplastic chemotherapy, and particularly those who receive high doses of corticosteroids are also at increased risk. Human immunodeficiency virus infection is also a risk factor but does not appear to be as important as organ transplantation or corticosteroid therapy.

Legionella pneumonia may be acquired in the community or in the hospital. Despite the fact that it is a respiratory tract disease that is transmitted by aerosols, person-to-person spread has not been documented.

The attack rate of the epidemic form of pneumonic illness is less than 5%, and the incubation period is usually between 2 and 10 days. In contrast, a nonpneumonic type of illness, known as *Pontiac fever*, has a very high attack rate and a very short incubation period. The explanation for the differing clinical and epidemiologic presentations is as yet unknown.

Pathophysiology

The only documented source of infection is water, and the predominant mode of transmission is by inhalation of a contaminated aerosol or possibly by aspiration of potable water. Direct contact with contaminated tap water may produce local infection if normal cutaneous defenses are abrogated by disease or trauma.

The major finding on pathologic examination is a lobular pneumonia, which may become so extensive that most of one or more lobes may be involved. The infiltrate spreads in the lung through bronchioles and by direct alveolar extension. Nodular consolidation occurs, and abscesses are present in as many as 20% of cases. Fibrinous or fibrinopurulent pleural effusions occur frequently, but empyema is rare. On microscopic examination, the alveolar infiltrate consists of neutrophils and, frequently, a large component of macrophages. Innumerable short bacilli can be demonstrated by the Dieterle stain in a typical case, both extracellularly and in phagocytic cells. Most of the bacteria are in the alveolar infiltrate. Some are present in the interstitium, and bacilli have been demonstrated in regional lymph nodes, Kupffer's cells of the liver, and sinusoidal cells of the spleen. In addition, a variety of other extrapulmonary inflammatory lesions, including intravascular infections, have been documented, but these are unusual complications.

L. pneumophila is a facultative intracellular bacterium. Alveolar macrophages and later blood macrophages that enter the air spaces are the initial site for bacterial replication. Complement receptors on alveolar macrophages serve as binding sites for *Legionella*, and enhanced opsonization occurs in the presence of specific antibody. Once phagocytized, *Legionella* evades phagolysosomal fusion and grows within the phagocytic vesicles of the macrophage. Cell-mediated immunity is the primary host defense against *Legionella* infection. Macrophages that have been activated by specifically sensitized T-lymphocytes inhibit intracellular growth, although significant bactericidal activity has been difficult to demonstrate in vitro. Immunoprotective antigens have been identified experimentally, but no single dominant virulence factor has been uncovered. Polymorphonuclear neutrophils do not support the growth of *Legionella* in vitro. Experimental studies suggest a protective role for neutrophils and for antibody, but they are secondary to cellular immunity in importance.

The participation of toxins in the pathogenesis of disease has been suggested because of the prominence of extrapulmonary symptoms and because of extensive cytolysis of the pulmonary inflammatory infiltrate in some cases. At least two cytotoxins, an endotoxin-like substance, and numerous extracellular enzymes have been described, but their roles in the production of disease are not yet clear.

CLINICAL DISEASE
Legionella pneumophila

L. pneumophila produces two distinct syndromes: Pontiac fever and Legionnaires' disease. Pontiac fever is a self-limited illness characterized by chills, fever, myalgias, and headache. The disease lasts 2 to 5 days, resolves without therapy, and leaves no sequelae. Pneumonia has not been associated with this syndrome.

Legionnaires' disease, the most common syndrome, is a pneumonic process that can be acquired in the community or the hospital. After an incubation period of 2 to 10 days, Legionnaires' disease begins with a prodrome of malaise, headache, and myalgia that lasts 1 to 2 days. The patient then becomes more acutely ill with chills, rigors, and prostration. Fever exceeds 40° C in 20% of patients. A more indolent onset is less common. The cough is initially dry or productive of only small amounts of mucoid sputum, but purulent sputum is eventually produced by 50% of patients. Dyspnea is common and 30% to 40% of patients report chest pain. Hemoptysis is rare, but blood-tinged sputum is not uncommon. Extrapulmonary symptoms may be dramatic, including nausea, vomiting, and abdominal pain in 10% to 20% and diarrhea in 50% of patients. One third of patients may have alterations in mental status, such as lethargy, confusion, agitation, and, less commonly, seizures, coma, or disturbances of gait.

On physical examination patients are usually moderately to severely ill. Relative bradycardia is present in 50% of patients. Physical examination of the chest reveals inspiratory crackles. Signs of consolidation may be present, especially late in the course of illness.

In 70% of patients, chest radiographs reveal a unilateral patchy alveolar infiltrate, usually in the lower lobes. Expansion of the infiltrate is common, more often to lobar consolidation or to adjacent lobes than to the contralateral lung. Pleural effusions occur in one third of patients. Hilar lymphadenopathy is unusual, and abscesses are rarely demonstrated on radiograph, although necrotizing inflammation and microabscesses are commonly demonstrated at postmortem examination. Other radiographic patterns include interstitial infiltrates and poorly defined rounded opacities that occur predominantly in the lower lobes and may suggest septic emboli. The chest radiograph may reveal a more extensive inflammatory process than would be suggested from physical examination. None of these symptoms, signs, or radiographic patterns absolutely distinguishes *L. pneumophila* pneumonia from other causes of community-acquired or hospital-acquired pneumonia.

Extrapulmonary inflammatory disease has been well documented but appears to be uncommon. Most dissemination probably occurs hematogenously, but direct extension could account for cases of pericarditis.

L. pneumophila has been reported as a cause of prosthetic and native valve endocarditis, myocarditis, pericarditis, infection of aneurysms and hemodialysis fistulas, sinusitis, pyelonephritis, pancreatitis, peritonitis, hepatic abscess, and postoperative wound infection. A leukocytosis of 10,000 to 20,000/mm³ is common, but the white blood cell count may be normal. Leukopenia is a poor prognostic sign.

Hyponatremia (serum sodium <130 mEq/L), which occurs in 50% of patients, is probably caused by salt and water loss rather than by inappropriate secretion of antidiuretic hormone as originally hypothesized. Hyponatremia occurs significantly more often in Legionnaires' disease than in other community-acquired pneumonias. Other less common laboratory abnormalities, which do not differentiate *Legionella* infections from other pneumonias, include hypophosphatemia, hematuria, proteinuria, myoglobinuria, thrombocytopenia,

hemolytic anemia, and elevations of serum aspartate aminotransferase, alkaline phosphatase, bilirubin, and serum creatine kinase.

Sputum frequently contains alveolar macrophages and polymorphonuclear leukocytes. The presence of many neutrophils and absence of bacteria in routine Gram stains of sputum is a useful clue to the possibility of Legionnaires' disease, especially if the patient has not responded as expected to therapy with β-lactam or aminoglycoside antibiotics.

A specific diagnosis can be made by culture of the organism from clinical specimens, by detection of a serologic response to *Legionella,* or by detection of bacterial antigen in body tissues or fluids. Recovery of the bacterium in culture is most definitive and should be attempted whenever possible. It is essential that the microbiology laboratory be notified that *Legionella* infection is suspected so that appropriate stains and media may be used when the specimens are processed. Screening of sputum specimens for purulence is not a valid method for selection of specimens. The medium of choice is buffered charcoal yeast extract agar supplemented with α-ketoglutarate (BCYE-α). Inoculation of an additional agar containing selective antimicrobial agents may increase the yield from sputum to 70%, but a nonselective agar must be included. Growth is usually detected within 3 to 5 days. Dual infections occur with other pathogens, including other *Legionella* species.

Blood can be cultured for *Legionella* using techniques that include inoculation of material onto BCYE-α agar. The lysis centrifugation system (Isolator, Wampole), broth systems with subculture including the BACTEC system (Becton Dickinson), and biphasic BCYE bottles have been inoculated successfully, but the sensitivity is not known.

Serum antibody to *Legionella* may be measured by microagglutination assays, by enzyme-linked immunoassays, or by indirect immunofluorescence (IFA) tests. The IFA test is the most readily available and the best studied serologic procedure for diagnosis of *Legionella* infections (Chapter 233).

A definitive diagnosis requires seroconversion, defined as a fourfold or greater increase in antibody titer to a minimum level of 1:128. A stable titer of 1:256 by IFA has been used to make a presumptive diagnosis when a compatible illness occurred in an epidemic setting. Most patients show seroconversion within 3 weeks of illness; some do not develop antibody until 6 weeks or later, and a few individuals never produce detectable antibody.

Antigen detection in clinical specimens has the advantage of providing prompt diagnosis. Organisms can be detected by direct immunofluorescence (DFA) examination of respiratory secretions, but the positive and negative predictive values are unacceptable, especially in populations with a low incidence of infection.

A moderately sensitive and highly specific enzyme immunoassay for serogroup 1 *L. pneumophila* antigen in urine is commercially available. Even with this assay, however, the predictive value of a positive test may be problematic if the incidence of infection is very low. Antigen may be excreted in the urine for weeks or months after an acute infection, so a positive test does not absolutely document the etiology of the acute illness. Latex agglutination tests, genetic probes for bacterial nucleic acid, and amplification assays are either not commercially available or are of unproved value.

The response to therapy is variable. Some patients defervesce soon after treatment is initiated and experience an increased sense of well-being within 24 to 36 hours. Others remain febrile and clinically ill for several days and then begin to improve slowly. The disease may progress radiographically in spite of overall clinical improvement.

The principal complication of Legionnaires' disease is respiratory failure, which may be associated with hypotension, shock, and renal failure. Thus appropriate antibiotic therapy often must be accompanied by aggressive, supportive care.

The prognosis of Legionnaires' disease is directly related to the presence or absence of underlying illness and to the use of appropriate or inappropriate antibiotics. Hospitalized patients who are otherwise in good health and who receive prompt erythromycin therapy have a mortality rate of less than 10%. On the other hand, the course of Legionnaires' disease has been fatal in more than three fourths of patients with significant underlying disease who did not receive erythromycin. Radiographic resolution of successfully treated *L. pneumophila* pneumonia often requires several months. Reinfection with a different strain of *Legionella* has been reported rarely; relapse of an

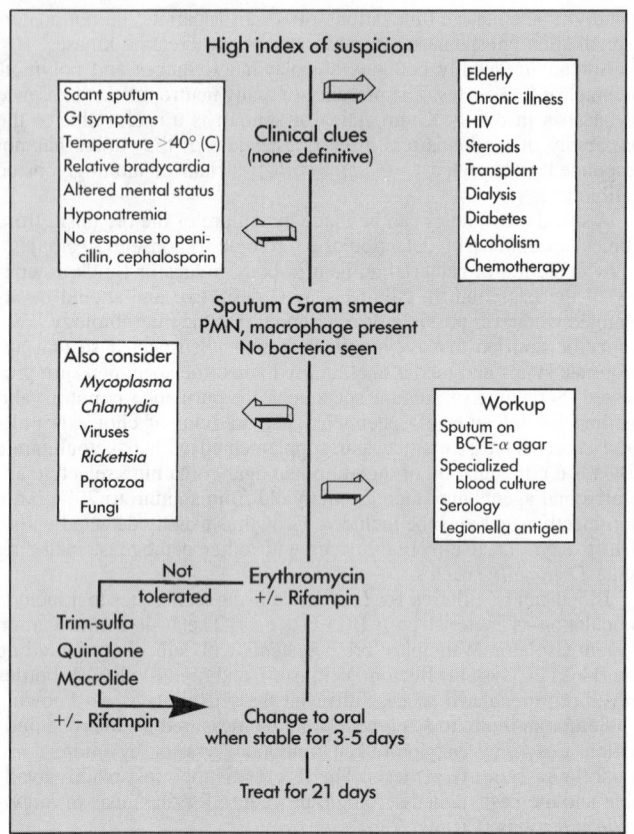

FIGURE 272-1 Diagnostic and therapeutic algorithm for *Legionella* pneumonia.

mg/kg for children other than neonates). The higher dose and the intravenous form should be used for moderate to severe infection and for immune-compromised hosts. Once the patient's clinical condition has stabilized for 3 to 5 days, oral erythromycin therapy (500 mg PO qid) can be substituted. Therapy should be continued for a combined duration of 3 weeks. Rifampin (600 mg PO bid) should be added for documented *Legionella* pneumonia or for severe pneumonia if *Legionella* is a very likely etiologic agent. Rifampin should not be used alone, because of the likelihood that resistance will develop.

Erythromycin can cause several troublesome side-effects, including painful venous sclerosis that may require central venous access, fluid overload in patients with cardiac disease, and gastrointestinal upset. If large intravenous doses are given, transient hearing loss may result (Chapter 231). Alternative therapy may, therefore, be needed. Trimethoprim-sulfamethoxazole has shown good activity in vitro, in animal studies, and in limited uncontrolled clinical use. The intravenous and oral forms are dosed at 10 mg/kg/day of the trimethoprim component in two to three divided doses. The new quinolones (ciprofloxacin, ofloxacin, and perfloxacin) have shown excellent in vitro activity, have been effective in animal models, and have been used successfully in very limited human studies. Therapeutic failures have also been described. Combination therapy with these quinolones and erythromycin needs further study.

The new macrolides (clarithromycin, azithromycin, and roxithromycin) also show promise in vitro, but experience with human infection is very limited. Imipenem-cilastatin, ticarcillin-clavulanic acid, amoxicillin-clavulanic acid, and clindamycin have shown clinical efficacy, but have not been tested sufficiently to employ in human infections. Variable success has been achieved in human subjects with tetracycline or doxycycline therapy.

Prevention. At present, little can be done to prevent sporadic, community-based Legionnaires' disease. Molecular analysis of bacterial isolates has been useful in epidemiologic assessment of environmental sites that are potential sources for dissemination of bacteria. Decontamination of these sources may abort epidemic or hyperendemic infection. In particular, chlorination or heat treatment of potable water systems has been associated with cessation of ongoing nosocomial outbreaks on several occasions. Epidemiologic and clinical surveillance should focus on the presence of human disease rather than environmental colonization because of the widespread distribution of these bacteria. All means of environmental decontamination identified to date have potential adverse effects on the physical integrity of the plumbing systems or on the safety of the individuals who use the system. Common-sense measures, such as using sterile water for wound care, for filling nebulizers and other aerosol generators, and possibly for any aqueous contact with extremely ill patients, are cheap and should be instituted in all hospitals.

incompletely treated primary infection is the more common cause of recurrent disease.

An approach to diagnosis and treatment of *Legionella* infections is outlined in Fig. 272-1. A high index of suspicion must be maintained for those patients with chronic underlying disease, immunosuppression, or advanced age, whether the infection is nosocomial or community acquired. Clinical clues should further raise suspicion, although there are no pathognomonic findings. The diagnostic evaluation should include culture of respiratory secretions, including sputum, and blood for *Legionella* and collection of acute and convalescent serum specimens for serologic testing. The enzyme immunoassay for serogroup 1 *L. pneumophila* antigen in urine should be considered, especially if the patient is unable to produce sputum for culture. Therapy with erythromycin should be started promptly after collection of diagnostic specimens and continued for 3 weeks. Initial therapy should be intravenous, and rifampin should be added for severe disease or extremely compromised patients. If erythromycin is not tolerated, alternative treatments may be used if the clinical response is monitored carefully.

Two important points must be considered when assessing antimicrobial efficacy against *L. pneumophila*. First, the bacterium lives and replicates intracellularly in macrophages. Second, it produces a β-lactamase that inactivates many β-lactam antibiotics. Effective antibiotics must resist enzymatic degradation and penetrate well into the cytoplasmic vacuoles where *Legionella* resides. Some antibiotics, such as aminoglycosides and cephalosporins, are active in vitro but are ineffective in vivo. Cell culture and animal models bring the testing process closer to in vivo reality, but ultimately clinical documentation of antimicrobial efficacy is required.

Erythromycin remains the antibiotic of choice for *Legionella* infections, based on in vitro, cell culture, animal model, and uncontrolled human studies. Erythromycin is concentrated within macrophages at 24 times the extracellular level and can kill phagocytized *Legionella*. The dose is 500 to 1000 mg every 6 hours (7.5 to 12.0

Legionella micdadei

Legionella micdadei (Pittsburgh pneumonia agent) was recognized initially as a cause of severe pneumonia in immunosuppressed patients. Pathologically, the pneumonia resembles that produced by *L. pneumophila*, but the bacilli may be partially or totally acid-fast in tissue. The bacterium is more fastidious than *L. pneumophila* but has been cultivated on BCYE-α medium. It is not acid-fast when grown on agar. *L. micdadei* is differentiated from its relatives by cell wall analysis, antigenic composition, and acid-fastness in tissue scrapings or sections. An identical bacterium (Tatlock bacillus) was isolated from the blood of a patient with Fort Bragg fever in 1943. The other cases of this nonfatal illness could not be linked to the bacterium, and the significance of the isolate remains unclear. Pontiac fever has been associated with *L. micdadei*. The bacterium has been isolated from multiple environmental sources, including tap water in respiratory therapy nebulizers.

Other Legionella Species

Infections with other species have been recognized infrequently or not at all. Pontiac fever has been caused by *Legionella feeleii* and *Legionella anisa*. *Legionella dumoffii* has produced clusters of nosocomial infection, including prosthetic valve endocarditis. Only *L.*

pneumophila, however, has been responsible for large, explosive outbreaks. Most patients infected by nonpneumophila species have had serious underlying diseases; all species of *Legionella* should be considered potentially pathogenic, given a sufficiently debilitated host. From the limited data available, the clinical disease, pathologic lesions, treatment, and prognosis do not appear to differ substantially from infections caused by *L. pneumophila.* Serologic documentation of these infections necessitates the demonstration of seroconversion in acute and convalescent specimens. Species other than *L. pneumophila* may be inhibited by antibiotics in selective media, so a nonselective agar must be inoculated.

BIBLIOGRAPHY

Balows A, Fraser DW, editors: International symposium on Legionnaires' disease, *Ann Intern Med* 90:491, 1979.

Barbaree JM, Breiman RF, Dufour AP, editors: *Legionella: current status and emerging perspectives,* Washington, DC, 1993, American Society for Microbiology.

Blander SJ, Horwitz MA: Vaccination with the major secretory protein of *Legionella* induces humoral and cell-mediated immune responses and protective immunity across different serogroups of *Legionella pneumophila* and different species of *Legionella, J Immunol* 147:285, 1991.

Edelstein PH: Legionnaires' disease, *Clin Infect Dis* 16:741, 1993.

England AC III et al: Sporadic legionellosis in the United States: the first thousand cases, *Ann Intern Med* 94:164, 1981.

Fang GD, Yu VL, Vickers RM: Disease due to the Legionellaceae (other than *Legionella pneumophila*): historical, microbiological, clinical, and epidemiological review, *Medicine* 68:116, 1989.

Fields BS, Fields SR, Loy JN, et al: Attachment and entry of *Legionella pneumophila* in *Hartmannella vermiformis, J Infect Dis* 167:1146, 1993.

Marston BJ, Lipman HB, Breiman RF: Surveillance for Legionnaires' disease: risk factors for morbidity and mortality, *Arch Intern Med* 154:2417, 1994.

Muder RR, Yu VL, Zuravleff JJ: Pneumonia due to the Pittsburgh pneumonia agent: new clinical perspective with a review of the literature, *Medicine* 62:120, 1983.

Nash TW, Libby DM, Horwitz MA: IFN-gamma-activated human alveolar macrophages inhibit the intracellular multiplication of *Legionella pneumophila, J Immunol* 140:3978, 1988.

Plouffe JF, File TM Jr, Breiman RF et al: Reevaluation of the definition of Legionnaires' disease: use of the urinary antigen assay. Community Based Pneumonia Incidence Study Group, *Clin Infect Dis* 20:1286, 1995.

Reinthaler FF, Sattler J, Schaffler-Dullnig K et al: Comparative study of procedures for isolation and cultivation of *Legionella pneumophila* from tap water in hospitals, *J Clin Microbiol* 31:1213, 1993.

Winn WC Jr: Legionnaires' disease: historical perspective, *Clin Microbiol Rev* 1:60, 1988.

Winn WC Jr, Myerowitz RL: The pathology of the *Legionella pneumonias:* a review of 74 cases and the literature, *Hum Pathol* 12:401, 1981.

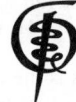

CHAPTER

273 Tuberculosis and Nontuberculous Mycobacterial Infections

Julie R. Brahmer and Peter M. Small

Three major categories of mycobacterial pathogens affect humans: the tuberculosis complex *(Mycobacterium tuberculosis, Mycobacterium bovis, Mycobacterium africanum,* and *Mycobacterium microti),* the nontuberculous mycobacteria, and *Mycobacterium leprae.* These bacteria are members of the family Mycobacteriaceae, order Actinomycetales, and share important characteristics: (1) after staining with certain dyes, they resist decolorization with an acid-alcohol mixture ("acid-fastness"); (2) their rates of growth are relatively slow; (3) they are obligate aerobes; and (4) under usual circumstances, they induce a granulomatous response in tissues of a susceptible host. In spite of these similarities, the organisms differ markedly in their ability to cause human disease and in the types of disease they may produce. Because *M. bovis, M. africanum,* and *M. microti* cause little human disease, they will not be considered. *M. leprae* is discussed in Chapter 275.

BOX 273-1

Classification of mycobacteria that may be human pathogens

Mammalian tubercle bacilli
  M. tuberculosis
  M. bovis (including strain BCG)
  M. africanum
  M. microti
  M. leprae
Nontuberculous mycobacteria
  Slow-growing potential pathogens
  M. avium complex
  M. scrofulaceum
  M. kansasii
  M. ulcerans
  M. marinum
  M. xenopi
  M. szulgai
  M. simiae
  M. hemophilium
  M. genovense
Rapid-growing potential pathogens
  M. fortuitum
  M. chelonei

Modified from Wolinsky E: Nontuberculous mycobacteria and associated disease, *Am Rev Respir Dis* 119:107, 1979.

TUBERCULOSIS

Characteristics of *M. tuberculosis*

M. tuberculosis is an acid-fast rod that typically is beaded or unevenly stained, is somewhat curved, and is approximately 0.3 to 0.6 μm in width and 1 to 4 μm in length. The acid-fast property is produced primarily by the lipid constituents of the mycobacterial cell wall and is usually demonstrated by the Ziehl-Neelsen staining procedure or a modification of this technique. The cell wall also has an affinity for the fluorescent dye, auramine O. Stains incorporating this reagent are used routinely by many laboratories. In Gram-stained preparations, *M. tuberculosis* may appear as gram-positive, although the staining is usually weak and varied. These staining characteristics are shared by all mycobacteria; thus no distinction can be made among *M. tuberculosis,* the nontuberculous mycobacteria, and *M. leprae* on a stained specimen. In addition, some *Nocardia* and *Actinomyces* species may be weakly acid-fast, and on rare occasions, be confused with mycobacteria.

Cultivation of the organism with examination of colonial appearance and determination of biochemical characteristics allows separation of *M. tuberculosis* from nontuberculous mycobacteria. The major categories of mycobacteria that may be pathogenic for humans are shown in Box 273-1. Mycobacteria typically are slow growing. Under optimal conditions, laboratory strains of *M. tuberculosis* undergo one replication in approximately 18 hours; this compares with 20 to 60 minutes for most other bacteria. Colonies are visible on agar-based (Middlebrook 7H10) media by 2 weeks, and on egg-based media (Löwenstein-Jensen) by 3 weeks. Rarely do colonies appear after 6 weeks of incubation. By using a liquid culture medium such as Middlebrook 7H11 and a radiometric detection system, mycobacterial growth can be detected in as short a time as 7 to 10 days.

Colonies of *M. tuberculosis* are buff colored and rough surfaced. Exposure to light causes no change in their pigmentation. The lack of pigment production and the rate of growth enable *M. tuberculosis* to be distinguished from most nontuberculous mycobacteria. The niacin test, a procedure in which niacin production by the organism is measured, usually enables distinction between *M. tuberculosis* and the nonpigmented, slow-growing mycobacteria, particularly *M. avium* complex, with *M. tuberculosis* nearly always showing a positive result. The finding of a strongly positive nitrate reduction test confirms

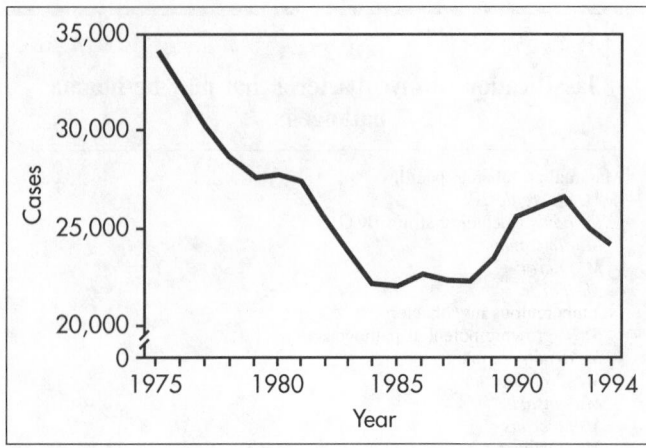

FIGURE 273-1   Numbers and rates of new cases of tuberculosis annually in the United States 1980 to 1991.
Courtesy MMWR.

the identification in the occasional niacin test–negative isolate of *M. tuberculosis.*

Epidemiology

Among infectious diseases, tuberculosis is the leading cause of death worldwide. The World Health Organization (WHO) estimates that approximately one third of the world's population is infected with *M. tuberculosis,* resulting in 8 million new cases of tuberculosis each year. The 2.9 million annual deaths from tuberculosis account for 6.7% of all deaths in developing countries and 26% of avoidable adult deaths. Furthermore, these numbers seem to be increasing because of the HIV pandemic.

Several lines of evidence demonstrate a significant increase in tuberculosis transmission over the past decade in many developed countries. In the United States, after decades of steady declines in the annual incidence of new cases of tuberculosis, the number of cases began increasing in 1985, and between then and 1991 the number of cases increased 18% nationwide, before resuming a downward trend (Fig. 273-1). In addition to this transient increase in the number of cases, this epoch of transmission has created a vast reservoir of latently infected individuals. Many of these individuals will likely progress to active tuberculosis for decades to come. The increase in cases was noted mainly within groups and in geographic areas where infection with human immunodeficiency virus (HIV) is prevalent, suggesting that a large proportion of these "excess cases" are occurring in individuals infected with HIV. However, other social factors such as homelessness, illicit drug use, and deteriorating public health infrastructure have also contributed significantly to the increase. Although composite data from the United States show low tuberculosis case rates, rates are high among specific groups. Case rates are particularly high among recent immigrants to the United States from countries having a high prevalence of tuberculosis, inner-city dwellers, men, and minority populations.

During this resurgence, tuberculosis caused by organisms resistant to antimicrobial agents also increased dramatically. This has been particularly marked in certain urban areas, such as New York City, where, in 1991, one third of all cases were resistant to at least one agent. The 1995 U.S. rates of resistance decreased from 1994. Of cases reported, the isoniazid-rifampin resistance rate is 1.4%.

A sensitive indicator of the seriousness of tuberculosis in a population is the age-specific prevalence of tuberculous infection as measured by tuberculin reactivity. According to the World Health Organization, in much of Asia and Africa 40% to 80% of children are infected by the age of 14 years. By comparing the age-specific infection prevalence during different periods, the effectiveness of tuberculosis control measures can be assessed precisely. For example, infection prevalence data clearly demonstrate the effectiveness of control measures in sharply reducing the amount of infectious tubercu-

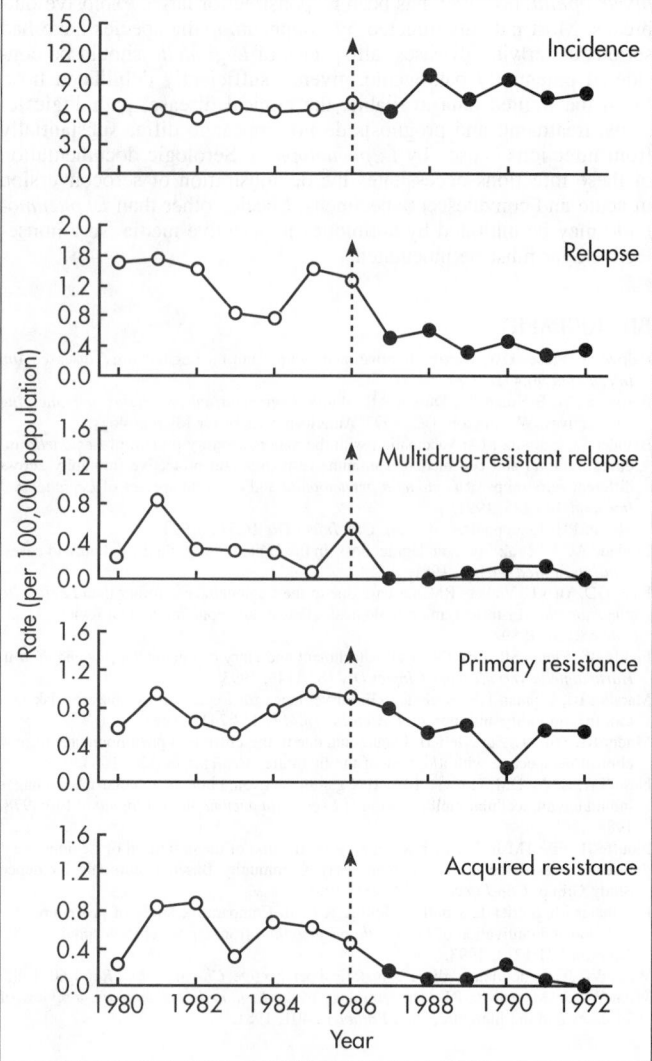

FIGURE 273-2   Incidence of *M. tuberculosis* infection and rates of relapse, relapse with multidrug-resistant tuberculosis (multidrug-resistant relapse), primary resistance, and acquired resistance from Tarrant County, Texas, from 1980 through 1992.
From *N Engl J Med* 330:1179-1184, 1994.

losis present in an area of Alaska; corresponding case rates (all ages combined) dropped from 1854 per 100,000 in 1950 to 141 per 100,000 in 1970.

One lesson learned from the resurgence of tuberculosis is the importance of a sustained commitment to basic tuberculosis control strategies and of ensuring that patients take their medication. The Centers for Disease Control and Prevention (CDC) now recommends that health care providers observe all tuberculosis patients taking their medication. The decrease in resistance rates is most likely due to induction of directly observed therapy, as seen in Texas in 1980 (Fig. 273-2). Data from China demonstrate that similar decreases can be achieved in developing countries.

Transmission of Tuberculous Infection.   The transmission of the tubercle bacillus from a communicable source to a potential new host nearly always takes place through the air. This route of transmission accounts for many epidemiologic features of the disease and is influenced by factors relating to the source of infection, the environment through which the infectious particle must travel, and the potential new host.

The vehicle for transmission of the tubercle bacillus is the droplet nucleus. Any exhalation of air from the lungs also expels water droplets. Once the droplet is outside the mouth, its water content quickly evaporates, leaving a solid nucleus. In persons whose respiratory secretions contain tubercle bacilli, the organism may be a part of this nucleus. Thus the determinants of droplet formation and expulsion in the respiratory tract greatly influence the potential for transmission of the organism. Coughing is the most efficient means of generating droplet nuclei; therefore the more symptomatic the person with pulmonary tuberculosis, the greater the infectious potential. Droplets are also generated by vocalization, sneezing, and normal breathing. The volume and viscosity of the pulmonary secretions also influence droplet formation, with a greater number of droplets being formed from thinner, more voluminous secretions.

The infectious potential of a given person also varies with the numbers of organisms that have access to the airway and are subject to aerosolization. The numbers of organisms being excreted can be quantified roughly by examination of an acid-fast stained sputum smear. Persons with organisms visible on a smear are shedding more bacilli than persons who have a negative smear and a positive culture. Persons with negative smears but positive cultures have a larger number of organisms than do those whose bacteriologic evaluation (smear and culture) does not demonstrate bacilli.

The radiographic severity of pulmonary tuberculosis correlates with both the number of organisms in the lung and the degree of infectivity. Cavitary lesions usually contain large numbers of organisms and, thus, usually are associated with positive sputum smears and high infectivity. At the other end of the spectrum, negative sputum smears and cultures occur quite commonly with solitary nodular lesions in the lung.

Extrapulmonary tuberculosis is generally not infectious; transmission of *M. tuberculosis* occurs only under unusual circumstances from extrapulmonary sites.

Effective antituberculosis drug therapy promptly reduces infectiousness, although patients may continue to have positive sputum smears and cultures. This phenomenon was noted initially in animal studies and subsequently has been confirmed in several clinical studies.

Environmental factors also exert considerable influence on transmissibility. The concentration of organisms in the air is determined not only by the number of organisms being expelled but also by the volume of the air into which the bacilli are dispersed. Thus exposures occurring in small, closed spaces are more likely to result in transmission than are those that take place in more open areas. Aerial transport of infectious particles is also dependent on particle size. Droplets produced from heavy, viscous, mucus-containing debris and clumps of bacilli settle out of the air quite rapidly; however, particles of 1 to 5 μm in diameter have little settling tendency and disperse throughout the air into which they are expelled. The majority of organisms do not survive more than a few minutes beyond the time of their expulsion, even though the particle remains suspended. Viability of the organisms is greatly reduced by exposure to ultraviolet light, either from the sun or from artificial sources. Ultraviolet lights that are correctly installed and maintained can effectively sterilize large volumes of air.

Removal of droplet nuclei from a closed environment by venting air to the outside likewise greatly reduces the concentration of organisms in a given volume of air. Present hospital isolation standards specify a minimum of six air changes per hour and no cross-circulation or recirculation of potentially contaminated air. Filters capable of screening out particles the size of droplet nuclei may be employed in air-cleaning systems, but are impractical for large-volume uses. A time-honored, though unproven, application of air filtration to decrease transmission is the use of masks. Although most masks are constructed from materials capable of excluding 1- to 5-μm particles, their loose fit permits the entrainment of unfiltered air between the mask and face. This problem may be reduced with well-fitted, disposable particulate respirators, but their long-term acceptability to patients or to persons in the patients' environment is limited.

There are also factors intrinsic to the potential recipient that influence his or her likelihood of acquiring a new tuberculous infection. The numbers of bacilli possibly inhaled by contact with a communicable source are determined by the duration of exposure and by the concentration of organisms in the air. Because tuberculous infection results in a specific cell-mediated immune response, further ex-

posures to the tubercle bacillus are far less likely to cause new infections. Thus tuberculin-positive persons are at lower risk of acquiring a new tuberculous infection than are tuberculin-negative persons. There have been, however, documented instances of exogenous reinfection of a previously infected person.

In immunocompromised persons, such as those with HIV infection, the protection afforded by prior infection with *M. tuberculosis* may not be sufficient to prevent a new infection, and reinfection may be more likely in this group.

Artificial infection by vaccination with bacille Calmette-Güerin (BCG) stimulates host defenses, although less specifically, and also reduces the proliferation of implanted organisms.

The transmission of tuberculosis can be minimized by adherence to basic principles. These include measures to promptly detect and treat persons with active tuberculosis and reduce microbial contamination of indoor air. Active surveillance for tuberculosis transmission is also needed. Compliance with these measures is particularly important in settings where tuberculosis is likely to be caused by organisms resistant to antimicrobial agents.

Pathogenesis

The fate of inhaled tubercle bacilli depends on a large number of factors, including the size of the inhaled particle (Chapter 229). Large droplets that are inhaled encounter a series of barriers in the nasal cavity and nasopharynx. Most particles larger than 8 to 10 μm in diameter are trapped in the upper airway. Particles between 5 and 10 μm enter the conducting airways, land on the mucociliary blanket that extends to the level of the terminal bronchiole, and are swept into the oropharynx. A substantial number of particles smaller than 5 μm in diameter penetrate beyond the ciliated epithelium and thus are retained in the lung.

Once in the alveolus, the tubercle bacillus encounters the second line of defense, the alveolar macrophage. Tubercle bacilli are chemotactic and attract macrophages, which ingest them. However, before the development of specific cellular immunity, the macrophage has only limited ability to kill the organism, and the bacillus proliferates within the cell. Depending on the number of infectious organisms inhaled and their rate of multiplication, an inflammatory response is generated in the area of implantation. At the same time, systemic hematogenous dissemination of the organisms occurs. The bacillemia usually does not cause symptoms but results in the seeding of other portions of the lungs and other organs with tubercle bacilli. Sufficient proliferation of organisms in either pulmonary or extrapulmonary sites may cause a clinically evident illness at this time. Immunosuppressed persons such as those with HIV infection are much more likely to develop tuberculosis soon after infection has occurred. In the vast majority of instances, however, the multiplication of organisms is held in check by nonspecific mechanisms until cellular immunity develops, usually 30 to 50 days after implantation. This is marked by the appearance of cutaneous reactivity to tuberculin. With the development of cellular immunity, sensitized T-lymphocytes produce and release lymphokines on exposure to the antigens of the tubercle bacillus. These lymphokines attract and activate macrophages, which in turn become much more potent in killing the organism. This specific defense mechanism is usually successful in halting the proliferation of organisms and in greatly reducing the numbers of, but not eliminating, viable bacilli.

It is estimated that in general, 3% to 5% of persons who acquire tuberculous infections develop clinically evident disease within 1 year after infection has taken place. In the remaining 95% to 97% of infected persons, the tuberculous infection is indicated only by a positive tuberculin skin test. Of this group of infected persons, approximately 5% develop clinically evident tuberculosis during their lifetimes. This risk varies considerably within the group, however. For example, tuberculin-positive persons who are also infected with HIV develop tuberculosis at a rate of 7% per year.

The factors responsible for endogenous reactivation of dormant tuberculous foci are largely unknown. Although it is possible to identify conditions that depress delayed hypersensitivity in most instances, these conditions are not evident in persons who develop tuberculosis. Thus it is nearly impossible to predict who among the estimated 15 million infected persons in the United States will develop tuberculosis.

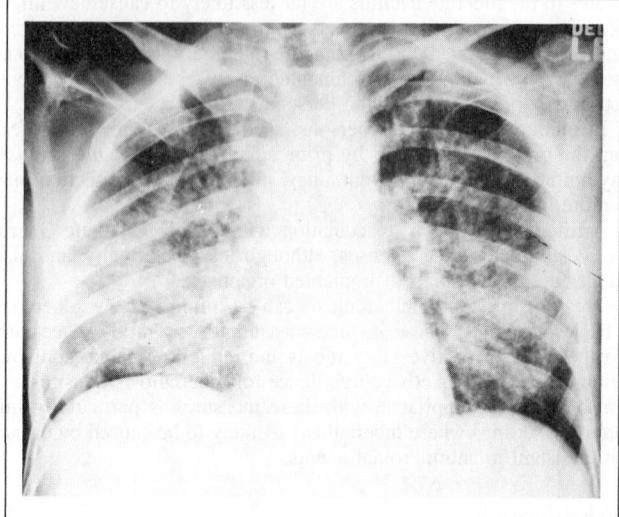

FIGURE 273-3   Chest radiograph showing diffuse pulmonary infiltration caused by tuberculosis in a 38-year-old alcoholic man. In this patient, the process was rapidly progressive and caused severe respiratory failure, disseminated intravascular coagulation, and death.

Clinical Spectrum

The clinical manifestations of tuberculosis span a broad range, from a subtle, indolent process that is only fortuitously detected to an explosive, life-threatening or fatal illness. The symptoms produced may be both systemic and local. The systemic manifestations are generally those of an infectious process, are often chronic, and include fever, weight loss, and fatigue. More specific symptoms are related to the location of the process.

While pulmonary disease accounts for the majority of cases of tuberculosis, extrapulmonary involvement (including lymphatic, pleural, genitourinary, bone, miliary, meningeal, and peritoneal tuberculosis) is increasingly common, particularly in individuals infected with HIV (Chapter 248).

Pulmonary Tuberculosis

Clinical Features.   The majority of newly discovered cases of tuberculosis involve the lungs. Thus, strictly from a numerical standpoint, pulmonary tuberculosis is the most important form of the disease. Moreover, because tuberculosis is an airborne infection, pulmonary lesions are nearly the only source of new infections.

Cough is the most common nonsystemic symptom of pulmonary tuberculosis. Although the cough may be nonproductive early in the process, as the lesions become more extensive and involve airways more directly, sputum is produced. Hemoptysis of significant amounts is generally uncommon as an early symptom but may occur when there is necrosis of lung parenchyma. Hemoptysis may also result from residual bronchiectasis or cavities from previous tuberculous disease (with or without mycetoma formation), and less commonly from calcified hilar lymph nodes eroding into the airway (broncholithiasis). Pleuritic chest pain may result from subpleural parenchymal inflammation with contiguous pleural membrane involvement or from tuberculous pleuritis without pulmonary parenchymal disease.

Abnormalities of respiratory function that are sufficiently severe to cause dyspnea are not common in tuberculosis. It should be emphasized, however, that extensive pulmonary tuberculosis may be the cause of acute respiratory failure that is occasionally accompanied by hypotension and disseminated intravascular coagulation (Fig. 273-3).

Laboratory Studies.   Patients with pulmonary tuberculosis may have abnormalities in routine laboratory studies, but these are not specific. Anemia is common in association with pulmonary tuberculosis but generally is caused by factors other than the lung infection itself. The syndrome of inappropriate secretion of antidiuretic hormone

(SIADH) may account for the hyponatremia seen in some patients with pulmonary tuberculosis. Hyponatremia that does not promptly respond to water restriction should be evaluated further with tests of adrenal function.

Radiographic Findings.   Pulmonary tuberculosis nearly always produces an abnormality on the chest radiograph. Rarely, an endobronchial lesion may be present without radiographically evident parenchymal involvement. In this situation and in recently infected persons, tubercle bacilli may be present in the sputum, but no detectable abnormalities will be present on the chest film.

The typical radiographic pattern of pulmonary tuberculosis in adults is that of an upper lobe process that may be accompanied by cavitation. Most commonly, the site of involvement is the apical or posterior portions of the upper lobes (Fig. 273-4). From these sites, infected material may spread within the airways to involve any other portion of the lungs and may cause pneumonic or cavitary lesions. Adults or children who have been infected recently and in whom clinically evident primary tuberculosis develops (Fig. 273-5) often have a lower lobe pneumonic process that nearly always in children and occasionally in adults is accompanied by hilar adenopathy. Atypical presentations occur commonly in patients with associated diseases that may alter host responsiveness. This has been noted especially in patients who have HIV infection. In these patients, tuberculosis is less likely to cause upper lobe cavitary lesions and more likely to have associated hilar or mediastinal adenopathy.

Spontaneous or drug-induced healing of tuberculous lesions generally leaves fibrotic or fibrocalcific residuals that are often associated with contraction of the involved area. Cavities also may persist after the active process has resolved. Changes in the appearance of these stable residual lesions may result from recurrence of the tuberculous process, superimposed bacterial infection, hemorrhage from old cavities or ectatic airways, or mycetoma formation in a preexisting cavity. In addition, there seems to be an increased frequency of carcinoma arising from scarred areas within the lung; thus new infiltrates or mass lesions should be evaluated with this in mind.

Bacteriologic Evaluation.   Confirmation of the diagnosis of pulmonary tuberculosis rests with the demonstration of *M. tuberculosis* by culture of pulmonary secretions or tissue. However, strong clinical evidence may be sufficient for a presumptive diagnosis, and in combination with the finding of acid-fast bacilli on a stained smear of sputum is highly predictive of tuberculosis. Nonetheless, confirmation by culture is essential because of the identical clinical picture that may be caused by nontuberculous mycobacteria and the lack of features on the smear that allow *M. tuberculosis* to be distinguished from nontuberculous mycobacteria.

The best source of material for bacteriologic evaluation is spontaneously expectorated sputum. The rate of positivity is usually greater and contamination with other bacteria is usually less when specimens are collected during a 1- to 2-hour period after the patient arises (as opposed to a 24-hour collection). Bacilli are likely to be seen on the smear when there are more than 10,000 organisms per milliliter of sputum. False-negative smears are caused by intermittent shedding of organisms or by errors in preparation or examination of the specimen. For this reason, multiple specimens should be collected. The optimum number of specimens for the organism to be isolated appears to be a minimum of three and a maximum of six; collecting more specimens does not increase the yield. False-positive smears may be produced by nontuberculous mycobacteria, although the capability of certain of these organisms to cause disease cannot be dismissed. Smears stained with the fluorescent auramine or rhodamine dyes are more likely to be false-positive because of staining artifacts and because of staining of nonviable bacilli. Positive fluorescent-stained smears therefore should be restained using the Ziehl-Neelsen technique or a related method. Because of the slow growth rate of *M. tuberculosis,* identification of the organism in culture using conventional methodologies may require up to 6 weeks. Sensitive radiometric techniques, which detect the liberation of radiolabeled byproducts of growing bacteria, can currently be combined with species-specific DNA probes to provide results within 10 to 14 days. The time required to detect and identify mycobacteria may soon be reduced to a few days using highly sensitive polymerase chain reaction

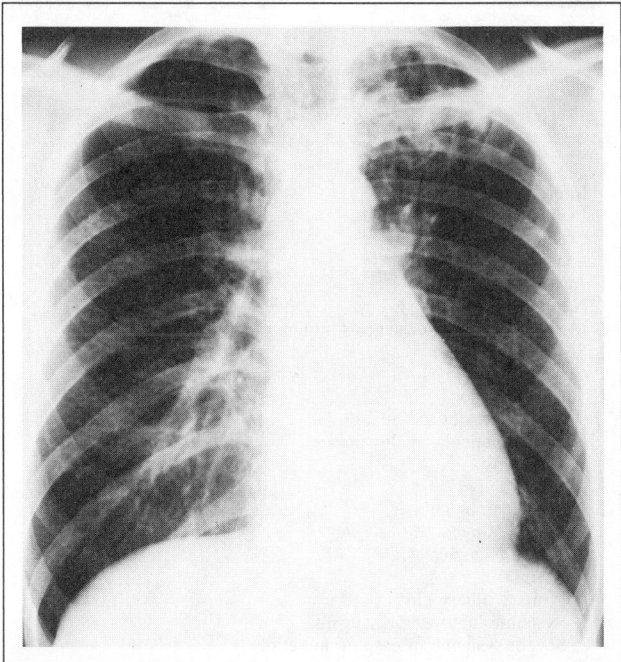

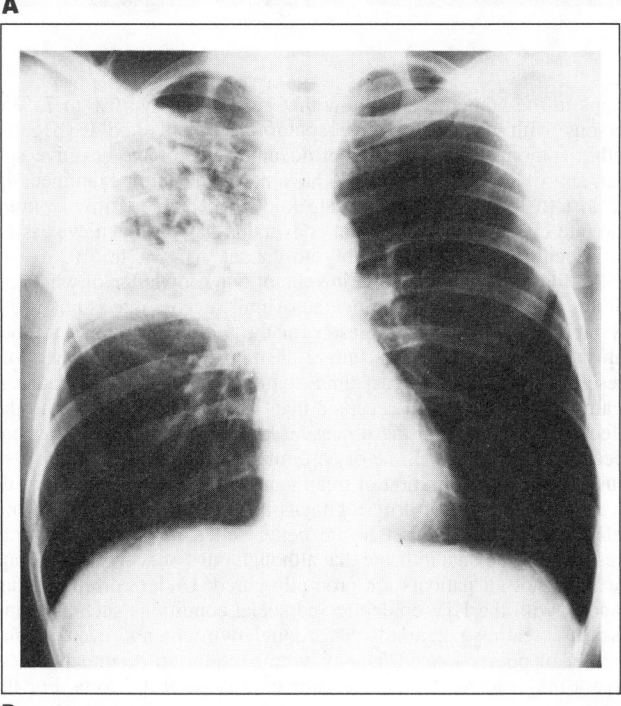

A

B

FIGURE 273-4 Typical chest radiographs showing pulmonary tuberculosis. **A,** Cavitary lesion with adjacent infiltration in the apical posterior segment of the left upper lobe. **B,** Extensive destruction with cavitation involving all segments of the right upper lobe.

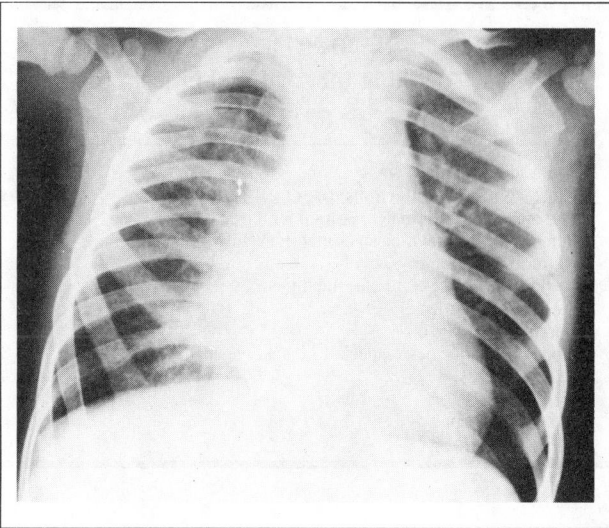

FIGURE 273-5 Chest radiograph of a 1-year-old child with primary tuberculosis. There is infiltration in the right middle lobe with associated loss of lung volume and enlargement of the right hilum.

(PCR) DNA amplification–based assays. The time required to detect and identify mycobacteria can be greatly diminished in smear-positive pulmonary cases by using recently introduced nucleic acid–based techniques. However, the performance characteristics of these assays in smear-negative and nonpulmonary cases remains to be determined, and they should be interpreted with caution in such patients.

There are several means of obtaining pulmonary secretions from persons who are not producing sputum. Sputum production may be induced by inhalation of hypertonic saline. Because these specimens look like saliva, they should be properly labeled so that they will not be discarded by the laboratory. Gastric lavage with saline also yields pulmonary secretions for examination. To be worthwhile this must be done early in the morning, before the patient has arisen. Once collected, the specimen should be processed promptly. The yield is less with gastric lavage than with induced sputum. Material also may be obtained by bronchoscopy with bronchial washing, bronchoalveolar lavage, and transbronchial biopsy.

Usually, patients who are severely ill with pulmonary tuberculosis have organisms present in their sputum smears, and therapy therefore can be started promptly. In patients who present more difficult diagnostic problems, therapy may be withheld until several specimens have been collected for bacteriologic evaluation. However, therapy usually does not reduce the isolation rate in the first several days of treatment.

Tuberculin Skin Testing. The only indication of tuberculous infection in persons who do not have tuberculosis is a positive cutaneous reaction to the tuberculin skin test. In immunologically competent persons, a positive tuberculin test can be elicited 2 to 10 weeks (average, 40 days) after infection occurs. Tuberculin purified protein derivative (PPD), is a protein precipitate obtained from filtrates of heat-sterilized cultures of tubercle bacilli. PPD is available on multiple-puncture devices and in solution for intradermal injection (Mantoux method). The activity of this material is measured in tuberculin units (TU) and is determined by comparison with a standard batch of PPD. Although multiple-puncture methods often are used for testing children, the Mantoux method, which uses 5 TU of PPD ("intermediate" strength), is the best way to identify tuberculous infection. Test strengths of PPD containing 1 TU per 0.1 ml ("first" test strength) and 250 TU per 0.1 ml ("second" test strength) are available but have no demonstrable usefulness in ordinary practice. The tuberculin test is administered by using a 26- or 27-gauge needle to inject 0.1 ml PPD into the skin on the volar surface of the forearm (although other sites may be used). The result is determined by measuring the diameter of induration 48 to 72 hours after injection. Most positive reactions remain positive for up to 7 days, however. Box 273-2 lists the American Thoracic Society/CDC classification for tuberculin skin test interpretations. Under most clinical circumstances, a reaction of 10 mm or more in diameter to a 5-TU test is considered indicative of tuberculosis infection. However, 5 mm is considered positive in certain high-risk individuals, such as foreign-born persons, or those likely to have suppressed immunity, such as persons infected with HIV. Because of the marked propensity of individuals infected with HIV who are exposed to tuberculosis to progress rapidly to active tuberculosis, it is important to know the HIV status of contacts to infectious cases and to begin isoniazid (INH) prophylaxis imme-

BOX 273-2
Criteria for defining tuberculin skin test reactions as positive

>5 mm induration
  Close contacts to infectious cases
  Persons with abnormal chest radiograph
  Persons with known or suspected HIV infection
>10 mm induration
  Residents of long-term care facilities
  Parenteral drug users
  Foreign-born persons
  High-risk minorities (especially blacks, Hispanics, and Native Americans)
>15 mm induration
  All other persons

BOX 273-3
Factors associated with false-negative tuberculin tests

Technical errors
  Improper administration
  Inaccurate reading
  Loss of potency of antigen
Patient-related factors
  Age
  Nutritional status
  Medications—corticosteroids, immunosuppressive agents
  Severe tuberculosis
  Coexisting diseases
    HIV infection
    Viral illness or vaccination
    Lymphoreticular malignancies
    Sarcoidosis
    Solid tumors
    Lepromatous leprosy
    Sjögren's syndrome
    Ataxia telangiectasia
    Uremia
    Primary biliary cirrhosis
    Systemic lupus erythematosus
    Severe systemic disease of any etiology

diately in HIV-seropositive contacts who have had significant exposure.

False-positive reactions may result from infections with nontuberculous mycobacteria, causing a lower grade tuberculin sensitization that usually produces reactions smaller than 10 mm. Vaccination with BCG also causes a reaction to the tuberculin test, although the history of prior vaccination should be ignored when interpreting skin test results in patients with a high likelihood of being infected with *M. tuberculosis.*

In persons who were infected some years in the past, tuberculin reactivity may diminish, causing the tuberculin test to become negative. However, the test itself may recall the sensitization and thus produce a subsequent positive test. This "boosted" reaction might be interpreted as the result of a tuberculous infection that took place between the two tests, when in fact the infection predated the first tuberculin test. This misinterpretation can be avoided if a so-called two-step test is performed. This approach is necessary only in persons who are likely to be retested at regular intervals, for example, hospital employees. In the two-step tuberculin test, the test is applied in the usual fashion but is read 7 days rather than the usual 2 to 3 days later. If the test is negative, a second test is applied at that time and is read in 2 or 3 days. A positive response to the second test would be the result of boosting, not of a new infection, and would reflect accurately the person's previous infection.

When the tuberculin test is used in the evaluation of patients suspected of having tuberculosis, the major concern is not with false-positive but with false-negative results. The possible causes of a false-negative tuberculin test are listed in Box 273-3.

The determination of true versus false negativity may be aided by administering, at the time of the second test, a battery of antigens to which most persons react. These include antigens made from mumps virus, *Candida,* tetanus toxoid, streptokinase streptodornase, and, depending on geographic considerations, *Histoplasma capsulatum* or *Coccidioides immitis.* Detectable induration in response to any of these antigens indicates that cellular immune mechanisms are intact and, thus, that the tuberculin test is probably truly negative; however, selective tuberculin anergy may occur. If there is no reaction to any of these antigens, the tuberculin test cannot be interpreted as either truly or falsely negative.

Chemotherapy

The development and application of specific antituberculosis chemotherapy in the late 1940s and early 1950s revolutionized the care of patients with tuberculosis. In theory, the initial treatment of tuberculosis should now be nearly uniformly successful. Under study conditions, it has been shown that cultures remain positive in 50% of patients at 1 month, in 15% at 2 months, and in less than 10% at 3 months. In practice, however, this is not the case. Success of therapy may be measured by the rates of sputum conversion and relapse after conversion. Data compiled by the CDC from tuberculosis control pro-

grams in the United States show that approximately 70% to 75% of persons with initially positive sputum had converted to negative within 6 months. Of patients not documented to have negative sputum, approximately 15% to 20% have not had sputum examined, 4% are lost to follow-up, and 4% are known to have positive sputum. The rate of relapse after sputum conversion has been achieved is not well documented but is probably no greater than 3% to 5%.

All these data indicate that in spite of our knowledge of what constitutes adequate chemotherapy, the overall success rate is not 100%. By far the most important reason for the failure of initial antituberculosis chemotherapy is the failure of the patient to comply with the prescribed regimen. At least three features of tuberculosis cause its treatment to be less well accepted than is usually the case with other infectious diseases: (1) the process is an indolent one and may produce few symptoms; (2) the disease must be treated with at least two drugs; and (3) the duration of treatment is lengthy. Thus much of the recent investigation of drug regimens has been directed toward providing treatment options that are better suited to patients' different lifestyles. These data indicate that although rates of successful therapy are high, not all patients are promptly cured. Under current circumstances, with the HIV epidemic and social conditions such as homelessness creating potentially hazardous environments, even a small number of poorly treated patients who continue to be infectious can have a major adverse effect on tuberculosis control efforts. For this reason, it is especially important that the details of therapy be carefully managed. In many instances directly observed therapy in which every dose of the drug is administered under direct supervision is necessary to ensure effectiveness.

The necessity for two drugs at least, and for lengthy treatment, reflects the microbiologic characteristics of the tubercle bacillus. First, in every group of tubercle bacilli there are naturally occurring drug-resistant mutants. Thus to kill all the organisms, more than one drug must always be used. Second, because the multiplication time for tubercle bacilli is 18 to 24 hours and because the organisms may have periods of dormancy interspersed with spurts of growth, it is necessary that drugs be administered for long periods.

Concurrent administration of agents with different antimicrobial mechanisms is also beneficial because bacilli reside in a variety of different microenvironments, such as within macrophages, where different antimicrobials have variable effects. These factors combine to make treatment a much more difficult and tiresome process for the patient. Fortunately, with the advent of rifampin, the total duration of

Table 273-1   Drugs used in the treatment of mycobacterial disease

| ANTITUBERCULOSIS DRUGS | ADULT DOSAGE | | MOST COMMON SIDE-EFFECTS | TESTS FOR SIDE-EFFECTS |
	DAILY	TWICE WEEKLY		
Primary				
Isoniazid	5-10 mg/kg, up to 300 mg PO or IM	15 mg/kg PO or IM	Peripheral neuritis, hepatitis, hypersensitivity	AST-ALT
Ethambutol	15-25 mg/kg PO	50 mg/kg PO	Optic neuritis (reversible with discontinuation of drug: very rare at 15 mg/kg), skin rash	Red-green color discrimination and visual acuity*
Rifampin	10-15 mg/kg, up to 600 mg PO	600 mg PO	Hepatitis, febrile reaction, purpura (rare), drug interactions	AST-ALT
Streptomycin	15 mg/kg, up to 1 g IM	15-25 mg/kg IM	Eighth nerve damage (vestibular), nephrotoxicity	Vestibular function, audiograms,* BUN, and creatinine
Pyrazinamide	25 mg/kg, up to 2 g PO		Hyperuricemia, hepatotoxicity	Uric acid, AST-ALT
Secondary				
Capreomycin	12-15 mg/kg, up to 1 g IM		Eighth nerve damage (auditory), nephrotoxicity, vestibular toxicity (rare)	Vestibular function, audiograms,* BUN, and creatinine
Kanamycin	12-15 mg/kg, up to 1 g IM		Eighth nerve damage (auditory), nephrotoxicity, vestibular toxicity (rare)	Vestibular function, audiograms,* BUN, and creatinine
Amikacin	15 mg/kg		Auditory, vestibulary, renal	Same as other aminoglycosides
Ethionamide	15 mg/kg, up to 1 g PO		GI disturbance, hepatotoxicity, hypersensitivity	AST-ALT
p-Aminosalicylic acid (aminosalicylic acid)	150 mg/kg, up to 12 g PO		GI disturbance, hypersensitivity, hepatotoxicity, sodium load	AST-ALT
Cycloserine	15 mg/kg, up to 1 g PO		Psychosis, personality changes, convulsions, rash	
Ofloxacin	600 mg		Rash, GI	
Ciprofloxacin	500-700 mg		GI, CNS	

BUN, Blood urea nitrogen; *AST,* serum aspartate aminotransferase; *ALT,* serum alanine aminotransferase.
*Determine at the start of treatment.

therapy necessary for successful treatment has been shortened substantially. In addition, twice-weekly regimens, both with and without rifampin, may be administered under direct observation to ensure that the patient receives the necessary amount of drug.

Antituberculosis Drugs. Currently there are 13 agents available in the United States for the treatment of tuberculosis (Table 273-1). The drugs are divided into two categories, primary and secondary. Agents in the primary group are those used in the initial treatment of tuberculosis. They represent the first choice because of their effectiveness, relatively low toxicity, and relatively low cost. The secondary agents are generally reserved for use in treating disease caused by organisms that are resistant to one or more of the primary drugs or in cases in which hypersensitivity or toxicity is caused by the primary drug. In general, the second-line drugs are less effective, more toxic, and more expensive than the primary agents.

Primary drugs. Isoniazid is the major drug in any initial treatment regimen. It is bactericidal and rapidly decreases the bacillary population in any lesion produced by tubercle bacilli that are susceptible to the drug. For this reason, it is probably the most important means of diminishing or abolishing the infectious potential of the patient with newly diagnosed tuberculosis. Because INH penetrates well into body tissues and fluids, it is equally effective in pulmonary and extrapulmonary disease. The drug is available in parenteral form and, thus, may be used in combination with an aminoglycoside antibiotic, usually streptomycin, in treating patients who cannot take oral medications.

Rifampin is also a potent bactericidal agent and is especially effective in eradicating organisms that grow in spurts. Rifampin is the agent that always should be used in patients who have INH-resistant organisms or have developed documented untoward effects from INH. In addition, as described below, the INH-rifampin combination forms

the core of current treatment regimens. Rifampin penetrates well into body fluids, including cerebrospinal fluid.

Both streptomycin and pyrazinamide are bactericidal under the proper pH conditions (streptomycin, alkaline; pyrazinamide, acid). Streptomycin is probably most effective in its early effect on rapidly proliferating organisms, but it is less effective in this regard than INH. On the other hand, pyrazinamide, because it is most efficient in an acid environment, is thought to inhibit or kill organisms that are contained within macrophages.

Ethambutol is not a particularly potent agent but is effective as a companion to the more potent agents because it diminishes the likelihood of proliferation of drug-resistant strains.

Secondary drugs. The other oral agents, ethionamide, cycloserine, and *p*-aminosalicylic acid, are bacteriostatic and are less efficacious than the first-line agents, and, in addition, are associated with frequent and serious toxic effects that greatly limit their use. The antibiotics kanamycin, capreomycin, and amikacin have properties similar to those of streptomycin; however, they tend to be more toxic (to kidneys and to the auditory component of the eighth cranial nerve) and are more expensive. Fluoroquinolones are another class of promising agents that have minimal toxicities.

Drug Regimens for Initial Treatment. A number of effective regimens can be fashioned using the primary agents described above. The overall goal is to use a regimen that combines optimal effectiveness with the shortest possible duration of administration. It is presumed that shorter durations of treatment foster patient compliance and thus allow resources to be focused on ensuring completion of treatment. Since the early 1950s, when truly effective treatment first became available, the necessary duration of therapy has been reduced from 24 months to 6 months. This reduction was largely

BOX 273-4
Considerations in choosing an antituberculosis drug regimen

History of previous therapy
Probability of primary isoniazid resistance
Assessment of patient compliance
Presence of coexisting diseases
Results of drug susceptibility studies
History of untoward reactions to antituberculosis drugs

brought about through the use of rifampin and, to a lesser extent, pyrazinamide. The regimen most widely used in the United States currently consists of INH, rifampin, pyrazinamide, sometimes supplemented by ethambutol for 2 months, followed by INH and rifampin for 4 months. Regimens shorter than 6 months have had an unacceptably high rate of unfavorable outcome and should not be used. If pyrazinamide is not used, INH and rifampin must be given for at least 9 months.

As discussed later, regimens of 6 to 9 months should be used only when susceptibility to INH and rifampin is proved or is highly likely. When there is resistance to one or both agents, regimens must be modified and given for a minimum of 12 months.

Special Considerations in Choosing a Drug Regimen. The important factors to be taken into account in deciding on an antituberculosis drug regimen are listed in Box 273-4.

History of previous therapy. Persons who have been treated previously with nonrifampin-containing regimens and have had subsequent recurrence of disease have a greater probability of having organisms that are resistant to the drugs they received previously. In a Public Health Service survey of 4017 patients who had received previous antituberculosis therapy and developed a subsequent recurrence of tuberculosis, 41% had organisms that were resistant to INH, streptomycin, or *p*-aminosalicylic acid, either alone or in combination. Previous therapy for tuberculosis in which a single agent, usually INH, was used was associated with a much greater frequency of resistance. In addition, the greater the length of therapy, the greater the likelihood of resistance. Patients who had received INH combined with one or more other agents for 1 to 6 months had a 23% incidence of resistance to INH. This increased to 53% with 1 to 2 years and to 72% with more than 2 years of therapy. Because of the likelihood of drug resistance, patients who have received previous therapy should be treated with at least two drugs that they have not been given in the past, preferably with at least one of the bactericidal agents. When the results of drug susceptibility testing are available, the regimen can be modified if necessary. In patients with INH-resistant organisms, a regimen of rifampin and ethambutol given for 12 months should be effective. If a rifampin-containing regimen was used, then it is likely that the organism will retain susceptibility to both INH and rifampin.

Probability of primary drug resistance. The frequency of resistance to INH occurring in patients who have not had previous INH therapy (i.e., primary resistance) has not appreciably increased in the United States during the past 15 to 20 years and remains low in many areas of the United States. There are, however, specific circumstances in which primary resistance is more common. In many parts of the world, the prevalence of primary INH resistance is much higher than in the United States. Persons likely to have acquired tuberculous infection in Southeast Asia, Korea, the Philippines, Hong Kong, Central America, Mexico, or Africa should have their initial chemotherapeutic regimens selected as if the organisms were resistant to INH. An appropriate regimen would consist of INH, rifampin, pyrazinamide, and ethambutol. Drug susceptibility studies should be obtained and the results used to modify the regimen. The same approach should be taken for patients thought to have acquired tuberculous infection from a person known to be excreting drug-resistant bacilli. Success rates with appropriate therapy for extended periods of time approximate those of tuberculosis that is sensitive to all agents.

Tuberculosis that is caused by organisms resistant to two or more primary agents (multidrug-resistant [MDR]) has become a major problem in areas such as New York City, where 19% of isolates from a 1-month period in mid-1992 were resistant to both INH and rifampin. MDR tuberculosis should be suspected in all patients who may have recently acquired their infections in the urban eastern United States, particularly if they are infected with HIV or have been treated previously for tuberculosis. Empiric therapy should be tailored to match the local drug resistance patterns. Generally regimens should include isoniazid and rifampin unless resistance to these agents is documented. Treatment should be based on in vitro drug susceptibilities of the isolate and should include three agents to which the isolate is sensitive. Even with optimal therapy, including judicious use of surgical resection of involved lung, treatment failure rates approach 50% in immunocompetent patients and are significantly higher in patients infected with HIV.

Patient compliance. The major reason for treatment failure in tuberculosis is failure of the patient to take medications as prescribed. This problem cuts across many demographic variables such as education, social class, occupation, age, and sex, making identification of patients who will be noncompliant a difficult task. For this reason, intensive efforts should be made at the outset of treatment to educate the patient about the disease and its treatment and to monitor compliance closely. If the patient shows a tendency toward noncompliance, he or she should be closely supervised for the duration of the treatment program, or directly observed biweekly therapy should be used.

Coexisting diseases. When possible, drugs having toxicities that may add to the effects of coexisting diseases should not be used. For example, the aminoglycoside antibiotics and capreomycin should be avoided in patients who have significant renal disease and in patients with impaired hearing or vestibular dysfunction. Ethambutol should not be given to patients with significant loss of vision.

An exception to the general rule stated previously is the use of INH and rifampin in patients with liver disease. Because of the central importance of these agents, they should not be considered to be contraindicated in the presence of liver disease. In general, in this situation they do not contribute to the further impairment of liver function. Although in this setting careful monitoring of liver function should be performed, it may be difficult to determine whether changes are caused by the underlying disease or the drugs.

Rifampin is a rather potent inducer of hepatic microsomal enzymes, which may accelerate the metabolism of certain drugs and thus decrease their effectiveness. Such interactions have been documented for oral contraceptives, cyclosporine, dapsone, corticosteroids, warfarin, methadone, oral hypoglycemic agents, and digoxin. The management of disorders for which these drugs are being used may be made more difficult by the use of rifampin but can be compensated for by adjusting their doses.

Drug susceptibility studies. Treatment of tuberculosis caused by organisms that are resistant to antituberculosis agents requires modification in treatment regimens. Therefore the recommendation now is to perform drug susceptibility tests on the initial isolate from all patients, and to repeat these tests if cultures remain positive for more than 3 months. The results of drug sensitivity testing may not be available until 8 to 12 weeks after submission of the specimen; thus initial therapy should be based on the considerations mentioned earlier. Subsequently, however, the results of such susceptibility studies can be used to modify the regimen. Susceptibility studies should be obtained for all previously treated patients and for patients with a high probability of primary drug resistance.

History of drug toxicity or hypersensitivity. If there is a clear history of a toxic reaction or an allergic reaction to a previously administered drug, the drug should be avoided and another agent substituted. It may be necessary to challenge the patient with the suspected drug under close observation to confirm the untoward effect. This is particularly true with INH and rifampin because of their central importance.

Management. Successful drug therapy using a combination of INH and rifampin should eradicate tubercle bacilli from the sputum of patients within 6 months. Patients whose sputum still contains organisms after 3 months of treatment should be carefully reevaluated to determine whether they are taking the drugs as prescribed and whether the organisms are susceptible to the agents being used. If the organisms are not resistant, strong consideration should be given to institution of a directly observed drug regimen. Patients who complete a 6-month regimen should have a follow-up evaluation approximately 6 months after completion of therapy. The relapse rate after therapy is completed is 1% to 2% and nearly all occur during the first 6 months after termination of treatment. Further routine follow-up evaluations are not necessary, but patients should be instructed to have any new respiratory symptoms evaluated promptly. Patients infected with HIV, who have tuberculosis caused by drug-sensitive *M. tuberculosis,* and who comply with therapy respond well to conventional therapy, although they do have a high incidence of adverse drug reactions.

In a patient who is receiving adequate chemotherapy, nonspecific factors such as rest, nutrition, and occupation have no effect on outcome. Activity should be regulated by symptoms, and diet by appetite. Patients whose symptoms allow it may resume working after adequate chemotherapy has been established.

Before the development of effective drug therapy, resectional surgery and collapse procedures were important in the treatment of pulmonary tuberculosis. Currently, however, surgical treatment has a very limited role. Resection may be considered when the tuberculosis is caused by organisms that are resistant to multiple drugs and there is a localized area of involvement. In addition, resection may be necessary because of massive hemoptysis originating either in an area of active tuberculous disease or in residual cavities or bronchiectasis left by previous tuberculosis.

The use of corticosteroid treatment in patients with pulmonary tuberculosis should be reserved for those who have extensive parenchymal infiltration with significant effects on respiratory gas exchange. Corticosteroids, by reducing the inflammatory response, may considerably improve arterial oxygen tension. Doses of 40 to 60 mg of prednisone or the equivalent of other corticosteroid preparations should be used, with the amount given being gradually reduced during a 1-week period before cessation, to decrease the likelihood of a sudden, "rebound" effect. Corticosteroids should not be used if the patient is not on effective chemotherapy.

There are several situations in which a physician may want to refer a patient with tuberculosis to an expert in tuberculosis management. These situations include: patients whose cultures fail to convert to negative by 3 months after the start of treatment, patients who do not respond to therapy, and patients with drug-resistant organisms. Patients who experience complicated drug toxicities secondary to their tuberculosis treatment regimen may also be referred.

Extrapulmonary Tuberculosis

The relative frequency of extrapulmonary tuberculosis was increasing before the HIV epidemic but has gone up considerably in association with HIV. In patients with advanced HIV infection and tuberculosis approximately 60% have extrapulmonary involvement with or without pulmonary disease. Extrapulmonary tuberculosis presents several important problems that differ from those presented by pulmonary disease.

1. Extrapulmonary tuberculosis is often a much more obscure process that is more difficult to diagnose than pulmonary tuberculosis.
2. Bacteriologic confirmation of the tuberculous nature of the process usually requires an invasive procedure.
3. Guidelines for chemotherapy and need for adjunctive measures are not as clear as with pulmonary tuberculosis.
4. Several forms of extrapulmonary tuberculosis may be life-threatening and if cured, may leave significant residual effects (disseminated tuberculosis, meningitis, pericarditis).

Compared with pulmonary tuberculosis, extrapulmonary disease is more common among younger persons, among ethnic groups other than blacks or whites, and among women. As with pulmonary tuberculosis, however, there is a progressive increase in case rates with increasing age. Exceptions to this trend include lymphatic and meningeal tuberculosis, for which the case rates are highest in the 0- to 4-year-old age-group.

The pathogenesis of most forms of extrapulmonary tuberculosis is the same as that of pulmonary tuberculosis. The sites are seeded at the time of initial dissemination, and organisms tend to persist in areas where the environment is favorable, probably where the oxygen tension is relatively high. Subsequently, because of some usually unidentifiable shift in the host-parasite relationship, the organism begins to proliferate, and clinical disease ensues. In some instances, direct invasion from contiguous sites may produce new foci of disease—pleuritis from subadjacent parenchymal involvement, pericarditis from rupture of adjacent lymph nodes. Distant sites may also be involved via spread through tubular structures—bladder, from renal foci; peritoneum, from female genital involvement; or gastrointestinal tract, from swallowed organisms originating in the lungs.

The definitive diagnosis of extrapulmonary tuberculosis depends on isolation of the organism. This is much more difficult than in pulmonary tuberculosis because there often is no ready source of specimens and, in addition, the numbers of organisms in extrapulmonary lesions are generally small. Of the 3850 cases of extrapulmonary tuberculosis reported in 1983, 92% had bacteriologic results, of which 77% (71% of the total) were positive. Ancillary diagnostic studies, for example, body fluid examination and histologic examination of biopsy specimens, provide important clues to the diagnosis of extrapulmonary tuberculosis. The tuberculin skin test has the same diagnostic value for extrapulmonary as for pulmonary disease. As previously stated, a negative tuberculin test does not exclude active tuberculosis. In patients with disseminated tuberculosis, because of the frequent severe systemic effects, the tuberculin test may be negative in as many as 50% of patients.

The basic principles of chemotherapy apply equally to extrapulmonary and pulmonary tuberculosis. Although few carefully designed studies that define optimum drug regimens and duration of treatment have been done, increasing experience has provided good evidence that 6- to 9-month regimens are equally effective in extrapulmonary tuberculosis. Thus the same regimens recommended for initial treatment of pulmonary tuberculosis can be recommended for extrapulmonary forms. In contrast to pulmonary tuberculosis, however, corticosteroid treatment and surgical interventions may play an important role in managing extrapulmonary tuberculosis.

Lymphatic Tuberculosis. The presenting manifestations of lymph node tuberculosis depend, in part, on the location of the involved nodes. By far the most frequent site of involvement is the neck, with mediastinal involvement being second; however, any lymph node in the body may be affected. Typically the process is first noted as a painless enlargement of one or more of a group of nodes. Although initially discrete and firm, they tend to become matted, inflamed, and fluctuant, and subsequently drain spontaneously if they are not treated. Mediastinal nodes may compress airways, causing cough, whereas abdominal adenitis may be associated with abdominal pain. Systemic symptoms are generally absent unless there is other involvement. The differential diagnosis can be extensive, ranging from cat-scratch disease to lymphoma. However, in a young, otherwise healthy patient with a positive tuberculin test, the diagnosis is usually apparent. When there is doubt, excisional biopsy or aspiration may be necessary. Cultures are positive in only 50% to 60% of cases thought to be tuberculous. In children, because of the greater frequency of adenitis caused by nontuberculous mycobacteria, culture of the organism is essential.

Chemotherapy is nearly always successful. However, resolution of the clinical findings is slow, and nodal enlargement and inflammation persist for many months. During the initial months of chemotherapy, the response is considered adequate if the condition does not worsen. Surgery rarely is needed, except to provide diagnostic material. If a fluctuant node appears to be ready to erode through the skin, however, aspiration is indicated. This minimizes the risk of chronic draining of sinus tracts that may result from spontaneous rupture.

Pleural Tuberculosis. Tuberculous pleuritis may present as a subacute or acute process with pleuritic pain and fever. As pleural fluid increases, the pain tends to decrease, and, in the majority of cases, the process resolves spontaneously. This form of pleural involvement is thought to be caused by rupture of an inapparent pulmonary parenchymal focus into the pleural space, with a subsequent hypersensitivity response to the tuberculoprotein of the organisms.

The fluid in a tuberculous effusion is serous and exudative, and typically has a white blood cell count of 1000 to 5000/μl, of which more than 80% are mononuclear cells. Very early in the course, however, the cells may be predominantly polymorphonuclear leukocytes. Only rarely are acid-fast bacilli seen on smears of pleural fluid. Cultures of the fluid yield the organism in approximately 40% to 50% of specimens. Closed-needle biopsy of the pleura, with culture of the biopsy specimen in addition to histologic examination, provides the diagnosis in 75% to 80% of cases. In spite of the relatively low yield of the standard bacteriologic procedures, the diagnosis can be established presumptively in the presence of compatible pleural fluid findings and a positive tuberculin test result. In this setting, even in the absence of bacteriologic confirmation, the patient should be treated for tuberculous pleuritis. Corticosteroids may cause more rapid resolution of the effusion and less residual pleural scarring, but such scarring only rarely presents a problem in any event.

Tuberculous empyema is a much less common form of pleural involvement. This is a more chronic, indolent process that is usually associated with evident pulmonary parenchymal tuberculosis. The empyema is produced by discharge of a large number of organisms into the pleural space, often via a bronchopleural fistula. The fluid produced is thick and frankly purulent and contains easily demonstrable acid-fast bacilli. Antituberculous chemotherapy alone is rarely successful in eradicating the infection, and surgical drainage procedures generally are required. If not drained, the empyema may erode directly through the chest wall (empyema necessitatis).

Genitourinary Tuberculosis.

The symptoms produced by genitourinary tuberculosis depend, in large part, on the specific site of involvement. Typically, urinary symptoms predominate over systemic symptoms, and dysuria, urinary frequency, hematuria, and, occasionally, flank pain are the most frequent complaints. In males with lower urinary tract involvement, epididymitis, orchitis, or prostatitis may be the causes of the initial manifestations. In women, infertility, pelvic pain, and menstrual irregularity may be presenting complaints. Involvement of the reproductive organs without concomitant renal tuberculosis is more common in women than in men. Constitutional symptoms also may occur but are more common when there is extragenitourinary involvement. In view of the indolent nature of tuberculosis, it is not surprising that the diagnosis is made in many cases by evaluating incidental findings such as an abnormal routine urinalysis in asymptomatic patients.

The urinalysis shows abnormalities in the vast majority of patients with genitourinary tuberculosis. The combination of pyuria in an acid urine without detection of pyogenic bacteria in culture is highly suggestive of tuberculosis. The results of urinalysis may be normal, however, in association with isolated genital lesions, especially in women, or when the drainage from a tuberculous kidney is blocked. When there is bladder involvement, pyogenic organisms also may be present and mask the tuberculous nature of the process.

When genitourinary tuberculosis is suspected, at least three first-voided morning urine specimens should be obtained. Smears of urine specimens from men occasionally show saprophytic acid-fast organisms and therefore should be interpreted cautiously. Cultures may be negative under the conditions previously described, with normal urinalysis results. Conversely, in patients with tuberculosis in other sites, especially the lung, urine cultures may grow *M. tuberculosis* in the absence of any evidence of genitourinary involvement. The diagnosis of isolated involvement of reproductive organs may require biopsy of the suspected site and culture of the tissue.

In most series of patients with genitourinary tuberculosis, 50% to 75% have chest radiographs indicative of old or current pulmonary tuberculosis. Other extrapulmonary sites may be involved as well.

Renal tuberculosis originates in the cortex of the kidney. Parenchymal destruction may occur, causing spread into the medulla and associated papillary necrosis or cavitation. The inflammation and scarring also may involve the collecting system and ureters, with subsequent stricture formation and hydronephrosis. Involvement of the bladder can cause marked scarring and contraction. The involved kidney or bladder may become nonfunctional. All these changes may be visualized on an intravenous pyelogram, retrograde pyelogram, or renal arteriogram. Calcified lesions may be seen on plain films and suggest the diagnosis.

As in other forms of tuberculosis, chemotherapy is highly success-

ful in the genitourinary type. Rarely, nephrectomy may be indicated because of intractable pain, chronic pyogenic infection in a nonfunctioning kidney, massive hematuria, or persistent tuberculous disease caused by organisms resistant to multiple drugs. Surgery also may be required to relieve symptomatic obstruction caused by ureteral stricture or to create an ileal bladder when the urinary bladder is nonfunctional. Patients who have evidence of ureteral stricture or extensive renal destruction should have repeat intravenous pyelograms at 4- to 6-month intervals during treatment, and annually for 5 years after completion of therapy. Performance of routine follow-up radiographic evaluation in uncomplicated cases is controversial and probably is unnecessary if there are no symptoms and the results of urinalysis are normal.

Bone and Joint Tuberculosis.

Skeletal tuberculosis most frequently involves the spine or weight-bearing joints, although any bone or joint in the body may be affected (Chapter 203). In most series of patients with skeletal tuberculosis, the spine is involved in 50% to 70%. Multiple lesions also may occur and may be difficult to distinguish from metastatic neoplasm solely by clinical or radiographic criteria. Pain is the usual presenting complaint, although the process is usually more indolent than is septic arthritis or osteomyelitis. Soft tissue swelling may also occur but usually fits the pattern of a "cold abscess" without apparent erythema or tenderness. In most instances, bone involvement occurs together with joint space invasion; thus arthritic symptoms may predominate. Spinal tuberculosis also may be associated with abscess formation in the paraspinous tissues and within the confines of the spinal canal. The latter occurrence can cause nerve root or spinal cord compression, sometimes with severe neurologic sequelae, including paraplegia.

On radiographic examination, skeletal tuberculosis cannot be distinguished with certainty from other chronic infectious processes and, as was noted earlier, it may occasionally mimic metastatic neoplastic lesions. Typically the radiographic picture is one of concurrent lysis and sclerosis of bone, with articular cartilage destruction indicated by narrowing of the joint space. In the spine, this is most commonly seen in the lower thoracic or upper lumbar vertebrae in adults, and in the thoracic vertebrae in children (Fig. 273-6). With progressive bone destruction, the anterior portions of adjacent vertebrae collapse, producing a gibbous deformity. A paraspinous abscess may be seen adjacent to the abnormality in the spine and is usually a spindle-shaped mass on anteroposterior views. Computed tomographic scanning of the spine is a more sensitive means of detecting both bone lesions and paraspinous abscesses than is conventional radiographic examination.

Although a strong presumptive diagnosis of skeletal tuberculosis may be made on the basis of radiographic findings, final diagnosis usually requires a positive tuberculin skin test, evident tuberculosis elsewhere, or biopsy confirmation. Aspiration of joint fluid and needle or open biopsy of bone lesions or synovium usually provide histologic and bacteriologic confirmation of the diagnosis.

The basic principles of chemotherapy for pulmonary tuberculosis apply to skeletal disease. Surgical intervention is usually unnecessary. Surgical decompression and debridement, sometimes accompanied by vertebral fusion, may be essential in spinal tuberculosis that is causing progressive neurologic abnormalities. Other involved joints should be immobilized and prevented from bearing weight.

Disseminated Tuberculosis.

Disseminated (miliary) tuberculosis is a multisystem process producing a complex of usually nonspecific symptoms including fever, anorexia, weight loss, weakness, and fatigue. More specific symptoms occur, depending on the sites of involvement. In children and immunosuppressed patients, disseminated tuberculosis is a direct result of progressive primary infection. In older persons, however, the pathogenesis is that of bloodstream seeding during recrudescence of previously dormant foci, usually within the lungs.

Physical findings are often nonspecific. Fever is documented in 75% to 80% of cases, with pulmonary findings, hepatomegaly, lymphadenopathy, and splenomegaly found in descending order of frequency. Neurologic findings and meningismus may dominate when there is meningeal involvement, and there may be detectable ascites when peritonitis is present. The only specific physical finding consists of tubercles in the choroidal coat of the retina, which are visible

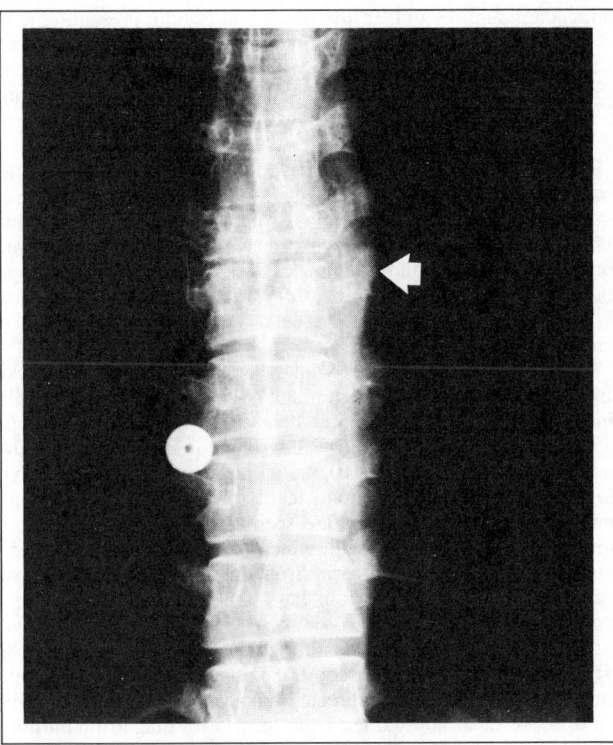

A

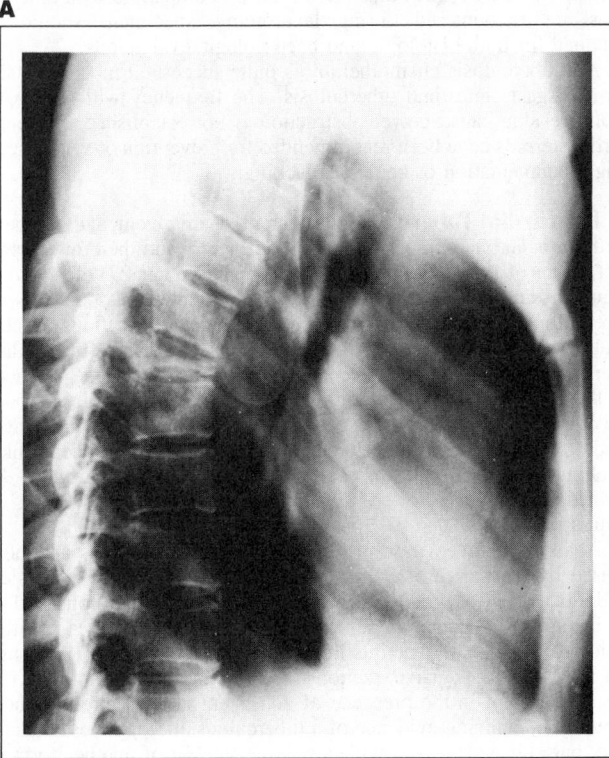

B

FIGURE 273-6   Anteroposterior **(A)** and lateral **(B)** views of the thoracic spine, showing total collapse of the sixth thoracic vertebra, narrowing of the intervertebral space, and early destructive changes in the seventh thoracic vertebra. In addition, there is a rounded density *(arrow)* on either side of the vertebral column at the level of the affected vertebrae, indicating a paraspinous abscess. This patient's complaints were back pain for 1 month and rapidly progressive weakness of the lower extremities.

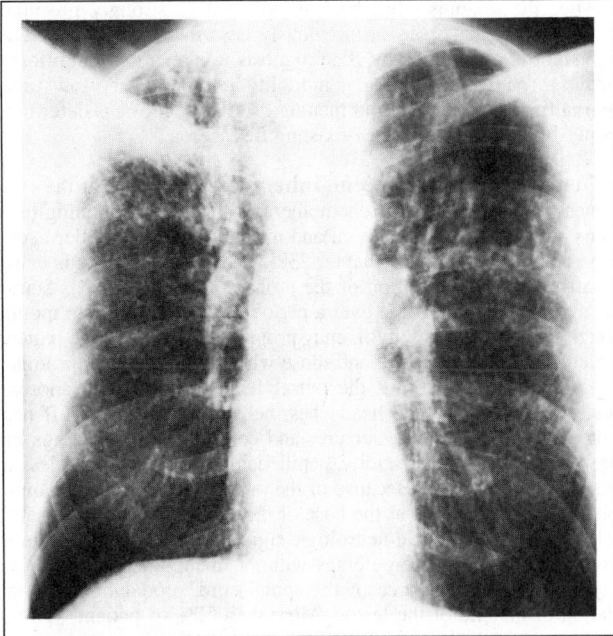

FIGURE 273-7   Chest radiograph showing diffuse pulmonary infiltration in a miliary pattern. There is also a cavitary process in the right upper lobe, from which the hematogenous spread probably occurred.

through an ophthalmoscope. The choroidal tubercles are usually multiple; about one fourth the diameter of the disc; gray, gray-white, or yellow; and most easily detected when the pupil is dilated.

Because of the nonspecific nature of presenting manifestations, disseminated tuberculosis often poses a difficult diagnostic problem. Although usually abnormal, the chest film may show no abnormalities until well after the onset of symptoms. The typical abnormality consists of uniformly distributed small nodular densities (Fig. 237-7). Additional findings suggestive of endogenous reactivation of tuberculosis may also be present, and pleural effusion may be seen.

Presumably because of more severe systemic effects of the disease, the tuberculin skin test is less frequently positive in miliary tuberculosis than in other forms of the disease. Most series report 50% to 55% of patients with an initial positive reaction to 5 TU of PPD.

Because the miliary lesions in the lungs are predominantly interstitial, sputum smears and cultures are less likely to demonstrate tubercle bacilli than in usual pulmonary tuberculosis. Acid-fast stains show organisms in 25% to 30% of patients, and *M. tuberculosis* is isolated in 50% to 70%. When sputum smears are negative, other sources of diagnostic material should be sought. Bronchoscopy with transbronchial biopsy has a high yield and in most instances should be the next step. In addition, joint, pleural, or peritoneal fluid should be aspirated, with subsequent biopsies as indicated; lumbar puncture should be performed if there are neurologic signs or symptoms. Biopsy of liver or bone marrow, with histologic examinations and culture, each has a 30% to 40% positive yield. Unfortunately, biopsies from both of these sources, particularly the liver, may show noncaseating granulomas and be bacteriologically negative, thus not substantiating the diagnosis.

Disseminated tuberculosis has been associated with a wide range of hematologic abnormalities. In some instances these are unusual enough to obscure the diagnosis. Anemia has been noted in 50% to 60% of patients with disseminated tuberculosis but is severe (hematocrit less than 30%) only in about 15%. The pattern is usually that of an anemia of chronic disease but may resemble aplastic anemia or myelofibrosis with pancytopenia. Abnormalities of the white blood cells also are encountered, and leukemoid reactions, agranulocytosis, and leukopenia are reported. In recent years, there have been several reports of disseminated intravascular coagulation, often accompanied by the adult respiratory distress syndrome, occurring in association with disseminated tuberculosis.

After the diagnosis has been established or strongly presumed, therapy should be based on previously described principles. Before the advent of chemotherapy, the prognosis was regarded as uniformly hopeless. With chemotherapy, mortality rates are very low unless meningitis is present. Without meningitis, the prognosis is determined mainly by patient age and co-existing diseases.

Central Nervous System Tuberculosis. In spite of the effectiveness of antituberculosis chemotherapy, tuberculous meningitis remains a highly lethal condition, and mortality rates in modern series range from 25% to 50% (Chapter 239). The poor prognosis is caused in part by the long duration of the process before therapy is started. The symptoms may evolve over a period of several weeks to months, though tuberculous meningitis may progress rapidly in some patients, particularly young children and those who are immunocompromised. Symptoms may include at the outset fever, malaise, and anorexia; these progress to include headaches, behavioral changes, stiff neck, photophobia, and, finally, seizures and coma. Physical findings may consist of fever, nuchal rigidity, papilledema, choroidal tubercles, and focal neurologic signs. Because of the predilection for the inflammation to be most marked at the base of the brain, cranial nerve palsies are fairly common. Focal neurologic signs also may be present in patients with isolated tuberculomas without meningitis. Tuberculomas may also involve any area of the spinal cord, producing symptoms relating to the site of the lesion. More than 50% of patients with tuberculous meningitis have evidence of tuberculosis elsewhere, whereas those with tuberculomas usually have no other evident sites of disease.

Lumbar puncture in patients with meningitis typically shows an increase in cerebrospinal fluid (CSF) pressure. The fluid itself usually contains 10 to 1000 white blood cells per microliter that are predominantly mononuclear leukocytes, an increased protein concentration, and a decreased glucose concentration. Protein concentrations may be extremely high, depending on the intensity and duration of the illness. Acid-fast staining of cerebrospinal fluid smears shows organisms in only a small number of patients, and the organism is isolated in cultures in 30% to 50%. The differential diagnosis of these clinical, neurologic, and cerebrospinal fluid findings is extensive. Often, however, the diagnosis can be strongly inferred if there is evidence of tuberculosis elsewhere.

There are no specific radiographic findings associated with tuberculosis of the central nervous system. In children, however, there may be radiologic evidence of intracranial hypertension. Rarely, the skull itself may be involved. Computed tomographic examination of the head is a sensitive means of detecting tuberculomas.

Treatment should be started promptly in all patients in whom central nervous system tuberculosis is proved or strongly suspected. Isoniazid and rifampin, and to a lesser extent streptomycin, ethambutol, and pyrazinamide, all penetrate inflamed meninges sufficiently to provide adequate cerebrospinal fluid concentrations. Intrathecal therapy is not necessary. Corticosteroids are especially beneficial in patients with more severe neurologic impairment, especially those with cerebral edema or high CSF protein concentration.

Surgical intervention in tuberculosis of the central nervous system is limited to two indications: (1) insertion of shunts to manage hydrocephalus as a sequela of meningitis, and (2) diagnosis of a tuberculoma and resection of the lesion if it is causing either intracranial hypertension or specific neurologic deficits because of compression of adjacent structures.

A poor prognosis in tuberculous meningitis correlates with increasing age, with the presence of coma or confusion at the time of diagnosis, and with increasing protein concentrations in the cerebrospinal fluid. The effects of these factors are reflected in both death rates and frequency of neurologic residua. Mortality continues to be 25% to 50%, and the frequency of persisting neurologic findings in survivors is 15% to 20%.

Gastrointestinal Tuberculosis. Although rarely encountered, tuberculosis of the gastrointestinal tract, abdominal organs, and peritoneum are forms of the disease that often are especially perplexing. Any portion of the alimentary tract from mouth to anus may be involved, although lesions proximal to the terminal ileum are extremely unusual. The sites of most common occurrence are the terminal il-

eum, cecum, and rectum. In the ileum and cecum, presenting manifestations are usually pain and/or intestinal obstruction, whereas rectal lesions may be manifested as fistulas, fissures, or abscesses. On radiographic examination, the lesion may be impossible to distinguish from neoplasm or inflammatory bowel disease, and in most patients, the diagnosis is made during surgery.

Tuberculous involvement of the peritoneum is manifested most frequently with abdominal pain, which often is accompanied by abdominal swelling. Fever, weight loss, and anorexia are also common. Some combination of these symptoms is usually present several months before the diagnosis is made. Radiographic evidence of pulmonary tuberculosis (current or old) varies in reported series from 6% to 80% but, when present, can lend weight to the diagnostic suspicion.

Ascitic fluid from patients with tuberculous peritonitis typically is exudative. It should be kept in mind, however, that when hypoalbuminemia is present, the protein content of the fluid may be less than 3.5 g/dl and yet be an exudate. White blood cell counts in the fluid range from as low as 50 to 10,000/μl and are predominantly lymphocytes, although polymorphonuclear lymphocytes occasionally predominate. Acid-fast organisms are seen rarely on stained smears of ascitic fluid. The frequency with which the organism is recovered in cultures varies in reported series from less than 10% to 83% and greater yields are obtained from large amounts of fluid (1 liter or more).

Histologic examination and culture of peritoneal tissue provide the best diagnostic yield. Laparoscopy or limited laparotomy is the preferred technique and allows directed biopsies. Because of abdominal pain or mass, laparotomy often is performed for diagnostic purposes. It should be emphasized that when findings compatible with tuberculosis are encountered during laparotomy, specimens should be obtained for both histologic and bacteriologic evaluations.

Antituberculosis chemotherapy is quite successful in treating any form of gastrointestinal tuberculosis. The frequency with which fibrotic residua cause bowel obstruction is not established. Although corticosteroids have been recommended for prevention of severe scarring, documentation of benefit is lacking.

Pericardial Tuberculosis. Tuberculous involvement of the pericardium is an uncommon (but potentially lethal and therefore important) form of extrapulmonary tuberculosis (Chapter 27). The symptoms, physical findings, and laboratory abnormalities associated with tuberculous pericarditis may be the result of the infectious process itself or of the pericardial inflammation causing pain, effusion, and eventually hemodynamic effects. The systemic symptoms produced by the infection are nonspecific. Fever, weight loss, and night sweats are common in reported series. Symptoms of cardiopulmonary origin tend to occur later and include cough, dyspnea, orthopnea, ankle swelling, and chest pain that occasionally mimics angina but is described as a dull ache; often it is affected by position and worsens on inspiration.

Apart from fever, the most common physical findings are those caused by the pericardial fluid and/or fibrosis, that is, the physical findings of some degree of either cardiac tamponade or constriction.

Definitive diagnosis of tuberculous pericarditis requires identification of the tubercle bacillus in pericardial fluid or tissue. Although not absolutely conclusive, demonstration of caseating granulomas in the pericardium in the presence of consistent clinical circumstances provides convincing evidence of a tuberculous etiology. Less conclusive, but still persuasive, evidence is the finding of another form of tuberculosis in a patient with pericarditis of undetermined origin. Still less direct and more circumstantial evidence of a tuberculous etiology is the combination of a positive intermediate-strength tuberculin reaction and pericarditis of unproved etiology.

Tubercle bacilli are identified in pericardial fluid in less than 25% to 30% (smear and culture combined). Biopsy of the pericardium with both histologic and bacteriologic evaluation is much more likely to provide a diagnosis, although a nonspecific histologic pattern and failure to recover the organisms do not exclude a tuberculous etiology. Approximately 25% to 30% of patients with tuberculous pericarditis have evidence of other organ involvement when the pericarditis is diagnosed.

Because of the potentially life-threatening nature of pericardial tuberculosis, treatment with antituberculosis agents should be instituted as soon as the diagnosis is made or strongly suggested. The likelihood of cardiac constriction is greater in patients who have had symptoms longer; thus early therapy may reduce the incidence of this complication.

Current data indicate that corticosteroids are valuable in treating tuberculous pericarditis. In a prospective randomized study, South African and British investigators reported a significantly lower mortality rate and need for subsequent surgical treatment in patients treated with corticosteroids. The benefits were seen both in patients with effusion and in those with constrictive pericarditis. The doses have been in the range of 60 to 80 mg of prednisolone or prednisone given daily for the first 4 weeks with a gradually decreasing dose during the next 6 to 8 weeks.

If hemodynamic compromise occurs, pericardiectomy may be necessary. Although pericardiocentesis generally improves the circulatory status, the improvement is usually temporary. Pericardial windows with drainage into the left pleural space often provide only temporary relief. The selection of patients for pericardiectomy is not clear cut except for those who have severe hemodynamic compromise. Persisting effusion, even with evidence of venous hypertension for as long as 6 months, has eventually responded to medical therapy alone. On the other hand, the longer the effusion persists, the thicker and more adherent is the pericardium, and the more difficult the procedure. In general, if venous hypertension persists beyond 6 months because of pericardial disease, pericardiectomy is indicated. Surgery also is indicated when there is decreasing heart size associated with increasing venous pressure, which indicates increasing constriction.

With proper therapy, mortality is probably in the range of 15% to 20%, and constriction occurs in about 15%. Constriction, if it is going to occur, is most likely to be apparent within 2 years and certainly within 5 years.

Prevention of Tuberculosis

Isoniazid Preventive Therapy. There is now a large body of data to substantiate the effectiveness of INH in preventing the progression of tuberculous infection to tuberculous disease. Presumably INH decreases the number of tubercle bacilli in (usually) inapparent foci formed at the time of the primary infection; the drug thereby decreases the likelihood that clinically evident disease will emerge from these foci. In a large series of studies of preventive therapy conducted by the Public Health Service involving some 70,000 participants, the case rate during the treatment year for those given INH was reduced by 84% compared with those given placebo. During subsequent years, there continued to be a greater number of cases in those who had received placebo. Overall, during a 10-year period of observation, INH preventive therapy resulted in a 61% reduction in tuberculosis cases.

Hepatitis is the major toxic effect of INH and must be balanced against the benefit of preventive therapy. The risk of INH-associated hepatitis increases with age: it is rare among persons under 20 years of age but occurs in approximately 2.3% of persons older than 49 years of age. Daily use of alcohol also increases the risk of hepatitis. Asymptomatic increases in serum transaminase levels are much more frequent than symptomatic hepatitis and occur in nearly 10% of all persons taking INH.

The indications for the use of INH preventive therapy are listed in Table 273-2. With each of these indications, the beneficial effect of INH in prevention of tuberculosis clearly outweighs the risk of hepatitis. It should be kept in mind, too, that the protective effect of INH is of extended (perhaps lifelong) duration, whereas the risk of hepatitis applies only during the medication year. Conversely, the risk of hepatitis during the treatment year may outweigh the risk of tuberculosis.

For preventive therapy in adults, a standard daily dose of 300 mg of INH should be given. For children, the dose is 10 mg/kg of body weight, up to a dose of 300 mg/day. The recommended minimum duration of INH administration is 6 months; however, persons with radiographic abnormalities suggestive of previous tuberculosis should be treated with INH for 12 months.

Persons receiving INH preventive therapy should be interviewed at monthly intervals to detect symptoms that may be caused by drug-

Table 273-2   Indications for use of isoniazid preventive therapy

GROUP	RISK OF TUBERCULOSIS
HIV-infected contact of infectious case	May exceed 30% with significant exposure
Recently infected persons (tuberculin convertors)	3%-5% during first year after infection
Positive tuberculin test associated with chest radiographic abnormalities suggestive of previous tuberculosis	1% per year for life
Tuberculin-positive close contact of newly discovered case	3.3% during first year after discovery
Household contacts who are tuberculin-negative at the time of initial evaluation	0.5% during first year after discovery
Tuberculin-positive adolescents	0.2% per year for 2-3 years
Tuberculin reactors in special clinical situations	Risk is not quantified
Prolonged corticosteroid or immunosuppressive therapy	
Hematologic or reticuloendothelial malignancies	
Insulin-requiring diabetes mellitus	
Pneumoconiosis	
After gastrectomy	
HIV infection	

related hepatitis. These symptoms are nonspecific and include anorexia, gastrointestinal complaints, fever, and myalgia. Complaints more specifically related to the liver, such as jaundice, dark urine, and abdominal discomfort in the right upper quadrant are relatively uncommon. Patients having these or other suggestive symptoms of hepatitis should have tests of liver function performed, and if they are abnormal, the drug should be discontinued. Routine measurement of liver function is not indicated except in persons who are at increased risk of hepatitis—those older than 35 years of age, alcohol users, and persons with preexisting, but stable, liver disease. Preventive therapy with INH should not be administered to persons with current unstable liver disease or to pregnant women. Persons with radiographically visible lesions or symptoms that could be tuberculous in origin must be fully evaluated, and current tuberculosis excluded before preventive therapy is started.

Preventive therapy in persons who have been exposed to INH-resistant organisms is an issue of increasing concern. Unfortunately, no other agents have been evaluated for use in this situation. Given the lack of data, the choice of treatment should be based on a case-by-case assessment that takes into account (1) the probability that infection with an INH-resistant organism has occurred, an analysis that can be derived in part from an evaluation of the previously listed factors that influence transmission; and (2) an estimation of the possible consequences of the infection—the probability of tuberculous disease and its severity. When the probability that transmission has occurred is thought to be small and the consequences not severe, INH may be used according to the usual criteria. When the risk of transmission is great and the consequences are possibly grave, rifampin is the agent of choice.

If the index case is also resistant to rifampin, multidrug preventive therapy should be strongly considered.

Immunization. The BCG vaccine was derived from a strain of *M. bovis* and attenuated through serial passage in culture. Artificial infection with the organism stimulates the immunologic response that was described earlier as occurring with natural tuberculous infection. The effect of this nonspecific response is to improve the ability of a person who has recently been infected with *M. tuberculosis* to contain the infection, thereby preventing early dissemination of the organism. No protection is provided for persons who are already infected when BCG is given. The reported effectiveness of BCG vaccination varies widely, probably because of variations in the potency of different strains of the organism and differing conditions and methods of administration of the vaccine. Indications for the use of BCG in developed countries are limited. Current recommendations in the United States state that BCG should be considered only for tuberculin-negative persons who are repeatedly exposed to untreated or ineffectively treated tuberculosis. Vaccination also may be considered for identified groups within the population that demonstrate an excessive rate of new infections (usually more than 1% per year) and in which the usual approaches to tuberculosis control have failed or have been shown not to be applicable.

In addition to the lack of consistent effectiveness of BCG immunization, administration of the vaccine usually produces a positive tuberculin skin test; the test therefore can no longer be used to identify tuberculous infection. This is a particular problem in immigrants to the United States from areas where BCG is commonly used. Because it is not possible to separate a BCG-induced tuberculin reaction from true infection, the history of BCG immunization is generally ignored, and the tuberculin reaction is interpreted and acted on according to standard criteria.

Public Health Considerations

Appropriate management of patients with tuberculosis must include attention to the public health aspects of this disease. Reporting of new cases of tuberculosis to public health authorities is generally mandatory. This ensures that cases are promptly and effectively treated, that the appropriate epidemiologic investigations are conducted, and that accurate data are collected. The most effective means of reducing the spread of tuberculous infection is prompt diagnosis and treatment of a patient with tuberculosis, which, as discussed previously, rapidly renders the person noninfectious. Thus tuberculosis is one of the few diseases in which treatment of the disease itself benefits not only the health of the patient but the health of the public as well.

These ends are served not only by instituting proper therapy but by monitoring the effects of therapy to ascertain that the response to treatment is as predicted and that the patient is not encountering adverse effects of the drug. Patients should be seen and evaluated at least at monthly intervals. Sputum specimens should be evaluated after 2 to 3 months of treatment to determine if sputum conversion has occurred. If conversion has not occurred, the use of public health personnel to directly supervise therapy should be considered. Sputum smear and culture should also be performed after 6 months of treatment to document the bacteriologic negativity. These examinations at 3 and 6 months should be regarded as part of the basic public health management of the patient.

The most effective tool for finding previously undetected cases of tuberculosis is the evaluation of contacts of newly identified cases. By incorporating an understanding of the factors that govern transmission of infection into the epidemiologic investigation, the investigation can be conducted in a prompt and efficient manner. Contacts should be evaluated using a "concentric circle" approach, starting with those persons in closest contact with the index case and working in progressively widening circles with decreasing levels of contact. Because tuberculosis can spread rapidly in populations that have a high incidence of HIV infection, special efforts must be made to rapidly investigate contacts in such settings. Contacts should receive a tuberculin test usually soon after being identified. Those with positive tests should have a chest film taken, and if there are radiographic abnormalities, a sputum examination should be performed. Children younger than 6 years of age should have a chest film taken even if the tuberculin test is negative because of the more severe nature of untreated tuberculosis in this age group. Contacts whose initial tuberculin test is negative should be retested approximately 8 weeks after contact is broken or the index case becomes noninfectious. This period allows sufficient time for tuberculin reactivity to develop if the contact was infected shortly before the index case was identified. As indicated previously, INH preventive therapy should be given to all household or other close contacts, particularly those infected with HIV. INH can be discontinued in those who remain tuberculin-negative on the 8-week tuberculin test.

The other major public health function with regard to tuberculosis is the collection and analysis of epidemiologic and program management data. Accurate information allows for proper priority assignment for tuberculosis control activities, identification of areas and groups in need of special attention, and evaluation of the effectiveness of control measures.

NONTUBERCULOUS MYCOBACTERIAL INFECTIONS

Although types of mycobacteria other than *M. tuberculosis* and *M. bovis* were recognized before the end of the nineteenth century, the potential pathogenic role of these organisms was not clearly appreciated until the early 1950s. Since that time, there has been increasing awareness of the spectrum of disease produced by these types of mycobacteria. Similarly, with advances in techniques for studying mycobacteria, their classification and taxonomy have become increasingly precise. Several important generalizations can be made regarding the nontuberculous mycobacteria.

1. They may produce pulmonary disease that is clinically, radiographically, and pathologically indistinguishable from tuberculosis, or they may exist as saprophytes in the lungs and cause no disease.
2. With the exception of *Mycobacterium kansasii,* they are usually resistant to antituberculosis agents.
3. Their epidemiology is largely unknown, but there are no proved instances of person-to-person transmission.

Characteristics of Nontuberculous Mycobacteria

As was stated earlier, the nontuberculous mycobacteria share many of the properties of the tubercle bacilli. They are nearly identical among themselves and to *M. tuberculosis* in their staining characteristics and in the tissue reaction produced. The major differences are in their cultural, biochemical, and antigenic features. Several classification schemes have been developed to allow grouping of like organisms; none has proved entirely satisfactory. Box 273-1 is a classification of potentially pathogenic mycobacteria that separates the nontuberculous mycobacteria only on the basis of their growth rates and emphasizes the need for species identification rather than grouping of the organisms.

The most frequently encountered mycobacteria are those of the *Mycobacterium avium* complex, *M. kansasii,* and *Mycobacterium scrofulaceum.* The *M. avium* complex contains a large number of serotypically distinct strains that are otherwise difficult to separate. Colonies of these organisms are usually buff colored and may resemble *M. tuberculosis. M. kansasii* generally produces colonies that acquire a yellow-orange color after exposure to light, whereas *M. scrofulaceum* colonies produce pigment without being exposed to light. These characteristics form the basis of the Runyon classification, which is as follows: group I, photochromogens *(M. kansasii);* group II, scotochromogens *(M. scrofulaceum);* group III, nonchromogens *(M. avium* complex); and group IV, rapid growers *(Mycobacterium fortuitum).*

Epidemiology. The epidemiology of the nontuberculous mycobacteria is largely unknown. There are, however, well-documented and striking foci of endemicity indicated by geographic distribution of reactors to skin tests with specific antigens and the distribution of disease. *M. avium* complex is highly endemic in the southeastern United States and is also found in western Australia and Japan, whereas *M. kansasii* is predominant in the westernmost midwestern states (Kansas and Nebraska), and in New Orleans, Dallas, and Chicago. Infection and disease caused by both organisms are found throughout the Midwest, and scattered pockets of disease caused by either *M. avium* complex or *M. kansasii* have been found throughout the United States.

In spite of the strikingly high prevalence of nontuberculous mycobacterial infection in many areas, the frequency with which clinically evident disease develops is much less than occurs after infection with *M. tuberculosis.*

Nontuberculous mycobacteria have been found in soil, seawater foam, tap water, pond water, milk, and bird feces. However, none of these sources or animals seems to serve as a reservoir.

The frequent occurrence of disease caused by *M. avium* complex in patients with AIDS does not fit with the pattern of distribution of organisms just described. Studies of the cumulative incidence of *M. avium* complex indicate that infection occurs in up to 24% of AIDS patients.

Clinical Features of Nontuberculous Mycobacterial Disease

In immunocompetent persons the nontuberculosis mycobacterial diseases are similar to tuberculosis in many ways, but they differ in several important respects: (1) the diseases tend to remain localized and progress extremely slowly, (2) constitutional symptoms are less prominent, (3) isolation of a nontuberculous mycobacterium from pulmonary secretions does not always confirm a diagnosis, (4) skin testing with tuberculins made from these organisms is of little value in making a diagnosis of disease resulting from a nontuberculous organism, and (5) with the exception of *M. kansasii,* response to chemotherapy is generally poor.

Pulmonary Disease. The lungs are the most frequent site of involvement for *M. kansasii* and *M. avium* complex; however, all the organisms have been associated with pulmonary disease. Disease occurs more commonly in men, and there is a definite association with preexisting lung disease, such as silicosis, bronchiectasis, or old tuberculosis. The following criteria must be met before pulmonary disease can be ascribed to a nontuberculous mycobacterium: (1) there must be a compatible pulmonary process visible on the chest radiograph; (2) colonies of the same organism must be isolated from several sputum specimens, or the organism must be isolated from biopsied lung tissue; and (3) tuberculosis must be excluded.

Treatment of pulmonary *M. kansasii* disease with a regimen of INH, rifampin, and ethambutol for 2 years is successful in more than 90% of patients, and surgery is indicated only rarely. *M. avium* complex and the other nontuberculous organisms that cause lung disease are much more difficult to treat. Regimens containing four, five, or six drugs sometimes supplemented by resectional surgery have been successful in only 41% to 77% of patients. Because of the potential toxicity and discomfort of regimens containing so many agents, the decision to treat disease caused by *M. avium* complex should not be made lightly and should take into account the disease's tendency to stabilize without treatment or to progress very slowly.

Lymphatic Disease. Disease of the lymph nodes is most commonly caused by *M. scrofulaceum.* In contrast, more than 90% of culture-proven mycobacterial lymphadenitis in adults is caused by *M. tuberculosis,* although *M. kansasii* and *M. avium* complex also cause adenitis.

When the diagnosis is suspected, excisional biopsy is the diagnostic procedure of choice. The major differential diagnosis is tuberculosis. The distinction can usually be made from epidemiologic features and the tuberculin skin test. Drug therapy is usually not indicated, and even partial excision of involved nodes is often successful.

Disseminated Disease in Immunocompromised Patients. Another indication of the low virulence of the nontuberculous mycobacteria is the infrequency with which disseminated disease occurs. The majority of patients who have had disseminated disease have also had serious hematologic or immunologic disorders. The mortality rate in these patients is extremely high.

The clinical manifestations of disease caused by the nontuberculous mycobacteria deserve special mention. As mentioned previously, a large proportion of patients with AIDS have disease caused by *M. avium* complex when their CD4 cell counts fall below 50. The involvement is largely extrapulmonary, with lymph node, blood, bone marrow, and a variety of viscera being the sources of positive cultures. Striking features of the illness are the nearly total absence of any granulomatous response to the organisms and the enormous numbers of bacilli present (Fig. 273-8).

The severity of systemic illness and the effects on organ function caused by *M. avium* complex are not clear. Patients commonly have a number of other infections that obscure the features of illness caused by any single organism. Weight loss of greater than 20 pounds, anorexia, abdominal pain, and diarrhea has been suggested as more common in patients with *M. avium* infection than in patients with other complications of HIV infection. Diagnosis is made by culturing the organism, usually from the blood.

Although early reports on the response to treatment of *M. avium* complex were discouraging, recent trials of multidrug regimens

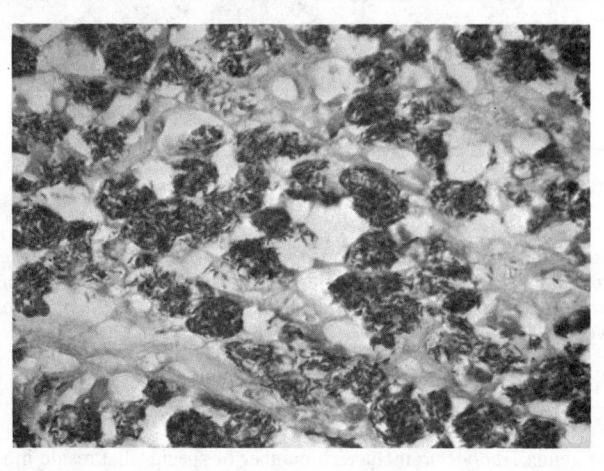

FIGURE 273-8   Photomicrograph of acid-fast stain of lymph node biopsy from patient with AIDS and disseminated *Mycobacterium avium* complex disease. Specimen is noteworthy for the large number of organisms present (more darkly staining areas) and the absence of an inflammatory response.

including ciprofloxacin, clofazimine, ethambutol, rifampin, and amikacin show symptomatic relief and improvement in microbiologic indicators.

Soft Tissue and Skeletal Disease. Soft tissue and skeletal sites of disease have been identified in association with a variety of nontuberculous mycobacteria. Common causes of these are cutaneous granulomas and ulcers from *Mycobacterium marinum.* The lesions usually are the result of a break in the skin contacting contaminated water, which is often, but not necessarily, inhabited by fish. Such infection may heal spontaneously, but if treatment is necessary, the lesion may respond to treatment with rifampin and ethambutol as well as other agents.

Injection-site abscesses caused by *Mycobacterium chelonei* have been reported in several large groups. More recently, *M. chelonei* has been reported as the etiologic agent in several cases of sternal osteomyelitis and mediastinitis after open heart surgery. *M. chelonei* does not respond to standard antituberculosis drugs but is susceptible to tetracyclines, cephalosporins, and sulfonamides. These agents plus debridement and drainage, with removal of infected tissue, are the only forms of treatment likely to succeed.

BIBLIOGRAPHY

American Thoracic Society/Centers for Disease Control: Treatment of tuberculosis and tuberculosis infection in adults and children, *Am J Respir Crit Care Med* 149:1359-1374, 1994.

Barksdale L, Kim K: *Mycobacterium, Bacteriol Rev* 41:217, 1977.

Barnes PF et al: Tuberculosis in patients with human immunodeficiency virus infection, *N Engl J Med* 324:1644, 1991.

Bloom BR, Murray CJL: Tuberculosis: commentary on a reemergent killer, *Science* 257:1055, 1992.

Dooley SW et al: Multidrug-resistant tuberculosis, *Ann Int Med* 117:257, 1992 (editorial).

Hopewell PC: Factors influencing the transmission and pathogenicity of *Mycobacterium tuberculosis:* implications for clinical and public health management of tuberculosis. In Sande MA, Hudson LD, Root RK, editors: *Contemporary issues in infectious diseases,* vol 5, *Respiratory infections,* New York, 1986, Churchill Livingstone.

Horsburgh CR: *Mycobacterium avium* complex infection in the acquired immunodeficiency syndrome, *N Engl J Med* 324:1332, 1991.

Rieder HL et al: Epidemiology of tuberculosis in the United States, *Am J Epidemiol* 11:79, 1989.

Tuberculosis morbidity—United States, 1994, *MMWR* 44(20):387-389, 395, 1995.

Tuberculosis morbidity—United States, 1995, *JAMA* 275(21):1629-1630, 1996.

Wallace RJ et al: Diagnosis and treatment of disease caused by nontuberculous mycobacteria, *Am Rev Respir Dis* 142:940, 1990.

Weis Stephen E et al: The effect of directly observed therapy on rates of drug resistance and relapse in tuberculosis, *N Engl J Med* 330:1179-1184, 1996.

Wolinsky E: Nontuberculous mycobacteria and associated disease, *Am Rev Respir Dis* 119:107, 1979.

274 Infections Caused by Spirochetes

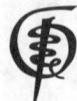

David Bangsberg and Michael F. Rein

Spirochetes that are pathogenic for humans include the genera *Treponema* (syphilis, yaws, pinta, and bejel), *Leptospira* (leptospirosis), *Borrelia* (Lyme disease and relapsing fever), and *Spirillum* (rat-bite fever).

INFECTIONS CAUSED BY *TREPONEMA* SPECIES (SYPHILIS, YAWS, PINTA, AND BEJEL)

The genus *Treponema* includes a number of species that reside in the gastrointestinal and genital tracts of humans. These organisms are culturable and frequently are isolated from mixed anaerobic (fusospirochetal) infections of the mucous membranes, but their specific pathogenic role is controversial. However, *T. pallidum, T. pertenue,* and *T. carateum,* which are human pathogens responsible for significant worldwide morbidity, are not cultivable by current techniques, and the diagnosis of a specific infection depends on clinical skills, pathologic specimens, and serologic tests.

The pathogenic treponemes are fine, spiral organisms approximately 0.15 mm wide and 6 to 15 mm long (Color Plate VIII-2). They have a trilaminar outer membrane similar to that of the gram-negative bacteria, but they have not been shown to possess a biologically active endotoxin. They are microaerophilic and survive poorly in atmospheric oxygen. Sensitive to drying and to extremes of temperature, they are transmitted almost uniformly by direct contact. Therefore syphilis is a sexually transmitted disease (STD), and the non-STD treponematoses are most prevalent in situations of overcrowding and poor hygiene.

Syphilis

Syphilis is a specific infection with *T. pallidum* and becomes evident as a chronic disease with subacute symptomatic periods separated by asymptomatic intervals during which the diagnosis can be made on serologic testing.

Epidemiology. The venereal nature of syphilis was recognized in the earliest descriptions of the disease. Infection develops in 30% to 50% of the sexual partners of patients with syphilitic lesions, but the risk of acquiring syphilis from a single sexual exposure to an infected partner is unknown. The average prevalence among sexual partners is so high that all patients presenting themselves for treatment because of such sexual contact within the past 90 days (the maximum incubation period for syphilis) should be given treatment, even in the absence of clinical or serologic evidence of disease. Such *epidemiologic treatment* is an important element of syphilis control.

Since 1985, the incidence of primary and secondary syphilis has been increasing. Syphilis is most prevalent in sexually active populations and age-groups, and the highest age-adjusted rates for reported early syphilis are found among 20- to 24-year-old men and women, although syphilis is also prevalent among 24- to 34-year-old men, particularly in heterosexual, drug-using populations and in the rural South.

The association of syphilis with human immunodeficiency virus (HIV) infection is striking, with HIV infection found in one fourth of syphilitics in some STD clinic populations. Patients with a diagnosis of syphilis should be carefully evaluated for the presence of other STDs, including HIV infection (Chapter 248).

Syphilis can be acquired by kissing a person with active oral lesions. Sexual abuse must be considered in any child with early-stage syphilis. Syphilis may be transmitted transplacentally to the fetus, and the risk of congenital syphilis is increased if syphilis is acquired during pregnancy. Women with multiple sexual partners should be screened for syphilis several times during pregnancy.

Pathophysiology. *T. pallidum* can penetrate intact mucous membranes or infect via tiny defects in cornified epithelium. Spirochetemia occurs very early in infection, even before the first lesions have appeared or the blood test result becomes reactive. This is particularly important in pregnancy, since pregnant women acquiring syphilis late in the third trimester may transmit the infection to the fetus but not manifest evidence of syphilis themselves until after delivery.

Syphilitic infection generally is characterized by an obliterative endarteritis resulting in impaired blood flow. The typical late manifestations of syphilis of the central nervous and cardiovascular systems largely result from vascular involvement in these areas.

Immune mechanisms contribute to the pathophysiology of syphilis. Late infection may elicit a granulomatous reaction called a *gumma*. The histopathologic features are nonspecific, and gummas may occur in any organ. Antigen-antibody complexes have been detected in the blood of patients with secondary syphilis and are responsible for the glomerulonephritis that may accompany this stage. At the same time, suppression of cell-mediated immunity in acquired immunodeficiency syndrome (AIDS) contributes to the greater severity and more rapid progression of disease in some patients.

Clinical Manifestations. The natural history of syphilis is generally divided into stages. After acquiring the organism, but before clinical or serologic manifestations develop, patients are said to have *incubating syphilis.* The incubation period usually lasts about 3 weeks but can range from 10 to 90 days. During this interval the diagnosis of syphilis cannot be made on clinical or serologic grounds. Therefore a patient who has had sexual exposure within the past 90 days to a person with infectious syphilis may have an undetectable infection. Such patients routinely should be given treatment.

Primary syphilis. At the end of the incubation period a lesion called a *chancre* develops at the point of initial inoculation and multiplication of the spirochete. Chancres are commonly located around the genitalia (Color Plate VIII-34) but may appear almost anywhere else on the body, and syphilis should be considered as part of the differential diagnosis of ulcerated lesions at any anatomic site. The chancre begins as a papule that erodes to form a gradually enlarging ulcer with a clean base and an indurated edge; generally it is relatively painless. Although the chancre usually occurs as a single lesion, multiple chancres are not rare.

Of patients with primary syphilis of the external genitalia, 50% to 70% subsequently develop relatively painless, usually bilateral, inguinal adenopathy *(satellite bubo).* Inguinal adenopathy is less common with the chancres involving the glans, the cervix, or the proximal portion of the vagina because these sites are drained by the iliac nodes, and regional adenopathy results from primary inoculation at other sites. Affected nodes usually are evident in a chain and are discrete, firm, and fairly movable.

Even without treatment, the chancre heals completely within about 4 to 6 weeks, and the regional adenopathy resolves.

Secondary syphilis. Two to 8 weeks (but occasionally as long as 6 months) after the appearance of the chancre the manifestations of secondary syphilis may develop. Sometimes, primary and secondary syphilis overlap, and the chancre is still obvious. On the other hand, some patients never notice the primary lesion and initially have the manifestations of secondary syphilis. This stage is a generalized illness that usually begins with symptoms suggesting a viral infection: headache, sore throat, low-grade fever, and, occasionally, a nasal discharge. Moderate leukocytosis and relative lymphocytosis are common, but atypical lymphocytes are not seen.

The disease progresses with development of lymphadenopathy and lesions of the skin and mucous membranes. Adenopathy is recognized in 75% of affected patients and is often generalized. Nodes most commonly involved include the inguinal, suboccipital, posterior auricular, and cervical. Epitrochlear adenopathy is common and should raise suspicions of secondary syphilis. The affected nodes are usually discrete, relatively nontender, firm, and freely movable. Suppuration, periadenitis, and lymphangitis are rare. Generalized lymphadenopathy in sexually active individuals should also raise the question of HIV infection.

Skin lesions are evident in 80% of the infected patients, but the lesions are highly variable and often closely imitate other conditions. Macular lesions (Color Plate VIII-46) are most common and are usually observed over the thighs, abdomen, and trunk, where they are generally bilaterally symmetric, tend to follow lines of skin cleavage, and have a coppery or "boiled ham" color. The lesions are sometimes *mildly* pruritic. The rash almost invariably involves the genitalia and often is prominent on the palms (Color Plate VIII-47) and soles, a distribution in itself highly suggestive of syphilis. Maculopapular lesions are also common, and follicular lesions may be present. Vesicles or bullae are distinctly rare in secondary syphilis in adults, although they may accompany congenital syphilis.

The mucous membranes are involved in more than half of cases, but the lesions may be subtle. In about one third of patients, mucous patches develop (painless, oval ulcerations usually covered with a gray or yellow membrane).

Condylomata lata are flat, hypertrophic lesions resembling warts and develop in moist areas. Frequently found around the anus or vagina, they do not indicate sites of inoculation but result from hematogenous dissemination of spirochetes.

Patchy, nonpruritic alopecia involving the scalp, beard, or eyebrows suggests secondary syphilis.

The central nervous system (CNS) is asymptomatically involved in about one third of patients with secondary syphilis, but CNS symptoms accompany only about 2% of the cases, which usually become evident as acute syphilitic meningitis. In these cases the cerebrospinal fluid (CSF) may contain up to 500 primarily mononuclear white blood cells/mm³ and, frequently, protein in excess of 100 mg/ml. The symptoms are those of a basilar meningitis and often include meningeal and cranial nerve signs. The CSF need not be examined in patients with secondary syphilis who do not have symptoms referable to the CNS. It may, however, be advisable to examine the CSF of *all* patients 1 year after they have been given treatment for early-stage syphilis to detect those with persistent CNS infection.

Hepatitis and immune complex glomerulonephritis occasionally accompany secondary syphilis. Uveitis and osteitis are rarely observed. Ulceronodular gastritis is increasingly reported and may be confused with gastric lymphoma.

Secondary syphilis usually resolves within 2 to 6 weeks, even without treatment. Some of the lesions may heal with scarring.

Latent syphilis. After untreated secondary syphilis resolves, the disease enters a latent stage in which the diagnosis can be made only on serologic testing. During the first 2 to 4 years of infection, but most commonly during the first year, at least 25% of patients have one or more mucocutaneous relapses in which the manifestations of secondary syphilis reappear. During these intervals, patients are once again contagious to sexual partners, and the underlying spirochetemia may result in transplacental transmission to the fetus. Such relapses are extremely rare after 4 years of latency.

About one third of patients entering latency are eventually spontaneously cured of the disease, with a gradual return of nontreponemal serologic test results toward nonreactive. Another third of patients remain infected but never develop further clinical manifestations of disease. In the remaining third of patients, manifestations of late syphilis eventually develop. Antibiotics administered for other infections may reduce the incidence of late syphilis.

Late syphilis. About 15% of untreated syphilitics, late-stage benign syphilis eventually develops. This disease becomes evident with destructive granulomas that typically involve the skin and the bones. These granulomas, or gummas, may produce lesions resembling segments of circles. Skin lesions characteristically heal at one edge and advance at others (serpiginous lesions). Gummas often heal with atrophic, superficial scarring. Bones are frequently affected; periostitis is characterized by localized increases in bone density or destructive lesions surrounded by sclerosis. The tibia is involved in about half of such patients, and the clavicle, skull, and fibula in about one fourth each. Biopsy findings are nonspecific and reveal granulomas. Organisms are rarely seen, and the pathogenesis of this stage may be largely hyperimmune.

Ten percent of untreated patients eventually have cardiovascular manifestations (Chapter 25). *T. pallidum* may directly affect the aortic endothelium, yielding an irregular intima reminiscent of tree bark. Involvement of the aortic valve cusps results in rolling and thickening and may lead to aortic insufficiency. The coronary ostia may also be involved in the endarteritis, leading to coronary occlusion. Involvement of the vasa vasora weakens the aortic media, and the aorta may

then develop an aneurysm. About half of syphilitic aneurysms occur in the arch, and another 40% involve other parts of the thoracic aorta. Dissection of syphilitic aortic aneurysms is rare.

Early evidence of cardiovascular involvement includes a localized aortic bulging on chest radiograph, an altered aortic second heart sound that is sometimes described as having a tambour quality, or precordial chest pain in a young person without other predisposing factors (Chapter 25). Later, symptoms of aortic insufficiency and congestive heart failure develop. Antisyphilitic therapy does not reverse existing cardiac damage, but appropriate therapy may slow the progression of the disease.

In about 8% of untreated patients, late syphilis involves the CNS. Mild CNS involvement affects 15% to 40% of patients with cardiovascular syphilis. Initially CNS disease is asymptomatic and can be detected only by examination of the CSF. The CSF should be examined in any patient with clinical or serological evidence of syphilis and neurologic signs or symptoms. Ideally, the CSF should also be examined in all patients being given treatment for syphilis of unknown duration or who have had syphilis for more than 1 year. This is particularly important for patients with a serum nontreponemal antibody titer of more than 1:16; patients who have other clinical evidence of active, late-stage syphilis (e.g., aortitis, gumma, iritis); or patients to whom one is planning to administer therapy with an antibiotic other than a β-lactam. Examination of the CSF should also be considered for all patients with syphilis who have a positive HIV antibody test result. The CSF should be evaluated in patients who have had a suboptimal response to therapy for early-stage syphilis because unsuspected asymptomatic neurosyphilis may account for some small percentage of apparent treatment failures. Indeed, observations on CNS involvement in early-stage syphilis support the recommendation that all patients with early-stage syphilis undergo examination of the CSF at least 1 year after completing therapy.

Meningovascular syphilis results from endarteritis and usually becomes evident as seizures or cerebrovascular accident. A stroke in a young person with no history of hypertension should prompt evaluation for meningovascular syphilis. Some patients exhibit a syndrome suggesting a basilar meningitis; such persons usually have a lymphocytic pleocytosis and increased protein in the CSF.

Spirochetes also may involve the brain substance directly, producing general paresis, which usually becomes evident as a disorder of higher cerebral functions. Affected individuals undergo personality changes; dementia and delusional states are common. Sometimes, the Argyll Robertson pupil is evident, which is small and further constricts with accommodation but does not react to light, a finding highly suggestive of neurosyphilis.

Tabes dorsalis results from involvement of the posterior columns and dorsal roots of the spinal cord. The disease becomes evident as a loss of vibration sense and proprioception that results in a characteristic broad-based gait. Affected patients also may note severe, sharp pains in any part of the body. Impotence and bladder dysfunction are relatively common. Optic atrophy is observed in one fourth of infected patients, and Argyll Robertson pupils are more common than in general paresis. Some patients with tabes have normal results of CSF and nonreactive nontreponemal tests for syphilis for both serum and CSF.

Syphilis and human immunodeficiency virus infection. Although anecdotal observations and small series of cases have suggested that immunodeficiency in AIDS may alter the course of syphilis, these observations have not been replicated in larger studies. Syphilitic patients with AIDS are relatively more likely to come to medical attention with secondary than with primary syphilis and are more likely to have the chancre persist into the secondary stage. Necrotizing lesions (*syphilis maligna*) may occur in secondary syphilis. Follow-up is essential.

Congenital syphilis. Congenital syphilis follows maternal spirochetemia and transplacental transmission of the organism. Since spirochetemia is more common in early-stage syphilis, babies born to women acquiring syphilis during pregnancy are more likely to have congenital syphilis than those whose mothers acquired syphilis before becoming pregnant. Consequent to the rise in the incidence of early-stage syphilis among heterosexuals, there has been a dramatic increase in congenital syphilis in some areas.

About three fourths of reported cases of congenital syphilis are diagnosed in patients over 10 years of age. Sometimes, the manifestations of congenital syphilis are recognized first by the internist. Patients with late-stage congenital syphilis may have the hutchinsonian triad, which includes Hutchinson's teeth: short, narrow, barrel-shaped incisors displaying a central notch. A second element of the triad is interstitial keratitis, which usually appears in patients between 5 and 20 years of age. The inflammation is expressed as photophobia, eye pain, blurred vision, and tearing. Nerve deafness completes the triad. Other late manifestations of congenital syphilis include fissuring around the mouth and anus (rhagades) and skeletal lesions that comprise anterior bowing of the tibia (sabre shin), enlargement of the medial end of the clavicle, perforation of the palate, or collapse of the nasal bones to produce a saddle-nose deformity.

Laboratory Diagnosis

Dark-field microscopy. The moist lesions of syphilis, including the chancre, mucous patches, and condylomata lata, usually contain sufficient numbers of spirochetes to permit their direct observation. The surface of a suitable lesion is cleaned with a gauze pad and is lightly abraded. Resulting blood is blotted away, and tissue fluid is expressed by squeezing the edges of the lesion. A small amount of fluid is transferred to a microscope slide and examined with the aid of a dark-field microscope. The dark-field condenser angles light through the specimen so that it does not directly enter the microscope objective. Therefore the background appears dark. Objects in the fluid are visualized because light reflecting from them enters the objective. *T. pallidum* is recognized by its characteristic morphologic appearance and movement (Color Plate VIII-2). Six to 14 regular spirals are maintained during its movements, and the organism is seen to rotate in corkscrew fashion around its long axis, to move forward and backward along this axis, and to bend at its midpoint. Dark-field examination of specimens from oral or intravaginal lesions is difficult because nonpathogenic spirochetes may closely resemble *T. pallidum*. The dry lesions of secondary syphilis are usually negative on dark-field examination.

Serologic diagnosis. A diagnosis of syphilis should be made or ruled out only after carefully considering all historical, epidemiologic, and clinical features of the case—not on the basis of serologic results alone. The serologic testing of syphilis is a far from perfect science. It has flowered because the organism cannot be cultured and the disease has long intervals devoid of clinical manifestations. All serologic test results can be nonreactive in patients with certain stages of active syphilis. In the setting of low prevalence the number of false-positive results increases relative to the number of true-positive results. All serologic test results for syphilis can be positive in patients without syphilis, and clinical judgment must enter into a decision to treat patients solely on the basis of serologic evidence of syphilis.

In patients with syphilis, antibodies usually develop that are directed against a poorly defined lipid that may be a component of the spirochete. Cross-reacting lipids are found in a variety of normal tissues and serve as the basis of the nontreponemal tests for syphilis, which employ a lipid extracted from beef heart (cardiolipin) as an antigen. Nontreponemal tests are easy to perform and inexpensive; they include the Venereal Disease Research Laboratory (VDRL) test, the rapid plasma reagin (RPR) test, and the automated reagin test (ART). Similar antibodies are produced in a variety of diseases other than syphilis. These include acute viral illnesses (e.g., varicella, hepatitis, and infectious mononucleosis), bacterial infections (e.g., leprosy, tuberculosis, and leptospirosis), and diseases associated with the formation of unusual immunoglobulins (e.g., intravenous drug abuse and collagen vascular diseases).

Nontreponemal test results may be quantitated, and results are usually expressed as the highest dilution of serum yielding a positive reaction. The RPR and ART may yield titers two to eight times as high as those obtained with the VDRL on the same serum. Because rising or falling titers have considerable clinical significance, patients followed over time should be studied with the same nontreponemal tests.

The titer of a nontreponemal test generally is expected to fall by a factor of at least four after adequate therapy of syphilis. This fourfold drop in titer generally occurs about 3 months after treatment of early-stage syphilis. With the RPR the fraction of patients reverting to nonreactive status after adequate treatment for primary syphilis is only 44% after 1 year and 60% after 2 years. After adequate treatment for secondary syphilis the percentage of seroreverting with the RPR is 22% after 1 year and 42% after 2 years. Patients having untreated syphilis for more than 2 years are unlikely to become nonreactive with the nontreponemal tests but should still show a fourfold drop in titer. Subsequent fourfold rises in titer suggest relapse or reinfection, and such patients should be reevaluated.

Patients with syphilis also develop antitreponemal antibodies, which can be detected by a variety of procedures that use *T. pallidum* as the antigen. In the fluorescent treponemal antibody-absorption (FTA-ABS) test, antitreponemal antibody is detected by indirect fluorescence of spirochetes. The microhemagglutination test for *T. pallidum* (MHATP) uses treponemal antigens attached to the surface of erythrocytes, which agglutinate when mixed with the serum from patients with syphilis. The MHATP is less sensitive than the FTA-ABS in primary syphilis (Table 274-1). Treponemal tests are generally used to confirm the diagnosis of syphilis in patients with reactive nontreponemal test results. The results are not routinely quantitated and usually remain reactive even many years after adequate treatment. False-positive treponemal test results but, surprisingly, not nontreponemal test results are seen in about 40% of patients with Lyme disease and some cases of rat-bite fever.

Certain facts regarding serodiagnosis should be borne in mind. Both treponemal and nontreponemal test results may be nonreactive in the patient who has just developed a chancre. Therefore a nonreactive test result for syphilis does not rule out the diagnosis in the patient whose lesion has just appeared.

In secondary syphilis all the serologic tests are reactive. Therefore a negative treponemal or nontreponemal serologic test result for syphilis essentially rules out secondary syphilis. This is particularly useful because the clinical diagnosis of secondary syphilis may be difficult. Rarely, antibody levels in secondary syphilis are so high that nontreponemal test results performed on undiluted serum may be false-negative. This so-called prozone phenomenon occurs in the setting of massive antibody excess. Quantitative test results, in which the serum is run at several dilutions, and treponemal test results remain reactive.

Nontreponemal test results for syphilis frequently become nonreactive in patients with late-stage syphilis. Patients having a workup for late-stage syphilis should have a treponemal test performed, even if the nontreponemal test results are nonreactive.

The treponemal test results usually remain positive for many years (possibly for life), even after adequate treatment for syphilis. Thus a persistently positive FTA-ABS test result is not an indication for retreating patients with a history of adequate therapy. An outline of the interpretation of serologic tests is given in Table 274-1.

Evaluation of cerebrospinal fluid. The laboratory diagnosis of neurosyphilis may be difficult. Evaluation should include a blood cell count, protein studies, and VDRL (not RPR) test. Each of these tests has relatively low sensitivity; negative results on any do not rule out the disease. Most patients with active neurosyphilis, however, have more than 5 white blood cells (usually lymphocytes)/mm^3 of CSF, although the counts are often less than 30 cells/mm^3. Protein levels may be slightly elevated. A reactive CSF-VDRL test result is considered diagnostic of neurosyphilis. Based on very few data, one might perform a CSF FTA-ABS test, recognizing that although the sensitivity for neurosyphilis is apparently very high, the specificity is low. The test result may be positive because a small amount of antitreponemal antibody has leaked into CSF from the systemic circulation. A negative test result probably rules out neurosyphilis to the extent possible by current means.

Therapy. Recommendations for the treatment of syphilis are summarized in Table 274-2. There is no evidence that *T. pallidum* has developed any resistance to penicillin. Some strains are highly resistant to erythromycin, which should be used only if no alternative can be found. Patients with syphilis and HIV infection should be given treatment with regimens that are effective against neurosyphilis.

More than half of the patients receiving treatment for early-stage syphilis with penicillin have a *Jarisch-Herxheimer reaction*. Usually beginning within 6 hours of treatment the reaction consists of fever, a transient exacerbation of skin lesions or adenopathy, occasional arthralgias, and, rarely, transient hypotension. The reaction is usually

Table 274-1 Interpretation of serologic test results for syphilis*

FINDING		INTERPRETATION OF FINDING: IS SYPHILIS PRESENT?*
NONTREPONEMAL TESTS	**TREPONEMAL TESTS**	
Nonreactive	Nonreactive	*Early primary syphilis is not ruled out by negative serologic test results.*
		Early syphilis is present in 13%-30% of patients who have a negative MHATP test result; in about 30% of patients who present with chancre but have a nonreactive reagin test; and in about 10% of patients who have a negative FTA-ABS test result.
		Late syphilis is present in a very small fraction of patients.
		Adequately treated syphilis in remote past may produce these results, but treponemal tests usually remain reactive.
	Reactive	Observed in about 10% of patients with chancre. The treponemal test results may turn positive shortly before the reagin tests. Reagin tests repeated after several days generally have positive results.
		In adequately treated early syphilis, the reagin test result may return to nonreactive within 1-2 years, whereas the treponemal test results generally do not.
		Late syphilis is not ruled out by a negative reagin test result. The sensitivity of the reagin tests is lower than that of treponemal tests in untreated late syphilis.
		In *secondary syphilis,* rarely, a highly reactive serum appears negative when tested undiluted with a reagin test because flocculation is inhibited by relative antibody excess. Not reported to occur with treponemal tests. Quantitative reagin test results are positive.
		False-positive treponemal test results occur in 40% of patients with Lyme disease.
Reactive	Nonreactive	Finding is not diagnostic of syphilis but constitutes a classic biologic false-positive reaction.
	Borderline (FTA-ABS)	Not diagnostic of syphilis: most patients (90%) with this pattern do not develop clinical or serologic evidence of syphilis. Repeat test is indicated. Chronic borderline results are associated with a variety of conditions other than syphilis.
	Beaded (FTA-ABS)	Not diagnostic of syphilis. Seen with collagen vascular disease.
	Reactive	Findings diagnostic of syphilis or other treponemal disease.
		In *adequately treated syphilis,* one would expect (1) a sustained fourfold drop in titer of reagin test, although reagin test result may remain positive after adequate therapy; (2) treponemal test results remain positive after adequate therapy.
		Concurrent false-positive results on both nontreponemal and treponemal tests could occur in rare instances. It may be impossible to rule out syphilis in an individual with this test profile.

*Serologic data must always be interpreted in the light of a total clinical evaluation. Diagnosis based on serologic criteria alone is fraught with error. Serologic tests apparently in conflict with clinical diagnosis should be confirmed by repetition or possibly referral to a reference laboratory.
FTA-ABS, Fluorescent trepomonal antibody-absorption test.

Table 274-2 Treatment of syphilis

DIAGNOSIS	RECOMMENDED TREATMENT	ALTERNATIVE PENICILLIN TREATMENT	IN PENICILLIN ALLERGY
Sexual contact to infectious syphilis (primary, secondary, early latent)	Benzathine penicillin G, 2.4 million U IM at a single treatment session	Procaine penicillin G, 600,000 U IM daily for 8 days	Tetracycline hydrochloride, 500 mg orally four times daily for 15 days or Doxycycline, 200 mg orally twice daily for 15 days or Ceftriaxone, 250 mg IM once*†
Early syphilis (primary, secondary, or latent of less than 1 year's duration)	Benzathine penicillin G, 2.4 million U IM at a single treatment session	Procaine penicillin G, 600,000 U IM daily for 8 days	Tetracycline hydrochloride, 500 mg orally four times daily for 15 days or Doxycycline, 200 mg orally twice daily for 15 days or Ceftriaxone, 250 mg IM once daily for 10 days*
Syphilis of more than 1 year's duration including latent, late benign, and cardiovascular	Benzathine penicillin G, 2.4 million U IM at weekly intervals for three doses	Procaine penicillin G, 600,000 U IM daily for 15 days	Doxycycline, 200 mg orally twice daily for 21 days or Ceftriaxone, 250 mg IM once daily for 14 days*
Neurosyphilis (asymptomatic paresis, tabes)	Aqueous crystalline penicillin G, 20 million U daily IV by continuous infusion or in divided doses, every 4 hours for 15 days‡	Procaine penicillin G, 600,000 U IM daily for 15 days	Doxycycline, 200 mg orally twice daily for 21 days or Ceftriaxone, 1 g IV once daily for 14 days*
Pregnancy	Regimen appropriate for stage of maternal syphilis	Regimen appropriate for stage of maternal syphilis	Ceftriaxone*§ or Consultation with an expert

*Ceftriaxone should not be used if there is a history of anaphylaxis to penicillin.
†This regimen appears to abort most but not all cases of incubating syphilis.
‡Some experts have suggested following this regimen with benzathine penicillin G as administered for syphilis of more than 1 year's duration.
§The treatment of syphilis in the penicillin-allergic pregnant patient is very difficult, and desensitization may be required. Consultation with an expert is recommended.
IM, Intramuscularly; *IV,* intravenously.

mild and abates in less than 24 hours. It is thought to result from the release of treponemal antigens on destruction of the organisms by penicillin or other antibiotics, and it can usually be managed with aspirin and reassurance.

The recommended treatment of early-stage syphilis in patients with HIV infection is the same as for other patients. Careful follow-up is critical. Serologic response to therapy is poorer among HIV-infected patients. However, it is not clear whether this is associated with worse clinical outcomes. Therapy for primary, secondary, or latent syphilis that achieves treponemocidal levels in the CNS does not alter disease progression compared with traditional regimens. A reactive CSF VDRL test result mandates treatment for neurosyphilis, but the presence of a low-level lymphocytic pleocytosis or low-grade elevation in the CSF protein level is often difficult to interpret. The conservative approach favors treatment of all patients with CSF abnormalities with regimens that are effective for neurosyphilis.

Nonvenereal Treponematoses

Spirochetes closely related to *T. pallidum* cause three non-STD infections that rarely are seen in the United States but are of great significance in other parts of the world. In these infections the skin or oral lesions contain large numbers of organisms that may be transmitted by personal, but not necessarily venereal, contact. Therefore, as one might expect, the diseases are most common in areas of poverty, poor hygiene, and overcrowding. Unlike venereal syphilis, these infections are generally acquired during childhood. Since the initial infection and spirochetemia occur before the childbearing years, congenital infection is essentially unknown. One theory holds that pinta is the oldest of the treponemal diseases and that the ancestral spirochete subsequently evolved to produce yaws, then bejel, and, finally, venereal syphilis. The organisms producing these diseases are morphologically identical to *T. pallidum,* and each infection elicits antibodies that are reactive in the nontreponemal and treponemal tests for syphilis. Thus, a reactive serologic test result for syphilis in a patient from an area endemic for any of these diseases should raise the possibility of the alternative diagnosis. All are treated successfully with long-acting penicillins.

Yaws. Yaws is common in the Caribbean, Latin America, Central Africa, and the Far East. In these tropical areas climate may contribute to dissemination by reducing the need for clothing. Three to 4 weeks after infection with *T. pertenue,* a papule develops that enlarges to form a raised, crusted lesion known as the *mother yaw.* As in syphilis, nontender regional adenopathy is common. Spirochetemia occurs, and 3 to 12 weeks later a diffuse papular eruption develops, with moist, raised, yellowish lesions that persist for 2 to 3 years and eventually become crusted. Involvement of the soles may make walking painful (crab yaws). In some colder climes, attenuated yaws may become evident as only a few lesions or even a single lesion. The skeletal system often is involved, and the resulting osteitis or periostitis may contribute to the pain. Late-stage yaws is quite similar to late-stage benign syphilis, with granulomatous lesions involving the skin and bones.

Pinta. Unlike the other treponematoses, pinta (infection with *T. carateum*) is limited to the skin. It is found only in Latin America. The initial, papular lesion appears 1 to 3 weeks after exposure and extends to become a scaly, flat, mildly pruritic patch accompanied by regional lymphadenopathy. Three to 9 months later, a generalized, scaly rash develops that may progress through a variety of changes of color including blue, violet, brown, and, finally, white. After 1 to 3 years depigmentation appears, usually on the extremities. Although the early lesions contain spirochetes, organisms rarely are demonstrated in the late-stage lesions.

Bejel. The spirochete of bejel is considered to be a variant of *T. pallidum.* It is found in saliva, and the infection is thought to be transmissible by kissing or by sharing eating utensils. Bejel is found in the eastern Mediterranean, the Balkans, and the cooler areas of northern Africa. Three weeks after infection a transient, painless oral lesion is occasionally recognized but often goes unnoticed. Spirochetemia occurs, and the usual initial presentation of bejel resembles that of secondary syphilis. Mucous patches, condylomata lata, and adenopathy develop. Unlike secondary syphilis, however, generalized rash and alopecia are quite rare. The late lesions of bejel resemble those of late-stage benign syphilis, and serpiginous skin lesions and bone pain are common.

Treatment. Nonvenereal treponematoses can all be treated with a single injection of 1.2 million U of benzathine penicillin G. As with the spirochete of syphilis, there is no evidence of increasing resistance to the penicillins on the part of other *Treponema* species. Penicillin-allergic patients presumably can be given treatment with tetracycline or erythromycin, but experience is limited.

INFECTIONS CAUSED BY LEPTOSPIRES (LEPTOSPIROSIS)
Organism

Leptospires are slender, tightly coiled, threadlike organisms with more than 200 serotypes. On dark-field microscopy leptospires appear actively motile, spinning rapidly about their long axis, and are distinguished by their terminal hooks.

Epidemiology

Leptospira interrogans is present worldwide but is more common in the tropics. In the United States, approximately 100 cases of leptospirosis are reported annually, either as sporadic cases or as small outbreaks. Most cases have occurred in Hawaii or the South Atlantic, Gulf, or Pacific coastal states.

Dogs, cattle, swine, mice, and rats are reservoirs for leptospires, usually as asymptomatic renal infection. Human infection occurs through exposure to contaminated urine. Outbreaks have been described in farm workers, veterinarians, rice field or sugarcane workers, and pet owners, either through direct contact with urine or indirect contact with contaminated soil or water. Household exposure has resulted from contact with domestic livestock, dogs, or rodent excreta, and outdoor recreational exposure is becoming more common.

Pathophysiologic Features

After penetrating the skin or mucous membrane the organisms disseminate throughout the body. Disease results from vasculitis leading to endothelial damage and hemorrhage. Liver failure is due to focal hepatocellular necrosis, renal failure is due to tubular epithelial necrosis and vasculitis, and pulmonary involvement includes patchy hemorrhagic pneumonitis. The pathophysiology of meningitis is unclear.

Clinical Manifestations

After an incubation period of 2 to 20 days (mean 10 days), the onset of illness is usually abrupt. Initial symptoms are nonspecific and include fever, chills, intense headache, myalgia, nausea, vomiting, and anorexia. Conjunctival suffusion, often in association with photophobia, occurs in 30% of cases and may be a valuable diagnostic clue. After initial symptoms human leptospirosis can be divided into two distinct clinical syndromes—anicteric leptospirosis and icteric leptospirosis.

Anicteric leptospirosis follows a biphasic course. Initially there is a septicemic phase associated with leptospiremia, which lasts approximately 7 days and is followed by a 2- to 3-day period of decreased fever. Recurrence of high fever marks the onset of the second, or immune, phase; it is temporally related to the appearance of immunoglobulin M (IgM) antibody and clearance of spirochetes from the blood. Aseptic meningitis is common in the immune phase. Early in the course of the meningitis neutrophils may predominate in the CSF, but, later, lymphocytes predominate. The CSF protein level may be elevated, but glucose level is normal. Uveitis, iritis, iridocyclitis, and chorioretinitis may also occur during the immune stage. Leptospiruria lasts for 1 to 3 weeks.

Icteric leptospirosis, also known as Weil's syndrome, is associated with hepatic, renal, and central nervous system (CNS) involvement. It comprises 10% to 15% of all cases of leptospirosis. The biphasic course of icteric leptospirosis may be obscured because of persistent fever. Jaundice and azotemia occur 3 to 7 days into the illness. Hepatic involvement may be mild or severe, with bilirubin levels reaching 60 to 80 mg/dl in extreme cases. The alkaline phosphatase, lactic dehydrogenase, serum aspartate aminotransferase, and serum alanine aminotransferase may all be elevated, usually two to three times normal and infrequently to the higher ranges typical of acute viral hepatitis. The hepatic lesions of leptospirosis are completely reversible.

Renal involvement can occur in both anicteric and icteric leptospirosis but is more severe in the icteric form. Renal insufficiency may begin 3 to 4 days into illness and peak at 2 weeks. Pyuria, hematuria, and proteinuria are common. Although the renal defect is usually reversible, anuria is associated with a poor outcome.

Skeletal muscle involvement occurs in 70% to 80% of cases in both forms of the disease and becomes evident as myalgia and elevated creatinine phosphokinase levels.

Other severe manifestations of icteric leptospirosis include vascular collapse, hemorrhagic pneumonitis, gastrointestinal tract hemorrhage, and myocarditis leading to congestive heart failure.

Laboratory Diagnosis

Leptospirosis is most often diagnosed on serologic testing by a fourfold rise in titer. Stable titers greater than or equal to 1:2000 are suggestive.

In the first 1 to 2 weeks after clinical onset leptospires can be cultured on special media from blood, urine, CSF, or tissue. Thereafter, urine provides the highest yield of positive cultures. Cultures may take up to 6 weeks to become positive.

Direct dark-field microscopy of urine or CSF specimens can sometimes be of value in the presumptive diagnosis of leptospirosis; however, misleading artifacts are commonly observed.

Treatment

Antibiotic therapy can shorten the duration of symptoms and reduce systemic, renal, and hepatic complications if started within 3 to 4 days of onset. Penicillin is the antibiotic of choice, and a dose of 1 million U intravenously every 6 hours has been recommended. As an alternative, tetracycline (250 to 500 mg orally every 6 hours) or doxycycline (100 mg orally twice a day) may be given. Therapy should continue for 7 to 10 days. The Jarisch-Herxheimer reaction has been reported with penicillin therapy and can be severe.

Prevention

Leptospirosis in prevented by personal protective measures, environmental sanitation, and vector control. Cases should be reported to public health authorities, since subsequent epidemiologic investigations have led to the discovery of large, common-source outbreaks. Doxycycline (200 mg orally once per week) can be given as chemoprophylaxis in individuals with significant exposure.

INFECTIONS CAUSED BY *BORRELIA* SPECIES (RELAPSING FEVER AND LYME DISEASE)

Borreliae are the causative agents of louse-borne relapsing fever (LBRF), tick-borne relapsing fever (TBRF), and Lyme disease. LBRF is caused by *Borrelia recurrentis*, TBRF is caused by over 15 borrelia species, and Lyme disease is caused by *Borrelia burgdorferi*.

Relapsing Fever

Epidemiology. Epidemic relapsing fever or LBRF is caused by *B. recurrentis* and is transmitted by the human body louse, *Pediculus humanus*. Humans are the only host for *B. recurrentis*. After a blood meal from an infected individual, *B. recurrentis* multiplies in the louse's hemolymph, and transmission to a new individual occurs when the fragile body of the louse is crushed during scratching, allowing the spirochetes to penetrate the skin of the new host. Epidemics of relapsing fever are usually associated with natural disasters,

wars, or famine. Although LBRF has been reported from all the inhabited continents except Australia, Africa is the only current major focus, with sporadic cases in Southeast Asia and South America. LBRF has not been reported in the United States during this century.

TBRF is caused by more than 15 borrelia species, which are categorized by their host-vector relationship. They are transmitted to man by ticks in the genus *Ornithodoros*. All tissues of the tick are infected, and transmission occurs through tick saliva or excrement during feeding. The disease occurs throughout the world, usually at higher altitudes in areas inhabited by small rodents. TBRF in the US occurs episodically in rural portion of the Western states. The largest US outbreak involved 62 campers in Arizona in 1973.

Pathophysiologic Features. Relapses are caused by the unusual ability of borreliae to change antigenic composition. This enables borreliae to escape lysis by antibody and phagocytosis by leukocytes, which are responsible for clearing spirochetes from the blood and thus for the clinical improvement between relapses. Clinical relapses occur when a new serotype proliferates, and clinical crises coincide with the appearance of antibody.

Clinical Features. Differences in clinical illness caused by the various *Borrelia* species, particularly those between LBRF and TBRF, are primarily differences in degree; LBRF tends to be a more severe illness than TBRF. After an incubation period of 5 to 9 days (range, 2 to 29 days), the spirochetes invade the bloodstream, and clinical illness begins suddenly with high fever, rigors, headache, myalgia, pain in small and large joints, nausea or vomiting, prostration, and, often, delirium. Eye pain, epistaxis, neck stiffness, nonproductive cough, and abdominal pain occur less commonly. Tachycardia and tachypnea are almost always present, whereas the frequency of other physical findings varies. These include jaundice, meningismus, and upper-quadrant abdominal tenderness with or without hepatomegaly or splenomegaly. Bleeding disorders, which can become evident as epistaxis or petechial rash, occur in up to half of patients. Neurologic manifestations, notably meningitis, encephalitis, or intracranial hemorrhage, may be prominent. A macular rash (usually occurring at the end of the first attack) has been described, and pulmonary edema attributable to myocarditis has been reported.

The first attack lasts, on average, 5 to 6 days in LBRF and 3 days in TBRF. Untreated, it ends by crisis, which becomes evident as sweating and an abrupt drop in temperature followed by hypotension and prostration. Rash, change in mental status, jaundice, and pulmonary edema suggest a poor prognosis. The overall mortality rate is 30% to 70% for untreated cases compared with 3% to 5% for treated ones. Death during treatment is often associated with the Jarisch-Herxheimer reaction leading to circulatory collapse. If untreated, zero to three relapses typically occur in LBRF, and three to five in TBRF. The interval between the first attack and the subsequent relapse is 5 to 6 days in LBRF and slightly longer in TBRF. Successive relapses become shorter and milder.

Spontaneous abortion occurs in 40% of infected pregnant women. Transplacental transmission may result in neonatal infection.

Laboratory Diagnosis. Diagnosis depends on demonstration of borreliae in the blood (or, rarely, CSF) or urine. The spirochetes can be visualized in fresh specimens by dark-field microscopy or, in stained smears, by light microscopy at a magnification of 400× to 1000×. Borreliae are the only spirochetes in the blood that are stainable with aniline dyes (Giemsa or Wright's); thin and thick smears are diagnostic in 70% of cases, and repeated smears may increase this yield (Fig. 274-1). The *Borrelia* index (number of spirochetes per white blood cell in a thick smear) provides a clue to the severity of illness; indices greater than two are associated with more severe complications. Organisms are rarely visualized in the blood between relapses and become increasingly difficult to find during subsequent relapses. Serologic tests are unreliable because of antigenic variation, and culture requires special techniques.

Other laboratory findings are nonspecific. The white blood cell count is usually normal but may be high or low; a left shift is common. Thrombocytopenia is common, particularly in patients with petechiae. Results of clotting studies are often abnormal, but disseminated intravascular coagulation is rare. The aspartate aminotransfer-

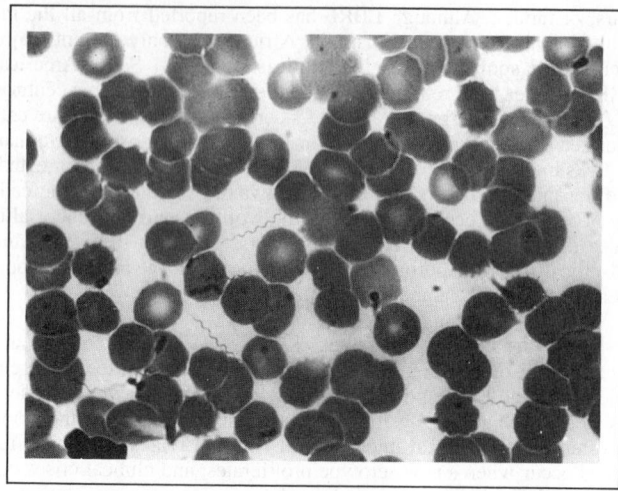

FIGURE 274-1   Giemsa stain of thin blood smear shows *Borrelia* spirochetes.

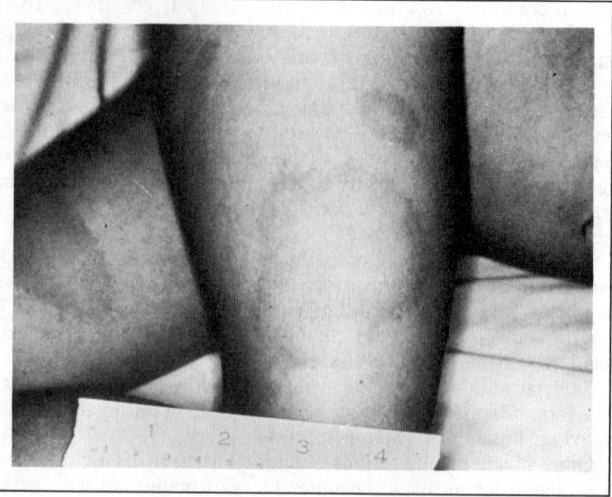

FIGURE 274-2   Multiple erythema migrans skin lesions.
From AC Steere et al: Erythema chronicum migrans and Lyme arthritis: the enlarging clinical spectrum, *Ann Intern Med* 86:685, 1977.

ase and bilirubin levels are usually mildly to moderately elevated. Nontreponemal test results for syphilis are occasionally reactive. The CSF contains primarily mononuclear cells during CNS involvement.

Treatment. Erythromycin, tetracycline, doxycycline, chloramphenicol, and penicillin are all employed. For TBRF, 500 mg of oral tetracycline every 6 hours for 5 to 10 days is recommended for adults. For LBRF a single oral dose of 500 mg of tetracycline or erythromycin, or 100 mg of doxycycline, has proved highly effective. In one study of LBRF, low-dose penicillin (100,000 U of procaine penicillin intramuscularly) was associated with more frequent relapses than either high-dose penicillin (200,000 or 400,000 U) or tetracycline (500 mg orally) but was also associated with lower mortality as a result of slower clearance of spirochetemia and a milder Jarisch-Herxheimer reaction.

All patients with LBRF should, if possible, be hospitalized and monitored for at least 24 hours after fluid resuscitation for hypotension or supportive measures for cardiac failure. The Jarisch-Herxheimer reaction can be treated with acetaminophen (650 mg orally) or hydrocortisone (500 mg intravenously) 2 hours before and 2 hours after the administration of antimicrobials.

Prevention. LBRF can be prevented by eliminating the poor hygienic conditions that favor the maintenance and spread of body lice. Emergency measures among groups at high risk, such as refugees, include providing a change of clothing and facilities for washing, as well as treating clothes with insecticidal agents. TBRF can be prevented by avoiding known habitats of *Ornithodoros* ticks, such as rodent-infested caves and cabins; removing rodent nests from dwellings; and rodent-proofing and applying acaricidal agents to known infested dwellings. Preparations containing N, N-diethyl-meta-toluamide (DEET) can be applied as tick repellents to skin and clothing, and permethrin-based acaricides can be applied to clothes and outer bedding in situations of high risk of exposure to infected ticks.

Lyme Disease

Lyme disease, first described in Lyme, Connecticut, in 1975, is a multisystem infection by *B. burgdorferi*. It begins with a characteristic skin lesion, erythema migrans (EM) (Fig. 274-2), which may be followed by neurologic, cardiac, and joint involvement.

Organism. *B. burgdorferi* is longer and more loosely coiled than other spirochetes. There are three genomic groups of the *B. burgdorferi sensu latu* complex. *B. burgdorferi sensu stricto* is most common in the United States, while *B. garinii* and *B. afzelii* are most common in Europe.

Epidemiology. *B. burgdorferi* is carried by hard ticks of the genus *Ixodes*. Different species have been described as vectors on each

continent where Lyme disease has been reported. In the United States Lyme disease occurs at highest incidence in three broad geographic areas: northeastern coastal states from Massachusetts to Virginia, the upper Midwest (especially Wisconsin and Minnesota), and northern California. The species of *Ixodes* in the United States include *Ixodes (dammini) pacificus* (along the Pacific coast) and *Ixodes scapularis* (northeastern, midwestern, southeastern and south-central states). Ixodes may also be infected with *Babesia* organisms (Chapter 279) in the Northeast and Midwest, which can lead to coinfection in 10% of individuals with Lyme disease.

The white-footed mouse (*Peromyscus leucopus*) in the East and the wood rat (*Neotoma fuscipes*) in California are reservoirs in the life cycle of *B. burgdorferi* infection, which involves transstadial transmission from larva to nymph and maintenance of adult tick populations by deer. Humans usually acquire Lyme disease from the bite of infective nymphs in the late spring and early summer. The rates of infection of *I. scapularis* with *B. burgdorferi* in endemic areas of the United States are in the range of 25% and 50%, respectively. In contrast, only 1% to 2% of *I. pacificus* ticks are infected with *B. burgdorferi* in the western United States.

Lyme disease has become the most frequently reported arthropod-borne disease in the United States. In 1994, 13,083 cases were reported to the Centers for Disease Control and Prevention (CDC), which is 58% more than 1993 and a 65 fold increase from the 497 cases reported in 1982 . The national incidence was 5.2 per 100,000 population in 1994, ranging from 0 in several states (Alaska, Hawaii, Arizona, Montana, North Dakota, and Mississippi) to 62.2 per 100,000 in Connecticut. The reported incidence in school-aged children in Connecticut has been as high as 10.1/1000 person-years for symptomatic disease and 3.8/1000 person-years for asymptomatic disease. Eighty-eight percent of cases were reported from Connecticut, Rhode Island, New York, New Jersey, Delaware, Pennsylvania, Wisconsin, and Maryland. Some of this increase may be due to rising rates of infection (15% to 25%) in *I. scapularis* in the Northeast. Most cases have onset of illness in the months of May to August, reflecting times of greatest human outdoor activity and nymphal tick activity.

Pathophysiologic Features. Direct tissue invasion by *B. burgdorferi* and host immunologic response are thought to interact in the production of the various clinical manifestations of the disease. Early in the infection, *B. burgdoferi* can be isolated from biopsy specimens of EM. The organism widely disseminates, with variable rates of isolation from other sites of involvement.

Immunoglobulin M antibodies to *B. burgdorferi* develop within 2 to 4 weeks after the onset of EM, peak after 6 to 8 weeks of illness, and disappear after 4 to 6 months of illness in most cases. Immunoglobulin G (IgG) antibodies are usually detectable within 6 to 8 weeks after the onset of EM, peak at 4 to 6 months after onset, and remain elevated indefinitely in adequately treated, asymptomatic patients and in patients with persistent infection. Antibiotic treatment of early-stage Lyme disease can abort a detectable antibody response.

Circulating immune complexes can be found in most patients with EM, and high levels are maintained in the blood of patients in whom neurologic or cardiac complications subsequently develop. Patients in whom these complications never develop or in whom only arthritis develops lose immune complexes from the blood, although high titers exist in the synovial fluid of patients with arthritis. It is unclear whether chronic arthritis is due to an autoimmune response involving autoreactive T cells and interleukin-1 or whether it is due to persistent infection.

Clinical Manifestations. Lyme disease is an acute and chronic, multisystemic inflammatory disease with protean manifestations. The disease has been divided into early and late stages, the manifestations of which often overlap but may also occur independently. In most patients all of the major manifestations do not develop, and asymptomatic infections may occur.

In most cases Lyme disease begins with the appearance of erythema at the site of the tick bite occurring 3 to 32 days (median, 7 days) after the tick bite; however, fewer than 25% of patients remember a tick bite. Over days to weeks spirochetes migrate outward in the skin, producing the characteristic large, expanding, annular lesion of EM. In as many as half of cases, secondary skin lesions occur elsewhere within a few days of the first, suggesting blood-borne dissemination of spirochetes. Most patients with EM have constitutional symptoms of low-grade fever, fatigue, myalgia, arthralgia, headache (occasionally excruciating), and stiff neck. In about 10% of patients symptoms of transient hepatitis develop. Lymphadenopathy, either regional or generalized, occurs in about one third of cases. In some patients signs of aseptic meningitis and meningoencephalitis develop. Conjunctivitis and endophthalmitis with impairment of vision may occur.

Untreated EM and associated early symptoms last about 3 weeks, but occasionally longer. Without treatment, neurologic abnormalities accompany EM in about 10% to 15% of patients. Four neurologic syndromes occur with acute dissemination of the spirochete: meningitis, cranial neuritis, radiculoneuropathy, and meningoencephalitis. Facial palsy occurs in 11% of cases and is bilateral in 23% of these. The most common neurologic symptom is headache, sometimes accompanied by signs of meningeal irritation and, less frequently, encephalitis. There are no specific neuroimaging findings. Patients with meningitic symptoms often have lymphocytic pleocytosis in CSF, and *B. burgdorferi* has been cultured from the fluid. Peripheral nervous system involvement most often becomes evident as motor and sensory radiculoneuritis, mononeuritis multiplex, or diffuse peripheral sensorimotor neuropathy in various combinations. Cardiac involvement, which becomes evident most commonly as prolonged first-degree atrioventricular block and, more rarely, as cardiomyopathy, occurs less frequently than neurologic abnormalities. Prolonged first-degree block (more than 0.30 milliseconds) appears particularly likely to progress, often precipitously, to higher degrees of heart block.

Arthritis usually begins somewhat later (median period, 4 weeks after onset of EM) than neurologic and cardiac manifestations. Initially, brief attacks (median, 8 days) of pain or swelling (or both) occur, usually in the large joints, separated by months of remission. Systemic symptoms (e.g., fever and malaise) may recur with attacks of arthritis. In about 10% of these patients chronic arthritis develops, which on clinical and pathologic examination resembles rheumatoid arthritis; alloantigen DRw2 occurs with increased frequency in patients with chronic Lyme arthritis.

Months to years after the initial infection with *B. burgdorferi*, patients with Lyme disease may have chronic encephalopathy, polyneuropathy, or less commonly, leukoencephalitis. Memory, mood, and sleep disturbances commonly occur in persons with encephalopathy.

Patients with encephalopathy usually produce intrathecal antibodies to the spirochete, may have evidence of continuing active infection, and usually improve with antibiotic therapy. Many of these patients also have peripheral nervous symptoms, either distal paresthesias or spinal or radicular pain. Electrophysiologic testing may reveal an axonal polyneuropathy. Chronic neurologic Lyme disease may be difficult to distinguish from multiple sclerosis or Alzheimer's

syndrome. Intrathecal antibody production, the presence of lesions in the periventricular white matter, and the absence of myelin basic protein or oligoclonal bands in CSF argue against a diagnosis of multiple sclerosis.

Laboratory Diagnosis. A diagnosis of Lyme disease should be based on compatible symptoms and signs in a patient with a reasonable probability of previous contact with ticks in an endemic area. Interlaboratory and serial testing of duplicate specimens has been highly variable in commercial laboratories. Current laboratory tests (with the exception of a positive culture for *B. burgdorferi*) are imperfect adjuncts only. Overdiagnosis based on serologic findings in the absence of characteristic clinical findings has led to overtreatment and severe antibiotic-related complications, including ceftriaxone-induced cholecystitis. In areas endemic for Lyme disease the diagnosis can be made on clinical grounds alone in the presence of classic EM. Diagnostic difficulty occurs with early-stage or atypical EM or when compatible systemic symptoms or signs occur in the absence of EM.

Culture of *B. burgdorferi* from infected tissues is highly specific but has low sensitivity and is only reliable from punch skin biopsy, which yields the organism in 50% to 80% of specimens.

The most commonly used serologic tests for Lyme disease include enzyme-linked immunosorbent assay (ELISA), immunofluorescent assay (IFA), and Western immunoblot. False-positive results may occur in 5% to 12% of specimens in low endemic areas and may be due to infections with other spirochetes (such as *T. pallidum* or normal oral flora), endocarditis, or other inflammatory conditions. Since false-positive results are common, ELISA and IFA tests should not be used as screening tests.

Because of the delayed antibody response, these test results are often negative in early-stage disease. Western immunoblots have higher specificity (>95%) but low sensitivity (30% to 40%) in early-stage infection. The sensitivity of the Western immunoblot increases in late-stage infections, and the test result can remain positive up to 3 years after adequate treatment. The Western immunoblot can be helpful in confirming a positive ELISA result in a two-step procedure. The CDC has recommended a two-test approach (similar to that for syphilis or HIV infection) using either ELISA or IFA followed by a Western immunoblot. Specimens that are negative on ELISA or IFA need not be confirmed by Western immunoblot. Both IgM and IgG procedures are required when Western immunoblot is performed in the first 4 weeks of illness, and the IgM response may be falsely negative in people with disease present for more than 1 month. For those with disease of greater than 1 month's duration, a positive IgM result by itself should not be used to diagnose active disease because of high rates of false-positive results with other infections. Two of three bands are necessary for a positive IgM result, and 5 of 10 bands are necessary for a positive IgG result with the Western immunoblot.

Clinical suspicion of CNS Lyme disease is an indication for lumbar puncture. Patients with CNS Lyme disease commonly have lymphocytic pleocytosis, and many have evidence of intrathecal production of antibodies to *B. burgdorferi*, as evidenced by higher titers in CSF than in serum. Polymerase chain reaction in the CSF is specific but insensitive (25% to 66%) in the diagnosis of neurologic disease.

Treatment. For early Lyme disease with EM and without evidence of CNS involvement the current drug of choice is doxycycline, 100 mg twice a day, or amoxicillin, 250 to 500 mg three or four times a day (with or without probenecid 500 mg three or four times a day) given orally for 10 to 21 days. Erythromycin (250 mg four times a day orally) can be used in penicillin-allergic patients for whom tetracyclines are contraindicated (e.g., pregnant or lactating women) but is generally considered inferior to amoxicillin or doxycycline. In double-blind randomized trials, doxycycline was equivalent to ceftriaxone and azithromycin was less likely to result in resolution of disease and had higher rates of relapse than amoxicillin.

Therapy for later stages and more severe manifestations of Lyme disease continues to be controversial. Few controlled clinical studies have been reported. For Lyme arthritis without evidence of CNS involvement oral doxycycline or amoxicillin with probenecid for 1 month appears to be effective. Ceftriaxone (2 g daily) and penicillin G (20 million U daily) for 2 to 3 weeks intravenously have also been used in those who fail to respond or relapse after oral therapy. Joint rest is indicated, and joint aspiration may have therapeutic benefit. Concurrent intraarticular corticosteroids may increase risk of antibiotic failure. Inflammation may persist for variable periods after successful antibiotic treatment of Lyme arthritis. If joint inflammation has not resolved after 1 month of antibiotic therapy, antiinflammatory agents and a waiting period of 3 months before retreatment may be warranted. Arthroscopic synovectomy may be of value in patients with persistent chronic arthritis that is not responsive to repeated courses of antibiotics.

Lyme disease of the CNS should be treated with intravenous antibiotics for at least 2 weeks. Ceftriaxone is preferred, but penicillin G has also been used. Lyme facial palsy without pleocytosis or evidence of intrathecal production of antibodies to *B. burgdorferi,* can be treated successfully with oral antibiotics (doxycycline alone or amoxicillin with probenecid).

Lyme carditis is generally a self-limited condition. Mild manifestations (e.g., first-degree atrioventricular block) may respond to oral antibiotics. Intravenous ceftriaxone or penicillin G has been used for more severe cardiac manifestations. Insertion of a temporary pacemaker may be necessary for some patients with complete heart block.

In general, therapy for Lyme disease in pregnant and lactating women is the same as in other adults. Tetracyclines, however, should not be used, and the safety of probenecid in pregnancy is unknown. Intravenous penicillin should be considered when there is evidence of disseminated disease.

Persistent levels of IgG and IgM antibodies to *B. burgdorferi* do not necessarily indicate persistent infection. Therefore the efficacy of antibiotic treatment should be judged on clinical response.

Prevention. Personal protection from bites of infective ticks is the principal prevention measure. The chance of a tick bite is reduced by avoiding tick-infested areas, wearing light-colored clothing so that ticks can be spotted more easily, and tucking pant legs into socks or boot tops. Insect repellents containing DEET can be applied to clothes and exposed skin other than the face, and permethrin compounds, which kill ticks on contact, can be sprayed on clothing. Application of acaricides to gardens, lawns, and the edge of woodlands near homes is being used to suppress vector ticks in some areas, as is the distribution of acaricide-impregnated cotton used by mice for nest building. One of the most important preventive measures is the early detection and proper removal by tweezers of ticks from the skin. Transmission of *B. burgdorferi* from an infected tick is unlikely to occur before 36 hours of attachment, and the risk of infection with *B. burgdorferi* after promptly removing an attached tick is only 1% to 3%, even in endemic areas. Therefore treatment of asymptomatic tick bites is not routinely indicated.

A recombinant vaccine has been developed against the outer-surface protein A (Osp-A). This vaccine has the highest potential benefit in the United States, where *B. burgdorferi* isolates are relatively uniform, whereas a polyvalent vaccine may be necessary to cover the more diverse isolates found in Europe. The Osp-A vaccine has shown high levels of protection in mice challenged with *B. burgdorferi.* Furthermore, spirochete numbers in ticks feeding on vaccinated mice are dramatically reduced or eliminated which suggests that the vaccine may have an effect in the vector before it is able to transmit the infection to the host. Phase I studies in humans have found good antibody response without serious toxicity, and efficacy studies are under way.

BIBLIOGRAPHY

Bakken LL, Case KL, Callister SM, et al: Performance of 45 laboratories participating in a proficiency testing program for Lyme disease serology, *JAMA* 268:891, 1992.

Brudge DR, O'Hanlon DP: Experience at a referral center of patients with suspected Lyme disease in an area of nonendemicity: first 65 patients, *Clin Infect Dis* 16:558, 1993.

Centers for Disease Control and Prevention: 1993 Sexually transmitted diseases treatment guidelines, *MMWR* 42(RR-14):27, 1993.

Centers for Disease Control and Prevention: Lyme disease: United States, 1994, *MMWR* 44:459, 1995.

Centers for Disease Control and Prevention: Recommendation for test performance and interpretation from the Second National Conference of Serologic Diagnosis of Lyme Disease, *MMWR* 44:591, 1995.

Dattwyler RL et al: Treatment of late Lyme borreliosis: randomized comparison of ceftriaxone and penicillin, *Lancet* 1:1194, 1988.

Dattwyler RJ, Luft BJ, Kunkel MJ et al: Ceftriaxone compared with doxycycline for the treatment of acute disseminated Lyme disease, *N Engl J Med* 337:289, 1997.

Farr RW: Leptospirosis, *Clin Infect Dis* 21:1, 1995.

Fiumara N: The diagnosis and treatment of infectious syphilis, *Compr Ther* 21:639, 1995.

Flores JL: Syphilis: a tale of twisted treponemes, *West J Med* 163:552, 1995.

Hutchinson CM et al: Altered presentation of early syphilis in patients with human immunodeficiency virus infection, *Ann Intern Med* 121:94, 1994.

Koff AB, Rosen T: Nonvenereal treponematoses: yaws, endemic syphilis, and bejel, *J Am Acad Dermatol* 29:519, 1993.

Larsen SA et al: Laboratory diagnosis and interpretation of tests for syphilis, *Clin Microbiol Rev* 8:1, 1995.

Meheus A, Antal GM: The endemic treponematoses: not yet eradicated, *World Health Stat Q* 45:228, 1992.

Meyer JC: Laboratory diagnosis of syphilis, *Curr Probl Dermatol* 24:1, 1996.

Nandwani R: Modern diagnosis and management of acquired syphilis, *Br J Hosp Med* 55:399, 1996.

Rahlenbeck SI, Gebre-Yohannes A: Louse-borne relapsing fever and its treatment, *Trop Geo Med* 47:49, 1995.

Rolfs RT: Treatment of syphilis 1993, *Clin Infect Dis* 20(suppl 1):S23, 1995.

Rolfs RT, Joesoef MR, Hendershot EF et al: A randomized trial of enhanced therapy for early syphilis in patients with and without human immunodeficiency virus infection, *N Engl J Med* 337:307, 1997.

Romanowski B et al: Serologic response to treatment of infectious syphilis, *Ann Intern Med* 114:1005, 1991.

Schofer H et al: Active syphilis in HIV infection: a multicentre retrospective survey, *Genitourin Med* 72:176, 1996.

Seboxa T, Rahlenbeck SI: Treatment of louse-bourne relapsing fever with low-dose penicillin of tetracycline: a clinical trial, *Scand J Infect Dis* 27:29, 1995.

Sigal LH: Lyme disease: *primum non nocere, J Infect Dis* 171:423, 1995.

Spach DH, Liles CW, Campbell GL et al: Tick-borne diseases in the United States, *N Engl J Med* 329:936, 1993.

---

275 Infection With *Mycobacterium leprae* (Leprosy)

Reuben Granich and Jonathan H. Mermin

Leprosy (Hansen's disease) is a chronic granulomatous disease caused by *Mycobacterium leprae*. The broad clinical spectrum of the disease reflects individual variation in cell-mediated immunity. Tuberculoid leprosy occurs in hosts with high immunologic resistance; lepromatous leprosy occurs in those with minimal resistance. Morbidity in leprosy results from host response rather than organism virulence and occurs by three major mechanisms: *M. leprae* skin and nerve infiltration causing a destructive tissue response, immune-complex formation resulting in generalized illness, and nerve obliteration leading to palsies and neurotropic injury.

Leprosy has been present in India and China since at least 600 BC. It was probably introduced into Mediterranean countries by Alexandrian armies returning from the Indian campaign in the 4th century BC. Peak prevalence occurred in Europe between AD1100 and AD1300 and declined thereafter, probably as a result of improvements in standards of living. The first case of leprosy in the United States occurred in 1758.

Persons with leprosy experience great social stigma. Historically they have been singled out for isolation, forced to wear clappers or bells, forbidden to marry, and buried alive. Discrimination remains a concern for many patients with leprosy. At the same time, marked changes have occurred in the prognosis and management of leprosy in the past two decades. The advent of multidrug therapy and improved leprosy control programs has resulted in better treatment, earlier diagnosis, and less discrimination.

MICROBIOLOGY

Gerhard A. Hansen identified *M. leprae* in 1873, making it the second known bacterium associated with human disease. *M. leprae* is a slender rod (1 to 8 μm long and 0.25 to 0.5 μm wide) that is indistinguishable on morphologic examination from other mycobacteria.

Table 275-1   Clinical, histologic, and immunologic features of leprosy

CLINICAL FEATURES	TUBERCULOID	BORDERLINE	LEPROMATOUS
Skin lesions			
Numbers	One to three	Several to many	Very many
Symmetry	Asymmetric	Asymmetric to symmetric	Symmetric
Anesthesia	Profound	Moderate	None
Neuropathy			
Thickening of sensory cutaneous nerves	Common	Absent	Absent
Thickening of nerves of predilection	0 to 2	Several, asymmetric	Delayed, symmetric
Histologic			
Granuloma cell	Epithelioid	Epithelioid or histiocyte	Foamy histiocyte
Lymphocytes	Plentiful	Moderate	Rare to absent
Bacilli	Absent	Present	Overwhelming
Lymph nodes	Normal	Epithelioid paracortical Infiltration	Paracortical replacement and germinal center hypertrophy
Immunologic			
Lepromin test	Strongly positive	Weakly positive or negative	Negative
In vitro cell-mediated immunity	Vigorous	Weak or absent	Absent
Hyperglobulinemia and false-positive serologic result	Absent	Absent	Common
Reactions			
Type I (lepra)	Rare	Very common	Rare
Type II (erythema nodosum leprosum)	Never	Possible	Common

It is an obligate intracellular parasite; however, it can remain viable outside the body for several days. *M. leprae* has not been cultured in vitro, but the organisms grow well when inoculated into the footpads of mice. This technique exploits the preference of *M. leprae* for cooler body parts and demonstrates its extremely long generation time of 12 to 14 days. *M. leprae* is acid- and alcohol-fast and easily stained in tissue sections or homogenates by the Ziehl-Neelsen technique. The cytoplasm of *M. leprae* is variably stained; a uniformly bright appearance indicates viablility; a beaded appearance indicates nonviability. This property is used to determine the *morphologic index* or percentage of viable organisms in tissue sections and skin smears. The *bacteriologic index,* a logarithmic measurement of the numbers of acid-fast bacilli in the dermis, is also used in evaluating patients and determining effectiveness of drug therapy. The cellular components responsible for pathogenicity and survival are not well understood. The best-characterized virulence factor is the surface lipid phenolic-glycolipid-I (PGL). PGL binds complement component C3 and protects the bacterium from oxidative killing. Primates and the nine-banded armadillo are the only known natural hosts.

EPIDEMIOLOGY

Leprosy is endemic in most of the tropical and warm-temperate countries of the world. Determinations of incidence and prevalence are often inaccurate because of limited resources for health care in the areas most affected and the stigma attached to the diagnosis. However, it is estimated that 1.8 million persons currently have active leprosy, compared with 5.5 million in 1992, and that 1 to 2 million are visibly disabled from the disease. Reductions in the prevalence of leprosy are due to leprosy control campaigns using multidrug treatment (MDT) regimens. The Indian subcontinent, South America, Africa, Southeast Asia, and the islands of the South Pacific are the most affected by the disease. India has 58% of the world's cases. Although rare, there are approximately 6000 cases in the United States with an annual incidence of about 200 cases, almost all acquired abroad. Endemic areas include Louisiana, Texas, California, and Hawaii. Only 25% of patients with imported disease were known to have leprosy at the time of immigration; 75% were first diagnosed in the United States. Immigrants with leprosy present no health risk to the U.S. population, since secondary transmission from imported cases does not seem to occur. The relative proportion of tuberculoid and lepromatous forms varies geographically; for example, 90% of cases are

tuberculoid in India and Africa, 50% in Southeast Asia, and 10% in Mexico.

The exact mechanism of leprosy transmission is not known, although inhalation of nasal secretions and skin contact are the most likely. Nasal secretions can contain more than 10^7 organisms/ml, and skin, 10^9 organisms/g; these mycobacteria remain viable for days. Few organisms are found or shed from unbroken epidermis. Trauma, secondary infection, and certain lepra reactions that cause epidermal exfoliation may increase risk of spread. The risk of infection is related to the closeness of contact, the bacillary burden of the index case, and the age of the exposed individual. Lepromatous leprosy, which is highly bacilliferous, is five times as contagious as the tuberculoid form, which is paucibacillary. Children are more susceptible than adults to the lepromatous form, and the prevalence in men is twice that in women. If a person in an endemic country contracts leprosy, there is a 10% chance that someone else in the house will become infected. However, in nonendemic countries such as the United States, leprosy develops in only 1% of household contacts.

PATHOPHYSIOLOGIC FEATURES

M. leprae is a highly infective organism with low pathogenicity; host factors are of paramount importance in determining morbidity. The organism enters through the skin or respiratory mucosa and, if not contained locally, disseminates hematogenously. The median incubation period is 3 to 5 years and, rarely, up to 40 years. The disease differentiates into one of its polar types (lepromatous or tuberculoid) or an intermediate or borderline form, depending on the cell-mediated immune competence of the host (Table 275-1). The manifestations of leprosy vary continuously from a form seen in patients with a vigorous cell-mediated response to that seen in patients with no effective reaction to infection. The Ridley-Jopling classification divides this spectrum into five groupings: tuberculoid, borderline tuberculoid, borderline, borderline lepromatous, and lepromatous. More recently, the World Health Organization devised a simplified classification based on numbers of *M. leprae* that patients harbor: paucibacillary (tuberculoid) and multibacillary (smear-positive borderline tuberculoid, borderline, borderline lepromatous, and lepromatous).

The forms of leprosy differ in prognosis, complications, and response to therapy. Patients with tuberculoid leprosy demonstrate vigorous granuloma formation, with recruitment of lymphocytes, epithelioid cells, and giant cells. Bacilli are rarely found; nerve damage is the result of inflammation and granuloma formation rather than mycobacterial destruction. Dermal nerve damage caused by granulomas is almost pathognomonic of leprosy and aids in distinguishing it from other granulomatous processes.

In contrast, patients with lepromatous leprosy have no effective cell-mediated response to *M. leprae*. It is unclear whether this lack of cell-mediated immunity is caused by or results from infection. Lepromatous disease is characterized by widespread dissemination of bacilli and by granuloma formation with foamy, vacuolated, fat-laden macrophages and few lymphocytes. Because of diminished host defense, nerve destruction is delayed, although bacillary infiltration may be more intense. There is, however, exuberant antibody production, which, although unable to control the infection, is responsible for the systemic, immune-complex–mediated complications of lepromatous leprosy. Both T-cell and macrophage defects have been described in patients with lepromatous leprosy. The lepromin test result is negative in lepromatous patients; however, they have normal immune responses to purified protein derivative if they are concomitantly infected with *Mycobacterium tuberculosis*.

The borderline forms of leprosy have intermediate histologic features and are immunologically unstable, shifting toward lepromatous disease with intercurrent infection or other stress, or toward the tuberculoid pole after treatment.

The earliest manifestations of leprosy are skin lesions. These hypopigmented, anesthetic patches can be single or multiple, have well- or ill-defined margins, and have a scaly or smooth surface. The lesions may heal without sequelae, or the disease may progress to any of the differentiated forms of leprosy.

CLINICAL FEATURES

Tuberculoid leprosy is characterized by one to three large (3 to 30 cm in diameter) annular macules or plaques with a raised erythematous edge and a depressed hypopigmented center. They are typically dry, hairless, scaly, and anesthetic and may occur anywhere, although the scalp, perineum, and skin folds tend to be spared. The face, extremities, and buttocks are most commonly affected. The sensory cutaneous nerves supplying the affected region are involved, and sensations of touch, pain, and temperature are completely lost. As the disease persists, thickening and, sometimes, tenderness of one or two of the larger neighboring peripheral nerves occur at typical locations: the ulnar nerve above the elbow, the posterior tibial nerve below the malleolus, the external popliteal nerve at the head of the fibula, and the facial and greater auricular nerves. The morbidity of the disease results from denervation leading to motor palsies and severe neuropathic damage to the extremities. Involvement of the facial nerve causes lagophthalmos and subsequent blindness.

Borderline leprosy is characterized by multiple skin lesions that are smaller than those of the tuberculoid form. Typically, they are red plaques or macules with a broad, irregular rim and a "punched out" center and are only minimally anesthetic. There is widespread, severe neuropathy involving both the small cutaneous nerves and many of the larger peripheral trunks. Neuritic leprosy is most often seen in patients with borderline infections and becomes evident with involvement of one or more of the major nerve trunks without cutaneous lesions. Patients with neuritic leprosy often have painful, enlarged nerves; regional anaesthesia; paresis; and muscular wasting.

The cutaneous features of lepromatous leprosy are multiplicity of skin lesions and marked bilateral symmetry, especially in the cooler body parts such as earlobes. The lesions take the form of nodules, papules, or plaques with hazy margins that blend into surrounding skin. The surface is smooth and shiny. Diffuse infiltration of the skin can cause facial coarsening that is referred to as leonine facies. The lateral one third of the eyebrows may be lost, and infiltration of the nasal mucosa and facial bones leads to nasal congestion, bleeding, and septal perforation. Atrophy of the anterior nasal spines and maxillary processes causes collapse. Extension of infection to the anterior ocular structures produces uveitis, keratitis, and blindness. Local induration results in subcutaneous mobile nodules of variable size, which are commonly found on the face and earlobes. Testicular damage leads to atrophy and gynecomastia. The liver, spleen, bone marrow, and kidneys may be involved. In pure lepromatous leprosy peripheral nerves are spared until late in the disease, but there may be a "stocking-glove" neuropathy as a result of dermal infiltration. In advanced lepromatous disease, peripheral nerve disease leads to widespread neuropathic deformities similar to complications from diabetes mellitus.

There are three types of reaction seen in patients with leprosy: lepra type I, lepra type II (erythema nodosum leprosum), and the Lucio phenomenon or reaction. Lepra type I reactions are seen in patients with nonpolar forms of leprosy and represent a delayed type IV hypersensitivity reaction. In some patients the reaction is followed by a shift toward the tuberculoid pole (reversal reaction); in others the reaction is followed by a permanent deterioration associated with lepromatous features, including a negative lepromin test result and increased numbers of bacilli in lesions (downgrading reaction). Type I reactions may be triggered by (1) multidrug therapy, especially those including dapsone; (2) vitamin A, iodides, or bromide; (3) intercurrent infections; (4) vaccinations; (5) pregnancy and lactation; or (6) other physiologic or psychologic stress. Skin lesions become erythematous and tender, and may ulcerate. Peripheral nerves swell, become tender, and may suffer rapid and permanent ischemic damage if constriction within the sheath occurs.

Erythema nodosum leprosum (ENL) is due to immune-complex deposition from a type III hypersensitivity reaction and occurs in almost half of lepromatous leprosy patients, usually after initiation of treatment. ENL, which also occurs in borderline lepromatous patients, is a systemic illness characterized by fever, malaise, anorexia, arthralgia, myalgia, increased skin and nerve disease, and a widespread erythematous nodular or papular rash that includes the face and proximal limbs. The nodules, usually located over the extensor surfaces of the body, may ulcerate to form erythema nodosum necroticans. Systemic involvement in the form of conjunctivitis, keratitis, iritis, uveitis, iridiocyclitis, hepatosplenomegaly, orchitis, polyneuritis, glomerulonephritis, and lymphadenopathy may also occur. Lepromatous leprosy patients should be warned of the signs and symptoms of ENL so that they can rapidly seek medical attention. Nerve abscesses may develop, necessitating urgent surgical decompression and drainage.

The Lucio reaction is a necrotizing vasculitis peculiar to Central and South America. The Lucio phenomenon is usually seen in patients with lepromatous leprosy, waxy skin, and absent eyebrows and eyelashes. The onset is characterized by gradually spreading purplish erythema followed by hemorrhagic infarct, blistering, and ulceration.

The deformities of leprosy have the following general causes: (1) direct tissue damage, (2) nerve paralysis, (3) lepra reactions, and (4) anesthesia and resulting injury. The ulnar nerve is most commonly involved; involvement leads to clawing of the fourth and fifth fingers and loss of interosseous musculature. Median nerve involvement leads to inability to oppose the thumb and grasp objects. Peroneal nerve damage results in foot drop. Loss of distal digits is due to insensitivity, trauma, secondary infection, and the osteolytic actions of lepromatous leprosy itself. Plantar ulceration under the bony heads of the metatarsals is particularly debilitating and can lead to osteomyelitis. Plantar ulcers require non–weight bearing, attention to the possibility of secondary infection, careful removal of calluses, and appropriate footwear. Although antibiotic treatment has made nasal collapse rare in the United States, it may still occur in some patients and can be corrected with cosmetic surgery.

DIAGNOSTIC TESTS

The diagnosis of leprosy is confirmed by the demonstration of acid-fast bacilli on slit-skin examination of skin plaques, cutaneous nodules, or nasal scrapings from patients with multibacillary forms of the disease. Slit-skin examination is used to establish the diagnosis, classify the patient for instituting MDT, and monitor for recurrence after completion of MDT. A scalpel is used to make a shallow slit in involved, unbroken skin. The edge of the wound is scraped with the scalpel blade, and the tissue pulp smeared on a slide and stained by the Ziehl-Neelsen method, as well as with hematoxylin and eosin. Generally, six smears are taken, each from a different site. Results of examination of the earlobe by this method are frequently positive, even in the absence of obvious lesions. Many patients with lepromatous leprosy are bacteremic, and organisms can be seen on buffy-coat examination. Because slit-skin examinations are rarely positive in paucibacillary leprosy, a skin biopsy may be necessary to demonstrate acid-fast organisms and characteristic granuloma of cutaneous nerves. The lepromin test and skin tests using soluble antigens of *M. leprae* are not useful in diagnosis.

DIFFERENTIAL DIAGNOSIS

The diagnosis of leprosy relies on clinical suspicion of hypopigmented macules, peripheral nerve abnormalities, chronic skin lesions, and nasal congestion, especially in patients from endemic areas. Sensory testing of skin lesions using cotton fibers or graded nylon fibers and evaluation for temperature discrimination are crucial in establishing the diagnosis. The differential diagnosis of tuberculoid and borderline tuberculoid leprosy includes lupus vulgaris, tinea corporis, discoid lupus erythematosus, and psoriasis. Indeterminate leprosy may be mimicked by vitiligo, superficial fungal infections, scars, nevi, cutaneous filariasis, postinflammatory hypopigmentation, and pityriasis rosea. Lepromatous leprosy may appear similar to dermal leishmaniasis, neurofibromatosis, myxedema, lymphoma, and sarcoidosis. Neuritic leprosy can be confused with peripheral neuritis, hypertrophic interstitial neuritis, primary amyloidosis of the nerves, meralgia paresthetica, lead intoxication, and diabetes mellitus.

TREATMENT

Long-duration monotherapy with diaminodiphenylsulfone (dapsone) had been, until the 1980s, the mainstay of leprosy treatment. However, the risk of relapse during monotherapy was high. MDT has been used since 1982 and has cured an estimated 6.7 million people. Antibiotic treatment of leprosy must contend with the increasing incidence of primary and secondary drug resistance, persistence of mycobacteria for years in patients with lepromatous leprosy, and problems with adherence to long-term therapy. Drugs used for treatment of leprosy include dapsone, rifampin, clofazimine, ethionamide, minocycline, clarithromycin, and fluoroquinolones. Dapsone is mycobacteriostatic and relatively nontoxic. Rifampin is rapidly bactericidal and well tolerated; however, its cost has precluded widespread use in some endemic countries. Clofazimine, a phenazine dye derivative, is particularly useful in patients who are prone to type I or II reactions. Side effects are reddish-brown skin pigmentation and abdominal discomfort.

The World Health Organization recommends that paucibacillary leprosy be treated with dapsone (100 mg daily) and rifampin (600 mg per month) for 6 months. Recommendations for multibacillary leprosy are both dapsone 100 mg and clofazimine 50 mg daily, plus rifampin 600 mg and clofazimine 300 mg once a month. If clofazimine produces unacceptable skin pigmentation, ethionamide (375 mg daily) may be substituted, with monitoring of liver enzymes. Treatment should be maintained for a minimum of 2 years and continued until skin-smear negativity is attained (usually 5 years). Some physicians in the United States treat lepromatous leprosy with both dapsone 100 mg and rifampin 600 mg daily for the first 3 years and daily maintainance therapy with dapsone for life.

Secondary drug resistance occurs in 2% to 8% of lepromatous patients. It may appear many years after therapy is started and is promoted by underdosing and irregular adherence. Minocycline (100 mg daily) has been shown to have bactericidal activity against *M. leprae* and has the possible advantage of dampening serious inflammatory reactions that are seen with other treatments. Clarithromycin and some fluoroquinolones have also shown bactericidal activity against *M. leprae*.

Effective chemotherapy should flatten plaques and nodules, although clinical improvement is slow and progress is measured in months and years. Occasionally, neuropathy improves, but usually neuronal degeneration has already occured.

Mild lepra type I reactions respond to analgesics, but severe reactions with neuritis, skin ulceration, or lesions on cosmetically important areas warrant clofazimine and systemic corticosteroids. Prednisone (40 to 60 mg daily) can be used initially and tapered over 2 to 3 months to prevent relapse. Mild ENL responds to analgesics and antipyretics, but severe disease also requires high-dose systemic corticosteroids, sometimes for months. Prednisone (60 mg daily) should be used at the outset. After the reaction is controlled, corticosteroids should be tapered slowly. Nerve paralysis accompanied by early nerve thickening and pain followed by painless loss of motor or sensory function should be aggresively treated with long-term high-dose cor-

✔ **WHEN TO REFER**

Consultation is essential in the management of leprosy. The extent of nerve involvement may be assessed with nerve conduction studies. Physical therapy and orthopedic, neurologic, and plastic surgical treatment are important adjuncts in the therapy of patients with significant neuropathic damage. Surgical consultation with a specialist may lead to relief for many of the deformities in leprosy. Consultation and assistance are available from the national treatment center in Carville, Louisiana (telephone: [800] 642-2477) and from regional clinics. Leprosy is a reportable disease, and the local health department should be notified.

ticosteroids for 3 to 6 months to prevent permanent nerve damage. Cold abscesses of a peripheral nerve require immediate surgical decompression. Thalidomide, 200 mg twice daily, tapering to 50 to 100 mg at night, is useful in patients in whom pregnancy is not a consideration. Thalidomide usually controls the reaction in 48 to 72 hours; however, side effects include tranquilization, transient mucosal dryness, skin rashes, constipation, and worsening of existing neuritis. Thalidomide is available as an investigational drug from the G.W. Long Hansen's Disease Center and a number of U.S. Public Health Service–sponsored regional ambulatory Hansen's Disease programs. Clofazimine has considerable antiinflammatory activity and is effective in doses of 100 to 300 mg daily, facilitating weaning from corticosteroids in chronic reactions. However, clofazimine takes 3 to 6 weeks to become fully effective. Since Lucio's phenomenon is thought to be the result of immune complexes, exchange transfusion has been recomended for severe cases.

BIBLIOGRAPHY

Gelber RH: Hansen's disease, *West J Med* 158:583-590, 1993.
Jakeman P, Smith WCS: Thalidomide in leprosy reaction, *Lancet* 343:432-433, 1994.
Ji B, Jamet P, Perani EG, Bobin P, Grosset JH: Powerful bactericidal activities of clarithromycin and minocycline against *Mycobacterium leprae* in lepromatous leprosy, *J Infect Dis* 168:188-190, 1993.
Mastro TD, Redd SC, Breiman RF: Imported leprosy in the United States, 1978–1988: an epidemic without secondary transmission, *Am J Public Health* 82:1127-1130, 1992.
Meyers WM: Leprosy, *Dermatol Clin* 10:73-96, 1992.
Ridley DS, Jopling WH: Classification of leprosy: a five-group system, *Int J Lepr Other Mycobact Dis* 34:255, 1966.
Sehgal VN: Leprosy, *Dermatol Clin* 12:629-644, 1994.
World Health Organization: Chemotherapy of leprosy: WHO technical report series, 847:1-24, 1994.
World Health Organization: Progress towards the elimination of leprosy as a public health problem. Part I. Weekly epidemiological record, 70:177-184, 1995.
World Health Organization: Leprosy disabilities: magnitude of the problem, Weekly epidemiological record, 70:269-276, 1995.

FUNGAL DISEASES

CHAPTER

276 Infections Caused by Common Fungi

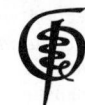

Thomas F. Patterson and John R. Graybill

Fungi, like mammalian cells, are eukaryotes, nonmotile cells with a nucleus containing several chromosomes and a nuclear membrane. Fungi also have a cell wall that is made up of chitin and polysaccharides, including α-glucans and β-glucans. The principal mammalian cell membrane sterol is cholesterol, whereas cell membranes of fungi contain ergosterol, a major target of antifungal agents. The cell wall

Table 276-1 Systemic dimorphic mycoses

MYCOSIS	GEOGRAPHIC REGION	EPIDEMIOLOGY	FORM/FREQUENCY
Blastomycosis	Scattered worldwide, parallels histoplasmosis	Soil, wood, beaver dams	Inhalation-acquired, skin lesions; uncommon in immunosuppression
Coccidioidomycosis	Southwestern United States	Soil, dust	Inhalation of highly infectious arthroconidia, meningitis life threatening
Histoplasmosis	Mississippi, Ohio river valleys, Latin America	Bird droppings, caves	Asymptomatic (normal hosts), valleys, disseminated/reactivated infection in AIDS
Paracoccidioidomycosis	Central, South America	Likely to be soil-associated, inhalation acquired	Most common infection in South and Central America; "mariner's wheel" of organisms, treated with trimethoprim-sulfamethoxazole or azoles
Penicilliosis	Southeast Asia, China	Bamboo rats	Geographically common invasive infection in AIDS patients; resembles histoplasmosis or tuberculosis
Sporotrichosis	Scattered worldwide	Vegetative material, rose thorns	Lymphangitic subcutaneous lesions, disseminated infection

Table 276-2 Opportunistic molds in systemic infection

MYCOSIS/ORGANISM	MAJOR RISK GROUPS	COMMENTS
Aspergillosis	Neutropenia, organ/bone marrow transplantation	Most common cause of invasive mold infection; requires early therapy and reversal of immunodeficiency
Pseudallescheriasis	Immunosuppression, trauma	Mimics aspergillosis on tissue sections; may be resistant to amphotericin B
Trichosporonosis	Leukemia, other malignancies	Tissues show septated hyphae and blastoconidia; antigenic cross-reactivity with *Cryptococcus* organisms
Fusariosis	Neutropenia	May be found in blood cultures; nodular skin lesions, therapeutic outcomes poor
Hyalohyphomycosis	Trauma, immunosuppression	General term for moniliaceous (lightly pigmented) molds; mimics aspergillosis on tissue sections
Zygomycosis	Diabetes, immunosuppression	Broad, rarely septated hyphae; resistant to azoles, requires surgical debridement and high-dose amphotericin B

is identified in tissues by specific stains including Gomori's methenamine silver and periodic acid–Schiff (PAS).

A few organisms that are not clearly classified as fungi have been characterized with RNA typing studies and molecular analysis. For example, RNA typing studies have classified *Pneumocystis carinii* as a fungus. *P. carinii* has been classified as a protozoan based on growth characteristics. It also has characteristics of a true fungus, such as chitin and β-glucans in its cell wall and a fungal-specific protein, elongation factor 3, but it differs from fungi because its cell membrane does not contain ergosterol and it is morphologically distinct. While molecular similarity of *P. carinii* to fungi exists, additional classification of such organisms is needed. Other organisms, such as *Loboa loboi* and *Rhinosporidium seeberi,* are presumed to be fungi but do not have in vitro culture systems. Molecular techniques are needed to establish the correct classification of such organisms.

Although there are thousands of fungi in nature, relatively few are human pathogens. However, the increasing numbers of immunosuppressed patients, such as those with malignancy, organ transplantation, and acquired immunodeficiency syndrome (AIDS), have resulted in a dramatic rise in fungal infections, since even less pathogenic fungi may cause infection in patients with abnormal host defenses. Most fungal pathogens, such as the dermatophytes, yeasts, and many molds, are present in a worldwide distribution. Other organisms are found within certain endemic areas. The endemic mycoses, which can occur in a patient with normal host defenses, include infection with *Coccidioides immitis, Histoplasma capsulatum, Blastomyces dermatitidis, Paracoccidioides brasiliensis,* and *Penicillium marneffei,* as well as sporotrichosis (Table 276-1). Although these organisms are found in a distinct geographic areas or specific epidemiologic settings, all are dimorphic, that is, they exist in nature as a mycelium, which is the infectious form, and in the host (37° C) as a yeast. Most cause infection through inhalation, but expression of infection depends on the immune status of the host. In normal hosts symptoms of infection may be minimal. In patients with abnormal host defenses, par-

ticularly those with altered cell-mediated immunity such as patients with AIDS, disseminated infection is common.

Other organisms are referred to as opportunistic pathogens. These ubiquitous organisms, including yeasts such as *Candida* species and opportunistic molds such as *Aspergillus* organisms and *Zygomycetes,* only rarely cause infection in normal hosts; but in patients with severely depressed host defenses they cause widely disseminated infection with high mortality rates (Table 276-2).

DIAGNOSIS

Culture of the fungal organism remains the standard for diagnosis of fungal infections. Improved sensitivity associated with standard blood culture techniques and use of special isolator blood cultures further enhances detection of many organisms, such as *H. capsulatum.* However, some organisms, particularly molds like *Aspergillus* and Zygomycetes, are rarely cultured from blood. Isolation of opportunistic pathogens from respiratory specimens may be associated with invasive infection, but respiratory tract cultures may also be positive in patients colonized with the organism. Thus the demonstration of organisms in tissue is needed to establish invasive disease.

Serodiagnosis can be used to establish a diagnosis of infection (Table 276-3). Serial rise in specific fungal antibody level is presumptive evidence of disease, but antibody testing of many mycoses in immunosuppressed patients is of limited value, since poor antibody responses may occur in these patients. Detection of fungal antigens or metabolites is also used in the diagnosis of infection and can be useful in management of some mycoses, such as histoplasmosis.

ANTIFUNGAL THERAPY

The increased number of systemic fungal infections has resulted in an increased number of antifungal agents to treat systemic mycoses (Table 276-4). Amphotericin B, a polyene antifungal, has remained the standard therapy for many systemic mycoses, despite more than

Table 276-3   Serodiagnosis of systemic fungal disease

MYCOSIS	TEST	COMMENT
Aspergillosis	Various antibody tests	Nondiagnostic for invasive disease; IgE may be useful for diagnosis/management of allergic bronchopulmonary aspergillosis
	ELISA/radioimmunoassay, latex agglutination	Antigen (usually galactomannan and related antigens) tests remain investigational; latex agglutination lacks sensitivity and specificity
Blastomycosis	Complement fixation; others	Lack specificity; identification of specific antigens may improve serodiagnosis
Candidiasis	Various antibody tests	Nondiagnostic
	Various antigen tests	Commercial tests lack sensitivity and specificity
Coccidioidomycosis	Complement fixation; complement fixation immunodiffusion	Specific; higher titers ($>1:8$) indicative of disseminated disease
	Tube precipitin	Specific; may revert to negative even with active disease
	Radioimmunoassay	Antigen tests; investigational
Cryptococcosis	Latex agglutination	Capsular polysaccharide; highly sensitive and specific for diagnosis; less useful for monitoring response
Histoplasmosis	Complement fixation	Titer $<1:8$ nonspecific
	Immunodiffusion	H band (more likely in active infection) and M band (may persist for years); cross-reactivity with other mycoses possible
	Radioimmunoassay/ELISA	Polysaccharide antigen; rapid diagnosis and monitoring of treatment response
Paracoccidioidomycosis	Immunodiffusion	Specific; not useful for monitoring response
	Complement fixation	Higher titers more likely to correlate with disease
Trichosporonosis	Cryptococcal latex agglutination	"False-positive" cross-reaction possible

ELISA, Enzyme-linked immunosorbent assay; *IgE,* immunoglobulin E.

Table 276-4   Antifungal agents for systemic mycoses

AGENT	MECHANISM	ACTIVITY
Amphotericin B	Binds ergosterol; cell leakage, rapid	Broad spectrum, few resistant organisms; dose-limiting nephrotoxicity; adverse reactions common
Fluconazole	Inhibition of ergosterol	Activity targeted to yeasts (particularly *Candida albicans* and *Cryptococcus*); very well tolerated; useful in long-term suppressive therapy, prophylaxis in certain high-risk patients
Itraconazole	Inhibition of ergosterol	Active against endemic mycoses, *Aspergillus* spp.; well tolerated, nausea with higher doses, erratic absorption; oral solution improves bioavailability
Ketoconazole	Inhibition of ergosterol	Indications limited to mucocutaneous candidiasis, non–life-threatening endemic mycotic infections; poor oral absorption, intolerance (nausea, vomiting, hepatic) with higher doses
Flucytosine	Inhibits protein synthesis	Use in combination with other agents in cryptococcosis, some candidiasis, other progressive infections; rapid resistance as single agent; neutropenia, gastrointestinal tract intolerance common, especially at higher doses

three decades. Major advantages of amphotericin B include its broad spectrum of activity, low rates of resistance, and rapid antifungal activity. However, for systemic infection amphotericin B must be administered intravenously and is associated with significant toxicity. Amphotericin B acts by rapidly binding to ergosterol in fungal cell membranes, causing cellular leak. Amphotericin B is insoluble in aqueous solutions, so it is commercially available as a deoxycholate, which is reconstituted in dextrose in water. It is usually administered in doses of 0.5 to 1.5 mg/kg per day over 2 to 4 hours with total doses of 15 to 30 mg/kg administered depending on specific mycoses and response. Adverse reactions are common. Phlebitis occurs in many patients when amphotericin B is administered peripherally and may be minimized with the addition of 500 to 1000 units of heparin to the infusion. Other infusion-related side effects include chills, fevers, and hypotension. Many clinicians administer a "test dose" of 1 mg of drug without premedication, to identify a potential anaphylaxis reaction. This dose can be conveniently administered by infusing 1 mg of the initial dose and observing for 15 minutes for a severe reaction before completing the initial infusion. Premedication with acetaminophen 650 mg and diphenhydramine 25 to 50 mg may ameliorate chills and fever. Severe rigors can be treated with meperidine 25 to 50 mg. The addition of hydrocortisone (25 to 50 mg) to each infusion may also help reduce these symptoms. The efficacy of these measures remains controversial. Other common side effects include nausea, malaise, weight loss, and anemia. Nephrotoxicity is the major dose-limiting side effect. Many patients have serum creatinine values that rise to 2.5 to 3.0 mg/dl, and do not require dose adjustment. Levels above those may require a decreased dose or discontinuation. Nephrotoxicity may be minimized with 1 L of normal saline admin-

istered before each dose. Renal tubular acidosis and electrolyte disturbances (hypokalemia and hypomagnesemia) are also common.

Lipid preparations of amphotericin B have been developed to allow administration of higher doses of amphotericin B with minimal nephrotoxicity. These preparations include amphotericin B lipid complex (ABLC, Abelcet), amphotericin B colloidal dispersion (Amphotec), and amphotericin B liposomes (Ambisome). These liposomal forms are associated with infusion reactions but are generally well tolerated at doses of 5 mg/kg or more and are effective in patients intolerant of or failing amphotericin B therapy. For example, amphotericin B lipid complex was shown to be less toxic and more effective in patients with invasive aspergillosis who had failed prior therapy with standard amphotericin B, although there are few direct comparative trials.

To reduce toxicity and allow oral therapy, the azole antifungals were developed. These compounds act to inhibit ergosterol synthesis through inhibition of a fungal demethylase enzyme. Early compounds included miconazole, which has few current indications for use, and ketoconazole, which continues to be used in mucocutaneous candidiasis and less severe infections. Newer triazole antifungals, itraconazole and fluconazole, have further enhanced efficacy and decreased toxicity. A number of newer azole compounds are also undergoing development. A comparison of the pharmacokinetics and activity of these agents is shown in Tables 276-5 and 276-6.

Ketoconazole and itraconazole have many similar pharmacokinetic properties. They are relatively water-insoluble, and both are available only in an oral formulation, although an intravenous preparation of itraconazole is undergoing evaluation. Both have decreased absorption in achlorhydric patients, including those on histamine

Table 276-5   Pharmacokinetic comparisons and major toxicities of azole antifungals

	KETOCONAZOLE	ITRACONAZOLE	FLUCONAZOLE
Route administered	Oral	Oral	Oral/IV
Achlorhydric effect	Marked	Significant	Minimal/none
Half-life	5-9 hours	30-42 hours	24-30 hours
Clearance	Hepatic	Hepatic	Renal, active metabolite unchanged
Usual, tolerated highest doses	400 mg/day	400-600 mg/day	800 mg/day
Drug interactions			
Increased azole clearance			
Phenytoin	+++	+++	0
Rifampin	++++	++++	++
Rifabutin		+++	+
Isoniazid	+++	0	0
Increased levels of other drug			
Phenytoin	++	++	+
Carbamazepine	++	++	+
Warfarin	++	++	+
Cyclosporine A	++	++	+
Terfenadine/astemizole	+++	++	+
Sulfonylureas	+	+	+
Digoxin	+	+	

Interaction: 0, none; +, almost none; ++, minimal; +++, significant; ++++, highly significant.

Table 276-6   Activity of azole antifungals in systemic infection

	KETOCONAZOLE	ITRACONAZOLE	FLUCONAZOLE
Yeasts			
Candida albicans	+++	+++	+++
Non-*albicans Candida*	+	++	++
Cryptococcus spp.	+	++	++++
Aspergillus spp.	0	+++	0
Other opportunistic molds	0	±	±
Zygomycetes	0	0	0
Endemic fungi	++	++++	++
Toxicity			
Nausea, vomiting	++++	++	+
Hepatic	++	+	+
Endocrine	+++	+	0
Rash	0	+	+

Activity: 0, none; +, almost none; ++, minimal; +++, significant; ++++, highly significant.

(H$_2$) blocking therapy. Absorption is improved with acid, such as cola; itraconazole has improved absorption with food. Itraconazole has significantly more activity against molds than ketoconazole or fluconazole. Interactions with other drugs metabolized through the P450 system are common. Side effects include hepatic toxicity, nausea, and vomiting. Itraconazole (at maximal doses of 400 to 600 mg/day) is associated with significantly less toxicity than ketoconazole. Itraconazole oral solution improves bioavailability.

Fluconazole is a water-soluble triazole that is available in both oral and intravenous preparations. Its absorption is not affected by acid or by food, and it is well tolerated at doses of 800 mg/day or more. Uncommon side effects include nausea, vomiting, hepatic toxicity, and cutaneous reactions, including Stevens-Johnson syndrome. Activity of fluconazole is primarily directed to yeasts, with limited activity against molds. Fluconazole has been particularly useful for treating uncomplicated candidemia, cryptococcosis, and oropharyngeal candidiasis. Both clinical and mycologic resistance to azoles has been associated with long-term therapy with subtherapeutic concentrations of the azoles.

Flucytosine is an orally administered pyrimidine analog. When the drug is used alone, resistance quickly develops, but it is used in combination with amphotericin B for cryptococcal meningitis and complicated candidal infections. Major toxicity includes leukopenia, thrombocytopenia, hepatitis, and colitis. The dose must be adjusted in patients with renal insufficiency. Additional agents with other fungal targets are undergoing development, including inhibitors of β-glucan (echinocandinins), chitin (nikkomycins), and cell wall formation.

DIMORPHIC FUNGI
Histoplasmosis

Microbiology and Epidemiology. The dimorphic fungus *Histoplasma capsulatum* is endemic to the Ohio and Mississippi river valleys. *H. capsulatum* exists in nature as a mycelium that includes 2- to 4-mm microconidia and larger macroconidia, the latter bearing rather characteristic tuberculate chlamydospores. The infectious mycelial phase of *H. capsulatum* is found in the excreta of chickens, certain other birds, and bats. At 37° C the mycelial form converts to the pathogenic yeast form, a characteristic that aids in identification. In tissues the yeast forms are usually found within giant cells or macrophages (Fig. 276-1) and may be visible on a buffy-coat blood or bone marrow smear. The organism grows slowly, taking up to 6 weeks to grow into visible colonies.

The growth of *H. capsulatum* in excreta found in bird roosts and bat-infested caves contributes to the association of epidemics with disturbances of nesting sites or spelunking. Many residents of the central United States have been infected with *H. capsulatum*, with initial infection, which is frequently asymptomatic, occurring in childhood. Outbreaks of histoplasmosis often occur on the periphery of the endemic areas, where there are more susceptible individuals during a point-source exposure. The intensity of exposure and the immune status of the host are closely linked to the clinical outcome of infection.

Infection may also result from disease reactivated many years after initial exposure in persons with abnormal cell-mediated immunity, including patients with AIDS. Such patients, even those living in nonendemic areas, may come to medical attention with symptomatic histoplasmosis as a result of recurrence from a latent foci of disease acquired many years earlier when residing in an endemic zone.

Pathophysiologic Features and Host Defenses. Infection occurs by inhalation of the microconidia, which convert into yeast cells. The organisms proliferate and are carried via lymphatics into the bloodstream, where hematogenous dissemination to the reticuloendothelial organs occurs. The onset of clinical symptoms of primary histoplasmosis is associated with a granulomatous response, which may later calcify. If there is failure of cell-mediated immunity, the organisms proliferate unchecked in macrophages and produce diffuse reticuloendothelial organ hyperplasia. An excessive host inflammatory response to primary infection or reinfection histoplasmosis probably contributes to the syndromes of fibrosing mediastinitis, broncholithiasis, histoplasmoma, and, possibly, chronic pulmonary

In contrast are forms of histoplasmosis that result from excessive host inflammatory response. These appear as either constrictive or mass lesions. The histoplasmoma is usually noticed as an asymptomatic "coin" lesion on radiographic examination, but erosion of a calcified granuloma into the airway may become a focus for obstruction and distal infection. Fibrosing histoplasma mediastinitis presumably is caused by strong fibrotic reaction to histoplasmal antigens. This produces a variety of entrapment syndromes involving the superior vena cava, major airways, and the aorta. Chronic pulmonary histoplasmosis, which occurs in only 1 in 2000 adults following acute exposure, has a striking predilection for patients with underlying lung disease and probably occurs from excessive immune response. Symptoms resemble other chronic granulomatous diseases and may last for several months. Radiographic patterns may include apical lung cavities and fibrosis. Progressive infection occurs in more than half of the patients.

Diagnosis. Histoplasmosis may mimic a variety of illnesses from influenza through lymphoma to tuberculosis, and diagnosis is often difficult. Cultures of sputum, urine, lymph node, liver, and bone marrow are frequently positive in disseminated disease, but since the organism grows slowly, results may be delayed for weeks. Lysis-centrifugation cultures may improve isolation of the organism. In patients with AIDS and histoplasmosis, more than half have positive peripheral blood or bone marrow stains (or both) for *H. capsulatum*.

The serologic tests for histoplasmosis antibodies include complement fixation and immunodiffusion (see Table 276-2). The complement fixation test is nonspecific at titers less than 1:8, is cross-reactive with other fungal pathogens, and may be negative in patients with disseminated disease. The immunodiffusion test to H and M antigens is positive in up to 90% of patients (probably less commonly with AIDS) and is specific. However, the most useful test is a radioimmunoassay developed by Wheat et al. to detect polysaccharide antigen, which is highly sensitive and specific in both urine and blood. In addition to being valuable in diagnosis, a declining titer of antigen is associated with response to therapy, whereas a rising titer may predict progression or relapse.

Therapy and Prognosis. Treatment depends on the form of the disease and the immunologic status of the host. Primary histoplasmosis need be treated only if a patient is severely symptomatic or hypoxic from a massive exposure. Although itraconazole has not been evaluated specifically for primary histoplasmosis, a course of 400 mg per day for 3 to 6 months may be as effective as and less toxic than amphotericin B. Corticosteroids may be used to reduce the inflammatory response but should not be given in the absence of antifungal therapy. Antifungal therapy is not indicated for broncholithiasis, histoplasmoma, or mediastinitis. Mediastinitis may require surgical decompression of vital mediastinal structures. Chronic pulmonary histoplasmosis may be treated with itraconazole or amphotericin B in patients with large cavities. Resection of large cavities may be of value in severely ill patients whose pulmonary function will tolerate surgery.

Disseminated histoplasmosis is most frequently seen in patients with AIDS, who may have an overwhelming course of infection. In severely ill patients amphotericin B at 50 mg per day should be used until the patient is clearly improving, usually for 1 to 2 weeks. Therapy can be continued with an azole, preferably itraconazole at 400 mg/day. Lifelong suppressive therapy is required in patients with AIDS, since relapse is common. In patients intolerant of itraconazole or in whom concomitant medications prohibit its use, fluconazole is an alternative agent.

Coccidioidomycosis

Epidemiology and Pathophysiology. *Coccidioides immitis* is a dimorphic fungus that is endemic to the southwestern United States, Mexico, and South America. In the United States more than 100,000 cases of coccidioidomycosis occur annually, with clinical manifestations ranging from asymptomatic or self-limited "valley fever" to widely disseminated infection including the central nervous system. The infectious mycelium is found in semiarid soil and is made up of intercalating arthroconidia and "ghost cells" (Fig. 276-2). The highly

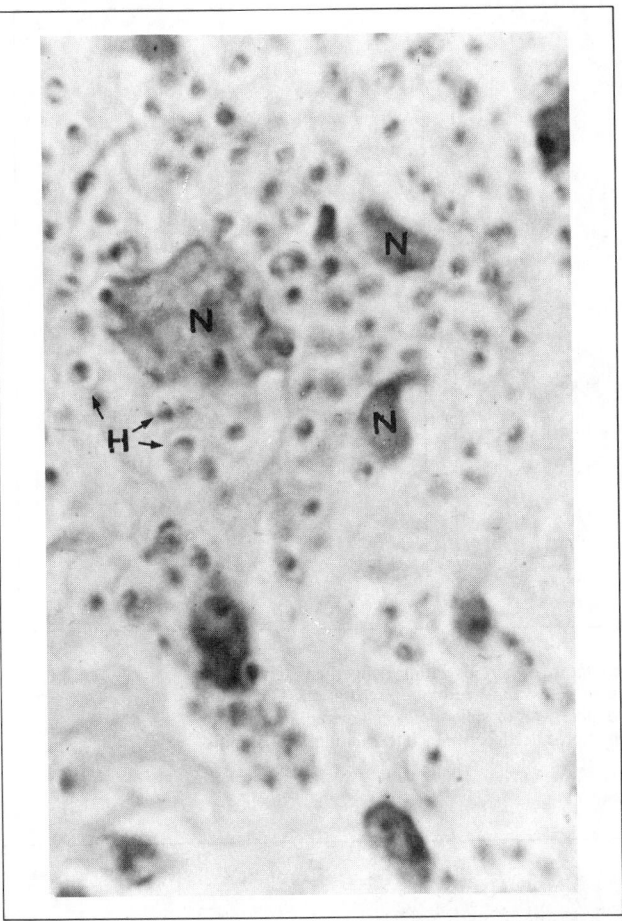

FIGURE 276-1 Morphologic appearance of *Histoplasma capsulatum*. Tissue form, with many small yeast cells *(H)* found with histiocytic cells, whose nuclei are indicated by *N*.

histoplasmosis. Immunity is not complete, particularly following heavy reexposure.

Clinical Manifestations. In the normal host, inhalation of small numbers of histoplasma microconidia is followed either by no symptoms or, a few weeks later, by symptoms resembling a viral syndrome. These symptoms of primary histoplasmosis are not specific and consist of cough, fever, myalgias, and, sometimes, pleuritic chest pain. After more intense exposure severe pulmonary illness can occur, with diffuse infiltrates, dyspnea, hypoxia, and acute respiratory distress. Pericarditis, arthritis, and widespread dissemination may also occur. Primary histoplasmosis usually subsides within 10 days, leaving an individual either no residua or punctate calcifications scattered throughout the lungs or spleen, or both. A massive exposure produces severe symptoms and a greater likelihood of disseminated disease.

Disseminated histoplasmosis results from failure of cell-mediated immunity. It may become evident as a fulminating illness, especially in infants, patients taking immunosuppressive medication, and patients with AIDS. The most common presentation is similar to other granulomatous disease, including fever, weight loss, nausea, vomiting, diarrhea, and anorexia. Evidence of lymph node enlargement, hepatosplenomegaly, oral mucosal ulcers, hypoadrenalism, or colonic masses should raise suspicion for this disease. Meningitis may occur in up to 20% of patients with disseminated disease and is especially common in patients with AIDS. Leukopenia and thrombocytopenia may reflect the often intense marrow infiltration. Chest radiographs usually show a diffuse interstitial infiltrate. A markedly elevated serum lactate dehydrogenase (LDH) level can be an important clue to the disease. In patients with AIDS, disseminated histoplasmosis may also become evident as a sepsislike syndrome with extremely high mortality.

A 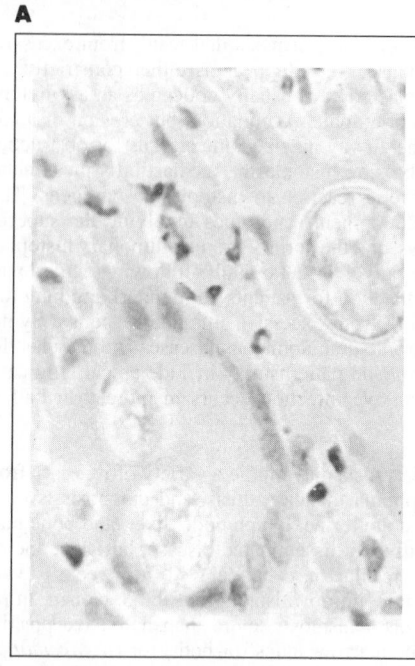 **B** 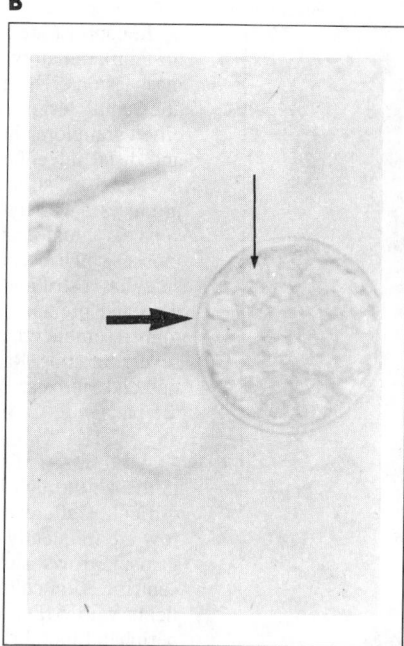 **C**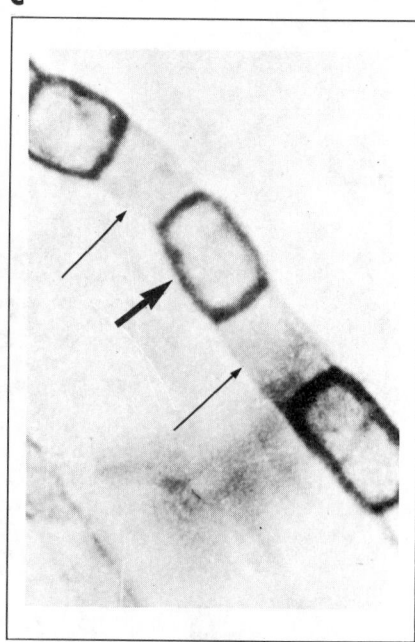

FIGURE 276-2 Morphologic appearance of *Coccidioides immitis*. **A,** Spherules within Langerhans' giant cells, shown by hematoxylin and eosin stain. **B,** Spherule in unstained potassium hydroxide preparation. The endospores within spherule *(small arrow)* and the clearly defined double wall of spherule *(large arrow)* are evident. **C,** Mycelial form with barrel-shaped arthroconidia *(large arrow)* spaced between intercalating "ghost cells" *(small arrows)*.

infectious arthroconidia are easily dispersed in wind and have been associated with epidemics of infection as a result of soil disturbances from construction or earthquakes. Cycles of drought and rain further enhance growth of the organism. Once inhaled by humans or animals, arthroconidia convert to spherules, which are progressively enlarging, round, chitinous structures up to 60 mm in diameter at maturity. These spherules spontaneously rupture, releasing many endospores. *C. immitis* thrives on most culture media, with growth within a week of culture.

Like histoplasmosis, the course of primary coccidioidomycosis depends largely on the immune status of the host. Once inhaled, arthroconidia convert to spherules. These spherules discharge endospores, which are ingested, but not killed, by neutrophils. Cell-mediated responses are critical to host defenses against the organism. If the host fails to develop an adequate cell-mediated immune response, the infection may produce fulminating coccidioidal pneumonia and widespread extrapulmonary abscesses. In a satisfactory host response, *C. immitis* stimulates formation of granulomas at each focus of infection. Factors such as intensity of exposure, racial susceptibility (heightened in blacks, Mexican Indians, and Filipinos), immunosuppressive medications, pregnancy, and AIDS adversely affect the course.

Clinical Manifestations. Primary coccidioidomycosis commences after an asymptomatic period of 1 to 2 weeks and produces an influenza-like syndrome in about half of the patients. A number of features, thought to be immunologic, are common in primary coccidioidomycosis, including erythema nodosum, erythema multiforme, and other rashes. Other primary symptoms include a dry cough, pleuritic chest pain, myalgias, arthralgia, fever, and sweats. Symptoms may last several weeks but usually resolve even without therapy. In approximately 5% of the patients, pulmonary findings including nodules and cavities persist. Chronic progressive pulmonary infection is characterized by the development of extensive thin-walled cavities that may rupture and cause fistula formation or empyema.

Disseminated coccidioidomycosis occurs in approximately 1 in 200 patients and primarily affects the skin and subcutaneous tissues, lymph nodes, bones, joints, and meninges. Cutaneous lesions may be nodular, ulcerative, or nondescript pigmented scars that irregularly break down and discharge small amounts of pus (Fig. 276-3). These

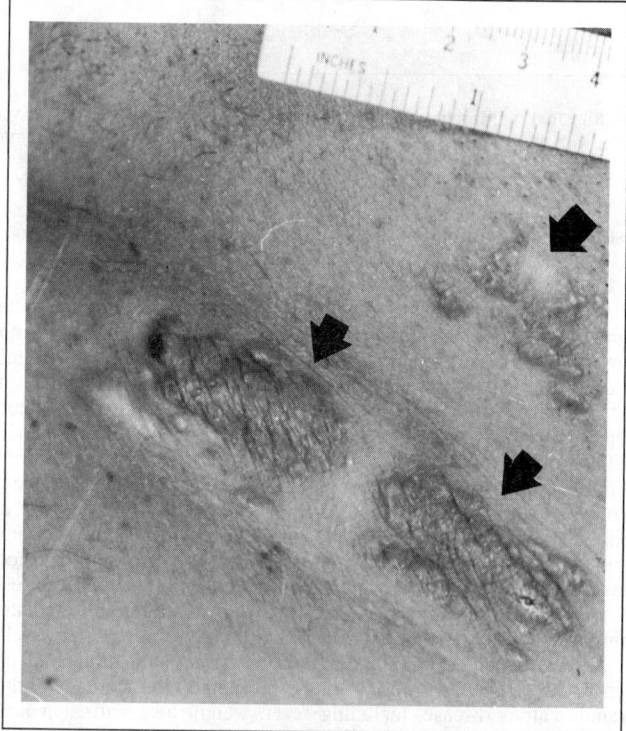

FIGURE 276-3 Nodular coccidioidal skin lesions that had persisted for more than 6 years on this man's neck.

lesions may be local or may represent extension of fistulous tracts from deep sites in muscles or viscera. They are not commonly painful. A common site for soft tissue invasion is the lymphatic system. Large paraspinous abscesses may produce radiculopathies and may be associated with vertebral osteomyelitis. Arthritis tends to involve the spine and weight-bearing joints. The most dreaded complication of coccidioidomycosis is the involvement of the central nervous system, which is most commonly a basilar meningitis. Untreated, coccidioidal meningitis progresses to involve cranial nerves and produce hydrocephalus. Patients with meningitis may have no other manifestations of coccidioidomycosis. The course is often chronic rather than acute. Cranial nerve impairments, personality changes, headaches, dulled mentation, and coma develop. Even with the most vigorous management, the mortality rate is 20% to 50%. Relapses are common.

Diagnosis. *C. immitis* can be readily cultured within a week often from sputum or infected tissues. Mycelial cultures are highly infectious and must be handled with extreme caution. The presence in tissue of a spherule is so characteristic that it can be easily seen on hematoxylin and eosin stains and may also be readily identified in potassium hydroxide preparations of purulent exudates. The result of a skin test with coccidioidin or spherulin is positive in many healthy persons living in endemic areas and converts to positive in most patients with primary coccidioidomycosis but does not indicate active disease. Results of serologic tests for immunoglobulin M (IgM) antibody may become positive by tube precipitin within the first few weeks of infection. The titer of immunoglobulin G (IgG) antibody, measured by the complement fixation test combined with immunodiffusion (IDCF), correlates with active disease and is associated with prognosis. A titer of 1:16 or higher is associated with disseminated disease. Serial titers are useful in management of infection but tend to change less in chronic pulmonary disease than in disseminated disease. Skin tests do not interfere with serologic studies, so both tests may be serially repeated to assess immune status and prognosis.

The diagnosis of coccidioidal meningitis is more difficult, since *C. immitis* is cultured from cerebrospinal fluid (CSF) in fewer than half of specimens. Lymphocytic pleocytosis and a depressed glucose level are found in about half of the initial CSF specimens. The presence of meningitis should be presumed if the CSF is abnormal and the organism is isolated from a nonmeningeal site. The precipitin test and latex agglutination tests are not of value in CSF testing, but a positive CSF complement fixation test result is diagnostic of coccidioidal meningitis.

Therapy and Prognosis. Of the major endemic mycoses, coccidioidomycosis has traditionally been the most refractory to amphotericin B and the most likely to relapse, sometimes years after completion of therapy. Amphotericin B has been used intravenously at 50 mg three times weekly up to a cumulative dose of 2.5 to 3 g, or 35 mg/kg. Both fluconazole and itraconazole have been successfully used for therapy and are clearly superior to ketoconazole in efficacy and tolerance for nonmeningeal disease.

Coccidioidal meningitis is a very difficult infection with frequent relapse and a high mortality rate, despite its chronic nature. Intrathecal amphotericin B has been used in many regimens but is associated with severe toxicity, and relapses are common. Fluconazole, which achieves excellent CSF levels following systemic administration, is a well-tolerated and highly effective treatment at 400 mg/day or higher, with remission occurring in more than 75% of patients. Itraconazole is also effective, but experience is more limited in meningeal disease. Lifelong therapy is required, since even late relapses may occur.

Blastomycosis

Epidemiology and Pathophysiology. *Blastomyces dermatitidis* is a dimorphic yeast that grows at room temperature as a mycelium, and at 37° C as a broad-based singly budding yeast. The organism is distinguished from *Cryptococcus neoformans* by the absence of a capsule and thick-walled buds to daughter cells, and from *Paracoccidioides brasiliensis* by its single buds. The organism can be isolated from moist soil of riverbanks and has been associated with beaver dams. Persons who engage in outdoor occupations such as highway construction and farming are more likely than city dwellers to become infected with blastomycosis. The endemic zone of blastomycosis is comparable to that of histoplasmosis.

Infection is thought to occur by inhalation of spores, which con-

vert to yeast forms and produce a primary flulike infection manifested by fever, cough, and chest pain. Lung infiltrates may clear or persist as fibrocavitary lesions. Hematogenous dissemination to the skin and bones occurred in two thirds of patients in one large series, and to the prostate, liver, spleen, and kidney in half. Less frequent is central nervous system and lymph node involvement. The adrenals are involved only occasionally.

Clinical Manifestations, Diagnosis, and Therapy. The characteristic clinical presentation is subacute or chronic, with fever, cough, weight loss, and an associated skin lesion. The skin lesions are often found to be several in number when carefully sought and may range from small acneiform pustules to large nodular or papulopustular lesions with heaped-up edges and small, black (pepperlike), pinpoint lesions in the central eschar (Color Plate VIII-48). They often are mistaken for carcinomas and appear on exposed surfaces of the body, infrequently involving mucosal surfaces. Skin lesions are accompanied by pulmonary and skeletal lesions in up to 40% of patients. Patients with AIDS have uncommonly become infected with the organism, with infection typically occurring as a late infection with widely disseminated disease.

Diagnosis of blastomycosis requires demonstration of the fungus by biopsy or potassium hydroxide preparation of a lesion specimen, with confirmation by culture. Urine and prostatic secretions may be positive for the organism even in the absence of symptoms. Serologic and skin tests cross-react with histoplasma antigens.

Therapy should be aimed at likely disseminated disease even if only a cutaneous lesion is identified. Itraconazole is the drug of choice in non–life-threatening disease, with response rates of greater than 90%. A dosage of 200 mg twice daily for at least 6 months is recommended. Fluconazole or ketoconazole is a less effective alternative therapy. Amphotericin B should be reserved for patients with life-threatening systemic infection and is usually given for a total course of 2 to 3 g.

Paracoccidioidomycosis

Paracoccidioides brasiliensis is a dimorphic fungus that produces a characteristic "pilot wheel" yeast form comprising a central cell surrounded by multiple buds. This fungus is the major endemic mycoses in South America. Appearance of disease in humans may occur many years after presumed inhalation exposure. There have been no epidemics to yield information on primary disease or natural reservoirs. The disease occurs sporadically. Men, particularly those engaged in outdoor occupations, are affected far more frequently than women.

Patients may seek medical attention with pulmonary disease or with the sequelae of hematogenous dissemination. On clinical examination the illness resembles chronic coccidioidomycosis, with a predominance of respiratory symptoms. Central and basilar infiltrates are common, whereas cavities are uncommon, and the apices are frequently spared. The lesions heal (in treated patients) with bullae and fibrosis, which may produce right-side ventricular failure. Mucosal or cutaneous ulcerated or nodular lesions can occur. Lymph node involvement is frequent, often leading to spontaneous drainage of purulent material. The genitourinary tract and adrenal glands may be involved. Like coccidioidomycosis, paracoccidioidomycosis may coexist with tuberculosis. This is uncommon in patients with AIDS.

Diagnosis is established by demonstration of the characteristic central cell with multiple bud complex on potassium hydroxide preparation or fungal strains and culture of the organism from tissue. Skin testing is unreliable, since false-negative reactions may occur. The diagnosis also can be established with serologic tests. Immunodiffusion is positive in 95% of patients and is highly specific. The complement fixation test also is specific.

Itraconazole is the drug of choice and can be given at even low doses of 100 mg/day for 6 months. An alternative is ketoconazole, which can be given at 200 or 400 mg/day for prolonged periods without toxicity. Adrenal insufficiency is common and should be considered on clinical examination. Sulfa drugs are also a cost-effective alternative regimen that is commonly used in South America, but treatment is prolonged and relapses are frequent.

Sporotrichosis

Sporothrix schenkii is a dimorphic fungus that causes sporadic disease in specific epidemiologic settings rather than endemic disease. *S. schenkii* may be cultured from the soil and a variety of vegetative material including straw, rose thorns, sphagnum moss, and wood. Traumatic inoculation of contaminated materials selects both the victims of cutaneous sporotrichosis (those who work in farming, plant nurseries, gardening) and the most common sites of primary lesions (extremities in adults, trunk and face in children).

More than three fourths of patients have locally inoculated lymphocutaneous disease. Disease develops weeks after inoculation and consists of a papular or ulcerated, painless lesion. Over succeeding weeks satellite lesions appear along the lymphatics draining the primary site (Color Plate VIII-49). Sporotrichosis uncommonly disseminates but may produce osteomyelitis and arthritis. It is uncertain whether pulmonary involvement is primary or secondary to hematogenous dissemination. Sporotrichosis is uncommonly associated with immunosuppression and is rare in patients with AIDS.

The clinical manifestations of sporotrichosis are usually mild and chronic. An appropriate history, together with the finding of the typical cutaneous lesion, should provide strong suggestive evidence. The peripheral lesion can be mimicked by mycobacterial infection *(Mycobacterium marinum, Mycobacterium chelonei, Mycobacterium fortuitum)*, nocardiosis, actinomycosis, or leishmaniasis. Bone and joint lesions must be distinguished from other forms of granulomatous osteomyelitis and arthritis. Pulmonary infiltrates and cavities may mimic coccidioidomycosis or tuberculosis. The diagnosis is most readily made by biopsies of infected tissues or sputum. The diagnosis is established by culture of the organism from the pus or cutaneous lesions. Growth of the organism may occur within 3 to 5 days. Histopathologic examination demonstrates the typical cigar-shaped yeasts that may be surrounded by a stellate, PAS-positive material known as an asteroid body. Serologic testing may be useful for extracutaneous infection such as meningitis, but antibodies may be present without the disease.

The least expensive form of treatment is saturated solution of potassium iodide, begun at 5 drops three times per day and progressively increased to 120 drops per day. This therapy is often poorly tolerated and is reliable only for lymphocutaneous disease. Therefore itraconazole has become the drug of choice for sporotrichosis. It may be given at 100 to 400 mg/day for 3 to 6 months, with the lower dose and shorter time for lymphocutaneous disease and the more intense courses for disseminated disease. Itraconazole is effective in more than 90% of patients with lymphocutaneous disease and about 75% of patients with extracutaneous disease. Fluconazole has also been used, but the response of lymphocutaneous disease, even at doses of 400 mg/day, appears to be less than with itraconazole.

Penicilliosis

Penicillium marneffei has emerged as an important dimorphic pathogen in Southeast Asia that produces a chronic disseminated infection in immunosuppressed hosts, particularly in patients infected with human immunodeficiency virus (HIV). The fungus is endemic to Southeast Asia and is associated with the bamboo rat. Infections have been reported in Northern Thailand and throughout China, and imported cases have been reported in Europe and Texas.

The organism is acquired through inhalation with the development of disseminated infection. Signs and symptoms mimic disseminated histoplasmosis or coccidioidomycosis, including fever, weight loss, cough, hepatosplenomegaly, lymphadenopathy, and skin lesions. Pulmonary infiltrates, anemia, and thrombocytopenia are common. The diagnosis is established by smears of bone marrow, buffy-coat smear of blood, or skin lesions that show elliptic yeasts that resemble *H. capsulatum* except that prominent cross-walls may be seen, which result from the organism dividing though fission. On culture the mold colony produces a distinctive red pigment.

Amphotericin B and itraconazole have been successfully used in therapy of this disease. Fluconazole is a less effective alternative. Long-term suppressive therapy appears to be necessary to prevent recurrence of infection.

Opportunistic Molds

Aspergillus Species

Epidemiology, Pathophysiology and Clinical Manifestations. *Aspergillus* species are ubiquitous organisms with septate branching at 45-degree angles. The fungus grows rapidly in vitro, and colonies appear in 3 to 7 days on most bacteriologic media. Exposure most commonly occurs through inhalation of the infectious conidia.

Aspergillus species produce three common pulmonary illnesses whose expression depends in large part on the status of the host. The first, bronchopulmonary allergic aspergillosis, occurs in atopic persons with preexisting asthma or cystic fibrosis. The disease is caused by the host response to the organism, with eosinophilia, pulmonary infiltrates, and bronchial plugging by secretions containing eosinophils and *Aspergillus* organisms. The condition may lead to bronchiectasis, but widespread invasion almost never occurs.

The second common manifestation of aspergillosis is pulmonary *Aspergillus* fungus ball. This usually results from colonization of a preexisting cavity produced by tuberculosis, histoplasmosis, or coccidioidomycosis. A central fungus ball is often freely movable within the cavity. This form of aspergillosis is rarely invasive.

The third form of pulmonary aspergillosis is a fulminating disease associated with widespread dissemination, with extensive pulmonary infection and extrapulmonary involvement, including the central nervous system. Disseminated aspergillosis usually begins in the setting of severe leukopenia or corticosteroid therapy. The disease progresses from local tissue invasion to a vasculitis caused by the mycelia. This vasculitis and plugging of pulmonary vessels may produce a clinical syndrome quite similar to that of pulmonary embolus, with similar radiographic changes. Sputum smears and cultures may be positive for *Aspergillus* organisms. Mortality is high in leukopenic patients and correlates closely with delays in initiation of treatment and with persistent leukopenia. Patients with persistent leukopenia have a diffuse aggressive disease, whereas those whose leukocytes return tend to develop pulmonary fungal balls that slowly resolve. In those of the latter group with cavitary disease there is a danger of severe hemoptysis.

Uncommon forms of aspergillosis include endocarditis, locally invasive disease, and madura foot. Endocarditis usually occurs on a prosthetic heart valve, possibly owing to contamination of the operative field by spores. The organisms tend to form very large vegetations, with frequent emboli to large vessels. Diagnosis is especially difficult, since blood cultures are almost always negative. The only clue to diagnosis may be obtained from histologic examination of embolus. Locally invasive disease may occur after traumatic inoculation of an otherwise healthy person. Necrotizing cutaneous ulcers may occur in leukopenic patients. Madura foot, or mycetoma, may have *Aspergillus* species contributing to the disease. Aspergilli may also form a mycetoma of the paranasal sinuses and cause chronic infiltrative pulmonary disease.

Diagnosis and therapy. Diagnosis of aspergillosis may be made presumptively from the characteristic septate hyphae seen in biopsy tissue specimens stained with Gomori's methenamine silver (Fig. 276-4). Because invasive procedures are often required, there has been a search for serologic tests for diagnosis. Results of tests for precipitating antibodies are almost always strongly positive in bronchopulmonary allergic aspergillosis, are usually positive in pulmonary mycetoma, and usually are negative in patients with disseminated disease. *Aspergillus* antigens may be detected in blood or bronchoalveolar lavage of patients with disseminated disease, but measurement of antigen is not commercially available. Other procedures, such as polymerase chain reaction (PCR), are undergoing evaluation as diagnostic tools.

Treatment of aspergillosis depends on the site of disease and the form it takes. Bronchopulmonary aspergillosis is effectively treated with corticosteroids. The goal is to reduce the host response (which produces most of the symptoms) without rendering the host severely immunosuppressed. Itraconazole may also be useful in reducing the fungal (antigen) burden. If progression of disease is documented, it may be necessary to treat local fungus balls of sinus and lung with excision. Because underlying cavitary disease is often severe enough to preclude surgery, little is usually done unless hemoptysis forces intervention. Amphotericin B penetrates poorly into the mass of

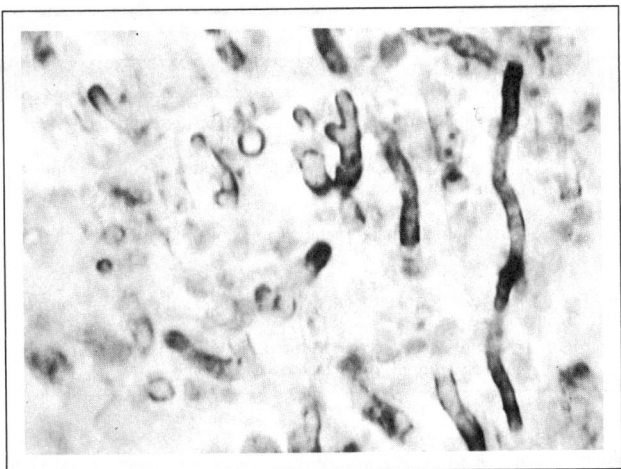

FIGURE 276-4   *Aspergillus fumigatus* hyphae from vegetation on an aortic valve showing the characteristic regular, septate branching hyphae. (Gomori's methenamine silver stain; original magnification ×1000.)

fungus in the mycetoma, and systemic treatment alone is rarely successful.

Disseminated disease should be treated promptly and aggressively with amphotericin B (1 mg/kg per day). Liposomal amphotericin B in high doses may offer benefit to patients who have intolerance or for whom standard amphotericin B therapy has failed. Duration of treatment is uncertain but should continue at least until manifestations appear to be subsiding. *Aspergillus* endocarditis requires surgery, and mortality is high. Combination therapy with itraconazole may offer improved efficacy. Itraconazole is useful in non–life-threatening infection and following an initial course of amphotericin B.

Zygomycetes
Epidemiology and Pathophysiology. The three genera *Absidia*, *Rhizomucor*, and *Rhizopus* account for most cases of zygomycosis. They can be readily distinguished from *Aspergillus* species and other hyalohyphomyces by broad, rarely septated hyphae that branch at right angles. Zygomycetes are found abundantly in nature and are common sources of bread mold contamination. Inhalation of the spores probably occurs repeatedly for most humans. Both acidosis and hyperglycemia, particularly, uncontrolled diabetes, are important predisposing factors for infection. Polymorphonuclear leukocytes readily kill the hyphae, and severe leukopenia is associated with lethal pulmonary disease.

The most common manifestation of zygomycosis is rhinocerebral disease. The fungus produces a necrotizing, locally invasive process of the palate or sinuses that directly invades and destroys adjoining structures. Vasculitis is frequent, with fungi invading and occluding arteries and veins. Symptoms begin with headache, eye irritation, and nasal stuffiness, sometimes with bloody discharge or a nasal eschar. Erosion into the orbit is associated with infraorbital numbness, proptosis, loss of vision, and both internal and external ophthalmoplegia. Ultimately, the fungi reach the brain, usually through the cribriform plate, and cause epidural and cerebral abscess, often complicated by cavernous sinus thrombosis. The course may be slow or fulminating.

Zygomycosis of the lungs may occur alone or as part of widely disseminated disease. This disease is similar to fulminating aspergillosis, with masses of fungi occluding blood vessels. Mortality is high, and the diagnosis is difficult to establish. Zygomycetes may invade denuded surfaces, especially burns or operative wounds. Outbreaks have been associated with contaminated dressings.

There are no serologic methods for diagnosis. Biopsies of deep specimens for histologic examination and culture are critically important. The treatment is amphotericin B, coupled with repeated, vigorous surgical debridement. The dosage must be rapidly accelerated to as high as 1.0 to 1.5 mg/kg per day and maintained until the pa-

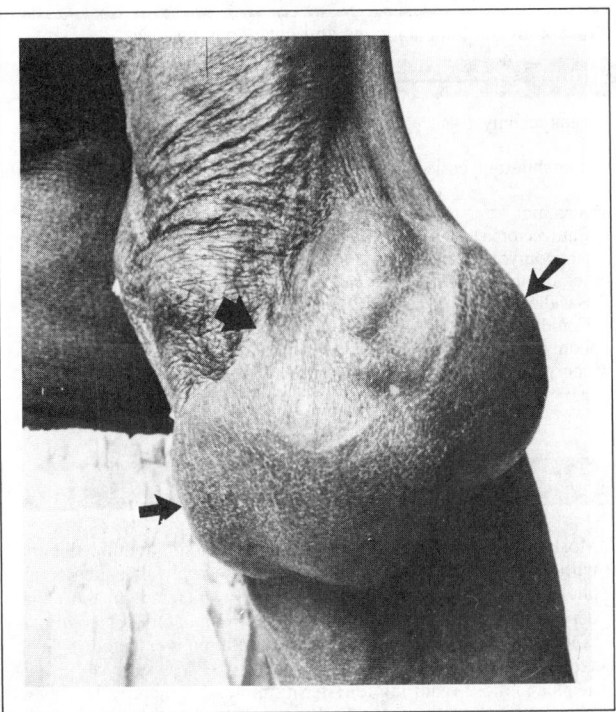

FIGURE 276-5   Chromoblastomycotic lesion of elbow.

tient is well on clinical examination. High doses of lipid forms of amphotericin B may improve the outcome. Another treatment factor is control of the underlying process, particularly diabetes mellitus or leukopenia.

Other Opportunistic Molds

A large number of molds have emerged as important pathogens in immunocompromised hosts. These organisms include *Fusarium*, *Pseudallescheria*, and *Trichosporon* spp.; *Pseudallescheria boydii*; and a variety of other rare fungi. These opportunistic organisms include dark-walled (dematiaceous) molds (e.g., *Bipolaris*, *Exoserohilum*, *Alternaria*, and *Dreschlera* spp.) and hyalohyphomycoses (hyaline mycelia) such as *Paecilomyces* and Penicillium spp. All these organisms very rarely cause infection in patients with normal host defenses, but in the presence of abnormal host defenses, such as patients with prolonged neutropenia, bone marrow transplantation, or advanced AIDS, overwhelming systemic infection may occur.

Subcutaneous and Cutaneous Mycoses

Chromoblastomycosis and Mycetoma. Chromoblastomycosis is a disease with many pathogens, mainly species of the genera *Fonsecaea*, *Exophiala*, and *Cladosporium* (Table 276-7). Infection is established after traumatic inoculation, usually into the extremities of barefoot farm workers of tropical countries. Lesions begin with papules and spread to nodules or large, cauliflower-like excrescences (Fig. 276-5). The disease is chronic, and rarely disseminates. The diagnosis is made by histologic and cultural demonstration of pigmented fungi in biopsy specimens. These organisms may be saprophytes or colonizers, so deep sampling of tissue is important.

The definitive treatment is surgical, with excision of local lesions; amputation may be required. Long-term therapy with itraconazole may produce responses in some patients. Treatment with amphotericin B and flucytosine has also been successful in selected cases.

Mycetoma is the name given to the destructive soft tissue and bone lesions caused by many fungi, including organisms of *Pseudallescheria*, *Exophiala*, *Aspergillus*, *Actinomyces*, *Streptomyces*, and *Nocardia* species. This disease was first described in India—hence the name madura foot. It occurs in the southern United States and tropi-

Table 276-7 Subcutaneous and cutaneous mycoses

MYCOSIS	ORGANISM(S)	COMMENT
Phaeohyphomycosis	*Exophiala jeanselmei, Phialophora* spp., *Cladosporium* spp., others	Dematiaceous fungi; subcutaneous or disseminated
Chromoblastomycosis	*Fonsecaea pedrosoi, Exophiala* spp., others	Cauliflower-like lesions; sclerotic bodies ("copper pennies") in tissue
Mycetoma		
Eumycetoma	*Pseudallescheria boydii, Madurella* spp., others	Granuloma, sinus, tracts, grains; endemic in India
Actinomycetoma	Actinomycetes	
Entomophthoramycosis		
Basidiobolomycosis	*Basidobolus ranarum*	Zygomycetes associated with reptiles, subcutaneous or nasal lesions
Conidiobolomycosis	*Conidiobolus coronatus*	
Lobomycosis	*Loboa loboi*	Keloid lesions, never cultured, dolphins also infected
Rhinosporidiosis	*Rhinosporidium seeberi*	Never cultured, nasal lesions

---

✔ WHEN TO REFER

Most patients with life-threatening mycoses still require therapy with amphotericin B. In many of those severely ill patients amphotericin B is not effective or is poorly tolerated. In those patients, liposomal amphotericin, immunomodulators, or combinations of antifungal agents may offer alternative therapies. The azoles offer particularly attractive options for less seriously ill patients and those requiring long-term suppressive therapy. However, some patients receiving azole therapy have "breakthrough" infection with less susceptible organism or have progressive symptoms. Many of these patients require more extensive mycologic and clinical evaluation and may need more aggressive antifungal therapies.

---

cal countries. Mycetoma begins after traumatic inoculation and progresses by formation of nodular granulomas and progressive destruction of tissues. Histologic and culture studies of involved tissues yield the pathogens. Definitive treatment is surgical. Itraconazole is of limited value in some patients.

Phaeohyphomycosis. Phaeohyphomycosis is a chronic necrotizing infection caused by any of a number of mycelial fungal species characterized by the presence of dark melanin pigment. The genera *Exserohilum, Phialophara,* and *Cladosporium,* are commonly involved, among others. Disease may follow traumatic inoculation (soft tissue, osteoarticular foci) or inhalation (sinusitis, chronic pneumonia). Disease is characteristically slowly progressive, destroying tissue over many months. An allergic form of sinusitis may occur and is characterized by the absence of tissue destruction and eosinophil-containing debris in sinus contents. Diagnosis is by direct demonstration of fungal hyphae and culture of the specific pathogen. The fungal pathogens are often but not always susceptible to amphotericin B or itraconazole.

BIBLIOGRAPHY

Anaissie E et al: New spectrum of fungal infections in patients with cancer, *Rev Infect Dis* 3:369-378, 1989.
Armstrong D: Treatment of opportunistic fungal infections, *Clin Infect Dis* 16:1-9, 1993.
Beck-Sague C, Jarvis WR: Secular trends in the epidemiology of nosocomial fungal infections in the United States, *J Infect Dis* 167:1247-1251, 1993.
Bradsher RW: Blastomycosis, *Clin Infect Dis* 14(suppl 1):S82-90, 1994.
Brummer E, Castenada E, Restrepo A: Paracoccidioidomycosis: an update, *Clin Microbiol Rev* 6:89-117, 1993.
Denning DW et al: NIAID Mycoses Study Group multicenter trial of oral itraconazole therapy for invasive aspergillosis, *Am J Med* 97:135-144, 1994.
Denning DW, Stevens DA: Antifungal and surgical treatment of invasive aspergillosis: review of 2,121 published cases, *Rev Infect Dis* 12:1147-1201, 1990.
Dismukes WE et al: Itraconazole therapy for blastomycosis and histoplasmosis, *Am J Med* 93:489-497, 1992.
Fader RC, McGinnis MR: Infections caused by dematiaceous fungi: chromoblastomycosis and phaeohyphomycosis, *Infect Dis Clin North Am* 2:925-938, 1988.
Galgiani JN, Ampel NM: Coccidioidomycosis in HIV-infected patients, *J Infect Dis* 162:1165, 1990.
Graybill JR: Future directions of antifungal chemotherapy, *Clin Infect Dis* 14:S17-181, 1992.
Hiemenz JW, Walsh TJ: Lipid formulations of amphotericin B: recent progress and future directions, *Clin Infect Dis* 22(suppl 2):S133-144, 1996.
Kauffman CA: Old and new therapies for sporotrichosis, *Clin Infect Dis* 21:981-985, 1995.
Kwon-Chung KJ: Phylogenetic spectrum of fungi that are pathogenic to humans, *Clin Infect Dis* 19:S1-7, 1994.
Kwon-Chung KJ, Bennett JE: *Medical mycology,* Philadelphia, 1992, Lea & Febiger.
Minamoto GY, Barlam TF, Vander Els NJ: Invasive aspergillosis in patients with AIDS, *Clin Infect Dis* 14:66-74, 1992.
Morrison VA, Haake RJ, Weisfort DJ: Non-*Candida* fungal infections following bone marrow transplantation: risk factors and outcome, *Am J Med* 96:497-503, 1994.
Patterson TF et al: The utility of antigen detection in the diagnosis of invasive aspergillosis, *J Infect Dis* 171:1553-1558, 1995.
Restrepo A: Treatment of tropical mycosis, *J Am Acad Dermatol* 31(3, pt 2):S91-102, 1994.
Stevens DA: Coccidioidomycosis, *N Engl J Med* 332:1077-1082, 1995.
Supparatpinyo K et al: *Penicillium marneffei* infection in patients infected with human immunodeficiency virus, *Clin Infect Dis* 14:871-874, 1992.
Wheat LJ et al: Disseminated histoplasmosis in AIDS: clinical findings, diagnosis and treatment, and review of the literature, *Medicine* 69:361-374, 1990.
Winn RE: Sporotrichosis, *Infect Dis Clin North Am* 2:899-911, 1988.

CHAPTER

277 Infections Caused by *Candida, Actinomyces,* and *Nocardia* Species

John E. Edwards, Jr.

CANDIDA SPECIES
Relevant Physiologic and Pathophysiologic Features

Candida species are small (4 to 6 μm in diameter), oval, thin-walled cells that reproduce by budding. Three morphologic forms are found in tissue: yeast, pseudohyphae, and hyphae. They can be identified in clinical specimens with warm 10% potassium hydroxide or Gram's stain. The organism is ubiquitous in nature and is a common human saprophyte. It grows well on most media used for routine recovery of microbial pathogens. Culturing from blood is facilitated with the lysis centrifugation technique. Although there are more than 100 species of *Candida,* those infecting humans are limited predominantly to *C. albicans, C. tropicalis, C. krusei, C. parapsilosis, C. guilliermondii, C. stellatoidea, C. pseudotropicalis, C. lusitaniae,* and *C. glabrata* (formerly *Torulopsis glabrata*). These species vary in their pathogenicity, epidemiology, organ predilections, and sensitivity to antifungal drugs.

Candida species are now among the most common nosocomial

pathogens, constituting 10% of isolates from blood cultures of hospitalized patients. Their emergence to this high level of prominence is a consequence of introducing modern therapeutic modalities into the treatment of patients who are seriously ill and require intensive therapy and monitoring for life support. Mucocutaneous candidal infections are among the most common opportunistic infections in patients with acquired immunodeficiency syndrome (AIDS).

Most frequently, candidal infections result from some form of compromise in the host defense mechanisms normally active against this saprophytic organism. Candidal infections that do not result from compromised host defenses include infections of the chorioretina and heart valves in heroin addicts, who inject the organism directly into their bloodstream. Also included is candidal vaginitis resulting mainly from local overgrowth of the organism after suppression of bacterial flora from antibiotic use. Two populations of patients susceptible to serious candidal infections are neonates with low birth weights and patients who require prolonged postoperative hospitalizations. These patients have some compromise of their normal defense mechanism but do not receive specific immunosuppressive therapy such as that given to patients with organ transplants.

Precisely what components of the normal host defense mechanisms are responsible for defense against the organism have not been defined. Clinical and in vitro observations suggest that cell-mediated immunity (CMI) (particularly lymphocyte function) is important in maintaining mucosal defense. For instance, patients with certain congenital abnormalities of the lymphocytic component of their CMI are prone to chronic mucocutaneous candidiasis. Patients with AIDS are also prone to candidal mucocutaneous infections, presumably as a result of their lymphocyte deficiency. Invasive candidiasis of the deep organs, usually initiated by hematogenous seeding, is considered to result from deficiencies in phagocytic mechanisms. Neutrophils and monocytes kill *Candida* organisms in vitro; neutropenia in patients treated with cytotoxic chemotherapeutic drugs for cancer is correlated with candidal infections. Complement and antibodies are opsonins for *Candida* organisms. The role of antibody in defense against *Candida* organisms is not clear; immunoglobulin G (IgG) anticandidal antibodies are present in nearly all normal individuals. Noncellular serum constituents other than complement and antibody may also have anticandidal properties.

Although *Candida* species are saprophytic, they have certain microbial characteristics that are likely to facilitate invasion once normal defense mechanisms are compromised. The organisms adhere to vaginal and oral epithelial cells, fibronectin, platelet-fibrin clots, acrylic, endothelium, plastics, and subendothelial matrix. They secrete proteases and phospholipases. *C. albicans* may be able to mechanically invade tissue with its tubular structures that form during germination. Certain *Candida* species have receptors on their surface that mimic human complement receptors and may facilitate their ability to invade tissue or escape host defense mechanisms.

Although the precise interactions between these potential pathogenicity factors and the specific defects in host defense mechanisms are not yet known, certain clinical circumstances are particularly prone to result in severe candidal infections. Generally, these clinical circumstances are characterized by iatrogenic compromise of the defense mechanisms. Therefore these organisms have evolved predominantly as a consequence of the advancement of medical therapeutics. The specific factors associated with severe candidal infections are the use of antibiotics, implantation of plastic indwelling intravascular catheters, cytotoxic chemotherapeutics for treatment of neoplastic diseases, corticosteroids, and immunosuppressive drugs for preventing transplanted organ rejection. The populations most often subjected to these factors are patients with cancer, organ transplants, or prosthetic material implants, patients undergoing complex surgical procedures (usually abdominal surgery), and low-birth-weight neonates who require intensive life support. The susceptibility of such a broad range of patients is the reason *Candida* species have emerged as such common nosocomial pathogens during the last two decades.

Clinical Manifestations

The term *thrush* refers to a form of candidiasis characterized by creamy white, curdlike patches on mucous membranes. When removed by scraping, they leave a raw, bleeding, ulcerative, painful surface. Thrush may occur in the mouth, esophagus, gastrointestinal tract, vagina, or bladder. The patches are pseudomembranes consisting of desquamated epithelial cells, leukocytes, bacteria, keratin, and necrotic tissue. The *Candida* organism can be visualized with 10% potassium hydroxide or Gram's stain. Simply culturing a plaque for *Candida* organisms is not sufficient to make a diagnosis, since the organisms may be present in the mouth without causing thrush. A specific diagnosis is necessary, since the patches of thrush are not distinctive in appearance and can be confused with other white lesions on mucous membranes, such as hairy leukoplakia in the mouth and the white plaques caused by gastric acid reflux in the esophagus. Thrush occurs most commonly in neutropenic patients, patients with diabetes, patients who have received antibiotics, patients with mucosal disruption from dentures, and patients who are generally severely debilitated by generalized illnesses or malnutrition. In patients who are neutropenic, cytomegalovirus and herpes viruses may cause lesions resembling thrush or may be present in thrush lesions concomitantly with the *Candida* organism. Esophagitis frequently occurs without obvious oral thrush. Candidal esophagitis may cause severe phagodynia. In its later stages it may become asymptomatic as a result of extensive involvement of the esophageal nerves. Identifying lesions consistent with candidal esophagitis, from which *Candida* species are recovered on plaque brushings, is sufficient reason to initiate therapy. To exclude other causes of the plaque or concomitant pathogens, biopsy is necessary. However, because the safety of biopsy is unclear, particularly with respect to dissemination, it should be reserved for special circumstances. Dissemination may occur from the esophagus in severe cases, and perforation may rarely occur. The presence of thrush of the mouth or esophagus, when there is no obvious reason for its occurrence, is a signal for a thorough evaluation for AIDS.

In addition to infecting the oral and esophageal mucosa, *Candida* species may infect the remainder of the intestinal tract. Gastric involvement may occur in patients with gastric ulcers that have become colonized and eventually infected with the organism, and in patients who are neutropenic from cancer chemotherapy. Infection of the mucous membranes of the gastrointestinal tract (including the stomach) occurs most commonly in neutropenic patients. The forms of infections are plaques of thrush, superficial erosions, ulcerations, and pseudomembrane formation. Perforation and, presumably, dissemination may occur. Diarrhea may be a consequence. Other organs within the abdomen that may become infected with *Candida* species are the gallbladder, liver, spleen, and pancreas. In the gallbladder a generalized cholecystitis may occur, or fungus balls that obstruct drainage may form. The extent of infection in the liver, spleen, and pancreas may range from small microabscesses and macroabscesses to large abscesses that cause extensive necrosis and organ failure. Hepatosplenic candidiasis, or chronic disseminated candidiasis, has emerged as an important problem in neutropenic patients. The latter term is preferable for describing this syndrome, since organs other than the spleen and liver are frequently involved, such as kidney. Usually, multiple microlesions and macrolesions are distributed throughout the involved organs from hematogenous seeding. The infection usually persists for many months and is generally refractory to therapy with the standard antifungals.

Candidal peritonitis has emerged as a serious problem in patients undergoing gastrointestinal tract surgery or sustaining trauma to the abdomen. Diagnosis is difficult without biopsy of the involved peritoneum. Frequently, *Candida* species are isolated from drainage of the peritoneum along with bacteria, so determining the precise role of the *Candida* organism is problematic.

Another important mucous membrane infection caused by *Candida* species is vaginitis. This infection is exceedingly common and occurs after a course of antibiotic treatment in the majority of patients. Either a thick, curdlike discharge or a scanty discharge may occur. Pruritus is almost always present. The urethra and the endometrium may become infected secondarily. Masses of hyphae, pseudohyphae, and leukocytes are present in the discharge. Some patients have frequent recurrences.

A large number of common cutaneous syndromes are caused by *Candida* species. Diaper rash in infants is frequently caused by *Candida* organisms. It usually starts in the perianal area and spreads over the distribution of the diaper. Wet diapers predispose to the infection.

Candida species are frequent causes of paronychia, especially in individuals who often immerse their hands in wash water. The lesion is a focal infection adjacent to the nail that becomes warm, glistening, and tense. It may extend under the nail. Candidal intertrigo is a common condition that begins as vesicopustules, which enlarge and rupture to cause maceration and fissures. It occurs in warm, moist areas of the skin surface that are in juxtaposition, such as under the breasts or in the inguinal areas. Satellite lesions may be present. It is associated with diabetes and obesity. Numerous organisms have been associated with pruritus ani; *Candida* species are commonly recovered when this condition is present. Marked erythema of the perianal skin occurs, maceration develops, and severe pruritus is present. The condition may spread extensively over the perineum or deep within the anal canal.

In addition to the common cutaneous conditions, a variety of less common conditions are caused by *Candida* species. Generalized cutaneous candidiasis is a widespread eruption of the trunk, thorax, and extremities. It usually becomes more pronounced in the genitocrural folds, anal region, axillae, hands, and feet. Both children and adults may be affected. *Erosio interdigitalis blastomycetica* is a term applied to the red-based, painful infection occurring in macerated skin between the toes and fingers. Candidal folliculitis is another cutaneous infection that occurs rarely. Candidal balanitis begins as vesicles on the distal end of the penis and frequently develops into patches. It may become extensive and spread beyond the genital area and is frequently associated with severe burning and itching. Chronic mucocutaneous candidiasis is a condition characterized by refractory infection of the skin, mucous membranes, and nails that is associated with a heterogenous group of immunologic abnormalities (Chapter 230). The major immune defect is failure of T-cell lymphocytes (thymus-derived) to respond to stimulation in vitro with candidal antigen. Cutaneous anergy occurs in half the patients. Patients are heterogenous in their deficiency of antigenic response both in vitro and cutaneously. Their immune deficiency is considered to be congenital. However, certain patients do not show evidence of the condition until their adult years. Whether the disease may be acquired in these patients, rather than congenital, remains unknown. Approximately half the patients have an associated endocrinopathy such as hypoparathyroidism, Addison's disease, hypothyroidism, or diabetes. Approximately half the patients also have autoantibodies to renal, thyroid, and gastric tissues. Additional associations with the syndrome are thymoma, dermatophytosis, dental dysplasia, vitiligo, polyglandular autoimmune disease, and autoantibodies to melanin-producing cells. Most patients survive for long periods. However, the disease may become severe and disfiguring. Death usually results from bacterial sepsis rather than disseminated candidiasis.

Infection of the blood and deep organs with *Candida* species is responsible for the substantial increase in frequency of nosocomial candidal infections and is the central problem of concern. The deep-organ infection usually occurs as a result of widespread hematogenous dissemination during conditions of relative immunocompromise. The populations usually acquiring widespread hematogenous infections are patients treated with cytotoxic chemotherapy for cancer, patients on immunosuppressive therapy after organ transplantation, patients sustaining burns, severely ill neonates with low birth weights, and patients having protracted postoperative courses (most frequently after gastrointestinal tract surgery). Iatrogenic factors common to these patients, other than cytotoxic immunosuppressive drugs and corticosteroids, are general debilitation, the use of antibiotics, the use of indwelling intravascular catheters for intravenous infusions or for monitoring cardiovascular status, and the use of hyperalimentation fluids for nutritional support. Precisely how the organism enters the blood stream is not clear. In some patients it may enter through intravenous access catheters. In others, probably the majority, it enters through the gastrointestinal tract, after it has proliferated to large numbers from iatrogenic factors promoting its growth. Once the vascular compartment has been invaded, the organism can disseminate to nearly any organ of the body. Those most commonly infected are the kidney, brain, heart, liver, spleen, skin, and eye. Those less commonly involved are skeletal muscle, bone marrow, spine, joints, and lung. Within these organs microabscesses and small macroabscesses develop that are generally diffusely spread throughout the organ. Except in the case of hepatosplenic involvement, the lesions rarely attain a size identifiable by currently available radiographic or radionucleotide imaging techniques.

After the organism has entered the intravascular compartment, it may trigger a shock syndrome in some patients. This syndrome is clinically indistinguishable from shock caused by gram-negative organisms. *Candida* species do not have an endotoxin that closely resembles that of the gram-negative organisms, and the syndrome is probably a result of cytokine production by the host. After infecting the deep organs, generalized organ failure may develop. Either extensive, diffuse cerebral infection or meningitis may develop from the central nervous system involvement. Heart failure and arrhythmias may be a consequence of the diffuse myocardial involvement and invasion of the cardiac conduction system. Liver failure and elevated hepatic enzyme levels may develop. Diminished renal function may be manifested by an elevation in blood urea nitrogen or serum creatinine level, and the glomerular filtration rate may decrease. Blindness may result from hematogenous candidal endophthalmitis. A miliary pattern may be present on chest x-ray in a small number of patients during the preterminal phase of the illness. Pain frequently accompanies the skeletal muscle infection. Small, macronodular skin lesions that contain the organisms on biopsy may develop. In rare instances bone marrow failure may be a consequence of severe marrow infection.

Management of patients with candidemia, who are predisposed by the iatrogenic factors associated with disseminated candidiasis, is highly challenging. No method exists to separate patients who have transient, catheter-associated candidemia from those with candidemia who have foci of infection in the deep organs. In the general hospitalized patient population, patients with candidemia have an overall mortality rate of approximately 50%. The mortality is attributable to *Candida* species in approximately 40%. An unknown number of patients have a delayed complication of the candidemia, such as hematogenous ocular, renal, or bone infection, that may become clinically overt days to even years after the initial candidemia. While extensive investigations have focused on the role of certain serodiagnostic techniques for separating patients with transient candidemia from those with visceral organ infection, no techniques are currently available for practical use that are widely accepted. The situation is complicated even more by the fact that approximately 40% of patients with widespread hematogenous infection do not have positive blood cultures. Therefore even blood cultures are relatively insensitive in detecting visceral organ infection. Because of the high mortality rates associated with candidemia, the lack of ability to distinguish patients with transient candidemia from those with deep organ infection, and the possibility of late complications of the candidemia, there is a strong consensus among certain clinical mycologists that all patients with candidemia should receive antifungal therapy, unless there is a contraindication to antifungal drugs (see Management).

Two forms of candidal infection associated with the candidemia–hematogenous dissemination syndrome deserve emphasis. They are hematogenous candidal endophthalmitis and the macronodular skin lesions resulting from dissemination to the skin. Both the skin lesions and the ocular infection are important in establishing the diagnosis of widespread hematogenous candidiasis, since they are both strongly correlated with involvement of multiple deep organs. Hematogenous candidal endophthalmitis is important not only for signalling the presence of infection in other deep organs, but also because the lesions may cause permanent blindness. Furthermore, in patients who are not neutropenic, involvement of the chorioretina may be a relatively common complication of candidemia caused by *C. albicans*. One prospective study has defined an incidence of 27% for the occurrence of hematogenous endophthalmitis in patients with candidemia. The lesions of hematogenous candidal endophthalmitis are round, cotton-ball–like lesions associated with vitreous haze. They may expand into a severe generalized endophthalmitis and may necessitate enucleation in some cases.

Several deep-organ candidal infections occur that are not complications of the candidemia–hematogenous dissemination syndrome. Candidal meningitis may occur as a complication of brain surgery or as a result of the implantation of prosthetic materials into the central nervous system. Rarely, candidal meningitis may occur de novo. Nearly all patients have a pleocytosis; in 50% it is predominately lymphocytic. Hypoglycorrhachia and elevated protein levels are present frequently, and the organism is seen on Gram's stain or wet preparation of the cerebral spinal fluid in 40% of patients. Two forms of candidal pneumonia exist. One is the diffuse miliary pattern associated with widespread hematogenous dissemination. It is almost always a preterminal event. The other form is that of a necrotic bronchopneumonia. It is rare and considered to be a result of a candidal superinfection of a bacterial pneumonic process. Care must be taken to avoid diagnosing candidal pneumonia in patients with a pulmonary infiltrate on chest x-ray and recovery of candida from the sputum. Biopsy evidence of candidal invasion of the pulmonary parenchyma is necessary to definitively establish this diagnosis. *Candida* organisms may infect prosthetic cardiac valves and the cardiac valves of drug addicts.

Candidal Infection of the Cardiovascular System. Rarely, native cardiac valves may become infected, especially in patients who have had a long-term intravenous catheter for parenteral fluid administration. Eradication of the infection from heart valves is exceptionally difficult; surgery is almost always required. In addition to occurring in the setting of widespread disseminated candidiasis, candidal pericarditis can complicate cardiac surgery, and candidal sternal osteomyelitis may occur at the surgical site. Candidal vascular infections occur most commonly at the site of intravascular catheter insertion. Thrombosis and infection caused by *Candida* organisms have been growing problems in recent years. Extensive infection of the thrombophlebitis caused by the catheter may develop, necessitating surgical removal of the clot. Fungus balls in the right atrium have been reported from indwelling subclavian catheters. Septic arterial emboli may also occur and cause mycotic aneurysms. They are usually a complication of candidal endocarditis. Candidal vascular infections occur most commonly at the site of intravascular catheter insertion. Candidal arthritis may occur as a result of joint trauma, surgery, intraarticular injections of corticosteroids, and heroin injection.

Candidal infections that have been reported but are not elaborated on include middle-ear infections, nasal ulcers, keratitis, lymphadenitis, sinusitis, laryngeal infection, diarrhea, the "drunken disease" (a syndrome described in Japan that is considered to be caused by alcohol absorption from fermentation by *Candida* organisms of carbohydrates in the gastrointestinal tract), and the yeast connection (fatigue and immune suppression postulated to result from overgrowth of *Candida* organisms on skin and mucous membranes).

Laboratory and Other Diagnostic Tests

Despite extensive investigations into antigen and antibody detection systems and detection of products secreted by the organism, there are no commercially available serodiagnostic tests for candidal infection of the deep organs that are considered to have acceptable true-positive and true-negative detection rates. With current techniques there is still approximately a 40% false-negative rate in culturing *Candida* organisms from the blood. The lysis-centrifugation technique both increases the sensitivity of blood cultures and reduces the time necessary for the organisms to grow. It is likely that a panel of serodiagnostic tests will be developed in the future to derive a probability for deep organ infection based on the number of positive test results and perhaps on quantitative aspects of their positivity.

Currently the only method to definitively diagnose deep organ infection is to demonstrate tissue invasion by *Candida* organisms on biopsy specimens. In certain clinical situations, however, a decision to initiate treatment may be made without definitive diagnosis. The two best examples are hematogenous candidal endophthalmitis and chronic hepatosplenic candidiasis. For instance, in a patient who is candidemic, who is known to have had a normal ocular fundus before the candidemia, and who develops lesions that are clinically compatible with the ocular lesions caused by *Candida* organism seeding, empiric therapy is initiated for treatment of the ocular disease. Similarly, in neutropenic patients who are candidemic and develop lesions in the liver compatible with hepatosplenic candidiasis, therapy may be initiated without biopsy of the lesions. As an alternative, an example for which a specific diagnosis is desirable is candidal pulmonary infection. A patient who has a pulmonary infiltrate on chest x-ray and has *Candida* organisms in the sputum may not have candidal pneumonia. Biopsy evidence of *Candida* organisms invading the pulmonary parenchyma is necessary to definitely establish the diagnosis of candidal pneumonia.

Management

The treatment of candidal infections must be directed at the specific form of infection, because of their varied nature and severity (Table 277-1). The majority of the cutaneous syndromes, such as candidal intertrigo, can be treated with topical imidazoles such as miconazole or clotrimazole. More severe cutaneous syndromes such as chronic mucocutaneous candidiasis require oral imidazoles such as ketoconazole or fluconazole for eradication. In especially severe circumstances, brief courses of amphotericin B may be necessary. Candidal vaginitis is usually responsive to topical imidazoles. In refractory cases oral ketoconazole or fluconazole may be necessary, but care should be taken to avoid its use in pregnancy. Fluconazole has now been approved by the U.S. Food and Drug Administration (FDA) for candidal vaginitis. For mild thrush, nystatin has been used for decades. However, it is being replaced by clotrimazole troches, which are considered more palatable by most patients. In refractory cases either ketoconazole or fluconazole may be necessary. In certain AIDS patients who have been given repeated treatment with azoles, organisms with relative azole resistance have been recovered. Candidal esophagitis can be treated successfully with oral ketoconazole or fluconazole. Recent studies in patients with AIDS have shown fluconazole to be more effective. It has the advantage of not requiring gastric acid for absorption; many patients with AIDS are relatively achlorhydric. In refractory cases brief courses of intravenous amphotericin B may be effective. Candidal infection of the gallbladder associated with obstruction usually requires surgery. Candidal peritonitis should be treated with intravenous amphotericin B in severely ill patients. Patients undergoing chronic peritoneal dialysis may benefit from fluconazole, although the data are limited at present. Whether removal of the dialysis catheter is necessary remains controversial; successes and failures have both been reported. However, if logistically feasible, it is probably better to replace the catheter. In general, infection of the deep organs such as the lung, heart, kidney, brain, bone, liver, spleen, and joints requires amphotericin B. (The role of fluconazole in these deep infections has not been clarified to date.) When comparative studies are performed, fluconazole may be found to be an effective alternative to amphotericin B. Because of the excellent penetration of fluconazole into the brain and its high level of excretion into the urine, the brain and kidneys will be of particular interest. Currently, candidal cystitis is treated successfully by removing the indwelling urinary bladder catheter, if present. If postcatherization candiduria persists in asymptomatic patients, it may resolve spontaneously. If not, a "washout" of the bladder with amphotericin B may be an alternative. 5-Fluorocytosine (5-FC) has been used successfully. However, de novo resistance to 5-FC may be present and resistance may develop during therapy. Fluconazole may be an effective alternative, and is more convenient to administer. Candidal endophthalmitis should be treated with intravenous amphotericin B. In patients whose lesions continue to progress under therapy or who have lesions in proximity to the macula, 5-FC should be added. The role of partial vitrectomy is highly important, and ophthalmologic consultation should be obtained for consideration of this procedure. The role of intravitreal antifungals remains controversial. Although fluconazole penetrates the intraocular structures, its use in patients with hematogenous candidal endophthalmitis is limited, and preliminary studies in animal models have shown it to be less effective than amphotericin B. More experience in humans is necessary to clarify its role. However, successful treatment with fluconazole alone has now been reported in patients, and use of fluconazole, once resolution begins following initial treatment with amphotericin B, is an attractive strategy.

The treatment of patients with candidemia deserves special emphasis. Because of the high mortality rate associated with candidemia, the high rates of attributable mortality to candidal infections complicating the candidemia, and the current lack of reliable methods to distinguish patients at high risk for widespread disseminated candidiasis from those with low risk, all patients with candidemia should be given treatment with antifungal agents unless there is a contraindication to the drugs. A multicenter cooperative study found no

Table 277-1   Treatment of candidiasis

FORM OF DISEASE	TREATMENT REGIMEN	COMMENTS
Uncomplicated mucosal disease	For thrush, clotrimazole troches or nystatin. For esophagitis, ketoconazole or fluconazole. For intertriginous disease or vaginal disease, topical miconazole, clotrimazole. For vaginal disease use topical azoles or oral fluconazole.	Fluconazole and ketoconazole are effective but should be reserved for severe or refractory infections. In AIDS patients, fluconazole has been more effective than ketoconazole.
Chronic mucocutaneous candidiasis	Ketoconazole 200 to 600 mg/day, PO Fluconazole 200 mg/day, PO	For control, intermittent IV amphotericin B may be necessary.
Upper urinary tract infection	Intravenous amphotericin B, 0.3-0.6 mg/kg/day until evidence of resolution. Fluconazole is under investigation.	
Cystitis	Remove catheter, amphotericin B bladder washout. 5-FC, 50-75 mg/kg/day, PO. Fluconazole under investigation. For severe cases, amphotericin B, IV.	Resistance to 5-FC may be present and also may develop during therapy.
Disseminated candidiasis and candidemia	Amphotericin B, 0.3-0.6 mg/kg/day for 1 to 3 weeks depending on severity. Flucytosine, 100 to 150 mg/kg/day, PO, may be added depending on severity. Patients with catheter-associated candidemia and a low probability of having disseminated candidiasis should receive fluconazole, 400 mg/day. All patients with candidemia, whether or not it is associated with a catheter, should be treated with an antifungal unless there is a contraindication.	A large, multicenter clinical trial comparing amphotericin B with fluconazole in candidemia has been completed in non-neutropenic patients. No statistically significant difference was seen.
Candida endophthalmitis	Amphotericin B at 0.3 to 0.6 mg/kg/day until evidence of resolution occurs. In severe cases or in cases where the macula is involved, 5-FC, 100-150 mg/kg/day, PO, should be added. Fluconazole is under investigation.	Partial vitrectomy should be considered with ophthalmologic consultation.
Candida endocarditis	Infected valve should be removed as soon as possible. After surgery, amphotericin B and 5-FC should be given for 6 weeks or more.	There are reports of rare cases of cure with amphotericin B therapy. They are the exception and the valve should be removed whenever possible.
Prosthetic implants infected with *Candida* spp.	Removal of implant is almost always necessary. Amphotericin B should be given after removal.	The role of fluconazole is not yet known.

AIDS, Acquired immunodeficiency syndrome; *5-FC*, 5-fluorocytosine; *IV*, intravenous; *PO*, orally.

statistically significant difference between amphotericin B and fluconazole (Itraconazole is not currently approved by the FDA in the United States for candidemia). However, most investigators believe that patients who are deteriorating or are in shock as a result of candidemia should be given treatment with amphotericin B or a combination of amphotericin B and 5-FC initially. If possible, if the candidemia is related to an intravascular catheter, the catheter should be removed. Certain clinical situations exist in which catheter removal is problematic and adjustments are necessary.

ACTINOMYCOSIS
Relevant Physiologic and Pathophysiologic Features

The organisms of the genus *Actinomyces* are true prokaryotic bacteria that cause indolent diseases that resemble fungal infection. These bacteria are gram-positive, filamentous (1 μm in diameter), and branching. They are either microaerophilic or anaerobic. Failure to culture clinical specimens in anaerobic conditions has caused serious delays in diagnosing actinomycosis. A hallmark of the species is its ability to form "sulfur" granules in tissue. These granules are amorphous masses of organisms that can become large enough to be seen without microscopy. Characteristic "bread crumb" colonies form in thioglycollate broth. On solid media early colonies are delicately branched. As they mature, they become large and heaped up with a lobulated surface. They resemble a molar tooth standing up from the agar's surface. The most important species causing human infections are *Actinomycetes israelii, Actinomyces naeslundii, Actinomyces viscosus,* and *Actinomyces odontalyticus.* A related organism, *Arachnia propionica,* is capable of causing classic lesions of actinomycosis. These organisms are human commensals found most commonly on the oral and pharyngeal mucosa.

Pathogenesis

Actinomyces organisms are saprophytes with a low level of virulence. Apparently, normal host defense mechanisms are highly efficient in protecting against them, since they are not common pathogens, even in patients with severe iatrogenic immunosuppression. However, in recent years a number of cases have been reported in patients who are immunocompromised because of AIDS. Generally, tissue trauma is necessary to provide a milieu conducive for invasion. Once established in a focus, the organisms proliferate to form the classic "sulfur" granules. Induration of the infected tissues is common. Another characteristic is the presence of other bacteria in addition to the *Actinomyces* species. These accompanying organisms are usually actinobacilli, *Haemophilus* species, and/or various oral anaerobes. These accompanying bacteria may facilitate the tissue invasion by the weakly pathogenic *Actinomyces* organisms.

On histopathologic examination, the lesions are characterized by numerous foamy macrophages, eosinophils, and giant cells, unlike the classic polymorphonuclear response seen with pyogenic bacteria. As chronicity increases, plasma cells appear, granules form, and extensive induration develops. A hallmark of the infection is its ability to cross anatomic barriers and to form sinus tracts extending to other organs or to the skin. When the sulfur granules become large enough to be visible without microscopy, they are yellow or dull white, hard, gritty structures that may be as large as 2 mm in diameter.

Clinical Manifestations

The most common infections of actinomycosis are cervicofacial, thoracic, abdominal, pelvic, and disseminated. Cervicofacial disease almost invariably begins as an extension from a peridental origin (Color Plate V-55). Frequently, minor trauma initiates the process. Although the most common form is an indolent, slowly evolving disease, a more rapidly progressive form occurs rarely. The disease process crosses

✔ *WHEN TO REFER*

Because of the complexities of establishing a diagnosis of hematogenously disseminated candidiasis and the intricacies of therapy, it is appropriate to refer nearly all patients in whom the disease is suspected. Identifying the patients at risk is critical to making an early diagnosis. Patients at risk are those who have had indwelling intravenous catheters, received multiple antibiotics, been treated with hyperalimentation fluids, and may be neutropenic from cytoxic chemotherapy for cancer treatment. Cancer chemotherapy patients, patients with prolonged postoperative hospitalization in intensive care units, low-birth-weight neonates, patients who have received organ transplants, and burn patients are particularly at risk. Usually these patients will have been treated with antibacterial antibiotics but remain febrile following treatment. It is appropriate to refer these patients to an infectious disease specialist for a thorough diagnostic evaluation and to determine appropriate definitive or presumptive therapy. In some populations prophylactic therapy may be warranted, but only after the epidemiology of the individual intensive care unit or hospital is surveyed. Since there are very few studies on the treatment of any form of candidal infection, assistance from an infectious disease consultant is helpful to derive the best treatment plan.

✔ *WHEN TO REFER*

Patients with facial, pulmonary, gastrointestinal tract, osseous, or pelvic infections that are chronic and have not been diagnosed through routine methods should be referred to an infectious disease specialist. Frequently, actinomycosis has not been considered in such patients and anaerobic cultures have not been performed. Once the diagnosis is established, the design of the therapeutic regimen should be made within the context of relatively long-term antimicrobial therapy.

anatomic boundaries and causes lumpy swelling of the face that may develop sinus tracts. The mandible is a much more frequent site of origin than the maxilla. However, almost any facial or cervical structure may become involved, including the tongue, sinuses, or thyroid. Rare complications are direct extension into the brain and hematogenous dissemination. The development of "cold" abscesses and draining sinus along the ramus of the mandible is the condition referred to classically as "lumpy jaw."

Thoracic actinomycosis is usually aspiration pneumonia, but it may result from extension into the thorax from adjacent anatomic sites such as the neck or abdomen. Rarely, it may be a result of hematogenous dissemination. The forms of pulmonary parenchymal involvement are nonspecific and include a bronchopneumonia or, rarely, a mass lesion. Empyema may develop. Extension through the lung parenchyma and pleural space into and through the chest wall may occur, resulting in a pulmonic-cutaneous sinus tract. An osteomyelitis of the rib may develop as the infection invades through the chest wall. The process may extend to the mediastinum or cross the boundary formed by the diaphragm into the abdominal cavity. As is characteristic of actinomycotic infections in general, the infection is indolent and may be relatively asymptomatic. Thoracic x-ray findings are not specific. Thoracic disease may resemble tuberculosis.

Abdominal actinomycosis is usually a complication of a primary nonactinomycotic process such as inflammatory bowel disease or surgery and, occasionally, complicates blunt trauma. *Actinomyces* infection may cause a chronic ileocecal inflammation resembling Crohn's disease or ileocecal tuberculosis. Virtually any portion of the gastrointestinal tract may be involved; gastric actinomycosis may resemble gastric ulcer disease. When the bowel is infected, secondary infection of the liver is relatively common. Sinus tracts may form, and the process may extend directly into the thoracic or pelvic cavities. Because of the indolent nature of the infection, diagnosis is invariably delayed.

Pelvic actinomycosis usually originates as an extension from an abdominal source. Virtually any pelvic organ may be involved. The ovaries and fallopian tubes are infected most commonly, although rare pelvic infection may result from the use of indwelling contraceptive intrauterine devices (IUDs). As many as 11% of women using IUDs have been found to have cervicovaginal colonization with *Actinomyces* organisms. In either case, the process may become extensive and involve nearly all the pelvic structures, including the urinary tract, by direct extension. Central nervous system actinomycosis occurs most commonly as a result of hematogenous spread from an abdominal or thoracic focus. Usually, solitary mass lesions occur. Meningitis or meningoencephalitis occurs less commonly. Extensive intracerebral infection may result from direct extension of a facial or cervical focus.

Osseous actinomycosis occurs either from direct extension or from hematogenous spread. Radiographic findings are nonspecific. Occasionally, trauma may be the cause.

Laboratory and Other Diagnostic Tests and Differential Diagnosis

Demonstration of invasion by the characteristic branched, grampositive filamentous structures on Gram's stain with confirmation by culture is necessary for definitive diagnosis. Proper processing of the specimen for anaerobic culturing is essential. Because of the similarities in the forms of clinical infection and similar appearance of the organisms on Gram's stain, it is desirable to distinguish actinomycosis from nocardiosis. The two diseases are treated with different antibacterials, so identifying the infecting agent facilitates early administration of the proper therapy. In contrast to *Nocardia* species, the *Actinomyces* organisms are not acid-fast. They form sulfur granules in tissues, a characteristic that *Nocardia* has only in exceptionally rare circumstances. Infection with the *Actinomyces* organism usually is accompanied by additional bacteria. The presence of the breadcrumb colonies in thioglycolate broth and the molar tooth colonies of *Actinomyces* organisms facilitate the early laboratory confirmation of the clinical and Gram's stain findings. There are no helpful skin or serodiagnostic tests.

Management

Nearly all cases respond to high-dose intravenous aqueous penicillin given for 4 to 6 weeks, followed by oral penicillin for months. In refractory cases surgery may be necessary. Surgery may be especially advantageous if the initial presentation is complicated by involvement of large masses of tissue. Alternatives to penicillin are tetracycline, erythromycin, and clindamycin. First-generation cephalosporins, third-generation celphalosporins, imipenem, ampicillin, and amoxicillin are also substitutes. There is no significant species variation in susceptibility to the agents.

NOCARDIOSIS
Relevant Physiologic and Pathophysiologic Features

The *Nocardia* species are classified in the family Actinomycetaceae. They are differentiated from organisms causing actinomycosis by being acid-fast and growing aerobically. They are related to mycobacteria. A special acid-fast stain is necessary using an aqueous sulfuric acid as the decolorizer rather than the acid alcohol used in the classic Ziehl-Neelsen stain, which decolorizes *Nocardia* species. The organisms are branched, filamentous, and gram-positive. *Nocardia* species are slow growing; in suspected cases, culturing specimens for a prolonged period may be helpful.

Nocardia organisms are ubiquitous saprophytes found in a large number of animal species and in decaying organic matter. They have been isolated from respiratory tract secretions of patients with chronic obstructive pulmonary airways disease who have no evidence of a *Nocardia* species infection.

The most common species of *Nocardia* infecting humans are *N. asteroides, N. brasiliensis,* and *N. otitidism-caviarum.* Other species rarely cause infection.

Nocardiosis is usually an opportunistic infection, although a significant number of infected patients have no recognizable immunocompromise. The most commonly infected immunocompromised patients are those receiving corticosteroids, patients with malignancies (especially lymphoreticular and chronic malignancy in general), patients receiving cytotoxic chemotherapy, and organ transplant recipients who are receiving immunosuppressive drugs. Patients with primary alveolar proteinosis have a particularly high propensity for nocardial infections, probably as a result of inadequately functioning pulmonary macrophages. Some *Nocardia* species can invade and replicate within macrophages. Acquisition of the disease is usually through inhalation of spores. Human-to-human transmission is possible, and outbreaks have been reported in transplantation units. Cutaneous forms of nocardial infection usually result from inoculation of soil harboring the organism.

The most common nocardial infection is pulmonary. After inhalation and establishment of infection, a necrotizing pneumonia develops that is usually not associated with an extensive inflammatory response of leukocytes. Once the necrotizing pneumonia begins, tissue destruction may occur, and the process becomes chronic. Like actinomycosis, in patients with nocardiosis sinus tracts may develop, extending through the chest wall onto the skin. Virtually any intrathoracic structure may become involved by direct extension. Hematogenous extension to the brain is not uncommon. Any patient with pulmonary nocardosis, whether or not they may be immunocompromised, should be evaluated carefully for the possibility of hematogenous dissemination to the brain. Hematogenous extension to nearly any organ is possible, and myriad hematogenous infections have been reported, including infections of the liver, spleen, kidney, adrenal gland, thyroid gland, prostate gland, and eye. X-ray and other radiologic findings are nonspecific. Hematogenous nocardial endophthalmitis has been specifically diagnosed with fine-needle retinal biopsy. In recent years the *Nocardia* organism has been one of many of the pathogens found in patients with AIDS. Infection in a variety of organs, including the lungs, brain, and esophagus, has been reported, in addition to suprarenal and paraspinal abscesses.

Laboratory and Other Diagnostic Tests and Differential Diagnosis

There are no diagnostic blood or skin tests. Blood cultures are not helpful. Diagnosis requires a biopsy specimen showing the characteristic organisms infecting tissue; positive cultures are confirmatory. Differentiation from actinomycosis is accomplished by demonstrating the acid-fast properties of *Nocardia* organisms, the lack of sulfur granules or other accompanying pathogens, aerobic growth, and the lack of "molar tooth" colony formation in cultures.

Management

Long-term therapy is necessary for virtually all forms of nocardiosis. Sulfonamides, most commonly sulfadiazine, are the first-line agents. Surgical intervention may be necessary, especially in central nervous system infection. Certain investigators prefer trimethoprim-sulfamethoxazole (TMP-SMX) to sulfadiazine as the first-line agent. The problems with TMP-SMX are treatment failure in some cases, lack of synergistic activity in approximately one third of species, and more toxicity in general than sulfadiazine alone. The increased toxicity is a particular problem in AIDS patients. Cycloserine has been advocated as an adjunctive therapy to the sulfadiazine. Additional agents that have been advocated include amikacin, cefotaxime, imipenem, ceftriaxone, and cefuroxime amoxicillin-clavulanic acid. Imipenem-cefotaxime, amikacin–TMP-SMX, and imipenem–TMP-SMX have all shown synergistic activity in vitro. Since the species of *Nocardia* vary in sensitivity, it is advisable to obtain sensitivity testing on clinical isolates for selection of the most effective therapeutic agent or combination of agents.

Most forms of nocardiosis require 4 to 6 weeks of treatment. In many instances an even longer period of therapy is necessary. Clini-

✔ **WHEN TO REFER**

Patients with infections resembling actinomycosis should be referred for appropriate diagnosis, differentiation from actinomycosis, and design of their therapeutic regimen. Changes in the therapy may be necessary according to the ability of the patient to tolerate long-term sulfa-containing regimens.

cal response to treatment does not occur early, and an initial delay of clinical response should be expected.

BIBLIOGRAPHY

Anaissie E: Opportunistic mycoses in the immunocompromised host: experience at a cancer center and review, *Clin Infect Dis* 14(suppl 1):S43, 1992.
Bodey GP: Azole antifungal agents, *Clin Infect Dis* 14(suppl 1):S161, 1992.
Bross JE, Gordon G: Nocardial meningitis: case reports and review, *Rev Infect Dis* 13:160, 1991.
Budren P: Actinomycosis, *J Infect Dis* 19:95, 1989.
Chatwani A, Amin-Hanjani S: Incidence of actinomycosis associated with intrauterine devices, *J Reprod Med* 39:585-587, 1994.
Cole GT, Halawa AA, Anaissie EJ: The role of the gastrointestinal tract in hematogenous candidiasis: from the laboratory to the bedside, *Clin Infect Dis* 22(suppl 2):S73-S88, 1996.
Edwards JE, Jr, Bodey GP, Bowden RA et al: International conference for the development of a consensus on the management and prevention of severe candidal infections. *Clin Infect Dis,* 25:43, 1997.
Edwards JE Jr, Filler SG: Current strategies for treating invasive candidiasis: emphasis on infections in nonneutropenic patients, *Clin Infect Dis* 14(suppl 1):S106, 1992.
Fife TD, Finegold SM, Grennan T: Pericardial actinomycosis: case report and review, *Rev Infect Dis* 13:120, 1991.
Goodman HM, Centeno BA: A 41-year-old woman with a swollen left leg, pelvic mass, and bilateral hydronephrosis: case records of the Massachusetts General Hospital, *N Engl J Med* 326:692, 1992.
Grieco MH, Kim J, Minamoto GY: Nocardial infection as a complication of AIDS: report of six cases and review, *Rev Infect Dis* 13:624, 1991.
Javaly K, Horowitz HW, Wormser GP: Nocardiosis in patients with human immunodeficiency virus infection: report of 2 cases and review of the literature, *Medicine (Baltimore)* 71:128-138, 1992.
Kaya E, Yilmazlar T, Emiroglu Z, Zorluoglu A, Bayer A: Colonic actinomycosis: report of a case and review of the literature, *Surg Today* 25:923-926, 1995.
Krone A et al: Nocardial cerebral abscess cured with imipenem/amikacin and enucleation, *Neurosurg Rev* 12:333, 1989.
Kwong JS et al: Thoracic actinomycosis: CT findings in eight patients, *Radiology* 183:189, 1992.
Lavy A, Militianu D, Eidelman S: Diseases of the intestine mimicking Crohn's disease, *J Clin Gastroenterol* 15:17-23, 1992.
Lecciones JA et al: Vascular catheter-associated fungemia in patients with cancer: analysis of 155 episodes, *Clin Infect Dis* 14:875, 1992.
Manfredi R, Mazzoni A, Marinacci G, Nanetti A, Chiodo F: Progressive intractable actinomycosis in patients with AIDS, *Scand J Infect Dis* 27:405-407, 1995.
Meunier F, Aoun M, Bitar N: Candidemia in immunocompromised patients, *Clin Infect Dis* 14(suppl 1):S120, 1992.
Miyamoto MI, Fang FC: Pyogenic liver abscess involving *Actinomyces*: case report and review, *Clin Infect Dis* 16:303-309, 1993 (comments).
Perelow JH et al: Disseminated pelvic actinomycosis presenting as metastatic carcinoma: association with the progesteasert intrauterine device, *Rev Infect Dis* 13:1115, 1991.
Pfaller MA: Nosocominal candidiasis: emerging species, reservoirs, and modes of transmission, *Clin Infect Dis* 22(suppl 2):S89-94, 1996.
Poland GA, Jorgensen CR, Sarosi GA: *Nocardia asteroides* pericarditis: report of a case and review of the literature, *Mayo Clin Proc* 65:819, 1990.
Sobel JD: *Candida* vulvovaginitis, *Semin Dermatol* 15:17-28, 1996.
Uttamchandani RB, Daikos GL, Reyes RR et al: Nocardiosis in 30 patients with advanced human immunodeficiency virus infection: clinical features and outcome, *Clin Infect Dis* 18:348-353, 1994.
Uzun O, Anaissie EJ: Problems and controversies in the management of hematogenous candidiasis, *Clin Infect Dis* 22(suppl 2):S95-101, 1996.
Walsh TJ et al: Experimental antifungal chemotherapy in granulocytopenic animal models of disseminated candidiasis: approaches to understanding investigational antifungal compounds for patients with neoplastic diseases, *Clin Infect Dis* 14(suppl 1):S139, 1992.
Yew WW et al: Two cases of *Nocardia asteroides* sternotomy infection treated with ofloxacin and a review of other active antimicrobial agents, *J Infect* 23:297, 1991.

278 *Cryptococcus neoformans* Infections

Thomas F. Patterson

Cryptococcosis is a systemic mycotic infection caused by the encapsulated yeast *Cryptococcus neoformans*. Primary infection usually occurs through inhalation and is most often asymptomatic. Disseminated infection, particularly to the central nervous system (CNS), may occur in patients with abnormal cellular immunity.

MICROBIOLOGY AND EPIDEMIOLOGY

Cryptococcal infection is almost always caused by the species *C. neoformans*, although infections with other *Cryptococcus* species may occur. The organism is a singly budding yeast that is characterized by its surrounding thick-walled polysaccharide capsule, which is easily visualized with India ink or nigrosin staining (Color Plate VIII-50). The species contains specific varieties and serotypes that cause infection in geographic regions. *C. neoformans* var. *neoformans* (serotypes A and D) is found throughout the United States and in most other areas of the world. In contrast, *C. neoformans* var. *gattii*, which comprises serotypes B and C, is geographically distinct for Australia and southern California.

On epidemiologic study, *C. neoformans* var. *gattii* has been linked to the eucalyptus tree, and *C. neoformans* var. *neoformans* is associated with pigeon droppings and soil. *C. neoformans* var. *gattii* is more likely to cause disease in immunocompetent hosts, whereas *C. neoformans* var. *neoformans* is the etiologic agent in patients with acquired immunodeficiency syndrome (AIDS).

Cryptococci are ubiquitous organisms that are inhaled via aerosols into the lung. In patients with human immunodeficiency virus (HIV) infection or those with other T-cell defects (such as patients undergoing organ transplants or receiving cytotoxic chemotherapy), meningeal disease may develop following pulmonary infection. Cryptococcal pneumonia preceding meningeal dissemination may be an early clue to the diagnosis.

In the United States, cryptococcal meningitis is associated with the diagnosis of AIDS in over 85% of cases. Despite the ubiquitous nature of the organism, before the AIDS epidemic, only 300 cases per year were estimated to occur in the United States. However, with the emergence of the *Cryptococcus* organism as a major pathogen complicating AIDS and with large numbers of other immunosuppressed patients, increasing numbers of patients with cryptococcosis are being reported worldwide. Cryptococcal disease has been reported in 6% to 7.5% of AIDS patients and comprises the most common life-threatening fungal infection in HIV-infected patients. Non–HIV-infected patients may have a variety of other immune defects attributable to malignancy, corticosteroid therapy, diabetes, chronic renal failure, organ transplantation, and other conditions. Patients with no immune defects constitute fewer than 5% of the cases; immune status should be assessed in patients with cryptococcal infection.

Risk factors for the development of cryptococcal meningitis in HIV-infected patients include decreased CD4 cells levels, but other specific risk factors remain poorly defined. Infection is associated with the outdoors or soil exposure, but geographic variation also occurs. The widespread use of fluconazole in patients with AIDS has been associated with a decrease in cryptococcal infection. Protective efficacy has been shown even in patients receiving intermittent courses of fluconazole therapy.

PATHOPHYSIOLOGY AND HOST DEFENSES

The major virulence factor identified for *C. neoformans* is synthesis of a polysaccharide capsule, which determines the serotype of the organism. *C. neoformans* produces no toxins and evokes a minimal inflammatory response in tissue. Acapsular mutants have reduced virulence or are avirulent in experimental animals. Relatively less virulent varients with small capsules have been reported from some patients with AIDS, suggesting that severely immunodeficient patients may exert little selective pressure for the production of capsule. Regulation of the encapsulation process may be adaptive for survival in the environment where encapsulation is suppressed and may favor growth or mating. In the host, however, encapsulation allows the organism to resist phagocytosis, induces T suppressor cell activity, and impairs leukocyte migration.

Capsular polysaccharides also suppress both specific and nonspecific antibody responses. A role of antibody in the phagocytosis and killing of cryptococci has been shown, but the clinical significance of antibody to cryptococci remains uncertain. Fewer than half the patients with cryptococcal meningitis produce antibody, but those who do seem to have a slightly improved prognosis. Capsular polysaccharide at serum levels associated with severe, disseminated disease causes specific immunoglobulin M and immunoglobulin G (IgM and IgG) antibody unresponsiveness. Those defects may persist up to 1 year after cure. Cryptococcal polysaccharide also inhibits phagocytosis, presumably by blocking recognition of the yeast cell. Neutrophils are present in the initial inflammatory response but, later, monocytes predominate. Cryptococcal polysaccharide can activate the alternative complement pathway in serum. C3-coated organisms are readily phagocytized by neutrophils but poorly by macrophages, which require activation for phagocytosis. In some patients with cryptococcal fungemia, C3 and factor B levels are depressed, presumably because of the alternative complement pathway activation by the heavy load of organisms.

Cell-mediated immunity appears to be the major defense against cryptococcal infection. The importance of cell-mediated immunity against *C. neoformans* is best supported by the predisposition of patients with impaired cell-mediated immunity to cryptococcosis. Defects in cell-mediated immunity can be identified in most patients with disseminated cryptococcosis; often the defects persist for years after the disease. The majority of apparently normal patients who are cured of cryptococcosis develop T-cell responsiveness and, presumably, immunity to the disease. In contrast, in patients with severe immunodeficiency, in vitro evidence of immunity usually fails to develop.

Host defense mechanisms against cryptococci are in part responsible for the neurotropic predilection of the organism. That is, normal cerebrospinal fluid (CSF) lacks immunoglobulins and complement and serves as a good growth medium for the organism. The inflammatory response is delayed in experimental infection and may be absent in human disease. On pathologic examination cryptococcal meningoencephalitis is characterized by basilar arachnoiditis, with clusters of yeasts in brain tissue associated with minimal inflammation.

CLINICAL MANIFESTATIONS

Primary cryptococcal disease of humans almost always occurs in the lungs. The disease can remain localized or disseminate to other tissues, most notably the CNS, even with resolution of the lung lesions. Central nervous system lesions are the most common and important clinical manifestations of cryptococcosis.

Central Nervous System

The clinical presentation of cryptococcal meningitis is nonspecific but includes headache, fever, nausea, vomiting, mental status changes, and neck stiffness. Less common are visual disturbances (such as blurred vision and photophobia), papilledema, cerebellar signs, seizures, and aphasia. In patients with AIDS the presentation of cryptococcal meningitis may be subtle as compared with non–HIV-infected patients and may include only headache and fever (Table 278-1). Fever and headache are common in AIDS patients who come to medical attention with cryptococcal meningitis. Meningismus and photophobia are strikingly less common (31%) in patients with AIDS than in non–HIV-infected patients, perhaps reflecting the poor host inflammatory response of HIV-infected patients. Both HIV-infected and

Table 278-1 Clinical presentation of cryptococcal meningitis in patients with and without acquired immunodeficiency virus (AIDS)

SIGN OR SYMPTOM	PATIENTS (%)	
	AIDS	NON-AIDS
Headache	87	81
Fever	60	88
Nausea, vomiting	53	38
Abnormal mental status	52	19
Meningismus	50	31
Photophobia	33	19
Seizures	15	8
No signs or symptoms	10	12

Data from Chuck SL, Sande MA: *N Engl J Med* 321:794-799, 1989; Patterson TF, Andriole VT: *Eur J Clin Microbiol* 8:457-465, 1989.

Table 278-2 Cerebrospinal fluid findings in cryptococcal meningitis in patients with and without acquired immunodeficiency syndrome (AIDS)

FINDING	PATIENTS (%)	
	AIDS	NON-AIDS
Opening pressure >200 mm H_2O	62	72
Glucose level <40 mg/dl	33	73
Protein level >45 mg/dl	58	89
White blood cell count >20 cells/mm^3	23	70
Positive India ink smear	74	60
Positive culture	95	96

Data from Chuck SL, Sande MA: *N Engl J Med* 321:794-799, 1989; Patterson TF, Andriole VT: *Eur J Clin Microbiol* 8:457-465, 1989.

non–HIV-infected hosts may have few clinical symptoms, so a high index of suspicion must be maintained to establish a diagnosis of CNS infection. Any patient with evidence of extraneural cryptococcosis should be evaluated for CNS disease. Likewise, symptoms of meningitis may be obscured by concurrent disease, especially in patients with AIDS. Altered mental status is an important predictor of a poor therapeutic outcome. Visual loss, which may be total in some patients, can result from optic tract involvement or from increased intracranial pressure. The late recrudescence of symptoms may result from relapse of infection or hydrocephalus.

Respiratory System

The lungs are the primary site of infection and in the majority of patients remain asymptomatic. Symptomatic patients most commonly seek medical care with a nonproductive cough, occasionally associated with scant blood-streaked sputum, dyspnea, and dull chest pain. Pulmonary findings may be nonspecific, ranging from mass lesions (with or without cavitation) to consolidation or airway colonization without parenchymal infiltration. The presence of respiratory symptoms may precede cryptococcal meningitis. Full identification of yeasts from respiratory samples should be made to evaluate for pulmonary cryptococcal infection. The isolation of cryptococci from respiratory secretions may occur in asymptomatic immunocompetent hosts and may not always indicate infection. However, patients with pulmonary cryptococcal infection should be evaluated for the presence of meningeal disease.

Other Sites of Infection

Cryptococcemia is the most common site for symptomatic extraneural infections and can be documented in more than half the HIV-infected patients with CNS disease. Cryptococcemia is a poor prognostic sign, particularly in non–HIV-infected patients. However, cryptococcemia may be present in the absence of meningitis in up to 30% of patients. Other extraneural sites of clinical infection include skin (frequently molluscum-like lesions, subcutaneous or mucosal lesions, pustules, and erythematous papules or cellulitis) and bone; urinary tract including the prostate; and endophthalmitis, endocarditis, pericarditis, orchitis, myositis, arthritis, bursitis, hepatitis, and peritonitis. Extraneural disease in patients with AIDS is common. Evaluation of extraneural sites, such as the prostate, for infection can be important in establishing a persistent focus of infection.

DIAGNOSIS

Examination of the spinal fluid in a patient with cryptococcal meningitis generally suggests a chronic, lymphocytic meningitis (Table 278-2). In non–HIV-infected patients the opening pressure is abnormally high (>180 mm H_2O) in 72%. CSF pleocytosis (usually lymphocytes) is common, although most patients have fewer than 150 leukocytes/mm^3. Low CSF glucose (<40 mg/dl) and elevated CSF protein (>45 mg/dl) concentrations are common. Organisms can be

detected in 60% of patients by means of India ink or nigrosin smears. Usually the organisms are easily cultured from the CSF. Occasionally, large volumes of CSF, cisternal puncture, or multiple samples are required to confirm the diagnosis.

Examination of the CSF in AIDS patients with cryptococcal meningitis produces findings similar to those seen in non-AIDS patients, with several notable exceptions (Table 278-2). Similar increased opening pressure is seen, as are hypoglycorrhacia and elevated protein concentrations. Rates of positive cultures are high, and the organism is seen on direct smear more frequently in HIV-infected patients than in those without HIV-infection. However, patients with AIDS often have a striking lack of inflammatory response to the disease: more than two thirds of patients have fewer than 20 leukocytes/mm^3.

Another area of contrast between AIDS and non-AIDS patients is in CSF cryptococcal antigen detection. In both groups, antigen detection using a commercial latex or enzyme-linked immunosorbent assay (ELISA) method is extremely sensitive, with positive results well over 90%. However, AIDS patients often have extraordinarily high antigen titers with values at times over 1:1,000,000. False-negative and false-positive reactions do occur, the latter most frequently in the past from rheumatoid factor cross-reactivity. Serum antigen levels are frequently higher than CSF antigen titers. Negative serum antigen reactions are uncommon in patients with cryptococcal meningitis. Serum antibody detection is not useful for diagnosis but may be useful in determining prognosis.

The use of CSF antigen tests, India ink smears, or cultures for *C. neoformans* should be performed on all CSF samples from patients with suspected cryptococcal infection, since positive results may be seen even in patients with a relatively normal CSF formula. Cultures are usually positive within 7 days, but late positive results (after 4 to 6 weeks of incubation) may occur, particularly in patients who have had prior therapy. Positive India ink smears may persist for weeks to months after diagnosis but may represent nonviable organisms.

Cultures from extraneural sites are commonly positive, especially in blood (up to 25% of non–HIV-infected patients and 50% or more of patients with AIDS), urine or prostatic secretions, skin lesions, and sputum. The detection of cryptococci in tissue samples can be confirmed with the use of a capsule-specific mucicarmine stain.

Radiographic procedures are generally nonspecific. Computed tomography (CT) of the head is generally indicated to evaluate for the possibility of other CNS mass lesions such as toxoplasmosis or CNS lymphoma in HIV-infected patients. Head CT scanning may reveal a cryptococcoma that may be enhanced with contrast. However, such lesions are rarely confused with the more typically ring-enhancing lesions of toxoplasmosis. Head CT scanning can also be used to evaluate for the presence of hydrocephalus (Fig. 278-1), although normal-sized ventricles may be present even in patients with elevated pressures.

Chest radiographs are also nonspecific. Findings range from asymptomatic pulmonary nodules to larger mass lesions with or without cavitation, segmental pneumonia, hilar adenopathy, pleural effu-

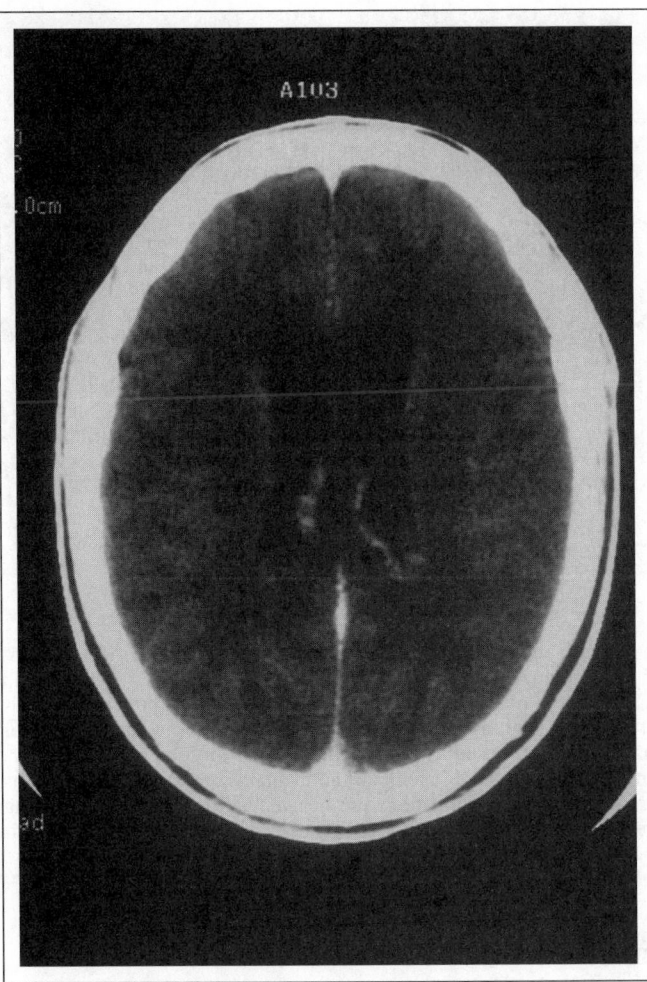

FIGURE 278-1 Computed tomography scan of a head, showing dilated ventricles in a patient with hydrocephalus associated with cryptococcal meningitis.

sions, and interstitial pneumonia (which may mimic pneumocystis pneumonia). Bone radiographs demonstrate lytic lesions.

THERAPY AND PROGNOSIS
Central Nervous System Infection

Before the advent of amphotericin B, cryptococcal meningitis was ultimately fatal in virtually 100% of patients, although long-term illnesses were reported. Even in the pre-AIDS era, mortality rates from cryptococcal infection ranged from 20% to 85% in patients with persistent immunosuppression but were extremely low in patients with no underlying immune defects. The use of low-dose amphotericin B (0.3 to 0.4 mg/kg per day) was evaluated to decrease amphotericin B toxicity. With those doses of amphotericin B, combination therapy with flucytosine improved the outcome by more rapidly sterilizing tissues. However, doses of 0.6 to 1.0 mg/kg per day of amphotericin B produced cure rates that were similar to combination therapy. Shorter courses of combination therapy could be given to patients with uncomplicated disease. In patients with AIDS amphotericin B (at an average dose of 0.4 mg/kg per day) was compared with fluconazole at doses beginning at 200 mg/day by the Mycoses Study Group. In this study both groups had similar but unacceptably low cure rates. Successful therapy, defined as negative CSF cultures at 12 weeks, occurred in 40% and 34% of the patients receiving amphotericin B or fluconazole, respectively. In addition, increased mortality approaching 40% occurred in a high-risk subset of patients.

Subsequent small studies demonstrated the utility of standard doses (0.7 mg/kg per day) of amphotericin B in reducing mortality, with response rates of 80% to 100%. This approach was evaluated in another clinical trial of over 400 patients conducted by the Mycoses Study Group, which used a 2-week "induction" of amphotericin at 0.7 mg/kg per day for 2 weeks with or without flucytosine, followed by 8 weeks of "consolidation" therapy using fluconazole or itraconazole at 400 mg/day. This regimen reduced mortality to 6% and resulted in negative culture rates at 2 weeks of 50% to 60%. Overall, the response rates were 70% to 80%, and the regimen was well tolerated.

The role of flucytosine remains controversial but may result in fewer longer-term relapses. Compliant patients without high risk factors can be successfully treated in some cases with fluconazole alone in doses of 400 mg/day or more. The use of higher doses of fluconazole or the addition of flucytosine to fluconazole to increase rates of culture sterilization has been advocated by some to increase the efficacy of primary fluconazole therapy. However, it is difficult to predict which patients will favorably respond to azole therapy; only selected patients should receive azoles alone for primary therapy.

The role of azoles in the therapy of non–HIV-infected patients is less established. In some non–HIV-infected patients the outcome using primary azole therapy has been poor, possibly because of the extent of infection present at diagnosis. The efficacy of fluconazole was compared with amphotericin B in a retrospective trial in non–HIV-infected patients; response rates of over 70% were found in both groups. Solid organ transplant patients and those without meningeal disease were more likely to have been selected to receive fluconazole. As in HIV-infected patients, treatment was more likely to fail in non–HIV-infected hosts who had more extensive disease or more pronounced immunosuppression.

The management of relapse or progressive infection in patients who have been given treatment with standard regimens remains difficult. It is important to document compliance with the prescribed antifungal regimens. In addition, antifungal susceptibility may be useful in predicting response. However, antifungal resistance to azoles or amphotericin B remains rare. In addition, presumably adequate serum and CSF antifungal levels have been demonstrated in some patients with progressive disease, with progression likely to be more related to host factors than to traditional antifungal drug failure.

Alternative regimens for cryptococcal meningitis include liposomal amphotericin B formulations. Successful use of these compounds, including amphotericin B lipid complex, AmBisome, and ABCD (Amphotec), have been reported in small clinical trials. Results of using liposomal doses of 5 to 7.5 mg/kg per day have been similar to those using amphotericin B. The role for these compounds appears to be primarily in patients intolerant of standard amphotericin B therapy.

Other azoles including itraconazole have also been advocated. Itraconazole has excellent in vitro activity against most cryptococci. However, its use in cryptococcal meningitis remains limited in part because of limited CSF penetration as compared with fluconazole and because the drug is poorly absorbed in many patients with AIDS.

Intraventricular amphotericin therapy has generally been reserved for very ill patients or those with recurrent or progressive disease, despite having received systemic amphotericin therapy. Intraventricular amphotericin B administered through a subcutaneous reservoir has been shown to possibly benefit seriously ill patients, but toxicity significantly limits its use. The newer azoles, such as fluconazole, which achieve excellent CNS concentrations when given systemically, have largely supplanted the use of intraventricular amphotericin B.

Adjunctive Therapy

Elevated CNS pressures are common in patients with AIDS and are responsible for much of the morbidity and mortality of the disease. Elevated pressures may be responsible for sudden deterioration or vision loss. Papilledema may occur in up to one third of patients and may be an important sign of elevated CSF pressures (Color Plate VIII-51). Patients with elevated CSF pressures (>20 cm H_2O) and associated clinical signs and symptoms such as headache and vomiting should be carefully monitored and aggressively managed to prevent

Table 278-3 Adjunctive therapy for management of elevated cerebrospinal fluid pressure in cryptococcal meningitis

ADJUNCTIVE THERAPY	COMMENT
Large-volume lumbar punctures	Frequent large-volume spinal taps (~30 ml); most commonly used therapy
Neurosurgical shunting	Not frequently required; may be effective when other measures are not successful
Acetazolamide	Pharmacologic intervention (250 mg four times daily) used to decrease spinal fluid production
Corticosteroids	Use remains controversial; not routinely recommended

complications (Table 278-3). Frequent (often daily) large-volume spinal taps may be required to manage the elevated pressures. Pharmacologic intervention with acetazolamide, which is aimed at decreasing CSF production, is advocated by some authorities. In addition, corticosteroids may also be effective, but their role remains controversial and they are not routinely recommended.

Suppressive Therapy and Prophylaxis

Suppressive therapy is required in persistently immunosuppressed patients to prevent relapse. Rates of recurrence in patients with AIDS range from 20% to 60% if therapy is not continued. Relapse may also occur in non–HIV-infected patients, particularly if they remain persistently immunosuppressed. In HIV-infected patients fluconazole at 200 mg/day was demonstrated to be superior to placebo and to weekly amphotericin B. A randomized trial comparing fluconazole 200 mg/day with itraconazole 200 mg/day in preventing relapse was stopped because relapse occurred in 24% of patients receiving itraconazole as compared with only 4% of those receiving fluconazole. The limited efficacy of itraconazole in that setting was, perhaps, related to inadequate absorption of itraconazole.

Prophylactic use of fluconazole at 200 mg/day significantly reduced the incidence of cryptococcal infection from a rate of approximately 7% in patients receiving clotrimazole troches to less than 1% in those receiving fluconazole. The major benefit of fluconazole was seen in patients with a CD4 cell count of less than 50/mm^3. Fluconazole prophylaxis for all AIDS patients is not routinely recommended, largely because of the cost associated with daily fluconazole use and the possibility of development of resistant thrush. Observational studies have suggested that intermittent fluconazole use can significantly reduce the rates of cryptococcal infection. This use is now being evaluated in clinical trials.

Extraneural Infection

Patients with pulmonary infection should be evaluated for the presence of meningeal infection. The role of amphotericin versus primary azole therapy in extraneural infection has not been established. Similarly, management of patients with positive serum cryptococcal antigen titers as the sole manifestation of infection is not well established. Clinical evaluation including lumbar puncture and smears and culture of secretions following prostatic massage may reveal a site of infection. A course of antifungal therapy is indicated, particularly in immunosuppressed patients.

Prognosis

Clinical and laboratory findings are useful to establish the prognosis of infection in both HIV-infected and non–HIV-infected hosts. In the pre-AIDS era, Diamond and Bennett showed increased mortality in patients with persistent immunosuppression, elevated CSF opening pressures, low glucose concentration, elevated CSF and serum antigen titers (>1:32), the lack of a CSF white blood cell response (<20

cells/mm^3) and a positive CSF smear. In patients with AIDS an abnormal mental status, elevated CSF or serum titers (>1:1024) and CSF white blood cell counts less than 20 cells/mm^3 predict a mortality rates as high as 40%, particularly if low-dose amphotericin B or azole therapy is used as primary therapy. Of those prognostic factors in patients with AIDS, an abnormal mental status at presentation was most predictive. Serum titers are not generally useful for predicting relapse or monitoring response to therapy. However, increasing antigen titers (particularly in the CSF) may occur in patients with relapse of infection.

✔ *WHEN TO REFER*

Most patients with cryptococcal meningitis respond to therapy with standard doses of amphotericin B at 0.7 mg/kg per day for 2 weeks followed by fluconazole at 400 mg/day for an additional 8 weeks. The addition of flucytosine may be useful for patients with severe disease. However, in the small number of patients who do not respond to this regimen, management may be difficult. Alterative regimens are not well established, and careful attention must be paid to aggressive management of elevated CSF pressures. In some patients CSF pressures remain elevated, despite intensive therapeutic efforts. Long-term maintenance therapy with fluconazole is generally effective in suppressing relapse of infection, but a large number of patients have now been maintained on suppressive therapy for several years. In patients whose infection relapses while they are on a maintenance regimen, therapeutic options are difficult because antifungal resistance may have developed. Newer antifungal agents and newer modes of antifungal delivery, such as combination antifungal therapy or liposomal amphotericin, offer additional options in patients with persistent disease.

BIBLIOGRAPHY

Bennett JE et al: A comparison of amphotericin B alone and combined with flucytosine in the treatment of cryptococcal meningitis, *N Engl J Med* 301:126-131, 1979.

Bozzette SA et al: A placebo-controlled trial of maintenance therapy with fluconazole after treatment of cryptococcal meningitis in the acquired immunodeficiency syndrome, *N Engl J Med* 324:580-584, 1991.

Chuck SL, Sande MA: Infections with *Cryptococcus neoformans* in the acquired immunodeficiency syndrome, *N Engl J Med* 321:794-799, 1989.

Denning DW et al: Elevated cerebrospinal fluid pressures in patients with cryptococcal meningitis and acquired immunodeficiency syndrome, *Am J Med* 91:267-272, 1991.

Diamond RD, Bennett JE: Prognostic factors in cryptococcal meningitis: a study in 111 cases, *Ann Intern Med* 80:176-181, 1974.

Dismukes WE et al: Treatment of cryptococcal meningitis with combination of amphotericin B and flucytosine for four as compared with six weeks, *N Engl J Med* 317:334-341, 1987.

Dromer F et al: Comparison of the efficacy of amphotericin B and fluconazole in the treatment of cryptococcosis in human immunodeficiency virus-negative patients: retrospective analysis of 83 cases, *Clin Infect Dis* 22(suppl 2):S154-160, 1996.

Larsen RA et al: Fluconazole compared with amphotericin B plus flucytosine for cryptococcal meningitis in AIDS: a randomized trial, *Ann Intern Med* 113:183-187, 1990.

Patterson TF, Andriole VT: Current concepts in cryptococcosis, *Eur J Clin Microbiol* 8:457-465, 1989.

Perfect JD: Cryptococcosis, *Infect Dis Clin North Am* 3:77-102, 1989.

Powderly WG et al: A controlled trial of fluconazole or amphotericin B to prevent relapse of cryptococcal meningitis in patients with the acquired immunodeficiency syndrome, *N Engl J Med* 326:793-798, 1992.

Powderly WG et al: A randomized trial comparing fluconazole with clotrimazole troches for the prevention of fungal infections in patients with advanced human immunodeficiency virus infection, *N Engl J Med* 332:700-705, 1995.

Powderly WG: Recent advances in the management of cryptococcal meningitis in patients with AIDS, *Clin Infect Dis* 22(suppl 2):S119-123, 1996.

Powderly WG: Editorial response: management of cryptococcal meningitis—have we answered all the questions? *Clin Infect Dis* 22:329-330, 1996.

Quagliarello VJ et al: Primary prevention of cryptococcal meningitis by fluconazole in HIV-infected patients, *Lancet* 345:548-552, 1995.

Saag MS et al: Comparison of amphotericin B with fluconazole in the treatment of acute AIDS-associated cryptococcal meningitis, *N Engl J Med* 326:83-89, 1992.

Sabetta JR, Andriole VT: Cryptococcal infection of the central nervous system, *Med Clin North Am* 9:333-344, 1985.

van der Horst CM et al: Treatment of cryptococcal meningitis associated with the acquired immunodeficicney syndrome, *N Engl J Med* 337:15-21, 1997.

PROTOZOAL DISEASES

CHAPTER

279 Infections Caused by Protozoa

Carolyn Petersen

Protozoa are unicellular, eukaryotic organisms consisting of membrane-bound organelles (nuclei, mitochondria, Golgi complexes, lysosomes, food vacuoles) within a cytosolic matrix. Most protozoa that infect humans are obligatory parasites and derive protection and nutrition from the host. However, *Naegleria* and *Acanthamoeba* are free-living amebae that can invade the human nervous system. Conversely, some parasitic protozoa, like *Dientamoeba fragilis* and *Blastocystis hominis,* may infect humans but rarely cause disease. These organisms are able to live in apparent harmony with the host.

Protozoa that infect humans are classified into phyla based on differences in morphologic features and life cycle (Table 279-1). A useful way to divide the pathogenic protozoa in clinical practice is by their means of entry—via the mucosa or the bloodstream—since these alternate portals of entry lead to primary mucosal or systemic immune responses that are important in the development of immunity. Many parasitic protozoa have developed mechanisms for evading the host's immune response, leading to persistent or repeated infections.

Clinicians need to have a broad general knowledge of protozoology for two reasons. First, some parasitic protozoa have worldwide distributions and can pose clinical and public health problems anywhere. For example, infections with *Toxoplasma, Cryptosporidium, Isospora, Cyclospora,* and microsporidium species typically occur in patients with acquired immunodeficiency syndrome (AIDS) (Chapter 248). Second, international travelers and refugees may bring protozoa ordinarily limited to the tropics to the notice of clinicians in developed countries (e.g., malaria and *Leishmania,* and *Trypanosoma* spp. Thus it is essential that clinicians recognize when protozoan diseases should be considered in the differential diagnosis. Referral is indicated for the rarely seen diseases that are due to *Leishmania* and *Trypanosoma* spp. Malaria in a nonimmune host that is due to *Plasmodium falciparum* should be seen by a consultant. Severe manifestations of protozoan diseases seen in AIDS patients may benefit from consultation. Giardiasis and trichomoniasis are usually handled by primary care physicians.

MALARIA

Human malaria is caused by four species of *Plasmodium: P. falciparum, P. vivax, P. ovale,* and *P. malariae.* Each species has its own characteristic epidemiologic, biologic, morphologic, and clinical manifestations. *P. falciparum* causes most of the morbidity and virtually all the mortality resulting from malaria and also presents the problem of drug resistance. The occurrence of *P. falciparum* in a nonimmune host (such as a traveler) is a medical emergency that demands hospitalization and prompt treatment with appropriate drugs. In some imported cases death attributable to falciparum malaria has resulted from delay in diagnosis or failure to institute proper treatment. *P. vivax, P. ovale,* and *P. malariae* can cause significant morbidity but rarely cause death and are generally sensitive to the most frequently used antimalarial drug, chloroquine. In the tropics and subtropics, malaria continues to be one of the most prevalent of all infectious diseases, despite the use of insecticides against the vector and antimalarial drugs for the treatment and prophylaxis of disease. The failure of these methods to eradicate malaria has led scientists to study other approaches to the control of malaria, including new approaches to treatment, malaria vaccines, and the biologic control of mosquitoes.

Table 279-1   Classification of parasitic protozoa

CLASSIFICATION	CHARACTERISTICS	EXAMPLES
Phylum Sarcomastigophora		
Subphylum Mastigophora	Trophozoites have one or more flagella; asexual reproduction	*Leishmania* *Trypanosoma* *Giardia* *Dientamoeba* *Trichomonas*
Subphylum Sarcodina	Locomotion by pseudopods	*Entamoeba* *Acanthamoeba* (free living) *Naegleria* (free living)
Phylum Apicomplexa	Invasive stages have apical organelles	
Class Sporozoa (Sporozoea)	Asexual (schizogony) and sexual (sporogony) reproductive cycles	*Isospora* *Toxoplasma* *Plasmodium* *Babesia* *Cryptosporidium* *Cyclospora* *Sarcocystis*
Phylum Microspora	Released into a cell from a spore by ejection from a long coiled polar tube	*Encephalitozoon* *Enterocytozoon* *Nosema* *Pleistophora* *Vittaforma*
Phylum Ciliophora	Simple cilia or compound ciliary organelles; asexual (binary) fission and sexual (conjugation) multiplication	*Balantidium*

Biology and Life Cycle

The parasite is maintained in nature by alternating between a sexual life cycle in mosquitoes and an asexual life cycle in humans. Female anopheline mosquitoes are the only insect vectors of human malaria. During a blood meal, mosquitoes inoculate sporozoites into the subcutaneous capillaries of the human host. In the exoerythrocytic cycle sporozoites rapidly invade hepatic parenchymal cells where they proliferate into intracellular merozoites. One week to 2 weeks after the initial mosquito bite, the merozoites rupture the hepatic cell and are released into the circulation, immediately invade erythrocytes, and begin the erythrocytic stage of the infection. The hepatic exoerythrocytic forms of *P. falciparum* and *P. malariae* rupture at the same time; none persist in the liver. With *P. vivax* and *P. ovale,* however, some hepatic forms remain dormant for months or years before they rupture and produce relapses of erythrocytic infection. Erythrocytic parasites never reinvade the liver. Therefore only *P. vivax* and *P. ovale* that are transmitted by mosquitoes can produce relapses.

After the merozoites invade the host's erythrocytes, most of the parasites develop asexually from young ring forms into larger, more cytoplasmic trophozoites. Trophozoites undergo asexual division and become schizonts, which contain 6 to 24 merozoites, the number varying with the species of plasmodia. When mature, the schizont ruptures the host erythrocyte and releases the merozoites, which rapidly invade fresh erythrocytes and begin the asexual life cycle again. The duration of the erythrocytic life cycle is 48 hours with *P. falciparum, P. vivax,* and *P. ovale* and 72 hours with *P. malariae.*

Some intraerythrocytic parasites do not develop asexually but differentiate into sexual parasites, the gametocytes. Gametocytes (male and female) can be distinguished in morphologic appearance from asexual parasites, and the gametocytes of different *Plasmodium* species can also be distinguished from each other. Once ingested by a mosquito, the gametocytes lyse the erythrocyte, become extracellular in the gut of the mosquito, and unite to form an oocyst, which develops into thousands of sporozoites over 9 to 14 days, depending on the ambient temperature. This process (sporogony) is more rapid at warm temperatures and ceases altogether at temperatures below 20°

C for *P. falciparum* and 16° C for *P. vivax.* Sporogony culminates with rupture of the oocyst and release of the sporozoites. The sporozoites migrate to the mosquito's salivary glands and are injected into a human or an animal during the next blood meal.

The invasion of hepatocytes by sporozoites and of erythrocytes by merozoites is mediated by specific ligands on the parasite surface that recognize determinants on the surface of the host cell. The circumsporozoite protein, merozoite surface antigen-1, erythrocyte binding antigen *(P. falciparum),* and Duffy binding protein *(P. vivax)* have been identified, cloned, sequenced, and found to contain ligands that participate in invasion of hepatocytes or erythrocytes. In addition, much has been learned about determinants on the erythrocyte surface that are involved in invasion. The Duffy blood group system appears to be required for invasion of erythrocytes by *P. vivax.* Blacks who are Duffy blood group negative (FyFy) are refractory to erythrocytic infection by *P. vivax.* The sialoglycoproteins (glycophorin and band 3) on the erythrocyte surface appear to be involved in invasion by *P. falciparum. P. vivax* and *P. ovale* can invade only reticulocytes, which limits the parasitemia to the number of circulating reticulocytes. *P. falciparum* invades reticulocytes preferentially but can infect erythrocytes of all ages, thereby producing infections with high-level parasitemias. *P. malariae* infects only mature erythrocytes.

Intraerythrocytic malaria parasites derive their energy from the anaerobic metabolism of glucose to lactic acid. Infected erythrocytes consume much more glucose than uninfected erythrocytes, and in some patients with very high-level parasitemias, this consumption of glucose may contribute to hypoglycemia. Malarial parasites obtain most of their amino acids for protein synthesis by ingesting hemoglobin from the host erythrocyte and digesting it within a food vacuole. A by-product of the hemoglobin digestion is malarial pigment (hemozoin), which consists of ferriprotoporphyrin IX, methemoglobin, and some malarial proteins.

Malarial parasites produce morphologic and functional changes in the membranes of infected erythrocytes. *P. falciparum* produces protrusions called *knobs* on the surface of erythrocytes containing trophozoites and schizonts. Knobs mediate attachment to venular endothelium via a recently cloned and sequenced ligand, PfEMP1. The parasites are thereby sequestered in the postcapillary venules of many organs. Because of sequestration, only ring forms of *P. falciparum* circulate in peripheral blood, a property that is helpful in distinguishing *P. falciparum* from other species of plasmodia. The mature parasites that are sequestered avoid circulating through the spleen, which is a major site of parasite destruction in malaria. In addition, the sequestered parasites may obstruct blood flow in cerebral vessels, leading to cerebral malaria. *P. vivax* and *P. ovale* produce indentations in the erythrocyte membrane called *caveolar-vesicle junctions,* which on Giemsa-stained blood smears produce the characteristic Schüffner's dots. The membrane of schizont-infected erythrocytes is more permeable to some small molecules than is the membrane of uninfected erythrocytes. This partial permeability may contribute to the increased uptake of glucose by infected erythrocytes and also leads to an increase in the intraerythrocytic sodium concentration and a decrease in the intraerythrocytic potassium concentration of infected erythrocytes. An excessive loss of potassium occurs with the *P. falciparum–* infected erythrocytes of individuals with hemoglobin S/A (Hb S/A) at low oxygen tensions. This loss of intracellular potassium is detrimental to the parasite and may be the mechanism for the protective effect of Hb S/A in falciparum malaria, since sequestration in postcapillary venules exposes the infected erythrocytes to low oxygen tension for 24 hours or longer.

Epidemiology

Most authorities estimate that there are more than 100 million cases of malaria per year worldwide and more than 1 million deaths resulting from malaria each year in Africa alone. Endemic malaria is largely a tropical disease, since mosquito transmission requires high relative humidity (>35%) for mosquito longevity and high ambient temperature (>16° C) for the sporogonic cycle of the parasite in mosquitoes. The degree to which *P. falciparum* is endemic within an area is determined by the intensity of mosquito transmission and by host immunity. Intense, year-round transmission results in a high prevalence (>75%) of infection and disease in young children, but those who

---

BOX 279-1
Geographic distribution of malaria*

Plasmodium falciparum
Sub-Saharan Africa
Southeast Asia
Haiti
New Guinea, Oceania
India, Pakistan
South America
Central America
Mexico
Middle East

Plasmodium vivax
India
Sri Lanka
Pakistan
Bangladesh
Southeast Asia
South America
Central America
Mexico
Asia
New Guinea
Oceania
Middle East

Plasmodium ovale
Africa

Plasmodium malariae
All malarious areas

*Areas where particular species of malaria are predominant. However, malaria must be considered as a potential cause of disease in travelers to all areas of the tropics and subtropics.

---

survive to adulthood have acquired immunity and generally have few or no symptoms. With intense seasonal transmission, adults as well as children have symptomatic infections because immunity wanes during the seasons when no transmission occurs. With less intense transmission the prevalence of infection falls, but the infections that occur often produce severe disease in children and adults.

Tropical Africa south of the Sahara is the major focus of malaria in the world (Box 279-1). *P. falciparum* is the predominant malarial parasite and causes high mortality in children. Those who survive to adulthood usually have a high degree of acquired immunity. *P. falciparum* is also prevalent in India, Southeast Asia, Haiti, New Guinea, Mexico, Central America, and South America. *P. vivax* can be transmitted at lower ambient temperatures than *P. falciparum* and thus has a range that extends further into the temperate-zone countries. *P. vivax* is the predominant malarial parasite in India, Sri Lanka, Pakistan, Bangladesh, and Central America and is also quite prevalent in Southeast Asia, South America, and Oceania. *P. ovale* has replaced *P. vivax* in West Africa and much of East Africa because most blacks in these areas have the Duffy blood group–negative phenotype and are resistant to *P. vivax. P. malariae* is cosmopolitan.

Most patients who are seen with malaria in Europe and the United States are refugees, travelers, or military personnel who acquired their infections in endemic areas. Other causes of malaria in nonendemic areas include congenital malaria, blood transfusion, and the sharing of needles by drug addicts. Malaria may occur among individuals residing near international airports because of the accidental importation of infected mosquitoes ("airport malaria"). In the central valley of California and along the U.S.-Mexican border occasional outbreaks of *P. vivax* malaria are transmitted by local *Anopheles* mosquitoes, which become infected by feeding on immigrants or migrant farm workers with malaria. Congenital malaria is transmitted at birth and should be considered in any infant born to a mother who has recently emigrated from an endemic area. The incidence of transfusion malaria has been greatly reduced by the exclusion of donors for 3 years after travel to or residence in an endemic area. However, since *P. vivax* and *P. ovale* may persist in the human host for 3 to 5 years and *P. malariae* for 50 years or more, an occasional case of transfusion malaria can still be expected to occur.

Pathophysiology and Immunity

The clinical manifestations of malaria are caused entirely by asexual, erythrocytic parasites. Symptoms, as well as morbidity and mortality, generally occur at lower levels of parasitemia in nonimmune hosts. The fundamental processes in the pathogenesis of malaria are (1) the rupture of schizont-infected erythrocytes, with release of merozoites; (2) destruction of host erythrocytes by the rupturing parasites; (3) changes in rheology produced by decreased deformability of infected erythrocytes and by the adherence of *P. falciparum*–infected erythrocytes to the endothelium of postcapillary venules; and (4) response of the host's immune and reticuloendothelial systems to malaria.

Malaria characteristically causes paroxysms of fever that occur when the schizonts rupture. Fever and malaise appear to be caused by a cascade that is initiated by release of a glycolipid with many of the properties of bacterial endotoxin on schizont rupture. Parasite products like endotoxon activate cytokines, particularly tumor necrosis factor (TNF) and interleukins (Il-1, Il-6 and Il-8). The fever pattern is determined by the degree to which the erythrocytic parasites are synchronized and rupture together. Thus highly synchronized infections produce a regular, intermittent fever pattern that occurs every 48 or 72 hours, depending on the species of plasmodia. However, infections are frequently asynchronous, especially with *P. falciparum*. When the erythrocytic parasites are not synchronized, the fever pattern may be irregular or even continuous. The fever of malaria is associated with peripheral vasodilation and a reduced effective intravascular volume.

Anemia is a common manifestation of malaria caused by all four species of plasmodia. The predominant mechanism is hemolysis resulting from the rupture of infected erythrocytes, although some children with chronic malaria may also have a dyserythropoietic state with low reticulocyte counts and recovery after treatment with antimalarial drugs. Hemolysis may also be the result of a Coombs test–positive hemolytic anemia induced by quinine or may be produced by the administration of oxidant drugs, (e.g., primaquine) to patients with glucose-6-phosphate dehydrogenase (G6PD) deficiency. With *P. falciparum*, high-level parasitemias or drug-induced hemolysis may produce marked intravascular hemolysis and hemoglobinuric renal failure ("blackwater fever").

The consequences of rheologic changes occur predominantly with *P. falciparum*. Erythrocytes containing trophozoites and schizonts have reduced deformability, which may lead to sluggish blood flow through the capillaries. In addition, infected erythrocytes adhere specifically to venular endothelium. Therefore blood flow may be obstructed, with resultant tissue anoxia, and changes also may occur in the permeability of the venular and capillary endothelium, allowing blood to extravasate into surrounding tissues. The principal target organs are the brain and intestines. A variety of cerebral symptoms may be produced in *P. falciparum* infections (cerebral malaria; see next section). On pathologic study the capillaries and venules of the gray matter of the cortex are filled with infected erythrocytes, ring hemorrhages develop around capillaries, and the brain is edematous. Sequestration and sludging in the intestinal capillaries and venules may lead to diarrhea and malabsorption.

Renal failure in *P. falciparum* malaria may result from hemoglobinuria, acute tubular necrosis, or ischemia of the renal cortex, perhaps related to splanchnic vasoconstriction. Pulmonary edema occurs in *P. falciparum* malaria, often as a terminal event. Increased permeability of the pulmonary-capillary membrane appears to occur, but the pathogenesis of this complication is not known.

Thrombocytopenia occurs frequently with all four species of plasmodia and may be due to increased consumption via accelerated coagulation cascade activity, bleeding, and splenic clearance. A chronic, immunecomplex glomerulonephritis that does not respond to antimalarial treatment occurs with *P. malariae*. The immune complexes contain antibody specific for *P. malariae* antigens as well as complement. Splenomegaly and, occasionally, hypersplenism are caused by hyperplasia of the reticuloendothelial system. Some patients who reside in

endemic areas of Africa, Indonesia, and New Guinea develop chronic, massive splenomegaly and a lymphocytic infiltrate in the sinusoids of the liver (tropical splenomegaly). Often these patients have high levels of antimalarial antibodies and no detectable parasites in their peripheral blood, but they respond to chronic antimalarial chemoprophylaxis. The pathogenesis of this syndrome is unknown. Malaria may prevent the host from developing a normal immune response to antigenic challenge, causing reduced response to some vaccines and a greater chance of intercurrent infection during malaria.

Acquired immunity to malaria develops only after repeated or prolonged infection and is predominantly directed against erythrocytic parasites. Immunity is usually not sterile, and individuals can be infected and may have circulating parasites, but the infection produces no symptoms. Immunity to malaria is species specific. With *P. falciparum* malaria, immunity has been shown to be strain specific, indicating that antigenic diversity exists among parasites. Although the passive transfer of antibody from immune individuals to nonimmune individuals protects against the symptoms of malaria, the renewed induction of immunity requires helper T cells. The spleen is the major site of parasite destruction in malaria and is of primary importance in the host's survival. Splenectomy may lead to a recurrence of disease or may render a previously immune individual susceptible to severe disease.

Besides acquired immunity, several genetically determined host factors influence host susceptibility to malaria. Hb S, thalassemia, and G6PD deficiency are associated geographically with the distribution of *P. falciparum* malaria. Direct evidence indicates that individuals who are heterozygous for the Hb S gene (Hb A/S) have a selective advantage against *P. falciparum* malaria compared with either homozygote (Hb A/A or Hb S/S). This has led to the persistence of the gene for Hb S as a balanced polymorphism in endemic areas. The mechanism of protection by Hb S appears to be the inhibition of parasite growth in Hb A/S erythrocytes at the low oxygen tensions that occur during sequestration in postcapillary venules. Other forms of genetically determined resistance include the Duffy blood group–negative phenotype (FyFy), which confers resistance to *P. vivax*, and ovalocytosis, which results in reduced invasion of erythrocytes by *P. falciparum*. The mutations that have been selected by malaria are an important legacy of the disease that will persist long after the disease is eradicated.

Clinical Manifestations

Patients infected by mosquito bite have an incubation period of 8 to 30 days before the onset of symptoms. However, chemoprophylaxis may prolong the incubation period to several months (all four species) or several years (*P. vivax, P. ovale*). Before the onset of fever many patients have a prodrome consisting of malaise, myalgia, cough, and headache that is often mistaken for a viral illness. The most characteristic symptom of malaria caused by all four species of plasmodia is the paroxysm of a shaking chill followed by fever and then sweating. The fever typically lasts for several hours and may reach 40° C or higher. With *P. falciparum* the fever may last longer or may be continuous. Many patients also have nausea, vomiting, diarrhea, headache, backache, abdominal pain, or delirium during the fever. Resolution of the fever is often accompanied by drenching sweats.

Periodicity of the fever is produced by synchronized infections in which all the schizonts rupture at the same time. Synchronized infections occur most often with *P. malariae* (paroxysms every 72 hours) and with relapses of *P. vivax* and *P. ovale* (paroxysms every 48 hours). Some patients may be quite asymptomatic between paroxysms. Fever is less likely to be periodic in *P. falciparum* infections or in the initial attack of *P. vivax*.

On physical examination many patients have splenomegaly and liver tenderness. Vigorous palpation of the spleen should be avoided because of the risk of splenic rupture. Scleral icterus, jaundice, and herpes labialis sometimes occur. During the rigor that initiates the malaria paroxysm, patients may have cold skin because of vasoconstriction. During the febrile stage, the skin is warm and postural hypotension may be caused by peripheral vasodilation.

Patients usually have a normochromic, normocytic anemia from hemolysis, a moderate leukopenia, and thrombocytopenia. The thrombocytopenia is rarely sufficient to cause bleeding. The peripheral smear may show monocytes containing malarial pigment. Malaria does not cause eosinophilia. Hyponatremia is common in *P. falciparum* malaria and is probably caused by sodium depletion and water retention. The urine should be examined for the presence of hemoglobinuria or evidence of acute tubular necrosis. The serum bilirubin level may be mildly elevated because of hemolysis, and there may be transaminase elevations to three to four times the normal values. More marked rise in the transaminase levels should raise the question of centrilobular necrosis (seen in severe malaria) or the possibility of another disease (e.g., viral hepatitis). The serum glucose level should be checked in patients with *P. falciparum* malaria, since hypoglycemia resulting from high levels of parasitemia or from quinine-induced insulin secretion sometimes occurs.

Complications in malaria are most common with *P. falciparum* because of the high-level parasitemias that occur. Patients with more than 100,000 parasitized erythrocytes/mm³ of blood are at great risk for severe hemolytic anemia and renal failure from hemoglobinuria (blackwater fever). Hemolysis and hemoglobinuric renal failure may also be produced by quinine sensitivity or by the treatment of G6PD-deficient patients with oxidant drugs. Renal failure in patients with malaria may also be caused by hypovolemia and acute tubular necrosis. Patients with malaria are extremely catabolic, and uremia may progress very rapidly.

Cerebral malaria occurs with *P. falciparum* and may become evident as alterations in the level of consciousness, organic psychosis, major motor seizures, or, rarely, as hemiparesis or a movement disorder. The cerebrospinal fluid (CSF) is usually normal, although a mild pleocytosis may occur. It must be emphasized that cerebral malaria is a diagnosis of exclusion, and it is imperative that other diseases (e.g., encephalitis, meningitis, brain abscess) be considered, even if the patient has circulating parasites. Pulmonary edema is usually a terminal event and is probably caused by increased capillary permeability. Rehydration is usually necessary because of fever and sweating, but it should be performed with great care in patients with high-level parasitemias.

Malaria in pregnancy may increase the chances of abortion or a low-birth-weight infant, especially in primiparous women. Malaria in children may be more indolent and chronic, becoming evident as a wasting disease with anemia and hepatosplenomegaly. Tropical splenomegaly with hypersplenism and Burkitt's lymphoma are two diseases associated with *P. falciparum* malaria.

Complications from nonfalciparum malaria occur infrequently. *P. vivax* produces rapid splenic enlargement and sometimes splenic rupture even after treatment has been started. *P. malariae* in children may cause a chronic, progressive glomerulonephritis that responds poorly to treatment with antimalarial drugs.

The duration of erythrocytic infection in untreated or inadequately treated patients with malaria varies with the species of *Plasmodium*. The mean duration of *P. falciparum* infection is about 100 days, and most infections are eliminated within 1 year. However, a few untreated or inadequately treated infections have lasted 3 to 4 years. Acquired immunity or partial treatment reduces parasitemia and symptoms. Periodic rises in the level of parasitemia can produce recurrent symptoms (recrudescence). *P. malariae* infections that are not treated persist for the life of the host. Patients with chronic *P. malariae* infection are usually asymptomatic, but they may have a recrudescence associated with surgery, splenectomy, or immunosuppressive therapy. *P. vivax* and *P. ovale* persist as latent forms in the hepatic parenchymal cells. Recurrences from hepatic forms are called *relapses*. Latent hepatic forms may persist for 3 to 5 years.

Diagnosis

Malaria should be suspected in any febrile patient who has traveled in an endemic area, who has abused intravenous drugs, or who has had a recent blood transfusion. In addition, the diagnosis of malaria should be considered in individuals with unexplained fevers who reside near international airports in the central valley of California or near the U.S-Mexico border.

Diagnosis requires demonstration of malarial parasites on Giemsa-stained blood smears. Blood smears should be examined immediately and every 12 hours until the diagnosis is confirmed or rejected be-

cause nonimmune patients may have symptoms at very low levels of parasitemia and because parasitemias (especially in *P. falciparum* malaria) may fluctuate. Thick smears permit more blood to be screened in less time but require greater experience on the part of the examiner. Once malarial parasites have been identified on the blood smear, the next step is to determine whether the patient has *P. falciparum* malaria because the species influences treatment. Patients with malaria who have recently returned from Africa or Haiti are very likely to have falciparum malaria, since *P. falciparum* is the predominant malaria parasite in these areas. The following morphologic criteria suggest falciparum malaria: the predominance of small ring forms and the occurrence of multiply infected erythrocytes; appliqué forms in which the ring parasite appears to be adjacent to the erythrocyte membrane; rings with two nuclei; and crescent-shaped gametocytes (Color Plate VIII-14). *P. falciparum* is also very likely if 5% or more of erythrocytes are infected. Morphologic criteria for *P. vivax* and *P. ovale* include the presence of trophozoites and schizonts as well as rings on the peripheral smear; enlargement of the infected erythrocytes (reticulocytes); and pink stippling of infected erythrocytes (Schüffner's dots) (Color Plate VIII-15). Other distinguishing characteristics are listed in Table 279-2. Serologic tests are not useful in the diagnosis of acute malaria.

Treatment

Patients with acute attacks of *P. vivax*, *P. ovale*, and *P. malariae* can be treated with chloroquine (Table 279-3). Outpatient therapy is appropriate if the patient does not vomit the medicine. With *P. vivax* and *P. ovale* the eradication of persistent hepatic forms (hypnozoites) requires treatment with primaquine phosphate, 26.3 mg daily for 14 days. The patient should first be checked for G6PD deficiency. Severe G6PD deficiency is a contraindication to primaquine, and such patients should be followed and any erythrocytic relapses treated with chloroquine. Patients with mild G6PD deficiency can be given treatment with primaquine at a reduced dosage of 45 mg weekly for 8 weeks. Primaquine is not indicated in patients with malaria acquired by transfusion or with congenital malaria, since erythrocytic parasites do not infect the liver.

The management of patients with *P. falciparum* malaria is more complicated because of the life-threatening nature of the infection and the possibility of drug resistance. Early diagnosis and rapid initiation of appropriate treatment are essential, and patients must be monitored closely to assess the response to treatment and to identify complications. The choice of initial treatment should be based on the severity of the infection and the possibility of drug resistance. Resistance to chloroquine is widespread and increasing, and there are only a few areas of the world from which chloroquine resistance has not been reported. Resistance to the combination of pyrimethamine plus sulfadoxine (Fansidar) has also been reported in Southeast Asia, Panama, South America, and East Africa. Fansidar has also been associated with severe allergic reactions (Stevens-Johnson syndrome, toxic epidermal necrolysis), with death occurring in approximately 1 in 20,000 persons taking the drug.

Patients with uncomplicated, chloroquine-sensitive *P. falciparum* malaria can be treated with chloroquine (Table 279-3). The reader is cautioned that resistance is spreading rapidly. Chloroquine-resistant *P. falciparum* infections occur in all malarious areas except Central America west of the Panama Canal Zone, Mexico, Haiti, the Dominican Republic, and most of the Middle East. However, chloroquine resistance has been reported in Yemen, Oman, and Iran. Patients who have uncomplicated falciparum malaria acquired in an area of known chloroquine resistance or who have transfusion malaria (source unknown) should be given treatment with quinine sulfate plus tetracycline or clindamycin (children, pregnant women) (Table 279-3). Quinidine can be substituted for quinine. Mefloquine at a dose of 1250 mg (750 mg or three tablets followed 6 to 8 hours later by 500 mg) is an alternative.

Severe or complicated *Plasmodium falciparum* malaria (parasitemia >100,000 organisms/mm³, hematocrit <30%, cerebral symptoms, or renal failure) is a medical emergency. Patients with these findings and patients who have severe and repeated vomiting or diarrhea should be given treatment with intravenous (IV) quinidine

Table 279-2   Clinical and diagnostic features in human malaria

	PLASMODIUM SPECIES			
	P. FALCIPARUM	*P. VIVAX*	*P. OVALE*	*P. MALARIAE*
Incubation period (days)*	8-25 (avg., 12)	8-27 (avg., 14)	9-17 (avg., 15)	15-30
Clinical features and complications	Fever often asynchronous, severe hemolysis, renal failure, pulmonary edema, cerebral malaria, thrombocytopenia, hypoglycemia	Anemia, thrombocytopenia, splenic rupture	Similar to *P. vivax*	Glomerulonephritis; erythrocytic infection persisting for years
Duration of erythrocytic cycle (hours)	48	48	48	72
Chloroquine resistance	Yes, widespread	Rare	No	No
Relapses from liver	No	Yes	Yes	No
Sequestration of trophozoites and schizonts	Yes	No	No	No
Morphologic characteristics	Rings predominate, thin cytoplasm, double nuclei, appliqué forms, multiply infected erythrocytes, crescent-shaped gametocytes	Enlarged erythrocytes, trophozoites with ameboid cytoplasm, Schüffner's dots	Oval erythrocytes, compact cytoplasm, Schüffner's dots	Erythrocytes not enlarged, compact cytoplasm (band forms)

*Incubation period may be prolonged by prophylactic medication. The incubation period of *P. vivax*, *P. ovale*, and *P. malariae* is occasionally months to years.

Table 279-3   Chemotherapy for patients with malaria

CLINICAL SETTING	DRUG TREATMENT
P. vivax, P. ovale, P. malariae, and chloroquine-sensitive *P. falciparum*	Chloroquine phosphate, 1 g orally followed by 500 mg in 6 hours and 500 mg daily for 2 days. For *P. vivax* and *P. ovale*, primaquine phosphate, 26.3 mg daily for 14 days, to eradicate persistent hepatic forms. Check G6PD level before treating with primaquine.
Chloroquine-resistant *P. falciparum*	Quinine sulfate, 650 mg orally every 8 hours for 3-7 days,* and tetracycline, 250 mg every 6 hours for 7 days, or clindamycin, 900 mg thrice daily for 3 days.
Severe or complicated *P. falciparum* (parasitemia >100,000 cells/mm³; hematocrit <30; renal failure; cerebral malaria; severe vomiting or diarrhea)	Quinidine, 10 mg/kg loading dose over 1 hour, then continuous infusion of 0.02 mg/kg/min until oral therapy can be started. Give slowly (over 4 hours) with continuous electrocardiographic monitoring. Begin oral medication with tetracycline or clindamycin when the patient's condition is stable.

*Relative resistance to quinine has developed in Southeast Asia and possibly in other areas, and treatment of relatively resistant strains should be continued for 7 days.

(Table 279-3). Vital signs should be monitored frequently, and the electrocardiogram (ECG) should be monitored continuously during IV quinidine administration. Quinidine, formerly a staple of hospital formularies for use as an antiarrhythmic, is no longer widely used for this indication. In the patient who requires IV therapy, the clinician should administer quinidine as rapidly as possible as this may prevent life-threatening delays in initiation of therapy. The maintenance dose of quinidine should be reduced in patients with renal failure. When the patient can take oral medication, quinine sulfate should be substituted and tetracycline or clindamycin added. All patients with cerebral symptoms should have a blood sample drawn for glucose assay, and 100 ml of 50% dextrose should be administered intravenously. Exchange transfusion has been reported to be efficacious in some patients with severe malaria and should be strongly considered

as an adjunct to antimalarial chemotherapy in patients with high-level parasitemias (>10%) or end-organ failure (renal failure, cerebral symptoms, pulmonary edema). Corticosteroids (dexamethasone) are not effective in the treatment of cerebral malaria and have been associated with a higher risk of complications, such as pneumonia and gastrointestinal tract bleeding.

Patients receiving treatment for *P. falciparum* should be monitored for at least 72 hours, since complications can occur even after therapy has been initiated. It is also important to demonstrate a decline in the level of parasitemia within 24 to 48 hours. The asexual parasitemia should be completely resolved in 4 to 5 days. Gametocytes are not affected by most antimalarial drugs, and their continued presence in the blood is not indicative of treatment failure. Patients must be warned about the possibility of a recrudescence 4 to 5 weeks (rarely, several months) after treatment.

Chloroquine has minimum toxicity. Its major toxicity occurs in Africans, who frequently have itching. Quinine or quinidine may produce symptoms resembling cinchonism (nausea, vomiting, tinnitus, vertigo), but this is not an indication to alter or discontinue treatment. Rarely, quinine causes severe Coombs-test–positive hemolytic anemia or an immune thrombocytopenia, requiring that the drug be stopped immediately. Mefloquine at treatment doses may cause nausea, vomiting, dizziness, diarrhea, toxic psychosis, and seizures.

Prevention in Travelers

Prevention of malaria in travelers is increasingly difficult because of the spread of chloroquine-resistant *P. falciparum* and the toxicity of some antimalarial drugs (Chapter 247). Physicians should warn travelers that fever occurring during or after travel in an endemic area may be caused by malaria even if chemoprophylactic drugs were used. Chapter 247 contains current recommendations for prophylaxis.

BABESIOSIS

Human babesiosis is a zoonotic, tick-borne infection of erythrocytes that is caused by two species of *Babesia*: *B. microti* and *B. divergens*. *Babesia* organisms are transmitted by *Ixodes* ticks during the course of a blood meal that must last for approximately 12 hours for transmission to occur. *Ixodes* ticks also transmit the spirochete that causes Lyme disease, and cotransmission of the two organisms may occur. *Babesia* infection may also be acquired by blood transfusion from an infected donor. In the vertebrate host, organisms invade erythrocytes and have an asexual, erythrocytic life cycle similar to that of *Plasmodium* species. There is no exoerythrocytic cycle. *Babesia* species have a wide host range, which includes a variety of wild and domestic animals. Humans are infected when they intrude on the habitat of the tick and the animal reservoir.

Epidemiology

Symptomatic human babesiosis occurs infrequently. Most reported cases have been caused by *B. microti* acquired along the northeastern coast of the United States (Nantucket Island, Martha's Vineyard, Long Island, Shelter Island). However, the range of the tick vector appears to be increasing, and human babesiosis has been described in Wisconsin, Minnesota, Georgia, Northern California, and Washington State. *B. divergens* infections have occurred only in individuals without spleens and have been reported from Europe and North America.

Pathogenesis and Immunity

Clinical consequences are produced by multiplication of organisms within erythrocytes and rupture of the infected erythrocytes. Infection may persist for months, perhaps because of antigenic variation by the parasite. Symptoms are more severe in elderly and splenectomized individuals. Whether infection confers immunity is unknown.

Clinical Manifestations

B. microti infections may be asymptomatic or may produce clinical manifestations ranging from mild to severe. The incubation period with *B. microti* is 1 to 4 weeks in tick-transmitted disease. There is usually a gradual onset of fever, chills, myalgias, and fatigue. Fever is irregular and not periodic. Physical examination may show hepatosplenomegaly. Patients usually have a moderate anemia, leukopenia, and elevated liver enzyme levels. Most reported cases of *B. microti* infection have been in immunocompetent persons who have not undergone splenectomy. Infections in this group are nonfatal, although malaise and fatigue often persist for several months. Noncardiogenic pulmonary edema has been described as an infrequent complication. Babesiosis has been reported as a chronic infection in patients with AIDS with or without splenectomy and should be considered in the differential diagnosis of fever or anemia in an HIV-positive individual from areas of the United States that are endemic for babesiosis.

B. divergens causes rapid onset of fever, chills, nausea, vomiting, and severe hemolysis in patients without spleens. Hemoglobinuria and renal failure are common. Most reported cases have been fatal. In northern California a *Babesia*-like organism that is phylogenetically similar to *Theileria* species has been identified as the cause of a febrile illness in patients with splenectomy.

Diagnosis

Babesiosis should be suspected in patients with fever and history of a tick bite, especially if the patient has been in the endemic area of the northeastern United States or if the patient lacks a spleen. Babesiosis should also be considered in patients who become ill following a blood transfusion. Diagnosis may be made by microscopic examination of Giemsa-stained blood smears. Repeat examinations may be required. *Babesia* organisms are morphologically similar to *P. falciparum*, but experienced microscopists can distinguish *Babesia* on the basis of formation of tetrads ("Maltese crosses"), absence of pigment granules in infected red blood cells (RBCs), and the presence of extracellular merozoites. Inoculation of gerbils or hamsters has also been used to establish the diagnosis. Recently the use of polymerase chain reaction (PCR) and indirect immunofluorescent antibody assays has increased the sensitivity of detection and strongly suggests that persistent microscopically undiagnosed infection may be a part of the clinical spectrum. These tests are not alternatives to the more rapid microscopic diagnosis in severe cases but may be beneficial in elusive cases.

Treatment and Prevention

Infection with *B. microti* is usually self-limited, but if symptoms are severe or persistent, treatment with a combination of clindamycin (1.2 g IV twice daily or 600 mg orally thrice daily for 7 days) and quinine (650 mg orally twice daily for 7 days) has been reported to reduce symptoms. Prolonged suppression of infection is indicated in

HIV-positive individuals after short-term treatment. Chemotherapy for patients with *B. divergens* has not been shown to be successful, but empiric treatment with pentamidine and cotrimoxazole was successful in one case with 5% parasitemia. Exchange blood transfusion may reduce the level of parasitemia and is a reasonable therapeutic maneuver in severely ill patients, followed by chemotherapy with clindamycin and quinine.

Infection can be prevented by avoiding exposure to ticks or by searching for and removing ticks, since prolonged feeding is required for transmission.

TOXOPLASMOSIS

Toxoplasmosis is caused by the sporozoan parasite *Toxoplasma gondii*. The organism is ubiquitous and infects more than 50% of individuals in some populations. Infection is often asymptomatic but may cause severe clinical consequences in immunocompromised hosts or if infection is acquired in utero. Central nervous system (CNS) toxoplasmosis is a common opportunistic infection in patients with AIDS (Chapter 248). Effective treatment is available for some forms of toxoplasmosis, but it may be impossible to eradicate the infection completely in patients with AIDS. In patients with congenital toxoplasmosis, irreversible sequelae may have occurred before therapy is initiated.

Biology and Life Cycle

T. gondii is an obligate intracellular parasite. The organism has a sexual cycle in the intestinal epithelium of cats (the definitive host) and an asexual extraintestinal cycle in the tissues of humans, most mammals, and birds (incidental hosts). Toxoplasma exist in three forms: trophozoites (or tachyzoites), cysts (which contain bradyzoites), and oocysts. *Trophozoites* invade cells and multiply intracellularly by asexual division. *Cysts* contain latent but viable trophozoites and are responsible for chronic infection. *Oocysts* are produced by sexual reproduction of toxoplasma in cats and, except for transmission, have no role in the pathogenesis of human disease. Human infection is acquired by five different routes: ingestion of oocysts in material contaminated by cat feces, including water; ingestion of tissue cysts in raw or undercooked meat; transplacental passage of trophozoites from an acutely infected pregnant woman to her fetus; transfusion of blood containing infected leukocytes; and transplantation of an infected organ.

The life cycle in humans is as follows. Ingested tissue cysts or oocysts are disrupted by digestive enzymes, and viable organisms are released. The organisms invade intestinal epithelium, multiply intracellularly to produce trophozoites, then disseminate throughout the body. Trophozoites are ovoid or crescent shaped and are stained by Giemsa. They can invade virtually any nucleated mammalian cell by endocytosis and multiply within the endocytic vesicle. Their intracellular survival in phagocytic cells is enhanced by the ability to prevent fusion of the host lysosomes with the endocytic vesicles containing trophozoites. In immunocompetent hosts the acute infection is terminated by a combination of humoral and cellular immunity, and the organisms form tissue cysts, which are resistant to destruction and are the hallmark of chronic infection. Tissue cysts may occur in any organ but are most often found in brain, heart, and skeletal muscle (especially the diaphragm). Trophozoites within cysts divide slowly (bradyzoites), producing about 300 viable organisms per cyst. Tissue cysts evoke minimum inflammatory response, despite the presence of parasite antigens in the cyst wall. The cyst wall can be stained with silver, and the bradyzoites stain strongly with periodic acid–Schiff. In immunodeficient hosts it is postulated that tissue cysts rupture, releasing trophozoites, which multiply rapidly (tachyzoites), disseminate, and produce disease.

Cats are also infected by the ingestion of oocysts or tissue cysts. The organisms released into the intestine may either develop asexually as just described or, as an alternative, may differentiate into male and female gametocytes. Fertilization occurs within the intestinal epithelial cells, and an oocyst is produced. The oocyst is released into the intestinal lumen and is excreted with the feces. Cats begin to excrete oocysts about 1 to 2 weeks after they are infected by eating tissue cysts or about 3 weeks after eating oocysts. Cats excrete 10 million oocysts per day for about 3 weeks; then their feces are no longer infectious. Although cats can be reinfected, oocyst excretion rarely occurs with the reinfections. Excreted oocysts must sporulate in the environment before they are infectious for other animals. Sporulation requires 1 to 21 days, depending on environmental factors. Infectious oocysts may survive in moist soil for more than 1 year and may contaminate fruits and vegetables.

Epidemiology

T. gondii is a zoonosis with a worldwide distribution, but the organism is more prevalent in areas with a warm, moist climate than in areas that are cold or arid. Serologic studies have demonstrated a high prevalence of antibody to toxoplasma in many populations. The antibody persists for life, and the prevalence of seropositivity increases with age. In many countries more than 50% of individuals are seropositive by the fourth decade of life. In most areas cats are the major source of transmission, but where raw or undercooked meat (especially mutton and pork) is eaten, infectious tissue cysts can transmit disease. Slaughterhouse workers may be at increased risk for infection.

The incidence of congenital toxoplasmosis is about the same in countries with high and low prevalence of seropositivity. Congenital infection occurs only if there is an acute infection during pregnancy, and only seronegative women are at risk of acute infection. Populations with a high prevalence of seropositivity contain a small group of seronegative women who are at high risk of acquiring infection during pregnancy. Populations with a low prevalence of seropositivity contain a large group of seronegative women at low risk of acquiring infection during pregnancy. Thus for both populations the proportion of women who acquire toxoplasmosis during pregnancy and transmit it to the fetus is about the same. The greatest risk of congenital infection probably occurs when a pregnant woman from a low-prevalence area travels to a high-prevalence area (e.g., El Salvador, Tahiti, France).

Pathogenesis and Immunity

Most manifestations of toxoplasmosis are caused by replicating trophozoites that disseminate throughout the body, destroying host cells and producing necrotic foci. Antibody and complement can kill extracellular trophozoites, but cell-mediated immunity and an effective oxidative burst by mononuclear phagocytes are required to stop the proliferation of intracellular organisms. Tissue cysts are not destroyed by the immune system but appear to persist in a latent but potentially infectious form for the life of the host. If the immune system is disturbed by intercurrent illness (e.g., AIDS, lymphoreticular malignancy) or by immunosuppressive therapy, tissue cysts may rupture and produce disseminated disease.

The pathologic changes of toxoplasmosis vary with the host's immune status. Most data on disease in immunocompetent hosts come from lymph node biopsies. *Toxoplasma* lymphadenitis produces a characteristic picture of follicular hyperplasia with clusters of epithelioid histiocytes invading the germinal centers. Trophozoites or tissue cysts are rarely seen. Toxoplasmosis in neonates and in patients with immunodeficiency may affect many organs, but the CNS is most often involved. The lesions in infants and adults are similar. Typically a meningoencephalitis occurs, which may be focal or diffuse and is characterized by necrosis and reactive microglial nodules. Trophozoites may invade the endothelium of blood vessels, producing ischemia and coagulation necrosis in the area supplied by the affected blood vessel. Lesions are usually multiple and may occur anywhere in the brain, although there is a predilection for the gray matter of the cortex and the basal ganglia. Patients with AIDS typically exhibit a mass lesion or lesions suggestive of a brain abscess. Trophozoites and tissue cysts can usually be identified on histologic examination. Infected infants often have a periventricular and periaqueductal vasculitis, which may lead to obstructive hydrocephalus and is responsible for the periventricular calcifications often seen on radiographs. Myocarditis, interstitial pneumonitis, pancreatitis, and skeletal myositis also occur frequently.

Ocular toxoplasmosis is usually a late manifestation of congenital infection. Tissue cysts that develop in the retina during acute infection release invasive trophozoites, which produce a necrotizing retinitis. Granulomatous inflammation of the choroid often follows, and with increasing tissue destruction there may be iridocyclitis, glaucoma, or cataracts.

Clinical Manifestations

In the normal adult most infections with *T. gondii* are asymptomatic. When symptoms occur (10% to 20% of infections), the most common manifestation is cervical lymphadenopathy, but any or all lymph node groups can be affected. The nodes are typically discrete, not matted together, and no overlying erythema or warmth and no suppuration occur. Retroperitoneal or mesenteric lymphadenopathy may produce abdominal pain. In addition to lymphadenopathy, some patients have headache, fever, malaise, myalgias, sore throat, or a maculopapular rash. Hepatosplenomegaly occurs occasionally, but the existence of a true *Toxoplasma* hepatitis has not been proved. Atypical lymphocytosis has been described, but toxoplasmosis is an infrequent cause of the infectious mononucleosis syndrome.

In the immunodeficient host, disseminated toxoplasmosis occurs most often by relapse of a chronic infection. The constellation of fever, unusual headaches, and mild neurologic findings should suggest the diagnosis of toxoplasma encephalitis in the immunocompromised host. CNS manifestations are the most frequent signs of toxoplasmosis in HIV-positive patients and occur in 5% to 10% of AIDS patients in the United States and in 10% to 40% of AIDS patients in Europe. Manifestations include focal neurologic signs of subacute onset and signs of generalized cerebral dysfunction (e.g., confusion, lethargy). Some patients have seizures, which may be generalized or focal. The manifestations of cerebral toxoplasmosis are not pathognomonic. The differential diagnosis includes chronic meningitis (especially from fungi or syphilis), herpes simplex encephalitis, encephalitis caused by human immunodeficiency virus (HIV) infections, drug toxicity, progressive multifocal leukoencephalopathy, and CNS malignancy. In patients with focal findings the possibility of cerebrovascular accident must also be considered. CSF abnormalities seen with toxoplasmosis are nonspecific and include mild mononuclear pleocytosis and elevated protein content with normal glucose level, but in some patients the CSF is entirely normal. Computed tomography (CT) of the brain frequently shows abnormalities. Multiple contrast-enhancing lesions with either a homogeneous density or ring enhancement are most common. Occasionally, only a single lesion is seen or the lesions are of low density and are not enhanced by contrast. Double-dose contrast administration appears to be superior to standard CT scanning. Some patients with normal CT scans have had focal abnormalities demonstrated by magnetic resonance imaging (MRI) scans. Retinitis is the second most common manifestation of *Toxoplasma* infection in AIDS patients. Although CNS findings predominate in immunocompromised patients, *Toxoplasma* interstitial pneumonitis is increasing in incidence in AIDS patients, perhaps because of improved diagnosis or increasing longevity of AIDS patients. The diagnosis is made by detection of *Toxoplasma* organisms in bronchoalveolar lavage fluid or lung biopsy specimens. Toxoplasmosis in the immunocompromised person may also become evident as fever of unknown origin or as a necrotizing myocarditis.

Congenital toxoplasmosis may occur when a previously uninfected (seronegative) woman has acute infection during pregnancy. The infection in the mother is usually asymptomatic but may produce fever and lymphadenopathy. Risk of fetal infection is lowest during the first trimester but results in the most severe disease. The risk of fetal infection is highest during the third trimester, but disease is less severe.

Toxoplasma infection during pregnancy may produce a variety of consequences. Spontaneous abortions occur, but their frequency is unknown. If the neonate has clinical evidence of infection at birth, sequelae are usually severe. Involvement of the CNS is always present and may include microcephaly, hydrocephalus, convulsions, deafness, and mental retardation. Intracranial calcifications may be apparent on radiographs after several months. Evidence of generalized infection may be present but is variable. Manifestations include lymphadenopathy, hepatosplenomegaly, jaundice, thrombocytopenia, anemia, fever, pneumonitis, and a rash. The differential diagnosis in neonates includes cytomegalovirus, rubella, and herpes encephalitis.

If congenital infection is subclinical at birth, clinical manifestations develop in most children observed into adolescence. Chorioretinitis is the most common late manifestation of congenital toxoplasmosis. The course of the disease consists of remissions and relapses. Patients may have intermittent unilateral blindness or pain in the eye. Microphthalmia, cataracts, and glaucoma also occur. During the initial stages funduscopy reveals clusters of elevated, yellowish-white patches. Later the lesions may be pale and contain black pigment. Other late sequelae of congenital infection include psychomotor retardation, seizures, cerebellar signs, and deafness.

Diagnosis

Two primary methods exist for the diagnosis of toxoplasmosis: histopathologic identification of the organism in biopsy material and serologic tests for antibodies to *Toxoplasma*. In addition, the histology of *Toxoplasma* lymphadenitis is very characteristic and in some hands diagnostic. Various serologic tests are available. The dye test is very specific and detects immunoglobulin G (IgG) antibodies that fix complement and lyse trophozoites. Indirect fluorescent antibody (IFA) tests detect IgG or immunoglobulin M (IgM) antibodies to *Toxoplasma*. IFA tests are easier to perform and more readily available than the dye test, but they are less reliable. Rheumatoid factors may cause false-positive results. IgM is detectable within a week of infection, rises rapidly to high titers ($>1:160$), then disappears within a few months. The IgG detected by IFA follows a pattern similar to that described for the dye test. An enzyme-linked immunosorbent assay (ELISA) that detects IgM antibodies is more sensitive than the IFA test and eliminates the false-positive results caused by rheumatoid factor, but this test is not routinely available. Other tests, including indirect hemagglutination, complement fixation, and direct agglutination, have been developed but are not in general use.

The approach to diagnosis should be determined by the clinical setting. In the immunocompetent host the diagnosis of acute acquired toxoplasmosis is confirmed by seroconversion from a negative to a positive dye test result or IFA test result or by a rise in titer of IgG antibody of two or more dilutions in sera drawn at 3-week intervals. A single high-titer dye test result or IFA test result is suggestive but not diagnostic of acute infection. An IgM antibody titer of 1:160 or higher by the ELISA test or by IFA is also diagnostic of acute infection.

Noninvasive diagnosis of acute toxoplasmosis in immunocompromised patients is difficult because antibody responses are depressed. Serum IgG antibody is detectable in 97% of patients at the time of diagnosis of *Toxoplasma* disease, since most cases of toxoplasmosis in immunocompromised hosts are caused by relapses or reactivation of chronic infection. Diagnostic changes in the titer of IgG antibody occur infrequently, even in biopsy-proven disease, and test results for IgM antibody are usually negative. Absence of detectable serum IgG mandates consideration of other diagnoses, since primary *Toxoplasma* encephalitis in AIDS patients is relatively rare. The diagnosis can be definitively made by demonstrating organisms in biopsy specimens from accessible lesions. However, if the CNS toxoplasmosis is strongly suspected on clinical grounds, it is reasonable to institute a therapeutic trial and observe an immunocompromised patient closely for evidence of a response consistent with the diagnosis. This is particularly true for the patient with AIDS and a positive *Toxoplasma* titer who has single or multiple ring-enhancing cerebral mass lesions. Since CNS toxoplasmosis is by far the most likely diagnosis, a 2-week trial of sulfadiazine and pyrimethamine with follow-up CT scanning is a common approach. If the patient does not have a positive *Toxoplasma* titer or lesions fail to improve, brain biopsy is recommended. If clinical or radiographic improvement is seen, chronic therapy (see next section) is indicated. Methods based on the detection of toxoplasma DNA by hybridization with specific probes or by amplification with PCR may soon provide more sensitive detection in immunocompromised persons but are not yet generally available.

The serologic diagnosis of congenital infection is complicated by the transplacental transfer of maternal IgG, which may persist in the infant for 6 to 12 months, and by the inability of infants to make antibodies to *Toxoplasma* until the second or third month of life. Serologic diagnosis of congenital toxoplasmosis requires persistent or rising titers of IgG antibody or the demonstration of IgM antibodies to *Toxoplasma*. Repeat tests should be performed monthly.

Table 279-4 Treatment of patients with toxoplasmosis

CLINICAL SETTING	SUGGESTED TREATMENT
Acute infection in immunocompetent patients	
Mild	No treatment
Severe or prolonged symptoms	Pyrimethamine, 200-mg loading dose in two divided doses followed by 25-75 mg/day, plus sulfadiazine, 100 mg/kg/day in three divided doses, plus folinic acid, 10 mg/day, for 3-4 weeks
Toxoplasmosis in immunodeficient patients	
Acute	Pyrimethamine, 200-mg loading dose followed by 75 mg/day, plus sulfadiazine, 100 mg/kg/day (to 8 g/day) in three divided doses, plus folinic acid, 10 mg/day, for 6 weeks (with clinical or radiologic response)
Acute, sulfa allergic	Pyrimethamine, 200-mg loading dose followed by 75 mg/day, plus clindamycin, 600-1200 mg IV every 6 hours or 600 mg PO every 6 hours, plus folinic acid, 10 mg/day, for 6 weeks (with clinical or radiologic response)
Maintenance	Pyrimethamine, 25 mg PO daily, plus sulfadiazine, 500 mg PO four times a day, or clindamycin, 1200 mg PO daily in divided doses
Ocular, congenital, and pregnancy associated	See text

IV, Intravenously; *PO,* orally.

The diagnosis of ocular toxoplasmosis is based on the observation of typical retinal lesions. A positive dye test result or IFA test result for IgG antibody is consistent with the diagnosis, and a negative IgG test result probably excludes the diagnosis. However, no characteristic changes occur in antibody titer because the acute infection is usually remote. Lesions that are not typical of toxoplasmosis should not be presumed to be caused by toxoplasmosis on the basis of a positive serologic finding.

Treatment and Prevention

Acute toxoplasmosis in the normal host is usually self-limited, and treatment should not be given unless symptoms are severe or persistent or the patient is pregnant.

Treatment is indicated for immunocompetent patients with severe or prolonged symptoms, for pregnant women, for immunocompromised individuals with disseminated toxoplasmosis, for patients with chorioretinitis caused by toxoplasmosis, and for those with congenital toxoplasmosis. The choice of drugs and the duration of treatment are determined by the clinical setting. Recommendations are given in Table 279-4. Steroids should be initiated with definitive therapy in patients with symptoms of raised intracranial pressure.

Pyrimethamine and sulfadiazine are active against *T. gondii* and are synergistic when given together. It is recommended that this combination be the regimen of first choice except during the first trimester of pregnancy, when pyrimethamine may be teratogenic. Some studies of toxoplasmosis in patients with AIDS suggest that higher daily doses of pyrimethamine (75 to 100 mg/day) may be beneficial. However, therapeutic recommendations for treatment of toxoplasmosis in AIDS patients have developed on the basis of consensus rather than clear-cut results of clinical studies and are frequently varied in patients with drug intolerance.

Folinic acid should generally be added because pyrimethamine is a folic acid antagonist and its use has been correlated with improved outcome. Blood cell counts should be checked frequently. Forty percent to 60% of AIDS patients who take pyrimethamine and sulfadiazine for CNS toxoplasmosis report toxic effects that necessitates discontinuation of the drugs, and some do not respond to this regimen. Clindamycin has been found to be effective in combination with pyrimethamine for the treatment of CNS toxoplasmosis in humans and can replace sulfadiazine in patients who are allergic to sulfa drugs, but is less effective for long-term prevention of relapses. Atovaquone and macrolides (clarithromycin, azithromycin) in special combination with pyrimethamine may be useful for treatment in selected cases, but their use has not been evaluated in large clinical trials.

Immunologically normal individuals with severe symptoms caused by acute toxoplasmosis should be given treatment for 3 to 4 weeks. The treatment of immunocompromised patients with disseminated (usually CNS) toxoplasmosis appears to result in improvement in about 80% of patients. Information from AIDS patients indicates that it is necessary to continue maintenance therapy indefinitely after clinical remission or improvement. In other immunocompromised patients, maintenance therapy should be continued as long as the immunocompromised state continues. Infants with congenital toxoplasmosis should be treated for 1 year. Various regimens have been suggested, and the reader is referred to specialty texts for details. Treatment of acute infection in pregnant women has the goal of preventing congenital disease. One recommended regimen is to treat the infection with pyrimethamine plus sulfadiazine in 5-week cycles consisting of daily treatment for 2 weeks followed by no treatment for 3 weeks; the cycle is continued until term. Pyrimethamine should be omitted during the first trimester, and sulfadiazine should be omitted near term because it increases the risk of kernicterus in neonates with hyperbilirubinemia. In a study from France, spiramycin (3 g/day) was used to treat maternal infections from the time of diagnosis until the end of the pregnancy, with some evidence of decreased sequelae in neonates. Ocular toxoplasmosis is treated for 1 month. A clinical response occurs in about 70% of patients.

Prevention is most important for seronegative women during pregnancy and for seronegative patients who are immunodeficient. Tissue cysts in meat are killed by temperatures over 66° C. Hands should be washed after handling raw meat. Cat feces should be avoided, gloves should be worn while gardening, and fruits and vegetables should be washed thoroughly. If a seronegative individual requires transfusion of leukocyte-rich blood products or an organ transplant, seropositive donors should be excluded if possible.

OTHER COCCIDIAN PARASITIC DISEASES

The coccidia have life cycles similar to that of *T. gondii,* with a sexual stage in the intestinal epithelium of the definitive host and an asexual stage in the gastrointestinal tract or the tissues. *Cryptosporidium, Isospora* and *Cyclospora* organisms have both sexual and asexual stages confined to the intestinal mucosa of a single host. *Sarcocystis* organisms have sexual and asexual cycles in different hosts and may involve the gastrointestinal tract or skeletal muscles of humans. Effective treatment of diarrhea that is due to coddician species, when it has been established, has included trimethoprim or pyrimethamine and a sulfa (Table 279-5).

Cryptosporidiosis

Infection with *Cryptosporidium* species in the immunocompetent as well as the immunodeficient host has been documented with increasing frequency since 1982, when it was recognized as a pathogen in AIDS patients. Ten percent to 15% of AIDS patients in the United States and up to 50% in developing countries are estimated to have cryptosporidiosis during the course of AIDS.

Biology and Life Cycle. Cryptosporidiosis is a zoonotic disease that frequently infects the young of many species, including calves, lambs, piglets, and children. *Cryptosporidium parvum,* the species that infects humans, has no host specificity among mammals and is thus readily passed between them. Asexual and sexual cycles of *C. parvum* occur in the epithelial cells of the small or large intestine, resulting in the development of fully sporulated oocysts that are shed into the environment. Infection occurs when oocysts are ingested and excystation occurs in the small bowel, releasing four motile sporozoites that invade the epithelial cells of the gastrointestinal tract and differentiate into merozoites. Merozoites may be released and reinvade adjacent cells to continue the asexual cycle or may develop into sexual forms that combine to form an oocyst. The oocyst may undergo excystation in the host of origin and repeat the cycle, or it

Table 279-5 Treatment of patients with intracellular gastrointestinal tract protozoa

SPECIES	SUGGESTED TREATMENT
Coccidians	
Cryptosporidium parvum	Nitazoxamide is available in open trial at 1000-3000 mg/day.* Nitazoxamide and bovine anti-*Cryptosporidium* colostral antibodies† are in phase II and III trials in some areas.
Cyclospora cayetanensis Immunocompetent hosts	Trimethoprim (160 mg)–sulfamethoxazole (800 mg) orally twice a day for 7 days.
AIDS patients	Trimethoprim (160 mg)–sulfamethoxazole (800 mg) orally four times a day for 10 days followed by trimethoprim-sulfamethoxazole prophylaxis three times a week to prevent relapse.
Isospora belli Immunocompetent hosts	Trimethoprim (160 mg)–sulfamethoxazole (800 mg) orally four times a day for 10 days, then twice a day for 3 weeks is effective. Pyrimethamine may be substituted for trimethoprim.
AIDS patients	Suppressive therapy is usually required after short-term therapy to prevent relapse.
Sulfa-allergic patients	Pyrimethamine alone at doses of 50 to 75 mg/day has been used in persons who are allergic to sulfonamides.
Microsporidium	
Enterocytozoon bieneusi and *Enterocytozoon intestinalis*	Albendazole 400 mg orally twice a day.‡

*UniMed Pharmaceuticals, Inc.
†Galagen, Inc.
‡May be more efficacious for *E. intestinalis* than for *E. bieneusi.*

may be excreted in an environmentally resistant form to continue the cycle in another host.

Epidemiology. Infection is most common in children, animal care workers, travelers, hospital personnel, and immunocompromised persons, especially transplant recipients and AIDS patients. Transmission is by the fecal-oral route, and person-to-person transmission of *Cryptosporidium* infection has been documented. The mean infectious dose (ID_{50}) for adult humans without serologic evidence of prior infection is 132 organisms. Contaminated water has been implicated in many outbreaks and is the suspected mode of transmission to travelers. Oocysts, the infecting stage, are difficult to remove by filtration because of their small size and are resistant to many disinfectants. Household pets or other domestic animals may constitute a reservoir for human infection.

Pathologic Features and Immunity. Histologic changes in the human small intestine associated with cryptosporidiosis have been described most thoroughly in patients with AIDS. They include villus atrophy and blunting, epithelial flattening, and inflammation of the lamina propria characterized by infiltration of plasma cells, lymphocytes, and macrophages. When infected, the pancreatic ducts, biliary tree, and gallbladder show moderate to severe epithelial hyperplasia and mural thickening. The cause of these histopathologic changes has not been determined; a toxin has not been identified. Lactose intolerance and fat malabsorption have been well documented in patients with cryptosporidiosis. Rarely, cryptosporidiosis of the bronchial epithelium or sinuses associated with gastrointestinal tract disease may develop in immunocompromised hosts.

Both the humoral and the cellular immune responses appear to be important in the control of cryptosporidiosis, but their relative importance and the mechanisms by which they do so have not been established.

Clinical Manifestations. Infection with *C. parvum* may be asymptomatic or may produce acute, self-limited, watery diarrhea in normal hosts. Low-grade fever may occur. Immunodeficient patients may have severe diarrhea with malabsorption, weight loss, and dehydration (Chapter 248). Profuse, watery diarrhea exceeding 20 L/day has been described. Severe, progressive disease occurs frequently in patients with AIDS, who may also have involvement of the biliary tract with symptoms of nausea, right upper quadrant abdominal pain, and elevated serum alkaline phosphatase levels.

Diagnosis. The diagnosis of cryptosporidiosis is often difficult because the oocysts in stool are very small and may be difficult to distinguish from yeast. It may be helpful to concentrate the organisms by sucrose flotation. Oocysts are not stained by periodic acid–Schiff or iodine but are acid-fast and can be stained with a modified Kinyoun or Ziehl-Neelsen stain (Color Plate VIII-33). A sensitive and specific fluorescein-labeled IgG monoclonal antibody and a stool antigen-capture ELISA are commercially available.

Treatment and Prevention. No effective treatment for cryptosporidiosis has been established. Experimental treatment with nitazoxanide, paromomycin, azithromycin, and bovine colostran antibodies directed against *Cryptosporidium* organisms is currently undergoing evaluation. Enteric precautions should be taken with infected individuals, especially in a hospital setting.

Cyclosporiasis

Cyclospora cayetanensis is a worldwide cause of diarrhea in immunocompetent persons and AIDS patients. Previously designated "big *Cryptosporidium*" or thought to be blue algae ("cyanobacterium-like bodies"), *Cyclospora cayetanensis* was recognized as a separate coccidian species in 1993. *Cyclospora* infections have been identified in otherwise healthy travelers to developing countries, in infants and children in developing countries, and in children in child care centers in the United States. *Cyclospora* infection may be associated with prolonged diarrhea in these populations. Epidemics in the United States have been associated with fecal-oral transmission through contaminated water and strawberries. Illness is characterized by watery diarrhea, abdominal cramping, decreased appetite and low-grade fever. Symptoms typically wax and wane for several weeks and may persist for several months. In Haiti the prevalence of *C. cayetanensis* (11%) in stools of AIDS patients with diarrhea approximates the incidence of *Isospora belli* (12%). Symptoms in the Haitian study of AIDS patients were indistinguishable from those reported in AIDS patients with isosporiasis or cryptosporidiosis. *Cyclospora* species, like *Cryptosporidium, Isospora,* and microsporidial species, may cause biliary tract disease in AIDS patients.

Microscopic examination of stool specimens using a modified Ziehl-Neelsen technique reveals abundant spherical bodies 8 to 10 microns in diameter that are similar in morphologic appearance to, but larger than, *Cryptosporidium* oocysts.

Immunocompetent patients have been successfully treated with trimethoprim-sulfamethoxazole (160 mg and 800 mg orally twice a day for 7 days). Patients with AIDS should receive treatment with higher doses of trimethoprim-sulfamethoxazole (160 mg and 800 mg orally four times a day for 10 days) followed by trimethoprim-sulfamethoxazole prophylaxis three times a week to prevent relapse.

Isosporiasis

Species of the genus *Isospora* have a single host, and all stages of the life cycle occur in the epithelium of the small intestine. Human disease is caused by *Isospora belli*. Infection is acquired by the ingestion of oocysts present in the feces of infected humans. Isosporiasis occurs infrequently in the United States but is endemic in some areas of Indochina, South America, and islands of the southwestern

Pacific. Infection may be asymptomatic or may cause watery diarrhea, abdominal cramping, nausea, and vomiting. Disease is usually self-limited and lasts 4 to 6 weeks but may be chronic and produce malabsorption and weight loss. In the United States, prevalence of infection in AIDS patients is highest in persons of Hispanic ethnicity. Rarely, disseminated extraintestinal tract disease has been reported in patients with AIDS.

Symptoms of *Isospora* infection are more severe in immunocompromised individuals, especially those with AIDS (Chapter 248). Isosporiasis has been an infrequent pathogen among AIDS patients in the United States but has been reported to occur in 15% of patients in Haiti. A leukocytosis with moderate eosinophilia (7% to 15%) is common. The diagnosis is made by identifying oocysts in stool samples (Color Plate VIII-1) or by identifying intracellular forms in small bowel biopsies. Trimethoprim (160 mg) and sulfamethoxazole (800 mg) orally four times a day for 10 days, then twice a day for 3 weeks is an effective regimen. Pyrimethamine plus a sulfonamide is also effective. Pyrimethamine alone at doses of 50 to 75 mg/day has been used in persons who are allergic to sulfonamides. Relapses are common in immunodeficient patients, and indefinite maintenance therapy may be necessary.

Sarcocystosis

Species of *Sarcocystis* have life cycles involving two hosts. Humans may be infected as definitive hosts by ingesting *Sarcocystis hominis*–infected tissue from cattle or *Sarcocystis suihominis*–infected tissue from swine. Infection is confined to the epithelium of the intestinal tract and may produce abdominal cramping, nausea, vomiting, and diarrhea of several days' duration. A relapse may occur several weeks later, during the peak of oocyst shedding. Spontaneous recovery follows. Diagnosis is made by identifying oocysts in the stool.

Humans probably can also be infected as incidental hosts by ingestion of oocysts of various species of *Sarcocystis*. Such infections are usually asymptomatic, but muscle involvement with swelling and weakness, fever, leukocytosis, and eosinophilia have been reported. Bronchospasm can occur. Diagnosis can be made only by biopsy of affected tissue, usually muscle. Antifolate drugs (e.g., sulfonamides, trimethoprim, pyrimethamine) appear to be effective.

MICROSPORIDIOSIS

Protozoan parasites of the phylum Microspora infect insects and a variety of wild and domesticated animals. They are small, spore-forming, obligate intracellular parasites that are found in the intestine, liver, kidney, cornea, brain, nerves, and muscles of their animal hosts. Microsporidiosis is recognized as a cause of gastrointestinal tract disease, renal disease, sinusitis, and keratitis in AIDS patients. Until recently, microsporidia have not been studied extensively as agents of disease because they are small, stain poorly, evoke little inflammation, and are difficult to diagnose in the absence of electron microscopy. Increasing study in the AIDS era has led to the discovery of new species and to the reclassification of old ones.

Biology and Life Cycle

Microsporidia multiply in the cytoplasm of host cells. Five genera, *Vittaforma, Nosema, Enterocytozoon, Encephalitozoon,* and *Pleistophora,* have been associated with human disease. Members of these genera have variable and complex structural relationships with the host cell cytoplasm. However, all are released into a cell from a spore by ejection from a long, coiled polar tubule, a characteristic microsporidian feature. Within the host cell development into schizonts (meronts), sporonts, sporoblasts, and spores occurs.

Epidemiology

The source of human infections is unknown, but both vertebrates and invertebrates may serve as reservoirs of infection. For example, *Encephalitozoon* organisms infect birds and mammals, and *Nosema* organisms infect insects. Spores, ingested after release from the gastrointestinal tract or in the urine of other infected animals, are thought to be the mode of transmission of disease. Serologic studies suggest that antibodies to *Encephalitozoon cuniculi* are widespread in animals and humans and are more frequently found in persons who have traveled to the tropics. *Enterocytozoon bieneusi* infection of AIDS patients may be as common as *Cryptosporidium* infection as a cause of diarrhea in AIDS patients. *Encephalitozooan intestinalis,* formerly called *Septata intestinalis,* also causes severe enteritis in AIDS patients and may disseminate to kidney.

Pathology and Immunity

Parasites may not evoke an inflammatory response in tissues, especially in immunocompromised patients, or may elicit moderate granulomatous inflammation with a mononuclear cell infiltrate. It is not known whether microsporidiosis in immunocompromised patients reflects activation of a latent infection.

Enterocytozoon bieneusi infection of the intestinal epithelium is confined to enterocytes covering the villi, especially those at the tip, and is associated with villous atrophy, cell degeneration, necrosis, and sloughing. The jejunum appears to be the preferred site of infection, the duodenum is less frequently infected, and the large intestine is relatively spared. *E. intestinalis* causes severe diarrhea and a granulomatous tubulointerstitial enteritis and may disseminate to lungs and sinuses. *Encephalitozoon cuniculi* infection may involve the kidneys and CNS in a wide range of mammals, including humans.

Clinical Manifestations

Although there are scattered reports of microsporidiosis in immunocompetent patients, disease caused by microsporidia is more widespread in immunocompromised hosts, especially those with AIDS. Infection of the intestinal epithelium with *E. bieneusi* is the most common manifestation of microsporidiosis in AIDS patients. Clinical manifestations of disease include wasting, chronic diarrhea, and cholangiopathy and are indistinguishable from the manifestations of isosporiasis and cryptosporidioisis in AIDS patients. Diarrheal stools are watery and are not accompanied by blood or fever. Routine laboratory test results are normal, with occasional hypokalemia and hypomagnesemia. Carbohydrate and fat malabsorption is present. *E. intestinalis* may be associated with hematuria and renal failure.

Two types of microsporidial ocular infection have been reported in AIDS patients. The first, corneal infection by organisms of the genus *Vittaforma corneae* following trauma, is seen in immunocompetent patients and may result in corneal perforation and blindness. The second type of infection, keratoconjunctivitis in AIDS patients, is caused by *Encephalitozoon hellem.*

Encephalitozoon organisms have also been reported in the peritoneum, and liver of AIDS patients; *Pleistophora* organisms have been reported in skeletal muscle. These genera and sites of infection do not appear to occur frequently.

Diagnosis

Encephalitozoon spores are gram positive, and some are acid fast, but spores of other genera stain unpredictably with these stains, and electron micrography may be required for identification. *E. bieneusi* may be identified on light microscopy of plastic sections of intestinal biopsy material stained with metheylene blue–azure II, basic fuchsin stain, or hematoxylin-eosin. Several groups have recently reported success with the use of Giemsa-stained stool specimens for diagnosis of *E. bieneusi* diarrhea, but these techniques have not come into common use. Giemsa-stained spores in the stool are oval, with the cytoplasm staining light gray-blue and the nucleus staining intensely purple. Ocular infection may be suspected on the basis of corneal scrapings and may be confirmed by electron microscopy. Most recently, modified trichrome and calcofluor stains have been examined and found to be useful for detecting microsporidia in a variety of specimens including conjunctival swabs and urine sediment. Refractory sinusitis may yield microsporidial species on electronmicrographic examination. Oligonucleotide probes specific for *E. cuniculi, E. hellem* and *E. intestinalis* have been developed.

Treatment

Albendazole (400 mg orally twice a day) may be useful for treatment of intestinal *E. bieneusi* or *Septata intestinalis.* Ocular lesions caused by *E. hellem* have responded to fumagillin eyedrops.

AMEBIASIS

Amebiasis is the disease caused by infection with the sarcodinian parasite *Entamoeba histolytica.* Infection is often asymptomatic but may cause diarrhea, severe colitis, a colonic mass, or extraintestinal disease, particularly abscess of the liver. The overall prevalence of amebiasis in the United States is low, but significant endemic foci exist and infection is common in homosexual men, immigrants, travelers, and refugees (Chapter 247). A major problem is the frequent failure of clinicians to consider the diagnosis of amebiasis. When the diagnosis is considered, many clinical laboratories lack expertise at identifying *E. histolytica* in the stool, leading to diagnostic errors. Serologic tests can detect antibodies to *E. histolytica,* but interpretation depends on the clinical setting. Effective therapy is available for most forms of amebiasis.

Biology and Life Cycle

The genus *Entamoeba* contains several species of human parasites (*E. histolytica, E. dispar, E. coli, E. hartmanni*) that may reside in the human colon. Identification of *Entamoeba* species is based on the number of nuclei in the cyst stage, the presence of erythrophagocytosis, and the size of the organisms. *E. histolytica* and *E. hartmanni* cysts contain four nuclei; *E. coli* cysts usually contain eight nuclei. *E. histolytica* produces larger cysts than *E. hartmanni* and phagocytizes erythrocytes. The presence of any of these organisms in stool indicates fecal-oral contamination, but only *E. histolytica* is able to invade the colonic mucosa. *E. hartmanni* and *E. coli* are generally considered to be nonpathogenic commensals. Recently Diamond and Clark have proposed, based on differences in enzymes, surface antigens, ribosomal genes and restriction length polymorphisms, that *E. histolytica* organisms, which are nonpathogenic for humans, be reclassified into a new species, *E. dispar,* which is morphologically identical to pathogenic *E. histolytica.* Invasive disease caused by pathogenic strains is prevalent only in certain geographic areas, principally the tropics, despite the organism's worldwide distribution.

E. histolytica has two stages (cyst and trophozoite) and multiplies asexually by binary fission. No sexual stage exists, and humans are the only hosts. Infection is usually transmitted by the ingestion of cysts present in feces or contaminated water or on fruits and vegetables. Trophozoites are killed by gastric acid and are not infectious when ingested orally. However, trophozoites inoculated into the rectum can transmit infection, and this may be one mechanism of transmission in homosexual men.

Ingested cysts are disrupted in the ileum, and trophozoites are released. Trophozoites are microaerophilic and localize in areas where enteric bacteria have created anaerobic conditions. They colonize the cecum first and then move distally through the colon, residing in the lumen or the glandular crypts. Trophozoites within the lumen of the intestine are protected from the host's immune system and may persist there for years. Pathogenic strains may penetrate the mucosal epithelium and invade the wall of the colon.

Cysts are produced in the lumen of the colon as the stool dehydrates. Therefore cysts are more frequently found in formed stools, and trophozoites in diarrheal stools. After evacuation, cysts can survive refrigeration but not prolonged freezing, and they can survive in cool water for weeks. They are not killed by chlorination of water at the concentrations used by most municipalities, but may be killed by dessication, boiling, or iodination. Most epidemics of amebiasis can be traced to contaminated water supplies, but where crowding or poor sanitation exists, direct fecal-oral transmission may occur.

Epidemiology

E. histolytica occurs in all climates throughout the world. The prevalence of infection may reach 50% in areas where there is contamination of drinking water or food crops with human feces. The prevalence of infection in most industrialized countries is 1% to 3%. In the United States, endemic foci have been identified on some Native American reservations with poor sanitation and in mental institutions, where fecal-oral transmission probably occurs. Some urban populations of homosexual men have a high prevalence of infection (20% or more) that is maintained by sexual transmission.

Pathogenesis and Immunity

E. histolytica within the lumen of the colon may provoke an increase in mucus secretion, a shortening of transit time for stool in the colon, or edema of the colonic mucosa. In general, however, the consequences of luminal infection are minimal.

Invasive disease requires a virulent strain of *E. histolytica*. Invasion usually begins in the glandular crypts of the cecum, appendix, or colon. Invasive amebae have a cytopathic effect on epithelial cells that is mediated by cysteine proteinases, collagenases, and cytotoxins, leading to lytic necrosis. The organisms penetrate the epithelial layer and burrow to the muscularis mucosa. They may spread laterally and produce a superficial ulceration or penetrate the muscularis and reach the submucosa, where there is little resistance to lateral spread. This process produces a flask-shaped lesion with a narrow neck at the portal of entry through the epithelium and a wide base in the submucosa. On histologic examination, lytic necrosis of host cells occurs, but there is little inflammatory cellular reaction. Amebae in the submucosa may coalesce and undermine the mucosa, producing shaggy ulcers with a diameter of several centimeters. Secondary bacterial invasion often occurs at this stage and is followed by infiltration of polymorphonuclear leukocytes. Trophozoites may continue to burrow through the wall of the colon, eventually penetrating the serosa and perforating the colon. Penetration of the intestinal wall is mediated by a proteolytic enzyme secreted by the parasite. Antibody to the protease appears to be predictive of invasive disease.

Amebomas are tumorlike lesions of the colon that are produced by an inflammatory reaction to the amebae and bacteria. On histologic examination, granulation tissue and fibrosis develop. Amebomas produce a localized thickening of the wall of the colon that may be mistaken for a malignant tumor on barium enema examination or on gross inspection at surgery.

Extraintestinal amebiasis is produced by perforation of the colon, by extension to the perianal skin, or by dissemination to the liver or other organs via the blood. Trophozoites in the wall of the colon penetrate mesenteric venules, enter the portal circulation, and are deposited in hepatic sinusoids, where they produce necrosis of the hepatic parenchyma and eventually an abscess. Amebic liver abscesses usually have a thin, fibrous wall and contain necrotic debris. Viable organisms are located at the periphery of the abscess cavity. Neutrophils are generally absent unless secondary bacterial invasion occurs, but most amebic liver abscesses are bacteriologically sterile. Liver abscesses may rupture into the peritoneum, the pleura, or the pericardium. Rarely, amebae gain access via the blood to other organs (e.g., the brain). The presence and the extent of extraintestinal amebiasis are not related to the severity of intestinal disease, and most patients with liver abscesses do not have parasites identified on stool examination.

Invasive amebiasis produces high levels of precipitating, agglutinating, and complement-fixing antibodies, some of which persist for years after infection. Cell-mediated immune responses have been demonstrated in some patients with amebic liver abscesses. Although protective immunity develops, the role of cell-mediated responses is not well defined. Recurrences of liver abscesses after successful treatment are extremely rare, however, suggesting that this form of disease produces at least partial resistance.

Clinical Manifestations

Intestinal amebiasis may be asymptomatic or may produce a spectrum of symptoms, from a slight loosening of the stool to severe colitis and dysentery. Amebiasis acquired in temperate countries is usually caused by nonpathogenic strains. Thus invasive colonic disease and liver abscess are rare in these areas. Acute infection with nonpathogenic strains does not result in morbidity, even in patients with AIDS.

The incubation period from infection to the appearance of organisms in the stool is 1 to 5 days. The clinical incubation period may be as short as 4 days or as long as several years. When amebae are limited to the lumen of the colon, patients may have intermittent increases in the frequency of stools and occasional, mild abdominal cramping. Invasive amebiasis that is limited to the rectosigmoid colon produces rectal tenesmus, crampy lower abdominal pain, and bloody mucoid stools. Patients usually have no fever. The liver may be diffusely enlarged, and liver function test results may be abnormal. In the absence of an abscess, however, there is no evidence of invasion of the liver by trophozoites. Symptoms may resolve spontaneously. Severe colonic involvement causes 20 or more bloody stools per day and constant, intense rectal tenesmus. Patients with extensive involvement of the colon are more likely to have vomiting, fever, intravascular volume depletion, and shock. Toxic megacolon or perforation of the colon may occur. The abdomen may be distended, and bowel sounds may be absent. A plain radiograph of the abdomen should be obtained and examined for evidence of perforation, cecal dilation, or toxic megacolon.

The presentation of a patient with ameboma may be more subtle, although the stools are usually bloody and abdominal pain is present. A colonic lesion can often be palpated, or the lesion may be identified on barium enema examination. Involvement of the cecum or appendix by *E. histolytica* produces right lower quadrant abdominal pain and rigidity and may be mistaken for appendicitis.

Amebic abscess of the liver is the most common extraintestinal manifestation of *E. histolytica* (Chapter 361). The abscess is usually solitary and in 80% of patients is located in the right lobe of the liver. Typically, abrupt onset of pain in the right upper quadrant of the abdomen and fever occur. Pain may be referred to the scapula or shoulder and is exacerbated by pressure or coughing; 50% of patients have a cough. On physical examination the liver is enlarged and tender; some patients are jaundiced. There is often respiratory splinting on the right side and dullness to percussion and decreased breath sounds at the base of the right-side lung field. A pleural or hepatic friction rub may be present. Abscesses in the left lobe of the liver produce epigastric or left shoulder pain. Some patients may have fever as the major symptom or may have a chronic course with anorexia and weight loss. Jaundice is present in about one third of patients. Patients usually have a neutrophilic leukocytosis; normochromic, normocytic anemia; and abnormal liver function test results. Amebiasis does not cause eosinophilia. Chest radiographs often show elevation of the right diaphragm, and a small, reactive pleural effusion may be seen if the abscess is superficial and near the diaphragm.

Complications of amebic liver abscesses include rupture and secondary bacterial invasion. Rupture from the right lobe of the liver may produce peritonitis or empyema. Amebae in the pleural space usually burrow into the bronchi, and trophozoites may be seen in the sputum. Abscesses in the left lobe of the liver may rupture into the pericardium and produce fulminant pericarditis or pericardial tamponade. Bacterial superinfection of an amebic abscess occurs in fewer than 5% of patients and is usually evident in rigors, spiking fever, positive blood cultures, and failure to respond to antiamebic chemotherapy.

Rarely, *E. histolytica* spreads hematogenously to the brain. Brain abscesses are usually solitary and in the cerebral cortex. Symptoms include fever, headache, and altered mental status. More than 90% of patients also have amebic liver abscesses. The course is rapidly progressive. Most of these cases have been diagnosed on postmortem examination.

Diagnosis

Amebiasis should be considered in the differential diagnosis of any patient with colonic disease, especially if there is chronic diarrhea with blood or blood-streaked mucus in the stool (Chapter 242). Compared with bacillary dysentery produced by *Shigella* or *Campylobacter* organisms, intestinal amebiasis has a more gradual onset and rarely produces vomiting, chills, or high fever (unless fulminant), and the stool contains few leukocytes. *Salmonella* enteritis is also more likely to cause fever and fecal leukocytes. Viral gastroenteritis tends to occur in seasonal epidemics and produces extraintestinal symptoms (e.g., coryza, myalgia, fever, headache). The distinction between inflammatory bowel disease (ulcerative colitis, regional enteritis) and amebic colitis may be difficult on clinical grounds. All patients in whom the diagnosis of inflammatory bowel disease is considered should have stool examined for *E. histolytica,* and a serologic test for amebiasis should be performed. Patients from endemic areas may have colonic disease of another origin, despite the presence of *E. histolytica* in the stool.

The diagnosis of amebiasis can be made in two ways: (1) by identification of trophozoites or cysts in feces or exudates and (2) by a positive serologic test result in a patient with clinical manifestations of invasive amebiasis. Intestinal amebiasis must usually be diagnosed by stool examination or by examination of aspirates obtained during sigmoidoscopy. Serologic test results are usually negative with mild intestinal disease but may be positive in patients with invasive amebiasis. The appearance of organisms in the stool follows a cyclic pattern, and the diagnostic yield is increased by examining multiple stool samples over several days. Examination of three stool samples yields the diagnosis in approximately 85% of infected individuals. Examination of a single stool sample may yield the diagnosis in only 40%. Amebae are more likely to be found in blood-tinged mucus than in fecal matter. A direct smear, examined while the stool sample is still warm, may reveal motile trophozoites. A direct smear should also be fixed and stained with iron hematoxylin or trichrome, and a concentrate (zinc-sulfate or formalin-ether) should be made (Color Plate VIII 52). The combination of these three procedures on three stool specimens gives the most accurate results. *E. histolytica* can also be identified on histologic examination in colonic mucosa. Biopsy specimens should be taken from the edge of an ulcer. False-negative results of stool examinations may occur if the microscopist is inexperienced or if interfering substances are present. Interfering substances include antibiotics, mineral oil, magnesium hydroxide, bismuth, kaolin, and barium. Tap water, saline, or soapsuds enemas may also interfere with diagnosis. False-positive results may occur if fecal leukocytes are misidentified as *E. histolytica.*

Diagnosis of extraintestinal amebiasis usually requires the combination of a compatible clinical syndrome and a positive serologic test result. Liver abscess is usually detected by radioisotope liver scanning, ultrasonography, or CT. A gallium scan may be of value in differentiating amebic liver abscess from pyogenic liver abscess. Fewer than 20% of patients with extraintestinal amebiasis have organisms in the stool. Various serologic tests are available, most frequently agar gel diffusion-precipitation or counterimmunoelectrophoresis. Results of these tests are positive only if invasive disease is present. Ninety-five percent of patients with liver abscess have positive serologic test results, and 80% to 90% of patients with severe intestinal tract disease have positive tests. Gel diffusion-precipitation and counterimmunoelectrophoresis results become negative several months after cure of the liver abscess; therefore these tests are useful in the assessment of treatment and the diagnosis of reinfection. Indirect hemagglutination is more sensitive, but the test result remains positive for years and is therefore more useful in patients from nonendemic areas.

Treatment and Prevention

The drugs that are effective in amebiasis can be classified according to their site of action. Those which act primarily in the lumen of the bowel include iodoquinol, diloxanide furoate, tetracycline, and paromomycin. Metronidazole is active both within the lumen of the bowel and in tissues. The choice of a drug or drugs should be based on the clinical setting and the potential toxic effects of the drugs. Table 279-6 presents treatment recommendations for patients with asymptomatic infection, mild intestinal tract disease, severe intestinal tract disease, and hepatic abscess.

Mild disease is defined as loose stool or diarrhea without blood and in the developed world is generally associated with nonpathogenic isolates *(E. dispar).* However, specific laboratory tests are not yet available to differentiate pathogenic and nonpathogenic isolates, so mild disease should be treated as potentially invasive. Severe disease means that there is evidence of tissue invasion (e.g., bloody stool or positive serologic finding). The regimen of metronidazole plus iodoquinol has proved effective in more than 90% of patients with intestinal tract disease. Occasional patients with extraintestinal amebia-

Table 279-6 Treatment of patients with amebiasis

CLINICAL SETTING	RECOMMENDED TREATMENT
Asymptomatic (cysts in stool)	Paromomycin, 10 mg/kg tid for 7 days, or iodoquinol, 650 mg tid for 20 days
Mild intestinal tract disease (no evidence of invasion)	Metronidazole, 750 mg PO tid for 7 days, followed by iodoquinol, 650 mg tid for 20 days, or paromomycin, 10 mg/kg tid for 7 days
Severe intestinal tract disease (evidence of invasion)	Metronidazole, 750 mg tid for 7 days (IV or PO), followed by iodoquinol, 650 mg tid for 20 days, or paromomycin, 10 mg/kg tid for 7 days; alternative regimen: dehydroemetine, 1 mg/kg IM daily for 10 days, followed by tetracycline, 500 mg four times a day for 10 days, plus iodoquinol, 650 mg tid for 20 days
Liver abscess	Metronidazole, 750 mg tid for 7 days (IV or PO), plus iodoquinol, 650 mg tid for 20 days; alternative regimen: dehydroemetine, 1 mg/kg IM daily for 10 days, followed by chloroquine phosphate, 1000 mg daily for 2 days then 500 mg daily for 21 days, plus iodoquinol, 650 mg tid for 20 days

PO, Orally; *IV,* intravenously; *IM,* intramuscularly; *tid,* three times a day.

sis have not responded to metronidazole for unknown reasons. However, they have usually responded to subsequent treatment with chloroquine or dehydroemetine. The vast majority of patients with amebic liver abscess respond to metronidazole therapy alone. Therapeutic needle aspiration of amebic liver abscesses is controversial. No data from controlled studies suggest that this procedure accelerates healing. However, some experienced clinicians recommend aspiration if concern exists about an impending rupture.

After treatment of intestinal tract disease, follow-up stool examinations should be performed at 1 month and at 6 months to ensure eradication. For patients with liver abscess a follow-up liver scan should be performed 2 to 4 months after treatment, when most lesions should have resolved. Occasionally, however, adequately treated liver abscesses may not resolve on radiograph examination for 12 months. Metronidazole is usually tolerated well but may cause nausea and abdominal fullness. Alcohol should be avoided because a disulfiram-like reaction may occur. Metronidazole is carcinogenic in rodents and mutagenic in bacteria; however, women inadvertently given treatment with metronidazole for trichomoniasis during pregnancy have not been shown to have adverse fetal effects. Thus pregnant women with severe disease should be given treatment with metronidazole because the risks to the fetus and mother from untreated severe disease are great. Iodoquinol has been associated with subacute myelooptic neuropathy in Japan. It may interfere with thyroid function tests for months following use.

The treatment of patients with amebiasis does little to interrupt transmission of infection, since reinfection can occur and most carriers are asymptomatic. In nonendemic areas it is useful to evaluate the household and sexual contacts of patients by performing three stool examinations. However, homosexual men with multiple sexual partners are likely to become reinfected. Prevention in endemic areas is difficult. Travelers may protect themselves by drinking only boiled or iodinated water. Fruits and vegetables must be washed with a strong detergent and rinsed with a dilute acid (e.g., vinegar) to eradicate infectious cysts.

INFECTIONS CAUSED BY FREE-LIVING AMEBAE (*NAEGLERIA* AND *ACANTHAMOEBA* SPECIES)

In contrast to the other protozoans that infect humans, the free-living amebae are not obligatory parasites; that is, they are able to survive and multiply in the environment in the absence of a host animal. Free-living amoebae cause three syndromes in humans: primary amoebic encephalitis, granulomatous amoebic encephalitis, and chronic acanthamoeba keratitis. Infection with the free-living ameba *Naegleria fowleri* causes an acute, primary meningoencephalitis that closely resembles bacterial meningitis on clinical examination, usually in persons who are immunologically normal. Several species of *Acanthamoeba* can also cause an acute primary meningoencephalitis, but subacute or chronic granulomatous disease, resembling a bacterial brain abscess, is more common. *Acanthamoeba* infection is more likely to occur in individuals who are immunosuppressed or debilitated, including persons with AIDS or diabetes, but otherwise healthy individuals may also be infected. Disseminated cutaneous acanthamobiasis without central system involvement occurs in some AIDS patients and may mimic cutaneous fungal disease. *E. histolytica* may also cause amebic meningoencephalitis, but only after secondary spread from other foci of disease, such as liver abscess or pulmonary disease. Some species of *Acanthamoeba* are also responsible for corneal ulceration.

Free-living amebae exist as trophozoites or cysts in fresh water or soil. Human infection usually occurs when there is contact with fresh water in aquariums, hydrotherapy pools, freshwater springs, lakes, ponds, or swimming pools.

Naegleria species invade the CNS by penetrating the nasal mucosa of the cribriform plate and then spreading through the fila olfactoria. *Acanthamoeba* species usually invade the CNS hematogenously after primary infection of the eye, skin, lung, prostate, or uterus. *Naegleria* organisms multiply rapidly and produce hemorrhagic necrosis of the gray matter of the cerebral cortex and then of the white matter and cerebellum. The subarachnoid space is also invaded. Most patients have a neutrophilic pleocytosis, and organisms can be identified in CSF. Some patients also have an inflammatory myocarditis, but *Naegleria* organisms are not usually identified in the myocardium.

Acanthamoeba infection may produce a pathologic and clinical picture identical to that of *Naegleria* infection or, more frequently, a chronic encephalitis with multiple brain abscesses. Whereas the cellular response to *Naegleria* infection involves primarily polymorphonuclear leukocytes, the response to *Acanthamoeba* infection usually involves lymphocytes, monocytes, and plasma cells. Invasion of the subarachnoid space occurs less frequently with *Acanthamoeba* infection, and organisms are rarely found in CSF.

The incubation period of acute amebic meningoencephalitis is 5 to 7 days. There is usually sudden onset of severe headache, fever, and meningismus. The diagnosis of *Naegleria* infection may be suggested by abnormal sensations of taste and smell because of olfactory involvement and by the presence of myocarditis. Examination of the CSF in acute disease usually reveals a high white blood cell count with a predominance of neutrophils. The concentration of glucose is usually low. Amebae may be identified in the CSF as highly motile trophozoites.

Subacute or chronic disease caused by *Acanthamoeba* organisms usually has a gradual onset. Headache, seizures, and focal findings on neurologic examination are common. MRI or CT scan of the brain may reveal multiple lesions, particularly in the white matter of the deep midline and midbrain structures. Examination of the CSF reveals an elevated white blood cell count with predominance of mononuclear cells but no organisms. The glucose level is usually normal.

The diagnosis of acute amebic meningoencephalitis is made by identifying trophozoites in the CSF in a patient with a history of exposure to fresh water (usually swimming or diving in a lake or pond). Active mononuclear white blood cells may be mistaken for amoebae, but amoebae may be distinguished by their progressive movement through extension of pseudopods. The diagnosis of chronic disease is more difficult. Brain biopsy usually reveals trophozoites and cysts. Several serologic tests are available. They may be helpful in patients with a compatible history and CSF abnormalities but with lesions not readily accessible for biopsy.

Most cases of amebic meningoencephalitis are fatal. Successful treatment of *N. fowleri* has followed early diagnosis accompanied by high-dosage amphotericin B (1 mg/kg per day). Intrathecal amphotericin B is recommended by some authorities. Miconazole and rifampin may also be active against the organism. There have been few survivors of cerebral disease caused by *Acanthamoeba* organisms. In vitro data suggest that polymyxin B and flucytosine may be useful and that they may act synergistically if given together. Pentamidine and ketoconazole have also been reported to possess in vitro activity.

Corneal ulcerations caused by *Acanthamoeba* organisms were originally thought to be associated with trauma to the cornea, but further evaluation of the marked increase in cases in the 1970s indicates that 85% are associated with the wearing of contact lenses without or without antecedent trauma. Acanthoamoeba keratitis is strongly linked to homemade saline solutions and the use of tap water for rinsing of contact lenses. Symptoms usually begin as a foreign-body sensation, followed by pain, photophobia, conjunctivitis, and blurred vision. Spontaneous remissions and relapses may occur as part of the natural history of the disease. The ulcers are shaggy, have an irregular border, and may resemble herpes. Other findings include iritis, a corneal ring infiltrate, cataracts, and breakdown of the corneal epithelium. Complete destruction of the cornea may occur. Diagnosis is made by histologic examination (10% potassium chloride [KOH] wetmount, calcifluor-stained smears) and culture of corneal scrapings. Treatment of corneal disease has been more successful than treatment of cerebral disease. The cornea should be surgically debrided and treated topically for 3 to 4 weeks with 1% miconazole nitrate, 0.1% propamidine isethionate, and neosporin. Frequent application of propamidine isethionate (every 15 to 60 minutes for the first 3 days) has been recommended.

GIARDIASIS

Giardiasis is caused by the luminal flagellate *Giardia lamblia*, which is the most common human protozoan enteropathogen throughout the world. Infection is frequently asymptomatic but may cause endemic or epidemic diarrhea. In children chronic infection may be associated with growth retardation. Effective treatment is available.

Biology and Life Cycle

The organism has two stages, trophozoite and cyst. Infection is acquired by the ingestion of as few as 10 cysts, which may be present in feces or contaminated water or food. Cysts rupture in the stomach and release trophozoites, which use their flagella to migrate to the duodenum and jejunum and attach to the brush border of intestinal epithelial cells. The parasite does not invade cells. No virulence factors have yet been identified, and the mechanism responsible for diarrhea is unknown. To complete the life cycle, cysts are produced in the lumen of the intestine and excreted in the feces. Cysts may survive in cold water for several months. There may be animal reservoirs of giardiasis. Cysts from beavers are infectious for humans.

Epidemiology

G. lamblia has a worldwide distribution. Prevalence rates in the developing world may be as high as 20% to 30%. *Giardia* organisms are a common pathogen in travelers and in epidemics of water-borne infectious diarrhea in the United States. Hikers may be infected by cysts in mountain streams. Person-to-person and food-borne transmission also occur. Epidemics have occurred in day-care centers and in custodial institutions. Some urban populations of homosexual men have a high prevalence of infection (20% or more) that is probably maintained by sexual transmission.

Pathogenesis and Immunity

The clinical consequences of infection are probably produced by heavy colonization of intestinal epithelium, disruption of the brush border, and interference with the bowel's absorptive capacity. Disaccharidase deficiencies, especially of lactase, occur. The parasite is not known to produce any toxins.

Repeated or prolonged exposure may produce a degree of protection, since residents of endemic areas seem to have a lower incidence of disease than nonimmune visitors. Hypogammaglobulinemia may predispose patients to more severe disease.

Clinical Manifestations

Infection with *G. lamblia* may be asymptomatic or may cause a spectrum of manifestations, from acute, self-limited diarrhea to chronic diarrhea with malabsorption and weight loss (Chapter 242). Epigastric cramping, anorexia, nausea, flatulence, and vomiting also occur.

Table 279-7   Treatment of patients with giardiasis

CLINICAL SETTING	RECOMMENDED TREATMENT
Immunocompetent or immuno- compromised patients	Metronidazole, 250 mg tid for 5 to 7 days
Pregnant women	Paromomycin, 10 mg/kg tid for 7 days

tid, Three times a day.

The acute illness usually lasts 3 to 4 days, but patients may have mild symptoms of epigastric fullness, flatulence, and loose stools for several weeks. Infection probably resolves spontaneously in many patients. Patients with chronic infection may have intermittent bouts of diarrhea and malaise or severe, persistent diarrhea with steatorrhea. Extraintestinal tract disease does not occur.

Few laboratory abnormalities are found. Blood cell counts, differential white blood cell count, and erythrocyte sedimentation rate are normal. Mild anemia may be present, more frequently in children than adults. Giardiasis does not cause fecal leukocytes, and usually no blood is seen in the stool. An upper gastrointestinal tract series may show mild dilation, reduced transit time, and thickening of mucosal folds. Patients with hypogammaglobulinemia and giardiasis may have small-bowel lymphoid nodules.

Diagnosis

Giardiasis should be suspected in all patients with diarrhea lasting more than a few days, especially if no fever and no fecal leukocytes are present. The diagnosis should also be considered in patients with malabsorption, especially if the patient is immunodeficient. The diagnosis can often be made by stool examination (Color Plate VIII-53). The yield is increased by examination of three stool samples in three forms (fresh wet mount for motile trophozoites, stained smear, and zinc-sulfate concentration on each stool sample).

As with *E. histolytica,* false-negative results may occur in the presence of interfering substances such as barium, antibiotics, or antidiarrheal compounds (kaolin, bismuth). If stool examination results are negative, the diagnosis may be made using commercial kits for detecting *G. lamblia* antigen in stools, a sensitive and specific method for diagnosis of giardiasis. The stool antigen test may ultimately replace other invasive tests, such as examination of duodenal material obtained by aspiration, string test (Enterotest, Hedeco, Palo Alto, Calif.), or biopsy. If biopsy is performed, specimens should be stained with Giemsa.

Serologic tests are available on a research basis.

Treatment and Prevention

Metronidazole has become the drug of choice in the United States at 250 mg PO four times a day for 5 days. Quinacrine (100 mg orally three times daily for 5 to 7 days) is an alternative drug, but its use is limited by nausea, vomiting, and mild diarrhea. Exfoliative dermatitis and delirium have occurred rarely. Paromomycin is less effective but is not systemically absorbed and may be used safely in pregnancy. Recommendations for treatment are given in Table 279-7.

The most important factor in preventing giardiasis is the proper treatment of water. Routine chlorination may not kill cysts; sedimentation, flocculation, and filtration should also be performed. Hikers can prevent giardiasis by boiling water for at least 1 minute or by adding halazone (5 tablets/L for 30 minutes) or iodine. Travelers to areas with contaminated water should drink only boiled or treated water and should not consume uncooked fruit or vegetables. Household and sexual contacts of infected individuals should have three stool examinations.

LEISHMANIASIS

Leishmaniasis is a general term for human disease caused by species of the genus *Leishmania.* Most human infections with *Leishmania* species are transmitted by sand flies from mammalian zoonotic reservoirs. Leishmaniasis usually takes one of three clinical forms: cu-

taneous, mucocutaneous, or visceral (kala-azar). The form is determined principally by the species of parasite, although the host's immune status and genetic background may also affect clinical manifestations. The taxonomy of the *Leishmania* organism is unsettled and is changing because new criteria are being proposed for the identification of species and subspecies. The classification of species in this chapter is based on clinical manifestations and epidemiology. *L. tropica* causes cutaneous disease in the Old World, *L. mexicana* and some subspecies of *L. braziliensis* cause cutaneous disease in the New World, other subspecies of *L. braziliensis* cause mucocutaneous disease, and *L. donovani* causes visceral leishmaniasis. Molecular research on *Leishmania* parasites promises to yield new approaches to taxonomy, diagnosis, and treatment.

Leishmaniasis is transmitted rarely in the southwestern United States, but most cases seen in the United States occur in travelers, immigrants, and refugees. The incubation period for mucocutaneous leishmaniasis may be months or years; therefore physicians must have a high degree of suspicion and inquire about travel over preceding years if the diagnosis is to be made. Diagnosis is made by identifying organisms in Giemsa-stained impression smears or biopsy specimens or by isolating the organism from infected tissues. A delayed hypersensitivity skin test and serologic tests may be helpful in some patients, and DNA hybridization probes have been developed. Effective chemotherapy is available for most clinical forms of leishmaniasis, but the drugs are toxic and they are often difficult to administer in less developed countries.

Biology and Life Cycle

Leishmania organisms have two forms: flagellated extracellular promastigotes in the sand fly vector and unflagellated intracellular amastigotes in mammalian hosts. All species of *Leishmania* are morphologically indistinguishable. The parasites multiply by asexual binary fission, and there is no sexual stage. *Leishmania* (and *Trypanosoma*) organisms have a DNA-containing organelle called the *kinetoplast* that stains intensely with Giemsa stain.

Leishmaniasis is transmitted to humans by the bite of infected female *Phlebotomus* sand flies or, rarely, by direct contact with infected cutaneous lesions. Promastigotes in the fly's proboscis are injected subcutaneously, where they bind to the surface of local tissue macrophages and are engulfed by phagocytosis. Recent studies indicate that the binding of promastigotes to macrophages is mediated by an intriguing example of molecular mimicry in which the promastigote becomes coated with the third component of complement, which then mediates binding of the promastigote to the C3 receptor on the macrophage. Once intracellular, the organisms transform into amastigotes, which multiply within phagolysosomes (Color Plate VIII-12). The biochemical basis for the parasite's ability to survive in the presence of lysosomal enzymes is unknown. After local proliferation at the site of inoculation, the organisms may remain localized or may metastasize to nasal mucous membranes or to the reticuloendothelial system, depending on the species of parasite. *L. tropica* and *L. mexicana* remain localized in the original site, the nearby skin, and the draining lymph nodes. *L. braziliensis* may metastasize to mucous membranes, but not to the viscera. *L. donovani* may spread through the blood to the reticuloendothelial system of multiple organs.

Sand flies that feed on infected humans or other mammals ingest dermal macrophages containing amastigotes. In the fly's gut the amastigotes exit from the macrophages and transform into flagellated promastigotes. The promastigotes multiply, migrate to the proboscis, and are injected into a human or an animal at the fly's next feeding.

Epidemiology

Leishmaniasis is primarily a disease of the tropics and subtropics because sand flies require a habitat with high humidity and high temperature. The incidence of cutaneous leishmaniasis has been estimated to be 1.0 to 1.5 million cases per year and of visceral disease, to be 500,000 cases per year. Sand flies breed in cracks of building walls, in rodent burrows, in piles of rubbish, and in shaded vegetation. With the exception of *L. donovani* in India, the disease is a zoonosis. The sand flies feed on human and animal blood, and dogs, rats, gerbils, and a variety of other mammals form a reservoir for human infec-

Table 279-8   Leishmaniasis: summary of epidemiologic and clinical features and treatment

SPECIES	GEOGRAPHIC LOCATION	RESERVOIR	CLINICAL FEATURES	TREATMENT
L. tropica				
L. tropica major	Desert areas of Central Asia, North Africa, Middle East	Desert rodents	Cutaneous: Acute, wet, ulcerated lesions on extremities	Pentostam,* 20 mg/kg/day IV or IM for 20 days; repeated courses may be needed; alternative drugs: amphotericin B, ketoconazole, or pentamidine
L. tropica minor	Urban areas of Middle East, Mediterranean littoral areas, India, Pakistan, Africa	Dogs	Cutaneous: Chronic, dry lesion that rarely ulcerates	Pentostam as for *L. tropica major*
L. mexicana	Yucatan peninsula, Belize, Guatemala, Venezuela, Dominican Republic, southern United States (rare)	Forest rodents	Cutaneous: Chiclero ulcer; single or limited number of skin lesions; may cause diffuse cutaneous leishmaniasis or, rarely, mucocutaneous leishmaniasis	Pentostam as for *L. tropica major;* most cases resolve spontaneously; if needed, Pentostam or amphotericin B in various doses for various lengths of time
L. braziliensis	Panama, Costa Rica, South America, including Brazil, Venezuela, Bolivia, Peru, northern Argentina	Forest rodents and dogs	Cutaneous and mucocutaneous (especially Brazil)	Pentostam as for *L. tropica major.* Addition of allopurinol, 20 mg/kg/day in four divided doses for 15 days increased cure rates compared with Pentostam alone. Allopurinol alone at the same dose was also effective.
L. donovani	Mediterranean littoral areas, Middle East, India, Pakistan, China, South and Central America *(L. chagasi),* Asia, Africa	Dogs, foxes, rodents; no animal reservoir in India	Visceral leishmaniasis	Pentostam as for *L. tropica major*

*Dosage of Pentostam is calculated as milligrams of antimony per kilogram. In the United States, Pentostam is available from the Drug Service of the Centers for Disease Control and Prevention (telephone: (404) 639-3670 or (404) 639-2888).
IV, Intravenously; *IM,* intramuscularly.

tion. In India, *L. donovani* is transmitted from person to person by anthrophilic (human-biting) sand flies. The geographic locations of disease and the local animal reservoirs are listed in Table 279-8. The epidemiology of mucocutaneous leishmaniasis is of practical importance, since the risk of subsequent mucous membrane involvement is affected by the locale where the primary infection occurred.

Pathogenesis and Immunity

The specific consequences of infection with *Leishmania* are determined by the tissue tropism of different species and by the host's immune response. The species that cause cutaneous or mucocutaneous disease may be limited in spread by temperature. With *L. tropica* and *L. mexicana,* amastigotes proliferate within macrophages at the site of the sand fly bite. An initial granulomatous reaction produces a papule that eventually breaks down and ulcerates. Cutaneous disease is usually self-limited and heals without chemotherapy. Antibody to leishmanial antigens is difficult to detect in patients with cutaneous disease and probably has little role in healing. Recovery depends on the development of cell-mediated immunity, which stops the intracellular multiplication of amastigotes and is evident on histologic examination as a lymphocytic infiltrate at the lesion. A delayed hypersensitivity skin test result (Montenegro test) is positive. Healing leaves a flat, atrophic scar and results in resistance to reinfection with the homologous parasite species. Some patients have an exuberant granulomatous reaction that produces persistent nodules at the edge of the primary lesion (leishmaniasis recidivans). In the absence of cell-mediated immunity, no lymphocytic infiltrate occurs, and parasites proliferate in the skin, producing diffuse cutaneous leishmaniasis. It is not known whether immunosuppression is caused by a parasite product or by an abnormality of the host immune system.

With some subspecies of *L. braziliensis,* lesions develop in the cartilage and mucous membranes of the nose months to years after the primary skin lesion has healed. Although patients usually have intact cell-mediated immune responses to leishmanial antigens, the

lesions progress and may be very destructive. Spontaneous recovery has not been reported.

L. donovani does not remain limited to the skin but disseminates and multiplies within the macrophages of the spleen, liver, bone marrow, and lymph nodes. Cell-mediated immune responses to leishmanial antigens are depressed, but high levels of antileishmanial antibodies can usually be detected. Cell-mediated immune responses develop after successful treatment, and patients who recover are usually immune to reinfection. It is postulated that suppressor cells or circulating immune complexes may have a role in the immunosuppression observed with visceral disease. Massive splenomegaly occurs frequently and is accompanied by sequestration of erythrocytes, leukocytes, and platelets in the spleen, leading to pancytopenia, which is compounded by decreased production by the infiltrated bone marrow. A polyclonal activation of B cells and hypergammaglobulinemia occur. Circulating immune complexes and rheumatoid factor can usually be detected, but their role in pathogenesis is not known. Many patients have a subclinical immune complex glomerulonephritis. After successful treatment, in some patients disseminated skin lesions develop that contain *L. donovani* (post–kala-azar dermal leishmaniasis).

Because of the protean manifestations of different leishmanial parasites in different hosts, the *Leishmania* organism has emerged as a model parasite for the study of cell-mediated immunity to intracellular organisms.

Clinical Manifestations

Infections with *Leishmania* can be acquired from a single sand fly bite, so only brief residence in an endemic area is needed. In addition, infection can be acquired by direct contact with infected skin lesions or, rarely, by blood transfusion. The incubation period for leishmaniasis varies from a few weeks to several years, but with *L. tropica* and *L. mexicana* it is usually 2 weeks to 3 months and with *L. donovani,* 3 to 8 months. *L. braziliensis* usually has an incubation period of 2 to 8 weeks for the cutaneous lesions. The time between the primary skin lesion and mucous membrane involvement is usually several years, although it may be as short as 1 month and as long as 25 years.

Cutaneous leishmaniasis may have some variation in clinical manifestations, depending on the parasite species and the geographic location where infection was acquired (Table 279-8). Typically there is, first, a papule, which enlarges, becomes crusted, and then (in *L. tropica major, L. mexicana,* and *L. braziliensis*) ulcerates. Ulcers have a diameter of about 2 cm and an indurated border. Satellite lesions may be adjacent to the primary skin lesion and along the draining lymphatics. Regional lymphadenopathy is common. Patients usually have no fever, and the lesions are painless unless secondarily infected by bacteria. Healing leaves a flat or depressed depigmented scar. Cutaneous lesions associated with particular geographic areas include chronic, dry, scaly solitary nodules on the face in *L. tropica minor* acquired in urban settings; acute, wet, ulcerated lesions on the extremities with *L. tropica major* acquired in rural locales; ulceration of the pinna of the ear (chiclero ulcer) with *L. mexicana* acquired by workers harvesting gum from chicle plants in Mexico, Belize, and Guatemala; hyperkeratotic or papillomatous lesions similar to yaws in Guyana, Surinam, and northern Brazil (forest yaws); and nodular lesions occurring in individuals residing in the Peruvian highlands (uta).

Diffuse cutaneous leishmaniasis has been observed in Ethiopia, Venezuela, Brazil, and the Dominican Republic. The lesions are widespread and typically remain as macules or papules without ulceration. The mucous membranes may be involved, but not the viscera. Lesions contain sparse lymphocytes, and there is cutaneous anergy to leishmanial antigens.

Mucocutaneous leishmaniasis (espundia) is caused by subspecies of *L. braziliensis* and is especially prevalent in Brazil south of the Amazon. In patients with cutaneous lesions the likelihood of subsequent mucous membrane involvement is about 80% if the infection was acquired in Brazil, 5% if acquired in Panama or Guyana, and less than 1% if acquired in Mexico. More than 90% of patients with espundia have scars of previous cutaneous involvement. Nasal lesions tend to destroy the cartilage of the septum and spread to the buccal mucosa, pharynx, and larynx. Isolated laryngeal involvement may occur. The initial manifestation of nasal involvement is usually nasal stuffiness. The disease is not self-limited and may progress to severe facial deformities. Complications include CSF leaks, meningitis, and cavernous sinus thrombosis.

Visceral leishmaniasis has similar clinical manifestations wherever it occurs. The onset of disease may be gradual or acute. There is usually fever, malaise, anorexia, cough, and weight loss. The liver and spleen are greatly enlarged, and some patients have diffuse lymphadenopathy. Pancytopenia resulting from hypersplenism and marrow infiltration is the most lethal complication of the disease. Light-skinned patients may be seen to develop a grayish discoloration of the skin, which led to the Indian name for the disease, *kala-azar,* which means "black fever." Death is usually caused by intercurrent bacterial infection, bleeding, or severe anemia. About 20% of Indian patients and 3% of African patients develop disseminated cutaneous lesions after treatment for visceral disease. The skin lesions may be nodular or flat and depigmented.

Diagnosis

A history of travel to or residence in an endemic area should lead to consideration of leishmaniasis in patients with skin lesions, nasal or oropharyngeal disease, or hepatosplenomegaly and pancytopenia. Visceral leishmaniasis epodemics have been reported in the last 10 years from India, Bangladesh, the Sudan, and northeastern Brazil, and sporadic cases have been reported in immunocompromised persons and American military troops who participated in Desert Storm in the Middle East. Visceral leishmaniasis must be differentiated from malaria (especially the tropical splenomegaly syndrome), schistosomiasis, and lymphoma. Cutaneous leishmaniasis may be found in travelers or military personnel as well as endogenous peoples in Latin America or the Middle East. Cutaneous disease must be differentiated from leprosy, atypical mycobacterial infection *(Mycobacterium marinum),* blastomycosis, histoplasmosis, sporotrichosis, nocardiosis,

syphilis, and yaws. Mucosal disease is primarily a problem in Latin America, especially Brazil. The differential diagnosis of mucocutaneous disease includes leprosy, syphilis, Wegener's granulomatosis, midline granuloma, paracoccidioidomycosis, and nasopharyngeal carcinoma. The potential for long incubation periods, especially in mucocutaneous disease, must be remembered.

The diagnosis of leishmaniasis can be made by identifying amastigotes in Giemsa- or Wright-stained impression smears or biopsy specimens or by culture of promastigotes in Novy-MacNeal-Nicole (NNN) or Schneider's *Drosophila* medium. In cutaneous disease organisms are most abundant at the periphery of ulcerated lesions or in nodular lesions. In mucocutaneous disease organisms may be obtained from scrapings or biopsy from the nasal mucosa, but usually few organisms are seen. In visceral leishmaniasis, bone marrow examination and culture are positive in more than 50%. Fine-needle splenic aspiration for culture and touch preparation is the most sensitive method, yielding a diagnosis in 88% to 96% of cases. Patients with concurrent HIV disease may have amastigotes in bronchoalveolar lavage or biopsy specimens from the gastrointestinal tract. An antigen for skin testing is available from the World Health Organization Leishmaniasis Reference Center, Hadassah Medical Center, Jerusalem, Israel. Serologic tests for antileishmanial antibodies are performed at the Centers for Disease Control and Prevention. Neither the skin test nor the serologic test is well standardized. Patients with cutaneous and mucocutaneous disease have positive delayed hypersensitivity skin test results. Patients with disseminated cutaneous leishmaniasis and visceral disease are anergic on the skin test but have high levels of circulating antibodies to leishmanial antigens. Some patients with mucocutaneous disease have positive serologic test results.

Treatment and Prevention

The pentavalent antimonial drug sodium stibogluconate (Pentostam) is active against all species of *Leishmania* and is available from the Centers for Disease Control and Prevention (Table 279-8). The dose of Pentostam recommended for all clinical forms of leishmanial disease is 20 mg/kg per day for 20 days. The maximum daily dose should not exceed 850 mg of pentavalent antimony. If clinical response has not occurred, longer treatment may be given. These large doses of Pentostam generally require IV administration. Clinical experience suggests that Pentostam causes few side effects, which are principally weakness, anorexia, mild reversible liver function abnormalities, and transient abnormalities of the T wave on ECG testing. With longer periods of treatment, leukopenia and thrombocytopenia may occur.

Repeated courses of Pentostam are often required for cure of mucocutaneous and visceral leishmaniasis. Evidence indicates that cutaneous or visceral disease acquired in East Africa may be more resistant to treatment. Alternative drugs include amphotericin B and pentamidine isothionate. Scientists are attempting to develop new drugs based on metabolic differences between the parasite and the host. Results with purine analogs and ketoconazole are promising. Allopurinol alone or in combination with Pentostam was recently shown to be more effective than Pentostam alone in curing American cutaneous leishmaniasis. Recombinant interferon-γ plus Pentostam has been used to successfully treat visceral leishmaniais that failed Pentostam therapy alone and may be useful in diffuse cutaneous disease.

Leishmaniasis is difficult to prevent. Neither vaccine nor effective chemoprophylaxis is available. Control of animal reservoirs is difficult. The prospects for a vaccine appear to be good, since cutaneous infection produces lifelong species-specific immunity. Travelers can obtain partial protection by the use of insect repellents and netting.

AFRICAN TRYPANOSOMIASIS

African trypanosomiasis is a zoonotic disease that is caused by two subspecies of *Trypanosoma brucei: T. brucei gambiense* and *T. brucei rhodesiense,* which differ in clinical manifestations, epidemiology, and vector habitat. Infection is transmitted by members of the genus *Glossina* (tsetse flies). A third subspecies, *T. brucei brucei,* is not infectious for humans but causes disease in livestock and has an im-

Table 279-9 African trypanosomiasis: clinical and epidemiologic features

TRYPANOSOMA SUBSPECIES	GEOGRAPHIC LOCATION	ANIMAL RESERVOIRS	CLINICAL FEATURES
T. brucei gambiense	Forested areas of West and Central Africa south of the Sahara	Possibly pigs, dogs, hartebeest, sheep, cattle	Acute systemic illness followed by chronic meningoencephalitic illness
T. brucei rhodesiense	Groups of trees in savanna areas of East Africa from Ethiopia and Uganda to Zambia and Zimbabwe	Antelope, hogs, cattle, sheep, goats, dogs, hartebeest, lions, hyenas	Acute systemic illness with early invasion of the central nervous system and prominent myocarditis

portant economic impact in Africa. Scientists have recently made rapid progress in understanding the biochemistry and molecular genetics of *Trypanosoma* species, but so far with little impact on the disease. Drug treatment is toxic and often ineffective, immunoprophylaxis has been frustrated by the parasite's capacity for antigenic variation, and vector control is extremely expensive for governments in endemic areas.

Biology and Life Cycle

T. brucei gambiense and *T. brucei rhodesiense* are morphologically identical, and the two subspecies are differentiated on the basis of epidemiology, vector habitat, and disease manifestations (Table 279-9). They are flagellated, extracellular organisms that multiply in the blood, tissue spaces, and CSF of mammalian hosts. They are ingested by the tsetse fly vector during a blood meal. Within the fly's midgut they shed their protective surface coat and transform into procyclic trypanosomes, which multiply and migrate to the salivary glands. Salivary gland organisms (called *epimastigotes*) multiply, then transform into nondividing metacyclic trypanosomes, which acquire a surface coat and are injected into a mammalian host during a fly's next blood meal. In the mammalian host the parasites transform into slender, blood-stage forms that circulate in the blood and divide rapidly by binary fission. Some of the blood parasites develop into short, stumpy forms that are adapted for uptake by the tsetse fly.

Trypanosomes have a central nucleus and, as with *Leishmania,* a densely stained kinetoplast at the base of the flagellum. The surface coat of blood-stage forms is composed of a single glycoprotein, the *variable surface glycoprotein* (VSG). The genome of African trypanosomes contains a multiplicity of genes for VSGs of different antigenic structure. The gene that is to be expressed is duplicated and transposed to a different region of the chromosome in such a way that cells usually express only one VSG at a time. The dividing organism can displace the VSG gene that was expressed and replace it with a new gene so that a VSG of different antigenic type is expressed. This process of gene switching results in antigenic variation. As the host makes antibody to a VSG of one type, trypanosomes bearing a different VSG appear.

Epidemiology

About 25,000 new cases of the disease are reported annually, and around 50 million people are classed as at risk of contracting the disease. Transmission by tsetse fly is limited to sub-Saharan Africa. *T. brucei gambiense* occurs in West and Central Africa, *T. brucei rhodesiense* in East Africa (Table 279-9). Infection can also be transmitted mechanically by blood-sucking insects, by blood transfusion, and congenitally from mother to child around the time of delivery.

Pathogenesis and Immunity

At the site of the tsetse fly's bite a mononuclear cell infiltrate produces a nodule (trypanosomal chancre). A systemic phase begins weeks to months after the tsetse bite and is characterized by recurrent waves of parasitemia, each consisting of serologically distinct parasites produced by antigenic variation of the VSG. Parasites eventually invade the CNS and produce a chronic meningoencephalitis. On histologic examination, perivascular infiltration by lymphocytes, monocytes, and plasma cells occurs. The plasma cells may be responsible for the high levels of IgM that occur in CSF. With *T. brucei*

rhodesiense the systemic phase is usually fulminant. Cardiac involvement dominates the pathologic and clinical picture, and the pathologic changes in the CNS may not occur.

The mechanisms by which the extracellular organisms produce disease are unknown. Patients typically have very high levels of serum and CSF immunoglobulins caused by polyclonal B-cell activation. These immunoglobulins do not produce immunity, and it has been proposed that the proliferating B cells may infiltrate tissues and produce disease.

Clinical Manifestations

The clinical manifestations of African trypanosomiasis are determined by the subspecies of parasite and may be different in travelers and expatriates compared with residents of the parasite's endemic area. With both subspecies the trypanosomal chancre is the first manifestation of disease. The chancre is typically on an exposed part of the body; is hard, red, and painful; and usually lasts 1 to 2 weeks. The systemic phase of illness is characterized by fever with a relapsing pattern, severe headache, and lymphadenopathy. Episodes of fever last 1 to 6 days. Afebrile remissions may last for several weeks. Posterior cervical nodes are classically enlarged (Winterbottom's sign). A nonpruritic, erythematous, macular rash may develop on the trunk. With West African trypanosomiasis *(T. brucei gambiense)* neurologic manifestations include changes in personality early in the course of disease, progressing to lassitude, indifference, and an uncontrollable urge to sleep during the day. In some patients a frank psychosis may develop. Hypertonicity, cerebellar ataxia, and movement disorders (most often, chorea and athetosis) may occur. Patients eventually become comatose. Splenomegaly is usually present during the later stages of disease. Death is often caused by intercurrent bacterial infection.

With East African trypanosomiasis *(T. brucei rhodesiense)* the disease is more acute. Neurologic manifestations are less prominent, and myocarditis or pericarditis is more frequently the cause of death.

Laboratory examination usually shows anemia, monocytosis, and hypergammaglobulinemia. The level of CSF protein (especially IgM) is elevated, and a lymphocytic pleocytosis occurs. The CSF glucose level is normal. Large, vacuolated plasma cells are occasionally observed in the CSF.

Diagnosis

Physicians in the United States are most likely to see African trypanosomiasis in travelers, returning expatriates, immigrants, and refugees. The possibility of congenital transmission should be kept in mind; the mother may be relatively asymptomatic. A careful travel history is essential and should elicit the type of terrain as well as the countries visited to determine the probability of exposure to the vector. Most travelers remember the painful trypanosomal chancre, even if it is no longer present. East African trypanosomiasis should be considered in individuals in whom fever, headache, myocarditis, or lymphadenopathy develops within a month after returning from an endemic area. West African trypanosomiasis is more indolent and requires a high index of suspicion if the diagnosis is to be made. The differential diagnosis includes malaria, tick-borne or louse-borne relapsing fever, typhoid fever, lymphoma, and other causes of chronic meningitis, encephalitis, or myocarditis.

The diagnosis is made by identifying organisms in Giemsa-stained blood smears, CSF, or lymph node aspirate (Color Plate VIII-16). The level of parasitemia in the blood varies with relapses and remissions, and multiple blood samples should be examined. When the para-

Table 279-10   Treatment of patients with African trypanosomiasis

CLINICAL SETTING	TREATMENT
Early (hemolymphatic stage) without meningeal involvement	Suramin, 100 mg test dose IV, then 1 g IV on days 1, 3, 7, 14, and 21; alternative regimens: eflornithine,* 400 mg/kg/day IV in four divided doses for 14 days followed by 300 mg/kg/day PO for 4 weeks, or pentamidine isethionate,* 4 mg/kg IV or IM daily for 10-14 days
Late stage with central nervous system involvement	Melarsoprol,† 3.6 mg/kg/day IV for 3 days, repeated after 7-day rest period and again after 10- to 14-day rest period; alternative regimens for patients who cannot tolerate melarsoprol: eflornithine as above or a combination of tryparsamide, 30 mg/kg IV (maximum, 2 g) every 5 days to a total of 12 injections, plus suramin, 10 mg/kg IV every 5 days to a total of 12 injections (regimen may be repeated after 1 month)

*Treatment with eflornithine is more effective against *T. brucei gambiense* than against *T. brucei rhodesiense*. Pentamidine is effective *only* against *T. brucei gambiense*.

†Melarsoprol is a highly toxic arsenical drug that frequently causes a reactive encephalopathy. It is available in the United States from the Drug Service of the Centers for Disease Control and Prevention (telephone: 404-639-3670 or 404-639-2888). The addition of corticosteroids to melarsoprol may prevent or reduce the symptoms of arsenical encephalopathy.

IV, Intravenously; *IM*, intramuscularly; *PO*, orally.

sitemia level is high, organisms may be observed on thick blood smears, but when the parasitemia level is low, diagnosis requires concentration techniques, such as examination of buffy-coat smears or filtration of blood through an ion-exchange column. A large volume of CSF (5 to 10 ml) should be centrifuged and stained if CNS disease is suspected. DNA hybridization probes and the PCR are being investigated for use in diagnosis.

Treatment and Prevention

Chemotherapy of African trypanosomiasis requires prolonged administration of toxic drugs and is complicated by the emerging resistance of some strains. Suramin is used to treat blood-stage disease. A test dose of 100 mg is given IV, followed by 1 g on days 1, 3, 7, 14, and 21. Toxicities include proteinuria (frequent) and hypotension, fever, and desquamative dermatitis (infrequent). Suramin is not effective against parasites in the CNS. Alternative drugs include eflornithine or pentamidine (Table 279-10).

Disease of the CNS is treated with arsenical drugs (melarsoprol or tryparsamide) given IV (Table 279-10). Toxic effects of arsenical drugs include encephalitis, exfoliative dermatitis, and peripheral neuropathy. Encephalopathy is more common in patients with heavy parasite burdens at the time of treatment. Adjunctive therapy with corticosteroids has been reported to prevent or ameliorate the symptoms of encephalopathy associated with arsenical treatment. Although it has generally been recommended that melarsoprol be given only if CNS disease is present, some authorities believe that CNS invasion occurs early in the disease and therefore recommend that a drug active in the CNS be given to all patients. Pentamidine has been effective in some cases of West African trypanosomiasis, and eflornithine has also been used successfully in a few patients.

Prevention of African trypanosomiasis is difficult. The most widely used approaches are vector control and the prospective searching for and treatment of infected individuals. However, the presence of animal reservoirs and the underground location of the tsetse pupal stage complicate control measures. The prospects for a vaccine are poor. An urgent need exists for development of new drugs. Selective inhibition of trypanosomal glyceraldehyde-3-phosphate dehydrogenase by compounds derived through protein structure-based design are the beginning of a new class of drugs for the treatment of sleeping sickness but are not clinically available. Travelers can partially protect themselves with insecticides, repellents, and netting and by keeping arms and legs covered while in endemic areas.

CHAGAS' DISEASE (AMERICAN TRYPANOSOMIASIS)

Chagas' disease is caused by *Trypanosoma cruzi,* a zoonotic organism that is transmitted between mammals and humans by triatomid insects (reduviid bugs.) The disease typically has an acute phase which may be asymptomatic, followed years or decades later by a chronic phase, in which the heart and the gastrointestinal tract are affected. The available drugs have low efficacy or high toxicity. No immediate prospect exists for a vaccine. The recent influx of Central American immigrants into the United States may result in more cases of Chagas' disease.

Biology and Life Cycle

T. cruzi is transmitted to humans by insects of the genera *Triatoma, Rhodnius,* and *Panstrongylus.* The most effective vectors have adapted to human dwellings, where they live in thatched roofs and in the crevices between bricks and maintain a cycle between humans and domestic animals. Infectious metacyclic trypomastigotes are excreted in the insect's feces during or immediately after a blood meal, and the organisms invade through the damaged skin or through mucous membranes. Although triatomids in the United States are infected with *T. cruzi,* transmission to humans rarely occurs because the U.S. insects do not defecate during or after their blood meal. Infection can also be transmitted by blood transfusion and congenitally. Several accidental laboratory-acquired infections have occurred among investigators studying Chagas' disease.

After invasion the *T. cruzi* organisms attach to macrophages and are internalized by phagocytosis. Once intracellular, they transform into amastigotes (no flagellum), lyse the phagosome, and multiply within the cytoplasm (Color Plate VIII-17). Intracellularly, some amastigotes differentiate into trypomastigotes (flagellated), which are released into the blood and disseminate to all host tissues. Triatomids feeding on infected animals or humans ingest trypomastigotes, which in the bug's intestinal tract transform into epimastigotes and multiply by asexual division. Within approximately 2 weeks they transform into metacyclic forms, which are excreted in the bug's feces.

As with *T. brucei* and the *Leishmania* species, *T. cruzi* has a DNA-rich kinetoplast that stains densely with Giemsa. No evidence indicates antigenic variation, and the chronicity of infection appears to result from the organisms' adaptation to intracellular life and their ability to evade the immune system.

Epidemiology

Chagas' disease afflicts more than 24 million individuals in South and Central America, producing a debilitating, lifelong disease. It is the leading cause of heart failure in many Latin American countries. The distribution of the infection corresponds to areas where the triatomid insects live close to humans. Proximity to humans occurs frequently when rural areas are opened up for agricultural development and the habitat of the vector and the animal reservoir is disrupted. In Latin America Chagas' disease is primarily a problem of poor persons in rural areas. Acute infection usually occurs in children, and the cardiac and gastrointestinal tract manifestations of chronic disease usually occur between ages 35 and 45 years of age. Cardiac and gastrointestinal tract disease is common in Brazil, but gastrointestinal tract disease rarely occurs in Venezuela, Colombia, and Panama. Studies indicate that 2% to 5% of Central American immigrants may be infected with *T. cruzi* and are at risk for developing Chagas' disease or for transmitting the parasite by blood transfusion. Occasional transmission to humans of *T. cruzi* by triatomid insects occurs in the southwestern United States. Immigrants from Latin America constitute a reservoir for the organism.

Pathogenesis and Immunity

T. cruzi is not known to produce any toxins or cytotoxic factors; it is likely that many of the consequences of infection result from the host's immune response. Frequently a local inflammatory response occurs at the site of infection, producing a painful nodule (chagoma). Trypomastigotes can be detected in the blood during the acute stage of disease. With chronic Chagas' disease the heart is most often affected. There are foci of fibrosis, which may be small or large and dense. When fibrosis is extensive, the heart is enlarged, the ventricular wall is thinned, and the fibrotic plaques may serve as the nidus for thrombosis. Fibrosis of the conducting system also occurs. The esophagus and colon may be greatly dilated and have hypertrophy of smooth muscle. On histologic study, involved tissues contain a mononuclear cell infiltrate. In the heart, myocardial fibers degenerate and fibrosis occurs. The number of neurons in the myenteric plexus may be reduced, which may contribute to the muscular hypertrophy and dilation of the esophagus and colon. Organisms are usually not apparent in the tissues in chronic disease, although they may be isolated from the blood by xenodiagnosis (see later discussion).

NK cells and IL-12–mediated mechanism of resistance to *T. cruzi,* which depends on interferon-γ and TNF-α and NO, have been reported to be important in the development of immunity.

Clinical Manifestations

The incubation period between infection and the onset of disease is not known but is probably longer than 1 week. The initial manifestation is usually the *chagoma,* a painful, red nodule at the site of infection. Conjunctival inoculation produces unilateral conjunctivitis and edema of the eyelids (Romaña's sign). The acute, intravascular stage of infection is usually asymptomatic, but fever, lymphadenopathy, hepatosplenomegaly, meningoencephalitis, myocarditis, or an erythematous rash may occur, especially in children. Some young patients may die with acute congestive heart failure during this stage of the illness, but most recover in 2 to 3 months and enter the prolonged, indeterminant stage of infection.

With chronic infection patients may remain asymptomatic or disease may develop years or decades later. The most frequent and most serious manifestation is Chagas' cardiomyopathy (Chapter 26). Patients usually have palpitations and may have symptoms of heart failure. The most common abnormalities are electrocardiographic: right bundle branch block in more than 60% of patients, left anterior hemiblock, atrioventricular block, premature ventricular contractions, and T-wave abnormalities. Atrial arrhythmias occur but are less common. ECG changes mimicking acute myocardial infarction have been reported. Fibrotic involvement of the myocardium produces biventricular failure, but the heart is usually not enlarged until late in the course of the disease. When cardiac involvement is extensive, mural thrombi and emboli typically occur.

Megaesophagus causes dysphagia, regurgitation, odynophagia, chest pain, cough, and frequent pulmonary aspiration. Barium swallow examination shows a spectrum of abnormalities, from retention of barium in the lower esophagus without dilation to a bulky, elongated, atonic esophagus. Megacolon causes constipation that may be extraordinarily severe, chronic abdominal distention, and pain. In patients with advanced disease, barium enema examination may show dilation, but in the initial stages of disease no abnormalities may be seen on radiographic examination. Colonic obstruction and perforation may occur.

Diagnosis

The most important consideration in the diagnosis of Chagas' disease is a history of travel to or residence in an endemic area. Transmission of *T. cruzi* in the United States has been reported but is exceedingly rare. The rapid diagnosis of acute Chagas' disease is best accomplished by identifying organisms in the blood, either by direct microscopic examination for motile trypomastigotes in the buffy coat or by Giemsa-stained blood smears. Organisms can be cultured on NNN medium in 1 to 2 weeks. Blood can be fed to reduviid bugs in the laboratory, and the intestinal contents of the bugs examined later for parasites *(xenodiagnosis).* Xenodiagnosis is very sensitive but requires 30 days. An immunofluorescence test that detects IgM antibodies to *T. cruzi* is available, but serologic testing has limited usefulness in the diagnosis of acute Chagas' disease because seroconversion often requires 3 to 4 weeks.

Patients in the indeterminant stage of infection have antibodies to *T. cruzi,* and parasites can be isolated by xenodiagnosis. Chronic Chagas' disease is diagnosed by identifying antibodies to *T. cruzi* in the serum of a patient with compatible clinical manifestations. Organisms are sparse and are not usually identified in tissue or isolated except by xenodiagnosis. Several serologic tests are available for the detection of antibody. False-positive results may occur with serum from patients with leishmaniasis or syphilis.

Treatment and Prevention

Nitrofurtimox (Lampit) is the only drug available in the United States for the treatment of Chagas' disease and can be obtained from the Centers for Disease Control and Prevention (telephone: (404) 639-3670 or (404) 639-2888). The drug reduces the duration of parasitemia and clinical manifestations in acute Chagas' disease, prevents seroconversion, and may occasionally cure infection. It is not known, however, whether cure of infection prevents chronic disease. No evidence indicates that nitrofurtimox reverses the manifestations of chronic disease. Use of the drug in the indeterminant stage of infection is controversial. The recommended dose is 8 to 10 mg/kg per day in four divided doses for 90 to 120 days. Side effects include nausea, vomiting, peripheral neuropathy, dermatitis, leukopenia, and delirium. As many as 50% of patients may have to discontinue the drug before completing the course. The addition of interferon-γ to nifurtimox for 20 days in a limited number of patients appeared to shorten the acute phase of the disease. An alternative drug, benzimidazole, is widely used in South America, but it does not appear to offer advantages over nitrofurtimox. Scientists are attempting to identify and develop other drugs for the treatment of Chagas' disease. D0870, a *bis*-triazole derivative, was able to prevent death and induced parasitologic cure in 70% to 90% of animals, in both the short- and long-term Chagas' disease. If these results are achievable in humans, D0870 will be an important new drug. A cysteine proteinase, cruzain, has been crystallized for development of specific anti–Chagas' disease therapy.

The treatment of patients with chronic Chagas' disease is supportive. Pacemakers may prolong the lives of patients with cardiac disease and conduction disturbances, but those with congestive heart failure respond poorly to inotropic agents. Megaesophagus can be treated by pneumatic dilation of the cardia of the stomach. Megacolon may respond to laxatives or enemas, or, if severe, to resection of the rectosigmoid and descending colon.

Strategies to prevent Chagas' disease include vector control with insecticides and improved housing in rural areas. To prevent transmission by transfusion, seropositive donors should be excluded. If this is not feasible, gentian violet can be added to blood to inactivate the organism. Travelers should avoid sleeping in dwellings with thatched roofs or in dilapidated buildings.

BALANTIDIASIS

Balantidiasis is a colonic disease caused by infection with the ciliated protozoon *Balantidium coli.* The disease is a zoonosis that affects a variety of domestic animals, especially pigs. Human infection is unusual but may occur with close contact with infected animals in tropical regions, especially Central and South America, Papua New Guinea, the Philippines, and Iran.

Biology and Life Cycle

Infection is transmitted by the ingestion of cysts in feces or contaminated food or water. Cysts rupture in the small intestine, and trophozoites localize in the colon. Trophozoites multiply asexually by binary fission and sexually by conjugation. The trophozoites use their cilia to invade the mucosal epithelium and may penetrate to all layers of the bowel wall. Some trophozoites undergo excystation in the lumen of the colon and are excreted in the feces.

Pathogenesis and Immunity

Trophozoite invasion of the colonic mucosa produces ulcerated lesions, most often in the rectosigmoid colon. The organism may penetrate the entire colon wall and cause perforation. Despite the invasion of blood vessels in the wall of the colon, extraintestinal tract disease does not occur.

Clinical Manifestations

Most infections are asymptomatic. Symptoms are more common in undernourished individuals. Patients may have recurrent episodes of diarrhea, which may be watery or may contain mucus and blood. Sigmoidoscopy reveals mucosal ulcerations with diameters of 1 to 2 cm.

Diagnosis

The diagnosis of balantidiasis should be suspected in individuals with colitis and a history of exposure to swine or other wild or domestic animals. Organisms can be identified in stool or in scrapings from ulcerations obtained during sigmoidoscopy. *B. coli* is a large organism (up to 150 μm long) and may be mistaken for debris.

Treatment and Prevention

Untreated balantidiasis may be fatal in malnourished or immunocompromised individuals. Tetracycline (500 mg four times a day for 10 days) is effective in most cases. The combination of iodoquinol (650 mg three times a day for 20 days) plus metronidazole (750 mg three times a day for 5 days) is also effective. Prevention requires reducing the contact between humans and infected animals and avoiding the contamination of food and water.

BLASTOCYSTIS HOMINIS

Blastocystis hominis is considered by most authorities to be a protozoan organism that can infect the human gastrointestinal tract, but its ability to cause disease is uncertain. The mechanism of transmission is unknown. Although *B. hominis* is frequently identified in fecal samples, its pathogenicity is controversial. No strong correlation has been found between *B. hominis* and gastrointestinal tract symptoms, and some patients have had resolution of symptoms, despite the continued presence of *B. hominis*. Most patients with *B. hominis* in their feces have another origin or cause for their symptoms. The organism is probably a commensal ("benign fellow traveler") in most persons, and other causes of intestinal tract disease, both infectious and noninfectious, should be sought, despite the identification of *B. hominis*. Patients with persistent diarrhea, repeated identification of *B. hominis* in the feces, and no other identifiable cause of disease may be treated with metronidazole (750 mg three times a day for 10 days) with or without the addition of iodoquinol (650 mg three times a day for 20 days). However, it is most important to conduct a thorough search for other causes of disease.

TRICHOMONIASIS
Biology and Life Cycle

Trichomoniasis is a genitourinary tract disease caused by the flagellate protozoon *Trichomonas vaginalis*. The organism has only a trophozoite stage and requires anaerobic, alkaline conditions for growth. It is transmitted only by direct contact, usually during sexual intercourse. Humans are the only hosts.

Epidemiology

T. vaginalis has a worldwide distribution. The prevalence of infection ranges from 5% to more than 50% in different populations. The factors associated with high prevalence include multiple sexual partners, poor personal hygiene, and low socioeconomic status. From 30% to 50% of women with gonorrhea have coexisting infection with *T. vaginalis*. From 66% to 100% of the female sexual partners of infected males become infected, and 30% to 80% of the male sexual partners of infected females become infected. Experimental data suggest that *T. vaginalis* can be transmitted by contaminated objects as well as by sexual intercourse.

Pathogenesis and Immunity

Infection may be chronic and asymptomatic or may produce vaginitis. Clinical manifestations in infected women may be produced by factors that raise vaginal pH (pregnancy, menses, anaerobic infection). With symptomatic infection, inflammation of the epithelium and submucosa of the vagina and cervix occurs. The cervix may have multiple petechiae (strawberry cervix). Desquamation of squamous epithelial cells plus an inflammatory exudate combine to produce a yellow-green discharge. Infection in men is more likely to be asymptomatic and to resolve spontaneously. Urethritis is the most common manifestation in men.

Clinical Manifestations

In women symptoms usually begin or worsen during the menstrual periods. The most common symptom is acute vaginal discharge (Chapter 244). Some women may have dysuria, vaginal itching, painful intercourse, and, rarely, abdominal pain. The severity of the symptoms correlates with the number of polymorphonuclear leukocytes in the discharge. Physical examination reveals a vaginal discharge. The vulva is usually erythematous and edematous and may be excoriated. The vaginal mucosa and cervix are red, and small punctate hemorrhages or ulcers may be seen. A few patients have cervical tenderness. Most infected men are asymptomatic. Men with symptoms most often have dysuria and a scant penile discharge. However, *T. vaginalis* is an infrequent cause of nongonococcal urethritis, and the identification of *T. vaginalis* in urethral smears does not prove that *T. vaginalis* is the cause of the urethritis. Other potential causes should be pursued (Chapter 244). Unusual complications include epididymitis and prostatitis.

Diagnosis

T. vaginalis infection should be considered in women with a vaginal discharge or with dysuria and a negative urine culture and in men with nongonococcal urethritis, prostatitis, or epididymitis that does not respond to standard therapy. Diagnosis is made by identifying *T. vaginalis* in wet mounts or Pap smears. The organism can be readily identified on fresh wet mounts by virtue of its motility. Wet mounts are more likely to be positive if the patient is symptomatic. Culture, if available, is the most sensitive diagnostic test. In men a swab of anterior urethral exudate should be examined for motile trophozoites, preferably in the morning before urination. Individuals (men or women) with *T. vaginalis* infection should be screened for the presence of other sexually transmitted diseases.

Treatment and Prevention

Most strains of *T. vaginalis* are sensitive to metronidazole, which can be given as a single oral dose of 2 g or in divided doses for 7 days (250 mg orally three times a day or 375 mg orally twice a day). The patient's sexual partners should also be treated. During the first trimester of pregnancy metronidazole should not be given. Twice-weekly vinegar douches or local application of clotrimazole may be effective. Women who remain infected should receive treatment with metronidazole before delivery to prevent transmission to the newborn.

DIENTAMOEBA FRAGILIS

Dientamoeba fragilis is a flagellate related to the trichomonads. Its pathogenicity has been controversial for years, but improvement in gastrointestinal tract symptoms has been reported with treatment. In one study of a semicommunal group, 56% of the adults carried the parasite and 85% of those infected had gastrointestinal tract symptoms, especially pain and flatus. Diarrhea occurred less frequently. Eosinophilia has been associated with infection. Treatment with iodoquinol at a dosage of 650 mg three times a day for 20 days eliminated the parasite in more than 80% of those who received treatment, but the number receiving treatment was small and no control group was reported. Tetracycline (500 mg four times a day for 10 days) and paromomycin (10 mg/kg per day for 7 days) also appear to be effective against *D. fragilis* infection.

NONPATHOGENIC PROTOZOA

Nonpathogenic protozoa, such as *Entamoeba hartmanni, Entamoeba coli, Endolimax nana,* and *Iodamoeba bütschlii,* have been reported to produce diarrheal disease in immunocompromised patients with AIDS and to respond to treatment. However, these reports do not contain control groups, and relapse often occurs. Thus it is likely that these patients have diarrhea as a result of HIV infection of enterocytes, *Cyclospora* organisms, microsporidial species, or as yet unrecognized pathogens. Nonetheless, appearance of any of the nonpathogenic protozoa in the stool is evidence of fecal-oral contamination and should alert the clinician to the possibility of undetected protozoan pathogens (e.g., *Giardia* organisms) that may respond to empiric treatment.

BIBLIOGRAPHY

Adams EP, MacLeod IN: Invasive amebiasis. II. Amebic liver abscess and its complications, *Medicine (Baltimore)* 56:325, 1977.
Boustani MR, Gelfand JA: Babesiosis, *Clin Infect Dis* 22:611, 1996.
Bryan RT: Microsporidiosis as an AIDS-related opportunistic infection, *Clin Infect Dis* 21(suppl 1):S62, 1995.
Daffos F et al: Prenatal management of 746 pregnancies at risk for congenital toxoplasmosis, *N Engl J Med* 318:271, 1988.
Dannemann B et al: Treatment of toxoplasmic encephalitis in patients with AIDS: a randomised trial comparing pyrimethamine plus clindamycin to pyrimethamine plus sulfadiazine, *Ann Intern Med* 116:33, 1992.
DeHovitz JA et al: Clinical manifestations and therapy of *Isospora belli* infection in patients with the acquired immunodeficiency syndrome, *N Engl J Med* 315:87, 1986.
Drugs for parasitic infections, *Med Lett Drugs Ther* 37:99, 1995.
Godwin TA: Cryptosporidiosis in the acquired immunodeficiency syndrome: a study of 15 autopsy cases, *Hum Pathol* 22:1215, 1991.
Goodgame R: Understanding intestinal spore-froming protozoa: cryptosporidis, microsporidia, isospora and cyclospora, *Ann Intern Med* 124:429, 1996.
Hagar JM, Rahimtoola SH: Chagas' heart disease in the United States, *N Engl J Med* 325:763, 1991.
Katlama C et al: Pyrimethamine-clindamycin vs. pyrimethamine-sulfadiazine as acute and long-term therapy for toxoplasmic encephalitis in patients with AIDS, *Clin Infect Dis* 22:268, 1996.
Kirchoff LV, Gam AB, Gilliam F: American trypanosomiasis (Chagas' disease) in Central American immigrants, *Am J Med* 82:915, 1987.
Leport C et al: Treatment of central nervous system toxoplasmosis with pyrimethamine/sulfadiazine combination in 35 patients with the acquired immunodeficiency syndrome: efficacy of long-term continuous therapy, *Am J Med* 84:94, 1988.
Lobel HO et al: Recent trends in the importation of malaria caused by *Plasmodium falciparum* into the United States from Africa, *J Infect Dis* 152:613, 1985.
Looareesuwan S et al: *Plasmodium falciparum* hyperparasitemia: use of exchange transfusion in seven patients and a review of the literature, *Q J Med* 277:471, 1990.
Ma P et al: *Naegleria* and *Acanthamoeba* infections: review, *Rev Infect Dis* 12:490, 1990.
Mahmoud AAF: The challenge of intracellular pathogens, *N Engl J Med* 326:761, 1992.
Marsden PD, editor: Intestinal parasites, *Clin Gastroenterol* 7:1, 1978.
McCabe RE et al: Clinical spectrum in 107 cases of toxoplasmic lymphadenopathy, *Rev Infect Dis* 9:754, 1987.
Miller KD, Greenberg CC, Campbell CC: Treatment of severe malaria in the United States with a continuous infusion of quinidine gluconate and exchange transfusion, *N Engl J Med* 321:65, 1989.
Miller LH: Strategies for malaria control: realities, magic, and science, *Ann N Y Acad Sci* 569:118, 1989.
Miller LH et al: Research toward malaria vaccines, *Science* 234:1349, 1986.
Miller RA, Minshew BH: *Blastocystis hominis:* an organism in search of a disease, *Rev Infect Dis* 10:930, 1988.
Millet V et al: *Dientamoeba fragilis:* a protozoan parasite in adult members of a semicommunal group, *Dig Dis Sci* 28:335, 1983.
Orenstein JM et al: Intestinal microsporidiosis as a cause of diarrhea in human immunodeficiency virus–infected patients: a report of 20 cases, *Hum Pathol* 21:475, 1990.
Pape JW et al: *Cyclospora* infection in adults infected with HIV: clinical manifestations, treatment and prophylaxis, *Ann Intern Med* 121:654, 1994.
Pearson RD: Clinical spectrum of leishmaniasis, *Clin Infect Dis* 22:1, 1996.
Pomeroy C, Filice GA: Pulmonary toxoplasmosis: a review, *Clin Infect Dis* 14:863, 1992.
Porter SB, Sande MA: Toxoplasmosis of the central nervous system in the acquired immunodeficiency syndrome, *N Engl J Med* 327:1643, 1992.
Reed SL: Amebiasis: an update, *Clin Infect Dis* 14:385, 1992.
Shadduck JA: Human microsporidiosis and AIDS, *Rev Infect Dis* 11:203, 1989.
White NJ et al: Severe hypoglycemia and hyperinsulinemia in falciparum malaria, *N Engl J Med* 309:61, 1983.
Wong B et al: Central nervous system toxoplasmosis in homosexual men and parenteral drug abusers, *Ann Intern Med* 100:36, 1984.

280 *Pneumocystis carinii* Infection

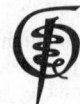

Sharon Safrin

THE ORGANISM

Despite the initial identification of the *Pneumocystis* organism in 1906 by Chagas and its recognition as a cause of pneumonia in humans in 1942, the inability to culture *Pneumocystis carinii* reliably in vitro has hindered our full understanding of its taxonomy and the development of optimal treatment.

Although *P. carinii* has been classified as a protozoan for many decades, there is greater than 90% homology of the 16S ribosomal ribonucleic acid (rRNA) of *P. carinii* with that of the fungus *Saccharomyces*. In addition, the properties of the dihydrofolate reductase enzyme of *P. carinii* (e.g., low molecular weight, absence of thymidylate synthetase activity) suggest a phylogenetic link with fungi. However, this organism's susceptibility to standard antifungal agents is poor, and many effective therapeutic agents (e.g., pentamidine, atovaquone) are antiparasitic.

EPIDEMIOLOGY

P. carinii has been visualized in the lungs of virtually all mammalian species (e.g., rats, guinea pigs, mice, rabbits, horses, and cats). Although the organisms found in animals and humans are morphologically identical, antigenic differences revealed by immunoblotting and molecular studies suggest infection by genetically distinct organisms.

Infection in humans is ubiquitous and occurs early in life. Serologic studies reveal the typical absence of serum antibody before the age of 1 year, with a rapid rise in seroprevalence rates to greater than 80% by 4 years of age in the general population. This high rate of prevalence suggests that episodes of *P. carinii* pneumonia may occur by reactivation of latent infection during periods of immunosuppression. However, small clusters of outbreaks in groups of individuals, as well as data from animal models, indicate that airborne transmission of the organism may result in acute disease. The recovery of genetically distinct isolates from recurrent episodes of *P. carinii* pneumonia in the same individual further supports the notion of acquisition of infection through exogenous sources rather than reactivation.

The vast majority of patients with *P. carinii* pneumonia have underlying immunosuppression, including infection with the human immunodeficiency virus (HIV), organ or bone marrow transplantation, and hematologic or solid organ malignancies (Box 280-1). At particular risk are patients with malignancies who are receiving corticosteroids or immunosuppressive chemotherapy.

BOX 280-1

Common predisposing factors to development of *Pneumocystis carinii* pneumonia

Primary immunodeficiency
Congenital: Cellular and/or humoral
Acquired

Secondary immunodeficiency
Prematurity
Malnutrition or starvation
Acquired immunodeficiency syndrome
Use of corticosteroid or immunosuppressive drug therapy
Lymphoreticular malignancy
Organ transplantation

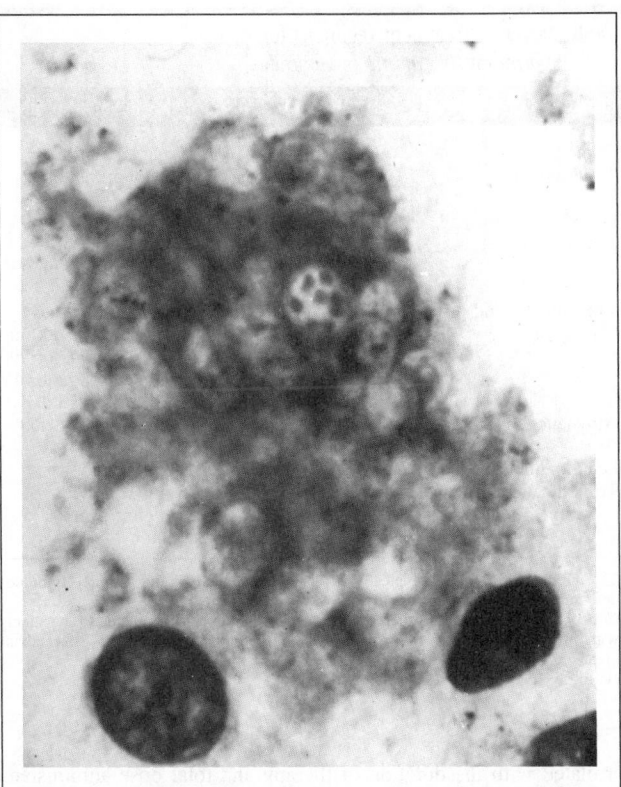

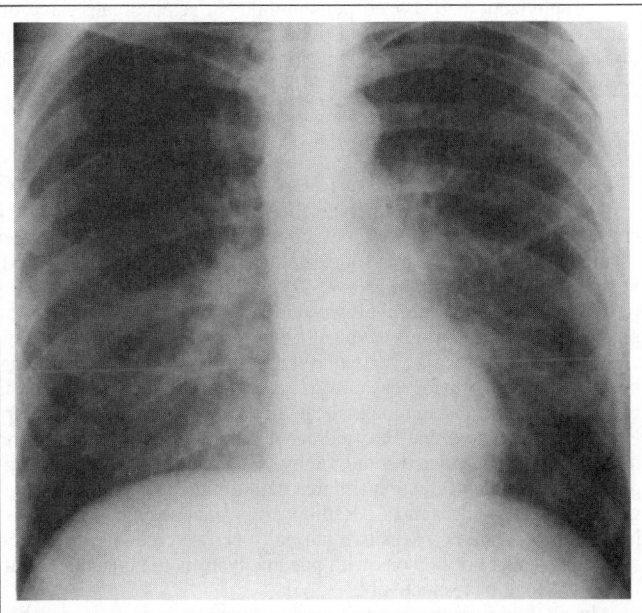

FIGURE 280-2   Diffuse interstitial infiltrates on chest radiograph of a patient with acquired immunodeficiency syndrome who has *Pneumocystis carinii* pneumonia.

FIGURE 280-1   *Pneumocystis carinii.* Giemsa-stained touch preparation of a transbronchial lung biopsy specimen from a patient with acquired immunodeficiency syndrome. A clump of eosinophilic proteinaceous material contains numerous cysts of *P. carinii,* including one with eight sporozoites.

Characteristics identifying HIV-infected patients at highest risk for development of *P. carinii* pneumonia include a CD4 cell count less than 200 cells/mm^3, the presence of HIV-associated clinical conditions such as oropharyngeal candidiasis or fever, and marked unintentional weight loss. Hazard rates for *P. carinii* pneumonia in AIDS patients are approximately twofold greater for men than for women and fourfold higher for whites than for blacks. Although it is estimated that approximately 5% of *P. carinii* infections occur in HIV-infected patients with CD4 cell counts above 200 cells/mm^3, other markers of high risk have yet to be elucidated.

PATHOPHYSIOLOGY

Depression in cell-mediated immunity appears to be the primary defect associated with the development of active *P. carinii* infection. However, the humoral immune system seems to play an important role as well, since pneumocystosis has occurred in patients with isolated congenital immunoglobulin deficiencies. Attachment of *Pneumocystis* organisms to type 1 alveolar epithelial cells, which are mediated by fibronectin and surface proteins, occurs by interdigitation of cell membranes. Resultant disruption of the alveolar-capillary membrane results in degeneration of type 1 alveolar cells and exudation of fluid into the alveolar space, with concomitant proliferation of *Pneumocystis* organisms. Accompanying changes include interstitial edema, decreased levels of surfactant, intrapulmonary shunting of blood with decreased lung compliance, and hypoxemia. The host inflammatory response may further compromise lung function.

On histopathologic examination, alveoli are filled with masses of eosinophilic material; these contain *Pneumocystis* cysts and trophozoites, as well as proteins such as surfactants (Fig. 280-1). Inflammatory cells in the alveoli are few, whereas the interstitial spaces contain variable numbers of plasma and mononuclear cells.

CLINICAL FEATURES

P. carinii pneumonia is generally manifested by fever, cough, and progressive shortness of breath (see Chapter 229). Although the onset of pneumocystosis in oncology patients is generally abrupt and rapidly progressive, it is often insidious and of prolonged duration in patients with AIDS. However, the tempo of the illness varies greatly from one individual to another. Fever, although usually present, is seldom high; shaking chills and pleuritic chest pain are distinctly infrequent. Cough is typically nonproductive, although superimposed infection with bacteria or other organisms may result in the production of mucus. Findings on auscultation of the lungs are often unremarkable. The chest radiogram typically shows symmetric, diffuse infiltrates with an interstitial pattern (Fig. 280-2). However, a wide spectrum of radiographic presentations have been described in patients with *P. carinii* infection, including coin lesions, focal consolidation, and cavitating nodules. Apical localization of infiltrates may be present, particularly in patients who develop *P. carinii* pneumonia while receiving prophylaxis with aerosolized pentamidine. Thin-walled cavities or cysts (pneumatoceles) are being recognized with increasing frequency. The chest radiograph may occasionally be within normal limits. Pleural effusion and mediastinal adenopathy are not typically present and should prompt consideration of alternative or additional diagnoses.

Laboratory studies (e.g., complete blood cell count, liver function studies) do not show distinctive abnormalities in patients with *P. carinii* pneumonia, although parameters such as white blood cell count and serum albumin level may be lowered as a reflection of underlying illness. The serum lactate dehydrogenase (LDH) level is elevated in approximately 85% of patients with *P. carinii* pneumonia, although this finding is more sensitive than specific. The degree of elevation in serum lactate dehydrogenase levels at initial evaluation correlates with prognosis, with patients having the highest levels demonstrating a poorer outcome. Rising serum LDH levels during therapy for *P. carinii* pneumonia are associated with decreased survival. Hypoxemia that becomes evident with a decreased arterial oxygen tension or an elevated arterial-alveolar oxygen gradient, or both, is typically present at the time of initial evaluation, although abnormalities may be less pronounced in patients with early-stage or less severe disease.

Most *P. carinii* infections are confined to the lungs. However, multiple foci of extrapulmonary infection have been described in the literature, particularly in HIV-infected patients who are receiving localized prophylactic aerosolized pentamidine. Infected organs have included the lymph nodes, spleen, liver, bone and bone marrow, skin, thyroid, choroid, adrenal gland, intestine, ear, meninges, pancreas, and perirectal area.

DIAGNOSIS

The initial evaluation of an at-risk patient who has nonproductive cough or shortness of breath typically consists of performance of a chest radiograph and assessment of arterial oxygenation by either oximetry or arterial blood gas measurements. Highly suggestive findings on chest radiograph (Fig. 280-2) should prompt attempts to confirm the diagnosis on morphologic study (see later discussion). In the patient with nonspecific or atypical findings on chest radiograph several adjunctive screening tests may be considered. A decreased carbon monoxide diffusing capacity (e.g., <75% of that predicted) is typically present and may signal the advisability of further workup. Recent data suggest that the finding of patchy nodular densities on high-resolution computed tomography (CT) scan of the lung is suggestive of *P. carinii* infection and that their absence may strongly suggest an alternative diagnosis. Radionuclide scanning of the lung using gallium citrate is a sensitive but nonspecific screening test based on the propensity of persons with pneumocystosis to concentrate gallium in their lungs selectively.

Morphologic diagnosis of *P. carinii* pneumonia is accomplished by microscopic examination of respiratory specimens derived either by induced sputum or bronchoscopy. Various histopathologic stains may be used for visual inspection. Stains such as modified methenamine silver and toluidine blue O enhance only the cyst wall, while Giemsa and modified Giemsa (e.g., Diff-Quik) stains enable visualization of both trophozoites and cysts (Fig. 280-1).

The sensitivity of diagnosis using induced sputa, while reported to be greater than 75% in some centers, seems, clearly, to depend on the expertise of both the respiratory therapist obtaining the specimen and the microbiologist examining the slide. The use of hypertonic saline nebulization for sputum induction, as well as sputum liquefaction using reducing agents such as dithioreitol, has helped to increase sensitivity. Both sensitivity and specificity are increased by using monoclonal antibodies directed against glycoproteins present in the cell walls of cysts and trophozoites. However, failure to detect *Pneumocystis* organisms in a specimen of induced sputa does not exclude the diagnosis (negative predictive value, approximately 60%). Bronchoalveolar lavage (BAL), when performed as a first-line test, has a sensitivity of 86% to 97%. In experienced centers, BAL is performed to confirm the diagnosis of *P. carinii* pneumonia when induced sputa examination is unrevealing. Transbronchoscopic biopsy is generally reserved for patients in whom the diagnosis remains in question after performance of initial studies.

Amplification of *Pneumocystis* nucleic acid through use of the polymerase chain reaction on serum or respiratory tract specimens is currently under evaluation as an alternative method of laboratory diagnosis. However, such methods carry the disadvantages of increased expense, increased technician labor, and risk of false-positive results. In addition, persistence of the organism for variable durations following clinical resolution of the infection may interfere with diagnosis in patients with recurrent episodes.

MANAGEMENT AND TREATMENT

Two treatment regimens, trimethoprim-sulfamethoxazole (TMP/ SMX) and pentamidine isethionate, have long been recommended for therapy for *P. carinii* pneumonia. However, several other treatment regimens are either in clinical use or actively under investigation (Table 280-1).

Most comparative trials performed to date have found TMP/SMX and parenteral pentamidine to be of equivalent efficacy in the treatment of *P. carinii* pneumonia; however, comparing the efficacies of these therapies is difficult because of the high rate of changes in therapy necessitated by adverse reactions in both groups. The most common side effects in patients receiving oral or intravenous TMP/ SMX therapy are rash, nausea, elevation of liver function values, and neutropenia; azotemia and anemia are less frequent. Parenteral pentamidine may cause renal dysfunction and hypoglycemia; both are

Table 280-1   Treatment regimens for patients with *Pneumocystis carinii* pneumonia

REGIMEN	FORMULATION	RECOMMENDED DOSAGE
Trimethoprim-sulfamethoxazole	Oral or IV	15 mg/kg/day of trimethoprim component
Dapsone and trimethoprim	Oral Oral	100 mg daily 15 mg/kg/day of trimethoprim component
Clindamycin and primaquine	Oral or IV Oral	600 mg three times daily, orally; 600 mg every 6 hours or 900 mg every 8 hours IV 15-30 mg (base) daily
Atovaquone	Oral (suspension)	750 mg (5 ml) twice daily
Pentamidine	IV	4 mg/kg/day
Trimetrexate and leucovorin (folinic acid)	IV Oral or IV	45 mg/m²/day 20 mg/m² every 6 hours

The duration of therapy is typically 14 days for patients without acquired immunodeficiency syndrome (AIDS) and 21 days for patients with AIDS.
Concomitant corticosteroid therapy (see text for dose) is recommended for patients with arterial oxygen tension less than 70 mm Hg or arterial-alveolar oxygen gradient greater than 35 mm Hg.
IV, Intravenous(ly).

correlated with the duration of therapy and total dose administered. Other potential side effects of pentamidine treatment include neutropenia, hypotension, nausea, elevation of liver function values, and acute or chronic hypoglycemia.

Several alternative agents are available for the treatment of patients with *P. carinii* infection (Table 280-1). Oral regimens include dapsone with trimethoprim, clindamycin with primaquine, and atovaquone. The combination of dapsone (100 mg daily) with oral TMP (15 mg/kg per day) was compared with oral TMP/SMX (15 mg/kg per day of the TMP component) in a randomized, double-blind multicenter study by the AIDS Clinical Trials Group of the National Institute of Allergy and Infectious Diseases (NIAID); no statistically significant differences in rates of therapeutic success (range, 88% to 91%) or dose-limiting toxicity (range, 24% to 36%) were found in 123 patients with mild to moderate disease. In this same study a third group of 58 patients randomized to receive clindamycin (600 mg three times daily) with primaquine (30-mg base/day) had similar rates of therapeutic success (93%) and dose-limiting toxicity (33%). Although rash was the most frequent cause of dose-limiting intolerance reported for all three treatment groups (range, 10% to 21%), other categories of toxicity varied. Patients receiving TMP/SMX had the highest frequency of elevated serum transaminase levels; those receiving clindamycin with primaquine had significantly more frequent neutropenia, anemia, and methemoglobinemia. Other categories of intolerance noted in previous studies include rash and nausea in association with administration of dapsone with trimethoprim and rash and diarrhea in association with the combination of clindamycin with primaquine. Dapsone and primaquine are contraindicated in patients with deficiency of the glucose-6-phosphate dehydrogenase or nicotinamide adenine dinucleotide (NADH) methemoglobin reductase enzymes, because of an increased risk of methemoglobinemia and hemolytic anemia.

The agent atovaquone is licensed in the United States as an alternative to oral TMP/SMX in intolerant patients. Two randomized, controlled trials found the pill formulation to be less efficacious but better tolerated than either oral TMP/SMX or intravenous pentamidine. A newer suspension formulation achieves substantially higher serum levels, however, and is expected to achieve higher efficacy rates.

Options for intravenous (IV) treatment regimens, in addition to TMP/SMX and pentamidine, include IV clindamycin (600 mg four times daily or 900 mg three times daily) with oral primaquine (15- to 30-mg base/day) and trimetrexate (Table 280-1). A randomized comparison of IV treatment with the dihydrofolate reductase inhibitor trimetrexate (45 mg/m^2/day) and TMP/SMX (20 mg/kg per day of the TMP component) in patients with moderate to severe *P. carinii* pneumonia demonstrated higher failure rates and decreased survival in patients receiving trimetrexate. Coadministration of high doses of folinic acid with trimetrexate prevents the occurrence of hematologic toxicities so that overall rates of dose-limiting toxicity are relatively low (approximately 8%). The drug has gained approval as an alternative therapy for patients intolerant of or refractory to TMP/SMX and is currently being reevaluated in combination with the sulfone dapsone.

Several other regimens are currently under study for treatment of pneumocystosis, including combinations of macrolides with sulfonamides, iron-chelating drugs, echinocandins and pneumocandins, 8-aminoquinolines, and antimicrotubule benzimidazoles.

The administration of adjunctive corticosteroid therapy has been shown to decrease the risk of respiratory failure and death in patients with moderate or severe *P. carinii* pneumonia (i.e., arterial oxygen tension <70 mm Hg or arterial-alveolar oxygen gradient >35 mm Hg). Such patients should receive prednisone (40 mg twice daily for 5 days, then 40 mg daily for 5 days, then 20 mg/day until completion of therapy) in conjunction with anti-*P. carinii* therapy. Early administration of corticosteroids appears to be important for maximal benefit.

PROGNOSIS

Response to therapy generally occurs within 5 to 7 days, whereas dose-limiting side effects most often appear in the second week of therapy. No therapy is wholly efficacious however, even if tolerated, and estimates of mortality range from 2% to 39%. The success of therapy depends on both the severity of infection at the time treatment begins and the presence of underlying pulmonary dysfunction. The two major complications during the course of illness are respiratory failure and the occurrence of pneumothorax.

Progression to extensive pulmonary consolidation, often requiring mechanical ventilation, may occur in patients with severe illness and is generally accompanied by extravasation of fluid into the lungs as a result of impairment of the alveolar-capillary membrane. Unilateral or bilateral pneumothoraces respond poorly to expansion or sclerotic therapy and thus carry a poor prognosis. An increased risk of pneumothorax in AIDS patients with *P. carinii* pneumonia is associated with aerosolized pentamidine treatment, the presence of pneumatoceles on chest radiograph, and a history of cigarette smoking.

PREVENTION

Anti-*P. carinii* chemoprophylaxis should be initiated in patients at highest risk for infection, that is, those undergoing intensive immunosuppressive therapy, AIDS patients who have had an episode of pneumocystosis, and HIV-infected patients ages 6 years or older in whom the CD4 cell count has fallen below 200 cells/mm^3. In patients who have had an episode of pneumocystosis, the risk of recurrent infection is high, approaching 35% in 6 months and 60% at 1 year after the acute episode. Therefore prophylaxis should be initiated immediately after completion of acute therapy.

TMP/SMX, dapsone, and aerosolized pentamidine are the three agents most frequently used for prophylaxis (Table 280-2), and recent controlled studies have compared them directly. In a recently completed multicenter randomized trial, the efficacy of TMP/SMX (one double-strength tablet twice daily), dapsone (50 mg twice daily), and aerosolized pentamidine (300 mg monthly) for primary prevention in patients with CD4 cell counts less than 200 cells/mm^3 did not differ significantly, with failure rates of approximately 20% associated with each regimen. However, in the subset of patients with CD4 cell counts less than 100 cells/mm^3 at the start of treatment, aerosolized pentamidine was less effective than the other two regimens. A secondary analysis evaluating failure rates during continued receipt of the initially assigned regimen favored TMP/SMX as most effective. Similarly, studies comparing TMP/SMX with aerosolized pentamidine for secondary prophylaxis in patients completing therapy for *P. carinii* pneumonia have demonstrated superiority of the former regimen.

Table 280-2   Drug regimens for prophylaxis of *Pneumocystis carinii* pneumonia

AGENT	FORMULATION	POSSIBLE DOSAGES
TMP/SMX	Oral	One DS tablet daily, one DS tablet thrice weekly, one SS tablet daily
Dapsone*	Oral	100 mg daily, 50 mg twice daily, 50 mg daily, 100 mg once or twice weekly
Pentamidine	Aerosolized	300 mg monthly

*In patients at risk of *Toxoplasma gondii* infection add pyrimethamine (dose, 25 to 50 mg once or twice weekly).
DS, Double strength; *TMP/SMX*, trimethoprim-sulfamethoxazole.

✔ WHEN TO REFER

Morphologic confirmation of the diagnosis of *P. carinii* pneumonia is desirable whenever feasible. Initial screening of the patient with physical examination, chest radiograph, and assessment of arterial oxygenation in most medical settings is followed by referral of the patient to a pulmonologist or respiratory therapist to obtain diagnostic specimens. Samples of induced sputum or those obtained by bronchoalveolar lavage are forwarded to the microbiology laboratory for visual examination. The initiation of empiric therapy while awaiting results of these tests is generally condoned in patients in whom a high level of suspicion of the diagnosis exists.

Limitations of current options for anti-*P. carinii* prophylaxis include both intolerance and imperfect efficacy. Efforts to increase tolerability of TMP/SMX, particularly in patients with AIDS, have focused on less frequent administration of the drug (e.g., thrice weekly) or on desensitization of patients with a history of intolerance through use of small, escalating dosages. Neither the efficacy nor the risk of TMP/SMX desensitization has been formally evaluated. The only identified predictor of failure of prophylaxis is profound T-helper lymphocytopenia (e.g., CD4 cell counts < 75 cells/mm^3). In addition to continued search for better tolerated or more effective anti-*P. carinii* prophylactic agents, identification of agents that are dually prophylactic against more than one opportunistic infection, particularly in patients with AIDS, continues to be sought. Potential candidates include atovaquone suspension, which has activity against both *P. carinii* and *Toxoplasma gondii*, and the addition of pyrimethamine to dapsone for combined anti-*Pneumocystis* and anti-*Toxoplasma* prophylaxis. The chronic use of pyrimethamine with sulfadiazine in AIDS patients with toxoplasmosis appears to incur a concomitant decreased risk of *P. carinii* pneumonia.

BIBLIOGRAPHY

Bozzette SA et al: The tolerance for zidovudine plus thrice weekly or daily trimethoprim-sulfamethoxazole with and without leucovorin for primary prophylaxis in advanced HIV disease, *Am J Med* 98:177-182, 1995.

Dohn MN et al: Oral atovaquone compared with intravenous pentamidine for *Pneumocystis carinii* pneumonia in patients with AIDS, *Ann Intern Med* 121:174-180, 1994.

Edman JC et al: Ribosomal RNA sequence shows *Pneumocystis carinii* to be a member of the fungi, *Nature* 334:519-522, 1988.

Hardy WD et al: A controlled trial of trimethoprim-sulfamethoxazole or aerosolized pentamidine for secondary prophylaxis of *Pneumocystis carinii* pneumonia in patients with the acquired immunodeficiency syndrome, *N Engl J Med* 327:1842-1848, 1992.

Hughes W et al: Comparison of atovaquone (566C80) with trimethoprim-sulfamethoxazole (TMP-SMZ) to treat *Pneumocystis carinii* pneumonia in patients with AIDS, *N Engl J Med* 328:1521-1527, 1993.

National Institutes of Health–University of California Expert Panel for Corticosteroids as Adjunctive Therapy for PCP: Special report: consensus statement on the use of corticosteroids as adjunctive therapy for *Pneumocystis* pneumonia in the acquired immunodeficiency syndrome, *N Engl J Med* 323:1500-1504, 1990.

Phair J et al: The risk of *Pneumocystis carinii* pneumonia among men infected with human immunodeficiency virus type 1, *N Engl J Med* 322:161-165, 1990.

Safrin S et al: Comparison of three regimens for treatment of mild to moderate *Pneumocystis carinii* pneumonia in patients with AIDS: a double-blind, randomized trial of oral trimethoprim-sulfamethoxazole, dapsone-trimethoprim, and clindamycin-primaquine, *Ann Intern Med* 124:792-802, 1996.

Sattler FR et al: Trimethoprim-sulfamethoxazole compared with pentamidine for treatment of *Pneumocystis carinii* pneumonia in the acquired immunodeficiency syndrome: a prospective, noncrossover study, *Ann Intern Med* 109:280-287, 1988.

Sattler FR et al: Trimetrexate with leucovorin versus trimethoprim-sulfamethoxazole for moderate to severe episodes of *Pneumocystis carinii* pneumonia in patients with AIDS: a prospective, controlled multicenter investigation of the AIDS clinical trials group protocol 029/031, *J Infect Dis* 170:165-172, 1994.

HELMINTHIC DISEASES

CHAPTER

281 Infections Caused by Helminths

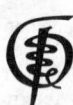

G. Richard Olds

Worms or helminths are the most common parasites of man, infecting almost half the world's population. Worms differ from other classes of infectious organisms in that they are large and multicellular; generally they are visible to the naked eye. Helminths have complex life cycles, often having several morphologically distinct forms (eggs, microfilaria, adult worms, and migrating larvae) within the infected host. Intermediate hosts (freshwater snails) or insect vectors (mosquitoes) are common. In general, helminths do not multiply in humans. Host immunity is directed toward the invasive larval forms of the parasite, whereas adult worms are resistant to the host's immune attack. Pathologic immune responses are often directed toward the progeny of adult worms (microfilaria or eggs). Helminths also distinguish themselves from other infectious agents of humans by their unique association with eosinophilic-staining polymorphonuclear leukocytes. Eosinophilia, however, is not universal among the helminth infections and is observed only when worms are present within host tissues. The mere presence of adult worms within the lumen of the intestine is not generally associated with peripheral blood eosinophilia. Clinically, most infected individuals are asymptomatic; symptomatic disease is associated with either heavy infections or an abnormal immune response to one or more stages of the parasite. Reinfections are common if not the rule. Treatment has vastly improved over the last decade but remains complicated and occasionally even toxic.

Taxonomists traditionally divide the helminths into nematodes (roundworms), trematodes (flukes), and cestodes (tapeworms). For the clinician, helminths may be divided into three major groups based on the life cycle and the severity of illness induced in humans. In this chapter worms whose entire life cycle in humans is confined to the gastrointestinal tract are discussed separately from those with a tissue migrating phase or those which reside entirely within host tissues.

STRICTLY INTESTINAL WORMS
Intestinal Nematodes

Several species of nematodes never invade host tissue. By analogy with a doughnut, these worms live their entire life within the doughnut hole (i.e., the alimentary tract of humans). Therefore they never cause eosinophilia. These parasites are common even in industrially developed countries. For example, more than 60 million Americans have pinworms. Such infections are rarely serious and are simple to treat medically. Reinfection remains the major obstacle to eradication (Table 281-1).

Enterobiasis. Pinworms are commonly found in families with small children or individuals confined to institutions where fecal-oral contamination is difficult to control. Adult worms reside in the large intestine and at night migrate to the rectal orifice, where the female deposits her eggs on the perirectal mucosa. Ova are quite irritative, leading to rectal and perineal pruritus. Intensive pruritus also helps the eggs to gain access to the fingers and fingernails, aiding human-to-human

transmission and autoinfection. Pinworm eggs remain viable for extended periods in the environment. People are easily reinfected and thus require repeated chemotherapy. Adult worms rarely cause more serious complications, although mechanical obstruction of the appendix has been reported. The diagnosis of enterobiasis is made by applying cellophane tape to the perianal skin and examining the tape for characteristic eggs under the microscope. Treatment with mebendazole is always curative. Reinfection is common; it is often advisable to treat all family members at the same time and repeat treatment 2 weeks later. Environmental manipulation (e.g., washing clothes in hot water) is best reserved for documented recurrent cases.

Trichuris trichiura. Whipworm is transmitted primarily in young children through fecal-oral contamination. Adult worms live in the colon where they attach to the colonic mucosa. Most individuals are asymptomatic. Rarely, very heavy infections are associated with bloody diarrhea and rectal prolapse. Children with minimal iron stores may become anemic, but this is uncommon in well-nourished children. Whipworm is easily diagnosed by finding the characteristic football-shaped ova in the stool. Treatment with mebendazole for 3 days or a single dose (400 mg) of albendazole is effective. Higher single doses of albendazole (600 mg) or repeated therapy (3 days) may be required for heavy infections. Follow-up stool examinations are recommended, since no treatment regimen is 100% effective.

Intestinal Cestodes

Three species of cestodes or multisegmental flatworms never invade beyond the intestinal mucosa. Disease is associated only with nutritional deprivation of the host or irritation of the intestinal mucosa. Infection is established through the ingestion of raw or undercooked meat that contains encysted larvae. After ingestion the head or scolex of the tapeworm attaches to the intestinal mucosa. The worm elongates, eventually producing egg-filled proglottids (individual segments) or free ova. A single worm infection is the rule. Because the larvae never penetrate tissue (the doughnut in the analogy), eosinophilia is not generally observed. Eosinophilia may be seen, however, with *Hymenolepis nana,* which invades the mucosa only. The pork tapeworm, *Taenia solium,* can cause both luminal infection and direct tissue invasion. Therefore this cestode is discussed both here and in another section on tissue invasive parasites (cysticercosis).

Taenia saginata. The beef tapeworm is uncommon in industrial countries. Humans become infected by ingesting meat containing cysticerci (the encysted larvae of cestodes). The adult worm can grow to 7 meters in length and generally lives in the upper small intestine. Most infected individuals are asymptomatic. Patients usually become aware of infection by passing proglottids in the stool. The diagnosis can be confirmed by direct examination of the stool for eggs and proglottids, or by adhesive tape examination for ova similar to that performed for pinworms. The specific species cannot be determined by the appearance of the ova. A closely related species, *Taenia solium* (see following discussion) can be reliably differentiated from *T. saginata* only by examination of passed proglottids, not by eggs. Since the treatment for all luminal tapeworms is niclosamide or praziquantel, determination of the specific species is not of great importance.

Taenia solium. The pork tapeworm causes two distinct diseases in humans. Luminal parasitism is caused by the ingestion of raw or undercooked pork. Adult *T. solium* worms cause few symptoms and are clinically indistinguishable from *T. saginatum* infection. Ingestion of viable ova (rather than raw pork) can lead to tissue infections through direct invasion by infective larvae, causing cysticerosis, a far more severe disease. Luminal parasitism and cysticercosis do not generally occur in the same individual; thus the latter is discussed later. As with *T. saginatum,* the diagnosis of intestinal tract infection is made by finding proglottids or eggs in the stool. Treatment with either niclosamide or praziquantel is curative, but the latter is preferred because it is effective against both the adults and the larvae.

Diphyllobothrium latum. The fish tapeworm is the largest of the human cestodes, reaching lengths of 10 meters. Humans are infected through the ingestion of raw or undercooked freshwater fish,

Table 281-1   Strictly intestinal helminths

FAMILY	SPECIES	TRANSMISSION	MAJOR CLINICAL PRESENTATION(S)	EOSINOPHILIA	DIAGNOSIS (ADULTS)	TREATMENT
Nematode	*Trichuris trichiura* (whipworm)	Fecal-oral	Diarrhea, rectal prolapse	No	Stool O&P	Albendazole* 400-600 mg/kg once *or* albendazole 400 mg/kg daily for 3 days *or* mebendazole 100 mg twice daily for 3 days
Nematode	*Enterobius vermicularis* (pinworm)	Fecal-oral	Perianal pruritus	No	Cellophane tape applied to rectum	Mebendazole 100 mg once (repeat in 2 weeks) *or* albendazole 400 mg/kg once (repeat in 2 weeks) *or* pyrantel pamoate 11 mg/kg (maximum, 1 g)
Cestode	*Taenia saginata* (beef tapeworm)	Ingestion of raw beef	Passage of proglottids	No	Proglottid in stool	Praziquantel* 5-10 mg/kg once *or* niclosamide 2 g once
Cestode	*Diphyllobothrium latum* (fish tapeworm)	Ingestion of raw fish	Vitamin B_{12} deficiency	No	Stool O&P	Same as *T. saginata*
Cestode	*Taenia solium* (pork tapeworm)	Ingestion of raw pork (see cysticercosis in text)	Passage of proglottids	No (yes in cysticercosis)	Stool O&P for intestinal infection	Praziquantel 5-10 mg/kg once for intestinal infection
Cestode	*Hymenolepis nana* (dwarf tapeworm)	Fecal-oral	Diarrhea, dizziness in children	Yes	Stool O&P	Praziquantel 25 mg/kg once
Trematode	*Fasciolopsis buski*	Ingestion of raw water chestnuts or bamboo	Diarrhea, intestinal or biliary tract obstruction	Yes	Stool O&P	Praziquantel 25 mg/kg three times daily for 1 day *or* niclosamide* 2 g once
Trematode	*Heterophyes heterophyes*	Ingestion of raw fish	Diarrhea, abdominal pain	Yes	Stool O&P	Praziquantel 25 mg/kg three times daily for 1 day
Trematode	*Metagonimus yokogawai*	Ingestion of raw fish	Diarrhea	Yes	Stool O&P	Praziquantel 25 mg/kg three times daily for 1 day
Trematode	*Echinostoma ilocanum*	Ingestion of raw fish	Diarrhea	Yes	Stool O&P	Praziquantel* 25 mg/kg three times daily for 1 day

*Considered an investigative drug for this indication by the United States Food and Drug Administration.
O&P, Ova and parasites.

particularly perch and pike. Because of unique ethnic dietary habits, infection is commonly found in individuals of Scandinavian, Japanese, Eskimo, and Jewish extraction. The life cycle in humans is similar to *Taenia saginata* except that the proglottids generally disintegrate in the small intestine. As a result, eggs rather than proglottids are passed in the stool in large numbers. In most infected individuals, symptoms do not develop as a direct result of parasitism. *D. latum* has a unique affinity for vitamin B_{12}, leading to deprivation in the host. As a result, megaloblastic anemia indistinguishable from that observed from other causes is occasionally found. The diagnosis can be made easily by examination of the stool for ova. Both niclosamide and praziquantel are curative.

Hymenolepis nana. With dwarf tapeworms, humans can be either the definite host (intestinal tract infection) or the intermediate host (tissue infection). In contrast to *T. solium,* however, tissue infection is confined to the intestinal wall; thus serious disease is almost never observed. The proglottids of *H. nana* autodigest in the small intestine, releasing viable ova that pass out in the stool, where they are transmitted from person to person by fecal-oral contamination. Children are commonly infected.

The life cycle of *H. nana* is unique among the helminths and shares with strongyloides the ability to cause internal autoinfection. This can lead to a large worm burden and clinical disease without reinfection from the environment. Although most infected individuals are asymptomatic, diarrhea and abdominal complaints are seen during autoin-

fection. Occasionally, dizziness and even seizures occur; these symptoms are the result of absorbed neurotoxic products of the parasite. Diagnosis is made by examination of the stool for ova. Niclosamide is effective, but praziquantel is the drug of choice, since it can kill both the adult worm and larval phases. The dose of praziquantel required for cure is higher than that needed for other luminal cestodes.

Intestinal Trematodes

Several trematodes that infect humans live their entire life cycle confined to the intestinal lumen. All have snail intermediate hosts, and infection occurs through the ingestion of raw food. Like *H. nana,* these helminths all cause injury to the columnar epithelium and therefore are associated with significant eosinophilia. Infection is diagnosed by stool examination for ova and is easily treated with praziquantel.

Fasciolopsis buski. This infection is common in Southeast Asia, China, and India and involves freshwater snails as an intermediate host. Humans become infected by ingesting raw water chestnuts or bamboo contaminated with cercariae. The fluke develops in the intestine and feeds on the columnar epithelial cells. Diarrhea may result and, rarely, adult worms may obstruct the common bile duct or intestines similarly to ascariasis. Characteristic ova are found in the stool. Infection can be prevented by proper sanitation. Treatment with praziquantel or niclosamide is curative. Oral hexylresorcinol and tetrachloroethylene have also been used.

Heterophyes heterophyes. This small intestinal fluke is common in the Orient, Africa, and the Middle East. Freshwater snails are the intermediate host and release cercariae into water. These organisms penetrate the skin of various species of fish, forming a resting stage of the parasite. Humans become infected by ingestion of the raw or undercooked fish. Adult worms can cause diarrhea and abdominal pain. On rare occasions tissue invasion by eggs can occur. The diagnosis is made by stool examination for ova. Praziquantel is the only effective drug.

Metagonimus yokogawai. This parasite has a similar life cycle and causes the same clinical disease as *H. heterophyges. M. yokogawai* is found in the Orient, Russia, and Southern Europe. Praziquantel is the drug of choice.

Echinostomas ilocanum. Infection is found primarily in the Philippines and Indonesia. Snails are the intermediate hosts; ingestion of raw freshwater mollusks leads to infection in humans. Diarrhea is the most common clinical symptom, and infection is easily diagnosed by stool examination for ova. Praziquantel is the drug of choice.

INTESTINAL HELMINTHS WITH TISSUE MIGRATORY PHASES

This class of parasites has a typical life cycle in humans—a larval stage where the parasite migrates through host tissues and an intestinal luminal phase where the adult worm resides. During migration (often through the lungs) these nematodes may cause fever and transient pulmonary infiltrates with eosinophilia (PIE) syndrome. During this stage the diagnosis cannot be made by examining the stool for ova and parasites, since the symptoms are produced by immature larvae. Serologic testing is the only reliable way of making the correct diagnosis. Symptoms are transient and normally do not require specific therapy (with the exception of strongyloides hyperinfection). The diagnosis and treatment of the adult intestinal stage are similar to those outlined for the strictly intestinal nematodes (Table 281-2).

Ascaris lumbricoides. These roundworms are one of the most common helminth infections of humans with over a billion individuals infected worldwide. Infection is found in individuals of all ages but is more common in children. Infection occurs from the ingestion of eggs through fecal-oral contamination. Ingested ova hatch in the intestine, and the larvae penetrate the intestinal mucosa. Larvae then migrate through the tissues to the lungs, penetrate into the alveolar spaces, migrate up the trachea, are swallowed, and finally arrive again in the intestinal lumen. Pulmonary symptoms (severe cough and allergic pneumonitis) are generally transient. Once the adult intestinal phase is reached, individuals are asymptomatic but heavily infected small children may have nutritional impairment. Rarely, adult worms obstruct the common bile duct or appendix or masses of worms lead to small bowel obstruction in small children. The diagnosis is easily made by examining the stool for ova. Mebendazole and piperazine citrate are very effective but require 2 to 3 days of treatment. Pyrantel pamoate and albendazole are both effective as single-dose drugs, but the former drug can cause gastrointestinal tract disturbances, dizziness, headache, and other systemic reactions. The combination of convenience and high efficiency makes albendazole the treatment of choice in most clinical settings.

Necator americanus and Ancylostoma duodenale. Hookworms infect half a billion individuals worldwide. Two species, *N. americanus* (New World hookworms) and *A. duodenale* (Old World hookworms) cause identical clinical symptoms in humans but differ slightly in their response to antihelminthic drugs. Hookworm larvae penetrate directly through intact skin on contact with contaminated soil. This can lead to a pruritic rash or ground itch. Maturing larvae have migratory patterns identical to those of Ascaris larvae and cause the same transient eosinophilic pneumonitis. Adult worms ultimately reside in the small intestine by attaching to the mucosa. Numerous ova are passed in the stool to complete the life cycle. Most individuals are asymptomatic. Since each adult worm ingests about 0.2 ml of blood per day, iron-deficiency anemia can develop in heavily infected children. The diagnosis of the intestinal phase of infection is easily made through examination of the stool for ova. Infection can be treated with pyrantel pamoate or mebendazole for 3 days or a single dose of albendazole.

Table 281-2   Intestinal helminths with a tissue migratory phase

FAMILY	SPECIES	TRANSMISSION	MAJOR CLINICAL PRESENTATION(S)	EOSINOPHILIA	DIAGNOSIS (ADULTS)	TREATMENT
Nematode	*Ascaris lumbricoides* (giant roundworm)	Fecal-oral	PIE, intestinal or biliary tract	During migration, obstruction	Stool O&P	Albendazole* 400 mg/kg once *or* pyrantel pamoate 11 mg/kg once *or* mebendazole orally, 100 mg twice daily for 3 days
Nematode	*Ancylostoma duodenale* (hookworm)	Skin penetration	PIE, iron-deficiency anemia, dermatitis	During migration	Stool O&P	Albendazole 400 µg/kg once *or* mebendazole orally, 100 mg twice daily for 3 days *or* pyrantel pamoate* 11 mg/kg (maximum, 1 g) for three days
Nematode	*Necator duodenale* (hookworm)	Skin penetration	PIE, iron deficiency anemia, dermatitis	During migration	Stool O&P	Same as above
Nematode	*Strongyloides stercoralis*	Skin penetration	PIE, diarrhea malabsorption Hyperinfection syndrome	Yes	Stool O&P	Thiabendazole 25 mg/kg twice daily for 2 days; 5 days for disseminated infection *or* ivermectin* 200 µg kg per day for 1-2 days *or* albendazole*† 400 mg every day for 3 days

*Considered an investigative drug for this indication by the United States Food and Drug Administration.
†Should be considered experimental treatment.
PIE, Pulmonary infiltrates with eosinophilia; *O&P,* ova and parasites.

Strongyloides stercoralis. Strongyloides have a life cycle similar to that of hookworms. Larvae live in fecally contaminated soil, penetrate through unbroken skin (ground itch), migrate through the lungs (pulmonary infiltrates with eosinophilia) and ultimately reside in the small intestine. One unique feature of the life cycle that is important to clinicians is that eggs released by adults can hatch in the small intestine and larvae can again penetrate the mucosa, causing autoinfection. Thus strongyloides can multiply in humans without reinfection from the environment; this means individuals can remain infected for life. Eosinophilia is commonly found during both the migratory and autoinfection phases of infection. Clinical symptoms are rare but can be associated with diarrhea and vague abdominal complaints.

Severe, even fatal dissemination of this parasite can be found in immunocompromised hosts. These include patients receiving high doses of steroids, patients with lymphoma and other malignancies, patients with severe malnutrition, and recently a patient with acquired immunodeficiency syndrome (AIDS). Disseminated strongyloides infection (hyperinfection) normally becomes evident as multiple gram-negative bacteremias and multiorgan involvement (renal, hepatic, pulmonary, and cardiac dysfunctions). Eosinophilia is commonly found in nonimmunosuppressed infected individuals but is almost never observed in disseminated infection because of the profound immunodepression of these at-risk patients. This often makes diagnosis difficult. Mortality rates are high even with appropriate therapy. In light of the severe and fatal nature of this complication, the diagnosis should be sought in patients with unexplained eosinophilia before the initiation of immunosuppressive therapy.

The diagnosis of infection with *Strongyloides* organisms may be difficult, since larvae are found in the stool in small numbers and standard direct examination techniques have very low yields. The modified Baermann technique of stool concentration is the direct method of choice and is almost four times more sensitive than other concentration techniques. However, it is not currently performed by many clinical laboratories. An alternate strategy is duodenal aspiration, but this approach is uncomfortable for the patient and may not increase the diagnostic yield over multiple stool examinations. In disseminated infection diagnosis by direct isolation of larvae has a much higher yield, since larvae are present in large numbers. Recently a specific serologic test has been developed that is clinically useful, particularly in the work-up of unexplained eosinophilia.

Because of the risk of dissemination, infected patients should always be given treatment. Thiabendazole is administered for 2 days for intestinal infections and is the drug of choice. Therapy is extended to 5 days when hyperinfection or dissemination is suspected. Thiabendazole may not kill tissue stage larvae, and repeat treatment may be necessary. Recently albendazole and ivermectin have been shown to be effective. Cyclosporine (3 mg/kg daily) has been shown to be effective in animal studies.

TISSUE HELMINTH INFECTIONS

Helminths that penetrate and live within human tissue are clearly the most important in clinical practice and the most difficult of the worm infections to diagnose and treat. The diagnosis is difficult, since examination of the stool for ova and parasites often does not suggest the diagnosis (trematodes are exceptions). Clinical manifestations are related to the intensity of infection as well as to the host's immune response to various stages in the parasite's life cycle. Diseases are typically chronic with symptoms developing months and usually years after a primary infection. All of these tissue infections are associated with eosinophilia, which often points the clinician in the right diagnostic direction. Recent drug developments (praziquantel, ivermectin and albendazole) make several previously untreatable infections curable.

Tissue Nematodes (Table 281-3)

Filaria. Almost half a billion people are infected with this family of tissue nematodes, mostly in tropical countries. Filariasis is transmitted by the bites of blood-sucking insects. During a blood meal the insect vector injects larvae into the definitive host (humans). Adult male and female worms mate, and the female releases larvae, called microfilaria, which migrate through the blood or tissues. These microfilaria are picked up by the insect vector during a blood meal to complete the life cycle. Migration of microfilaria is often timed to maximize uptake of the parasite by the insect vector (nocturnal or diurnal). Clinical evidence of disease is generally related to an over-exuberant host response to dead or dying adult worms or microfilaria; live worms are generally resistant to host immune attack. The location and severity of inflammation gives rise to the clinical syndromes unique to each species of filariae. In general, eosinophilia is prominent in all patients with filariasis. In fact, it is the most common cause of eosinophilia in whites returning from sub-Saharan Africa. The specific diagnosis of filariasis, however, is difficult and often requires the aid of a specialist. The treatment of most forms of filariae still remains less than satisfactory, but promising studies are currently under way using either ivermectin to kill microfilaria or high-dose albendazole to kill adult worms.

Wuchereria bancrofti **and** ***Brugia malayi.*** Lymphatic filariasis infection is transmitted to humans by mosquitoes. Infections are commonly found in tropical regions of Africa, South America, Southeast Asia, and several Pacific islands. Mature male and female worms reside in the lymphatics of the legs, scrotum, arms, and thorax. Females release microfilaria into the bloodstream with a pronounced nocturnal periodicity (11:00 PM to 1:00 AM). In some strains found in the South Pacific maximal microfilaria blood concentrations are found at noon.

Adult worms are resistant to host immune attack but secrete metabolic products that can cause local inflammation and induce thickening of the lymphatic walls. Some infected individuals are asymptomatic for years. Others never develop symptoms, despite years of documented microfilaremia. When adult worms die, they become highly antigenic and evoke a sudden, severe local inflammatory reaction. Lymphangitis and lymphadenitis are usually the first clinical symptoms of infection and last several days to weeks (a single episode normally resolves without sequelae). Inflammation is normally associated with fever, adenopathy, and eosinophilia. Repeated episodes of lymphangitis lead to permanent obstructions to lymph drainage and chronic lymphedema. Hydroceles, chylous ascites, elephantiasis, and megascrotum are common chronic sequalae. Microfilaria, whether dead or alive, do not elicit any immunologic responses except in the unusual syndrome, tropical pulmonary eosinophilia, which is discussed later.

The diagnosis of lymphatic filariasis can be difficult. The definitive diagnosis is made by finding the characteristic microfilaria in the blood. The highest yields occur in blood obtained between 11:00 PM and 1:00 AM. Circulation of microfilaria can also be induced by administration of diethylcarbamazine (DEC) and blood collection 1 hour later. Serologic tests may be suggestive but cross-react with all human and animal filarias and even with many other helminth infections. Recently, better serologic tests have been developed that may allow improved diagnosis and quantification of the adult worm burden.

Treatment remains unsatisfactory. DEC kills microfilaria, but daily therapy is required and can induce significant toxic effects such as fever, severe pruritis, postural hypotension, nausea, and vomiting. These result from host immune reactions to dead and dying microfilaria rather than direct toxicity of the drug. Gradually increasing doses of DEC is often required in an attempt to limit this toxicity. DEC is then continued for 3 weeks. DEC does not kill adult worms, and the microfilaria levels may return to pretreatment values several months later. Ivermectin appears in preliminary trials to be quite effective when used in higher doses than those currently used in onchocerciasis (400 μg/kg) and may kill adult worms with repeated doses. Treatment with albendazole (400 mg daily for 3 weeks) also appears in preliminary studies to kill adult worms. Both of these treatments, however, should still be considered investigational. Treatment of chronic lymphedema is largely unsuccessful, but occasionally the condition is correctable by surgery.

Onchocerca volvulus. River blindness is caused by the filarial worm endemic in central and South America and tropical Africa. Infection is spread by the bite of a blackfly of the genus *Simulium*. Since the vector breeds in fast-flowing water, transmission is often seasonal

Table 281-3   Tissue nematode infections

SPECIES OR CONDITION	EPIDEMIOLOGY	TRANSMISSION	MAJOR CLINICAL PRESENTATION(S)	DIAGNOSIS	TREATMENT
Wuchereria bancrofti (lymphatic filariasis)	Tropics and subtropics	Mosquito	Lymphatic obstruction	Night blood	DEC* 50 mg 1st day, 50 mg tid 2nd day, 100 mg tid 3rd day, 2 mg/kg tid for 20 days, *or* ivermectin†‡§ 400 µg/kg *or* albendazole†‡§ 400 mg for 21 days
Brugi malayi (lymphatic filariasis)	South and Southeast Asia	Mosquito	Lymphatic obstruction	Night blood	Same as above*
Loa loa (eyeworm)	West and Central Africa	Deerfly, Horsefly	Calabar swellings	Day or night blood	DEC as above* *or* ivermectin†‡§ as above
Onchocerca volvulus (river blindness)	Central and South America	Blackfly	Dermatitis blindness	Skin snips	Ivermectin§ 150 µg/kg once every 3-12 months
Tropical pulmonary eosinophilia	All of the above areas	Unknown	Eosinophilia pneumonitis	Serologic tests, clinical picture	DEC 2 mg/kg tid for 7-21 days *or* ivermectin†‡§ *or* albendazole†‡ as outlined for *Wucheria bancrofti*
Dracunculus medinensis (guinea worm)	Africa	Step-wells	Painful boil in legs	Visualization of worm	Niridoazole† 25 mg/kg for 10 days *or* metronidazole† 250 mg tid for 10 days
Angiostrongylus cantonensis	Southeast Asia and Pacific	Raw mollusks or crustaceans	Eosinophilia meningitis	Clinical picture	Surgical removal
Angiostrongylus costaricensis	Same	Same	Same	Same	Surgical removal plus mebendazole 100 mg bid for 5 days *or* ?thiabendazole†‡ 25 mg/kg tid for 3 days
Gnathostoma spinigerum	Thailand and Japan	Raw fish	Eosinophilia, meningitis, subcutaneous swellings	Serologic tests	Surgical removal plus mebendazole‡ 200 mg every 3 hours for 6 days
Anisakis specus	Japan and Scandinavia	Raw fish	Benign stomach "tumor"	Endoscopy with biopsy, serologic tests	Surgical removal
Visceral larva migrans	Worldwide	Ingestion of soil (pica)	Fever, abdominal pain, optic involvement, diarrhea	Serologic tests	Albendazole† 400 mg bid for 3-5 days *or* DEC† 2 mg/kg bid for 10 days *or* mebendazole† 100-200 mg for 5 days *or* thiabendazole† 25 mg/kg bid for 5 days (maximum, 3 g per day) all with steroids‡
Cutaneous larva migrans	Worldwide	Skin penetration	Creeping eruption	Clinical picture	Thiabendazole topically or 50 mg/kg per day (maximum, 3g per day) for 2-5 days *or* albendazole† 200 mg bid for 3 days *or* ivermectin†§ 150-200 µg/kg once
Trichinella spiralis	Worldwide	Raw meat, periorbital edema	Fever, myalgias	Serologic tests, muscle biopsy	Thiabendazole†‡ 25 mg/kg for 5 days (maximum, 3 g per day) *or* mebendazole†‡ 200-400 mg tid for 3 days, 400-500 mg tid for 10 days *or* albendazole†‡ 400 mg bid for 10 days; ?steroids
Strongyloidosis	Worldwide, immunosuppressor	Fecal-oral	Gram-negative bacteremia, multiple organ involvement	Stool ova and parasites, tissue biopsy	Thiabendazole 25 mg/kg bid for 2 days, 5 days for dissemination *or* albendazole† 400 mg/day for 3 days *or* ivermectin†§ 200µg/kg per day for 1-2 days†§

*May precipitate severe reactions in heavily infected individuals.
†Considered an investigative drug for this indication by the United States Food and Drug Administration.
‡Effectiveness not clearly established.
§Not available in the United States. (Available through the Centers for Disease Control and Prevention.)
DEC, Diethylcarbamazine; *tid*, three times daily; *bid*, twice daily.

and generally confined to the proximity to rivers and streams. Adult *O. volvulus* worms live in subcutaneous nodules. The female releases microfilaria that migrate through connective tissues and skin.

Although both adult worms and microfilaria can evoke an immunologic response from the host, microfilaria are primarily responsible for the morbid sequelae of infection. Microfilaria in the skin or eye induce a low-grade inflammation leading to chronic pathologic sequelae. Most individuals have no symptoms early in infection. Painless subcutaneous nodules can be palpated over bony prominences. These are usually found in the lower extremities and buttocks in individuals in Africa and around the head and neck in individuals in South and Central America. Recurrent pruritic rashes or conjunctivitis is the first clinical manifestation of disease. During the chronic stages of infection the skin may become thickened and lichenified ("crocodile skin"). Blindness may ultimately occur as a result of recurrent punctate keratitis, corneal fibrosis, and chorioretinitis with or without glaucoma. Retinal involvement including optic neuritis can also be found.

The diagnosis is often suspected if there is a high level of eosinophilia and a history of travel to an endemic area. The definitive diagnosis is made by direct identification of microfilaria in skin snips (2 to 4 mm^2 bloodless superficial pieces of skin incubated in saline) or by visualization of microfilaria during a slit-lamp examination of the eye. Excision of the characteristic subcutaneous nodules can also make the diagnosis. Occasionally the diagnosis can be made by observing the rapid development of a severe pruritic rash following a single test dose of DEC (Mazzotti test). A specific serologic test is currently available from the Centers for Disease Control and Prevention (CDC) in Atlanta and is helpful in making the diagnosis.

DEC has been used for many years to treat onchocerciasis but is often associated with severe reactions in infected patients (see preceding discussion of lymphatic filiariasis) and must be administered daily for 14 days. Furthermore, DEC does not kill adult worms and may accelerate blindness. Treatment with intravenous suramin is necessary to eradicate adult worms but is quite toxic and now rarely used. As a result, it is no longer acceptable to use these medications now that newer drugs are available. Ivermectin is currently the drug of choice, but it has not been approved by the U.S. Food and Drug Administration (FDA). It can be obtained in the United States from the CDC. A single 150-μg/kg oral dose is used. This eradicates microfilaria for almost a year, with a marked reduction in adverse side effects. Minor side effects include rash, pruritus, and fever and are a manifestation of the dying microfilaria. A complete ophthalmologic examination should be performed before treatment. The dose of ivermectin is repeated every 6 to 12 months. Recent studies suggest that treatment every 3 to 4 months with ivermectin slowly reduces the viability of adult worms, but this more aggressive use of ivermectin is still investigational.

Loa loa. Loaiasis is endemic in eastern and central tropical Africa. Infection is transmitted by the bites of deerflies and horseflies. Adult worms migrate through subcutaneous tissues releasing microfilaria into the bloodstream.

In *L. loa* infection only the adult organism is involved in the disease. Adult worms release antigenic secretions as they pass over bony prominences or joints, particularly the wrists. These antigens evoke intense local reactions called calabar swellings. Localized areas of inflammation are intensely pruritic and generally bring the patient to the attention of a physician. In industrialized countries this condition is often misdiagnosed as chronic urticaria or as a pyogenic infection. Eosinophilia is prominent. Rarely, an adult worm is seen migrating across the conjunctiva or sclera of the eye, producing intense inflammation.

The diagnosis of *L. loa* infection is made largely on clinical grounds, since the patient may have calabar swellings and intense eosinophilia months before microfilaria can be found in the blood. Since microfilaria are released with a diurnal periodicity blood specimens should be collected at noon and midnight. No serologic test is completely reliable, but serologic testing may point the clinician in the right diagnostic direction.

DEC kills microfilaria and, often, adult worms in this disease. Treatment may, however, precipitate calabar swellings in locations where adult worms are migrating and often causes systemic allergic reactions, particularly in individuals with documented microfilaremia.

Coadministration of antihistamines or corticosteroids is often indicated to blunt the severe allergic reactions observed in individuals with microfilaremia. When adult worms are present in the eye, surgical excision is advised. Preliminary studies suggest that both high-dose ivermectin and albendazole can be effective but are still investigational.

Other Human Filariases. A variety of other human filariases have been described but are of limited pathogenicity in man. These include *Dipetalonema perstans*, *Dipetalonema streptocerca* and *Mansinella ozzardi*. Normally these organisms are of importance only because they can be confused with other, more serious filarial pathogens of humans. These infections are treated with DEC, mebendazole or Ivermectin.

Nonhuman-Host Filarial Infections. A variety of nonhuman filariae can occasionally infect humans but the life cycle is not completed. The most common are *Dirofilaria immitis* and *Dirofilariasis tenuis* in North America. Dogs are the normal definitive host. Infected humans are almost always asymptomatic but seek medical treatment for isolated pulmonary or subcutaneous nodules. Treatment is by excision.

Tropical Pulmonary Eosinophilia. Tropical pulmonary eosinophilia (TPE) is a syndrome that includes cough, dyspnea, and pulmonary infiltrates associated with intense eosinophilia in patients from areas endemic for lymphatic filariasis.

The exact pathogenic mechanism of TPE is unknown but is believed to be an overexuberant host response to microfilaria. Microfilaria are not found in the blood but have occasionally been found in lymph node or lung biopsy specimens. Adult worms have not been identified.

The syndrome is typically seen in young men. Initial symptoms include a dry cough, wheezing, dyspnea, low-grade fever, and, occasionally, diffuse lymphadenopathy and hepatosplenomegaly. The chest radiograph generally suggests diffuse patchy infiltrates. Occasionally, hemoptysis occurs. Pathologic specimens of the lung demonstrate an intense eosinophilic bronchopneumonia. Untreated, the syndrome can be quite prolonged, with frequent exacerbations and remissions. Pulmonary fibrosis can be a late complication.

The diagnosis depends on the correct combination of symptoms in an individual from an area endemic for lymphatic filariasis and exclusion of other likely diagnoses (generally tissue migration of other helminths, which are usually transient). Eosinophil counts are often quite high, as are serum immunoglobulin E (IgE) levels. Patients generally have elevated antibody titers to a wide variety of filarial antigens.

Patients with TPE normally respond to DEC (3 mg/kg three times daily for 14 to 21 days) without recurrence. Treatment with albendazole or high-dose ivermectin is still experimental.

Dracunculiasis. Guinea worm is an infection now found almost exclusively in Africa and is maintained in locations where humans must walk through or step into their sources of drinking water.

Dracunculus larvae infect microscopic crustaceans that contaminate drinking water. After copepods are ingested, infective larvae are released into the small intestine. Parasites penetrate the intestinal wall and migrate through subcutaneous tissue to the lower extremities. A painful boil develops over the gravid female worms. On immersion of the limb in water, the boil ruptures. The uterus of the female is prolapsed through this ulceration, releasing larvae into the water, where they complete the life cycle.

The first symptom of infection is normally an intense pruritus associated with formation of a painful papule. Multiple papules are not uncommon and are usually found on the legs and feet. Occasionally, ulcers are found on the upper extremities and trunk. Diarrhea, urticaria, and pruritus are not uncommon before ulceration.

The diagnosis can be made by immersion of the ulcer into water. This normally allows visualization of the adult female worm or demonstration of the larvae in the water after centrifugation.

Patients receive treatment with niridazole followed by mechanical removal of the worm. Infection can be prevented by sieving of drinking water or the elimination of open step-in wells.

Trichinella spiralis. Trichinosis infection is distributed worldwide. People become infected by the ingestion of viable larvae encysted in raw or undercooked meat. After passage through the stomach, larvae mature into adult worms in the small intestine. Females produce larvae that penetrate the intestinal wall and migrate throughout the body, eventually encysting within striated muscle.

When the adult worms are in the intestine (first 2 to 3 weeks), they may cause enteritis. During the migrating phase larvae attempt to penetrate a variety of host cells, generally leading to cell death. This is a particular problem when larvae penetrate into the brain, heart, or eye. Successful penetration occurs only in striated muscle tissue where they encyst. Penetration, however, still results in edema and myositis for 7 to 14 days.

Early symptoms are often mistaken for nonspecific gastroenteritis or flu. In the intestinal phase of infection diarrhea, vomiting, and abdominal pain are common. The penetration of larvae can rarely be associated with gram-negative bacteremia (similar to disseminated strongyloides). In classic cases patients become ill 1 to 2 weeks after ingestion of undercooked meat with periorbital edema, petechial hemorrhages, fever, myalgias, and a prominent eosinophilia. The severity of symptoms usually relates to the size of the inoculation dose. Deaths (2% of cases) generally occur as a result of cardiac, central nervous system, or pulmonary involvement.

The diagnosis of trichinosis can be aided by a recent history of ingestion of undercooked meat. Several species have been implicated, including sources of beef and pork and a variety of wild animals. The total eosinophil count is very high, as are serum levels of creatine phosphokinase (CPK) and serum glutamate oxaloacetate transaminase (SGOT) from damaged muscles. Several serologic tests exist, but results may be negative in early stages of the disease. Skeletal muscle biopsy of the deltoid or gastrocnemius muscle allows for the definitive diagnosis of the disease.

The therapy for trichinosis is less than satisfactory. Thiabendazole kills adult worms but has little effect on migrating larvae. Mebendazole and albendazole have also been used. Mild antipyretics and analgesics help with symptoms. Corticosteroids should be reserved for patients with severe or life-threatening infections.

It is easier to prevent than treat trichinosis. Cooking (59° C for 10 minutes) or freezing (−20° C for 3 days) kills *T. spiralis* larvae. Most infections occur as a result of ingestion of smoked, salted, or dried raw meat, particularly pork.

Angiostrongyliasis *(Angiostrongylus cantonensis* and *Angiostrongylus costarcensis).* These parasites cause eosinophilic meningitis and abdominal pain and originate in Southeast Asia and the Pacific or Central America, respectively. Infection is acquired by the ingestion of raw or undercooked mollusks and crustaceans. The disease is generally self-limiting, but rare fatalities do occur. No specific diagnostic test or therapy is available, although some authors suggest that the clinical course is shortened by thiabendazole. Albendazole, levamisole, and ivermectin have all been effective in animals.

Gnathostoma spinigerum. Gnathostomiasis occurs in Thailand and Japan through the ingestion of raw fish. In humans larvae penetrate the wall of the intestines and migrate through the body until they die. Although migratory subcutaneous swellings and, occasionally, eosinophilic meningitis can occur, illness is normally self-limiting. Surgical removal plus albendazole, 400 to 800 mg a day for 21 days, is effective.

Anisakiasis. Infection with a variety of ascaris-like marine nematodes can cause disease in humans following the ingestion of raw fish. Therefore disease is common in Japan, Thailand, and Scandinavia. Larvae attempt to penetrate the intestinal mucosa but die. Inflammation around dead larvae produces an intense granulomatous reaction, which can resemble carcinoma of the stomach. The definite diagnosis is made with endoscopic biopsy. No specific therapy exists except surgical removal.

Visceral Larva Migrans. Visceral larva migrans is caused by the accidental ingestion of dog or cat ascaris eggs. Typically, small children ingest contaminated soil (pica). The larvae penetrate the in-testinal mucosa and migrate through the liver, brain, eyes, and lungs. Eventually the larvae die, leading to massive inflammation with eosinophilic granulomatous reactions.

Patients have a wide variety of symptoms ranging from minor abdominal complaints to multiorgan system involvement with high fever and eosinophilia. Hepatic and pulmonary involvement is quite common. Involvement of the eye causes endophthalmitis and is commonly seen in children 5 to 8 years of age. The diagnosis can be made on the basis of serologic findings. Illness is usually self-limited. Corticosteroids are used in severe cases. DEC (2 mg/kg three times daily for 10 days), albendazole (400 mg twice daily for 5 days) and mebendazole (100 to 200 mg twice daily for 5 days) have been used.

Cutaneous Larva Migrans. Cutaneous larva migrans is caused by the skin penetration of canine or feline hookworms or strongyloides infection. The condition is most frequently found in the United States along the southern coast. The migrating larvae are unable to penetrate below the stratum germinativum of the skin and cause pruritic serpentine inflammatory lesions in the skin, particularly in areas of the body with direct contact with the ground. Eventually the larvae die, but thiabendazole is often used either topically or systemically. Thiabendazole can be used topically. Recently albendazole (200 mg twice daily for 3 days) has been reported to be effective, as has ivermectin (150 to 200 μg/kg as a single dose).

Tissue Trematodes

Tissue trematodes are among the most important of the helminths that cause infection in humans. Freshwater snails, the intermediate hosts for all trematode infections, and the geographic distribution of the specific snail species generally determine the location of human disease. In the past, many tissue trematode infections were either untreatable or cured only through the use of very toxic drugs. The recent development of praziquantel has allowed safe, effective treatment of all these infections with the exception of *F. hepatica* (Table 281-4).

Schistosomiasis (Bilharziasis). An estimated 300 million people throughout the world are infected with one of the four species of schistosomes. *Schistosoma mansoni* is endemic in Africa, the Middle East, South America, and the Caribbean (including Puerto Rico). *S. haematobium* is commonly found throughout Africa and the Middle East. The Far Eastern strain, *S. japonicum,* is endemic in China, the Philippines, and Indonesia, while *S. mekongi* is found in Southeast Asia and the Middle East.

Infected freshwater snails release cercariae that penetrate human skin on contact with fresh water. Larvae migrate through the body (including the lungs) and mature into adult male and female worms. The precise location of adult worm pairs varies with the species. Adult *S. mansoni, S. japonicum,* and *S. mekongi* worms live on the mesenteric venules, whereas *S. haematobium* worms reside in the vesical venules. Female adult worms release 200 to 300 eggs per day, most of which pass out of the body in the urine or stool (depending on the species) to complete the life cycle.

Initial contact with cercariae can induce an intensely pruritic dermatitis (swimmer's itch). During migration of the larvae symptoms include fever and pulmonary infiltrates with eosinophilia (PIE). In individuals with a heavy inoculum a serum sickness–like syndrome termed Katayama fever can develop that is occasionally fatal.

Most individuals have chronic infection with schistosomes, and the disease depends on the specific species. In *S. mansoni, S. japonicum,* and *S. mekongi,* eggs are passed in the stool. Chronic intestinal infections can lead to intermittent diarrhea, dysentery, and vague somatic complaints. Some eggs are carried upstream with the portal blood flow, where they become lodged in the presinusoidal spaces of the liver. There they evoke granulomatous inflammatory reactions that result in enlargement of the liver and spleen. Hepatic fibrosis and a permanent obstruction to portal blood flow are late sequelae. The hepatic fibrosis induced by schistosomiasis is unique. Early fibrosis is confined to the portal tracts, hepatic architecture is preserved, and normal hepatocellular functions are maintained until very late in infection. Bleeding esophageal varices are the leading cause of death in

Table 281-4   Tissue trematode infections

SPECIES	EPIDEMIOLOGY	TRANSMISSION	LOCATION	MAJOR CLINICAL ADULT WORMS	DIAGNOSIS PRESENTATION	TREATMENT
Schistosoma species						
S. mansoni	Africa, South America, Middle East, Carribbean	Contact with fresh water	Mesenteric vasculature	Portal hypertension, hepatosplenomegaly	Stool O&P, rectal snips	Praziquantel 20 mg/kg bid for 1 day *or* praziquantel 40 mg/kg once *or* oxamniquine 10 mg/kg bid for 1 day
S. japonicum	China, Philippines, Indonesia	Contact with fresh water	Mesenteric vasculature	Same as above plus seizures	Stool O&P, rectal snips	Praziquantel 20 mg/kg tid for 1 day
S. mekongi	Thailand, Laos, Cambodia	Contact with fresh water	Mesenteric vasculature	Same as *S. japonicum*	Stool O&P, rectal snips	Praziquantel 20 mg/kg tid for 1 day
S. haematobium	Africa, Middle East	Contact with fresh water	Vesical venules	Hematuria, hydronephrosis, bladder carcinoma	Urine O&P	Praziquantel 20 mg/kg bid for 1 day *or* praziquantel 40 mg/kg once
Clonorchis sinensis	Japan, China, Korea	Raw fish	Biliary tree	Cholangitis, portal hypertension, cholangiocarcinoma	Stool O&P	Praziquantel* 25 mg/kg tid for 2 days
Fasciola hepatica	Worldwide where sheep are raised	Raw watercress	Bile ducts and biliary	Right upper quadrant pain and fever, liver tissue, obstruction, hepatic fibrosis	Stool O&P, serologic tests	Albendazole* 10 mg/kg for 7 days or bithionol† 30-50 mg/kg
Paragonimus westermani	Orient, India, Central Africa	Raw crab	Lungs	Cough, sputum production (looks like tuberculosis)	Sputum and Stool O&P	Praziquantel* 25 mg/kg tid for 2 days *or* bithionol† as above
Opisthorchis viverrini	Europe, Asia and Southeast Asia	Raw freshwater fish	Biliary tree	Same as *Clonorchis* species	Stool O&P	Praziquantel* 25 mg/kg tid for 1 week

*Considered an investigative drug for this indication by the United States Food and Drug Administration.
†Available only from the Centers for Disease Control and Prevention in the United States.
O&P, Ova and parasites; *bid,* twice daily; *tid,* three times daily.

intestinal schistosomes. Intestinal schistosomiasis may predispose the patient to both hepatocellular carcinoma and carcinoma of the colon, but this association remains controversial.

Adult *S. haematobium* worms live in the vesicle venules, and eggs are passed in the urine. Chronic granulomatous inflammation of these organs leads to hematuria, hydronephrosis, and subsequent renal failure. Long-standing infection with urinary schistosomiasis is a documented risk factor in the development of carcinoma of the bladder.

Schistosomiasis can also cause several other clinical syndromes. Erratic migration of adult worms in *S. japonicum* (and, rarely, *S. mansoni*) can lead to deposition of ova in the brain or spinal cord, resulting in focal epilepsy or transverse myelitis. *Salmonella* organisms can also live within the adult worms. This may lead to recurrent bouts of salmonellosis, including typhoid fever.

The diagnosis of schistosomiasis is generally made by finding schistosome ova in the stool or urine. Biopsy specimens of the rectal mucosa (rectal snips) are often positive in light intestinal infections. Serologic testing is available and may be of value with central nervous system involvement. The liver fibrosis induced by schistosomiasis gives a characteristic pattern on ultrasound and computed tomography (CT) scans. The bladder frequently calcifies late in *S. haematobium* infection.

Treatment is now greatly simplified, since praziquantel (40 mg/kg given as a single or a divided dose) is very effective for *S. mansoni* and *S. haematobium* and is currently the drug of choice for all schistosome species of humans. The Asian species (*S. japonicum* and *S. mekongi*) require 60 mg/kg in three divided doses. Oxaminiquine is also effective in *S. mansoni;* metriphonate is effective against *S. haemotobium.* Praziquantel is useful in the treatment of central nervous system infection.

Clonorchis sinensis. Chinese liver fluke infection is common in individuals from China, Japan, Southeast Asia, and Hawaii. People become infected by ingestion of infected raw freshwater fish.

Larvae encyst in the intestine and migrate up the biliary tract, where they mature into adult worms. Migration of these larvae is associated with fever, eosinophilia, liver enlargement, and, occasionally, cholangitis. The chronic presence of adult worms causes dilation and inflammation along the biliary tree. Tissue damage with subsequent fibrosis can also occur in the liver parenchyma. Light infections are generally asymptomatic, but long-standing infections can lead to periportal fibrosis, cirrhosis, and obstruction of portal blood flow. Patients with chronic infection are also at risk for the development of cholangiocarcinoma.

The diagnosis is made by examining the stool for ova or through biliary tract aspirates in cases of light infection. Praziquantel is the drug of choice in higher doses than used for schistosomes (75 mg/kg in three divided doses). Albendazole (10 mg/kg for 7 days) has also been effective. Care must be taken during treatment, however, since dead worms may precipitate biliary tract obstruction leading to suppurative cholangitis.

Fasciola hepatica. The liver fluke *F. hepatica* causes a disease known as sheep liver rot. This disease is found in sheep- and cattle-raising areas of the world. Infection is maintained in the environment by sheep and freshwater snails. Humans become accidentally infected through the ingestion of watercress contaminated with metacercariae. Larvae penetrate the small intestine into the peritoneum and migrate toward the liver. This acute phase of infection is associated with fever, pain in the right upper quadrant of the abdomen, myalgias, and, occasionally, urticaria. Adult worms live in the bile ducts and within

Table 281-5   Tissue cestoid infections

SPECIES	EPIDEMIOLOGY	TRANSMISSION	MAJOR CLINICAL PRESENTATION(S)	DIAGNOSIS	TREATMENT
Taenia solium (cysticercosis)	Worldwide	Ingestion of eggs or autoinfection from tapeworm	Seizures, focal neurologic symptoms, hydrocephalus	Serologic tests, characteristic head CT, x-ray, of soft tissues	Albendazole 5 mg/kg tid for 8-28 days, repeated as necessary *or* praziquantel 20 mg/kg tid for 15 days; both treatments with or without steroids
Echinococcus granulosus (hydatid)	Sheep- and cattle-raising areas of the world	Association with dogs, ingestion of contaminated dog excreta	Single mass in liver or lungs, anaphylactic shock after blunt trauma	Characteristic abdominal CT, serologic tests	Surgery *or* surgery *and/or* albendazole 400 mg bid for 28 days, repeated as necessary *or* ?albendazole plus Praziquantel*†
Echinococcus multilocularis	Northern latitudes, North America, Europe and Asia	Associated with infected animals or ingestion of food contaminated with dog excreta	Alveolar mass in liver	Characteristic abdominal CT, serology tests	Surgery or surgery plus albendazole*† 400 mg bid for 28 days

*Considered an investigative drug for this indication by the United States Food and Drug Administration.
†Effectiveness not clearly established.
CT, computed tomography; *tid,* three times daily; *bid,* twice daily.

the liver parenchyma. Eggs leave the liver through the common bile duct to be passed in the stool. Chronic infection may lead to fibrosis or necrosis of the liver. Adult worms may also obstruct bile ducts.

A unique clinical syndrome is caused by an unusual migration of the adult worms to the oral pharynx. This condition, known as halzoun, causes intense pain in the throat, edema, and, occasionally, laryngeal obstruction and death. Other ectopic migrations of the worms can cause focal neurologic symptoms.

The diagnosis is generally made by finding the characteristic eggs in the stool. However, results of stool examinations are negative if adult worms are present only in ectopic locations. Abdominal CT scans are very helpful in visualizing fascioliasis in the liver, and serologic tests are available to diagnose ectopic infections. *F. hepatica* is unique among the flukes in that infections do not respond to praziquantel. Bithionol* is the drug of choice. Recently triciabendazole (Fasinex), a veterinary fasciolide, has been used effectively as single-dose treatment. In cases of halzoun, surgical removal of the fluke is indicated.

Paragonimus westermani. This lung fluke is commonly found throughout the Orient but can rarely occur in the United States. Humans become infected by the ingestion of raw freshwater crabs or crayfish. Larvae encyst in the duodenum, penetrate the intestinal wall, and migrate to the lungs. Adult worms live in fibrotic cysts located near the periphery of the lungs. Female worms deposit eggs that penetrate through the bronchioles and are coughed up with sputum.

Most individuals are asymptomatic during this migration. Chronic infection is characterized by persistent cough, intermittent hemoptysis, and pleuritic chest pain. The clinical symptoms and chest radiographs are similar to and often confused with those of tuberculosis. Paragonimiasis can rarely be complicated by bacterial infection, pleural effusions, and clubbing of the fingers and toes. Ectopic foci of adult worms in the brain can be confused with tumors.

The diagnosis can be made by finding eggs in the sputum or stool (ova are frequently swallowed). Eosinophilia is normally present. Serologic tests are available but cannot distinguish present from past infection. High-dose praziquantel (75 mg/kg divided into three doses over a day) is effective in treatment. Bithionol has also been used.

Opisthorchis viverroni and ***Opisthorchis felineus.*** In Southeast Asia these two species infect humans and cause opisthorchiasis. This disease is indistinguishable from clonorhiasis and responds to praziquantel.

*Available through the CDC Drug Service: (404) 639-3670.

Tissue Cestodes

Tapeworms confined to the intestines of humans cause little morbidity and almost no mortality (see earlier discussion). In contrast, significant clinical evidence of disease and mortality are observed when cestodes invade tissues. Patients are frequently asymptomatic during dissemination of the larvae. The diagnosis is also difficult because eosinophilia is uncommon and negative serologic test results are the rule in early stages of infection. With death or rupture of the larval stage an inflammatory response occurs, resulting in clinical evidence of disease (Table 281-5).

Cysticercosis. Cysticercosis is the disseminated larval stage of the pork tapeworm, *T. solium.* The condition is common worldwide and is the world's leading cause of seizures. Humans become infected by ingestion of eggs of the adult tapeworm. This is in contrast to intestinal infection (pork tapeworm), which is caused by ingestion of raw pork. Autoinfection (infection caused by a person's own tapeworm) can occur. In general, most people with cysticercosis do not harbor adult tapeworms in their intestines.

After being ingested, the larva migrate throughout the body and form fluid-filled cysts that are 0.5 to 1 cm in diameter. Cysticerci remain viable for 3 to 5 years and evoke little host response. Cysticerci can develop in almost any tissue in the body; the central nervous system is commonly infected. When they degenerate they evoke a massive eosinophilic reaction. Calcified lesions are a late effect. On clinical examination, headache, seizures, focal neurologic symptoms, and alterations in mental states are seen. Untreated, symptoms subside in weeks to months, then recur when another cysticercus dies.

The diagnosis of cysticercosis should be suspected in any individual with new onset of seizures. Characteristically a contrast head CT scan shows multiple or single-ring enhancing lesions. Nuclear magnetic resonance (NMR) scans are superior and may reveal cysticerci that are not apparent on CT. Radiographs of the skull and extremities may show calcified cysticerci. Cerebrospinal fluid (CSF) and serum indirect hemagglutination assays are not helpful because significant false-positive and false-negative results are obtained. The test of choice is an immunoblot assay available through the CDC and from some commercial laboratories. This test is almost 100% specific and 98% sensitive. Rarely patients have a negative test result early in the natural history of the disease. In these cases a therapeutic trial with praziquantel is probably more benign than craniotomy.

Praziquantel (50 mg/Kg a day in three divided doses for 15 to 30 days) effectively kills the cysticerci but can also exacerbate neurologic symptoms through associated inflammation around other dying cysticerci. This can be used diagnostically during therapeutic trials, since treatment can induce new lesions on CT and NMR brain scans. When the diagnosis is known, however, the concurrent use of steroids is strongly advised because they reduce the blood levels of praziquantel; it is unknown whether this reduces the cure rate. Albendazole appears to be at least equally effective and, in at least one study, more efficacious; 15 mg/kg per day in three divided doses for 8 to 28 days has been used successfully. Repeated treatment may be necessary. Steroids do not appear to decrease albendazole blood levels, whereas taking the drug with a fatty meal enhances blood levels.

***Echinococcus granulosus* (Hydatid disease).** *E. granulosus* is a tapeworm of dogs and is common in the cattle- and sheep-raising areas of the world. People become infected by ingestion of the eggs, generally from intimate contact with dogs. Larvae encyst in the small intestine where they penetrate the intestinal wall and are carried by the mesenteric vasculature to various sites within the body including the liver, lung, and, rarely, the brain. A single fluid-filled cyst forms, which contains multiple protoscolices (one protoscolex is capable of forming a new cyst). Over the next several years the cysts slowly enlarge. Symptoms develop when the cyst becomes a large, space-occupying mass. The liver is the most common location, and abdominal pain and signs of cholestasis may occur. In the lungs pleuritic pain and cough are common. Rupture of the cyst may occur spontaneously or following blunt trauma, precipitating an anaphylactic reaction. The spillage of protoscolices into the abdominal cavity also leads to multiple daughter cysts, which develop months to years later.

The diagnosis is generally suspected on physical examination when the cyst is felt as a large, nontender intrahepatic mass. Abdominal CT scans show the cystic nature of the lesion with the characteristic hydatid "sand" in dependent areas. Older cysts may calcify and be visible on plain radiographs. Several serologic tests are helpful in confirming the diagnosis.

Surgical removal of the cyst is curative, but spillage during the procedure may cause either an anaphylactic reaction or dissemination of daughter cysts. The cyst can be sterilized during surgery by instilling hypertonic saline into it. Medical treatment with mebendazole has been disappointing, although some cures have been documented. Albendazole appears to be the current drug of choice (400 mg twice daily for 28 days). Repeated treatments are often necessary. Blood levels can be increased by giving the medication with a fatty meal. The combination of praziquantel and albendazole kills protoscolices and should be tried if rupture or spillage occurs and if advocated before surgery.

Echinococcus multilocularis. *E. multilocularis* is similar to *E. granulosus* in its pathogenesis but usually infects wild canines such as foxes or wolves. Domestic dogs are occasionally infected. Humans become infected by association with canines or fecally contaminated foods. Infection is common in Alaska, Canada, Siberia, and northern parts of the continental United States and Europe. The cysts of *E. multilocularis* are alveolar and invade adjacent tissue. No specific limiting capsule is found, and infection may spread to adjacent sites. The cyst grows much like a malignant tumor dissecting into the liver parenchyma. As a result, surgical removal is difficult if not impossible. Occasionally, mebendazole is effective. Albendazole appears to be the best clinical choice in surgical patients, particularly if combined with praziquantel, but this treatment should be considered investigational.

PARASITE-INDUCED EOSINOPHILIA

Most of this chapter presents specific helminthic infections. However, the clinician often encounters a patient with unexplained eosinophilia in which there is a strong clinical suspicion of a parasite cause. These patients include recent immigrants or visitors from developing countries, travelers returning from extended stays overseas, or indigenous patients in which other causes (e.g., drug reaction, connective tissue diseases, malignancies, fungal infections) seem very unlikely or have been ruled out.

It is important to confirm that eosinophilia is actually present. Since the eosinophil is a relatively rare cell in the peripheral blood smear, significant errors can be made using the differential to estimate eosinophilia. Therefore an absolute eosinophil count should al-

✔ WHEN TO REFER

The treatment of intestinal helminths is generally straightforward and normally handled entirely by primary care physicians. Appropriate consultation regarding diagnosis and management should probably be sought when patients have more "exotic diseases," although in many cases this does not require a specific referral. Many issues can be dealt with over the phone with a knowledgeable consultant. However, treatment of more serious helminth infections, such as cysticercosis or disseminated strongyloidiasis, as well as the management of parasitic infections with unusual side effects or complications, such as *Loa loa* infection, is probably best referred to an individual with previous clinical experience.

In contrast to most other areas of medicine, clinical experience and expertise in parasitic diseases is often found in unusual places. Many infectious disease experts lack personal experience or are relatively unfamiliar with non–U.S.-based parasitic diseases. However, individuals with less background in this specialty but with significant experience overseas are often very helpful. For example, a general surgeon with previous experience with hydatid disease is often instrumental in successful surgical management of this condition. Similarly, an individual with previous missionary experience in Central Africa might be very skilled in the treatment of *Loa loa* infection. The American Society of Tropical Medicine and Hygiene maintains a register of physicians who are skilled in clinical tropical diseases and parasitology, which could be helpful to the practitioner who is caring for patients with these more "exotic" parasitic diseases.

ways be performed. This value is also useful to confirm a therapeutic response to empiric trials with antiparasitic drugs.

An initial evaluation should include at least three stool examinations for ova and parasites. These results, however, may be misleading. A few helminths do not cause eosinophilia (Table 281-1) but are commonly found in the stool. In addition, with the exception of trematodes, adult worms that produce eggs in the stool are not the stage of the life cycle responsible for eosinophilia; the migrating larvae generally stimulate eosinophilia. Since *Ascaris* or hookworm ova can be found in a fourth of the world's population, one should be careful to consider other possible causes.

Total IgE levels are generally elevated in parasitic infections. Other useful laboratory tests include SGOT, alkaline phosphotase, CPK levels, and erythrocyte sedimentation rate; chest and thigh radiographs may also be useful. An accurate travel history can generally suggest or exclude many of the potential pathogens.

A knowledge of the likely parasitic causes of eosinophilia is often helpful in directing the choice of further diagnostic tests. For example, in whites returning from Africa, filariasis is the most likely cause, whereas among Southeast Asian immigrants strongyloidiasis is typically the causative infection. If three stool examinations do not reveal a pathogen, day and night blood samples and skin snips for microfilaria or rectal snips for schistosome ova are indicated (depending on the appropriate travel history). Serologic tests may also be useful. Among the most useful are serologic tests for *Strongyloides stercoralis,* since it is frequently missed in the stool. Newer culture techniques increase the diagnostic yield but are not generally available. A *Dirofilaria immitis* (dog heartworm) serologic test result is positive in a variety of human filarial infections including tropical pulmonary eosinophilia. Although not diagnostic of any specific disease if the titer is high, the test can help direct further investigation. Other more specific serologic tests, such as the new serologic tests for onchocerciasis and cysticercosis that are available from the CDC, the National Institutes of Health, and a variety of private laboratories, are quite helpful when used in the proper clinical setting.

A specific diagnosis is not found in up to 40% of patients with eosinophilia of presumed parasitic origin. Therefore therapeutic trials with mebendazole, albendazole, thiabendazole, praziquantel or DEC are often indicated. An immediate response to DEC is pathognomonic for filarial infection. When ivermectin is available in the United States for human use, it would appear to be useful in empiric trials as well. Generally 2 to 3 months is required to document a decrease in the total eosinophil count in response to empiric drug treatment.

If eosinophilia persists, despite these empiric trials, serious consideration should be given to the diagnosis of hypereosinophilic syndrome.

BIBLIOGRAPHY

Apt W, Aguilera X, Vega F et al: Treatment of human chronic fascioliasis with triclabendazole: drug efficacy and serologic response, *Am J Trop Med Hyg* 52(6):532, 1995.

Caumes E, Carriere J, Datry A, et al: A randomized trial of ivermectin versus albendazole for the treatment of cutaneous larva migrans, *Am J Trop Med Hyg* 49(5):641, 1993.

Coulared JP, Rossignol JF: Albendazole: a new single-dose antihelminthic: study in 1455 patients, *Acta Trop (Basel)* 41(1):87, 1984.

Drugs for parasitic infections, *Med Lett Drugs Ther* 37:961, 1995.

Gann PH, Neva FA, Gam AA: A randomized trial of single- and two-dose ivermectin versus thiabendazole for treatment of strongyloidiasis, *J Infect Dis* 169:1076, 1994.

Greene BM, Taylor HR, Curp EW et al: Comparison of ivermectin and diethylcarbamazine in the treatment of onchocerciasis, *N Engl J Med* 313:133, 1985.

Grove DI: Strongyloidiasis: a conundrum for gastroenterologists, *Gut* 35:437, 1994.

Hao W, Pei-Fan Z, Wen-Guang Y et al: Albendazole chemotherapy for human cystic and alveolar echinococcosis in northwestern China, *Trans R Soc Trop Med Hyg* 88:340, 1994.

Harries AD, Myers B, and Chattacharrya D: Eosinophilia in Caucasians returning from the tropics, *Trans R Soc Trop Med Hyg* 80:327, 1986.

Jones SK, Reynolds NJ, Oliwiecki S, Harman RRM: Oral albendazole for the treatment of cutaneous larva migrans, *Br J Dermatol* 122:99-101, 1990.

Kar SK, Patnaik S, Mania J, Kumaraswami V: Ivermectin in the treatment of bancroftian filarial infection in Orissa, India, *SE Asian J Trop Med Public Health* 24(1):80, 1993.

Khuroo MS, Dar MY, Yattoo GN, et al: Percutaneous drainage versus albendazole therapy in hepatic hydatidosis: a prospective, randomized study, *Gastroenterology* 104:1452, 1993.

Kumaraswami U, Ottesen EA, Vigayasekaren V et al: Ivermectin for the treatment of *Wuchereria bancrofti* filariasis: efficacy and adverse reactions, *JAMA* 259(21):3150, 1988.

Mahmoud AAF, editor: Praziquantel for the treatment of helminthic infections, *Advan Inter Med* 32:193, 1987.

Martin-Prevel Y, Cosnefroy J-Y, Tshipamba P et al: Tolerance and efficacy of single high-dose ivermectin for the treatment of loiasis, *Am J Trop Med Hyg* 48(2):186, 1993.

Nutman TB, Ottesen EH, Ieng S et al: Eosinophilia in Southeast Asian refugees: evaluation at a referral center, *J Infect Dis* 155:309, 1987.

Perry JL, Mathews JS, Miller GR: Parasite detection efficiencies of five stool concentration systems, *J Clin Microbiol* 28(6):1094, 1990.

Peterson PK, Verhoef J, editors: Diethylcarbamazine and ivermectin, *Antimicrob Agents Chemother* 2:253, 1987.

Seidel JS, editor: Symposium on parasitic infections, *Pediatr Clin North Am* 32:4, 1985.

Sturchler D, Schubarth P, Gualzata M et al: Thiabendazole vs. albendazole in treatment of toxocariasis: clinical trial, *Ann Trop Med Parasitol* 83(5):473-478, 1989.

Takayanagui OM, Jardin E: Therapy for neurocysticercosis: comparison between albendazole and praziquantel, *Arch Neurol* 49:290, 1992.

Tompkins RK: Management of echinococcal cysts of the liver, *Mayo Clin Proc* 66:1281-1282, 1991 (editorial).

Warren KS, Mahmoud AAF, editors: *Tropical and geographic medicine*, ed 2, New York, 1990, McGraw-Hill.

Wilson ME: *A world guide to infections,* New York, 1991, Oxford University.

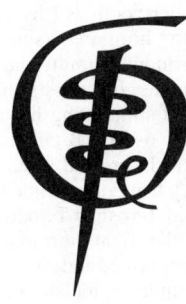

PART NINE

Endocrinology, Metabolism, and Genetics

CHAPTER

282 Principles of Endocrine Physiology

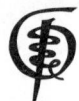

Richard M. Jordan and Peter O. Kohler

Traditionally *hormones* are defined as secretory products that travel through the blood to affect distant tissues and organs. It is now apparent that these concepts are too restrictive. Some hormones such as testosterone and estradiol have important local effects on their secretory organs in addition to the tissues they reach via the circulation. Such localized action, known as *paracrine function,* is also characteristic of several other classes of chemical mediators not usually considered hormones. These include mediators of the inflammatory response (histamine, bradykinin, slow-reacting substance) and a host of neurotransmitters. Overlap of function further blurs the distinction between neurotransmitters and hormones. Norepinephrine functions both as a neurotransmitter and as a hormone. Likewise, small peptides manufactured in the hypothalamus (thyrotropin-releasing hormone and somatostatin) appear to serve as neurotransmitters and hormones.

A single hormone can be manufactured in several different organs. For example, proopiomelanocortin, the precursor for corticotropin (ACTH) endorphins and β-lipotropin, is synthesized not only in the anterior pituitary but also in the brain, placenta, gastrointestinal tract, and reproductive organs. Other small peptides have been found common to the brain and the gastrointestinal tract. Thus the identity of separate specific organs constituting an endocrine system is no longer adequate because organs not normally considered endocrine are now known to secrete hormones important for maintaining the body's homeostasis. This is true for the gastrointestinal tract, kidney, liver, and lungs, which are all sites of hormone synthesis.

CLASSES OF HORMONES

One scheme of categorizing hormones is based on their chemical structure. Four major classes are generally recognized: peptides, amines, iodothyronines, and steroids. Peptide hormones are the largest class and are divided into smaller peptides (thyrotropin-releasing hormone, gonadotrophin-releasing hormone, somatostatin, etc.), larger peptides (insulin, growth hormone, parathyroid hormone, etc.), and glycoproteins (luteinizing hormone, follicle stimulating hormone, chorionic gonadotropin, and thyroid stimulating hormone). Structurally glycoproteins are composed of α- and β-chains. Glycosylation may be necessary for interaction of the α- and β-subunits.

Iodothyronines (l-thyroxine [T_4], triiodothyronine [T_3]) are derivatives of a single aromatic amino acid, tyrosine. Two iodinated tyrosine molecules are attached to form the final hormone product. Catecholamines (norepinephrine, epinephrine, and dopamine) are enzymatic modifications of tyrosine. Similarly, melatonin is formed from tryptophan. Steroid hormones are derived from cholesterol, and all have a similar core known as the *cyclopentanoperhydrophenanthrene nucleus.* Variations in bond saturation and side chain modifications of this core give a unique biologic action to each steroid hormone.

HORMONE SYNTHESIS
Peptide Hormones

Peptide hormone synthesis proceeds in the same manner as that of other proteins. This process is illustrated in Figs. 282-1 and 282-2. A typical gene (Fig. 282-1) responsible for hormone synthesis includes a strand of deoxyribonucleic acid (DNA) containing the base sequence responsible for transcription of the complementary nucleotide sequence of premessenger ribonucleic acid (RNA) (pre-mRNA). Interspersed in the transcription unit are base sequences that are not translated (introns). Their function, if any, is unknown. Exons are the

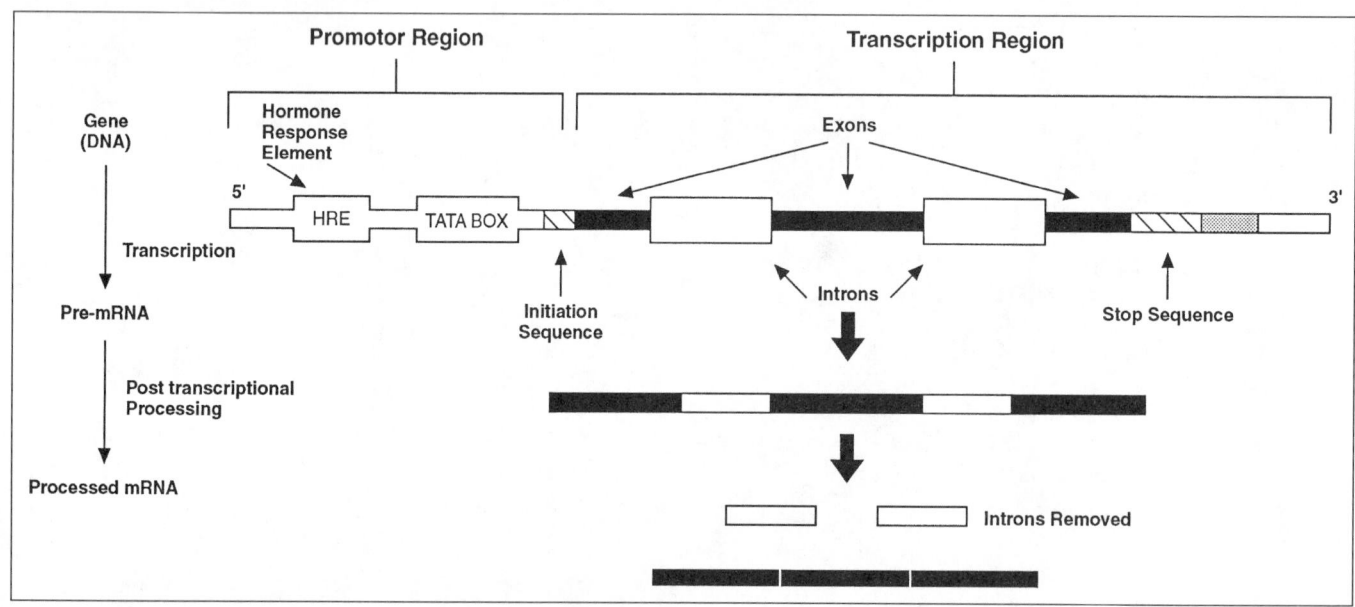

FIGURE 282-1 Gene structure and the steps involved in encoding a polypeptide. Exons contain the complementary base sequence that forms the processed mRNA. Some base sequences (introns) are transcribed into pre-mRNA from the gene but are removed during posttranscriptional processing and do not contribute to the translated amino acid sequence of a protein. Hormone response elements interact with steroid hormone–receptor complexes to affect the transcription product. The TATA box (thymine-adenine, thymine-adenine) is a base sequence that promotes the action of RNA polymerase, the enzyme responsible for polymerization of RNA into complementary base sequences from the DNA template. *HRE,* Hormone response element; *mRNA,* messenger ribonucleic acid; *DNA,* deoxyribonucleic acid.

base sequences that dictate the formation of a specific protein. The entire transcription is flanked by a promoter region at the 5′ end that determines where the transcription coding sequence begins and has regions that respond to regulatory influences such as steroid hormones. The 3′ end of the gene contains the signal sequence that terminates transcription.

The pre-mRNA formed contains the sequences derived from both introns and exons. The intron-derived sequences are removed during RNA processing, leaving mature mRNA. More than one mRNA can be formed from a single pre-mRNA. The mRNA is exported from the nucleus into the cytoplasm, where it becomes associated with ribosomes (Fig. 282-2). Ribosomes function as the machinery of protein synthesis and perform the process of elongating peptide chains (see later discussion). The ribosome-cytoplasmic mRNA complex is called the *polyribosome*. Amino acids from the cytoplasm are carried to this complex by transfer RNA (tRNA) and are attached to a growing peptide chain as the ribosome moves along the mRNA from the 5′ to the 3′ end. All 20 amino acids have one or more species of tRNA specific for the amino acid. The specific amino acid is attached to the peptide chain because the tRNA has a complementary three-base sequence (anticodon) on its active end that recognizes a triplet nucleotide sequence (codon) on the mRNA. As the newly synthesized protein emerges from the ribosome, a sequence of 15 to 30 mostly hydrophobic amino acids (the signal peptide) is exposed to the cytoplasm. The signal peptide binds to a cytoplasmic molecule called *signal recognition peptide* (SRP). This association blocks further translation until the SRP binds to a signal receptor on the endoplasmic reticulum. There is also a receptor on the endoplasmic reticulum for the ribosome. This binding process frees the signal peptide from the

SRP, and the elongation of the protein resumes, thereby pushing it through the membrane to the interior of the endoplasmic reticulum. As long as the hormone precursor molecule has the signal peptide attached, it is called a *preprohormone*. The signal peptide, however, is quickly cleaved by a trypsinlike enzyme residing in the membrane of the endoplasmic reticulum, changing the precursor to a prohormone. When a termination sequence on the mRNA is reached, translation stops and the peptide chain is released. The ribosome then dissociates into its two subunits and drifts off into the cytoplasm. The prohormone is transfered via transport vesicles to the Golgi apparatus, where further posttranslational modifications occur such as glycosylation and cleavage of amino terminal residues. In the Golgi apparatus, the peptide hormones are packaged into microvesicles or secretory granules and are either stored or immediately secreted into the extracellular fluid. The entire process from the beginning of synthesis to hormone secretion or storage can occur in less than 1 hour.

Steroid Hormones

The various steroid hormones are derived from enzymatically induced alterations of a cholesterol core. In the adrenals and gonads, pituitary trophic hormones stimulate these changes. Unlike peptide-secreting cells, the precursor (cholesterol) is supplied by plasma lipoproteins or is synthesized directly by the cell. Inside the mitochondria, cholesterol is converted to pregnenolone. Further transformation of pregnenolone occurs after it leaves the mitochondria and enters the endoplasmic reticulum. It is here that side chain modifications occur. These biosynthetic processes occur in the adrenal cortex, testis, ovary, and, to some extent, fat.

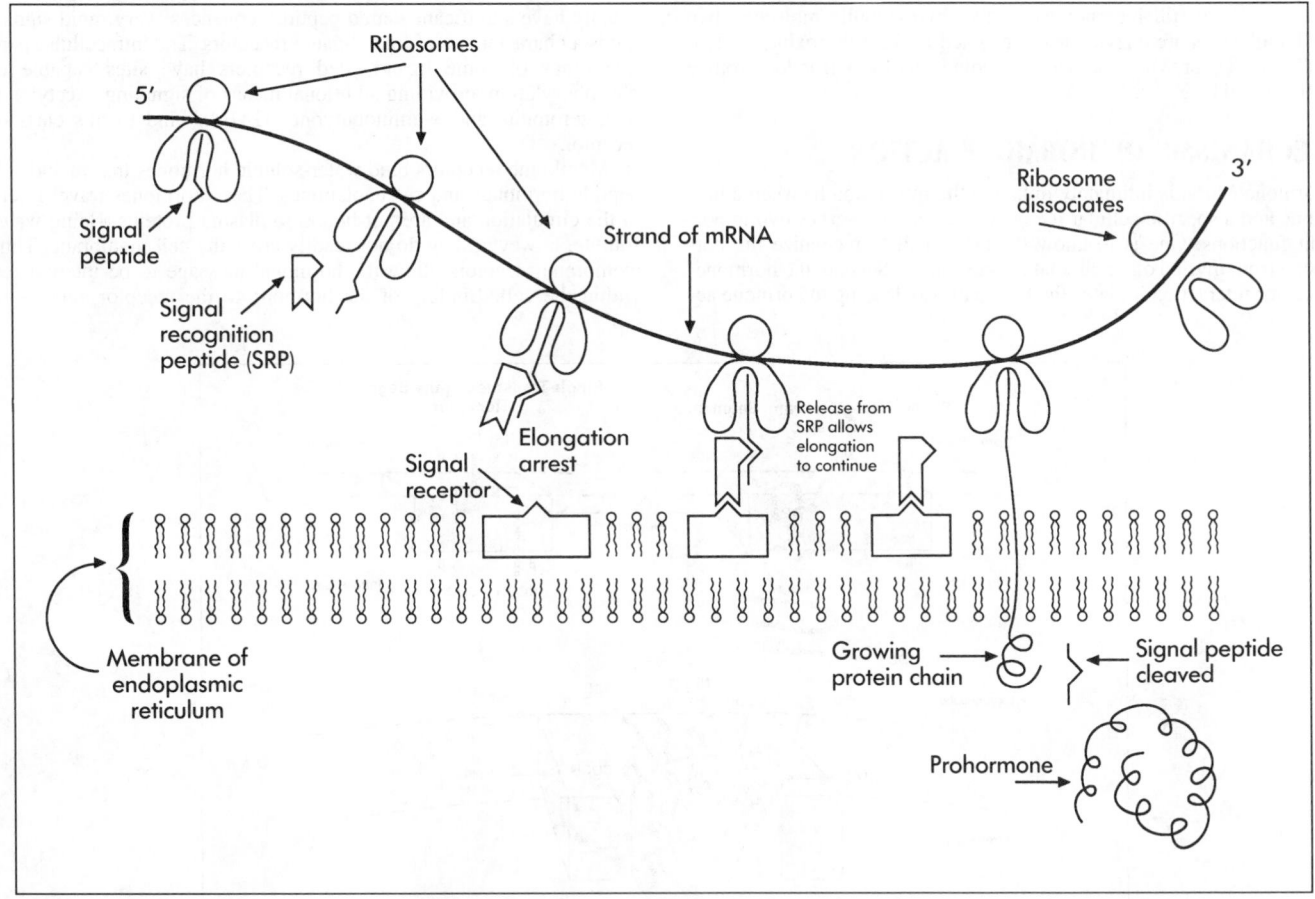

FIGURE 282-2 Process of peptide hormone synthesis. The protein chain is extruded from the ribosome complex until signal peptide combines with signal recognition peptide (SRP). This stops further elongation until SRP binds to the signal receptor on the surface membrane of the endoplasmic reticulum. This frees the peptide chain, allowing it to resume elongation. Signal peptide leads the protein chain through the membrane, and once it reaches the interior of the endoplasmic reticulum, signal peptide is cleaved. *SRP,* Signal recognition peptide.

The synthesis of the steroid vitamin D differs considerably from that of other steroid hormones in that transformation occurs in several different organs. Cholecalciferol (vitamin D) is either initially synthesized in the skin nonenzymatically by the action of ultraviolet radiation on 7-dehydrocholesterol or absorbed from the intestine. Vitamin D then is transported to the liver, where it is converted to a 25-hydroxylated product. This product is the major circulating form of the vitamin. Conversion to the most active vitamin D metabolite, 1,25-hydroxyvitamin D, occurs in the kidney.

Catecholamines

Catecholamines are synthesized from the amino acid tyrosine in nerves and in the adrenal medulla. The synthetic process involves hydroxylation and decarboxylation (removal of a COOH group) of tyrosine (Chapter 299). Tyrosine is first converted to dihydroxyphenylalanine by the rate-limiting enzyme tyrosine hydroxylase and then to dopamine by a decarboxylase. Dopamine enters granulated vesicles and is transformed to norepinephrine by dopamine β-hydroxylase. Tissues that contain phenylethanolamine N-methyl transferase (adrenal medulla, organ of Zuckerkandl, and some central nervous system neurons) are capable of converting norepinephrine to epinephrine.

Thyroid Hormone

Thyroglobulin is a large, 660,000-dalton protein produced by the thyroid follicular cell. This molecule contains more than 100 tyrosine residues that have a spatial orientation that makes them susceptible to iodination. Iodide is actively trapped by the follicular cell, oxidized to iodine, and then attached to tyrosine residues (*organification*). Either monoiodotyrosine (MIT) or diiodotyrosine (DIT) is formed, depending on whether one or two molecules are added to the tyrosine moiety. While still incorporated in the thyroglobulin molecule, two DIT molecules are enzymatically coupled to form thyroxine (DIT + DIT → T_4), or MIT and DIT are joined to form triiodothyronine (DIT + MIT → T_3).

MECHANISMS OF HORMONE ACTION

Hormone action is intimately linked to the interaction between a hormone and a specific cellular receptor. The receptor serves two important functions: One is to allow the target cell to recognize the hormone from myriad other circulating substances. Second, the hormone-receptor interaction initiates the final pathway leading to hormone action. At present, two broad categories of hormone receptors are recognized: receptors that reside on the cell membrane surface and receptors found in the interior of the cell.

Membrane Receptors

There are three general structural classes of glycoprotein cell surface membrane receptors (Fig 282-3). The largest family, with more than 100 species known, is the seven–transmembrane segment receptors. They are characterized by seven hydrophobic transmembrane segments that loop through the cell membrane, forming three intracellular loops and three extracellular loops. The N-terminus of the receptor protein is extracellular, whereas the C-terminus resides in the cytoplasm of the cell. The C-terminus region contains the domain capable of phosphorylation. The multiple extracellular loops form sites for stimulation and inhibition by circulating hormones. Glucagon, calcitonin, TSH, ACTH, LH, and FSH are hormones that signal through this class of receptors.

Another class of receptor contains only a single hydrophobic transmembrane component. These receptors are highly mobile and "float" on the lipid bilayer of the cell. Some are capable of being internalized. The external portion may have dual units connected by a disulfide bond or an IgG-like structure. The intracellular domain may have intrinsic tyrosine kinase activity (insulin, epidermal growth factor), serine-threonine kinase activity (inhibin, activin), or guanylate cyclase activity (atrial natriuretic peptide). Some receptors have no intrinsic enzymatic activity but become associated with a cytoplasmic tyrosine kinase (prolactin, growth hormone, erythropoietin).

The third class of surface receptors have four transmembrane segments. Several such subunits form a ligand-gated ion channel across a membrane, which facilitates the passage of Na^+, K^+, Ca^{2+}, and anions. The subunits forming the channel are not always identical but usually have significant shared peptide sequences. Very rapid signaling is a characteristic of ligand-gated receptors. The intracellular peptide loops of some ligand-gated receptors have sites capable of phosphorylation, providing additional means of signaling. Acetylcholine, serotonin, and γ-aminobutyrate (GABA) bind to this class of receptor.

Membrane receptors bind water-soluble hormones that include all peptide hormones and catecholamines. These hormones travel freely in the circulation and are not bound to plasma proteins. Being water soluble, however, they do not readily cross the cell membrane. Thus membrane receptors allow the hormonal message to be internalized within the cell. Binding of the hormone to the receptor appears to

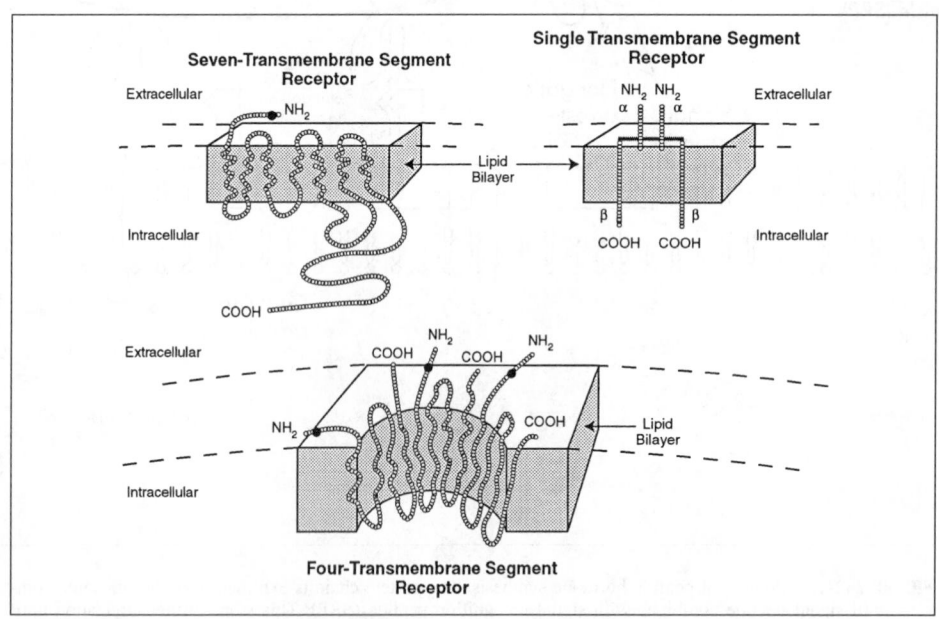

FIGURE 282-3   Structure of the three major classes of cell surface receptors. The four–transmembrane segment receptors may have several segments grouped together to form the boundaries of the membrane channel.

involve both hydrophobic and electrostatic interactions. This process is reversible, so receptors may be recycled and used more than once. In some instances the receptor-hormone complex is internalized, and at that point it is subject to degradation by cytoplasmic proteases.

Activation of Adenyl Cyclase

The translation of hormone messages involves a cascade of complex events illustrated in Fig. 282-4. The initial steps are hormone recognition by the receptor and formation of the hormone-receptor complex. This interaction increases the affinity of the hormone complex for a family of guanosine triphosphate (GTP) regulatory proteins called *G proteins* that bind and hydrolyze guanosine triphosphate (GTP). There are stimulatory (G$_s$) and inhibitory (G$_i$) G proteins. Both classes are heterotrimers composed of α-, β-, and γ-subunits. The β- and γ-subunits are identical in the stimulatory and inhibitory systems, whereas the α-subunits differ. In the absence of hormone being bound to the receptor, the G protein is kept inactive by the α-subunit binding guanosine diphosphate (GDP). When the hormone occupies the receptor, the α-subunit binds GTP and dissociates from the β-γ complex. The α-GTP stimulatory subunit then activates adenyl cyclase (the second messenger). The β-γ subunit also may activate other second messengers.

Once adenyl cyclase is activated, it catalyzes the conversion of adenosine triphosphate (ATP) to cyclic 3′5′-adenosine monophosphate. In the cytoplasm of the cell, cyclic AMP combines with regulatory subunits of cyclic AMP–dependent protein kinases, causing the subunits to dissociate from the enzyme, thereby activating the protein kinase. Activated protein kinase in turn catalyzes the phosphory-

lation of other enzymes or proteins by ATP, and this leads to an alteration of cell function in a hormone-specific fashion. Cyclic AMP activity is in part regulated by the cytoplasmic enzyme phosphodiesterase, which deactivates cyclic AMP by converting it to 5′-adenosine monophosphate.

The G$_i$ protein complex works in a parallel fashion and is activated by a separate hormone-receptor interaction. When the α-inhibitory subunit dissociates from the G$_i$ protein complex, however, it inhibits adenyl cyclase. This additional mechanism gives precise control over regulation of hormone action.

Calcium Mediation of Hormone Action

Not all hormones use adenyl cyclase as their intracellular messenger. Influx of Ca^{2+} plays an important role as an effector of hormone action (Fig. 282-5). One means by which intracellular Ca^{2+} concentration increases is by the hormone-receptor complex opening Ca^{2+} channels of the plasma membrane and allowing influx of extracellular Ca^{2+} into the cell along an electrochemical gradient. It is also possible that intracellular calcium bound by organelles is released. The increase in intracellular Ca^{2+} activates protein kinases and causes subsequent phosphorylation of protein as described for cyclic AMP. Although Ca^{2+} may directly activate some enzymes, most of the effects of Ca^{2+} are mediated through a low-molecular-weight, ubiquitous, intracellular protein called *calmodulin*. Calmodulin is a single-chain peptide structure with four binding sites for Ca^{2+}. After Ca^{2+} is bound to calmodulin, the protein undergoes conformational changes and becomes activated. Activated calmodulin becomes associated with calmodulin-sensitive enzymes such as protein kinases, and this

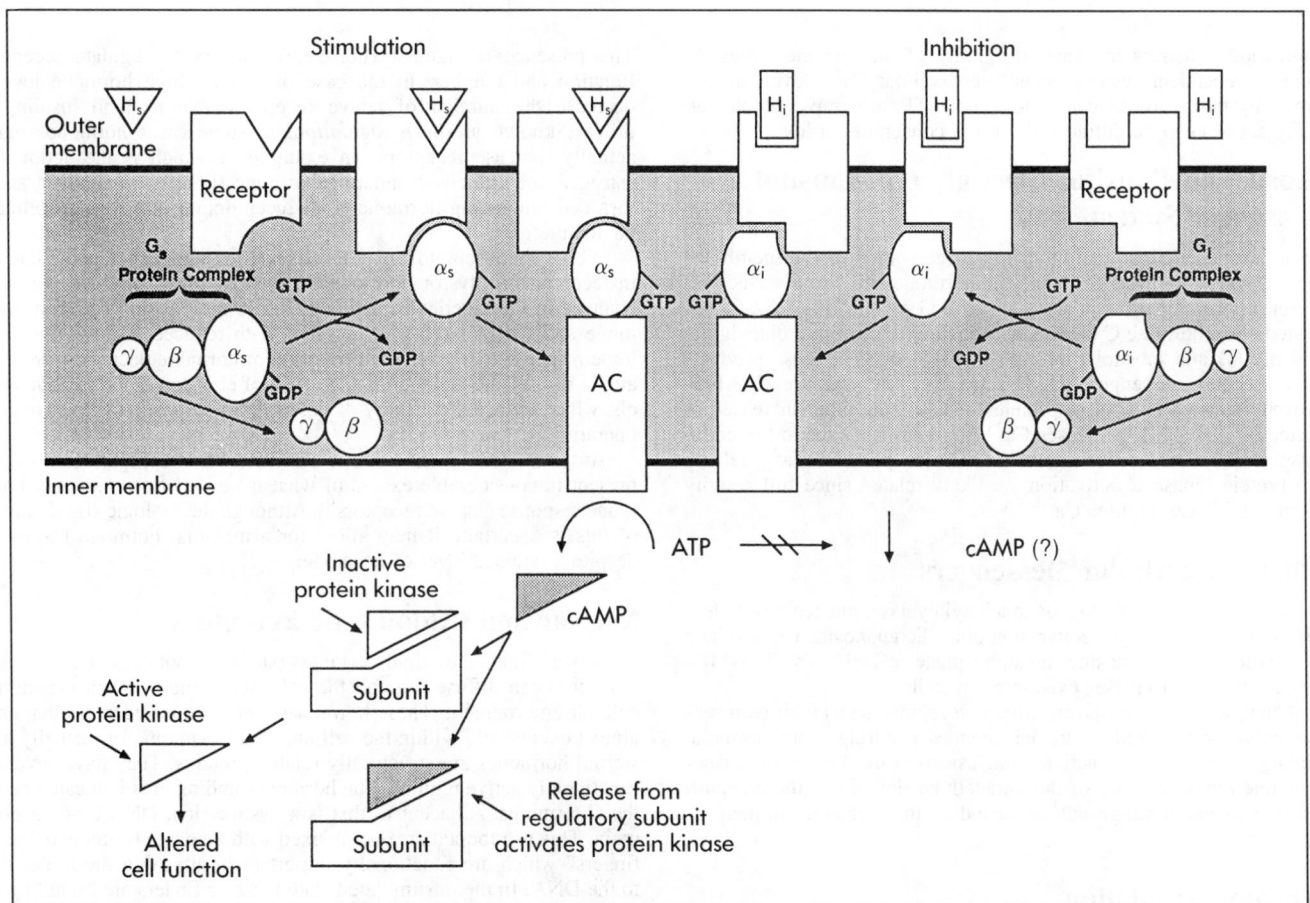

FIGURE 282-4   The multiple steps leading to stimulation and inhibition of adenyl cyclase and subsequent altered cell function (see text for discussion). The α-subunit of stimulatory G protein complex stimulates adenyl cyclase, whereas the α-subunit of inhibitory G protein complex decreases cyclic AMP formation. H$_s$, stimulatory hormone; H$_i$, inhibitory hormone; G$_s$, stimulatory G protein; G$_i$, inhibitory G protein complex; *AC*, adenyl cyclase.

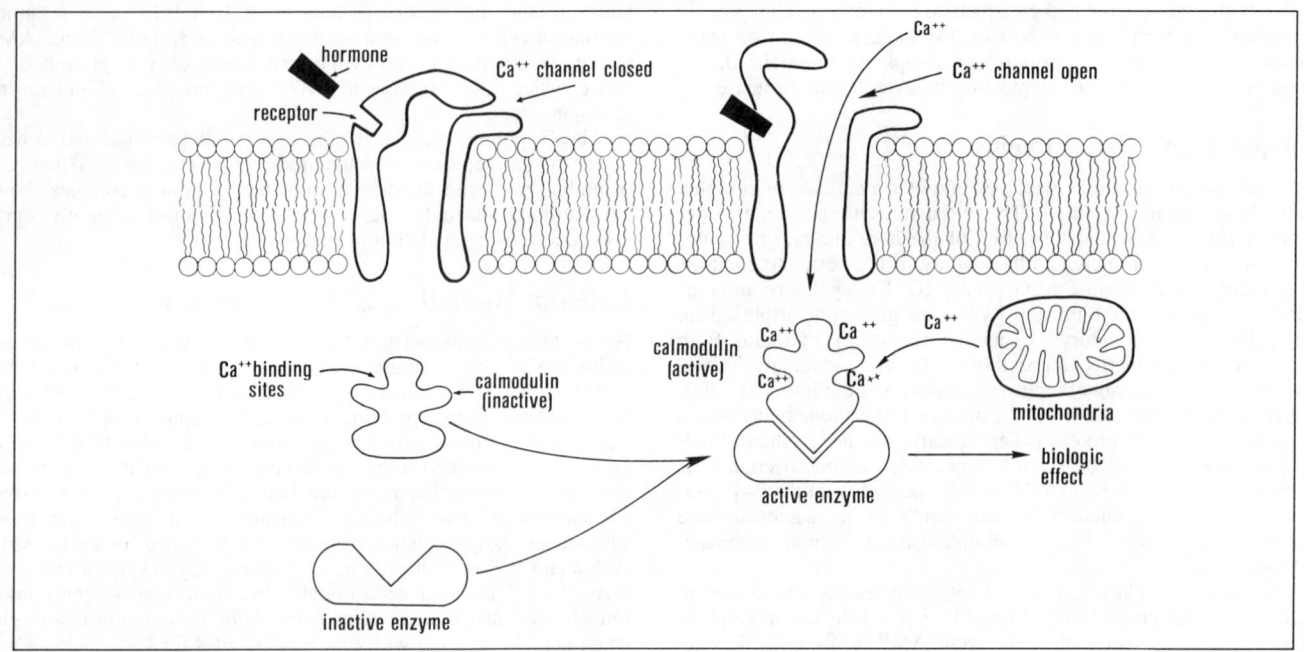

FIGURE 282-5 Schematic diagram showing a hormone stimulating calcium entry into the cell. Once inside the cell, calcium may bind to a ubiquitous regulatory protein, calmodulin, and activate it, which in turn activates protein kinase enzymes (see text for details).

From Kohler PO, Jordan RM, editors: *Clinical endocrinology,* New York, 1986, Wiley.

interaction enhances the catalytic ability of the enzyme. After the calcium-dependent activity occurs, intracellular Ca^{2+} levels are restored by the action of calcium-sodium ATPase pumps, which normally act to keep the intracellular Ca^{2+} concentration low.

Phosphatidylinositol-Diacylglycerol-Inositol Messenger System

Some hormones signal activity through activation of the membrane enzyme, phospholipase C. When the hormone binds to a surface receptor, phospholipase C is activated by a G protein (Fig. 282-6) Activated phospholipase C cleaves phosphatidylinositol into diacylglycerol (DAG) and inositol triphosphate (IP_3). Both of these products act as second messengers. DAG activates protein kinase C, which phosphorylates a number of proteins, resulting in either increased or decreased activity. IP_3 releases Ca^{2+} from storage sites in the endoplasmic reticulum and mitochondria. The coupling of Ca^{2+} release and protein kinase C activation are likely related since full activity of protein kinase requires Ca^{2+}.

Other Intracellular Messengers

Guanylate cyclase is analogous to adenyl cyclase, but seemingly less common. It catalyzes the conversion of cyclic guanosine triphosphate (cGTP) to cyclic guanosine monophosphate (cGMP). Cyclic GMP–dependent protein kinases exist in many cells.

A number of single transmembrane receptors act as their own second messengers. Conformational changes resulting from hormone binding to the receptor activate intrinsic tyrosine kinase or serine-threonine kinase activity of the intracellular domain of the receptor. Insulin and epidermal growth factor induce these changes in their receptors.

Receptor Regulation

Regulatory processes controlling the concentration of cell surface receptors are being elucidated. Receptors are proteins synthesized on the rough endoplasmic reticulum and processed in the Golgi apparatus and are transported via secretory vesicles to the plasma membrane. Because they are integral membrane proteins, receptors are subject to recycling processes and are continuously synthesized and degraded.

The presence of agonist (hormone) appears to regulate receptor function and number. In the case of insulin, high hormone levels decrease the number of active receptors able to bind insulin, a process known as *down regulation.* In some cases hormones may actually increase receptors, an example of which is the action of estrogen and follicle-stimulating hormone (FSH) to increase granulosa cell luteinizing hormone (LH) receptors during ovarian follicular maturation.

A concept different from reduced receptor number is that of change in receptor affinity for hormone. Alterations of affinity involve true changes in the kinetics of association and dissociation between hormone and receptor (H + R ~ HR). With reduced affinity, the biologic response to a given concentration of hormone decreases. An example of this phenomenon is the effect of elevated blood insulin levels, which reduce the affinity of the receptor for insulin (negative cooperativity).

An interesting observation is that membrane receptors are often present in considerable excess of what is needed for a maximal hormone response ("spare receptors"). Although the biologic significance of this is uncertain, it may allow for a maximal hormone response despite a reduced level of hormone.

Nuclear and Cytoplasmic Receptors

Hormones that are lipid soluble (steroids, vitamin D, thyroid hormone) can diffuse through the cell membrane to reach the intracellular environment. These hormones then bind to receptors that are almost exclusively within the cell nucleus. Receptors for virtually all steroid hormones are structurally related proteins. They have several functionally active regions. The hormone-binding area is located near the C-terminus. Adjacent to this is a cystine-rich, DNA binding domain. This is a looped area complexed with zinc and forms two "zinc fingers" which are functionally important in attaching the molecule to the DNA. In the unstimulated state the zinc fingers are bound by a specific protein. When the receptor binds a hormone, conformational changes occur, displacing the protein and the zinc fingers extend to bind with DNA. There are also areas that stimulate or repress gene transcription. The areas on the chromatin that respond to the hormone-receptor complex are called *hormone responsive elements* (HREs). The movement of this hormone-receptor complex to the nucleus is called *translocation.* In some manner the interaction of the hormone-

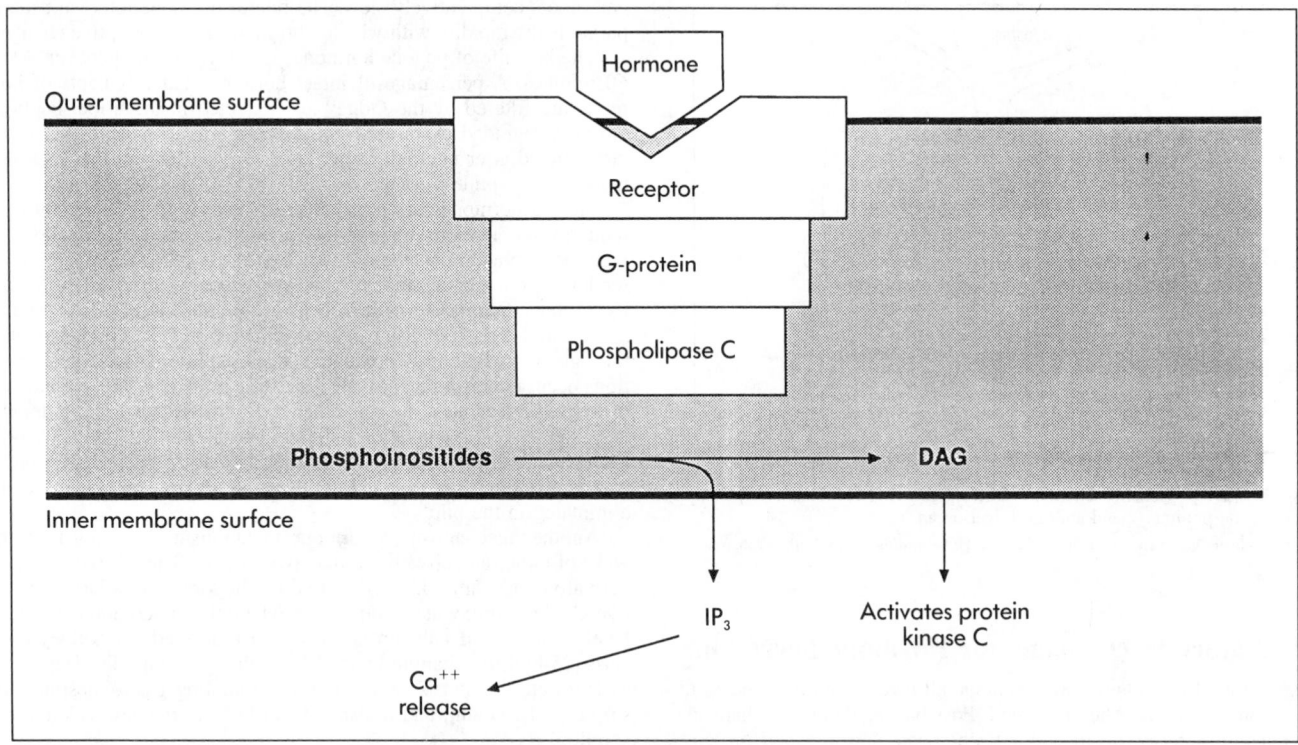

FIGURE 282-6   Activation of inositol triphosphate and diacylglycerol from phosphoinositides. Both IP₃ and DAG act as second messengers. *IP₃,* Inositol triphosphate; *DAG,* diacylglycerol.

receptor complex with the HREs facilitates transcription, possibly by making the specific gene more accessible to mRNA.

The nuclear receptors for thyroid hormone are similar to the steroid hormone receptors; however, these receptors are bound to chromatin while inactive. Triiodothyronine then displaces a co-repressor protein, inducing conformational changes, thereby activating the receptor-hormone complex leading to transcription and new protein synthesis. These receptors have high-affinity but low-capacity binding properties and bind T_3 better than T_4.

Our understanding of the regulatory processes governing nuclear and cytoplasmic receptors is incomplete. However, we know that progesterone is capable of reducing the concentration of its receptor. Progesterone also reduces the number of estrogen receptors. Estrogen, on the other hand, increases the synthesis of its own and progesterone receptors. Recycling and degradation mechanisms are poorly understood.

HORMONE SECRETION

Endocrine cells that store peptide or amine hormones in granules have a readily releasable pool of hormone. Granules are discharged in close temporal relationship with the appropriate stimulus *(stimulus-secretion coupling)* regardless of whether the stimulus is neural or hormonal. The process of secretion is dependent on an influx of calcium into the cell. In some cells the entry of ionic calcium causes contraction of a microfilament system that appears to be important in guiding hormone granules to the cell surface. At the surface, the storage vesicle surrounding the granule fuses with the plasma membrane, and the granule is expelled at the cell-capillary interface (exocytosis). For a number of endocrine cells, the stimulus for secretion causes new hormone synthesis. This phenomenon results in a biphasic release, an early pulse of stored hormone followed by a more sustained release of newly synthesized hormone.

In contrast to peptides and amines, steroids are secreted by simple bulk transfer, down concentration gradients from the gland to the blood. Steroid-producing cells store very little of their final product, and therefore, the stimulus for hormone release is linked to the stimulus for accelerated hormone synthesis.

Thyroid hormone secretion is unique. Substantial amounts of thyroid hormone are stored within the thyroid follicles attached to the colloid protein. Follicular colloid-containing thyroglobulin is engulfed by the projections from the follicular cells. Thyroglobulin isolated in this fashion is subjected to proteolysis with release of thyroid hormone. The thyroid hormone then diffuses out of the cell. In this case, the secretory process does not respond rapidly to a stimulus, distinguishing it from the stimulation-release relationship seen with peptide and amine hormones.

Hormone secretion does not occur at a uniform rate. Peptide and catecholamines in particular are released episodically. Feeding, fasting, or nonspecific stress may have stimulatory or inhibitory effects on hormone secretion. Sleep-related hormone release occurs with many hormones, including growth hormone and prolactin. Circadian variation, which is a self-sustaining repetitive fluctuation with a period of approximately 24 hours, is characteristic of ACTH release. In many clinical situations a knowledge of these variations may be crucial for accurate interpretation of blood hormone concentration levels.

Transport

Most hormones are transported at least some distance to their target organs. Usually transport occurs in blood, but lymph and cerebrospinal fluid may also be important transport media. Peptide hormones and catecholamines are water soluble and travel freely in these fluids. Lipid-soluble hormones (thyroid hormone and all steroid hormones), however, are transported in association with plasma carrier proteins. Many carrier proteins such as cortisol-binding globulin, thyroid-binding globulin, sex hormone–binding globulin, and vitamin D–binding globulin have a high affinity for a single hormone. Nonspecific, low-affinity binding also occurs, because most of the lipid-soluble hormones bind to albumin. The physiologic function of carrier proteins is uncertain. Binding is not necessary for hormone action to occur. In fact, it is the free hormone that initiates hormone-mediated activity. Carrier proteins possibly act to buffer sudden increases in hormone availability or serve as a reservoir by preventing rapid hormone degradation. Despite such plausible theories of function, an absence or excess of carrier proteins does not cause any apparent clinical disease.

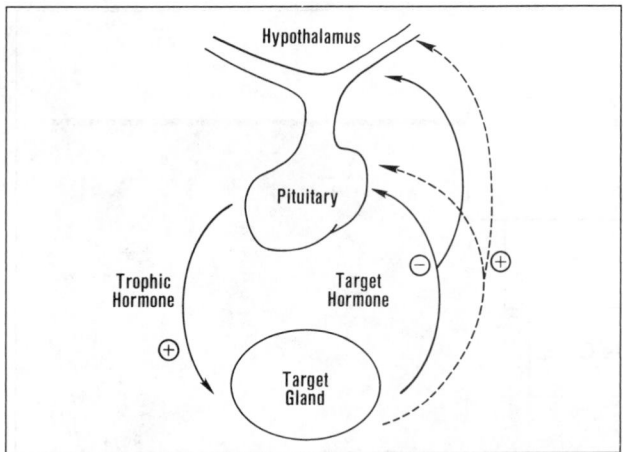

FIGURE 282-7 General schematic drawing showing feedback relationships between the pituitary gland and the target organ.
From Kohler PO, Jordan RM, editors: *Clinical endocrinology,* New York, 1986, Wiley.

Regulatory Mechanisms for Hormone Secretion

Regulation of hormone action occurs at all levels from the process of secretion to action at the target cell. Possible regulatory mechanisms by receptor activity, postreceptor phenomena, and transport proteins were mentioned in preceding sections.

Influences that directly stimulate hormone secretion can be divided into two broad categories: neural discharge and feedback regulation responding to changing blood levels of hormone or other chemical mediators. Although either variety of stimulus may occur independently of the other, more often they are coupled to control secretion.

Examples of neural-mediated hormone secretion are stress-induced release of pituitary hormones (ACTH, growth hormone, prolactin) via action of hypothalamic peptides, circadian release of ACTH, sleep patterns of growth hormone secretion, and nocturnal gonadotropin release during puberty. Vasopressin release after hypotension and oxytocin secretion after suckling are mediated by neural stimuli.

The most familiar example of a changing hormone level causing hormone secretion is that of feedback regulation (Fig. 282-7). In most instances, active secretion of a trophic hormone is inhibited by feedback suppression from the target hormone. There are numerous examples of this type of servomechanism in endocrinology, including regulation of thyroid-stimulating hormone (TSH), ACTH, and the gonadotropins by their respective target cell hormones. A nonhormonal mediator of feedback inhibition is calcium. Small changes in extracellular ionic calcium are quickly followed by reciprocal changes in parathyroid hormone secretion.

A more complex example of feedback regulation is the relationship between glucose and insulin. Elevation of the blood glucose level causes insulin release, which acts to return the glucose level to normal. Conversely, hypoglycemia decreases insulin secretion. Hypoglycemia, however, also triggers the release of insulin counterregulatory hormones (glucagon, epinephrine, cortisol, and growth hormone), which stimulate either glycogenolysis or glyconeogenesis, or both, in an active effort to increase the blood glucose concentration.

Feedback may be positive or negative. An example of positive feedback is the effect of estradiol on gonadotropin secretion at a specific time during the follicular phase of the human menstrual cycle. At this point in the cycle, estradiol levels reach a critical level for a sustained period, causing the midcycle LH and FSH surge. At other times estradiol feedback is negative. The exact mechanism by which such dual feedback occurs is not known.

Degradation of Hormone

To make adaptive changes to the environment, the endocrine system must be able to dispose of hormone as well as secrete it. Several mechanisms for hormone degradation exist, some of which are rapid

and others comparatively slow. The rate of hormone removal usually parallels the rapidity with which a hormone effects adaptive changes.

The half-life of peptide hormones is short, varying between 8 and 60 minutes. A percentage of intact hormone and fragments of hormone are filtered by the kidney and excreted in the urine. Peptides are also degraded by proteases and peptidases in plasma and at the target gland after internalization. Other organs such as the liver also metabolize peptides.

Steroid hormones are metabolized primarily in the liver through reductions, oxidations, hydroxylations, side chain cleavages, and conjugation to glucuronates and sulfates. These transformations not only render the compounds inactive but also increase their water solubility, thereby facilitating excretion in urine and bile. Catecholamines are cleared very rapidly from the circulation and are inactivated through methylation and oxidative deamination. These transformations occur either intraneuronally or extraneuronally. The degradation of thyroid hormone is accomplished by iodine removal via a deiodinase and also by conjugation with glucuronates and sulfates. Deiodinated metabolites are excreted in urine, whereas most of the conjugated metabolites are excreted in bile. Vitamin D metabolites also are eliminated in the bile.

Another mechanism of hormone metabolism is routing to pathways of either an active or an inactive product. The 25-hydroxylated derivative of vitamin D is converted by the kidney to a largely inactive 24,25-hydroxylated compound when the blood ionic calcium level is normal. If calcium conservation is needed, the kidney converts 25-hydroxyvitamin D to 1,25-hydroxyvitamin D. The 1,25-hydroxylate product is very active in promoting gastrointestinal absorption of calcium, and it also acts on bone to increase calcium resorption.

BIBLIOGRAPHY

Ascoli M, Segaloff DL: On the structure of the luteinizing hormone/chorionic gonadotropin receptor, *Endocr Rev* 10:27, 1989.

Brown MS, Anderson RGW, Goldstein JL: Recycling receptors: the round-trip itinerary of migrant membrane proteins, *Cell* 32:663, 1983.

Exton JH: Phosphinositide phospholipids and G proteins in hormone action, *Annu Rev Physiol* 56:349, 1994.

Goodman MH: *Basic medical endocrinology,* ed 2, New York, 1994, Raven.

Herbert E, Uhler M: Biosynthesis of polyprotein precursors to regulatory peptides, *Cell* 30:1, 1982.

Means AR, Chafouleas JG: Calmodulin in endocrine cells, *Annu Rev Physiol* 44:667, 1982.

O'Malley BW: Steroid hormone action in eukaryotic cells, *J Clin Invest* 74:307, 1984.

Rasmussen H: The calcium messenger system, *N Engl J Med* 314:1094, 1164, 1986.

Roth J, Taylor SI: Receptors for peptide hormones: alterations in disease of humans, *Annu Rev Physiol* 44:639, 1982.

Schulman H: The multifunctional Ca^{2+}/calmodulin-dependent protein kinase, *Curr Opin Cell Biol* 5:247, 1993.

Strader CD, Fong MF, Tota MR et al: Structure and function of G protein–coupled receptors, *Annu Rev Biochem* 63:101, 1994.

Tsai M-J, O'Malley BW: Molecular mechanisms of action of steroid/thyroid hormone receptor superfamily members, *Annu Rev Biochem* 63:451, 1994.

CHAPTER

283 Physiology of Bone and Mineral Homeostasis

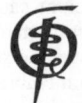

Gregory R. Mundy and Charles A. Reasner II

FUNCTIONS OF THE SKELETON

Bone is a unique mineralized connective tissue that comprises cortical or compact bone and trabecular or cancellous bone. Cortical bone makes up approximately 80% of the total skeleton and trabecular bone 20%. Conversely, trabecular bone is responsible for 80% of bone turnover, and cortical bone, which is metabolically much less active, accounts for only 20% of bone turnover. Cortical bone is present in the

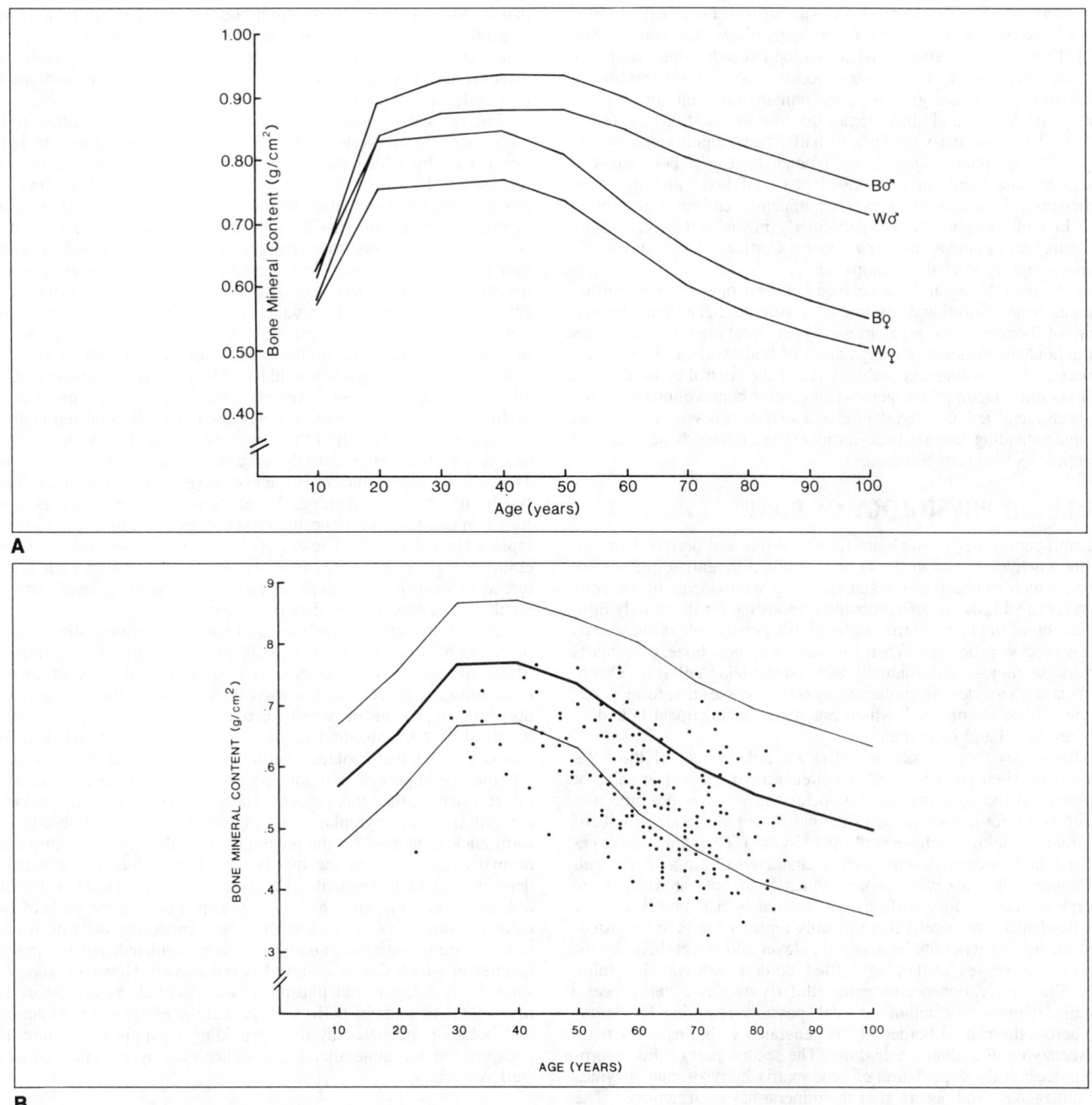

FIGURE 283-1   A, Relationship between bone mineral content (radial midshaft) and age. Note that males have higher bone mineral content than females and blacks have higher bone mineral content than whites; decline in bone mineral content is accelerated in females in the immediate post-menopausal years. **B,** Bone mineral content in white females with osteoporosis plotted in relation to age. The solid center line is the mean value for normal white females, and the outer line marks the 95% confidence limits. Each point represents an individual patient. Note that there is considerable overlap between normal individuals and patients with osteoporosis, although the majority of patients have a value below the mean normal value.

shafts of the long bones, whereas cancellous bone occurs in the vertebrae, ends of the long bones, and ribs. Bone not only provides structural support for the body but is the storehouse for 99% of the body's calcium, 80% of the phosphate, and substantial amounts of magnesium, sodium, and carbonate. Because the skeleton is a source of these ions, they are available when systemic deficiencies occur. When calcium deficiency occurs, bone resorption maintains the serum and tissue calcium supply but weakens the skeleton. Bone also provides a defense mechanism against systemic acidosis and assists renal and respiratory systems in maintaining acid-base balance. Bone resorp-

tion leads to release of additional phosphate and carbonate to buffer systemic acidosis.

NATURAL HISTORY OF THE SKELETON

Figure 283-1 illustrates the changes that occur in bone with aging. Throughout life bone is continually being resorbed and reformed at discrete sites throughout the skeleton. This process is known as *bone turnover* or *bone remodeling*. The total bone mass depends on the closely associated processes of bone resorption and bone formation, which are under the control of specialized bone cells called *osteoclasts* (for bone resorption) and *osteoblasts* (for bone formation). During adolescence, bone formation exceeds bone resorption, and an increase in bone mass occurs. Bone mass reaches a maximum after linear growth stops, remains constant for approximately 10 years, and then begins to fall in the third or fourth decade. The bone mass declines to half its maximum value by age 80 or 90 (age-related bone loss). Women have less bone mass at maximum and show an accelerated phase of bone loss just after menopause. This loss involves predominantly endosteal resorption with loss of cancellous bone, particularly in the vertebrae, without adequate replacement by new bone. Cortical bone mass also declines rapidly after the menopause.

Bone remodeling and the balance between rates of bone formation and bone resorption determine bone volume. Because the remodeling of bone occurs asynchronously at local and discrete sites throughout the skeleton, the regulation of bone volume, particularly trabecular bone volume, is probably under the control of local rather than systemic factors. The factors that control bone volume have not yet been identified. Clearly, their characterization is vitally important for understanding normal bone turnover, age-related bone loss, and osteoporosis (see later discussion).

CELLULAR PHYSIOLOGY OF BONE

Osteoprogenitor cells, which are fibroblast-like and derived from local mesenchymal cells in the bone marrow, differentiate into *osteoblasts,* which synthesize collagen and other components of the bone matrix. Osteoblasts are also probably responsible for the orderly mineralization of the bone matrix, although the precise role of these cells in this process is unclear. When surrounded by new bone, osteoblasts become *osteocytes* and gradually stop synthesizing collagen. Osteoblasts and osteocytes are connected by cell processes that form a continuous "bone membrane," which establishes a functional boundary between blood and bone mineral.

Osteoclasts (bone-resorbing cells) are independent of the bone membrane. Their precursor cell is a circulating mononuclear cell that originates in the bone marrow. Osteoclasts arise from the same precursor as the formed elements of the blood (colony-forming units of the granulocyte-macrophage series [CFU-GM]). They are highly specialized multinucleated cells with a characteristic area of the cell membrane called a *ruffled border,* which is the site at which bone resorption occurs. Bone surfaces are covered by a flattened layer of spindle-shaped lining cells that probably represent cells in the osteoblast lineage. Osteoclasts lie above this layer and resorb bone by insinuating processes containing ruffled borders between the lining cells. Bone resorption occurs extracellularly as a two-step process. Initially, it involves calcium removal, possibly requiring H^+ secretion across the ruffled border. H^+ is generated within osteoclasts by an isoenzyme of carbonic anhydrase. The second part of this resorption process is the degradation of bone matrix by lysosomal enzymes and collagenase and occurs after the mineral has been removed. The number and activity of osteoclasts are under hormonal regulation. Osteoclast formation and activity is stimulated by parathyroid hormone (PTH); parathyroid hormone–related protein (PTH-rP); vitamin D metabolites, prostaglandins E; cytokines, such as interleukin-1, interleukin-b, and tumor necrosis factor; thyroid hormones; and growth factors such as epidermal growth factor and the transforming growth factors. Osteoclast activation involves an increase in size and number of ruffled borders. Osteoclast activity is inhibited by calcitonin transiently, glucocorticoids (depending on the stimulus), plicamycin, oral phosphate, and the bisphosphonates. Osteoclast-like cells also resorb calcified cartilage and dentin.

MATRIX FORMATION AND CALCIFICATION

Bone organic matrix consists predominantly of type I collagen (about 95%), but it also contains acidic glycoproteins, sulfated proteoglycans, and a calcium-binding protein that contains γ-carboxyglutamic acid residues (called the *bone Gla protein* or *osteocalcin*). The function of the bone Gla protein is unknown, but its measurement is now being used as a marker of bone turnover (Chapter 286). It is synthesized by a cell in the osteoblast lineage, and it has been suggested

that its function may be to inhibit and thereby regulate bone matrix mineralization. The bone Gla protein constitutes about 20% of the noncollagen protein in bone. Other similar noncollagen proteins are osteonectin, osteopontin, and bone sialoprotein II. Their functions are also under investigation.

The cellular mechanisms by which bone is formed differ in different parts of the skeleton. Intramembranous bone formation is the mechanism by which the flat bones of the calvarium and face are formed and by which the width of the long bones is determined. In this process, bone formation begins with a condensation of an island of mesenchymal cells that differentiate into osteoblasts and produce surrounding new bone that enlarges circumferentially and gradually mineralizes. As the osteoblasts become buried in the new bone matrix, they become osteocytes. The mechanism of bone formation is entirely different in the long bone shafts. In these bones, bone formation begins on an anlage of cartilage. A collar of bone develops around this cartilage anlage to form the midshaft of the bone *(diaphysis).* The cartilage is formed by chondroblasts. The cartilage anlage is eventually penetrated by blood vessels and is gradually resorbed by multinucleated cells to form the marrow cavity. Specialized areas of the anlage near each end of the long bone contain hypertrophic chondrocytes and are known as the *epiphyseal plates* or *growth plates.* This area is responsible for continued increase in length of the bone. As the resorption of cartilage by multinucleated cells occurs, bone forms on cartilaginous trabeculae and is remodeled by osteoclasts and replaced by osteoblasts. The origin of these osteoblasts is unclear. This entire process is known as *endochondral bone formation.* It is disturbed in states of vitamin D deficiency, so that the growth plate expands and matrix mineralization is impaired.

One of the unique qualities of bone that distinguishes it from other connective tissues is that its protein matrix is mineralized. Mineralization of bone occurs only after several days of *osteoid maturation,* a process that involves secretion of the collagen and noncollagen proteins of bone by active osteoblasts. The precise steps involved in mineralization of this matrix are unclear, but cell-free matrix vesicles that contain alkaline phosphatase and other enzymes that may be important in producing increased local concentrations of mineral may initiate this process. These matrix vesicles are probably derived from the cytoplasm of osteoblasts and chondroblasts and form nucleation sites for the precipitation of the mineral required for normal calcification of the matrix. The bone mineral is eventually deposited as hydroxyapatite $[Ca_{10}(PO_4)_6(OH)_2]$ crystals within the *hole zones* of collagen, which are the gaps between the ends of two collagen molecules. It is clear that these processes of bone formation and mineralization must be carefully regulated, but the precise manner in which this is achieved is not known. However, adequate supplies of calcium and phosphate are essential, as are the active metabolites of vitamin D. It is likely that the effect of the vitamin D metabolites is mediated by their providing a supply of calcium and phosphate at the mineralizing site rather than by affecting mineralization directly.

STRESS AND COUPLING

Rates of skeletal growth are influenced by stress, and in particular by weight bearing. This may be mediated through a piezoelectric effect, which can be generated by compression or tension on collagen. Bone growth is also dependent on a number of hormones including growth hormone, insulin-like growth factor I (also called *somatomedin C*), insulin-like growth factor II, transforming growth factor B, bone morphogenetic proteins, the fibroblast growth factors, thyroid hormones, vitamin D metabolites, corticosteroids, and sex hormones.

Once the skeleton is formed, it is remodeled continuously by resorption of old bone in haversian canals and on the endosteal (trabecular) surfaces and by formation of new bone, which is deposited at these sites of resorption. The mechanism of this "coupling" of bone formation to bone resorption is unknown. This process of coupling of bone formation to bone resorption is the key event in bone that controls skeletal mass. Age-related bone loss is due to a relative increase in bone resorption over bone formation. When the factors and events that regulate this coupling are understood, it may be possible to understand the pathogenic events involved in age-related bone loss and other metabolic bone diseases.

CALCIUM METABOLISM
Distribution

Extracellular fluid calcium is a tightly controlled variable that has a number of vital functions. About 40% of the total calcium in the extracellular fluid is ionized or free and is closely regulated by homeostatic mechanisms. Of the total body calcium, 99% is distributed in bone, with the rest in soft tissue and the extracellular fluid. Ionized calcium in the extracellular fluid is regulated at the sites of calcium flux, which occur across the gastrointestinal tract, bone, and kidney. Precise regulation of extracellular ionized calcium concentration is necessary because ionized calcium influences a number of important metabolic processes including (1) cellular secretion of secretory proteins, hormones, and other products including neurotransmitters; (2) coupling between cell excitation and contraction, in the case of muscle cells, or secretion by secretory cells; (3) cell growth and division; (4) blood coagulation mechanisms, by acting as a cofactor for the enzymes involved in clotting; (5) maintenance of cell membrane stability and permeability; (6) regulation of enzyme activity including enzymes involved in glycogenolysis, gluconeogenesis, and protein kinases, which are calcium dependent; and (7) mineralization of newly formed bone. The mechanisms by which calcium influences these processes are unclear. However, movement of calcium ions into or out of the cytosol by regulated processes is clearly important.

The necessity for a precise regulatory mechanism to maintain the serum ionized calcium concentration between narrow limits is clear. When variations in the serum calcium concentration outside the normal range occur, disturbances in cell function result that can be anticipated from knowledge of the effects of ionized calcium on cell metabolic processes. For example, hypocalcemia is associated primarily with nerve conduction disturbances. Common symptoms include paresthesias, tetany, and convulsions. Hypercalcemia is also associated with disturbances in neuronal function. In severe hypercalcemia, patients may suffer from lethargy and impaired mental status; gastrointestinal disturbances including nausea, vomiting, and constipation; and disturbances in neuromuscular function characterized by muscle weakness and hypotonicity.

Intracellular calcium is distributed in subcellular compartments in a unique manner. Extracellular fluid calcium concentration is similar to the intramitochondrial calcium concentration (approximately 10^{-3}M). In contrast, the concentration of calcium in the cytosol is 1000 to 10,000 times less (10^{-6} to 10^{-7}M). It appears likely that there are separate active transport mechanisms responsible for pumping calcium from the cytosol into the extracellular fluid, into mitochondria, and possibly into microsomes. The mechanisms that are responsible for controlling fluxes of calcium across the plasma membrane and across the mitochondrial membrane are unclear but are clearly important for regulation of many important cellular events. Calcium is present in relatively high concentrations in the endoplasmic and sarcoplasmic reticula and is important for muscle contraction. During muscle excitation, the initial event is depolarization of the plasma membrane, which leads to release of calcium from the sarcoplasmic reticulum into the cytosol. Increases in cytosolic calcium in the muscle cell lead to conformational change in the protein troponin, which subsequently initiates the actin-myosin interaction, the basis of muscle contraction. Only small changes in cytosolic calcium concentration are required for excitation-response coupling in secretory cells. Excitation and depolarization of the plasma membrane are associated with entry of calcium from the exterior to the cytosol and with release of proteins stored within secretory granules. This may involve interactions with cyclic nucleotides and subsequent events, including facilitation of binding and fusion of secretory granules with the plasma membrane; activation of the tubulin-microtubule system, causing movement of secretory granules toward the cell exterior; and activation of specific adenosine triphosphatase (ATPase) enzymes involved in release of secretory granule contents to the exterior. In the gut and kidney, and possibly in bone, calcium is transported across cells to the extracellular fluid. The molecular mechanisms involved in entry of calcium into the cell, transcellular calcium transport, and exit from the cell are not clear. Calmodulin is a ubiquitous calcium-binding protein with a molecular mass of 7000 daltons that is present in all cells. It is an intracellular receptor protein for calcium that may be responsible for delivering calcium to spe-

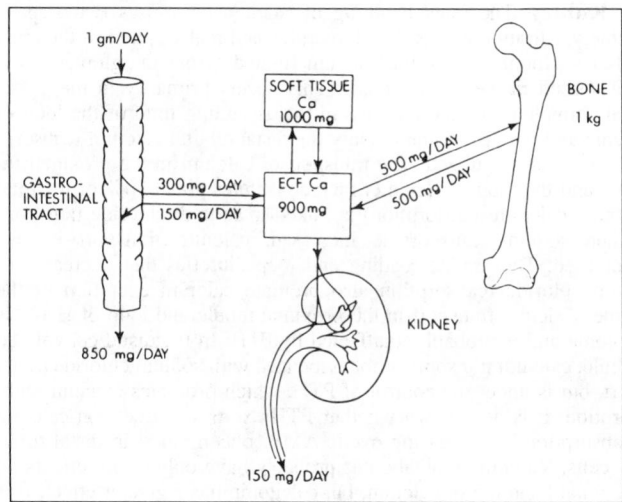

FIGURE 283-2 Major sites of calcium regulation and control of calcium homeostasis. Values are for a normal adult at zero calcium balance. Younger growing individuals show a higher percentage of absorption from the gut and bone resorption with net positive calcium balance.

From Mundy GR, Canalis EM, Raisz LG: *Conn Med* 40:680, 1976.

cific intracellular sites where calcium-regulated metabolic events occur. It is likely that the binding of calcium to calmodulin leads to specific conformational changes in the calmodulin molecule that in turn influence the way calmodulin interacts with specific target proteins, leading to changes in their activity.

Major Systems Controlling Extracellular Calcium Homeostasis

Extracellular fluid calcium is a closely guarded variable that is regulated within 5% of mean by hormonal control of calcium fluxes that occur across the gut, renal tubules, and bone (Fig. 283-2).

Gastrointestinal Tract. In the gastrointestinal tract, calcium is absorbed predominantly in the small bowel and excreted via the bile and pancreatic ducts. Calcium absorption from the gut occurs by two regulated processes, active calcium transport and facilitated diffusion. Secretion of calcium in the intestinal juices is probably unregulated but takes place mostly proximal to the sites of calcium absorption. The amount of calcium absorbed can vary from 20% to 70%, depending on the amount of calcium in the diet and vitamin D status. This adaptation of calcium transport to the available dietary calcium is probably mediated by 1,25-dihydroxyvitamin D. The variation in calcium absorption is less than the variation in dietary supply of calcium. The average American diet contains approximately 1000 mg calcium per day, although many elderly people ingest less. The highest rate of absorption of calcium occurs in the duodenum. However, calcium absorption also occurs in the ileum and jejunum, and because these segments of intestine are longer, the major part of calcium absorption takes place in these segments. Active calcium transport is associated with synthesis of a calcium-binding protein in intestinal cells whose activity is regulated by 1,25-dihydroxyvitamin D and that is probably important in the translocation of calcium across the gut wall. The active transport of calcium requires metabolic energy and is a saturable process. This indicates that a point can be reached when the addition of more calcium will yield no further increase in calcium transport. Calcium transport across the gut is inhibited by corticosteroids and by dietary components such as oxalate and phytate. It is decreased in patients with chronic renal failure and vitamin D deficiency. Parathyroid hormone (PTH) increases calcium absorption in the gut indirectly by increasing the synthesis of 1,25-dihydroxyvitamin D. Calcium absorption is increased in patients with vitamin D intoxication and the absorptive form of idiopathic hypercalciuria. Calcium absorption is also increased by dietary sugars such as lactose, and fatty acids.

Kidney. The renal handling of calcium comprises two steps—namely, filtration across the glomerulus and reabsorption in the renal tubules. About 99% of the calcium filtered across the glomerulus is reabsorbed in the renal tubules. This occurs primarily in the proximal convoluted tubule but also in the ascending limb of the loop of Henle and the distal tubule. Only the distal tubular calcium reabsorption is finely regulated. The transport of calcium in the proximal tubule and the loop of Henle (which constitutes about 90% of the total tubular calcium reabsorption) is linked to sodium chloride transport. When sodium transport is increased, calcium transport is also increased. Thus saline loading and loop diuretics that decrease sodium chloride reabsorption also promote calcium excretion in the urine. Calcium transport in the proximal tubule and loop of Henle is isotonic and is probably unaffected by PTH. In the distal convoluted tubule, calcium transport is not associated with sodium chloride transport, but is under the control of PTH, which promotes calcium reabsorption. It is not known whether PTH exerts its effects on calcium reabsorption by increasing cyclic AMP concentration in distal tubular cells. Vitamin D metabolites probably have only minor effects on the renal handling of calcium, but calcitonin has a greater effect. It is likely that part of the effect of calcitonin to lower serum calcium in hypercalcemic patients is due to increased renal calcium excretion. Thiazide diuretics decrease calcium excretion, probably by direct effects on increasing calcium reabsorption in the loop of Henle and the distal segments.

Bone. Increases in osteoclast activity cause release of bone calcium into the extracellular fluid. This process is stimulated by PTH and 1,25-dihydroxyvitamin D and is inhibited by calcitonin. The effects of these three systemic hormones are regulated by negative feedback controls. There are other hormonal factors that stimulate or inhibit bone resorption, but the effects of these factors on bone do not appear to be regulated. The effects of bone resorption and bone formation on maintenance of extracellular fluid calcium concentration are considered in more detail later.

Parathyroid Hormone

Synthesis and Secretion. Parathyroid hormone is an 84–amino acid, single-chain polypeptide hormone that is secreted by the chief cells of the parathyroid glands. The PTH gene product is a larger precursor molecule called *prepro-PTH* composed of 110 amino acids and having a molecular weight of about 13,000. This precursor is rapidly processed in the rough endoplasmic reticulum to a smaller molecule known as *pro-PTH*, which is a linear peptide of 90 amino acids with a molecular weight of approximately 10,000. Within the Golgi zone, pro-PTH is further processed to native PTH (1-84), which is stored in secretory granules in the parathyroid cells and released from the parathyroid cells in response to a fall in the ionized calcium concentration bathing the parathyroid glands. The hormone that is secreted by the glands is further cleaved in the periphery by the kidneys and liver into smaller fragments. The amino-terminal (or N-terminal) fragments comprise the biologically active moiety of the molecule. The first 34 amino acids of the molecule are required for biologic activity. The carboxyl-terminal (C-terminal) fragments are biologically inert.

Biosynthesis and release of PTH are regulated by the extracellular fluid calcium concentration. A fall in calcium concentration stimulates PTH secretion, and an increase inhibits it. The molecular mechanism responsible for sensing extracellular fluid calcium concentration has recently been identified as a G protein–linked 7-membrane spanning protein (the calcium sensor). PTH secretion is also stimulated by adrenergic agonists, prostaglandins of the E series, and, acutely, by falls in magnesium ion concentration. The physiologic significance of these latter stimuli is unknown. PTH secretion is inhibited by severe magnesium depletion of chronic duration and by active vitamin D metabolites.

Biologic Effects. Parathyroid hormone affects calcium and phosphate fluxes in the bone, kidneys, and gastrointestinal tract. In *bone*, the major effect of PTH in vivo is to increase bone turnover, to stimulate osteoclastic bone resorption, and to increase new bone formation. In vitro, PTH inhibits bone collagen synthesis, so that the effects observed in vivo may be indirect and secondary to the effects

on osteoclastic bone resorption. It is likely that the effects of PTH to increase bone resorption are not mediated directly by an action on the osteoclasts but through an intermediate cell. Although the effects of PTH on the osteoblast may be mediated by cyclic AMP, it is still not clear that PTH acts on osteoclastic bone resorption through this second messenger. When PTH is administered intermittently in pharmacologic doses, it causes an increase in bone formation on trabecular bone surfaces. This "anabolic" effect is being utilized experimentally as a potential therapy for diseases of bone loss such as osteoporosis.

In the kidney, PTH increases renal tubular reabsorption of calcium and decreases urinary calcium excretion relative to the filtered load. It also decreases renal tubular reabsorption of phosphate, leading to renal phosphate wasting. Both of these effects are probably mediated by cyclic AMP. The major regulatory effect of PTH on calcium and phosphate handling by the renal tubules occurs at the distal tubule site. Parathyroid hormone has other effects on the kidneys, including inhibition of renal tubular bicarbonate reabsorption in the proximal tubule and stimulation of the complex renal 1-hydroxylase enzyme, which leads to increased production of 1,25-dihydroxyvitamin D.

Parathyroid hormone's effects on the *gut* are indirect. PTH causes increased absorption of calcium from the gut indirectly through its effects on the kidney to increase synthesis of 1,25-dihydroxyvitamin D.

PTH mediates its effects on target organs via a receptor that has recently been identified and molecularly cloned. The receptor is a transmembrane protein that appears to be related to the calcitonin receptor structurally and activates both adenylate cyclase and the phosphoinositol pathway signaling mechanisms.

The overall effect of PTH therefore is to increase the serum calcium concentration and decrease the serum phosphorus level because of its combined effects on the gut, kidney, and bone.

Calcitonin

Synthesis and Secretion. Calcitonin is a 32–amino acid peptide that is synthesized and secreted by the parafollicular cells of the thyroid. In birds, fish, and reptiles, these cells form a separate organ known as the *ultimobranchial gland.* The calcitonin gene encodes a larger molecular species than the secreted form known as *procalcitonin.* In humans, this molecule has a molecular weight of about 17,500. The calcitonin molecule has a proline-amide group at the carboxyl-terminal and a disulfide bridge linking amino acids 1 and 7 from the amino-terminal, which is necessary for biologic activity. The major circulating form is the calcitonin monomer or 32–amino acid molecule. It is metabolized predominantly in the kidney. The plasma half-life of calcitonin is approximately 5 minutes.

The calcitonin gene also encodes another recently described peptide known as *CGRP* (the *calcitonin gene-related peptide*), whose physiologic function at the present time is unknown, but which is secreted mole for mole with calcitonin. CGRP has potent effects on vascular smooth muscle. It also inhibits bone resorption but is much less potent than calcitonin. Cells other than the thyroid parafollicular cells can synthesize calcitonin. Biologically inert calcitonin may be synthesized by certain nonthyroid tumors, and there is some evidence for calcitonin secretion in the brain. The physiologic significance of extrathyroidal calcitonin production is unknown.

Calcitonin is released from the thyroid parafollicular cells in response to an increase in extracellular fluid calcium or by the action of gastrointestinal hormones including gastrin, glucagon, secretin, and cholecystokinin-pancreozymin. Gastrin is the most potent of these secretagogues. Calcitonin release from the parafollicular cells is inhibited by a fall in serum calcium concentration.

Biologic Effects. The precise physiologic role of calcitonin is still unknown. Calcitonin's most prominent effect is to inhibit osteoclastic bone resorption, which it does rapidly and effectively. Calcitonin inhibits all stages of osteoclast differentiation from its precursors, decreases the activity of preformed osteoclasts, and causes the dissolution of osteoclasts into mononuclear cells. Calcitonin's effects on inhibiting osteoclastic bone resorption are transient, and this loss of responsiveness in the continued presence of calcitonin (known as the *escape phenomenon*) may be due to *down regulation* (decreased calcitonin receptor number or binding of calcitonin in the continued presence of calcitonin). Therefore in patients with an absence of calcitonin-secreting cells (after thyroidectomy) and in patients with medullary thyroid carcinomas who have markedly increased circulating concentrations of calcitonin, there are no clear abnormalities in either bone cell function or in calcium homeostasis.

It has been postulated that calcitonin is required to protect the body against postprandial hypercalcemia and to protect the growing or maternal skeleton from continued bone resorption when calcium is being absorbed from the gut after a calcium-rich meal. Calcitonin has no major effects on bone formation, on vitamin D metabolism, or on absorption of calcium from the gut. Patients with medullary thyroid carcinoma and excess calcitonin secretion may have diarrhea caused by increased secretion of fluid and electrolytes in the small intestine. The precise mechanism is unclear.

The gene for the calcitonin receptor has also recently been molecularly cloned. The calcitonin receptor belongs to the same family of receptors as PTH; it is a transmembrane receptor protein that mediates its effects through adenylate cyclase.

Calcitonin receptors have been described on many cells outside bone including many tumor cells, lymphocytes, and neuronal cells. The physiologic or pathologic significance of these extraosseous receptors is entirely unknown. Calcitonin has been used as a therapeutic agent in diseases associated with increased bone resorption, including Paget's disease, hypercalcemia, and osteoporosis. It is a very useful agent in Paget's disease, is effective in hypercalcemia when used in association with glucocorticoids (which inhibit bone resorption), and may be of slight benefit in some patients with osteoporosis and increased rates of bone resorption. The form of calcitonin that has been most widely used in treatment is salmon calcitonin, which is biologically very potent. Eel and human calcitonin are also now used in different countries and have similar biologic effects.

Vitamin D

Synthesis and Metabolism. The vitamin D metabolites are a group of steroid-like compounds known as *sterols* that are derived exogenously from plant ergosterol in the diet or endogenously from 7-dehydrocholesterol in the skin.

Vitamin D_3 is synthesized in the skin by the action of ultraviolet light on 7-dehydrocholesterol (previtamin D_3) in epidermal cells. This process occurs in several intermediate steps that are not enzyme controlled. Vitamin D_3 synthesized in the skin is absorbed in the small intestine and is transported in the plasma bound to a carrier protein known as the *vitamin D–binding protein.* An additional major source of vitamin D in humans is the diet. Plant ergocalciferol (previtamin D_2) is analogous to 7-dehydrocholesterol and is converted to vitamin D_2 by exposure to ultraviolet irradiation. The subsequent metabolism and biologic activity of the active forms of vitamin D_2 (from plant origins) and vitamin D_3 (from synthesis in the skin) are identical in humans. In the liver, vitamin D undergoes the first metabolic step that involves biologic activation. Here it is hydroxylated in the 25 position to 25-hydroxyvitamin D, which is the major circulating form of the sterol. 25-Hydroxyvitamin D is transported in the plasma bound to the vitamin D–binding protein to the kidney, where it undergoes a number of further hydroxylation steps. The major biologically active metabolite produced by the kidney is 1,25-dihydroxyvitamin D, which is the most potent and rapid acting of all the vitamin D metabolites. The other major renal metabolite of vitamin D metabolism is 24,25-dihydroxyvitamin D. Whether it has any important biologic effects is still controversial.

Vitamin D metabolism is carefully regulated. Synthesis in the skin is influenced by sunlight exposure, and there are seasonal variations in the circulating concentrations of 25-hydroxyvitamin D. Synthesis in the skin is greatest in summer in persons exposed to the sun. However, it is not clear whether degree of skin pigmentation has a major effect on vitamin D_3 production. The 25-hydroxylation process in the liver is not well understood. This activation process does not appear to be tightly regulated. When availability of substrate vitamin D is high (excess sunlight exposure, excess vitamin D ingestion), there is increased production of 25-hydroxyvitamin D, and when substrate availability is low, production is decreased. Thus measurement of circulating 25-hydroxyvitamin D is a reliable index of vitamin D supply.

In contrast, 1-hydroxylation in the kidney is carefully controlled by ambient phosphate concentration and PTH. In addition, there possibly is regulation by sex hormones and prolactin. However, the major regulators of 1-hydroxylation are PTH and phosphate. Dietary phosphate deprivation causes increased activity of the 1-hydroxylase reaction by mechanisms that are unclear. Parathyroid hormone stimulates the 1-hydroxylation mechanism by a direct effect. Thus the effect of a decrease in dietary phosphate or serum phosphate concentration is to increase production of 1,25-dihydroxyvitamin D. The renal 1-hydroxylase is a complex mitochondrial p450 cytochrome enzyme system that is present in the proximal convoluted tubule of the kidney. Other extrarenal 1-hydroxylation enzyme systems have been described in the placenta, bone, and chronic inflammatory cells. The physiologic significance of extrarenal 1-hydroxylation is not clear, but this mechanism is probably important in diseases such as sarcoidosis in which 1-hydroxylation does occur outside the kidney and leads to hypercalcemia.

The 24-hydroxylase system is much less well described. It is present in the proximal convoluted tubule and is stimulated by 1,25-dihydroxyvitamin D. 25-Hydroxyvitamin D is metabolized in the kidney and possibly other sites to 24,25-dihydroxyvitamin D. Whether 24,25-dihydroxyvitamin D has a physiologic role remains unknown. It may merely represent an alternative inactivation pathway to the 1-hydroxylase pathway. Both 1,25-dihydroxyvitamin D and 24,25-dihydroxyvitamin D are converted to 1,24,25-trihydroxyvitamin D. 1,24,25-Trihydroxyvitamin D is further metabolized by removal of a side chain to form calcitroic acid. How these degradation pathways are controlled is presently unknown, but the overall process resembles the formation of bile acids from cholesterol.

The vitamin D metabolites are bound to serum proteins in the circulation, like other steroids and sterols. The major serum transport protein is an α_2-globulin known as the *vitamin D–binding protein,* the *group-specific component,* or *Gc protein.* 1,25-Dihydroxyvitamin D is also probably bound to glycoproteins in the circulation. The circulating forms of the sterols are more than 99% bound to transport proteins. The concentration of the metabolites of vitamin D_3 is higher than that of vitamin D_2 in human subjects. Vitamin D_3 and vitamin D_2 probably have identical biologic activity. Vitamin D_2 and vitamin D_3, 25-hydroxyvitamin D, 1,25-dihydroxyvitamin D, and 24,25-dihydroxyvitamin D are all conjugated in the liver to form glucuronides and sulfates that have enterohepatic circulation.

Biologic Effects. 1,25-Dihydroxyvitamin D is the major active metabolite of vitamin D. 25-Hydroxyvitamin D is biologically active but has only one thousandth the activity of 1,25-dihydroxyvitamin D. Vitamin D itself is inactive biologically and can be regarded as a prohormone. The vitamin D metabolites increase the absorption of calcium and phosphate from the gut into the blood by active transport. They also increase bone resorption by stimulating osteoclast activity. The overall effect is to increase serum concentrations of calcium and phosphorus. In the absence of vitamin D or in conditions of impaired vitamin D metabolism, there is a failure of mineralization of newly formed bone with subsequent development of the metabolic bone disease known as *rickets* (children) or *osteomalacia* (adults). 1,25-Dihydroxyvitamin D corrects this failure to mineralize newly formed bone. It is still controversial whether it does this solely by providing a supply of calcium and phosphate that is available at the mineralizing site or whether the active metabolites of vitamin D are also required to stimulate the osteoblast to mineralize bone normally. However, recent data suggest that the former is the more likely mechanism.

1,25-Dihydroxyvitamin D causes the kidney to stimulate calcium and phosphate reabsorption. It also increases 24-hydroxylase activity, which may be a major step in inactivation. The renal effects of 1,25-dihydroxyvitamin D are probably relatively unimportant compared with its bone and gut effects.

Recent studies have shown that 1,25-dihydroxyvitamin D affects osteoclast activation differently than other hormonal stimulators of bone resorption such as PTH or the prostaglandins. 1,25-Dihydroxyvitamin D seems to be an important factor in stimulating fusion and differentiation of osteoclast progenitors into mature osteoclasts, in addition to causing activation of preformed osteoclasts. It also has significant local effects in the bone marrow microenvironment on modulating immune responses and inhibiting lymphocyte activation. It inhibits lymphocyte mitogenesis and production of the lymphokine interleukin 2 but can stimulate production of the bone-resorbing monokine interleukin 1 in some systems. These local inter-actions between the vitamin D metabolites, immune cells, and oste-oclasts and their progenitors may be very important factors in our understanding of normal bone cell metabolism and function and con-stitute an active area of current research.

The vitamin D receptor has recently been characterized and mo-lecularly cloned. It belongs to the same family of receptors as all of those for the steroid hormones, as well as those for retinoic acid and thyroid hormones. Recent observations have shown that point muta-tions in the vitamin D receptor are responsible for some inherited forms of rickets associated with vitamin D resistance. More recent studies have suggested that polymorphisms in the vitamin D receptor are a major genetic determinant of bone mass, which in turn is a de-terminant of risk of osteoporosis.

OTHER HORMONES AFFECTING CALCIUM HOMEOSTASIS AND THE SKELETON

1. *Growth hormone and somatomedin C.* Growth hormone acceler-ates skeletal growth, partly through somatomedin C (also called *insulin-like growth factor I*), which stimulates protein synthesis and sulfation in cartilage. Somatomedin C also stimulates bone collagen synthesis directly.

2. *Thyroxine and triiodothyronine.* The thyroid hormones stimulate bone turnover and are required for normal skeletal growth and bone remodeling. They have a direct effect on bone similar to that of PTH, which probably explains the osteopenia and hypercalce-mia that occasionally occur in hyperthyroidism. Patients with hy-perthyroidism have increased renal tubular phosphate reabsorption and may have hyperphosphatemia, increased serum alkaline phos-phatase concentration, and increased urine hydroxyproline excre-tion.

3. *Glucocorticoids.* Glucocorticoids can inhibit both bone formation and bone resorption directly in pharmacologic doses; this charac-teristic may explain their causing osteoporosis when used chroni-cally. Their inhibitory effect on osteoclastic bone resorption ex-plains the lowering of the serum calcium level seen in some pa-tients with hypercalcemia of malignancy treated with these agents. However, bone resorption may be increased in humans with prior normal calcium homeostasis who are treated with glucocorticoids because of (1) impaired calcium absorption in the gut, which leads to secondary hyperparathyroidism, and (2) direct stimulation of PTH secretion. The effect on the intestinal mucosa in inhibiting calcium absorption may be direct or may be due to impaired me-tabolism of vitamin D. The overall increase in bone resorption and decrease in bone formation cause decreased bone mass and osteo-porosis.

4. *Estrogens and androgens.* The sex steroids, especially estrogens if they are given to females around the time of menopause, stimu-late skeletal maturation and epiphyseal closure at puberty and can prevent loss of bone mass in adults. Inhibition of bone resorption by estrogens and androgens has been postulated but has never been demonstrated directly. Their effects on bone may be indirect and may be mediated by changing the concentrations of other hormones such as PTH or cytokines such as interleukin 1 and in-terleukin 6.

5. *Insulin.* Insulin stimulates bone collagen synthesis in vitro. In pa-tients with diabetes mellitus, osteopenia frequently develops and this may be due in part to insulin lack. It is likely that these ef-fects of insulin are mediated through the insulin-like growth fac-tor I receptor.

6. *Epidermal growth factor and related peptides.* Epidermal growth factor and a family of related peptides produced by tumors and some normal tissues have important effects on bone. The tumor-derived growth factors, platelet-derived growth factor (PDGF), and transforming growth factor-α (TGFα) stimulate bone resorption in vitro and may play a role in bone destruction associated with some solid tumors. In addition, these factors are present in the normal embryo and may be important for skeletal modeling during growth and remodeling during wound and fracture repair.

7. *Growth regulatory factors stored in bone.* Recent observations have shown that the bone matrix is a repository for a number of powerful bone growth regulatory factors. These include transform-

ing growth factor-β (TGF-β), insulin-like growth factors I and II, the fibroblast growth factors (FGF), and a newly described family of growth factors that are related to TGF-β called the *bone mor-phogenetic proteins* (BMP). These factors cause the formation of new bone when injected into subcutaneous tissue in vivo and may be important in endochondral bone formation, fracture repair, and repair of bone defects. The expression of the BMP family by bone cells is important in normal osteoblast differentiation, and in em-bryonic life for determining skeletal shape and size. Observations in mice have shown that in particular BMP-5 and GDF-5 (another member of the BMP family) are important for normal skeletal pat-terning, but it seems likely that other members of this family will also be implicated as further research is performed. Recent obser-vations in mice and patients with rare skeletal diseases have also shown that the FGF family is required for normal skeletal devel-opment. In achondroplasia, which is a common disorder of limb development, there is a mutation in one of the receptors for the FGF family, FGF receptor 3. Other less common inherited diseases of skeletal development such as Jackson-Weiss disease and Crou-zon syndrome are associated with point mutations in other FGF receptors.

8. *Local hormones* (cytokines).

   a. *Prostaglandins* produced by chronic inflammatory cells stimu-late bone resorption and may mediate localized bone loss in periodontal disease, rheumatoid arthritis, and certain neo-plasms. These locally acting factors are produced by cells found at sites of chronic inflammation such as macrophages.

   b. *Osteoclast-activating factor (OAF)* is a potent stimulator of bone resorption that is produced by activated lymphocytes. OAF does not represent one molecule but is probably composed of the cytokines interleukin 1, interleukin 6, lymphotoxin, and tumor necrosis factor, which have recently been purified and molecularly cloned. These cytokines are potent bone-resorbing factors in vitro and in vivo. In multiple myeloma, which is usu-ally associated with bone destruction and often with hypercal-cemia, the malignant cells secrete these and related cytokines.

   c. *Parathyroid hormone–related protein (PTH-rP)* is a peptide produced by many squamous cell carcinomas associated with the hypercalcemia of malignancy. PTH-rP activates the PTH re-ceptor and has many of the same biologic effects on bone and kidney in patients with cancer as PTH. However, PTH-rP also has an important role at the growth plate in normal embryonic life. Absence of PTH-rP expression in mice is associated with abnormally increased rates of endochondral ossification caused by enhanced cartilage cell differentiation. Activating mutations of the PTH-PTH-rP receptor in humans (Janssen disease) is also associated with growth plate abnormalities and disturbances of limb growth.

   d. Other local factors in the bone cell microenvironment may play a role in osteoclast generation and activity. These include γ-interferon and transforming growth factor-β (TGF-β), which inhibit osteoclast activity, and monocyte-macrophage colony-stimulating factor (M-CSF), which increases osteoclast forma-tion. Deficient M-CSF production has been shown to cause os-teopetrosis in mice during the neonatal period. In this regard, it is possible that 1,25-dihydroxyvitamin D can also be consid-ered a local hormone. There have been indications (not yet con-firmed) that it could be produced by cells in the bone marrow microenvironment. If this turns out to be true, this sterol may also be important in controlling local osteoclast differentiation as well as in modulating immune function.

BIBLIOGRAPHY

Agus ZS, Goldfarb S, Wasserstein A: Calcium transport in the kidney, *Rev Physiol Bio-chem Pharmacol* 90:155, 1981.

Eisman J: Vitamin D metabolism. In Mundy GR, Martin TJ, editors: *Physiology and phar-macology of bone: handbook of experimental pharmacology, Berlin, 1993,* Springer-Verlag.

Erlebacher A, Filvaroff EH, Gitelman SE et al: Toward a molecular understanding of skeletal development, *Cell* 80:371-378, 1995.

Garrett IR et al: Production of the bone resorbing cytokine lymphotoxin by cultured hu-man myeloma cells, *N Engl J Med* 317:526, 1987.

Hauschka PV et al: Growth factors in bone matrix, *J Biol Chem* 261:12665, 1986.

Hirsch PF, Munson PL: Thyrocalcitonin, *Physiol Rev* 49:548, 1969.

Hughes MR et al: Point mutations in the human vitamin D receptor gene associated with hypocalcemic rickets, *Science* 242:1702, 1988.

Juppner H et al: A G-protein linked receptor for parathyroid hormone and parathyroid hormone related peptide, *Science* 254:1024, 1991.

Karaplis AC, Luz A, Glowacki J et al: Lethal skeletal dysplasia from targeted disruption of the parathyroid hormone–related peptide gene, *Genes Dev* 8:277-289, 1994.

Klahr S, Hruska K: Effects of parathyroid hormone on the renal reabsorption of phosphorus and divalent cations. In Peck WA, editor: *Bone and mineral research: annual 2,* Amsterdam, 1983, Excerpta Medica.

Kronenberg HM: Parathyroid hormone—molecular biology, chemistry and actions. In Mundy GR, Martin TJ, editors: *Physiology and pharmacology of bone: handbook of experimental pharmacology,* Berlin, 1993, Springer-Verlag.

Lin HY et al: Expression cloning of an adenylate cyclase-coupled calcitonin receptor, *Science* 254:1022, 1991.

Morrison NA, Qi JC, Tokita A et al: Prediction of bone density from vitamin D receptor alleles, *Nature* 367:284-287, 1994.

Moseley JM et al: Parathyroid hormone–related protein purified from a human lung cancer cell line, *Proc Natl Acad Sci USA* 84:5048, 1987.

Mundy GR: Bone resorption and turnover in health and disease, *Bone* 8:S9, 1987.

Mundy GR: The hypercalcemia of malignancy revisited, *J Clin Invest* 82:1, 1988.

Mundy GR, Martin TJ: Hypercalcemia of malignancy—pathogenesis and treatment, *Metabolism* 31:1247, 1982.

Mundy GR, Roodman GD: Osteoclast ontogeny and function. In Peck WA, editor: *Bone and mineral research V,* Amsterdam, 1987, Elsevier.

Nordin BEC: Plasma calcium and plasma magnesium homeostasis. In Nordin BEC, editor: *Phosphate and magnesium metabolism,* Edinburgh, 1976, Churchill-Livingstone.

Rousseau F, Bonaventure J, Legeai-Mallet L et al: Mutations in the gene encoding fibroblast growth factor receptor-3 in achondroplasia, *Nature* 371:252-254, 1994.

Schipani E, Kruse K, Juppner H: A constitutively active mutant PTH-PTHrP receptor in Jansen-type metaphyseal chondrodysplasia, *Science* 268:98-100, 1995.

Suva LJ et al: A parathyroid hormone–related protein implicated in malignant hypercalcemia: cloning and expression, *Science* 237:893, 1987.

Yates AJP et al: Effects of a synthetic peptide of a parathyroid hormone–related protein on calcium homeostasis, renal tubular calcium reabsorption and bone metabolism, *J Clin Invest* 81:932, 1988.

Wozney JM et al: Novel regulators of bone formation: molecular clones and activities, *Science* 242:1528, 1988.

CHAPTER

284 Principles of Genetic Disorders

Robb E. Moses and R. Ellen Magenis

Medical genetics is a cross-discipline specialty in which patient care may extend to other areas of medicine. The tools available for diagnosis and treatment in medical genetics apply not only to inherited disorders but also to diseases that reflect an alteration of the function or structure of the genome and its expression during the life of an individual. Gene therapy or modification of the expression of genes is part of future medical practice.

Both intuitive and a practical knowledge of genetics have been of long-standing benefit to medical practice. Traits such as polydactyly and color-blindness were described in the eighteenth century with regard to patterns of inheritance. In the nineteenth century, the characteristics of X-linked recessive inheritance for hemophilia were recognized by Otto in New England. Autosomal recessive inheritance was also described in the nineteenth century. The use of twins for separating environment and heredity in analysis of human disease was another nineteenth century development.

These observations were placed on a rational basis with the mid-nineteenth century work of Mendel. The core contribution of Mendel's work was to recognize that inheritance can be viewed as a unit or packet of information, passed from parent to offspring. The term *gene* refers to this unit of inheritance. The definition of what constitutes a gene has changed with increasing refinement of knowledge. Mendel established the principle of *segregation,* that is, that genes encoding the same function (alleles) in diploid organisms pass through generations separately, and the effect of these genes can be monitored in subsequent generations. This observation led to the concepts of *dominance* and *recessiveness,* which refer to the expressed traits (phenotypes) and not to the genes themselves. The dominant

phenotype is a trait that is expressed in the heterozygote; the recessive trait is not noted in heterozygotes. Today a phenotype may be analyzed at the molecular level. An individual may demonstrate the dominant trait with a variable *expressivity.* Indeed the appearance of the dominant trait may even be so low as to be absent, referred to as *nonpenetrant.*

Independent assortment refers to the observation that unrelated genes behave in an independent matter. Alleles segregate; nonalleles (independent genes) assort. Genes that assort completely independently are unlinked. *Linkage* refers to the observation that genes on the same chromosome may be close enough to travel together at meiosis. This linkage is a reflection of physical distance. A new combination of genes after meiosis is referred to as *recombination.* Because humans carry two copies of each gene, 50% recombination is equivalent to independent assortment and shows that the two *loci* (physical locations of the gene) are either on different chromosomes or so far apart on one chromosome that recombination is frequent enough to produce independent assortment. Units of recombination are *morgans;* 1 centimorgan (cM) equals approximately one megabase of DNA.

DNA is the physical basis for inheritance. The symmetry of the double helix model gives a rationale for transmission of genes. The mesh between the two DNA strands implies that genetic information is encoded in a linear array that can be duplicated by template function. The linear array is composed of a variable sequence of only four basic repeating units.

Within the past 20 years the number of defined genetic syndromes that can be assigned to a single gene with characterized inheritance has gone from several dozen to more than 4000. Of equal importance has been the recognition of *multifactorial* or *polygenic* traits, in which multiple genes interact with the environment to produce a disease. Patients in this category may state to the physician that "hypertension runs in my family." An appreciation of the interaction of the genome of an individual and the environment will become increasingly important.

MOLECULAR GENETICS OF THE HUMAN GENOME

Genes are organized in the DNA double helix. This helix is composed of two chains of deoxynucleotides in antiparallel; the polarity of each strand follows the 5′ to 3′ phosphodiester linkage between the deoxyribose moieties. Deoxyribonucleic acid (DNA) and ribonucleic acid (RNA) are synthesized only in the 5′ to 3′ direction. One strand of DNA is recognized as the "sense" or coding strand. The gene is "read" or transcribed from the 3′ to 5′, so the messenger RNA can be synthesized in the permissible 5′ to 3′ direction. The initiation of transcription typically occurs at a significant distance before the start of the coding region of the gene. Coding regions of genes are frequently separated by long stretches or spacers of apparently noninformative DNA. The intervening stretches are termed *introns;* the coding regions, *exons.* The primary RNA message from the coding unit of the gene contains RNA complementary to both exons and introns in a continuous fashion. At the 3′ end of the RNA transcript, there is a polyadenylation signal. The initial RNA transcript is processed into mature RNA by the removal of introns by the RNA splicing process and addition of adenosine residues at the 3′ end. This process is dependent on ribozymes, catalytic RNA molecules. The processed messenger RNA is translated into the protein product (Fig. 284-1). There are several steps at which the expression of the gene product might be regulated: transcription, splicing, translation, and modification or activation of the protein product. In addition, the transport of the protein product to the appropriate site for action in the cell is required. If transport signals are not encoded and processed appropriately, failure of transportation of the protein to the proper location for activity may result.

DNA is notable for its chemical stability. It is a good repository for the genetic information of a cell. The replication of DNA is accomplished and monitored by accurate enzymes. The overall mistake level is approximately 1 in 10^{10} nucleotide addition events. The cellular processes responsible for this very low error rate include the accuracy of enzymes responsible for synthesis of the DNA. These enzymes appear to have an overall mistake frequency of about 1 in

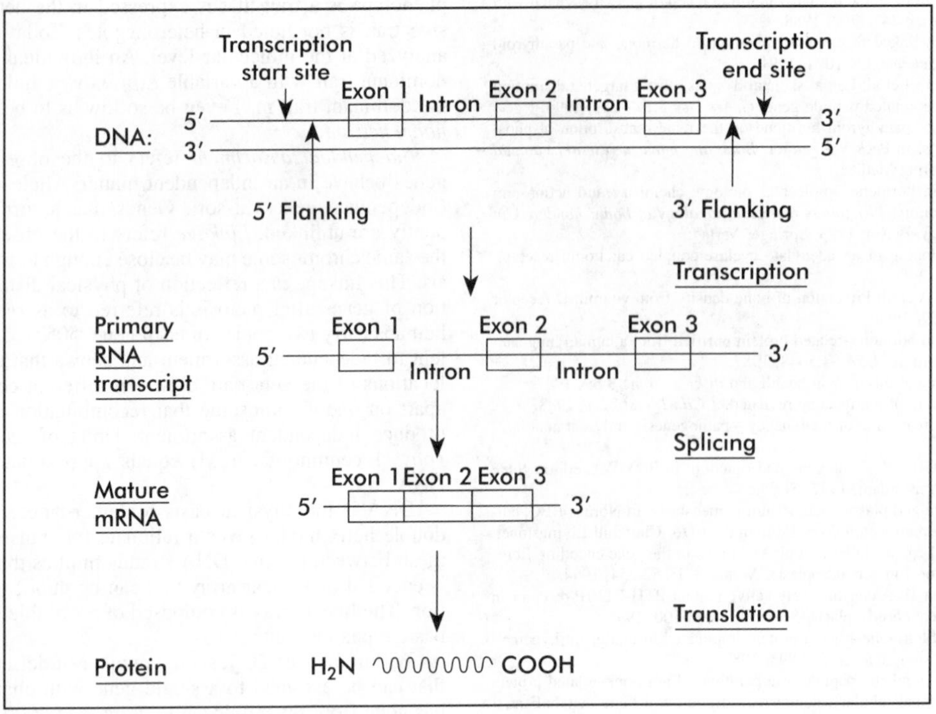

FIGURE 284-1   Processing of genomic information.

10^5 to 10^6. DNA polymerases are associated with a "proofreading" or "editorial" $3'$ exonuclease activity, which removes mismatched nucleotides preferentially and reduces the error rate an additional 100-fold. Finally, newly incorporated bases are screened for mismatches by an elaborate correction system. These systems have the ability to recognize the correct or parental strand of DNA that serves as a template. Corrections are preferentially made in the newly synthesized DNA strand. Mismatch correction lowers the overall mistake frequency an additional 100-fold.

However, the genome is not a static entity. The very low mistake level resulting from DNA replication provides a degree of variability in newly synthesized DNA. Mutations can also result from physical agents such as high energy radiation or from chemical agents. Cells have processes for recognition and repair of damage to the DNA. Damage or alteration to the DNA must be passed by the replication complex in the synthesis of new DNA in order to "fix" the mutation in the genome. A point mutation may be "silent" because of degeneracy in the code, in which case the alteration in the nucleotide still permits coding for the same amino acid that was previously encoded. Amino acid incorporation is encoded in a triplet code and the third position is particularly tolerant of change. Alternatively, a mutation may be silent because of a conservative substitution of an amino acid with similar physical characteristics to the original amino acid and no alteration in the properties of the resulting gene product. An additional reason for a silent mutation is a nonconservative amino acid change in a portion of the protein that is not required for function. Finally a silent mutation may occur in an intron and thus cause no alteration in the resulting protein product.

On the other hand, several types of mutations may significantly alter the function of the gene product. In one case, the mutation may alter the junction sites between introns and exons in such a way that splicing is altered. Such a mutation may result in the omission of an entire exon from the coding RNA. Another result that produces noticeable change in the gene product can be the substitution of a dissimilar amino acid in the portion of the gene encoding the active site of the protein or required for formation of required tertiary structure. A mutation may also produce a "stop" codon that is recognized by the cellular machinery as a signal to cease synthesis of protein. Occurrence of such a mutation early in the coding sequence for the protein can lead to the production of a truncated peptide without func-

tion. In addition to point mutations resulting from single base substitutions, large deletions and rearrangements may result from recombination. Indeed, such events may be large enough to be recognizable in chromosome analysis.

The sexual process also provides for a rich genetic diversity. With independent assortment of genes on separate chromosomes and random reassociation of chromosomes during meiosis, there are 2^{23} combinations for the 46 chromosomes in each fertilized egg as a result of spermatogenesis and oogenesis and fertilization to form a diploid individual.

Multiple alleles existing at the same locus are the result of independent mutational events. If a given allele reaches a level of 1% in the population, it is a *polymorphism*. Sometimes polymorphisms can be recognized at the protein level, as in the case of a number of erythrocyte enzymes. However, variation at the nucleotide sequence level qualifies equally well as a polymorphism. Such polymorphisms are useful in DNA diagnostic procedures. In addition, nucleotide sequence variation may occur at sites outside the gene but close enough to the gene to be tightly linked and therefore unlikely to be subject to recombination. If such a variance outside a gene is associated with an allele of the gene, the extragenic variation or polymorphism is said to be in *disequilibrium* with the allele. The linkage of detectable nucleotide polymorphisms constitutes a *haplotype*. Through the use of *restriction endonucleases* that recognize and cleave DNA only at sites of specific sequence, diseases have been associated with recognized nucleotide polymorphisms either inside or outside the gene. Thus significant detectable molecular diversity is present in the human genome, and this diversity may serve as a signature for detection of an allele and tracking of that allele through a family with inherited disease.

Variations in the nucleotide sequence that are detected as a result of the infrequent cutting by restriction endonucleases are termed *restriction fragment linked polymorphisms* (RFLPs). These reflect the variation in the size of the product after digestion of the DNA with a given restriction enzyme and detection with a "probe" of DNA, a labeled fragment known to lie within the region (Fig. 284-2). By the process of hybridization on a solid matrix, a variation in size can be detected. This process, the *Southern blot,* serves as a basis for detection of polymorphisms at the nucleotide level. This is the basic study for establishing linkage of a nucleotide polymorphism with an allele.

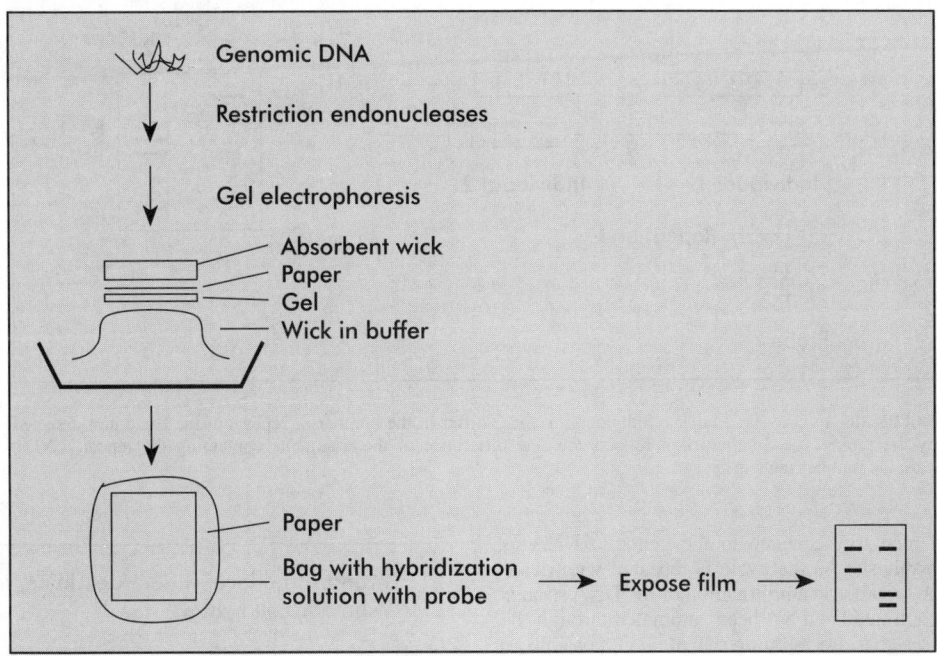

FIGURE 284-2   Southern hybridization. Flow of method for detecting polymorphism at restriction sites.

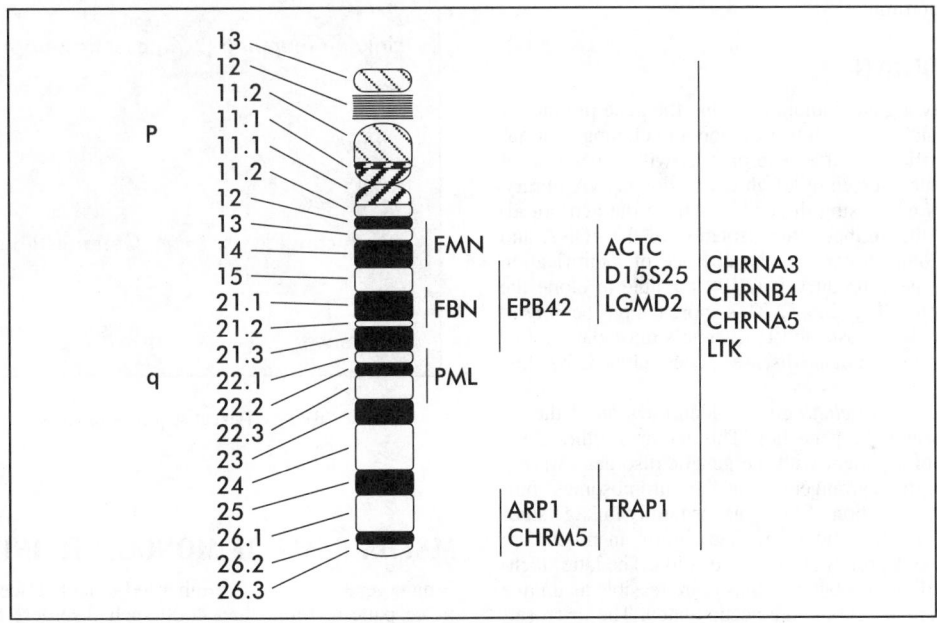

FIGURE 284-3   Ideogram of chromosome 15. The abbreviations denote DNA fragments known to be on chromosome 15, and the vertical bars indicate localization of the markers.

A rapid accumulation of markers has been assigned to each of the human chromosomes, which has allowed construction of a linkage map for human chromosomes (Fig. 284-3). The Human Genome Project accumulates the information in centralized fashion. The information is available on the internet in continuously updated format (http://www.ncbi.nlm.nih.gov/).

As analysis of the genome of higher organisms proceeded, it became clear that there were frequently occurring patterns of repeat sequences that took place as often as a million times in the genome. The size of the repeating unit is a continuum from two nucleotides *(micro-satellite DNA)* to dozens of nucleotides. Such repeats are random in occurrence but are relatively stable in location. One of the frequently occurring repeated sequences in the human genome can

be cleaved by the restriction endonuclease Alu I. These *Alu sites* serve as convenient anchor points in the genome for molecular analysis. There is variation from individual to individual in the number of times the unit is repeated at a given site. Thus through cleavage by restriction enzymes, it is possible to detect variation (polymorphism) between individuals. Variation in length of the tandem repeat units forms the basis for DNA fingerprinting of individuals and is useful from both a diagnostic and a forensic standpoint (Fig. 284-4). Because the *variable number tandem repeats* (VNTRs) are extremely polymorphic, use of several probes will establish identity with a high probability.

The *polymerase chain reaction* (PCR) utilizes synthesis across a region of DNA using oligonucleotides of known sequence that hy-

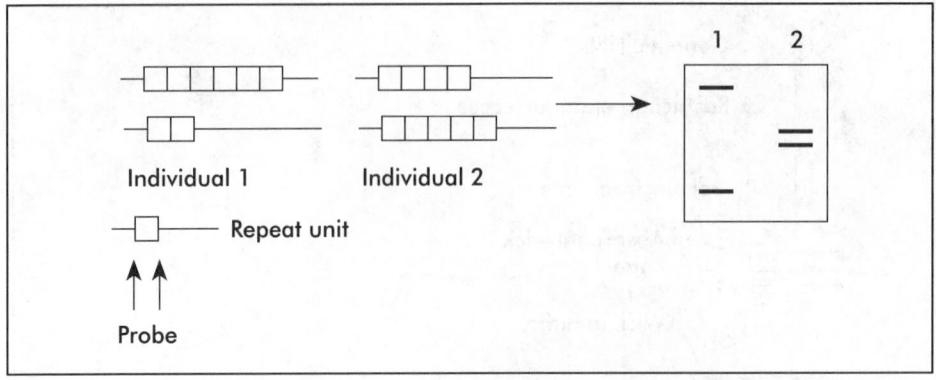

FIGURE 284-4   VNTR analysis. Individuals 1 and 2 differ in the number of repeats of the basic unit detected by the probe. The Southern blot reflects the size difference of the fragments containing the repeat. *VNTR*, Variable number tandem repeat.

bridize to their complementary sequence in the genomic DNA as primers for the DNA synthesis. As the cycle is repeated with denaturation and renaturation, geometric amplification of the DNA strands occurs. The process is facilitated and has been automated through the use of DNA polymerases that are thermoresistant. It is possible to detect the presence of normal or mutated alleles in amplified regions through the use of *allele specific oligonucleotide* (ASO) *probes* and hybridization or restriction fragment length polymorphism (RFLP) analysis. Thus it is now possible to analyze directly at the molecular level for certain common mutations.

POSITIONAL CLONING

It is possible to identify a gene without knowing the gene product or its function. The "classic" approach to isolation and cloning of a human gene involves purification of a gene product with generation of antibodies to that product, screening of an expression cDNA library, identification of clones expressing the epitopes from the gene product by screening with the antibody, and isolation of the cDNA and hybridization to a genomic library. In the absence of identification and purification of the gene product, it is still possible to clone the gene by positional cloning (Fig. 284-5). This approach has been used successfully for the cystic fibrosis and Duchenne's muscular dystrophy genes, among many human disease genes cloned by this approach.

A critical step in *positional cloning* is the identification of the region of the genome where the gene lies. This requires either good fortune in recognition of a patient with the genetic disorder carrying a recognizable deletion or rearrangement in the chromosomes, pinpointing an area of likely position of the gene, or family linkage studies in which several affected and unaffected family members are screened with unique DNA probes of known location. The latter technique requires many individuals but becomes more feasible as unique DNA probes for the human genome are accumulated. The microsatellite repeats are valuable for localization.

Linkage analysis consists of tracking a DNA polymorphism with affected and unaffected individuals until a high likelihood that a polymorphism is in disequilibrium with the disease-causing gene is established. The *logarithm of the odds of disequilibrium* (LOD) is accepted as being significant at a level of 3, meaning that the odds that the association will occur by random chance are only 1:1000. Once a high LOD score to linked markers is established, then recombinational mapping may be pursued by screening of libraries containing large genomic inserts. *Yeast artificial chromosomes* (YACs) are capable of containing 800 kilobases or more of DNA. Vectors containing such large fragments of genetic material permit analysis of larger segments of the intact genome structure. Once YACs containing regions of interest are identified, they can be used to derive linkage analysis with affected family members. As specific cDNA probes become available from these studies, the linkage analysis can proceed to cDNA and cloning in phage or plasmids and eventually to direct sequencing of the gene.

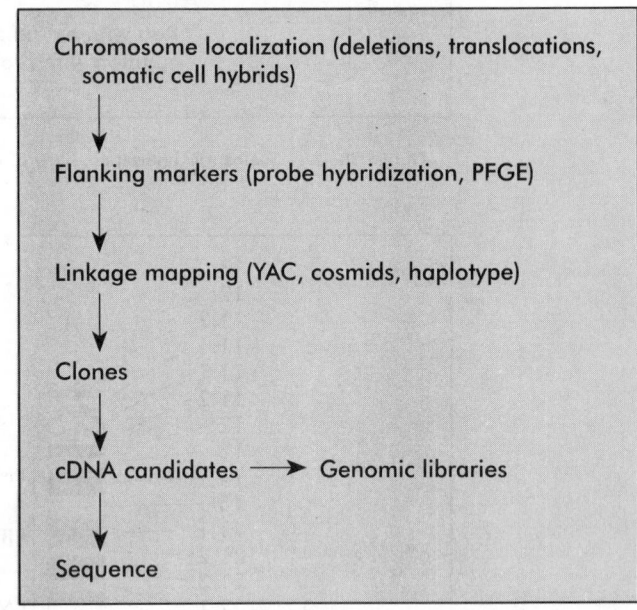

FIGURE 284-5   Typical sequence of steps in positional cloning.

MECHANISMS OF MONOGENIC INHERITANCE

Single gene disorders are inherited defects traceable in a unit inheritance pattern. More than 4000 such disorders are recognized. Individually they tend to be rare, but overall they represent a significant health burden on the population (several percent of all birth defects).

If an individual has one defective allele, he or she is described as being *heterozygous* for that gene. An individual completely defective in both alleles or completely normal in both alleles is described as being *homozygous*. In reality, as a result of variability, individuals differ in alleles at any given locus. However, the concept of homozygous and heterozygous is useful. Dominance and recessiveness relate to the function of the gene product and not to the gene. *Dominance* refers to the observable gene-related trait seen in an individual who is heterozygous for a given gene function, and *recessiveness* refers to the trait observed in the individual who is completely defective in that gene function. In many instances, the function of the gene product is not completely dominant or recessive, and therefore *codominant* and *incompletely dominant* refer, respectively, to traits that are simultaneously expressed or appear to be masked in the presence of the function of an additional gene product. In the case of many metabolic enzymes, a relatively modest level of activity is sufficient to

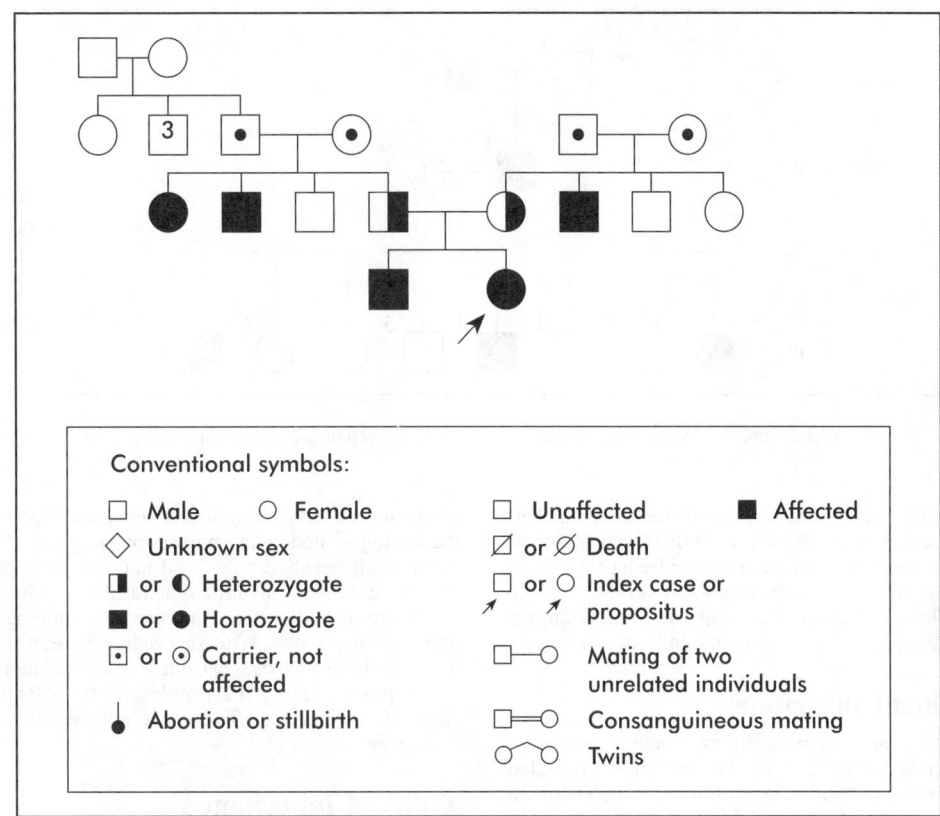

FIGURE 284-6 Autosomal recessive pedigree.

supply the requirements. Individuals who are phenotypically normal may be demonstrated to be partially deficient in the enzymatic activity. In some instances it is possible to identify such individuals as genetically heterozygous by biochemical tests.

Autosomal Recessive Inheritance

The pedigree of a typical autosomal recessive inheritance pattern is illustrated in Fig. 284-6 for the disease cystic fibrosis. This is one of the most common genetic diseases and has a carrier frequency of about 1 in 25 among the white population in North America.

In the case of cystic fibrosis, heterozygotes show no defect and are detectable only by detailed molecular analysis. Therefore the defective gene is not detected in the population at large. However, affected individuals carry a life-threatening burden with digestive problems, thick secretions, and impaired pulmonary function. The isolation of the cystic fibrosis gene was a triumph of positional genetics. The gene is a membrane protein responsible for a "channel" function.

There are several characteristics of the pedigree analysis for a typical autosomal recessive disorder (Fig. 284-6).
- The pattern of inheritance is "horizontal." The hallmark is that several siblings are affected when neither parent is affected.
- Males and females are equally affected.
- The parents are carriers and may be demonstrated as such if testing is available. This is the notorious "silent" gene disease.
- Consanguinity of the parents becomes more common with increasing rarity of the disease.

The autosomal recessive inheritance pattern demonstrates the principles of segregation. Each of the parents, who are normal, carries one normal and one defective allele and therefore has a 50% chance at meiosis of donating a defective allele to the gamete. It follows that the offspring will have genotypes in the ratio of $1:2:1$ and a ratio of $3:1$ for phenotype. That is, 75% of the offspring of such a mating will appear normal and 25% will show the recessive or disease phenotype. Note that "normal" offspring have a two-

thirds risk of being carriers for the defective gene. Think of each parent as (Ff), where F represents the normal gene and f represents the deficient gene encoding the cystic fibrosis gene product. With a 50% chance of F or f in gamete cells for each parent, inspection shows that (FF) will occur in one fourth of the pregnancies, (Ff) will occur in half of the pregnancies, and (ff) will occur in one fourth of the pregnancies.

Diseases that are burdensome but not lethal before reproductive age are not "genetic lethal." Defective alleles frequently may be inherited, but also arise by new mutation. Variant alleles can be maintained stably in the population. The equilibrium for two alleles is described by the Hardy-Weinberg formula:

(EQ. 1)

$$p^2 + 2pq + q^2 = 1$$

where p = frequency of one (normal) allele (A), q = frequency of other (abnormal) allele (a), and p + q = 1.

Several major deficient alleles may exist in the population for a recessive disease. Therefore the presence of a disease does not connote the presence of a specific allele. An autosomal recessive disease phenotype also may result from deficiencies in any of several genes. Multiple genes may be involved in a metabolic pathway, and homozygous deficiency in any of the genes may produce the same "terminal phenotype." A good example is the DNA repair diseases such as xeroderma pigmentosum, where more than one gene is involved, but the ultimate phenotype in the disease is the same. Thus in a sequential multigenic biochemica! pathway, a deficiency in any one of the genes may produce the same disease.

In the case of autosomal recessive diseases, it is important for the clinician to consider the possibility of consanguinity, or incest. The likelihood increases as the rarity of the disease increases. Decreasing carrier frequency makes the chance of mating with a heterozygote less likely. As heterozygotes become increasingly rare in the population, the likelihood of consanguinity or incest increases proportion-

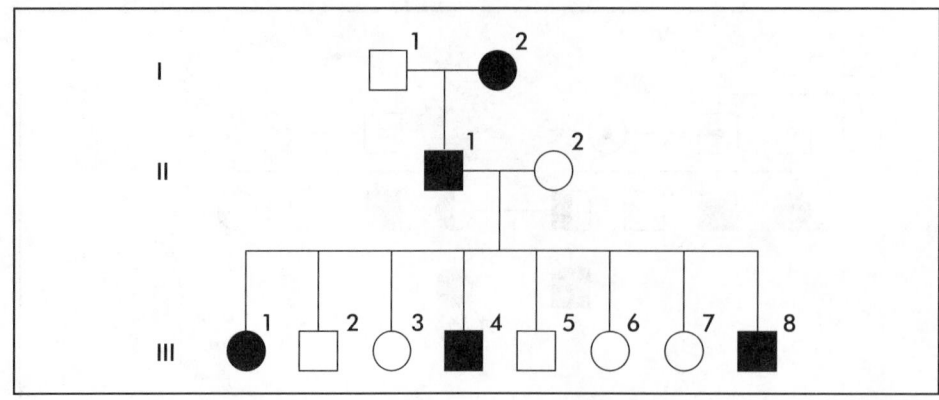

FIGURE 284-7   Autosomal dominant pedigree. The symbols are as in Figure 284-6.

ately. In the case of cystic fibrosis, the likelihood that a carrier (heterozygote) will marry a carrier is about 1 in 900. However, in the case of a disease that is more rare and has a carrier frequency of, for example, 1 in 100, the chance of heterozygotes marrying is 1 in 10,000. When such a disease appears in a family, it is important for the clinician to assess the possibility of consanguinity carefully.

Autosomal Dominant Inheritance

Autosomal dominant inheritance shows a different pattern than autosomal recessive inheritance (Fig. 284-7). The pedigree illustrated demonstrates the inheritance pattern for neurofibromatosis. There are several hallmarks of autosomal dominant inheritance patterns:

- A "vertical" transmission pattern.
- Male-to-male transmission.
- Males and females equally affected.
- A 50% risk for the disease in each child of an affected parent.

Particularly intriguing aspects of autosomal dominant disorders are *variable expressivity* and *penetrance*. Partial or complete effect of the genetic defect in individuals carrying a single mutated allele is the result of variable expressivity. Nonpenetrance is no observable phenotype in an individual known to have the defective allele. Individuals who bear the disease have one normal and one affected allele. Because an individual has a 50% chance of donating either allele to a gamete at meiosis, there should be a 50% probability that the offspring of an affected individual will demonstrate the genetic defect. For example, in the case of neurofibromatosis, expression is variable. It is not uncommon to encounter a patient who manifests a number of the findings of neurofibromatosis, including neurofibromas, multiple café-au-lait spots, altered pigmentation patterns, and intracranial tumors, but has "normal" parents. On inspection, one parent may manifest no more findings than axillary freckling, a hallmark of neurofibromatosis. Although the deficient allele is clearly present in the parent, it had not caused disease.

Autosomal dominant inheritance patterns may reflect new mutations. If two individuals who are normal have an affected child with an autosomal dominant disease, the offspring may well represent a new mutation. In such an instance, the likelihood that additional offspring will be affected is low for that couple, with established paternity. The certainty with which the clinician can make this prediction is linked to the likelihood of high penetrance and high expressivity for the defective gene; a disease with such a high expressivity is achondroplasia. A secondary consideration is that the mutation rate may increase with the age of the parents, best demonstrated with paternal age. Thus if an older normal couple have an achondroplastic child, it is a relatively safe conclusion that the offspring represents a new mutation. In this case, the recurrence risk for subsequent children with achondroplasia is low.

As in the case of autosomal recessive diseases, more than one gene defect may be involved in producing the same terminal phenotype in autosomal dominant diseases. This is the case in tuberosis sclerosis, in which two individual genes cause a similar phenotype.

Recently a particular class of mutations has been identified in some autosomal dominant diseases. The defect arises as the result of expansion of a repeating triplet sequence. The expression may be in the coding or noncoding portion of the gene. The affected allele has a dominant negative effect and may represent a "gain of function." The diseases so far identified as resulting from this type of mutation are neurologic diseases, for example, Huntington's syndrome and myotonic dystrophy. With succeeding generations the number of repeats tends to increase, causing earlier and more severe appearance of symptoms. This gives a molecular basis for the clinical phenomenon of *anticipation*. The exact number of repeats varies wildly among the diseases.

X-linked Inheritance

X-linked inheritance involves genes that are on the X chromosome. Several points are important in consideration of X-linked inheritance. First, in females two X chromosomes are present, but one is inactivated. The inactivation process is random. Thus females are mosaic for X chromosome alleles. A few genes on the X chromosome have been shown to escape inactivation. X inactivation occurs at an early stage in embryologic development, at about 16 days after fertilization. Once inactivated, a given X chromosome remains inactivated in that somatic cell line and all cells derived from that cell line. Random inactivation means that females can carry X chromosomes that contain deficient alleles that may or may not be inactivated, thus giving them partial activity for a number of enzymes. If a female has a gene for an X-linked recessive disorder on one of her X chromosomes, cells may express the deficient allele or the normal allele. Because X inactivation is random, females carry approximately equal numbers of active paternal and maternal X chromosomes. Should a number of X chromosomes bearing the normal gene be inactivated, the female may express or partially express the deficiency. On this basis the occasional female who is a carrier of Duchenne's muscular dystrophy shows some impairment of muscular function. Rarely a female who is homozygously defective for an X-linked disorder occurs. Presumably such an occasion arises from a nondisjunction event or in a situation in which mutant alleles are common in the population. An X-linked pedigree (Fig. 284-8) shows a different inheritance pattern from either recessive or dominant autosomal characteristics:

- No male-to-male transmission.
- All daughters of an affected male are carriers.

The X-linked fragile-X syndrome is notable as an example of a disease caused by expansion of a triplet repeat sequence (CGG). An increase in the number of times the triplet is repeated in the maternal X chromosome predisposes sons to fragile-X syndrome. Expansion appears to occur in the mother. Depending on X inactivation, daughters may be affected as well as sons, but only at decreased frequency because of the randomness of X inactivation.

MULTIFACTORIAL (COMPLEX) INHERITANCE

It is readily recognized that height, skin color, hair color, and intelligence are related to characteristics common to each parent. A number of frequently occurring diseases, such as diabetes mellitus, hypertension, coronary artery disease, schizophrenia, metabolic disor-

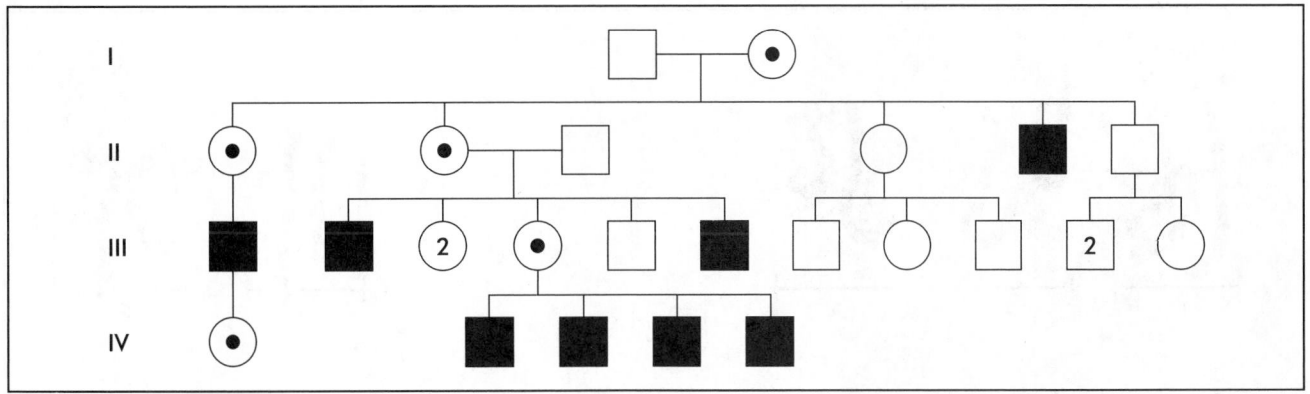

FIGURE 284-8   X-linked pedigree. The symbols are as in Figure 284-6.

ders, neural tube defects, and facial defects, are known to be polygenic or multifactorial disorders. These are the disorders that are recognized as "running in the family." A feature of multifactorial disorders is that the pattern of inheritance is not simple and cannot be demonstrated to fit a mendelian pattern. The appearance of these disorders may be dependent on the interaction of the environment and the genotype of the affected individual.

HUMAN CHROMOSOMES

At the beginning of cell division the apparently homogeneous nuclear material condenses into discrete elements, called *chromosomes* because of the color obtained with various stains. The distribution of chromosomes in germ cell division was noted by Sutton and Boveri in 1902 to be similar to the transmission of hereditary characteristics. They surmised that chromosomes are physical carriers of hereditary traits. Though it was known that the number and structure of these chromosomes were characteristic for each species examined, the chromosome number for humans was disputed until 1956, when Tjio and Levan established the number as 46.

The discipline of human cytogenetics has expanded rapidly since 1956 to include many areas, several of which have clinical relevance:
- The delineation of numerous congenital malformation syndromes caused by chromosome aberration.
- The detection of specific chromosome *aneuploidies* (incorrect number) and rearrangements associated with specific leukemias and solid tumors.
- The investigation of the possibility that viruses, chemicals, radiation, drugs, and other environmental agents that have a direct effect on chromosomes may be responsible for some congenital anomalies and neoplasias.

The Human Karyotype

The human *karyotype* is a standardized way of arranging metaphase chromosomes that facilitates their classification and identification and aids in the detection of chromosome anomalies. The normal human karyotype has 23 pairs of chromosomes representing the *diploid* complement of 46 chromosomes. Twenty-two of these pairs are the *autosomes*; the remaining pair consists of the *sex chromosomes*, which are morphologically distinctive in males and females. A normal karyotype is noted as 46,XX (female) or 46,XY (male). The longer arm of the chromosome is termed *q*, the other *p*.

In females the sex chromosomes are identical in size and are called the "Xs." Although the Xs in females are genetically homologous chromosomes (as in the case of autosomes), in the normal diploid interphase cell, one of the Xs forms a condensed *heterochromatic* body in interphase called the *Barr body*. The Barr body represents the inactive X. This process is important with regard to X chromosome *dosage compensation* (more genetic material in XX females than XY males).

In males, one of the sex chromosomes is smaller and is called the *Y*; it is not strictly homologous, except at the end of the short arm, to the X. The Y contains genes specific for male sex determination.

Chromosome Identification and Chromosome Staining Techniques

Chromosome banding techniques have provided the means of distinguishing each of the 22 pairs of autosomes and the X and Y chromosomes. A nomenclature that assigns a number for each band according to distance from the centromere and location on the long or short arm has been devised. The occurrence of staining *heteromorphisms* (normal inherited variations) usually located at the centromere region allowed further distinction between homologues, and in some cases, their parental origin.

The most informative stage of the cell cycle for examination of chromosomes is early metaphase/late prophase. Cells for tissue culture can be obtained from several sources, most commonly peripheral blood, skin biopsy specimens, amniotic fluid, chorionic villi, bone marrow, and solid tumors. Peripheral blood is the most convenient source of cells for chromosome analysis. The lymphocytes are normally in a resting stage but can be stimulated to transform into actively growing cells by addition of a mitogen such as phytohemagglutinin. During the last 1 to 2 hours of culture a mitotic arresting agent, colchicine, is added to the culture to prevent cell entry into metaphase.

There are now many techniques for staining human chromosomes. Commonly employed techniques can display routine banding or reverse banding, centromeric regions, and heteromorphisms. Methods to increase the band number *(high-resolution chromosomes)* have been devised. The detailed chromosome morphology can be correlated with gene or specific DNA sequences and presented as a combined ideogram. This information is continuously updated and can be obtained from the genetic databases on the internet (Fig. 284-9).

CHROMOSOME ABNORMALITIES
Types of Chromosome Abnormalities

There are two major types of human chromosome abnormalities: numerical and structural. Numerical abnormalities may involve extra or missing chromosomes *(aneuploidy)*, an extra set of chromosomes *(triploidy)*, or extra sets of chromosomes *(polyploidy)*. Structural aberrations include partial loss of a chromosome or addition of chromosomal material on a chromosome (partial aneuploidy), such as terminal and interstitial deletions, duplications, rings, and isochromosomes. In addition, translocations or rearrangements of material within a chromosome or between chromosomes may occur. Each of the structural abnormalities may be familial or sporadic in origin.

Mechanism of Formation and Parental Origin of Abnormalities

Aneuploidy most often results from a meiotic segregation error *(nondisjunction)* in meiosis I or II. Such errors occur in both male and female meiosis, but more often in meiosis I in the female, and incidence increases with age. Postmeiotic or mitotic nondisjunction can also occur. The result is then *mosaicism* (e.g., 45,X/46,XX) and the

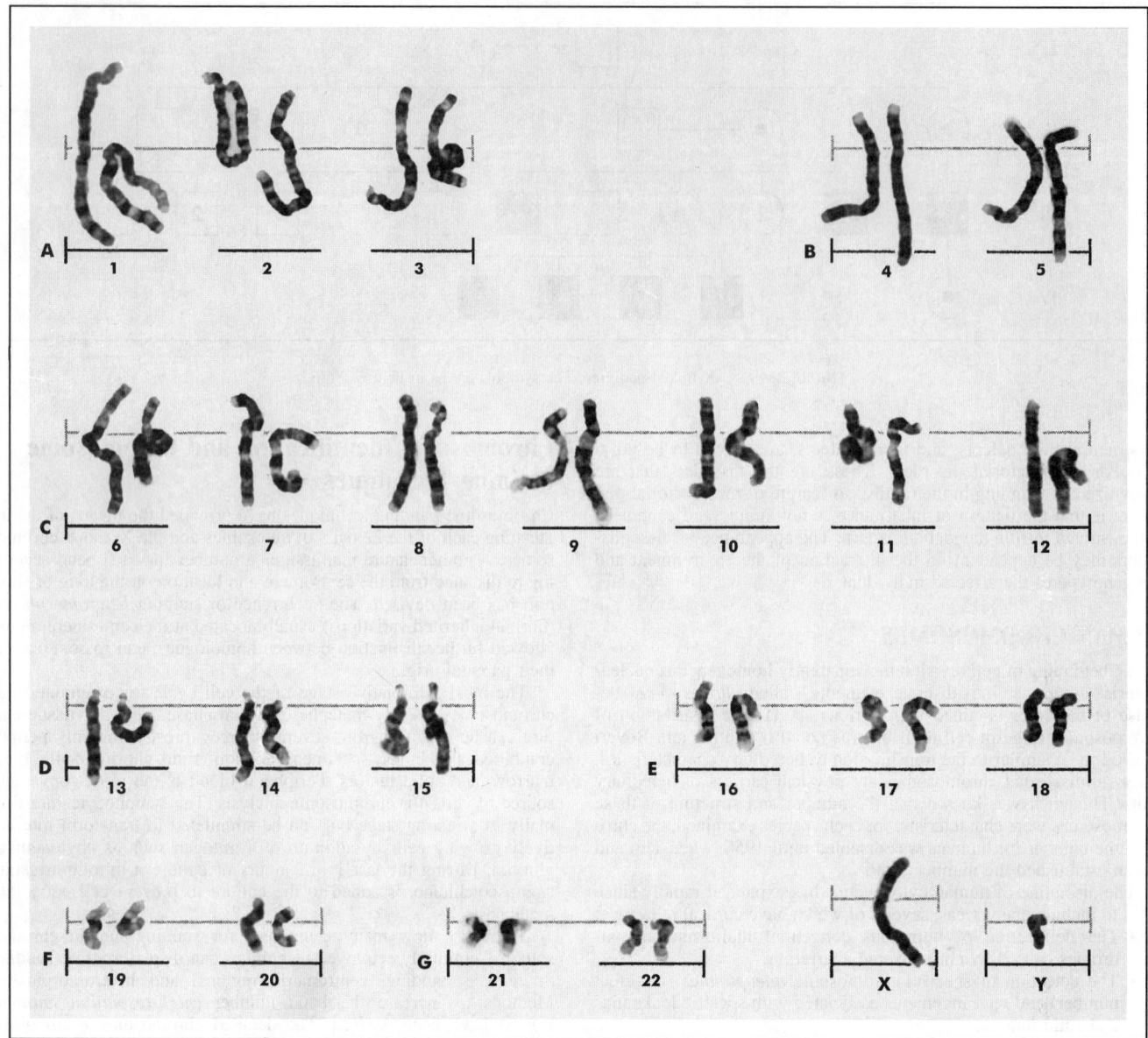

FIGURE 284-9   G-banded male karyotype at the approximate 650-band stage according to the International System for Human Cytogenetic Nomenclature (ISCN) (1995).

individual has two distinct cell populations. The origin of the error can be determined by use of microsatellite DNA.

In trisomy 21, the most common chromosome aneuploidy, a maternal age effect has been demonstrated. The cause is unknown, but the errors appear to occur primarily in meiosis I.

Partial deletions, duplications, or aneuploidy may result from balanced *translocations* between chromosomes in a parent. By far the most frequent translocation is the robertsonian type, in which two chromosomes fuse at their centromeres, thus reducing the number of chromosomes. Affected individuals, when balanced carriers, are themselves normal but have a higher risk for abnormal offspring. Balanced reciprocal exchange between two chromosomes in a parent may result in unbalanced or balanced as well as normal products, but the chance of having chromosomally unbalanced offspring is relatively high. *Inversion* refers to the reorientation of a part of a chromosome within the chromosome. Inversions also may be balanced or unbalanced. When they are balanced, chromosome imbalance occurs only if there is an odd number of crossovers in meiosis.

Somatic chromosome aberrations, including aneuploidy, deletion,

duplication, and translocation, have also been associated with human disease. These abnormalities are presumably not inherited because they are localized only to specific tissues. The molecular basis is known for some of these abnormalities, for example, the *Philadelphia chromosome* (a chromosome 9/22 translocation), which is usually present in chronic myelogenous leukemia. However, the precipitating event for the translocation is not known.

Chromosome Syndromes

Approximately 50% of first trimester spontaneous abortions are chromosomally abnormal. Abnormalities in early abortuses tend to differ from those found later in gestation and include trisomy for all the chromosomes except chromosome 1. The two most common abnormalities, occurring in about 25% of the chromosomally abnormal abortuses, are triploidy and 45,X Turner's syndrome. Triploidy is characterized by cystic degeneration of the placenta, sometimes appearing as hydatidiform mole; there is usually an accompanying fetus. The fetus is small for gestational age and has low-set ears and syndactyly. About 0.5% to 1% of all liveborns have chromosome abnormalities, and 7% to 10% of stillbirths and neonatal deaths are due to chromosome imbalance.

Autosomal trisomies in fetuses who survive to term include trisomies 13, 18, and 21. Of these, only trisomy 21 cases survive beyond infancy. These trisomies are also found in early spontaneous abortions. About 70% of trisomy 21 conceptuses are lost before term.

There are an almost unlimited number of different ways in which the 46 chromosomes can be broken with pieces lost (deletions) or reattached (translocation/duplications). Numerous described syndromes are due to imbalance of such chromosome segments.

Sex chromosome abnormalities have less severe phenotypic consequences than those produced by autosomal imbalance. This may be caused by lyonization (inactivation) of the excess X chromosomes, and paucity of genes affecting the brain or body structure on the Y. 45,X *Turner's syndrome* individuals who survive to term are relatively mildly affected. The patients are females who are short and infertile and have variable somatic abnormalities. Typically the individual has a short, wide or webbed neck; downslanted eyes; shield chest; and short fourth metacarpals. Mosaicism is frequent; the other cell line may be normal XY or XX or an X long-arm rearranged chromosome. Less often other structural rearrangements occur. 45,XO occurs in 1/2500 live female births.

Triple X females (47,XXX) occur in about 1/1000 births; they are phenotypically normal females with varying degrees of mental retardation and behavioral difficulties. XXY patients (Klinefelter's syndrome), on the other hand, are tall and may be mildly mentally retarded. The occurrence is 1/800 male births. These individuals are almost always infertile as a result of hypogonadism (Chapter 301).

Several *microdeletion* syndromes have been described. They may appear to have a sporadic inheritance. The deletions generally include only a single chromosome band. An example is the *WAGR syndrome* (Wilms' tumor, aniridia, genital abnormalities, and mental retardation). There are multiple anomalies, predisposition to Wilms' tumor, and generally loss of the lactic dehydrogenase A gene. A dominant disease gene for aniridia maps to the same region.

Microdeletions on chromosome 22 are associated with several diseases with some features shared. The several diseases are now combined into the "catch-22" syndrome (cardiac defect, abnormal facies, thymus hypoplasia, cleft palate, and hypocalcemia). The evidence for microdeletion in a high percentage of the patients was established by the use of *FISH* (fluorescent in situ hybridization). In this technique, DNA probes located in the region are modified to bind fluorescent reporter molecules. After chromosome preparation the probes are hybridized. A microdeletion leads to failure of the fluorescent signal. A control probe must be used to show that the chromosome is present (Color Plate IX-1).

The recognizable phenotypic abnormalities of the various syndromes associated with chromosome imbalance must be due to the actions or loss of actions of the genes located in the involved segments that alter development. Though a number of known genes have been shown to have dose effects in patients with unbalanced chromosomes, these genes are unlikely to be causative factors; the genes crucial to the phenotype may be genes expressed during embryogenesis and then "turned off."

Imprinting

Imprinting is the differential expression of maternal and paternal genomes in mammalian development. Several lines of evidence favor the occurrence of differential expression, that is, genes from one parent must be "turned off." For example, nuclear transplantation experiments in mice have shown that a parthenogenetically produced egg develops to birth only when a male-derived genome is introduced by fusion of karyoplasts. Thus a maternally and a paternally derived genome are necessary for mammalian development. The suspected mechanism of imprinting appears to be differential methylation.

In humans, the Prader-Willi and Angelman's microdeletion syndromes are examples of imprinting. A small deletion of the proximal long arm of chromosome 15 is found in approximately 85% of Prader-Willi patients, with normal chromosomes in the parents (Fig. 284-10). Parental origin studies show in all cases

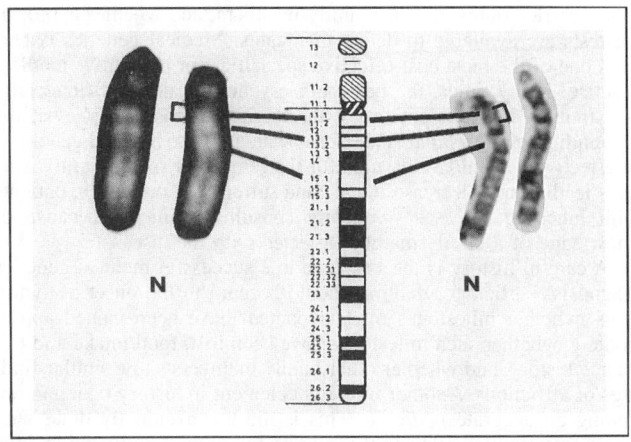

FIGURE 284-10   Chromosome 15 showing the deletion of the proximal long arm typical of Prader-Willi and Angelman's syndromes. The left chromosome pair is R-banded; the region that is deleted in the far-left chromosome is bracketed on the normal chromosome. The right chromosome pair is G-banded; the far-right chromosome has the deletion, and brackets on the normal chromosome indicate the region deleted. Lines to the idiogram indicate specific bands and their assigned members. Short arm bands p11.2, stalk p12, and satellite p13 are highly variable among unrelated individuals but are stably inherited and useful for parental origin studies. *N,* Normal chromosome.

examined that the deletion occurred as a de novo event in the father. Angelman's syndrome includes characteristic minimally dysmorphic facies, small hands, but normal growth, severely delayed development, ataxic gait, seizures, and frequent unprovoked laughter. Feeding problems provided by incoordination of suck and swallow, sleep difficulties, hyperactivity, tremulousness, and seizures generally develop in infancy. A deletion of the same region of chromosome 15 as in Prader-Willi syndrome is found in these patients, but chromosomes of the parents are normal. However, in all cases of Angelman's syndrome in which parental origin studies were performed, the affected chromosome was from the mother. A small ribonucleoprotein (SNRPN) appears to be the critical genetic component. In cases of Prader-Willi where there is not a deletion, molecular analysis indicates a methylation pattern compatible with silencing of the paternal gene.

Uniparental disomy, or two copies of a chromosome from one parent, has been noted in most of the Prader-Willi patients who do not have a cytogenetic or molecular deletion, providing further evidence for the role of imprinting in this region of chromosome 15. In these cases there are two copies of the maternal chromosomes (most frequently both of the mother's 15s, but occasionally two copies of the same chromosome 15) and no chromosome 15 from the father. Though uniparental disomy is unusual in Angelman's syndrome, there are the expected findings of two chromosome 15s from the father and no chromosome 15 from the mother.

Uniparental disomy may produce a "loss of heterozygosity." This can result from a nondisjunction event in meiosis or in somatic tissue. It is important in human cancers, since it can lead to loss of tumor suppressor genes with subsequent tumor development. A good example is retinoblastoma.

DIAGNOSIS AND MANAGEMENT OF GENETIC DISORDERS
Approach to the Patient

Medical genetics is a cross-discipline field with an interesting combination of tertiary and primary care. In evaluating patients, the clinical geneticist may interact with specialists in several areas of medicine. Counseling and ability to communicate, particularly with regard to accurate historical information, are requisites. Since medical genetics is a family-oriented specialty, the physician should view the patient as a member of a group and not as an isolated case with a potentially important inherited problem. Consideration must be given to the carrier status of other family members, and whether appropriate tests are available to detect that status. Medical genetics is perhaps one of the most cost-effective specialties for preventive medical practice. Many times, the cost both psychologically and financially is extremely high for patients with inherited diseases. However, the recognition of a *proband* (index case) can alert the medical geneticist to effective screening measures for the remainder of the family, perhaps leading to a decrease in cost and suffering. Conversely, patients with inherited diseases frequently consult a clinician because of knowledge of a family member affected with the disease.

A careful history is the keystone to a successful medical genetics diagnosis. Particular attention should be paid to the onset of symptoms, whether milestones of development have been gained appropriately, whether such milestones have been lost, food intake and tolerance history, and whether other family members show similar findings or afflictions. Another important element in history taking is obtaining an accurate *pedigree*. This is most conveniently done with forms that readily delineate the generations in the family and include adequate space for annotation with names. Two important points with regard to pedigree analysis are last names before marriage and ethnic and locale origins of families. Frequently, such information can be a clue to consanguinity. Attention should be given to individuals who die suddenly or in an unexplained manner or who manifest certain phenotypic features that may be associated with the disease of interest. A good example is Marfan's syndrome, in which sudden death produced by aortic rupture is associated with numerous phenotype findings. The age at onset of symptoms should be noted. In history taking, it is important to obtain details of the obstetric history for any pregnancies involving affected individuals, with attention to intercurrent infections, unexplained fevers, and drug or teratogen exposures for the mother. It is also important to note a history of any spontaneous miscarriages. Medical records to substantiate the diagnosis and photographs of other affected family members, when they cannot be present, can be invaluable.

The physical examination in the practice of medical genetics should note the symmetry of the body and its parts as well as relative size and conformation compared to those of the normal population. Available tables of height, weight, head circumference, interocular distance, and other parameters are indispensable in evaluating dysmorphology and establishing a base for diagnosis. Diagnosis in medical genetics frequently begins with an orderly listing of abnormal physical findings followed by a systematic comparison to listings of associations of abnormalities and photographs of patients from recognized syndromes. Such dysmorphology data bases are available in computer software.

Testing and Diagnosis: Referrals to Genetics

Referrals to genetics are appropriate on several bases:

- Failure of normal development
- Loss of developmental milestones
- Mental retardation
- Dysmorphology
- Family history of a disease
- Maternal age greater than 35 at delivery
- Coma in newborn

Failure of an infant to achieve normal development or losses of function (e.g., coordination) in an adult may herald inherited disease. With the advent of molecular testing, referrals for mental retardation are uniformly appropriate. Establishing a diagnosis in patients with abnormal appearance and the risk of recurrence are the domain of clinical genetics. Recognition of a family disease or hallmark of disease (e.g., sudden death in family member in middle age) calls for a genetics evaluation. Specific circumstances such as a maternal age of greater than 35 or coma in a newborn require prenatal counseling or metabolic evaluation, respectively, to meet normal standards of care.

After history taking and physical examination, the physician faces the decision of ordering additional tests to establish a diagnosis or to evaluate the relative severity of the disease in the individual. The decision is based on the physical findings and the suggestions from the history. During the evaluation of patients, psychometric testing to establish development and intelligence level is appropriate. With infants, developmental testing and comparative evaluation in relation to normal milestones are as significant as in older children and adults. Where appropriate, psychologic evaluation can be very helpful.

The use of consultations is critical in medical genetic diagnosis. For example, an ophthalmologic consultation is routinely used for patients who manifest mental retardation because many inherited diseases have ocular features that are helpful, if not pathognomonic. For a number of inherited diseases, radiologic studies can be definitive—for example, vertebral films in the mucopolysaccharidoses, and three-dimensional radiologic techniques to evaluate central nervous system development, as well as standard films. Ultrasonography both for diagnosis and for monitoring is appropriate in a number of inherited disorders. Establishing the diagnosis is the keystone to successful family counseling.

With regard to laboratory testing, it is helpful to divide the approach into three categories: metabolic, karyotype analysis, and DNA or molecular testing (Fig. 284-11). Metabolic testing is appropriate in the case of mental retardation as a screening test using the urine or serum. It is good practice to include evaluation of levels of organic acids and amino acids, especially with the presence of seizures. If the patient in the perinatal period has seizures, evaluation of levels of organic acids and blood ammonia is appropriate. If symptoms appear to be related to dietary history, metabolic evaluation is also suggested. Loss of developmental milestones is a hallmark of storage disease and should alert the physician to that possibility.

Karyotype analysis is indicated when a patient exhibits dysmorphology, multiple anomalies, and/or mental retardation. In some situations it is appropriate to request a specialized karyotype analysis, for example, fluorescent in situ hybridization (FISH) when a microdeletion is suspected.

The number of tests to which DNA diagnosis can be advantageously applied is growing rapidly. This technique is most promising when a disease has a low new mutation frequency, no available metabolic test exists, but the defective gene has been identified. This permits focused testing of the common mutations. For example, with cystic fibrosis about 85% to 87% of cases can be detected with molecular techniques. None of the testing methods should be viewed as operating in isolation from the others. It is likely that tests that are now performed at the DNA level may be performed at the "metabolic" level once the gene product and its function have been further assessed.

COUNSELING AND PRENATAL DIAGNOSIS

Medical genetics is unusual in its requirement for and reliance on patient and family counseling. In this respect, the physician frequently uses the services of genetic counselors who are trained in gathering information and explaining heritable disorders to patients. Counseling is an integral part of diagnosis and treatment and must be adjusted to the needs of the patient: that is, does the patient require primarily recurrence risk data or outlook for his or her own disease? The salient points of genetic counseling follow.

- Basis for and certainty of the diagnosis
- Burden of the disease
- Recurrence risk
- Treatment

The first step in genetic counseling is to inform the patient of the diagnosis, the basis of the conclusions regarding the diagnosis, and the level of certainty. It is important at this step to be thorough. It is also important not to attach a label to a patient if the diagnosis is uncertain. During this phase of the counseling, pictures are frequently helpful. For example, in chromosomal disorders, the basis for the diagnosis can be established more clearly if the clinician uses diagrams or actual pictures of chromosomes, if possible, of the disorder under discussion. Are any additional tests required? The level of certainty of the diagnosis justifies the administration of additional tests. The burden of the diagnosis is the physical, emotional, and financial load the diagnosis implies. Some diagnoses, such as malformations, have a relatively light impact in regard to viability of the patient but a significant psychologic impact, as well as implications for reconstructive surgery. Recurrence risk is important to establish with regard to future childbearing, risk for the offspring who already exist, and implications for other family members. Here the counselor must be circumspect.

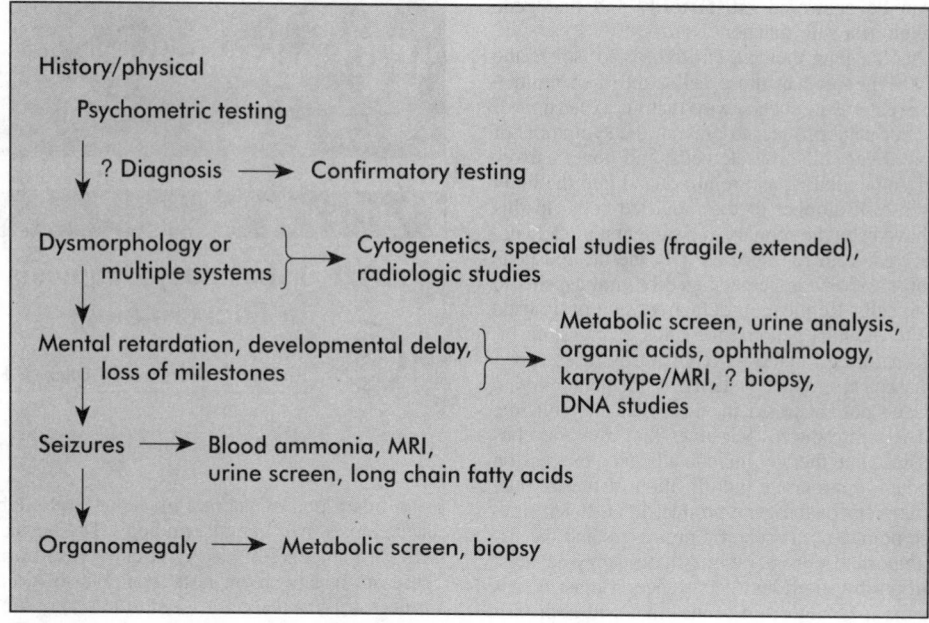

FIGURE 284-11 Diagnostic testing. Flow chart for patient evaluation with regard to laboratory procedures.

Sensitivity to both the patient's and other family members' privacy must be considered. The physician is dependent on the goodwill of family members and the action of the patient or the patient's relatives for identifying additional affected family members, obtaining specimens for further diagnostic tests, and collecting additional historical information. Many times, information about other family members is helpful in forming a basis for diagnosis. For example, a history of family members' dying suddenly of aneurysms is compatible with a history of Marfan's syndrome in the family and implies that the patient under consultation does not represent a new mutation.

Treatment options and outlooks are important considerations for the patient. Can the recurrence risk for a couple be lowered by prenatal diagnosis or by artificial insemination? Are these alternatives acceptable to the patient? In genetic counseling, the physician must provide information that the patient will use to make decisions within his or her ethical framework. Will termination after prenatal diagnosis be an acceptable alternative? If not, is the cost of the prenatal diagnostic procedures worthwhile? What is the level of certainty for prenatal diagnostic procedures? These are significant points that should be considered by the counselor in talking with the family.

Prenatal diagnosis and counseling are usually based on a couple's desire for prenatal diagnosis because of an empiric risk for disease or a patient's desire for prenatal diagnosis because of a familial history. In the first category, advanced maternal age, with increased risk of chromosomal aneuploidy, is the most common reason for counseling. In the latter category, a typical reason for prenatal diagnosis would be screening tests that indicate that the couple are carriers for Tay-Sachs disease, an autosomal recessive disease with a high burden. Other common reasons for prenatal diagnosis and counseling are a family history of chromosomal disorders, multifactorial disorders, or a disease manifesting dysmorphic features. In the latter case, the diagnosis can occasionally be established in utero by ultrasound. For example, achondroplasia can be observed in utero in an ultrasound given on a routine basis.

In counseling, it is useful to inform the patient of the general population risk of birth defects (approximately 3%), with the exact level depending on where the boundaries are set for a "birth defect." This risk places the increasing chance of chromosomal abnormality with increasing maternal age in perspective. It is important to inform the patient of what prenatal diagnosis cannot rule out, and the physician should emphasize that a normal result in a given test does not represent a clean bill of health for the pregnancy. The statements of the counselor should be couched in terms of risk estimates and percentage of chances.

TREATMENT

Treatment of individuals with genetic disorders is not a new field. The psychologic and social support requirements of the patient, although not curative, are an integral part of treatment. For example, in Prader-Willi syndrome patients regularly require psychologic counseling and evaluation and considerable monitoring for eating disorders. Although not representing a cure, such elements can be effective in controlling the results of the abnormal gene. Phenylketonuria (PKU) offers an example of biochemical treatment, in which the dietary restriction of phenylalanine is critical to the patient's achieving normal or nearly normal intelligence. There seems little doubt that early institution of and strict adherence to the dietary regimen are required for normal function. In other instances, supplying a cofactor can be remarkably effective. For example, in biotinidase deficiency, pharmacologic doses of biotin prevent the appearance of disease.

Enzyme therapy has been an attractive goal in the treatment of inherited disorders. Important considerations in this regard still include the blood-brain barrier and the half-life or duration of the infused enzyme in the bloodstream. Several promising examples are the treatment of Gaucher's disease with sphingomyelinase and Fabry's disease with α-galactosidase. Enzyme replacement therapy is feasible when the metabolic defect can be corrected by circulating enzymes available in large amounts of high purity. Production of human enzymes in mammalian expression systems avoids antigenic stimulus and proper modification to permit "targeting" for uptake by specific tissues.

Therapy by substituting normal functional genes for deficient genes seems an attainable goal. It is useful to distinguish somatic cell gene therapy from germ cell gene therapy. In the former, the goal would be to cure the defect in a patient, and in the latter, an additional goal would be to prevent a defect in the offspring of the patient. The ethical implications are viewed by society as somewhat different: in the former, the net effect would be little different from that of treating a patient with a dietary supplement; in the latter, the result is that future generations may be affected in terms of permanent alteration. In either instance the question of adverse risk produced by derepression or repression of a gene product remains open. Is it possible, for example, to inactivate a tumor suppressor gene and increase the risk of cancer in a patient? Evidence seems to indicate that, in fact, such questions can be answered satisfactorily and that gene therapy can be undertaken in a safe manner.

One of the approaches to gene therapy, ex vivo, is to isolate the patient's cells, modify the genome in those cells, and then reintroduce those cells into the patient in such a way that an expansion of the cells supplies sufficient gene product to prevent the symptoms of the disease. For example, liver cells, muscle cells, and bone marrow cells can all be isolated, manipulated, and reintroduced into the body with a subsequent increase in number of the modified cells. In this approach, retroviruses have been the primary experimental model vector. Cloning vectors derived from retroviruses with the desired gene inserted in an expression cassette can be packaged in viral capsids to allow infection of human cells. Replication-defective vectors are used to "force" integration into the host genome for stable expression, indexed by a selectable trait for cell marking. RNA retroviruses carrying a drug-resistance marker are model systems. If adequate expression can be monitored and demonstrated in vitro, then the cell line that has been modified is reintroduced. Variables that must be controlled to ensure successful gene therapy include adequate expression of the gene and its product, appropriate modification of the product to allow function, and delivery of the gene product in sufficient levels. With regard to these points, tissue-specific promoters and the tissue of production are important considerations. If the enzyme must be modified to allow proper transport and persistence, it must be ensured that the altered gene is produced in tissues that will appropriately carry out such functions.

Alternative gene delivery systems have been developed. Vectors derived from adenoviruses capitalize on the virus's efficient uptake by cells.

Adequate means of delivering and monitoring the expression of genes are therefore at hand. Other essential needs for routine application of gene therapy include mechanisms for tissue targeting on a routine basis, vectors with promoter-enhancer systems active in a given tissue over a long time frame, possible controllable expression, and, most importantly, safety. Meeting each of these needs appears feasible.

The potential applications for gene therapy are much broader than in "genetic" diseases. It seems likely that gene therapy will not be limited to rare inherited disorders but will find use in other areas such as immune dysfunction and cancer. The cost-effectiveness and range of usefulness promise to make gene therapy the treatment of choice in a broad array of disorders. We may expect to see application of this technology in a variety of situations within the next decade.

BIBLIOGRAPHY

Blau HM, Springer ML: Molecular medicine gene therapy: a novel form of drug delivery, *N Engl J Med* 333:18, 1995.
Boguski MS, Schuler GD: Establishing a human transcript map, *Nat Genet* 10:4, 1995.
Collins FS: Positional cloning: let's not call it reverse anymore, *Nat Genet* 1:3, 1992.
Emery A, Rimoin D: *Principles and practices of medical genetics,* ed 2, New York, 1990, Churchill Livingstone.
Glover TW: Catching a break on 22, *Nat Genet* 10:3, 1995.
Gorlin RJ et al: *Syndromes of the head and neck,* ed 3, New York, 1990, Oxford.
Jennings C: How trinucleotide repeats may function, *Nature* 378:6553, 1995.
McKusick VA: *Mendelian inheritance in man,* ed 11, Baltimore, 1995, Johns Hopkins University Press.
Patterson M, Todd JA: A complex issue, *Trends Genet* 11:12, 1995.
Scriver CR et al: *The metabolic basis of inherited disease,* ed 8, New York, 1995, McGraw-Hill.
Thompson MS, McInnes RR, Willard HP: *Thompson and Thompson genetics in medicine,* ed 5, Philadelphia, 1991, Saunders.

II LABORATORY TESTS

285 Laboratory Diagnosis in Endocrinology

Richard M. Jordan and Peter O. Kohler

In no other area of internal medicine is the laboratory more crucial for diagnosis than in endocrinology. The physician, however, faces a difficult challenge in making effective use of laboratory technology. There are usually more tests available to evaluate a condition than are necessary to diagnose it, and the diagnostic procedures often involve complex and expensive manipulations. Thus the clinician needs a thorough understanding of endocrine pathophysiology, not only to interpret results but also to know which tests to order. Without this knowledge, it is inevitable that time and resources will be wasted.

GENERAL PRINCIPLES OF ENDOCRINE TESTING
General Categories of Endocrine Tests

Endocrine evaluation can be divided into two broad categories: testing in the basal state and testing designed either to increase or to decrease hormone secretion (stimulation and suppression tests).

Basal Tests. Basal testing should be done when the patient is resting and has fasted for approximately 8 to 12 hours. Ideally the patient should not be acutely ill, and medication should be withdrawn. The last stipulation is often difficult to meet.

Stimulation Tests. Stimulation testing is used primarily to assess the adequacy of hormone reserve. Direct testing uses a specific trophic hormone or an agent known to induce a target gland hormone response. The patient's response is then compared with standards derived from normal individuals. Stimulation testing is also used to elicit an inappropriate secretory response. An example is the secretion of calcitonin after pentagastrin injection in patients with medullary carcinoma of the thyroid. A calcitonin response is not seen in normal individuals, thus the anomalous response becomes a diagnostic marker for disease.

Another variety of stimulation testing involves tests that inhibit feedback suppression. There are two general mechanisms by which this can be accomplished. The testing agent can block target gland hormone secretion, which then results in increased trophic hormone release. This occurs as a result of diminished feedback inhibition caused by a lower concentration of target gland hormone. Metyrapone stimulation utilizes this physiologic principle. A testing agent can also inhibit feedback suppression by blocking the action of the target hormone at the site of trophic hormone secretion. In this instance, the agent employed usually occupies the receptors for the target hormone but has little or no ability to decrease trophic hormone release. Clomiphene stimulation is an example of this form of feedback inhibition.

Suppression Tests. Suppression testing is commonly used in the evaluation of endocrine hypersecretory disorders. Usually these testing procedures inhibit physiologic hormone secretion. With autonomous hormone secretion there is loss of feedback to signals that normally suppress hormone secretion. Failure of appropriate suppression to occur offers strong evidence for loss of normal control mechanisms and associated glandular abnormality.

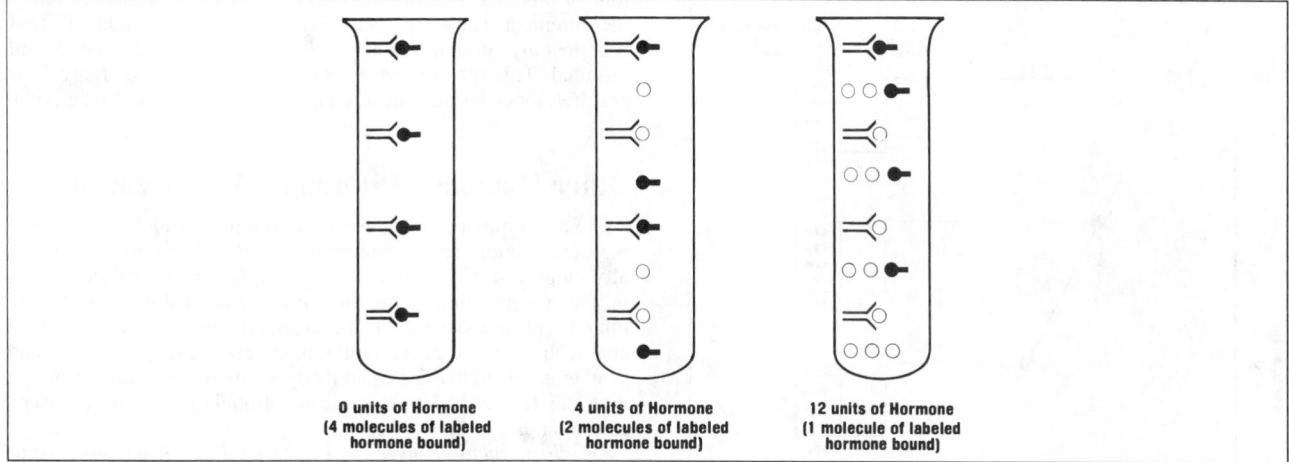

FIGURE 285-1   The principles of radioimmunoassay *(see text)*. With no endogenous hormone, all of the labeled *(radioactive)* hormone is bound by antibody specific for the hormone. A precipitate of antibody and hormone would then show increased radioactivity. With very high levels of endogenous hormone, the great majority of antibody is bound by endogenous hormone. In this case, very little radioactivity would be detected in the hormone-antibody precipitate.   Antibody;   , labeled hormone ○, endogenous hormone.

Measurement of Hormone Concentration in Blood

Many hormones are released episodically. Fortuitous determination at either the height of a secretory burst or its nadir may therefore give misleading results. To obviate this problem, it is helpful to obtain three blood specimens at intervals of 15 minutes or more. Equal aliquots from the specimens are pooled into a single combined specimen. The value obtained should closely approximate the average hormone concentration, and the patient is charged for only a single hormone determination. It is especially important to obtain pooled specimens when measuring gonadotropins, estrogens, and testosterone; it is not necessary for most other hormones. The difficulty of collecting several blood specimens is greatly lessened by using an indwelling catheter kept patent with a heparin-saline solution.

Hormones also are subject to biologic variations and rhythms that reflect either influences from the environment or regular oscillations originating from within the patient *(endogenous rhythms)*. External stimuli causing a stress reaction may cause acute release of several hormones including adrenocorticotropic hormone (ACTH), cortisol, growth hormone, prolactin, and epinephrine. The endogenous rhythmic oscillations of hormone concentration may have a 24-hour periodicity *(circadian)* or exhibit cyclicity of more than 24 hours *(infradian)*. These factors must be considered when interpreting hormone concentrations in blood.

Many hormones are transported in plasma partly bound to binding proteins and partly unbound or free. It is only the free portion that is active; however, in some cases (e.g., thyroid hormone), the great majority exists in the bound form. Routine testing techniques are not capable of separating the bound from the free portions of the hormone and measure only the total hormone concentration. Thus conditions that greatly alter protein binding of hormones may lead to an inaccurate estimate of the active hormone level. When conditions exist that alter binding (see later discussion), the clinician should request that the free hormone concentration be measured.

Measurement of Hormone Concentration in Urine

The measurement of a hormone or its metabolites in urine theoretically corrects for fluctuating blood levels and integrates the concentration over a longer period (usually 24 hours). To assess whether a urine collection is complete, creatinine excretion in the urine should be measured. The creatinine content in an adult sample is usually 1 g or more per day. For testing procedures requiring multiple urine collections during a series of diagnostic manipulations, such as dexa-

methasone suppression for Cushing's syndrome, it is essential to save a small aliquot from each total volume until all testing is completed and results are returned to the physician. This will allow retrieval and retesting of specimens that are lost or improperly handled by laboratory personnel. Many hormones measured in the urine are metabolic products of conjugation. Their measurement commonly utilizes laborious extraction procedures or chromatography. Very large and dilute urine volumes make total extraction and accurate measurement of the products difficult.

Immunoassay

No single technologic development has advanced endocrinology further than the immunoassay. It allows investigators to understand the pathophysiology of many diseases and provides a powerful tool for diagnosing endocrine disorders. Despite its importance, the principles of immunoassay are relatively simple (Fig. 285-1). It consists of the following major components.

1. An antibody that is specific for the particular hormone being measured.
2. A fixed and specific amount of the hormone that is labeled with a radioactive marker.
3. A specimen that contains an unknown amount of hormone.

To perform the assay, the antibody and the labeled hormone are added to the specimen with the unknown amount of hormone. The endogenous hormone (the hormone originally present in the specimen) and the labeled hormone (the hormone added in the laboratory) compete for binding sites on the antibody. If there is a large concentration of endogenous hormone, most of the antibody will be bound to it and little antibody remain to bind the labeled hormone. Thus the antibody-hormone complex will contain only a small amount of labeled hormone and therefore little radioactivity. Conversely, if the concentration of endogenous hormone is small, the antibody will bind relatively more labeled hormone, and the antibody-hormone complex will contain considerable radioactivity. To measure the amount of radioactivity that is bound, the hormone bound to the antibody and the unbound hormone must be separated, and there are a variety of techniques for accomplishing this. One method commonly used employs a "second antibody," which binds the hormone-specific "first antibody" and facilitates the precipitation of the hormone-antibody complex. Determining the unknown hormone level is possible by comparing the amount of binding in the unknown specimen to a standard curve (Fig. 285-2). Standard curves are established by adding known quantities of unlabeled hormone and determining the percentage of radiolabeled hormone bound.

The immunoassay is usually sensitive and reliable. Different anti-

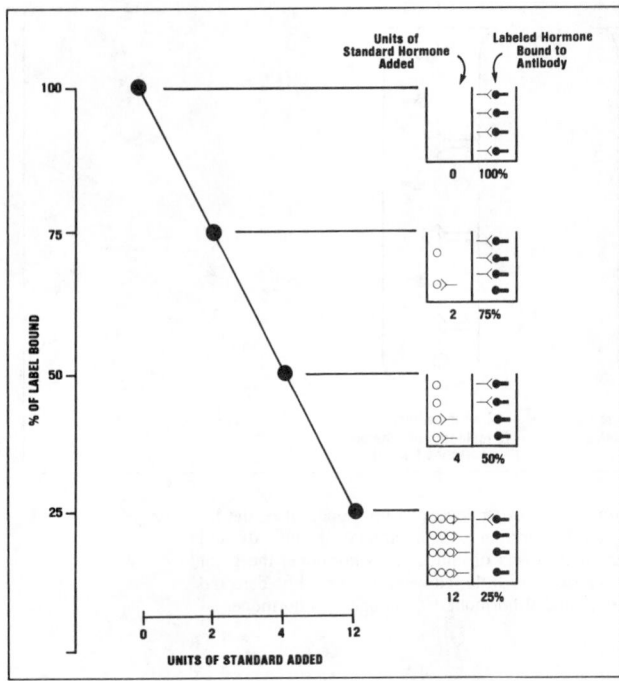

FIGURE 285-2 Standard curve for radioimmunoassay. As the amount of standard *(unlabeled)* hormone is increased, less of the labeled hormone is bound by antibody specific to the hormone. Thus knowledge of the amount of radioactivity bound by antibody when a known amount of hormone is added allows determination of the amount of endogenous hormone in an unknown sample. For accurate measurement, the same quantity of antibody and label must be used in unknown samples as is used in plotting the standard curve. The standard curve illustrated here is linear and therefore is idealized. Most standard curves show considerable flattening and less sensitivity at the lower and upper limits of assay detectability. This is not a problem at the upper limits of detectability (high levels of endogenous hormone) because such samples can be diluted and reassayed. ⌒ Antibody; ●─, labeled hormone; ○, standard (unlabeled) hormone.

bodies to the same hormone, however, can vary in *specificity* (degree of binding to other proteins in addition to the one being measured) and *affinity* (concentration of antibody needed to bind a given amount of hormone). Therefore results of laboratories employing different assay systems often are not strictly comparable. It is also important to realize that an antibody may bind prohormones or hormone fragments (which often are not active), so the value determined is not necessarily a measurement of biologically active hormone.

Newer techniques that increase sensitivity and specificity of the immunoassay are being used by commercial laboratories. Use of monoclonal antibodies (a single clone of antibody with affinity for only a single antigenic site on a hormone) improves the specificity of an assay and diminishes interlaboratory variation of results.

Chemiluminescence immunoassay may offer an alternative to immunoassay. It is similar to the classic immunoassay except that it employs the antigen labeled with a chemiluminescent compound (acridinium esters) as the tracer. When acridinium is oxidized, it emits photons of approximately 430-nm wavelength that are detected by a photomultiplier. The photon strikes are counted and converted to counts in a way similar to that of a γ-counter that quantitates radioactivity.

Immunometric assays, employed to measure intact parathyroid hormone (iPTH), use two separate antibodies to PTH. One binds to the amino-terminal and the other to the carboxyl-terminal of the hormone. The carboxyl-terminal antibody is coupled to a solid support matrix. The antibody–solid support complex binds all the intact PTH (which has both a carboxyl- and an amino-terminal) and the carboxyl end fragments (which have only the carboxyl-terminal). Amino end fragments are not bound by the solid phase as the serum filters through it. A second antibody, which reacts only to the amino-terminal, is then added to the solid phase. It is labeled with radioio-

dine or linked to a chemiluminescent substance to allow detection and measurement. The second antibody binds only to the intact PTH since it is the only substance attached to the solid phase that has an amino-terminal. This type of assay results in enhanced specificity for several hormones because of a reduction in nonspecific background activity.

Other Methods of Hormone Measurement

Although immunoassay is presently the most widely used means of measuring hormone concentration, other methods are still occasionally employed. *Competitive protein binding* is a displacement assay in which a specific binding protein and a labeled tracer hormone are mixed with the substrate to be measured. Its principles are entirely analogous to those of the radioimmunoassay except that the binding protein is substituted for an antibody. Cortisol is sometimes measured with this technique by using a cortisol-binding globulin (transcortin) as the binding protein.

Radioenzymatic conversion is a technique that employs the addition of radiolabeled hormone to a specimen and then, with a fixed amount of an added enzyme, causes conversion of a portion of the hormone to metabolites that are radiolabeled. The quantity of labeled metabolites is then measured. If the endogenous concentration of hormone is large, the enzyme will convert relatively little labeled hormone to metabolite. If the endogenous hormone concentration is low, more of the added labeled hormone will be converted, thereby increasing the total labeled metabolites. This technique is helpful when the hormone metabolites are easier to measure than the hormone, as in the case of catecholamines.[3]

Radiographic and Isotopic Studies in Endocrinology

Computed tomography has had a great impact on the neuroradiologic evaluation of patients with suspected hypothalamic-pituitary disease. High-resolution scanners demonstrate abnormalities as small as 1.5 mm within the pituitary gland. Small hypothalamic tumors can be seen but may be hard to distinguish from normal tissues if the tumor is a well-differentiated neural cell neoplasm. Computed tomography is a very sensitive means of detecting suprasellar calcifications in patients with craniopharyngiomas. Adrenal tumors as small as 0.5 cm can be seen if they lie in the lateral wings of the adrenal gland. The adrenal gland, however, thickens considerably where the lateral wings join, and if a tumor is located there it must be larger than 1.5 cm to be identified consistently. Adrenal tumors may not be detected if there is little fat surrounding the adrenal glands. Fat outlines the adrenal borders, and its absence obscures abnormalities in adrenal gland contour.

Computed tomography of the pancreas is sometimes helpful in detecting insulinomas. However, the tumor must be larger than 2 cm to be identified. Another application of this technique includes evaluation for extraocular muscle enlargement or a retroorbital mass in patients with unilateral exophthalmos. Less common uses of computed tomography are the evaluation of thyroid and parathyroid tumors and detection of early osteoporosis. The place of computed tomography in the evaluation of these disorders, however, is not yet established.

Ultrasonography is an increasingly important tool in endocrine evaluation. Ultrasonography may reveal a thyroid gland to have multiple nodules and a low risk of malignancy. Also, isolated nodules that are predominantly cystic nodules are very unlikely to be malignant. In patients with exophthalmic Graves' disease, the orbital contents can be visualized by this technique and distinguished from tumors causing exophthalmos. Ultrasound is also valuable for evaluating ovarian structure in patients with hirsutism. Although it is a sensitive means of detecting polycystic ovaries, ultrasound does have some limitations in detecting ovarian tumors. In thin patients, tumors as small as 1 cm can be identified. Adipose tissue, however, is echogenic and makes interpretation of the study very difficult in obese patients, in whom tumors as large as 5 cm can be missed. This is unfortunate because physical examination of the ovaries is most likely to be inadequate in obese patients.

Radioisotope studies are particularly important in the evaluation of thyroid disease. An iodine-123 tracer is given to patients with suspected hyperthyroidism; if hyperthyroidism is present, the 24-hour thyroid uptake of this isotope is usually greater than 30%. The test is not useful for diagnosing hypothyroidism because iodine is present in ever-increasing quantities in our diet, effectively abolishing a lower normal limit to the uptake. Functional characteristics of thyroid nodules can also be studied with thyroid scans. Areas with autonomous function often show increased uptake, whereas hypofunctional areas show diminished uptake. Technetium-99, which delivers very little radioactivity to the thyroid, also can be used for this purpose. Technetium, however, is trapped but not organically bound to thyroglobulin and may make some nonfunctional nodules appear functional. This may inappropriately lower the suspicion of cancer because functioning nodules are very unlikely to be cancerous. Metaiodobenzylguanidine (MIBG) resembles norepinephrine and is taken up by chromaffin tissue. MIBG, when labeled with iodine-131, detects primary pheochromocytoma and metastasis from malignant pheochromocytomas. Islet cell tumors and carcinoids often contain somatostatin receptors. Administration of radiolabeled octreotide, a somatostatin analog, will sometimes detect these tumors.

Magnetic resonance imaging (MRI) is not invasive and does not use ionizing radiation. It delivers anatomically detailed images of the pituitary and hypothalamus. Tumors to 0.3 cm in diameter can be seen. The neck and mediastinum can be visualized well in searching for metastatic thyroid cancer, substernal goiter, or parathyroid adenoma after an unsuccessful surgical exploration. It also holds promise for ovarian imaging because it delivers a negligible amount of radiation. MRI may be superior for detection of pheochromocytoma since the T2-weighted signals show a characteristic high signal intensity.

Selective venous catheterization with hormone measurement in venous effluent can be a useful means of locating the source of hormone hypersecretion. The technique is most widely employed in the study of primary hyperaldosteronism after other localizing techniques have failed to determine whether a single adenoma is present or both glands are hyperplastic. The right adrenal vein cannot always be entered because of its small size and variable anatomic position. Venous catheterization is also used to locate a parathyroid adenoma in patients with a previously failed parathyroidectomy or in those with difficult-to-diagnose Cushing's syndrome in which selective catheterization of the inferior petrosal vein and measurement of ACTH concentration can establish the presence of pituitary-dependent Cushing's syndrome. Occasionally these studies are used to localize pheochromocytoma, insulinoma, and carcinoid.

SPECIFIC ENDOCRINE TESTS
Hypothalamic-Pituitary Testing

Many tests are available for evaluating the reserve of specific anterior pituitary hormones (Fig. 285-3) (Chapter 295). Stimulatory agents increase secretion either by hypothalamic pathways or by direct stimulation of the anterior pituitary. Some testing agents cause release of multiple hormones.

Thyrotropin-releasing Hormone. In normal individuals thyrotropin-releasing hormone (TRH) causes the release of thyroid-stimulating hormone (TSH) and prolactin (PRL). In theory, the test can distinguish between hypothalamic and pituitary deficiency. Unfortunately, there is overlap between the responses observed in these two disease states because some patients with pituitary disease have a normal TSH response (the expected response with hypothalamic disease), and patients with hypothalamic disease may demonstrate a subnormal TSH response (the expected response for pituitary disorders). These paradoxical responses and the fact that PRL reserve rarely needs to be tested limit the usefulness of TRH testing for pituitary disease. The test is used to evaluate patients for suspected hyperthyroidism because an even slightly excessive thyroid hormone concentration suppresses the TSH response to TRH. Thus an absent or blunted TSH response to TRH is supportive evidence for hyperthyroidism in patients with an equivocally elevated thyroid hormone level in blood. For evaluation of most cases of hyperthyroidism, however, a finding of a suppressed TSH level using the newer, sensitive assay has largely replaced the TRH test. TRH testing remains useful in the evaluation of hyperthyroidism with a normal or elevated TSH

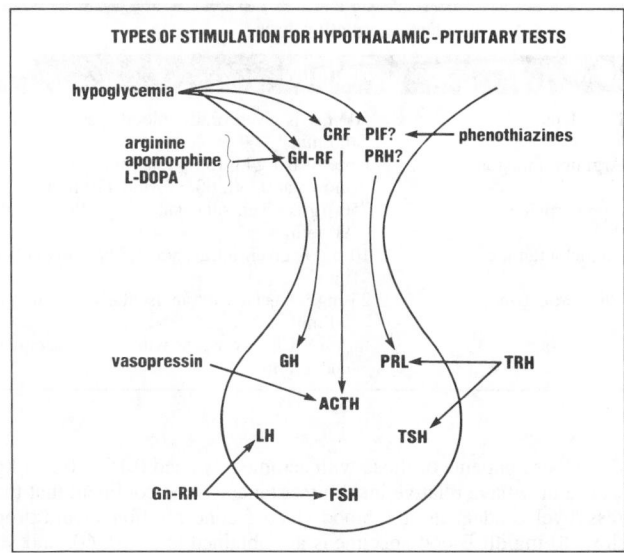

FIGURE 285-3 Stimulatory agents cause increased anterior pituitary hormone secretion either by hypothalamic pathways or by direct stimulation of the anterior pituitary gland. The level at which these stimulatory agents exert their effects is shown. *GH-RF,* Growth hormone–releasing factor; *PIF,* prolactin-inhibiting factor; *PRH,* prolactin-releasing hormone.

concentration. Patients with TSH-secreting pituitary tumors rarely show any TSH responsiveness to TRH, whereas those with pituitary resistance to thyroid hormone feedback do have a TSH response to TRH. To perform this test, 500 μg of TRH is administered intravenously, and blood for TSH is collected at 0, 15, 30, and 60 minutes. The TSH level should show increments of at least 5 μU/ml. Age blunts the TSH response, and the increase may be less than 2 μU/ml in normal men over 50 years of age.

Gonadotropin-releasing Hormone. Both luteinizing hormone (LH) and follicle-stimulating hormone (FSH) are released by gonadotropin-releasing hormone (GnRH). In adults, the LH response is greater than the FSH response. In children, the responses of LH and FSH are approximately equal except during puberty, when the FSH response exceeds that of LH. As with TRH, a single injection of GnRH may not distinguish between a hypothalamic origin and a pituitary origin of gonadotropin deficiency. However, with intermittent injections (over at least 2 weeks), virtually all patients with a hypothalamic defect will respond to GnRH. Patients are given 100 μg of GnRH intravenously, and blood is collected at 0, 30, and 60 minutes. In adults the LH level increases by at least 20 mIU/ml. The FSH concentration is much less responsive, and an increase of less than 2 mIU/ml is seen in some normal individuals.

Corticotropin-releasing Hormone. In identifying the cause of Cushing's syndrome, corticotropin-releasing hormone (CRH) may be useful. Patients with pituitary-dependent Cushing's syndrome have an ACTH response to CRH. Those with ectopic ACTH syndrome do not show an ACTH increase. However, there is overlap of the ACTH response between these disorders, and CRH does not always distinguish between them. Measurement of simultaneously obtained ACTH specimens from the inferior petrosal sinus and a peripheral vein after CRH administration is a more reliable means to separate pituitary-dependent Cushing's syndrome from ectopic ACTH secretion. CRH (1 μg/kg) is given by bolus, and blood samples for ACTH are obtained at 0, 15, 30, and 60 minutes. The maximum ACTH response occurs at 15 minutes and the cortisol peaks at 30 to 60 minutes.

Insulin-induced Hypoglycemia. In response to the stress of hypoglycemia, ACTH, PRL, and GH (growth hormone) are secreted. Stimulation occurs via activation of hypothalamic pathways; therefore a subnormal hormone response occurs with either hypothalamic or pituitary disease. Regular insulin is administered at a dose of 0.1

Table 285-1 Pituitary stimulation tests

AGENT	PROTOCOL	NORMAL RESPONSE
Levodopa	500 mg is given orally; blood specimens are obtained at 0, 30, and 60 min	GH level should exceed 7 ng/ml
Arginine infusion	Dose of 0.5 g/kg (30 g maximum) is infused over 30 min; blood is drawn at 0, 30, 60, 90, and 120 min	GH level should exceed 7 ng/ml
Apomorphine	750 μg is given subcutaneously. Blood is obtained at 0, 30, 60, and 90 min	GH level should exceed 7 ng/ml
Metoclopramide	10 mg is given intravenously; blood is collected at 0, 30, 60, and 90 min	PRL level exceeds 100 ng/ml
Chlorpromazine	25 mg is injected intramuscularly; blood is obtained at 0, 30, 60, and 90 min	PRL level increases 2 times baseline level or achieves an absolute value >20 ng/ml
Vasopressin	Infuse 2 U/hr over 2 hr with blood specimens collected at 0, 30, 60, and 120 min	Plasma cortisol should exceed 20 μg/dl

U/kg. Obese patients or those with acromegaly need 0.15 to 0.2 U/kg because they have relative insulin resistance. To be confident that the stress level is adequate, the blood glucose concentration should drop below 40 mg/dl. Blood specimens are obtained at 0, 30, 60, and 90 minutes. If symptoms of hypoglycemia are excessive, the patient can be given intravenous glucose without fear of compromising the test's accuracy because the hypoglycemic stress will have already occurred. In a normal response, GH exceeds 7 ng/ml, and cortisol exceeds 20 μg/dl. PRL usually increases to 30 ng/ml or more, but there is rarely a need to measure it during dynamic testing. The presence of seizure disorders or coronary artery disease is a contraindication for the test. The test also should be avoided in elderly people. Subnormal increments in GH without pituitary disease are seen in obese patients and in those with long-standing hypothyroidism and hypogonadism.

Other Stimulation Tests. GH is released by a number of pharmacologic agents including *levodopa, arginine,* and *apomorphine* (Table 285-1). All work through activation of hypothalamic pathways. Obesity blunts the GH response to hypoglycemia. *Chlorpromazine* and *metoclopramide* are antidopaminergic drugs that stimulate PRL secretion (Table 285-1). These PRL stimulatory tests do not aid in the diagnosis of PRL-secreting pituitary tumors. Lysine vasopressin directly stimulates the pituitary to release ACTH (Table 285-1). This agent directly tests the pituitary-adrenal axis whereas it bypasses the hypothalamus. It is best given by intravenous infusion but can also be given as an intramuscular injection. Side-effects are abdominal pain, nausea, defecation, and occasional attacks of angina. Side-effects have limited the clinical application of vasopressin stimulation, and the test is obviously contraindicated in patients with coronary artery disease or hypertension.

Tests Using Feedback Inhibition. *Metyrapone* inhibits the adrenal enzyme 11-β-hydroxylase, thereby blocking the conversion of 11-deoxycortisol to cortisol (Fig. 285-4). Cortisol levels fall, and because 11-deoxycortisol is not an effective inhibitor of ACTH, ACTH levels increase. This stimulates the production of more 11-deoxycortisol, which is measured directly in the blood by radioimmunoassay or in the urine as a 17-hydroxycorticosteroid. The test should not be done in patients with suspected adrenal insufficiency because the reduced cortisol production can precipitate adrenal crisis. The test is very helpful in identifying patients with pituitary-dependent Cushing's syndrome because this is the only variety of Cushing's syndrome in which the urinary 17-hydroxycorticosteroid level increases after administration of metyrapone. There are two varieties of the metyrapone test, an overnight test and a 3-day test. To perform the overnight test, metyrapone, 30 mg/kg, is given orally at midnight. At 8:00 AM, blood is drawn for 11-deoxycortisol and cortisol level determinations. The 11-deoxycortisol level should increase to more than 8 μ/dl in patients with a normal pituitary-adrenal axis, and the cortisol concentration should be less than 5 μ/dl (a low cortisol level indicates that the block of 11-β-hydroxylase is adequate). The 3-day test is accomplished by measuring a baseline urinary 17-hydroxycorticosteroid value and then administering 750 mg of metyrapone every 4 hours for six doses. The urinary 17-hydroxycorticosteroid concentration should increase two to three

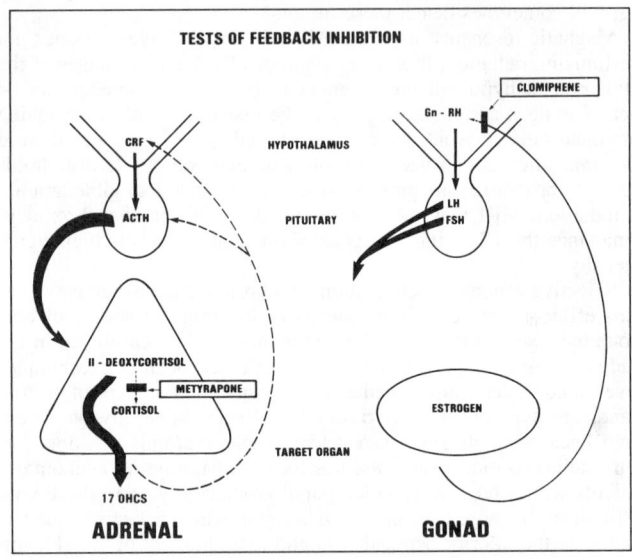

FIGURE 285-4 Metyrapone and clomiphene cause increasing trophic hormone secretion by blocking feedback inhibition. Metyrapone blocks the conversion of 11-deoxycortisol to cortisol by inhibiting the enzyme 11-β-hydroxylase. Cortisol levels fall, thereby diminishing feedback inhibition, which results in increased ACTH secretion. Clomiphene, a weak estrogen analog, binds to hypothalamic estrogen receptors and blocks estrogen feedback inhibition, resulting in increased gonadotropin secretion. *ACTH,* Adrenocorticotropic hormone.

times over the baseline value on day 2 or day 3. Several drugs (diphenylhydantoin, phenobarbital, primidone, and phenylbutazone) may accelerate the clearance of metyrapone and cause the urinary 17-hydroxycorticosteroid response to be blunted or absent.

Clomiphene is an estrogen analog that blocks estrogen effect. Loss of estrogen feedback activity at the hypothalamus causes gonadotropin secretion to increase, allowing evaluation of the hypothalamic-pituitary axis (Fig. 285-4). To conduct the test, pooled specimens of LH and FSH are obtained on day 1, and then clomiphene is given orally, 50 mg twice daily, for 10 days. The maximum gonadotropin response is usually seen approximately 10 days after beginning the drug. FSH and LH should increase by at least 50% over baseline levels when measured at day 10. Depression is the only major side-effect. Ovulation may be induced in a previously infertile woman.

Suppression Tests. The *dexamethasone suppression test* measures the intactness of glucocorticoid-ACTH feedback regulation. Patients with a higher setpoint of ACTH secretion or autonomous cortisol secretion are resistant to dexamethasone suppression. The test is used for the diagnosis of Cushing's syndrome. There are two types of dexamethasone suppression tests, an overnight screening test and a 6-day test used for definitive diagnosis. The overnight screening test is performed by giving 1 mg of dexamethasone at 11:00 PM and obtaining an 8:00 AM plasma cortisol level. This amount of glucocorticoid is sufficient to suppress ACTH (cortisol) secretion in normal individuals but not in patients with Cushing's syndrome regardless of type. Normal individuals suppress the cortisol level to less than 5 μg/dl. In patients with Cushing's syndrome the level remains greater than 5 μg/dl and is often above 10 μg/dl. The 6-day test, when coupled with an accurate 8:00 AM plasma ACTH level determination, allows the physician to distinguish between the different types of Cushing's syndrome. The 6-day test is divided into two parts. Initially, a "low dose" (0.5 mg q6h) and then a "high dose" (2 mg q6h) of dexamethasone are administered. The low dose suppresses ACTH secretion (and therefore cortisol level) in normal individuals but not in patients with Cushing's syndrome. Patients with pituitary-dependent Cushing's syndrome, however, show ACTH suppression when they are given sufficiently high doses of dexamethasone. This higher threshold of suppression occurs because of an altered feedback mechanism to glucocorticoids. Patients with other varieties of hypercortisolism such as ectopic ACTH secretion and adrenal tumors show no change in cortisol secretion regardless of the dosage of dexamethasone given. Thus the differential response to low-dose dexamethasone is used to separate normal individuals from patients with Cushing's syndrome, and the high-dose test separates patients with pituitary-dependent Cushing's syndrome from those with adrenal tumors or ectopic ACTH secretion. Adrenal tumors suppress ACTH concentration to undetectable levels, allowing them to be distinguished from the ectopic ACTH syndrome, which has a high ACTH concentration. False-positive results may result from accelerated metabolism of dexamethasone induced by certain drugs such as diphenylhydantoin, phenobarbital, primidone, and phenylbutazone. Thyrotoxicosis also increases the clearance of dexamethasone and may cause a false-positive result.

Glucose suppression of GH is used to evaluate autonomous GH secretion. In normal individuals GH secretion is suppressed to less than 2 ng/ml 60 to 120 minutes after 100 g of oral glucose is given. In contrast, acromegalic patients rarely show a decrease to less than 5 ng/ml, and in some instances a paradoxic increase of GH occurs. To perform this test, 100 g of glucose is given orally, and GH level is measured 90 minutes later. It is not helpful to obtain a baseline GH level.

Basal Pituitary Hormone Measurements. A basal level of PRL is useful in the evaluation of hyperprolactinemia. A concentration of greater than 200 ng/ml almost always indicates a PRL-secreting pituitary tumor. Values less than this are not discriminatory because they may be due to tumors or other causes of hyperprolactinemia (Chapter 295).

In patients with suspected hypothyroidism a basal *TSH* concentration should always be obtained with the initial battery of thyroid function studies. A low or normal TSH level in patients with established hypothyroidism indicates that hypothalamic or pituitary disease is responsible because with even mild primary hypothyroidism the TSH level is elevated. Figure 285-5 illustrates the principle of loss of feedback inhibition with increased secretion of trophic hormone. A caveat is the "sick euthyroid syndrome" (Chapter 297), in which a low total thyroxine (T_4) level is seen with a normal TSH level. These patients are not clinically hypothyroid and have normal levels of free T_4.

The same principle applies to *LH* and *FSH* measurements as that described for TSH. A low or normal concentration in the presence of low gonadal steroid levels suggests hypothalamic or pituitary disease (Table 285-2). In women, such information must be interpreted in conjunction with the menstrual cycle because in the early follicular phase both gonadotropin and gonadal steroid levels may normally be low. As a rule, however, women with normal menstruation rarely need evaluation for hypogonadism.

Basal ACTH levels are helpful in the diagnosis and differentiation of Cushing's syndrome. High levels are seen with ectopic ACTH syndrome, and undetectable levels are observed with adrenal tumors.

There is, however, considerable overlap of ACTH levels in normal individuals and patients with pituitary-dependent Cushing's syndrome. It is not necessary to measure ACTH to document that hypocortisolism is primary rather than secondary. Normal ACTH levels

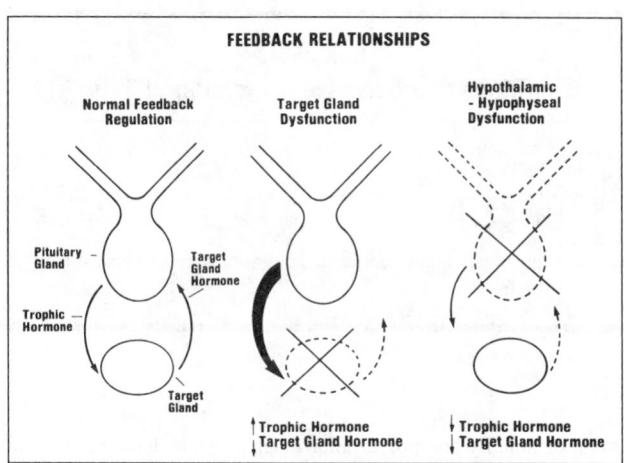

FIGURE 285-5   Normally the endocrine target hormone causes feedback suppression of its anterior pituitary trophic hormone. With loss of target gland function, feedback inhibition decreases, causing increased trophic hormone secretion. Hypothalamic-hypophyseal dysfunction results in both decreased trophic hormone level and target hormone secretion.

Table 285-2   Gonadotropins

CLINICAL STATE	LH mIU/ml	FSH ImU/ml
Prepubertal	2-6	1-3
Adult	6-25*	4-20*
Menopausal, castrate	>25	>20

*Midcycle peak of LH is 2 to 3 times baseline value and for FSH is approximately 2 times baseline value.

Table 285-3   Normal age-related changes in IGF-I

| | IGF-I CONCENTRATION (mcg/L) | |
AGE IN YEARS	MALE	FEMALE
3 to 12	80-940	110-462
13 to 18	180-836	120-660
Adult	140-390	140-390

vary widely between 20 and 110 pg/ml. Higher concentrations are seen in normal individuals in response to stress.

Determination of a basal *GH* level is rarely helpful in evaluation of either GH deficiency or GH excess. In contrast, measurement of *insulin-like growth factor I (somatomedin C, IGF-I)* level by radioimmunoassay gives useful information about both of these conditions. Insulin-like growth factor I is the mediator of GH action. In acromegaly an elevated IGF-I is a sensitive marker for even mild hypersecretion of GH. GH deficiency is suggested by values lower than the age-related lower limits listed in Table 285-3. There are several serum proteins that bind insulin-like growth factors. Insulin-like growth factor binding protein 3 (IGFBP-3) is growth hormone dependent and is low in GH deficiency and elevated in acromegaly. Normal values are from 2000 to 4000 mcg/L.

Posterior Pituitary Testing (Chapter 296)

Plasma Vasopressin Concentration. Measurement of the plasma vasopressin concentration with a simultaneously performed plasma osmolality evaluation is an accurate method of diagnosing diabetes insipidus. A low vasopressin concentration with elevated plasma osmolality is virtually diagnostic of central diabetes insipidus. Patients with elevated vasopressin concentration in the face of an elevated

---

BOX 285-1

Conditions that decrease conversion of T_4 to T_3

Caloric restriction
Acute febrile illness
Liver disease
Renal insufficiency*
Burns
Drugs (propranolol, glucocorticoids, propylthiouracil, iodinated contrast agents)

---

*T_4 level also may be low.

---

plasma osmolality and polyuria have nephrogenic diabetes insipidus, assuming that hypotension, diabetes mellitus, and salt-wasting nephropathy are excluded. Unfortunately, few reliable assays are available to the clinician. There also is a delay of days to weeks before the results of the assay are available and a diagnosis established.

Water Deprivation The water deprivation test assesses the urine-concentrating ability of a patient and the effect of exogenously administered vasopressin on urine osmolality. In patients with diabetes insipidus, urine is not concentrated during water deprivation despite developing hyperosmolality. Vasopressin is then given, to decrease free water clearance and allow the urine to become concentrated in patients with central diabetes insipidus. Patients with nephrogenic diabetes insipidus do not respond to vasopressin, and the urine remains dilute. In patients with primary polydipsia the urine is concentrated during water deprivation, although not always to normal values. These patients do not respond to vasopressin if water deprivation has been continued to the point of maximum urine osmolality. The testing procedure protocol is outlined in Chapter 296.

Water Loading. Most cases of inappropriate vasopressin secretion (SIADH; inappropriate secretion of antidiuretic hormone) can be diagnosed on the basis of the history, physical examination, serum and urine electrolyte levels, and plasma and urine osmolality. Occasionally, however, it is necessary to subject a difficult-to-diagnose patient to water loading. Most individuals excrete 50% of an administered water load (20 ml/kg body weight of tap water given over 30 minutes) within 4 hours. Failure to do so is presumptive evidence of SIADH if hypocortisolism and hypothyroidism are excluded. Drugs such as chlorpropamide, clofibrate, diphenylhydantoin, and procainamide may decrease water clearance and cause false-positive results. As a precautionary measure, hourly serum osmolarity should be determined.

Tests of Thyroid Function (Chapter 297)

Radioimmunoassay of Thyroid Hormone. Thyroid hormone radioimmunoassays (RIAs) routinely measure the total thyroxine level (T_4-RIA) and the total triiodothyronine concentration (T_3-RIA). Because most of the circulating T_4 and T_3 is bound to thyroglobulin (99.95% and 99.5%, respectively), the assay results are greatly affected by drugs and clinical conditions that alter thyroid-binding globulin (TBG) concentration (Chapter 297). The normal T_4-RIA is 5.5 to 11.5 μg/dl. The normal T_3-RIA concentration is 80 to 195 ng/dl. A number of conditions decrease the conversion of T_4 to T_3 and subsequently cause low total levels without hypothyroidism (Box 285-1). For this reason and also because the T_3 level often remains normal despite mild hypothyroidism, the T_3-RIA is an unsuitable screening test for hypothyroidism.

Free Thyroid Hormone Concentration. Measurement of the free thyroid hormone level is more difficult and expensive than assays that measure the total thyroid hormone concentration. Generally the free T_4 or the free T_3 concentration is determined by equilibrium dialysis. Newer, less time-consuming methods have appeared, including kits that measure the free T_4 by radioimmunoassay. The reliabil-

ity of these faster methods, however, is still in question. The advantage of determining the free thyroid level is that changes in TBG do not affect the result. The normal free T_4 concentration is 0.8 to 2.4 ng/ml, and the normal free T_3 level is less than 350 pg/ml.

Thyroid-stimulating Hormone. The use of monoclonal antibodies has increased the sensitivity of the TSH assay to the degree that low TSH levels can be distinguished from normal. Conventional TSH assays are only capable of discriminating high levels from normal. The sensitive TSH assay is useful as a screening test for hyperthyroidism. Suppressed TSH levels coupled with borderline or elevated thyroid hormone levels are indicative of primary hyperthyroidism. Not all commercially available assays are uniformly accurate, however, and some euthyroid patients have suppressed sensitive TSH levels. An elevated TSH level with high thyroid hormone levels suggests the rare disorder of secondary hyperthyroidism from a pituitary or hypothalamic source. High TSH levels, however, are usually indicative of primary hypothyroidism. A value of less than 0.4 μU/ml is low or suppressed, values 0.5 to 5 μU/ml are normal, and values greater than 7 μU/ml are elevated.

Thyroid Hormone-binding Globulin, T_3 Resin uptake. TBG level is assessed indirectly by the T_3 resin uptake test (Fig. 285-6). This test measures the capacity of a resin to bind radioactive T_3 in the presence of TBG. The key to understanding the test is the realization that TBG binds radiolabeled T_3 preferentially compared with the resin. In hyperthyroidism, excess thyroid hormone occupies the TBG, leaving few sites for the radiolabeled T_3 to be bound. Thus most of the added radiolabeled T_3 is bound by the resin, giving a high resin uptake. In hypothyroidism, there are many unoccupied thyroid hormone–binding sites on TBG; therefore most of the T_3 is bound by TBG and little is taken up by the resin, resulting in a low resin uptake. Confusing results may be obtained in the presence of conditions that either increase or decrease TBG level (Fig. 285-6). Estrogens, for example, increase TBG level and cause more thyroid hormone to be bound, thus increasing the total thyroid hormone concentration. A new equilibrium is reached, however, and the free thyroid hormone level remains normal. Because of excess TBG, more radiolabeled T_3 is bound, causing the resin uptake to be low. Thus a paradoxical situation results in which the total T_4 (or total T_3) level is elevated, but the T_3 resin uptake is low. Conversely, if TBG levels are reduced, the total thyroid hormone level is low, but the resin uptake is elevated. The normal T_3 resin uptake value varies among laboratories. A common normal range is 25% to 35%. TBG can be measured directly by radioimmunoassay. In most instances, however, this offers little advantage compared with the less expensive T_3 resin uptake test. The normal TBG concentration is 1 to 15 mg/dl.

Corrected Thyroxine Concentration. A simple calculation can be performed to correct for alterations in the total T_4 concentration induced by changes in TBG.

$$\text{Corrected total } T_4 = \text{patient's } T_4 \times \frac{\text{patient's } T_3 \text{ resin uptake}}{\text{average } T_3 \text{ resin uptake}}$$

For example, if the patient's T_4 concentration is elevated to 14 μg/dl but the T_3 resin uptake value is low at 20%, it is unclear whether hyperthyroidism is present. Using the equation, the corrected T_4 is 9.3 μg/dl.

$$14 \text{ μg} \times \frac{20}{30} = 9.3 \text{ μg/dl}$$

The average T_3 resin uptake value is the midpoint between the upper and lower limits of the particular T_3 resin uptake assay being used. The normal range for the corrected T_4 concentration is the same as that of total T_4. A similar calculation is used to determine a corrected total T_3 level.

Antithyroid Peroxidase Antibodies and Antithyroglobulin Antibodies. Circulating antibodies to these antigens imply inflammation and destruction of thyroid tissue. High titers of either an-

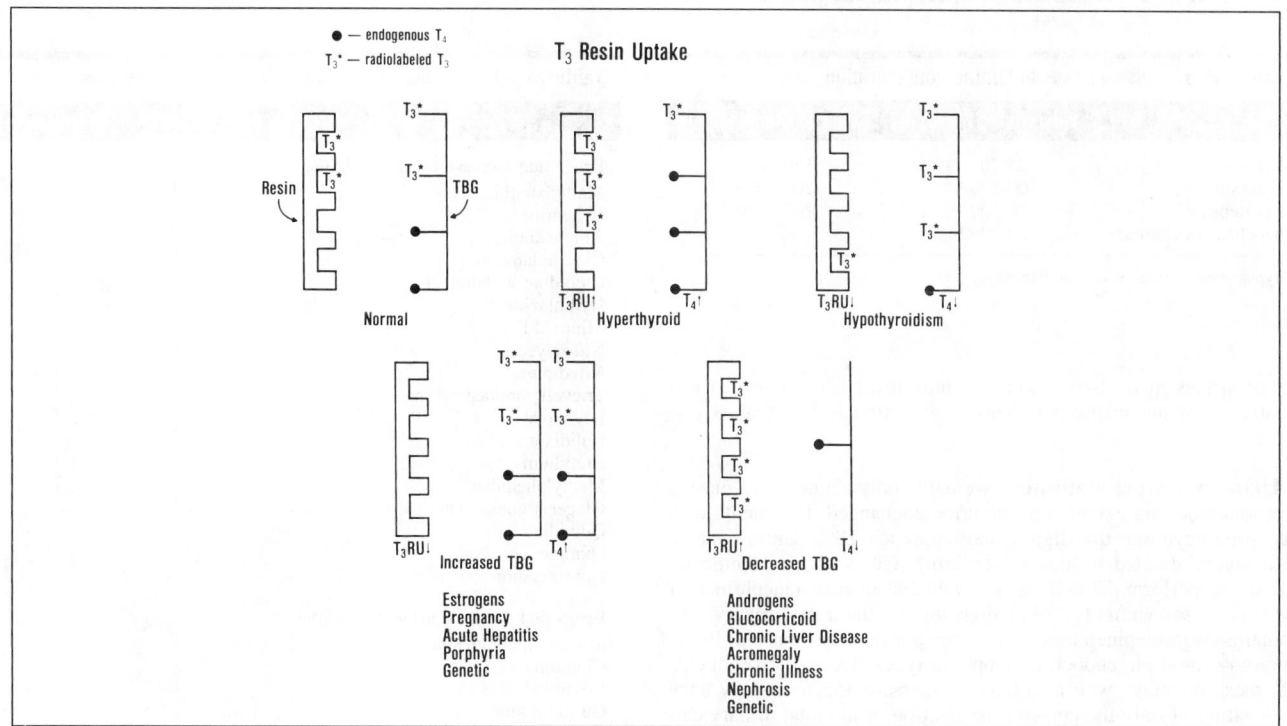

FIGURE 285-6   The effects of hyperthyroidism, hypothyroidism, increased TBG, and decreased TBG on the T₃resin uptake. Clinical states that either increase or decrease TBG concentrations are listed

tibody strongly suggest autoimmune lymphocytic thyroiditis (Hashimoto's thyroiditis). It is unusual, however, for knowledge of these antibody titers to influence the management of a patient.

Serum Thyroglobulin Level. Normal individuals usually have low but readily detectable levels of thyroglobulin in serum. After a total thyroidectomy, however, thyroglobulin levels should be undetectable while taking replacement amounts of thyroid hormone. This relationship makes thyroglobulin level a useful index to follow in patients with thyroid cancer. Detectable levels after thyroidectomy for thyroid cancer or the subsequent development of titers usually indicates the presence of metastatic disease. Thyroglobulin is also helpful for differentiating between "painless" subacute thyroiditis and factitious hyperthyroidism (Chapter 297). Patients with subacute thyroiditis should have high levels, reflecting thyroid gland damage and release of its products into the circulation, whereas patients taking thyroid hormone have low or undetectable thyroglobulin levels. In normal individuals thyroglobulin levels vary from 5 to 25 ng/ml.

T₃ Suppression Test. In normal individuals, exogenously administered T₃ suppresses TSH secretion, which in turn decreases the thyroid uptake of radioiodine. Resistance to suppression indicates either autonomous thyroid hormone secretion, as occurs in Graves' disease, or toxic multinodular goiter. The test is accomplished by performing a 24-hour radioiodine uptake determination and then administering 75 μg of T₃ for 10 days. On the tenth day the 24-hour uptake test is repeated (the tracer dose is given on the ninth day). Most normal persons suppress the uptake to less than 2%. Patients with autonomous thyroid hormone secretion show less than 50% suppression of the baseline radioiodine uptake. The test is helpful in patients who have symptoms that suggest hyperthyroidism but show equivocal results in thyroid function testing. Thyrotoxic symptoms may develop during the period of T₃ administration; therefore concurrent administration of a β-blocking agent increases patient tolerance of the test. The test is contraindicated in individuals with coronary disease and in the elderly.

TSH Stimulation Test. The TSH stimulation test measures the ability of the thyroid gland to incorporate radioiodine in response to exogenously administered TSH. The test can determine whether primary hypothyroidism is present in a patient taking thyroid hormone, although it is a somewhat impractical means of accomplishing this

end. A response to TSH does not exclude hypothyroidism secondary to hypothalamic or pituitary disease. Its major use is to distinguish silent subacute thyroiditis from factitious hyperthyroidism. The damaged gland in the former condition prevents uptake of iodine, whereas patients taking thyroid hormone, even to the point of hyperthyroidism, still have normal uptake (>10%) in response to TSH. Bovine TSH, 10 units daily, is administered for 3 days, and the radioiodine uptake test is performed on the third day. Occasionally, severe allergic reactions occur, so patients should be skin-tested with TSH before testing.

Thyroid-Stimulating Immunoglobulin. Thyroid-stimulating immunoglobulin (TSI) is an antibody to the TSH receptor. TSI is usually detectable in patients with Graves' hyperthyroidism. It should not be routinely measured, although it is sometimes helpful when the diagnosis or etiology of hyperthyroidism is unclear. The presence of TSI also may confirm the diagnosis of Graves' euthyroid opthalmopathy.

Pentagastrin and Calcium Stimulation Tests of Calcitonin. Patients with medullary thyroid cancer secrete calcitonin after the administration of pentagastrin or calcium to a much greater extent than normal individuals. Pentagastrin is given at a dose of 0.5 μg/kg, or 150 mg/kg of calcium chloride is infused over 10 minutes and blood is collected at 0, 2, 5, and 10 minutes. Basal levels are normally less than 20 pg/ml in women and less than 30 pg/ml in men. With a tumor, stimulated values almost always exceed 425 pg/ml. Normal individuals may show some increase, but it is considerably smaller.

Adrenal Medullary Hormones (Chapter 299)

Metanephrines. Metanephrine and normetanephrine are formed when epinephrine and norepinephrine, respectively, are methylated by the enzyme catechol-O-methyltransferase. Together, these urinary catecholamine metabolites are termed *metanephrines*. A 24-hour urine collection for metanephrines is an accurate, reliable, simple, and cost-effective screening test for the diagnosis of pheochromocytoma. Normal values are less than 1.3 mg/24 hr.

Vanillylmandelic Acid. Vanillylmandelic acid (VMA) is a metabolic product formed by the action of monoamine oxidase on

Table 285-4 Plasma catecholamine concentration

	EPINEPHRINE (pg/ml)	NOREPINEPHRINE (pg/ml)
Basal	25-70	150-400
Major stress*	100-500	200-2000
Hypertension	20-100	200-5000
Pheochromocytoma	50-2000	>2000

*Hypoglycemia, surgery, cardiac ischemia.

Table 285-5 Agents interfering with catecholamine assays

	METANEPHRINES	VMA	CATECHOLAMINES
Drugs that increase urine metabolites			
Methylxanthine	↑	↑	↑
Ephedrine	↑	↑	↑
Amphetamines	↑	↑	↑
Catecholamines	↑	↑	↑
Clonidine withdrawal	↑	↑	↑
Hydralazine	↑	↑	↑
Minoxidil	↑	↑	↑
Nitroglycerin	↑	↑	↑
Nifedipine	↑	↑	↑
Tricyclic antidepressants*	↑	↑	↑
Levodopa	↑	↑	↑
Nalidixic acid	—	↑	—
Bretylium	—	—	↑
Methylphenidate	—	—	↑
Glyceryl guaiacolate	—	↑	—
Quinidine	—	—	↑
Quinine	—	—	↑
Isoproterenol	—	—	↑
Drugs that decrease urine metabolites			
α-Methylparatyrosine	↓	↓	↓
Clonidine	↓	↓	↓
Reserpine	↓	↓	↓
Guanethidine	↓	↓	↓
Clofibrate	—	↓	—
Disulfiram	—	↓	—
Sodium diatrizoate	↓	—	—
Drugs that have a mixed effect on urine metabolites			
Ethanol	↑	↓	↑
Methyldopa	↑	↓	↑
Methenamine mandelate	—	↓	↑
MAO inhibitors	↑	↓	↑
Chlorpromazine	—	↓	↑

*Acute effect.

metanephrines. It is also a good screening test but is somewhat less sensitive than metanephrines. Normal excretion is less than 8 mg/24 hr.

Urinary Catecholamines. Normally, only about 1% of plasma catecholamines are excreted in the urine unchanged. In patients with pheochromocytoma, this figure may approach 10%. Unfortunately, the assay is affected by many interfering agents and is technically difficult to perform. Thus it is less valuable than metanephrines or VMA as a screening test. Fractionation of the total urinary catecholamines into epinephrine or norepinephrine may be useful in patients with multiple endocrine neoplasia types IIA and IIB. Patients with these disorders who also have a pheochromocytoma may have an elevation of only the epinephrine fraction of the total urinary catecholamines. Normal adults excrete 20 to 70 μg of norepinephrine and 0 to 15 μg of epinephrine during a 24-hour period.

Plasma Catecholamines. A carefully collected and meticulously measured plasma catecholamine determination is a very sensitive method for diagnosing pheochromocytoma. At present, however, few commercially available assays can duplicate the sensitivity of the expensive and technically difficult research assays. We therefore reserve plasma catecholamine level measurement for cases in which clinical suspicion is very high but results of repeated urine studies are normal. The clinician should take special care to choose a laboratory that has an assay of proven reliability. When the measurement is made, the patient should be medication free and fasting. Dihydrocaffeic acid (found in all coffees and some colas) may cause a false-positive test. An indwelling, heparinized catheter should be inserted, and the patient should remain supine for 30 minutes before collection. This will reduce the chance of stress-induced plasma catecholamine elevation. Total catecholamine level is usually greater than 2000 pg/ml in patients with pheochromocytoma. Normal values are listed in Table 285-4.

Clonidine Suppression. If results of urine and blood studies are equivocal for pheochromocytoma or if suspicion remains high despite normal testing results, clonidine suppression of plasma norepinephrine levels may be helpful. Clonidine is a central α-adrenergic stimulant that ultimately results in diminished sympathetic outflow and a fall in norepinephrine levels. If norepinephrine production is autonomous, as it is with a pheochromocytoma, norepinephrine levels remain elevated and unchanged 3 hours after 0.3 mg of oral clonidine. Norepinephrine levels generally fall into the normal range if another cause is generating the hypertension even if the basal level is elevated. However, false-negative and false-positive results occasionally occur.

Agents Interfering With Catecholamine Assays. In general, interfering agents are most likely to cause spurious elevation of the urinary and plasma catecholamine levels. Metanephrines are least likely to be affected, although x-ray contrast media such as sodium diatrizoate (Renografin) depress values for as long as 1 week. VMA colorimetric assays that rely on a diazotized *p*-nitroaniline reaction are sensitive to interference with numerous dietary substances such as coffee, tea, chocolate, bananas, cheese, and vanilla. This method is now used infrequently, and dietary restriction before VMA measurement is usually not necessary. Clinical conditions, including acute myocardial infarction, diabetic ketoacidosis, burns, and shock, all may cause elevations of catecholamine levels and those of their urine me-

tabolites. Table 285-5 lists the drugs that may interfere with each of the assays.

Adrenal Cortex (Glucocorticoids) (Chapter 298)

Plasma Cortisol. Blood cortisol levels are measured by radioimmunoassay. Because it is released in a pulsatile fashion, random measurements are rarely diagnostic of either hypocortisolism or hypercortisolism. An exception, however, is the acutely ill patient with adrenal crisis. Major stress causes the cortisol level to exceed 20 μg/ml in normal persons. A concentration significantly less than this is strong evidence of adrenal insufficiency. Patients receiving estrogens may have extremely elevated plasma cortisol levels (>60 μg/ml) without Cushing's syndrome because of an estrogen-induced increased production of cortisol-binding globulin. Some clinicians measure morning and evening cortisol levels as a screening test for Cushing's syndrome because there is a loss of circadian cyclicity in this disorder. Normal 8:00 AM levels are 6 to 22 μg/ml. The PM cortisol level should be measured between 10:00 PM and midnight, when the concentration is less than 5 μ/dl. Values obtained earlier than 10:00 PM may still approach morning levels and may therefore be misleading.

Urinary 17-Hydroxycorticosteroids. The urinary 17-hydroxycorticosteroid test measures the 17,21-dihydroxy-20-keto metabolites of cortisol and cortisone and, when the formation of these compounds is inhibited by metyrapone testing, the metabolites of 11-deoxycortisol. Like plasma cortisol, 17-hydroxycorticosteroid levels are seldom helpful as an isolated measurement. The advantage of this measurement over a plasma cortisol measurement is that secretion is evaluated over a 24-hour period. Normal values are 3 to 10 mg/24 hr (or 2.5 to 7.0 mg/g of creatinine).

Urinary Free Cortisol. Less than 1% of cortisol is excreted unchanged in the urine. Measurement of the free cortisol level is particularly valuable as a screening test for Cushing's syndrome because more than 90% of patients have elevated values. Urine free cortisol is not a reliable screening test for adrenal insufficiency. Acute illness and pregnancy may cause false elevations. Normal levels vary greatly from laboratory to laboratory depending on the extraction procedure used to remove cortisol. A common normal range is 20 to 90 μg in 24 hours.

ACTH Stimulation Tests. ACTH directly stimulates the adrenal gland to secrete cortisol. The lack of an increase of cortisol or urinary 17-hydroxycorticosteroid level (if they are low at onset) demonstrates primary adrenal insufficiency. The test does not reliably detect secondary adrenal insufficiency. There are two varieties of tests, a rapid test and a prolonged test. Most cases of adrenal insufficiency are adequately demonstrated with the rapid test. To perform the rapid test, 250 μg of cosyntropin is administered either intramuscularly or intravenously. After 1 hour the injection is repeated. One hour after the second injection, blood is drawn for cortisol measurement. Administering cosyntropin twice eliminates the occasional equivocal result obtained with the standard single dose test. In normal individuals the cortisol level increases to an absolute value of greater than 20 μ/ml. Although a baseline cortisol value at 0 minute is often obtained, it rarely adds useful information to the patient's evaluation.

To demonstrate primary adrenal insufficiency definitively, the long ACTH stimulation test is used. This test is conducted by measuring baseline urinary 17-hydroxycorticosteroids on day 1 and day 2. On days 3, 4, and 5, 250 μg of cosyntropin is administered intravenously for 8 hours each day while urine collection for 17-hydroxycorticosteroids continues. By day 5, in normal individuals 17-hydroxycorticosteroid levels increase to greater than 25 mg in 24 hours. Patients with hypopituitarism have a stepwise increase of the urinary 17-hydroxycorticosteroid level even if the value on day 5 is less than 25 mg in 24 hours. Patients with primary adrenal insufficiency show little or no increase at any time during the test. Patients can be treated with dexamethasone 0.5 mg twice daily to prevent the development of symptomatic adrenal insufficiency during the 5-day test. Dexamethasone does not cross-react with assays for cortisol or 17-hydroxycorticosteroid level.

Adrenal Cortex (Androgens)

Urinary 17-Ketosteroids. Androgens such as androstenedione, dehydroepiandrosterone, and androsterone are metabolized to 17-ketosteroids. All of these compounds have a keto group at C-17. Although measurement of the 17-ketosteroids provides an assessment of both adrenal and ovarian androgen production, testosterone normally forms less than 1% of this metabolite. Thus patients with testosterone-secreting tumors may have normal levels of urinary 17-ketosteroids. Very high 17-ketosteroid levels are seen in androgen-secreting adrenal tumors (especially adrenal carcinoma) and congenital adrenal hyperplasia. Women normally excrete 5 to 15 mg in 24 hours and men 5 to 17 mg in 24 hours. Because 24-hour urine collections can be cumbersome, a single determination of a blood dehydroepiandrosterone sulfate level (discussed later) has largely replaced measurement of 17-ketosteroids.

Plasma Dehydroepiandrosterone and DHEA-Sulfate. Approximately 80% of dehydroepiandrosterone (DHEA) is formed by the adrenal gland. DHEA-sulfate is a sulfated conjugate and is present in higher quantities than is DHEA. Also, a somewhat higher percentage of total DHEA-sulfate is of adrenal origin than is the total percentage of circulating DHEA. However, either can be used to evaluate adrenal androgen secretion, and in many laboratories measurement of one or the other hormone has replaced 17-ketosteroid values because of the test's ease of collection. Normal concentrations of DHEA and DHEA-sulfate in women are 3 to 6 ng/ml and 850 to 4300 ng/ml, respectively. DHEA in men ranges from 4 to 7.5 ng/ml and DHEA-sulfate from 1100 to 5600 ng/ml.

Plasma 17-Hydroxyprogesterone. 17-Hydroxyprogesterone is the precursor of 11-deoxycortisol in the cortisol synthetic pathway.

Table 285-6 Plasma renin activity

	NG/ML/HR
Normal diet (Na intake 100 mEq/day)	
Supine	1.1 ± 0.8
Upright	1.9 ± 1.7
Low-salt diet (Na intake 10 mEq/day)	
Supine	2.7 ± 1.8
Upright	6.6 ± 2.5
Diuretic and low-salt diet	10.0 ± 3.7

Its conversion to 11-deoxycortisol is dependent on the enzyme 21-hydroxylase. Thus patients with the 21-hydroxylase deficiency variety of congenital adrenal hyperplasia (the most common type) and 11-hydroxylase deficiency have elevated basal levels of 17-hydroxyprogesterone that may be 5- to 50-fold higher than normal. Patients with mild deficiency of 21-hydroxylase may have elevated levels only after ACTH stimulation. Unstimulated levels in normal women are 25 to 85 ng/ml in the follicular phase, and 100 to 275 ng/ml in the luteal phase. In men, normal levels are less than 25 ng/ml. One hour after administration of 250 μg of cosyntropin, in normal individuals 17-hydroxyprogesterone levels rarely increase to greater than 300 ng/ml. In congenital adrenal hyperplasia, levels increase to greater than 1000 ng/ml even in mild deficiency states when the basal 17-hydroxyprogesterone concentration is normal.

Adrenal Cortex (Mineralocorticoids)

Plasma Aldosterone. The concentration of aldosterone in blood is highly dependent on posture and salt intake. With normal salt intake (approximately 110 mEq/day), the supine plasma aldosterone level is 5 to 15 ng/dl, and the 2-hour upright level is 20 to 75 ng/dl. To diagnose primary hyperaldosteronism, it is necessary to demonstrate poor suppressibility of aldosterone with salt administration; this can be done with the *saline infusion test*. The test is performed by infusing 2 L of saline solution over a 4-hour period with the patient recumbent. In patients with an aldosterone-secreting tumor, the plasma aldosterone concentration is usually not suppressed to less than 10 ng/ml, although levels occasionally fall below this in patients with bilateral hyperplasia of the zona glomerulosa.

18-Hydroxycorticosterone. Measurement of this mineralocorticoid is useful to separate patients with an aldosterone-secreting adenoma from those with bilateral hyperplasia. The 18-hydroxycorticosterone concentration is less than 60 ng/dl in patients with hyperplasia, whereas patients with an adenoma have values greater than 100 ng/dl.

11-Deoxycorticosteroid. The level of 11-deoxycorticosteroid (DOC) is elevated in patients with congenital adrenal hyperplasia from 11- and 17-hydroxylase deficiency. It also is elevated in some patients with ectopic ACTH syndrome and adrenal carcinoma. The normal concentration is 4 to 12 ng/dl.

Plasma Renin Activity. Plasma renin activity (PRA) is not a direct measurement of plasma renin concentration. Rather, it is a determination of the ability of plasma to generate angiotensin I from renin substrate. Normal levels are highly dependent on volume status, posture, and salt intake (Table 285-6). Patients with primary mineralocorticoid excess almost invariably have subnormal PRA even under conditions that stimulate renin. One stimulating procedure is to maintain a low-salt diet for 4 days and then measure PRA. Another means of evaluating PRA is to institute a low-salt diet for 2 days and then administer 80 mg of furosemide, then have the patient maintain upright posture for 4 hours (Table 285-6).

Captopril Test. Captopril, an angiotensin converting enzyme inhibitor, causes a fall in the plasma aldosterone level to below 15 ng/dl in patients with essential hypertension. In primary hyperaldosteronism, aldosterone secretion is not dependent upon the renin-angiotensin axis and there is little response of aldosterone to captopril. The test is performed by giving 25 mg of captopril orally on an ad libitum salt diet. Plasma aldosterone and PRA are measured before and 120 minutes after captopril. A plasma aldosterone/PRA ratio of over 50 makes primary aldosteronism very likely.

Urinary Aldosterone Excretion. As with plasma aldosterone, the urinary aldosterone level depends on volume status and salt intake. During high-normal sodium intake (greater than 120 mEq/day) aldosterone excretion ranges between 4 and 17 μg/24 hours. Values higher than 17 μg/24 hours during salt loading suggest a diagnosis of primary aldosteronism. After 4 days of salt restriction (10 mEq/day), the urinary aldosterone excretion should be 20 μg/24 hours. Patients with isolated aldosterone deficiency generally have values of less than 15 μg/24 hours during salt restriction.

Tests of Male Gonadal Function (Chapter 301)

Testosterone. Testosterone level is measured by radioimmunoassay. Its determination should be accompanied by gonadotropin level measurement. Low testosterone levels with low gonadotropin values suggest pituitary-hypothalamic disease, whereas with primary testicular disease gonadotropin concentrations are high with a low testosterone level. Acute or chronic stress also may lower the testosterone level in the absence of gonadal disease. The normal adult male concentration is 350 to 1200 ng/dl.

Estradiol. Estradiol level should be measured in men with gynecomastia and other feminizing conditions. Elevated levels are seen with neoplasms, liver disease, and hyperthyroidism and in older men. In normal men, the estradiol level should not exceed 45 pg/ml.

β-Subunit Human Chorionic Gonadotropin. β-Subunit human chorionic gonadotropin, placental hormone, is produced by trophoblastic tumors, germinal cell neoplasms, and nongerminal cell cancers such as adenocarcinoma of the lung, gastric cancer, and islet cell tumors. The presence of β-human chorionic gonadotropin in a man with gynecomastia or impotence of recent onset is an indicator of serious disease. Normally, levels should be undetectable or very low (less than 5 ImU/ml).

Chorionic Gonadotropin Stimulation. During the onset of puberty it may be necessary to assess the capacity of the testis to secrete testosterone, because at this time low gonadotropin secretion may normally exist with low testosterone levels. A dose of 1500 U of human chorionic gonadotropin is injected intramuscularly, and testosterone level is measured 48 hours later. Values should clearly increase, often into the normal adult male range (300 to 1200 ng/dl), thereby indicating that the testosterone secretory capacity of the testis is normal.

Semen Analysis. Semen analysis is an excellent test of gonadal function. Normal parameters indicate that gonadal function is normal without the need to perform hormonal analysis (which is generally more expensive). A normal sperm count is 20 to 50 million sperm per milliliter with 60% of the sperm demonstrating normal structure and at least 50% should be motile. Fertility, however, has been documented in men with counts of less than 10 million/ml. The normal volume of the ejaculate is between 2 and 6 ml. It is sometimes helpful to test for the presence of seminal fructose. Fructose is the product of the seminal vesicles, and its absence in azoospermic men implies blocked ejaculatory ducts or congenital absence of the vas deferens. Specimens for semen analysis should be collected by masturbation after at least 48 hours of sexual abstinence and should be examined within 1 hour of collection.

Tests of Female Gonadal Function (Chapter 300)

Estradiol. Estradiol concentration varies widely during the normal human menstrual cycle (Table 285-7). In amenorrheic patients, estradiol levels may be needed to evaluate ovarian secretory capac-

Table 285-7 Estrogen and progesterone concentration in women

PHASE OF CYCLE	ESTRADIOL ((pg/ml)	PROGESTERONE (ng/dl)
Early follicular	10-30	—
Late follicular	30-70	2-90
Luteal	100-300*	600-3000
Menopausal	5-25	<30

*Midcycle estradiol peak may be up to 600 pg/ml.

ity. Gonadotropin levels also should be obtained to allow separation of primary and secondary deficiency states.

Progesterone. In some women, progesterone secretion is inadequate to maintain the corpus luteum and may account for infertility. Normal levels are listed in Table 285-7.

Total Testosterone. Testosterone level is often elevated in women with anovulation or hirsutism. Mild elevations are seen in polycystic ovarian disease and other nonneoplastic virilizing disorders. Patients with testosterone-secreting tumors generally have levels that are greater than 200 ng/dl. Normal values are 20 to 90 ng/dl.

Unbound Testosterone. Approximately 99% of testosterone is bound in women. In some women with hirsutism, the total testosterone concentration is normal, but the unbound fraction is elevated. Normal unbound levels range from 0.09 to 1.2 ng/dl.

Androstenedione. Androstenedione is a relatively weak androgen that originates from the ovary, adrenal glands, and by conversion in peripheral tissues. Although it has several sources, its level is commonly elevated in women with an ovarian cause (e.g., polycystic ovarian disease) of hyperandrogenization. Normal levels are 50 to 250 ng/dl.

Dihydrotestosterone. Testosterone is converted to the potent androgen dihydrotestosterone (DHT) by the enzyme 5-α-reductase. DHT is the major androgen that affects hair follicles. Elevated levels indicate increased 5-α-reductase activity, although the level of androstanediol glucuronide (see later discussion) is probably a better measure of this activity. Normal DHT levels range from 5 to 30 ng/dl.

Androstanediol Glucuronide. Androstanediol glucuronide is a tissue metabolite of DHT, and serum levels correlate well with 5-α-reductase activity and androgen cellular activity. Absolute increases in level of this metabolite are often found in hirsute women with normal levels of total and unbound testosterone. The finding of an elevated androstanediol level, however, does not often affect therapy, and the test should not routinely be done for the diagnosis of hirsutism. Normal adult female levels are 60 to 800 ng/dl.

Progesterone Withdrawal Test. The progesterone withdrawal test evaluates whether there is sufficient estrogen secretion to cause endometrial development in women with amenorrhea. If estrogen effect is present, a normal menstrual period will occur after administration of progesterone. Withdrawal bleeding indicates that the hypothalamic-pituitary-gonadal-uterine axis is intact. Lack of bleeding gives no information about the level of the defect. To perform the test, 10 mg of oral medroxyprogesterone is administered for 5 days. As an alternative, 100 mg of progesterone-in-oil as a single dose can be given intramuscularly. Vaginal bleeding should occur within the following 14 days.

Sequential Estrogen-Progesterone Stimulation. Patients who do not have vaginal bleeding after progesterone withdrawal should be treated with sequential estrogen and progesterone to exclude a primary endometrial disorder as the cause of amenorrhea. If, despite adequate hormonal stimulus, there is no bleeding, an endometrial cause of the amenorrhea is likely. If bleeding occurs, the lesion is at a level higher than the endometrium. The test is completed

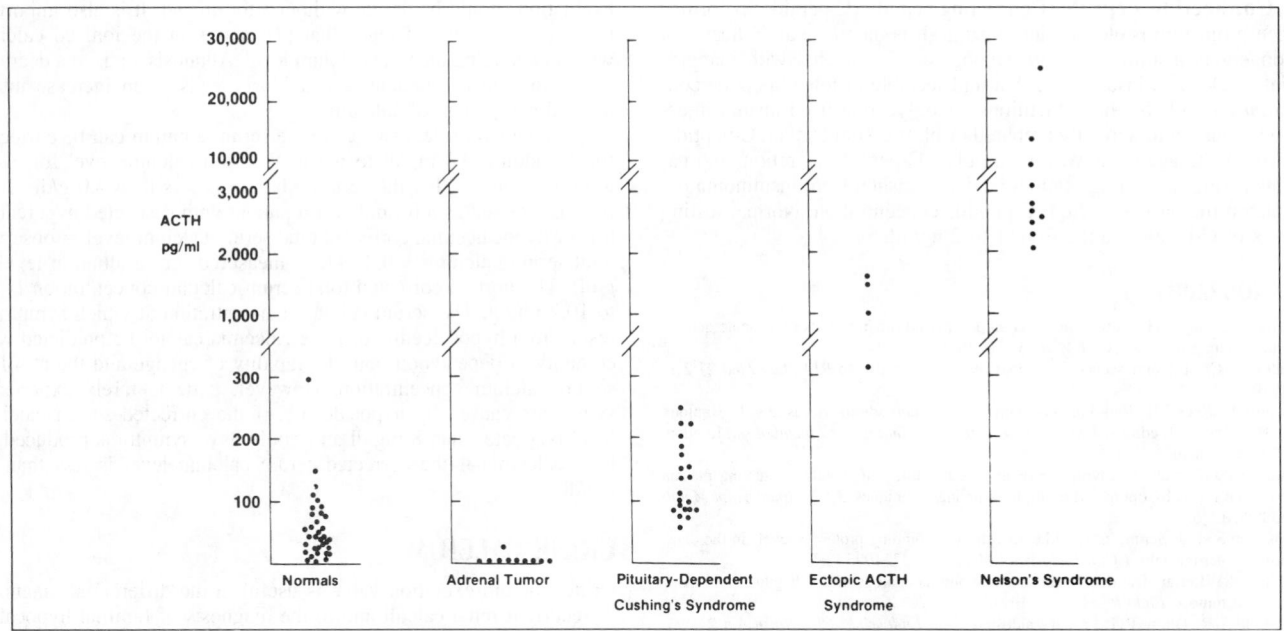

FIGURE 285-7   Plasma ACTH concentration in patients with Cushing's syndrome. From Cook et al: *West J Med* 132:111, 1980.

by administering either 2.5 mg of conjugated estrogens or 0.2 mg of ethinyl estradiol for 21 days. On day 16, 10 mg of medroxyprogesterone is added and continued until day 21. In the following 10 days, menstrual bleeding should appear. For the test result to be conclusively abnormal, the cycle of medication should be repeated three times without the occurrence of vaginal bleeding.

Basal Body Temperature. Basal body temperature is measured to determine whether ovulation has occurred. The temperature is taken for 5 minutes before the woman gets out of bed in the morning. Normally, temperatures are stable during the follicular phase, but just before ovulation, a dip is seen. If ovulation occurs and progesterone secretion is sufficient to maintain the corpus luteum, the basal body temperature increases by at least 1° F.

Genetic Studies

Buccal Smear. Cells with more than one X chromosome have detectable chromatin (Barr body) on the nuclear membrane. In normal women, 20% to 40% of somatic cells have Barr bodies. In men the total is less than 5%. To obtain cells, the inside of the cheek is scraped with a metal spatula, and the cells are smeared on a glass slide and then placed in a fixative. The slide is then stained and read by a technician experienced in cytologic analysis.

Chromosomal Analysis. Chromosomal analysis is very expensive and as a rule does not need to be done for confirmation of disorders such as Turner's syndrome, Klinefelter's syndrome, XX sex reversal syndrome, and XYY syndrome. Women with gonadal dysgenesis and virilization, however, should have a karyotype. In this case, the finding of a Y chromosome indicates that testicular elements are probably present in the gonad. This abnormality requires surgical intervention because such gonads are at increased risk for malignant degeneration.

Miscellaneous

Urinary 5-Hydroxyindoleacetic Acid. 5-Hydroxyindoleacetic acid (5-HIAA) is a product of serotonin metabolism. Its excretion is above normal in almost all patients with the carcinoid syndrome. Dietary products that contain serotonin must be excluded before measurement; these include walnuts, bananas, avocados, chocolate, and red plums. Cough preparations that contain glyceryl guaiacolate falsely elevate 5-HIAA level, and phenothiazines falsely depress 5-HIAA level. Reserpine releases serotonin and can cause a mild elevation. False elevations are also seen in nontropical sprue. Normal excretion is from 5 to 9 mg/24 hours; however, most patients with carcinoid excrete more than 50 mg/24 hours. Modest elevations of less than 25 mg/24 hours are often due to one of the factors mentioned other than carcinoid.

Gastrointestinal Hormones. A basal *gastrin* level of more than 500 pg/ml in a patient with acid hypersecretion is highly suggestive of a gastrinoma (Zollinger-Ellison syndrome). Gastrin values between 250 and 500 pg/ml are equivocal and require evaluation with the *secretin stimulation test*. It is performed by administering 2 IU/kg of secretin intravenously and collecting blood at 0, 2, 5, and 10 minutes. The gastrin level increases by at least 200 pg/ml in patients with a gastrinoma. Duodenal ulcer, gastric outlet obstruction, retained antrum, G cell hyperplasia or hypertrophy, and renal insufficiency may cause elevations of basal gastrin levels but do not show an increase after secretin. *Somatostatin* is produced by somatostatinomas and can be measured in blood. Patients with somatostatinomas have somatostatin levels that range from 150 to 100,000 pg/ml. Normal individuals have levels of less than 80 pg/ml. Patients with WDHA syndrome (watery diarrhea, hypokalemia, achlorhydria) have VIP (vasoactive intestinal peptide) levels of greater than 30 pmol/L. Normal is less than 20 pmol/L.

Insulin. Measurement of insulin is useful in evaluating a patient with fasting hypoglycemia. During a fast, when the plasma glucose concentration is less than 40 mg/dl, the plasma insulin level should be less than 5 to 10 µU/ml. Values higher than this are very suggestive of insulinoma if connecting peptide level is also elevated (see later discussion). Higher fasting insulin levels are seen in obese patients without insulinoma as a result of insulin resistance. In thin and normal-weight persons, the insulin/glucose ratio should be less than 0.25 when the plasma glucose level is less than 40 mg/dl. Proinsulin levels of greater than 25% of the total immunoreactive insulin activity are suggestive of an insulinoma.

Connecting Peptide. Connecting peptide (C-peptide) is formed when proinsulin is cleaved into insulin. It is therefore an indicator of endogenous insulin secretion. Hypoglycemic patients with inappropriately elevated insulin level but undetectable or low C-peptide concentration probably have factitious hypoglycemia from insulin injection because commercially prepared insulins do not contain C-peptide. Sulfonylurea agents, however, stimulate C-peptide secretion, and patients taking these drugs cannot be distinguished from insulinoma patients on the basis of a high C-peptide concentration. Normal fasting levels of C-peptide range from 1 to 2 ng/ml.

BIBLIOGRAPHY

Degroot LJ, Mayor G: Admission screening by thyroid function tests in an acute general care teaching hospital, *Am J Med* 93:558, 1993.

Dudley R: Chemiluminescence immunoassay: an alternative to RIA, *Lab Med* 21:216, 1990.

Edwards R, Rees LH: Radioimmunoassay and immunoradiometric assays. In Bouloux P-MG, Rees LH, editors: *Diagnostic tests in endocrinology and metabolism,* London, 1994, Chapman & Hall.

Goldzieher JW et al: Improving the diagnostic reliability of rapidly fluctuating plasma hormone levels by optimized multiple sampling techniques, *J Clin Endocrinol Metab* 43:824, 1976.

Grinspoon S et al: Serum insulin-like growth factor-binding protein-3 levels in the diagnosis of acromegaly, *J Clin Endocrinol Metab* 80:927, 1995.

Lamberts SWJ et al: The role of somatostatin and its analogs in the diagnosis and treatment of tumors, *Endo Rev* 12:450, 1991.

Litchfield WR, Dlugy RG: Primary aldosteronism, *Endocrinol Clin North Am* 24:593, 1995.

Nakamura T et al: The value of paramagnetic contrast agent gadolinium-DTPA in the diagnosis of pituitary adenomas, *Neuroradiology* 30:481, 1988.

Nicoloff JT, Spencer CA: The use and misuse of the sensitive thyrotropin assays, *J Clin Endocrinol Metab* 71:553, 1990.

Sheps SG et al: Recent developments in the diagnosis and treatment of pheochromocytoma, *Mayo Clin Proc* 65(1):88, 1990.

CHAPTER

286   Diagnostic Approach to Bone and Mineral Disorders

Gregory R. Mundy and Charles A. Reasner II

SERUM CALCIUM

The total serum calcium level has three components. About 45% is protein bound (predominantly to albumin) and is biologically inert, about 5% is complexed or chelated to citrate and is also biologically inert, and about 50% belongs to the ionized or free component, which is metabolically active. Measurements of the ionized calcium component are not generally available except in special laboratories and as a special procedure. The autoanalyzers used in most laboratories measure total serum calcium level accurately and reproducibly, although probably not as accurately as the atomic absorption spectrophotometer. The normal total serum calcium concentration is between 8.5 and 10.2 mg/dl of serum unless there are abnormalities in the serum proteins. The serum calcium level is a remarkably well guarded variable, but it should be appreciated that the only component of the total serum calcium level that is regulated by calciotropic hormones is the ionized calcium. Clinicians should not base decisions on the total serum calcium concentration without considering changes in concentrations of plasma proteins, particularly albumin. The ionized calcium component is more difficult to measure than the total serum calcium, and, provided the serum protein concentrations can be measured, measurements of ionized calcium are rarely necessary. One possible exception occurs in patients with myeloma in whom the total serum calcium concentration is occasionally increased as a result of excessive binding of calcium to the myeloma protein, whereas the ionized calcium level may be normal. In these patients, the ionized calcium determination would be useful. The blood for serum calcium

evaluation should be drawn without a tourniquet. It is also important to be aware of the changes that pH causes in the ionized calcium without changing the total calcium level. Alkalosis leads to a decrease in the ionized component, and acidosis leads to an increase in the ionized component of calcium.

As a general rule, changes in the serum albumin can be corrected for by adding 0.8 mg/dl to the total serum calcium level for every gram of albumin that the serum albumin is less than 4.0 g/dl of serum. Expressed as a formula for a patient with suspected hypercalcemia or hypocalcemia, corrected total serum calcium level = observed total serum calcium − 0.8 (4.0 − measured serum albumin level in g/dl). The normal corrected total serum calcium concentration is 8.5 to 10.2 mg/dl. The serum calcium concentration at which symptoms result from hypocalcemia or hypercalcemia cannot be predicted with certainty. It depends on both the rapidity of change and the absolute serum calcium concentration. However, patients rarely experience symptoms caused by hypocalcemia if the corrected serum calcium level is greater than 8 mg/dl and rarely have symptoms produced by hypercalcemia if the corrected serum calcium level is less than 11 mg/dl.

URINE CALCIUM

Urine calcium excretion value is useful in the differential diagnosis of recurrent renal calculi and in the diagnosis of familial hypocalciuric hypercalcemia, a condition readily confused with asymptomatic primary hyperparathyroidism. Urine should be collected for 24 hours in containers with an acid preservative, and creatinine should be determined on the same specimen to ensure adequacy of the collection. Urine calcium concentration is an important variable to follow in patients with hypoparathyroidism who are being treated with vitamin D and calcium supplementation. In this condition, the concentration of calcium in the urine may be markedly elevated because the effect of parathyroid hormone (PTH) to increase calcium reabsorption is absent. The dose of vitamin D should be titrated against the urine calcium level so that urine calcium does not rise over 350 mg/day. This is usually accomplished with a serum calcium level that is below the normal range but still high enough to keep the patient asymptomatic. In the differential diagnosis of idiopathic hypercalciuria, it is important to know the calcium intake because normal calcium excretion varies considerably with dietary calcium level. Although any absolute criterion for the diagnosis of hypercalciuria is arbitrary and is likely to include some normal individuals and overlook some patients with abnormal calcium homeostasis or abnormal renal tubular calcium handling, on an average daily intake of 600 to 1000 mg of elemental calcium, most normal men have urine calcium excretion of less than 300 mg/day, and women have less than 250 mg/day. In idiopathic hypercalciuria, values are higher. On a restricted calcium diet (400 mg/day), most normal men have urine calcium excretion of less than 250 mg/day, and normal women have less than 200 mg/day. In familial hypocalciuric hypercalcemia, urine calcium excretion is usually less than 100 mg/day despite hypercalcemia.

SERUM ALKALINE PHOSPHATASE

Alkaline phosphatase is an enzyme found in and released by active osteoblasts. Its precise physiologic role is still a mystery, although it is likely to be involved in bone mineralization. An increased serum alkaline phosphatase concentration is associated with increases in bone formation. The concentration of this enzyme in the serum reflects bone turnover and is usually elevated when bone resorption is increased, for example, during childhood and in hyperthyroidism, because bone formation and bone resorption are linked or coupled. The enzyme is secreted from cells into the blood and is measured routinely on small samples of serum in an autoanalyzer. The most striking increases in serum alkaline phosphatase concentration occur in Paget's disease and occasionally in osteoblastic metastases caused by metastatic carcinoma. Alkaline phosphatase level is also usually increased in patients with osteolytic metastases from metastatic solid tumors. However, it is often normal in patients with myeloma, reflecting the fact that bone formation is usually not increased in this disorder. The total serum alkaline phosphatase concentration is composed of a number of isoenzymes produced by both the liver and the bone. These may be distinguished by electrophoresis or by the relative heat lability of the bone fraction at 56° C for 15 minutes (bone alkaline phosphatase burns). In the near future, bone-specific alkaline phosphatase level is likely to be measured by using monoclonal antibodies. Liver alkaline phosphatase concentration is increased in biliary tract obstruction and in hepatocellular disease. Elevation of the concentration of alkaline phosphatase of liver origin is accompanied by increases in other serum enzymes of hepatic origin, including γ-glutamic pyruvic transaminase and 5′ nucleotidase.

URINE HYDROXYPROLINE

Hydroxyproline is an amino acid that is almost unique to collagen and is a breakdown product of collagen degradation. Its urinary excretion can be measured, and it reflects increased collagen turnover from any source including bone. However, urinary hydroxyproline level varies with the diet. For accurate assessment of collagen turnover, the patient should be on a gelatin-free diet. This limits the usefulness of the test. Urinary hydroxyproline is increased in any condition associated with increased collagen turnover such as Paget's disease, thyrotoxicosis, or acromegaly. It has limited clinical use but has been a reasonable marker of response to therapy in patients with Paget's disease. In patients with Paget's disease who are being treated with bisphosphonates or calcitonin, the fall in urinary hydroxyproline level appears several weeks before the fall in alkaline phosphatase level, suggesting that the reduction in bone formation is due to the inhibition of osteoclastic bone resorption caused by the drug therapy.

URINARY EXCRETION OF COLLAGEN PYRIDINIUM AND DEOXYPYRIDINIUM CROSSLINKS

Pyridinoline (Pyr) and deoxypyridinoline (D-pyr) are two nondigestible pyridinium crosslinks present in the mature form of collagen. D-pyr is present only in significant amounts in the type 1 collagen of bone. Thus its measurement in the urine is a reflection of rates of bone resorption. Because its urinary excretion is not altered by diet, it has potential as a much more helpful measure of rates of bone resorption than urine hydroxyproline level. Preliminary information indicates that urinary D-pyr is increased in all states of increased bone resorption, including the postmenopausal period in women. Other markers are currently being developed. These include the amino- and carboxy-terminal propeptides of Type 1 collagen. Some of these measurements can be readily determined by enzyme-linked immunosorbent assay (ELISA).

SERUM PHOSPHORUS

Serum phosphorus concentration is determined in most laboratories by autoanalyzer. It is not as tightly regulated as the serum calcium level and can vary by 50% in the normal individual with changes in diet, fasting, vomiting, or renal function. The serum phosphorus value may fall by 30% 2 hours after a carbohydrate-rich meal, and this should be considered when serum phosphorus level measurements are being assessed. It also varies with age and sex and is slightly higher in females than in males at any age but is clearly higher in childhood and adolescence when bone turnover is high. The measurement of phosphate excretion and its expression as the tubular reabsorption of phosphate (TRP), fractional excretion of phosphate, or tubular maximal reabsorption of phosphate as a fraction of the glomerular filtration rate (GFR [TmP/GFR]) are useful in patients with hypophosphatemia in whom renal phosphate loss is suspected; however, it is less useful in the differential diagnosis of hypercalcemia, because patients with primary hyperparathyroidism or malignancy may have increased urinary phosphate excretion. The presence of hypercalcemia and hyperphosphatemia suggests excess vitamin D activity.

IMMUNOREACTIVE PARATHYROID HORMONE

Parathyroid hormone (PTH) level is now readily measurable in the serum by radioimmunoassay. For many years this assay was beset

with problems, but these problems have been largely resolved. Prior difficulties were caused by fragmentation of PTH that occurs in the circulation that yielded multiple circulating fragments varying both in biologic activity and in immunoreactivity. PTH measurements by the newer immunoradiometric assays (IRMAs) are valuable because they measure the complete intact molecule (Table 286-1).

The biologically active portion of the PTH molecule resides in the first 34 amino acids from the amino- or N-terminal end. The carboxy-terminal (C-terminal) end of the molecule is biologically inert. Unfortunately, the portions of the PTH molecule that have been most readily measured by immunoassay in the past are not biologically active. Most of the earlier assays used antibodies that cross reacted with fragments that included the carboxy-terminus of the PTH molecule, called *C-terminal assays*. Results from these assays are difficult to interpret in patients with impaired renal function because the C-terminal fragments of PTH depend on the kidneys for clearance. Immunoreactive plasma PTH concentrations increase according to these assays when the serum creatinine level is greater than 2 mg/dl. The amino-terminal or N-terminal assays more closely reflect minute-to-minute secretion by the parathyroid gland and measure the biologically active portion of the molecule. The amino-terminal assays were more useful in patients with renal failure or in those in whom it was necessary to localize abnormal parathyroid tissue using selective sampling of veins draining the neck and mediastinum.

There is probably no point in measuring PTH unless the serum calcium level is abnormal. By and large, measurement of immunoreactive PTH is most useful in making the differential diagnosis of hypercalcemia and in particular distinguishing patients with primary hyperparathyroidism from those with other causes of hypercalcemia. Patients who have a PTH concentration that is 30% greater than the top of the normal range in any assay can be confidently diagnosed as having primary hyperparathyroidism in the absence of renal failure. A PTH measurement in the normal range is difficult to distinguish from low values in most of the commonly available assays, and probably in all assays some patients with proven primary hyperparathyroidism have values in the normal range. Nomograms comparing serum PTH values with serum calcium values have been widely used but have often been overinterpreted. In the differential diagnosis of hypocalcemia, measurement of PTH should distinguish patients with pseudohypoparathyroidism from those with primary hypoparathyroidism. In the latter condition, secretion of PTH does not occur and the immunoreactive serum concentrations are low. In patients with pseudohypoparathyroidism (peripheral tissue resistance to PTH), the serum concentrations are increased secondary to hypocalcemia. Another use of the PTH assay is to follow patients with chronic renal failure and secondary hyperparathyroidism.

In using PTH assays it should be emphasized that only one assay

Table 286-1 Disorders of calcium metabolism—use of circulating measurements of calcium, phosphorus, and PTH concentrations

SERUM CA	SERUM P	PLASMA PTH	DISORDER
↑	↑	↓ or Nl	Increased gut absorption of calcium (vitamin D intoxication, sarcoidosis, milk-alkali syndrome)
↑	↑	↑	Hypercalcemia of any cause and renal failure
↑	↓	↑	Primary hyperparathyroidism
↑	↓	↓ or Nl	Humoral hypercalcemia of malignancy
↓	↓	↑	Vitamin D deficiency, hypomagnesemia*
↓	↑	↑	Pseudohypoparathyroidism, renal failure, acute pancreatitis
↓	↑	Nl or ↓	Primary hypoparathyroidism

*PTH release is stimulated by acute hypomagnesemia. In contrast, chronic hypomagnesemia is associated with low serum PTH. *Nl*, Normal.

should be used in following one patient, because assays are likely to vary in terms of the tracer, the standard, and the antisera.

VITAMIN D METABOLITES

Two biologically active metabolites of vitamin D, 25-hydroxyvitamin D and 1,25-dihydroxyvitamin D, are frequently measured in the blood. The serum 25-hydroxyvitamin D measurements are more useful clinically. This metabolite is the major circulating form of the vitamin and reflects vitamin D intake. It is particularly valuable if the physician suspects either vitamin D intoxication or vitamin D lack caused by dietary deficiency or malabsorption. The 25-hydroxyvitamin D level is measured by competitive protein-binding assay, and normal values are in the range of 10 to 80 ng/ml. Levels are higher in patients living in sunny climates and during the spring and summer. Concentrations of less than 5 ng/ml are seen in vitamin D deficiency.

1,25-Dihydroxyvitamin D is the most active metabolite of vitamin D, but it is more difficult to measure, and knowledge of the serum concentration has limited clinical usefulness. This hormone is increased in patients with hypercalcemia produced by sarcoidosis and other granulomatous diseases, in those with primary hyperparathyroidism, and in some patients with lymphomas. However, the 1,25-dihydroxyvitamin D level provides only slightly more information than measurement of the serum calcium in these situations. Possibly one situation where it is clearly indicated is the rare patient with rickets caused by tissue resistance to 1,25-dihydroxyvitamin D (vitamin D–dependent rickets type II). In this syndrome, the serum 1,25-dihydroxyvitamin D concentrations are markedly increased.

SERUM CALCITONIN

Serum immunoreactive calcitonin concentration is easier to measure than PTH level, and there are better correlations from laboratory to laboratory in the results. Unfortunately, it has limited clinical usefulness. Calcitonin levels are increased in patients with medullary carcinoma of the thyroid and are used in such patients for making the diagnosis and for monitoring response to therapy or for recurrence. Calcitonin measurement can also be used for localizing the site of tumor by selective venous sampling. In patients with early disease or with familial medullary thyroid carcinoma when the disease is still occult, abnormal calcitonin level measurements may be recognized only after provocative testing with pentagastrin or calcium infusion. Both of these agents are calcitonin secretagogues, and patients with excess calcitonin-secreting cells usually show an exaggerated calcitonin response after their administration. Of these two secretagogues, pentagastrin is the more reliable. Serum calcitonin level is lower in women than in men at all ages, but recent data suggest that there is no age-related decrease, despite earlier reports to the contrary. Some patients with nonthyroid malignancies may have high circulating calcitonin levels produced by ectopic secretion. Ectopic calcitonin is usually biologically inert.

URINARY CYCLIC ADENOSINE MONOPHOSPHATE

The measurement of urinary cyclic adenosine monophosphate (AMP) level gives information similar to that yielded by PTH assays, and its concentration in urine depends mainly on biologically active PTH. As with the PTH immunoassay, measurements are difficult to interpret in the presence of renal failure. Urinary cyclic AMP values have been used in the differential diagnosis of the subtypes of idiopathic hypercalciuria, but the clinical usefulness in this situation is doubtful. In the differential diagnosis of hypercalcemia, many patients with hypercalcemia of malignancy also have an increase in urinary cyclic AMP level. Therefore the efficacy in distinguishing malignancy from primary hyperparathyroidism as the cause of hypercalcemia is limited. The major use of urinary cyclic AMP level in the past has been to distinguish pseudohypoparathyroidism from primary hypoparathyroidism. In the latter condition, there is a sharp rise in urinary cyclic AMP level after PTH infusion, whereas in the former condition there is tissue insensitivity to PTH. Nephrogenous cyclic AMP level has been measured by many workers in investigative studies but probably does not give more useful clinical information than the simpler

---

> ### BOX 286-1
> ### Biochemical markers of bone turnover
>
> **Markers of bone formation**
> Serum total and bone-specific alkaline phosphatase
> Serum osteocalcin (bone Gla protein)
> Serum procollagen 1 extension peptides
>
> **Markers of bone resorption**
> Total and dialyzable urine hydroxyproline
> Urine pyridinoline and deoxypyridinoline (collagen crosslinks)
> Serum tartrate–resistant acid phosphatase

measurement of urinary cyclic AMP level. The urine collection should be made in the same way as that for urinary calcium determination. Ideally, the measurement should be expressed in terms of the glomerular filtration rate, that is, as nanomoles per deciliter of glomerular filtrate.

STEROID SUPPRESSION TEST

The steroid suppression test now has a limited place in the differential diagnosis of hypercalcemia, because plasma PTH measurements have improved. In this test 100 mg of cortisone acetate or its equivalent is given per day for 10 days, and the serum calcium level is measured on alternate days. Patients with primary hyperparathyroidism essentially never show a decrease in serum calcium concentration in response to glucocorticoids. However, the serum calcium level in patients with sarcoidosis or other causes of hypercalcemia produced by increased calcium absorption from the gut is almost invariably suppressed. About 30% of patients in whom malignant disease is responsible for hypercalcemia show suppression of the serum calcium level during the steroid suppression test. These tests are most useful in the asymptomatic patient in whom the plasma PTH determination is not diagnostic, and the possibility that sarcoidosis or occult malignancy is responsible for the hypercalcemia needs to be excluded.

BIOCHEMICAL MARKERS OF RATES OF BONE RESORPTION AND BONE FORMATION

Accurate measurements of overall rates of bone resorption and bone formation would be very helpful in clinical practice. For example, to assess efficacy of therapies that inhibit bone resorption, an inexpensive measurement of resorption rates such as a biochemical value that can be determined by noninvasive techniques would be very useful (Box 286-1). Biochemical markers are not useful for diagnosis, because they are not specific for the different disease states. An exception may be Paget's disease of bone, in which rates of bone resorption and bone formation may greatly exceed those of other conditions, and markers such as urine hydroxyproline or serum alkaline phosphatase level may be so markedly increased that the diagnosis is apparent. As indicated earlier, there is great interest currently in the development of new and better markers of bone formation and bone resorption.

It should be remembered that the techniques of measurement of bone mineral density, bone histomorphologic characteristics, and biochemical markers of rates of bone resorption measure essentially different things. The biochemical markers reflect bone turnover in the whole skeleton but give no information about local or regional changes. In contrast, bone histomorphometry limits assessments to a localized area of the skeleton but does provide morphologic information on the nature of the abnormality. Bone mineral density provides a static measurement at one point in time but gives no information on structure or relative rates of bone resorption or bone formation. These techniques are thus complementary. Some workers believe that patients in later life can be categorized into fast bone losers and slow bone losers by measurement of some of the biochemical markers and that the use of these markers in combination with bone mass measurements is useful in deciding a therapeutic plan.

SERUM BONE GLA PROTEIN

The bone Gla protein (also called *osteocalcin*) is a major protein constituent of the bone matrix whose function is unclear. It may function as an inhibitor of normal bone mineralization. It composes 20% of the noncollagenous protein in bone. It can be measured in the serum by radioimmunoassay as a measurement of increased bone turnover, and in particular as a value of osteoblastic activity. Recently developed sandwich assays using monoclonal antibodies may improve the sensitivity and specificity. Circulating concentrations do not correlate perfectly with serum alkaline phosphatase concentration, and it is likely that these two proteins are the products of different cells in the osteoblast lineage. This measurement is primarily an investigative tool currently, and its clinical usefulness remains to be determined.

BONE HISTOMORPHOMETRY

Quantitative bone histomorphometry data obtained from nondecalcified biopsy specimens from the iliac crest are now frequently used to make an accurate diagnosis of the nature of a metabolic bone disease. Bone biopsies are particularly useful in the differential diagnosis of osteopenia. The technique is to take a through-and-through section of bone from the iliac crest by percutaneous needle biopsy after the patient takes two short courses of tetracycline separated by a known number of days, usually 10. Tetracycline is laid down at the site of mineral deposition, and this technique allows measurement of rates of bone formation in terms of the mineral apposition rate. Tetracyclines can be identified in nondecalcified bone sections because these antibiotics have a characteristic fluorescence in ultraviolet light. A suitable labeling regimen is to give tetracycline (500 mg po bid) for 2 days, wait 10 days, and then give demethylchlortetracycline (demeclocycline 300 po bid) for 4 days. The biopsy is taken 2 to 4 days after cessation of the demeclocycline. Drugs that interfere with absorption of tetracyclines such as phosphate binders or antacids should be avoided while the tetracyclines are being administered.

The bone biopsy specimen must be nondecalcified so that evaluation of the amount of mineralized bone relative to unmineralized bone can be assessed. This is necessary for the diagnosis of osteomalacia. The bone biopsy also allows evaluation of the surfaces involved in osteoclast activity, but unlike bone formation, no measurement of the rate of bone resorption is possible. The biopsy needle must be of sufficient size and diameter to permit the core of bone to be removed without compression or distortion, which would make it impossible to assess the relative trabecular bone volume. The procedure is generally well tolerated and is associated with low morbidity. Bone histomorphometry is most useful clinically in the differential diagnosis of osteopenia, particularly in distinguishing osteomalacia from osteoporosis (Box 286-2). Bone biopsy is also useful in assessing bone abnormalities in patients with renal osteodystrophy.

Although this technique provides valuable information, there are problems with sampling, because cellular events occurring in the iliac crest may not be representative of those in the thoracic or lumbar vertebrae. It allows the diagnosis of osteomalacia to be excluded, but it does not give a precise measurement of total bone mass because of the imprecision of the technique and the potential sampling error between the iliac crest and the spine. For the same reasons, it is not a useful technique for monitoring therapy. The most important parameters that can be determined are trabecular bone volume, mineral apposition rate, and percentages of the total bone surfaces involved in osteoclastic bone resorption and bone formation. In osteoporosis, there is a decrease in bone volume but no increase in unmineralized bone (osteoid tissue). In osteomalacia, there is an increase in osteoid tissue with a decrease in the mineral apposition rate. The osteoid tissue is assessed by the percentage of total bone surfaces covered with osteoid tissue and the width of the osteoid seams. In states of high bone turnover such as primary hyperparathyroidism, hyperthyroidism, or Paget's disease, there is increased osteoid tissue, but this can be distinguished from osteomalacia because in these conditions the mineral apposition rate is increased.

BOX 286-2
Possible assessments with bone biopsy

Osteoporosis
Volume of trabecular bone relative to volume of tissue

Osteomalacia
Area of bone surface covered by osteoid tissue
Width of osteoid seams
Volume of osteoid tissue
Mineral appositional rate (requires serial biopsies and tetracycline markers)
Calcification front (requires tetracycline marker or special stains)

Others
Area of bone surface involved in resorption (scalloped margins with or without osteoclasts)
Area of bone surface involved in formation (lined by osteoblasts)

MEASUREMENT OF BONE MINERAL CONTENT

During the past 20 years, a number of techniques for measuring bone mineral density have been introduced. The technology for measurement of bone mineral density and evaluation of patients with osteoporosis is continuing to evolve. These techniques have improved because of the growing interest in osteoporosis and have now become part of routine medical practice. Moreover, the great demand for these instruments together with improvements in technical performance have made the measurements less expensive. These instruments now make it possible not only to evaluate the total skeleton but also to evaluate bone mineral density in specific regions of the skeleton separately and thus provide information on the independent status of cortical and cancellous bone. These measurements also allow estimation of bone strength and prediction of future fracture risk. However, it should be appreciated that they do not make a diagnosis of specific bone diseases and do not distinguish the nature of the bone disease responsible for a decline in bone mineral density. Four techniques are widely used currently: single-beam photon absorptiometry, dual-beam photon absorptiometry (DPA), quantitative computed tomography (QCT), and dual-energy x-ray absorptiometry (DEXA). Newer noninvasive techniques, ultrasound and magnetic resonance imaging (MRI), are also currently being investigated.

The *T-Score* is used to describe the bone mass in an individual patient. The numeric value reflects the standard deviation above or below the peak bone mass of young normal controls. For example, a 60-year-old woman with a T-Score of -3, has a bone mass 3 standard deviations below a normal 35-year-old woman. For each standard deviation decline in bone mass, there is slightly more than a doubling in the fracture risk.

A task force of the National Osteoporosis Foundation has recommended the following clinical indications for bone mass measurements: (1) estrogen-deficient women, (2) the presence of vertebral abnormalities on plain x-rays, (3) patients requiring glucocorticoid therapy, and (4) patients with primary hyperparathyroidism. Patients with T-Scores of less than -2 should receive therapy. Patients with T-Scores greater than $+1$ have a very low risk of fracture. Individuals with T-Scores between -2 and $+1$ may be candidates for intervention based on other risk factors for osteoporotic fractures and their overall health assessment.

Single-Beam Photon Absorptiometry

The single-beam photon absorptiometry technique uses iodine-125 (^{125}I) and a scintillation detector to measure bone mineral content in the forearm bones. The reproducibility and precision of the determination (approximately 2% to 3%) are impaired because of the difficulty of repositioning the forearm precisely in successive measurements. It gives information only on bone mineral densities in the distal extremities and cannot determine the nature or extent of diseases of generalized bone loss. This technique measures cortical bone predominantly, and correlations between changes in the bone mineral content in the cortical bone of the forearm and the bone mineral content of the cancellous bone of the vertebrae are often poor. For example, about 30% of persons with clinical osteoporosis have normal forearm bone mineral density according to some investigators. However, in individual patients with abnormal findings, this method may be useful for monitoring changes in bone mineral densities during a long period of observation. This is more likely to be valuable in primary hyperparathyroidism, in which beneficial therapeutic intervention is possible, than in osteoporosis, in which treatment is difficult for established disease. Because many patients with vertebral body collapse produced by osteoporosis have normal forearm bone mineral density measurements according to this technique, it is obviously inadequate as a screening test to select patients at risk for the development of osteoporosis. The radiation exposure is minimal, and recent technical advances using rectilinear scanning have improved both precision and sensitivity.

Dual-Beam Photon Absorptiometry

The dual-beam photon absorptiometry (DPA) technique utilizes a multienergy isotope, gadolinium-135. It allows measurement of bone mineral content in the lumbar spine. It measures all the bone (both cortical and trabecular) in the vertebral body, with a precision of 2% to 3%. An on-line computer image is used to assess results. Modifications in the technique also allow measurement of bone mineral content in the femoral neck. This technique is still relatively new, and variations in results are reported by different groups. It has the advantage of measuring bone mineral density in the bones that are primarily affected in osteoporosis and age-related bone loss. The radiation exposure is minimal, but DPA scanning is time-consuming.

Computed Tomography

The computed tomography (CT) technique uses CT scanners operated in a quantitative rather than an imaging mode. It measures a defined amount of trabecular bone in the vertebrae and compares it with a known standard. Bone in the femoral neck can also be examined. The precision and sensitivity of the current measurements are greatly improved, although there is still controversy about how reproducible and how accurate they are. Many investigators feel that the current techniques are not precise enough to allow meaningful sequential measurements. A major problem is that intramedullary fat and subcutaneous tissue can make the results difficult to interpret. Patients with dorsal kyphosis may find this procedure less acceptable than the other techniques because of discomfort in positioning the patient during the performance of the test.

Dual-Energy X-Ray Absorptiometry

In the dual-energy x-ray absorptiometry (DEXA) technique, a dual x-ray source replaces the isotope source used in DPA. This technique has the advantage of greater accuracy and precision than DPA and can be performed much more rapidly. Moreover, radiation exposure is even lower. It is used for the same measurements and in the same situations as DPA. This is the current state-of-the-art method. Newer applications such as lateral spine scanning (which may provide better measurements of cancellous bone) and body composition analysis are now possible with this technique.

Newer Techniques

The potential of ultrasound for measurement of bone mineral density is currently under evaluation. Ultrasound is a simple noninvasive technique that is being used to assess bone mineral density in the patella, cortical bone of the femur and radius, and os calcis. Ultrasound has the advantage of being less expensive and therefore potentially more accessible to patients, and in addition is radiation free. Magnetic resonance imaging (MRI) provides indirect measurements of bone mineral density and is still in the early stages of investigation.

BIBLIOGRAPHY

Bijvoet OLM: Kidney function in calcium and phosphate metabolism. In Avioli LV, Krane SM, editors: *Metabolic bone disease,* vol 1, New York, 1977, Academic Press.

Delmas PD: Clinical use of biochemical markers of bone remodeling in osteoporosis. In Christiansen C, Overgaard K, editors: *Osteoporosis 1990,* Third International Symposium on Osteoporosis, Copenhagen, Denmark, 1990, Osteopress.

Delmas PD et al: Urinary excretion of pyridinoline crosslinks correlates with bone turnover measured on iliac crest biopsy in patients with vertebral therapy, *J Bone Min Res* 6:639, 1991.

Dent CE: Cortisone test for hyperparathyroidism, *Br Med J* 1:230, 1956.

Eastell R, Riggs BL: Diagnostic evaluation of osteoporosis, *Endocrinol Metab Clin North Am* 17:547, 1988.

Epstein S: Serum and urinary markers of bone remodeling: assessment of bone turnover, *Endocr Rev* 9:437, 1988.

Eyre D: Collagen crosslinking amino-acids, *Methods Enzymol* 144:115, 1987.

Genant HK et al: Non-invasive bone mineral analysis: recent advances and future directions. In Christiansen C, Overgaard K, editors: *Osteoporosis 1990,* Third International Symposium on Osteoporosis, Copenhagen, Denmark, 1990, Osteopress.

Hui SL, Slemenda CW, Johnston CC Jr: Baseline measurement of bone mass predicts fracture in white women, *Ann Intern Med* 111:355-361, 1989.

Johnston CC Jr, Melton LJ III, Lindsay R et al: Clinical indication for bone mass measurement, *J Bone Min Res* 4(suppl 2):1-28, 1989.

Meunier PJ: Histomorphometry of the skeleton. In Peck WA, editor: *Bone and mineral research annual 1,* Princeton, 1983, Excerpta Medica.

Mundy GR: Differential diagnosis of osteopenia, *Hosp Pract* 11:65, 1978.

Mundy GR: Anatomy, physiology and function of bone: bone resorbing cells. In Favus MJ, editor: *Primer on the metabolic bone disease and disorder of mineral metabolism,* Kelseyville, Calif, 1990, American Society for Bone and Mineral Research.

Parfitt AM, Oliver I, Villanueva AR: Bone histology in metabolic bone disease: the diagnostic value of bone biopsy, *Orthop Clin North Am* 10:329, 1979.

Robins SP et al: Measurement of the cross linking compound, pyridinoline, in urine as an index of collagen degradation in joint disease, *Ann Rheum Dis* 45:969, 1986.

Uebelhart D et al: Urinary excretion of pyridinium crosslinks: a new marker of bone resorption in metabolic bone disease, *Bone Mineral* 8:87, 1990.

Uebelhart D et al: Effect of menopause and hormone replacement therapy on the urinary excretion of pyridinium crosslinks, *J Clin Endocrinol Metab* 72:367, 1991.

Watson L, Moxham J, Fraser P: Hydrocortisone suppression test and discriminant analysis in differential diagnosis of hypercalcemia, *Lancet* 1:1320, 1980.

III CLINICAL SYNDROMES

CHAPTER

287 Weight Loss

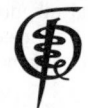

Richard M. Jordan and Peter O. Kohler

Severe loss of weight in the absence of intentional dietary restriction is virtually always a sign of serious systemic or psychiatric disease. In the elderly, rapid weight loss is highly correlated with morbidity and mortality.

Weight loss can be separated into two broad categories (Box 287-1). The first group of patients have weight loss with normal or excessive food intake. The second group of patients have weight loss with diminished food intake. Some patients in this category have disease processes that actually cause increased caloric needs despite decreased intake. The disease states most notable for causing weight loss and the mechanisms by which weight loss is produced are briefly discussed later (Chapters 334 and 347).

ENDOCRINE DISORDERS

Endocrine diseases are almost always a consideration in the differential diagnosis of weight loss. Although important, these disorders are less frequently responsible for weight loss than are gastrointestinal disease, malignancy, and depression.

BOX 287-1
Causes of weight loss

I. Weight loss with normal to increased food intake associated with unimpaired appetite
   A. Insulin-dependent diabetes mellitus
   B. Thyrotoxicosis
   C. Pheochromocytoma
   D. Carcinoid
   E. Malabsorption and maldigestion
   F. Intestinal parasite infestation
   G. Diencephalic syndrome
   H. Malignancy (uncommon)
   I. Luft's syndrome
II. Weight loss with normal or decreased food intake
   A. Impaired appetite that in some cases may be coupled with an increased caloric requirement
      1. Malignancy
      2. Psychiatric disorders (including anorexia nervosa)
      3. AIDS
      4. Liver disease
      5. Addison's disease
      6. Uremia
      7. Chronic infection
      8. Chronic lung disease
      9. Chronic inflammatory disease
      10. Cardiac cachexia
      11. Diabetic neuropathic cachexia
      12. Hypothalamic tumor (very rare)
   B. Unimpaired appetite but decrease of food intake secondary to other factors
      1. Gastric ulcer
      2. Duodenal ulcer with outlet obstruction
      3. Postgastrectomy syndrome
      4. Regional enteritis
      5. Ulcerative colitis
      6. Food faddism
      7. Social isolation

Insulin-dependent diabetes mellitus, especially in young persons, often causes weight loss. This is in part a consequence of fluid and calorie loss secondary to glycosuria. Although many patients manifest polyphagia and polydipsia, some are anorectic. In patients with long-standing diabetes mellitus, additional factors may contribute to weight loss. The chronic debilitating nature of the disease may cause depression and anorexia. A few patients have gastric atony with greatly delayed gastric emptying (gastroparesis diabetacorum), causing nausea, vomiting, and painful abdominal distention. These symptoms discourage regular or adequate food ingestion and lead to poor diabetic control and undernutrition. Many diabetic patients develop a diarrhea that is commonly accompanied by steatorrhea, although uncomplicated diabetic steatorrhea is usually not a primary cause of weight loss. True malabsorption from celiac disease or pancreatic exocrine insufficiency, however, occasionally is associated with diabetes mellitus and must be considered in the diabetic patient with weight loss. Rarely, in older diabetic male patients profound weight loss is combined with autonomic and peripheral neuropathy (diabetic neuropathic cachexia). The cachexia is so impressive that malignancy is usually suspected. The pathophysiologic features of the disorder are unknown, but patients usually recover spontaneously after approximately 1 year.

Thyrotoxicosis and pheochromocytoma cause hypermetabolism and produce weight loss. In both diseases weight loss may be prominent despite excessive caloric intake. Usually, either disorder is easy to recognize. In elderly patients, however, hyperthyroidism may occur with very few of the classic symptoms (apathetic thyrotoxicosis). Thus unexplained weight loss in an older patient should always prompt the physician to measure the thyroid hormone concentrations. Luft's syndrome is a rare disease of skeletal muscle mitochondria in which there are excessive respiration and uncoupling of oxidative phosphorylation. Although not actually an endocrine disorder, the hy-

permetabolism present suggests the diagnosis of hyperthyroidism. The carcinoid syndrome may increase the metabolic rate, and when this is coupled with diarrhea and malabsorption (features that are often present), considerable weight loss can occur. Almost 50% of patients with carcinoid suffer a significant loss of body weight.

When Addison's disease presents insidiously, weight loss is a prominent manifestation. Weakness, fatigue, nausea, and abdominal cramping are all additive factors that cause anorexia and weight loss. Dehydration may also contribute. Hypothalamic tumors, although more commonly associated with marked obesity, can interfere with appetite generation and cause cachexia. Such patients have been diagnosed mistakenly as having anorexia nervosa. In early childhood, an anterior hypothalamic tumor sometimes causes a poorly understood disorder in which cachexia occurs despite increased food intake (diencephalic syndrome).

GASTROINTESTINAL DISEASE

Gastrointestinal disease causes weight loss through anorexia, distressing symptoms that discourage eating, and malabsorption. Chronic liver disease—especially chronic active hepatitis or alcoholic liver disease with cirrhosis—may cause anorexia and weight loss (Chapters 355 and 357).

In esophageal disorders, gastric ulcers, duodenal ulcers with outlet obstruction, postgastrectomy syndromes, and chronic pancreatitis, the ingestion of food may cause such discomfort that patients severely limit oral intake. Abdominal pain and bloody diarrhea initiated by eating may cause patients with regional enteritis and ulcerative colitis to experience significant weight loss. The edentulous patient may be incapable of mastication and lose weight.

Malabsorption or maldigestion can result from many diseases (Chapter 340). Although malabsorption is usually symptomatic and clinically quite evident, it can occasionally be subtle in presentation. Protein-losing enteropathy may also cause weight loss. The edema and ascites resulting from hypoalbuminemia may overshadow any gastrointestinal symptoms present.

PSYCHIATRIC DISORDERS

Anorexia nervosa is always a consideration when a young woman has unexplained weight loss (Chapter 334). The disorder is rare in men. Although there are differing theories concerning the psychiatric aspects of the disorder, virtually all patients demonstrate some degree of psychologic abnormality. Pathologic interrelationships between mother and daughter are commonly present. The conflict in many cases is the parent's need to stay in control, opposing the child's desire for independence. In some patients depression is present. This disorder has several endocrine manifestations, and some evidence suggests that anorexia nervosa may be associated with a hypothalamic disorder. Many (if not all) of the endocrine abnormalities, however, are also seen in simple starvation without anorexia nervosa.

In moderate to severe depressive illness, 70% to 80% of patients experience diminished appetite and weight loss. Because depression is present in up to 4% of the U.S. population, it is probably the single most overlooked disease in a medical practice. Schizophrenia, manic-depressive disorders, and chronic anxiety states may also be associated with weight loss. Drug dependence, especially alcoholism and narcotic addiction, commonly results in weight loss. The mechanism is complex and involves primary effects of the drugs, decreased intake of food, associated chronic illnesses, and depression. Rarely, transient weight loss occurs in patients who surreptitiously ingest thyroid hormones and amphetamines. Weight loss results primarily from induced hypermetabolism and muscle wasting and, in the case of amphetamines, from anorexia. Weight usually stabilizes, however, in spite of continued ingestion of these agents. Extremely heavy tobacco abuse also is a cause of anorexia and weight loss.

CANCER

The possibility of cancer is always a major concern in any unexplained weight loss. The cause of weight loss is usually multifactorial. The basal metabolic rate is often elevated, with values of +35% to +74% being reported (+15% is the usual upper limit in normal persons). Patients with leukemia and lymphoma tend to have the highest metabolic rates. Rapid cell growth is in part responsible. The patient's nutrients are used by the tumor, and a considerable amount of energy is expended by the neoplastic cells in maintaining such functions as active transport, synthesis of new proteins, and other processes of cell growth. One specific metabolic abnormality that has been identified is excessive activity of the Cori cycle. The Cori cycle (which consumes considerable energy) involves the conversion of glucose to lactate by the liver and kidney and then the resynthesis of glucose from these substrates. Studies indicate that cancer patients with the greatest weight loss also have the highest activity of the Cori cycle. Alterations in taste and production of an anorexigenic substance are other likely contributing factors. Cachectin or tumor necrosis factor is a polypeptide produced by mononuclear macrophages. It is capable of producing both weight loss and fever and may be a cofactor causing weight loss in some cancer patients, as well as in chronic infections. Depression on learning that cancer is present also contributes to anorexia. Local tumor factors such as mechanical obstruction can interfere with assimilation of nutrients, and malabsorption may be present in pancreatic cancer. The treatment to which many cancer patients are subjected (surgery and chemotherapy) may increase metabolic demands and cause anorexia.

INFECTIONS

Acquired immunodeficiency syndrome (AIDS) or AIDS-related complex is now an important consideration in any patient who experiences weight loss. Often other symptoms or signs (fatigue, fever, lymphadenopathy, night sweats, or diarrhea) are present to suggest this possibility. Weight loss in patients with AIDS is often multifactorial, with malabsorption-malnutrition, psychiatric factors, and hormonal abnormalities all contributing. Tuberculosis and other insidious infections such as subacute bacterial endocarditis and brucellosis should be considered in patients with low-grade fever and weight loss. For each degree of fever (Fahrenheit), the patient's metabolic rate increases 7%. Besides anorexia and fever, there is evidence that acute and chronic infections have primary metabolic effects on the cell, contributing to the patient's negative nitrogen balance. Cachectin (see earlier discussion of cancer) may play a role in the pathogenesis of the weight loss.

All of these factors operating together have the potential to cause weight loss of significant proportion. Infestation with intestinal parasites that consume host nutrients is rare in Western countries but should be considered when weight loss occurs despite normal caloric intake.

MISCELLANEOUS DISORDERS

Uremia from any cause can be responsible for decreased appetite and weight loss. Chronic inflammatory disease, especially rheumatoid arthritis and lupus erythematosus, also should be considered, although usually the presence of either disease is obvious. Likewise, cardiac cachexia is rarely occult. Loss of weight in severe congestive heart failure results from anorexia coupled with increased metabolic demands of the hypertrophied myocardium and respiratory muscles. In advanced cases of chronic lung disease, the work of breathing increases caloric needs; however, the effort of eating may become so taxing that food intake actually decreases, thereby causing loss of weight. A cause of malnutrition and weight loss that appears to be increasing in frequency is food faddism. Occasionally, distance-running enthusiasts who have greatly increased caloric requirements follow unusual diets that are calorically and nutritionally inadequate. Social isolation in elderly or debilitated individuals also can contribute to weight loss.

APPROACH TO THE PATIENT WITH WEIGHT LOSS

Several factors deserve emphasis when a patient with weight loss is evaluated. The starting weight, final weight, and period over which weight was lost are obviously important. The patient's weight should then be expressed as a percentage of the ideal body weight to quantify the degree of weight loss and malnutrition. Rapid loss of more

than 10% of normal weight may compromise the patient, whereas the same loss over a prolonged period may have few deleterious effects. A weight loss of approximately 20% in the nonobese patient is indicative of moderate malnutrition. Loss of 35% to 50% of normal body weight represents severe malnutrition and is virtually always life-threatening.

A history of increased or depressed appetite suggests conditions in one of the two major categories listed in Box 287-1. Dietary composition also should be known because foods of low nutritive value (snack foods) or alcohol abuse may mask the presence of protein malnutrition. Symptoms of diarrhea, bulky malodorous stools, nausea, and vomiting suggest a gastrointestinal cause of the weight loss. The presence of anorexia may indicate depression or other psychiatric disturbance that may be revealed by a detailed social and personal history. Anorexia and associated symptoms of hemoptysis, fever, lymph node swelling, hematuria, change in bowel habits, or abdominal pain may provide evidence for the possibility of cancer or an infectious process.

In addition to the physical findings specific to the disease entities listed in Box 287-1, general physical manifestations that indicate severe malnutrition may occur with weight loss. Dermal changes of perifollicular hyperkeratotic papules, pellagrous dermatitis, petechiae, and ecchymoses may occur, although these changes are most common in children. Cheilosis, glossitis, and stomatitis with superficial ulcerations may be found. The presence of edema, either from malnutrition or secondary to a disease associated with weight loss, may camouflage the wasting and weight loss.

Usually the differential diagnosis is apparent at the conclusion of the history and physical examination. Laboratory and radiologic studies should be used to confirm the diagnosis. However, if weight loss remains unexplained, the patient must have thorough testing for cancer. This may require a full complement of gastrointestinal radiography, abdominal computed tomography scans, intravenous pyelography, ultrasonography, and bone marrow examination. Although virtually any neoplasm may cause weight loss, tumors that are especially associated with this sign are pancreatic cancer, gastrointestinal malignancies, renal cell cancer, lung cancer, lymphomas, and leukemias.

BIBLIOGRAPHY

Andres R et al: Body weight changes and all-cause mortality: a review, *Ann Intern Med* 119:737, 1993.

Berkman B et al: Failure to thrive: paradigm for the frail elderly, *Gerontologist* 5:654, 1989.

Beutler B, Cerami A: Cachectin: more than a tumor necrosis factor, *N Engl J Med* 316:279, 1987.

Grunfeld C, Feingold KR: Metabolic disturbances and wasting in the acquired immunodeficiency syndrome, *N Engl J Med* 327:329, 1992.

Holroyde CP et al: Altered glucose metabolism in metastatic carcinoma, *Cancer Res* 35:3710, 1975.

Marton KI, Sox HC Jr, Krupp JK: Involuntary weight loss: diagnostic and prognostic significance, *Ann Intern Med* 95:568, 1981.

Pamuk ER et al: Weight loss and subsequent death in a cohort of U.S. adults, *Ann Intern Med* 119:744, 1993.

Warren MP: Anorexia nervosa. In DeGroot LJ, editor: *Endocrinology*, ed 3, Philadelphia, 1995, WB Saunders.

Weiss RJ: Unexplained weight loss in an elderly patient: delayed diagnosis of thyrotoxicosis, *Postgrad Med* 86:177, 1989.

CHAPTER

288 Obesity

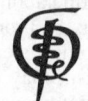

Edward S. Horton

Obesity is a condition in which there is an excess of body fat. It is usually, but not always, associated with being "overweight" when compared to population norms for body weight related to age, gender, height, and frame size. The increased fat mass may be due to an increase in the lipid content of individual fat cells, an increase in to-

---

BOX 288-1
Classification of obesity

Familial
  Onset usually in childhood
  Prevalence in first-degree relatives
  Genetic and cultural determinants
  Potential association with other diseases such as non–insulin de-
    pendent diabetes mellitus, hyperlipidemias, hypertension, gout
Isolated
  Onset usually in adolescence or adulthood
  Common contributing factors
    Increased food intake
    Decreased physical activity
    Withdrawal from smoking
    Estrogens
    Drugs affecting energy intake or expenditure
      Phenothiazines, serotonin antagonists, tricyclic antidepres-
        sants, marijuana, sulfonylureas
  Commonly associated diseases
Hypothalamic disorders
  Tumors—craniopharyngioma, glioma, cyst, etc.
  Inflammation—sarcoidosis, tuberculosis, eosinophilic granuloma,
    encephalitis, leukemia
  Trauma—after head injury
  Benign intracranial hypertension
Endocrine disorders
  Cushing's syndrome
  Insulinoma
  Hypothyroidism
  Hypogonadism
  Polycystic ovary syndrome
  Growth hormone deficiency
Congenital disorders
  Prader-Willi syndrome
  Laurence-Moon-Biedl syndrome
  Alstrom's syndrome
  Familial partial lipodystrophy

tal fat cell number, or a combination of the two. The distribution of body fat may be generalized or localized to specific regions. Thus obesity is not a single disease entity but a syndrome with many causes, including combinations of genetic, nutritional, environmental, and sociologic factors. This results in a varied picture of obesity with regard to its natural history, complications, association with other diseases, and response to treatment.

No completely satisfactory classification of the various forms of obesity has been developed, although attempts have been made to categorize obesity according to the distribution of body fat (central vs. peripheral), proposed pathogenetic mechanisms (metabolic vs. regulatory), age at onset (childhood, early adulthood, gestational, middle age), cellular character of the adipose tissue (hypertrophic vs. hyperplastic), and cause (genetic, hypothalamic, dietary, physical inactivity, and endocrine disease) (Box 288-1). Recent studies have focused on the possibility that low resting metabolic rates and decreased spontaneous physical activity may be predisposing factors to the development of obesity in some individuals. Another area of active investigation is focused on understanding the several factors that regulate food intake, including central nervous system, gastrointestinal, and hormonal mechanisms.

Leptin, a recently discovered hormone synthesized and secreted from adipose tissue, has been shown to be a potent regulator of food intake in rodents, and its role in human obesity is now under investigation. In normal animals, leptin decreases food intake, apparently by binding to hypothalamic receptors that inhibit the synthesis and release of neuropeptide-Y, a substance involved in regulation of appetite. The genetically obese mouse (ob/ob) has a defect in the synthesis of leptin and the administration of leptin to these animals rapidly normalizes their body weight. In contrast, the obese diabetic mouse (db/db) has a defect in hypothalamic leptin receptors, is resistant to the hormone, and develops obesity despite high plasma leptin concentrations.

Human obesity is usually associated with increased plasma leptin concentrations and increased leptin expression in fat cells. Leptin resistance may also be present, but it is not known if this is a primary abnormality causing obesity or an adaptive response to the elevated plasma leptin levels. The discovery of leptin has stimulated much new research on the regulation of food intake and the molecular mechanisms of obesity. These investigations may lead to a better understanding of the cause and pathogenesis of the various forms of obesity and an improved classification system. Currently, however, the classification in Box 288-1 may be useful in developing an approach to the diagnosis and treatment of the obese patient.

DIAGNOSIS

Just as there has been difficulty in classifying obesity, there has also been a lack of uniformity in defining diagnostic criteria. This is due, in part, to the fact that methods for accurately measuring body fat content are not readily available in clinical practice. Often the diagnosis is obvious clinically. Examination of the patient may reveal large amounts of subcutaneous adipose tissue that can be demonstrated by the "pinch test" or measured as skinfold thickness by specially designed calipers. In general, approximately 50% of body fat is in subcutaneous tissue, so measurement of skinfold thickness at one or more sites can be used to estimate total body fat. The upper limit of normal for skinfold thickness over the triceps area is considered to be 23 mm in adult men and 30 mm in adult women, with somewhat lower values in children. Others have correlated the sum of skinfold thickness measured at several sites (e.g., biceps, triceps, subscapular, and suprailiac) with measurements of total body fat content, and from these data have developed predictive tables for adult men and women.

Perhaps the most common method for diagnosing obesity is by the use of tables of desirable weights for sex and height, such as those developed by the Metropolitan Life Insurance Company in 1959 and revised in 1985. The patient's weight compared to "desirable weight" is usually expressed as the *percent overweight,* with the upper limit of normal considered to be 20% above the standard. What is actually determined by the use of these tables is the body weight of an individual relative to an arbitrary standard and not the degree of body fatness. Thus a person who has a large skeletal and muscle mass may be "overweight" by the tables but not obese.

Several other measurements of height and weight have been used to diagnose obesity, the most commonly used being the body mass index (BMI), which is the ratio of weight in kilograms to height in meters squared (kg/m^2). This is now the preferred method of expressing body size and correlates well with more precise measurements of body composition. The normal range for BMI is 20 to 25; 25 to 30 indicates mild obesity, 30 to 40 moderate obesity, and more than 40 severe obesity.

Where available, estimates of total body fat by body density measurements, isotope dilution, potassium-40 counting, or total body electrical conductivity or electrical impedance methods can be used to diagnose obesity with greater accuracy. Current practice is to consider a fat content of greater than 20% in men and 28% in women to indicate obesity. However, such a definition is arbitrary and does not consider the anatomic character, distribution, or health consequences of the obesity.

Measurement of the waist to hip circumference ratio (WHR) as an index of upper body (abdominal) obesity versus lower body (buttocks and thighs) obesity is also useful, because an increase in intraabdominal fat is associated with an increased risk for metabolic abnormalities and adverse health consequences. The WHR is determined by measuring the circumference at the navel and the maximum circumference of the hips and buttocks. It is normally greater in men than in women and tends to increase somewhat with increasing age in both sexes. Precise upper limits of normal have not been defined, but a WHR more than 1.0 in men and more than 0.85 in women is associated with an increased risk of metabolic abnormalities.

PATHOPHYSIOLOGY

Regardless of the underlying cause, the final common pathway for the development of obesity is an excess of energy intake over energy expenditure leading to deposition of body fat. In humans, very little de novo lipogenesis occurs in adipose cells. Lipids, either derived directly from the diet or synthesized in the liver from excess carbohydrates, are transported to adipose tissue as chylomicrons or very-low-density lipoproteins (VLDLs). The triglycerides in these particles are hydrolyzed by lipoprotein lipase located in capillary endothelium, taken up in adipose cells, and then reesterified into cellular triglycerides. During periods of negative energy balance, stored triglycerides are released from adipose cells as glycerol and free fatty acids and metabolized for energy production. When energy intake exceeds energy expenditure over a long period, obesity results.

It is now clear that many factors regulate both energy intake and energy expenditure and that defects in one or more of these factors may play a significant role in the pathogenesis of obesity. Energy intake is regulated by internal factors governing hunger, satiety, and appetite; by the efficiency with which ingested food is digested, absorbed, and metabolized; and by external factors such as the availability of food, composition of the diet, social pressures, and environmental conditions. Energy expenditure is determined by factors that regulate the basal metabolic rate, thermic response to food ingestion, energy used during physical activity, and responses to environmental conditions such as exposure to cold temperatures. Changes in thyroid hormone metabolism, sympathetic nervous system activity, and insulin sensitivity all affect energy expenditure.

The concept that obesity is always associated with hyperphagia is no longer tenable. Daily energy intake may be the same or less than in lean subjects if energy expenditure is also reduced. This may occur if the resting metabolic rate is low or if the subject is physically inactive. However, in most patients, total daily energy expenditure correlates well with the fat-free mass when corrected for levels of physical activity.

DIFFERENTIAL DIAGNOSIS

By far the most common forms of obesity are those that occur in adolescence or adulthood in association with one or more contributing factors such as excessive food intake, decreased physical activity, withdrawal from smoking, use of oral contraceptives, or use of medications that affect the regulation of food intake or energy expenditure. Familial forms of obesity are also common, although onset is usually during childhood and a positive family history of lifelong obesity is present. To assess these patients a detailed history is required to determine the age of onset, rate of progression, prior treatments, and present status of the obesity. In addition, the presence or absence of associated diseases and any identifiable contributing factors, including medications, diet, physical activity, and psychologic, social, and environmental characteristics, should be determined. The physical examination should include an assessment of the severity of the obesity and the anatomic distribution of body fat. Both the BMI and the WHR should be calculated and recorded.

Hypothalamic disorders associated with obesity are characterized by hyperphagia and, in some cases, decreased physical activity. Other signs of hypothalamic dysfunction such as altered temperature regulation and fluid balance, as well as signs of neurologic disease, are often present. Endocrine disorders associated with obesity should be considered if other characteristic signs and symptoms are present.

The various congenital syndromes associated with obesity are rare but should be considered if the characteristic stigmata are present. Prader-Willi syndrome is suggested by a combination of muscle hypotonia in infancy, short stature, delayed bone maturation, cryptorchidism, and mental retardation. Other manifestations may include small hands and feet, strabismus, and dental enamel hypoplasia. The Laurence-Moon-Biedl syndrome is characterized by retinitis pigmentosa, polydactyly or syndactyly, mental retardation, and hypogonadism. Nerve deafness and abnormalities of the heart and kidneys may also occur. Alstrom's syndrome is similar to Laurence-Moon-Biedl syndrome and includes atypical retinitis pigmentosa, nerve deafness, hypogonadism, and diabetes mellitus. Familial lipodystrophy is a variable disorder characterized by a marked decrease in subcutaneous fat in one segment of the body and hypertrophy of fat in another. It is more frequent in women, and a familial pattern of fat distribution is common. For example, several members of one family may have a marked decrease in fat over the torso and upper extremities and a marked increase in the hips, buttocks, and legs, whereas another family may exhibit the opposite pattern.

ASSOCIATED DISEASES

Taken as a group, the obese have an increased overall mortality rate when compared to a normal-weight population. The mortality ratio increases with increasing severity of obesity. At a BMI of 30, the relative risk is approximately 1.3, and with a BMI of 40 the risk is increased to 2.5, compared to that of a normal-weight population. Obesity is also associated with several other diseases that may result in significant morbidity or may be the primary cause of death. These include a cluster of metabolic abnormalities commonly referred to as the *syndrome of insulin resistance* (SIR), which includes hyperinsulinemia, insulin resistance, non–insulin dependent diabetes mellitus (NIDDM), hyperlipidemia, hypertension, and gout. In women, hyperandrogenism may also be present. Other diseases associated with obesity include coronary artery disease, cerebral and peripheral vascular disease, biliary tract disease, osteoarthritis, and gout. In addition, menstrual irregularities and diseases of the reproductive tract, particularly endometrial carcinoma, are more common in obese women.

Many of these conditions are improved significantly by weight reduction, and treatment of obesity plays a major role in their prevention and management. It is particularly important in the management of NIDDM, hyperlipidemia, and hypertension. In these conditions, even modest degrees of weight reduction may result in marked improvements in blood glucose and VLDL concentrations, moderate decreases in cholesterol level, and significant fall in blood pressure.

Metabolic abnormalities that lead to the development of one or more of the associated diseases are not present in all obese individuals. A population of "healthy" obese exists, and epidemiologic data suggest that in the older age groups life expectancy may actually be increased when a moderate degree of obesity is present. This may represent a "selected" population and reemphasizes that obesity is not a single entity but a group of conditions with various causes and prognoses.

Psychologic and social handicaps may be a major problem for the obese and should be considered in evaluating the patient. Discrimination against obese individuals in several sectors of society, including acceptance into universities and professional schools, job promotion, and fashion design, has been demonstrated in a variety of studies, and the obese are frequently treated as if they are lazy or lack will-power to control their weight. Depression, lack of self-confidence, and a sense of guilt are common in patients with obesity and may constitute barriers to successful treatment.

TREATMENT

The basic goal of treatment is to reduce the excess adipose tissue mass by creating a negative net energy balance. Ideally, this should be accomplished with the least possible loss of lean body mass and without impairment of vital organ functions. Once the desired body weight is achieved, a new steady state of energy balance should be maintained by balancing caloric intake with energy expenditure. Nutritional adequacy of the diet with regard to vitamins, minerals, and other essential nutrients should be maintained as much as possible during weight loss and is a major goal during weight maintenance. If the obesity is caused by another disease process, treatment of the underlying condition may be sufficient to improve or cure the condition without specific dietary interventions.

The vast majority of patients with obesity should be treated by a program combining reduction in energy intake, increased physical activity, and attention to correcting identified factors contributing to the obesity. Support systems to promote modifications in lifestyle are particularly important for long-term success of weight reduction and weight maintenance programs.

A negative energy balance of 500 kcal/day can usually be maintained over many weeks or months. This is safe and can be expected to result in an average rate of weight loss of 1 lb/wk. If more rapid weight loss is desired, diets ranging from 600 to 1000 kcal/day can be used but require careful monitoring and supplementation of essential nutrients. These very low calorie diets are not generally recommended for long-term use. Daily energy intakes of less than 600 kcal/day have been associated with sudden death, most likely caused by cardiac arrhythmias associated with electrolyte imbalance or myocardial degeneration. They also result in significant negative nitrogen balance and loss of lean body mass. For these reasons they should rarely be used.

Medications that suppress appetite or stimulate energy expenditure are commonly used to potentiate weight loss, but their effects are often transient. Many have undesirable side-effects and/or potential for habituation. New compounds are currently being developed that may be more effective and prevent these problems.

A number of surgical procedures have been developed for the treatment of severe, life-threatening obesity. Of these, the most common in current use are gastric bypass and gastroplasty procedures. Complications of these procedures, although fewer than those of some of the other surgical treatments, are still troublesome and include development of stomal ulcers, obstruction of the anastomosis, reflux esophagitis, recurrent vomiting, diarrhea, and dumping syndrome.

In general, patients seeking treatment for severe obesity for the first time should be considered for medical therapy including appropriate dietary, physical exercise, and behavior modification regimens and support. Gastric restrictive or bypass procedures could be considered for well-informed and motivated patients with acceptable operative risks, provided they are selected carefully after evaluation by a multidisciplinary team with medical, surgical, psychiatric, and nutritional expertise. Regardless of the therapeutic approach selected, obesity is a chronic disease and long-term management and surveillance are necessary.

BIBLIOGRAPHY

Bogardus C et al: Familial dependence of the resting metabolic rate, *N Engl J Med* 315:96, 1986.

Bray GA: Complications of obesity, *Ann Intern Med* 103:1052, 1985.

Bray GA: Obesity, *Dis Mon* 35:451, 1989.

Fujioka S et al: Contribution of intra-abdominal fat accumulation to the impairment of glucose and lipid metabolism in human obesity, *Metabolism* 36:154, 1987.

Gastrointestinal Surgery for Severe Obesity NIH Consensus Development Conference Consensus Statement, Volume 9(1) March 25–27, 1991.

King AC et al: Diet vs. exercise in weight maintenance: the effects of minimal intervention strategies on long-term outcomes in men, *Arch Intern Med* 149:2741, 1989.

Kissebah AH et al: Relation of body fat distribution to metabolic complications of obesity, *J Clin Endocrinol Metab* 54:254, 1982.

Landin K et al: Importance of obesity for the metabolic abnormalities associated with an abdominal fat distribution, *Metabolism* 38:572, 1989.

Maffei M et al: Leptin levels in human and rodent: measurement of plasma leptin and ob RNA in obese and weight-reduced subjects, *Nat Med* 1:115, 1995.

Pelleymounter MA et al: Effects of the obese gene product on body weight regulation in ob/ob mice, *Science* 260:540, 1995.

Ravussin E et al: Determinants of 24-hour energy expenditure in man: methods and results using a respiratory chamber, *J Clin Invest* 78:1568, 1986.

Ravussin E et al: Reduced rate of energy expenditure as a risk factor for body-weight gain, *N Engl J Med* 318:467, 1988.

Roberts SB et al: Energy expenditure and intake in infants born to lean and overweight mothers, *N Engl J Med* 318:461, 1988.

Sims EAHS, Danforth E Jr: Expenditure and storage in man, *J Clin Invest* 79:1019, 1987.

Stephens TW et al: The role of neuropeptide Y in the antiobesity action of the obese gene product, *Nature* 377:530, 1995.

Stunkard AJ et al: The body-mass index of twins who have been reared apart, *N Engl J Med* 322:1483, 1990.

Williamson DF et al: The 10-year incidence of overweight and major weight gain in U.S. adults, *Arch Intern Med* 150:665, 1990.

Woo R, Kush-Daniels R, Horton ES: Regulation of energy balance, *Annu Rev Nutr* 5:411, 1985.

Zhang Y et al: Positional cloning of the mouse obese gene and its human homologue, *Nature* 372:425, 1994.

289 Weakness

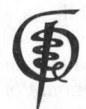

David L. Vesely

Weakness, fatigue, and *loss of energy* are all terms used by patients to describe similar subjective symptoms. On closer questioning, *fatigue* usually refers to a loss of power or strength associated with exertion. *Loss of energy,* on the other hand, more often refers to a generalized feeling of inability to begin movement not associated with exertion. *Weakness* usually relates to a loss of strength in one or more muscle groups. Weakness becomes a more objective finding when decreased muscular power is demonstrated. Objective weakness may be divided into several groups based on where the majority of the patient's weakness is located anatomically (Box 289-1).

BOX 289-1
Differential diagnosis of muscle weakness

I. Primary proximal weakness
  A. Muscle
     1. Endocrine: hyperthyroidism, hypothyroidism, subacute thyroiditis, hyperparathyroidism, acromegaly, Addison's disease (acute adrenal insufficiency), primary aldosteronism, steroid myopathy (Cushing's syndrome; iatrogenic), and male hypogonadism
     2. Metabolic: diabetes mellitus, insulin-induced hypoglycemia, glycogen storage diseases (acid maltase deficiency, muscle phosphorylase deficiency, muscle phosphofructokinase deficiency), lipid storage disease (carnitine deficiency), and alcoholic myopathy
     3. Muscular dystrophies: limb-girdle, Duchenne's, Becker's
     4. Inflammatory myopathies: polymyositis, dermatomyositis, other collagen vascular diseases including rheumatoid arthritis, sarcoidosis, human immunodeficiency virus
     5. Hypercalcemia, hypophosphatemia, hypokalemia, and hyperkalemia of any cause
     6. Drug induced: colchine, chloroquine, cimetidine, amidarone, β-blockers, D-penicillamine, cyclosporine, suramin
  B. Neuromuscular junction: myasthenia gravis, Eaton-Lambert, botulism, organophosphate poisoning
  C. Peripheral nerve: diabetic proximal neuropathy, Guillain-Barré syndrome, acute intermittent porphyria, tick paralysis, and arsenic poisoning
  D. Anterior horn cell: poliomyelitis, chronic spinal muscular atrophy
II. Primary distal weakness
  A. Muscle: myotonic dystrophy
  B. Peripheral nerve: beriberi, diphtheria, lead, porphyrins, carcinomatous neuropathy, chronic progressive demyelinating neuropathy, peroneal muscle atrophy (Charcot-Marie-Tooth), Guillain-Barré syndrome, Refsum's disease, compressive lesions (root, plexus, nerve)
  C. Anterior horn cell: poliomyelitis, motor neuron disease
III. Generalized weakness
  A. Decreased cardiac output (mitral stenosis, tricuspid stenosis, mitral regurgitation)
  B. Acute infectious diseases and chronic infectious diseases such as tuberculosis, brucellosis, and trichinosis
  C. Chronic glomerulonephritis and other causes of uremia, including generalized rhabdomyolysis
  D. Pernicious anemia (and other anemias)
  E. Hepatitis
  F. Neurosyphilis
  G. Psychiatric illnesses such as depression
  H. Multiple sclerosis
  I. Mitochondrial myopathy—genetic, zidovudine
  J. L-tryptophan (eosinophilia-myalgia)

DIFFERENTIAL DIAGNOSIS

The mode of onset and progression of the weakness are helpful in distinguishing particular disorders in the differential diagnosis of weakness. Several disorders are associated with rapid onset of weakness, including the Guillain-Barré syndrome, botulism, organophosphate poisoning, severe electrolyte imbalance, diphtheria, and acute polymyositis. A history of relapses and remissions could suggest myasthenia gravis, a relapsing peripheral neuropathy, one of the periodic paralyses, exogenous potassium depletion, or a collagen-vascular disease. Other disorders are slow in onset, with a progressive deterioration of strength that should suggest one of the muscular dystrophies. Any consideration of differential diagnosis must take into account associated signs such as atrophy or muscle wasting. It is important to note whether the muscle wasting follows the distribution of any particular nerve; this can provide a clue to the neurologic basis of the wasting. Careful note should be made of the way a patient walks into a room, sits down, or gets up from a chair. A patient who has no difficulty in removing a shirt over the head but gives way when formal muscle testing of the shoulders is attempted may not have organic weakness. The diagnosis of hysterical weakness or malingering depends chiefly on the discovery of inconsistencies when all the clinical signs are considered as a whole.

ENDOCRINE CAUSES

Of the various causes of muscle weakness, endocrine myopathies currently represent the most easily correctable of the neuromuscular disorders (Chapter 148). Weakness as a symptom of hyperthyroidism was reported by Graves as early as 1835 and is found on physical examination in approximately 80% of hyperthyroid patients. Usually the proximal limb muscles are involved, and the shoulder girdle muscles are involved more often than the muscles of the pelvic girdle. As with other types of proximal muscle involvement described later, these patients have difficulty in walking up stairs, getting up from a chair, and combing their hair without resting. With increasing severity of the thyrotoxic myopathy, the distal musculature often becomes involved, and occasionally bulbar weakness also occurs. After successful treatment of hyperthyroidism, the patient usually fully recovers muscular strength, as with other endocrine myopathies described later. With respect to weakness in hyperthyroid patients, it should be remembered that there is also a 30-fold increase in incidence of myasthenia gravis in Graves' disease patients compared with the incidence in the general population. Periodic paralysis is also associated with Graves' thyrotoxicosis but differs from familial hypokalemic periodic paralysis (which it closely resembles) in that 95% of thyrotoxic patients have no familial pattern and periodic paralysis attacks disappear without recurrence after the patient becomes euthyroid. Asians are especially prone to thyrotoxic periodic paralysis.

Weakness is also present in up to 40% of all hypothyroid patients but is generally less marked than in hyperthyroid patients. Weakness is likewise a presenting symptom of hyperparathyroidism, and 20% to 30% of these patients have objective signs of proximal muscle weakness in the lower extremities on neurologic testing. In addition to hyperparathyroidism, hypercalcemia and hypophosphatemia of any cause are also causes of proximal muscle weakness.

Weakness is a major symptom in approximately 40% of patients with acromegaly and is related to a combination of myopathy and neuropathy. A large percentage of patients with acromegaly are still clinically weak a year or more after treatment. Muscle weakness is a common symptom in Addison's disease. It appears to be closely related to the hyperkalemia because, when potassium levels are normalized, weakness usually disappears. Hyperkalemia or hypokalemia (e.g., primary aldosteronism) of any cause may produce proximal muscle weakness.

Cushing's syndrome typically becomes manifest with proximal muscle weakness in 80% to 90% of these patients. Steroid myopathy, including that produced by exogenous steroids, may be the most common endocrine cause of weakness. Noticeable muscle weakness resulting from corticosteroid administration usually occurs 3 to 20 months after starting the respective steroid. Male hypogonadism is sometimes associated with a generalized weakness.

METABOLIC CAUSES

Of the metabolic causes of weakness, poorly controlled diabetes mellitus is the most common. Severe hypophosphatemia in the diabetic or nondiabetic patient may cause weakness. Weakness is one of the symptoms of marked hyperglycemia and acute hypoglycemia of any cause. The glycogen storage and lipid storage diseases are relatively rare, but proximal muscle weakness is one of their prominent features. Proximal muscle atrophy and weakness, mainly of the lower limbs, occur in the chronic alcoholic patient.

MUSCULAR, NEUROMUSCULAR, AND NEURAL CAUSES

The progressive muscular dystrophies are among the genetic causes of marked proximal muscle weakness. Thus Duchenne's pseudohypertrophic pelvifemoral muscular dystrophy and Becker's pseudohypertrophic (milder course) muscular dystrophy are inherited as X-linked recessive diseases. Limb-girdle dystrophy is usually inherited as an autosomal recessive trait, but it occasionally follows an autosomal dominant pattern of inheritance.

The inflammatory myopathies are characterized by (1) the relatively common polymyositis, which is a symmetric, painless weakness of the proximal limb and trunk muscles without any clinically apparent skin lesions, and (2) dermatomyositis, which has a similar distribution of proximal muscle weakness accompanied by skin lesions, the most pathognomonic of which is the heliotrope (lilac-colored) rash over the eyelids, nose, forehead, and fingernails. All the collagen-vascular diseases and sarcoidosis can cause a myopathy that is similar to polymyositis.

Human immunodeficiency virus type 1 (HIV-1) may cause a proximal myopathy usually of the nemaline rod type or an inflammatory myopathy similar to polymyositis. A far more common myopathy in individuals infected with HIV-1 is due to treatment with zidovudine (AZT). This myopathy usually presents after more than a year of therapy and is characterized by wasting of the buttock muscles with associated leg weakness, which is usually reversible with cessation of AZT treatment. Other drugs that induce myopathies are colchicine, chloroquine, D-penicillamine, cimetidine, amiodarone, β-blockers, cyclosporin, and suramin. The eosinophilia-myalgia syndrome is usually caused by the ingestion of L-tryptophan.

Myasthenia gravis in its advanced stages causes a weakness of the proximal muscles of the limbs. True myasthenia gravis rarely occurs without weakness of the muscles innervated by the cranial nerves. The weakness of myasthenia gravis is episodic and is characterized by partial recovery of strength after a period of rest and after administration of anticholinesterase drugs. Eaton-Lambert syndrome is a myasthenia-like condition associated with cancer, such as small-cell carcinoma of the lung. The weakness in this syndrome usually involves the pelvic, thigh, and shoulder muscles and spares the ocular and bulbar muscles.

With peripheral nerve involvement, weakness may advance during a period of days to involve the proximal and distal limb muscles, as in the Landry-Guillain-Barré syndrome, tick paralysis, and acute intermittent porphyria, or it may develop rather slowly, over a period of weeks, as in arsenic or lead poisoning or the diabetic neuropathies. Diabetic mononeuropathy may, however, develop rapidly. If proximal muscle weakness is asymmetric and is accompanied by atrophy, hyperreflexia, and fasciculations, diseases of the anterior horn cell should be suspected.

Distal muscle weakness gives rise to difficulty with fine coordinating movements and with grip, causing problems with performing such daily activities as buttoning a shirt or tying a shoelace. Severe distal symmetric weakness that rapidly advances to the point where the patient is confined to a wheelchair is seen with the carcinomatous and uremic polyneuropathies. An exception to the general rule that muscle disease becomes manifest with proximal weakness is the profound distal weakness seen in patients with myotonic dystrophy, in which hand, facial, and neck muscles are usually affected. Genetic causes of distal weakness include Charcot-Marie-Tooth (peroneal muscle) atrophy and Refsum's disease (chronic polyneuropathy with ichthyosis, deafness, and retinitis pigmentosa). Compression of a nerve against the underlying bone also results in distal weakness; mild cases recover fairly rapidly (2 to 12 weeks). All of the polyneuropa-

✔ *WHEN TO REFER*

If the muscle weakness is distal and due to a peripheral nerve problem and/or a muscular dystrophy, then patients should be referred to a neurologist. If the muscle weakness is secondary to an endocrine and/or metabolic disease, an endocrinologist may be invaluable in the management of these patients. A valvular heart lesion causing the weakness is usually best managed by a cardiologist. Each of the other causes of weakness can usually be managed in an excellent fashion by an internal medicine primary care physician.

thies caused by diphtheria, diabetes, and lead intoxication also can lead to distal muscle weakness.

MISCELLANEOUS CAUSES

A general weakness is seen in disorders of decreased cardiac output such as mitral stenosis, tricuspid stenosis, and mitral regurgitation. Acute and chronic infectious diseases such as brucellosis, tuberculosis, and trichinosis may show weakness frequently accompanied by fever. All severe anemias, including acute blood loss and hepatitis, may cause a generalized feeling of fatigue. A generalized weakness is often associated with chronic glomerulonephritis. Uremia of any cause may lead to a generalized weakness in addition to the distal muscle weakness discussed earlier. If the patient has weakness in only one limb, and that is associated with optic neuritis and an alteration in emotional response, multiple sclerosis should be considered. A generalized weakness in an individual or family may be due to mitochondrial dysfunction, which has been reported in more than 100 cases. Finally, neurosyphilis and psychiatric illnesses that mimic many disease states should be considered in patients with a generalized weakness.

APPROACH TO DIAGNOSIS

Diagnostic aids for determining the cause of weakness include serum enzyme levels. Of the serum enzymes, creatine phosphokinase (CPK) shows the largest increase in neuromuscular disease, so this enzyme level is routinely obtained. Other intramuscular enzymes whose levels are elevated in the serum in the conditions described earlier are aldolase, glutamic oxaloacetic transaminase, glutamic pyruvic transaminase, and lactic dehydrogenase. Another diagnostic aid is electromyography, which suggests denervation of muscle if fasciculations are seen, or anterior horn cell disease if fibrillations are present. With this technique, myasthenia gravis with a progressive decrement in muscle response to tetanic stimulation can be differentiated from the Eaton-Lambert syndrome, which has a terminal increase in response. At rest, patients with myopathies generally show no electrical activity. Muscle biopsies with ultrastructural studies are often helpful if the above studies plus the history and physical examination do not reveal the diagnosis. Thus muscle biopsies help make the diagnosis in denervation atrophy, in muscle dystrophies, and in the glycogen storage diseases. Lumbar puncture with examination of the spinal fluid is also helpful in diagnosing certain causes of weakness such as the Guillain-Barré syndrome and neurosyphilis.

MANAGEMENT

Management depends upon the specific cause of weakness determined in the earlier described diagnostic tests. Thus if the cause is endocrine or infectious, correction of the underlying endocrine condition or infection usually results in a remission of the weakness. If the cause, on the other hand, is due to a peripheral neuropathy or primary muscular dystrophy, the weakness may not be reversible. Inflammatory myopathies may have a dramatic response to treatment with corticosteroids.

BIBLIOGRAPHY

Brew BJ: Central and peripheral nervous system abnormalities, *Med Clin North Am* 76:63, 1992.

Espinoza R et al: Characteristics and pathogenesis of myositis in human immunodeficiency virus infection: distinction from azidothymidine-induced myopathy, *Rheum Dis Clin North Am* 17:117, 1991.
Johnston W et al: Late onset mitochondrial myopathy, *Ann Neurol* 37:16, 1995.
Links TP et al: Familial hypokalemic periodic paralysis: clinical, diagnostic, and therapeutic aspects, *J Neurol Sci* 122:33, 1994.
Vesely DL: Recognition and managing acute adrenal insufficiency, *J Crit Illness* 3:101, 1988.

CHAPTER

290 Hirsutism

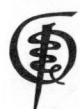

D. Lynn Loriaux

The human body, except the palms of the hands, the soles of the feet, and the lips, is covered with hair follicles. Two kinds of hair grow from these follicles: vellous hairs and terminal hairs. Terminal hairs are typified by the hairs of the scalp. Vellous hairs are typified by the facial hairs of children. The relative distribution of terminal and vellous hair differs between men and women. This results from the effect of androgens. Androgens change vellous hairs to terminal hairs in certain *androgen-sensitive* areas such as the face, upper back and shoulders, chest, and, to some extent, the arms and legs. *Androgen-dependent* hirsutism is a disorder of women in which the hair distribution acquires a male pattern. Hirsutism in any other pattern is referred to as *non–androgen dependent* hirsutism. It is most commonly an untoward side-effect of some medication. Examples of drugs that cause non–androgen dependent hirsutism include diazoxide, minoxidil, phenytoin, glucocorticoids, and cyclosporin A. The following discussion applies only to the androgen-dependent form of the disorder.

SYMPTOMS

Most patients with hirsutism complain of increased hair growth on the face. In particular, the need to remove the hair leads to a feeling of "defeminization." Many women with hirsutism complain of oligoamenorrhea and infertility. Symptoms of virilization are uncommon. When present, they include deepening of the voice, increasing muscle bulk, and qualitative changes in libido that can be characterized as masculine.

SIGNS

Terminal hairs in a masculine distribution define the condition. Less than 5% of normal women have terminal hairs on the cheeks, less than 3% have terminal hairs over the sternum, and, for practical purposes, normal women never have terminal hair over the shoulders, upper back, and upper abdomen. The quantity and quality of the hair distribution over the arms and legs are not in themselves useful in establishing the diagnosis. Signs of virilization include temporal balding, deepening of the voice, and clitoromegaly.

ETIOLOGY

The cause of androgen-dependent hirsutism is increased androgen effect. This can result from the overproduction of androgens or from increased sensitivity to their action. In women, androgens arise from two organs: the ovary and the adrenal gland. Thus most of the disorders that result in hirsutism are disorders of one or both of these organs (Box 290-1). When an abnormality of the ovary or adrenal gland cannot be identified, the disorder is called *idiopathic hirsutism*. The ovary is usually the source of increased androgen secretion in these cases.

The adrenal causes of hirsutism include adrenal cancer, virilizing adrenal adenoma, and the virilizing forms of congenital adrenal hyperplasia; 21-hydroxylase deficiency, 11-hydroxylase deficiency, and 3-hydroxysteroid dehydrogenase deficiency.

BOX 290-1
Causes of androgen-dependent hirsutism

I. Ovarian
  A. Neoplastic
    1. Tumors of gonadal stroma
      a. Sertoli-Leydig tumors (arrhenoblastoma)
      b. Granulosa-theca tumors
      c. Sertoli cell tumor
      d. Lipid cell tumor
      e. Gynandroblastoma
    2. Germ cell tumors
      a. Teratoma
    3. Mixed stroma and germ cell tumors
      a. Gonadoblastoma
  B. Nonneoplastic
    1. Idiopathic hirsutism
    2. Polycystic ovary syndrome
    3. Insulin resistance
II. Adrenal
  A. Neoplastic
    1. Adrenal carcinoma
    2. Virilizing adrenal adenoma
  B. Nonneoplastic
    1. Congenital adrenal hyperplasia
      a. 21-Hydroxylase deficiency
      b. 11-Hydroxylase deficiency
      c. 3-β-Hydroxysteroid dehydrogenase deficiency
    2. Cushing's disease
III. Iatrogenic or factitious
  A. Androgens
    1. Synthetic androgens
    2. Parenteral testosterone esters
  B. "19-nor" Progestins

The ovarian causes of hirsutism include ovarian neoplasms, idiopathic hirsutism, polycystic ovary, insulin resistance, and persistent corpus luteum of pregnancy.

Iatrogenic and factitious forms exist. Synthetic *impeded androgens* currently are used to treat disorders such as endometriosis, fibrocystic breast disease, and hereditary angioneurotic edema. This treatment is usually accompanied by some degree of hirsutism. The attempt to improve athletic performance through the use of androgens has also led to many cases of hirsutism.

DIAGNOSIS

The physician evaluating a hirsute patient should have the possibility of serious underlying disease foremost in mind. Points that tend to separate the serious causes of hirsutism from the benign should be emphasized in the evaluation.

History

The benign forms of hirsutism usually have their onset in the peripubertal period. Hirsutism having its onset distinctly before or after puberty suggests a serious underlying disorder. Benign hirsutism usually develops over a course of 2 or 3 years and then becomes relatively stable. Hirsutism that is progressive is worrisome. Oligoamenorrhea and amenorrhea are found in both benign and malignant forms of hirsutism. Virilization, manifest by deepening of the voice, temporal balding, and changes in libido, is an ominous finding. A family history of hirsutism or a history of medication use that has hirsutism as an untoward side-effect suggests benign disease.

Physical Examination

A careful quantitation of the distribution of terminal hair is of primary importance. This assessment will be used to evaluate the extent to which the patient deviates from the normal distribution of terminal hair growth in women, the rate of progression of hirsutism, and its response to therapy if and when initiated. "Soft" findings of virilization include increased skin thickness, acne, increased muscle bulk, and a masculine pattern of fat distribution. A more objective measure of masculinization is clitoral size. This can be assessed conveniently by the method described by Tagatz and colleagues. A careful search should be made for pelvic and abdominal masses. Truncal skin creases, the axillae, and the wrinkles of the neck should be examined carefully for acanthosis nigricans. Signs of other diseases associated with hirsutism, including Cushing's syndrome and acromegaly, should be noted.

Laboratory Evaluation

The measurement of plasma testosterone concentration plays a central role in the laboratory evaluation of the disorder because the process is androgen mediated. Ideally, the concentration of plasma testosterone should be measured at least three times to provide a more reliable estimate of the "true" concentration of the hormone. Testosterone concentrations greater than 200 ng/dl are rarely seen in the benign forms of hirsutism. Thus testosterone concentrations of this magnitude require a thorough evaluation for adrenal and ovarian neoplasms using pelvic ultrasound and imaging of the adrenal glands. On the other hand, testosterone concentrations in the normal range are rarely associated with serious abnormality.

Low testosterone concentrations in association with a "benign" history suggest the diagnosis of idiopathic hirsutism or the polycystic ovarian syndrome. These conditions have a benign course and a good outcome. Plasma testosterone values between the upper limit of normal and 200 ng/dl can have any cause. Patients with attenuated congenital adrenal hyperplasia usually fall into this range. This disorder should be excluded with the "short" adrenocorticotropic hormone (ACTH) stimulation test. After intravenous administration of synthetic ACTH, 250 μg over 1 minute, the plasma concentrations of several steroid biosynthetic intermediates are measured at 45 and 60 minutes. The most common form of congenital adrenal hyperplasia, the 21-hydroxylase deficient form, can be diagnosed by measuring the plasma concentration of 17-hydroxyprogesterone, the steroid intermediate just before the enzyme block. The concentration of 17-hydroxyprogesterone should not exceed 350 ng/dl in normal subjects after the administration of ACTH. The plasma concentration of 17-hydroxyprogesterone usually exceeds 2000 ng/dl in subjects with the disease. 11-Deoxycortisol and 17-hydroxypregnenolone are the appropriate steroid intermediates to measure for the diagnosis of the 11-hydroxylase and 3-β-hydroxysteroid dehydrogenase forms of the disorder, respectively.

If congenital adrenal hyperplasia is excluded, the possibility of neoplasm remains. Pelvic ultrasound and adrenal computed tomography are the best tests for this evaluation.

TREATMENT

The treatment of adrenal and ovarian neoplasms is surgical extirpation. The treatment for the attenuated forms of congenital adrenal hyperplasia is administration of exogenous glucocorticoids. The preparation of choice is hydrocortisone at a dose of 12 to 15 mg/m^2/day given once a day in the morning. The treatment of virilization associated with insulin resistance is gonadotropin suppression using either the gonadotropin-releasing hormone superagonists or a combination of estrogen and progesterone in a dose sufficient to suppress luteinizing and follicle-stimulating hormone secretion (the standard birth control pill is usually adequate for this purpose).

The choice of treatment for the benign forms of hirsutism, idiopathic hirsutism, and the polycystic ovary syndrome is less clear. Because the pathophysiology of these disorders is still in an imperfect stage of understanding, rational therapy remains elusive. The general guide should be to intervene, if necessary, in the least noxious way acceptable to both patient and physician.

The available therapeutic modalities for hirsutism are shown in Box 290-2. Briefly, shaving is always effective. It is usually rejected because of feelings of defeminization. Wax depilatories and electrolysis are more acceptable; electrolysis is the more effective and expensive of the two. Birth control pills result in improvement in about 70% of treated subjects but expose the patient to the risks of sys-

---

BOX 290-2
Treatment modalities for hirsutism

Physical removal
   Shaving
   Wax depilatories
   Electrolysis
Suppression of androgen secretion
   Ovary
      Birth control pills
      Gonadotropin-releasing hormone superagonists
   Adrenal
      Glucocorticoids
      Synthesis inhibitors (ketoconazole)
Androgen antagonists
   Cyproterone acetate
   Spironolactone

---

temic estrogen therapy. These risks become more frequent and severe with advancing age. Glucocorticoids improve symptoms in about 50% of subjects but expose the patient to the risk of adrenal suppression, a potentially lethal condition.

In the author's view, exogenous glucocorticoids are only indicated in the treatment of hirsutism when the diagnosis of attenuated congenital adrenal hyperplasia is unequivocal. Finally, antiandrogens such as cyproterone and spironolactone have recently gained popularity for the treatment of idiopathic hirsutism and polycystic ovary syndrome. Most studies show success rates approaching 100%, but the long-term consequences of treatment with these agents remain unknown.

It should be noted that improvement in hirsutism is a slow process, and final judgment on the success or failure of a given intervention should not be made before at least 6 months has elapsed.

BIBLIOGRAPHY

Burkman RT Jr: The role of oral contraceptives in the treatment of hyperandrogenic disorders, *Am J Med* 98(1A):130S-136S, 1995.

Conway GS, Jacobs HS: Clinical implications of hyperinsulinaemia in women, *Clin Endocrinol* (Oxf) 39(6):623-632, 1993.

Franks S: Polycystic ovary syndrome, *N Engl J Med* 333(13):853-861, 1995 (published erratum appears in *N Engl J Med* Nov 23, 333[21]:1435), 1995.

Knochenhauer ES, Azziz R: Advances in the diagnosis and treatment of the hirsute patient, *Curr Opin Obstet Gynecol* 7(5):344-350, 1995.

Richards RN, Meharg GE: Electrolysis: observations from 13 years and 140,000 hours of experience, *J Am Acad Dermatol* 33(4):662-666, 1995.

Rittmaster RS: Use of gonadotropin-releasing hormone agonists in the treatment of hyperandrogenism, *Clin Obstet Gynecol* 36(3):679-689, 1993.

Rittmaster RS: Finasteride, *N Engl J Med* 330(2):120-125, 1994.

Rittmaster RS: Clinical review 73: medical treatment of androgen-dependent hirsutism, *J Clin Endocrinol Metab* 80(9):2559-2563, 1995.

Wild RA: Obesity, lipids, cardiovascular risk, and androgen excess, *Am J Med* 98(1A):27S-32S, 1995.

CHAPTER

291 Amenorrhea

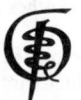

William F. Crowley, Jr.

Amenorrhea rarely fails to get a woman's attention and evoke concern. In adolescence, amenorrhea raises the possibility of reproductive inadequacy in adulthood. In women of reproductive years, it suggests the possibility of pregnancy—a cause of joy or distress, depending on the woman's situation. In older women, the possibility of the menopause and with it the end of reproductive capability represents yet another of life's transitions with which the patient must cope. Thus the appearance of amenorrhea usually evokes strong feelings in the patient and frequently leads to an interaction with the physician.

When consulted by a patient with amenorrhea, physicians must use all resources at their command. In almost no other area of endocrinology does the physician use every aspect of the history and physical examination, especially the social and dietary history, the concurrent use of medications, the exercise history, a careful examination of body weight versus height, and a skin examination. Evidence from each of these lines of inquiry is critical to the generation of a differential diagnosis, which, when combined with carefully targeted laboratory testing, can identify most of the organic causes of amenorrhea and permit a presumptive diagnosis of the functional causes. Thus in the evaluation of amenorrhea, there is no substitute for a detailed history and physical examination to focus laboratory testing and make the evaluation cost effective and accurate.

Amenorrhea can be classified into four anatomic, functional, and etiologic categories: disorders of the hypothalamus, the pituitary gland, the ovary, and/or the uterus. The initial evaluation of a patient with amenorrhea is aimed at localizing the defect to one of these four areas, and then, once the defect has been localized to a given anatomic level, generating a differential diagnosis that employs the previously gleaned historic and physical examination information. In this sense, the approach to a patient with amenorrhea is similar to the intellectual thrust of the evaluation of a patient with a neurologic lesion because the anatomic localization precedes and focuses the subsequent generation of a differential diagnosis and the initiation of therapy.

HYPOTHALAMIC CAUSES

The hypothalamus, the site of the most common defect in a population of women with amenorrhea, secretes gonadotropin-releasing hormone (GnRH) in an episodic fashion. This hypothalamic secretion of GnRH is modulated by many factors. Suspension of GnRH secretion, for example, is a mechanism by which reproductive processes can be suppressed by environmental stresses such as malnutrition and/or weight loss. A residual of this normal adaptive mechanism so necessary from an evolutionary view is commonly seen in women suffering from anorexia and/or bulimia. In both of these circumstances the hypothalamic input to the reproduction system is altered, depending on the metabolic signals arriving at the hypothalamus from the periphery. Similarly, stress exerts its primary impact on hypothalamic GnRH secretion and is a frequent cause of amenorrhea in young women. When seen in this perspective, many of the circumstances that are encountered in a clinical setting and deemed pathologic are really adaptive responses to environmental stress. Most of these challenges mediate their effect on the reproductive system primarily through extinction or alteration of the pattern of the GnRH secretion.

Because GnRH cannot be easily measured in the systemic circulation, clinicians must rely on gonadotropin measurements for inferential information about the status of the hypothalamic secretion of GnRH. When extensive studies are undertaken using frequent sampling of peripheral luteinizing hormone (LH) and follicle-stimulating hormone (FSH) measurements as an index of GnRH secretion, it is clear that the vast majority of patients with a defect in the hypothalamic secretion of GnRH (termed *hypothalamic amenorrhea*) really represent the clinical consequences of a spectrum of neuroendocrine abnormalities of GnRH secretion. These vary from a totally apulsatile pattern of GnRH release, to defects of its amplitude or frequency, to a persistently pubertal pattern termed a *developmental arrest* (Fig. 291-1). Because two thirds to three fourths of all patients with amenorrhea have a hypothalamic cause to their amenorrhea, an understanding of the spectrum of the abnormalities of GnRH secretions and their various modes of clinical and biochemical presentation is essential to any coherent understanding of a patient with amenorrhea.

The clinical circumstances in which hypothalamic amenorrhea most frequently occurs are those of psychologic stress. These include recent loss of a loved one, change of residence or job, or affective disorders such as depression. Previously referred to as *stress-related* amenorrhea or *boarding-school* amenorrhea, these terms all describe the ensemble impact of a series of psychologic stresses on the central nervous system, which are, in turn, meted out in abnormalities of

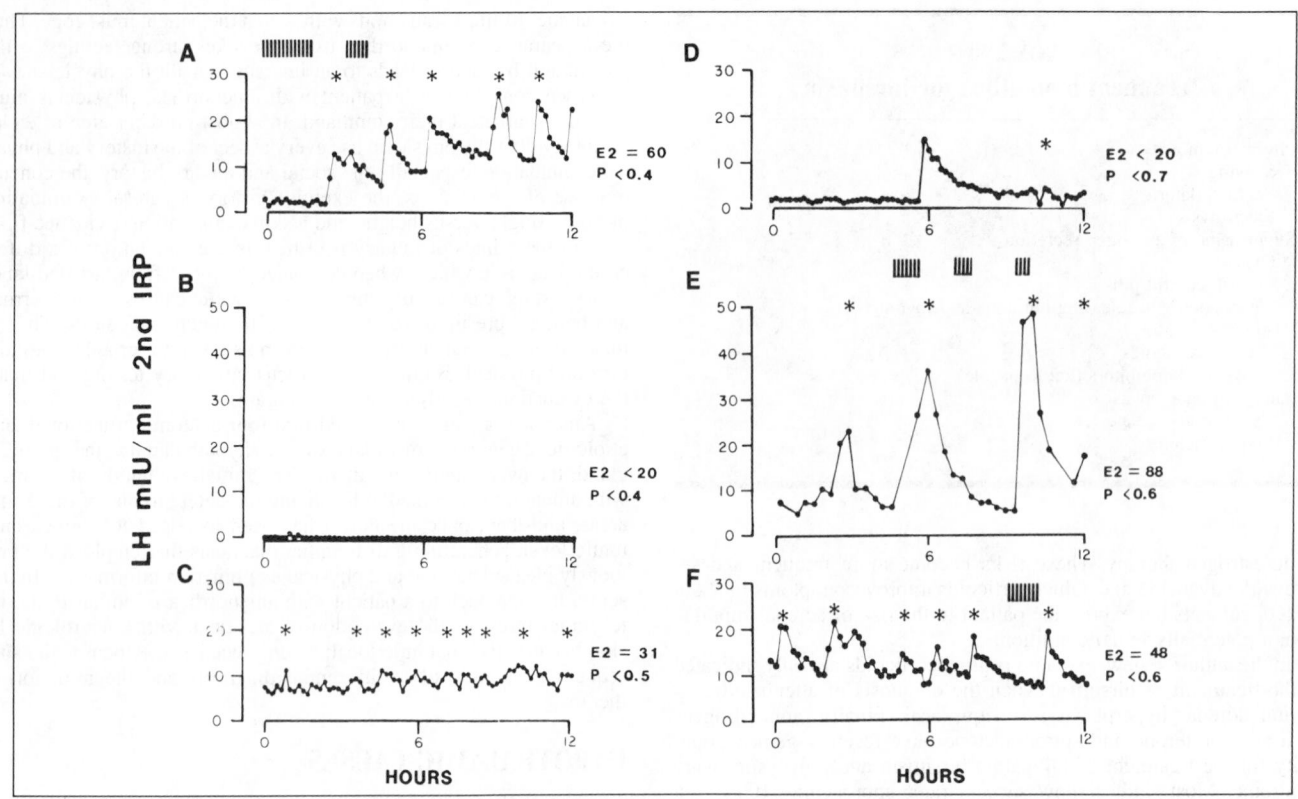

FIGURE 291-1   GnRH secretion in women with hypothalamic amenorrhea. Luteinizing hormone secretion in normal women and women with hypothalamic amenorrhea, demonstrating the spectrum of GnRH-induced LH secretory patterns seen. **A,** Normal women. **B-F,** Women with hypothalamic amenorrhea. **B,** Apulsatile pattern. **C,** Disordered amplitudes. **D,** Disordered frequency. **E,** Sleep-entrained pattern *(developmental arrest)*. **F,** Unclassified pattern. *LH,* Luteinizing hormone; *GnRH,* gonadotropin-releasing hormone.

GnRH secretion. More often, however, the individual psychologic stresses are more subtle and frequently not manifest during the initial visits to the physician. As the physician comes to know the patient better, these individual stresses often reveal themselves during repeated interactions. Similarly, there is a wide degree of personal variability in the responsiveness to a given stress such that no two women may respond in a similar fashion.

One of the puzzling features of patients with hypothalamic amenorrhea is the wide spectrum of biochemical abnormalities of gonadotropin and sex steroid levels these patients may have. If the patients are completely deficient in endogenous GnRH secretion (often the case in severe anorexia nervosa), randomly drawn levels of LH and FSH are very low, often with the LH level being much lower than the FSH level. This discrepancy relates to the fact that LH secretion is largely determined by GnRH secretion alone, whereas FSH secretion is supported by both GnRH and local activin production in the gonadotrope. Since the latter is less affected by GnRH abnormalities, FSH secretion is often sustained out of proportion to that of LH. In addition, the profound estrogen deficiency that accompanies such a complete absence of GnRH-induced gonadotropin secretion is likely a partial explanation for the relative preservation of FSH secretion in these patients because of the absence of estrogen-induced negative feedback. Thus the pattern of low-level LH with normal follicular phase levels of FSH is a frequent occurrence in the most profound type of hypothalamic amenorrhea. The attendant hypoestrogenemia is often apparent on physical examination as vaginal dryness and pallor. Such patients frequently have vaginal dryness and complain of dyspareunia. Despite these manifestations of severe peripheral estrogen deficiency, hot flashes are absent in patients with hypothalamic amenorrhea, as opposed to those patients with a primary ovarian defect who exhibit severe hot flashes, sometimes with considerably less clinical evidence of estrogen deficiency.

Although these clinical and biochemical findings suggest a com-

plete form of total GnRH deficiency, more frequently patients with hypothalamic amenorrhea experience only a partial defect in endogenous GnRH secretion such that the peripheral levels of gonadotropins vary, depending on the particular period of random sampling. Should the patient have recently experienced an isolated burst of GnRH-induced gonadotropin secretion, the plasma LH levels may exceed those of FSH (Fig. 291-1, *D*), producing a pattern that can suggest other disorders such as polycystic ovarian disease. However, on repeated testing during multiple office visits or during a prolonged period of sampling during an inpatient evaluation (generally reserved for a research setting), mean LH and FSH levels are generally documented to be in the normal, follicular phase range. Thus the total daily pattern of gonadotropin pulsations is aberrant and insufficient to initiate and sustain folliculogenesis and to mount an ovulatory LH surge in these patients. This combination of random levels of gonadotropins and sex steroids within the follicular phase ranges in an otherwise amenorrheic subject is often puzzling to the physician unless he or she keeps in mind that the pattern of GnRH-induced gonadotropin secretion over longer periods is defective in such patients. As a consequence, most diagnoses of hypothalamic amenorrhea are made on a presumptive basis in which the history and physical examination are compatible; the biochemical testing fails to reveal specific evidence of primary ovarian failure or hyperprolactinemia, and other anatomic causes of amenorrhea have been eliminated.

Given the presumptive diagnosis of hypothalamic amenorrhea, the therapeutic considerations must be tailored to individual circumstances. For example, if the environmental stress is soon to be removed, the disorder will be self-limited and may not require any therapy other than educating the patient. If prolonged amenorrhea is present, hypoestrogenemia, with attendant decreases in bone density, may prompt the institution of estrogen replacement therapy. It is important to remember that other specific causes of amenorrhea (such as a prolactin-secreting pituitary tumor) must be eliminated before undertaking estrogen replacement therapy because estrogen therapy can induce growth of such tumors in certain circumstances.

Should the patient wish to conceive, clomiphene, an antiestrogen capable of blocking endogenous estrogen receptors and stimulating GnRH secretion, may be administered in increasing doses to induce ovulation and allow attempts at conception. It is important to reserve this form of therapy for women who have some evidence of endogenous GnRH secretion as witnessed clinically by estrogen effects on examination or direct measurement and who wish to conceive because the obvious attendant dangers of pregnancy must be prevented, unless specifically desired. Should clomiphene fail to induce ovulation or result in a conception, then administration of graded doses of menotropins (Pergonal) (human FSH and LH) or Menotropin (isolated human FSH) can be undertaken. However, this should be done only under circumstances in which careful monitoring of both peripheral levels of estradiol and ovarian ultrasound evaluations, as well as prior experience with menotropins, are available to the clinician.

More recently, the administration of pulsatile GnRH in a physiologic pattern using portable infusion pumps has been demonstrated to restore a normal pattern of gonadotropin secretion, induce the growth of a single follicle, and stimulate ovulation in more than 90% of patients with hypothalamic amenorrhea. The ability of pulsatile GnRH to limit attempts at ovulation induction to single folliculogenesis represents a significant achievement. Such a physiologic hypothalamic replacement schedule has several advantages over the other regimens of clomiphene and menotropins, with their inherent risks of hyperstimulation and multiple gestation, as well as the high costs inherent in such outcomes.

Finally, the literature has suggested that progestin-induced menstrual bleeding can be used either as a diagnostic test for patients with hypothalamic amenorrhea or, when administered monthly, as an alternative therapy. However, this test is neither sensitive nor specific because the response to progestin administration ultimately depends on the degree of endogenous GnRH-induced gonadotropin secretion, which, in turn, is stimulating ovarian sex steroid production. Should the patient be completely deficient in GnRH, then progestin administration invariably results in the absence of any withdrawal bleeding. Conversely, should sufficient endogenous GnRH secretion be present, then a progestin-induced menstrual period occurs. However, the same patient, at various times during the natural history of recovery or relapse from hypothalamic amenorrhea, may differ in her responses to this intervention. Thus this test is not helpful diagnostically in this clinical setting.

PITUITARY CAUSES

Pituitary defects, particularly prolactinomas, make up approximately 20% of cases of amenorrhea. Although patients with prolactin-secreting tumors may exhibit the more typical presentations of a pituitary tumor, including headache, visual field defects, and other hormonal deficiencies, such clinical presentations are increasingly rare (Chapter 295). In fact, amenorrhea is usually the earliest symptom of a prolactin-secreting microadenoma, which was classified as a cause of hypothalamic amenorrhea before the ability to determine prolactin levels in the peripheral circulation. This historical misclassification attests to the similarity of biochemical presentation of some pituitary prolactinomas and hypothalamic amenorrhea. Although the anatomic defect in prolactinomas is at the level of the pituitary gland, the cause and pathologic characteristics of the amenorrhea occurring in this clinical setting generally result from the ability of prolactin to disrupt endogenous GnRH secretion. As a consequence, the biochemical and clinical presentations of prolactinomas are often indistinguishable from those of hypothalamic amenorrhea.

The fact that the defect in prolactinoma patients is not in the pituitary is suggested by several observations. First, many prolactinomas are so small that they are undetectable by conventional radiographic techniques. Thus their mass effect cannot account for the associated disruption of the accompanying menstrual cyclicity. Second, institution of bromocryptine therapy promptly restores menstrual cyclicity in the vast majority of such patients, demonstrating the functional integrity of their residual gonadotroph population. Finally, when prolactinoma patients have been examined with intensive sampling of their gonadotropin levels, a spectrum of GnRH-induced patterns of gonadotropin release indistinguishable from that of subjects with hypothalamic amenorrhea can be observed.

Consequently, once the anatomic considerations of diagnosing a prolactinoma by nuclear magnetic resonance scanning and/or computed tomography in a patient demonstrating hyperprolactinemia have been addressed, these patients generally revert to a normal menstrual cyclicity, with reinstitution of normal prolactin levels via administration of a long-acting dopamine agonist such as bromocryptine. Because dopamine serves as the natural prolactin-inhibiting factor, patients with prolactinoma may represent an example of endogenous catecholamine defect, giving rise to reduced dopaminergic inhibition of prolactin secretion. After initial surgical removal of the tumor, a 30% to 50% recurrence rate has been noted despite apparent cure. This observation supports the notion that the basic defect is indigenous to the hypothalamus. Therefore, surgery is now generally reserved for those cases in which there is an anatomic defect secondary to the tumor size, such as headaches, visual field compression, or extraocular movement paralysis. Radiotherapy has been used rarely in this circumstance and is generally reserved for those patients in whom tumor size rather than menstrual irregularity is the major symptom.

Finally, it is important to remember that other pituitary defects such as acromegaly, Cushing's syndrome, and gonadotropin-secreting tumors, as well as postpartum pituitary infarction, also can cause amenorrhea. These are rare causes and should be treated on an individual case basis, depending on tumor size and/or biochemical function. In most of these circumstances, the appearance of amenorrhea is but one of several symptoms heralding the onset of the process and therefore of secondary concern.

OVARIAN CAUSES

Ovarian causes of amenorrhea can be divided into two broad categories: those associated with hyperandrogenic dysfunction of ovarian secretion and those associated with premature failure of ovarian secretion.

Androgen-secreting defects of the ovary can be either benign (such as polycystic ovarian disease and/or hyperthecosis) or neoplastic (such as Sertoli-Leydig cell tumors, lipoid cell tumors, and other hormonally functioning ovarian tumors that secrete androgens, estrogens, or, more typically, a combination of both).

Polycystic ovarian disease (PCOD) and/or hyperthecosis is a condition that is part of a spectrum of benign hyperandrogenic lesions of the ovary, presenting with recurrent anovulation, oligoamenorrhea, signs and symptoms of hyperandrogenemia, ovarian enlargement in most cases, and an abnormally high LH/FSH ratio in the peripheral circulation. The presumed pathophysiologic characteristics of polycystic ovarian disease represent a vicious cycle in which ovarian androgen hypersecretion is associated with an abnormally high LH/FSH ratio. This abnormal gonadotropin ratio thwarts adequate follicular growth and ovulation, results in an overstimulation of the thecal component of the ovary, and, in turn, begets further hyperandrogenemia. This cycle seems to be multifactorial, as suggested by the accompanying features of polycystic ovarian disease occurring in the setting of several other conditions. In addition, it is clear that the majority of these patients have both abnormalities of insulin secretion and resistance to its peripheral action, perhaps as a primary abnormality. The other conditions associated with PCOD include insulin resistance, attenuated congenital adrenal hyperplasia, and acanthosis nigricans. Although these patients typically have irregular menstrual periods, they often experience amenorrhea. Physical examination often reveals hirsutism, acne, and excessive oiliness of the skin—all manifestations of hyperandrogenemia. The treatment of this condition depends on the wishes of the patient but generally requires ovarian suppression to ameliorate the hyperandrogenic symptoms. When fertility is desired, ovulation induction with clomiphene and/or gonadotropins is required. Hyperthecosis is generally viewed as a variant of the polycystic ovarian syndrome in which the number of follicles is reduced and the thecal component is increased. Both of these conditions must be differentiation from tumors of the ovary, and this differentiation can usually be made by a combination of the extreme levels of hyperandrogenemia present in tumors (i.e., plasma testosterone concentrations in excess of 200 ng/dl) and unilateral ovarian enlargement by ultrasound examination.

✔ WHEN TO REFER

Following the initial history, physical examination, and screening of serum gonadotropins (LH and FSH), prolactin, estradiol, and (if indicated) androgen levels (testosterone and/or androstenedione), an initial determination can be made by the primary physician as to the anatomic level and presumed etiology of the amenorrhea. At that point, a referral may well be in order, depending upon the further work-up and therapy of the patients. For example, women with prolactinomas are best handled by endocrinologists. Those requiring ovulation induction and/or in vitro fertilization (IVF) services should be referred to specialists in those areas. Hormonal replacement of premature ovarian failure can be undertaken by internists and/or gynecologists. Polycystic ovarian disease should be referred for endocrine follow-up and management by endocrinologists, gynecologists, and cosmeticians. One critical feature that determines the pathway of subsequent management and referral should be the wishes of the patient—hormonal replacement, fertility, or cosmetic considerations each have different implications for referral.

Premature ovarian failure represents the other group of ovarian disorders that are characterized by amenorrhea and symptoms typical of menopause. Thus hot flashes, vaginal dryness, elevated FSH and LH levels, and "castrate" ranges of estradiol are the typical biochemical findings of this condition. The causes of this group of conditions include a familial syndrome of unknown origin; karyotypic abnormalities, particularly those of the X chromosome; autoimmune variations of ovarian failure; the "resistant ovary" syndrome, in which the ovary is insensitive to gonadal stimulation but retains primordial follicles; and those following exposure to environmental toxins or chemotherapy. More recently, genetic deletions on the X chromosome and mutations in the FSH receptor have been documented as causes of ovarian failure. Treatment for premature ovarian failure includes sex steroid hormone replacement to alleviate the symptoms of estrogen deficiency and to prevent diminution of bone density with time. Pregnancy is now possible with fertilized donor egg insemination into the uterus.

UTERINE CAUSES

Uterine sources of amenorrhea, particularly Asherman's syndrome, in which severe endometrial scarring obliterates the endometrial lining, are the most frequently overlooked causes of amenorrhea by internists. The clinical history of these patients is usually characterized by a prior pelvic infection, recent uterine manipulation such as dilation and curettage, and/or uterine packing after excessive hemorrhaging with abortion. Intrauterine devices can cause endometrial scarring, which, over time, can also lead to this condition. Usually there is a history of antecedent, gradual decreases in menstrual flow, often with increasing cramping and abdominal pain produced by cervical stenosis. This diagnosis is best considered by a thoughtful history and examination of the basal body temperature charts, which demonstrate a biphasic pattern typical of ovulatory periods but are not accompanied by endometrial bleeding at the end of the menstrual period. In fact, cyclic monthly pain may replace normal endometrial withdrawal bleeding, indicating a hematocolpos. Transvaginal ultrasound examinations can be relied on to make this diagnosis. The use of estrogen followed by progesterone withdrawal bleeding also results in the lack of menstrual withdrawal bleeding, providing the patient takes an adequate dose of the sex steroid hormone replacement therapy.

SUMMARY

A careful history and physical examination can usually localize the cause of amenorrhea to one of four anatomic locations. Specific blood testing can then eliminate the anatomic causes of amenorrhea, focus the differential diagnosis to a given level, and often foreshadow rational therapy of that condition.

BIBLIOGRAPHY

Fries H et al: Epidemiology of secondary amenorrhea. II. A retrospective evaluation of etiology with special regard to psychogenic factors and weight loss, *Am J Obstet Gynecol* 118:473, 1974.
Kleinberg DL et al: Galactorrhea: a study of 235 cases, including 48 with pituitary tumors, *N Engl J Med* 296:589, 1977.
Santoro N et al: Hypogonadotropic disorders in men and women: diagnosis and therapy with pulsatile GnRH, *Endocr Rev* 7:11, 1986.

CHAPTER

292 Impotence and Altered Libido

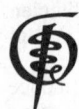

John C. Marshall

Impotence is the inability to achieve or maintain a penile erection that is adequate to allow satisfactory sexual intercourse. Penile erection is due to vascular engorgement of the corpora cavernosa. This process is incompletely understood but results from complex mechanisms involving emotional, neurologic, vascular, and hormonal components. Present data indicate that central nervous system (CNS) signals are transmitted via the thoracic sympathetic and sacral parasympathetic outflows through nerves adjacent to the prostate and rectum. Parasympathetic and nonadrenergic, noncholinergic (NANC) stimuli effect release of vasoactive polypeptide and acetyl choline and generation of nitric oxide (NO), which cause relaxation of arterial and sinusoidal smooth muscle in the corpora cavernosa. Sympathetic α_2 adrenergic activity decreases during erection, reducing penile smooth muscle tone, which allows the increased blood flow to engorge the corpora cavernosa. Abnormalities of any of these systems can result in impotence. Impotence is a common complaint in middle-aged men, and previous estimates suggested that psychogenic causes were responsible in 50% to 90% of cases. Recent evidence has indicated that this view may be incorrect, and the presence of defined pathologic abnormalities has been emphasized in several studies. Medications, psychogenic causes, and endocrine abnormalities each accounted for approximately 25% of cases in these studies, with diabetes, other neurologic diseases, urologic abnormalities, and miscellaneous causes accounting for the remaining 25% of patients. Thus psychogenic impotence is a diagnosis of exclusion, and impotence should be formally evaluated by history, clinical examination, and appropriate laboratory tests.

CLINICAL ASSESSMENT

Disorders commonly associated with impotence are shown in Table 292-1; specific endocrine causes are shown in Table 292-2.

History

The history should document the onset of impotence (acute or gradual) and establish whether impotence is complete or whether erections still occur at night or in response to a full bladder. Sexual desire or libido may be normal or reduced. A careful history of past and present medications and their relationship to the onset of symptoms should be established. Detailed questions should evaluate the presence of neurologic disease (both central and peripheral), and symptoms of vascular insufficiency such as angina or claudication should be assessed. Vascular insufficiency may be present in the absence of large vessel disease because lesions of the blood vessels in the penis may contribute significantly to a reduced ability to increase penile blood flow. In particular, the presence of polyuria and polydipsia may indicate diabetes mellitus, and a family history of non–insulin dependent (type 2) diabetes suggests the possibility of subclinical diabetes. Abdominal or pelvic surgery, particularly radical prostatectomy or rectal surgery, may be important. The patient's mental status should be evaluated, especially the presence of depression

Table 292-1 Disorders associated with impotence

DISORDER	MECHANISMS AND CLINICAL FEATURES	SERUM HORMONES
Medications/substance abuse Antihypertensives, diuretics, tranquilizers, antidepressives, phenothiazines, spironolactone, cimetidine, estrogens, chemotherapeutic agents, marijuana, opiates, alcohol	Medication history: Most antihypertensive agents can interfere with autonomic nervous function. Spironolactone and cimetidine act as peripheral androgen antagonists	LH, FSH, and testosterone concentrations usually normal LH, FSH, and testosterone concentrations suppressed by estrogens Prolactin concentration increased by phenothiazines, opiates, and some antidepressive agents
Psychogenic	Diagnosis of exclusion. Impotence with only one partner. Erections may occur at night or with a full bladder	Normal
Neurologic Depression, peripheral neuropathy, parkinsonism, syphilis, demyelinating diseases, spinal cord section, pelvic nerve section	Abnormalities of autonomic and/or somatic innervation. Detailed examination essential including peripheral and perineal sensation and anal sphincter tone. History of radical prostatectomy or pelvic surgery. Diabetic neuropathy is the most common problem and may precede marked elevation of blood glucose level	Normal
Vascular Atherosclerosis, sickle cell disease, thrombotic disorders	Impaired blood flow to the corpora cavernosa. Claudication and evidence of lower limb ischemia may be present	Normal Testosterone concentration may be low and LH and FSH concentrations elevated if severe testicular ischemia is present.
Endocrine* Hypothalamic-pituitary disorders, primary testicular disease	Usually caused by reduced testosterone secretion. Onset is gradual and associated with reduced libido. Clinical evidence of hypogonadism (pale soft skin, reduced beard growth) may be present. Testes may be slightly reduced in size and of soft consistency	Testosterone concentration low LH and FSH concentrations elevated in testicular disease and normal or low in hypothalamic-pituitary disorders Prolactin concentration may be elevated
Cirrhosis Alcoholic, hemochromatosis	Probably related to abnormal estrogen metabolism. Stigmata of liver disease (spider nevi). Gynecomastia is often present, and the testes are soft and reduced in size	Testosterone concentration low or low normal Estradiol concentration elevated or upper normal LH and FSH concentrations variable—normal or low
Uremia	Multifactorial causes, related to endocrine and other metabolic abnormalities. Anemia present and clinical evidence of renal failure	Testosterone concentration low LH and FSH concentrations normal or elevated Prolactin concentration elevated
Penile abnormalities Peyronie's disease, congenital vascular abnormalities	Impaired blood flow resulting from local causes. Erections may be painful in Peyronie's disease. Chordee or fibrous plaques may be present in the penis	Normal

*A detailed listing of endocrine disorders causing impotence is given in Table 292-2.

or emotional lability. A detailed history of the marital relationship is essential, and the attitudes of both partners to sexual relations should be established. A history relating to family stability, recent family bereavement, or evidence of alcohol or other substance abuse should be obtained.

Physical Examination

Physical examination should emphasize the neurologic, vascular, and endocrine systems. Detailed examination of the external genitalia is essential. Examination of the vascular system should include auscultation and palpation of peripheral pulses, particularly in the lower limbs, and evidence of ischemia (cold feet, skin changes, ulceration) should be sought. Neurologic examination should include gait and coordination, and assessment of peripheral motor and sensory function in the legs is particularly important. Genital and perineal sensation should be assessed and the presence of a normal cremasteric reflex and anal sphincter tone determined. Autonomic nervous system function can be assessed by means of changes in heart rate and blood pressure during a Valsalva maneuver or isometric hand grip. Endocrine evaluation should include a careful search for the presence of hypogonadism with its associated skin changes (thin, pale skin) and diminished sexual hair growth. The penis should be examined both for normal pubertal development and for presence of chordee or fibrous plaques in the corpora cavernosa. Testicular size and consistency should be documented together with the presence or absence of gynecomastia. Additionally, evidence of hypothyroidism or hyperthyroidism should be sought.

DIFFERENTIAL DIAGNOSIS

The differential diagnosis of impotence should focus on determining whether impotence is a manifestation of an underlying disease process or simply a functional disturbance. In some instances the temporal relationship of symptoms (i.e., to previous prostate surgery or to initiation of medications) points to the cause. Similarly, the occurrence of impotence only with a specific partner, or the presence of spontaneous erections at night or with a full bladder, suggests a psychologic basis. Additionally, reduced libido together with impotence suggests an endocrine disorder, depression, or a systemic disease as opposed to vascular or peripheral neuropathic causes.

In many cases, the exact cause remains uncertain after clinical examination, and hormonal measurements are required to exclude endocrine disease. The usual hormonal changes are shown in Tables 292-1 and 292-2. Laboratory assessment of gonadal function is indicated in all patients for two reasons. First, hypogonadism may coexist with other disorders such as diabetic neuropathy or vascular insufficiency. Second, the clinical manifestations of hypogonadism are subtle and develop slowly in adult men over months to years. In men who have undergone spontaneous puberty, diminished testosterone secretion may be manifest initially by reduced libido and impotence, and only months to years later will clear clinical evidence of hypogonadism be found. Postpubertally, penile size does not decrease in the absence of testosterone. Testicular size and consistency mainly reflect seminiferous tubule mass, and this only partly regresses with reduced secretion of pituitary follicle-stimulating hormone (FSH) and luteinizing hormone (LH). Thus diminished testosterone secretion may not be evident from clinical examination, and the serum testosterone level should be measured in all impotent men.

Table 292-2 Endocrine disorders causing impotence and decreased libido

DISORDER	MECHANISMS AND CLINICAL FEATURES	HORMONAL AND RADIOLOGIC ABNORMALITIES
Hypothalamic—tumor or cyst, granuloma (sarcoid, tuberculosis, histiocytosis X), trauma, idiopathic	Reduced secretion of gonadotropin-releasing hormone (GnRH) or interrupted hypothalamic-portal blood flow. Clinical evidence of TSH or ACTH deficiency may be present as a result of failure of hypothalamic-releasing factors. Diabetes insipidus is often present. Prolactin may be elevated because of reduced dopamine secretion	Testosterone level low, LH and FSH levels low Prolactin level may be elevated but not above 150 ng/ml CSF cytologic and/or culture abnormal in granulomatous disease Normal sellar radiographic, but CT scan shows hypothalamic abnormality
Pituitary Tumors—chromophobe adenoma, prolactinoma, Cushing's disease, acromegaly	Hypopituitarism is due to a mass effect in chromophobe tumors. Hyperprolactinemia inhibits GnRH secretion, which is reversible. Glucocorticoids inhibit gonadotropin secretion. Clinical evidence of hypogonadism is usually present with soft testes. Signs of Cushing's syndrome or acromegaly may be present. Variable degrees of TSH and ACTH deficiency may be present, more commonly in chromophobe tumors	Testosterone level low, LH and FSH levels low or low normal Prolactin levels >200 ng/ml indicate a prolactinoma Variable degrees of hormone deficiency on pituitary reserve testing Sellar radiographic often normal in Cushing's disease CT scan or MRI shows pituitary tumor in almost all cases
Carotid artery aneurysm	Compression of pituitary by the aneurysm with variable degrees of pituitary failure	Hormonal abnormalities similar to tumors. CT scan with contrast usually reveals diagnosis, but carotid angiography may be needed to distinguish from a chromophobe adenoma
Hemochromatosis	Deposition of iron in pituitary. Variable degrees of hypogonadism and hypopituitarism are seen clinically. May be associated with cirrhosis and diabetes mellitus	Testosterone level low, LH and FSH levels low or low normal Variable hormonal deficiencies revealed by pituitary reserve testing Radiographic and CT scan findings normal
Testicular Klinefelter's syndrome	Presence of extra X chromosome and 47, XXY karyotype. Most men have partial pubertal development and eunuchoidal habitus. Testes are small (<2 cm) and firm. Mosaicism may occur, and some men have normal secondary sex characteristics with small testes. These patients usually are infertile	Testosterone level low, LH level elevated, FSH markedly elevated Testosterone and LH levels occasionally normal and only FSH level may be elevated 47, XXY karyotype
Tumors—Leydig's cell, embryonal cell, teratoma, choriocarcinoma	Leydig's cell tumors secrete estradiol, which suppresses LH, FSH, and testosterone secretion. Embryonal cell tumors and teratomas may secrete hCG, which stimulates estradiol secretion. A testicular nodule is usually palpable, and gynecomastia is commonly present	Leydig's cell—testosterone level low, LH and FSH levels low, and estradiol level elevated Teratomas—testosterone levels often normal, estradiol level elevated, LH and FSH levels low or low normal; hCG may cross-react in LH assays
Hemochromatosis	Iron deposition in the testes. Variable degrees of hypogonadism are seen, and the testes are usually small and soft	Testosterone level low. LH and FSH levels are variable because iron may also be deposited in the pituitary, producing gonadotropin deficiency
Orchitis—mumps, venereal disease, tuberculosis	Usually results in infertility caused by seminiferous tubule damage, but rarely Leydig's cell failure and hypogonadism also occur. Testes are small and soft and often asymmetrically affected	Testosterone level low, FSH level markedly elevated, LH level elevated
Radiation therapy or chemotherapy—alkylating agents	The germinal epithelium is damaged, but Leydig's cell involvement may occur. Seminiferous tubule damage may be reversible over months to years. Testes are usually small and soft	Testosterone level may be low, FSH level markedly elevated, LH level may be elevated
Idiopathic	Testicular degeneration affecting both the seminiferous tubules and Leydig's cells. The patient is clinically hypogonad, and the testes are small and soft	Testosterone level low, LH and FSH levels elevated
Thyroid disease Hypothyroidism, hyperthyroidism	Mechanisms are uncertain. In hypothyroidism LH, FSH, and testosterone secretion may be reduced. Hyperthyroidism increases sex hormone–binding globulin levels, and increased amounts of testosterone are protein bound. Peripheral conversion of androgens to estrogens may also be increased. Gynecomastia may be present in hyperthyroidism	Hypothyroidism—testosterone level low or low normal. LH and FSH levels low or normal; prolactin level elevated in severe hypothyroidism Hyperthyroidism—testosterone level normal or elevated, estradiol level normal or elevated, LH and FSH levels normal or elevated
Other disorders—chronic disease, usually associated with weight loss (malignancy, infections, gastrointestinal granulomatous disorders)	Chronic weight loss is associated with reduced GnRH secretion, which is reversible if weight regain occurs	Testosterone level low, LH and FSH levels low

Clinical evidence can provide important clues to the diagnosis. The presence of gynecomastia (in the absence of medication use) suggests estrogen excess or testosterone lack. Testosterone-deficient men are more sensitive to the effects of estradiol, and gynecomastia may occur in the presence of a normal serum estradiol level. Estrogen excess can occur as a result of testicular tumors (Leydig's cell tumors; secretion of estradiol, choriocarcinoma or teratomas secreting human chorionic gonadotropin [hCG]), and rarely adrenal tumors. Testosterone insufficiency may be secondary to hypothalamic-pituitary disease or may result from primary testicular disorders (Table 292-2). In hypothalamic-pituitary disease, LH and FSH secretion is reduced, resulting in a low serum testosterone concentration. In primary testicular disease, a low serum testosterone level is accompanied by elevated levels of LH and FSH caused by the absence of testosterone-negative feedback. Evidence of hypothyroidism or adrenal insufficiency together with hypogonadism suggests a pituitary tumor as the underlying cause. Galactorrhea, rarely present in men, suggests the presence of a prolactinoma. Signs of Cushing's syndrome or acromegaly may indicate a pituitary tumor.

Small, soft testes may reflect prolonged reduction of gonadotropin secretion or primary testicular disease. The testes may be soft and small after mumps orchitis, but very small testes (less than 2 cm in length) of firm consistency suggest Klinefelter's syndrome. In this disorder, most men are clinically hypogonadal with low levels of testosterone, but 20% have a normal or low-normal testosterone level and infertility. Polyuria and polydipsia may be manifestations of diabetes insipidus resulting from hypothalamic disorders. More commonly, however, polyuria, especially when associated with weight loss, suggests diabetes mellitus. Diabetes mellitus is the most common endocrine disorder causing impotence, and in approximately 50% of diabetic men impotence develops. The underlying abnormality is usually a diabetic autonomic neuropathy, and this may be indicated by a history of nocturnal diarrhea, bladder dysfunction, postural hypotension, or abnormal pulse rate changes after a Valsalva maneuver. Less often, diabetic impotence is due to vascular insufficiency, which may be clinically evident as lower limb ischemia.

Thyroid disease, both hypothyroidism and hyperthyroidism, may be associated with impotence, although the mechanisms are not fully understood. In hyperthyroid men, serum estradiol and testosterone concentrations may both be increased as a result of elevated levels of sex hormone–binding globulin (TeBG). TeBG has a higher affinity for testosterone than estradiol, and more testosterone is bound to protein, which can reduce the concentration of biologically active "free" testosterone. In addition, peripheral conversion of androgens to estrogens is increased by thyroid hormone, which may result in increased serum estradiol concentration. In hypothyroidism, gonadotropin secretion may be impaired, and in severe hypothyroidism hyperprolactinemia may contribute to reduced gonadotropin and testosterone secretions. Hyperprolactinemia also occurs in chronic renal failure. Serum estradiol level may be elevated in cirrhosis of the liver caused by impaired metabolism of estrogen, and estradiol may inhibit gonadotropin secretion, resulting in soft testes and low testosterone secretion rates. Cirrhosis may be a manifestation of hemochromatosis, and iron deposition may also be present in the pituitary and in the gonad, leading to hypogonadism of pituitary and/or testicular origin. Impotence together with hypogonadism may be present in many chronic diseases, particularly those associated with marked weight loss such as malignancy or Crohn's disease. Severe weight loss results in reduced hypothalamic secretion of gonadotropin-releasing hormone (GnRH) and consequent reduced gonadotropin secretion from the pituitary.

LABORATORY INVESTIGATION

Laboratory screening should include a complete blood count, assessment of hepatic and renal function, and measurement of a fasting serum glucose level. A borderline fasting glucose level or family history of non–insulin dependent diabetes (type 2) may occasionally need to be pursued by a glucose tolerance test. If thyroid disease is suspected, TSH, thyroxine, and T$_3$-resin uptake should be measured, particularly in the elderly because clinical signs of hyperthyroidism may be absent. In view of the subtle clinical presentation of hypogonadism, serum testosterone level should always be measured and used

---

BOX 292-1
Laboratory investigation of impotent men

1. Complete blood count; BUN, creatinine clearance; bilirubin, SGOT, SGPT, alkaline phosphatase; fasting glucose level (postprandial glucose or GTT if borderline). Serum TSH, thyroxine, and T$_3$-resin uptake if clinically indicated
2. Serum testosterone
   If normal: no endocrine diseases (pursue other causes—see Table 292-1)
   If low or low normal*: Measure LH and FSH levels

If LH and FSH levels are low or low normal	*If LH and FSH levels are elevated*
Hypothalamic-pituitary disease, chronic illness, or weight loss	Primary testicular failure Pursue etiology (Table 292-2)
Serum prolactin Thyroxine, T$_3$-resin uptake CT or MRI scan of pituitary Pituitary reserve function tests (insulin hypoglycemia and releasing hormones)	Chromosome karyotype if hypogonad or small, firm testes

*Serum testosterone level may be low in marked obesity as a result of decreased levels of sex hormone–binding globulin. LH, FSH, and prolactin levels are normal. BUN, blood urea nitrogen; SGOT, serum glutamicoxaloacetic transaminase; SGPT, serum glutamic-pyruvic transaminase; GTT, glucose tolerance test; CT, computed tomography; MRI, magnetic resonance imaging.

---

as the basis on which to pursue further endocrine evaluation. The need for subsequent testing depends on the serum testosterone level and is summarized in Box 292-1. Additional laboratory tests may be indicated by the clinical findings. The presence of gynecomastia indicates that serum estradiol level should be measured. Similarly, if a testicular tumor is suspected, measurement of β-hCG and α-fetoprotein levels may reveal the presence of a teratoma. A normal serum testosterone value usually precludes the need for further endocrine evaluation, and other causes of impotence should be sought (Table 292-1). If serum testosterone level is normal and a psychogenic cause of impotence is suspected, measurement of nocturnal penile tumescence using a strain gauge may be indicated. The presence of nocturnal erections indicates normal function and helps to support the diagnosis of psychogenic impotence. If suspected, vascular insufficiency can be established by measurement of penile blood pressure by Doppler ultrasound. A penile/brachial blood pressure index of 0.6 or less suggests impairment of arterial blood flow.

MANAGEMENT

Wherever possible, management of impotence should be directed toward the underlying cause. If medications are suspected, the feasibility of stopping the drug or changing to an alternative form of therapy should be considered. This is particularly important in patients receiving treatment for hypertension. With the exception of prolactinomas, resection of pituitary tumors is not usually associated with a return of gonadotropin secretion, and replacement therapy with androgens is required. Treatment of prolactinomas, however, particularly medical therapy with bromocriptine, often results in a return of normal gonadal function, although this process is slow and occurs over several months. Removal of estrogen-secreting Leydig's cell tumors is usually followed by recovery of reproductive function. Primary testicular failure should be treated by replacement of testosterone, using transdermal patches or intramuscular injections of a long-acting testosterone ester (testosterone enanthate or cypionate). A dose of 200 mg at 2- to 3-week intervals maintains serum testosterone level in the normal range. In patients with psychogenic impotence, marital or psychologic counseling of both partners may be helpful. When impotence is due to neuropathy, libido is often normal, and failure to achieve an erection may be a cause of considerable marital disharmony. In this situation, a penile prosthesis may be considered as a means of alleviating symptoms. Alternatives to a penile prosthesis include intracavernosal self-injection of papaverine or a combination of prostaglandin E_1 and phentolamine. This results in a penile erection that persists for 30 to 40 minutes and allows intercourse. Complications include priapism and fibrosis of the corpora cavernosa, and the long-term safety and efficacy of this treatment remain to be established.

BIBLIOGRAPHY

Diagnostic and therapeutic technology assessment: vasoactive intracavernous pharmacotherapy for impotence: papaverine and phentolamine, *JAMA* 264:752, 1990 (editorial).
Kelly TM et al: Hypogonadism in hemochromatosis: reversal with iron depletion, *Ann Intern Med* 101:629, 1984.
Korenman SG: Advances in the understanding and management of erectile dysfunction, *J Clin Endocrinol Metab* 80:1985, 1995.
Korenman SG et al: Secondary hypogonadism in older men: its relation to impotence, *J Clin Endocrinol Metab* 71:763, 1990.
Kursh ED et al: Injection therapy for impotence, *Urol Clin North Am* 15:625, 1988.
Nickel JC et al: Endocrine dysfunction in impotence: incidence, significance and cost-effective screening, *J Urol* 132:40, 1984.
Rajfer J et al: Nitric oxide as a mediator of relaxation of the corpora cavernosa in response to non-adrenergic, non-cholinergic neurotransmission, *N Engl J Med* 326:90, 1992.
Slag MF et al: Impotence in medical clinic outpatients, *JAMA* 249:1736, 1983.
Sparks RF, White RA, Conolly PB: Impotence is not always psychogenic—new insights into hypothalamic pituitary gonadal dysfunction, *JAMA* 243:750, 1980.
Steers WD: Neural control of penile erection, *Semin Urol* 8:66, 1990.
Whitehead ED et al: Diagnostic evaluation of impotence, *Postgrad Med* 88:123, 1990.
Whitehead ED et al: Treatment alternatives for impotence, *Postgrad Med* 88:139, 1990.

293 Gynecomastia

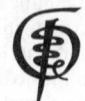

John C. Marshall

Gynecomastia is an increase of breast tissue in males. True gynecomastia consists of proliferation of both ductal and stromal tissue and results from conditions that cause imbalance of levels of serum androgens and estrogens—either estrogen excess or testosterone deficiency. Estrogen excess occurs infrequently as a result of estrogen-secreting tumors. More commonly a relative excess of estrogens is present when serum testosterone concentration is reduced. In adult men, approximately 10% of serum estradiol level is from secretion by the testis; 40% is from peripheral conversion of testosterone to estradiol (aromatization), which occurs predominantly in fat cells, liver, and muscle; and 50% is derived from peripheral conversion of estrone to estradiol. Estrone itself is primarily derived from peripheral aromatization of adrenal androstenedione. The testes are the source of virtually all testosterone in plasma. Thus disorders that reduce testicular hormone secretion remove the major source of plasma testosterone but have much less effect on circulating estradiol, producing a situation of relative estrogen excess.

CLINICAL ASSESSMENT

Conditions commonly associated with gynecomastia and the mechanisms involved are shown in Table 293-1. In patients with gynecomastia, the etiology is idiopathic in 25%, persistent since puberty (25%), due to medications in 15%, associated with cirrhosis or malnutrition (10%), or testicular failure (10%). The remaining 15% of cases are due to uncommon causes (1% to 4% each) including testicular tumors, hyperthyroidism, gonadotropin deficiency, or renal failure.

History and Physical Examination

In addition to documenting the onset and duration of gynecomastia, a careful history of pubertal maturation and a detailed medication history should be obtained. A family history of hypogonadism or infertility may be helpful, and the presence of infertility or anosmia in

family members may point to a diagnosis of isolated gonadotropin deficiency. Gynecomastia is usually bilateral, but because marked asymmetry is often present, it may appear unilateral. True gynecomastia consists of concentric hypertrophy of breast tissue and is usually palpable as a discrete plaque of tissue beneath the areola. Commonly the plaque is 3 to 5 cm in diameter, but in severe cases it may be similar to a normal female breast. Gynecomastia should be distinguished from lipomastia, a diffuse increase in adipose tissue. Palpation of the breast over tensed pectoralis major muscles (by apposition of the hands) allows delineation of gynecomastia and differentiation from lipomastia. A hard nodule fixed to underlying tissues or to skin suggests male breast cancer (rare) and should be biopsied. Evidence of cirrhosis, renal failure, or marked weight loss, and presence or absence of a goiter should be sought on physical examination. Secondary sexual characteristics, including those of skin (thin, soft, and pale with reduced sebum secretion in testosterone deficiency), sexual hair and beard growth, and genital development, should be assessed. Examination of the genitalia is most important. The penis and testicles should be measured and the presence of developmental abnormalities noted. Hypospadias or partial scrotal fusion together with other evidence of incomplete masculinization suggests a partial form of an androgen-resistance syndrome. Testicular nodules or a marked inequality in testis size may indicate the presence of a testicular tumor.

DIFFERENTIAL DIAGNOSIS

Gynecomastia is present in the majority (up to 75%) of boys during pubertal maturation and is usually transient, lasting from 6 to 18 months. Breast enlargement may be associated with breast tenderness and reflects the initial transient stage of gonadotropin stimulation of an immature testis when estrogen secretion exceeds that of testosterone. Rarely, gynecomastia fails to regress during the later stages of normal puberty, but persistence of gynecomastia should initiate a search for other pathologic factors. Medications may be important, and the use of marijuana may be associated with persistence of gynecomastia. Gynecomastia occurs with increased frequency in elderly men, and its cause is probably multifactorial. Many elderly patients take medications for other disorders. Additionally, serum testosterone level tends to fall, and sex hormone–binding globulin level rises after the sixth decade, which may reduce biologically available testosterone and produce a relative estrogen excess.

Gynecomastia may be present in hypogonadism as a result of hypothalamic-pituitary or gonadal disorders, but it is more common in gonadal disorders. Klinefelter's syndrome is important in this regard, and 50% of men have gynecomastia in addition to small, firm testes. Abnormalities of the genitalia, partial masculinization, and development of gynecomastia at adolescence suggest an androgen-resistance syndrome. These men have a normal 46, XY karyotype, and genital abnormalities vary from small testes and hypospadias (Reifenstein's syndrome) to failure of scrotal fusion and abnormal descent of the testes (partial forms of testicular feminization). Serum hormone level measurements in these patients vary but usually include elevated levels of gonadotropins and estradiol. A similar clinical presentation may result from abnormalities of testosterone metabolism (deficiency of the 5-α-reductase enzyme that converts testosterone to dihydrotestosterone).

The presence of a testicular nodule indicates a possible testicular tumor, which may secrete estradiol (Leydig's cell tumor) or human chorionic gonadotropin (hCG) (teratoma, choriocarcinoma). The diagnosis of a Leydig's cell tumor is suggested by an elevated serum estradiol concentration and low levels of luteinizing hormone (LH), follicle-stimulating hormone (FSH), and testosterone. hCG-secreting tumors may be associated with normal or elevated levels of estradiol and testosterone, but measurement of the β-subunit of hCG in serum confirms the diagnosis. Rarely, the source of hCG is an extratesticular tumor of the lungs, stomach, pancreas, or liver.

Gynecomastia occurred in many newly released prisoners of war after World War II when food was made available. Starvation or severe weight loss from any cause results in reduced hypothalamic gonadotropin-releasing hormone (GnRH) secretion and consequent low serum levels of gonadotropins and testosterone. Weight gain is associated with a return of GnRH secretion, and the pattern of increased gonadotropin and sex steroid levels is similar to that seen dur-

Table 293-1   Causes of gynecomastia

CAUSE	MECHANISMS AND CLINICAL FEATURES
Physiologic	
Puberty	Gonadotropin stimulation of the prepubertal testis initially produces estradiol secretion. Later, testosterone secretion is dominant and gynecomastia is consequently transient
Senescence	Uncertain mechanisms but probably related to decreased serum testosterone and increased sex hormone–binding globulin (TeBG), resulting in a reduction in biologically available testosterone. Peripheral aromatization is also increased
Pathologic	
Hypogonadism Primary testicular disease or secondary to hypothalamic-pituitary disorders	Reduced testosterone secretion. Estrogens from the adrenal and from peripheral conversion of androstenedione produce a relative estrogen excess. Gynecomastia is usually present in Klinefelter's syndrome and less commonly in hypothalamic-pituitary disease
Androgen-resistance syndromes Testicular feminization, complete and partial forms; Reifenstein's syndrome	Abnormalities of the cytosolic androgen receptor, which is absent in testicular feminization and is reduced in number or has abnormal function in partial syndromes. Testosterone action is absent or reduced. Elevated LH and FSH levels stimulate testosterone and estradiol secretion, but only estradiol has peripheral effects. Gynecomastia is usually present. The phenotype may be female in testicular feminization, and varying degrees of abnormal scrotal fusion or hypospadias are present in partial forms
Tumors Testicular—Leydig's cell	Estradiol secreted by Leydig's cell tumors
Teratoma or choriocarcinoma	hCG secretion may be present
Adrenal	Some adrenal carcinomas secrete estradiol, which also suppresses LH and FSH secretion
Other—adenocarcinomas of lung and stomach, hepatoblastomas	Secretion of gonadotropins or hCG by tumors
Starvation and refeeding	Weight loss caused by starvation, malabsorption, or chronic illness is associated with gonadotropin-releasing hormone (GnRH) deficiency. With recovery, GnRH secretion increases, hormonal changes resemble those seen in normal puberty, and transient gynecomastia may occur
Hyperthyroidism	Mechanisms uncertain. Thyroid hormones increase TeBG synthesis, and testosterone binding is increased. Peripheral conversion of androgens to estrogen is increased and leads to a relative estrogen excess
Cirrhosis	Reduced estradiol metabolism. Increased serum estrogen concentrations suppress LH and FSH levels and also increase TeBG levels. Testosterone binding is increased, and a state of relative estrogen excess results
Renal failure	Mechanisms are uncertain, but serum testosterone level is reduced and levels of gonadotropins are usually elevated. Prolactin level is elevated but the significance is uncertain
Carcinoma of the male breast	Rare tumor. Gynecomastia is unilateral and may be very tender
Medications	
Spironolactone, cimetidine, cyproterone, flutamide, ketoconazole	Compete for androgen receptors. Spironolactone and ketoconazole decrease testosterone secretion and displace estrogens from TeBG
Marijuana, digitalis	Weak intrinsic estrogen effects. Marijuana may also compete for androgen receptors
Chemotherapy (alkylating agents)	Predominant effect is on germinal epithelium, but Leydig's cells may be involved
Estrogens, testosterone, hCG	Testosterone treatment of hypogonadism is initially associated with transient gynecomastia produced by peripheral conversion to estradiol. hCG stimulates estradiol secretion in addition to testosterone secretion
Methyldopa, reserpine tricyclic antidepressants	Unknown mechanisms. Serum prolactin level may be elevated, but significance is uncertain

ing normal puberty. Thus gynecomastia results from the same mechanisms that occur during pubertal maturation.

Abnormalities of sex hormone–binding globulin (TeBG) concentrations may play a role in the gynecomastia associated with alcoholic cirrhosis and hyperthyroidism. In cirrhosis, impaired estrogen metabolism leads to upper normal or elevated serum estradiol levels, which inhibit gonadotropin secretion and increase TeBG production. Testosterone binding is increased, and as gonadotropin secretion is inhibited, levels of unbound biologically active testosterone fall. Similarly, excess thyroid hormone directly stimulates TeBG synthesis, which may explain the gynecomastia seen in some thyrotoxic men.

Medications that may cause gynecomastia are shown in Table 293-1 together with their presumed mechanism of action. Gynecomastia is commonly associated with use of drugs that increase serum estradiol levels (directly or indirectly) and drugs that interfere with testosterone synthesis or binding to its intracellular receptor. Many medications have been associated with gynecomastia, but in most instances the exact mechanisms are unknown.

LABORATORY INVESTIGATION AND MANAGEMENT

In pubertal adolescents with normal genitalia, the presence of gynecomastia is assumed to be normal unless it is very severe or does not regress spontaneously. In some cases, however, severe gynecomastia may occur in the absence of demonstrable hormonal abnormalities and may require excision to spare the adolescent undue emotional

trauma. In adult men, the appearance of gynecomastia should always be investigated unless it is clearly related to the use of a medication such as spironolactone. Initial investigation should include a complete blood count and assessment of hepatic and renal function. If thyroid disease is suspected, TSH, serum thyroxine, and T_3-resin uptake measurements should be obtained, especially in elderly men because clinical manifestations of thyrotoxicosis may be absent. Hormonal measurements should include serum estradiol, testosterone, LH, FSH, and β-hCG levels. A low testosterone level with elevated LH and FSH values points to primary gonadal disease. A chromosome karyotype may be indicated, particularly if the testes are small and firm or if clinical evidence of abnormal penile and scrotal development is present. Low testosterone, LH, and FSH values indicate hypothalamic-pituitary disease. In these patients, serum prolactin level should be measured and a computed tomography (CT) scan performed. Elevated serum estradiol levels may indicate a testicular tumor, and the level of the β-subunit of hCG should be measured. In the absence of a testicular nodule and β-hCG, an increased serum estradiol value may indicate an adrenal feminizing tumor. Urinary 17-ketosteroid or serum dehydroepiandrosterone sulfate level may be elevated, but a CT or magnetic resonance imaging (MRI) scan of the adrenals should be performed to exclude an adrenal tumor (Box 293-1).

Management should be directed at the cause whenever possible. Medication-related gynecomastia usually regresses after the drug is stopped. Gynecomastia associated with the use of hCG or testosterone for treatment of hypogonadism is transient and should simply be

BOX 293-1
Investigation of gynecomastia

1. Complete blood cell count, hepatic and renal function
   TSH if clinically indicated
2. Plasma T, E₂, β-hCG*

   If T is low:
   LH, FSH
   High value
   Testicular failure
   Low value
   Hypothalamic/pituitary disease, chronic illness, or weight loss
   Prolactin, CT, or MRI of pituitary, pituitary function tests

   If T is elevated:
   LH
   High value suggests hyperthyroidism or androgen insensitivity

   If E₂ or β-hCG is elevated:
   Testicular ultrasound
   If negative, chest and abdominal CT scan, adrenal CT or MRI

   If all normal:
   Idiopathic gynecomastia

*T, testosterone; E₂, estradiol; β-hCG, β-subunit of human chorionic gonadotropin.

observed. If tenderness is severe or the patient excessively embarrassed, tamoxifen 10 mg bid given for 1 to 3 months is often effective. In most cases, removal of a testicular or adrenal tumor will result in regression of gynecomastia, but if gynecomastia is severe, complete regression may not occur. In such cases, or when the exact cause is not known, the breast tissue should be excised if the degree of gynecomastia is sufficient to cause the patient embarrassment.

BIBLIOGRAPHY

Bardin CW, Wright W: Androgen receptor deficiency: testicular feminization, its variants and differential diagnosis, *Ann Clin Res* 12:236, 1980.

Berkovitz GD et al: Familial gynecomastia with increased extraglandular aromatization of plasma C¹⁹ steroids, *J Clin Invest* 75:1763, 1985.

Braunstein GD: Gynecomastia, *N Engl J Med* 328:490, 1993.

Carlson HE: Gynecomastia, *N Engl J Med* 303:795, 1980.

Casey RW, Wilson JD: Antiestrogenic action of dihydrotestosterone in mouse breast; competition with estradiol for binding to the estrogen receptor, *J Clin Invest* 74:2272, 1984.

Kim I, Young RH, Scully RE: Leydig cell tumors of the testis: a clinicopathological analysis of 40 cases and review of the literature, *Am J Surg Pathol* 9:177, 1985.

McDermott MT, Hofeldt FD, Kidd GS: Tamoxifen therapy for painful idiopathic gynecomastia, *South Med J* 83:1283, 1990.

McDonald PC et al: Origin of estrogen in normal men and in women with testicular feminization, *J Clin Endocrinol Metab* 49:905, 1979.

Moore DC et al: Hormonal changes during puberty. V. Transient pubertal gynecomastia and abnormal androgen/estrogen ratios, *J Clin Endocrinol Metab* 58:492, 1984.

Parker LN et al: Treatment of gynecomastia with tamoxifen: a double-blind cross-over study, *Metabolism* 35:705, 1986.

Webster DJT: Benign disorders of the male breast, *World J Surg* 13:726, 1989.

Wilson JD, Aiman J, McDonald PC: The pathogenesis of gynecomastia, *Adv Intern Med* 25:1, 1980.

294 Disorders of Adolescent Growth and Development

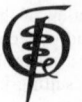

H. Verdain Barnes

Adolescence is characterized by dramatic physical, psychologic, and social growth and development. For the physician to provide optimal comprehensive medical care, each feature must be considered in evaluating, diagnosing, and treating the adolescent. This chapter discusses the normal physical growth and development characteristics of puberty, their assessment, and selected abnormalities of height, weight, and secondary sexual development.

PUBERTY

For clinical purposes, *puberty* can be defined as the interval from the earliest prepubertal changes in adrenal steroid secretion to the attainment of adult height, weight, and secondary sexual characteristics. Puberty is the concluding segment of normal physical growth. This continuum of growth begins in utero with sexual differentiation and the ontogeny of the adrenals, hypothalamus-pituitary, and gonads. The result is a physically mature adult with the capacity to reproduce. Consequently human puberty is best viewed as a part of this continuum of maturation rather than an isolated event. The *primum movens* that initiates puberty remains unknown, although much is known about the process.

Hormone Changes

The endocrine system provides the first measurable evidence that puberty has begun. The primary endocrine systems involved include the adrenals, hypothalamic-pituitary unit, and gonads. The first identifiable changes occur in the adrenal: adrenarche. Histologically the medullary capsule begins to disappear, and the zona reticularis develops. Accompanying these changes is a substantial increase in the microsomal enzymes 17, 20-desmolase and 17-α-hydroxylase, and sulfokinase activity appears. The result is a substantial increase in circulating dehydroepiandrosterone (DHEA) and its sulfate (DHEAS), along with modest increases in δ-4-androstanedione and androsterone. In both sexes DHEA and DHEAS concentrations begin to rise between the ages of 7 and 9 years. Both hormones are produced almost entirely (>90%) by the adrenal gland and rise progressively during puberty to adult concentrations. The initiator of normal adrenarche is unknown.

The next identifiable event occurs within 1 to 2 years when both sexes appear to have a progressive decrease in the sensitivity of the hypothalamic-pituitary unit to the negative feedback by the prepubertal levels of the gonadal steroids. The result is an increase in the production and episodic release of gonadotropin-releasing hormone (GnRH) by the hypothalamus. Initially major pulsatile releases of GnRH occur only during non–rapid eye movement (REM) sleep. The resulting sleep-related increases in gonadotropin secretion are accompanied by a rise in circulating gonadal steroid levels.

Additional evidence of decreasing sensitivity of the hypothalamic-pituitary unit includes an increased luteinizing hormone (LH) response to a single intravenous bolus of GnRH. During the prepubertal period the LH response is small compared to the response seen at the onset of puberty. With the onset of puberty, there also appears to be a change in gonad sensitivity to stimulation by human chorionic gonadotropin (HCG). This change may in part be explained by an increased number of gonadotropin receptor sites on the gonad, a change that may be induced by follicle-stimulating hormone (FSH).

During puberty there is a progressive increase in DHEA, DHEAS, GnRH, LH, FSH, testosterone, dihydrotestosterone, and estradiol concentrations in both sexes. The progression generally correlates with the Tanner stages of secondary sexual development.

Table 294-1   Actions of selected hormones during puberty

HORMONE	SEX	ACTIONS
Gonadotropin-releasing hormone (GnRH)	M/F	Stimulates pituitary secretion of LH and FSH
	F	Stimulates midmenstrual cycle LH surge
Growth hormone–releasing hormone (GHRH)	M/F	Stimulates pituitary secretion of GH
Growth hormone (GH)	M/F	Stimulates bone and lean body mass growth
Insulin-like growth factor I (IGF-I)	M/F	Is necessary for growth hormone action
Luteinizing hormone (LH)	M	Stimulates Leydig's cell production and secretion of testosterone
	F	Stimulates theca cells to production and secretion of estrogens; induces ovulation by midcycle surge; initiates and maintains the corpus luteum and may stimulate the release of progesterone
Follicle-stimulating hormone (FSH)	M	Stimulates late stages of gametogenesis, maintains normal spermatogenesis, and may influence seminiferous tubule growth
	F	Stimulates cyclic growth and development of primary ovarian follicle, stimulates theca cell transformation
Testosterone	M	Stimulates phallus, scrotum, prostate, and seminal vesicle growth; accelerates linear growth; hastens epiphyseal fusion; increases pubic axillary and facial hair growth, skin oiliness, libido, red cell mass, muscle mass, and larynx size
	F	Accelerates linear growth; increases pubic and axillary hair
Estrogen	M	Hastens epiphyseal fusion; stimulates breast development
	F	Stimulates labia, uterus, vagina, and ductal breast development; increases areolar pigmentation; markedly hastens epiphyseal fusion; increases fat mass and distribution; triggers midcycle LH surge
Adrenal androgens (DHEA, DHEAS)	M/F	Initiates pubic hair and linear growth
Progesterone	F	Converts proliferative to secretory endometrium; stimulates lobuloalveolar breast growth

M, male; F, female.

As female puberty progresses, a positive hypothalamic-pituitary-gonad feedback system develops. Near the time of menarche, the hypothalamus and pituitary begin to respond to estrogen feedback with a pulsatile release of GnRH followed by LH when the critical level of circulating estradiol is reached. This monthly occurrence produces the LH peak that heralds ovulation. When this positive feedback mechanism is fully developed, regular ovulatory menstrual cycles occur (typically 2 to 5 years postmenarche).

Growth hormone (GH) plays a significant role in pubertal growth. The regulation of growth hormone (GH) production and secretion is complex. The central nervous system, hypothalamus, and pituitary are all involved. Growth hormone–releasing hormone (GHRH) and somatotropin release–inhibiting hormone (SRIH) are secreted by the hypothalamus. The secretion of GHRH and SRIH appears to be modulated by adrenergic, dopaminergic, cholinergic, nutrition, and emotional factors. GHRH appears to be the major controller of GH secretion from the pituitary and somatostatin the controller of the frequency and duration of GH pulses from the pituitary. Once secreted by the pituitary, GH binds to the target cell's surface via a specific GH receptor. Many of the dominant effects of GH on pubertal growth appear to be mediated by a group of insulin-like growth factors, particularly IGF-I. These proteins circulate bound to an insulin-like growth factor binding protein (IGFBP), primarily IGFBP-3, which appears to transport and regulate some of IGF-I's actions. GH and IGF-I peak during the normal pubertal growth spurt. The higher levels of 24-hour integrated concentrations of GH seen in adolescents compared to prepubertal children and young adults are due to increased GH pulse amplitudes. During puberty there is an IGF-I peak that coincides with the maximum pubertal increase in lean body mass, height, and weight. This temporary rise in the IGF-I level usually begins at about 10 years of age in the average female and 12 to 24 months later in the average male. These changes in GH and IGF-I levels appear to be sex steroid–dependent. The peak levels of GH and IGF-I typically occur during Tanner stage 2 to 4, being earlier in the female adolescent and later in the male. In addition to appropriate gonadal steroid levels, adequate nutrition, especially protein, is required for normal pubertal growth.

There is no convincing evidence that the concentrations of thyroxine, triiodothyronine, cortisol, glucagon, or parathyroid hormone change significantly during normal puberty. Prolactin levels do not change in the male and change only after menarche in the female. On the other hand, some and perhaps all of these hormones may have a permissive or facilitating role in normal pubertal growth and development. For example, it is known that low or elevated levels of thyroid hormone and cortisol, low insulin and parathyroid hormone lev-

els, and elevated prolactin levels can significantly alter linear growth and/or secondary sexual development.

The level of inhibin, produced by Sertoli (testes) and granulosa (ovary) cells, also rises progressively during puberty and may play an important role in the negative feedback control of FSH secretion. The level of anti-mullerian hormone, also produced by the Sertoli and granulosa cells, decreases during puberty, but no precise role in the normal physiology of puberty has been elucidated. The primary hypothalamic, pituitary, adrenal, and gonadal hormones of puberty, along with their primary actions in pubertal growth and development, are shown in Table 294-1.

GROWTH DURING PUBERTY

All body components except the thymus, tonsils, and adenoids normally increase in size during puberty. The most obvious changes occur in height, weight, and the sex organs.

Normal Linear Growth

The height increase that follows adrenarche usually accounts for 20% to 25% of the final adult height in both sexes. The majority of the growth occurs during a 36-month span within which the pubertal growth spurt, the peak height velocity (PHV) year, occurs. PHV in the female precedes the male by 12 to 24 months. Although there is substantial normal variability in linear growth velocity in this age group, there is minimal variability for a given individual. Consequently the norm is for the adolescent to remain near his or her own established percentile of linear growth velocity until he or she reaches adult height.

Normal Weight Growth

The adolescent's gain in weight after the onset of adrenarche accounts for about 50% of his or her adult weight. More than half of this weight gain occurs during a 36-month period within which the peak weight velocity year (PWV) occurs. In general, the PWV year coincides with the PHV year, but tends to follow PHV in the female. In the female, menarche usually occurs within the 6 to 12 months following PWV. Each individual normally remains near his or her established percentile for weight gain from about 6 years of age until the onset of puberty.

The major contributors to adolescent weight increase are muscle, fat, and bone masses. The increase in lean body mass (for practical purposes, muscle mass) begins near the onset of adrenarche and peaks at the time of PHV and PWV. The total gain in lean body mass is quantitatively and qualitatively greater in males than in females with comparable stages of secondary sexual development. On the other hand, nonlean body mass (for practical purposes, fat) increases considerably in females and minimally in males during puberty. The percentage of body weight as fat in the male decreases to about 9% by the completion of the adolescent "growth spurt," whereas in the female it typically increases to about 20%.

Bone mass increases in parallel to muscle mass. Importantly, skeletal maturation or bone age can be assessed radiographically by evaluating the relative shape, position, and degree of epiphyseal fusion of the hand, wrist, and knee. Bone age has been pictorially defined in the standard Greulich and Pyle atlas. In general, the hand and wrist epiphyses are completely fused by the age of 17 years in the female and 19 years in the male. Once fusion has occurred, there is little chance for a significant increase in height.

Normal Secondary Sexual Development

The development of adult secondary sexual characteristics is a major milestone for the body-conscious adolescent. During puberty the normal male experiences about a seven-fold increase in the size of the testes, epididymis, and prostate, as well as about a two-fold increase in phallus size. The normal female has a five- to seven-fold increase in the size of the uterus and ovaries, as well as a substantial increase in the size of the vagina, fallopian tubes, labia, clitoris, and breasts. In both sexes, pubic hair and areola size progressively increase during puberty, axillary hair develops, and, in the male, the voice lowers and beard growth appears.

SELECTED DISORDERS OF PUBERTAL GROWTH AND DEVELOPMENT

The most common concerns and problems of adolescent growth and development seen by the physician are constitutional delay of pubertal growth and/or development, idiopathic (familial) short stature, exogenous obesity, and gynecomastia. Less frequent but notable are familial tall stature, the chronic diseases associated with a delay in growth and/or development, and the gonadal dysgenesis syndromes. Of the chronic diseases, the most common are Crohn's disease and hypothyroidism, which in this age group may have an occult presentation.

Constitutional Delay of Pubertal Growth and/or Development

Constitutional growth or developmental delay is estimated to occur in up to 5% of adolescents. Because a delay for the male tends to carry more cultural stigmata, males tend to seek help earlier and more frequently. Constitutional delay of pubertal growth and/or development, often referred to as *constitutional delay of puberty* (CDP), is the most common cause (90% to 95%) of growth and development concerns in adolescents. Consequently, physicians need to be knowledgeable about its diagnosis and management.

CDP patients usually seek medical attention between ages 14 and 16 years (mean = 14.9 years). The cause of this normal variation in growth and development is unknown. CDP patients ultimately achieve full adult secondary sexual characteristics, ability to reproduce, and height compatible with their genetic background. The diagnosis of this growth variant remains provisional until adult maturation is achieved, a process that may extend into the patient's middle 20s. Typically, however, the delay is about 3 years compared to peers of the same sex. In all published studies the number of females is small.

The typical male patient has an uneventful medical history including an uncomplicated birth and a normal birth length. When the adolescent seeks medical attention his height is usually at or below the 5th percentile (15% to 25% above the 5th percentile). His average linear growth velocity is typically between 4.0 and 5.5 cm/yr. Over half of these patients have a family history of delayed puberty. When present, this can often be used to reassure the adolescent and his or her parents. Finally, these patients typically exhibit some degree of impaired self-image and/or body image that may be severe enough to produce an arrest of his psychosocial development.

BOX 294-1

Guidelines for a provisional diagnosis of constitutional delay of pubertal growth and development

---

Required features
1. Detailed negative review of the endocrine, neurologic, cardiorespiratory, gastrointestinal, renal, and musculoskeletal systems
2. Evidence of appropriate nutrition and eating habits
3. Linear growth rate of at least 4.0 cm/yr (average about 5 cm/yr)
4. Normal physical examination including the genital anatomy, smell, and body proportions
5. Normal hemoglobin, erythrocyte sedimentation rate, renal profile, urinalysis, thyroid profile including TSH (third generation); negative stool for blood, and a noncastrate level of urinary or serum LH (IRMA) and FSH
6. 1.5 to 4.0 year delay in bone age compared to chronologic age

Supportive features
1. Family history of constitutional delay of growth and development
2. Height near 5th percentile for chronologic age
3. Normal sella turcica by CT or MRI if neurologic history and/or manifestations are present

---

TSH, thyroid stimulating hormone; LH, luteinizing hormone; FSH, follicle-stimulating hormone.

The physical examination findings are normal for a prepubertal male. In most studies the mean presenting height is about 145.0 cm and weight around 39.7 kg. This results in a derived height age of about 11.3 years and weight age of 12.0 years. The mean bone age is about 12.0 years, or a delay of about 2.7 years compared to chronologic age.

The subsequent growth and development pattern in these patients is variable. The most common is a relatively normal rate of progression to maturity once puberty begins. Next in frequency is a slow rate of progression with maturity attained in the early 20s. The remaining few patients have a very slow progression and reach maturity in the middle 20s.

In the differential diagnosis, idiopathic (familial) short stature and five other entities merit special consideration.

A confident provisional clinical diagnosis of CDP can be made by using the guidelines detailed in Box 294-1. A variety of laboratory tests and procedures have been reported to distinguish hypogonadotropic hypogonadism from constitutional delay of puberty. Unfortunately no simple, reproducible single test has proven to be sensitive or specific enough provide a clean separation of these diagnoses. Presently the gonadotropin-releasing hormone agonist (Nafarelin) test appears to have the most promise. For the moment the confirmation of the onset of puberty by the presence of testes with a length of greater than 2.5 cm or volume greater than 3 ml by orchidometer, serum testosterone level above 50 mg/dl, increase in LH (IRMA) to intravenous GNRH stimulation by more than 7.6 IU/L, or pubertal pattern of nocturnal LH (IRMA) pulsatility are the best correlates available for a diagnosis of CDP.

Crohn's Disease

In about 30% of Crohn's disease patients there is a delay in secondary sexual development and/or growth (Chapter 341). In up to 20% of adolescents with Crohn's disease, abdominal and bowel complaints may be subtle with no history of diarrhea. In most, one or more of the following laboratory abnormalities is present: elevated erythrocyte sedimentation rate in 84%, decreased serum albumin level in 64%, or iron deficiency anemia in 50%.

Hypothyroidism

In the adolescent, thyroid hormone deficiency may be occult and is often insidious in onset. A delay in secondary sexual development may be less pronounced than the retardation of linear growth. Of the author's last 59 hypothyroid adolescents, less than 50% had such common manifestations as lethargy, excess weight gain, dry or coarse skin, constipation, cold intolerance, bradycardia, weakness, or facial edema, and one quarter did not have an obvious goiter. The most common cause is chronic lymphocytic thyroiditis (Hashimoto's) (Chapter 297). The laboratory test of choice is a third-generation TSH.

Turner's Syndrome

Gonadal dysgenesis is the most common cause of hypergonadotrophic hypogonadism in phenotypic females. The classic 45, XO chromatin pattern is found in roughly half of these patients and a mosaic pattern (XX/XO) in the remainder (Chapter 284). The mosaic patient may have few and occasionally no somatic stigmata other than short stature (i.e., well below the 1st percentile for chronologic age) to suggest Turner's syndrome.

In males with very short stature for chronologic age and delayed secondary sexual development, Noonan's syndrome, although rare, is a consideration. This syndrome can occur in both sexes.

Klinefelter's Syndrome

Klinefelter's syndrome is the most common form of male primary hypogonadism. Adolescent males with normal or tall stature who have an abnormal delay in the onset or progression of secondary sexual development should be evaluated for this diagnosis, particularly if the testes are relatively small and firm, fat distribution is eunuchoid, and/or gynecomastia is present (Chapter 301).

The second most common cause of eunuchoidism is a classic or variant form of Kallmann's syndrome. This type of hypogonadotrophic hypogonadism is usually a X-linked recessive or autosomal dominant disorder. The syndrome typically manifests as delayed puberty. In the classic form, the patient has eunuchoid features with anosmia or hyposmia (Chapter 301).

Idiopathic (Familial) Short Stature

Second in frequency to CDP among adolescents with growth concerns is idiopathic (familial) short stature. Shortness is often a major concern to an adolescent and his or her parents regardless of whether the adolescent is lagging behind peers in secondary sexual development. These adolescents usually have a benign medical history and normal physical examination including body habitus and proportions. Secondary sexual development is typically not abnormally delayed. They typically have a bone age that is commensurate with chronologic age and a height age (height age = the age found when the patient's actual height is placed on the 50th percentile of a longitudinal growth chart) that is less than the bone age. The family history of short stature is often impressive.

Growth Hormone Deficiency

The classic form of pituitary GH deficiency is usually diagnosed in childhood. The congenital causes include a deletion of the GH gene, idiopathic GHRH deficiency, or developmental anomalies such as pituitary aplasia/hypoplasia or midline brain abnormality. These patients have low basal levels of GH, an abnormal response to standard GH provocative tests (exercise, levodopa, arginine, and/or insulin), a low basal level of IGF-I, a decreased 24-hour integrated GH concentration, and a low nocturnal GH peak. In gene deletion or developmental anomalies, there appears to be an abnormal response to GHRH, whereas in idiopathic GHRH deficiency there is a near-normal response to the intravenous administration of GHRH. The former patients respond to GH therapy and the latter to GH or GHRH therapy. These congenital causes occur in only a small number of patients with GH-related short stature. Patients with documented GH deficiency usually respond to GH therapy, but the adult heights achieved have clearly been less than expected. Only recombinant DNA–derived GH should be prescribed.

A larger, less clearly defined, and more controversial group of patients appear to have GHRH, GH, IGF-I, IGF binding protein-3 (IGFBP-3), and/or GH-receptor gene problems. These patients may present during puberty with short stature for their chronologic age.

They may or may not have accompanying pubertal delay. A spectrum of laboratory features may be seen in these patients: (1) a normal response to provocative GH stimulation tests, low basal IGF-I levels for chronologic age, low 24-hour integrated GH concentration, and low nocturnal GH peak (i.e., GH neurosecretory dysfunction), (2) a normal basal IGF-I level and an apparent target cell resistance to IGF-I, (3) an excessive level of somatostatin, which inhibits GH release, (4) a normal GH test with low IGF-I levels with an apparently abnormal GH molecule or increased GH degradation, (5) a mutation of the cell surface receptor for GH, or (6) a deficiency of IGFBP-3. Growth hormone neurosecretory dysfunction (GHND) is the most common. Patients with the first two types of laboratory characteristics may respond in varying degrees to GH therapy, but there are no convincing studies that this response results in an increase in predicted adult height. The routine use of GH therapy in these patients is not recommended.

Familial Tall Stature

Normal adolescents who are above the 95th percentile for height for their chronologic age may seek medical attention. Most often the patient is a tall female with a tall mother and/or father. These adolescents have a normal health history and physical examination including body habitus. The predicted adult height can be estimated on the basis of midparental height (see later discussion) and/or bone age. If the predicted adult height is more than 5 cm above the midparental height, or the parents and family are not tall, constitutional early normal maturation, acromegaly, giantism (cerebral or lipodystrophic), hyperthyroidism, Marfan's syndrome, tumor of the ovary (granulosa cell) or testicle (interstitial cell), and homocystinuria enter the differential diagnosis. In males, an XYY chromosome abnormality and Klinefelter's syndrome should also be considered. For those with constitutional early normal maturation, the adult height is usually within 5 cm of the midparental height. There is no proven therapy for individuals with familial tall stature.

Weight Abnormalities

The desire to control body weight and its distribution is a fanatic concern of many adolescents in the United States. The most common weight problems (eating disorders) encountered by physicians are obesity and anorexia nervosa.

Among overweight adolescents, exogenous obesity is the primary type (approximately 95%). An accentuation of long-standing obesity or the onset of excessive weight gain during puberty is relatively common. The former is typically familial. The families of these patients often have several obese first-order relatives including one or both parents. The problem begins in childhood. Fat distribution tends to follow that of obese family members. Hyperplasia of the adipose tissue is a common finding. A rare adolescent patient has an associated type II diabetes mellitus or hyperlipidemia.

Those in whom the onset of obesity occurs during puberty also tend to have a family history of obesity. Their dietary history typically demonstrates an excess calorie intake that is often accentuated by stress, depression, and/or boredom.

In both groups caloric intake typically exceeds the expenditure of calories. No definite metabolic or endocrine dysfunction has yet been proven to be the cause of these conditions. The other causes of obesity in adolescents are rare; however, the possibility of an identifiable hypothalamic, adrenal, thyroid, pancreatic, or gonadal cause should not be overlooked. When one of these rare causes is present, there is usually ample evidence in the history and physical examination to suggest the diagnosis.

Anorexia nervosa should be considered in females (female/male ratio >19:1) who are underweight and have delayed or normal secondary sexual development associated with primary amenorrhea, particularly if they are rapidly losing weight. Most are white, middle- to upper-class, intelligent teenagers. Virtually all have a fear of being fat and a distinctly distorted perception of their body. Without these latter two characteristics, some other diagnosis is more likely. Most also have a history of physical hyperactivity, usually including a preoccupation with exercise, a strong appetite, constipation, cold intolerance, depression, and/or anxiety. They are typically obsessive-compulsive and perfectionistic. Frequent and at times dramatic mood swings are common. On physical examination bradycardia, systolic hypotension, hypothermia, dry carotenemic skin, and lanugo hair are common findings (Chapter 334).

Adolescent Breast Growth Abnormalities

The most common breast abnormality brought to the physician's attention is gynecomastia. In a third to a half of adolescent males, 1 to 3 cm of breast tissue below the areola, *benign adolescent gynecomastia,* develops. It is typically bilateral and nontender but may be unilateral and/or sporadically tender. The age of onset is usually between 12.5 and 14 years of age during Tanner gonad stage 3 and before the PHV year. This gynecomastia tends to develop over 1 to 6 months. In the majority, resolution occurs spontaneously over the ensuing 6 to 18 months. When it persists for longer than 2 years, spontaneous regression is rare. Gynecomastia should be suspected in the adolescent male who refuses to be seen at home or at school without his upper body covered, or refuses to attend or shower in physical education classes, or voices a concern about his masculinity (Chapter 293).

In the adolescent female a variety of breast growth problems may occur. In descending order of frequency they are: breast asymmetry, polythelia, areolar overgrowth, inverted nipple, massive breast(s), breast hypoplasia, virginal hypertrophy, and amastia. The most common concern called to the attention of the physician is breast asymmetry. This is a normal finding in breast development but is usually minimal by breast stage 5. About 5%, however, continue to have a noticeable difference. Polythelia is a normal variant seen in about 2% of adolescent females. Areolar overgrowth usually occurs in early puberty but typically resolves or becomes substantially less prominent as the breasts develop. The failure of the nipple to extend beyond the surface of the areola may be a concern to the adolescent female but is a normal variant that rarely has medical significance.

The development of massive breasts that produce physical discomfort because of their weight is rare, as is virginal hypertrophy. The former condition is usually symmetric and develops progressively over the duration of pubertal breast growth, whereas the latter is typically rapid in onset and progression and is more likely to be unilateral. The presence of large, heavy, pendulous breasts in this age group may result in a negative self-image and body image resulting in a withdrawal from social and sports activities.

EVALUATING PUBERTAL GROWTH AND DEVELOPMENT

Virtually all adolescents have a degree of concern about whether their personal growth and secondary sexual development are normal. Their questions in these areas are often indirectly stated or not verbalized at all. Consequently the physician should be aware that such concerns are normal and common. Any adolescent's growth and development concern should be seriously and carefully considered by the physician, regardless of whether the concern is medically justified.

A complete medical history is crucial, including an assessment of the adolescent's diet and exercise. Inadequate nutrition, especially protein, can adversely affect growth. Unusual or bizarre eating habits may signal the presence of an eating disorder such as anorexia nervosa, bulimia, or obesity. Excess, little, or no exercise may also adversely affect weight growth.

The adolescent's psychosocial function at home, with peers, and in school should be carefully assessed. A real or perceived abnormality in growth and/or development may arrest or impede function in one or more of these areas. For example, an underdeveloped adolescent may refuse to attend or shower after physical education class. A detailed review of systems for subtle as well as overt endocrine, neurologic, cardiac, respiratory, gastrointestinal, renal, or musculoskeletal signs and symptoms is essential to assess for clues of an occult chronic disease that may affect growth and/or development (hypothyroidism, Crohn's disease, etc.).

A complete physical examination is mandatory, including an accurate assessment of height, weight, and secondary sexual development. Such an examination cannot be adequately performed when clothing covers the area to be examined. If there is a possibility of

inflammatory bowel disease, a rectal examination and stool sample for occult blood are required. A pelvic examination in the adolescent female is necessary if delayed secondary sexual development and/or primary amenorrhea is being evaluated. Finally, adolescents are almost invariably apprehensive about the examination. Consequently the outcome of the examination may be optimized by a brief explanation of the specific components of the examination before beginning. This is preferably done with the patient still clothed.

Assessing Height and Weight

Because height is genetically determined, the adolescent's height and linear growth velocity should be considered in the context of the mother's and father's and family heights. An accurate measurement of height without shoes using a stable measuring scale with a right-angle device to extend from the crown of the head to the scale is important for both initial evaluation and follow-up of growing adolescents. This is particularly critical in those suspected of having a growth problem.

Weight, its distribution, and body composition appear to be polygenetically determined, although they can be significantly modified by the environment. From current data it is not possible to confidently predict an "ideal" body weight for age. Likewise, it is not possible to state a precise weight at which medically significant undernutrition or unhealthy overnutrition begins.

The adolescent's current height and weight and all known previous values should be plotted by chronologic age on a longitudinal growth chart (Tanner and Whitehouse, or 1976 National Center for Health Statistics) and/or a growth velocity chart (Tanner and Whitehouse). These graphs provide a simple and useful method of (1) following the patient's rate of growth, (2) establishing the individual patient's own growth percentile, and (3) determining his or her height age and weight age. The latter are easily derived from a longitudinal growth chart by drawing a line from the patient's current height or weight to the 50th percentile and a perpendicular line to the age axis. Since the 5th and 95th percentiles represent two standard deviations from the mean for a given chronologic age, they can be used as clinically acceptable limits for normal variability. For an adolescent in a tall (adult male heights greater than 188 cm or female >174 cm) or short (adult male height <166 cm, for female <149 cm) family, his or her established linear growth velocity can be used as the basis for assessing growth during the pre-PHV years. Distinct deviations from a patient's own growth percentile merit evaluation. If the patient's weight percentile is well below his or her linear growth percentile, a careful search for an underlying chronic process such as Crohn's disease or anorexia nervosa is warranted.

Although no absolute criteria for recognizing abnormal linear growth and weight gain can be applied to all adolescents, the following guidelines have proved clinically useful. The guidelines for abnormal height are (1) a linear growth rate that is less than 4.5 cm or more than 9.0 cm in the years before the PHV year, (2) an acceleration of linear growth velocity that is equivalent to the individual's velocity for his or her PHV year before age 11.5 years in males and 9.5 years in females, (3) no PHV year by age 16 years, or (4) a distinct plateau or deceleration from the individual's established linear growth velocity. The latter is best assessed by using a linear growth velocity chart because longitudinal growth curves are based on cross-sectional height for chronologic age rather than individual longitudinal data. The guidelines for abnormal weight are (1) a distinct acceleration (>7 kg/yr) before the PWV year or deceleration (<1 kg/yr) in weight gain, or (2) an unexplained weight loss of more than 2 kg during the peripubertal or pubertal years.

Those adolescents identified as potentially abnormal by these guidelines should, at a minimum, have a careful and complete history and physical examination to search for those disorders known to affect pubertal growth and development adversely (Table 294-2).

Assessing Secondary Sexual Development

The changes in the adolescent male's gonads, phallus, and scrotum and in the female's breast (areola and papilla) along with pubic hair growth in both sexes provide an important index of secondary sexual development. A descriptive staging system developed by Tanner and colleagues is the current standard for assessment. A clinically useful

Table 294-2 Selected disorders associated with growth and/or development problems in the adolescent

CAUSES	PUBERTAL DELAY ALONE	PUBERTAL DELAY AND SHORT STATURE	SHORT STATURE ALONE
Normal variants*			
Constitutional delay of puberty	X	X	—
Idiopathic short stature	—	X	X
Growth hormone deficiency disorders			
Classic isolated pituitary GH	—	X	X
Idiopathic GHRH/GH	—	—	X
Neurosecretory dysfunction	—	X	X
Panhypopituitarism	—	X	—
Gonadotropin deficiency disorders			
Idiopathic isolated LH and/or FSH	X	X	—
Idiopathic GnRH	X	X	—
Acquired LH and/or FSH	X	X	—
Acquired GnRH	X	X	—
Gonad deficiency disorders			
Idiopathic gonadal steroid	X	X	—
Acquired gonadal steroid	X	X	—
Congenital syndromes			
Klinefelter's	X	—	—
Kallmann's	X	—	—
Turner's	—	X	X†
Noonan's	—	X	X
Pure or mixed gonadal dysgenesis	—	X	—
Chronic diseases‡			
Diabetes mellitus	X	X	X
Crohn's disease	X	X	X
Ulcerative colitis	X	X	X
Renal tubular acidosis	—	X	X
Hypothyroidism	X	X	X
Hyperthyroidism	X	—	—
Anorexia nervosa	X	X	X
Malnutrition	—	X	X
Sickle cell disease	X	X	X

X, reported; —, not reported, GH, growth hormone; GHRH, growth hormone-releasing hormone; LH, luteinizing hormone; FSH, follicle-stimulating hormone; GnRH, gonadotropin-releasing hormone.
*Most common.
†Mosaic.
‡Variable incidence of linear growth retardation and/or pubertal delay.

Table 294-3 Staging guidelines for secondary sexual development

MALE			
GENITAL STAGE	SIZE OF TESTES	SCROTUM	PHALLUS (LENGTH)
G1	<2 cm	Prepubertal	Prepubertal (4-8 cm)
G2	2-6 cm	Becomes reddened and thinner	Minimal or no enlargement (4-10 cm)
G3	6-12 cm	Greater thinning and enlargement	Increased length (6-14 cm)
G4	12-18 cm	Color darkens and further enlargement	Increased length, circumference, and gland size (8-15 cm)
G5	>18 cm	Adult	Adult (10-18 cm)

FEMALE		
BREAST STAGE	BREAST	AREOLA AND PAPILLA (NIPPLE DIAMETER)
B1	Prepubertal	Prepubertal (1.3-4.5 mm)
B2	Budding-elevation above chest wall by mound of subareolar breast tissue	Areola widens Papilla erect
B3	Larger and more elevation	Further widening of areola (1.5-6.7 mm)
B4*	Larger and more elevation	Areola and papilla form a mound projecting from the breast contour (4.50-10.9 mm)
B5	Adult (size variable)	No mound; areola and breast in same plane (7.1-12.7 mm)

MALE AND FEMALE			
PUBIC HAIR STAGE	AREA	AMOUNT	TYPE
PH1	Male	0	
	Female	0	
PH2	Male—base of phallus and/or scrotum	+	Long (straight or curly), slightly pigmented, and downy
	Female—labia majora and/or mons veneris	+	
PH3	Male—spread to mons veneris	++	Increased curl, coarseness, and pigmentation
	Female—increased area of mons veneris		
PH4	Male—greater areas of mons veneris	+++	Greater curl and coarseness
	Female—almost entire mons veneris	+++	
PH5	Male and Female—entire mons veneris and medial aspect of the thighs	++++	Adult

Modified from Barnes HV. In Moss AJ, editor: *Pediatrics update,* New York, 1979, Elsevier.
*Does not occur in all individuals.

modification of their system is shown in Table 294-3. Such staging affords the physician objective parameters by which to assess the onset, status, and progression of an adolescent's sexual maturation.

Because the correlation between gonad or breast and pubic hair is variable, each should be assessed independently. The use of a Prader orchidometer improves accuracy and reproducibility when quantitating testicular volume. There are no standards for female breast size; therefore, size per se is not evaluated in staging.

The age of onset for secondary sexual development and the duration of the intervals between stages vary considerably within as well as between the sexes. Although there are no absolute criteria for recognizing abnormal secondary sexual development that apply to all adolescents, clinically useful guidelines can be stated by using the mean plus or minus two standard deviations or the 5th and 95th percentiles. Guidelines for the age of onset and rate of progression are shown in Table 294-4. Those adolescents who vary beyond these limits should be carefully evaluated (Table 294-2) for hypothalamic, pituitary, or gonadal disorders, as well as the chronic diseases known to affect pubertal growth and development.

For adolescents with short or tall stature and/or a delay in secondary sexual development, a hand or wrist radiograph for bone age should be obtained. For those being evaluated for CDP, a bone age delayed by more than 4.5 years suggests a more serious diagnosis, such as an underlying chronic disease, or, if delayed less than 1.5 years, familial short stature. The Greulich and Pyle bone age tables for height and chronologic age can also be used to make a reasonable prediction of

the anticipated adult height. Patients with short stature and/or pubertal delay may require a focused computed tomography (CT) of the head to assess the size and structure of the sella turcica and pituitary.

In these patients a hemoglobin, erythrocyte sedimentation rate, renal profile, urinalysis, third generation measurement of thyroid-stimulating hormone (TSH), and blood or urine LH (IRMA) and FSH evaluation are recommended. If the patient's erythrocyte sedimentation rate is elevated and he or she has anemia, hypoalbuminemia, or

Table 294-4 Mean age of onset and interval between pubertal events

EVENT	MEAN AGE OF ONSET*	STAGE AND INTERVAL BETWEEN STAGES (YR)†
Males		
G2	11.9 ± 2.2	
PH2	12.3 ± 1.6	G2-3 0.4-2.2
G3	13.2 ± 1.6	PH2-3 0.1-1.0
PHV	13.8 ± 2.2	G3-4 0.2-1.6
PWV	13.9 ± 1.8	PH3-4 0.3-0.5
PH3	13.9 ± 1.8	G4-5 0.4-1.9
AH	14.0 ± 2.2	PH4-5 0.2-1.5
VC	14.1 ± 1.8	
G4	14.3 ± 1.6	G2-5 1.9-4.7
PH4	14.7 ± 1.8	
FH	14.9 ± 2.2	
G5	15.1 ± 2.2	
PH5	15.3 ± 1.6	
Females		
B2	11.2 ± 3.2	
PH2	11.9 ± 3.0	B2-3 0.2-1.0
PHV	12.5 ± 3.0	PH2-3 0.2-1.3
PWV	12.4 ± 2.8	B3-4 0.1-2.2
B3	12.4 ± 2.4	PH3-4 0.2-0.9
PH3	12.7 ± 1.0	B4-5 0.1-6.8
AH	13.1 ± 1.6	PH4-5 0.6-2.4
B4	13.1 ± 1.4	
Menarche	13.3 ± 2.6	B2-5 1.5-9.0
PH4	13.4 ± 2.4	
B5	14.5 ± 3.2	
PH5	14.6 ± 2.2	

*Data derived from Lee PA: *J Adolesc Health Care* 1:26, 1980; mean $\pm$ 2 standard deviations.
†Data from Marshall WA et al: *J Arch Dis Child* 44:291, 1969; 45:13, 1970; and Tanner JM et al: *Arch Dis Child* 51:170, 1976, 5th to 95th percentiles.
G, Genital stage; *PH,* pubic hair stage; *AH,* axillary hair; *VC,* voice change; *FH,* facial hair; *B,* breast stage; *SD,* standard deviation.

a stool positive for blood, a thorough evaluation for Crohn's disease is in order. If only anemia and/or hypoalbuminemia is present, anorexia nervosa should also be considered.

When familial short stature is considered the likely diagnosis, a helpful adjunct in the initial assessment is a calculation of the adolescent's expected adult height based on midparent height. The determination of midparent height using Tanner and colleagues' method for calculation can provide a realistic final adult height range for the adolescent. The value is calculated for males by plotting the father's and mother's height on the right coordinate of a standard growth chart, adding 13 cm to the mother's height to correct for the difference in the mean heights of adult men and women, then calculating the mean of the father's and mother's (corrected) heights. This midparent height is then used as the midpoint for the target adult height for the adolescent. A clinically useful approximation of the 3rd and 97th percentiles is obtained by subtracting or adding 10 cm, respectively, to the midparent height. The midparent height for females is similarly derived, but here 13 cm is subtracted from the father's height with no adjustment to the mother's height. The respective percentiles for females are approximated by subtracting or adding 9 cm to the midparent height. These values are useful in adolescent and parent counseling. If the extrapolated height of the adolescent is more than 5 cm below the midparent height, a comprehensive evaluation for possible endocrine dysfunction or occult chronic disease is warranted.

THERAPY

Therapeutic intervention may be aggressively sought by a distraught adolescent and/or his or her parents. Consequently the physician should be prepared to provide a measured discussion of the diagnosis, as well as effective patient and parent counseling.

The vast majority (80% to 90%) of patients who have CDP require only supportive counseling. Stress should be placed on the fact that the patient is normal but slow in developing to his or her full adult maturation and reproductive capability. Follow-up observation is needed about every 6 months. Some males, however, experience a

✔ WHEN TO REFER

When the diagnosis is questionable or the adolescent requests further evaluation, the patient's GH status may merit evaluation. Since the testing for GH abnormalities requires rigorous conditions for testing and interpretation, it is typically beyond the expertise of the primary care generalist. Therapy with GH also requires careful monitoring and experience. Consultation and follow-up by an endocrinologist, who is expert in growth disorders, should be the standard.

When Turner's or Klinefelter's syndrome is suspected, a chromosome analysis with banding should be performed. If confirmed, the Turner's syndrome patient should have hormone therapy designed and initiated by a physician with expertise in managing both the psychosocial and the hormone components of therapy. If anorexia nervosa is suspected, the patient should have psychiatric evaluation and care. Patients with Klinefelter's syndrome should have an endocrinology consultation and be treated with an oral or intramuscular testosterone preparation (Chapter 301).

Adolescents with a chronic disease that retards linear growth may or may not have a delay in the onset of sexual development. Controlling the disease process as quickly and completely as possible is important to ensure maximum linear growth. Once secondary sexual development is complete, catch-up growth cannot occur. If the disease requires the use of a growth-retarding medication such as glucocorticoids, it is critical to use the smallest possible dose to control the disease so that appropriate linear growth can occur. In general, alternate-day doses of 30 mg of prednisone or its equivalent among the intermediate-acting steroids allow greater linear growth than a 5 to 10 mg daily dose. For example, most Crohn's disease patients with growth retardation grow about 2.0 to 3.0 cm per year. If secondary sexual development and epiphyseal closure occur at the expected time, such a patient may lose close to 21.0 cm (8.4 inches) in height. When the disease is controlled with 15 mg of prednisone a day, growth is similar, whereas twice that dose every other day allows 70% to 80% of normal linear growth. Chronic disease patients with growth and development retardation should be managed jointly with a physician knowledgeable about adolescent growth and development.

profound arrest in psychosocial maturation or are so psychologically distraught that pharmacologic intervention is an appropriate consideration. In such cases, the patient and parents should be made aware of the pros and cons of hormone therapy. The adolescent, in conjunction with the parents, should make the decision to have or not to have hormone therapy. If such therapy is warranted and chosen, 200 mg of testosterone enanthate in oil administered intramuscularly once a month for a maximum of 4 to 6 months will typically produce a progression of pubic hair and phallus development by a mean of 1.6 stages and 3.4 cm, respectively, plus an acceleration of linear growth by a mean of 9.8 cm. For most, these changes have a dramatic positive effect on body perception and psychosocial maturation. This regimen, according to several studies, does not compromise final adult height. Similar results can be achieved with oral testosterone or oxandrolone administration, but intentional overdosing by an elated adolescent is often problematic. Currently no accepted hormone therapy can be recommended for females with constitutional delay of growth and development.

Patients with secondary hypothyroidism should be treated with L-thyroxine in doses sufficient to maintain the third-generation TSH level in the normal range. For most adolescents, this dose ranges from 0.125 to 0.175 mg daily.

Benign pubertal gynecomastia often resolves spontaneously and requires no therapy. When there is major psychologic dysfunction regardless of the amount of breast tissue present or when the amount of breast growth is considerable, surgical therapy is indicated. Simple mastectomy is immediately successful and continues to be the only effective method of therapy if the amount of breast tissue is large or the gynecomastia has persisted 2 years or longer. About 70% of adolescents with small to moderate gynecomastia, when treated within 6 to 12 months of onset, appear to respond to 200 to 300 mg of danazol a day for 4 to 6 months.

BIBLIOGRAPHY

Barnes HV: Recognizing normal and abnormal growth and development during puberty. In Moss AJ, editor: *Pediatrics update*, New York, 1979, Elsevier.

Bercu BB et al: Growth hormone neurosecretory dysfunction, *Clin Endocrinol Metab* 15:537, 1986.

Cara JF: Growth hormone in adolescence: normal and abnormal, *Endocrinol Metab Clin North Am* 22:533-552, 1993.

Genentech Collaborative Study Group: Idiopathic short stature: results of a one-year controlled study of human growth hormone treatment, *J Pediatr* 115:713, 1989.

Ghai K et al: Gonadotropin releasing hormone agonist (Nafarelin) test to differentiate gonadotropin deficiency from constitutionally delayed puberty in teen-age boys: a clinical research center study, *J Clin Endocrinol Metab* 80:2980-2986, 1995.

Goddard AD et al: Mutations of the growth hormone receptor in children with idiopathic short stature, *N Engl J Med* 333:1093-1098, 1995.

Goldstein S et al: The physiology of puberty. In Moss AJ, editor: *Pediatrics update*, New York, 1984, Elsevier.

Hamill PV et al: Physical growth: National Center for Health Statistics percentiles, *Am J Clin Nutr* 32:602, 1979.

Kletter GB et al: Disorders of puberty in boys, *Endocrinol Metab Clin North Am* 22:455-477, 1993.

Lee PA: Normal ages of pubertal events among American males and females, *J Adolesc Health Care* 1:26, 1980.

Rosenfeld RG et al: A prospective, randomized study of testosterone treatment of constitutional delay in growth and development in male adolescents, *Pediatrics* 69:681, 1982.

Rosenfeld RL: Diagnosis and management of delayed puberty, *J Clin Endocrinol Metab* 70:559, 1990.

Schuh R et al: Breast disorders of adolescence. In Kreutner AK, Reycroft-Hollingsworth D, editors: *Adolescent obstetrics and gynecology*, Chicago, 1978, Year Book.

Smith CP et al: Relationship between insulin, insulin-like growth factor I, and dehydroepiandrosterone sulfate concentrations during childhood, puberty and adult life, *J Endocrinol Metab* 68:932, 1989.

Spagnoli A et al: Characterization of a low molecular mass form of insulin-like growth factor binding protein-3 (17.7 kilodaltons) in urine and serum from healthy children and growth hormone (GH)-deficient patients: relationship with GH therapy, *J Clin Endocrinol Metab* 80:3668-3676, 1995.

Tanner JM et al: Clinical longitudinal standards for height and velocity for North American children, *J Pediatr* 107:317, 1985.

Wu FCW et al: Patterns of pulsatile luteinizing hormone secretion before and during the onset of puberty in boys: a study using an immunoradiometric assay, *J Clin Endocrinol Metab* 70:629, 1990.

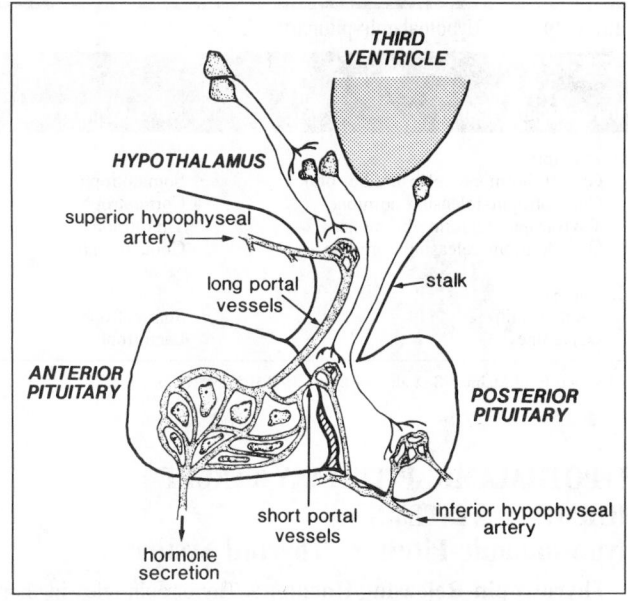

FIGURE 295-1 Hypothalamic-pituitary axis. Diagram showing sites of hypothalamic nuclei that synthesize releasing and inhibiting hormones and hypothalamic closed portal system impinging on specific target cells types in the anterior pituitary gland. The anterior pituitary hormones, GH, PRL, ACTH, TSH, FSH, and LH, are secreted into the systemic circulation through the pituitary veins and inferior petrosal sinuses into the internal jugular vein. The posterior pituitary (neurohypophysis) derives hypothalamic signaling by direct neural extension of the nuclei synthesizing antidiuretic hormone and oxytocin. *GH*, Growth hormone; *PRL*, prolactin; *ACTH*, adrenocorticotropic hormone; *TSH*, thyroid-stimulating hormone; *FSH*, follicle-stimulating hormone; *LH*, luteinizing hormone.

IV DISORDERS OF THE ENDOCRINE GLANDS

SPECIFIC ENDOCRINE, METABOLIC, AND GENETIC DISORDERS

CHAPTER

295 Disorders of the Hypothalamus and Anterior Pituitary

Shlomo Melmed and Glenn D. Braunstein

ANATOMY AND PHYSIOLOGY OF HYPOTHALAMIC-PITUITARY AXIS
Anatomy of the Pituitary Gland

The pituitary gland, weighing between 500 and 1000 mg, lies in the sella turcica within the sphenoid bone. The roof of the sphenoid sinus forms the floor of the sella, allowing direct surgical approach to the anterior pituitary gland via the transsphenoidal route. The cavernous sinus, containing the carotid arteries and third, fourth, and sixth cranial nerves, bounds the pituitary gland laterally; the optic chiasm lies over the superior aspect of the pituitary fossa. The diaphragma sella, the dural roof of the pituitary, separates the pituitary gland from the optic chiasm and cerebrospinal fluid. The soft tissue structures surrounding the pituitary gland may be compressed by superior or lateral extension of sellar or parasellar space-occupying lesions, resulting in cranial nerve palsies or visual field defects. The bone surrounding the pituitary gland may also be eroded by an expanding pituitary mass, resulting in the thinning and erosion of bony structures such as the clinoids.

The hypothalamus, extending from the margin of the optic chiasm to the mammillary bodies posteriorly, contains cell bodies that synthesize the specific hypothalamic-releasing and -inhibiting hormones, as well as the neurohypophyseal hormones.

Blood is supplied to the anterior pituitary primarily through the hypothalamus from the internal carotid arteries and superior hypophyseal arteries. The hypothalamic-pituitary-portal circulation consists of a rich venous connection between the hypothalamus and the pituitary, constituting the major blood supply of the anterior lobe. A secondary and less important blood supply to the anterior lobe is derived directly from the superior hypophyseal artery, whereas the inferior hypophyseal artery directly supplies the posterior pituitary gland. The primary blood supply to the pituitary therefore facilitates the transport of hypothalamic peptides to the anterior pituitary lobe (Fig. 295-1).

The hypothalamus synthesizes and secretes releasing or inhibiting hormones into the hypophyseal-portal blood supply. These hormones impinge directly on the anterior pituitary gland and regulate synthesis and secretion of the pituitary trophic hormones from specific cells that exhibit distinctive immunohistochemical and specific morphologic characteristics (Table 295-1). Somatotroph cells secrete growth hormone (GH); prolactin (PRL) is secreted by lactotrophs; corticotrophs secrete adrenocorticotropic hormone (ACTH) as well as opiate derivatives of its precursor, proopiomelanocortin (POMC); gonadotrophs secrete follicle-stimulating hormone (FSH) as well as luteinizing hormone (LH). Thyrotropin is secreted by thyrotrophs.

Table 295-1   Hypothalamic-pituitary axis

		HORMONE EXPRESSION	
HYPOTHALMIC HORMONE	PITUITARY TARGET CELL	TROPHIC	PERIPHERAL
Stimulatory			
Growth hormone–releasing hormone	Somatotroph	Growth hormone	Insulin-like growth factor I
Corticotropin–releasing hormone	Corticotroph	ACTH and related peptides	Cortisol
Thyrotropin–releasing hormone	Thyrotroph	Thyrotropin	Thyroid hormones
Gonadotropin–releasing hormone	Gonadotroph	Luteinizing hormone	Gonadal steroids
		Follicle-stimulating hormone	Inhibin
Inhibitory			
Somatostatin	Somatotroph	Growth hormone	
Dopamine	Lactotroph	Prolactin	

Modified from Melmed S et al: *Ann Intern Med* 105:238, 1986.

HYPOTHALAMIC-PITUITARY TARGET HORMONE SYSTEMS

Hypothalamic-Pituitary Thyroid System

Thyrotropin-Releasing Hormone. Thyrotropin-releasing hormone (TRH), a tripeptide (pyroglutamyl histidylprolinamide), interacts with receptors on the thyrotroph, where it stimulates thyroid-stimulating hormone (TSH) secretion. In addition, TRH also stimulates the lactotroph cell to secrete PRL.

Thyroid-Stimulating Hormone. Thyroid-stimulating hormone (TSH) is a glycoprotein hormone synthesized in the thyrotroph cell of the anterior pituitary. The alpha subunit of TSH is common to each of the glycoprotein hormones including TSH, FSH, LH, and human chorionic gonadotropin (hCG). The biologic specificity of these hormones is conferred by their unique beta subunits. Thyroid-stimulating hormone stimulates the thyroid gland to synthesize and secrete thyroid hormones. The secretion of TSH is stimulated by hypothalamic TRH and is inhibited by a potent negative feedback system mediated by peripheral thyroid hormones. Hypothalamic somatostatin (SRIF) and dopamine also inhibit TSH secretion. Nevertheless the negative feedback inhibition of TSH secretion by thyroid hormone overrides positive input from the hypothalamus. For example, hyperthyroid patients with mildly elevated T_4 levels do not respond by releasing TSH after an injection of TRH.

Testing of thyroid-stimulating hormone reserve. To test for pituitary TSH reserve, TRH (200 µg) is administered intravenously. Normal response is a two- to threefold increase in TSH levels occurring within 30 minutes after injection. Hypothyroidism caused by thyroid failure results in an exaggerated TSH response to TRH. Thyroid-stimulating hormone response is blunted in hyperthyroidism, exogenously administered thyroid hormone, and pituitary failure. Pituitary hypothyroidism is also characterized by low basal TSH levels in the face of thyroid failure, whereas hypothalamic hypothyroidism may have normal, low, or slightly elevated TSH level with low serum thyroxine level. In the latter situation, the TSH may have reduced biologic activity.

Hypothalamic-Pituitary Adrenal System

Corticotropin-Releasing Factor. Corticotropin-releasing factor (CRF) is a 41 amino acid hypothalamic peptide that stimulates the release of ACTH from the corticotrophs of the anterior pituitary. Corticotropin-releasing hormone is synthesized in the paraventricular nucleus of the hypothalamus as well as in higher brain regions.

Adrenocorticotropic Hormone. The corticotroph cell of the anterior pituitary contains a large polypeptide molecule, POMC, which is the precursor for beta lipotropin, beta endorphin, and ACTH. Adrenocorticotropic hormone, a 39 amino acid single-chain polypeptide, stimulates adrenal steroidogenesis. Adrenal cortisol participates in the negative feedback regulation of both pituitary ACTH and hypothalamic CRF release. Loss of cortisol inhibition in patients with primary adrenal failure results in extremely high ACTH levels. The circadian rhythm of ACTH secretion results in peak levels in the early morning; the lowest levels are attained in the late evening. Stress overrides both the negative feedback regulation of cortisol and the circadian rhythm of ACTH secretion.

Testing for adrenocorticotropic hormone reserve. Testing for ACTH reserve is potentially hazardous in patients with compromised adrenal function and should be performed under careful supervision.

Insulin hypoglycemia. Regular insulin should be administered intravenously, 0.05 to 0.1 units per kilogram. The blood sugar level should fall to 50% of baseline within 30 minutes. Normal ACTH reserve is confirmed by a plasma cortisol response of 7 µg per deciliter above the baseline, a doubling of the baseline cortisol level, and a peak value of at least 20 µg per deciliter. The peak cortisol response occurs approximately 30 to 45 minutes after hypoglycemia develops. Insulin hypoglycemia is contraindicated in patients who have primary adrenal insufficiency or who are elderly, suffer from heart disease, or are susceptible to seizures.

Metyrapone. 3 g Metyrapone is given orally at 11 PM with a snack. Serum compound S (11-deoxycortisol) and cortisol levels are measured at 8 AM the following morning. The metyrapone causes a block in the conversion of 11-deoxycortisol to cortisol, blocking the major negative feedback inhibitor of ACTH secretion. The resultant surge in ACTH secretion stimulates production of compound S, which should be at a level greater than 8 µg per deciliter in individuals with a normal pituitary adrenal axis. Plasma cortisol levels must fall to less than 5 µg per deciliter for the result of this test to be valid.

Cortrosyn stimulation test. As an indirect test of pituitary ACTH reserve, adrenal cortisol reserve may be evaluated. Injection of synthetic ACTH 1 to 24 (cortrosyn 250 µg) intravenously or intramuscularly is followed by measuring serum cortisol levels after 30 and 60 minutes. Normally cortisol levels should double, rise at least 7 µg per deciliter, or have peak levels of more than 20 µg per deciliter. A blunted response indicates either impaired pituitary ACTH level reserve or primary adrenal failure.

Corticotropin-releasing hormone test. As a direct test of corticotroph function, corticotropin-releasing hormone, 1 µg per kilogram, is administered intravenously. Plasma and/or serum cortisol responses are measured frequently during the next 60 minutes. Hypopituitary patients show a blunted response to CRF. Interestingly, patients harboring a corticotroph cell adenoma causing Cushing's disease often have an exaggerated ACTH response to CRF. Patients with ectopic ACTH-secreting tumors do not demonstrate a further rise in ACTH levels in response to CRF.

Test for adrenocorticotropic hormone hypersecretion. Dexamethasone suppression test should be performed to rule out a corticotroph-secreting adenoma resulting in Cushing's disease. Details of this test are provided in Chapter 298.

Hypothalamic-Pituitary Gonadal System

Gonadotropin-Releasing Hormone (GnRH). Hypothalamic gonadotropin-releasing hormone (GnRH), a 10 amino acid peptide, is synthesized in the preoptic region of the hypothalamus and regulates the secretion of both LH and FSH by pituitary gonadotrophs.

The synthesis of this decapeptide appears to be under positive feedback control by peripheral estrogens. It is secreted in a pulsatile fashion every 60 to 120 minutes.

Gonadotropins. The two gonadotrophic hormones, LH and FSH, are glycoprotein hormones produced by the gonadotroph cell. Like TSH, the specific beta subunit confers biologic specificity on each of these hormones. In women, LH appears to mediate ovulation and maintenance of the corpus luteum; in men, LH controls testosterone synthesis and secretion by the Leydig cell. In women, FSH regulates the development and maturation of the ovarian follicle and stimulates the secretion of ovarian estrogen. In men, FSH is responsible for the development of seminiferous tubules and stimulates spermatogenesis. Feedback regulation of gonadotropin secretion is complex with both positive and negative components mediated by levels of gonadal steroids, especially estradiol, and gonadal polypeptide inhibitory (inhibins) or stimulatory (activins) hormones.

Testing for luteinizing hormone and follicle-stimulating hormone reserve

Gonadotropins. The best diagnostic test of gonadotropin deficiency is the concurrent measurement of peripheral serum gonadotropin and gonadal steroid concentrations. Circulating testosterone or estradiol levels are low in patients with pituitary gonadotropin deficiency. Three pooled serum samples drawn 20 minutes apart are used to measure serum LH and FSH levels to compensate for the neurosecretory pulses of gonadotropin release. The normal values are 4 to 20 mIU per milliliter for the gonadotropin hormones. Normal testosterone levels are above 280 ng per deciliter. Normal estradiol levels vary with the menstrual cycle but should be greater than 30 pg per milliliter in postpubertal premenopausal women.

Gonadotropin-releasing hormone test. To stimulate the gonadotrophs to secrete gonadotropins directly, 100 μg GnRH is administered intravenously. Luteinizing hormone levels usually peak within 30 minutes, whereas FSH levels plateau after 1 hour. Normal responses vary according to the menstrual cycle, age, and sex of the patient. Generally, LH levels increase about threefold; the FSH increase is somewhat more blunted. A normal response does not exclude the presence of pituitary hypogonadism, just as an absent response cannot reliably distinguish pituitary from hypothalamic causes of hypogonadism.

Hypothalamic-Pituitary Growth Hormone System

Growth Hormone–Releasing Hormone. Growth hormone–releasing hormone (GHRH), a 44 amino acid peptide, is synthesized in the hypothalamus and stimulates the release of GH from the somatotrophs. It was originally characterized from an ectopic pancreatic tumor and has potent GH-releasing activity when administered intravenously.

Somatostatin. Somatotropin release–inhibiting factor (SRIF) is synthesized in the medial preoptic area of the hypothalamus. This hypothalamic hormone inhibits the secretion of pituitary GH. It participates together with GHRH in a dual control system for the regulation of GH secretion. Interestingly, SRIF is also found in many extrahypothalamic tissues, including the central nervous system, gastrointestinal system, and pancreas.

Growth Hormone. Growth hormone, quantitatively the main hormone secreted by the pituitary, is composed of 191 amino acids and has a molecular weight of 22,000 daltons. This polypeptide mediates linear growth together with other hormones and growth factors. Hypothalamic stimulatory and inhibitory peptides regulate GH secretion. Secretion is stimulated by GHRH and inhibited by SRIF. The pulsatile secretion of GH appears to involve a tonic balance between GHRH and SRIF. The secretion of these two peptides appears to be out of phase, which results in sequential peaks and troughs of GH secretion. Peak secretory bursts occur between 11 PM and 1 AM. Physical exercise, emotional stress, and nutritional status all appear to regulate GH secretion at the level of the hypothalamus.

Growth hormone binds to receptors in the liver and induces insulin-like growth factor I (IGF-I) production, which has been shown to mediate most of the growth-promoting actions of GH. Acting by way of a negative feedback loop, IGF-I suppresses GH secretion. Insulin-like growth factor I is also produced by extrahepatic tissues and may play a role in local tissue growth.

In the circulation, IGF is bound to a family of structurally homologous binding proteins (IGFBPs). Six distinct IGFBPs have been identified. IGFBP-3 acts as the main reservoir of circulating IGF, and its molar concentration corresponds to the concentration of total IGF peptide. IGFBP levels are low in states of growth hormone deficiency, liver disease, and malnutrition. In fact, measurements of serum IGFBP-3 concentrations may be useful as reflections of growth hormone deficiency. Smaller IGF binding proteins may also act to regulate the accessibility of IGF-I to target tissues.

Testing for growth hormone reserve. Tests of GH reserve have classically involved the indirect stimulation of the somatotroph to secrete GH.

Insulin hypoglycemia. Insulin is administered 0.05 to 0.1 unit per kilogram intravenously. Blood glucose concentration should be reduced to at least 40 mg per deciliter or to at least 50% of the patient's initial blood glucose levels. Serial blood samples are drawn for measurement of GH and glucose levels. Peak response of GH occurs between 60 and 90 minutes and should be at least 7 ng per milliliter in 90% of normal patients.

Arginine infusion. Arginine infusion, 0.5 g per kilogram administered intravenously over 30 minutes, normally results in peak GH response at 60 to 90 minutes of at least 7 ng per milliliter.

L-Dopa and clonidine. L-Dopa (500 mg) or clonidine (0.025 mg), administered orally, may also be used to stimulate GH secretion. These oral tests are far safer than insulin tests and are preferred for elderly patients. Blood is drawn every 30 minutes and peak GH levels are found between 60 and 90 minutes.

Growth hormone–releasing hormone test. To test somatotroph secretory capacity directly, GHRH (1 μg/kg) is administered intravenously and serial blood samples drawn. Growth hormone levels usually peak within the first hour after injection. Patients with GH deficiency caused by hypopituitarism do not respond to GHRH. A GH response after repeated GHRH stimulation may indicate the presence of a hypothalamic disorder and defective synthesis or release of endogenous GHRH. Obesity and type II diabetes also cause a flattened GH response to GHRH.

Testing for growth hormone hypersecretion. After the oral administration of 75 g of glucose, GH normally is suppressed to less than 1 ng per milliliter within 120 minutes. Paradoxic GH responses to glucose are seen in about 75% of patients with acromegaly. A similar paradoxic decline may be found with L-dopa. Furthermore, a GH response to TRH may be seen in about 50% of patients with acromegaly.

Basal IGF-I levels are useful for the screening of GH excess because IGF-I levels do not fluctuate rapidly and they reflect the integrated secretion of GH over time. Levels above 2.2 units per milliliter are usually found in patients with acromegaly or gigantism. However, IGF-I levels are not as useful for screening for hypopituitarism, because the levels in hypopituitary patients may overlap with those of normal individuals.

Hypothalamic-Pituitary Prolactin System

Prolactin-Inhibiting Factor. The primary hypothalamic prolactin inhibitory factor is dopamine, which is a potent inhibitor of pituitary lactotroph prolactin synthesis and release. This tonic inhibition of prolactin by dopamine can be blocked by dopamine antagonists. Administration of potent dopamine antagonist drugs such as metoclopramide which do not cross the blood-brain barrier and which impinge directly on the anterior pituitary gland, result in enhanced basal prolactin secretion. Furthermore, depletion of hypothalamic dopamine by drugs, including the phenothiazines, causes hyperprolactinemia and even galactorrhea. This observation of the dopaminergic inhibition of prolactin secretion has allowed the design of therapeutic agents such as bromocriptine to suppress excessive secretion of prolactin.

Although no hypothalamic prolactin-releasing factor has been proved conclusively, vasoactive intestinal polypeptide (VIP) appears to be an important stimulator of prolactin synthesis and secretion by the pituitary.

Table 295-2 Administration of hypothalamic-releasing hormones as a combined anterior pituitary function test*

HYPOTHALAMIC HORMONE	RADIOIMMUNOASSAY OF PITUITARY HORMONE	VENOUS SAMPLING TIME AFTER INFUSION (MIN)
TRH 200 μg	TSH	15, 30
	PRL	10, 15
CRF 1 μg/kg	ACTH	10, 45, 60
GHRH 1 μg/kg	GH	45, 60
GnRH 100 μg	FSH	45, 60, 90
	LH	15, 30

Modified from Sheldon WR et al: *J Clin Endocrinol Metab* 60:623, 1985.
*Basal (zero time) samples are initially drawn for each hormone measurement. All four hypothalamic-releasing hormones are administered intravenously sequentially over 60 seconds, then followed by venous sampling for specific hormone radioimmunoassay at the indicated times.

Prolactin. Prolactin has a molecular weight of 21,500 daltons, contains 199 amino acids, and has a high degree of homology with GH and placental lactogen concentrations. Prolactin secretion is directed by inhibitory hypothalamic control. Dopamine inhibits whereas TRH and VIP stimulate PRL secretion. However, the physiologic role of TRH is unclear, because the level of TSH, which is released by TRH, does not rise during lactation when PRL levels are high. Prolactin secretion is also stimulated by estrogen, which may be the most important peripheral regulator of PRL secretion. Prolactin levels are often elevated in hyperestrogenemic states.

Testing for prolactin reserve. Thyrotropin-releasing hormone (200 μg intravenously by bolus) is administered. The peak PRL response after 10 to 20 minutes should be three- to fivefold above the baseline. Normal basal PRL levels are less than 20 ng per milliliter. Metoclopromide, 10 mg intramuscularly, may also be used as a stimulator of PRL release. The normal response is a doubling of PRL levels after 1 hour.

Testing for prolactin hypersecretion. A basal PRL level greater than 200 ng per milliliter strongly suggests the presence of a PRL-secreting adenoma. Although responses to TRH, metoclopromide, and L-dopa may be variable in patients harboring PRL-secreting adenoma, these tests are of limited utility in diagnosing the presence of such adenomas.

Quadruple-bolus testing. To provide an efficient and sensitive method for comprehensive testing of anterior pituitary reserve function, all four hypothalamic-releasing hormones may be administered simultaneously (Table 295-2) (Fig. 295-2). Although often not practical, this comprehensive test serves to define the trophic hormone axes.

CLINICAL SYNDROMES
Hypothalamic Dysfunction

The hypothalamic nuclei surrounding the third ventricle are essential for the normal physiologic regulation of water metabolism, temperature control, appetite and food intake, the sleep-wake cycle, visceral (autonomic) functions, and control of anterior pituitary function. In addition, emotional expression, behavior, and short-term memory are influenced by this region. Small lesions in the hypothalamus therefore may give rise to several clinical abnormalities.

Several disease processes may involve the hypothalamus, including primary intracranial tumors, infiltrative disorders, trauma, vascular abnormalities, and developmental malformations. Over half of these patients have neuroophthalmologic abnormalities, pyramidal tract or sensory nerve involvement, headaches, and extrapyramidal cerebellar signs. Approximately one third exhibit recurrent vomiting, diabetes insipidus, somnolence, dysthermia, appetite dysfunction, and hypogonadism or precocious puberty.

Specific signs and symptoms of hypothalamic clinical syndromes have been localized to nuclear lesions (Fig. 295-3). Slow-growing lesions generally remain asymptomatic for substantially longer periods than acute insults. Destruction of a single unilateral nucleus usually does not result in a clinical syndrome as the remaining intact con-

tralateral nucleus is sufficient to maintain appropriate physiologic homeostasis. Lesions arising from the third ventricle or basal hypothalamus or diffuse infiltrative conditions are most likely to lead to symptoms resulting from involvement of both homologous nuclei. Clinical manifestations also depend on whether a lesion involving a nucleus is stimulatory or destructive. For example, a tumor invading and destroying the tuberal area may result in hypogonadism, whereas a hamartoma in the same region may lead to precocious puberty. Systemic diseases such as sarcoidosis or histiocytosis that involve the hypothalamus usually have extrahypothalamic manifestations that may provide a clue to the underlying cause of the hypothalamic disorder.

Hypopituitarism

The clinical manifestations of hypopituitarism depend on the degree of pituitary hormone deficiency. The deficiency of anterior pituitary hormones may be isolated or may result from a combination of several hormone deficiencies. Generally, the pattern of hormone loss in a destructive pituitary lesion results in initial loss of GH, followed by gonadotropin, TSH, and finally ACTH secretion.

Causes. The causes of hypopituitarism are outlined in Box 295-1. Congenital conditions such as septo-optic dysplasia, Prader-Willi syndrome, and Laurence-Moon-Biedl syndrome usually are apparent in childhood. Isolated GH deficiency is an important cause of short stature. Cysts of the base of the brain impinging on the hypothalamus may also cause pituitary failure. The vascular causes of hypopituitarism include pituitary apoplexy, Sheehan's syndrome, carotid aneurysm, as well as connective tissue disease and arteritides including systemic lupus erythematosus.

Autoimmune lymphocytic hypophysitis is a recently recognized cause of pituitary failure. This condition has been described in association with pregnancy. The pituitary failure usually involves all the trophic hormones. The magnetic resonance image (MRI) of this condition may be difficult to differentiate from that of a pituitary tumor. Although the treatment of patients with this disorder does not require surgery, the diagnosis may be difficult and may only become evident on histologic examination of a surgical specimen. Other inflammatory causes of pituitary failure include histiocytosis, sarcoidosis, and chronic infection giving rise to granulomatous disease of the hypothalamus or pituitary including tuberculosis, syphilis, and various mycoses.

Damage to the hypothalamus or hypothalamic-pituitary unit cause pituitary failure. Trauma to the base of the brain may result in a stalk section and hemorrhage in the pituitary fossa. Ionizing radiation, especially with doses above 4000 rad, and surgery are iatrogenic causes of pituitary damage. Hemochromatosis, amyloidosis, and metastatic carcinoma are important lesions that may infiltrate the hypothalamus, and sometimes the pituitary itself, and cause pituitary failure. Interestingly, metastatic carcinoma is relatively rare in the anterior pituitary and is more commonly found in the posterior pituitary. This may be explained by the blood supply of the anterior pituitary, which comes primarily from the hypothalamic portal system, whereas the posterior pituitary has a direct blood supply from the internal carotid and the inferior hypophyseal arteries. The important tumors that metastasize to the pituitary are breast and bronchial carcinomas.

Tumors of the hypothalamus and pituitary are important causes of destruction and compression of the anterior pituitary, frequently resulting in its failure. The most common hypothalamic tumor is craniopharyngioma; this nonfunctioning mass may damage the hypothalamic neurons responsible for releasing factor production or may disrupt the vascular or neural connections between the hypothalamus and pituitary, resulting in growth failure and other features of hypopituitarism. Hypothalamic gliomas, germinomas, and hamartomas may impinge on the normal hypothalamic function through their mass effects, and there may also be functional and elaborate excessive amounts of hypothalamic-releasing hormones. Both functioning and nonfunctioning pituitary adenomas may compress normal surrounding pituitary tissue, resulting in pituitary failure. Usually the destruction of local pituitary tissue has to be fairly significant for pituitary failure to occur. Finally, idiopathic pituitary failure is occasionally

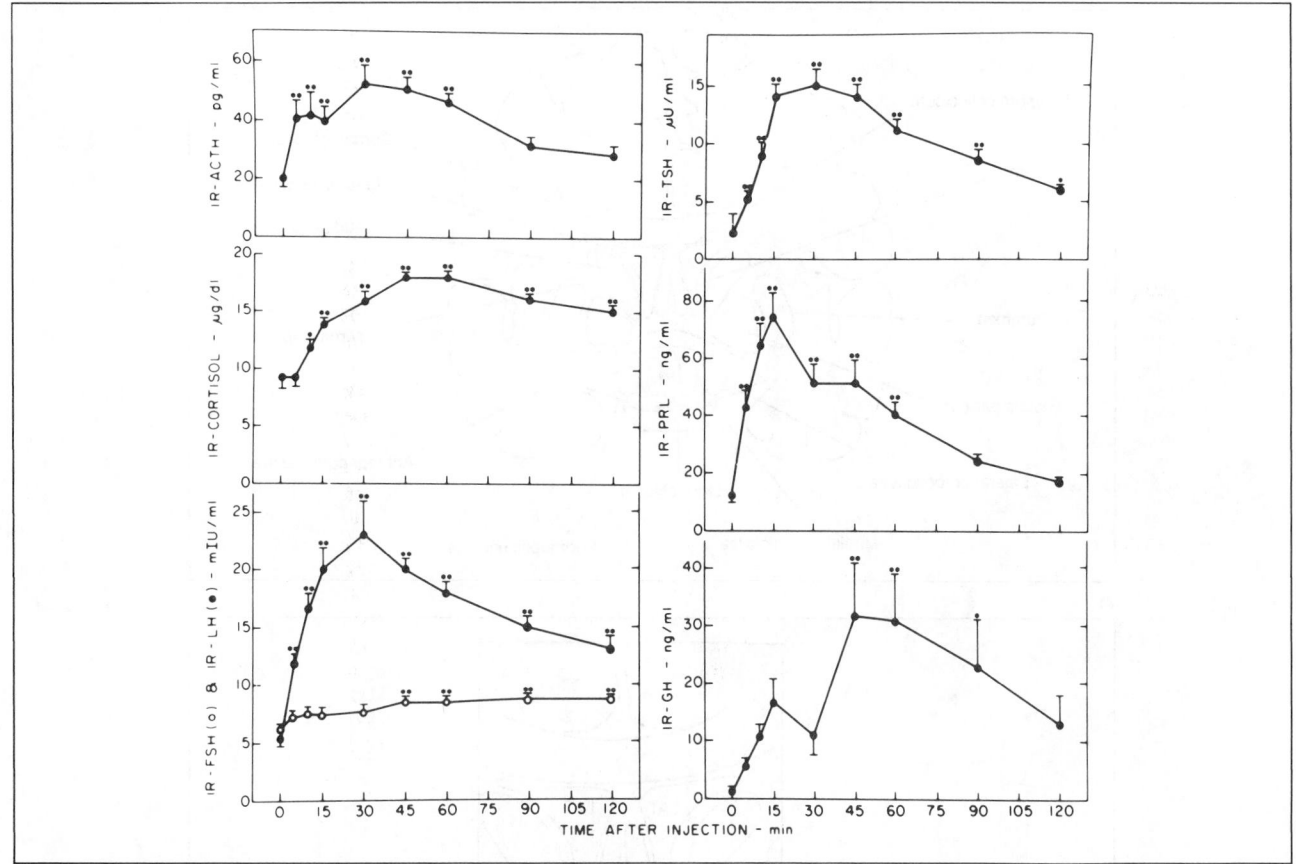

FIGURE 295-2   Quadruple bolus test of anterior pituitary hormone reserve. Mean plasma or serum ($\pm$SEM) levels of hormones at intervals after administration of all four hypothalamic-releasing hormones in 26 normal subjects. $P < 0.05$; $**P < 0.01$ (compared to baseline value). All four hypothalamic-releasing hormones are administered as depicted in Table 295-2. *SEM,* Standard error of the mean.

From Sheldon WR et al: *J Clin Endocrinol Metab* 60:623, 1985.

seen in patients with primary empty sella and with idiopathic diabetes insipidus.

Signs and Symptoms of Pituitary Failure. Any combination of single or multiple hormone loss may occur in lesions of the pituitary gland. Isolated deficiency of a single hormone may also occur.

Growth hormone deficiency. Growth retardation, short stature, and fasting hypoglycemia are the clinical hallmarks of GH deficiency during infancy and childhood. Delayed puberty may also be present. Children with this deficiency, which may be isolated, are usually round faced with a chubby appearance and lack good muscular development. Adults may not have any manifestations of GH deficiency, unless combined with ACTH deficiency, which may result in fasting hypoglycemia. Currently, adult GH replacement is being evaluated for efficacy and safety.

Gonadotropin deficiency. Central hypogonadism during childhood results in failure to enter normal puberty. Breast development is delayed, and pubic and axillary hair do not develop normally, although some sexual hair growth takes place if ACTH secretion is intact and stimulates adrenal androgen production. In females, primary amenorrhea is also present. In boys, small testes and phallus and sparse body hair are evident. If the gonadotropin deficiency is isolated, growth may be delayed but continues as a result of failure of long-bone epiphyseal closure. Therefore isolated hypogonadism causes adolescents to be tall and have eunuchoidal proportions. In these individuals, the upper/lower segment ratio is less than 1. Their arm span is usually greater than their height by 5 cm or more. In postpubertal women, hypogonadism is manifested as secondary amenorrhea, breast atrophy, and loss of pubic and axillary hair. In men, testicular atrophy, decrease in body hair growth, decrease in libido, impotence, and infertility are present.

Thyroid-stimulating hormone secretion deficiency. Deficiency of TSH secretion causes failure of thyroid function. The thyroid gland becomes involuted, and clinical features of hypothyroidism including lethargy, cold intolerance, constipation, bradycardia, delayed reflex relaxation time, and hoarseness become apparent. These patients may be differentiated from those who have primary hypothyroidism by a low circulating level of TSH in the presence of low thyroid hormone levels. The low TSH levels do not respond to exogenously administered TRH because of the pituitary lesion.

Adrenocorticotropic hormone deficiency. Deficiency in ACTH results in adrenal failure with a spectrum of presentations including orthostatic hypotension, weakness, hypothermia, nausea, vomiting, dehydration, lethargy, coma, and even death. Hypokalemia is usually not seen because of the maintenance of mineralocorticoid secretion through the renin-angiotensin-aldosterone system.

Vasopressin deficiency. Vasopressin (ADH) deficiency occurs when lesions involve the posterior pituitary. Damage to the hypothalamic nuclei or the posterior pituitary extensions of their axons results in diminished release of ADH. The symptoms of diabetes insipidus include polyuria, polydypsia, and nocturia.

Pituitary Apoplexy

Acute massive infarction of the pituitary gland (apoplexy) is a rare, life-threatening disorder that requires prompt diagnosis and treatment.

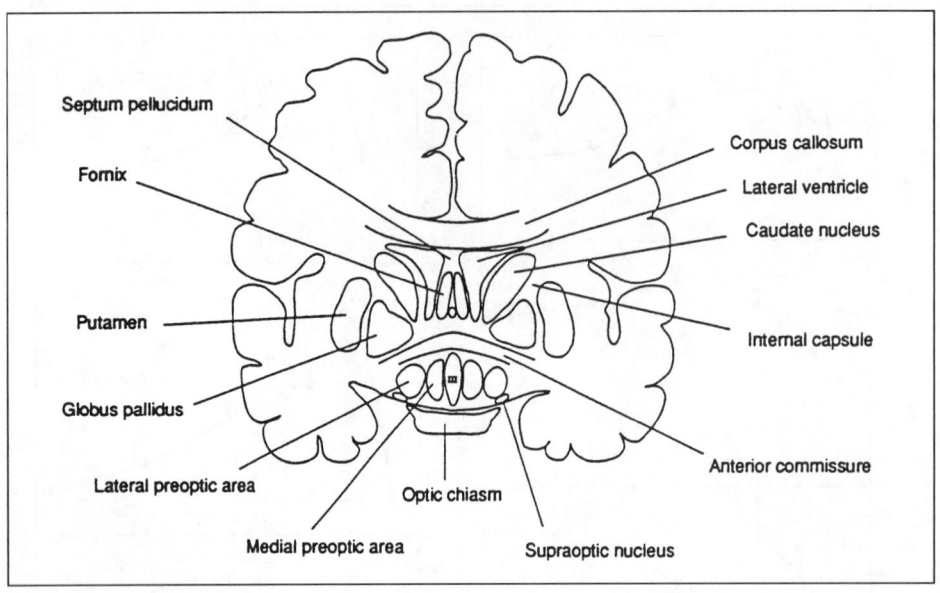

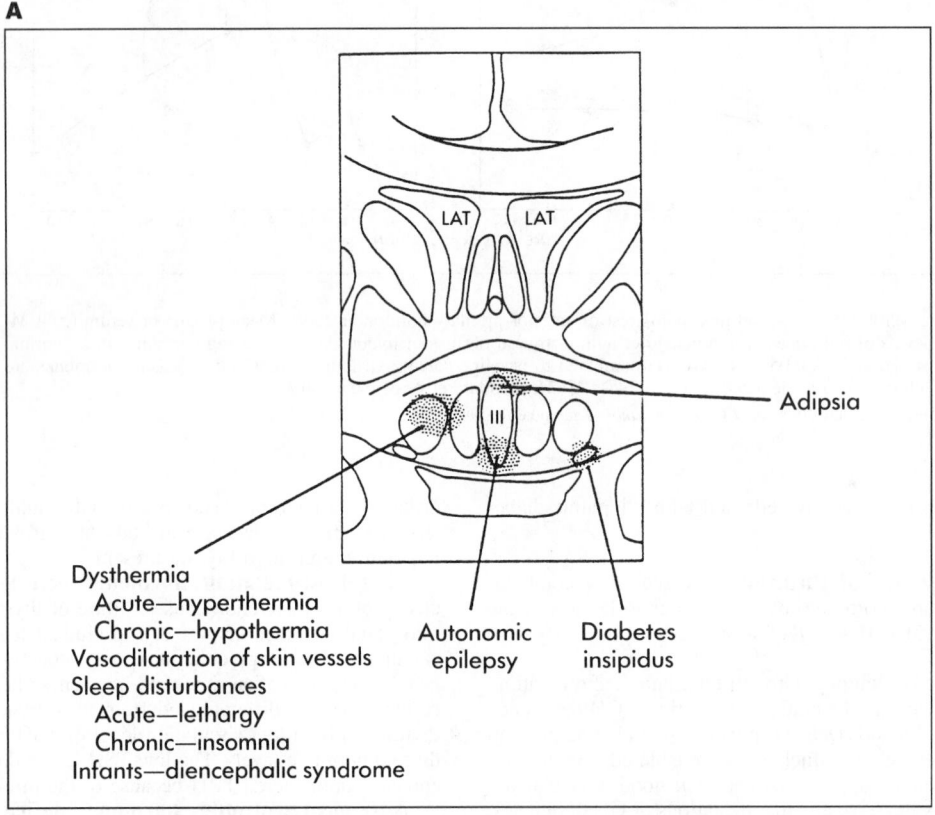

FIGURE 295-3   **A,** Frontal section of the preoptic region of the hypothalamus. **B,** Clinical findings associated with lesions affecting the preoptic region.

Causes. Predisposing factors that may lead to occlusion or severe spasm of the arteries supplying the anterior lobe and pituitary stalk include pregnancy, pituitary tumor, acquired or hereditary bleeding or clotting disorders, trauma, carotid angiography, radiation therapy of pituitary tumors, artificial respiration, increased intracranial pressure, diabetes, and atherosclerosis. Pathogenesis of this condition results from total ischemia associated with initial acute arterial spasm. This is followed by vascular congestion and thrombosis.

Signs and Symptoms. The clinical presentation of pituitary apoplexy includes a wide range of symptoms and signs including sudden death. Retro-orbital or frontal headache occurs most commonly and is usually severe in nature and of very sudden onset. This may be accompanied by diplopia caused by compression of the cranial nerves (especially III and VI) supplying the extraocular muscles as a result of increased cavernous sinus pressure. Impaired visual acuity, photophobia, and visual blurring may precede the other clinical manifestations of apoplexy. Neurologic features of apoplexy commonly include alteration in consciousness, drowsiness, coma, and death. These signs may be accompanied by hemiparesis, hemianesthesias, signs of meningeal irritation, nausea, vomiting, and diabetes insipidus. Hyperpyrexia is also commonly seen. Less common physical findings include seizures, aphasia, dementia, and lower cranial nerve palsies. Systemic alterations in temperature, respiratory

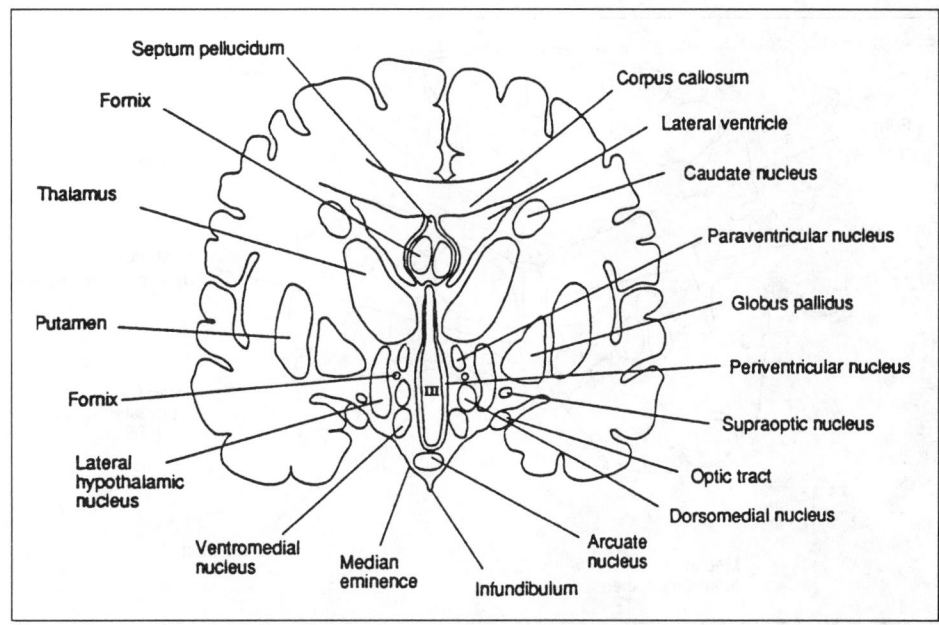

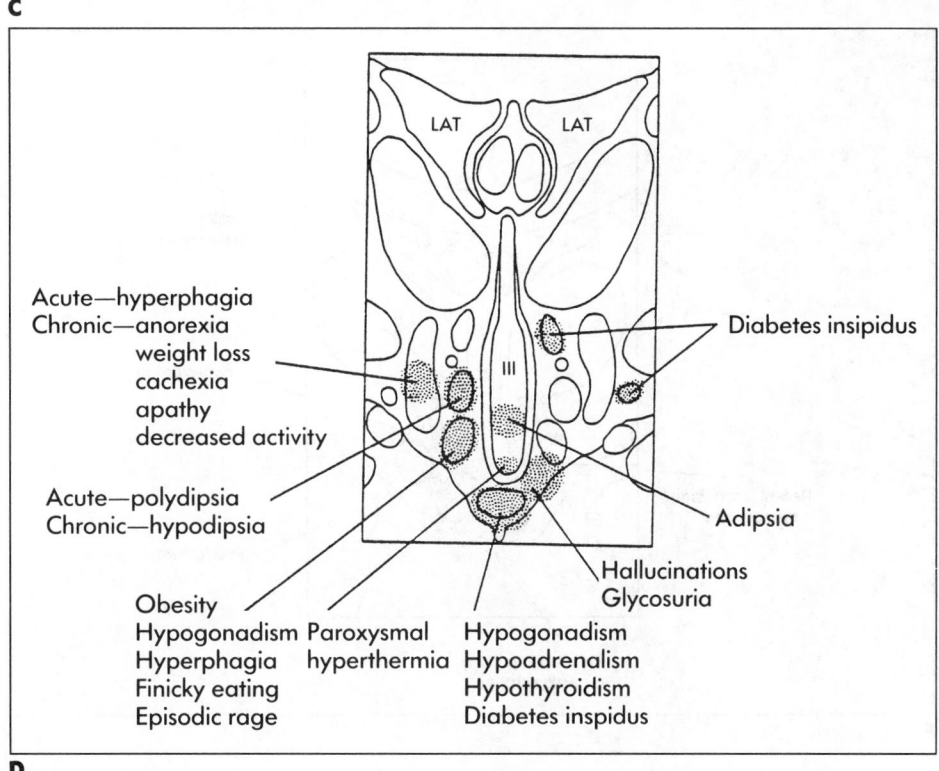

FIGURE 295-3, CONT'D. **C,** Frontal section of the supraoptic region of the hypothalamus. **D,** Clinical findings associated with lesions in the supraoptic region.

rates, and blood pressure may occur if hypothalamic compression is significant. The clinical manifestations of apoplexy usually reflect the anatomic focus of the lesion. Accompanying adrenal insufficiency caused by pituitary failure may also contribute to the clinical picture.

Examination of the cerebrospinal fluid (CSF) usually reveals xanthochromia or fresh blood. Cerebrospinal fluid pressure and protein levels are usually elevated, and peripheral blood may show a leukocytosis. Computed tomography (CT) scan or MRI of the pituitary may identify a pituitary mass with or without suprasellar extension and associated perisellar bleeding.

Differential Diagnosis. Differential diagnosis of this condition must be made quickly to ensure lifesaving intervention. The

conditions to be considered in the differential diagnosis include ruptured intracranial aneurysm, acute meningitis, infarction of the base of brain, degenerative encephalopathy, and supratentorial herniation.

Treatment of Hypopituitarism
Adrenocorticotropic hormone replacement. The usual adult replacement dose of hydrocortisone is 20 mg in the morning and 10 mg at night. Alternatively, 25 mg cortisone acetate can be administered in the morning and 12.5 mg at night. Patients should be advised to increase the amount of medication to two to three times the normal replacement level before minor stresses such as dental procedures and to carry a Medi-Alert (Turlock, California) identification

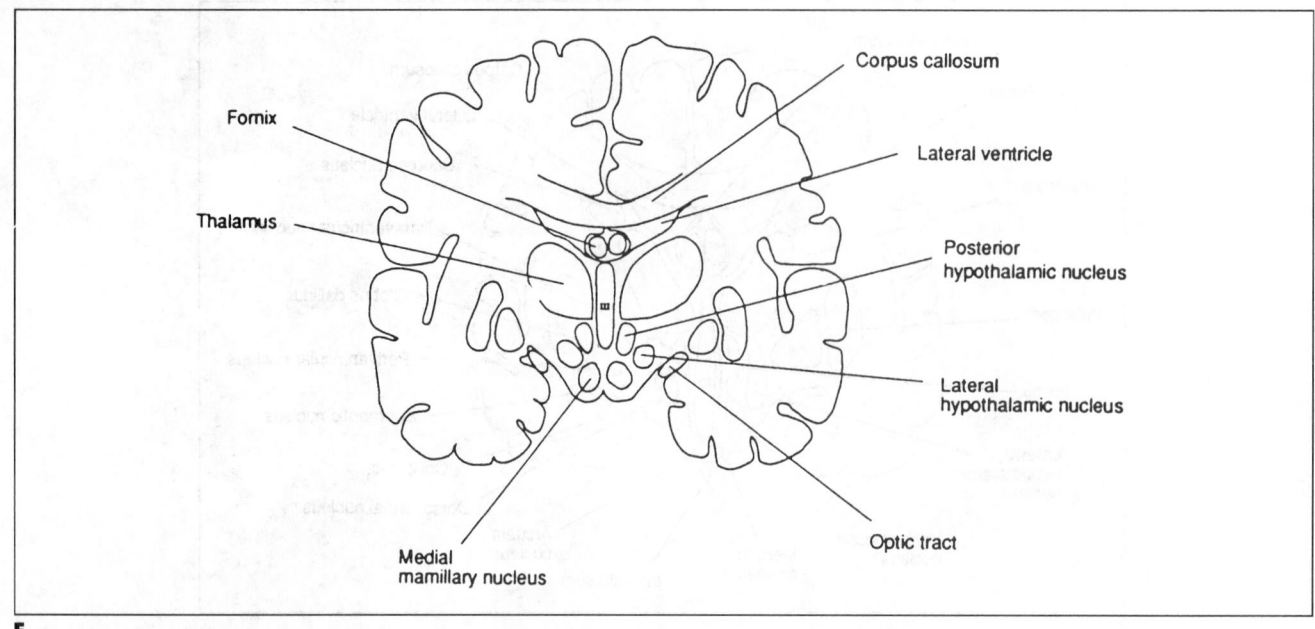

E

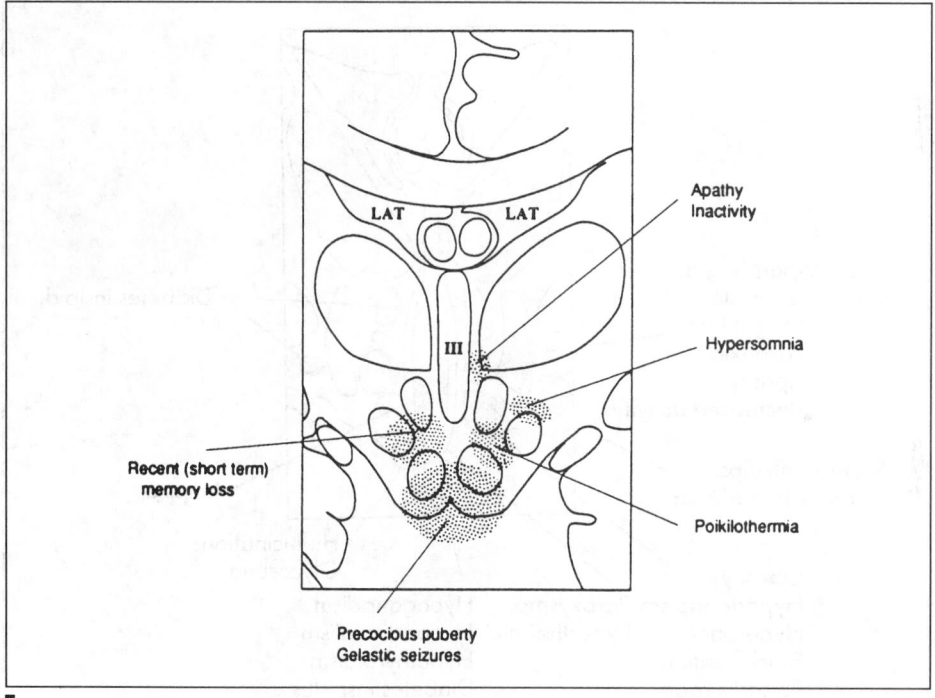

F

FIGURE 295-3, CONT'D. **E,** Frontal section of the mammillary region of the hypothalamus. **F,** Clinical findings associated with lesions involving the mammillary region. *III,* Third ventricle; *LAT,* lateral ventricle.

From Braunstein GD. In Melmed S, editor: *The pituitary,* Cambridge, Mass, 1993, Blackwell Scientific.

explaining the necessity to administer cortisol during any accident or other stress.

Thyroid-stimulating hormone replacement. The usual recommended replacement of thyroid hormone is in the form of synthetic L-thyroxine. This should be given in doses ranging from 0.075 to 0.15 mg once daily. Peripheral conversion of T_4 to T_3 provides physiologic amounts of T_3, as the majority of circulating T_3 is normally derived from peripheral hepatic conversion from T_4.

Gonadotropin replacement. In males, testosterone enanthate or cypionate injections, 200 mg intramuscularly every 2 weeks, may be given to testosterone-deficient men. Androgen replacement may also be accomplished transdermally, either through the scrotal skin (Testo-

derm 4 mg/day or 6 mg/day patches, Alza Pharmaceuticals, Palo Alto, Calif) or through another system that can be worn on the upper arms, thighs, back or abdomen (Androderm, two 2.5 mg patches applied daily, SmithKline Beecham Pharmaceuticals, Philadelphia, Penn). In females there are several regimens that are equally effective. Estrogen replacement therapy is accomplished by administering ethinyl estradiol 0.02 to 0.5 mg, or conjugated equine estrogens 0.625 to 1.25 mg daily or application of estradiol skin patches containing 4 or 8 mg of estrogen twice weekly. In order to facilitate cyclic uterine shedding and prevention of endometrial carcinoma, medroxyprogesterone acetate 5 to 10 mg is added on days 1 to 15 of each month. As an alternative, the estrogen may be administered along with medroxy-

---

BOX 295-1
Causes of hypopituitarism

Congenital or acquired
  Septo-optic dysplasia
  Hypogonadotropic hypogonadism
  Prader-Willi syndrome
  Laurence-Moon-Biedl syndrome
  Isolated GH deficiency
  Basal encephalocele
Vascular
  Pituitary apoplexy
  Sheehan's syndrome
  Arteritides
  Carotid aneurysm
Inflammatory
  Autoimmune lymphocytic hypophysitis
  Histiocytosis
  Sarcoidosis
  Tuberculosis
  Syphilis
  Mycoses
Physical agents
  Cranial trauma and hemorrhage
  Ionizing radiation
  Stalk section
  Surgery
Infiltrations
  Hemochromatosis
  Metastatic carcinoma (breast and bronchus)
  Amyloidosis
Tumors
  Hypothalamic
    Craniopharyngioma
    Glioma
    Germinoma
    Meningioma (sphenoidal ridge)
    Hamartoma
    Leukemia and lymphoma
  Pituitary
    Functioning macroadenomas
    Nonfunctioning macroadenomas
Idiopathic
  Empty sella
  Diabetes insipidus

---

progesterone acetate 2.5 to 5 mg daily. This latter regimen usually results in irregular bleeding during the first year and then amenorrhea afterward. In both sexes, if fertility is desired, then gonadotropin therapy with menopausal gonadotropins and hCG should be instituted to induce ovulation or spermatogenesis. Alternatively, synthetic GnRH may be given in pulsatile fashion via an infusion pump.

Growth hormone replacement. Children with short stature caused by GH deficiency or GH neurosecretory defect are treated with synthetic human GH derived from molecular recombinant techniques. The hormone is administered intramuscularly or subcutaneously at a dose of 0.04 mg/kg/day by daily subcutaneous injection until fusion of the long-bone epiphyses takes place. Growth hormone therapy is currently being evaluated in adults who are in catabolic states including those who have burns and respiratory insufficiency, and for postoperative recovery. The hormone is also being tested for use in the management of osteopenia and loss of lean body mass associated with aging.

Vasopressin replacement. ADH is provided by intranasal desmopressin (DDAVP) at a dose of 0.05 to 0.1 ml twice daily but must be titrated in each patient. An oral tablet form of this hormone has recently been approved.

Treatment of pituitary apoplexy. The treatment of pituitary apoplexy is a medical emergency. Intravenous fluid and oxygen should be administered immediately with intravenous hydrocortisone (200 mg). Intravenous hydrocortisone boluses should be repeated as

required during the initial phase of recovery. Intravenous thyroxine should not be administered until the hydrocortisone has been given. The increased metabolic demands of the administered thyroid hormone may precipitate adrenal crisis if the patient has not had adequate cortisone replacement. The dose of intravenous thyroxine is usually 500 μg administered as an intravenous bolus. Thereafter up to 100 μg intravenously daily is continued, as required. Blood glucose level should also be carefully monitored during the acute phase of apoplexy as these patients may be acutely hypersensitive to insulin because of the absence of the pituitary hormones that usually antagonize insulin action (e.g., GH, ACTH). These patients may therefore require intravenous glucose administration in addition to their initial acute hormonal replacement.

Pituitary Tumors

Sensitive and specific immunotechniques have provided insight into the cellular pathophysiology of the anterior pituitary tumors. Each of the anterior pituitary cells as well as their putative primitive stem cell precursors, either singly or in combination, may give rise to pituitary adenomas that express functional hormones. Prolactin, GH, and POMC-expressing adenomas account for the vast majority of adenomas removed surgically. Prolactin-secreting adenomas account for at least one third of all pituitary adenomas. Gonadotropin- and TSH-secreting tumors account for less than 5% of all pituitary tumors. Recent studies have shown that some "nonfunctioning" tumors that do not secrete biologically active hormones may contain and/or secrete the common glycoprotein hormone alpha subunit.

Diagnosis. The mass effects or hormonal aberrations induced by pituitary tumors lead to the signs and symptoms that alert the patient and clinician. These manifestations may appear initially as a result of compression of adjacent neurologic structures while causing systemic effects by way of excess peripheral hormonal action. Depending on its structure, a tumor may cause hyposecretion of one hormone and hypersecretion of another. Hypersecretion of a pituitary trophic hormone can cause acromegaly, amenorrhea-galactorrhea, impotence, or Cushing's disease. Hyposecretion may result in hypogonadism, hypothyroidism, or hypoadrenalism.

Diagnosis of pituitary adenomas has been aided by the advent of sophisticated imaging techniques: CT and MRI (Fig. 295-4). These noninvasive procedures have many advantages over multidirectional polytomograms, pneumoencephalograms, angiograms, and venograms because they eliminate morbidity, decrease the cost of preoperative evaluation, and lessen the length of hospital stay. In addition, MRIs have the ability to detect microadenoma masses smaller than 3 mm that might otherwise be missed by less advanced techniques and also provide the best visualization of the hypothalamus.

Local Neurologic Effects. Nearly one half of all patients with pituitary tumors larger than 1 cm experience severe headache. Although the cause of the headache is unknown, it may result from pressure on the diaphragma sella by the tumor mass.

The optic chiasm, which lies above the sella turcica of the pituitary, is frequently impinged on by the encroaching tumor, causing visual field defects, initially beginning with loss of red perception. Approximately one half of patients with pituitary tumors before 1972 had evidence of a bitemporal hemianopsia or a superior bitemporal defect. Today, because of the ready availability of hormone assays and sensitive sellar and parasellar imaging techniques, pituitary masses can be diagnosed much earlier, and the incidence of ophthalmologic lesions has declined.

Hypothalamic involvement by pituitary tumors can result in diabetes insipidus, as well as sleep or appetite disorders. In addition, changes in autonomic nervous system function, fluid output, temperature regulation, and behavior can occur.

When macroadenomas invade the cavernous sinus, the third, fourth, and sixth cranial nerves, as well as the ophthalmic and maxillary divisions of the fifth cranial nerve, can be affected. These neurologic changes may result in ptosis, ophthalmoplegia, or diplopia; they may also cause decreased facial sensation. Hemorrhage into the tumor may result in pituitary apoplexy or acute necrosis. When this occurs, severe headache, visual impairment, paralysis, lethargy, coma,

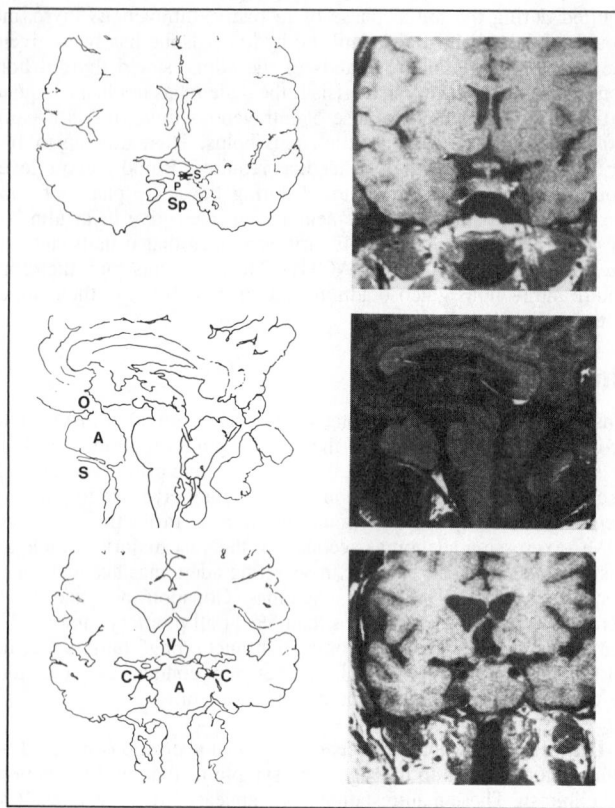

FIGURE 295-4 MRI scans of head showing the normal anatomic relations of the pituitary gland *(top)* and a large GH-cell pituitary macroadenoma enlarging the sella and extending ventrally *(middle and bottom)*. Bony and soft tissue structures are clearly identified. *A,* Adenoma; *C,* internal carotid arteries; *O,* optic tract; *P,* normal pituitary; *Sp,* sphenoid sinus; *S,* pituitary stalk; *V,* fourth ventricle; *MRI,* magnetic resonance imaging.

or evidence of meningeal irritation or increased intracranial pressure may follow.

Growth Hormone-Secreting Pituitary Tumors

Hypersomatotropism may be caused by pituitary or extrapituitary tumors (Box 295-2). Hypersecretion of GH can manifest itself in different ways, depending on the age of the patient. In children or adolescents whose epiphyseal growth centers have yet to fuse in the long bones, hypersomatotropism can cause gigantism. In adults, this excessive secretion results in acromegaly.

Acromegaly

Clinical manifestations. The clinical features of acromegaly occur slowly and are often only noticed after many years of gradual change (Fig. 295-5). Tumor size tends to be larger in younger acromegalic patients. The clinical presentation reflects the response to local tumor growth, the effects of peripheral tissue changes, and the indirect and direct effects of continuous GH hypersecretion (Box 295-3).

Clinical manifestations of acromegaly include visceromegaly of the kidney, heart, and, rarely, liver and spleen. Cardiac abnormalities such as asymmetric septal hypertrophy and left ventricular hypertrophy also result from acromegaly. The excessive growth of soft tissues results in the characteristic coarsening of the facial features. In addition, the hands, feet, and tongue become larger, and excess skin develops around the neck and axillae; skin tags are prominent. The changes in bone, cartilage, and skin can result in prognathism, frontal bossing, kyphosis, and dental malocclusion. A further complication of acromegaly occurs when the median nerve becomes entrapped in the carpal tunnel; this leads to acroparesthesia. Hyper-

---

BOX 295-2
Causes of hypersomatotropism

Pituitary
  Eutopic
    Densely or sparsely granulated GH cell adenoma
    Mixed GH cell and PRL cell adenoma
    Mammosomatotroph cell adenoma
    Acidophil stem cell adenoma
    Plurihormonal adenoma
  Ectopic
    Sphenoid sinus or parapharyngeal GH cell adenoma
Extrapituitary
  Ectopic GH-secreting tumor
    Pancreas, breast, lung
  Excess GHRH secretion
    Eutopic
      Hypothalamic hamartoma
    Ectopic
      Bronchial and intestinal carcinoid tumors
      Pancreatic islet-cell tumors
  Acromegaloidism

Modified from Melmed S et al: *Endocr Rev* 4:271, 1983.

tension may develop, as well as colonic polyps, which may become carcinomatous.

Insulin-like growth factor I, which is secreted under the influence of GH rather than the presence of the GH itself, is responsible for the acral enlargement seen in acromegaly. On the other hand, GH has direct anti-insulin effects, which can lead to insulin resistance and hyperinsulinism. However, although glucose intolerance is common at presentation, clinical diabetes mellitus is present in only approximately 15% of cases.

Menstrual disturbances are common in women with acromegaly. Similarly, males frequently have hypogonadism. The gonadotrophs can be destroyed by macroadenomas, which may cause hypogonadotropic hypogonadism. When tumors secrete both GH and PRL, hyperprolactinemia can result. This may also occur when a macroadenoma compresses the pituitary stalk, resulting in the disruption of dopamine transmission from the hypothalamus to the adenohypophysis. In both instances, hypersecretion of PRL can inhibit the normal cyclic discharge of GnRH, which in turn inhibits gonadotropin release and gonadal steroid secretion, resulting in hypogonadism.

Recently extrapituitary causes of acromegaly have been documented (see Box 295-2). Immunoreactive GH has been found in lung adenocarcinoma, breast cancer, and ovarian tissue extracts in vitro, and ectopic GH production has been documented in a patient with intramesenteric islet-cell tumor. Hypothalamic tumors, including hamartomas, choristomas, gliomas, and gangliocytomas, may be associated with acromegaly, resulting from the somatotroph hyperplasia or adenomas with excessive pituitary GH secretion stimulated by the GHRH elaborated by these tumors. Ectopic GHRH secretion has also been documented in pancreatic islet-cell, lung, and intestinal carcinoid tumors. Regardless of the tumor's location, patients with acromegaly have the classic clinical features of acromegaly, along with elevated circulating levels of GH and GHRH. The structure of GHRH was originally derived from extracts of pancreatic islet-cell tumors.

In contrast to classic acromegaly, acromegaloidism is a rare abnormality in which the clinical features of acromegaly are present in the absence of a pituitary or extraadenohypophyseal tumor. In fact, acral enlargement can occur in the absence of elevated GH levels. It has been speculated that in such cases, the patient has a unique growth factor distinct from the known growth factors that promote in vitro erythroid growth.

Diagnosis. Although elevated GH levels are the hallmark of acromegaly, evidence of these increased levels does not necessarily mean an exclusive diagnosis of the disease. Elevated GH levels of more than 10 ng per milliliter, although found in more than 95% of

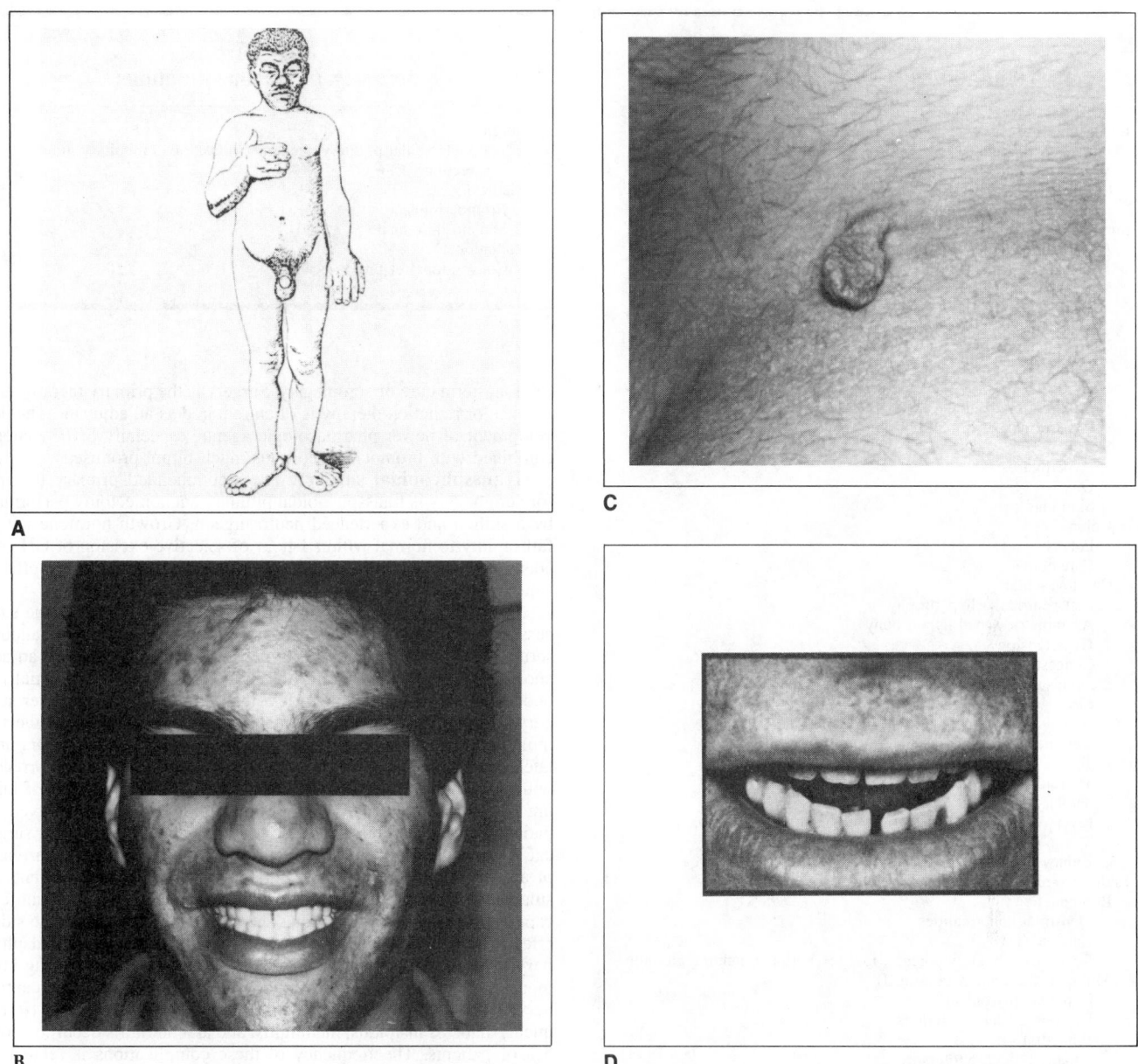

FIGURE 295-5   Clinical signs of hypersomatotrophism seen in acromegaly. **A,** Original figure depicting earliest illustration of clinical features of acromegaly by Minkowski in 1887. Note acromegalic facies, fleshy fingers and toes, and frontal bossing. **B,** Young male acromegalic with active perspiration, oily skin, acne, and widened tooth gap. **C,** Prominent skin tags are important signs of acromegaly and may be associated with the presence of colon polyps. **D,** Increased overbite and widening of spaces between incisors caused by mandibular growth in acromegaly.

A from Minkowski: *Berliner Klinische Wochenschrift,* May, 1887.

all acromegalics, can also occur in patients with anorexia nervosa, malnutrition, diabetes, renal failure, porphyria, cirrhosis, or stress. For a conclusive diagnosis of acromegaly, an oral glucose tolerance test must be administered. This test usually demonstrates a failure to suppress GH. Nearly one third of patients who have acromegaly exhibit no change in their GH levels after a glucose tolerance load. Twenty to forty percent experience a paradoxic increase of GH secretion, and 5% to 7% show normal suppression. Abnormalities of GH secretion may also occur in response to other stimuli (e.g., dopamine agonists, TRH, GnRH, and VIP).

As mentioned previously, increased IGF-I levels are responsible for the classic acral enlargement that clinically defines acromegaly. Biochemical evidence of IGF-I hypersecretion correlates well with a diagnosis of active acromegaly, perhaps even better than do fasting or glucose-suppressed GH levels. Thus the first step in screening for

acromegaly should entail measuring the patient's serum concentration of IGF-I; there is virtually no overlap in these levels between patients with acromegaly and normal individuals. When an elevated IGF-I level is detected, the patient should be evaluated further with an MRI or CT scan of the anterior pituitary and a postglucose GH determination. If no pituitary mass is detected, then further imaging should be performed to establish the location of an ectopically secreting GHRH or GH tumor. Measurements of immunoreactive serum GHRH levels may help to distinguish between these latter entities.

Therapy of Acromegaly. Management of patients harboring pituitary tumors is aimed at reducing or ablating the tumor mass, correcting visual and neurologic defects, preserving anterior pituitary function, and preventing progression or recurrence of the condition.

BOX 295-3
Clinical features of acromegaly

Local tumor effects
  Pituitary enlargement
  Visual field defects
  Cranial nerve palsy
  Headache
Somatic
  Acral enlargement
    Thickening of soft tissue of hands and feet
  Musculoskeletal
    Prognathism
    Malocclusion
    Arthralgias
    Carpal tunnel syndrome
    Acroparesthesia
    Proximal myopathy
    Hypertrophy of frontal bones
  Skin
    Hyperhydrosis
    Oily
    Skin tags
  Colon
    Polyps
    Carcinoma
  Cardiovascular
    Left ventricular hypertrophy
    Asymmetric septal hypertrophy
    Hypertension
    Congestive heart failure
  Sleep disturbances
    Sleep apnea
    Narcolepsy
  Visceromegaly
    Tongue
    Thyroid
    Salivary gland
    Liver
    Spleen
    Kidney
Endocrine-metabolic
  Reproduction
    Menstrual abnormalities
    Galactorrhea
    Decreased libido, impotence, low sex hormone-binding globulin
  Multiple endocrine neoplasia (I)
    Hyperparathyroidism
    Pancreatic islet-cell tumors
  Carbohydrate
    Impaired glucose tolerance
    Insulin resistance and hyperinsulinemia
    Diabetes mellitus
  Lipids
    Hypertriglyceridemia
  Mineral
    Hypercalciuria, increased 1,25 $(OH)_2D_3$
    Urinary hydroxyproline
  Electrolyte
    Low renin
    Increased aldosterone
  Thyroid
    Low thyroxine-binding globulin

Modified from Melmed S and Fagin J: *West J Med* 146:328, 1985.

BOX 295-4
Acromegaly: treatment options

Surgical
  Transsphenoidal pituitary adenomectomy or extrapituitary tumor
    resection
Medical
  Bromocriptine
  Somatostatin analog
Radiation
  Conventional or proton beam

---

ful, long-term cure of acromegaly. Surgery is the primary therapy, and medical or radiation therapy is often required as an adjuvant. The development of newer pharmacologic agents, especially SRIF analogs combined with bromocriptine, holds much future promise.

Transsphenoidal surgery. The recommended primary therapy for acromegaly is transsphenoidal pituitary adenomectomy performed by a skilled and experienced neurosurgeon. Growth hormone levels fall rapidly to normal within 1 hour of selective excision of GH cell adenomas, and the amelioration of soft tissue and metabolic effects caused by elevated GH levels begins almost immediately.

Several clinical and biochemical features usually predict the success of surgery. Almost 90% of patients with preoperative random serum GH levels less than 40 ng per milliliter and harboring an adenoma totally confined within the pituitary fossa have an initial reduction in serum GH levels to less than 5 ng per milliliter after surgery. Normal postoperative pituitary function is expected if the tumor is well encapsulated. Long-term follow-up results (5 years and later) in these patients, however, are less favorable. Tumor recurrence with or without clinical features of acromegaly and evidence of failure to suppress GH levels after oral glucose has been observed in patients who had initially met the criteria of cure. Incomplete surgical resection of tumor tissue may result in postoperative recurrence of acromegaly. Although GH cell adenomas are usually well encapsulated, functioning tumor cells may be seeded in the dura and escape visualization and resection. The most important endocrine side-effects of surgery are damage to the remainder of the normal pituitary gland, resultant pituitary failure, and necessity for lifelong hormone replacement. Cerebrospinal fluid leaks, sinusitis, central nervous system damage, hemorrhage, transient or permanent (infrequent) diabetes insipidus, meningitis, and arachnoiditis occur in about 5% of patients. The frequency of these complications is related to the size of the tumor. Postoperatively, an empty sella may rarely lead to impingement of the optic chiasm. A mortality rate of about 1% is seen, especially with large invasive tumors.

Radiation therapy. Irradiation is recommended as an adjuvant form of therapy in acromegaly. A total dose of 5000 rad is administered over 4 to 6 weeks. The time required to lower GH levels effectively by 50% is usually at least 2 years. After 10 years, GH levels are normalized in about 75% of acromegalics. The arrest of tumor growth is almost universal, and most GH cell adenomas eventually shrink after irradiation.

Radiation damage to the surrounding tissues may occur, especially if more than 5000 rad is administered. Some degree of hypopituitarism develops in approximately one half of all patients after 10 years. Hypocortisolism and hypogonadism are the usual hormone deficits; isolated hypothyroidism occurs in about 20% of these patients. Proton beam therapy has the advantage over conventional radiotherapy in that the patient can receive the total radiation dosage in only one or two visits without resulting skin damage. Radiation damage to cranial nerves and other surrounding structures, however, is a significant side-effect of this form of radiation. Radiation therapy is an inappropriate option for young patients because of the slow decrease in GH concentration.

Medical treatment of acromegaly
Bromocriptine. Bromocriptine (bromo-alpha-ergocryptine), a lysergic acid ergot derivative with dopamine agonist properties, may

---

Pituitary secretion of GH should be totally suppressed to stop the progression of physical signs caused by hypersomatotropinemia. In addition, any other pituitary trophic hormone disorders should also be corrected. Criteria for absolute cure of acromegaly include GH suppressibility after administration of oral glucose (<1 ng/ml), reappearance of normal circadian rhythm of GH secretion, normal GH increase after provocative stimulation, normal circulating IGF-I levels, and, finally, disappearance of paradoxic GH responses. By these criteria, no single therapeutic option (Box 295-4) really offers a 100% success-be used to treat acromegaly. Because neoplastic somatotrophs respond inappropriately to dopamine agonists by suppression of GH secretion in more than 50% of acromegalics, bromocriptine is useful as both primary and adjuvant medication for acromegaly. The doses of bromocriptine used in acromegaly are usually higher than those required to suppress PRL secretion. If a beneficial effect of bromocriptine is observed, it is usually seen with up to 30 mg of bromocriptine daily. Basal serum GH levels are decreased to less than 10 ng per milliliter in about 50% of cases. A GH level of less than 5 ng per milliliter has been observed in 20% of reported cases; shrinkage of tumor size probably only occurs in about 10% to 20% of cases. Most patients report a significant improvement in clinical symptoms, including reduction of perspiration, decreased soft tissue swelling, and decreased ring size. Bromocriptine therefore causes clinical improvement in many patients despite persistently raised GH and/or IGF-I levels.

Because bromocriptine is a dopamine agonist and possesses ergotlike properties, side-effects involving the cardiovascular, nervous, and digestive systems are anticipated. Although the incidence of adverse reactions to bromocriptine is quite high, these are usually transient in nature and mild or moderate in degree. Nausea, headache, dizziness, fatigue, lightheadedness, vomiting, abdominal cramps, nasal congestion, constipation, diarrhea, and drowsiness have been reported. Furthermore a mild hypotensive effect may result in postural orthostasis when therapy is initiated. Tolerance to these effects generally develops within 2 to 3 weeks of continued usage. Less frequent reactions include gastrointestinal bleeding, dizziness, exacerbation of Raynaud's syndrome, hair loss, alcohol potentiation, and visual hallucinations. These side-effects may be ameliorated by temporarily reducing the dosage of the medication and by increasing the dose by intervals no more frequent than every 3 days or longer. Gastrointestinal side-effects may be eased by prescribing the medication with meals. Nevertheless, the drug is remarkably free of major side-effects and has been used successfully for many years in patients with hyperprolactinemia, acromegaly, and Parkinson's disease.

Somatostatin analog. The physiologic inhibitor of GH secretion, SRIF, was a natural candidate as a pharmacologic agent in acromegaly. An octapeptide SRIF analog (octreotide, D-Phe-Cys-Phe-D-Tryp-Cys-Thr-[OH]) with high potency and prolonged inhibition of GH secretion has been used successfully to lower GH levels in most acromegalic patients and to shrink some GH cell adenomas.

The octapeptide SRIF analog (Octreotide) because of its prolonged half-life inhibits growth hormone secretion for 6 to 8 hours after a subcutaneous injection. Octreotide (100 μg every 8 hours subcutaneously) lowers growth hormone levels in most acromegalic patients and suppresses integrated growth hormone secretion over 6 hours to less than 5 ng/ml in about two thirds of patients. Similarly, IGF-I levels are normalized in about two thirds of the patients. The drug shrinks about 30% of growth hormone cell adenomas and also alleviates soft tissue swelling, excessive perspiration, joint pains, and headache. Side-effects include transient gastrointestinal upset and loose stools during the first 2 weeks of treatment. Intestinal malabsorption and asymptomatic gallstones occur in up to a third of patients receiving the medication long term. This promising new drug may be effective as a primary therapy of acromegaly (especially in elderly patients), as a presurgical drug to shrink tumors, or in postoperative treatment of recurrent acromegaly.

Hyperprolactinemia

Causes. Among the various physiologic states that influence PRL secretion are exercise, pregnancy, lactation, nipple stimulation, diet, and female orgasm (Box 295-5). Serum PRL levels are elevated by 60% within 2 hours of sleep onset, resulting in a circadian diurnal variation in PRL levels. Stress such as surgery or acute myocardial infarction can also result in hyperprolactinemia. Various pharmacologic agents have the ability to influence PRL secretion. These include dopamine receptor antagonists (e.g., metoclopramide), tricyclic antidepressants, reserpine, estrogens, opiates, and cimetidine. Hypothalamic and pituitary disorders are among the pathologic causes of hyperprolactinemia; diseases of the hypothalamus may lead to a reduction in dopamine secretion, resulting in disinhibition of PRL secretion. Lactotroph microadenomas or macroadenomas directly secrete PRL; pathologic processes directly involving the pituitary stalk may disrupt the hypothalamohypophyseal portal system and prevent

---

> ## BOX 295-5
> ## Causes of hyperprolactinemia
>
> Physiologic
> Pregnancy and lactation
> Sleep
> Stress
> Exercise
> Chest wall stimulation or trauma
> Coitus
> Pathologic
> Hypothalamic
>   Inflammation
>   Tumor
> Pituitary
>   Lactotroph microadenoma or macroadenoma
>   Acromegaly
>   Stalk section caused by pituitary or parasellar mass
>   Empty sella syndrome
> Peripheral
>   Hypothyroidism
>   Chronic renal failure
> Pharmacologic
> Psychotropic agents
>   Phenothiazines
>   Tricyclic antidepressants
>   Opiate alkaloids
> Antiemetics and antihistamines
>   Metoclopramide
>   Sulpiride
>   Cimetidine
> Antihypertensives
>   Methyldopa
>   Reserpine
> Hormones
>   Estrogens
>   Thyrotropin-releasing hormone

Modified from Melmed S et al: *Ann Intern Med* 105:238, 1986.

---

dopamine from reaching the lactotrophs. Primary hypothyroidism may be associated with hyperprolactinemia, especially in children, presumably through enhanced TRH stimulation of the lactotroph.

Thus hypersecretion of PRL may be accounted for by a factor that impedes dopamine synthesis or release, or by an increase in the release of a putative PRL-releasing factor. Similarly, factors that antagonize dopamine receptors may also account for elevated serum PRL levels.

Prolactin-Secreting Pituitary Tumors

Clinical presentation. Prolactinomas are the most common pituitary tumors. Although the tumorigenesis of prolactinomas is incompletely understood, the high rate of postsurgical recurrence implies that hypothalamic dysfunction is an important pathophysiologic factor. These tumors are diagnosed more often in women than men, possibly as a result of the difference in clinical manifestations between women and men (Table 295-3). Microadenomas are more common in women, and macroadenomas are more frequent in men. This may reflect a different natural history for these tumors in men and women. Only a small percentage of microadenomas in women appear to become macroadenomas. Furthermore, prolactinomas frequently cause menstrual disturbances, and thus tumors in women are generally discovered earlier than are the analogous tumors found in men. The presenting symptoms in men include decreased libido and impotence; these problems tend to become clinically manifest 10 to 15 years later than the presenting symptoms in women. By the time of diagnosis, the macroadenomas found in men may also have caused visual field abnormalities, secondary hypogonadism, hypothyroidism, and adrenal insufficiency.

The frequency of hyperprolactinemia correlates well with reproductive abnormalities in women. Approximately 15% of women with amenorrhea have elevated levels of serum PRL. In addition, 28% of women with galactorrhea without amenorrhea have hyperprolactine-

Table 295-3   Clinical features of patients with prolactin-secreting pituitary adenomas

	WOMEN (%)	MEN (%)	P VALUE
Mean age, years	28.4	43.3	<0.001
Amenorrhea	83	—	—
Primary amenorrhea	6	—	—
Oligomenorrhea	10	—	—
Galactorrhea	81	6	<0.001
Headaches	38	36	NS
Weight gain	25	22	NS
Visual abnormalities	10	38	<0.001
Decreased libido or impotence	14	71	<0.001
Fatigue	12	12	NS
Acne or hirsutism	8	—	—
Gynecomastia	—	21	—
Delayed sexual development	—	14	—
Macroadenoma	36	91	<0.001
Microadenoma	64	9	<0.001

Modified from Melmed S et al: *Ann Intern Med* 105:238, 1986.
NS, Nonsignificant.

mia. Of women who have both problems, more than three fourths have increased PRL levels. Infertility is found in many women with PRL-secreting tumors and is the result of anovulation or an insufficient luteal phase.

Elevated PRL levels have the potential to impede the cyclic release of gonadotropins. In addition, they may interrupt the peripheral activity of gonadotropins on the gonads. Thus women frequently suffer from estrogen deficiency, which in turn may lead to osteopenia and to decreased vaginal secretions causing dyspareunia. Hyperprolactinemia can also cause elevated androgen levels. In women, this can lead to hirsutism and acne. In men, however, serum testosterone levels are depressed in at least two thirds of patients with prolactinomas. When the tumor is detected and treated early, testosterone levels may ultimately increase back to normal. In other instances, irreversible damage to the pituitary gonadotrophs may prevent the normalization of testosterone levels. Furthermore elevated PRL levels may impede the peripheral action of testosterone, perhaps by interfering with the conversion of testosterone to dehydrotestosterone. Clinically, this condition can manifest as impotence.

Diagnosis. The first stage of diagnosis of PRL-secreting pituitary tumors involves measuring basal serum PRL concentrations. When levels exceed 200 ng per milliliter (upper limit of normal is 20 to 25 ng per milliliter), a pituitary tumor is very likely. Prolactinomas are invariably present when levels surpass 300 ng per milliliter. Levels below 200 ng per milliliter might be caused by a variety of conditions, including drug-induced hyperprolactinemia, renal failure, and thyroid or hypothalamic disorders. To confirm the presence of a tumor, CT or MRI scanning of the pituitary-hypothalamic region should be performed when several serum samples show persistent hyperprolactinemia.

Unfortunately, no definitive test determines whether elevated PRL levels result from pituitary tumors or from other causes. Nevertheless, TRH stimulation tests are commonly administered. In controls, serum PRL concentrations more than double during this test; most patients with PRL-secreting tumors exhibit no, or very little, change; however, this lack of response occurs despite the source of elevated PRL.

Medical management of hyperprolactinemia. Bromocriptine is the treatment of choice for hyperprolactinemia associated with amenorrhea, galactorrhea, and infertility. The initial dose of bromocriptine is 2.5 mg daily. An additional 2.5 mg tablet should be added every week until therapeutic response is achieved. The therapeutic dosage required to suppress PRL level and to reverse the signs and symptoms of hypogonadism ranges from 2.5 to 15.0 mg per day. Women should be counseled to use a mechanical contraceptive device to prevent unwanted pregnancy during bromocriptine treatment, because ovulatory menstrual cycles generally resume within 2 to 3 months. If menstruation does not occur within 3 days

of the expected period once ovulatory cycles are established, treatment with bromocriptine should be discontinued and a pregnancy test performed.

Bromocriptine is used for initial therapy in patients with PRL-secreting macroadenomas or persistent postsurgical hyperprolactinemia. The drug is also indicated to attempt shrinkage of large tumors before surgery. A number of studies have demonstrated the efficacy of bromocriptine as primary therapy for macroadenomas in treating visual and neurologic impairments as well as normalizing PRL levels. In a multicenter prospective study, tumor size was reduced by 50% or more in two thirds of patients harboring a PRL-secreting macroadenoma. In about a third of patients, tumor size was reduced by 10% to 25%. Even with dramatic reductions in PRL secretion and tumor size, pituitary function generally remains intact. Long-term postsurgical treatment prevents tumor regrowth and hyperprolactinemia. Bromocriptine treatment extending over 4 to 6 years has been continued with sustained benefits and few adverse effects. The drug lowers PRL levels, restores reproductive function in males and females, shrinks tumor size, and restores visual field deficits. Bromocriptine therefore offers safe and effective long-term therapy for prolactinomas. If, however, the bromocriptine is discontinued, the tumor may rapidly return to its original size.

Cushing's Disease

The clinical presentation of hypercortisolism is discussed elsewhere (Chapter 298). The primary therapy of Cushing's disease is surgical removal of the ACTH-secreting corticotroph cell adenoma. Because this tumor may be very small, in some patients no pituitary tumor is visualized even by current imaging techniques. In others, postsurgical recurrence of the excessive ACTH secretion occurs. The major causes of patient morbidity and mortality resulting from Cushing's disease include arteriosclerosis, infection, and depression leading to suicide. Because of these deleterious effects on patient morbidity and a 5 year mortality rate of 50%, aggressive therapeutic intervention is warranted.

Medical Management

Neuropharmacologic. As several brain and hypothalamic neurotransmitters that regulate POMC secretion have now been recognized, several neuropharmacologic agents have been used to control excessive ACTH secretion.

Serotonin is a potent stimulator of ACTH release. Cyproheptadine, an antiserotoninergic agent that acts to block ACTH release at the level of the hypothalamus, has been used to treat recurrent or primary Cushing's disease when surgery is contraindicated. Clinical and biochemical remission occurs in a small percentage of patients after about 3 months of medication. The drug has also been used as an adjuvant to pituitary irradiation. The initial dose of 4 mg three times a day is increased gradually to 4 mg every 4 hours. Side-effects of cyproheptadine include hyperphagia and somnolence. Excessive ACTH secretion invariably recurs after the drug is discontinued.

Although bromocriptine is not primarily indicated for treating corticotroph cell adenomas, it may acutely suppress ACTH secretion in some patients. Bromocriptine nonresponders often harbor relatively easily excisable ACTH-secreting adenomas. Patients who suppress ACTH levels with bromocriptine appear to have a less favorable response to surgical resection of the adenoma.

Steroidogenesis inhibitors. The biosynthesis of adrenal steroids is a complex posttranslational event, involving several key enzymes. *Ketoconozole,* an antifungal agent, inhibits steroidogenesis and has been used successfully to suppress urinary cortisol excretion during long-term treatment with 400 to 800 mg daily. Because gonadal steroidogenesis may also be blocked, some patients may require sex steroid replacement. Limited evidence suggests that ketoconozole inhibits ACTH secretion at the pituitary or hypothalamic level. *Metyrapone,* an inhibitor of 11-beta-hydroxylase as well as of pregnenolone production, suppresses cortisol synthesis and secretion within a week of starting treatment. The side-effects of the drug include exacerbation of hirsutism, nausea, and gastrointestinal discomfort. Although long-term treatment effectively inhibits steroidogenesis, hypertension and hypokalemia may result from the accumulation of mineralocorticoids above the enzymatic block. *Aminoglutethimide* blocks the conversion of cholesterol to pregnenolone. Within 3 to 5 days of administration (up to 1.5 g/day), adrenal steroidogenesis is suppressed, but the resultant increased release of ACTH may override the enzyme block and continue to stimulate cortisol production. Side-effects include skin rash and lethargy. Combination therapy with metyrapone may allow lower doses of aminoglutethimide to be used. Mitotane is a potent inhibitor of adrenal steroidogenesis, and its long-term use results in a "medical" adrenalectomy. The doses used in Cushing's disease (5 to 12 g daily) are lower than those usually used for adrenal carcinoma. Significant lowering of cortisol levels occurs in approximately 50% of patients within 6 months. Side-effects of mitotane include hypotension and secondary hypercholesterolemia. Mifepristone (RU-486), a peripheral glucocorticoid antagonist, acutely lowers cortisol levels, but its long-term efficacy is not proved.

Gonadotropin-Secreting Pituitary Tumors

Clinical Presentation. Gonadotropin-secreting pituitary tumors are rare pituitary tumors that occur mainly in male patients. They usually appear as a result of local pressure signs, for example, visual impairment. The patient also may have hypogonadism caused by down regulation of the pituitary gonadal axis by the high levels of secreted gonadotropins, although some patients may actually have longstanding primary hypogonadism resulting in gonadotroph hyperplasia and adenoma formation.

The majority of these patients have increased circulating levels of FSH and LH with respective discordant increases of the beta LH and beta FSH subunits, as compared to the alpha subunit. Most patients respond to GnRH by enhanced secretion of gonadotropins. Some patients may retain a degree of normal feedback regulation by showing suppression of gonadotropin levels with administration of sex steroids.

Gonadal function is usually suppressed in these patients with low or normal testosterone levels, or low or normal sperm counts. Rarely, excessive production of LH alone by a tumor may result in increased levels of testosterone.

Differential Diagnosis. The diagnosis is difficult to make in females because of the associated high gonadotropin levels of postmenopausal women. Primary gonadal failure or menopausal failure may result in secondary pituitary enlargement, further confounding the differential diagnosis.

Treatment. Treatment of these tumors is primarily surgical. The large pituitary mass should be resected. Adjuvant treatment with bromocriptine has been successful in several patients who have shown suppression of the elevated gonadotropin levels. The drug is especially useful for recurrences of the excess gonadotropin secretion after surgery.

Thyroid-Stimulating Hormone-Secreting Tumors

The thyroid-stimulating hormone-secreting tumors are extremely rare and are often plurihormonal and secrete GH, PRL, and alpha glycoprotein subunits as well as TSH. Approximately one half of the patients with these tumors have associated acromegaly or hyperprolactinemia. Thyroid-stimulating hormone-secreting tumors exhibit the signs and symptoms of hyperthyroidism. The cardinal features include inappropriately elevated TSH levels in the presence of elevated thyroid hormone levels. Interestingly, about a third of patients treated for TSH-secreting pituitary tumors have TSH levels less than 10 μU per milliliter. New ultrasensitive TSH radioimmunoassay should therefore be used to discriminate between low and inappropriately "normal" circulating TSH levels in patients with hyperthyroidism.

Treatment. The treatment of these tumors is primarily surgical excision. Bromocriptine and SRIF analog may be used as adjuncts to surgical management. Octreotide also effectively controls the hypersecretion of TSH and the associated hyperthyroidism in some patients as well as shrinking tumor size.

Empty Sella Syndrome

Acquired or congenital anatomic defects in the diaphragma sella may allow arachnoid herniation into the pituitary fossa, leading to formation of an empty sella. The sella becomes partially filled by arachnoid membrane, CSF, and the compressed pituitary gland. The empty sella syndrome is fairly common and accounts for about one third of radiologically demonstrable pituitary sella abnormalities.

Causes. A primary empty sella probably results from a congenital weakness in the diaphragma sella. This has been associated with obesity in females, increased intracranial pressure, multiparity, and hypertension. Other primary causes include intracranial tumors, pseudotumor cerebri, hydrocephalus, and hypoventilation with or without associated congestive heart failure. Several conditions may lead to a secondary empty sella. These include damage to the pituitary gland after pituitary surgery, radiation, hemorrhage, and infarction. The infarction may occur spontaneously in a normal pituitary gland (e.g., Sheehan's syndrome) or in a pituitary adenoma.

Clinical Presentation. The empty sella is usually asymptomatic and is detected on routine imaging of the head. Approximately 10% of patients with the empty sella syndrome, however, have a history of chronic headaches. Visual field disturbances are rare and may result from herniation of the optic chiasm into the CSF compartment within the sella.

Endocrine function in such patients is usually normal, although partial hypopituitarism may be present in a minority. A blunting of the GH or cortisol response to insulin-induced hypoglycemia may be a subtle indication of pituitary failure in patients primarily affected by empty sella syndrome. The presence of isolated or multiple trophic pituitary hormone deficiencies in association with the empty sella suggests that the lesion may have been caused by infarction of a pituitary adenoma. Acromegaly, hyperprolactinemia, and Cushing's disease have also been described in the presence of an empty sella.

Differential Diagnosis. The primary diagnosis of empty sella is made by sensitive imaging techniques including MRI and CT scanning. The classic radiologic picture is the infundibulum "sign," in which the pituitary stalk is clearly identified with the flattened pituitary tissue. The density of the CSF occupying the sella is also clearly distinguishable from normal pituitary density by MRI. Finally, herniation of the optic chiasm may be noted in the sella. It is important to distinguish intrasellar pituitary lesions from empty sella syndrome. The MRI and CT imaging may usually help make this distinction. Nevertheless, the presence of a microadenoma in the remnant pituitary tissue may pose a difficult radiologic diagnostic dilemma.

Treatment. Corrective surgery may be required for persistent CSF rhinorrhea, visual field defects, or prolapse of the optic chiasm. Endocrine deficits should be treated by replacement with specific hormones, and endocrine hyperfunction should be treated in relation to the specific hormone being hypersecreted by the concurrent adenoma.

BIBLIOGRAPHY

Greenman Y, Melmed S: Diagnosis and management of non-functioning pituitary tumors, *Annu Rev Med* 47:95, 1996.

Herman VS and Braunstein GD: Gonadotropin secretory abnormalities, *Endocr Metab Clin* 20:519, 1991.

Iranmanesh A et al: Low basal and persistent pulsatile growth hormone secretion in normal and hyposomatotrophic men studied with a new ultrasensitive chemiluminescence assay *J Clin Endo Metab* 78:526, 1994.

Jorgensen JOL: Human growth hormone replacement therapy: pharmacologic and clinical aspects, *Endocr Rev* 12:189, 1991.

Kohler PO: Treatment of pituitary adenomas, *N Engl J Med* 317:45, 1987.

Lamberts S et al: Octreotide, *N Engl J Med* 334:246, 1996.

Loriaux L: Treatment of Cushing's syndrome and adrenal cancer, *Endocr Metab Clin* 20:767, 1991.

Melmed S: Acromegaly, *N Engl J Med* 322:966, 1990.

Melmed S et al: Recent advances in pathogenesis, diagnosis and management of acromegaly, *J Clin Endo Metab* 80:3395, 1995.

Neely EK, Rosenfeld RG: Use and abuse of human growth hormone, *Annu Rev Med* 45:407, 1994.

✔ *WHEN TO REFER*

The patient harboring a functional or nonfunctional pituitary tumor should be referred to an endocrinologist to confirm the diagnosis and to initiate therapeutic measures. Once the initial therapy has been determined, patients will require long-term endocrine follow-up, including imaging, biochemical, visual, and systemic clinical testing. As treatment choices often entail weighing relative benefits and risks, the patient will often benefit from the combined counsel of the referring physician, the consulting endocrinologist, and the neurosurgeon.

For patients diagnosed with pituitary failure, after initial evaluation and therapeutic stabilization by an endocrinologist the referring physician may continue to manage the patient and should be alert for potential complications or changing treatment requirements (e.g., pregnancy, surgery, or other illness).

Novel treatment such as octreotide, growth hormone, or oral DDAVP should initially be started under the auspices of an endocrinologist.

Sheldon WR et al: Rapid sequential intravenous administration of four hypothalamic releasing hormones as a combined anterior pituitary function test in normal subjects, *J Clin Endocrinol Metab* 60:623, 1985.

Vance ML: Hypopituitarism, *N Engl J Med* 330:1651, 1994.

CHAPTER

296 Disorders of the Posterior Pituitary

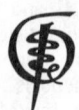

Gary L. Robertson

BASIC PRINCIPLES
Anatomy

The *posterior pituitary,* or *neurohypophysis,* is an extension of the ventral hypothalamus that penetrates the diaphragma sellae and attaches to the dorsal and caudal surfaces of the adenohypophysis. The part above the diaphragm is variously referred to as the *infundibulum* or *median eminence,* and that below as the *infundibular process* or *pars nervosa.* The posterior pituitary is supplied with blood by the superior and inferior hypophyseal arteries, which arise from the posterior communicating and intracavernous portion of the internal carotid. The arterioles divide in the pars nervosa into localized capillary networks that drain directly into the jugular vein via the sellar, cavernous, and lateral venous sinuses. In the infundibulum, the capillary networks coalesce into the portal veins, which supply blood to the adenohypophysis.

On histologic examination, the neurohypophysis appears as a network of capillaries, pituicytes, and nonmyelinated nerve fibers containing numerous electron-dense neurosecretory granules. The neurons terminate as bulbous enlargements juxtaposed to capillary networks scattered throughout all levels of the neurohypophysis. Those that reach the pars nervosa appear to originate primarily in nuclei of the supraoptic and, to a lesser extent, the paraventricular regions of the hypothalamus. Those neurons that terminate more proximally, particularly in the median eminence, probably arise in other hypothalamic areas, primarily the paraventricular nucleus (Fig. 296-1). Neurosecretory neurons from this nucleus also project to other parts of the brain, most notably the nucleus tractus solitarius and/or vasomotor center in the medulla.

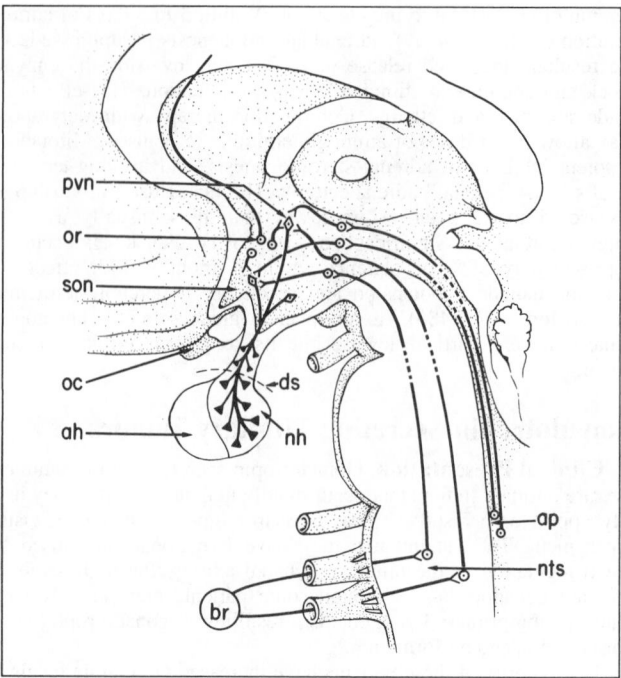

FIGURE 296-1   The neurohypophysis and its principal regulatory afferents. *nh,* Neurohypophysis; *ah,* adenohypophysis; *ds,* diaphragma sellae; *oc,* optic chiasm; *son,* supraoptic nucleus; *pvn,* paraventricular nucleus; *or,* osmoreceptor; *br,* volume and baroreceptor; *nts,* nucleus tractus solitarius; *ap,* area postrema (emetic center).

Modified from Robertson GL. In Ingbar SH, editor: *The year of endocrinology 1977,* New York, 1978, Plenum.

Biochemistry

Chemistry. Vasopressin and oxytocin are the major if not the only hormones secreted by the neurohypophysis in adult humans. Both hormones are nonapeptides composed of a six-membered disulfide ring and a three-membered tail, on which the terminal carboxyl group is amidated (Fig. 296-2). Vasopressin differs from oxytocin in that phenylalanine is substituted for isoleucine in the ring, and arginine for leucine in the tail. These two changes confer markedly different biologic properties on the peptides.

Both vasopressin and oxytocin are stored in the posterior pituitary as insoluble complexes with specific proteins known as *neurophysins.* Two distinct types of neurophysin have been identified in humans. One is found exclusively in granules containing oxytocin, the other in association with vasopressin. Both neurophysins appear to be single-chain polypeptides of approximately 10,000 molecular weight (MW). Each neurophysin binds oxytocin and vasopressin equally well, indicating that the specific hormonal associations found in vivo are a function of cellular compartmentalization as well as a common biosynthesis.

Synthesis and Hormone Release. Vasopressin and oxytocin are synthesized in the supraoptic and paraventricular nuclei, packaged in granules with neurophysins, and transported down the axons to terminal dilations, where they are stored until release. Each hormone is produced by a different population of neurons. However, the biosynthetic mechanisms appear to be similar. Synthesis of vasopressin occurs via a macromolecular precursor that also contains the sequence for neurophysin and a glycoprotein. The gene that codes for this precursor is located on chromosome 20 and is composed of three exons. The precursor is cleaved during transport to yield the active hormone, neurophysin, and other still unidentified peptides. Stimuli, such as dehydration, increase synthesis as well as secretion of the hormone. Mutations in the gene that codes for the vasopressin precursor recently have been linked to the inherited form of neurogenic diabetes insipidus (discussed later).

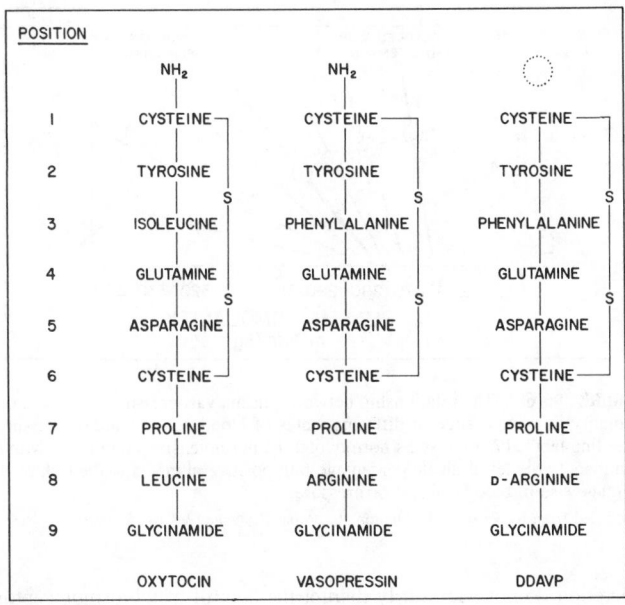

FIGURE 296-2   The structure of oxytocin, vasopressin, and a synthetic analog, 1-desamino-8-D-arginine vasopressin (DDAVP).

Vasopressin secretion, together with that of its associated neurophysin, probably occurs through a calcium-dependent process of exocytosis similar to those described for other neurosecretory systems. In plasma, the neurophysin-hormone complex dissociates completely, and most if not all plasma vasopressin circulates in the free or unbound state. However, platelets contain relatively large amounts of vasopressin that is taken up from plasma and released or metabolized very slowly.

Physiology

Control of Secretion. Vasopressin secretion is influenced by a number of different factors. Probably the most important influence under physiologic conditions is the osmotic pressure of body water. This effect is mediated by osmosensitive neurons located in the anterior hypothalamus near the supraoptic nuclei (Fig. 296-1). Osmoregulatory function can be examined by measuring plasma vasopressin level in healthy adults during various states of hydration (Fig. 296-3). At plasma osmolalities below a certain minimum or "threshold" value, plasma vasopressin is uniformly suppressed to low or undetectable levels. Above the threshold, plasma vasopressin level rises in direct proportion to osmolality. A plasma osmolality change of only 1% is sufficient to cause a measurable change in plasma vasopressin level. This extreme sensitivity enables the osmoregulatory system to play a dominant role in mediating the vasopressin response to changes in water balance.

The response of this osmoregulatory system is also remarkably precise. Although there is a relatively large scatter in the relationship between plasma vasopressin level and plasma osmolality in the normal adult population (Fig. 296-3), this variation is due principally to large individual differences in the set and sensitivity of the system. The basis for these individual differences in osmoregulatory function is not completely known. Aging is associated with some increase in sensitivity but cannot be the only cause, because even among young adults, sensitivity may differ by more than 10 times. Recent studies indicate that these individual differences are relatively constant and are determined to a great extent by heredity. The function of the osmoregulatory system is similar in males and females, although the threshold or set of the system is reduced during pregnancy and the luteal phase of the menstrual cycle.

The sensitivity of the osmoreactor is not the same for all plasma solutes (Fig. 296-4). Sodium and associated anions, which normally constitute more than 95% of the total osmotic pressure in plasma, are the most effective solutes in stimulating vasopressin secretion. Sug-

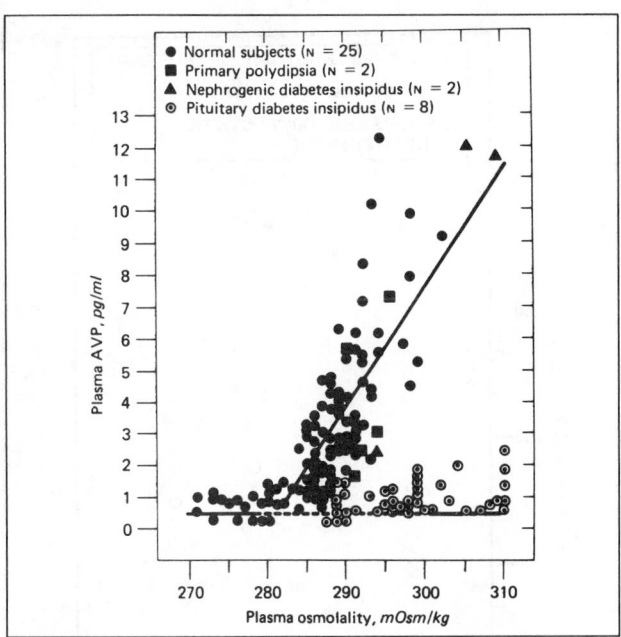

FIGURE 296-3   The relationship of plasma vasopressin (AVP) to plasma osmolality in healthy adults and patients with polyuria of diverse causes. *AVP,* plasma vasopressin.

From Robertson GL et al: *J Clin Invest* 52:2340, 1973.

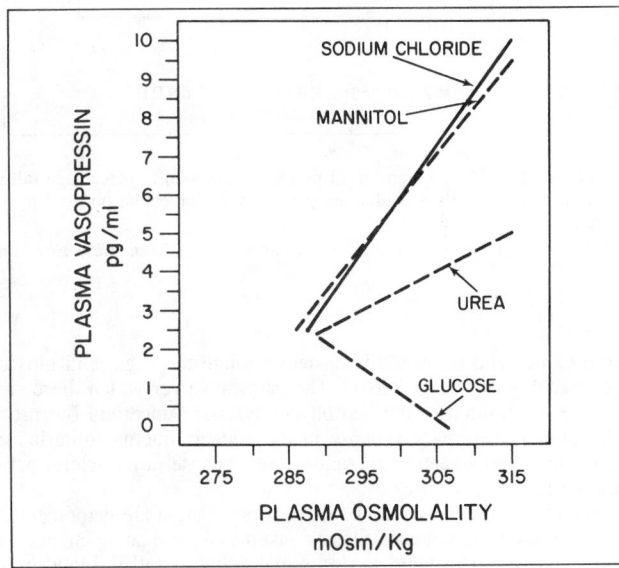

FIGURE 296-4   The relationship of plasma vasopressin to plasma osmolality in healthy adults during the infusion of hypertonic solutions of various solutes.

ars, such as mannitol and sucrose, are also very potent when given intravenously. In contrast, an increase in plasma osmolality produced by urea or glucose causes minimal or no stimulation of vasopressin secretion in healthy persons. In patients with insulin-deficient diabetes mellitus, however, hyperglycemia is moderately stimulatory. The mechanism by which the osmoreceptor discriminates between different solutes or the same solute under different conditions is not known with certainty, but it is thought to be based on the differences in cellular permeability.

Vasopressin secretion also can be influenced by acute alterations in blood volume or pressure. These effects are mediated primarily by afferent fibers that arise in baroreceptors in the heart, aortic arch, and

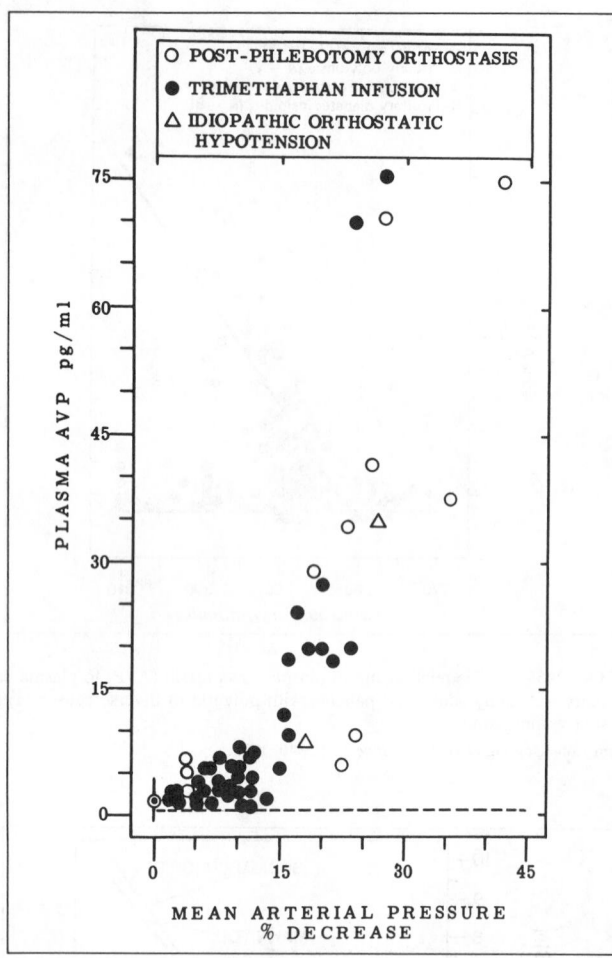

FIGURE 296-5 The relationship of plasma vasopressin to percentage fall in blood pressure in healthy adults and patients with idiopathic postural hypotension.

From Robertson GL: In Felig P et al, editors: *Endocrinology and metabolism,* New York, 1981, McGraw-Hill.

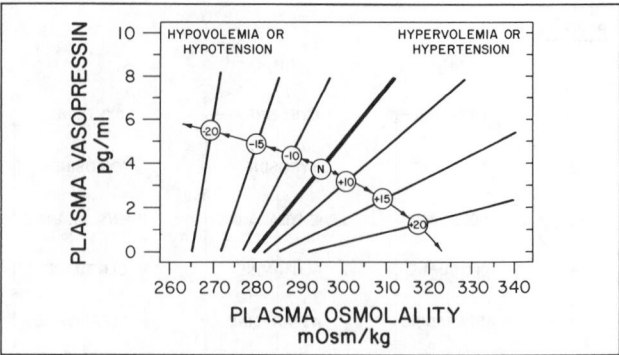

FIGURE 296-6 The relationship between plasma vasopressin and plasma osmolality in the presence of differing states of blood volume and/or pressure. The line labeled *N* represents normovolemic, normotensive conditions. Minus numbers to the left indicate percentage fall; positive numbers to the right, percentage rise in blood volume or pressure.

Modified from Robertson GL, Shelton RL, Athar S: *Kidney Int* 10:25, 1976.

carotid sinus and reach the brainstem through the vagal and glossopharyngeal nerves (Fig. 296-1). The pathways over which these signals are transmitted to the neurohypophysis are uncertain but probably involve a primary synapse in the nucleus tractus solitarius of the medulla and a secondary, opioidergic synapse in the lateral parabrachial nucleus.

The characteristics of the baroregulatory system are demonstrated by the relationship between plasma vasopressin and acute changes in arterial pressure (Fig. 296-5). In normal adults, a fall in blood pressure increases plasma vasopressin level by an amount that is roughly proportional to the degree of hypotension. However, because this relationship is exponential or curvilinear, there is little or no effect on vasopressin until blood pressure falls by more than 10%, which usually evokes a very large response. The volume control of vasopressin secretion in humans appears to respond in a similar manner. Thus upright posture, which acutely lowers central or effective blood volume by 8% to 15%, usually has minimal effects on vasopressin in healthy adults, whereas upright posture superimposed on acute diuretic-induced volume depletion significantly increases plasma vasopressin in direct proportion to the absolute level of hypovolemia achieved. The relative insensitivity of vasopressin secretion to small changes in blood volume is considerably different from the extreme potency of osmotic stimuli. This difference in sensitivity is important for understanding both the physiologic processes of water balance and the mechanism of action of certain commonly used diagnostic tests for vasopressin activity.

Blood volume or pressure changes sufficient to affect vasopressin secretion do not necessarily disrupt the control of the osmoreceptor. In fact, they appear to shift the set of the system in such a way as to increase or decrease the effect of a given osmotic stimulus (Fig. 296-6). Therefore, even during significant hypovolemia and/or hypotension, plasma vasopressin level can still be suppressed or stimulated appropriately by changes in plasma osmolality. This type of interaction indicates that osmotic and hemodynamic stimuli ultimately converge and act on the same population of neurosecretory neurons. Moreover, the vasopressin response to acute hypotension and/or hypovolemia appears to decrease with sustained stimulation. The mechanism of this attenuation has not been ascertained but appears to involve "resetting" of the baroregulatory system. However, it may be important for understanding the abnormalities in vasopressin secretion in patients with congestive heart failure or other chronic abnormalities in hemodynamic function.

Vasopressin secretion also may be stimulated by nonosmotic and nonhemodynamic factors. In humans one potent stimulus is nausea. The pathway mediating this response has not been defined but appears to involve the chemoreceptor trigger zone in the area postrema of the medulla (Fig. 296-1). Drugs and procedures, including apomorphine, morphine, nicotine, and alcohol and chemotherapy, can activate this pathway. The effect on vasopressin secretion is potent and immediate. Vasopressin levels elevations up to 100 to 1000 times basal levels may occur even when the nausea is transient and no vomiting or blood pressure changes are noted. Fluphenazine, haloperidol, or promethazine in doses sufficient to prevent nausea prevents the vasopressin response.

Acute insulin-induced hypoglycemia is a less potent stimulus for vasopressin release. The receptor and pathway mediating this effect are unknown but appear to be different from those for osmotic, hemodynamic, and emetic stimuli. The degree of hypoglycemia required to evoke vasopressin release has not been defined precisely but appears to be similar to that for other hormones responding to hypoglycemia. A 50% fall in plasma glucose level induced by insulin increases plasma vasopressin two- to fourfold. Whether other forms of hypoglycemia have similar effects on vasopressin level is unknown, but 2-deoxyglucose, which produces intracellular glucopenia, is also stimulatory.

Angiotensin II also has been implicated in the control of vasopressin secretion. Its mode of action is uncertain but appears to involve one or more sites in the central nervous system. The levels of plasma renin and/or angiotensin required to stimulate vasopressin release are probably quite high. Most of the studies have reported infusion of angiotensin in pressor doses with two- to fourfold increases in plasma vasopressin level. Whether the endogenous renin-angiotensin system plays an important role in the pathophysiology of vasopressin secretion has not been established.

Acute hypoxia or hypercapnia also stimulates vasopressin release. The pathways that mediate these effects have not been well defined but appear to involve peripheral as well as central chemoreceptors.

BOX 296-1

Drugs and hormones that affect vasopressin secretion

Stimulatory	Inhibitory
Acetylcholine	Norepinephrine
Nicotine	Fluphenazine
Apomorphine	Haloperidol
Morphine (high doses)	Promethazine
Epinephrine	Oxilorphan
Isoproterenol	Butorphanol
Histamine	Morphine (low doses)
Bradykinin	Alcohol
Prostaglandins	Carbamazepine
Beta-endorphin	Glucocorticoids
Cyclophosphamide (iv)	? Phenytoin
Vincristine	Clonidine
Insulin	Muscimol
2-Deoxyglucose	
Angiotensin	
Lithium	
? Chlorpropamide	
? Clofibrate	

The "thresholds" for these stimuli in humans are also uncertain, but, in the case of acute hypoxia, a fall in PaO$_2$ to less than 40 torr appears to be necessary. This mechanism probably is responsible for the osmotically inappropriate secretion of vasopressin that occurs in many patients with acute respiratory failure.

Pain, emotion, physical exercise, or other forms of nonspecific stress have long been thought to cause the release of vasopressin. However, it is unknown whether the response to stress is specific or due simply to some secondary stimulus such as the hypotension and/or nausea that often accompanies a vasovagal reaction to pain or intense emotion. In humans as well as rats, pain or other noxious stimuli of an intensity sufficient to activate the pituitary adrenal axis and sympathetic nervous system do not stimulate vasopressin secretion unless they also produce nausea and/or hypotension. Elevations in temperature are also reported to stimulate vasopressin release, but again, it is unclear whether the effect is primary or secondary to changes in blood volume and pressure. Resolution of these issues is necessary for understanding the pathogenesis of the inappropriate secretion of the hormone that occurs in a variety of clinical conditions (Chapter 112).

Many drugs and hormones also influence the secretion of vasopressin (Box 296-1). Stimulants, such as isoproterenol, nicotine, and apomorphine, probably act, at least in part, by producing nausea or lowering blood pressure. Agents such as histamine, bradykinin, the prostaglandins, beta-endorphin, morphine, and cyclophosphamide may act by the same mechanisms. Vincristine and lithium may stimulate by a direct effect on the neurohypophysis. The increase of vasopressin caused by chlorpropamide, clofibrate, and carbamazepine is still controversial, and a mechanism of action has not been proposed.

Pressor agents such as norepinephrine inhibit vasopressin release indirectly by raising arterial pressure. Dopaminergic antagonists, including fluphenazine, haloperidol, and promethazine, appear to act through suppression of the chemoreceptor trigger zone because they inhibit vasopressin release to emetic but not to osmotic or hemodynamic stimuli. Glucocorticoids appear to inhibit vasopressin secretion in healthy adults as well as in patients with adrenal insufficiency. However, it is still unclear whether these steroids act centrally or by raising blood volume and pressure. Intravenous phenytoin may inhibit vasopressin release, but the effect is inconsistent and the mechanism has not been defined. Opiates, including oxilorphan, butorphanol, and low doses of morphine, inhibit vasopressin secretion by raising the osmotic threshold. Carbamazepine inhibits vasopressin by decreasing the sensitivity of the osmostat.

The regulation of oxytocin secretion is understood less well because assays with the requisite sensitivity and specificity were not developed until very recently. However, secretion is known to be stimulated by breast-feeding. In humans, it is not stimulated by hyperosmolality or nausea but may be increased slightly by acute hypoglycemia.

Distribution and Clearance. After release into the systemic circulation, vasopressin is rapidly distributed throughout the extracellular fluid. Equilibration between the intravascular and extravascular compartments occurs within 15 minutes. This rate is consistent with the molecular size and absence of binding to macromolecular components of plasma. After achieving equilibrium, vasopressin is cleared more slowly from the plasma. This slower disappearance probably reflects irreversible or metabolic clearance. The rate of this clearance varies considerably from person to person; average half-time is about 16 minutes.

Most of the vasopressin clearance in vivo appears to take place in the liver and kidney. These organs appear to inactivate vasopressin through reduction of the disulfide bridge followed by cleavage of the bond between residues 1 and 2. In pregnant women, the metabolism of vasopressin is increased slightly by a proteolytic enzyme known as *vasopressinase,* which appears in plasma by the second trimester and does not disappear until the second to fourth postpartum week. Because the activity of the enzyme is increased by contact with plastic or glass, reliable measurement of vasopressin level in pregnancy plasma requires the use of special proteolytic inhibitors during collection and processing of the samples.

Some undegraded vasopressin is excreted intact in urine. The amount varies considerably, but in normally hydrated healthy adults, it is rarely more than about 1% to 5% of the total metabolic clearance rate. Although the mechanisms involved in vasopressin excretion are not known, it probably is filtered at the glomerulus and reabsorbed to varying degrees by the tubules. This readsorption seems to be linked in some way to the renal clearance of sodium, because the urinary clearance of vasopressin varies markedly in close association with changes in solute clearance. Therefore measurements of urinary vasopressin do not always provide a reliable guide to changes in plasma vasopressin, particularly when there are changes in glomerular filtration and/or solute excretion.

Oxytocin distribution and clearance appear to be similar to those of vasopressin. Almost nothing is known about the metabolism or clearance of neurophysin except that it too can be recovered from urine.

Action. The major function of vasopressin is conservation of body water by reduction of urine output. This antidiuretic effect is achieved by promoting the reabsorption of solute-free water in the distal and/or collecting tubules of the nephron (Chapters 101 and 112). The degree of urinary concentration varies as a function of the plasma vasopressin level (Fig. 296-7). In healthy adults, this relationship is quite sensitive, because maximum urinary concentration occurs at a plasma vasopressin level of only about 5 pg per milliliter. At similar concentrations, vasopressin also reduces the rate of extrarenal water loss.

In addition to its effects on water output, vasopressin also causes contraction of smooth muscle in blood vessels and the gastrointestinal tract, secretion of adrenocorticotropic hormone (ACTH) by the anterior pituitary, hepatic glycogenolysis, platelet aggregation, release of factor VIII by endothelium, and alterations in firing by a variety of brain neurons. The concentration of vasopressin required to affect these systems is not known, but it appears to be many times greater than those found in systemic plasma under physiologic conditions. It is conceivable, however, that the marked increases in vasopressin secretion produced by such stimuli as hypotension or nausea reach levels sufficient to affect vascular tone, gastrointestinal tract motility, portal blood flow, or clotting. The cellular mechanisms involved in the extrarenal actions of vasopressin are still undefined. It has been found, however, that the vascular, pituitary, and renal tubular effects of the hormone are mediated by different receptors (V1A, V1B, and V$_2$) with affinities for different parts of the vasopressin molecule. Structural modifications that abolish pressor activity do not decrease, and may even enhance, its antidiuretic activity. Analogs capable of antagonizing selectively the pressor and antidiuretic actions of vasopressin have been developed and used effectively in experimental studies in human volunteers. However, they are not yet available in

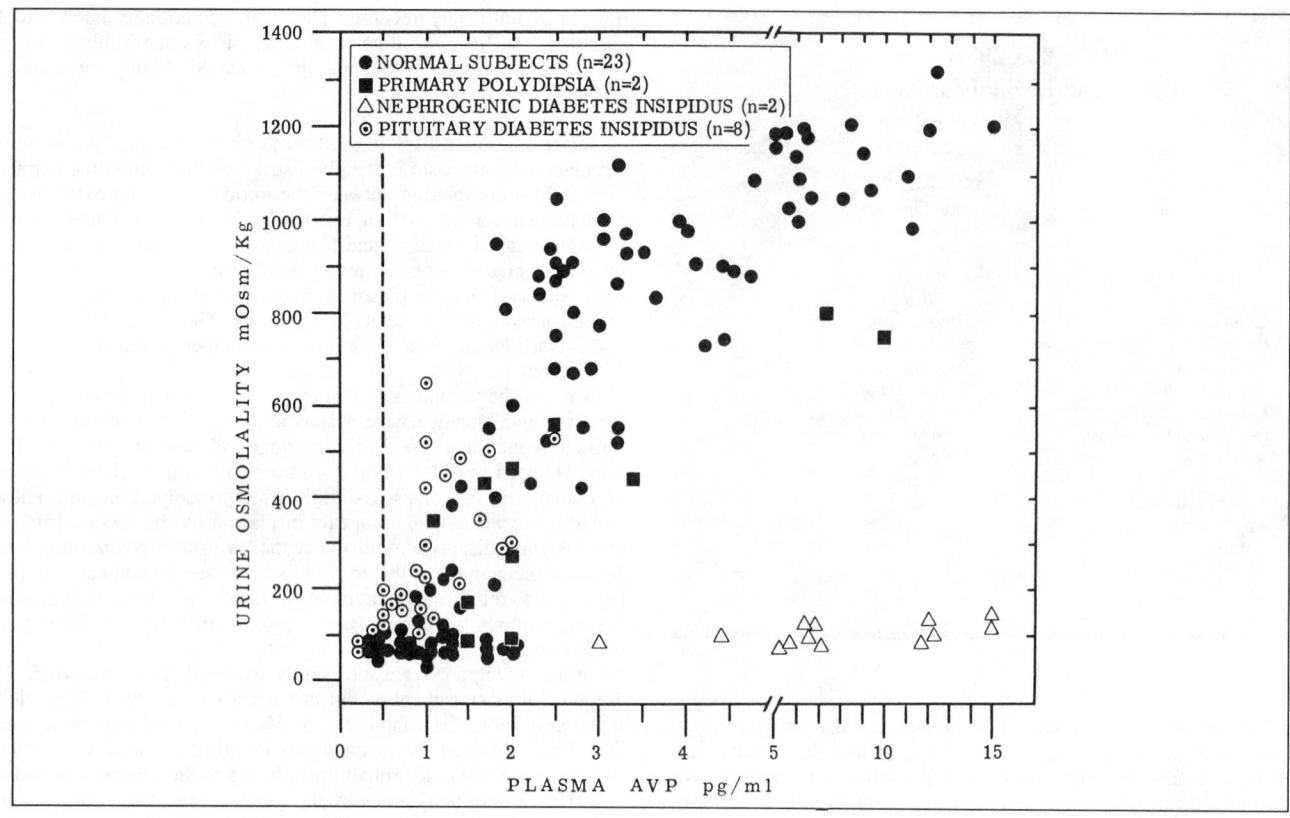

FIGURE 296-7   The relationship of urine osmolality to plasma vasopressin concentration in healthy adults in various states of hydration and in patients with polyuria of diverse causes.
From Robertson GL et al: *J Clin Invest* 52:2340, 1973.

the United States for treating disorders caused by excessive production of vasopressin.

A major biologic action of oxytocin is to facilitate breast-feeding by causing the ejection of milk. This effect occurs through stimulation of contractile epithelial cells in the lactating mammary gland. Oxytocin appears to stimulate contraction of the uterus at parturition. Whether the hormone has any significant effect in males is unknown. Recently it has been shown that oxytocin has significant antidiuretic effects in some patients with neurogenic diabetes insipidus, suggesting that a chronic deficiency of vasopressin alters the V_2 receptor to enhance its receptivity and/or responsiveness to oxytocin.

The neurophysins have no recognized biologic action apart from complexing oxytocin and vasopressin in neurosecretory granules. Although present in plasma, they do not serve as binding or transport proteins because, in blood, the higher pH and lower concentration of the reactants favor complete dissociation.

Extrarenal Water Output. The volume of water lost by evaporation from skin and lungs varies markedly, depending on such factors as dress, humidity, environmental temperature, activity, and vasopressin secretion. Under conditions typical of modern, sedentary urban life, insensible water loss in a healthy 70-kg man or woman approximates urine output (1 L/day). However, if vasopressin is absent or activity or temperature increases, the rate of insensible water loss also rises and, under extreme conditions, may approach the maximum rate of water excretion by the kidney (20 L/day). Hence, in quantitative terms, insensible water loss and the factors that influence it are just as important to the economy of water balance as are the factors that regulate urine output.

Water Intake. The thirst mechanism provides an indispensable adjunct to the antidiuretic mechanism in controlling water balance. In physiologic usage, *thirst* is defined as a consciously perceived need for water. This drive must be distinguished from dietary, social, psy-

chogenic, and other environmental causes of drinking. Thirst is stimulated by many of the factors that cause vasopressin release. Hypertonicity of the plasma appears to be the most potent stimulus. Normally, an increase in plasma osmolality of only 2% to 3% above basal levels results in a strong desire to drink. The absolute level of plasma osmolality at which thirst develops varies somewhat from person to person but averages about 295 mOsm per kilogram. This level is considerably above the osmotic threshold for vasopressin release and closely approximates that at which maximum concentration of the urine normally occurs. Water intake can also be osmotically inhibited. This inhibitory control manifests as a sense of satiation and a reduction in the basal rate discretionary fluid intake when healthy adults are treated with saturating doses of antidiuretic hormone. It occurs with reductions in plasma osmolality and sodium of only 1% to 3% and is normally sufficient to prevent water intoxication even if antidiuresis is fixed at maximum levels.

Although the neuronal pathways that mediate thirst and satiation have not been totally defined, they appear to involve osmoreceptors located in the anterolateral hypothalamus near, but not totally coincident with, the osmoreceptors that regulate vasopressin release. The specificities of the two systems appear to be similar. Thus plasma solutes such as sodium or mannitol are potent dipsogens, whereas plasma urea or glucose has little or no effect on thirst.

A decrease in blood volume or pressure is also dipsogenic. The degree of hypovolemia and/or hypotension required to produce thirst is not well defined for humans but again appears to be greater than that needed to effect vasopressin release. Therefore it appears unlikely that hemodynamic variables have an important influence on water intake, except under pathologic conditions. The mechanism by which hypovolemia and/or hypotension produces thirst is unknown but may involve a resetting of the osmoregulatory system via the same or similar pathways as vasopressin release. Recent evidence suggests that thirst may also be influenced by receptors in the oropharynx, but their role in water intake regulation has not yet been clarified.

VASOPRESSIN DEFICIENCY: DIABETES INSIPIDUS
(see also Chapter 112)
Clinical Features

Neurogenic diabetes insipidus is a disorder characterized by the excretion of large amounts of dilute urine. The polyuria varies considerably from patient to patient, ranging from as little as 3 to as much as 20 L/day. It must be distinguished from simple *urinary frequency,* a disorder in which total output may be normal. Thirst and polydipsia are also prominent features of diabetes insipidus. In correlation with the polyuria, they also vary in severity from patient to patient.

Apart from polyuria and increased thirst, diabetes insipidus is associated with few other symptoms or complaints. Fatigue and irritability are sometimes mentioned, but these symptoms are mild and rarely, if ever, prompt the patient to seek medical care. Even the polyuria and polydipsia are remarkably well tolerated and often are not even mentioned to a physician until they become severe. As often as not, they come to light only during a careful examination for some other complaint such as headache, loss of vision, or symptoms referable to a deficiency of some other pituitary hormone. The scant attention paid to symptoms of polyuria and polydipsia is unfortunate because they can be treated quite easily and are often the harbinger of a more serious disorder.

Diabetes insipidus also is associated with relatively few physical signs. Except in unusual cases associated with damage to the thirst mechanism, dehydration is not sufficiently severe to be evident on physical examination. The only other physical signs are those caused either by the underlying disease itself (Box 296-2) or by concurrent damage to other pituitary hormones or neighboring neuronal systems. The latter may be manifested as visual field defects, obesity, hypogonadism, hypothyroidism, secondary adrenal insufficiency, and, in children, retarded growth or delayed pubescence.

Except for hyposthenuria, results of routine laboratory tests are usually normal in uncomplicated neurogenic diabetes insipidus. As with symptoms and physical signs, all other laboratory abnormalities are due to the underlying disease itself or to concurrent damage to neighboring hormonal and/or neuronal systems. Plasma osmolality and/or sodium concentration is not appreciably elevated unless the patient's thirst mechanism is also damaged or the ability to drink is otherwise impaired.

Differential Diagnosis

Neurogenic diabetes insipidus must be differentiated from other causes of polyuria and polydipsia (Box 296-2). The most common is the *solute diuresis* that accompanies severe uncontrolled diabetes mellitus or other conditions associated with deficient reabsorption of salt and water in the proximal nephron. It is characterized by a greatly increased rate of total solute excretion, an abnormality that is useful in distinguishing it from other causes of polyuria and polydipsia. Besides neurogenic diabetes insipidus, the latter include *nephrogenic diabetes insipidus* (resulting from an impaired response to the antidiuretic effect of vasopressin) and *primary polydipsia* (caused by excessive ingestion of water) (Chapters 112 and 122).

Pathogenesis and Pathophysiology

Neurogenic diabetes insipidus is caused by insufficient amounts of plasma vasopressin. This deficiency results in a decrease in the hydroosmotic permeability of the distal and collecting tubules of the kidney. As a consequence, dilute urine formed in more proximal parts of the nephron is excreted essentially unchanged. The resultant loss of solute-free water causes mild dehydration, a rise in plasma osmolality, and the stimulation of thirst. The net effect is that water intake rises to a level sufficient to balance output, and the osmotic pressure of body fluid is stabilized at a new level, slightly above normal.

The magnitude of the polyuria and polydipsia depends on several variables, including the severity of vasopressin deficiency, the integrity of the thirst mechanism, the solute load, and the state of renal function. As a general rule, clinically significant polyuria does not

---

BOX 296-2

Causes of diabetes insipidus

I. Vasopressin deficiency (neurogenic or central diabetes insipidus)
  A. Decreased secretion
    1. Idiopathic
      a. Sporadic (? autoimmune)
      b. Familial (autosomal dominant inheritance)
    2. Traumatic (accidental or surgical)
    3. Malignancy
      a. Primary (craniopharyngioma, germinoma, meningioma, pituitary adenoma with suprasellar extension)
      b. Metastatic (lung, breast, leukemia)
    4. Granuloma (sarcoid, histiocytosis, xanthoma dissemination)
    5. Infectious (meningitis, encephalitis, syphilis)
    6. Vascular (aneurysm, Sheehan's syndrome, cardiac arrest, vasculitis)
    7. Psychobiologic (anorexia nervosa)
    8. Toxic (carbon monoxide)
    9. Congenital malformations
  B. Increased metabolism
    1. Pregnancy
II. Vasopressin resistance (nephrogenic diabetes insipidus)
  A. Idiopathic
    1. Sporadic
    2. Familial (X-linked recessive inheritance)
  B. Postobstructive
  C. Malignancy (retroperitoneal fibrosarcoma)
  D. Granuloma (sarcoid)
  E. Infectious (pyelonephritis)
  F. Vascular (sickle cell disease or trait)
  G. Metabolic (hypokalemia, hypercalciuria)
  H. Toxic (lithium, demeclocycline, methoxyflurane, methicillin)
  I. Malformations (polycystic disease)
  J. Pregnancy
III. Excessive water intake (primary polydipsia)
  A. Psychogenic (schizophrenia, affective disorders)
  B. Dipsogenic
    1. Idiopathic
    2. Traumatic
    3. Granuloma (neurosarcoidosis)
    4. Infectious (meningitis)
    5. Other (multiple sclerosis)

---

occur until the secretory capacity of the neurohypophysis has been reduced by more than 50%. Because many patients with neurogenic diabetes insipidus retain some capacity to release vasopressin in response to osmotic stimulation, the concentration of hormone that circulates under basal conditions is determined by the level of plasma osmolality at which thirst occurs. If this limit is raised or abolished (e.g., by damage to the osmoreceptor or by externally imposed water deprivation), plasma osmolality may rise sufficiently to stimulate the release of vasopressin in amounts adequate to produce urinary concentration. This interplay between the factors that determine water intake and output explains the seeming paradox that *many patients with neurogenic diabetes insipidus concentrate their urine during a standard dehydration test.* Vasopressin release also can be effected by nonosmotic stimuli. Because it is so potent, nausea or orthostatic hypotension may evoke significant increases in plasma vasopressin level even in patients who fail to respond to hypertonicity. In some patients, smoking has a similar effect. Hence these and other variables known to influence vasopressin level must always be kept in mind when interpreting the antidiuretic response to diagnostic or therapeutic procedures.

Changes in renal function also influence the severity of polyuria in patients with neurogenic diabetes insipidus. For any given level of plasma vasopressin, a rise or fall in solute excretion results in a proportionate increase or decrease in the volume of filtrate delivered to the collecting tubules. Hence the volume of urine excreted is influenced appreciably by changes in salt intake or other factors that alter solute load. In addition, neurogenic diabetes insipidus often results in two changes in the antidiuretic response to vasopressin. First, many such patients appear to be supersensitive to the antidiuretic effect of very low plasma concentrations of the hormone. The mechanism of this change is unknown, but it may involve increased affinity and/or number of renal vasopressin receptors, as occur with chronic deficiency of certain other hormones. Second, the hypersensitivity to very low concentrations of vasopressin is usually accompanied by a reduction in maximum urinary concentrating capacity. As a result, raising plasma vasopressin to normal or even supranormal levels increases urine osmolality less in patients with neurogenic diabetes insipidus than it does in healthy adults. This diminution in maximum concentrating response is thought to be due to "washout" of the medullary concentration gradient caused by chronic polyuria. It is not sufficiently severe to interfere with treatment of the polyuria and quickly resolves when antidiuresis is re-established; however, in conjunction with the changes in receptor affinity noted, it complicates the interpretation of certain commonly used diagnostic procedures (discussed later).

Nephrogenic diabetes insipidus is caused by deficient renal response to the antidiuretic actions of vasopressin (Box 296-2). Vasopressin secretion is normal. In other respects, the pathophysiology of nephrogenic and neurogenic diabetes insipidus is similar. Increased excretion of solute-free water results in mild hypertonic dehydration and stimulation of thirst. The degree of polyuria also depends to a great extent on the rate of solute excretion. Two distinct forms of nephrogenic diabetes insipidus have now been recognized. In one, the renal resistance is complete, and urine remains dilute even when there are marked increases in plasma vasopressin (type I). In the second, the renal resistance is partial or relative and urinary concentration does occur if plasma vasopressin level is elevated to more than 20 times normal (type II). As might be expected, there are important differences in the clinical behavior of these two forms of disorder. Unlike those with type I, patients with type II nephrogenic diabetes insipidus concentrate their urine in response to marked elevations in plasma vasopressin level produced either by prolonged water deprivation or by administration of vasopressin in standard diagnostic doses (0.05 to 0.1 U/kg). Hence in conventional indirect tests, they behave like patients with neurogenic diabetes insipidus yet respond inadequately to the standard therapeutic doses of the hormone.

Primary polydipsia is caused by excessive water intake. It results in a slight fall in plasma osmolality and an appropriate decrease in vasopressin secretion and urine concentration. As a result, water excretion rises to balance intake, and plasma osmolality stabilizes at a new level, only slightly below normal. In some cases, the polydipsia is associated with inappropriate vasopressin secretion, which, by retarding water excretion, leads to a marked reduction in plasma osmolality and/or sodium concentration. In some patients, the excessive intake of water appears to be due to an abnormality in the osmoregulation of thirst (dipsogenic). In many others, however, thirst is denied, and the excessive drinking appears to be due to more generalized cognitive dysfunction caused by serious mental illness (psychogenic). Like other forms of chronic polyuria, primary polydipsia results in a reduction in maximum urinary concentrating capacity. Whether primary polydipsia also causes supersensitivity to the antidiuretic action of small amounts of vasopressin is unclear.

Solute diuresis causes polyuria by overwhelming the distal diluting and concentrating mechanisms. As a consequence, large volumes of nearly isotonic urine are excreted, regardless of the plasma vasopressin level. Because water is lost in excess of sodium, the effective osmotic pressure of plasma tends to rise, and thirst is stimulated. The severity of the polyuria depends primarily on the rate of solute excretion. At high flow, it is largely independent of vasopressin secretion, water intake, or type of solute present. Thus increased excretion of sodium, mannitol, urea, or glucose has essentially the same diuretic effect.

Diagnosis

Evaluation of the patient with polyuria and polydipsia should begin with a check for solute diuresis. In most cases, testing the urine for glucose suffices. If the test result is negative, other forms of solute diuresis can be ruled out simply by calculating the osmolar excretion rate. Depending on diet, healthy adults normally excrete somewhere

---

BOX 296-3
Evaluation of suspected diabetes insipidus

1. Measure plasma osmolality and/or sodium concentration under conditions of ad libitum fluid intake. If they are above 295 mOsm/kg and 143 mEq/L, the diagnosis of primary polydipsia is excluded, and the testing should proceed directly to step 3 to distinguish between neurogenic and nephrogenic diabetes insipidus

2. If basal plasma osmolality and/or sodium is not elevated, perform a dehydration test. If urinary concentration does not occur before plasma osmolality and/or sodium reaches 295 mOsm/kg or 143 mEq/L, the diagnosis of primary polydipsia is again excluded, and the evaluation should proceed to step 3

3. Inject aqueous vasopressin (Pitressin) in a dose of 10 mU/kg body weight and collect urine every 30 minutes for the next 2 hours. If urine osmolality rises more than 50% above the value obtained at the end of the dehydration test, neurogenic diabetes insipidus is established. If not, administer a larger dose of vasopressin (50 mU/kg) to distinguish partial from complete nephrogenic diabetes insipidus

4. If dehydration results in urinary concentration, measure plasma vasopressin level and relate it to the levels of plasma and urine osmolality by using suitable nomograms (e.g., Figs. 296-3 and 296-7). If the level of plasma osmolality achieved is insufficient to permit a clear distinction between normal and subnormal vasopressin response (>292 mOsm/kg), infuse 3% saline solution at a rate of 0.1 ml/kg/min for 2 hours, and repeat the measurements of plasma osmolality and vasopressin level

5. If vasopressin level measurements are not available, admit the patient and perform a closely monitored therapeutic trial with intranasal desmopressin, 25 µg every 12 hours. If the trial corrects polydipsia as well as polyuria, and hyponatremia does not occur, the diagnosis of neurogenic diabetes insipidus is established. If the trial reduces polyuria, but not polydipsia, or produces other evidence of water intoxication, primary polydipsia is likely, and therapy should be discontinued until definitive diagnosis can be made by vasopressin assay. If desopressin does not reduce either polyuria or polydipsia, the diagnosis of nephrogenic diabetes insipidus is established. In some patients, repeat tests with higher doses of the drug may be indicated to distinguish between the complete and incomplete forms of the disorder

---

between 500 and 1000 mOsm per day. If the product of urine volume in liters per day and urine osmolality in milliosmoles per kilogram exceeds 1500, solute diuresis is likely, and efforts to identify and correct it should be undertaken before proceeding with testing for diabetes insipidus. If the product is less than 1500 mOsm per day, solute diuresis is unlikely, and further tests to differentiate among the other three causes of polyuria are indicated (Box 296-3).

The next step is to assess the state of hydration by measuring plasma osmolality during ad libitum intake of fluids. To be meaningful, this measurement must be made on fresh plasma with the use of a carefully calibrated osmometer. Serum should not be used for this purpose because it can result in relatively large artifacts. If these requirements cannot be met or if plasma glucose or urea level is abnormal, it may be preferable to rely on measurements of plasma sodium. If basal plasma osmolality and/or sodium concentration is above the normal range and the patient is still excreting increased volumes of dilute urine, the polyuria almost certainly is not due to primary polydipsia, and the testing can proceed directly to the vasopressin (Pitressin) test to differentiate between neurogenic and nephrogenic diabetes insipidus. The drug should be given parenterally, and urine osmolality measured before administration and at half-hour intervals for 2 hours after injection. Under these conditions, a maximum rise in urine osmolality of 50% or more is almost invariably diagnostic of neurogenic diabetes insipidus. A smaller increase or no change indicates nephrogenic diabetes insipidus.

In most patients plasma osmolality and sodium level are within normal limits under basal conditions (Fig. 296-8). In this case, a dehydration test should be performed. All liquids are withheld, and body weight as well as plasma and urine osmolality are measured hourly as dehydration develops. If urinary concentration does not occur be-

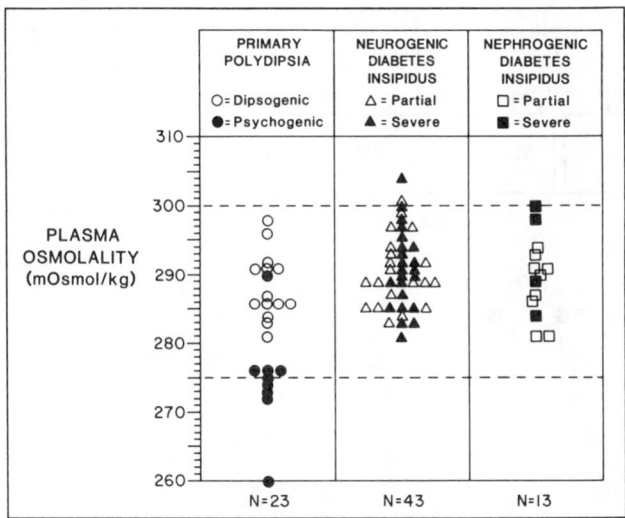

FIGURE 296-8 Basal plasma osmolality in patients with polyuria of diverse causes.

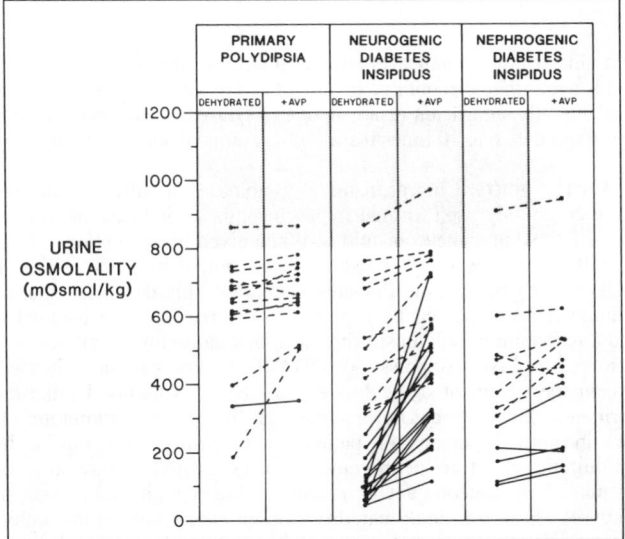

FIGURE 296-9 Urine osmolality after a standard dehydration test and administration of vasopressin in patients with polyuria of diverse causes. In the category of primary polydipsia, the solid line indicates the values obtained in a patient with severe psychogenic polydipsia. The broken lines indicate the values obtained in 13 patients with dipsogenic polydipsia. In the categories of neurogenic and nephrogenic diabetes insipidus, the solid and broken lines indicate the values obtained in patients with severe or partial defects, respectively. *AVP*, vasopressin.

fore body weight falls by 5% or plasma osmolality and sodium level rise to 295 mOsm per kilogram and 143 mEq per liter, respectively, primary polydipsia is excluded, and the vasopressin test described previously can be used to differentiate between neurogenic and nephrogenic diabetes insipidus.

However, if fluid deprivation leads to urinary concentration, this indirect test does not distinguish reliably among primary polydipsia, "partial" neurogenic diabetes insipidus, and "partial" nephrogenic diabetes insipidus because all three conditions can manifest identical changes in urine osmolality (Fig. 296-9). Hence some other diagnostic approach must be used. The simplest, safest, and most reliable method is to measure plasma vasopressin as well as plasma and urine osmolality at the end of the dehydration test (Box 296-3). By plotting urine osmolality as a function of the concurrent plasma vasopressin level on a suitable nomogram, almost all patients with type I

or II nephrogenic diabetes insipidus can be identified (Fig. 296-7). A similar plot of plasma vasopressin level as a function of plasma osmolality serves to differentiate patients with neurogenic diabetes insipidus from those with primary polydipsia (Fig. 296-3). In a few cases in which the level of plasma osmolality achieved is insufficient to permit unambiguous interpretation of the vasopressin concentration values, repeat assay after infusion of hypertonic (3%) saline solution (0.1 ml/kg per minute for 2 hours) almost always clarifies whether secretion of the hormone is normal or subnormal.

If a vasopressin assay suitable for diagnosing diabetes insipidus is not available, the best alternative is to perform a closely monitored therapeutic trial with standard doses of desmopressin. If treatment for 1 or 2 days has no effect, the patient probably has nephrogenic diabetes insipidus. On the other hand, if the polyuria and polydipsia are abolished without producing significant hyponatremia, the diagnosis of neurogenic diabetes insipidus is indicated. If treatment reduces polyuria but not polydipsia, or produces other signs of water intoxication, the diagnosis of primary polydipsia should be strongly suspected. In such a case, however, other evidence should be sought because an occasional patient with unequivocal neurogenic diabetes insipidus also responds in this way.

Recent studies suggest that magnetic resonance imaging (MRI) may also permit diagnosis of neurogenic diabetes insipidus. On T1-weighted images, the normal posterior pituitary emits a high-intensity signal or "bright spot" which is not eliminated by fat suppression techniques and is often absent in patients with neurogenic diabetes insipidus. However, this approach to the differential diagnosis can be misleading because the signal is also absent in 20% to 40% of normal adults and may be present in some patients with familial or idiopathic forms of neurogenic diabetes insipidus that result from highly selective destruction of vasopressinergic neurons.

Because of possible involvement of neighboring structures, other diagnostic studies are indicated in patients with neurogenic diabetes insipidus. Besides radiographic evaluation by computed tomography or MRI of the sella and hypothalamus, visual fields and anterior pituitary function should also be thoroughly tested. In addition, other studies to determine the underlying disease process may be indicated.

SPECIFIC DISEASE ENTITIES

Deficiency of vasopressin secretion results from destruction of the neurohypophysis by any of several different pathologic processes. The most common cause before the advent of transsphenoidal approaches was surgical removal of pituitary tumors. Because the neurohypophyseal neurons originate in the hypothalamus and have many fibers that terminate above the sella turcica, pituitary adenomas that are confined to the sella turcica usually do not destroy enough of the gland to cause clinically apparent diabetes insipidus. However, tumors such as craniopharyngioma or germinoma that arise in the hypothalamus often manifest first as diabetes insipidus. Metastases from cancer of the lung or breast, leukemic infiltrates, and extramedullary hematopoiesis can also cause the syndrome. Certain granulomatomas or lipid storage diseases, such as sarcoidosis, histiocytosis, or, more rarely, xanthoma disseminatum, cause diabetes insipidus by infiltrating the pituitary or meninges at the base of the brain. These diseases are usually systemic, and, by the time they cause diabetes insipidus, usually have manifested themselves elsewhere (e.g., in lung, bone, or skin). Acute infections occasionally involve the neurohypophysis. Perhaps because the neurohypophysis has such a large secretory reserve and a bilateral blood supply, vascular disease is an unusual cause of diabetes insipidus. For reasons not altogether clear, some patients with anorexia nervosa have a mild form of neurogenic diabetes insipidus that disappears when the malnutrition is corrected.

Much, if not most, of the neurogenic diabetes insipidus now seen in an office practice is idiopathic. The few histologic studies done in such patients reveal extensive loss of neurosecretory neurons in the supraoptic and, to a lesser extent, paraventricular nuclei. Idiopathic neurogenic diabetes insipidus can occur in sporadic or familial patterns. The familial form begins in childhood and is inherited in an autosomal dominant mode. It is due to a missense mutation in the part of the vasopressin precursor gene that codes for the signal peptide (exon 1) or the central, highly conserved structure of the neurophysin moiety (exon 2) (Fig. 296-10). By some as yet to be determined mechanism, these mu-

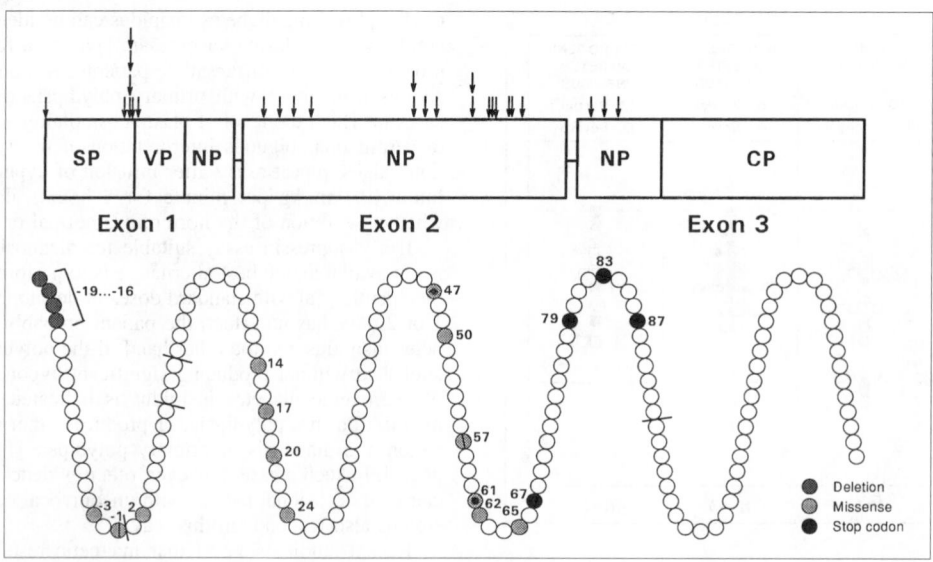

FIGURE 296-10   Schematic diagram of the vasopressin neurophysin gene showing the location of missense or nonsense mutations that have been identified in patients with familial neurogenic diabetes insipidus. *SP,* signal peptide; *VP,* vasopressin; *NP,* neurophysin; *CP,* copeptin. Vertical arrows indicate location of mutations.

tations cause postnatal degeneration of the neurons that express the gene, leading to severe deficiency of vasopressin.

Primary polydipsia is often associated with schizophrenia or other psychiatric illnesses. The pathogenic link is unknown, but, in many cases, the polydipsia seems to be prompted not so much by true thirst as by other motives, such as a desire to cleanse the body of poisons or other harmful substances. Primary polydipsia can also be due to an abnormality in the osmoregulation of thirst. Most of these cases are idiopathic, but the syndrome also is associated frequently with neurosarcoidosis and has been observed with trauma, tuberculous meningitis, and multiple sclerosis.

Renal resistance to the antidiuretic action of vasopressin can also result from a variety of diseases and drugs (Box 296-1). Nephrogenic diabetes insipidus is discussed in Chapters 112 and 122.

Treatment

Vasopressins. For many years, the only practical therapy for neurogenic diabetes insipidus was injection of Pitressin tannate in oil. Intramuscular injection of 5 to 10 units every 48 to 72 hours gives satisfactory relief of the polyuria and polydipsia in most patients but could also result in inadequate or erratic response caused by failure to emulsify the mixture adequately by shaking and warming the vial before use. Recently, this preparation of vasopressin was withdrawn from the market. Because its duration of action is only a few hours, aqueous vasopressin is not suitable for long-term treatment of diabetes insipidus and therefore is used primarily for diagnostic purposes.

Desmopressin or DDAVP (Fig. 296-2) is a synthetic analog of vasopressin. This preparation possesses many advantages in the treatment of diabetes insipidus. Modifications in positions 1 and 8 of the molecule double its antidiuretic potency, eliminate its pressor actions, and increase the resistance to metabolic degradation. Desmopressin has much longer antidiuretic action than does native vasopressin. Administration of 10 to 25 μg by nasal insufflation twice daily affords complete relief of polyuria in most adults. Rhinitis and/or sinusitis may interfere with its absorption, but resistance caused by antibody production has not been reported. DDAVP is also available in a form suitable for parenteral use. A dose of 1 to 4 μg administered once daily by intramuscular injection usually provides complete relief of polyuria and polydipsia in patients with neurogenic diabetes insipidus. Recently, an oral form of DDAVP has been approved for use in the United States. The doses required for control of diabetes insipidus range from 100 to 200 μg orally twice to three times daily. DDAVP has few side-effects. Excess water retention may occur, but the effect is usually transient even if therapy is continued. Sustained hyponatre-

mia almost always indicates an abnormality in the thirst mechanism and is a reason to discontinue treatment and repeat the diagnostic studies. The only significant disadvantage of DDAVP is its cost, which is approximately 6 to 10 times that of other forms of antidiuretic therapy.

Oral Agents. Chlorpropamide (Diabinese), a sulfonylurea drug more commonly used to treat hyperglycemia in diabetes mellitus, is also effective in diabetes insipidus. When given in conventional doses of 250 to 500 mg a day, it reduces urine output by 30% to 70% in patients with neurogenic diabetes insipidus. This decrease in urine volume is accompanied by a proportionate rise in urine osmolality and a reduction in polydipsia similar to that caused by small doses of vasopressin. Like vasopressin or DDAVP, chlorpropamide is ineffective in the treatment of nephrogenic diabetes insipidus. Unlike the hormones, however, chlorpropamide has little or no antidiuretic effect in normal persons or patients with primary polydipsia. Its antidiuretic effect in neurogenic diabetes insipidus may also be attenuated by concomitant or recent treatment with vasopressin or DDAVP. These seemingly paradoxic observations suggest that chlorpropamide acts via a mechanism similar to that of vasopressin itself but does so only if there has been a prolonged deficiency of the hormone. Studies in the toad bladder and rats suggest that chlorpropamide acts by potentiating the renal tubular effects of small, subthreshold amounts of vasopressin. Other mechanisms may also be involved because, in contrast to earlier impressions, the antidiuretic effect of the drug is as great in patients with severe deficiency as in those with partial deficiencies of vasopressin. The side effects of chlorpropamide therapy include hypoglycemia and alcohol-induced flushing. The former is rare and usually can be prevented by avoidance of prolonged fasting or exercise. The latter is more common but is usually mild and may subside with repeated exposure. Other sulfonylurea drugs do not have a significant antidiuretic effect in patients with diabetes insipidus and, in some cases, may even have a mild diuretic action.

Clofibrate (Atromid-S), which is commonly used to treat hyperlipidemia, also may reduce polyuria and polydipsia in patients with diabetes insipidus. At conventional doses of 0.5 to 1.0 g three times daily, its antidiuretic effect is usually less than that of chlorpropamide, although in some patients clofibrate is more effective. The mechanism of action is not known. Clofibrate is also ineffective in nephrogenic diabetes insipidus and has only minimal antidiuretic action in normal subjects and patients with primary polydipsia. Clofibrate has not been shown to potentiate the renal actions of vasopressin. Major side effects include myalgia, increased transaminase level, and gastroenteritis. These abnormalities often subside with continued treatment but in some cases may necessitate discontinuation of the drug.

Carbamazepine (Tegretol) also reduces or eliminates polyuria and polydipsia in patients with neurogenic diabetes insipidus. Its mechanism of action is also unclear but probably does not involve increased secretion of vasopressin. Its use in the treatment of diabetes insipidus is limited by the seriousness of some of its side effects.

Thiazide diuretics also reduce polyuria in patients with diabetes insipidus. Unlike chlorpropamide and clofibrate, the thiazides are equally effective in patients with nephrogenic diabetes insipidus, indicating that they work by a different mechanism. By inhibiting sodium reabsorption in the ascending limb of Henle's loop, the thiazides interfere with maximum urinary dilution. At the same time, they contract the extracellular fluid volume and increase salt and water reabsorption in the proximal tubule. The net effect is a slight rise in urine osmolality and a proportionately larger reduction in urine volume. At conventional doses, thiazide diuretics significantly potentiate the antidiuretic effect of chlorpropamide in neurogenic diabetes insipidus and are most useful in conjunction with one of the other oral agents. Other than occasional hypokalemia, serious side effects are rare. Because thiazides reduce the ability to excrete a water load in all persons, they may produce water intoxication in patients with primary polydipsia.

The appropriate role of the oral drugs in the management of diabetes insipidus is not clear. Used alone or in combination with thiazide diuretics, chlorpropamide or clofibrate can reduce polyuria to asymptomatic levels in most patients. Oral drugs have the advantage of convenience and relatively lower cost. This form of treatment is associated, however, with a greater incidence of undesirable side effects, and there are unresolved questions about their long-term safety. Moreover, oral drugs probably should not be used in pregnancy, because of possible teratogenic effects. These medications also are potentially hazardous to young children. In these situations, desmopressin appears to provide the safest and most effective form of therapy.

Several other measures may be helpful in reducing polyuria in either nephrogenic or neurogenic diabetes insipidus. Salt restriction reduces urine output by increasing the volume of filtrate reabsorbed isosmotically in the proximal nephron. Caffeine and other methylated xanthines have exaggerated diuretic effects in patients with diabetes insipidus. Often elimination of coffee or tea from the diet substantially improves control of polyuria.

BIBLIOGRAPHY

Barron WM: Water metabolism and vasopressin secretion during pregnancy. In Lindheimer MD, Dawson JM, editors: *Baillier's clinical obstetrics and gynecology,* vol 1, Renal disease in pregnancy, Philadelphia, 1987, Lea & Febiger.

Iwasaki Y, Gaskill MB, Robertson GL: Adaptive resetting of the volume control of vasopressin secretion during sustained hypovolemia, *Am J Physiol* 268(Regulatory Integrative Comp Physiol 37):R349, 1995.

Ohnishi A, Orita Y, Okahara R et al: Potent aquaretic agent: a novel nonpeptide selective vasopressin 2 antagonist (OPC-31260) in men, *J Clin Invest* 92:2653, 1993.

Rittig G, Robertson GL, Giggaard C et al: Identification of 13 new mutations in the vasopressin-neurophysin II gene in 17 kindreds with familial autosomal dominant neurohypophyseal diabetes insipidus, *Am J Hum Genet* 58:107, 1996.

Robertson GL: Thirst and vasopressin function in normal and disordered states of water balance, *J Lab Clin Med* 101(3):351, 1983.

Robertson GL: Disorders of thirst in man. In Ramsey D, editor: *Thirst: physiological and psychological aspects.* London, 1991, Springer-Verlag.

Robertson GL: Diabetes insipidus. *Endocrinol Metab Clin North Am* 24(3):549, 1995.

Robertson GL, Aycinena P: Neurogenic disorders of osmoregulation, *Am J Med* 72:339, 1982.

Robertson GL, Berl T: Pathophysiology of water metabolism. In Brenner BM, Rector FC, editors: *The kidney,* ed 5, Philadelphia, 1995. Saunders.

Schmale H, Fehr S, Richter D: Vasopressin synthesis: from gene to peptide hormone, *Kidney Int* 8(suppl S):13, 1987.

Zerbo RL, Miller JZ, Robertson CL: The reproducibility and heritability of individual differences in osmoregulatory function in normal human subjects, *J Lab Clin Med* 117(1):51, 1991.

297 Disorders of the Thyroid

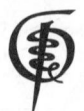

Gerald S. Levey and Irwin Klein

THYROID GLAND ANATOMY

The thyroid gland arises from embryonic endoderm and migrates caudad during development to its adult position at the base of the neck. Occasionally, accessory thyroid tissue can be found along this path of descent either at the base of the tongue or along the thyroglossal duct. By the 12th week of gestation the thyroid gland is morphologically and functionally intact and the thyroid epithelial cells have formed small, intact colloid-containing follicles. The thyroid also contains C cells known to secrete calcitonin.

The normal thyroid gland weighs approximately 20 g and is composed of two lateral lobes and an isthmus. The isthmus lies just below the cricoid cartilage anterior to the trachea, and the lateral lobes extend superiorly and somewhat laterally in the jugular groove for approximately 4 to 5 cm (Fig. 297-1). Inspection and palpation of the thyroid allow identification of symmetric or asymmetric enlargement of the lateral lobes (goiter), discrete nodules, thyroid tenderness, or changes in consistency of the normally fleshy gland. Various methods have been recommended for the proper palpation of the thyroid, but no single technique is necessarily superior and each examiner should employ the approach that best suits the individual case.

THYROID HORMONE FORMATION AND METABOLISM

The formation of the thyroid hormones thyroxine (T_4) and triiodothyronine (T_3) depicted in Fig. 297-2 requires an adequate supply of exogenous iodine. Iodine is usually provided by the ingestion of food, water, or dietary supplements. Once absorbed, the iodine is converted to inorganic iodide and then concentrated by the thyroid gland by a trapping process that requires an intact membrane, sodium-potassium-adenosinetriphosphatase (Na^+-K^+ATPase), adenylate cyclase, and specific membrane lipids. Inorganic iodide is converted to organic iodine by a membrane-bound peroxidase enzyme, which in the presence of hydrogen peroxide incorporates the newly organified iodine into tyrosine molecules in thyroglobulin, a glycoprotein in the colloid within the thyroid follicle. The iodination of the tyrosines occurs at either one (monoiodotyrosine [MIT]) or two (diiodotyrosine [DIT]) sites. MIT and DIT are in turn coupled, probably by an enzymatic reaction, in which two molecules of DIT would yield T_4 and one molecule each of MIT and DIT would yield T_3. The reaction producing T_4 is the major one, because the T_4/T_3 ratio in thyroglobulin is about 13:1. Most T_3 is produced by deiodination of T_4 in peripheral tissues. After the coupling reaction, the nascent thyroid hormones are still bound to thyroglobulin in the colloid follicle.

In order to make thyroid hormone available for transport to the bloodstream, pieces of thyroglobulin are removed from the follicle by endocytosis, resulting in the formation of vesicles known as colloid droplets. Within the cell, lysosomes containing proteases fuse with the colloid droplets and hydrolyze thyroglobulin, causing the release of free T_3 and T_4. Although some of the free thyroidal T_3 and T_4 is deiodinated in the thyroid gland with the iodine reentering the thyroid iodine pool, most of the T_3 and T_4 diffuses into the bloodstream, where it is bound to specific serum transport proteins.

The major thyroid transport protein for T_4 is thyroxine-binding globulin (TBG), a glycoprotein that normally accounts for about 80% of the bound serum thyroid hormone. T_4 is also bound by transthyretin (TTR, formerly known as thyroxine-binding prealbumin [TBPA]) and to a much more limited extent by albumin. T_3 is mostly bound by TBG and to a minor degree by albumin. TBG has about a 10-fold higher affinity for T_4 than T_3; therefore approximately *0.05%* of the total serum T_4 and *0.5%* of the total serum T_3 are in an unbound (free) state, although in reversible equilibrium with the bound

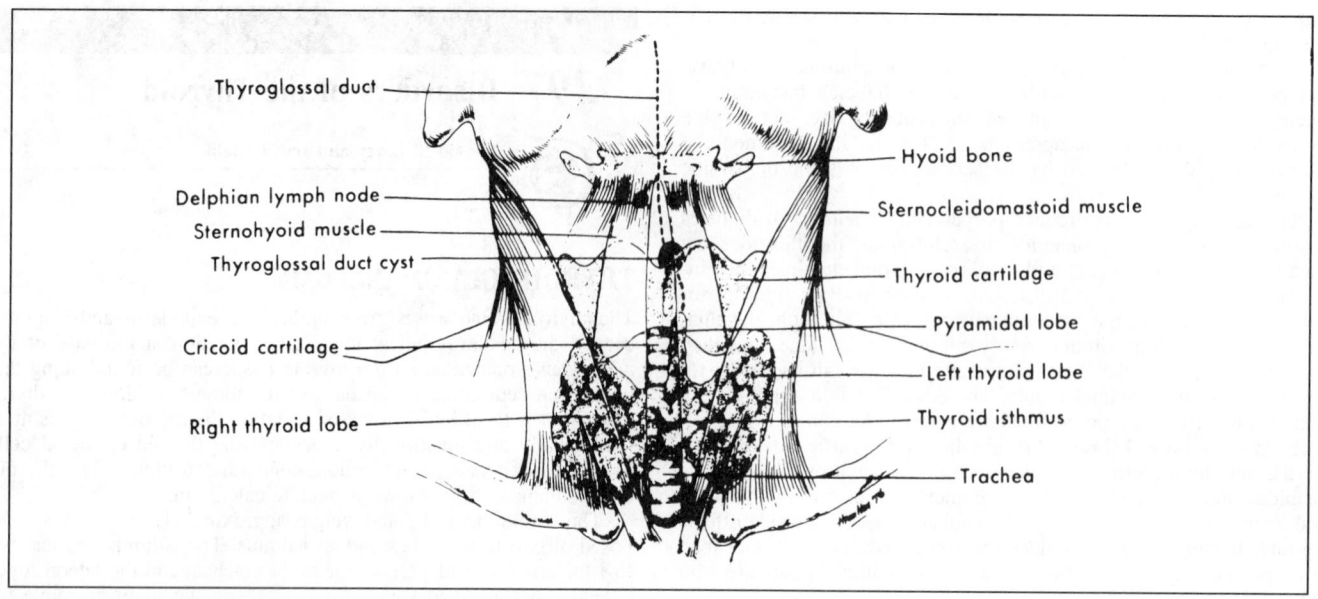

FIGURE 297-1   Normal thyroid gland anatomy.
From Prior JA, Silberstein JS: *Physical diagnosis: the history and examination of the patient,* ed 7, St Louis, 1981, Mosby.

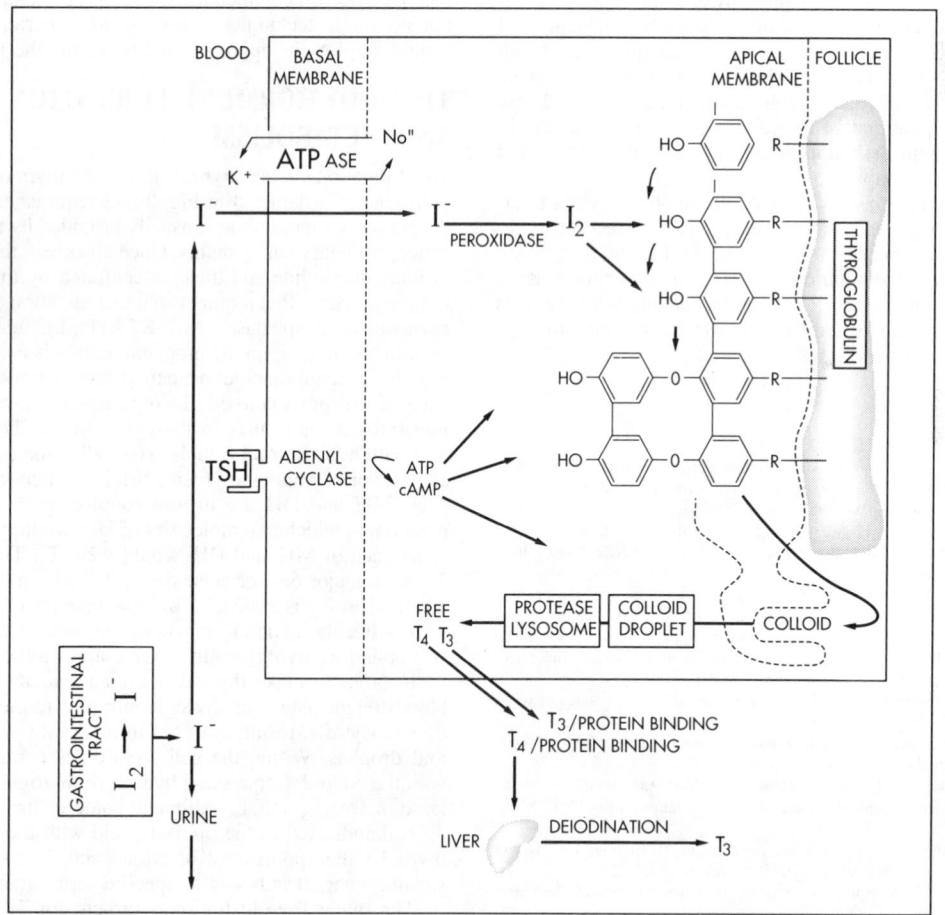

FIGURE 297-2   Formation of thyroid hormone within the thyroid epithelial cell. *ATP,* Adenosine triphosphate; *cAMP,* cyclic adenosine monophosphate; *TSH,* thyroid-stimulating hormone.
Modified from Berkow R, editor: *The Merck manual of diagnosis and therapy,* ed 16, Rahway, NJ, 1992, Merck.

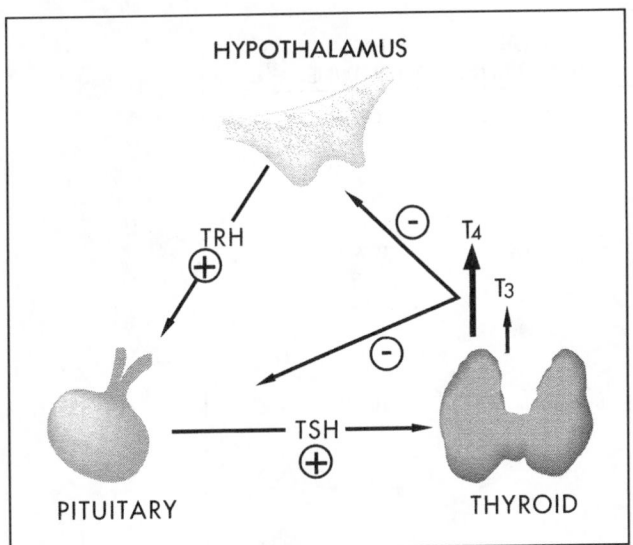

FIGURE 297-3   Schematic representation of the regulation of thyroid gland function by the hypothalamus and the pituitary gland. *TRH*, thyroid-reducing hormone.

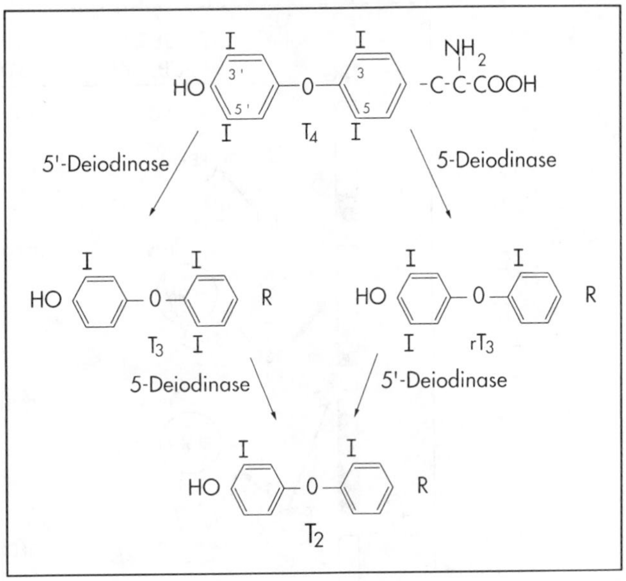

FIGURE 297-4   Enzymatic metabolism of thyroxine.

hormone. The concentration of free hormone is a function of this equilibrium and the number of occupied and unoccupied binding sites on TBG. This characteristic assumes particular importance in interpreting the laboratory tests (described later) measuring the concentrations of thyroid hormone in serum.

Thyroid-stimulating hormone, thyrotropin (TSH), is the major regulator of thyroid gland growth and function. All of the reactions necessary for the intrathyroidal formation of T_4 and T_3 are under the influence and control of TSH, a glycoprotein formed and secreted by the thyrotroph cells of the anterior pituitary. TSH is composed of two distinct subunits; the alpha subunit is common to three other glycoprotein hormones including follicle-stimulating hormone, luteinizing hormone, and human chorionic gonadotropin and is responsible for adenylate cyclase activation in the thyroid cell membrane. The beta subunit confers binding specificity to the hormone for its cell surface receptor. Once the TSH binds to its thyroid plasma membrane receptor on the external cell surface, it activates the enzyme adenylate cyclase, increasing the formation of cyclic adenosine monophosphate (AMP), the nucleotide that serves as an intracellular messenger to mediate the effects of TSH on the thyroid cell. The control of TSH secretion and synthesis is complex and involves local mechanisms within the pituitary as well as the hypothalamus. Within the pituitary regulation is primarily modulated by the intrapituitary T_3 concentration derived from both circulating free T_3 and intrapituitary conversion of T_4 to T_3. Elevation of the circulating levels of free thyroid hormones inhibits TSH secretion from the pituitary, and more sustained elevation of the levels of free thyroid hormone decreases the biosynthesis of TSH in the thyrotroph cell. Conversely, decreased circulating levels of free thyroid hormone result in increased synthesis and release of TSH from the pituitary and subsequent rise in the circulating TSH.

TSH secretion from the pituitary is also influenced by thyrotropin-releasing hormone (TRH), a 3 amino acid peptide (pyro-Glu-His-Pro-NH) synthesized primarily in the paraventricular nuclei in the hypothalamus and stored in the median eminence (Fig. 297-3). TRH is released into the portal venous system between the hypothalamus and pituitary, binds to the thyrotroph cells of the anterior pituitary, increases the entry of extracellular calcium into the thyrotroph cells, and increases both synthesis and release of TSH. The precise regulation of TRH has not been completely elucidated, although it appears to be a classic endocrine feedback mechanism with excess thyroid hormone depressing and deficient thyroid hormone stimulating its production and release.

It is now clear that thyroidal production of T_3 accounts for only about 15% to 20% of the circulating T_3. The remainder (80% to 85%) is produced by monodeiodination of the outer ring of T_4 by the

membrane-bound enzyme 5'-deiodinase (Fig. 297-4). It is also clear that T_3 is at least 3 and perhaps as much as 10 times more potent than T_4 in its biologic activity. T_3 exerts its cell-specific effect by binding to a discrete set of nuclear proteins. The proteins are part of the c-erbA family of protooncogenes and interact with thyroid hormone response elements, which are DNA elements residing in the promoter region of certain genes. T_4 binds to the nuclear receptor with a much lower affinity than T_3 and, therefore, may be regarded as a prohormone serving mainly as a substrate for the all-important peripheral conversion to T_3 in the liver, pituitary, kidney, and other organs.

Monodeiodination of the inner ring of T_4 yields a metabolite known as reverse T_3 (rT_3), which has no significant metabolic activity. rT_3 is present in normal human serum, and, in trace amounts, in thyroglobulin. From 15 to 40 weeks of fetal life, amniotic fluid concentrations of T_3 are low and rT_3 levels are much higher than the corresponding values in maternal serum. The rT_3 in amniotic fluid is derived primarily from the fetus via the action of the 5-deiodinase enzyme. At delivery, the deiodination pattern is switched to the normal adult pattern, and rT_3 levels fall rapidly and T_3 levels rise. Subsequent deiodinations of T_3 and rT_3 shown in Fig. 297-4 result in a series of metabolites probably having no biologic activity. Thyroid hormone metabolism can be altered by various pathologic states including infection, trauma, starvation, and heart failure. To understand the changes in serum levels of T_4, T_3, and rT_3 that occur in the patients, it is necessary to have knowledge of the fundamental biochemistry and cellular biology of the deiodinases. The 5'-deiodinase has two distinct forms: 5'-deiodinase type I and 5'-deiodinase type II. Type I is located predominantly in liver and kidney; its activity is decreased in the fasted state and hypothyroidism and increased in hyperthyroidism; is inhibited by propylthiouracil, amiodarone, and the contrast agents iopanoic acid (Telepaque) and ipodate (Oragrafin); and has a substrate preference for rT_3. The 5'-deiodinase II is located predominantly in pituitary and brain; its activity is increased in hypothyroidism, unchanged by fasting, and decreased in hyperthyroidism; is inhibited by amiodarone, iopanoic acid, and ipodate but not by propylthiouracil; and has a substrate preference for T_4, which enables the pituitary thyrotroph cell to metabolize T_4 independently.

About 80 to 90 μg of T_4 is produced each day, and deiodination is the major pathway by which it is metabolized. Approximately 80% of T_4 secreted by the thyroid is deiodinated in the periphery, half to T_3 and half to rT_3, and eventually to the other metabolites shown in Fig. 297-4. T_4 that is not deiodinated is eliminated by fecal excretion.

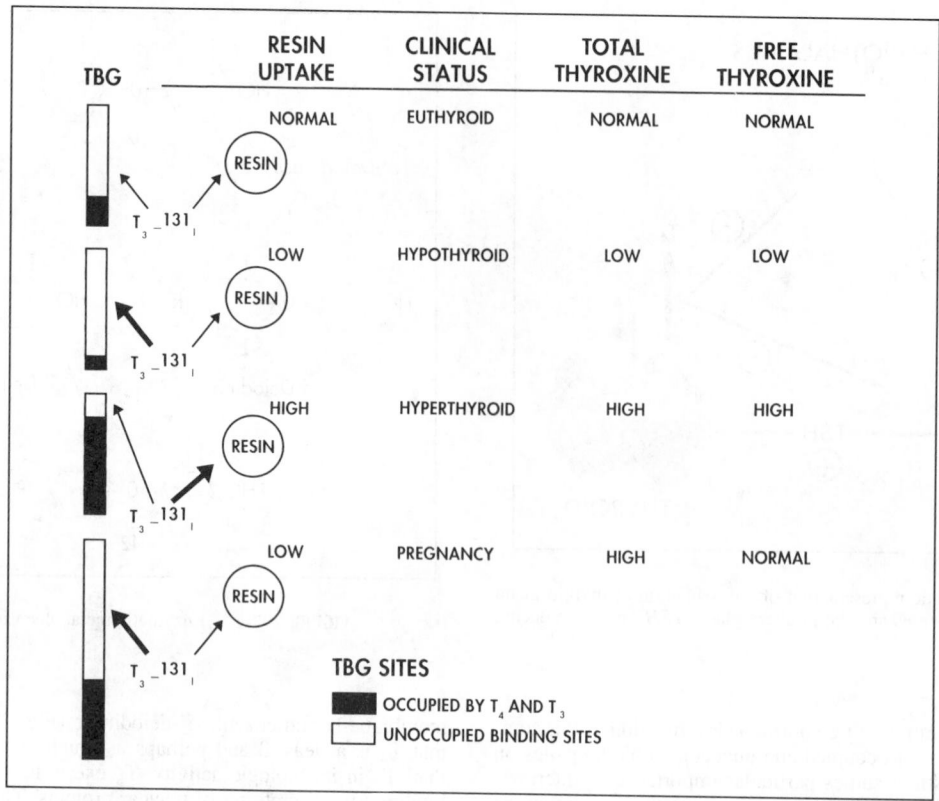

TBG	RESIN UPTAKE	CLINICAL STATUS	TOTAL THYROXINE	FREE THYROXINE
	NORMAL	EUTHYROID	NORMAL	NORMAL
	LOW	HYPOTHYROID	LOW	LOW
	HIGH	HYPERTHYROID	HIGH	HIGH
	LOW	PREGNANCY	HIGH	NORMAL

TBG SITES

■ OCCUPIED BY T_4 AND T_3
□ UNOCCUPIED BINDING SITES

FIGURE 297-5 Schematic representation of the T_3 resin uptake test. *TBG*, thyroxine-binding globulin. Modified from Berkow R, editor: *The Merck manual of diagnosis and therapy,* ed 16, Rahway, NJ, 1992, Merck.

LABORATORY TESTS TO ASSESS THYROID FUNCTIONAL STATUS AND ANATOMY

There are a number of readily available laboratory tests to assess a patient's thyroid functional status and anatomy. Numerous complexities and pitfalls pose a distinct challenge to the clinician who must interpret the results and employ the findings to arrive at a diagnostic conclusion. Each of the commonly used tests is discussed, and the inherent problems in interpretation noted.

Serum Total T_4 and T_3 Levels

Serum total T_4 and T_3 levels have been classically measured by radioimmunoassays and more recently by nonisotopic enzyme linked immunosorbent assay (ELISA). The tests are highly sensitive and specific, are reasonably inexpensive, and accurately measure the total concentrations of T_4 and T_3. T_4 is often used to assess thyroid functional status. Normal serum levels in most laboratories are about 5 to 11 μg/dl for T_4 and 80 to 160 ng/dl for T_3. Measurement of total T_4 is unaffected by contaminating non-T_4 iodine. In most cases changes in thyroid gland function result in a corresponding change in T_4 and T_3 levels. It must be remembered that over 99% of the T_4 and T_3 are protein-bound and that the free hormone, which is biologically active, is only a fraction of the total T_4 and T_3 levels. Therefore changes in serum binding protein (most commonly TBG, but occasionally TTR or albumin) levels produce elevations or depressions of total T_4 level. Thus a patient with an increase or decrease in the concentration of TBG may have normal thyroid gland function despite serum total T_4 and total T_3 levels equivalent to what is found in hyperthyroidism or hypothyroidism. In hyperthyroidism or hypothyroidism, the concentration of the free hormone changes, whereas isolated changes in TBG, TTR, or albumin leave the free T_4 or free T_3 at normal levels (changes in thyroid binding proteins in euthyroid patients are discussed later).

Measures of Thyroid Hormone Protein Binding

The T_3 resin uptake is used to circumvent the problem of alterations in amount of serum TBG and is only useful in conjunction with a simultaneous measure of total T_4 or T_3. The T_3 resin uptake reflects the unsaturated thyroid hormone binding sites on TBG (Fig. 297-5) and is not a measure of circulating T_3. In the normal subject 25% to 35% of the TBG binding sites are occupied by thyroid hormone. In hypothyroidism, characterized by decreased levels of circulating thyroid hormone, there are decreased numbers of occupied and increased numbers of unoccupied TBG binding sites. Increased amounts of the ^{125}I-T_3 are bound to TBG, resulting in a decreased uptake of ^{125}I-T_3 by the resin. In hyperthyroidism, the converse pertains.

The T_3 resin uptake is most useful for interpreting alterations of serum total T_4 when there is an increase or decrease in the amount of TBG without any actual change in thyroid gland function. For example, when TBG is increased in hyperestrogenemic states, there are increased numbers of both occupied and unoccupied binding sites on TBG (see *lower panel,* Fig. 297-5). The total T_4 is increased because the actual number of TBG sites binding T_4 or T_3 is increased. However, as in the euthyroid state with normal free T_4 levels, only about 25% to 35% of the total sites are occupied, leaving an increase in unoccupied sites to bind ^{125}I-T_3, resulting in a decreased resin uptake. In settings where the TBG is decreased, the opposite is found. To aid in standardization, some laboratories report the T_3 resin uptake as a ratio (thyroid hormone binding ratio [THBR]; normal, 0.085:1.10) of the patient's serum to a normal control population. Many laboratories also report additional results known as the free thyroxine index (FTI), or T_7, which are simply mathematically derived figures based on the values for T_4 and T_3 resin uptake that, although theoretically correct, have only modest accuracy.

Table 297-1 Serum thyroid-stimulating hormone (TSH) concentrations in various thyroid disease states

	SERUM TSH (MU/ML) RANGE
Normal*	0.1-5.0
Hyperthyroid	<0.1
Hypothyroid	
Subclinical	6-16
Overt primary	20-200
Secondary	0.1-5.0
Euthyroid sick syndrome	0.1-5.0
Recovery phase	0.1-15

*Varies with the specific assay employed; values <0.01 reported with highly sensitive assays.

Free T₄ and Free T₃ Determinations

Theoretically, free T_4 and free T_3 determinations would be the ideal test because they most accurately reflect thyroid status. However, the concentrations of free T_4 and free T_3 are low and difficult to measure. The methods used, including radioimmunoassay and equilibrium dialysis, are fraught with technical pitfalls and expensive. Equilibrium dialysis gives the most reliable results.

Serum Thyroid-Stimulating Hormone Concentration

The measurement of serum TSH concentration is the single best test for evaluation of thyroid function. In primary hypothyroidism the TSH level is uniformly elevated; however, in the unusual setting of secondary hypothyroidism caused by pituitary or hypothalamic failure the TSH level may be normal or low (Table 297-1).

In hyperthyroidism the normal feedback mechanism of T_4 on the pituitary leads to suppression of TSH synthesis and release. Using standard "first-generation" TSH radioimmunoassays did not allow for the discrimination between low normal and the suppressed levels characteristic of hyperthyroidism. This limitation led to the development of second- and third-generation assays using ELISA and chemiluminescent methodologies with greater sensitivity, specificity, and speed. At present, the basal serum TSH level measured by a highly sensitive (second-generation) and specific method can reliably discriminate hyperthyroid from euthyroid patients. The basal serum TSH level measured by such an assay is now the preferred alternative to the TRH stimulation test in assessing hyperthyroidism. The normal range in most assays is 0.1 to 5.0 µU/ml. A detectable serum TSH level has the same significance as a normal response to TRH and excludes hyperthyroidism except in rare cases of TSH-producing thyrotroph tumors of the pituitary. An undetectable basal TSH level has the same significance as a subnormal response to TRH and indicates either subclinical or overt hyperthyroidism. As a result the measurement of basal serum TSH level now provides a reliable index of thyrotroph activity across the entire spectrum of thyroid disease from primary hypothyroidism to hyperthyroidism.

Thyrotropin-Releasing Hormone Test

The sensitive TSH test has decreased the usefulness of the TRH stimulation test. The TRH test measures serum TSH levels after synthetic TRH is injected intravenously or intramuscularly. Normally, there is a rapid rise in TSH level of 5 to 25 µU/ml, reaching a peak in 30 minutes. In men older than 40 years of age, the release of TSH in response to TRH declines. The release of TSH in response to TRH is exaggerated in primary hypothyroidism: maximal stimulated values of TSH exceed 30 µU/ml. In hyperthyroidism TSH release is suppressed in response to injected TRH by the inhibitory effects of elevated intrapituitary free T_3 and T_4 levels on the pituitary thyrotroph cell.

The TRH test is useful in distinguishing thyroid dysfunction caused by pituitary disease that results from failure to release TSH in response to TRH in the clinical setting of hypothyroidism. Patients who are hypothyroid as a result of hypothalamic failure (a rare entity) and deficient TRH level have either normal or delayed release of TSH.

Antithyroid Antibodies

The most common determinations of antithyroid antibodies are antimicrosomal and antithyroglobulin. Both tests are highly organ specific and sensitive; however, the antimicrosomal antibodies are most useful because they most frequently yield positive findings in the two thyroid autoimmune diseases of major concern to the clinician, Hashimoto's thyroiditis and Graves' disease.

Antimicrosomal antibodies are directed primarily against the membrane-bound thyroid peroxidase. The antibody levels are elevated, often in very high titers, in the majority of patients with Hashimoto's thyroiditis and frequently in patients with Graves' disease. In contrast, antithyroglobulin antibodies are present in a smaller percentage of patients with Hashimoto's thyroiditis and less than half of those with Graves' disease.

Thyroid-Stimulating Hormone Receptor Antibodies

The thyroid goiter and autonomous hyperfunctioning of the thyroid characteristic of Graves' disease is due to an antibody directed against the thyroid TSH receptor. The antibody, which is an immunoglobulin G (IgG) can be detected in more than 90% of patients with Graves' disease. Because Graves' disease has characteristic clinical manifestations and diagnosis is usually not difficult, TSH receptor antibody (TRAb) determination is unnecessary in most cases. Measurement is most useful in women who are pregnant because high titers are associated with a greater risk of development of thyrotoxicosis in the neonate—key information for the obstetrician and pediatrician. Measurement of TRAb is also of some value in establishing the diagnosis of euthyroid Graves' disease in patients with ophthalmopathy and normal thyroid function.

Serum Thyroglobulin

Thyroglobulin is present in low serum concentrations in the normal population. Concentrations are elevated in pregnancy (normal finding) and in a number of thyroid disorders including nontoxic goiter, hyperthyroidism, subacute thyroiditis, thyroid adenoma, and differentiated (usually metastatic) thyroid cancer of the papillary and follicular types. Determination of serum thyroglobulin is of greatest use in follow-up care of patients who have had treatment for differentiated thyroid cancer. After successful treatment and institution of thyroid hormone in suppressive doses, serum thyroglobulin level is usually well within the normal range (<5 ng/ml). Elevations of serum thyroglobulin level in this setting indicate the presence of residual or recurrent thyroid cancer.

THYROID IMAGING TECHNIQUES
Radioisotopic Scintiscanning

Scintiscanning has been used as an important tool for the evaluation of thyroid function and the noninvasive assessment of thyroid anatomy for many years. Originally the isotope used for scanning was [131]I. More recently, ^{123}I has superseded ^{131}I as the isotope of choice. Technetium (^{99m}Tc) pertechnetate, an anion concentrated by the thyroid, is also used to assess thyroid anatomy. In scintiscanning studies, the radiation emitted by the isotopes is recorded by a scanner and scintillation detectors on x-ray film or on a fluorescent screen that can be directly viewed and photographed. In addition, the use of ^{131}I or ^{123}I permits the quantitation of the thyroidal uptake of iodine over a fixed period and can be selectively used to assess the functional state of the thyroid gland.

At present, ^{123}I is the isotope of choice for scanning procedures. It has a much shorter half-life than ^{131}I and because of the absence of beta radiation gives a significantly smaller radiation dose to the thyroid. [99m]Tc has a short half-life and delivers a low dose of radiation to the thyroid but does not readily permit the calculation of a functional uptake and is not organically bound, thus creating its own technical and interpretive problems.

There are a number of indications for thyroid imaging studies. One is the assessment of thyroid nodules to define whether they are functional (hot or warm nodules) or nonfunctional (cold nodules). Warm or hot nodules are rarely malignant, and almost all thyroid cancers are cold on scintiscanning. Specificity is not ideal because most benign thyroid nodules are also cold on scintiscan. A second indication for scanning techniques is to permit localization of the thyroid, which is of particular importance in patients with substernal goiters. A third is the localization of metastatic deposits of differentiated thyroid cancer or of residual normal thyroid tissue after surgery. A fourth indication is the anatomic evaluation of the thyroid, important in differentiating agenesis of one lobe of the thyroid vs. a hyperfunctioning nodule that has suppressed the opposite lobe of the thyroid. Scintiscanning helps in distinguishing a multinodular goiter from other goitrous enlargements of the thyroid.

For functional assessment, the uptake of ^{123}I or ^{131}I is measured at two time intervals, 6 and 24 hours. Normal individuals vary somewhat from laboratory to laboratory but in general, normal 24-hour uptake ranges from 2% to 35%. Because of the high iodine content of the diet in the United States, the lower limit of ^{123}I or ^{131}I uptake in normal individuals has declined; therefore the radioiodine uptake is no longer useful in the assessment of hypothyroidism. The 24-hour uptake is most useful in diagnosing hyperthyroidism of the Graves' disease type in which it is uniformly elevated and therefore can serve in distinguishing some of the various types of hyperthyroidism described later.

In addition to radiation exposure, the use of these tests has disadvantages in terms of high cost and time inconvenience for the patient. In addition, myriad factors increase or decrease the uptake. Therefore scintiscanning should only be used in a cost-effective and discriminating approach to medical care.

Ultrasonography

The ultrasound technique provides a sensitive assessment of thyroid anatomy including a reasonably accurate estimation of size. It has the advantage of not requiring radioactive isotopes, so there is no radiation exposure to the patient. The main use of ultrasound is to determine whether a nodule is solid, cystic, or a mixture of the two. A purely cystic nodule has a greatly reduced chance of being malignant. The main disadvantages of ultrasound are that it does not allow discrimination of benign and malignant nodules solely on the basis of solid or cystic characteristics, an overall lack of specificity in identifying discrete nodules, and the cost.

INVASIVE TECHNIQUES

Thyroid biopsy provides the most useful and specific tool for deciding whether a thyroid nodule is benign or malignant and therefore is the routine procedure of choice for the evaluation of a solitary thyroid nodule. There are two basic biopsy techniques. The more commonly employed is fine-needle (22 to 27 gauge) aspiration. It is simple and safe, requiring only local anesthesia. The needle is inserted into the nodule, suction is applied at various angles, cells are drawn into the barrel of the needle, and the aspirate is placed on a microscopic slide for cytologic examination. Closed percutaneous biopsy using a Vim-Silverman needle is highly effective as a diagnostic tool but is more difficult to perform and occasionally associated with complications such as hemorrhage.

Fine-needle aspiration is highly sensitive and specific and has decreased the need for surgical removal of thyroid nodules by at least 50%. As a result of biopsy technology, the prevalence of thyroid cancer in a surgically removed nodule has risen from about 5% to 15% to 35% to 50%.

Thyroid biopsy is not reliable for diagnosing follicular cancer because histologic evidence of capsular or blood vessel invasion must be demonstrated to establish the diagnosis. Biopsy can confirm the clinical and/or serologic evidence for Hashimoto's thyroiditis; however, if lymphoma of the thyroid is a consideration, cutting-needle (core) or open biopsy may be required. The problem of the management of nodules whose aspirates are interpreted as suspicious or in-

determinate has not been resolved. Depending on the clinical setting, surgical removal or observation during suppression therapy with thyroxine is the usual course of action.

ALTERATIONS OF THYROID FUNCTION TESTS IN EUTHYROID PATIENTS
Euthyroid Sick Syndrome

The occurrence of both elevated and low concentrations of total T_4 and total T_3 in clinically euthyroid patients is well established. Patients with a variety of acute or chronic nonthyroidal illnesses, other stresses, or abnormal nutritional states may have abnormal thyroid function test results. Although serum total T_4 levels may vary, the hallmark of the euthyroid sick syndrome is a low serum T_3 level. In large part, the decreased serum total T_3 level is a result of decreased peripheral conversion of T_4 to T_3, secondary to a decrease in the activity of the 5'-deiodinase. This leads in turn to decreased metabolism (outer-ring deiodination) of rT_3 with consequent rise in serum rT_3 level. In acute and severe stress there is a decrease in binding of thyroid hormone to TBG, thereby altering the distribution and serum levels of both T_4 and T_3. Thus, while measured total T_4 and T_3 levels may be low, the serum free hormone (especially for T_4) levels are commonly within the normal range. The serum TSH level is usually normal, although in the recovery period from the euthyroid sick syndrome, the TSH level may be moderately elevated. Box 297-1 shows the wide variety of conditions and diseases commonly associated with this syndrome, including fasting, protein-calorie malnutrition, trauma, myocardial infarction, heart failure, cardiopulmonary bypass surgery, chronic renal failure, diabetic ketoacidosis, cirrhosis, and sepsis.

The interpretation of thyroid function test result abnormalities observed in the euthyroid sick syndrome may be further complicated by the effects of a variety of drugs frequently used in acute and chronic illness that impair the peripheral conversion of T_4 to T_3 in liver and kidney (propranolol, dexamethasone) and in liver, kidney, and pituitary (amiodarone, iodinated contrast agents).

The diagnostic dilemma usually confronting the clinician in euthyroid sick syndrome is whether the patient is hypothyroid or euthyroid. The most sensitive indicator of hypothyroidism caused by primary thyroid gland failure is a marked elevation of serum TSH level; patients with the euthyroid sick syndrome have normal levels of serum TSH. In some cases of cirrhosis and in the recovery phase of euthyroid sick syndrome modest increases in TSH level may be found. However, corticosteroids and dopamine, which are frequently used in seriously ill patients, may lower TSH levels and can complicate the interpretation of the thyroid tests. Hypothyroidism in the patient with a coexistent acute or chronic systemic illness is suggested by a low or low-normal serum rT_3 level because rT_3 level should otherwise be increased in the euthyroid sick syndrome.

The laboratory diagnosis of hyperthyroidism may also be obscured in the euthyroid sick syndrome by the often dramatic lowering of the serum total T_3 concentration. In this situation, clinical signs of hyperthyroidism, presence of a goiter and/or exophthalmos and elevated radioiodine uptake serve as key determinants establishing the underlying presence of thyrotoxicosis.

Because of the many pitfalls in the interpretation of thyroid function test results in the euthyroid sick syndrome, there is no substitute

---

BOX 297-1
Euthyroid sick syndrome (nonthyroidal illness)

Fasting	Thermal injury
Starvation	Heart failure
Protein-calorie malnutrition	Hypothermia
Sepsis	Myocardial infarction
Trauma	Chronic renal failure
Cardiopulmonary bypass	Diabetic ketoacidosis
Widespread malignancy	Cirrhosis

for sound clinical judgment based on a meticulous history and physical examination when attempting to interpret thyroid function test result abnormalities in the acutely or chronically ill patient.

Euthyroid Hyperthyroxinemia

Since the advent of the routine assays of serum T_4 level, a number of conditions have been recognized to increase the level in euthyroid patients (Box 297-2) producing a state called euthyroid hyperthyroxinemia. Elevation in the concentration of TBG is recognized as the most common cause of elevation of the serum total T_4 level in the euthyroid patient. TBG level is most commonly increased by pregnancy and use of oral contraceptives; in the acute phase of infectious hepatitis; and on a genetic or idiopathic basis (Box 297-3). It is occasionally increased in hypothyroidism, acute intermittent porphyria, and prolonged therapy with perphenazine. Hyperestrogenemic states, such as those produced by pregnancy and oral contraceptive therapy, are the most common cause of increased TBG levels, and treatment with the antiestrogen tamoxifen can also increase TBG. Because hyperthyroidism and hypothyroidism are commonly found in women between the ages of 20 and 50, it is important that the clinician be aware of the effects of estrogens on TBG level. Recently it has been shown that estrogens do not increase TBG level by increasing its synthesis, but rather prolong its half-life by increasing the sialic acid content of TBG.

Other causes of an elevated T_4 level in the euthyroid state, in addition to TBG elevation, include abnormalities of the other binding proteins, TTR and albumin; autoantibodies that bind T_4; generalized thyroid hormone resistance; drugs such as amiodarone and the contrast agents ipodate and iopanoic acid; acute psychiatric illness; acute nonthyroidal medical illness; and ingestion of synthetic thyroxine.

Abnormalities in T_4 binding to albumin and TTR, although rare, provide useful insights into these binding proteins. A recently described condition known as familial dysalbuminemic hyperthyroxinemia (FDH) is associated with serum total T_4 levels two to three times normal. FDH is an inherited disease transmitted as an autosomal dominant trait and appears to be more common in Hispanic populations. In the affected patients, the defect results from the presence of an abnormal binding site for T_4 on one quarter to half of the circulating albumin molecules, which have an affinity for T_4 about 50 times normal. T_3 levels are normal because albumin binds T_3 only weakly. The T_3 resin uptake is usually normal; free thyroxine index is elevated; and serum free T_4 level, serum TSH level, and TSH response to TRH are normal, confirming the euthyroid state despite the marked elevation of T_4 level.

Euthyroid hyperthyroxinemia is also found in two rare syndromes characterized by increased binding of T_4 to TTR. One syndrome was described in a family in which the TTR was characterized by an abnormally high binding affinity of prealbumin for T_4. The other syndrome was described in two patients with a glucagonoma in which an increased amount of TTR was synthesized by the alpha cells of the pancreatic tumor. Serum T_3 level, T_3 resin uptake, TSH level, and TSH response to TRH are normal in these syndromes.

Rarely hyperthyroxinemia may be the result of anti-T_4 antibodies. These autoantibodies may cause an assay artifact or an actual increase in bound circulating T_4 level. Other thyroid function test findings are normal.

In recent years, the sporadic or familial occurrence of generalized resistance to thyroid hormones has been described; it is characterized by elevated total and free T_4 and T_3 levels and inappropriately elevated levels of TSH for the measured levels of T_4 and T_3. Some patients have a goiter, and selected young patients show signs of thyroid hormone deficiency such as growth retardation, delayed bone maturation, and deaf-mutism. Patients with generalized thyroid hormone resistance are most often clinically euthyroid. The generalized defect in cellular thyroid hormone action is a result of a mutation in the T_3-binding domain of the nuclear thyroid hormone receptor protein c-erbA beta. The mutations are family specific, and both heterozygous and homozygous individuals have been described.

Rare patients have selective pituitary resistance to thyroid hormone and often exhibit the symptoms and signs of hyperthyroidism, increased serum total and free T_4 and T_3 levels, increased TSH level, and a normal TSH response to TRH. This organ-selective resistance to T_3 action probably results from the tissue-specific distribution of multiple types of the c-erbA nuclear-binding protein isoforms. Pituitary resistance to thyroid hormone can be distinguished from hyperthyroidism secondary to a TSH-producing pituitary adenoma by the finding that TSH produced by the adenoma is unresponsive to TRH stimulation and the serum level of the alpha subunit of TSH is increased.

Amiodarone and the radiographic contrast agents iopanoic acid (Telepaque) and ipodate (Oragrafin) inhibit 5'-deiodination in liver and kidney and therefore impair the peripheral conversion of T_4 to T_3, resulting in a decrease in serum T_3 levels and increase in rT_3 levels (Fig. 297-4). In addition, these drugs inhibit the 5'-deiodinase II found in the pituitary, decreasing intrapituitary T_4 to T_3 conversion and causing a rise in TSH. Serum T_4 levels may be elevated, either secondary to the TSH elevation or as a result of decreases in the T_4 clearance rate. It should be noted that these drugs contain high concentrations of iodine and may also result in either iodide-induced hypothyroidism or, rarely, iodide-induced hyperthyroidism. The beta-adrenergic blocking drug propranolol, when given in high doses, occasionally is associated with elevated T_4 levels. The mechanism appears to be secondary to an inhibition of T_4 to T_3 conversion and decrease in the disposal rate of T_4, a property that is specific for the d-isomer of propranolol. Other beta-adrenergic blockers do not exert this effect.

Acute Psychiatric Illness

Acute psychiatric illness is associated with an increased incidence of T_4 level elevation, especially in patients having unipolar or bipolar depression, hyperemesis gravidarum, or paranoid schizophrenia. Although the patients are invariably euthyroid clinically, they frequently have a blunted to absent TSH response to TRH. The T_4 values and TRH responsiveness usually return to normal with treatment or resolution of the underlying condition. The mechanism of the abnormality is unknown.

L-Thyroxine Therapy

Patients treated with oral L-thyroxine may occasionally have elevated T_4 levels, despite being clinically euthyroid and having normal T_3 levels. The mechanism of the increase is unclear; however, it seems to be

---

BOX 297-2
Euthyroid hyperthyroxinemia

Elevated thyroxine-binding globulin level
Thyroid hormone resistance state
Iodine and iodine-containing drugs (amiodarone, ipodate)
High-dose propranolol
Acute psychiatric illness
Familial dysalbuminemic hyperthyroxinemia
Hyperemesis gravidarum

BOX 297-3
Alterations in thyroxine-binding globulin levels

Increased	Decreased
Estrogens	Androgens
Pregnancy	Glucocorticoids
Oral contraceptives	L-Asparaginase
Tamoxifen	Nephrotic syndrome
Perphenazine	Acromegaly
Clofibrate	Severe illness
Acute hepatitis	Starvation
Acute intermittent porphyria	Chronic hepatitis
Genetic	Genetic

BOX 297-4
Euthyroid hypothyroxinemia

Nonthyroidal illness
Decreased thyroxine-binding globulin level
Drugs
    Carbamazepine (Tegretol)
    Phenytoin
    Salicylates
    Triiodothyronine
Genetic

BOX 297-5
Causes of thyrotoxicosis

Common	**Uncommon**
Graves' disease	Pituitary adenoma
Subacute thyroiditis	Struma ovarii
Silent	Metastatic thyroid cancer
Painful	Embryonal carcinoma of the
Toxic adenoma	testes
Toxic multinodular goiter	Choriocarcinoma
Excessive thyroxine hor-	Hyperemesis gravidarum
mone replacement	Isolated pituitary resistance
Iodide (Jodbasedow syn-	to thyroid hormone
drome)	

BOX 297-6
Common symptoms and signs of thyrotoxicosis

Tachycardia	Goiter
Anxiety	Tachycardia
Tremulousness	Widened pulse pressure
Increased appetite	Tremor
Weight loss	Warm smooth skin
Heat intolerance	Lid lag
Excessive sweating	Stare
Proximal muscle weakness	Exophthalmos*
Emotional lability	Infiltrative dermopathy*
Increased defecation	Hyperreflexia
Decreased sleep time	

*Specific for Graves' disease.

---

greater 2 to 4 hours after ingestion of the dose. Thus it is probably best to obtain the blood sample for testing before the daily dose is administered. The serum T_3 level is normal if the patient is euthyroid. The supersensitive TSH appears to be the preferred test to assess the patient's metabolic state and to guide thyroxine replacement dosing.

Euthyroid Hypothyroxinemia

A decrease in serum total T_4 level in euthyroid patients is known as euthyroid hypothyroxinemia. It is most commonly due to a decrease in the major binding protein, TBG. A decrease in TBG level is seen in a number of conditions (Box 297-4). Pharmacologic doses of glucocorticoids and testosterone, high levels of growth hormone as found in active acromegaly, and loss of large amounts of protein in the urine of patients with the nephrotic syndrome are among the more common causes of TBG deficiency and euthyroid hypothyroxinemia. A decrease in TBG level may also occur on a genetic basis and is X-linked; males are more severely affected than females. The deficiency of TBG on a genetic basis may be found in as many as 1 in 2000 people and is much more common than the genetic condition producing an increase in TBG. Because transthyretin and albumin are minor binding proteins for T_4, decreases in these proteins alone do not lower T_4 to below-normal levels.

Two types of drugs, phenytoin and salicylates, cause euthyroid hypothyroxinemia. Phenytoin appears to decrease the binding of T_4 to TBG and, most important, accelerates T_4 degradation and disposal. Salicylates inhibit the binding of T_4 and T_3 to TBG.

Severe systemic illness in a euthyroid patient may be associated with a decreased serum total T_4 level secondary to endogenous inhibitors of T_4 binding to TBG.

THYROTOXICOSIS

Thyrotoxicosis is a complex pathophysiologic state secondary to excessive concentrations of free, biologically active thyroid hormone (T_4/T_3) in the blood and tissues. The term *thyrotoxicosis* is frequently used interchangeably with *hyperthyroidism*. However, in the strictest sense, *hyperthyroidism* comprises conditions in which the excessive amounts of thyroid hormone are derived from an overactive, hyperfunctional thyroid gland; *thyrotoxicosis* applies more broadly and includes all causes of excess thyroid hormone, whether they are intrinsic or extrinsic to the thyroid gland.

Causes

There are many causes of thyrotoxicosis (Box 297-5). The most common are Graves' disease, toxic multinodular goiter, toxic adenoma, thyrotoxicosis factitia, subacute thyroiditis, silent thyroiditis, excessive thyroid hormone replacement therapy, and iodide (Jodbasedow syndrome). Uncommon causes include TSH-producing tumor of the pituitary, metastatic embryonal carcinoma of the testis, choriocarcinoma, struma ovarii, metastatic follicular thyroid cancer, and isolated pituitary resistance to thyroid hormone.

Signs and Symptoms

The general signs and symptoms of thyrotoxicosis may be among the most dramatic found in clinical medicine or conversely may be subtle.

The more overt signs and symptoms tend to occur most frequently in the young, whereas in elderly patients, many of the typical findings may be masked and are more likely to be misdiagnosed. The general clinical features of thyrotoxicosis are extraordinarily diverse because thyroid hormone affects virtually every organ system in the body. Some of the signs and symptoms are associated with all forms of thyrotoxicosis and some are found only in specific types. The expression of the various signs and symptoms is also influenced by the duration of the thyrotoxicosis. The most frequent signs and symptoms associated with thyrotoxicosis are shown in Box 297-6. The signs and symptoms are common to all forms of thyrotoxicosis with notable exceptions such as ophthalmopathy and infiltrative dermopathy, which are specific representatives of the immunologic aspects of Graves' disease (discussed later). Goiter is present in most, but not all, types of thyrotoxicosis. Symptoms and signs referable to the cardiovascular system are regularly present in all cases and include sinus tachycardia, palpitations, widened pulse pressure with an elevated systolic blood pressure, hyperdynamic precordium, and brisk carotid upstrokes. Patients may have supraventricular arrhythmias, classically atrial fibrillation. Elderly patients with low serum TSH levels and normal serum T_4 levels may exhibit this arrhythmia as the only clue to the presence of subclinical thyrotoxicosis.

The skin is usually smooth, warm, and moist with increased sweating. The hair is fine and grows faster than normal. Areas of depigmentation (vitiligo) or increased pigmentation are characteristic of Graves' disease. Patients complain of hypersensitivity to heat and may feel uncomfortably warm even in winter. Appetite is often dramatically increased and classically associated with a significant weight loss because of the increased metabolic rate. Patients complain of excessive nervousness and anxiety and many describe it as feeling as though they have had "too much caffeine." A tremor of the hands, which may interfere with fine movements such as writing or using utensils, is regularly found and is most easily demonstrated with the hands outstretched. Patients usually have excessive energy and frequently complain of decreased sleep time, although fatigue and proximal muscle weakness are associated with longer-duration disease. Complaints suggesting proximal muscle weakness include exercise intolerance and difficulty in lifting or carrying heavy objects, combing hair, climbing stairs, or arising from a chair. Gastrointestinal tract complaints include an increased number of bowel movements and occasionally frank diarrhea. Women may notice a decrease in frequency of menstrual periods; men may note mild gynecomastia. Eye signs common to all types of thyrotoxicosis include stare, lid lag, and lid retraction. Exophthalmos and extraocular muscle palsies are potentially more serious developments and are specific for Graves' disease.

Many of the symptoms and signs of thyrotoxicosis are secondary to excessive adrenergic hormone stimulation. Although the hyperadrenergic state characteristic of thyrotoxicosis has been recognized for most of the 20th century and subjected to numerous investigations, the precise mechanism of increase in adrenergic tone is unclear. Direct measurements of serum catecholamine levels yield normal or low findings. Despite the lack of understanding of this clinical finding, drugs that counteract adrenergic hormones such as beta blockers are highly effective, improving a number of the signs and symptoms of thyrotoxicosis.

The role of the adrenergic nervous system is further emphasized when considering the differential diagnosis of thyrotoxicosis. Anxiety states and pheochromocytoma can produce many of the same clinical findings. Meticulous history and physical examination are usually sufficient to rule out these diagnoses. Patients with anxiety states have cool skin, cool and moist palms of the hands, normal sleeping pulses, and, unless fortuitously present, no goiter. Patients with pheochromocytoma have paroxysmal symptoms and usually manifest diastolic hypertension. Goiter is absent. If history and physical examination are insufficient to establish the diagnosis, routine thyroid function tests including a sensitive TSH assay should be used to rule out thyrotoxicosis.

Graves' Disease

Graves' disease, also known as diffuse toxic goiter, Basedow's disease, or Parry's disease, is an immunologic disorder characterized by the presence of one or more of the following: goiter, hyperthyroidism, ophthalmopathy, and infiltrative dermopathy. The typical patient has goiter and hyperthyroidism and often has either overt or subtle ophthalmopathy. Infiltrative dermopathy is much less common. Graves' disease occurs more commonly in women in a ratio of about 8:1 and has a prevalence as high as 2% of the female population. There is a strong genetic component with an increased frequency of HLA-B8 and HLA-DR3 in Europeans, HLA-BW35 in Japanese, and HLA-BW46 in Chinese. Families may have some members with Graves' disease and some with Hashimoto's thyroiditis. Graves' disease occurs at all ages and is the most common form of hyperthyroidism, particularly in patients less than 50 years of age; hyperthyroidism secondary to nodular goiter assumes increasing importance in older patients, although some of these may have Graves' disease variants.

Graves' disease is an autoimmune disease. Patients and their families have an increased frequency of other autoimmune diseases such as myasthenia gravis, lupus erythematosus, insulin-dependent diabetes mellitus, pernicious anemia, Sjögren's syndrome, Addison's disease, and autoimmune thrombocytopenic purpura. There is a high frequency of thyroid-antimicrosomal antibodies. In some patients with Hashimoto's thyroiditis, Graves' disease may ultimately develop, and in some patients with Graves' disease Hashimoto's thyroiditis and later hypothyroidism evolve.

Graves' disease is well established as one of several diseases secondary to antibodies to a cell surface receptor. The antibody in Graves' disease is directed at the TSH receptor (TRAb). The antibody may be a family of antibodies directed against different domains of the TSH receptor, one being stimulatory of all the thyroid hormone biosynthetic processes within the thyroid, one predominantly an inhibitor of TSH binding, and another perhaps a stimulator of thyroid cell growth. TRAbs are present in more than 90% of all patients with Graves' disease. They are immunoglobulins (IgG) that may arise secondary to defects in T-lymphocyte suppressor (CD 8+) cell function. The role of the thyrocyte as the source of one or more cell surface antigens, which are crucial in the autoimmune diathesis that leads to

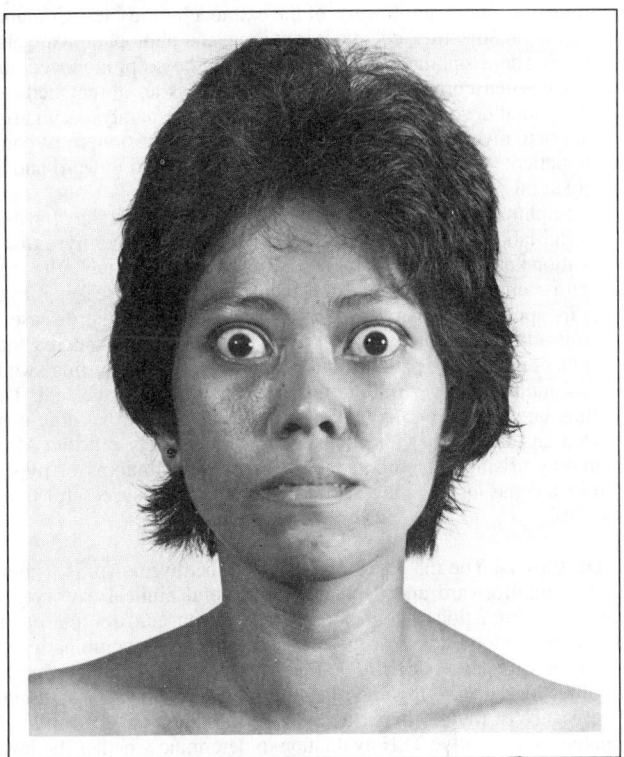

FIGURE 297-6   Graves' disease manifesting as hyperthyroidism and ocular involvement with significant proptosis and stare.

Graves' disease, is currently under investigation. Whether it is a major histocompatability complex (MHC) class II antigen or non-MHC epitope that is essential to this disease remains to be determined.

The clinical picture of a patient with Graves' disease serves as the prototype for all patients with thyrotoxicosis with notable exceptions unique to Graves' disease. The plethora of symptoms and signs can be categorized into three basic components. The first are those produced by adrenergic stimulation, including tachycardia, palpitations, nervousness, anxiety, depression, irritability, tremor, ocular stare, lid lag, increased systolic blood pressure, widened pulse pressure, and increased cardiac contractility and output. These are characteristically dependent on the continuing presence of adrenergic stimulation and are amenable to acute therapeutic intervention with antiadrenergic agents and relatively easily reversed. A second component are those signs caused by excess thyroid hormone, including increased oxygen consumption, hyperphagia, increased synthesis of a variety of structural and enzymatic proteins, myopathy, some psychologic disturbances, and possibly some component of the tachycardia, arrhythmias, and cardiac hypertrophy. Because thyroid hormone effects are mediated at the nuclear level by changes in specific protein synthesis, the alterations produced by thyroid hormone excess tend to be prolonged and therefore slower to reverse with therapy, which must be directed first at achieving normal levels of thyroid hormone.

The third or immunologic component is unique to patients with Graves' disease and is not part of the symptoms and signs found with the other causes of thyrotoxicosis. The most constant sign in this component is a diffuse goiter that is secondary to the growth stimulation of the thyroid provided by TRAb. The goiters of Graves' disease are of variable size, ranging from the minimum enlargement so common in elderly patients to the symmetrically enlarged, prominent thyroid glands of younger patients. Lymphadenopathy, splenomegaly, and vitiligo are present in a small but significant percentage of patients.

Two prominent manifestations of the immunologic component deserve special mention. Ophthalmopathy (Fig. 297-6), including exophthalmos and extraocular muscle inflammation, results from a complex, apparently antigen- and organ-specific immunologic reaction. The immunologic process is characterized by proliferation of retroorbital tissue, producing exophthalmos, lymphocytic infiltration, edema, inflammation, and, later, fibrosis of the extraocular muscles. Conjunctival irritation, injection, edema, lacrimation, and photophobia are also observed. The exophthalmos can occasionally be so pronounced and progressive that corneal irritation and visual loss are threatened, requiring orbital decompression. Extraocular muscle paralysis can arise secondary to myositis and produce disabling double vision; most commonly patients manifest difficulty in convergence and upward and/or superolateral gaze.

The ophthalmopathy may occur before the onset of signs, symptoms, and laboratory abnormalities characteristic of hyperthyroidism, a condition known as euthyroid Graves' disease. Ophthalmopathy may worsen or improve during the treatment of Graves' disease; it may make its appearance many years after the treatment of the disease.

Infiltrative dermopathy, also known as pretibial myxedema, occurs in less than 5% of patients. It is characterized by nonpitting swelling and induration over the pretibial area and dorsa of the feet. The swelling and induration may be localized to plaques or be more generalized and is usually violaceous and often intensely pruritic. Most commonly arising contemporaneously with the symptoms of hyperthyroidism, the lesions may also appear years after successful treatment.

Diagnosis. The diagnosis of Graves' hyperthyroidism is usually quite straightforward and depends on a careful clinical history and physical examination, a high index of suspicion, and routine determinations of blood levels of the thyroid hormones. A combination of serum total T_4 level, THBR, or free thyroxine index is appropriate initial testing because together they are highly accurate for assessing the presence of thyroid hyperfunction. A useful and cost-effective alternative is a sensitive TSH evaluation to determine whether the level is suppressed. The sensitive TSH determination is also very useful when the diagnosis of hyperthyroidism remains unclear after the initial T_4 and THBR evaluations. Such a circumstance occurs in selected cases of Graves' hyperthyroidism, in which the serum total T_3 level is elevated and the T_4 level normal (T_3 toxicosis). The suppressed TSH level confirms the thyroid overactivity.

Radioiodine scanning should not be considered a routine test in Graves' disease and should generally be used to discriminate among the various forms of thyrotoxicosis when this distinction may guide therapy (e.g., Graves' disease vs. toxic multinodular goiter). Radioiodine uptake is useful in the diagnosis and plays a particularly helpful role in distinguishing Graves' disease from silent thyroiditis and in the calculation of the dose of ^{131}I when the latter is selected as the treatment modality. Radioiodine scanning and uptake should not be performed in women in the childbearing years until pregnancy has been ruled out.

Treatment. A number of highly effective therapeutic agents and approaches are used for the treatment of Graves' disease, including propylthiouracil and methimazole, ^{131}I, surgery, adrenergic blocking drugs, and iodide. The selection is determined primarily by the clinical setting and the preference of the physician.

Propylthiouracil and methimazole are thionamides that inhibit thyroid hormone biosynthesis and are most commonly used in younger patients. They act to decrease organification and impair the coupling reaction in a dose-dependent manner. At high doses (>600 mg/day) propylthiouracil, but not methimazole, inhibits the peripheral conversion of T_4 to T_3. Both drugs may exert some of their effects via the immune system. There is clinical evidence that they decrease activated helper T cells and increase activated suppressor T cells as well as lower TRAb levels.

The usual starting dose for propylthiouracil is 100 to 150 mg orally every 8 hours and for methimazole 30 to 45 mg orally in one daily dose. When the patient becomes euthyroid, the dose is decreased to the lowest possible total daily dose to maintain normal thyroid function. Complications of these agents include nausea, loss of taste, and, in less than 0.5% of patients, agranulocytosis. After treatment with these drugs for periods up to 1 to 2 years, a variable number of patients (15% to 40%) with Graves' disease enter remission. Evidence that a patient with Graves' disease is undergoing remission is provided by a marked decrease in size of the goiter, a fall in TRAb levels, and the return of a normal TSH level. Relapses are frequent and unpredictable.

In comparing these two drugs, both have relative advantages in different situations. Methimazole has a long duration of action, enabling it to be given in one daily dose enhancing patient compliance. Propylthiouracil crosses the placenta and crosses into breast milk much less than methimazole and is the preferred drug, if antithyroid drug therapy must be used in pregnancy or during breast-feeding. It also decreases T_4 to T_3 conversion, which is of theoretic advantage in emergency situations such as the treatment of thyroid storm.

Radioiodine. Radioiodine therapy has received widespread acceptance as the treatment of choice for Graves' disease. It is safe, is economical over the long range, and effectively ablates functioning thyroid tissue. Its limitation in treatment of younger patients stems from the persistent concern about its potential effect on the progeny of patients treated with this isotope. Experience in more than 500,000 patients has indicated that there is no evidence of any increased genetic damage in the offspring. There has been no increased incidence of leukemia, carcinoma of the thyroid, or other tumors in the patients or their progeny. Hypothyroidism is the major undesired effect of ^{131}I therapy. It is difficult to gauge the dose even after measurements of iodine uptake and thyroid size, and there is no way to predict the response of the gland. One year after ^{131}I therapy, at least one fourth of the patients are hypothyroid, and this percentage further increases with time. On the other hand, if smaller doses are used, there is a higher incidence of recurrence of hyperthyroidism.

Surgery. Subtotal thyroidectomy is no longer a preferred treatment for patients with Graves' disease. It is reserved for young patients with the disease who do not enter remission with propylthiouracil or methimazole therapy and who are not candidates for radioiodine therapy. Surgery may be used for patients who have a clinically palpable, cold nodule in the Graves' disease goiter.

Iodide. Iodide is mainly used for the emergency management of thyroid storm and for thyrotoxic patients about to undergo surgery, because of its rapid effect and ability to decrease the vascularity of the thyroid gland. In pharmacologic doses (>5 mg per day), iodide rapidly inhibits the release of T_3 and T_4 from the thyroid gland. It also inhibits the organification of iodine, a transitory effect in almost all patients, lasting a few days to a week. Iodide is not used for routine treatment of hyperthyroidism and frequently complicates treatment because it greatly expands glandular iodide stores, making it more difficult to treat with antithyroid drugs and subsequent ^{131}I administration.

Complications of iodide therapy include inflammation of the salivary glands, conjunctivitis, and skin rashes. Rarely, administration of iodide to a euthyroid patient may precipitate hyperthyroidism (discussed later).

Beta-Adrenergic Blockade. Beta-adrenergic blocking agents are very effective in the short-term treatment of many of the most acute and prominent symptoms of hyperthyroidism. Propranolol is the beta-adrenergic blocking drug used most frequently. Within hours it improves palpitations, tachycardia, anxiety, and tremor. Associated depression may improve, and proximal myopathy occasionally improves significantly. Beta-blocking drugs do not affect the nonadrenergically mediated symptoms or signs of hyperthyroidism such as goiter, heat intolerance, ophthalmopathy, or weight loss.

Beta blockers are indicated in the following settings: (1) the short-term management of tachycardia or other debilitating cardiovascular symptoms, especially in older patients with no history of congestive heart failure; (2) symptomatic relief of severe anxiety or tremor; (3) with self-limited hyperthyroidism such as that found in subacute and silent thyroiditis; and (4) in thyroid storm, in which they produce a very rapid decrease in heart rate (in 2 to 3 hours when given orally; in minutes when given intravenously) that may be critical in management. The usual daily dose of propranolol taken orally is 40 to 160 mg in four divided doses.

Contraindications to the use of propranolol and other beta blockers include chronic lung disease (asthma, emphysema, bronchospasm) wherein abolition of the beta-adrenergic mechanisms responsible for bronchodilation may lead to severe bronchospasm and respiratory failure, sinus bradycardia or greater than second-degree heart block,

BOX 297-7
Causes of thyrotoxicosis with a low radioiodine uptake

Thyrotoxicosis factitia
Subacute thyroiditis
Iodine
Struma ovarii

in treatment of patients receiving other myocardial depressants such as quinidine or procainamide, and in congestive heart failure. If a patient has heart failure that is heart rate–related, in conjunction with proper monitoring, propranolol may be given with other cardiotropic drugs cautiously by intravenous (IV) titration to decrease the heart rate; shorter-acting beta blockers such as esmolol may be preferable. Propranolol is also contraindicated in patients receiving monoamine oxidase inhibitors, and care should be exercised in patients prone to spontaneous hypoglycemia, such as insulin-dependent diabetics.

Toxic Nodular Goiter (Plummer's Disease)

Autonomous, hyperfunctioning nodules may develop in a setting of a single-nodule or multinodule goiter. The reason for the hyperfunction is unknown, but there seems to be a clear progression from a nontoxic to a toxic state with time. In a single nodule of sufficient size the excess levels of T_4 and T_3 suppress the remainder of the thyroid gland. Multinodular goiters may have one or more hyperfunctioning nodules. Toxic nodular goiters are more common in older patients. The symptoms and signs are typical of hyperthyroidism, are usually milder than those seen in Graves' disease, and have no immunologic component. The diagnosis is established by routine thyroid blood tests. There is a high frequency of T_3 toxicosis. Radioiodine scanning is necessary to define the anatomy of the thyroid. Radioactive iodine and surgery are the usual treatment options. Many toxic nodular glands are relatively resistant to ^{131}I therapy and require high doses for successful treatment.

Thyrotoxicosis Factitia

The syndrome of thyrotoxicosis factitia usually results from deliberate, surreptitious administration of thyroid hormone or inadvertent overdose during thyroid hormone treatment. The physician should have a high index of suspicion for this diagnosis in thyrotoxic patients who do not manifest a goiter. If T_4 is ingested in excess, the laboratory findings consist of high total T_4 and T_3 levels, high THBR level, a low radioiodine uptake, and absent goiter. If T_3 is ingested in excess, the laboratory findings consist of a low total T_4 level, high total T_3 level, low to low-normal THBR level, low radioiodine uptake, and absent goiter (Box 297-7).

Subacute (DeQuervain's) Thyroiditis

Subacute, or DeQuervain's, thyroiditis, or inflammatory disease of the thyroid characterized by a tender goiter, is discussed in more detail in the section Thyroiditis. During the acute inflammatory stage of several weeks' duration preformed stores of thyroid hormone within thyroglobulin are released into the bloodstream and the thyroid hormone is made available to the tissues after hydrolysis of the thyroglobulin. The thyrotoxicosis is self-limited, lasting only as long as the preformed stores of hormone are released by the inflammatory process. Serum total T_4 and T_3 levels are elevated, TSH level is suppressed, and classically the radioiodine uptake is 0% or only 1% to 2%.

Silent Thyroiditis

Silent thyroiditis, an autoimmune disorder, is discussed in more detail in the section Thyroiditis. Although silent thyroiditis occurs in both women and men, it is more common in women, particularly in the postpartum period. The thyrotoxic stage of this thyroiditis is usually quite mild, generally seen in the first few weeks to months after delivery, and self-limited. There is only a mild degree of thyroid enlargement and the gland is nontender. Serum total T_4 and T_3 levels are elevated, TSH level is suppressed, and radioiodine uptake is normal or low. Thyroid antimicrosomal antibodies are present in many patients.

Thyroid Hormone Therapy

In the course of thyroid hormone replacement therapy, patients may be euthyroid clinically and have normal or high normal total T_4 and T_3 concentrations but suppressed TSH concentration indicated by sensitive assay. These patients have subclinical hyperthyroidism. It is important to adjust the replacement dose downward because patients such as these are at risk for increased bone turnover and cardiac effects including atrial fibrillation and ventricular hypertrophy.

Iodine-Induced Thyrotoxicosis (Jodbasedow Syndrome)

Iodine-induced thyrotoxicosis (Jodbasedow syndrome) usually occurs when large doses of iodine are administered to patients with underlying thyroid disease such as nontoxic multinodular goiter or iodine-deficient goiter and was originally described in patients with a diffuse goiter. The source of excess iodine is frequently provided in the course of a diagnostic test using iodinated-contrast agents but occasionally is derived from dietary supplements or from drugs such as amiodarone that are 30% (by weight) iodine. The hyperthyroidism is generally of short duration, lasting several days to several weeks. Total T_4 and/or T_3 level is elevated, and radioiodine uptake is low. Definitive therapy may be required, depending on the underlying thyroid abnormality.

Rare Causes of Thyrotoxicosis

The hyperthyroidism secondary to a TSH-producing tumor of the pituitary is due to overproduction of T_4 and T_3 after sustained stimulation of the thyroid by TSH. The goiter is usually small, and the condition may not be suspected unless a TSH level is obtained and found to be inappropriately elevated. Hyperthyroidism secondary to choriocarcinoma is due to the ability of human chorionic gonadotropin (HCG) to bind to thyroid TSH receptors weakly and stimulate the gland. Struma ovarii is an ovarian teratoma containing functioning thyroid tissue; radioiodine scanning reveals uptake in the ovarian tumor and suppression of thyroid uptake of radioiodine. Widely metastatic follicular thyroid cancer of substantial mass may have enough functional thyroid tissue to produce either T_4 or T_3 toxicosis. Treatment is surgical removal of the tumor, appropriate chemotherapy, or, in the case of metastatic follicular cancer, administration of ^{131}I.

Special Problems

Thyrotoxic Storm. Thyrotoxic storm is a dreaded complication of Graves' disease characterized by abrupt onset of florid symptoms of thyrotoxicosis, with some additional symptoms and signs not typical of uncomplicated Graves' disease including fever, hypotension, marked weakness, extreme restlessness, confusion, psychosis or even coma, cardiovascular collapse, and shock. These signs and symptoms are a manifestation of the loss of the normal ability to regulate heat dissipation, maintain circulatory hemodynamics, and control oxygen consumption in a severely hypermetabolic state. Thyroid storm occurs in untreated or inadequately treated Graves' disease and may be precipitated by infection, trauma, surgery, diabetic acidosis, stress, toxemia of pregnancy, labor and delivery, or discontinuance of antithyroid medication.

The patients have obvious signs of Graves' disease and almost always have large goiters. The presence of fever is a sine qua non for the diagnosis, which is made by the usual tests. Radioiodine uptake is particularly useful because 2-hour uptake of ^{123}I or ^{131}I is markedly elevated, helping to establish the diagnosis very quickly. Total

BOX 297-8
Treatment of thyroid storm

Propranolol: 160 mg/day orally in four divided doses; or 1 mg
  slowly IV every 4 hours under careful monitoring
IV glucose solutions
Correction of dehydration and electrolyte imbalance
Iodide-30 drops: Lugol's solution daily orally in three or four di-
  vided doses; or 1 to 2 g sodium iodine slowly by IV drip
Propylthiouracil: 900 to 1200 mg/day orally or by gastric tube
Cooling blanket for hyperthermia
Plasmapheresis to lower T_4 and T_3 levels (in selected cases)
Digitalis if necessary
Treatment of underlying disease (e.g., infection)
Corticosteroid: 100 mg hydrocortisone IV every 8 hours
Definitive therapy after control of the crisis: ablation of the thyroid
  gland with ^{131}I or surgery.

BOX 297-9
Causes of hypothyroidism

Autoimmune (atrophic)
Postablative
Goitrous (iodine or synthetic defect)
Athyreotic
Nonautoimmune thyroiditis

T_4 and T_3 levels are elevated to the same degree observed in uncomplicated Graves' disease.

Acute treatment of thyroid storm consists of administration of propranolol orally or intravenously, intravenous sodium iodide, and an antithyroid drug such as propylthiouracil (900 to 1200 mg daily) (Box 297-8). Supporting measures including administration of intravenous fluids, oxygen, a cooling blanket, and glucocorticoids are usually required. Plasmapheresis may be required to lower T_4 and T_3 levels rapidly. Historic mortality in thyroid storm is about 20%; however, prompt recognition and treatment should lead to a satisfactory result. Improvement should be expected within 24 hours and recovery within a few days to a week. Ultimate definitive therapy after recovery should consist of treatment with ^{131}I.

T_3 Toxicosis. In general, T_3 and T_4 concentrations are regularly increased in patients with hyperthyroidism. In Graves' disease, increases in serum T_3 concentrations are usually somewhat greater on a proportional basis compared with T_4 concentrations, probably as a result of both increased thyroidal secretion of T_3 and increased peripheral conversion of T_4 to T_3. Occasional patients early in the course of Graves' disease may demonstrate all or most of the signs and symptoms of hyperthyroidism but normal values for serum total T_4 level, THBR, and radioiodine uptake. When measurement of serum total T_3 level is shown to be elevated, and the TSH level is suppressed, the condition is called T_3 toxicosis. In these patients eventually the classic laboratory abnormalities of hyperthyroidism develop when the state of T_3 toxicosis continues untreated. In addition to Graves' disease, the incidence of T_3 toxicosis appears to be increased in areas where dietary intake of iodide is lowest and in patients with nodular goiter or a toxic adenoma. Because T_3 toxicosis is merely an early manifestation of thyrotoxicosis when it is discovered, it should be treated by the usual means.

Thyrotoxicosis in Pregnancy. Graves' disease may arise de novo during pregnancy, or the patient may have Graves' disease, treated or untreated, and become pregnant. In any case, thyrotoxicosis in pregnancy is often a significant diagnostic and management challenge. Diagnosis is difficult because in pregnant women a small degree of thyroid enlargement and symptoms and signs of hypermetabolism such as anxiety, irritability, polyphagia, heat intolerance, increased sweating, and warm, moist skin develop. By the fourth to fifth month of pregnancy, total T_4 and T_3 levels are normally elevated about twofold and T_3 resin uptake or THBR is low secondary to TBG level elevation. Therefore the presence of a normal or high normal T_3 resin uptake or THBR is suggestive of hyperthyroidism. Discovery of suppressed TSH level by a sensitive TSH assay is diagnostic. Serum TRAb level should be determined to alert the pediatrician to the possibility of neonatal thyrotoxicosis. Radioiodine uptake and scanning are absolutely contraindicated because radioiodine crosses the placenta and can destroy the fetal thyroid gland, which is formed and functioning by the 12th week of pregnancy.

Treatment should be initiated with propylthiouracil in the usual starting dosage; methimazole is relatively contraindicated because it crosses the placenta to a greater extent than propylthiouracil. Propylthiouracil should be decreased to the lowest effective dose necessary to control the hyperthyroidism as soon as possible to minimize the risk of fetal goiter and/or hypothyroidism. If necessary, surgical treatment of the hyperthyroidism can be performed in the second trimester, but it is best to avoid surgery and the attendant risks of anesthesia and operative complications to the fetus. Surgery is contraindicated in the first and third trimesters because of a high risk of induction of premature labor and miscarriage. The fact that Graves' disease is difficult to manage adds a compelling reason to treat the disease definitively in any woman in the childbearing years to prevent potential complications of hyperthyroidism and its therapy in pregnancy.

Thyrotoxicosis in Adolescence. The most common cause of thyrotoxicosis in adolescence is Graves' disease. Its general clinical features in adolescence are similar to those in adulthood. Additional considerations arise in selection of therapy. Treatment options include antithyroid drugs, radioiodine, and surgery. Posttreatment hypothyroidism should be promptly treated to prevent the disruptive effects of hypothyroidism on growth and development.

HYPOTHYROIDISM

Deficiency in the amount of biologically active thyroid hormone at the tissue level is called hypothyroidism. Hypothyroidism is generally classified into two major groups: (1) primary hypothyroidism caused by thyroid gland failure and (2) secondary or central hypothyroidism produced by failure of the pituitary or hypothalamus in which the defect is a deficiency of TSH. Hypothyroidism caused by hypothalamic failure is also referred to as tertiary hypothyroidism because TRH deficiency causes inadequate TSH secretion from an otherwise functional thyrotroph cell of the anterior pituitary.

Causes

The most common type of hypothyroidism is that due to primary thyroid gland failure. Within this group are five basic causes of primary hypothyroidism (Box 297-9): autoimmune (atrophic), which includes chronic lymphocytic thyroiditis (Hashimoto's thyroiditis) and silent thyroiditis; postablative (^{131}I, thyroidectomy, head and neck irradiation); goitrous, athyreotic, and nonautoimmune thyroiditis (such as Riedel's thyroiditis); and subacute thyroiditis. The hypothyroidism of silent thyroiditis and subacute thyroiditis is usually but not always transient.

The most common cause is the atrophic autoimmune type, which is most likely a late stage of Hashimoto's (autoimmune) thyroiditis because the majority of the cases have significant elevations of thyroid antimicrosomal antibody levels. It is more common in women than men and is often associated with other autoimmune diseases of the endocrine system, including autoimmune hypoparathyroidism, adrenal failure, hypogonadism, and insulin-dependent diabetes mellitus. Recent studies have identified the presence of TSH receptor blocking antibodies as an important and potentially reversible cause of hypothyroidism in a subset of patients. Postablative primary thyroid gland failure is quite common and is usually found after ^{131}I treatment of thyrotoxicosis or subtotal or near-total thyroidectomy for thyroid cancer, Graves' disease, or toxic multinodular goiter. External mantle irradiation for Hodgkin's disease may also lead to thyroid gland failure; this generally evolves over a period of 5 to 10 years.

In goitrous hypothyroidism, goiter ensues because of decreased ability of the thyroid gland to synthesize thyroid hormone, leading to increased TSH secretion, which results in an increase in the size of the thyroid gland. Among the causes of goitrous hypothyroidism are endemic goiter, which occurs in regions of iodide deficiency such as the mountainous areas of Europe and South America. Children born of parents having an endemic goiter may be born with goitrous hypothyroidism (endemic cretinism). Drugs can produce goitrous hypothyroidism. The chronic administration of large doses of iodides as in expectorants sometimes results in goiter and hypothyroidism because of an inhibition of the organification step within the thyroid and an absence of the normal escape mechanism. Propylthiouracil and methimazole used for the treatment of hyperthyroidism may produce hypothyroidism and goiter. When used in pregnant women, they cross the placenta, occasionally causing goitrous hypothyroidism in the fetus. Lithium, which inhibits thyroid hormone synthesis and release, commonly produces a goiter and in a small subset of patients (primarily those with antimicrosomal antibodies) can induce hypothyroidism. Some vegetables, such as cassava, rutabaga, and white turnips, contain natural goitrogens. Drugs and natural goitrogen-induced causes are completely reversible when the offending agent is removed. A variety of genetic defects affecting thyroid hormone biosynthesis causes goitrous hypothyroidism. These genetic defects can affect transport of iodide, organification of iodide (with sensory nerve deafness and Pendred's syndrome), coupling of iodinated tyrosines, and intrathyroidal deiodination of thyroid hormone.

Athyreotic cretinism is found in children born with an absence of the thyroid gland. The various forms of thyroiditis which can result in atrophic or goitrous hypothyroidism are described in the section Thyroiditis. Hashimoto's thyroiditis may be the most common form of hypothyroidism if it is in fact the cause of end-stage, atrophic thyroid gland failure. In the early stages of Hashimoto's thyroiditis, the thyroid gland is typically enlarged, firm and rubbery in consistency, and infiltrated with lymphocytes. Although the production of thyroid hormone may remain normal, a subset of patients develop an inability to synthesize thyroid hormone. Defects in iodide organification with maintenance of iodide trapping are characteristic of Hashimoto's thyroiditis.

Riedel's thyroiditis is characterized by a dense fibrosis of the thyroid gland. Silent thyroiditis and subacute thyroiditis usually evolve through a hyperthyroid stage before the hypothyroid stage, and the hypothyroidism is usually transient.

Secondary forms of hypothyroidism are unusual, and the tertiary subgroup (hypothalamic) are rare in ordinary practice. Secondary and tertiary forms include pituitary tumors, vascular anomalies, infections, granulomatous disease, and other causes.

Symptoms and Signs

The symptoms and signs of primary thyroid gland failure are extraordinarily varied as a result of the multiple physiologic and biochemical effects of thyroid hormone on virtually every organ system. The symptoms and signs stand in stark contrast to those found in thyrotoxicosis and may be equally dramatic in their clinical presentation, which comprises the syndrome known as myxedema. On the other hand, they may be so subtle and insidious that the diagnosis may be overlooked for many months or even years unless the physician has a high index of suspicion and the patient or family is alert to the changes. The most common and characteristic symptoms and signs of hypothyroidism (myxedema) are listed in Box 297-10. The patients complain of weakness, fatigue, and general lack of energy. The voice is hoarse, and speech is dysarthric and slow. The facial expression is dull, and puffiness and periorbital swelling are caused by infiltration with the mucopolysaccharides hyaluronic acid and chondroitin sulfate. Patients frequently complain of cold intolerance and constipation.

Eyelids droop because of decreased adrenergic tone; hair is sparse and coarse; the skin is dry, scaly, and thick and has a definite pallor. There is often carotenemia, which is particularly notable on the palms and soles because of deposition of carotene in the lipid-rich epidermal layers. Patients are forgetful and show other evidence of intel-

---

> **BOX 297-10**
> ## Common symptoms and signs of hypothyroidism
>
> | | |
> |---|---|
> | Weakness | Eyelid droop |
> | Fatigue | Facial puffiness |
> | Cold intolerance | Periorbital edema |
> | Constipation | Hoarse voice |
> | Weight gain | Dry skin and hair |
> | Snoring | Bradycardia |
> | Menorrhagia | Diastolic hypertension |
> | Muscle cramps and stiffness | Delayed deep tendon reflex |
> | Paresthesias in hands and feet | Hypothermia |

lectual impairment, with a gradual change in personality. There may be frank psychosis ("myxedema madness").

Deposition of a proteinaceous material as well as an increase in muscle fiber diameter in the tongue may produce macroglossia, thick speech, and snoring. Bradycardia is found, and diastolic hypertension occurs in approximately 20% of patients. The heart may appear to be enlarged, usually as a result of the accumulation of a serous effusion of high protein content in the pericardial sac. There may also be pleural or abdominal effusions. The pericardial and pleural effusions develop slowly and only infrequently cause respiratory or hemodynamic distress. Paresthesias of the hands and feet are common, produced by carpal-tarsal tunnel syndromes caused by deposition of proteinaceous fluid in the ligaments around the wrist and ankle, producing nerve compression. Neuromuscular manifestations are varied, ranging from reflexes that are characterized by a slow relaxation to muscle hypertrophy, percussion myoedema, and myotonia. There is often menorrhagia, in contrast to the hypomenorrhea of hyperthyroidism. Hypothermia is often noted if the temperature is measured rectally.

It is important to differentiate secondary or central hypothyroidism from primary. There are a number of clinical clues, which usually result from secondary involvement of other endocrine organs when the pituitary and/or hypothalamus fails. These clues include amenorrhea rather than menorrhagia in a woman with known hypothyroidism; atrophic breasts; skin and hair that are thin and not coarse; skin depigmentation, diastolic hypotension, and a small heart without pericardial effusion.

Laboratory Diagnosis

The laboratory diagnosis of primary hypothyroidism is reasonably straightforward. Serum total T_4 and T_3 levels and THBR are low and the sine qua non is an elevated serum TSH level, usually to values above 20 μU/ml. The TSH level is the single best test for the diagnosis of primary thyroid gland failure for several reasons. The serum concentration of TSH rises early in the disease when serum concentrations of T_4 and/or T_3 may still be in the low-normal range. The TSH allows primary and secondary hypothyroidism to be distinguished, is normal in cases of euthyroid hypothyroxinemia, and plays the key role in the complex differentiation of hypothyroidism from the euthyroid sick syndrome.

Thyroid antimicrosomal antibodies can be useful in the laboratory assessment of hypothyroidism because they are present in most cases of hypothyroidism caused by Hashimoto's thyroiditis and also in the atrophic form of primary hypothyroidism. Radioiodine uptake is of no value in the diagnosis of primary thyroid gland failure.

Other laboratory abnormalities present in primary hypothyroidism may occasionally be the precipitating reason to diagnose hypothyroidism. These include elevation of serum cholesterol level and unexplained anemia, which may be normochromic-normocytic, hypochromic-microcytic, or, occasionally, macrocytic; increased serum levels of creatine kinase with a normal percentage of the CK-MB isoenzyme; elevation of other muscle enzymes, including aldolase, lactic dehydrogenase, and serum glutamic–oxaloacetic acid (SGOT); and hyperuricemia and hyponatremia. The electrocardiogram (ECG) classically shows a sinus bradycardia with low voltage in the precordial leads. Chest radiograph may show an enlarged heart, which on echocardiogram is usually noted to be secondary to a pericardial effusion.

The laboratory assessment of secondary hypothyroidism reveals several important differences from primary hypothyroidism. Most significantly serum TSH levels are low or normal, despite low serum total T_4 and T_3 levels. The TRH test is useful in confirming the diagnosis of secondary vs. primary hypothyroidism and pivotal in distinguishing between pituitary failure and hypothyroidism resulting from hypothalamic failure. In the former, TSH is not released in response to the injection of TRH, whereas in the latter it is released, albeit usually more slowly and with a delayed peak. Cholesterol levels are often not increased by secondary or tertiary hypothyroidism. Other abnormalities noted are consistent with the associated failure of other pituitary hormones such as growth hormone (GH), luteinizing hormone (LH), follicle-stimulating hormone (FSH), and adrenocorticotropic hormone (ACTH).

Differential Diagnosis

The fully expressed picture of hypothyroidism (myxedema) is classic, and the diagnosis usually obvious to the clinician. Many of the clinical features can be suggestive of chronic renal failure, nephrotic syndrome, or severe anemia. Patients who have euthyroid sick syndrome can pose a significant diagnostic challenge because of the degree of illness and the complexity of changes in the thyroid function tests. The euthyroid hypothyroxinemias require an understanding of thyroid function tests to prevent misdiagnosis as hypothyroidism. More subtle or subclinical presentations of hypothyroidism require a high index of suspicion based on the clinical setting such as age, sex, family history, postpartum history, associated autoimmune disease, or the finding of the other laboratory changes noted.

Treatment

The treatment of hypothyroidism is usually relatively simple and begins to produce highly satisfactory relief of symptoms within several days to several weeks. A variety of thyroid hormone preparations are available for replacement therapy, including synthetic preparations of T_4 and T_3, combinations of the two in purified thyroglobulin, and desiccated animal thyroid. Synthetic preparations of pure T_4 (L-thyroxine) are preferred and should be used for the routine treatment of all cases of hypothyroidism. Synthetic L-thyroxine is given once per day, generally in the morning. The average maintenance dose is 100 to 125 μg/day orally. In general, the maintenance dose decreases in the elderly and may increase in pregnant women. A wide variety of incremental dosages are available to accommodate those requiring maintenance doses significantly above or below the average. Absorption is fairly constant at about 75% of the administered dose. T_3 is generated by peripheral conversion of T_4, preventing the chemical and clinical T_3 toxicosis found in the administration of T_3 or T_3-T_4 combinations. The dose used should be the minimum that restores TSH levels to normal. The induction of subclinical hyperthyroidism as demonstrated by a suppressed TSH level by the sensitive assay should be prevented in the replacement therapy for hypothyroidism. This is important from a long-term perspective to prevent cardiac- and possibly bone-related complications.

Most patients under the age of 50 tolerate the initiation of full thyroid hormone replacement therapy without any difficulty. However, in older patients and in hypothyroid patients with known coronary artery disease the initiation of thyroid hormone therapy with full replacement doses may precipitate angina pectoris caused by the increase in myocardial oxygen consumption and heart rate and the demand this places on the coronary artery blood supply. Therefore in older patients with or without known coronary artery disease it is prudent to begin replacement therapy with a low dose. A reasonable scheme would be to begin with 25 μg T_4/day orally and increase by 25 μg T_4/day orally every 4 weeks, the time required for thyroid hormone to exert its maximum effects. Serum TSH level should be determined before each additional increase, until the desired replacement dose is attained. Smaller increments in dose may be required in some patients.

Patients with hypothyroidism and coexistent adrenal insufficiency

---

> **BOX 297-11**
> **Treatment of myxedema coma**
>
> Thyroid hormone administration
>   I-thyroxine 300 to 500 μg IV, then 100 μg daily
> or
>   Triiodothyronine 25 to 50 μg IV then 25 μg every 8 hours
> Intravenous fluids
> Gentle warming
> Glucocorticoid 50 to 100 mg hydrocortisone every 8 hours
> Antibiotics for suspected infection
> Respiratory support

---

caused by either primary adrenal gland or secondary pituitary (ACTH) failure should receive replacement therapy with corticosteroids before or at the time of replacement with thyroid hormone. Such treatment prevents the potential induction of acute adrenal insufficiency by the increase in cortisol metabolism imposed by thyroid hormone therapy.

T_3 should not be used alone for long-term replacement because its rapid turnover usually requires that it be taken at least twice daily. Some clinicians occasionally use T_3 as starting therapy because of the potential for more rapid onset of action. With the exception of myxedema coma, the chronic nature of hypothyroidism does not require rapid reversal of the metabolic and clinical changes. In addition, administering standard replacement amounts of T_3 (25 to 75 μg/day) results in rapidly increasing serum T_3 concentrations to potentially supranormal levels that return to normal or below normal by 24 hours. Therefore patients who receive T_3 are subject to varying therapeutic effects as a result of the short half-life (24 hours) of this preparation. Similar patterns of serum T_3 concentrations are seen when mixtures of T_3 and T_4 are taken orally. As noted, replacement regimens with synthetic preparations of T_4 reflect a different pattern of serum T_3 response with increases in serum T_3 to normal levels that occur gradually over 4 to 6 weeks.

Desiccated animal thyroid preparations are too variable in potency to be reliable and should not be used.

Special Problems

Myxedema Coma. Myxedema coma is a life-threatening but uncommon complication of hypothyroidism. It occurs most commonly but not exclusively in colder weather. Myxedema characteristically is found in patients with long-standing untreated primary hypothyroidism. Patients have a combination of altered mental status or coma, extreme hypothermia (temperatures 24° to 32.2° C [75.2° to 90° F]) hyporeflexia or areflexia, seizures, CO_2 retention, bradycardia, hypoxemia, and respiratory depression caused by decreased cerebral blood flow. Severe hypothermia may be overlooked unless special low-reading thermometers are used. Precipitating factors include exposure to cold, infection, trauma, and drugs such as sedatives that suppress the central nervous system (CNS). Rapid diagnosis based on clinical judgment, history, and physical examination is imperative because early death is likely if the diagnosis is overlooked. Once the diagnosis is seriously considered, treatment needs to be instituted before the return of the laboratory test results because the usual delay in the reporting of these tests is too long under these circumstances. It is preferable to initiate therapy and terminate it if thyroid function test results rule out the diagnosis rather than delay therapy and discover too late that the patient had myxedema with coma.

The treatment of myxedema coma is outlined in Box 297-11. The cornerstone is the administration of an intravenous bolus of thyroxine (300 to 500 μg) to saturate the unoccupied binding sites on TBG, making free hormone available for response, followed by daily intravenous doses of 50 to 100 μg of synthetic L-thyroxine. Because T_3 is now commercially available for parenteral use, this may provide more rapid metabolic responses in the treatment of myxedema coma. Supporting measures consisting of gentle warming and administration of

IV fluids, glucocorticoids, and antibiotics as necessary are lifesaving. The patient should not be rewarmed rapidly because it may precipitate cardiac arrhythmias. If alveolar ventilation is compromised, mechanical ventilation should be instituted.

Subclinical Hypothyroidism. The entity of subclinical hypothyroidism is characterized by normal serum total T_4 and T_3 concentrations and modest elevations of serum TSH level to between 6 and 15 μU/ml in patients who either are clinically euthyroid or have only subtle signs of hypothyroidism. The disorder is more common in women: overall prevalence estimates range from 5% to as high as 20% of women over the age of 60. Subclinical hypothyroidism appears to be part of the spectrum of autoimmune thyroiditis because of the frequent association of increased levels of thyroid antimicrosomal antibodies. The diagnosis is usually made in the course of general screening of patients, particularly elderly patients, for nonspecific complaints such as mild fatigue, lack of energy, mild depression, and constipation.

The decision whether to treat a patient with normal serum T_4 and T_3 levels and modest elevations of serum TSH level is a difficult one. In younger patients the tendency is to treat any reproducible TSH level elevation, especially in the setting of autoimmune thyroiditis (positive antibodies). In elderly patients the issue is less clear, and in the absence of information from randomized clinical trials, therapy should be reserved for patients with both elevated TSH and thyroid antimicrosomal antibody concentrations ($>1:1600$). In the absence of these antibodies the rate of progression to overt hypothyroidism is low. The metabolic complications of the milder, subclinical forms of hypothyroidism remain unresolved.

Once therapy has been initiated, it is important to ensure that the TSH concentration is normalized and not suppressed. Otherwise, subclinical hypothyroidism is exchanged for subclinical hyperthyroidism with its attendant risks.

Cardiac Surgery. Patients undergoing coronary artery bypass surgery have a fall in serum T_3 level during and after surgery. Although most studies have failed to show a clinical benefit from treatment of the low T_3 (nonthyroidal illness) level syndrome, a recent study of high-risk cardiac surgery patients has demonstrated improved hemodynamics and decreases postoperative arrythmias in T_3-treated compared with control patients. These observations support the important role of thyroid hormone in regulating cardiovascular performance.

THYROIDITIS
Hashimoto's Thyroiditis (Chronic Lymphocytic Thyroiditis, Autoimmune Thyroiditis)

Hashimoto's thyroiditis is characterized by a modest-sized goiter, lymphocytic infiltration of the thyroid, presence of organ-specific autoantibodies in a majority of patients, and hypothyroidism. It is one of the three major causes of primary thyroid gland failure. Hashimoto's thyroiditis is more common in women (8:1), is most frequent between the ages of 30 to 50, is frequently familial, and tends to be chronic and progressive.

Substantial evidence suggests that Hashimoto's thyroiditis is an autoimmune disease. Thyroid antimicrosomal and antithyroglobulin antibodies are commonly present; however, the thyroid inflammation is a cellular-mediated immune response. Occasionally the hypothyroidism is due to the presence of thyrotropin-blocking antibodies that block the binding of TSH to its receptor. In some patients Hashimoto's thyroiditis may evolve into the classic thyrotoxicosis of Graves' disease, and Graves' disease may have certain features in common with Hashimoto's thyroiditis, such as the presence of antimicrosomal and antithyroglobulin antibodies. Hashimoto's thyroiditis frequently coexists with other autoimmune diseases such as Sjögren's syndrome, pernicious anemia, rheumatoid arthritis, lupus erythematosus, progressive systemic sclerosis, myasthenia gravis, autoimmune hepatitis, primary biliary cirrhosis, Addison's disease (adrenal insufficiency), hypoparathyroidism, and insulin-dependent diabetes mellitus.

The incidence of Hashimoto's thyroiditis is increased in patients with chromosomal disorders including Turner's, Down, and Klinefelter's syndromes. There may be an increased incidence of papillary cancer of the thyroid, and there is a high concordance with thyroid lymphoma (see the section Thyroid Cancer). The early stages of the disease, which may last months to several years, are characterized by a nontender goiter of variable size that is firm and rubbery. Other features are lymphocytic infiltration of the thyroid, elevated levels of antithyroid antibodies (antimicrosomal and antithyroglobulin), normal or decreased serum T_4 level, and increased serum TSH level. Thyroid radioiodine uptake is increased with a patchy distribution caused by abnormalities within the thyroid epithelial cell that permit trapping of iodide but disrupt normal organification. About 20% of patients are frankly hypothyroid in the early stages.

The late stage of Hashimoto's thyroiditis is most likely represented in part by the typical adult atrophic, thyroid gland failure. The thyroid gland at this stage is fibrotic in addition to being atrophic and may no longer be palpable. However, many patients have a modestly enlarged, irregular, firm thyroid gland. Elevated levels of antithyroid antibodies may spontaneously decline with time. Serum T_4 and T_3 levels are generally below normal and serum TSH level is markedly elevated in the late stages of the disease, although some patients maintain normal thyroid function throughout. The hypothyroidism of classic Hashimoto's thyroiditis is almost always permanent; however, hypothyroidism associated with the presence of thyrotropin-blocking antibodies may be transient and remit.

Histopathologic examination of the gland reveals diffuse infiltration with lymphocytes, disruption of follicle architecture, and some degree of fibrosis. Epithelial cells demonstrating oxyphilic changes in the cytoplasm, called Askanazy cells, are pathognomonic of Hashimoto's thyroiditis.

The differential diagnosis is quite limited, and the laboratory abnormalities usually clearly distinguish Hashimoto's thyroiditis from nontoxic, euthyroid goiter. The most difficult differential is between Hashimoto's thyroiditis and thyroid lymphoma, which may also be associated with markedly elevated levels of thyroid antimicrosomal antibodies. Open biopsy may be required to obtain enough tissue to establish the diagnosis.

Thyroid hormone is provided to correct hypothyroidism and to attempt to decrease the size of the goiter or prevent its further growth. Surgical resection of the thyroid is reserved for large, cosmetically unattractive glands or in the unusual circumstance when compressive symptoms of the trachea or esophagus develop. Thyroid hormone replacement is given after surgery.

Subacute Thyroiditis (Granulomatous, Giant Cell, or DeQuervain's Thyroiditis)

Subacute thyroiditis is an inflammatory disease of the thyroid that may be caused by a virus. Mumps and viruses associated with upper respiratory tract infections are suspected etiologic agents. The clinical features are characteristic and the diagnosis straightforward. Patients usually experience sudden onset of "sore throat" (neck pain) with progressive tenderness in the neck and low-grade fever (37.8° to 38.3° C). The neck pain shifts characteristically from side to side and finally settles in one area, frequently radiating to the jaw and ears. It is often confused with dental problems, pharyngitis, or otitis and is aggravated by swallowing or turning the head. There are profound lassitude and fatigue not seen in other thyroid disorders. Symptoms and signs of thyrotoxicosis regularly occur in the first few weeks of the disease because of preformed hormone release from the markedly inflamed gland. Physical examination reveals a thyroid that is asymmetrically enlarged, very firm to hard in consistency, and exquisitely tender.

Histologic studies show destruction of follicles, a characteristic giant cell infiltration surrounding a central core of colloid, inflammation, and mild fibrosis. Laboratory findings early in the disease include an increase in T_4 level, a suppressed TSH level, a decrease in radioiodine uptake (often to 0%), leukocytosis, and a markedly elevated sedimentation rate. After several weeks, the T_4 level is decreased, the TSH level remains suppressed, and the radioiodine uptake remains low. At this stage symptoms of hypothyroidism may develop. Once the TSH level begins to rise and inflammation disappears, thyroid function test results normalize. Subacute thyroiditis is self-limiting, generally subsiding in a few months, and full recovery is the rule. Occasionally the thyroiditis recurs, and rarely it results in permanent hypothyroidism. Because the disease is self-limited, treatment should be conservative, consisting of administration of beta blockers for disturbing symptoms of thyrotoxicosis, aspirin 650 mg every 4 hours, and, only as a last resort, glucocorticoids such as prednisone 5 mg orally every 6 hours. On discontinuance of the latter, there is often a severe rebound in symptoms.

Subacute thyroiditis most frequently must be differentiated from hemorrhage into a nodule or cyst. This is best accomplished by the normal sedimentation rate and thyroid function test results associated with hemorrhage into a nodule or cyst. Pyogenic thyroiditis, although rare, also must be differentiated. The thyroid in this case is reddened, fever and leukocytosis are very high, and a specific septic site extrinsic to the thyroid is evident. *Pneumocystis carinii* can cause painful nodular thyroiditis in patients with acquired immunodeficiency syndrome (AIDS).

Silent Thyroiditis

Silent thyroiditis is an autoimmune disorder more common in women, often in the postpartum period. It is characterized by a variable but mild degree of thyroid enlargement and absence of thyroid tenderness. There is a self-limited hyperthyroid phase of several weeks to several months, often followed by a period of hypothyroidism (postpartum hypothyroidism) lasting weeks to months.

Many of the patients have elevated antimicrosomal antibody levels. This disease may be an autoimmune variant of Hashimoto's thyroiditis because biopsy results show lymphocytic infiltration. Diagnosis requires a high index of suspicion based on the clinical setting and generally mild symptoms. Total T_4 and T_3 levels are elevated, and the radioiodine uptake normal or low. The white blood cell count and sedimentation rate are normal.

Because silent thyroiditis is a self-limited, transient disorder that lasts 1 to 6 months, treatment is conservative. The thyrotoxic stage usually requires only adrenergic blockade with propranolol. Surgery and radioactive iodine therapy are contraindicated, and thionamides ineffective. The transient phase of hypothyroidism may require thyroid hormone replacement therapy if the patient is symptomatic. Most patients recover normal thyroid function; however, in some permanent hypothyroidism develops. Relapses may occur, particularly in cases of postpartum thyroiditis in which subsequent pregnancies may be followed by additional attacks. Some evidence suggests that thyroid hormone treatment before pregnancy can prevent these relapses.

Riedel's Thyroiditis

Riedel's thyroiditis, a rare form, is most common in women above age 50 and is characterized by an intense fibrosis of the thyroid gland and surrounding tissues in the neck. The thyroid is enlarged, nontender, and fixed in position and feels woody-hard on palpation. The thyroiditis may progress to clinical hypothyroidism. Frequently, Riedel's thyroiditis results in compression of adjacent structures producing respiratory distress and/or dysphagia. Surgical resection of the thyroid gland may be required to preserve and restore tracheal and esophageal function. A cine esophagram or flow-volume loop can give objective confirmation of clinical symptoms of dysphagia or dyspnea. The administration of synthetic L-thyroxine corrects any hypothyroidism but does not result in regression of the goiter.

EUTHYROID GOITER

Euthyroid (nontoxic) goiter is a common endocrine disease that may be defined as an enlargement of the thyroid gland without clinical hypothyroidism or hyperthyroidism. There are two general classes of euthyroid goiter: endemic and sporadic.

Endemic goiter is for all intents and purposes synonymous with iodine deficiency. The optimum intake of iodine for adults is about 100 to 150 μg daily. About 800 million people live in iodine-deficient areas of the world, including the mountainous regions of Central Europe, Asia, and South America, as well as lowland regions of Greece, the Netherlands, and Finland. In these population groups, endemic goiter occurs in at least 10% of the population, and there may be as

many as 200 million endemic goiters worldwide. There are no iodine-deficient areas in the United States, although in the early part of the 20th century there were several areas, most notably the Great Lakes region. Iodine prophylaxis achieved by the supplementation of table salt and foods such as bread and cereal eliminated the problem of iodine-deficient goiter.

Sporadic goiter occurs in less than 10% of any population group. Its prevalence is about 4% in the United States. It is more common in women than men (8:1), and onset is frequently noted at the time of puberty, pregnancy, and menopause. Euthyroid goiters may be subclassified as either diffuse or nodular, and nodular goiters may be characterized by either single or multiple nodules. Nodular goiters are more frequent in women than men (4:1), and the prevalence increases with age. The nodular goiters pose specific and significant diagnostic and therapeutic challenges for the clinician. Decisions must frequently be made as to whether a nodule is benign or malignant or whether a patient with a multinodular goiter having areas of autonomous function is hyperthyroid.

Pathogenesis

Endemic goiter is clearly related to iodine deficiency, which leads to a sequence of events characterized by impaired production of thyroid hormone, increased TSH secretion, enlargement of the thyroid to a clinically evident goiter, and increased ability of the hyperplastic thyroid gland to trap iodide, permitting synthesis of adequate amounts of thyroid hormone to maintain the euthyroid state. Failure to trap enough iodide results in inability to maintain the euthyroid state and ultimately in the endemic form of goitrous hypothyroidism.

The pathogenesis of either the diffuse or nodular type of sporadic goiter is not completely understood. In some cases there may be an inherent enzymatic defect in thyroid hormone biosynthesis that impairs the production of thyroid hormone, leading to increased TSH secretion and thyroid gland size. Defects at any of the biosynthetic steps such as trapping, organification, or coupling presumably may be congenital or acquired. Obvious congenital defects are rare; sporadic, acquired defects are largely unproved. If they exist, they theoretically should be associated with demonstrable increases in serum TSH concentrations. However, most if not all patients with nontoxic goiter have normal serum TSH concentrations, raising serious questions as to the validity of this theory. Over the past decade immunologic growth factors that may play a role in the development of sporadic goiter have been identified. These factors, called thyroid growth immunoglobulins (TGIs), in contrast to TRAb found in Graves' disease, stimulate growth but not biosynthesis of thyroid hormone and probably bind to a different domain of the TSH receptor.

The evolution of a nontoxic, diffuse goiter to a multinodular goiter remains unexplained. Neither TSH nor TGI stimulation seems to explain the heterogeneity of the multinodular goiter, characterized by areas of autonomous function and hypofunction and areas of hyperplasia and involution.

Histopathologic Features

Endemic goiters are hyperplastic and show a significant reduction in the amount of intrafollicular colloid and a decrease in size of columnar epithelial cells. Microscopic areas of papillary cancer may be found in long-standing endemic goiter. Sporadic goiter has a normal histologic appearance except for slight hyperplasia. Multinodular goiters have areas of hyperplasia, involution, cystic degeneration, fibrosis, hemorrhage, and, late in the disease, areas of calcification. Hyperplastic areas are presumably functionally autonomous and may be hyperfunctional, leading to clinical or subclinical hyperthyroidism.

Clinical Presentation

Endemic or sporadic goiters are of variable size, are diffusely enlarged, and may be quite firm on palpation. Nodular goiters are irregular on palpation; nodules may be soft, firm, and even stone hard. Patients are generally asymptomatic, and the goiter incidentally detected by the patient, a family member, or the physician on routine physical examination. Patients may note a tightness, tickling, or irritation in the throat, precipitating frequent dry cough or clearing of the throat. Large goiters may produce tracheal and/or esophageal compression, leading to respiratory distress and/or dysphagia. Infrequently, these large benign goiters may result in superior vena cava obstruction. Narrowing of the thoracic inlet produces obstruction of venous return from the head, neck, and arms, which is accentuated by raising the arms; this may cause lightheadedness or dizziness. The goiters may also be of sufficient size to compress the recurrent laryngeal nerve, producing hoarseness. Hemorrhage into one of the nodules of a multinodular goiter produces exquisite tenderness and enlargement of a nodule that may be confused with subacute thyroiditis.

Laboratory Assessment

Thyroid function testing in patients with endemic goiter usually reveals a low or low-normal serum total T_4 level, normal serum total T_3 level, and mildly elevated TSH levels. The 24-hour radioiodine uptake is elevated, reflecting the avidity of the iodine-deficient thyroid gland for iodide. Scanning reveals a homogeneous distribution of iodide. Serum total T_4, T_3, and TSH levels and 24-hour radioiodine uptake are generally normal in sporadic diffuse and multinodular goiter. Radioiodine scanning of multinodular goiters reveals a patchy distribution of the isotope with areas of hyperfunction and hypofunction corresponding to the various autonomously functioning macronodules and micronodules. The picture of the multinodular goiter provided by the scintiscan and the irregularity of the gland on palpation can be confused with Hashimoto's thyroiditis. Determination of serum thyroid antimicrosomal and antithyroglobulin antibody levels should differentiate the two conditions because uncomplicated multinodular goiter is not associated with the presence of these antibodies.

Treatment

The cornerstone of treatment of endemic goiter is the provision of supplementary dietary iodine. Most, but not all, long-standing goiters regress in size. Prevention is the ideal treatment, and population groups in iodine-deficient areas should receive iodide supplementation in their diet. Therapeutic amounts of iodide given to a patient with iodine deficiency may in selected cases precipitate thyrotoxicosis. The iodine-deprived thyroid gland has developed a highly efficient trapping and biosynthetic pathway that is sufficiently autonomous that it may transiently overproduce thyroid hormone when provided with excess iodide. This mechanism is similar to what may occur when excess iodide is provided to patients with sporadic or multinodular goiters when receiving iodinated contrast agents or expectorants containing iodide (see Iodine-Induced Thyrotoxicosis [Jod-basedow Syndrome]).

The treatment of sporadic goiter is individualized. In the cases where drugs or goitrogens are etiologic, discontinuing their use leads to regression of the goiter. In the minority of patients with a sporadic goiter and elevated serum TSH level, the judicious use of L-thyroxine replacement may lead to a decrease in gland size. Some nontoxic diffuse goiters shrink rapidly within several weeks to several months, others regress in size slowly, and some remain unchanged, providing the insight that TSH may be only partly or not at all responsible for the goitrous enlargement of the thyroid in some patients. Multinodular goiters usually do not decrease in size in response to synthetic L-thyroxine administration because of the functional autonomy of many areas of the thyroid gland. The existence of autonomously functional areas frequently results in the induction of thyrotoxicosis when exogenous thyroid hormone is provided because it is in effect additive to the autonomous endogenous production. Therefore when using synthetic L-thyroxine therapy in patients with a multinodular goiter the physician must be careful to initiate therapy with lower doses, 25 to 50 μg daily. Therapy should probably be reserved for patients with an elevated serum TSH level and not given to those patients who already manifest a suppressed TSH level from the autonomously functioning areas of the goiter.

Surgical therapy should be reserved for diffuse or nodular euthyroid goiters that cause objectively confirmed significant obstructive symptoms and signs. Thyroid hormone replacement is provided after surgery.

THYROID NEOPLASMS
Benign Neoplasms

Benign neoplasms of the thyroid are classified as adenomas. Most adenomas are seen to be nonfunctional (cold nodule) on scintiscan of the thyroid (Fig. 297-7), although occasionally they may demonstrate normal function (warm nodule) or hyperfunction (hot nodule), thereby suppressing the remainder of the thyroid tissue and causing thyrotoxicosis.

Thyroid adenomas are of greatest concern clinically because they must be differentiated from follicular thyroid cancer, which can be a significant diagnostic challenge. History and physical examination provide useful but generally inconclusive insights as to whether a nodule is malignant. Fig. 297-8 shows a suggested schema to differentiate benign from malignant nodules. Certain factors increase clinical suspicion of malignancy. A history of radiation exposure to head, neck, or upper chest during childhood is perhaps the single most im-

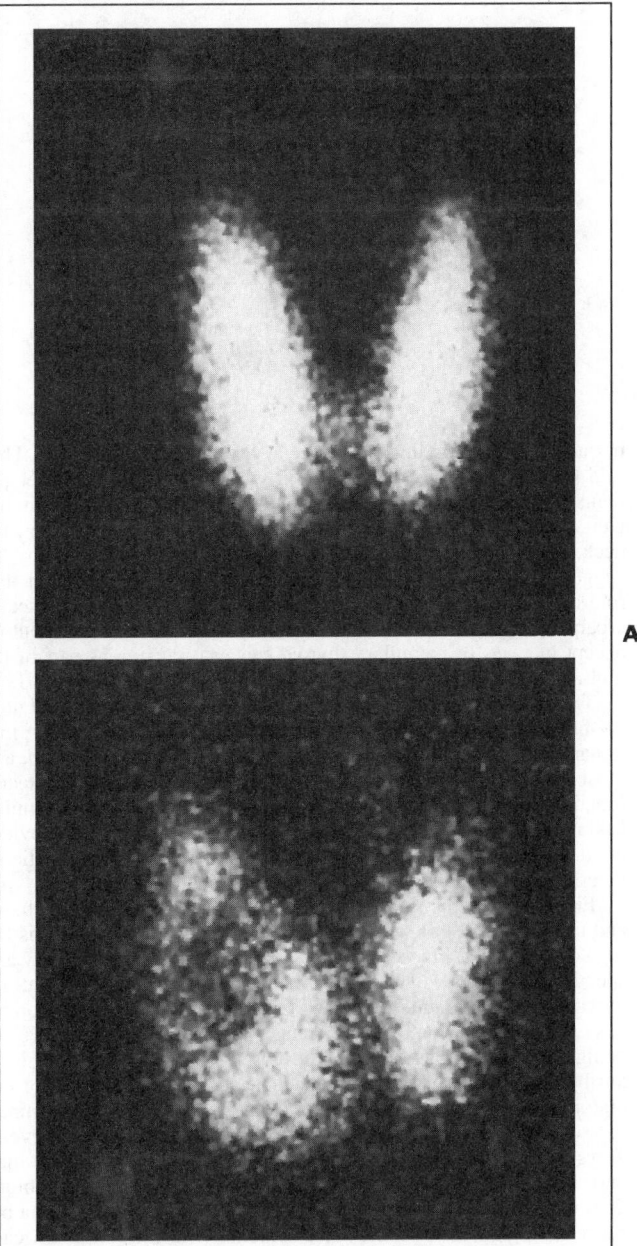

FIGURE 297-7   Radioactive iodine scanning of the thyroid gland. **A,** Normal thyroid. **B,** Cold (nonfunctional) area in the right lobe.

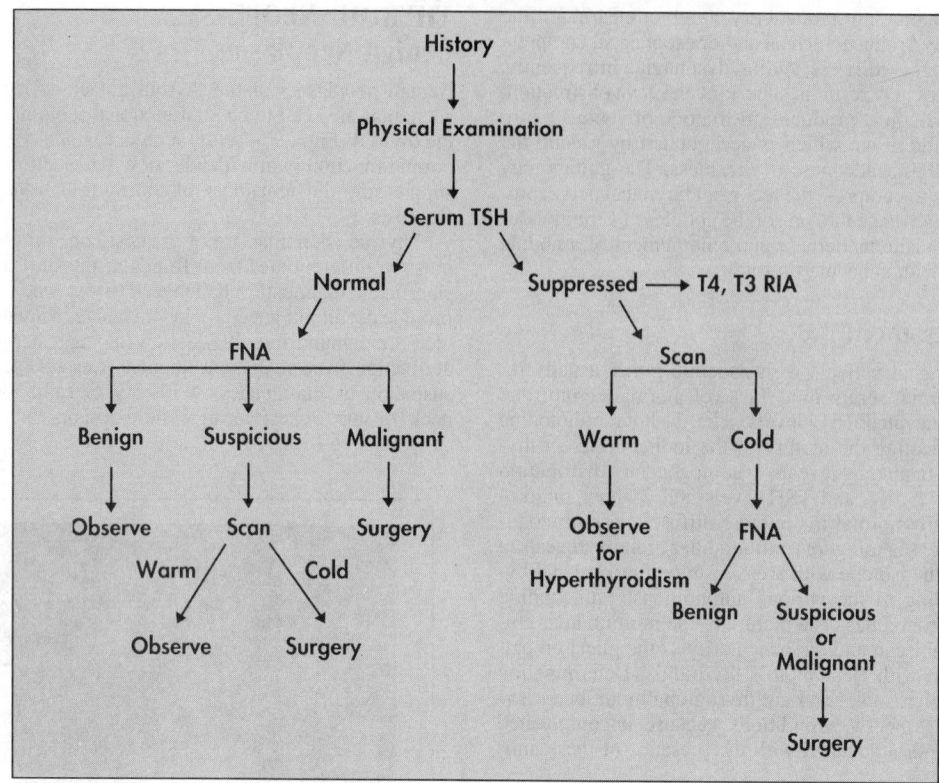

FIGURE 297-8 Evaluation of a patient with a palpable thyroid nodule. *FNA*, Fine-needle aspiration; *RIA*, radioimmunoassay.

portant historical finding (see Special Problem, in the section Thyroid Cancer). Nodules developing in young (<age 20) or older patients (>age 60) or in males (any age) are more likely to be malignant. Rapid growth of the nodule, fixation to local structures in the neck, stony-hard consistency, and associated lymphadenopathy all suggest thyroid cancer. Occasional patients with differentiated thyroid cancer may have anterior cervical adenopathy in the absence of a palpable thyroid nodule. Family history is usually not contributory except in cases of medullary thyroid cancer occurring as part of the multiple endocrine neoplasia (MEN) syndrome types 2A and 2B.

The traditional laboratory evaluation procedures for a thyroid nodule fail to discriminate between benign and malignant lesions. A malignant thyroid nodule is almost always cold on radioiodine scan, and most adenomas are cold nodules. However, a nodule that is clearly functional (warm or hot) is rarely a cancer; therefore, scintiscanning has a selective role in diagnostic testing. Ultrasonography provides good information about size and cystic elements but cannot reliably identify a malignancy and should not be used routinely.

Fine-needle aspiration (FNA) thyroid biopsy is the most reliable and useful diagnostic technique for assessing whether a nodule is benign or malignant. Fine-needle aspiration has excellent sensitivity and specificity, thereby significantly decreasing the indiscriminant removal of thyroid nodules. Nodules read as benign after aspiration biopsy have only a small chance (range, <1% to as high as 10%) of being malignant in actuality. These false-negative results have been attributed to sampling errors, inadequate specimens, and lack of operator experience. Fine-needle aspiration also assists in discriminating solid from cystic nodules. When the fine-needle aspirate reveals a cyst, the fluid should be examined cytologically because a small percentage of cysts are associated with thyroid cancer. The technique does not distinguish follicular adenoma from follicular carcinoma because the diagnosis of follicular carcinoma is largely based on capsular or vascular invasion, and cannot be discerned on a cytologic preparation from an aspiration biopsy. Biopsy findings of nodules that are interpreted to be malignant should prompt surgical removal. Biopsy results read as suspicious, significantly atypical, or indetermi-

nate present a further problem. The nodule can be evaluated by radioiodine scanning, and functioning nodules observed over time or, if cold, surgically removed.

Treatment. The medical treatment of a benign thyroid nodule is currently controversial. Historically such nodules are treated with suppression by synthetic L-thyroxine to decrease TSH level. A serum TSH level should be determined to prevent subclinical hyperthyroidism. Patients should be reexamined at 6-month intervals to determine changes in the size of the nodule. A variable percentage of warm and cold nodules regresses; similarly a variable percentage of thyroid nodules regress without L-thyroxine therapy. Therefore the decision to use L-thyroxine must take into account this diversity of information, and perhaps pending updated clinical trials. Hyperfunctioning benign nodules may be treated with ^{131}I or surgery. Usually ^{131}I therapy is preferred because it is simple, safe, noninvasive, and less expensive than surgery and does not entail significant complications. Hypothyroidism usually does not ensue, in contrast to ^{131}I treatment of Graves' disease, because the hyperfunctioning nodule has suppressed TSH and the rest of the gland does not incorporate ^{131}I and is not destroyed.

Malignant Neoplasms

Thyroid cancer is the most common endocrine cancer; however, among all types of cancers in the general population it is distinctly uncommon. There are about 10,000 to 12,000 new cases diagnosed in the United States and about 1100 deaths per year. In its occult form thyroid cancer is much more common because routine autopsy studies reveal that as many as 5% to 20% of normal thyroid glands may have foci of malignant thyroid tissue, the clinical significance of which is unclear. The general term *thyroid cancer* incorporates different types of cancer ranging from well-differentiated, slow-growing tumors having an excellent prognosis to aggressive, poorly differentiated cancer with a poor prognosis. The facts that thyroid cancer represents less than 1% of all cancer deaths and less than 10% of patients with thyroid cancer die of the disease have promoted the repu-

BOX 297-12
Types of primary thyroid cancer

Papillary
Follicular
Anaplastic
Medullary
Lymphoma

tation of thyroid cancer as a relatively benign malignancy. Because many patients who have the common thyroid malignancies are disease free 20 to 30 years after diagnosis, various surgical and medical approaches may claim a certain success. Accepted therapies for the various thyroid cancers are discussed in the section devoted to each tumor.

The various types of primary thyroid cancers are listed in Box 297-12. Three of the types are derived from follicular epithelium: papillary, follicular, and anaplastic. The other primary cancers of the thyroid are thyroid lymphoma and medullary cancer. The latter arises from the parafollicular or C cells and has distinctive biochemical manifestations.

Thyroid cancers, similar to other malignancies, are thought to arise from a series of mutational events leading to the abnormal growth of genetically modified cells. Recent studies have identified increased expression of the ras, myc, and fos oncogenes in follicular thyroid neoplasms, with a mutation of the p53 tumor suppressor gene linked to anaplastic tumors. The RET oncogene is closely linked to the familial form of medullary thyroid cancer.

Papillary Carcinoma. Papillary carcinoma is the most common of the primary thyroid cancers, accounting for about 60% to 70% of all thyroid cancer in adults. It is more common in women than men (2:1 to 3:1), has a peak incidence in the third and fourth decades of life, may occur at any age, and is more aggressive in older patients. Most patients have an asymptomatic neck mass, occasionally several nodules are palpable, and in about one third of patients palpable cervical lymph nodes are present. Patients with papillary cancer may have a history of irradiation of the head, neck, or upper chest during childhood.

Papillary carcinoma is the slowest growing thyroid cancer. The tumor is unencapsulated and may infiltrate surrounding tissue, spreading by lymphatics to the cervical lymph nodes. In as many as 5% of patients an isolated cervical metastasis (formerly known as a lateral aberrant thyroid) may be the dominant finding and the thyroid gland may have only a microscopic focus of papillary cancer. Vascular invasion is rare. Distant metastases occur in about 10% of adults and are most frequent in lung, bone, and brain.

The tumor has a characteristic histopathologic picture consisting of folds of columnar epithelium, papillary projections (fronds), and scattered, concentrically layered deposits of calcium called psammoma bodies. Most tumors are mixtures of papillary and follicular tumor elements. This characteristic has important therapeutic implications because follicular tumor tissue concentrates radioiodine, whereas papillary tissue does not.

Several factors are associated with a poorer prognosis for patients with papillary carcinoma, including age greater than 50, male sex, local tumor invasion at the time of surgery, and presence of distant metastases. Unlike that in primary cancers found in other organs, the presence of local lymph node metastases does not adversely affect the prognosis. The overall mortality rate of papillary carcinoma is quite low: survival rates of 90% or more at 20 or 30 years are the rule influenced by the risk factors noted earlier. The cause of death produced by this tumor is usually local tumor invasion involving the trachea and/or esophagus. Rarely, the tumor undergoes an anaplastic change, becoming more virulent and metastasizing widely.

Follicular Carcinoma. Follicular carcinoma is a primary thyroid cancer that accounts for about 15% of all thyroid carcinoma. It

is more common in women than men (2:1 to 3:1) and more common in patients over the age of 40. Many patients have a history of irradiation of the head, neck, or upper chest. There are a number of important differences between well-differentiated follicular and papillary carcinomas. Follicular carcinomas are encapsulated and usually spread by vascular invasion and not to regional lymph nodes. Patients with follicular cancer tend to have smaller thyroid tumors and may have distant metastasis. Bone metastases may occur early, are very destructive, and respond poorly to radioiodine therapy. Liver and lung are other common sites of distant metastases. Follicular tumor tissue has the ability to concentrate radioiodine, albeit less efficiently than normal thyroid tissue, and to synthesize thyroid hormone in minor amounts. Therefore widespread metastatic follicular carcinoma of substantial mass can occasionally produce enough thyroid hormone to induce thyrotoxicosis, most commonly T_3 toxicosis.

Follicular carcinoma, like papillary carcinoma, is a slow-growing tumor; however, follicular carcinoma has a less favorable prognosis. The age of the patient, size of the tumor, and the degrees of capsular and vascular invasion influence the prognosis.

An uncommon variant of follicular carcinoma is the Hürthle cell carcinoma. This tumor is characterized by increased amounts of acidophilic cytoplasm, which on electron microscopy is shown to contain an abundance of mitochondria. These tumors may also metastasize widely. However, unlike follicular carcinoma, they rarely concentrate radioiodine.

Treatment. The surgical treatment of well-differentiated papillary and follicular carcinomas remains controversial; however, certain generalities can be stated. A papillary carcinoma less than 1.0 cm (microcarcinoma) in size is usually treated by lobectomy and isthmusectomy and examination of ipsilateral lymph nodes with removal of grossly involved nodes. Cure rates are high, and postoperative radioiodine treatment unnecessary. Synthetic L-thyroxine should be given postoperatively in doses that lower TSH, but at the same time prevent thyrotoxicosis. TSH suppression is important because the growth or recurrence of papillary (and follicular) cancers are thought to be in part TSH dependent.

Papillary carcinoma greater than 1.0 cm in size or infiltrative into surrounding tissues requires an operation that safely removes all thyroid tissue without associated complications of hypoparathyroidism or nerve paralysis. Surgery may be either a total thyroidectomy or a lobectomy on the involved side and near-total lobectomy on the contralateral side. In the higher-risk patient thyroid hormone is withheld postoperatively until the patient has become hypothyroid, at which time radioiodine scanning is performed. Residual normal thyroid and tumor tissue is destroyed using high doses of ^{131}I. One week after this treatment a whole-body scan is performed in an attempt to determine the presence of any distant, functional metastases. On completion of the postoperative diagnostic and therapeutic maneuvers, synthetic L-thyroxine therapy is begun in doses adequate to suppress TSH as described. After surgery and adjunctive treatment yearly follow-up evaluation is required; this entails careful neck examination and serum thyroglobulin level determinations that provide a sensitive indicator for residual or recurrent tumor tissue, because normal tissue has been destroyed by the ^{131}I. Selected patients require follow-up radioiodine scanning.

Follicular cancer, regardless of size, is treated by total thyroidectomy or a procedure modified to perform a total lobectomy on the involved side and near-total lobectomy on the contralateral side. Unlike papillary carcinoma, there is no relationship of size to the aggressive behavior of the tumor. ^{131}I is administered, and follow-up evaluation is conducted as described.

Anaplastic Carcinoma. About 5% of thyroid cancers are anaplastic. The tumor is slightly more common in women than men and may arise from preexisting papillary carcinoma or multinodular goiter. It has a peak incidence in the sixth and seventh decades of life, although it has been reported in patients less than 40 years old, including some children. The clinical picture is usually that of a rapidly growing thyroid mass that may be associated with dysphagia, hoarseness, hemoptysis, and respiratory distress. The mass is very firm to stony-hard on palpation and is fixed to surrounding structures. This aggressive clinical course must be differentiated from that of thyroid lymphoma (discussed later), which is treatable and generally has a more favorable prognosis. Most patients with anaplastic carcinoma die within months after the diagnosis is made, and few survive more than 1 year.

Histopathologic examination of needle biopsy specimens reveals anaplastic spindle and multinucleated giant cells with many mitoses; areas of necrosis and inflammation are prominent. Islands of papillary and/or follicular carcinoma may be present, supporting the likelihood of a precursor role for these tumors in some cases.

Treatment is palliative. Surgery is best used to relieve tracheal and esophageal obstruction. Chemotherapy and radioiodine therapy are usually ineffective; radiotherapy can in some cases slow disease progression.

Lymphoma. Thyroid lymphoma accounts for only a small percentage of thyroid cancer cases. It is more common in women than men (3:1) and has a peak incidence in the seventh or eighth decade of life but may occur as early as the third decade. The history is usually one of a rapidly enlarging mass in the thyroid associated with varying degrees of pain and tenderness. There may be hoarseness and respiratory distress. The tumor is very firm to stony-hard on palpation.

Findings of histopathologic examination are most often consistent with a diffuse histiocytic lymphoma. Importantly, there is almost always histologic evidence of Hashimoto's thyroiditis and many patients are hypothyroid. Many thyroid lymphoma patients have markedly elevated levels of thyroid antimicrosomal antibodies. The relation of Hashimoto's thyroiditis to thyroid lymphoma appears to be more than coincidental. Although the actual number of cases of thyroid lymphoma arising in patients with Hashimoto's thyroiditis is small, the risk of development of thyroid lymphoma is higher in patients with Hashimoto's thyroiditis, as is the risk of development of other lymphoproliferative or myeloproliferative syndromes.

The diagnosis of thyroid lymphoma is usually made by large (core)-needle biopsy, and occasionally, open biopsy. Large-needle biopsy or open biopsy results may be more reliable than fine-needle aspirates because the specimens obtained provide an opportunity to assess intact histologic features that are critical to distinguishing lymphoma from Hashimoto's thyroiditis. Evidence for associated Hashimoto's thyroiditis and the biopsy results serve to distinguish thyroid lymphoma from anaplastic carcinoma, which has similar clinical features.

The prognosis is improved by early diagnosis. When lymphoma is confined to the thyroid gland, 5-year survival rates are as high as 75% to 85%; extension into the neck has a 5-year survival rate of about 35% to 40%, and widely disseminated lymphoma a 5-year survival rate of only about 5%. Patients below the age of 65 and men have significantly longer median survival rates.

The treatment of thyroid lymphoma usually consists of radiotherapy and chemotherapy alone or in combination. Surgery is only performed to relieve tracheal obstruction or occasionally to stage for more extensive disease.

Medullary Carcinoma. Approximately 5% to 10% of all new cases of thyroid cancer are medullary carcinomas. The tumor arises from the parafollicular C cells, which produce the polypeptide hormone calcitonin. It is slightly more common in women than men and has a peak incidence in the fifth and sixth decades of life. There are four forms of medullary thyroid cancer: sporadic, that associated with MEN type 2A (Sipple's syndrome), that associated with MEN type 2B, and a familial form without other associated endocrine tumors (familial medullary thyroid cancer [FMTC]). Patients usually have a clinically apparent thyroid mass that is cold on scintiscan. When associated with MEN type 2A, there may be a history of pheochromocytoma or hyperparathyroidism; with type 2B there may be a history of pheochromocytoma and a clinical picture of marfanoid habitus and diffuse ganglioneuromas most evident on the tongue.

The sporadic form is more common (about 4:1), occurs in older age-groups (above age 40), and is usually unilateral. The familial forms are inherited as an autosomal dominant trait with variable penetrance; the tumor is almost uniformly bilateral in distribution, occurring in patients less than 35 years of age, and occurs in three forms. Medullary carcinoma associated with FMTC has the overall best prognosis, that associated with MEN 2B the worst; the prognosis for

the sporadic form and MEN 2A is intermediate. Disease prognosis is directly related to the degree of tumor calcitonin as measured by immunohistochemistry. Medullary carcinoma spreads via lymphatics to lymph nodes in the neck and mediastinum. It also regularly metastasizes to distant sites, most commonly lung, bone, and liver.

Medullary thyroid carcinoma has demonstrable genetic and biochemical markers and may be associated with several paraneoplastic syndromes.

Recent studies have shown that mutations in the RET protooncogene exist in the familial forms of medullary thyroid cancer. The presence of these mutations can be determined and are predictive for both C-cell hyperplasia and medullary cancer even before serum calcitonin levels are abnormal. Calcitonin level is the biologic marker for this tumor and is elevated in the basal state or with stimulation by pentagastrin or calcium infusion in most cases. Serum calcitonin levels provide the most useful tool for detecting the existence of residual tumor tissue postoperatively. Despite its role in downward regulation of serum calcium, the elevated level of calcitonin associated with this tumor only rarely results in hypocalcemia.

Medullary thyroid carcinoma is also associated with classic Cushing's syndrome or carcinoid syndrome caused by the ectopic production of ACTH or serotonin by the tumor. Ectopic production of prostaglandins, kinins, and vasoactive intestinal peptide leads to watery diarrhea in certain patients. The tumor also produces histaminase, which is a useful marker for metastatic disease, and carcinoembryonic antigen, another potential tumor marker.

Diagnosis of medullary carcinoma of the thyroid can be made by the determination of a specific mutation in the RET oncogene in familial cases or by measurement of basal and/or stimulated levels of calcitonin. In the familial forms a diagnostic evaluation for pheochromocytoma is imperative before any surgical intervention. Patients with MEN type 2A should also have determinations of serum calcium and parathyroid hormone levels.

Tissue diagnosis is readily made by large-needle or open biopsy, most commonly at the time of surgery. The tumor consists of large aggregates of C cells, epithelial cells, fibrous tissue, and deposits of amyloid. Deposits of calcium salts account for the occasional observation of dense, homogeneous conglomerate calcifications on routine radiographs of the primary or metastatic tumor.

Treatment of medullary carcinoma of the thyroid consists of total thyroidectomy with prophylactic central lymph node dissection. Lateral cervical lymph nodes are sampled, and if the result is positive, additional lymph node dissection is performed. Normal-appearing nodes are usually not removed. Most surgeons do not perform aggressive, radical neck dissection as its utility in producing longer survival rates and cures is uncertain. Radiotherapy, radioiodine therapy, and chemotherapy are generally ineffective. In the familial forms determination of RET oncogene mutations and basal and stimulated calcitonin levels is essential to detect the precursor of medullary carcinoma, C-cell hyperplasia, because thyroidectomy at this stage is likely to be curative.

Risk factors associated with poor prognosis include male sex, lymph node involvement, extrathyroidal extension, and association with MEN type 2B. Five- to 10-year survival rates of 67% to 80% are not uncommon in the various reported series with FMTC and tumors associated with MEN type 2A.

Special Problem: External Irradiation of the Head, Neck, and Upper Thorax in Infancy and Childhood. External irradiation of the head, neck, or upper thorax was administered in the past to treat a variety of conditions, including recurrent tonsillitis, adenoiditis, acne, tinea capitis, and thymic enlargement. The thyroid was incidentally irradiated by these procedures. Although not appreciated at the time, relatively small doses of radiation (between 90 and 900 R) during infancy and childhood increase the risk of developing benign and malignant thyroid neoplasms. Another demonstration of the effects of external irradiation has been a consequence of the atomic bomb blasts (Japan and Marshall Islands), which resulted in an increased incidence of both benign and malignant thyroid nodules.

It requires a latency of approximately 5 years after exposure to develop a thyroid tumor, but the patient remains at increased risk for neoplasia for at least 30 to 40 years after exposure and possibly for life. A thyroid neoplasm develops in no more than half of those irradiated, and most cases are benign. However, in about 5% of the irradiated group differentiated thyroid carcinoma develops. The tumors are generally slow-growing, relatively nonaggressive, and frequently multicentric, and thyroid scintiscanning does not always reflect areas of involvement. Microscopic foci of cancer have been observed in areas indicated to be normal by scintiscanning. The significance of this finding remains unclear.

The initial evaluation of all patients who have received external irradiation to the thyroid gland should include examination of the thyroid gland for any palpable abnormality. In the absence of any abnormality, some physicians recommend physiologic replacement therapy with thyroid hormone, with the aim of suppressing TSH secretion to decrease the chance of developing a thyroid neoplasm. Whether this desirable goal can be accomplished is uncertain. Any palpable thyroid nodule is a candidate for open surgical biopsy, but perhaps FNA cytologic evaluation can be used to guide therapy. All patients should have a determination of thyroid autoantibody levels in the initial evaluation because a scan abnormality or a diffuse or irregular enlargement of the thyroid gland may be due to Hashimoto's thyroiditis. Parathyroid adenomas producing hypercalcemia are also more common in these patients. Physical examination of the neck should be performed yearly.

Total or near-total thyroidectomy is the treatment of choice for thyroid cancer in this setting followed by ablation of residual thyroid tissue with radioiodine. The overall prognosis is no different from that described for differentiated thyroid cancer.

BIBLIOGRAPHY

Brent GA: The molecular basis of thyroid hormone action, *N Engl J Med* 331:847, 1994.

Cooper DS: Thyroxine suppression therapy for benign modular disease, *J Clin Endocrinol Metab* 80:331, 1995.

Demeure MJ, Clark OH: Surgery in the treatment of thyroid cancer, *Endocrinol Metab Clin North Am* 19(3):663, 1990.

Fagin JA et al: High prevalence of mutations of the p53 gene in poorly differentiated human thyroid cancer, *J Clin Invest* 91:179, 1993.

Hamburger JI: The various presentations of thyroiditis: diagnostic considerations, *Ann Intern Med* 104:219, 1986.

Helfand M, Crapo LM: Monitoring therapy in patients taking levothyroxine, *Ann Intern Med* 113:450, 1990.

Klein I et al: Treatment of hyperthyroid disease, *Ann Intern Med* 121:281, 1994.

Klemperer JD et al: Thyroid hormone treatment after coronary-artery bypass surgery, *N Engl J Med* 333:1522, 1995.

Lips CJM et al: Clinical screening as compared with DNA analysis in families with multiple endocrine neoplasia type 2A, *N Engl J Med* 331:828, 1994.

Maniotti S: The aging thyroid, *Endocr Rev* 16:686, 1995.

Mazzaferri EL, Jhiang SM: Long-term impact of initial surgical and medical therapy on papillary and follicular thyroid cancer, *Am J Med* 97:418, 1994.

Refetoff S: Resistance to thyroid hormone: a historical review, *Thyroid* 4:345, 1994.

Sawin CT et al: Low serum thyrotropin levels as a risk factor for atrial fibrillation in older persons, *N Engl J Med* 33:1249, 1994.

Spencer CA et al: Thyrotropin (TSH)-releasing hormone stimulation test responses employing third and fourth generation TSH assays, *J Clin Endocrinol Metab* 76:494, 1993.

Van Herle AJ et al: The thyroid nodule, *Ann Intern Med* 96:221, 1982.

Weetman AP, McGregor AM: Autoimmune thyroid disease: further developments in our understanding, *Endocr Rev* 15:788, 1994.

CHAPTER

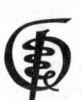

298   Disorders of the Adrenal Cortex

John Kendall and D. Lynn Loriaux

STRUCTURE AND FUNCTION OF THE ADRENAL GLANDS

The adrenal cortex, like the steroid-producing cells of the gonads, arises from the splanchnic mesoderm during the second month of fetal life. The adrenal medulla is derived from the neuroectoderm and joins the cortical cells during the sixth week of fetal life. The adrenal glands are in the retroperitoneal space adjacent to the upper pole of the kidney and derive their blood supply from small arteries arising from the aorta, the inferior phrenic, and the renal arteries. The venous drainage of the left adrenal gland is into the left renal vein; the right adrenal gland empties directly into the inferior vena cava. The glands are conical and have a combined weight of 6 to 10 g. The cortical portion of the gland is divided into three zones, each with special functional properties. The outermost zone, *zona glomerulosa,* is composed of clusters of lipid-poor cells that primarily synthesize aldosterone and 18-hydroxy-corticosterone. The intermediate layer, *zona fasciculata,* is thicker and primarily synthesizes cortisol and its precursors. The innermost zone, *zona reticularis,* primarily synthesizes the weak adrenal androgens, dehydroepiandrosterone (DHEA) and androstenedione. Both of these inner zones are lipid rich.

The adrenal medulla occupies the central core of the gland and is composed of chromaffin cells that synthesize and secrete norepinephrine and epinephrine. The conversion of norepinephrine to epinephrine is a cortisol-dependent reaction, and the location of the adrenal medulla inside the cortisol-producing adrenal cortex facilitates this reaction.

BIOSYNTHESIS OF ADRENOCORTICAL HORMONES

The core structure of all adrenal steroids is the four-ring cyclopentanoperhydrophenanthrene nucleus. It is composed of 17 carbon atoms. Modifications, primarily at positions 11, 17, and 18, lead to a series of compounds with glucocorticoid, mineralocorticoid, androgenic, and estrogenic activities (Fig. 298-1).

Adrenal steroid biosynthesis begins with cholesterol. Cholesterol can be synthesized in the adrenal gland *de novo,* or taken up from the circulating plasma. The first step in steroid biosynthesis occurs in the mitochondria where the cholesterol desmolase enzyme system removes six carbons of the cholesterol side chain yielding pregnenolone. Most of the remaining biosynthetic steps occur in the microsomes. Certain enzymatic modifications are specific to the different zones of the adrenal cortex. For example, in the zona glomerulosa, pregnenolone is converted to progesterone and then to a series of aldosterone precursors. In the zonae fasciculata and reticularis, pregnenolone and progesterone are hydroxylated at the 17-position to form precursors of all other adrenal steroids. Cortisol accounts for about 50% of the total adrenal steroid secretion. The "adrenal androgens," DHEA and androstenedione, account for most of the remainder. Small amounts of estrogen and testosterone are derived from the adrenal androgens.

REGULATION OF ADRENOCORTICAL SECRETION

The adrenal cortex is under the control of two stimulatory peptides, adrenocorticotropic hormone (ACTH) and angiotensin II. Other factors such as serum sodium and potassium can modulate aldosterone secretion. The principal modulator of adrenocortical steroid biosynthesis, however, is ACTH. ACTH is a 39-amino-acid polypeptide. A synthetic derivative, Cortrosyn, contains the first 24 amino acids of the native molecule and is commercially available for the clinical evaluation of adrenocortical function.

ACTH binds to cell surface receptors and stimulates cell growth and the biosynthesis of steroid hormones. ACTH increases the adrenal cellular uptake of cholesterol and stimulates the first rate-limiting step in steroid biosynthesis, the conversion of cholesterol to pregnenolone. ACTH is secreted by pituitary corticotrophs that are regulated in turn by two hypothalamic hormones, corticotropin-releasing hormone (CRH) and vasopressin. ACTH secretion is episodic. There are about 10 secretory "bursts" during each day, the majority clustered between 6:00 AM and 10:00 AM. The nadir of ACTH secretion occurs during the early hours of sleep. Cortisol secretion is entrained to ACTH secretion, leading to the familiar diurnal pattern of plasma cortisol concentration: high cortisol levels in the early morning, low cortisol levels in the evening.

Stresses such as trauma, infection, fear, and volume depletion lead to increased cortisol secretion. This increase in secretion usually is sustained for the duration of the stress. With the termination of stress it subsides in a matter of hours. Circulating concentrations of cortisol

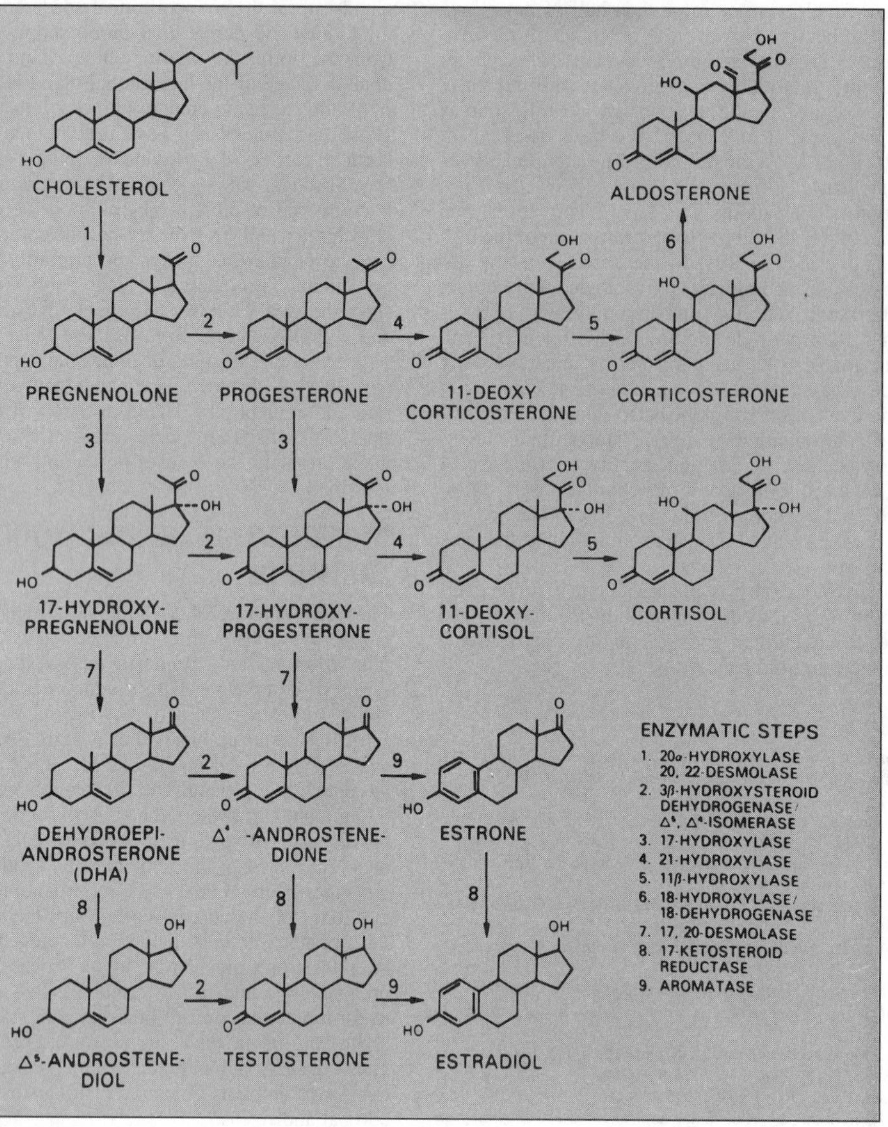

FIGURE 298-1 The steroid biosynthetic cascade from cholesterol to the four classes of steroid hormones of adrenal origin: glucocorticoids, mineralocorticoids, androgens, and estrogens.

are maintained in the "normal" range by a negative feedback system. Cortisol restrains its own secretion by inhibiting CRH secretion and by inhibiting the ability of CRH to stimulate ACTH secretion from the anterior pituitary gland. This effect of cortisol is blunted by stress and is absent in some diseases such as Cushing's disease. As expected, glucocorticoid administration can suppress ACTH secretion. If glucocorticoids are administered in supraphysiologic amounts for a prolonged period, pituitary-adrenal axis suppression can be clinically significant. There is gradual recovery of the pituitary-adrenal axis following withdrawal of corticosteroids. It can require more than a year if the duration of treatment is prolonged.

Aldosterone secretion is regulated primarily by the renin-angiotensin system. Renin is secreted by the juxtaglomerular cells in response to decreased "effective" blood pressure in the afferent arterioles of the kidney. Renin in turn converts angiotensinogen, a polypeptide prohormone of hepatic origin, to angiotensin I, a decapeptide. Angiotensin I in turn is converted to angiotensin II, the bioactive octapeptide, by angiotensin-converting enzyme (ACE) in vascular endothelial cells. Angiotensin II acts directly on the zona glomerulosa to stimulate aldosterone biosynthesis and secretion. Like ACTH, its primary action is on the rate-limiting biosynthetic step that converts cholesterol to pregnenolone. Aldosterone and the less potent mineralocorticoid precursors, desoxycorticosterone, corticosterone,

and 18-hydroxycorticosterone, act principally on the kidneys to retain sodium and expand extracellular fluid volume. As volume expands, the stimulus for renin secretion is reduced, angiotensin II production is diminished, and mineralocorticoid secretion slows. In addition to the important role in regulating aldosterone secretion, angiotensin II has multiple effects on normal circulating fluid volume and blood pressure. Angiotensin II stimulates vascular smooth muscle contraction and renal tubular sodium reabsorption and decreases free water clearance.

Potassium and sodium also can modulate aldosterone secretion. Potassium and angiotensin II both increase free calcium in zona glomerulosa cells. It has been proposed that the final common pathway for both of these effects, and perhaps for that of ACTH as well, is through a calcium-mediated "second messenger" transduction system. Sodium also affects zona glomerulosa function, but its regulatory effects appear to be mediated through changes in vascular volume. Other suggested modulators of aldosterone production include dopamine (inhibitory), proopiomelanocortin derivatives (stimulatory), and atrial natriuretic hormone (stimulatory).

Circulating cortisol is bound to plasma proteins. At normal plasma cortisol concentrations, only 10% is free. ("Free" cortisol has two meanings in adrenal parlance. "Urinary free cortisol" refers to excreted unmetabolized hormone. Circulating cortisol not bound to

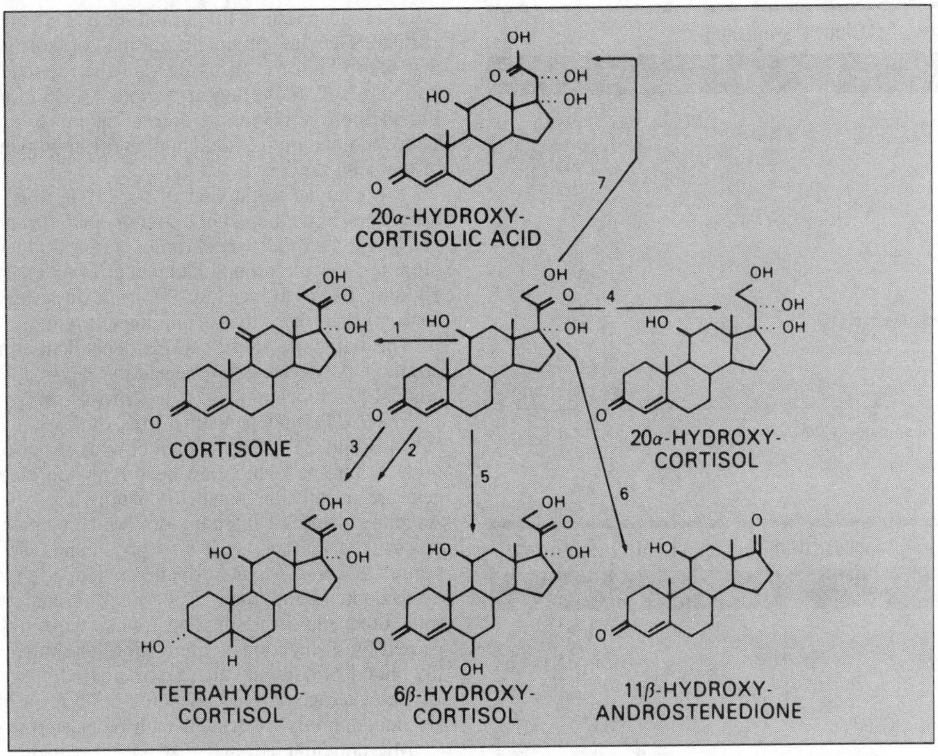

FIGURE 298-2 The products of metabolism of cortisol.

plasma proteins is also referred to as free cortisol.) The protein bound fraction is divided between transcortin, a high-affinity, low-capacity alpha globulin, and albumin, a low-affinity, high-capacity transport protein. At greater than normal plasma concentrations, cortisol is increasingly bound to albumin. Transcortin concentrations are increased by estrogen. The birth control pill and pregnancy both elevate transcortins in this way. Elevated resting plasma cortisol concentrations in women must be interpreted in conjunction with the estrogen "status." Aldosterone is weakly bound to circulating plasma proteins and circulates in the plasma primarily in the free form.

Both hormones are metabolized in the liver. Hepatic extraction removes virtually all free hormone in one "pass." This rapid clearance accounts in part for the lability of plasma concentrations of both aldosterone and cortisol. The urinary excretion of unmetabolized (free) cortisol and aldosterone constitutes less than 1% of total urinary metabolites of these hormones. Nonetheless, the measurement of urinary free cortisol is the best available clinical index of the cortisol secretion rate.

Urinary tetrahydroaldosterone is the most commonly employed index of adrenal aldosterone secretion. There are more than a dozen metabolites of cortisol in urine. The largest fraction, 25%, is tetrahydrocortisol (Fig. 298-2). This metabolite is conjugated with glucuronide making it water soluble. It accounts for most of the urinary "17-hydroxysteroids" (Porter-Silber chromogens). Drugs and diseases that affect the hepatic metabolism of cortisol can alter the urinary concentrations of tetrahydrocortisol. The conversion of cortisol to cortisone is a metabolic step of increasing clinical interest. This conversion is dependent upon 11-β-steroid dehydrogenase (11-β-HSD). Enhanced activity of this enzyme reduces the bioavailability of cortisol, diminished activity increases its bioavailability. Several disorders are thought to be due to alterations in 11-β-HSD activity, for example, the "pseudo-Cushing's" syndrome associated with alcoholism. The pseudohyperaldosteronism of licorice ingestion, formerly attributed to a steroid agonistic effect of glycyrrhizic acid, also seems to be explained by an inhibition of 11-β-HSD.

ADRENAL HYPERFUNCTION
Cushing's Syndrome

Cushing's syndrome was first described by Harvey Cushing in 1910. He called the disorder the polyglandular syndrome. The first patient, a 23-year-old woman, had centripetal obesity, hypertension, proximal muscle weakness, abdominal striae, hirsutism, thinning of the scalp hair, purpura, insomnia, and backache. In discussing the case, Cushing noted that similar clinical findings had been reported in association with adrenal tumors, and closed by saying:

> It will thus be seen that we may perchance be on the way toward the recognition of the consequences of "hyperadrenalism." Heretofore, the only recognizable clinical state associated with primary adrenal disease has been the syndrome of Addison, and the grouping of these cases may possibly add one more to the series of clinical conditions related to primary maladies of the ductless glands.*

The syndrome was codified 20 years later in his now classic monograph, which appeared in the *Johns Hopkins Medical Journal* in 1932. He had, by this time, recognized the trophic influence of the pituitary "basophils" on the adrenal glands and shown that basophilic tumors of the pituitary gland can cause the same clinical syndrome as tumors of the adrenal gland. Thus, the stage was thus set for our current classification of Cushing's syndrome into ACTH-dependent and ACTH-independent forms.

Clinical Manifestations. The adrenal cortex produces three classes of steroid hormones: glucocorticoids, mineralocorticoids, and sex steroid (androgen and estrogen) precursors. Hyperfunction of the gland can produce clinical signs of increased activity of one or all of these steroid hormone types. Cushing's syndrome is the clinical expression of the overproduction of glucocorticoid.

Increased glucocorticoid action can be thought of as "antianabolic." The biochemical mechanism can be conceptualized as energy

---

*Cushing H: *The pituitary body and its disorders*, 1912, Philadelphia, JB Lippincott, p 219.

Table 298-1 Causes of Cushing's syndrome

CAUSE	RELATIVE INCIDENCE
ACTH dependent	75%
Cushing's disease	60%
Ectopic ACTH secretion	15%
Ectopic CRH secretion	<1%
ACTH independent	25%
Endogenous	
Adrenal cancer	15%
Adrenal adenoma	10%
Micronodular adrenal disease	<1%
Exogenous	
Factitious	<1%
Iatrogenic	Very common

ACTH, Adrenocorticotropic hormone; *CRH*, corticotropin-releasing hormone.

Table 298-2 Tumors associated with the ectopic ACTH syndrome

TUMOR	FREQUENCY (%)
Oat cell carcinoma	50
Tumors of foregut origin	35
Thymic carcinoma	
Islet cell tumor	
Medullary carcinoma of thyroid	
Bronchial carcinoid	
Pheochromocytoma	5
Other	10
Gonadal	
Prostate and cervical carcinoma	
Tumors of unknown origin	

ACTH, Adrenocorticotropic hormone.

deprivation resulting from a glucocorticoid-mediated antagonism of insulin action. The concept, although an oversimplification, explains why so many cell types diminish "specialized" activity as a consequence of glucocorticoid excess. As a prime manifestation, protein wasting occurs, so muscles become weak, bones become thin, and skin is rendered unable to sustain the stresses of normal activity, leading to striae and poor wound healing. The vasculature becomes fragile, and ecchymoses result. The immune system is less efficient, encouraging opportunistic infection. Insulin resistance leads to glucose intolerance.

Most patients with Cushing's syndrome gain weight; some lose it. As expected, the difference appears to depend on food intake. A good appetite in the presence of hypercortisolism leads to truncal obesity with a characteristic accentuation of fat deposition in a yokelike distribution over the clavicles and around the neck. Failure of appetite prevents this. Thus cancer and other wasting illnesses, when associated with hypercortisolism, can manifest only the "antianabolic" features of the illness.

To the extent that sex steroid precursors are produced, women manifest some degree of masculinization and men manifest some degree of feminization. To the extent that mineralocorticoids are produced, arterial hypertension and hypokalemic alkalosis occur. Laboratory findings associated with hypercortisolism are confined mainly to the complete blood-cell count in which erythrocytosis, granulocytosis, and lymphocytopenia are prominent manifestations.

Causes. There are six recognized causes of Cushing's syndrome. They can be divided into ACTH-dependent and ACTH-independent types (Table 298-1). ACTH-dependent Cushing's syndrome has two causes: the ACTH-secreting pituitary adenoma and the non-pituitary ACTH-secreting tumor. ACTH-secreting pituitary tumors are referred to as Cushing's disease, the most common cause of Cushing's syndrome. For reasons yet unknown, the small tumors that cause this

disorder are resistant in variable degree to the "feedback" effects of cortisol. Thus they maintain plasma cortisol "homeostasis" in a range that is too high for all tissues but the microadenoma itself. Like the normal gland, these tumors secrete ACTH in a pulsatile fashion. Unlike the normal gland, the diurnal pattern of cortisol secretion is lost. These tumors are usually small and rarely alter the bony architecture of the sella turcica.

The ectopic production of ACTH is most commonly caused by neoplasms of the lung. Other tumors include endocrine tumors of foregut origin and the pheochromocytoma (Table 298-2). These tumors often process the proopiomelanocortin parent protein differently than pituitary tissue. Hence, ACTH from these tumors frequently can be distinguished from that of pituitary origin.

The hallmark of the ACTH-dependent forms of Cushing's syndrome is the presence of measurable plasma ACTH in a patient with clinical and biochemical "hypercortisolism."

The ACTH-independent forms of Cushing's syndrome are adrenal in origin. (This excludes factitious or iatrogenic causes of Cushing's syndrome, which are becoming more common.) Adrenal cancers are usually large when Cushing's syndrome becomes evident. As many as half of these tumors can be palpated through the abdominal wall at the first visit to a physician. The average size of these tumors is about 6 cm in diameter, rendering them easily detectable by computed tomography (CT) scan. Adrenal cancers can produce steroids other than cortisol. Thus, when Cushing's syndrome is accompanied by virilization, feminization, or mineralocorticoid excess, the likelihood of adrenal cancer is increased.

The average adrenal adenoma is 3 cm in diameter. These tumors are uncommonly associated with other steroid-mediated syndromes.

Micronodular adrenal disease is a disorder of children, adolescents, and young adults. The adrenal glands contain numerous small (<3 mm) pigmented nodules that secrete cortisol in sufficient quantity to suppress pituitary ACTH secretion. The cortex between the micronodules is atrophic, in contrast to the ACTH-mediated processes. The biochemical pathogenesis of this disorder is unknown. It can occur in sporadic or familial form. Multiple pigmented lentigines, cardiac myxomas, and other neoplasms can be associated with it. Bilateral macronodular adrenal disease is a comparatively rare disorder of adults. The adrenal glands contain nodules up to several centimeters in diameter and their total combined weight may exceed 100 g. Biochemical responses are quite variable. The etiology is not clear, but in some instances may represent an evolution from an ACTH-dependent hyperplasia to an ACTH-independent disorder.

The most common cause of ACTH-independent Cushing's syndrome is iatrogenic. Glucocorticoids in pharmacologic quantities are used to treat many diseases with an inflammatory component. Given enough time, this will lead to Cushing's syndrome with all of its attendant untoward sequelae. Rarely, glucocorticoids are taken surreptitiously, a difficult diagnostic challenge for the clinician.

Diagnosis and Differential Diagnosis. The diagnosis of Cushing's syndrome requires the clinical picture of the disorder in association with supporting biochemical evidence of glucocorticoid excess. There are two biochemical abnormalities of Cushing's syndrome: an increased secretion rate of cortisol and a disordered circadian pattern of cortisol secretion. In addition, there are two important caveats. First, these abnormalities can have a periodic variation in intensity or can even be intermittent. Second, these abnormalities are found in most cases of factitious or iatrogenic Cushing's syndrome.

The most useful clinical test for assessing the cortisol production rate is the urinary free cortisol excretion. Values consistently in excess of 250 μg/day are virtually diagnostic of Cushing's syndrome. Depression, alcoholism, hypoglycemia, and psychic or physical stress can produce urinary free cortisol excretion rates above normal, but these values are rarely greater than 250 μg/day. Thus in the "gray" zone between normal (<100 μg/day) and 250 μg/day will be many patients with pseudo-Cushing's syndrome and a few with "true" Cushing's syndrome.

Characteristic of the pseudo-Cushing's disorders, however, is a "normal" diurnal pattern of cortisol secretion. This contrasts with patients with Cushing's syndrome in whom that rhythm is lost. Thus a clear demonstration of the loss of normal diurnal variation is strong evidence for the diagnosis of Cushing's syndrome. Since cortisol is secreted in a pulsatile fashion in normal and abnormal states, single morning and evening values are inadequate for this demonstration. We recommend sampling blood at 30-minute intervals between 6:00 AM and 8:00 AM, and 10:00 PM and 12:00 AM (midnight) for the measurement of cortisol. The rule of thumb is that the mean evening value should be less than half of the mean morning value, assuming a "normal" sleep-wake cycle. This approach allows the diagnosis of Cushing's syndrome in some patients who are excreting urinary free cortisol in amounts less than 250 μ/day.

Once the diagnosis of Cushing's syndrome has been established, effective therapy depends on an accurate differential diagnosis of the underlying cause. The traditional approach to this problem employs the dexamethasone suppression test. Exogenous dexamethasone at a dose of 2 mg/day for two days suppresses the urinary excretion of Porter-Silber chromogens to less than 2 mg/day in virtually all normal people. The same qualitative phenomenon occurs in patients with Cushing's disease, but the necessary dose is greater. Between 80% and 90% of patients with Cushing's disease reduce the excretion of Porter-Silber chromogen by more than 50% of "baseline" at a dose of dexamethasone of 8 mg/day. Patients with other causes of Cushing's syndrome usually fail to suppress the excretion of Porter-Silber chromogens with this dose of dexamethasone. Since Cushing's disease accounts for 70% of patients with Cushing's syndrome, the majority of patients can be classified in this way. Failure to suppress the excretion of Porter-Silber chromogens with dexamethasone should lead to a careful search for primary adrenal disease with adrenal CT scan and, if absent, a thorough search for an ectopic source of ACTH secretion. This search should concentrate on the chest, where more than 90% of these lesions are found. Full lung CT and magnetic resonance imaging (MRI) scans are the procedures of choice.

This approach to the differential diagnosis of Cushing's syndrome, however, misclassifies as many as 15% of patients with Cushing's disease. In addition, certain ACTH-secreting tumors, notably the bronchial carcinoid, can meet the criteria in as many as 40% of cases. Patients with "periodic" Cushing's syndrome are easily misclassified with this traditional approach.

Recent improvements in ACTH measurement technique have allowed a new approach to the differential diagnosis of Cushing's syndrome based on the measurement of plasma ACTH and the response of ACTH to corticotropin-releasing factor (CRF).

The concept underlying this approach is that if ACTH is measurable in the plasma of a "hypercortisolemic" patient, the process is ACTH dependent. This categorizes patients into ACTH-dependent and ACTH-independent forms of Cushing's syndrome. The precise localization of the site of ACTH production can be accomplished with the technique of inferior petrosal sinus sampling for plasma ACTH.

Inferior petrosal sinus sampling allows the measurement of ACTH concentrations in blood immediately draining the pituitary gland. The average ratio of ACTH concentration, central to peripheral blood, is 20:1. The lower limit of this range in patients with a pituitary ACTH source is a ratio of 2. If the gradient is measured 3 to 5 minutes after CRF administration, the lower bound is 3. The maximum gradient seen in subjects with an ectopic source of ACTH is 2 in either circumstance. Thus the test has immense power for localizing disease "to" or "away from" the pituitary gland.

The test has the added benefit of allowing the preoperative localization of the ACTH-secreting microadenoma to the right or left hemisphere of the anterior pituitary gland. A right-to-left gradient of greater than 1.5 has been associated with correct localization in 85% of surgically confirmed cases. The gradient can be attributed to the almost complete lateralization of the venous drainage from the right to left halves of the pituitary gland into the right- or left-inferior petrosal sinus.

This information allows the surgeon, in the absence of an identifiable tumor, to remove the "hemipituitary" suspected of harboring the lesion. It should be noted that the interpretation of apparent lateralization in samples obtained by inferior petrosal sinus sampling is reliable only if the sella turcica has not been surgically explored previously. Once operated on, the venous drainage of the pituitary gland is so altered that interpretation of relative (right to left) ACTH concentrations has no diagnostic value.

When ACTH cannot be measured in the plasma, the search for primary adrenal disease or a factitious cause of Cushing's syndrome should proceed as outlined under the traditional approach to differential diagnosis.

If either the traditional approach or the contemporary "ACTH directed" approach discloses contradictory or inconsistent results, periodic or intermittent hypersecretion of cortisol should be suspected. This can be verified only by serial urine collections for the measurement of urinary free cortisol or Porter-Silber chromogens. Once established, however, inferior petrosal sinus sampling during a "hypersecretory" period is a powerful approach to differentiated diagnosis.

Treatment

Cushing's disease. The rediscovery of the transsphenoidal approach to the pituitary fossa, coupled with modern optics and image intensification, has moved neurosurgical treatment of Cushing's disease into the forefront of the treatment options for this disorder. In the hands of a skilled surgeon the success of this approach exceeds 90% on the first attempt. If the first attempt fails, and it can be documented that there is still a central gradient of ACTH, a second surgical attempt has a success rate of about 50%. The advent of inferior petrosal sinus sampling for ACTH has provided the surgeon with a rational procedure in the event that a pituitary tumor cannot be found: hemihypophysectomy. The current estimate of the recurrence rate of Cushing's disease is about 5%. Transsphenoidal microadenectomy is not without occasional complications. The mortality rate is about 1%. Infection in these immune-compromised patients is a common cause of death. Morbidity such as cerebrospinal fluid (CSF) leak, sinusitis, and diabetes insipidus (usually transient) occurs in about 5% of patients.

When surgery is not a viable therapeutic option, irradiation coupled with mitotane should be considered. A congener of dichlorodiphenyltrichloroethane (DDT), this drug is an adrenolytic agent that has variable efficacy against adrenal cancer. The drug is very fat-soluble, so changes in dose are reflected slowly in changes in the circulating concentrations of the compound. The urinary excretion of mitotane continues for months after cessation of its administration. Conventional x-ray, 4500 rads over a 6-week period, is given in association with mitotane at a dose of 3 g/day. Most cases can be controlled with this regimen. When "control" has been maintained for 1 year, mitotane should be discontinued. If the disorder recurs, mitotane therapy is reinstated for another year. Most patients, with time, can discontinue mitotane permanently as the effects of irradiation become established. This approach has no known mortality and a high rate of success. Morbidity includes the nonspecific effects of sella turcica irradiation: hypopituitarism in variable degree and nonspecific cognitive changes. In addition, the long-term consequences of mitotane therapy are unknown.

Bilateral adrenalectomy is the final option for patients refusing or failing treatment with the first two approaches. Although almost always curative, bilateral adrenalectomy is associated with a high mortality rate, approaching 5% in some series. The requirement for lifelong treatment with glucocorticoid and mineralocorticoid should also be taken into consideration. Patients with Cushing's disease run the risk of subsequent pituitary tumor enlargement and pigmentation, Nelson's syndrome. The extent of this risk has been estimated at 5% to 10%.

Ectopic ACTH secretion. Surgical ablation of the ectopic ACTH source is the preferred treatment for this disorder. When the source of ACTH cannot be localized or is too advanced or widespread for an effective surgical approach, blockade of adrenal steroidogenesis is the treatment of choice. The availability of ketoconazole for this purpose has considerably facilitated this therapeutic option. Ketoconazole blocks adrenal steroidogenesis at several levels, the most important being the 20-22 desmolase step that catalyzes the conversion of cholesterol to pregnenolone. Because this is the earliest step in the steroid biosynthetic cascade, the accumulation of troublesome intermediates such as 11-deoxycorticosterone, which can worsen hypertension, is avoided. Patients with a "fixed" ACTH secretion rate (i.e., without an intact feedback axis) usually respond well to this agent at doses ranging from 400 to 1200 mg/day. Effective blockade in patients with an occult source of ACTH often can be maintained for years. In this setting, regular reevaluation in search of the responsible neoplasm can successfully identify the source and allow definitive surgical treatment. The primary toxicity of ketoconazole is hepatocellular. Rising plasma liver enzyme concentrations necessitate cessation of the drug. This is an uncommon occurrence. When it does occur, other blocking agents are available and can be used singly or in combination. These include metyrapone, aminoglutethimide, and trilostane.

Adrenal adenoma and carcinoma. The primary treatment for these disorders is surgical. The prognosis for malignant behavior based on gross and microscopic pathologic examination is unreliable. On clinical examination lesions greater than 6 cm in diameter tend to have malignant behavior. Failure to image with iodocholesterol also has bad prognostic implication.

Small tumors can be removed through a unilateral flank incision. Large tumors must be removed via the transabdominal approach to allow careful examination of the liver, the pararenal structures, and the great veins.

Benign lesions are cured by surgery. Hence, with continued absence of local spread or metastases, watchful waiting should be emphasized. Evidence for malignancy, be it local recurrence or distant spread, calls for the addition of chemotherapy.

Chemotherapy for adrenal cancer is little changed from the early 1960s, when mitotane was first introduced. When used to treat adrenal cancer, the drug traditionally has been pushed to toxicity. Recent studies support this practice and suggest that success may relate to dose and plasma levels of mitotane achieved. The common toxicities of the drug are nausea, somnolence, ataxia, and reduced attention span. When encountered, reduction of the dose by increments of 20% usually halts the progression of side effects. Liver and bone marrow toxicity are not problems with this drug.

Treated this way, about 25% of patients have an objective remission that becomes evident in shrinkage of a measurable lesion. The average duration of these remissions is 7 months. Throughout the course surgically negotiable disease should be removed, even though it is clear that the operation will not be curative. The rationale behind this approach is that hemorrhagic or septic episodes associated with large tumor masses are a common and serious complication in this disease and, theoretically, can be prevented by early surgical intervention. Using this approach, these patients follow a survival curve with a half-time of about 4 years.

The drug mitotane alters the pathway of adrenal metabolism, so in the absence of significant tumor effect the excretion of Porter-Silber chromogens or 17-ketosteroids is reduced. This does not equate with nor should be confused with, a "true" remission. Urinary free cortisol is free of this artifact and, if a chemical parameter of progress is deemed essential, this should be the chosen one.

Micronodular adrenal disease. The treatment for this disorder is bilateral adrenalectomy.

Recovery. A final word about the treatment of Cushing's syndrome: successful intervention invariably makes patients feel worse, leading to an occasional "credibility gap." This should be anticipated: recovery to a usual state of good health can require a year or more. Foreknowledge of this can prevent anxiety and depression and work as a positive force in the rehabilitation process.

MINERALOCORTICOID EXCESS

In humans, aldosterone is the major mineralocorticoid. It is a product of the zona glomerulosa of the adrenal gland. Aldosterone exchanges sodium ions for potassium and hydrogen ions in the proximal tubule of the kidney. Since sodium is primarily an extracellular ion, its balance is reflected in vascular volume. Vascular volume in turn regulates the secretion of aldosterone via the renin-angiotensin system. Thus the metabolic picture of mineralocorticoid excess is a hypokalemic metabolic alkalosis in association with a suppressed plasma renin activity. When aldosterone is the offending mineralocorticoid, plasma aldosterone levels are normal or high. When some other mineralocorticoid is the offending agent, aldosterone levels are suppressed.

Causes of Mineralocorticoid Excess

The mineralocorticoid excess syndromes can be thought of as primary or secondary. The primary causes are those in which the secretion of excess mineralocorticoid is the fundamental lesion. The secondary

---

> **BOX 298-1**
> ## Common causes of mineralocorticoid excess
>
> I. With hypertension (primary mineralocorticoid excess)
>   A. Due to aldosterone
>   1. Aldosterone secretion the *primary* lesion
>   a. Aldosterone-secreting adenoma
>   b. Idiopathic hyperaldosteronism
>   c. Dexamethasone-suppressible hyperaldosteronism
>   d. Adrenocortical carcinoma
>   2. Aldosterone secretion *secondary* to another lesion
>   a. Renal artery stenosis
>   b. Renin-secreting tumor
>   c. Malignant hypertension
>   d. Chronic renal disease
>   B. Due to some other mineralocorticoid
>   1. Adrenal cancer
>   2. 11-Beta hydroxylase deficiency
>   3. 17-Hydroxylase deficiency
>   4. Liddle's syndrome
>   5. 11-Beta hydroxysteroid dehydrogenase deficiency
>   6. Licorice ingestion
> II. With normal blood pressure
>   A. Chronic renal disease
>   B. Hepatic cirrhosis
>   C. Cardiac failure
>   D. Covert vomiting
>   E. Covert diuretic use
>   F. Covert laxative use
>   G. Familial chloride diarrhea

causes are those in which the excess secretion of mineralocorticoid occurs in response to another fundamental lesion. Examples of primary disease are the aldosterone-secreting adenoma and adrenal cancer. Examples of secondary mineralocorticoid excess are cirrhosis of the liver and congestive heart failure. The primary syndromes of mineralocorticoid excess are usually associated with hypertension and require treatment. The secondary syndromes of mineralocorticoid excess are usually associated with normotension or hypotension and usually do not require specific therapy other than that directed toward the underlying lesion. The common causes of mineralocorticoid excess are listed in Box 298-1.

Diagnosis and Differential Diagnosis

The symptoms most frequently reported by patients with primary mineralocorticoid excess are headache, easy fatigability, and weakness. Hypertension is the most common sign. The finding of hypokalemia and a metabolic alkalosis in a hypertensive patient should lead to further evaluation. The first step in this evaluation is to measure a *stimulated* (with 4 hours of upright posture) plasma renin activity. Values less than 2 ng/ml per hour strongly indicate the presence of mineralocorticoid excess. A plasma aldosterone concentration measured at the same time categorizes the mineralocorticoid excess syndrome into that caused by aldosterone versus that caused by some other mineralocorticoid. A plasma aldosterone concentration greater than 14 ng/dl is virtually diagnostic of primary hyperaldosteronism. Lower levels are compatible with the diagnosis but must be shown to be "non-suppressible" with an infusion of 2 L of normal saline over 4 hours to confirm the diagnosis. At the conclusion of the infusion, plasma aldosterone concentration should be greater than 5 ng/dl and usually exceeds 10 ng/dl in proven cases of primary aldosterone excess.

Patients with aldosterone excess require localization of the source of aldosterone secretion before definitive therapy can be planned. Localization depends on determining whether aldosterone is being secreted by one or by both adrenal glands. Unilateral aldosterone secretion is almost always from an aldosterone-secreting adenoma and can be cured by adrenalectomy on that side. Bilateral secretion of aldosterone is the result of bilateral hyperplasia of the zona glomerulosa, and this condition responds poorly to adrenalectomy. The most reliable way to localize the source of excess aldosterone secretion is by bilateral adrenal vein catheterization. Thirty minutes after the intravenous injection of 250 μg cosyntropin, aldosterone and cortisol are measured in blood samples drawn simultaneously from each adrenal vein. In patients with bilateral disease the aldosterone/cortisol ratio is the same. In patients with unilateral disease there is marked asymmetry in the ratios, the larger of the two identifying the gland harboring the adenoma. Treatment can be planned on the basis of these findings.

In patients with hypertension and mineralocorticoid excess attributable to a mineralocorticoid other than aldosterone, adrenal cancer should be suspected. The single best test for identifying this cause of mineralocorticoid excess is the adrenal CT scan. Since adrenal cancers are nearly always large at the time of discover, usually greater than 6 cm in diameter, the CT scan can be counted on to identify nearly all such lesions. The remaining causes of nonaldosterone mineralocorticoid excess, aside from licorice ingestion, require the measurement of steroids (biosynthetic intermediates) that are not widely available, and this evaluation should be pursued in a specialty center.

Treatment

Aldosterone-mediated mineralocorticoid excess syndromes usually require treatment. Aldosterone-secreting adenomas usually can be managed successfully with surgery. An ongoing puzzle in the management of these disorders is the well-established observation that bilateral adrenal secretion of aldosterone does not respond well to surgery. The metabolic changes can be reversed, but the associated hypertension is rarely improved.

The mineralocorticoid excess syndromes associated with normal blood pressure (the "secondary" syndromes) are best treated with therapy directed at the underlying disorder. These patients are best given treatment with a combination of an aldosterone antagonist, spironolactone, to control hypokalemia, and a standard drug regimen for the associated hypertension.

The therapy for adrenal cancer is primarily surgical, with the addition of mitotane in cases of metastatic disease. The enzyme deficiency disorders, 11-beta hydroxylase deficiency, and 17-hydroxylase deficiency, are treated with exogenous glucocorticoid, and 11-beta hydroxy steroid dehydrogenase deficiency is treated with spironolactone.

ADRENAL HYPOFUNCTION

Adrenal hypofunction results from destruction of the adrenal cortex (primary adrenal insufficiency) or from ACTH deficiency (secondary adrenal insufficiency). In both instances, lack of glucocorticoid and mineralocorticoid account for the major clinical manifestations.

The clinical manifestations of chronic adrenal insufficiency include weakness, fatigue, weight loss, hypotension, anorexia and, occasionally, diarrhea. Cutaneous hyperpigmentation is characteristic of primary adrenal insufficiency and is a useful differential diagnostic sign. The hyperpigmentation is typically located over the elbows, knuckles, in axillary folds, and in the buccal mucosa. Areas of existing pigmentation such as the palmar creases, the areolae, and the lip margins can become strikingly hyperpigmented. It is useful to inquire about recent injuries or surgical procedures, since healing tissues can exhibit transient hyperpigmentation. Hyperpigmentation can be difficult to assess in dark-skinned people and in "weathered" individuals. In these instances, examination of the oral mucosa, especially the buccal mucosa, tongue, and gingival margins, is important, since these are frequently hyperpigmented in primary adrenal insufficiency and only rarely so otherwise.

Pubic and axillary hair in women depend on weak adrenal androgens and can be absent or sparse in women with chronic adrenal insufficiency. Diminished or absent axillary hair is a frequent finding in men with hypopituitarism and reflects diminished secretion of adrenal and gonadal androgens. Sexual hair is present in men with primary adrenal insufficiency, since the gonadal secretion of androgens is not materially affected by hypocortisolism.

Acute adrenal insufficiency often is first recognized during a stressful event such as surgery or infection. The hallmark of this dis-

---

BOX 298-2
Causes of adrenocortical insufficiency

Primary adrenocortical insufficiency
Acquired disorders (Addison's disease)
  Idiopathic autoimmunity
  Infectious causes (tuberculosis, AIDS, fungal infections, sepsis)
  Metastic or invasive disorder (tumors, sarcoidosis, amyloidosis)
  Adrenal hemorrhage (trauma, shock, coagulopathies)
  Iatrogenic (surgery, adrenal inhibitors, anticoagulation)
Congenital and familial
  Congenital adrenal hyperplasia (enzymatic deficiencies)
  Congenital adrenal hypoplasia
  Congenital unresponsiveness to ACTH
  Adrenoleukodystrophy
  Adrenomyeloneuropathy

Secondary adrenocortical insufficiency
Hypothalamopituitary suppression by glucocorticoids
  Exogenous glucocorticoid or ACTH administration
  Endogenous suppression by adrenal or pituitary hyperfunction
    (Cushing's syndrome)
Hypothalamopituitary disease
  Invasive neoplasms (pituitary tumor, craniopharyngioma, eosinophilic granuloma, lymphoma, leukemia)
  Infections (tuberculosis, fungal)
  Surgery and trauma

ACTH, Adrenocorticotropic hormone; *AIDS*, acquired immunodeficiency syndrome.

order is hypotension resistant to correction with "volume" and pressor agents. Common laboratory tests often provide the first clues of adrenocortical hypofunction. The combination of hyponatremia, hyperkalemia, mild metabolic acidosis, and slight elevation of the blood urea nitrogen and hematocrit are classic findings.

Causes of Adrenal Insufficiency

Primary adrenal insufficiency (Addison's disease) is most commonly due to autoimmune destruction of the adrenal cortex (Box 298-2). This accounts for 80% of cases. Tuberculosis is cited as the second leading cause, accounting for about 10% of cases. The balance is made up by fungal infections (blastomycosis, histoplasmosis), hemorrhage into the gland (coagulopathies, iatrogenic anticoagulation, surgery), metastatic neoplasms, sarcoidosis, amyloidosis, acquired immunodeficiency syndrome (AIDS), adrenal leukodystrophy, and congenital adrenal hypoplasia. Autoimmune adrenocortical destruction spares the adrenal medulla, whereas all other destructive origins can involve both the adrenal cortex and the adrenal medulla.

Autoimmune adrenalitis is associated with several other endocrine autoimmune glandular disorders. Most notable among these are thyroiditis and diabetes mellitus. The triad of adrenalitis, thyroiditis, and diabetes mellitus is also known as Schmidt's syndrome. Other, less common autoimmune associations include pernicious anemia, vitiligo, hypoparathyroidism, and mucocutaneous candidiasis. The autoimmune disorders of the endocrine system do not always become evident simultaneously.

Secondary adrenal insufficiency is more common than primary adrenal insufficiency. Secondary adrenal insufficiency is caused by a lack of ACTH stimulation of the gland and most commonly follows prolonged glucocorticoid therapy. Intrinsic or metastatic hypothalamic and pituitary disease is uncommon.

Diagnosis

The diagnosis can be confirmed definitively by demonstrating an impaired adrenal response to exogenously administered ACTH. A single injection of 250 μg of the synthetic ACTH (cosyntropin) should produce a plasma cortisol concentration of at least 20 μg/dl 45 minutes after administration. A diminished or absent response establishes the diagnosis of adrenal insufficiency but does not distinguish primary from secondary causes of the disorder. In primary adrenal insufficiency, plasma ACTH values are elevated, and the combination of an impaired cortisol response to cosyntropin challenge and a high plasma ACTH level is strong evidence for the diagnosis of primary adrenal insufficiency.

Treatment

The therapy for adrenal insufficiency is straightforward: replace the deficient hormones (cortisol and aldosterone). The cortisol replacement dose is 12 to 15 mg cortisol/m^2 body surface area per day. The total dose ranges between 20 and 30 mg/day for most adults. Traditionally, cortisol is given as a divided dose, two thirds in the morning and one third in the afternoon. A recent randomized, double-blind study of three dosing regimens (taking all of the daily cortisol in the morning vs. all in the afternoon vs. the traditional two-thirds:one-third mode) showed a statistically significant subjective patient preference for the traditional regimen. In the authors' opinion, a single daily dose in the morning is sufficient and advantageous for compliance and convenience. Compliance is enhanced by this regimen. Patients with primary adrenal insufficiency require both cortisol and fludrocortisone (Florinef). Orally administered aldosterone is not readily absorbed from the gastrointestinal tract. A synthetic analog of aldosterone, fludrocortisone, is orally active and is given in doses ranging from 0.05 to 0.2 mg daily. Generally an oral dose of 0.1 mg daily suffices. Measurable indices of therapeutic efficacy include changes in body weight and postural blood pressure. Laboratory measures of adrenal function such as of serum electrolyte values and plasma ACTH, renin, and urinary cortisol concentrations can be reserved for resolving issues such as questions of compliance or lack of response to traditional maintenance therapy. Of particular note, the plasma ACTH concentration is not a useful tool for monitoring primary adrenal insufficiency, since it frequently remains high in the face of adequate treatment.

Acute adrenal insufficiency is usually evident as shock that is poorly responsive to volume and pressor therapy. This condition requires emergency treatment. Infusion of isotonic saline should be started immediately. Intravenous cortisol, 100 mg as a bolus injection, should be given immediately after blood is taken for the measurement of cortisol and ACTH. This should be repeated every 6 hours thereafter for the first 48 hours. When the crisis is past, a return to the usual oral replacement dose can be accomplished over 48 hours. This diagnosis is often suspected in seriously ill patients. Therapy should be initiated without waiting for laboratory confirmation with the decision to continue dependent on the results of pretherapy tests.

Patients receiving long-term treatment with systemic corticosteroids can require replacement therapy if the treatment is terminated abruptly or tapered too quickly. Withdrawal from long-term therapy can be associated with fatigue, weakness, arthralgia, and occasional desquamation mimicking—in part, the symptoms of chronic adrenal insufficiency. Suppression of the pituitary-adrenal axis rarely occurs in patients given treatment with corticosteroids for less than 2 or 3 weeks. If the suppression has been prolonged, however, recovery can require up to 1 year. Patients receiving long-term corticosteroid therapy are thought to require an increase in cortisol dose during periods of acute stress. It is traditional to "cover" such periods of stress by doubling the cortisol dose on the "day of" and the "day after" the stressful event. Some experts recommend "tapering" the dose back to maintenance levels over several days. In the authors' opinion, this is unnecessary. If the patient has been given treatment with adequate replacement therapy before the stress, poststress tapering can be conducted very rapidly.

Isolated mineralocorticoid deficiency causes urinary retention of potassium, resulting in hyperkalemia, retention of hydrogen ions, and urinary sodium wasting. Hyperkalemia, although usually asymptomatic, can cause muscle weakness and life-threatening cardiac arrhythmias. Classic sodium wasting becomes evident as orthostatic hypotension. However, in the most common presenting form of hypoaldosteronism the sodium wasting can be offset by the sodium retention associated with severe renal disease. Hyporeninemic hypoaldosteronism is the most common form of isolated mineralocorticoid defi-

ciency. The disorder is frequently associated with diabetes mellitus and usually appears late in the course of that disease.

The hyporeninemic hypoaldosteronism of diabetes is usually accompanied by asymptomatic hyperkalemia and mild acidosis. The renal complications of diabetes, including glomerulopathy and nephropathy, can predominate and result in seemingly paradoxical sodium retention and the absence of orthostatic hypotension. In other circumstances, however, the sodium-depleting effect of hypoaldosteronism predominates and leads to the expected orthostatic hypotension. This form of hypoaldosteronism is most likely the result of impaired renin secretion caused by the complications of diabetes in the afferent arterioles of the kidney. Although the resultant hyperkalemia of hypoaldosteronism would be expected to stimulate aldosterone synthesis, the stimulus is not sufficient to overcome the absence of renin.

Other causes of isolated mineralocorticoid deficiency are intrinsic nondiabetic renal disease and, more rarely, congenital adrenal hyperplasia.

The objectives of treatment of isolated mineralocorticoid deficiency are to reduce hyperkalemia and, if sodium wasting predominates, to expand effective blood volume. Fludrocortisone can be used to replace deficient mineralocorticoid. Serum potassium concentration falls and fluid volume expands as sodium is retained. In hyporeninemic hypoaldosteronism the effective blood volume may be increased because of advanced diabetic renal disease. In this instance a combination of dietary potassium restriction, potassium-binding agents, and diuretics may be required to maintain appropriate potassium levels and an effective blood volume. It should be noted that asymptomatic mild elevations of serum potassium concentration may necessitate only close clinical observation rather than therapy.

CONGENITAL ADRENAL HYPERPLASIA
Categories

There are five enzymatic steps between cholesterol and cortisol that, when attenuated, lead to specific syndromes of congenital adrenal hyperplasia (CAH). All are transmitted as autosomal recessive traits. The affected enzymes, in order from cholesterol to cortisol, are 20-22 desmolase, 3-beta-hydroxy-steroid dehydrogenase (3-β-HSD), 17-hydroxylase, 21-hydroxylase, and 11-hydroxylase (Fig. 298-3). The most common of these, 21-hydroxylase deficiency, accounts for 85% of cases. 11-Hydroxylase deficiency and 3-β-HSD deficiency account for most of the remainder.

A convenient way to categorize these disorders is into virilizing and feminizing forms. 21-Hydroxylase deficiency and 11-hydroxylase deficiency are virilizing forms; 20-22 desmolase deficiency and 17-hydroxylase deficiency are feminizing forms. 3-β-HSD is virilizing in females and feminizing in males. All forms of CAH can adversely affect reproductive competence by altering sex-steroid synthesis and secretion. The most common form of CAH to do this, by far, is the 21-hydroxylase–deficient form of the disease.

21-Hydroxylase deficiency occurs in two major clinical forms: "classic" and "attenuated." The classic form is usually evident in neonatal life or early in childhood. It has two clinical presentations, roughly equal in prevalence: the "simple virilizing" form and the "salt-wasting" form. The simple virilizing form is the most common cause of heterosexual precocious puberty in girls and isosexual precocity in boys. It usually becomes evident after the neonatal period. The salt wasting form of the disorder occurs when the synthesis and secretion of both cortisol and aldosterone are impaired. These children are usually discovered in the neonatal period because of failure to thrive. Infant girls with both forms of the disease can have ambiguous genitalia; several different mutations of the 21-hydroxylase gene have been associated with the classic form of 21-hydroxylase deficiency. These include gene deletions, gene conversion events, and point mutations.

The attenuated form of the disorder is usually detected in the peripubertal period of life. The usual manifestations are those of idiopathic hirsutism and the polycystic ovary syndrome. Hirsutism, oligomenorrhea, and infertility dominate the clinical picture. There is only one form of the attenuated variety of 21-hydroxylase deficiency, but there is great variability in severity. "Salt loss" is not a feature, but mild impairment of mineralocorticoid secretion can be demon-

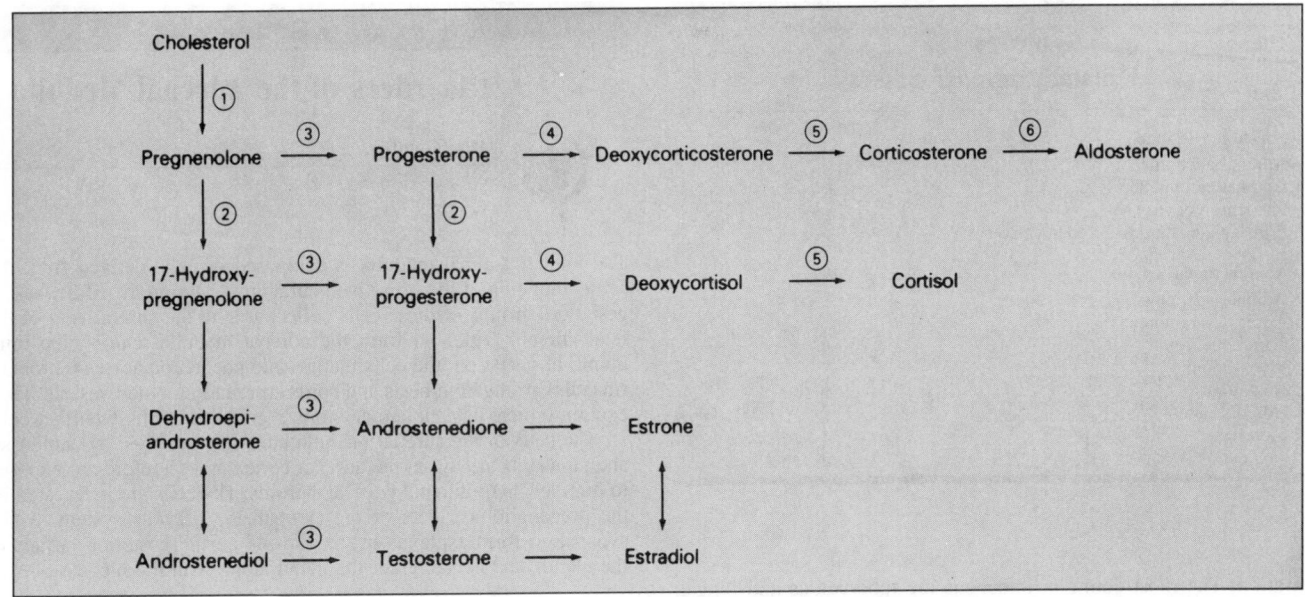

FIGURE 298-3   The sites of the five enzyme blocks leading to the various syndromes of congenital adrenal hyperplasia. *1*, 20-22 desmolase; *2*, 17-hydroxylase; *3*, 3-β-hydroxy-steroid dehydrogenase; *4*, 21-hydroxylase; and *5*, 11-hydroxylase.

strated in most cases. There is an association with the human leukocyte antigen HLA-B14 and the HLA-DR1 haplotypes. In these cases there is a single base change in the 21-hydroxylase gene.

The incidence of the attenuated form of the disease varies widely depending on the specific population under study. For example, it occurs in 1 in 27 Ashkenazi Jews, 1 in 53 Hispanics, 1 in 63 Yugoslavs, and 1 in 333 Italians. Other studies show "carrier" rates ranging between 1% and 6%. The disorder can vary in severity from hirsutism, oligomenorrhea, and infertility at one extreme to phenotypically normal women at the other extreme with no abnormality other than the characteristic biochemical markers of the disease.

Diagnosis

The disorder should be considered in all cases of hirsutism, oligomenorrhea, or unexplained infertility. If plasma testosterone concentrations are in the normal range, attenuated CAH is unlikely. At the other extreme, plasma testosterone levels above 200 ng/dl are rarely associated with the attenuated forms of CAH. Plasma testosterone levels between 65 and 150 ng/dl, however, are characteristic of attenuated CAH. The appropriate diagnostic test is a plasma 17-hydroxy-progesterone measurement 45 minutes after the administration of 250 μg cosyntropin. In normal subjects, 17-hydroxy-progesterone levels do not exceed 350 ng/dl after an ACTH challenge. The 17-hydroxy-progesterone value following administration of cosyntropin is virtually always in excess of 1000 ng/dl in patients with attenuated CAH.

Treatment

Since the basic lesion is an inefficient production of cortisol caused by an altered 21-hydroxylase enzyme, the process can be reversed by supplying cortisol from an exogenous source. The production rate of cortisol ranges from 6 to 9 mg/m² body surface area per day; reductions in bioavailability attributable to absorption and metabolism result in a recommended oral dose of 12 to 15 mg/m² body surface area. Supplying this amount by mouth, once a day, effectively reduces the increased testosterone production rate. In most instances, hirsutism improves and cyclic menses return.

"INCIDENTAL ADRENAL MASS"

Adrenal tumors are being discovered with increasing frequency as a by-product of improved radiologic imaging of the abdomen. Since

---

> ### BOX 298-3
> ### Bilateral adrenal masses
>
> A. Functional lesions
>   1. ACTH-dependent Cushing's syndrome
>   2. Congenital adrenal hyperplasia
>   3. Pheochromocytoma
>   4. Conn's syndrome, hyperplastic variety
>   5. Micronodular adrenal disease
>   6. Idiopathic bilateral adrenal hypertrophy
> B. Nonfunctional lesions
>   1. Infection (tuberculosis, fungi)
>   2. Infiltration (leukemia, lymphoma)
>   3. Replacement (amyloidosis)
>   4. Hemorrhage
>   5. Bilateral metastases

ACTH, Adrenocorticotropic hormone.

these tumors are found by diagnostic procedures carried out for another purpose, they have been termed the "incidental adrenal mass." Once discovered, they pose a diagnostic and therapeutic dilemma, since a judgment must be made about the clinical significance of the mass and how it can be managed cost effectively.

The differential diagnoses of unilateral and bilateral incidental adrenal masses are listed in Boxes 298-3 and 298-4.

All lesions must be evaluated for function. The history and physical features are important guides in this determination. Features of glucocorticoid excess are those of Cushing's syndrome. Hypertension associated with an adrenal mass suggests Cushing's syndrome, hyperaldosteronism, or pheochromocytoma. Hirsutism of recent onset, particularly if associated with signs of virilization such as temporal balding, deepening of the voice, and clitoromegaly, suggests androgen secretion.

The syndrome of adrenal insufficiency has already been mentioned. Unilateral disease, of course, is not associated with adrenal insufficiency. Said another way, the diagnosis of primary adrenal insufficiency implies bilateral disease. When bilateral masses are present, the differential diagnosis includes infection and neoplastic in-

---

BOX 298-4
Unilateral adrenal masses

Functional lesions
Adrenal adenoma
Adrenal carcinoma
Pheochromocytoma
Primary aldosteronism, adenomatous type

Nonfunctional lesions
Adrenal adenoma
Adrenal carcinoma
Ganglioneuroma
Myelolipoma
Hematoma
Adrenolipoma
Metastasis

---

filtration. The most common infections are tuberculous and fungal. The most common tumors are breast and lung.

The laboratory evaluation of the incidentally discovered adrenal mass should concentrate on the best screening tests for disorders of hormone excess or deficiency. The best screening test for Cushing's syndrome is the 24-hour urinary free cortisol; for primary aldosteronism, the upright plasma renin activity; for pheochromocytoma, plasma catecholamines after clonidine; and for sex-steroid–secreting adenomas, plasma testosterone in women, and estrone in men. In bilateral disease congenital adrenal hyperplasia should be excluded by measuring 17-hydroxy-progesterone and 11-deoxycortisol 45 minutes after administration of 250 μg of intravenous cosyntropin. Adrenal insufficiency can be identified by an absent or subnormal response of plasma cortisol to the standard 250-μg intravenous injection of cosyntropin. A single plasma ACTH measurement differentiates primary from secondary adrenal insufficiency in patients "failing" the cosyntropin test.

Functional lesions other than congenital adrenal hyperplasia must be treated surgically. Congenital adrenal hyperplasia is treated with exogenous glucocorticoid and, when indicated, mineralocorticoid. All unilateral adrenal lesions should be evaluated by fine-needle biopsy. All adrenal lesions that represent disease metastatic "to" the adrenal gland should be treated as part of the therapy for the underlying neoplasm. Incidental masses of adrenal origin that are greater than 3 cm in diameter should be excised. Masses of adrenal origin that are less than 3 cm in diameter are rarely malignant and can be safely managed conservatively. Unequivocal growth, however, is generally considered an indication for surgical intervention.

Although surgical treatment is palliative when the cancer is metastatic, surgery can be helpful in "debulking" the mass to reduce symptoms of hormone excess. The only effective medical treatment for adrenocortical carcinoma is op′DDD, which is not curative. The side effects of this drug are serious, and the disadvantages of its use can outweigh the symptomatic benefits to the patient.

BIBLIOGRAPHY

Aron DC, Tyrrell BT, editors: Cushing's syndrome. *Endocrinol Metab Clin North Am* 23(3):451-698, 1994.

Blumen JD, Sealey JE, Schussel Y et al: Diagnosis and treatment of primary aldosteronism, *Ann Intern Med* 121:877-855, 1995.

Miller WL: Congenital adrenal hyperplasias, *Endocrinol Metab Clin North Am* 20:721-749, 1991.

Riedel M, Wiese A, Schurmeryer TH, Brabant G: Quality of life in patients with Addison's disease: effects of different cortisol replacement modes, *Exp Clin Endocrinol* 101:106-111, 1993.

Vallotton MB: Endocrine emergencies: disorders of the adrenal cortex, *Baillieres Clin Endocrinol Metab* 6:41-56, 1992.

Wilson RC, Mercado AB, Cheng KC, New MI: Steroid 21-hydroxylase deficiency: genotype may not predict phenotype, *J Clin Endocrinol Metab* 80:2322-2329, 1995.

---

299 Disorders of the Adrenal Medulla

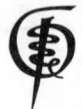

Alan Goldfien

The human adrenal medulla is composed of cells derived from the sympathogonia of the primitive neural crest. During the fifth week of gestation, groups of these cells collect around the central vein of the fetal adrenal cortex to form the adrenal medulla. During the third month of gestation, the cells mature into pheochromacytes (chromaffin cells) arranged in nests and cords surrounding blood vessels. They contain typical catecholamine storage granules by the twelfth week.

The cells of the adrenal medulla are richly supplied by capillaries and sinusoids arising in the adrenal cortex and therefore are exposed to high levels of adrenal cortical steroids. The cells are innervated by the preganglionic fibers of the sympathetic nervous system, which synapse to form a plexus in the capsule on the posterior surface of the gland. The nerves enter the gland along with the blood vessels.

HORMONES OF THE ADRENAL MEDULLA

The adrenal medulla synthesizes and secretes catecholamines as well as enkephalins. Special techniques indicate that other active peptides—such as dynorphins, vasoactive intestinal peptide, somatostatin, and substance P—can be found in chromaffin cells of various species. The physiologic significance of these findings is unknown.

Catecholamines: Biosynthesis and Metabolism

The catecholamines—epinephrine and norepinephrine—are normally produced in the adrenal medulla, brain, and sympathetic neurons. In peripheral adrenergic neurons, L-tyrosine entering the cell from the circulation is converted to dihydroxyphenylalanine (dopa) by the mitochondrial enzyme tyrosine hydroxylase. Dopa decarboxylase converts dopa to dopamine, which is taken up by specific storage granules. Dopamine in the granule is converted to norepinephrine by dopamine β-hydroxylase. In the adrenal medulla, in some neurons in the brain, and in tumors producing epinephrine, norepinephrine is converted to epinephrine by the action of the enzyme phenylethanolamine N-methyltransferase (PNMT). This process is summarized in Fig. 299-1. In the adrenal medulla and sympathetic nerve endings, catecholamines are stored in granules that appear to contain and release a number of active peptides, including adrenocorticotrophic hormone (ACTH), vasoactive intestinal peptide (VIP), and the enkephalins. Adrenomedullin, a peptide originally isolated from pheochromocytoma tissue, is also produced in the adrenal medulla. It exhibits potent depressor and vasorelaxant activity. It has also been found in the heart, lung, kidney and brain as well as vascular endothelium. The N-terminal 20–amino acid peptide of proadrenomedullin, from which adrenomedullin is derived, is found in the same tissues. This peptide exerts hypotensive effects by inhibiting neural transmission at sympathetic nerve endings. Recent studies indicate that peptides derived from the chromogranins are physiologically active and may modulate catecholamine release.

In the basal ganglia, in some hypothalamic nuclei, and in other central and peripheral neurons, dopamine is the final product and neurotransmitter. Dopamine is also secreted by some tumors.

When norepinephrine is released at nerve endings, 85% to 90% is taken up by the neuron and reutilized or metabolized there by monoamine oxidase (MAO). Amines not taken up by the neuron or bound to the adrenergic receptor are taken up at other sites on the effector cell and metabolized by catechol-O-methyltransferase (CMT). A small amount of the norepinephrine enters the circulation. The catecholamines released by tumors enter the circulation and are metabolized in the same manner as those released by the adrenal medulla. They circulate bound to albumin or a closely associated protein and act by binding to the adrenergic receptors in the membranes of cells. Catecholamines not bound to the receptor are metabolized by CMT

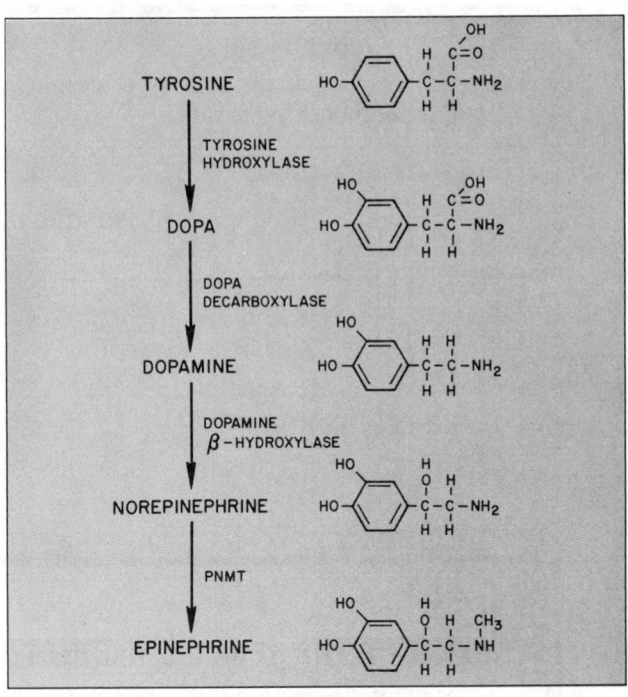

FIGURE 299-1   Biosynthesis of the catecholamines. *PNMT*, Phenylethanolamine N-methyltransferase.

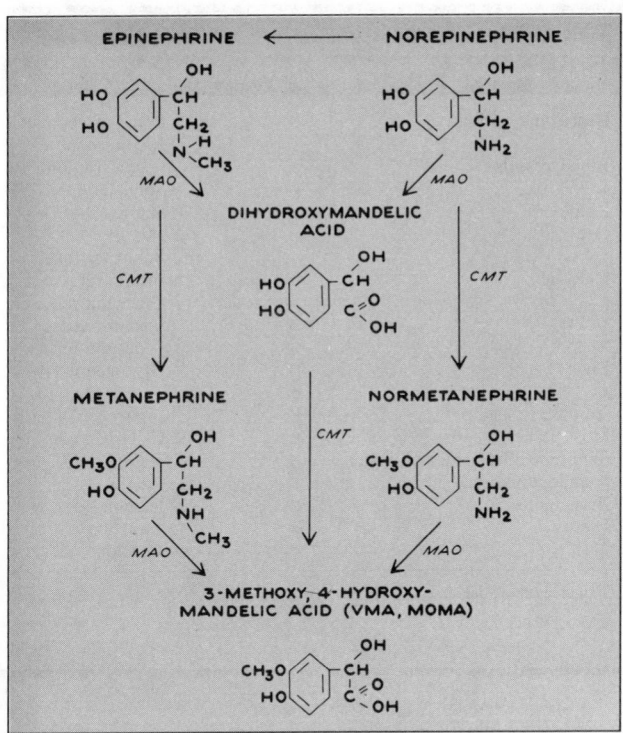

FIGURE 299-2   Metabolism of epinephrine and norepinephrine by monoamine oxidase (MAO) and catechol-O-methyltransferase (CMT).

or MAO. A single passage through the liver or kidney removes two thirds of the free amine. Normally, only a few percent of these amines appear in the urine unchanged or conjugated to glucuronic or sulfuric acid. About half of the catecholamine released is acted on by both enzymes and excreted in the urine as vanillylmandelic acid (VMA). These pathways of metabolism are summarized in Fig. 299-2. The plasma concentration of epinephrine and norepinephrine and the amounts of catecholamines and metabolite excreted daily are shown in Table 299-1.

Release of these hormones at synaptic clefts and into the circulation regulates many important cellular functions and organ responses. These responses are mediated by specific adrenergic receptors in the cell membrane.

There are two classes of adrenergic receptors—alpha and beta—each of which has several subtypes. These receptors were classified by the relative potencies of a series of adrenergic agonists and antagonists. Each of the subtypes is now known to be coded by one or more separate genes.

These receptors are proteins with seven membrane-spanning groups of amino acids. They are coupled to intracellular processes by trimeric G proteins, which consist of α-, β-, and γ-subunits. When hormone binds to the receptor, the β- and γ-subunits dissociate from the α-subunits, allowing GDP to be replaced by GTP. The α-subunit is then able to activate postreceptor pathways. The α_1-subtype are postsynaptic receptors that typically mediate vascular and other smooth muscle contraction. When agonist binds to this receptor, the alpha subunit of the guanyl nucleotide-binding protein G_q activates phospholipase C, which acts on phosphatidylinositol bisphosphonate to produce 1,4,5-inositol trisphosphate and diacylglycerol. These second messengers mediate intracellular effects of the agonist. Epinephrine and norepinephrine are potent agonists for this receptor, whereas isoproterenol is weakly active. The α_2-subtype is found on sympathetic nerve terminals, where it acts to inhibit the release of norepinephrine. It is also found in platelets and at many postsynaptic sites. The binding of agonist to α_2-receptors releases G_i alpha, which inhibits the enzyme adenylyl cyclase and reduces the formation of cyclic adenosine monophosphate (cAMP). Prazosin is a selective antagonist at the α_1-receptor and yohimbine is selective for the α_2-receptor, whereas phentolamine and dibenzyline act at both.

Table 299-1   Normal plasma levels of catecholamines, their urinary excretion rates, and their major metabolites

CATECHOLAMINE OR METABOLITE	NORMAL SUBJECTS	
	AT REST	MARKED ACTIVITY OR STRESS
Plasma		
Epinephrine	20-50 pg/ml	150 pg/ml
Norepinephrine	100-400 pg/ml	1000 pg/ml
Urine		
Epinephrine	5-20 μg/24 hr	100 μg/24 hr
Norepinephrine	20-60 μg/24 hr	200 μg/24 hr
Metanephrines	<1.3 mg/24 hr	
VMA	<7.0 mg/24 hr	

There are several β-receptor subtypes. Agonist binding to these receptors activates adenylyl cyclase via the G_s α-subunit to increase the production of cAMP, which in turn converts protein kinase A to its active form. The β-receptor, which mediates the direct cardiac effects, is more responsive to isoproterenol than to epinephrine or norepinephrine, whose potencies are similar. At the β_2-receptor—which mediates vascular, bronchial, and uterine smooth muscle relaxation—isoproterenol is also most potent; but epinephrine is much more potent than norepinephrine. The β_3-receptors are found in adipose tissue. Some of the physiologic effects of the catecholamines are listed in Table 299-2.

HYPOFUNCTION OF THE ADRENAL MEDULLA

Hypofunction of the adrenal medulla is most often the consequence of bilateral adrenalectomy. In these patients, when adrenal corticoid replacement therapy is instituted, careful studies show only minor delays in recovery from insulin-induced hypoglycemia. The loss of this response is of no clinical significance, except in patients with diabe-

Table 299-2   Adrenergic responses of selected tissues

ORGAN OR TISSUE	RECEPTOR	EFFECT
Heart (myocardium)	β_1	↑ Force of contraction
		↑ Rate of contraction
Blood vessels	α	Vasoconstriction
	β_2	Vasodilatation
Kidney	β	Renin release
Gut	α, β	↓ Motility
		↑ Sphincter tone
Pancreas	α	↓ Insulin release
		↓ Glucagon release
	β	↑ Insulin release
		↑ Glucagon release
Liver	β	↑ Glycogenolysis
	α	
Adipose tissue	β	↑ Lipolysis
Most tissues	β	↑ Calorigenesis
Skin (apocrine glands on hands, underarms, etc.)	α	Sweating
Bronchioles	β_2	Dilatation
Uterus	α	Contraction
	β_2	Relaxation

↑, Increased; ↓, decreased

BOX 299-1

Causes of orthostatic hypotension

Functional	Neurogenic (autonomic insufficiency)
Reduction in effective blood volume	Familial dysautonomia
Hemorrhage	Shy-Drager syndrome
Prolonged bed rest	Parkinson's disease
Adrenal insufficiency	Tabes dorsalis
Pregnancy	Syringomyelia
Drugs altering vascular reactivity or nervous system function	Cerebrovascular disease
	Peripheral neuropathy caused by diabetes
Antihypertensives	Idiopathic orthostatic hypotension
Adrenergic antagonists	Sympathectomy
Ca^{2+} channel blockers	
Antidepressants	
Alcohol and depressants	

---

tes mellitus in whom the glucagon response is also deficient, leaving them more susceptible to severe bouts of hypoglycemia. Adrenal medullary deficiency occurring as part of a more generalized autonomic insufficiency is associated with severe orthostatic hypotension; however, the role of the adrenal medulla is difficult to assess. Causes of orthostatic hypotension are shown in Box 299-1.

Autonomic insufficiency is associated with disorders of nervous system function (Box 299-1). In normal individuals, assuming the upright position allows pooling of blood in the lower extremities. The initial fall in blood pressure stimulates baroreceptor activity, which activates central reflex mechanisms causing arterial and venous constriction, increased cardiac output, and release of renin and vasopressin. In patients with autonomic insufficiency, however, the interruption of afferent, central, or efferent components of this reflex results in failure to compensate for the fall in blood pressure and blood supply to the brain. This result leads to lightheadedness, syncope, and/or convulsions.

The most effective treatment of these symptoms is volume expansion using fludrocortisone. However, simple measures such as raising the head of the bed at night and using support garments may be sufficient to control the symptoms in some patients. Chronic constriction of the vascular bed using sympathomimetic agents has also been used but is not as effective as volume expansion.

BOX 299-2

Common symptoms in patients with hypertension due to pheochromocytoma

Symptoms during or following a paroxysm
Headache
Sweating
Forceful heartbeat ± tachycardia
Anxiety or fear of impending death
Tremor
Fatigue or exhaustion
Nausea and vomiting
Abdominal or chest pain
Visual disturbance

Symptoms noted between paroxysms
Increased sweating
Cold hands and feet
Weight loss
Constipation

HYPERFUNCTION OF THE ADRENAL MEDULLA

Increased production of catecholamines occurs during severe stress. The physiologic role of the adrenal medulla differs from that of the remainder of the peripheral sympathetic nervous system. Whereas the sympathetic nerves provide fine regulation of cellular function, the medulla secretes large amounts of catecholamines when deviations from homeostasis are extreme. Abnormal increases in circulating catecholamines are most commonly seen in patients with tumors derived from chromaffin tissue (pheochromocytomas). However, levels may be elevated in patients undergoing severe mental or physical stress or illness.

PHEOCHROMOCYTOMAS

Pheochromocytomas are tumors arising from chromaffin cells in the sympathetic nervous system. They release epinephrine and norepinephrine into the circulation, causing hypertension and other signs and symptoms. It is estimated that 0.1% of patients with diastolic hypertension have pheochromocytomas. These tumors are found at all ages and in both sexes and are most commonly diagnosed in patients in the fourth and fifth decades of life.

Although uncommon, the disorder is important to diagnose. If they remain undetected in pregnant women, these tumors often can cause death during delivery. They also can be fatal in patients undergoing surgery for other disorders and in patients with hypertension and its complications. When such tumors are recognized early and properly managed, almost all the patients recover completely following removal of benign tumors (Chapter 32).

Clinical Manifestations

Although the majority of patients with functioning tumors have symptoms most of the time, they vary in intensity and are perceived to be episodic or paroxysmal in most patients. Most patients with persistent hypertension also have superimposed paroxysms. A small number of patients are entirely free of symptoms and hypertension between attacks and may give no evidence of excessive catecholamine release during these intervals.

In patients with paroxysmal release of catecholamines, the symptoms resemble those produced by the injection of epinephrine or norepinephrine, and the symptom complex is far more consistent than is suggested by the variability of patients' complaints (Box 299-2). An episode usually begins with a sensation of "something happening" deep inside the chest, and a stimulus to deeper breathing is noted. The patient then becomes aware of a pounding or forceful heartbeat caused by the β_1-receptor–mediated increase in cardiac output. This throbbing spreads to the rest of the trunk and head, causing a headache. The intense α-receptor–mediated peripheral vasoconstriction causes cool hands and feet and pallor in the face. The combination of increased cardiac output and vasoconstriction causes marked elevation of the blood pressure when large amounts of catecholamines are released. The decreased heat loss and increased metabolism may cause a rise in temperature. These factors also cause reflex sweating. This sweating may be profuse and usually follows the cardiovascular effects, which begin in the first few seconds of the attack. The increased glycolysis and α-receptor–mediated inhibition of insulin release cause an increase in blood sugar levels. Patients experience marked anxiety with all but the mildest attacks, and, when episodes are prolonged, severe nausea, vomiting, visual disturbances, chest or abdominal pain, and paresthesias or seizures can occur. A feeling of fatigue or exhaustion usually follows.

In patients with paroxysmal symptoms, attacks may occur at intervals of months or as frequently as 25 times daily and may last from minutes to days. Usually they occur several times weekly or more often and last for 15 minutes or less. As time passes, the attacks usually increase in frequency but do not change much in character. They often are precipitated by activities that compress the tumor—such as changes in position, exercise, lifting, defecation, or eating—and by emotional distress or anxiety.

Patients with persistently secreting tumors also may experience the symptom complex described earlier when transient increases in the release of catecholamines are provoked by the same stimuli. In addition, the increased metabolic rate usually causes weight loss or, in children, a lack of weight gain, as well as heat intolerance and increased sweating. The effects on glycogenolysis and insulin release can produce hyperglycemia and glucose intolerance.

Chronic constriction of the arterial and venous bed leads to a reduction in plasma volume in most of these patients. The inability to further constrict this bed on arising and the down regulation of receptors and desensitization cause the postural hypotension that is characteristically observed. Chronic exposure to increased levels of circulating catecholamines produces a diffuse myocarditis in some patients. Unfortunately, specific electrocardiographic changes may be absent or may be attributable to left ventricular hypertrophy, and heart failure under cardiovascular stress may be the first clinical manifestation. Retinal and renal vascular lesions commonly associated with hypertension may be found.

A few patients with tumors secreting large amounts of dopamine rather than epinephrine or norepinephrine have been described and found to be normotensive.

In addition to the catecholamines, pheochromocytomas produce a wide variety of active peptides. These include somatostatin, substance P, adrenocorticotropin, β-endorphin, lipotropin, vasoactive intestinal peptide, interleukin-6, parathyroid hormone-related protein, neuropeptide Y, calcitonin, calcitonin gene-related peptide, metenkephalin, serotonin, gastrin, neurotensin, pancreastatin, galanin, and IGF-II. Secretion of large amounts of these substances may result in atypical clinical presentations.

Familial Syndromes and Other Tumors

These tumors occur sporadically or as a heritable disorder, either alone or, more commonly, in association with other endocrine tumors. In multiple endocrine neoplasia (MEN) type II or type IIa, or Sipple's syndrome, the patient may also have a calcitonin-producing adenoma of the parathyroid. In MEN type IIb or III, pheochromocytomas occur in association with mucosal neuromas, which are numerous and small and are found around the mouth. The transmission of these disorders follows the pattern of an autosomal dominant gene with incomplete penetrance. Mutations in the RET protooncogene are responsible for inherited multiple endocrine neoplasia type II (MENII) syndromes. The RET protooncogene is normally expressed in the adrenal medulla and cerebellum. Levels of RET mRNA may be overexpressed in some sporadic pheochromocytomas. These tumors may be preceded or accompanied by hyperplastic changes in the adrenal medulla, thyroid, and parathyroid glands and are multicentric in origin. Pheochromocytomas in these patients are bilateral, and additional tumors may be found outside the adrenal glands, and bilateral adrenalectomy may be advisable. It is necessary to screen the families of these patients for evidence of tumors. In families with

suspected MENII, DNA analysis for RET protooncogene mutations provides unambiguous identification of individuals at risk. The diagnosis of medullary carcinoma of the thyroid and tumors of the parathyroid glands is discussed in Chapters 297 and 322, respectively.

Pathology

Pheochromocytomas occur wherever chromaffin tissue is found. The adrenal medulla contains the largest collection of chromaffin cells. In the fetus, the organ of Zuckerkandl is also very large, but it is gradually replaced by fibrous tissue after birth and is small in the adult. Chromaffin cells also are found in association with sympathetic ganglia, nerve plexuses, and nerves.

More than 95% of pheochromocytomas are found in the abdomen and 85% are in or near the adrenal. Common extraadrenal sites are near the kidney and in the organ of Zuckerkandl. Those in the chest are in the posterior mediastinum. The intracranial lesions reported are thought to be metastatic in origin. The tumors may be multicentric in origin, particularly when familial. Although fewer than 10% of adults have multiple tumors, they are found in about one third of children with pheochromocytomas.

Pheochromocytomas vary in weight from under 1 g to several kilograms; however, they are usually small, most weighing well under 100 g. They are vascular tumors and commonly contain cystic or hemorrhagic areas. The cells tend to be large and contain typical catecholamine storage granules like those in the adrenal medulla. Multinucleated cells, pleomorphic nuclei, mitoses, and extension into the capsule and vessels are sometimes seen but do not indicate that the tumor is malignant.

Adrenal medullary hyperplasia also has been described as the cause of an indistinguishable clinical picture and has been suggested to be a precursor of the tumors seen in the MEN syndrome, as well as occurring sporadically.

Diagnosis

Although the pattern of the manifestations described earlier can be elicited in almost all patients with functioning tumors who are capable of clear communication, the variability of presenting complaints may be confusing and is sometimes misleading. Women whose episodes are first noted around the time of the menopause may be thought to be experiencing "hot flashes." The diagnosis may be made only when hormonal therapy has failed to alleviate the symptoms or the episode is observed and the blood pressure taken during the attack. When a pheochromocytoma causes hypertension late in pregnancy, it may be confused with preeclampsia. Other causes of increased sympathetic activity that must be distinguished from pheochromocytomas are listed in Box 299-3.

On physical examination, hypertension is usually present. Wide fluctuations of blood pressure are characteristic, and marked increases may be followed by hypotension and syncope. When pressure is elevated, postural hypotension is present. Typically, the hypertension does not respond to commonly used antihypertensive regimens, and

---

BOX 299-3

Differential diagnosis of hypertension secondary to other causes

Severe anxiety attacks
Paroxysmal tachycardias
Coronary insufficiency
Hypertensive crises associated with paraplegia
Acute porphyria
Autonomic epilepsy
Monoamine oxidase inhibitors
Tyramine in patients on monoamine oxidase inhibitors
Menopausal "hot flashes"
Hyperdynamic β-adrenergic states

such drugs as guanethidine and ganglionic blockers can induce paradoxical pressor responses. These patients, usually thin, have a forceful heartbeat, which is often visible and easily palpable. They feel warm, may have pallor of the face and chest, perspire, have cool and moist hands and feet, and prefer a cool room. Patients with long-standing and persistent symptoms and hypertension may have retinopathy. Rarely, a mass may be palpable in the abdomen or neck, and deep palpation of the abdomen may produce a typical paroxysm.

The diagnosis of pheochromocytoma should be considered in all patients with paroxysmal symptoms; in children with hypertension; in adults with severe hypertension that does not respond to therapy; in hypertensive patients with diabetes and/or hypermetabolism; in patients with hypertension in whom symptoms resemble those described earlier or can be evoked by exercise, position change, emotional distress, or antihypertensive drugs such as guanethidine and ganglionic blockers; and in patients who become severely hypertensive or go into shock during anesthesia, surgery, or delivery. Patients who have disorders sometimes associated with pheochromocytomas (neurofibromatosis, mucosal adenomas, von Hippel's disease, or medullary carcinoma of the thyroid) or first-order relatives with a pheochromocytoma should be investigated.

Ganglioneuromas (which are usually small, well-differentiated tumors arising from ganglion cells) and neuroblastomas (highly malignant tumors arising from more primitive sympathoblastic cells) can produce catecholamines and present a similar clinical picture. Dopamine is usually the major active catecholamine produced and leads to elevation of plasma, dopamine, and homovanillic acid levels in the urine.

Diagnostic Tests and Procedures. The assay of catecholamines and their metabolites has markedly simplified the diagnosis of this disorder. Surgical exploration of a patient for this disorder should not be undertaken without chemical confirmation of the diagnosis.

In patients with continuous hypertension or symptoms, levels of plasma or urine catecholamines and their metabolites usually are clearly increased. A reliable assay of the catecholamines, metanephrines, or vanillylmandelic acid (VMA) is usually sufficient to confirm the diagnosis. Patients with large tumors may excrete disproportionately greater amounts of catecholamine metabolites because the amines can be metabolized by enzymes in the tumor cells before their release. Malignant tumors may release large amounts of dopamine, increasing plasma dopamine and leading to the excretion of large amounts of homovanillic acid in the urine. It is important to eliminate drugs and dietary substances that interfere with these assays or to choose an appropriate assay procedure so that results are not misleading.

In patients having brief and infrequent paroxysms with symptom-free intervals, confirmation of the diagnosis may be more difficult. Although large amounts of catecholamines are produced during the brief episode, the total amount excreted during a 24-hour urine-collection period may not be clearly abnormal; this is in contrast to values in patients whose tumors secrete continuously. The latter group will accumulate larger amounts of catecholamines and metabolites even though secretion rates are lower and symptoms are less severe. Therefore sampling of blood or timed urine collections during a carefully observed episode may be necessary to confirm the diagnosis.

In patients with typical symptoms, provocative tests with glucagon or histamine are rarely needed; however, the possibility of a pheochromocytoma may be strong enough, or its presence dangerous enough (e.g., in pregnancy or before surgery), to require the use of these testing procedures to rule out the presence of such a tumor.

Assays for catecholamines and their metabolites are used to screen patients at high risk. Indications for screening patients are listed in Box 299-4. When blood cannot be obtained from patients at rest, the administration of 0.3 mg of clonidine given 2 to 3 hours before sampling reduces the neurogenic contribution to norepinephrine levels.

In the occasional patient in whom the chemical tests are inconclusive, it may be useful or more convenient to institute therapy with phenoxybenzamine over 1 to 2 months to observe effects both on the nature and frequency of attacks and on the blood pressure. A salutary effect will sometimes be observed for a few weeks but seldom lasts longer in the absence of a pheochromocytoma. A good response indicates the need for reappraisal of the patient.

BOX 299-4
Patients to be screened for pheochromocytoma

Hypertensive patients with symptoms in Box 299-2
Young hypertensives, particularly with:
    Weight loss
    Seizures
    Orthostatic hypotension
    Unexplained shock
Family history of pheochromocytoma or medullary carcinoma of
    thyroid
Hypertension associated with:
    Neurofibromatosis and other neurocutaneous syndromes
    Mucosal neuromas
    Hyperglycemia
    Severe uncontrollable hypertension
Shock or severe pressor responses to:
    Induction of anesthesia
    Delivery
    Antihypertensive drugs
    Incidentally discovered adrenal tumors

Localization of Tumors. When the diagnosis has been established, the tumor must be located. Computed tomography (CT) and magnetic resonance imaging (MRI) are of great value in localizing these tumors (Fig. 299-3). MRI is somewhat more successful in locating extraadrenal tumors and has the advantage of producing brighter images with T_2-weighting in contrast to most other adrenal tumors. Sonography also has proved to be safe and useful. Central venous sampling of blood for catecholamine assay via percutaneous venous catheter has been of great value in cases in which radiographic procedures fail, in which multiple tumors or metastases are suspected, or in which previous exploration has not disclosed all the tumor tissue.

Although not as widely available, scintigrams following the injection of ^{131}I-labeled metaiodobenzylguanidine (MIBG) are quite specific for identifying masses producing catecholamines, including neuroblastomas and pheochromocytomas. Administration of MIBG in these patients results in detectable images in 48 to 72 hours. It is particularly useful in identifying extraadrenal tumors and metastases. It has also been used in the treatment of malignant tumors not amenable to surgical removal (see later discussion).

Incidentally Discovered Tumors (Incidentalomas). As noted earlier, the use of CT and MRI to localize these tumors is indicated only after the diagnosis has been confirmed. Because these procedures are frequently used diagnostic tools, tumors in the region of the adrenal gland are found in about 2% of patients having CT or MRI scans. These patients should be screened for pheochromocytomas clinically and chemically as part of their workup.

Management

Optimal management of patients with pheochromocytomas requires an understanding of the pathophysiology produced by excessive catecholamines and an acquaintance with the action of adrenergic antagonists and other drugs used in the treatment of these patients (Chapter 32).

As soon as the diagnosis has been confirmed, therapy with adrenergic antagonists should be instituted. Appropriate treatment is directed toward reducing the patient's symptoms, lowering of blood pressure, and amelioration of the paroxysms that either occur spontaneously or are induced by studies undertaken to localize the tumor or tumors. Such treatment will allow expansion of the vascular bed and plasma volume and will reduce the amount of transfused blood required for the maintenance of blood pressure after surgical removal of the tumor.

Although only a few days of this therapy are required for the preoperative study and preparation of these patients for surgery, prolonged medical therapy is advantageous in patients who have had

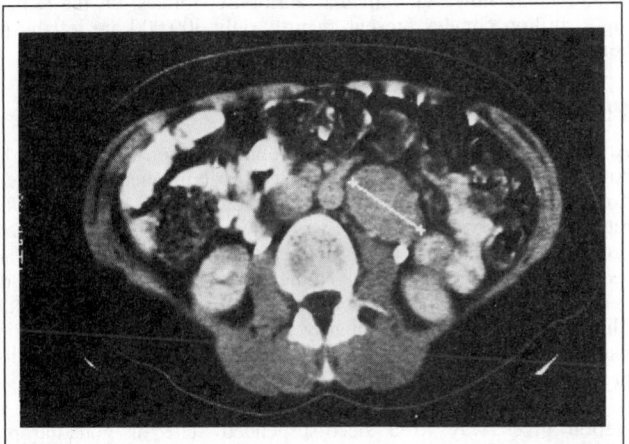

A

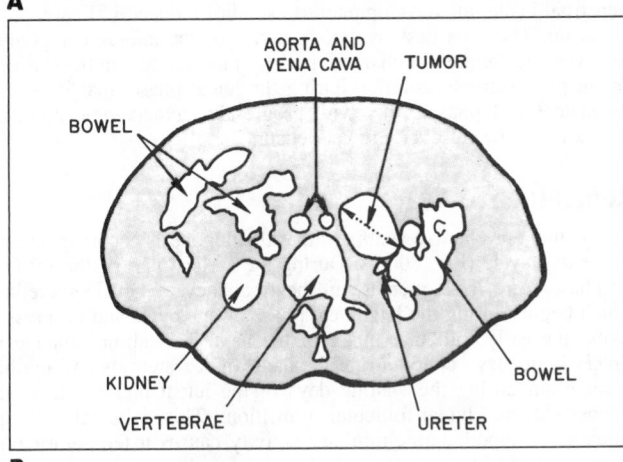

B

FIGURE 299-3 **A,** An extraadrenal pheochromocytoma localized to the left infrarenal area of the sympathetic chain by computed axial tomography. **B,** Identification of the important features of the scan.

From Goldfien A: Diseases of the adrenal medulla. In Greenspan FA, Baxter JD, editors: *Basic and clinical endocrinology,* Los Altos, Calif, 1982, Lange.

recent myocardial infarctions, who have clinical evidence of catecholamine cardiomyopathy, or who are in their last trimester of pregnancy. They can be maintained on medical therapy until surgical removal of the tumor is undertaken.

Agents that commonly have been used in therapy include phentolamine and phenoxybenzamine. In patients with persistent paroxysms, phenoxybenzamine—a noncompetitive α-adrenergic antagonist with a prolonged effect—is indicated. Treatment is begun with dosages of 20 to 40 mg/day and can be increased by 10 to 20 mg every 1 to 2 days until the desired effect is achieved. Completely normal blood pressure (lower than 140/90) may not be achieved and is not required. A dosage of 60 to 80 mg daily is usually adequate, but two to three times as much may be necessary. When marked tachycardia or arrhythmias occur, small doses of propranolol may be required but should only be given after α-receptor blockade is established.

Patients with infrequent paroxysms and an absence of interval manifestations can be treated similarly. Rapid titration of the dose may be difficult using phenoxybenzamine, however, because of its long half-life (36 hours). Prazosin, an α-antagonist, has also been found to be effective in these patients.

Preparation of the patient in this manner minimizes the hazards of anesthesia and surgery. The patient's blood pressure and cardiogram should be monitored continuously, and phentolamine and/or nitroprusside, propranolol, and other antiarrhythmic agents should be available. When multiple intraabdominal tumors are suspected, they should be approached through a transabdominal incision to allow exploration of the adrenals, sympathetic ganglia, bladder, and other pelvic structures. These tumors have been successfully removed by laparoscopic surgery. This approach can significantly reduce postopera-

tive morbidity. When bilateral adrenal tumors are found and the adrenals removed, adrenocortical steroid replacement is required (Chapter 298).

When the tumor is removed, the blood pressure usually falls to levels of about 90/60 mm Hg. A lower pressure or poor peripheral perfusion may indicate the need for blood volume expansion with whole blood, plasma, or other fluids. Pressor therapy is not usually required and should not be substituted for volume expansion.

The lack of a fall in pressure at the time of tumor removal (even in the presence of adrenergic blockade) suggests the presence of additional tumor tissue.

In patients with tumors producing persistent hypertension, the initial fall in blood pressure may be followed by an elevation of blood pressure postoperatively. The accompanying symptoms of sympathetic stimulation disappear, however, and the blood pressure and catecholamine levels return to normal over the next few weeks. If the blood pressure remains elevated, but the patient is otherwise asymptomatic, another cause for the elevated blood pressure should be considered. The presence of a renal vascular lesion or other coexistent causes of hypertension have been reported in several patients with pheochromocytomas. These tumors may be silent, secreting only small amounts of hormone. When these tumors are resected, the patient may show little change, and hypertension, if present, may persist.

Patients with nonresectable malignant tumors, metastases, or those who for other reasons are not amenable to successful surgical treatment can be managed medically for prolonged periods. Phenoxybenzamine can be used chronically as described. Patients with malignant tumors have also benefited symptomatically from treatment with α-methyl metatyrosine, an inhibitor of tyrosine hydroxylase, the rate-limiting enzyme in the biosynthetic process.

The incidence of malignant tumors in reported studies varies from less than 5% to more than 10%. These tumors can be recognized during surgery when there is significant local infiltration or metastases are identified. About 5% to 10% of patients thought to have been cured later experience recurrence of the tumor. Patients with extraadrenal tumors and those whose tumors cells contain increased amounts of nuclear DNA are at higher risk of recurrence and should be screened at regular intervals after surgery. Although some patients with malignant pheochromocytomas die early because of disseminated disease, there are long-term survivors. The most common site of metastases is the skeleton, and these lesions may respond well to radiation therapy. The use of combination chemotherapy, alone or in combination with radiation, for soft tissue lesions has been successful in reducing the size and activity of metastases in some patients. The therapeutic use of ^{131}I-metaiodobenzylguanidine is being explored. Preliminary reports indicate that half of the patients treated experience partial remissions.

BIBLIOGRAPHY

Averbuch SD et al: Malignant pheochromocytoma: effective treatment with a combination of cyclophosphamide, vincristine, and dacarbazine, *Ann Intern Med* 109:267, 1988.
Clutter WE et al: Epinephrine plasma metabolic clearance rates and physiologic thresholds for metabolic and hemodynamic actions in man, *Clin Invest* 66:94, 1980.
Cryer PE: Physiology and pathophysiology of the human sympathoadrenal neuroendocrine system, *N Engl J Med* 303:436, 1980.
Freier DT, Thompson NW: Pheochromocytoma and pregnancy: the epitome of high risk, *Surgery* 114:1148, 1993.
Goldfien A: The adrenal medulla. In Greenspan FA and Baxter JD, editors: *Basic and clinical endocrinology,* Norwalk, Conn, 1995, Appleton & Lange.
Hollister AS: Orthostatic hypotension: causes, evaluation, and management, *West J Med* 157:662, 1992.
Krempf M et al: Use of m-[131I]Iodobenzylguanidine in the treatment of malignant pheochromocytoma, *J Clin Endocrinol Metab* 72:455, 1991.
Ledger GA et al: Genetic testing in the diagnosis and management of multiple endocrine neoplasia type II, *Ann Intern Med* 122:218, 1995.
Manger WM and Gifford RW: *Pheochromocytoma,* New York, 1977, Springer.
Osella G et al: Endocrine evaluation of incidentally discovered adrenal masses (incidentalomas), *J Clin Endocrinol Metab* 79:1532, 1994.
Ross NS, Aron DC: Hormonal evaluation of the patient with an incidentally discovered adrenal mass, *N Engl J Med* 323:1401, 1990.
Satoh F et al: Adrenomedullin in human brain, adrenal glands and tumor tissues of pheochromocytoma, ganglioneuroblastoma, and neuroblastoma, *J Clin Endocrinol Metab* 80:1750, 1995.
Shimosawa T et al: Proadrenomedullin NH_2-terminal 20 peptide, a new product of the adrenomedullin gene, inhibits norepinephrine overflow from nerve endings, *J Clin Invest* 96:1672, 1995.

300 Disorders of the Ovary

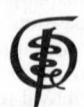

William F. Crowley, Jr.

BASIC PHYSIOLOGY

The human ovary is divided functionally and morphologically into two separate compartments. The first, composed of the granulosa and thecal cells, is responsible for steroidogenesis. In concert, the cells of this compartment secrete the sex steroids that initiate the appearance of secondary sexual characteristics at puberty, sustain cyclic estrogen and progesterone secretion throughout the reproductive years, and maintain low-level estrogen and androgen secretion after the menopause. These steroidogenic cells also secrete numerous peptides and growth factors into the follicular milieu to sustain the maturing oocyte.

The second ovarian compartment, which is responsible for gametogenesis, consists of the germinal epithelium, or the oocyte population. There is an intimate dialogue between these two ovarian compartments that orchestrates the coordinate steroid secretion, development, and maturation of the follicle each month. The steroidogenic constituents of the ovary support the final stages of development of these oocytes and ensure their timely preparation for ovulation and possible fertilization (Fig. 300-1).

Ovarian function can be viewed developmentally in four distinct periods: the neonatal period, puberty, the reproductive years, and the menopause.

Neonatal Period

Throughout early development the ovary undergoes a continual attrition of its germ cell population, initially in the absence of follicle-stimulating hormone (FSH) but by the middle of gestation in its presence. The peak population of 7 million oocytes is attained by the fifth month of embryonic development, whereas only 2 million remain at birth. Thus fetal development is associated with a progressive, relentless loss of germ cells. The steroidogenic compartment is also generally inactive until the final trimester of pregnancy.

By the time of delivery, pulsatile gonadotropin secretion occurs with a predominance of FSH over luteinizing hormone (LH) secretion. This gonadotropin secretion initiates steroidogenesis and early folliculogenesis, both of which are maintained during the neonatal period. After this brief developmental window of hypothalamic-pituitary-ovarian activity the ovary undergoes a quiescence that is accompanied by a decrease in steroidogenesis during the ovarian latency

of childhood; however, follicular attrition continues. Of the remaining 2 million oocytes present at birth, only 300,000 are left by puberty.

Puberty

At puberty, sleep-entrained gonadotropin secretion (Fig. 300-2) becomes manifest, initially with a marked predominance of FSH secretion in the female. The gonadotropins secreted with a high FSH/LH ratio reinitiate ovarian function with subsequent steroidogenic secretion from the granulosa cells, the secretion of inhibins A and B, and secondary sexual maturation. Numerous ovarian follicles also develop, but the vast majority of these early follicles do not ovulate. This early anovulation is primarily related to the failure of estradiol-induced positive feedback and consequent lack of an orderly LH surge in response to estradiol.

By late puberty, the sleep-entrained pattern of gonadotropin secretion gives way to a sleep-suspended state of gonadotropin-releasing hormone (GnRH) release in the early follicular phase of the menstrual cycle, the development of estradiol-induced LH surge, and ovulation. These earliest ovulatory cycles of the adolescent period, however, are frequently characterized by inadequate length or insufficient progesterone secretion during the luteal phase, that is, an inadequate luteal phase. Only with progressive gynecologic maturity does a fully normal ovarian cycle occur.

Reproductive Years

During the reproductive years cyclic folliculogenesis occurs in a regular 28-day cycle (Fig. 300-3). During the earliest part of the follicular phase there is an increase in the frequency of GnRH secretion, which begins during the late luteal phase of one cycle and progresses across the early follicular phase of the next. This abrupt change in GnRH frequency occurs during the nadir of sex steroids and inhibin A secretion during the waning days of the luteal phase, which are reached at the luteal-follicular transition. This relatively abrupt increase in hypothalamic-pituitary activity causes a temporary predominance of FSH secretion, which subsequently recruits a new wave of folliculogenesis in the ovaries. By days 5 to 7 into a given menstrual cycle, the dominant follicle's destiny is manifest. Enhanced estradiol secretion from this follicle can be documented by ovarian vein sampling as early as day 7. Soon thereafter, the dominant follicle becomes visible on ultrasonograph, eventually reaching a diameter of approximately 1.5 to 2.5 cm by midcycle.

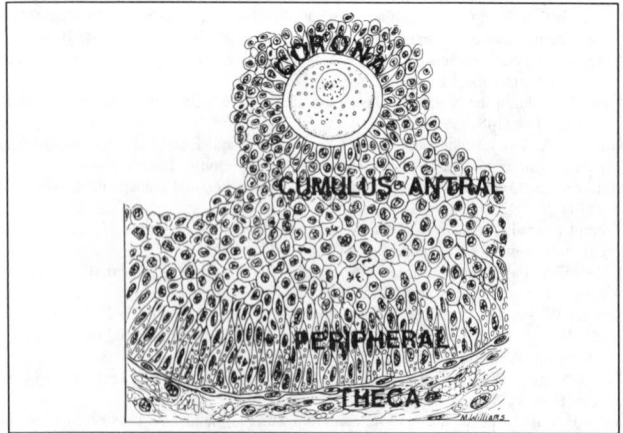

FIGURE 300-1   A section through a graafian follicle. Granulosa cells surround the oocyte and secrete estradiol.

Courtesy Dr L. Zoller, Department of Anatomy, Boston University School of Medicine.

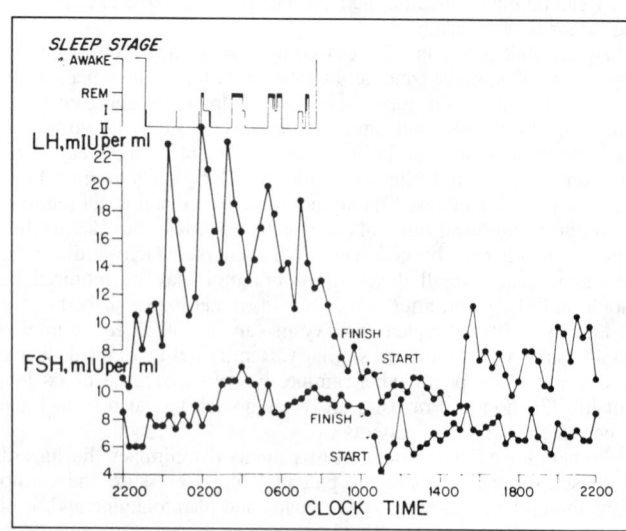

FIGURE 300-2   Serial blood luteinizing hormone (LH) and follicle-stimulating hormone (FSH) concentrations obtained every 20 minutes during sleep and wakefulness in a 13-year-old pubertal girl.

From Boyar RM et al: *N Engl J Med* 289:282-286, 1973.

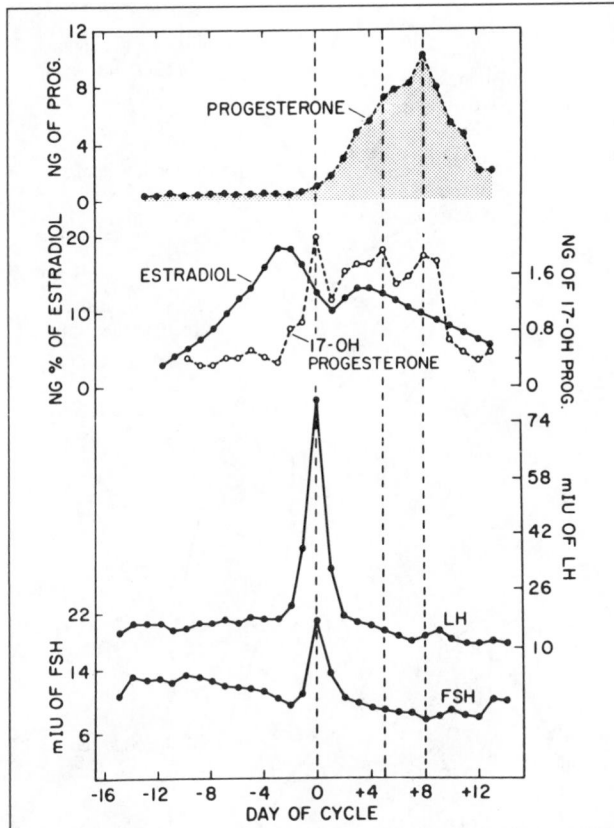

FIGURE 300-3   Mean plasma LH, FSH, and steroid concentrations in apparently normally cycling young women. Levels are synchronized about the midcycle or periovulatory surge of LH.

From Vaitukaitis JL, Ross GT: *Pharmacol Ther* 1:317-329, 1976.

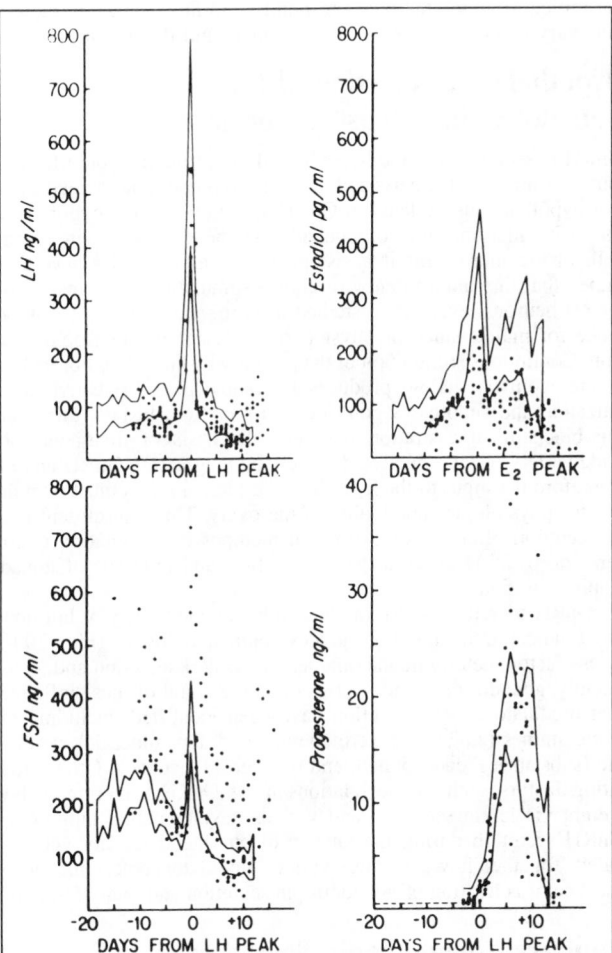

FIGURE 300-4   Circulating levels of LH, FSH, estradiol, and progesterone among perimenopausal women. The 95% competence limits for gonadotropin and sex steroid levels among women during their earlier years of reproduction are encompassed by the connected line.

From Sherman BM, West JH, Korenman SG: *J Clin Endocrinol Metab* 42:629-636, 1976.

During the subsequent follicular phase of the menstrual cycle the development of the dominant follicle is associated with a coordinated atresia of the remaining cohort of recruited follicles, which is associated with gradually declining FSH levels. Eventually the rising tide of estradiol secreted from the emerging dominant follicle evokes an LH surge from the pituitary. This LH secretion causes rupture of the follicle, permitting release of the mature oocyte. Thereafter, the corpus luteum secretes progesterone, estradiol, and inhibin A, which act in concert to slow GnRH secretion and suppress pituitary FSH secretion across the luteal phase until the next luteal-follicular transition. This combination of biochemical events results in a nadir of circulating gonadotropin levels by the midluteal phase, a marked slowing of the GnRH pulse generator, and eventually, luteolysis. After dissolution of the corpus luteum, the frequency of GnRH secretion increases abruptly once again, with levels of FSH rising more rapidly than those of LH, and the next wave of folliculogenesis ensues. Should fertilization have occurred in the cycle, the corpus luteum of pregnancy is sustained by human chorionic gonadotropin (hCG) and other, as yet undescribed, factors that support the corpus luteum of pregnancy until the time of placentation.

Menopause

Commencing in the fifth decade of life, the ovarian complement of oocytes begins to approach exhaustion. As this relentless loss of germ cells occurs, there is an initial decline in inhibin A levels and a consequent isolated rise of FSH followed by increased LH levels (Fig. 300-4). After the complete disappearance of oocytes a marked atrophy of the ovaries ensues, with a consequent rise of both gonadotropins to castrate levels. However, a persistent secretion of androstenedione remains, as well as low levels of estrogen from the menopausal ovary. Although insufficient to sustain menstrual cyclicity and prohibit symptoms of estrogen deficiency, these hormone levels are

significant, since symptoms occur if the postmenopausal ovary is removed. At menopause, symptoms of estrogen deficiency such as hot flashes, vaginal dryness, atrophy of the secondary sexual characteristics, and decreased bone density may appear after the decrease in steroidogenesis is complete.

Summary

The ovary undergoes a programmed series of specific developmental and physiologic changes over the life span of the female that reflect a delicate balance of steroidogenesis and gametogenesis. Sex steroid secretion from the ovary initiates sexual maturation, maintains the sex steroid–dependent target organs in a state of readiness for implantation, and eventually decreases at the menopause. Gametogenesis occurs in the milieu of this carefully coordinated sex steroid environment, permits fertility, and ensures the reproductive capability of the individual as well as the propagation of the species.

MODULATION OF GONADOTROPIN SECRETION

Ovarian function is principally determined by the timing, relative ratios, and pattern of gonadotropin secretion from the anterior pituitary gland. These in turn are modulated by both hypothalamic GnRH secretion and ovarian sex steroid and peptide secretion. The relative influences of these predominantly positive (hypothalamic input) and negative (ovarian feedback) inputs to the gonadotroph then determine the milieu to which the ovary responds, and the changes in these inputs vary dynamically across development and the menstrual cycle.

Hypothalamic Secretion of the Gonadotropin-Releasing Hormone

GnRH is secreted into the hypophyseal-portal blood supply from the nerve terminals of the parvocellular neurons predominantly in the anterior hypothalamus. Release of GnRH secretion into the hypophyseal-portal circulation, and consequently on the gonadotropin-secreting cells of the anterior pituitary, is episodic. Classic studies have determined that this intermittency of GnRH stimulation is intrinsic to the GnRH neurons, even when studied in vitro, and is of critical importance for maintenance of physiologic levels of gonadotropin secretion. Continuous stimulation of the pituitary by GnRH and/or its long-acting agonistic analogs produces a paradoxical and selective desensitization and suppresses gonadotropin secretion. In fact, this resulting biochemical castration has been the basis of treatment for a wide variety of reproductive disorders by long-acting GnRH analogs. Therefore the input to the hypothalamic-pituitary axis must be pulsatile for physiologic functioning of the ovary. This intermittent mode of secretion offers several different methods of modulating ovarian function by differences in patterns, ratios, and intervals of gonadotropin secretion.

GnRH secretion is also modulated by a wide variety of hormonal, environmental, metabolic, and developmental inputs (Fig. 300-5). These factors determine the ontogeny of GnRH secretion and, consequently, gonadotropin and ovarian output. Several of these influences that modulate GnRH secretion have been identified, including biogenic amines (adrenergic, serotonergic, and dopaminergic), peptidergic (substance P endorphins), and sex steroid feedback. Other modulating factors such as the relationship of GnRH secretion to body weight via leptin secretion and various developmental inhibitors of GnRH secretion during the latency of childhood are not yet elucidated. Together, however, these various modulators determine the quiescence or activation of gonadotropin secretion and ovarian function.

Pituitary Gonadotropin Secretion

The pituitary gonadotropins LH and FSH are glycoproteins comprising common alpha subunit and a unique beta subunit (Chapter 295). The frequency of secretion of these gonadotropins depends solely on the frequency of antecedent GnRH secretion from the hypothalamus. The amplitude of their secretion, however, is determined by the quantity of GnRH secreted within a given episode of hypothalamic secretion, as well as by negative feedback of sex steroids and other ovarian products. Thus by a combination of varying the amount and frequency of GnRH secretion from the hypothalamus, as well as the sex steroid and peptide secretion from the ovarian follicle, the anterior pituitary gonadotroph is essential in determining both the paracrine hormonal milieu within the ovary and the intensity of gonadotropin secretion to the ovary. The combined feedback mechanisms of estradiol, progesterone, and the inhibins modulate the level of FSH secretion, such that only a single, dominant follicle develops each month.

Ovarian Feedback Mechanisms

The major sex steroids that exert feedback effects on gonadotroph are estradiol and progesterone. Estradiol, secreted by the granulosa cells of the growing follicle, initially exerts a negative feedback effect on LH and FSH secretion by two different mechanisms. The initial feedback effects of estradiol on the pituitary gonadotroph are to decrease LH and FSH secretion and increase GnRH pulse frequency across the follicular phase of the cycle. However, the negative feedback exerted by estradiol on FSH secretion is the predominant effect. This, in turn, limits the quantity and possibly the bioactivity of the FSH available to the growing follicle in such a manner that only a single follicle is cultivated. The hormonal support for other, nondominant follicles of the cohort is insufficient, and they become atretic. The dominant follicle has aquired an increased number of FSH receptors and therefore is relatively protected from the effects of a serial decline in circulating FSH. The dominant follicle is thus capable of surviving the progressively lower amounts of FSH occurring across

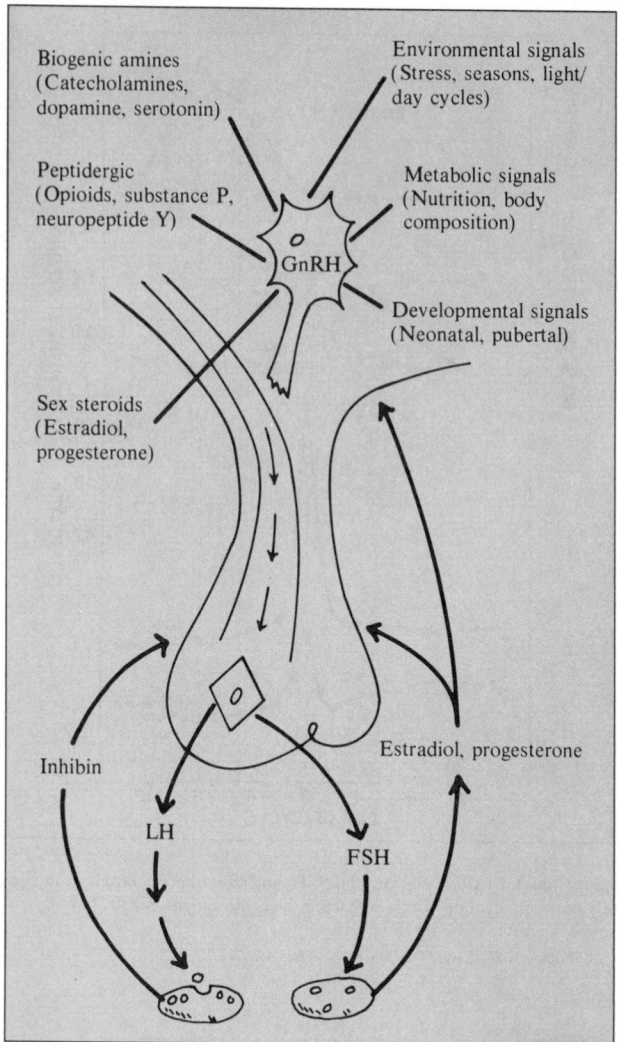

FIGURE 300-5 Overview of the hypothalamic-pituitary-ovarian axis. Gonadotropin-releasing hormone (GnRH) is secreted episodically from the hypothalamus and causes pulsatile release of LH and FSH.

the middle-to-late follicular phase of the cycle from the negative feedback effects of increasing estradiol levels. Atretic follicles do not have this capability and therefore involute during this period.

In addition to estradiol's early negative feedback on gonadotropin secretion, it has a later, positive feedback effect on the quantity of GnRH secreted at the midcycle but not its frequency. This feedback, combined with the positive effects of estradiol on the pituitary, culminates in the midcycle LH and FSH surge. These ovarian feedback effects, taken in combination with the serial changes in inhibin A, which increases across the follicular phase, dictate the declining FSH levels across the follicular phase with progressive increases in LH levels and culminate in the midcycle surge of both gonadotropins, which ruptures the dominant follicle and releases the egg.

At the uterine level, estradiol secretion across the follicular phase induces growth in the glandular elements, an increase in the width of the endometrium, and initiation of a number of secretory events designed to result in successful implantation of the subsequently fertilized ovum.

Commencing at the time of ovulation, progesterone becomes the dominant ovarian sex steroid. Progesterone has a marked, negative feedback effect on the frequency of GnRH secretion from the hypothalamus, resulting in progressive and near-total cessation of GnRH secretion over the ensuing 14 days of the luteal phase. Progesterone also halts the progressive proliferation of the endometrium that occurred during the estrogen-dominant follicular phase of the cycle and causes differentiation of the glandular epithelium into a secretory pattern with the appearance of glycogen at the base of the endometrial cells. With declining levels of progesterone across the last half of the luteal phase, there is a gradual withdrawal of steroid support, resulting in a series of microinfarctions of the glandular element and culminating in sloughing of the endometrium at the time of the menstrual period.

The granulosa cells of the ovarian follicle also produce inhibin A and B, dimeric proteins composed of an alpha subunit covalently linked with a beta subunit to form a biologically active dimer, which exert a potent and relatively selective inhibition of FSH secretion, both basally and in response to GnRH, at the level of the anterior pituitary gland. The two inhibins appear to have a reciprocal relationship in their secretion pattern from the granulosa cells of the ovary, whereas inhibin B secretion rises dramatically from the luteal-follicular transition through the early and midfollicular phase, when inhibin A levels are quite low. During the late follicular phase, however, inhibin B levels decline, whereas A levels rise just before the midcycle surge, when FSH levels are the lowest during the follicular phase. Inhibin A continues to be secreted across the luteal phase in a pattern reminiscent of that of progesterone, whereas inhibin B remains low until the luteal-follicular transition. The selective inhibition of FSH secretion is particularly evident in the midluteal phase of the cycle, during which inhibin A combines with the midluteal peaks of estradiol and progesterone to achieve a maximal suppression of FSH secretion. Inhibin levels subsequently decline by the late luteal phase, thus permitting a rise in FSH to occur, which reinitiates the next wave of folliculogenesis. Ovarian cells also appear capable of making a beta/beta homodimer termed *activin,* which has opposing actions to those of inhibin; however, it appears that most of circulating activin is bound to follistatin, its binding protein, which completely neutralizes its effect. Thus, whereas inhibin suppresses basal FSH and GnRH-stimulated FSH secretion from the anterior pituitary, activin's role in the stimulation of FSH secretion as a circulating hormone remains dubious. However, the intrapituitary role of activin to stimulate and sustain FSH beta-subunit biosynthesis is clearly the most important one in maintaining releasable pools of FSH for GnRH to release.

In addition to the ability to secrete these modulatory peptides, developing granulosa cells of the follicle contain both estrogen and androgen receptors, which permit a local response to secreted sex steroids. Moreover, the mechanisms of action of these sex steroids are often in opposition, thus providing a local set of modulators of follicular growth. Estrogen increases the number of FSH receptors on the follicle and thus contributes importantly to the emerging dominance of one follicle. In contrast, androgens binding to their receptors inhibit this process in the soon-to-be-atretic follicle. Estrogens also increase the number of LH receptors on the granulosa cells and thus further prepare the dominant follicle for responding to the ensuing LH surge. Androgens oppose this mechanism of action.

Thus it is clear that there are several active autocrine and paracrine systems at work within the ovary. These ensure the achievement of dominance and ovulation of that dominant follicle at the time of the midcycle, while opposing forces induce atresia of the competing follicles.

LABORATORY TESTS AND DIAGNOSTIC PROCEDURES
Gonadotropin Levels (Chapter 295)

Because the secretion of gonadotropins is intermittent, randomly obtained LH levels are of somewhat limited value in assisting with the diagnosis of various conditions that are likely to affect the ovary. Since FSH has a longer serum half-life than LH (3 hours vs. 20 minutes), a random determination is of considerably more diagnostic value. Given these limitations, the diagnosis of certain ovarian dysfunctions can be greatly facilitated by random gonadotropin determinations. For example, premature ovarian failure is uniformly characterized by a striking elevation of the serum FSH levels into the menopausal ranges (Table 300-1). In this circumstance FSH levels are often the first gonadotropin levels to be elevated, in addition to being elevated to a greater degree than LH levels, thereby becoming a sine

qua non for this diagnosis. Similarly, patients with polycystic ovarian disease (Fig. 300-6) have a remarkable elevation of the LH/FSH ratio as a result of an increased frequency and amplitude of gonadotropin pulsations when compared with normal levels. Consequently, random samples of gonadotropins are often useful in assisting with this diagnosis because they demonstrate consistently high LH/FSH ratios.

It is crucial to interpret all gonadotropin determinations in view of the patient's menstrual history, including both the preceding and the subsequent menstrual period, because dramatic changes occurring across the menstrual cycle can often mimic the changes seen in various diseases. In addition, any gonadotropin determinations must be viewed in relation to their accompanying sex steroid levels. For example, if LH and FSH levels are elevated in a random sample, one needs to know whether the patient is cycling and therefore if these values were possibly obtained at midcycle, or whether the patient was amenorrheic with hot flashes and low estradiol levels, in which case a diagnosis of premature ovarian failure is more appropriate. Therefore a good menstrual cycle history and accompanying sex steroid levels are critical for the interpretation of random gonadotropin levels.

Most gonadotropin assays are increasingly specific for the dimeric form or beta subunit of each of the gonadotropins. Because no pure standard exists for gonadotropin determinations, however, the measured levels are by necessity referenced to an international reference preparation, most often the *Second International Reference Preparation of Human Menopausal Gonadotropin (hMG).* Perhaps more important than the individual reference standard that is used is the need for the clinician to be familiar with the laboratory and its normal ranges. To achieve this goal, the physician must communicate with the laboratory to determine the confidence in the normative ranges. Table 300-1 demonstrates normal gonadotropin and sex steroid levels performed on the basis of daily blood values across 80 ovulatory cycles; thus the levels are reasonably precise determinations of the normal range for this particular reference laboratory.

With the recent widespread availability of recombinant gonadotropins and monoclonal antibodies, it will soon become possible to make more precise and universally applicable determinations of gonadotropins based on molar equivalents. In addition, the specific epitopes recognized by these antibodies will be determined; thus the combination of improved measurements and pure standards will address many of the previous methodologic problems inherent in gonadotropin determinations.

Sex Steroid Levels

Estradiol and progesterone levels are usually measured by radioimmunoassay following organic solvent extraction of plasma to eliminate sex steroid binding to testosterone-estrogen binding globulin (TEBG) and cortisol-binding globulin (CBG), which bind estradiol and progesterone, respectively. Such binding globulins obscure direct plasma measurements and therefore often necessitate either a preassay extraction step or the addition to the assay buffer of several substances capable of dissociating the sex steroids from their binding proteins prior to assay. Normative values for each of these levels are listed in Table 300-1 and do not vary as much from laboratory to laboratory as do gonadotropins because pure standards and relatively specific antisera are now widely available.

Inhibin/Activin Levels

Only recently have widely validated assays for the dimeric forms of inhibin and activin become available. Such assays will become more widely available in the near future for use in diagnosing various infertility states.

Ultrasonographic Studies

With the advent of transvaginal ultrasonography it has now become simple to define the anatomic detail of the ovary in considerable detail by this noninvasive method, including total ovarian size, number and size of developing ovarian follicles, and the stroma/theca ratio. Thus it is relatively easy to distinguish a neonatal ovary from one that is inactive during the latency of childhood. The pubertal ovary

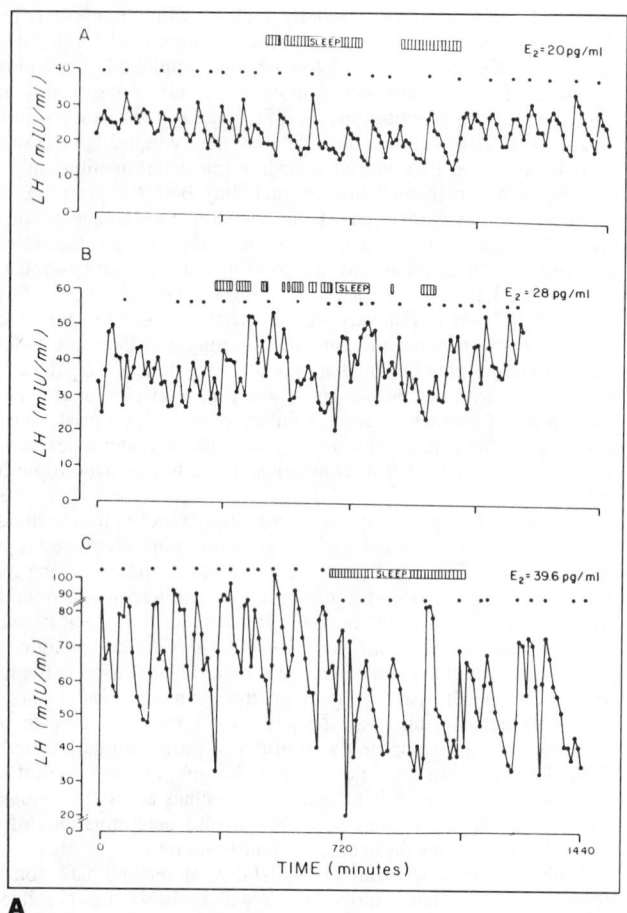

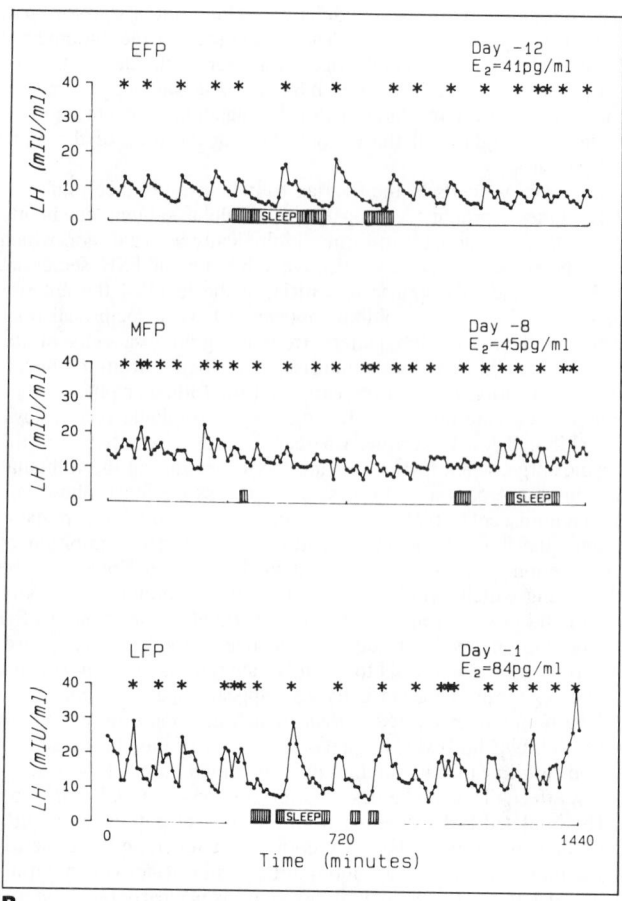

FIGURE 300-6.   A, Gonadotropic pulsations in three women with polycystic ovarian disease. Compare with **(B)** pulsations in three normal women from early follicular phase (EFP) *(upper right),* midfollicular phase (MFP) *(middle right),* and late follicular phase (LFP) *(lower right)* of a normal ovulatory cycle. The increase in both the frequency and amplitude of GnRH-induced gonadotropin pulsations in women with polycystic ovarian disease is apparent.

From Waldstreicher et al: *J Clin Endocrinol Metab* 66:165-172, 1988.

Table 300-1   Normative data: female reproductive hormones

| | | MENSTRUAL CYCLE* | | | |
	PREPUBERTY	EF	MIDCYCLE	LF	MENOPAUSE
Estradiol (pg/ml)	<10	23-56	115-500	68-180	<20
Progesterone (ng/ml)	<0.2	0.2-0.6	0.3-3.5	6.5-32	<0.2
LH (mIU/ml)	<0.8-5.0	5-26	43-187	2-35	30-150
FSH (mIU/ml)	1-10	5-28	13-41	5-15	30-170
Testosterone (ng/dl)	<50	—	<90	—	<70

*Based on 80 ovulatory cycles.
EF, Early follicular phase; *FSH,* follicle-stimulating hormone; *LF,* late follicular phase; *LH,* luteinizing hormone.

also has been identified to have a distinct morphologic appearance with numerous large cysts, very similar to that of some patients with polycystic ovarian disease. However, pubertal patients show a change in this morphologic appearance over time, whereas patients with polycystic ovarian disease show an increasing tendency to subcortical cysts, nonovulatory follicles, an increase of stromal/cortex ratio, and an increased ovarian size over time. Similar studies of postmenopausal women reveal the absence of follicular structure and small ovaries, although this is very difficult to distinguish from a relatively inactive ovary in an amenorrheic patient. Serum gonadotropin levels, however, can be helpful in distinguishing primary gonadal failure from that resulting from a hypogonadotropic state. Thus pelvic ultra-sonography can serve as an increasingly effective alternative for laparoscopic visualization of ovarian size and morphologic appearance in the future.

PATHOPHYSIOLOGIC DISORDERS

Ovarian disorders may be differentiated into two broad classes. The first includes disorders whose pathophysiology stems from inappropriate input to the ovary by the hypothalamic-pituitary axis. These include primary amenorrhea attributable to GnRH deficiency, "hypothalamic amenorrhea" attributable to an impaired secretion of GnRH, and polycystic ovarian disease. In the second group of ovarian disorders there is an intrinsic disorder within the ovary itself. Typical examples include Turner's syndrome, in which the gametogenic portion of the ovary is exhausted before menarche, and premature ovarian failure. In both disorders there are elevated gonadotropin levels as a result of an intrinsic ovarian abnormality.

Ovarian Disorders Associated With Abnormal Hypothalamic-Pituitary Input

Hypothalamic Amenorrhea. As described in detail in Chapter 291, the clinical presentation of patients with hypothalamic amenorrhea can occur before puberty (primary amenorrhea) or after menarche (secondary amenorrhea). The usual clinical associations with hypothalamic amenorrhea include stress, recent medical illness, exercise, severe weight loss (anorexia nervosa), bulimia, or other medical disorders that are usually accompanied by an alteration of body weight or other metabolic stress.

The central pathophysiologic abnormality of hypothalamic amenorrhea relates to disordered endogenous secretion of GnRH from the hypothalamus. These abnormal patterns of GnRH secretion (Fig. 300-1) occupy a spectrum of abnormalities of GnRH secretion, varying from the total absence of GnRH secretion to disorders of its frequency or amplitude. Correction of this condition can result from mere removal of the stress to the hypothalamic-pituitary-gonadal axis. For example, in the vast majority of cases, instituting nutritional rehabilitation, decreasing exercise, removal of stress, and so forth result in a restoration of menstrual cycles with ovulation. If menses do not resume spontaneously and fertility is the goal of the patient, a variety of agents can be used to induce ovulation, including clomiphene citrate, pulsatile GnRH, or exogenous gonadotropin administration. It should be recalled that hypothalamic amenorrhea is always a diagnosis of association and exclusion. Therefore anatomic defects of the hypothalamic-pituitary axis, prolactin-secreting tumors, and polycystic ovarian disease must be excluded on the basis of history, physical examination, appropriate anatomic studies, and measurement of serum prolactin and androgen levels.

Polycystic Ovarian Disease and Hyperthecosis. Polycystic ovarian disease (PCOD) can have myriad presentations, including oligoamenorrhea, hirsutism, amenorrhea, or, rarely, frank virilization. The most typical presentation is oligoamenorrhea in association with a slowly progressive hirsutism having its onset in the peripubertal period. These clinical features are often combined with variable elevations of androgen secretion, abnormally high LH/FSH ratios, and recurrent anovulation. More recently, sensitive ultrasonographic visualizations of the ovary have revealed enlarged ovaries, a very high stroma/follicle ratio, and a peripheral array of numerous small follicles underlying a thickened capsule. These changes are in sharp distinction to the typical changes in the ovary during the peripubertal period, in which a lesser degree of ovarian enlargement occurs. During puberty a consistent array of large follicles are interspersed throughout the ovary, and there is a lack of consistent demonstration of a thecal hyperplasia to the ovaries. Pathologic examination confirms what is seen on ultrasonograph, that is, a number of peripherally arrayed and luteinized follicles without evidence of recent ovulation and marked thecal and interstitial hyperplasia of the ovary itself.

Hyperthecosis is believed to be a variant of PCOD in which the number of follicles is even more dramatically reduced, with a corresponding increase in the hyperplastic theca associated with normal-sized ovaries. This dense thecal involvement is also accompanied by higher degrees of hyperandrogenemia.

Undoubtedly, the polycystic ovary can be produced by several pathophysiologic mechanisms. In this regard, it is much akin to an end-stage kidney. Most certainly, one of the pathophysiologic schemas involves an increase in the amplitude and frequency of endogenous GnRH secretion, resulting in an abnormally high LH/FSH ratio. This abnormal ratio in turn results in an overstimulation of the thecal components of the ovary by LH, insufficient stimulation of folliculogenesis by FSH, and a recurrent anovulatory state associated with thecal hyperplasia and hyperandrogenemia from the ovary. It is unclear whether this abnormality of hypothalamic-pituitary secretion is primary or merely a result of hyperandrogenemia elsewhere. However, pituitary

suppression by oral contraceptive agents or GnRH analogs results in a complete reversion of the biochemical abnormalities and the reduction in size of the ovaries during serial follow-up studies.

Yet another mechanism of production of PCOD disease syndrome seems to occur in its association with insulin resistance. The clinical marker of this pathophysiologic subset of PCOD patients is acanthosis nigricans, which serves as the dermatologic marker of severe insulin resistance. It appears that the theca of the ovary has receptors for somatomedin-C that are stimulated by the high circulating insulin levels, which, in conjunction with the high LH levels, results in an overresponsiveness of the ovary with androgen secretion. Undoubtedly, further pathophysiologic pathways to the production of PCOD will be uncovered.

Treatment of this condition depends on the patient's complaint. For patients merely requiring regular menstrual periods and/or relief of their hirsutism, suppression of the pituitary-ovarian axis with birth control pills or GnRH analogs results in an orderly shedding of the endometrium, reduction of endometrial hyperplasia, institution of regular menses, and a decrease of ovarian production of androgens with their attendant hirsutism. For patients desiring fertility, induction of ovulation with clomiphene citrate, pulsatile GnRH, or exogenous gonadotropin administration can be undertaken. Special care should be given to patients with PCOD, since they are particularly prone to ovarian hyperstimulation and multiple gestation by each of these methods of ovulation induction. For the rare subset of patients with PCOD in association with congenital hyperplasia or mild hyperprolactinemia, correction of the underlying defect results in restoration of normal menstrual cycles and fertility. In vitro fertilization is playing an increasing role in the fertility wishes of patients with PCOD.

Disorders of the Ovary With Intrinsic Ovarian Disease

Turner's Syndrome. Patients with Turner's syndrome demonstrate a complete deletion of their second X chromosome and thus most commonly have a karyotype of XO. Usually this is a lethal defect, and approximately 99% of Turner's syndrome karyotypes are associated with early fetal loss. Approximately 1% of patients with the Turner's syndrome karyotype survive; this number is even greater when one considers subtle mosaicism of the X chromosome with more variable clinical abnormalities that resemble Turner's syndrome. Typically, children with Turner's syndrome come to medical attention with various dysmorphic features such as hypertelorism, widely spaced nipples, increased carrying angles of the elbow, cardiac abnormalities, and, most commonly in early childhood, lymphedema. By midchildhood, their growth deficiency becomes evident, multiple cutaneous nevi appear, and many of the other skeletal features such as increased carrying angles of the elbows become more apparent. For individuals with mosaicism, all of these manifestations are attenuated.

The ovarian morphology in Turner's syndrome consists of an ovary that is generally similar to that of a postmenopausal ovary. Although the disease may be recognized at birth or during early childhood, most typically Turner's syndrome patients come to medical attention at menarche with primary amenorrhea in association with short stature at puberty. Some patients with retention of a portion of the second X chromosome and consequent mosaicism can retain sufficient numbers of ovarian follicles to have a normal puberty, secondary amenorrhea, and even conception if the presentation of the syndrome is sufficiently attenuated. The mechanism by which this accelerated atresia of ovarian follicles in childhood occurs in patients with the absence of an X chromosome is unknown. It is quite clear, however, that the presence of a second X chromosome is protective against this rapid depletion of the follicles in early childhood, which produces menopause before the age of menarche in the XO patients.

Therapy is generally supportive in childhood, although the combination of growth hormone plus nonaromatizable androgens now appears to offer promise for increasing midchildhood growth velocities and, perhaps, adult stature. During puberty, estrogen administration promotes secondary sexual characteristics at the appropriate time. Should fertility become a request, in vitro fertilization with donor eggs can be explored.

Gonadal Dysgenesis in Phenotypically and Karyotypically Normal Women. A small subset of women have hypergonadotropic amenorrhea with a normal karyotype evident at puberty. Whereas some of these women may have subtle deletions of the X chromosome not demonstrable by usual karyotypic methods, others may also have had in utero or neonatal viral infections such as mumps that may have destroyed the germinal cell epithelium before puberty. Generally these patients come to medical attention with primary amenorrhea and elevated gonadotropin levels quite similar to patients with Turner's syndrome, but lack the other dysmorphic features suggestive of deletion of the other X chromosome. In general, these patients grow normally during childhood but lack a pubertal growth spurt. Because they do not exhibit sex steroid secretion from the gonads at puberty, however, their epiphyses do not fuse until early in adult life; thus they may have eunucoidal body proportions, their span exceeding their height by several inches. The upper/lower segment ratio is also increased in these individuals, depending on the time of diagnosis.

Premature Ovarian Failure. Approximately 10% of patients presenting at a reproductive clinic with secondary amenorrhea demonstrate a hypergonadotropic condition, *premature ovarian failure,* if it occurs before age 35 years. This syndrome has many causes and typically becomes evident with a history of a waxing and waning course characterized by periods of hot flashes, elevated gonadotropin levels, and amenorrhea alternating with periods of breast tenderness, remission of hot flashes, and ovulation with spontaneous pregnancy. Such a course is quite similar to that occurring during the normal perimenopausal period immediately before the completion of the menopausal process in women ages 40 to 45 years.

Conditions associated with the menopausal process, suggesting an autoimmune basis in a subset of patients, include autoimmune thyroiditis and adrenal failure in conjunction with premature menopause (Schmidt's syndrome). In other women onset follows chemotherapy in early life for childhood malignancies, abdominal irradiation, or toxic exposures such as mumps or oophoritis. Other subsets have a familial pattern and have been determined to have subtle deletions of an otherwise normal X chromosome so that only premature ovarian failure is manifest. Other subjects with premature ovarian failure have been demonstrated to have "resistant" ovaries in which follicles are evident on histologic examination in their ovaries, despite hypergonadotropic hypogonadism. In this subset an antibody to the FSH receptor, suggesting an autoimmune origin, has been demonstrated in several cases.

The waxing and waning nature of this condition makes interpretation of any treatments particularly problematic. Thus pregnancies have been reported with low-dose estrogen, high-dose glucocorticoid, oral contraceptive, and GnRH analog suppression of this condition. Whether any of these are truly effective or are merely temporarily associated with a natural remission of the process remains unclear. From a practical viewpoint, in vitro fertilization with donor egg insemination is an alternative for patients seeking fertility.

Swyer's Syndrome. A rare form of XY gonadal dysgenesis, Swyer's syndrome, is an uncommon disorder in which patients are usually phenotypically normal females who come to medical attention with amenorrhea and bilateral streak ovaries. They may exhibit some sign of Turner's syndrome such as wide carrying angles of their elbows and short stature. However, they differ from Turner's syndrome patients in that they have some signs of androgen excess that typically only appear at the time of pubertal activation of gonadotropin secretion. This hyperandrogenicity correlates with the presence of a portion of the Y chromosome; such findings are often associated with gonadal tumors on pathologic review and are an indication for removal of the gonad in these cases as soon as the diagnosis is made.

Because the gonads of patients with Swyer's syndrome are quite dysgenetic and have a high incidence of neoplastic transformation beginning in the second decade of life, their gonads should be removed as soon as the diagnosis is made. These tumors are often malignant, and gonadoblastoma or dysgerminoma can become evident in adolescence. Therefore prompt attention to this aspect of their care is mandatory.

Ovarian Tumors. Most tumors of the ovary, including follicular cysts, corpus luteum and theca lutean cysts, and endometrial cysts, are benign. Functional ovarian tumors account for only 1% to 3% of all ovarian tumors. The granulosa cell tumors are usually small and unilateral and secrete estrogens. They may become evident in childhood as isosexual precocity or in older women as postmenopausal bleeding. During the reproductive years, the most common endocrine presentation is prolonged, irregular bleeding. However, it is the ovarian enlargement that is most generally evident in the reproductive years.

Androgen-secreting tumors of the ovaries include Sertoli-Leydig cell tumors, which are often small but can reach 8 to 10 cm in diameter. These rare tumors secrete androgen, which usually calls attention to them with varying degrees of hirsutism and virilization from their elevated serum testosterone levels, which may achieve adult male ranges. This diagnosis is suspected on the basis of an unusually high serum testosterone concentration, which exceeds levels seen in patients with PCOD (generally <150 ng/dl in patients with PCOD). The weaker androgens may also exhibit elevated levels, depending on the individual tumor type. Levels of urinary 17-ketosteroids, however, which measure the metabolites of these weak androgens, are almost always elevated and should always be determined in the presence of an ovarian mass with hirsutism. Tumors secreting either estrogens or androgens may be very small and difficult to identify on most imaging procedures, although transvaginal ultrasonography has recently been quite helpful in identifying even small tumors.

The treatment for all of these ovarian tumors is surgical removal. Ultrasonographic evaluation is quite useful when followed by laparotomy for removal and determination of cell type.

BIBLIOGRAPHY

Engel E, Forbes AP: Cytogenetic and clinical findings in 48 patients with congenitally defective or absent ovaries, *Medicine* 44:139, 1965.

Filicori M, Santoro N, Merriam GR, Crowley WF: Characterization of the physiologic pattern of episodic gonadotropin secretion throughout the human menstrual cycle, *J Clin Endocrinol Metab* 62:1136-1144, 1986.

Hall JE, Schoenfeld DA, Martin KA, Crowley WF: Hypothalamic donadotropin-releasing hormone secretion and follicle-stimulating hormone dynamics during the luteal-follicular transition, *J Clin Endocrinol Metab* 74:600-607, 1992.

Hodgen G: The dominant ovarian follicle, *Fertil Steril* 38:281-300, 1982.

Lambert-Messerlian GM, Hall JE, Sluss PM et al: Relatively low levels of dimeric inhibin circulate in men and women with polycystic ovarian syndrome, *J Clin Endocrinol Metab* 79:45-50, 1994.

McKenna TJ: Pathogenesis and treatment of polycystic ovary syndrome, *N Engl J Med* 318:558-562, 1988.

Richards JS: Maturation of ovarian follicles: actions and interactions of pituitary and ovarian hormone on follicular cell differentiation, *Physiol Rev* 60:51-89, 1980.

Stouffer RL, editor: *The primate ovary,* New York, 1987, Plenum.

CHAPTER

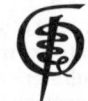

301 Disorders of the Testis

Richard J. Santen

ANDROGEN METABOLISM

The Leydig or interstitial cells of the testis secrete testosterone in response to luteinizing hormone (LH), a glycoprotein that binds to high-affinity, G protein–coupled receptors. Production of testosterone approximates 7000 μg daily with a diurnal variation causing peak serum levels at 4:00 AM to 8:00 AM and nadir concentrations 20% to 30% lower at 4:00 PM to 8:00 PM. A small percentage of testosterone (approximately 2%) circulates in a nonbound state in plasma, whereas the remainder is bound either to testosterone-estrogen–binding globulin (TEBG) or to albumin (Fig. 301-1). Only TEBG binds testosterone with sufficiently high affinity to retard entry into tissues. Several

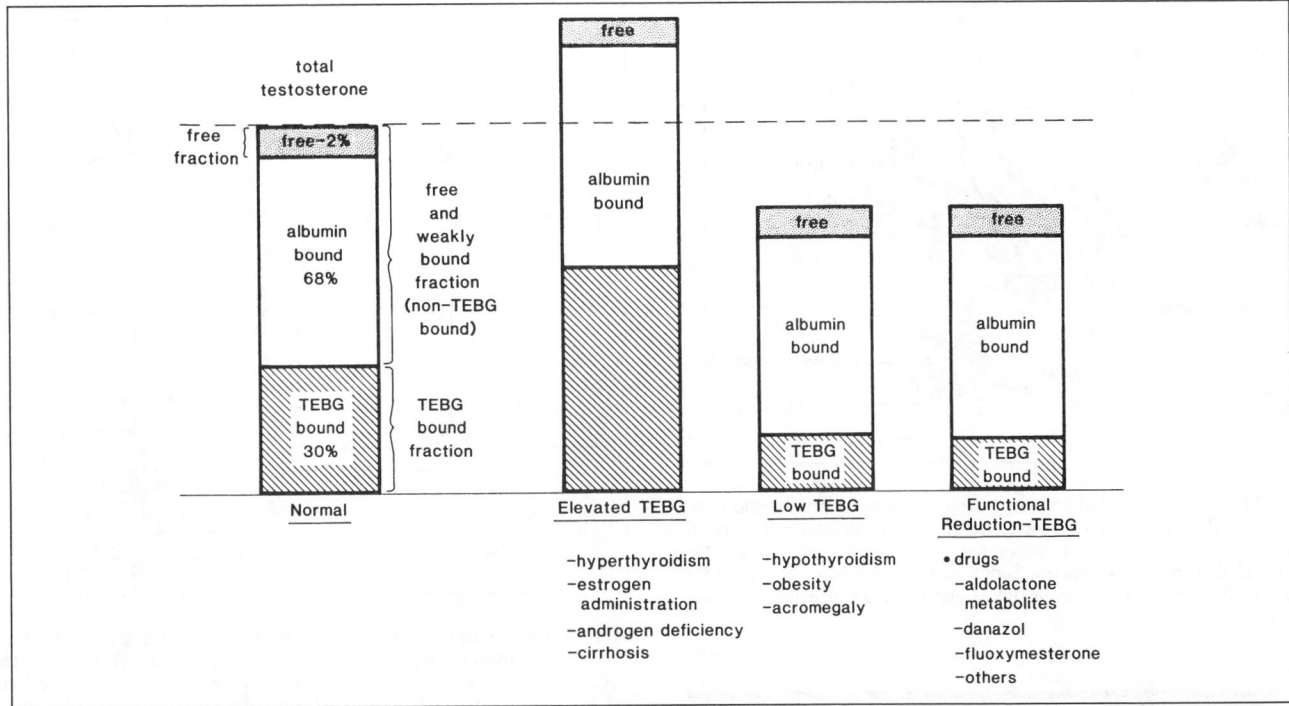

FIGURE 301-1   Fractions of bound, weakly bound, and free testosterone in normal men with disorders producing high or low levels of the sex hormone–binding protein, also known as *testosterone-estrogen–binding globulin* (TEBG).

clinicopathologic events alter the absolute levels of TEBG in plasma (Fig. 301-1).

Testosterone serves predominantly as a prehormone and undergoes conversion to more potent metabolites through two activation pathways. One results in the aromatization of testosterone to estradiol, a compound with 200-fold greater gonadotropin-suppressive potency on a mass basis. The second catalyzes the 5α reduction of testosterone to dihydrotestosterone, the androgen that binds to nuclear receptors in most androgen-responsive tissues. Two isozymes of 5α-reductase, type I and type II, have been identified, and the separate genes cloned. In prostate the type II isozyme predominates; in seminal vesicles, sebaceous glands, kidney, skin, hair, and other tissues variable amounts of both isozymes are present.

After metabolic activation, androgens induce their hormonal effects (Box 301-1) through binding to the androgen or estrogen receptors. In tissues such as muscle and hypothalamus, testosterone interacts directly with receptors without undergoing conversion to dihydrotestosterone. Androgen inactivation also occurs in liver and peripheral tissues either by modification to inactive free steroids or by conjugation to glucuronide or sulfate.

GERM CELL PRODUCTION

Seminiferous tubules, which are tightly coiled and up to 70 cm long, provide a continuous pathway for delivery of sperm from the testes to the rete testis, caput epididymis, and vas deferens. The seminiferous tubules are lined by a basal laminar layer and by myoid cells, which impart the ability for propulsion of fluids within the lumen (Fig. 301-2). Immature stem cells called *spermatogonia* lie along the basal lamina, interspersed between the supporting cells, called Sertoli cells (Fig. 301-2). Follicle-stimulating hormone (FSH) binds to specific receptors in the Sertoli cell and modulates the process of spermatogenesis. Testosterone, whose concentrations in the testis are 100 times those in peripheral plasma, acts in concert with FSH. Testosterone stimulates the spermatogonia and primary spermatocytes to complete meiotic divisions, and FSH facilitates maturation of spermatids to spermatozoa during the process of spermatogenesis. The human testis manufactures $123 \pm 18 \times 10^6$ sperm daily. The full process of spermatogenesis requires 74 ± 5 days, whereas transport through the epididymis and further maturation there take another 12 days.

HYPOTHALAMUS-PITUITARY

Gonadotropin secretion represents a discontinuous process characterized by a series of discrete, self-limited pulses (Fig. 301-3, *A* and *B*). Two steroids, testosterone (T) and estradiol (E_2) independently regulate this process. Negative feedback, the primary mechanism of LH control, can be mediated by a modulation in pulse frequency or amplitude. The control of FSH secretion is more complex. Testosterone and estradiol both inhibit FSH through a reduction in gonadotropin-releasing hormone (GnRH) secretion. In addition, a polypeptide heterodimer with alpha and beta subunits, a product of the testes (Fig. 301-3, *B*) called *inhibin*, exerts suppressive effects on FSH exclusively, acting primarily at the level of the pituitary. FSH (and also LH) stimulates increments in plasma inhibin, thus providing an ancillary negative feedback control system for FSH. Beta-beta subunit homodimers of inhibin called activin stimulate FSH secretion and may also participate in FSH regulation.

AGE-DEPENDENT PHYSIOLOGIC CHANGES IN TESTICULAR FUNCTION

During the first 2 months of life LH and testosterone levels approach those of adult life. After this brief period the hypothalamic-pituitary-testicular axis becomes quiescent, and LH and testosterone levels remain low (i.e., <1 mIU/ml and <20 ng/dl, respectively) during childhood. Testicular size is stable from birth until age 6 years, at which time the testes gradually enlarge in proportion to somatic growth. The pubertal process begins on average at age 11 in boys (95% confidence limits, 9 to 13 years), when an increase in LH, FSH, and testosterone secretion occurs. The first physical evidence of puberty, rapid testicular enlargement, appears approximately 6 months later, when the testes increase to greater than 2.9 cm on the long axis or 6 ml in volume. Once the process begins, pubertal testosterone increases

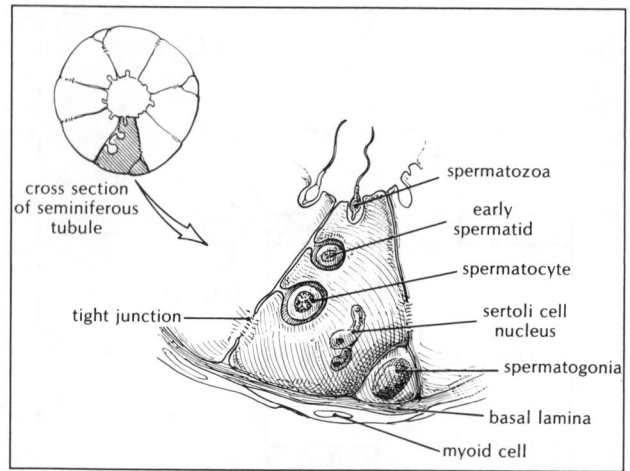

FIGURE 301-2   Diagrammatic representation of a seminiferous tubule to illustrate the relationship between the lining membrane structures (i.e., basal lamina and myoepithelial cells), Sertoli cell cytoplasm, and germinal cells. Specialized tight junctions between Sertoli cells form a blood testis barrier and create the outer or basal compartment and the inner or adluminal compartment.

BOX 301-1
Clinical actions of androgen

Androgen-receptor mediated

In utero
  External genitalia development.
  Wolffian duct development.
Prepubertal: Possible male behavioral effects.
Pubertal
  External genitalia: Penis and scrotum increase in size and become pigmented, and rugal folds appear in scrotal skin
  Hair growth: Mustache and beard develop, and scalp line undergoes recession. Pubic hair develops. Axillary, body, extremity, and perianal hair appears.
  Linear growth: Pubertal growth spurt appears. Androgens interact with growth hormones to increase IGF-1 levels.
  Accessory sex organs: Prostate and seminal vesicles enlarge, and secretion begins.
  Voice: The pitch is lowered because of enlargement of larynx and thickening of vocal cords.
  Psyche: More aggressive attitudes are evident, and sexual potential develops.
  Muscle mass: Muscle bulk increases, and positive nitrogen balance is demonstrable.
Adult
  Hair growth: Androgenic patterns are maintained. Male baldness may be initiated.
  Psyche: Behavioral attitudes and sexual potency are maintained.
  Spermatogenesis: Interaction with FSH modulates Sertoli cell function and stimulates spermatogenesis.
  Hematopoiesis: Stimulates erythropoietin and has direct marrow effect on erythropoiesis.

Estrogen-receptor mediated*

Pubertal
  Bone: Closure of the epiphyses.
Adult
  Bone: Prevention of bone loss and osteoporosis.

*After conversion of testosterone to estradiol.

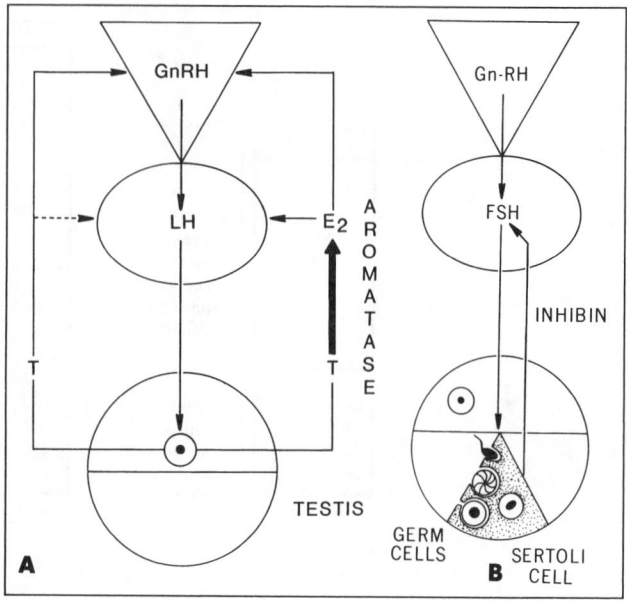

FIGURE 301-3   Diagrammatic representation of the feedback interactions between the hypothalamus *(triangle)*, pituitary *(ovoid)*, and testis *(circle)*. **A,** The Leydig cells of the testis secrete testosterone *(T)*, which exerts negative feedback effects on LH secretion at the hypothalamic level and through conversion to estradiol on the pituitary. Testosterone is converted into estradiol *(E₂)* by the enzyme aromatase, which is present in fat, muscle, and liver. Estradiol exerts negative feedback effects at both hypothalamic and pituitary levels. Because estradiol and testosterone both lower gonadotropin-releasing hormone (GnRH) levels, sex steroids also inhibit follicle-stimulating hormone (FSH) secretion (not shown). **B,** An additional control mechanism exists for FSH whereby the Sertoli cells of the testis secrete inhibin. This protein product is thought to act at the pituitary to inhibit FSH secretion.

rapidly over a 10- to 12-month period and reaches levels 20-fold higher than those observed in the prepubertal period.

After puberty the hypothalamic-pituitary-testicular axis remains stable until approximately the fourth decade. Thereafter, the efficiency of Leydig cell steroidogenesis declines variably as a function of aging and illness. The number of adult Leydig cells progressively falls as a function of age from 432 million ± 45 million per testis to 243 million ± 27 million in men older than 50, and each Leydig cell decreases in size. Consequently, LH levels gradually rise and responsiveness to human chorionic gonadotropin (hCG) diminishes. Despite this process, free testosterone levels may be maintained in certain healthy men, but in most, a fall in levels occurs with aging. Total testosterone level declines to a lesser extent than free levels because TEBG concentrations increase with age.

ASSESSMENT OF CLINICAL STATUS

An understanding of the normal actions of androgens in utero, during puberty, and in adulthood (Box 301-1) facilitates a logical approach to evaluation. Patients with *congenital hypogonadism* come to medical attention with sexual infantilism and retarded growth for age. The history and physical examination should focus on external genitalia, hair growth, linear growth, accessory sex organs, voice, psyche, and muscle mass. *Acquired hypogonadism* results in a loss of androgen-mediated effects (Box 301-1) and directs attention toward patterns of hair growth, testis size, sexual potential, behavioral patterns, maintenance of bone density, spermatogenesis, and hematopoiesis.

ASSESSMENT OF HORMONAL STATUS
Basal Levels

Pulsatile gonadotropin secretion introduces an error in estimates from single samples that approximates ±60% for LH and ±20% for FSH. Recent developments in technology involving two-site immunoflu-

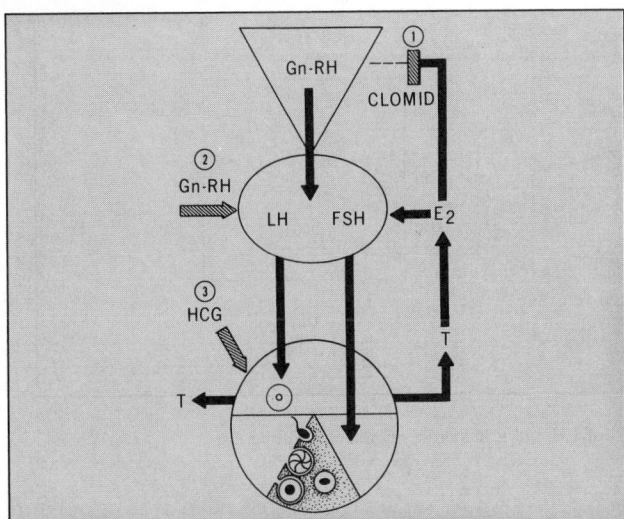

FIGURE 301-4   Diagrammatic representation of sites of action of stimulation tests of the testis. Hypothalamus *(triangle)*, pituitary *(ovoid)*, and Leydig and germ cell compartments of the testis *(circle)*. *hCG,* Human chorionic gonadotropin.

orometric assays have markedly enhanced the sensitivity and specificity of gonadotropin measurements. Based on cost and precision, a practical recommendation for gonadotropin assessment includes obtaining a single measurement of LH and FSH in plasma and confirming results by repeat measurements in a pool of four samples taken at 20-minute intervals if the initial level is borderline high or low. Single samples are usually adequate for clinical assessment of testosterone and dihydrotestosterone levels. The diurnal rhythm of testosterone necessitates obtaining early morning (i.e., 8:00 AM to 10:00 AM) samples and using normative values for that time of day. When abnormal values for total testosterone are detected, attention should be directed toward the possibility of TEBG abnormalities (Fig. 301-1), and non-TEBG–bound testosterone values should be specifically requested.

Dynamic Tests

Interruption of the estrogen-negative feedback axis with the antiestrogen clomiphene citrate (Clomid) (Figs. 301-4 and 301-5; Table 301-1) stimulates both LH and FSH and secondarily testosterone and estradiol. Exogenous GnRH administration releases LH and FSH from the pituitary. Direct provocative testing of the testes requires administration of hCG and assessment of plasma testosterone increments at various time intervals (Figs. 301-4 and 301-5).

GENETIC ANALYSIS

Karyotype analysis, which has superseded use of the buccal smear, provides a direct method for assessing chromosomal abnormalities and is performed on blood lymphocytes, skin fibroblasts, and gonadal tissues. Oligonucleotide sequences on the Y chromosome that control testicular development can now be probed by complement DNA (cDNA) hybridization to determine the presence of this portion of the Y chromosome.

DISORDERS AFFECTING ANDROGEN PRODUCTION
Hypogonadotropic Syndromes (Box 301-2)

Organic Hypogonadotropism
Multiple tropic hormone deficiencies. Patients with multiple tropic hormone deficiencies commonly come to medical attention with severe growth retardation if prepubertal and with delayed adolescence when older. Adults seek attention because of impotence,

---

BOX 301-2
Classification of hypogonadotropic hypogonadism

I. Organic causes
  A. Multiple tropic hormone deficiencies
    1. Idiopathic
    2. Secondary to tumor
    3. Miscellaneous causes
      a. Histiocytosis X
      b. Tuberculosis
      c. Sarcoidosis
      d. Collagen vascular diseases
      e. Hypophysitis
  B. Secondary to hyperprolactinemia
  C. Isolated gonadotropin deficiency
    1. Hypogonadotropic eunuchoidism (Kallmann's syndrome)
      a. Complete
      b. Partial (predominant LH deficiency—fertile eunuch syndrome)
      c. Variant form (isolated FSH deficiency)
    2. Specific genetic syndromes
      a. Prader-Labhart-Willi
      b. Laurence-Moon-Biedl
      c. Möbius
      d. Other rarer disorders
  D. Acute and chronic illness
    1. Malnutrition
    2. Miscellaneous acute illnesses
    3. Emotional disorders
    4. Liver disease (one subgroup)
    5. Renal disease (one component)
    6. Hemochromatosis
    7. Human immunodeficiency virus infection
II. Functional cause: Physiologic delayed puberty

FSH, Follicle-stimulating hormone; *LH,* luteinizing hormone.

headaches, or visual disturbance. Testosterone, LH, and FSH levels are low in patients with each of these disorders. Deficiencies of growth hormone, thyroxine, or cortisol focus the differential diagnosis toward pathologic processes of the pituitary or hypothalamus.

Hyperprolactinemia. A functional defect in gonadotropin secretion attributable to elevated prolactin levels may cause delayed puberty or adult-onset hypogonadotropism. Prolactin acts on the hypothalamus to increase dopamine turnover and thereby inhibit GnRH release. Hyperprolactinemia may be related to use of centrally acting drugs such as the phenothiazines or to the presence of a prolactin-producing tumor.

Isolated Gonadotropin Deficiency. Gonadotropin deficiency without loss of other anterior pituitary hormones results from a number of genetic disorders (Box 301-2). Subjects with these conditions come to medical attention with sexual infantilism or incomplete sexual development.

Kallmann's syndrome. Hypogonadotropic eunuchoidism, or Kallmann's syndrome, is the most common cause of isolated gonadotropin deficiency and is inherited either as an autosomal dominant, X-linked recessive or non-X–linked recessive disorder. The X-linked form represents a defect in the Kalig-1 gene localized at XP22.3. An adhesion molecule coded for by Kalig-1 mediates the early embryonic migration of GnRH neurons from the nasal plate to the hypothalamus. Genetic defects in this molecule prevent migration and result in absence of GnRH neurons in the hypothalamus. Depending on the relative degree of reduction of these hypothalamic neurons, GnRH secretion can be absent or blunted. Associated abnormalities may include hyposmia or anosmia, cryptorchidism, cleft lip or cleft palate, and congenital deafness. When anosmia is present, atrophy or absence of the olfactory sulcus or bulbs can be demonstrated on magnetic resonance imaging (MRI) studies. When genes contiguous with Kalig-1 are deleted or defective, unilateral renal agenesis and a variety of neurologic abnormalities may be present.

The degree of either LH or FSH deficiency in patients with Kall-

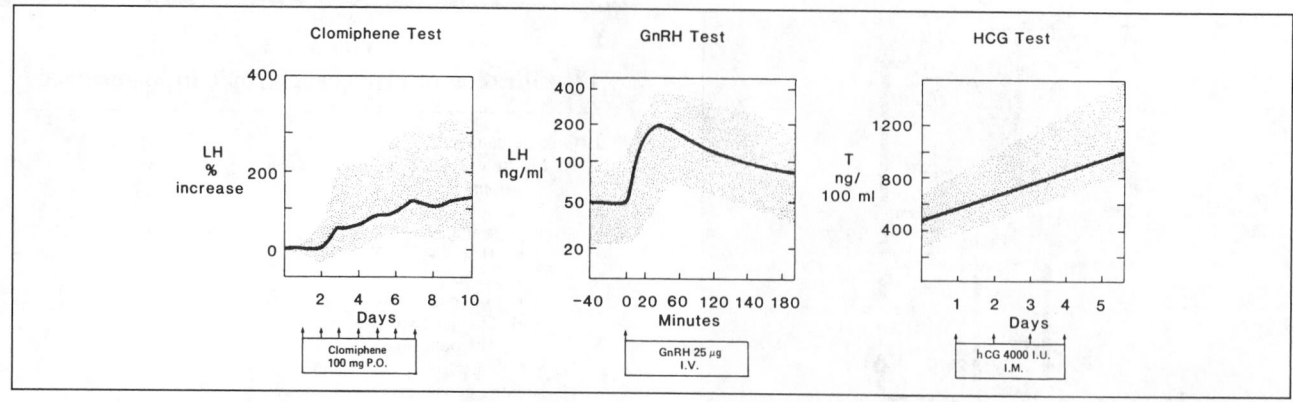

FIGURE 301-5   Mean *(solid lines)* and ranges *(shaded areas)* of LH and testosterone increments during clomiphene, GnRH, and hCG tests.

Table 301-1   Normal basal and stimulated hormone levels

| | BASAL | STIMULATED MEAN % INCREASE (RANGE) | | |
		CLOMIPHENE	GNRH	HCG
Plasma				
LH	4-20 mIU/ml	100 (30-400)	450 (50-1200)	—
FSH	4-20 mIU/ml	50 (20-200)	70 (9-176)	—
Testosterone	300-1200 ng/dl	(0-65)	No rise	100 (50-200)

Test protocols:
Clomiphene test: 100 mg clomiphene citrate (Clomid) daily by mouth for 7 days; draw blood sample before and on day 8.
GnRH test: 25 µg GnRH intravenously with collection of blood before and 30, 60, 90, and 120 minutes after administration.
hCG test: 4000 IU hCG on day 1; draw blood sample before and on day 5.

FSH, Follicle-stimulating hormone; *GnRH*, gonadotropin-releasing hormone; *hCG*, human chorionic gonadotropin; *LH*, luteinizing hormone.

mann's syndrome may vary, and clinical presentations range from absent sexual maturation to incomplete sexual development to nearly normal adult phenotype. Gonadotropin measurements can range from exceedingly low to the lower limit of adult normal values, and full spermatogenesis and normal testicular size may occur in some patients (fertile eunuch syndrome).

The major problem in diagnosis of isolated gonadotropin deficiency in boys under 18 years of age is to differentiate patients with an organic defect from those with delayed puberty on a functional basis. While a test examining responses to a long-acting GnRH analog has been reported as relatively discriminatory, no means are available to absolutely distinguish between these two groups of patients. Demonstration of associated somatic abnormalities such as anosmia or hyposmia, an abnormal olfactory sulcus on MRI, or a cleft lip or palate provides the best means of confirming the diagnosis of Kallmann's syndrome. Approximately 80% of boys with hypogonadotropic hypogonadism exhibit either anosmia or hyposmia; therefore this clinical finding is useful. If no associated congenital anomalies are present or there is no family history of the condition, the only definitive means of making the diagnosis of hypogonadotropic eunuchoidism may be to restudy the patient at 18 to 20 years of age when most boys with physiologic delay will have undergone pubertal changes.

Patients with Kallmann's syndrome have low levels of LH, FSH, and testosterone under basal conditions and during provocative testing. Measurement of growth hormone, thyroxine, prolactin, and adrenal hormones and MRI of the pituitary may be necessary to rule out multiple tropic hormone deficiencies and structural causes.

Specific Genetic Syndromes With Predominant Hypogonadotropism. The *Prader-Labhart-Willi syndrome* (HHHO) is an inherited disorder characterized by *h*ypotonia (especially in infancy), *h*ypogonadism, *h*ypomentia or mental retardation, *o*besity, short stature, and adult-onset diabetes mellitus. A defect in chromosome 15 has been described in nearly half the cases studied. The *Laurence-Moon-Biedl syndrome* is characterized by retinitis pigmentosa, obesity, mental retardation, and polydactyly and is associated with hypogonadism in 50% of affected patients and delayed adolescence in another 30%. Retinal degeneration occurs between 4 and 10 years of age, and obesity somewhat earlier.

Systemic Illness. Acute and chronic illness represents the most common cause of hypogonadotropic hypogonadism encountered in clinical practice. Associated malnutrition often is present as an underlying pathogenetic feature. Intestinal disease with malabsorption, recurrent infections, neoplastic disease, fasting, or primary malnutrition may lower testosterone levels in adults or cause poor growth and delayed pubertal progression in adolescents. Severe burns, coma, acute myocardial infarction, elective surgery, and critical illness may produce a reduction of LH and testosterone, similar to the well-known reductions in TSH and thyroxine production in the "euthyroid sick syndrome."

Emotional Disorders. Adult men with anorexia nervosa come to medical attention with gonadotropin deficiency and hypogonadism in association with weight loss. In adolescents psychiatric illness or emotional stress may cause inhibition of gonadotropin secretion and delay the pubertal process. An increase in corticotropin-releasing factor, activating the opiatergic neurons and lowering gonadotropin secretion, has been suggested as a potential mechanism.

Obesity. Massive obesity is associated with low testosterone levels and low to low-normal LH levels. Reductions in TEBG levels are partially responsible for the lowering of total testosterone level, but free or weakly bound testosterone levels are often low as well. Increased aromatization of testosterone to estradiol is present, but the

BOX 301-3
Hypergonadotropic hypogonadism

I. Gonadal defects
  A. Genetic
    1. Klinefelter's syndrome
    2. Myotonic dystrophy
    3. Syndrome of webbed neck, ptosis, hypogonadism, congenital heart disease, short stature
    4. XYY syndrome
    5. Down syndrome
    6. Miscellaneous
  B. Anatomic: Functional prepubertal castrate
  C. Gonadal toxins
    1. Drugs
    2. Ionizing irradiation
  D. Enzyme defects
    1. 17α-Hydroxylase deficiency
    2. 17-Ketoreductase deficiency
  E. Viral: Mumps orchitis
  F. Diabetes mellitus
  G. Associated with aging
II. Hormone resistance
  A. Androgen insensitivity
  B. 5α-Reductase deficiency

testosterone levels can be returned to normal with weight loss of insufficient degree to lower estradiol levels.

Liver Disease. Hypogonadism, gynecomastia, and testicular atrophy are commonly observed in men with hepatic cirrhosis; two subgroups of patients are described. In the hypogonadotropic subgroup LH and FSH levels are suppressed because of associated malnutrition or because of enhanced aromatization of testosterone to estradiol and increased estrogen-negative feedback. The hypergonadotropic subgroup has primary gonadal disease as a result of the direct toxic effects of alcohol. LH levels are elevated, and testosterone responses to exogenous hCG are diminished. Additional effects of alcohol on the liver to increase testosterone metabolic clearance rate may also lower circulating androgen concentrations.

Other Chronic Diseases. *Chronic renal failure* is associated with hypogonadism and hyperprolactinemia. Gonadotropin levels, although normal to slightly elevated, are reduced relative to the level of circulating testosterone. *Hemochromatosis* may involve the pituitary with resultant gonadotropin deficiency and hypogonadism. *Isolated gonadotropin deficiency* and fractional panhypopituitarism may be caused by lymphocytic hypophysitis. Nearly 50% of men with *acquired immunodeficiency syndrome* (AIDS) and some with AIDS-related complex (ARC) have low plasma testosterone levels. In the majority (75%), gonadotropin levels are inappropriately low. *Narcotic analgesics* reduce the secretion of LH and testosterone, resulting in a reversible form of hypogonadotropin hypogonadism.

Physiologic Delayed Puberty (Constitutional Delay)

From an early age, boys with physiologic delayed puberty lag 1 to 3 years behind their peers in statural growth and bone age and may fall as low as the first percentile on growth charts. The diagnosis is suspected in a short, adolescent-aged boy of 14 years or older with testes of prepubertal size whose father, brothers, or cousins initiated puberty between the ages of 14 and 18. The major problem in diagnosis is the differentiation of boys with physiologic delayed puberty from those with complete or incomplete forms of hypogonadotropic eunuchoidism. If anosmia or hyposmia is absent, there is no definite means of establishing the diagnosis of delayed puberty other than careful, prolonged observation. Measurement of gonadotropin levels with ultrasensitive assays at 6-month intervals over 1 to 2 years provides reassurance if levels rise appreciably during the period of observation.

Hypergonadotropic Hypogonadism

Primary disorders of testicular function result in incomplete sexual maturation, hypogonadism, and elevated gonadotropin levels (Box 301-3). The defect in testosterone secretion is often partial, and androgen-related somatic changes occur at puberty but are incomplete. Testicular growth is diminished because of the dysgenetic nature of the gonad. The gynecomastia that frequently develops during puberty is more severe than that observed in normal boys. In adults testicular failure produces impotence as an early symptom and loss of secondary sex characteristics as a late finding, often taking 5 to 10 years to develop.

Genetic Disorders. *Klinefelter's syndrome* is characterized by the presence of one or more supernumerary X chromosomes (Table 301-2). The classic (XXY) form occurs in approximately 1 in 500 males (0.21%, infants and 0.15% to 0.24%, adults; Table 301-2). This disorder is highly suspected in an adult with firm testes of less than 2 cm in length who has clinical signs of androgen deficiency of variable degree. Gynecomastia occurs in 85% of patients. Epiphyses close late, resulting in a slight increase in height over that predicted. Large prospective surveys indicate a decrease in mean intelligence test scores and educational level achieved in men with Klinefelter's syndrome compared with controls of similar age. A slightly increased proportion may have frankly subnormal intelligence. Personality disorders are reported to occur more commonly in men with Klinefelter's syndrome than in the normal population.

The degree of Leydig cell dysfunction in Klinefelter's syndrome is variable. Mean testosterone concentrations in patients as a group are approximately half (i.e., 300 ng/dl) those in normal men (600 ng/dl); however, 40% of patients have total testosterone levels in the normal, albeit low-normal, range. Plasma estradiol level is twofold higher in patients with Klinefelter's syndrome because of an increased conversion of testosterone into estradiol. Plasma TEBG levels rise in response to the overproduction of estradiol, and the fraction of non–TEBG-bound testosterone is reduced. Consequently, some patients with normal total testosterone levels exhibit low "free and weakly bound" testosterone concentrations (Fig. 301-1). The diagnosis of Klinefelter's syndrome of any type is confirmed by karyotype analysis of blood lymphocytes. Elevation of plasma FSH is uniform, and of LH nearly uniform. Response to exogenous hCG is blunted, indicating decreased testicular reserve function.

Other Syndromes. *Mumps* involves the testes and produces an acute, highly painful, inflammatory disorder in 15% to 25% of pubertal or postpubertal patients with acute infection. Germ cells degenerate, and Leydig cell dysfunction develops gradually over a period of years. Patients then come to medical attention with symptoms of androgen deficiency or infertility. A history of painful orchitis distinguishes these patients from those with Klinefelter's syndrome, who otherwise can have similar complaints.

Myotonic dystrophy is a familial disorder characterized by cataracts, baldness, muscle weakness, and hypogonadism in 80% of affected males. *Noonan's syndrome,* a condition associated with webbed neck, ptosis, hypogonadism, congenital heart disease, and short stature, is also called male Turner's syndrome. Additional clinical findings include facies typical of Turner's syndrome in girls, low-set ears, shieldlike chest, cryptorchidism, diminished spermatogenesis, decreased Leydig cell function, cubitus valgus, and cardiovascular anomalies (especially pulmonic stenosis). The *XYY syndrome, Down syndrome, sickle cell disease,* and *autoimmune disorders* may also be associated with testicular failure and other endocrine deficiency states. Patients with the *functional prepubertal castrate syndrome* (anorchia) come to medical attention with signs and symptoms of severe androgen deficiency and lack anatomically demonstrable or functioning testes, but exhibit normal external genitalia. Bilateral testicular torsion, which occurs sometime after embryologic development is completed, probably explains the loss of testes in these patients. Bilateral cryptorchidism is often suspected in these patients but practically ruled out when castrate levels of gonadotropins are found in association with prepubertal levels of testosterone.

Table 301-2   Clinical features of Klinefelter's syndrome

| | | VARIANT FORMS* | | |
PARAMETER	CLASSIC FORM	XX	MOSAIC FORMS*	POLY X + Y
Incidence	1/500	1/9000	Unknown	Unknown
Clinical features	Testes <2 cm and firm	Shorter in stature	Testis may be normal sized	Increased incidence of cryptorchidism
	Eunuchoidal proportions	Hypospadias		Radioulnar synostosis
	Gynecomastia			
	Personality disorder			
	Androgen deficiency of variable degree			
Laboratory determinations	LH elevated			
	FSH extremely elevated			
	Testosterone lowered (in 50%)			
	Barr body present			
Karyotype	47, XXY	46, XX	XXY/XY; XXY/XX	XXXY, XXXXY, XXXXXX
Spermatogenesis	Azoospermia		Impairment less severe	
Testis biopsy	Hyalinized tubules		Less severe damage	
	Relative Leydig cell hyperplasia			

*Only divergent features are listed.
Modified from Bardin CW, Paulsen CA. In Williams RH, editor: *Textbook of endocrinology,* ed 6, Philadelphia, 1981, WB Saunders.
FSH, Follicle-stimulating hormone; *LH,* luteinizing hormone.

Gonadal Toxins. Cytotoxic drugs used as treatment of the nephrotic syndrome or of neoplastic disease commonly produce testicular damage. The alkylating agents are particularly common offenders. In nearly 100% of patients receiving MOPP (mechlorethamine, vincristine, procarbazine, prednisone) chemotherapy, azoospermia and compromised androgen production develop. Radiation therapy that includes the gonads also results in testicular failure. Spermatogenic elements are more sensitive to these effects than are Leydig cells. Polychlorinated insecticides, dibromochloropropane, and marijuana may also cause a reduction in sperm count and motility.

Enzyme Defects. Genetic males with complete 17α-hydroxylase and 17-ketosteroid reductase deficiencies come to medical attention as phenotypic females with partial virilization at puberty. Incomplete defects result in lack of full pubertal development, hypospadias, and gynecomastia in phenotypic males.

Diabetes Mellitus. Impotence, which occurs in 50% of diabetic men, is usually multifactorial, with evidence of vascular, neurologic, or psychogenic factors. A subgroup of men with organic impotence without vascular disease has diminished testosterone but elevated LH levels, suggesting a primary gonadal defect. Impotence improves with testosterone therapy if candidates for therapy are carefully selected.

Male Climacteric. The hormonal changes associated with aging reflect a gradual 50% decrease in the number of Leydig cells occurring after the age of 50 years. As a result, hCG responsiveness is blunted, free testosterone levels diminish gradually, and gonadotropins increase. Less than expected reflex gonadotropin elevations are observed, which reflects a component of diminished hypothalamic pituitary reserve. Replacement of testosterone may be warranted as a therapeutic trial in highly selected patients after a clear demonstration of low androgen levels. Further study is required to develop clear guidelines in the evaluation and treatment of such patients.

Hormone Resistance. Syndromes of androgen insensitivity may be complete or incomplete. In the complete form affected men come to medical attention as phenotypic females with primary amenorrhea and breast development. With incomplete insensitivity the defect ranges from mild to severe, and patients may exhibit diminished body hair, gynecomastia, hypospadias, bifid scrotum, cryptorchidism, or only azoospermia. Elevated LH levels in such patients reflect resistance to androgens at the hypothalamic-pituitary level. FSH titers are usually normal. Genetic mutations of the androgen receptor gene are reported that result in absent receptor function and explain the complete form of this disorder. Other mutations only impair receptor function and produce incomplete androgen insensitivity.

Deficiency of the enzyme 5α-reductase produces a form of androgen resistance resulting from a lack of conversion of testosterone to dihydrotestosterone. These patients exhibit ambiguous genitalia at birth and are usually reared as females. At puberty, partial virilization with penile growth and increase in muscle mass ensue. Facial hair, acne, and frontal balding are lacking, whereas spermatogenesis may be normal. In primitive cultures these individuals take on a male role at puberty. Resistance to LH produces a picture of more complete androgen deficiency with sexual infantilism resulting from a functional lack of stimulation of the Leydig cells to make testosterone.

Treatment

Approaches to treatment differ depending on the clinical circumstances and desires of the patient (Table 301-3). In *delayed adolescence* major psychological effects may result from a delay in adolescent sexual development. These considerations favor treatment empirically in patients over 14 years of age when clinical circumstances warrant. With *adult hypogonadotropic hypogonadism* the treatment goal is to maintain plasma testosterone levels in the adult normal range (300 to 1200 ng/dl) over a prolonged period. Injectable testosterone (Table 301-3) or transdermal patches are preferred unless fertility is an immediate goal. In that instance, hCG is given until testosterone levels are normal for at least 6 months; then FSH preparations such as menotropins (Pergonal) may be added. When gonadotropin deficiency is incomplete, hCG alone often initiates adequate degrees of spermatogenesis. In patients with *adult hypergonadotropic hypogonadism* direct replacement of androgen provides the only effective therapy.

Disorders Affecting Spermatogenesis

Germinal cell dysfunction occurs in 3% to 5% of the male population and produces infertility. Initial evaluation of the infertile man involves documentation of low sperm counts in at least three semen analyses obtained at monthly intervals. If quantitative counts are consistently below 20 million sperm/cm³ or 50 million total count, germinal cell dysfunction is highly suspect. A workup is then initiated to identify possible etiologic causes. Disorders of germinal cell function can be classified as hypogonadotropic, hypergonadotropic, and eugonadotropic.

When germinal cell mass or Sertoli cell function is sufficiently reduced, plasma or urinary FSH levels increase, often without a concomitant rise in LH. A current hypothesis attributes this monotropic FSH rise to a reduction in testicular inhibin with partial interruption

Table 301-3   Treatment of testis disorders

GROUP	GOAL OF TREATMENT	TREATMENT MODALITY	DOSAGE
Delayed adolescence	• Initiate androgenic effects with subreplacement doses of testosterone to maintain plasma levels of 100-200 ng/dl • Promote secondary sex characteristics and normal linear growth • Observe for spontaneous maturational changes during periods off medication	• Testosterone enanthate or cypionate	• 50-100 mg every 3-4 weeks IM • Treat for 3-month periods alternating with no therapy for 3 months over a 1-2 year period if physiologically delayed puberty suspected • After 2 years, if no spontaneous pubertal rise in testosterone, increase to adult replacement levels of testosterone
Adult hypogonadotropic hypogonadism	• Long-term maintenance of testosterone levels at 300-1200 ng/dl	• Trans-Derm patch • Testosterone enanthate or cypionate • Human chorionic gonadotropin • Gonadotropin-releasing hormone • Testosterone undecanoate	• One scrotal patch per day *or* one patch on back per day • 100 mg every 7 days IM or • 200 mg every 10-14 days IM or • 300 mg every 21 days IM • 1000-4000 IU two-three times per week • 2-20 μg subcutaneously two-three times per hour • 200 mg orally four times daily (not available in the United States)
Adult hypergonadotropic hypogonadism	• Long-term maintenance of testosterone levels at 300-1200 ng/dl	• Trans-Derm patch • Testosterone enanthate or cypionate • Testosterone undecanoate	• One scrotal patch per day *or* one patch on back per day • 100 mg every 7 days IM or • 200 mg every 10-14 days IM or • 300 mg every 21 days IM • 200 mg orally four times daily (not available in the United States)
	• Provide subreplacement doses of androgen	• Fluoxymestrone • Methyltestosterone	• 5-10 mg orally daily • 25 mg daily by linguet

IM, Intramuscularly.

of FSH-negative feedback, although other explanations are possible. The degree of plasma FSH elevation can be used as a marker for the severity of germinal cell dysfunction. The availability of this measurement has largely obviated the need for testicular biopsy, since the specific histologic pattern does not usually influence patient management decisions.

Many hormonal therapies have been proposed to enhance sperm production in men with germinal cell failure. Although uncontrolled studies report benefit, carefully randomized, placebo-controlled trials do not demonstrate the efficacy of these approaches. However, a newly developed method for microinjecting single sperm into oocytes represents an advance in the treatment of oligospermic males and results in in vitro fertilization rates as high as 70%.

Hypergonadotropic Disorders. The *Sertoli-cell–only syndrome* is a disorder in which all germinal cell elements in the testis except Sertoli cells are lost, but Leydig cell function is relatively preserved. Clinical examination reveals normal pubic and axillary hair but small soft testes averaging 2 to 4 cm on their long axes (10 to 20 ml). FSH levels are uniformly elevated, and azoospermia is found on semen analysis. Half of the patients exhibit subclinical Leydig cell dysfunction characterized by elevated LH levels with normal or slightly reduced testosterone concentrations and blunted responses to hCG.

Idiopathic seminiferous tubular failure with hyalinization is diagnosed on testicular biopsy in men with oligospermia or azoospermia whose FSH levels are elevated. Testis size may be reduced to below adult normal limits of 3.5 cm on the long axis or 20 ml.

Eugonadotropic Disorders. Patients with oligospermia but normal FSH levels are considered to have eugonadotropic germinal cell failure. Two subtypes are described: arrest of germinal cell maturation at a specific step and generalized hypospermatogenesis affecting all germ cell elements. Clinical examination reveals no abnormal-

ity, and testis size is usually normal. On testis biopsy, only minimal peritubular hyalinization or normal peritubular elements are present.

Incompetence of the left or, less commonly, the right testicular vein results in the formation of dilated veins in the scrotum, a condition called *varicocele.* Empirical observations suggest an etiologic association between varicocele and infertility. Varicocele can be palpated during Valsalva's maneuver in approximately 40% of men with oligospermia or azoospermia. The majority of reports indicate improved semen quality in 60% to 70% and fertility in 30% to 40% of men after high venous ligation to correct the varicocele; however, no definitive study including a control group conclusively establishes the validity of this treatment.

A thorough search for infectious agents has identified a variety of organisms in the seminal fluid of men with oligospermia or with decreased sperm motility. Mycoplasma infection, particularly *Ureaplasma urealyticum,* has been suggested as a causative agent in infertility, but this theory remains controversial. The presence of an excess number of leukocytes in the seminal fluid suggests the possibility of infection. A cause-and-effect relationship between the documented infection and the associated infertility has not yet been established. Most large infertility clinics, however, routinely recommend antibiotics such as doxycycline when infection is suspected by the presence of pus cells on several seminal fluid examinations or when cultures are positive.

The sinopulmonary-infertility syndrome is diagnosed in patients with recurrent sinopulmonary infections, defective sperm motility, and dysfunction of cilia in the respiratory tract and on the spermatozoa. Cystic fibrosis and Young's syndrome (azoospermia in association with inspissated secretions in the vas deferens) represent two well-defined subtypes.

Genetic Syndromes. Fifteen percent of men with azoospermia have genetic abnormalities, including XY and XYY karyotypes, reciprocal autosomal and other translocations, and a variety of other abnormalities. The frequency of these disorders in oligospermic men with counts of 1 to 20 million sperm/cm³ is 1.65%. Recent studies detect DNA microdeletions on the long arm of the Y chromosome in 18% of men with azospermia or severe oligospermia.

Autoimmunity. Infertility and oligospermia occur in association with certain autoimmune disorders such as Addison's disease and the familial autoimmune endocrine deficiency syndrome. The presence of autoantibodies against the testis has been demonstrated in these patients and in other patients with oligospermia or azoospermia.

Heat. Exposure to heat reproducibly reduces sperm production temporarily in a number of animal species. Although this effect has been incompletely documented in men, studies suggest that the heat encountered in a sauna may be sufficient to temporarily reduce sperm production.

Hypogonadotropic Syndromes. These disorders are uniformly associated with androgen deficiency and are described with disorders of androgen production.

BIBLIOGRAPHY

Adler RA: Clinically important effects of alcohol on endocrine function, *J Clin Endocrinol Metab* 74:957, 1992.

Bhasin S: Androgen treatment of hypogonadal men, *J Clin Endocrinol Metab* 74:1221, 1992.

Bhasin S et al: Measurement of circulating inhibin levels: revisiting the inhibin hypothesis, *J Clin Endocrinol Metab* 81:1318, 1996 (editorial).

Bhasin S, De Kretser DM, Baker HWG: Pathophysiology and natural history of male infertility, *J Clin Endocrinol Metab* 79:1525, 1994.

De Bellis A et al: Characterization of mutant androgen receptors causing partial androgen insensitivity syndrome, *J Clin Endocrinol Metab* 78:513, 1994.

Dobs AS et al: Endocrine disorders in men infected with human immunodeficiency virus, *Am J Med* 84:611, 1988.

French FS et al: Molecular basis of androgen insensitivity, *Recent Prog Horm Res* 46:1, 1990.

Green JS et al: The cardinal manifestations of Bardet-Biedl syndrome, a form of Laurence-Moon-Biedl syndrome, *N Engl J Med* 321:1002, 1989.

Grumbach MM, Conte FA: Disorders of sexual differentiation. In Wilson JD, Foster DW, editors: *Textbook of endocrinology,* ed 8, Philadelphia, 1992, WB Saunders.

Illingworth PJ et al: Inhibin-B: a likely candidate for the physiologically important form of inhibin in men, *J Clin Endocrinol Metab* 81:1321, 1996.

Meikle AW et al: Enhanced transdermal delivery of testosterone across nonscrotal skin produces physiological concentrations of testosterone and its metabolites in hypogonadal men, *J Clin Endocrinol Metab* 74:623, 1992.

Murray FT et al: Gonadal dysfunction in diabetic men with organic impotence, *J Clin Endocrinol Metab* 65:127, 1987.

Prager D, Braunstein GD: X-Chromosome-linked Kallmann's syndrome: pathology at the molecular level, *J Clin Endocrinol Metab* 76:824, 1993 (editorial).

Rogol AD, Yesalis CE III: Anabolic-androgenic steroids and athletes: what are the issues? *J Clin Endocrinol Metab* 74:465, 1992.

Rosenfield RL: Diagnosis and management of delayed puberty, *J Clin Endocrinol Metab* 70:559, 1990.

Santen RJ: The testis. In Felig P et al, editors: *Endocrinology and metabolism,* ed 3, New York, 1995, McGraw-Hill.

Smith BR et al: Adrenal and gonadal autoimmune diseases, *J Clin Endocrinol Metab* 80:1502, 1995 (editorial).

Snyder PJ: Clinical use of androgens, *Annu Rev Med* 35:207, 1984.

Spratt DI et al: The spectrum of abnormal patterns of gonadotropin-releasing hormone secretion in men with idiopathic hypogonadotropic hypogonadism: clinical and laboratory correlations, *J Clin Endocrinol Metab* 64:283, 1987.

Spratt DI et al: Reproductive axis suppression in acute illness is related to disease severity, *J Clin Endocrinol Metab* 76:1548, 1993.

Tenover JS: Effects of testosterone supplementation in the aging male, *J Clin Endocrinol Metab* 75:1092, 1992.

Veldhuis J: The hypothalamic-pituitary-testicular axis. In Yen SSC, Jaffe RB, editors: *Reproductive endocrinology,* ed 3, Philadelphia, 1991, WB Saunders.

Veldhuis J et al: Amplitude suppression of the pulsatile mode of immunoradiometric luteinizing hormone release in fasting-induced hypoandrogenemia in normal men, *J Clin Endocrinol Metab* 76:587, 1993.

Veldhuis J et al: Evidence for attenuation of hypothalamic gonadotropin-releasing hormone impulse strength with preservation of GnRH pulse frequency in men with chronic renal failure, *J Clin Endocrinol Metab* 76:648, 1993.

Vermeulen A, et al: Attenuated luteinizing hormone (LH) pulse amplitude but normal LH pulse frequency, and its relation to plasma androgens in hypogonadism of obese men, *J Clin Endocrinol Metab* 76:1140, 1993.

Vermeulen A, Kaufman JM: Role of the hypothalamo-pituitary function in the hypoandrogenism of healthy aging, *J Clin Endocrinol Metab* 75:704, 1992 (editorial).

Whitcomb RW: The approach to the oligoazoospermic male, *Endocrinologist* 1:125, 1991.

302 Benign Breast Disease

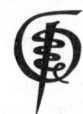

Richard J. Santen and Joann Pinkerton

ANATOMY AND PATHOPHYSIOLOGY

During embryologic development epithelial cells from the anlage of the nipple invaginate into the breast connective tissue to form a series of ducts. These structures branch several times before terminating in lobular buds. Later, during pubertal development, estrogen levels increase and stimulate further proliferation of ductal tissue. With the onset of ovulatory cycles progesterone enhances proliferation of the lobular end bud. During pregnancy, prolactin increases and stimulates the lobular cells to produce milk protein. Growth hormone, cortisol and thyroxine, while not directly influencing mammary cell growth and differentiation, act permissively, whereas testosterone blocks the stimulatory effects of estrogen and progesterone.

The mature breast is not a static organ but undergoes cyclic change during the menstrual cycle. The rate of proliferation of breast cells increases during the luteal phase and decreases during the follicular phase. Progesterone, in conjunction with estrogen, stimulates proliferation and differentiated function of ductular and lobular cells. Consequently, the breast may increase in size by 10% to 15% during the late luteal phase. These changes are responsible for the increase in localized pain in breast nodules or in global breast tenderness experienced during this phase of the menstrual cycle.

Benign breast disease represents a spectrum of disorders characterized by exaggerated growth of breast elements. Several of these conditions impart no increased risk of developing breast cancer on prolonged follow-up (Fig. 302-1). The most common condition, *fibrocystic changes,* consists of an increased number of cysts or fibrous tissue in an otherwise normal breast (Fig. 302-2). Current terminology considers that fibrocystic changes do not constitute a disease state, since these lesions occur in 60% of North American women. Page and Dupont considered *fibrocystic disease* to consist of fibrocystic changes in conjunction with pain, nipple discharge, or a degree of lumpiness sufficient to cause suspicion of cancer in an individual lesion. Cysts, which form as a result of blockage or dilation of ducts, are of two types: small cysts lined by flattened cells and larger cysts with an apocrine cell layer. *Duct ectasia* is characterized by distention of subareolar ducts and presence within them of yellowish-orange material with crystalline oval and round structures. This material is thought to be lipid in origin. Penetration of the duct wall by this material produces inflammatory changes in the surrounding tissues. Spontaneous resolution may occur, but residual fibrosis and nodule formation may persist. Isolated *fibrous change* results from stromal proliferation in the areas surrounding the cysts. Duct ectasia and stromal fibrosis may occur in concert or as isolated entities. Solitary *papillomas* consist of a monotonous array of papillary cells that grow out from the cyst wall. These are quiescent and solitary and have a single stalk. *Simple fibroadenomas* are benign neoplasms containing glandular and fibrous tissue.

Certain other benign lesions are associated with a 1.5- to 2-fold greater risk of breast cancer development over a 20-year period of follow-up. The lesions in this category are diverse but characterized by an increased rate of cellular proliferation. *Ductal hyperplasia* without atypia represents the most common type. Epithelial cells lining the basement membrane of ducts increase but retain typical benign cellular features and vary in size and shape. Lobular tissue can also undergo hyperplastic change with increased fibrous tissue and interspersed glandular cells: a lesion called *sclerosing adenosis.* When multiple areas of papilloma form, *diffuse papillomatosis* is present. *Complex fibroadenomas* are defined as lesions containing cysts greater than 3 mm in diameter, sclerosing adenosis, epithelial calcification, or papillary apocrine changes. This entity imparts an increased risk when surrounded by proliferative changes in the surrounding glandular tissue.

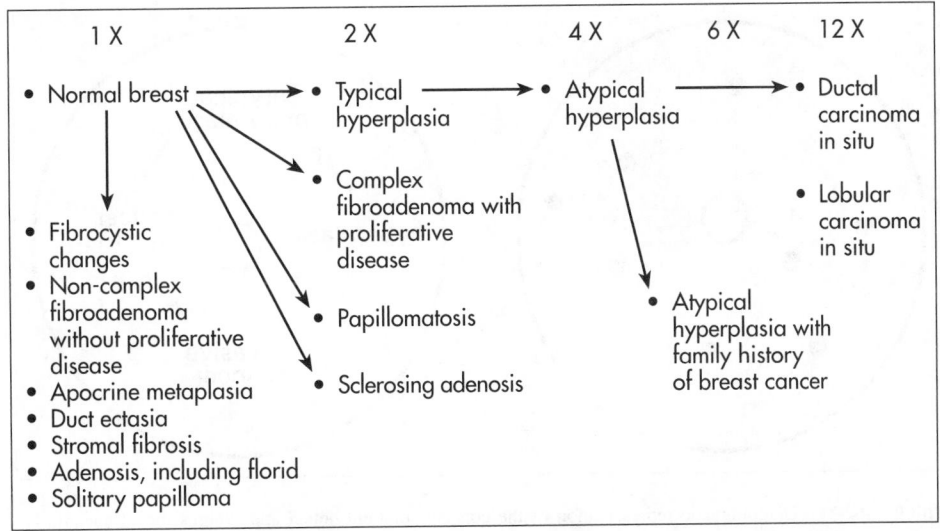

FIGURE 302-1   The relative risk of the later development of invasive breast cancer with specifically defined benign breast lesions and carcinoma in situ. Interestingly, with each of these lesions, the breast cancer that develops many years later usually involves a different area of the breast than that of the initial lesion.

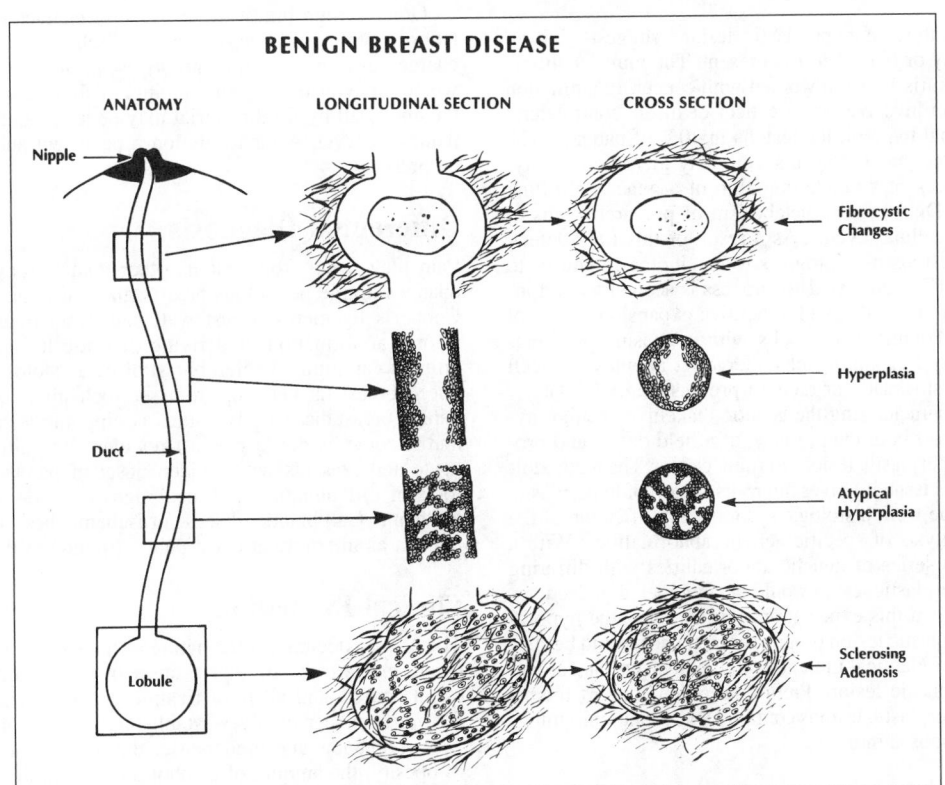

FIGURE 302-2   Diagrammatic representation of the types of benign breast lesions that are commonly observed.

The spectrum of benign lesions extends to those with an even higher risk of later breast cancer development. *Atypical hyperplasia* of either ductular or lobular elements imparts a fourfold increased risk of breast cancer if sporadic and a sixfold greater risk in patients with a strong family history of breast cancer. When the degree of atypia progresses even further, the lesions are no longer called benign but are classified as *carcinoma in situ* and consist of both ductal and lobular subtypes. The risk of development of invasive cancer when these lesions are present is 10- to 12-fold over a period of 20 years (Fig. 302-1).

Etiologic Factors

Few studies have addressed the potential causes of fibrocystic changes. A limited number of observations suggest that ingestion of caffeine with consequent inhibition of phosphodiesterase and increased tissue cyclic adenosine monophosphate (cAMP) levels may cause fibrocystic changes. Other studies do not support this still controversial hypothesis. Experimental iodine deficiency in rodents can cause lesions that are similar to fibrocystic disease in patients. Symptomatic improvement in patients with fibrocystic disease has been re-

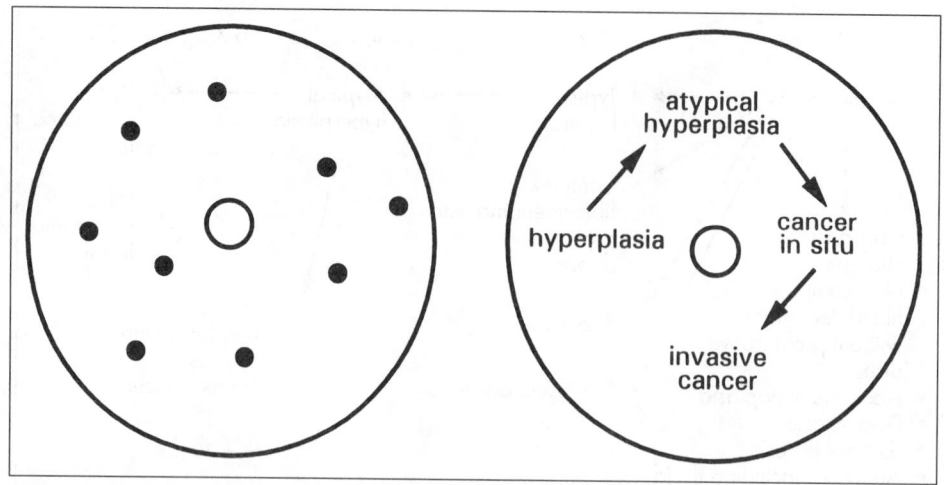

FIGURE 302-3   Diagrammatic representation of the concepts of field defect and progression of specific lesions to invasive cancer.

ported with iodine administration, suggesting an etiologic association. Clearly, definitive studies of the causes of fibrocystic decease are lacking at present.

The multicentric nature of hyperplastic lesions suggests that an underlying abnormality or *field defect* is present. The multifocality is most apparent in breast tissue from women with cancer. Examination of tissue adjacent to an invasive breast cancer or in the contralateral breast reveals additional hyperplastic lesions in 40% of patients. The nature of the field defect has not been specifically identified but hypothetically could represent a single mutation of a gene controlling cellular proliferation, DNA repair, metabolism of procarcinogens or carcinogens, or other cellular events. As a result of this field defect, one of the resulting lesions may progress to carcinoma in situ or to frank invasive cancer (Fig. 302-3). This process is sequential and involves multiple mutational "hits" with repetitive expansion of parent and daughter clones. Populations of cells with increasing proliferative potential or reduced capability of undergoing apoptosis or cell death result from this stochastic or random process (Fig. 302-4).

Preliminary data characterizing the genetic makeup of benign hyperplastic lesions support both the presence of a field defect and progression of specific hyperplastic lesions to frank cancer. The methodology used to address this issue involves microdissection of hyperplastic and normal breast tissue from histologic sections, amplification of the DNA present, and analysis of specific genetic abnormalities. With a field defect, a random series of genetic abnormalities with differing mutations in each hyperplastic lesion would be anticipated; indeed, recent observations confirm this expectation. Furthermore, the hypothesis that a single hyperplastic lesion progresses to cancer would be supported by the finding of identical mutations in the invasive cancer and its neighboring hyperplastic lesion. Preliminary data support this as well, since 90% of hyperplastic lesions contain DNA mutations similar to those in the contiguous tumors.

Clinical Symptoms

Patients with fibrocystic changes or hyperplastic lesions as well as normal women can have increased breast tenderness during the luteal phase of the menstrual cycle. Other women have constant pain as a result of the breast lesions. Some clinicians differentiate clinical syndromes attributable to fibrocystic changes into those of *mazoplasia, adenosis,* and *cystic* phases. Mazoplasia occurs in the 20s and becomes evident with upper outer-quadrant breast pain and an indurated axillary tail primarily as a result of stromal proliferation. Women in their 30s have multiple breast nodules 2 to 10 mm in size as a result of glandular cell proliferation. Women in their 30s and 40s come to medical attention with solitary or multiple cysts. Acute enlargement of cysts may cause severe, localized pain of sudden onset. Because breast ducts are usually patent in the presence of benign lesions, breast

discharge is common, and pale to green/brown/black discharge may be present.

Other benign breast diseases cause characteristic clinical presentations. With *papillomas,* bloody discharge is common. Milk discharge may be present with *hyperprolactinemia,* although normal women may also have this finding. With *duct ectasia,* penetration of the duct wall by lipid material may be associated with acute redness, pain, and fever. After resolution a persistent subareolar nodule may be present.

Differential Diagnosis

Pain may result from lesions other than fibrocystic or hyperplastic changes. Large pendulous breasts may cause pain from stretching of Cooper's ligaments. Chest wall pain from trauma, costochondritis, prior scar formation, underlying pleuritic lesions, or thoracic spine arthritis can mimic benign breast disease. Motor vehicle accident–induced breast fat necrosis from seat belt injury also masquerades as benign breast disease. Hydradenitis suppurativa can involve the breast and become evident as breast nodules and pain. Mastitis is usually acute and presents with sudden onset of pain with systemic symptoms of inflammation and local signs of tenderness, induration, and erythema. Gall bladder disease or ischemic heart disease may become evident as intermittent chest pain attributed to the breast.

Clinical Evaluation

The history documents the nature of the pain and its relationship with cyclic menses, the timing of onset of breast lumps and their subsequent course, and all prior treatments. Determination of risk factors for breast cancer involves establishing the age of onset of menarche, first pregnancy, and menopause; the degree and rate of progression of obesity; the amount of alcohol intake; and the number and ages of family members with breast cancer. During the perimenopausal transition, breast symptoms may fluctuate in parallel with the intermittent secretion of estradiol. Consequently, women in their 40s and early 50s should be questioned regarding irregularity of menses and intermittent vasomotor symptoms.

The physical examination seeks to delineate breast nodules and elicit breast discharge or localized pain. Ideally, the examination is performed when the breasts are least stimulated—7 to 9 days after the onset of menses. The four breast quadrants, the subareolar area, and the axilla are systematically examined with the patient in the lying and sitting positions. With fibrocystic changes the breasts may have a doughy consistency but lack well-defined, palpable lesions. Fibroadenomas are usually discrete and firm with distinctly marginated borders. Hyperplastic areas or cysts may also be discrete and mimic the findings expected with small malignant lesions. Suspicious

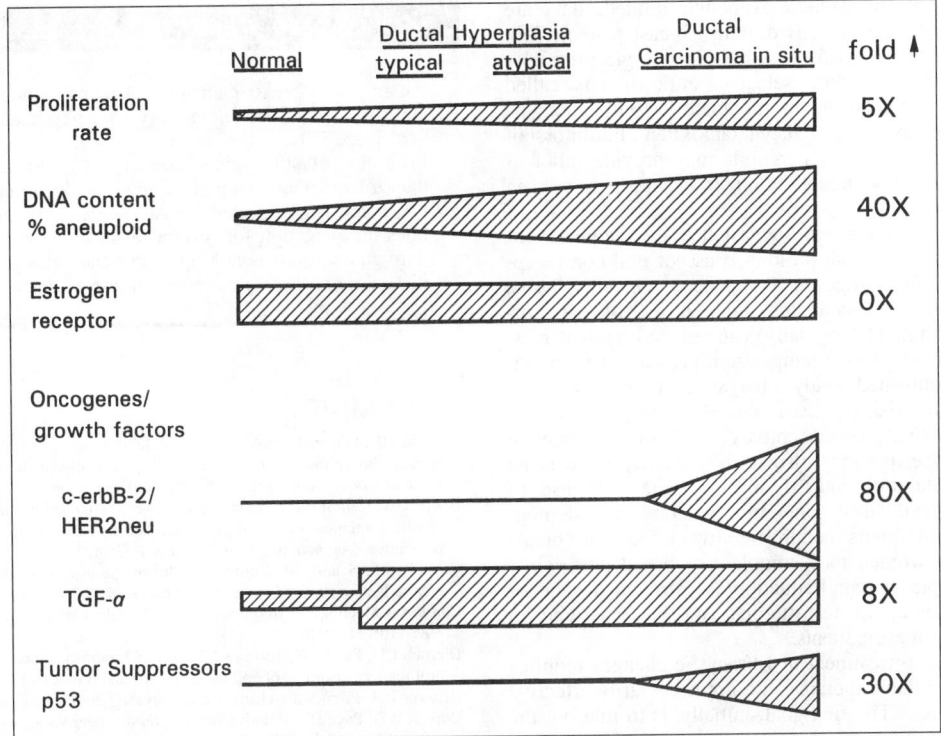

FIGURE 302-4 Progression from a benign to a malignant lesion probably represents the accumulation of an increasing number of genetic mutations. The proliferation rate increases fivefold when comparing benign breast tissue with carcinoma in situ. The DNA content, as represented by aneuploidy (i.e., DNA with greater or less DNA than expected for the presence of 46 chromosomes) increases 40-fold between normal breast tissue and carcinoma in situ. Estrogen receptor does not appear to change greatly. The oncogene TGF-α increases concomitantly with the appearance of hyperplasia. The oncogene c-erb b-2/HER2neu and mutations of the tumor suppressor p53 increase only in ductal carcinoma in situ.

areas can be marked with a BB and tape to correlate with mammographic changes. The axillae should be examined carefully for the presence of suspicious enlargement of solitary or multiple nodes. Uncommonly, breast cancer can be detected by axillary node involvement in the absence of palpable or radiographic abnormality in the breast.

Diagnostic Studies

Mammography is useful for evaluation of suspected palpable lesions in patients that come to medical attention with a history suggestive of benign breast disease. Women in their 20s to early 50s have benign breast disease in the presence of palpable lesions nearly 10 times more frequently than neoplasms. Consequently, the goal of mammography is to provide reassurance to the patient and physician that the risk of neoplasm is low. Round, dense lesions on mammography often represent cystic fluid. Ultrasonography in conjunction with mammography allows discrimination of solid from cystic lesions. Needle aspiration under ultrasound guidance further documents the cystic nature of the lesion. Microcalcifications may suggest cancer, particularly when small, numerous, clustered, and variously shaped. Repeat mammography in 6 months is recommended if the risk of cancer is thought to be less than 2%. If the risk is believed to be greater, core biopsy is recommended. Radiographically directed core biopsy provides highly discriminative information regarding the presence or absence of malignancy. If this technique is not available, insertion of a wire into the lesion or radiographic examination followed by surgical excision or merely removal of clearly palpable lesions is appropriate. The exact role of magnetic resonance imaging (MRI) in evaluating breast lesions is currently being determined and digital mammography appears promising for evaluation of dense breasts. Ideally a team including a radiologist experienced in mammography, ultrasound, and core needle biopsy, as well as a surgeon with expertise in breast cancer, should be involved in the evaluation of patients with suspected breast malignancy.

TREATMENT
Fibrocystic Changes

Therapeutic choices for symptomatic fibrocystic changes exist but generally lack validation based on definitive, randomized, controlled clinical trials. Avoidance of caffeine has been proposed as a specific means of controlling breast pain. Support for this approach has been conflicting, with the majority of double-blind studies showing no benefit. On the other hand, case control studies suggest that individuals ingesting caffeine have a higher prevalence of fibrocystic breast changes than women not ingesting caffeine. Experienced clinicians believe that patients may benefit from limiting caffeine as well as tobacco. This therapeutic approach, often recommended to patients, is not detrimental and could be beneficial. Vitamin E has also been used as a therapeutic measure to relieve pain. Data demonstrating the efficacy of this approach are also conflicting, but advocates recommend doses of 400 IU twice daily as a means of reducing breast pain. Clinical trials demonstrate the benefit of linoleic acid given in the form of evening oil of primrose capsules, 500-1000 mg three times daily.

Hormonal therapies are based on the rationale that proliferation of breast tissue depends on hormonal stimuli. Danazol, an impeded androgen, lowers levels of luteinizing hormone (LH) and follicle-stimulating hormone (FSH) and, consequently, estrogen levels. In addition, the androgenic effects of danazol block the effects of estrogen on breast tissue. Doses starting with 100 mg daily with escalation to 200 mg twice daily are recommended. Double-blind studies provide evidence of efficacy for this approach with decreased pain and nodule size occurring in two thirds of patients. Common side effects include weight gain, acne, hirsutism, a sensation of bloating, and amenorrhea in more than half of women. Although limited, data are available to suggest that antiestrogens diminish breast pain in 70% of patients. This approach is based on sound physiologic principles but requires further testing. More selective antiestrogens called SERMs (selective estrogen receptor modulators) will soon be available and may be more useful thean tamoxifen. Inhibitors of prolactin such as bromocriptine or pergolide may provide relief of pain to some patients, but double-blind trials have not been consistently positive.

Observations from a decade ago suggest that the frequency of fibrocystic changes decreases with prolonged use of oral contraceptives, as a result of the progestin component. On this basis, European investigators suggested that high doses of 19 nor-progestins such as norlutate (10 mg daily) can reduce breast pain, as well as the degree of breast tissue temperature present on thermography. A recent, unconfirmed study also suggests that 19 nor-progestins can reduce the risk of breast cancer in patients receiving long-term treatment. Oral contraceptives containing moderate amounts of 19 nor-progestins may also be beneficial for the same reason, but further data are required on this issue. The use of progestins is controversial since some investigators have demonstrated proliferative and others nonproliferative effects on breast tissue. Postmenopausal women may complain of breast pain while receiving hormonal replacement. Reduction in estrogen dosage or addition of small amounts of testosterone can be beneficial in relieving breast pain in these patients.

A practical approach to treatment of fibrocystic changes requires a balanced view that available therapies are not necessarily effective but are generally not toxic. The first goal, initially, is to rule out the presence of cancer in dominant lesions using mammography, ultrasonography, and core or excisional biopsy. Recommendations include use of a soft bra and mild analgesics such as acetaminophen, nonsteroidal antiinflammatory agents, or aspirin for breast pain; mild diuretics late in the menstrual cycle for pain related to breast engorgement; and aspiration for painful cysts. With continued symptoms, avoidance of caffeine or addition of primrose oil at 500-1000 mg three times daily or vitamin E at 400 IU twice daily is reasonable, since neither are harmful and benefits, although potentially resulting from a placebo effect, may ensue. After observation for 3 months on these regimens, patients requiring danazol therapy will be apparent because of continued severe pain. With nonresponders to danazol, tamoxifen 10 mg twice daily, bromocriptine 5 mg daily, pergolide 50 µg daily, or high-dose progestins (norlutate, 5 to 10 mg daily) may be used. As pregnancy may occur during administration of tamoxifen, bromocriptine, or pergolide, patients should be advised to use barrier contraception. Careful diaries correlating severity of pain with phase of the menstrual cycle aid in assessment of response to therapy.

Proliferative Lesions

Treatment of proliferative lesions with and without atypia is similar to that of fibrocystic changes. The increased risk of breast cancer imparted by the presence of hyperplasia requires yearly mammographic follow-up and greater attention to breast self examination. In postmenopausal women with proliferative lesions the question of breast cancer risk from hormone replacement therapy arises. Some studies showed no increased risk. Others suggested that after 10 years of estrogen replacement, in one additional woman in 100, breast cancer will develop as a result of taking estrogens. Data in women with proliferative breast disease suggest no incremental risk beyond that imparted by the lesion itself. For this reason, many experts believe that estrogen replacement therapy is not contraindicated in postmenopausal women with proliferative breast lesions.

The presence of bloody discharge with or without associated nodules suggests intraductal papillomatosis. Contrast galactography with insertion of dye into the appropriate duct at the nipple allows demonstration of space-occupying lesions in the duct. If present, surgical exploration allows removal and cessation of discharge. Galactorrhea, on the other hand, requires measurement of plasma prolactin and evaluation of the cause of hyperprolactinemia if present.

✔ **WHEN TO REFER**

Patients with breast pain without palpable nodules are appropriately managed by their primary care physicians. Referral should take place if continued pain is present on stopping caffeine and institution of other minor measures. Consideration of the use of danazol or other major measures should initiate a referral. The presence of a suspected breast nodule on mammography constitutes an indication for referral to a team experienced in core or wire-guided excisional biopsy. Presence of a palpable breast nodule with a negative mammogram also warrants referral.

BIBLIOGRAPHY

Berardo MD, O'Connell P, Allred DC: Biological characteristics of premalignant and pre-invasive breast disease. In Pasqualini JR, Katzenellenbogen BS, editors: *Hormone dependent cancer,* New York, 1996, Marcel Dekker, pp. 1-23.

Boone CW, Kelloff GJ, Freedman LS: Intraepithelial and postinvasive neoplasia as a stochastic continuum of clonal evolution, and its relationship to mechanisms of chemopreventive drug action, *J Cell Biochem* 17G:14, 1993.

Connolly JL, Schnitt SJ: Clinical and histologic aspects of proliferative and nonproliferative benign breast disease, *J Cell Biochem* 17G:45, 1993.

Consensus Meeting: Is "fibrocystic disease" of the breast precancerous? *Arch Pathol Lab Med* 110:171, 1986.

Dietrich CU, Pandis N, Teixeira MR et al: Chromosome abnormalities in benign hyperproliferative disorders of epithelial and stromal breast tissue, *Int J Cancer* 60:49, 1995.

Drukker BH: Fibrocystic change of the breast, *Clin Obset Gynecol* 37(4):903, 1994.

Dupont WD, Page DL: Relative risk of breast cancer varies with time since diagnosis of atypical hyperplasia, *Hum Pathol* 20(8):723, 1989.

Dupont WD, Page DL, Parl FF et al: Long-term risk of breast cancer in women with fibroadenoma, *N Engl J Med* 331(1):10, 1994.

Dupont WD, Page DL, Rogers LW, Parl FF: Influence of exogenous estrogens, proliferative breast disease, and other variables on breast cancer risk, *Cancer* 63:948, 1989.

Eskin BA, Grotkowski CE, Connolly CP, Ghent WR: Different tissue responses for iodine and iodide in rat thyroid and mammary glands, *Biol Trace Elem Res* 49:1, 1995.

Fiorica JV: Fibrocystic changes, *Obstet Gynecol Clin North Am* 21(3):445, 1994.

Ghent WR, Eskin BA, Low DA, Hill LP: Iodine replacement in fibrocystic disease of the breast, *Can J Surg* 36(5):453, 1993.

London SJ, Connoly JL, Schnitt SJ, Colditz GA: A prospective study of benign breast disease and the risk of breast cancer, *JAMA* 267(7):941, 1992.

Micale MA, Visscher DW, Gulino SE, Wolman SR: Chromosomal aneuploidy in proliferative breast disease, *Hum Pathol* 25:29, 1994.

O'Connell P, Pekkel V, Fuqua S et al: Molecular genetic studies of early breast cancer evolution, *Breast Cancer Res Treat* 32:5, 1994.

Page DL, Dupont WD: Anatomic markers of human premalignancy and risk of breast cancer, *Cancer* 66:1326, 1990.

Plu-Bureau G, Le MG, Sitruk-Ware R et al: Progestogen use and decreased risk of breast cancer in a cohort study of premenopausal women with benign breast disease, *Br J Cancer* 70:270, 1994.

Potten CS, Watson RJ, Williams GT et al: The effect of age and menstrual cycle upon proliferative activity of the normal human breast, *Br J Cancer* 58:163, 1988.

Slovak ML, Wolman SR: Breast cancer cytogenetics: clues to genetic complexity of the disease, *Breast J* 2(2):124, 1996.

CHAPTER

303 Diabetes Mellitus

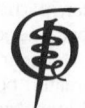

Alan J. Garber

Diabetes mellitus is a disease complex characterized primarily by relative or absolute insufficiency of insulin secretion and concomitant insensitivity or resistance to the metabolic action of insulin on target tissues. Hyperglycemia results as a consequence of the defects in insulin secretion and action. Ultimately, in the diabetic process, there may be widespread involvement of virtually every organ system. This involvement is characterized by microvascular disease with capillary basement membrane thickening, macrovascular disease with accelerated atherosclerosis, neuropathy involving both the somatic and autonomic nervous systems, neuromuscular dysfunction with muscle wasting, embryopathy, and decreased resistance to infection. Hyperglycemia may be undetected before the development of such chronic complications of diabetes mellitus as nephropathy, retinopathy, myocardial infarction, or gangrene of the lower extremities.

Although diabetes mellitus was recognized as a clinical entity 2000 to 3000 years ago, clearly effective long-term treatment was unavailable until insulin was extracted from pancreatic tissues in 1921 by Banting and Best. Since the development of crystalline insulin, refinements in therapy have sought to make use of the improvements in insulin pharmacology that have resulted from complexing insulin with other proteins such as protamine or from producing crystalline zinc precipitates of insulin. Research based on the hypoglycemic effects of sulfonamide antibiotic derivatives has resulted in a class of orally administered hypoglycemic agents, the sulfonylureas. These drugs are useful in the treatment of diabetic patients who secrete inadequate amounts of endogenous insulin. Despite the clinical availability of insulin since the mid-1920s, patients have continued to die of diabetes mellitus and its complications. In contrast to the situation in the preinsulin era, patients may now easily survive multiple episodes of diabetic ketoacidosis or hyperosmolar nonketotic coma only to succumb slowly to the chronic complications of diabetes mellitus.

Diabetes mellitus is the fourth leading cause of death by disease in the United States and the leading cause of irreversible blindness and chronic renal failure. The estimated prevalence ranges from 3% to 10% of the population, and it is increasing at a rapid rate within the United States. Accelerated atherosclerosis produces 80% of all diabetic mortality, three fourths of it owing to coronary disease. The socioeconomic impact of diabetes is devastating to individual patients and society as a whole. Although inheritance and obesity are major risk factors for the development of diabetes mellitus, particularly the type 2 non–insulin-dependent form, the disease is found throughout the world and is seemingly independent of the carbohydrate content of the local diet.

PHYSIOLOGY
Regulation of Human Carbohydrate and Fuel Metabolism

In the resting or postprandial state, normal humans have an absolute requirement for approximately 180 g of carbohydrate per day to meet the energy requirements of the central nervous system and other tissues, such as erythrocytes, which are devoid of mitochondrial oxidative metabolism. This daily requirement is usually met by the ingestion of foodstuffs containing at least this quantity of carbohydrate. Increased glucose concentrations after eating stimulate pancreatic beta-cell insulin secretion while simultaneously reducing pancreatic alpha-cell glucagon secretion. These changes are amplified by the simultaneous secretion of enteric hormones that augment the insulin response to orally ingested glucose. The ingested carbohydrate is taken up by the liver and is also passed through to peripheral tissues for subsequent utilization. Initially, glucose is phosphorylated and stored in the form of hepatic glycogen, which may contain as much as 125 g of glucose (Fig. 303-1). Glycogen synthesis in the liver is stimulated by insulin activation of hepatic glycogen synthetase activity as well as by a possible inhibition of phosphorylase activity. This activity is reinforced by the declining glucagon level. The increased insulin and decreased glucagon concentrations combine to increase the rate of flux in the pathway of anaerobic glycolysis in the liver by activating key enzymes of glycolysis. By these mechanisms, glucose, once phosphorylated as glucose 6-phosphate, may be stored as glycogen and also may be catabolized to the important three-carbon pyruvate within the liver.

When the sites available for further glycogen synthesis have been saturated, excess carbohydrate in the liver can then be transformed and subsequently stored in the form of fatty acids. The increased insulin and decreased glucagon concentrations provide an activation of pyruvate dehydrogenase. This substance, combined with pyruvate carboxylation to form oxalacetate, supplies both substrates required for net citrate formation. The large quantities of reducing equivalents gen-

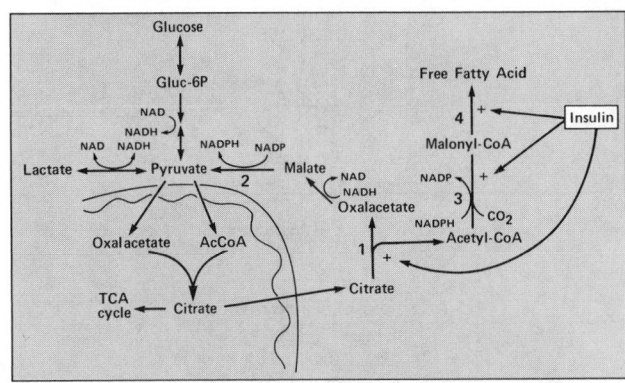

FIGURE 303-1 Mitochondrial-cytosolic interactions for lipogenesis and gluconeogenesis. *1,* Citrate cleavage enzyme; *2,* malic enzyme; *3,* acetyl coenzyme A carboxylase; *4,* fatty acid synthetase.

erated by glycolysis at the level of glyceraldehyde-3-phosphate dehydrogenase are transported within the inner mitochondrial membrane and tend to shift the oxidation reduction potential of the mitochondria to a more reduced state.

In the absence of substantial energy demands, adenosine triphosphate (ATP) levels remain high, and reduced nicotinamide-adenine dinucleotide (NADH) levels relative to NAD levels are also elevated. For these reasons, citrate oxidation and forward flow of the citric acid cycle are inhibited, most notably at isocitrate dehydrogenase (Fig. 303-1). Citrate efflux from the mitochondria occurs, and hydrolytic cleavage catalyzed by citric cleavage enzyme produces acetyl coenzyme A (acetyl CoA) and oxalacetate. Insulin induces fatty acid synthetase and acetyl CoA carboxylase activities. Acetyl CoA is carboxylated to form malonyl-coenzyme A (malonyl CoA), which is the first committed substrate for fatty acid synthesis and is also a key intermediate that inhibits fatty acid oxidation in liver. This regulation of fatty acid oxidation results from the potent inhibition by malonyl CoA of carnitine acetyltransferase I activity in the liver mitochondrial membrane. As a result, synthesized fatty acids cannot reenter the mitochondria for subsequent degradation via the beta oxidation sequence. By these mechanisms, fatty acid accumulation follows the ingestion of large quantities of carbohydrate. These fatty acids are esterified to form triglycerides and are subsequently exported from the liver as very-low-density lipoprotein (VLDL) particles. Owing to the activation by insulin of peripheral lipoprotein lipase activity in the capillary vasculature surrounding adipose tissue, the secreted VLDL particles are hydrolyzed. The fatty acids are taken up by human adipose tissue and subsequently reesterified and stored as triglycerides. Insulin facilitates the latter process (1) by increasing glucose transport and glycolysis in the adipocyte, thereby increasing alpha-glycerolphosphate availability for triglyceride synthesis, and (2) by an antagonism of cyclic adenosine monophosphate (cAMP)–mediated processes of triglyceride hydrolysis.

Metabolic Fate of Ingested Protein

Ingestion of a pure protein meal produces an amino acidemia that stimulates the secretion of both glucagon and insulin. The increased glucagon concentration stimulates amino acid utilization by the liver, primarily to supply substrate for hepatic gluconeogenesis. Many amino acids are catabolized wholly or in part to compounds that ultimately form oxalacetate, aspartate, or malate. Oxalacetate is the substrate for phosphoenolpyruvate carboxykinase, a key gluconeogenic enzyme (Fig. 303-2). Amino acid carbon skeletons forming pyruvate require the enzymatic action of pyruvate carboxylase to synthesize oxalacetate. Glucagon induces the synthesis of phosphoenolpyruvate carboxykinase messenger RNA. Glucagon also stimulates the gluconeogenic enzyme fructose-1,6-diphosphatase activity.

After protein feeding, insulin also stimulates amino acid uptake and protein synthesis in peripheral tissues. Amino acids taken up by the liver are used for hepatic protein synthesis as well as for hepatic

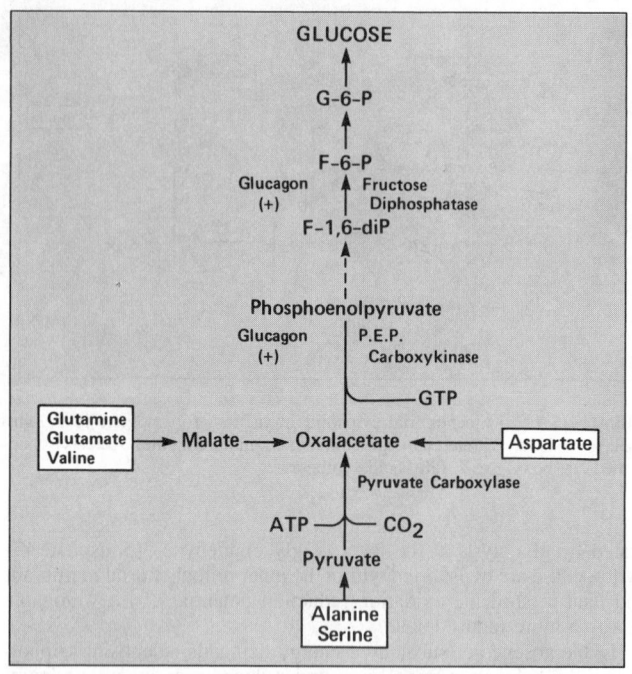

FIGURE 303-2 Hepatic gluconeogenesis in humans.

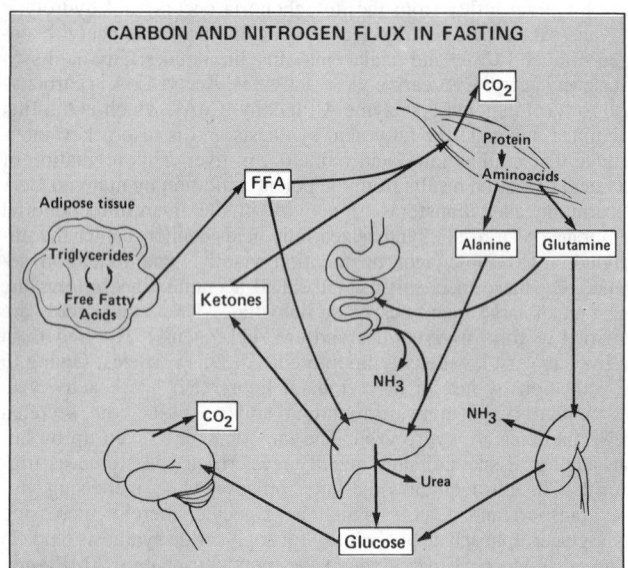

FIGURE 303-3 Organ-organ interactions for glucose homeostasis during fasting.

gluconeogenesis. The latter is critical in the absence of adequate carbohydrate intake.

Glucose Homeostasis During Fasting

Because the liver stores only about 100 to 125 g of glucose as glycogen, maintenance of circulating glucose concentrations, even after an overnight fast, must depend on gluconeogenesis (Fig. 303-3). Lactate is the principal precursor for hepatic gluconeogenesis in humans, generating approximately 50 g/day of glucose. Lactic acid must be recycled to glucose within the liver, or lactic acidosis will ensue. This cyclic pathway is called the *Cori cycle.*

To meet the continuing loss of glucose carbon during fasting or in periods of carbohydrate deprivation, which is oxidized to carbon dioxide in the central nervous system, large quantities of carbon from

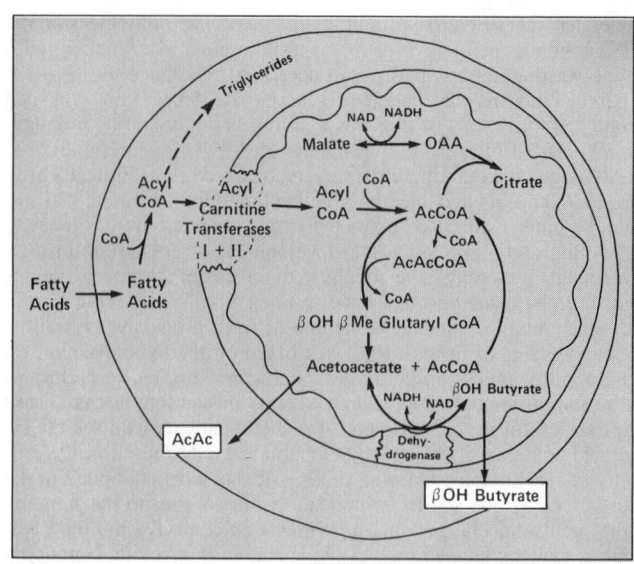

FIGURE 303-4 Hepatic ketogenesis.

nonglucose sources must be mobilized and converted to glucose. Some of this requirement may be supplied by recycling of glucose-derived glycerol, which is liberated by triglyceride hydrolysis in adipose tissue. However, only amino acids derived from protein may provide the bulk of the precursor requirement for hepatic glucose production because a net synthesis of carbohydrate cannot be supported by fat oxidation. Of all amino acids studied, only alanine is taken up significantly by the liver. Indeed, the utilization of alanine is second only to the uptake and utilization of lactate by the liver. The source of this alanine is muscle. Alanine and glutamine synthesized largely from other amino acids account for the bulk of amino acid carbon released from skeletal muscle (Fig. 303-3). The amino acid precursors are liberated by the degradation of skeletal muscle proteins. Muscle protein homeostasis is modulated in part by insulin, which facilitates muscle protein synthesis and retards muscle protein degradation. Glutamine released from skeletal muscle is oxidized in the small intestinal mucosa leading in part to a net formation of alanine and lactate. Both these compounds are released into the portal venous circulation as fuels for subsequent hepatic glucose production. Muscle protein mass may be preferentially mobilized and delivered as gluconeogenic precursors to the liver for maintenance of hepatic glucose production in the fasting state (Fig. 303-3).

Regulation of Hepatic Ketogenesis

Despite the availability of relatively large quantities of muscle protein, the obligate glucose need would require that more than 1 kg of muscle/day be degraded to meet the glucose requirement of fasting. Because the skeletal muscle mass accounts for 40% to 50% of body weight, it is apparent that no more than 10 days of starvation could be endured before substantial impairment of muscle function would occur from muscle wastage (Fig. 303-3). To meet the energy requirements of the central nervous system during starvation without impaired muscle function, alternative fuels are utilized. Because the bulk of excess ingested calories are stored as triglycerides, fatty acids become a primary source of energy for most tissues under conditions of starvation. Thus skeletal muscle, heart, liver, and most other tissues sharply increase their metabolism of fatty acids for energy production. The central nervous system, however, is unable to oxidize large quantities of free fatty acids. Instead, keto acids are used.

During fasting, rapid rates of hepatic fatty acid oxidation are accompanied by high glucagon and low insulin levels, which increase hepatic mitochondrial carnitine acyltransferase activity owing to a marked diminution of malonyl-CoA concentrations in the fasted state (Fig. 303-4). At the same time, mitochondrial oxalacetate also may be depleted by hepatic gluconeogenesis (removal by phosphoenolpyruvate carboxykinase) (Fig. 303-2). Acetyl-CoA accumulation oc-

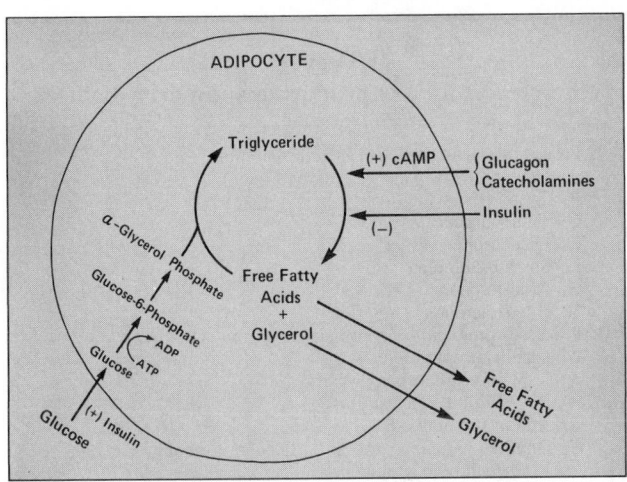

FIGURE 303-5   Triglyceride turnover in the adipocyte.

curs because the compound cannot be cleared by condensation with oxalacetate to form citrate. Disposal of the accumulated, excess hepatic acetyl-CoA occurs via condensation to form beta-hydroxy beta-methylglutaryl CoA, which is subsequently cleaved to form acetoacetate and acetyl CoA (Fig. 303-4). Acetoacetate is secondarily reduced by β-hydroxybutyrate dehydrogenase to form its hydroxy analog, β-hydroxybutyrate. These two compounds are referred to jointly as *ketone bodies* or *keto acids*.

During fasting, rates of hepatic ketogenesis increase rapidly, and keto acids accumulate in blood, to concentrations of 3 to 5 mM. Because of this, ketonuria develops within 48 hours in females and 72 hours in males. At concentrations of 3 mM or greater, circulating keto acids become an important and competitive substrate for central nervous system oxidative metabolism. Keto acids are utilized in the brain, heart, and skeletal muscle. Through this use of keto acids, central nervous system glucose consumption may be reduced dramatically. Thus in prolonged starvation, total glucose requirements can be decreased to between 50 and 80 g/day; muscle wastage is thereby reduced to less than 0.2 kg/day. This prevents significant muscle dysfunction during fasting.

Fatty Acid Metabolism During Fasting

Triglyceride turnover in adipose tissue is controlled by a variety of hormones and cyclic nucleotides. Storage of triglycerides is promoted by insulin, which induces lipoprotein lipase. This enzyme is necessary for triglyceride hydrolysis and to clear circulating chylomicrons and VLDL of free fatty acids, for subsequent uptake by adipose tissue. Esterification of these free fatty acids requires insulin together with availability of intracellular glucose. The adipocyte is dependent on insulin for glucose transport. Glucose-derived α-glycerophosphate is the essential substrate for fatty acid esterification (Fig. 303-5). Because of the absence of glycerol kinase in adipose tissue, reutilization of glycerol liberated by triglyceride hydrolysis does not occur.

Triglyceride hydrolysis to fatty acids is regulated by both cyclic adenosine monophosphate–dependent and –independent mechanisms. Catecholamines and, to a lesser extent, glucagon stimulate adenylyl cyclases on the plasma membrane of the adipocyte. As a consequence, both of these hormones may greatly stimulate triglyceride hydrolysis. Although cyclic AMP–associated mechanisms are important for the regulation of triglyceride hydrolysis in adipose tissue, growth hormone and cortisol also influence triglyceride breakdown in adipose tissue via noncyclic nucleotide–dependent mechanisms. Most of the antiinsulin hormones increase net free fatty acid delivery from adipose tissue so that oxidative fuel can be made available for all tissues of the body during physical or metabolic stress. In diabetes mellitus, increased triglyceride turnover and increased net triglyceride hydrolysis produce high levels of free fatty acids in blood, and these tend to accelerate rates of hepatic ketogenesis. Because blood levels of free fatty acids can increase 10- to 20-fold during periods of maxi-

mal glucagon and catecholamine stimulation, they are oxidative fuels for energy generation in peripheral tissues. Indeed, free fatty acids are so well utilized that they effectively compete with keto acids for oxidation in the citric acid cycle and thereby block the disposal of keto acids when their concentration would have otherwise been sufficient to induce rapid rates of keto acid utilization. By this competition, free fatty acids contribute significantly to the development of ketoacidosis in patients with diabetes mellitus.

Integrated Fuel Homeostasis

From the preceding discussion it can be seen that the blood glucose level is a closely regulated, finely controlled parameter. Because of the obligate requirement for glucose maintained by the central nervous system, numerous metabolic systems have been evolved and organized to maintain blood glucose levels in all circumstances.

Insulin is the major anabolic hormone regulating the metabolism of virtually all body fuels and substrates. It promotes the storage of carbohydrate, initially in the form of hepatic glycogen, as well as skeletal muscle glycogen. The latter is available primarily as an emergency fuel for skeletal muscle contraction during periods of severe hypoxia or anoxia. Insulin is also strongly anabolic for the long-term storage of fuels in the form of triglycerides, the most efficient form of fuel storage available to humans. Insulin also promotes the net synthesis of free fatty acids in liver. The free fatty acids formed from excess carbohydrate ingestion are then stored in peripheral adipose tissue. Insulin plays a primary anabolic role in skeletal muscle, as it facilitates amino acid uptake as well as protein synthesis by independent mechanisms, and it retards the degradation of skeletal muscle proteins.

Glucagon, cortisol, and catecholamines are the major catabolic hormones in humans. The importance of glucagon is focused primarily on maintenance of blood glucose concentrations during fasting or periods of inadequate carbohydrate intake. To reduce the total body requirement for glucose, glucagon facilitates hepatic ketogenesis so that an alternative fuel, namely keto acids, may be produced for central nervous system energy requirements. Glucagon does not play a major role in the mobilization of substrates from peripheral tissue for subsequent metabolism in the liver. Glucagon is without effect on the mobilization of skeletal muscle proteins, which provide the ultimate carbon source for the bulk of glucose formed from amino acids during short-term starvation. Furthermore, glucagon plays only a secondary role in the regulation of triglyceride hydrolysis and free fatty acid mobilization from adipose tissue. In these peripheral tissues, a combination of high glucagon and especially low insulin levels appears to make available the amino acid and free fatty acid substrates for hepatic metabolism. Reinforcement of these effects of glucagon by catecholamines occurs in adipose tissue and by cortisol in both skeletal muscle and adipose tissue.

CLASSIFICATION

Over the years, a variety of classifications and diagnostic criteria for diabetes mellitus have been proposed. Although diabetes mellitus is primarily a disease of inadequate insulin secretion and action, measurements of abnormal insulin action in terms of serum or blood glucose are used almost exclusively to diagnose diabetes mellitus. In most formulations, basal euglycemia in the fasting state and an unimpaired ability to dispose of a carbohydrate load have been most widely used to assess the presence or absence of diabetes. Conditions other than diabetes mellitus also are associated with abnormal carbohydrate metabolism, carbohydrate intolerance, and even fasting hyperglycemia. A recent attempt has been made to resolve these differences and to organize the available clinical data to provide a scientific basis for interpretations of fasting serum or plasma glucose concentrations and also of serum glucose responses during glucose tolerance tests. Three major types of patients with diabetes mellitus are now recognized.

Type 1 Diabetes Mellitus

Patients with type 1 diabetes mellitus have little or no endogenous insulin secretion. The onset of the disease is usually clinically abrupt, with marked polyuria, polydipsia, polyphagia, weight loss, and fatigue. These patients are highly prone to ketosis and frequently may present themselves for treatment in an initial episode of diabetic ketoacidosis. In other classifications, this form was termed *juvenile-onset diabetes mellitus,* or *ketosis-prone diabetes mellitus.* These patients generally have lost weight and are frequently at or below ideal body weight. As a result, there is marked sensitivity or brittleness to exogenous insulin administration, particularly with regular insulin.

This form of diabetes mellitus can occur at any age. Incidence most commonly peaks in the middle of the first decade and again at the time of the growth acceleration of adolescence. A prodromal phase of polyuria, polydipsia, and weight loss may precede the development of ketoacidosis by a period of days to months, but it most commonly is noted for only 2 to 4 weeks before onset of ketoacidosis. As with all other forms of primary diabetes mellitus, a genetic predisposition appears to underlie the pathogenesis of type 1 diabetes mellitus, although the family history is less strongly associated than in type 2. Patients with type 1 disease have in common one of several human leukocyte antigen histocompatibility antigens (e.g., B8, B15, DW3, DW4), and islet cell antibodies, especially one directed against glutamic acid decarboxylase (GAD) frequently observed before or at the time of diagnosis. A viral etiology involving one of several enteroviruses such as coxsackievirus B_4 and mumps has been proposed in these patients. Recently, evidence has been developed to suggest that an ongoing, autoimmune T-cell–mediated destruction of pancreatic beta cells may underlie type 1 diabetes mellitus. Clinical trials with immunosuppressive medications or with low-dose insulin have demonstrated some efficacy in prolonging the honeymoon phase of type 1 diabetes and in arresting the loss of residual insulin secretion in newly diagnosed patients. A brief period of early, aggressive glucose control, as with a biostator, may prolong residual, endogenous insulin secretory capacity and improve long-term glucose control in newly diagnosed patients.

Type 2 Diabetes Mellitus

Patients with type 2 diabetes mellitus maintain some endogenous insulin secretory capability, despite the overt abnormalities of glucose homeostasis, including fasting hyperglycemia and/or carbohydrate intolerance. Unlike type 1 patients, patients with type 2 diabetes mellitus are relatively resistant to the development of ketosis in the basal state because of the retention of endogenous insulin secretory capabilities. These patients generally demonstrate marked resistance or insensitivity to the metabolic actions of endogenous as well as exogenous insulin, in part as the result of decreased insulin receptors. A failure of postreceptor coupling and of intracellular insulin action is a more important cause of insulin resistance. In offspring of type 2 patients, insulin resistance appears inherited and is present at maturity. This resistance may also be the best predictor of a future diabetic state. A syndrome of insulin resistance (syndrome X) has been proposed to explain the frequent association of hypertension, hyperuricemia, carbohydrate intolerance, abdominal obesity, dyslipidemia, and accelerated atherosclerosis. Mild to marked obesity is present in approximately 80% of type 2 diabetic patients at the time of diagnosis. Obesity is a major risk factor for the development of this type of diabetes mellitus, owing in part to the associated insulin resistance. Nevertheless, it is clear that a primary insufficiency of insulin secretion is the pathologic essential for the clinical development of type 2 diabetes mellitus.

Although there can be limitations on insulin secretory capacity in type 2 diabetes, together with the presence of insulin insensitivity, these patients do not have an absolute dependence on injectable insulin for their survival. The clinical presentation of patients with type 2 disease varies greatly. These patients may manifest diabetes only after the development of complications such as retinopathy or nephropathy. On the other hand, type 2 patients may also seek treatment because of significant polyuria, polydipsia, easy fatigability, and irritability. In patients having one or more of the chronic complications of diabetes, marked abnormalities of carbohydrate metabolism are generally not observed, and these patients may even have normal fasting glucose levels. The frequency of vascular complications in diabetes is also amplified synergistically by common comorbid illnesses such as hypertension and dyslipidemia.

Most patients with type 2 diabetes mellitus are diagnosed after the

---

BOX 303-1
Pathologic processes producing secondary diabetes

I. Processes causing reduced insulin secretion
   A. Pancreatitis or pancreatectomy
   B. Cystic fibrosis
   C. Hemochromatosis
   D. Pheochromocytoma
   E. Somatostatinoma
   F. Aldosteronoma
   G. Hypokalemia
II. Processes producing impairment of insulin action
   A. Insulin receptor defects
      1. With acanthosis nigricans
      2. Insulin receptor antibodies
   B. Antiinsulin antibodies
   C. Diseases producing excess antiinsulin hormones
      1. Pheochromocytoma
      2. Cushing's syndrome
      3. Acromegaly
      4. Glucagonoma
      5. Thyrotoxicosis
III. Diseases producing secondary diabetes by unknown mechanisms
   A. Muscular dystrophies
   B. Myotonic dystrophy
   C. Acute intermittent porphyria
   D. Glycogen storage disease, type I
   E. Hyperlipidemia
   F. Friedreich's ataxia
   G. Laurence-Moon-Biedl syndrome
   H. Syndrome of progeria
   I. Prader-Willi syndrome
   J. Chromosomal aberrations
      1. Klinefelter's syndrome
      2. Turner's syndrome
      3. Down syndrome
   K. Sexual ateliotic dwarfism

---

age of 40 years. This form of diabetes often is called *adult-onset* or *ketosis-resistant diabetes mellitus.* Nevertheless, the onset of type 2 diabetes mellitus, including the so-called maturity-onset diabetes mellitus of the young (MODY), can occur at any age. Most forms of type 2 disease show strong heritable influences in their transmission. In MODY, an autosomal dominant inheritance of an abnormal glucokinase has been established. In other forms of type 2 diabetes mellitus, the mode of transmission is less clear; however, a dominant inheritance is suspected. Nevertheless, because of the relationship between preexisting obesity and the development of type 2 disease, environmental influences clearly play a strong role in the development of the disease.

Secondary Diabetes Mellitus

Secondary diabetes mellitus is a category that constitutes a heterogeneous grouping of patients for whom a designation of either of the traditional forms of diabetes mellitus appears inappropriate. Although abnormal glucose metabolism may be demonstrated by fasting hyperglycemia or an impaired ability to dispose of a carbohydrate load, genetically determined inadequacies of insulin secretion or action are not the primary pathogenic abnormality in secondary diabetes. The age of onset and clinical presentation may vary according to the etiology of the secondary diabetes. In general, any disease producing an impairment of insulin secretion or resulting in antagonism to insulin action can be associated with secondary diabetes mellitus. These primary diseases may include endocrine pancreatic insufficiency following chronic recurrent pancreatitis or cystic fibrosis. Other diseases, such as acanthosis nigricans, may be associated with antibodies to the insulin receptor. These may block the metabolic actions of insulin and therefore produce marked insulin resistance and secondary diabetes mellitus (Box 303-1).

A large number of diseases may interfere with the metabolic ac-

BOX 303-2
Drugs producing impaired glucose tolerance and/or hyperglycemia

Diuretics and antihypertensive agents
Thiazide diuretics
Clonidine
Furosemide

Agents with hormonal activity
Glucocorticoids
Oral contraceptives
Thyroid hormone
Progestins

Neuroactive agents
Haloperidol
Lithium carbonate
Phenothiazines
Tricyclics
Adrenergic agonists

Antiinflammatory agents
Indomethacin

Miscellaneous
Isoniazid
Nicotinic acid
Cimetidine
Heparin

tions of insulin at the post–insulin-receptor level. These diseases include endocrinopathies such as acromegaly, glucagonoma, Cushing's syndrome, pheochromocytoma, and thyrotoxicosis. In addition, carbohydrate intolerance and fasting hyperglycemia have been observed in a variety of metabolic disorders, such as the muscular dystrophies, glycogen storage disease (type I), and lipoatrophic diabetes mellitus, and in several chromosomal diseases such as Klinefelter's and Down syndromes. A variety of drugs also has been associated with carbohydrate intolerance and secondary diabetes mellitus. Some diuretics and antihypertensives such as diazoxide have direct antagonistic effects on endogenous insulin secretion, whereas others produce hypokalemia, which reduces insulin output. Neuroactive agents such as phenytoin, lithium carbonate, and tricyclic antidepressants also can impair glucose tolerance. A more complete listing of drugs that induce secondary diabetes mellitus is provided in Box 303-2.

Diagnostic Criteria for Diabetes Mellitus

In most normal subjects mean fasting serum glucose concentrations of approximately 80 mg/dl with a maximal increase in the postprandial state to approximately 140 mg/dl are routinely observed. However, considerable variability among individuals has been observed in large-scale patient population studies. There also may be considerable variation in group mean data for fasting circulating glucose concentrations between ethnic groups such as the Pima Indians as compared with white Americans. Individual variations may reflect the influence of age and metabolic and hormonal states, which can profoundly influence fasting glucose concentrations in otherwise normal subjects. Physical or emotional stress, infection, undernutrition, bed rest, and trauma are some of the more common causes of transient carbohydrate intolerance. Marked variation among multiple glucose tolerance tests on the same individual has been observed without subsequent deterioration of fasting glucose levels. For this reason, fasting hyperglycemia or abnormal carbohydrate tolerance should be reproducible on two or more occasions before the diagnosis of diabetes mellitus or impaired carbohydrate metabolism is made.

Because of the complexity of glucose tolerance testing and the variability encountered among tests, glucose tolerance testing is not advisable as a routine screening measure for diabetes mellitus unless there is a reason to establish this diagnosis. Standardization of glucose tolerance tests seems essential for their interpretation. In an otherwise healthy, unstressed ambulatory patient, at least 3 days of a relatively high carbohydrate diet (a minimum of 150 g of carbohydrate per day) are required for study of normal insulin secretory dynamics. The glucose tolerance test should always be performed in the morning, after 10 to 12 hours of overnight fasting, and the patient should refrain from significant caffeine or nicotine use during this period. A load of 75 g of glucose or of rapidly absorbed dextrins (e.g., Glucola) should be ingested and plasma glucoses determined at 0, 0.5, 1.0, 1.5, and 2.0 hours after initiation of the test.

There are two major reasons to perform glucose tolerance tests. First, patients with multiple borderline fasting serum glucose levels (110-125 mg/dl) should be evaluated further with glucose tolerance tests to establish the degree of hyperglycemia. Second, patients with symptoms that may be clearly related to diabetes mellitus, or those with overt disease that may be a complication of diabetes mellitus (e.g., an otherwise unexplainable neuropathy) must have the possible diagnosis of abnormal carbohydrate metabolism clearly established or refuted. In the latter group, a complete workup for other causes of symptoms or disease consistent with diabetes mellitus also should be initiated. A second glucose tolerance test may be necessary to establish firmly the diagnosis of diabetes mellitus in these patients.

The 2-hour postprandial glucose level is of questionable value as a screening test for diabetes mellitus. The quantity of carbohydrate ingested, the other constituents of the meal, and the prior nutritional state of the patient may all combine to produce a false-negative, as well as false-positive, result. Such an outcome usually is not acceptable for any screening test. For these reasons, glucose tolerance screening is better performed by measuring a 2-hour sample after proper preparation and a defined glucose load.

Specific Diagnostic Criteria. The diagnosis of diabetes mellitus is made by a reproducible demonstration of fasting hyperglycemia. Fasting serum glucose levels of 126 mg/dl or greater on two or more occasions are diagnostic of diabetes mellitus in the adult, and this finding obviates the need for a glucose tolerance test in the absence of other causes of hyperglycemia. Increased certainty in the diagnosis is produced by such concomitant symptoms of classic diabetes mellitus as polyuria, polydipsia, polyphagia, weight loss, fatigue, and ketonuria. When one is testing glucose tolerance for diagnosis, a 2-hour venous plasma or serum glucose value must exceed 200 mg/dl. Other criteria have been used to evaluate and diagnose diabetes by glucose tolerance testing. However, because of the relative absence of retinal and renal microvascular complications in those patients having a 2-hour plasma glucose value less than 200 mg/dl, the less stringent criteria indicated earlier are more appropriate for the diagnosis of type II diabetes mellitus. Otherwise, a large group of patients with only abnormal carbohydrate tolerance 2-hour, >140 and ≤199 mg/dl) may be misdiagnosed as having diabetes mellitus, and they may thereby experience unnecessary difficulties with employment and insurability. Based on large population surveys, it seems that only patients with marked hyperglycemia (fasting ≥140 mg/dl and 2-hour postglucose, ≥200 mg/dl) are subject to the development of diabetic macrovascular and microvascular complications such as retinopathy and nephropathy. On the other hand, patients with less marked hyperglycemia (fasting, 110 to 125 mg/dl; postglucose peak, ≥200 and 2-hour postglucose, between 140 and 199 mg/dl), although not subject to the development of microvascular complications, do have accelerated macrovascular disease.

Impaired glucose tolerance is a functional diagnosis that represents an intermediary state in the evolution of clinical diabetes mellitus. A proportion of patients with abnormal glucose tolerance tests will progress to overt diabetes mellitus if a sufficient period of time elapses (5%/year or 30% after 10 years) or if endogenous or exogenous stress factors develop. A diagnosis of impaired or abnormal glucose tolerance assumes a fasting plasma glucose concentration of 125 mg/dl or less. If, on glucose tolerance testing, a patient has a 2-hour serum or plasma glucose level ranging between 140 and 200 mg/dl, the diagnosis of probable impaired glucose tolerance may be entertained.

Table 303-1   Criteria for diagnosis of gestational diabetes*

SAMPLE TIME	VENOUS PLASMA (MG/DL)	VENOUS WHOLE BLOOD (MG/DL)
Fasting	105	90
1-hour	190	170
2-hour	165	145
3-hour	145	125

*Values obtained from glucose tolerance testing must be equal to or greater than at least two of the values above.

Table 303-2   Recommended standards of glucose control for patients with diabetes mellitus*

INDEX	GOOD	ACCEPTABLE	FAIR	POOR
Fasting-serum (capillary)†	≤115(100)	≤140(120)	≤200(170)	>200
2-hour postprandial-serum (capillary)†	≤140(120)	≤175(150)	≤235(200)	>235
Glycosylated hemoglobin	≤6%	≤8%	≤10%	>10%

*Standards set by the American Diabetes Association and the US Department of Public Health Service, 1986.
†Each value expressed as mg/dl.

From these criteria, it can be seen that the diagnosis of diabetes mellitus and that of impaired glucose tolerance is somewhat similar. The only difference between these two diagnoses lies in the result obtained for the 2-hour sample, which ranges between 140 and 199 mg/dl for a diagnosis of impaired glucose tolerance, whereas values of 200 mg/dl or greater are diagnostic of diabetes mellitus. Of course, these results must be reproducible if either diagnosis is to be established by glucose tolerance testing alone.

Gestational Diabetes

Pregnant women with no previous history of abnormal carbohydrate metabolism may develop impaired glucose tolerance or overt diabetes mellitus during pregnancy, particularly during the third trimester of the pregnancy when substantial resistance to the metabolic actions of insulin becomes apparent. A diagnosis of gestational diabetes implies that carbohydrate metabolism was normal before pregnancy. Most patients will return to normal glucose tolerance or impaired glucose tolerance in the postpartum state. Less commonly, such patients may maintain an overt diabetic state and therefore must be reclassified as having type 2 diabetes mellitus. Because of the increased risk of perinatal fetal morbidity and mortality, it is essential to establish a diagnosis of gestational diabetes as early as possible. Because approximately one third to half of patients with gestational diabetes develop, most commonly, type 2 diabetes mellitus after 5 to 10 years, careful characterization of the diagnosis again is essential.

The incidence of gestational diabetes is approximately 1% to 2% of all pregnancies and increases with maternal age and parity. It must be suspected in any patient having glycosuria, a positive family history of diabetes mellitus, a history of unexplained stillbirth or prior abortion, a previous history of possible diabetic embryopathy, or previous congenital abnormalities. Because of the metabolic stress of pregnancy, independent values for interpretations of glucose tolerance tests are essential for the diagnosis of gestational diabetes (Table 303-1). All women should be screened with either a 2-hour glucose test after a 50-g glucose load or a 100-g oral glucose tolerance test (OGTT). Considerably lower fasting and 2-hour values must be exceeded for a diagnosis of gestational compared with type 2 diabetes mellitus. In addition, the criteria of O'Sullivan and Mahan require only that two or more of the values be met or exceeded, of the fasting and 1-, 2-, and 3-hour samples drawn after a 100-g oral glucose challenge. Because other criteria for the diagnosis of gestational diabetes are presently unavailable for evaluation, the dissimilarity between those of O'Sullivan and Mahan and the diagnostic criteria presented for nonpregnant adults must remain. Because of the improved fetal viability in mothers given adequate treatment for gestational diabetes, the diagnostic criteria shown previously must be applied carefully. A high index of suspicion must be maintained for patients with any major risk factor that may lead to a deterioration of carbohydrate tolerance in the third trimester. To avoid fetal loss, proper therapy must be established during this period.

MANAGEMENT

The two basic forms of diabetes mellitus (type 1, insulin-dependent, and type 2, non–insulin-dependent) both require intensive patient education and management by the physician; however, the patient must also assume a major proportion of responsibility for management of the disease. Education by trained professionals is essential for all newly diagnosed patients. The physician should assume the posture of a counselor or advisor who can best outline treatment modalities or options and counsel the patient regarding therapeutic decisions. It is essential that the patient actively participate in these therapeutic decisions, particularly because successful implementation of such decisions frequently is determined by the patient's sense of responsibility for treatment.

Motivational and behavioral approaches to management are especially important in adolescent diabetic patients, who may experience enormous adjustment difficulties owing to disturbances of their self-image produced by diabetes mellitus. Rebellious, defiant, and self-destructive behavior; manipulative maneuvers for secondary gain; and depressive episodes are common in the adolescent patient newly diagnosed with diabetes mellitus. However, similar psychological disturbances may occur in any patient who has been diagnosed as having insulin-dependent diabetes mellitus. In obese adults with type 2 diabetes mellitus, equally difficult, but far more subtle, problems relating to weight reduction are frequently encountered. Habitual overeating, together with a lack of appropriate physical activity, results in obesity, which the patient maintains despite strong societal and peer pressures. Therefore considerable effort must be initiated and maintained to negate the secondary gain that these patients obtain from continuing their excessive food intake. A third major area requiring a thoughtful, motivational approach is the introduction of insulin therapy to patients who object to self-injection. This problem with the acceptance of insulin therapy is compounded by the relative dietary rigidity imposed by pharmacologic preparations of insulin. Total deletion of meals or a complete revamping of dietary intake on impulse can produce disastrous acute hypoglycemic episodes or periods of profound hyperglycemia. The induction of guilt in the patient by an admonishing physician can produce counterproductive behavior that ultimately results in a vicious circle of even greater difficulty in management. As patients become increasingly frustrated and made to feel guilty by their maladaptive behavior, they may become depressed and self-destructive. As a consequence, a further deterioration in diabetic control results. An agreed on consensus for standards of diabetic control and the degree of control are shown in Table 303-2.

Other medical approaches to diet therapy, including behavioral modification, insight psychotherapy, and supportive psychotherapy, may be required to supplement the counseling and advice provided by the physician caring for the patient with diabetes mellitus. A supportive and conciliatory role on the part of the practitioner will usually prove far more rewarding than admonitions in the long-term management of the patient's diabetes.

Dietary Management

The first and essential treatment for all patients with diabetes mellitus is diet management. Diet therapy is aimed at achieving four major goals:

1. Maintenance or establishment of ideal body weight
2. Distribution of the caloric intake into many small loads taken through the widest possible interval during the day
3. Avoidance of rapidly absorbed carbohydrate loads
4. Maintenance of proper, long-term nutritional balance

In prescribing a diet, the prescription must be arrived at rationally and with the patient's understanding. Capricious estimations of patients' caloric requirements to lose or gain weight can become puni-

Table 303-3   Approximate caloric requirements to maintain body weight in adults

ACTIVITY LEVEL	CALORIES/KG/DAY
Basal (bed rest)	20-25
Sedentary (desk work)	30
Vigorous (postal worker)	35
Extraordinarily active (lumberjack)	40-50

tive and therefore are unlikely to produce desirable outcomes. For the vast majority of patients with type 2 diabetes mellitus, weight reduction is necessary. On the other hand, a minority of patients with type 2 and a majority of patients with type 1 diabetes are already at or near ideal body weight, and weight maintenance is all that is required. A minority of patients with type 1 diabetes may be substantially underweight. Such individuals show extreme sensitivity to pharmacologic injections of insulin, and this sensitivity considerably complicates the induction and maintenance of good control of blood glucose concentrations. To calculate the caloric prescription required for patients with diabetes mellitus, the patient's present body weight and an estimation of his or her customary degree of physical activity are required. Most of the calories are consumed by the basal metabolic rate, and only about 25% to 40% more calories are required in any sedentary lifestyle (Table 303-3).

Thus the 70-kg sedentary subject (e.g., office worker) consumes approximately 2100 calories per day to maintain that weight. At most, a 20% variance can be attached to this number. For this patient, a caloric prescription ranging between 1700 and 2500 calories per day should be adequate. To prevent weight gain, particularly during the initial phases of insulin administration, a diet containing slightly fewer than the calculated required number of calories is advisable. It is particularly important to emphasize to the patient the need to determine carefully the portion size during the initial phase of therapy. Most patients consistently underestimate the sizes and quantities of the foods they consume.

A more frequent consideration in the dietary prescription is the need to adjust the patient's present weight to the estimated ideal body weight. Most commonly, this requires weight reduction. Behavioral modification approaches that attempt to elucidate the underlying causes of compulsive overeating in each patient may provide good long-term results. A successful weight-reducing diet must provide a sufficiently attractive and pleasant food experience for the patients so that they can follow modified diets for the rest of their lives. This requirement cannot be met by unbalanced, markedly hypocaloric, semistarvation diets, which produce excessive ketosis and wastage of lean body mass. A weight reduction greater than 1.0 to 1.5 kg per week is usually inadvisable. An even slower rate of weight reduction is advisable for the older patient.

Because a pound of fat represents approximately 3500 calories, a 1-kg weight loss per week amounts to a caloric deficit of 1000 calories per day. Thus a 100-kg obese, active woman who eats approximately 2500 to 3000 calories per day to maintain her weight should receive a caloric prescription for not more than 1500 to 2000 calories if she is to lose 1 kg per week. Some adjustment for individual metabolic differences and overestimations of portion size may be necessary, thereby justifying an initial prescription of 1200 to 1800 calories per day. As the patient's weight and caloric expenditure decline, downward readjustment of the caloric prescription will be necessary to reflect the decreased caloric needs. For example, when the patient has reduced to 90 kg, the diet must be reduced by 250 to 300 calories to maintain the same rate of weight loss. Periodic reevaluation requires periodic downward adjustments of the caloric intake. At 70 kg, this same active woman would need to consume about 1750 to 2100 calories per day to maintain that weight. A continuing weight loss of 1 kg per week would require a caloric prescription of about 1000 calories to maintain constant weight loss. As the diet progresses, the patient becomes both more familiar with and accepting of the diet. An initial prescription of 1000 calories will not be as well tolerated by the patient because of inadequate secondary benefit from food ingestion. The slower approach substitutes secondary benefit from weight reduction and the resultant improved body image for that derived from food intake. This dietary approach requires periodic supervision and monitoring by the physician and, perhaps, by a nutritionist, of calories ingested, with considerable advice regarding the pitfalls of portion size, food tasting while preparing the family meals, and unprescribed snacks. If increased physical activity is also a component of the weight-reducing regimen, appropriate increases in caloric intake have to be considered (see also Chapter 347).

Exchange Lists. The most commonly used dietary prescriptions are obtained from the exchange lists developed by the American Diabetes Association. Although considerable variation can be produced in the caloric content per day, diets derived from these lists distribute daily calorie intake as about 20% for breakfast, 30% for lunch, 40% for dinner, and about 10% for a snack (usually given at bedtime). The diet contains approximately 15% to 20% protein, 30% to 35% fat, and 50% to 60% carbohydrate. Most of the carbohydrate is in the form of complex starches that do not produce accentuated peaks of hyperglycemia similar to those produced by equal quantities of refined sugars such as sucrose. Modifications of these diets may be made easily by moving bread, fruit, or meat exchanges from one meal to another or by substituting exchanges, as each exchange contains a known amount of calories in the form of protein, fat, or carbohydrate. A diet high in fiber should be prescribed to further reduce postprandial hyperglycemia. Although detailed dietary instruction regarding the implementation of an exchange list diet usually requires counseling from a dietitian, the physician should be familiar with the prescribed diet to counsel patients properly. Allowances should be made for ethnic food preferences and occasional off-diet food consumption.

Considerable care and forethought are required in using exchange lists. The use of these lists may not be practical for some patients because of financial, occupational, or uncommon dietary preferences. For such patients, a constant carbohydrate diet is frequently prescribed in which the amount of carbohydrate, particularly that in the form of rapidly absorbed carbohydrate, is controlled, and less attention is paid to the distribution of protein and fat. It also should be noted that for patients with hyperlipidemias secondary to poorly controlled diabetes mellitus, the American Diabetes Association diet is usually sufficient for control of types IV and V hyperlipidemia. However, modifications of the American Diabetes Association diet must be made for the less frequently occurring type IIB hyperlipidemia (Chapter 306). It must be emphasized that food consumption must be modified in accordance with gross changes in physical activity, especially for type I diabetic patients in whom, if hypoglycemic reactions are to be avoided, ingestion of concentrated carbohydrates such as candy and sweetened beverages may be needed before, during, and sometimes after strenuous exercise.

Oral Hypoglycemic Agents

Four major classes of oral hypoglycemic agents are currently available for use in patients with type 2 diabetes mellitus. The largest and only class available until recently in the United States was the sulfonylureas. During the initial phase of treatment, sulfonylureas increase the quantity of insulin secreted in response to a given glucose concentration. With prolonged use, however, additional effects of the sulfonylureas tend to maintain lower blood sugars. These effects may be at the level of tissue insulin-receptor density or of the coupling of insulin receptors to metabolic processes in target cells. Sulfonylureas may diminish hepatic glucose production and gluconeogenesis from alanine. Sulfonylureas also diminish or abolish the delayed insulin release in response to glucose noted in patients with type II diabetes. For this reason, sulfonylureas may be particularly useful in the treatment of that form of reactive hypoglycemia caused by early diabetes mellitus.

The second major class of oral antidiabetic agents are biguanides such as metformin, which exerts its antidiabetic action by mechanisms not dependent on insulin secretion. Metformin is as effective in reducing fasting blood glucose levels as a second-generation sulfonylurea. Either agent generally reduces fasting glucose level 60 to 80 mg/dl, and each may be used alone or in combination with each other, since both agents have complementary rather than overlapping mechanisms of action. Of note, metformin also acts to improve dyslipidemias. These include reductions of triglycerides by 15% to 25%, total and low-density lipoprotein (LDL) cholesterol by 8% to 10%, and modest increases in high-density lipoprotein (HDL) cholesterol. Because metformin appears to improve the apparent efficiency of insulin action, its use is generally associated with a modest decline in circulating insulin levels. Metformin usage is also associated with minimal weight gain or even with weight loss. The effect is unique to metformin and is in marked contrast to the rather substantial weight gain associated with initiation of sulfonylureas. A prospective, double-blinded, multicenter study has demonstrated synergy with regard to glycemic control when both metformin and a second-generation sulfonylurea are used in combination. Although metformin monotherapy alone is not associated with documented hypoglycemia, when used in combination with agents elevating insulin levels, such as sulfonylureas, metformin addition can be associated with hypoglycemic events as glycemic control improves.

Metformin should be taken with meals to minimize its potential for gastric irritation. One third of patients have benign, self-limited diarrhea lasting 1 to 2 weeks. Because metformin is excreted unchanged in the urine, it should not be given to azotemic patients, and its use should be discontinued when creatinines exceed 1.5 mg/dl in males and 1.4 mg/dl in females. It should be discontinued 1 to 2 days before major surgery or angiographic dye studies to eliminate any potential drug accumulation. If azotemia results from the procedure, the major toxicity of metformin is lactic acidosis. The incidence of fatal lactic acidosis with metformin is the same as or less than with sulfonylureas. In acute cardiovascular or pulmonary decompensation, both of which are also associated with lactic acidosis, metformin should be withheld until vascular or pulmonary stability is achieved.

A third class of antidiabetic oral agents is available in the United States. α-Glucosidase inhibitors such as acarbose produce significant reductions of postprandial hyperglycemia but only modest improvements in fasting hyperglycemia. Whereas metformin or sulfonylureas generally improve hemoglobin A_{1c} (HbA_{1c}) levels by approximately 1.8% to 2.0% in multicenter trials performed in the United States, acarbose improves HbA_{1c} levels by 0.7% to 0.8%. Since insulin levels decline with acarbose use, hypoglycemia is not likely with acarbose monotherapy. Acarbose can be used alone or in combination with metformin, sulfonylureas, or insulin, or in any combination of these. The incremental improvement expected from acarbose addition in a combination therapy program is a reduction in HbA_{1c} of 0.5%. The decrement is markedly less than the results of metformin addition in patients whose condition is inadequately controlled on a regimen of sulfonylureas alone in whom a HbA_{1c} reduction of 1.9% was observed.

Although acarbose itself is not absorbed, one third of an administered dose is absorbed as acarbose metabolites and these are excreted in the urine. Thus this drug should not be given to azotemic patients (creatinine level, $\geq$2.0 mg/dl). Because acarbose retards polysaccharide hydrolysis in the small bowel, these carbohydrates are presented more distally, producing bloating, distention and notable flatulence. With continued administration, these side effects improve.

A fourth class of antidiabetic agents has recently been approved: the thiazolidinediones. The first of these is troglitazone. It is most effective when used in combination with insulin or other oral agents, producing HbA reductions of 1.4% to 1.7% from baseline. It is seemingly less effective as monotherapy. Troglitazone is an insulin sensitizer, producing reductions in triglycerides and insulin levels but increasing LDL cholesterol levels and weight gain. A significant minority of patients do not respond to this agent. It is not associated with hypoglycemia or with observed long-term toxicities. The mechanism of insulin sensitization may involve the PPAR γ nuclear receptor and the slow induction of insulin-regulated enzymes, particularly in fat cells.

It now seems apparent that the management of patients with type 2 diabetes involves incremental responses beginning with pharmacologic monotherapies, much as the management of hypertension has evolved over the preceding 40 years. The choice of first-line pharmacologic management for patients failing an adequate trial of diet and exercise depends on the individual patient profile. That profile should be matched to the pharmacodynamic profile of the four major available classes of oral antidiabetic agents. For example, obese patients, dyslipidemic patients, or those prone to or fearful of hypo-glycemia might be good candidates for primary monotherapy with a biguanide such as metformin, since the latter tends to produce minimal weight gain, may improve dyslipidemias, and is not associated with documented hypoglycemia when used alone. Troglitazone may be an alternative, particularly if azotemia is present. On the other hand, patients who are not obese may harbor an underlying element of insulin insufficiency. Therefore they may be better candidates for long-term sulfonylurea therapy, since the latter is generally associated with an augmentation of insulin secretory response, and this weight gain with such therapy is often well tolerated. Regardless of the specific choice of antidiabetic agents, either sulfonylureas or metformin would be expected to lower fasting glucose levels 60 to 80 mg/dl. This is likely to be adequate for approximately 35% to 50% of the diabetic population failing diet and exercise therapy alone. The remainder may require combination therapy with both metformin and a sulfonylurea or troglitazone therapy. A combination of sulfonylureas with metformin has the capability of producing an additional 75-mg reduction in fasting hyperglycemia value or an additional HbA_{1c} reduction of 1.9%. In patients failing combinations of two agents the addition of a third oral agent—troglitazone or acarbose—may be useful. Because of patient reluctance regarding insulin therapy, multiple oral antidiabetic therapies may be preferable to combination therapies of oral agents such as sulfonylureas or metformin with insulin.

Seven major sulfonylureas are presently available in the United States for the treatment of diabetes mellitus. Of these, tolbutamide, acetohexamide, tolazamide, and chlorpropamide are so-called first-generation agents, whereas glyburide, glipizide, and glimeperide are second-generation agents. The principal differences among these sulfonylureas lie in their ability to induce hypoglycemia, in their adverse effects profile, and in their duration of action. Tolbutamide (Orinase) has a relatively low potency/weight ratio and a short biologic effect. Chlorpropamide (Diabinese) has a considerably prolonged biologic action and increased potency/weight ratio; but has the disadvantage of producing hypoglycemia if a meal is delayed or omitted, or if the drug is taken in an excessive dose.

Differences among these agents result from variations in their means of metabolism and disposal. Second-generation agents have the highest potential efficacy of all sulfonylureas. Neither agent potentiates antidiuretic hormone action, increases water retention, potentiates congestive heart failure, nor results in hyponatremia as does chlorpropamide. Glipizide, now available in a once-daily, controlled delivery system, appears primarily to increase the quantity and rapidity of insulin secretion and secondarily to potentiate insulin action. It is therefore most useful in normal-weight to moderately obese patients with type 2 diabetes mellitus, as these patients may be relatively insulopenic. On the other hand, glyburide, now available in a microcrystalline, fine form, is most efficacious in severely obese patients with diabetes, as they have relative hyperinsulinism and marked insulin resistance.

Although the oral antidiabetic agents are appropriate therapy for patients with type 2 diabetes mellitus, they are not appropriate for patients with type 1 diabetes mellitus, as the latter group has markedly reduced or wholly absent endogenous insulin secretory capabilities. This may not entirely exclude acarbose or metformin, since the existing data are inadequate for a full evaluation.

Because type 1 diabetes is associated with episodic ketosis, any patient in whom significant weight loss or ketosis has occurred is generally not a candidate for exclusive oral therapy.

Insulin Therapy

Animal insulin preparations have varying quantities of immunoassayable glucagon, pancreatic polypeptide, vasoactive intestinal peptide, somatostatin, and proinsulin. In general, human insulin preparations are relatively pure, containing less than 50 contaminating protein molecules per million (ppm).

Both conventional and modified analogs of human insulin are now available. Because of self-association, human regular insulin has a prolonged duration and slow onset of action. Reversal of B28-PRO-B29 LYS to lyspro insulin prevents this binding, speeds absorption,

Table 303-4   Selected clinical characteristics of insulin preparations

ONSET OF ACTION	INSULIN	DURATION OF ACTION (H)		PEAK EFFECT (H)		COMPATIBLE MIXED WITH
		INITIAL	CHRONIC USE	INITIAL	CHRONIC USE	
Fast	Lyspro analog	3	3	1	1	All intermediate and long-acting
Rapid	Crystalline zinc (CZI, regular crystalline soluble actrapid)	6	16	2-3	5-6	All insulin
	Semilente	12		3-6		Lente
Intermediate	Neutral protamine (isophane, NPH)	14-24	24	6-12	10-12	Regular insulin
	Globin	18		6-8		
	Lente	18-24	24	8-14	10-12	Regular insulin and semi-Lente
Long	Protamine zinc (PZI)	36		16-24		
	Ultralene	36		20-30		Regular insulin and semi-Lente

and reduces the duration of insulin action to 3 rather than 6 hours. Less hypoglycemia and greater convenience result. In general, the use of purified monospecies human insulin is preferred for new patients and for all patients who have localized or systemic reactions or allergies to subcutaneous insulin of animal origin.

There is a wide variety of pharmacologic insulin preparations including relatively rapid-acting and intermediate-acting insulin; specially marketed mixtures of NPH (isophane insulin USP) and regular insulins; intermediate-acting insulins such as NPH and Lente insulin; and prolonged-acting insulins such as ultra-Lente and protamine zinc insulin (Table 303-4). Despite this variety of preparations, their use either alone or in combination, even with multiple daily injections, does not in any way reproduce the exquisite physiologic regulation of the blood glucose level observed in nondiabetic patients. This no doubt reflects the absence of finely regulated endogenous insulin secretion. Greater than normal levels of circulating insulin are required to suppress the gluconeogenic, glycogenolytic, and ketogenic potential of the pathologic hyperglucagonemia in patients with diabetes, perhaps as the result of systemic rather than portal insulin delivery.

Subcutaneous injections of insulin commit the patient to an organized and predictable lifestyle with respect to both food ingestion and exercise patterns. Continuous subcutaneous insulin infusion by a portable pump has shown promise in selected patients, particularly those who are pregnant. These pumps infuse a relatively small hourly dose of insulin, with much greater increments administered immediately before and during each meal. Although better, near-normal control of blood glucose levels has been demonstrated in these patients, there is some question as to whether this route of insulin delivery is routinely applicable to all patients with insulin-dependent (type 1) diabetes mellitus. As an alternative to infusion pump usage, intensive, multidose regular insulin therapies have been proposed. These rely on the use of subcutaneous regular insulin before meals together with one or two small daily doses of ultralente to suppress ketogenesis. Glycemic control with this paradigm is fundamentally identical to that produced by continuous pump infusion. Either technique allows more variability in meal timing than does the use of one or two doses of intermediate-acting insulin. Intensive research work is also presently ongoing regarding nasal insulin administration, glucose sensors to be used with automated insulin pump systems, as well as islet cell transplantation. Routine clinical application of the latter would appear to be years in the future, if ever. Segmental pancreas transplantation, performed simultaneously with transplantation of a kidney in patients with renal failure, offers promise of improved glycemic control and may require little or no exogenous insulin.

Types of Insulin Therapy. A number of approaches to the use of insulin therapy are presently used. In one, multiple small doses of lyspro or regular insulin are administered before meals together with a small evening dose of intermediate-acting (NPH or Lente) or long-acting (ultra-Lente) insulin to prevent nocturnal glycosuria and early morning hyperglycemia and ketosis. This method of insulin administration tends to produce good to excellent control of the blood glucose concentrations, but it has several major disadvantages. First, pa-

tients must be willing to accept three or four injections of insulin per day and must be prepared to give these injections before meals. Second, patient self-reliance in judging meal size and regular insulin requirements is necessary, as type 1 patients tend to be sensitive to small changes in the dose of regular insulin administered. Further, these dose schedules depend on knowing the premeal glucose level by self-monitoring before each meal. The patient must therefore be willing and able largely to self-regulate therapy. Many physicians believe that this method of insulin administration produces the best control of blood glucose concentrations and the lowest incidence of the development of the chronic complications of diabetes mellitus. However, adequate studies comparing this method of insulin administration with the use of intermediate-acting insulin, alone or in combination with regular insulin, are presently unavailable. A consensus also has developed that the attainment of true euglycemia with insulin administration is a difficult, if not impossible, goal using presently available means of insulin administration. Nevertheless, normalization of the glucose level to the degree possible without inducing multiple episodes of serious hypoglycemia is the most prudent long-term management goal for patients with type 2 diabetes. Combination oral agent insulin therapy may also produce superior glycemic control. One or two doses of intermediate or long-acting insulin coupled with metformin or troglitizone may produce excellent preprandial and postprandial control in mild to moderately obese type 2 patients. Metformin is associated with weight loss; troglitizone is associated with weight gain.

Evaluation of Antidiabetic Therapy. Available means of evaluating the extent of diabetic control include multiple fasting and spot serum glucose determinations and HbA_{1c} determinations.

The development of assays for determining the extent of glycosylation of hemoglobin resulting in the formation of HbA_{1c} in red blood cells permits a general assessment of the overall extent of hyperglycemia experienced by patients with diabetes mellitus. The nonenzymatic addition of glucose to hemoglobin A appears to occur in approximate proportion to the extent of hyperglycemia. In normal subjects 6% or less of hemoglobin A is glycosylated, whereas in patients with diabetes, glycosylated hemoglobin A may be as great as 20%.

The American Diabetes Association believes that a level of HbA_{1c} of 7.0% or less is the goal of diabetes management and that levels greater than 8% are unacceptable because of the risk of microvascular complications. It should be noted, however, that the rate of formation of HbA_{1c} is considerably faster than its rate of disappearance. Thus HbA_{1c} may be useful in monitoring diabetic outpatients during periods of stable and rapidly deteriorating control but is not suitable to detect rapid metabolic improvement. Because of the relatively long half-life of hemoglobin in the circulation, glycosylation of other proteins may be more useful for assessments of improving or deteriorating control. One such protein is serum albumin, which is also glycosylated but has a much shorter life span in blood. The fructosamine reaction is a crude assessment of primarily glycosylated albumin levels and therefore reflects diabetes control in the prior 2-week period. Another shortcoming of HbA_{1c} measurements is the many technical

Table 303-5   Efficacy of assessments of antidiabetic therapies

VALUE	GOAL LEVEL	ACCEPTABLE LEVEL
Hemoglobin A_{1c}	≤7.0%	≤8.0%
Fasting glucose	≤115 mg/dl	≤140 mg/dl
2-hour postprandial glucose	≤140 mg/dl	≤200 mg/dl
Total cholesterol	≤180 mg/dl	≤200 mg/dl
LDL cholesterol	≤130 mg/dl	≤160 mg/dl
Triglyceride	≤150 mg/dl	≤200 mg/dl

difficulties only recently recognized by the most sophisticated research laboratories.

Fasting hyperglycemia with values in excess of 140 mg/dl is clearly associated with an increased risk of microvascular complications of diabetes, such as retinopathy and nephropathy. This is also true for 2-hour postprandial glucose levels persistently in excess of 200 mg/dl. Therefore these levels are the outer limits of "acceptable" hyperglycemia in patients with diabetes. These levels correspond roughly to a level of HbA_{1c} of 8% or better. The virtual elimination of microvascular risk requires fasting glucose levels persistently below 115 mg/dl and 2-hour postprandial levels below 140 mg/dl. This corresponds to HbA_{1c} target levels of less than 7%. These levels should also be accompanied by improvements in rates of macrovascular disease or atherosclerosis. The latter seems to be relatively more sensitive to minor degrees of hyperglycemia, particularly postprandial hyperglycemia, and, to a lesser extent, fasting hyperglycemia. On the other hand, abnormalities of lipid levels as well as lipoprotein structure may be more important vectors for accelerated atherosclerosis than hyperglycemia in patients with diabetes. To that end, any evaluation of the adequacy of antidiabetic therapies must include an assessment of total and LDL cholesterol levels, as well as triglyceride levels (Table 303-5). Hypertriglyceridemia may be the best predictor of coronary mortality in patients with diabetes; nonetheless, low HDL cholesterol levels are also an ominous sign. Levels less than 35 mg/dl are clearly poor prognostic indicators in males, as are levels less than 45 or 55 mg/dl in females, if one is to mitigate the increased cardiovascular risk attendant to low levels of HDL cholesterol. In most patients with diabetes, low HDL levels rarely respond to enhanced glycemic control. Good glycemic control improves triglyceride levels, although not to normal. Pharmacologic therapies may be necessary to reverse diabetic dyslipidemias. Acceptable and target levels of total and LDL cholesterol and triglyceride levels are provided in Table 303-5.

Home monitoring of blood glucose by using glucose oxidase-based strip technology with or without electronic monitoring devices has virtually revolutionized diabetes management. Aside from the ability to assess blood glucose directly at any time desired, home glucose monitoring has generally produced vastly improved patient compliance. Home glucose monitoring provides an instantaneous, direct assessment of the blood glucose concentration, which has immediacy and impact on the patient's awareness. Correlation of medication or dietary errors follows as the natural consequence. Home monitoring should be used for all patients taking insulin and has even proved quite useful for diet- or diet- and oral agent–controlled patients. In the latter instances, negative feedback of dietary indiscretions tends to reduce or eliminate maladaptive behavior. In patients on weight reduction programs, the early and rapid fall in glucose levels, which is disproportionate to the extent of weight loss, tends to reinforce the beneficial effects of diet and to compensate for the reduced secondary gain to the patient resulting from reduced food intake. In general, preprandial and postprandial capillary glucose levels for an entire day provide a pattern of glucose control that otherwise would represent unavailable data for patient and physician alike.

Insulin Dosage. Therapy is begun by administering a comparatively small dose of intermediate insulin such as NPH or Lente insulin. This dose should be approximately 40% of the estimated daily insulin requirement for the patient. At ideal body weight, most patients require 30 to 50 units per day of exogenously administered, highly purified insulin, whether given as a single preparation or in combination with another insulin preparation. With increasing weight, however, higher insulin dosage is required. In general, the greater the body weight of the patient, the greater the insulin requirement. Thus in an average-sized adult, an initial dose of 15 to 20 units of intermediate insulin is usually given; this is raised over the next several days to weeks by 4- to 6-unit increments until a good therapeutic effect is attained. Administered insulin behaves somewhat differently from patient to patient, and the time of occurrence of peak action must be determined for each person. Some patients experience a relatively rapid onset of peak effects of NPH or Lente insulin, occurring 4 to 6 hours after injection, whereas most patients have peak effects from a morning injection of NPH or Lente insulin coincident with, or immediately before, the evening meal. A third group of patients have peak biologic effects of insulin at considerably later periods, perhaps many hours after the evening meal. If hyperglycemia is not easily controlled, the approximate time of the biologic peak should be determined. In subjects having a peak action of NPH or Lente insulin occurring at the time of the evening meal, blood glucose concentrations should be reduced to approximately 80 to 100 mg/dl immediately before the meal, so that the resulting caloric surge may be well controlled.

In a minority of patients hyperglycemia will be well controlled throughout the day and night on one dose of intermediate-acting insulin. Even though excellent control can be obtained before the evening meal, noticeable hyperglycemia may persist before breakfast or in the late morning hours after breakfast. In most instances, a second dose of NPH insulin may be necessary to normalize fasting glucose levels in these subjects. This second dose of insulin should be considerably less than the morning dose and should be administered immediately before the evening meal or occasionally at bedtime. When the second dose of insulin is begun, it is usually necessary to continue the same total insulin dosage to prevent hypoglycemia before the evening meal.

Changes in the amounts of insulin administered should be made no more frequently than every other day in outpatients and should usually not be more than 10% to 20% of the total insulin dose. If marked hyperglycemia is observed after breakfast and before lunch, a mixture of regular together with NPH (or Lente) insulin may be necessary, instead of solely NPH insulin in the morning. The addition of regular insulin in the morning usually requires a proportional reduction of the intermediate-acting insulin dosage. Mixtures of rapid- and intermediate-acting insulins will broaden the duration of peak actions of NPH and Lente insulins and will tend to make peak biologic effects of insulin injections coincident with postprandial hyperglycemia after the evening meal. This approach is recommended for patients with an idiosyncratic late peak action of NPH or Lente insulin. The mixed-insulin morning dose plus a second evening dose produces improved control of difficult to manage diabetic hyperglycemia. Aside from idiosyncratic biologic responses to insulin, most patients tend to show progressive lengthening of the interval between the time of insulin injection and the appearance of peak hyperglycemic action as the dosage of intermediate-acting insulin is increased, particularly for doses of NPH or Lente insulin greater than 40 units per day. Thus in patients with obesity or other reasons for insensitivity to pharmacologic preparations of insulin, dosages in excess of 40 to 60 units per day may show peak biologic activity occurring considerably later than the evening meal, and, in many circumstances, in the early morning hours. Such patients must either be treated with mixtures of rapid- and intermediate-acting insulin or, alternatively, switched to human insulin of recombinant DNA origin. The latter tends to produce more rapidly appearing and more pronounced peak biologic effects regardless of the pharmacologic nature of the preparations. This effect may result from the lower antigenicity of human insulin and its reduced antibody binding. As a consequence, human insulin is preferred in most clinical settings in which large insulin doses are used and in which delayed insulin responsiveness is noted.

The pattern of delayed responsiveness toward large dosages (>40 U/day) is a consequence of the depot nature of subcutaneous insulin injection. Diminishing the morning dose of NPH or Lente insulin by approximately 10 units and adding equal amounts of regular or semi-Lente insulin produces a faster onset of activity, assuming that human insulin is already being used. It may also be necessary to split the total dose of insulin into a morning dose containing two thirds to three fourths of the total and a smaller evening dose containing one fourth to one third of the total when the single morning dose is in excess of 40 to 60 units per day. Splitting the total dose of intermediate-acting insulin results in significantly greater overall hypoglycemic action for the total dose of insulin administered, and therefore it should not be accompanied by a large increase in the total dose prescribed. Indeed, a small reduction in total insulin administered per day may be wise if dose splitting is considered on an outpatient basis. Evening doses of insulin of between 8 and 20 units of NPH or Lente given with the evening meal or at bedtime are usually adequate to produce fasting euglycemia in these subjects. Rarely, a "dawn phenomenon," characterized by insulin hypersensitivity from midnight through 4:00 AM followed by rising insulin resistance from 4:00 AM onward, may complicate insulin therapy in adolescents and young adults. Administration of the evening insulin dosage at bedtime is usually effective treatment, as the peak insulin action is then shifted to the point of rising relative insulin resistance, without producing antecedent hypoglycemia during the phase of insulin hypersensitivity. If residual hyperglycemia remains at the time of the noon meal, larger morning doses of regular or semi-Lente insulin should be used. These approaches may be summarized into the following sequential guidelines:

1. Control blood glucose level before the evening meal (single dose of intermediate-acting insulin or a mixed dose of rapid plus intermediate insulin for late peak action).
2. Control residual fasting hyperglycemia (split dose of intermediate-acting insulin).
3. Control late-morning hyperglycemia (mix rapid-acting with morning intermediate-acting insulin).
4. Control bedtime hyperglycemia (mix rapid-acting with evening intermediate-acting insulin).
5. Use enough insulin in appropriate mixtures to maintain near-normal fasting venous glucose concentrations (<115 mg/dl) and postprandial venous blood glucose concentrations below values that appear to be associated with microangiopathies (<140 to 200 mg/dl).

Insulin allergy and the so-called honeymoon effect are two relatively common complications noted soon after starting insulin therapy. In type 1 subjects having severe hyperglycemia or ketoacidosis, insulin requirements may decrease dramatically, and the patient may no longer appear to require insulin, as hyperglycemia is no longer present. This honeymoon period may last from days to months and is invariably accompanied by a subsequent deterioration in metabolic control, after which the patient is usually left insulin dependent. Despite this seeming lack of need for insulin, these injections should never be totally discontinued, but the dose should be reduced to the smallest amount not producing hypoglycemia. Even if 1 unit per day is given, this dose should be sufficient to prevent an anamnestic response in which increased doses are required later.

Approximately 5% to 20% of patients begun on insulin therapy will show some manifestation of local or systemic insulin allergy. Most commonly, local reactions include erythema and dysesthesias at the injection site. Continued insulin together with antihistamine therapy should be efficacious, and most cases clear spontaneously within 6 to 12 months. More serious, but less common, generalized and systemic reactions to insulin may also occur, including local and generalized urticaria, angioneurotic edema, and anaphylaxis. Changing insulin preparations to highly purified monocomponent, monospecies insulin, particularly human insulin, is generally helpful. Desensitization may be necessary, but it is not always permanent and may therefore need to be repeated if symptoms recur. Angioneurotic edema and anaphylaxis must be treated immediately with glucocorticoids, antihistamines, and epinephrine if necessary.

Somogyi and Dawn Phenomena.

Episodic hypoglycemia, usually nocturnal, followed by rebound hyperglycemia, with or without mild ketosis, may occur in patients receiving excessive quantities of insulin. In most instances, this Somogyi phenomenon develops in response to excess insulin administration. The pathogenesis of this effect has been attributed to the adrenergic and glucagon response and, to a lesser extent, cortisol and growth hormone hypersecretion caused by hypoglycemia. These hormones increase glycogenolysis and gluconeogenesis, and epinephrine diminishes glucose uptake by peripheral tissues. Collectively, these events cause hyperglycemia.

These hormones also increase free fatty acid mobilization from adipose tissue and favor hepatic ketogenesis, thereby causing ketosis.

Most commonly, the hypoglycemic episode occurs in the early morning hours and may be attributed to an evening dose of insulin that is in excess of the patient's needs or to a late peak hypoglycemic action of the morning dose of insulin. As a consequence, such patients have bedtime urinary glucose and ketone body spillages that are usually absent, yet awaken the next morning with substantial glycosuria, and perhaps ketonuria, before breakfast. The presence of ketonuria is a helpful point for the differential diagnosis in this setting, as the patient must be clearly and substantially underinsulinized or substantially overinsulinized for ketosis to develop in the morning. If the total dose of insulin administered to the patient is in excess of what might be expected, then the Somogyi effect should be suspected. Confirmation of these suspicions can be obtained by hospitalizing the patient and sampling blood for glucose concentrations at frequent (1- to 4-hour) intervals during a 24-hour period. The Somogyi phenomenon is documented by wide fluctuations in blood glucose concentrations (40 to 400 mg/dl) despite a lack of food intake. Alternative evidence for this effect can be obtained by determinations of blood glucose at 3:00 AM and 5:00 AM; however, this requires accurate home glucose monitoring technique for the outpatient management of diabetes. Treatment of the Somogyi effect is straightforward once the diagnosis is made. The offending insulin injection should be reduced until the rebound hyperglycemia clears. Modification of a morning intermediate-acting insulin dose with rapid-acting insulin or a complete change to a shorter-acting insulin such as semi-Lente may be necessary. The dawn phenomenon is morning hyperglycemia and insulin resistance, not as the result of antecedent hypoglycemia, but instead owing to predawn surges in growth hormone and, to a lesser extent, other counterregulatory hormones. This phenomenon occurs primarily in younger, generally type 1 patients and requires 3:00 AM glucose monitoring for verification. Treatment consists of moving evening intermediate insulin shots to bedtime (10:00 PM), thereby producing peak morning hyperinsulinism at 6:00 AM, the peak time of insulin resistance.

Insulin Resistance.

Insulin resistance was traditionally defined as the requirement for more than 200 units of insulin per day to control hyperglycemia. By definition, this requirement must be exceeded in the absence of diabetic ketoacidosis, sepsis, and other causes of acute and transient insensitivity to the metabolic actions of insulin. In view of the more recently noted lower need for exogenous insulin in completely depancreatized patients, however, definitions of insulin resistance have been reconsidered, and it is now thought to be present when the exogenous insulin requirement exceeds 100 units per day. Clinically, insulin resistance was recognized in patients with overt hyperglycemia who responded inappropriately to conventional insulin doses and were found to have neutralizing antibodies to circulating insulin, but both the spectrum and subsequent recognition of insulin-resistant states have undergone a major expansion in recent years. It is now known that insulin resistance may occur independent of overt glucose intolerance with hyperglycemia. Thus insulin resistance may be present despite a euglycemic status, provided that supranormal concentrations of insulin are present. On the other hand, persistent hyperglycemia may be present even though pharmacologic quantities of exogenous insulin are administered.

In the majority of patients with true insulin resistance, resistance is the result of obesity, antiinsulin antibodies, malignancies, associated endocrinopathies, lipodystrophy, an immune dysfunction characterized by antireceptor antibodies (type B) or a reduction in receptor concentration (type A), acanthosis nigricans, a variety of autoimmune disorders, primary ovarian abnormalities with and without features of lipodystrophy, pregnancy, or the secretion of endogenous abnormal insulins. To discern the cause of insulin resistance, it is important to recognize that the first step in the action of insulin is its binding to insulin-receptor molecules on the external surface of the target cell plasma membrane. Therefore for simple convenience, it is easy to categorize insulin resistance as resulting from events occurring before, at, or after the point of hormone-receptor interaction.

The presence of substantial quantities of antiinsulin antibodies to animal (or human) insulin preparations can produce considerable wastage of insulin and also successfully compete with the insulin receptor for available circulating insulin. Practically all insulin-treated patients develop low concentrations of immunoglobulin G (IgG) antiinsulin antibodies, but in less than one patient per thousand do the antiinsulin antibody titer and affinity become sufficient to cause clinically apparent insulin resistance. Most commonly, antibody-mediated insulin resistance develops in a patient previously exposed for a period of time to exogenous insulin that is then discontinued and subsequently readministered. The repeated challenge with insulin induces an immunologic reaction similar to the anamnestic responses observed to other antigens.

Substantial antibody titers to insulin can be detected by modifications of the radioimmunoassay techniques for measuring insulin in serum or plasma. The titer of antiinsulin antibody present and the degree of clinical insulin resistance, however, are not closely correlated. Beef insulin has three amino acid residues that differ from those of human insulin; pork insulin has only one such differing amino acid residue. Thus most antibodies to pharmacologic preparations of insulin have higher affinities for beef than for pork or human insulin. As a consequence, switching the patient to a purified pork or human regular insulin generally proves effective in reducing the quantities of insulin required for controlling acute hyperglycemia. As much as 100,000 units of regular insulin has been administered to overcome the insulin-antagonistic action of antibodies in patients having diabetic ketoacidosis. If purified human regular or Lente insulin does not reduce the high insulin requirements of patients with antibody-mediated insulin resistance, prednisone therapy as an immunosuppressive measure often will be efficacious, despite its relative antagonism to insulin action.

The lowest possible steroid dose producing acceptable and predictable insulin requirements should be given. Prednisone should be started at doses of 60 to 100 mg/day and continued until the insulin dosage decreases, usually within several days. A daily tapering of the prednisone should then be initiated. Maintenance prednisone dosage is generally 10 to 30 mg/day. The natural history of antibody-mediated insulin resistance is characterized by a spontaneous remission of this phenomenon 6 to 18 months after its presentation. As a consequence, marked hypoglycemia can result at the time of remission if the patient is maintained on large quantities of subcutaneous insulin.

A relatively rare cause for prereceptor insulin resistance results from the secretion of an abnormal insulin molecule that binds with less affinity to insulin receptors and has a diminished biologic activity. Another nonimmune form of insulin resistance noted very rarely in insulin-dependent diabetic patients (type I) derives from a reduced bioavailability of insulin after subcutaneous, but not intravenous, injections. This phenomenon is thought to be the result of local destruction or sequestration of insulin in its subcutaneous depot. Some investigators believe that this syndrome results from compliance failures or from occult infection and is not a unique pathologic entity.

Obesity, particularly abdominal obesity, is associated with the most common and best studied form of insulin resistance. This resistance is a heterogeneous disorder that is not directly proportional to the degree of obesity. In mildly hyperinsulinemic but resistant obese patients, the density of insulin receptors is reduced, and the resistance is primarily the result of the decreased receptor density. A postreceptor defect in coupling to metabolic processes may also be present. Weight reduction is the only effective therapy for the insulin resistance of obesity because the loss of receptors is reversible with weight reduction, and insulin responsiveness usually reverts toward normal.

Insulin resistance syndromes. Other forms of insulin resistance occur in three recently recognized syndromes. One syndrome, *type A*, occurs in females and is usually characterized by hyperglycemia, acanthosis nigricans, and polycystic ovaries. Various degrees of virilization have been observed, and serum testosterone concentrations may be increased slightly. The concentration of insulin receptors on circulating monocytes is reduced, and the receptor defect is not improved by dietary restriction as it is in obesity. In addition, some of these patients seem to have a postreceptor defect in coupling to insulin-responsive metabolic pathways.

Another of these syndromes, *type B,* is an autoimmune disease characterized by hyperglycemia, acanthosis nigricans, and diminished binding of insulin to its cellular receptor owing to the presence of circulating antireceptor antibodies. This syndrome may be associated with several accompanying disorders such as lupus erythematosus,

Sjögren's syndrome, and ataxia telangiectasia. Antiinsulin-receptor antibody titers may fall after immunosuppressive therapy.

The *type C* syndrome of insulin resistance is characterized by the familial occurrence of insulin resistance coupled with acanthosis nigricans, acral hypertrophy, and muscle cramps. Ovarian dysfunction may occur in females, although testicular function may be normal in males. Fasting euglycemia or hyperglycemia may be present, but patients are resistant to the hypoglycemic effects of intravenous insulin injection at customary doses. Endogenous hyperinsulinemia is present, and insulin-receptor density on circulating monocytes is reduced.

Endocrinopathies such as Cushing's syndrome, pheochromocytoma, acromegaly, thyrotoxicosis, and profound hyperlipidemias are all associated with increased insulin requirements for diabetic control. Glucocorticoid excess is associated with reduced affinity of insulin receptors, but insulin requirements are usually not increased in patients taking less than the equivalent of 20 mg of prednisone daily. Epinephrine induces peripheral and hepatic insulin insensitivity through beta-adrenergic receptor mediation. As a result, peripheral tissues are insensitive to incremental changes in plasma insulin concentrations. The mechanism of this catecholamine effect is unclear. Medical or surgical management for hyperthyroidism, Cushing's disease, and acromegaly is indicated before good control of carbohydrate disturbances can be obtained.

The *syndrome of insulin resistance* or *syndrome X,* as it is also termed, describes the frequent association as comorbid illnesses of carbohydrate intolerance, essential hypertension, dyslipidemia, abdominal obesity, and accelerated atherosclerosis. Hyperuricemia may also occur. The hyperinsulinemia and dyslipidemia may account, at least in part, for the accelerated atherosclerosis of these disease entities. Both insulin resistance and dyslipidemia tend to antedate the subsequent appearance of diabetes or hypertension by years or decades. The precise etiologic significance of these associations is unclear at present and may not occur in all racial and ethnic groups equally. Nevertheless, the postulation of insulin resistance as a unifying mechanism linking many associated atherogenic illnesses has proved extremely attractive to many investigators.

Lipoatrophic diabetes mellitus is an insulin-resistant state characterized by the lack of subcutaneous fat and by hyperlipidemia and an elevated metabolic rate. In some patients, lipoatrophy is associated with acanthosis nigricans and a variety of autoimmune disorders. This rare and complex disease appears to consist of a spectrum of disorders that at one extreme is associated with circulating antiinsulin-receptor antibodies or with altered insulin binding to receptors and at the other extreme with reversible hyperlipidemia with normal insulin-receptor number. There may be a primary disturbance of receptor coupling that produces rapid insulin desensitization. Therapy is limited primarily to dietary manipulations, including a low-carbohydrate diet and exogenous insulin administration.

ACUTE METABOLIC COMPLICATIONS OF DIABETES MELLITUS

Among the acute metabolic consequences of diabetes mellitus or its treatment are four distinctly different forms of coma. These are (1) diabetic ketoacidosis, (2) hyperosmolar nonketotic coma, (3) lactic acidosis, and (4) hypoglycemia. Diabetic patients are also subject to the other causes of coma found in the nondiabetic patient population including alcohol-induced ketosis. Certain features of the history and physical examination, as well as selected laboratory determinations, are extremely useful for the rapid differentiation of the forms of diabetic coma. For example, insulin hypoglycemia is a fulminant disorder generally precipitated by vigorous exercise, omission of food intake, or overdosage with either insulin or sulfonylureas. In addition, the patient is usually profusely diaphoretic, tachycardic, tremulous, and hypothermic. The specific clinical presentations and the diagnostic and therapeutic maneuvers pertaining to each of these comas are discussed in the following pages.

Diabetic Ketoacidosis

Diabetic ketoacidosis is a life-threatening metabolic disorder characterized by accelerated rates of hepatic glycogenolysis, gluconeogenesis, ketogenesis, and impaired glucose and ketoacid utilization, all

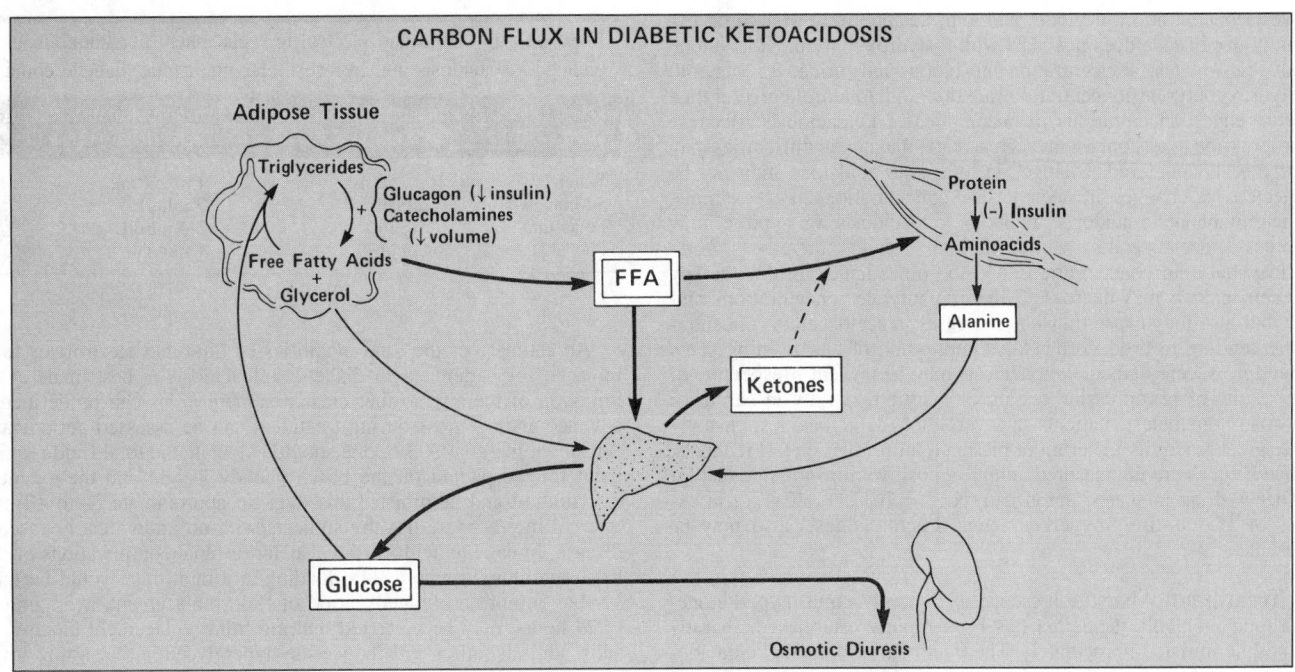

CARBON FLUX IN DIABETIC KETOACIDOSIS

FIGURE 303-6   Metabolic alterations in diabetic ketoacidosis.

of which result in elevated concentrations of glucose and keto acids in blood. These disturbances, coupled with increased fatty acid mobilization from adipose tissue and increased muscle proteolysis, flood the bloodstream with an overabundance of fuels for hepatic glucose and ketone overproduction (Fig. 303-6).

The major hormonal abnormalities are an insufficient quantity of circulating insulin to restrain catabolism and profound hyperglucagonemia. Hyperglycemia produces an osmotic diuresis and thereby causes intravascular volume depletion, which in turn stimulates sympathetic outflow and catecholamine release. The increased catecholamines dramatically increase free fatty acid mobilization from adipose tissue. Increased levels of epinephrine and glucagon in the blood augment hepatic gluconeogenesis, glycogenolysis, and ketogenesis. In addition, epinephrine diminishes any residual endogenous insulin secretion. The hypoinsulinemia and hyperglucagonemia decrease hepatic malonyl CoA concentrations and may increase hepatic carnitine concentrations. Both effects facilitate fatty acylcarnitine translocation across the liver inner mitochondrial membrane so that increased free fatty acid oxidation results in accelerated hepatic ketogenesis. The markedly increased free fatty acid levels also diminish ketone-body oxidation in peripheral tissues, thereby producing a marked hyperketonemia and massive ketonuria. The release of other stress hormones such as cortisol and growth hormone reinforces these pathogenic developments in diabetic ketoacidosis, as these hormones generally exhibit antiinsulin activity. Even though glucose and ketone bodies have no maximal renal tubular reabsorption rates, glycosuria and ketonuria during diabetic ketoacidosis occur because less than 100% of these filtered compounds are reabsorbed by the renal tubules. Massive renal glucose and keto acid excretion with the resultant osmotic diuresis produces large losses of sodium, potassium, calcium, phosphate, ammonium, and other ions in the urine. These severe losses of water and electrolytes, combined with the marked acidemia, may ultimately produce cardiovascular failure and death.

Diabetic ketoacidosis is usually accompanied by a history of several days of polyuria and polydipsia but can appear as a fulminant disorder within a few hours, especially in cases of insulin pump failure. It occurs in lean or obese patients and may be found in younger, as well as older, patients. Contrary to popular opinion, there are more new cases of diabetes presenting with ketoacidosis in adults than in children. Morbid cardiovascular events, infections, trauma, pregnancy, emotional stress, excessive alcohol ingestion, and omission of prescribed insulin are frequent precipitating causes of diabetic ketoacidosis. On occasion, there may be no obvious precipitating cause.

The physical findings of tachypnea, dehydration, and some degree of acetone halitosis (a fruity odor to the breath) are usually present. Abdominal pain with or without findings consistent with pancreatitis also may occur. Kussmaul respirations are usually present when the arterial pH is less than 7.3, but these finally may disappear owing to patient exhaustion. The central nervous system may no longer respond to severe acidosis when the arterial pH values are less than 6.9. These patients may have marked hyperlipidemia in serum or blood since type IV and type V hyperlipidemias are common in ketoacidosis. Lipemia retinalis is present when the plasma triglyceride concentration is greater than 2000 to 5000 mg/dl.

Laboratory confirmation of diabetic ketoacidosis should be made rapidly. Criteria for the diagnosis—hyperglycemia, hyperketonemia, and metabolic acidosis—may be present to varying degrees. For example, in a young, pregnant, insulin-dependent diabetic patient with a propensity for excreting urinary glucose, severe hyperketonemia and metabolic acidosis may be present despite a plasma glucose concentration of 200 mg/dl or less. On the other hand, in an insulin-dependent diabetic patient with prerenal azotemia, plasma glucose concentrations can be greater than 1000 mg/dl, and arterial pH less than 7.2, with only modest hyperketonemia; however, patients with advanced renal failure are generally resistant to the development of ketoacidosis. The finding of metabolic acidosis in these patients may be the result, instead, of lactic acidosis. Rarely, an insulin-dependent diabetic patient with protracted vomiting may manifest severe hyperglycemia, hyperketonemia and yet have a paradoxic metabolic alkalosis, owing to the marked gastric loss of hydrochloric acid in vomitus.

Patients with diabetic ketoacidosis usually urinate profusely, and thus urine demonstrating 4+ glycosuria and intense ketonuria can be obtained readily. In patients with neurogenic bladder atony, catheterization may be necessary. An adequate intravenous route for administering saline should be established; simultaneously, blood should be drawn for determinations of glucose, urea, creatinine, and electrolyte (Na^+, K^+, Cl^-, and HCO_3^-) levels. If available, Dextrostix or Chemstrips can be used to determine rapidly the presence of hyperglycemia while awaiting the more accurate plasma glucose concentration from the clinical laboratory. Arterial blood gas values should be obtained if possible. Additional plasma or serum should be obtained for semiquantitative determinations of circulating ketone bodies. The routinely used reagent for ketoacid detection in blood and urine is nitroprusside (Ketostix, Acetest).

Nitroprusside reacts with acetoacetate, the ketone body with the lowest concentration in blood, and with acetone only to a slight extent. Nitroprusside does not react with β-hydroxybutyrate, the ketone body in greatest concentration in blood and urine. In general, β-hydroxybutyrate concentrations are threefold to tenfold greater than acetoacetate concentrations in uncomplicated ketoacidosis. Because nitroprusside reacts only with acetoacetate, diagnostic difficulties may rarely be encountered. Changes in total keto acid load may not be reflected by changes in acetoacetate concentrations. For example, concomitant lactic acidosis, alcoholic ketoacidosis, or hypoxia may depress acetoacetate concentrations and increase beta-hydroxybutyrate concentrations. On the other hand, insulin therapy for ketoacidosis may decrease β-hydroxybutyrate concentrations rapidly but also may cause transient increases in acetoacetate concentrations, tending to produce the false impression of a worsening state. Therefore severe diabetic ketoacidosis may be present irrespective of the results of nitroprusside testing of ketone reactivity in serum or plasma. Nonetheless, patients in severe diabetic ketoacidosis usually have great reactivity of serum or plasma to nitroprusside test reagents. Since ketones are unmeasured anions, a positive nitroprusside test together with an increased anion gap ($Na^+ - [Cl^- + HCO_3^-]$) in excess of 15) confirms hyperketonemia. Lactic acidosis also may be present.

Treatment. After the presence of hyperglycemia, hyperketonemia, and metabolic acidemia has been rapidly established, therapy should be initiated immediately. The treatment of diabetic ketoacidosis must be tailored to the individual patient. Five general areas of treatment can be broadly differentiated: (1) constant patient monitoring and reevaluation, (2) fluid and electrolyte replacement, (3) rapid-acting insulin administration, (4) glucose supplementation as necessary, and (5) therapy for the precipitating cause. The patient should be weighed and the degree of dehydration assessed. The patient's state of consciousness, respiratory and heart rates, blood pressure, and temperature should be recorded at frequent intervals on a clinical flow sheet. This record also should contain notations of all fluid, electrolytes, and insulin administered as well as the laboratory data (including serial values for glucose, electrolytes, urea, creatinine, arterial or venous gases and pH, and urinary glucose and acetoacetate reactivities). Because hypothermia is an occasional finding, the presence of even a mild temperature elevation suggests an underlying infection. Parenteral and oral intake and urinary output should be recorded hourly on the flow sheet. In the unconscious patient with a history of vomiting or apparent gastric dilation, nasogastric aspiration should be performed.

Having established the diagnosis, one should begin fluid and electrolyte replacement immediately. Intravascular volume depletion and a diminished glomerular filtration rate usually will be present. To expand the contracted intravascular volume rapidly and thereby improve tissue perfusion, normal saline should be first administered. Such expansion will also reduce adrenergic outflow and thereby diminish free fatty acid mobilization. Rates of saline administration should approximate 1 L/hr, and at least 1 to 2 L of normal saline should be administered, except to patients with marked cardiovascular disease in whom slower rates of fluid administration may be necessary.

For patients with arterial pH levels less than 6.9 or in whom Kussmaul's respiration has ceased because of physical exhaustion, bicarbonate administration is advisable. Otherwise, for pH values greater than 7.0, sodium bicarbonate in itself is usually not necessary or even desirable. Diabetic ketoacidosis tends to be a self-correcting acidosis because complete oxidation of the accumulated strong organic acids (acetoacetate and beta-hydroxybutyrate) will restore arterial pH to normal. If excess quantities of bicarbonate are administered, rebound peripheral alkalosis with paradoxic central nervous system acidosis may occur because of differential transport of carbon dioxide, but not bicarbonate, across the blood-brain barrier. These changes can then produce obtundation and the appearance of secondary relapse or coma in patients seemingly cured of diabetic ketoacidosis. Excessive sodium bicarbonate administration to patients increases the sodium load dramatically and therefore may lead to hypernatremia and the subsequent development of a hyperchloremic metabolic acidosis (normal anion gap). This development is of particular consequence in patients with known cardiovascular disease, a major complication of long-standing diabetes mellitus.

Table 303-6 Fluid and electrolyte replacement per kilogram in diabetic ketoacidosis and hyperosmolar nonketotic diabetic coma

REPLACEMENT SUBSTANCES	DIABETIC KETOACIDOSIS (PER KG)	HYPEROSMOLAR NONKETOTIC DIABETIC COMA (PER KG)
Water	100-150 ml	150-200 ml
Sodium	7 mEq/L	7 mEq/L
Potassium	5 mEq/L	2-4 mEq/L
Phosphate	1 mmol	1 mmol

An estimate of the total quantities of fluid and electrolytes to be replaced for patients with diabetic ketoacidosis is best made at the initiation of therapy so that clear treatment goals can be defined in advance and progress during treatment can be assessed periodically. As shown in Table 303-6, one should calculate the total fluid requirement for the patient on the basis of body weight and the extent of dehydration and administer this over an approximate 8- to 12-hour interval in otherwise healthy subjects with no known cardiovascular disease. In patients with cardiovascular or renal complications of diabetes mellitus, in whom fluid loading at a rapid rate would be inadvisable, a more prolonged period of fluid replacement, averaging 16 to 24 hours, may be preferred. During fluid replacement therapy, insulin administration will reduce the hyperglycemia, but not to levels sufficient to prevent the continuation of some degree of osmotic diuresis. Thus during the initial period of fluid replacement, one fourth to half of fluids administered are usually excreted in the urine. Replacement of urinary losses by 0.5 N saline should be performed for a second 8- to 12-hour period after the initial 1 to 2 L of saline are administered. For rapid expansion of intravascular volume, fluid and sodium replacement should consist exclusively of normal saline for the first 1-2 liters. Thereafter, fluid replacement should rely on 0.5 N saline until the blood glucose level falls to 250 to 300 mg/dl. As glucose levels fall, 5% dextrose should be added.

Patients having ketoacidosis are frequently oliguric as a result of the markedly diminished glomerular filtration rate caused by hypovolemia. Despite the marked potassium losses observed in these patients, they are usually normokalemic or hyperkalemic at the time of presentation. For this reason, an admitting electrocardiogram is frequently useful. In patients without signs of hyperkalemia and in whom reasonable urine output can be observed, potassium administration should be initiated early in the course of fluid therapy for diabetic ketoacidosis. Otherwise, profound hypokalemia will be observed 4 to 8 hours after initiation of therapy for ketoacidosis. This development is a result of H^+-K^+ shifts that occur with rising blood pH and with transport of potassium intracellularly during glucose uptake by cells. After the development of a satisfactory urinary output, approximately 20 to 40 mEq/L of potassium should be added to replacement solutions of half normal saline as they are administered to patients, generally at a rate of 0.50 to 1.0 L/hour. Potassium administration in patients with diabetic ketoacidosis should be continued as long as fluid replacement is ongoing.

Hypophosphatemia often develops in patients with severe diabetic ketoacidosis and marked dehydration. This hypophosphatemia initially may not be apparent because of phosphate shifts from intracellular to extracellular compartments. Phosphate is primarily an intracellular anion, and levels of phosphate in blood may not provide an adequate assessment of the extent of intracellular phosphate depletion. In general, phosphate must be given judiciously to patients with renal failure because of the potential for intravenous phosphate to produce marked hypocalcemia and hypomagnesemia. Although phosphate losses may be as high as potassium losses in patients with diabetic ketoacidosis, phosphate replacement by continuous intravenous infusion should deliver approximately 20 mmol of phosphate per liter of 0.5 N saline. Intravenous phosphate should be given to markedly dehydrated, severely hyperglycemic patients or to those with serum phosphate levels less than 1.5 mMol/L. Serious hypophosphatemia (<1 mMol/L) may produce late-developing complications of diabetic ketoacidosis, most notably rhabdomyolysis. As a secondary result of the destruction of skeletal muscle, oliguric renal failure may be produced. Other complications of hypophosphatemia include hemolysis and cardiac conduction abnormalities. Mild hypophosphatemia may be repleted by oral ingestion of foodstuffs after reversal of ketosis.

Insulin administration must be initiated early in the management of diabetic ketoacidosis. It may be given by four major therapeutic modes, including intermittent intravenous boluses, intermittent split-dose subcutaneous and intravenous injection, intermittent intramuscular injection, and continued intravenous infusion. Each method of administration possesses its own unique advantages and disadvantages, and no single method is appropriate for all patients with diabetic ketoacidosis.

The route of administration should be chosen with a prior knowledge of insulin pharmacokinetics. Several major guiding principles for insulin therapy can be outlined. First, intravenous administration alone should be considered for all patients in whom marked hypotension or hypovolemia is observed. Absorption of subcutaneous insulin may be impaired as a result of poor tissue perfusion in these patients. Second, if intermittent bolus intravenous administration is chosen, the frequency of boluses should be sufficient to maintain adequate serum insulin levels of at least 200 to 400 $\mu U/ml$ throughout the course of treatment of diabetic ketoacidosis. Because the half-life of intravenous insulin is approximately 4 minutes, boluses of insulin should be administered at 30- to 60-minute intervals to maintain adequate peripheral levels of insulin. Intermittent intravenous boluses of insulin in usual dosages of 0.5 to 2.0 units/kg produce hypoglycemia more frequently than any other method of insulin administration. Continuous intravenous insulin administration has the advantage of producing a predictable rate of decline in blood glucose levels and a satisfactory response in most patients with diabetic ketoacidosis. The recognition and management of insulin-antibody–mediated diabetic ketoacidosis, however, is considerably more complicated in patients receiving continuous intravenous insulin infusions. In general, infusion rates that would be sufficient to saturate the insulin–antibody-binding capacities are far greater than the customary rates of infusion used to treat uncomplicated ketoacidosis.

For continuous intravenous administration, a priming dose of approximately 0.1 unit/kg should be administered, followed by a continuous infusion of 0.1 unit/kg per hour. This dose may be given by infusion pump or by an independent intravenous drip system. Higher rates of infusion may be necessary for markedly obese patients or for patients in whom extraordinarily high levels of antiinsulin hormones might be encountered, such as patients with sepsis. Doses for bolus intravenous insulin administration should approximate 0.5 unit/kg administered at half-hour intervals.

At any time that urine glucose spillage becomes less than 4+ and blood glucose levels fall below 250 mg/dl, a change in fluid administration to include 5% dextrose will be necessary. This dose will prevent symptomatic hypoglycemia and facilitate the reversal of ketosis, because glucose is essential for free fatty acid reesterification in adipose tissue. Doses of 25 to 100 units of regular insulin administered both subcutaneously and intravenously at 2-hour intervals are also appropriate therapy for most patients with diabetic ketoacidosis. Higher doses may be necessary in patients with insensitivity to insulin action, as might be expected in obese or septic subjects. Regardless of the route of insulin administration, only regular insulin should be administered to patients in diabetic ketoacidosis.

Each patient must be reevaluated at 1- to 2-hour intervals to ensure improved metabolic status. A failure of improvement can be inferred from a lack of arterial or venous pH changes or from the lack of reduction of glucose levels. Initially, hemodilution produced by administration of normal saline will result in a falling blood glucose level because of renal glucose excretion. Increases in arterial pH, however, generally are not produced by rehydration to any significant extent; pH thus may be the best guide to treatment in patients with diabetic ketoacidosis. This guideline is particularly important as it is the acidosis itself that is generally the most life-threatening component of the syndrome of diabetic ketoacidosis.

In general, patients presenting with diabetic acidosis in the late afternoon or early evening may be started on intermediate insulin the next morning because this interval should be sufficient to change arterial pH to values greater than 7.35 and to improve bicarbonate levels to normal. If the patient is capable of maintaining adequate food intake, the usual and customary dose of intermediate-acting insulin

should be given. For patients in whom severe metabolic stress secondary to infection has precipitated the episode of diabetic ketoacidosis, additional insulin, in the form of small doses of regular insulin, may be necessary to prevent recurrent ketosis. This dose may be administered on the basis of a supplementary sliding scale based on double voided urines at 4- to 6-hour intervals or by the judicious use of regular insulin using serum glucose determinations before meals and bedtime. Although sliding scales that give 10 to 25 units for 4+ glucosuria are in common use, routine coverage for acetonuria should be avoided. The latter requires physician reevaluation. In patients never previously managed on insulin, a starting dose of 20 to 25 units of intermediate-acting insulin may be given and supplemented with small quantities of regular insulin, as indicated earlier. These doses should be adjusted on a daily basis so that the patient is ultimately discharged on one or two doses of intermediate insulin, alone or in combination with short-acting insulin.

During the initial phase of management for patients with diabetic ketoacidosis, the precipitating cause of the ketoacidosis must be identified. Thus urinary tract infections or other (occult as well as more obvious) bacterial or viral illnesses must be identified and treated appropriately to successfully manage the ketoacidosis. Lumbar puncture should be considered in all patients with evidence of serious, unexplained infection or with disturbances in their level of consciousness, particularly if there are other neurologic findings. Antecedent or intercurrent myocardial infarction and cerebrovascular accident also must be considered in the evaluation of potential precipitating causes of diabetic ketoacidosis. Because diabetic subjects tend to evolve asymptomatic or atypical angina and myocardial infarction, electrocardiographic evaluation at the time of admission and after reversal of diabetic ketoacidosis seems essential. One must deal with such antecedent or intercurrent conditions appropriately, in addition to giving treatments designed to reverse ketoacidosis.

Alcoholic Ketosis

Ketoacidosis may be noted in clinical circumstances other than diabetes mellitus, (e.g., acute ethanol intoxication in a fasted patient). These patients are generally suffering from chronic hypocaloric malnutrition and chronic ethanol abuse. Pertinent clinical features of alcoholic ketoacidosis include dehydration, vomiting, and the presence of associated manifestations of alcoholism, particularly pancreatitis, gastrointestinal tract bleeding, hepatitis, cirrhosis, and delirium tremens. At the time of presentation, serum glucose concentrations may vary greatly but are usually less than 200 mg/dl. Nitroprusside reactivity in serum varies from "trace" to "strong," but there is usually a moderate reactivity even though a fulminant hyperketonemia and a large anion gap are present. This discordance occurs because of the high β-hydroxybutyrate/acetoacetate ratio produced by high rates of ethanol oxidation to acetate in the liver. The arterial pH may reveal either an acidemia or alkalemia, the latter occurring because these patients tend to lose hydrogen ions during vomiting. Concentrations of lactate, uric acid, bilirubin, urea, triglycerides, transaminases, alkaline phosphatase, and amylase are generally elevated. In most instances, rehydration with normal saline and parenteral nutrition with glucose is the only treatment necessary. Only occasionally will insulin be required because of underlying diabetes or because of the impaired insulin release of starvation. Potassium and phosphate supplements are needed. Rarely, bicarbonate therapy may also be necessary. When treating alcoholic ketosis, it should be recognized that diabetic patients also may suffer from alcoholism. Thus a patient in alcoholic ketoacidosis with a low blood glucose concentration, a high blood β-hydroxybutyrate concentration, and moderate acidemia can become overtly diabetic in hyperglycemic coma if glucose is infused intravenously unaccompanied by adequate amounts of insulin. Therefore the same degree of cautious clinical monitoring and repeated examinations of blood glucose, electrolytes, gases, and pH are required for these critically ill patients as for patients in diabetic ketoacidosis (Chapter 115).

Hyperosmolar Nonketotic Coma

This form of diabetic coma occurs less frequently than diabetic ketoacidosis. It is most common in the elderly diabetic person and is only rarely observed in younger patients. Hyperosmolar nonketotic diabetic coma is characterized by marked hyperglycemia, which is usually greater than that accompanying diabetic ketoacidosis. Initial serum glucose concentration ranges from 600 to 2400 mg/dl. The greater hyperglycemia in hyperosmolar nonketotic coma as compared with ketoacidosis is the result, in part, of more severe dehydration. In the past, it has been associated with a mortality of 30% to 80%. Hyperosmolar coma is defined by values of serum osmolality greater than 325 mOsm/L. (Osmolality may be determined directly or may be approximated by mathematical formulas such as $2[Na^+ + K^+]$ + glucose/18 + BUN/2.8.) These patients are, most typically, nonacidotic at the time of presentation; but mild to moderate metabolic acidosis may be observed, with arterial pH levels as low as 7.2. This acidosis may result in part from a concurrent element of lactic acidosis from the impaired tissue perfusion due to marked hypovolemia. Frequently, a small degree of ketosis is found in undiluted sera in patients whose primary disorders are hyperglycemia and hyperosmolality.

Factors precipitating hyperosmolar nonketotic coma are generally similar to those precipitating diabetic ketoacidosis. Often this disorder develops in a patient not previously known to have diabetes mellitus. Precipitating causes include administration of fluids high in glucose content either intravenously or during peritoneal dialysis or hemodialysis. Other causes are administration of glucocorticoids, diuretics, and phenytoin. The hyperosmolar state, in contrast to diabetic ketoacidosis, is preceded by a more prolonged period of polyuria, polydipsia, and increasing progressive dehydration. This period may range from 5 to 21 days and is often accompanied by a history of increasing enfeeblement, mental confusion, somnolence, and, ultimately, coma. The early phases of the hyperosmolar coma also may be marked by urinary incontinence secondary to a profound osmotic diuresis, which combined with the mental symptoms, may be confused with primary cerebrovascular disease by friends and relatives. This comparatively slow and progressive deterioration of the patient, together with a high mortality rate, stands in marked contrast to the dramatic presentation and relatively low morbidity and mortality of diabetic ketoacidosis.

Because of the relative absence of ketosis in patients with hyperosmolar nonketotic coma, it has been postulated that there must be more circulating insulin activity in this condition than in diabetic ketoacidosis. Clinical studies, however, have failed to discern any significant difference in insulin levels between these two forms of diabetic coma. The essential biochemical difference between the two syndromes is that free fatty acid levels in hyperosmolar nonketotic coma are normal in contrast to the tenfold or greater elevation of free fatty acid levels in diabetic ketoacidosis. This difference may be the result of a relative failure of adrenergic nervous system adaptation to hypovolemia. In the elderly, the lack of a volume-dependent augmentation of free fatty acid mobilization from adipose tissue because of a diminished catecholamine output could thus explain the absence of ketosis in these persons.

Thrombotic events are the principal cause of death in patients with hyperosmolar nonketotic coma. These may be the result of increased platelet coagulability combined with the more extensive atherosclerotic vascular disease in the elderly. Patients initially may appear with antecedent myocardial infarctions, cerebrovascular accidents, or acute renal failure. Any or all of these also may develop during the course of treatment for hyperosmolar nonketotic coma. Because the fluid deficit in these patients is extremely severe (ranging from 10% to 20% of body weight), extreme care must be taken to avoid precipitating congestive heart failure or pulmonary edema after rapid rehydration in patients already having compromised myocardial function.

Treatment of the Hyperosmolar State. Treatment of the hyperosmolar nonketotic state should be directed first to fluid and electrolyte replacement, as this is undoubtedly the most dangerous element of the syndrome. An average net fluid deficit of 150 ml/kg has been observed, but with extremely severe hyperglycemia, greater fluid losses (up to 200 ml/kg body weight) can be expected. The estimated fluid loss should be replaced in the first 18 to 24 hours of therapy, and rates of intravenous infusion should be adjusted every 2 to 4 hours, with frequent reassessments of the patient's cardiovascular status and electrolyte balance. As in diabetic ketoacidosis, water is lost in excess of sodium. Saline 0.5 N will generally adequately replace the salt and water deficit in these patients.

Early in the course of treatment, a more rapid expansion of intravascular volume and correction of prerenal azotemia is accomplished by the use of normal saline rather than 0.5 N saline. Furthermore, normal saline is hypotonic compared to the marked hypertonicity of the hyperosmolar state. Thus extracellular tonicity can be reduced and free water obtained even using normal saline. Lastly, normal saline has the additional advantage of producing smaller volume or fluid shifts in tissue compartments such as the central nervous system, which have maintained intracellular volume status by the creation of intracellular idiogenic osmols. These osmotically active equivalents may be generated by the uncovering of charge groups on intracellular proteins, and they must be allowed to be recovered during the period of fluid replacement so as to avoid marked brain edema. For these reasons, 1 to 2 L of normal saline given at a rate of 0.5 to 1.0 L/hour should be used as early fluid therapy. After initiation of a urinary output or other clinical improvement in tissue perfusion, 0.5 N saline should be utilized for the remainder of volume replacement.

Potassium replacement should also be initiated after urinary output is ensured, since hypokalemia will occur during insulin treatment of the hyperglycemia. The extent of the hypokalemia in untreated patients is, however, somewhat less than that observed in patients with diabetic ketoacidosis, as no hydrogen-potassium ion exchange secondary to acidosis has usually occurred. Because acute oliguric renal failure is a common concomitant of hyperosmolar nonketotic coma, intravenous potassium therapy must be given judiciously and with monitoring of serum potassium concentrations. It may also be advisable in the presence of anuria to maintain electrocardiographic surveillance of T-wave configuration in such patients. Phosphate depletion also may be observed in patients with hyperosmolar nonketotic coma, particularly during successful rehydration and normalization of serum glucose concentrations. Therapy with intravenous phosphate should be undertaken under the same circumstances as outlined for diabetic ketoacidosis.

Insulin therapy of the hyperglycemia in patients with the hyperosmolar nonketotic coma also must be approached carefully and with frequent monitoring of blood glucose concentrations. Choices regarding the route and manner of insulin delivery in the hyperosmolar nonketotic coma are similar to those for insulin delivery in diabetic ketoacidosis. A relatively high proportion of patients, however, demonstrates poor tissue perfusion secondary to the marked hypovolemia. Therefore subcutaneous, and even intramuscular, insulin may be inappropriate in these persons. Intermittent boluses of 5 to 10 units of rapid-acting insulin at 30- to 60-minute intervals should be sufficient to produce steady decreases in blood glucose concentrations in these patients. As an alternative, a priming injection of 0.1 unit/kg followed by continuous intravenous infusion of 0.05 to 0.10 unit/kg per hour of rapid-acting insulin will produce a sufficiently rapid decline in circulating glucose concentrations.

Rapid correction of the hyperglycemia is ill advised in these patients because such a rapid glucose reduction may be accompanied by unwarranted shifts of water from extracellular to intracellular compartments, including the brain. Throughout the course of therapy for hyperosmolar nonketotic coma, appropriate treatment for any underlying precipitating cause, such as infection, sepsis, or myocardial infarction, must be undertaken. Unlike the case in ketoacidosis, glucose or insulin infusion after reduction of hyperglycemia to concentrations below 200 mg/dl may not be necessary. Adequate fluid replacement, however, may not have been achieved by this time in the course of therapy. If such is the case, then small doses of intermediate-acting or rapid-acting insulin, followed by surveillance of blood glucose concentrations, may be necessary while rehydration continues. After resolutions of the acute disorder, maintenance therapy for diabetes mellitus obviously is needed.

Lactic Acidosis

In normal humans at rest, lactate is produced as the end product of glycolysis, primarily by tissues devoid of mitochondrial oxidative metabolism. However, under anaerobic conditions, virtually all tissues can produce lactate, including the central nervous system, muscle, and skin. Of these tissues, skeletal muscle may be the major site of lactic acid production, particularly during vigorous or hypoxic exercise. On the other hand, the liver is the major organ extracting lactic acid from the blood, although in certain states lactate is utilized by the kidney, the heart, and even skeletal muscle. Indeed, lactate is the predominant substrate for hepatic gluconeogenesis. When rates of peripheral lactic acid production and hepatic lactate extraction are balanced and equal, acid-base balance is unchanged. Lactic acidosis develops only when lactic acid production exceeds lactate utilization (Chapter 115).

Both accelerated production and diminished utilization occur as consequences of decreased tissue oxygenation. This may result from tissue hypoperfusion secondary to occlusive vascular disease or congestive cardiomyopathy. Hyperglycemia and dehydration are also important mechanisms predisposing patients to the development of lactic acidosis. For these reasons, it is not surprising that about half of the patients who develop lactic acidosis are diabetic. Sepsis, hemorrhage, overdose with ethanol, methanol, salicylates, or biguanides may also cause lactic acidosis. Accumulations of biguanides to toxic levels increase the risk of lactic acidosis, in part owing to biguanide inhibition of electron transport. Thus neoplastic tissue that depends on anaerobic glycolysis for energy may greatly increase lactate production but will not produce lactic acidosis unless lactate extraction by the liver is diminished, perhaps as the result of hepatic metastases. A variety of enzymatic defects—such as a depressed pyruvate dehydrogenase activity (which can develop in diabetes mellitus or in thiamine deficient states) or congenital enzyme defects in glucose-6-phosphatase, fructose-1,6-diphosphatase, pyruvate carboxylase, or pyruvate dehydrogenase—can also result in lactic acidosis. A relatively large proportion of patients, however, develop acute lactic acidosis with no discernible cause; these must be termed *idiopathic*.

Patients with lactic acidosis generally are acutely ill; they may be stuporous or obtunded, tachypneic, or hypotensive. The diagnosis of lactic acidosis should be suspected in patients with a metabolic acidosis that is not accounted for by drug ingestion, uremia, or ketoacidosis. The finding of an increased anion gap should arouse suspicion. The diagnosis may be confirmed by the demonstration of an arterial pH of less than 7.3 and a blood lactate concentration of greater than 5 to 10 mMol/L. In practice, however, the diagnosis is usually made on clinical grounds by exclusion of all other causes of metabolic acidosis. Confirmation of the diagnosis of lactic acidosis is difficult because lactate is not easily or rapidly measured in most laboratories. Specific enzymatic assays for lactate are available, but these are time-consuming and not routinely offered in most hospitals.

The initial therapy for lactic acidosis should include intravenous sodium bicarbonate in sufficient amounts to buffer the acidemia. Half of the measured bicarbonate deficit in total body water should be replaced in the first hour of treatment. Arterial pH should then be measured, and further bicarbonate administered if necessary. Unless the specific precipitating cause of the lactic acidosis is identified and treated, continued bicarbonate infusions will be necessary. If metformin accumulation owing to renal failure is suspected, dialysis may be used to remove the biguanide. Intravenous regular insulin should be infused to reverse hyperglycemia and to activate pyruvate dehydrogenase in the diabetic patients. Glucose infusion should be initiated concurrently with insulin once the hyperglycemia is corrected. Identifying and treating the initiating or predisposing cause of the lactic acidosis are essential. Hemorrhagic hypovolemia requires fluid and/or blood replacement. Sepsis requires appropriate antibiotic therapy, pharmacologic doses of glucocorticoids, and fluids. Myocardial infarction and congestive heart failure require inotropic agents and diuretics. Peritoneal dialysis may rarely be needed in renal failure to treat salt overload after sodium bicarbonate administration or to remove drugs. Serial arterial blood gases and pH values are needed in monitoring the patient's responses. Vasoconstrictive drugs increase lactate concentrations and should be avoided.

Hypoglycemic Coma

There are two major forms of hypoglycemic symptoms. The first group is adrenergic-mediated events including profuse sweating, tachycardia, tremulousness, and nervousness. The second group of symptoms is attributable to central nervous system fuel deprivation and includes slurred speech, diplopia, headache, confusion, somnolence, coma, and seizures. Although sensitivity to hypoglycemia among patients varies greatly, adrenergic reactions and mechanisms usually become apparent with acute falls of blood glucose levels to less than 40 mg/dl. The most notable exception is in patients on beta-blocking drugs or with long-standing diabetes mellitus and central or peripheral adrenergic autonomic neuropathy. Cerebral symptoms also begin at blood glucose levels less than 50 mg/dl, with initial symptoms generally consisting of headache. Disorientation frequently is observed at blood glucose levels less than 30 mg/dl; seizures and coma generally appear at blood glucose levels less than 25 mg/dl.

Hypoglycemia always should be considered in any patient brought to the emergency room in coma. In known diabetics on insulin or sulfonylurea therapy, hypoglycemia is an even more likely cause of coma. The absence of Kussmaul's respiration and dehydration and a significant lack of acetone in the breath should increase the suspicion of hypoglycemia. The presence or recent history of grand mal seizures or of focal seizures in elderly persons having underlying cerebrovascular disease should further increase the suspicion of hypoglycemic coma. A history of a missed meal or of unusually vigorous exercise also may be obtained. Confirmation of this diagnosis can be obtained rapidly by Chemstrip analysis of blood glucose levels. Values less than 50 mg/dl should be considered as representing hypoglycemic coma until it is proved otherwise.

Therapy with 50% glucose solution should be initiated at once. Of this solution, 50 to 100 ml may have to be given to revive patients in hypoglycemic coma. Patients with long-standing hypoglycemia may not respond to this amount of glucose. Factors such as body weight and the amount of insulin or hypoglycemic agent ingested will determine the quantity of dextrose required for normalization of blood glucose concentrations. Many patients will awaken immediately when adequate circulating glucose concentrations are achieved. A significant proportion of these patients will show temporary or persistent features of residual neurologic deficit.

In small children or in subjects with veins difficult to access for 50% glucose administration, glucagon (0.5 mg) may be given intramuscularly, followed by a second dose within 15 minutes. Failure to respond to this dose of glucagon can be observed in patients with preexisting depletion of hepatic glycogen stores, as might occur in a patient after severe and prolonged exercise. In no instance should the patient be regarded as cured simply because an improved state of consciousness is produced. If an overdose of large quantities of insulin or of sulfonylureas has occurred, relapse into hypoglycemia can be anticipated if no effort is made to ensure a continued intake of carbohydrate. The latter may be achieved by having the patient ingest orange juice or tea with added sucrose or glucose. Intravenous glucose administration using 10% glucose and water may be necessary. This is of some consequence in patients with sulfonylurea overdosage in whom a vigorous insulin secretory response to 50% glucose infusion will be observed. In these subjects, a prolonged course of therapy using a progressive reduction in the rate of infusion of 10% glucose and water is necessary to prevent relapse into hypoglycemia. Rarely, patients may require glucocorticoids to raise the blood glucose concentration to acceptable levels. This therapy should extend generally over two and preferably three half-lives for the ingested sulfonylurea. Focal seizures or residual neurologic deficit that does not clear in a conscious patient after hypoglycemia should prompt the physician to investigate potential abnormalities of cerebrovascular supply or central nervous system structure.

Reevaluation of diabetes management should be initiated in patients having serious hypoglycemic episodes. In particular, attention must be focused on the manner in which hypoglycemic agents are being self-administered and on the nature of diet regulation in these subjects. Other potential problems causing a marked increase in insulin sensitivity, such as that produced by adrenal insufficiency, renal insufficiency, liver disease, and pituitary dysfunction, also should be considered.

Prevention of Diabetic Comas

In addition to control of blood glucose, other aspects of diabetic care are important in the prevention of acute complications. Control of infections is particularly important. Hyperglycemia in patients with diabetes mellitus impairs a number of aspects of leukocyte function. These include leukocyte chemotactic response, phagocytosis, and bacterial killing. These impairments, together with the predilection of diabetic patients to microvascular and macrovascular disease, which impairs regional blood flow, tend to increase both the frequency and severity of acquired infectious processes. Staphylococcal pyoderma, gram-negative and anaerobic infections of the extremities, and pyelonephritis with papillary necrosis all occur more commonly in patients with diabetes mellitus. Mucormycosis of the paranasal sinuses is a rare infection, found almost only in patients with diabetes. Often, patients with severe bacterial infections develop bacterial sepsis. Such a state leads to a marked deterioration in the degree of diabetic control and may even precipitate diabetic ketoacidosis or hyperosmolar nonketotic coma. The worsening hyperglycemia tends in turn to facilitate a more severe bacterial infection because of further impairment in white cell function owing to hypovolemia with impaired tissue perfusion. For these reasons, serious infections in patients with diabetes mellitus must be treated vigorously and early in their course. Therapy with bactericidal antibiotics, preferably with combinations of therapeutic agents having synergistic interactions, should be instituted immediately after cultures are obtained. Control of the blood glucose level cannot be achieved in this setting by using routine or preexisting dosage of insulin or of oral sulfonylureas. Under these circumstances, particularly with sepsis, continuous intravenous infusion of insulin in relatively low doses (0.05 to 0.4 unit/kg/hour) should be considered as an initial treatment. For patients with marked obtundation or inability to ingest food, intravenous glucose may be administered concurrently with insulin. At least 150 to 200 g/day of carbohydrate should be given in the form of glucose in order to suppress starvation ketosis. This method is generally preferable to the use of intermittent sliding-scale urinary glycosuria coverage, which allows intervals of 6 hours or more to pass before supplementary insulin is administered. The disadvantages of sliding-scale coverage include failures to obtain a urine specimen so that coverage can be given, potential variance between urinary glucose spillage and blood glucose concentrations, and interfering agents that can yield either false-positive or false-negative test results. In patients with severe sepsis, more frequent intervals for the administration of relatively small doses of insulin by sliding scale may yield acceptable results. In most instances, the blood glucose levels should be monitored at 1- to 4-hour intervals. The glucose levels should be held to 100 to 150 mg/dl in patients with severe infection.

CHRONIC COMPLICATIONS OF DIABETES MELLITUS

Chronic complications of diabetes mellitus are divided into three major categories: macrovascular disease, microvascular disease, and the neuropathies. Treatment of these disorders is not satisfactory. Prevention or at least a retardation of the progression of these complications is the goal of the physician. Although the mechanisms accounting for the development of diabetic complications are probably multifactorial, most authorities accept a correlation between the degree and duration of hyperglycemia and the frequency of complications. These relationships are probably valid for the macrovascular lesions as well as the microvascular and neuropathic lesions.

Macrovascular Disease

Occlusive coronary artery disease and concomitant congestive heart failure account for more than 70% of mortality in all patients with diabetes. Although this phenomenon is generally noted after 15 or more years of diabetes, it may be the initial finding in some patients with diabetes mellitus. Atherosclerosis occurs at a frequency nearly twofold to fourfold greater in males and females, respectively, than that in the nondiabetic population. At least three major elements of the diabetic process together accelerate the complex mechanism(s) of atherosclerosis. First, the insulin-resistant state, which appears years to decades before clinical hyperglycemia, produces hyperinsulinemia; the latter clearly predicts coronary morbidity and mortality in multiple widely disparate populations. Second, a dyslipidemia in patients with diabetes and in the prediabetic, insulin-resistant state is frequently apparent. Such a dyslipidemia is characterized by elevated concentrations of triglyceride as VLDL and depressed levels of high-density lipoprotein (HDL) cholesterol; this is seen in patients either with poorly controlled type 1 insulin-dependent disease or type 2 non–insulin-dependent disease, whether in males or females. Indeed, the depression of HDL cholesterol levels in females with diabetes mellitus is greater than that seen in males and accounts, in part, for the differentially greater acceleration of atherosclerosis in diabetic

females, particularly premenopausal females, as compared to diabetic males of the same age. Depressed HDL cholesterol levels are a clear and well-characterized risk factor for coronary atherosclerosis. The hypertriglyceridemia may itself be atherogenic or may lead to the formation of atherogenic precursors such as modified LDL cholesterol particles known as LDL subclass B, or small, dense LDL. The latter appears in most insulin-resistant states and has been shown to be three times more atherogenic than ordinary, unmodified LDL. The latter is generally replaced by smaller, denser LDL when triglyceride concentrations are well in excess of 150 mg/dl. Third, hyperglycemia accelerates atherogenesis by way of protein glycation. Such glycation modifies endothelial basement membrane permeability and function, so as to allow greater rates of lipoprotein deposition in the arterial wall. The glycation simulates the production of a macrophage chemotaxis factor, thereby recruiting cells responsible for the early foam cell phase of atherosclerosis.

Glycation also generates growth factors capable of accelerating the cellular proliferation characteristic of the fibrous plaque. These factors include platelet-derived growth factors and other advanced glycosylation product growth factors. Glycation modifies the function of a number of lipoprotein particles, including LDL particles. When glycated, Apo B 100, the receptor-binding protein on LDL, shows greater cellular uptake of LDL particles. Glycation also modifies the tendency towards oxidation of LDL lipids. Oxidized LDL is more readily taken up by macrophages in the so-called scavenger pathway. Glycation of HDL is also observed. When glycated, HDL binds less well to its cellular and tissue receptors and catalyzes processes related to reverse cholesterol transport at rates only about half those seen with the unglycated lipoprotein. Other aspects of the diabetic state contribute to accelerated atherosclerosis, including potential modifications of VLDL particles themselves in such a fashion as to produce smaller, denser VLDL. These modified particles appear to interact with vascular endothelium to produce increased levels of thromboxane and reduced PGF_1a, thereby explaining, in part, an increased tendency toward thrombosis in patients with diabetes. Atherosclerotic macrovascular disease appears to be histologically similar in both diabetic and nondiabetic subjects, despite the rapid and occasionally fulminant progression of the disorder in diabetics. Thus patients in their late teens and early 20s may begin to be symptomatic from severe atherosclerosis, particularly in type 1 (insulin-dependent) diabetes.

The precise pathogenesis of the accelerated atherosclerosis is unclear. Although qualitatively similar in diabetic and nondiabetic patients, atherosclerosis in diabetes mellitus has several unique aspects. Coronary atherosclerosis in diabetic patients can involve the whole of the right and left coronary circulation and may not be limited primarily to proximal lesions as noted in nondiabetic patients. Such diffuse coronary artery disease frequently is accompanied by marked left ventricular dysfunction, which is frequently out of proportion to the degree of reduction in coronary blood flow. In the absence of previous myocardial infarction, a hypokinetic left ventricle in patients with diabetes has been interpreted to suggest a diabetic cardiomyopathy. Whether such cardiomyopathy exists independent of either macrovascular or microvascular disease is somewhat open to question, although it should be suspected in all poorly controlled diabetic patients with marked protein wasting.

Treatment for diabetic cardiomyopathy is similar to that of other forms of congestive cardiomyopathy. If there is impaired runoff in the distal coronary circulation of a patient, coronary artery bypass surgery may be more hazardous and less satisfactory in its overall outcome. Nevertheless, patients having high risk for myocardial infarction or demonstrating moderate to severe left ventricular impairment to exercise are still good candidates for coronary artery revascularization procedures.

Atypical angina and atypical symptomatology of myocardial infarction occur in diabetic persons. Some patients will not experience the usual degrees of pain during episodes of myocardial ischemia or infarction. The absence of severe chest pain or pressure in postoperative subjects must therefore be compensated for by a higher index of suspicion in the attending physician. Diabetic patients may have a greater tendency to manifest atypical symptoms of coronary insufficiency such as epigastric distress or heartburn. Neck pain or pain radiation to both shoulders is also more common. Lastly, patients with diabetes mellitus also tend to manifest coronary artery insufficiency

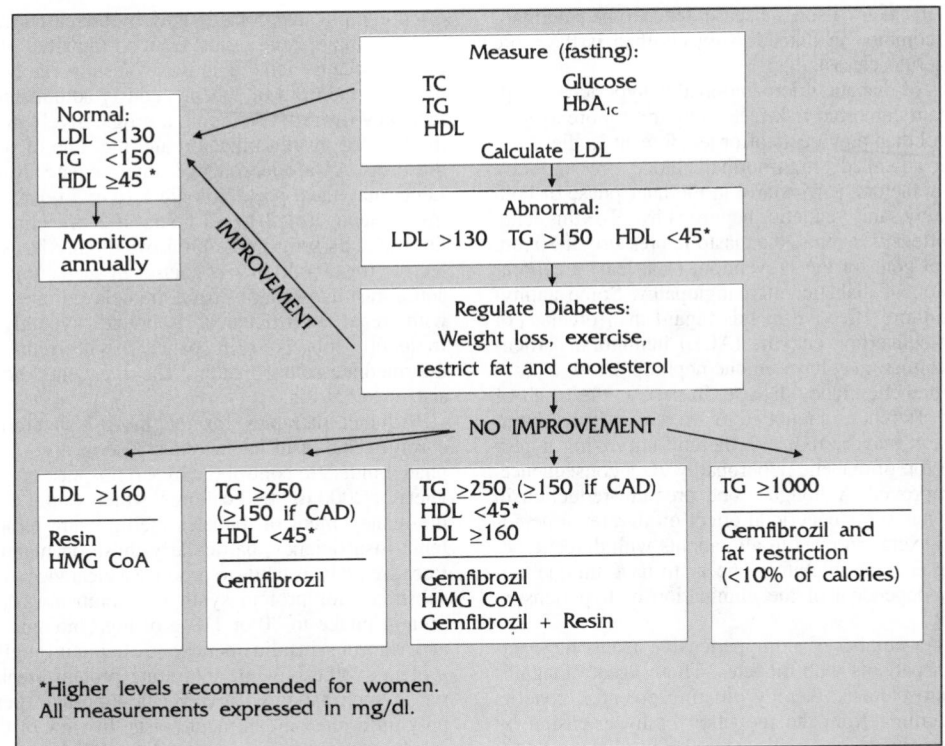

FIGURE 303-7 Management of dyslipidemia in patients with diabetes.
From *Diabetes Care* 15:1068, 1992.

by the episodic development of painless congestive heart failure with exercise or stress.

Medical management of coronary artery disease, as well as peripheral vascular disease, should aim at normalizing the hyperglycemia and eliminating obesity and dyslipidemias. Exercise and weight loss, with reduced fat intake and avoidance of alcohol consumption, is the preferred form of therapy for type 2 diabetes mellitus in patients with mild to moderate dyslipidemia or hyperlipidemia. Insulin is required in hypoinsulinemic patients. With insulin lack, the lipid disturbances are characterized by an excess accumulation of VLDL triglyceride-rich particles in blood and by an increase of substrate delivered to the liver for VLDL synthesis. This process leads to an acquired type IV hyperlipidemia. In more severe cases, a type V hyperlipidemia characterized by the presence of chylomicrons in addition to VLDL particles also may be observed. In general, these patients have triglyceride levels greater than 1500 mg/dl and manifest lipemia retinalis at triglyceride levels of 2000 or greater. Virtually all types of hyperlipidemia, with the possible exception of type IIa hypercholesterolemia alone, may occur in uncontrolled diabetes mellitus.

The treatment of the acquired hyperlipidemia of diabetes mellitus should be directed initially toward control of the blood glucose concentration by using exercise and diet therapy, and insulin if necessary. Patients with hyperlipidemia and hyperglycemia require greater than normal quantities of insulin. Insulin requirements of 100 to 200 units per day may be encountered, and these may not necessarily decrease as the hyperlipidemia is improved. Appropriate diet therapy such as an American Diabetes Association or American Heart Association diet for hyperlipidemia must be instituted. Caloric restriction to achieve ideal weight is essential. For most patients, these therapies will not completely control hypertriglyceridemia. Additional therapies using gemfibrozil may also be indicated, but only after attempts to control the hyperglycemia have been made. Nicotinic acid tends to worsen diabetic control and therefore should only be instituted in selected patients with careful monitoring of the patient (Chapter 306). An overall approach to the management of hyperglycemia and dyslipidemia in diabetic patients is provided in Fig. 303-7. For patients with familial combined or mixed dyslipidemias characterized by high LDL cholesterol, high VLDL triglyceride and low HDL cho-

lesterol levels, a combination of lipid-lowering agents may be necessary. Ideally, double therapy should use gemfibrozil plus a bile salt resin or an HMG-CoA reductase inhibitor with reduced skeletal muscle toxicity such as pravastatin. Furthermore, two or three agents may be useful in patients with advanced coronary disease in whom regression of atherosclerosis may be possible, particularly if a low-fat diet can be followed.

As with coronary artery disease, peripheral vascular disease in diabetic patients tends to be qualitatively similar, but quantitatively greater, than that observed in nondiabetic patients. However, the frequency of distal involvement, particularly of the lower limb, is far higher in diabetic subjects, especially in those who smoke. As a consequence of the impaired distal runoff in the circulation below the popliteal fossa, peripheral vascular bypass surgery for distal lower extremity ischemia is often less rewarding in diabetic than nondiabetic patients. If relatively isolated aneurysms or occlusions of the distal aorta or the common iliac or femoral artery can be demonstrated, then resection and graft or bypass surgery may prove helpful in ameliorating symptoms such as claudication and in improving the muscle dysfunction of diabetic patients with severe peripheral vascular disease. In the more common syndromes of peripheral vascular insufficiency such as the Leriche syndrome, bypass surgery has proved helpful, although not totally satisfactory, in diabetic subjects. Lumbar sympathectomy is sometimes helpful in relieving mild rest pain but probably does not alter the long-term course of atherosclerosis. Little evidence, however, suggests that sympathectomy produces a lasting improvement in peripheral vascular blood flow; sympathectomy does not appear to reverse gangrenous complications or prevent amputations in patients with severely impaired circulation either. Attempts aimed at reducing risk factors such as obesity, cigarette smoking, and a lack of exercise should be encouraged.

Microvascular Disease

Capillary basement membrane thickening or the accumulation of periodic–acid Schiff–positive material within the microvasculature of diabetic subjects is a characteristic lesion of diabetes (Chapter 117). In the kidney, the formation of nodular areas of intercapillary glomerulosclerosis (Kimmelstiel-Wilson's disease) tends to be pathognomonic, but it is less common in diabetic subjects than is the more frequent diffuse glomerulosclerosis.

In almost all forms of diabetic microangiopathy, hypertension appears to be an important comorbid risk factor requiring more aggressive attention to control than previously afforded. Recent studies have clearly indicated that so-called "high-normal" blood pressures are clear, independent risk factors, particularly in the later phase of both proliferative retinopathy and diabetic nephropathy. To this end, therapy with antihypertensive agents to a diastolic pressure of 80 mm Hg or less is a general goal for the prevention, or at least amelioration, of the progression of diabetic microangiopathy. Some antihypertensive agents are more effective in this regard than others. For example, angiotensin-converting enzyme (ACE) inhibitors, particularly short-acting inhibitors, may have unique nephroprotective properties with regard to diabetic kidney disease. In part, as the result of preferential action on efferent as compared to afferent arterials, intraglomerular hypertension may be reduced, thereby improving hyperfiltration, an initial lesion of diabetic nephropathy. As a consequence, proteinuria is also improved. Although blood pressure reduction in hypertensive patients has some beneficial effect on intrarenal hemodynamics and protein excretion rates in all patients with diabetic nephropathy, converting enzyme inhibitors appear to have unique, additional advantages independent of the elimination of hypertension per se.

On the other hand, a number of antihypertensive agents have untoward side effects in patients with diabetes. These agents magnify the potential for atherosclerosis, thereby vitiating potential benefits on atherosclerosis accruing from the reduction of hypertension by worsening such concomitant abnormalities as the insulin resistance and hyperglycemia of diabetes or the dyslipidemia of diabetes. Thiazide diuretics may more likely be associated with an increased mortality in hypertensive diabetic patients than other forms of antihypertensive therapy. They certainly have not proved satisfactory, either alone or in combination with beta blockers, in reducing the accelerated atherosclerosis of patients treated for hypertension. Additionally, each agent alone and in combination, appears to increase the risk of becoming diabetic substantially. Some calcium slow channel entry antagonists also have untoward effects on the calcium-potassium channel in beta cells. As a consequence of their use, impaired insulin secretion and hyperglycemia have been reported. In contrast, alpha₁-adrenergic antagonists appear to improve the dyslipidemia in patients with diabetes while producing effective, hypertensive therapy. There is evidence for synergy between alpha-adrenergic antagonists and converting enzyme inhibitors in patients requiring multiple drug therapies or for step therapy protocol in patients with diabetes.

Diabetic Nephropathy

Diabetic nephropathy (Chapter 117) becomes clinically apparent (initially as albuminuria) approximately 15 years after the onset of diabetes mellitus in at least 50% of type 1 diabetic patients. Nephropathy may be predicted by the early development of microalbuminuria (>30 μg/min) in patients years before clinical macroproteinuria is seen. The disease has a slowly progressive course over a 10-year interval, at which point azotemia generally becomes apparent. A small fraction of diabetic patients with proteinuria develop an overt nephrotic syndrome. The appearance of obvious proteinuria often is correlated with the appearance of overt diabetic retinopathy, although the two do not necessarily appear simultaneously. Impairment of urinary bladder emptying because of diabetic autonomic neuropathy may aggravate advancing renal insufficiency.

Management of diabetic nephropathy focuses on preventing further deterioration by using low-protein diets, ACE inhibitors, and vigorous glucose and hypertension control. A reduction of glomerular hyperfiltration by decreased protein intake and especially by ACE inhibition with captopril, in particular, will tend to arrest the long-term decline in glomerular filtration rates. Hypertension must be normalized in all diabetic patients, as it increases the incidence, severity, and progression of all microvascular and macrovascular complications. A mean arterial pressure of less than 93 mm Hg (<120/<80 mm Hg) is required to arrest progression of nephropathy.

The management of diabetic patients with renal insufficiency is often complicated considerably by increased insulin sensitivity. This increase may result in part from an impaired glomerular clearance of insulin because renal disposal of insulin can account for the removal of up to one third of subcutaneously administered insulin. There is a tendency toward developing a progressively greater interval between the time of insulin injection and the time of peak biologic action of the drug. As a consequence, intermediate insulins such as NPH or Lente may have peak biologic activity in diabetic patients with renal insufficiency at 18 to 30 hours after injection. Shorter-acting insulins, such as semi-Lente on a twice-daily basis, may prove more effective for blood glucose control in such subjects. The delay in peak action results primarily from the delayed rates of removal in patients with renal insufficiency. Rebound hyperglycemia also may be frequently observed in patients with renal failure treated with intermediate-acting insulin. These patients, however, are highly resistant to ketosis.

Adjunct therapies for the more characteristic abnormalities of chronic renal insufficiency must also be used, such as the use of phosphate binders to control the hyperphosphatemia of renal insufficiency. Diets of 2000 to 3000 calories, which would otherwise be unusual in the management of diabetes mellitus, are indicated in patients with renal insufficiency, particularly those on maintenance hemodialysis. Because dialysis tends to produce a clearance of numerous amino acid substrates for protein synthesis, compensatory increases in dietary protein intake to 80 or 110 g of high biologic value protein per day and rigorous insulin therapy to maintain euglycemia and stimulate protein synthesis while inhibiting protein breakdown may be essential in such patients. However, low-protein diets are preferred when only mild renal impairment exists. In view of the accelerated atherosclerosis and metabolic instability of diabetic patients on hemodialysis, renal transplantation is a better mode of therapy for chronic azotemia.

Diabetic Retinopathy

Diabetic retinopathy is a progressive deterioration in the microcirculation to the retina observed in patients with diabetes mellitus. Deterioration in intimal integrity, as evidenced by fluorescein leakage from retinal capillaries, can be observed within weeks of the development of flagrant hyperglycemia. After approximately 10 years of poorly controlled diabetes mellitus, microaneurysms are present in at least 50% of patients. Retinal microaneurysms, saclike excrescences of intimal basement membrane from the extended walls of the capillaries, are best seen by using fluorescein angiography. Evidence has been presented that vigorous control of glucose concentrations is associated with a diminished rate of microaneurysm formation in type 1 diabetic patients compared with patients having relatively less well-controlled hyperglycemia. Retinopathy is present in 90% of patients with diabetes for over 30 years.

After the appearance of microaneurysms, the course of diabetic retinopathy may progress to the development of punctate hemorrhages together with hard, waxy-appearing exudates. The triad of hemorrhages, exudates, and microaneurysms is frequently called *background retinopathy* (Plate IX-2). This type can be accompanied by fluffy, so-called cotton wool exudates over the retina, which result from microinfarcts and retinal scarring. Hard exudates are the extravasation of proteinaceous and lipid-rich intravascular fluid that appear because of the increased permeability of retinal capillaries and are analogous to the proteinuria of the glomerular disease of diabetes mellitus (Plate IX-3).

In most patients, background retinopathy tends to remain relatively stable, although slowly progressive. In a minority of patients, retinal hemorrhages on a much larger scale develop from the weakened membranes of the dilated and tortuous retinal vessels. After resorption of much of the blood-containing material, progressive scarring develops. New retinal vessels that form in the scar area (a process termed *neovascularization*) appear to penetrate into the vitreous. In later stages, the vascular tufts contract toward the vitreous, producing a secondary retinal detachment. This process of proliferative retinopathy causes the profound loss of vision and ultimate blindness in patients with diabetes mellitus (Plate IX-4). Recent well-controlled studies have demonstrated that photocoagulation with argon laser light or retinal coagulation with a xenon lamp may prevent retinal detachment and preserve sight. Laser therapy may be used to accurately photocoagulate the contents of a dilated and tortuous vessel. Much of the stimulus to neovascular proliferation is the apparent result of the production of an angiogenesis factor by an ischemic retina. A decreased production of this factor by the destruction of portions of the retina using peripheral retinal photocoagulation ameliorates this proliferation by reducing angiogenesis. In patients with advanced vitreous involvement, surgical vitrectomy and vitreous replacement may offer some restoration of vision. For these reasons, ophthalmologic consultation and follow-up of all patients having moderate to advanced background retinopathy should be obtained at least annually.

Other parts of the eye also may be involved by diabetes mellitus. Chronic hyperglycemia may lead to temporary changes in lens shape that may result in marked fluctuations of visual acuity. Approximately 6 to 8 weeks of glucose control is required to reestablish lenticular curvature. Cataracts develop in patients with diabetes mellitus more frequently than in the normal population. In patients with galactosemia, the role of polyol formation has been clearly demonstrated in the hydration cataract. Similar mechanisms also have been postulated to explain the excessive rate of cataract formation in diabetic subjects. Chronic hyperglycemia may lead to excess sorbitol formation in the diabetic lens, thereby causing an osmotic gradient along which extracellular waste may flow into the lens. As a consequence, lens protein architecture may be disrupted, thereby generating a cataract. There is no evidence to demonstrate that good control of the blood glucose level prevents the development of cataracts in diabetic subjects. Once developed, reversal of cataract formation by nonsurgical means appears to be futile. Glaucoma also occurs with increased frequency in diabetic subjects. Presumably, the mechanisms of glaucoma development in such patients relates to posthemorrhagic fibrosis and scarring of the outflow tract for fluids (the canal of Schlemm) as the result of stimulated anterior chamber angiogenesis by the same factor(s) produced by the ischemic retina.

Diabetic Neuropathy

Diabetic neuropathy is a troublesome consequence of diabetes mellitus. Unlike many of the other chronic consequences of diabetes, the neuropathy may occur early in the disease. Nevertheless, the frequency and severity of diabetic neuropathy increase proportionately with the duration and severity of the hyperglycemia in diabetes mellitus. In some patients, an acute loss of diabetic control may be accompanied by abrupt manifestations of diabetic neuropathy, most commonly distal paresthesias and dysesthesias.

Although diabetic neuropathy does not contribute substantially to mortality in patients with diabetes mellitus, it does contribute to high morbidity and impairment of lifestyle. Of all the chronic complications of diabetes, neuropathy appears to be the most responsive to therapies that normalize circulating glucose concentrations.

Virtually every aspect of the peripheral nervous system can be involved in diabetic neuropathy. Such neuropathy may be classified according to the area of peripheral nervous system involvement. For example, the most commonly encountered form of diabetic neuropathy is that of symmetric distal polyneuropathy, usually affecting the lower extremity more commonly than the upper extremity. Diabetic neuropathy also may present as a radiculopathy or as a mononeuropathy of either a single nerve or multiple nerve trunks. Spinal cord and visceral involvement also may be evidenced in syndromes such as the tabetic-like neuropathy mimicking tertiary syphilis. In this neuropathy, lancinating pains of the abdomen or distal lower extremity may be excruciating. Charcot's joints also may be observed in patients with diabetes mellitus and usually involves the foot, although, rarely, involvement of the knee and upper extremity has been observed.

Virtually any cranial nerve, alone or in combination, may be involved in an acute presentation of diabetic neuropathy. Cranial nerves III, IV, and VI are most frequently affected. Other cranial nerves, however, such as VII, VIII, and XII may also be involved by the diabetic neuropathic process. Finally, almost every aspect of autonomic nervous system function may be seriously impaired by diabetic neuropathy. Such neuropathy may be patchy and incomplete in nature and may involve either a single aspect of autonomic function or a broad spectrum of functions.

The pathogenesis of diabetic neuropathy is unclear. Multiple mechanisms may be involved. Acute mononeuropathies alone (simplex), or in combinations (multiplex) in which nearly total dysfunction of whole nerve trunks can be observed, may result from a relatively sudden infarction of one or more branches of the vasa nervorum (the penetrating arteries delivering and maintaining circulation to nerve trunks). On the other hand, the slowly progressive deterioration of peripheral nervous system function seen in the systematic distal polyneuropathies may not be attributed to an infarction process. With progressive deterioration, axonal and nerve cell death may occur, accounting for the sensory anesthesia observed in these patients. Chronic hyperglycemia may lead to excess sorbitol formation in Schwann cells of nerve trunks. The enzyme responsible for sorbitol formation, aldose reductase, has a relatively low affinity for glucose, the concentration of which is the primary rate-controlling event for sorbitol formation. Clearance of osmotically active sorbitol depends on diffusion of the hexatol to the axon, where reoxidation to fructose may occur via sorbitol dehydrogenase. In diabetic nerve, sorbitol content is increased. Consequently, the increased osmotically active substances in the Schwann cell may produce an extracellular-to-intracellular fluid shift resulting in Schwann cell swelling and disruption. Because these cells are responsible for the maintenance of axonal integrity, axonal dysfunction and death may be observed.

Distal Polyneuropathies. These complications are the most commonly encountered complaints of diabetic patients related to diabetic neuropathy. The distal paresthesias and dysesthesias may occur insidiously or may be acute during loss of diabetic control secondary to infection or other forms of severe stress. In the lower extremities, the involvement is usually bilateral, symmetric, and accompanied by severe pain. In individual subjects the pain may be perceived differently (e.g., as cramping, burning, or lancinating). The painful polyneuropathies of diabetes are often experienced with increased intensity at night. Paresthesias are most commonly expressed as numbness, tingling, or pins-and-needles sensations. The physical examination is generally unremarkable because neurologic functioning, including vibratory sensation, may be preserved. However, the sensational pain and light touch, particularly differentiation of sharp from dull objects, may be impaired. The most common concomitant of symmetric polyneuropathy in diabetic subjects is the bilateral absence of ankle and/or knee jerks. Indeed, diabetes mellitus is the most common explanation for bilaterally absent ankle jerks. Other explanations must be sought for unilaterally absent reflexes in the lower extremity, even in diabetic patients.

Treatment of diabetic polyneuropathy is usually unsatisfactory. Initial therapy should be directed toward establishing good control of the serum glucose concentrations in patients with diabetes mellitus. Treatment of residual symptoms has been attempted by using a combination of vitamin B therapies including thiamine (100 mg three times a day), folic acid (3 mg daily), vitamin B_{12} (1000 μg intramuscularly daily for 5 days), and a broad spectrum of other vitamins.

Initial expectations of this type of therapy were somewhat more enthusiastic and positive than subsequent results have warranted; however, there is increased protein and B-vitamin catabolism in diabetic subjects, and such patients do have lower serum vitamin concentrations than comparable diabetic patients without diabetic neuropathy. Additional therapy with either phenytoin or carbamazepine may be tried. Both agents have been reported to improve diabetic paresthesias in one third to half of subjects studied. These pharmacologic agents may act by stabilizing axonal transmembrane potentials, thereby blocking pain and paresthesias. Carbamazepine is associated with a higher incidence of side effects than is phenytoin. The latter should be tried initially at full anticonvulsant doses. These agents are most effective for pseudotabetic symptoms. Amitriptyline and fluphenazine are also useful in the treatment of diabetic neuropathy. The effectiveness of aldose reductase inhibitors is presently being assessed.

Advanced sensory loss producing peripheral anesthesia in the lower extremity results in the development of a Charcot's joint. Destruction of the cartilaginous joint lining occurs from repeated trauma incurred as a result of loss of sensation. Abnormalities of chondrocyte metabolism and function also have been suggested as being involved in the pathogenesis. With continued use of the joint, destruction of the normal architecture and the attendant appearance of loose bodies within the joint may be observed on radiographic examination. Ultimately, a total destruction of the normal joint architecture and a loss of normal function occur. Treatment of Charcot's joints of the lower extremity often requires combined surgical and rehabilitative efforts.

A more frequent concomitant of distal anesthesia is the development of neurotropic ulceration, particularly on the plantar aspect of the foot. Anesthesia leads to a worsening of any minor injury because of the absence of protective painful stimuli. This problem, in addition to preexisting microvascular and macrovascular circulatory impairments, characterizes the underlying mechanisms that may lead to rapid gangrene after foot injury.

All patients with diabetes mellitus should perform careful self-examination of their feet. Foot hygiene should be maintained with particular attention to the care and trimming of toenails and calluses. Extreme care should be taken in selecting footwear. Because diabetic patients have an early tendency toward hyperhidrosis and subsequent anhidrosis, the use of all-leather shoes is advised, as leather maintains an adequate rate of evaporation of perspiration. Absorbent socks also should be worn at all times. In the diabetic patient, shortening of the flexor tendons may occur, leading to hammer-toe deformities. This problem produces maldistribution of the weight on the foot and causes callosities. Therefore correction of maldistributed weight to prevent pressure on ulcerated lesions is important. Vigorous treatment of any form of ulceration of the diabetic foot is essential in preventing gangrene and ultimate amputation of the extremity. Prevention of infection in moderate- to large-sized ulceration initially should be attempted by topical antibiotic therapy. Advanced infected ulcerations require large doses of bactericidal antibiotic, generally given intravenously. Frequent debridement of the ulcerated area, particularly to prevent undermining of the ulcer margin by the spreading necrotic process, is also essential. Rest and elevation of the foot and frequent soaks in warm, but not hot, Betadine-water mixtures are also useful.

In diabetic patients with advanced microvascular and macrovascular circulation to the foot, amputation may be required if progressive unremitting infection or gangrene occurs. An obvious line of demarcation should develop. In all instances, amputation should be performed well above this line. Transtarsal amputation for infected ulcerations of the diabetic metatarsal area usually is not successful. To provide maximum rehabilitation of these patients, however, amputation below major joints such as the ankle or knee is more advisable than amputation above these joints. In particular, below-the-knee amputations almost always provide greater patient mobility and rehabilitation than do above-the-knee amputations. In the acutely infected patient, surgical therapies, such as vascular bypass procedures, aimed at increasing regional blood flow rarely prevent the need for amputation. In all instances, osteomyelitis should be considered in cases of persistent, nonhealing diabetic foot ulceration with consistent evidence of bacterial infection.

Diabetic Neuromuscular Disease

Diabetic neuromuscular disease can be differentiated into several different syndromes. In the upper extremity, painless atrophy of the intrinsic muscles of the hand can be observed. This is most obvious for the thenar and hypothenar eminences as well as the interosseous spaces. The atrophy may progress to a point of nearly total loss of intrinsic musculature. This process is always accompanied by a loss of motor power in the upper extremity, particularly the distal muscles. This form of peripheral neuropathy may or may not be accompanied by sensory anesthesia in the upper extremity. Upper-extremity diabetic neuromuscular disease appears to be more common in the elderly and in males. Many of these patients have mild to moderate hypertriglyceridemia. Control of hyperglycemia and hypertriglyceridemia may be accompanied by improvement of the neuromuscular disease after a period of 6 to 12 months.

Diabetic neuromuscular disease of the lower extremity, more commonly referred to as *diabetic amyotrophy,* resembles a progressive weakness and wasting of proximal lower-extremity muscles involving the pelvic girdle and anterior thigh compartments, most commonly the quadriceps femoris. This condition is usually accompanied by severe pain, although anesthesia may be observed. Unlike upper-extremity diabetic neuromuscular disease, lower-extremity disease may be asymmetric in distribution and generally heals spontaneously in 2 to 4 months from time of diagnosis. A similar, but less painful, variant of diabetic amyotrophy occurs in the upper extremity and is associated with progressive wasting of the intrinsic musculature of the shoulder girdle. In many patients, a combined defect involving the proximal musculature of both upper and lower extremities may also be observed. In these subjects, vigorous control of the blood glucose level by insulin therapy may provide the only beneficial form of therapy.

Acute Mononeuropathies

Acute mononeuropathies may manifest themselves in virtually any single nerve trunk. Most commonly encountered are acute mononeuropathies of the cranial nerves, although other mononeuropathies such as acute foot drop also may be observed. Diabetic mononeuropathies may manifest themselves as acute, painful extraocular muscle palsies. In general, pain precedes the development of palsy by 5 to 10 days. Although the pain may be trigeminal in distribution, the diplopia and subsequent clinical involvement of the cranial nerves III, IV, or VI alone or in combination soon provide the basis for a diagnosis. When the third cranial nerve is involved, there is characteristic sparing of the pupillary fibers in more than 80% of cases, which provides a point of important differential significance because aneurysms or intracranial mass lesions generally involve both the pupillary fibers and the myelinated fibers to the extraocular muscles.

Specific therapies for diabetic extraocular palsy do not exist. Rest and local supportive measures generally will suffice until there is regression of the self-limited condition. Approximately 2 to 3 months is required for relatively complete healing. Other cranial nerves may be involved, producing considerable concern regarding the underlying diagnosis. Most commonly, extraocular involvement affects the seventh and eight cranial nerves and may manifest itself initially with a Bell's palsy–like syndrome together with equilibrium or hearing impairment. On occasion, patients with diabetes mellitus may also have isolated primary pupillary abnormalities such as anisocoria with diminished reactivity to light but generally not accommodation. This may resemble an Argyll Robertson pupil.

Diabetic Autonomic Neuropathy

The autonomic neuropathies of diabetes may be manifested as a heterogeneous and complex combination of disorders involving virtually every organ system. The autonomic neuropathies are discussed here in terms of the organ system involved.

Gastrointestinal Tract Neuropathies. Virtually every aspect of gastrointestinal dysfunction may be produced by diabetic neuropathy. This may range from disordered esophageal motility to diabetic gastroparesis with impaired gastric emptying and may even include impaired peristalsis with diabetic diarrhea. Most common and distressing of the neuropathies affecting gastrointestinal tract function is that of diabetic diarrhea. The patient complains of explosive diarrhea, seemingly worse at night, although daytime hyperactivity is fairly common. The diarrhea is not preceded by cramps and may be sufficiently severe and sudden as to produce the appearance of fecal incontinence. Characteristic roentgenographic patterns of disordered small bowel motility are sometimes observed in patients with diabetic diarrhea. Control of diabetic hyperglycemia is effective in improving the diarrhea in a small proportion of patients. Anticholinergics such as diphenoxylate (Lomotil) and stool-bulking agents have limited utility. Therapies using oral antibiotics such as tetracycline for relative bacterial overgrowth in the small intestinal lumen may be efficacious. Clonidine (0.2 to 0.3 mg/day) appears to be the most successful treatment to date.

Diabetic gastroparesis leads to early satiety and unpredictable gastric emptying accompanied by nausea and vomiting. This is a relatively distressing concomitant of diabetic visceral autonomic neuropathy. Gastroparesis tends to produce unpredictable losses in diabetic control owing to the inconstancy of food absorption. Multiple small feedings of a predominantly liquid, low-fat diet may be effective in maintaining nutrition. Approximately 1 to 3 months of rigorous euglycemia is essential before the symptoms of this disorder will disappear. Cisapride or secondarily metoclopramide may be very useful in facilitating gastric emptying; cholinergic agonists in general have limited utility.

Genitourinary Neuropathies. Mild to severe urinary bladder dysfunction occurs in more than 50% of patients with diabetes mellitus of more than 20 years' duration. Decreased bladder propulsive power and increased residual volume may be observed on voiding cystometrogram studies. As a consequence of the increasing residual volume, there is a deterioration in the utility of double-voided urines as indices of diabetic control. Therapy with cholinergic agonists is only partially effective. Because of the impairment of the sensation of the need for micturition, a reasonably successful strategy has been to urge patients with this complication to perform timed voidings regardless of the perceived need to void. As increasing paresis of the detrusor muscle occurs, increasing residual volume develops. Proportional to the degree of residual volume, there is early asymptomatic bacteriuria and, ultimately, overt cystitis. In more advanced cases, bladder neck resection may be attempted to reduce the amount of detrusor power required for bladder emptying. Urinary diversion may become necessary in a few patients.

Impotence and impairment of sexual function occur in more than 50% of men with long-standing diabetes and may be the first manifestation of the disease. Psychogenic causes for impotence should be excluded because diabetes does not preclude the relatively more common, psychologic etiology of impotence. A characteristic history of progressive loss of penile tumescence, diminution of morning erection, and inability to masturbate despite preservation of libido is highly suggestive of diabetic impotence. Serum testosterone concentrations are usually normal. Cystometrograms should be performed to establish whether bladder neuropathy coexists in these patients. Sleep laboratories that determine organic penile dysfunction may be helpful in establishing the diagnosis.

If mild to moderate impotence has occurred for only a brief time, rigorous control of the blood glucose concentrations may occasionally reestablish penile function. Hormone replacement therapy with testosterone, vitamins, or other medications is largely unsuccessful. In advanced cases, surgical implantation of penile prostheses may be the only available treatment. Sexual dysfunction in women with diabetes mellitus is rarely observed.

Cardiovascular Neuropathy. Autonomic neuropathy manifested by orthostatic hypotension is relatively common in patients with diabetes mellitus and may be disabling. This is associated with an increased risk of sudden death, as well as silent ischemia and infarction. These patients may not be able to rise from a supine position without a period of 10 to 30 minutes of adaptation to an increasingly upright posture. The diagnosis is made by demonstrating a decrease of approximately 25 mm Hg in systolic or 10 mm Hg in diastolic pressure after 2 minutes of upright posture without a compensatory increase of the heart rate. Other entities to be considered are adrenal insufficiency, Shy-Drager syndrome, and primary autonomic dysfunction. In the Shy-Drager syndrome central nervous system dysfunction, particularly extrapyramidal and cerebellar dysfunction, should be demonstrable. Irregularity of sweating may also accompany diabetic autonomic dysfunction. Partial or total anhidrosis may be observed. A patchy distribution of sweating may be particularly evident in the face. An unusual variant of autonomic instability may be manifested by the profuse, drenching perspiration observed in certain diabetic patients after meal ingestion (gustatory sweating).

Treatment of orthostatic hypotension can be difficult. A high-salt diet will increase intravascular volume and thereby tend to maintain central nervous system perfusion despite excessive pooling of venous blood in the legs on standing. Expansion of intravascular volume using fludrocortisone (Florinef) in doses of 0.1 to 0.5 mg/day may also be used. Both of these therapies must be used judiciously in patients with concomitant cardiovascular disease, as volume overload and supine hypertension may result. Jobst stockings or even antigravity suits may be useful in reducing the severity of venous pooling of blood. The use of adrenergic pressors such as ephedrine may be hazardous and should be avoided as an initial therapy.

Diabetic Dermopathy

A variety of complex and poorly understood lesions of the skin have been reported in patients with diabetes mellitus. Most common of these is the change in color and consistency of the skin, particularly over the anterior pretibial area in both type I and type II diabetic patients. The skin becomes mildly atrophic, waxy in consistency, and has a pale, almost translucent appearance. This is accompanied by hair loss, to a level at least as high or higher than the change in skin consistency. These changes begin in the dorsum of the foot and ascend slowly with time. Treatment generally yields less than encouraging results, with the principal effort directed at good diabetic control. Necrobiosis lipoidica diabeticorum is a far more dramatic lesion but is observed in less than 5% of patients with diabetes mellitus. It may occur before or coincident with the diagnosis of diabetes. Necrobiosis produces a focal area of atrophic scarring in the anterior pretibial area bordered by a painful margin of erythematous, maculopapular, almost xanthomatous-like eruptions. Subsidence of the inflammatory process is accompanied by enlargement of the atrophic scarring, which itself is painless. There may be areas of telangiectasia at the margin. Therapy is nonspecific, focusing on control of diabetic hyperglycemia. Corticosteroids have been advocated for necrobiosis but do not appear to stop the progression of this self-limited disease. Less dramatic than necrobiosis diabeticorum are the more darkly pigmented shin spots seen in diabetic subjects. These macular areas of hyperpigmentation are painless and proliferate slowly with increasing duration of diabetes mellitus.

The patient with diabetes may have lipoatrophy or lipohypertrophy at insulin injection sites. The pathogenesis of these phenomena is unclear. Lipohypertrophy may be up to 5 to 10 cm in diameter. Highly purified preparations of insulin, such as single-component insulin, cause the disorders less commonly. Treatment of a preexisting lipoatrophy by injection of the purer insulin into the margin of the lesion appears to be one reasonably successful therapeutic approach. In patients not responding to these maneuvers, insulin administration should be restricted to areas of less cosmetic importance.

Diabetes and Pregnancy

Pregnancy considerably accelerates several of the chronic complications of diabetes mellitus and is accompanied by a high incidence of fetal wastage. Therefore pregnancy is not advisable for diabetic patients with microvascular disease. With considerable patient effort and attention to self-management, successful pregnancies can be achieved in patients with advanced, noncardiac complications. To reduce the fourfold incidence of fetal malformation in the infants of diabetic mothers, a period of 6 to 12 months of excellent control of the hyperglycemia before pregnancy seems indicated. Based on the experience of a number of investigators, multiple insulin doses containing primary regular or at least two doses of intermediate-acting insulin with rapid-acting insulin as needed will be essential for excellent diabetic control. As an alternative, mechanical insulin delivery systems such as the insulin infusion pump may improve diabetic control. Regardless of the mode of insulin administration, frequent home monitoring by using Dextrostix with a reflectance meter or Chemstrip BG will greatly improve diabetic control, especially during the last half of pregnancy.

During pregnancy, an early decreased insulin requirement is followed by later insulin resistance and insensitivity. In the first trimester, insulin requirements may be observed to decrease concomitantly with the growth of the fetal-placental unit, which acts to consume glucose and other nutrients. It should be remembered that the central nervous system consumes the largest portion of the obligate daily glucose requirement in the healthy adult. In the pregnant patient, the growth of a second central nervous system increases the carbohydrate demand dramatically. This development is particularly important during the third trimester, when an unusual form of ketosis may develop without striking hyperglycemia. It may be that the fetal-placental unit accounts for rapid glucose utilization but still allows for ketosis owing to insulin insufficiency.

Because of the antagonism to insulin action produced primarily by placental hormones (human placental lactogen, estrogen, and progesterone), insulin insensitivity develops during the second half of pregnancy. These patients therefore may precipitously develop diabetic ketoacidosis with glucose levels unusually low for that condition. Excessive fetal wastage is produced either by extreme hypoglycemia or by an episode of ketoacidosis. The necessary reduction of insulin requirements in the first trimester can be easily accomplished if multiple serum glucose determinations and double-voided urine glucose assessments are made routinely. By the second trimester the increasing antagonism to insulin action becomes apparent, necessitating a return to approximately that dose of insulin used in the antegravid period. By the beginning of the third trimester, insulin requirements rise. Immediately after delivery the insulin requirement may again drop precipitously. During the third trimester there is an increased glomerular filtration rate in the mother, with a resulting decrease in the renal tubular reabsorption of glucose. At this point, glycosuria may also contribute to a significant reduction of serum glucose levels disproportionate to the degree of insulinization of the patient.

Although the patient in the third trimester is extremely prone to develop ketoacidosis, monitoring of urinary glucose levels may provide an overestimation of insulin requirements. For these reasons, early admission to the hospital of third-trimester patients may markedly increase fetal survival in infants of type I diabetic mothers. Excellent control of the blood glucose concentration must be maintained up to week 34 to 36 of the pregnancy. At this point, determinations of the fetal lung maturity become a paramount guide to the course of the pregnancy. If difficulties are encountered in maintaining diabetic control or if toxemia in the mother or macrosomia in the fetus develops, elective cesarean section should be considered when fetal lung maturity has occurred. The goals of management of the pregnant diabetic patient should be (1) rigid control of fasting glucose to between 80 and 100 mg/dl, (2) avoidance of glucosuria, and (3) adherence to weight schedules. Although multiple injections of mixed insulins or of regular insulin generally are adequate therapy, better results may be obtained from continuous subcutaneous insulin infusion pumps (see also Chapter 372).

BIBLIOGRAPHY

Adrogue HJ et al: Plasma acid-base patterns in diabetic ketoacidosis, *N Engl J Med* 307:1603, 1982.

Bailey CJ: Biaguianides and NIDDM, *Diabetes Care* 16:755-772, 1992.

Bierman EL: Atherogenesis in diabetes, *Arterioscler Thromb* 12:647-656, 1992.

Bolli GB, Gerlich JE: The "dawn phenomenon": a common occurrence in both non–insulin-dependent and insulin-dependent diabetes mellitus, *N Engl J Med* 310:746, 1984.

Bolli GB et al: Glucose counterregulation and waning of insulin in the Somoyogi phenomenon (posthypoglycemic hypercemia), *N Engl J Med* 311:1214, 1984.

Chiasson J-L, Josso RG, Hunt JA et al: The efficacy of acarbose in the treatment of patients with non–insulin dependent diabetes mellitus: a multicenter controlled clinical trial, *Ann Intern Med* 121:928-935, 1994.

DeFronzo RA, Goodman AM, the Multicenter Metformin Study Group: Efficacy of metformin in patients with non–insulin-dependent diabetes mellitus, *N Engl J Med* 333:541-549, 1995.

DeFronzo RA, Ferrannini E: Insulin resistance: a multifaceted syndrome responsible for NIDDM, obesity, hypertension, dyslipidemia, and atherosclerotic cardiovascular disease, *Diabetes Care* 14:173-194, 1991.

Fontbonne AM, Eschwége EM: Insulin and cardiovascular disease: Paris prospective study, *Diabetes Care* 14:461-469, 1991.

Garber AJ, Vinik A, Crespin SR: Detection and management of lipid disorders in diabetic patients: a commentary for clinicians, *Diabetes Care* 15:1068, 1992.

Haffner SM, Stern MP, Hazuda HP et al: Cardiovascular risk factors in confirmed prediabetic individuals: does the clock for coronary heart disease start ticking before the onset of clinical diabetes? *JAMA* 263:2893-2898, 1990.

Hermann LS, Scherstén B, Bitzén P-O et al: Therapeutic comparison of metformin and sulfonylurea, alone and in various combinations: a double-blind controlled study, *Diabetes Care* 17:1100-1109, 1994.

Horton ES: Exercise. In Lebovitz HE editor: *Therapy for diabetes mellitus and related disorders,* ed 2, Alexandria, Va, 1994, American Diabetes Association.

Kitabachi AE, Fisher JN, Murphy MB, Rumbak MJ: Diabetic ketoacidosis and the hyperglycemic, hyperosmolar nonketotic state. In Kahn CR, Weir GC, editors: *Joslin's Diabetes Mellitus,* ed 13, Philadelphia, 1994, Lea & Febiger.

Klein R, Klein BEK, Moss SE, Cruickshanks KJ: Relationship of hyperglycemia to the long-term incidence and progression of diabetic retinopathy, *Arch Intern Med* 154:2169-2178, 1994.

Kreisberg RA: Diabetic ketoacidosis: new concepts and trends in pathogenesis and treatment, *Ann Intern Med* 88:681, 1978.

Kuusisto J, Mykkanen L, Pyorala K, Laakso M: NIDDM and its metabolic control predict coronary heart disease in elderly subjects, *Diabetes* 43:960-967, 1994.

Liang JC, Goldberg MF: Treatment of diabetic retinopathy, *Diabetes* 29:841, 1980.

Nathan DM: Long-term complications of diabetes mellitus, *N Engl J Med* 328:1676-1685, 1993.

National Institute of Diabetes and Digestive and Kidney Diseases: Diabetes statistics, Pub No 949-3822, Betheseda, Md, 1994, US Department of Health and Human Services, National Institutes of Health.

Polonsky K et al: Relation of counterregulatory responses to hypoglycemia in type I diabetes, *N Engl J Med* 307:1106, 1982.

Roy N, Chou MYC, Field JB: Time-action characteristics of regular and NPH insulins in insulin-treated diabetics, *J Clin Endocrinol Metab* 50:475, 1980.

Suter SL, Nolan JJ, Wallace P et al: Metabolic effects of new oral hypoglycemic agent CS-045 in NIDDM subjects, *Diabetes Care* 15:193-203, 1992.

The Diabetes Control and Complications Trial Research Group: the effect of intensive treatment of diabetes on the development and progression of long-term complications in insulin-dependent diabetes mellitus, *N Engl J Med* 329:977-986, 1993.

United Kingdom Prospective Diabetes Study Group: United Kingdom Prospective Diabetes Study (UKPDS) 13: relative efficacy of randomly associated diet, sulfonylurea, insulin, or metformin in patients with newly diagnosed non-insulin dependent diabetes followed for three years, *Br Med J* 310:83-88, 1995.

---

304 Hypoglycemia

William E. Clutter and Philip E. Cryer

PHYSIOLOGY

Certain human tissues such as the brain have an obligate requirement for glucose; even brief glucose deprivation causes severe cerebral dysfunction. Other tissues, such as muscle, fat, and liver, utilize glucose when it is plentiful (e.g., after a carbohydrate-containing meal) but can utilize other metabolic fuels. The glucose taken up by these tissues may be metabolized or stored in the form of glycogen.

In view of the obligate glucose requirements of the central nervous system, prevention of a low plasma glucose concentration (hypoglycemia) is critical to survival. Normally the plasma glucose concentration is maintained within narrow limits by a tightly regulated balance between glucose efflux from and influx into the circulation. Moreover, entry of glucose from ingested carbohydrate normally is intermittent; the postprandial period is a state of enhanced glucose metabolism and storage and suppressed endogenous glucose production. In contrast, the postabsorptive period is a state of partially suppressed glucose utilization and enhanced glucose production. The latter is the result of the breakdown of glycogen (glycogenolysis) and the formation of new glucose (gluconeogenesis). Under most circumstances the liver is the predominant source of endogenous glucose production, although the kidneys become a major source of glucose during prolonged fasting. After an overnight fast most endogenous glucose production is from glycogenolysis, but after approximately 24 hours of fasting virtually all the glucose produced is by gluconeogenesis.

The prevention of hypoglycemia between meals requires (1) a structurally and enzymatically intact liver; (2) adequate hepatic glycogen stores and an adequate supply of gluconeogenic precursors (lactate, pyruvate, glycerol, and gluconeogenic amino acids such as alanine); and (3) appropriate regulatory signals.

The major regulatory signals involved in transition between the fed and the fasted state are insulin and glucagon. Insulin, secreted from pancreatic beta cells into the portal circulation in response to a meal, suppresses hepatic glucose production and stimulates glucose utilization by insulin-sensitive tissues. Glucagon stimulates hepatic glucose production by both glycogenolysis and gluconeogenesis. Its secretion from pancreatic alpha cells is suppressed after a carbohydrate meal, which favors glucose conservation. In the postabsorptive state, insulin secretion is suppressed and glucagon secretion increases. This combination of low insulin and high glucagon hormonal signals results in accelerated hepatic glucose production and diminished glucose utilization. In addition to glucagon, the hormones epinephrine, cortisol, and growth hormone also promote glucose production and limit glucose utilization. Glucagon, epinephrine, cortisol, and growth hormone are often referred to as glucose counterregulatory hormones.

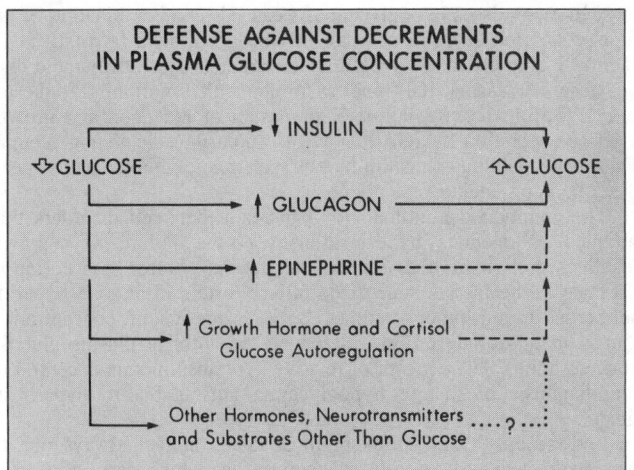

FIGURE 304-1   Normal glucose counterregulation. The hierarchy of the redundant glucoregulatory factors involved in prevention or correction of hypoglycemia during decrements in plasma glucose counterregulation in normal humans.

From Cryer PE, Gerich JE. In Rifkin H, Porte D, editors: *Ellenberg and Rifkin's diabetes mellitus,* ed 4, New York, 1989, Elsevier.

Physiologic studies have shown that the following principles (summarized in Fig. 304-1) govern glucose counterregulation and the prevention or correction of hypoglycemia:

1. Decreased insulin secretion plays an important role in prevention or correction of hypoglycemia. However, glucose counterregulation is not due solely to dissipation of insulin but rather to coordinated dissipation of insulin and activation of redundant glucose counterregulatory systems.
2. Glucagon plays a primary counterregulatory role.
3. Epinephrine is not normally required for glucose counterregulation but compensates to a large degree when glucagon secretion is deficient (e.g., during insulin-induced hypoglycemia in type I diabetes mellitus). Hypoglycemia occurs or progresses only when both glucagon and epinephrine are deficient and insulin is present, or when insulin action is excessive.
4. Cortisol and growth hormone are not critical to correction of hypoglycemia or to prevention of hypoglycemia after an overnight fast. Nevertheless, patients with chronic deficiencies of these hormones occasionally develop fasting hypoglycemia.
5. Although other hormones, neural mechanisms, or glucose autoregulation may be involved in counterregulation, they are not sufficiently potent to prevent or correct hypoglycemia when both glucagon and epinephrine are deficient and insulin is present.

The glycemic threshold for suppression of insulin secretion in response to declining plasma glucose level lies well within the physiologic range for plasma glucose. In keeping with their role in prevention as well as correction of hypoglycemia, the glycemic thresholds for release of counterregulatory hormones lie just below the physiologic plasma glucose range and well above the threshold for symptoms of hypoglycemia.

PATHOPHYSIOLOGY
Clinical Manifestations

The symptoms caused by hypoglycemia can be divided into the following categories: (1) neurogenic (autonomic) symptoms attributable to the sympathoadrenal and parasympathetic discharge triggered by a falling plasma glucose level and (2) neuroglycopenic symptoms attributable to cerebral dysfunction caused by glucose deprivation. Neurogenic manifestations include tachycardia, palpitations, anxiety, tremor, sweating, and hunger. The magnitude of the sympathoadrenal and parasympathetic response to decrements in plasma glucose is inversely related to the glucose nadir, so the lower the plasma glucose concentration, the more intense the neurogenic symptoms. However, the neuroendocrine response is not altered by the rate of plasma glu-

cose decline. Awareness of hypoglycemia is largely due to recognition of neurogenic symptoms.

Neuroglycopenic manifestations range from subtle mental impairment to coma and death. Symptoms may include lethargy, drowsiness, faintness, confusion, blurred vision, difficulty speaking, abnormal behavior, incoordination and seizures. Both hypothermia during hypoglycemia and posthypoglycemic fever have been described.

During a fall in plasma glucose level, normal individuals develop symptoms at a plasma glucose concentration of 50 to 55 mg/dl (2.8 to 3 mmol/L), below the thresholds for suppression of insulin secretion and activation of counterregulatory hormone secretion. The threshold for cerebral dysfunction that becomes evident as impaired cognition is 45 to 50 mg/dl (2.5 to 2.8 mmol/L). Thus the normal sequence of responses to a fall in plasma glucose level is (1) decreased insulin secretion, (2) increased counterregulatory hormone secretion, (3) symptoms, and (4) impaired cognition.

These glycemic thresholds are not fixed but may be altered by antecedent plasma glucose levels. Even a single episode of hypoglycemia shifts the glycemic thresholds for counterregulatory hormone secretion and hypoglycemic symptoms to a lower value. This phenomenon accounts for the occurrence of hypoglycemia with only minor symptoms in some patients with fasting hypoglycemia. Although cognitive dysfunction generally correlates with the degree of hypoglycemia, some patients tolerate low plasma glucose concentrations relatively well. The mechanism by which hypoglycemia alters glycemic thresholds appears to involve increased transport of glucose across the blood-brain barrier.

Hypoglycemic symptoms typically clear rapidly after the plasma glucose concentration is restored to normal. More gradual clearing of neuroglycopenic symptoms over hours, or even days, sometimes follows profound hypoglycemia. Prolonged, severe hypoglycemia can cause permanent cerebral damage.

Causes

Hypoglycemia has conventionally been classified into two categories: fasting (or postabsorptive) hypoglycemia and reactive (or postprandial) hypoglycemia. However, with very rare exceptions, all patients with clinically important hypoglycemia have a disorder that causes fasting hypoglycemia. In some cases hypoglycemia also develops in these patients shortly after meals, but the differential diagnosis remains that of fasting hypoglycemia.

Although once widely used for the diagnosis of reactive hypoglycemia, the oral glucose tolerance test is unreliable and should not be used to diagnose suspected hypoglycemia. Patients given the diagnosis of reactive hypoglycemia based on this test rarely have hypoglycemia during daily life (after ordinary meals or during spontaneous symptoms).

The major causes of fasting hypoglycemia are outlined in Box 304-1. Hypoglycemia occurs when glucose use exceeds glucose production. Fasting hypoglycemia in patients with the various forms of hyperinsulinism and in those with tumors secreting insulin-like hormones is due to suppressed hepatic glucose production coupled with inappropriately high rates of glucose utilization. Impaired hepatic glucose production with ongoing obligate glucose utilization (e.g., by the brain) is believed to be the predominant mechanism of fasting hypoglycemia attributable to drugs, hormonal deficits, hepatic dysfunction, chronic renal failure, and the childhood hypoglycemic disorders. Clearly, accelerated glucose utilization in conditions such as vigorous exercise and pregnancy could exacerbate fasting hypoglycemia attributable to any of the disorders listed. However, accelerated glucose utilization alone seldom results in fasting hypoglycemia because of the normal capacity to increase glucose production.

By far the most common cause of hypoglycemia is therapy of diabetes mellitus with insulin or sulfonylureas. Although hypoglycemia is a major therapeutic limitation in diabetes, it seldom presents a diagnostic problem. These drugs may also be used to produce factitious hypoglycemia, however, especially among medical personnel and others with knowledge of diabetes. Ethanol inhibits gluconeogenesis but not glycogenolysis. Thus it causes hypoglycemia only when hepatic glycogen is depleted in fasting or malnourished individuals. Salicylates cause hypoglycemia in children by an unknown mecha-

BOX 304-1
Causes of fasting hypoglycemia

Drugs
Insulin
Sulfonylureas
Ethanol
Salicylates
Pentamidine
Quinine

Critical organ failure
Renal failure
Hepatic failure
Cardiac failure
Sepsis
Malnutrition

Hormonal deficiencies
Cortisol
Growth hormone
Glucagon plus epinephrine

Extrapancreatic tumors
Endogenous hyperinsulinism

Pancreatic beta-cell disorders: Neoplastic (insulinoma), hyperplastic, or functional
Insulin secretagogues (e.g., sulfonylureas)
Autoimmune hypoglycemias: Antibodies to insulin, antibodies to insulin receptors

Hypoglycemias of infancy and childhood
Neonatal hypoglycemias
Congenital deficiencies of glucogenic enzymes
Ketotic hypoglycemia of childhood

nism. Pentamidine and quinine stimulate insulin release and presumably cause hypoglycemia by this means. A number of other drugs have been associated with hypoglycemia, but in most cases other potential causes of hypoglycemia were present and a clear causal relationship was not established.

Renal insufficiency is a major factor associated with hypoglycemia in hospitalized patients. The mechanisms are not known, although the majority of patients who develop hypoglycemia are malnourished. The development of renal failure in diabetes mellitus often reduces insulin requirements and increases the risk of hypoglycemia. Hepatic disease can cause hypoglycemia as a result of inadequate glucose production. Because the liver is normally able to increase glucose output several-fold, only severe hepatic dysfunction causes hypoglycemia. Hypoglycemia in patients with cardiac failure or sepsis is probably a result of impaired hepatic and renal function. Hypoglycemia has rarely been attributed to malnutrition without other disorders.

Adrenocortical insufficiency commonly leads to anorexia and weight loss. Further, cortisol is required to maintain normal levels of hepatic gluconeogenic enzymes and to mobilize gluconeogenic precursors; it also antagonizes the effects of insulin. Deficiency of growth hormone produces enhanced insulin sensitivity. Despite these effects, in most adults with cortisol or growth hormone deficiency, or both, hypoglycemia does not develop. On the other hand, hypoglycemia is an important manifestation of these disorders in children. Combined deficiency of glucagon and epinephrine occurs in some patients with insulin-dependent diabetes mellitus and greatly increases the risk of insulin-induced hypoglycemia. Deficiency of either glucagon or epinephrine alone, however, would not be expected to produce hypoglycemia; indeed, hypoglycemia that is due to deficiency of either or both has not been shown convincingly in nondiabetic patients.

Fasting hypoglycemia occurs in some patients with large extrapancreatic tumors, especially mesenchymal tumors such as mesotheliomas and retroperitoneal sarcomas, and hepatic and adrenal carcino-

mas. In many cases hypoglycemia is caused by a combination of tumor production of a precursor of insulin-like growth factor II (IGF-II) and increased access of IGF-II to target tissues attributable to a decrease in plasma IGF-binding proteins that normally sequester IGF-II within the circulation. Suppression of glucagon and growth hormone secretion by IGF-II may also contribute to hypoglycemia. Ectopic production of insulin by extrapancreatic tumors has not been described convincingly.

The common denominator of pancreatic beta-cell disorders that produce endogenous hyperinsulinism is the failure to suppress insulin secretion normally when the plasma glucose concentration declines in the fasting state. This failure results in relative hyperinsulinemia during hypoglycemia (i.e., a plasma insulin concentration that is inappropriately high relative to the ambient plasma glucose concentration). The concept of relative hyperinsulinemia is central to the diagnosis of fasting hypoglycemia attributable to hyperinsulinism.

Endogenous hyperinsulinism in adults is almost always due to pancreatic beta-cell tumors or insulinomas, which can occur anywhere in the pancreas. In about 80% of cases there is a single benign adenoma, whereas about 10% of cases are due to multiple benign adenomas and 5% to 10% are due to carcinomas. Insulinomas occur in all age-groups, although two thirds are diagnosed between the ages of 30 and 60 years. Approximately 60% of reported cases have been in women. Islet cell tumors, often multiple and including beta-cell tumors, are one component of the multiple endocrine neoplasia type I syndrome, along with hyperparathyroidism and pituitary tumors. This familial disorder is inherited as an autosomal dominant trait.

Most infants with persistent hyperinsulinism do not have insulinomas or other detectable pathologic lesions. A genetic defect of the sulfonylurea receptor of beta cells appears to cause excessive insulin secretion in these patients. Nesidioblastosis (islet cells interspersed among pancreatic exocrine cells), once believed to be the basis for hyperinsulinism, is a normal finding in infants and is not associated with hypoglycemia.

Intermittent hypoglycemia with inappropriately high serum free insulin concentrations has been recognized in a few patients found to have serum autoantibodies to insulin. It is presumed that insulin periodically dissociates from these antibodies, causing hyperinsulinism and hypoglycemia. Most of these patients have other evidence of autoimmune disease. Autoantibodies to the insulin receptor usually produce insulin resistance, but in rare patients they may cause hypoglycemia, presumably by mimicking the effects of insulin.

A number of hypoglycemic disorders are unique to or typically present in infancy or childhood. Transient neonatal hypoglycemia in infants of diabetic mothers is thought to be due to chronic fetal hyperglycemia with resultant fetal hypersecretion of insulin that persists for a time after birth. Many neonates who are small for gestational age have transient hypoglycemia, which appears to be due to delayed induction of one or more gluconeogenic enzymes.

Ketotic hypoglycemia of childhood is a poorly understood syndrome that becomes evident between the ages of 1 and 5 years, remits before the age of 10 years, and is characterized by fasting hypoglycemia with normal suppression of insulin secretion. Because normal children develop hypoglycemia during fasts, these patients may simply represent one extreme of the normal distribution of glucose production during fasting.

Reactive hypoglycemia has been described in patients who have undergone gastrectomy or gastric bypass. Rapid absorption of ingested carbohydrate, together with enhanced secretion of gut factors that act as insulin secretagogues, is believed to cause marked hyperinsulinemia followed by hypoglycemia. Most descriptions of this disorder have relied on the oral glucose tolerance test for diagnosis. Whether, and how often, hypoglycemia after ordinary meals develops in such patients is unclear.

Patients with the rare enzymatic defects galactosemia and hereditary fructose intolerance have vomiting and reactive hypoglycemia after meals containing these sugars. Other manifestations include hepatomegaly and jaundice. These disorders usually become apparent in childhood. With these rare exceptions, the existence of reactive hypoglycemia, as a disorder distinct from fasting hypoglycemia, has not been convincingly shown.

CLINICAL AND LABORATORY DIAGNOSIS
Confirmation of Hypoglycemia

The presence of hypoglycemia is often suspected on the basis of a history compatible with neurogenic or neuroglycopenic symptoms. Although sometimes compelling, the history is more often only suggestive, since such symptoms are common in a variety of other disorders. Thus the diagnosis of hypoglycemia is suspected much more often than it is confirmed. Symptoms of hypoglycemia usually occur more than several hours after meals, often after exercise. However, as noted above, patients with disorders that cause fasting hypoglycemia, may also develop hypoglycemia within several hours of a meal. Occasionally, a hypoglycemic disorder is first suspected because of a low glucose level in a plasma sample obtained for other reasons.

Once suspected, the diagnosis of hypoglycemia is most convincingly established when it is based on Whipple's triad: symptoms consistent with hypoglycemia, a concomitant low plasma glucose concentration, and relief of symptoms after the glucose level is raised to normal. The diagnosis of a hypoglycemic disorder is seldom tenable in the absence of consistent symptoms.

Patients with fasting hypoglycemia may have plasma glucose levels below 45 mg/dl (2.5 mmol/L) after a 10- to 12-hour overnight fast, especially with repeated measurements. Thus the first diagnostic step in suspected fasting hypoglycemia is to measure the plasma glucose concentration after an overnight fast, on several days if necessary. A value less than 45 mg/dl documents the presence of fasting hypoglycemia. If plasma glucose level is greater than 45 mg/dl after an overnight fast, the fast should be prolonged until symptomatic hypoglycemia with a plasma glucose level less than 45 mg/dl occurs, or for a maximum of 72 hours. Plasma glucose should be measured at least every 4 hours (more frequently as plasma glucose level falls) and when symptoms occur. Bedside glucose monitoring devices may be used for rapid estimation but are not accurate enough for definitive diagnosis; laboratory measurements should be performed. Symptomatic hypoglycemia usually occurs within the first 24 hours of a diagnostic fast in affected patients. A period of exercise at the end of a prolonged fast may precipitate hypoglycemia in an affected patient, in contrast to the normal stability of plasma glucose during exercise.

When symptomatic hypoglycemia with a plasma glucose level less than 45 mg/dl occurs, certain tests should be performed to distinguish among possible causes. Plasma insulin and C-peptide should be measured, preferably on several samples, before the fast is ended, and a plasma or urine assay for sulfonylureas should be performed.

Failure of the plasma glucose concentration to fall below 50 mg/dl during a prolonged fast, particularly if a period of exercise is included, excludes the diagnosis of fasting hypoglycemia. In men, fasting plasma glucose values below 50 mg/dl document the presence of fasting hypoglycemia. The same statement cannot be made for women or children, in whom plasma glucose concentrations commonly fall below 50 mg/dl in the absence of symptoms during a prolonged fast. If values below 50 mg/dl are associated with unequivocal symptoms in a woman or a child, fasting hypoglycemia has been documented. If not, convincing biochemical evidence is required for diagnosis of a fasting hypoglycemic disorder (see later discussion).

The differential diagnosis of fasting hypoglycemia can be narrowed rapidly with standard clinical data. A history of the use of insulin or other offending drugs may be obtained. Surreptitious use of hypoglycemic drugs, however, may be difficult to detect and requires screening of urine or plasma for such agents. Sulfonylureas may be inadvertently substituted for another drug, so the identity of each of the patient's medications should be confirmed by inspection. Critical organ dysfunction severe enough to cause hypoglycemia becomes apparent on clinical examination and with routine laboratory tests. Extrapancreatic tumors associated with hypoglycemia generally are large and clinically evident. The hypoglycemias of childhood are self-limited except in patients with congenital enzymatic defects in whom associated findings suggest the diagnosis. In the absence of these causes the differential diagnosis is limited to excessive insulin secretion or deficient glucose counterregulatory hormone secretion.

Hypoglycemia stimulates the secretion of cortisol, growth hormone, glucagon, and epinephrine. Thus the finding of elevated plasma concentrations of these hormones during spontaneous (or insulin-induced) hypoglycemia excludes deficiencies. It is conventional to assess the adequacy of growth hormone and cortisol secretion in patients with fasting hypoglycemia (Chapter 285). Because deficiencies of glucagon or epinephrine rarely if ever cause hypoglycemia except in patients with insulin-dependent diabetes, these hormones usually are not measured.

Diagnosis of hyperinsulinism requires the demonstration of an inappropriately elevated plasma insulin level during hypoglycemia. Plasma insulin concentrations are often not elevated above the fasting reference range. Because normal insulin secretion nearly ceases when the plasma glucose concentration falls to less than 45 mg/dl, plasma insulin concentrations should be measured when the fasting plasma glucose level falls below this level. In such samples a plasma insulin concentration greater than 6 μU/ml (36 pmol/L) is diagnostic of hyperinsulinism.

Measurement of plasma C-peptide (the connecting peptide cleaved from proinsulin during conversion to insulin) can distinguish endogenous hyperinsulinism from surreptitious insulin administration. When plasma glucose level is less than 45 mg/dl, a plasma C-peptide level greater than 0.6 ng/ml (0.2 nmol/L) confirms that hyperinsulinism is of endogenous origin. Because C-peptide levels are also elevated in factitious hypoglycemia attributable to sulfonylureas, plasma or urine should be tested for these drugs. C-peptide levels are suppressed below these values in patients with exogenous hyperinsulinism (except in the presence of insulin antibodies; see later discussion). In an adult, fasting hypoglycemia that is due to hyperinsulinism implies the presence of an insulinoma if factitious hypoglycemia has been excluded.

Most patients with pancreatic beta-cell neoplasms have increased plasma levels of proinsulin during hypoglycemia. Specific proinsulin immunoassays have a high degree of sensitivity for insulinomas and may be useful when insulin and C-peptide levels during a diagnostic fast are equivocal. Other conditions, however, produce elevated proinsulin levels, so the diagnosis cannot be made on this basis alone.

The presence of circulating antibodies to insulin in patients with no history of insulin use suggests surreptitious insulin injection or autoimmune hypoglycemia. Such antibodies produce artifactually high values for plasma insulin in double-antibody immunoassays, and by binding endogenous proinsulin, which contains the C-peptide sequence, they also elevate plasma total C-peptide immunoreactivity. Methods are available for measuring free insulin and C-peptide levels in the presence of insulin antibodies. Injection of human insulin produces a much smaller immune response than animal insulins, and surreptitious use of human insulin may produce hypoglycemia in the absence of detectable antibodies to insulin. This diagnosis is still evident, however, from the combination of elevated plasma insulin and suppressed plasma C-peptide levels.

Evaluation of a patient with fasting hypoglycemia should include a diagnostic fast, with measurement of plasma insulin and C-peptide when the plasma glucose is less than 45 mg/dl (and preferably several such measurements), along with assay for sulfonylureas and antibodies to insulin. The differential diagnosis of hyperinsulinism is summarized in Table 304-1.

The preceding discussion assumes accurate measurement of the plasma glucose concentration. Artifactual lowering of the measured glucose level (pseudohypoglycemia) can occur if separation of the plasma from the formed elements of the blood is delayed for several hours, especially if glucose utilization by the formed elements is excessive (e.g., marked leukocytosis). This can be avoided by prompt centrifugation of the blood sample or by the use of special sampling tubes containing an inhibitor of glycolysis.

As noted earlier, patients with disorders that cause fasting hypoglycemia (such as insulinoma) may also have postprandial hypoglycemia. If hypoglycemia is suspected in a patient with symptoms that regularly occur within a few hours of a meal, plasma glucose should be measured during fasting as described earlier. If fasting does not provoke hypoglycemia, a hypoglycemic disorder is very unlikely. If strong clinical suspicion persists, plasma glucose should be measured frequently after ordinary mixed meals, while the patient records all symptoms and their time of occurrence. Unless typical symptoms occur and both coincide with low plasma glucose values and abate as plasma glucose levels rise (Whipple's triad), the diagnosis of reactive hypoglycemia can be confidently excluded. Blood glucose self-monitoring devices are not sufficiently reliable for such testing and

Table 304-1   Differential diagnosis of hyperinsulinism

	POSTABSORPTIVE VENOUS PLASMA GLUCOSE <45 MG/DL			
	INSULIN	C PEPTIDE	INSULIN ANTIBODIES	OTHER
Exogenous hyperinsulinism	↑	↓*	+	
Endogenous hyperinsulinism				
Insulinoma	↑	↑	—	↑ Proinsulin
Sulfonylurea	↑	↑	—	Positive sulfonylurea assay
Autoimmune hypoglycemia				
Antibodies to insulin	↑ ↑ ↑†	↓*	+	
Antibodies to insulin receptor	↑	?	—	Insulin receptor antibodies present; associated autoimmune disorder

*Free C-peptide levels are low, but total C-peptide levels may not be because of cross reactivity with antibody-bound proinsulin.
†Insulin antibodies artifactually increase insulin levels measured by double-antibody radioimmunoassay.

should not replace plasma glucose measurements by a clinical laboratory. The oral glucose tolerance test should not be used for diagnosis of suspected hypoglycemia, since plasma glucose concentrations reach nadirs less than 50 mg/dl after glucose ingestion in 10% of normal asymptomatic persons.

TREATMENT
Fasting Hypoglycemia

Management of fasting hypoglycemia requires urgent treatment, diagnosis, and long-term prevention. The short-term treatment of hypoglycemia is the oral or intravenous administration of glucose. If the patient is unable to take carbohydrate by mouth, 25 to 50 g of glucose (in the form of a 50% glucose solution) should be given by intravenous injection immediately after drawing a sample for glucose determination and a sample to be saved for additional diagnostic studies. Glucagon (1.0 mg intramuscularly), which promotes hepatic glucose release, can be used when immediate glucose administration is impractical. However, the effect of glucagon is transient and exogenous glucose administration should be started as soon as possible. The plasma glucose concentration is followed to ensure that hypoglycemia does not recur; continuous glucose infusions may be required to prevent recurrent hypoglycemia in some disorders.

After initial treatment the mechanism of hypoglycemia should be determined. Drug-induced hypoglycemia can be treated with glucose infusion and drug withdrawal. Documented hormonal deficits can be treated by hormone replacement. Hypoglycemia associated with extrapancreatic tumors may improve with reduction in tumor size achieved through surgery, chemotherapy, or radiotherapy. Hepatic dysfunction extensive enough to cause hypoglycemia is generally fatal unless it is either reversible or treated with hepatic transplantation. Recurrent fasting hypoglycemia associated with inanition, as in chronic renal failure, may respond to a high-caloric intake with frequent feedings.

The primary treatment of fasting hypoglycemia attributable to endogenous hyperinsulinism is surgical excision of the beta-cell abnormality. Solitary pancreatic tumors can be enucleated. Multiple tumors should be resected as much as possible, and sufficient pancreatic tissue to preserve function should be left. Because reduction of total tumor mass, even without cure, may render the patient euglycemic, total pancreatectomy should not be the primary procedure. In a collected series, 95% of patients with benign insulinomas were euglycemic after surgery. Complications include pancreatitis, pancreatic fistulas, and infections. Permanent diabetes may follow extensive pancreatic resection.

Computed tomography of the abdomen should be performed before surgery for insulinoma, since it can locate a minority of beta-cell tumors and can detect hepatic metastases from malignant insulinomas. Many other preoperative localization procedures have been proposed, but none has more than limited sensitivity, in part because insulinomas are usually small (median diameter, 1 to 2 cm). In patients with a clearly established diagnosis of endogenous hyperinsulinism, palpation by an experienced surgeon combined with intraoperative ultrasonographic examination of the pancreas allows successful removal of an insulinoma in the great majority of patients. This

✔ *WHEN TO REFER*

The diagnosis and treatment of hypoglycemia that is due to drugs, critical organ failure, or endocrine deficiency is usually straightforward. Referral of patients to an endocrinologist is warranted if they have documented fasting hypoglycemia and the diagnosis is not clear after a diagnostic fast with measurement of plasma insulin and C-peptide. Patients with endogenous hyperinsulinism should be referred to a surgeon with experience in treatment of these disorders.

high success rate suggests that invasive preoperative localization studies are not warranted, since negative results do not eliminate the need for surgery and positive results have not been shown to improve the outcome of surgery. If a pancreatic tumor cannot be located at laparotomy, it is preferable to forego extensive resection and pursue further localizing studies.

Medical palliation of hyperinsulinism that is not surgically correctable includes frequent oral feedings. Diazoxide, a drug that suppresses insulin secretion, may ameliorate hypoglycemia. Side effects include edema, nausea, and hypertrichosis. The somatostatin analog octreotide ameliorates hypoglycemia in some patients but is ineffective or worsens hypoglycemia in others. Chemotherapy may palliate symptoms in some patients with metastatic islet cell carcinomas; a combination of streptozocin and doxorubicin appears most effective.

Patients with reactive hypoglycemia attributable to galactosemia or hereditary fructose intolerance should avoid foods containing those sugars.

BIBLIOGRAPHY

Cryer PE: Glucose counterregulation: prevention and correction of hypoglycemia in humans, *Am J Physiol* 264:E149-155, 1993.
Daughaday WH: The pathophysiology of IGF-II hypersecretion in non–islet cell tumor hypoglycemia, *Diabetes Metab Rev* 3:62, 1995.
Doherty GM et al: Results of a prospective strategy to diagnose, localize, and resect insulinomas, *Surgery* 110:989-997, 1991.
Grunberger G et al: Factitious hypoglycemia due to surreptitious administration of insulin: diagnosis, treatment and long-term follow-up, *Ann Intern Med* 108:252-257, 1988.
Heerden JA et al: Occult functioning insulinomas: which localizing studies are indicated? *Surgery* 112: 1010-1015, 1992.
Heller SR, Cryer PE: Reduced neuroendocrine and symptomatic responses to subsequent hypoglycemia after one episode of hypoglycemia in nondiabetic humans, *Diabetes* 40:223-226, 1991.
Kao PC et al. Proinsulin by immunochemiluminometric assay for the diagnosis of insulinoma, *J Clin Endocrinol Metab* 78:1048-1051, 1994.
Mitrakou A et al. Reversibility of unawareness of hypoglycemia in patients with insulinomas, *N Engl J Med* 329:834-839, 1993.
Moertel CG et al: Streptozocin-doxorubicin, streptozocin-fluorouracil, or chlorozotocin in the treatment of advanced islet-cell carcinoma, *N Engl J Med* 326:519-523, 1992.
Service FJ: Hypoglycemic disorders, *N Engl J Med* 332:1144-1152, 1995.
Service FJ et al: Functioning insulinoma: incidence, recurrence and long-term survival of patients—a 60-year study, *Mayo Clin Proc* 66:711-719, 1991.
Snorgaard O, Binder C: Monitoring of blood glucose concentration in subjects with hypoglycemic symptoms during everyday life, *Br Med J* 300:16-18, 1990.

Thomas PM et al: Mutations in the sulfonylurea receptor gene in familial persistent hyperinsulinemic hypoglycemia of infancy, *Science* 268:426-429, 1995.

Towler DA et al: Mechanism of awareness of hypoglycemia: perception of neurogenic (predominantly cholinergic) rather than neuroglycopenic symptoms, *Diabetes* 42:1791-1798, 1993.

CHAPTER

305 Heritable Disorders of Carbohydrate Metabolism

Alan J. Garber

NONDIABETIC MELLITURIAS

The nondiabetic melliturias comprise a heterogeneous group of disorders united solely by the presence of a reducing sugar in the urine. False-positive urine testing that can result from drug administration must be excluded. A variety of pharmacologic preparations such as levodopa, excessive quantities of salicylates, ascorbic acid, chloral hydrate, and x-ray contrast media can produce false-positive urine sugar testing using the Clinitest copper reduction method for reducing substances in urine. On the other hand, these same agents are capable of producing false-negative results in the presence of glucose when glucose oxidase enzyme strips are used, as they interfere with the coupling of the peroxide generated by glucose oxidase to the color-developing system in the enzyme strips. False-positive results with glucose oxidase testing generally result from oxidizing agents such as hypochlorite and peroxides. In all instances, the finding of glucosuria or glycosuria requires a careful evaluation to firmly exclude the diagnosis of diabetes mellitus.

Renal Glucosuria

See Chapter 360.

Pentosuria

Pentosuria originally was described more than 90 years ago; since then, over 200 cases of patients with pentosuria have been reported in the literature. In all instances, the pentose excreted appears to be xylulose, although small amounts of L-arbitol have been isolated from the urine in some patients. In all patients thus far examined, the excretion of L-xylulose ranges between 1 and 4 g/day. This amount is virtually constant on a daily basis within the same patient and is largely unaffected by dietary pentose intake. The inheritance pattern of this autosomal recessive disease is largely confined to patients of Eastern European Jewish extraction and to a lesser number of Lebanese origin.

A diagnosis of pentosuria should be suspected in all patients having positive reducing substances in their urine that are consistently negative for glucose using glucose oxidase enzymatic strips. Diabetes mellitus also should be excluded in these patients. Further chemical testing of the reducing substance in the urine must demonstrate substantial quantities of L-xylulose. Pentosuria was originally classified as an inborn error of metabolism by Garrod in 1908. Subsequent studies have demonstrated that the metabolic defect arises from a deficiency of L-xylitol dehydrogenase (NADP$^+$). This enzyme catalyzes the reduction of xylulose to xylitol, an important step in the metabolism of glucuronic acid. Heterozygous states may be detected by using glucuronic acid loading with subsequent assessments of serum xylulose levels. As an alternative, the activity of the NADP-L-xylulose dehydrogenase may be assayed directly in red blood cells of the patient suspected of having this metabolic defect. Because this abnormality is harmless and individuals manifest no symptomatology, no treatment is necessary.

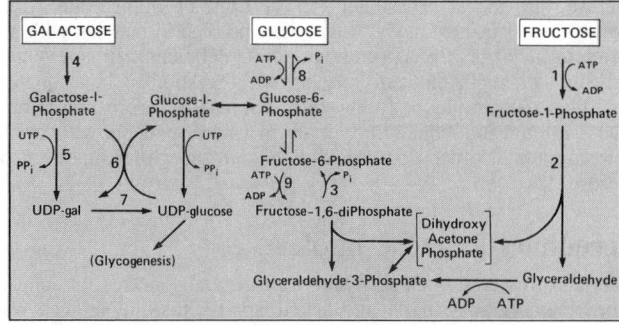

FIGURE 305-1   Pathways of hexose metabolism in humans.

Enzyme	Deficiency state
1 Fructokinase	Essential fructosuria
2 Fructose-1-phosphate aldolase	Hereditary fructose intolerance
3 Fructose-1,6-diphosphatase	Fructose-1,6-diphosphatase deficiency
4 Galactokinase	Galactosemia
5 UDP galactose pyrophosphorylase	Galactosemia
6 Gal-1-phosphate uridyltransferase	Galactosemia
7 UDP glucose epimerase	Galactosemia
8 Glucose-6-phosphatase	Glycogen storage disease (GSD) type I (hepatorenal)
9 Phosphofructokinase	GSD type VII

Essential Fructosuria

In addition to pentoses such as L-xylulose, nonglucose-reducing sugars such as fructose also may be found in the urine of otherwise asymptomatic patients. Patients having essential fructosuria excrete variable amounts of fructose, depending on the dietary intake of that sugar. Fructosuria is a relatively rare, genetically transmitted, inborn error of metabolism and is most probably an autosomal recessive disorder in patients having the fully developed expression of the defect. Although fructosuria is somewhat more common in patients of Jewish ancestry, the proportion of Jewish subjects to the total number of cases reported is lower than that with pentosuria. Fructosuria should be suspected in all nondiabetics having a nonglucose-reducing substance in the urine. However, specific enzymatic or chromatographic techniques are necessary for further elucidation of the reducing sugar present in the urine.

Fructosuria is believed to result from a relative or absolute deficiency in the activity of the first enzyme of hepatic fructose metabolism, fructokinase (Fig. 305-1). This enzyme, which rapidly phosphorylates fructose to form fructose 1-phosphate, is absent in essential fructosuria. Fructose excretion depends largely on the amount of fructose ingested. Renal disposal of ingested fructose may account for the clearance of 20% to 25% of the total ingested fructose. Fructosuria is an entirely benign condition. Unlike the more serious inborn error of fructose metabolism (hereditary fructose intolerance), benign fructosuria does not produce any other disturbance of intermediary metabolism. For this reason, no treatment is necessary.

Other Forms of Nondiabetic Mellituria

A variety of other monosaccharides and disaccharides may appear in the urine of patients because of impaired or absent enzymatic function necessary for the disposal of these sugars or because of a vast dietary intake that exceeds the capacity of normal enzyme activities to dispose rapidly of these sugars. In almost all instances, these forms of nondiabetic mellituria are not of clinical significance. Galactosuria may be noted occasionally in normal subjects ingesting large quantities of this monosaccharide. More commonly, galactosuria is seen in concert with galactosemia.

Mannoheptulose is a seven-carbon monosaccharide found in relatively large quantities in avocados. Accordingly, mannoheptulosuria may be observed in normal individuals after the ingestion of large amounts of this fruit. This condition is of no clinical consequence.

Lactose may appear occasionally in the urine of women late in the third trimester of pregnancy. It also may be seen in patients with severe intestinal tract disease without lactase deficiency. In no event is lactosuria of major clinical consequence. Ingestion of large quantities of cane sugar may be followed occasionally by sucrosuria in otherwise normal individuals. In certain instances, patients with cystic fibrosis have also been described with sucrosuria after ingestion of sucrose.

Hereditary Fructose Intolerance

Although this autosomal recessive trait generally makes its appearance clinically at an early age, hereditary fructose intolerance was first diagnosed in an adult patient.

Hereditary fructose intolerance has two major clinical manifestations. In previously undiagnosed adults, a relatively characteristic history of nausea, vomiting, and cerebral symptoms of hypoglycemia after ingestion of fructose-containing foods is obtained. Often, these patients will report a spontaneously developed aversion to fructose-containing fruits and other foods prepared with cane sugar as a sweetener. Most notably, this symptom develops into a childhood pattern of aversion to candy and sweets, and is maintained throughout adult life.

Despite the repeated episodes of hypoglycemia, adults with hereditary fructose intolerance generally show normal intelligence and suffer no residual effect, provided they have successfully managed to avoid ingesting large quantities of fructose. In marked contradistinction to this relatively benign presentation in adults, children with hereditary fructose intolerance frequently manifest nausea, vomiting, cerebral dysfunction, and generalized failure to thrive. On occasion, the attacks of hypoglycemia can be so severe that they produce unconsciousness and tonic seizures. Physical examination may show hepatosplenomegaly and perhaps icterus. There may be ascites and marked liver dysfunction. Initial screening laboratory data in children with hereditary fructose intolerance may be markedly abnormal, with moderately severe elevations of serum glutamic-oxalacetic transaminase and serum pyruvate-oxalacetic transaminase. There may be hyperbilirubinemia and other findings of liver dysfunction as well as phosphaturia, glycosuria, bicarbonate wasting, and aminoaciduria. In contrast, adults may manifest few, if any, detectable biochemical abnormalities under routine screening procedures. In all instances, fasting blood sugar and serum phosphate levels are normal.

The key biochemical defect in hereditary fructose intolerance is the virtual absence of fructose 1-phosphate aldolase (aldolase B) activity owing to nonsense, missense, or splice site mutations. This second enzyme of fructose metabolism catalyzes the cleavage of fructose 1-phosphate into dihydroxyacetone phosphate and glyceraldehyde. The latter two compounds are subsequently degraded within the glycolytic pathway, ultimately to form pyruvic acid. Thus an absence of fructose 1-phosphate aldolase results in the accumulation of substantial quantities of fructose 1-phosphate in liver and in other tissues having a significant activity of fructokinase. After fructose ingestion, fructose 1-phosphate levels rise rapidly in the hepatocyte, thereby serving as a sink for inorganic phosphate and ultimately resulting in a relative depletion of adenosine triphosphate (ATP) in the hepatocyte. Because inorganic phosphate is a major determinant of the rate of oxidative phosphorylation by mitochondria, its depletion, together with a resulting loss of ATP, results in hypoglycemia, owing to a failure of hepatic glycogenolysis and gluconeogenesis. Additional direct effects of the accumulated excess fructose 1-phosphate on hepatic phosphorylase also may account for the lack of responsiveness of patients to exogenous glucagon during a hypoglycemic episode. The defect in fructose 1-phosphate aldolase appears to be an autosomal recessive trait. Asymptomatic carrier states having approximately half of normal enzymatic activities have been identified. In these carriers, recent studies using phosphorous nuclear magnetic resonance (NMR) have shown abnormal hepatic energy metabolism on fructose loading and a clear tendency to hyperuricemia.

A diagnosis of hereditary fructose intolerance can be made by the demonstration of characteristic hypoglycemia and hypophosphatemia after fructose administration. Fructose may be given orally or, preferably, intravenously at a dose of 0.5 g/kg of body weight. This dose may be excessive for a relatively malnourished child or infant, but it is appropriate for adults or well-nourished children. Hypoglycemia in adults is observed 60 to 90 minutes after fructose ingestion, whereas in children the hypoglycemia occurs somewhat earlier, generally by 45 minutes after fructose administration. Concurrent with hypoglycemia or shortly preceding it, serum phosphate levels fall dramatically, generally to levels 60% or less of the initial serum phosphate level. Symptoms of hypoglycemia that may occur 15 to 30 minutes after fructose administration are largely due to the initial phases of hypoglycemia and reflect, initially, adrenergic responses, and, later, central nervous system responses to the hypoglycemia. A careful examination of the urine during a fructose tolerance test will demonstrate the presence of aminoaciduria; rising serum levels of hepatic enzymes also may be observed before the conclusion of the test. Treatment for hereditary fructose intolerance, elimination of fructose from the diet, is highly effective.

GLYCOGEN STORAGE DISEASES

The glycogen storage diseases are a heterogeneous group of metabolic disorders affecting many different tissues. Their common characteristic is the excessive accumulation of glycogen, usually with organ dysfunction. They are logically considered as defects at several points in the cycle of glycogen synthesis and breakdown.

Glycogen synthesis begins with phosphorylation of glucose to form glucose 6-phosphate, which is subsequently rearranged by the action of phosphoglucomutase to form glucose 1-phosphate (Fig. 305-2). This glucose 1-phosphate condenses with uridine triphosphate (UTP) to generate an active form of glucose, uridine diphosphate-glucose (UDP-glucose). This activated form of glucose is subsequently condensed with priming chains of preexisting glycogen to produce chain lengthening by alpha-1,4-glucosyl linkage formation. The enzyme catalyzing this condensation, glycogen synthase or UDP-glucose-glycogen-alpha,1,4-glucosyltransferase, is the first major control point for the regulation of glycogen formation in mammalian liver. The enzyme exists in two forms. The independent, or dephosphorylated, form of the enzyme is fully active with respect to glycogen formation. Agents increasing muscle cyclic adenosine monophosphate (cyclic 3',5',AMP) levels, such as epinephrine and glucagon, accelerate glycogen degradation. Increased cyclic AMP levels also stimulate that kinase, which phosphorylates glycogen synthase to form the D, or relatively inactive, form of the enzyme. The enzyme glycogen-synthase kinase, which phosphorylates glycogen synthase, is found in close association with the synthase as part of the glycogen particulate complex of mammalian liver and muscle. Glucose, vagal stimulation, and insulin tend to increase the activity of glycogen synthase, most probably by dephosphorylating the enzyme.

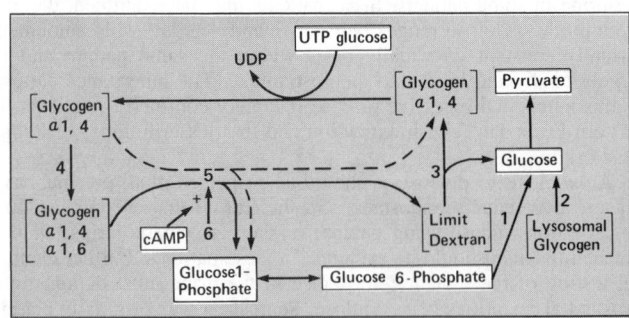

FIGURE 305-2 Pathways of hepatic glycogen synthesis and degradation.

Enzyme	Deficiency state
1 Glucose 6-phosphatase	Glycogen storage disease (GSD) type I (hepatorenal)
2 Acid maltase	GSD type II (Pompe's disease)
3 Debranching enzyme	GSD type III
4 Branching enzyme	GSD type IV
5 Phosphorylase	Muscle: GSD type V (McArdle's disease)
	Liver: GSD type VI (Hers' disease)
6 Phosphorylase kinase	GSD type VIII

To maintain efficient storage of glucose as glycogen, long chains of alpha-1,4-glucosyl linkages must be modified so that alpha-1,6 branch points interrupt the linear array of glucose residues. The branching enzyme (alpha-1,4-glucan:alpha-1,4-glucan-6-glucosyltransferase) is responsible for rearranging alpha-1,4 linkages so that the linear array spans no more than six to ten glucose residues before a branch point occurs. This multibranched nature of glycogen structure results in a more rapid acceleration of glucose liberation by phosphorolysis than would otherwise occur using a much smaller number of linear alpha-1,4 sequences.

The second major point of hormonal regulation of glycogen metabolism is exerted on the enzyme catalyzing the primary step of glycogen degradation, phosphorylase. As is the case with glycogen synthase, glycogen phosphorylase exists in two forms—a phosphorylated form, which is active, and a dephosphorylated form, which is inactive. Phosphorylation of the inactive phosphorylase is catalyzed by the enzyme phosphorylase b kinase. This kinase itself exists in both active and inactive forms, which are phosphorylated and dephosphorylated, respectively. Regulation of phosphorylase b kinase by phosphorylation is catalyzed by cyclic AMP modifications of cyclic AMP–dependent protein kinase. Dissociation of the regulatory subunit from the catalytic subunit of cyclic AMP–dependent protein kinase rapidly accelerates the ATP-dependent phosphorylation of phosphorylase b kinase. Phosphorylase b kinase in turn phosphorylates the subunits of phosphorylase b, using ATP as substrate. Phosphorylase alone is not sufficient to maintain maximal rates of glycogenolysis in mammalian liver or muscle. Although phosphorylase cleaves alpha-1,4-glucosyl linkages to form glucose 1-phosphate, phosphorylase is without substantial activity on alpha-1,6-glucosyl linkages. Without further enzymatic activity, phosphorolysis of glycogen results in the formation of a limit dextran composed of peripheral alpha-1,6 linkages with interior, and a few exterior, alpha-1,4 linkages. Continuation of glycogenolysis then requires the action of debrancher enzyme (amylo-1,6-glucosidase), which hydrolyzes these linkages to form free glucose rather than glucose 1-phosphate. An intermediary enzyme responsible for continuing glycogenolysis is the oligo-1,4→1,4-glucan transferase, which rearranges the initial two or three alpha-1,4 linkages before the alpha-1,6 branch point to another locale in the glycogen molecule in such a way that the alpha-1,6 linkage is exposed to the catalytic site of the debrancher enzyme. Regulation of glycogenolysis by factors altering debrancher enzyme or the alpha-1,4-glucantransferase has not been described.

The glucose 6-phosphate formed by the action of phosphoglucomutase on the resulting glucose 1-phosphate is hydrolytically cleaved by the action of microsomal glucose 6-phosphatase in kidney and liver. Cleavage of the glucose ester results in the formation of free inorganic phosphate. The activity of the enzyme shows some hormonal regulation by agonists such as glucocorticoids. Direct effects of glucagon and of falling insulin levels, as during fasting, also have been postulated, although the precise biochemical mechanism for these effects has not yet been defined.

Type I Glycogen Storage Disease

Glucose-6-phosphatase deficiency is an inborn error of metabolism, known originally as *von Gierke's disease*. It results from a lack of hepatic and renal glucose-6-phosphatase activity. As a consequence, these patients have a characteristic history of hypoglycemia from infancy onward. Massive hepatomegaly is usually present. Splenomegaly is rare. Enlargement of the kidneys is also described. Characteristic symmetric, yellowish paramacular lesions are found in the retina in about half of the patients with von Gierke's disease. Osteoporosis is common, as are tendinous xanthomas on the extensor surfaces of the extremities. Many subjects have tophi because hyperuricemia accompanies this condition. Generalized platelet dysfunction, with a tendency to persistent bleeding after trauma or surgery, is described, as is inflammatory bowel disease. Hypoglycemia is present to a highly variable extent. The disorder is more common and much more serious in infants than in older children and adults. Metabolic acidosis often is found because lactic acidemia occurs, presumably as a consequence of impaired hepatic lactate clearance that is due to a failure of hepatic gluconeogenesis. Ketosis frequently occurs in patients with this disease, although careful study has not substantiated this as a central element. On the contrary, infants and children with hypoglycemia and ketosis should be investigated more carefully for the presence of other disorders such as fructose diphosphatase deficiency. A Fanconi-like syndrome is rare in patients with type I glycogen storage disease. These patients also have marked hyperlipidemia, most probably due to the inability to store glucose as glycogen; this causes an increased flux of ingested carbohydrate toward hepatic triglyceride and cholesterol metabolism. There is, in addition, a reduction in the activity of lipoprotein lipase in these patients. The hyperuricemia described in patients with type I glycogen storage disease was initially attributed to chronic metabolic acidosis with a resulting diminution in urinary uric acid clearance, but more recent study has shown that uric acid formation is increased. The precise biochemical mechanism producing the increased biosynthesis is not understood. There is also reactive hyperinsulinemia, and polycystic ovaries are often noted. These findings suggest underlying insulin resistance, perhaps as the result of the dyslipidemia.

A diagnosis of type I glycogen storage disease should be suspected when hypoglycemia is unresponsive to epinephrine or glucagon administration. In the absence of glucose-6-phosphatase activity, significant amounts of free glucose cannot be released to the circulation after phosphorolysis of liver or kidney glycogen. The enzymatic assays of glucose-6-phosphatase activity in kidney or liver biopsies are an essential requisite for the diagnosis. The disease is inherited as an autosomal recessive trait, and carriers may have a reduced activity of the enzyme in liver, kidney, or intestinal mucosal biopsies. Carriers are asymptomatic.

Treatment of glycogen storage disease type I is relatively straightforward. The hypoglycemia requires frequent feedings. Treatment of the nocturnal hypoglycemia by continuous infusion via nasogastric tube has been effective. Approximately 10 mg/kg per minute of carbohydrate must be administered. Recently, oral feedings of uncooked cornstarch at 6-hour intervals have been equally effective and better tolerated in children and adults but not in infants. Diminished insulin release may be produced by the use of diazoxide, which thereby reduces the tendency of the liver to store large quantities of glucose in the form of glycogen. Further amelioration of the hepatomegaly may be achieved by the somewhat more drastic use of portal diversionary procedures so that less glucose is stored as glycogen. Orthotopic liver transplantation may provide the best long-term therapy.

Type II Glycogen Storage Disease

Alpha-1,4-glucosidase deficiency, also known as *Pompe's disease,* results in a glycogenosis most commonly noted in infancy. It primarily affects the heart, although other forms of the disease affecting primarily skeletal muscle also have been described. Pompe's disease manifests itself as generalized cardiac dysfunction with cardiomegaly, congestive heart failure, cyanosis, and ultimately death within the first year of life. The skeletal muscle form of the disease presents later in childhood or in adult life, tends to resemble a lysosomal storage disease or generalized myopathy, and must be differentiated carefully from such. The glycogenosis results from a failure of lysosomal hydrolysis of glycogen particles. In most mammalian tissues, cells are in a constant state of turnover in which older constituents are degraded and replaced by newly synthesized protein, lipid, and carbohydrate components of the cell. This remodeling process depends largely on lysosomal degradation of cellular constituents and organelles. Glycogen degradation in lysosomes requires an acid maltase enzyme, an alpha-1,4-glucosidase, having an acid pH optimum. This enzyme activity is deficient in patients with Pompe's disease. As a result, the lysosomes become engorged with ingested glycogen that cannot be digested; this ultimately results in cellular swelling, cellular dysfunction, and cellular death.

Type II glycogen storage disease is generally accepted to be an autosomal recessive genetic disease, and a diagnosis can be made only by the demonstration of the acid maltase deficiency in leukocytes or tissue biopsies of patients suspected of the diagnosis. Other biochemical tests generally are normal in these patients, except those resulting from the organ dysfunction produced. No treatment for this condition exists, and its inexorable course cannot be modified.

Type III Glycogen Storage Disease

In *amylo-1,6-glucosidase deficiency,* also known as *debrancher enzyme deficiency,* a limit dextran glycogenosis results from the ongoing action of phosphorylase, but not of debrancher, activity. Thus as in type I glycogen storage disease, the patient has hepatomegaly (but less kidney enlargement) and, more commonly, splenomegaly. Although severe hypoglycemia and convulsions may occur in this condition, these tend to be generally milder than in patients with type I glycogen storage disease. Skeletal muscle and cardiac enlargement has also been described, but kidney enlargement is not common. Mild hyperlipidemia, but not hyperuricemia, may be anticipated, and biochemical abnormalities characteristic of liver dysfunction are observed frequently. The disease appears to be inherited as an autosomal recessive trait, and the treatment is similar to that of type I glycogen storage disease. Multiple small feedings may be used to ameliorate the hypoglycemia, and portal diversionary procedures may be necessary for the hepatomegaly and glycogenosis. Unlike the situation in type I glycogen storage disease, patients with type III glycogenosis frequently have a long and relatively asymptomatic life.

Type IV Glycogen Storage Disease or Branching Enzyme Deficiency

This relatively rare form of glycogen storage disease is also known as *amylopectinosis* or *Anderson's disease.* As with other forms of glycogen storage disease, growth retardation and failure to thrive are common in the early childhood period. Hepatomegaly, hypotonia, and splenomegaly also may be observed. The disease follows an inexorable course that is associated with cirrhosis, hepatic failure, and death within the first few years of life. Although the liver contains normal concentrations of glycogen, the biochemical nature of this glycogen is abnormal. Relatively long chains of alpha-1,4-amyloselike glycogen particles are synthesized. Because of the enzymatic deficiency, there is a markedly reduced number of branch points in each glycogen molecule. Consequently, glycogen solubility is reduced and phosphorylase activity becomes insufficient. An autosomal recessive inheritance has been described. No treatment for this condition is available.

Type V Glycogen Storage Disease or Muscle Phosphorylase Deficiency

In this disorder, originally described by McCardle, there is a prominent and unusual history of severe muscle cramps and a limitation of muscle function during exercise. The metabolic defect, which is the absence of glycogen phosphorylase in skeletal muscle, is undoubtedly present from birth but produces few if any symptoms during childhood. The disease becomes prominent in early adulthood, when severe muscle cramps and secondary myoglobinuria develop. Later, muscle wasting and weakness become increasingly severe as the myoglobinuria diminishes. Physical examination of these patients is generally unremarkable, as are most routine biochemical determinations. The normal postexercise rise in venous lactate levels does not occur in patients with this glycogen storage disease owing to a failure of muscle glycogenolysis. This block in glucose mobilization during anoxic exercise thereby limits muscle ATP formation by anaerobic glycolysis. As a result of the diminished availability of high-energy phosphate, gross muscle dysfunction and cell leakage become apparent, causing myoglobinuria. Continued injury results in cell death and gross signs of muscle wasting. Muscle energy metabolism during aerobic states is otherwise intact owing to mitochondrial preservation and function. Phosphorous NMR studies clearly show normal work capacity provided that muscle atrophy has not occurred. This disorder is inherited as an autosomal recessive trait; the diagnosis is proved only by muscle biopsy and direct assays of the enzymes. Treatment with a variety of agents such as glucose, fructose, and isoproterenol to raise free fatty acid levels has been advocated. None of these provide consistent or long-lasting benefits. In all instances, strenuous exercise should be avoided.

Type VI Glycogen Storage Disease

Recently, patients with increased hepatic glycogen levels and a 75% to 80% reduction of hepatic phosphorylase activity have been noted. Clinically, these patients resemble those with mild forms of type I glycogen storage disease. Owing to the intrinsic difficulties in the assay of liver phosphorylase activity, the precise biochemical defect, as well as its existence as a separate clinical entity, remains open to question.

Type VII Glycogen Storage Disease or Muscle Phosphofructokinase Deficiency

Phosphofructokinase is the key regulatory enzyme of the glycolytic pathway. The deficiency of this enzyme results in a diminished glycolytic clearance of glucose taken up by cells having an insulin-facilitated or insulin-requiring mechanism for glucose uptake. The glycogen storage in this condition results from the overaccumulation of fructose 6-phosphate and glucose 6-phosphate, which cannot be cleared by the usual pathways of anaerobic glycolysis. As a consequence, glucose 6-phosphate is converted to increased amounts of glycogen. An autosomal recessive inheritance seems apparent for this condition. Treatment is generally unavailable, although a low-carbohydrate diet with frequent small feedings may ameliorate the overaccumulation of glucose in the form of stored glycogen in skeletal muscle.

Type VIII Glycogen Storage Disease or Hepatic Phosphorylase b Kinase Deficiency

As discussed earlier, phosphorylase activation requires at least two other enzymatic activities. Thus the findings of a low phosphorylase activity may suggest a diminished phosphorylase mass or a diminished activation mechanism regulating phosphorylase activity. In patients with a diminished phosphorylase b kinase activity, hepatomegaly and glycogenosis have been reported. Phosphorylase activation (conversion of phosphorylase b to phosphorylase a) is markedly slowed compared to that in normal persons. There is normal responsiveness to glucagon, however, and chronic glucagon administration produces a diminution of the hepatomegaly. This disease appears to follow an X-linked inheritance pattern. The patients have only mild symptoms, which are generally linked to the hepatomegaly, and they exhibit mild hypoglycemia on exertion. Treatment is not fully satisfactory at the present time.

GALACTOSEMIA

As is the case with the metabolism of most other hexoses in mammalian tissues, galactose is initially phosphorylated by a relatively specific galactokinase found in mammalian liver and, to a lesser extent, in other tissues. Galactokinase phosphorylates galactose in the presence of ATP to form galactose 1-phosphate and ADP (Fig. 305-1). Subsequently, the galactose 1-phosphate must be activated by transfer to a uridylyl group catalyzed by the galactose-1-phosphate-uridylyltransferase. In this reaction, galactose 1-phosphate condenses with UDP-glucose to form UDP-galactose + glucose 1-phosphate. The resulting UDP-galactose is converted to UDP-glucose by the action of UDP-galactose-4'-epimerase. Subsequently, the UDP-glucose is hydrolyzed by a pyrophosphorylation reaction such that UTP + glucose 1-phosphate is subsequently generated. The glucose 1-phosphate formed from galactose metabolism may be utilized directly for glycogen biosynthesis or, alternatively, may be converted to glucose 6-phosphate by the action of phosphoglucomutase and subsequently metabolized by anaerobic glycolysis or released as free glucose, depending on the fuel and energy requirements of the organism. Reduction of galactose to galactitol (a hexitol) is an alternative means of galactose disposal.

Two relatively specific and different presentations of galactosemia have been described. In the first and more serious of these inborn errors of metabolism, there is a near absence of the UDP-glucose-galactose-1-phosphate-uridylyltransferase. This absence most commonly manifests itself as a failure to thrive in infancy. Vomiting, diarrhea, and abnormal liver function with jaundice or hepatomegaly are generally present within the first week of life or at any time after milk ingestion. Because the predominant sugar of milk is lactose, a disaccharide composed of glucose and galactose, the infant is exposed to large quantities of galactose early in life. Severe hemolysis, ascites, and cataracts within a few days of birth have all been reported in a large proportion of patients who have the transferase form of galactosemia. If the disorder is left untreated, severe mental retardation and a failure of neurologic development will become apparent after the first few months of life. On occasion, failure to thrive and vomiting may be relatively less in some patients, and, after 3 to 6 months, these patients may manifest motor retardation, neurologic deficits, hepatic enlargement, and cataracts. In rare instances this presentation may not occur until the second to fourth year of life.

Routine laboratory testing usually will reveal a hyperchloremic metabolic acidosis, albuminuria, aminoaciduria reminiscent of Fanconi's syndrome, and, occasionally, lower-than-normal fasting glucose levels. The specific tests for galactose in blood will reveal substantial elevations in all patients studied. A diagnosis of galactosemia may be suspected on the basis of the appearance of a nonglucose reducing sugar in the urine.

Because the toxicity resulting from galactosemia is produced by accumulations of large quantities of intracellular galactose 1-phosphate or galactitol, therapy for this state must be directed toward producing a galactose-free diet for these patients. Initially, this means an elimination of milk and milk products from the diet. More commonly, Nutramigen and soy bean milks are used. Because of the difficulties of dietary adherence, this therapy is not always successful. Nevertheless, rapid relief of all symptoms will be observed in patients ingesting minimal quantities of galactose. Even the cataracts will regress, although they may not clear completely in most circumstances. Reversal of the mental retardation or, indeed, its prevention depends on an early initiation of a diet free of galactose. Mothers known to have produced galactosemic infants in the past should be kept on a galactose-free diet throughout subsequent pregnancies. This appears to be most helpful in preventing mental retardation and leads to early diagnosis in subsequent offspring with galactosemia. The diagnosis may be suspected in patients having galactose in blood or urine, but confirmation is required by direct assay of the activity of the uridylyltransferase in leukocytes, skin fibroblasts, or liver biopsies of these patients.

More recently, a second form of galactosemia has been described in which the biochemical defect appears to be an absence or deficiency of galactokinase. This condition was initially described in a 44-year-old adult. In general, these persons have milder involvement of the liver and spleen. Cataracts are considerably smaller, although they occur at remarkably young ages in galactosemic, as compared to nongalactosemic, patients. Most commonly, these findings should make the clinician suspicious of galactosemia. Screening tests for nonglucose-reducing sugars in the urine should be performed. Specific enzymatic assays should be used to confirm the diagnosis. In general, toxicity produced by the galactokinase deficit results primarily from the reduction of excessive quantities of galactose to galactitol in tissues such as the lens. The resulting hexitol produces premature cataracts by osmotic swelling and disruption of lens architecture. Similar mechanisms may occur in neuronal tissue, and it is possible that part of the central nervous system toxicity associated with more severe deficiency of the uridylyltransferase may result from galactitol formation. Treatment, as with the other form of galactosemia, rests primarily on the institution and maintenance of a galactose-free diet. Symptoms may resolve and cataracts may improve, although they do not disappear completely.

BIBLIOGRAPHY

Bondy PK, Rosenberg LE, editors: *Diseases of metabolism,* ed 8, Philadelphia, 1980, WB Saunders.

Buiman D, Holton JB, Pennock CA, editors: *Inherited disorders of carbohydrate metabolism,* Baltimore, 1980, University Park.

Burmeister LA, Valdivia T, Nuttall FQ: Adult hereditary fructose intolerance, *Arch Intern Med* 151:773, 1991.

Chen YT, Cornblath M, Sidbury JB: Cornstarch therapy in type I glycogen-storage disease, *N Engl J Med* 310:171, 1984.

Couper R, Kapelushnik J, Griffiths AM: Neutrophil dysfunction in glycogen storage disease Ib: association with Crohn's-like colitis, *Gastroenterology* 100:549, 1991.

Greene HC et al: Continuous nocturnal intragastric feeding for management of type I glycogen-storage disease, *N Engl J Med* 294:423, 1976.

Kirschner BS, Baker AL, Thorp FK: Growth in adulthood after liver transplantation for glycogen storage disease type I, *Gastroenterology* 101:238, 1991.

Schwenk WF, Haymond MW: Optimal rate of enteral glucose administration in children with GSD-I, *N Engl J Med* 314(11):682, 1986.

Seegmiller JE et al: Fructose-induced aberration of metabolism in familial gout identified by 31P magnetic resonance spectroscopy, *Proc Natl Acad Sci U S A* 87:8326, 1990.

Stanbury JB, Wyngaarden JB, Fredrickson DS, editors: *The metabolic basis of inherited disease,* ed 5, New York, 1983, McGraw-Hill.

306 Disorders of Lipids and Lipoproteins

Scott M. Grundy

This chapter describes common disorders of lipid metabolism, particularly those leading to accelerated coronary atherosclerosis. Certain rarer abnormalities of lipid metabolism also are considered because their clinical recognition is essential and because they provide insights into key steps of lipid regulation. Before considering abnormal states, however, lipid metabolism under normal circumstances is reviewed.

LIPID METABOLISM

The major lipids of the body are triglycerides, cholesterol, and phospholipids. The predominant phospholipid is lecithin, but others—sphingomyelin and cephalins—also are important for cellular function and transport of lipids. The chemical structures of the major lipids, including representative fatty acids, are presented in Fig. 306-1.

Triglycerides consist of three fatty acid molecules esterified to glycerol. Fatty acids vary in chain length and degree of saturation. The most common fatty acids of the saturated series are palmitic acid (16:0)* and stearic acid (18:0); they are the primary constituents of most hard fats, whether of animal or plant origin. The major monounsaturated fatty acid is oleic acid (18:1ω9); it is the most prevalent fatty acid consumed in most diets. Oleic acid can be synthesized by both animals and plants.

Plants, but not animals, can synthesize two types of polyunsaturated fatty acids: they are ω6 and ω3 fatty acids. The major ω6 fatty acid, linoleic acid (18:2ω6), has 18 carbon atoms with two double[2]

---

*(chain length: double bonds)

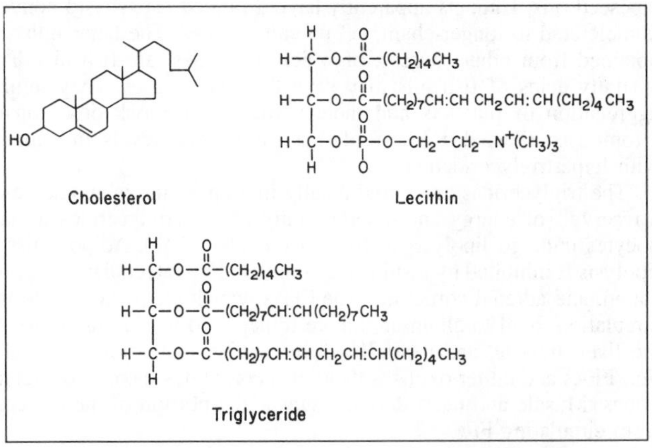

FIGURE 306-1   The major lipids of plasma: cholesterol, lecithin, and triglyceride. Typical fatty acids are shown esterified to the latter two lipids.

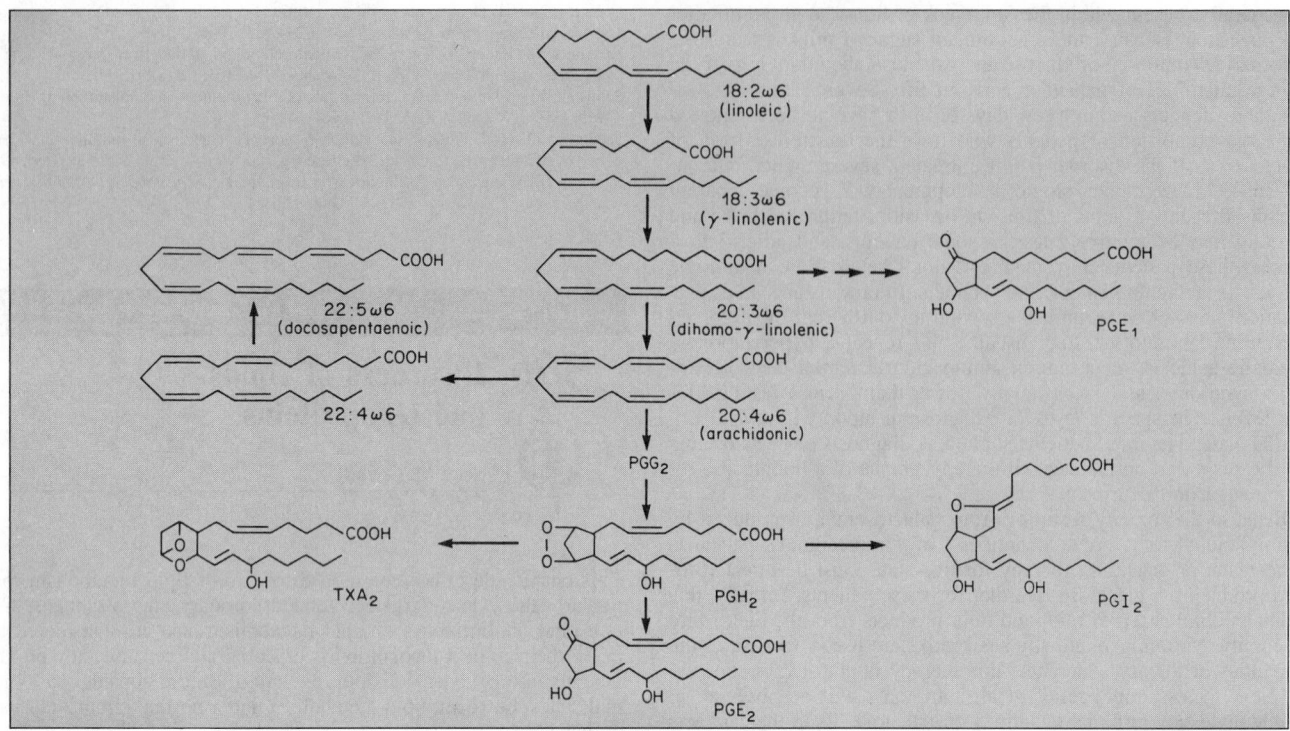

FIGURE 306-2   Synthesis of prostaglandin of the 1 series *(PGE₁)* and prostanoids of the 2 series, prostaglandin *(PGE₂)*, thromboxane *(TXA₂)*, and prostacyclin *(PGI₂)*. Also, docosapentaenoic acid is synthesized from the key intermediate, arachidonic acid.

bonds, the second being six carbon atoms removed from the terminal methyl group. Linoleic acid occurs mainly in plant oils; it comprises 77% and 56% of the fatty acids of safflower oil and soybean oil, respectively. Linoleic acid is an essential dietary fatty acid for humans because it cannot be made by the body but is required for normal metabolism. It is an important constituent of cell membranes and a precursor for longer-chain fatty acids that are transformed into prostaglandins, thromboxanes, and prostacyclins of the 1 and 2 series (Fig. 306-2).

The parent ω3 fatty acid is linolenic acid (18:3ω3); it, too, cannot be synthesized by the body. A deficiency of linolenic acid uniquely leads to abnormalities in retinal function; thus it appears to be an essential fatty acid. It can be converted to fatty acids of longer-chain length and move double bonds, which become precursors to prostaglandins, thromboxanes, and prostacyclin of the 3 series. Linolenic acid occurs in substantial amounts in soybean and rapeseed oils. Humans apparently have a limited capacity to convert linoleic acid to longer-chain, ω3 polyunsaturates. The latter must be obtained from other sources, of which the richest are fish oils. The ω3 fatty acids of fish oils may have therapeutic uses. They inhibit aggregation of platelets and thereby may reduce risk of coronary thrombosis; they also lower plasma triglyceride levels in patients with hypertriglyceridemia.

The triglycerides are stored mainly in adipose tissue and serve as a reservoir of energy and essential fatty acids. Triglycerides in adipocytes undergo lipolysis to free fatty acids (FFAs). Adipose tissue lipolysis is inhibited by insulin and stimulated by catecholamines, glucagon, and adrenal corticoids. The FFAs, which are released into the circulation, bind to albumin and are transported to various tissues—the liver, muscle, and heart. The liver extracts a portion of circulation FFAs and either oxidizes them or incorporates them into triglycerides. Muscle and heart derive a substantial portion of their energy from circulating FFAs.

Cholesterol is an important lipid, playing a key role in maintaining the integrity of cellular membranes. It is the sole source of steroid hormones and bile acids. Cholesterol is produced in most tissues but mainly in the liver and intestinal mucosa. It is synthesized from

acetate by a series of about 20 reactions (Fig. 306-3). In the synthetic sequence, acetate is condensed to acetoacetate, which takes another acetate residue to form hydroxy-methyl-glutaryl coenzyme A (HMG CoA). The conversion of HMG CoA to mevalonic acid, catalyzed by the enzyme HMG CoA reductase, is a rate-limiting step in the synthesis of cholesterol. Mevalonic acid undergoes a series of condensation reactions, resulting in a straight-chain hydrocarbon, squalene, which cyclizes to a sterol, lanosterol; the latter is converted to cholesterol. The rate of cholesterol synthesis is influenced by the concentration of cholesterol within cells. For example, a rise in cellular cholesterol content suppresses the activity of HMG CoA reductase. Thus feedback control maintains cellular cholesterol at optimum levels. As cells accumulate excessive amounts of cholesterol, a portion is esterified with a fatty acid, a reaction that is catalyzed by the enzyme acylcholesterol acyltransferase (ACAT); the product is stored temporarily as cholesterol ester until needed by the cell.

The liver promotes the excretion of cholesterol in two ways. First, a portion of hepatic cholesterol is converted into the "primary" bile acids, cholic acid and chenodeoxycholic acid; second, cholesterol is secreted directly into bile. Direct secretion is made possible by the solubilizing power of bile acids. Both cholesterol and bile acids enter the intestine through the biliary tract. About 40% to 60% of intestinal cholesterol is reabsorbed; the remainder is excreted into feces. Cholesterol is absorbed almost exclusively in the upper small intestine. Normally, almost all of the bile acids (approximately 98%) are reabsorbed, mainly in the distal small intestine. Only a very small fraction of bile acids entering the intestine reaches the colon and is excreted in feces.

The bile acids return in portal blood to the liver, where they are extracted almost completely in their first pass. They are resecreted rapidly into bile to complete the enterohepatic circulation. In the liver the bile acids inhibit the conversion of cholesterol into bile acids by suppressing the rate-limiting reaction in bile acid synthesis, the 7-alpha-hydroxylation of cholesterol. The rate of flux of bile acids through the liver thus regulates cholesterol catabolism and indirectly influences hepatic concentrations of cholesterol.

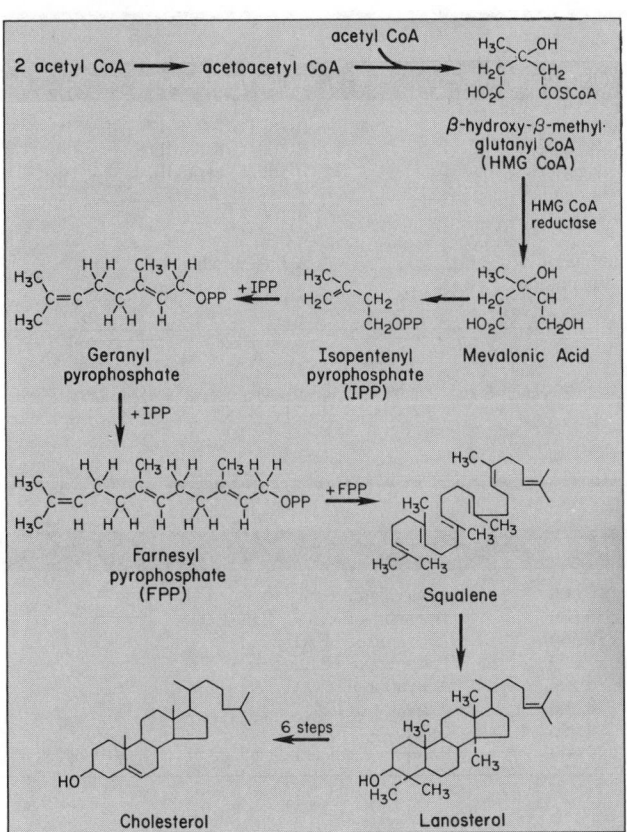

FIGURE 306-3 Key steps in synthesis of cholesterol.

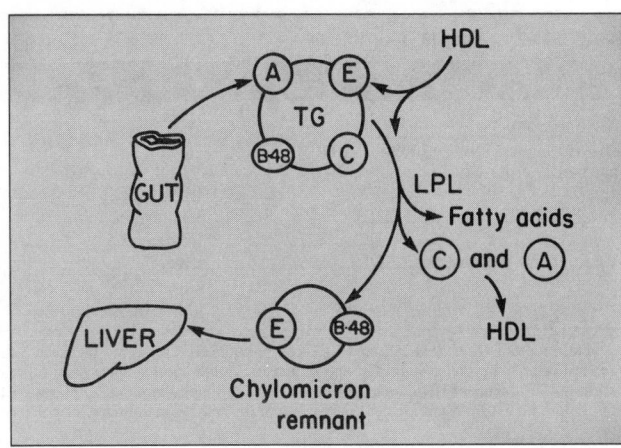

FIGURE 306-4 Formation and catabolism of chylomicrons. The chylomicrons are produced by the intestine and contain mainly triglycerides *(TG)* in their lipid core. The surface coat contains apoprotein (apo) As (A-I, A-II, A-IV), Es, Cs, and B-48. The apo Es and Cs are derived in part from high-density lipoprotein (HDL). Triglycerides undergo lipolysis by lipoprotein lipase (LPL) to release fatty acids. Simultaneously, apo Cs and apo As are released and enter HDL. The residual lipoproteins, chylomicron remnants, retain apo E and apo B-48 and are taken up by the liver.

LIPOPROTEIN METABOLISM

Lipids are insoluble in aqueous solutions, and they cannot circulate freely in plasma. Instead, they are complexed with specialized proteins called *apolipoproteins,* or *apoproteins.* Lipid-apoprotein complexes are named lipoproteins. They have a central core of nonpolar lipids (cholesterol ester and triglycerides) and a surface coat of more polar constituents—unesterified cholesterol, phospholipids, and apoproteins. Lipoproteins are produced by the gut and liver but are modified extensively in plasma. The major function of lipoproteins is to transport lipids (i.e., triglycerides, cholesterol, and lipid-soluble vitamins) from one site to another. They also help to stabilize the plasma membranes of cells that are bathed by plasma and lymph. The major lipoproteins of plasma and their constituents are listed in Table 306-1.

Apolipoproteins

The apoproteins of lipoproteins possess unique sequences of amino acids that allow them to bind to lipids and yet be dissolved in aqueous plasma. Each apoprotein has one or more specific functions, including (1) solubilizing lipids for secretion from cells, (2) transporting lipids in plasma, (3) activating enzymes responsible for hydrolysis of lipids, (4) accepting lipids through exchange reactions, and (5) binding to specific cell-surface receptors that provide a mechanism for cellular uptake and degradation of lipoproteins. The major apoproteins, along with their sites of origins, molecular weights, and general functions, are listed in Table 306-2.

Chylomicrons

After dietary lipids are digested and absorbed, they are transported away from the intestinal tract by lipoproteins called chylomicrons (Fig. 306-4). The triglycerides are the major class of lipids in the diet, and as they enter the upper small intestine, they undergo lipolysis by pancreatic lipase, being degraded to fatty acids and monoglycerides;

the latter are taken up by the intestinal mucosa and resynthesized into triglycerides. Simultaneously, unesterified cholesterol of dietary and biliary origin enters mucosal cells and is esterified. Newly formed triglycerides and cholesterol esters are incorporated into chylomicrons, which are secreted into chyle. Chylomicrons are the largest of the plasma lipoproteins. More than 95% of their weight is triglyceride; only 1% is cholesterol ester. Apoproteins also constitute only about 1% by weight. The major apoprotein of chylomicrons is apoprotein B-48 (apo B-48), a highly insoluble protein with a molecular weight of approximately 250,000. Other apoproteins—the apo Cs, apo Es, and apo As—also are present; they are either secreted with chylomicrons or transferred from high-density lipoproteins (HDLs).

Chylomicrons enter the bloodstream through the thoracic duct and pass into peripheral capillary beds. At the surface of capillary endothelial cells they come in contact with an enzyme, lipoprotein lipase (LPL). This enzyme is activated by one of the C apoproteins, apo C-II. The triglycerides of chylomicrons are hydrolyzed to fatty acids and glycerol. The rate of lipolysis may be modulated by apo C-III, an apoprotein that apparently inhibits LPL. During lipolysis the soluble apoproteins (apo Cs and apo As) are released into the circulation and loosely attach to HDL; here they are held in reserve for reutilization by very-low-density lipoprotein (VLDL).

When lipolysis of chylomicrons is almost complete, smaller lipoproteins, called *chylomicron remnants,* return to the circulation. These partially degraded lipoproteins contain only small amounts of triglyceride but retain almost all of the newly absorbed cholesterol esters. Chylomicron remnants are cleared rapidly by the liver. Thus fatty acids originating in dietary triglycerides are released in peripheral tissues, whereas dietary cholesterol passes directly to the liver with chylomicron remnants.

Very-Low-Density Lipoproteins

The liver also secretes triglyceride-rich lipoproteins called VLDLs (Fig. 306-5). In the fasting state, almost all plasma triglycerides are present in VLDLs. Newly secreted, or nascent, VLDLs contain little cholesterol ester. The major apoprotein of VLDL is apo B-100, which is a very large molecule (molecular weight, about 550,000) and is highly insoluble. Nascent VLDLs also contain apo E, and as they circulate, they acquire apo Cs and more apo E from HDL. VLDLs also accept cholesterol esters from HDL. In contrast to chylomicrons, VLDLs have no apo A-I or apo A-II. Circulating VLDLs are smaller than chylomicrons and have less triglycerides but more cholesterol esters.

As VLDLs enter the peripheral circulation, they, too, come in con-

Table 306-1   Plasma lipoproteins

LIPOPROTEIN	ORIGIN	MAJOR LIPID CONSTITUENTS(S)	MAJOR APOLIPOPROTEINS
Chylomicrons	Gut	Triglycerides	B-48, E, C-II, C-III, A-I, A-II, A-IV
Very-low-density lipoproteins (VLDL)	Liver	Triglycerides	B-100, C-II, C-III, E
Intermediate-density lipoproteins (IDL)	VLDL catabolism	Triglycerides	B-100, C-11, C-III, E
	Liver (?)*	Cholesterol	
Low-density lipoproteins (LDL)	IDL catabolism	Cholesterol	B-100
	Liver (?)*		
High-density lipoproteins (HDL)	Liver	Cholesterol	A-I, A-II, others†
	Gut	Phospholipids	
	Other lipoproteins‡		

*Several reports suggest that IDL and LDL can be secreted directly by the liver, although this has not been proved.
†Several other apoproteins—apo Cs, apo E, apo A-IV, and apo D—have been reported in HDL.
‡Various constituents of HDL are acquired as these lipoproteins circulate in plasma. HDL may obtain phospholipids and apoproteins C-II, C-II, and E during lipolysis of triglyceride-rich lipoproteins. Cholesterol can be derived from the plasma membranes of cells.

Table 306-2   Major apolipoproteins of plasma lipoproteins

APOLIPOPROTEIN	ORIGIN	LIPOPROTEIN SOURCE(S)	MOLECULAR WEIGHT	FUNCTION
B-48	Gut	Chylomicrons	260,000	Chylomicron transport
B-100	Liver	VLDL, IDL, LDL	550,000	Transport of VLDL, IDL, LDL
A-1	Gut, liver	Chylomicrons, HDL	28,300	Activator of LCAT
A-II	Gut, liver	Chylomicrons, HDL	17,000	Transport of HDL
C-I	Liver	VLDL, IDL, HDL	6,500	Activation of LCAT
C-II	Liver	VLDL, IDL, HDL	8,800	Activator of LPL
C-III	Liver	VLDL, IDL, HDL	8,750	Unknown
E	Liver	VLDL, IDL, HDL	35,000-39,000	Receptor-mediated clearance of remnant lipoproteins

LCAT, Lecithin-cholesterol acyltransferase; *LPL,* lipoprotein lipase.

tact with LPL, and their triglycerides undergo lipolysis. The soluble apo Cs are released, but apo B-100 and much of apo E remain attached to the residual lipoproteins, which are called VLDL remnants. The latter have been largely depleted of triglyceride but remain enriched in cholesterol ester. VLDL remnants can have two fates. In normal persons, at least 60% of circulating VLDL remnants are removed by the liver, and their uptake is mediated by receptors that recognize apo E. More than one receptor may be involved in this process. VLDL remnants not removed by the liver are converted to low-density lipoproteins (LDLs). The precise mechanisms by which conversion to LDL occurs are unknown, although the liver may be involved. A hepatic enzyme, *hepatic triglyceride lipase,* located on the surface of liver cells, may hydrolyze the remaining triglycerides of VLDL remnants, which results in loss of essentially all apoproteins except apo B.

Low-Density Lipoproteins

The LDLs normally transport most of the cholesterol in plasma; they originate from catabolism of VLDL through intermediate-density lipoproteins (IDLs) or VLDL remnants (Fig. 306-6). LDLs contain mostly cholesterol esters in their nonpolar cores and carry very little triglyceride. Each particle of LDL has approximately 17,000 molecules of cholesterol ester. The only apoprotein of LDL is apo B-100, which is retained after catabolism of VLDL. Most LDLs are cleared from the circulation by LDL receptors. These receptors are the same as those which remove VLDL remnants. Both the liver and many extrahepatic tissues express LDL receptors, but LDLs are removed principally by the liver. Most LDLs are cleared by LDL receptors, but smaller amounts leave by nonreceptor pathways, either in the liver or in extrahepatic tissues. Normally, 10% to 15% of the circulating pool of LDL is taken up each day by nonreceptor pathways. Another 15% to 30% of the pool is eliminated daily by LDL receptors. In total, 30% to 45% of the plasma pool of LDL is cleared from the circulation every day.

A cell commonly used for study of LDL receptors is the fibroblast (Fig. 306-7). In tissue culture each fibroblast expresses 20,000 to 50,000 receptors. The LDL receptor is a protein molecule that resides on the surface of cells in specialized regions of the plasma membrane called coated pits. The latter are indentations in the membrane. These pits are covered by a protein, *clathrin,* which gives the pits a fuzzy-coated appearance. These "coated" pits cover only about 2% of the cell surface, but they contain almost all LDL receptors. When LDLs (or VLDL remnants) bind to the receptor, the resulting complexes of receptor and lipoprotein are internalized. This process occurs by invagination of the coated pit to form endocytic vesicles. These vesicles, containing the coated surface, pass through the cytoplasm until they fuse with lysosomes. In lysosomes the components of LDL undergo hydrolytic degradation. Apo B is degraded to amino acids, and cholesterol esters to unesterified cholesterol. Cholesterol passes out of the lysosome, where it inserts into membranes or remains in cytoplasm to regulate the cell's synthesis of cholesterol.

The number of LDL receptors synthesized by cells is adjusted by feedback regulation, and when intracellular concentrations of unesterified cholesterol rise, synthesis of receptors diminishes; on the contrary, when the concentration of cholesterol drops, synthesis of receptors escalates. Thus cellular concentrations of cholesterol couple inversely with the quantity of LDL receptors fabricated by the cell.

Small numbers of LDL particles are dispatched by other varieties of receptors. The macrophage, for example, maintains only few receptors for normal LDL, but it has numerous receptors for chemically modified LDL. Derivatives of LDL can be created in vitro that bestow recognition by these other macrophage receptors. One such derivative is acetyl LDL. Each macrophage has 20,000 to 40,000 receptors that bind to acetyl LDL, whereas these same receptors do not recognize native LDL. One attribute of the acetyl LDL receptor is that it is not under feedback regulation by intracellular cholesterol. Macrophages can acquire large amounts of cholesterol via modified LDL receptors, yet the number of receptors per cell remains constant. Macrophages also express receptors for another lipoprotein called beta-VLDL, a variant of the VLDL remnant. If VLDL remnants are delayed in their clearance from plasma, they become enriched in cholesterol esters and the product, beta-VLDL, is recognized by the macrophage. Macrophage uptake of lipoproteins could be important in atherogenesis because once LDLs enter the arterial wall, they may become chemically modified, and uptake of this modified LDL could transform macrophages into foam cells.

Recent evidence suggests that oxidation of LDL within the arte-

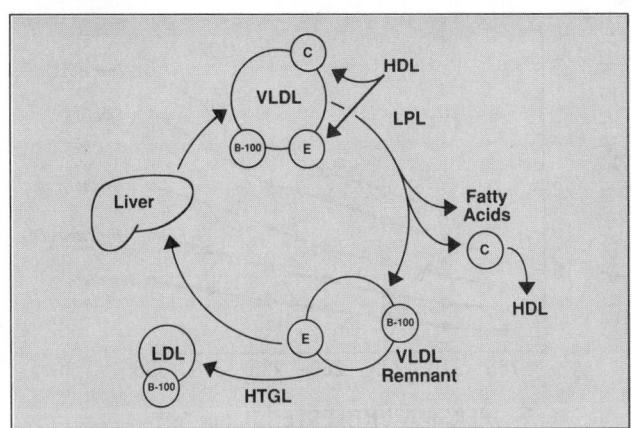

FIGURE 306-5   Metabolism of very-low-density lipoprotein (VLDL). The liver secretes VLDL, which contain triglycerides as its major core lipid. Nascent VLDL contain apo B-100 and some apo E, and as these lipoproteins circulate they acquire apo Cs, possibly more apo Es, and cholesterol esters from HDL. The VLDL are degraded by LPL with release of fatty acids and apo Cs, the latter returning HDL. The product of lipolysis, VLDL remnants, contain both cholesterol esters and smaller amounts of triglycerides as core lipids, and mainly apo-100 and apo Es as surface apoproteins. VLDL remnants can be taken up by the liver, or they can be degraded to LDL. The latter may be mediated in part by hepatic triglyceride lipase (HTGL). Normally, about 60% of VLDL remnants are removed by the liver, whereas the remainder are converted to LDL.

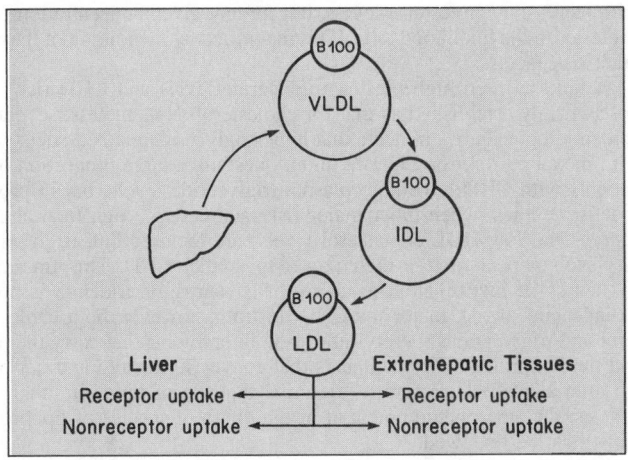

FIGURE 306-6   Metabolism of LDL. The sole apoprotein of LDL is apo B-100. LDLs contain mainly cholesterol esters in their lipid core. LDLs are derived from the catabolism of VLDL and intermediate-densty lipoprotein (IDL). LDLs can have several fates. About 70% of LDLs are removed by the liver, and the remainder by extrahepatic tissues. About 50% to 75% of LDLs are cleared by LDL receptors (receptor uptake), either in the liver or in extrahepatic tissues. The remaining LDLs are removed by nonreceptor pathways, either in liver or extrahepatic tissues. Thus the major pathway of clearance of LDL is receptor uptake in the liver, but other pathways are involved.

rial wall may be one of the critical modifications leading to uptake by macrophages. Oxidized LDL not only is susceptible to macrophage uptake, but also may promote atherosclerosis in other ways (e.g., as a chemoattractant for macrophages and a cytotoxin).

High-Density Lipoproteins

Cholesterol can enter extrahepatic tissues either by uptake of LDL cholesterol or by new synthesis within these cells. Because cholesterol cannot be degraded in extrahepatic tissues, it must be returned to the liver for excretion, a process called *reverse cholesterol trans-*

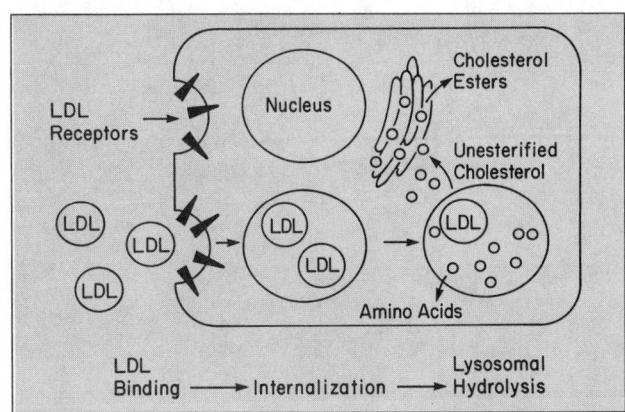

FIGURE 306-7   Cellular metabolism of LDL. The plasma LDL bind to LDL receptors located in coated pits of cells. The LDL are then internalized, and the components undergo hydrolysis in lysosomes. The protein moiety of LDL is degraded to amino acids, and unesterified cholesterol is released to the cell cytoplasm. In the cytoplasm it can inhibit the cell's own synthesis of cholesterol, or it can be stored as cholesterol ester.

port. Although the mechanisms for reverse cholesterol transport are not fully understood, another lipoprotein, HDL, may play an important role. The metabolism of HDL is complex and remains to be elucidated fully, but a general outline has emerged and can be reviewed.

The core lipids of HDL are mainly cholesterol esters. The HDLs are relatively small particles, and their surface-coat constituents—apoproteins, phospholipids, and unesterified cholesterol—predominate over core lipids. Several apoproteins (A-I, A-II, Cs, and Es) reside in HDL. The major apoproteins are A-I and A-II. Apo A-I is a single polypeptide chain of 243 amino acid residues. Apo A-II is a dimer of two identical chains, each chain having 77 amino acids; the chains are linked by a disulfide bond. Lesser amounts of other apoproteins—apo Cs and apo Es—are sequestered in HDL for transfer later to triglyceride-rich lipoproteins. HDLs consist of relatively small particles, ranging in diameter from 40 to 100 Å. More particles of HDL are in circulation than any other type of lipoprotein. HDLs can be divided into two major subfractions, HDL_3 and HDL_2, the former being more dense than the latter.

The components of HDL have multiple origins. The apoproteins stem from both liver and gut. The liver apparently secretes apo A-I and apo A-II complexed with phospholipids. These complexes are called nascent HDL (Fig. 306-8). The intestine also secretes nascent HDL containing apo As. As nascent HDLs circulate, they undergo transformation into mature HDL. Additional phospholipid is acquired by transfer from the surface coats of both chylomicrons and VLDL. Unesterified cholesterol translocates to HDL from the surfaces of cells or from other lipoproteins. This cholesterol undergoes esterification, catalyzed by the action of an enzyme called lecithin-cholesterol acyltransferase (LCAT); this enzyme transfers a fatty acid residue from lecithin to cholesterol. As cholesterol esters are synthesized, they begin to form a core in the lipoprotein, forcing it to assume a spheric shape. This spheric particle goes by the name HDL_3; as HDL_3 acquires more new cholesterol, it grows into a still larger particle, HDL_2.

The outcomes for whole HDL particles and their constituents are multifarious. Some HDL may enter the liver unchanged, possibly via a receptor for apo As. Some components of HDL also can be eliminated piecemeal. The cholesterol esters of HDL can be transferred to VLDL in exchange for triglycerides. Thereafter, VLDL cholesterol esters can reach the liver via hepatic uptake of the products of VLDL catabolism, namely, VLDL remnants and LDL. Further, some of the phospholipids of HDL may be lost on the surface of liver cells during interaction with hepatic triglyceride lipase; this reaction may convert HDL_2 back into HDL_3. An HDL-binding protein apparently resides on the surface of cells, which transfers HDL cholesterol esters directly into cells; the residual HDL particles then return to the circulation. This return of cholesterol from peripheral tissues to the liver occurs by several different pathways.

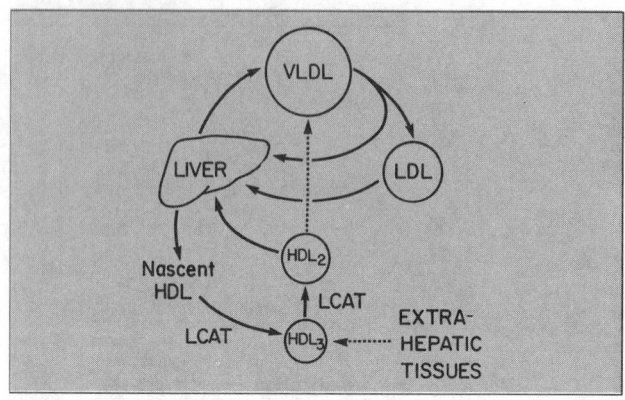

FIGURE 306-8 Metabolism of HDL. The liver secretes nascent HDLs, which are converted to HDL₂ by incorporation of cholesterol esters into the lipid core of the lipoprotein. The formation of cholesterol esters is catalyzed by the enzyme lecithin-cholesterol acyltransferase (LCAT). Unesterified cholesterol for incorporation into HDL can be derived from extrahepatic tissues. The dashed lines indicate the flow of cholesterol molecules. HDL₃ is converted to HDL₂ by further incorporation of cholesterol esters. HDL₂ may be removed intact by the liver, but HDL₂ also can transfer some of its cholesterol ester to VLDL. This cholesterol can return to the liver with either VLDL remnants or LDL.

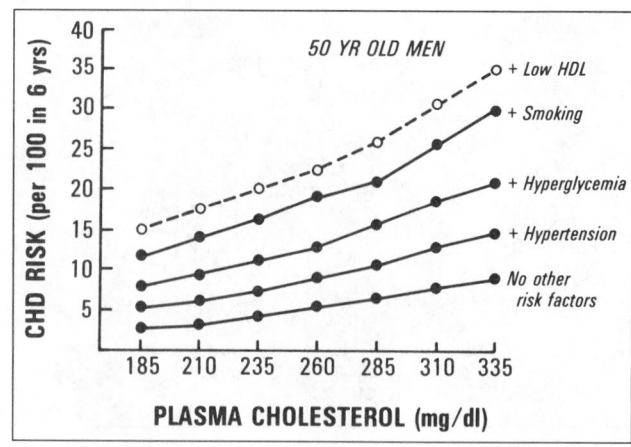

FIGURE 306-10 Risk for CHD at various levels of plasma cholesterol in the presence or absence of other risk factors. Risk is expressed as number of new cases of CHD per 100 men at age 50 years over a 6-year period. Data were obtained from the Framingham Heart Study. The addition of risk factors progressively increases risk for CHD at any level of cholesterol.

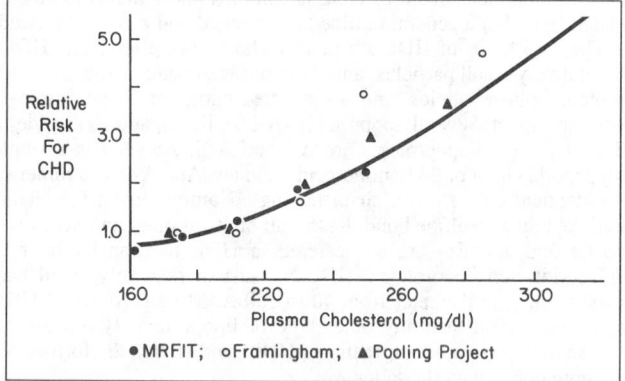

FIGURE 306-9 Relative risk for coronary heart disease (CHD) at various levels of plasma cholesterol. Data are shown for the Multiple Risk Factor Intervention Trial (MRFIT), the Framingham Heart Study, and the Pooling Project.

LIPOPROTEINS AND ATHEROSCLEROSIS

A major component of atherosclerotic plaques is cholesterol; this cholesterol is believed to be derived largely from plasma cholesterol. Multiple lines of evidence implicate elevated plasma cholesterol levels as a cause of atherosclerosis. For example, in several species of animals, high-cholesterol diets induce marked hypercholesterolemia and atherosclerosis. Likewise, in patients with genetic forms of severe hypercholesterolemia premature atherosclerotic disease frequently develops. Furthermore, the level of plasma cholesterol is positively correlated with the risk for coronary heart disease (CHD). Many epidemiologic surveys have demonstrated that this correlation holds over a broad range of cholesterol levels. This link exists both within and between populations. Several studies in the United States (e.g., the Framingham Heart Study, the Pooling Project, and the Multiple Risk Factor Intervention Trial [MRFIT]) have demonstrated a positive, curvilinear relationship between plasma cholesterol and relative risk for CHD (Fig. 306-9). As cholesterol levels increase, particularly above 200 mg/dl, the risk for CHD begins to rise more steeply. At 240 mg/dl, risk is much higher than at 200 mg/dl; and at 300 mg/dl risk is raised threefold to fourfold.

Because of the strong relationship between plasma cholesterol and CHD, an elevated cholesterol level must be considered a major risk factor for CHD; however, it is only one of several other proved risk factors, the latter including hypertension, diabetes mellitus, cigarette smoking, and low levels of plasma HDL. The Framingham Heart Study has shown that coronary risk at any given level of cholesterol is compounded when several risk factors exist concurrently (Fig. 306-10). Even in the absence of other risk factors, the risk for CHD rises with increasing cholesterol levels, but for any given concentration of cholesterol, the likelihood of CHD is magnified by the joining of these other risk factors.

A link between high plasma triglyceride levels and CHD risk is not as firmly established as that for cholesterol. Nonetheless, several epidemiologic studies indicate that hypertriglyceridemia is associated with increased risk for CHD. Without question, a large proportion of patients with CHD have high plasma triglyceride levels, but in prospective studies, when other major risk factors (e.g., high total cholesterol and low HDL cholesterol levels) are factored out, triglyceride levels appear to lose their power to predict CHD. This finding has led some investigators to claim that hypertriglyceridemia is not an independent risk factor for CHD. In truth, however, both cholesterol and triglycerides merely reflect the lipoproteins that carry them, and the lipoproteins are the agents that convey lipids into and out of the arterial wall. Therefore, to describe the role of lipids in atherogenesis, the atherogenic potential of the different species of lipoproteins must be reviewed.

Chylomicrons

The chylomicron lipoproteins in their native form may not be atherogenic. Their major constituent, triglycerides, contributes little to the lipid component of atherosclerotic plaques. Chylomicrons are large particles and seemingly filter poorly through the endothelium and into subintimal spaces; this lack of penetration probably minimizes their atherogenic capability. This fact could explain why severe hyperchylomicronemia, attributable to a deficiency of LPL, does not induce premature atherosclerosis. Nevertheless, some investigators believe that chylomicrons are indirectly atherogenic. When these particles interact with endothelial-surface LPL, cholesterol may be released, which then passes through the intima and into the arterial wall. If so, more cholesterol may infiltrate the arterial wall when high cholesterol intakes enrich chylomicrons with cholesterol.

Chylomicron Remnants

Lipolysis of triglycerides of chylomicrons spawns smaller, cholesterol-enriched particles, chylomicron remnants. Thus chylomicron remnants presumably are more atherogenic than native chylomicrons. However, plasma concentrations of chylomicron remnants generally are low, even after a fatty meal, because they are cleared rapidly by the liver. Consequently, it is not known whether chylomicron remnants contribute to atherosclerosis under normal circumstances.

Very-Low-Density-Lipoproteins

The atherogenic potential of VLDLs, like that of chylomicrons, is uncertain. Elevated levels of VLDL often are found in patients having premature CHD; nonetheless, VLDLs are relatively large particles, contain mainly triglycerides, and probably filter poorly through the endothelial lining of the arterial wall. Furthermore, some patients with high VLDL levels seem remarkably free of atherosclerosis. Despite these factors, under some circumstances VLDLs may deliver cholesterol into the arterial wall. If the protective endothelium becomes disrupted, VLDLs could penetrate the intima and thus be atherogenic. One cause of endothelial injury may be smoking, and our clinical experience suggests that most hypertriglyceridemic patients with CHD are smokers. In addition, there are growing signs that the hypertriglyceridemic state may predispose to coronary thrombosis; several elements of the clotting system have been reported to be abnormal in patients with elevated triglycerides levels.

VLDL Remnants

The VLDL-remnant lipoproteins are probably the most atherogenic of the various forms of VLDL. They are the smallest particles in the VLDL fraction, have the least triglycerides, and are relatively enriched in cholesterol esters. Indeed, patients displaying high concentrations of VLDL remnants seem to be at risk for premature CHD. Some types of remnants, specifically beta-VLDL, are particularly susceptible to uptake by macrophage receptors and appear to be highly atherogenic.

Low-Density Lipoproteins

The LDLs are thought to be the most atherogenic of all lipoproteins. Elevated concentrations of LDL definitely accelerate atherosclerosis, and when their levels are very high, CHD often occurs prematurely. LDLs are relatively small particles, are rich in cholesterol ester, and readily penetrate the arterial intima. LDLs contain the highly insoluble apo B-100, which may be responsible for entrapment of LDL in the subintimal space. Indeed, intact particles of LDL can be identified in most atherosclerotic plaques. The passage of an excess of LDL into the arterial wall is considered by many authorities to be the major factor responsible for atherosclerosis. The lack of CHD in countries where levels of LDL are low, despite a relatively high prevalence of other risk factors (e.g., smoking, hypertension, diabetes mellitus), supports the concept that excessive filtration of LDL into the artery is a necessary condition for atherogenesis.

High-Density Lipoproteins

Although HDLs contain a high percentage of cholesterol, they are not atherogenic; indeed, high plasma levels of HDL may protect against atherosclerosis. This protection could be due to HDL's role in reverse cholesterol transport; that is, HDL may remove excess cholesterol from the arterial wall. This function may occur maximally when circulating levels of HDL are high, and reverse cholesterol transport may be retarded by low levels. This concept agrees with the inverse correlation between HDL levels and CHD risk. Limited studies suggest that HDL_2 is more protective against CHD than is HDL_3. Recent data suggest that the most protective form of HDL is that in which apo A-I is the exclusive apoprotein of the HDL particle. It has been shown that the HDL_2 fraction is enriched with this type of particle.

Agreement that reverse cholesterol transport explains the inverse correlation between HDL levels and CHD risk is not universal. High HDL concentrations may merely reflect a "healthy" transport system for plasma lipids; for instance, when plasma total cholesterol and triglyceride levels are high, HDL levels frequently are low. Thus increased atherogenicity might reside more in an elevation of apo B–containing lipoproteins than in HDL per se. In addition, low-HDL levels frequently occur in the presence of other CHD risk factors (e.g., smoking, obesity, and lack of exercise). Thus the low-HDL level–CHD link may be the result of several factors beyond the action of HDL to promote reverse cholesterol transport. In recent years a lipoprotein Lp(a) has come into prominence as a definite risk factor for CHD.

EFFECTS OF DIETARY FACTORS ON LIPOPROTEIN METABOLISM

Several dietary factors influence the plasma lipoproteins. Because the diet has been implicated in atherogenesis, a review of dietary effects on lipoprotein metabolism seems appropriate. Each of the major dietary constituents is considered separately.

Saturated Fatty Acids

The American diet typically is rich in saturated fatty acids. These acids come from animal meats (beef and pork), dairy products (milk, butter, and cheese), eggs, tropical oils (coconut oil, palm oil, cocoa butter, and hard margarines), and baked goods. Many Americans consume from 15% to 18% of their total calories as saturated fatty acids. Three types of saturated fatty acids—lauric acid, myristic acid, and palmitic acid—raise the plasma total cholesterol level; a fourth, stearic acid, does not. For every 1% of total calories consumed as cholesterol-raising saturated acids, the plasma total cholesterol level increases by about 2.7 mg/dl. This response is relative to a baseline of carbohydrate, which is considered to have no effect on cholesterol levels; in other words, when the diet contains 18% of its calories as cholesterol-raising saturated fatty acids, the plasma total cholesterol level will be 45 mg/dl higher than when the diet is completely free of saturated acids and carbohydrates are consumed in their place.

Most of the rise in plasma cholesterol level caused by saturated fatty acids occurs in LDL, but the cholesterol level in VLDL and HDL may rise slightly. The major action of the saturated acids is to impair the clearance of LDL, most likely by suppressing the synthesis of LDL receptors. They probably free increased amounts of unesterified cholesterol in the liver to inhibit LDL-receptor synthesis.

Polyunsaturated Fatty Acids

The polyunsaturated fatty acid, linoleic acid, lowers the plasma cholesterol level when substituted for saturated fatty acids. Every 1% of calories of linoleic acid, when exchanged for carbohydrate, reduces the plasma cholesterol levels by about 1 mg/dl. The major reduction occurs partly in LDL, but levels of VLDL and HDL also fall. Whether linoleic acid has an inherent plasma LDL–lowering property compared with carbohydrate has not been determined.

In the past, relatively high intakes of linoleic acid were recommended. In recent years, however, concern has been mounting about possible harmful effects of excessive intakes of linoleic acid. No large population has ever consumed high amounts of linoleic acid for prolonged periods; consequently their safety has not been proved. Moreover, several additional adverse effects for polyunsaturates have been postulated. High intakes of linoleic acid may increase the risk of gallstones, potentiate chemical carcinogenesis, or suppress the immune system. Beyond these effects, they can alter the composition of membrane phospholipids, the consequences of which are unknown. Thus it is now recommended that intakes of linoleic not exceed the current intake of 7% of total calories.

Monounsaturated Fatty Acids

The major monounsaturated fatty acid of the diet is oleic acid. When oleic acid replaces dietary saturated acids, plasma total cholesterol level falls. The percentage of reduction in LDL levels with oleic acid is similar to that for linoleic acid. Oleic acid, however, does not reduce the HDL level as much as does linoleic acid. A major advantage of oleic acid is that large amounts of olive oil, containing mainly oleic acid, have been consumed in the Mediterranean region for many years without evidence of side effects, nor does it produce the adverse effects in animals that have been noted for linoleic acid. Furthermore, populations consuming large amounts of olive oil have a low prevalence of CHD. Thus oleic acid-rich diets appear preferable to those high in linoleic acid in preventing coronary disease.

Carbohydrates

Dietary carbohydrates can be considered neutral in their effect on total cholesterol and LDL levels. Therefore, when they are substituted for dietary saturated fatty acids, the plasma cholesterol levels fall. The degree of fall in LDL levels may be slightly less than when linoleic acid or oleic acid is substituted for saturates, but in practical terms the differences are small. However, a sudden increase in carbohydrate intake may raise plasma triglyceride levels and lower HDL concentrations. If the carbohydrate intake is gradually increased and is in the form of fiber-containing foods, such induced hypertriglyceridemia may be avoided. Thus the neutrality of carbohydrates extends only to LDL levels.

High-carbohydrate diets by definition are low in fat. Low-fat diets are consumed in many regions, particularly in developing countries where prevalence of CHD is low. No adverse effects of low-fat diets are known, provided intakes of protein and other essential nutrients are adequate. Both simple and complex carbohydrates (i.e., starch) have similar effects on lipoprotein metabolism, although complex carbohydrates are thought to be preferable for a variety of other reasons. They cause fewer dental caries, and they contain more fiber and usually are consumed with fruits and vegetables that contain various vitamins and minerals.

Cholesterol

American adults typically consume 350 to 500 mg of cholesterol per day, about half of which is absorbed. The influence of dietary cholesterol on plasma lipoproteins is variable. Cholesterol in the diet can raise concentrations of cholesterol in all lipoprotein fractions—VLDL, LDL, and HDL. The dietary cholesterol effect on LDL is enhanced when saturated fatty acids are present. Dietary cholesterol raises LDL levels by suppressing synthesis of LDL receptors in the liver.

Protein

In some species the type of protein in the diet can influence levels of plasma lipids. For example, in rabbits casein raises the cholesterol level, and vegetable proteins lower it. In humans, even if serum cholesterol responses to different types of proteins are not identical, differences are relatively small. In general, animal proteins do not raise cholesterol levels relative to vegetable proteins.

Alcohol

Alcohol stimulates the synthesis of hepatic triglycerides, promoting secretion of VLDL triglycerides. The latter raises serum triglyceride levels, especially in obese people or in those having a lipolytic defect. In the latter, ingestion of alcohol, even in moderate quantities, can cause a striking hypertriglyceridemia. Alcohol also raises HDL-cholesterol concentrations, leading some authorities to postulate benefit. In truth, however, the consequences of this change as they pertain to coronary risk are not known. In contrast, alcohol ingestion has almost no effect on the metabolism of LDL.

Caloric Restriction and Weight Loss

The obese state, characterized by a high caloric intake, has several effects on lipoprotein metabolism, most notably, increasing synthesis of VLDL and raising serum triglyceride levels. Even in obese patients who do not develop frank hypertriglyceridemia, secretion rates of VLDL are high; these patients are protected from elevated VLDL concentrations only by enhanced efficiency of their lipolytic system. Overproduction of VLDL in turn increases conversion of VLDL to LDL; consequently, LDL levels often rise. Again, however, concentrations of LDL are not invariably boosted in obese people, suggesting that some people compensate by increasing their clearance of LDL. Obesity, in general, is associated with low HDL levels; as might be expected, weight reduction tends to restore levels to normal. Fur-

thermore, weight reduction lowers plasma triglyceride levels. In contrast, changes in LDL levels consequent to weight reduction are less constant; in some patients levels of LDL fall; in others there is no change, and in a few there is even an increase in LDL level.

EFFECTS OF DRUGS ON LIPOPROTEIN METABOLISM

Several drugs can be used to treat abnormalities in lipoprotein metabolism. They differ in their actions and are classified here according to their major mechanisms.

Drugs That Enhance the Clearance of LDL

Levels of LDL can be reduced by promoting the clearance of LDL from plasma. This process is usually accomplished by stimulating the activity of LDL receptors. The liver is the major site of clearance of LDL. As indicated before, the expression of LDL receptors on liver cells depends in part on hepatic cholesterol content. Of most importance for drug therapy, a fall in cholesterol content in the liver enhances the synthesis of LDL receptors. The potential for drug action to effect this change exists at several sites of metabolic control: synthesis of cholesterol, secretion of cholesterol into bile, intestinal reabsorption of cholesterol, and conversion of cholesterol into bile acids (Fig. 306-11, *A*). Therapeutic modification of these key pathways affects hepatic cholesterol concentration, thereby modifying LDL-receptor synthesis (Fig. 306-11, *B*). Thus receptor synthesis can be amplified by hindering reabsorption of cholesterol, restricting synthesis, or upgrading conversion of cholesterol into bile acids; the latter response is customarily achieved by barring the reabsorption of bile acids.

Bile Acid Sequestrants. These agents act entirely within the gastrointestinal tract to block the reabsorption of bile acids. Two available agents are cholestyramine and colestipol. These nonabsorbable resins have quaternary amine groups that bind to the acidic group of bile acids, lessening their reabsorption and return to the liver. Consequently, their feedback repression on transformation of cholesterol into bile acids disengages; secondarily, as more cholesterol converts into bile acids, hepatic concentrations of cholesterol are reduced, LDL-receptor synthesis is augmented, and plasma levels of LDL and VLDL remnants fall. Bile acid sequestrants also modestly spur the synthesis of VLDL triglycerides, causing mild hypertriglyceridemia in some patients.

Currently available sequestrants are not highly proficient for binding of bile acids in the intestine; therefore large doses (e.g., 16 to 30 g/day) are required for a maximal reduction of LDL level. Many patients cannot abide such high doses. In these individuals lower doses (e.g., 8 to 10 g/day) can be tried and may yield a sufficient response. The sequestrants constipate many patients by preventing the normal laxative action of bile acids. They can give other gastrointestinal tract symptoms (heartburn, abdominal pain, bloating, belching, and nausea); however, these usually dissipate after several weeks of therapy. The sequestrants have no untoward effect outside the gastrointestinal tract, other than raising triglyceride levels in some patients, nor have they been shown to be carcinogenic.

Bile acid sequestrants were demonstrated to reduce the risk for CHD in the Lipid Research Clinics (LRC) Coronary Primary Prevention Trial (CPPT). In this large clinical trial, cholestyramine therapy produced a 10% reduction in plasma cholesterol level, compared with placebo. This change gave a 19% decrease in rate of new-onset CHD in middle-aged, hypercholesterolemic men. The results of this trial provided strong evidence for efficacy of cholesterol lowering in prevention of CHD.

Cholesterol-Absorption Blockers. This class of drug inhibits cholesterol reabsorption in the intestine and reduces amounts of cholesterol reaching the liver. This action reduces hepatic cholesterol and enhances LDL-receptor activity. The ideal drug for blocking the reabsorption of cholesterol has yet to be discovered and developed. The most potent agent currently available is neomycin. At 2 g/day, it effectively blocks the absorption of cholesterol. The drug has potential side effects. It alters the flora of the bowel, which theoretically can

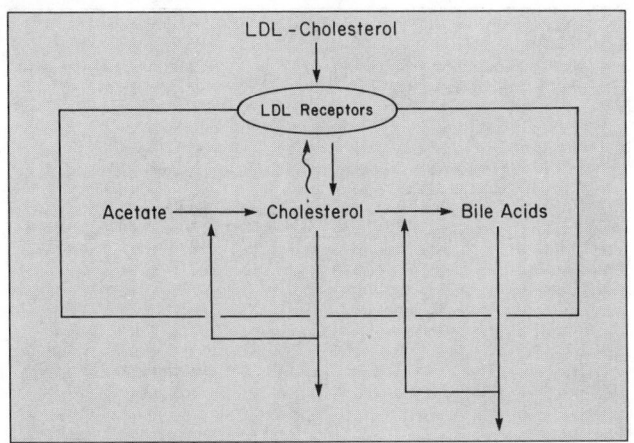

A

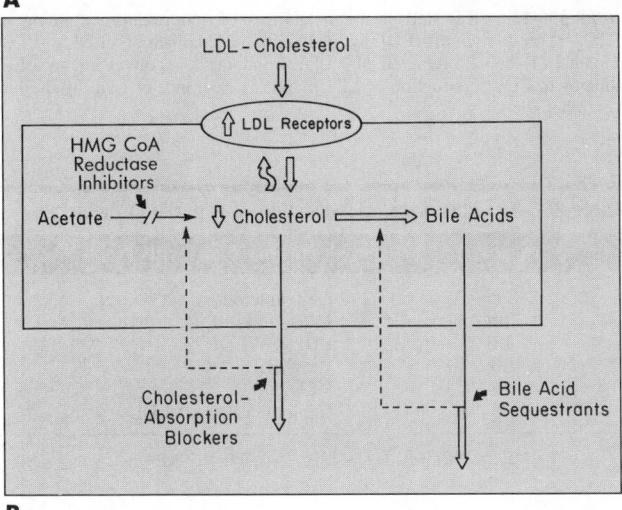

B

FIGURE 306-11   Relationship between LDL receptors and the enterohepatic circulation (EHC) of cholesterol and bile acids. **A,** In the liver cell, cholesterol is formed from acetate and is partially converted to bile acids. Both cholesterol and bile acids are secreted into the intestine and are partially reabsorbed to complete the EHC. The return of cholesterol to the liver causes feedback inhibition on cholesterol synthesis, and the return of bile acids inhibits the conversion of cholesterol into bile acids. Both processes regulate the amount of cholesterol in the liver cell. This quantity of hepatic cholesterol determines the number of LDL receptors synthesized, which in turn regulates the uptake of LDL cholesterol. Thus the EHC plays an important role in modulating the activity of LDL receptors. **B,** Effects of induced alterations in the EHC on the activity of LDL receptors. The quantity of cholesterol in the liver cell can be reduced in three ways: (1) by blocking the reabsorption of bile acids, (2) by blocking the reabsorption of cholesterol, and (3) by inhibiting the synthesis of cholesterol (with hydroxy-methyl-glutaryl coenzyme A [HMG CoA] reductase inhibitors). The fall in hepatic cholesterol due to any of these mechanisms stimulates the synthesis of LDL receptors, which in turn causes increased hepatic uptake of LDL and a fall in plasma LDL levels.

induce a resistant infection. It also has a toxic potential, and prolonged usage might impair hearing, although this response has not been proved for low oral doses. The Food and Drug Administration (FDA) has not approved neomycin for treatment of hypercholesterolemia, and its use for routine management of high LDL levels cannot be recommended. Other drugs that interfere with absorption of cholesterol are beta-sitosterol and the nonabsorbable fat substitute, olestra. Beta-sitosterol, a plant sterol, is a relatively weak cholesterol-absorption blocker. Olestra was recently approved by the FDA to be used in snack foods; at present it is not available as a drug to be used to block cholesterol absorption. Thus effective drugs to inhibit cholesterol reabsorption to lower plasma cholesterol levels are lacking.

HMG CoA Reductase Inhibitors (Statins). This class of drug inhibits cholesterol synthesis in the liver. In so doing, it enhances LDL receptor activity and lowers plasma LDL levels.

Five agents in this class have been approved by the FDA: lovastatin, pravastatin, simvastatin, fluvastatin, and atorvastatin. All drugs have the same mechanism of action and similar side effects. However, doses of the statins differ. For example, 40 mg/day of lovastatin and pravastatin are equivalent in cholesterol-lowering action to 20 mg simvastatin, 80 mg fluvastatin, and 10 mg of atorvastatin. At these doses, LDL cholesterol levels are reduced by about 20% to 30%. Higher doses of all drugs are more efficacious, although increments in response decline at increasing doses. Side effects also tend to increase with rising dose. Side effects are infrequent but can include myopathy (myalgia, muscle weakness, elevations of serum creatine kinase levels, and sometimes, hemoglobinuria) and mild hepatotoxicity. These side effects are reversible by discontinuation of the drug.

Statins not only have been found to be highly efficacious for treatment of elevated serum cholesterol, but they also have been invaluable for proving the "lipid hypothesis": that cholesterol lowering will reduce the risk for CHD. Two types of studies have been carried out with the statins. One kind of study tests whether cholesterol lowering will retard the development of atherosclerosis or reverse existing coronary plaques. For this purpose, quantitative coronary angiography is used. Several angiographic trials have employed statins or other efficacious therapies for cholesterol lowering. Results showed that changes in plaque size are relatively small, despite marked cholesterol lowering. During the course of these trials, acute coronary events (unstable angina or acute myocardial infarction) were recorded. Unexpectedly, cholesterol-lowering therapy produced a marked reduction in acute coronary events, many more than would be predicted from the change in lesion size. This important observation gave rise to the concept of the unstable coronary plaque. Other investigations have demonstrated that acute coronary events are the result of rupture of plaques with a superimposed thrombosis. Plaque rupture occurs at unstable regions where lipid accumulation is pronounced; apparently cholesterol-lowering therapy stabilizes these regions and reduces the risk for acute coronary events.

The efficacy of statin therapy for reducing coronary morbidity and mortality has been amply demonstrated in recent, large clinical trials. Two of these trials—the Scandinavian Simvastatin Survival Study (4S) and the Cholesterol and Recurrent Events (CARE) study—demonstrated a striking decrease in recurrent coronary events and coronary deaths in patients with established CHD. Another trial, the West of Scotland Coronary Prevention Study (WOSCOPS), gave similar results in high-risk, hypercholesterolemic patients without clinical evidence of CHD. These beneficial results of statin therapy were observed with a minimum of side effects. Thus they provide a strong rationale for use of statin therapy in high-risk patients.

Thyroid Hormones. Thyroid hormones enhance clearance of circulating LDL. This action accounts for the low level of plasma cholesterol in hyperthyroidism and the opposite in hypothyroidism. Thyroid hormones apparently enhance LDL-receptor activity. In the past, D-thyroxine was used to treat hypercholesterolemia; however, because of its cardiac side effects, the use of D-thyroxine was abandoned for this purpose.

Probucol. The lipid-soluble antioxidant probucol promotes the clearance of LDL and lowers LDL levels. Probucol either enhances the affinity of LDL for LDL receptors or promotes removal of LDL by nonreceptor pathways. The drug apparently does not alter hepatic metabolism of cholesterol, as do statins, and seemingly does not increase LDL-receptor activity; nevertheless, it lowers levels of LDL by 10% to 20%. However, probucol also lowers HDL levels. A recent clinical trial found no efficacy of probucol in reducing progression of peripheral atherosclerosis; this finding combined with a lesser efficacy for cholesterol lowering compared with statins has largely eliminated its clinical use.

Drugs That Inhibit the Synthesis of Lipoproteins

Nicotinic acid inhibits hepatic secretion of VLDL particles and thereby lowers both VLDL and LDL levels. It effectively reduces elevated plasma lipid levels in several types of hyperlipidemia. Nicotinic acid further causes a pronounced increase in HDL cholesterol levels. Side effects preclude its use in many patients. Common side effects include gastrointestinal tract distress, flushing and itching of the skin, elevation of plasma glucose level, rise in uric acid level, hepatic dysfunction, and skin rash. Peptic ulcer disease may be exacerbated or reactivated. For maximum lipid lowering, nicotinic acid must be given in relatively large doses—3.0 to 4.5 g/day. However, a lower dose, 1.5 g/day, can be moderately efficacious. To minimize flushing, initial small doses (i.e., 100 mg three times daily with meals) are indicated; the dose is then increased gradually as tolerated. Flushing also may be lessened by low-dose aspirin.

Drugs That Potentiate Lipoprotein Lipase

Fibric acids seemingly enhance the activity of LPL. Two such agents, clofibrate and gemfibrozil, are currently available in the United States, and two others, bezafibrate and fenofibrate, are used in Europe. Enhancement of LPL activity accelerates catabolism of triglyceride-rich lipoproteins—chylomicrons, VLDL, and VLDL remnants—and lowers triglyceride levels.

The fibric acids may influence lipoprotein metabolism in other ways too. They frequently cause a modest rise in HDL cholesterol levels; however, this may be a result of lowering triglyceride levels. In hypertriglyceridemic patients lowering of triglyceride levels commonly is accompanied by a rise in LDL cholesterol levels. However, in hypercholesterolemic patients fibric acids moderately lower LDL cholesterol levels. Side effects occur uncommonly but can include abdominal discomfort, cholesterol gallstones, or myopathy, the latter being accompanied by a high creatine kinase level. Risk for myopathy is highest in patients with renal impairment. The fibric acids predispose to cholesterol gallstones by increasing output of biliary cholesterol and reducing synthesis of bile acids; the result is bile supersaturated with cholesterol. Fibric acids must be given in low doses to patients with renal insufficiency; they are contraindicated in liver disease. One clinical trial suggested that clofibrate may raise the risk of gastrointestinal tract cancer, although convincing proof is lacking. In another trial gemfibrozil therapy reduced the risk for CHD in hypercholesterolemic patients without incurring serious side effects. In the latter study the major benefit for CHD prevention was observed in patients who had elevated plasma triglyceride levels accompanying hypercholesterolemia. The major use of these agents at present, however, is for treatment of severe hypertriglyceridemia, not for prevention of CHD.

HYPERLIPIDEMIA

Hyperlipidemia means an increase in either plasma cholesterol or plasma triglyceride levels. Causes of hyperlipidemia fall into three categories: dietary, genetic, and the result of other conditions. Dietary hyperlipidemias tend to be mild, whereas some genetic hyperlipidemias are severe. Frequently, moderate hyperlipidemia is the result of dietary excesses combined with several less critical gene polymorphisms. Secondary hyperlipidemias result from various metabolic disorders or certain drugs. Various hyperlipidemias commonly accelerate atherosclerosis and predispose to CHD.

Hyperlipidemia is synonymous with hyperlipoproteinemia (HLP), an increase in plasma lipoprotein levels. HLP results from defects at any of several regulatory steps in lipoprotein metabolism (Fig. 306-12), including (1) production of VLDL, (2) lipolysis of VLDL (or chylomicrons), (3) removal of VLDL remnants, (4) conversion of VLDL remnants to LDL, and (5) clearance of LDL. HLP has been categorized into *phenotypes,* or patterns of elevations of the different lipoproteins (Table 306-3). This classification is merely a shorthand notation for the types of lipoproteins that are present in excess. The phenotype alone does not reveal the underlying metabolic defect; several different abnormalities can produce the same phenotype. The phenotype classification, although still used by some authorities, has fallen out of favor. For greater simplicity, HLP can be divided into hypercholesterolemia or hypertriglyceridemia.

Hypercholesterolemia

The term *hypercholesterolemia,* high plasma cholesterol level, has undergone an evolution in meaning. Previously, hypercholesterolemia

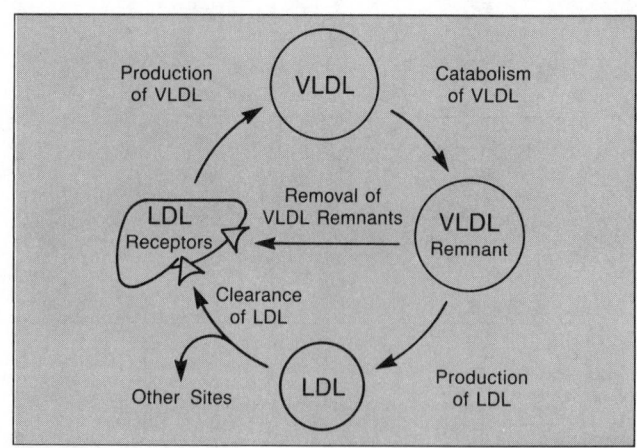

FIGURE 306-12   Key steps in the metabolism of lipoproteins containing apo B-100: (1) production of VLDL by the liver, (2) catabolism of VLDL to VLDL remnants, (3) hepatic removal of VLDL remnants, (4) conversion of VLDL remnants to LDL (production of LDL), and (5) clearance of LDL by the liver or extrahepatic sites.

Table 306-3   Phenotypic classification of hyperlipoproteinemia

PHENOTYPE	LIPOPROTEIN PRESENT IN EXCESS
I	Chylomicrons
IIa	LDL
IIb	LDL + VLDL
III	Beta-VLDL
IV	VLDL
V	Chylomicrons + VLDL

LDL, Low-density lipoprotein; *VLDL,* very-low-density lipoprotein.

was defined as a plasma cholesterol level above the 95th percentile cut-point for the population distribution. More recently, it has been redefined by its relation to CHD risk. For example, the National Cholesterol Education Program classifies the serum total cholesterol into three categories: desirable cholesterol level (<200 mg/dl), borderline-high cholesterol level (200 to 239 mg/dl), and high cholesterol level (>240 mg/dl). The current distribution of total cholesterol levels in the American population is approximated in Table 306-4. For all adults (ages 20 to 74 years) 20% to 25% have cholesterol levels exceeding 240 mg/dl. For many persons the total cholesterol level is a fairly good indicator of the LDL cholesterol level, but for some it is not. Therefore measurement of LDL cholesterol can be helpful. The distributions of LDL cholesterol levels for American men and women are given in Table 306-5. In the present discussion, hypercholesterolemia is classified as mild, moderate, or severe. The approach outlined for management of these categories of hypercholesterolemia is consistent with that recommended by the National Cholesterol Education Program.

Mild hypercholesterolemia (borderline-high cholesterol level) is defined as a total cholesterol level in the range of 200 to 239 mg/dl. This range corresponds to LDL cholesterol of 130 to 159 mg/dl. Epidemiologic studies indicate that risk for CHD at a level of 240 mg/dl is substantially above that for levels below 200 mg/dl; within the borderline zone (200 to 239 mg/dl) coronary risk rises progressively (Fig. 306-9). Other risk factors compound the risk imparted by mild hypercholesterolemia (Fig. 306-10). Therefore patients with cholesterol levels in the range of 200 to 239 mg/dl (LDL cholesterol level, 130 to 159 mg/dl) should be evaluated carefully for the risk factors shown in Fig. 306-10. A man who exceeds age 45 years can be considered to be at increased risk through the combination of aging and male sex. Postmenopausal women also are regarded at increased risk. If a patient with mild hypercholesterolemia has two CHD risk factors, but not established CHD, lower LDL cholesterol levels to below 130 mg/dl. In most patients without CHD whose LDL levels are in this range,

Table 306-4 Population distribution of plasma total cholesterol levels (mg/dl)*

| | WHITE MEN | | | | WHITE WOMEN | | | | |
| | PERCENTILES | | | | PERCENTILES | | | | |
AGE (yr)	5	50	75	95	5	50	75	90	95
20-24	118	159	179	212	121	165	186	220	237
25-29	130	176	199	234	130	178	198	217	231
30-34	142	190	213	258	133	178	199	215	228
35-39	147	195	222	267	139	186	209	233	249
40-44	150	204	229	260	146	193	220	241	259
45-49	163	210	235	275	148	204	231	256	268
50-54	157	211	237	274	163	214	240	267	281
55-59	161	214	236	280	167	229	251	278	294
60-64	163	215	237	287	172	226	251	282	300
65-69	166	213	250	288	167	233	259	282	291
70+	144	214	236	265	173	226	249	268	280

*Modified from the Lipid Research Clinics Population Studies Data Book: the prevalence study, Bethesda, Md, 1979, National Institutes of Health Publication No. 79-1527.

Table 306-5 Population distribution of plasma low-density lipoprotein cholesterol levels (mg/dl)*

| | WHITE MEN | | | | WHITE WOMEN | | | |
| | PERCENTILES | | | | PERCENTILES | | | |
AGE (yr)	5	50	75	95	5	50	75	95
20-24	66	101	118	147	57	102	118	159
25-29	70	116	138	165	71	108	126	164
30-34	78	124	144	185	70	109	128	156
35-39	81	131	154	189	75	116	139	172
40-44	87	135	157	186	74	122	146	174
45-49	98	141	163	202	79	127	150	186
50-54	89	143	162	197	88	134	160	201
55-59	88	145	168	203	89	145	168	210
60-64	83	143	165	210	100	149	168	224
65-69	98	146	170	210	92	151	184	221
70+	88	142	164	186	96	147	170	206

*Modified from the Lipid Research Clinics Population Data Book: the prevalence study, Bethesda, Md, 1979, National Institutes of Health Publication No. 79-1527.

BOX 306-1

American Heart Association recommended diet (Step I)

Composition

Limit intakes of total fat to 30%, saturated and polyunsaturated fatty acids to 10%, and monounsaturated fatty acids to 15% of total calories; limit dietary cholesterol to 300 mg/day.

General description

Limit meat to no more than 7 oz/day
    Include only chicken and turkey with skin removed, and use lean cuts of fish, veal, beef, pork, or lamb.
Restrict eggs to two per week, including those used in cooking.
Restrict milk products to 1% fat milk, ice milk, sherbet, low-fat frozen yogurt, low-fat cheese, and low-fat cottage cheese.
Avoid hard fats; use only vegetable oils, olive oil, or margarines.
All vegetables and fruits are allowed except for coconut.
Bread, cereals, pasta, potatoes, and rice are allowed except when made with eggs; limit starchy foods to prevent weight gain.
Avoid whole-milk products, marbled meats, fish eggs, organ meats, bakery goods made with hard fats and eggs, and rich desserts.

---

nondrug therapy is indicated. If CHD is present, the goal of LDL lowering should be a level less than 100 mg/dl.

The predominant cause of mild hypercholesterolemia (and borderline–high-risk LDL cholesterol level) is an excessive intake of saturated fatty acids, cholesterol, and total calories, the latter causing obesity. Current eating habits and lack of physical activity among American adults probably raise the plasma cholesterol level by 40 to 50 mg/dl above levels that would occur on a diet low in saturated fatty acids and cholesterol combined with desirable body weight and a habit of vigorous exercise. Therefore the primary therapy of mild hypercholesterolemia is modification of the diet, combined with weight control and regular exercise. Diet modification aims primarily to decrease intakes of saturated fat and cholesterol. This can be achieved by the Step I diet of the American Heart Association and the National Cholesterol Education Program; this diet restricts intake of fat to about 30% of total calories, saturated fatty acids to less than 10% of calories, and dietary cholesterol to less than 300 mg/day (Box 306-1).

Moderate hypercholesterolemia is a plasma cholesterol level in the range of 240 to 300 mg/dl. This definition requires an LDL cholesterol level in the range of 160 to 220 mg/dl. Within this range the risk for CHD rises progressively from approximately twofold to fourfold above baseline. Although dietary excesses contribute to moderate hypercholesterolemia, genetic influences increasingly are at play. Moreover, some genetic factors may enhance sensitivity to dietary excesses (i.e., they produce an accentuated rise in LDL cholesterol level). Genetic factors affecting regulation of LDL-receptor activity probably are particularly influential in determining sensitivity of LDL

cholesterol levels to dietary excesses. Moreover, defective regulation of LDL-receptor activity may act independent of the diet to increase LDL cholesterol levels. Effects of a deficiency of LDL receptors on lipoprotein metabolism are shown in Fig. 306-13. Occasionally, suppression of LDL-receptor synthesis is caused by hypothyroidism; thus reduced thyroid function should be sought in any hypercholesterolemic patient. An appreciable number of hypercholesterolemic patients apparently have an abnormality in LDL apolipoprotein B-100—an abnormality that interferes with the normal binding between LDL and LDL receptors. Other causes for elevated LDL levels are overproduction of VLDL particles by the liver and an abnormally high conversion of VLDL to LDL.

Because LDL cholesterol levels in the range of 160 to 220 mg/dl impart a distinct increase in coronary risk, institution of LDL-lowering therapy is warranted. In patients without clinical CHD, nondrug therapy should be employed first and in all patients. This means reducing intake of saturated fatty acids, cholesterol, and total calories (if obesity is present). The Step I diet should be instituted by the physician and immediate staff (Box 306-1). A lipoprotein profile should be checked at 6 weeks and 3 months; if the LDL cholesterol level has not fallen to below 160 mg/dl (in the absence of two other risk factors) or to below 130 mg/dl (in the presence of two other risk factors), saturated fatty acids and cholesterol in the diet should be further curtailed. A registered dietitian can help modify the diet to achieve this goal. In patients who are not otherwise at high risk for

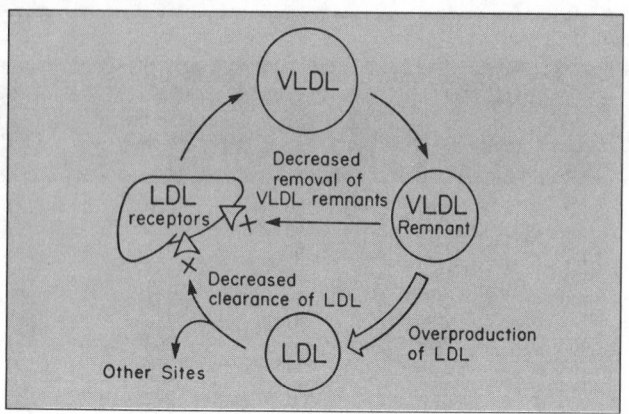

FIGURE 306-13 Effects of a deficiency (or reduction) of LDL receptors on lipoprotein metabolism. First, hepatic clearance of VLDL remnants is reduced and, consequently, more VLDL remnants are converted to LDL; second, clearance of LDL is reduced. The net result of both changes is an increase in LDL concentrations.

CHD, dietary therapy should be continued for another 3 months before considering use of cholesterol-lowering drugs. For high-risk, middle-aged, or elderly patients, earlier institution of drug therapy may be warranted.

If the therapeutic goals for LDL lowering are not achieved by nondrug therapy, drugs can be considered. The decision to use drugs depends on a variety of factors, including an estimate of the patient's overall risk status, age, motivation, and general health. The preferable drug for moderate hypercholesterolemia in patients without CHD is a bile acid sequestrant. These agents are especially useful in younger adults (up to age 45 years) who are not at high, short-term risk for CHD. Some patients, however, cannot tolerate bile acid sequestrants, and alternative drugs must be considered. Nicotinic acid is another effective cholesterol-lowering drug; it has proved effective for reduction of coronary mortality. However, nicotinic acid is accompanied by side effects in some patients that prevent its use. Statins are the most effective for reducing LDL levels in patients with moderate hypercholesterolemia. Fibric acids cause only moderate reductions of LDL cholesterol. Probucol decreases LDL concentrations somewhat more than fibric acids; however, it also reduces HDL cholesterol levels. Neither fibric acids nor probucol seem appropriate for treatment of moderate hypercholesterolemia because better choices are available.

If a patient with moderate hypercholesterolemia has established CHD, the goal of therapy is to reduce the LDL level to below 100 mg/dl. Very often, this level cannot be achieved by dietary therapy alone; thus it is frequently necessary to turn to drug therapy. Moreover, drug therapy can be instituted simultaneously with nondrug treatment in CHD patients with moderate hypercholesterolemia. Among the drugs, statins are particularly attractive for reducing LDL cholesterol levels in patients with established CHD. In moderate hypercholesterolemia, however, LDL cholesterol levels often cannot be reduced to below 100 mg/dl with statin therapy alone. If that is the case, combining a bile acid sequestrant with a statin can be highly effective for achieving the goals of LDL lowering.

A special case is the postmenopausal woman with moderate hypercholesterolemia (and elevated LDL cholesterol). LDL levels rise after the menopause because of loss of estrogens, which curtails their action to stimulate the synthesis of LDL receptors. The risk for CHD rises progressively after the menopause; this increased risk may be due in part to higher LDL levels. One approach to postmenopausal hypercholesterolemia is to institute estrogen replacement therapy. A reduction of LDL levels of 10% to 15% occurs in many patients. If LDL lowering is not sufficient by estrogen replacement therapy alone, or if the woman has established CHD or other CHD risk factors, statin therapy can be considered.

Severe hypercholesterolemia consists of plasma cholesterol level over 300 mg/dl (LDL cholesterol over 220 mg/dl). Risk for CHD above this level exceeds that at baseline at least four-fold. The most severe elevations of plasma cholesterol occur in patients with hereditary defects in the gene encoding the LDL receptor. Several different genetic defects in the primary structures of the receptor have been delineated, ranging from complete absence to aberrant receptor protein. Collectively, these defects cause the syndrome called *familial hypercholesterolemia*. Their effects on LDL metabolism are shown in Fig. 306-13. Because one gene for the LDL receptor is inherited from each parent, the disease usually occurs in the heterozygous form. One in 500 persons has heterozygous familial hypercholesterolemia; the homozygous form is much rarer (1 per 1,000,000). Heterozygous familial hypercholesterol is evident as plasma total cholesterol levels in the range of 300 to 500 mg/dl, tendon xanthomas, and premature CHD. In men CHD frequently develops in their 30s or 40s, or even earlier, whereas in women CHD often develops in their 50s and 60s.

About 1% of adult Americans have cholesterol levels that consistently exceed 300 mg/dl. Some of these patients have undetected familial hypercholesterolemia, but in most a monogenic inheritance cannot be demonstrated. Nonetheless, most of them appear to have a reduced activity of LDL receptors, possibly attributable to a metabolic suppression of LDL receptor synthesis. Such patients rarely have tendon xanthomas, and coronary events generally do not occur as early as in patients with familial hypercholesterolemia; nevertheless, they are at high risk for CHD and should be given appropriate treatment. First, however, secondary forms of elevated LDL cholesterol level should be ruled out. Hypothyroidism can cause severe hypercholesterolemia, as can biliary obstruction. In the latter condition the excess plasma cholesterol is mainly unesterified, and the increased serum cholesterol is not found in LDL per se but in an abnormal lipoprotein called *lipoprotein X*. The nephrotic syndrome also causes severe hypercholesterolemia; it may be accompanied by hypertriglyceridemia.

Because primary severe hypercholesterolemia imparts a high risk for CHD, LDL levels should be lowered. Maximal dietary therapy should be initiated; for most patients, this means taking a diet very low in saturated fatty acids (less than 7% of calories) and cholesterol (less than 200 mg/day). Although dietary therapy helps in management, cholesterol-lowering drugs may be needed to bring the LDL cholesterol to acceptably low levels. Statins have become the preferred agents for treatment of severe hypercholesterolemia. However, statins alone often do not normalize serum cholesterol levels. In most patients a second drug, usually a bile acid sequestrant, is needed to bring cholesterol levels to the normal range. In some patients with severe hypercholesterolemia, the combination of a statin and nicotinic acid can effectively lower cholesterol levels; however, this combination has been largely superseded by a statin plus sequestrant.

Hypertriglyceridemia

Hypertriglyceridemia is defined here as a plasma triglyceride level that exceeds 200 mg/dl. In its pure form the plasma total cholesterol level is less than 240 mg/dl. Most patients with pure hypertriglyceridemia have an increase in VLDL triglyceride levels—hence the term *endogenous hypertriglyceridemia,* also called type IV HLP. In most patients serum triglyceride levels are in the range of 200 to 400 mg/dl. An elevation of endogenous triglycerides can be due to either a hepatic overproduction or a defective lipolysis of VLDL triglycerides (Fig. 306-14). Either defect produces several metabolic consequences for the metabolism of other lipoproteins: an increased concentration of VLDL cholesterol, abnormalities in the composition of VLDL particles, increased concentrations of VLDL remnants and intermediate-density lipoprotein (IDL), increased conversion of VLDL to LDL, enhanced catabolism of LDL, reduction in particles of reduced size, and decreased concentrations of HDL cholesterol. Any or all of these metabolic consequences of hypertriglyceridemia may be responsible for an increased rate of atherogenesis accompanying the hypertriglyceridemic state. The more common forms of hypertriglyceridemia are considered here.

Diet-Induced Endogenous Hypertriglyceridemia. Certain dietary factors (e.g., excessive intakes of total calories, carbohydrates, and ethanol) stimulate the production of VLDL triglycerides. In some persons high secretion rates of VLDL triglycerides do not induce hy-

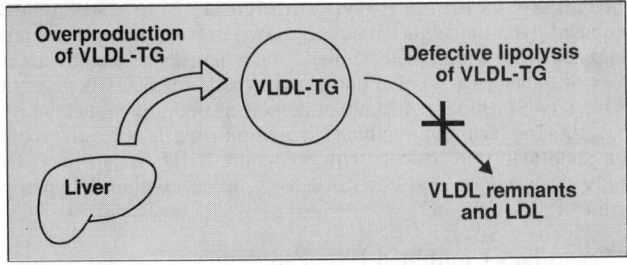

FIGURE 306-14   Mechanisms of primary hypertriglyceridemia. An increase in VLDL triglyceride concentrations can be the result of either of two mechanisms: (1) hepatic overproduction of VLDL triglycerides (VLDL-TG) or (2) defective lipolysis of VLDL triglycerides.

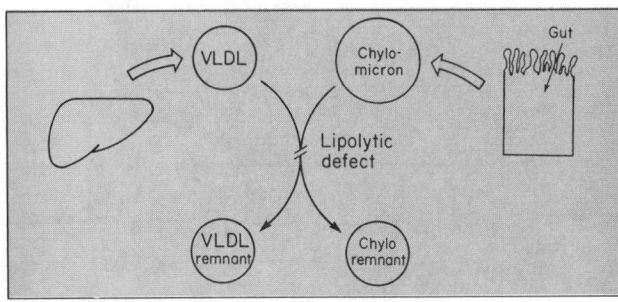

FIGURE 306-15   Mechanism of type V hyperlipoproteinemia (HLP). An elevation of both VLDL and chylomicron levels in type V HLP is the result of two metabolic defects: (1) overproduction of VLDL and (2) a lipolytic defect for triglyceride-rich lipoproteins including both VLDL and chylomicrons.

pertriglyceridemia because of a concomitant high activity of LPL. In others, however, LPL fails to compensate adequately, so overproduction of VLDL triglycerides causes mild hypertriglyceridemia; in this case, triglyceride levels rise to 200 to 400 mg/dl. In obese patients the number of VLDL particles entering the plasma is increased; consequently, more VLDL particles are converted to LDL. Regardless of whether lipoprotein concentrations are elevated in obese patients, the transport of an excessive number of lipoproteins through the plasma compartment may contribute to an increased risk for CHD. In contrast, high-carbohydrate diets and high intakes of ethanol increase the triglyceride content of each VLDL particle, but they do not raise the number of VLDL particles secreted into plasma. A higher flux of VLDL triglycerides, attributable to an excess of dietary carbohydrates or alcohol, appears to be less atherogenic.

Primary Endogenous Hypertriglyceridemia. This disorder can result from either overproduction of VLDL triglyceride or defective lipolysis of VLDL triglycerides (Fig. 306-14). When several members of a single family have elevated serum triglyceride levels, the condition is called *familial hypertriglyceridemia*. Primary overproduction of VLDL triglycerides is analogous to the high secretion of VLDL triglycerides induced by dietary carbohydrates or alcohol. The number of VLDL particles secreted into plasma is not increased; only the quantity of triglycerides per particle is raised. The cause of primary overproduction of VLDL triglycerides is unknown; in some cases it may be due to resistance to the peripheral action of insulin. The causes of defective lipolysis of VLDL triglycerides are poorly understood. Most patients probably have a mild deficiency of LPL. Some, however, may have defects in the chemical composition of VLDL, making the lipoprotein a poor substrate for LPL. Defective lipolysis of VLDL triglycerides is difficult to distinguish from overproduction of VLDL triglycerides, but for clinical purposes it is sufficient to recognize the presence of primary endogenous hypertriglyceridemia. Either cause of hypertriglyceridemia can give rise to the metabolic consequences mentioned previously. Increasing evidence suggests that elevated triglyceride levels raise the risk for CHD, possibly because of these secondary metabolic changes in lipoprotein metabolism.

For patients with primary endogenous hypertriglyceridemia, changes in lifestyle (control of weight, increased physical activity, and restriction of excess carbohydrates and alcohol) are the first modes of therapy. If dietary therapy is not successful for normalizing triglyceride levels, drug therapy can be considered, especially if the patient has CHD or other coronary risk factors outlined in Fig. 306-10. Nicotinic acid is the drug of choice; if it is not tolerated, gemfibrozil is a good alternative. If the patient does not have CHD or other risk factors, it may be prudent to withhold drug therapy and to attempt to control elevated triglyceride levels by diet modification and exercise.

Secondary Hypertriglyceridemia. An increase in VLDL triglycerides without a concomitant increase in cholesterol levels can be produced by certain diseases or drugs: (1) poorly controlled diabetes mellitus, (2) chronic renal failure, (3) rare dyslipoproteinemias, (4) oral contraceptives, and (5) beta-adrenergic blocking agents. Com-

monly, these secondary causes accentuate a latent primary hypertriglyceridemia.

A common cause of secondary hypertriglyceridemia is non–insulin-dependent diabetes mellitus (NIDDM). This condition induces both overproduction of VLDL triglycerides and reduced lipolysis of triglyceride-rich lipoproteins. The high output of VLDL triglycerides may be caused by two factors: increased serum FFA and hyperglycemia; it also can be accentuated by obesity. Reduced lipolysis of plasma triglycerides may be the result of a decrease of LPL activity caused by an impaired action of insulin. Hypertriglyceridemia may be one factor responsible for the increased risk for CHD associated with NIDDM. Treatment should be directed, first, toward improving glycemic control, reducing weight in obese patients, and increasing exercise. Lipid-lowering drugs have not been investigated extensively in NIDDM. Nicotinic acid can worsen hyperglycemia and raise uric acid levels in diabetics. Gemfibrozil lowers triglyceride levels but may increase the LDL cholesterol level. Statins show promise for serum cholesterol lowering in diabetic patients. Secondary prevention trials (4S and CARE) showed that statins will reduce recurrent coronary events in diabetic patients with established CHD.

Combined Hyperlipidemias

Combined hyperlipidemias are defined as an increase in plasma lipids, total cholesterol (<240 mg/dl), and plasma triglyceride (>250 mg/dl) levels. Combined hyperlipidemia is identified when a lipoprotein profile is determined in a patient found to have high levels of plasma cholesterol. It can be the result of several primary and secondary disorders in lipoprotein metabolism; not uncommonly, primary and secondary disorders are present in the same individual. The major forms of combined hyperlipidemia can be considered.

Marked Hypertriglyceridemia with Elevated Cholesterol Levels. When triglyceride levels exceed 500 mg/dl, increases in both VLDL and chylomicrons typically are present (type V HLP). Cholesterol levels usually exceed 240 mg/dl. Raised concentrations of cholesterol usually are limited to triglyceride-rich lipoproteins; LDL cholesterol levels typically are normal or even reduced. Type V HLP usually results from combined overproduction of VLDL and reduced lipolysis of triglyceride-rich lipoproteins (Fig. 306-15). These two abnormalities together can result from any combination of dietary, primary, or secondary hypertriglyceridemia, as discussed in the previous section. The most immediate danger of severe type V HLP is acute pancreatitis. Many, but not all, older patients with type V HLP also have premature atherosclerotic disease; the latter is more likely to occur when other risk factors such as smoking or diabetes mellitus are present.

When triglyceride levels are in the range of 500 to 1000 mg/dl, the principles of therapy are similar to those described previously for endogenous hypertriglyceridemia. For severe type V HLP, treatment frequently requires a combination of diet and drug therapy. The intake of fat should be curtailed to reduce the formation of chylomicrons. Clearance of chylomicrons can be promoted in some patients by a fibric acid such as gemfibrozil. If the fibric acid does not clear

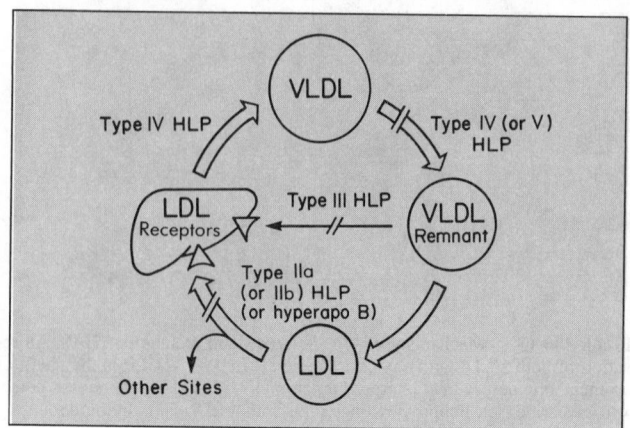

FIGURE 306-16 Factors contributing to multiple lipoprotein phenotypes. Type IV HLP can result from either overproduction or defective clearance of VLDL. When both defects are present, the patient may have type V HLP. The E-2/2 genotype delays clearance of VLDL remnants and, when combined with another defect in triglyceride metabolism, results in type III HLP. A defective clearance of LDL in association with other defects can produce either hyperapobetalipoproteinemia (hyperapo B) or type II HLP (IIa or IIb).

chylomicronemia, elevated triglyceride levels may respond to nicotinic acid, a drug that inhibits the synthesis of VLDL. Recent reports indicate that high intakes of fish oil also inhibit synthesis of VLDL; Therefore, fish oil supplementation may be used as an adjunct to therapy in some patients with type V HLP. If a patient has a dietary component to overproduction of VLDL (e.g., obesity or excessive alcohol intake), emphasis should be on dietary modification; if a second disorder is the major factor, treatment should be aimed at eliminating this disorder.

Familial Combined Hyperlipidemia. A common form of combined hyperlipidemia is familial combined hyperlipidemia. This disorder was first defined as a monogenic hyperlipidemia characterized by multiple lipoprotein phenotypes (types IV, V, III, IIA, and/or IIB) in a single family. Some family members may have elevations in both cholesterol and triglyceride levels; others have isolated hypercholesterolemia or hypertriglyceridemia. Moreover, fluctuating patterns of hyperlipidemia within a single individual are common. Familial combined hyperlipidemia has been estimated to occur in approximately 1% of the population. The metabolic defect responsible for this disorder is unknown; several investigators postulate that the liver synthesizes an excess of lipoproteins containing apolipoprotein B-100. Such a defect could account for multiple lipoprotein abnormalities in a single individual or family. Regardless of which lipoprotein phenotype is present, the risk for CHD appears to increase.

An alternate explanation for multiple lipoprotein phenotypes within a single family might be that several lipoprotein defects are inherited simultaneously (Fig. 306-16). Such defects could include overproduction of lipoproteins, defective lipolysis of triglyceride-rich lipoproteins, defective clearance of remnant lipoproteins, or reduced activity of LDL receptors, or a combination of these. Considering the relatively high prevalence of all of these abnormalities among American adults, coinheritance of metabolic defects should be relatively common.

Treatment of combined elevations of cholesterol and triglyceride levels, evident as elevated levels of VLDL and LDL, requires attention to both types of lipids. Elevated serum cholesterol and triglyceride levels can be treated together or separately. Weight reduction, increased exercise, and reduced intakes of saturated fatty acids may lower both serum cholesterol and triglyceride levels. If drug therapy seems appropriate, either because of inadequate response to dietary therapy or the presence of CHD or other risk factors, nicotinic acid is the drug of choice because it acts to reduce levels of all lipoproteins. If nicotinic acid is not effective or tolerated, various combinations of drugs can be tried. The combination of fibric acid and a statin can be highly effective but is associated with an increased risk for drug-induced myopathy. A fibric acid and bile acid sequestrant is another effective, relatively safe combination.

Primary Combined Hyperlipidemia. Most patients with combined hyperlipidemia cannot be shown to have multiple lipoprotein phenotypes within their families. Some patients belong to the category of undetected familial combined hyperlipidemia, whereas others have two or more concomitant defects in lipoprotein metabolism (Fig. 306-16). Primary combined hyperlipidemia is a relative common abnormality in patients with premature CHD. Treatment is basically the same as that described for familial combined hyperlipidemia.

Secondary Combined Hyperlipidemia. A common cause of combined hyperlipidemia is NIDDM. In most NIDDM patients, weight reduction and better control of hyperglycemia reduces both cholesterol and triglyceride levels; cholesterol lowering can be enhanced by use of statins. In the nephrotic syndrome, hypercholesterolemia and increased serum triglycerides often coexist; one abnormality responsible for the combined hyperlipidemia may be an overproduction of lipoproteins by the liver, although the hypertriglyceridemia may be due in part to a defective lipolysis of VLDL triglycerides. The hyperlipidemia of the nephrotic syndrome has proved difficult to treat successfully; even so, statin therapy has proven to be moderately effective. Limited data suggest that nephrotic patients are at increased risk for CHD if they have prolonged hyperlipidemia. Thus cholesterol-lowering drug therapy can be justified in patients with chronic forms of the nephrotic syndrome.

HYPOALPHALIPOPROTEINEMIA (LOW LEVELS OF HIGH-DENSITY LIPOPROTEIN)

The HDL cholesterol level should be measured along with total cholesterol when a patient is being tested for CHD risk. The distributions of HDL cholesterol levels in Americans are given in Table 306-6. For patients with high-normal or elevated LDL cholesterol levels, an HDL cholesterol level below 35 mg/dl definitely is a cause for concern. A reduced HDL level can be caused by one or more factors, many of which are reversible (Box 306-2).

Whether specific treatment of low HDL cholesterol levels will reduce CHD risk is uncertain. Clinical trials aimed primarily at raising levels of HDL cholesterol have never been carried out. Moreover, the mechanisms underlying the association between low HDL levels and increased CHD risk are not fully understood. The best approach to management of patients with low HDL levels probably is to modify factors that influence both HDL metabolism and other risk factors. For example, HDL cholesterol concentrations can be increased by weight reduction in obese persons, by smoking cessation, by aerobic exercise, and by correction of elevated cholesterol and triglyceride concentrations. More controversial is whether regular consumption of alcohol for the purpose of raising the HDL level is advisable; its utility in preventing CHD has not been proved, and serious social and physical consequences of excessive intake of alcohol cannot be ignored.

Some regimens that reduce LDL (or total cholesterol) levels also may lower the HDL level. For example, diets high in polyunsaturated fatty acids or carbohydrates reduce the level of plasma HDL, as does the cholesterol-lowering drug probucol. The argument has been made that the decrease in the plasma LDL accompanying these regimens more than offsets any reduction in HDL because in populations in which levels of LDL and rates of CHD are low, the HDL cholesterol level may be low as well. Thus the concept thus has arisen that the total cholesterol/HDL cholesterol ratio may be a better indicator of coronary risk than either the total cholesterol or HDL cholesterol level alone. The risk ratios for varying total cholesterol/HDL cholesterol ratios for American men are listed in Table 306-7, and these ratios can be used to predict coronary risk. It should be kept in mind, however, that a high level of HDL does not completely negate the risk imparted by an elevated level of LDL.

RARE DISORDERS OF LIPID METABOLISM

Because the metabolism of lipids and lipoproteins is complex, defects can occur at multiple sites. Most defects result from abnormalities in the synthesis of a key protein or lipid. Some defects can produce hyperlipidemia, but other abnormalities cause low levels of lipoproteins or bizarre defects in lipoprotein metabolism. Although

Table 306-6 Population distribution of plasma high-density lipoprotein cholesterol (mg/dl)*

	WHITE MEN						WHITE WOMEN					
	PERCENTILES						PERCENTILES					
AGE(yr)	5	10	25	50	75	95	5	10	25	50	75	95
0-4												
5-9	38	42	49	54	63	74	36	38	47	52	61	73
10-14	37	40	46	55	61	74	37	40	45	52	58	70
15-19	30	34	39	46	52	63	35	38	43	51	61	74
20-24	30	32	38	45	51	63	33	37	44	51	62	79
25-29	31	32	37	44	50	63	37	39	47	55	63	83
30-34	28	32	38	45	52	63	36	40	46	55	64	77
35-39	29	31	36	43	49	62	34	38	44	53	64	82
40-44	27	31	36	43	51	67	34	39	48	56	65	88
45-49	30	33	38	45	52	64	34	41	47	58	68	87
50-54	28	31	36	44	51	63	37	41	50	62	73	91
55-59	28	31	38	46	55	71	37	41	50	60	73	91
60-64	30	34	41	49	61	74	38	44	51	61	75	92
65-69	30	33	39	49	62	78	35	38	49	62	73	98
70+	31	33	40	48	56	75	33	38	48	60	71	92

*Modified from the Lipid Research Clinics Population Studies Data Book: the prevalence study, Bethesda, Md, 1979, National Institutes of Health Publication No. 79-1527.

BOX 306-2
Causes of reduced plasma high-density lipoprotein cholesterol

Obesity
Tobacco use
Lack of exercise
Hypertriglyceridemia
Hypercholesterolemia
Genetic factors (poorly defined)
Drugs
    Progestational agents
    Anabolic steroids and androgens
    Beta-adrenergic blocking agents
    Thiazide diuretics
Some cholesterol-lowering regimens
    Diets (low-fat, low-cholesterol, high–polyunsaturated fat diets)
    Drugs (probucol)

Table 306-7 Relation of total cholesterol/HDL cholesterol ratio to risk for coronary heart disease (men aged 50-70 years)

TOTAL CHOLESTEROL/HDL CHOLESTEROL RATIO	CORONARY HEART DISEASE RISK RATIO
3.0	0.5
4.4	1.0
6.2	2.0
7.7	3.0
9.5	4.0

Castelli WP, Abbott RD, McNamara PM: *Circulation* 67:730, 1983.
HDL, High-density lipoprotein.

---

these disorders are rare, they can be devastating to the affected patient.

Abnormalities in the Synthesis of Apolipoproteins

Apolipoprotein B. A failure to synthesize lipoproteins containing apo B is responsible for the disorder called abetalipoproteinemia. In the most common form of this disorder both apo B-100 and apo B-48 are absent, but one patient has been reported who had apo B-48 but no apo B-100. Classic abetalipoproteinemia is characterized by a lack of chylomicrons, VLDL, and LDL. A failure to synthesize chylomicrons causes malabsorption of fat, and absence of VLDL and LDL results in severe reductions in plasma triglyceride and cholesterol levels. Low levels of plasma cholesterol induce deformities of red blood cells (acanthocytosis), and after several years, progressive neurologic involvement develops—retinitis pigmentosa and ataxic neuropathy. Failure to transport vitamin E in LDL probably is responsible for neurologic signs; progression of neurologic defects apparently can be retarded by parenteral administration of large doses of vitamin E.

A congenital reduction in synthesis of apo B–containing lipoproteins causes hypobetalipoproteinemia, or a very low level of LDL. Synthesis of defective forms of the apo B molecules produces a similar clinical picture. Although the LDL concentration is markedly reduced in these disorders, it is not absent. Patients with hypobetalipoproteinemia generally are spared the severe sequelae of abetalipoproteinemia, although occasionally these may occur when LDL reduction is severe.

Recently, a familial defective form of apo B-100 has been reported. The defect prevents the binding of LDL apo B to LDL receptors and results in hypercholesterolemia.

Apolipoprotein A. A rare disorder resulting from a defect in metabolism of apo A is Tangier disease. This disorder appears to be the result of enhanced catabolism of HDL. Both apo A-I and apo A-II levels in plasma are greatly reduced, but neither apoprotein has been shown to be structurally abnormal. Patients with Tangier disease accumulate large amounts of cholesterol esters in reticuloendothelial tissues, most notably in the tonsils; they commonly have a relapsing neuropathy and corneal opacities. Tangier disease follows autosomal recessive inheritance, and consanguinity is common. The disease may not accelerate atherosclerosis, despite the marked reduction in HDL levels.

Another disorder in metabolism of apo A is characterized by a familial deficiency of both apo A-I and apo C-III and severe coronary atherosclerosis. In this disorder xanthoma of skin and tendons and corneal clouding are present. The reason for the presence of premature atherosclerosis with combined deficiency of apo a-I and apo C-III, but not Tangier disease, is unclear. Certain abnormal forms of apo A-I, such as one called A-I Milano, cause relatively low levels of HDL but not premature atherosclerosis.

Apolipoprotein E. A point mutation in the synthesis of apo E produces an abnormal isoform of this apo E. Two normal isoforms of apo E, apo E-3 and apo E-4, bind tightly to hepatic receptors for chylomicron remnants and LDL. In so doing, they promote hepatic uptake of chylomicron remnants and VLDL remnants. The abnormal isoform of apo E is called apo E-2, and it binds poorly to LDL receptors. Every person inherits two genes encoding for apo E. Six genotypes thus are possible: E-3/3, E-3/4, E-3/2, E-4/4, E-4/2, and E-2/2. The E-2/2 genotype occurs in about 1 in 100 Europeans and Americans, and its presence in the absence of other defects of lipoprotein metabolism causes hyperlipidemia. The E-2/2 pattern, however, occasionally contributes to a unique form of hyperlipidemia called familial dysbetalipoproteinemia or type III HLP. This disorder is characterized by accumulation of remnant-like lipoproteins called beta-VLDLs. Affected patients frequently have tuberous or tuberoeruptive xanthoma; yellow discolorations of palmar and digital creases; and premature atherosclerosis of coronary arteries, internal carotids, and abdominal aorta. Beta-VLDLs are VLDL remnants enriched in cholesterol esters; they are identified by a cholesterol/triglyceride ratio in VLDL exceeding 0.3. Most patients with dysbetalipoproteinemia have the E-2/2 genotype combined with overproduction of VLDL (Fig. 306-16). The overproduction of VLDL may be primary or secondary to diabetes mellitus and/or obesity. Recently, a new kindred of patients has been described who have no plasma apo E. This disorder, which also may be characterized by dysbetalipoproteinemia, presumably represents a complete failure to synthesize apo E.

Apolipoprotein C. As indicated previously, a deficiency of apo C-III can occur with a lack of apo A-I; low levels of HDL but not hyperlipidemia result. In another rare condition, apo C-II, the apoprotein required for activation of LPL, is genetically absent. Its absence causes severe hypertriglyceridemia and chylomicronemia. Affected patients are prone to repeated bouts of acute pancreatitis and, sometimes, chronic pancreatitis. Premature atherosclerosis accompanying deficiency of apo C-II has not been reported.

Abnormalities in Enzymes Affecting Lipoprotein Metabolism

Lipoprotein Lipase. A familial deficiency of LPL is a rare autosomal recessive condition. It results in a severe lipolytic defect for chylomicrons and, consequently, severe chylomicronemia (type I HLP). Levels of VLDL are relatively normal, and apparently atherosclerosis is not accelerated. Severe chylomicronemia is present from birth, and skin xanthomas and pancreatitis may occur in infancy or childhood. The plasma creams with chylomicrons, but the infranatant remains relatively clear because VLDL levels are only mildly elevated. Treatment requires a marked reduction of dietary fat, if possible to less than 10% of total calories. Medium-chain triglycerides can provide a partial replacement of dietary fat, but because these cause ketosis when given in large doses, their intake must be limited. Lipid-lowering drugs are of no value in treatment of type I HLP.

Lecithin-Cholesterol Acyltransferase. A genetic deficiency of LCAT occurs rarely as an autosomal recessive disease. It is characterized by failure to form cholesterol esters in plasma. Clinical manifestations include multiple defects in metabolism of lipoproteins, corneal opacities, anemia, renal failure, and premature atherosclerosis. The absence of cholesterol esters in plasma results in an array of abnormalities in lipoproteins. The LDL are unusually large and disk-shaped. HDL also are abnormal in size and shape, and various abnormalities are present in VLDL.

Abnormalities in Enzymes Affecting Sterol Metabolism

Lysosomal Acid Lipase. This enzyme hydrolyzes both the triglycerides and cholesterol esters that enter lysosomes with LDL. The absence of this lipase causes either a severe disease or a more benign one. The former, called Wolman's disease, is usually fatal before the age of 1 year. Features of Wolman's disease include massive accumulation of lipids in liver and spleen and a generalized failure to thrive. In the less severe form, cholesterol ester storage disease, patients often live to adulthood. Nonetheless, they have hepatomegaly because of accumulation of cholesterol esters in the liver. These patients frequently have hypercholesterolemia and premature atherosclerosis.

Defective Bile Acid Synthesis. A defect in the side chain oxidation of cholesterol in its conversion to bile acids causes a disease called cerebrotendinous xanthomatosis. The primary defect in this disease appears to reside in mitochondrial 26-hydroxylation, a key reaction in the conversion. Consequently, the synthesis of the primary bile acids, cholic acid and chenodeoxycholic acid, is reduced. The resulting deficiency of bile acids causes a loss in the feedback regulation of bile acid synthesis, and increased amounts of cholesterol begin to be converted into bile acids. Because of the block in this conversion, however, intermediate steroids are shunted into other products including complex bile alcohols and cholestanol (dehydrocholesterol). Cholestanol becomes incorporated into plasma lipoproteins and, because of its unique physicochemical properties, promotes deposition of both cholesterol and cholestanol into tendons, brain tissue, and the arterial wall. The result is tendinous xanthomatosis, progressive neurologic dysfunction including dementia, spinal cord paresis and cerebellar ataxia, and premature atherosclerosis. A recent report indicated that the neurologic components of cerebrotendinous xanthomatosis can be reversed by oral administration of chenodeoxycholic acid, which inhibits the rapid catabolism of cholesterol, reduces the formation of cholestanol, and apparently reverses tissue deposition of sterols.

BIBLIOGRAPHY

Brown BG, Zhao X-Q, Sacco DE, Albers JJ: Lipid lowering and plaque regression: new insights into prevention of plaque disruption and clinical events in coronary disease, *Circulation* 87:1781-1791, 1993.

Brown MS, Goldstein JL: A receptor-mediated pathway for cholesterol homeostasis, *Science* 232:34-47, 1986.

Buchwald H, VBarco RL, Matts JP et al: Effects of partial ileal bypass surgery on mortality and morbidity from coronary heart disease in patients with hypercholesterolemia: report of the Program on the Surgical Control of the Hyperlipidemias (POSCH), *N Engl J Med* 323:946-955, 1990.

Consensus Development Conference: Lowering blood cholesterol to prevent heart disease, *JAMA* 253:2080-2086, 1985.

Expert Panel on Detection Evaluation, and Treatment of High Blood Cholesterol in Adults: National Cholesterol Education Program: second report of the expert panel on detection, evaluation, and treatment of high blood cholesterol in adults (Adult Treatment Panel II), *Circulation* 89:1329-1345, 1994.

Frick MH et al: Helsinki Heart Study: primary-prevention trial with gemfibrozil in middle-aged men with dyslipidemia: safety of treatment, changes in risk factors, and incidence of coronary heart disease, *N Engl J Med* 317:1237-1245, 1987.

Grundy SM: Cholesterol and coronary heart disease: a new era, *JAMA* 256:2849-2858, 1986.

Grundy SM: HMG CoA reductase inhibitors for treatment of hypercholesterolemia, *N Engl J Med* 319:24-32, 1988.

Grundy SM, and Denke MA: Dietary influences on serum lipids and lipoproteins, *J Lipid Res* 31:1149-1172, 1990.

Lipid Research Clinics Coronary Primary Prevention Trial Results. I. Reduction in incidence of coronary heart disease, *JAMA* 251:531-564, 1984.

Lipid Research Clinics Primary Preventtion Trial Results. II. The relation of reduction in incidence of coronary heart disease to cholesterol lowering, *JAMA* 251:365, 1984.

Report of the Expert Panel on Population Strategies for Blood Cholesterol Reduction: National Cholesterol Education Program, *Circulation* 83:2154-2232, 1991.

Ross R: The pathogenesis of atherosclerosis: an update, *N Engl J Med* 314:488-500, 1986.

Rossouw JE, Lewis B, Rifkind BM: The value of lowering cholesterol after myocardial infarction, *N Engl J Med* 323:1112-1119, 1990.

Scandinavian Simvastatin Survival Study Group: Randomised trial of cholesterol lowering in 4444 patients with coronary heart disease: the Scandinavian Simvastatin Survival Study (4S), *Lancet* 344:1383-1389, 1994.

Shepherd J, Cobbe SM, Ford I et al for the West of Scotland Coronary Prevention Study Group: Prevention of coronary heart disease with pravastatin in men with hypercholesterolemia, *N Engl J Med* 333:1301-1307, 1995.

Stary HC: The histological classification of atherosclerotic lesions in human coronary arteries. In Fuster V, Ross R, Topol EJ, editors: *Atherosclerosis and coronary heart disease,* Philadelphia, 1996, Lippincott-Raven.

CHAPTER

307 Lipodystrophies

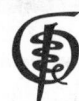

M. Joycelyn Elders

The lipodystrophies are a group of rare metabolic disorders characterized by abnormalities in adipose tissue, generalized or partial loss of body fat, abnormalities of carbohydrate and lipid metabolism, severe resistance to endogenous and exogenous insulin, and immunologic dysfunction. These disorders differ in the anatomic distribution of the dystrophic tissue and are associated with variable degrees of multiple system involvement. The lipodystrophies may be divided into three major categories: total, partial, and localized, based on the anatomic distribution of the lipodystrophic change.

Total lipodystrophy consists of congenital or acquired complete loss of adipose tissue, usually associated with hepatomegaly, hyperglycemia, hyperlipidemia, and hypermetabolism. Other associations include acanthosis nigricans, acromegalic gigantism, generalized hyperpigmentation, renal disease, central nervous system disorders, cardiomegaly, hypertrichosis, hypertrophy of external genitalia, and advanced bone age. Partial lipodystrophy is usually manifest as symmetric or asymmetric loss of adipose tissue with or without facial involvement and with or without atrophy of the extremities or the trunk. This syndrome has also been associated with renal disease, diabetes, hyperpigmentation, hirsutism, hepatomegaly, and hyperlipemia. Localized lipodystrophy is usually manifest as well-demarcated, multifocal atrophic lesions with or without other associated diseases. In each of these categories there are several syndromes that have distinguishable physical, genetic, immunologic, or biochemical characteristics.

A classification of this heterogeneous group of disorders is shown in Box 307-1. Whether each of these disorders is a distinct entity or whether they together represent a spectrum of disease has not been completely determined. The specific pathophysiology is not clear; however, the clinical syndromes are fairly distinct.

LEPRECHAUNISM

Leprechaunism is a rare inherited syndrome that includes characteristic facial features, intrauterine growth retardation, phallic enlargement, marked deficiency of subcutaneous fat stores, and striking cutaneous abnormalities (Figs. 307-1 and 307-2). Biochemical alterations have included postprandial hyperglycemia, hyperinsulinism, insulin resistance, abnormalities of the insulin receptor, fasting hypoglycemia, and increased gonadotropins.

The high frequency of consanguinity and familial occurrence suggests that leprechaunism is transmitted by an autosomal recessive

---

BOX 307-1

Classification of the major lipodystrophic syndromes

I. Total lipodystrophy
   A. Leprechaunism
   B. Congenital
   C. Acquired
II. Partial lipodystrophy
   A. Acquired
   B. Familial
   C. Lipoatrophic diabetes mellitus
III. Localized lipodystrophy
   A. Mesenteric
   B. Membranous
   C. Centrifugal

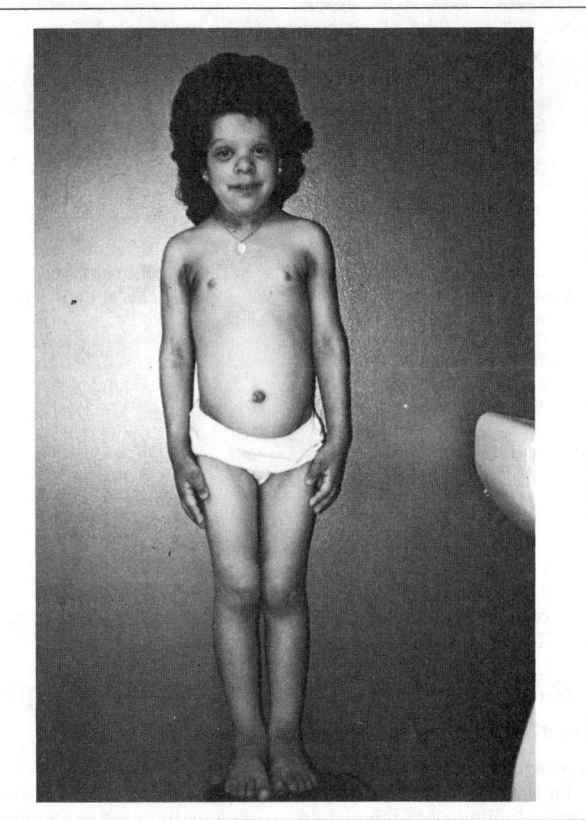

FIGURE 307-1   Patient with leprechaunism. Characteristic facies, absence of subcutaneous tissue, acanthosis nigricans, and hypertrichosis are evident.

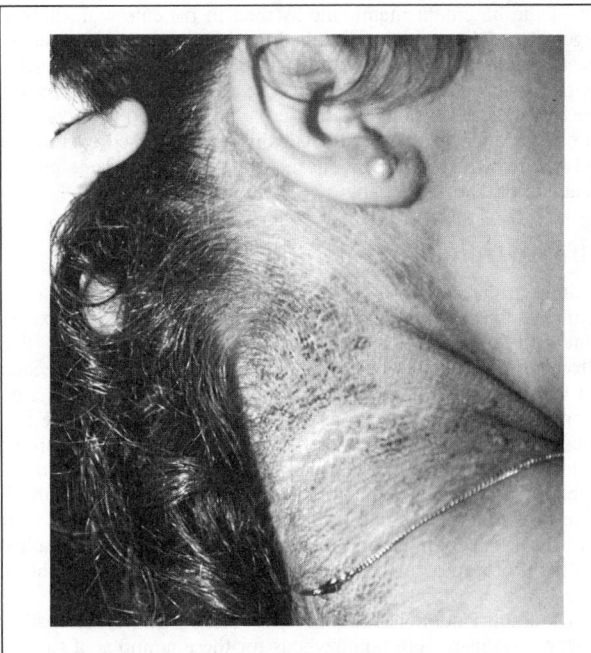

FIGURE 307-2   Same patient as shown in Figure 307-1.

Table 307-1   Clinical comparison of the major lipodystrophic syndromes

| CLINICAL FINDINGS | TOTAL LIPODYSTROPHIES | | | PARTIAL LIPODYSTROPHIES | |
	LEPRECHAUNISM	CONGENITAL	ACQUIRED	ACQUIRED	FAMILIAL
Inheritance	Autosomal recessive	Autosomal recessive	Sporadic	Usually sporadic	Always familial More than one genera- tion affected Autosomal dominant
Age at recognition	Infancy	Infancy	Childhood-adult	Childhood-adult	Puberty
Sex incidence	Female/male (2:1)	Female/male (2:1)	Female predominance	Female predominance	Female predominance
Sites of lipoatrophy	Generalized	Face, trunk, limbs	Face, trunk, limbs	Face, upper trunk, upper limbs	Trunk and limbs
Prominence of muscles	Absent	+	Absent	Absent	Absent
Genital enlargement	+++	+	+	Absent	Common
Hepatomegaly/cirrhosis	±	Common	Common	Usually absent	Absent
Acanthosis nigricans	+++	++	+	Rare	+
Hypertension	±	+→++	+	Absent	Common
Associated abnormalities	Absent	Hepatic, renal, neuro- logic, cardiac	None	Renal, neurologic	None

+, Mild; ++, moderate; +++, severe.

mode of inheritance. There is a 2:1 female/male ratio, and most of the infants manifest severe failure to thrive and early death.

Carbohydrate Metabolism and Insulin-Receptor Abnormalities

All patients with leprechaunism studied thus far have shown evidence of abnormal glucose homeostasis. Fasting hypoglycemia has been a frequent finding and is thought to be secondary to an accelerated response to fasting or to decreased glycogen synthesis during feeding with decreased glycogen stores. Excessive elevations of the blood glucose level are frequent in association with elevated blood insulin levels and pancreatic islet cell hyperplasia. Pathologic findings have included enlarged kidneys with enlargement of the glomeruli and thickening of the basement membrane as seen in patients with diabetes; enlargement of the ovaries and granulosa cell tumors; enlargement of the testes; increased iron deposition in the liver; calcific deposits in the kidneys; decreased lymphoid tissue; marked ductal hyperplasia of the breast; severe acanthosis nigricans; and marked hyperkeratosis of the skin. Some of these patients exhibited increased excretion of epidermal growth factor (EGF) in the urine, suggesting one possible mechanism for the skin changes (Chapter 303).

Pathophysiology

Mutations in the insulin receptor or in the regulatory region of the insulin receptor can cause genetic syndromes associated with extreme insulin resistance. The severe insulin resistance seen in these syndromes is more likely due to abnormalities of the insulin receptor rather than an abnormal insulin molecule. Studies have shown a correlation between point mutations of a single amino acid in the insulin receptor and severe insulin resistance. In some patients a homozygous leucine-proline mutation at amino acid position 233 in the alpha chain of the insulin receptor is found. In others an arginine for glycine substitution at amino acid position 31 has been found in the alpha-beta proreceptor. In both instances the mutation blocks cleavage of the proreceptor and transport from intracellular sites to the cell surfaces.

DNA amplification techniques have demonstrated that patients with leprechaunism were homozygous for these amino acid substitutions, whereas the parents and grandparents studied were heterozygous for these amino acid substitutions. Heterozygous family members had mild to moderate in vitro binding defects, but no clinical manifestations. Both the leucine to proline mutation at amino acid 233 in the alpha chain of the insulin receptor and the glycine to arginine substitution at amino acid 31 in the proinsulin receptor alter conformation of the receptor such that transport to the Golgi compartment where proteolytic processing occurs is inhibited. In other cases mutations in exon 13 of the insulin receptor have been found. This mutation shifts the reading frame and introduces a premature chain termination codon. This mutant allele is predicted to be a null allele that encodes a truncated receptor lacking both transmembrane and tyrosine kinase domains.

These mutant insulin receptors are associated with the following: (1) decreased insulin binding to the receptor, (2) decreased insulin-stimulated 2-deoxy glucose uptake, (3) decreased autophosphorylation of the beta subunit of the insulin receptor, and (4) decreased half-life and a lack of recognition of the receptor by monoclonal antibodies directed against conformation-dependent epitopes. Further study may detect other amino acid mutations that will explain the similarities between leprechaunism, congenital lipodystrophies, other lipodystrophies, and insulin-resistant syndromes.

CONGENITAL TOTAL LIPODYSTROPHY

Congenital total lipodystrophy is a rare disorder of carbohydrate and lipid metabolism. In the majority of cases it has an autosomal recessive inheritance pattern. The disease is characterized anatomically by a generalized and extreme lack of fat in subcutaneous tissue, clinically by extreme insulin resistance and diabetes mellitus, and biochemically by hyperglycemia and triglyceride hyperlipidemia. In addition to the lack of adipose tissue, a number of clinical features are observed from birth or early infancy.

Clinical Manifestations

Congenital total lipodystrophy is a very rare syndrome (Table 307-1) that affects twice as many females as males. The onset is usually about the time of birth. The most striking feature of this condition is total lipodystrophy. There is virtual absence of fat from all subcutaneous tissue, including the distal portions of the body. The musculature is prominent, giving the patient a herculean appearance (Fig. 307-3). It is thought that these patients have an actual increase in muscle mass; however, some data suggest that the muscles are not truly hypertrophic but only appear to be so because of the lack of subcutaneous tissue.

The facies are very distinct. The masseters are prominent. The cheeks appear sunken owing to the lack of buccal fat pads, and the forehead is wrinkled, giving the patient an appearance of senility. The bony prominences and muscles are clearly outlined, and most patients have a very prominent abdomen.

Skeletal growth and maturation appear to be accelerated. There is mild to moderate hypertension, and the liver is always enlarged but not enough to account for the very prominent abdomen. These patients frequently develop acanthosis nigricans, which may be observed at any age but is most prominent in pubertal patients. It most frequently involves the neck, axillary, and inguinal areas, but it can have a generalized distribution. Other dermatologic features include hir-

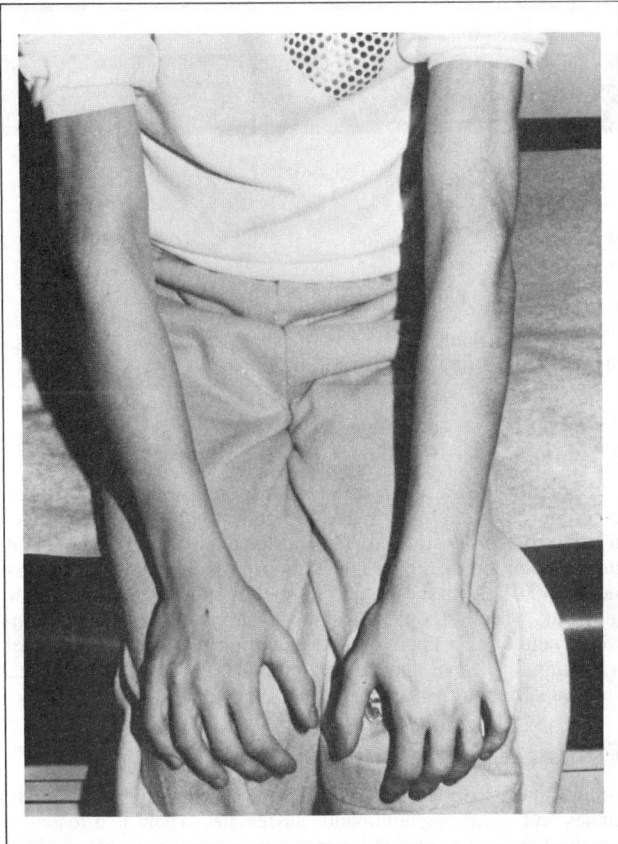

FIGURE 307-3 Patient with acquired total lipodystrophy. Prominent triceps muscles and absence of subcutaneous tissue are evident.

sutism, eruptive xanthomas, and marked thickening of the skin. Genital hypertrophy is frequently observed.

Developmental milestones in children are usually normal, but mental retardation has been associated with total lipodystrophy in some instances. There are usually very few symptoms until the onset of diabetes, which usually appears during the pubertal years. Ketosis is rare, despite the lack of dietary therapy or insulin treatment. Renal disease may occur. The most common cause of death at any time from infancy to the fourth decade is hepatic failure.

Laboratory Findings

The laboratory findings in generalized lipodystrophy are dominated by marked disturbance in fat and carbohydrate metabolism and, in most patients, by an increased basal metabolic rate (Table 307-2). The glucose tolerance and fasting insulin levels are normal early but may be slightly elevated. Early in the disease the insulin response to glucose is exaggerated and prolonged, with mild insulin resistance. From the ages of 8 to 10 years, glucose tolerance decreases rapidly, with grossly elevated insulin levels. The insulin responses to oral and intravenous glucose and to tolbutamide are exaggerated. Insulin resistance is marked and increases with age. After 12 years, there is a cessation of growth and onset of frank diabetes, with fasting hyperglycemia and diabetic glucose tolerance curves. A decreased insulin response to glucose stimulation occurs, suggesting the partial exhaustion of the beta cells. Hyperlipidemia, present in a majority of patients, is a constant feature in older patients, but the younger child may have normal lipid fractions.

An increased metabolic rate has been encountered in some patients with total lipodystrophy; however, thyroid, adrenal, and gonadal function studies have been normal. There is an exaggerated luteinizing hormone (LH), follicle-stimulating hormone (FSH), thyroid-stimulating hormone (TSH), and prolactin response to exogenously administered releasing hormones, suggesting lesions in the target or-

gans. Although rapid growth is observed and the bone age is advanced in children, growth hormone and somatomedin levels are normal.

Liver function test results may be abnormal, especially in the late stages of the disease, when liver fibrosis occurs. All of the liver enzyme levels are frequently elevated. Alkaline phosphatase levels may demonstrate transient increases secondary to the increase in triglyceride levels. Renal function is usually normal in children; however, there is a progressive decline with increasing age of the patient. The intravenous pyelogram may reveal kidney enlargement. The ventriculogram and pneumoencephalogram frequently reveal ventricular dilation. Pathologic findings are related to the complete lack of fat in the subcutaneous tissues and to hepatomegaly. This histologic appearance of the liver is that of marked fatty changes, congestion, and fibrosis, with abundant glycogen. Microscopic study of the muscle demonstrates hypertrophy associated with areas of degenerative fibrosis or infiltration with adipose tissue. The heart and kidneys are usually enlarged.

Pathophysiology

The origin of this disorder is unknown. Insulin-receptor binding in a patient with total lipodystrophy is decreased. When these patients fast for 48 to 72 hours, however, insulin-receptor binding improves. Other studies have suggested a reversible loss of coupling of normal insulin receptors to metabolic pathways. The receptor loss is thought to be tissue specific, involving only adipose tissue and liver.

The mechanism of insulin resistance in total lipodystrophy is unknown. Previous studies that have attempted to determine whether there is an abnormality in receptor function have produced varying results. In some patients there is a quantitative receptor defect, in which there is a decrease in the number of receptors, but the residual receptors appear to be normal in all respects. The quantitative defect in receptor number persists in cell culture in vitro, suggesting that this defect is genetic. In other patients there appears to be a qualitative defect in the insulin receptor, in which insulin may bind to its receptor with a different affinity, or there may be a lack of insulin binding to the high-affinity receptor component. In still other patients, receptors are abnormally insensitive to changes in temperature and pH.

Along with qualitative and quantitative receptor defects, some patients are considered to have postreceptor defects or an abnormality in the insulin receptor that interferes with the coupling of insulin binding to insulin action. The biochemical defect resides at a step distal to the hormone receptor. No insulin antibodies or insulin receptor antibodies have been found. Some patients have entirely normal insulin binding to erythrocytes, monocytes, and cultured fibroblasts. Heterogeneity of insulin receptor interaction has been reported even in the same family of patients with lipodystrophy.

The mechanism of the lipemia is not understood but has been postulated to be related to (1) excessive secretion of "adipokinin," (2) somatotropin action, (3) intact lipogenesis from carbohydrate, owing to lack of an unknown enzyme necessary for the deposition of subcutaneous fat, or (4) absence of functional adipose tissue and saturation of other storage sites (e.g., liver). None of these postulates has been substantiated.

Differential Diagnosis

Total lipodystrophy can usually be differentiated from other disorders by the generalized absence of fat tissue and the "athletic" appearance and prominent abdomen of affected children.

Congenital generalized lipodystrophy has many features of leprechaunism, including genital hypertrophy, acanthosis nigricans, and hypertrichosis (Table 307-1). However, the disease differs from leprechaunism because it is associated with increased growth and muscle mass and hepatosplenomegaly. Acanthosis nigricans with insulin resistance type B has antiinsulin-receptor antibodies, not found in leprechaunism, whereas acanthosis nigricans and insulin resistance type A have defective insulin receptors and are associated with accelerated growth and virilization (Chapter 291). The typical triglyceride hyperlipidemia and insulin-resistant diabetes further substantiate the diagnosis.

Partial lipodystrophy has many features in common with total li-

Table 307-2 Laboratory comparison of the major lipodystrophic syndromes

	TOTAL LIPODYSTROPHIES			PARTIAL LIPODYSTROPHIES	
	LEPRECHAUNISM	CONGENITAL	ACQUIRED	ACQUIRED	FAMILIAL
Hypertriglyceridemia	—	+++	++	±	++
Hypoglycemia	+++	—	—	—	—
Ketosis	—	—	—	—	—
Insulin resistance	+++	+++	++	+	+
Hyperinsulinemia	+++	+++	++	—	—
Insulin receptor abnormal	++	Affinity	—	—	—
Glucose intolerance	+++	++	++	++	++
Liver dysfunction	—	++	++	—	—
Hypothalamic-pituitary function	Normal	Normal	Normal	Normal	Normal
Bone age	Retarded	Accelerated	Normal	Normal	Normal

—, Absent; ±, mild; ++, moderate; +++, severe.

podystrophy (e.g., the facial appearance and well-outlined musculature of the involved areas). The muscles in partial lipodystrophy, however, are not hypertrophied, and the fat tissue remains intact in distal portions of the extremities. Some patients with hypothalamic lesions may present a clinical picture resembling that of total lipodystrophy. For example, patients with diencephalic syndrome of early infancy have neither complete loss of adipose tissue nor accelerated growth. They usually have markedly increased appetites, increased motor activity, abnormal cerebrospinal fluid findings, skin pallor with normal hemoglobin concentrations, decreased pituitary reserve, and inadequate thyroid function.

The masculine appearance, advanced growth, clitoral or penile enlargement, and hirsutism seen in lipodystrophy may be confused with the appearance of patients with congenital adrenal hyperplasia. Adrenal function in patients with total lipodystrophy, however, is normal.

Treatment

There is no known specific drug treatment for the lipodystrophies. Pimozide, a dopamine-receptor blocker, has been reported to be useful, but long-term clinical trials have shown no effect.

Fenfluramine, another dopamine-receptor blocker, blocks the synthesis of triglycerides, reduces intestinal absorption of triglycerides, increases carbohydrate utilization in vivo, and decreases brain serotonin, suggesting a possible defect in serotonin metabolism in the central nervous system. Despite reports of its usefulness, long-term use of this drug has also been ineffective.

Diet therapy is of some value in the control of hyperglycemia and hyperlipidemia. The use of small, frequent feedings and partial substitution of medium-chain triglycerides for polyunsaturated fats appears beneficial.

Plastic surgery with implants of monolithic silicon rubber for correction of the deficient soft tissue of the face is an effective therapy. Dental prostheses may be useful in some instances. Long-term management is usually related to therapy for the renal and endocrine dysfunctions that occur.

PARTIAL LIPODYSTROPHY

The partial lipodystrophies, like the total lipodystrophies, may be inherited or acquired and may have a symmetric or asymmetric distribution. The origin of partial lipodystrophy is unknown. Postulated etiologic factors include familial or genetic disease, infections, immunologic disorders, or neurogenic dysfunctions. Partial lipodystrophy has been documented to occur in successive generations and to be associated with a genetically determined hypocomplementemia.

Hypocomplementemia and C3 nephritic factor are known to occur in partial lipodystrophy. Abnormalities of the complement system are thought to precede the development of the dystrophy. However, the occurrence of partial lipodystrophy without complement and C3 nephritic factor has been documented. Partial lipodystrophy is also known to be associated with other autoimmune disorders, such as systemic lupus erythematosus, Sjögren's syndrome, idiopathic thrombocytopenic purpura, thyrotoxicosis, and myasthenia gravis.

In addition to the genetic, infectious, and immunologic hypotheses proposed as etiologic in partial lipodystrophy, a neurogenic origin has also been postulated. This postulate is based on the (1) anatomic distribution of the atrophic adipose tissue, (2) autonomic dysfunction, (3) fatty tissue transplant studies showing atrophy of normal graft when transplanted into dystrophic areas and normal development of dystrophic tissue when implanted into a normal field, (4) abnormalities of hypothalamic-pituitary function, and (5) headache as a common manifestation.

ACQUIRED PARTIAL LIPODYSTROPHY

Acquired partial lipodystrophy is the most common of the lipodystrophies and occurs predominantly in females. There is a loss of fat from the face and trunk, with normal or excessive deposition in the pelvic girdle or lower limbs. This disorder is usually progressive and has been called cephalothoracic progressive lipodystrophy. Occasionally, only one side is affected, although some authors have suggested that unilateral partial lipodystrophy is a separate disorder.

Partial lipodystrophy has its onset from age 2 to 40 years, but the majority of patients are younger than 16 years. Clinical manifestations associated with this disease include a sensation of coldness of involved areas, vague abdominal complaints or vomiting, frequent defecation, headache, nervousness, and fatigue. Some of the signs are tachycardia, Raynaud's phenomenon, and excessive sweating. Various pathologic conditions have been associated with partial lipodystrophy, including central nervous system dysfunction, hyperthyroidism, diabetes mellitus, menstrual disorders, ovarian abnormalities, and hypogonadism. Hepatomegaly has been observed in some patients, but the most serious pathologic association is renal dysfunction. Proteinuria is much more frequent in partial lipodystrophy than in the other syndromes. The complement system is abnormal, with decreased levels of C3. Treatment of this condition is symptomatic.

LIPOATROPHIC DIABETES

Classically, this disease has been divided into congenital and acquired forms. The congenital forms of lipoatrophic diabetes are rare. The lipodystrophies may be generalized (transmitted as an autosomal recessive trait) or partial (transmitted as an autosomal dominant trait). The acquired form may develop in children or adults and may be generalized or partial. It often develops after an acute illness but may have an insidious onset. Both congenital and acquired lipoatrophic diabetes are associated with abnormalities in carbohydrate metabolism, manifested by hyperglycemia, glucosuria, increased plasma insulin levels, and insulin resistance. Patients usually do not develop ketoacidosis, but it has been known to occur. Familial lipoatrophic diabetes is a syndrome that appears to have a dominant mode of inheritance and is characterized by fat atrophy of the limb and trunk with sparing of the face, which may actually be rounded. The neck may also be spared. The disease usually begins at puberty but may not appear until middle age. It primarily involves females; males are rarely affected. Insulin resistance and hyperglycemia are usual, with severe hypertriglyceridemia and eruptive xanthomas. The vaginal labia are hypertrophied, and polycystic ovaries may be seen. Acanthosis nigricans is usually present. Liver and renal disease usually does not occur. The pattern of inheritance is consistent with an autosomal dominant transmission with variable expression.

Laboratory findings reveal a mild type V hyperlipidemia, chemical diabetes, and high plasma insulin levels. This disease has to be distinguished from the partial or total absence of subcutaneous fat as well as from the congenital lipodystrophies.

Acquired lipoatrophic diabetes usually begins in adolescence or early adult life. It shares certain features with congenital lipodystrophy such as acanthosis nigricans, hyperlipidemia, and hepatosplenomegaly, leading in some cases to frank cirrhosis. Insulin-resistant diabetes mellitus is almost invariably present, but neurologic, cardiac, and renal abnormalities are usually absent.

PARTIAL LIPODYSTROPHY ASSOCIATED WITH OTHER ANOMALIES

This autosomal dominant form of partial lipodystrophy involves the face and buttocks and is nonprogressive. It has its onset in infancy or early childhood and is associated with Rieger's anomaly, short stature, midface hypoplasia, hypotrichosis, and insulinopenic diabetes. Rieger's anomaly is a nonspecific defect associated with variable eye and tooth abnormalities. Eye anomalies include hypoplasia of iris stroma, prominent Schwalbe's ring, iridocorneal synechiae, microcornea or megalocornea, strabismus, and a predisposition to glaucoma. Tooth abnormalities include hypodontia, microdontia, enamel hypoplasia, atypically shaped teeth, and malocclusion. This condition differs from familial autosomal lipodystrophy in that onset occurs in infancy, other anomalies are associated, and the face is involved.

LOCALIZED LIPODYSTROPHY

The localized lipodystrophies have well-demarcated, multifocal lesions and often are associated early with a lymphocytic panniculitis, suggestive of an inflammatory mechanism.

MESENTERIC LIPODYSTROPHY

This isolated lipodystrophy of the fatty tissue surrounding the small intestine has also been called mesenteric panniculitis, lipogranuloma of the mesentery, and other names. Whatever the terminology, histologic findings are uniform in all cases: abundant adipose tissue interspersed with fibrous tissue. Forty-two percent of patients develop mesenteric thickening, 32% show a large single tumor, and 26% have multiple tumors. Clinical symptoms vary from an acute condition of the abdomen to vague nonspecific abdominal pain. Displacement of the gastrointestinal tract, a frequent finding on on x-ray film, is believed to be caused by enlarged mesenteric fat arising from the celiac axis.

MEMBRANOUS LIPODYSTROPHY

This condition is a rare inherited disease characterized by symmetric multiple cystic bone lesions and progressive neuropsychiatric symptoms including progressive dementia, seizures, ataxia, tremors, and loss of consciousness. The neuropsychiatric symptoms are considered to be related to a sclerosing leukoencephalopathy of the cerebrum. These patients may also have ischemic necrosis of the lens.

CENTRIFUGAL LIPODYSTROPHY

This rare discrete condition is characterized by a localized cutaneous depression enlarging in a centrifugal distribution. The depression is due to a marked dystrophic change of the subcutaneous adipose tissue. The findings in this condition must be distinguished from changes resulting from long-standing insulin administration that are seen in patients with type I diabetes.

BIBLIOGRAPHY

Aarskog D et al: Autosomal dominant partial lipodystrophy associated with Rieger anomaly, short stature, and insulinopenic diabetes, *Am J Med Genet* 51:29, 1983.

✔ *WHEN TO REFER*

Patients who come to medical attention with absence of subcutaneous fat or lipoliptrophy, unless this is known to be a result of the administration of subcutaneous insulin, should be referred to a center where a specific diagnosis can be made. Infants who come to medical attention with evidence of intrauterine growth retardation, hypoglycemia, or hyperglycemia and elevated insulin levels should also be referred. This is no specific treatment for this group of disorders, but various therapies are being tried, including recombinant human growth hormone and insulin-like growth factor I.

Backeljauw PF et al: Effect of intravenous insulin-like growth factor I in two patients with leprechaunism, *Pediatr Res* 36(6):749-754, 1994.
Bier DM et al: Glucose kinetics in leprechaunism: accelerated fasting due to insulin resistance, *J Clin Endocrinol Metab* 51:988, 1980.
Grunberger G et al: Insulin receptors in normal and disease states, *Clin Endocrinol Metab* 12:191, 1983.
Haruta T et al: Amplification and analysis of promoter region of insulin receptor gene in a patient with leprechaunism associated with severe insulin resistance, *Metabolism* 44(4):430-437, 1995.
Hone J et al: Homozygosity for a null allele of the insulin receptor gene in a patient with leprechaunism, *Hum Mutat* 6(1):17-22, 1995.
Keenan BS et al: The effect of diet upon carbohydrate metabolism, insulin resistance, and blood pressure in congenital total lipoatrophic diabetes, *Metabolism* 29:1214, 1980.
Krook A et al: Molecular scanning of the insulin receptor gene in syndromes of insulin resistance, *Diabetes* 43(3):357-368, 1994.
Longo N et al: Impaired growth in Rabson-Mendenhall syndrome: lack of effect of growth hormone and insulin-like growth factor I, *J Clin Endocrinol Metab* 79(3):799-805, 1994.
Rossini AA et al: Metabolic and endocrine studies in a case of lipoatrophic diabetes, *Metabolism* 26:637, 1977.
Suzuki Y et al: Insulin resistance associated with decreased levels of insulin-receptor messenger ribonucleic acid: evidence of a de novo mutation in the maternal allele, *J Clin Endocrinol Metab* 80(4):1214-1220, 1995.
Wachslicht-Rodbard H et al: Heterogeneity of the insulin-receptor interaction in lipoatrophic diabetes, *J Clin Endocrinol Metab* 52:416, 1981.

V   METABOLIC DISORDERS IN ADULTS

CHAPTER

308 Disorders of Amino Acid Metabolism

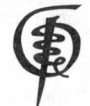

Jess G. Thoene

Disorders of amino acid metabolism, transport, and storage constitute a heterogeneous group of conditions whose clinical impact ranges from mild (e.g., cystathioninuria) to severe (e.g., propionic acidemia) with death occurring during infancy or childhood. Most disorders of amino acid metabolism are associated with mental retardation and decreased life span. Those resulting from disorders of amino acid transport or storage (cystinosis, Hartnup's disease, iminoglycinuria, cystinuria, Lowe's syndrome) have a varied clinical presentation. Though each disease is rare in the general population, with incidences ranging from 1:10,000 to 1:200,000 live births, collectively they impose a substantial disease burden. They are inherited, with a few exceptions, as autosomal recessive conditions. In the diseases that manifest themselves in infancy, rapid and accurate diagnosis is essential

Table 308-1 Disorders of amino acid metabolism that may be encountered in adults

CONDITION	AGE OF PRESENTATION	MAJOR SYMPTOMS
PKU	Infancy	Seizures, retardation (untreated)
Cystinuria	Adolescence, young adult	Kidney stones
Citrullinemia (adult form)	Childhood	Mental retardation
Vitamin-responsive organic acidemias	Infancy	Variable
Homocystinuria	Childhood	Thromboses
Cystathioninuria	Variable	Variable
Cystinosis (benign form)	Childhood	Keratopathy
Hartnup's disease	Childhood	Dermatitis, neurologic abnormalities
Alkaptonuria	Adult	Arthritis, pigmentary changes
Gyrate retinal atrophy	Adolescence	Visual loss
Partial OTC deficiency	Intrapartum Postpartum	Hyperammonemia coma

PKU, Phenylketonuria; *OTC*, ornithine transcarbamylase.

Table 308-2 Amino acids of clinical interest and some related diseases

AMINO ACID	RELATED DISEASES	AVAILABLE THERAPY
Glycine	Nonketotic hyperglycinemia	+
	Ketotic hyperglycinemia	+
Alanine	Lactic acidoses	+
Valine	Hypervalinemia	+
	MSUD	+
	Methylmalonic aciduria	+
Isoleucine	Propionic acidemia	+
	MSUD	+
Leucine	Isovaleric acidemia	+
	MSUD	
Methionine	Hypermethioninemia	NI
Cysteine	—	NI
Cystine	Cystinosis	+
	Cystinuria	+
Serine	Hyperoxaluria II	–
Threonine	Hyperthreoninemia	–
Phenylalanine	PKU	+
	Atypical PKU and variants	
Tyrosine	Hereditary tyrosinemia	+
Asparagine	—	NI
Glutamine	—	NI
Tryptophan	Tryptophanuria	—
Proline	Hyperprolinemia I and II	NI
Aspartic acid	—	NI
Glutamic acid	Pyroglutamic acidemia	–
Histidine	Histidinemia	+
Arginine	Hyperargininemia	+
Lysine	Hyperlysinemia	+
Arginisuccinic acid	Argininosuccinic aciduria	+
Ornithine	Hyperornithinemia	+
	Ornithine aminotransferase deficiency	+
Citrulline	Citrullinemia	+
Homocystine	Homocystinuria	+
Cystathionine	Cystathioninuria	NI
Pipecolic acid	Hyperpipecolatemia	—
	Zellweger's syndrome	
Beta-alanine	Beta-alaninemia	—

*+, Potential or proved therapy; –, no effective therapy; NI, therapy not indicated; MSUD, maple syrup urine disease; PKU, phenylketonuria.

because, in some instances, therapy is highly effective if instituted early. In all cases, genetic counseling can be offered. Until recently, most patients with disorders of amino acid metabolism have not survived to young adulthood; however, the development of effective therapies for some previously lethal disorders (see Disorders of the Urea Cycle and Disorders of Branched-Chain Amino Acid Metabolism) has permitted greatly improved life expectancy. In the near future, therefore, these conditions will assume a practical significance for internists as they previously have for pediatricians. A list of some disorders of amino acid metabolism that may be encountered in the adult population is given in Table 308-1.

The amino acids known to be associated with human disease and the availability of therapy are listed in Table 308-2. The listing is not exhaustive, and the reader is referred to the general references at the end of the chapter for more detailed discussions. Although the structures of the 20 amino acids required for protein synthesis and the urea-cycle intermediates have been known for approximately 50 years, new amino acids continue to be discovered (e.g., gamma-carboxyglutamic acid, beta-carboxyaspartic acid). It is reasonable to assume that new inborn errors of amino acid metabolism will continue to be described as knowledge concerning normal amino acid metabolism and genetic regulation accumulates.

The diagnosis of disorders of amino acid metabolism can be difficult because of the nonspecific modes of presentation, the nature of the analytic instruments required in establishing the diagnosis, and the relative scarcity of these diseases in the general population. Accumulation of significant clinical experience in this field requires a wide referral area and sufficient laboratory resources to permit rapid and reliable diagnosis.

Because the alpha-amino group of amino acids reacts with ninhydrin to form colored compounds, the diagnosis of amino acidopathies has relied on detection through the use of this reagent. Indeed, the number of known inborn errors of amino acid metabolism increased dramatically during the 20 years after the introduction of the automatic amino acid analyzer. Amino acids in plasma and urine also may be estimated qualitatively via one- or two-dimensional chromatography and also by high-voltage electrophoresis. Interpretation of these patterns requires familiarity with normal variants and artifacts; newborn and premature infants may show a physiologic aminoaciduria due to relative immaturity of the tubular reabsorption mechanism for amino acids. Certain antibiotics also stain with ninhydrin and cause false-positive test results.

After transamination, amino acids become "invisible" to methods that rely on the ninhydrin reaction for visualization and quantitation. Thus those inborn errors resulting from defects after transamination generally require means other than the amino acid analyzer for iden-

tification. This group, known collectively as *organic acidemias,* has been delineated by a variety of techniques, the most universal of which is gas chromatography-mass spectrometry (GC-MS). GC-MS instrumentation can provide unambiguous identification of nanogram amounts of all volatile metabolites present in a given sample. Commercially available computerized data systems have greatly facilitated the reduction of the enormous amount of information each plasma or urine sample analyzed produces. GC-MS analysis, however, has some drawbacks. It requires relatively extensive sample preparation, and the instruments are expensive and not generally available in clinical laboratories.

Because of the severity of presentation of many inborn errors of metabolism and lack of pharmacotherapy, patients are likely to be candidates for the initial trials of gene therapy. The objectives for gene therapy, in addition to successfully isolating the working gene for the disease in question, include developing a delivery system directed at the tissue(s) of interest and generating expression of sufficient activity to produce clinical improvement. Some diseases (ornithine transcarbamylase deficiency; see later discussion) are known to be clinically asymptomatic when only a few percentages of residual activity are present. Achievement of this level of activity by exogenous gene therapy appears possible.

HYPERPHENYLALANINEMIA

Classic phenylketonuria (PKU) was described in 1937 and is perhaps the most widely studied aminoacidopathy. The incidence of PKU in the North American population is 1:14,000. A number of other con-

Table 308-3 Hyperphenylalaninemias

CONDITION	CLINICAL ASPECTS	PRESUMED DEFECT	BLOOD PHENYLALANINE
PKU	Mental retardation, hypopigmentation	Phe hydroxylase absent	>20 mg/dl on regular diet
Persistent hyperphenylalaninemia	Normal	Decreased Phe hydroxylase	May be same as PKU early; later 4-20 mg/dl on regular diet
Transient mild hyperphenylalaninemia	Normal	Maturational delay of hydroxylase	May be same as PKU early; progressively declines toward normal
Transaminase deficiency	Normal	Phe transaminase deficiency	Varies with dietary protein intake
Dihydropteridine reductase deficiency	Initially normal; seizures, abnormal development evident within first year of life	Deficiency of dihydropteridine reductase	Variable, may be as in type I
Abnormal dihydropteridine reductase function	Myoclonus, uncontrolled movements, tetraplegia, greasy skin, recurrent hyperthermia	Unknown; functional abnormality of dihydropteridine reductase	May be >20 mg/dl

Phe, Phenylalanine; *PKU*, phenylketonuria.
Modified from Stanbury J, Wyngaarden JB, Fredrickson DS, editors: *The metabolic basis of inherited disease*, ed 5, New York, 1983, McGraw-Hill.

ditions producing hyperphenylalaninemia have since been described (Table 308-3), reinforcing the need for precise diagnosis in this as in other amino acidopathies.

Classic PKU is an autosomal recessive condition resulting from deficiency of hepatic phenylalanine hydroxylase, which converts phenylalanine to tyrosine. It requires tetrahydrobiopterin as a cofactor. Untreated classic PKU produces clinical symptomatology that includes severe mental retardation, hypopigmentation of skin and hair, eczematoid rash, seizures, microcephaly, and electroencephalographic abnormalities. The plasma phenylalanine concentration is sustained at greater than 20 mg/dl. Urinary excretion of alternative metabolites of phenylalanine (phenylpyruvic, phenylacetic, and phenyllactic acids) is responsible both for the musty odor associated with these patients and also for the characteristic green color produced in the urinary ferric chloride test.

The specific mechanism responsible for mental retardation in these patients has not yet been identified, although direct cerebral toxicity from elevated levels of phenylalanine and its keto analogs has been postulated. Deficits resulting from decreased production of neurotransmitters derived from tyrosine are also possible. Artificially produced hyperphenylalaninemia in experimental animals has led to disruption of cerebral polyribosomes, defective cerebral protein synthesis, decreased brain cerebroside and sulfatide content, and decreased DNA content of cerebrum and cerebellum. Additionally, depletion of certain amino acids from the brain has been proposed as a result of sustained hyperphenylalaninemia.

Dietary treatment of classic PKU has proved to be one of the most effective means of ameliorating the inborn errors of metabolism. Diets low in phenylalanine were first used to treat PKU in the 1950s. It has since been demonstrated that, if the diet is begun early in life (ideally less than 1 month of age), the mean intelligence quotient (IQ) of the treated PKU patients is very close to 100. This is in marked contrast to the IQ of untreated PKU patients, which is always less than 50 and is generally around 20. Because of the need for early intervention, most states have initiated mandatory infant PKU screening during the nursery stay to ensure rapid detection and early treatment. The diet consists of a semisynthetic formula low in phenylalanine, and it is supplemented with natural foods low in phenylalanine. The amount of dietary phenylalanine is adjusted on an individual basis to maintain the plasma phenylalanine level between 2 and 12 mg/dl. This is usually achieved at an average daily intake of 250 to 500 mg of phenylalanine throughout childhood. The question of when to terminate the diet is currently unresolved. However, most workers in the field agree that maintenance of a low-phenylalanine diet is desirable through at least 8 years of age.

A number of children have been born to mothers with PKU. These offspring have had abnormalities thought to result from intrauterine hyperphenylalaninemia. They include a variety of congenital anomalies, growth retardation, and mental retardation (over 90%). These findings clearly indicate a need for effective management of maternal PKU, including maintenance of the mother on a low-

phenylalanine diet throughout pregnancy. Available data are too limited at present to judge the effectiveness of this therapy.

TYROSINEMIA

Plasma tyrosine level is elevated in several conditions, including hereditary tyrosinemia, transient tyrosinemia, tyrosine aminotransferase deficiency, "tyrosinosis," and generalized liver dysfunction, as well as in other unrelated conditions. In all instances, significant tyrosinemia leads to excessive urinary excretion of phenolic metabolites, producing a positive urinary nitrosonaphthol test result.

Hereditary tyrosinemia is an autosomal recessive condition that is very rare in the general population; however, it is concentrated in a certain French-Canadian community where the carrier frequency is approximately 1 in 30 individuals. The genetic defect is now known to be deficiency of hepatic fumarylacetoacetate lyase. The primary clinical manifestations of this condition are hepatocellular dysfunction progressing to nodular cirrhosis, associated with a renal tubular nephropathy producing the renal Fanconi syndrome and hypophosphatemic rickets. Deficiency of p-hydroxyphenylpyruvic acid oxidase produces elevated urinary excretion of the phenolic compounds p-hydroxyphenylacetic acid, p-hydroxyphenyllactic acid, and p-hydroxyphenylpyruvic acid. Detection of succinylacetone in the urine is virtually diagnostic of this condition. Treatment with a diet low in tyrosine is reported to improve renal function. Recently the drug NTBC 2 (2-nitro-4-trifluoromethylbenzoyl)-1, 3-cyclohexanedione) has been introduced as treatment for tyrosinemia type 1. This compound acts as an inhibitor of 4-hydroxyphenylpyruvate dioxygenase and prevents the formation of maleylacetoacetate and fumarylacetoacetate, which are the toxic metabolites responsible for the cirrhosis and presumably the hepatocellular carcinoma. The drug is well tolerated and results in rapid normalization of liver function assays and alphafetoprotein. Clinical investigation is ongoing.

Transient tyrosinemia of the newborn is the most commonly encountered defect of tyrosine metabolism and has been found in up to 30% of premature infants. It is characterized by marked elevation in plasma tyrosine level (up to 36 mg/dl; normal, less than 1.3 mg/dl), tyrosyluria, no consistent abnormal clinical findings, and rapid response to both protein restriction and vitamin C supplementation. It is thought to result from delayed maturation of p-hydroxyphenylpyruvic acid oxidase, which requires vitamin C as a cofactor. It appears not to be a hereditary disorder and is important chiefly in distinguishing this benign condition from other, more serious disorders of tyrosine metabolism that are heritable.

Tyrosine aminotransferase deficiency has been reported in a small number of patients characterized by striking elevations in plasma tyrosine (30 to 50 mg/dl) and tyrosyluria accompanied by a constellation of clinical findings, including mental retardation, palmar-plantar keratosis, microcephaly, seizures, and corneal clouding. In contrast to patients with hereditary tyrosinemia, liver and kidney diseases are absent in these patients. A defect in hepatic cytosol tyrosine aminotransferase has been reported in one such patient. Amelioration of the skin lesions has been reported to result from a diet low in phenylalanine and tyrosine.

Generalized hepatic dysfunction is known to lead to aberrations in tyrosine metabolism, including elevation in plasma tyrosine and tyrosyluria. Associated pathologic conditions reported to induce tyrosinemia include viral hepatitis, cirrhosis, neonatal giant-cell hepatitis, and cytomegalovirus infection. Other illnesses that have been associated with tyrosinemia include fructose-1,6-diphosphatase deficiency, galactosemia, cystic fibrosis, and hypothyroidism.

HISTIDINEMIA

Histidinemia results from a deficiency of the enzyme histidine-alpha-deaminase, which converts histidine to urocanic acid. It is inherited as an autosomal recessive trait. Elevated histidine in plasma is associated with excessive urinary excretion of alternative histidine metabolites, primarily imidazole pyruvic acid, which produces a green color on reaction with ferric chloride. The clinical features of this condition include mental retardation (50%) and speech defects. Diets low in histidine are effective in lowering plasma histidine in this condition; however, clinical improvement has not been documented. Because mental retardation is an inconstant finding in this condition, neonatal screening for histidinemia has not been adopted widely.

DISORDERS OF THE UREA CYCLE

The urea cycle is the primary mechanism in mammalian tissues for the disposal of nitrogen waste generated primarily from protein metabolism. The urea cycle intermediates and their interrelationships are shown in Fig. 308-1. For each "turn" of the cycle, 2 moles of ammonia are excreted in the form of 1 mole of urea. Ammonia enters the cycle, both as free ammonium in the first reaction in the cycle, and as aspartic acid in the third reaction. Both carbamylphosphate synthetase (CPS) and ornithine transcarbamylase (OTC) are located within mitochondria; the remaining three enzymes, argininosuccinate synthetase (AS), argininosuccinate lyase (AL), and arginase (ARG), occur in the cytosol. Citrulline and ornithine shuttle between the mitochondrial interior and the cytosol. Understanding of the regulation of urea cycle activity has recently been advanced with the description of N-acetylglutamate as a positive modulator of CPS activity. N-acetylglutamate is formed via the action of N-acetylglutamate synthetase which is itself positively modulated by arginine. Thus conditions leading to elevated arginine, such as dietary protein load, also enhance activity of the urea cycle, tending to preserve homeostasis.

Interruption of the urea cycle due to an enzymatic deficiency impairs the organism's ability to excrete waste nitrogen and leads to a common complex of clinical findings, which usually include marked hyperammonemia, mental retardation, protein intolerance, seizures, coma, and death in infancy if untreated. All known genetic disorders of the urea cycle are inherited as autosomal recessive conditions, except ornithine transcarbamylase (OTC) deficiency, which is X-linked.

The approaches to short-term therapy of ammonia intoxication due to a urea cycle defect are similar, regardless of the particular defect involved. Ammonia removal may be accomplished by exchange transfusion, peritoneal dialysis, or hemodialysis. Hemodialysis appears to be the most effective short-term means of ammonia removal. In addition to general supportive care, which usually requires circulatory and respiratory support, patients with urea cycle disorders require protein-restricted diets to reduce the total nitrogen load. This diet can be accomplished by diluting a standard infant formula in such a way that appropriate fluid and caloric needs are supplied together with a total daily protein intake of approximately 1 g/kg of body weight. Long-term measures to assist in nitrogen removal have included administration of keto acid analogs of essential amino acids, arginine supplementation, and sodium benzoate. A drug comprising sodium benzoate and sodium phenylacetate (Ucephan, Kendall McGaw) has received Food and Drug Administration (FDA) approval for the treatment of urea cycle disorders.

Some older children with disorders of the urea cycle have demonstrated recurrent hyperammonemic episodes that are unresponsive to therapy. In these instances orthotopic hepatic transplantation has been accomplished with satisfactory results.

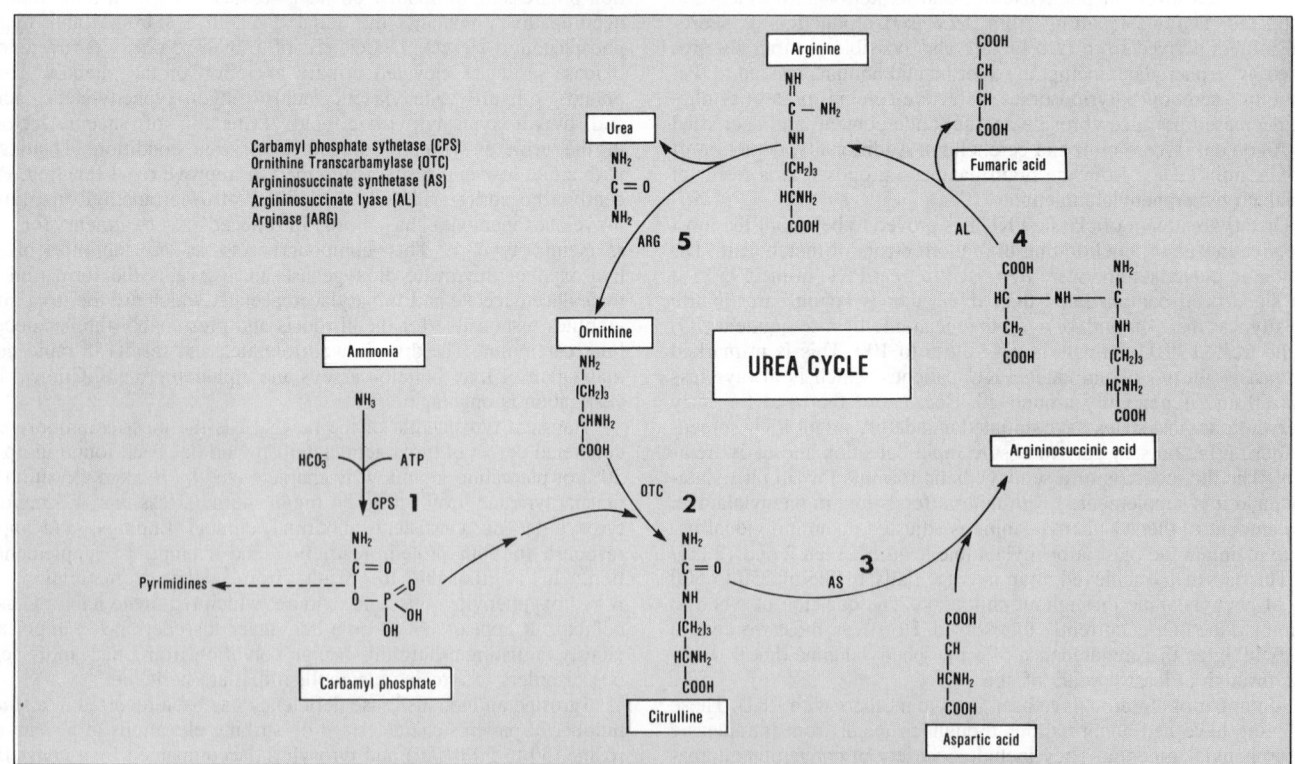

FIGURE 308-1   The urea cycle. Enzymes: *1*, carbamylphosphate synthetase *(CPS)*; *2*, ornithine transcarbamylase *(OTC)*; *3*, argininosuccinate synthetase *(AS)*; *4*, argininosuccinate lyase *(AL)*; *5*, arginase *(ARG)*.

Differential diagnosis of hyperammonemia requires knowledge of the patient's blood ammonia concentration, plasma amino acid and volatile fatty acid pattern, and urinary orotic acid concentration (Table 308-4). Utilization of these data to specify the site of interruption of the urea cycle is described for each condition.

Carbamylphosphate synthetase (CPS) deficiency interrupts the first step in the classic urea cycle and leads to hyperammonemia, vomiting, protein intolerance, lethargy, and seizures. Patients with this condition have manifested symptoms from as early as 1 day of age to as late as several weeks. Hyperammonemia may be moderate (300 to 600 μg/dl; normal is less than 120 μg/dl). Because no other urea cycle intermediates are formed, no specific pattern of metabolites is found on analysis of plasma or urine. Lysine, glutamine, and alanine levels may be elevated as a nonspecific response to hyperammonemia. Urinary orotic acid level is normal or low. Because N-acetylglutamate synthetase activity is inhibited by propionylcoenzyme A (propionyl-CoA), a similar pattern may be seen in propionic acidemia; hence plasma volatile fatty acid determination should be made to rule out this and related conditions. The enzymatic defect should be confirmed in liver.

Ornithine transcarbamylase deficiency is manifested in a manner similar to that of CPS deficiency, except that only males are usually severely affected, owing to the X-linked nature of the disorder. Clinically affected females with a milder course, characterized primarily by protein intolerance, have been described, are thought to represent instances of unfavorable lyonization (inactivation of the normal X chromosome), and may demonstrate only minimal (1% to 5%) residual activity for OTC. Recent studies have shown that some heterozygote females develop hyperammonemic coma during the intrapartum period. One death and several catastrophic episodes of hyperammonemia have been reported from this previously unrecognized condition.

Carbamylphosphate is shunted into the pyrimidine pathway and results in a markedly elevated urinary excretion of orotic acid, distinguishing this condition biochemically from CPS deficiency. Pronounced hyperammonemia (>1000 μg/dl) occurs, accompanied by elevations in plasma alanine, glutamine, and lysine levels, with a reduced concentration of plasma citrulline. Confirmation should be made of the enzymatic deficiency in the liver.

Citrullinemia results from deficiency of argininosuccinic acid synthetase and is inherited as an autosomal recessive disorder. It is characterized by high blood levels of ammonia (1000 to 3000 μg/dl) and citrulline. Urinary orotic acid excretion is also elevated. Clinical symptomatology in the neonatal type of citrullinemia is very similar to the previously described urea cycle disorders with protein intolerance (characterized primarily by vomiting of protein meals) and obtundation occurring early in life. Genetic heterogeneity has been described, including variants with reduced ammonia concentrations and mild or intermediate symptomatology.

Argininosuccinic aciduria results from deficiency of argininosuccinase. It occurs in approximately 1:60,000 live births and presents clinically with seizures, coma, mental retardation, and hyperammonemia. A large proportion of affected patients do not survive infancy. There is marked elevation of argininosuccinic acid in plasma, cerebrospinal fluid, and urine. Fifty percent of patients have demonstrated a characteristic friability of the hair called *trichorrhexis nodosa*. As

in citrullinemia, there is heterogeneity in the clinical expression of this condition. Subacute and late-onset variants have been described, as well as the classic neonatal type that is lethal if untreated. The condition is inherited as an autosomal recessive trait. Biochemical explanation for the variable clinical severity is lacking.

Hyperargininemia results from arginase deficiency and is distinguished from the preceding diseases in that it results in mental retardation but appears not to share the lethal neonatal expression characteristic of the other disorders. It is characterized by marked elevations of arginine in the blood, spinal fluid, and urine, whereas hyperammonemia is variable. The available data are consistent with an autosomal recessive mode of inheritance.

Organic acidemias may cause severe hyperammonemia as a result of inhibition of N-acetylglutamate synthetase by acylcoenzyme A (acyl-CoA) esters. Levels of acyl-CoA esters are elevated in various disorders of branched-chain amino acid metabolism. Any infant with hyperammonemia should have plasma fatty acids measured early in the diagnostic workup to avert use of inappropriate therapy designed for urea cycle disorders.

DISORDERS OF LYSINE METABOLISM

A variety of conditions characterized by elevations in the concentration of lysine in the plasma are known.

Periodic hyperlysinemia associated with hyperammonemia has been described, in which the ammonia level approaches 600 μg/dl. In this condition, oral lysine loading leads to a pronounced elevation in the concentration of ammonia in the blood. A reduced level of hepatic lysine dehydrogenase has been found.

Persistent hyperlysinemia is clinically different from the preceding disorder in that ammonia is not elevated. Mental retardation has been an inconstant finding.

Hyperpipecolatemia has been described in a small number of patients characterized clinically by hypotonia, hepatomegaly, and mental retardation. All known patients with this disorder are males, suggesting an X-linked inheritance pattern. Pipecolic acid is an alternative degradation product of lysine; however, lysine-loading tests in these patients have not produced elevation in the plasma pipecolic acid concentration. The biochemical defect is unknown, and effective therapy for this condition is lacking. Some, but not all, patients with Zellweger's syndrome also have manifested elevation in plasma pipecolate concentration. Patients with Zellweger's syndrome have hypotonia, mental retardation, hepatomegaly, renal cortical cysts, and early death.

DISORDERS OF BRANCHED-CHAIN AMINO ACID METABOLISM

Disorders of the branched-chain amino acids (leucine, isoleucine, and valine) account for the bulk of the organic acidemias, as the majority of defects in the metabolic pathways are located distal to an irreversible decarboxylation that occurs after transamination and thus all subsequent metabolites lack amino groups. Much of the clinical symptomatology is similar within this group of disorders. In the newborn period, symptoms may include protein intolerance and vomiting, lethargy, seizures, profound metabolic acidosis, coma, and death. Some

---

Table 308-4   Laboratory aids in the differential diagnosis of hyperammonemia

CONDITION	AMMONIA	URINARY OROTIC ACID	CITRULLINE	ARGININOSUCCINATE	ARGININE	OTHER
			METABOLIC ABNORMALITY			
CPS deficiency	↑↑↑	N to ↓	Absent to low	N	N	↑ Glutamine and alanine
OTC deficiency	↑↑↑	↑↑	Absent to low	N	N	↑ Glutamine and alanine
Citrullinemia	↑↑↑	↑	↑↑↑	N	N	—
Argininosuccinic aciduria	↑↑	N	↑	↑↑↑	↑	—
Hyperargininemia	↑ to N	↑	N	N	↑↑	—
Transient hyperammonemia	↑↑↑	N	N	N	N	—
Organic acidemias	↑↑	N	N	N	N	Abnormal organic acid excretion

↑↑↑, Marked elevation; ↑↑, moderate elevation; ↑, mild elevation; *N*, normal; *CPS*, carbamylphosphate synthetase; *OTC*, ornithine transcarbamylase.

Table 308-5 Disorders of branched-chain amino acid metabolism

LEUCINE	ISOLEUCINE	VALINE
Hyperleucine-isoleucinemia	Hyperleucine-isoleucinemia	Hypervalinemia
Maple syrup urine disease (MSUD)	MSUD	MSUD
Isovaleric acidemia	Beta-ketothiolase deficiency	Propionic acidemia
Beta-methylcrotonylglyc-inuria	Propionic acidemia	Methylmalonic acid-uria
Beta-hydroxy-beta-methylglutaric acid-uria	Methylmalonic acid-uria	Multiple carboxylase deficiency
Multiple carboxylase deficiency	Multiple carboxylase deficiency	—

of the disorders may also be manifested with hyperammonemia, unusual odors, and hypoglycemia. Survival of the initial episode may be followed by failure to thrive, mental retardation, recurrent attacks of severe ketoacidosis, thrombocytopenia, and neutropenia. All known disorders are inherited as autosomal recessive conditions. Because of the common clinical presentation, identification of the specific defect requires laboratory measurement of the abnormal metabolites that accumulate in blood and urine. This process entails analysis by gas chromatography, GC-MS, and/or high-performance liquid chromatography. Precise identification is essential, as some of these disorders are completely reversible with appropriate dietary therapy and/or vitamin supplementation. The metabolism of these three amino acids proceeds in a series of analogous reactions such that, in one instance, they share a common enzyme (branched-chain keto acid-decarboxylase) and, in others, they feed into a common metabolite (e.g., both valine and isoleucine are metabolized via propionyl-CoA). The disorders associated with each amino acid are given in Table 308-5. The following discussion is limited to the more widely characterized disorders. Many of those disorders lead to a secondary carnitine deficiency due to renal excretion of acyl-carnitine esters. Therapy with 100 to 300 mg/kg/day of L-carnitine can dramatically reduce the episodes of metabolic acidosis.

Maple syrup urine disease (MSUD) is due to a deficiency of the enzyme branched-chain keto acid-decarboxylase, which is common to all three degradation pathways. The disease has a frequency of about 1:220,000 live births and is characterized by a peculiar sweet smell to the urine, which gives this condition its name. This enzymatic deficiency gives rise to accumulation of the branched-chain amino acids and the corresponding keto acids. Leucine concentration is grossly elevated and may reach concentrations 50-fold above normal. As in other inborn errors, the disease has variable clinical expression. The neonatal form manifests itself in the first week of life with vomiting, lethargy, hypertonicity, seizures, and, without appropriate therapy, death in the newborn period. These patients require a special diet low in branched-chain amino acids. Because of its severity and its responsiveness to early treatment, some states have included this condition in newborn screening programs. Milder variants have been described that have later onset of symptoms and intermittent acute episodes that correlate with the stress of infections or protein excess. A thiamine-responsive variant has also been described. This condition shows marked resolution of amino acid and keto acid elevations as well as clinical improvement on doses of thiamine of 10 to 150 mg/day.

Isovaleric acidemia results from a deficiency of isovaleryl-CoA dehydrogenase. It is characterized clinically by overwhelming neonatal illness, with vomiting, ketoacidosis, lethargy, coma, seizures, and a characteristic odor of "sweaty feet." These patients also may demonstrate thrombocytopenia and leukopenia. Isovaleric acid is elevated in plasma several hundredfold during acute episodes but may be only 10- to 50-fold elevated during stable intervals. Urinary isovalerylglycine excretion is relatively constant and provides a helpful diagnostic aid. Short- and long-term management is similar to that

for the other disorders in this pathway. Oral glycine therapy also has been advocated to assist in clearance of isovaleric acid via enhanced excretion of isovalerylglycine. Glycine (100 to 200 mg/kg/day) appears to be an effective treatment.

Propionic acidemia results from deficiency of propionyl-CoA carboxylase, the enzyme that catalyzes conversion of propionate to D-methylmalonate. The enzyme requires biotin as a cofactor. Clinically, these patients manifest overwhelming illness in the neonatal period that may resemble neonatal sepsis. They are lethargic, with metabolic acidosis, ketosis, and hypotonia. Coma and seizures may supervene, with early death occurring in the majority of the untreated patients. Because of inhibition of synthesis of N-acetylglutamate by propionyl-CoA, these patients may have marked hyperammonemia and resemble patients with urea cycle defects. Propionic acid is markedly elevated in plasma as well as urine. Other elevated urinary metabolites include methylcitrate, beta-hydroxypropionate, and propionylglycine. Glycine is characteristically elevated in plasma and urine as well, a finding that led to the original term, *kerotic hyperglycinemia,* for this condition as well as methylmalonic aciduria. The glycine elevation may be due to inhibition of the glycine cleavage enzyme system by the accumulation of branched-chain amino acid metabolites proximal to propionyl-CoA. Short-term care requires cardiorespiratory support, correction of the severe metabolic acidosis, and removal of the excess accumulation of propionic acid and ammonia. This approach is usually accomplished by either peritoneal dialysis or exchange transfusions. Because some patients have been described who responded to biotin, a therapeutic trial of 1 to 5 mg/day of biotin should be performed. Long-term care involves maintenance of a diet low in protein or use of special formulas low in the branched-chain amino acids. These patients can exhibit good metabolic control and acceptable growth and development on diets supplying 1.0 to 1.5 g/kg/day of protein.

Methylmalonic aciduria results from an enzymatic defect in the conversion of D-methylmalonic acid to succinic acid, or from a defect in the pathway for vitamin B_{12} transport and activation. These patients are clinically similar to patients with propionic acidemia, but they also may demonstrate hypoglycemia, neutropenia, thrombocytopenia, hyperammonemia, perammonemia, and hyperglycinemia. The diagnosis rests on demonstration of methylmalonic acid in plasma or urine. Because methylmalonic acid can decarboxylate to propionic acid during gas chromatographic analysis, it is important to assay each supposed propionic (acidemic) directly for methylmalonic acid by a colorimetric or other assay. Several variants of this condition are known, some of which are vitamin B_{12}-responsive. Again, an early therapeutic trial to determine vitamin responsiveness is indicated. Other disorders of branched-chain amino acid metabolism are listed in Table 308-5. They generally are rare in the newborn population and require extensive diagnostic evaluation.

Biotinidase deficiency deserves discussion because of the gratifying response biotin produces in these patients (Figs. 308-2 and 308-3). This disorder is not truly a defect in branched-chain amino acid metabolism per se; rather, it results from an inability to properly metabolize the vitamin biotin. Because four carboxylases require biotin as a cofactor (propionyl-CoA, acetyl-CoA, beta-methylcrotonyl-CoA, and pyruvate carboxylase), many metabolic ramifications result from this defect. Patients demonstrate ketosis, lactic acidosis, alopecia, ataxia, and developmental delay. The condition results from a defect in biotinidase, which releases biotin from the lysine moieties of dietary protein. A striking clinical response to 1 to 10 mg/day of oral biotin is found. Some states have now instituted newborn screening programs for biotinidase deficiency.

DISORDERS OF METABOLISM OF SULFUR-CONTAINING AMINO ACIDS

Homocystinuria may result from the following causes: a deficiency of cystathionine synthetase (which catalyzes the conversion of methionine to cystathionine), from a block in the metabolism of N^5-methyltetrahydrofolate (the methyl donor in the above reaction) or from deranged vitamin B_{12} metabolism. Classic homocystinuria resulting from cystathionine synthetase deficiency is characterized by elevations in plasma homocystine and methionine up to 100 times normal. This enzymatic deficiency shows autosomal recessive inheritance, and the clinical phenotype includes failure to thrive, light com-

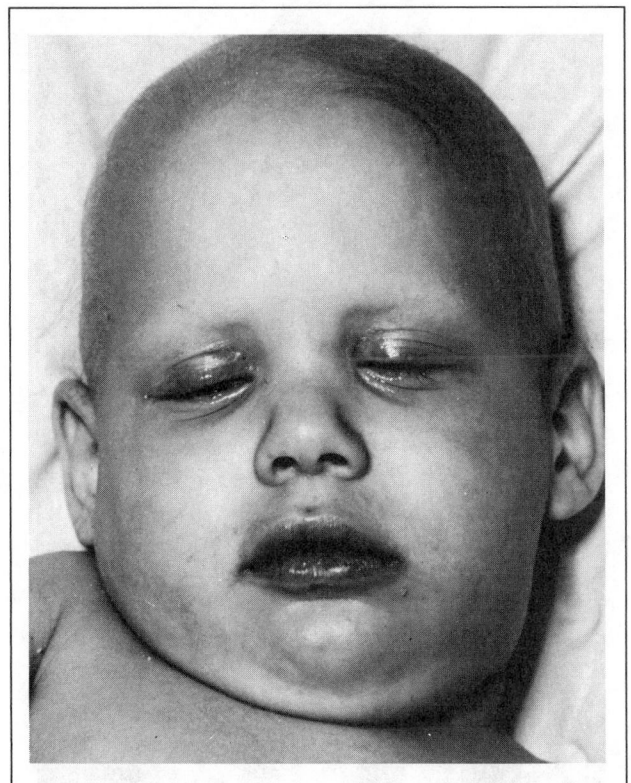

FIGURE 308-2   A girl (2 years, 9 months old) with biotinidase deficiency at the time of diagnosis.

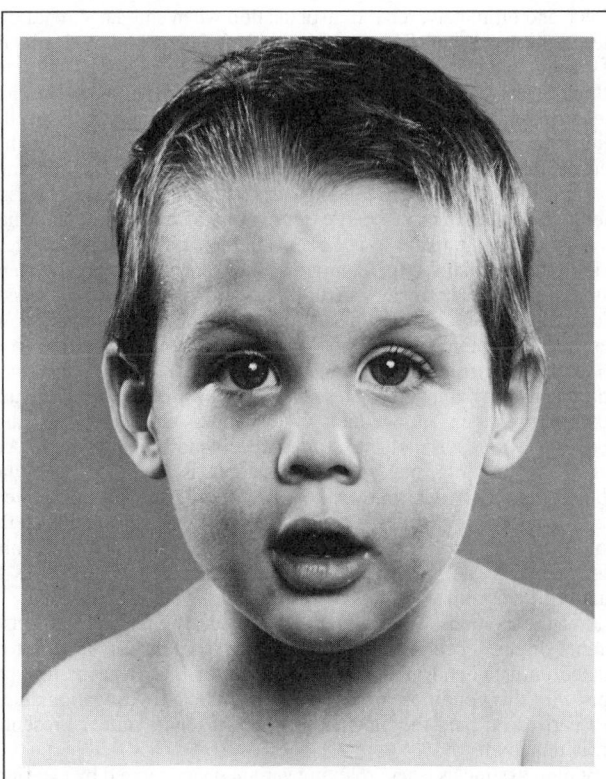

FIGURE 308-3   The same patient as in Fig. 308-2 after 4 months of oral biotin, 10 mg/day.

plexion, and mental retardation. Patients also may demonstrate marfanoid habitus, and ectopia lentis develops by 3 years of age. The primary clinical disabilities are life-threatening venous and arterial thromboses, the biochemical explanation for which has not been elucidated. Therapeutic measures advocated include diets low in methionine and supplemented with cystine to avert the abnormal biochemical consequences of this block. Proof of effectiveness of this therapy is still accumulating. Some patients respond to large doses of vitamin B₆.

Cystathioninuria results from deficiency of cystathionase, which catalyzes the conversion of cystathionine to cysteine; the disorder appears to be the result of an autosomal recessive trait. A consistent clinical pattern in this condition has not been observed. Some patients are retarded, whereas others have normal intelligence.

Other disorders of sulfur-containing amino acid metabolism include sulfite oxidase deficiency, beta-mercaptolactate-cysteine disulfiduria, glutathionuria, and taurinuria. These patients generally are discovered as a result of either mass screening programs in retarded populations or a specific metabolic evaluation in a retarded patient.

MISCELLANEOUS DISORDERS OF AMINO ACID METABOLISM

Nonketotic hyperglycinemia results from a defect in the glycine cleavage enzyme system. It appears to be transmitted as an autosomal recessive trait and is manifested either as overwhelming disease in the newborn period, with coma, seizures, and death, or more gradually as failure to thrive and mental retardation. It is characterized clinically by massive elevation in the concentration of glycine in plasma, cerebral spinal fluid, and urine, without other abnormal metabolic findings. These signs distinguish the condition from the hyperglycinemia that accompanies propionic acidemia and methylmalonic aciduria. Effective therapy for this condition has not been devised, although some beneficial results have been reported from the use of sodium benzoate and/or dextromethorphan.

Retinal gyrate atrophy is the result of ornithine-delta-amino-

transferase deficiency. It produces a characteristic atrophic degeneration of retina and choroid and results initially in night blindness, followed by loss of peripheral vision leading to blindness during the fifth decade. The patients have a characteristic hyperornithinemia that responds to a diet low in arginine. Stabilization of visual function has been achieved on a low-protein diet.

DISORDERS OF AMINO ACID STORAGE
Cystinosis

The term *cystinosis* refers to disorders whose major biochemical characteristic is intralysosomal storage of the disulfide amino acid cystine in most body tissues. Cystine crystals may be seen in the cornea by slit-lamp examination as an aid to diagnosis. These crystals also are found in bone marrow aspirates and biopsies of rectal mucosa. There is marked heterogeneity of clinical expression, but all forms appear to be inherited as autosomal recessive traits. The clinical categories that have been distinguished are termed *infantile nephropathic, juvenile,* and *benign.*

Infantile nephropathic cystinosis is characterized by the onset within the first year of life of the renal Fanconi syndrome (aminoaciduria, glycosuria, proteinuria, phosphaturia, polyuria); failure to thrive; and photophobia, retinopathy, and keratopathy. Children with this condition have fair skin and blond hair if they are white. Nonwhites generally appear to have lighter skin coloration than other family members. At about the fourth or fifth year of life, failure of glomerular filtration occurs, progressing to end-stage renal disease by the end of the first decade of life. Renal rickets also occurs concomitantly with the renal failure. Many patients also develop hypothyroidism by 10 years of age (Chapter 297).

The cause of cystine accumulation within cystinotic lysosomes is now known to be a defective lysosomal transport system for cystine. In normal lysosomes, the transport system removes cystine residues from the lysosomal compartment. The relationship between lysosomal cystine storage and clinical symptomatology has not been established.

Therapy for this disorder has traditionally included salt and water replacement, treatment with vitamin D for the vitamin D–resistant rickets, and ultimately, renal transplantation when end-stage renal disease has been reached. The transplanted kidney parenchymal cells do not accumulate cystine, and the transplantation experience in patients with cystinosis is parallel to that in patients of similar age who have received transplanted kidneys for other causes. Attempts at specific therapy for cystinosis have included a cystine-free diet, which has been demonstrated to be unhelpful and perhaps harmful, and a variety of agents directed at reducing intralysosomal cystine. The first among these agents to be tried extensively was dithiothreitol, which has been demonstrated to lower circulating leukocyte cystine concentrations. Unfortunately, the compound has considerable toxicity and is unpleasant to administer. Ascorbic acid has been tried because it reduces the cystine content of cystinotic fibroblasts in culture; however, a double-blind clinical trial revealed no beneficial effect from this agent. Subsequently, a clinical trial of cysteamine therapy was undertaken in cystinosis, because it is the most efficient compound known for reducing intracellular cystine in tissue culture. Cysteamine therapy for nephropathic cystinosis received FDA approval in August 1994. The drug, marketed as Cystagon, is produced by Mylan Laboratories, Inc (Morgantown, WV). The drug has been relatively free of side effects except for nausea and vomiting attributable to the thiol odor and taste. When provided early and consistently, ideally before age 2 years, Cystagon preserves renal function and leads to enhanced linear growth.

Juvenile cystinosis is an intermediate variety in which the onset of renal disease occurs later, and end-stage renal disease may not be reached until the end of the second decade of life. Because few patients with this condition are known, few clinical investigations have been carried out and the biochemical reason for its milder presentation is unknown.

Benign cystinosis is a perplexing variant characterized by eye findings similar to those of the other forms, but no other clinical signs or symptoms. These patients are usually discovered during routine ophthalmologic examinations. The inheritance pattern is autosomal recessive, and the biochemical abnormality that permits heterogeneity in this condition has not yet been determined.

Alkaptonuria

Alkaptonuria was described in 1908 by Garrod. Inherited as an autosomal recessive condition, it is due to inability to further metabolize homogentisic acid, a tyrosine metabolite, to maleylacetoacetic acid. Homogentisic acid in urine oxidizes spontaneously to dark pigmentary material, drawing its presence to medical attention. The condition is usually asymptomatic until the fourth decade of life, when accumulation of homogentisic acid leads to ochronosis with pigmentary deposits in the sclera, ears, and other exposed cartilage. Ultimately, the joints and tendons become generally involved and degenerative arthritis occurs (Chapter 209). No effective treatment for the degenerative changes has been described.

DISORDERS OF AMINO ACID TRANSPORT
Cystinuria

Cystinuria is an autosomal recessive condition characterized by marked hyperexcretion of the amino acids cystine, lysine, ornithine, and arginine (Chapter 111). These amino acids share the structural characteristics of two amino groups separated by four to six intervening atoms and also share a common epithelial transport mechanism. Cystinuria results from a disorder of epithelial transport for these compounds, both in the intestinal mucosa and in the renal tubule. The clinical symptomatology, however, results solely from the hyperexcretion of cystine, the least-soluble amino acid. Precipitation of cystine in situ leads to the formation of renal and bladder calculi, which produce the potential for obstruction and infection and lead patients to seek medical attention. Pure cystine calculi are visible on x-ray films because of high sulfur content but are more radiolucent than calcium-containing stones. The diagnosis may be suspected by the nitroprusside test, which gives a pink color reaction in urine containing more than approximately 100 μg of cystine per milligram of urinary creatinine. The diagnosis is confirmed by qualitative or quantitative assessment of the other amino acids in urine. In the United States, the incidence is estimated at approximately 1 in 7000, mak-

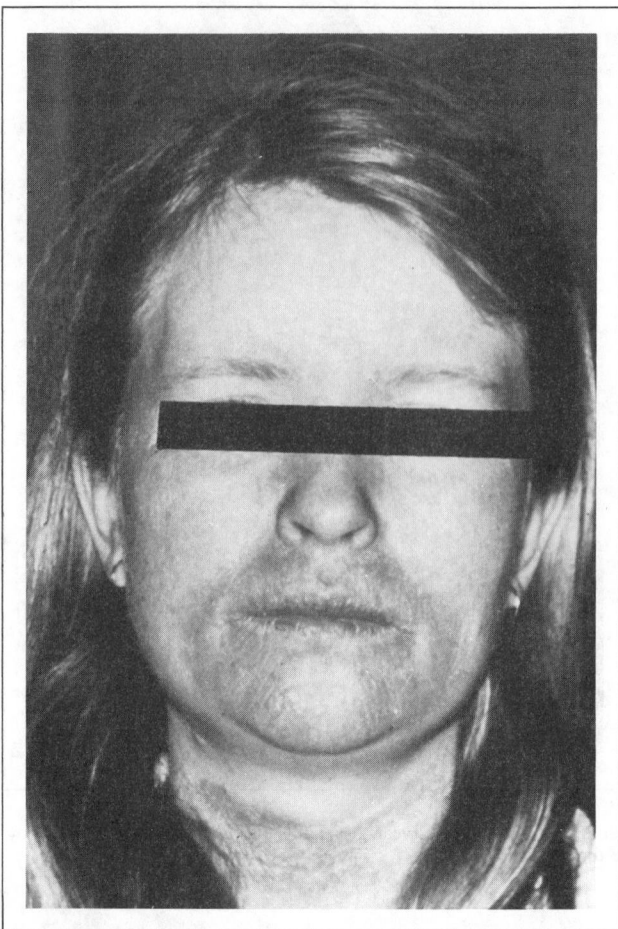

FIGURE 308-4　A patient with Hartnup's disease. Eczematoid rash is present on face and neck.
Courtesy Dr. F. Navab.

ing this one of the most common inborn errors. Therapy is directed toward maintaining cystine in solution, a goal that can be accomplished by maintaining a neutral or basic urinary pH and increasing urine flow. A usual regimen requires treatment with alkalinizing agents and maintaining fluid intake between 4 and 8 L per day. Additionally, penicillamine has been proposed for enhancing the solubility of cystine because penicillamine forms a mixed disulfide with cystine that is markedly more soluble than cystine itself. Treatment with 1 to 3 g D-penicillamine per day has been demonstrated to enhance cystine excretion and to prevent renal calculi formation. Existing calculi also may be dissolved. However, penicillamine therapy may produce adverse side effects, primarily in the form of fever, erythematous skin rash, and arthralgias. These side effects usually reverse when therapy is stopped, and, in many instances, penicillamine may then be reintroduced at a slower rate of administration without recurrence of adverse reactions.

Other Amino Acid Transport Disorders

Hyperdibasic aminoaciduria results from an apparently isolated defect in renal and intestinal transport of lysine, arginine, and ornithine. Its existence indicates that there is an alternative transport system for these three amino acids that is not shared by cystine, and absence of increased cystine excretion distinguishes this disorder from cystinuria. Clinically, the disease is characterized by diarrhea, intestinal malabsorption, and growth retardation with, in a few instances, mental retardation. The disease appears to respond to treatment with a low-protein diet.

Familial iminoglycinuria results in the excretion of increased

✔ *WHEN TO REFER*

Disorders of amino acid metabolism produce a wide spectrum of clinical disabilities. For this reason, referral needs range from urgent to elective. Patients with cardiovascular catastrophe incident to homocystinuria require emergent referral for treatment of the cardiovascular accident, as well as dietary management to attempt to reduce the risk of future thromboses. Patients with well-managed disorders require referral for genetic counseling as they contemplate reproduction. Appropriate referral for the numerous rare disorders encompassed in this chapter requires access to information on a wide variety of topics. One such compendium is listed in the references *(Physicians' Guide to Rare Diseases)*. Additional sources may be found by contacting the National Organization for Rare Disorders (1(800) 447-NORD).

quantities of glycine and hydroxyproline. This observation gave rise to the hypothesis, since confirmed, that these two amino acids share a common transport system in the kidney. No clinical abnormalities have been reported, and it appears to be inherited as an autosomal recessive trait.

Hartnup's disease results from a defect in transport of the "neutral" amino acids, which include alanine, serine, threonine, valine, leucine, isoleucine, phenylalanine, tyrosine, tryptamine, and histidine. These compounds are elevated fivefold to tenfold above normal in the urine of these patients. The condition is inherited as an autosomal recessive trait. Clinical features include a pellagra-like eczematoid, photosensitive rash of the extremities and face (Fig. 308-4); some inconstant neurologic symptoms including nystagmus, ataxia, tremor, and diplopia; and psychiatric disturbances ranging from emotional lability to frank hallucinations. Mental retardation is also an inconstant finding. The clinical features appear episodically and have been precipitated by sulfonamide therapy, exposure to sunlight, fever, or other stress. There is considerable similarity between this condition and pellagra, which results from dietary nicotinamide deficiency. Therapy with nicotinamide has resulted in improvement in both the skin and neurologic abnormalities.

Lowe's syndrome results in the renal Fanconi syndrome and is accompanied by X-linked inheritance, congenital cataracts, buphthalmos, failure to thrive, severe mental retardation, and hypotonia. The biochemical defect in this condition has not been identified.

BIBLIOGRAPHY

Brusilow S et al: Treatment of episodic hyperammonemia in children with inborn errors of urea synthesis, *N Engl J Med* 310:1630, 1984.

Buchanan D, Thoene J: Dual-column high-performance liquid chromatographic urinary organic acid profiling, *Anal Biochem* 124:108, 1982.

Chalmers R, Lawson A: *Organic acids in man,* London, 1982, Chapman and Hall.

Gahl W et al: Cysteamine therapy for children with nephropathic cystinosis, *N Engl J Med* 316:971-977, 1987.

Hamosh A et al: Dextromethorphan and high-dose benzoate therapy for nonketotic hyperglycinemia in an infant, *J Pediatr* 121(1):131-135, 1992.

Lindstedt S et al: Treatment of hereditary tyrosinaemia type I by inhibition of 4-hydroxyphenylpyruvate dioxygenase, *Lancet* 340:813-817, 1992.

Msall M et al: Neurologic outcome in children with inborn errors of urea synthesis, *N Engl J Med* 310:1500, 1984.

Nyhan W: *Abnormalities in amino acid metabolism in clinical medicine,* Norwalk, Conn, 1984, Appleton-Century-Crofts.

Scriver C et al, editors: *The metabolic basis of inherited disease,* ed 7, New York, 1995, McGraw-Hill.

Thoene J, editor: *Physician's guide to rare diseases,* ed 2, Montvale, NJ, 1995, Dowden.

Thoene J, Wolf B: Biotinidase deficiency in juvenile multiple carboxylase deficiency, *Lancet* 1:398, 1983.

309 Lysosomal Storage Diseases

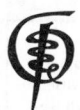

Alan J. Garber

Cellular composition is determined by the balance of degradation and resynthesis of intracellular components. Cells must adapt to changing internal and external demands by altering their structural and functional composition. The process of component turnover not only salvages damaged or degraded components but is essential to redirect ongoing processes toward new needs. For example, protein degradation rates are increased in both regenerating liver and hypertrophying muscle. Although in these states there is overall net synthesis, substantial redirection and adaptation are required. Lysosomes, cytoplasmic organelles containing hydrolytic enzymes, are the major site for the degradation of structural and functional cellular components; therefore, defects in lysosomal function impair cellular adaptive change and ultimately induce a loss of cellular function.

LYSOSOMAL PHYSIOLOGY

Lysosomes contain a host of degradative enzymes that are maximally active at an acid pH. The interior of the lysosome is maintained at about pH 4.5 by an adenosine triphosphate–dependent proton pump. Lysosomal enzymes are synthesized on the rough endoplasmic reticulum and processed as they pass through the endoplasmic reticula. A crucial step in this pathway is the addition of mannose 6-phosphate residues. This addition is generated by a two-step process. N-acetylglucosamine-1-phosphate is transferred to mannose residues, generating a phosphodiester. N-acetylglucosamine is then removed, leaving the mannose 6-phosphate residue as a lysosomal enzyme recognition marker. Receptors for mannose 6-phosphate reside on the specialized areas of the smooth endoplasmic reticulum that are destined to become the lysosome. These receptors bind the mannose 6-phosphate-labeled enzymes. As the new organelle is formed, it thereby incorporates lysosomal enzymes within it. Lysosomes internalize and subsequently degrade endogenous or exogenous materials. In addition to the ongoing degradation of endogenous cellular constituents, lysosomes are important to metabolize low-density lipoproteins (LDLs) and some hormones via endocytosis and subsequent incorporation.

The concept of a lysosomal storage disease was first formulated by Hers to explain the pathogenesis of Pompe's disease, in which the histologic appearance of intracellular organelles filled with amorphous material results from a deficiency in lysosomal acid maltase. These findings correlate with progressive muscular dysfunction as described in Chapter 305. Lysosomal storage diseases were originally defined as a deficiency of a single lysosomal enzyme activity that causes undegraded material to accumulate within the lysosomes, leading to progressive disease. Subsequently, other lysosomal storage diseases were identified in which defects of lysosomal physiology cause multiple enzymatic defects (see ML II).

GENERAL CONSIDERATIONS

Dozens of lysosomal storage diseases have been identified. The most common have been grouped according to similarities in their clinical presentation, the biochemistry of the accumulated materials, and the enzymatic deficiencies involved. The schema in Fig. 309-1 attempts to guide the clinician toward a discrete group of diagnostic possibilities from among the many diseases described.

First, a reasonable index of suspicion is necessary. In infants and children, the classic findings of coarse facies with organomegaly, immobile joints, skeletal changes, and mental retardation suggest a mucopolysaccharide storage disease or mucolipidosis. Neurologic signs such as loss of developmental milestones, hypotonia or spasticity, exaggerated startle reflexes, or seizures are also indicative of lysosomal storage diseases, particularly the lipidoses. Clinical findings may be

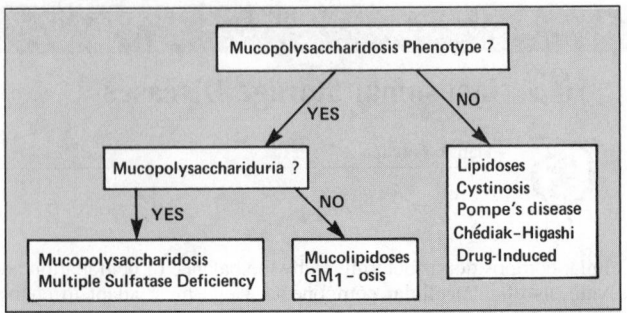

FIGURE 309-1   Approach to the diagnosis of lysosomal storage diseases.

more subtle in adults, but progressive organomegaly, skeletal anomalies, mental retardation, affective disorders, and visual or auditory deficits all suggest a lysosomal disorder. The hallmark of lysosomal storage disease is the engorged lysosome. Circulating leukocytes, conjunctival biopsy specimens, and cultured cells may all show cytoplasmic inclusions. The inclusions may display distinct morphology in light and electron microscopy and thus lead to a specific diagnosis. The biochemical demonstration of a specific enzyme deficiency is required for definitive diagnosis. Most lysosomal diseases may be diagnosed by assay of enzymes in circulating leukocytes, biopsy material, or cultured fibroblasts. The latter is often used for prenatal diagnosis by amniocentesis.

The great clinical heterogeneity seen within these diseases may occur for many reasons. Different isoenzyme deficiencies may produce different functional losses with the same observed total activity. Different mutations within the same structural gene may produce total or partial defects in enzymolysis; partial blocks produce lower activity but may also produce different substrate affinities. The loss of an activating factor may also impair enzymatic activity, without a mutation in the enzyme itself.

The impact of the loss of enzymatic activity will be serious when the enzymatic activity is crucial for cellular function. Disorders of mucopolysaccharides affect virtually all tissues. Gangliosidoses primarily affect the brain, and cystinosis affects the kidney, in which sulfhydryl exchange is active. Additionally, these diseases affect the young, in whom turnover and remodeling are great. Diseases mild enough to spare the patient until adulthood manifest more subtle lesions and are perhaps the greatest diagnostic challenges among the lysosomal storage diseases.

MUCOPOLYSACCHARIDOSES

The mucopolysaccharidoses constitute a class of diseases characterized by an inability to completely degrade mucopolysaccharides. Mucopolysaccharides are nitrogenous polysaccharides that, when conjugated to core proteins, form the glycosaminoglycans. Enzymatic defects lead to the accumulation of mucopolysaccharides and chemically similar substrates within the lysosome. Because mucopolysaccharides are found throughout the body, it is understandable that most organ systems are affected by these diseases.

The organ systems most commonly affected include bone, viscera, connective tissue, and brain. Dysostosis multiplex denotes the characteristic bony abnormalities of widening of the medial clavicle, widening and shortening of the long bones, flattening of the ribs, beaking of the vertebrae with lumbar kyphosis, and enlargement of the sella turcica. Dysostosis multiplex is fully expressed in Hurler's disease and is present to some degree in most of the mucopolysaccharidoses. Hepatosplenomegaly is a frequent finding, as is asymptomatic carpal tunnel syndrome. Coarse facies, a depressed nasal bridge, corneal clouding, retinal disease, optic nerve swelling, and later atrophy, joint stiffness, deafness, cardiovascular anomalies, and neurologic abnormalities may all be present to a variable extent (Fig. 309-2). In particular, the degree of skeletal dysplasia and the presence or absence of corneal clouding or mental retardation may be useful in the differential diagnosis (Table 309-1). All mucopolysaccharidoses follow an

autosomal recessive inheritance except for the X-linked mucopolysaccaridosis (MPS) II (Hunter's disease) and may be diagnosed in utero by enzyme assay of cultured amniotic fibroblasts or through chorionic villus sampling. The detection of the carrier state of MPS types I, III, IV, and VI has not been reliable, owing to the overlapping of enzymatic activity values with those from normal individuals. MPS II heterozygotes may be diagnosed by the assay of cloned fibroblasts. Roughly half of the clones will be enzyme deficient by virtue of the random deactivation of X chromosomes in the carrier female.

MPS IH (Hurler's Syndrome)

MPS IH is the prototypic mucopolysaccharidosis. After the first few months of life, physical and mental abnormalities become obvious and usually prove fatal within the first decade. Physical changes include dysostosis multiplex; hepatosplenomegaly; joint stiffness with claw hands; and a large head with coarse, thickened features (Fig. 309-2, *A*). Corneal clouding is a constant feature in this disease. Mental development slows and regresses after the first year. Cardiovascular abnormalities with valvular heart disease, pulmonary hypertension, and pulmonary insufficiency all lead to early mortality. The specific defect in alpha-L-iduronidase prevents normal catabolism of dermatan sulfate and heparan sulfate. Urinary mucopolysaccharides contain dermatan sulfate and heparan sulfate in a ratio of about 7:3.

MPS IS (Scheie's Syndrome)

MPS IS is also caused by a defect in alpha-L-iduronidase, the same enzyme activity lacking in MPS IH. Although it seems likely that MPS IH and MPS IS are allelic mutations at the same locus, it remains to be explained how MPS IS also can have no demonstrable enzyme activity but display much less clinical severity than MPS IH. These patients enjoy a nearly normal life span and intelligence. Physical findings include corneal clouding, cardiovascular disease, and normal stature despite stiff joints and genu valgum (Fig. 309-2, *B*). The face is coarse, with a broad mouth. Retinitis pigmentosa may develop. Diagnosis rests with the demonstration of alpha-L-iduronidase deficiency in the presence of only moderate physical abnormalities. Urinary mucopolysaccharides contain dermatan sulfate and heparan sulfate in a ratio of about 3:2.

MPS I (Iduronidase Deficiency)

A third MPS I, alpha-L-iduronidase-deficient phenotype has been reported. These patients present with physical features intermediate between MPS IH and MPS IS, with fair preservation of intelligence. This phenotype, termed *Hurler-Scheie syndrome* (MPS IH/IS), has been considered a compound of Hurler and Scheie alleles. However, reports of several patients from consanguineous parentage suggest the existence of a third independent allele.

MPS II (Hunter's Syndrome)

MPS II is an X-linked disorder that produces a phenotype similar to, but less severe than, MPS IH. The lack of corneal clouding is a useful feature for differentiation. MPS II derives from a deficiency in iduronate sulfatase that causes urinary excretion of equal proportions of dermatan sulfate and keratan sulfate. The occurrence of enzymatically proved MPS II in females may be due to rare homozygosity, codominance, or an autosomal variant. Heterozygous females may be detected by enzyme assay of cloned fibroblasts. Two clinically distinct subtypes may be distinguished within this syndrome: severe and mild. Both subtypes segregate as an X-linked disorder.

The severe form of MPS II is distinguished by the development between the second and sixth year of life of physical defects including deafness, stiff joints, coarse facies, and skeletal abnormalities (Fig. 309-2, *C*). Mental deterioration follows. Death from respiratory and cardiovascular disease usually occurs in the second decade. The mild form of MPS II causes only mild physical abnormalities, which may include joint stiffness, carpal tunnel syndrome, short stature, deafness, and retinal dystrophy. Mental status may be normal or mildly retarded. Most patients survive between three and six decades.

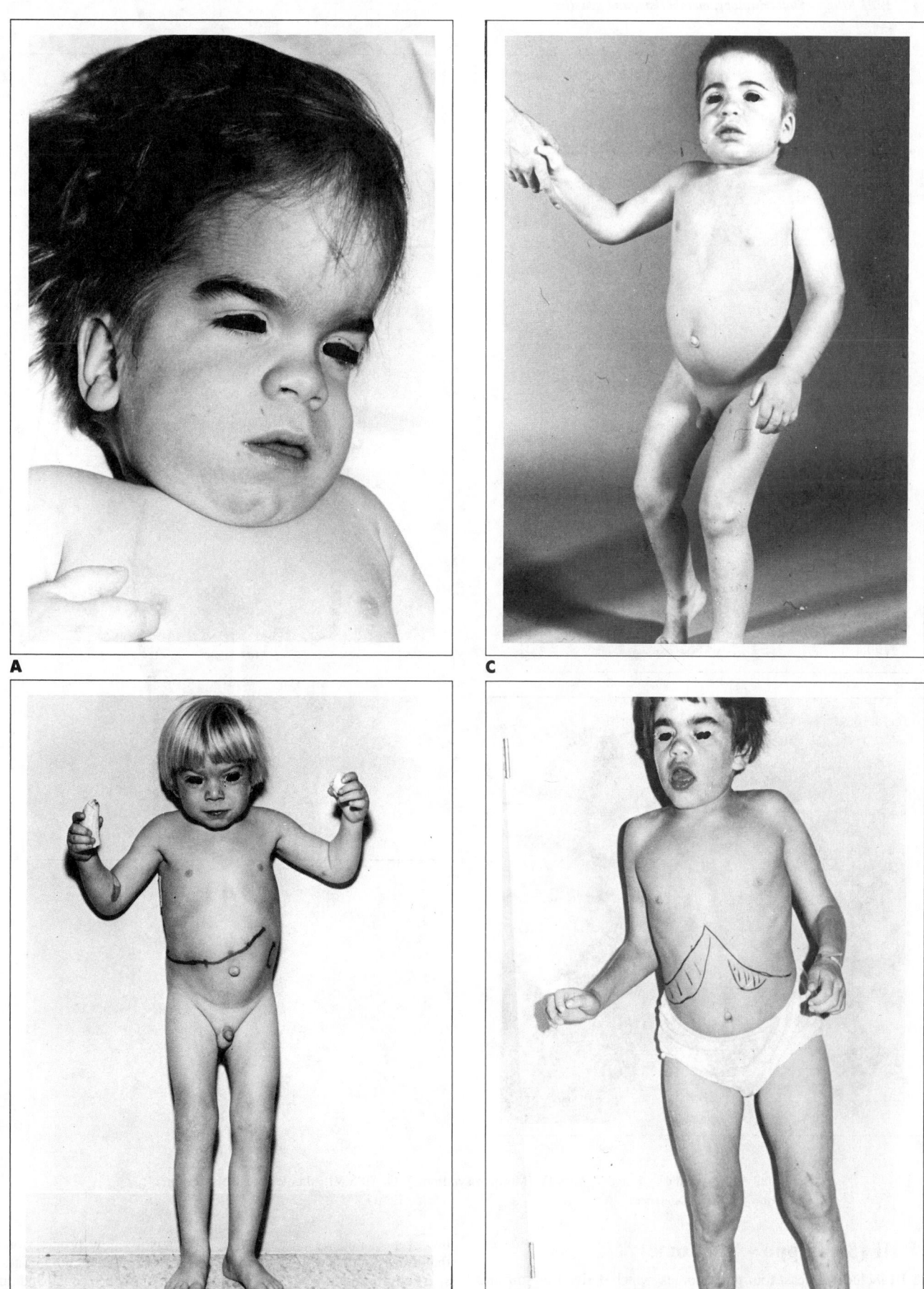

FIGURE 309-2 Physical characteristics of patients with mucopolysaccharidosis (MPS). **A,** MPS IH (Hurler's disease). **B,** MPS IS (Scheie's syndrome). **C,** MPS II (Hunter's syndrome). **D,** MPS III (Sanfilippo's syndrome).

Continued

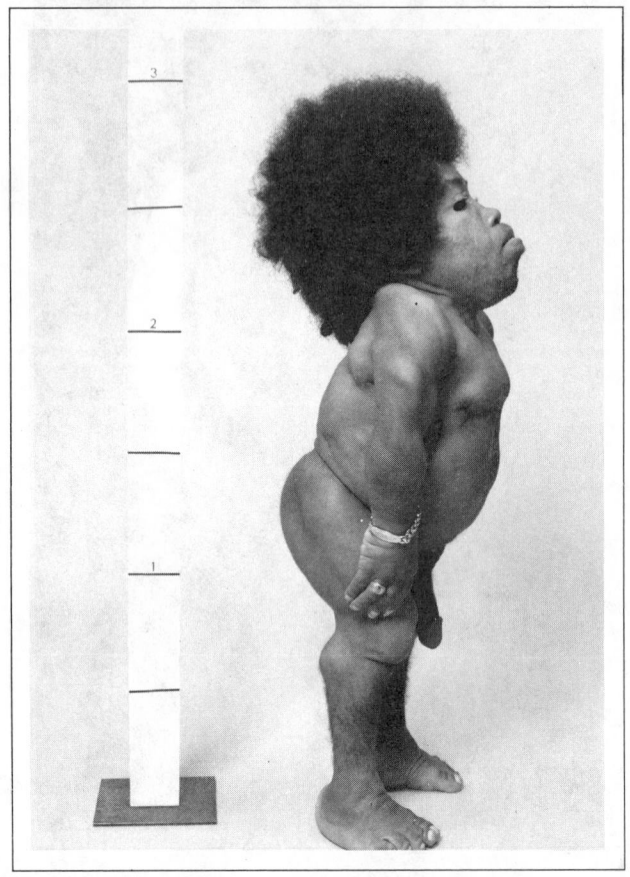

E

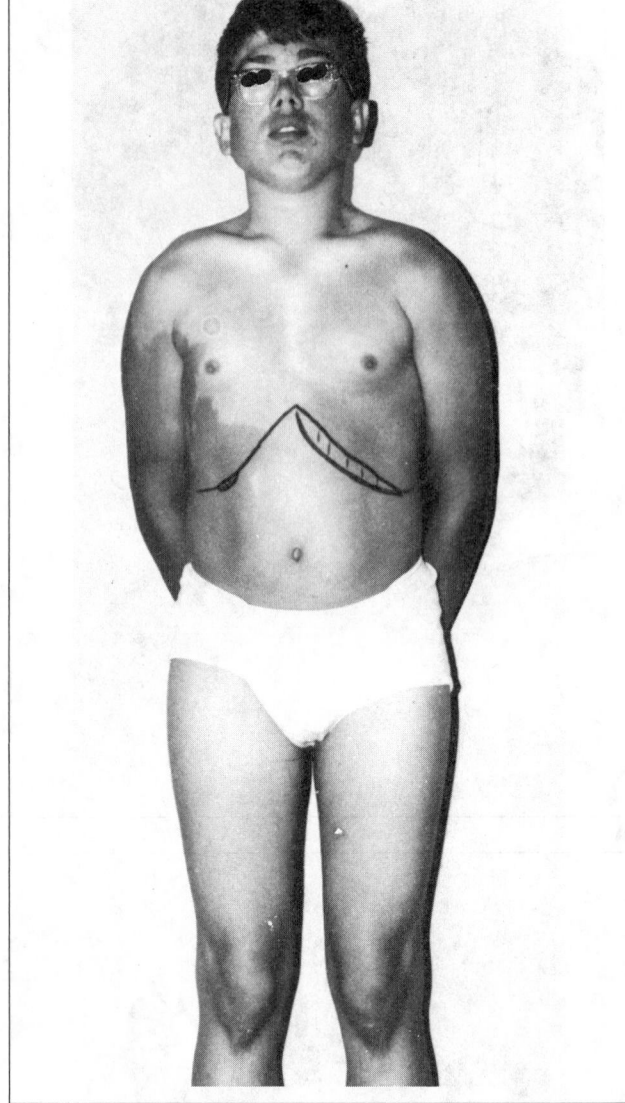

G

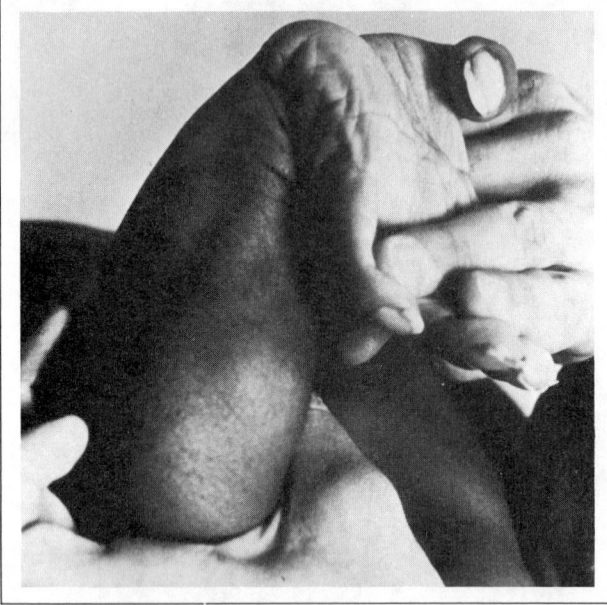

F

FIGURE 309-2—cont'd **E** and **F,** MPS IV (Morquio syndrome). **G,** MPS VI (Maroteaux-Lamy syndrome). Courtesy Dr. Nicola Diferrante.

MPS III (Sanfilippo's Syndrome)

MPS III includes at least four phenocopies, which derive from different enzymatic defects. The clinical presentation begins between 2 and 4 years of age. First, there is loss of neurologic milestones, and this is followed by facial coarsening (Fig. 309-2, *D*), joint stiffness, and mild organomegaly reminiscent of mild MPS I. Corneal clouding,

however, is notably absent. There is relatively slow progression of the disease, with severe neurologic deficits, severe mental retardation, spasticity, and seizures. Death is most common in the second and third decades. MPS III is currently divided into subtypes A, B, C, and D, each with a unique enzyme deficiency. All types show mild to moderate mucopolysacchariduria, with a predominance of heparan sulfate. Type A results from a deficiency of heparan-N-sulfatase; type B, from

Table 309-1   The mucopolysaccharidoses

DESIGNATION	DISTINGUISHING CHARACTERISTICS	URINARY MPS	EPONYM	ENZYME DEFICIENCY
MPS IH	Severe MPS phenotype, mental retardation, corneal clouding, early death (first decade)	Dermatan sulfate Heparan sulfate	Hurler	Alpha-L-iduronidase
MPS IS	Mild MPS involvement with nearly normal intelligence and stature, corneal clouding, normal life span	Dermatan sulfate Heparan sulfate	Scheie's	Alpha-L-iduronidase
MPS II	Mild: Mild MPS, short stature, mental retardation with nearly normal life span, X-linked, clear corneas	Dermatan sulfate Heparan sulfate	Hunter's	Iduronate sulfatase
	Severe: Moderate MPS with mental retardation, deteriorating in second decade, X-linked, clear corneas			
MPS III	Mild MPS with clear corneas, severe mental retardation with neurologic decay	Heparan sulfate	Sanfilippo's	Type A: heparan-N-sulfatase Type B: N-acetylglucosaminidase Type C: acetyl-CoA glucosamide-N-acetyltransferase Type D: N-acetyl-alpha-D-glucosamine-6-sulfatase
MPS IV, A, B	Severe skeletal involvement with odontoid hypoplasia, lax joints, corneal clouding, normal intelligence	Keratan	Morquio	A: N-acetylgalactose sulfatase B: Beta-galactosidase
MPS V	Vacant			
MPS VI	Mild: Mild MPS phenotype, short stature, normal intelligence, corneal clouding, striking metachromatic inclusions	Dermatan sulfate	Maroteaux-Lamy	N-acetylhexosamine-4-sulfate sulfatase (arylsulfatase B)
	Severe: Moderate MPS phenotype with mortality in second decade, odontoid hypoplasia, normal intelligence, corneal clouding, striking metachromatic inclusions			
MPS VII	MPS phenotype with odontoid hypoplasia and corneal clouding, mild to moderate retardation (very heterogeneous)	Dermatan sulfate	Sly	Beta-glucuronidase

N-acetyl-alpha-glucosaminidase deficiency; type C, from a deficiency of acetyl-CoA-alpha-glucosamide-N-acetyltransferase; and type D from N-acetyl-alpha-D-glucosamine-6-sulfatase. Diagnosis depends on the clinical presentation of characteristic physical changes, severe mental degeneration, urinary excretion of heparan sulfate, and the identification of a specific enzyme deficiency.

MPS IV (Morquio's Syndrome)

Morquio's syndrome displays unique physical findings among the mucopolysaccharidoses. Skeletal abnormalities predominate (Fig. 309-2, *E*), with prominence of the lower ribs after the first year of life, spatulate ribs, flattening of the vertebra with kyphosis, and later osteoporosis. A constant and striking feature is hypoplasia of the odontoid process. This anomaly often leads to cervical compression and myelopathy, which may be a major source of morbidity. Corneal clouding and aortic valve disease are frequent findings. In contradistinction to MPS types I to III, the joints are lax with notable wrist instability (Fig. 309-2, *F*). Intellectual development is normal in MPS IV. The major sources of morbidity and mortality are respiratory insufficiency, cord compression, and cardiovascular disease. Two enzyme defects have been associated with the Morquio phenotype. Morquio A (MPS IVA) was originally described with deficiency of N-acetylgalactose sulfatase activity. A more recently described phenocopy, denoted Morquio B (MPS IVB), reveals a deficiency in beta-galactoside in which some residual activity toward GM$_1$ ganglioside avoids the presentation of frank GM$_1$ gangliosidosis.

MPS V

This classification, formerly held by Scheie's syndrome, is vacant since the discovery that Scheie's and Hurler's syndromes result from defects at the same gene locus.

MPS VI (Maroteaux-Lamy Syndrome)

The clinical picture of MPS VI shows great heterogeneity. The severe form manifests in the second or third year of life and resembles MPS I, with kyphosis, anterior sternal protrusion, restricted joints, corneal clouding, and coarse facies (Fig. 309-2, *G*). Hydrocephalus and cervical cord compression may also develop owing to odontoid hypoplasia. Mortality often occurs in the second decade. A mild form characterized by corneal clouding, short stature, and inguinal hernia has been identified. This form seems compatible with a normal life span and may be distinguished from MPS IS by the inevitable short stature that it engenders. A normal intelligence seems to be preserved in all forms. Diagnosis relies on the clinical presentation, urinary excretion of dermatan sulfate, and the demonstration of a deficiency of N-acetyl-hexosamine-4-sulfate sulfatase activity.

MPS VII

First described as a separate disease in 1973, MPS VII is associated with characteristic mucopolysaccharidotic facies, dysostosis multiplex, and psychomotor retardation within the first year of life. Hypoplasia of the odontoid process and gibbous deformity are also present. The limited number of patients described thus far show significant heterogeneity in the severity of physical and mental abnormalities. Beta-glucuronidase activity is deficient in this disease, which leads to urinary excretion of heparan sulfate and dermatan sulfate.

MUCOLIPIDOSES

The mucolipidoses are grouped together on the basis of clinical similarities, but recent work has shown wide divergence in their pathogeneses. The key finding in this group of diseases is an MPS-type

Table 309-2   The mucolipidoses

DESIGNATION	DEFECT	DISTINGUISHING FEATURES
ML I	Alpha-N-acetlneuraminidase	Moderate MPS phenotype, moderate retardation, neural degeneration in later years.
ML II	N-acetylglucosamine-phosphotransferase	Severe MPS phenotype and retardation, clear corneas, neural decay by first decade
ML III	N-acetylglucosamine-phosphotransferase	Moderate MPS phenotype, mild retardation, corneal clouding
ML IV	Ganglioside sialidase	No MPS phenotype except corneal clouding, hypotonia, and hyperflexia; mild retardation
Mannosidosis	Alpha-mannosidase + packaging defect	Moderate MPS phenotype, severe retardation, clear corneas
Fucosidosis	Fucosidase	Type I: Moderate MPS phenotype, retardation with progressive decay to death in first decade
		Type II: Slight MPS phenotype with moderate retardation and slow neural deterioration, angiokeratoma corporis diffusum
Aspartylglucosaminuria	N-aspartyl-beta-glucosaminidase	Mild MPS phenotype; usually Finnish ancestry; pigmentation abnormalities with acne; severe retardation with affective disorders

ML, Mucolipidosis; *MPS*, mucopolysaccharidosis.

phenotype despite normal urinary mucopolysaccharides. Mucolipidosis (ML) types I and VI, mannosidosis, fucosidosis, and aspartylglucosaminuria result from classic single-enzyme defects that lead to the accumulation of glycosylated proteins. Mucolipidosis (ML) II and III result from the abnormal packaging of lysosomal enzymes in the organelle (Table 309-2). Chorionic villus sampling may be used in fetal diagnosis; however, care must be exercised to avoid contamination by maternal tissue.

ML I (Sialidosis I)

These patients develop an MPS-like phenotype during the first year of life and progress to mild somatic involvement with moderate mental retardation. There is considerable heterogeneity within this syndrome, and there are reports of cherry-red spots and corneal opacities. The findings of a mild MPS phenotype, mental retardation, normal urinary mucopolysaccharides, and leukocyte inclusions point toward ML I and suggest further enzymatic analysis. This syndrome is associated with a deficiency in alpha-N-acetylneuraminidase. Two subtypes have been identified, and these have different clinical courses. The fusion of cells from these subtypes reconstitutes enzyme activity. Thus at least two alpha-N-acetylneuraminidase deficiency diseases seem to reside within ML I.

ML II (I Cell Disease)

Striking skeletal involvement coupled with respiratory difficulties brings these patients to attention within the first month of life. Progressive mental deterioration, heart disease, and respiratory failure occur within the first decade. Fibroblasts from ML II display numerous coarse inclusions, hence the denotation of "I"-cell disease. A number of lysosomal enzyme activities are lacking in ML II cells; however, culture medium from such cells contains high enzyme activities. This disease, and probably ML III as well, derives from defects in the pack-

aging of certain lysosomal enzymes. Instead of clustering within primary lysosomes, the enzymes are secreted from the cell. The biochemical defect resides in the labeling of lysosomal enzymes with mannose 6-phosphate. ML II and ML III are now known to be deficient in N-acetylglucosamine-phosphate transferase, producing a defect in mannose 6-phosphate labeling of lysosomal enzymes. Without this marker, receptors in the endoplasmic reticulum membrane are unable to accumulate the enzymes for packaging into primary lysosomes. Thus in distinction to defects in lysosomal enzyme catalysis, these diseases stem from the disruption of general lysosomal physiology.

The diagnosis of ML II rests with the severe clinical presentation described above, the absence of mucopolysacchariduria, and a deficiency of N-acetylglucosamine-1-phosphotransferase. Plasma lysosomal enzyme activities are elevated, whereas cultured fibroblasts are deficient in several enzyme activities.

ML III (Pseudo-Hurler Dystrophy)

Although this syndrome is biochemically similar to type II ML, the clinical manifestations are less severe. Physical abnormalities begin during the first few years of life with the development of stiff joints that progress to claw-hand deformities. There are slightly coarsened facies, corneal clouding, and mild mental retardation. Although these findings suggest an MPS, urinary mucopolysaccharides are normal. Plasma lysosomal enzymes are elevated and cultured fibroblasts show multiple lysosomal enzyme deficiencies. The molecular defect in ML III leads to aberrant packaging of lysosomal enzymes. Current studies implicate considerable genetic heterogeneity in ML II and ML III, suggesting that multiple loci may reside within these clinical syndromes. Diagnosis depends on clinical presentation, the presence of normal urinary mucopolysaccharides, disproportionate changes in plasma and cellular lysosomal enzyme levels, and a deficiency in N-acetylglucosamine-1-transferase.

ML IV

A recently recognized syndrome, ML IV includes the clinical findings of corneal clouding, hypotonia, and developmental delay. Histologic studies show lysosomal inclusions; tissue analysis has indicated an increase in gangliosides GM_3 and GD_3. Recent reports implicate ganglioside sialidase as the deficient enzyme activity in this disorder.

Alpha-Mannosidosis

This syndrome is typified by the early development of a mildly Hurler-like physical appearance. A broad skull with prominent jaw and forehead development is a nearly constant finding. These patients may die within the first decade of life, but studies also report that some survive into adulthood. Mental retardation is usually severe. Fibroblast studies show that large quantities of alpha-mannosidase are secreted into the culture medium. Coculture with ML II cells causes restoration of intracellular alpha-mannosidase activities. Thus it appears that this disease may be caused by improper incorporation of alpha-mannosidase into the primary lysosome. The diagnosis depends on an MPS-like phenotype without mucopolysacchariduria and is confirmed by finding a deficiency of lysosomal alpha-mannosidase activity.

Fucosidosis

Patients with fucosidosis display a wide diversity of clinical presentations, ranging from rapid progression and death in the first years of life to slow deterioration with survival into adulthood. In the type I infantile form, the first year of life brings muscular hypotonia, excessive sweating, Hurler-like disease phenotype, mental retardation, and death between 4 and 6 years of age. In the juvenile type II form, there is a slower progression, with a high incidence of angiokeratoma corporis diffusum, which formerly was thought unique to Fabry's disease. Diagnosis may be difficult in this heterogeneous disease. If there is a suspicion of this ML, the presence of high levels of sweat electrolytes and angiokeratoma corporis diffusum may suggest type II. Definite diagnosis requires a determination of fucosidase activity in leukocytes or cultured fibroblasts. Thus far, no relationship be-

Table 309-3   The lipidoses

SYNDROME	DISTINGUISHING FEATURES	DEFECT
Farber lipogranulomatosis	Joint swelling, stiffness, and pain in first year; widespread granuloma in dermis and pulmonary tree	Ceramidase
Niemann-Pick	Acute: Failure to thrive, cachexia, neurologic signs, and cherry-red spots in the macula	Sphingomyelinase
	Juvenile: Gait changes and ataxia in first year	
	Chronic: Adult hepatosplenomegaly and respiratory disease with normal intellect	
Gaucher's	Infantile: Failure to thrive, hypertonia, and neurologic signs with death in first 2 years; Gaucher's cells	Glucocerebrosidase
	Juvenile: As in infantile, with slower progression and survival into first decade; Gaucher cells	
	Chronic: Adult hepatosplenomegaly, osteoporosis; Gaucher cells	
Krabbe's	Increased startle reflex, progressing to hyperreflexia and opisthotonos to vegetative state in first year; globoid cells	Galactocerebrosidase
Metachromatic leukodystrophy (MLD)	Infantile: Gait changes progress to weakness and psychomotor disability and blindness in first years	Arylsulfatase A
Multiple sulfatase deficiency	MLD-like presentation in presence of MPS phenotype with urinary mucopolysaccharides	Arylsulfatase A, B, C
Fabry's	Angiectasis corporis diffusum, renal pain, renal and cardiac failure	Alpha-galactosidase
GM₁ gangliosidosis	Infantile: MPS-like phenotype with failure to thrive progressing to decerebrate rigidity and respiratory failure	Beta-galactosidase
	Juvenile: Mild or no MPS features, psychomotor retardation in first decade	
	Adult: Ataxia and seizures	
GM₂ gangliosidosis	Infantile (Tay-Sachs, Sandhoff): Cherry-red retinal spots, exaggerated startle reflex progressing to hyperactivity, psychomotor retardation, and a vegetative state with death in first years	Tay-Sachs: hexosaminidase A
	Juvenile (Tay-Sachs): Delayed progression of infantile form through first and second decades	Sandhoff's hexosaminidase A and B.
	Adult (Tay-Sachs): Dystonia and spinocerebellar degeneration	

MPS, Mucopolysaccharidosis.

tween the severity of disease and residual enzyme activity has been established.

Aspartylglucosaminuria (N-Aspartyl-Beta-Glucosaminidase Deficiency)

This disease is considered with the mucolipidoses because of its MPL-like phenotype in the absence of mucopolysacchariduria. Aspartylglucosaminidase cleaves carbohydrate-protein linkages from many glycolipids; its deficiency allows the accumulation of mucopolysaccharide-like materials within the lysosomes. These patients, almost exclusively of Finnish ancestry, come to attention because they miss developmental milestones and remain severely retarded. Most show no gross neurologic deficits but display aggressive or affective psychologic disorders. Coarse facies, a broad nose, moderate dysostosis multiplex, and dermatologic abnormalities may suggest a mucopolysaccharidosis. Respiratory and gastrointestinal tract disorders also are reported. Circulating leukocytes have prominent inclusions. Urinalysis shows overexcretion of 2-acetamido-1-(beta-1-L-aspartamido)-1,2, dideoxy-beta-D-glucose in the urine. Definitive diagnosis depends on enzymatic assays in plasma leukocytes or circulating fibroblasts.

LIPID STORAGE DISEASES

Lipid storage diseases are associated with the finding of high levels of lipid compounds in the tissues of affected patients. Most of these patients lack the striking skeletal and soft-tissue abnormalities common to mucopolysaccharidoses and mucolipidoses. They do, however, commonly manifest severe derangements in central nervous system development (Table 309-3). Except for the X-linked Fabry's disease, these diseases are inherited in an autosomal recessive manner (Chapter 284).

Chemistry

Aside from acid lipase deficiency, the lipid storage diseases involve defects in sphingolipid metabolism. The sphingolipids are derived

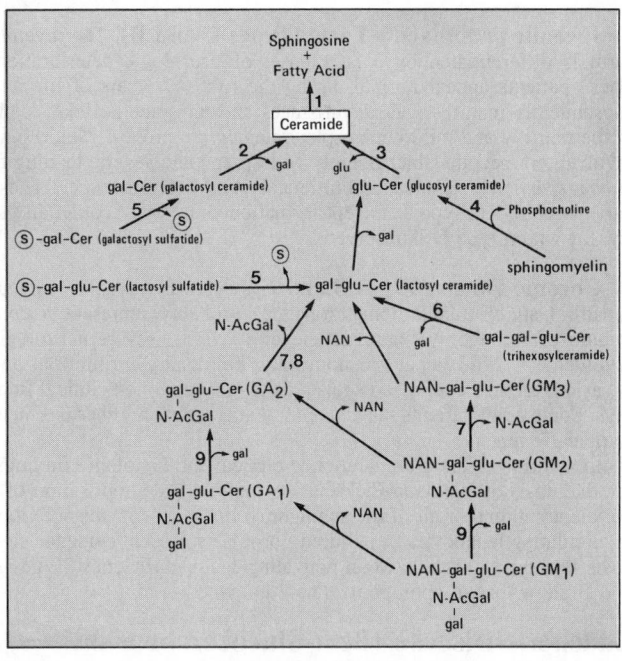

FIGURE 309-3   Pathways of sphingolipid catabolism and disorders produced by enzyme deficiencies. *NAN,* N-acetyl neuraminic acid; *N-AcGal,* N-acetyl galactose; *gal,* galactose; *glu,* glucose.

from sphingosine—fatty acid conjugates termed *ceramides* (Fig. 309-3). Ceramide may be conjugated with phosphocholine to form sphingomyelin, a widespread membrane component. Ceramide also may be sulfated to form sulfatides, glycosylated to form ceramide-n-hexoses, or further conjugated with sialic acid to form the gangliosides.

Farber Lipogranulomatosis (Acid Ceramidase Deficiency)

This disease presents a characteristic clinical syndrome. Although clinically normal at birth, within 2 to 4 months infants with Farber disease develop joint swelling and stiffness in their extremities. Superficial nodules and thickenings appear on the joints, which become painful. Flexion contractures result. Laryngeal swelling, stridor, and pulmonary consolidation lead to significant morbidity and mortality within the first 2 years. In a milder form of this disease, patients survive into their second decade. These patients accumulate subcutaneous nodules on extensor surfaces of the extremities and spinal column. Mental status has been reported as ranging from normal to slightly retarded. Widespread granulomatous infiltration of the dermis, respiratory tract, and other organs is a constant and characteristic finding. These granulomas are composed of histiocytes, lymphocytes, and giant cells around a core of foam cells. Enzymatic diagnosis may be performed on washed leukocytes or cultured fibroblasts.

Niemann-Pick Disease (Sphingomyelinase Deficiency)

Niemann-Pick disease includes a number of disorders that differ in clinical presentation and may be due to differences in sphingomyelinase isoenzyme activities. All patients with Niemann-Pick disease show organomegaly and foamy histiocytes on marrow biopsy. They often demonstrate retinal cherry-red spots. The most common forms are accompanied by severe neurologic disorder, but some chronic forms have mild or unappreciable neuropathology.

Acute Infantile Form (Type A). This most common subtype manifests itself within the first months of life. Infants feed poorly, fail to thrive, and show slow neurologic development and hepatosplenomegaly. Retinal cherry-red spots occur in half of all patients. Cachexia, central neurologic decay, and death occur within the first few years of life.

Juvenile or Subacute Form (Types C and D). The juvenile form is differentiated by a later onset of neurologic deterioration. These patients appear normal during the first few years of life and subsequently manifest gait disturbances and mild ataxia. Foam cells in the marrow and mild hepatosplenomegaly are present. Neurologic involvement becomes increasingly widespread and severe, leading to ataxia, spasticity, seizures, and ultimately to a vegetative state. These patients belong to type C, except for patients of Nova Scotian ancestry, for whom type D is reserved.

Chronic Forms (Types B and E). Types B (juvenile nonneuropathic) and E (adult nonneuropathic) probably represent a continuum of sphingomyelinase deficiencies without severe neurologic involvement. Mild hepatosplenomegaly, pulmonary infiltration, and occasional retinal cherry-red spots are the most common clinical findings. Some adult patients may have mild ataxia but are otherwise neurologically intact.

In addition to the aforementioned clinical and histologic findings, the diagnosis of Niemann-Pick disease requires a demonstration of a deficiency in one or all of the sphingomyelinase isoenzyme activities in circulating leukocytes or cultured fibroblasts. Recent evidence suggests that type C is due to an activating-factor deficiency. Types A and B show loss of sphingomyelinase enzyme.

Gaucher's Disease (Beta-Glucocerebrosidase Deficiency)

Most common of the sphingolipidoses, Gaucher's disease manifests itself in three distinct subtypes. The infantile neuropathic form (type II) becomes clinically apparent within the first months of life. Hepatosplenomegaly, failure to thrive, feeding difficulties, respiratory disease, and neurologic damage generally are found. Neurologic involvement proceeds to hypertonia, spasticity, and laryngeal stridor. Death occurs during the first year of life, usually owing to pulmonary failure. The infrequent juvenile neuropathic form (type III) displays many of the type II characteristics in a delayed form. In the first decade, hepatosplenomegaly, with easy bruisability, bone pain, abdominal

pain, hyperreflexia, and spasticity, all develop. These patients often die in the second decade.

The most common form, chronic nonneuropathic (type I), may manifest itself in adulthood with hepatosplenomegaly, easy bruisability, anemia, and bone pain. No neurologic abnormalities are evident. Major findings include osteoporosis or necrosis of the vertebrae and proximal femur, hepatosplenomegaly, and an increased serum acid phosphatase level. All patients have diagnostic "Gaucher" cells on marrow biopsy. By phase microscopy, there is wrinkled cytoplasm with fibrillar inclusions. The nucleus is acentric; inclusions are periodic acid–Schiff (PAS)–positive. The definitive diagnosis rests with increased tissue glucosylceramide levels and a deficiency of beta-glucocerebrosidase in circulating leukocytes or cultured fibroblasts.

Krabbe's Disease (Beta-Galactocerebrosidase Deficiency

This rare sphingolipidosis presents with acute central nervous system degeneration in the first few months of life; mortality usually occurs within the first year. Clinically, there are the findings of irritability, exaggerated startle reflex, and limb stiffening. Rapid deterioration follows, with the development of hypertonicity, opisthotonos, and blindness within months. The antemortem phase consists of a decerebrate vegetative state. Several late-onset cases have been described. Conjunctival biopsy reveals characteristically ballooned Schwann cells. The cerebral white matter shows a complete loss of myelin and a proliferation of globoid cells (histiocytes with PAS-positive inclusions). Animal models as well as human material show the accumulation of galactosylsphingosine, a potentially cytotoxic metabolite. Definitive diagnosis is made by the demonstration of beta-galactocerebrosidase deficiency in circulating leukocytes or cultured fibroblasts.

The Sulfatidoses

Metachromatic Leukodystrophy (Sulfatide Lipidosis). This disease also may be divided into subtypes according to the time of onset and progression of disease. The most common infantile form is manifested within the first few years of life in behavioral abnormalities, gait disturbances, weakness, and hypotonia. Hypertonia may then follow, together with cerebellar signs, quadriplegia, and blindness. These severely disabled patients may live for a decade or more. A less frequent juvenile form begins within the first decade of life and is manifested in behavioral or visual problems. These problems may be subtle initially but gradually progress to major deficits. This form may progress for decades, only to be terminated by a fatal infection.

The adult form is protean in presentation; initial symptoms suggest a psychiatric disorder. Beginning in the second to fourth decades, these patients exhibit thought disorders, disorientation, and bizarre behavior; they frequently are misdiagnosed as schizophrenic. A subsequent loss of intellectual function, with the appearance of ataxia, paresis, and seizures, indicates the true nature of this disorder. The diagnosis requires an assay of leukocyte or cultured fibroblasts for arylsulfatase A activity. Conjunctival biopsy shows dense metachromatic inclusions within Schwann cells. Brain histology shows demyelination with metachromatic staining of intracellular inclusions. Sulfatide levels are greatly increased in brain, kidneys, and liver.

Multiple Sulfatase Deficiency. This rare disease has clinical findings similar to those of late infantile metachromatic leukodystrophy; however, some findings are identical to those of the mucopolysaccharidoses, such as hepatosplenomegaly, flared ribs, and a J-shaped sella turcica. Urinary mucopolysaccharides show increased levels of dermatan sulfate and heparan sulfate. Cultured fibroblasts and peripheral leukocytes show deficiencies in arylsulfatases A, B, and C and in steroid sulfatase as well. This differentiates the disease from Maroteaux-Lamy and metachromatic leukodystrophies in which only arylsulfatases B and A, respectively, are deficient.

Fabry's Disease (Ceramide Trihexoside Lipidosis)

An X-linked disorder, Fabry's disease becomes apparent in the first decade of life with the onset of a characteristic skin lesion and pain. Female carriers manifest a full spectrum of involvement, from mild to severe. Angiokeratoma corporis diffusum begins as clusters of dark red, punctate angiectases grouping symmetrically over the hips, buttocks, thighs, lower abdomen, and lumbar region. Only fucosidosis type II exhibits this same lesion. Attacks of excruciating pain affect the digits and may radiate proximally to include the abdomen. These attacks are accompanied by fever and an increased erythrocyte sedimentation rate. Paresthesias or nagging pain in the extremities also may develop. Dysfunction of cardiovascular tissue leads to significant cardiovascular disability, with coronary artery disease and congestive failure. Renal failure leads to uremia and hypertension in the third to fifth decade. Cerebrovascular involvement may be evidenced by seizures and sensory or motor dysfunction. Whorl-like opacities in the superficial layers of the cornea provide a distinctive finding. This disease is diagnosed by the characteristic clinical presentation and the finding of alpha-galactosidase deficiency.

The Gangliosidoses

GM₁ Gangliosidoses (Beta-Galactosidase Deficiency). This disease is divided into two forms: infantile (type I) and juvenile (type II). However, there is likely to be a spectrum from infantile to adult forms. Beta-galactosidase deficiencies lead to the accumulation of GM_1 and glycosaminoglycans. This leads to an MPS-like appearance in the acute infantile form without mucopolysacchariduria. The infantile form manifests itself at birth in peripheral edema, hypotonia, poor appetite, respiratory insufficiency, frontal bossing, and depressed nasal bridge. These patients commonly develop hepatosplenomegaly and dysostosis multiplex. A retinal cherry-red spot is often present. Retardation and hyperreactivity progress to decerebrate rigidity, blindness, and death from respiratory failure by the age of 2 years. The juvenile form shows intellectual and motor decline by 1 year of age. Hepatosplenomegaly and dysostosis multiplex are mild or absent. An adult form has been reported, which entails the development of ataxia and seizures in early adulthood. Coarse features, skeletal anomalies, and mild retardation are variable findings in this group. A diagnosis depends on the demonstration of an accumulation of GM_1 ganglioside in the brain or on the lack of beta-galactosidase activity.

GM₂ Gangliosidoses. Tay-Sachs disease (hexosaminidase A deficiency) and Sandhoff disease (hexosaminidase A and B deficiencies) produce nearly identical clinical courses. The patients are notable for their doll-like features and pink, translucent skin. At 3 to 6 months of age, feeding difficulties, listlessness, motor weakness, and exaggerated startle reflex are noted. Retinal cherry-red spots in the macula are almost always present. Later, progressive motor weakness, macrocephaly, deafness, blindness, and convulsions ensue. Death from pneumonia is usual by age 2 years. Much rarer juvenile forms of these diseases involve deterioration of intellectual and motor functions in the first decade, which progresses to retardation and decerebrate rigidity by the second decade. An adult form has been reported, with slow deterioration from childhood. Muscle atrophy, dystonia, and dysarthria suggest spinocerebellar degeneration, whereas visual and intellectual capacities remain intact.

Tay-Sachs disease is carried in high frequency by Ashkenazi Jews (0.033 carrier rate). Definitive diagnosis is by assay of hexosaminidase isoenzyme activities; heterozygotes show a 50% diminution of activity, whereas some patients with late-onset disease show an apparently less severe defect. In Tay-Sachs disease, GM_2 gangliosides accumulate in brain; in Sandhoff disease, GM_2 gangliosides accumulate in other viscera as well.

Acid Lipase Deficiencies

Two diseases stem from an inability to hydrolyze lysosomal triglycerides and cholesteryl esters. Wolman disease manifests itself within the first month of life in forceful vomiting, diarrhea, anemia, and thrombocytopenia. Massive hepatosplenomegaly and adrenal calcifications are characteristic findings. Neurologic development appears normal. The ensuing cachexia leads to death by 6 months of age. Cholesteryl ester storage disease is a more benign chronic condition, characterized by hepatosplenomegaly, accelerated cardiovascular disease, cholesteryl ester and triglyceride accumulation, and elevated levels of circulating LDL. This causes a pattern similar to Fredrickson's

class II hyperlipidemia. These diseases stem from deficiencies in the same enzyme activity and are best diagnosed by the demonstration of low levels of acid lipase in circulating leukocytes or cultured fibroblasts.

OTHER LYSOSOMAL STORAGE DISEASES
Chédiak-Higashi Syndrome

This childhood disease is manifested in photophobia and hypopigmentation of skin, hair, and eyes. Repeated severe bouts of infection precede the later onset of central and peripheral neuropathy, mental retardation, and seizures. Many patients survive into their teens, only to develop a lymphoreticular malignancy. The hallmark of this disease is giant peroxidase-positive granules in circulating leukocytes. Lysosomal inclusions also are found in Schwann cells, liver, and spleen. Abnormally large melanosomes are found in areas of cutaneous depigmentation.

Cystinosis

The acute nephropathic form of cystinosis is manifested in the first year of life with failure to thrive, polyuria, and polydipsia. Metabolic acidosis, Fanconi-like syndrome, and vitamin D–resistant rickets ensue. These eventually result in dwarfism. Characteristic eye changes include patchy retinal hypopigmentation and fine corneal crystalline deposits demonstrable by slit lamp. Most patients have a light complexion and blond hair. Less acute forms have been reported, in which the patients have little or no nephropathy. Crystalline inclusions occur in conjunctiva, cornea, and leukocytes. A diagnosis depends on the clinical presentation, the histology, and the demonstration of high cystine content in leukocytes or cultured fibroblasts.

Drug-Induced Lysosomopathies

Chlorpromazine, tricyclic antidepressants, chloroquine, and the aminoglycoside antibiotics all interfere with lysosome function in cultured cells. Clinically, chloroquine and the aminoglycosides demonstrate toxicities that may result from an inhibition of lysosomal action. Chloroquine in moderate to high doses produces corneal opacities and myopathy characterized by intracellular lamellar inclusion bodies containing acid phosphatase. Retinal dysfunction also may be linked to chloroquine, which, in animal studies, produces lamellar inclusion bodies in retinal ganglion cells. Since chloroquine is an amphiphilic cationic drug, it concentrates in lysosomes, is protonated, and may then interfere with acidification or with enzyme-substrate interactions. The aminoglycosides concentrate in renal tubular lysosomes, where they may interfere with component turnover by inhibiting phospholipases and thus produce phospholipid accumulation in lamellar inclusion bodies and subsequent cell toxicity. No histologic findings currently support a similar mechanism in aminoglycoside-mediated ototoxicity.

TREATMENT

The lysosomal storage diseases are presently incurable. The only area of therapy currently practicable consists of medical support and intervention when complications occur. Prevention rests with contraception or prenatal diagnosis and therapeutic abortion.

Several experimental therapies have attempted to restore the deficient enzyme activities within the affected organ systems. The most commonly used technique has been enzyme infusion. Since the liver accumulates and degrades infused enzymes, additional techniques have attempted to direct enzymes into other affected organs. Acid maltase has been linked to LDL to promote muscle uptake in patients with Pompe's disease. Enzymes have been encapsulated in liposomes, red blood cell ghosts, and synthetic polymers in order to maintain their circulating levels. Liposomes incorporating glycoproteins may serve to direct the liposomal contents to tissues with specific glycoprotein receptors. Intrathecal administration has been attempted in Tay-Sachs disease. These types of therapy have often shown short-term beneficial effects in reducing organomegaly and increasing peripheral substrate clearance.

Transplantation affords an indwelling source of circulating enzyme activity and may provide a site of peripheral substrate clearance. Fibroblast and amniotic membrane transplantation in MPS, kidney transplantation in Fabry's disease, and spleen or kidney transplantation in Gaucher's disease have all been attempted. Again, short-term improvement has been noted in tissue levels and plasma clearance of accumulated substrate.

Bone marrow transplantation has now been used in many of the lysosomal storage diseases. Because of host-versus-graft disease and because the host may produce antibodies to the new lysosomal enzymes, displacement bone marrow transplants have been used with ablation of the host marrow before transplantation. With the significant morbidity and mortality attendant to this strategy, transplantation has been used primarily in fatal diseases. Significant improvement in soft tissue involvement has been seen, particularly in the mucopolysaccharidoses and Gaucher's disease. Although some patients with MPS I have exhibited slowed mental decay with transplantation, little central nervous system improvement is seen in the lipid storage diseases. Skeletal abnormalities appear fixed in these patients by the time of transplantation. Current work in this area involves decreasing the risk of transplantation and of modulating blood-brain barriers to enzyme passage.

With the cloning of many lysosomal enzymes, gene-specific reconstitution has become a realistic endeavor. Human gene replacement will be used first in tissue-specific diseases, such as severe combined immunodeficiency. Later, however, gene insertion may be used in fibroblasts or perhaps in other tissues with wider distribution. Successful implantation of human beta-glucoronidase in animal systems has been observed. Gene therapy of the lipid storage disorders will be most difficult because of central nervous system involvement. Retroviral targeting techniques or transplantation of fetal tissues will likely be used in this setting.

BIBLIOGRAPHY

Adinolfi M, Brown S: Strategies for the correction of enzyme deficiencies in patients with mucopolysaccharidosis, *Dev Med Child Neurol* 26(3):404, 1984.

Ben-Yoseph Y, Mitchell DA, Nadler HL: First trimester prenatal evaluation for I-cell disease by N-acetylglucosamine 1-phosphotransferase assay, *Clin Genet* 33:38, 1988.

Durand P: Recent progress in lysosomal diseases, *Enzyme* 38:256, 1987.

Fortuin JJH, Kleijer WJ: Hybridization studies of fibroblasts from Hurler, Scheie, and Hurler/Scheie compound patients: support for the hypothesis of allelic mutants, *Hum Genet* 53:155, 1980.

Gijsbertus TJH et al: Morquio B syndrome: a primary defect in β-galactosidase, *Am J Med Genet* 16:261, 1983.

Glew RH et al: Mammalian glucocerebrosidase: implications for Gaucher's disease, *Lab Invest* 58(1):5, 1988.

Hobbs JR: Experience with bone marrow transplantation for inborn errors of metabolism, *Enzyme* 38:194, 1987.

Holton JB, editor: *The inherited metabolic diseases,* New York, 1987, Churchill Livingstone.

Igisu H, Suzuki K: Progressive accumulation of toxic metabolite in a genetic leukodystrophy, *Science* 224(4650):753, 1984.

Kolodny EH: Early detection of lysosomal storage diseases, *Ann N Y Acad Sci* 477:312, 1986.

Libert J: Diagnosis of lysosomal storage diseases by the ultrastructural study of conjunctival biopsies, *Pathol Annu* 1:37, 1980.

Lüllman-Rauch R: Lysosomes in applied biology and therapeutics, *Front Biol* 48:49, 1979.

Muenzer J: Mucopolysaccharidoses, *Adv Pediatr* 33:269, 1981.

Stanbury JB, Wyngaarden JB, Fredrickson DS, editors: *The metabolic basis of inherited disease,* ed 5, New York, 1983, McGraw Hill.

CHAPTER

310 Phakomatoses

Thomas D. Gelehrter

Phakoma, from the Greek *phako,* for lentil, is an ophthalmologic term for the small intraocular tumors found in neurofibromatosis and tuberous sclerosis. The term *phakomatoses* is sometimes used to describe a group of neurocutaneous diseases including neurofibromato-

sis, tuberous sclerosis, and von Hippel-Lindau disease, diseases we now understand to be inherited, multisystem disorders resulting from mutations in putative tumor suppressor genes.

NEUROFIBROMATOSIS

Neurofibromatosis 1 (NF1), or von Recklinghausen's neurofibromatosis, is a relatively common inherited hamartomatous disorder characterized by pigmented skin lesions, multiple cutaneous and subcutaneous tumors, and a variety of other manifestations affecting multiple organ systems. The severity of the disease varies widely among affected persons even within the same family. Because of its frequency (approximately 1 in 3000) and protean manifestations, NF1 is seen by every physician.

Clinical Features

The clinical features of neurofibromatosis are extremely varied and are different by patient age. The most characteristic findings are café-au-lait spots and multiple neurofibromas, but neither finding alone is diagnostic of neurofibromatosis.

Café-au-lait spots are hyperpigmented macules that are distributed randomly on the body, though relatively few appear on the face. They are often present at birth or very early in life and tend to increase in number, size, and pigmentation over time. Approximately 10% of normal adults have one to five café-au-lait spots, usually less than 1.5 cm in greatest diameter; more than six spots greater than 1.5 cm in diameter are considered a diagnostic sign of neurofibromatosis and are found in 75% to 85% of affected patients. Less than 1% of normal children have more than two such spots; more than five spots greater than 0.5 cm in diameter are considered diagnostic in children. Axillary freckling is a characteristic though less frequently observed sign. Freckles are also found in other flexural, intertriginous areas, including the groin, antecubital, and inframammary regions. Such freckling is virtually never seen in unaffected individuals. Other forms of hyperpigmentation may be observed; occasionally, large dark macules may overlie plexiform neurofibromas.

Multiple neurofibromas affect the skin of most patients, but may also be found in deeper tissues and internal organs innervated by the autonomic nervous system. Pedunculated dermal neurofibromas are rare in childhood but increase in number at puberty and frequently increase in women during pregnancy. These benign multiclonal lesions contain a mixture of cells including fibroblasts, Schwann cells, and often mast cells. Although these skin neurofibromas virtually never undergo malignant transformation, they may be cosmetically disfiguring when present in large numbers and may cause pruritus. Subcutaneous neurofibromas frequently develop along the course of peripheral nerves. When present in the spinal canal or its foramina, they can produce significant neurologic symptoms because of compression. The most serious type of neurofibroma is the highly vascular, infiltrating plexiform neurofibroma, which is responsible for major disfigurements such as localized gigantism and overgrowth of extremities or the face.

The most characteristic ocular findings in neurofibromatosis are Lisch nodules, which are smooth, dome-shaped, tan nodules on the iris surface. These hamartomatous lesions are not neurofibromas and can be distinguished on slit-lamp examination from the common flat iris freckles or nevi. Lisch spots are found in more than 90% of adult patients but appear to be less frequent in childhood. Whether they are seen in unaffected individuals is disputed. Other eye findings include choroidal hamartomas, myelinated corneal nerves, optic nerve tumors, and characteristic lesions of the eyelid caused by plexiform neurofibromas.

The central nervous system is also prominently affected in neurofibromatosis. Learning disabilities affect approximately 50% of children with this disease and are a significant problem in this age-group. A variety of central nervous system tumors are found more frequently in neurofibromatosis than in the general population. Optic gliomas are a characteristic finding in NF1. It is now recognized that 15% to 20% of patients have such tumors detectable by computed tomography (CT); however, only about 1% of these patients are symptomatic. Therefore it is not recommended that patients with NF1 undergo routine CT or magnetic resonance imaging (MRI) scanning. If the patient's vision is not compromised, these tumors should simply be watched; therapy is indicated only if vision deteriorates. In a young child with NF1, decreased visual acuity or disconjugate gaze should suggest further evaluation for optic glioma. Acoustic neuromas do not occur with increased frequency in NF1; bilateral acoustic neuromas should suggest a separate and distinct entity, neurofibromatosis 2 (NF2) (see later discussion). Other tumors such as astrocytomas and meningiomas are pathologically like those seen in patients without neurofibromatosis but appear to occur more frequently in patients with neurofibromatosis. Approximately half of patients complain of headaches. Most headaches respond similarly to those in patients without NF1 and, if stable, need not raise concern. If the headaches are new or have changed in pattern, however, they should be carefully evaluated. Seizures and frank mental retardation are found only in a minority (<10%) of patients with neurofibromatosis.

Musculoskeletal involvement is common in neurofibromatosis, indicating an important mesodermal component of this disease. Mild short stature is usual, and macrocephaly is very frequent, especially in the second decade of life. Macrocephaly does not correlate with intellectual impairment or other central nervous system abnormalities. The most common orthopedic problem is kyphoscoliosis. In addition to the usual form of scoliosis found in about one third of children with neurofibromatosis, there is an uncommon but characteristic acute anterior angulation of the lower cervical and upper thoracic spine. Congenital bowing of the tibia and/or fibula, and less frequently of the radius and/or ulna, is a characteristic lesion in neurofibromatosis and a difficult one to manage orthopedically. Although the bowing may remain static, it can progress to pathologic fractures and pseudarthrosis. Growth abnormalities including asymmetry and localized gigantism secondary to infiltrating plexiform neurofibromas may be a major source of morbidity, particularly in children.

Malignancy is generally considered a part of the clinical picture of neurofibromatosis. There does not appear to be an increase in the frequency of common cancers in patients with this disease; however, there is clearly a higher frequency of certain rare malignancies such as neurofibrosarcoma, malignant schwannoma, and pheochromocytoma, and probably of Wilms' tumor, rhabdomyosarcoma, and Ph[1]-negative leukemia. The risk of sarcomatous degeneration of preexisting neurofibromas is unknown. It is unlikely that pedunculated skin neurofibromas ever undergo malignant transformation; however, internal plexiform neurofibromas and schwannomas, especially those in the posterior mediastinum, apparently can undergo such change.

Hypertension is common in neurofibromatosis and is usually of the essential variety. Pheochromocytomas occur in less than 5% of patients with neurofibromatosis, far more frequently than in the general population. Rarely does this tumor occur before the age of 20 years in neurofibromatosis patients. Children with neurofibromatosis have a higher than usual frequency of renal artery stenosis. The lesions are usually located at the origin of the artery, are frequently bilateral, and are the result of vascular dysplasia rather than compression by neurofibromas.

Constipation occurs commonly, reflecting involvement of Auerbach's plexus of the colon. Gastrointestinal and genitourinary tract bleeding may be encountered because of neurofibromas in the lumen of the colon or bladder. Disorders of sexual development including precocious puberty may also occur more frequently in neurofibromatosis than in the general population.

In the neonatal and early childhood period, most affected patients will be asymptomatic and have only café-au-lait spots. A minority will have severe involvement, including plexiform neurofibromas of the face, limb overgrowth, or congenital pseudarthrosis. Later in childhood, learning and behavioral problems, scoliosis, or central nervous system tumors such as optic glioma may bring the patient to medical attention. Cutaneous neurofibromas begin to appear at puberty. Although the majority of patients will not have severe problems resulting from this disease, patients cannot be reassured with any certainty. There appears to be no difference in the severity of manifestations between sporadic and familial cases.

Genetics and Pathophysiology

Neurofibromatosis is inherited as a simple autosomal dominant trait that affects both sexes with equal frequency and severity. The gene

appears to have a high penetrance; that is, an individual carrying the gene virtually always shows some manifestation of the disease by adulthood. However, the nature and severity of the pathologic manifestations vary widely, even within families. The causes of this variability are unknown. Neurofibromatosis occurs in approximately 1 in 3000 individuals and affects all races. Approximately half of cases are sporadic and presumably represent new mutations. Estimates of the mutation rate for the neurofibromatosis gene are approximately 10^{-4} per gamete per generation, the highest for any human gene.

The gene for NF1 has been mapped to the centromeric region of chromosome 17 (17q11.2) and has been cloned. The gene for NF1 spans approximately 300 kb of genomic DNA and encodes a 13-kb mRNA that is ubiquitously expressed. There is no evidence of locus heterogeneity; that is, all cases of NF1 can be mapped to this single genetic locus. More than 90 distinct mutations have been described in the *NF1* gene and range from large deletions to missense and nonsense mutations. There is no correlation between specific mutations and a particular disease phenotype. The *NF1* gene product is a cytoplasmic protein called neurofibromin, which is associated with microtubules. A portion of the *NF1* gene shares sequence similarity with a GTPase activating protein (GAP). GAP proteins accelerate the hydrolysis of *ras*-guanosine triphosphate to *ras*-guanosine diphosphate, converting the protooncogene protein *ras* from the active to the inactive form. Thus neurofibromin may act as a tumor suppressor by regulating the function of *ras,* which plays an important role in growth and proliferation. In addition, somatic mutations in *NF1* resulting in absence of neurofibromin have been described in a variety of tumors, further supporting this hypothesis.

Diagnosis

The diagnosis of NF1 rests on clinical observations, history, family history, and physical examination. Because none of the clinical features is found in every patient with the disease, no single clinical feature is absolutely diagnostic. The National Institutes of Health consensus diagnostic criteria for NF1 include the presence of two or more of the following: (1) six café-au-lait spots over 1.5 cm in greatest diameter in postpubertal individuals or 0.5 cm in children, (2) two or more neurofibromas of any type or one plexiform neurofibroma, (3) axillary or inguinal freckling, (4) optic glioma, (5) two or more Lisch nodules, (6) a distinctive bony lesion such as sphenoid dysplasia or thinning of long-bone cortex with or without pseudoarthrosis, and (7) a first-degree relative with NF1. The large size of the *NF1* gene makes direct DNA diagnosis exceedingly difficult. Protein truncation assays, however, can detect approximately 70% of causative mutations. Given the great variability in clinical phenotype among affected individuals in a family with NF1, analysis of DNA mutations will most likely not be very helpful in predicting the patient's phenotype.

Management

Treatment of patients with NF1 is directed at education and genetic counseling, surveillance for the appearance of complications of this condition, and early detection of malignancy. All patients with neurofibromatosis and their families should be offered accurate and sensitive genetic counseling. The risk for each offspring of a patient with neurofibromatosis is 50%, regardless of sex. This risk is the same whether the proband represents a familial or a sporadic case. Nevertheless, it is important to determine whether the patient represents a sporadic or familial case because in the latter circumstance other family members (e.g., siblings) are at risk. Therefore parents and siblings of a patient with neurofibromatosis should be evaluated through a careful history and physical examination. A postpubertal individual at risk of neurofibromatosis who has no signs of the disease is very unlikely to be carrying this gene, and the risk for his or her offspring should be no higher than that in the general population. Genetic counseling must also include a detailed explanation of the clinical spectrum of the disease, possible complications, and available therapy. The extremely variable expression of the disease should be clearly discussed. Because the disease can be very mild and benign in some patients and disfiguring and incapacitating in others, the genetic counselor must attempt to balance creating undue anxiety about the future with an unrealistically optimistic forecast for the patient and offspring.

✔ *WHEN TO REFER*

Because the protean manifestations of neurofibromatosis require the services of multiple medical and surgical specialties, there is considerable risk that the patient's care can become fragmented. Patients with neurofibromatosis require considerable supportive care and should be provided with accurate and understanding genetic counseling. Thus the medical geneticist is well situated to coordinate care for patients with NF1. A network of specialized neurofibromatosis treatment centers around the country has been established for the care of patients with this condition. The National Neurofibromatosis Foundation* provides information and support for patients, families, and physicians dealing with this disease.

*95 Pine St, 16th Floor, New York, NY 10005.

Dermal neurofibromas can be removed by surgery, dermabrasion, or carbon dioxide laser treatment. Patients should be seen on at least a yearly basis, and evidence of complications should be sought. Particular attention should be paid to blood pressure and possible neurologic, ophthalmologic, and orthopedic problems, with appropriate specialized evaluations as needed.

Neurofibromatosis 2

In addition to NF1, a separate and distinct entity known as bilateral acoustic neurofibromatosis, or neurofibromatosis 2 (NF2), is also an autosomal dominant trait, occurring in approximately 1 per 1,000,000 individuals. It is characterized by bilateral acoustic neuromas (actually, vestibular schwannomas) with onset of symptoms in the second and third decade, other central nervous system tumors, and, in 50% of patients, by posterior subcapsular cataracts. Multiple café-au-lait spots, multiple neurofibromas, Lisch nodules, and other manifestations of NF1 are uncommon. The gene for NF2 has been mapped to chromosome 22q 12.2 and cloned. Relatives at risk for NF2 who are more than 15 years old should be followed by regular MRI, ophthalmologic examination, and audiologic evaluation, including brainstem auditory evoked response (BAER).

TUBEROUS SCLEROSIS

Tuberous sclerosis (TSC) is a dominantly inherited hamartomatous disorder with an incidence of 1:6000 that is characterized by seizures, mental retardation, and skin and eye lesions. The name reflects the characteristic subependymal hamartomas and cortical tubers that are the pathologic hallmark of the disease. Like neurofibromatosis, tuberous sclerosis is extremely variable in its manifestations and severity.

The classic picture of TSC consists of the triad of mental retardation, seizures, and adenoma sebaceum. The seizures, found in 60% of patients, include characteristic myoclonic jerks and infantile spasms (hypsarrhythmia). Mental retardation is found in about half of patients, especially in children with seizures, and is variable in degree. Behavioral abnormalities are also frequent, including attention deficit disorder and autism. Cranial CT scans reveal periventricular calcification and/or tubers in 60% to 90% of patients. Cortical tubers are thought to disrupt and displace normal cortical architecture, causing the neurologic problems in TSC. In addition, large giant cell astrocytomas may cause obstruction of cerebrospinal fluid flow.

The best-known skin findings are adenoma sebaceum, which are actually facial angiofibromas, commonly occurring in the nasolabial region and over the cheeks. These lesions usually do not appear until the age of 3 to 5 years and blossom at about puberty, when they may be mistaken for acne. Facial angiofibromas, found in 75% of patients, are considered pathognomonic of TSC, as are subungual and periungual fibromas. Hypomelanotic skin macules, often oval (hence the name "ash leaf spots"), are an even more frequent skin manifestation but are not diagnostic. They are best seen with a Wood's lamp, and may be apparent in the newborn period. Other skin lesions include

forehead fibrous plaques and shagreen patches. Retinal astrocytic hamartomas or phakomas (including both white plaques and mulberry lesions) are seen in approximately half of patients with TSC and are diagnostic of this disease.

Other characteristic lesions include gingival fibromas, renal angiomyolipomas and cortical cysts (best detected by CT scans or ultrasound), cardiac rhabdomyomas (found in 50% of affected infants), and, rarely, pulmonary cystic lesions that may be associated with spontaneous pneumothorax. The renal angiomyolipomas and cysts usually do not cause functional impairment, but hemorrhage and progressive renal failure have been reported.

Diagnosis of tuberous sclerosis is straightforward in severe cases with classic manifestations on the basis of history, examination of the skin and eyes, and confirmatory studies such as electroencephalography, CT, and histologic confirmation of clinical lesions. Diagnosis in mildly affected individuals, especially in adults who have neither retardation nor seizures, can be difficult. Parents and other first-degree relatives of an affected child should have a careful examination of the nailbeds and skin, including Wood's lamp examination, and examination of the retina through a dilated pupil. CT or MRI scans and renal ultrasound may be necessary to detect mildly affected individuals. Consensus diagnostic criteria for TSC have been developed.

There are no specific laboratory tests for this disease, and prenatal diagnosis is not available, although fetuses have been diagnosed by echocardiographic demonstration of a rhabdomyoma.

Genetics

Tuberous sclerosis is inherited as an autosomal dominant trait with high penetrance and markedly variable expressivity. In about half of families with TSC the disease has been mapped to a locus on the long arm of chromosome 9 (*TSC1* at 9q34). In the remaining families there is linkage to a locus on chromosome 16 (*TSC2* at 16p13.3). *TSC2* has been cloned and encodes a protein, tuberin, which, like neurofibromin, shows homology to a GTPase activating protein. Loss of heterozygosity at *TSC2* in hamartomas from patients with TSC, presumably a result of somatic mutation, is also consistent with *TSC2* acting as a tumor suppressor.

Approximately 60% of cases are sporadic and probably represent new mutations. Because a parent may be very mildly affected, however, it is necessary to evaluate carefully parents and other first-degree relatives of patients with diagnosed cases of TSC to distinguish new mutations from familial cases.

Management

Treatment of TSC is directed at treatment of seizures and management of learning disorders and behavior difficulties. In addition, surveillance for and management of complications and patient education and genetic counseling are mainstays of therapy. Genetic counseling should be offered to families with affected members. It is clear that a mildly affected parent may have a severely affected child, and there is considerable variation in severity even within families. Thus it is impossible to predict whether an affected child will have severe or mild manifestations. On the other hand, a mildly affected young adult is unlikely to develop more serious complications later in life. The National Tuberous Sclerosis Association* is available to help affected patients and families.

VON HIPPEL-LINDAU DISEASE

Von Hippel-Lindau (VHL) disease is a relatively rare (1:36,000), dominantly inherited, complex tumor disorder characterized by retinal angiomatosis and cerebellar hemangioblastoma. Retinal angiomas usually appear by the third decade of life. Angiomatous tumors, characteristically found in the cerebellum but also in other parts of the brain, spinal cord, adrenals, lungs, and liver, tend to develop later in life. Renal cell carcinoma is a particularly frequent cause of death. Polycythemia, pheochromocytoma, and pancreatic carcinoma are ad-

*8181 Professional Place, Suite 110, Landover, MD 20785-2226.

✔ *WHEN TO REFER*

Because VHL disease is a precancerous disorder and some of the manifestation are amenable to treatment and cure when detected early, genetic counseling and careful screening and follow-up of relatives at risk are mandatory. Ophthalmologic testing should be done on a yearly basis and continue to at least the age of 60 years. Enhanced MRI of brain and spine are recommended every other year, at least, after the age of 11 years, and abdominal CT or ultrasound yearly after the age of 11. As in the case of the other phakomatoses, patient education and genetic counseling are essential parts of management. Also, like these other conditions, multiple specialties are involved in the care of patients with VHL disease; thus coordination of care by a medical geneticist is highly recommended. Two support groups for patients and families with VHL disease that are good sources of information and support are the VHL Family Alliance* and the von Hippel-Lindau Syndrome Foundation.†

*VHL Family Alliance, 171 Clinton Road, Brookline, MA 02146.
†Von Hippel-Lindau Syndrome Foundation, 32 Beaverson Blvd., Building 2, Suite B, Brick, NJ 08723.

ditional features of the disease, as are cysts of the pancreas, kidneys, and epididymis.

Genetics

VHL disease is inherited as an autosomal dominant disorder with considerable intrafamilial variation in age of onset and expression. The gene for VHL disease has been mapped to chromosome 3 (3p25) and cloned. The product of this gene interacts with a cellular transcription factor, elongin, to regulate elongation of gene transcription and is thus thought to act as a putative tumor suppressor gene. Consistent with this view, mutations in the *VHL* gene have been described in 80% of sporadic cases of clear cell renal cancers.

Two major clinical types of VHL disease have been described. In the more common type 1 VHL disease patients typically have retinal and central nervous system hemangioblastomas, renal cysts and cancers, and pancreatic cystic disease, but not pheochromocytoma. In families with type 2 VHL disease, pheochromocytomas are a part of the disease picture. Both types of families map to the same genetic locus; that is, there is no locus heterogeneity. More than 90% of type 2 families (with pheochromocytoma) have missense mutations in the VHL gene, with two common mutations accounting for 46% of these. Direct DNA diagnostic tests are now available; approximately 65% of mutations can be identified. Diagnosis by linkage analysis can also be performed in families with multiple living affected family members. In families in which DNA tests are diagnostic, only genetically affected members need to be screened, thus sparing unaffected relatives from frequent, costly tests.

BIBLIOGRAPHY

Choyke PL, Glenn GM, McClellan MW et al: von Hippel-Lindau disease: genetic, clinical and imaging features, *Radiology* 194:629-642, 1995.
Gutmann DH, Collins FS: von Recklinghausen neurofibromatosis. In Scriver CR, Beaudet AL, Sly WS, Valle D, editors: *The metabolic and molecular bases of inherited disease*, New York, 1995, McGraw-Hill.
Heim RA, Kam-Morgan LNW, Binnie CG et al: Distribution of 13 truncating mutations in the neurofibromatosis 1 gene, *Hum Mol Genet* 4:975-981, 1995.
Kwiatkowski DJ, Short MP: Tuberous sclerosis, *Arch Dermatol* 130:348-354, 1994.
Webb DW, Osborne JP: Tuberous sclerosis, *Arch Dis Child* 72:471-474, 1995.
Zbar B, Kishida T, Chen F et al: Germline mutations in the Von Hippel-Lindau disease (*VHL*) gene in families from North America, Europe, and Japan, *Hum Mutat* 8:348-357, 1996.

311 Disorders of Porphyrin Metabolism

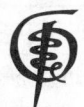

Joseph R. Bloomer

The porphyrias are metabolic disorders in which excess accumulation and excretion of porphyrins and porphyrin precursors occur. The principal clinical manifestations are cutaneous lesions, neurologic dysfunction, and hepatic disease.

PATHOGENESIS OF BIOCHEMICAL ABNORMALITIES

Since the biochemical abnormalities in each of the porphyrias reflect an enzyme abnormality in the pathway of heme biosynthesis (Fig. 311-1; Table 311-1), a knowledge of the pathway is necessary to understand the chemical findings.

Heme is synthesized by eight enzymatically controlled steps. The first and last steps take place within the mitochondria; the intervening steps occur in the cytosol or at the mitochondrial membrane.

The first step is catalyzed by the enzyme δ-amino-levulinic acid (ALA) synthase. The reaction involves the condensation of glycine with succinyl coenzyme A. The product is a β-keto acid (2-amino-3-oxoadipate), which spontaneously decarboxylates to form ALA. The enzyme requires pyridoxal phosphate, which "activates" the glycine molecule toward attack by the succinyl coenzyme A. As a branch point enzyme, ALA synthase is predictably the primary control point for the pathway. In liver its synthesis is repressed by the end product of the pathway, heme; its transport into the mitochondrion is inhibited by heme; and heme is an allosteric inhibitor of the enzyme reaction. The forms of porphyria that cause attacks of neurologic dysfunction have increased production of ALA as a result of induction of hepatic ALA synthase activity.

The second step of heme biosynthesis results in the condensation of two molecules of ALA with the elimination of two molecules of water, forming the monopyrrole porphobilinogen (PBG). The reaction occurs in the cytosol and is catalyzed by the enzyme ALA dehydrase.

The third and fourth steps in the reaction series are catalyzed in concert by the enzymes PBG deaminase (or hydroxymethylbilane synthase) and uroporphyrinogen III synthase (formerly cosynthase). The first of these catalyzes the head-to-tail condensation of four PBG molecules (eliminating four molecules of ammonia) to produce a noncyclized tetrapyrrole called *hydroxymethylbilane*. Because of the structure of PBG, this intermediate has alternating acetate and propionate substituents on the pyrrole units. Uroporphyrinogen III synthase catalyzes a cyclization reaction with the concomitant "inversion" of the fourth pyrrole unit, resulting in the formation of the asymmetric uroporphyrinogen III. In the absence of uroporphyrinogen III synthase, hydroxymethylbilane spontaneously cyclizes to form the symmetric, but biologically inactive, uroporphyrinogen I.

The fifth step in the pathway is catalyzed by uroporphyrinogen decarboxylase. The cytosolic enzyme sequentially removes the carboxylate groups of the four acetate substituents of uroporphyrinogen, leaving behind methyl substituents and producing coproporphyrinogen III. This enzyme also decarboxylates uroporphyrinogen I to form coproporphyrinogen I.

The sixth step converts two of the four propionate substituents of coproporphyrinogen III into vinyl groups by way of oxidative decarboxylation. The product is protoporphyrinogen IX. The enzyme responsible for this is coproporphyrinogen oxidase.

The penultimate step of heme biosynthesis results in the controlled six-electron oxidation of protoporphyrinogen to form protoporphyrin. The enzyme, protoporphyrinogen oxidase, is located within the inner mitochondrial membrane. The fate of the six electrons is unknown.

The eighth step of heme biosynthesis, catalyzed by ferrochelatase,

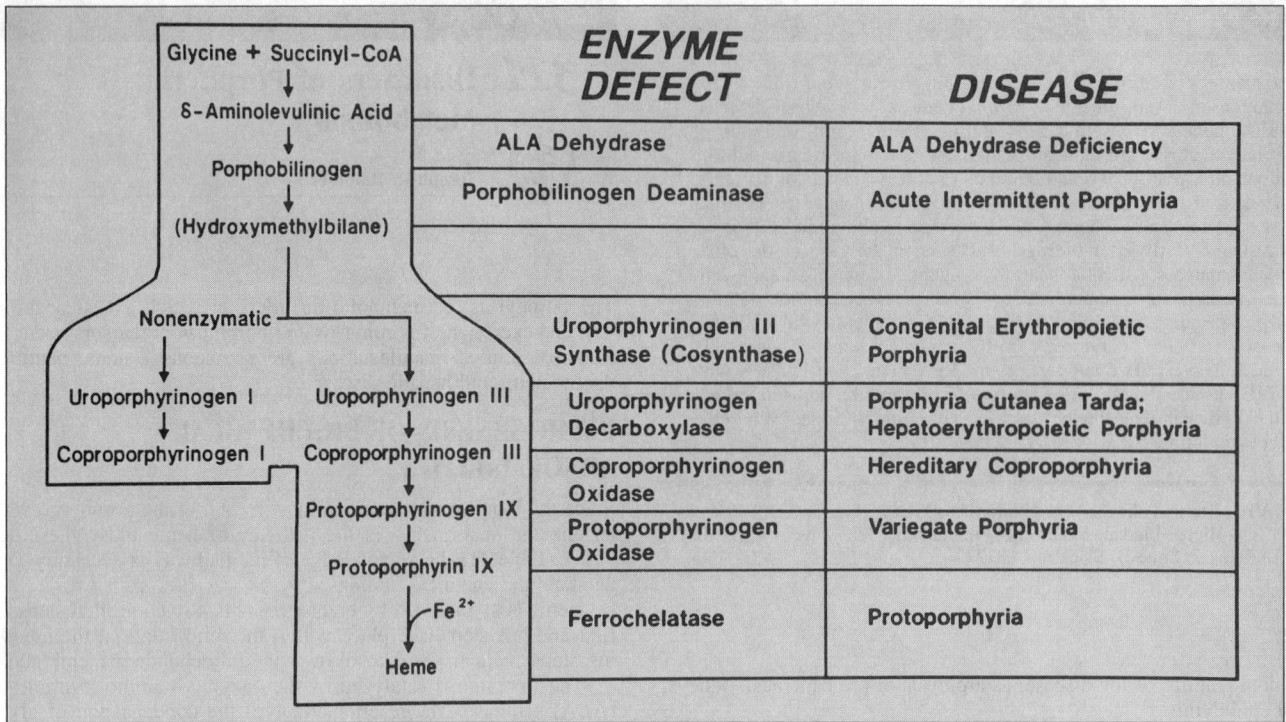

FIGURE 311-1   Heme biosynthesis, showing the sites of enzyme defects in the different porphyrias. As a consequence of the enzyme defects, porphyrins and porphyrin precursors are accumulated and excreted in excessive amounts. *ALA,* Aminolevulinic acid.

From Bloomer JR, Bonkovsky HL: *Dis Mon* 35:1, 1989.

Table 311-1   Principal clinical and biochemical manifestations in the porphyrias

DISORDER	CUTANEOUS LESIONS	NEUROLOGIC DYSFUNCTION	HEPATIC DISEASE	MAJOR SITE OF PORPHYRIN OVERPRODUCTION	ERYTHROCYTES	URINE	FECES
Congenital erythropoietic porphyria	+	0	0	Bone marrow	↑ Uroporphyrin	↑ Uroporphyrin	↑ Uroporphyrin and coproporphyrin
Protoporphyria	+	0	+	Bone marrow and liver	↑ Protoporphyrin	—	↑ Protoporphyrin
Porphyria cutanea tarda	+	0	+	Liver	—	↑ Uroporphyrin	Isocoproporphyrin
Hepatoerythropoietic porphyria	+	0	+	Bone marrow and liver	↑ Zn-protoporphyrin	↑ Uroporphyrin	Isocoproporphyrin
Acute intermittent porphyria	0	+	0	Liver	—	↑ ALA and PBG	—
Variegate porphyria	+	+	0	Liver	—	↑ ALA, PBG, and coproporphyrin	↑ Protoporphyrin
Hereditary coproporphyria	+	+	0	Liver	—	↑ ALA, PBG, and coproporphyrin	↑ Coproporphyrin
ALA dehydrase deficiency	0	+	0	Liver	—	↑ ALA	—

ALA, δ-aminolevulinic acid; *PBG,* porphobilinogen.
This table does not list all of the biochemical abnormalities and only serves as a guide to indicate which measurements are most critical in the evaluation of the porphyrias.

results in the insertion of divalent iron into the center of the porphyrin nucleus with the displacement of two protons, forming heme. The reaction occurs at the inner face of the inner mitochondrial membrane.

All tetrapyrrole intermediates before protoporphyrin are at the oxidation state of a porphyrinogen, which consists of four pyrrole units separated by methylene groups. Porphyrinogens are nonplanar, nonaromatic, colorless compounds. In vitro they are susceptible to spontaneous oxidation, resulting in the conversion of the porphyrinogen to the porphyrin. The latter results from the formal loss of six hydrogen atoms, four from the methylene bridge carbons and two from pyrrole nitrogens. The resulting porphyrin, a cyclic compound composed of four pyrroles separated by methene bridges, is a planar aromatic compound that is deeply colored and fluorescent.

Defects in these enzymatic steps underlie the biochemical abnormalities that characterize the different porphyrias. In keeping with the importance of heme biosynthesis to aerobic cells, any inborn error of the pathway must cause only a partial reduction in the synthesis of heme. Thus it is not surprising that most of the porphyrias are autosomal dominant traits (i.e., one normal and one mutant gene). The porphyrias that are autosomal recessive traits (congenital erythropoietic porphyria, ALA dehydrase deficiency, and hepatoerythropoietic porphyria) result in the production of enzymes with greatly reduced but not totally absent activities.

Whereas the enzyme defects may be expressed in any heme-forming tissue of a patient with porphyria, only the bone marrow and liver are quantitatively important in the overproduction of porphyrins and porphyrin precursors (Table 311-1). This formed the basis for the classification of the porphyrias as either erythropoietic or hepatic, depending on which tissue is the major site of expression of the biochemical abnormality.

Reduction in the activity of an enzyme may result from decreased synthesis of the enzyme protein, a structural defect leading to an unstable protein, or a structural defect resulting in altered enzyme function. The first two mechanisms reduce the amount of protein, which, when evaluated using an antibody against the protein, cause a reduction in cross-reactive immunologic material (CRIM) and are said to be *CRIM-negative*. The latter mechanism may also cause CRIM-negative mutations if the structural alterations are major or at the sites of immunologic determinants. However, the amount of CRIM may be unaffected. This is called *CRIM-positive* mutation.

Both CRIM-positive and CRIM-negative mutations occur in specific types of porphyria, indicating that genetic heterogeneity exists for these disorders (i.e., more than one class of gene mutation causes the phenotype of the disease). For example, in acute intermittent porphyria (AIP), in which there is a deficiency of PBG deaminase activity, four classes of mutations have been identified by comparing the amount of CRIM with enzyme activity. Two of these mutations are CRIM-negative and two CRIM-positive. Similarly, both CRIM-positive and CRIM-negative mutations have been described in hepatoerythropoietic porphyria and in protoporphyria.

Advances in molecular biology techniques have enabled the sequences for the human genes encoding the enzymes of heme biosynthesis to be determined. As a consequence, it has been possible to identify specific genetic lesions present in many porphyria patients and their families. Specific gene defects have been described in all types of porphyria and show that the porphyrias are genetically heterogeneous disorders. In AIP alone, approximately 70 distinct mutations have been found, which include point mutations leading to missense, nonsense, and splice site (exon deletions) errors and insertion and deletion (frameshift) mutations leading to truncated or nonsense protein sequences. Any of the mutations that result in altered immunologic determinants or unstable protein products lead to CRIM-negative phenotypes. It is expected that this pattern of genetic heterogeneity will be the rule rather than the exception in most heritable disorders.

PATHOGENESIS OF MAJOR CLINICAL MANIFESTATIONS

The signs and symptoms most commonly seen in the porphyrias are cutaneous and neurologic (Table 311-1). In some types, both manifestations occur, whereas in others only one feature is present. Cutaneous lesions result from the photosensitizing effects of porphyrins, which are deposited in the skin or are circulating in dermal blood vessels. Light with a wavelength of approximately 400 nm excites electrons of the porphyrins to elevated energy levels, causing the formation of compounds that react with molecular oxygen to form reactive oxygen species. The reactive oxygen may then damage tissue through peroxidation of membrane lipids and cross-linking of membrane proteins.

Neurologic dysfunction occurs in the types of porphyria that are termed *acute* or *inducible* and may cause life-threatening complications such as respiratory paralysis. The pathogenesis of neurologic dysfunction has not been precisely determined, but one consideration is that ALA, which is overproduced in the liver as a consequence of the induction of hepatic ALA synthase activity, acts as a neurotoxin. A second possibility is a heme deficiency state. Experimental studies support both possibilities, and neurologic dysfunction may be caused by a combination of these factors.

Hepatic disease is an important feature of some types of porphyria. The descriptions and pathogenesis of the hepatic disease are discussed in the individual sections that follow.

TYPES OF PORPHYRIA
Congenital Erythropoietic Porphyria (Günther's Disease)

The very rare disease of congenital erythropoietic porphyria is transmitted in an autosomal recessive manner. It results from a deficiency of uroporphyrinogen III synthase (cosynthase) activity. In the absence of uroporphyrinogen III synthase, PBG is converted to uroporphyrinogen I, which cannot be used and is excreted mainly in the urine.

The clinical manifestations involve the skin and erythron. Photosensitivity may begin in infancy. Vesicles or bullae occur on exposed portions of the body and, through the process of ulceration and healing, lead to scarring. Repeated episodes of ulceration and scarring cause severe deformity of the fingers, ears, and nose. Conjunctivitis, keratitis, changes in pigmentation, alopecia, and hypertrichosis of the face and limbs are other complications.

The excess uroporphyrin originates in developing erythrocytes in the bone marrow. Hematologic findings include a shortened red blood cell life span, reticulocytosis, and circulating normoblasts. Splenomegaly is often present. Although slight elevation of serum bilirubin level may be present, clinically evident jaundice is rare. In addition to hemolysis, ineffective erythropoiesis may play a role in causing anemia. In some patients increased red blood cell production is sufficient to prevent anemia.

Pathologic findings include normoblastic hyperplasia in the marrow, fluorescence of a variable fraction of marrow normoblasts and circulating erythrocytes, increase of the pulp and follicular hyperplasia in the spleen, increased melanin in the epidermis, and fibroblast proliferation in the skin. The liver may be enlarged with an increase of hemosiderin, but histologic changes are nonspecific.

The diagnosis is indicated by severe cutaneous photosensitivity beginning in infancy or childhood, dark ("port wine") urine, erythrodontia, and hemolytic anemia. Confirmation comes from measurement of urinary uroporphyrin and demonstration of fluorescence of circulating erythrocytes and marrow normoblasts. Cells exhibit characteristic red fluorescence when irradiated with light of 400-nm wavelength (Soret band). Fluorescence of the teeth may also be found.

Treatment is directed to prevent skin lesions and manage the hemolytic anemia. Protection from sunlight is important. The creams and lotions used for standard sunburn protection are of no value because they do not absorb the long wavelengths that cause skin damage. Beta-carotene (Solatene) may be administered but has less efficacy than in protoporphyria (further details are presented under the treatment of protoporphyria). Secondary skin infections are treated with antibiotics.

Since excessive porphyrin production is augmented by the stimulation of erythropoiesis that results from hemolytic anemia, splenectomy has been used in treatment. In some cases hemolysis has been reduced, and this has been associated with lessening of photosensitivity. Urinary and fecal porphyrin excretion often decrease after splenectomy. Transfusions inhibit erythropoiesis and decrease porphyrin excretion. Intravenous administration of hematin has also been shown to decrease erythrocyte and urinary uroporphyrin levels in a few patients.

Patients with congenital erythropoietic porphyria rarely survive beyond middle age. Although the cause of death has not always been clearly defined, renal failure or hepatic failure has sometimes been the terminal event.

Protoporphyria (Erythrohepatic Porphyria and Erythropoietic Protoporphyria)

Protoporphyria is transmitted as an autosomal dominant disorder with variable expression. It perhaps occurs in 10 to 20 individuals per 100,000 population. A deficiency of ferrochelatase activity has been demonstrated. As a consequence of the ferrochelatase defect, protoporphyrin accumulates in excessive amounts. This causes high levels of protoporphyrin in erythrocytes, bile, and feces. There is no increase of porphyrins in the urine. The absence of abnormalities in the urine is probably the reason the disease was not recognized as a type of porphyria until 1961.

Cutaneous symptoms usually begin in childhood. Burning or itching of the skin occurs after a variable period of exposure to sunlight (sometimes within a few minutes). Light that has passed through window glass may evoke symptoms. Burning is often accompanied by erythema and edema of exposed areas. The latter may persist for weeks. Chronic lesions cause thickening and scarring of the skin of the nose, cheeks, back of the hands, and fingers. An amorphous periodic acid–Schiff–positive material is often demonstrable in and around capillary walls in skin that is exposed to light. This has also been found in variegate porphyria and porphyria cutanea tarda.

The other major clinical manifestation in protoporphyria is hepatobiliary disease. Protoporphyrin-rich gallstones are present in some patients. Liver biopsy specimens from patients frequently show mild abnormalities in the form of portal inflammation and fibrosis, along with deposition of brown pigment. In a few individuals (less than 10% of patients) severe liver disease develops that can lead to death from hepatic failure. The livers of these patients have been black and cirrhotic. The black appearance is caused by massive deposits of pigment in hepatocytes, Kupffer's cells, portal macrophages, and bile canaliculi and small bile ducts. When examined by polarization microscopy, the pigment deposits are birefringent, and by electron microscopy they are shown to contain crystals. Isolation and characterization of the pigment crystals indicate that they are composed of protoporphyrin, and it is currently thought that hepatic protoporphyrin deposition is the cause of the liver disease.

Approximately 20% to 30% of patients have mild anemia with hypochromic microcytic indices. A variable fraction of marrow erythroid cells and circulating erythrocytes have red fluorescence. The bone marrow morphologic appearance is normal.

Acute photosensitivity reactions, with or without objective skin changes, suggest the diagnosis. Confirmation requires the demonstration of increased erythrocyte protoporphyrin. In contrast to lead poisoning and iron-deficiency anemia, the increased protoporphyrin in erythrocytes occurs as free protoporphyrin and not the zinc chelate.

Oral administration of beta-carotene is of value in increasing tolerance to light. This benefit may not be evident for 1 to 3 months after starting therapy. A yellowish discoloration of skin appears to be the only side effect. Methods to prevent and reverse hepatic protoporphyrin accumulation in patients with liver disease include attempts to suppress excess protoporphyrin production by means of red blood cell transfusions and intravenous administration of hematin, and interruption of the enterohepatic circulation of protoporphyrin by oral administration of cholestyramine or activated charcoal. Liver transplantation has been done successfully in several patients with advanced liver disease who failed to respond to medical therapy.

The prognosis depends on whether liver disease develops. Other manifestations probably do not affect life span.

Acute Intermittent Porphyria

The autosomal dominant disorder of AIP has an estimated prevalence of 5 to 10 cases per 100,000 population. Many cases exist in latent form. The manifest disease is more frequent in women. The fundamental defect is a deficiency of PBG deaminase activity.

The defect in PBG deaminase causes increased excretion of ALA and PBG in urine. When an acute attack of neurologic dysfunction occurs, excretion of these compounds increases because of induction of hepatic ALA synthase activity. Recovery is associated with a decline in their excretion, but values almost always remain above normal.

The disease may exist in latent form indefinitely, but several factors precipitate acute attacks. These include drugs (barbiturates and sulfonamides, most commonly), starvation or excessive dieting, female sex hormones, and infections. Patients should not have pentobarbital for dental extractions or surgery.

The acute attack can involve any portion of the nervous system. The abdominal pain that frequently occurs during acute attacks is thought to result from imbalance in the autonomic innervation of the gut. Other manifestations of autonomic neuropathy are sinus tachycardia, labile hypertension, sweating, and vascular spasm (e.g., retina or skin). When peripheral neuropathy occurs, it is usually preceded by abdominal pain. The peripheral neuropathy may be sensory or motor. There may be pain in the back and legs or paresthesias. Motor neuropathy can involve any peripheral nerve and may be symmetric or asymmetric with a variable rate of progression. Complete flaccid paralysis can develop over a period of days. Respiratory paralysis sufficient to require assisted ventilation is a grave prognostic sign. In severe attacks some patients are unable to speak, breathe, or swallow. Central nervous system manifestations include seizures, hallucinations, coma, hypothalamic dysfunction, cerebellar and basal ganglion manifestations, and bulbar paralysis. Depression and organic brain syndrome are the two most characteristic psychiatric problems.

The profound hyponatremia that develops in some patients results from gastrointestinal tract loss of sodium, inappropriate release of antidiuretic hormone, and, possibly, primary renal sodium loss. Hypercholesterolemia, hyperamylasemia, and increased serum thyroxinbinding globulin occur in some patients.

During the acute attack the diagnosis is made by demonstrating increased PBG in the urine. Positive screening tests for PBG, such as the Watson-Schwartz or Hoesch test, should be confirmed by quantitative measurement of PBG. Since increased urinary PBG also occurs during acute attacks of variegate porphyria and hereditary coproporphyria, specific diagnosis is made by demonstration of decreased erythrocyte PBG deaminase activity.

Treatment involves prophylaxis, symptomatic management, and reversal of the fundamental disease process. All patients should be instructed to avoid the known precipitating factors. The abdominal pain often can be controlled with phenothiazines, but meperidine may be necessary. Propranolol has been used to control autonomic manifestations such as tachycardia and hypertension. A high-carbohydrate intake (400 g/day or more if possible) causes a decrease of porphyrin precursor excretion and produces clinical improvement in some patients. The reason for the spectrum of responsiveness (from spectacular recovery to little or no effect) is unknown. Since this therapy has virtually no risk, it should be instituted in all acute attacks. Although the value of intravenous hematin administration has not been proved by double-blind studies, it does lower porphyrin precursor excretion and is useful in the treatment of acute attacks, particularly if started early. Hematin therapy has little effect on established neuropathy, in which nerve regeneration is the rate-limiting factor in recovery. Since hematin affects blood clotting, caution should be exercised in patients with coagulopathies or in those receiving anticoagulants.

In previous studies the mortality rate for serious paralytic attacks was 40% to 60%. Modern management of critically ill patients has reduced this rate, but death still occurs.

Variegate Porphyria

The prevalence of the autosomal dominant disorder of variegate porphyria is unknown in the United States, but it is undoubtedly lower than that of AIP. A deficiency of protoporphyrinogen oxidase activity is the fundamental defect. During acute attacks the excretion in the urine of ALA and PBG is increased. During asymptomatic periods porphyrin precursor excretion is often normal, but urinary uroporphyrin and coproporphyrin may be increased, the latter usually exceeding the former. Fecal protoporphyrin is increased during both symptomatic and asymptomatic periods.

Cutaneous or neurologic manifestations (or both) occur. Increased skin fragility with formation of bullae, erosions, scarring, and pigmentation occur in skin exposed to sunlight. Facial hypertrichosis and chronic thickening of skin also occur. The acute attacks of neurologic dysfunction can be precipitated by the same factors as in AIP, and the manifestations are the same.

The diagnosis during the acute attack is suggested by demonstration of increased ALA and PBG in the urine. Since this finding also occurs in attacks of AIP and hereditary coproporphyria, it is not specific for variegate porphyria. So far as prophylaxis and treatment of the acute attack are concerned, however, distinction among these three disorders is academic. During asymptomatic periods or the presence of cutaneous symptoms alone, an increase of urinary uroporphyrin and coproporphyrin may be demonstrable, but these findings may be confused with those of porphyria cutanea tarda. The increase of fecal protoporphyrin that occurs in variegate porphyria allows the differentiation of these disorders.

Therapy of the acute attack of neurologic dysfunction is the same as for AIP. Treatment of cutaneous manifestations is difficult. Betacarotene therapy, as described for protoporphyria, has not been of value.

Hereditary Coproporphyria

Like the other two acute types of porphyria, this dominantly transmitted disease can remain latent indefinitely or attacks can be precipitated by the same factors that activate AIP. Decreased coproporphyrinogen oxidase activity causes increased excretion of fecal coproporphyrin. Urine coproporphyrin may be increased. An increase of urinary coproporphyrin without other urine findings is not specific for porphyria, since secondary coproporphyrinuria is seen in a number of hepatic, hematologic, malignant, and toxic diseases. During acute attacks urinary excretion of ALA and PBG is increased, but it may be normal during asymptomatic periods.

Hereditary coproporphyria can cause both neurologic dysfunction and cutaneous manifestations. Treatment is the same as for AIP and variegate porphyria.

Porphyria Cutanea Tarda

This disease can occur sporadically, as a familial disease, and also as a toxic disorder caused by exposure to hexachlorobenzene and related compounds. The disease is the most common of the porphyrias.

A deficiency of uroporphyrinogen decarboxylase activity is the basic defect. In the familial form of the disorder, this deficiency is found in all tissues, whereas in the toxic and sporadic forms, enzyme deficiency appears to be restricted to the liver.

Uroporphyrin and coproporphyrin are increased in the urine, with the former exceeding the latter. Urinary ALA may be minimally increased, but PBG is not. A group of tetracarboxyl porphyrins known as *isocoproporphyrins* are excreted in the feces.

Three factors that may activate the disease are increased ingestion of iron, alcoholism, and estrogen use. There are no neurologic manifestations. Minor trauma to skin causes vesicles or bullae that develop on sun-exposed areas, but acute photosensitivity reactions are not frequent. Vesicles and bullae rupture and are followed by erosions and scarring. Over time, hirsutism, milia, areas of pigmentation and depigmentation, and sclerodermoid changes develop. Iron overload is present, and serum iron levels are often increased. Liver biopsy usually shows hepatocellular injury, along with fatty infiltration and hemosiderosis, and patients with long-standing untreated disease may develop cirrhosis and hepatocellular carcinoma. In the United States fewer than 10% of patients develop cirrhosis. Alcoholism may be in part responsible for the hepatic damage. Recent studies have shown that patients with this disease also frequently have chronic hepatitis C.

The diagnosis should be considered when vesicles or bullae appear on exposed areas of skin. The disease is more frequent in men and usually appears after age 35. Young women have developed the cutaneous lesions while taking oral contraceptives, particularly when this has accompanied significant alcohol intake. During cutaneous symptoms urinary uroporphyrin excretion usually exceeds that of coproporphyrin in porphyria cutanea tarda, whereas the opposite is generally seen in variegate porphyria. The high fecal protoporphyrin level seen in variegate porphyria is also useful in distinguishing the two diseases. Decreased erythrocyte uroporphyrinogen decarboxylase activity can be used to diagnose porphyria cutanea tarda in its familial form.

Removal of body iron by repeated phlebotomy causes a decrease of urinary porphyrin excretion and clinical remission. Removal of 5 to 10 L is usually required. Therapy is monitored by urinary uroporphyrin excretion. Chloroquine in low doses (125 to 250 mg three times a week) may also be used in treatment, particularly if the patient is intolerant of phlebotomy.

Hepatoerythropoietic Porphyria

Hepatoerythropoietic porphyria is a rare form of porphyria, having been described in only about 20 patients. The disease becomes evident within the first year of life as a skin disease resembling porphyria cutanea tarda. Patients are severely affected and develop excess facial hair, scarring of the hands and face, sclerodermoid changes, and acrosclerosis. The cutaneous symptoms improve somewhat as patients grow older, but hepatic disease supervenes. There are often slight to modest increases in serum transaminase and γ-glutamyl transpeptidase levels. The liver shows red fluorescence and a nonspecific hepatitis or portal inflammation. This may progress to cirrhosis. Adults usually have mild normochromic anemia, and fluorescent normoblasts are found in the bone marrow.

The abnormalities in porphyrin metabolism resemble those of porphyria cutanea tarda, with the additional feature that zinc protoporphyrin levels in erythrocytes are increased.

Hepatoerythropoietic porphyria is caused by a severe deficiency

in the activity of uroporphyrinogen decarboxylase (5% to 10% of normal). The parents of such patients have approximately a 50% decrease in activity. Thus hepatoerythropoietic porphyria is the homozygous form of decarboxylase deficiency, whereas familial porphyria cutanea tarda is the heterozygous form.

There have been few reports of therapy. The methods outlined for porphyria cutanea tarda seem rational, although iron removal is not likely to be of benefit. Administration of hematin or hypertransfusion, or both, may be considered when the bone marrow appears to be an important source of porphyrin overproduction.

Aminolevulinic Acid Dehydrase Deficiency

A few patients who had acute porphyria-type symptoms were shown to have a 98% to 99% deficiency of ALA dehydrase activity. Their parents had 50% of normal activity. These findings suggest that rare instances of homozygous deficiency of ALA dehydrase activity produce acute attacks of porphyria.

Management is the same as that for the other acute types of porphyria.

BIBLIOGRAPHY

Anderson KE: The porphyrias. In Zakim D, Boyer TD, editors: *Hepatology: a textbook of liver disease,* Philadelphia, 1996, WB Saunders.

Bloomer JR, Straka JG, Rank JM: The porphyrias. In Schiff L, Schiff ER, editors: *Diseases of the liver,* Philadelphia, 1993, Lippincott.

Kappas A et al: The porphyrias. In Scriver CR et al, editors: *The metabolic basis of inherited disease,* New York, 1989, McGraw-Hill.

Lamon JM et al: Hematin therapy for acute porphyria, *Medicine (Baltimore)* 58:252, 1979.

Schmid R, Schwartz S, Watson CJ: Porphyrin content of bone marrow and liver in the various forms of porphyria, *Arch Intern Med* 93:167, 1954.

With TK: A short history of porphyrins and the porphyrias. *Int J Biochem* 11:189, 1980.

CHAPTER

312   Hypercalcemia

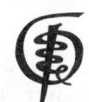

John P. Bilezikian

CAUSES AND DIFFERENTIAL DIAGNOSIS

The causes of hypercalcemia are listed in Box 312-1. Primary hyperparathyroidism and malignant neoplasms, the most common causes of hypercalcemia, are covered separately in Chapters 322 and 323. Despite the fact that in the great majority of patients with hypercalcemia (approximately 90%), one of these two causes is responsible, it is important to consider other causes of hypercalcemia in the course of a diagnostic evaluation.

The differential diagnosis of hypercalcemia depends on the history, the physical examination, and appropriate laboratory tests. If a malignancy is present, it is usually readily discovered. The malignant disorders most frequently associated with hypercalcemia are multiple myeloma; carcinoma of the lung, breast, esophagus, kidneys, ovary, or bladder; and lymphoma. The mechanisms for the elevated level of serum calcium in malignant disease are covered in Chapter 323. Primary hyperparathyroidism is distinguished from hypercalcemia of malignancy on clinical grounds and by obtaining a parathyroid hormone level (see Chapter 323). The concurrence of hypercalcemia and an elevated parathyroid hormone level, in the absence of renal failure, establishes the diagnosis of primary hyperparathyroidism. It is very rare for a malignant disorder, regardless of the mechanism of the hypercalcemia, to be associated with an elevated level of parathyroid hormone. In the syndrome of humoral hypercalcemia of malignancy, the parathyroid hormone–like protein (PTHRP) elaborated by the tumor does not cross-react in any of the commercially available radioimmunoassays or immunoradiometric assays for parathyroid hormone. Thus even when PTHRP is responsible for the hypercalcemia, the parathyroid hormone level is not elevated (see Chapter

---

BOX 312-1
Causes of hypercalcemia

Primary hyperparathyroidism
Cancer
    Parathyroid hormone-related protein
    Ectopic production of 1,25-dihydroxyvitamin D
    Other factors produced ectopically
    Lytic bone metastases
Nonparathyroid endocrine disorders
    Thyrotoxicosis
    Pheochromocytoma
    Adrenal insufficiency
    Vasoactive intestinal polypeptide hormone-producing tumor
Granulomatous diseases (1,25-dihydroxyvitamin D excess)
    Sarcoidosis
    Tuberculosis
    Histoplasmosis
    Coccidioidomycosis
    Leprosy
Medications
    Thiazide diuretics
    Lithium
    Estrogens and antiestrogens
Milk-alkali syndrome
Vitamin A intoxication
Vitamin D intoxication
Familial hypocalciuric hypercalcemia
Immobilization
Parenteral nutrition
Acute and chronic renal insufficiency

---

322). Somewhat more difficult is the situation in which the concentration of parathyroid hormone is low and the diagnosis of malignancy cannot be made. The less common causes of malignancy must then be considered.

Nonparathyroid Endocrine Disorders

Hypercalcemia occurs in approximately 5% to 10% of patients with hyperthyroidism, caused presumably by rapid bone turnover. The calcium level is usually less than 11.5 mg/dl and is readily reversible after successful therapy for the hyperthyroid state. Hypercalcemia associated with pheochromocytoma may occur in the syndrome of multiple endocrine neoplasia type II, in which case primary hyperparathyroidism is concurrent. Alternatively, and analogous to humoral hypercalcemia of malignancy, some pheochromocytomas may elaborate a hypercalcemic factor. The proper approach to the patient with a pheochromocytoma and hypercalcemia is to remove the adrenal tumor first. Pancreatic islet cell tumors that secrete vasoactive intestinal polypeptide (VIP) can be associated with severe hypercalcemia. Similar to the situation with pheochromocytoma, the VIPoma may coexist with hyperparathyroidism as part of a multiple endocrine neoplasia syndrome (in this case, type I), but there are other patients in whom the hypercalcemia remits after removal of the pancreatic tumor. Addison's disease is another rare endocrine cause of hypercalcemia. The mechanism may be due to loss of the antagonistic properties of glucocorticoids on calcium absorption. Several decades ago, tuberculosis used to be the most common cause of adrenal insufficiency. In view of the presence of hypercalcemia in some patients with tuberculosis (see later discussion), this possible cause of the adrenal insufficiency should be borne in mind when hypercalcemia and adrenal insufficiency are seen together.

Vitamin D

Vitamin D toxicity can induce hypercalcemia among patients being treated for chronic hypoparathyroid states. When the parent compound, vitamin D, is responsible, hypercalcemia can persist for months because of the large potential storage depots for the vitamin in fat tissue. The levels of serum calcium and phosphate are both elevated, as is the 25-hydroxyvitamin D level. The level of active metabolite, 1,25-dihydroxyvitamin D, is not usually elevated unless ingestion of this active metabolite is responsible for the hypercalcemia. The list of granulomatous diseases associated with hypercalcemia is long; the hypercalcemia in these diseases is caused, in many instances, by the granulomatous tissue producing 1,25-dihydroxyvitamin D. Sarcoidosis is the best example of a granulomatous disease that can induce hypercalcemia, but other noteworthy examples are tuberculosis, histoplasmosis, coccidioidomycosis, leprosy, berylliosis, candidiasis, eosinophilic granuloma, and silicone implantation. Ectopic production of 1,25-dihydroxyvitamin D by malignant lymphomas also occurs. Causes of hypercalcemia in acquired immunodeficiency syndrome (AIDS) may relate to malignant lymphomatous processes to which these patients are predisposed.

Medication-Induced Hypercalcemia

Thiazide diuretics may be responsible for hypercalcemia in the absence of any intrinsic abnormality in calcium metabolism. Thiazide-induced hypercalcemia is one of those situations in which the parathyroid hormone level may be elevated as a result of a nonparathyroid cause. The hypercalcemia remits after withdrawal of the thiazide in a substantial number of patients, although it is also possible that primary hyperparathyroidism will be unmasked. The determination of cause of hypercalcemia, when it surfaces during thiazide therapy, cannot be made with confidence until 2 or 3 months after the diuretic is discontinued. Patients receiving lithium carbonate may develop hypercalcemia. Here again, the medication should be discontinued, if possible, to determine whether the lithium is responsible for the altered parathyroid sensitivity to calcium or whether primary hyperparathyroidism is present. Estrogens and antiestrogens (tamoxifen) have been reported to result in hypercalcemia in a significant number of patients with breast carcinoma. Usually these patients have known, extensive bone metastases. Very unusual examples of medication-induced hypercalcemia are milk-alkali syndrome and vitamin A toxicity.

Unusual Causes

Familial hypocalciuric hypercalcemia (FHH) is an important consideration in the differential diagnosis of hypercalcemia because it can easily be mistaken for primary hyperparathyroidism. The distinction between FHH and primary hyperparathyroidism rests on several features: genetics (autosomal dominance) with early penetrance in childhood; normal parathyroid hormone level; low urinary calcium excretion (Ca/Cr clearance <0.01); and lack of typical clinical features of primary hyperparathyroidism (see Chapter 322). Recent studies have shown that FHH is due to a mutation in the gene that codes for the plasma membrane–associated calcium-sensing receptor. Immobilization hypercalcemia does not usually occur, despite the negative calcium balance to which all immobilized individuals are subject, unless there is an underlying abnormality in calcium metabolism such as Paget's disease or malignancy. Hypercalcemia, however, may regularly occur in growing children who have been immobilized because of a fracture or some other reason. Hypercalcemia in patients receiving parenteral nutrition may develop when administered calcium is greater than 300 mg per day and when renal function is impaired. Hypercalcemia after long-term parenteral nutrition also occurs, but its mechanism is obscure. It is likely to be related to the osteomalacia that frequently develops in these individuals. Hypercalcemia may occur in the setting of acute or chronic renal failure.

CLINICAL FEATURES

Hypercalcemia is associated with signs and symptoms that are independent of its causes. When therapy for hypercalcemia per se is considered, these particular features should be assessed and not confused with signs and symptoms that may be caused more specifically by the patient's underlying disorder. Measures to reduce the serum calcium concentration do not ameliorate aspects of the patient's symptoms that are not a result of hypercalcemia. Admittedly, when symptoms are rather general (e.g., weakness, lethargy), a specific cause may be exceedingly difficult to pinpoint. In such cases, empiric but

BOX 312-2
Clinical features of hypercalcemia

General
  Weakness
  Dehydration
  Metastatic calcification
Central nervous system
  Impaired concentration
  Increased sleep requirement
  Altered states of consciousness (confusion, lethargy, stupor, coma)
Gastrointestinal tract
  Polydipsia
  Anorexia
  Nausea
  Vomiting
  Constipation
  Pancreatitis
  Peptic ulcer
Renal
  Polyuria
  Decreased function
  Decreased concentrating ability
  Nephrolithiasis
  Nephrocalcinosis
Cardiovascular
  Hypertension
  Electrocardiographic changes (shortened QT interval)
  Increased sensitivity to digitalis

Table 312-1   Management of hypercalcemia

GENERAL	SPECIFIC
Rehydration	Bisphosphonates
Saline administration	Plicamycin
Diuresis with furosemide	Calcitonin
	Gallium nitrate
Dialysis	Phosphate
Mobilization	Glucocorticoids
	Therapy of underlying cause

judicious therapy for the hypercalcemia may be warranted. The reported value for the serum calcium should always be interpreted with knowledge of the serum albumin value, the major circulating calcium-binding protein. When the serum albumin is normal, approximately 50% of the total calcium value reflects the physiologically active, free ionized form. If the serum albumin level is low, as is often the case in sick patients, the ionized calcium level is greater than 50% of the measured value, and the hypercalcemia is actually greater than that indicated by the total serum calcium level. For every gram per deciliter of reduction in the serum albumin level, the measured total serum calcium concentration should be adjusted upward by 0.8 mg/dl to appreciate more accurately the degree of true hypercalcemia (see Chapter 286).

If the serum calcium level is only mildly elevated (<11.5 mg/dl), there are few if any signs or symptoms of hypercalcemia. If the serum calcium level is between 11.5 and 13.5 mg/dl, patients may or may not be symptomatic. Invariably, symptoms are present if the serum calcium is greater than 13.5 mg/dl. The rate at which the serum calcium level rises is also a factor that helps to determine the degree of symptomatology. For a given calcium level, the patient who experiences the more rapid rise is the more symptomatic. A list of signs and symptoms of hypercalcemia is presented in Box 312-2. Included in the list is a set of problems that can make relatively mild hypercalcemia a medical emergency. Polyuria not accompanied by adequate oral fluid replacement can lead to decreased intravascular volume, thus increasing the severity of hypercalcemia. Worsening hypercalcemia in turn can lead to decreased fluid intake, because of anorexia, and more marked polyuria. Ensuing diminished renal function, because of dehydration, eventually leads to reduced clearance of the serum calcium. This cycle can rapidly lead to a hypercalcemic emergency. Such patients are invariably symptomatic both because of the level of the serum calcium and the rapidity of its rise. This pathophysiologic mechanism can be operative in virtually any underlying cause of hypercalcemia.

TREATMENT

Therapeutic agents for hypercalcemia can lower the serum calcium level in virtually all cases. The range of therapeutic options provides the opportunity to tailor treatment to the patient's condition. If the serum calcium level is mildly elevated and not accompanied by any of the clinical features described above, therapy should be tempered

accordingly. On the other hand, life-threatening hypercalcemia requires a much more aggressive approach. An important principle of therapy is to take into account the underlying cause of the hypercalcemia. In patients with mild, asymptomatic primary hyperparathyroidism, the approach is much different from that in the patient who presents in parathyroid crisis. In thyrotoxicosis, the hypercalcemia is best approached by treating the hyperthyroidism. In familial hypocalciuric hypercalcemia, patients are not treated. In hypercalcemia that develops late in the course of an incurable malignancy, the physician must consider the stark reality of the patient's prognosis. Severe hypercalcemia in the patient with terminal malignancy is sometimes best left untreated.

General measures to treat hypercalcemia are applicable to all hypercalcemic states, independent of their underlying etiology (Table 312-1). Hydration is a key approach because the pathophysiologic events induced by the hypercalcemia lead invariably to dehydration. The serum calcium level declines simply by restoration of intravascular volume and improved renal glomerular filtration. Rehydration with intravenous saline has an additional advantage in that the saluresis so induced is associated with an obligatory increase in renal excretion of calcium. The use of a loop diuretic such as furosemide facilitates the loss of sodium and calcium and may be particularly valuable in patients whose cardiovascular tolerance to saline administration is limited. Diuresis with furosemide should be employed only after fluid therapy has first restored intravascular volume. Depending on the patient's capacity to handle the volume load, it is reasonable to administer judicious doses of furosemide (10 to 20 mg intravenously every 6 to 12 hours). If fluid tolerance is not viewed with concern, furosemide should not be used but rather reserved for signs of fluid overload, should they become evident. Thiazide diuretics should never be used because they may actually worsen the hypercalcemia. Peritoneal or hemodialysis should be considered if the hypercalcemia is severe and associated with renal failure. Although the patient with hypercalcemia may not be ambulatory at the time of admission to the hospital, every effort should be made to mobilize the patient as soon as possible. Mobilization helps to reduce the negative calcium balance associated with loss of weight bearing.

Specific measures to reduce severe hypercalcemia are often indicated. Most pathophysiologic mechanisms responsible for severe hypercalcemia lead to accelerated calcium mobilization from bone caused by activation of the osteoclast, the bone cell responsible for bone resorption. Specific therapies inhibit this process by impairing osteoclast-mediated bone resorption.

The bisphosphonates are pyrophosphate analogs that effectively inhibit osteoclast-mediated bone resorption. Three bisphosphonates are available worldwide: ethane hydroxy 1,1-diphosphonic acid (etidronate), dichloromethylene diphosphonate, and aminohydroxypropylidene diphosphonate (pamidronate). Etidronate and pamidronate are available at this time in the United States. Parenteral etidronate reduces the serum calcium level effectively. An oral form may help to maintain reduced calcium levels. Concerns about a potential adverse side effect of etidronate, impaired bone formation, are not important when the drug is used acutely and in a limited way.

Pamidronate is a more potent bisphosphonate than etidronate, but it has a similar time course of action, the serum calcium declining within 48 hours after the first dose. Adverse effects of parenteral pamidronate are limited to a transient temperature elevation (less than 2° C), transient leukopenia, and a small reduction in serum phosphate concentration. The effective intravenous dosage range for pamidronate is 30 to 90 mg. The highest recommended dose, 90 mg, has been associated with protracted hypocalcemia ("overshoot") and thus should be reserved for those with truly life-threatening hypercalcemia or hypercalcemia refractory to lower doses.

Plicamycin (mithramycin) is a specific osteoclast inhibitor and thus is effective in any hypercalcemic condition associated with accelerated osteoclast-mediated bone resorption. Potential side effects of plicamycin include nephrotoxicity, hepatotoxicity, and platelet dysfunction. These adverse effects and the need for parenteral administration limit the use of plicamycin to the acute therapy of hypercalcemia. It has no role as a chronic therapy.

Calcitonin should theoretically be an ideal therapy for hypercalcemia because it not only inhibits osteoclast function but also increases urinary calcium excretion. Although calcitonin is not as potent as the bisphosphonates or plicamycin, it nevertheless reduces the calcium transiently and may be of use as adjunctive therapy when the serum calcium level is extremely high. Combinations of calcitonin and other agents have been employed to amplify and prolong the hypocalcemic effects of calcitonin. Combination therapy with glucocorticoids or bisphosphonates does not appear to be more effective than the additive effects of each agent alone. But combination therapy with calcitonin and a bisphosphonate, for example, can be very useful, taking advantage of the more rapid effect of calcitonin and the more potent effect of the bisphosphonate. Calcitonin occasionally causes mild transient nausea, abdominal cramps, and flushing.

Gallium nitrate, another inhibitor of bone resorption, reduces the serum calcium level with a time course similar to that of the bisphosphonates. It should not be used when the serum creatinine level is elevated or with other potential nephrotoxic agents. Clinical experience with gallium nitrate has been somewhat disappointing.

Glucocorticoid administration may be efficacious in certain malignant disorders such as multiple myeloma, lymphoma (especially that associated with human T-lymphotropic virus type 1 [HTLV-1] associated infection), and some breast cancers. In other disorders characterized by excessive absorption of calcium from the gastrointestinal tract (vitamin D intoxication, sarcoidosis, milk-alkali syndrome), glucocorticoids can also be useful. In these settings, glucocorticoids act directly on gut epithelial cells to inhibit calcium transport. These forms of hypercalcemia are also ameliorated by limiting the amount of calcium in the diet.

Phosphate inhibits bone resorption, limits gastrointestinal tract absorption of calcium, and complexes circulating calcium. This last mechanism may lead to an adverse side effect, ectopic deposition of calcium phosphate salts in soft tissues. Because of this concern, parenteral phosphate is not used except in the most dire situations. Oral phosphate has no useful role in the therapy of life-threatening hypercalcemia because it is relatively weak and may not be tolerated by the patient who is likely to be suffering from the gastrointestinal tract manifestations of hypercalcemia.

An important consideration in the hypercalcemic patient is the underlying cause. Specific therapy, if available, for the cause of the hypercalcemia may be as effective in lowering the serum calcium level as the approaches outlined above.

BIBLIOGRAPHY

Bilezikian JP: Management of acute hypercalcemia, *N Engl J Med* 326:1196, 1992.

Bilezikian JP, Singer FR: Acute management of hypercalcemia due to parathyroid hormone and parathyroid hormone-related protein. In Bilezikian JP, Marcus R, Levine MA, editors: *The parathyroids,* New York, 1994, Raven.

Blind E, Nissenson R, Strewler GJ: Parathyroid hormone related protein. In Becker KL, editor: *Principles and practice of endocrinology and metabolism,* Philadelphia, 1995, JB Lippincott.

Broadus AE et al: Humoral hypercalcemia of cancer: identification of a novel parathyroid hormone-like peptide, *N Engl J Med* 319:556, 1988.

Fatemi S, Singer FR, Rude RK: Effect of salmon calcitonin and etidronate on hypercalcemia of malignancy, *Calcif Tissue Int* 50:107-109, 1992.

Grill V, Martin TJ: Parathyroid-hormone-related protein as a cause of hypercalcemia of malignancy. In Bilezikian JP, Marcus R, Levine MA, editors: *The parathyroids,* New York, 1994, Raven.

Nussbaum SR et al: Highly sensitive two-site immunoradiometric assay of parathyrin, and its clinical utility in evaluating patients with hypercalcemia, *Clin Chem* 33:1364, 1987.

Nussbaum SR, Potts JT Jr: Advances in immunoassays for parathyroid hormone. In Bilezikian JP, Marcus R, Levine MA, editors: *The parathyroids,* New York, 1994, Raven.

Pollak MR, Brown EM, Chou Y-HW et al: Mutations in the human Ca^{2+}-sensing receptor gene cause familial hypocalciuric hypercalcemia and neonatal severe hyperparathyroidism, *Cell* 75:1297, 1993.

313 Hypocalcemia

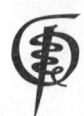

John P. Bilezikian

Disorders associated with hypocalcemia include a long list of causes as noted in Box 313-1. The first consideration in any individual whose total serum calcium level is below normal is to ascertain that hypocalcemia is actually present. The total serum calcium level reflects the contribution of calcium bound to albumin (about 50%) as well as the physiologically active free calcium concentration. When the serum albumin value is below normal, a relatively common feature in the very ill patient, the total serum calcium level is low. If the serum ionized calcium were measured in patients with hypoalbuminemia, it would be normal. Because a direct determination of ionized calcium is not always available, the same correction factor indicated previously in consideration of hypercalcemia (Chapter 312) is made for hypocalcemia. The acid-base status of the patient is another factor that may influence the degree to which a patient may be symptomatic from hypocalcemia. In alkalosis, more calcium is bound to albumin. The change in equilibrium, favoring calcium in its inactive, bound form, gives rise to more symptoms for a given level of the total serum calcium when alkalosis is present. On the other hand, acidosis leads to a greater amount of free calcium and thus favors fewer symptoms for a given level of total serum calcium. Another factor that has only recently been recognized as potentially important in

---

BOX 313-1
Differential diagnosis of hypocalcemia

Situational
  Hypoalbuminemia
  Alkalosis
  Elevated concentrations of free fatty acids
  Intensive care unit–associated
Hypoparathyroidism
  Postsurgical hypoparathyroidism
  Autoimmune hypoparathyroidism
    Isolated
    Multiple glandular failure
  Genetic
Magnesium deficiency, severe
Hypermagnesemia
Infiltrative diseases of parathyroid glands
  Hemochromatosis
  Thalassemia
  Wilson's disease
  Metastatic carcinoma
  Amyloidosis
Ionizing radiation or chemotherapy
Congenital disorders (DiGeorge's syndrome, Kearns-Sayre syndrome)
Neonatal hypocalcemia
Relative hypoparathyroidism
  Acute pancreatitis
  Acute release of cellular phosphate
    Rhabdomyolysis
    Chemotherapy
    Toxic shock syndrome
  Osteoblastic metastases
  Multiple, citrated blood transfusions
  States of 1,25-dihydroxyvitamin D deficiency
  Some vitamin D resistant states
Resistance to parathyroid hormone
  Pseudohypoparathyroidism
    Type Ia and type Ib
    Type II

shifting the partition ratio between bound and free calcium is circulating free fatty acids. Free fatty acids can permit more calcium binding to albumin and thus may lead to a reduced ionized calcium concentration. Despite these considerations and the underlying medical disorder, the presence of hypocalcemia in an acutely ill patient is not always easily explained. It is often obscure and not clearly related to abnormalities in parathyroid hormone or to 1,25-dihydroxyvitamin D.

DIFFERENTIAL DIAGNOSIS
Hypoparathyroidism

Hypoparathyroidism is defined as a state of hypocalcemia that occurs in association with deficient parathyroid glandular function. In all true hypoparathyroid states the parathyroid hormone concentration is low. The coexistence of hypocalcemia and abnormally low parathyroid hormone levels differentiates the hypoparathyroid states from those hypocalcemic disorders caused by nonparathyroid abnormalities in which there is a compensatory increase in parathyroid hormone levels. The widespread availability of sensitive, reliable assays for parathyroid hormone permits one to rely on this assay for establishing the diagnosis of hypoparathyroidism. The serum phosphate level tends to be in the upper range of normal, perhaps because of the loss of the phosphaturic actions of parathyroid hormone. The 1,25-dihydroxyvitamin D concentration may be low both because parathyroid hormone, a major stimulus to the formation of 1,25-dihydroxyvitamin D, is low and because elevated phosphate level suppresses formation of the active vitamin D metabolite.

Postsurgical Hypoparathyroidism. Hypoparathyroidism develops in a small percentage of patients who have undergone neck surgery. Following the removal of parathyroid tissue for hyperparathyroidism, a transient hypoparathyroid state may develop owing to several possible factors. These factors include interference with the vasculature of the remaining parathyroid tissue; a brief period is required for the suppressed normal glands to recover function, or for rapid remineralization of bone in patients with hyperparathyroid bone disease (hungry bone syndrome). In this latter instance, calcium in the intravascular space is rapidly exiting, to be deposited into the remineralizing skeleton. Management of the hypocalcemia in these patients is designed to cover the period before normal mineral homeostasis is reestablished, usually a matter of days. Some patients, however, develop permanent hypoparathyroidism following neck surgery. This condition is more likely to occur if the operation has been associated with major local anatomic dissection. Occasionally, all normal parathyroid tissue is inadvertently removed or, in patients who have already undergone previous parathyroid surgery, normal parathyroid tissue may have been removed at an earlier time. Postsurgical hypoparathyroidism does not always occur in the days to weeks after surgery but rather may develop years later. In this situation, it is believed that functional parathyroid tissue, left with a marginal blood supply at the time of surgery, is rendered hypofunctional with further compromise of vascular integrity over the years. Postsurgical hypoparathyroidism can develop after any neck surgery, not just following parathyroid surgery.

Autoimmune Hypoparathyroidism. Autoimmune hypoparathyroidism (formerly called idiopathic hypoparathyroidism) encompasses a rather heterogeneous group of syndromes in which parathyroid hormone secretion is deficient. The most common form is not associated with a family history or with other glandular deficiencies. It can occur at any age, although it becomes apparent most commonly in children. Females are affected twice as often as males. Parathyroid antibodies are usually present in isolated, autoimmune hypoparathyroidism. These antibodies may be directed against the secretion of parathyroid hormone itself or against parathyroid tissue. In other cases of isolated, autoimmune hypoparathyroidism the parathyroid glands are infiltrated with fat and replaced by fibrosis.

Autoimmune hypoparathyroidism also occurs as a component of the multiple end-organ endocrine deficiency syndrome. When familial, the transmission pattern is most compatible with autosomal recessive inheritance. It may also be seen sporadically without a familial background. The most classic combination of endocrine glands involved is the parathyroids and the adrenals. Mucocutaneous candidiasis is usually also present. Gonadal failure, hypothyroidism, and diabetes mellitus may also be seen. Nonendocrine abnormalities, besides mucocutaneous candidiasis, such as pernicious anemia, chronic active hepatitis, alopecia, vitiligo, or malabsorption, may be present or develop over time. The clinical presentation of this form of auto-immune hypoparathyroidism varies with respect to the sequence of glandular involvement and also to the number of different glands affected in the course of the patient's life. Virtually every combination of end-organ deficiencies with or without the aforementioned nonendocrine manifestations of the syndrome has been described. Antibodies directed against specific endocrine tissues and T-cell abnormalities suggest an autoimmune origin. The multiple end-organ endocrine deficiency syndrome has also been described in connection with a constellation of developmental abnormalities.

Genetic Hypoparathyroidism. Hypoparathyroidism can occur, although much more rarely than the autoimmune form, as a familial syndrome. In this form of the disorder parathyroid antibodies are absent. Genetic studies have shown that the structural gene for parathyroid hormone is present in these individuals. Several mutations have been described for an autosomal dominant and autosomal recessive forms of familial hypoparathyroidism. The point mutations are found in the region of the preproPTH gene. Altered trafficking of the preproPTH molecule through the cell or altered processing of the messenger RNA (mRNA) for preproPTH leads in each case to defective parathyroid hormone secretion. Another genetic form of hypoparathyroidism has been described in which there is an activating mutation of the gene that codes for the calcium sensing receptor. Familial hypoparathyroidism also has been described as an X-linked disorder. The gene defect in this syndrome is not related to the parathyroid hormone gene but rather to events that are required for parathyroid cell development and function.

Magnesium. Severe hypomagnesemia is associated with hypocalcemia caused in part by impaired secretion of parathyroid hormone. The functional hypoparathyroidism in severe magnesium deficiency is discussed in detail elsewhere (Chapter 315). Hypermagnesemia can also be associated with functional hypoparathyroidism and hypocalcemia. In this case the parathyroid glands are inhibited in a normal physiologic way by the elevated magnesium level. Clinically, the setting in which this is most likely to occur is when magnesium is used to control premature labor. In most obstetric patients, however, the reduction in serum calcium is mild and usually not associated with symptoms.

Rare Causes of Hypoparathyroidism. Infiltration of the parathyroids by heavy metals such as iron (hemochromatosis, thalassemia) or copper (Wilson's disease) can lead, in rare instances, to hypoparathyroidism. Infiltration of the parathyroid glands can also occur, but very rarely, in metastatic carcinoma, in sarcoidosis, and in amyloidosis. Even more uncommon are reported examples of hypoparathyroidism in patients who have received previous irradiation to the head and neck. Similarly, parathyroid gland function has unusually been reported to be compromised following therapy with cytotoxic chemotherapeutic agents such as doxorubicin, cytosine arabinoside, asparaginase, and WR2721.

Neonatal and Congenital Disorders. A transient period of mild hypocalcemia is normal during the first 3 weeks of life, a normal consequence of immature parathyroid glands that are unable to compensate for the expected decline in the neonatal calcium concentration. Transient neonatal hypoparathyroidism may be more severe in the offspring of hyperparathyroid mothers. After feedings have begun, during the fourth through sixth week of life, neonatal hypocalcemia may be caused by the high phosphate content of foods, especially cow's milk. A milk mixture with a high calcium/phosphate ratio (4:1) is helpful until the parathyroid glands develop adequate maturity.

Hypoparathyroidism occurs as a component of anomalies associated with maldevelopment of the branchial pouches. The best known of these congenital causes of hypoparathyroidism is DiGeorge's syndrome, in which the absence of the third and fourth branchial pouches leads to absence of the parathyroid and thymus glands. Deficient T-cell–mediated immunity caused by agenesis of the thymus is the most devastating part of this disorder, leading to death from severe viral and fungal infections within the first few years of life. When the first and fifth branchial pouches do not develop, hypoparathyroidism may be seen in association with a host of physical anomalies such as hypertelorism, antimongoloid slant, micrognathia, and aortic arch abnormalities. Hypoparathyroidism is also associated with other rare developmental abnormalities such as familial nephrosis, nerve deafness, lymphedema, prolapsing mitral valve, brachydactyly, and the Kearns-Sayre syndrome.

Relative Hypoparathyroidism

Hypocalcemia can develop in patients who have normal parathyroid gland responsiveness. In this setting the parathyroid glands react to the hypocalcemia, associated with a host of different primary disorders (see Box 313-1), by secreting more hormone. The secondary hyperparathyroidism is an attempt to overcome the hypocalcemia induced by the pathophysiologic mechanisms involved in these various disorders. It is important to recognize the difference between primary hyperparathyroidism, a hypercalcemic disorder due to excessive secretion of parathyroid hormone (Chapter 322), and secondary hyperparathyroidism, an appropriate compensatory response to hypocalcemia. Primary hyperparathyroidism is virtually always associated with hypercalcemia, whereas secondary hyperparathyroidism is associated with hypocalcemia, if compensatory secretion of parathyroid hormone is inadequate (i.e., relative hypoparathyroidism). If compensatory secretion of parathyroid hormone is adequate, the patient's calcium concentration may be in the low-normal range, at the expense of deleterious effects of elevated parathyroid hormone levels on bone and other target tissues.

Vitamin D Deficiency or Resistance. A major category of hypocalcemia associated with secondary increases in parathyroid hormone is deficiency of 1,25-dihydroxyvitamin D. A long list of gastrointestinal tract and renal diseases account for the majority of patients with 1,25-dihydroxyvitamin D deficiency. Defective mineralization of bones in adults gives rise to a clinical hallmark of vitamin D deficiency: osteomalacia. In these patients, the four parathyroid glands are hyperplastic. With appropriate management of the underlying disease, normal parathyroid function can sometimes be reestablished. Certain forms of vitamin D resistance may also be associated with a secondary hyperparathyroidism. These disorders are all considered in detail elsewhere (Chapter 316).

Pseudohypoparathyroidism. This classic disorder of calcium metabolism has an unmistakable physical appearance characterized by short stature, round facies, short neck, and foreshortened metacarpal and metatarsal bones (Albright's hereditary osteodystrophy or pseudohypoparathyroidism type Ia; Fig. 313-1). It is a genetic disease with several different transmission patterns: sex-linked dominant, autosomal recessive, and autosomal dominant. Patients usually have low-normal to frankly retarded intelligence. There may be a history of childhood seizures. Radiologically evident calcifications in the basal ganglia and cataracts are common. The serum calcium level is low and the serum phosphate level is elevated. In contrast to true hypoparathyroidism, the parathyroid hormone level is elevated, hence the designation *pseudohypoparathyroidism*. The salient biochemical feature of pseudohypoparathyroidism is resistance to the actions of parathyroid hormone. There is neither a phosphaturic nor a cyclic adenosine monophosphate (AMP) response to parathyroid hormone in the classic (type Ia) syndrome (Fig. 313-2). The typical patient with pseudohypoparathyroidism type Ia may show resistance to the actions of other hormones besides parathyroid hormone. Hypothyroidism, hypogonadism, glucagon resistance, defective olfaction, and prolactin deficiency have all been reported in pseudohypoparathyroidism. Pseudohypoparathyroidism type Ib is identical to type Ia except for the fact that Albright's hereditary osteodystrophy is not present and other hormone resistant states are not seen. Patients do have the biochemical abnormalities. In contrast, after Albright described pseudohypoparathyroidism, he observed a patient with the typical body habitus but without evidence for hypocalcemia or target organ resistance. In his attempt to distinguish this variant from classic pseudohypoparathyroidism, Albright dubbed it *pseudopseudohypoparathyroidism*. Pseudohypoparathyroidism and pseudopseudohypoparathyroidism clearly belong to the same genetic family as evidenced by family trees that contain both forms of the disorder, by selected patients whose biochemical profile has been known to cross over to the other, and by the molecular basis of the disorder (see later discussion). Even other variants of pseudohypoparathyroidism exist such as those characterized by resistance to the renal actions of parathyroid hormone but sensitivity to its skeleton actions. Equally uncommon, some patients demonstrate a normal cyclic AMP response to parathyroid hormone but no phosphaturia (type II).

Important clues to the defect in pseudohypoparathyroidism were gained by observations related to the fact that the constellation of hormone resistance that is included in the syndrome involves the adenylyl cyclase messenger system. A site common to all hormones that use adenylyl cyclase is the guanine nucleotide binding protein, G_s, that links their different receptors to the catalytic unit of adenylyl cyclase. Patients with Albright's hereditary osteodystrophy (pseudohypoparathyroidism type Ia) demonstrate a 50% reduction in G_s (Fig. 313-3). Levels of the inhibitory guanine nucleotide–binding protein, G_i, are normal. Despite the importance of this observation, reduced G_s levels do not entirely account for the syndrome. Patients with pseudopseudohypoparathyroidism in which the typical physiognomy is not accompanied by hormone resistance, nevertheless, do have reduced G_s levels. Only patients with the classic disorder, but not all, have the reduction in G_s. Patients with type Ib and parathyroid resistance in the absence of any other hormone resistance have normal levels of G_s, implying that this isolated hormone-resistant state might be caused by a defect in the parathyroid hormone receptor per se or some non–G protein-related postreceptor abnormality. There is even evidence for a circulating parathyroid hormone–like inhibitor in pseudohypoparathyroidism. These points suggest that reduced levels of G_s are not necessarily causally related to hormone resistance in pseudohypoparathyroidism and also that the underlying mechanisms for the various forms of pseudohypoparathyroidism are likely to be heterogeneous.

Acute Pancreatitis. When acute pancreatitis is severe, it is associated with hypocalcemia, a very poor prognostic sign. It is still not known why patients may become so markedly hypocalcemic, but current evidence continues to focus on deposition of calcium soaps in conjunction with fatty acid lipolysis in pancreatitis. Although most patients have a secondary elevation of parathyroid hormone level, there is debate about whether the parathyroid hormone response is sufficiently vigorous with respect to the extent of the hypocalcemia.

Other Causes. Other causes of relative hypoparathyroidism may be the result of rapid release of phosphate from cells. Chemotherapy for acute leukemia or Burkitt's lymphoma, acute rhabdomyolysis, and toxic shock syndrome may all be associated with massive release of cellular phosphate into the circulation. Another mechanism is operative in the hypocalcemia associated with osteoblastic metastases in breast and prostatic carcinoma. The extremely rapid influx of calcium from blood to bone in these examples of osteoblastic metastatic bone disease is believed to be responsible for the hypocalcemia. Multiple, citrated blood transfusions can lead to complexing of free ionized calcium with citrate sufficiently great to reduce the ionized calcium concentration.

CLINICAL FEATURES

The presence of signs and symptoms of hypocalcemia is a function of the absolute level of the calcium concentration as well as the rate of its fall. Chronic hypocalcemia is much less likely to be associated with classic clinical features than acute hypocalcemia in which the serum calcium concentration is reduced rapidly. The neuromuscular system is affected most often, giving rise to latent or frank excitability. The patient may complain of paresthesias of the extremities or a feeling of numbness, especially if the extremity is left in a resting position. Chvostek's sign is elicited by gently tapping the facial nerve anterior to the ear. Twitching of the proximate facial muscles indicates latent neuromuscular excitability. Mere contraction at the lip is a less reliable sign because it may be found in as many as 10% of normal subjects. Another classic sign of latent tetany is Trousseau's

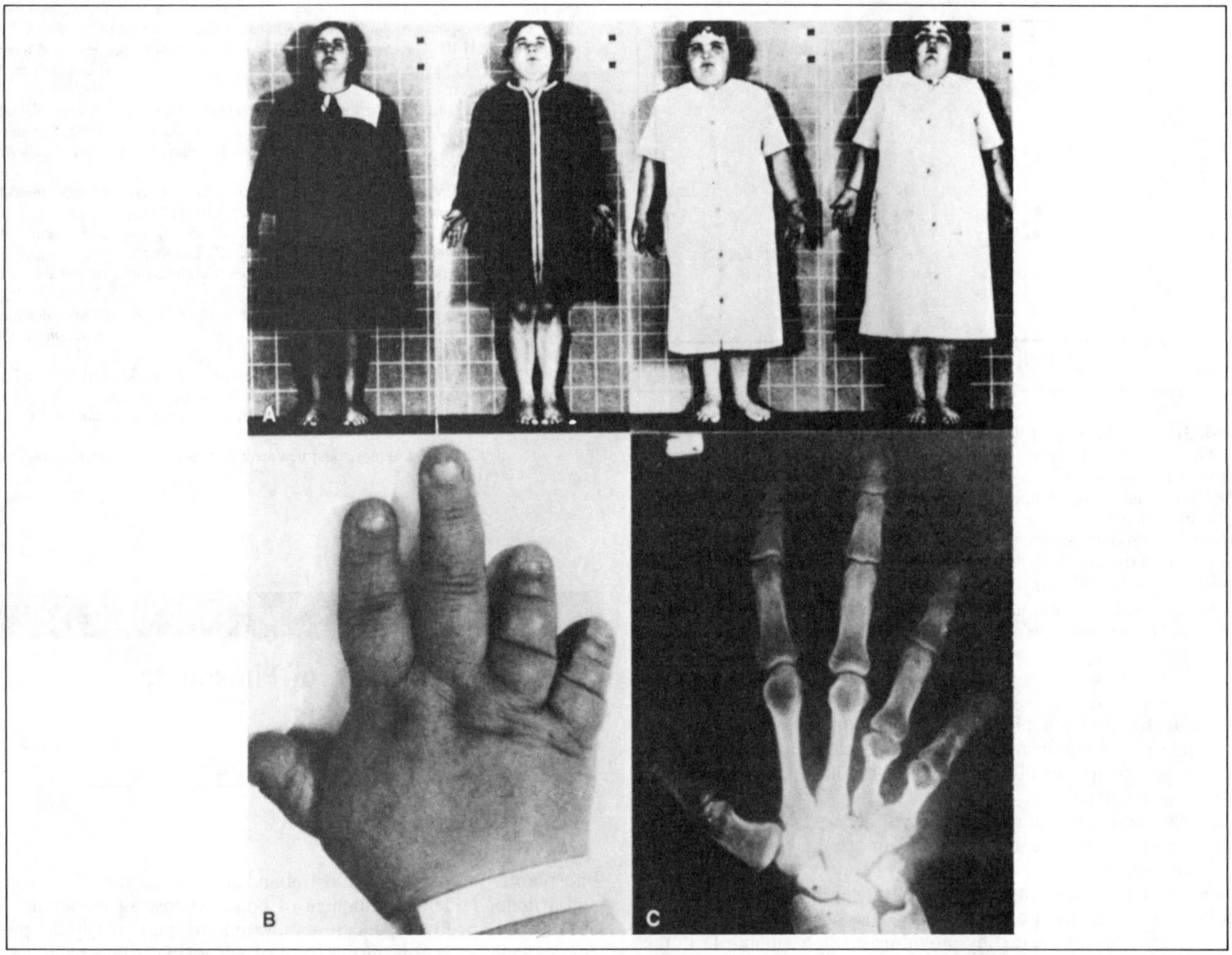

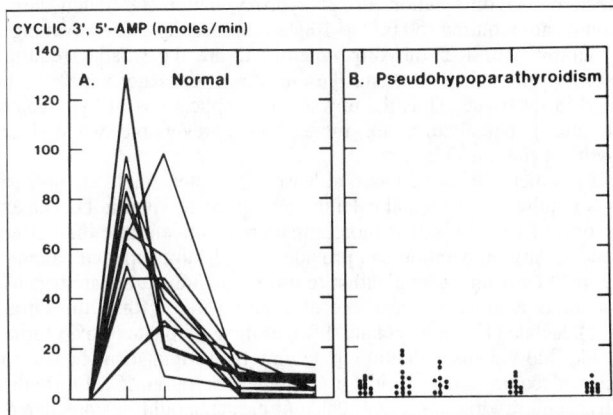

FIGURE 313-1   The physical features of four sisters with pseudohypoparathyroidism. **A,** Short stature, round facies, and shortened neck are evident. **B,** The metacarpal bones of the fourth and fifth digits are foreshortened, giving this characteristic appearance to the knuckles. **C,** Radiograph demonstrating the shortened metacarpal bones.

A from Kinard RE et al: *Arch Intern Med* 139:204, 1979; **B** and **C** from Levine MA et al: *Johns Hopkins Med J* 151:137, 1982.

sign, elicited by carpal spasm after inflation of the blood pressure cuff to just above systolic blood pressure for 2 minutes. Carpal spasm consists of flexed elbow, flexed wrist, adducted thumb, flexed metacarpophalangeal joints, and extended interphalangeal joints. In acute hypocalcemia, spontaneous carpal-pedal spasm may be present. The QT interval on the electrocardiogram may be prolonged. Laryngospasm is a rare but life-threatening manifestation of hypocalcemia. Frank convulsions may be observed, especially in individuals with an underlying seizure disorder. A few examples of reversible congestive heart failure due to hypocalcemia have been reported.

In chronic hypocalcemia associated with hypoparathyroid states, long-term complications include ectopic calcium deposition in soft tissues, cataracts, and basal ganglia calcifications. Rarely, extrapyramidal signs suggestive of parkinsonism are observed. Papilledema and intestinal malabsorption with steatorrhea are also seen occasionally.

TREATMENT

The major aim of therapy is to alleviate signs and symptoms of hypocalcemia or, if possible, to prevent their appearance. There is no urgent need to treat the patient with mild hypocalcemia who is asymptomatic. Patients with marked hypocalcemia (less than 6.5 mg/dl) are a greater problem because symptoms can develop rapidly. Acute hypocalcemia is treated by the intravenous administration of calcium.

FIGURE 313-2   Parathyroid hormone resistance in pseudohypoparathyroidism. **A,** Normal patients respond to an infusion of parathyroid hormone with a rapid, marked increase in the urinary excretion of cyclic adenosine monophosphate (AMP). **B,** In pseudohypoparathyroidism this response to parathyroid hormone is markedly blunted.

Modified from Chase LW et al: *J Clin Invest* 48:1832, 1969.

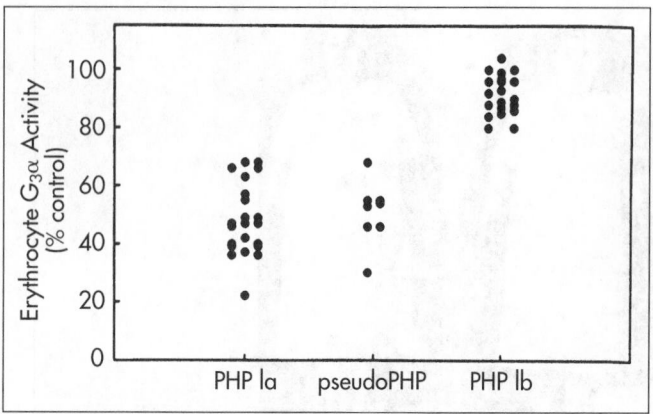

FIGURE 313-3   Activity of the stimulatory guanine nucleotide binding protein, G_s, in different forms of pseudohypoparathyroidism. G_s activity in complementation assays with S49 cyc$^-$ membranes, which genetically lack G_s but retain all other components necessary for hormone-responsive adenylyl cyclase activity. Activity was reduced by approximately 50% in patients with classic pseudohypoparathyroidism (PHP 1a) and in pseudopseudohypoparathyroidism (pseudoPHP) but was normal in patients with pseudohypoparathyroidism type Ib (PHP1b).

From Streeten EA, Levine MA. In Becker KL, editor: Principles and practice of endocrinology and metabolism, Philadelphia, 1995, JB Lippincott.

As is true for infusion of any electrolyte solution, administration should be slow and deliberate. The goal of acute therapy is to control the signs and symptoms of hypocalcemia, not necessarily to normalize the serum calcium.

The chronic hypoparathyroid states require long-term therapy. Vitamin D and calcium are the mainstays of treatment. Theoretically, any of the preparations of vitamin D can be used to treat any of the chronic hypocalcemias. Knowledge of the state of vitamin D metabolism helps to adapt the treatment more specifically. Simple vitamin D deficiency is easily treated by providing enough vitamin D in the diet (400 to 1000 IU daily). For diseases of the gastrointestinal tract, larger amounts (50,000 IU twice weekly) are required. 25-Hydroxyvitamin D (25 to 50 µg daily) overcomes the initial hydroxylation defect in severe liver disease. The disorders associated with impaired conversion of 25-hydroxyvitamin D to 1,25-dihydroxyvitamin D (hypoparathyroidism, pseudohypoparathyroidism, renal disease, vitamin D–dependent rickets type I) can be treated with near physiologic doses of 1,25-dihydroxyvitamin (0.25 to 0.5 µg daily). If the parent form of vitamin D is used in these disorders associated with defective 1-hydroxylation of 25-hydroxyvitamin D, much larger amounts are required (50,000 to 100,000 units daily). The advantages of therapy with 1,25-dihydroxyvitamin D are the smaller required dose, its shorter half-life, and the fact that it does not appear to be stored in fat tissue. Thus the unwanted complications of hypercalcemia and hypercalciuria are more readily reversible when 1,25-dihydroxyvitamin D is used.

If the diet does not contain at least 1 g of elemental calcium, patients require supplemental calcium in addition to vitamin D. The exact form of calcium salt is more a matter of convenience than effectiveness. Any preparation can provide enough supplemental calcium. The most convenient preparation to use is calcium carbonate because it contains a greater percentage of calcium (40%) than the citrate (21%), lactate (13%), gluconate (9%), or the glubionate (6.6%) forms. In older individuals, calcium citrate may be advantageous because it does not require gastric acid for efficient absorption. If achlorhydria or hypochlorhydria is present, calcium citrate should be considered.

BIBLIOGRAPHY

Albright F et al: Pseudohypoparathyroidism: an example of Seabright-Bantam syndrome, *Endocrinology* 3:922, 1942.

Arnold A, Horst SA, Gardella TJ et al: Mutation in the signal peptide-encoding region of the preproparathyroid hormone gene in familial, isolated hypoparathyroidism, *J Clin Invest* 86:1084, 1990.

Chase LW, Melson GL, Aurbach GD: Pseudohypoparathyroidism: defective excretion of 3',5'-AMP in response to parathyroid hormone, *J Clin Invest* 48:1832, 1969.

Eastell R, Heath H III: The hypocalcemic states: their differential diagnosis and management. In Coe FL, Favus MJ, editors: *Disorders of bone and mineral metabolism,* New York, 1992, Raven.

Eisenbarth GS, Jackson RA: The immunoendocrinopathy syndromes. In Wilson JD, Foster DW, editors: *Williams textbook of endocrinology,* Philadelphia, 1992, Saunders.

Guise TA, Mundy GR: Evaluation of hypocalcemia in children and adults, *J Clin Endocrinol Metab* 85:1473, 1995.

Pollak MR, Brown EM, Estep HL et al: Autosomal dominant hypocalcemia caused by a Ca^{2+}-sensing receptor gene mutation, *Nat Genet* 8:303, 1994.

Rude RK: Magnesium metabolism. In Becker KL, editor: *Principles and practice of endocrinology and metabolism,* Philadelphia, 1995, JB Lippincott.

Stewart AF et al: Hypocalcemia due to calcium soap formation in a patient with a pancreatic fistula, *N Engl J Med* 315:496, 1986.

Streeten EA, Levine MA: Hypoparathyroidism and other causes of hypocalcemia. In Becker KL, editor: *Principles and practice of endocrinology and metabolism,* Philadelphia, 1995, JB Lippincott.

Thakker RV: Molecular genetics of hypoparathyroidism. In Bilezikian JP, Marcus R, Levine MA, editors: *The parathyroids,* New York, 1994, Raven.

Thakker RV: Molecular genetics of parathyroid disease, *Curr Opin Endocrinol Diabetes* 3:521, 1996.

Tohme JF, Bilezikian JP: Diagnosis and treatment of hypocalcemic emergencies, *Endocrinologist* 6:10, 1996.

314   Disorders of Phosphate Homeostasis

Fuad N. Ziyadeh and Stanley Goldfarb

Phosphorus is among the most abundant constituents of all tissues and a major mineral component of bone. Almost all metabolic processes are critically dependent on phosphorus, particularly the provision of cellular energy in the form of adenosine triphosphate (ATP) and the phosphorylation of various enzymes such as protein kinases that express hormone action. In addition, phosphorus may influence the oxygen-carrying capacity of hemoglobin through regulation of 2,3-diphosphoglycerate (2,3-DPG) synthesis. Phosphorus is also an important constituent of membrane phospholipids that play an essential role in cell membrane integrity and in regulation of the phosphoinositide system, a critical regulatory system in cell homeostasis.

The total body content of phosphorus is about 1000 g, of which approximately 85% is in bone and most of the remainder is intracellular. Of the total plasma inorganic phosphorus, about 10% is protein-bound and about 5% is complexed. The remainder is in the form of orthophosphates. It has been customary to express concentrations in terms of elemental phosphorus but to refer to it as phosphate. The normal fasting serum phosphate level in adults is 3.0 to 4.5 mg/dl. This value is higher in children and postmenopausal women. There is a diurnal variation of serum phosphate level with a morning nadir. In addition, ingestion of carbohydrate lowers phosphate concentration by enhancing cellular uptake; ingestion of phosphate-rich food results in elevation of serum phosphate level. Thus it is important for the interpretation of serum and urinary levels that samples be obtained in the fasting state.

The average daily intake of phosphorus in the United States is about 1000 mg, mostly provided by dairy products, meats, eggs, and to a lesser extent, vegetables and grains. The mechanism of small intestinal absorption is complex, but the largest component is absorbed by passive diffusion. A smaller but significant component is absorbed actively under the influence of 1,25-dihydroxycholecalciferol (1,25-DHCC). The net amount of phosphate that is absorbed from the gastrointestinal tract is approximately 700 mg per day. The gastrointestinal tract also secretes a relatively fixed amount of phosphate of about 200 mg per day that appears in stools. At steady state, adults must excrete in the urine an amount equal to net intestinal absorption every day to maintain normal external balance. This underscores the role of the kidney as the most important regulatory organ of serum phosphate and total body content of phosphorus.

Phosphate is freely filtered at the glomerulus. Approximately 80% of the filtered load is reabsorbed along the proximal tubule, 10% in the distal nephron, and the remainder appears in the final urine. Tubular phosphate transport is a result of a membrane carrier activated by cell sodium entry (sodium-phosphate cotransport) as well as the cellular use of phosphate in metabolic pathways. Parathyroid hormone (PTH) and dietary phosphate intake are the two most important regulators of urinary phosphate excretion. A rise in serum PTH depresses tubular reabsorption of phosphate by a process involving stimulation of proximal tubular cyclic adenosine monophosphate (AMP) and phosphoinositide production, and leads to phosphaturia. Renal phosphate transport is also directly influenced by dietary intake of phosphate. If the diet is deficient in phosphate, normal individuals demonstrate an immediate and profound reduction in urinary phosphate excretion. The mechanism of this enhanced renal phosphate retention is unclear, but suppression of PTH secretion is not the primary factor. In experimental animals, the same acute response to reduction of dietary phosphate is observed despite PTH infusion or parathyroidectomy. Urinary phosphate excretion is also a function of the filtered load of phosphate, the product of serum phosphate and the glomerular filtration rate (GFR). As the filtered load increases, the capacity to reabsorb phosphate increases until a maximum rate of transport for phosphate is reached. If the filtered phosphate load is above the maximum rate of transport for phosphate, urinary phosphate excretion is augmented; if the filtered load is below the maximum rate of transport, virtually no phosphate appears in the urine.

Movement of phosphorus between the extracellular and intracellular compartments (internal balance) occurs continuously, and enhanced shifts of phosphate between these compartments may produce marked changes in the serum phosphate concentration, which is discussed later.

HYPOPHOSPHATEMIA

Hypophosphatemia (Box 314-1) is defined as a low concentration of phosphate in the serum. Whether hypophosphatemia results in symptomatic and clinically important cellular phosphate depletion or not is a complex function of the level of cellular phosphate stores and the metabolic activity of the tissue, as discussed below. Hypophosphatemia may occur with or without a reduction in total body phosphate content, that is, phosphate depletion. Three major mechanisms may underlie hypophosphatemia: decreased intestinal absorption, enhanced urinary excretion, and enhanced uptake of phosphate from the extracellular to the intracellular compartment or bone. At times, more than one mechanism may be involved in causing hypophosphatemia.

Etiology

Gastrointestinal Tract Causes. Since phosphate is ubiquitous in foods, hypophosphatemia secondary to a selective decrease in phosphate intake is unusual. The kidney responds to dietary restriction of phosphate almost immediately in such a way that urinary phosphate excretion falls within the first 24 hours (and probably within the first few hours) and negative phosphate balance is prevented. (The signal for this acute response is likely to be the acute fall in serum phosphate level that results from dietary phosphate restriction.) However, since obligate intestinal secretion of phosphate persists, prolonged dietary phosphate deficiency may lead to phosphate depletion and a negative phosphate balance. Prolonged starvation can also lead to a negative phosphate balance, but the catabolic effects of a calorie-protein malnutrition result in increased breakdown of cells and release of large amounts of intracellular phosphate. This process may lead to normalization of serum phosphate and occasionally even to frank hyperphosphatemia, despite severe total body phosphate depletion. An important cause of hypophosphatemia is the intake of large amounts of aluminum-, magnesium-, or calcium-containing antacids. In the intestinal lumen, these antacids bind both dietary and secreted phosphates and render them unabsorbable. Most syndromes of general intestinal fat malabsorption are also associated with hypophosphatemia. Although increased fecal excretion of phosphate does contribute to the negative phosphate balance, the predominant mecha-

---

BOX 314-1
Causes of hypophosphatemia

I. Decreased gastrointestinal tract absorption of phosphate
  A. Starvation, malnutrition
  B. Malabsorption
  C. Phosphate-binding antacids
II. Increased renal excretion of phosphate
  A. Primary hyperparathyroidism
  B. Secondary hyperparathyroidism
  C. Fanconi's syndrome
  D. Familial hypophosphatemia
  E. Oncogenic osteomalacia
  F. Diuretic phase of acute tubular necrosis
  G. Postrenal transplantation
  H. Idiopathic hypercalciuria
  I. Glycosuria
  J. Acute volume expansion
  K. Acetazolamide therapy
III. Enhanced cellular uptake
  A. Glucose-insulin infusions
  B. Catecholamine infusions
  C. Respiratory alkalosis
  D. Treatment of ketoacidosis
  E. Recovery phase of malnutrition
  F. Total parenteral nutrition
  G. Hungry bone syndrome
  H. Alcohol withdrawal
  I. Fructose intolerance
  J. Theophylline overdose
  K. Severe hyperthermia
IV. Abnormalities in vitamin D metabolism*

*The predominant mechanism is secondary hyperparathyroidism, but decreased intestinal absorption also contributes to hypophosphatemia.

---

nism is the enhanced phosphaturia that develops as a result of secondary hyperparathyroidism (secondary to concomitant calcium and vitamin D malabsorption).

Renal Causes. Decreased renal tubular phosphate reabsorption is generally caused either by an intrinsic defect in tubular transport or, more commonly, by extrinsic factors that inhibit phosphate reabsorption. In all these disorders, the urine contains significant amounts of phosphate despite hypophosphatemia. Intrinsic tubular defects of phosphate transport may be a component of Fanconi's syndrome (glycosuria, generalized aminoaciduria, bicarbonaturia, uricosuria, and phosphaturia). Decreased renal tubular phosphate reabsorption is responsible for hypophosphatemia in familial hypophosphatemic rickets and oncogenic osteomalacia (see Chapter 317).

The most common cause of renal phosphate wasting is primary or secondary hyperparathyroidism (see Chapter 322). Other conditions associated with increased renal wasting of phosphate include the diuretic phase of acute tubular necrosis, postrenal transplantation, and idiopathic hypercalciuria. Hyperglycemia with glycosuria may promote renal phosphate excretion and contribute to phosphate depletion in uncontrolled diabetes. This effect may result from competition between glucose and phosphate for transport across the brush border of the proximal tubule. Acute volume expansion with saline, high-dose glucocorticoids, acetazolamide therapy, hyperthermia, and chronic metabolic acidosis are also known to promote urinary phosphate excretion.

Redistribution of Phosphate. Increased cellular phosphate uptake may lead to various degrees of hypophosphatemia. In hospitalized patients, glucose infusions are the most common cause of hypophosphatemia. It is thought that glucose-induced insulin release promotes phosphate entry from the extracellular space into the cellular pool. Therapy of diabetic ketoacidosis can precipitate varying degrees of hypophosphatemia. Prior to therapy, patients with diabetic ketoacidosis may already be in marked negative phosphate balance because of glycosuria, metabolic acidosis, and poor intake of phosphate. However, serum phosphate is often normal, presumably as a result of the enhanced catabolic rate. On administration of large amounts of insulin, the serum phosphate level may rapidly fall, reaching between 1 and 2 mg/dl in the majority of patients within the first 24 to 48 hours. If insulin is administered at more physiologic rates, only mild reductions of serum phosphate are seen. During this time, urinary phosphate level becomes very low, reflecting enhanced anabolism and insulin-stimulated tubular reabsorption of phosphate.

Acute respiratory alkalosis has been frequently associated with hypophosphatemia. However, experimental studies of this phenomenon were complicated by concurrent glucose infusions to the subjects; only mild hypophosphatemia develops in uncomplicated respiratory alkalosis in the absence of concomitant glucose infusions. The hypophosphatemia that develops in gram-negative septicemia and liver disease is presumably caused in part by respiratory alkalosis, but other factors may also be operative.

Stimulation of the beta-adrenergic system or catecholamine infusions may also be responsible for redistribution of phosphate from the extracellular to the intracellular compartment similar to the effects of insulin and respiratory alkalosis. Regimens of total parenteral nutrition that do not include phosphate may lead to profound hypophosphatemia. This effect may be caused in part by absence of phosphate supplementation, but the major cause of hypophosphatemia is the rapid cellular uptake of phosphate during refeeding. Rapid mineralization of bone after parathyroidectomy for primary hyperparathyroidism, after treatment of renal osteodystrophy by parathyroidectomy, or after renal transplantation may all be associated with severe hypophosphatemia, a situation often termed the *hungry bone syndrome*. Osteoblastic metastases, particularly in prostatic cancer, may have a similar effect whereby phosphate is taken up by bone from the extracellular space. Patients with rapidly growing malignancies such as Burkitt's lymphoma have recently been described in whom tumor uptake of phosphate has led to persistent hypophosphatemia. Eventual hyperphosphatemia occurred when tumor breakdown was induced by chemotherapy.

Several of the aforementioned mechanisms may be simultaneously present in the individual patient presenting with severe hypophosphatemia and phosphate depletion. Perhaps the most common clinical conditions are chronic alcoholism and alcohol withdrawal. Serum phosphate levels may be normal when patients are first admitted to the hospital but subsequently decline when withdrawal ensues and therapy is administered. Poor intake, malabsorption from concomitant pancreatic insufficiency, and increased urinary losses from the generalized catabolic state may all contribute to chronic phosphate depletion in alcoholic patients. On alcohol withdrawal, serum phosphate level falls precipitously because of respiratory alkalosis, intravenous glucose infusions, refeeding, and therapy with oral antacids.

Patients with burn injury often develop hypophosphatemia, the lowest levels being reported on the fifth hospital day. Multiple causes are identified such as respiratory alkalosis, catecholamine release, total parenteral nutrition with rapid tissue deposition, and administration of large doses of antacids. Recent studies also suggest that hyperthermia-associated hypophosphatemia may be severe (serum phosphate level of less than 1.0 mg/dl) and clinically important. Renewed interest in hyperthermia as an adjunctive therapy for treatment of malignancy makes this an important observation.

Clinical Manifestations

Hypophosphatemia is commonly encountered in clinical practice. Approximately 2% of all patients admitted to a general hospital may have a serum phosphate level of less than 2 mg/dl. The incidence rises sharply in patients suffering from various debilitating illnesses such as malnutrition, malabsorption, alcoholism, burns, and sepsis. Glucose infusions and antacid ingestion, especially in the postsurgical patient, often result in further lowering of serum phosphate concentration.

Hypophosphatemia may be associated with the syndrome of symptomatic phosphate depletion. Clinical manifestations may be totally absent in mild hypophosphatemia but may be life threatening in prolonged severe hypophosphatemia (serum phosphate concentration less than 1 mg/dl). Significant complications of hypophosphatemia and phosphate depletion may involve many organic functions.

Two fundamental biochemical abnormalities may underlie the manifestations of hypophosphatemia: depletion of intracellular ATP and decreased levels of erythrocyte 2,3-DPG. These abnormalities may lead to organ dysfunction and tissue hypoxia. Typically, acute hypophosphatemia in a previously normal individual is not associated with any specific symptoms, since cellular stores are adequate to prevent critically low concentrations. If long-standing negative external phosphate balance has occurred and cell glycolysis and glycogen formation are then stimulated, for example by insulin, then critical cell phosphate deficits occur. ATP formation falls while use rises, and 2,3-DPG production falls. Enzymatic production of ATP and 2,3-DPG requires adequate cell inorganic phosphate.

Common symptoms of persistent hypophosphatemia include anorexia, dizziness, bone pain, paresthesias, proximal muscle weakness, and waddling gait. In general, neuromuscular symptoms predominate in acute hypophosphatemia, and skeletal symptoms in chronic hypophosphatemia. With extreme hypophosphatemia (serum phosphate level less than 0.5 mg/dl), an encephalopathy may develop with irritability, nervousness, dysarthria, confusion, stupor, seizures, and coma. In the alcoholic patient, these manifestations may mimic delirium tremens. Hallucinations, however, do not occur in hypophosphatemia. Skeletal muscle may be acutely affected by hypophosphatemia with resultant rhabdomyolysis. This entity is recognized by an abnormal elevation of creatinine phosphokinase and aldolase levels in serum. Alcoholics may be most vulnerable to development of rhabdomyolysis, especially during the first few days of hospitalization, when acute hypophosphatemia is superimposed on underlying chronic phosphate deficits.

Chronic hypophosphatemia is usually associated with musculoskeletal manifestations. Proximal muscle weakness and damage can develop, but the most serious consequence of this myopathy is respiratory muscle failure. Cardiac muscle may also be involved in severe hypophosphatemia, but frank congestive heart failure is rarely observed unless significant underlying myocardial disease is also present. A recent study has documented that acute, glucose-induced hypophosphatemia produces no detrimental effects on myocardial function in patients with no underlying heart disease.

Abnormalities in mineral metabolism are often noted in long-standing chronic hypophosphatemia. Rickets and osteomalacia develop as a result of impairment of osteoid mineralization. Bone pain, pathologic fractures, rheumatic complaints, and proximal muscle weakness are common features in adults with osteomalacia. Correction of phosphate deficiency results in striking bony healing.

Hypercalciuria is often associated with mild degrees of hypophosphatemia and phosphate depletion. The major cause of hypercalciuria is a specific defect in calcium reabsorption in the distal nephron. Other mechanisms involved in the genesis of hypercalciuria include the direct stimulation of bone resorption by hypophosphatemia and the effect of hypophosphatemia to increase 1,25-DHCC. This compound stimulates both intestinal calcium absorption and bone resorption. All these effects tend to increase serum calcium and promote urinary losses of calcium. Interestingly, the syndrome of idiopathic hypercalciuria seen in approximately 50% of patients with calcium urolithiasis is often associated with a mild chronic hypophosphatemia and renal phosphate wasting.

Hematologic manifestations of hypophosphatemia involve disturbances in erythrocyte, leukocyte, and platelet functions. Since phosphate is a substrate for the generation of the high-energy phosphate bonds in ATP that are necessary for the initial phases of glycolysis, hypophosphatemia causes a reduction in red blood cell 2,3-DPG and a shift of the dissociation curve for oxyhemoglobin to the left. This results in decreased tissue delivery of oxygen and tissue hypoxia. In addition, hemolytic anemias may also be present because ATP deficiency produces enhanced membrane fragility and decreased erythrocyte survival. Hemolysis is rare unless profound degrees of hypophosphatemia develop (serum phosphate level less than 0.2 mg/dl). Depressed leukocyte phagocytic activity and migration may be observed in severe hypophosphatemia. This has been implicated as a contributory factor in the increased susceptibility to infection in critically ill patients. Defective aggregation and shortened survival of platelets have been observed in severe hypophosphatemia induced in laboratory animals. These defects were also implicated in specific bleeding abnormalities in a few patients.

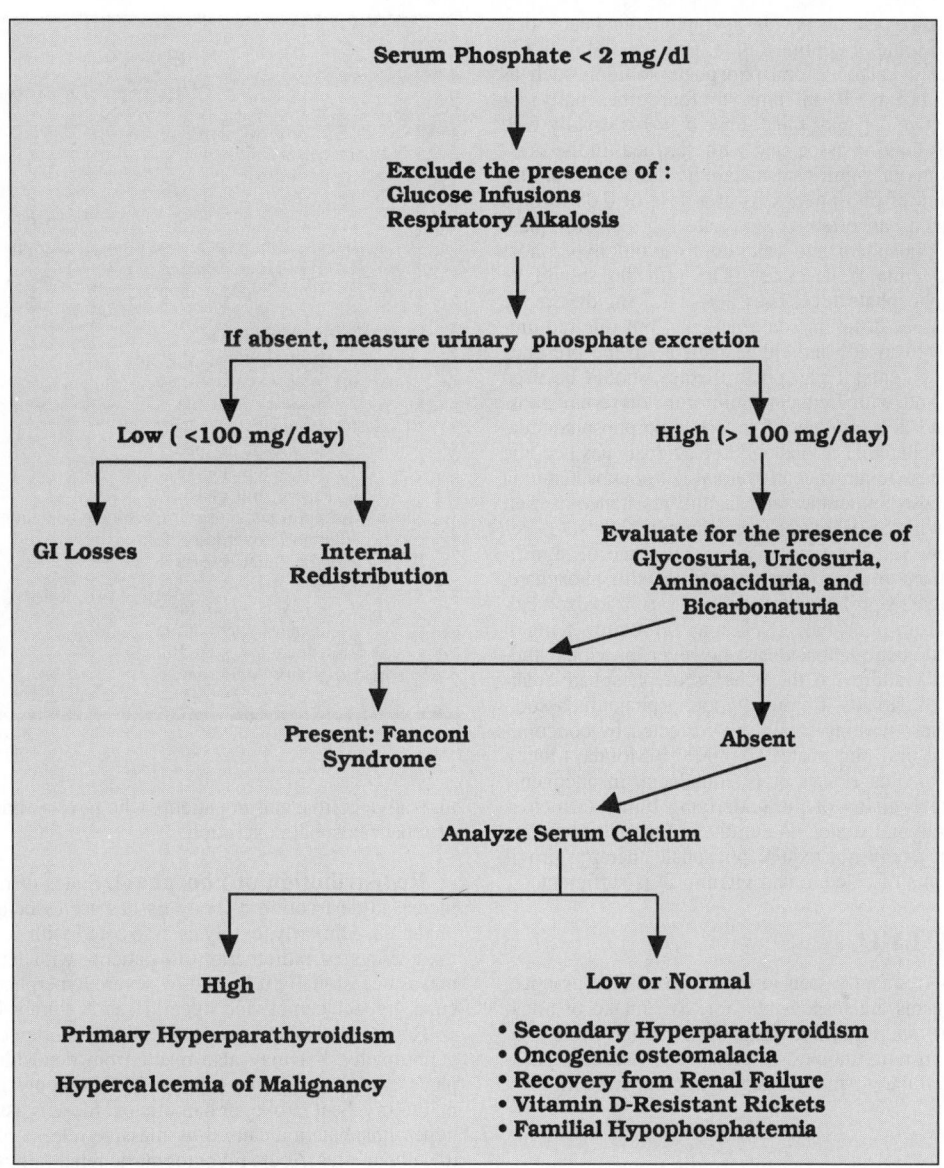

Serum Phosphate < 2 mg/dl

↓

Exclude the presence of :
Glucose Infusions
Respiratory Alkalosis

↓

If absent, measure urinary phosphate excretion

Low (<100 mg/day)   **High (> 100 mg/day)**

GI Losses   **Internal**   **Evaluate for the presence of**
                       Redistribution   **Glycosuria, Uricosuria,**
                                             Aminoaciduria, and
                                             Bicarbonaturia

Present: Fanconi   **Absent**
Syndrome

Analyze Serum Calcium

High   **Low or Normal**

Primary Hyperparathyroidism   • **Secondary Hyperparathyroidism**
                                              • **Oncogenic osteomalacia**
Hypercalcemia of Malignancy   • **Recovery from Renal Failure**
                                              • **Vitamin D-Resistant Rickets**
                                              • **Familial Hypophosphatemia**

FIGURE 314-1   Diagnostic workup of hypophosphatemia.

Diagnostic Approach

In the majority of patients with hypophosphatemia, the underlying cause is usually apparent from the history (Fig. 314-1). The most common causes of acute hypophosphatemia in hospitalized patients are glucose infusions and respiratory alkalosis. In other patients, additional diagnostic workup may be required. The measurement of urinary phosphate can be helpful in many situations. Hypophosphatemia caused by deficient intake or antacid use leads to a marked decrease in urinary phosphate excretion (less than 100 mg/day). Inappropriately increased urinary phosphate excretion in the face of hypophosphatemia is usually caused by hyperparathyroidism or primary renal tubular defects. Measurement of serum calcium is very helpful in this setting. If serum calcium level is high, primary hyperparathyroidism is the most likely diagnosis. If serum calcium level is low, a form of secondary hyperparathyroidism is often present. Most patients with hypophosphatemia, hypocalcemia, and secondary hyperparathyroidism have a disorder in vitamin D metabolism such as occurs with poor nutritional intake, malabsorption, or postgastrectomy. When serum calcium and PTH levels are normal, hypophosphatemia associated with increased renal phosphate wasting denotes a defect in renal tubular function. The concomitant findings of bicarbonaturia, glycosuria, or aminoaciduria establish the diagnosis of Fanconi's syndrome.

In the absence of these associated findings, however, the diagnosis is either familial hypophosphatemic rickets or oncogenic osteomalacia. The latter requires a careful search for an underlying neoplasm.

Prevention and Treatment

In patients receiving total parenteral nutrition, prevention of hypophosphatemia can be achieved by supplementation with 10 to 15 mMol of potassium phosphate for every 1000 calories provided. Early resumption of oral feeding in the hospitalized patient and judicious use of antacids may decrease the incidence and severity of hypophosphatemia. In general, therapy for hypophosphatemia depends on its severity and acuteness, underlying causes, and the presence or absence of significant clinical symptoms of phosphate depletion. In most cases of mild to moderate acute hypophosphatemia (serum phosphate level of 1.5 to 2.5 mg/dl), especially in the absence of significant symptoms, parenteral therapy is not indicated. In fact, such therapy may be complicated by secondary hypocalcemia. Correction of the underlying disorder (e.g., glucose infusions, respiratory alkalosis, sepsis) and restoration of an adequate diet may be sufficient. Most patients with severe hypophosphatemia (serum phosphate level of less than 1 mg/dl) should be treated with adequate phosphate replacement therapy. Occasionally, such patients may be asymptomatic; hence, oral therapy is the preferred route of administration. Provision of milk (33 mMol phosphate/L) or a balanced oral phosphate solution such as Fleet's Phospho-Soda (15 to 30 ml three to four times daily) or Neutra-Phos capsules (two capsules three times daily) is usually well tolerated. Higher doses may be associated with diarrhea. In the presence of severe symptoms or significant metabolic derangements, intravenous administration of phosphate salts at a dose of 0.08 to 0.16 mMol/kg over 6 hours is an effective and safe regimen. Frequent monitoring of serum phosphate and calcium to avoid hyperphosphatemia and hypocalcemia is necessary. The infusion should be stopped when serum phosphate level rises above 1.5 mg/dl. Severe deficits may require larger doses in some patients, but this requirement cannot be predicted in any individual patient. In the presence of renal insufficiency, parenteral phosphate therapy should be used with extreme caution and with frequent monitoring of serum phosphate to avoid the rapid development of severe hyperphosphatemia. Treatment of hypophosphatemia in diabetic ketoacidosis has become popular, but its usefulness remains controversial. Hypophosphatemia may contribute to glucose intolerance and insulin resistance as well as to tissue hypoxia owing to decreases in erythrocyte 2,3-DPG. Recent clinical trials, however, did not show any evidence of significant clinical benefit from routine supplementation with phosphate, and many patients showed significant reduction in serum ionized calcium levels. Rarely, serum phosphate levels may fall below 1 mg/dl in patients treated for diabetic ketoacidosis; however, previous studies have not specifically addressed the benefits of phosphate treatment in this subgroup of patients. Chronic hypophosphatemia associated with renal phosphate wasting should be corrected by concomitant supplementation of oral phosphates (30 to 90 mMol/day) and a vitamin D metabolite to treat rickets or osteomalacia. In oncogenic osteomalacia, adequate excision of the underlying tumor (which is often a benign mesenchymal tumor) is curative. Hypophosphatemia of vitamin D deficiency may not require phosphate therapy; provision of adequate amounts of calcium and vitamin D is sufficient.

HYPERPHOSPHATEMIA

Hyperphosphatemia is frequently seen in clinical medicine practice. Three general mechanisms are responsible: massive intake of phosphate, impaired renal excretion resulting from renal failure or impaired PTH action on renal tubules, or enhanced release of phosphate from the intracellular to the extracellular compartment (Box 314-2).

Etiology

Renal Causes. Renal failure is the most common cause of hyperphosphatemia. With reduction of GFR below 30 ml per minute, phosphate excretion is impaired, despite marked degrees of secondary hyperparathyroidism. Acute renal failure is commonly associated with variable degrees of hyperphosphatemia. Trauma and rhabdomyolysis often lead to further elevations in serum phosphate concentration in acute renal failure. Impaired renal excretion of phosphate is uniformly seen in hypoparathyroidism and related disorders. Excess renal phosphate reabsorption is also seen in acromegaly and thyrotoxicosis because growth hormone, through increased insulin-like growth factor-1 (IGF-1) production, and thyroid hormone also elevate the maximum rate of transport for phosphate. Renal tubular phosphate reabsorption is also increased in sickle cell anemia, tumoral calcinosis, and treatment with some bisphosphonates. Tumoral calcinosis is a rare congenital disorder characterized by hyperphosphatemia, normocalcemia, normal PTH levels, and large calcified masses around large joints. The primary defect is an elevation in the maximum rate of phosphate transport/GFR manifesting as increased tubular phosphate reabsorption (Chapter 122).

Gastrointestinal Tract Causes. Excess intake of phosphate may lead to transient hyperphosphatemia. Rapid increases in urinary phosphate excretion often normalize the serum phosphate level unless significant reductions in GFR are also present. Administration of phosphate-containing laxatives or enemas may lead to acute elevations in serum phosphate concentration in otherwise normal individuals, but this effect is more marked in patients with an atonic colon or

---

BOX 314-2
Causes of hyperphosphatemia

I. Renal causes
  A. Renal failure
    1. Acute
    2. Chronic
  B. Increased tubular reabsorption of phosphate
    1. Hypoparathyroidism
    2. Pseudohypoparathyroidism
    3. Acromegaly
    4. Thyrotoxicosis
    5. Bisphosphonate therapy
    6. Tumoral calcinosis
    7. Sickle cell anemia
II. Gastrointestinal tract causes
  A. Acute phosphate load
    1. Intravenous therapy
    2. Excess oral intake
  B. Surreptitious abuse of phosphate-containing laxatives
  C. Vitamin D overdose
III. Increased cellular release
  A. Rhabdomyolysis
  B. Tumor lysis syndrome
  C. Malignant hyperthermia
  D. Transfusion of stored blood
  E. Respiratory acidosis

---

ulcerative colitis, and in patients who have a concomitant impairment of renal phosphate excretion.

Redistribution of Phosphate. States of rapid catabolism with increased destruction of body tissues are associated with hyperphosphatemia. Similarly, cytolysis associated with administration of cytotoxic drugs or radiotherapy to patients with leukemia and lymphomas is occasionally followed by severe hyperphosphatemia, hyperkalemia, hypocalcemia, and hyperuricemia (tumor-lysis syndrome).

Renal insufficiency in these patients is often caused by acute urate nephropathy, but may also result from deposition of calcium phosphate complexes in the kidney. Rhabdomyolysis after trauma, thermal injury, heat stroke, or narcotic overdose is associated with marked hyperphosphatemia caused by massive release of phosphate from intracellular sites. Acute myoglobinuric renal failure may supervene and impair renal phosphate excretion, further aggravating the hyperphosphatemia. Respiratory acidosis may cause hyperphosphatemia, presumably through cellular shifts of phosphate into the extracellular fluid.

Clinical Manifestations

The clinical effects of hyperphosphatemia are primarily related to associated disorders of calcium metabolism. Secondary hypocalcemia, ectopic soft tissue calcifications, reduced bone resorption, and suppression of renal 1α-hydroxylation of 25-DHCC are prominent manifestations. It seems likely that when hyperphosphatemia develops and the calcium-phosphate product in the serum exceeds 70, the chances of ectopic calcifications increase. Common sites of soft tissue calcification include blood vessels, cornea, lung, skin, kidney, and periarticular areas. Hyperphosphatemia may also play a role in the development of secondary hyperparathyroidism of renal failure. Moreover, the severity of renal osteodystrophy correlates well with the severity of hyperphosphatemia in chronic renal failure. It is also possible that uncontrolled calcium-phosphate deposition in the kidney may contribute to the inexorable progression of renal injury in chronic renal failure.

Diagnostic Approach

In most situations, the cause of hyperphosphatemia is easily identified from examining the clinical situation. A reduction in the GFR below 30 ml per minute is the most common cause. The serum level of phosphate rarely exceeds 12 mg/dl even if severe renal failure supervenes, unless excessive amounts of phosphate are added to the circulation. Surreptitious abuse of phosphate-containing laxatives may pose some difficulty in diagnosis. In other conditions associated with hyperphosphatemia, measurements of urinary excretion of phosphate are helpful in making a diagnosis. Twenty-four-hour urinary excretion of phosphate is elevated (above 1000 mg/day) in association with excess phosphate loads and is depressed and reflects intake if the individual is in external balance (often below 1000 mg/day) in situations characterized by enhanced renal tubular reabsorption. In the latter disorders, determinations of serum calcium and PTH levels offer helpful clues to the underlying process. Serum PTH level is low in idiopathic or postsurgical hypoparathyroidism but is elevated in pseudohypoparathyroidism or in secondary hyperparathyroidism, whereas serum calcium level is often low in these conditions.

Treatment

Acute severe hyperphosphatemia with symptomatic hypocalcemia requires prompt treatment. If renal failure is not present, urinary phosphate excretion can be increased with the use of isotonic saline or sodium bicarbonate, 1 to 2 L over 2 hours, and acetazolamide, 500 mg every 6 hours. When renal failure is present, institution of hemodialysis can promptly remove substantial amounts of phosphate and correct the hyperphosphatemia and the hypocalcemia. When very rapid control is required, glucose and insulin infusions promote cell phosphate uptake and may ameliorate hyperphosphatemia until dialysis is begun. The chronic hyperphosphatemia seen in chronic renal failure, hypoparathyroidism, or tumoral calcinosis is treated primarily by a low-phosphate diet and calcium-containing antacids.

BIBLIOGRAPHY

Agus ZS: Oncogenic hypophosphatemic osteomalacia, *Kidney Int* 24:113, 1983.

Delmez JA, Slatopolsky E: Hyperphosphatemia: its consequences and treatment in patients with chronic renal failure, *Kidney Int* 29:303, 1992.

Fisher NJ, Kitabachi AE: A randomized study of phosphate therapy in the treatment of diabetic ketoacidosis, *J Clin Endocrinol Metab* 57:177, 1983.

Gravelyn TR et al: Hypophosphatemia-associated respiratory muscle weakness in a general inpatient population, *Am J Med* 84:870, 1988.

Halevy I, Bulvik S: Severe hypophosphatemia in hospitalized patients, *Arch Intern Med* 148:153, 1988.

Knochel JP: Hypophosphatemia in the alcoholic, *Arch Intern Med* 140:613, 1980.

Knochel JP, Agarwal R: Hypophosphatemia and hyperphosphatemia. In Brenner BM, editor: *The kidney*, ed 5, Philadelphia, 1996, Saunders.

Lentz RD, Brown DM, Kjellstrand CMM: Treatment of severe hypophosphatemia, *Ann Intern Med* 82:941, 1978.

Ritz E: Acute hypophosphatemia, *Kidney Int* 22:84, 1982.

Rubin M, Narins RG: Hypophosphatemia: pathophysiological and practical aspects of therapy, *Semin Nephrol* 10:536, 1990.

Ryan EA, Reiss E: Oncogenous osteomalacia: review of the world literature of 42 cases and report of two new cases, *Am J Med* 77:501, 1984.

Shilo S, Werner P, Hershko G: Acute hemolytic anemia caused by severe hypophosphatemia in diabetic ketoacidosis. *Acta Haematol (Basel)* 73:s5, 1985.

Wilson HK et al: Phosphate therapy in diabetic ketoacidosis, *Arch Intern Med* 142:517, 1982.

315 Disorders of Magnesium Homeostasis

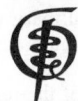

Sidney Kobrin and Stanley Goldfarb

The total body magnesium content is approximately 25 mEq/kg. (One millimole of magnesium is synonymous with 2 mEq and 24 mg.) Of this amount only about 1% is extracellular, resulting in a normal plasma magnesium concentration of between 0.75 and 1.0 mmol/L. Magnesium is the second most abundant intracellular ion. About 20% to 30% of plasma magnesium is protein-bound, mainly to albumin. The rest exists in free ionized form or in complexes. In clinical prac-

tice corrections of plasma magnesium concentrations are not made for alterations in protein (albumin) concentration, and no routine method exists for determining ionized magnesium concentration.

The bulk of total body magnesium is distributed between bone (approximately two thirds) and the intracellular compartment (approximately one third), primarily in muscle tissue. Bone magnesium is not readily available for defense against hypomagnesemia. In chronic magnesium depletion states it is the skeletal pool that is most consistently diminished and is the most useful guide to total body magnesium stores.

NORMAL MAGNESIUM METABOLISM
Intestinal Magnesium Handling

The Food and Nutrition Board of the National Academy of Sciences recommends a daily dietary intake of 12 to 14 mMol of magnesium. This requirement may increase during pregnancy, lactation, and adolescence. The average American diet contains approximately 10 to 15 mMol/day, which is very close to the recommended amount. This suggests that magnesium deficiency may develop if dietary intake or intestinal absorption is modestly decreased or magnesium losses are slightly greater than normal. Gastrointestinal tract absorption of magnesium varies depending on the amount ingested. When dietary magnesium intake is typical (12 mmol/day), 30% to 40% of ingested magnesium is absorbed (Fig. 315-1). Under conditions of low magnesium intake (1 mmol/day), approximately 80% is absorbed; only 25% is absorbed when magnesium intake is high (25 mmol/day). Presumably, only ionized magnesium is available for transport. Increased luminal phosphate or fat may precipitate with magnesium, decrease the amount of available ionized magnesium, and reduce intestinal magnesium absorption.

Although somewhat controversial, the majority of evidence suggests that two additional factors may play a role in the regulation of intestinal magnesium absorption. Vitamin D $(1,25[OH]_2D_3)$ directly increases intestinal magnesium absorption, whereas parathyroid hormone probably increases magnesium absorption indirectly by increasing $1,25(OH)_2D_3$ synthesis.

Renal Handling of Magnesium

Since magnesium absorption and secretion by the gastrointestinal tract are largely unregulated and little shift occurs in the various pools of magnesium on a day-to-day basis, the kidney serves as the major regulator of magnesium balance. Under normal conditions the non–protein-bound plasma magnesium is freely filtered at the glomerulus. About 20% to 30% of filtered magnesium is reabsorbed in the proximal tubule, and the major portion (60% to 65% of filtered load) is absorbed in Henle's loop. The distal nephron absorbs about 5% of magnesium, leaving about 5% of filtered load to be excreted in the urine. Both sodium loading and calcium loading decrease magnesium reabsorption in Henle's loop, thereby enhancing magnesium excretion. Parathyroid hormone may directly increase magnesium reabsorption in Henle's loop, opposing the indirect decrease in reabsorption as a result of hypercalcemia. An important factor regulating renal magnesium excretion is plasma magnesium level. As a result of the slow equilibration between extracellular and intracellular magnesium, the plasma magnesium concentration falls rapidly with negative magnesium balance. The reduction in plasma magnesium leads to a marked reduction in renal magnesium excretion unless urinary magnesium wasting is present. Conversely, magnesium infusions or hypermagnesemia, or both, lead to prompt increases in urinary magnesium excretion, even in previously magnesium-depleted patients.

MAGNESIUM DEFICIENCY AND HYPOMAGNESEMIA

The plasma magnesium level may not be a reliable indicator of total body magnesium stores. However, except in a few clinical situations, persistent hypomagnesemia represents total body magnesium deficiency. Isolated primary magnesium deficiency as a result of dietary deficiency is extremely uncommon because of the ubiquity of magnesium in all foods and renal magnesium conservation. Therefore magnesium deficiency usually occurs because of large losses from

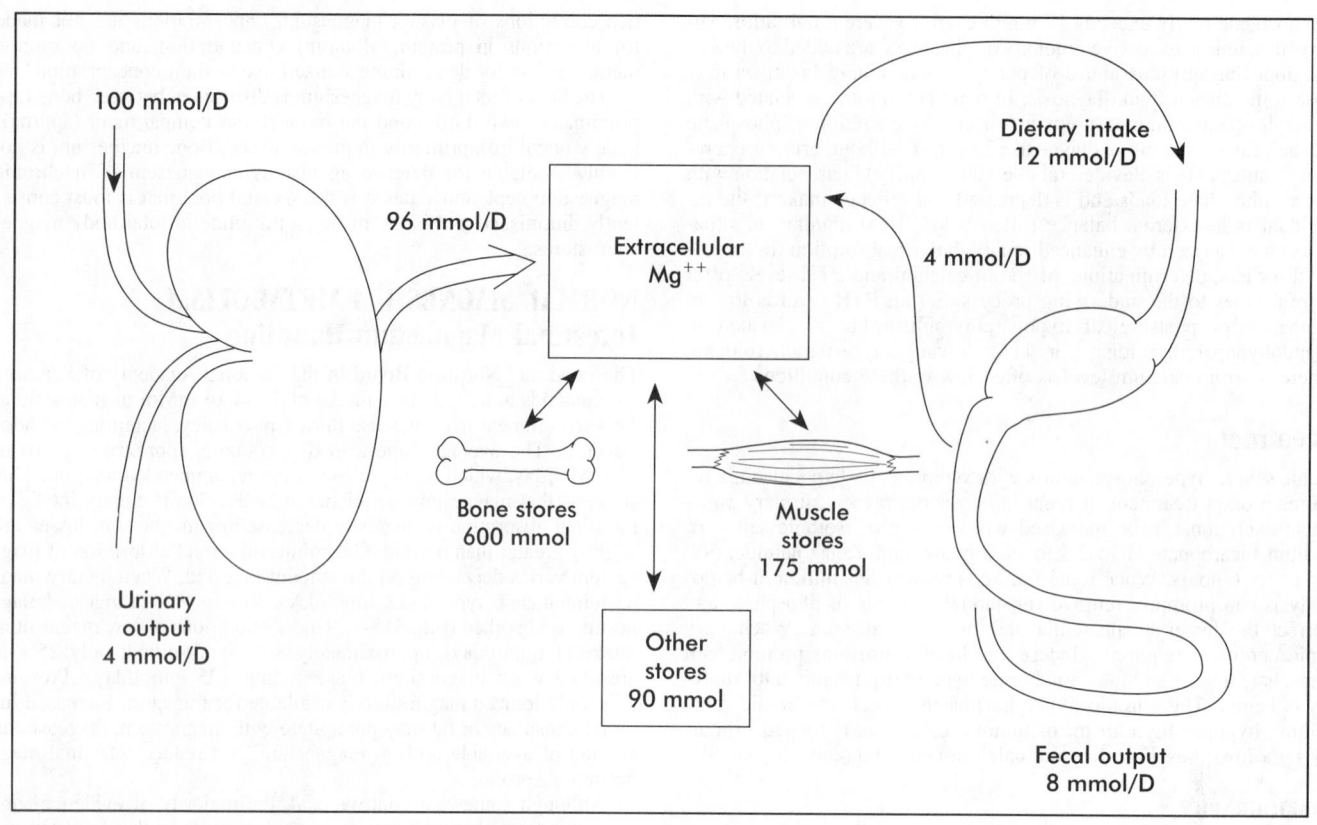

FIGURE 315-1   Distribution of magnesium in the body and daily fluxes of magnesium between diet, gastrointestinal tract, kidney, and various body pools.

the gastrointestinal tract or the kidney. The causes of hypomagnesemia are listed in Box 315-1.

Etiology

Internal Redistribution. Acute decreases in serum magnesium may occur with normal total body levels. Such redistribution may be seen with large infusions of intravenous glucose and during refeeding in children with protein-calorie malnutrition. Redistribution has also been reported with insulin therapy of diabetic ketoacidosis, during acute alcohol withdrawal, and in association with acute respiratory alkalosis. Hyperadrenergic states may also cause intracellular shifting of magnesium. In addition, catecholamines may increase circulating levels of free fatty acid that combine with free plasma magnesium. In acute pancreatitis, formation of magnesium-soap complexes has been postulated as contributing to hypomagnesemia. After parathyroidectomy for hyperparathyroidism a significant decrease in serum magnesium may be seen in association with hypocalcemia and hypophosphatemia as part of the "hungry bone syndrome."

Gastrointestinal Tract Causes. During prolonged starvation magnesium depletion may be seen as a consequence of decreased intake and persistent renal losses caused by associated ketoacidosis. Magnesium deficiency is more readily seen in a variety of intestinal conditions associated with markedly diminished absorption and/or enhanced secretion. These include inflammatory bowel diseases such as ulcerative colitis and regional enteritis, extensive resections of small bowel (particularly involving the terminal ileum), and other conditions associated with generalized malabsorption. Formation of poorly soluble magnesium complexes with fat diminishes intestinal magnesium absorption. A rare syndrome of primary intestinal malabsorption of magnesium exists and is usually seen in association with hypocalcemia and seizures early in infancy. Large losses of magnesium may be associated with prolonged upper or lower intestinal tract

fluid losses. The concentrations of magnesium in upper gastrointestinal tract (bile, gastric, pancreatic) fluid range between 0.2 and 0.5 mmol/L. In the lower gastrointestinal tract the magnesium concentration may be as high as 7 mmol/L.

Renal Losses. Urinary losses are usually reduced to less than 1 mEq per day shortly after institution of a magnesium-deficient diet. This efficient conservation may be diminished in the presence of various intrinsic or extrinsic renal disorders. These include the recovery phase of acute tubular necrosis, postobstructive diuresis, and postrenal transplantation. Renal tubular acidosis and Bartter's syndrome may also be associated with renal magnesium wasting. The associated potassium depletion or hyperaldosteronism, or both, in several of these states may contribute to impaired tubular reabsorption of magnesium. A primary renal magnesium-wasting syndrome exists in association with hypokalemia and nephrocalcinosis.

Use of drugs, particularly loop diuretics (furosemide, bumetanide, and ethacrynic acid), constitutes the largest single cause of renal magnesium wasting. These diuretics cause a greater fractional inhibition of magnesium than of sodium reabsorption in Henle's loop. Thiazides cause a much smaller increase in magnesium excretion. Multiple courses of high-dose aminoglycoside therapy have resulted in a tubulopathy characterized by hypomagnesemia, increased urinary potassium losses, hypokalemia, and hypocalcemia. *cis*-Platinum treatment for malignancy has been associated with a high frequency of hypermagnesuria and hypomagnesemia. The mechanism of the renal magnesium wasting has not been elucidated, although it probably results from damage to the ascending limb of Henle's loop.

Plasma volume expansion and osmotic diuresis induced with glucose, mannitol, or urea cause large renal losses of magnesium. Phosphate depletion has been associated with diminished tubular reabsorption of magnesium. Calcium loading and a variety of causes of hypercalcemia are associated with renal magnesium wasting and hypomagnesemia. The mechanism in each of these conditions is related to

---

BOX 315-1
Causes of magnesium deficiency

Redistribution
Insulin administration
Hungry bone syndrome
Catecholamine excess states
(?) Acute respiratory alkalosis
Acute pancreatitis
Miscellaneous
  Excessive lactation and sweating

Gastrointestinal tract causes
Reduced intake
  Starvation
  Postoperative
Reduced absorption
  Specific magnesium malabsorption
  Generalized malabsorption syndrome
  Extensive bowel resections
  Diffuse bowel disease or injury
  Chronic diarrhea, laxative abuse

Renal causes
Primary tubular disorders
  Primary renal magnesium wasting
  Welt's syndrome
  Bartter's syndrome
  Renal tubular acidosis
  Diuretic phase of acute tubular necrosis
  Postobstructive diuresis
  Post–renal transplantation status
Extrarenal factors that increase magnesuria
  Drug-induced losses
    Diuretics, aminoglycosides, digoxin, *cis*-platinum, foscarnet,
      pentamidine, tacrolimus, and cyclosporine
  Hormone-induced magnesuria
    Aldosteronism, hypoparathyroidism, hyperthyroidism
  Ion- or nutrient-induced tubular losses
    Hypercalcemia
    Extracellular fluid volume expansion
    Glucose, urea, mannitol diuresis
  Phosphate depletion
  Alcohol ingestion

Complex causes
Alcoholism
Diabetic ketoacidosis

BOX 315-2
Clinical manifestations of magnesium deficiency

Definitely associated with magnesium deficiency
Metabolic
Refractory hypocalcemia responsive only to magnesium therapy
Refractory hypokalemia responsive only to magnesium therapy
Cardiovascular
Increased susceptibility to digoxin-related arrhythmias
Peripheral nervous system
Tremor of extremities and tongue
Myoclonic jerks
Chvostek's sign (common)
Trousseau's sign (rarely)
Tetany (rarely unless concomitant hypocalcemia)
General muscular weakness (particularly respiratory muscles)
Paresthesias
Central nervous system
Apathy, depression
Some or all facets of delirium, seizures
Coma, vertigo, nystagmus, and (rarely) movement disorders

Probably associated with magnesium deficiency
Cardiovascular
Ventricular arrhythmias: premature ventricular contractions, ventricu-
  lar tachycardia, torsades de pointes
Ventricular fibrillation
Atrial arrhythmias (rare): Atrial fibrillation and atrial tachycardia
Hypertension
Coronary artery spasm
Sudden death
Miscellaneous
Increased urolithiasis
Hemolysis
Gastrointestinal tract: Esophageal spasm, anorexia, nausea, and ady-
  namic ileus
Osteomalacia

---

an inhibitory action on magnesium reabsorption in Henle's loop. The effect of alcohol is discussed later. Organic acidoses (lactic and ketoacids) are associated with increased renal magnesium losses.

The major effects of hormones on magnesium balance may be indirect. Thus, although parathyroid hormone enhances renal magnesium absorption, hyperparathyroidism may be associated with magnesuria because of the more potent counteracting effect of hypercalcemia on magnesium transport in the ascending limb of Henle's loop. Hypomagnesemia in hyperaldosteronism may be related to volume expansion or potassium depletion, or both, although the possibility of a direct alteration of aldosterone on magnesium absorption has not been eliminated.

Complex Causes

Alcoholism. Alcoholism is the clinical condition in which hypomagnesemia is seen most frequently. Multiple factors may contribute to the magnesium deficiency with or without hypomagnesemia in alcoholic patients. Poor nutrient intake in combination with increased losses from bouts of diarrhea produce external losses. Renal conservation may be impaired by associated starvation ketoacidosis. Acute ethanol administration also increases urinary magnesium excretion by a direct tubular effect. During acute illness, acute withdrawal from alcohol, acute respiratory alkalosis, and intravenous glucose administration may all cause intracellular shifts of magnesium with hypomagnesemia. Acute pancreatitis may cause further internal redistribution and hypomagnesemia. Other associated electrolyte disorders such as hypocalcemia and hypokalemia may contribute to significant neuromuscular symptoms in the alcoholic patient. Chronic pancreatitis and liver disease are common in alcoholic patients and may lead to fat malabsorption and decreased magnesium absorption as described earlier.

Diabetic Ketoacidosis. Hypomagnesemia develops in 7% of patients who come to medical attention with severe diabetic ketoacidosis. Renal magnesium wasting occurs because of the osmotic diuresis induced by hyperglycemia, ketoaciduria, and the catabolic effect of insulin deficiency, which leads to breakdown of intracellular organic compounds and release of magnesium from cells. During therapy the anabolic effects of insulin drive magnesium back into cells, and 50% to 60% of patients become transiently hypomagnesemic after 12 hours of treatment.

CLINICAL CONSEQUENCES OF MAGNESIUM DEFICIENCY

Whether the clinical effects of hypomagnesemia reflect total body deficiency or the low serum level is not well established. Clinical effects have been seen in acute hypomagnesemic states presumably not associated with total body magnesium deficiency, and magnesium administration may improve some clinical neuromuscular symptoms even in the absence of hypomagnesemia. Clinical interpretation of these effects is usually confounded by other coexisting electrolyte disturbances, mainly hypocalcemia and hypokalemia. The clinical spectrum of the consequences of magnesium deficiency are listed in Box 315-2.

Biochemical Effects

Various plasma and total body electrolyte abnormalities are seen frequently with magnesium deficiency. In experimental magnesium deficiency, hypokalemia and increased urinary potassium excretion occur. When hypokalemia coexists with hypomagnesemia, it is relatively refractory to potassium infusion unless the magnesium deficiency is corrected. It is unclear whether the defect reflects primary renal tubular losses or alterations at the cellular membrane level leading to net cellular losses of potassium.

Hypocalcemia is also frequently seen in hypomagnesemic states. This may be related to decreased parathyroid hormone levels through a direct failure of secretion in the parathyroid gland or diminished bone response to the hormone in the presence of hypomagnesemia. Vitamin D fails to correct the hypocalcemia. Associated hypocalciuria and positive calcium balance suggest that decreased skeletal release is the predominant cause of the hypocalcemia.

Neuromuscular Effects

The neuromuscular effects of hypomagnesemia occur commonly in association with hypocalcemia or hypokalemia, or both. However, the symptoms and signs may be seen in the absence of any other electrolyte abnormalities. Moreover, when hypomagnesemia and hypocalcemia coexist in the face of neuromuscular symptoms, infusion of magnesium, but not calcium alone, may reverse the effects.

Cardiac Effects

Arrhythmias are the most serious complications of magnesium deficiency. They frequently occur in association with digitalis therapy or hypokalemia, or both. Even in the absence of other associated conditions, hypomagnesemia may predispose to arrhythmias. Atrial premature contractions and sinus or nodal tachycardia may occur. The PR and QT intervals may be prolonged, and flattening of T waves may be seen. Ventricular premature contractions and in extreme cases ventricular tachycardia and fibrillation may be caused by magnesium deficiency. Treatment with antiarrhythmic drugs may be ineffective unless magnesium deficiency is corrected. In some situations magnesium infusions alone have abolished ventricular premature contractions. The American Heart Association's *1992 Guidelines for Cardiopulmonary Resuscitation and Emergency Cardiac Care* include a recommendation that magnesium sulfate be added for the management of torsade de pointes, severe hypomagnesemia, or refractory ventricular fibrillation. There is still major concern as to whether mild magnesium depletion predisposes individuals to cardiac arrhythmias. There is conflicting data as to whether this occurs in otherwise healthy individuals. However, the data suggest that mild hypomagnesemia may predispose to arrhythmias in the setting of acute ischemic heart disease or congestive heart failure, after cardiopulmonary bypass, or in the acutely ill patient in the intensive care unit. Studies aimed to determine whether magnesium repletion in these situations reduces the development of arrhythmias or improves patient survival have been poorly designed or have shown conflicting results.

Magnesium deficiency and cardiac glycosides interact to maximize cardiac toxicity. Magnesium deficiency increases the uptake of digoxin by myocardial cells, and both magnesium deficiency and cardiac glycosides decrease the activity of the sodium-potassium adenosine triphosphatase (ATPase) pump and may cause a reduction in intracellular potassium content.

ASSESSMENT OF MAGNESIUM STATUS

The majority of patients with clinical manifestations of magnesium deficiency have hypomagnesemia. Measurement of the serum magnesium concentration is relatively easy and has become the method of choice for estimating body magnesium content, although there are limitations to its usefulness in evaluating total body magnesium stores. The normal serum magnesium concentration in humans is 0.9 $\pm$ 0.07 mmol/L. Symptoms of magnesium deficiency are generally not seen unless serum values are 0.25 to 0.35 mmol/L below the normal value.

There are two caveats to be considered when serum magnesium determination is used to diagnose magnesium deficiency. First, most methods of serum magnesium determination measure total magnesium concentration, but only free magnesium is biologically active. Because 25% to 30% of serum magnesium is bound to albumin and therefore inactive, measuring total serum magnesium may provide a spuriously low value in hypoalbuminemic states. Knoll et al. have reported a formula to correct serum magnesium for hypoalbuminemia:

$$\text{Corrected serum Mg}^{++} \text{ (mmol/L)} = \text{measured total serum Mg}^{++} \text{ (mmol/L)} + 0.005 \text{ (40} - \text{grams of albumin per liter)}$$

Serum contains only 0.3% of total body magnesium and may not always accurately reflect the intracellular magnesium status. It is possible for patients to be normomagnesemic but be depleted of intracellular magnesium and exhibit clinical manifestations of magnesium deficiency. There is no quick, simple, and accurate test to measure intracellular magnesium concentration.

A surrogate for direct intracellular magnesium concentration is the measurement of magnesium retention after acute magnesium loading. Patients undergoing this test should not be receiving medication that affects renal excretion of magnesium. This method is useful only when there is a strong clinical suspicion of magnesium deficiency in the setting of normomagnesemia (e.g., unexplained electrocardiographic and neuromuscular disorders). Individuals with a magnesium deficit retain a significant fraction of the injected magnesium. The method described by Bohmer *et al* is widely used in this regard.

The first step is to collect a 24-hour urine specimen and measure the magnesium content. If the content is less than 1 mmol/day, the magnesium load is administered. Thirty millimoles of magnesium sulfate are infused intravenously in 0.5 L of 5% dextrose water over a period of 8 to 12 hours. Once this infusion is initiated, a second 24-hour urine specimen should be collected and the magnesium-content determined. Patients excreting less than 50% of the administered load are total body magnesium–deficient; those with normal total body magnesium stores excrete more than 60% of the administered load. This test should be performed with great caution in patients with renal failure and cardiac conduction disturbances.

TREATMENT

Therapy depends on the severity of the hypomagnesemia and the associated clinical conditions. With mild hypomagnesemia, and in the absence of severe clinical symptoms or signs, no specific treatment other than institution of a normal diet is required. When malabsorption is present, decrease in dietary fat intake may improve magnesium absorption. With severe deficits supplemental oral and parenteral magnesium is needed. Renal reabsorption is complete only when hypomagnesemia is present; acute infusions transiently raise the level of serum magnesium, and up to 50% of the replacement dose may be excreted in the urine. The presence of renal insufficiency requires a reduction in the replacement dose, as well as very close observation of serum levels and deep tendon reflexes. Several different oral salts are available. At high doses they induce catharsis. In general, the replacement dose should be less than that needed to induce diarrhea. Magnesium chloride may have advantages over other magnesium salts. Relatively insoluble salts may require conversion to the more soluble chloride form in the presence of gastric acid. This conversion may be impaired in elderly individuals or patients receiving medication that reduces or neutralizes gastric acid. Absorption of the anion present in some magnesium salts may lead to metabolic alkalosis. Absorption of chloride does not lead to metabolic alkalosis. Because of the relatively efficient gastrointestinal tract absorption of magnesium chloride, diarrhea may be less common than that associated with other magnesium salts. The sustained-release preparations (e.g., SlowMag TM, 3.5 mmol per tablet) may be advantageous. Avoiding high peaks in plasma magnesium levels may reduce urinary magnesium wasting as described previously. Six to eight tablets should be taken daily in divided doses for severe magnesium depletion; two to four tablets per day may suffice for mild asymptomatic disease. Magnesium gluconate is well tolerated, but it provides less elemental magnesium per gram consumed than other salts. Magnesium oxide is also well tolerated and may be given in doses of 250 to 500 mg (6.25 to 12.5 mmol magnesium) four times daily, with up to 25% to 50% absorption.

The potassium-sparing diuretics such as amiloride may decrease

---

BOX 315-3
Causes of hypermagnesemia

I. Decreased renal excretion
   A. Renal failure: Glomerular filtration rate less than 30 ml/min
   B. Hyperparathyroidism
   C. Hypothyroidism
   D. Addison's disease
   E. Lithium intoxication
   F. Familial hypocalciuric hypercalcemia
II. Other causes: Usually in association with decrease in glomerular filtration rate
   A. Endogenous loads
      1. Diabetic ketoacidosis
      2. Severe tissue injury: Burns
   B. Exogenous loads
      1. Gastrointestinal tract
         a. Magnesium-containing laxatives and antacids
         b. High-dose vitamin D analogs
      2. Parenteral: Management of toxemia of pregnancy

✔ *WHEN TO REFER*

Many of the causes of hypomagnesemia and hypermagnesemia are reversible and may be obvious following a detailed history, physical examination, and simple laboratory tests. Referral to a nephrologist interested in disorders of magnesium metabolism should be considered when this process fails to determine the underlying cause of the magnesium disorder. Referral should also be considered when therapy instituted by the primary physician fails to restore normomagnesemia or resolve the abnormality precipitated by the derangement in magnesium metabolism.

---

urinary magnesium excretion by increasing its reabsorption in the cortical collecting tubule. These drugs should be considered in patients with persistent urinary magnesium wasting, especially when magnesium repletion alone does not restore normomagnesemia.

In the presence of severe deficits (usually equal to 37.5 to 50 mmol), major neuromuscular or cardiac findings, or large gastrointestinal tract losses, parenteral administration is required. Magnesium sulfate is available in a 50% solution in 2-ml ampules (4.06 mmol). Twelve milliliters (24.5 mmol) may be diluted in 1 L of 5% dextrose solution and infused over a 3-hour period. Another 40 mmol may be infused in 2 L for the remainder of the first 24-hour period; thereafter, 24.5 mmol per day is given over the next 3 to 4 days. In patients who cannot tolerate the excess volume the 50% magnesium sulfate solution may be given intramuscularly in divided doses although the injection is usually painful. It is to be stressed that the presence of renal insufficiency of any degree requires significant reduction in dose. Serum level should be kept between 1.0 and 1.25 mmol/L during replacement. When hypokalemia or hypocalcemia coexists with hypomagnesemia, the magnesium deficits must be corrected before adequate potassium or calcium replacement can be achieved.

HYPERMAGNESEMIA

Hypermagnesemia is an uncommon clinical disorder in the absence of renal insufficiency. In a normal individual up to 80% of an exogenous load is excreted by the kidney. As glomerular filtration falls, the fractional excretion of magnesium per nephron rises. Normal magnesium balance may be maintained until the glomerular filtration rate falls below about 30 ml per minute.

The causes of hypermagnesemia are listed in Box 315-3. They may be subdivided into endogenous and exogenous sources and appear almost invariably in association with acute or chronic impairment in renal function. Decreased renal excretion may be seen with hyperparathyroidism, hypothyroidism, adrenal insufficiency, and lithium intoxication. In hyperparathyroidism the direct tubular effect of parathyroid hormone is usually counteracted by the magnesuric effect of hypercalcemia. Familial hypocalciuric hypercalcemia, in contrast to primary hyperparathyroidism, is characterized by a high serum magnesium level.

Causes

Exogenous Loads. Magnesium-containing antacids and enemas given in the presence of moderate to severe impairment in renal function represent the typical setting for hypermagnesemia. Large amounts of magnesium may be absorbed from colonic enemas. Although vitamin D normally plays no major role in magnesium metabolism,

large doses of the active metabolites given to patients with chronic renal failure may increase absorption of magnesium. Not infrequently, mild to moderate or even severe hypermagnesemia may be seen during therapy for toxemia of pregnancy, when large doses of intravenous magnesium sulfate are used. Neonatal and maternal hypermagnesemia may occur.

Clark and Brown have recently suggested that magnesium absorption may be increased in elderly patients with gastrointestinal tract disorders such as colitis, gastritis, and active ulcer disease. These patients may develop hypermagnesemia while ingesting relatively modest doses of magnesium salts, even in the presence of relatively normal renal function.

Clinical Consequences

Clinical effects are usually not seen until the serum magnesium level exceeds 4 mEq/L. The major effects are inhibition of neuromuscular transmission and cardiac electrical conduction. With a serum magnesium level of more than 4 mEq/L, deep tendon reflexes are abolished. Lethargy is seen at levels approaching 7 mEq/L. Paralysis of voluntary muscles and respiratory failure may occur at levels of 10 mEq/L. Cardiovascular effects include hypotension and prolongation of the PR and QT intervals, as well as QRS interval duration at levels of 5 to 10 mEq/L. At levels of 15 mEq/L, complete heart block or asystole may occur.

Moderate acute hypermagnesemia after parenteral infusions may cause hypocalcemia. The mechanism has recently been investigated in pregnant women receiving magnesium and is the result of direct suppression of parathyroid hormone secretion. Renal phosphate excretion may be reduced and mild hyperphosphatemia may be seen, probably as a consequence of decreased parathyroid hormone levels.

Treatment

Mild hypermagnesemia without major neuromuscular or cardiac disturbance requires no specific therapy other than withdrawal of magnesium-containing salts. During treatment with large doses of magnesium-containing salts, deep tendon reflexes should be monitored closely. If they are absent, magnesium administration should be withheld. Magnesium-containing antacids and enemas should be avoided in patients with chronic renal failure.

When severe hypermagnesemia exists with neuromuscular or cardiac depression, or both, ventilatory assistance and cardiac electrical pacing may be required. Intravenous calcium acutely antagonizes the inhibitory effects of magnesium. Calcium gluconate or calcium chloride may be infused over a 5-minute period in a dose calculated to give 100 to 200 mg of elemental calcium. Intravenous glucose and insulin may be given to shift magnesium transiently into cells. Definitive therapy with hemodialysis is necessary.

BIBLIOGRAPHY

Agus ZS, Wasserstein A, Goldfarb S: Disorders of calcium and magnesium homeostasis, *Am J Med* 72:473, 1982.

Aikawa JK: Biochemistry and physiology of magnesium, *World Rev Nutr Diet* 28:112, 1978.

Aurbach GD, Marx SJ, Spiegel AM: Calcium homeostasis. In Wilson JD, Foster DW, editors: *Textbook of endocrinology*, Philadelphia, 1985, Saunders.

Bar RS, Wilson HE, Mazzaferri EL: Hypomagnesemic hypocalcemia secondary to renal magnesium wasting: a possible consequence of high-dose gentamicin therapy, *Ann Intern Med* 82:646, 1975.

Clark BA, Brown RS: Unsuspected morbid hypermagnesemia in elderly patients, *Am J Nephrol* 12:336, 1992.

Cohen LF et al: Acute tumor lysis syndrome: a review of 37 patients with Burkitt's lymphoma, *Am J Med* 68:486, 1980.

Elin RJ: Magnesium metabolism in health and disease, *Dis Mon* 34:161, 1988.

Gonin RE, Knochel JP: Magnesium deficiency, *Adv Intern Med* 28:509, 1983.

Grillo JA, Gonzalez ER: Changes in the pharmacotherapy of CPR, *Heart Lung* 22:548, 1993.

Iseri LT, Freed J, Barres AR: Magnesium deficiency and cardiac disorders, *Am J Med* 58:837, 1975.

Kobrin S, Goldfarb S: Magnesium deficiency, *Semin Nephrol* 10:525, 1990.

Kroll MH, Elin RJ: Relationships between magnesium and protein concentration in serum, *Clin Chem* 21:224-246, 1985

Massry SG: Pharmacology of magnesium, *Ann Rev Pharmacol Toxicol* 17:67, 1977.

Parfitt AM, Kleerekoper M: Clinical disorders of calcium, phosphorus, and magnesium metabolism. In Maxwell MH, Kleeman CR, editors: *Clinical disorders of fluid and electrolyte metabolism*, ed 3, New York, 1980, McGraw-Hill.

Rude RK, Singer FR: Magnesium deficiency and excess. *Annu Rev Med* 32:245, 1981.

Seller RH et al: Digitalis toxicity and hypomagnesemia, *Am Heart J* 79:57, 1970.

Shils ME: Experimental human magnesium depletion, *Medicine (Baltimore)* 48:61, 1969.

CHAPTER

316 Osteoporosis

Lawrence G. Raisz

Osteoporosis is by far the most common metabolic disorder of bone. It is estimated that in the United States about 40% of women over the age of 50 years and 12% of older men will sustain an osteoporotic fracture during their lifetime. In the past, osteoporosis has been diagnosed only after the fracture has occurred, but this is clearly not optimal. As pointed out by a recent Consensus Development Conference, the definition of osteoporosis should be *"a disease characterized by low bone mass and architectural deterioration of bone tissue leading to enhanced bone fragility and a consequent increase in fracture risk."* Recently a World Health Organization Study Group recommended diagnostic categories for osteoporosis, based on measurements of bone mass or density (Box 316-1). This approach is still not fully applied in clinical practice because of the high cost and limited availability of these measurements. Nevertheless, this approach is optimal, since prevention of fractures is the major goal in management of the disease. Most patients are postmenopausal women or older men. In these patients osteoporosis is often termed "primary," "postmenopausal," "senile," or "involutional," to distinguish them

---

BOX 316-1

Diagnostic categories for osteoporosis based on measurements of bone mineral density or bone mineral content

1. Normal: A value for BMD or BMC within 1 standard deviation of the young adult reference mean.
2. Low bone mass (osteopenia): A value for BMD or BMC more than 1 standard deviation and less than 2.5 standard deviations below the young adult mean.
3. Osteoporosis: A value for BMD or BMC 2.5 standard deviations below the young adult mean.
4. Severe osteoporosis (established osteoporosis): A value for BMD or BMC more than 2.5 standard deviations below the young adult mean in the presence of one or more fragility fractures.

From the World Health Organization Technical Report Series 843: Assessment of fracture risk and its application to screening for osteoporosis, Geneva, 1994, The Organization.
BMC, Bone mineral content; *BMD,* bone mineral density.

---

from patients with secondary forms and diseases that mimic or aggravate osteoporosis. The latter are less common but are important to recognize because they can often be treated effectively (Box 316-2).

CLINICAL DESCRIPTION

Osteoporosis can be recognized on clinical examination either by measurement of bone density or by identification of a fragility fracture, that is, fractures that occur spontaneously or after minimal or moderate trauma. The most common are vertebral compression fractures, fractures of the neck or greater trochanter of the femur, and fractures of the distal radius (Colles'). However, fragility fractures can occur at other sites including the pelvis, the ribs, and the shafts of the long bone. The incidence of the common osteoporotic fractures in both men and women is illustrated in Fig. 316-1. The term "type I" osteoporosis has been applied to patients with Colles' or vertebral compression fractures, which occur most often in postmenopausal women. The term "type II" osteoporosis has been used to describe hip fractures, which tend to occur later in life. Since these syndromes overlap extensively, it may be more useful simply to characterize osteoporotic patients by the specific site of their fractures.

Vertebral Crush Fracture

The clinical course of vertebral crush fractures is highly variable. At one extreme are patients in whom anterior wedging of the vertebrae

---

BOX 316-2

Classification of osteoporosis and related disorders

Primary osteoporosis

Postmenopausal, senile, or involutional
    Vertebral crush fracture syndrome
    Fracture of the proximal femur
    Colles' fracture
Idiopathic osteoporosis
Juvenile osteoporosis

Endocrine osteoporosis

Hyperparathyroidism
Cushing's syndrome
Hyperthyroidism
Hypogonadism
Diabetes mellitus

Nutritional osteoporosis

Scurvy
Malnutrition
Calcium deficiency
Malabsorption

Secondary osteoporosis

Alcoholism
Liver disease
Renal disease

Hematopoietic osteoporosis

Myeloma
Lymphoma
Leukemia
Mastocytosis
Thalassemia

Congenital osteoporosis

Osteogenesis imperfecta
Homocystinuria

Osteomalacia

Nutritional
Malabsorptive
Renal
Vitamin D–resistant
Anticonvulsant

develops with little or no progression; at the other extreme are patients who have multiple vertebral collapse with marked pain and deformity. Anterior wedging alone may not be due to osteoporosis but may represent deformation attributable to Scheuermann's disease or osteoarthritis. Most patients with vertebral compression fractures have an acute onset of back pain with minimal or no trauma. The vertebrae from the 5th thoracic to the 5th lumbar positions (T5-L5) are most frequently affected. Lumbar compressions are more likely to be associated with trauma. The subsequent course is quite variable. Progression of existing fractures with further loss of vertebral height probably occurs more frequently than new fractures. Vertebral crush fracture leads to kyphosis and loss of lumbar lordosis and may impair chest wall function. Protuberance of the abdomen is disfiguring and uncomfortable. Ultimately the ribs impinge on the iliac crest, producing additional pain. It is common to find other musculoskeletal disorders in these patients, including spondylolisthesis, disk disease, and osteoarthritis. Although patients with severe osteoarthritis are less likely to have osteoporosis, osteoarthritic changes in the spinal facets are common in osteoporotic patients, possibly related to their compression deformities.

Colles' Fracture

A fracture of the distal radius caused by a fall on the outstretched hand occurs at all ages in both men and women but shows an increased incidence in women beginning as early as age 40 years. This is probably related to loss of trabecular bone mass in the distal radius beginning before menopause. Patients with Colles' fractures should have bone density measurements and be put on an appropriate preventive regimen, since they are at higher risk for additional fragility fractures. Colles' fractures usually heal uneventfully, but local deformity and impaired function can occur if they are not well managed.

Fractures of the Proximal Femur

The lifetime risk of femoral fracture is somewhat less than that of vertebral fracture, but the morbidity and mortality are much greater. The incidence increases markedly with age. This is related to the frequency and type of falls, as well as to bone fragility. Bone loss in the proximal femur continues and may even accelerate in older individuals. Risk factors for falls, including neuromuscular deficits and the use of medications that affect balance and gait, also increase with age. Intertrochanteric fractures are more closely associated with trabecular bone loss than are fractures of the neck of the femur, but low bone density in the femoral neck is predictive of hip fracture at both sites.

OTHER FORMS OF PRIMARY OSTEOPOROSIS

Juvenile osteoporosis is a relatively rare disorder that usually develops before the pubertal growth spurt. In these patients there may be a dissociation between linear growth and the ability to consolidate and strengthen the skeleton. Thus vertebral and other fractures may occur. The disorder appears to be self-limited, and treatment is conservative, consisting of minimizing trauma, maintaining nutrition, and using a physiotherapy program that stimulates muscle and bone without causing injury. Antiresorptive therapy has been used in these patients, but no controlled studies have been made to prove its efficacy.

Idiopathic osteoporosis is a term applied to premenopausal women or younger men with osteoporosis for which there is no identified secondary cause. It is rare and clinically heterogeneous. Biopsy specimens may show increased or decreased bone turnover. The disease is often self-limited, but antiresorptive or anabolic therapy should be considered in severe cases. Bone biopsy may be indicated to rule out unusual causes such as mastocytosis and to guide therapy.

SECONDARY OSTEOPOROSIS

There are a large number of disorders associated with decreased bone mass in which the clinical picture may resemble primary osteoporosis. In some the histologic appearance is different. For example, in primary and secondary hyperparathyroidism and in some cases of hyperthyroidism there is increased turnover with osteitis fibrosa cystica; in osteogenesis imperfecta there may be abnormal collagen patterns; and in myeloma and mastocytosis characteristic abnormal cells are found. In Cushing's syndrome there is marked inhibition of osteoblastic function, but there may also be increased bone resorption. In patients with gastrointestinal tract, liver, and renal disease osteoporosis may occur, but there may also be osteomalacia because of impairment of calcium absorption and vitamin D metabolism. Severe osteomalacia that is due to vitamin D deficiency or abnormal vitamin D activation usually produces characteristic biochemical changes, but in many cases the histologic picture is difficult to predict from clinical data.

The separation among these disorders and primary osteoporosis may be indistinct, and they may coexist. It is important to consider secondary forms of osteoporosis and osteomalacia not only in patients whose presentation is atypical, but also in patients who appear to have

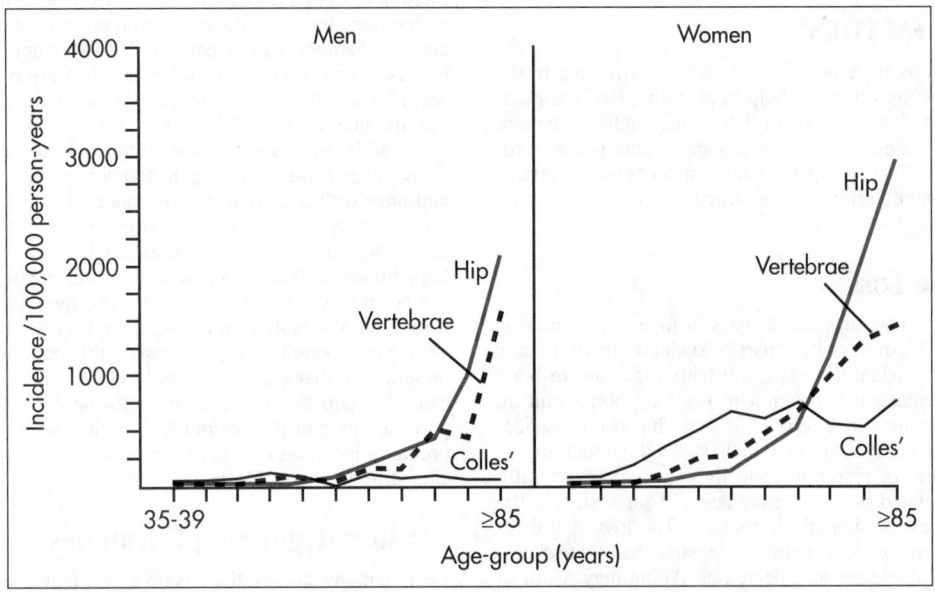

FIGURE 316-1   Age-specific incidence rates for hip, vertebral, and Colles' fractures in men and women living in Rochester, Minnesota.
From Cooper C, Melton LJ III: *Trends Endocrinol Metab* 3:224, 1992.

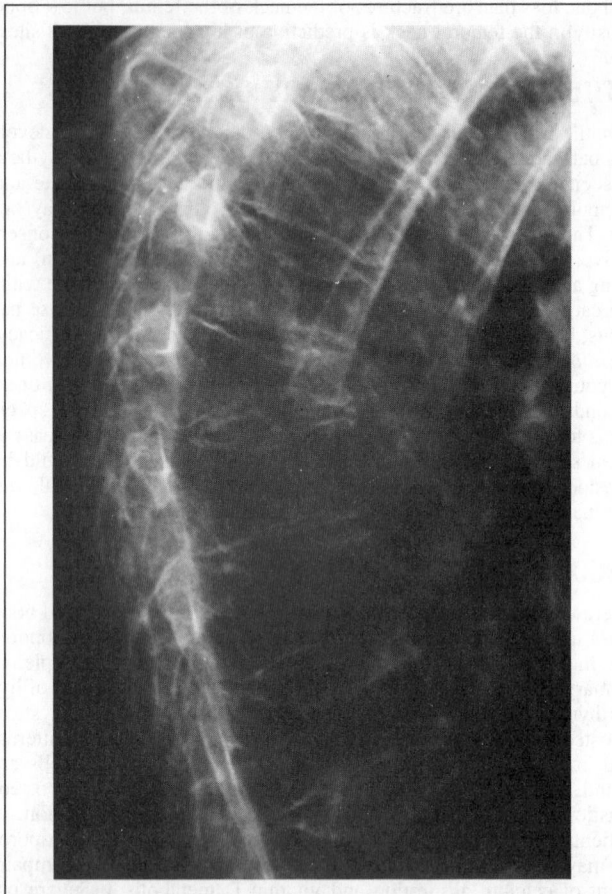

FIGURE 316-2   Vertebral crush fractures. Radiograph of the lateral spine shows multiple compression and wedge fractures of the thoracic vertebrae that occurred without trauma between the ages of 60 and 70 years in a patient with severe postmenopausal osteoporosis.

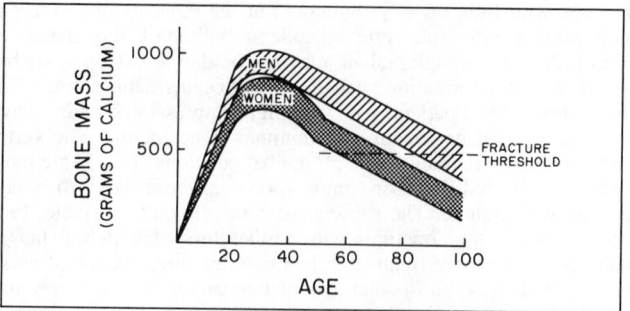

FIGURE 316-3   Changes in bone mass with age. Bone mass is higher in men than in women, and age-related loss occurs in both sexes but is accelerated in women at menopause. The concept of a fracture threshold is indicated by the dashed line. By the World Health Organization Criteria these individuals can be considered osteoporotic (see Box 316-1).

linking, and decreased content of water can all contribute to increased bone fragility.

Genetic and Constitutional Factors

Certain populations, such as Northern European and Asian women, are at higher risk for the development of osteoporosis. The lower prevalence of osteoporosis in blacks may be related to greater bone and muscle mass and also to decreased bone turnover. Osteoporotic patients often have a positive family history, and first-degree relatives of these patients are likely to have a decreased bone mass. Patients with osteoporosis tend to be thinner and have a lighter frame with narrower bones than patients with osteoarthritis. However, osteoporosis with vertebral crush fractures can still occur in women who have osteoarthritis. Recent studies have suggested that different alleles of the vitamin D receptor gene can determine peak bone mass and bone turnover. The results are controversial, but it seems likely that a number of genetic determinants of bone mass and turnover will be identified in osteoporosis. Genetic analysis could provide a basis for more accurate prognosis and more focused prevention programs.

Menopause

Accelerated bone loss associated with withdrawal of ovarian hormones is clearly a major pathogenetic factor (Fig. 316-3). Although there is extensive evidence that estrogen withdrawal results in accelerated bone loss and that estrogen replacement can prevent it, the precise mechanism is not clear (Fig 316-4). Alterations in systemic hormones have been described, but the data are not consistent. Hence it seems more likely that estrogen affects bone metabolism by altering the production of local factors.

In addition to menopause, either natural or following oophorectomy, other forms of estrogen deficiency such as Turner's syndrome and amenorrhea associated with anorexia nervosa or intense athletic training may result in decreased bone mass. Androgen and estrogen deficiency in men are also associated with bone loss and increased bone turnover. There is an increase in the rate of bone resorption when sex hormones are withdrawn, followed by a delayed increase in bone formation, probably as a result of the increased number of resorption sites. Since bone loss is progressive, the amount of bone formed must be less than that required to replace the bone resorbed. This could be caused in part by loss of template for new bone formation because of perforations and discontinuities, particularly in trabecular bone, but probably indicates that sex hormones not only inhibit osteoclasts, but also stimulate osteoblasts.

Calcium-Regulating Hormones

Despite many studies, there is no agreement about the role of calcium-regulating hormones in the pathogenesis of osteoporosis. To establish such a role, there should be a substantial difference in the level of or response to a particular hormone in osteoporotic patients compared

primary osteoporosis, since identification of a specific cause or aggravating factor may result in more effective treatment.

PATHOGENETIC FACTORS

A large number of factors have been identified as contributing to the development of osteoporosis that can help in assessing risk and planning treatment. Nevertheless, we cannot determine whether a patient will have osteoporosis based on these factors and cannot predict progression of the disease. Thus the pathogenetic mechanisms, particularly in severe progressive vertebral crush fracture syndrome, remain largely unknown.

Age-related Bone Loss

The pattern of gain and loss of skeletal mass in men and women is illustrated in Fig. 316-2. An important part of skeletal growth occurs during and after puberty when there is a substantial increase in bone mass. This involves endosteal apposition in the long bones and an increase in trabecular bone. Once peak bone mass has been reached, there is presumably a period during which skeletal remodeling is tightly coupled and rates of resorption and formation are essentially equal. However, age-related bone loss may begin at some sites in the third and fourth decades, particularly in women. The loss of trabecular bone, which turns over more rapidly, is greater than that of cortical bone, but cortical thickness also decreases. Aging may result in other changes that affect bone strength. Loss of continuity of trabecular structure, accumulation of microfractures, death of osteocytes with hypermineralization of lacunae, changes in collagen cross-

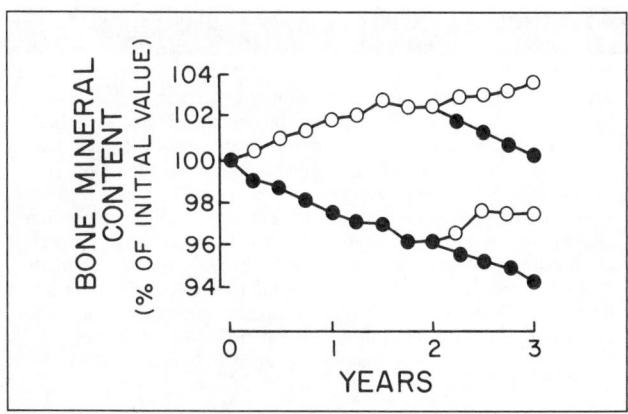

FIGURE 316-4   Bone loss at menopause. Bone mineral content of the distal radius was measured serially in postmenopausal women. Women who did not have treatment showed progressive bone loss *(closed circles);* women who received treatment with estrogen maintained or had increased bone mass *(open circles).* If estrogen therapy was begun in previously untreated women at the end of 2 years, there was a positive effect on bone mass; if estrogen was discontinued at this time, bone loss occurred. However, the gains achieved during the prior 2 years of treatment were maintained.
Modified from Christiansen C et al: *Lancet* 1:459, 1981.

with age-matched controls. Of course, some overlap is expected, since some control patients may have asymptomatic osteoporosis. Parathyroid hormone levels are not elevated in vertebral crush fracture patients, and some data suggest a decrease in parathyroid responsiveness. A small decrease in 1,25-dihydroxyvitamin D has also been reported, but there is a substantial overlap of osteoporotic patients with normal individuals. Most studies do not show a difference in calcitonin levels. The role of these hormones in the pathogenesis of hip fracture is also difficult to evaluate. There is an age-related increase in parathyroid hormone levels, and the increase of 1,25-dihydroxyvitamin D in response to calcium deprivation or parathyroid hormone administration may be blunted. There may also be an age-related decrease in calcitonin levels. These changes could be a result of the decreases in renal mass and intestinal calcium transport associated with aging. These may combine with decreased intake of calcium and vitamin D to produce secondary hyperparathyroidism and decreased stimulation of parafollicular cells that secrete calcitonin.

One difficulty with assigning a role for calcium-regulating hormones in osteoporosis is uncertainty concerning their long-term effects on bone formation. Parathyroid hormone and 1,25-dihydroxyvitamin D inhibit collagen synthesis acutely. However, prolonged, intermittent administration of parathyroid hormone can increase trabecular bone mass. The vitamin D metabolites may have a similar effect, but this is not as well documented.

Other Humoral Factors

In addition to the calcium-regulating hormones, other systemic factors, as well as local factors produced by bone cells or adjacent marrow, can influence bone resorption and formation and may be involved in the pathogenesis of osteoporosis. Insulin-like growth factors (IGFs) stimulate bone growth, whereas glucocorticoids inhibit it. There is little evidence that the systemic levels of these hormones are altered in osteoporosis, except for glucocorticoid-induced osteoporosis, but cellular responses or local production of IGFs and the binding proteins that modulate their activity could be altered.

Bone turnover depends on local mechanisms that initiate resorption at particular sites and regulate the coupled formation response. Prostaglandins are produced by bone and may mediate the response of bone to mechanical forces. Increased prostaglandin production has been implicated in inflammatory bone loss. Prostaglandins may also be involved in the response to estrogen withdrawal, since bones from oophorectomized rats can produce an increased amount of prostaglandin E_2. Interleukins 1 and 6 and tumor necrosis factor α are cyto-

kines that can stimulate bone resorption and inhibit bone formation. Blocking these cytokines has been reported to prevent bone loss in oophorectomized animals. Bone cells can produce other macromolecular factors that stimulate formation, including transforming growth factor β, bone morphogenetic proteins, fibroblast growth factors, and platelet-derived growth factors. Until we are able to measure the local concentrations of these cytokines and growth factors in bone in humans, we cannot determine their potential pathogenetic role in osteoporosis.

Nutritional Factors

Calcium plays a role in the prevention and treatment of osteoporosis. Low calcium intake early in life may result in a decrease in peak bone mass. Age-related bone loss cannot be abrogated by calcium supplements but can be slowed. Although excessive intakes of protein and phosphate can produce negative calcium balance, it is not clear that these are important in the pathogenesis of osteoporosis. Ascorbic acid deficiency and excessive intakes of vitamins A and D can cause bone loss but are rarely encountered in clinical practice.

Activity and Lifestyle

Bone requires mechanical stimulation to maintain its mass and strength. Immobilization results in rapid bone loss as a result of both increased resorption and decreased formation. Moreover, moderate exercise may increase bone mass in postmenopausal women. The effects of intense exercise appear to depend on whether sex hormone function is altered. In women who exercise intensely and have amenorrhea, particularly if this begins early after puberty, bone mass is lower than in age-matched controls. Other aspects of lifestyle that may reduce bone mass are cigarette smoking and a high alcohol intake. The mechanism of decreased bone mass in alcoholics is not known, but poor nutrition and direct effects of alcohol on bone have been implicated.

DIAGNOSIS
Bone Densitometry

Bone densitometry can be used to make the diagnosis of osteoporosis and determine the probability of future fractures. The most widely used system is dual-energy x-ray absorptiometry of the lumbar spine or proximal femur. Measurements of the distal radius by dual- or single-energy x-ray absorptiometry and of trabecular bone density in the spine by computerized tomography are also used to make the diagnosis and predict fracture risk. Screening procedures using ultrasound with no radiation exposure are being evaluated.

There is considerable debate about the indications for bone densitometry. Densitometry is indicated when it will have an effect on clinical decision making, for example, to help in deciding for or against hormone replacement therapy at menopause. In patients who already have fractures, densitometry can be used to confirm the diagnosis of osteoporosis and to provide baseline data for assessing the response to therapy. Densitometry is useful in assessing patients at risk for secondary osteoporosis, particularly patients receiving glucocorticoids. With increased options for treatment and prevention the use of bone densitometry is likely to increase, and this should decrease the cost.

Biochemical Markers

There is great interest in the use of new biochemical markers to assess bone turnover and guide therapy in osteoporosis. Markers of bone resorption, such as pyridinoline cross-links or other cross-linked peptides derived from collagen degradation and of bone formation, such as bone-specific alkaline phosphatase, osteocalcin, and procollagen peptides, are more informative than the older tests, such as serum total alkaline phosphatase, urinary calcium, and urinary hydroxyproline levels. Studies using these new measurements suggest that high bone turnover is associated with low bone mass and rapid bone loss. However, the values show a wide scatter and are not reliable for individual diagnosis. Markers may be useful in individual patients to assess the response to therapy.

Differential Diagnosis

In patients with vertebral crush fracture the diagnosis of primary osteoporosis is made by exclusion. In the typical case of a postmenopausal woman with a crush fracture a careful history and physical examination and limited laboratory studies are usually sufficient to rule out diseases that mimic or aggravate primary osteoporosis. The most important of these are primary hyperparathyroidism, osteomalacia, hyperthyroidism, multiple myeloma, and Cushing's syndrome. Gastrointestinal tract and renal disease may predispose a patient to osteomalacia or secondary hyperparathyroidism, as well as osteoporosis.

Routine laboratory studies in otherwise healthy patients with low bone mass should include a measurement of serum calcium, preferably as ionized calcium or as total calcium, together with a measurement of serum albumin to correct for any protein abnormalities. In patients with established osteoporosis, serum calcium, phosphorus, creatinine, and alkaline phosphatase levels; protein electrophoresis; fasting urine calcium/creatinine ratio; a blood cell count; and a serum thyroid-stimulating hormone (TSH) level are sufficient to rule out the most common secondary causes. Measurement of 25-hydroxyvitamin D should be obtained if there is a suggestion of vitamin D deficiency, and 24-hour urinary free cortisol measurement if there are clinical signs or symptoms pointing to Cushing's syndrome. Bone biopsy specimens obtained after double tetracycline labeling can be used to assess bone mineralization and can be useful in atypical or severe cases to diagnose unusual causes such as mastocytosis or a lymphoproliferative disorder.

Prevention

Once fractures have occurred, osteoporosis is often progressive, despite therapy. The goal of treatment is to reduce the incidence of further fractures. Because of this, there has been considerable emphasis on initiating prevention programs before fractures occur. Efforts at prevention should begin in childhood and be reinforced in young adults. An adequate calcium intake of approximately 1200 mg/day in adolescents and 1000 mg/day in adults, combined with a program of physical activity that maintains muscle strength and bone mass, might reverse the current trend toward an increasing incidence of osteoporotic fractures in individuals in industrialized countries.

The most important time for considering additional preventive measures is at menopause. Estrogen replacement therapy (ERT) has been shown to decrease the frequency of both vertebral and hip fractures. Although the advantages and disadvantages of hormone replacement have been much debated, the benefits probably outweigh the risks in patients who have low bone mass and are likely to develop osteoporotic fractures. Since estrogen also can decrease the risk of cardiovascular disease and reduce overall mortality, many physicians recommend it universally unless there is a contraindication. However, many women either refuse estrogen or discontinue it unless they are clearly at risk and are monitored. For this reason, measurement of bone mass in perimenopausal women may be cost-effective.

There are contraindications to hormone replacement. Patients who have had breast cancer or serious thromboembolic complications from prior estrogen therapy should not be treated with hormone replacement. Patients with disseminated lupus erythematosus may relapse on a regimen of estrogen. There are relative contraindications, including a family history of breast or endometrial carcinoma, fibrocystic breast disease, and gallbladder disease. Unopposed estrogen therapy increases the risk of endometrial carcinoma, but this is prevented by adding a progestin to the regimen. The effective dose of estrogen is probably 0.625 mg/day of conjugated estrogen or its equivalent. Estradiol can be given transdermally as well as orally. When the uterus is present, medroxyprogesterone or its equivalent can be given either for 10 to 14 days of each month in doses of 5 to 10 mg/day or continuously at doses of 2.5 to 5 mg/day. The former regimen results in regular menses, which many patients find difficult to accept. With continuous combined therapy, patients may have a few initial episodes of bleeding that then stop. Patients should have a mammogram before being placed on hormone therapy and yearly thereafter. Endometrial biopsy should be performed yearly if unopposed estrogen is used or whenever there is atypical bleeding. When estrogen is con

✔ **WHEN TO REFER**

The diagnosis, prevention, and treatment of osteoporosis should be in the hands of the primary care physician. Referrals are indicated in complex cases, particularly when the possibility of a bone biopsy is being considered. The patients most likely to be referred include men with severe osteoporosis and premenopausal women. Primary care physicians also need assistance in the interpretation of bone densitometric measurements and in developing appropriate nutrition and exercise programs. Referrals can often be made to an osteoporosis center, many of which have teams of physical therapists, nutritionists, and other ancillary personnel to help the patient cope with osteoporosis. Information on such centers can be obtained from the National Osteoporosis Foundation, 1150 17th St. NW, Suite 500, Washington, DC 20036.

traindicated in high-risk patients, other antiresorptive agents should be considered.

The preventive regimen should not be limited to hormone replacement therapy. Calcium supplementation and an exercise program that includes 3 to 4 hours of weight-bearing exercise weekly should be part of the program. Patients should be advised to discontinue smoking, reduce their intakes of alcohol and caffeine, and avoid excessive intake of protein. An adequate vitamin D intake of 400 units/day or its equivalent in sun exposure should be maintained. Compliance with a prevention program depends on patient motivation. Monitoring the patients with bone density measurements at 1- to 3-year intervals and maintaining exercise programs through group activities can help achieve good compliance.

Treatment

Patients who have had a fracture of a vertebra, distal radius, proximal femur, or any other site with minimal trauma should be evaluated for osteoporosis and put on the same conservative regimen used for prevention. Because most patients have limited mobility after fracture, the exercise regimen must be carefully tailored to their capacity and carried out under supervision. Although many patients improve on hormone replacement therapy, calcium supplementation, and exercise, some show progressive bone loss and continue to have fractures, and in others ERT is not tolerated or is contraindicated. In these individuals alternative therapies are indicated. Calcitonin can be used to inhibit bone resorption and increase bone mass. It is reported to be most effective in patients with high turnover of bone. Calcitonin has been given by subcutaneous injection, but this is uncomfortable and can produce anorexia and nausea. A nasal preparation is now available that appears to be better tolerated. The relative efficacy of nasal calcitonin compared with other treatment modalities has not been established, but it appears to be safe.

Bisphosphonates can also be used to decrease bone resorption. These agents have been used in the treatment of Paget's disease and hypercalcemia of malignancy for many years. Recently one bisphosphonate, alendronate, was approved for the treatment of osteoporosis in the United States based not only on evidence of an increase in bone mass, but also of a decrease in the incidence of vertebral fractures.

Sodium fluoride has been used extensively in patients with vertebral crush fracture. High doses can cause side effects, and even though bone mass is increased, this may not result in a decrease in the incidence of fractures. Recently, a slow-release, low-dose intermittent regimen of sodium fluoride was found to decrease the incidence of new vertebral fractures. A number of other agents are being tested, including calcitriol and other vitamin D metabolites as well as parathyroid hormone given intermittently. Treatment options for osteoporosis are continuing to increase in number and effectiveness. In most patients, bone mass can be preserved given a comprehensive regimen, adequate encouragement, and appropriate follow-up.

BIBLIOGRAPHY

Bilezikian JP, Raisz LG, Rodan GA: *Principles of bone biology,* San Diego, 1996, Academic.

Eriksen EF et al: Cancellous bone remodeling in type I (postmenopausal) osteoporosis: quantitative assessment of rates of formation, resorption and bone loss at tissue and cellular levels, *J Bone Miner Res* 5:311, 1990.

Grisso JA et al: Risk factors for falls as a cause of hip fracture in women, *N Engl J Med* 324:1326, 1991.

Kanis JA et al: The diagnosis of osteoporosis, *J Bone Miner Res* 9:1137, 1994.

Liberman UA et al: Effect of oral alendronate on bone mineral density and the incidence of fractures in postmenopausal osteoporosis, *N Engl J Med* 333:1495, 1995.

Marcus R, Feldman D, Kelsey J editors: *Osteoporosis,* San Diego, 1996, Academic.

Raisz LG: Local and systemic factors in the pathogenesis of osteoporosis, *N Engl J Med* 318:818, 1988.

Riggs BL, Melton LJ: The prevention and treatment of osteoporosis, *N Engl J Med* 327:620, 1992.

Silverberg SJ et al: Abnormalities in parathyroid hormone secretion and 1,25-dihydroxyvitamin D_3 formation in women with osteoporosis, *N Engl J Med* 320:277, 1989.

Tosteson ANA et al: Cost-effectiveness of screening postmenopausal white women for osteoporosis: bone densitometry and hormone replacement therapy, *Ann Intern Med* 113:594, 1990.

CHAPTER

317 Osteomalacia and Disorders of Vitamin D Metabolism

L. Lyndon Key, Jr., and Norman H. Bell

DEFINITION

Osteomalacia is a skeletal disorder in which mineralization of the newly formed osteoid or organic matrix of bone is defective. In children the disease is rickets. In this condition defective mineralization of cartilage that affects the epiphyseal growth plate leads to an alteration in the maturation and pattern of cellular growth and development of epiphyseal plates, widening of the ends of long bones, retardation of growth, and the skeletal deformities described below.

PHYSIOLOGY OF BONE FORMATION

The normal sequence of bone formation first requires the production of an organic matrix or osteoid, which is then mineralized. The process of calcification is complex and still not well understood. Calcium and phosphate in the extracellular fluid are supersaturated, and metastatic calcification is prevented by pyrophosphate and possibly other substances that include peptides. Initially, bone mineral is deposited as amorphous calcium phosphate that is later converted to hydroxyapatite $[Ca_{10}(PO_4 6(OH)_2]$ (see Chapter 283).

The rate of bone formation and calcification can be measured by histomorphometric techniques that employ tetracycline labeling. Tetracycline antibiotics have the fortuitous property of being deposited in a fluorescent, bandlike pattern at the mineralization front. As a consequence, they are readily visualized on histologic sections under a fluorescent microscope. Short-term administration of tetracycline in two series of doses with a timed interval allows appositional growth rate of the skeleton to be estimated by measuring the distance between the two fluorescent bands. In normal adult subjects this distance averages approximately 1 μm per day. In osteomalacia and rickets the distance is reduced. In severe cases of rickets and osteomalacia the mineralization defect may be so marked that it is possible to discern only a single band of fluorescence (Plate IX-5). When the newly formed matrix mineralizes either poorly or not at all, it appears as a wide osteoid seam. The two distinguishing diagnostic features of osteomalacia on bone biopsy are wide osteoid seams and diminished mineralization. Both findings are essential to establish the diagnosis with certainty because an increase in width of osteoid seams

is found in states of high bone turnover such as primary hyperparathyroidism, hyperthyroidism, and Paget's disease.

CLINICAL FEATURES

In children with rickets growth is often retarded and the skeleton is subject to deformities and fractures, regardless of pathogenesis. Defective mineralization of cartilage and the skeleton produces the greatest abnormalities in the bones with the most rapid growth. Just as the rate of growth of different parts of the skeleton varies with age, the clinical findings of rickets also vary with age and often provide an indication of the age of onset of the disease. At birth and during the first year of life, softening of the cranium or craniotabes commonly occurs as a consequence of rapid growth of the skull. This results in widening of the cranial sutures, frontal bossing, and posterior flattening of the skull. In infancy and early childhood thickening of the forearm at the wrist and of the costochondral junctions (the rachitic rosary) is the consequence of rapid growth of the arms and ribcage, respectively. Indentation of the lower ribs at the site of attachment of the diaphragm, Harrison's groove, may be apparent. Dental eruption is frequently delayed, and abnormalities in dentition, as well as an increased frequency of caries, occur. In later childhood and adolescence bowing of the lower extremities, especially around the knees, may result from rapid growth of the legs.

In infants and children listlessness and irritability are common. In infants myopathy is indicated by generalized hypotonia, whereas in older children proximal muscle weakness is observed.

In adults the clinical manifestations of osteomalacia are frequently subtle and may be overlooked, and the patients may be asymptomatic. When present, symptoms include diffuse skeletal pain and proximal muscular weakness. The pain is characteristically dull and aching, present in the lower back or hips or at sites where fractures have taken place; the pain is worsened by activity. Bone tenderness may be present on palpation. Fractures of the vertebrae, ribs, and long bones may occur, often with little trauma. Muscular weakness may be severe and is frequently associated with wasting. Since weakness usually involves the proximal muscle group, particularly the lower extremities, it may contribute to the waddling gait, a characteristic finding.

Hypocalcemia is sometimes found in patients with rickets and osteomalacia. As a result, lethargy, diarrhea, laryngeal stridor, grand mal seizures, cataracts, and increased intracranial pressure may ensue. Headaches and papilledema occur as a result of the increased intracranial pressure. In children mental retardation sometimes results from chronic hypocalcemia.

LABORATORY FINDINGS

In osteomalacia the serum calcium level is normal or low, and serum phosphorus level is normal or low depending on the absence or presence of secondary hyperparathyroidism and defects in phosphate handling. An elevation of serum alkaline phosphatase level is the most consistent finding. Serum immunoreactive parathyroid hormone is often increased. Reduction of the filtered load of calcium and increased circulating parathyroid hormone combine to produce a low urinary calcium. Increases in urinary cyclic adenosine monophosphate (AMP) and hydroxyproline result from increased secretion of parathyroid hormone and enhanced bone resorption, respectively. Levels of serum 25-hydroxyvitamin D and 1,25-dihydroxyvitamin D are normal, reduced, or elevated depending on the cause of the underlying disease.

RADIOGRAPHIC AND NUCLEAR MEDICINE FINDINGS

The radiographic findings in rickets and osteomalacia are manifestations of the histopathologic abnormalities. In rickets there is a widening of the epiphyseal growth plate, and the ends of the growing metaphyses are irregular or cupped. Loss of the trabecular pattern of the metaphyses, thinning of the cortices of the diaphyses, and bowing of the long bones may be present.

The most common radiographic finding in osteomalacia is a reduction in skeletal density, a nonspecific change that is of little value

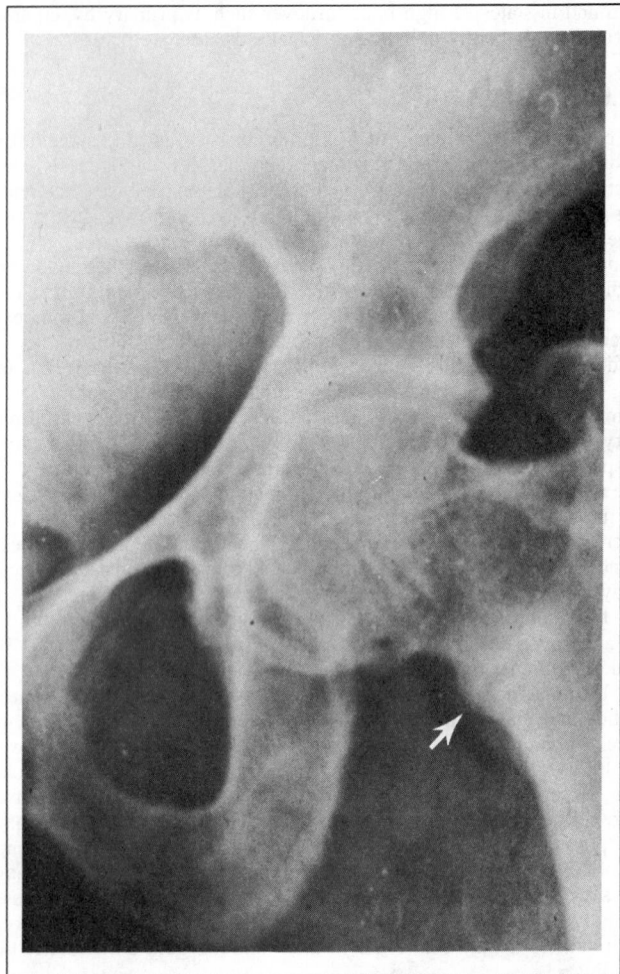

FIGURE 317-1   Radiograph showing a pseudofracture of the femoral neck in a patient with osteomalacia.

Courtesy Dr. Robert Weinstein.

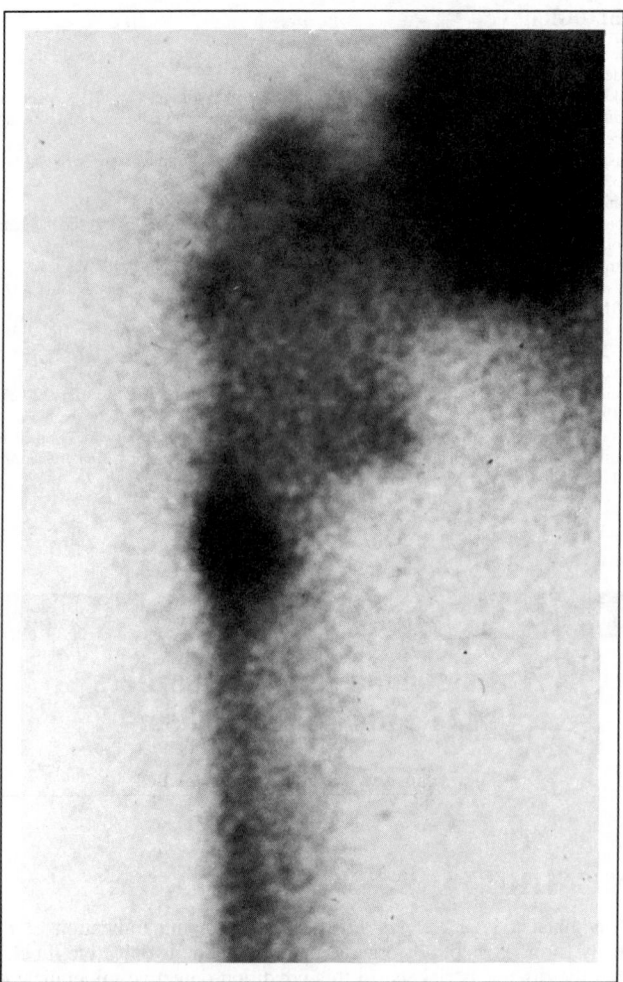

FIGURE 317-2   Technetium-99 pyrophosphate bone scan of a femur showing a hot spot at the site of a pseudofracture in a patient with osteomalacia.

Courtesy Dr. Robert Weinstein.

diagnostically, since it is seen in other conditions such as osteoporosis. More helpful in this regard are the less frequently occurring coarsening of the trabecular pattern and the presence of pseudofractures. The pseudofractures or Looser's zones are narrow lines of radiolucency that usually transect and lie either at right angles or obliquely to the cortical margins of bones (Fig. 317-1). They are often bilateral and symmetric, and they commonly occur where major arteries cross bones. Sites include the axillary margins of the scapula, lower ribs, superior and inferior pubic rami, inner margins at neck of the proximal femora, and posterior margins of the proximal ulna. Multiple bilateral and symmetric pseudofractures in a patient with osteomalacia are called Milkman's syndrome.

The pathogenesis of Looser's zone is thought by some authors to represent a stress fracture that is repaired by laying down of osteoid that is inadequately mineralized. Since pseudofractures often lie adjacent to arteries, other authors attribute the lesion to mechanical erosion caused by arterial pulsations. This possibility is strengthened by arteriographic demonstrations that arteries frequently overlie sites of pseudofractures. Further, true fractures can occur at these weakened areas.

Another distinctive radiographic finding in osteomalacia is the "rugger jersey" appearance of the spine. This results from such changes in advanced disease that the vertebral bodies become concave as a result of softening of the bone. In contrast, the vertebral disks are large and biconvex. In osteomalacia the incidence of compression fractures of the spine is lower than in osteoporosis.

In rickets and osteomalacia skeletal changes sometimes result from secondary hyperparathyroidism. These include subperiosteal resorption of the phalanges and resorption of the distal ends of the long bones such as the clavicle and humerus. In some instances radiographic features of excess parathyroid hormone may be more prominent than those of rickets or osteomalacia.

In patients with osteomalacia bone scans show increased uptake of technetium-99 pyrophosphate by long bones and wrists and prominence of the calvarium and mandible. Less evident are beading at the costochondral junctions and marked uptake of the tracer by the sternum and its margins, the so-called "tie sternum." In addition, pseudofractures appear as hot spots (Fig. 317-2). In some instances pseudofractures may be evident only on radiographs, and in other instances only on bone scan. Hot spots can be diagnosed erroneously as metastatic lesions.

In osteomalacia bone mineral density determined by single- and dual-photon absorptiometry may be diminished.

DIFFERENTIAL DIAGNOSIS

Mineralization is impaired by deficiencies of calcium, phosphate, or alkaline phosphatase. Rickets and osteoporosis can result from a number of causes that include abnormalities in the metabolism of vitamin D, deficiencies of calcium or phosphate, deficiencies of alkaline phosphatase, or defects in mineralization (Box 317-1). The pathogenesis and clinical laboratory findings in selected individual diseases are described later.

BOX 317-1
Causes of osteomalacia and rickets

I. Abnormalities in vitamin D metabolism
  A. Vitamin D deficiency
    1. Nutritional deficiency
    2. Lack of exposure to sunlight
    3. Malabsorption syndromes
      a. Postgastrectomy, partial or total
      b. Small bowel disease
      c. Pancreatic insufficiency
  B. Defective dermal production of vitamin D₃
    1. Chronic renal disease
    2. Aging
  C. Defective hepatic 25-hydroxylation of vitamin D
    1. Primary biliary cirrhosis
    2. Biliary atresia
    3. Biliary fistula
  D. Defective renal 1α-hydroxylation of 25-hydroxyvitamin D
    1. Hypoparathyroidism
    2. Pseudohypoparathyroidism
    3. Chronic renal insufficiency
    4. Vitamin D–dependent rickets type I
    5. Hypophosphatemic rickets
    6. Tumor-induced osteomalacia
    7. Age-related osteomalacia
  E. Defective target-organ response to 1,25-dihydroxyvitamin D
    1. Vitamin D–dependent rickets type II
    2. Anticonvulsant therapy
  F. Renal loss of vitamin D–binding protein
    1. Nephrotic syndrome
II. Phosphate deficiency
  A. Diminished intake
    1. Neonatal rickets
    2. Excess aluminum hydroxide ingestion
  B. Impaired renal tubular phosphate reabsorption
    1. Primary renal tubular defects
      a. X-linked hypophosphatemic osteomalacia

      b. Adult-onset hypophosphatemic osteomalacia
      c. Sporadic acquired hypophosphatemic osteomalacia
      d. Fanconi's syndromes
        (i) Wilson's disease
        (ii) Lowe's disease
        (iii) Tyrosinemia
        (iv) Glycogen storage disease
        (v) Cystinosis
        (vi) Ifosfamide therapy
    2. Secondary renal tubular "defects"
      a. Primary hyperparathyroidism
      b. Secondary hyperparathyroidism
      c. Renal tubular acidosis
      d. Tumor-induced osteomalacia
III. Mineralization defects
  A. Enzyme deficiency
    1. Hypophosphatasia
  B. Circulating inhibitor(s) of calcification
    1. Chronic renal failure
    2. Hypophosphatasia (increased pyrophosphate)
  C. Drugs and ions
    1. Diphosphonates
    2. Fluoride
    3. Aluminum intoxication
  D. Abnormal bone collagen or matrix
    1. Chronic renal failure
    2. Osteogenesis imperfecta
    3. Fibrogenesis imperfecta ossium
IV. States of rapid bone formation
  A. Postoperative primary hyperparathyroidism with osteitis fibrosa cystica
  B. Osteopetrosis
V. Miscellaneous
  A. Parenteral alimentation

NUTRITIONAL DEFICIENCIES

In children in the United States rickets and osteomalacia resulting from deficiency of vitamin D are uncommon. When they do occur, they are usually caused by lack of sunlight and the resultant diminished dermal synthesis of vitamin D₃. Lack of dietary intake is an infrequent factor, since milk and dairy products are fortified with vitamin D. In contrast, rickets and osteomalacia are more common in other parts of the world, particularly in underdeveloped countries. Rickets sometimes results from dietary deficiencies of vitamin D and calcium, even in tropical climates. In the United Kingdom rickets and osteomalacia occur in immigrant Indians and Pakistanis. Several factors are contributory. Endogenous production of vitamin D₃ is limited in women who remain indoors and wear traditional clothing because of diminished exposure to sunlight. Dietary practices such as the use of chupputti flour are also a factor. This flour is derived from wheat that has a high content of phytate and binds calcium, resulting in increased fecal excretion of the ion. Lignin, a component of wheat flour, binds to bile acids and prevents their absorption. Vitamin D, which normally forms micelles with bile acids, a requirement for its absorption by the intestine, is bound by the lignin–bile acid complex instead and is not absorbed. Removal of chupputti flour from the diet corrects abnormal vitamin D and mineral metabolism. Deficiency of vitamin D can be prevented by fortification of the diet with the vitamin. In women dietary deficiency of the vitamin is often so profound that it causes rickets and hypocalcemia in their nursing infants.

In developed countries elderly individuals are at greatest risk for osteomalacia. The reason is multifactorial. There is an age-related decline in the dermal synthesis of 7-dehydrocholesterol, so the production of vitamin D₃ declines. In addition, impaired production of 25-

hydroxyvitamin D in the liver, diminished synthesis of 1,25-dihydroxyvitamin D in the kidneys, and a decline in the transport of calcium in response to 1,25-dihydroxyvitamin D occurs in aging individuals. These abnormalities in vitamin D metabolism and function, coupled with inadequate exposure to ultraviolet light in individuals who are housebound and chronically institutionalized, as well as inadequate dietary intakes of vitamin D and calcium, provide the background for the development of osteomalacia.

GASTROINTESTINAL TRACT AND HEPATIC DISORDERS

Since vitamin D is absorbed in the proximal small intestine, a process that requires bile acids, and since vitamin D and its metabolites undergo an enterohepatic circulation, deficiency of the vitamin can result from gastrointestinal tract diseases that impair the intestinal absorption or interfere with the enterohepatic circulation of vitamin D. Diseases associated with osteomalacia include nontropical sprue, regional enteritis, scleroderma, blind-loop syndrome, multiple jejunal diverticulae, and idiopathic steatorrhea. Osteomalacia is also a complication of a number of surgical procedures, including subtotal gastric resection with gastroenterostomy, small bowel resection, and intestinal bypass for the treatment of morbid obesity. The incidence of osteomalacia in these various conditions differs. For example, bone disease is common in patients who have the Billroth-II procedure, which is used to treat peptic ulcer, but is uncommon in patients with sprue. Impaired intestinal absorption of calcium and vitamin D contribute to the development of osteomalacia.

Osteomalacia and rickets also occur as a complication of hepatocellular, biliary, and pancreatic disorders. Biliary obstruction, which produces parenchymal disease of the liver, can diminish the synthesis of 25-hydroxyvitamin D and interfere with the intestinal absorption of vitamin D and calcium. Some patients can be improved by increasing their exposure to sunlight and the subsequent endogenous production of vitamin D_3. In others, a defect in synthesis of 25-hydroxyvitamin D is so severe that vitamin D is ineffective and 25-hydroxyvitamin D_3 or 1,25-dihydroxyvitamin D_3 must be administered. In a patient with a defect in bile acid synthesis, replacement of the bile acid, chenodeoxycholic acid (125 mg twice a day), corrected the abnormal absorption of vitamin D and healed the rickets. Thus bile acid administration could be an alternative or supplemental means of treatment in patients with liver disease.

HYPOPARATHYROIDISM AND PSEUDOHYPOPARATHYROIDISM

Two diseases that infrequently result in osteomalacia are hypoparathyroidism and pseudohyperparathyroidism. Patients may seek medical attention with complaints of bone pain, and the diagnosis is made definitively by histomorphometric analysis of a bone biopsy specimen. Radiographs of the skeleton are sometimes unremarkable and therefore may not be helpful in diagnosis.

In hypoparathyroidism, hypocalcemia and low or low-normal serum 1,25-dihydroxyvitamin D levels are usually present and are important in the pathogenesis of the bone disease. Since parathyroid hormone is the major regulator of the renal synthesis of 1,25-dihydroxyvitamin D, low levels of serum 1,25-dihydroxyvitamin D and hypocalcemia in hypoparathyroidism result from deficiency of the hormone. Patients with hypoparathyroidism often can be given effective treatment with vitamin D, but some require more specific treatment with 1,25-dihydroxyvitamin D_3.

Pseudohypoparathyroidism is a disorder in which resistance to parathyroid hormone leads to hypocalcemia, retention of phosphate, and low levels of serum 1,25-dihydroxyvitamin D. Impaired production of 1,25-dihydroxyvitamin D results from defective synthesis of cyclic adenosine 3′,5′-monophosphate, since values are increased by administration of dibutyryl cyclic adenosine 3′,5′-monophosphate. In addition, in patients with pseudohypoparathyroidism skeletal manifestations of secondary hyperparathyroidism can develop because of hypocalcemia and increased circulating parathyroid hormone. Some patients can be given effective treatment with vitamin D; others may require 1,25-dihydroxyvitamin D_3.

VITAMIN D–DEPENDENT RICKETS, TYPE I

Vitamin D dependent rickets is an inborn error of vitamin D metabolism that is genetically transmitted as an autosomal-recessive trait. Typically infants with this disorder appear normal at birth, and the characteristic clinical and biochemical features of rickets develop during the first year of life. Biochemical features include hypocalcemia, normal or low levels of serum phosphate, elevation of serum alkaline phosphatase levels, and increased serum immunoreactive parathyroid hormone. The disease results from an absence or inactive form of renal 25-hydroxyvitamin D-1-α-hydroxylase. As a result, serum 25-hydroxyvitamin D level is normal and the level of serum 1,25-dihydroxyvitamin D is markedly reduced. Patients sometimes can be given treatment successfully with large doses of vitamin D or 25-hydroxyvitamin D_3 but readily respond to physiologic doses of 1,25-dihydroxyvitamin D_3.

HYPOPHOSPHATEMIC OSTEOMALACIA

Hypophosphatemic rickets is usually an X-linked dominant familial disorder but is occasionally sporadic. The onset is between 1 and 1½ years of age and is associated with delayed or abnormal dentition. Screening studies in families indicate that fasting hypophosphatemia is the most common manifestation of the disorder. Serum immunoreactive parathyroid hormone and serum calcium levels are usually normal. There is a broad clinical spectrum of disease that varies from individuals who have hypophosphatemia and no apparent bone disease, usually females, to individuals who are symptomatic and have severe bone disease. The degree of hypophosphatemia and severity of bone disease are not correlated, although the diminished growth rate in these individuals is attributed to hypophosphatemia.

Hypophosphatemia in this condition results from impaired reabsorption of filtered phosphate by the proximal renal tubule. Available evidence indicates that two separate mechanisms exist for phosphate transport in the renal tubule, a parathyroid hormone–dependent component that is responsible for two thirds of the tubular reabsorption of phosphate and a parathyroid hormone–independent component that is regulated by the serum calcium and is responsible for the remaining third of net tubular reabsorption of the ion. The parathyroid hormone–dependent component is completely lacking in men with hypophosphatemia and is partially deficient in women with hypophosphatemia. Defective phosphate transport is also present in the intestinal mucosa, indicating that the deficit is generalized and not restricted to the kidney.

Renal production of 1,25-dihydroxyvitamin D is also impaired and serum values are inappropriately low for the degree of hypophosphatemia. In addition, circulating 1,25-hydroxyvitamin D responds poorly to exogenously administered parathyroid hormone. The defect appears to be coupled to the abnormality in renal phosphate transport. As shown in Fig. 317-3, plasma 1,25-dihydroxyvitamin D varies directly with the renal tubular maximum for the absorption of phosphorus per liter of glomerular filtrate (TmP/GFR) in patients with X-linked hypophosphatemia, normal individuals, and patients with other defects in phosphate transport, including tumor-induced osteomalacia. Although it is quite likely that the renal production of 1,25-dihydroxyvitamin D and renal tubular reabsorption of phosphate are linked, treatment with 1,25-dihydroxyvitamin D_3 does not reverse the renal phosphate wasting and restoration of serum phosphate to normal levels does not enhance the renal production of 1,25-dihydroxyvitamin D.

Of interest is the fact that tumoral calcinosis appears to be the mirror image of X-linked hypophosphatemia and tumor-induced osteomalacia (Fig. 317-3). In tumoral calcinosis the renal tubular reabsorption of phosphate and plasma 1,25-dihydroxyvitamin D are both abnormally increased.

A type of hypophosphatemic rickets has been described—hereditary hypophosphatemic rickets with hypercalciuria—that is characterized by an elevation in levels of circulating 1,25-dihydroxyvitamin D and hypophosphatemia. In this disorder phosphate repletion alone results in healing of osteomalacia. In other forms of hypophosphatemic rickets and osteomalacia treatment requires both phosphate and 1,25-dihydroxyvitamin D_3, which must be administered lifelong. If therapy is adequate, the bone disease can be almost completely reversed. Occasional complications of therapy include hypercalcemia and soft tissue calcification, including nephrocalcinosis, calcification at tendon attachments to bone, and cardiac valves. Although soft tissue calcifications are widely believed to be a result of increased calcium absorption and the resultant hypercalciuria in response to 1,25-

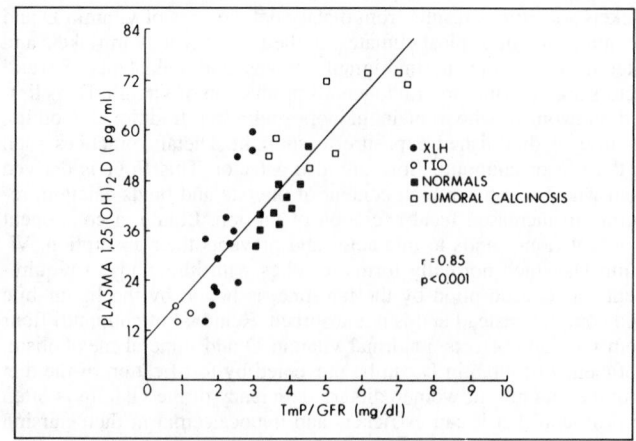

FIGURE 317-3 Relationship between plasma 1,25-dihydroxyvitamin D and TmP/GFR in normal subjects, patients with hypophosphatemic rickets *(XLH)*, tumor-induced osteomalacia *(TIO)*, and tumoral calcinosis.

From Drezner MK. In Zackson DA, editor: *A CPC series: cases in metabolic bone disease,* New York, 1987, Triclinica Communications.

dihydroxyvitamin D$_3$, there is evidence that complications correlate more strongly with the amount of phosphate administered.

TUMOR-INDUCED OSTEOMALACIA

Tumor-induced osteomalacia is a disorder similar to hypophosphatemic rickets in that the osteomalacia is associated with renal phosphate wasting and an inappropriately low level of serum 1,25-dihydroxyvitamin D. It is seen with a variety of benign or malignant neoplasms, such as sarcomas, hemangiomas, giant cell tumors of the colon, and carcinoma of the breast and prostate. Complete remission occurs with removal or irradiation of the tumor.

The clinical and biochemical features are typical of osteomalacia. Patients often have generalized muscle weakness and bone pain. Serum calcium level is usually normal to slightly reduced. Serum phosphate level is low, and serum alkaline phosphatase and urinary calcium levels are elevated.

It is likely that the hypophosphatemia results from one or more factors produced by the tumors that alter the renal tubular reabsorption of phosphate in the proximal tubule and interfere with the renal production of 1,25-dihydroxyvitamin D. Treatment of the disorder is resection or irradiation of the lesion. If this is not possible, treatment with phosphates and vitamin D or 1,25-dihydroxyvitamin D$_3$ may be used.

VITAMIN D–DEPENDENT RICKETS, TYPE II

Vitamins D-dependent rickets, type II, results from end-organ resistance to 1,25-dihydroxyvitamin D. The clinical, biochemical, and skeletal findings of the disorder may appear during infancy, childhood, or adolescence. The disease is sporadic or familial and is transmitted as an autosomal-recessive trait. Infants with the familial disease may have permanent alopecia, usually a sign of severe disease. Studies with cultured skin fibroblasts from patients with the disorder demonstrate a wide variety of abnormalities in the uptake and nuclear binding of radiolabeled 1,25-dihydroxyvitamin D$_3$, indicating genetic heterogeneity in the disorder. More recent studies show mutations in the vitamin D receptor gene. In children with the most profound defects the disorder is difficult to treat, and sometimes these children die of pneumonia. Patients with severe disease often respond poorly even to large doses of 1,25-dihydroxyvitamin D$_3$ but respond favorably to long-term infusions of calcium.

ANTICONVULSANT-INDUCED OSTEOMALACIA

Osteomalacia can be seen in patients with epilepsy who are receiving anticonvulsant therapy, especially phenobarbital and phenytoin (Dilantin). The clinical spectrum ranges from asymptomatic individuals with a reduction in bone mass to patients with hypocalcemia, clinically apparent bone disease, fractures, and pseudofractures. The incidence of bone disease is higher in patients who receive more than one anticonvulsant drug.

Anticonvulsant drugs induce hepatic microsomal mixed-function oxidase activity. This results in increased hepatic conversion of vitamin D and 25-hydroxyvitamin D to more polar, biologically inactive metabolites. As a consequence, serum 25-hydroxyvitamin D level is reduced. Since the level of serum 1,25-dihydroxyvitamin D is normal, however, the bone disease may not be caused by abnormal vitamin D metabolism. In experimental animals phenytoin inhibits the intestinal absorption of calcium, and both phenytoin and phenobarbital inhibit mobilization of calcium from bone in vitro. Inhibition of the peripheral actions of 1,25-dihydroxyvitamin D is apparently responsible for the bone disease.

Administration of vitamin D corrects and prevents biochemical and radiographic abnormalities of osteomalacia and decreases the incidence of fractures in patients who are being given treatment with anticonvulsants.

RENAL DISEASE

Patients with renal disease develop rickets and osteomalacia based on three mechanisms: diminished renal production of 1,25-dihydroxyvitamin D, abnormal mineralization caused by aluminum

toxicity, and formation of abnormal collagen or matrix (Box 317-1). Metabolic bone disease encountered in uremic patients includes osteitis fibrosa, osteomalacia, and mixtures of both of these disorders. With progressive renal failure there is an inability to rapidly excrete phosphate, leading to a reciprocal reduction in serum calcium and increases in the secretion of parathyroid hormone. Phosphate retention, however, suppresses the renal production of 1,25-dihydroxyvitamin D, and the reduction is reversed or prevented by phosphate restriction. With advancing renal insufficiency the kidney loses its capability to synthesize 1,25-dihydroxyvitamin D, and rickets and osteomalacia may occur. Osteomalacia may also develop as a result of phosphate depletion induced by dialysis or as a result of renal phosphate wasting following kidney transplantation.

Aluminum is implicated in the defective mineralization seen in renal osteodystrophy. Evidence for this stems from several epidemiologic and experimental observations. First, it was noted that there was a high prevalence of dialysis-dependent bone diseases in patients undergoing hemodialysis with a water of high aluminum content. There was also a decreased incidence of these diseases after removal of aluminum. In addition, patients with dialysis-dependent osteodystrophy seem to have higher plasma aluminum concentrations that correlate with bone aluminum content. Histomorphometric examination of bone reveals that aluminum is deposited along the mineralization front. Use of desferrioxamine in affected patients has resulted in clinical improvement of bone disease, as well as decreased plasma and bone aluminum concentrations. Animal studies demonstrate that aluminum loading in rats and dogs is associated with the development of osteomalacia. The severity of impairment in mineralization was increased in uremic animals. Inappropriately low or decreased serum parathyroid hormone levels resulting from parathyroidectomy seem to put patients at risk for the development of this entity.

On the other hand, several theoretical and experimental observations question the pathogenic role of aluminum in this disorder. It is not clear that aluminum is the only metal contaminating dialysis fluid that was removed with water purification. It is also noted that aluminum deposition at the mineralization front does not imply causality and may instead represent an epiphenomenon. Animals made osteomalacic by vitamin D depletion and given aluminum demonstrated aluminum deposits at the mineralization site in a pattern and to an extent that was identical to the dialysis-dependent patients with osteomalacia. In addition, vitamin D repletion resulted in normal calcification even in the face of continued aluminum administration. Staining of the normally mineralized bone indicated that calcification had occurred at sites where aluminum had previously been deposited.

Chronic acidosis associated with renal disease such as renal tubular acidosis without renal insufficiency has also been associated with the development of osteomalacia. Treatment with alkali may suffice in these patients and avert the possible complications of vitamin D therapy.

MINERALIZATION DEFECTS

Bisphosphonates are protein-seeking agents that have the structure -P-C-P, are derivatives of pyrophosphate, and can impair mineralization. One of them, disodium etidronate, is effective in producing remission of Paget's disease. However, in high doses (20 mg/kg of body weight) etidronate produces osteomalacia and fractures. At lower doses (5 to 7.5 mg/kg of body weight) it corrects the biochemical and skeletal abnormalities of Paget's disease without impairing mineralization.

Fluoride, when taken long-term in large doses (more than 20 mg of fluoride intramuscularly per day), produces skeletal fluorinosis. This syndrome is characterized by periosteal new bone formation, osteophyte formation, arthralgias, and abnormal hardening of the bone. Total osteoid surface area and width are increased. New periosteal bone formation may be abnormal and demonstrates a disordered lamellar structure.

Aluminum was implicated in the pathogenesis of osteomalacia and fractures that occur in patients receiving total parenteral nutrition who receive amino acids in the form of casein hydrolysate. High concentrations of aluminum were found in the casein hydrolysate and in skeletal tissue. In individuals in whom osteomalacia develops during treatment with total parenteral nutrition, the level of serum immunoreactive parathyroid hormone was either abnormally low or in the lower range of normal. The pathogenesis is thought to be similar to that of aluminum-related osteomalacia that occurs in patients with renal insufficiency.

HYPOPHOSPHATASIA

Hypophosphatasia is a rare disease characterized by low activity of serum and bone alkaline phosphatase. Abnormal mineralization of the skeleton resulting in rickets and osteomalacia is found, together with premature loss of deciduous teeth and increased phosphoethanolamine and pyrophosphate in blood and urine. The disease is transmitted as an autosomal-recessive trait and is prevalent in inbred populations.

Three types of hypophosphatasia are recognized based on the age of onset and clinical severity: infantile, childhood, and adult. Infantile hypophosphatasia usually develops before 6 months of age and can be diagnosed in utero. It is the most common form of this disorder and is associated with severe rickets and failure to thrive. Increased intracranial pressure, hypercalcemia, hypercalciuria, and nephrocalcinosis are found. The skeletal disease is so severe that less than 50% of infants survive. Childhood hypophosphatasia develops after 6 months of age and is characterized by premature loss of deciduous teeth, increased susceptibility to infection, and retarded growth. Radiographic findings include deossification with a coarse trabecular pattern, bowing deformities, and fractures. Irregular epiphyses and islands of radiolucency are present in the shafts of long bones. Spontaneous healing of rachitic skeletal changes occurs, but permanent teeth are lost early.

Adult hypophosphatasia is quite rare. Patients often have a history of rickets, loss of deciduous teeth in childhood, and early loss or extraction of permanent teeth. Radiographs may show a coarse trabecular pattern, Looser's zones, and subperiosteal bone formation. The diagnosis is established by findings of low levels of serum alkaline phosphatase and elevated levels of serum and urine phosphoethanolamine. There is no effective form of treatment, although vitamin D has produced some improvement in a few patients. In a number of patients vitamin D intoxication has developed. Treatment with phosphate improved mineralization of the skeleton in some instances when given in doses of 1.25 to 3.0 g of neutral phosphate. Some clinical improvement has been observed when purified alkaline phosphatase is infused intravenously into patients with hypophosphatasia, but experience is limited.

TREATMENT

The goals of treatment of rickets or osteomalacia are to correct hypocalcemia if it is present; to prevent symptoms and sequelae of hypocalcemia including seizures and cataracts; to prevent or correct the skeletal deformities of rickets and osteomalacia and those of secondary hyperparathyroidism; to prevent hypercalcemia, hypercalciuria, and their consequences; and to produce normal growth and development of the skeleton in children. Vitamin D and a number of its derivatives are available in the United States. Vitamin D is available as capsules (50,000 international units [IU] or 1.25 mg) for oral administration, in sesame oil (500,000 IU or 12.5 mg/ml) for injection, and in propylene glycol (250 IU or 6.25 µg per drop) for oral administration. The advantages of vitamin D therapy are that the cost is modest and that it is often effective, even in patients with abnormal vitamin D metabolism. The disadvantages of vitamin D therapy are that several weeks may be required to achieve optimal therapeutic effectiveness, the therapeutic dose is near the toxic dose, and biologic activity persists after its administration is stopped.

25-Hydroxyvitamin D_3 is available in capsules of 20 and 50 µg. The drug may be particularly useful in patients with hepatic disease and impaired synthesis of 25-hydroxyvitamin D. The onset of action of the drug is more rapid than that of vitamin D. The disadvantages are much the same as those of vitamin D. However, the half-life of the drug (2 to 3 weeks) may be shorter than that of vitamin D, which is stored in fat, so in the event of toxicity the biologic effects after cessation of administration may not be as long-lasting as those of vitamin D.

1,25-dihydroxyvitamin D_3 is marketed as capsules of 0.25 and 0.50 µg and an intravenous preparation of 1 or 2 µg/ml. The advantages of the drug are its rapid onset of action and the rapid disap-

pearance of its biologic effect after discontinuation. The half-life of the drug is less than 6 hours. One disadvantage is that hypercalcemia may occur after long-term treatment during which the abnormal calcium metabolism is stabilized. Hypercalcemia can be treated by stopping the drug and prevented by decreasing the dose. Hypercalcemia occurs fairly frequently, so patients must be closely monitored. 1,25-Dihydroxyvitamin D_3 is most useful in diseases in which its synthesis by the kidney is impaired. It is sometimes of value in disorders in which resistance to its effects occurs at the cellular level. In the latter instance, higher doses are required.

Dihydrotachysterol is available in tablets of 0.125, 0.2, and 0.4 mg. The drug has a rapid onset of action and a relatively short duration of biologic action after cessation of administration. The 180-degree rotation of the A ring permits the hydroxyl group in the free position to act as a pseudohydroxyl group. The drug becomes biologically active after it undergoes 25-hydroxylation in the liver. Since it does not need to be hydroxylated in the 1α position, the drug is of potential value in treating the same diseases as those for which 1,25-dihydroxyvitamin D_3 is indicated.

Calcium supplements should be administered in divided doses, since calcium absorption is abnormally low in most patients with osteomalacia. Administration of calcium decreases the amount of vitamin D or its analogs that are required for treatment. The content of elemental calcium varies among preparations, so the amount that provides 1 g of elemental calcium also varies. One to two grams per day of elemental calcium should be administered to adults in divided doses. The dose should be modified depending on the severity of the disease. Children should receive 30 to 60 mg/kg body weight per day. The dose should be modified depending on the severity of the disease.

Deficiency of vitamin D in adults is treated by the daily administration of 5000 IU (125 µg) to 10,000 IU (250 µg) of vitamin D_2 until healing of bone disease occurs. Children should be given treatment with 1000 IU (25 µg) per day. This low dose does not mask vitamin-resistant syndromes and rarely results in the hypocalcemia seen in the "hungry bone" syndrome associated with the initiation of vitamin D therapy. In noncompliant patients a single, high dose (500,000 IU or 12.5 mg) of vitamin D (the "stoss treatment") delivered either as an intramuscular injection or by mouth is frequently effective. After the bone disease is healed, 400 IU (10 µg), the recommended daily requirement, prevents recurrence. Larger doses of 50,000 IU (1.25 mg) to 100,000 IU (2.5 mg) may be required in patients with gastrointestinal tract, renal, or hepatic disease. As already noted, treatment with 25-hydroxyvitamin D_3 is indicated when there is marked impairment of hepatic vitamin D-25-hydroxylase.

Vitamin D, 50,000 IU (1.25 mg) to 100,000 IU (2.5 mg) per day or more, is often effective in treating osteomalacia resulting from diseases that are associated with renal insufficiency, hypoparathyroidism, and pseudohypoparathyroidism but may not be effective in the treatment of bone diseases associated with vitamin D–dependent rickets type I, hypophosphatemic rickets, and tumor-induced osteomalacia. In these disorders 1,25-dihydroxyvitamin D_3, 0.5 to 3 µg per day, is usually effective. The dose of vitamin D, 25-hydroxyvitamin D_3, and 1,25-dihydroxyvitamin D_3 varies from patient to patient and in a given individual must be determined by trial and error for the treatment of hypophosphatemic rickets. Phosphate supplements of 2 to 4 per day in divided oral doses and as much as 4 µg per day of 1,25-dihydroxyvitamin D_3 are essential to heal the bone disease. Lifelong treatment is required. Removal or irradiation of tumor is required to treat tumor-induced osteomalacia.

Osteomalacia associated with vitamin D–dependent rickets type II sometimes responds to treatment with vitamin D. However, in instances of a more profound target-organ defect, 1,25-dihydroxyvitamin D_3 is necessary. Doses as high as 15 to 20 µg per day are sometimes required and, even then, may not be effective. Under these circumstances long-term parenteral administration of calcium can be used to heal the bone disease.

Osteomalacia associated with renal tubular acidosis is treated initially with 5000 IU (1.25 mg) to 10,000 IU (2.5 mg) of vitamin D. The acidosis is corrected by treatment with sodium bicarbonate. Once the bone disease heals, however, vitamin D is not required.

Hypercalcemia and hypercalciuria sometimes occur during treatment with vitamin D and its metabolites. Individuals may be asymptomatic or have anorexia, nausea, vomiting, weight loss, headache, constipation, polyuria, polydipsia, and altered mental status. The abnormal calcium metabolism is characterized by increased intestinal absorption and enhanced release of calcium from skeletal tissue. Decline of renal function, nephrocalcinosis, nephrolithiasis, urinary tract infections, and even death may ensue. Patients who are receiving long-term treatment with vitamin D and its analogs require careful follow-up at intervals of 4 to 6 weeks with measurement of serum and urinary calcium levels and serum creatinine level. Careful evaluation of patients is important, since there is no way of predicting when or in whom vitamin D intoxication will develop. Of interest, vitamin D intoxication is almost never seen when the "stoss treatment" is used in children. The most effective means of treatment of these side effects and complications is prevention. When intoxication does occur, the drug and calcium supplements should be stopped, and fluids (3 to 4 L per day) should be given. Either the dose of vitamin D or its derivatives should be reduced, or another drug should be substituted. When intoxication is severe, treatment with prednisone or salmon calcitonin may be required.

BIBLIOGRAPHY

Balsan S, Tieder M: Linear growth in patients with hypophosphatemic vitamin D–resistant rickets: influence of treatment regimen and parental height, *J Pediatr* 116:365, 1991.

Bell NH, Stern PH: Hypercalcemia and increases in serum hormone value during prolonged administration of 1α,25-dihydroxyvitamin D, *N Engl J Med* 298:1241, 1978.

Drezner MK: Understanding the pathogenesis of X-linked hypophosphatemic rickets: a requisite for successful therapy. In Zackson DA, editor: *A CPC series: cases in metabolic bone disease,* New York, 1987, Triclinica Communications.

Epstein S et al: 1α,25-Dihydroxyvitamin D₃ corrects osteomalacia in hypoparathyroidism and pseudohypoparathyroidism, *Acta Endocrinol* 103:241, 1983.

Gazit D et al: Osteomalacia in hereditary hypophosphatemic rickets with hypercalciuria: a correlative clinical-histormorphometric study, *J Clin Endocrinol Metab* 72:229, 1991.

Hodsman AB et al: Bone aluminum and histomorphometric features of renal osteodystrophy, *J Clin Endocrinol Metab* 54:539, 1982.

Hutchinson FN, Bell NH: Osteomalacia and rickets, *Semin Nephrol* 12:127, 1992.

Lobaugh B, Burch WM Jr, Drezner MK: Abnormalities of vitamin D metabolism and action in the vitamin D–resistant rachitic and osteomalacia disease. In Kumar R, editor: *Vitamin D: basic and clinical aspects,* Boston, 1984, Martinas Nijhoff.

Ott SM et al: Aluminum is associated with low bone formation in patients receiving chronic parenteral nutrition, *Ann Intern Med* 98:910, 1983.

Pratt CB et al: Ifosfamide, Fanconi's syndrome, and rickets, *J Clin Oncol* 9:1495, 1991.

Verge CR et al: Effects of therapy in X-linked hypophosphatemic rickets, *Am J Dis Child* 145:1165, 1991.

CHAPTER

318 Paget's Disease of Bone

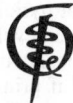

Frederick R. Singer

In 1876, Sir James Paget, a remarkable English surgeon, described a focal disorder of bone that produced slowly progressive enlargement and deformity of the skeleton. He believed this was a rare disorder, but in the ensuing years the application of biochemical testing and x-rays to clinical medicine made it apparent that this disease was not uncommon.

Paget's disease has been estimated to be present in 2% to 3% of the population over 50 years of age in countries where it is commonly found. Perhaps the population most affected by this condition is the Lancashire region of England, where the prevalence is estimated to be more than 8%. The disease follows patterns of English migration to Australia, New Zealand, South Africa, and the United States and is relatively common on the continent of Europe and in cities in South America with heavy European immigration. Paget's disease is strikingly uncommon in Scandinavia, China, Japan, and India. The disease shows no clear predilection for either sex. Up to 40% of patients have at least one other family member affected by the disease. Examination of familial patterns of the disease suggests an autosomal dominant pattern of inheritance with incomplete penetrance.

Studies in England have suggested that exposure to dogs may be a risk factor, but this has not proven a universal finding.

PATHOLOGIC FEATURES

Generally, Paget's disease affects one or several bones, most often the skull, vertebrae, pelvis, femur, and tibia. It is believed that a focal increase in osteoclasts initiates an osteolytic process, which must evolve over decades before a bone such as the femur is totally involved. The osteoclasts in Paget's disease are sometimes quite large and may be found to have many more nuclei than normal. Behind the advancing front of osteoclasts into normal bone, there is evidence of great cellular activity. Osteoblasts have proliferated and line bony trabeculae that have undergone partial resorption by the osteoclasts. Fibroblasts, connective tissue, and blood vessels have replaced most of the hematopoietic cells of the marrow. The bone matrix has assumed a "mosaic" pattern with irregular cement lines instead of the normal symmetry of the collagen fibers in parallel. Sometimes a "burned-out" stage of Paget's disease is found in which cellular activity is reduced or absent but the abnormal matrix persists.

The ultrastructure of the osteoclast in Paget's disease is characterized by the presence of abnormal nuclear and cytoplasmic inclusions, which closely resemble the nucleocapsids of viruses of the Paramyxoviridae family. Immunocytochemical studies have demonstrated that the osteoclasts harbor measles virus and/or respiratory syncytial virus nucleocapsid antigens. Measles virus and canine distemper virus messenger RNA (mRNA) transcripts have been found in pagetic bone specimens, but their relevance to the origin of the disease is unclear.

CLINICAL COURSE

Paget's disease is not usually discovered until middle age. It is not known precisely what percentage of patients with Paget's disease are symptomatic. In a study in Germany it was estimated that less than 1% of affected individuals had symptoms. Although this may be an underestimate of symptomatic patients, it is clear that many individuals are discovered to have this disease only when an abnormal x-ray or laboratory test is encountered during the course of a routine examination or while another disorder is being evaluated. In symptomatic patients the most common complaints are skeletal deformity and musculoskeletal pain.

On physical examination the skull, the clavicles, or the long bones of the lower extremities may be seen to be abnormal in an asymmetric distribution. Gross enlargement of these bones may be obvious, and deformity of weight-bearing bones is also quite prominent. If the skull is involved, hearing loss is quite common in the later stages. Vertigo, tinnitus, and less commonly, headaches, may also be present. Basilar impression may be associated with neurologic syndromes related to compression of the spinal cord, the brainstem, the cerebellum, and the basilar and vertebral arteries. A common site of involvement is the spine, the thoracic and lumbar vertebrae most often being affected. Multiple vertebrae or a solitary vertebra may be abnormal.

Back pain is a common complaint and may be caused by Paget's disease, but degenerative arthritis of the spine is quite common. Less often, spinal stenosis may result in severe pain. Vertebrae affected by Paget's disease are also susceptible to compression fractures. A common site of involvement is the pelvis and femurs. When disease is present in these areas, degenerative arthritis of the hip is a major problem, leading to pain and impaired mobility. Bowing of the femur or tibia is also a cause of difficult ambulation. Degenerative arthritis in the knees and ankles may be associated with lower-extremity deformities.

Pathologic fractures sometimes occur in the femur and tibia of patients with Paget's disease. Nonunion is relatively infrequent but more likely to occur if the femur is fractured. A useful physical finding suggesting Paget's disease in the lower extremities is the observation of increased skin temperature over an affected bone. This is a consequence of increased blood flow not only to the bone but to the surrounding cutaneous region.

Examination of the fundus may reveal angioid streaks in about 10% of patients. This finding reflects defects in Bruch's membrane of the retina. This finding is seldom associated with impaired vision. Patients in whom more than 15% of the skeleton is affected by Paget's disease have increased cardiac output. This could predispose an indi-

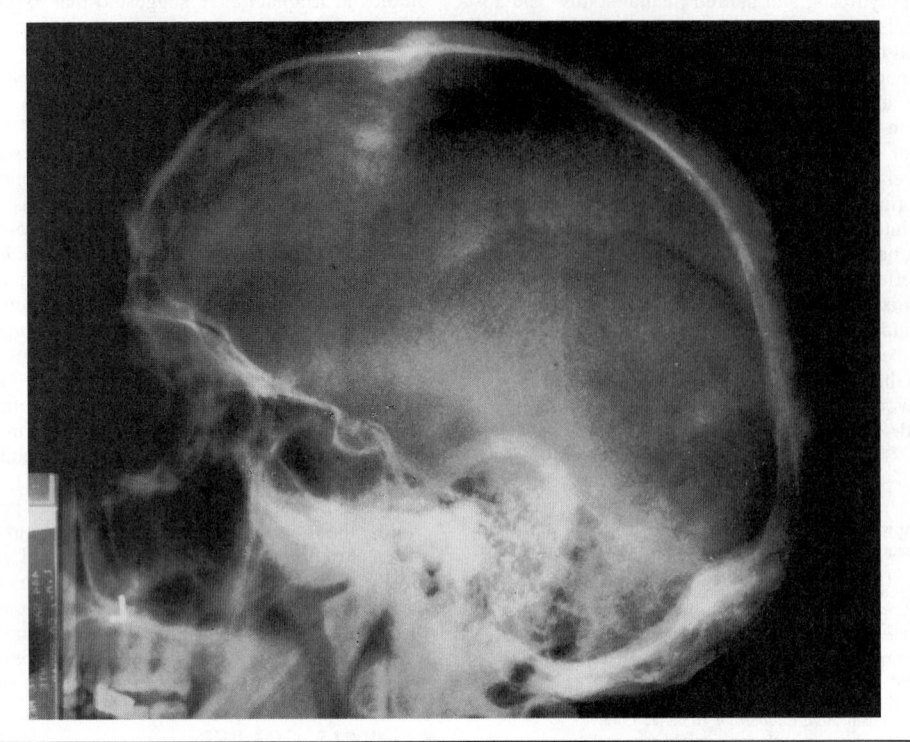

FIGURE 318-1   Lateral x-ray of the skull demonstrating large radiolucent areas termed *osteoporosis circumscripta*. Early sclerotic lesions are also apparent.

vidual to congestive heart failure, but high-output cardiac failure is not a common feature, even in patients with very extensive disease.

The most deadly complication of Paget's disease is the development of a sarcoma in a preexisting lesion of Paget's disease. The prognosis in such patients is quite poor, probably because of the difficulties in early diagnosis. A relatively rapid increase in skeletal deformity or sudden worsening of bone pain suggests an underlying tumor. Sarcomas occur in fewer than 1% of patients. Even less common are benign giant cell tumors, which can also arise in the pagetic bone.

RADIOLOGIC FINDINGS

The diagnosis of Paget's disease is primarily made by radiographic examination, since its features are so characteristic that a bone biopsy is seldom necessary. The early phases of the disease are most readily recognized in the skull and long bones. The initial lesion is a radiolucent area, which in the skull has been termed *osteoporosis circumscripta* (Fig. 318-1). In a long bone the radiolucent lesion usually begins at either end of the bone and progresses with a sharply defined V shape either proximally or distally. The average rate of progress of such lesions has been measured to be approximately 1 cm per year. Uncommonly this osteolytic phase may result in an expansile lesion resembling a cyst at the end of a long bone such as the tibia.

After many years the osteolytic phase is transformed into an osteoblastic or osteosclerotic phase. Chaotic new bone formation leads to striking enlargement of the calvarium, which has a "cotton-wool" appearance (Fig. 318-2). It is likely that patients with severe enlargement of the skull have had the disease since childhood. The osteolytic lesions in the long bones evolve into lesions with thickened bone and irregular trabeculations. In the pelvis a classic sign of Paget's disease is thickening of the iliopectineal line, the "brim sign." The vertebral bodies are generally noted to be sclerotic rather than radiolucent, at the time of diagnosis (Fig. 318-3). At times, a sclerotic vertebra from Paget's disease may be difficult to distinguish from a malignant lesion. However, in Paget's disease the vertebral body is often larger than adjacent normal vertebrae (Fig. 318-3). In patients with back pain computed tomography and magnetic resonance imaging of the spine are useful techniques to help evaluate the cause of the pain.

The most sensitive means of detecting Paget's disease is by utilizing radioactive tracers that localize in bone. Occasionally, lesions that are difficult to visualize on radiographic examination may be strongly positive on a bone scan.

BIOCHEMISTRY

Routine biochemical screening in patients with Paget's disease usually results in an isolated abnormality, elevation of serum alkaline phosphatase activity. The level of this index of osteoblastic activity correlates quite well with the extent and activity of the disease. Another index of osteoblastic activity, the blood level of the vitamin K–dependent protein osteocalcin, inexplicably is less useful. Indices of bone matrix resorption such as urinary hydroxyproline or pyridinoline cross-links excretion are usually not needed for clinical evaluation unless liver disease or pregnancy complicates the clinical course. Hypercalcemia may occur if patients are immobilized or if primary hyperparathyroidism or a malignancy develops. Hyperuricemia in the presence or absence of gout may be found and, perhaps, reflect high turnover of nucleic acids.

TREATMENT

Until the origin of Paget's disease is determined, definitive therapy is not possible. Nevertheless, during the past 20 years it has become possible to deal effectively with many of the manifestations of the disease using appropriate medical and surgical treatment.

Many patients require no treatment, since they are asymptomatic and do not have disease in weight-bearing bones. The main indications for drug treatment are relief of bone pain, preparation for orthopedic surgery, prevention of progression of osteolytic lesions in weight-bearing bones, and prevention or stabilization of hearing loss.

Calcitonin

Salmon calcitonin is an inhibitor of osteoclast activity that reduces both bone resorption and, secondarily, bone formation when given

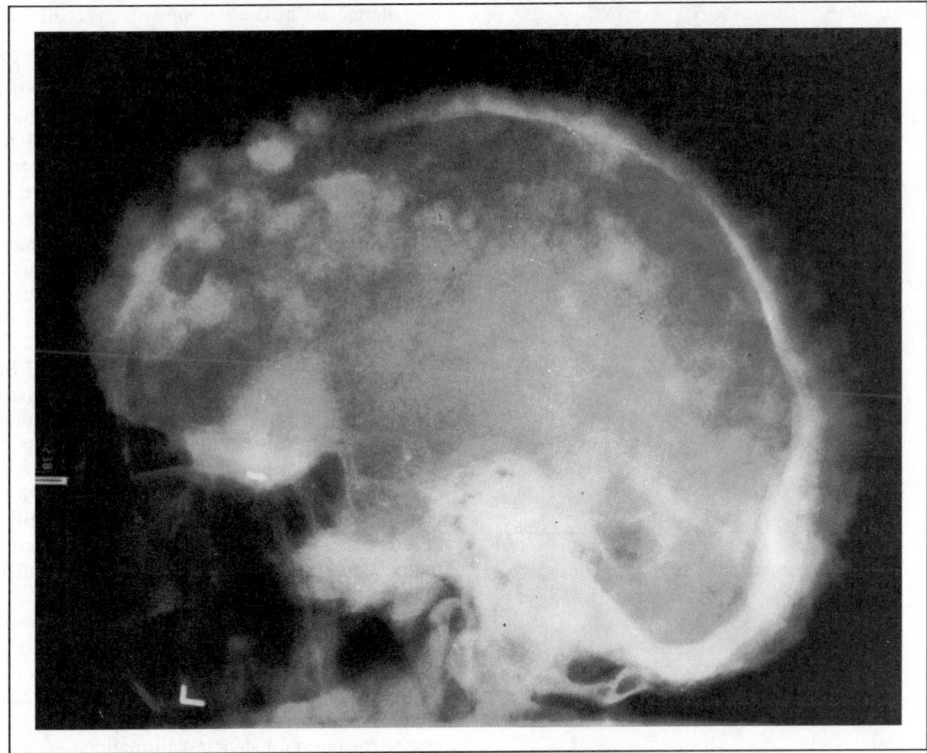

FIGURE 318-2   Lateral x-ray of the skull of a patient with advanced Paget's disease. There is generalized thickening of the calvarium with patchy sclerosis exhibiting a "cotton-wool" appearance.

long-term by subcutaneous injection. Treatment results in relief of bone pain, resolution of osteolytic lesions, reduction of increased cardiac output, stabilization of hearing, and reversal of neurologic deficits in some patients. Subcutaneous treatment with 50 units of salmon calcitonin daily or on alternate days usually decreases serum alkaline phosphatase activity by 50%. Side effects include nausea and facial flushing, which usually are tolerable. Antibodies develop in about 50% of patients receiving treatment with salmon calcitonin and may produce clinical resistance. These patients respond well to other agents. If calcitonin treatment is discontinued, the disease becomes more active within months.

Bisphosphonates

The bisphosphonates, analogs of pyrophosphoric acid, are agents that localize to the surface of bone and inhibit bone resorption. Etidronate disodium, the seminal bisphosphonate, is administered orally at a dose of 5 mg/kg body weight daily for 6-month courses. It produces clinical benefits quite similar to those of calcitonin. The main differences are that etidronate is ineffective in healing osteolytic lesions and doses greater than 5 mg/kg may induce osteomalacia. In recent years more potent bisphosphonates have been approved for Paget's disease. Intravenous pamidronate disodium and oral alendronate sodium are highly effective in reducing disease activity, even in patients with extensive disease.

Surgery

Drug therapy cannot reverse the structural abnormalities found to produce significant morbidity in some patients with advanced Paget's disease. Patients with neurologic problems resulting from basilar impression require occipital decompression, and patients with spinal stenosis may need surgical intervention. The severe pain and impaired ambulation caused by degenerative arthritis of the hip can be effectively relieved by a total hip replacement. Impaired ambulation and knee or ankle pain caused by severe tibial bowing usually respond well to a high-level tibial osteotomy. Before elective surgery it is wise to administer medical therapy for up to 3 months to minimize intra-

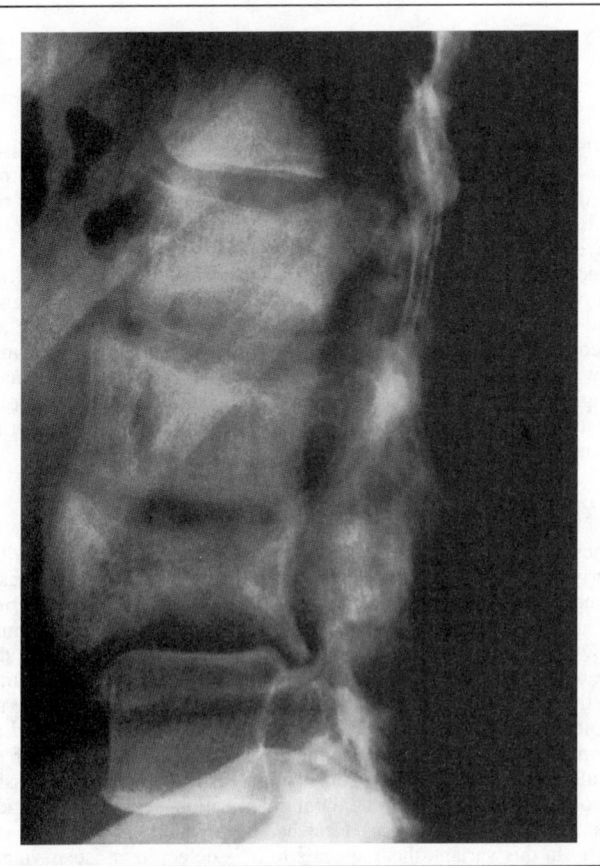

FIGURE 318-3   Lateral x-ray of the lumbar spine demonstrating three enlarged vertebral bodies. The distal vertebral body is compressed and encroaching on the spinal canal.

✔ *WHEN TO REFER*

The majority of patients with Paget's disease probably do not need referral to a specialist. The most common occasions for referral are when there is a consideration of surgery and when standard medical therapy proves ineffective.

operative and postoperative bleeding and prevent hypercalcemia caused by immobilization.

BIBLIOGRAPHY

Kanis JA: *Pathophysiology and treatment of Paget's disease of bone,* Durham, NC, 1991, Carolina Academic.
McDonald DJ, Sim FH: Total hip arthroplasty in Paget's disease, *J Bone Joint Surg Am,* 69:766, 1987.
Meyers M, Singer F: Osteotomy for tibia vara in Paget's disease under cover of calcitonin, *J Bone Joint Surg Am,* 60:810, 1978.
Singer FR: Paget's disease of bone. In De Groot LJ, editor: *Endocrinology,* ed 3, Philadelphia, 1995, Saunders.
Singer FR, Minoofar PN: Bisphosphonates in the treatment of disorders of mineral metabolism, *Adv Endocrinol Metab* 6:259, 1995.

CHAPTER

319 Osteopetrosis

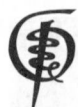

Gregory R. Mundy and Charles A. Reasner II

Osteopetrosis is the name given to a number of inherited bone disorders characterized by an increase in bone mass that impairs normal medullary hematopoiesis and obstructs osseous foramina. These disorders are characterized by a generalized increase in radiodensity and have been called *marble bone disease.* They are rare congenital disorders caused primarily by defective bone resorption. There is impaired remodeling of bone and a subsequent increase in trabecular and cortical bone matrix, usually with disorganized architecture and incomplete mineralization. The excess bone may obliterate the marrow cavity and encroach on nerve foramina. The bones are usually fragile, despite their increased radiodensity, and fracture easily. It has been suggested that *chalk bone disease* would be a more appropriate name than *marble bone disease.*

PATHOPHYSIOLOGY

There are several different types of osteopetrosis, but the primary underlying mechanism is the same—a failure of normal osteoclastic bone resorption. A particularly malignant childhood form, inherited as an autosomal recessive trait, is characterized by severe bone marrow failure and usually a poor prognosis. The more benign form that presents during adult life is inherited as an autosomal dominant trait. In this adult variety, bone marrow failure does not occur, but the patient may have an increased susceptibility to fracture, increased radiodensity, and encroachment on cranial nerves at the base of the skull. There is a third form in humans, a rare autosomal recessive disorder characterized by cerebral calcification, renal tubular acidosis, and osteopetrosis. This form has been called *marble brain disease.* In this variant, there appears to be a defect in an isoenzyme of carbonic anhydrase (carbonic anhydrase II), which is apparently necessary for normal osteoclastic bone resorption. This enzyme is present in the osteoclast and is probably essential for the normal osteoclast

to generate an acid environment under its ruffled border, which is required in bone resorption.

There are a number of animal models of osteopetrosis in the mouse, rat, and rabbit. Much has been learned about normal bone resorption from studies of these models. Some variants can be cured by inoculation of normal mononuclear cells from the bone marrow or spleen of a littermate that presumably contain osteoclast precursors. In some variants osteoclast numbers are increased and in others they are decreased. Recent observations have shed considerable light on two murine models of osteopetrosis. These are the op/op variant, in which it has been shown that osteopetrosis is caused by impaired formation of osteoclasts. This occurs because stromal cells in this condition are unable to produce biologically active monocyte-macrophage–colony-stimulating factor (M-CSF). The disease in this case can be reversed by treatment with M-CSF. In another recently described variant of murine osteopetrosis, there is deficiency in expression of the src protooncogene. This protooncogene encodes an intracellular tyrosine kinase. Unlike op/op osteopetrosis, in src-deficient osteopetrosis the osteoclasts are formed but ineffective. This disorder can be cured by transplantation with normal osteoclast precursors. Thus osteopetrosis is caused primarily by incompetent osteoclasts that are nonresponsive to hormones and other factors that normally regulate their activity, with subsequent impairment of normal bone resorption and bone remodeling.

In more recent gene knockout experiments it has been shown that failure of expression of the c-fos protooncogene is also associated with osteopetrosis.

The different types of osteopetrosis are caused by a spectrum of abnormalities in the osteoclast, its precursor cells, or the factors necessary for normal osteoclast formation.

CLINICAL FEATURES

The common childhood form of the disease is severe and usually results in death during the first 2 years of life. In contrast, the adult form is mild and does not usually impair life expectancy. The rare childhood form of the disorder associated with carbonic anhydrase II deficiency is not characterized by bone marrow failure, and although it is compatible with long survival, renal tubular acidosis may shorten life expectancy.

Bone marrow failure is the critical feature of the childhood form; it is characterized by persistence of bony trabeculae, which almost completely fill the marrow cavity (Fig. 319-1). The consequences are anemia, leukopenia, and thrombocytopenia. As a result, extramedullary hematopoiesis may occur, but the children frequently die during infancy from the consequences of bone marrow failure such as infection or bleeding. If patients with this form of the disease survive into adult life, they suffer from anemia, recurrent fractures, and hepatosplenomegaly. Some have symptoms caused by encroachment of bone on cranial nerves, such as deafness or blindness, and most who survive have growth retardation. In the more benign adult form of the disease, sufficient marrow cavity is present for normal hematopoiesis, and the major symptomatology in these patients comes from their increased susceptibility to fracture. Many of these patients are asymptomatic, however, and the disease may be recognized accidentally when an x-ray is taken for some reason unrelated to the disease.

Despite their increased radiologic density, the bones are more likely to fracture because of poor organization of the bony architecture and the relative increase in woven bone. There is a failure of both primary modeling and subsequent haversian and trabecular remodeling. Although the bones are more susceptible to fracture, healing appears to proceed normally.

Despite the changes in bone histology and the propensity to fracture, deformity is usually not prominent. When it does occur, it is characterized by thickening of the shafts of the long bones so that the bones develop broad or club-shaped ends. The disease may be patchy in some bones, with some segments of bone appearing normal and some sections sclerotic on x-rays. This occurs most frequently in the vertebral bodies and the metacarpals. The skull and pelvis show a uniform increase in bone density, and the long bones show obliteration of the marrow cavity by dense compact bone.

Failure of resorption of cortical bone may result in obliteration of osseous foramina and entrapment of nerves, particularly the cranial

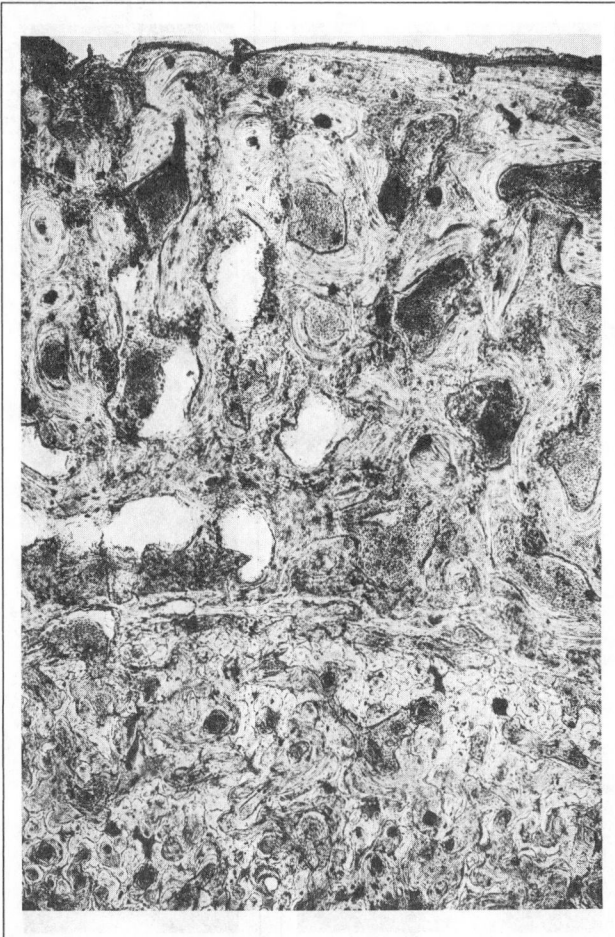

FIGURE 319-1 Osteopetrosis. This illustration at low magnification reveals a densely calcified bone producing a pattern called *helter-skelter arrangement.* There is no peculiar pattern.

A syndrome of acquired osteosclerosis associated with deep aching in the pelvis and legs, elevated skeletal turnover, and high vitamin D levels has recently been reported in young adults. Interestingly, these patients have serologic evidence of infection with hepatitis C. The relationship between the viral infection and bone disorder is unknown.

Excess fluoride ingestion for many years causes generalized osteosclerosis, the formation of osteophytes, and calcification of ligaments. Endemic fluorosis is seen in some parts of the world where the drinking water contains enormous amounts of fluoride, such as India and South Africa. It does not occur with the much smaller amounts that are added to drinking water to prevent dental caries in many communities in the United States. It occurs occasionally in patients with osteoporosis who are treated with fluoride therapy. Fluorotic bone is radiologically dense but is poorly mineralized and characterized on histologic examination by excess osteoid. Fluoride stimulates osteoblast activity, but the mineral phase of bone is defective, and the bone is brittle.

TREATMENT

The benign adult form of osteopetrosis requires no treatment. Autosomal recessive infantile osteopetrosis has been treated recently with bone marrow transplantation, which has resulted in good responses in the short term in a few patients. The mortality caused by transplant complications is high, but in some of those who do survive there is evidence, at least for a few years, of normal osteoblastic bone resorption. This procedure was first tried only a few years ago, so the long-term results are not yet known.

Several children with severe osteopetrosis have been treated with 1,25-dihydroxyvitamin D in an effort to provoke the nonresorbing osteoclast to resorb bone or to cause differentiation of mononuclear cell precursors to mature normal osteoclasts. Although there has been no improvement clinically, in one patient there was evidence in a bone biopsy specimen of increased osteoclastic bone resorption. This therapy is also experimental at the present time.

Another form of experimental therapy recently used, which seems to produce excellent results in at least some patients, is gamma interferon. Interferon therapy either improved or stabilized the condition of all of the 11 patients who completed 18 months of treatment.

BIBLIOGRAPHY

Coccia PF: Cells that resorb bone, *N Engl J Med* 310:456, 1984.
Coccia PF et al: Successful bone marrow transplantation for infantile malignant osteopetrosis, *N Engl J Med* 302:701, 1980.
Felix R, Cecchini MG, Fleisch H: Macrophage colony stimulating factor restores in vivo bone resorption in the op/op osteopetrotic mouse, *Endocrinology* 127:2592, 1990.
Fischer A et al: Bone-marrow transplantation for immunodeficiencies and osteopetrosis: European survey, 1968-1985, *Lancet* 2:1080, 1986.
Grigoriadis AE, Wang ZQ, Cecchini MG et al: c-fos: A key regulator of osteoclast-macrophage lineage determination and bone remodeling, *Science* 266:443, 1994.
Key L et al: Treatment of congenital osteopetrosis with high-dose calcitriol, *N Engl J Med* 310:409, 1984.
Key LL, Rodriguez RM, Willi SM et al: Long-term treatment of osteopetrosis with recombinant human interferon gamma, *N Engl J Med* 332:1594, 1995.
Kodama H et al: Congenital osteoclast deficiency in osteopetrotic (op/op) mice is cured by injections of macrophage colony stimulating factor, *J Exp Med* 173:269, 1991.
Mundy GR, Raisz LG: Disorders of bone resorption. In Bronner F, Coburn JW, editors: *Disorders of mineral metabolism,* New York, 1981, Academic.
Nordin BEC: *Metabolic bone and stone disease,* Baltimore, 1973, Williams & Wilkins.
Raisz LG et al: Studies on congenital osteopetrosis in microphthalmic mice using organ culture: impairment of bone resorption and response to physiologic stimulators, *J Exp Med* 145:857, 1977.
Sly WS et al: Carbonic anhydrase II deficiency in 12 families with the autosomal recessive syndrome of osteopetrosis with renal tubular acidosis and cerebral calcification, *N Engl J Med* 313:139, 1985.
Sorell M et al: Marrow transplantation for juvenile osteopetrosis, *Am J Med* 70:1280, 1981.
Soriano P et al: Targeted disruption of the c-src proto-oncogene leads to osteopetrosis in mice, *Cell* 64:693, 1991.
van Buchem FSP: Hyperostosis corticalis generalisata, *Acta Med Scand* 189:257, 1971.
van Buchem FSP, Hadders HN, Hansen W: Hyperostosis corticalis generalisata: report of 7 cases, *Am J Med* 33:387, 1962.
Walker DG: Bone resorption restored in osteopetrotic mice by transplants of normal bone marrow and spleen cells, *Science* 90:784, 1975a.
Whyte PW, Murphy WA, Villareal DT et al: Diffuse osteosclerosis in intravenous drug abusers, *Am J Med* 95:661, 1993.

nerves. As indicated above, this is characteristic of the severe childhood variant.

DIFFERENTIAL DIAGNOSIS

A number of other diseases may be associated with an increase in bone density. This is usually more localized than it is in most patients with osteopetrosis, and it does not date back to childhood. Some tumors are associated with focal osteoblastic metastases, which occur around metastatic tumor deposits. This is most common in patients with carcinoma of the prostate or breast, but it also occurs occasionally in patients with hematologic neoplasms such as Hodgkin's disease or myeloma. Most patients with myeloma have discrete osteolytic lesions. Bones affected by osteoblastic metastases are also more fragile and susceptible to fracture than normal bones, despite the increase in radiologic density. Pycnodysostosis is a very rare autosomal recessive disorder in which, although there is increased remodeling of the trabecular bone, cortical bone may be of increased density. There is frequently hypoplasia of the mandible and clavicle and resorption of the terminal phalanges of the fingers. The patients are usually very short, and the bones are susceptible to fracture. The x-ray appearance of many of the bones resembles that of osteopetrosis. van Buchem's disease, or hyperostosis corticalis generalisata, is characterized by thickening of cortical bone and is probably caused by increased bone formation rather than impairment of bone resorption. This condition is also inherited, although the mode of transmission is unclear. The skull is primarily involved. Engelmann's disease, or progressive diaphyseal dysplasia, is characterized by localized cortical thickening and is a rare autosomal dominant disorder.

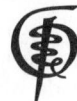

320 Fibrous Dysplasia

Gregory R. Mundy

Fibrous dysplasia is a disorder of expanding benign lesions occurring in either one or multiple sites in the skeleton. The condition is unusual but not rare. Occasionally, multiple bone lesions may be associated with cutaneous pigmented macules and endocrine dysfunction. This triad of physical signs is also known as the *McCune-Albright syndrome*. Approximately half of all patients have the classic triad, and most of the rest have two of the physical signs. The pattern of bones involved, the age of onset, and the natural history vary enormously from patient to patient. The bone disorder represents a developmental abnormality of bone-forming mesenchyma. The bone lesions are present in early childhood, but the diagnosis may not be apparent until later in life. Recently, it has been shown that in all affected tissues there is an activating mutation of the alpha subunit of the G protein ($G_s\alpha$) that couples hormone receptors to adenylate cyclase, resulting in constitutive activation of adenylate cyclase in those tissues. The condition is recognized at least three times as commonly in females as it is in males.

The McCune-Albright syndrome usually becomes evident in childhood with spontaneous fracture or fracture after trivial injury, or premature vaginal bleeding in girls. The bone lesions may be monostotic or polyostotic. Fibrous tissue in the marrow proliferates, and the adjacent cortical bone is eroded. The bones most frequently affected are the femur and tibia, skull, facial bones, and ribs. The clinical features are pain, deformity, pathologic fracture, and epiphyseal growth changes. Frequent deformities include leg-length discrepancies and bowing of the lower extremities. The characteristic deformity of the femur results in the "shepherd's crook," which causes a lateral or outward bowing of the femoral neck and shaft (Fig. 320-1). The tibia tends to bow inwards. The bone lesions may be multiple, but they are focal and discrete. The facial lesions may cause facial asymmetry with severe distortions. The maxillary bones are frequently involved. The bone lesions are usually multifocal but unilateral, and on the same side of the body as the skin lesions. The natural history of the bone lesions varies enormously. In most patients the frequency of fractures is greatly increased during childhood but decreases after puberty.

Skin lesions are the most common extraskeletal manifestations. The lesions occur most frequently on the sacrum, buttocks, and upper spine. They are hairless, flat, melanotic areas that do not cross the midline and have serrated margins. Because they may be confused with the lesions of neurofibromatosis, Albright claimed that their margins were like the coast of Maine (rough border), whereas the margins of neurofibromatosis were more like the coast of California (smooth border). However, dermatologists have been unable to distinguish the lesions on these grounds, and there are no characteristic differences in the histologic features of the lesions in the two conditions. These pigmented macules may be present at birth.

A number of abnormalities of endocrine function have been described in Albright's syndrome. The most common has been precocious puberty, which may cause vaginal bleeding in infants or in young girls. Precocious puberty in girls can lead to rapid bone maturation, early epiphyseal closure, and subsequent short stature. This feature of the condition is characterized by autonomous ovarian function and undetectable levels of circulating gonadotropins. Other endocrine conditions have been associated with Albright's syndrome, including acromegaly, primary hyperparathyroidism, hyperthyroidism, Cushing's syndrome, and hypophosphatemia associated with vitamin D–resistant rickets.

The hyperfunction of multiple endocrine organs in this syndrome results from an activating mutation in the $G_s\alpha$ gene, which results in the constitutive activation of adenylate cyclase in these tissues. The $G_s\alpha$ mutations are present in all affected endocrine tissues, as well as the café au lait skin lesions. Similar defects are not found in normal

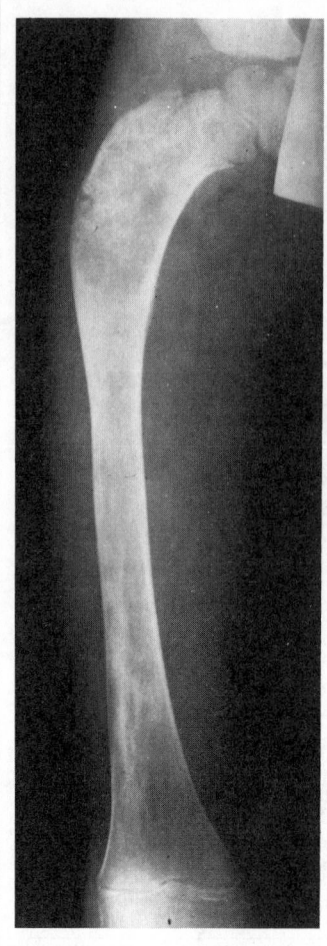
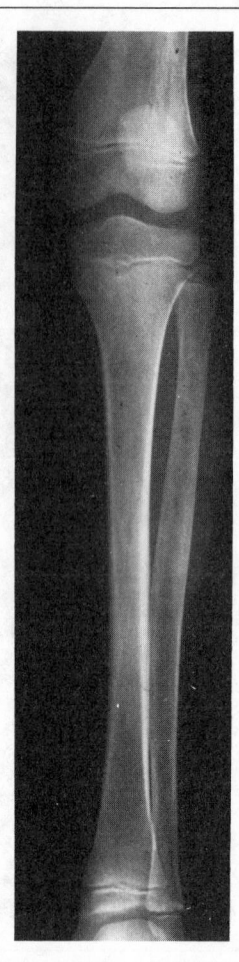

FIGURE 320-1   Deformity of femur caused by fibrous dysplasia.

tissue from these patients. The relationship between these conditions and the bone lesions is unknown.

The x-ray appearance of the bone lesions of fibrous dysplasia is frequently diagnostic. In the long bones there is characteristic thinning of the cortical bone caused by endosteal erosion (Fig. 320-1). This thinning produces the appearance of a cyst, but in fact the lesions contain solid masses of fibroosseous tissue. The lesion may be radiolucent or have a ground-glass appearance if osseous trabecular bone is present. X-rays of the skull frequently show increased density at the base with thickening of the occiput (this is the most common radiologic sign) and lateral displacement of the orbital cavity. The lesions may be confused with those of Paget's disease, but the thinning of the cortical bone, absence of marked evidence of new bone formation in the long bones, and the younger age of the patient help to make the diagnosis of fibrous dysplasia.

The serum alkaline phosphatase level is usually normal in patients with fibrous dysplasia, but it may be slightly elevated, particularly after a pathologic fracture. The serum calcium is not increased unless the patient has coexistent primary hyperparathyroidism.

Treatment of this condition is primarily surgical. No medical therapy has been found to be valuable. Calcitonin has been tried and has been unsuccessful. Radiation therapy has also been used but has not produced any benefit and has been associated with later development of malignant transformation. When this rare complication occurs, it may be in the form of osteosarcoma, fibrosarcoma, chondrosarcoma, or mixed mesenchymal tumors. Treatment of the bone lesions of fibrous dysplasia is usually limited to correction of deformity or treatment of fracture. Curettage and grafting of the lesions do not necessarily lead to improvement.

BIBLIOGRAPHY

Albright F et al: Syndrome characterized by osteitis fibrosa disseminata, areas of pigmentation and endocrine dysfunction, with precocious puberty in females, *N Engl J Med* 216:727, 1937.

Dockerty MB et al: Albright's syndrome, *Arch Intern Med* 75:357, 1945.

Falconer MA, Cope CL: Fibrous dysplasia of bone with endocrine disorders and cutaneous pigmentation (Albright's disease), *Q J Med* 11:121, 1942.

Fibrous dysplasia of bone, *Br Med J* 1:685, 1971, (editorial).

Gibson MJ, Middlemiss JH: Fibrous dysplasia of bone, *Br J Radiol* 44:1, 1971.

Harris WH, Dudley HR, Barry RJ: The natural history of fibrous dysplasia, *J Bone Joint Surg Am* 44:207, 1962.

Hunter D, Turnbull HM: Hyperparathyroidism: generalized osteitis fibrosa, *Br J Surg* 19:203, 1931.

Lee PA, Van Dop C, Migeon CJ: McCune-Albright syndrome, *JAMA* 256:2980, 1986.

Lichtenstein L: Polyostotic fibrous dysplasia, *Arch Surg* 36:874, 1938.

Nordin BEC: *Metabolic bone and stone disease*, Baltimore, 1973, Williams & Wilkins.

Schwindinger WF, Francomano CA, Levine MA: Identification of a mutation in the gene encoding the alpha subunit of the stimulatory G protein of adenylyl cyclase in the McCune-Albright syndrome, *Proc Natl Acad Sci U S A* 89:5152, 1992.

Weinstein LS, Shenker A, Gejman PV et al: Activating mutations of the stimulatory G protein in the McCune-Albright syndrome, *N Engl J Med* 325:1688, 1991.

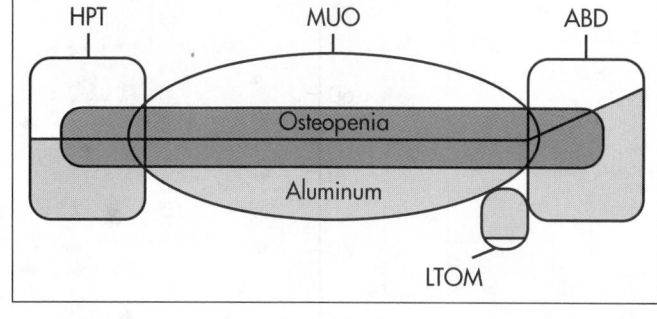

FIGURE 321-1   Schematic representation of the four main histologic groups of renal osteodystrophy: predominant hyperparathyroid bone disease *(HPT)*, mixed uremic osteodystrophy *(MUO)*, low-turnover osteomalacia *(LTOM)*, and adynamic bone disease *(ABD)*.

CHAPTER

321 Renal Bone Disease

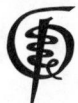

Hartmut H. Malluche and Marie-Claude Monier-Faugere

Bone changes are associated with various diseases of the kidney. They are seen mainly in patients with kidney diseases resulting in impaired glomerular filtration. However, they also occur after kidney transplantation, with normal glomerular filtration rate and defects in tubular function, with renal stone disease, with nephrotic syndrome with or without loss of glomerular filtration, and with oxalosis.

The most prominent bone disease occurs in patients with partial or complete loss of glomerular filtration and are discussed in detail here.

PREVALENCE

Histologic abnormalities of bone are found in virtually all patients with reduction in kidney function requiring chronic maintenance dialysis. The earliest histologic changes are seen after a relatively mild reduction in glomerular filtration rate (creatinine clearances between 70 and 40 ml/min). The histologic abnormalities at these early stages are usually not associated with clinical symptoms. They include mild to moderate secondary hyperparathyroid bone disease with or without defective bone mineralization. In patients with end-stage renal failure, a combination of both occurs, but one or the other lesion may predominate.

PATHOGENETIC FACTORS

Several interrelated and independent factors have been recognized in the pathogenesis of renal osteodystrophy. These factors include alterations in phosphate and calcium homeostasis, vitamin D metabolism, and parathyroid gland activity; accumulation of aluminum in bone and other organs; and dialysis-related factors. There is still considerable controversy about the sequence of pathogenetic events in the early stages of renal osteodystrophy.

Increased reduction in nephron mass results in phosphorus load presented to the remaining nephrons, which may result in reduced activity of the renal C_1-α-hydroxylase and consequently in relative or absolute deficiency of the active vitamin D metabolite calcitriol. Other potential pathogenetic factors in early renal failure include resistance to vitamin D, which is probably related to abnormal interaction between vitamin D receptor and its gene response elements, and alterations in the calcium/parathyroid hormone axis. Diminished vitamin D activity leads to secondary hyperparathyroidism. If the compensatory capacity of the kidney can no longer increase the excretion of phosphate through the remaining nephrons to compensate for advanced nephron loss (glomerular filtration rate <25% of normal), frank hyperphosphatemia ensues, which is usually associated with hypocalcemia. Thus advanced renal osteodystrophy becomes evident with hyperparathyroid bone disease and abnormal bone mineralization.

During the last decade, aluminum has been identified as an additional factor contributing to the severity of renal bone disease. Accumulation of aluminum in bone and other organs such as parathyroid glands used to be a frequent complication in patients receiving dialysis. It is now observed at a decreasing rate, currently in approximately 20% of chronic dialysis patients. Accumulation of aluminum in parathyroid glands results in decreased secretion of parathyroid hormone and suppression of bone turnover. In addition, aluminum inhibits renal and intestinal C_1-α-hydroxylase activity and may thus further reduce levels of calcitriol. Aluminum accumulation in bone is associated with abnormal mineralization and reduction in bone formation and resorption with a disproportionately greater effect on formation, which leads to negative bone balance, ultimately causing osteomalacia, adynamic bone disease, and osteopenia. Several sources of aluminum have been identified in dialyzed patients and include high concentrations of aluminum in water used for dialysis and aluminum-containing phosphate binders. The use of reverse osmosis and substitution of aluminum-containing phosphate binders by calcium salts have greatly reduced exposure of dialysis patients to aluminum. However, aluminum is ubiquitous in nature and is often present in drinking water, other drinking fluids, processed food, and medications. Also, its intestinal absorption may be aggravated by oral citrate intake and possibly other substances. Recently, it has been observed that end-stage renal patients newly enrolled in a dialysis program and never exposed to aluminum-containing phosphate binders may develop aluminum-related bone disease. This worrisome observation indicates that aluminum intoxication will not completely disappear.

The contribution of acidosis to the pathogenesis of renal bone disease in patients with reduced kidney function has not been fully elucidated and awaits further studies.

Institution of chronic maintenance dialysis may alter the course of renal bone disease. Dialysate calcium concentrations should be sufficient to counteract a negative calcium balance. Patients receiving peritoneal dialysis may have episodes of peritonitis, which may result in losses of vitamin D–binding protein.

HISTOLOGIC PATTERNS

Renal bone disease in patients with reduced kidney function can be subdivided into three major histologic groups: (1) predominant hyperparathyroid bone disease, (2) low-turnover renal bone disease including osteomalacia and adynamic bone disease, and (3) mixed uremic osteodystrophy consisting of mild to moderate hyperparathyroid bone disease and defective mineralization (Fig. 321-1). The histologic pattern is determined by the major pathogenetic factor responsible,

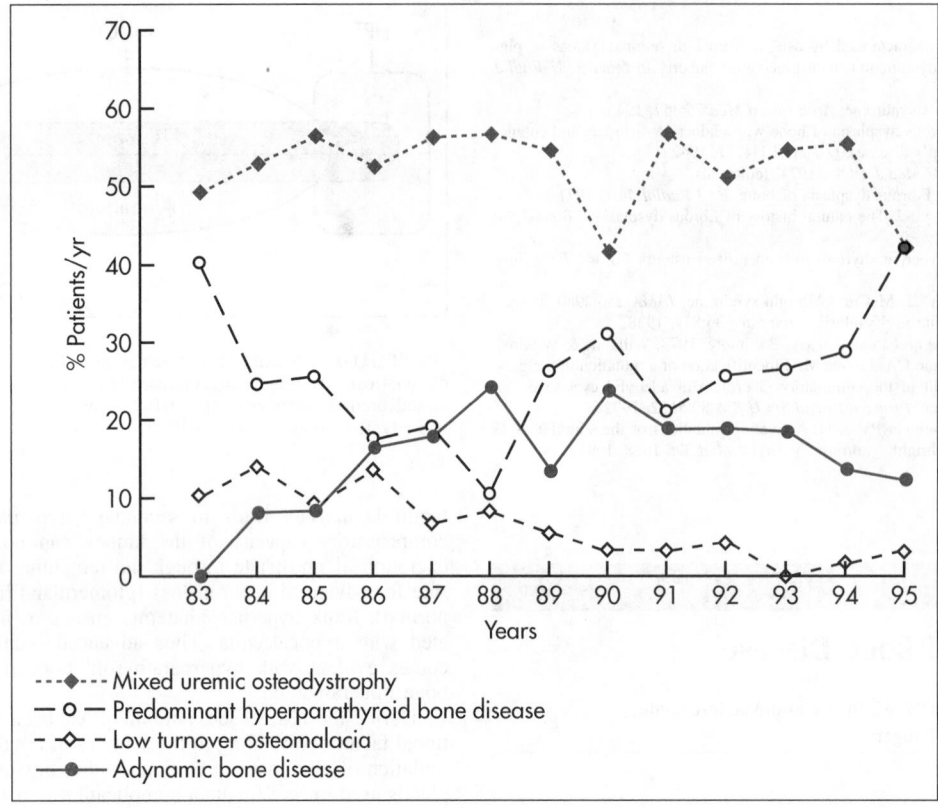

FIGURE 321-2 Evolution of the four histologic groups of renal osteodystrophy from 1983 to 1995.

namely, secondary hyperparathyroidism, deficiency of the active vitamin D metabolite, or accumulation of aluminum in bone. Even though these groups do not represent fully separate entities, it is worthwhile to distinguish them because therapy can be tailored according to the predominant histologic findings. Transformation from one form to another can occur. The prevalence of the different forms may vary depending on geographic factors, aluminum exposure, therapy with vitamin D metabolites, dietary intake, and dialysis-related factors. Approximately 45% to 90% of unselected patients with end-stage renal failure have mixed uremic osteodystrophy, 5% to 30% predominant hyperparathyroid bone disease, and 5% to 35% low-turnover renal bone disease. Over the past few years, the incidence of adynamic bone disease has increased gradually (Fig. 321-2). The factors associated with the growing occurrence of adynamic bone disease include (1) the persistence of aluminum accumulation, (2) the increasing age of the patients, (3) the increased number of diabetics undergoing dialysis, (4) chronic ambulatory peritoneal dialysis, (5) high intake of calcium salts as phosphate binders, and (6) overzealous calcitriol therapy. Possible clinical problems arising from adynamic bone disease include tendency toward hypercalcemia, soft tissue calcifications and possibly calciphylaxis, and delayed healing of microfractures and macrofractures. Virtually all patients with mild to moderate renal failure have mild hyperparathyroidism or mixed renal osteodystrophy.

Predominant Hyperparathyroid Bone Disease
(Fig. 321-3; Color Plate IX-5)

Histologic changes represent the effects of excess parathyroid hormone on the skeleton. There is an abundance of osteoclasts, osteoblasts, and osteocytes.

Disturbed osteoblastic activity results in disorderly production of collagen, which is deposited not only toward the trabecular surface but also into the marrow cavity, causing peritrabecular and marrow fibrosis. The nonmineralized component of bone, that is, osteoid, is increased, and the normal three-dimensional architecture of osteoid

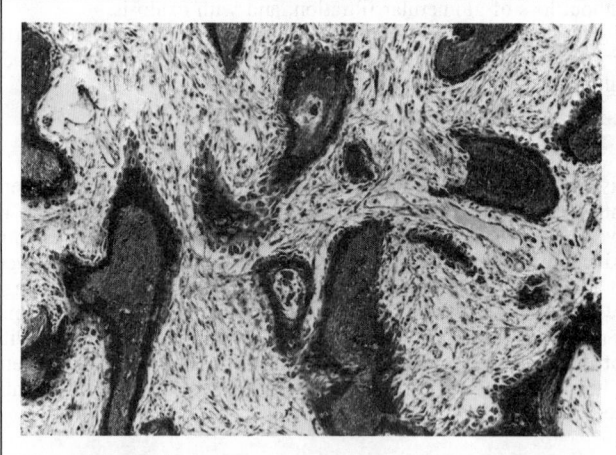

FIGURE 321-3 Predominant hyperparathyroid bone disease. Undecalcified 3-μm thick section of anterior iliac bone from chronically dialyzed patient. Abundance of osteoclasts, osteoblasts, and osteocytes. Marrow fibrosis. Irregular trabecular surface and tunneling resorption of mineralized bone underneath osteoid. Modified Masson-Goldner stain. Original magnification ×8.

From Malluche HH, Faugere MC: *Atlas of mineralized bone histology,* New York, 1986, Karger.

is frequently lost—that is, osteoid seams no longer exhibit their usual birefringence under polarized light; instead, a disorderly arrangement of "woven osteoid" and "woven bone" with a typical criss-cross pattern under polarized light is seen. The mineral apposition rate and number of actively mineralizing appositional sites are increased, as documented under fluorescent light after administration of time-

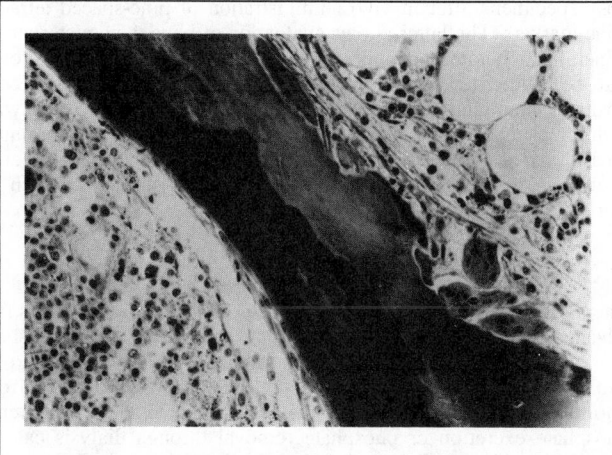

FIGURE 321-4   Mixed uremic osteodystrophy. Undecalcified 3-μm thick section of anterior iliac bone from chronically dialyzed patient. Presence of multinucleated osteoclasts resorbing bone and new bone apposition at the opposite side of the trabeculum. Increased osteoid seam thickness. Mild peritrabecular fibrosis. Modified Masson-Goldner stain. Original magnification ×20.

From Malluche HH, Faugere MC: *Atlas of mineralized bone histology,* New York, 1986, Karger.

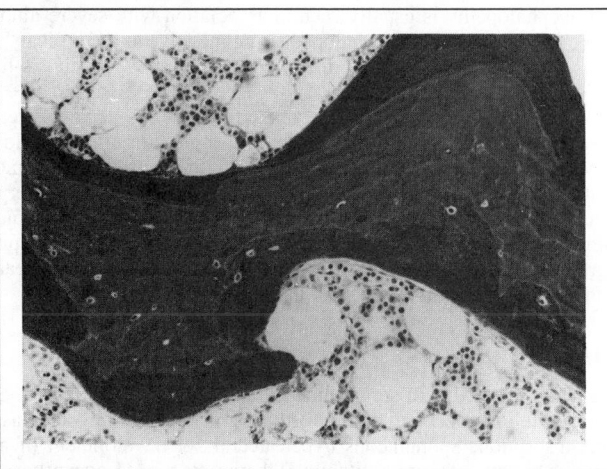

FIGURE 321-5   Low-turnover osteomalacia. Undecalcified 3-μm thick section of anterior iliac bone from chronically dialyzed patient. High osteoid volume caused by increased fraction of trabecular surface covered by osteoid seams and increased osteoid seam width. Irregular interface between osteoid and mineralized bone, reflecting previously enhanced resorptive activity. Absence of peritrabecular and marrow fibrosis. Paucity of bone-forming and bone-resorbing cells. Modified Masson-Goldner stain. Original magnification ×12.5.

From Malluche HH, Faugere MC: *Atlas of mineralized bone histology,* New York, 1986, Karger.

spaced tetracycline markers. There is a tendency for cancellous bone mass to rise with increasing levels of parathyroid hormone. Approximately 25% of patients with predominant hyperparathyroid bone disease do have stainable bone aluminum.

Mixed Uremic Osteodystrophy (Fig. 321-4; Color Plate IX-5)

This form of renal osteodystrophy becomes evident with two major abnormalities: hyperparathyroid bone disease and defective mineralization. Both histologic features may coexist at varying degrees in different patients. Cancellous bone volume is usually within the normal range. Factors that cause bone mass to decrease in dialyzed patients with mixed uremic osteodystrophy include accumulation of aluminum in bone, prolonged immobilization, and malnutrition. The major histologic abnormalities consist of accumulation of lamellar and woven osteoid with normal or increased thickness of osteoid, high-normal or increased number of osteoclasts and osteoblasts, and mild to moderate peritrabecular fibrosis. Evaluation of bone under fluorescent light after time-spaced tetracycline administration reveals a decrease in doubly labeled lamellar osteoid seams.

Approximately 50% to 65% of patients with mixed uremic osteodystrophy come to medical attention with stainable bone aluminum at the mineralization front. Aluminum in this location is associated with reduced osteoblastic activity, resulting in a decrease in bone formation and mineralizing activity.

Low-Turnover Renal Bone Disease (Fig. 321-5)

The histologic hallmark of low-turnover osteomalacia is a dramatic reduction in the number of bone-forming and bone-resorbing cells associated with an accumulation of lamellar osteoid that occupies most of the trabecular surface and represents a considerable fraction of the trabecular bone volume. Total cancellous bone volume may be increased, mainly as a result of the excessive accumulation of osteoid. This is not infrequently accompanied by a reduction in mineralized trabecular bone mass. The smooth contour of the osteoid-marrow interface is in striking contrast to the irregular interface between osteoid and mineralized bone, which reflects past resorbing activity. More than 90% of patients with low-turnover osteomalacia have histologically stainable aluminum deposits at the bone-osteoid interface. When signs of low bone turnover are found combined with paucity

of bone-forming and bone-resorbing cells, and osteoblastic dysfunction without accumulation of osteoid, the histologic abnormality is called *adynamic renal bone disease.*

CLINICAL FEATURES

Patients with mild or moderate renal insufficiency are rarely clinically symptomatic. Patients with end-stage renal disease requiring dialysis are liable to develop (1) mechanical insufficiency of the skeleton such as fractures of tubular bones, crush fractures of the vertebrae, and rib fractures and epiphysiolysis in children (slipping of the epiphyses due to impaired transformation of growth cartilage into regular metaphyseal spongiosa) and (2) soft tissue and vascular calcifications.

Approximately 20% of dialyzed patients have bone pain and pseudogout and/or palpable extraosseous calcifications. Periarticular calcifications and soft tissue calcifications are preferentially seen in patients with predominant hyperparathyroid bone disease, whereas loss of height and spontaneous fractures occur mainly in patients with low-turnover osteomalacia. Clinical problems caused by soft tissue and vascular calcifications are seen earlier in the course of the disease, whereas orthopedic skeletal problems arise with increasing duration of dialysis. The "red eye syndrome" resulting from inflammatory reactions and irritation caused by conjunctival calcifications is seen in approximately 10% of dialyzed patients. If calcifications occur in the cornea, band keratopathy can be demonstrated by slit-lamp examination. Soft tissue calcifications—that is, tumoral calcifications, pseudogout, and skin calcifications in adult dialysis patients—are clearly related to the magnitude of the calcium-phosphate product and are responsive to its lowering. In contrast, vascular calcifications are unrelated to the calcium-phosphorus product and do not respond to its normalization. In long-term dialysis patients, carpal tunnel syndrome and arthralgias are often associated with β2-microglobulin amyloid deposition in articular and periarticular structures. No specific therapy is known for this abnormality.

Renal osteodystrophy in children and growing individuals may have a different clinical picture. Although bone pain, pseudogout, soft tissue calcifications, conjunctival calcifications, and serum biochemical changes are generally not strikingly different from those seen in adults, vascular calcifications are quite infrequent in children receiving chronic maintenance dialysis.

Encephalopathy is usually seen in association with severe aluminum intoxication. The encephalopathy might evolve as the typical "dialysis dementia" with waxing and waning or as acute psychosis-like clinical presentation.

Morbidity and mortality are related to the severity of renal osteodystrophy. Severe hyperparathyroid bone disease and low-turnover renal bone disease are associated with a high degree of morbidity and mortality. Toxic effects of parathyroid hormone on the peripheral and central nervous system have been implicated in clinical complications such as pruritus, muscle weakness, and electroencephalographic disturbances. Morbidity, disability, and mortality are clearly increased when aluminum accumulation in bone is found.

DIAGNOSIS

The diagnostic value of serum biochemical parameters is limited. Serum calcium is poorly related to histologic parameters of osteoclastic bone resorption. Spontaneous hypercalcemia or development of hypercalcemic episodes with vitamin D therapy is more frequently seen in patients with predominant hyperparathyroid bone disease and in patients with adynamic renal bone disease. Serum alkaline phosphatase level is directly related to the amount of osteoid in the skeleton (regardless of the type). Therefore alkaline phosphatase level indicates the severity but not the quality of the bone disease. Serum parathyroid hormone levels are higher in the group of patients with predominant hyperparathyroid bone disease and lower in those with low-turnover renal bone disease, but there is a considerable overlap. Patients with normal or low serum parathyroid hormone levels (measured by immunoradiometric assay) usually have adynamic bone disease, and patients with more than nine times elevated levels of parathyroid hormone have predominant hyperparathyroid bone disease. Serum parathyroid hormone concentrations between these levels are not predictive of underlying type of bone disease. Serum levels of calcitriol are decreased or low in most patients with renal osteodystrophy. Serum levels of osteocalcin reflect bone turnover and particularly bone formation, but further studies are needed to establish the place of this measurement. Measurements of serum concentrations of aluminum do not have a predictive value for aluminum accumulation in bone. Measurements of serum aluminum before and 24 to 48 hours after a single intravenous infusion of deferoxamine (Desferal, 5 to 15 mg/kg body weight infused at a rate not to exceed 15 mg/kg body weight per hour) can be used as a screening test. In combination with low serum parathyroid hormone levels the test has good specificity but low sensitivity.

Information obtained from skeletal x-rays has to be interpreted with an understanding of the underlying histologic changes. In nondialyzed patients there is a notable discrepancy between cancellous and cortical bone, that is, cancellous bone mass may be increased and cortical bone may be normal or decreased. In dialyzed patients, normal, decreased, or increased cancellous bone mass may be found. The erosion of cortical bone by osteoclastic resorption accounts for the roentgenologic finding of subperiosteal resorption, periosteal and endosteal resorption cavities, cortical striation, and cortical thinning. These changes may be represented radiologically by erosive cortical defects in the skull ("pepper pot skull"), acroosteolysis of the clavicula, and erosion of the terminal finger phalanges. A "rugger jersey" appearance of the spine and a ground-glass appearance of the skull, ribs, pelvis, and metaphysis of tubular bones reflect cancellous changes. In advanced hyperparathyroid stages, "pseudocysts" or "brown tumors" may be observed. Looser's zones that are straight bands of radiolucency abutting onto the cortex and running perpendicular to the long axis of bone are of relatively low sensitivity and low specificity for the diagnosis of osteomalacia. The combination of hyperparathyroid bone disease and defective mineralization renders interpretation of the x-ray findings particularly difficult, since signs of increased bone resorption may be seen on x-rays reflecting past resorbing activity, which may have been succeeded by accumulation of osteoid. Since osteoid is radiolucent, the superimposed osteomalacia is missed by x-ray examination. Similar limitations apply to the measurement of bone mineral content by dual photon absorptiometry techniques.

Currently, the only unequivocal tool for diagnosis of renal osteodystrophy is histologic examination of nondecalcified bone biopsy specimens after in vivo administration of time-spaced tetracycline markers. The latter allows evaluation of bone dynamics such as mineralization rate and bone turnover. The bone specimens should also be stained for aluminum because histochemically stainable deposits of aluminum at the bone-osteoid interface correlate better with histologic abnormalities in bone than concentrations of aluminum measured by atomic absorption spectrophotometry. Further specific histochemical stains may be necessary if other substances such as iron, lead, or amyloid are suspected.

PREVENTION AND THERAPY

Therapeutic intervention should begin before the patient develops far-advanced bone disease, that is, not later than at the time of institution of dialysis. Secondary hyperparathyroidism can be prevented by avoiding deviations of serum calcium and phosphorus levels from normal. An imbalance between dietary phosphate intake and renal phosphate excretion or phosphate removal through dialysis can be avoided by reducing dietary phosphate intake and intestinal phosphate absorption.

Even though prescription of phosphate-restricted diet appears logical in patients with reduced kidney function, it is often difficult to obtain full compliance. Therefore phosphate binders are customarily prescribed to reduce intestinal absorption of phosphate. Most available potent intestinal phosphate binders contain aluminum. Calcium salts such as calcium acetate and calcium carbonate are at this time the preferred first-line preventive or therapeutic approach to hyperphosphatemia. The clinical efficacy and safety of other phosphate binders await further study.

Persistent hyperphosphatemia despite therapy using phosphate binders may not always be related to lack of compliance. Excess circulating levels of parathyroid hormone may enhance release of phosphate from bone, thus maintaining hyperphosphatemia that is unresponsive to oral phosphate binders.

Serum calcium levels can be kept in the normal range by avoiding hyperphosphatemia, by oral administration of calcium salts such as calcium carbonate (0.5 to 1.5 g/day), or by therapy using the active vitamin D metabolite calcitriol (0.25 to 2.0 μg/day, Rocaltrol). It is advisable to start with low doses, increasing the daily dose in steps of 0.25 μg if serum calcium levels do not increase (at least 0.5 mg/dl) after 2 weeks of therapy.

More recently, intravenous administration of calcitriol (1 to 4 μg three times per week, Calcijex) is used as therapy for hypocalcemia and elevated parathyroid hormone levels in dialysis patients. The intravenous administration has been shown to be associated with less frequent episodes of hypercalcemia; this is apparently related to the relatively higher concentrations reached in the target organ parathyroid gland compared to the intestine. As an alternative, pulse oral calcitriol can be used in lieu of calcitriol injections.

Prospective clinical studies show that early administration of calcitriol can reverse the histologic bone abnormalities, and administration of pharmacologic doses of the drug is beneficial in patients with mixed uremic osteodystrophy. However, doses less than 0.5 μg per day should be used in early to moderate renal failure (with close monitoring of serum and urine calcium levels) to avoid overcorrection, that is, suppression of bone turnover. Also, the positive response to calcitriol is reduced if there is accumulation of aluminum in bone.

In patients with predominant hyperparathyroid bone disease and those with low-turnover renal bone disease, vitamin D therapy frequently leads to hypercalcemia. Concomitantly elevated serum phosphorus levels may raise the calcium phosphorus product to critical levels (more than 70 mg/dl) associated with deposition of calcium salts in soft tissues. The hypercalcemia seen in patients with predominant hyperparathyroid bone disease receiving vitamin D therapy is caused in part by the effect of the active vitamin D metabolite on bone. In contrast, hypercalcemia in patients with low-turnover osteomalacia receiving vitamin D therapy results most probably from the positive effect of vitamin D on intestinal calcium absorption while the capacity of bone to incorporate calcium is reduced owing to low bone turnover and lack of excretory kidney function.

Intravenous therapy with deferoxamine is beneficial for patients with aluminum accumulation in bone. Deferoxamine is a potent drug for removal of aluminum from bone. However, it should be borne in mind that removal of aluminum from bone may transform the histologic findings of low-turnover osteomalacia to those of mixed uremic osteodystrophy and those of mixed uremic osteodystrophy to predominant hyperparathyroid bone disease. Deferoxamine should be given intravenously one to three times per week, preferably during dialysis, at a dose of 5 to 15 mg/kg body weight and at a rate not to exceed 15 mg/kg per hour. Considering the dialysance of the deferoxamine-aluminum complex and the total amount of aluminum that may accumulate in bone and other organs, long-term therapy is required for most patients.*

Predominant hyperparathyroid bone disease without aluminum accumulation in bone requires surgical reduction of parathyroid gland mass if administration of intravenous calcitriol is ineffective. The exact threshold at which intravenous calcitriol is no longer able to suppress parathyroid gland overactivity and when surgery remains the only tool awaits further study. Total parathyroidectomy with transplantation of parathyroid tissue to the forearm or subtotal parathyroidectomy is the preferred choice for patients who need surgery. However, recurrent severe gland hyperplasia and invasive cell growth have been described. Thus some authors advocate total parathyroidectomy. Other clinical indications for surgical reduction of parathyroid gland mass include pruritus and progressive extraosseous calcifications. Treatment with orally administered calcitriol should be considered postoperatively to avoid further hyperplasia of the transplanted gland. Withholding calcitriol replacement after surgery for days or a few weeks allows the transplanted gland to assume its function more rapidly at the new site and to mobilize soft tissue calcifications.

The occurrence of severe osteomalacia after parathyroidectomy in patients with bone aluminum and the finding of enhanced aluminum uptake by bone after parathyroidectomy call for careful documentation of the absence of stainable aluminum by bone histology before parathyroidectomy is contemplated. Lowering the serum parathyroid hormone levels is usually an effective therapy for pruritus. Before surgery, antipruritic medications such as diphenylhydramine (Benadryl) and/or activated charcoal may be helpful. Periarticular and soft tissue calcifications and symptoms of periarthritis respond to the lowering of the calcium-phosphorus product by parathyroidectomy.

BIBLIOGRAPHY

Baker LRI et al: 1,25(OH)$_2$D$_3$ administration in moderate renal failure: a prospective double-blind trial, *Kidney Int* 35:661, 1989.

Faugere MC, Malluche HH: Stainable aluminum and not aluminum content reflect histologic changes in bone of dialyzed patients, *Kidney Int* 30:717, 1986.

Faugere MC et al: Loss of bone resulting from accumulation of aluminum in bone of patients undergoing dialysis, *J Lab Clin Med* 107:481, 1986.

Malluche HH, Faugere MC: *Atlas of mineralized bone histology,* New York, 1986, Karger.

Malluche HH, Faugere MC: Renal bone disease 1990: an unmet challenge for the nephrologist, *Kidney Int* 38:193, 1990.

Malluche HH, Faugere MC: Uremic bone disease: current knowledge, controversial issues and new horizons, *Miner Electrolyte Metab* 17:281, 1991.

Malluche HH et al: Bone histology in incipient and advanced renal failure, *Kidney Int* 9:355, 1976.

Malluche HH et al: The use of deferoxamine in the management of aluminum accumulation in bone in patients with renal failure, *N Engl J Med* 311:140, 1984.

Malluche HH et al: Bone biopsies in patients with renal failure: why, when and how—short course, *J Am Soc Nephrol* 4:11, 1993.

Monier-Faugere MC, Malluche HH: Trends in renal osteodystrophy: a survey from 1983 to 1995 in a total of 2,248 patients, *Nephrol Dial Transplant* 11(suppl 3):110-120, 1996.

Ott SM et al: Prevalence of bone aluminum deposition in renal osteodystrophy and its relation to the response to calcitriol therapy, *N Engl J Med* 307:709, 1982.

Qi Q et al: Predictive value of serum parathyroid hormone levels for bone turnover in patients on chronic maintenance dialysis, *Am J Kidney Dis* 26:622, 1995.

Smith AJ et al: Aluminum-related bone disease in mild and advanced renal failure: evidence for high prevalence and morbidity and studies on etiology and diagnosis, *Am J Nephrol* 6:392, 1986.

Teitelbaum SL: Renal osteodystrophy, *Hum Pathol* 15:306, 1984.

*Note: Approval by the Food and Drug Administration for the use of calcitriol and deferoxamine in the management of bone abnormalities of patients with renal osteodystrophy is pending.

322 Primary Hyperparathyroidism

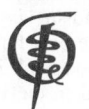

John P. Bilezikian

Primary hyperparathyroidism is a common endocrine disorder caused by the excessive secretion of parathyroid hormone from one or more parathyroid glands. The major actions of parathyroid hormone—to mobilize calcium from bone and to conserve calcium in the kidney—account for hypercalcemia, a hallmark of the disease. In some cases an additional action of parathyroid hormone, to facilitate the conversion of 25-hydroxyvitamin D to the active metabolite, 1,25-dihydroxyvitamin D, leads to increased absorption of calcium from the gastrointestinal tract. Despite the remarkable variability in clinical and biochemical features of primary hyperparathyroidism, the serum calcium level is virtually always elevated. As noted in Chapter 312, primary hyperparathyroidism, along with hypercalcemia of malignancy, is the cause of hypercalcemia in the vast majority of cases. It should always be seriously considered as a potential cause of hypercalcemia.

PREVALENCE

Estimates of prevalence of primary hyperparathyroidism range from 1 in 500 to 1 in 1000. This prevalence is markedly higher than estimates in the 1930s and 1940s when primary hyperparathyroidism was considered uncommon. The dramatic increase in recognized cases coincides with the widespread introduction of the multichannel autoanalyzer in clinical medicine in the 1970s. Primary hyperparathyroidism is now most often discovered incidentally when the patient is being evaluated by the physician for a set of complaints that are completely unrelated to hypercalcemia. Primary hyperparathyroidism occurs at all ages with a peak incidence in the sixth decade of life; women are affected more commonly than men by a ratio of 3:2. The disorder is relatively unusual in children.

PATHOLOGY AND ETIOLOGY

The vast majority of patients with primary hyperparathyroidism, 80% to 85%, have a single adenoma that varies in size from relatively small (less than 0.5 g) to very large (over 10 g). Even the modest parathyroid adenoma is much larger than the normal gland, which is only approximately 25 mg. Most adenomas are less than 1 g in size. They appear histologically as a confluence of encapsulated chief cells with a rim of normal tissue at the margin. It is unusual for a patient to harbor more than one adenoma. Cystic elements in an adenomatous gland may call attention to a rare familial variant, cystic parathyroid adenomatosis. Although the parathyroid adenoma is most commonly found at one of the usual locations of parathyroid tissue (the four poles of the thyroid gland), the tumor may be found at unusual locations in up to 10% of patients with adenomatous disease. Ectopic sites include the lateral area of neck, the retroesophagus, within the thyroid gland itself, and the mediastinum.

Approximately 20% of patients with primary hyperparathyroidism have a pathologic process involving all four glands with hyperplasia. Four-gland hyperplasia may occur sporadically but is seen also in conjunction with multiple endocrine neoplasia (MEN) type I or II. The extent to which each gland is involved varies in that some hyperplastic parathyroids appear to be abnormal only because of diminished fat content, whereas others are grossly enlarged. Involvement of all parathyroid glands in hyperplastic disease contrasts markedly with the normal appearance of three parathyroid glands when the pathologic condition is adenoma. This distinction is important because the surgical approach to the patient is defined in part by the pathologic features of primary hyperparathyroidism.

The rarest presentation of primary hyperparathyroidism is parathyroid carcinoma, occurring in well under 1% of patients. As is the case for many endocrine neoplasms, it is difficult to distinguish on pathologic grounds benign from malignant disease. Several histologic features such as mitoses, vascular invasion, and fibrous trabeculae are important clues. In addition, metastases to contiguous (thyroid, neck muscles, esophagus) or more distant sites (cervical lymph nodes, lung, liver) help to establish the diagnosis of parathyroid malignancy.

The underlying cause of primary hyperparathyroidism is not known. Most patients develop the disease in the absence of a family history or possible predisposing factors such as childhood neck irradiation. Molecular analysis of adenomatous parathyroid tissue indicates that the disease is most likely monoclonal in origin.

Several patients with primary hyperparathyroidism have been described in whom strong enhancer elements of the parathyroid hormone (PTH) gene are rearranged to be in close proximity to the PRAD 1 protooncogene. The result of this rearrangement is overexpression of PRAD 1, thus converting it to an oncogene and stimulating parathyroid growth. This is the only oncogene implicated to date in parathyroid neoplasia, accounting for only a small percentage of patients with primary hyperthyroidism. Perhaps more important is the association of genetic alterations in a number of tumor suppressor genes. Heterogeneity of this general molecular mechanism is underscored by a large number of different tumor suppressor genes that have been implicated.

SYMPTOMS AND SIGNS

The manifestations of primary hyperparathyroidism include potential involvement of many organ systems. They are caused either by the effects of excess parathyroid hormone on its target tissues or by the major biochemical consequences of hypercalcemia. Certainly, hypercalcemia may give rise to its own set of signs and symptoms such as shortened QT interval on the electrocardiogram, polyuria, polydipsia, anorexia, constipation, and depressed central nervous system function (see Chapter 312). These features are specific for hypercalcemia; they are not specific for primary hyperparathyroidism. The extent to which manifestations of hypercalcemia are present is related to the level of the elevated serum calcium, the rate of its rise, and the chronicity of the problem. In addition to hypercalcemia, primary hyperparathyroidism causes systemic abnormalities, some of which are classic manifestations of the disease. The designation *disorder of bones and stones* illustrates two specific organ systems at risk for damage or dysfunction from primary hyperparathyroidism.

Bone Disease

The classic bone disease of primary hyperparathyroidism is *osteitis fibrosa cystica*. Clinically, patients have bone pain and occasional pathologic fractures. Resorption of bone caused by excessive secretion of parathyroid hormone is associated with several typical radiologic signs. Subperiosteal resorption of the distal phalanges is the most specific sign of primary hyperparathyroidism. It is appreciated best on the radial side of the middle phalanges. Similar radiologic changes may be present in the skull, where a moth-eaten or salt-and-pepper pattern is evident. The distal third of the clavicles may demonstrate tapering of bone density. Locally destructive lesions appearing as bone cysts or "brown tumors" in the long bones and pelvis constitute another skeletal manifestation of primary hyperparathyroidism (Fig. 322-1). Brown tumors are collections of osteoclasts intermixed with poorly mineralized woven bone. Nonspecific generalized demineralization is sometimes evident in the absence of obvious hyperparathyroid bone disease. Osteitis fibrosa cystica was always uncommon in primary hyperparathyroidism, never composing more than 10% of the hyperparathyroid population. It is even more uncommon now. However, in populations without ready access to medical care, overt parathyroid bone disease is still seen.

Although the milder form of primary hyperparathyroidism seen today suggests that patients are discovered before radiologic signs develop, this does not mean that most patients are spared skeletal involvement. Approaches more sensitive than conventional radiography demonstrate the presence of bone involvement in a greater percentage of patients. Noninvasive densitometry of the skeleton, in fact, shows that many patients without overt radiologic hyperparathyroid bone disease have evidence of demineralization. The particular distribution of reduced bone mineral density in primary hyperparathy-

roidism appears to be preferential to cortical bone (long bones) as compared with cancellous bone (spine). Involvement of cortical bone with preservation of cancellous bone is compatible with the physiologic actions of parathyroid hormone.

The ability to measure bone mineral density in primary hyperparathyroidism has become an important tool in the evaluation of patients, in decisions about management, and in monitoring. Subclinical involvement of cortical bone in primary hyperparathyroidism is confirmed with even greater sensitivity by histomorphometric analysis of the percutaneous bone biopsy specimen. Among many asymptomatic patients, cortical width, formation, and resorption surfaces, as well as bone formation rates, are affected. Consistent with data obtained from bone densitometry, cancellous bone volume does not appear to be reduced in primary hyperparathyroidism. Scanning electron microscopy of bone biopsy specimens illustrates this point well (Fig. 322-2).

Renal Disease (also see Chapter 111)

Kidney stones are one of the classic complications of primary hyperparathyroidism. Before the clinical profile of primary hyperparathyroidism began to change approximately 20 years ago, nephrolithiasis occurred in approximately one third of all patients with the disorder. The incidence of nephrolithiasis is now closer to 15% to 20%. In the occasional patient a symptomatic kidney stone is the first manifestation of primary hyperparathyroidism. It is thus still strongly advisable to investigate the possibility of primary hyperparathyroidism in any patient who comes to medical attention with a kidney stone, although fewer than 1 in 20 is ultimately shown to have the disease. Besides stones, the kidney may be affected in other ways, such as deposition of calcium-phosphate crystals throughout the renal parenchyma. This process, nephrocalcinosis, may be associated with diminished renal function. Some patients with primary hyperparathyroidism demonstrate a decreased rate of creatinine clearance without nephrocalcinosis or other obvious cause. Perhaps the most common association between primary hyperparathyroidism and the kidney is hypercalciuria. Urinary calcium excretion over 250 mg daily is seen in 20% to 25% of patients with primary hyperparathyroidism. The hypercalciuria is caused by the greater load of filtered calcium, which exceeds the capacity of the kidney to conserve it, despite the conserving actions of parathyroid hormone. It is not clear whether hypercalciuria in this setting predisposes patients to nephrolithiasis and/or nephrocalcinosis.

Other Organ Involvement

The hyperparathyroid syndrome includes the potential for involvement of organ systems besides the skeleton and the kidneys. The common complaints of weakness and easy fatigability may be associated with a particular neuromuscular syndrome characterized by atrophy of type II muscle fibers. More recent experience suggests that the neuromuscular component of primary hyperparathyroidism is more likely to consist of a less specific set of neurologic manifestations. In fact, the weakness and easy fatigability of primary hyperparathyroidism is typically not associated now with any clinical neurological findings.

The gastrointestinal tract may also appear to be a target of the hyperparathyroid state. Historically, peptic ulcer disease was regarded as a frequent complication. It is now seen predominantly with MEN syndrome type I in which primary hyperparathyroidism and peptic ulcer may coexist. Otherwise, there is debate over whether there is a pathophysiologic association between these relatively common disorders. Similarly, the association between primary hyperparathyroidism and acute pancreatitis remains to be established on pathophysiologic grounds.

The articular system is affected in primary hyperparathyroidism, with gout and pseudogout both being seen. In the absence of symptoms older patients with chondrocalcinosis of the knees and wrists may be at risk for the development of pseudogout. A well-known anemia of primary hyperparathyroidism is characterized by normocytic and normochromic indices. It is an unusual finding, occurring only when other systemic manifestations of primary hyperparathyroidism are present. The anemia is completely reversible after successful removal of the parathyroid adenoma. Hypertension has been thought for many years to be a complicating feature of primary hyperpara-

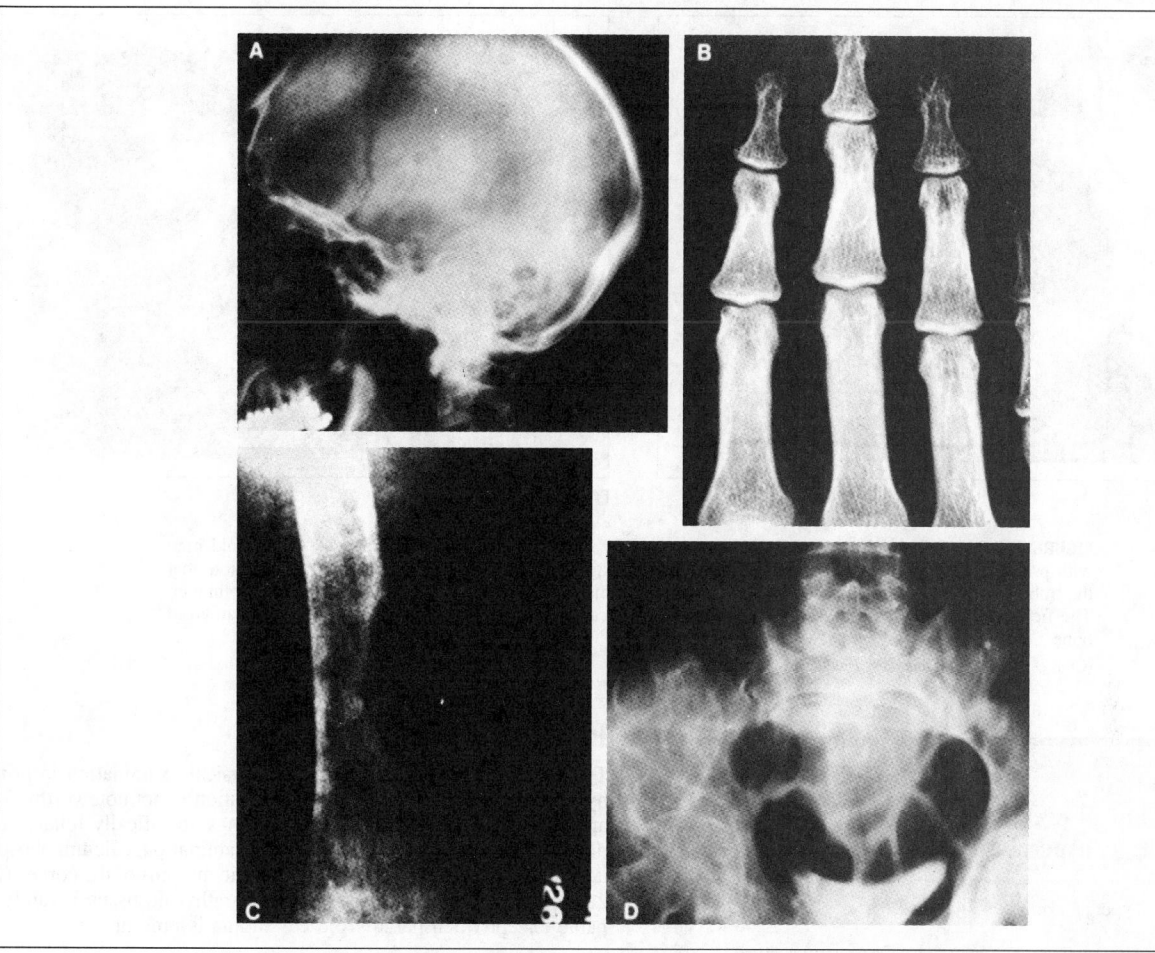

FIGURE 322-1   Osteitis fibrosa cystica in primary hyperparathyroidism. **A,** Note the salt-and-pepper appearance of the skull. **B,** Subperiosteal bone resorption can be appreciated along the radial margins of the distal phalanges. **C,** The lytic lesion on the lateral border of the femur is a brown tumor that subsequently healed after successful parathyroidectomy. **D,** Confluent cystic bone disease in the pelvis of a woman with severe primary hyperparathyroidism.

thyroidism. However, in only a very small minority of patients (less than 10%) is the blood pressure significantly lowered after surgery. As with the association with peptic ulcer disease, it is unclear whether hypertension and hyperparathyroidism are linked pathophysiologically or whether the incidence of both disorders together more likely reflects the expected coincidence of two common diseases. In yet another nonspecific association, a host of neuropsychiatric syndromes has been described in patients with primary hyperparathyroidism, the most common being depression. More subtle features include lack of concentrating ability and a sense of intellectual weariness.

DIAGNOSIS
Forms of Clinical Presentation

Given the extremely wide range of potential organ involvement in primary hyperparathyroidism, it is not surprising that the disease may become evident with one or more of the previously mentioned complications (Box 322-1). Isolated stone or bone disease or virtually any other potential target organ can be a focus of concern that accompanies the diagnosis. The most common presentation of primary hyperparathyroidism, however, is asymptomatic primary hyperparathyroidism, in which hypercalcemia is present in the absence of any specific signs or symptoms commonly or clearly attributed to the disease. Most often, patients have serum calcium values not more than 1 mg/dl above the upper limits of normal. Asymptomatic primary hyperparathyroidism dominates the modern clinical presentation of the disease.

In this large cohort of asymptomatic patients, management decisions are imprecise and therapeutic guidelines are uncertain.

In marked contrast to the most common presentation of primary hyperparathyroidism as an asymptomatic disorder, primary hyperparathyroidism presents rarely as life-threatening hypercalcemia with very high calcium values. Some of the highest serum calcium levels, up to 25 mg/dl, have been reported in patients with primary hyperparathyroidism. A history of mild hypercalcemia is present in approximately 25% of these patients. Acute primary hyperparathyroidism (parathyroid poisoning, parathyroid crisis) usually develops in patients who have an intercurrent illness for which they are immobilized or bedridden. Dehydration is another etiologic factor. Under these conditions, a state of further negative calcium balance ensues, parathyroid hormone levels increase markedly, and the serum calcium rises accordingly. Anorexia and polyuria lead to further dehydration and higher levels of serum calcium, and a worsening cycle of escalating hypercalcemia is established. Acute primary hyperparathyroidism is an important consideration in acutely hypercalcemic individuals because it is curable and readily reversible. On clinical grounds it may be difficult, if not impossible, to distinguish acute primary hyperparathyroidism from parathyroid carcinoma.

On the extreme other hand, there are occasional patients with normal serum calcium values who are suspected of having primary hyperparathyroidism because of nephrolithiasis or other well-known complications. The term *normocalcemic hyperparathyroidism* has been applied to these patients. It is a misnomer because the calcium

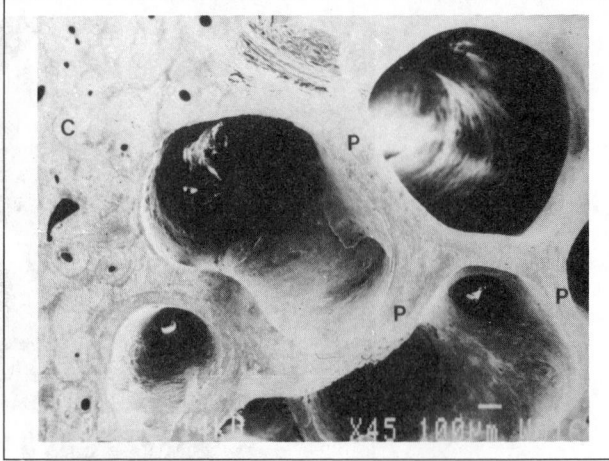

FIGURE 322-2 Primary hyperparathyroidism as seen by scanning electron microscopy. A 45-year-old man with primary hyperparathyroidism **(A)** is compared to an age- and sex-matched normal subject **(B).** Note that the trabecular plates *(P)* are conserved in hyperparathyroidism, but that the cortex *(C)* is considerably thinner. The field width is 2.4 mm in each case, and the magnification is the same for normal and hyperparathyroid bone.

(Courtesy Dr. David Dempster, Helen Hayes Hospital.)

BOX 322-1
Clinical presentations of primary hyperparathyroidism

Asymptomatic hypercalcemia
Bone or stone disease
Other recognized complications (neuromuscular, gastrointestinal tract, articular, hematologic, central nervous system)
Acute primary hyperparathyroidism
Parathyroid carcinoma
Familial primary hyperparathyroidism
Primary hyperparathyroidism in pregnancy
Neonatal hyperparathyroidism
Multiple endocrine neoplasia type I or II

---

level can be shown to become abnormal in these patients at periodic intervals.

Primary hyperparathyroidism may be associated with MEN type I (parathyroid, pituitary, pancreas) or type II (medullary thyroid cancer, pheochromocytoma; see Chapter 299). Primary hyperparathyroidism can also occur rarely as an isolated familial disease involving only the parathyroids. A pathologic variant of familial primary hyperparathyroidism is cystic parathyroid adenomatosis, characterized by recurrent parathyroid disease over years as glands become sequentially involved.

Primary hyperparathyroidism can develop during pregnancy. The diagnosis may be suspected in retrospect after delivery when neonatal hypocalcemia and tetany occur in the offspring. The neonatal hypocalcemia is believed to be caused by suppression of neonatal parathyroid function by the maternal hypercalcemia. Primary hyperparathyroidism can become evident as life-threatening hypercalcemia discovered soon after birth. These children display a characteristic hypotonia and can be managed only by emergency parathyroidectomy. At operation, all four glands are involved in a hyperplastic process. Kindreds of families with neonatal primary hyperparathyroidism have been described in which familial cystic adenomatosis and/or familial hypocalciuric hypercalcemia are also present. The molecular basis of this syndrome is a single (familial hypocalciuric hypocalcemia [FHH]) or double (neonatal primary hyperparathyroidism) mutation in the gene that encodes for the calcium-sensing receptor.

Physical Findings

The most noteworthy aspect of the physical examination in primary hyperparathyroidism is that the examination is not noteworthy. There are usually no abnormal physical findings specifically related to the disease. By ophthalmologic slit-lamp examination, calcium phosphate deposition in the medial and lateral limbic margins of the cornea (band keratopathy) is seen rarely. Enlarged parathyroid tissue is rarely palpable except when parathyroid carcinoma is present.

Laboratory Findings and Differential Diagnosis

Hypercalcemia is a sine qua non of the disease. The serum phosphorus is usually in the lower range of normal, but in approximately one third of patients it may be frankly low. If the serum alkaline phosphatase activity (bone-derived) is elevated, it usually reflects active bone disease and is accompanied by elevations in serum osteocalcin level (a marker of osteoblast activity) and urinary hydroxyproline or collagen cross-links (markers of osteoclast activity). 1,25-Dihydroxyvitamin D levels may be elevated, although this is not specific for primary hyperparathyroidism. 1,25-Dihydroxyvitamin D levels are elevated in a number of other conditions associated with hypercalcemia such as sarcoidosis, other granulomatous diseases, certain lymphomas, and vitamin D toxicity (see Chapter 312). The actions of parathyroid hormone to alter acid-base handling in the kidney lead sometimes to mild hyperchloremia and metabolic acidosis. Urinary calcium excretion is elevated in approximately one fourth of all patients. Phosphaturia, a major physiologic action of parathyroid hormone, may also be demonstrated.

The most useful test for the diagnosis of primary hyperparathyroidism is the parathyroid hormone measurement per se. The most useful assays are those that measure intact hormone or fragments with specificity for mid- or carboxy-terminal regions of parathyroid hormone. These assays show frank elevations in parathyroid hormone in 85% to 90% of patients with surgically proved primary hyperparathyroidism (Fig. 322-3). The urinary cyclic adenosine monophosphate (AMP) level, another marker of parathyroid hormone activity, does not usually add much to the diagnostic evaluation in view of the utility of the assays for parathyroid hormone. The diagnosis of primary hyperparathyroidism is made by the simultaneous presence of hypercalcemia and an elevated level of parathyroid hormone (see Chapter 312). The only exceptions to this general rule are the hypercalcemias associated with the use of thiazide diuretics and lithium. The history usually points out these two possibilities fairly readily. In these situations, the only way to determine the cause of the hypercalcemia is

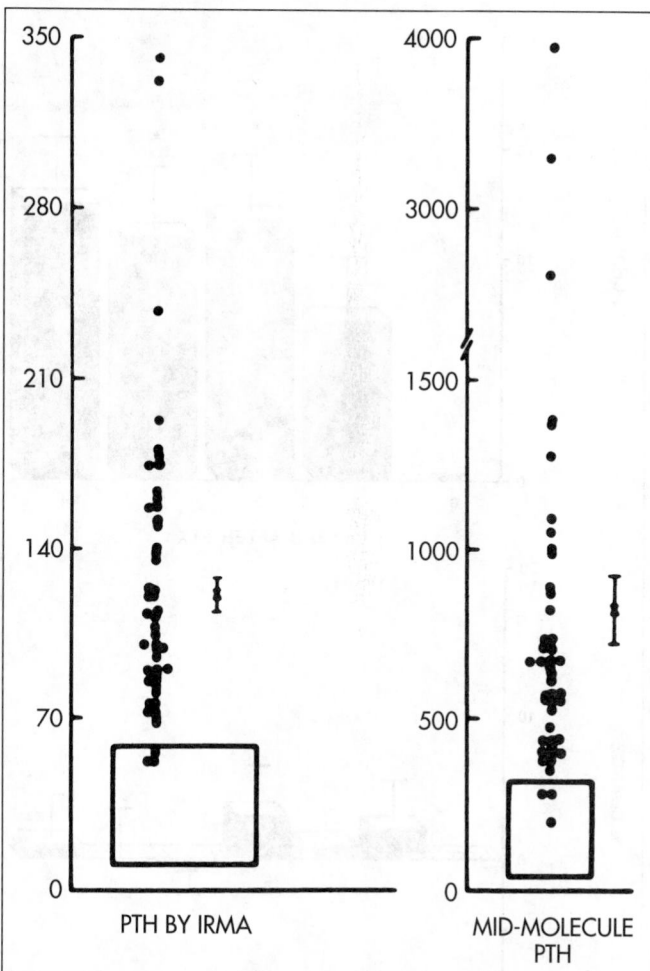

FIGURE 322-3 Usefulness of intact and middle region immunoassays for parathyroid hormone in patients with primary hyperparathyroidism.
Modified from Silverberg et al: *J Bone Miner Res* 4:283, 1989.

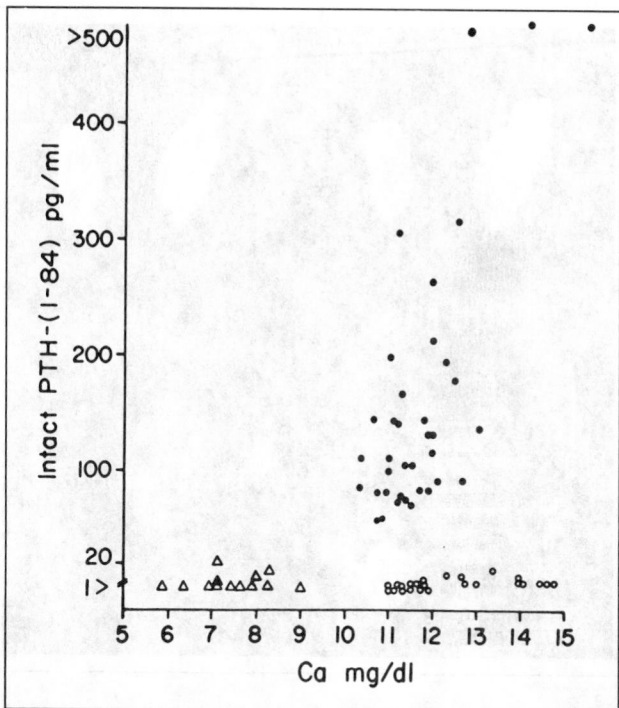

FIGURE 322-4 Usefulness of the immunoradiometric assay for parathyroid hormone in the differential diagnosis of hypercalcemia. Patients with surgically proved primary hyperparathyroidism show elevations (>65 pg/ml) in virtually all cases. Patients with malignancy show levels that are below or at the lower limit of normal (12 pg/ml).

From Nussbaum SR et al: Highly sensitive two-site immunoradiometric assay of parathyrin and its clinical utility in evaluating patients with hypercalcemia, *Clin Chem* 33:1364, 1987.

to withdraw the suspected medication, if possible, and to repeat the tests in 2 to 3 months.

Another important reason why the immunoassays for parathyroid hormone have become so useful in establishing the diagnosis of primary hyperparathyroidism relates to our better understanding of some of the other causes of hypercalcemia. In malignant disease, parathyroid hormone levels are not elevated. The parathyroid hormone–like protein, implicated in the syndrome of humoral hypercalcemia of malignancy, does not cross-react in the available immunoassays for parathyroid hormone (Fig. 322-4). Thus, virtually all malignant disorders, except for parathyroid carcinoma and the exceedingly rare example of ectopic production of authentic parathyroid hormone by a malignant tumor, show suppressed levels of parathyroid hormone. Similarly, in those malignancies and granulomatous disorders associated with hypercalcemia and elevated levels of 1,25-dihydroxyvitamin D, the parathyroid hormone level is suppressed. Where multiple, local factors in bone are responsible for malignancy, here too, the parathyroid hormone level is not elevated.

Familial hypocalciuric hypercalcemia should be considered in patients who appear to have primary hyperparathyroidism. FHH is a disorder characterized by mild hypercalcemia, very low urinary calcium excretion (calcium/creatinine clearance less than 0.01), and mild hypermagnesemia. Parathyroid hormone levels are not elevated. Although the high penetrance of the disorder causes hypercalcemia in childhood, it may not be recognized until early adulthood. Patients with FHH are remarkably free from complications associated with primary hyperparathyroidism, an observation that has given rise to

the description *benign familial hypercalcemia*. Adults with FHH need no treatment. Subtotal parathyroidectomy does not cure the disease. As noted earlier, the molecular basis for FHH is due to a mutation in the gene that controls the calcium^{2+}-sensing receptor; thus FHH is fundamentally a different disorder from primary hyperparathyroidism.

TREATMENT
Surgery

The definitive treatment for primary hyperparathyroidism is surgical removal of the abnormal gland(s). In the days when primary hyperparathyroidism was often accompanied by signs and symptoms, the case for parathyroid surgery was relatively straightforward. Now, however, the typical patient is asymptomatic. We do not know and cannot yet predict who among the asymptomatic patients will develop complications of parathyroid disease. Nevertheless, recent advances in our knowledge of primary hyperparathyroidism have let to a set of guidelines that are used widely in deciding whether a patient should be recommended for surgery.

Current surgical guidelines include patients with any of the following six features: (1) a serum calcium level greater than 1 mg/dl above the upper limits of normal; (2) signs or symptoms of primary hyperparathyroidism, regardless of the actual serum calcium value; (3) markedly reduced cortical bone density; (4) age, under 50 years; (5) an episode of acute primary hyperparathyroidism; and (6) hypercalciuria (greater than 400 mg/day). When these guidelines are applied to patients with primary hyperparathyroidism, approximately half become surgical candidates. About two thirds of these patients are asymptomatic but by virtue of age, hypercalciuria, or reduced bone density fall into the group for whom surgery is recommended.

Parathyroidectomy should be performed by an expert neck surgeon who is intimately familiar with the difficult aspects of the procedure. Parathyroid surgery tends to be difficult because abnormal glands are still rather small. In addition, they do not always have the

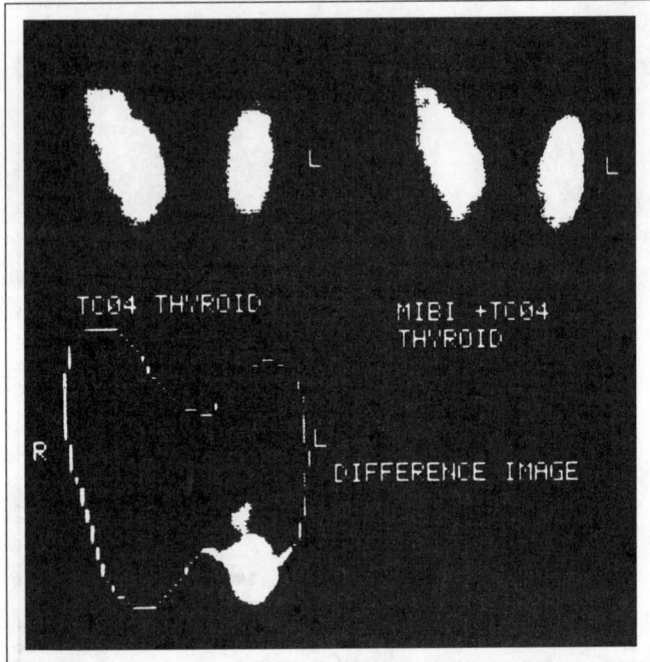

FIGURE 322-5 Localization of parathyroid tissue by imaging with technetium-99m-Sestamibi. Tc-99m pertechnetate *(upper left),* TC-99m sestamibi *(upper right),* and change detection image *(bottom)* in a patient with a pedunculated left upper pole parathyroid adenoma.

From Johnston LM, Carrol MJ, Critton KE et al: The accuracy of parathyroid gland localization in primary hyperparathyroidism using sestamibi radionuclide imaging, *J Clin Endocrinol Metab* 81:346-352, 1996.

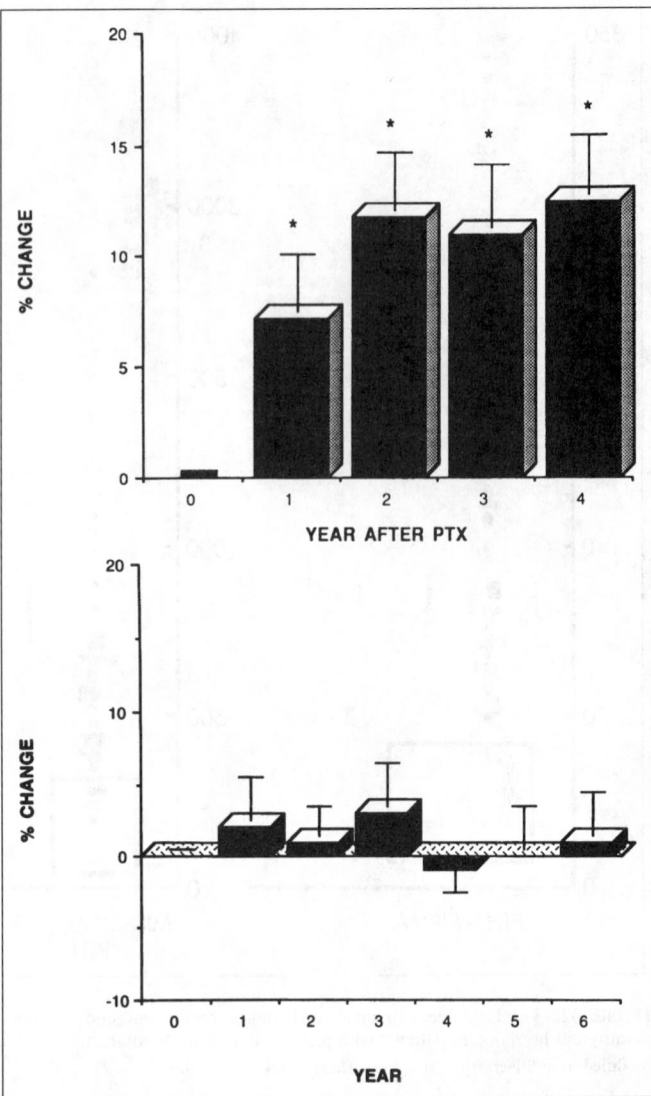

FIGURE 322-6 The course of bone density in postmenopausal women with primary hyperthyroidism with or without parathyroid surgery. Bone density was measured for 4 years in two groups of patients: those who underwent successful parathyroid surgery **(A)** and those who did not meet any surgical criteria and therefore were followed conservatively **(B).** The data are shown for the lumbar spine, but similar results were obtained at the hip region (femoral neck) and at the distal radius. Bone density increases impressively in those who had surgery and was essentially stable among those who did not have surgery.

From Silverberg SJ, Gartenberg F, Jacobs TP et al: Increased bone mineral density after parathyroidectomy in primary hyperparathyroidism, *J Clin Endocrinol Metab* 80:729-734, 1995.

characteristic red-brown color and oval cigarlike configuration and may look very much like a fat globule. Moreover, they are occasionally found in ectopic sites. If an adenoma is discovered, an attempt is usually made to locate all other parathyroid glands to ascertain that they are normal. Pathologic features are checked during the operation by examination of frozen sections of tissue. If parathyroid hyperplasia is discovered, removal of 3½ glands is performed, leaving sufficient residual parathyroid tissue to maintain normal parathyroid function. Some surgeons remove all four hyperplastic glands and transplant remnants of parathyroid tissue into the forearm. Tissue from an adenomatous gland is not transplanted as a rule. When parathyroid surgery is successful, which should occur approximately 90% to 95% of the time, patients usually have a transient 1- to 2-day period of mild hypocalcemia followed by a return of the serum calcium level to normal as the suppressed normal glands regain function. In patients with overt skeletal disease, there may be a prolonged period of hypocalcemia caused by rapid reversal of the negative state of calcium balance and deposition of calcium into bone (hungry bone syndrome). A more permanent complication of parathyroid surgery is hypoparathyroidism. In the patient who has had previous neck surgery and removal of some parathyroid tissue already, postoperative hypoparathyroidism may be evident soon after surgery and documented by monitoring the lack of return of parathyroid function. However, hypoparathyroidism does not develop, sometimes, until months to years after surgery. In this situation, it is possible that the remaining parathyroid tissue is left with marginal vasculature and that with age, there is further reduction in vascular integrity. Another permanent complication of parathyroid surgery is recurrent laryngeal nerve damage with resultant hoarseness and loss of voice volume.

In patients who have had previous neck surgery, localization techniques are usually indicated. Among the noninvasive approaches to localization, interest centers around ultrasonography, computed tomography, magnetic resonance imaging, and scintigraphy. For all procedures, limitations include their resolving power, making adenomas smaller than 200 mg difficult to delineate, and an appreciable inci-

dence of false-positive localization. These approaches, nevertheless, are destined to improve with advancing technology (Fig. 322-5). For example, the imaging agent technetium-99m Sestamibi has become the agent of choice in the radionuclide imaging of parathyroid tumors.

The invasive techniques of arteriography and selective venous catheterization can provide definitive anatomic and functional identification of parathyroid tissue, but they are time-consuming, operator-dependent, and expensive procedures. Nevertheless, they should be used in patients with previous neck surgery for whom it is vitally important to identify the location of the adenoma preoperatively. Most medical centers do not routinely perform these procedures. Patients in need should therefore be referred to those few hospitals in the United States that have the requisite expertise to conduct these tests successfully.

Medical Therapy

There are several groups of patients with primary hyperparathyroidism in whom surgery is not a clear option. The large cohort of patients with asymptomatic primary hyperparathyroidism illustrates the problem faced by the physician. It is not known which patients will eventually develop complications of the disease and which will remain asymptomatic. There are no clinical or laboratory criteria by which risks or probabilities of complications can be established. The variable natural history of primary hyperparathyroidism often leaves the clinician undecided between a surgical approach and a more conservative medical one. Many clinicians, however, do not recommend surgery unless the patient meets one of the surgical guidelines. Approximately 50% of patients meet one or more surgical guidelines. In addition to the asymptomatic hyperparathyroid patient who does not meet surgical guidelines, medical management is often reserved for patients who refuse surgery and for patients who are no longer surgical candidates because of coexisting medical problems. Also included in this group are patients with persistent hyperparathyroidism who had unsuccessful previous neck operations and failed attempts at preoperative localization.

General guidelines for the patient with primary hyperparathyroidism follow from a consideration of the hypercalcemia per se. The management of acute hypercalcemia associated with primary hyperparathyroidism follows the same guidelines as those presented in Chapter 312. For routine primary hyperparathyroidism in which calcium levels are only mildly elevated, adequate hydration and ambulation are always to be encouraged, as well as avoidance of diuretics such as thiazides that may actually worsen the hypercalcemia. Dietary recommendations for calcium intake should be moderate. A rationale to recommend high dietary calcium intake in order to suppress parathyroid glandular activity might be associated with worsening hypercalcemia, especially if the 1,25-dihydroxyvitamin D level is elevated. On the other hand, low dietary calcium intake could theoretically lead to further stimulation of parathyroid hormone secretion. Oral phosphate therapy may lower the serum calcium level and is a reasonable mode of therapy. Chronic administration could conceivably predispose patients to ectopic calcium phosphate deposition and further elevation of parathyroid hormone levels. Postmenopausal women may be helped by estrogen therapy, although parathyroid hormone levels do not decline and phosphate levels may be further reduced. A newer generation of pyrophosphate analogs known as *bisphosphonates* might be shown in the next several years to be useful in primary hyperparathyroidism.

A new class of agents that function as cellular calcimimetics is being developed. This class of compounds interacts with the calcium^{2+}-sensing receptor to alter its functioning and to lead to increases in intracellular calcium. Such increases in cellular calcium in the parathyroid cell reduce secretory and synthetic processes of the cell, resulting in a reduction in extracellular parathyroid hormone.

Course of Medical and Surgical Therapy for Primary Hyperparathyroidism

Patients who undergo successful parathyroid surgery are cured of the hypercalcemia with normalization of serum and urinary indices of the disease. Moreover, they have, in general, a substantial increase in bone mineral density over the ensuing 4 years (Fig. 322-6). The increase in bone density is of particular note because it indicates that to a certain extent, at least, this is a reversible process. On the other hand, patients who are not surgical candidates and are followed conservatively seem to show a very stable course with respect both to biochemical and densitometric indices. These observations suggest that it is important to determine by a complete evaluation whether a patient is a surgical candidate and to follow the aforementioned guidelines in making the decision about surgical intervention.

BIBLIOGRAPHY

Bijvoet OLM, Fleisch HA, Canfield RE, Russell RGG, editors: *Bisphosphonates on bones,* Amsterdam, 1995, Elsevier.
Bilezikian JP, Silverberg SJ: Usefulness of bone mass measurements in primary hyperparathyroidism, *Curr Opin Endocrinol Diabetes* 3:514-520, 1996.

Bilezikian JP, Silverberg SJ, Gartenberg F et al: Clinical presentation of primary hyperparathyroidism. In Bilezikian JP, Marcus R, Levine MA editors: *The parathyroids,* New York, 1994, Raven.
Endres DB, Villanueva R, Sharp DR Jr, Singer FR: Measurement of parathyroid hormone, *Endocrinol Metab Clin North Am* 18:611-629, 1989.
Fitzpatrick LA, Bilezikian JP: Acute primary hyperparathyroidism, *Am J Med* 82:275, 1987.
Heath H III, Hodgson SF, Kennedy MA: Primary hyperparathyroidism: incidence, morbidity, and potential economic impact in a community, *N Engl J Med* 302:189, 1980.
Hendy GN, Arnold A: Molecular basis of PTH overexpression. In Bilezikian JP, Raisz LR, Rodan GA, editors: *Principals of bone biology,* San Diego, 1996, Academic.
Johnston LM, Carroll MJ, Britton KE et al: The accuracy of parathyroid gland localization in primary hyperparathyroidism using sestamibi radionuclide imaging, *J Clin Endocrinol Metab* 81:346-352, 1996.
Nemeth EF: Calcium receptors as novel drug targets. In Bilezikian JP, Raisz LR, Rodan GA, editors: *Principles of bone biology,* San Diego, 1996, Academic.
Potts JT Jr, editor: Proceedings of the National Institutes of Health Consensus Development Conference on Diagnosis and Management of Asymptomatic Primary Hyperparathyroidism, *J Bone Min Res* 6(suppl 2):S1, 1991.
Shane E, Bilezikian JP: Parathyroid carcinoma. In Williams CJ et al, editors: *Textbook of uncommon cancer,* New York, 1988, Wiley.
Silverberg SJ, Gartenberg F, Jacobs TP et al: Longitudinal measurements of bone density and biochemical indices in untreated primary hyperparathyroidism, *J Clin Endocrinol Metab* 80:723-728, 1995.
Silverberg SJ, Gartenberg F, Jacobs TP et al: Increased bone mineral density after parathyroidectomy in primary hyperparathyroidism, *J Clin Endocrinol Metab* 80:729-734, 1995.

CHAPTER

323 Malignant Disease and the Skeleton

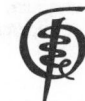

Gregory R. Mundy and Charles A. Reasner II

BONE METASTASES

Tumors frequently involve the skeleton. They may metastasize to bone to form either lytic (destructive) or blastic (formative) lesions (Fig. 323-1). Lytic metastases are much more common than blastic metastases, although most tumors that metastasize to bone have both lytic and blastic elements. The cellular and molecular mechanisms responsible for causing these increases in bone resorption and bone formation are undergoing intense investigation. As described in Chapter 283, bone that is resorbed is usually replaced by newly formed bone. However, in some tumors the increase in bone formation is too pronounced to be accounted for simply by the physiologic coupling mechanism that normally links bone formation to bone resorption. These tumors produce bone growth factors that stimulate adjacent osteoblasts to form new bone. The tumors that are most frequently associated with osteoblastic metastases are carcinomas of the prostate and breast. Metastatic prostatic cancer frequently shows osteoblastic bone formation around metastatic deposits in bone, whereas this effect is less common in metastatic breast cancer.

Most tumors that metastasize to bone cause osteolytic bone destruction. These metastases may be associated with hypercalcemia. The molecular mechanisms responsible for osteolytic metastases and bone destruction are unclear but comprise both the migration of tumor cells toward bone surfaces and then local destruction of bone when tumor cells are housed within the bone marrow cavity adjacent to endosteal bone margins. The destruction of bone is primarily mediated by osteoclasts.

The mechanism of osteoclast activation is complicated. It may involve local mediators of osteoclastic bone resorption that are produced by the tumor within the bone marrow cavity, including cytokines and prostaglandins. It also probably involves the tumor peptide parathyroid hormone–related peptide (PTH-rP), which is produced by some tumors such as breast cancers when they metastasize to bone.

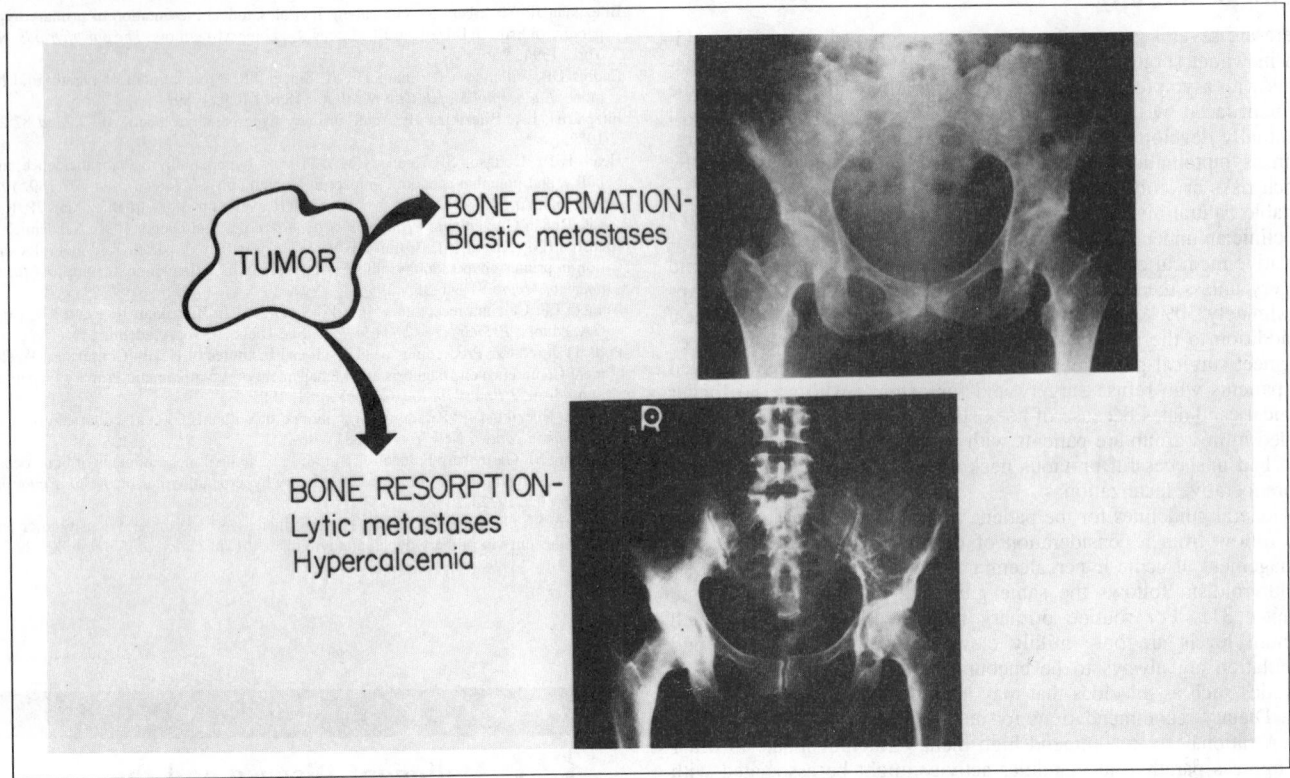

FIGURE 323-1 Tumor products may cause increases in osteoblast activity (blastic metastases) or increases in osteoclast activity (lytic metastases and/or hypercalcemia).

Table 323-1 Malignancies associated with hypercalcemia

TYPES OF MALIGNANCY	PERCENTAGE OF TOTAL
Lung	35
Breast	25
Hematologic (myeloma, lymphoma)	14
Head and neck	6
Renal	3
Prostate	3
Unknown primary	7
Others	8

Modified from Mundy GR, Martin TJ: *Metabolism* 31:1247, 1982.

CLINICAL CONSEQUENCES OF MALIGNANT INVOLVEMENT OF THE SKELETON

The clinical consequences of malignant involvement in the skeleton include bone pain, fracture, and hypercalcemia (discussed later). Once tumors involve the skeleton, they are usually incurable and only palliative therapy is possible. Bone metastases are frequently complicated by severe pain and occasionally by fracture after trivial injury. The most effective current form of therapy for localized tumor involvement of the skeleton is radiation therapy.

Hypercalcemia of Malignancy

Although hypercalcemia is a frequent complication of malignant disease, there is a clear association between certain tumors and hypercalcemia. Hypercalcemia occurs most commonly in patients with squamous cell carcinomas of the lung, head, and neck, breast cancer, and hematologic malignancies such as myeloma and T-cell lymphomas. The tumors most frequently associated with hypercalcemia are shown in Table 323-1.

Pathogenesis. For convenience we can classify hypercalcemia into three clinical categories, since a different pathogenetic mechanism is likely to be responsible in each case, and therapy differs in each of these categories.

Solid tumors without bone metastases. This group probably accounts for 30% to 40% of patients with hypercalcemia of malignancy. It has been designated *humoral hypercalcemia of malignancy,* since it appears likely that a humoral factor (or factors) released by the tumor cells is responsible for stimulating bone resorption and renal tubular calcium reabsorption, thereby causing hypercalcemia. Humoral hypercalcemia of malignancy is also often (but not always) associated with renal phosphate wasting and hypophosphatemia, increased nephrogenous cyclic adenosine monophosphate (AMP) generation, and increased immunoreactive PTH-rP. Immunoreactive parathyroid hormone concentrations are suppressed. These features are depicted in Fig. 323-2. The condition occurs most frequently in patients with squamous cell carcinomas of the lung, head, and neck and carcinoma of the ovary, pancreas, and kidney.

The mechanisms by which tumor cells cause an increase in serum calcium have been clarified recently. Hypercalcemia occurs because of an increase in osteoclastic bone resorption and an increase in the reabsorption of calcium in the renal tubules. Most but not all patients with this syndrome of humoral hypercalcemia of malignancy (HHM) have increased circulating concentrations of the tumor peptide PTH-rP. This factor has homology with parathyroid hormone (PTH) at the N-terminal end, binds tightly to the PTH receptor, and shares with PTH the capacity to increase osteoclastic bone resorption, increase calcium reabsorption in the renal tubules, and increase the plasma calcium. Whether it has additional effects distinct from those of PTH is still not clear. However, the clinical syndromes of PTH excess (primary hyperparathyroidism) and PTH-rP excess (HHM) are not identical (Table 323-2). The reasons may be that PTH-rP has effects distinct from those of PTH, or that other factors produced in HHM modify the effects of PTH-rP mediated through the PTH receptor. Since there are other factors produced by tumors associated with HHM that profoundly affect bone cells and calcium homeostasis in patients with cancer, the latter explanation seems likely. These other

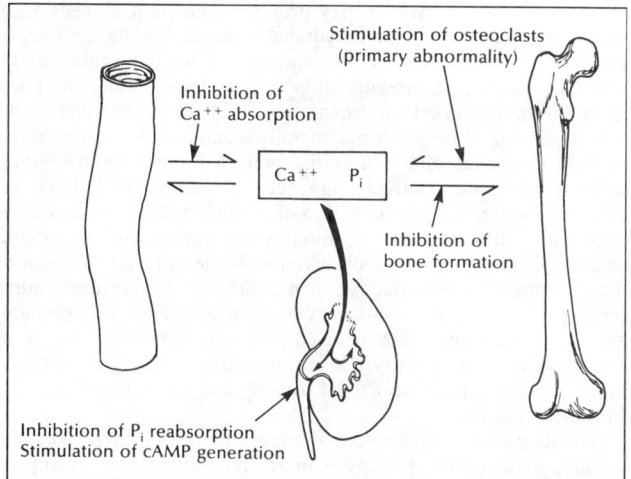

FIGURE 323-2 Tumor products cause the syndrome of humoral hypercalcemia of malignancy by causing the illustrated effects on calcium and phosphate homeostasis.

Table 323-2 Comparison of clinical features in primary hyperparathyroidism and humoral hypercalcemia of malignancy

CLINICAL FEATURE	PRIMARY HYPERPARATHYROIDISM	HUMORAL HYPERCALCEMIA OF MALIGNANCY
Serum calcium	Increased	Increased
Serum phosphorus	Decreased	Decreased
Serum alkaline phosphatase	N or increased	N or increased
Serum chloride	>103 mEq/liter	<98 mEq/liter
Serum bicarbonate	<25 mEq/liter	>25 mEq/liter
Plasma parathyroid hormone	Increased	N or decreased
Plasma PTH-rP	N or increased	Increased
Serum 1,25-dihydroxyvitamin D	N or increased	N or decreased
Gut absorption of calcium	Increased	Decreased
Urine phosphate excretion	Increased	Increased
Urine calcium excretion	Increased	Increased

N, normal.

factors include tumor necrosis factor (TNF), which is produced by normal host cells stimulated by the presence of the tumor and has been shown to cause hypercalcemia in some human tumors, and interleukin-1α, interleukin-6, and transforming growth factor α, which are powerful bone resorbing factors that cause hypercalcemia and are frequently produced by solid tumors in association with PTH-rP.

Solid tumors with metastasis. The most common tumor in this group is carcinoma of the breast. This group accounts for about 40% of all patients with hypercalcemia of malignancy. The mechanism of hypercalcemia is presumably related to the excessive osteolytic bone destruction that accompanies the metastatic process. The cellular events involved in the development of an osteolytic metastasis have been examined using in vitro techniques.

Liotta has described a multistep process by which tumor cells metastasize to different organs. The initial event is shedding of tumor cells from the primary tumor site followed by their entry into the bloodstream. After this, the tumor cells spread to vascular organs such as the red bone marrow and, provided the situation is appropriate, form secondary tumors in these organs. Their escape from the vascular channels in the bone marrow to the interstitial tissue involves adherence to the basement membrane of the capillary walls, the disruption of the capillary walls by the production of degradative proteolytic enzymes by the tumor cells, and the migration of tumor cells through these breaks in the endothelium to the interstitial space. Tumor cells are then attracted to the endosteal bone surface, possibly by chemoattractant factors in bone or at the bone surface. Once at the endosteal surface, tumor cells cause bone destruction by stimulating osteoclasts. They do this by several mechanisms, including the production of tumor factors such as PTH-rP, transforming growth factor α, or interleukin-1, or by provoking host immune cells to release cytokines that stimulate osteoclastic bone resorption.

Hematologic malignancies. Hematologic malignancies such as myeloma are frequently associated with bone destruction. This type of bone destruction is osteoclastic and appears to be caused by the release of a family of lymphokines called *osteoclast-activating factors* by the malignant lymphoid cells. Recently, osteoclast-activating factor has been shown to consist of several purified and molecularly cloned proteins, including lymphotoxin, tumor necrosis factor, interleukin-6, and interleukin-1. In myeloma, lymphotoxin, interleukin-1, and interleukin-6 have all been implicated. Myeloma is almost invariably associated with osteoclastic bone resorption, and 20% of patients also develop hypercalcemia. Hypercalcemic patients with myeloma usually have impaired renal function.

A human type C retrovirus (human T-cell lymphotrophic virus type I [HTLV-I]) has been a consistent finding in a particular form of T-cell lymphoma. The patients universally have a paraneoplastic syndrome characterized by increased bone turnover, abnormal bone scans, and hypercalcemia. Many of these patients produce PTH-rP. It has also been found that some patients with T-cell lymphomas and hypercalcemia have high circulating 1,25-dihydroxycholecalciferol concentrations. This is a result of metabolism of 25-hydroxyvitamin D to 1,25-dihydroxyvitamin D stimulated by the HTLV-infected cells.

Clinical Features. The clinical features of patients with hypercalcemia of malignancy may be confused with the terminal features of malignant disease. Thus many of the symptoms of hypercalcemia such as nausea, vomiting, weight loss, confusion, and lethargy could be ascribed to the malignant disease itself, to the chemotherapy or irradiation therapy that many of these patients receive, or to hypercalcemia. It is important to distinguish these because hypercalcemia is potentially reversible.

There is a rough relationship between the absolute concentration of the serum calcium and symptoms caused by hypercalcemia. In patients with malignant disease, hypercalcemia usually develops fairly rapidly, so symptoms may become apparent at relatively lower serum calcium levels than in primary hyperparathyroidism, in which the patient may become adjusted to a high level of serum calcium and be relatively asymptomatic with much higher serum calcium concentrations. The symptoms depend on the rapidity of the rise in serum calcium level, as well as the absolute serum calcium concentration.

Differential Diagnosis. In considering the differential diagnosis of hypercalcemia, one must consider all the other causes of hypercalcemia and their relative frequencies. Malignant disease and primary hyperparathyroidism are responsible for almost 90% of all causes of hypercalcemia, so that in any patient with hypercalcemia the cause is likely to be one of these two conditions. It is also important to note that primary hyperparathyroidism is a very common disease and may occur coincidentally in a patient with malignant disease. There are many case reports of the coexistence of these two conditions. It is particularly important to consider this possibility in patients with tumors that are rarely associated with hypercalcemia, such as carcinoma of the uterine cervix, or with cancers that may be frequently associated with hypercalcemia but not in the particular clinical situation in which it is being observed, for example, in early carcinoma of the breast without evidence of bone metastasis. In general, occult malignancy is an unusual cause of hypercalcemia. Since primary hyperparathyroidism is so common in the elderly female population, when an elderly woman comes to medical attention with asymptomatic hypercalcemia without obvious malignant disease, the most likely diagnosis is primary hyperparathyroidism.

As indicated earlier, a number of diagnostic tests can be used to distinguish the hypercalcemia of malignancy from other causes of hypercalcemia. Of course, it is important initially to determine whether the patient has malignant disease or metastatic bone disease by a careful history and physical examination and possibly by the use of bone scans and skeletal x-rays. The differential diagnosis has become much more straightforward with introduction of the PTH IRMA assay. In the great majority of patients this assay clearly distinguishes patients with primary hyperparathyroidism from those with non–PTH-mediated causes of hypercalcemia such as malignancy, in which the serum PTH concentrations are suppressed.

The other tests that may be used to separate hypercalcemia of malignancy from primary hyperparathyroidism and other causes of hypercalcemia include measurement of the serum chloride level (usually less than 100 mEq/L in patients with malignant disease but greater than 103 mEq/L in patients with primary hyperparathyroidism); the serum phosphorus level (usually less than 3.5 mg/dl in patients with primary hyperparathyroidism, but it may be less or more in patients with malignant disease); urinary or nephrogenous cyclic AMP (which is increased in patients with primary hyperparathyroidism and may be increased, normal, or suppressed in patients with malignant disease); and the steroid suppression test, which essentially never decreases the serum calcium in patients with primary hyperparathyroidism but does suppress the serum calcium in about one third of patients with hypercalcemia or malignancy and in all patients with hypercalcemia caused by increased absorption of calcium from the gastrointestinal tract.

Sometimes the cause of hypercalcemia can be determined from a careful clinical history. For example, progressive increase in the serum calcium usually occurs fairly rapidly in patients with malignant disease, whereas in patients with primary hyperparathyroidism careful review of the patient's records may indicate that mild hypercalcemia has been present for many years. It is also important to appreciate that hypercalcemia may worsen very rapidly in patients with malignant disease after treatment with estrogen or antiestrogen therapy if the patient has metastatic breast cancer, after volume depletion caused by diuretic therapy, or after vomiting subsequent to treatment with cytotoxic drugs or radiation therapy.

The differential diagnosis of hypercalcemia is also considered in Chapter 312.

Treatment. The indication for treatment of patients with malignant disease is an increased serum calcium level in the symptomatic patient. Although it is controversial whether to treat patients who are asymptomatic, a reasonable approach is to treat all patients with definite hypercalcemia of malignancy. Even if patients are asymptomatic, the serum calcium may increase very rapidly, which could lead to the patient's rapid demise.

The treatment of hypercalcemia has been discussed elsewhere (Chapter 312). The agents available for urgent treatment include saline to correct dehydration and promote a calcium diuresis; calcitonin and glucocorticoids, which rapidly reverse increased bone resorption; and furosemide, which may promote a calcium diuresis when used in large doses in fully rehydrated patients. For the less urgent treatment of hypercalcemia, the currently available agents in the United States are pamidronate, etidronate, gallium nitrate, and plicamycin (mithramycin). Pamidronate and etidronate are bisphosphonates. Both should be given parenterally. Pamidronate is more effective than etidronate and is now the preferred agent. Both of these bisphosphonates are relatively slow acting, with maximal effects unlikely to be observed before 4 days of treatment. There is less experience with gallium nitrate, but initial response rates are encouraging and possibly similar to those observed with pamidronate. Gallium nitrate is probably more effective than etidronate. Unlike these other agents, plicamycin has been available for many years. It is probably more toxic and should now be used only when the other agents are ineffective. It is particularly dangerous to use in patients with renal failure because it has direct renal toxicity and the kidney is responsible for its clearance.

Patients with osteolytic bone disease who are not hypercalcemic may also benefit from therapy with an inhibitor of bone resorption such as one of the new-generation bisphosphonates. These drugs may prevent progression of bone disease or even prevent the skeletal complications of malignancy such as hypercalcemia and intractable bone pain. They have recently been approved by the U.S. Food and Drug Administration for this indication.

BIBLIOGRAPHY

Case records of the Massachusetts General Hospital: case 15-1971. *N Engl J Med* 284:839, 1971.

Garrett IR et al: Production of the bone resorbing cytokine lymphotoxin by cultured human myeloma cells, *N Engl J Med* 317:562, 1987.

Liotta LA: Tumor invasion: role of the extracellular matrix, *Cancer Res* 46:1, 1986.

Moseley JM et al: Parathyroid hormone-related protein purified from a human lung cancer cell line, *Proc Natl Acad Sci U S A* 84:5048, 1987.

Mundy GR: The hypercalcemia of malignancy revisited, *J Clin Invest* 82:1, 1988.

Mundy GR: Pathophysiology of skeletal complications of cancer. In Mundy GR, Martin TJ, editors: Physiology and pharmacology of bone, *Handbook of experimental pharmacology,* Springer (in press).

Mundy GR, Martin TJ: Hypercalcemia of malignancy: pathogenesis and treatment, *Metabolism* 31:1247, 1982.

Mundy GR et al: The hypercalcemia of malignancy: clinical implications and pathogenic mechanisms, *N Engl J Med* 310:1718, 1984.

Mundy GR et al: Tumor products and the hypercalcemia of malignancy, *J Clin Invest* 76:391, 1985.

Myers WPL: Hypercalcemia in neoplastic disease, *Arch Surg* 80:308, 1960.

Powell D et al: Non-parathyroid humoral hypercalcemia in patients with neoplastic disease, *N Engl J Med* 289:176, 1973.

Sporn MB, Todaro GJ: Autocrine secretion and malignant transformation of cells, *N Engl J Med* 303:878, 1980.

Suva LJ et al: A parathyroid hormone-related protein implicated in malignant hypercalcemia: cloning and expression, *Science* 237:893, 1987.

Yates AJP et al: Effects of a synthetic peptide of a parathyroid hormone-related protein on calcium homeostasis, renal tubular calcium reabsorption and bone metabolism, *J Clin Invest* 81:9232, 1988.

PART TEN

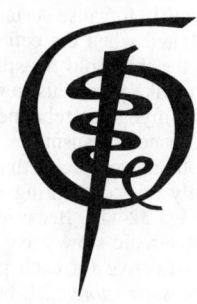

Alimentary Tract, Liver, Biliary Tree, and Pancreas

ALIMENTARY TRACT

324 Alimentary Tract Motor Function

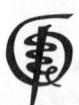

Raj K. Goyal

The motor activity of the alimentary tract helps to prepare the food for digestion and facilitate absorption as the residues are carried caudally for final expulsion. The alimentary tract consists of functionally distinct segments such as the esophagus, the stomach, and the small and large intestines, each of which possesses distinctive motor activity. Despite major differences in function and motor control, the different segments have a similar overall structural organization. The wall of the alimentary tube consists of an outer layer of longitudinal muscle and an inner layer of circular muscle. Internal to these muscle layers is the submucosa, which is delimited by the muscularis mucosa. The mucosa lines the lumen and is separated from the muscularis mucosa by the lamina propria.

The motor activity of each part of the gut is designed to provide propulsion appropriate for the particular physical character and viscosity of food at its level of the alimentary canal. The distinctive motor activities of the different segments of the gut also permit performance of certain specialized functions. For example, the esophagus transports small chunks of swallowed food, whereas the stomach temporarily stores, digests, and grinds solid food into small particles and delivers them to the small bowel. The small bowel functions to allow digestion and absorption. The large bowel acts to retain food residues for several hours or days. Its motor activity allows absorption of water, so that watery food residues are converted to a semisolid or solid consistency. The large bowel also "turns over" residues, of which a small portion is expelled daily during defecation.

Various sphincters separate different segments of the alimentary tract. The sphincters act as one-way valves, normally allowing only forward flow. In addition to directing flow, some sphincters regulate the flow of volume and physical character of contents from one segment to another. Gastrointestinal motility is controlled by *myogenic, neural,* and *hormonal factors.* The distinctive motor activities of different segments of the gut and the sphincters are due to the heterogeneity and specializations of these controlling factors.

CONTROL SYSTEMS OF MOTOR ACTIVITY
Myogenic Factors

Muscles are the ultimate mediators of motor function. Whereas striated muscles have no myogenic tone, the smooth muscle of the gut possesses an intrinsic ability to generate tone or cause phasic contractions. Smooth muscle cells are normally in an electrically polarized state (i.e., the inside of the cell is negative in relation to the outside). The potential difference across the smooth muscle plasma membrane is called the *resting membrane potential* and is due to asymmetric distribution of charged cations and anions across the cell membrane. Muscle contraction is usually associated with depolarization, and inhibition of contraction is associated with hyperpolarization of the smooth muscle membrane. There is, however, marked heterogeneity in the specific electrical and mechanical behavior of smooth muscle in different regions of the gut.

The excitability of smooth muscle is determined by the resting membrane potential. Smooth muscles that have a less negative mem-

brane potential *(depolarized)* are more excitable than those with a more negative membrane potential *(hyperpolarized).* Smooth muscles in several regions of the gut exhibit oscillatory changes in the resting membrane potential. These oscillatory changes are called *slow waves.* Slow waves are not found in the esophagus but occur with remarkable consistency and regularity in the stomach and the small bowel. Slow waves occur irregularly and inconsistently in the colon.

The electrical activity associated with a contraction is called an *action potential.* The most obvious electrical activities associated with muscle contraction are rapid transient depolarizations called *spike potentials.* The spike potentials occur in bursts to cause phasic contractions, and they may occur continuously to cause sustained tonic contractions. Spike potentials are initiated when the cell membrane depolarizes to a value that is above the threshold for spike generation. Depolarization with superimposed spike potentials in many gastrointestinal smooth muscles occurs as a myogenic rebound following the hyperpolarizing action of inhibitory neurotransmitter substances released from the nerves. In smooth muscle cells that exhibit slow waves, spike bursts are more likely to occur during the depolarization phases of the slow wave (Fig. 324-1). Because each smooth muscle segment has its own characteristic slow wave frequency, the maximal rate of spike bursts is distinctive for each part of the gut. The slow waves are also called *pacesetter potentials* because they set the pace at which spike bursts will occur. They are also called *electrical control activities,* because they determine the occurrence of a spike burst. The pacemaker activity is provided by specialized cells called the *interstitial cells of Cajal.* Development of these cells depend upon a tyrosine kinase, cKit. Mutations in the cKIT gene are associated with intestinal motility disorders. The spike potentials in turn are called *electrical response activity.* An intense excitatory stimulus is associated with a large depolarization that may overwhelm the effect of a slow wave. With such stimuli, spike burst activity can occur regardless of the phase of the slow wave and can be prolonged to cover several slow wave cycles. The frequency and amplitude of the spikes and the duration of spike bursts determine the amplitude and duration of contractions. A weak spike burst may not be associated with contraction.

Smooth muscle contraction can also occur in association with electrical activities other than spikes. Slow waves themselves may cause a small degree of contraction during their depolarization phases. In the stomach, excitatory agents may cause an increase in the amplitude of slow wave depolarizations, which in turn are associated with contractions. These depolarizations in the stomach are therefore also called *action potentials.* In the esophagus, spike bursts occur without an underlying slow wave. In colonic smooth muscle a prolonged spike burst covering several slow waves induces long-duration contractions.

Depolarization of gastrointestinal smooth muscle membrane results from influx of positively charged (Na^+ and Ca^{2+}) ions or efflux of negatively charged (Cl^-) ions. Depolarization also results from the inhibition of K^+ efflux. On the other hand, hyperpolarization results from either an increase in K^+ or a decrease in Cl^- efflux. Depolarization in the membrane leads to opening of the voltage sensitive Ca^{2+} channels and Ca^{2+} influx. Hyperpolarization serves to inhibit the voltage-dependent Ca^{2+} channels and, thus, inhibit Ca^{2+} entry into the cells. The coupling between electrical depolarization and muscle contraction is called *electromechanical coupling* and is caused by depolarization-induced increase in intracellular Ca^{2+}.

Sometimes, smooth muscle contraction or relaxation can occur without any associated electrical events. Such mechanical phenomena are due to the direct action of endogenous neurotransmitters and hormones or exogenous pharmacologic agents on intracellular Ca^{2+} or other mediators of contraction. This phenomenon is called *pharmacomechanical coupling.* Because Ca^{2+} plays a critical role in the contraction of smooth muscles, calcium channel blockers serve as effective agents in inhibiting contractions of gastrointestinal smooth muscle. Intracellular messengers such as cyclic adenosine monophosphate (cAMP), cyclic guanosine monophosphate (cGMP), and phosphoinositols are involved in the actions of hormones and neurotransmitters in the smooth muscle. These messengers act by modulating various ion channels and intracellular Ca^{2+} concentrations in the smooth muscles. In general, intracellular increases in both cAMP and cGMP lend to relaxation, and activation of the PI pathway leads to contraction of the muscles. However, there is marked heterogeneity

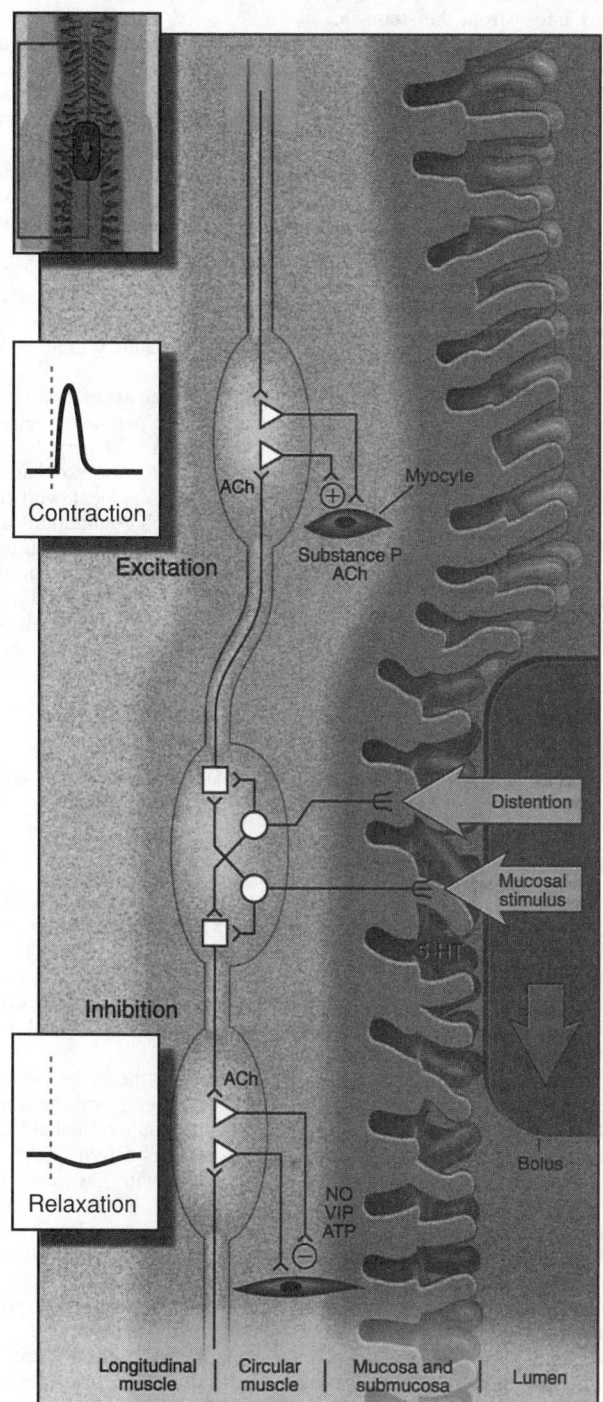

FIGURE 324-1   Peristalsis is the result of a series of local reflexes, each consisting of a contraction of intestinal muscle above an intraluminal stimulus and a relaxation of muscle below the stimulus (inset, upper-left-hand corner). The release of 5-HT by mucosal stimulation or mechanical distention of the gut lumen (main panel) triggers activity in the intrinsic afferent neurons (◯). Above the site of the stimulus, ascending cholinergic interneurons (▢) relay this signal to excitatory motor neurons (▷) containing acetylcholine (Ach) and substance P. As a result, the circular-muscle layer above the stimulus contracts. At the same time, below the stimulus site, descending cholinergic interneurons activate inhibitory motor neurons that contain nitric oxide (NO), vasoactive intestinal polypeptide (VIP), and ATP, causing relaxation. The resultant forces propel the bolus in an antegrade direction. As the bolus moves, it triggers similar local peristaltic reflexes at successive sites along the gut. The symbol ⫤ represents afferent-nerve endings; ⅄, efferent-nerve endings; ⊕, excitatory influence; and ⊖, inhibitory influence.

From Goyal RK and Hirano I: The enteric nervous system, *N Engl J Med* 334:1106-1115, 1996.

in the cellular mechanisms of contraction in the different gastrointestinal smooth muscles.

Of the several muscle layers in the alimentary canal, contraction of the circular muscle is largely responsible for luminal occlusion and movement of food through the gut. These contractions occur either as a single monophasic contraction or as a train of contractions and may be either propagated or nonpropagated. The propagated waves may move forward (that is, caudally *[peristaltic contractions]*) or backward (that is, orally *[antiperistaltic contractions]*). The nonpropagated waves may occur as simultaneous contractions along a portion of the alimentary canal *(spastic contractions)* or as isolated contractions that occur randomly in time and space *(segmental contractions)*. Nonpropagated contractions help in digestion by facilitating mixing and absorption. Measurements that merely document the presence of intestinal contractions without indicating their propagational properties give no information about the movements of the intestinal contents. When contractions are spastic or segmental or when there are no contractions, there is little movement of intestinal contents. Only peristaltic contractions are associated with significant caudal movement of intestinal contents. In turn, antiperistaltic contractions cause retrograde movement.

The longitudinal muscle contractions also play an important role in the movement of luminal contents by sliding the intestine over the food in the lumen, just as one slides a pillowcase over a pillow. Contractions of the muscularis mucosa may be important both in the mixing of food and enzymes and in the expulsion of glandular secretions into the bowel lumen.

Neural Control

The skeletal muscles at either end of the gastrointestinal tract connect directly with the central nervous system (CNS) through the lower motor neurons. The nervous system exerts total mastery over these muscles. When the nerves are destroyed, these muscles become paralyzed. The lower motor neurons cause muscle contractions by releasing acetylcholine at the motor end plate. Acetylcholine acts on the striated muscles via nicotinic acetylcholine receptors.

The neural control system for smooth muscle consists of extrinsic nerves composed of motor sympathetic and parasympathetic nerves, and intrinsic or "intramural" enteric nerves, which include the myenteric and submucous plexuses. The intrinsic nerves of the gut constitute the *enteric nervous system,* which can integrate and execute gastrointestinal function independent of the central nervous system. The neurons in the enteric nervous system exhibit morphologic, chemical, and functional characteristics that are similar to those of the central nervous system. The enteric nervous system represents the "local brain" of the gut, whereas the sympathetic and parasympathetic pathways provide connections between the central and enteric nervous systems. There are major differences in the anatomic details, chemical nature of transmitters, and organization of neural functions in the different regions of the gut.

Sympathetic nerves exert their effect by releasing norepinephrine and other catecholamines. The sympathetic nerves in general exert an inhibitory effect on the motor activity of the gut except in sphincters, which contract in response to sympathetic stimulation. Sympathetic overactivity may produce *adynamic ileus,* which is sometimes erroneously called *paralytic ileus,* a misnomer because there is no true muscular paralysis involved. On the other end of the spectrum, pharmacologic or surgical sympathectomy may cause diarrhea resulting from the increased propulsive activity in the gut.

Parasympathetic nerves exert a more discrete effect on the motor activity of the gut than do sympathetic nerves. Parasympathetic nerves have both excitatory and inhibitory effects on gastrointestinal smooth muscle. The vagus nerves mediate esophageal peristalsis and control gastric emptying. Vagal denervation impairs esophageal peristalsis and delays gastric emptying. Because the influence of parasympathetic nerves on the small bowel and colon is relatively small, nearly normal function continues in their absence. Sacral parasympathetic nerves exert an important influence on anorectal activity, and their lesions cause disorders of defecation. Neuronal pattern generators in central nervous system provide programmed patterned activation of vagus splanchnic nerves to produce complex motor activities such as swallowing and defecation and other reflexes that express the motility changes in stress behavioral alterations.

There are separate sets of excitatory and inhibitory enteric motor nerves. The muscle inhibition and excitation work in concert to produce a wide spectrum of motor activity that is seen in different parts of the gut, including the peristaltic reflex (Fig. 324-1). The intramural neurons coordinate and organize activities such as peristalsis, sphincter relaxation, and more complex motor activities. Contractions can occur in smooth muscles in the absence of neural control; however, they are purposeless. Because extrinsic nerves exert their effects via the enteric neurons, lesions of enteric neurons may mimic some of the effects of extrinsic denervation in addition to producing some effects that are characteristic of lesions of the enteric nerves alone. Chagas' disease, which is due to the involvement of myenteric neurons by *Trypanosoma cruzi,* causes widespread derangement in gastrointestinal motility. This disease results in the loss of peristalsis in the esophagus as well as impaired relaxation of the lower esophageal sphincter, together producing the clinical picture of achalasia (Chapter 333), gastric stasis (Chapter 337), small intestinal pseudo-obstruction syndrome (Chapter 342), and megacolon resembling that of Hirschsprung's disease (Chapter 339). Many nerve growth factors and receptors with tyrosine kinase activity participate in development and caudal migration of the enteric nerves in the gut. Mutations in the genes for endothelin-3 or its receptor or RET protooncogene are associated with Hirschsprung's disease.

Hormonal Control

Almost two dozen circulating hormones have been shown to modify gastrointestinal motility, although their physiologic importance is not fully known. For example, gastrin increases lower esophageal sphincter pressure and delays gastric emptying. Secretin, VIP, somatostatin, and opioids delay gastric emptying and may decrease small bowel transit time. Calcitonin gene-related peptide may be involved in both the sensory and motor neural pathways. Although opioids cause constipation, motilin increases gastric emptying and enhances transit through the small intestine. Motilin induces and coordinates interdigestive migrating motor complex (MMC) activity in the stomach and small bowel.

MOVEMENT OF FOOD THROUGH VARIOUS GUT SEGMENTS
Oral Cavity and Pharynx

After food enters the mouth, it is prepared and formed into a bolus and is transported to the esophagus through the pharynx. The oral phase of swallowing is completely under voluntary control. As the bolus enters the oropharynx, an involuntary swallowing reflex is initiated by activation of sensory receptors on the posterior part of the oral cavity. The bolus enters the oropharynx, the nasal and laryngeal passages are occluded, and a wave of peristalsis sweeps the bolus ahead of it. The upper esophageal sphincter opens in anticipation of the arriving bolus. The pharynx and the upper esophageal sphincter are composed of striated muscles. They are innervated by lower motor neurons that accompany vagal and other cranial nerves. A pattern generator for the complex swallowing activity is in the so-called swallowing center in the brain stem. The activity of the swallowing center is modulated by cortical neurons. Neuromuscular disorders that involve these nerves or muscles cause pharyngeal paralysis. Pharyngeal paralysis produces the characteristic symptoms of dysphagia, nasal regurgitation, and tracheobronchial aspiration.

Esophagus

The peristaltic wave that starts in the pharynx continues through the esophagus at a speed of 3 to 4 cm per second, carrying the food bolus ahead of it. The normal transit time of a bolus of food through the esophagus is 5 to 6 seconds. The lower esophageal sphincter opens well before the arrival of the peristaltic wave so that food can pass into the stomach. When the bolus enters the stomach, the lower esophageal sphincter resumes the resting, contracted state.

Peristaltic contractions that occur in response to a swallow are called *primary peristalsis* and are always initiated in the pharynx. *Secondary peristalsis* occurs in response to esophageal distention and is not initiated by pharyngeal activity. The role of secondary peristalsis is to help clear the esophagus of food residue and materials that may reflux into it from the stomach.

The cervical esophagus is composed of striated muscle that is directly innervated by lower motor neurons. Primary as well as secondary peristalsis in the cervical esophagus are due to sequential activation in the brain stem of lower motor neurons that supply the progressively caudally placed musculature of the cervical esophagus.

The thoracic esophagus is composed of smooth muscle that is innervated by myenteric neurons, which are in turn innervated by vagal parasympathetic preganglionic fibers. In the thoracic esophagus, primary peristalsis involves a vagally mediated central mechanism as well as a peripheral mechanism that involves myenteric neurons. Secondary peristalsis, however, is due entirely to local myenteric reflexes. The inhibitory neurotransmitters VIP and NO are involved in lower esophageal sphincter relaxation and the latency gradient of peristalsis.

Peristaltic contractions in the smooth muscle consist of a wave of hyperpolarization followed by depolarization. The peristaltic behavior is due to a progressive increase in the duration of hyperpolarizations aborally along the esophagus. In disease states the esophageal contractions may lose their peristaltic behavior coincident with the loss of aborally increasing hyperpolarizations. Such contractions are called *nonperistaltic* or *tertiary* contractions. The specific neurotransmitters that participate in peristalsis are not fully known, but it appears that multiple inhibitory and excitatory transmitters—including acetylcholine, substance P, and NO—are involved. Weak or absent esophageal contractions (as occur in esophageal scleroderma) cause dysphagia, whereas strong but nonperistaltic contractions (as occur in diffuse esophageal spasm) cause dysphagia and chest pain. Defective relaxation of the lower esophageal sphincter (as in achalasia) also causes dysphagia, whereas inappropriate relaxation or basal hypotension of the sphincter causes gastroesophageal reflux and esophagitis (Chapter 333).

Stomach

As swallowed food fills the stomach, the proximal stomach relaxes to accommodate the contents without causing an increase in luminal pressure. The distal stomach also becomes quiet, and any ongoing motor activity is inhibited. These responses are mediated by the vagus nerve along with intramural inhibitory neurons. Impaired gastric accommodation leads to symptoms of early satiety and enhanced gastric emptying of liquids.

A short time after a meal, peristaltic waves in the body and antrum of the stomach resume and then become stronger, carrying small bits of gastric contents into the terminal antrum. The terminal antrum contracts as a whole against a closed pylorus. This activity helps to grind coarse food into finer particles and mix it with gastric secretions. In the early phase of this activity the pylorus is partially open, allowing passage into the duodenum of small quantities of liquids and solid particles less than 2 mm in diameter. However, such passage of food into the small bowel occurs only if small intestinal contractions at that precise time are inhibited. This requires coordination of antral and duodenal contractions. As the antrum continues to contract, larger particles of food are retropulsed into the main cavity of the stomach. The antrum then relaxes until the next peristaltic wave brings in another portion of food. Thus the antrum and the pylorus act in a coordinated fashion to limit as well as to achieve the emptying of gastric contents. This mechanism is of primary importance in the grinding of digestible solid food and its eventual emptying from the stomach. Vagal inhibitory and excitatory pathways are involved in mediating these responses.

The rate of gastric emptying of liquids and small particulate solids (less than 2 mm) is dependent on the volume of gastric contents. The larger the volume is, the faster the initial emptying rate. Gastric emptying is also regulated by the physicochemical properties of the chyme that enters the duodenum. The duodenal mucosa possesses sensory receptors that activate neurohumoral reflexes that influence gastric emptying. If the chyme coming out of the pylorus is drained so that it does not come in contact with the duodenum, gastric emptying increases markedly. Emptying is inhibited by increasing osmolarity, pH below 3.5, and products of fat digestion. Products of carbohydrate and protein digestion have only a small inhibitory effect. During the digestive period, only liquids and small particles of ground digestible solids leave the stomach, whereas large pieces of indigestible food are retained. One or two hours after a meal, all liquids and digestible solids leave the stomach. At this time, trains of contractions appear that occur at a rate of three to five per minute (which is the rate of gastric slow waves) and move across the stomach. Vagal nerves play an important role in these migratory contractions. Normally the stomach is emptied of all food materials in 2 to 4 hours.

Delayed gastric emptying occurs in a variety of disorders involving myogenic, neural, or hormonal control systems. Myopathic diseases of the gastric smooth muscle (e.g., scleroderma or visceral myopathy) and abnormalities of gastric slow waves such as tachygastria (fast rate of gastric slow waves) or gastric arrhythmia (disorganized gastric slow waves) lead to gastric stasis and symptoms of postprandial fullness, nausea, and vomiting. Similarly, bilateral vagotomy or a vagal neuropathy such as diabetic neuropathy also leads to gastric stasis. Stasis of indigestible solids in the stomach can lead to formation of gastric bezoars (Chapter 337). In diabetic gastroparesis the intradigestive migrating activity front is particularly abnormal, leading to delayed emptying of indigestible solids as an early manifestation of the disease. Disruption of neuronal nitric oxide synthase gene leads to gastric stasis and dilation. Gastric prokinetic agents such as metoclopramide, domperidone, or cisapride improve delayed gastric emptying by increasing the amplitude of antral contractions, improving antroduodenal coordination, and initiating "migrating activity fronts." Macrolide antibiotics such as erythromycin act on motilin receptors to initiate migrating motor complexes and to improve gastroduodenal coordination to enhance gastric emptying.

Other factors can also lead to delayed gastric emptying such as sympathetic overactivity or increased levels of most of the gastrointestinal hormones, particularly cholecystokinin, secretin, glucagon, VIP, and somatostatin. On the other hand, motilin causes enhanced gastric emptying. Rapid gastric emptying can also occur after gastrectomy and may lead to symptoms of dumping syndrome (Chapter 336). The pyloric sphincter also acts to prevent duodenogastric reflux. An increased duodenogastric reflux may contribute to gastritis (Chapter 337) and gastric ulcer.

Small Intestine

Liquids and finely ground food particles enter the small bowel with antral contractions. The pattern of small bowel motor activity observed when food is present in the small intestine is called the *fed pattern* and is characterized by segmental contractions. The segmental contractions are monophasic contraction waves that occur at different sites along the small bowel in a random fashion. Segmental contractions do not propagate in either an aboral or oral direction. These contractions are responsible for the mixing of food with digestive enzymes in intestinal, pancreatic, and biliary secretions. Additional stirring and mixing of the intestinal secretions and food are provided by the muscular activity movement of the villi. Mixing and stirring of intestinal contents are necessary not only for digestion but also for absorption of food. If segmental contractions are inhibited, as in certain disease states such as scleroderma or hollow visceral myopathy, intestinal digestion and absorption are impaired. In the absence of stirring, water layers develop between the intestinal mucosa and the food that is present in the lumen. The unstirred water layers impose a barrier between molecules of digested food and the intestinal mucosa.

Interspersed among the abundant segmental contractions during the fed pattern are also some contractions that propagate aborally for distances of several centimeters. These contractions help gradually to move the food as it is being digested and absorbed. Impaired transit of food throughout the small intestine has been shown to cause reflex inhibition of gastric emptying and may therefore contribute to early satiety, bloating, and anorexia.

After the digestion and absorption of food are completed, the pattern of small bowel motor activity is replaced by patterns of cyclic motor activity called *interdigestive migrating motor complexes*. Each migrating motor complex consists of periods of inactivity alternating with segmental or propulsive contractions (Fig. 324-2). The period of inactivity, which lasts around 20 to 60 minutes, is called *phase I*. Phase I inactivity is followed by irregular segmental contractions that last for a variable period and are called *phase II* activity. Phase II is

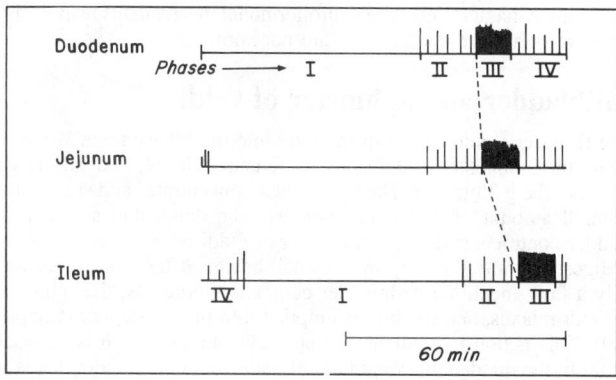

FIGURE 324-2 Periodic activity in the small bowel in the resting state. Note aboral migration of phase III, also called the *activity front*. The migrating motor complex is present at rest and is interrupted promptly by feeding.

followed by regular contractions of the activity front, which is designated *phase III*.

The activity front that is the hallmark of the migrating motor complex consists of an 8- to 10-minute cluster of regularly occurring contractions (Fig. 324-2). The rate of contraction varies in different parts of the small bowel and is determined by the intrinsic frequency of the slow wave in that segment of the intestine. The contraction rate in the activity front is around 12 per minute in the human duodenum. This rate decreases distally along the intestine, so that in the ileum the rate of contraction is 3 to 5 per minute. The activity front migrates toward the terminal ileum at a rate of 4 to 6 cm per minute and gradually decreases to 1 to 2 cm per minute as it approaches the terminal ileum. The activity front reaches the terminal ileum in 1½ hours, triggering a new activity front to begin in the duodenum. Activity fronts are inhibited by ingesting a meal and are thought to be initiated by the hormone motilin. The migrating motor complexes are responsible for the slow propagation of food residues through the small bowel and have been called the *interdigestive housekeepers* of the small intestine. Somatostatin can initiate migrating motor complexes; however, its overall effects on small bowel motility are not well understood. Somatostatin delays intestinal transit in normal subjects, but in patients with intestinal pseudo-obstruction a stable analogue of somatostatin has been shown to enhance small bowel transit.

Another type of propulsive contraction in the small bowel is the *giant peristaltic contraction,* which normally occurs periodically and only in the distal small intestine and the colon. These contractions are called *giant* because their amplitude is 1.5 to 2.0 times larger and their duration 4 to 6 times longer than the usual intestinal contraction. The electrical correlate of giant contractions is not known. Giant peristaltic contractions involve simultaneous contractions of a large (20 to 30 cm) segment of small intestine, and they propagate uninterrupted and aborally at a speed of 1 cm per second. Thus a giant peristaltic contraction can sweep food residues through the whole length of the intestine in a few minutes.

In certain disease states, giant peristaltic contractions can originate in the proximal small bowel and proceed aborally uninterrupted. These peristaltic contractions in the small intestine can be induced by intraluminal administration of agents such as vinegar or shortchain fatty acids. They can also be induced by administration of antibiotics such as erythromycin. Irradiation therapy and parasitic infections have been reported to cause an increase in the frequency as well as being a more proximal origin of these contractions in the small bowel. Most of the manipulations that induce giant peristaltic contractions also cause diarrhea, and therefore it is reasonable to assume that these contractions may be involved in the pathogenesis of diarrhea. One of the interesting features of giant peristaltic contractions is their potential for producing painful abdominal cramps. These cramps are presumably related to vigorous, long-duration contraction involving large segments of the intestine. The occurrence of giant peristaltic contractions in the ileum is often associated with the perception of abdominal pain and cramps in patients with irritable bowel syndrome (Chapter 339). The neurohormonal mechanisms responsible for giant peristaltic contractions are not known.

Gallbladder and Sphincter of Oddi

Bile flows continuously from the liver into the biliary tract. Between meals the sphincter of Oddi largely remains closed, and bile is directed to the gallbladder. The gallbladder concentrates and stores bile. A small amount of bile is emptied into the duodenum as the gallbladder contracts and as the sphincter of Oddi relaxes during the interdigestive motor activity in the small bowel. After a meal, particularly a fatty meal, the gallbladder contracts vigorously, the sphincter of Oddi relaxes, and the bile is emptied into the duodenum (Chapter 349). This action is mediated by cholecystokinin, which is released by fat in the duodenum. Weakness of gallbladder contraction leads to enlargement of the gallbladder and stasis, which may predispose toward formation of gallstones. Impaired relaxation of the sphincter of Oddi may be responsible for biliary dyskinesia associated with pain and liver function abnormalities (Chapter 365).

The purpose of the motor activity of the colon is to mix, store temporarily, and propel food residues of semisolid to solid consistency very slowly. The main role of the ascending colon is to receive and store mostly liquid contents discharged through the ileocecal valve. The role of the left side of the colon is to store food residues for periodic expulsion into the rectum. Colonic motor activity is quite complex and promotes stasis and retropulsion in addition to infrequent but vigorous aboral propulsion of fecal material. Colonic motor activity consists of segmental contractions of either short (less than 10 seconds) or long (around 1 minute) duration. The short-duration contractions occur as a result of spike bursts in association with colonic slow waves. Because colonic slow waves occur irregularly at a frequency of 3 to 12 minutes, these contractions have a similar rate of repetition. The long-duration contractions occur without respect to slow waves and are associated with either long-duration spike bursts or oscillating potentials. The short- and long-duration contractions may occur singly, but more often they occur in trains. These trains of mostly nonpropulsive but sometimes retropulsive activity constitute a large portion of the motor activity of the colon. Segmental contractions in the left side of the colon are also associated with haustral contractions. The haustra are formed by thin, annular contractions that produce transitory septa, breaking up the lumen into saccules. Segmental contractions in the left colon provide resistance to distal movements of the contents; these contractions are increased in patients with constipation and are decreased in patients with diarrhea.

Slow and rapid caudal shifts of colon contents occur during its propulsive motor activity. Slow shifts of colonic contents occur with migrating trains of short- or long-duration contractions, which migrate at rates of 4 to 6 cm per minute and 0.5 to 2 cm per minute, respectively. The mean duration of these trains of contractions is 10 minutes, and they recur every 30 minutes. These migratory contractions move caudally over half the length of the colon. The migratory trains of contractions are separated by a period of quiescence, which may be interrupted by nonmigratory trains of short- or long-duration contractions. Rapid shifts of large volumes of colonic contents from the proximal colon to the middle or distal colon occur secondary to motor activity called *mass movement* or *giant peristaltic contractions* of the colon. Mass movements can occur without defecation or during defecation depending on their propagation through either a part or the entire length of the colon. The giant migrating contraction is two to three times larger in amplitude than are other colonic contractions, and its duration is around 1 minute. It propagates at a fast velocity of 0.2 to 3 cm per second. These contractions can occur singly or in trains of two or more contractions.

Mass movements are induced in the left colon as a reflex response to certain stimuli, such as eating (gastrocolic reflex) or rising in the morning (orthocolic reflex). During these movements, distal segments of the colon are relaxed to accommodate food residues that are pushed forward by the contractions. These reflexes are mediated by neurohumoral mechanisms and are affected by conditioning, but the precise role of neurohumoral control factors in the production of colonic motor activity is not fully understood. The gastrocolic reflex is heightened in some patients with the irritable bowel syndrome (Chapter 339). Weak colonic contractions lead to colonic stasis, megacolon,

and constipation. Diminished mass movements also lead to constipation, whereas frequent mass movements may lead to frequent defecation. Increased segmental contractions may lead to abdominal pain and constipation. Prolonged haustral contractions may mold feces into fecal pellets like rabbit stools, which sometimes occur in patients with the irritable bowel syndrome. Defective relaxation of distal colonic segments also leads to functional obstruction of the passage of fecal contents and megacolon.

Defecation

The rectum is normally empty. Mass movement of the left side of the colon displaces feces into the rectum. When the rectum is distended with fecal matter, the defecation urge is experienced. It is associated with reflex relaxation of the internal anal sphincter and reflex contraction of the external anal sphincter. This urge may be suppressed, in which case both of the anal sphincters become contracted. Contraction of the rectum then propels the feces back into the colon, or the rectum simply accommodates the feces. However, if the subject decides to answer the call, the defecation reflex is activated. Intraabdominal pressure is increased by contractions of the abdominal muscle and diaphragm. The external and internal anal sphincters remain relaxed, and feces are expelled.

In Hirschsprung's disease the internal anal sphincter and the aganglionic segment of the colon fail to relax, causing constipation and megacolon (Chapter 339). Fecal incontinence occurs when liquid feces appear in the rectum, and the anal sphincters, particularly the external anal sphincter, are paralyzed. This may also occur when the threshold of rectal sensations becomes greater than the threshold of rectosphincteric inhibitory reflex, as may happen in patients with diabetic neuropathy.

BIBLIOGRAPHY

Goyal RK, Hirano I: The enteric nervous system, *N Engl J Med* 334:1106, 1996.

Hamdy S et al: The cortical topography of human swallowing musculature in health and disease, *Nature Med* 2:1217, 1996.

Janssens J et al: Improvement of gastric emptying in diabetic gastroparesis by erythromycin, *N Engl J Med* 322:1028, 1990.

Kellow JE, Phillips SF: Altered small bowel motility in irritable bowel syndrome is correlated with symptoms, *Gastroenterology* 92:1885, 1987.

Mayer E. Physiology of gastric storage and emptying. In Johnson LR, editor: *Physiology of the gastrointestinal tract,* ed 3, New York, 1994, Raven Press, pp. 929-976.

Sanders KM: Electrophysiology of dissociated gastrointestinal muscle cells. In Wood JD, editor: *Handbook of physiology: the gastrointestinal system—motility and circulation,* vol I, Bethesda, Md, 1989, American Physiologic Society.

Sanders KM: A case for interstitial cells of Cajal as pacemakers and mediators of neurotransmission in the gastrointestinal tract, *Gastroenterology* 111:492, 1996.

Sarna SK: Physiology and pathophysiology of colonic motor activity, *Dig Dis Sci* 36:827,998, 1991.

Soudah A, Hasler W, Owyang C: Effect of octreotide on intestinal motility and bacterial overgrowth in scleroderma, *N Engl J Med* 325:1461, 1991.

Tonini M: Recent advances in the pharmacology of gastrointestinal prokinetics, *Pharmacol Res* 33:217, 1996.

Wald A, Tunngunkla AK: Anorectal sensorimotor dysfunction in fecal incontinence in diabetes mellitus: modification with biofeedback therapy, *N Engl J Med* 310:1282, 1984.

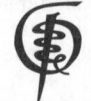

CHAPTER

325   Gastric Secretion

Jean-Pierre Raufman

Gastric secretion represents a highly coordinated, complex process that results in the delivery of a variety of materials into the gastric lumen and the bloodstream. Secretion into the gastric lumen of hydrogen ion and pepsinogen, a proenzyme that is rapidly converted to the acid protease *pepsin,* assists in the digestion of food. Mucus secretion protects the surface epithelium and increases the viscosity of gastric contents. Secretion of intrinsic factor, the only gastric function that is essential to life, aids the ileal absorption of vitamin B$_{12}$. Endocrine cells release hormones, such as gastrin and somatostatin, into the circulation. These agents help to coordinate the release of materials into the gastrointestinal lumen and to regulate cell growth and differentiation.

Proper timing of stimulation and inhibition of acid and pepsinogen secretion in relation to ingestion of a meal is critical for appropriate digestion and absorption of nutrients and for protection of surface epithelium. Cephalic, gastric, and intestinal regulation of gastric secretion is a highly integrated process that involves neuronal, hormonal, paracrine, and autocrine input to secretory cells. Current concepts regarding the regulation of this process are derived from a combination of in vivo studies using a variety of animal and human models and in vitro studies using isolated gastric glands or dispersed mucosal cells. It is only by combining information obtained from these experimental approaches that an understanding of the physiologic regulation of gastric secretion can be achieved.

As illustrated in Fig. 325-1, the stomach can be divided into anatomic and functional regions. The glandular (exocrine) stomach, comprising the fundus and body, contains epithelial cells that line the mucosal surface and secrete mucus and bicarbonate. Studding the mucosal surface are gastric pits that are the outlet into the lumen of gastric glands (Fig. 325-2). Gastric glands contain parietal (also referred to as *oxyntic*) and chief cells that secrete acid and pepsinogen, respectively. Moreover, these glands contain endocrine cells, including enterochromaffin-like (ECL) cells, that contribute to paracrine regulation of parietal and chief cell function.

The endocrine stomach, comprising the antrum, contains cells that secrete chemical messengers. Foremost among these are G and D cells, which release gastrin and somatostatin, respectively. D cells are particularly interesting because the inhibitory peptide somatostatin can act in a hormonal (via secretion into the bloodstream), paracrine (via release from dendritic processes extending from D cells to neighboring cells), or autocrine (via interaction of somatostatin with receptors on D cells) manner.

The anatomic distinctions shown in Fig. 325-1 are somewhat arbitrary because, as shown in Fig. 325-2, small numbers of endocrine cells that regulate parietal and chief cell function are sprinkled throughout the gastric glands of the fundus and body. Moreover, evidence indicates that the glandular elements of the fundus and body may be heterogeneous. Nevertheless, these anatomic distinctions are helpful in understanding the coordination of gastric secretion following ingestion of a meal.

ACID SECRETION
Regulation of Gastric Acid Secretion

Acid secretion by parietal cells represents an integrated response to (1) stimuli from the central and enteric nervous systems and (2) gastric and intestinal elements (Fig. 325-3). Although previous literature refers to "phases" in the regulation of secretion, it is now clear that these processes are highly interactive and overlapping.

In the central nervous system (CNS), areas of the brain stem—including the area postrema, the nucleus tractus solitarius, and the dorsal motor nucleus of the vagus—are activated by the smell, taste, chewing, or swallowing of food (Fig. 325-3, *A*). Nutritional stimuli, particularly hypoglycemia detected by hypothalamic glucose sensors, also activate the dorsal motor nucleus of the vagus. The dorsal motor nucleus integrates this sensory, cognitive, and nutritional information and modulates vagal stimulation of gastric secretion, which can be interrupted by truncal vagotomy. Transmission of secretory signals from the brain stem is mediated by vagal secretory efferent fibers that synapse with ganglion cells of the enteric nervous system (ENS). Hence the central nervous system does not stimulate acid secretion directly, but instead modulates the activity of the ENS, a dense network of glial cells containing as many neurons as the spinal cord. Projections from ganglion cells in the enteric nervous system release acetylcholine and various peptide neurotransmitters and biogenic amines that bind to specific receptors on parietal or enterochromaffin-like cells. Projections from the enteric nervous system onto antral G cells may indirectly promote acid secretion by stimulating gastrin release.

Gastric regulation of acid secretion occurs when food enters the stomach (Fig. 325-3, *B*). Two major factors are responsible for acti-

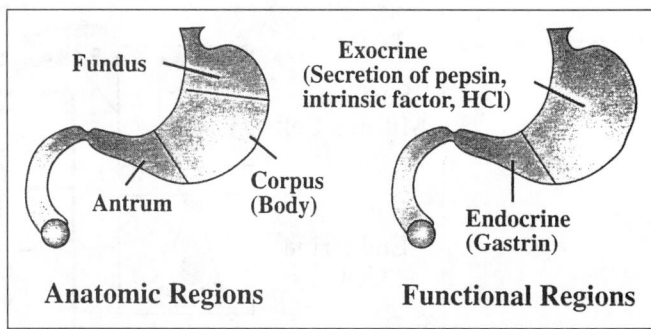

FIGURE 325-1   Anatomic and functional regions of the stomach. The glandular proximal stomach (fundus and body) contains parietal and chief cells that secrete acid and pepsinogen, respectively. The distal stomach (antrum) contains G and D cells that release gastrin and somatostatin, respectively.
From Chang EB, Sitrin MD, and Black DD: *Gastrointestinal, Hepatobiliary, and Nutritional Physiology,* Philadelphia, 1996, Lippincott-Raven, p. 54.

vating intragastric stimulation of acid secretion: distention of the stomach and the presence of the products of protein digestion in the antrum. Minimal levels of gastric distention stimulate the neurons of the ENS and, in turn, vagal afferent fibers, thereby further increasing efferent vagal tone via the dorsal motor nucleus of the vagus. Further distention activates ENS neurons that stimulate parietal cells directly, inhibit somatostatin release from D cells, and stimulate the release of gastrin from antral G cells and histamine from ECL cells. G cells are also stimulated by the presence of large peptides (peptones) and aromatic amino acids (phenylalanine and tryptophan) in the antral lumen. Unlike products of protein digestion, fats and carbohydrates are not important stimulants of gastric acid secretion.

Intestinal regulation of acid secretion, a minor component of this process, starts when food enters the duodenum (Fig. 325-3, *C*). As in the stomach, luminal distention and the presence of amino acids are the major stimulants of this aspect of gastric secretory control.

Parietal Cell Receptors and Signal Transduction Mechanisms

In recent years a great deal has been learned regarding the receptors and mechanisms that mediate acid secretion at the cellular level. Although it was recognized for many years that parietal cells express receptors for acetylcholine, histamine, and gastrin, it is only recently that the relative roles of these receptors in mediating secretion have been appreciated. Binding of acetylcholine to muscarinic (M$_3$) receptors on parietal cells stimulates phospholipid turnover and an increase in cellular calcium (Fig. 325-4). Histamine (H$_2$) receptors on parietal cells are coupled to secretion via activation of adenylyl cyclase and the generation of cyclic AMP. The intracellular steps leading from increases in cellular calcium and cyclic AMP to H$^+$ secretion remain to be elucidated. As discussed in the next section, although gastrin (CCK-B) receptors are expressed on parietal cells, activation of these receptors does not directly stimulate acid secretion but may have more to do with potentiation of acid secretion caused by other mechanisms or with cellular growth and differentiation. Moreover, gastrin has trophic effects on progenitor cells in fundic mucosa and on ECL cells.

Regulation of Parietal Cell Function by ECL Cells

Current understanding of the regulation of gastric acid secretion indicates the interaction of many mucosal cellular elements. The importance of histamine as a stimulant of acid secretion from parietal cells assigns the ECL cell a central role in integrating stimulatory and inhibitory stimuli from various sources and determining the rate of secretion.

As described in the previous section, after a meal, gastrin is released from antral G cells into the circulation and is transported to the gastric glands in the fundus and body of the stomach. Although gastrin binds to parietal cell receptors, the major part of its secretory actions is mediated by interaction with an intermediary, the ECL cell.

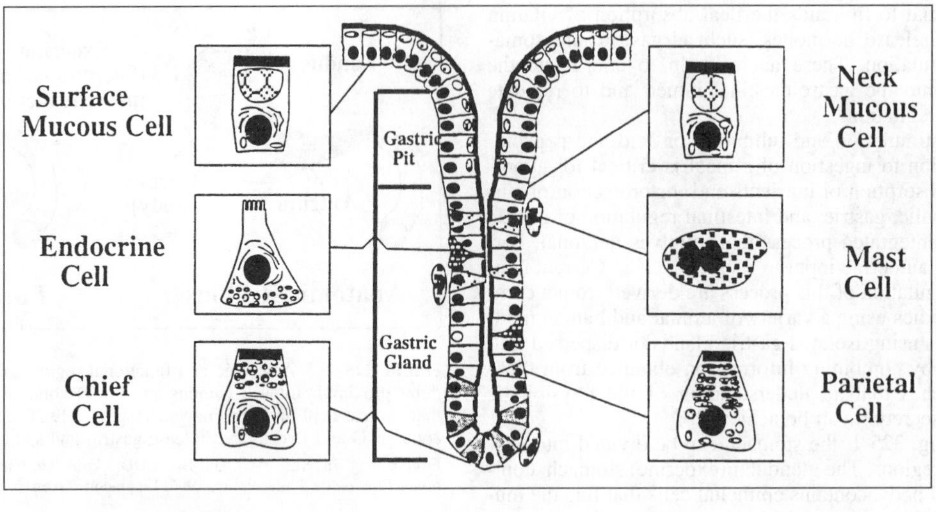

FIGURE 325-2 Side view of representative gastric pit and gland. These secretory units stud the mucosa of the fundus and body of the stomach.

Modified from Chang EB, Sitrin MD, and Black DD: *Gastrointestinal, Hepatobiliary, and Nutritional Physiology,* Philadelphia, 1996, Lippincott-Raven.

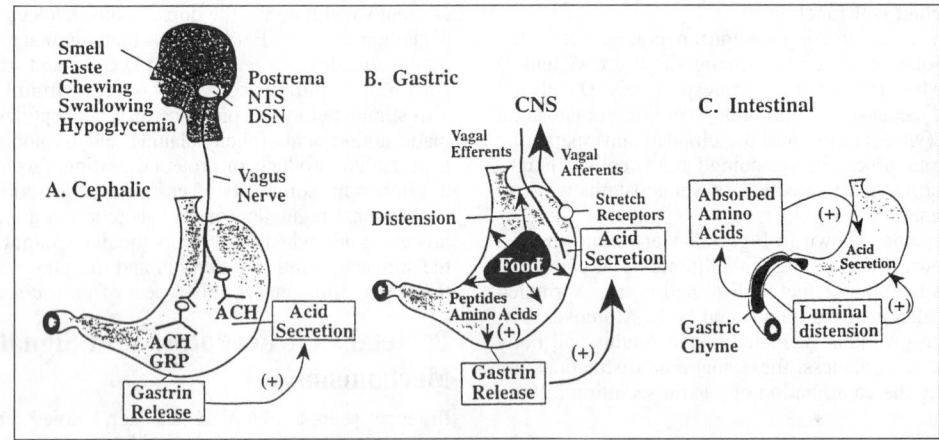

FIGURE 325-3 Regulation of gastric acid secretion. Acid secretion represents an integrated response to **A,** Cephalic, **B,** Gastric, and **C,** Intestinal stimuli. NTS, nucleus tractus solitarius; DSN, dorsal nucleus of vagus nerve; ACh, acetylcholine; GRP, gastrin-releasing peptide.

Modified from Chang EB, Sitrin MD, and Black DD: *Gastrointestinal, Hepatobiliary, and Nutritional Physiology,* Philadelphia, 1996, Lippincott-Raven.

Gastrin binds to gastrin (CCK-B) receptors on ECL cells and stimulates the release of histamine, which, in turn, binds to H_2 receptors on parietal cells, thereby stimulating acid secretion (Fig. 325-4, *right*). Likewise, acetylcholine, released from neurons of the ENS as described earlier, binds to M_1 receptors on ECL cells to cause the release of histamine. Hence the ECL cell plays a pivotal role in regulating acid secretion, and, as proposed by Code and others many years ago, histamine is a "final common pathway" for acid secretion. Evidence from in vitro models indicates a potentiating interaction between acetylcholine and histamine. That is, acid secretion with a combination of acetylcholine and histamine is greater than would be expected from adding the responses observed with these agents acting alone.

Inhibitory Mechanisms

Less is known regarding inhibitory mechanisms that modulate or "shut off" acid secretion. The apical surface of antral G cells is in contact with the gastric lumen, enabling the cells to measure the pH of gastric contents. As gastric pH falls below 3, gastrin release from G cells decreases. Failure of feedback inhibition of gastrin secretion in patients with decreased acid secretion (gastric atrophy or antisecretory therapy) may result in elevated levels of circulating gastrin.

Somatostatin released from mucosal D cells can inhibit gastrin and histamine release. D cells located in the gastric fundus release somatostatin in response to circulating gastrin and to neural (ENS) stimulation by calcitonin gene-related peptide (CGRP). Somatostatin released from these cells interacts with somatostatin type-2 receptors on ECL cells, thereby inhibiting the secretion of histamine. Antral D cells can be stimulated by the ENS and, like G cells, have the ability to sense gastric pH. Hence, as luminal pH falls below 3, somatostatin is released from the ends of long dendritic processes that abut G cells, interacts with specific receptors on these cells, and inhibits gastrin secretion. Antral somatostatin release can also be stimulated by enteric neurons containing peptide neurotransmitters and inhibited by neurons containing acetylcholine. Evidence indicates continuous inhibition of acid secretion by antral somatostatin. It is likely that acetylcholine release stimulates acid secretion, in part, by decreasing the inhibitory influence of somatostatin.

Finally, ECL cells possess inhibitory histamine type-3 (H_3) receptors that allow histamine to act in an autocrine manner. That is, as the concentration of histamine in the pericellular space rises, increased occupation of ECL H_3 receptors inhibits further release of histamine.

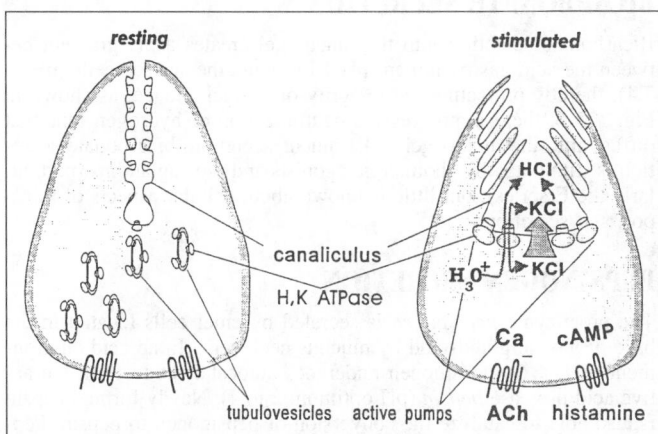

FIGURE 325-4   Activation of gastric parietal cells by acetylcholine (ACh) interacting with M_3 muscarinic receptors and histamine with H_2 histamine receptors on basolateral membranes. In resting parietal cells *(left)* the secretory canaliculus is collapsed and the H^+-K^+-ATPase (proton pump) is present in cytoplasmic tubulovesicles. When the cell is activated *(right)* by acetylcholine and histamine, membranes of tubulovesicles merge with canalicular membranes. The canaliculus expands, as do microvilli on the canalicular surface. The presence of K^+ on the extracytoplasmic aspect of the proton pump is sufficient to activate H^+ (H_3O^+) secretion.

(From Hersey SJ and Sachs G: Gastric acid secretion, *Physiol Rev* 75:155-189, 1995.

Parietal Cell Hydrogen-Potassium-ATPase (H^+-K^+-ATPase)

The secretion of concentrated hydrochloric acid and proteases into the stomach requires cells with unique structural and functional features. With the exception of left ventricular myocytes, gastric parietal cells contain more mitochondria than any other cells in the body, implying an extemely high oxidative capacity. Moreover, numerous interconnecting canaliculi, lined by microvilli, course through the cytoplasm and open to the apical cell surface (Fig. 325-4, *right*). In resting parietal cells the region adjacent to the apical secretory canaliculus contains many tubulovesicles. Stimulation of gastric acid secretion is associated with a decrease in the number of cytoplasmic tubulovesicles and an increase in the size and microvillus surface of the canaliculi, thereby increasing the surface area of the cell some six- to tenfold (Fig. 325-4). Based on these histologic observations Golgi proposed that parietal cells were the source of gastric acid. It is now apparent that the movement and function of the H^+-K^+-ATPase accounts for the morphologic features of gastric parietal cells.

The parietal cell has the unique ability to pump 0.16 N hydrochloric acid across a 10^5- to 10^6-fold concentration gradient (approximately cellular pH 7.4; gastric luminal pH 1 to 2). The membrane-bound H^+-K^+-ATPase, commonly referred to as the *proton pump,* mediates this astonishing feat. This heterodimer consists of an approximately 100-kDa α-subunit and a 34-kDa β-subunit. Evidence indicates that the α-subunit, containing 10 transmembrane segments, is responsible for the ion transport and catalytic properties of the H^+-K^+-ATPase, whereas the β-subunit has a structural and membrane-targeting function.

The driving force for proton transport by the pump appears to be potassium ion. In the resting parietal cell the inactive H^+-K^+-ATPase is found in tubulovesicle membranes that are separate from the secretory canaliculus and do not provide sufficient amounts of K^+ to the luminal surface of the pump (Fig. 325-4, *left*). In contrast, in the activated cell (Fig. 325-4, *right*), the H^+-K^+-ATPase is transported to the apical canalicular membrane, where an active K^+ and Cl^- conductance maintains sufficient K^+ on the extracytoplasmic surface of the pump to activate proton secretion (Fig. 325-5). K^+ is exchanged for H^+ coupled to a cycle of phosphorylation and dephosphorylation of the α-subunit of the enzyme, with magnesium-ATP as the phosphate donor. This process results in the extrusion of 160 mM hydronium ion (H_3O^+) into the membrane-enclosed canaliculus in ex-

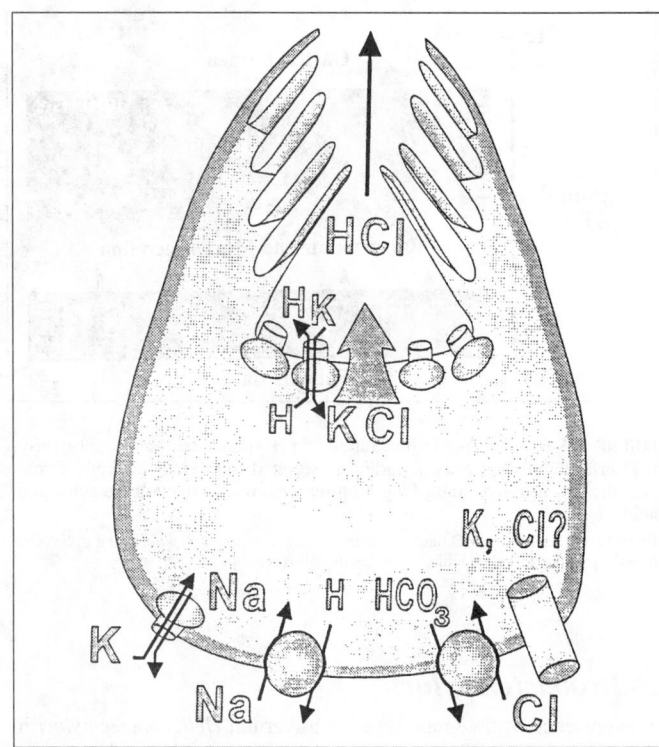

FIGURE 325-5   Model of ion fluxes involved in acid secretion from activated parietal cells. Canalicular membranes contain a KCl transporter that provides suffient K^+ on the extracytoplasmic face of the H^+-K^+-ATPase to drive H^+ secretion. Basolateral membranes contain a variety of K^+ channels, Na^+/H^+ and Cl^-/HCO_3^- exchangers, and a Na^+-K^+-ATPase.

From Hersey SJ and Sachs G: Gastric acid secretion, *Physiol Rev* 75:155-189, 1995.

change for internalization of 140 mM K^+. The availability of K+ in the canalicular lumen is the major, if not only, factor that controls proton transport by the H^+-K^+-ATPase. Finally, pumping of acid (pH $\approx$ 0.8) from the canaliculus through an apical pore into the gastric lumen is apparently mediated solely by hydrostatic forces.

ABNORMALITIES OF GASTRIC ACID SECRETION
Increased Gastric Acid Secretion

Gastric acid hypersecretion (fasting acid secretion >10 mEq/hour) is observed in Zollinger-Ellison syndrome, systemic mastocytosis, and basophilic leukemia. Nevertheless, the most common form of gastric acid hypersecretion is idiopathic. That is, the stimulant for excess acid secretion in these patients is unknown.

In Zollinger-Ellison syndrome a gastrin-secreting tumor (gastrinoma), usually located in the pancreas or duodenum, releases gastrin into the blood stream in an autonomous fashion. Hypergastrinemia results in gastric acid hypersecretion (mediated by histamine release from ECL cells); gastric fold hypertrophy (increased parietal cell mass); and varying gastrointestinal manifestations, including diffuse mucosal ulceration, diarrhea, and esophagitis. Acid hypersecretion in systemic mastocytosis and basophilic leukemia is a consequence of parietal cell stimulation by histamine release from proliferating mast cells and basophils, respectively.

Decreased Gastric Acid Secretion

Gastric atrophy may result in the disappearance of parietal and chief cells, with a consequent decrease in acid and pepsinogen secretion. Moreover, in these patients the absence of intrinsic factor secretion results in pernicious anemia. Although a hyposecretory state had been reported in patients infected with the human immunodeficiency virus, recent studies indicate that this is uncommon.

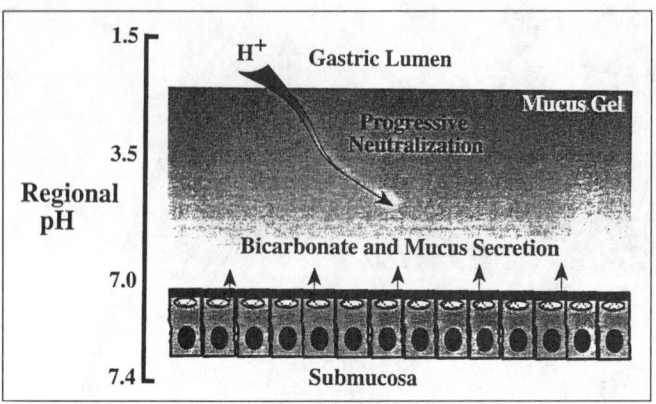

FIGURE 325-6   Schematic illustration of pH gradient in mucus gel overlying surface epithelial cells. Bicarbonate secreted from epithelial cells permeates the gel, thereby establishing a buffer zone that protects these cells from acid.

From Chang EB, Sitrin MD, and Black DD: *Gastrointestinal, Hepatobiliary, and Nutritional Physiology,* Philadelphia, 1996, Lippincott-Raven, p. 67.

Helicobacter pylori

The presence of the gram-negative bacterium *Helicobacter pylori* in the mucus layer of the stomach is strongly associated with the presence of duodenal and gastric ulcers. Moreover, in the United States, approximately 50% of the population harbors this microbe. Hence many investigators have examined the effect on acid secretion of colonization or infection of the stomach with this organism.

Depending on the stage of infection, *H. pylori* may be associated with hyposecretion, normal secretion, or hypersecretion of gastric acid. Acute infection has been associated with profound hypochlorhydria that may facilitate growth of the organism in the stomach. Basal secretion generally returns to normal several months after infection, despite persistence of the microorganism. Nonetheless, acid secretion in response to a meal or stimulation with gastrin-releasing peptide (GRP) may be 2- to 3-fold greater than normal. Finally, over years, the extension of gastritis proximally from the antrum to the fundus may result in gastric mucosal atrophy with a reduction in acid secretory capacity.

Hypochlorhydria associated with acute *H. pylori* infection may be caused by direct effects on parietal cells by bacterial lipopolysaccharides and cytokines (e.g., interleukin (IL)-1β, IL-6, IL-8, and tumor necrosis factor) that are part of the inflammatory response, or by an acid inhibitory factor released by the bacterium. Chronic *H. pylori* infection is associated with increased basal gastrin secretion, increased meal- or GRP-stimulated gastrin release, and decreased expression of somatostatin. These findings may account for the exaggerated acid response and the loss of normal inhibitory controls observed in patients infected with *H. pylori*.

MUCUS SECRETION

Generally, gastric mucus is a clear viscid secretion—consisting of mucin, epithelial cells, leukocytes, bicarbonate, and inorganic salts suspended in water—that protects the surface epithelium (Fig. 325-6). Mucin is composed of hydrophilic glycopeptides that form a gel that is 95% water. The glycosidic portion, attached at serine and threonine residues, makes up 85% of the molecular weight (>500 kDa) of mucin. The nonglycosylated portion of mucin serves as a site for disulfide cross-linkages, thereby creating an insoluble gel.

The insoluble mucus gel covers most of the mucosal surface of the stomach. Degradation of mucus by gastric peptic activity results in the formation of soluble mucin, which lubricates partially digested food in the stomach. Although it appears that mucus secretion occurs continuously, little is known regarding the cellular regulation of mucous cells. Nevertheless, cholinergic agonists and prostaglandins are known to stimulate mucus secretion.

BICARBONATE SECRETION

Bicarbonate secretion into the mucus gel creates a pH gradient between the acid gastric lumen (pH 1 to 3) and the surface cells (pH ≈ 7.4), thereby protecting the integrity of the gel. Hence, as shown in Fig. 325-6, there is progressive neutralization of hydrogen ions that diffuse into the mucus gel. Like mucus secretion, bicarbonate secretion is stimulated by cholinergic agonists and prostaglandins (particularly the E series), but little is known about cellular aspects of transport and secretion.

PEPSINOGEN SECRETION

The proenzyme *pepsinogen* is secreted by chief cells located in the base of gastric glands and by mucous neck cells. In an acid environment (pH < 6), pepsinogen undergoes autocatalysis to form the active acid protease *pepsin* (pH optimum 2 to 4). Newly formed pepsin is also able to catalyze the conversion of pepsinogen to pepsin. Peptic digestion of proteins results in the formation of large peptide fragments, *peptones,* that are futher digested in the small intestine. In the gastric antrum and duodenum, peptones stimulate the release of gut hormones, such as gastrin and cholecystokinin.

Chief Cell Receptors and Signal Transduction Mechanisms

Current concepts regarding receptors on gastric chief cells and signal transduction pathways that are activated when these receptors are activated by their respective ligands are shown in Fig. 325-7. Two major pathways mediate pepsinogen secretion. Agents such as cholecystokinin (CCK), gastrin, and cholinergic agonists (acetylcholine) interact with CCK-A, CCK-B (gastrin), and M_3 muscarinic receptors, respectively, thereby activating phospholipase C, phospholipid turnover, and the production of inositol trisphosphate (IP_3) and diacylglycerol (DAG). IP_3 stimulates the release of calcium from intracellular stores. Calcium interacts with calmodulin to regulate the activity of several kinases and phosphatases. DAG directly activates different isoforms of protein kinase C.

Agents such as vasoactive intestinal peptide (VIP) and secretin interact with specific chief cell receptors to activate adenylyl cyclase, thereby causing an increase in cellular levels of cyclic AMP. Cyclic AMP activates a cAMP-dependent protein kinase (protein kinase A). Although it seems clears that prostaglandins of the E and A series interact with receptors that are linked to adenylyl cyclase, the effects of this interaction are concentration-dependent and differ depending on the prostaglandin concentration and the species examined. Whereas low concentrations of prostaglandins appear to inhibit pepsinogen secretion, high concentrations may actually stimulate secretion. The actions of histamine, a weak stimulant of pepsinogen secretion, appear to be mediated by the adenylyl cyclase system.

Inhibitory peptides, peptide-YY (PYY), neuropeptide-Y (NPY), and somatostatin interact with chief cell receptors linked to adenylyl cyclase. Nevertheless, it has not been demonstrated in vivo that these inhibitory peptides play a role in modulating pepsinogen secretion.

The phospholipase and adenylyl cyclase pathways share common features. In both, cellular receptors are linked to effector enzymes by guanine nucleotide binding (G) proteins: G_q for activation of the phospholipase C pathway, G_s for activation of the adenylyl cyclase pathway, and G_i for inhibition of the adenylyl cyclase pathway. Moreover, both signaling cascades result in the activation of kinases or phosphatases that cause phosphorylation or dephosphorylation, respectively, of presently undefined protein substrates. "Cross-talk" between these signaling pathways may further modulate proenzyme secretion. Ultimately, these phosphorylation events lead to migration of proenzyme-laden zymogen granules to the luminal surface of the cell, fusion of granule membranes with the plasma membrane, and release of pepsinogen into the lumen of the gastric gland.

Regulation of Pepsinogen Secretion

Despite the scheme shown in Fig. 325-7, little is known about in vivo regulation of pepsinogen secretion. Direct determination of chief cell responses in vivo are masked by fluid fluxes from the cells of the

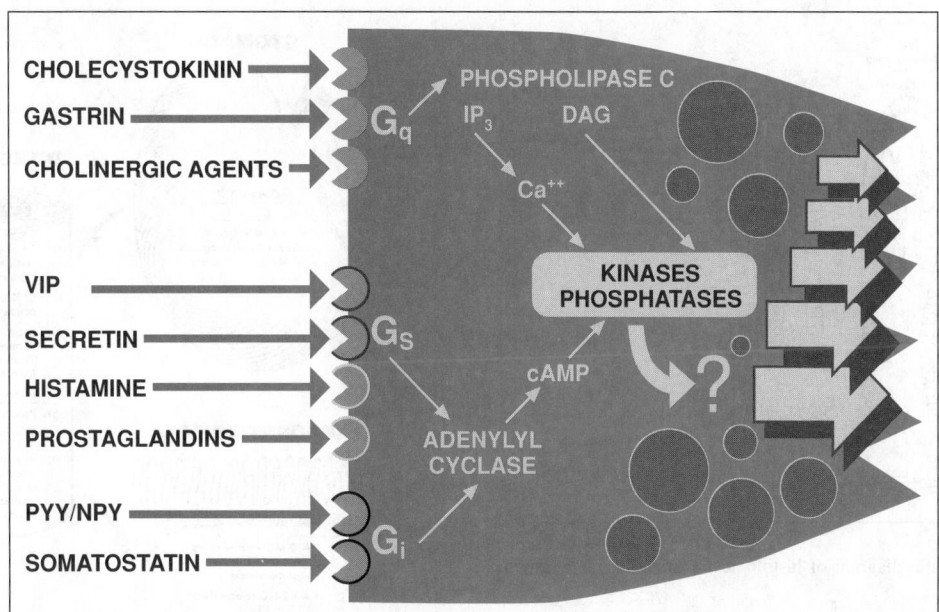

FIGURE 325-7 Cartoon illustrating receptors and signal transduction mechanisms in gastric chief cells. Details represent information obtained from experiments using chief cells from various mammals, including humans. The question mark indicates that protein substrates for activated kinases and phosphatases are currently unknown. *VIP*, Vasoactive intestinal peptide; *PYY*, peptide-YY; *NPY*, neuropeptide-Y; *IP$_3$*, inositol trisphosphate; *DAG*, diacylglycerol.

Modified from Raufman JFP, *Yale J Biol Med*, 69(1):85-90, Jan/Feb 1997.

gastric pit. Hence it is difficult to determine the actual responses of chief cells to in vivo stimuli.

BIBLIOGRAPHY

Helander HF, Keeling DJ: Cell biology of gastric acid secretion, *Bailliere Clin Gastroenterol* 7:1, 1993.

Hersey SJ, Sachs G: Gastric acid secretion, *Physiol Rev* 75:155, 1995.

McGowan CC et al: *Helicobacter pylori* and gastric acid: biological and therapeutic implications, *Gastroenterology* 110:926, 1996.

Raufman JP: Gastric chief cells: receptors and signal transduction mechanisms, *Gastroenterology* 102:699, 1992.

Sachs G et al: The pharmacology of the gastric acid pump: the H^+, K^+ ATPase, *Ann Rev Pharmacol Toxicol* 35:277, 1995.

Schubert ML, Makhlouf GM: Neural, hormonal, and paracrine regulation of gastrin and acid secretion, *Yale J Biol Med* 65:553, 1992.

CHAPTER

326 Intestinal Absorption

Jerry S. Trier

The complex processes of digestion and absorption that take place in the stomach, small intestine, and colon of normal human beings are remarkably efficient. An adult who eats an average Western diet ingests approximately 100 g of fat, 400 g of carbohydrate, 100 g of protein, and 1.5 to 2.0 L of fluid per day. This diet also contains substantial amounts of sodium, chloride, potassium, and calcium as well as small amounts of other essential elements and vitamins. An additional load of roughly 7 L of endogenous fluids—including biliary, gastric, and pancreatic secretions—enters the intestine. These endogenous secretions contain substantial quantities of ions, protein, cholesterol, phospholipids, and bile salts. Normally this massive load is reduced by absorption in the small intestine to a volume of 1.0 to 1.5 L, which enters the colon. Further water and ion absorption in the colon results in a stool mass of less than 200 g per day that contains 2 to 6 g of fat, 1 to 2 g of nitrogen, and less than 20 mEq each of sodium, potassium, chloride, and bicarbonate. In this chapter, intestinal digestion and absorption are reviewed briefly, because an understanding of these processes is helpful in assessing alimentary tract diseases in which normal digestion and/or absorption is perturbed.

Because the intestine is a relatively narrow but long tube (12 to 20 ft) with many redundant loops, it uses its allocated space within the abdomen efficiently. Moreover, the surface specializations of the small intestine—which include circular or spiral folds (plicae circulares), microscopic mucosal villi, and ultrastructurally apparent apical microvilli on absorptive cells—amplify the surface presented to the luminal contents to approximately 1000 times that of a cylindrical tube with a flat surface (Fig. 326-1).

Digestion and absorption of most dietary lipids, proteins, and carbohydrates occur with remarkable efficiency in the duodenum and jejunum; therefore these nutrients are usually absorbed before the residual intestinal chyme reaches the ileum. However, substantial absorption of fats, carbohydrates, peptides, and amino acids may occur in the distal small intestine when digestion and absorption in the proximal intestine are compromised by disease. Absorption of calcium, food iron, and folic acid is most efficient in the proximal intestine, whereas absorption of most bile salts and vitamin B$_{12}$ occurs in the ileum. The colon absorbs water, sodium, chloride, and bicarbonate efficiently. In patients with carbohydrate malabsorption, and, to a lesser degree, in normal individuals, the colon also conserves carbohydrate by absorbing more than 50% of the breakdown products of bacterial carbohydrate metabolism.

During absorption, the end-products of digestion must first traverse the intestinal epithelial barrier to gain access to the terminal capillaries and lymphatics in the core of the villus for distribution to distant sites. This is accomplished by two major transport mechanisms: passive diffusion and active transport (Box 326-1). Substances absorbed by *passive diffusion* follow either a chemical gradient from a high to low concentration or, if the molecule is charged, an electrical gradient. Neither energy nor a membrane carrier is required for

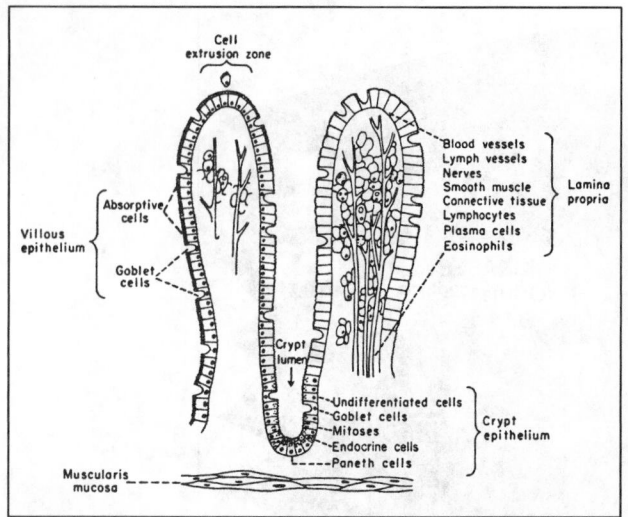

FIGURE 326-1 Schematic diagram of histologic organization of the small intestinal mucosa.

BOX 326-1

Primary mechanism of absorption of some specific nutrients*

Active transport	Diffusion
Glucose	Short- and medium-chain
Galactose	fatty acids
Amino acids	2-Monoglycerides
Di- and tripeptides	Lysophospholipids
Na^+	Cholesterol
Cl^-	Vitamin D, carotenoids
Iron	K^+
Vitamin B_{12}	H_2O
Ca^{2+}	Fructose (facilitated diffusion)

*There is also substantial passive diffusion of Na^+ and Cl^-, especially in the upper small intestine.

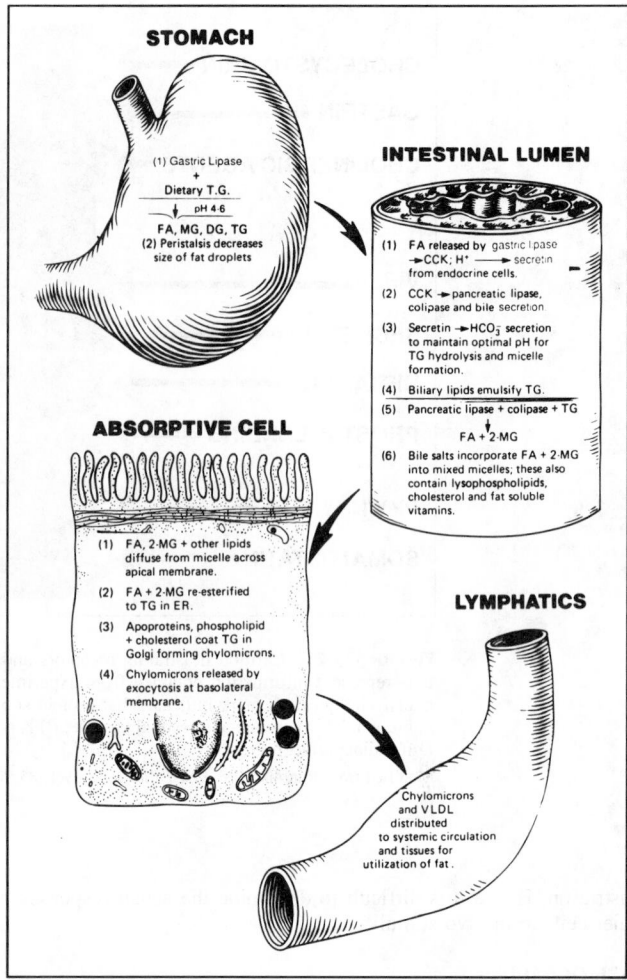

FIGURE 326-2 The location of major events of dietary fat absorption. *FA*, Fatty acid; *MG*, monoglyceride; *DG*, diglyceride; *TG*, triglyceride; *CCK*, cholecystokinin; *ER*, endoplasmic reticulum; *VLDL*, very-low-density lipoprotein.

---

passive diffusion. Examples of substances absorbed by this mechanism include the products of triglyceride hydrolysis and, in the small intestine, potassium. Substances absorbed by *active transport* move against osmotic or chemical gradients from low to high concentrations and, if charged, against electrical gradients. During active transport, energy is expended, and selective carriers or pumps, membrane proteins that facilitate transport across membranes against gradients, are required.

Two other transport mechanisms are facilitated diffusion and endocytosis. *Facilitated diffusion,* like passive diffusion, requires no energy and follows osmotic and chemical gradients but occurs more rapidly than passive diffusion, presumably because a carrier is present. Fructose appears to be absorbed by facilitated diffusion. *Endocytosis* permits bulk or receptor-mediated transport of large molecules such as intact proteins. During endocytosis, small regions of the apical plasma membrane first indent the absorptive cell cytoplasm. These regions then pinch off, forming small, membrane-bounded vesicles containing luminal contents that are then processed in the cell or that may traverse and then leave the cell cytoplasm by subsequent fusion of the vesicle membrane with the basolateral membrane. Endocytosis is important in transcellular calcium transport and in intestinal transport of colostral immunoglobulin in some neonatal mammals. Endocytosis also plays a role in sampling of luminal antigens in adults. Receptor-mediated endocytosis of regulatory peptides such as vasoactive intestinal peptide by the basolateral membrane of intestinal epithelial cells may be important in the regulation of certain intestinal transport processes, such as electrolyte transport.

ABSORPTION OF LIPIDS

Normally, most dietary fats consist of long-chain triglycerides, which, if not hydrolyzed and dispersed, are not absorbed by the small intestine. The steps involved in triglyceride digestion and absorption are summarized in Fig. 326-2. Triglyceride digestion begins in the stomach, where gastric peristalsis reduces the size of triglyceride droplets and facilitates contact with a lipase secreted by gastric chief cells. This gastric lipase is acid-stable, with a pH optimum that ranges from 2.2 to 6. It releases fatty acids from triglycerides in the stomach. Initial intragastric lipid digestion is probably of substantial physiologic importance, since it appears responsible for hydrolysis of 10% to 30% of dietary triglyceride. The fatty acids released by the process emulsify triglycerides and stimulate the release of cholecystokinin from the duodenal mucosa, which in turn stimulates secretion of pancreatic lipase and bile into the duodenal lumen. Gastric lipase is normally ineffective in the lumen of the intestine because its pH optimum is exceeded and the enzyme is inhibited by bile salts. In patients with pancreatic exocrine insufficiency, it appears to account for the majority of intraluminal lipid hydrolysis.

As gastric contents enter the duodenum, hydrogen ions release secretin from the duodenal mucosa. Secretin stimulates pancreatic and bile duct bicarbonate secretion. Secretion of bicarbonate normally maintains the intraluminal pH at approximately 6.5, an optimum level for intraluminal fat digestion and dispersion. Bile salts, together with biliary lecithin and cholesterol, emulsify dietary fats to small droplets, increasing their surface area. Emulsification is important because pancreatic lipase works only at the surface of the fat droplet. Pancreatic lipase hydrolyzes long-chain triglycerides at the α-ester linkages, releasing a mixture of free fatty acids and 2-monoglycerides. Colipase, a small protein also secreted by the pancreas, is necessary for this hydrolysis; it facilitates attachment of pancreatic lipase to the surfaces of the triglyceride droplets and blocks bile salt inhibition of pancreatic lipase. Dietary and biliary phospholipids such as lecithin are hydrolyzed intraluminally by phospholipase A_2 at their 2-ester linkage, whereas sphingolipids appear to be hydrolyzed by a specific brush border enzyme. Cholesterol esters and several other lipids are hydrolyzed by a bile salt–stimulated carboxyl ester lipase secreted by the pancreas. These reactions add additional fatty acids, 1-lysophospholipids, and absorbable unesterified cholesterol to the intraluminal contents.

Bile salts synthesized in the liver and secreted in the bile as glycine and taurine conjugates of cholic and chenodeoxycholic acid play a crucial role in dispersing this complex mixture of lipolytic products for intestinal absorption. These detergents have both hydrophilic and hydrophobic domains and, at their normal intraluminal concentration of 5 to 10 mM, form water-soluble micelles. The micelles then incorporate the products of fat digestion and other lipids, such as fat-soluble vitamins, forming a clear solution of mixed micelles. The hydrophobic (nonpolar) molecular domains are located inside the mixed micelle; the hydrophilic (polar) molecular domains are at the aqueous interface on their surface. Larger vesicles that are composed of mixed lipids saturated with bile salts are up to ten times the diameter of mixed micelles and also form in the proximal intestine during postprandial fat digestion. Vesicles require less bile salt than do micelles for solubilizing the products of lipid digestion; therefore they may be of great importance in maintaining fat absorption in bile salt–deficient patients.

Mixed micelles and vesicles shuttle the products of intraluminal digestion through the unstirred water and mucous layers to the apical surfaces of intestinal absorptive cells. Although for years it was assumed that the lipid components of mixed micelles and liposomes diffused across the lipid-rich plasma membrane, recent studies suggest the presence of a carrier that is specific for long-chain fatty acids in the brush border membrane. The majority of conjugated bile salt molecules remain in the lumen to be absorbed subsequently in the ileum by an efficient Na^+-dependent active transport mechanism. Bile salts are returned via the portal circulation to the liver, where they are again secreted in the bile. This enterohepatic circulation of bile salts recycles the major portion of the 4-g bile salt pool approximately six to eight times daily with such efficiency that less than 0.4 g normally passes into the colon for excretion in the stool (Chapter 349).

Once in the absorptive cell cytoplasm, fatty acids bind to a fatty acid–binding protein that facilitates their rapid transfer to the cisterns of the endoplasmic reticulum. There, the long-chain fatty acids, monoglycerides, and diglycerides are enzymatically esterified to triglycerides. Next, nascent chylomicra are formed largely in the Golgi material of the absorptive cells, where specific apoproteins synthesized in the endoplasmic reticulum, phospholipids, and cholesterol coat the triglyceride droplet. Chylomicra leave the absorptive cells by exocytosis after migrating to the basolateral membrane in vesicles derived from the Golgi material. The chylomicra then enter the intestinal mucosal lymphatic lacteals for distribution to the general circulation.

Because absorption of dietary fat is a complex phenomenon, it is not surprising that it can be impaired by diverse disease processes. For example, the intraluminal phase of fat digestion can be altered (1) after partial or total gastric resection, which would interfere with gastric lipase digestion; (2) in pancreatic insufficiency, which would result in lipase and colipase deficiency; (3) in states with massive gastric acid hypersecretion or bicarbonate hyposecretion, which result in too low a pH in the intestinal lumen for optimal lipolysis and lipid dispersion; (4) in hepatobiliary disease, which results in impaired delivery of conjugated bile salts to the intestinal lumen; and (5) in extensive ileal disease, which results in interruption of the enterohepatic circulation of bile salts. The uptake of properly digested fat by the intestinal mucosa can be impaired by the reduction of the absorptive surface by massive intestinal resection or by mucosal diseases such

as celiac sprue. Intracellular triglyceride reesterification is impaired in mucosal diseases that cause absorptive-cell damage, such as celiac sprue. Exit of dietary fat from absorptive cells is defective in abetalipoproteinemia, in which chylomicron formation or secretion is defective. Finally, distribution of absorbed lipid to the general circulation is defective in disease states, such as retroperitoneal neoplasm or primary intestinal lymphangiectasia, that are associated with lymphatic blockage.

Triglycerides composed of medium-chain fatty acids (6 to 10 carbon atoms) are more readily hydrolyzed by pancreatic lipase. In addition, the intestine can absorb intact medium-chain triglycerides to some degree. Unlike long-chain fatty acids, medium-chain fatty acids are not resynthesized after uptake by absorptive cells, but enter the intestinal capillaries and then the portal vessels as free fatty acids. This simpler absorptive process for medium-chain triglycerides has led to their use as effective, albeit expensive, dietary supplements for patients with diseases associated with impaired fat assimilation.

ABSORPTION OF CARBOHYDRATES

Dietary carbohydrates consist largely of polysaccharide starch, the disaccharides sucrose and lactose, and small amounts of the monosaccharides glucose and fructose. Starch has two components, amylose and amylopectin. These are efficiently digested intraluminally by salivary and pancreatic amylases to α-limit dextrans, composed of 4 to 10 glucose molecules, and to the disaccharide maltose and the trisaccharide maltotriose.

Dietary disaccharides and the products of intraluminal starch digestion do not cross the intestinal epithelial barrier, but must first be digested to their constituent monosaccharides glucose, galactose, and fructose. This occurs at the level of the microvillus, where the enzymes glucoamylase, maltase, sucrase, and lactase form an integral part of the microvillus membrane. Hydrolysis of disaccharides is more rapid than uptake of monosaccharides, except for lactose, which is hydrolyzed at a slower rate than the released monosaccharides are absorbed.

Glucose and galactose are absorbed by an energy-requiring active transport process that involves an integral membrane 75 kD protein Na^+/glucose cotransporter that has been cloned and sequenced. Glucose and galactose are then transported out of the cell by GLUT2, a transporter that is not Na^+-coupled. Sodium is transported out of the cell by a sodium-potassium-adenosine triphosphatase (Na^+-K^+-ATPase) in the basolateral membrane, which also provides energy for the process. Fructose absorption is by facilitated diffusion utilizing a transporter designated GLUT5 on the apical cell surface and GLUT2 on the basolateral cell surface and does not require energy.

Because the amount of amylase secreted normally by the pancreas greatly exceeds what is needed for normal polysaccharide digestion, malabsorption of carbohydrates in disease states usually involves defective digestion or transport at the level of the intestinal mucosa. Examples include primary disaccharidase deficiency (lactase deficiency); a defect in the Na^+/glucose cotransporter (glucose-galactose malabsorption); or a reduction in the absorptive surface, resulting in secondary disaccharidase deficiency and impaired monosaccharide transport (celiac sprue).

ABSORPTION OF PROTEIN

Intraluminal digestion of dietary protein begins in the stomach, although only a small fraction of dietary protein is hydrolyzed by gastric pepsin. However, the amino acid and polypeptide products of intragastric protein hydrolysis release cholecystokinin, the major stimulus for secretion of pancreatic proteases, from the duodenal mucosa. Pancreatic proteases are secreted as inactive precursors that must be activated by hydrolysis of a peptide bond in each enzyme molecule. Such activation is initiated through the conversion of trypsinogen to trypsin by enterokinase, an enzyme adherent to the microvillus membrane of duodenal absorptive cells. Trypsin activates additional trypsinogen, as well as all other pancreatic proteolytic proenzymes. Some of the pancreatic proteases are endopeptidases (trypsin, chymotrypsin, and elastase), which hydrolyze peptide bonds in the interior of the protein molecule; others are exopeptidases (carboxypeptidases), which hydrolyze peptide bonds at the carboxyl terminus of protein molecules. The products of pancreatic protease digestion include neutral and basic amino acids and small peptides composed of two to six amino acid residues.

Like disaccharidases, some peptidases are located within the microvillus membrane as integral membrane proteins. Other peptidases are located within the cytoplasm of the epithelial cells. The microvillus membrane peptidases hydrolyze some of the small peptide products of pancreatic protease digestion to dipeptides and amino acids at the surfaces of absorptive cells. In contrast to disaccharides, which must all be hydrolyzed to monosaccharides before absorption, certain dipeptides and tripeptides (such as diglycine, glycylleucine, and triglycine) are efficiently absorbed by an energy-requiring peptide transporter that appears also to transport protons. Because the portal effluent from the intestine mainly contains amino acids, after absorption these small peptides are hydrolyzed by cytosolic peptidases to their constituent amino acids.

There are several transport mechanisms for the absorption of the different classes of amino acids. Most are energy requiring, at least partially sodium-dependent, and selective for the L-stereoisomers. Three transport neutral amino acids (the neutral brush border transporter, the phenylalanine carrier, and the imino carrier). There is also some transport of leucine by facilitated diffusion. Acidic and basic amino acids are each handled by separate carriers. Thus genetic defects in amino acid transport mechanisms, as occur in cystinuria and Hartnup disease, result in defective transport of only those selected amino acids that use the specific carrier that is absent or abnormal.

The absorption of certain dipeptides, such as glycylleucine, is more efficient than the absorption of equimolar mixtures of their constituent free amino acids. This has clinical implications in nutrition therapy, because not only are dipeptides more readily absorbed but they also present less of an intraluminal osmotic load, a characteristic that is especially desirable in patients with intestinal mucosal diseases.

There is evidence that very small amounts of intact proteins breach the epithelial barrier of the intestine. Much of this transport probably occurs via M cells in epithelium overlying lymphoid follicles (Chapter 327) and is important to the afferent limb of the intestinal immune response.

WATER AND ION ABSORPTION

Transport of water and the major ions Na^+, K^+, Cl^-, and HCO_3^- in the human intestine is complicated and not yet fully understood. This is not surprising, because the gut is lined by heterogeneous populations of epithelial cells whose capacity for absorption of ions and water varies. For example, whereas the major function of villus absorptive cells is to absorb, there is evidence that the less differentiated crypt cells secrete water and ions into the gut lumen. Net fluid and ion transport in the gut depends on the balance between absorption and secretion. Absorption predominates under normal conditions; however, in certain toxigenic enteric bacterial infections, with certain hormone-secreting tumors, and in some primary intestinal mucosal diseases, secretion may greatly exceed absorption, with devastating consequences.

There are two pathways by which small molecules, such as water and ions, may cross the mucosa: the paracellular and transcellular pathways. *Paracellular transport* requires penetration only of the tight junctions that connect adjacent epithelial cells at the apex of the lateral membrane, with subsequent diffusion along the lateral intercellular space. There is evidence that the tight junctions connecting adjacent small intestinal epithelial cells are quite permeable, especially to cations, and that the paracellular pathway is a major site of transepithelial water transport and also some ion transport. Transport via the paracellular pathway is passive and therefore follows electrochemical, osmotic, and hydrostatic gradients. Intestinal permeability is greater in the proximal than in the distal intestine. Recent studies suggest that tight junction permeability increases when the mucosa is exposed to an osmolar load, as occurs during normal alimentation. *Transcellular transport* of ions requires their passage through two membrane barriers—the apical plasma membrane and the basolateral plasma membrane—as well as through the cytosol. Because plasma membranes are predominantly lipoidal, diffusion of hydrophilic molecules is limited, and membrane transporters facilitate transcellular ion movement.

Na^+ transport is both active and passive along the length of the small intestine and the colon. Several mechanisms are involved: (1) coupled neutral NaCl entry, which may involve Na^+-H^+ and Cl^--HCO_3^- exchange at the apical surface in the small intestine and colon; (2) Na^+ cotransport with sugars and amino acids in the small intestine, the basis for oral rehydration solutions for the treatment of infectious diarrhea; and (3) electrogenic Na^+ absorption at all levels of the small and large intestine that use Na-K-ATPase, which is located in the epithelial cell basolateral membrane. Unlike Na^+ transport, K^+ transport appears passive in the small intestine, but there is active absorption and secretion in the colon, with secretion predominating. HCO_3^- appears to be secreted actively by the duodenum, ileum, and colon, whereas Cl^- is normally absorbed actively in the ileum and colon. Water movement is by passive diffusion throughout the intestine and follows osmotic and hydrostatic gradients. Water transport can contribute to ion transport by the mechanism of solvent drag. During this process the solutes not filtered out by the cell membrane or tight junctions are carried along by the moving stream of solvent.

ABSORPTION OF IRON

To maintain iron balance, the healthy adult male must absorb 0.5 to 1.0 mg per day, whereas the healthy adult female requires 1.5 to 2.0 mg per day during her reproductive years. Because normal iron intake in the Western diet averages 10 to 20 mg, the absorption of iron is a highly regulated process in which the gastrointestinal tract plays a major role in maintaining homeostasis, because intake exceeds needs. In iron deficiency, iron absorption increases; in iron excess, except in idiopathic hemochromatosis, iron absorption decreases. Heme iron from animal tissues is absorbed by the intestine more effectively than iron from cereals and vegetables. Inorganic iron is less avidly absorbed than food iron, but divalent ferrous ion is absorbed more efficiently than trivalent ferric ion.

Absorption of iron, especially of inorganic iron, is most efficient in the duodenum. Heme iron and nonheme iron are absorbed by distinctive mechanisms. During the absorption of hemoglobin iron, the heme moiety is split from globin by intraluminal proteolytic hydrolysis and is absorbed intact after binding to a membrane receptor. Heme is then degraded within the absorptive cell, releasing inorganic iron into the portal circulation.

Within the gut lumen, inorganic iron forms chelates with ascorbic acid, amino acids, and sugar. In the case of ferric ion, this process is enhanced by hydrochloric acid in the stomach. Such chelation enhances the solubility of iron in the more alkaline environment of the duodenum. Inorganic iron then enters absorptive cells via a saturable process. The regulation of mucosal iron absorption remains incompletely understood but may involve a specific 56-kD iron-binding protein on the brush border, mucosal iron content, ferritin, transferrin receptors and transferrin saturation, and erythropoietin.

Acute or prolonged excessive iron intake can overwhelm the mucosal regulatory process and result in acute iron toxicity or iron overload. Moreover, in patients with idiopathic hemochromatosis, the mucosal regulatory process may be defective, and amounts of iron greater than the body needs are absorbed. The importance of the duodenum in iron absorption is underscored by the high prevalence of iron deficiency in patients with mucosal lesions involving the proximal intestine (such as in celiac sprue) or in patients in whom the duodenum has been surgically bypassed (e.g., after partial gastrectomy with gastrojejunostomy).

ABSORPTION OF CALCIUM

Of the 1 g of calcium ingested daily in the average Western diet and the 300 mg added by endogenous secretions, 900 mg is excreted in the stool, resulting in a net normal gain of approximately 100 mg per day via the gut. In individuals who are not increasing or decreasing total body calcium, this 100 mg is excreted in the urine. Calcium is absorbed most avidly by the duodenum by an active transport mechanism, but substantial absorption that is adaptable to body needs also occurs in the small bowel distal to the duodenum. Thus the intestine is important in maintaining calcium homeostasis.

Vitamin D plays a key role in regulating calcium absorption. After its absorption from the gut or its production in the skin, vitamin D is hydroxylated in the 25 position in the liver and in the 1 position in the kidney to 1,25-dihydroxycholecalciferol. This active form of vitamin D then binds to a specific receptor in the small intestinal epithelium. There it stimulates calcium transport by mechanisms that are not fully understood. After carrier-mediated uptake across the apical membrane, calcium binds to calbindin D for transport through the absorptive cell cytoplasm and is extruded across the basolateral membrane by Ca^{2+}-ATPase. There is also evidence that there may be some transport of calcium via the paracellular pathway by a process that is not saturable or vitamin D–dependent, especially in the distal small intestine.

Mucosal lesions of the small intestine may result in direct impairment of calcium transport. Impaired intraluminal digestion and mucosal lesions also result in impaired vitamin D absorption. Steatorrhea facilitates formation of insoluble calcium soaps of fatty acids, decreasing the availability of soluble calcium for intestinal absorption.

ABSORPTION OF VITAMIN B₁₂

Although the requirement for vitamin B_{12} (cobalamin) is less than 2 μg per day, its absorption by the intestine is complex. After its release from foodstuffs of animal origin, vitamin B_{12} binds to several glycoproteins, or R-binders, found in saliva, gastric juice, and bile. In the upper small intestine, pancreatic proteases hydrolyze the R-binders, releasing vitamin B_{12}, which then binds to intrinsic factor (IF), a 44,000-dalton protein secreted in humans by gastric parietal cells. IF-B_{12} complex is resistant to intraluminal proteolysis and arrives intact in the distal ileum, where it binds to a specific receptor present only on the microvillus membrane of ileal absorptive cells. The mechanism involved in the subsequent transfer of vitamin B_{12} into and across the ileal epithelium and the mechanism of its release from IF are poorly understood. However, several hours after IF-B_{12} binds to the apical surface of ileal absorptive cells, B_{12} appears in the circulation complexed to transcobalamin II. Transcobalamin II delivers vitamin B_{12} to tissues and is the most important circulating B_{12} transport protein. A substantial amount of vitamin B_{12} is stored in the liver, normally enough to meet the body's needs for 4 to 5 years. Therefore factors inducing impaired B_{12} assimilation may be present for several years before B_{12} deficiency becomes evident.

Because of the complexity of vitamin B_{12} assimilation, abnormalities in several alimentary tract organs can impair its absorption. These include (1) gastric mucosal atrophy, which results in IF deficiency; (2) pancreatic exocrine insufficiency, which may, because of impaired intraluminal proteolysis, decrease B_{12} release from R-binders; (3) ileal mucosal disease, which results in decreased absorptive cell receptors for IF-B_{12}; and (4) conditions that result in long-term intraluminal bacterial overgrowth in the small intestine because bacteria in the small intestine may competitively bind and absorb B_{12}, reducing its availability for ileal absorption.

ABSORPTION OF FOLATES

Fruits, vegetables, liver, and yeast are important dietary sources of folates, of which roughly 90% are polyglutamate conjugates. Because pteroylmonoglutamate is absorbed much more effectively than pteroylpolyglutamates, deconjugation is an essential step in folate absorption. Folate conjugase is present in the microvillus membrane of duodenal and jejunal absorptive cells. The monoglutamate is then transported by the absorptive cell largely by a saturable process that appears to involve monoglutamate: OH^- exchange. The rate of hydrolysis greatly exceeds that of transport, which is rate limiting. The capacity for folate absorption is greatest in the duodenum and jejunum; consequently, the diseases in which mucosal lesions are most severe in the proximal intestine (e.g., celiac sprue) are frequently associated with folate deficiency. Unlike vitamin B_{12}, liver stores are usually sufficient to sustain body folate needs for only 2 to 3 months.

BIBLIOGRAPHY

Alpers DH: Digestion and absorption of carbohydrates and proteins. In Johnson LR, editor: *Physiology of the gastrointestinal tract,* ed 3, vol 2, New York, 1994, Raven Press, p. 1723.

Chang EG, Rao MC: Intestinal water and electrolyte transport mechanisms of physiological and adaptive responses. In Johnson LR, editor: *Physiology of the gastrointestinal tract,* ed 3, vol 2, New York, 1994, Raven Press, p. 2027.
Gray GM: Dietary protein processing: intraluminal and enterocyte surface events. In Schultz SG, editor: *Handbook of physiology,* vol 4, Bethesda, Md, 1991, American Physiological Society, p. 411.
Hamosh M: Gastric and lingual lipases. In Johnson LR, editor: *Physiology of the gastrointestinal tract,* ed 3, vol 2, New York, 1994, Raven Press, p. 1239.
Madara JL, Trier JS: The functional morphology of the mucosa of the small intestine. In Johnson LR, editor: *Physiology of the gastrointestinal tract,* ed 3, vol 2, New York, 1994, Raven Press, p. 1577.
Nemere I, Norman AW: Transport of calcium. In Schultz SG, editor: *Handbook of physiology,* vol 4, Bethesda, Md, 1991, American Physiological Society, p. 337.
Schron CM: Vitamins and minerals. In Yamada T, editor: *Textbook of gastroenterology,* Philadelphia, 1995, JB Lippincott, p. 467.
Tso P: Intestinal lipid absorption. In Johnson LR, editor: *Physiology of the gastrointestinal tract,* ed 3, vol 2, New York, 1994, Raven Press, p. 1867.
Wright, EM: The intestinal Na⁺/glucose contransporter, *Ann Rev Physiol* 55:575, 1993.

CHAPTER

327 Intestinal Immunity

Martin F. Kagnoff

The gastrointestinal tract contains approximately 25% of the lymphoid tissue in the body. Gut-associated lymphoid tissue (GALT) is exposed continually to materials from the external environment such as food antigens, bacteria, bacterial products, viruses, and parasites. In addition, the GALT is a key component of the more generalized mucosal immune system, which includes lymphoid tissue in the respiratory tract, genitourinary tract, and mammary glands. Intestinal immune reactions normally play an important role in host protection. However, abnormalities in intestinal mucosal immune function may contribute to allergic and autoimmune disorders and to specific intestinal diseases such as ulcerative colitis, Crohn's disease, and celiac disease (Chapters 340 and 341). The importance of the intestinal immune system in host protection is perhaps best highlighted in the clinical syndromes that involve deficiencies in either immunoglobulin production (e.g., selective IgA deficiency, common variable immunodeficiency syndromes) or T-cell function (e.g., acquired immunodeficiency syndrome).

GUT-ASSOCIATED LYMPHOID TISSUE

The immune system in the intestine has three major lymphoid components. These components are the Peyer's patches, the lamina propria lymphoid cells, and the intraepithelial lymphocytes. These three components are anatomically distinct and differ in their content of B- and T-lymphocyte subsets. Nonetheless, it is important to note that these three components are interrelated in terms of function.

Peyer's Patches and Lymphocyte Migration

Peyer's patches are instrumental in the generation of the intestinal mucosal immune response. These lymphoid structures contain collections of lymphoid follicles and are present predominantly in the distal small intestine. Lymphocytes in Peyer's patches are separated from the intestinal lumen by epithelial cells that include specialized cells, termed *M cells,* that are scattered throughout the gut epithelium overlying the follicles of the Peyer's patch (Fig. 327-1). The M cells facilitate the transport of macromolecules from the intestinal lumen into the Peyer's patch.

B and T lymphocytes in Peyer's patches are activated by antigenic materials that enter from the intestinal lumen. Some of these cells then exit from this lymphoid structure, enter the lymphatic system, and undergo a migratory path that includes entry into the mesenteric lymph nodes, subsequent passage into the thoracic duct lymph and systemic circulation, and ultimate lodging in the intestinal mucosa.

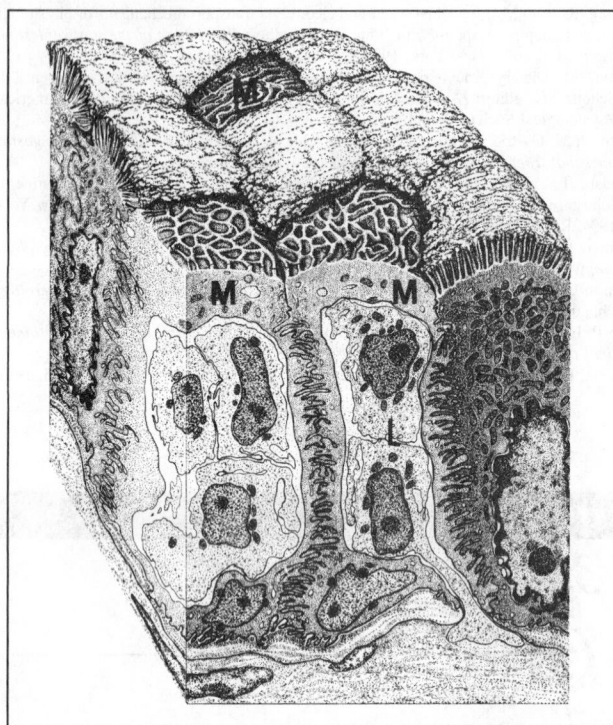

FIGURE 327-1 M cells in the epithelium overlying a human Peyer's patch. Three M cells with luminal surface microfolds are schematically shown interdigitating with adjacent columnar cells over a Peyer's patch. The mononuclear lymphoid cells directly beneath the M cells may approach to within 0.3 μm of the intestinal lumen. *M*, M cells; *L*, lymphoid cells.

From Owen RL, Nemanic P: *Scan Electron Microsc* 2:367, 1978.

Many B lymphocytes that originate from Peyer's patches ultimately lodge in the lamina propria region of the intestinal mucosa. T lymphocytes lodge either in the lamina propria or between epithelial cells lining intestinal villi. Other B and T lymphocytes lodge in extraintestinal sites such as the salivary glands, mammary gland, female genital tract, and respiratory tract (Fig. 327-2).

Intraepithelial Lymphocytes

Intraepithelial lymphocytes (IELs) are located between the intestinal epithelial cells close to the basement membrane (Fig. 327-3). These lymphocytes are abundant within the intestine. Thus normally there is approximately one IEL for every six intestinal epithelial cells. The majority of IELs are T lymphocytes, most of which have the CD8 marker on their surface. Of IELs, 90% to 95% belong to the alpha/beta lineage of T lymphocytes, whereas approximately 5% to 10% belong to the gamma/delta T cell lineage. Many IELs contain large cytoplasmic granules. IELs produce cytokines, but generally their other functions are not well characterized. However, IELs appear to be increased in diseases such as celiac disease and during infection with parasites such as *Giardia lamblia,* and, in the former, there is a marked increase in the proportion of IELs belonging to the gamma/delta T-cell lineage. Nonetheless, knowledge of the ontogeny of IELs, the types of antigens they recognize, and the role of IELs in normal immune defense and possibly in tissue-damaging mechanisms in disease is incomplete.

Lamina Propria Lymphoid Cells

The lamina propria within intestinal villi contains B cells, plasma cells, and lymphocytes as well as other important mononuclear cells (macrophages, eosinophils, and mast cells) interspersed in a vascular and lymphatic-rich connective tissue (Fig. 327-3). Seventy to ninety percent of plasma cells in the intestinal lamina propria produce antibody of the IgA immunoglobulin class. Of note, the distribution of T-cell subsets in the lamina propria differs markedly from that in the

intraepithelial region. Thus the ratio of T cells in the lamina propria that have the CD4 marker usually associated with helper/inducer T cells to those having the CD8 marker is similar to that seen in the peripheral circulation (i.e., a CD4/CD8 ratio of greater than 1.0).

One additional point regarding the relationship between the intestinal lymphoid compartments warrants mention. A large proportion of Peyer's patch B cells is committed to the ultimate expression of the IgA immunoglobulin class. Thus B cells that migrate out of Peyer's patches and lodge in the intestinal lamina propria and in other secretory sites (e.g., lungs, mammary gland) produce IgA in those sites after activation. This explains the predominance of IgA-producing cells in the intestinal lamina propria and at other secretory sites. Lymphocyte migration from the gut to the female breast explains why IgA antibodies in colostrum and milk can be directed against antigens encountered in the intestinal tract. Consistent with this, breast feeding is known to protect the newborn against infection with enteric pathogens.

SECRETORY IGA
Structure

IgA secreted by the plasma cells in the intestinal lamina propria comprises the major immunoglobulin class in intestinal secretions. The adult human small intestine has as many as 10^{10} IgA-producing cells per meter and secretes more than 3 g of IgA per day into intestinal secretions. IgA in intestinal secretions differs from serum IgA in several important respects and is termed *secretory IgA (sIgA)*. Unlike monomer IgA, which has two heavy and two light chains and is produced largely in the bone marrow and other nonmucosal sites, IgA secreted into the intestinal juice is dimeric (four heavy and four light chains). In addition, sIgA has two extra polypeptide chains termed *secretory component* and *J chain* (Fig. 327-4).

Secretory component, also known as the *polyimmunoglobulin receptor,* is a transmembrane glycoprotein that is found on the basal and lateral surfaces of intestinal epithelial cells. This molecule functions as a receptor for the uptake and transport of dimeric IgA and other polymeric immunoglobulins (i.e., IgM) across the intestinal epithelial cell and into the intestinal secretions. During the transport process, secretory component binds covalently to IgA. Once in the intestinal lumen, the association between secretory component and IgA appears to stabilize the IgA molecule, making it less susceptible to proteolytic digestion (Fig. 327-5).

The J chain protein is produced by plasma cells in the lamina propria and is a component of all polymeric immunoglobulin (both IgA and IgM). This protein appears to be important in the process of immunoglobulin polymerization. Thus IgA in intestinal secretions is a product of two different cell types—the plasma cell (IgA and J chain) and the intestinal epithelial cell (secretory component).

Function

The biologic functions of sIgA reflect its ability to bind antigen in the intestine. By binding to gut bacteria, sIgA can prevent bacterial attachment and penetration of intestinal epithelial cells. IgA also can bind to viruses and prevent viral colonization, and IgA can bind to macromolecules from food substances and prevent their passage across the intestinal mucosa.

Different immunoglobulin classes differ structurally and mediate different effector functions. IgA is not efficient at activating cell-damaging lytic mechanisms (e.g., complement activation) and in general does not participate in inflammatory reactions. However, the intestinal mucosa is exposed to a wide variety of antigenic materials that may enter the lamina propria of the normal or damaged intestine. Therefore it is important not to produce in the gut significant amounts of immunoglobulin isotypes such as IgG, which can participate in tissue-damaging immune reactions. Consistent with this, normally the intestinal tract contains few IgG-producing cells. However, in inflammatory bowel disease and celiac disease, IgG-producing cells are significantly increased in the intestinal mucosa and appear to play an important role in intestinal inflammation. Of note, there are increased numbers of IgE-producing cells in the normal intestinal tract relative to other sites. Although the function of those cells is not clear, IgE in the gut is known to be involved in host interactions with para-

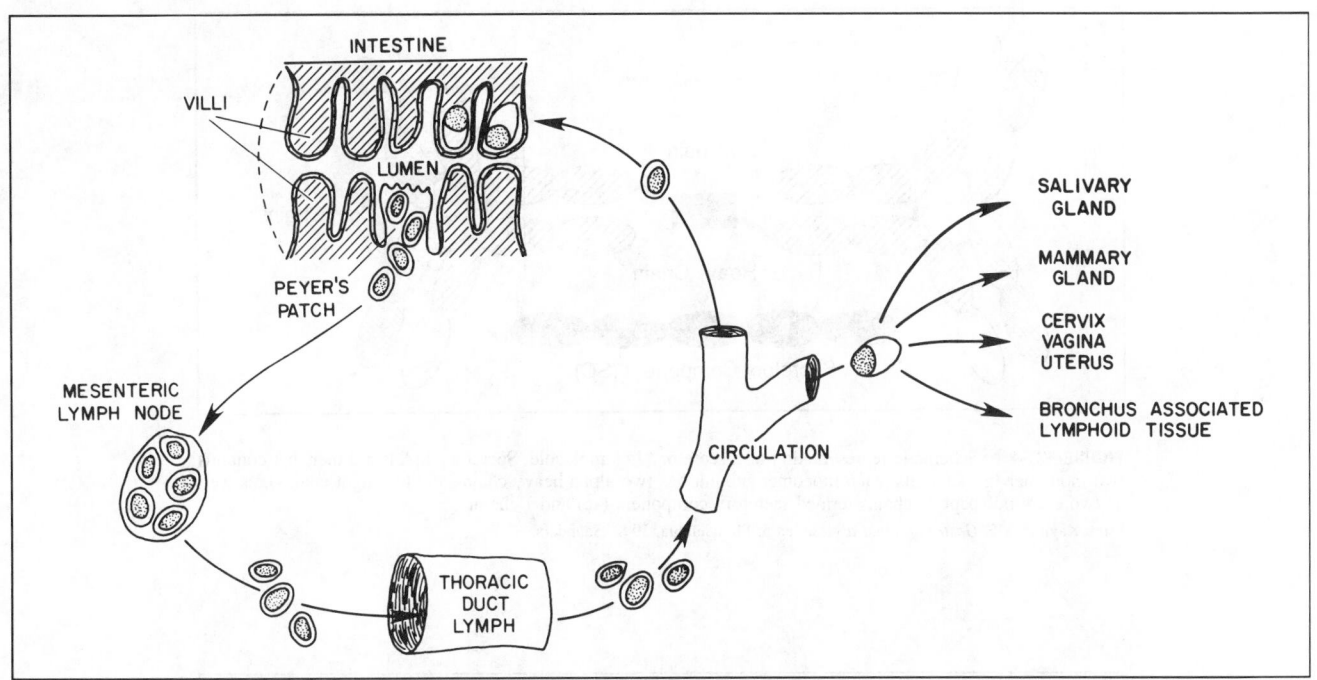

FIGURE 327-2   Lymphocytes activated by antigen in Peyer's patches migrate to the mesenteric lymph node and thoracic duct lymph before entering the circulation. B cells disseminate to the lamina propria and T cells to the lamina propria and intraepithelial region of the intestine. Other cells leave the circulation and lodge in extraintestinal lymphoid tissues, including the salivary glands, mammary glands, female genital tract, and respiratory tract.

From Kagnoff MF: *Gastrointestinal disease,* ed 5, Philadelphia, 1992, Saunders.

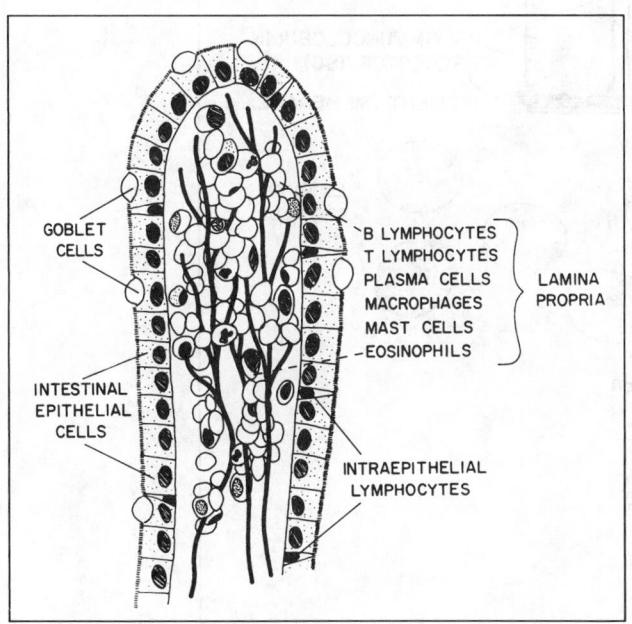

FIGURE 327-3   Schematic representation of an intestinal villus demonstrating intraepithelial lymphocytes situated near the basement membrane between intestinal epithelial cells. The lamina propria within villi is rich in vasculature and lymphatics, and it contains B lymphocytes, T lymphocytes, and plasma cells, as well as macrophages, mast cells, and eosinophils. Intraepithelial T lymphocytes have predominantly the CD8 phenotype, whereas in the lamina propria, CD4 T lymphocytes are more abundant than CD8 T lymphocytes.

From Kagnoff MF: *Physiology of the gastrointestinal tract,* New York, 1987, Raven.

sites and in intestinal allergic reactions. Further, IgE, acting through the release of mast cell mediators, may play a role in some diarrheal disorders by increasing intestinal fluid and electrolyte secretion.

IgA Deficiency

Humans have two subclasses of IgA: IgA1 and IgA2. Selective IgA deficiency is the most commonly recognized immunodeficiency (occurring in 1 in 500 to 1 in 700 of the population) and is usually associated with decreased levels of both IgA1 and IgA2. In addition, IgA deficiency may be accompanied by low levels of IgG2 and IgG4, is a frequent component of common variable immunodeficiency syndromes, and can be found along with abnormal cell-mediated immunity or IgE deficiency in diseases such as ataxia telangiectasia. IgA1 and IgA2 are coded for by separate genes on chromosome 14. Rare individuals having selective IgA2 deficiency caused by a deletion of the IgA2 gene have been described.

In patients with celiac disease there is approximately a tenfold increase in selective IgA deficiency over the numbers expected among the general population. Further, individuals with selective IgA deficiency have an increased prevalence of (1) autoimmune and connective tissue disease, (2) autoantibodies in the absence of overt autoimmune disease, (3) allergic disorders, and (4) malignancy. Such individuals frequently have circulating antibodies to food proteins and circulating immune complexes. This circumstance supports the notion that intestinal IgA plays a physiologic role in limiting the absorption of antigenic material from the gut.

Gastrointestinal manifestations vary among the different immunodeficiency syndromes. Gastrointestinal infections are not characteristic of selective IgA deficiency, a disorder in which increased numbers of IgM-producing cells often compensate for the IgA deficiency. When these individuals develop infections, the infections tend to be sinopulmonary. In contrast, gastrointestinal manifestations are frequent in the common variable immunodeficiency syndromes. This group of disorders is characterized by a low level of IgG along with diminished IgM or IgA levels. Diarrhea occurs in as many as 60% of these individuals, and 20% to 30% have mild to moderate malab-

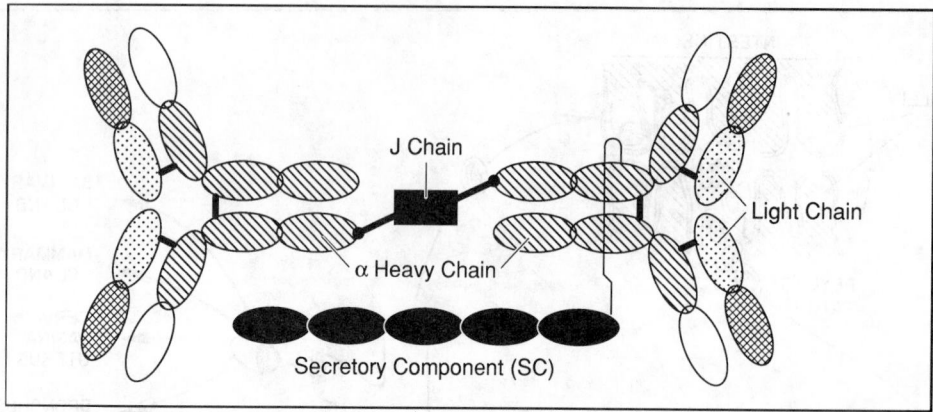

FIGURE 327-4 Schematic representation of a secretory IgA molecule. Secretory IgA is a dimer that contains two monomer IgA subunits (each monomer subunit has two alpha heavy chains and two light chains), as well as two extra polypeptide chains termed secretory component (sc) and J chain.

From Kagnoff MF: *Gastrointestinal disease*, ed 5, Philadelphia, 1992, Saunders.

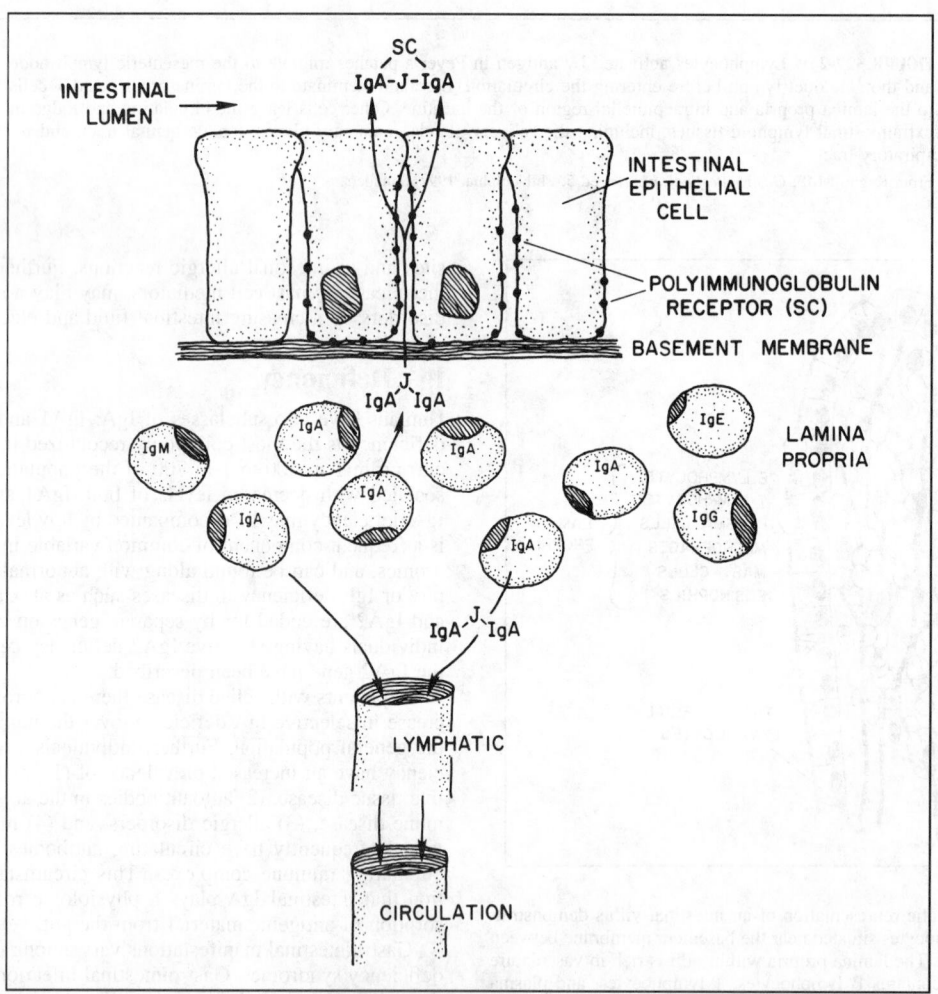

FIGURE 327-5 Transport of IgA into intestinal secretions. Dimer IgA containing the J chain is secreted by plasma cells in the lamina propria. This molecule couples with the polyimmunoglobulin receptor (also known as *SC*) on the basal and lateral surfaces of the intestinal epithelial cell. The IgA-SC complex is endocytosed and transported through the intestinal epithelial cell and secreted into the intestinal lumen as sigA (dimer IgA plus J chain and SC). IgA produced in the lamina propria also can enter the draining lymphatics and circulation, and IgA-producing cells can disseminate to extraintestinal secretory sites. *IgA,* Immunoglobulin A.

From Kagnoff MF: *Gastrointestinal disease*, ed 5, Philadelphia, 1992, Saunders.

sorption, often associated with infection with the protozoan parasite *Giardia lamblia*. Common variable immunodeficiency syndromes may be accompanied by nodular lymphoid hyperplasia of the small intestine and occasionally of the stomach, colon, and rectum, as well as by abnormalities in intestinal villous architecture. T cells also are important in host mucosal immunity. For example, persistent gastrointestinal infections with protozoan parasites such as *Cryptosporidium* spp. or *Isospora belli* are seen with systemic and mucosal T-cell deficiencies like those that occur in the acquired immunodeficiency syndrome (Chapter 346).

Food Allergy

Food allergy is a pathologic reaction that results from an immunologic response to ingested food antigens. As such, food allergy must be clearly differentiated from a broad spectrum of food intolerances. The latter represent adverse reactions to foods that are nonimmunologically mediated (e.g., reactions to toxins or pharmacologic mediators in foods, lactose intolerance). The diagnosis of food allergy frequently rests on the demonstration that clinical symptoms disappear when an offending food protein is eliminated from the diet and appear after ingestion of the food, ideally tested in a double-blind fashion. Unfortunately, tests commonly used to diagnose food allergy such as skin tests and radioallergosorbent (RAST) tests do not always correlate with clinical disease.

Immune reactions to foods such as milk and soy are relatively common in infancy and early childhood. However, food allergies also occur in adults and may result in a combination of gastrointestinal, respiratory, and cutaneous complaints. Colitis-like symptoms, protein-losing enteropathies, malabsorption syndromes, skin reactions such as urticaria and eczema, respiratory symptoms such as asthma and rhinitis, and acute anaphylactic reactions have all been attributed to food allergies. Allergy to cow's milk is the best studied example of food protein allergy. Other food substances frequently associated with allergy include eggs, chicken, fish, shellfish, nuts, and wheat products. Allergic reactions are caused by an IgE-mediated mechanism wherein mast cells coated with IgE degranulate and release biologically active mediators that act on local tissues to produce vasodilation, contraction of smooth muscle, and, at mucosal surfaces, secretion of mucus. Little is known about immune reactions to food proteins that are mediated by immunoglobulin classes other than IgE or by cell-mediated immune mechanisms.

ENTERIC IMMUNIZATION AND ORAL TOLERANCE

The nature of the immune response evoked after immunization by the intestinal route depends on several factors, including the type and dose of the immunizing antigen. Most enterically administered proteins are not effective at stimulating local mucosal IgA responses. In contrast, antigens that persist in the intestinal tract (e.g., attenuated virus) and antigens that can bind to the mucosal surface (e.g., cholera toxin, cholera toxin B subunit) are very effective at stimulating mucosal IgA responses. In addition, mucosal immune responses to proteins that are otherwise poorly immunogenic in the intestine can be substantially increased when the proteins are coadministered with adjuvants such as cholera toxin. Immunization with viruses and bacteria that invade across mucosal surfaces (e.g., poliovirus, *Shigella* spp.) can stimulate immune responses that mediate local protection in the intestinal tract, as well as systemic immune responses. Antibody responses tend to be restricted to the region of the intestine that was exposed to the immunizing antigen rather than be generalized throughout the entire intestinal tract.

Decreased systemic immune responsiveness to a specific antigen following exposure to that antigen by the enteric route is termed *oral tolerance*. Oral tolerance is revealed when attempts are made to parenterally immunize an individual to the same antigen that was previously administered by the enteric route. A similar phenomenon is seen following antigen exposure via the nasal route. There has been marked interest in oral tolerance and how to optimize this host response because of its potential as a modality for preventing and treating organ-specific autoimmune and inflammatory diseases. Moreover, the factors that determine whether an individual develops oral tolerance or

systemic immunity to an antigen administered by the enteric route are of considerable importance when considering the development of mucosal vaccines. Recent studies indicate that protein antigens linked to the cholera toxin B subunit are potent activators of oral tolerance.

BIBLIOGRAPHY

Kagnoff MF: Celiac disease. In Yamada T et al, editors: *Textbook of gastroenterology*, ed 2, Philadelphia, 1995, Lippincott.
Kagnoff MF: Immunology and inflammation of the gastrointestinal tract. In Feldman M, Scharschmidt BF, Sleisenger MH, editors: *Sleisenger and Fordtran's gastrointestinal and liver disease*, ed 6, Philadelphia, 1997, Saunders.
Kagnoff MF, Kiyono H, editors: *Essentials of mucosal immunology*, San Diego, 1996, Academic Press.
Kiyono H, Ogra PL, McGhee JR: *Mucosal vaccines*, San Diego, 1996, Academic Press.
Ogra PL et al: *Handbook of mucosal immunology*, San Diego, 1994, Academic Press.
Weiner HL, Mayer LF, editors: Oral tolerance: mechanisms and applications, *Ann NY Acad Sci*, vol 778, New York, 1996.

II DIAGNOSTIC PROCEDURES AND TESTS

CHAPTER

328 Gastrointestinal Endoscopy

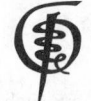

Bret T. Petersen

Gastrointestinal endoscopy is designed to provide direct visual examination of the inside of the gastrointestinal tract. The original fiberoptic endoscopes use bundles of small, flexible glass fibers to transmit light to and carry images back from the gastrointestinal tract; these endoscopes have largely been replaced by video endoscopes, which transmit the images electronically from a small video chip at the tip of the instrument through a processing unit to a television screen. These instruments have controls that move the tip of the instruments in different directions and open channels for suction; insufflation of air and water; and insertion of a variety of accessory instruments for obtaining mucosal biopsies, application of cautery, or other therapeutic purposes.

GENERAL INDICATIONS AND CONTRAINDICATIONS

Both the referring physician and the endoscopist have responsibility for the appropriate selection of gastrointestinal endoscopy for evaluation of clinical problems. In recent years many centers have adopted a practice of open-access endoscopy scheduling, wherein all general and specialty physicians can schedule routine upper and lower endoscopy to be performed by the gastroenterologist. This has increased utilization with perhaps some decline in appropriateness.

Endoscopy is costly and carries with it some risk for the patient. Therefore diagnostic or therapeutic procedures should be planned only when the information gained will materially affect the decisions regarding the clinical management or when the anticipated therapeutic benefit exceeds the relative risk of the procedure.

Most procedures are performed without any discomfort to the patient and are safe. Relative contraindications to the performance of elective endoscopy include inability of the patient or family to provide informed consent, uncontrolled bleeding diatheses, severe cardiorespiratory compromise, recent acute myocardial infarction, known gastrointestinal perforation, and complete bowel obstruction. Many anticoagulated patients require elective endoscopy for symptom evaluation. Decisions to proceed while the patient is still antico-

---

BOX 328-1

Indications for esophagogastroduodenoscopy (EGD)

Esophagus
Persistent esophageal pain despite therapy
Dysphagia
Suspect Barrett's esophagus
Barrett's esophagus—for surveillance biopsies
Suspect or confirm portal hypertension by identification of varices
Varices—for endoscopic therapy
Caustic ingestion
Dilation of stricture or stoma

Gastroduodenum
Persistent dyspepsia or pain despite therapy
Persistent nausea or vomiting
Early satiety, anorexia
Unexplained weight loss
History of gastric polyps—for surveillance
Familial polyposis—surveillance of duodenum with side-viewing endoscope
Gastric ulcer—biopsy or follow-up

Gastrointestinal bleeding
Hematemesis and/or melena
Iron deficiency anemia
Positive fecal blood test

Abnormal x-ray of esophagus or gastroduodenum
Thickened folds, ulceration, mass lesion, stricture

---

agulated should be guided by anticipated need for therapy, such as polypectomy, sphincterotomy, and control of gastrointestinal bleeding. Such procedures should be performed only after reversal of the anticoagulated state.

CONSCIOUS SEDATION AND ANALGESIA

Most endoscopic procedures are performed after administration of systemic sedation or analgesia. The most commonly used parenteral agents are the benzodiazepines midazolam (Versed) and diazepam (Valium) administered alone or in combination with a narcotic such as meperidine (Demerol) or fentanyl (Sublimaze). Requirements for sedation vary greatly by the individual patient, the patient population, and the procedure type and goals.

Systemic sedation contributes a major part of the cost and the risk of gastrointestinal endoscopy. Administration of "conscious sedation" requires intravenous access, monitoring of vital signs, availability of resuscitative equipment, and facilities for adequate postprocedure recovery. Occasional patients carry such significant risk for sedation that anesthesia consultation and perhaps endotracheal intubation are advisable. This pertains particularly to those patients with airway compromise, risk of blood or food aspiration, or significant cardiorespiratory disease who are scheduled to undergo upper gastrointestinal tract endoscopy.

UPPER GASTROINTESTINAL ENDOSCOPY

Endoscopic examination of the esophagus, stomach, and duodenum (esophagogastroduodenoscopy = EGD) is performed after a 6- to 8-hour fast. Survey EGDs can be completed in 5 to 10 minutes. The risk of upper endoscopy to a patient in good general health is negligible. Most complications occur in patients with serious underlying cardiac or respiratory disease. Complications may be estimated at a morbidity of 0.13% and mortality of 0.004%.

Endoscopy is now the preferred initial study for the evaluation of most upper gastrointestinal tract symptoms (Box 328-1). As a general rule, elective surgery should not be performed for disease of the upper gastrointestinal tract without prior endoscopic confirmation.

Symptoms and Signs

The symptoms of *odynophagia* and *dysphagia* are best evaluated by upper endoscopy in all patients, young and old. Specific visual and cytologic or histologic diagnoses may lead to specific therapies for esophagitis caused by acid or by candida or viral infections. Endoscopy allows confident exclusion of malignancy when strictures are identified, as well as definitive or palliative therapy of all varieties of strictures, webs, rings, or achalasia.

Dyspepsia and *heartburn* should prompt endoscopy when they fail to respond to a limited several-week trial of medical therapy. Similarly, endoscopy should be employed to clarify the etiology of *persistent vomiting, unexplained weight loss,* or *anorexia.* Indications for endoscopy are stronger in older patients, in whom malignancy is a greater risk.

Gastrointestinal bleeding of almost all degrees is most efficiently evaluated with endoscopy. The site of bleeding can be accurately localized in more than 90% of patients presenting with *melena* or *hematemesis.* Identification of active bleeding or high-risk stigmata, such as protruding visible vessels or adherent clots with fresh blood present, usually prompts application of endoscopic therapy to stop bleeding and to prevent recurrent bleeding. Usual techniques include injection of epinephrine or saline as vasoconstricting or tamponading agents and thermal coagulation using bipolar electrical probes, the thermal "heater probe," or neodymium:yttrium-aluminum-garnet (Nd-YAG) laser therapy. Variceal bleeding can be arrested with endoscopic injection sclerotherapy or with rubber band ligation.

Iron deficiency anemia and *occult gastrointestinal bleeding* are indications for upper endoscopy when colonic lesions have been excluded. Clinically silent mucosal erosions and ulcers may be found in patients taking nonsteroidal antiinflammatory agents and in those with unrecognized chronic reflux. Erosions at the lower end of large diaphragmatic hernias where the stomach rides over the diaphragmatic hiatus may be found.

Abnormal Radiologic Findings

Endoscopy is also indicated to diagnose or exclude malignancy and to achieve a pathologic diagnosis whenever solitary *ulcers* are identified radiographically in the esophagus or stomach. Healing of gastric ulcers that are considered to be benign should be confirmed by a follow-up endoscopy to fully exclude a malignancy. More than 90% of malignant ulcers are correctly identified by combined visual and biopsy characterization. Endoscopic evaluation is not needed for duodenal ulcers because they are rarely malignant. Endoscopy is optimal for diagnosing active ulcer disease in the symptomatic patient with radiographic evidence of past scarring.

Endoscopy is essential for both diagnosis and treatment of *esophageal strictures.* Optimal pathologic results are obtained when both endoscopic biopsy and brush cytologic examination are used together. Benign and malignant strictures can be palliated by endoscopic passage of guide wires through to the stomach, followed by passage of rigid or balloon dilators using either endoscopic or fluoroscopic guidance. Esophageal obstruction can be further palliated by endoscopic placement of large, semiflexible plastic stents or smaller, self-expanding metallic stents. Obstruction from bulky intraluminal cancers can be palliated also by tissue coagulation using Nd-YAG lasers, BICAP tumor probes, or alcohol injection. Photodynamic therapy can induce flat or bulky lesions to slough by selective tissue photostimulation with lasers after administration of sensitizing dyes.

Mass lesions of the esophagus or stomach should be further evaluated with upper endoscopy and biopsy prior to definitive management. Identification of lymphoma or rare inflammatory lesions will prompt further characterization or systemic staging and potentially nonsurgical management. Submucosal masses may be best characterized by the addition of endoscopic ultrasonography, and some polypoid lesions can be definitively managed endoscopically.

Radiographic identification of enlarged or abnormal gastric folds is an indication for EGD. At endoscopy, normal folds will efface or flatten as the stomach is distended with air. The differential diagnosis for a nondistensible stomach or noneffacing folds includes infiltrating carcinoma, lymphoma, gastric varices, hypertrophic gastropathies such as Ménétrier's disease, and hypersecretory conditions such as Zollinger-Ellison syndrome. The visual appearance alone is often not diagnostic, and it may be necessary to perform deep biopsy of the mucosa using snare excision of a bulky fold. Endoscopic ultrasonography may clarify many of the potential diagnoses, improving the safety and yield of deep biopsy. Occasionally it is necessary to obtain full-thickness biopsies by laparoscopic or open surgical means.

Cancer Surveillance

Upper endoscopy is recommended for cancer surveillance in two primary groups in the United States. In patients with long-standing or severe reflux esophagitis, normal squamous lining may be replaced by metaplastic columnar epithelium called *Barrett's mucosa.* These patients are at an increased risk for the development of esophageal adenocarcinoma. Screening examination with aggressive biopsy sampling for cancer or dysplasia is widely practiced. The optimal frequency of surveillance examination remains undefined. Patients with familial adenomatous polyposis syndromes are at increased risk for development of periampullary carcinoma. They are advised to have screening examinations of the duodenum performed with a side-viewing scope every 2 to 3 years.

Food Impaction, Foreign Body Removal, and Substance Ingestion

Endoscopy is also employed to remove food or foreign bodies that lodge in the esophagus and large or sharp foreign bodies that enter the stomach. A variety of grasping devices can be passed through the biopsy channel of the endoscope to remove such items. Often the endoscope is passed through an overtube to protect the airway and to remove sharp or multiple foreign bodies from the stomach more safely. Delayed removal of food impactions can lead to progressive esophagitis, aspiration, or trauma from retching. Following food impaction removal, many patients have no demonstrable pathologic condition other than disproportion between the ingested food and the lumen caliber. Strictures or rings noted at the time of endoscopy can be dilated if the mucosa is not overly inflamed.

Careful early endoscopy has been used as a means of staging the severity of injury from ingestion of caustic alkaline or acidic substances. The presence and location of erythema, ulceration, or sloughing mucosa can guide intensity of subsequent care.

Feeding Tube Placement

Full enteral nutrition can be provided via tubes placed into the stomach or small intestine via the anterior abdominal and gastric walls. Percutaneous endoscopic gastrostomy (PEG) provides an excellent alternative to nasogastric or nasojejunal tube feeding when long-term enteric tube feeding is required. Nasoenteric tubes can be placed by endoscopic or radiographic means, whereas gastrostomy tubes can be placed endoscopically, radiographically, or surgically.

Small-Bowel Biopsy and Aspiration

Endoscopy is also used for obtaining small-bowel biopsy and aspiration of the luminal contents. They are very useful in the investigation of patients with chronic diarrhea or malabsorption caused by small-bowel mucosal diseases and by parasitic infection such as giardiasis. Endoscopic duodenal aspiration is also used to look for cholesterol crystal to help in the diagnosis of idiopathic pancreatitis or right upper quadrant pain.

ENTEROSCOPY

Occasional patients with occult gastrointestinal bleeding or abnormal small-bowel contrast studies benefit from endoscopic examination of the jejunum or ileum (Box 328-2). Standard EGD accomplishes examination of the entire second portion and often the third portion of the duodenum. Examination beyond the ligament of Treitz can be accomplished by either push-type extended upper endoscopy or passive Sonde enteroscopy. In push enteroscopy a pediatric colonoscope or a dedicated longer and more slender instrument with full endoscopic steering and therapeutic capabilities is advanced 50 to 100 cm into the jejunum. Use of an overtube extending from mouth to duodenum facilitates deeper intubation by preventing looping in the greater curvature of the stomach.

BOX 328-2

Indications for enteroscopy

Abnormal small-bowel roentgenogram
Chronic blood loss anemia
Recurrent upper intestinal bleeding of uncertain source

Sonde enteroscopy utilizes a 6-foot-long and even more slender instrument fitted with a balloon at the distal tip. Balloon insufflation and administration of prokinetic agents to stimulate motility facilitate advancement well into the ileum over 4 to 6 hours. The examination is accomplished during gradual, semicontrolled withdrawal over approximately 30 minutes. Regions of abnormality can be noted and localized with radiographic assistance, but sampling and therapy are not possible.

Push enteroscopy has become a routine study in the evaluation of occult bleeding, since many vascular malformations extend into the upper small intestine. Sonde enteroscopy is reported to yield important findings in as many as one fourth of patients studied, but its use has been limited by the lack of traditional endoscopic biopsy and therapy capabilities.

Intraoperative enteroscopy is occasionally employed as the last and most definitive mucosal examination of the small intestine in patients with blood loss anemia who have become transfusion-dependent. The endoscope is introduced via a sterile sheath into a mid-gut enterotomy, and examination is accomplished segmentally 1 foot at a time as the surgeon clamps and unclamps the bowel to avoid overdistention of the entire lumen. The surgeon examines the transilluminated bowel in a darkened room as the endoscopist examines the interior. Vascular lesions are treated endoscopically or surgically, depending on their number and location.

RIGID PROCTOSCOPY

Rigid proctoscopy provides a direct view of the rectum extending up to 20 to 25 cm above the anal verge. The proctoscope is a hollow, metal or plastic tube that is passed into the rectum with the assistance of a smooth-tipped obturator for plugging the leading end. Preparation is usually with a phosphosoda or gentle tap-water enema. The procedure is performed with the patient in the knee-chest or left lateral Sim's position, or on a special table that elevates the hips and places the patient in a head-down position. Proctoscopy is an easy technique to learn. Most specialists in general surgery and family or general medicine perform the procedure. No sedation is required.

Rigid proctoscopy is indicated in the evaluation of anal, perianal, and perineal pain or pruritus, palpable masses, bright red bleeding per anus, fecal incontinence, and for therapy or follow-up of hemorrhoids and anorectal tumors. Proctoscopy provides easy access for rectal biopsy for amyloidosis. Rigid proctoscopy has been used as a screening examination for rectal carcinoma; however, since the regional distribution of colorectal cancers has migrated proximally, it has largely been supplanted by flexible sigmoidoscopy. Rigid proctoscopy provides a cost-effective distal examination for combination with barium enema examination of the more proximal colon.

FLEXIBLE SIGMOIDOSCOPY

Examination of the rectum and sigmoid colon is readily achieved with a flexible 30- or 60-cm fiberoptic or video endoscope. The longer version is generally preferred because it often provides an examination to the splenic flexure. The procedure takes about 5 minutes and generally requires no sedation. Preparation is the same as for rigid proctoscopy.

Indications for flexible sigmoidoscopy are very similar to those for rigid proctoscopy (Box 328-3), but it also provides adequate depth of insertion to view or biopsy the sigmoid colon for diverticular stricture assessment and diarrhea assessment with histologic exclusion of collagenous or microscopic colitis. Flexible sigmoidoscopy every 3

BOX 328-3

Indications for rigid and flexible sigmoidoscopy

Rectal, anal, or perianal bleeding*,†
Rectal, anal, or perineal pain
Palpable rectal or anal mass*,†
Rectal biopsy for amyloid
Sigmoid biopsy for collagenous colitis*
Cancer screening and follow-up after therapy*,†
Evaluation of inflammatory bowel disease†
Change in bowel pattern—constipation or diarrhea*
Fecal incontinence
Abdominal pain, bloating, or swelling*
Assessment of colostomy, ileostomy, or ileal pouch
For therapy of rectal polyp, hemorrhoids, enlarged anal papillae, fulguration of bleeding sites in rectum

---

*Often combined with barium enema
†Colonoscopy may be preferable study

BOX 328-4

Indications for colonoscopy

Polyps or cancer
Known polyp or cancer, to rule out synchronous lesion
History of colorectal polyps: usually every 3 to 5 years
History of colorectal cancer: usually at 1 year, then every 3 years
Strong family history of colorectal cancer: usually every 3 to 5 years

Inflammatory bowel disease
Chronic colitis to diagnose, evaluate severity and extent
Chronic ulcerative colitis (CUC) surveillance for dysplasia

Gastrointestinal bleeding
Hematochezia likely not from perianal or rectal area
Melena of unknown origin
Iron deficiency anemia
Positive fecal blood test

Unexplained diarrhea
Abnormal colon roentgenogram

---

to 5 years is recommended as a screening measure for colorectal carcinoma in patients over 50 years of age.

COLONOSCOPY

Colonoscopy is performed with 130- to 180-cm-long endoscopes designed with a combination of flexibility and torque stability to facilitate passage through the entire colon. Colonoscopy is a difficult technique that requires extensive experience for proficiency. A competent colonoscopist should be able to pass the instrument to the cecum in more than 90% of examinations in 10 to 45 minutes.

Patients are prepared for colonoscopy either by 1 or 2 days of liquid diet, laxatives, and enemas or by ingestion of a large volume of isotonic electrolyte lavage solution (Golytely and others). Parenteral sedation and analgesia are generally required. The major hazards are perforation, hemorrhage, and cardiorespiratory complications. The overall complication rate is 0.07% to 0.2% for diagnostic procedures and 1% for therapeutic procedures.

Polyps and Cancers

A major use of colonoscopy is to diagnose and treat colonic polyps. Patients are usually referred for colonoscopy because a polyp or cancer is found on barium enema radiography or flexible sigmoidoscopic examination (Box 328-4). Colonoscopy is indicated to remove the index polyp and to screen the remainder of the colon for synchronous lesions. Polyps are removed either by a wire-loop electrosurgical snare or by "hot-biopsy" forceps, which sample and ablate small lesions simultaneously. Following endoscopic or surgical removal of polyps or surgical resection for cancer, patients should be reexamined at regular intervals so that new "metachronous" polyps can be detected and removed as they appear. The risk for identification of future polyps or cancers varies by adequacy of the initial examination and by size, number, and histologic characteristics of the index lesions. The optimal interval between such surveillance examinations is still being defined. Current practice favors reexamining the colon 1 year after a cancer resection and 3 to 5 years after polypectomy.

Inflammatory Bowel Disease

Colonoscopy is very helpful in the evaluation of patients with inflammatory bowel disease. The severity and extent of inflammatory bowel disease are more accurately determined by colonoscopy than by radiographic examination. Patients suspected of having either ulcerative colitis or Crohn's disease and who have had negative radiographic and proctosigmoidoscopic examination results sometimes may have the diagnosis established by colonoscopy. The ileocecal valve and the terminal ileum can usually be entered when Crohn's disease of that area is suspected. Colonoscopy is often helpful in planning surgical therapy in patients with Crohn's disease. Surveillance colonoscopy is often performed at 1- to 3-year intervals in patients with ulcerative

colitis of 8 to 10 years or longer duration. Findings of dysplasia or overt malignancy prompts recommendations for proctocolectomy, or surgical removal of the entire colon and rectum. Full colonoscopy is contraindicated in severe acute colitis.

Gastrointestinal Bleeding

Colonoscopy is indicated primarily for diagnosis and occasionally for therapy when patients present with positive fecal blood tests, iron deficiency anemia without apparent cause, melena of unknown origin, or hematochezia likely not from the rectum or perianal area. Assuming an outlet or perianal cause for positive stool tests or anemia, without excluding the possibility of proximal cancer, is risky in individuals over 40 to 50 years of age. Colonoscopy is difficult in the presence of massive bleeding. A rapid 2-hour lavage preparation facilitates the examination. Vigorous bleeding is often best evaluated by angiography, whereas moderate rates of bleeding can sometimes be localized before colonoscopy or surgery by isotope-labeled red blood cell (RBC) scans.

Other Indications

Another indication for colonoscopy is diverticulosis, which is a very common finding in older patients. When the disease process is severe, radiographic diagnosis of polyp or cancer within the involved segment of bowel is very difficult. Such lesions are much more easily recognized during colonoscopic examination. Acute diverticulitis is a contraindication for colonoscopy, but the procedure can be helpful in chronic cases.

Diagnosis in the patient with worrisome symptoms and an indeterminate or unsatisfactory barium enema examination is often facilitated by colonoscopy. This situation frequently occurs in elderly or disabled patients, who can be quite difficult to prepare for either examination. Under these circumstances, colonoscopy may be preferable to repeated attempts to perform a radiographic study.

Chronic or severe acute diarrhea can be evaluated with colonoscopy and biopsy when more limited endoscopic examinations are normal. Pseudomembranous colitis is occasionally found in a proximal segmental distribution. Collagenous or microscopic colitis is usually evident in left-sided biopsies, but proximal sampling may be indicated for significant long-standing diarrhea without prior diagnosis.

The isolated finding of abdominal pain is not a good reason to perform colonoscopy. A lesion large enough to produce pain usually does so by partially obstructing the colon. Such lesions are almost always detected by radiographic examination. Most patients with colonic pain and a negative radiographic examination result suffer from spasm secondary to an irritable colon. Colonoscopy is not needed to confirm this diagnosis.

BOX 328-5
Indications for ERCP

Biliary indications
Abdominal pain suggesting biliary disease (usually with abnormal laboratory findings or imaging)
Jaundice or cholestasis
Acute cholangitis
Known or suspected biliary fistula or leak
Known biliary stricture
Known or presumptive papillary stenosis
Known primary sclerosing cholangitis with complications

Pancreatic indications
Abdominal pain suggesting pancreatic disease (usually with abnormal laboratory findings or imaging)
Suspect pancreatic cancer: when imaging studies (CT, US) not diagnostic
Pancreatic insufficiency or malabsorption
History of idiopathic acute pancreatitis
Severe acute gallstone pancreatitis
Painful chronic pancreatitis: for therapy or preoperative study
Pancreatic pseudocyst: for therapy or preoperative study
Pancreatic fistula or leak: for therapy or preoperative study

ERCP, Endoscopic retrograde cholangiopancreatography; *CT,* computed tomography; *US,* ultrasonography.

BOX 328-6
Indications for endoscopic ultrasonography

Staging known esophageal, pancreatic, and rectal cancer
Biopsy of mediastinal and retroperitoneal masses or adenopathy
Evaluation of obstructive jaundice in cases of suspected pancreatic cancer
Evaluation of thickened gastric folds
Evaluation and biopsy of submucosal mass lesions in any location

---

BOX 328-7
Indications for diagnostic laparoscopy

Chronic abdominal or pelvic pain
Suspicion of recurrent, partial small-bowel obstruction with negative contrast studies
Idiopathic ascites
Suspicion of peritoneal disease
Staging intraabdominal malignancy before laparotomy

ENDOSCOPIC RETROGRADE CHOLANGIOPANCREATOGRAPHY

Endoscopic retrograde cholangiopancreatography (ERCP) is a combined endoscopic and radiologic procedure for evaluation and therapy of the biliary and pancreatic ducts (Box 328-5). A lateral-viewing endoscope is positioned in the second portion of the duodenum opposite the papilla of Vater. A small, 1.5-mm catheter passed through the instrument channel is selectively advanced into the common bile or main pancreatic duct. Injection of contrast material then allows fluoroscopic and radiographic visualization of the ducts. Preparation requires 6 to 8 hours of fasting, as well as cleaning of any contrast in the gut, which may hinder imaging of the ducts. Prophylactic antibiotics are administered for procedures in patients with jaundice, known or anticipated duct obstruction, or pseudocysts. The procedure is technically demanding; however, skilled endoscopists should achieve a cannulation success rate of 90% to 95% or better.

The alternative to ERCP for evaluation of the bile duct is *percutaneous transhepatic cholangiography* (PTC). ERCP is preferred in patients with ascites or coagulopathy and when findings may require concurrent therapy, such as duct stone removal. PTC is performed when ERCP fails to adequately image the bile duct or when altered upper gut anatomy precludes access to the papilla.

Cholangiography is indicated when symptoms, laboratory findings, or imaging suggest large bile duct disease. Most common are cholestasis, jaundice, or dilated bile ducts on ultrasonography or computed tomography (CT) scanning, with or without abdominal pain.

When therapeutic measures are indicated, the ampulla of Vater can be incised by electrosurgical current (sphincterotomy). This facilitates tissue sampling, stone removal, stricture dilation, and stent placement.

Indications for pancreatography include situations in which pancreatic disease is suspected but cannot be completely characterized by CT or ultrasonography. This includes obstructive duct lesions of pancreatitis or cancer, acute recurrent pancreatitis, and chronic pancreatitis. Pancreatography provides guidance for surgical management of chronic pancreatitis, pancreatic pseudocysts, and other cystic tumors or masses. A rapidly evolving application of endoscopy is pseudocyst drainage via direct puncture through a contiguous wall of the stomach or the duodenum. The role of urgent ERCP for sphincterotomy and gallstone removal in severe acute biliary pancreatitis remains incompletely defined.

The major risks of ERCP include development of pancreatitis in 1% of diagnostic procedures and in 5% to 15% of therapeutic procedures, bleeding in 2% of patients undergoing sphincterotomy, and secondary cholangitis or pseudocyst infection in 1% of patients with duct obstruction or cyst filling.

ENDOSCOPIC ULTRASONOGRAPHY

Endoscopic ultrasonography represents the newest and most rapidly progressing application of gastrointestinal endoscopy. By advancing ultrasound probes into the lumen of the gastrointestinal tract, it is possible to place them very close to or in direct contact with organs or tissues of interest. This yields much greater spatial resolution than can be accomplished transcutaneously. Most useful to date have been the dedicated systems that incorporate ultrasound scanners into endoscopes. Contact with the mucosa is ensured by filling the stomach with water or using a water-filled balloon attached to the endoscope. One instrument utilizes a rotating sector scanner that provides a radial image encompassing 360 degrees around the tip of the endoscope. Another uses a linear array scanner aligned in parallel with the biopsy channel of the endoscope. This allows for real-time, ultrasound-guided access to deep tissues for aspiration biopsy, fluid sampling, or injection therapy. Ultrasound probes that are passed through the biopsy channel of a standard endoscope have also been developed for use during standard endoscopy and for passage into the biliary and pancreatic ducts during ERCP. Endoscopic ultrasonography is most useful for evaluating submucosal lesions, for determining the extent of invasion by tumors, and for imaging adjacent organs such as the pancreas or bile ducts (Box 328-6).

LAPAROSCOPY

Laparoscopy (peritoneoscopy) visualizes the peritoneal cavity by means of a short, rigid scope passed through the anterior abdominal wall. Initial access is gained by puncture with a special blunt-tipped needle. Following distention of the abdominal cavity with carbon dioxide or nitrous oxide, trochars are placed to facilitate repeated passage of the endoscope and grasping or sampling tools. Both lobes of the liver, the spleen, the gallbladder, and the peritoneal surfaces can be seen.

Laparoscopy came into use in the United States in the 1970s, primarily for gastroenterologists to obtain visually directed biopsy of focal liver lesions. It has been largely replaced for this indication by biopsy with either ultrasound or computed tomography guidance. Gynecologists have used laparoscopy for many years to visualize and treat pelvic disease. Current diagnostic applications of laparoscopy include evaluation of chronic abdominal pain potentially related to adhesions and evaluation of unexplained ascites (Box 328-7). Since the introduction of laparoscopic cholecystectomy in the late 1980s, many general surgical procedures—including fundoplication, herniorrhaphy, and appendectomy—have been adapted to laparoscopic approaches.

BIBLIOGRAPHY

Blackstone MO: *Endoscopic interpretation,* New York, 1984, Raven.
Cotton PB, Williams CB: *Practical gastrointestinal endoscopy,* ed 3, Oxford, UK, 1990, Blackwell.
Schiller KRF et al: *A color atlas of gastrointestinal endoscopy,* Philadelphia, 1987, Saunders.
Silverstein FE, Tytgat NJ: *Atlas of gastrointestinal endoscopy,* Philadelphia, 1987, Saunders.
Silvis S: *Therapeutic endoscopy,* ed 2, New York, 1990, Igaku-Shoin.
Sivak MV: *Gastroenterologic endoscopy,* Philadelphia, 1987, Saunders.

CHAPTER

329 Evaluation of Esophageal Disease

Konrad S. Schulze-Delrieu and Robert W. Summers

MANIFESTATIONS OF ABNORMAL SWALLOWING AND OF ESOPHAGEAL DISEASE

A careful consideration of symptoms can provide specific information about many functional and structural abnormalities of the swallowing mechanism. After a detailed history the physician can formulate the principal diagnostic possibilities and assess the need for specific diagnostic tests and treatments. Abnormalities of the swallowing structures in the head, neck, and chest lead to difficulties with swallowing. The tongue collects the bolus and drives it through the pharynx; atrophy, resection, or incoordination of the tongue impairs the initiation of the swallow and the propulsion of the bolus into the esophagus. The larynx occludes the airway during swallowing and coughing. Paralysis of the vocal cords, laryngeal anesthesia, or laryngectomy increases the likelihood for aspiration to occur or for failure of aspirated material to be cleared by adequate coughing. The esophagus accepts the bolus from the pharynx and moves it from the vicinity of the airways to the stomach. Delayed bolus passage or gastric regurgitation into the esophagus may expose the pharynx and airways when they are unprotected. Most local diseases produce unique and discrete deficits that are easily corrected or compensated for. Systemic diseases, such as diseases of the cranial motor nerves that control the pharyngeal and esophageal musculature, may impair too many swallowing functions for treatment or rehabilitation to be effective.

The purpose of the history is to relate swallowing difficulties to a specific anatomic site or disease process: to reconstruct the sequence in which specific difficulties arose: and to establish their association with pain, loss of muscle strength or sensation, and disturbances of speech or voice. Oral disease processes interfere with the initiation of the swallow. Pharyngeal disorders manifest themselves immediately after swallow initiation, often through frightening sensations such as choking. If neurologic disease impairs the coordination of oropharyngeal structures, boluses with the consistency of pudding may pose no problems, whereas carbonated beverages might. Sensations from esophageal disorders are experienced several seconds after swallow initiation. Mechanical obstruction of the esophagus leads to difficulty with solids first; motor abnormalities of bolus affect liquids and solids equally.

Dysphagia, Odynophagia, and the Globus Sensation

Dysphagia is the sensation experienced when the passage of a bolus from the mouth to the stomach is slowed or arrested. Oropharyngeal dysphagia implies difficulty in propelling a bolus from the mouth into

the gullet; it is often associated with coughing, choking, or nasal regurgitation of swallowed material. Weakness or incoordination of the musculature of the tongue, pharynx, and larynx is frequent in neurologic disease, especially after cerebrovascular accidents. Preparation of an oral bolus may become nearly impossible in such situations, and this dysphagia may be accompanied by nasal speech, dysphonia, or dysarthria. (See Chapter 140 for additional information on dysarthria and pharyngeal paralysis.)

Esophageal dysphagia is the sensation provoked when a bolus sticks in the esophageal body. Symptoms may occur in the neck or the retrosternal region, but the level of the sensation is not an accurate guide to the level of the lesions. Motility disorders of the esophagus usually interfere with the swallowing of both liquids and solids. Partial mechanical obstructions caused by mucosal webs, peptic strictures, and tumors primarily produce difficulty with the swallowing of solid boluses; patients adapt by changing to a soft diet, and they learn to wash foods down with liquids. Dysphagia that progresses over weeks or months from difficulties with solids to difficulties with liquids is typical of esophageal cancer. Progression is slower with peptic stricturing.

Pain on swallowing, or *odynophagia,* denotes a disruption of the mucosal lining of the oropharynx or esophagus. Odynophagia occurs mainly with opportunistic infections, caustic lesions, and cancers. Such diseases may cause continuous substernal pain that is markedly increased during swallowing. Opportunistic infections occur in diabetes, in AIDS, and following chemotherapy and immunosuppression. Common causative organisms are herpes simplex virus, cytomegaloviruses, and *Candida* spp. Odynophagia is rare in uncomplicated reflux esophagitis; a penetrating esophageal ulcer, superimposed caustic or infectious lesions, or malignant transformation need to be considered. Dysphagia, especially if progressive or accompanied by odynophagia, signals serious disease and calls for detailed radiographic and endoscopic examination of the pharynx and esophagus.

A chronically sore throat or a tightness or fullness in the neck that is not specifically aggravated by swallowing is often labeled as the globus sensation (also called *globus melancholicus* or *globus hystericus*), or pseudodysphagia. Subtle abnormalities in or around the upper esophageal sphincter (UES) may be responsible and may be associated with strenuous swallowing, the need to double-swallow or clearing of the throat excessively. Symptomatic relief may come through simple measures, including reflux precautions or cessation of smoking. The globus sensation may also be experienced in choledocholithiasis, in cardiovascular disease, and in emotional distress.

Regurgitation, Aspiration, Drooling, and Water Brash

Regurgitation is characterized by the unexpected, effortless appearance of gastrointestinal contents in the mouth, when both the upper and the lower esophageal sphincters fail. Regurgitation is often confused with vomiting; it differs from the latter in that it is not preceded by nausea. It does not involve forceful retching and is often postural. Regurgitation of undigested food indicates the accumulation of material in an area proximal to the stomach; this occurs in Zenker's diverticula, esophageal diverticula, and achalasia of the esophagus. A sour taste suggests mixture of the food with gastric acid; bitterness suggests mixture with bile from duodenal contents.

When patients have severe reflux, regurgitation of sour or bitter fluids occurs most frequently when they lie down or increase their abdominal pressure. Patients with easily provoked reflux and regurgitation are prone to severe esophagitis and should undergo diagnostic evaluation. These patients are at risk of nocturnal aspiration and should be specifically questioned about recurrent pneumonias, dyspnea, and cough during recumbency. Reflux may induce bronchospasm and asthma attacks through aspiration or reflex mechanisms. Hoarseness, otitis media, and dental etching are lesser known sequelae of reflux. Regurgitation that occurs only in the context of eructation after large meals is less serious and by itself is not an indication for full diagnostic testing. Coughing and choking with drinking of liquids but without dysphagia suggest the possibility of an esophageal-bronchial fistula.

Water brash is the outpouring of salivary secretions in response to gastroesophageal reflux. Acidification of the esophagus stimulates oropharyngeal secretions through a vagal reflex. Hypersalivation is also triggered by esophageal obstruction and bolus impaction. Paralysis of the pharynx leads to retention of saliva and food, to drooling, and to spillage into the airway. Mumbled speech and nasal voice are other common features. Drooling caused by facial weakness and poor labial closure is less serious than drooling caused by pharyngeal dysfunction.

Heartburn and Food Intolerance

Heartburn (pyrosis) is common even with mild gastroesophageal reflux. It is a less reliable indicator of demonstrable disease than is dysphagia. Burning or pressure associated with heartburn may be described as "sour stomach" or "gas." Heartburn may occur only after big meals as a barely perceptible retrosternal warmth, gnawing, or pressure, which is promptly relieved by antacids or other liquids. It may be provoked along with regurgitation by bending at the waist, lifting, or the supine position. Alternatively, esophagitis may cause pain as intense as myocardial ischemia and may respond poorly to antacids (see discussion of chest pain in next section).

Poor tolerance of large meals and of specific foods (or dyspepsia) is shared by esophageal disease with peptic ulcer disease, gallstone disease, and many other gastrointestinal diseases. Frequently blamed for esophageal symptoms are acidic foods (e.g., orange or spicy tomato juice); and foods of high osmolarity (candy, chocolate, pastry); or foods with a high fat content, especially if fried.

Chest Pain of Esophageal Origin

Esophageal chest pain is thought to relate to mucosal injury and altered motility. Esophageal colic is a common manifestation of diffuse esophageal spasm and other motility disorders characterized by the excessive force of esophageal contractions (i.e., the hypertensive or "nutcracker" esophagus). Of hiatal hernias, only the rare paraesophageal type is currently accepted as a direct cause of esophageal pain. Esophageal stretch can also cause chest pain: in bolus impaction the esophagus proximal to the obstruction dilates and contracts vigorously. The ingestion of ice-cold liquids can cause esophageal colic-like distress, but the esophagus is actually wide and flaccid in this situation. Esophageal pain may abate in response to smooth muscle relaxants such as nitroglycerin.

Because of the prevalence, morbidity, and mortality associated with coronary artery disease, a cardiac origin must always be the first consideration in chest pain. Cardiovascular causes include aortic aneurysm and atypical angina; local tenderness may suggest costochondritis. Diseases of mediastinum, pleura, or lungs might also be the cause of chest pain, especially if esophageal symptoms are absent and changes in esophageal structure or function changes are minor.

Esophageal disease is common and frequently coexists with cardiac disease; it is probable that esophageal reflux can induce cardiac pain in patients who have coronary disease, as well as those who do not. Because of the common innervation of the heart and the esophagus, over half of patients with substernal pain are unable to distinguish which is the origin of their symptoms. Therapy with vasodilators (e.g., nitrates and calcium channel blockers) may trigger symptomatic reflux by lowering sphincter pressure. Like cardiac pain (see Chapter 16), esophageal pain may radiate to the epigastrium, the neck, or the left arm; it may be exercise induced; and it may respond to nitrates. A history of pyrosis, regurgitation, dysphagia, or relief with antacids may be a clue to an esophageal source.

Patients with these symptoms should undergo endoscopic and histologic or at least radiologic examination of the esophagus. If the diagnosis remains unclear, 24-hour pH monitoring, noting periods of chest pain, may be helpful. Even if symptoms are not clearly related to the esophagus, a trial of antireflux measures may be helpful. Additional attempts to implicate the esophagus in noncardiac chest pain rely on 24-hour recordings of esophageal pressures or provocation of abnormal contractions or of cardiac ischemia, as described later. The indications for these tests await clearer definition, particularly in the absence of esophageal symptoms.

PHYSICAL EXAMINATION

Alertness and physical and social independence are prerequisites to food intake. Heavy sedation and processes impairing cognitive func-

tions interfere with swallowing. Intubation of the esophagus and trachea, recumbency, and other restraints interfere with sensory feedback, laryngeal ascent, and other important swallowing functions. Laryngeal ascent places the larynx in a safe position during swallowing, inverts the epiglottis, and pulls the UES open. Laryngeal ascent is mediated by the external laryngeal musculature; it can be assessed by placing an index finger above the thyroid cartilage while the patient swallows; the thyroid should impart its upward thrust on the finger. The function of the internal laryngeal musculature is assessed by asking the patient to speak and to cough. If the voice is hoarse and the cough is weak, laryngoscopy may reveal vocal cord paralysis. If the voice is wet and gurgly, pharyngeal retention and aspiration must be suspected. The tongue should be inspected for bulk and mobility. Its force may be judged by having it press onto the examiner's finger outside the cheek.

The oral cavity is assessed for moisture. Salivary secretions are essential for formation of the bolus, for lubrication of the bolus passage, and for clearance and neutralization of the esophagus. Diminished salivary secretion, or *xerostomia*, is an effect of many drugs, of dehydration, and of destruction of salivary glands by radiation or autoimmune inflammation (in the "sicca syndrome"). Xerostomia may lead to altered taste, painful mucosal fissures, and poor oral intake. Xerostomia also increases the residue of food and debris, which sticks in the oropharynx and becomes contaminated. This increases the risks from aspiration.

Swallowing should be tested only after the patient's underlying condition has stabilized. Respiratory reserve should be adequate and the risk of aspiration small. Once ice chips and pasty materials have been swallowed without difficulty in the upright position, challenges may be increased. Dry crackers may be tested and the oral cavity be inspected after several minutes of chewing or swallowing. Alternatively, the patient may be placed in the recumbent position to test the ability of the esophagus to propel the bolus to the stomach when gravity has been eliminated. The arrival of the bolus causes a hissing sound in the epigastrium within 10 seconds of laryngeal ascent. Testing the gag reflex serves little purpose in the assessment of swallowing functions. Many individuals hardly gag but swallow normally. The gag reflex is very active in pseudobulbar palsy; yet pseudobulbar palsy is virtually synonymous with severe abnormalities of oropharyngeal swallowing.

Local processes are best assessed by visualization of the mucosal structures through direct inspection, laryngoscopy, and esophagoscopy. When mucosal disease is suspected, samples should be obtained for histologic or other examinations. Functional deficits are assessed by a neurologic examination of the head and neck, with particular emphasis on the movements of the tongue and of the larynx, and by listening to the volume and character of voice and speech. If safe, functional deficits can then be further assessed by testing of swallowing by bedside and radiographic examinations. Dehydration, weight loss, and aspiration all call for rehabilitation through dietary modification or compensatory techniques of swallowing where possible and institution of nonoral feeding where needed.

DIAGNOSTIC TESTS
Barium Contrast Studies and Fluoroscopic Examination of Deglutition

The structural integrity of the oropharynx and the esophagus is comprehensively assessed by barium contrast examination. The mucosa of the oropharynx and the esophagus should be smooth. The shape and bulk of the tongue, the size and symmetry of the pharyngeal recesses, and the distensibility of the pharynx and esophagus should be noted. The site and size of diverticula, strictures, webs, hernias, and other abnormalities should be recorded. Chronic injury may shorten the esophagus; shortening is recognized by the formation of transverse mucosal folds in the distal esophagus or by a persistent hiatal hernia. Webs and rings produce indentations of the barium column. Webs are delicate and occur mostly in the cervical esophagus. Strictures are segments in which the walls indent the normal esophageal lumen or lack normal distensibility. Most "peptic" strictures (strictures that complicate gastroesophageal reflux) occur in the distal esophagus and are fairly short and concentric. "Lye" strictures follow the ingestion of corrosives and may be long and tortuous. Lye strictures may give rise to malignancies. Carcinomas may cause strictures, irregular filling defects, disruption of the mucosal pattern, and ulcerations. Tumors originating deep in the esophageal wall (e.g., leiomyomas) or outside the esophagus form smooth mounds that indent the lumen. Computed tomography and endoscopic ultrasonography can help determine the intramural and extramural extent of tumors and their resectability.

Dynamic contrast radiography is the standard diagnostic test to study all stages of swallowing. Small barium boluses ("cookie swallow") are used to assess oropharyngeal functions, including the rotary movements of the jaws, the initiation of the swallow, the completeness of laryngeal ascent with the inversion of the epiglottis, and the effectiveness of peristalsis in clearing the valleculae and pyriform sinuses. Penetration of contrast into the larynx or its aspiration into the trachea should lead to immediate measures to prevent its recurrence. This can often be achieved by a change in the size or consistency of the bolus, by a change in the position of the head, or by a special swallow maneuver. The study should be performed after patients have recovered from acute incidents (cerebrovascular accidents or surgical resection). The information should be used for rehabilitation to produce effective and safe swallows or for decisions about alternative feeding modes. The assessment of peristalsis by videofluoroscopy reveals most motility disorders of the esophagus. In a recumbent person, the peristaltic wave produced by swallowing should sweep the entire barium bolus from the pharynx through the esophagus into the stomach in under 10 seconds; esophageal contractions should produce a sharp coning of the tail of the barium column. With ineffective peristalsis, the tail of the barium column becomes fuzzy and residual barium remains in the esophageal body; with obstruction, the bolus may shoot back proximally ("bolus escape"). A barium-soaked marshmallow or piece of bread or a 12-mm barium tablet aids in the demonstration of subtle strictures or motor abnormalities. In diffuse spasm, disordered contractions squeeze the barium column into discrete segments or propel it in an orad direction. In achalasia the sphincter forms a smoothly tapered stricture at the gastroesophageal junction ("bird beak"). The esophageal body above it may be distended by residue or may be tortuous ("sigmoid esophagus"). Peristalsis is weak or absent below the level of the aortic arch.

Other imaging studies may contribute to the understanding of esophageal problems. The scintigraphic evaluation of deglutition with the use of radioisotope-labeled boluses provides some quantitative information about esophageal transit and gastroesophageal reflux. However, the technique provides insufficient detail to detect anatomic abnormalities. It represents only one point in time and is not a reliable screening procedure. Computed tomography and magnetic resonance imaging are most useful to detect inflammatory or neoplastic processes in the head, neck, or mediastinum that impinge on the oropharynx or esophagus.

Esophageal Endoscopy, Brushings, Biopsies, and Ultrasonography

Many lesions are difficult to diagnose by radiography alone. Direct visualization of the oropharynx, larynx, and the esophagus is superior to radiographic examination for the detection of small mucosal lesions and should be performed if the radiographic examination suggests a tumor, a stricture, or a mucosal change with long-term implications (Barrett's mucosal metaplasia, Chapter 333). The hypopharynx and larynx can be viewed by a mirror held in the posterior pharynx or by a fiberendoscope introduced through the nose. Specimens can be removed by biopsy or brushing for histologic, cytologic, or microbial examination. Information relevant to pharyngeal and laryngeal function may be readily apparent: excessive mucus in the pharyngeal recesses signals poor pharyngeal peristalsis; erosions along the posterior aspects of the vocal folds may imply reflux injury; inadequate adduction of vocal cords may imply vocal cord paralysis and poor protection from aspiration. These examinations can be performed under local anesthesia in an office chair. Esophagoscopy is typically performed under conscious sedation using a video endoscope that allows simultaneous inspection of the stomach and duodenum. Esophagoscopy also serves to obtain samples for histologic or microbial examination. Especially in debilitated and immunosuppressed patients with esophageal symptoms, viral, bacterial, and fungal cultures should be obtained from abnormal mucosa and planted immediately on appropriate culture or transport media. Esophagoscopy serves also to treat esophageal lesions through dilatation of strictures, placement of lumen-expanding stents, obliteration of esophageal varices, and other procedures (Chapter 333). Emergency endoscopy should be performed when food or a foreign body is impacted in the esophagus and sedation and spasmolytics have been to no avail. If the impaction is in the distal esophagus, food can often be carefully pushed into the stomach. Caution must be exercised, however, because the impaction may have occurred because of a stricture or tumor. Indigestible material can be removed through an overtube. Objects in the proximal esophagus are better removed under general anesthesia using a rigid esophagoscope. Details of endoscopic technique are described in Chapter 328.

Heartburn alone is not an indication for esophagoscopy. If pyrosis is severe, progressive, or refractory to antireflux therapy or if other symptoms such as bleeding, dysphagia, or odynophagia are present, endoscopy should be done. Any stricture, ulcer, or mass involving the esophagus that is demonstrated radiologically should be visualized and biopsy specimens taken. Benign-appearing strictures may be malignant; achalasia may be mimicked by carcinomas infiltrating the gastroesophageal junction.

Esophageal lesions from reflux occur first at the gastroesophageal squamocolumnar junction, an irregular but sharply demarcated border where the salmon-colored gastric mucosa meets the more pearly pink esophageal mucosa. Erosions and exudate occur on the crests of the folds, spread proximally, and become confluent. The severity of esophagitis is reflected in the longitudinal and the circumferential extent of the esophageal erosions. Mucosal metaplasia (Barrett's epithelium) appears where erosions have healed; it forms salmon-pink islands or tongues of columnar mucosa. The length of the metaplastic esophageal segment above the lower sphincter should be noted and multiple biopsies obtained. In the absence of gross lesions, biopsy specimens should be taken 5 cm proximal to the lower sphincter if it is critical to determine the likelihood of symptoms relating to chronic reflux. Chronic esophagitis causes a characteristic change in mucosal structure with increased relative height of papillae and basal cell layer. Histologic evidence of esophagitis may be present in the absence of visible abnormalities.

Follow-up endoscopy for uncomplicated reflux esophagitis is unnecessary unless symptoms do not respond to medical therapy, complications arise, or surgical therapy is contemplated. On the other hand, surveillance endoscopy is probably indicated for all patients with Barrett's esophagus, as the risk of esophageal adenocarcinoma appears to be increased at least fortyfold in this condition. Multiple biopsies at multiple levels are necessary to detect dysplasia or early cancer.

Endoscopic ultrasonography is increasingly used to evaluate submucosal lesions such as leiomyomas, and to determine the extent of spread of esophageal cancers. The depth of neoplastic infiltration can be assessed with 90% accuracy and the spread to lymph nodes with 80% accuracy. The addition of transesophageal aspiration biopsies enhances the diagnostic confidence and may eliminate the need for exploratory surgery. Through the use of Doppler probes, endoscopic ultrasound allows assessment of blood flow in varices and the need for further treatment.

Esophageal Manometry

In esophageal manometry the mechanical activity of the esophagus and of its sphincter is revealed by luminal pressure sensors. The normal human esophagus generates pressures of 60 to 100 mm Hg in response to swallowing, the highest pressures being generated in the middle of the esophagus (Fig. 329-1). Pressure waves have a sequential progression from proximal to distal, and at any individual sensor a single contraction wave does not normally last more than 7 seconds. Manometric pressures reflect *bolus* (cavity, luminal) *pressures* and *contact* (squeeze) *pressures*. In the normal esophageal body the amplitude of the contact pressure at any one site well exceeds that of its preceding bolus pressure. If the gradient between bolus and contact pressure falls below 30 mm Hg, it is likely that the contraction does not effectively clear the lumen and that *bolus escape* as described under the radiographic examination will occur. Most swallows lead

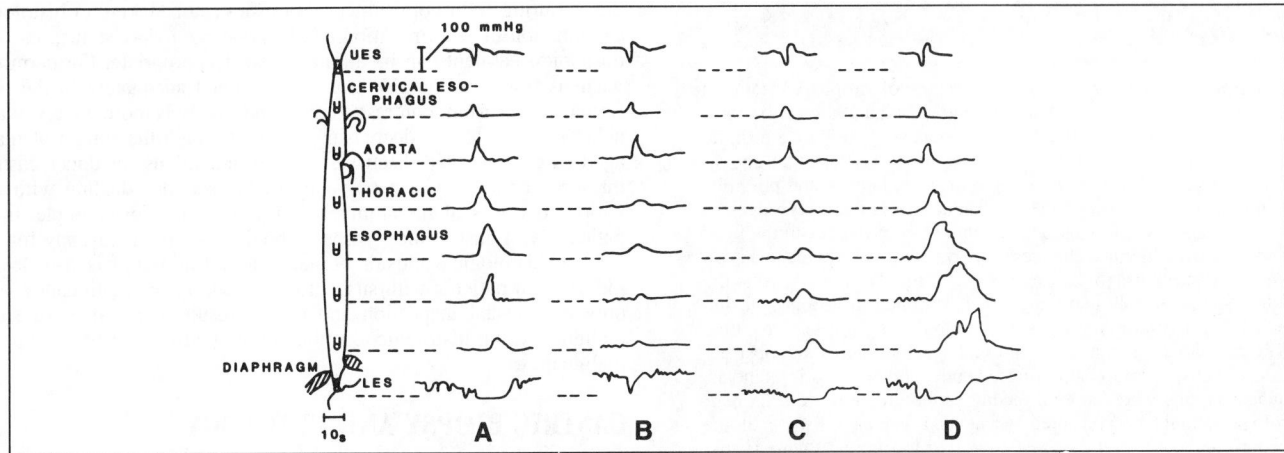

FIGURE 329-1   Patterns of esophageal motility. In this semischematic drawing, the pressure sensors span the entire esophagus from the upper esophageal sphincter to the lower esophageal sphincter. **A,** In the normal state *(first panel),* both sphincters maintain a high-pressure zone in which respiratory movements lead to pressure undulations. Swallowing leads to a brief relaxation of the upper esophageal sphincter and a longer relaxation of the lower esophageal sphincter. A contraction wave travels through the esophageal body; its amplitude is around 100 mm Hg and its duration about 4 seconds. Pressure patterns are abnormal in the distal two thirds of the esophagus in achalasia, systemic sclerosis, and esophageal spasm. **B,** In achalasia *(second panel)* the lower esophageal sphincter pressure is high and fails to disappear for an appropriate length of time on swallowing. Contractions in the esophageal body are weak and nonsequential. **C,** In systemic sclerosis *(third panel),* lower esophageal sphincter pressure is low; esophageal contractions are weak but generally sequential. Similar abnormalities are often seen in erosive esophagitis and Barrett's esophagus. **D,** In esophageal spasm *(fourth panel),* esophageal contractions last more than 7 seconds and generate pressures above 150 to 200 mm Hg. Contractions may also be repetitive and nonsequential. *UES,* Upper esophageal sphincter; *LES,* lower esophageal sphincter.

to a complete peristaltic sequence, and repetitive esophageal contractions do not occur.

The resting pressure generated by the normal lower esophageal sphincter (LES) is 20 to 40 mm Hg, and it relaxes to near zero pressure with the onset of a swallow. The sphincter is located at the point of respiratory reversal. In achalasia and some cases of esophageal spasm, sphincter pressure tends to be higher and the sphincter fails to relax. In patients with severe esophagitis and sclerodermatous esophagus, the high-pressure zone may be virtually abolished. A "common cavity phenomenon" (identical simultaneous waves at several sites) is observed with incompetence of the LES: increases of intragastric pressure are transmitted to the esophagus. Otherwise, manometry does not distinguish reliably between a competent and an incompetent LES. Similar waves may occur with straining, retching, or coughing.

Esophageal manometry is useful in the evaluation of achalasia, diffuse spasm, scleroderma, and other motility disorders. It is sometimes the only test that demonstrates those esophageal disorders that are characterized by excessive or reduced force of esophageal contractions. Abnormal contractions may not occur during short recording periods. Abnormal esophageal motor function on manometry is considered by many surgeons at least a relative contraindication to fundoplication.

Measurements of pH

Gastroesophageal reflux can be monitored by introducing a pH probe into the distal esophagus and continuously recording luminal pH. Acid reflux is defined as a sudden drop of intraluminal pH to 4 or less, which is followed by stepwise increases in pH. At pH values above 4, pepsin is inactive; activity of pepsin is a factor in the corrosiveness of the refluxate. Reflux episodes are recorded and compared with normative data derived from cohort studies. The timing of heartburn and chest pain may also be noted. Parameters that are processed by most commercial programs include the frequency and the duration of reflux episodes, the total number of reflux episodes lasting more than 5 minutes, and the total or relative time of esophageal acidification. Data may be further broken down between times of meals, sleep, and other activity. The pH parameter that best correlates with esophageal

lesions on endoscopic examination is the total time the pH is <4. Times below 5% pose a low risk and times well above 10% pose a high risk. Individual reflux profiles do not necessarily predict the presence of endoscopic esophagitis. This may be explained by factors such as the volume or the composition (bile salts, pancreatic enzymes), which are not assessed by the pH profile. Other variables include prior treatment and individual variations of mucosal resistance. A pH profile within the range of this group of normals does not exclude the possiblity that reflux contributes to a disease manifestation, nor does a pH profile outside this group of norms by itself constitute gastroesophageal reflux disease (GERD) or the need for reflux treatment.

In the presence of classic reflux symptoms and erosive esophagitis, all information required to guide therapy is at hand. Reasonable indications for 24-hour pH include the following:

1. To determine the role of gastroesophageal reflux with atypical symptoms and with chest pain not related to ischemic heart disease.
2. To identify the role of reflux in respiratory symptoms including asthma and laryngitis; this may require the placement of a second pH probe in the cervical esophagus or the pharynx. (pH values for upper esophageal or pharyngeal acid exposure are different from those of the lower esophagus; normative data remain to be established.)
3. To assess whether medical or surgical therapy controlled reflux adequately if symptoms persist.
4. To predict the necessity and duration for antireflux therapy over the long term.

BIBLIOGRAPHY

Baehr PH, McDonald GB: Esophageal infections: risk factors, presentation, diagnosis, and treatment, *Gastroenterology* 106:9, 1994.

Behar J, Biancani P: Pathogenesis of simultaneous esophageal contractions in patients with motility disorders, *Gastroenterology* 105:111, 1993.

Bell NJV, Hunt RH: Role of gastric acid suppression in the treatment of gastroesophageal reflux disease, *Gut* 33:118, 1992.

Benjamin SB: The relationship between esophageal motor disorders and microvascular angina, *Med Clin North Am* 74:1135, 1991.

Bonacini M, Young T, Laine L: The causes of esophageal symptoms in human immunodeficiency infection: a prospective study of 110 patients, *Arch Intern Med* 151:1567, 1991.

Breumelhof R et al: Analysis of 24-hour esophageal pressure and pH data in unselected patients with noncardiac chest pain, *Gastroenterology* 99:1257, 1990.

Browning TH: Diagnosis of chest pain of esophageal origin, *Dig Dis Sci* 35:289, 1990.

✔ *WHEN TO REFER*

Referral for a comprehensive assessment of oropharyngeal and esophageal structures by barium contrast examination is recommended whenever remediable local lesions are likely to contribute to the problems. Progressive dysphagia or odynophagia should prompt referral for endoscopic examination, biopsy, and possibly, cytologic examination. If the dysphagia affects the early stages of swallowing—as if it is associated with pain or masses in the head and neck or with voice changes—referral should be made to a head and neck specialist (otolaryngologist); if the dysphagia affects the late stages of swallowing, a physician trained in esophageal diseases (most commonly a gastroenterologist) should be consulted. Referral should be made for all esophageal strictures and obstructions (webs, symptomatic rings, peptic and neoplastic stenosis, achalasia) and when nonoral feeding is required long-term. A neurologist should be consulted whenever a primary disease of the central nervous system, cranial nerves, or local musculature is suspected. Neurologic diseases may be eminently treatable (Parkinson's disease, myasthenia) or preventable (cerebrovascular thrombosis). Rehabilitation for oropharyngeal dysphagia following operative resection and following cerebrovascular accidents can often be achieved by compensation and through special swallowing maneuvers. Referral to a speech pathologist trained in the management of oropharyngeal dysphagia may be rewarding.

Cannon RO et al: Coronary flow reserve, esophageal motility, and chest pain in patients with angiographically normal coronary arteries, *Am J Med* 88:217, 1990.

Cook IJ et al: Pharyngeal (Zenker's) diverticulum is a disorder of upper esophageal sphincter opening, *Gastroenterology* 103:1229, 1992.

Ghillebert G et al: Ambulatory 24-hour intraoesophageal pH and pressure recordings vs provocation tests in the diagnosis of chest pain of esophageal origin, *Gut 31:738, 1990.*

Groher ME: The detection of aspiration and videofluroscopy, *Dysphagia* 9:147, 1994.

Hewson EG et al: 24-hour esophageal pH monitoring: the most useful test for evaluating noncardiac chest pain, *Am J Med* 90(5):576, 1991.

Jacob B, Kahrilas PJ, Herzon G: Proximal esophageal pH-metry in patients with reflux laryngitis, *Gastroenterology* 100:2, 305-310, 1991.

Kahrilas PJ, Clouse RE, Hogan WY: American Gastroenterological Association technical review on the clinical use of manometry, *Gastroenterology* 107:1865-1884, 1994.

Massey BT et al: Abnormal esophageal motility: an analysis of concurrent radiographic and manometric findings, *Gastroenterology* 101:344, 1991.

Reid BJ et al: Endoscopic biopsy can detect high-grade dysplasia or early adenocarcinoma in Barrett's esophagus without grossly recognized neoplastic lesions, *Gastroenterology* 94:81, 1988.

Shaker R et al: Esophagopharyngeal distribution of refluxed gastric acid in patients with reflux laryngitis, *Gastroenterology* 109:1575, 1995.

Tio TL et al: Esophagogastric carcinoma: preoperative TNM classification with endosonography, *Radiology* 173:411, 1989.

CHAPTER

330 Evaluation of Gastroduodenal Diseases

Walter L. Peterson

VISUALIZATION OF THE STOMACH AND DUODENUM

Barium contrast radiographic examination of the stomach and duodenum (upper gastrointestinal [UGI] series) and endoscopy of the UGI tract have been the most frequently utilized procedures for evaluation of gastroduodenal diseases. The major indications for these techniques are UGI hemorrhage, upper abdominal pain, and symptoms of delayed gastric emptying. For several reasons, it is reasonable to suggest that, in 1997, barium contrast studies are almost obsolete. Endoscopy is generally regarded as the more accurate of the two procedures; during endoscopy, mucosal biopsies can be taken for histologic examination or determination of *Helicobacter pylori* status, and endoscopic treatment can be administered if appropriate. Furthermore, whereas fewer radiologists are being trained adequately in the performance of barium contrast studies, endoscopy is more widely available than ever and is decreasing in cost through the spread of managed care. A detailed discussion of the indications for upper gastrointestinal endoscopy can be found in the sections dealing with the various diseases of the stomach and duodenum. For example, most patients with gastric ulcer disease should undergo endoscopy for visual and histologic exclusion of malignancy. Endoscopy is also clearly indicated in patients with suspected gastroduodenal malignancy. Not only may visual inspection and biopsy results confirm or rule out malignancy, but histologic examination may also identify the type of malignancy.

GASTRIC BIOPSY AND CYTOLOGY

An important aspect of UGI endoscopy is its use in obtaining tissue for histologic and cytologic examination. Tissue is routinely obtained from patients with gastric ulcers or mass lesions to exclude or confirm malignancy. The procedure's usefulness in diagnosing malignancy depends primarily on three factors: (1) the number of specimens obtained, (2) the care with which they are collected and processed, and (3) the expertise of the pathologist examining the specimens. In most instances, if six to eight endoscopic biopsy specimens are obtained, malignant lesions of the stomach can be detected with 80% to 90% accuracy. In cases where the biopsy result is benign, cytologic examination ("touch-preps" or brushings) increases accuracy to 95%. However, accurate cytologic findings depend on the expertise of the cytologist, and many institutions do not have such experts. In these situations, false-positive and false-negative results become a problem. In centers without expert cytologists, it appears prudent to rely on visual inspection of the lesion and perhaps more biopsy procedures than would otherwise be performed. Lavage cytologic examinations, done infrequently in the past, offer no advantage over endoscopically directed brush cytologic examinations.

Submucosal or nonulcerated lesions present a special problem, because often only normal mucosa is obtained by endoscopic pinch biopsies. In these instances it may be helpful to perform suction biopsies, such as are obtained in the small bowel, or to use the "lift-and-cut" snare technique to obtain a large piece of gastric tissue (see Chapter 328). This technique may be especially helpful in evaluating patients with large gastric folds if the differential diagnosis includes lymphoma or Ménétrier's disease (Chapters 337 and 338). If this technique is not diagnostic and if the index of suspicion for infiltrative neoplasm is high, full-thickness biopsies of the stomach should be obtained by laparotomy.

GASTRIC ANALYSIS

Gastric analysis is becoming a lost art, and there are fewer and fewer indications for the procedure. However, it is still of potential benefit in three clinical conditions. First, patients with hypergastrinemia should have gastric analysis to differentiate between states of low acid secretion (i.e., gastric atrophy) and autonomous production of gastrin (i.e., Zollinger-Ellison syndrome). Second, some experts believe patients with Zollinger-Ellison syndrome should be treated with increasing doses of drugs until basal acid secretion falls below a certain level (e.g., 10 mmol/hr). If this approach is taken, basal acid output should be measured during the hour just preceding the next scheduled dose of medication. Third, gastric analysis may be of use to determine the adequacy of vagotomy in patients who have postsurgical recurrent ulceration.

Measurement of Gastric Acidity and Secretion

Gastric juice is collected in 15-minute samples through a sump-type nasogastric tube. Systemic medications designed to reduce acid secretion should be stopped 36 hours before gastric analysis, and no food or antacid is ingested for the prior 10 hours. (See Chapter 325 for special instructions in patients with suspected Zollinger-Ellison syndrome.) Gastric acidity of the samples may be determined either by a pH electrode or by titration to pH 7.0 with a base such as sodium hydroxide. Acid secretion in millimoles (or milliequivalents) per 15 minutes is calculated by multiplying the acidity (mmol/L) times the volume (liters/15 min).

Basal Acid Output

Basal acid output (BAO) is the sum of acid secretion rates during four 15-minute collections, expressed as millimoles (or milliequivalents) per hour. BAO fluctuates from day to day but, in normal subjects, ranges from 0 to 12 mmol/hr, with a mean of 2 to 4 mmol/hr (Chapter 325).

Stimulated Acid Output

The stimulants most often used to determine the maximum ability of parietal cells to secrete acid are histamine, betazole hydrochloride (Histalog), and pentagastrin. Because pentagastrin has fewer side effects than histamine and because it elicits its effects more quickly than betazole hydrochloride, it is now the stimulant of choice. After determination of BAO, pentagastrin (6 µg/kg) is injected subcutaneously and gastric contents are collected during four 15-minute periods. Results may be expressed as maximum acid output (MAO) or peak acid output (PAO). MAO is the sum of the four 15-minute values. PAO is the sum of the two highest consecutive 15-minute values multiplied by 2. The PAO can be reproduced with repeated testing and in normal subjects ranges from about 10 to 80 mmol/hr, with a mean of 33 mmol/hr (Chapter 325).

Interpretation of Basal Acid Output and Peak Acid Output in Disease

Acid secretory values in patients with duodenal ulcer are, on average, higher than those in normal subjects. However, only approximately one third of patients with duodenal ulcer have basal or peak acid outputs above the upper limit of normal. Patients with Zollinger-Ellison syndrome virtually always have a BAO greater than 12 to 15 mmol/hr and a BAO/PAO ratio of more than 60%.

Patients with gastric ulcers secrete, on average, less acid than normal subjects, but again there is overlap. Achlorhydria is defined by many as a PAO of 0, with pH of gastric contents never falling below 6.0 after stimulation. Benign peptic ulcer disease rarely occurs in achlorhydric patients. Thus a diagnosis of gastric carcinoma is suspected until disproved by endoscopy, biopsy, or cytologic examination.

Gastric Analysis After Ulcer Surgery

An especially difficult clinical problem in which gastric analysis may provide useful information is the evaluation of patients with recurrent ulcers after gastric surgery. Most surgical procedures involve some form of vagotomy, and regardless of a patient's acid-secretory status, the crucial question usually revolves around the completeness of the vagotomy. If there is evidence that a vagotomy has been incompletely performed, a repeat vagotomy might be considered. If the vagotomy is judged adequate, some form of gastric resection may be in order. For many years the only way of testing the adequacy of vagotomy was by insulin-induced or 2-deoxyglucose–induced hypoglycemia. These procedures are hazardous and may induce acid secretion by means other than vagal stimulation alone. Modified sham feeding—in which patients see, smell, taste, and chew (but do not swallow) food—is safe and is believed to stimulate acid secretion solely via the vagus nerve. Studies indicate that, in the presence of a complete vagotomy, the 60-minute acid output by aspiration during 30 minutes of modified sham feeding plus 30 minutes after sham feeding is less than 10% of a patient's PAO. Values higher than this suggest that the vagus nerve is intact. This test may be useful in planning additional surgery for patients who have postoperative ulcer recurrence.

SERUM GASTRIN LEVELS

Normal fasting serum gastrin levels vary among different laboratories, but in most laboratories fasting values greater than 100 to 200 pg/ml are considered to be abnormal. The two most common causes of hypergastrinemia are the Zollinger-Ellison syndrome and atrophic gastritis (Chapters 325 and 337), two conditions that may readily be distinguished by gastric analysis. Other disorders reported to produce elevated fasting gastrin values include renal insufficiency and the short bowel syndrome.

Although a serum gastrin value above 1000 pg/ml in a patient who is not achlorhydric is virtually diagnostic of Zollinger-Ellison syndrome, values between 200 and 1000 pg/ml may be found in patients with duodenal ulcer with and without Zollinger-Ellison syndrome. In the postoperative patient the differential diagnosis also includes post-vagotomy hypergastrinemia and the retained-antrum syndrome. In patients with only modest elevations in serum gastrin levels, the secretin infusion test may help differentiate among these conditions.

Two clinical units of GIH secretin per kilogram of body weight is injected intravenously over a 30- to 60-second period. Serum gastrin determinations are obtained twice just before secretin injection and at 2, 5, 10, 15, and 20 minutes after secretin injection. In all but patients with Zollinger-Ellison syndrome, secretin has little effect on serum gastrin levels. Rises of 200 pg/ml or more above basal levels are reported to be diagnostic of Zollinger-Ellison syndrome, although a few patients with proved Zollinger-Ellison syndrome may not exhibit a positive response to secretin.

TESTS TO DETECT THE PRESENCE OF *Helicobacter pylori*

Tests to detect the presence of *H. pylori* may be broadly grouped into those that require gastric tissue, usually obtained at the time of endoscopy, and those that do not.

Tests That Require Gastric Tissue

The most specific test for the presence of *H. pylori* is culture of the organism from gastric mucosal biopsy sections. However, the organism is quite fastidious, culture takes several days, and many routine hospital laboratories do not offer this test. As antibiotic resistance becomes more common, culture of *H. pylori* will likely become more readily available. A more sensitive test is histologic examination of mucosal biopsies, in which even small numbers of organisms can be seen with routine hematoxylin and eosin or Giemsa stains. These tests are modestly expensive and also time consuming. The presence of *H. pylori* in tissue can be diagnosed indirectly by tests that detect the presence of urease, an enzyme produced by the organism. Mucosal biopsy specimens are placed onto a urea-containing medium. If urease is present, the urea will be hydrolyzed into carbon dioxide and ammonia, the latter of which raises the pH of the medium and produces a color change of a pH-sensitive indicator. The first such test was a gel test, which required up to 24 hours to be read. Newer membrane-based tests can be read at 1 hour. The most cost-effective way to diagnose *H. pylori* using gastric tissue is to "bank" several biopsies and send them for histologic assessment only if the rapid urease test is negative.

Tests That Do Not Require Gastric Tissue

Another means of detecting the presence of urease is a breath urea test. Urea labeled with ^{13}C or ^{14}C is ingested with a liquid meal. If urease is present, labeled carbon dioxide is split off, absorbed into the circulation, and expired into the breath, which is collected and analyzed. The easiest and least expensive test for *H. pylori* is determination of serum IgG antibodies to the organism. This is a very specific test for the presence of *H. pylori* infection at some time in a person's life, but it may be less sensitive for current infection.

GASTRIC EMPTYING

Delayed gastric emptying can usually be diagnosed by means of a careful history and physical examination. If the patient reports vomiting recognizable food long after a meal and if a succussion splash is heard on examination, delayed gastric emptying may be the diagnosis. Response to therapy is best determined by resumption of the patient's ability to eat without discomfort or vomiting. Three tests—

the saline load test, gastric isotopic scanning, and emptying of radiopaque markers—are available to provide objective confirmation of the diagnosis of delayed emptying and the response to therapy. Each test has its limitations, however, and none enables the clinician to differentiate between an obstructing lesion of the antral pyloric region, such as peptic ulcer or cancer, and primary motor disorders of the stomach, such as postvagotomy paresis. This differentiation must be accomplished by a UGI series or, preferably, endoscopy.

The saline load test is simple to perform and does not require expensive equipment. It has been validated only in patients with organic outlet obstruction and measures only the emptying of liquids, and therefore has limited clinical importance. Gastric isotopic scanning measures the emptying of both solids and liquids and is especially helpful in cases of suspected primary motor disorders. The radiopaque marker study measures the emptying of indigestible solids and may be more sensitive in some situations than isotopic scanning.

Gastric Isotopic Scanning

Gastric isotopic scanning accurately quantitates the ability of the stomach to empty its contents and is especially useful when endoscopy discloses no organic obstruction to explain delayed emptying. For example, patients with suspected diabetic gastroparesis or postvagotomy paresis may have a motility disorder that can be confirmed and quantitated by means of this test. Response to nasogastric suction or motility-enhancing drugs such as bethanechol chloride (urecholine chloride) or metoclopramide may also be assessed.

Isotopic scanning involves administration of a liquid or solid meal to which a radioisotope has been added. Isotopes employed include chromium (^{51}Cr), indium (^{113m}In), and technetium (^{99m}Tc). The isotope present at any time after administration of the meal is measured by a scintillation counter or a gamma camera. Although liquids are rather easily labeled with isotope, ingenuity has been required to label solids. One technique involves injecting chickens with ^{99m}Tc, which is rapidly incorporated into the liver. The harvested chicken liver is cooked, diced, and eaten by the patient. Because liquids and solids empty at different rates, investigators are now using meals with both liquid and solid components, with separate isotopes for each component. The major drawbacks to the procedure are that it requires expensive equipment and special expertise.

Emptying of Solid Radiopaque Markers

A recent study suggests that the emptying of 1-cm segments of radiopaque plastic tubing (0.2-cm diameter), acting as indigestible solids, may be a simple and inexpensive means of detecting abnormal gastric motility. When 10 such markers are given with a meal to normal subjects, all the markers will be emptied (as determined by a plain abdominal radiograph) within 6 hours. In patients with diabetes mellitus, markers often are present in the stomach after 6 hours. Early studies suggest that this technique may be more sensitive than the more expensive gastric isotopic scan. Further work is needed to determine the clinical utility of this test.

OTHER TECHNIQUES

Patients with gastrointestinal bleeding are sometimes evaluated with ^{99m}Tc sulfur colloid or ^{99m}Tc-labeled red blood cells to detect the site of blood loss. Although sometimes useful in patients with obscure bleeding below the ligament of Treitz, these techniques have almost no value in patients with gastroduodenal bleeding.

Experimental modalities that may, in the future, be of benefit in the evaluation of gastroduodenal diseases include endoscopic Doppler studies to evaluate the patency (i.e., potential for further bleeding) of arteries eroded by peptic ulcers and endoscopic ultrasound techniques.

BIBLIOGRAPHY

Brady CE: Secretin provocation test in the diagnosis of Zollinger-Ellison syndrome, *Am J Gastroenterology* 86:129, 1991.
Cutler AF et al: Accuracy of invasive and noninvasive test to diagnose *Helicobacter pylori* infection, *Gastroenterology* 109:136, 1995.
Feldman M, Richardson CT, Fordtran JS: Experience with sham feeding as a test for vagotomy, *Gastroenterology* 79:792, 1980.
Feldman M, Smith HJ, Simon TR: Gastric emptying of solid radiopaque markers: studies in healthy subjects and diabetic patients, *Gastroenterology* 87:895, 1984.
Goldschmiedt M, Feldman M: Gastric secretion in health and disease. In Sleisenger MH, Fordtran JS, editors: Gastrointestinal disease, ed 5, Philadelphia, 1993, Saunders.
Horowitz M, Dent J: Clinical relevance of disordered gastric emptying, *Baillierse Clin Gastroenterol* 5:371, 1991.
Morrisey JF, Reichelderfer M: Gastrointestinal endoscopy, *N Engl J Med* 325:1142, 1214, 1991.
Peterson WL: *Helicobacter pylori* and peptic ulcer disease, *N Engl J Med* 324:1043, 1991.

331 Evaluation of Intestinal Disease

Nicholas O. Davidson

INTRODUCTION

In the evaluation of diseases of the small and large intestine, the clinician must be aware of the complexity and multidimensional nature of this process. As with any multisystem disorder, important clues may be provided by the presence of extraintestinal manifestations of disease. By extension, as with any investigation of human disease, the starting point is the history and physical examination. This chapter will give an overview of the approach to investigating intestinal diseases, with emphasis on the pertinent diagnostic tests available to assist in reaching a diagnosis.

Throughout the history, it is especially useful to make note of features that may favor a particular etiology of disease. A helpful, general classification of such an algorithm would include consideration of the following major groupings of fundamental processes:

Drug induced
Infectious
Inflammatory or immunologic
Vascular
Neoplastic
Neuromuscular
Metabolic
Iatrogenic (from trauma, surgery, or radiation)

Continuous, thoughtful referral to this list during the interview process will lead the physician to the most productive evaluation of the historical features of the particular disease. Of special relevance to the evaluation of intestinal diseases are the characteristics of the stool, in particular, the presence of diarrhea and its associated features. For instance, above and beyond the general characterization of the diarrhea itself—in particular, its periodicity, color, consistency, and other physical attributes—there are several important features to elicit. Is the diarrhea accompanied by pain? Does it wake the patient at night? Is blood present within the stool or found on the toilet tissue? In regard to the evaluation of intestinal diseases, it is important to bear in mind that the major function of these organs is the digestion and absorption of nutrients. Accordingly, a hallmark of intestinal disease tends to be malabsorption, with the associated features of weight loss and malnutrition. For instance, eliciting a history of alterations in the skin complexion and painful cracking of the areas around the mouth or tongue may suggest deficiencies of vitamin A and C or other micronutrient deficiency. Altered taste or olfactory sensation of food within the mouth is common in zinc deficiency, which accompanies some cases of malabsorption.

In the physical examination it is important to pay attention to the presence of signs of extraintestinal manifestations of disease, such as (1) clubbing, which is associated with several chronic intestinal diseases, including Crohn's disease and ulcerative colitis; and (2) koilonychia (iron deficiency) and other changes in the appearance of the finger nails, such as transverse ridging, which are associated with nutritional deficiency. In addition, the presence of follicular keratosis suggests vitamin A deficiency and angular stomatitis of the mouth is associated with numerous vitamin deficiencies, including deficiencies in folate, pyridoxine, riboflavin, and niacin. The presence of peripheral edema may be associated with extreme protein wasting states resulting from exudative enteropathy. Also, a variety of neurologic manifestations exist in association with deficiencies of distinct micronutrients, including peripheral neuropathies (thiamine, pyridoxine); dementia with or without subacute combined degeneration (vitamin B_{12}); tetany and hyperreflexia (calcium and magnesium deficiency states associated with vitamin D–deficient states); and nystagmus and external ophthalmoplegia (thiamine). Many of the detailed historical and physical features of specific intestinal diseases are discussed in the relevant chapters dealing with individual diseases.

STUDIES OF THE FORMED BLOOD ELEMENTS

Disorders of nutrient absorption or diseases associated with intestinal blood loss may be accompanied by abnormalities of the peripheral blood. These will be considered in turn.

Red Blood Cell Abnormalities

Anemia is very common in intestinal diseases and has many contributing causes. Chronic blood loss leads to iron deficiency and microcytic anemia. However, as discussed in a later section, with or without anemia the presence of occult blood in a stool examination warrants further investigation. Microcytic anemia is associated with disorders of iron absorption, which may accompany diffuse disease of the upper small bowel, such as celiac sprue. Macrocytic anemia may arise from either folate or vitamin B_{12} deficiency. Vitamin B_{12} deficiency can arise from defects in any of several critical steps in its absorption, including defective production of intrinsic factor by the stomach (atrophic gastritis; abnormally low small intestinal luminal pH (Zollinger-Ellison syndrome); the presence of bacterial overgrowth; diseases of the terminal ileum (Crohn's disease); or surgical resection. Folate deficiency can arise from diseases of the proximal small intestine, such as celiac or tropical sprue. This feature distinguishes bacterial overgrowth, where folate levels are increased. In addition, it is important to remember that vitamin B_{12} deficiency can in turn lead to folate malabsorption. Furthermore, it is not infrequently observed that several of these deficiencies (iron, folate, and B_{12}) coexist in the same patient, producing a mixed microcytic and macrocytic picture on peripheral blood smear. In addition, other abnormalities of red cell morphology may point to specific diseases; Howell-Jolly bodies, for example, are found in some patients with celiac sprue.

White Blood Cells

Increased numbers of peripheral blood neutrophils are associated with infections caused by many of the enteroinvasive pathogens, often in association with features of a systemic inflammatory process such as fever. Examples of such organisms include *Salmonella* spp., *Shigella* spp., *Campylobacter jejuni, Vibrio parahaemolyticus,* enteroinvasive *Escherichia coli, Yersinia* spp., *Aeromonas* spp., and *Clostridium difficile.* Leukocytosis and fever may also arise in association with intraabdominal abscess formation, for example, from an appendiceal or diverticular collection. In addition, fever and leukocytosis are features equally consistent with idiopathic inflammatory bowel diseases, such as Crohn's disease and ulcerative colitis.

In addition to intestinal diseases associated with leukocytosis, intestinal diseases associated with immune deficiency states—particularly acquired immunodeficiency syndrome (AIDS) and acquired immunodeficiency associated with prolonged chemotherapy and immunosuppressive regimens—now appear to be of emerging importance. Such patients are at risk for infections with *Cryptosporidium* spp., microsporidians, *Giardia lamblia,* cytomegalovirus, *Entamoeba histolytica,* and other organisms. In addition, patients with prolonged neutropenia are more susceptible to *Clostridium difficile* infections.

The presence of elevated eosinophils in the peripheral blood should alert the clinician to the possibility of parasitic or helminthic infestation. Infestations with roundworm and tapeworms are notorious in this regard. Patients who are receiving corticosteroid therapy

or who have impaired cellular immunity are susceptible to life-threatening hyperinfection with strongyloides, and thus the presence of eosinophilia in these subjects should prompt an examination of the stool and appropriate serologic examination. Finally, peripheral eosinophilia may be associated with diarrhea in subjects with eosinophilic gastroenteritis.

The presence of lymphopenia may be found in exudative enteropathies such as celiac sprue and may be a prominent feature in diseases of intestinal lymphatic drainage, such as primary intestinal lymphangiectasia. Secondary intestinal lymphangiectasia, such as accompanies radiation damage or diffuse infiltrative diseases, may also produce lymphopenia.

STUDIES OF SERUM ELECTROLYTES AND OTHER CHEMICAL FACTORS

Abnormalities in serum electrolytes are common in diarrheal diseases and usually reflect predictable disturbances resulting from fluid loss. Hypokalemia is common in this setting and is frequently accompanied by alkalosis. Patients with large villous adenomas frequently present with diarrhea and isolated hypokalemia. In addition, the presence of severe hypokalemia in association with diarrheal disease refractory to investigation, should lead to a search for potential laxative abuse, particularly if there is evidence of other psychiatric illness. As alluded to earlier, malabsorption of vitamin D may lead to a low serum calcium and magnesium concentration. In this regard, it is important to determine ionized calcium, since hypoalbuminemia may itself produce low total serum calcium levels. Hypoalbuminemia may reflect disturbances in protein losses from the intestinal tract, as with celiac sprue or idiopathic inflammatory bowel diseases. Subjects with congenital or acquired hypogammaglobulinemia are predisposed to infections that cause diarrhea, particularly giardiasis.

Abnormalities in the delivery or effective intraluminal concentration of bile salts are frequently associated with fat maldigestion and malabsorption, which, in turn, produces a constellation of disturbances in blood chemistry. Serum cholesterol concentrations are invariably decreased from the patient's baseline, and serum carotene concentrations are usually low. As a result of the disturbances in fat absorption, there is a decreased absorption of the fat-soluble vitamins (A, D, E, and K). Defects in absorption of vitamins A and D have been alluded to earlier. Defects in vitamin K absorption affect the synthesis of factors II, VII, IX, and X and lead to prolongation of the prothrombin time and a bleeding diathesis. Defects in vitamin E absorption are of great significance in neural development in childhood.

Low serum iron and elevated total iron binding capacity are associated with iron deficiency states. Similarly, reduced serum and red cell folate levels may be seen in malabsorption states, as well as in chronic starvation and malnutrition states, such as chronic alcoholism. Serum vitamin B_{12} levels are reduced in bacterial overgrowth states and in the presence of ileal disease or resection. Serum zinc levels are reduced in chronic diarrheal conditions and in association with prolonged malnutrition. Low serum zinc levels may be associated with defects in wound healing and repair; thus attention to zinc status is important in patients recovering from surgical procedures, particularly those with idiopathic inflammatory bowel disease.

In the evaluation of chronic diarrheas, it may become important to determine the circulating levels of certain hormones, some of which may function as autonomous secretagogues. These include gastrin, vasoactive intestinal polypeptide (VIP), calcitonin, substance P, thyroxine, and histamine. Gastrinomas are occasionally associated with protracted diarrhea and malabsorption, but this tumor most commonly presents as severe intractable ulcer disease. The etiology of the diarrhea in this setting is multifactorial, with contributions from the direct toxic effect of acidic pH on the small intestinal mucosa and the irreversible acidic denaturation of pancreatic lipase leading to fat maldigestion. VIP-omas of the pancreas produce a dramatic diarrheal condition, usually of high volume, that is invariably associated with severe hypokalemia. Calcitonin levels may be elevated with medullary carcinoma of the thyroid; this syndrome is frequently complicated by severe diarrhea. Diarrhea may occasionally be seen in both multiple endocrine neoplasia syndromes (MEN) I and IIA. In addition, isolated disturbances of thyroid function, particularly hyperthyroidism, may be associated with diarrhea and malabsorption. Diarrhea is also a feature of glucagonomas and somatostatinomas. Studies of urinary 5-hydroxyindole acetic acid (5-HIAA) may indicate the presence of carcinoid syndrome, whereas the levels of histamine may be elevated in subjects with systemic mastocytosis, another rare cause of diarrhea.

EXAMINATION OF THE STOOL

An indispensable component of the physical examination, regardless of an underlying suspicion of intestinal disease, is the careful inspection of the patient's stool. It is estimated that each year 60,000 people in the United States die from colon cancer; it has been suggested that careful screening could reduce this figure by up to one third. The examination of a patient's stool for the presence of occult blood is thus a vital component of the physical examination. In addition, recent developments in the technology for evaluating the presence of occult blood in the stool may improve the sensitivity of this test.

Direct visual examination of the stool is also helpful in establishing the potential etiology of intestinal diseases. Foul smelling, greasy stools that tend to be difficult to flush suggest the presence of steatorrhea. In addition, the response of the diarrhea to fasting—in conjunction with measurement of stool osmolality—is useful in establishing a diagnosis of osmotic diarrhea. Alkalinization of the stool may be helpful in establishing a diagnosis of laxative abuse. Some commercially available laxatives contain phenolphthalein, which turns red after alkalinization, whereas bisacodyl-containing laxatives turn the stool a bluish purple after alkalinization. Other tests to help establish the diagnosis of laxative abuse are discussed in a later section.

In regard to the evaluation of both acute and chronic diarrheas, examination of the stool for the presence of leukocytes, ova and parasites, and *Clostridium difficile* toxin is a very useful component of the algorithm used to establish a diagnosis. This examination should be conducted on freshly isolated samples and should ideally be conducted at least three times. In addition, this examination should precede the administration of enemas in preparation for endoscopic or radiologic examination of the bowel, since this may preclude the identification of organisms for several days.

The presence of *inflammatory cells* in the stool is of central importance in establishing the diagnosis and etiology of acute infectious diarrheas. In considering the diseases in which fecal leukocytes (pus) are present, organisms such as *Salmonella* spp., *Shigella* spp., *Campylobacter jejuni*, enteroinvasive *E. coli*, and *Clostridium difficile* should be considered strongly. Fecal leukocytes may be found in subjects with amebic dysentery, but this is not invariable. An experienced observer may identify trophozoites in the stool of patients with amebic colitis. In subjects with acute diarrheal disease and no detectable fecal leukocytes, organisms such as *Vibrio cholerae*, toxigenic *E. coli*, *Clostridium perfringens*, *Bacillus cereus*, *Giardia lamblia*, *Cryptosporidium* spp., and viral agents (Norwalk and rotavirus) should be considered.

Pus cells are anticipated in the stool of patients with chronic diarrheas resulting from idiopathic inflammatory bowel disease but are absent from the stool of subjects with diarrhea caused by celiac sprue. The evaluation of subjects with chronic diarrhea should also include serial examinations for the presence of ova and parasites, as well as stool culture.

In the evaluation of chronic diarrheas, a component of the investigation that is often useful is the *response to fasting*. Watery diarrheas that tend to resolve following this maneuver include those with an osmotic precipitant. This group includes the ingestion of nonabsorbable solutes (including magnesium-containing laxatives) or nonabsorbable carbohydrates (including sorbitol, which is often inadvertently consumed in the form of sugar-free gum) and the presence of various forms of carbohydrate malabsorption. Bile salt–induced diarrhea, although not produced by an osmotic effect, may also respond to fasting by virtue of the reduction in enterohepatic recycling. By contrast, diarrhea produced by the autonomous synthesis of secretagogues (including calcitonin, gastrin, VIP, pancreatic polypeptide, substance P, and histamine) is unresponsive to fasting.

Measurement of stool osmolality may assist in the differentiation of secretory from osmotic causes of diarrhea. However, it is important to bear in mind that the ingestion of sodium sulfate or sodium

phosphate, often in the form of laxatives, does not produce an osmotic gap, since the stool sodium content is also high. In this situation the simultaneous determination of stool electrolytes, including chloride concentrations, can be useful.

Measurement of stool pH is also useful, since carbohydrate malabsorption syndromes and many of the osmotic causes of diarrhea associated with the use of nonabsorbable carbohydrates generate increased quantities of intraluminal short-chain fatty acids, which lower stool pH. In the evaluation of suspected maldigestion and malabsorption syndromes, one of the benchmark determinations is the presence of increased amounts of *fecal fat*. In this regard, it is important to distinguish both by history and direct examination between steatorrhea (the presence of fatty stool) and diarrhea. The usual method for establishing the presence of steatorrhea is the collection of stools for quantitative fecal fat. This is usually performed for 72 hours and optimally requires that the subject consume a diet containing at least 75 g of fat per day. A quick estimate of the presence of steatorrhea can often be obtained by examination of a stool sample following mixing with alcohol and water, followed by the addition of Sudan III, which stains triglyceride an intense red color.

SPECIFIC TESTS FOR THE PRESENCE OF MALABSORPTION
Xylose Absorption Test

The sugar d-xylose is a pentose sugar that is absorbed without further processing by the small intestinal enterocyte, through both active and passive routes, and is not subsequently metabolized. Accordingly, the cumulative excretion of d-xylose in the urine or its peak serum concentration following the administration of a known quantity of the sugar by mouth is an extremely useful test of the integrity of the small bowel mucosa. The patient is usually fasted overnight and challenged with a 25-g bolus of d-xylose, followed by ample fluids to maintain good urine output. Normally, excretion of at least 5 g occurs over a 5-hour period, and serum levels at 1 to 2 hours exceed 25 mg/dl. Values less than these indicate mucosal disease, providing that none of the following exclusionary criteria exist:

> Presence of delayed gastric emptying, common in diabetics and the elderly.
> Presence of small intestinal bacterial overgrowth, in which case the sugar is metabolized by the bacteria.
> Presence of ascites, which increases the volume of distribution.
> Abnormalities in renal function, which diminish the excretion of d-xylose into the urine.

Hydrogen Breath Test

The diagnosis of carbohydrate malabsorption can often be made following a period of fasting, but the addition of a hydrogen breath test may help to discriminate between small intestinal mucosal disease and pancreatic insufficiency in the further evaluation of carbohydrate malabsorption. The test relies on the fermentation of unabsorbed carbohydrates by the colonic flora, with the consequent production of hydrogen, usually 3 to 5 hours following challenge with an oral carbohydrate load. One particularly informative modification of the test is to use a challenge of carbohydrate in the form of rice cakes, a substrate that has been found to generate large amounts of hydrogen when unabsorbed. The utility of this test can be further enhanced by repeating the examination following the administration of pancreatic supplements, a source of amylase. A decrease in breath hydrogen production following pancreatic supplementation points to pancreatic insufficiency as the likely cause of carbohydrate malabsorption. An early peak of breath hydrogen production (within 1 to 2 hours) is consistent with bacterial overgrowth of the small intestine and reflects abnormal intraluminal fermentation of dietary carbohydrate.

^{14}C-Triolein Breath Test

In some test centers the evaluation of fecal fat by chemical analysis of stool has been replaced by the examination of exhaled, radiolabeled CO_2 following administration of radiolabeled triolein. The principle of the test is that intraluminal lipolysis of triglyceride releases radiolabeled fatty acid, which is absorbed and transported to the liver, where it is ultimately metabolized, releasing $^{14}CO_2$, which is exhaled and measured. The test obviates the collection and analysis of stool, but its interpretation is subject to a number of reservations. Like the d-xylose test, it requires normal gastric emptying and assumes a normal volume of distribution (i.e., no ascites). In addition, the test is unreliable in subjects with liver failure or in the presence of obstructive lung disease.

^{14}C-Cholylglycine Absorption Test

There are two restricted functions of the ileal enterocyte, namely, the active absorption of bile salts and the absorption of vitamin B_{12}. In the assessment of bile salt malabsorption, subjects are given an oral dose of radiolabeled cholylglycine, the conjugated form of cholic acid. Under normal conditions, virtually the entire dose (~95%) is absorbed and undergoes enterohepatic recycling, with less than 5% entering the colon. The small quantities that enter the colon undergo deconjugation, and the radiolabeled glycine moiety is absorbed, returned to the liver, and metabolized to $^{14}CO_2$. Thus under normal circumstances, less than 5% of the dose is excreted on the breath at 8 hours. Under conditions of small intestinal bacterial overgrowth, which lead to deconjugation of the tracer within the upper small bowel, or in the presence of ileal disease, bypass, or resection, which leads to increased quantities of the tracer being delivered to the colon and subsequently absorbed, there is a correspondingly increased quantity of $^{14}CO_2$ detected on the breath.

Absorption of Vitamin B_{12}

As alluded to earlier, the absorption of vitamin B_{12} occurs only in the ileum. Various modifications of the Schilling test are available to determine the absorption of vitamin B_{12} with or without supplementation with intrinsic factor. The results of this test establish the diagnosis of vitamin B_{12} malabsorption and may point to a lack of intrinsic factor or to the presence of ileal disease (inflammation, infiltration, resection, or bypass) or bacterial overgrowth as a cause. To assist in the further evaluation of suspected bacterial overgrowth, the test may be conducted before and after the administration of a course of broad-spectrum antibiotics. In addition, the important role of pancreatic trypsin in cleaving gastric R proteins has been implicated in the malabsorption of vitamin B_{12} in some patients with pancreatic insufficiency. Another variant of the Schilling test is now available in which the differential urinary excretion of cobalamin bound to extrinsic R proteins is compared with that of cobalamin administered with intrinsic factor. Subjects with pancreatic insufficiency are able to absorb normally vitamin B_{12} conjugated to intrinsic factor, since ileal function is intact. In contrast, these subjects are unable to cleave the exogenous cobalamin–R protein complex, which consequently precludes its association with endogenous intrinsic factor and thereby leads to defective absorption. The absorption of vitamin B_{12} in relation to specific diseases is considered in greater detail in Chapter 326 of this text.

Demonstration of *enteric protein loss* can be accomplished by means of the α_1-antitrypsin clearance test, which determines the extent of intestinal loss of a protein synthesized exclusively in the liver through the simultaneous measurements of serum and fecal concentration. An alternative approach, based on the same principle, involves measurement of the clearance of radiolabeled serum albumin.

RADIOLOGIC STUDIES

An overview of some of the available radiologic studies is presented in this chapter; however, detailed discussion of the interpretation is found in the chapters dealing with specific diseases. General features of importance in the interpretation of the plain supine and erect abdominal radiograph include (1) the presence of distension of localized loops of bowel and the presence of air-fluid levels, features consistent with intestinal obstruction; (2) free air under the diaphragm, suggesting perforation of a hollow viscus; and (3) the presence of gas in the bowel wall, a feature compatible with intestinal ischemia and pneumatosis intestinalis. Nodularity or disturbance of the mucosal architecture and disturbances such as "thumb-printing" suggest the presence of ischemic bowel disease. The presence of pancreatic calcification may assist in the evaluation of suspected malabsorption.

Contrast radiology is also of use in regard to the evaluation of small intestinal diseases. Barium contrast studies can be performed by several techniques, including an oral small-bowel follow-through series or enteroclysis, the latter approach requiring intubation of the patient. Enteroclysis offers significant advantages over the oral small-bowel series in that controlled luminal distension can be achieved along with significantly less flocculation of barium, the net result of which is a considerable enhancement of either single or double contrast imaging. Enteroclysis is particularly useful in the evaluation of intermittent small-bowel obstruction, Crohn's disease, and small-bowel tumors. Meckel's diverticulum, which may occasionally be diagnosed by this approach, is more readily diagnosed by technetium-99 (^{99}Tc) scintigraphy. In addition, useful preliminary information is often gathered from enteroclysis in the evaluation of patients with suspected malabsorption.

Radiologic examination of the colon may offer valuable information, particularly in defining the extent and severity of idiopathic inflammatory bowel disease and diverticular disease and in the assessment of colonic polyps and carcinomas. In addition, patients with pelvic malignant disease in whom progression into adjacent structures is considered often benefit from barium contrast examination of the rectosigmoid to define extrinsic compression or displacement.

Angiography is useful in the evaluation of intestinal bleeding, often demonstrating the presence of unsuspected tumors or one of the different forms of angiodysplasia. Generally, the rate of blood loss must approach 1 ml per minute to demonstrate extravasation of contrast. Angiography is also used to establish a diagnosis of mesenteric ischemia. Finally, angiography is useful in establishing the diagnosis of small-bowel leiomyomas, which are usually hypervascular, and in the staging of intestinal carcinoid tumors.

Computed tomography (CT) is useful in the evaluation of inflammatory bowel disease, particularly in the discrimination of inflammatory masses and abscesses and in the diagnosis of intraabdominal fistulas. CT is also a reliable method for demonstrating intussusception. The applications of CT scanning in the evaluation of liver and pancreatic diseases are discussed elsewhere.

Other imaging modalities, including magnetic resonance imaging, have limited utility in the diagnosis of intestinal diseases as a result of motion artifacts produced by peristalsis.

ENDOSCOPY AND BIOPSY

Endoscopic examination of the upper gastrointestinal tract for evaluation of intestinal diseases may assist in the diagnosis of duodenal tumors (such as ampullary carcinoids) and localized inflammatory bowel disease (such as duodenal Crohn's disease) and is a useful means of obtaining aspirates for examination in cases of suspected malabsorption. With a sufficiently long instrument, it is possible to obtain biopsies from the distal portion of the duodenum as part of the evaluation of malabsorption. The interpretation of data provided by small intestinal biopsy is analyzed in Box 331-1.

Flexible sigmoidoscopy is of immense utility in the evaluation of diarrhea and in the initial approach to the patient with lower intestinal bleeding. In the evaluation of diarrhea, flexible sigmoidoscopic examination of the rectum and distal large bowel may identify ulceration and the presence of exudates, from which samples can be taken for microscopic identification and culture of organisms, including ova and parasites. The presence of pseudomembranes may provide a clue to infection with *Clostridium difficile*. In addition, the appearance of the mucosa in patients with chronic, unexplained diarrhea may provide clues to laxative abuse in the event that melanosis coli is identified.

The applications of colonoscopic examination in the evaluation of lower gastrointestinal tract malignancy, ischemia, diverticular disease, acute and chronic bleeding, inflammatory bowel disease, and infectious colitis are discussed in the relevant chapters dealing with these diseases.

EVALUATION OF MOTILITY

Colonic dysmotility is considered to be a major factor in the etiology of the symptoms associated with irritable bowel syndrome and some cases of chronic constipation. Clinical investigation of these disorders by means of evaluating the progress of nonabsorbable radionu-

---

BOX 331-1
Information provided by mucosal biopsy of small intestine

I. Disorders in which biopsy result is diagnostic: diffuse lesions
  A. Whipple's disease (Trophyerema whippelii)
    1. Lamina propria infiltrated with PAS-positive macrophages
    2. Characteristic bacilli in mucosa
  B. *Mycobacterium avium-intracellulare* enteritis: similar to Whipple's disease but bacilli are acid fast
  C. Severe immunoglobulin deficiency
    1. Mucosal architecture from normal to flat
    2. Plasma cells absent or markedly diminished in lamina propria
    3. Giardia trophozoites often present
  D. Abetalipoproteinemia
    1. Mucosal architecture normal
    2. Lipid-laden absorptive cells appear vacuolated
II. Disorders in which biopsy result may be diagnostic: patchy lesions
  A. Intestinal lymphoma
    1. Villi widened, shortened, or absent
    2. Malignant lymphoma cells in lamina propria and submucosa
  B. Intestinal lymphangiectasia
    1. Mucosal architecture normal
    2. Dilated lymphatics in lamina propria and submucosa
  C. Eosinophilic enteritis
    1. Mucosal architecture from normal to flat
    2. Patchy infiltration of lamina propria with eosinophils and neutrophils
  D. Mastocytosis
    1. Mucosal architecture from normal to flat
    2. Patchy infiltration of lamina propria with mast cells, eosinophils, and neutrophils
  E. Amyloidosis
    1. Mucosal architecture normal
    2. Amyloid in lamina propria and submucosa shown with Congo red stain
  F. Crohn's disease
    1. Mucosal architecture variable
    2. Noncaseating granulomata and inflammation in lamina propria and submucosa

G. Giardiasis
    1. Mucosal architecture from normal to flat
    2. Trophozoites in lumen and on surface of absorptive cells
    3. Minimal to severe inflammation in lamina propria
  H. Coccidiosis
    1. Villi shortened
    2. Crypts hyperplastic
    3. Coccidial forms on surface of (cryptosporidosis) or within *(Isospora)* absorptive cells
    4. Inflammation of lamina propria
III. Disorders in which biopsy result is abnormal but not diagnostic
  A. Celiac sprue
    1. Villi shortened or absent
    2. Crypts hyperplastic
    3. Severe absorptive cell damage
    4. Inflammation of lamina propria
  B. Unclassified sprue: indistinguishable from celiac sprue
  C. Tropical sprue
    1. Mucosal architecture from nearly normal to flat mucosa (as in celiac sprue)
    2. Absorptive cell damage mild
    3. Inflammation of lamina propria
  D. Viral gastroenteritis: indistinguishable from mild to moderate tropical sprue lesion
  E. Intraluminal bacterial overgrowth: may be normal or indistinguishable from mild to moderate tropical sprue lesion
  F. Folate and/or B_{12} deficiency, acute radiation enteritis
    1. Shortened villi
    2. Hypoplastic crypts
    3. Megalocytic epithelium
    4. Diminished mitoses
    5. Inflammation of lamina propria

PAS, Periodic acid-Schiff.

---

clides is currently confined to referral centers with expertise in nuclear medicine.

Anorectal manometry, on the other hand, is a useful adjunct to the investigation of patients with chronic constipation and incontinence and may provide information concerning the function of the internal and external sphincter muscles. In particular, the evaluation of anal sphincter tone can be used in combination with biofeedback techniques to improve the coordination of sensation and muscle contraction in some patients, particularly those with neurogenic causes of constipation.

BIBLIOGRAPHY

Allison JE et al: A comparison of fecal occult-blood tests for colorectal-cancer screening, *N Engl J Med* 334:155, 1996.
Donowitz M, Kokke FT, Saidi R: Evaluation of patients with chronic diarrhea: a review, *N Engl J Med* 332:725, 1995.
Guerrant RL, Bobak DA: Bacterial and protozoal gastroenteritis: a review, *N Engl J Med* 325:327, 1991.
Halsted CH: The importance of malnutrition in a patient with malabsorption, *Gastrointest Dis Tod* 3(6):1, 1994.
Kerlin P et al: Rice, flour, breath hydrogen, and malabsorption. *Gastroenterology* 87:578, 1984.
Levine MS et al: Contrast radiology. In Yamada T, editor: *Textbook of gastroenterology,* ed 2, Philadelphia, 1995, Lippincott, p. 2627.
Morrisey JF, Reichelderfer M: Gastrointestinal endoscopy, *N Engl J Med* 325:1142, 1214, 1991.
Ransohoff DF, Lang CA: Improving the fecal occult-blood test, *N Engl J Med* 334:189, 1996.
Trier JS: Intestinal malabsorption: differentiation of cause, *Hosp Pract* 23(5):195, 1988.

III CLINICAL SYNDROMES AND SPECIFIC DISEASE ENTITIES

CHAPTER

332 Gastrointestinal Bleeding

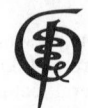

Gregory L. Eastwood

Throughout most of the gastrointestinal (GI) tract, the lumen of the gut is separated from the capillary blood supply by only a single layer of epithelial cells. Thus even minor injury to the epithelial lining may result in gastrointestinal bleeding.

Gastrointestinal bleeding ranges in severity from acute massive hemorrhage to chronic, intermittent, or nearly inconsequential blood loss. For the purposes of the following discussion, however, gastrointestinal bleeding is categorized as acute or chronic.

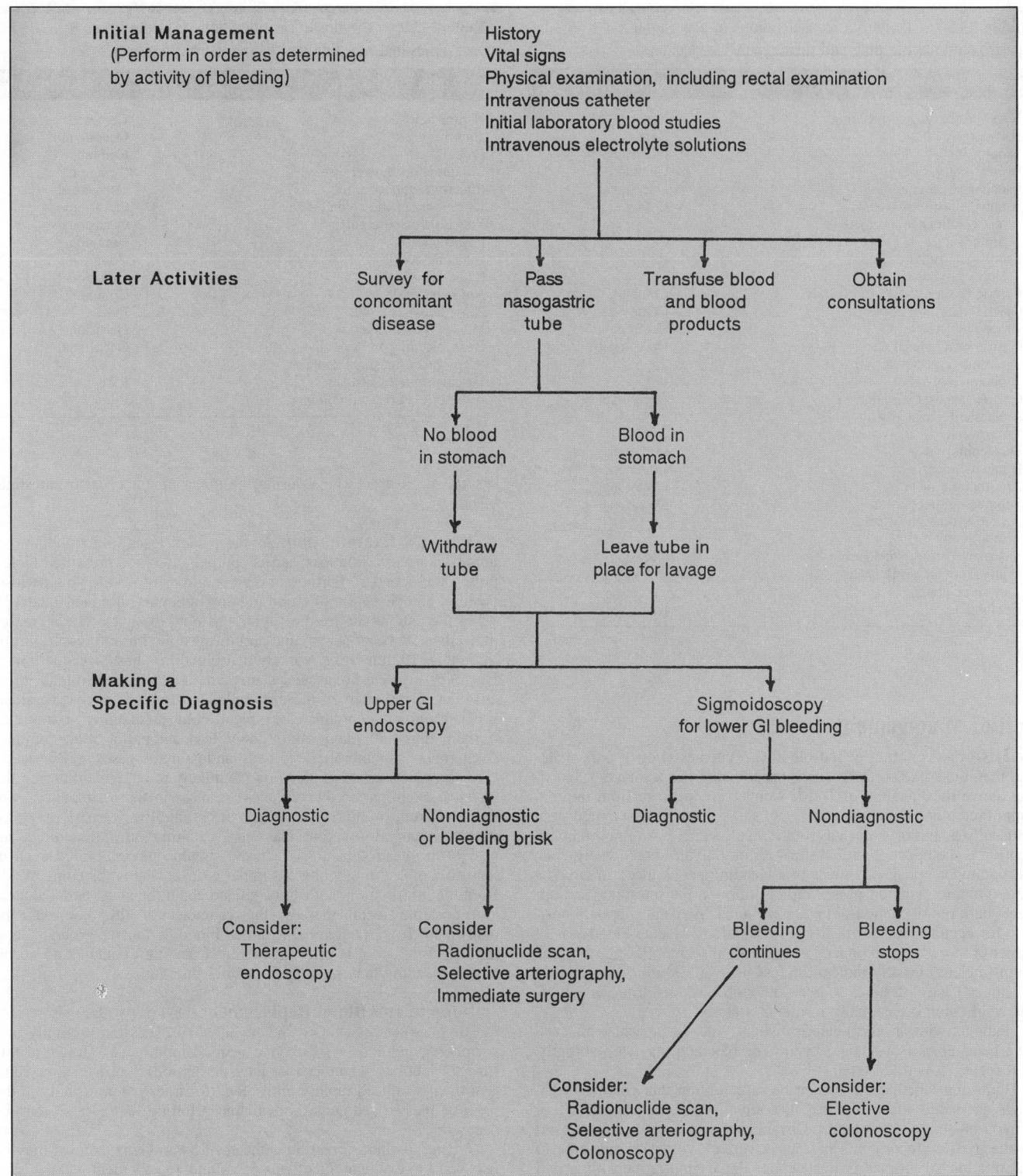

FIGURE 332-1   Management of acute gastrointestinal bleeding.

ACUTE GASTROINTESTINAL BLEEDING

Gastrointestinal bleeding generally is classified as either upper or lower in origin (Tables 332-1 and 332-2) because its source is only rarely in the "middle," that is, in the jejunum or ileum, and also because the presenting symptoms and signs frequently are characteristic of either an upper or lower gastrointestinal source. Although diagnostic methods and specific therapies may differ for upper and lower gastrointestinal bleeding, the principles of initial management of all patients with acute gastrointestinal bleeding are the same (Fig. 332-1). The orderly sequence of history taking, physical examination, diagnostic evaluation, and treatment frequently is readjusted to meet immediate demands, and the important aspects of each step often comingle in the first critical moments of managing the acutely bleeding patient.

Table 332-1   Diagnostic considerations in acute upper gastrointestinal bleeding and their relative frequencies

DIAGNOSTIC CONSIDERATION	RELATIVE FREQUENCY
Nasal or pharyngeal bleeding	Rare
Hemoptysis	Rare
Esophagitis	Occasional
Esophageal varices	Common
Esophageal carcinoma	Occasional
Esophagogastric mucosal tear (Mallory-Weiss syndrome)	Common
Esophageal rupture (Boerhaave's syndrome)	Rare
Gastric erosions	Common
Gastric ulcer	Common
Gastric varices	Common
Gastric or duodenal neoplasms (carcinoma, lymphoma, polyps)	Occasional
Gastric mucosal vascular ectasia associated with cirrhosis	Occasional
Duodenitis	Occasional
Duodenal ulcer	Common
Anastomotic ulcer	Occasional
Submucosal neoplasms (leiomyoma, most common)	Occasional
Vascular-enteric fistula (usually from an aortic aneurysm or graft)	Occasional
Hemobilia	Rare

Table 332-2   Diagnostic considerations in acute lower gastrointestinal bleeding and their relative frequencies

DIAGNOSTIC CONSIDERATION	RELATIVE FREQUENCY
Hemorrhoids	Common
Anal fissure	Occasional
Proctitis	Common
Inflammatory bowel disease	Common
Infectious enterocolitis	Occasional
Carcinoma of the colon	Occasional
Rectal or colonic polyps	Occasional
Diverticulosis	Common
Ischemic colitis	Common
Radiation colitis	Occasional
Angiodysplasia	Common
Amyloidosis	Rare
Meckel's diverticulum	Occasional
Brisk bleeding from an upper gastrointestinal source	Occasional
Vascular-enteric fistula	Rare
Antibiotic-associated colitis	Rare

essary, surgical decisions during the management of gastrointestinal bleeding.

Physical Examination. As the patient loses intravascular volume because of blood loss, cardiac output and blood pressure fall and pulse rate increases. Further, under conditions of severe volume loss, postural compensation of blood pressure and pulse are inadequate. If, when the patient sits from a supine position, the pulse rate increases more than 20 beats per minute and the systolic blood pressure drops more than 10 mm Hg, it is likely that blood loss has exceeded 1 liter. However, age, cardiovascular status, and rate of blood loss all influence the development of these so-called postural signs. Peripheral vasoconstriction may produce the typical "cold and clammy" extremities of the patient with major abrupt blood loss, and pallor of the conjunctivae, mucous membranes, nailbeds, and palmar creases may be seen.

The precise cause of bleeding is unlikely to be evident during the physical examination. Nevertheless, a mass in the abdomen, an abdominal bruit, or the physical signs of chronic liver disease may provide relevant information. The rectal examination allows direct access to the gastrointestinal tract and should not be omitted even in instances of seemingly obvious upper gastrointestinal bleeding. Aside from the information that can be gained about the anus, perianal area, and possible rectal masses, the character of the stool can be confirmed. If the patient has vomited blood or "coffee-grounds" material, yet the stool is brown, or even if the stool contains no occult blood, bleeding may have been of brief duration.

Volume and Blood Replacement. One or two large-bore (14- to 16-gauge) intravenous catheters should be inserted promptly into peripheral, jugular, or subclavian veins. Blood can be drawn at this time for laboratory studies (see later discussion). Normal saline solution then is infused rapidly until blood for transfusion, usually in the form of packed red cells, is available. Clotting factors also may be necessary.

A central venous pressure catheter or Swan-Ganz catheter may be necessary to evaluate the effects of volume replacement and the need for continued infusion of blood, particularly in elderly patients or those with cardiovascular disease. Finally, monitoring urine output provides a reasonable indication of vital organ perfusion. In severely ill patients a urinary catheter may be necessary.

Nasogastric Intubation and Gastric Lavage. A nasogastric (NG) tube should be passed in all patients with acute gastrointestinal bleeding unless the source is obviously the lower GI tract. Blood from an esophageal or gastric source pools in the stomach, and, in more than 90% of bleeding duodenal ulcers, the blood refluxes across the pyloric channel into the stomach. If the aspirate is clear or clears readily with lavage, the nasogastric tube may be removed. If there is fresh blood or a large amount of old blood or retained material, the

Initial Management

History. Vomiting of red blood (hematemesis) or of dark material that looks like coffee grounds usually signifies a source of bleeding above the ligament of Treitz. Conversely, passage from the rectum of red blood (hematochezia) or of a dark, mahogany-colored stool is usually a sign of lower gastrointestinal bleeding. An important exception is the upper gastrointestinal lesion that bleeds profusely, such as ruptured esophageal varices or a bleeding peptic ulcer, in which a large volume of blood passes rapidly through the intestines and appears dark red or even bright red at the anus. Stools may remain positive for occult blood for nearly 2 weeks after an acute blood loss of 1 liter or more from an upper gastrointestinal source. Passage of black stool (melena) usually indicates a loss of over 100 ml of blood from an upper gastrointestinal source, although bleeding from as low as the right colon occasionally results in melena.

Patients with an aorto-enteric fistula typically present with massive hematemesis or hematochezia. The bleeding may stop abruptly. If it recurs, it is often fatal.

Inquiring whether the patient has a condition that could bleed—such as peptic ulcer disease, ulcerative colitis, diverticulosis, or polyposis—may be important. Cirrhotics may have vascular ectasias of the gastric mucosa and, of course, varices. However, this type of information sometimes is misleading. For example, more than half of acutely bleeding patients with known esophageal varices have another lesion in the upper gastrointestinal tract.

Recent ingestion of aspirin or other nonsteroidal antiinflammatory drugs or alcohol raises the possibility that gastric erosions may be the cause of upper gastrointestinal bleeding. With respect to lower gastrointestinal bleeding, if the patient is over age 60, the four most common causes of lower gastrointestinal bleeding are diverticulosis, ischemic bowel disease, angiodysplastic lesions of the colon, and carcinoma. None of these diagnoses is common in the young patient, in whom colonic polyps, ulcerative colitis, Crohn's disease, and enteric bacterial and parasitic bowel disease are more likely.

Knowledge of concomitant illness—such as heart, liver, renal, or neurologic disease—may be valuable in guiding medical and, if nec-

stomach should be lavaged by means of a large-bore sump tube (20 to 24 French) or an Ewald tube in which additional side holes have been cut. Emptying the stomach facilitates subsequent endoscopy and may contribute to hemostasis by allowing the gastric musculature to contract.

The duration of nasogastric intubation must be individualized. The uses of the NG tube are to document the presence of blood, monitor the rate of bleeding, identify recurrence of bleeding after initial control, lavage and decompress the stomach, and remove gastric acid. However, there are a number of adverse effects. The NG tube is uncomfortable for the patient and may predispose to gastroesophageal reflux and aspiration. Moreover, the tube may irritate the esophagogastric junction and the gastric mucosa, creating mucosal artifacts and aggravating existing lesions. Because of its adverse effects, the NG tube should be removed promptly when it no longer fulfills a useful purpose.

Laboratory Studies. Initial blood studies should include a complete blood cell count (CBC); assessment of electrolytes, blood urea nitrogen (BUN), creatinine, glucose, calcium, phosphate, and magnesium levels; and blood for typing. Hemoglobin and hematocrit are usually low, and their level may have some relation to the degree of blood loss. However, some patients bleed so rapidly that there is not sufficient time for the blood volume to equilibrate, and the hemoglobin and hematocrit are normal or only slightly reduced. In the acutely bleeding patient, changes in blood pressure and pulse and direct evidence of massive bleeding are better indicators than hemoglobin and hematocrit for replacement of blood and administration of electrolyte solutions.

A low mean cell volume may mean that the patient is iron deficient and that the duration of blood loss has been prolonged. Elevated mean cell volume may indicate folate or vitamin B_{12} deficiency and raises the possibility of ethanol abuse, chronic liver disease, gastric cancer in association with pernicious anemia, or regional enteritis involving the terminal ileum.

Clotting status should be assessed with platelet count, prothrombin time, and partial thromboplastin time. If a defect in clotting exists, prompt correction of the deficiency is crucial. Extensive transfusion dilutes platelets and clotting factors, particularly factors V and VII. This problem can be treated by infusion of fresh-frozen plasma and platelets as necessary. Also, a high proportion of patients who bleed while taking therapeutic anticoagulants do so from a clinically significant lesion. Thus it is important to evaluate these patients for gastrointestinal pathologic condition in addition to correcting their clotting status.

Leukocytosis may accompany acute gastrointestinal bleeding, but it usually is not in excess of 15,000 white blood cells per cubic millimeter. However, leukocytosis should not be attributed to acute blood loss without first seeking sources of infection.

An elevated BUN level in a patient whose BUN has recently been normal or whose serum creatinine concentration is normal suggests an upper gastrointestinal bleeding source. The rise in BUN usually is due to the hypovolemia of acute blood loss, but digestion of blood proteins in the small intestine and the absorption of nitrogenous products also can contribute. In patients with impaired liver function, the increased protein load from the hemoglobin in blood may be sufficient to induce hepatic encephalopathy. Thus gastric lavage and control of the bleeding are especially important in these patients.

Because of rapid fluid shifts during gastrointestinal bleeding and subsequent infusion of blood, blood products, and other fluids, frequent assessment of serum electrolyte, calcium, phosphate, and magnesium levels is necessary.

Most patients who receive blood transfusions do not need calcium supplements, although hypocalcemia as a result of binding of calcium by anticoagulants in banked blood may occur after massive transfusion. Patients who receive more than 100 ml of blood per minute may be given 0.2 g $CaCl_2$ via another intravenous line during the time the blood is infusing. Measurement of the ionized calcium and monitoring of the electrocardiogram Q-T interval are recommended during the rapid infusion of anticoagulated blood.

Depending on the clinical presentation, other blood studies may also be important, such as serum amylase, liver, and cardiac enzyme tests. In severely ill patients, arterial blood gases should be monitored.

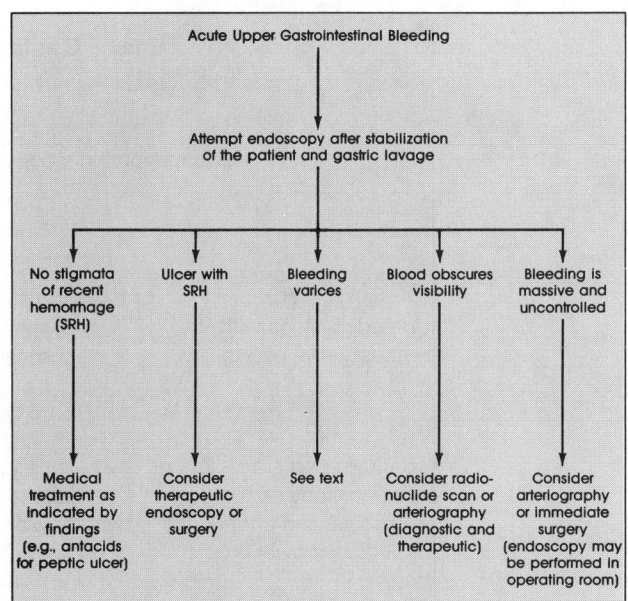

FIGURE 332-2   Scheme for the diagnostic evaluation of acute upper gastrointestinal bleeding. Stigmata of recent hemorrhage are a visible vessel, fresh blood clot, black slough, and active bleeding.

Team Approach. The appropriate management of acute gastrointestinal bleeding typically involves a team of physicians. Specific diagnostic studies, discussed later, usually require the expertise of a gastroenterologist or a radiologist. Further, a surgeon who has been involved with the patient from the outset is in a much better position to make a decision regarding operative intervention.

Diagnostic and Therapeutic Studies

After the patient with acute gastrointestinal bleeding has been stabilized, specific diagnostic studies can be undertaken to identify the source of bleeding (Figs. 332-1, 332-2, and 332-3). Some diagnostic procedures, such as endoscopy and arteriography, also have therapeutic capabilities.

Endoscopy. Endoscopy usually is recommended as the initial diagnostic procedure in patients with acute upper gastrointestinal bleeding because knowledge of a specific diagnosis may dictate a specific treatment regimen. For example, treatment of bleeding esophageal varices (see later discussion) is different from treatment of peptic ulcer, gastric erosions, or a Mallory-Weiss mucosal tear of the esophagogastric junction. Further, the endoscopic identification of active bleeding or evidence for recent bleeding—such as oozing or spurting blood, a protruding visible vessel, an adherent clot, or a black slough—may have prognostic and therapeutic significance. Patients with these findings are more likely to have uncontrolled bleeding or recurrent bleeding and to require intervention by therapeutic endoscopic methods or by surgery.

A number of reliable methods of treating patients endoscopically have been developed over the past decade. Endoscopic injection sclerotherapy of esophageal varices and variceal ligation are as effective as or better than surgical procedures, such as portosystemic shunts and esophageal transection, in controlling acute variceal bleeding. The question remains whether surgical or nonsurgical procedures improve survival. With regard to endoscopic treatment of bleeding ulcers (Table 332-3), the following statements can be made: (1) multipolar electrocoagulation, laser photocoagulation, and injection of sclerosants or epinephrine appear to be capable of controlling acute bleeding; (2) laser photocoagulation and electrocoagulation may reduce the need for emergency surgery and improve survival; (3) laser therapy is the most difficult to learn, whereas injection therapy is the least

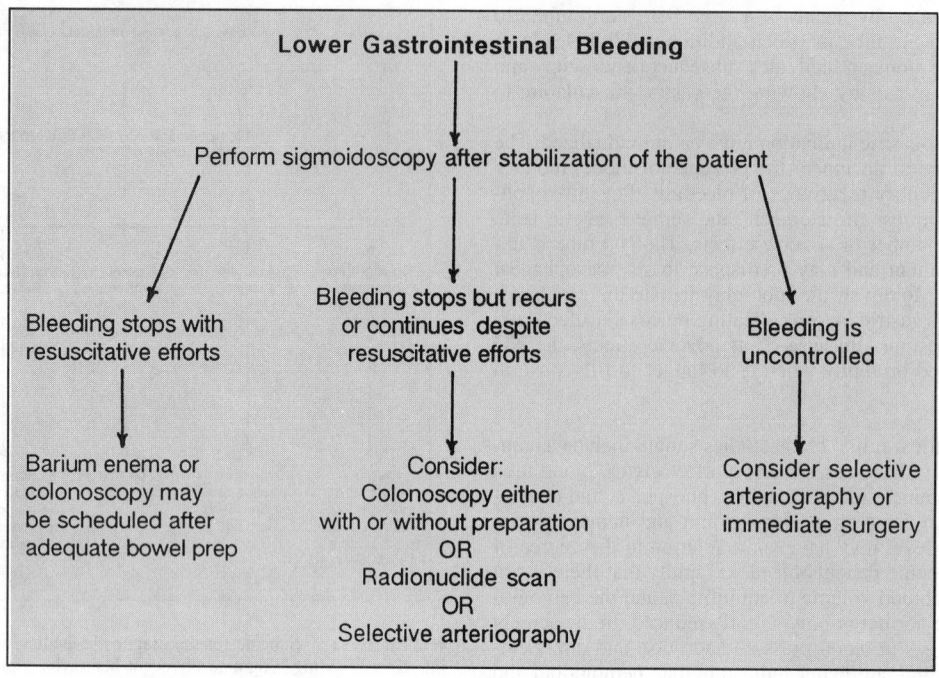

FIGURE 332-3   Scheme for the diagnostic evaluation of acute lower gastrointestinal bleeding.

Table 332-3   Endoscopic treatment of bleeding ulcers

	ELECTROCOAGULATION	LASER PHOTOCOAGULATION	INJECTION THERAPY
Control of bleeding	Yes	Yes	Yes
Reduction in need for surgery	Yes	Yes	?
Reduction in mortality	Yes	Yes	?
Difficulty to learn	Intermediate	Most	Least
Safety	Intermediate	Least	Most
Expense	Intermediate	Most	Least

difficult; and (4) injection therapy appears to be the safest and the least expensive.

Because bleeding from upper gastrointestinal lesions stops spontaneously in 75% to 90% of patients, endoscopic treatment should not be used indiscriminately. In general, patients with actively oozing or spurting ulcers are candidates for endoscopic treatment. Most endoscopists would also treat a visible vessel, and, although the procedure is controversial, some would even advocate dislodging an adherent clot to apply their method of endoscopic hemostasis. In all instances the application of endoscopic therapy is dependent on accessibility. Thus some bleeding ulcers, particularly those within the duodenum, are in positions that are not readily amenable to endoscopic treatment.

The initial diagnostic procedure for acute lower gastrointestinal bleeding is proctosigmoidoscopy using either a rigid or a flexible instrument. This procedure should be performed while the patient is bleeding actively to maximize the chance of making a diagnosis (see Fig. 332-3).

The role of fiberoptic colonoscopy in massive lower gastrointestinal bleeding remains controversial. Blood and stool tend to obscure visibility. Some endoscopists advocate that an emergency colonoscopy be performed after cleaning the colon with osmotically balanced electrolyte solutions or saline solution, administered orally or by nasogastric tube. Others prefer initial selective arteriography, saving colonoscopy as an elective procedure. (For a detailed discussion of endoscopy see Chapter 328.)

Radionuclide Scanning. Scanning the abdomen after intravenous injection of sulfur colloid or red blood cells labeled with technetium 99m (^{99m}Tc) may indicate the site of bleeding and lead to more definitive diagnostic or therapeutic procedures. The radionuclide scan appears to be more sensitive than selective arteriography in detecting active bleeding because a positive scan requires a lower rate of bleeding (less than 0.5 ml per minute). However, the radionuclide scan is considerably less specific than arteriography in locating the site of bleeding.

Selective Arteriography. Selective arteriography of the celiac axis, superior mesenteric artery, inferior mesenteric artery, or their branches can be both diagnostic and therapeutic. A focal collection of extravasated dye indicates a bleeding arterial lesion. It has been estimated from animal studies that, for this to occur, the rate of blood loss must be at least 0.5 ml per minute (750 ml/day). In hemorrhagic gastritis, a diffuse blush in the region of the stomach may appear. During the venous phase, esophageal, gastric, or small intestinal varices may be seen, although actual variceal bleeding usually cannot be documented by arteriography.

Infusion of vasopressin, 0.1 to 0.5 unit per minute into the artery supplying the bleeding site, has been effective in controlling arterial bleeding (Fig. 332-4). Diffuse hemorrhagic gastritis has been treated by vasopressin infusion into the left gastric artery. Even variceal bleeding may be controlled by vasopressin infusion into the superior mesenteric artery, thereby diminishing splanchnic blood flow and reducing portal venous pressure. Infusion of vasopressin into a peripheral vein at a rate of 0.3 to 1.2 units per minute has been shown to be as effective as intraarterial vasopressin infusion in the control of bleeding from esophageal varices, and the frequencies of cardiovascular side effects after peripheral and arterial vasopressin infusion are similar. In patients at risk for ischemic cardiovascular disease, venous infusion of nitroglycerin may reduce the hazard of va-

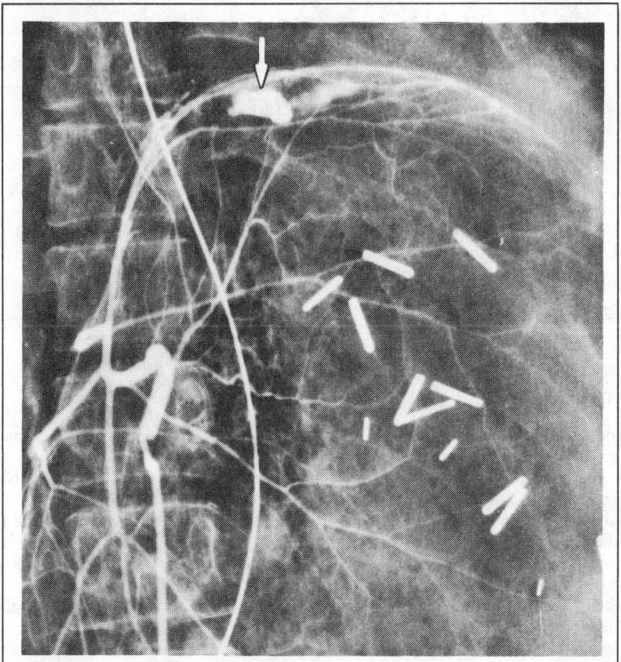

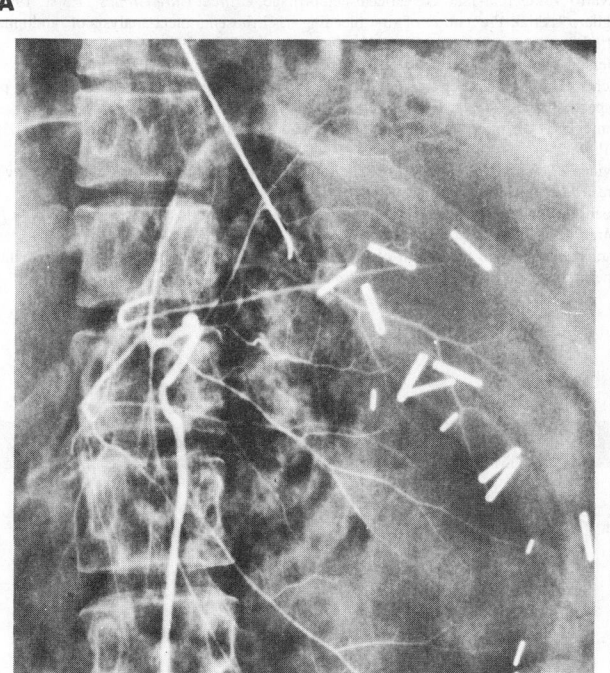

FIGURE 332-4 Selective arteriogram from a woman with acute upper gastrointestinal hemorrhage. Endoscopy revealed a gastric ulcer of the fundus. **A,** Extravasation of dye in the fundus of the stomach *(arrow).* **B,** Infusion of vasopressin into the left gastric artery at 0.2 U per minute has resulted in a cessation of bleeding, manifested by disappearance of the extravasated dye.

Arteriograms courtesy of Frederick Keller, M.D.

sopressin. Injection of autologous clot or small pieces of gel foam to embolize arteries supplying localized bleeding sites also has controlled bleeding in diverticulosis, angiodysplasia, and, occasionally, peptic ulcer disease.

Barium Contrast Radiography. Barium contrast studies of the upper or lower gastrointestinal tract usually are not recom-

mended in the initial diagnostic evaluation of patients with acute gastrointestinal bleeding. Such studies have a lower diagnostic yield than endoscopic methods, and barium in the stomach or intestine can hinder endoscopic visualization and render an arteriogram uninterpretable.

Antacids and Antisecretory Agents

The reduction of intragastric acid in patients with upper gastrointestinal bleeding is helpful in two ways. First, the direct harmful effects of acid and pepsin on the bleeding site are diminished. Second, a less acid environment promotes platelet aggregation and clotting.

After the acute bleeding has abated and gastric lavage is no longer necessary, an appropriate initial regimen is administration of 30 ml of antacid by nasogastric sump tube every 2 hours. The tube is clamped for the first hour and suctioned for the second hour. Measurement of intragastric pH just before the next antacid dose indicates whether the frequency and dose of antacid should be increased. The intent is to maintain the intragastric pH above 4. Whether intravenous H_2 antagonists are as efficacious as antacids for the control of gastric acid in acute upper gastrointestinal bleeding is controversial. After the nasogastric tube has been removed, the patient may be treated with oral antacids and an acid-antisecretory agent.

Treatment of Bleeding Esophageal Varices

For a more detailed discussion see Chapter 354.

Management of Acute Bleeding. The treatment of bleeding esophageal varices differs substantially from the treatment of most other bleeding lesions of the upper gastrointestinal tract. Moreover, patients with esophageal varices typically have severe liver disease and thus are likely to suffer from poor nutrition, blood clotting disorders, and encephalopathy, all of which can adversely affect morbidity and mortality.

In most institutions, endoscopic injection sclerosis or endoscopic ligation by means of rubber O-rings (banding) is the initial choice of treatment. Some endoscopists prefer to control bleeding first by peripheral venous vasopressin (discussed earlier) or balloon tamponade before attempting sclerosis. Endoscopic ligation is as effective as sclerosis in controlling bleeding. Ligation eradicates the varices more rapidly than sclerosis and reduces the adverse side effects—such as fever, chest pain, esophageal ulceration, and pleural effusion—that have been associated with sclerosis.

The triple-lumen Sengstaken-Blakemore (SB) tube is representative of several tubes that can compress gastroesophageal varices by balloon tamponade. One lumen is used to evacuate the stomach. The second and third lumens lead to the gastric and esophageal balloons, respectively. Some newer tubes have a fourth lumen that allows suction of blood and secretions from the esophagus. If the fourth lumen is not present, an accessory sump tube should be passed alongside the SB tube into the midesophagus.

The SB tube has been associated with serious complications, including occlusion of the airway by the esophageal balloon, pulmonary aspiration of secretions and blood from the esophagus, and ischemic necrosis of the esophageal mucosa caused by prolonged compression by the balloon. Appropriate use of the SB tube, as described by Pitcher, minimizes these risks.

Because the surgical mortality is so high in patients with bleeding esophageal varices, emergency surgery (portacaval anastomosis or esophageal transection and reanastomosis) is an unwelcome last resort in the treatment of acute variceal bleeding.

Long-Term Management. After acute variceal bleeding has been controlled by endoscopic injection sclerosis, balloon tamponade, or vasopressin infusion, a decision regarding long-term management of the varices must be made because the risk of rebleeding is high. Beta-blockade therapy to reduce portal hypertension in patients with mild liver disease and little or no ascites may be effective. However, because enthusiasm for beta-blockade has waned and long-term survival of some patients may be increased after either chronic endoscopic sclerosis or portasystemic shunt surgery, most patients should be considered for one of those treatments. The risk of encephalopathy is lower and the risk of rebleeding is higher in sclerosed patients than in shunted patients, but the short- and long-term survival and total health care costs are about the same with both methods of treatment. Chronic endoscopic sclerosis, consisting of repeated injections separated by 1 to 4 weeks, is a reasonable first choice. Complications include perforation of the esophagus, mucosal ulceration and necrosis, and stricture formation. Repeated endoscopic ligation of varices until they are obliterated appears to be associated with fewer complications and may be as effective as sclerosis. Patients who have recurrent variceal bleeding despite sclerotherapy or ligation and are acceptable operative risks may benefit from portasystemic shunt surgery.

CHRONIC GASTROINTESTINAL BLEEDING

Most lesions that cause acute bleeding also can cause chronic bleeding from the gastrointestinal tract. Chronic bleeding usually is slow and may be intermittent, sometimes making diagnosis difficult.

If the history and physical examination do not strongly suggest an upper gastrointestinal site of bleeding, the usual first diagnostic study is a colonoscopy. When colitis is suspected, a balanced electrolyte bowel preparation or no preparation at all is preferred to a cathartic.

If no lesion of the large bowel is identified, upper gastrointestinal endoscopy should be performed to examine the esophagus, stomach, and proximal duodenum. Further evaluation is accomplished by radiologic examination of the small bowel by means of either a small-bowel series or a small-bowel enema (enteroclysis). The latter sometimes yields more diagnostic information than a conventional small-bowel series and is performed by passing a tube by mouth into the proximal small intestine and then injecting barium and methylcellulose.

A small number of patients continue to bleed, usually intermittently, from a source that defies location, even after repeated hospital admissions. Unusual causes of bleeding must be considered in these patients, and sometimes extraordinary measures are required to make the diagnosis.

A ^{99m}Tc sulfur colloid scan may show a Meckel's diverticulum that contains gastric mucosa. Although only about 20% of Meckel's diverticula contain gastric mucosa, these are the diverticula that ulcerate and bleed. Thus a scan that reveals a Meckel's diverticulum in a bleeding patient who has no other identifiable site of bleeding is strong evidence that the diverticulum is the source.

Selective arteriography usually is not helpful in a chronically bleeding patient because the rate of bleeding is too slow to visualize the lesion. However, arteriography may suggest a tumor or an angiodysplastic lesion by showing an abnormal vascular pattern. Vascular lesions of the bowel, particularly in the ascending colon, are an important cause of gastrointestinal bleeding. These vascular lesions occur in all age groups but more frequently in the elderly and perhaps in patients with aortic stenosis. Arteriovenous shunts appear to develop as a normal consequence of aging and thus may occur in asymptomatic elderly people. Telangiectatic lesions anywhere within the gastrointestinal tract also may occur spontaneously, or they may be associated with hereditary telangiectasia (Osler-Weber-Rendu disease).

In some instances, obscure small intestinal lesions may be identified by passing an endoscope from above or below into the small intestine at the time of laparotomy. The surgeon advances the endoscope with ease throughout the small intestine by direct manipulation. Lesions can be visualized directly through the instrument by the endoscopist or may be transilluminated through the bowel wall and discovered by the surgeon.

Factitious gastrointestinal bleeding must be considered in some chronically bleeding patients. Self-injury, surreptitious phlebotomy, ingestion of blood, and rectal instillation of blood have all been used to simulate disease. Of such patients 90% are women, and they typically have worked in a medically related field. Close supervision of the patient, alertness to unexplained needle marks, and a careful watch for hidden needles and syringes may suggest the diagnosis.

✔ *WHEN TO REFER*

As discussed earlier, the management of the patient with gastrointestinal bleeding usually is a team effort. Thus, in a practical sense, most patients with gastrointestinal bleeding are referred by the physician with primary responsibility to colleagues for gastroenterologic, radiologic, and surgical consultation and for specific diagnostic tests as part of the appropriate management. If endoscopic, radiologic, or surgical expertise is not available, the patient with acute gastrointestinal bleeding should be stabilized and referred to a center where such expertise is available.

BIBLIOGRAPHY

Bentley DE, Richardson JD: Role of tagged red blood cell imaging in the localization of gastrointestinal bleeding, *Arch Surg* 126:821, 1991.

Caos A et al: Colonoscopy after golytely preparation in acute rectal bleeding, *J Clin Gastroenterol* 8:46, 1986.

Eastwood GL: Endoscopy in gastrointestinal bleeding: are we beginning to realize the dream? *J Clin Gastroenterol* 14:187, 1992.

Grande JP, Ackermann DM, Edwards WD: Aortoenteric fistulas: a study of 28 autopsied cases spanning 25 years, *Arch Pathol Lab Med* 113:1271, 1989.

Luk GD, Bynum TE, Hendrix TR: Gastric aspiration in localization of gastrointestinal hemorrhage, *JAMA* 241:576, 1979.

Maglinte DDT et al: Enteroclysis in the diagnosis of chronic unexplained gastrointestinal bleeding, *Dis Colon Rectum* 28:403, 1985.

Navarro VJ, Garcia-Tsao G: Variceal hemorrhage, *Critical Care Clinics* 11:391, 1995.

Pagliaro L et al: Prevention of first bleeding in cirrhosis: a meta-analysis of randomized trials of nonsurgical treatment, *Ann Intern Med* 117:59, 1992.

Peterson WL: Clinical risk factors, *Gastrointest Endosc* 36:S14, 1990.

Pitcher JL: Safety and effectiveness of the modified Sengstaken-Blakemore tube: a prospective study, *Gastroenterology* 61:291, 1971.

Pointer R et al: Endoscopy treatment of Dieulafoy's disease, *Gastroenterology* 94:563, 1988.

Savides TJ, Jensen DM: Endoscopic therapy for severe gastrointestinal bleeding, *Adv Intern Med* 40:243, 1995.

Skeens J, Semba C, Dake M: Transjugular intrahepatic portosystemic shunts, *Annu Rev Med* 46:95, 1995.

Wara P: Endoscopic prediction of major rebleeding: a prospective study of stigmata of hemorrhage in bleeding ulcer, *Gastroenterology* 88:1209, 1985.

CHAPTER

333 Esophageal Diseases

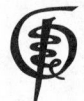

Robert W. Summers and Konrad S. Schulze-Delrieu

Clinical problems arise commonly because of inflammation of the esophageal mucosa, tumors, or neuromuscular abnormalities that interfere with esophageal transit. Esophageal inflammation is often due to the reflux of corrosive gastrointestinal secretions and is sometimes caused by the ingestion of caustic agents or drugs. Viral or fungal infections may involve the esophagus, particularly in association with oropharyngeal or systemic infections. Esophageal dysmotility may be caused by systemic diseases that interfere with esophageal neuromuscular function (e.g., scleroderma, diabetes, Parkinson's disease) or by primary abnormalities in the intrinsic esophageal nerves and muscle (e.g., achalasia, spasm).

SYNDROMES OF CHRONIC GASTROESOPHAGEAL REFLUX AND REFLUX ESOPHAGITIS

The terms *hiatal hernia, reflux,* and *esophagitis* are often used interchangeably. The term *reflux* refers to the regurgitation of gastrointestinal contents into the esophagus without associated retching and vomiting. The contents may be gas, food, or gastrointestinal secretions. Belief episodes of reflux are common, particularly in the postprandial period, but rarely cause symptoms in healthy individuals. Abnormal reflux may manifest itself by ease of provocation (e.g., the regurgitation of gastric contents on stooping or lying down) or by frequency (e.g., the occurrence of heartburn after each meal). Long-term monitoring of esophageal pH (Chapter 329) is the best current means to document an abnormal reflux profile. *Gastroesophageal reflux disease* refers to manifestations of esophageal, laryngeal, or pulmonary injury related to the reflux of gastrointestinal contents. The most common manifestation is *reflux esophagitis;* the term should be reserved for instances in which reflux-related changes in esophageal structure have been documented. Other problems in which gastroesophageal reflux disease has been implicated include sore throat, earache, dental deterioration, laryngitis, aspiration pneumonia, asthma, and interstitial pulmonary fibrosis.

Etiology and Pathogenesis

The severity of gastroesophageal reflux disease depends on (1) the severity of the mechanical dysfunction, (2) the composition of the refluxate, and (3) the resistance of the target organ. Variations in these individual factors probably contribute to the development of laryngeal or respiratory tract complications from reflux in some patients in the absence of esophageal lesions.

Mechanical Abnormalities. Abnormalities of lower esophageal sphincter (LES) function, of esophageal peristalsis and clearance, and of gastric motility are common in gastroesophageal reflux disease. Because the esophageal abnormalities may themselves be worsened by esophagitis and may improve as the esophagitis improves, it is at times difficult to distinguish cause from effect. In a few instances, abnormal reflux can be tracked to a specific cause such as gastric intubation; pregnancy; or removal or destruction of the gastric cardia by operation, tumor, or systemic sclerosis. In some families, reflux complications occur at an early age in several individuals; it is possible that this reflux is due to an inherited defect in the antireflux barrier. An *incompetent LES* as defined by the virtual absence of a high-pressure zone and the presence of the "common cavity phenomenon" (Chapter 329) occurs in patients with scleroderma and severe esophagitis but otherwise is an inconstant finding in gastroesophageal reflux disease. Most episodes of gastroesophageal reflux occur across a competent sphincter that relaxes intermittently; the relaxation of the LES in these instances is thought to relate to inhibitory reflexes that can be triggered by gastric distention.

Esophageal clearance is impaired in many patients with gastroesophageal reflux disease. When there is significant inflammation of the esophageal mucosa, many swallows do not lead to the normal sequential contraction of the esophagus known as *primary peristalsis.* Swallowing ceases during sleep; combined with the horizontal position, this characteristic increases the time during which any refluxate is in contact with the esophageal mucosa.

Abnormalities of gastric emptying often compound the motility problems occurring with gastroesophageal reflux. Gastric retention from any cause aggravates reflux by increasing the volume of secretions available for reflux. Conditions that reduce the gastric storage capacity and increase postprandial intragastric pressure, such as partial gastric resections, also seem to increase the risk of reflux.

Corrosiveness of the Refluxate. The composition of the refluxate is another determinant of injury. If the refluxate consists entirely of air and gas, the resulting belching would be considered harmless. It is also likely that neutral solutions refluxing back from the stomach would be of little importance to the esophagus but could have undesirable effects if aspirated into the respiratory tract. The hydrochloric acid and pepsin produced by the stomach are held primarily responsible for the corrosiveness of the gastric refluxate. Gastric secretions attack intercellular junctions and produce patchy, superficial lesions. Although acid is the most important factor causing injury, the rate of gastric secretion is no greater than in normal individuals; injury is caused by the increase in the time of mucosal exposure to acid. Bile salts damage plasma membranes, thereby potentiating the corrosiveness of gastric secretions. Particularly severe esophageal injury can be produced by deconjugated bile salts in combination with tryp-

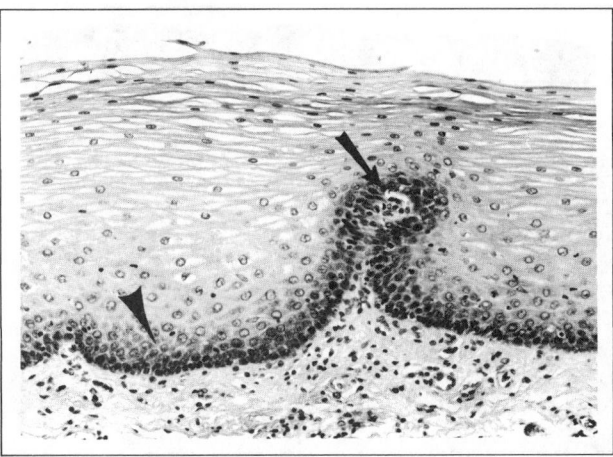

FIGURE 333-1   Normal histologic appearance of the esophageal mucosa *(original magnification, ×50).* The squamous epithelium is many layers thick and is supported by the lamina propria. Extensions of the lamina propria form papillae in the epithelium; the tips of the papillae reach about half the total epithelial height *(arrow).* The germinative cells are recognized by their dark-staining nuclei. They are found in the basal cell layer, which contributes less than 15% of the total epithelial height *(arrowhead).*
Photomicrograph courtesy of Frank Mitros, M.D., Department of Pathology, University of Iowa.

sin. High gastric concentrations of bile salts have indeed been found in some patients with severe reflux esophagitis, and pancreaticobiliary secretions are held responsible for the esophageal reflux lesions that may occur in patients with achlorhydria or after total gastrectomy.

Resistance of the Esophageal Mucosa. The resistance of the esophagus to damage relates largely to the barrier functions of its mucosa. Important components of the barrier are (1) the glycoconjugate matrix in the extracellular space of the superficial layers of the squamous mucosa and (2) an antiport in the squamous cells that prevents cellular acidification and swelling. Alkaline mucosal and salivary secretions contribute to esophageal resistance by flushing the esophagus of residue and by neutralizing acid adherent to the esophageal mucosa. This function is impaired in the "sicca syndrome."

Indirect Consequences of Gastroesophageal Reflux. Not all clinical manifestations of reflux are mediated by the direct exposure of tissues to the refluxate; gastroesophageal reflux stimulates esophageal nerves, which mediate reflex responses. Oropharyngeal secretions are triggered by esophageal acidification (leading to water brash). Esophageal distention and acidification lead to forceful contraction of the upper esophageal sphincter (cricopharyngeal spasm or globus sensation). Reflex responses as well as aspiration of refluxate are thought to be responsible for the bronchospasm, laryngospasm, and cricopharyngeal spasm that occur in some patients with gastroesophageal reflux.

Pathology of Reflux Esophagitis

Reflux can cause a variety of morphologic changes. Acute injury is characterized by edema and necrosis, particularly of cells in the more basal layers of the squamous epithelium. The initial lesions occur in the distal esophagus; as the disease progresses, lesions spread to more proximal esophageal segments, and chronic changes may develop in the distal esophagus. The major changes are (1) epithelial erosions; (2) squamous cell hyperplasia; (3) mucosal metaplasia (Barrett's esophagus); and (4) esophageal scarring (short esophagus, peptic esophageal stricture).

Esophageal Erosions. Esophageal erosions are circumscribed areas of epithelial desquamation (compare Figs. 333-1 and 333-2). The mucosal blood vessels become congested, and the lamina propria and surrounding epithelium are infiltrated by leukocytes, many

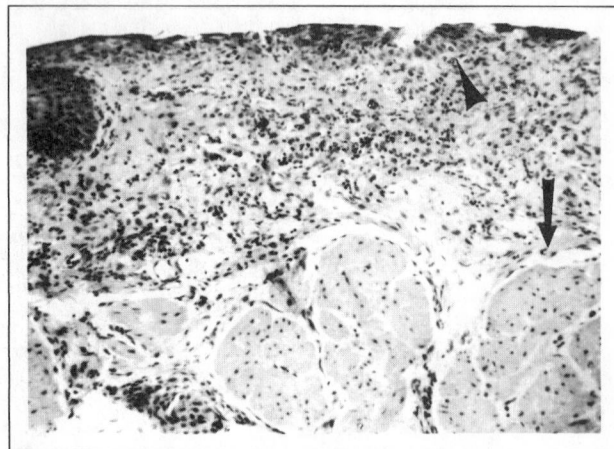

FIGURE 333-2 Histologic abnormalities in reflux esophagitis *(original magnification, ×30)*. Esophageal erosion caused by esophageal reflux. Most layers of the epithelium have sloughed off, and only the basal cells remain *(arrowhead)*. The lamina propria is infiltrated by many inflammatory cells. The arrow points to the muscularis mucosae *(×100)*.

Photomicrograph courtesy of Frank Mitros, M.D., Department of Pathology, University of Iowa.

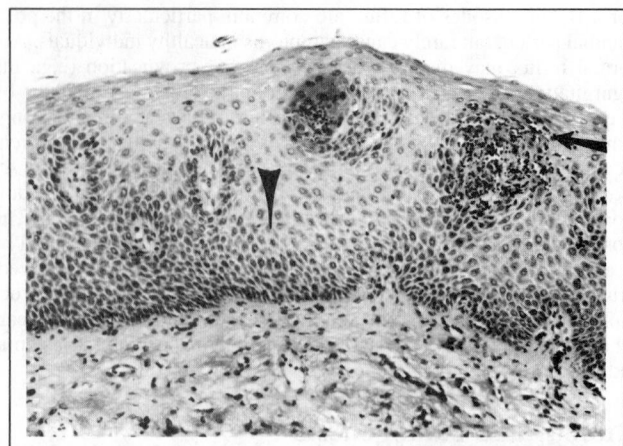

FIGURE 333-3 Epithelial hyperplasia *(original magnification, ×40)*. There is proliferation of basal cells *(arrowhead)*, and the papillae reach through more than 75% of the total epithelial height *(arrow)*. The blood vessels in the papillae are congested.

Photomicrograph courtesy of Frank Mitros, M.D., Department of Pathology, University of Iowa.

of which are eosinophils. Acute erosions are covered by a fibrinous exudate and have an erythematous margin. Erosions progress by involving ever-larger areas of the mucosal surface but do not penetrate the submucosa.

Squamous Cell Hyperplasia. The loss of superficial cells provokes regeneration in the basal cell layer, or *acanthosis* (Fig. 333-3). Basal cells proliferate into the lamina propria, and the papillae remain covered only by relatively few layers of mature squamous cells. With long-standing recurrent injury the bases of the papillae become narrow, and some papillae branch. *Epithelial hyperplasia* of the esophagus is present if the basal cells compose more than 30% of total epithelial height and the papillae more than 75%. Precise diagnosis depends on the histologic examination of biopsy specimens; the diagnosis should be suspected in patients with severe heartburn whose esophageal mucosa appears grossly intact on endoscopy but shows a linear hyperemia from ectatic blood vessels.

Mucosal Metaplasia (Barrett's Esophagus). Replacement of the normal squamous epithelium by columnar epithelium is known as *Barrett's esophagus,* or intestinal metaplasia of the esophageal mucosa (Fig. 333-4). True peptic esophageal ulcers may develop in the metaplastic columnar epithelium. Ulcers form round-to-oval craters that reach the submucosa. Chronic injury leads to peptic esophageal strictures and may cause shortening of the esophagus. Peptic strictures are concentric and less than 1 cm long.

The most common type of epithelium in Barrett's esophagus is the so-called specialized columnar epithelium. This epithelium resembles intestinal mucosa because it forms villi and contains intestinal-type goblet cells. It is most often found immediately adjacent to the squamocolumnar junction, and it is the usual site for dysplasia. Less common types of metaplastic epithelium resemble the epithelium from the gastric cardia and from other parts of the stomach and do not require surveillance.

Most adenocarcinomas of the esophagus arise in metaplastic specialized columnar epithelium. Dysplasia, similar to that seen in long-standing ulcerative colitis, is thought to be the intermediate stage between metaplasia and neoplasia. It has been claimed that malignant transformation occurs in as many as 10% of cases of Barrett's esophagus, but this reported high incidence has recently been challenged.

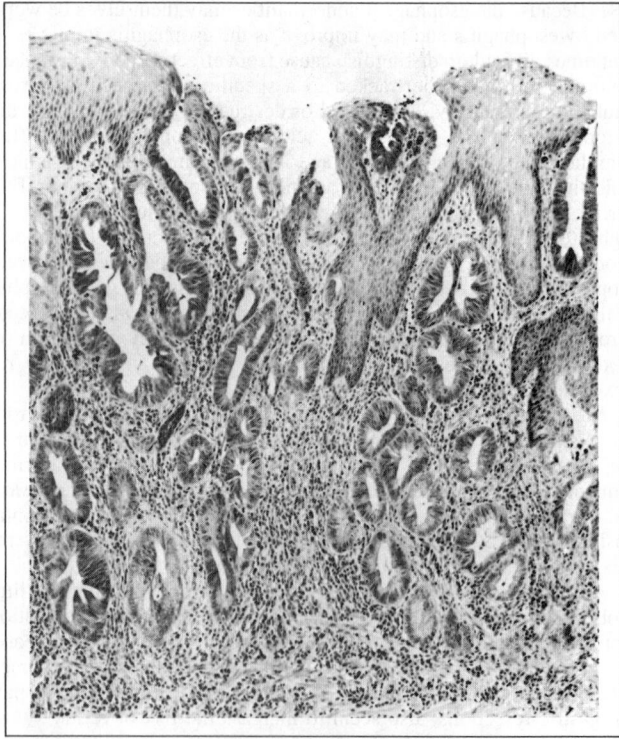

FIGURE 333-4 Epithelial metaplasia *(original magnification, ×16)*. The esophageal mucosa consists of columnar epithelium (Barrett's esophagus) intermixed with squamous epithelium.

Photomicrograph courtesy of Frank Mitros, M.D., Department of Pathology, University of Iowa.

Clinical Presentation and Diagnosis

Three syndromes are associated with chronic gastroesophageal reflux: (1) chronic postprandial dyspepsia with minimal esophageal involvement, (2) erosive esophagitis, and (3) Barrett's esophagus (esopha-geal metaplasia). Individual syndromes may evolve one from the other during the course of the disease and overlap.

Gastroesophageal Reflux With Minimal Esophageal Changes (Esophageal Hypersensitivity, Chronic Esophagitis). Postprandial dyspepsia is a common complaint in middle-aged men and women; most have experienced heartburn and food intolerance since adolescence or early adulthood. Some patients become

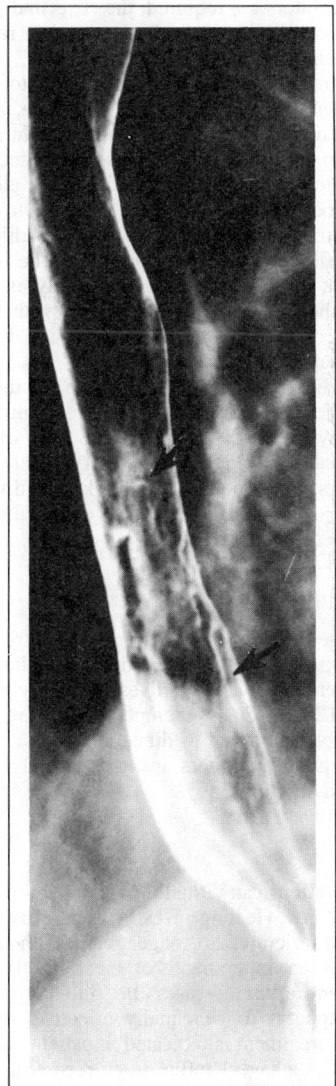
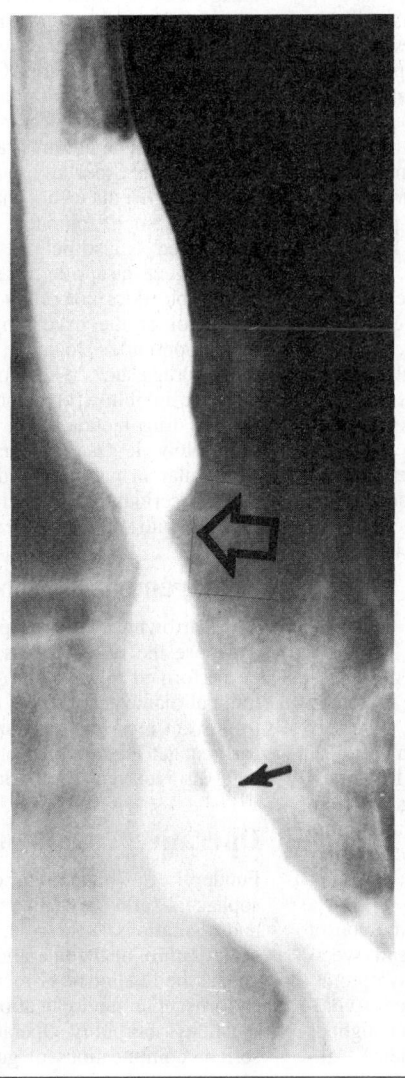
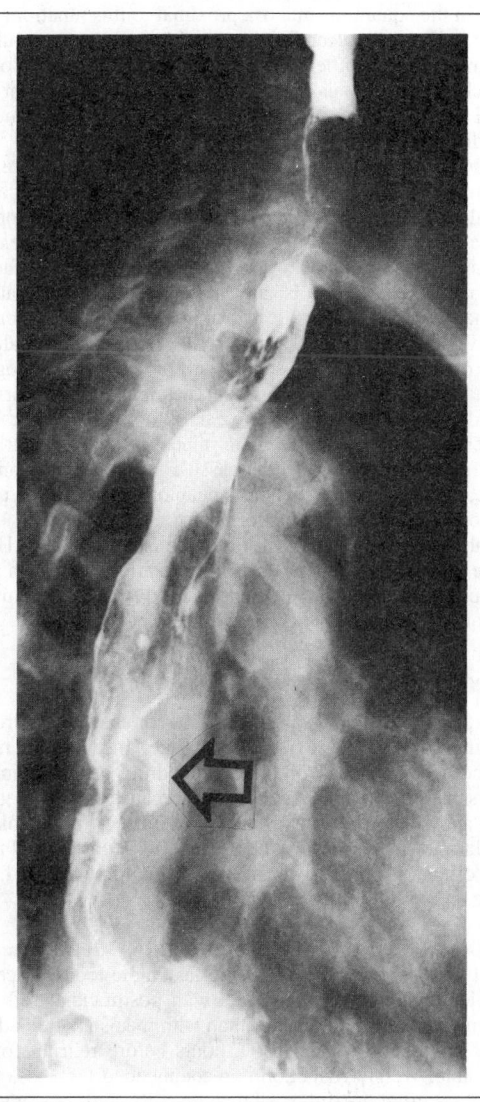

FIGURE 333-5   **A,** Radiographic appearance of reflux esophagitis. This barium contrast study shows a linear erosion *(lower arrow)* and a circumscribed erosion *(upper arrow)*. **B,** Shortened esophagus with peptic stricture. Peptic strictures are fairly concentric, smooth, and narrow *(large arrow)*. Esophageal shortening has led to herniation of the stomach. The small arrow indicates the gastroesophageal junction. **C,** Peptic esophageal ulcer. The occurrence of an ulcer crater *(arrow)* in the esophagus is indicative of Barrett's esophageal mucosal metaplasia.

Radiographs courtesy of Charles C. Lu, M.D., Department of Radiology, University of Iowa.

symptomatic especially after voluminous, greasy, or spicy meals. Epigastric pressure is often relieved by belching; thus the term *daytime bloaters*. In others, reflux symptoms may be triggered by mechanical factors, including exercise and recumbency *(night burners)*.

Acid perfusion of the esophagus (the Bernstein test) reproduces symptoms in most affected individuals (Chapter 329). LES pressure and esophageal contractions are typically normal. Increased frequency of reflux events is common during nighttime or postprandial recording periods. Endoscopic and histologic examination of esophageal mucosa shows erythema and basal cell hyperplasia only. This is the most common and least serious form of esophageal reflux disease.

Gastroesophageal Reflux Complicated by Erosive Esophagitis. Erosive esophagitis is apparently about as common as peptic ulcer disease. Many of these patients experience not simply heartburn but also high epigastric and substernal pain and regurgitation even when fasting. Dysphagia may result from muscle spasm or eventually from scarring with stricture formation. Occult blood loss is common, and severe bleeding occurs occasionally. Shortening of the esophagus with a persistent axial hiatal hernia may be present. LES pressure is low or normal, and esophageal contractions are often weak

and abortive. The pH profile is severely abnormal, particularly for the increased duration of reflux periods during recumbency. The severity of esophagitis is best assessed by endoscopic examination of the longitudinal and circumferential extent of erosive changes (Plate X-1). Endoscopy is indicated for patients with dysphagia to exclude malignancy.

Gastroesophageal Reflux Complicated by Esophageal Metaplasia (Barrett's Esophagus). Although most common in the middle-aged and elderly, Barrett's esophagus can be present in all age groups, including infants. This condition manifests itself most often as dysphagia from an esophageal stricture or, less commonly, as a bleeding esophageal ulcer. The absence of heartburn despite a highly abnormal reflux profile in many of these patients may be linked to the special properties of the metaplastic epithelium.

Diagnostic studies reveal severe reflux and poor esophageal clearance. On radiographic examination the esophagus may appear shortened, poorly distensible, and often strictured or ulcerated. Strictures are located at the junction of squamous and columnar epithelium, which is displaced proximally (thus the term *midesophageal stricture*) (Fig. 333-5, *C*). Typical erosive esophagitis with superficial ulcers is seen in the squamous mucosa proximal to this junction, whereas deep peptic "Barrett's ulcers" that resemble peptic gastric ulcers occur in the metaplastic epithelium distal to the junction. A "short esophagus" (brachyesophagus) is recognized by the formation of a permanent axial (or "sliding") hiatal hernia or by transverse mucosal folds in the distal esophagus.

Endoscopy, biopsy, and cytologic examination are essential for examination of the epithelial changes. Columnar cell metaplasia should be suspected when the esophageal mucosa appears salmon-red and velvety instead of glistening smooth and pearly-pink with proximal displacement of the squamocolumnar interface. In columnar metaplasia there is a risk of recurrent ulceration, stricture formation, and neoplastic transformation. Effective medical or operative treatment that controls reflux is thought to halt the progression of metaplasia. Endoscopy with biopsy and cytologic evaluation for the early detection of dysplasia or cancer is currently recommended about every other year, although whether this is cost-effective remains to be determined. Other biomarkers may be helpful in suggesting an increased risk of progression to dysplasia and adenocarcinoma such as aneuploidy on flow cytometry, chromosomal abnormalities such as p_{53} mutations or microsatellite instability, or an increase in ornithine decarboxylase. However, until these have been studied in more detail to establish their clinical usefulness, histologic evidence of dysplasia remains the most important finding for decision making.

Treatment

Avoidance of esophageal injury is paramount. Many drugs, including calcium channel blockers, theophylline, and nitrates, may adversely affect the esophagus. Anticholinergic drugs are contraindicated in patients with gastroesophageal reflux because they decrease LES pressure and delay gastric emptying. Abstinence from smoking and from drinking of alcohol and coffee is helpful. Nonsteroidal antiinflammatory drugs are probably harmful and should be avoided, because they increase susceptibility to acid injury.

Dietary and Other Symptomatic Measures. Reduction of meal size and a diet that is low in fat, acidic foods, spices, and sweets provide relief in many patients with postprandial reflux symptoms. Taking fluids between rather than with meals is often advised. Avoidance of food or liquids for 2 hours before retiring for the night is desirable. Weight reduction is recommended for obese patients. Antacids are often helpful to alleviate heartburn or postprandial fullness. Alginic acid preparations are also popular, but their effectiveness is not established.

Postural Measures. Esophageal clearance through gravity can be facilitated during sleep by elevating the head of the bed, which is best done by placing 4- to 6-inch blocks under the legs at the head of the bed; foam wedges long enough to elevate the entire chest can also be used. Postural measures are particularly helpful in patients with manifestations of recumbent reflux (i.e., nocturnal aspiration and cricopharyngeal spasm). Because of their inconvenience, postural measures are unlikely to be executed unless sleeping partners as well as patients understand their purpose.

Drugs
Antisecretory drugs (histamine H_2-receptor antagonists or proton pump inhibitors). For mild to moderate symptoms with mild histologic changes, H_2-receptor antagonists are usually adequate in standard twice-daily dosage (cimetidine, 400 mg; ranitidine and nizatidine, 150 mg; and famotidine, 20 mg). For more severe symptoms with erosive esophagitis the antihistamine should be given at 1.5 to 2 times the standard dose for at least 2 months. However, the proton pump inhibitors omeprazole 20 mg/per day or lansoprazole 30 mg/per day are more effective in relieving symptoms and decreasing the severity of esophagitis (80% healed with standard dose, 96% healed with double dose for 2 months). Efficacy in relieving symptoms and healing may be increased by doubling the dose of either agent. Relapse is the rule after the drugs are discontinued. Long-term medical treatment is moderately effective in controlling symptoms and inflammation. Attempts should be made to reduce the dosage and/or frequency to control symptoms, but if high-dose H_2-receptor

antagonists or proton pump inhibitors are required, the costs and potential risks of long-term medical therapy must be weighed in relation to operative therapy, especially in younger patients.

Gastrokinetic drugs. Gastrokinetic drugs (bethanechol, metoclopramide, cisapride) stimulate salivation, increase LES pressure, and improve esophageal clearance in the supine but not in the upright position. Nighttime administration in conjunction with use of antisecretory agents is especially indicated in conditions of nocturnal or alkaline reflux. Bethanechol may be gradually increased from 10 to 40 mg at bedtime if tolerated. Metoclopramide, 10 to 20 mg at bedtime if tolerated, is also helpful to alleviate nausea or vomiting. The preferred agent, cisapride, taken at 10 to 20 mg four times daily, is effective but does not produce the visceral cramps common with bethanechol or the psychologic or dystonic reactions common with metoclopramide. However, cisapride should not be used with antifungal drugs such as ketoconazole or miconazole, selective serotonin reuptake inhibitors or macrolide antibiotics, all of which inhibit the hepatic drug–metabolizing enzyme cytochrome P_{450} and raise cisapride blood levels. This may cause prolonged Q-T interval, serious ventricular arrhythmias, and torsades de pointes. The prokinetic drugs deserve serious consideration in maintenance therapy, especially in patients with mild to moderate symptoms.

Management of Esophageal Strictures

Any narrowing of the esophageal lumen may compromise nutrition and pose the risk of bolus impaction. Esophageal dilatation should be performed to the point where dysphagia resolves, generally at a luminal diameter in excess of 12 mm. Every attempt should be made to prevent recurrent stricture formation and to dilate strictures at an early stage. High-dose proton pump inhibitors are most effective in delaying recurrent acid-induced strictures.

Operative Treatment

Fundoplication and similar operations can virtually eliminate gastroesophageal reflux and its symptoms. Healing of esophageal erosions and ulcerations is the rule, and strictures no longer recur. Although initial failure of the operation is rare in the hands of experienced surgeons, the likelihood of recurrent reflux increases after 5 to 10 years. Laparoscopic fundoplication appears to be equally effective, with much less morbidity. Operative treatment is indicated in patients with serious complications of gastroesophageal reflux (e.g., recurrent aspiration pneumonia, peptic strictures, bleeding esophageal erosions or ulcers, and intractable symptoms that fail to respond to rigorous medical management). Pyrosis alone may occasionally become an indication for fundoplication in patients who do not wish to depend on long-term use of acid-suppressing drugs. The use of fundoplication is controversial in patients with scleroderma and other diseases that permanently impair esophageal motility and clearance.

Dysplasia

The finding of dysplasia in Barrett's epithelium requires action to reduce the risk of progression to adenocarcinoma. If it is low grade, intense medical therapy should be instituted and the frequency of endoscopic surveillance should be increased to 3 to 6 months. If high-grade dysplasia is confirmed by a second biopsy or is associated with a raised lesion, the entire segment should be resected. Preliminary studies have shown that destruction of the mucosa by laser or by thermal or photodynamic therapy results in replacement of the transformed mucosa by squamous epithelium if acid is greatly suppressed by high-dose proton pump inhibitors. It is hoped that the squamous mucosa can be maintained and the progression to adenocarcinoma arrested, but the long-term benefits remain to be established.

CHEMICAL AND PHYSICAL ESOPHAGEAL INJURY

As the first segment of the digestive tract, the esophagus is particularly prone to thermal, mechanical, and caustic injury. Drinking steaming hot beverages can produce serious esophageal injury and has caused the sloughing of entire mucosal casts. Sharp objects such as plastic or glass fragments, fish bones, or even corn chips can lacerate the esophageal mucosa or become embedded in its wall. Accidental ingestion of acids and alkalis by children and ingestion of such substances with suicidal intent by depressed persons cause severe esophageal injury. Iatrogenic esophageal injury ("pill esophagitis") results if certain drugs reside in the esophagus for an undue amount of time.

Esophageal Injury From Lye and Related Agents

Many household and industrial products, such as lye, contain sodium hydroxide, potassium hydroxide, ammonia, or various acids. Esophageal damage occurs in stages; in the immediate stage, liquefaction necrosis destroys the tissue and may produce perforation and mediastinitis. At the end of the first week, scarring begins as fibroblasts lay down collagen. Subsequently, mucosal reepithelialization and scar retraction occur. Lye strictures usually develop within the first 3 months after the injury.

Ingestion typically leads to immediate burning of the mouth and attempts to spit out the material. Chest pain and odynophagia follow if the esophagus is injured. Not all patients who have ingested caustic agents and suffered oropharyngeal burns have esophageal or gastric lesions. The presence and extent of esophageal and gastric lesions should be assessed by early endoscopy. The procedure is safe provided that the endoscope is not advanced beyond the first caustic lesion.

If esophageal injury is present, food should be withheld and intravenous fluids administered. Antibiotics are indicated primarily for the treatment of septic complications, such as mediastinitis. Corticosteroids are often administered to prevent or reduce stricture formation, but proof of their efficacy is lacking. The best way to deal with strictures is by early detection and dilation. Esophagograms should be made regularly between the second week and the third month after esophageal injury, and bougienage should be started as soon as a stricture is demonstrated. Caustic strictures may involve long esophageal segments and consist of dense collagen, making dilation difficult. Long-term follow-up observation is recommended because of the risk of recurrent stricture formation and, eventually, esophageal cancer.

Esophageal Injury Caused by Drugs (Pill Esophagitis)

Particularly when esophageal transit is delayed, bulky tablets or capsules may remain in the esophagus long enough to disintegrate and cause lesions. Patients who take pills while recumbent and without adequate liquids are at particular risk. Pills are most likely to lodge at the level of the aortic arch or the left main bronchus or proximal to the lower sphincter or an enlarged left atrium. Drug-induced esophageal lesions are manifested by sudden onset of odynophagia and retrosternal discomfort shortly after drug ingestion.

Doxycycline, other tetracyclines, and clindamycin are commonly implicated. Other responsible preparations include wax-matrix potassium chloride tablets, dental cleansing tablets, ascorbic acid, ferrous sulfate, quinidine, slow-release theophylline, and nonsteroidal antiinflammatory agents. The acidity or alkalinity of a medication is a major factor in its caustic action. Doxycycline, tetracycline, and ferrous sulfate dissolved in water form solutions with pH values of 3.0 or less. At endoscopy a circumscribed ulcer surrounded by normal mucosa is seen, typically in the midesophagus. Perforation and severe hemorrhage are rare. Treatment is symptomatic with antisecretory agents and local anesthetics, such as lidocaine, but it may take weeks.

Caustic esophageal injury by drugs is preventable. Patients should always remain upright while taking tablets or capsules, and they should swallow medication with adequate amounts of fluids (75 to 100 ml). Some patients prefer applesauce, bananas, or similar semisolid foods as carriers. Patients who have difficulty swallowing should be assisted into a sitting position and instructed to take sips of water even before swallowing the drug. The use of liquid preparations or crushed tablets is advisable in high-risk patients.

Radiation Esophagitis

The esophagus may receive damaging doses of irradiation as part of radiotherapy for mediastinal tumors. Radiation injury is dose related but is enhanced by such chemotherapeutic agents as doxorubicin, bleomycin, and actinomycin D. Epithelial necrosis and mucosal ul-

ceration and inflammation occur. They may be followed by superinfection with opportunistic organisms (especially candidiasis) and transmural inflammation. The mucosa becomes reepithelialized 3 to 4 weeks after radiation is stopped. Motor abnormalities or strictures may occur months to years after the insult.

In the early stages of radiation esophagitis, patients experience odynophagia and substernal pain. Barium esophagram and esophagoscopy reveal fine serrated ulcers and edema of the mucosa. Local anesthetics, liquid diets, or parenteral fluid administration may be temporarily needed. Dysphagia occurs in the later stages because strictures form; these strictures should be dilated.

Bolus Impaction and Foreign Bodies

Foreign bodies or poorly masticated food may become impacted in the esophagus. Infants and intoxicated or mentally ill individuals may swallow coins, pins, or batteries. At special risk for food impaction are edentulous individuals or patients with a Schatzki's ring or other type of esophageal stricture. Patients experience substernal pain, excess salivation, and regurgitation. A chest radiograph is often sufficient to locate radiopaque objects. If the object is radiolucent, a contrast esophagram is required.

If the impaction is recent and caused by digestible food, spontaneous passage may occasionally be facilitated through the use of anticholinergic agents, glucagon, or carbonated beverages. Endoscopy can be used with gentle pressure to push a digestible bolus into the stomach. If that fails, the bolus and all indigestible material should be removed with airway protection to prevent esophageal necrosis or obstruction elsewhere. To prevent recurrent impactions, patients must be evaluated and treated for any predisposing esophageal disease.

Mallory-Weiss Laceration and Boerhaave's Syndrome

A mucosal laceration at the gastroesophageal junction leading to acute gastrointestinal hemorrhage is known as the *Mallory-Weiss syndrome*. This syndrome accounts for 5% to 15% of all upper gastrointestinal hemorrhages (Chapter 332). Severe retching and vomiting after an alcoholic binge are the most common causes of the laceration. Orogastric intubation, lifting and straining, abdominal trauma, and cardiopulmonary resuscitation have also been implicated. Most tears occur at the gastroesophageal junction. Lesions are rarely detected radiographically, and esophagoscopy is the preferred means of diagnosis.

Bleeding from Mallory-Weiss tears stops spontaneously in most cases. Endoscopic interventions (epinephrine injection or electrocautery), vasopressin infusion, or arterial embolization may obviate surgical intervention in patients who cease to bleed spontaneously.

Boerhaave's syndrome is an esophageal rupture caused by severe vomiting after excessively large meals. Esophageal rupture can also be produced by physical trauma, including forceful epigastric compression to dislodge boluses impacted in the upper airway (Heimlich maneuver). Acute epigastric and substernal pain, dyspnea, tachycardia, cyanosis, and subcutaneous and mediastinal emphysema follow esophageal rupture. Mortality is high, even if the problem is promptly recognized and treated with surgical repair and antibiotics.

INFECTIOUS ESOPHAGITIS
Etiology and Predisposing Factors

Immunosuppression predisposes to esophageal infections. Those at most risk are patients with malignancies and the acquired immunodeficiency syndrome (Chapter 346) and those undergoing chemotherapy, organ transplantation, or treatment with corticosteroids. Infections also occur in patients with diabetes mellitus, after broad-spectrum antibiotic therapy, and with severe debilitating disease or advanced age. As a rule, infectious esophagitis differs by its diffuse involvement of the entire esophagus from reflux esophagitis, which leads primarily to circumscribed linear lesions of the distal esophagus.

Herpes viruses and the *Candida* fungal organisms account for most cases of infectious esophagitis. Mixed infections are common, and lesions are often secondarily infected with bacteria. In the herpes family, herpes simplex, varicella zoster, and cytomegalovirus (CMV) may

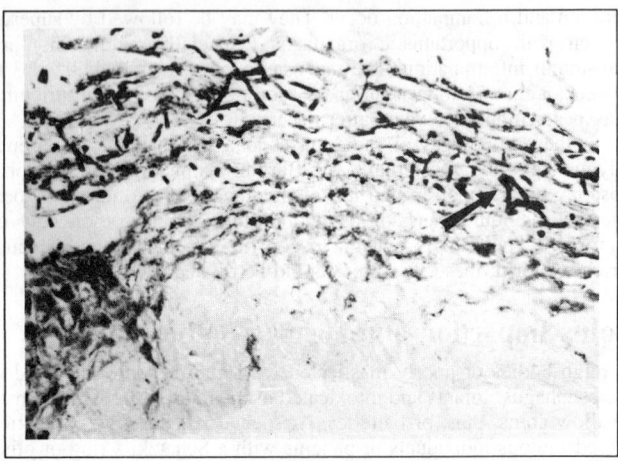

FIGURE 333-6 This debris from a candidal ulcer shows mycelia stained with a silver stain *(arrow) (original magnification, ×100).*
Photomicrograph courtesy of Frank Mitros, M.D., Department of Pathology, University of Iowa.

all cause esophagitis. Herpes simplex is commonly carried by human hosts. Human immunodeficiency virus type 1 (HIV-1) may itself cause one or more oral and esophageal ulcerations. *Candida* species are found in the mouths of as many as 50% of normal individuals. *C. albicans* is the most important fungal species causing esophagitis, although *C. krusei, C. tropicalis, Torulopsis glabrata, Histoplasma capsulatum,* and *Aspergillus* species have also been reported. Tuberculosis is the most common chronic bacterial infection of the esophagus; acute streptococcal infections may also involve the proximal esophagus.

Clinical and Laboratory Findings

The most prominent symptom is odynophagia (painful swallowing), which is often severe enough to interfere with eating and drinking. Dysphagia and continuous substernal pain are common. Bleeding is usually absent or occult, but hematemesis and melena develop in a few patients. Serious complications include esophageal obstruction, aspiration pneumonitis, esophageal perforation, and systemic dissemination.

The oropharynx should be examined for vesicles, ulcers, or thrush indicative of herpes or candidiasis. The barium esophagram in candidiasis typically reveals ragged mucosal ulcerations and plaques. Endoscopic examination plus mucosal biopsies, brushing, and cultures of biopsy tissue are necessary to determine the cause. Widely scattered vesicles or shallow discrete ulcers with a clean granular base and slightly raised margins are suggestive of herpes. CMV ulcerations are usually well demarcated, large, solitary, hemorrhagic, and often in the distal esophagus. Yellowish white "cheesy" pseudomembranes over shaggy hemorrhagic ulcers are suggestive of candidiasis. Ulcers devoid of pathogens are likely to be due to HIV-1 itself unless biopsy shows Kaposi's sarcoma or lymphoma or the history suggests pill-induced ulceration. The endoscopic changes are not always typical, and nonspecific mucosal erythema, viability, erosions, or confluent ulcerations with exudate may be seen. Debris from either the ulcer base or the plaques often contains *Candida* pseudohyphae and other yeast forms that can be demonstrated microscopically by potassium hydroxide preparations or Gram stains from mucosal scrapings. In tissue sections, silver methenamine stains clearly demonstrate the yeast forms among desquamated epithelial cells (Fig. 333-6). The characteristic Cowdry type A inclusion, seen in cells from the margin of herpetic ulcers, is an eosinophilic intranuclear inclusion surrounded by a clear halo and a rim of chromatin. Both intranuclear and cytoplasmic inclusions occur with cytomegalovirus, and infected cells are characteristically related to inflamed blood vessels in the granulation tissue of the ulcer base. Immunostaining, in situ hybridization, and polymerase chain reaction (PCR) amplification are increasingly sensitive for CMV. Cultures for *Candida* fail to

distinguish commensal organisms from pathogens; results of serologic tests are nonspecific. A rise in titer to complement-fixing antibody in patients with suspected herpetic esophagitis is helpful.

Treatment

Local anesthetics such as viscous lidocaine are useful to diminish odynophagia. If patients are unable to swallow, nutrition must be provided via enteral or parenteral feedings. Mild oropharyngeal and esophageal candidiasis in immunocompetent patients usually responds to treatment with an oral nystatin suspension (500,000 to 1,000,000 units three to five times daily) or clotrimazole troches (10 mg five times daily). If local treatment fails or in immunosuppressed patients, ketoconazole (200 mg per day) or, preferably, fluconazole (100 to 200 mg daily) should be given. In more severe infections and in systemic disease, amphotericin B in an intravenous dosage of 0.3 to 0.5 mg/kg/day for 7 days is effective.

Acyclovir taken orally at 200 mg five times daily for 2 weeks is beneficial in systemic herpes infections and should be tried in patients with severe herpes esophagitis. In patients with mild herpes esophagitis, improvement often occurs when the immunosuppressive drug dosage is reduced. Ganciclovir at 5 mg/kg IV twice daily for 2 to 3 weeks or foscarnet at 60 mg/kg three times daily for 2 to 3 weeks suppress cytomegalovirus esophagitis.

ESOPHAGEAL WEBS, RINGS, AND DIVERTICULA
Cervical Webs and Schatzki's Rings

Esophageal rings and webs are thin membranous structures that cause focal narrowing of the esophageal lumen. They are a common cause of intermittent dysphagia for solids. In the cervical esophagus, single webs occur most commonly just below the cricoid muscle. They originate from the anterior wall of the esophagus opposite C6 or C7 (Fig. 333-7, *A*).

The formation of membranous webs is part of an inflammatory response. Irradiation of the esophagus can produce multiple esophageal webs. The triad of iron deficiency anemia, glossitis, and postcricoid web is known as either the *Plummer-Vinson Syndrome* or the *Patterson-Kelly syndrome*. It occurs mostly in menstruating women of northern European descent. Patients with this syndrome are at risk for carcinoma of the pharynx and cervical esophagus.

Mucosal diaphragms in the distal esophagus are referred to as *Schatzki's rings.* They are located at the squamocolumnar junction and thus typically lie within the high-pressure zone generated by the LES and above the diaphragmatic hiatus. Rings 1.2 cm or less in diameter usually produce dysphagia, whereas those 2.0 cm or more in diameter rarely cause symptoms. Radiographic demonstration of even large-diameter Schatzki's rings is common if the esophagus is well distended (Fig. 333-7, *B*). Schatzki's rings are easily demonstrable endoscopically if the distal esophagus is observed carefully during air insufflation (Plate X-2).

Symptomatic cervical webs and Schatzki's rings should be dilated or ruptured with an endoscope with bougies. Iron deficiency, if present, should be evaluated and treated.

Esophageal Diverticula

Most esophageal diverticula are acquired and hence are more common in the elderly. Most diverticula do not contain any muscularis propria and probably form because of increased luminal pressure (i.e., they are pulsion diverticula). Esophageal diverticula are classified according to their location as (1) those occurring at the pharyngoesophageal junction (Zenker's diverticula); (2) those occurring in the vicinity of the tracheal bifurcation (midesophageal diverticula); and (3) those occurring close to the diaphragmatic hiatus (epiphrenic diverticula).

Zenker's Diverticula. The muscle fibers of the pharynx and of the upper esophageal sphincter (UES) leave between them a weak area through which hypopharyngeal herniations can occur. These herniations occur most commonly on the left side, less commonly posteriorly and in the midline, and rarely on the right side. Hypertrophy of the UES is often associated with Zenker's diverticulum and is rec-

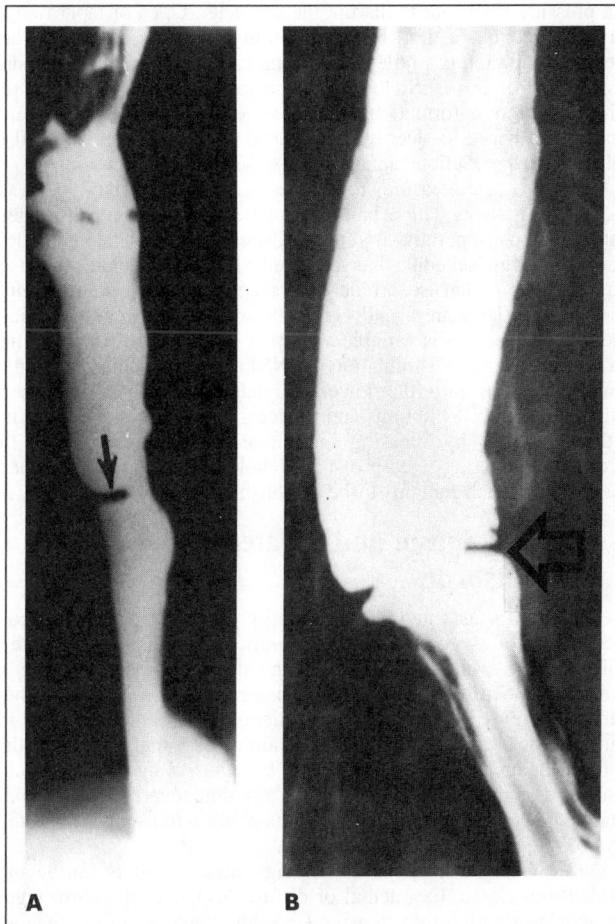

FIGURE 333-7   A, Cervical web *(arrow)*. Cervical webs indent the lumen from the anterior esophageal wall at the level of the lower cervical spine. **B,** Schatzki's ring *(arrow)* is a thin diaphragm at the gastroesophageal junction above a hiatal hernia.

Radiographs courtesy of Charles C. Lu, M.D., Department of Radiology, University of Iowa.

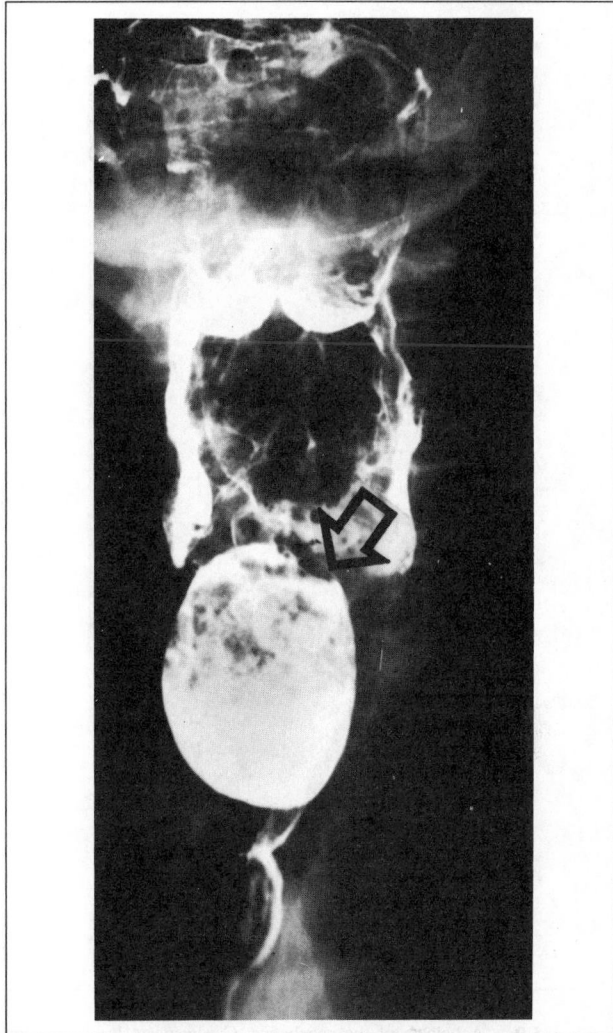

FIGURE 333-8   This Zenker's diverticulum *(arrow)* is partially filled with food and impinges in the lumen of the cervical esophagus. It is in a posterior location. The most common location is left lateral.

Radiograph courtesy of Charles C. Lu, M.D., Department of Radiology, University of Iowa.

ognized radiographically as a smooth persistent indentation at the esophageal inlet. The "cricoid achalasia" syndrome is the pharyngeal dysphagia and globus sensation often observed in this setting. Hypertrophy interferes with the sphincter's compliance and hence its full opening during pharyngeal deglutition.

Most patients with Zenker's diverticula are male and 50 years or older. Patients usually describe an insidious onset of cervical dysphagia for solids and liquids. They may regurgitate undigested food several hours or days after meals and complain of cough or bad breath. Many patients try to empty the sac by manipulation of the neck or some bodily contortion. Patients are at risk for aspiration, and impaired nutrition is common.

On physical examination, gurgling and a lump may be found on palpation of the neck. Careful videoradiographic examination of deglutition with lateral views is mandatory (Fig. 333-8). An endoscopic search for coexistent treatable lesions such as reflux esophagitis is valuable, but care must be taken to prevent perforating the thin-walled diverticulum. Resection of the diverticular sac is recommended when it is more than 5 cm in diameter and causes compression and regurgitation. Sectioning of the cricopharyngeal muscle is often added to diverticulectomy and is sometimes the only treatment needed when the diverticulum is small.

Midesophageal Diverticula. Midesophageal diverticula occur over the bifurcation of the trachea. In the past they were associated with traction from inflamed mediastinal lymph nodes caused by tuberculosis or histoplasmosis. At present, most midesophageal diver-

ticula are associated with esophageal spasm and related motility disorders of the esophagus. Midesophageal diverticula rarely cause symptoms and should not be resected unless hemorrhage, impaction of food, or fistulization has occurred.

MOTILITY DISORDERS OF THE ESOPHAGUS
Achalasia

In achalasia the LES fails to relax in response to swallowing, and the smooth muscle of the esophageal body fails to generate peristaltic contractions. Food and secretions accumulate in the esophagus. With time the esophagus dilates and becomes tortuous. Stasis esophagitis may result, and there is an increased risk for the development of squamous cell carcinoma.

Esophageal achalasia is associated with destruction of nerve ganglia in the myenteric plexus of the esophagus. In South America, megaesophagus occurs as a consequence of infection by *Trypanosoma cruzi* (Chagas' disease), but in other parts of the world this etiology is virtually unknown. Occasionally, infiltrating carcinomas or lymphomas produce an achalasia-like syndrome.

Achalasia develops at any age. Occurrence in members of the same family has been described, but most cases are isolated and idiopathic. Patients note dysphagia with both solids and liquids; they often swal-

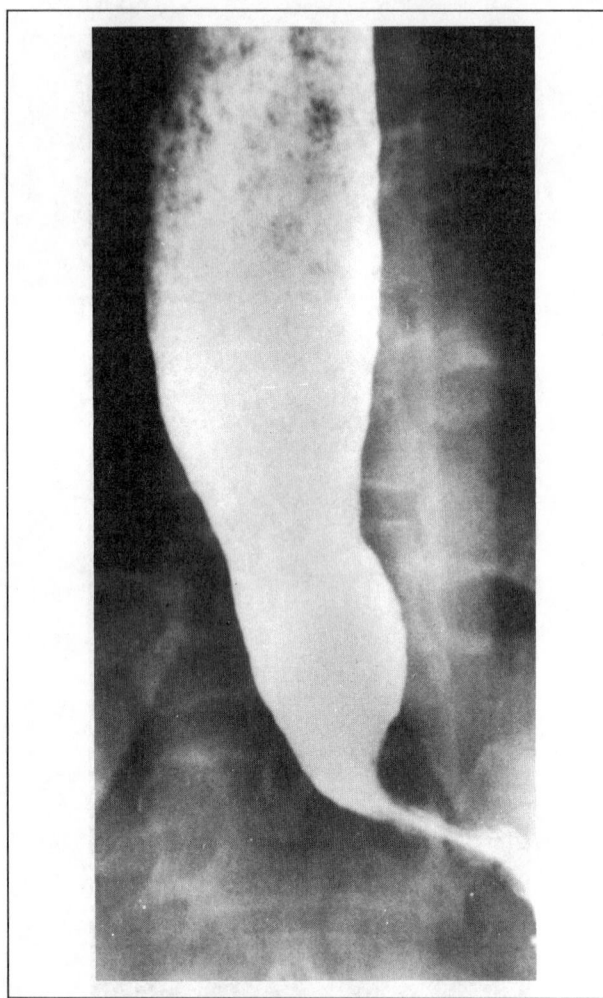

FIGURE 333-9   Achalasia of the esophagus. Cardiospasm leads to a long, horizontal stricture *(beak)* at the gastroesophageal junction. The body of the esophagus is dilated and filled with food.

Radiograph courtesy of Charles C. Lu, M.D., Department of Radiology, University of Iowa.

low air and go through Valsalva's maneuver to empty their gullet. A substernal pressure sensation and weight loss are common. Chest pain is rarely severe. Regurgitation and aspiration dominate the clinical presentation in some patients.

Radiographic examination characteristically shows absence of the gastric air bubble and a long concentric narrowing at the gastroesophageal junction, with a variable degree of dilation and elongation of the esophagus (Fig. 333-9). Poor clearance of barium paste when the patient swallows in the supine position is also characteristic. Esophageal manometry is helpful; the resting pressure of the LES is normal or high; swallows fail to produce complete and lasting reductions of LES pressure. Contractions of the distal two thirds of the esophageal body are of low amplitude and are nonsequential. Administration of a cholinergic agent leads to high-amplitude esophageal contractions (denervation hypersensitivity).

Because the motor abnormality in achalasia is occasionally the first manifestation of a tumor at the gastroesophageal junction, a careful endoscopic examination with biopsy is mandatory in all cases of esophageal achalasia. In uncomplicated achalasia the endoscope passes into the stomach easily, without resistance.

Treatment is aimed at lowering the resistance to passage of esophageal contents through the LES. In most cases this can be achieved by forceful dilation of the LES; a 30 to 40 mm balloon is placed in the gastric cardia under endoscopic or fluoroscopic control and inflated

to a pressure sufficient to disrupt the sphincter. Open or laparoscopic operative section of the LES (Heller's myotomy) is indicated when pneumatic dilation has failed or is technically not feasible. Such successful abolition of LES closure is associated with the risk of esophagitis or stricture formation from gastroesophageal reflux. Patients should be advised to sleep with the head of the bed elevated and to follow other precautions against reflux (see earlier discussion).

Pharmacologic measures to decrease LES pressure have been advocated for patients with achalasia who are poor candidates for pneumatic dilation or operative myotomy. Unfortunately, to date no widely successful drug schedule has emerged. The most commonly used drugs are sublingual isosorbide dinitrate, 5 to 10 mg, or nifedipine, 10 to 30 mg. They are usually given 30 to 45 minutes before meals. Their rate of success is variable and often short lived. Low-frequency transcutaneous nerve stimulation (TENS) and endoscopic injection of botulinum toxin into the lower esophageal sphincter have been claimed to relieve symptoms and reduce sphincter pressure. The first is thought to act by releasing vasoactive intestinal peptide and the second by inhibiting release of acetylcholine. The long-term benefit of either approach remains to be established.

Esophageal Spasm and Related Motility Disorder

In esophageal spasm and related motility disorders, esophageal contractions are of excessive force and duration. Esophageal clearance is typically poor even though no mechanical obstruction or organic lesion can be identified. Patients have intermittent dysphagia or chest pain, which may be intense. Some patients avoid eating in public for fear of being interrupted by bouts of pain or by forceful regurgitation of food. In most patients the pain is brought on by meals or emotional stress, although it may occur at any time, even during sleep. A detailed discussion of chest pain and its relation to esophageal pathophysiology is provided in Chapter 329.

On the basis of manometric findings these disorders can be subdivided into classic (segmental or diffuse) esophageal spasm, vigorous achalasia with a hypertensive LES, and "nutcracker esophagus." It is not known whether these manometric subdivisions correspond to different disease entities or whether they represent different expressions of the same disease.

Classic esophageal spasm is characterized by the nonprogressive nature of esophageal contractions. Contractions involve long segments of the esophageal smooth muscle at the same time (thus the term *diffuse* or *segmental esophageal spasm*). There is hyperplasia of esophageal smooth muscle, which may be recognized radiographically as thickening of the esophageal wall. Other radiographic features of esophageal spasm are irregular "tertiary contractions" that are unrelated to swallowing (Fig. 333-10) and may give the esophagus a corkscrew appearance. On radiographic studies or radionuclide scanning, ineffective esophageal clearance resulting from to-and-fro movements of the bolus may be appreciated.

Manometric criteria for esophageal spasm include the presence of simultaneous contractions, repetitive contractions, and contractions of excessive force and duration (Chapter 329 and Fig. 329-1). LES function is normal in most patients with esophageal spasm, but distinguishing it from achalasia is occasionally rendered difficult by the presence of a hypertensive sphincter that fails to relax (a condition referred to as *vigorous achalasia*).

Segmental esophageal spasm and vigorous achalasia are rare disorders. More common than segmental esophageal spasm is a variant of esophageal spasm, the so-called nutcracker esophagus. In this disorder, dysphagia is not a problem because esophageal contractions are progressive but are of excessive force or duration (Chapter 329). One problem with the diagnosis of esophageal spasm and its variants is that esophageal motility may be normal at the time of manometry, although provocative testing (Chapter 329) may demonstrate manometric abnormalities. Recent data suggest that the pain is related to hypersensitivity of the visceral afferent pathway associated with contractile hyperactivity and reduced esophageal compliance.

A search must be made to determine whether the motility disorder is precipitated by esophageal reflux, inflammation, or obstruction. Even if no discrete stricture is identified, esophageal bougienage may

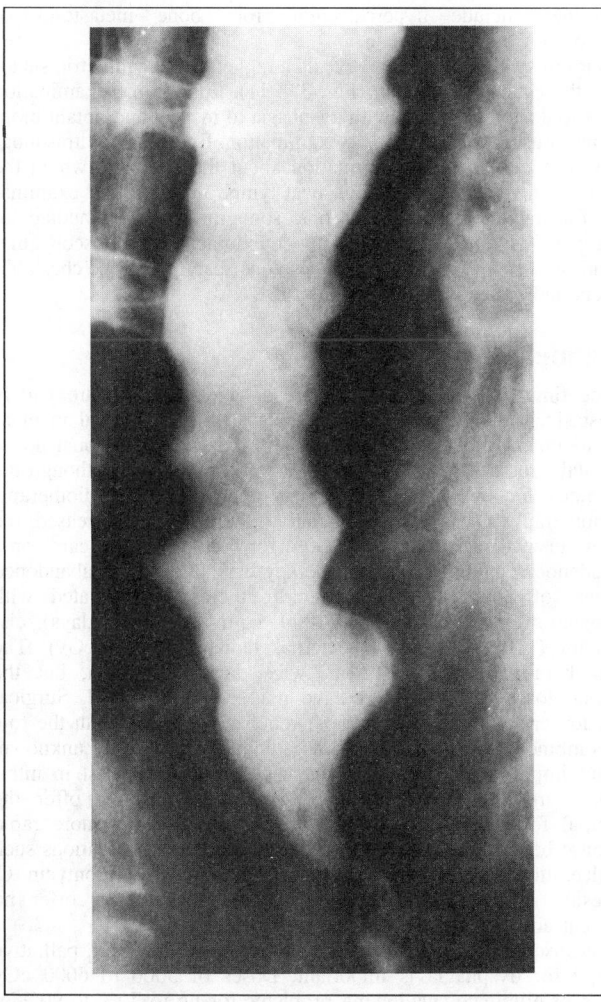

FIGURE 333-10 Corkscrew esophagus characteristic of diffuse esophageal spasm. Tertiary contractions of the esophagus lead to the formation of many pseudodiverticula.

Radiograph courtesy of Charles C. Lu, M.D., Department of Radiology, University of Iowa.

improve dysphagia. Similarly, measures to prevent reflux or reduce acid, even if this does not seem to be a severe problem, might prove more rewarding than pharmacologic manipulation of esophageal contractile activity. Tranquilizers, smooth muscle relaxants, nitroglycerin, and calcium antagonists provide some relief. No effective therapy for the chest pain of nutcracker esophagus exists, although some patients obtain some benefit with the tricyclic antidepressant agents. Pneumatic dilation of the LES should be reserved for conditions associated with a hypertensive LES. Long surgical myotomy is occasionally advocated when nutrition is impaired but carries the risk of severe reflux esophagitis.

Esophageal Motility Disorders Produced by Systemic Disease

Patients with progressive systemic sclerosis are particularly prone to severe reflux esophagitis and often develop recurrent esophageal strictures at a young age. Incompetence of the LES, poor esophageal clearance, and delayed gastric emptying contribute to reflux esophagitis. The mechanical abnormalities result from replacement of esophageal smooth muscle by collagen. This esophageal fibrosis is a consequence of the underlying vascular disease.

Barium swallows show ineffective esophageal peristalsis. On manometry, contractions in the esophageal body are shown to be weak,

and the gastroesophageal high-pressure zone may be absent (see Fig. 329-1). Endoscopic examination often reveals extensive esophageal erosions.

Patients with systemic sclerosis and reflux esophagitis should observe strict reflux precautions and be maintained on antisecretory drugs, at least at night. It is doubtful that they can be helped by gastrokinetic drugs or operative treatment.

Poor LES pressure and weak, nonsequential esophageal contractions are common in patients with *diabetes mellitus* and diabetic neuropathy. Symptoms may be inconspicuous, yet treatment of an associated reflux esophagitis may be needed.

Dysphagia, both pharyngeal and esophageal, is a common problem in *Parkinson's disease*. Up to half of the patients have findings consistent with esophageal spasm; gastroesophageal reflux and poor esophageal clearance are common in the rest. Treatment of the Parkinson's disease with anticholinergics and levodopa often aggravates the dysphagia.

BENIGN TUMORS

Leiomyomas are the most common of the benign esophageal tumors. They are usually small and asymptomatic and are often discovered incidentally on a barium esophagram as smooth, round filling defects. Large tumors may cause dysphagia and rarely ulcerate and bleed. Endoscopically, they appear as firm, rounded mounds that usually have an intact overlying mucosa. Surgical resection of esophageal leiomyomas is indicated for severe pain, dysphagia, bleeding, compression of a vital structure, or progressive enlargement. Similar presentations may occur with other, less common benign tumors (lipomas, fibromas, and neurofibromas). Ultrasonic endoscopy is helpful to distinguish these benign lesions from invasive carcinoma or lymphoma.

MALIGNANT NEOPLASMS
Incidence and Risk Factors

It is estimated that 12,300 new esophageal cancers will be discovered in 1996 and that 11,200 will die of the disease. The incidence of esophageal carcinoma varies greatly among geographic regions. The risk is particularly high in northern Iran, central Asia, and southeastern Africa. The incidence in the United States is about 4 per 100,000 population per year, with a male predominance of approximately 3:1. The incidence is several times higher in blacks than in whites. This great variation in the incidence of esophageal carcinoma suggests that environmental factors are of great importance in its origin.

Alcohol and tobacco are risk factors for the development of squamous cell esophageal cancer in the Western world. In other regions, ingestions of hot beverages, mycotoxins from moldy or pickled food, combustion products of opium, or N-nitrosyl compounds appear to be associated with high rates of esophageal cancer. In addition, deficiencies of vitamins A, C, and riboflavin; trace minerals; and other nutrients may increase susceptibility. Peptic and lye strictures, webs, achalasia, and diverticula cause esophageal stasis and have been implicated as risk factors for esophageal cancer. The familial condition of tylosis (hyperkeratosis of the hands and feet), celiac sprue, and the Plummer-Vinson syndrome are associated with a high incidence of esophageal squamous cell carcinoma. The progression of reflux lesions to esophageal metaplasia and neoplasia is well recognized, and the presence of tylosis palmeris or Barrett's metaplasia requires regular screening with endoscopy and biopsy every 1 to 3 years.

Pathology

Of primary esophageal cancers throughout the world, 90% are squamous cell cancers. However, the proportion of adenocarcinomas is increasing dramatically. Adenocarcinomas that involve the gastroesophageal junction are often considered extensions of primary gastric cancers, but more than half of these cancers actually arise in dysplastic Barrett's epithelium.

The development of squamous cell carcinoma is thought to be preceded by dysplasia of the squamous epithelium, whereas the development of adenocarcinoma is probably preceded by dysplasia of the specialized columnar epithelium. In squamous cell dysplasia the basal zone shows increased mitotic activity, increased nuclear size, and hyperchromatism. In invasive carcinoma, cells break through the muscularis mucosae and form nests in the submucosa. Invasive squamous cell carcinoma produces a fungating (polypoid), ulcerating, or infiltrating pattern.

Because the esophagus has rich submucosal lymphatics, spread to the regional nodes occurs early in the course of the disease. Tumor cells spread to paraesophageal and upper abdominal lymph nodes from the distal esophagus, and to the posterior mediastinal, tracheobronchial, and deep cervical nodes from in the proximal esophagus. Metastasis to the liver is common, but spread also occurs to the lung and pleura, aorta and pericardium, adrenal glands, kidneys, bone, pancreas, and thyroid.

Clinical and Laboratory Findings

Dysphagia is the most common symptom for which patients seek medical attention. The dysphagia is progressive: over a few weeks to a few months, patients adopt a soft and then a liquid diet. Weight loss is prominent. Dull retrosternal and (sometimes) back pain occurs as the tumor enlarges. Bleeding occurs when the tumor ulcerates, but massive hemorrhage is rare. Aspiration caused by esophageal obstruction or tracheoesophageal fistula may cause coughing, other respiratory symptoms, and pneumonia or sepsis. Cervical lymph nodes and the liver are enlarged when the disease is advanced. Hoarseness arises from laryngeal nerve involvement. Paraneoplastic syndromes include hypercalcemia from bone metastases or parathormone-like expression.

Barium swallow typically reveals a ragged and asymmetric stenosis of the esophageal lumen (Fig. 333-11). Endoscopic examination is essential for all patients with dysphasia to inspect and obtain biopsies and brushings for cytologic examination. Endoscopic ultrasonography provides essential information about the extent to which the tumor has invaded the wall and local lymph nodes. Other examinations for staging include endoscopic sonography and computed tomography (CT) of the thorax and upper abdomen. Bronchoscopy, mediastinoscopy, laparoscopy, or radioisotope scanning of the chest, abdomen, and bones may also be helpful.

Treatment

At the time of presentation, most esophageal cancers are widely metastasized and beyond cure; accurate staging is critical in planning treatment. Local extension through the wall to regional nodes and vital structures makes surgical therapy impossible. Although the cure rates are low, a multidisciplinary approach with radiotherapy, chemotherapy, and possibly operative therapy has increased the 5-year survival rate from 5% to 30% for both squamous carcinoma and adenocarcinoma. Unimodal therapy has largely been abandoned because of poor results. Commonly, therapy is initiated with combinations of 5-fluorouracil (1000 mg/m^2/day for 4 days), cisplatinum (100 mg/m^2), and external radiation (5000 cGy). The chemotherapy is usually given twice during radiation, but the optimal doses and schedules have not been established. Surgical resection can provide a more rapid relief of symptoms, but the role of combined surgery and chemoradiotherapy is still unknown. Recent improvements in technique have renewed interest in intracavitary irradiation or high-dose brachytherapy. They offer the potential for better local control of the tumor and a more rapid response but may also increase treatment-related complications such as ulcerations, fistulas, and strictures. Bleomycin, mitomycin C, vindesine, and adriamycin have been used, but they offer no clear-cut advantage over other agents.

Because the disease is often advanced at the first visit, palliative therapy for dysphagia is important. Doses of 5000 to 6000 cGy reduce or eliminate swallowing problems for up to 70% to 90% of patients for variable periods of time. Dysphagia may recur because of tumor regrowth or stricture, but this can be treated with dilation, laser therapy, or electrocautery. Alternatively, improved coated prosthetic stents can be used for recurrent tumor or for fistulas between the esophagus and trachea or bronchi. Maintenance of a lumen for secretions, fluid, and nutrition is a high priority of palliative therapy. If this is not possible, a feeding gastrostomy is necessary. Because of the complex problems encountered and the need for a multidisciplinary approach, referral to a specialized center is recommended to plan and carry out therapy.

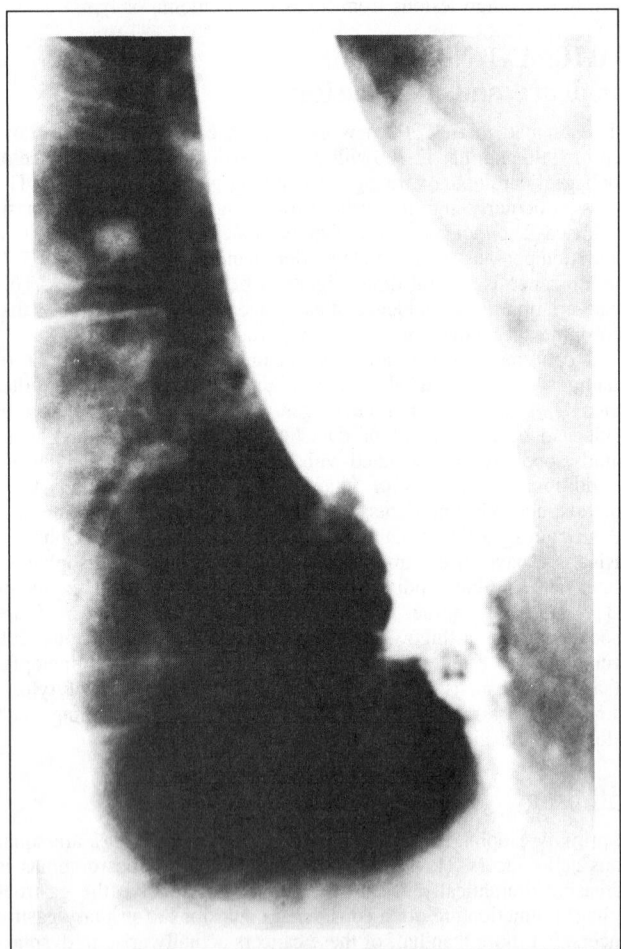

FIGURE 333-11   Esophageal carcinoma. The tumor has led to an asymmetric, long stricture in the distal esophagus. The mucosal outline is shaggy.
Radiograph courtesy of Charles C. Lu, M.D., Department of Radiology, University of Iowa.

BIBLIOGRAPHY

Castell DO: *The esophagus,* Boston, 1992, Little, Brown.
Dodds WJ: The pathogenesis of gastroesophageal reflux disease, *AJR,* 151:49, 1988.
Harding SM, Richter JE: The role of gastroesophageal reflux in chronic cough and asthma, *Chest* 111:1389, 1997.
Ilson DH, Kelsen DP: Management of esophageal cancer, *Oncology* 10:1385, 1996.
Kahrilas PJ: Gastroesophageal reflux disease, *JAMA* 276:983, 1996.
Parkman HP et al: Pneumatic dilatation or esophagomyotomy treatment of idiopathic achalasia: clinical outcomes and cost analysis, *Dig Dis Sci* 38:75, 1993.
Pera M et al: Barrett's disease: patholophysiology of metaplasia and adenocarcinoma, *Ann Thorac Surg* 56:1191, 1993.
Rao S et al: Unexplained chest pain: the hypersensitive, hyperreactive, and poorly compliant esophagus, *Ann Intern Med* 124:950, 1996.
Richter JE: Motility disorders of the esophagus. In Yamada T, Alpers DH, Owyang C et al, editors: *Textbook of gastroenterology,* Philadelphia, 1995, JB Lippincott.
Schmidtt CM, Brazer SR: Clinical aspects of esophageal cancer. In Rutstgi AK, editor: *Gastrointestinal cancers: biology, diagnosis and therapy,* Philadelphia, 1995. Lippincott-Raven.
Smith PD: Esophageal infections in HIV-1 disease. In Bluser MJ, Smith PD, Ravidin JI et al, editors: *Infections of gastrointestinal tract,* New York, 1995, Raven.
Spechler SJ, the Department of VA Gastroesophageal Reflux Disease Study Group: Comparison of medical and surgical therapy for complicated gastroesophageal reflux disease in veterans, *N Engl J Med* 326:786, 1992.
Vigneri S et al: A comparison of five maintenance therapies for reflux esophagitis, *N Engl J Med* 333:1106, 1995.

CHAPTER

334 Nausea, Vomiting, and Anorexia

Irfan Soykan and Richard W. McCallum

Nausea, vomiting and anorexia can be serious conditions that occur frequently as a result of a variety of disorders, some of the gastrointestinal tract, but also including more generalized disturbances involving the central nervous system, endocrine and metabolic problems, and psychiatric illnesses. Although nausea, vomiting, and anorexia frequently coexist, they are discussed separately in this chapter.

NAUSEA AND VOMITING

The word *nausea* is derived from the Greek word for *ship* and can be defined as an unpleasant sensation, usually felt in the upper abdomen, associated with the desire to vomit. Unlike vomiting, which is a mechanical act that can be reproduced in experimental animals and therefore studied in the laboratory, nausea is a subjective symptom. Thus very little is known about the neural pathways that mediate nausea. A better understanding of nausea requires the use of quantitative physiologic indices. Recent studies in human volunteers indicate that plasma vasopressin levels (10 to 20 times those required for maximal antidiuresis), β-endorphin and adrenocorticotropic hormone (ACTH) levels are markedly increased after nausea is induced by motion, parenteral apomorphine, or chemotherapeutic agents. Specifically in motion sickness, the link between vasopressin and the central release of β-endorphin suggests a vasopressin–β-endorphin–ACTH response that is subject to feedback control by

glucocorticoid action. In this respect, an integrated paraventricular system that acts as a coordinator for the body's autonomic and endocrine responses to stressful stimuli, including nausea, has been proposed. Antral arrythmias (such as antral tachygastria) are well described in nauseated subjects. The close association between tachygastria and nausea strongly suggests a linkage between gastric antral arrythmias and epigastric symptoms and/or nausea. In general, a stimulus that produces nausea, if sufficiently intense or prolonged, results in vomiting.

Vomiting is defined as the forceful expulsion of gastric contents out of the mouth. The act of vomiting is usually preceded by retching. Vomiting is an important symptom for two major reasons. First, it can be the initial or predominant presentation in a number of major medical diagnoses (e.g., gastric or intestinal obstruction, myocardial infarction, pregnancy, appendicitis, uremia, diabetic ketoacidosis, Addison's disease). Second, regardless of its cause, it can lead to life-threatening complications.

Vomiting is coordinated by a medullary control system rather than by a unique, well-defined "vomiting center." Neurons involved in coordinated vomiting are embedded in an arc of neurons radiating from the area postrema and nucleus solitarius through the intermediate reticular zone of the lateral tegmental field to the ventrolateral medulla. The vomiting reflex involves a complex integration of signals from both the somatic and autonomic nervous systems (Fig. 334-1). Emetic stimuli can cause vomiting by at least two mechanisms. First, an emetic stimulus can activate afferent neural pathways that act directly on the vomiting center in the dorsal portion of the medulla oblongata. Orally ingested copper sulfate or certain toxins cause vomiting by this mechanism. In experimental animals, ablation of the vagus nerves and sympathetic pathways within the abdomen prevents vomiting induced by orally administered copper sulfate. It is likely that afferent impulses from parts of the body other than the gastrointestinal tract (e.g., the pharynx and the heart) can also cause vomiting by directly activating the vomiting center.

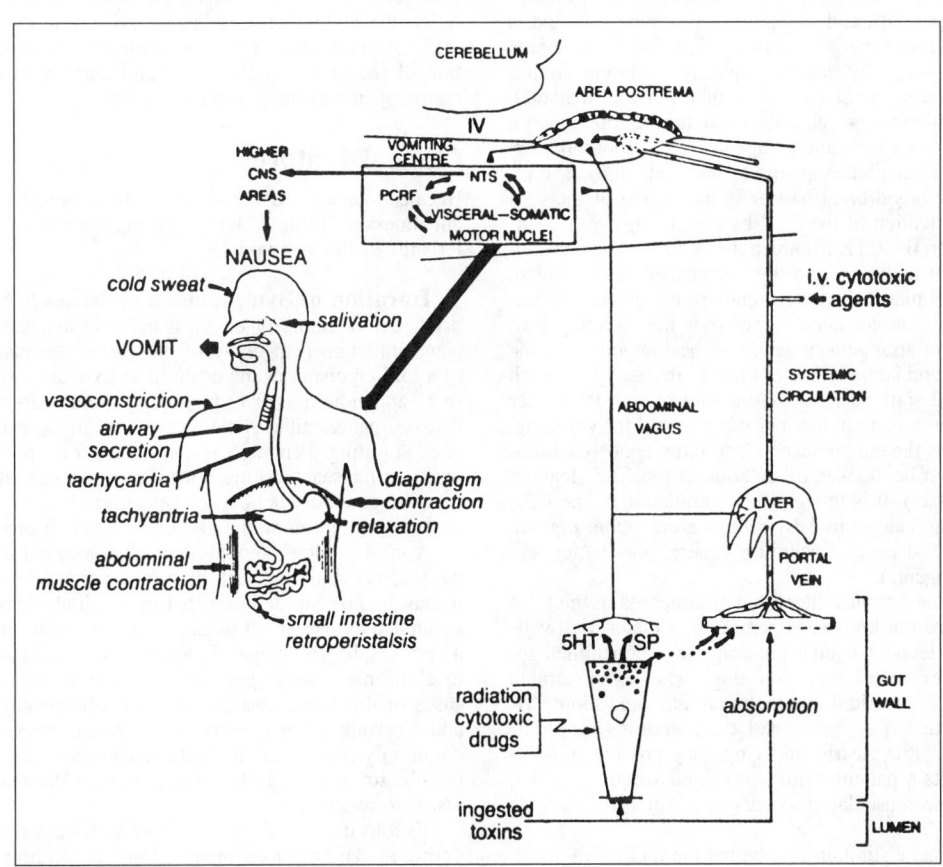

FIGURE 334-1   Major components of the emetic reflex believed to be involved in emesis evoked by cytotoxic therapy or by orally ingested toxins.

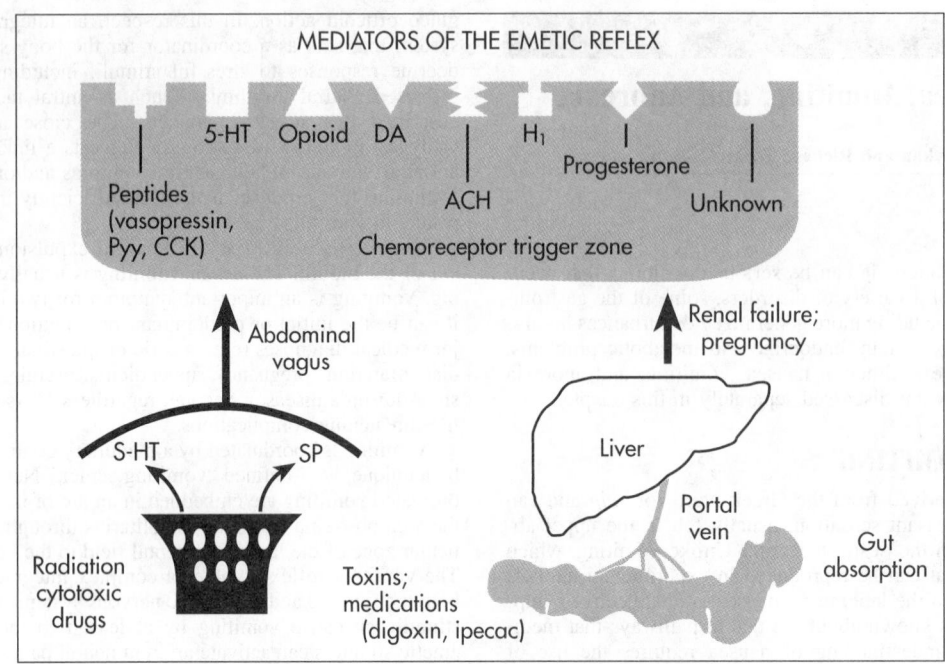

FIGURE 334-2   Mediators of the emetic reflex.

A second mechanism by which an emetic stimulus can lead to vomiting is activation of the chemoreceptor trigger zone (CTZ), which is located in the area postrema of the medulla in the floor of the fourth ventricle. The area postrema is a special sensory organ rich in dopaminergic (D2), serotoninergic (SHT3), histaminergic (H1), muscarinic (acetyl choline, or *ACh*), and vasopressinergic receptors and is a chemoreceptive area for triggering vomiting (Fig. 334-2). The area postrema may be stimulated by vagal or splachnic afferent stimuli (e.g., copper sulfate, visceral pain, gastrointestinal mucosal irritants), by endogenoeus conditions (e.g., chronic renal failure, pregnancy), or by exogenously circulating emetic agents (e.g., apomorphine, L-dopa, digitalis, ipecac, chemotherapeutic agents, radiation). The incomplete nature of the blood-brain barrier in the region of the area postrema facilitates activation of the CTZ by circulating agents. Unlike the vomiting center, the CTZ is unresponsive to electrical stimulation. Its main efferent pathway is to the nucleus solitarius, which, along with the parvicellular reticular formation and several medullary visceral and somatic motor nuclei, composes the vomiting center. This close anatomic arrangement seems to be important for the integration of visceral and somatic nuclei that are necessary for such a complex visceral and somatic reflex. Communication with higher centers may play a role in nausea, but it is not required for vomiting. In experimental animals the emetic response to intravenously administered apomorphine can be blocked by ablation of the CTZ (leaving the vomiting center intact). It is thought that stimulation of the CTZ is important in vomiting caused by labyrinthine stimulation, uremia, diabetic ketoacidosis, and drugs (including general anesthetics and certain antineoplastic agents).

Although the exact neurotransmitters that are released in the CTZ and vomiting center are not known, dopamine is a major and well-studied mediator. Thus levodopa and bromocriptine (a dopamine agonist) commonly cause nausea and vomiting, whereas dopamine antagonists—such as haloperidol, metoclopramide, and domperidone—are effective antiemetics. Since the latter two drugs are prokinetics as well and accelerate gastric emptying, they provide an additional advantage in certain patients with nausea and vomiting caused by gastrointestinal neuromuscular disorders (e.g., diabetic patients with gastroparesis).

Regardless of the emetic stimulus or whether the CTZ is involved, the vomiting center is the anatomic location from which the act of vomiting is initiated and coordinated. The vomiting sequence can be summarized as follows. During nausea, gastric tone is reduced, in as-

sociation with gastric electrical arrhythmias, whereas the tonus in the duodenum may increase, leading to reflux of duodenal contents into the stomach. During retching, there is to-and-fro movement of gastric contents into a dilated esophagus. The antrum and pylorus are contracted; the lower esophageal sphincter is relaxed; and, temporarily, the abdominal esophagus and gastric cardia herniate into the thorax. Vomiting occurs as a result of a forceful sustained contraction of the abdominal muscles and diaphragm while the cardia remains open and the pylorus contracted.

Clinical Features

Because nausea and vomiting can be manifestations of many different illnesses (Table 334-1), it is important to discern certain characteristics of the symptoms.

Duration of Symptoms. If symptoms have been present for a brief period (hours or days), it is likely that the illness is due to an acute infection (especially of the gastrointestinal tract); to ingestion of a toxin, poison, or medication; to an acute inflammatory condition (e.g., appendicitis); or to pregnancy. Some patients with peptic ulcer disease, pancreatitis, cholecystitis, and myocardial infarction experience vomiting. Peptic ulcer and nonulcer dyspepsia patients may experience nausea resulting not from a gastric obstruction but because they are generally helicobacter-positive. This organism may promote nausea through ammonia and other toxins it produces.

A viral etiology should also be considered in patients where the nausea and vomiting is chronic in duration (>3 months). By history, it may be possible to elicit that their initial illness was characterized by an acute onset of an illness consistent with viral gastroenteritis. In a very small percentage of patients, this viral gastroenteritis can lead to a chronic state of gastroparesis lasting months to years. In adult cases of this type, Epstein-Barr virus, herpesvirus, cytomegalovirus, and Norwalk agent have been suspected, whereas rotavirus is more commonly considered in children. This chronic gastroparesis can take months to years to fully resolve and for the neuromuscular mechanisms to regenerate.

Various drugs and chemicals are well known to induce nausea and vomiting. The most encountered one is alcohol; chronic alcohol users experience nausea and vomiting as a part of their daily life. Cardiotonic agents such as digitalis and quinidine and many of the drugs used in cancer chemotherapy cause nausea and vomiting. Among

Table 334-1   Medications and dosing schedules for nausea and vomiting

AGENT	MECHANISM OF ACTION	DOSAGE AND ADMINISTRATION
5-HT$_3$ antagonists Ondansetron Granisetron	5-HT$_3$ blockade	IV: 32 mg or 150 mcg/kg (8 mg tid); PO: 8 mg bid-tid
Substituted benzamides Metoclopramide Trimethobenzamide	Dopamine receptor blockade, 5-HT$_3$ blockade	IV: 1-2 mg/kg q2h (chemotherapy) or 10 mg q3-4h (vomiting); SC: 5-10 mg qid; PO: 10-20 mg qid IM: 200 mg tid-qid; PO: 250 mg tid-qid
Phenothiazines Prochlorperazine Perphenazine Promethazine Thiethylperazine Triflupromazine Chlorpromazine	Dopamine receptor blockade	IV, IM, PO: 5-10 mg q3-4h (max: 40 mg/day); rectally: 25 mg bid PO: 8-24 mg/day; IM: 5 mg daily PO, IM: 25 mg, then 12.5-25 mg as needed q4-6h PO, IM: 10 mg bid-tid PO: 25-30 mg daily; IM: 5-15 mg q4h as needed (max: 40 mg) PO: 10-25 mg q4-6h; IM: 25 mg then 25-50 mg; rectally: 50-100 mg tid-qid
Corticosteroids Dexamethasone Methylprednisolone	Unclear	IV: 20 mg IV: 125-500 mg qid for total of four doses
Benzodiazepines Lorazepam Diazepam	Anxiolytic amnesic	PO, IV: 1-2 mg q4-6h PO, IV: 2-5 mg q4-6h
Cannabinoids Dronabinol Nabilone	Central psychotropic action	PO: 5-10 mg repeated at 2- to 4-hour PO: 1-2 mg bid
Anticholinergics Scopolamine	Cholinergic blockade	Topical: 1 patch behind ear several hours before travel; PO, SC: 0.6-1 mg
Benzimidazole derivative Domperidone	Dopamine receptor blockade	PO: 10-30 mg qid; rectally: 20 mg qid
Butyrophenones Haloperidol Droperidol	Dopamine receptor blockade	IV: 1-2 mg; IM, PO: 1, 2, or 5 mg q2h as needed IV: 1.25-2.5 mg
Antihistamines Diphenhydramine Hydroxyzine Meclizine Dimenhydrinate Cyclizine hydrochloride Buclizine hydrochloride	H$_1$ receptor antagonism	PO: 50 mg 30 min before travel; IM, IV: 10 mg increased to 25-50 mg q2-3h if needed, max: 400 mg daily PO, IM: 25-100 mg tid-qid PO: 25-50 mg before travel IV: 50 mg diluted in 10 mg saline; IM: 50 mg; PO: 50-100 mg q4h; Rectally: 10 mg tid PO: 50 mg before travel PO: 50 mg before travel

IV, Intravenously; *PO*, orally; *IM*, intramuscularly; *SC*, subcutaneously.

other commonly used agents, nonsteroidal antiinflamatories, antiarrhythmics, aminophylline, ipecac, colchicine, L-dopa, oral contraceptives, opiates, and the somatostatin analogue octreotide may also cause nausea and vomiting.

Another condition associated with nausea and vomiting mainly in children and young adults is Münchausen's syndrome–by–proxy. This is a psychiatric disorder in which a parent overreports or produces illness in her/his child. Münchausen's syndrome–by–proxy may be suspected when symptoms given by history are not confirmed on direct observation, or when the degree of symptom disability is out of proportion to objective evidence of impaired GI motility.

Nausea and vomiting that have been present for weeks or months may suggest partial mechanical obstruction of the stomach or small intestine, carcinoma (especially of the stomach or pancreas), intracranial abnormality (e.g., brain tumor), or a psychogenic process. It is also always important to consider a nonmechanical or functional disorder otherwise referred to as a GI motility disturbance, such as gastroparesis diabeticorum and idiopathic intestinal pseudoobstruction.

Timing of Vomiting in Relation to Meals. Vomiting during or shortly after a meal is seen in patients with psychogenic vomiting and sometimes in patients with a peptic ulcer in the pyloric channel. Patients with psychogenic vomiting rarely vomit in public; they usually control their urge to vomit until safely in the privacy of a toilet. These patients sometimes self-induce emesis. Self-induced emesis is

a component of bulimia nervosa (Box 334-1). Regurgitation of undigested food shortly after eating can also be seen in patients with esophageal disorders (stricture, cancer, Zenker's diverticulum, achalasia, and gastroesophageal reflux). In these latter patients, regurgitation is not usually preceded by nausea; instead, the patient often experiences dysphagia. In addition, in the latter conditions, reflux of gastric contents can occur at night in the lying position or when the patient is sleeping.

Rumination syndrome, which is often confused with a gastric motility disorder, should be kept in mind in patients with vomiting of unknown etiology. Vomiting of rumination syndrome is effortless and occurs within 15 minutes of eating and involves liquids, even water, as well as solids. Patients with rumination syndrome generally do not lose weight and have minimal nausea, and psychologic contributory factors can be identified. The diagnosis of rumination syndrome can be confusing and is possible only if one is aware of this condition.

Vomiting that occurs an hour or more after eating is characteristic of gastric outlet obstruction or a gastric motor disorder. Physical findings can include a succussion splash and visible peristalsis. An emesis of long-retained gastric contents does not always mean obstruction at the pylorus or duodenum. It simply means impaired gastric emptying, and this is seen also in cases of gastroparesis, a motility disorder, in the absence of gastric outlet obstruction.

Vomiting upon arising in the morning is characteristic of vomit-

---

BOX 334-1

Criterial for bulimia nervosa and anorexia nervosa

Diagnostic criteria for 307.51 bulimia nervosa

A. Recurrent episodes of binge eating. An episode of binge eating is characterized by both of the following:
　1. Eating, in a discrete period of time (e.g., within any 2-hour period), an amount of food that is definitely larger than most people would eat during a similar period of time and under similar circumstances.
　2. A sense of lack of control over eating during the episode (e.g., a feeling that one cannot stop eating or control what or how much one is eating).
B. Recurrent inappropriate compensatory behavior in order to prevent weight gain, such as self-induced vomiting; misuse of laxatives, diuretics, enemas, or other medications; fasting; or excessive exercise.
C. The binge eating and inappropriate compensatory behaviors both occur, on average, at least twice a week for 3 months.
D. Self-evaluation is unduly influenced by body shape and weight.
E. The disturbance does not occur exclusively during episodes of anorexia nervosa.

Specify type

Purging type: during the current episode of bulimia nervosa, the person has regularly engaged in self-induced vomiting or the misuse of laxatives, diuretics, or enemas.

Nonpurging type: during the current episode of bulimia nervosa, the person has used other inappropriate compensatory behaviors, such as fasting or excessive exercise, but has not regularly engaged in self-induced vomiting or the misuse of laxatives, diuretics, or enemas.

Diagnostic criteria for 307.1 anorexia nervosa

A. Refusal to maintain body weight at or above a minimally normal weight for age and height (e.g., weight loss leading to maintenance of body weight less than 85% of that expected; or failure to make expected weight gain during a period of growth, leading to body weight less than 85% of that expected).
B. Intense fear of gaining weight or becoming fat, even though underweight.
C. Disturbance in the way in which one's body weight or shape is experienced, undue influence of body weight or shape on self-evaluation, or denial of the seriousness of the current low body weight.
D. In postmenarcheal females, amenorrhea (i.e., the absence of at least three consecutive menstrual cycles). A woman is considered to have amenorrhea if her periods occur only following hormone (e.g., estrogen) administration.

Specify type

Restricting type: during the current episode of anorexia nervosa, the person has not regularly engaged in binge eating or purging behavior (e.g., self-induced vomiting or the misuse of laxatives, diuretics, or enemas).

Binge eating/purging type: during the current episode of anorexia nervosa, the person has regularly engaged in binge eating or purging behavior (e.g., self-induced vomiting or the misuse of laxatives, diuretics, or enemas).

---

ing in pregnancy but may also be seen in uremia; alcoholism; increased intracranial pressure (including brain tumors); narcotic withdrawal syndromes; and gastroparesis of neuromuscular etiology, particularly in diabetic gastopathy with or without hyperglycemia on awakening.

Content and Odor of the Vomitus. The presence of old food suggests gastric retention, assuming achalasia and Zenker's diverticulum are excluded. The presence of bile in the vomitus is often not as significant as it may seem. Normally, bile regurgitates from the duodenum into the stomach sufficiently to stain vomitus from almost any cause. An absence of bile in retentive vomitus might suggest obstruction at or proximal to the pylorus. An unusually heavy concentration of bile in postprandial vomitus is present in gastroparesis following antral resections and also might suggest the afferent loop syndrome

in a patient who has had a gastrojejunostomy. The presence of blood in the vomitus is of obvious importance, although it must be remembered that vomiting of any cause may lead to a Mallory-Weiss laceration of the gastric or esophageal mucosa and thus to hematemesis or a bloody nasogastric aspirate (see later discussion). The odor of the vomitus may be feculent as a result of bacterial overgrowth secondary to gastric or small bowel stasis, obstruction, or ischemia.

Associated Symptoms. Fever, weight loss, abdominal mass, menstrual irregularity, history of prior abdominal surgery, jaundice, migraine headache, chest pain, and many other factors influence the clinical impression in a patient with vomiting. Paraneoplastic syndomes may present with nausea and vomiting, thought to be mediated by antineuronal antibodies that induce a bowel neuropathy usually in the setting of small cell cancer of the lung.

Consequences

The most common consequence of vomiting is the loss of water and electrolytes (especially chloride, hydrogen, potassium, and sodium ions) from the body. The result is a hypochloremic, hypokalemic, metabolic alkalosis. As the extracellular fluid volume shrinks, the concentration of bicarbonate in plasma increases, and as a result the renal threshold for bicarbonate reabsorption can be exceeded. This may lead to a transient sodium bicarbonaturia, which exacerbates sodium depletion. Thus a low urine chloride concentration (<10 mEq/L) is a more sensitive index for assessing the degree of salt depletion than the urine sodium concentration. In addition, the kidney may contribute to potassium losses and hypokalemia as a result of secondary hyperaldosteronism. In some patients, vomiting may be surreptitious or concealed. Also, in patients with eating disorders, laxatives and diuretics may be simultaneously taken to lose weight, and this contributes to hypokalemia. Thus the presence of a hypochloremic, hypokalemic, metabolic alkalosis should arouse suspicion that a patient has been vomiting. In addition to the loss of water and electrolytes, loss of ingested nutrients by vomiting contributes to weight loss and malnutrition. In specific cases, relevant drug levels should be obtained. Tests for occult alcohol or drug use (i.e., surreptitious use of narcotics and ipecac) can be helpful.

Another serious sequela of vomiting is pulmonary aspiration, which usually occurs in patients with neurologic problems, such as head trauma, drug overdose, or cerebrovascular accident. Aspiration also can occur as a complication of vomiting during general anesthesia. The presence of hydrochloric acid in the terminal airways leads to an intense chemical pneumonitis. In addition, acid in the proximal airway can lead to laryngospasm and bronchospasm.

Mallory-Weiss syndrome is a complication of retching and vomiting. The lesion is a mucosal tear or tears, usually on the gastric side of the gastroesophageal junction, although the tear may extend to the esophagus. Many patients with Mallory-Weiss syndrome have hiatal hernias. Although intraluminal bleeding stops in most cases, some patients require transfusions, endoscopic hemostatic therapy, or surgery. On rare occasions, bleeding may dissect into the wall of the esophagus, leading to a hematoma that may cause difficulty in swallowing or chest pain. Postemetic esophageal hematomas resolve spontaneously in 5 to 7 days.

Vomiting may lead to life-threatening rupture of the esophagus (Boerhaave's syndrome) or proximal stomach. The usual presentation of esophageal rupture is severe epigastric pain, cyanosis, dyspnea, left pleural effusion on chest roentgenogram, and mediastinal or subcutaneous emphysema. Treatment usually consists of thoracotomy to repair the damaged esophagus.

Treatment

If vomiting has been severe enough to lead to volume depletion and electrolyte disturbances, intravenous fluid and electrolyte replacement is warranted. When the cause of vomiting can be ascertained, this should be remedied if possible. For example, gastric outlet obstruction or small bowel obstruction may require tube decompression or surgical intervention; adrenal (Addisonian) crisis requires hydrocortisone; and drug-induced vomiting requires a reduction in dosage or cessation of the medication. A variety of drugs have antiemetic prop-

---

BOX 334-2
Differential diagnosis of nausea and vomiting

Central nervous system disorder

Trauma
Intracranial mass
Intracranial bleeding
Meningitis
Labyrnthitis
Meniere's disease
Acoustic neuroma
Classic migraine
Motion sickness

Esophageal diseases

Achalasia
Stricture
Zenker's diverticulum

Psychogenic

Rumination
Self-induced

Gastrointestinal diseases

Hepatitis
Peptic ulcer disease
Pancreatitis
Cholecystitis
Peritonitis
Obstruction of any cause
Infectious agents
Inflammatory bowel disease
Gastric malignancy

Gastrointestinal neuropathy

Diabetic gastroparesis
Parneoplastic syndrome
Idiopathic pseudoobstruction
Idiopathic gastroparesis
Postvagotomy syndrome
Tachygastria

Gastrointestinal myopathy

Amyloidosis
Idiopathic pseudoobstruction

Drugs

Antiarrythmics
Alcohol
Aminophylline
Bromocriptine chemotherapy
Colchicine
Digoxin
Erythromycin
Ipecac
L-Dopa
Nonsteroidal antiinflammatory drugs
Nicotine
Opiates
Oral contraceptives
Salicylates

Systemic disorders

Severe pain
Progressive systemic sclerosis
Diabetic ketoacidosis
Addison's disease
Thyrotoxicosis
Seizure disorders
Uremia
Amyloidosis
Acute infection
Myocardial infarction
Radiation sickness hyponatremia
Hypercalcemia
Acidosis
Hyperglycemia

Pregnancy

Morning sickness
Hyperemesis gravidarum

---

erties, including anticholinergics, antihistamines, benzodiazepines, cannabinoids, corticosteroids, dopamine antagonists, and newly described serotonin antagonists (Box 334-2). Antiemetic drugs may be helpful for temporary control of symptoms, but they should not be used in place of early definitive therapy. When the cause of nausea or vomiting is not known or when specific treatment is not available (e.g., viral gastroenteritis), it is often necessary to employ an antiemetic drug.

Antihistamines are useful in vomiting that is secondary to motion sickness and other vestibular disturbances. Phenothiazines and butyrophenones help vomiting caused by radiation, gastroenteritis, or drugs. Because phenothiazines can cause blood dyscrasias, jaundice, or extrapyramidal reactions, they should be used cautiously. Prokinetic agents, such as metoclopramide, domperidone, cisapride, and erythromycin, may be useful in patients with nausea and vomiting produced by gastroparesis syndromes. Tetrahydrocannabinol (dronabinol), a component of marijuana, is effective in prevention of vomiting induced by anticancer chemotherapy agents but also in other nausea-vomiting states not responding to conventional therapy. Metoclopramide, domperidone, and dexamethasone are also effective in this setting. Selective 5-hydroxytryptamine₃ receptor antagonists, such as ondansetron and granisetrone, have recently been shown to be highly effective in controlling chemotherapy-induced emesis as well as other causes of vomiting refractory to conventional therapy. Benzodiazepines (e.g., lorazepam) or behavior modification can be employed to reduce anticipatory nausea and vomiting that may precede anticancer chemotherapy.

Pregnancy is a specific consideration. Reassurance should be provided for "morning sickness," because the syndrome usually abates after the sixteenth week. In the second or third trimester, metoclopramide can be administered intravenously in 10-mg doses every 6 hours; this dosage may be used orally as well. Intravenous or oral ondansetron has an important role also and could be continued with metoclopramide.

For nausea and vomiting caused by gastrointestinal motility disorders, combining a peripherally acting prokinetic agent (i.e., cisa-

pride) with a centrally acting adjunctive antiemetic (i.e., domperidone) should be considered. This approach of using a combination of pharmacologic agents probes different mechanisms of disease and may help address the different patient subgroups.

ANOREXIA

Anorexia can be defined as the lack of or loss of appetite. It is not to be confused with early satiety, in which patients experience hunger but, because of a problem with gastric filling or gastric emptying, stop eating prematurely. Anorexia is also not to be confused with sitophobia, in which a patient fears eating because pain or other unpleasant sensations are likely to occur (e.g., abdominal angina).

Very little is known about what regulates hunger and appetite. The control of feeding appears to involve a "feeding center" in the lateral hypothalamus and the "satiety center" in the ventromedial hypothalamic nuclei. The anatomic location and functional contributions of these centers are predicated on observations of the effects of destructive lesions produced experimentally in these regions. It is likely that the brain, liver, gastrointestinal tract, and ingested nutrients are important. Psychologic factors are also important in food intake. Thus persons with profound depression may lose their appetite despite appropriate signals from the gut, liver, and bloodstream. There is also evidence to suggest that patients with cancer may develop learned aversions to specific foods eaten during the phase of tumor growth and/or nausea-producing chemotherapy.

Virtually any disorder of the gastrointestinal tract, liver, pancreas, or biliary tree can be associated with anorexia. In addition, many drugs, especially antineoplastic agents, lead to anorexia. There are many extraintestinal illnesses in which anorexia is a major feature. These include cancer; infections; endocrine disturbances (Addison's disease, panhypopituitarism, hyperparathyroidism); collagen vascular diseases; renal disease; pulmonary disorders (especially chronic obstructive lung disease); congestive heart failure; and psychiatric illness (especially depression). How these diseases cause anorexia is incompletely understood. Anorexia, if prolonged, leads to weight loss;

protein-calorie malnutrition; and, eventually, death. To be noted in this regard is that anorexia, with or without prominent weight loss, may exist for some time before a serious organic digestive disease, such as cancer, becomes apparent. Therapy for anorexia should be directed to the underlying cause.

Anorexia Nervosa

The disorder of anorexia nervosa is characterized by a distorted, implacable attitude toward eating that overrides hunger warnings and threats. As a result of decreased caloric intake, weight loss is profound and death may result. In most cases the patient is a female below the age of 25 years. Because of a distorted body image, the patient strives to become thin, and thus avoids food. Recently there has been increasing concern of physical and/or sexual abuse in the family or personal settings of the patients presenting to the physician as just "an eating disorder." There is evidence that these patients experience hunger but that they suppress the sensation because not eating is more pleasurable. Thus the term *anorexia nervosa* is a misnomer. During the disease, amenorrhea develops, sometimes before weight loss occurs. Criteria for diagnosis are summarized in Box 334-1.

Patients with anorexia nervosa may maintain an interest in food by becoming gourmet cooks or dietitians. Yet they will hoard food or throw it out rather than eat it. Intake of carbohydrate and fat is especially reduced. Some patients also have features of bulimia nervosa (Box 334-1). Thus patients may present with weight loss and a hypokalemic, hypochloremic alkalosis caused by vomiting and/or secret use of laxatives, diuretics, and amphetamines. Other patients, who vomit more frequently and conspicuously, may be referred for evaluation of vomiting and weight loss. The majority of patients with anorexia nervosa (80% in one report) have slower than normal gastric emptying, although the connection between slow gastric emptying and anorexia and vomiting is unclear. The patients who have been reported to have impaired gastric emptying have lost more than 20% of their ideal body weight and, when trying to eat and regain their weight, they experience satiety, bloating, nausea, and abdominal pain. It is believed that antral motility is impaired by the sustained lack of significant oral intake. Moreover, the antrum is very sensitive to any distention and produces symptoms when attempts at eating resume. By slowly increasing consistency and size of meals, retraining of the stomach will occur and gastric emptying will slowly improve.

The cause of anorexia nervosa is not known, although most consider it a primary psychiatric disorder. The disease can be diagnosed after other diseases that lead to decreased food intake and weight loss have been excluded. It is important to exclude cancer and endocrine disturbances (especially panhypopituitarism and hypoadrenalism). Patients with anorexia nervosa are usually alert, active, and unaware that there is a problem. They may be exercise fanatics and deny that they are ill. Patients with panhypopituitarism are weak and lethargic and freely admit that they are not well.

Therapy for anorexia nervosa is both nutritional and psychiatric. In some cases, malnutrition may be so advanced that parenteral hyperalimentation may be necessary temporarily. Enteral feedings involving placement of nasogastric or nasoenteric tube may be required. As soon as possible, attempts should be made to supply calories, protein, and vitamins orally. Gastric prokinetic agents may help in initiating oral intake by accelerating the slowed gastric emptying and reducing the discomfort, bloating, and fullness that limit attempts to eat. Early in the course, psychiatric consultation should be sought. In some cases it may be helpful to institute a behavior modification program with rewards for weight gain. Family group therapy sessions may be useful. The prognosis is generally good, although relapses are common and approximately 1 in 20 patients dies of the disease.

BIBLIOGRAPHY

Berk JE: Anorexia. In Berk JE, Haubrich WS, editors: *Gastrointestinal symptoms: clinical interpretation*, Philadelphia, 1991, BC Decker, pp. 233-240.

Feldman M, Samson WK, O'Dorisio TM: Apomorphine-induced nausea in humans: release of vasopressin and pancreatic polypeptide, *Gastroenterology* 95:721, 1988.

Grundy D, Reid K: The physiology of nausea and vomiting. In Johnson LR, editor: *Physiology of the gastrointestinal tract*, New York, 1994, Raven, pp. 879-902.

Halmi KA: Anorexia nervosa and bulimia, *Annu Rev Med* 38:373, 1987.

Haubrich WS: Nausea and vomiting. In Berk JE, Haubrich WS, editors: *Gastrointestinal symptoms: clinical interpretation*, Philadelphia, 1991, BC Decker, pp. 91-103.

Hyman PE: Chronic intestinal-pseudoobstruction. In Hyman PE, editor: *Pediatric gastrointestinal motility disorders*, New York, 1994, Academy Professional Information Services.

Janssens J et al: Improvement of gastric emptying in diabetic gastroparesis by erythromycin, *N Engl J Med* 322:1028, 1990.

Koch K: Approach to the patient with nausea and vomiting. In Yamada T, editor: *Textbook of gastroenterology*, Philadelphia, 1995, JB Lippincott.

Kurtzman FD et al: Eating disorders among selected student populations at UCLA, *J Am Diet Assoc* 89:45, 1989.

Lee M, Feldman M: Nausea and vomiting. In Sleisenger MH, Fordtran JS, editors: *Gastrointestinal disease*, ed 5, Philadelphia, 1993, WB Saunders.

Marty M et al: Comparison of the 5-hydroxytryptamine₃ (serotonin) antagonist ondansetron (GR38032F) with high-dose metoclopramide in the control of cisplatin-induced emesis, *N Engl J Med* 322:816, 1990.

McCallum RW: Cisapride: a new class of prokinetic agent, *Am J Gastroenterol* 86:135, 1991.

McCallum RW: Nausea and vomiting. In Friedman G, Jacobson ED, McCallum RW, editors: *Gastrointestinal pharmacology & theraputics*, Philadelphia, 1997, Lippincott-Raven, pp. 603-610.

McCallum RW, Grill BB, Lange R et al: Definition of a gastric emptying abnormality in patients with anorexia nervosa, *Dig Dis Sci* 30:713-722, 1985.

Miller AD, Nonaka S, Jakus J: Brain areas essential or non-essential for emesis, *Brain Res* 647:255-264, 1994.

Muraoka M et al: Psychogenic vomiting: the relation between patterns of vomiting and psychiatric diagnoses, *Gut* 31:526, 1990.

Tortorice PV, O'Connell MB: Management of chemotherapy-induced nausea and vomiting, *Pharmacotherapy* 10:129, 1990.

Worsley A et al: The weight control practices of 15-year-old New Zealanders, *J Paediatr Child Health* 26:41, 1990.

335 Abdominal Pain

T. Edward Bynum

Abdominal pain is a common presenting complaint. It may be the symptom of a variety of intraabdominal diseases or the major expression of diseases that reside primarily outside the abdominal cavity. The variety of diseases that cause abdominal pain and the tendency for both the location and the character of abdominal pain to be nonspecific make abdominal pain difficult to evaluate in some patients. This difficulty is compounded by unusual or bizarre types of abdominal pain that do not seem to have an organic basis (and may be psychosomatic), by "chronic pain syndrome," and by a less than discrete separation of functional and organic mechanisms in the generation of abdominal pain. This chapter presents current concepts relating to abdominal pain, an approach to evaluation of the patient who has abdominal pain, and an attempt to identify those types of abdominal pain most difficult to understand and diagnose.

CLASSIFICATION, CAUSES, AND PATHOPHYSIOLOGY

Abdominal pain is categorized as *visceral, somatic* (or *parietal*), and *referred*. The distinctions are somewhat artificial neurophysiologically, but they are useful clinically and conceptually. Visceral pain arises from an abdominal viscus; it is most commonly dull, cramping, or gnawing in quality, and not well localized to a specific region within the abdomen (usually midline). Pain is felt at the midline because bilateral dermatome innervation takes place at a stage in embryologic development in which the abdominal organs are a simple midline tube. This stage precedes the budding out that produces liver, biliary tree, and pancreas and precedes the elongation and rotation of the gastrointestinal tract. Somatic pain arises in the parietal peritoneum or structures of the body wall in the region of the abdomen. It is localized, aggravated by movement, and often characterized as sharp and discrete. Referred pain is perceived in areas remote from where it originates, usually because the diseased organ shares a neu-

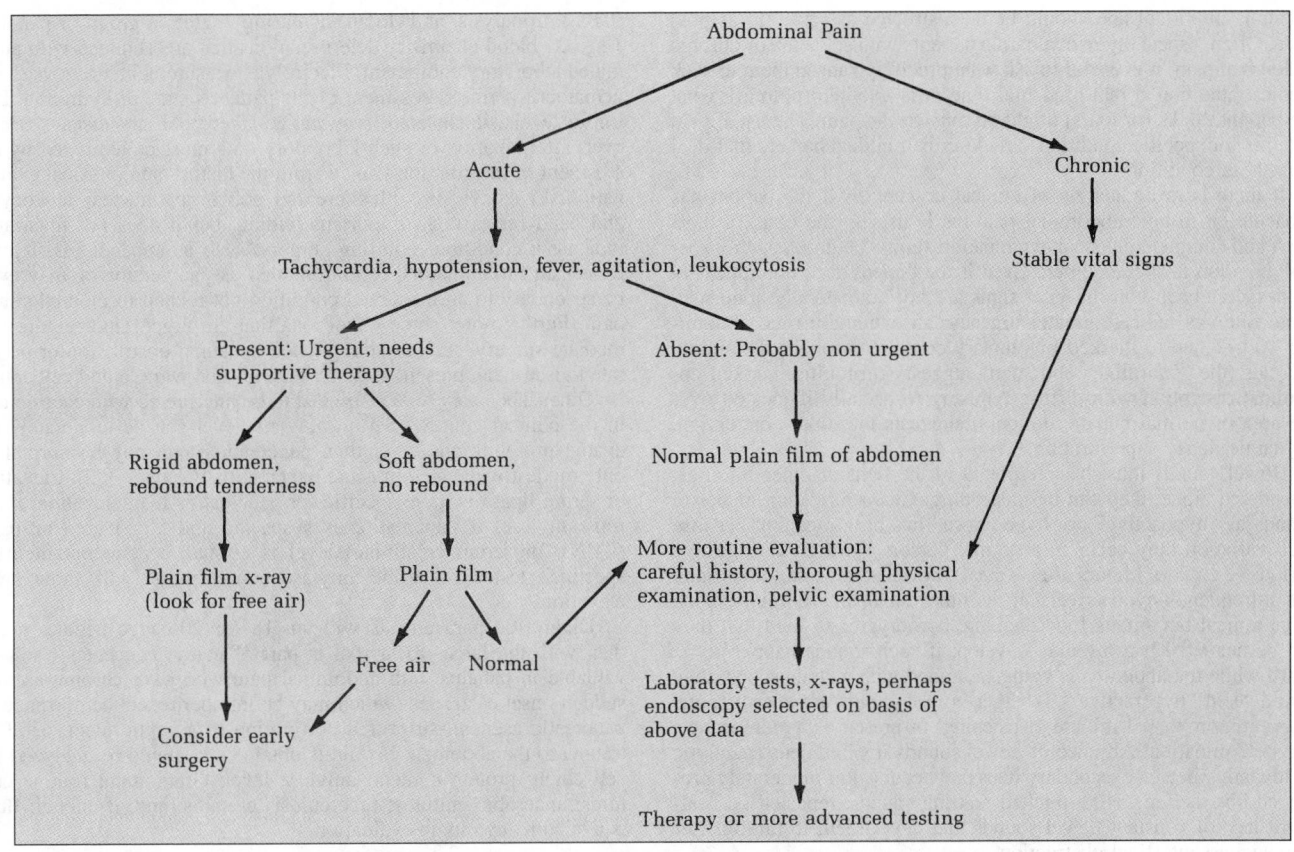

FIGURE 335-1   Evaluation of patients with abdominal pain.

ral segment with the area where pain is felt. Its character is usually similar to that of somatic pain.

Rapidly developing distention, stretching, or traction of an abdominal viscus and/or mesentery is the principal cause of visceral pain. Inflammation increases the sensitivity (lowers the threshold) of pain receptors, probably by releasing mediators such as histamine, prostaglandins, kinin polypeptides, substance P, serotonin, and potassium. Abdominal pain commonly occurs when normal or increased motor contractions affect an inflamed lesion. Thus distention, stretching, and traction generate pain in intraabdominal organs in which obstruction, ulceration, ischemia, infection, or mass lesions exist.

The mechanisms involved in some causes of abdominal pain are not well understood. Metabolic or toxic disorders such as porphyria and lead poisoning may be accompanied by severe and persistent abdominal pain but no demonstrated distention, altered contractions, or inflammation. Familial Mediterranean fever is characterized by severe abdominal pain, often with evidence for nonspecific peritonitis as part of a more general polyserositis, but the cause is not known beyond its geographic and genetic associations.

It is not clear whether patients who experience psychogenic (or psychosomatic) abdominal pain have markedly enhanced perceptions of normally occurring motor functions, which they perceive as "pains," or whether such patients have centrally mediated abnormalities in motor contractions, with or without transient local distention. Perhaps other, as yet unidentified phenomena may be involved. Diseases of the nerves—such as diabetic neuropathy, herpes zoster, and advanced syphilis—may cause the patient to perceive pain in the abdomen when there is no actual disease of intraabdominal organs, peritoneum, or abdominal wall.

PATIENT EVALUATION

The first step in evaluating a patient with abdominal pain is to assess the severity and urgency of his or her situation and determine whether there may be associated conditions that represent a major threat to the patient. If the situation is urgent and potentially ominous, addi-

tional evaluation must be tailored to the patient's needs and to the clinical circumstances. Some therapy or management may be necessary before or during further evaluation. Fig. 335-1 summarizes the approach to the evaluation of patients with abdominal pain.

The initial assessment should establish whether the abdominal pain is acute or chronic. If pain is acute, the clinician must determine whether the situation is urgent. If pain is chronic, the clinician must determine whether there has been an acute (and perhaps urgent) exacerbation of the chronic condition. The perceptive clinician may pick up clues early in the evaluation that suggest a psychogenic basis for the abdominal pain. Early determination of psychogenic pain can eliminate costly, unnecessary, and perhaps risky procedures and enable the clinician to switch to an approach in which sympathetic listening and support are emphasized.

The signals of urgency are similar to those in other severe acute illness. At the extreme, they include coma, shock, and cardiac or respiratory arrest. Short of that, mental confusion, restlessness, sweating, pallor, and clamminess should cause concern. Careful attention should be given to the vital signs: greater clinical urgency is suggested by tachycardia, orthostatic hypotension, or high fever, which suggest massive hemorrhage or sepsis and require immediate therapeutic intervention. If the patient is free of these signs, a more systematic and standard approach to the evaluation is appropriate.

The history (as obtained from all available sources, including the patient or relatives, old medical records, and referring physicians) is extremely important. The history alone may allow functionally accurate diagnosis in a majority of patients, as high as 80% by some estimates. It often provides more essential information than do laboratory tests, radiographs, and other special tests. If the patient does not volunteer information about specific aspects of the pain, it must be elicited. Important aspects include intensity; character (dull, sharp, intermittent, constant, throbbing, burning, etc.); location; radiation; timing and setting; association with gastrointestinal functions (eating, defecation) or body positions; factors or events that contribute to exacerbation or relief; associated symptoms; use of narcotics or other medications; and relation to menstrual periods. The sequence of events is important and should be reconstructed as carefully as possible. Often, especially in evaluating patients with subacute or chronic abdominal pain, it is useful to ask what precisely caused them to seek medical attention at that particular time. It is also helpful to ask what the patient thinks (or fears) might be causing the pain. The usual pain patterns for specific conditions are described in the chapters that deal with these conditions.

If there is no indication of clinical urgency or if the patient has subacute or chronic abdominal pain (as is usually the case), a thorough and complete physical examination should be done, paying special attention to the abdomen. Even if the patient does not appear to be desperately ill and the vital signs are not dramatically abnormal, some findings indicate greater urgency: an extremely rigid abdominal wall related to marked involuntary contraction of the abdominal muscles (the "boardlike" abdomen) suggests peritonitis; marked abdominal distention with diffuse tympany (especially if located over the area of normal hepatic dullness) suggests intestinal obstruction, adynamic ileus, or perforation.

Bowel sounds must be interpreted in the light of other findings; considered alone, they can be misleading. Characterization of bowel sounds as "hypoactive" or "hyperactive" has little meaning because such variation may occur in a normal person. During interdigestive periods (e.g., 2 to 3 hours after a meal), bowel sounds are often quiet and infrequent—hypoactive. On the other hand, if a normal person skips a meal but smells food cooking, borborygmi so loud that they can be heard 10 ft away may develop; if such sounds happen to be heard while the abdomen is being examined with a stethoscope, they would seem "hyperactive." Whether bowel sounds are absent (none heard in more than 1 minute of listening) or present is a more important determination. Absence of bowel sounds implies ileus (paralytic or adynamic ileus, or secondary ileus that occurs after moderately prolonged obstruction). High-pitched tinkling sounds, repeated peristaltic rushes, or constant bowel sounds that never seem to diminish or stop suggest intestinal obstruction.

Percussion of the abdomen is the best technique for eliciting signs of peritoneal inflammation. A deep push into the abdomen followed by sudden release, as traditionally taught, will cause discomfort and distress for the patient, who may then jeopardize further evaluation by resisting future attempts at abdominal examination.

Rectal examination may help localize the site of pain, as, for example, in acute appendicitis or diverticulitis. Careful examination of the regions where hernias can occur (inguinal, femoral, umbilical, at the site of previous surgery, etc.) is essential for all patients who experience abdominal pain. Pelvic examination should not be neglected or deferred in female patients, particularly if the cause of abdominal pain is not apparent from the history and examination of the abdomen, because pelvic inflammatory disease and diseases of the ovaries often produce abdominal pain.

Potent analgesics (particularly narcotics and sedatives) should not be administered before initial history taking and physical examination, because they may considerably alter physical findings and the patient's ability to give verbal information. If feasible, such medication should be withheld if confirmation or elaboration of the physical examination by a senior colleague or surgical consultant is indicated. When appropriate, pain relief should be provided parenterally with, for example, meperidine (Demerol), 100 mg, or morphine, 10 mg. These medications must be used cautiously if there is any indication of decreased respiratory reserve.

If surgery is a possibility but not immediately necessary or certain, it is wise to obtain a surgeon's consultative participation at an early stage in the evaluation. Should the patient's condition suddenly deteriorate, the surgeon who has seen the patient earlier will better know how to proceed. If the patient is ill but the advisability of surgery is unclear, reevaluation at the bedside at frequent intervals is essential.

LABORATORY TESTS

In many emergency rooms and other primary care facilities, a number of "routine" or standard blood tests are performed, sometimes before a physician has seen the patient and often without regard for the nature of the clinical problem or findings obtained during history taking and physical examination. Such tests are the complete blood count

(CBC), urinalysis, and (to an increasing degree) a group or panel of 12 to 24 blood chemistry determinations that are obtained with automated laboratory equipment. Electrolyte measurement, urinalysis, and hematocrit permit assessment of the patient's state of hydration. Bilirubin levels, if elevated, may suggest hepatobiliary disease. However, interpretation of such laboratory data must be tempered by assessment of information gained from the history and physical examination. Leukocytosis with increased polymorphonuclear leukocytes and band forms is an important finding, but it does not invariably indicate a condition requiring surgery, such as appendicitis. It may reflect an inflammatory condition such as pancreatitis or may even be secondary to an incidental condition not related to the abdominal pain. Furthermore, some conditions that are urgent and require immediate surgery, such as strangulated intestinal obstruction or perforated viscus, can present at first with a normal white blood cell count.

Other laboratory tests also need to be interpreted with caution and in the clinical context. Serum amylase level can be moderately elevated in conditions other than pancreatitis and may be normal or only modestly elevated in acute pancreatitis (Chapter 352). Elevation of serum lipase is more specific for pancreatitis than elevation of serum amylase. If pancreatitis is suspected and blood urea nitrogen (BUN) (or serum creatinine) level is normal, a concomitant urine specimen tested for urine amylase concentration will show great elevation.

Diagnostic paracentesis with an 18- or 20-gauge needle, rather than with the large trocar that is part of many paracentesis sets, is valuable in patients with abdominal pain who have chronic ascites, sudden onset of ascites (which may be intraperitoneal hemorrhage or pancreatic ascites), suspected perforation of a peptic ulcer, or blunt trauma to the abdomen. If fluid is obtained, it should be analyzed for cell count; protein content; amylase level; Gram stain; routine cultures; anaerobic cultures; tuberculosis cultures; and, if enough fluid is available, cytologic evaluation.

RADIOGRAPHY

Plain flat and upright radiographs are the most valuable tests, beyond the history and physical examination, in evaluation of patients with acute abdominal pain. The major radiographic findings pertinent to acute abdominal pain are free intraperitoneal air (Fig. 335-2) and dilated loops of intestine. In addition, an astute radiologist may be able to identify other pertinent findings, such as air-fluid levels, abscess, ascites, enlarged intraabdominal organs, masses, gallstones, air in the biliary tree, probable level of intestinal obstruction, intraluminal or extraluminal foreign bodies, calcifications, aneurysms, renal calculi, and possibly related bone fractures.

Free intraperitoneal air indicates perforation of a hollow viscus, provided the patient has not had abdominal surgery within the preceding 6 days or an even more recent laparoscopy (peritoneoscopy), or tubal insufflation test. If dilated loops of intestine are present, usually with air-fluid levels, the distinction between paralytic ileus and intestinal obstruction can be very difficult. In ileus the entire bowel, both large and small intestines, is usually dilated. If this is so and if there is air in the rectum, the diagnosis is quite likely to be ileus. Both small and large bowel are dilated in distal sigmoid obstruction as, for example, in sigmoid volvulus or in distal sigmoid stricture from cancer or diverticulitis, but air is usually absent from the rectum. If the patient has ileus to a degree that shows obviously dilated loops of bowel on plain film, bowel sounds are almost always absent. If the patient has obstruction that has not been present for a prolonged period, abnormal bowel sounds usually are present or, less commonly, bowel sounds may be normal.

Contrast radiographic studies infrequently have a role in the evaluation of acute abdominal pain. If intestinal obstruction is a possibility, a gentle barium enema examination should be the initial contrast study. It may localize the site of obstruction in the colon or may clear the colon so that the small bowel can be examined safely. In some rare instances the situation may be sufficiently confusing and the need for information sufficiently great that water-soluble contrast material, meglumine diatrizoate (Gastrografin), is given orally (or by nasogastric tube) to elucidate possible perforation. Barium can be given orally to localize the level of small bowel obstruction if colonic obstruction and visceral perforation have been excluded. If indicated by previ-

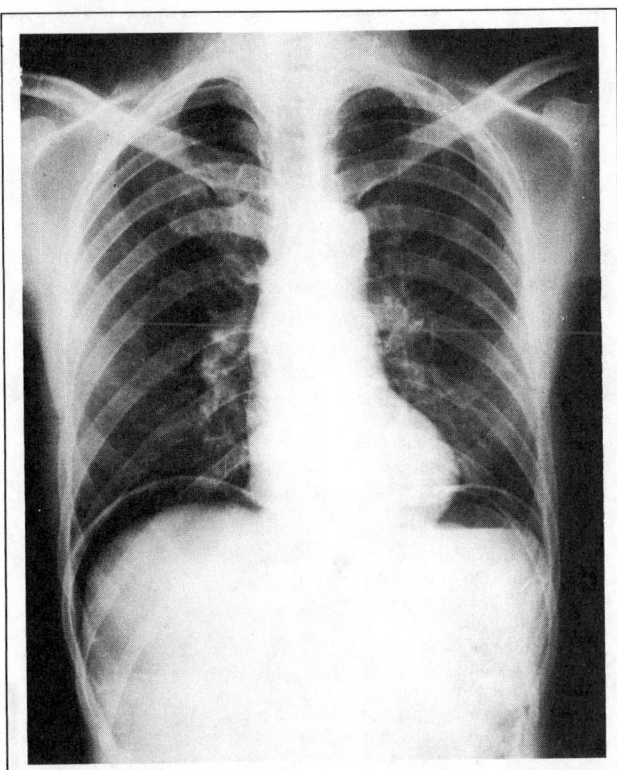

FIGURE 335-2   Upright radiograph of the chest showing free intraperitoneal air beneath both sides of the diaphragm. The patient had a perforated peptic ulcer.

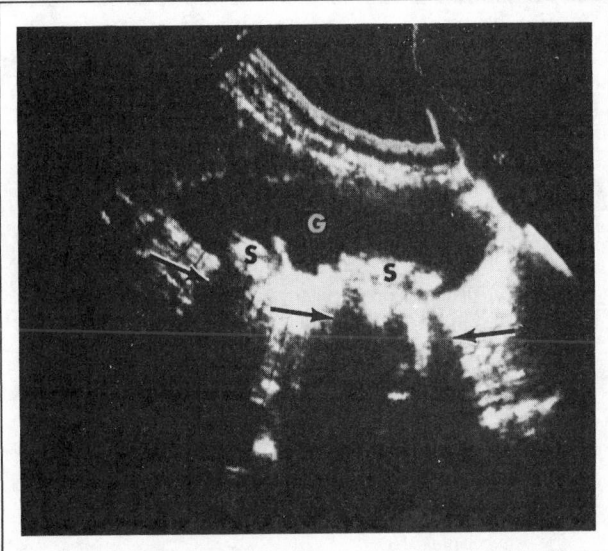

FIGURE 335-3   Ultrasound view (sonogram) of right upper quadrant of the abdomen showing the gallbladder, which contains filling defects. The presence of acoustic shadows *(arrows)* confirms that these filling defects are gallstones. *G,* Gallbladder; *S,* filling defects.

ously accumulated information, an intravenous pyelogram may reveal the cause of pain.

Standard barium swallow radiography (the upper gastrointestinal series) has its greatest utility in evaluating patients with nonurgent acute or chronic abdominal pain. With regard to the patient with chronic or chronically recurrent abdominal pain, it is unlikely that repeated barium contrast studies will reveal any additional information if findings of earlier studies done for the same indication were negative. Certainly, such studies should generally not be repeated if the same study has been performed competently within the preceding 6 months.

OTHER STUDIES
Sonography

Abdominal sonography (ultrasonography) is particularly appealing in that, in addition to being noninvasive, it does not expose the patient to radiation. Sonography is valuable and reliable in detecting stones in the gallbladder (Fig. 335-3) and abdominal aortic aneurysms. A skilled examiner often is able to detect dilated intrahepatic bile ducts; a thickened gallbladder wall; a dilated proximal common bile duct; intrahepatic, intraabdominal, and pelvic abscesses; periappendiceal fluid; splenic hematomas; hydronephrotic kidneys; and masses greater than 2 to 3 cm in diameter. The value, reliability, and reproducibility of sonography are functions of the skill and experience of the sonographer.

Computed Tomographic Scan

Abdominal computed tomographic (CT) scans expose the patient to radiation but give excellent views of remarkably high resolution that are readily understood by anyone familiar with sagittal section anatomy. The CT scan is usually superior to sonography for evaluation of the pancreas (Fig. 335-4) and kidneys and for assessment for intraabdominal or pelvic abscesses; sonography is more sensitive for detecting gallstones in the gallbladder.

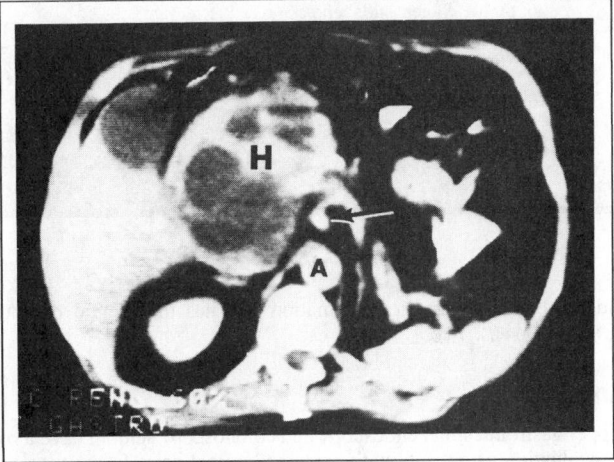

FIGURE 335-4   CT scan of the abdomen in a patient with acute and chronic pancreatitis complicated by pancreatic pseudocysts. Cystic defects are evident in a massively enlarged pancreatic head. The aorta and superior mesenteric artery (arrow) are evident. H, head; A, aorta.

The advent of sonography and CT scanning (as well as endoscopic retrograde cholangiography and percutaneous transhepatic cholangiography) has sharply reduced the role of radioisotope scans in the evaluation of abdominal disorders. In the patient with abdominal pain in whom acute cholecystitis is suspected but not established, failure to visualize the gallbladder during a ^{99m}Tc HIDA scan helps establish the diagnosis of acute cholecystitis (Chapter 364).

Arteriography

Abdominal arteriography is most useful in evaluating patients with abdominal pain secondary to blunt trauma. If an abdominal aortic aneurysm is suspected as the cause of the patient's pain (especially if there is clinical evidence of dissection), arteriography is often done to obtain additional, more detailed information before surgical therapy. Arteriography should be considered early in the evaluation of patients with suspected ischemic bowel disease because it may pro-

---

BOX 335-1
Classification of acute abdominal pain

A. Urgent condition
  1. Appendicitis
  2. Abdominal aortic aneurysm
    a. Ruptured aneurysm
    b. Dissecting aneurysm
  3. Perforation
    a. Peptic ulcer (stomach, duodenum)
    b. Diverticulum of colon
    c. Meckel's diverticulum
    d. Diverticulum of duodenum, small intestine
    e. Duodenal stump (after gastric resection)
    f. Surgical anastomosis
    g. Boerhaave's syndrome
    h. Crohn's disease
    i. Ingested foreign body (chicken bone, straight pin, etc.)
    j. Cecal volvulus
    k. Nonspecific ulcers of jejunum or ileum
    l. Lymphoma (especially *after* therapy)
    m. Gallbladder
    n. Ulcerative colitis (with toxic dilation)
  4. Obstruction with strangulated loop of bowel
    a. Adhesions
    b. Hernias
    c. Cecal or sigmoid volvulus
    d. Gastric volvulus
  5. Ischemia of small intestine
    a. Occlusive ischemia
    b. Nonocclusive ischemia
  6. Acute cholecystitis, cholangitis
  7. Ruptured ectopic pregnancy
  8. Bacterial abscess of liver
  9. Pancreatic abscess
  10. Ruptured hepatic adenoma, hepatoma, or hemangioma
  11. Ruptured spleen
B. Less urgent condition
  1. Viral gastroenteritis

  2. Staphylococcal toxin gastroenteritis
  3. Peptic ulcer
  4. Hepatitis
    a. Viral
    b. Toxic
    c. Ischemic
  5. Spontaneous bacterial peritonitis
  6. Acute pancreatitis
  7. Diabetic neuropathy
  8. Crohn's disease
  9. Ulcerative colitis
  10. Pelvic inflammatory disease
  11. Infectious enterocolitis
  12. Mesenteric lymphadenitis
  13. Nephroureterolithiasis
  14. Budd-Chiari syndrome
  15. Venoocclusive disease of liver
  16. Splenic infarction
  17. Twisted ovarian cyst
  18. Hemorrhage into uterine fibroid
  19. Fitz-Hugh-Curtis syndrome
  20. Endometritis
  21. Psychogenic
  22. Diverticulitis
  23. Intestinal obstruction
  24. Skeletal muscle spasm, hematoma, tear
C. Deceptive causes of abdominal pain
  1. Myocardial infarction
  2. Pulmonary embolus
  3. Adrenal insufficiency
  4. Herpes zoster
  5. Acute pyelonephritis
  6. Pneumonia
  7. Trauma to testicle
  8. Familial Mediterranean fever
  9. Porphyria

---

vide essential diagnostic information and has therapeutic potential (Chapter 344).

Endoscopy

Upper gastrointestinal endoscopy and colonoscopy seldom have a role in evaluation of patients with acute abdominal pain. In patients with nonurgent acute, subacute, or chronic abdominal pain that has not been diagnosed by the tests mentioned so far, endoscopy of the upper gastrointestinal tract may reveal an ulcer of the stomach or duodenum in 10% to 15% of patients in whom barium contrast radiograph results were negative. Only rarely can the endoscopist identify a colonic source of abdominal pain not seen on barium enema. An exception is the unusual patient with Crohn's disease whose diagnosis was not established by radiographs.

Laparoscopy

Laparoscopy is rarely used in evaluating abdominal pain. However, in selected cases of acute abdominal pain, such as blunt trauma, stab wounds, suspected ruptured ectopic pregnancy, or acute pelvic inflammatory disease, laparoscopy can give information not otherwise available that may reduce the need for exploratory surgery, thus reducing the cost of health care.

Surgery

Abdominal surgery (exploratory laparotomy) is required in some patients to establish the cause of acute abdominal pain, especially when the condition is urgent and disease that requires surgical therapy may be present. There is little if any role for exploratory surgery in the

diagnosis of chronic abdominal pain. Unfortunately, many such patients have had previous abdominal surgery, which only complicates the evaluation and its interpretation. Adhesions by themselves do not cause pain. Adhesions may cause obstruction, which causes pain, and which would be evident on a plain x-ray film of the abdomen.

DIFFERENTIAL DIAGNOSIS

The clinical features, laboratory test results, and data from other tests and procedures that enable the specific distinction of one disease from another in the patient presenting with abdominal pain are not discussed here. The reader is referred to chapters dealing with specific disease entities and Boxes 335-1 and 335-2. The most common urgent causes of abdominal pain are appendicitis, perforated viscus, diverticulitis, small bowel ischemia or infarction (including intestinal obstruction with strangulation of a loop of bowel), cholecystitis and cholangitis, fulminant pancreatitis, and fulminant ulcerative colitis (often with toxic dilation of the colon). The most common extraabdominal diseases that are urgent and can present as abdominal pain are atypical myocardial infarction, pulmonary embolus, ruptured ectopic pregnancy, and dissecting aortic aneurysm.

PSYCHOGENIC ABDOMINAL PAIN

In some patients with acute abdominal pain and in more with chronic abdominal pain, extensive evaluation fails to identify an organic lesion or definite malfunction that accounts for the pain. Such a negative evaluation represents "diagnosis by exclusion," which (although controversial) might be more appropriately labeled *failure of diagnosis,* in which all common and most rare or exotic diseases that can cause abdominal pain have been excluded. In this circumstance the

---

BOX 335-2
Causes of chronic abdominal pain

I. Inflammatory causes
  A. Chronic pancreatitis
  B. Pelvic inflammatory disease
  C. Crohn's disease
  D. Chronic ulcerative colitis
  E. Tuberculous peritonitis
  F. Chronic cholecystitis
II. Neoplastic causes
  A. Adenocarcinoma of pancreas
  B. Carcinoma of stomach
  C. Carcinomatosis peritonei
  D. Primary hepatocellular carcinoma
  E. Mesothelioma of peritoneum
  F. Carcinoma of kidney
  G. Intraabdominal or retroperitoneal lymphoma
  H. Carcinoma of ovary
III. Metabolic causes
  A. Porphyria
  B. Lead poisoning
  C. Adrenal insufficiency
IV. Vascular causes
  A. Aortic aneurysm
  B. Mesenteric vascular insufficiency ("abdominal angina")
V. Other causes
  A. Irritable bowel syndrome
  B. Distended urinary bladder
  C. Fecal impaction
  D. Hydronephrosis
  E. Mesenteric cyst
  F. Endometriosis
  G. Ovarian cyst
  H. Psychogenic

pain is interpreted as malingering, hysterical, imaginary, or psychogenic. Such a sequence or process may not be entirely invalid, but the interpretation and its connotations rarely, if ever, help the patient. Furthermore, it behooves physicians to keep in mind the fallibility of any diagnostic test as well as their own fallibility and at least to consider the possibility that some pain-generating disease has been overlooked because of a laboratory error or because the disease is in too early a stage to be identified by current methods. If that possibility seems remote, in lieu of extending the evaluation to expensive and/or risky procedures or senselessly repeating tests, the physician might seek or become aware of positive evidence of psychologic disturbance or emotional maladjustment. Such evidence is usually subjective and is often vague, but its presence allows the clinician to incorporate more "diagnosis by inclusion" into the evaluation. Depression is commonly a precursor of chronic abdominal pain. In actual clinical encounters, however, the dilemma may be whether the patient has abdominal pain because of depression or whether the patient has become depressed because of chronic abdominal pain for which no physician can find the cause and for which there has been no effective therapy.

If the abdominal pain is crampy, intermittent, exacerbated by stress, and associated with alternating constipation and diarrhea, it is reasonable to assume that the cause is irritable bowel syndrome. Irritable bowel syndrome is the most common gastrointestinal affliction in the United States and probably in all the industrialized nations (Chapter 339).

Organic disease subjects patients to social, occupational, and psychologic complications and manifestations. This is particularly true for patients with pain. If, after evaluation, a patient's abdominal pain is not diagnosed, the physician must consider the pain to be real (even if psychogenic) and give that patient the same psychologic support that is given the patient who has a diagnosed organic disease. The negative evaluation should be discussed gently but frankly, and the patient should be given the opportunity to react to this information. Then, while acknowledging the reality of the pain, the physician

should suggest to the patient the possibility that it could be the manifestation of emotional disturbance, maladjustment, or stress rather than cancer or some other organic disease. If the patient has no insight or is at risk for narcotic dependency, the physician should consider referral to a unit or center that specializes in pain.

BIBLIOGRAPHY

Avorn J et al: The neglected medical history and therapeutic choices for abdominal pain, *Arch Intern Med* 151:694, 1991.
Bugliosi TF et al: Acute abdominal pain in the elderly, *Ann Emerg Med* 19:1383, 1990.
Drossman DA: Patients with psychogenic abdominal pain, *Am J Psychiatry* 139:1549, 1982.
Goyal RK, Hirano I: The enteric nervous system, *N Engl J Med* 334:1106, 1996.
Graham A et al: Laparoscopic evaluation of acute abdominal pain, *J Laparoendosc Surg* 1:165, 1991.
Gray DW, Collin J: Nonspecific abdominal pain as a cause of acute admission to hospital, *Br J Surg* 74:239, 1987.
Irwin TT: Abdominal pain: a surgical audit of 1190 emergency admissions, *Br J Surg* 76:1121, 1989.
Lee PWR: The plain x-ray in the acute abdomen, *Br J Surg* 63:763, 1976.
Nauta RJ, Magnant C: Observation versus operation for abdominal pain in the right lower quadrant: roles of the clinical examination and the leukocyte count, *Am J Surg* 151:746, 1986.
Nemcek AA Jr: CT of acute gastrointestinal disorders, *Radiol Clin North Am* 27:773, 1989.
Saclarides T et al: Abdominal emergencies, *Med Clin North Am* 70:1093, 1986.
Shafer N: Psychophysiologic diagnosis, *Med Counterpt* 5:42, 1973.
Silen W: *Cope's early diagnosis of the acute abdomen,* rev ed, New York, 1983, Oxford University Press.
Way LW: Abdominal pain. In Sleisenger MH, Fordtran JS, editors: *Gastrointestinal disease,* ed 4, Philadelphia, 1989, WB Saunders.
Wolf S, editor: *Abdominal diagnosis,* Philadelphia, 1979, Lea & Febiger.

CHAPTER

336 Peptic Ulcer Disease

Juan-R. Malagelada

A peptic ulcer is a circumscribed mucosal breach that extends deeply into the submucosa. This depth measure is a clear-cut distinction with erosions that represent mucosal breaches extending up to, but not through, the muscularis mucosa. Erosions may, however, constitute a phase of ulcer development or accompany some forms of peptic ulcer.

A peptic ulcer may develop in any part of the gastrointestinal (GI) tract exposed to acid and pepsin. The most common locations are the stomach and duodenal bulb, but peptic ulcers may also develop in the esophagus, in the small bowel, and in a Meckel's diverticulum with heterotopic gastric mucosa. Peptic ulcer is a disease typically characterized by a cyclic pattern of healing and relapses, unless appropriate preventive or therapeutic measures are adopted. Therefore active ulcers, erosions, partially healed ulcers, scars, and secondary deformity of the gut wall may coexist or be observed at different stages in the same patient.

The incidence of peptic ulcer in the Western world is decreasing, most likely because of a change in the prevalence of *Helicobacter pylori* infection, which is a major etiopathogenic factor. However, peptic ulcer remains a very common disease. About 10% of the population may develop the condition sometime during their life. Duodenal ulcer is most common in young and middle-aged adults, whereas gastric ulcer is most prevalent in the fourth to sixth decades of life. Men and women are equally affected.

RELEVANT PHYSIOLOGY AND PATHOPHYSIOLOGY

Nowadays most peptic ulcers originate as a complication of either *Helicobacter pylori* infection or consumption of nonsteroidal antiinflammatory drugs (Fig. 336-1). This assertion represents a substan-

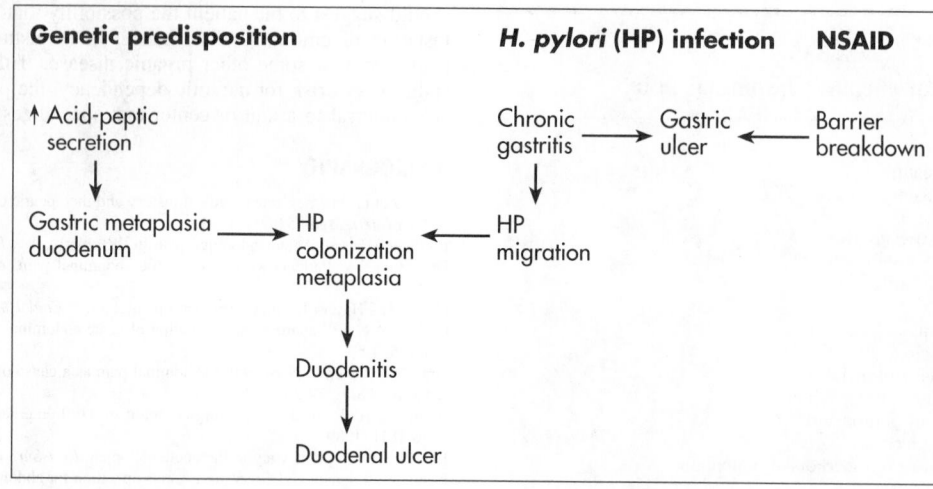

FIGURE 336-1   The pathogenesis of ulcer disease.

tial departure from the previously long-held view that acid hyperse-cretion was the fundamental pathogenetic factor, particularly of duo-denal ulcer.

Helicobacter pylori (HP) is a flagellate bacterium that colonizes the gastric mucosa and causes chronic mucosal inflammation. The in-fection is predominantly antral, apparently on account of the predi-lection of the germ for non–acid-secreting epithelium, particularly when acid secretory rates are normal or high, as is often the case in duodenal ulcer. Antral gastritis associated with HP infection may ham-per endocrine D-cell function, decreasing somatostatin counterregu-lation of antral G cells, which secrete gastrin. The resulting hyper-gastrinemia may both stimulate basal acid secretion and trophically expand parietal cell mass and, hence, acid secretory capacity. To what extent genetic predisposition is important in determining the interplay among various interacting factors remains unknown, but HP infec-tion appears to play a primary role since it is uncommon for duode-nal ulcer to develop in the absence of HP infection (probably less than 20%). Moreover, longitudinal studies show that HP-associated gastritis is associated with a fivefold to tenfold increase in the prob-ability of developing duodenal ulcer disease within the next 10 years, and eradication of HP infection effectively prevents relapse of duo-denal ulcer disease.

Some uncertainty remains, however, as to how HP-associated gas-tritis causes an ulcer located in the duodenal bulb. A sensible expla-nation is that chronically increased duodenal acid load (be it second-ary to hypergastrinemia or genetically determined) induces islands of metaplastic gastric-like mucosa in the duodenal bulb. When these metaplastic areas themselves become colonized by HP, they become inflamed, bicarbonate secretion diminishes, and these and other fac-tors weaken the resistance of the epithelium to luminal content. Thus the mucosa becomes susceptible to ulceration. Some authors even speculate that the site in the duodenal bulb that ulcerates corresponds to the area preferentially hit by the acid-peptic jet that squirts through the pylorus with each peristaltic wave. The relapsing nature of duo-denal ulcer disease would be hypothetically explained by cycles of ulcerative destruction of the susceptible metaplastic epithelium in the bulb, followed by regrowth of new foci, themselves susceptible to eventual damage and ulceration.

As reported in the medical literature, 60% to 80% of all gastric ulcers are also associated with HP infection. However, a substantial percentage of gastric ulcers is secondary to nonsteroidal antiinflam-matory drugs (NSAIDs), with or without concomitant HP infection. In gastric ulcer the cytotoxic properties of the bacterium and the host mucosal inflammatory response disrupt the normal resistance of the gastric mucosa to acid-peptic activity, thus leading to ulceration (Fig. 336-2). As the gastritis progresses, it extends from the antrum into the corpus, reducing the acid-secretory cell mass of the stomach, but at the same time it renders the mucosa more susceptible to luminal aggressions and ulceration. This process probably explains why most

patients with gastric ulcer caused by HP infection have normal or even decreased acid secretory rates.

In gastric ulcer the crater tends to develop preferentially, though not exclusively, on the lesser curvature near the junction between the non–acid-secreting and the acid-secreting mucosa, apparently because this is the most vulnerable area. As years go by, the gastritic mucosa begins to develop atrophic patches that extend and eventually may reduce the acid secretory capacity of the stomach to nonulcerating levels. Ulcer relapses abate, but the gastric mucosa is now prone to development of intestinal metaplasia and malignant transformation.

In practice, the sequence of gastritis to gastric ulcer to neoplasia is rarely documented in the same patient. More common is the coex-istence of a gastric ulceration with malignant transformation—one of the reasons why it is mandatory to check every gastric ulcer for dys-plastic changes.

As indicated earlier, a substantial proportion of gastric ulcers, and an undetermined but smaller proportion of duodenal ulcers, are sec-ondary to ingestion of NSAID. The gastrointestinal toxicity of these agents is mostly manifested acutely with erosive or ulcerative lesions that may be clinically silent or manifest with symptoms, hemorrhage, or perforation. However, chronic ulcers may also be induced. The point prevalence of gastroduodenal ulceration among patients reg-ularly ingesting NSAID for rheumatologic conditions is quite high, although many of these lesions belong to the clinically silent cate-gory. The risk of bleeding is highest within the first month of NSAID treatment.

The pathophysiology of NSAID-induced ulcers is only partially understood. It involves inhibition of the tissular enzyme cyclooxyge-nase, which normally participates in the synthesis of protective pros-taglandins. Other factors may also be important, particularly recruit-ment of circulating cytotoxic neutrophils that further expand tissue injury. Infection with HP is an independent risk factor. Thus infec-tion with HP apparently neither increases nor diminishes the risk of gastroduodenal ulceration in NSAID users (Table 336-1).

CLINICAL PRESENTATION; LABORATORY AND OTHER DIAGNOSTIC TESTS
Symptomatology

Ulcer disease may first manifest clinically in different ways. Ulcers may be silent and recognized incidentally by a diagnostic test per-formed for other reasons. Some ulcers present abruptly with a com-plication, most commonly perforation or hemorrhage. The typical pre-sentation of ulcer disease, however, is with recurrent episodes of pain. The pain is almost invariably located in the epigastrium and may ra-diate through to the dorsum. The quality of the pain is variable. Some patients describe it as burning; others describe it as an uncomfortable

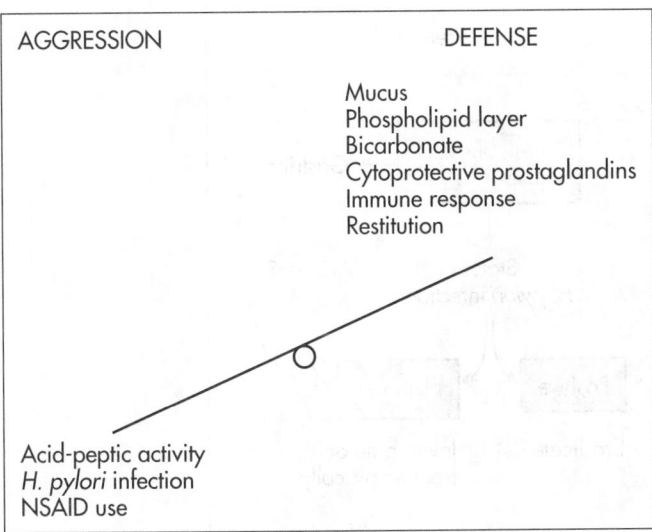

FIGURE 336-2   The pathophysiology of peptic ulcer.

Table 336-1   Prevalence of gastroduodenal lesions associated with chronic use of NSAID drugs

| | SITE | | | |
TYPE OF LESION	GASTRIC	DUODENAL	BOTH SITES	TOTAL
Superficial mucosal lesions (petechial, erosions)	25%	9%	4%	37%
Ulcers	15%	10%	—	24%

Modified from Geiss GS, Stead H, Walcermirck CB: *J Rheumatol* 18(suppl 28):11-14, 1991.

feeling of emptiness of the stomach, referred to as painful hunger. Indeed, the pain may improve with ingestion of food, only to return in the postprandial period. The timing of the pain in relation to meals as well as the soothing effects of food, however, are quite nonspecific and may also occur in patients with functional dyspepsia without ulcer. Only the night pain that wakes patients several hours after a late meal has a substantial probability of representing ulcer pain. When ulcers penetrate through the gastroduodenal wall into adjacent structures, the pattern and radiation of pain tend to change. In untreated patients, symptoms tend to conform to a relapsing pattern with bouts of daily pain lasting 2 to 8 weeks and separated by longer periods of symptomatic remission.

Besides the pain, during symptomatic ulcer episodes, patients may complain of retrosternal burning (pyrosis) or acidic regurgitation into the throat. These symptoms may reflect concomitant gastroesophageal reflux aggravated by hyperacidity or delayed gastric emptying. Nausea and vomiting may be associated symptoms but, again, these are quite nonspecific and common in patients with functional dyspepsia. Presence of significant diarrhea, not ascribable to drugs such as magnesium-containing antacids, raises the possibility of a Zollinger-Ellison syndrome. In between bouts of ulcer relapse, patients may feel well and may be able to eat even heavy, spicy meals without any apparent discomfort. This is a useful hint, because in functional dyspepsia, the occurrence of suggestive symptomatology and of food intolerance is usually less well circumscribed to defined periods, as is the case in ulcer relapse.

Physical examination is usually unrevealing. If bleeding occurs as a complication, the patient may present with pallor or, acutely, signs of hypovolemia. It is important to check the color of the stools. Bleeding may manifest very obviously, as hematemesis, but also as melena (black feces). When there is acute perforation, the epigastric pain is severe, the patient appears distressed, and characteristically there isintense contracture of the abdominal muscles apparent on palpation, together with a rebound sign of peritoneal irritation.

In chronic pyloric stenosis, nowadays rare, there may be a noticeable splash on palpation of the upper abdomen, reflecting a dilated stomach full of fluid and gas.

Diagnostic Work-Up

The diagnosis of ulcer disease must follow two parallel and complementary paths (Fig. 336-3). The imaging path has as its main objective to establish the presence of the ulcer and, in the case of gastric lesions, to exclude malignancy. The other path is directed at establishing the cause of the ulcer disease to achieve cure. This second path involves tests for detection of HP infection and tests for the di-

agnosis of hypersecretory syndromes, including Zollinger-Ellison syndrome. The two paths will be analyzed separately.

The *imaging diagnostic path* is appropriate for most patients with suspected ulcer disease. In the context of primary care medicine it has been proposed that patients younger than 45 years with epigastric pain consistent with ulcer disease, but without alarm symptoms or signs (bleeding, weight loss, etc.), the imaging part of ulcer diagnosis may be skipped in favor of an empiric therapeutic trial. The trial would consist of 4 to 6 weeks of treatment with an antisecretory agent (H_2-blocker or a proton pump inhibitor). Only patients whose pain persists or who experience early relapse would be selected for imaging diagnostic tests. This approach has the potential disadvantage of not being as efficient as it initially appeared to be, because in many instances the diagnostic endoscopic or radiologic work-up is just delayed, not avoided, and additional costs in drugs and visits have to be taken into account.

Perhaps a recently proposed more sensible approach is to evaluate HP status before the patient undergoes endoscopy. Patients with ulcer symptoms and negative HP who are not ingesting NSAIDs and without complicating symptoms have a low probability of ulcer disease and perhaps may be spared the cost and discomfort of imaging tests, chiefly endoscopy.

Leaving aside the aforementioned simplifying options, it appears reasonable to begin in most patients by establishing the presence of ulcer. Two imaging tests are suitable: barium contrast radiologic testing and endoscopy. Ordinarily, endoscopy is preferred because it is far more accurate, particularly for duodenal ulcer, and it facilitates checking for HP status by obtaining antral biopsies for bacterium identification. Most important, if a gastric ulcer is discovered at endoscopy, it can be biopsied to verify the absence of dysplastic or neoplastic changes. Nevertheless, whether ulcer biopsy should be routinely performed is arguable. Experienced endoscopists are capable of visually identifying most benign ulcers (superficial, nitid borders, multiple ulcerations, etc.) and can then skip biopsy. However, given the grave potential consequences of delaying diagnosis of small ulcerative neoplasias, biopsy should, in principle, be performed. Ecoendoscopy is a useful adjuvant when there are submucosal lesions or the ganglionar status needs to be determined.

Radiologic studies for ulcer diagnosis, once the cornerstone of the diagnostic process, are infrequently indicated today. They are less reliable than endoscopy (particularly for bulb ulcers) and do not permit biopsy of suspicious gastric lesions, thus forcing an endoscopic procedure to be performed subsequently. Computed tomography (CT) of the abdomen may be a useful adjunct to evaluate wall thickness and surrounding planes, but it should be used only for such specific indications.

As indicated earlier, the *second diagnostic path* focuses on establishing the cause of the ulcer disease. Establishing the presence of HP infection is key, via one of three possible approaches:

1. HP serologic testing, which is a simple, accurate blood test; however, after HP eradication with antibiotics, it may take 6 to 8 months for HP antibodies to fall to undetectable levels.
2. ^{13}C-urea breath test, which is based on detection of HP urease activity. It is a noninvasive and relatively simple test, but it is more expensive than serologic testing. Its main advantage is that it becomes negative as soon as HP is eradicated, although a minimum 1-month interval after antibiotic treatment should be observed to reduce false negatives.

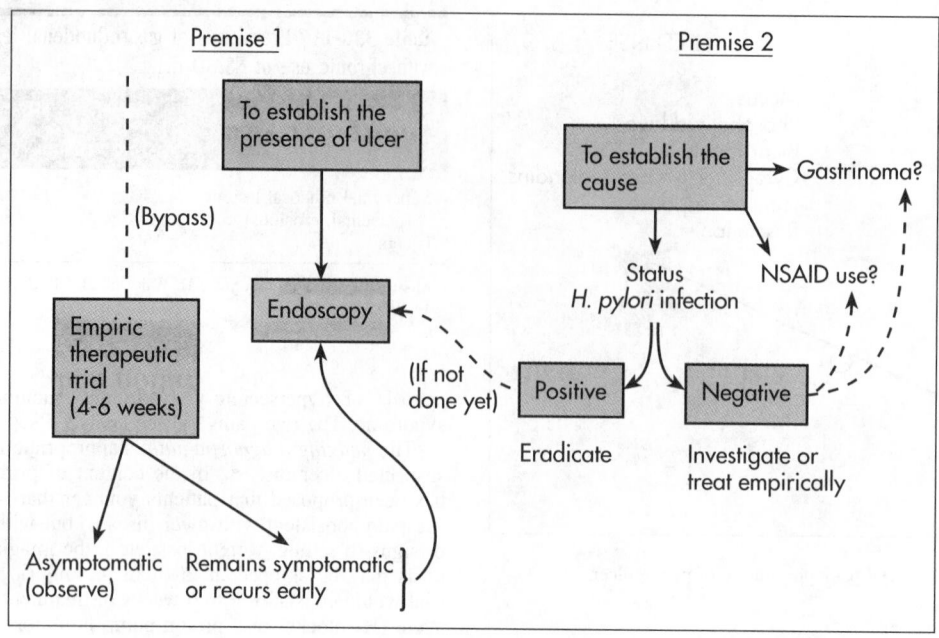

FIGURE 336-3 The diagnostic process in ulcer disease.

Table 336-2 NSAID-related gastropathy: relation between gastroduodenal lesions and symptoms

CLINICAL STATUS	ENDOSCOPIC FINDINGS
Chronic dyspeptic symptoms (20%-30%)	No visible lesions (20%)
	Erosions or petechial findings (50%)
	Ulcer crater (30%)
Asymptomatic (75%-80%)	No visible lesions (50%)
	Erosions or petechial findings (45%)
	Ulcer crater (5%)

Modified from Barrier CH, Hirschowitz BS: Controversies in the detection and management of nonsteroidal antiinflammatory drug–induced side effects on the upper gastrointestinal tract, *Arthritis Rheum* 32:926-932, 1989.

BOX 336-1
The differential diagnosis of ulcer disease

- Functional dyspepsia
- Gastric neoplasia
  Adenocarcinoma
  Lymphoma
- Gastroesophageal reflux disease (not rarely associated with ulcer)
- Neuropathic gastroparesis (pain and delayed emptying)
- Giant fold gastritis (Ménètrier's disease, other)
- Other upper abdominal conditions associated with pain (pancreatic disease, biliary disease, etc.)

---

3. Histological examination of gastric mucosal biopsies, which is the standard procedure when endoscopy is first performed for diagnosis.

Besides HP infection, hypersecretory conditions are a possible cause of ulcer disease. Hypergastrinemic syndromes (gastrinoma, antral G-cell hyperplasia) are best detected via determination of serum gastrin levels, basal and poststimulus (IV secretin, meal). Gastrin determinations are usually requested when ulcer disease is associated with certain symptoms and signs suggestive of marked gastric hypersecretion (diarrhea, ulcers extending distally beyond the bulb, enlarged gastric folds), or in ulcers refractory to conventional therapy. The most important aspect is not to miss a small gastrinoma that could be resected early. (About 50% of all gastrinomas are associated with spread, chiefly regional or to the liver.) NSAID-related ulcers are usually anticipated by the information obtained by anamnesis, although it should be understood that NSAID-related gastric lesions may also be asymptomatic (Table 336-2).

Gastric analysis—that is, gastric intubation for quantification of gastric acid output, basal and poststimulation (usually subcutaneous (SC) pentagastrin)—is at present rarely indicated. However, it may be performed in two specific circumstances: (1) in some patients with raised gastrin and equivocal provocative responses, in whom it is important to establish whether there is hypersecretion associated with hypergastrinemia; and (2) in patients with clinical and indirect (i.e., enlarged folds, abundant clear fluid at endoscopy) evidence of gastric hypersecretion, normal gastrin levels, and negative provocative tests, to determine whether they are truly hypersecretors, and the magnitude of acid output. This latter situation arises particularly in patients with recurrent ulcer disease after a prior ulcer operation (vagotomy or vagotomy and antrectomy). In some patients with ulcerative lesions and surreptitious consumption of NSAIDs, blood drug levels may be determined by specific analysis.

Differential Diagnosis

The most important differential diagnosis of ulcer disease is with gastric neoplasias and functional dyspepsia (also referred to as nonulcer dyspepsia). This section will deal primarily with the differential diagnosis of these two key conditions, and describe afterwards other less common possibilities (Box 336-1).

Gastric neoplasia may present with a clinical picture indistinguishable from that of benign ulcer disease. In fact, some forms of gastric neoplasia appear to overlap with ulcer disease from a pathogenetic and pathophysiologic standpoint. A mucosal form of B-cell gastric lymphoma (MALT) is consistently associated with HP infection. MALT lymphoma may be clinically silent and discovered incidentally (for instance, a CT scan shows thickening of gastric folds) or manifest with ulcer-like symptoms leading to endoscopy, biopsy, and identification of the typical infiltrative lesion. Early identification is critical because in the initial stages a substantial proportion of MALT lymphomas regress with HP eradication by appropriate antibiotic therapy and may even be permanently cured.

Gastric adenocarcinoma may also present with clinical manifestations compatible with ulcer disease, and some forms of gastric cancer may even resemble morphologically benign ulcer disease. In the preendoscopic era of radiologic diagnosis the potential confusion between a benign and a malignant gastric ulcer was a matter of great concern. The practice of endoscopy and of obtaining with multiple biopsies of the ulcer crater has greatly reduced the probability of a diagnostic mix-up. Thus the standard recommendation in gastric ulcer is to repeat endoscopy about 1 month after therapy and verify complete healing. A special form, early gastric cancer, that may present as a small superficial lesion with good prognosis after surgical excision is specially important to recognize. The possibility of an ulcerative malignant lesion developing in the duodenal bulb and being confused with benign duodenal ulcer is remote. Hence duodenal ulcers are not customarily biopsied at endoscopy.

Functional dyspepsia is quite common in the general population and sometimes difficult to separate from ulcer disease. The clinical manifestations are quite similar, although, as stated earlier, night pain is more typical of ulcer disease. Since many patients with ulcer disease are nowadays treated (by self or by their primary physician) with antisecretory drugs, the morphologic pictures of the two conditions at deferred endoscopy may not differ much. HP-positive gastritis and erosions in the prepyloric region or in the duodenal bulb, for instance, would not allow reliable separation. Conversely, an active ulcer, a healing crater, or evident scarring would allow definite diagnosis of ulcer disease. Nevertheless, the two conditions are common and may coexist in the same patient, so a well-healed scar from a former ulcer crater is no guarantee that the patient's current symptoms do not represent functional dyspepsia.

Another condition likely to be confused with or sometimes coexisting with ulcer disease is symptomatic gastroesophageal reflux. (Pyrosis is the cardinal complaint.) Relatively rare gastric disorders such as Ménètrier's disease or gastroparesis secondary to neuropathy may sometimes present with a clinical picture manifesting with epigastric pain that may be confused with peptic ulcer.

Management

Management of ulcer disease is best considered under three possible scenarios: (1) acute or first symptomatic presentation, (2) chronic symptomatic disease, and (3) complicated disease.

Acute or First Symptomatic Presentation. Patients presenting with an initial bout of ulcer disease ordinarily describe epigastric pain or discomfort of several weeks' duration that leads to elective medical consultation. Rarely, ulcer disease manifests with a severe and more abrupt picture of severe unremitting pain, nausea and vomiting, and inability to ingest food that would require emergency consultation. The clinician seeing for the first time a patient with the common presentation may consider two common but opposite alternative possibilities: functional dyspepsia or gastric neoplasia. Functional dyspepsia in a patient younger than 45 years old who presents without alarm signs may be treated with a 4- to 6-week therapeutic trial with either a proton pump inhibitor, a prokinetic, or both. Alternatively, the clinician may request an HP serologic test and, if positive, either try eradication antibiotic therapy or perform endoscopy to firmly establish the diagnosis. If the HP test is negative and the patient is not on NSAIDs, ulcer disease is possible but not too likely. Patients with clinical features suggestive of ulcer disease rather than functional dyspepsia and those patients with alarm signs suggesting complicated or neoplastic disease should undergo immediate upper gastrointestinal endoscopy. Biopsies should then be obtained for assessment of HP status (if not known already from prior HP serologic testing) and also from areas (large folds, gastric ulcer borders, atypical scarred mucosa, etc.) that may harbor dysplastic, metaplastic, or neoplastic tissue. Ordinarily, no further diagnostic procedures are needed, except in specific instances when serum gastrin and provocative tests or gastric analysis is required.

Chronic Symptomatic Disease. This usually entails a history of relapsing epigastric pain and associated symptoms that may have been punctuated by episodes of complications, such as bleeding,

failed medical or surgical therapies, and general dissatisfaction with the course of events. Management of these patients requires, first, a reassessment of diagnosis. Endoscopy is mandatory, along with verification of HP status. If the patient has recently received HP eradication therapy, it should be remembered that serologic testing takes 6 months to normalize even if treatment has been successful. Either morphologic assessment of infection or a ^{13}C urea breath test may be more appropriate in the time window between 1 month after antibiotics and half a year, when serologic test results usually (but not invariably) become negative.

Complicated Disease. The three major complications of ulcer disease are perforation, hemorrhage, and stenosis.

Perforation is almost invariably an acute event whereby gastric contents spill into the peritoneal cavity. Sometimes perforation may develop slowly with penetration of the ulcer crater into adjacent tissues, most commonly the pancreas. Acute free perforation should be managed as an emergency. Typical clinical symptoms and signs (abrupt onset of severe abdominal pain, abdominal muscular contraction, and manifestations of peritoneal irritation) are helpful in establishing the presumptive diagnosis. This should be confirmed by obtaining an abdominal roentgenogram (with the patient standing, sitting up, or lying on the left side, depending on the hemodynamic status) that shows free air inside the peritoneal cavity. Treatment is surgical unless there is a specific contraindication. Formerly the surgeon would suture the ulcer and perform an acid-reducing operation such as proximal gastric vagotomy or vagotomy and resection. Current success in long-term cure of ulcer disease via HP eradication has led many medical-surgical teams to advise surgical closure only, followed by appropriate antisecretory-antibiotic treatment.

Hemorrhage is a common complication of ulcer disease, occuring in 5% to 10% of all patients over the total time span of their ulcer activity (Fig. 336-4). Hemorrhage may occur as a serious acute event associated with hemodynamic shock and high mortality, or as a slow or intermittent blood loss that leads to chronic anemia with relatively modest clinical repercussion. Management varies accordingly. Serious acute events are best managed by admission into a medical facility, particularly if the institution is provided with a "GI bleeding unit" specialized in management of gut hemorrhage. Once the hemodynamic status is stabilized, endoscopy should be performed to ascertain the origin of the bleeding. Often it is convenient to obtain antral biopsies, away from the ulcer crater, to ascertain HP status, although serological testing is a valid alternative. Endoscopy may have prognostic and cost-containment value in that "clean base" ulcers carry a significantly lower risk of rebleeding during the succeeding 24 to 72 hours than either oozing ulcers, ulcers with a fresh clot, or ulcers with the "visible vessel" sign. Hence the former may be discharged early from the hospital at an acceptable risk. Acute endoscopy may also have an important therapeutic role because it would allow argon beam laser treatment or direct injection of vasoconstrictive or sclerosing substances into the base of a bleeding ulcer or one with signs of high risk of rebleeding. These procedures, if performed skillfully, are capable of stopping the hemorrhage in a substantial proportion of cases. Blood transfusion should be considered early but judiciously in the management of a bleeding ulcer. If there are not additional risk factors (e.g., angina pectoris, pulmonary hypoxemia), it is acceptable not to transfuse unless the hematocrit drops to 22 or lower. However, in cases with rapid bleeding the hematocrit may not reflect the hemodynamic situation, and transfusion is then indicated on the basis of clinical signs (pallor, systolic blood pressure below 90 mm Hg, pulse >100/min) to prevent collapse. Volume expanders are an alternative, and artificial blood substitutes may need to be used for patients, such as Jehovah's Witnesses, whose religion forbids transfusion of human blood.

Rebleeding within the first 72 hours carries an even greater risk of mortality than the initial bleeding, particularly in patients older than 55 years. Endoscopic hemostatic procedures, as described earlier, have greatly facilitated management of acutely bleeding ulcers, but surgery is still required for patients whose hemorrhage does not stop or recurs soon thereafter. Thus, in general, rebleeders in the older age-group and failed hemostatic procedures constitute a strong indication for surgery.

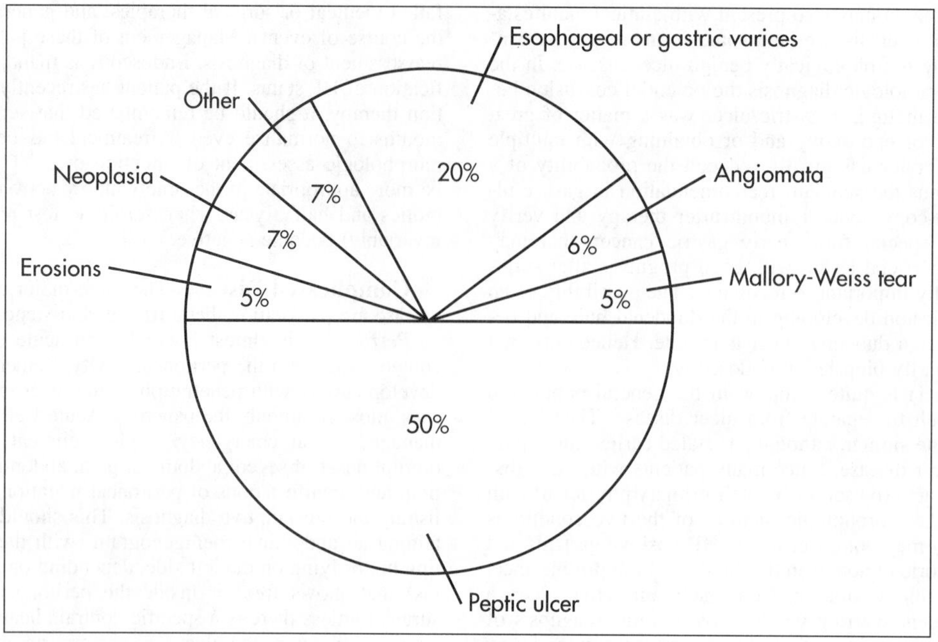

FIGURE 336-4   Causes of severe upper gastrointestinal bleeding.

Bleeding patients who recover should be managed like ordinary ulcers. Eradication of HP in infected patients provides good protection against both ulcer recurrence and rebleeding. NSAID-induced ulcers should be managed either by withdrawal of the culprit drug or by the use of adjuvant antisecretory agents (e.g., the more potent H_2 blockers and proton pump inhibitors) or prostaglandin derivatives.

Gastric outlet obstruction is a complication of ulcer disease that has become now relatively rare because of early detection and treatment. As would be anticipated on an anatomic basis, gastric outlet obstruction results most often from chronic, scarring pyloric and bulbar ulcers. Edema and inflammation play an important role, and occasionally the clinical picture of outlet obstruction, essentially nausea and vomiting, may develop in a patient with active disease without severe stenosis. Management should therefore should involve three steps: (1) endoscopy (with prior aspiration and lavage if food retention is significant) for diagnosis; (2) intense antisecretory treatment (IV in severe obstruction) with or without nasogastric suction (if persistent vomiting); and (3) eventually, conventional therapy of ulcer disease or surgery (in case of unresolving or tight obstructive scarring). Endoscopic dilation with appropriate balloons is another alternative to surgery, but reliable long-term follow-up results are lacking.

SPECIFIC THERAPY FOR ULCER DISEASE

Dietary measures have become largely unnecessary, except for simple logical norms in the acute phase, such as avoiding large quantities and greasy and spicy foods (particularly uncomfortable if there is associated gastroesophageal reflux); excess alcohol; and smoking, if applicable. The latter measure is particularly relevant in terms of reducing probability of ulcer recurrence if all other medication is stopped. Avoidance of NSAIDs and other offending drugs is necessary.

The cardinal therapeutic measure in acute ulcer disease is antisecretory therapy. Nowadays H_2-receptor blockers and proton pump inhibitors are the drugs of choice, depending on availability and cost. In general, the more intense the reduction in acid secretion is, the more quickly the patient becomes asymptomatic, and the shorter time it takes to achieve complete ulcer healing. Omeprazole (20 mg daily), famotidine (40 mg daily), cimetidine (1200 mg daily), and ranitidine (300 to 600 mg daily) are acceptable regimens. However, antisecretory therapy is best used, in most instances, in conjunction with HP eradication. Triple therapy combining a proton pump inhibitor, clar-

ithromycin (500 mg), and amoxycillin (1 g twice daily for 10 to 14 days) gives eradication rates of greater than 90% and is most acceptable. For specific allergies, substitution of tinidazole (500 mg twice daily) or tetracyclin (1.5 g daily in divided doses) is also adequate. The new combination of ranitidine and bismuth is also a valid alternative to the proton pump inhibitor in the multiple-agent regime.

HP-negative patients with idiopathic ulcer disease (a minority) and ongoing NSAID-treated patients may require long-term maintenance antisecretion with low-dose (usually 50% of the acute dose) of the H_2-receptor antagonist or proton pump inhibitor initially used. NSAID-related ulcers with known positive HP status should probably also undergo eradication to prevent the long-term complications of chronic gastritis.

An alternative to the treatment and prevention of NSAID ulcers is the use of prostaglandin derivatives such as misoprostol, but diarrhea and abdominal cramping are annoying side effects.

Recurrent ulcers, after appropriate initial treatment, must be investigated to establish the cause of the recurrence. The main possibilities are as follows:
1. Failure of HP eradication or reinfection. This would warrant retreatment, and most authors advise using a somewhat different antibiotic combination, to use four rather than three agents, and to include a bismuth-containing preparation in the program.
2. Continuing ingestion of NSAIDs without concomitant antisecretory or prostaglandin treatment. In this case it is advisable to increase the level of protection by shifting to a stronger agent or increasing the dose.
3. A hypersecretory syndrome with or without hypergastrinemia, whereby identification and, if possible, correction of the cause of hypersecretion is ideal, and, if not possible, providing adequate protection with a proton pump inhibitor.

Today, surgery has a limited role in the treatment of ulcer disease (except in acute complicated situations), largely because of the success of medical treatment. Surgery is stil indicated for free perforation, life-threatening hemorrhage, or unremitting outlet obstruction.

Chronic ulcer resistant to medical therapy is exceptional, but there are patients who are unable to ingest or comply with medication. For those, it may still be appropriate to perform surgery. In theory, a proximal gastric vagotomy (excising individual vagal branches that innervate the proximal acid-secreting portion of the stomach and leaving antral branches intact) is the ideal procedure because of high therapeutic success and reduced chance of long-term postoperative sequelae. However, the results of this procedure are linked to surgi-

✔ *WHEN TO REFER*

Ulcer disease is a medical condition that may be managed by a broad spectrum of clinical practitioners. Uncomplicated early disease tends to be seen first by primary care physicians, who may appropriately undertake the initial steps: office evaluation, check for HP status, and consideration of an empiric trial along the lines described previously. Current medical systems tend to favor that endoscopy be requested on an ad hoc basis without prior consultation by a gastroenterologist. This is fine when the clinical features meet the standard presentation. Patients with alarming signs (e.g., anemia, weight loss, atypical pain referral, protracted vomiting) are best managed in consultation with a gastroenterologist early on, since prior knowledge of the case may allow the subspecialist to better assess or manage features at endoscopy, for instance, by performing endoscopic sclerosis of an oozing ulcer or perhaps obtaining an alternative test such a CT scan before endoscopy. Medical treatment and follow-up of peptic ulcer may be competently conducted by the primary care physician. However, early or frequent recurrence of symptoms would warrant gastroenterologic consultation. Surgical treatment of uncomplicated ulcers is nowadays rarely required, but clearly a decision on whether to submit a patient to gastric surgery would be best taken in consultation with both the gastroenterologist and the abdominal surgeon.

cal skills and experience, which is now minimal for a younger generation of surgeons. Thus a more traditional vagotomy and pyloroplasty or drainage procedure (with or without antrectomy) offers greater probability of therapeutic success, albeit with a higher chance of unpleasant postoperative symptomatic sequelae such as dumping, diarrhea, and gastroparesis.

CHAPTER

337 Gastritis and Other Gastric Diseases

Gregory L. Eastwood

The term *gastritis* applies to a wide variety of hemorrhagic or inflammatory conditions of the gastric mucosa that differ in pathogenesis and clinical manifestations.

ACUTE GASTRITIS

Acute gastritis ranges from inflammation of the mucosa to multiple erosions and subepithelial hemorrhage throughout the stomach, with consequent loss of blood and tissue fluid. Erosions and subepithelial hemorrhages are defects that are confined to the mucosa. If erosions extend through the muscularis mucosae, frank ulcers are formed. Acute gastritis may involve the mucosa of the entire stomach, it may be limited to the fundic or antral mucosa only, or it may appear in a patchy distribution anywhere within the stomach. Predisposing conditions to acute gastritis are indicated in Box 337-1.

Hydrochloric acid appears to be a requisite to the pathogenesis of acute erosive gastritis, regardless of what other agent or predisposing condition may be present. Aspirin, a weak organic acid, is nonionized and lipid soluble when it is in an acid milieu below its pK_a of 3.5. Consequently, aspirin, like other weak organic acids, diffuses rapidly into the gastric mucosa under these conditions and causes mucosal injury. Because prostaglandins are believed to be important in protecting the gastric mucosa, the inhibition of prostaglandin synthesis by aspirin also may contribute to the pathogenesis of aspirin-

---

BOX 337-1

Conditions that cause acute gastritis

Aspirin and other nonsteroidal antiinflammatory drugs (NSAIDs)
Bile, pancreatic secretions, and other duodenal contents
Ethanol
Helicobacter pylori
Irradiation
Ischemia
Physiologic stress (e.g., shock, sepsis, burns, multiple organ system failure)
Psychologic stress?
Trauma (e.g., nasogastric suction, therapeutic endoscopic techniques, large hiatal hernia)

---

induced gastritis. Ethanol, which is lipid soluble at any pH, does not depend on acid to exert its harmful effects on the gastric mucosa, although an acid environment augments the injury caused by ethanol. Ingestion of the nonsteroidal antiinflammatory agents, such as indomethacin and ibuprofen, also may be associated with acute gastritis.

Focal, but sometimes extensive, gastritis can develop as a result of trauma from nasogastric tubes; therapeutic endoscopic techniques, such as laser and electrocoagulation; and local mucosal irritation from movement within a hiatal hernia. *Helicobacter pylori* is also recognized as a cause of acute gastritis.

In addition to the exogenous agents indicated, several endogenous conditions predispose the gastric mucosa to acute gastritis. Reflux of bile and other duodenal contents may result from a poorly functioning pyloric sphincter and appears to be more common in patients with gastric ulcer disease. Free reflux of bile also occurs after pyloroplasty or antrectomy with gastroenterostomy and is believed to predispose the gastric mucosa not only to acute erosive gastritis but also to the chronic gastritis that develops after gastric surgery (see later discussion). Further, in patients who are under severe stress with sepsis; shock; burns; or renal, hepatic, or respiratory failure, erosions or frank ulcers of the stomach may develop. Alterations in mucosal blood flow, inhibition of gastric epithelial renewal, or impairment of the gastric mucosal defense mechanisms may play a major role in these conditions. Although acid continues to be an important pathogenic factor, many patients with acute gastritis secrete only small amounts of acid. The major complication of acute erosive gastritis is bleeding, which may be mild or severe and life threatening but is not often associated with pain.

Because the erosions and subepithelial hemorrhages of acute gastritis are superficial, barium contrast radiographic studies are seldom helpful. The definitive diagnosis of acute erosive gastritis is best made by early gastroscopy, which allows direct inspection and biopsy of the gastric mucosa.

The gastric mucosa is capable of rapid healing. Thus most patients who suffer the effects of acute gastritis recover promptly when the offending agent is removed. If the gastritis is related to a predisposing condition, that condition should be treated. Antacid therapy is indicated in addition to the other measures employed in the management of upper gastrointestinal bleeding (Chapter 332). H_2-receptor antagonists, proton pump inhibitors, and sucralfate also have been used. Some patients, particularly those with severe predisposing disease, respond poorly to treatment, continue to bleed from gastric erosions in spite of appropriate medical therapy, and require emergency surgery. Most patients improve after antrectomy and vagotomy; rarely is total gastrectomy necessary to control bleeding.

CHRONIC GASTRITIS

Chronic gastritis typically is not erosive and thus is not necessarily the consequence of long-standing acute gastritis. The histopathology of chronic gastritis involving fundic mucosa, which lines the body and fundus of the stomach, is a continuum that can be separated into three categories: chronic superficial gastritis, chronic atrophic gastri-

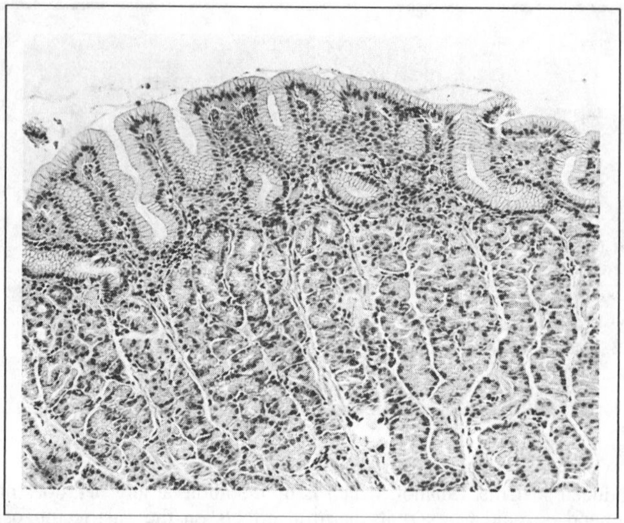

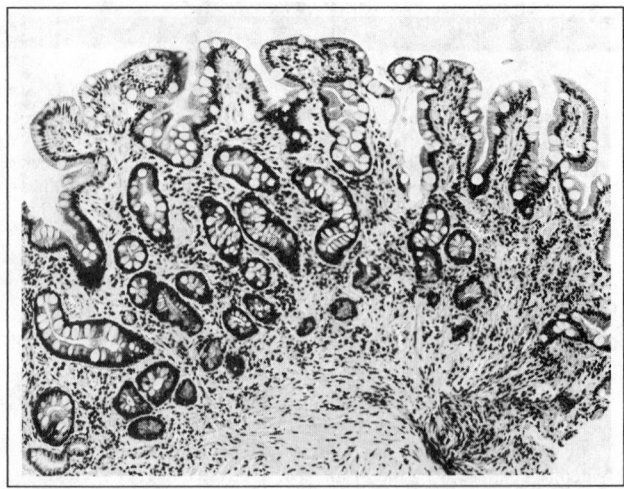

FIGURE 337-1　Photomicrograph of normal human gastric fundic mucosa. Mucus-secreting epithelial cells cover the surface of the mucosa and extend down into the gastric pits. Beneath the pits and emptying into them are long, convoluted glands lined by acid- and intrinsic factor–secreting parietal cells and pepsinogen-secreting chief cells. The lamina propria between the pits and glands contains mononuclear cells and blood vessels.

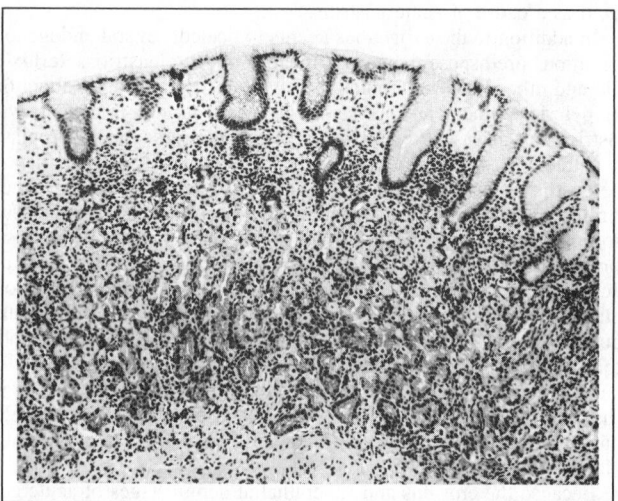

FIGURE 337-2　Photomicrograph showing chronic superficial gastritis. The density of mononuclear cells within the lamina propria is increased throughout the mucosa, particularly in the upper third.

FIGURE 337-3　Photomicrograph showing intestinal metaplasia of atrophic gastric mucosa. Villiform appearance and numerous goblet cells are characteristic. The number of gastric glands is diminished, parietal and chief cells are absent, and the thickness of the mucosa is reduced.

tis, and gastric atrophy. A photomicrograph of normal fundic mucosa is shown in Fig. 337-1 for comparison with subsequent examples showing chronic gastritis.

In *chronic superficial gastritis* the lamina propria is infiltrated with plasma cells, lymphocytes, and, in some instances neutrophils and eosinophils (Fig. 337-2). This process may occur throughout the mucosa but typically is localized to the upper third in the region of the gastric pits. Below the pits the lamina propria between the gastric glands often appears normal, except when the inflammation is extensive. The surface epithelial cells may be flattened, and some cells are necrotic.

Chronic atrophic gastritis is characterized by infiltration of plasma cells, lymphocytes, and, if severe, neutrophils. This infiltration is similar to that seen in chronic superficial gastritis, but it extends down to involve the fundic glands and the interglandular spaces. The glands become atrophic, so the spaces between them widen and the number of parietal and chief cells is reduced. The mucosal thickness decreases, although the muscularis mucosae becomes hypertrophied.

In some instances pseudopyloric or intestinal metaplasia develops. In pseudopyloric metaplasia the glands lose their parietal and chief cells and become lined by mucus-secreting cells similar to those in normal pyloric (antral) mucosa. Intestinal metaplasia occurs when the glands become lined by intestinal-type absorptive cells, goblet cells, and Paneth's cells (Fig. 337-3).

In *gastric atrophy* the fundic glands have undergone pyloric or intestinal metaplasia so that few or no parietal or chief cells are visible. The mucosa is thin, and only minimal inflammatory cell infiltration is seen in the lamina propria, although some lymphoid aggregates may be present.

Chronic gastritis also develops in antral mucosa, but its appearance is somewhat different from that in fundic mucosa. Normal antral mucosa has deeper pits than fundic mucosa so that the pits occupy as much as half of the mucosal thickness, although total mucosal thickness in the antrum is less than in the fundus. In addition, normally there is more cellular infiltration in the lamina propria of the antrum than in the fundus. Thus classification of the severity of gastritis based on the degree of inflammation is difficult. Antral gastritis may be graded as mild, moderate, or severe on the basis of an evaluation of the degree of obliteration of the pyloric glands, the degree of infiltration of the lamina propria by inflammatory cells, and the presence and extent of intestinal metaplasia.

In some patients, superficial gastritis, atrophic gastritis, and gastric atrophy represent different stages in the same disease. In other patients, atrophic gastritis or gastric atrophy seems to arise without prior progression through a stage of superficial gastritis. These differences in presentation may be explained by the diverse causes of chronic gastritis, which include immunologic mechanisms as well as chronic exposure of the gastric mucosa to harmful agents.

Chronic gastritis that involves the body and fundus of the stomach and is associated with atrophic changes has been called *type A*. Patients with pernicious anemia have type A gastritis, although most patients with type A gastritis do not have pernicious anemia. Type A gastritis may be an autoimmune disorder. Humoral antibodies to the microsomal fraction of parietal cells are present in 20% to 50% of patients who have idiopathic atrophic gastritis and in up to 95% of patients with pernicious anemia, and antibodies to intrinsic factor are found frequently in patients with pernicious anemia. Defects in cell-mediated immunity also may be important in the development of chronic gastritis.

Type B gastritis, which is the more common type, primarily involves the antrum but may progress proximally to include fundic mucosa. *H. pylori* has been implicated as the cause of most cases of type B gastritis. *H. pylori* is in adherent mucus overlying antral mucosa in almost all individuals with type B gastritis yet is found only rarely in individuals with normal antral mucosa. The prevalence of *H. pylori,* like that of type B gastritis, increases with age in populations studied to date. Most patients with duodenal ulcers have *H. pylori*–associated gastritis (Chapter 336). On the other hand, the vast majority of individuals with *H. pylori*–associated gastritis, a very common entity, do not have peptic ulcer disease. Chronic gastritis of varying degrees increases with normal aging, as does the prevalence of *H. pylori.* Whether *H. pylori* is in any way related to the atrophic changes associated with type A gastritis is not known.

Patients who have chronic gastritis typically have no symptoms that can be related directly to the gastric lesion. Hence treatment with antibiotics to eliminate *H. pylori* is not indicated in the absence of associated refractory duodenal ulcer disease. The diagnosis of gastritis is made by biopsy of the gastric mucosa. Most patients with atrophic gastritis who are achlorhydric do not have vitamin B_{12} malabsorption or pernicious anemia, although in some patients symptomatic associated conditions—such as pernicious anemia, iron deficiency anemia, gastric polyps, or gastric cancer—may develop. The diagnosis and treatment of these complications constitute the management of patients with chronic gastritis. Patients who have vitamin B_{12} deficiency with or without pernicious anemia should receive monthly 100 μg injections of vitamin B_{12}. Because patients with atrophic gastritis or gastric atrophy are at higher than normal risk of gastric cancer, they should see a physician periodically to determine whether new signs or symptoms have developed. A special subgroup of atrophic gastritis patients are those who underwent partial gastrectomy 20 or more years previously. Current evidence is conflicting as to whether these patients are at higher risk for gastric cancer.

OTHER TYPES OF GASTRITIS
Hypertrophic Gastritis

Hypertrophic gastritis is characterized by large mucosal folds in all or part of the stomach. This condition is composed of two entities, Ménétrier's disease and hypersecretory gastropathy, but some patients show features of both. In Ménétrier's disease, hyperplasia of the gastric pits and superficial epithelium is the predominant histologic abnormality. Epigastric pain, vomiting, and upper gastrointestinal bleeding are common complaints. Massive loss of tissue protein from the gastric mucosa may lead to hypoproteinemia and edema. Acid secretion is normal or low. In the related condition, hypersecretory gastropathy, the hypertrophic mucosal folds are composed primarily of enlarged fundic glands that may contain increased numbers of parietal cells. High acid secretion is typical, whereas loss of protein is not.

The diagnosis of hypertrophic gastritis is made by obtaining full-thickness mucosal biopsies of the gastric body. The hypoproteinemia of Ménétrier's disease is treated with a high-protein diet. Acid hypersecretion may respond to H_2-receptor antagonists or omeprazole. When these measures fail, surgical excision of the involved portion of the stomach may be indicated. Although the relationship between hypertrophic gastritis and gastric cancer has been debated, they appear to be associated in less than 10% of cases.

Other conditions that cause large gastric folds include carcinoma, lymphoma, and granulomatous disease. Parietal cell hyperplasia caused by the trophic effect of gastrin also produces large folds in the fundic mucosa of patients with Zollinger-Ellison syndrome.

Granulomatous Gastritis

Virtually any disorder that is associated with granuloma formation can cause granulomatous involvement of the stomach. The most frequent causes of granulomatous gastritis are tuberculosis, sarcoidosis, gastric Crohn's disease, and syphilis. Also, eosinophilic granulomas may develop as a result of infestation with the nematode larvae of *Anisakis marina,* or they may be idiopathic. Idiopathic eosinophilic granulomas of the stomach, which usually are nodular lesions of the antrum and are not associated with peripheral eosinophilia, should not be confused with eosinophilic gastroenteritis, in which the gastrointestinal tract may be infiltrated diffusely with eosinophils and in which peripheral eosinophil counts are high.

Patients with granulomatous gastritis may have epigastric pain,

vomiting, and gastric outlet obstruction as well as the signs and symptoms of the underlying disease. Treatment depends on the cause. When the cause of the underlying disease is itself unknown—as in sarcoidosis, Crohn's disease, and idiopathic eosinophilic granuloma—corticosteroids may be beneficial. Occasionally, surgical removal of an obstructing or ulcerating lesion is necessary.

Eosinophilic Gastritis

Eosinophilic gastritis is usually part of a more generalized eosinophilic infiltration of the gastrointestinal tract that is of unknown cause (Chapter 340). Peripheral eosinophilia is usually prominent. Patients have attacks of abdominal pain, vomiting, and diarrhea and may have protein-losing enteropathy. When the primary involvement is in the stomach, the radiologic appearance may resemble that of carcinoma, and symptoms may reflect gastric outlet obstruction. Endoscopic biopsy of the stomach may establish the diagnosis, although surgical biopsy is occasionally necessary. Treatment with corticosteroids results in dramatic improvement in most patients, whereas elimination diets, from which foodstuffs suspected of causing an allergic response have been omitted, generally are unsuccessful (Chapter 340).

Corrosive Gastritis

A wide variety of agents, if swallowed, can cause extensive injury to both the stomach and the esophagus (Chapter 333). Chief among these are lye, other strong alkalis, strong acid, and formaldehyde, as well as numerous household and commercial cleaners and solvents. The degree of injury depends on the amount and concentration of the substance swallowed and whether the stomach contains food. Patients generally experience severe abdominal pain and may have massive gastric bleeding. Perforation of the stomach or proximal bowel may occur. Fibrous stricture of the lumen of the stomach is a late complication. A cautious endoscopic examination is indicated to assess the extent of injury and to suction any remaining corrosive material (Chapter 333). Treatment consists of fluid, electrolyte, and blood replacement; antacid administration; and nasogastric suction. The efficacy of steroids in preventing late strictures is not established. Antibiotics may be indicated for complications such as aspiration. Indications for surgery include development of uncontrolled bleeding, gangrene, perforation, and obstruction caused by stricture during healing.

Infectious Gastritis

Acute infection of the stomach may produce a diffuse phlegmonous, or suppurative, gastritis. This rare condition probably arises from preexisting disease of the stomach, such as damage by ethanol or noxious agents, chronic gastritis, trauma, or upper gastrointestinal surgery. The α-hemolytic streptococcus is the most common organism involved, although *Escherichia coli,* staphylococci, pneumococci, *Clostridium perfringens, Proteus vulgaris,* and *Bacillus subtilis* also have been implicated. Suppurative gastritis is a medical emergency with a high mortality and may require surgical resection after appropriate treatment with fluids, electrolytes, and antibiotics.

H. pylori also causes acute gastritis of less severity and is recognized as the major cause of type B chronic gastritis that involves the antrum (see earlier discussion).

Fungal infection, notably candidiasis, can involve the stomach in patients who take immunosuppressive medication, steroids, or antineoplastic agents or who are receiving radiotherapy. Gastric candidiasis also has been described as a superinfection in some patients who have been treated with cimetidine, as well as in association with chronic gastric ulcers, although its significance in these conditions is unclear.

Irradiation Gastritis

Irradiation causes both acute and chronic injury to the gastric mucosa. Within days or months after exposure to irradiation, varying degrees of mucosal inflammation, necrosis, and ulceration may occur in a dose-dependent fashion. Later, arterioles become narrowed as a result of swelling of the vessel walls and endarteritis. The mucosa usually regenerates, but submucosal fibrosis and edema and endarteritis often persist. A chronic gastric ulcer that is indistinguishable from

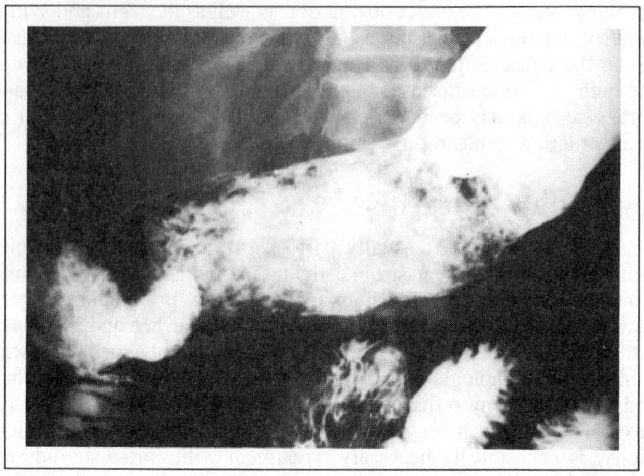

FIGURE 337-4   Upper gastrointestinal radiograph series showing a large bezoar of the body of the stomach. The barium does not penetrate completely through the mass, resulting in an amorphous mottled appearance.
Radiograph courtesy of Murray Janower, M.D.

a chronic peptic ulcer except for the presence of antral fibrosis and obliterative endarteritis may develop.

MISCELLANEOUS DISORDERS OF THE STOMACH
Bezoars and Foreign Bodies

A *gastric bezoar* is a firm aggregation of nondigestible material that fails to pass into the small intestine. Bezoars are of two general types: trichobezoars, which are composed of hair, and phytobezoars, which are composed of plant products. Some bezoars contain elements of both. Bezoars can be associated with nausea, vomiting, abdominal pain, and a sensation of epigastric fullness, or they may be asymptomatic. Bezoars occur rarely in normal stomachs; they are most often associated with vagotomy and partial gastric resection or other conditions that induce gastric stasis, such as diabetic visceral neuropathy.

The diagnosis of gastric bezoar can be suspected if an upper gastrointestinal series shows an irregular mass in the stomach into which there is variable penetration of barium (Fig. 337-4). Upper gastrointestinal endoscopy with biopsy yielding hair or vegetable matter confirms the diagnosis. Bezoars may be disrupted by endoscopic manipulation. Phytobezoars may respond to cellulase, papain, or acetylcysteine enzyme treatment. A liquid diet and gastric lavage are also helpful. Phytobezoars that remain after medical therapy and nearly all trichobezoars require surgical removal.

Hypertrophic Pyloric Stenosis

Hypertrophy and edema of the pyloric muscle is a condition most often seen in infants within the first month of life, but it also may occur in adults. In infants the cause is obscure, whereas in adults the disease may be idiopathic or associated with peptic ulcer disease, antral gastritis, or carcinoma.

In newborns with hypertrophic pyloric stenosis, projectile vomiting develops, either immediately with the ingestion of food or after the stomach is filled. Because so little of what is ingested reaches the intestine, constipation is a frequent complication and the infant fails to gain weight. Visible peristalsis, a firm mass in the right upper abdomen before the patient has eaten, and a distended epigastrium in response to feeding are typical findings on physical examination. An abdominal roentgenogram taken with the infant in the upright position shows a large gastric air bubble and little or no air in the bowel. Upper gastrointestinal series shows a long, narrow pyloric channel, and the duodenal bulb and prepyloric antrum may be indented by the mass. The treatment of infantile hypertrophic pyloric stenosis is surgical division of the pyloric muscle from the serosa to the mucosa.

The signs and symptoms of adult hypertrophic pyloric stenosis are similar to those in the infant, except that a pyloric mass is rarely felt. Although surgical division of the pylorus is usually effective, the need to differentiate idiopathic disease from pyloric channel ulcer or gastric carcinoma makes local resection a more appropriate operation for most patients.

Diverticula

Seventy-five percent of gastric diverticula occur on the posterior wall within 2 cm of the esophagogastric junction. They are thought to be congenital. Diverticula that develop either as a result of peptic or neoplastic disease or as a result of surgery for those conditions are usually found in the prepyloric antrum. Rarely is a diverticulum, either idiopathic or acquired, located between these two extremes. Gastric diverticula are typically discovered as incidental findings on barium contrast studies. The vast majority are asymptomatic. Symptoms of pain, pressure, or dyspepsia, when they do occur, probably are related to other disease. However, bleeding and perforation of gastric diverticula have been reported and are treated surgically. Otherwise, no treatment is indicated.

Volvulus

Rarely the stomach may twist on itself and cause either acute symptoms with severe pain, vomiting, and shock or the chronic, more subtle symptoms of mild pain and early satiety. Lengthy or lax ligaments are the major factors that predispose the stomach to gastric volvulus. Other predisposing factors include paraesophageal hernia, intrinsic lesions of the stomach, and adjacent masses or enlarged organs, which can distort the stomach and allow it to twist.

The diagnosis is suggested on abdominal roentgenogram, which shows two air-fluid levels in the left upper abdomen. Barium fails to pass into the stomach or, if it does, shows the twisted appearance of the organ. Decompression and relief of the volvulus can sometimes be accomplished by gentle passage of a nasogastric tube or endoscope and gastric suction. Acute strangulation of the stomach or recurrent or refractory volvulus must be treated surgically by gastropexy and repair of predisposing conditions.

Gastroparesis

Failure of the stomach to empty produced by a disturbance in gastric motility constitutes *gastroparesis*. The major causes are inflammatory conditions within the abdomen, scleroderma, diabetic neuropathy, vagotomy, and anticholinergic medications. Gastric emptying also can be delayed after gastric surgery and may be due to a combination of tissue swelling, vagotomy, and removal of the antrum, which is responsible for the major portion of gastric motility. Patients complain of epigastric fullness, and reflux or vomiting of gastric contents may occur. Obstructing lesions should be ruled out by barium contrast studies or gastroscopy. The treatment of gastroparesis begins with the treatment of the associated condition. Nasogastric suction may be necessary to decompress the stomach. Postoperative gastroparesis may not respond until nasogastric suction has been performed for several weeks. The smooth muscle agonist metoclopramide and the antibiotic erythromycin have been useful in promoting gastric emptying in some patients, provided mechanical obstruction is not present.

BIBLIOGRAPHY

Blaser MJ: Hypotheses on the pathogenesis and natural history of *Helicobacter pylori*–induced inflammation, *Gastroenterology* 102:720, 1992.

Hansson L-E et al: *Helicobacter pylori* infection: independent risk indicator of gastric adenocarcinoma, *Gastroenterology* 105:1098, 1993.

Lundegardh G et al: Stomach cancer after partial gastrectomy for benign ulcer disease, *N Engl J Med* 319:195, 1988.

National Institutes of Health Consensus Development Panel: *Helicobacter pylori* in peptic ulcer disease, *JAMA* 272:65, 1994.

Parsonnet J et al: *Helicobacter pylori* infection and the risk of gastric carcinoma, *N Engl J Med* 325:1127, 1991.

Weinstein WM: The diagnosis and classification of gastritis and duodenitis, *J Clin Gastroenterol* 3(suppl 2):7, 1981.

CHAPTER

338 Tumors of the Stomach

Robert C. Kurtz

INCIDENCE AND EPIDEMIOLOGY OF GASTRIC ADENOCARCINOMA

Gastric carcinoma is the third most common gastrointestinal cancer in the United States and the second most common cancer worldwide. In the United States, carcinoma of the stomach is rare in persons under 20 years of age but the incidence rises gradually to more than 110 cases per 100,000 per year in those above 50 years old. The disease occurs preponderantly in males; the male/female incidence is as high as 2:1 in certain age groups. The death rate from gastric cancer has been declining in the United States over the past several decades. Incidence data from the National Cancer Institute's Surveillance, Epidemiology, and End Results (SEER) program have revealed sharply rising rates of adenocarcinoma of the gastric cardia and esophagus. Among white, middle-class males, adenocarcinoma of the cardia of the stomach accounts for about one half of the gastric cancers. In Japan, gastric cancer is a leading cause of cancer death. Other areas of the world in which there is a high prevalence of gastric cancer include Thailand, Finland, and the mountainous regions (but not the coastal regions) of Colombia. However, even in these countries the incidence has declined in recent years. Studies have shown that Japanese who emigrate reduce their chances of development of gastric cancer by 25%. Incidence in second-generation Japanese in the United States is reduced even further, by more than 50%. Variations in incidence of gastric cancer in different geographic locations and in migratory populations strongly suggest that environmental factors are important in the development of the disease. Such environmental factors may be carcinogens in food, but no one food that is common to all of the high-risk areas has been identified. Types of foods incriminated include cereal, dried foods, smoked fish, salted foods, and cured foods. Fresh fruits and vegetables are thought to be protective.

Studies suggest a correlation between dietary nitrate intake and gastric cancer incidence. Nitrosamines are potent carcinogens in a number of animal species. These substances could play a role in the development of gastric cancer either by their presence in ingested food or by their in vivo production in the stomach of persons affected by nitrosation of secondary amines with nitrite. Human gastric juice contains a significant amount of amines that may be converted to nitrosamines in acid pH by nonenzymatic means or in neutral pH by certain bacteria. The previously widespread practice of salting foods and meats with a combination of sodium chloride and nitrate may have led to the substantially higher rate of gastric cancer seen in the United States before the widespread use of refrigeration. In addition, the nitrate content of the soil is much higher in high-incidence geographic areas; for example, in Colombia the nitrate content is higher in the mountains than near the coast.

Polycyclic hydrocarbons are another important group of compounds found in foods as well as in the environment. Studies of smoked foods in Iceland have shown that these foods contain large amounts of benzopyrene.

A number of molecular genetic studies have been performed to see if specific abnormalities could be reproducibly detected in gastric adenocarcinoma. Typically, mutations or allelic loss of adenomatous polyposis coli (APC) and p_{53} genes have been described. What role these abnormalities play, as well as their sequence in cancer development and other critical molecular abnormalities, awaits elucidation.

Familial aggregations of gastric cancer have been reported, but the influence of heredity in the development of the disease is not well understood. In one inbred Virginia family, 12 patients with gastric cancer were identified in four generations. In relatives of patients with gastric cancer the disease develops at a substantially higher rate.

Whether these family members have a genetic predisposition to gastric cancer or whether the persons affected have been exposed to common environmental factors is unknown. Interestingly, gastric cancer represents the most common extracolonic gastrointestinal tract cancer in the hereditary nonpolyposis colon cancer syndrome (HNPCC).

In a large population-based study in Shandong, China, the risk of developing gastric cancer was influenced not only by dietary factors and cigarette usage, but also by heredity. This risk rose by 80% among those with gastric cancer in a family member. Studies of the ABO blood groups show that blood type A is most commonly associated with gastric cancer. About 50% of patients with the diffuse type of gastric cancer have type A blood, whereas only 38% of the general population have this blood type. The reason for this difference is not known.

PREMALIGNANT CONDITIONS
Atrophic Gastritis (Chapter 337)

Chronic atrophic gastritis is frequently seen in patients who have concurrent gastric cancer. Chronic gastritis is also associated with pernicious anemia, and it increases in frequency with increasing age. In severe chronic atrophic gastritis with hypochlorhydria or achlorhydria, "intestinalization" of the mucosa may occur. If gastric cancer later develops in these patients, it is usually the intestinal type.

Cell kinetic studies have shown that atrophic gastritis represents a hyperproliferative state in which the rapidly replicating proliferative compartment of the gastric gland has moved up to the luminal surface from its usual location in the gland neck. Although such early changes may be reversible, decrease in acid production, colonization by bacteria, and endogenous formation of nitrosocompounds with potential mutagenicity may eventually lead to the development of cancer. However, although all patients with gastric cancer have underlying atrophic gastritis, the vast majority of people with atrophic gastritis never develop gastric cancer.

Pernicious anemia falls into the category of autoimmune chronic atrophic gastritis with associated "extragastric" features such as thyroiditis, diabetes mellitus, Addison's disease, and vitiligo. In 1955 a large study was published that followed more than 1200 patients with pernicious anemia at Boston City Hospital and found 28 patients with gastric cancer. This rate was considerably higher than the rate of gastric cancer in the general population in Massachusetts at that time. More recent studies have suggested that the previously observed risk of gastric cancer in pernicious anemia is no longer seen. It is likely that the association of gastric cancer and pernicious anemia initially observed was a reflection of the high incidence of gastric cancer at that time.

Studies using a serologic test for *Helicobacter pylori* infection associated with chronic atrophic gastritis have shown that *H. pylori* infection is associated with an increased risk of gastric cancer and may represent a cofactor in its pathogenesis. How chronic infection with *H. pylori* causes gastric cancer is not known, but several investigators have suggested an increase in cellular proliferation, intestinalization (metaplasia), dysplasia, and then cancer.

There have been a number of reports both supporting and rejecting the relationship between previous subtotal gastrectomy for peptic ulcer disease and later development of cancer in the gastric stump. These cancers have generally developed 20 years or more after the subtotal gastrectomy. The risk appears greater after a Billroth II than after a Billroth I anastomosis and may be etiologically related to the reflux of bile and pancreatic juice through the gastrojejunostomy. Because the risk of gastric cancer in the gastric remnant is low in areas where the incidence of gastric cancer is low, as in the United States, periodic endoscopic surveillance of these patients is not recommended.

Gastric polyps

There are a number of different types of gastric polyps, some of which are associated with gastric cancer. About 75% to 90% of gastric polyps are hyperplastic. Hyperplastic polyps seem to be related to a regeneration of the gastric mucosa after injury and are not premalignant lesions. About 10% to 25% of gastric polyps are adenomatous.

Adenomatous polyps are most commonly found in the antrum of the stomach and have malignant potential. Reported incidence of gastric cancer occurring in gastric adenomatous polyps greater than 2 cm in diameter varies widely (average incidence, about 40%). Several syndromes of generalized polyposis of the gastrointestinal tract include gastric polyps. In the Peutz-Jeghers syndrome, hamartomatous gastric polyps occur with some frequency. Though their premalignant potential is low, Peutz-Jeghers syndrome polyps in the stomach and duodenum have occasionally developed into carcinomas. In adenomatous polyposis coli and Gardner's syndrome, adenomatous polyps of the stomach have been described, and the development of gastric cancer in this setting has recently been reported.

When a gastric polyp is found, upper gastrointestinal endoscopy should be performed. The appearance of the polyp is often helpful. Hyperplastic polyps are covered by normal-appearing mucosa; adenomatous polyps appear redder. If a biopsy specimen shows hyperplasia, no further therapy need be considered. If the polyp is adenomatous, biopsy findings may be misleading and the polyp should be removed by endoscopic polypectomy or surgery.

Immunodeficiency Disorders

Gastric cancer has been described most commonly in patients who have common variable immunodeficiency. Approximately 50% of patients who have common variable immunodeficiency have achlorhydria, atrophic gastritis, and a pernicious anemia–like syndrome without autoantibodies to intrinsic factor and parietal cells. Gastric cancer has also been noted in patients with selective immunoglobulin A (IgA) deficiency.

PATHOLOGY

Gastric adenocarcinoma has been classified into diffuse and intestinal types (Table 338-1). The intestinal type resembles small bowel mucosa. Cell cohesion is described as the morphologic cement that causes the neoplastic cells to attach to each other and form glandlike structures. When this cohesive element is absent, the malignant cells infiltrate the stomach wall, the so-called diffuse type of gastric adenocarcinoma. In high-risk areas of the world the intestinal type of gastric cancer predominates. The diffuse cancer has a poorer prognosis, is more common in women and younger patients, and generally is not associated with the premalignant conditions noted previously. Because of the stomach's rich lymphatic supply, gastric cancer rapidly spreads to the regional lymph nodes.

Early gastric cancer, confined to the mucosa, is identified in more than one third of cases of gastric cancer in Japan. This is probably attributable to aggressive screening programs in that country. In Europe and the United States, early gastric cancer is found in only 5% to 10% of patients with gastric cancer. In Japan, more than 90% of patients with early gastric cancer can be expected to survive 5 years. Improved survival is also seen in Europe and the United States with early gastric cancer, but not yet to the levels in Japan.

Carcinoma of the stomach may occur as a superficial spreading tumor and may be difficult to diagnose. Superficial spreading gastric cancer involves only the mucosal surface and imparts to it a granular appearance. Occasionally, in more advanced cases, superficial spreading carcinoma can infiltrate the muscularis mucosae. Regional lymph nodes may show metastasis despite the superficial distribution.

CLINICAL FEATURES OF GASTRIC CARCINOMA

Most gastric cancers in the United States are at an advanced stage when diagnosed. Weight loss seems to be the most predictable symptom and is seen in 70% to 80% of patients. The second most common symptom is pain. This may be epigastric, substernal, or back pain, and it occurs in 70% of patients. Abdominal pain may mimic that of benign peptic ulcer disease, with relief obtained by ingesting antacids, H₂-receptor antagonists, proton pump inhibitors, and food. In other patients, pain is worse after eating, and anorexia and vomiting are present, especially if distal tumors cause pyloric obstruction. Patients frequently report a distaste for foods containing

Table 338-1   Gastric adenocarcinoma pathologic classification (Lauren)

	INTESTINAL TYPE	DIFFUSE TYPE
Incidence	50%-85%	15%-35%
Sex	Men > women	Men = women
Age	Older patients	Young patients
Environment	High risk	Lower risk ?
Blood group A	No	Yes
Helicobacter pylori	Common	Rare

beef. Because of reduced dietary intake, constipation is common. Both acute and chronic upper gastrointestinal bleeding may occur, with hematemesis and melena, although frank hemorrhage occurs infrequently, usually in less than 10% of patients. Weakness and fatigue related to decreased dietary intake, weight loss, and anemia are also common complaints. Worsening angina pectoris and dyspnea may be related to progressive anemia. Dysphagia is an important symptom of adenocarcinoma of the fundus of the stomach, which involves the cardioesophageal junction. Jaundice may be present secondary to liver metastasis or extension of the cancer into the porta hepatis. Large bowel involvement by metastasis spreading through the gastrocolic ligament may be mistaken for primary colonic cancer and may cause large intestinal obstruction. Bone pain or neurologic symptoms of cord compression signal metastatic disease.

Physical examination may not reveal abnormality except in advanced disease. The physician may find signs of anemia, recent weight loss with temporal wasting and loss of muscle mass, and lymph node enlargement, particularly in the left supraclavicular area (or Virchow's signal node) or the left side of the neck. Physical findings may also include a palpable abdominal mass if the cancer is large, hepatic enlargement related to metastatic disease, gastric dilation, and a succussion splash. Jaundice may be present if liver metastases are extensive or positioned at the porta hepatis. Malignant ascites can occur with metastatic gastric cancer. Rectal examination may reveal a rectal "shelf" (Blumer's shelf). Metastases are thought to spread by gravity to the true pelvis and form the shelf noted on rectal examination. Umbilical nodules indicate the presence of metastatic disease. Rarely, acanthosis nigricans may be found on examination of the patient's skin, particularly in the axillae or other body folds.

LABORATORY STUDIES IN GASTRIC CANCER

Between 40% and 50% of patients with gastric cancer are anemic at the time of presentation, usually as a result of chronic blood loss. The anemia is usually microcytic (iron deficiency), but it may be megaloblastic (pernicious) or mixed in type. Microangiopathic anemia has also been reported. The result of the stool test for occult blood is frequently positive, and melena occurs occasionally. Patients with atrophic gastritis, with or without gastric cancer, may have hypochlorhydria or achlorhydria. Decreased production of gastric acid occurs in some individuals during the aging process. Thus gastric secretory function should not be used as a diagnostic tool in gastric cancer detection. In patients who have chronic gastritis involving the proximal portion of the stomach but not the antrum, serum gastrin levels may be high. When gastritis involves the entire stomach, including the antrum, gastrin levels may be low or normal. Because they are so variable, serum gastrin levels are not useful as a screening test for gastric cancer.

DIAGNOSIS

A high index of suspicion is important in diagnosing gastric cancer. Early evaluation of patients for the possibility of gastric cancer is recommended if the family history reveals gastric cancer, gastric polyps, immunodeficiency, atrophic gastritis, pernicious anemia, or gastric ulcer disease. Barium radiographic examination of the upper gas-

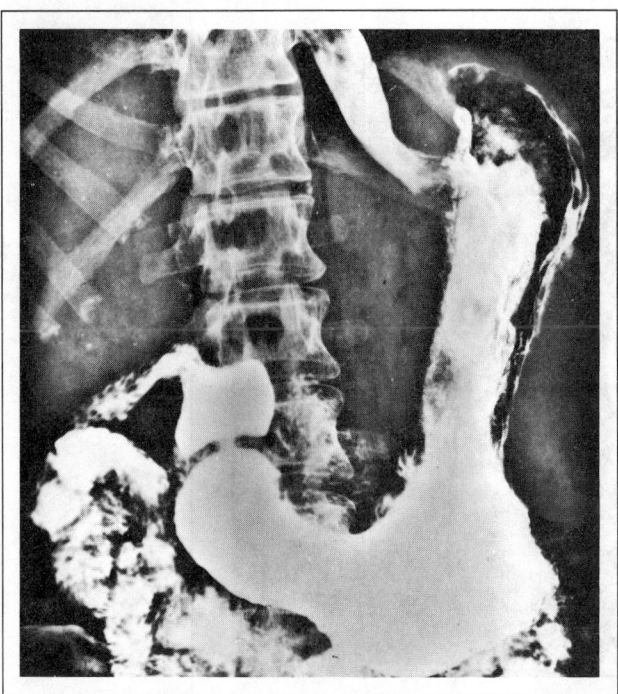

FIGURE 338-1   Adenocarcinoma of the proximal stomach. Note the apparent rigidity and narrowing of the stomach with multiple filling defects.

trointestinal tract enables the physician to suspect the appropriate diagnosis in 75% to 80% of patients (Fig. 338-1). Abnormalities seen on radiographic examination include lack of distensibility of the stomach, an ulcerated mass or mass effect surrounding an ulcer, a mass in any portion of the stomach, enlarged gastric folds, and obstructing lesions at the cardioesophageal junction or at the pylorus.

Generally, the location of an ulcer is not important in assessing the possibility of malignancy, although ulcers within 1 cm of the pylorus are usually benign and fundic ulcers are more likely to be malignant. Malignant ulcers may occur on both the greater and lesser curvatures.

Endoscopy, Biopsy, and Cytology

Upper gastrointestinal endoscopy provides the best overall method of diagnosing gastric cancer (see Plate X-3 and Chapter 328). Both biopsy and brush cytologic evaluation should be performed because they are complementary. In general, the more biopsies obtained, the higher the diagnostic yield. At least four to six biopsy specimens should be obtained from each separate lesion for maximum yield. For suspected submucosal lesions, multiple biopsy specimens can be obtained from the same site, with each successive sample being slightly deeper. In diagnosing exophytic gastric cancers the combination of brush cytologic evaluation and biopsy is accurate in more than 90% of patients. When cancers are infiltrative, the accuracy of endoscopic brush cytologic evaluation and biopsy falls to about 50%. A technique using endoscopic needle aspiration cytologic study may further increase the diagnostic yield. Overall, the diagnostic accuracy resulting from use of radiographic examination, endoscopy, biopsy, and cytologic evaluation is greater than 90%.

Endoscopy is superior to diagnostic radiographic examination in differentiating benign from malignant gastric ulcers on the basis of appearance alone, and this advantage is substantially improved with the addition of biopsy and cytologic study techniques (Chapter 328). Should all patients with gastric ulcers undergo endoscopy? In one series, 3.3% of radiologically identified benign gastric ulcers were seen by endoscopy to be carcinomas. Other studies have demonstrated that up to 7% of radiologically benign gastric ulcers are

actually malignant. Radiologic evidence of gastric ulcer healing with medical management is not sufficient to exclude the possibility that the ulcer is malignant. Early performance of endoscopy and biopsy is the best way to evaluate gastric ulcers. Even if the initial endoscopic examination reveals a benign gastric ulcer, it should be followed endoscopically at 6- to 8-week intervals until complete healing occurs. If the ulcer persists (Chapter 328), a repeat biopsy should be performed.

Computed Tomography

Barium upper gastrointestinal radiography, endoscopy, and biopsy are almost always performed before gastric cancer surgery. These diagnostic procedures give little information about the preoperative stage of this disease. Computed tomography (CT) has been successfully used to evaluate gastric wall thickness, direct extension of tumor into adjacent organs, regional and retroperitoneal lymph node enlargement, ascites, and liver metastases. CT has been shown to predict with reasonable accuracy which patients can undergo curative surgery and which tumors are unresectable. A substantial savings in time and resources should be realized as this modality is used more frequently for gastric cancer staging.

Endoscopic Ultrasonography

Endoscopic ultrasonography (EUS) is an endoscopic technique that combines visual endoscopy and ultrasonography. High-frequency EUS can produce detailed images of the stomach wall, allowing an accurate assessment of depth of tumor invasion (Fig. 338-2). CT produces only a measurement of total wall thickness and contour to estimate depth of tumor invasion. The accumulating data indicate that EUS represents a significant advance in the clinical staging of gastric cancer. Because of its limited depth of field, EUS cannot replace CT for detection of distant metastases. However, it is more accurate in assessing depth of cancer invasion and also appears to be more accurate in determining cancer spread to regional lymph nodes. CT and EUS can judge nodal metastases by the size of imaged structures consistent with lymph nodes. EUS can image much smaller nodes (2 to 3 mm) and in addition can provide diagnostically helpful echo patterns. Malignancy is suggested if imaged lymph nodes are round, sharply demarcated, and hypoechoic. With new linear array endoscopic ultrasound equipment, biopsy of suspect regional lymph nodes is possible. However, surgery is frequently performed even if adjacent lymph nodes are positive. If the cancer has spread to more distant lymph nodes, such as those in the area of the celiac axis, surgical cure is unlikely.

In a study from Memorial Sloan-Kettering Cancer Center, EUS and CT were compared to surgical pathologic evaluation for staging gastric cancer preoperatively in 50 patients. Results showed that EUS agreed with surgical pathology in 88% versus 35% for CT in staging depth of tumor wall penetration ($p < 0.00005$), and in 72% versus 45% in staging nodal disease ($p < 0.02$). Endoscopic ultrasonography is also useful in identifying extraluminal recurrence of gastric cancer.

Other Diagnostic Tests

Evaluation of the bilirubin, alkaline phosphatase, and 5'-nucleotidase may indicate metastatic liver disease. If imaging studies suggest metastases, liver biopsy can confirm their presence. Carcinoembryonic antigen (CEA) concentration may be elevated in patients with gastric cancer, usually with advanced disease. If CEA level is elevated preoperatively and becomes normal after surgery, it can be used in follow-up evaluations. As in colonic cancer, CEA level frequently rises in recurrent gastric cancer months before the development of clinical recurrence. β-Subunit human chorionic gonadotropin (HCG) level is elevated in 20% of patients with gastrointestinal cancers, including gastric cancer. A few patients with gastric carcinoma have elevations of serum α-fetoprotein level. Fetal sulfoglycoprotein antigen has been detected in the gastric juice of patients with gastric cancer. The sulfoglycoproteins of carcinomatous gastric juice have often been associated with blood group A activity.

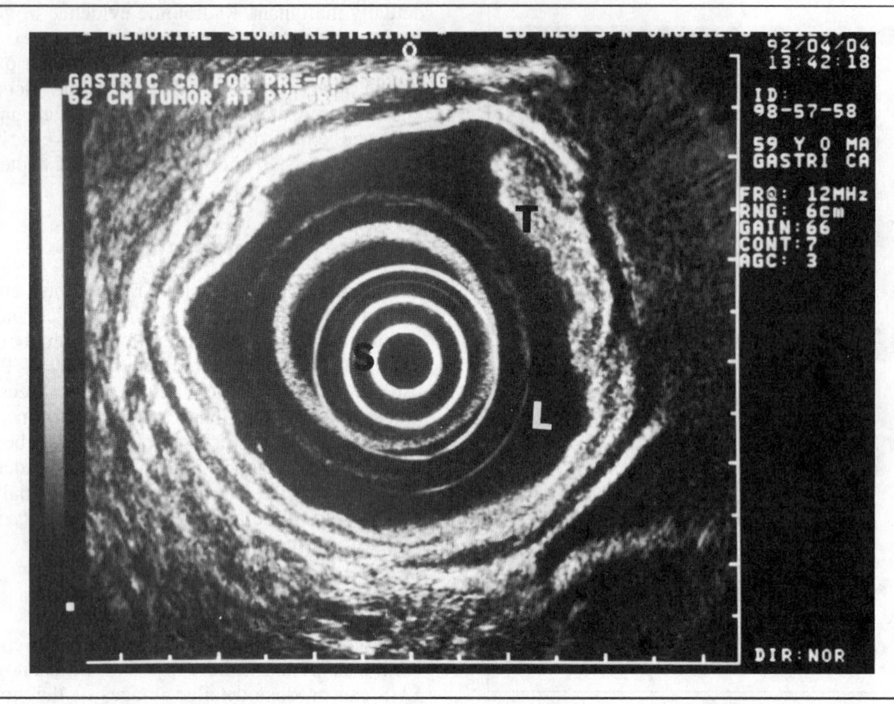

FIGURE 338-2   An endosonogram of an early stage gastric cancer that does not penetrate the stomach wall. The lumen contains the endoscope with its associated sonographic artifact. *T,* Early stage gastric cancer; *L,* lumen; *S,* endoscope.

Courtesy of Charles J. Lightdale, M.D.

TREATMENT

Surgery is the primary therapy for gastric cancer. If cancer is confined to the stomach, with extension only to the regional lymph nodes, curative procedures should be considered. If there is extension of the cancer beyond the stomach—for example, to the spleen—the spleen should be removed. If the cancer involves the upper third of the stomach, total gastrectomy and splenectomy is considered by many to be the procedure of choice. In Japan, with the use of radical surgery, including extensive lymph node dissection, even patients with advanced gastric cancer have a 5-year survival rate greater than 40%. Total gastrectomy is rarely indicated for palliation. Instead, the bulk of the cancer is removed to control bleeding, obstruction, or pain. When a curative resection cannot be performed, distal gastric exclusion or gastroenterostomy may relieve obstruction. Prosthetic tubes can be inserted to bypass obstructing lesions in the esophagus, at the cardioesophageal junction, and even farther distally in the stomach and small bowel. Laser therapy is useful to open obstructing cardioesophageal cancers. Feeding jejunostomy or gastrostomy is rarely indicated. Operative mortality varies, depending on the type of surgery performed, from approximately 7% with distal subtotal gastric resection to 23% for extended total gastrectomy.

Generally, conventional external radiation therapy has not been effective because of the radioresistance of gastric cancer. Implantation of radioactive materials into remaining tumor areas during surgery has met with varying results. Intraoperative radiation therapy (IORT) to the tumor bed is also being studied after curative and palliative surgical resection. In one report the 5-year survival of patients who received IORT with advanced stage gastric cancer was better than that of patients who did not.

Chemotherapy with 5-fluorouracil (5-FU), doxorubicin hydrochloride (adriamycin), and mitomycin-C or methyl-CCNU (chloroethyl cyclohexyl nitrosourea) may be useful in the management of patients with either residual, postsurgical disease or recurrent gastric cancer. Chemotherapeutic agents can be given as adjuvants to patients at high risk for recurrent disease. In North America the Gastrointestinal Tumor Study Group (GITSG), in a randomized prospective trial, investigated the benefit of adjuvant chemotherapy using 5-FU plus methyllomustine given postoperatively for 2 years, compared with no postoperative therapy. An improvement of survival was noted, but three similar trials failed to confirm the positive results. Because of lack of proven efficacy and the potential toxicity of these drug regimens, adjuvant chemotherapy for gastric carcinoma remains investigational. Drugs capable of producing higher response rates and more durable, complete tumor responses as shown in patients with unresectable or recurrent gastric cancers will be needed for future adjuvant trials. Using chemotherapy before surgery is now being studied (neoadjuvant chemotherapy), as is intraperitoneal chemotherapy. It is hoped that administering anticancer drugs into the peritoneal cavity will prevent or delay a common pattern of gastric cancer recurrence.

Numerous clinical trials of chemotherapy of advanced gastric carcinoma have appeared in the literature. The FAM regimen (5-FU, doxorubicin, and mitomycin-C) received most of the attention in the 1980s. Although the initial experiences suggested an objective response rate of 37% to 63%, more recently the responses obtained have been about 20%, with complete response rates below 5%. Other chemotherapy protocols have yielded higher response rates. One such protocol consists of 5-FU, doxorubicin, and methotrexate, with leucovorin rescue (FAMTX protocol), and another of etoposide, doxorubicin, and cisplatin (EAP protocol). Drug toxicities are moderately severe.

The patient undergoing surgery coupled with chemotherapy or radiation therapy is at a tremendous disadvantage if nutrition is not maintained. Enteral nutrition is preferable, but if it is not possible, other measures, including intravenous hyperalimentation, must be made part of the treatment plan (Chapter 347).

PROGNOSIS

Early diagnosis affects the prognosis because if a long period elapses from the onset of symptoms to diagnosis, lymphatic spread is more likely. If the cancer is limited to the mucosa, a 90% to 95% cure rate

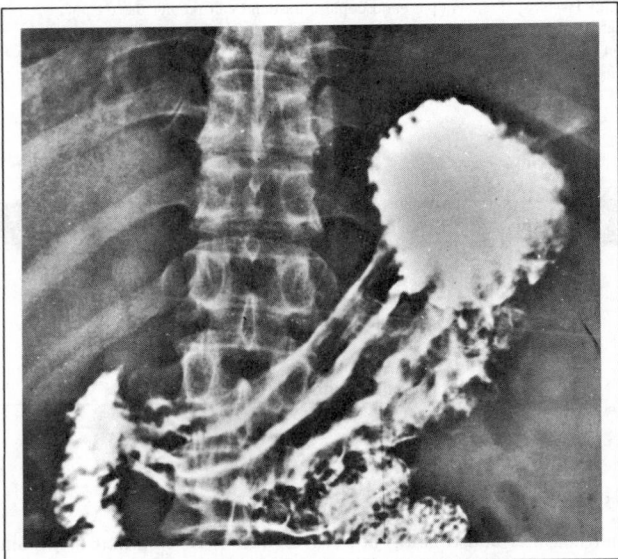

FIGURE 338-3 Gastric lymphoma. Large rugal folds run through the body of the stomach. This is suggestive but not diagnostic of gastric lymphoma. Hypertrophic gastropathy (Ménétrier's disease) may also present this radiographic picture.

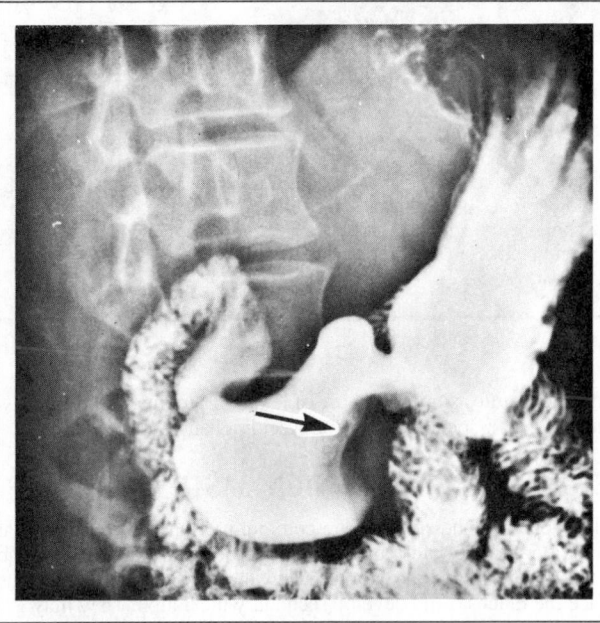

FIGURE 338-4 Leiomyosarcoma of the body of the stomach. This tumor originates in the wall of the stomach *(arrow)* and has a characteristic radiologic appearance. It frequently has a central ulceration. It is often not possible to differentiate the benign from the malignant form of this tumor.

is possible. Resection of gastric cancer limited to the mucosa and submucosa has almost a 70% cure rate. If perigastric lymph nodes are involved with tumor, the 5-year survival rate is less than 15% despite resection. Linitis plastica and infiltrating lesions have a very poor prognosis compared with that of polypoid or exophytic lesions. Gastric cancer presenting as a peptic ulcer is associated with a 5-year survival rate of 25% to 35%.

LYMPHOMA OF THE STOMACH

Lymphomas of the stomach are less common than gastric adenocarcinomas and account for about 5% of gastric malignant lesions. Non-Hodgkin's lymphoma involves the stomach much more commonly than does Hodgkin's disease. The stomach can be involved by primary lymphoma or it may be involved secondarily, in conjunction with disseminated intraabdominal or systemic lymphoma. The average age of patients with lymphoma is about a decade less than that of those with gastric adenocarcinoma. Males are affected more frequently than females. A nested, case-control study using stored serum specimens suggested that *H. pylori* may be associated with non-Hodgkin's gastric lymphoma. This may be especially true with a type of B-cell lymphoma known as mucosa-associated lymphoid transformation (MALT). Reports of complete regression of the MALT lymphomas with antibiotic eradication of *H. pylori* are of interest.

The most common symptom of gastric lymphoma is pain, but bleeding, obstruction, and perforation may also occur, mimicking the manifestations of peptic ulcer disease. A palpable epigastric mass is a common presenting feature. Gastric lymphoma often presents radiographically with bulky or prominent mucosal folds (Fig. 338-3). A mass may be seen, with ulceration and nodularity. Gastric lymphoma may be difficult to differentiate from adenocarcinoma, since gastric lymphoma may resemble linitis plastica or superficial spreading carcinoma. Many but not all gastric lymphomas can be diagnosed by gastroscopy with biopsy and brush cytologic evaluation. Lymphomatous involvement of the stomach may be confused with Ménétrier's disease (Chapter 337). Full-thickness surgical biopsy specimens obtained at the time of laparotomy may be needed to distinguish Ménétrier's disease from lymphoma. Endoscopic mucosal biopsy specimens are often inadequate, since the physician can never be sure that no underlying lymphoma or cancer is present.

Another gastric lesion that may confuse the diagnosis of gastric lymphoma is pseudolymphoma. This lesion accompanies some benign gastric ulcers and may represent an atypical inflammatory response in the region of the ulcer. Differentiating this lesion from true lymphoma, even in excised tissue, may be difficult for the pathologist.

Patients with lymphomas of the stomach have a significant incidence of nonneoplastic gastric lesions such as stress ulcers, erosive gastritis, and candidal gastritis (Chapter 337).

With a diagnosis of gastric lymphoma, the patient should undergo a thorough evaluation to determine the extent of the disease. In addition to the standard evaluation, chest and abdominal CT scan, bone marrow biopsy, and immunoglobulin analysis are performed. The results of these studies allow a tentative clinical staging of the disease into stomach involvement alone or stomach plus extragastric disease categories. This staging has implications for management because patients with extragastric disease would be candidates for chemotherapy in addition to surgery and radiotherapy. The 5-year survival rate for patients with primary lymphoma of the stomach after surgery is about 50% for non-Hodgkin's lymphoma and less for Hodgkin's disease because Hodgkin's disease, involving the stomach is almost never localized. The best prognosis is for small, well-differentiated lesions confined to the stomach, without lymph node involvement, and with only superficial infiltration of the gastric wall.

OTHER MALIGNANT STOMACH TUMORS

Metastatic disease to the stomach from other primary tumor sites is uncommon. It occurs most often in lung cancer, breast cancer, and malignant melanoma. Adrenocortical steroids used in the treatment of breast cancer have been implicated in the spread of this disease to the stomach. Half the patients with ulcerated metastatic gastric lesions have severe gastric bleeding.

Leiomyosarcoma of the stomach constitutes about 1% of gastric tumors and may present with a large intramural mass with central ulceration (Fig. 338-4). Massive bleeding or a palpable mass of which the patient is aware may be the presenting complaints. The tumor may be slow growing. After resection the 5-year survival rate for patients with leiomyosarcoma of the stomach is about 50%. Metastases to the liver and nodes are common, but these patients have a better prognosis than those with most other metastatic tumors. Hepatoma, fibrosarcoma, myxosarcoma, and neurogenic sarcoma are extremely rare

Smith JW et al: Preoperative endoscopic ultrasound can predict the risk of recurrence after operation for gastric carcinoma, *J Clin Oncol* 11:2380, 1993.
You WC et al: Diet and high risk of stomach cancer in Shandong, *Chin Cancer Res* 48:3518, 1988.

✔ WHEN TO REFER

Tumors of the stomach generally require management by specialists. It is important to act promptly to evaluate patient symptoms that fail to resolve with a brief course of therapy. Diagnostic evaluations may be initiated by the primary care physician based on the patient's signs and symptoms and often include contrast barium radiographs. If a gastric tumor is strongly suspected, the patient should be referred to a gastroenterologist for upper endoscopy and then to either a surgeon or a medical oncologist, depending on tumor staging.

and have features similar to those of leiomyosarcoma. Neurogenic sarcoma can be associated with von Recklinghausen's disease.

LEIOMYOMAS AND BENIGN GASTRIC TUMORS

Leiomyomas of the stomach are commonly found at postmortem examination and are rarely of clinical significance. They usually occur in the distal half of the stomach and may encroach on the lumen, efface the mucosa, and develop secondary ulceration. They may grow in the direction of the serosa, producing a mass that is predominantly extrinsic. Simultaneous inward and outward growth results in a dumbbell shape. This shape is also characteristic of leiomyosarcomas, and differentiation by radiographic examination (Fig. 338-4) or gastroscopy is difficult. Bleeding can occur, and epigastric pain may simulate peptic ulcer disease. Gastroscopic examination reveals effaced but normal mucosa overlying the mass. Biopsy is often unrewarding. Small, asymptomatic leiomyomas need not be removed, but symptomatic lesions, or those more than 3 cm in diameter, should be removed by surgery.

Neurofibromas, which are occasionally associated with von Recklinghausen's disease; neuromas, lymphangiomas; ganglioneuromas; lipomas; and carcinoids can involve the stomach. Multiple gastric carcinoid tumors have been seen in a few patients with pernicious anemia or atrophic gastritis. One possible mechanism for the development of these tumors is achlorhydria and subsequent hypergastrinemia with stimulation of the enterochromaffin-like cells in the gastric mucosa.

BIBLIOGRAPHY

Ajani JA et al: Resectable gastric carcinoma: an evaluation of preoperative and postoperative chemotherapy, *Cancer* 68:1501, 1991.
Blot WJ et al: Rising incidence of adenocarcinoma of the esophagus and gastric cardia, *JAMA* 265:1287, 1991.
Botet JF et al: Preoperative staging of gastric cancer: comparison of endoscopic ultrasound and dynamic CT, *Radiology* 181:426, 1991.
Brooks JJ, Enterline HT: Primary gastric lymphomas: a clinicopathologic study of 58 cases with long-term follow-up and literature review, *Cancer* 5:701, 1983.
Bucholtz TW, Welch CE, Malt RA: Clinical correlates of resectability and survival in gastric carcinoma, *Ann Surg* 188:711, 1978.
Carter DC: Cancer after peptic ulcer surgery, *Gut* 28:921, 1987.
Correa P: The epidemiology of gastric cancer, *World J Surg* 15:228, 1991.
Erickson RA: Impact of endoscopy on mortality from occult cancer in radiographically benign gastric ulcers: a probability analysis, *Gastroenterology* 93:835, 1987.
Hermans J et al: Adjuvant therapy after curative resection for gastric cancer: meta-analysis of randomized trials, *J Clin Oncol* 11:1441, 1993.
Kelsen DP: Adjuvant and neoadjuvant therapy for gastric cancer, *Semin Oncol* 23(3):379-389, 1996.
Kurtz RC et al: Upper gastrointestinal neoplasia in familial polyposis, *Dig Dis Sci* 32:459, 1987.
Kurtz RC, Sherlock P: The diagnosis of gastric cancer, *Semin Oncol* 12:11, 1985.
LaCave A et al: An EORTC Gastrointestinal Group phase III evaluation of combinations of methyl-CCNU, 5-fluorouracil, and adriamycin in advanced gastric cancer, *J Clin Oncol* 5:1387, 1987.
Lundegardh G et al: Stomach cancer after partial gastrectomy for benign ulcer disease, *N Engl J Med* 319:195, 1988.
Parsonnet J et al: *Helicobacter pylori* infection and the risk of gastric cancer, *N Engl J Med* 325:1127, 1991.
Remine WH: Gastric sarcomas, *Am J Surg* 120:320, 1970.
Robertson CS: A prospective randomized trial comparing R_1 subtotal gastrectomy with R_3 total gastrectomy for antral cancer, *Ann Surg* 220:176, 1994.
Shiu MH et al: Management of primary gastric lymphoma, *Ann Surg* 195:196, 1982.
Shiu MH et al: Influence of the extent of resection on survival after curative treatment of gastric carcinoma: a retrospective multivariate analysis, *Arch Surg* 122:1347, 1987.

CHAPTER

339 Diarrhea, Constipation, and Irritable Bowel Syndrome

Robin D. Rothstein

DIARRHEA AND CONSTIPATION

Diarrhea and constipation are two of the most common complaints encountered in clinical medicine. An organized approach to these problems requires an understanding of normal and abnormal bowel habits in the general population and in the individual patient. The definitions of diarrhea and constipation used by the physician may not be those used by the patient. Because diarrhea and constipation are nonspecific symptoms, further evaluation is often necessary to determine their underlying causes.

Diarrhea means a greater-than-normal stool output, often largely water, which is usually accompanied by increased stool frequency. Approximately 9 L of fluid enter the duodenum on a daily basis. Most of the fluid is absorbed in the jejunum and ileum. Approximately 1 L of fluid enters the colon, where all but about 150 ml is absorbed. Average daily adult stool weights are less than 200 g/day. Diarrhea is usually perceived by the patient as any change in bowel habits in which stool frequency or volume (or both) has increased or in which stool consistency has become more fluid.

The definition of *constipation* is often based on patient's symptoms. Constipation has been defined as two or fewer bowel movements per week; stool weight <35 g/d; or a sensation of straining, incomplete evacuation, or hard, lumpy stools on >25% of occasions.

Diarrhea

Pathogenesis. Increased fecal water content can result from either a decrease in the amount of fluid absorbed or an increase in the secretion of fluid sufficient to overwhelm the absorptive capacity of the bowel distal to the secretory site. Decreased absorption of fluid can occur as a result of (1) inability to absorb osmotically active solutes, which subsequently retain water in the lumen of the gut; (2) lack of contact between intraluminal contents and absorptive surfaces; (3) change in active ion transport; and (4) increase in tissue hydrostatic pressure. A change in net active intestinal ion transport causing diarrhea results from a combination of decreased sodium absorption and increased chloride secretion. These changes are mediated by increases in intracellular cyclic adenosine monophosphate (cAMP), cyclic guanosine monophosphate, or calcium, by either a direct action on the intestinal epithelial cell or via intermediate steps.

The contribution of alteration in motility to the pathogenesis of diarrhea is less well understood. Many agents that cause diarrhea have been shown, experimentally, to be associated with changes in the motor activity of the bowel. Examples include the effects, in animals, of cholera toxin, enterotoxigenic *Escherichia coli*, ricinoleic acid, and prostaglandins. The importance of motor disturbances relative to the secretory effects of agents that cause diarrheal disease in human beings is not known.

Acute Diarrhea

Diarrhea is considered acute if of less than 2 to 3 weeks' duration in a patient without a prior history of similar complaints. Most episodes of acute diarrhea are self-limited and are infectious or toxin-mediated

BOX 339-1
Pathogenetic mechanisms of diarrhea

I. Decreased fluid absorption
  A. Inability to absorb osmotically active solutes
    1. Oral intake of poorly absorbable solutes (laxatives, some oral alimentation fluids)
    2. Maldigestion and malabsorption
      a. Diffuse mucosal disease (sprue, Whipple's disease, lymphoma, amyloidosis, ischemia)
      b. Patchy mucosal disease (viral, protozoal)
      c. Pancreatic insufficiency (chronic pancreatitis, pancreatic carcinoma, pancreatic resection, cystic fibrosis)
      d. Enzyme deficiencies (lactase, sucrase-isomaltase)
      e. Bile salt deficiency (biliary obstruction, bacterial overgrowth, ileal resection, Crohn's disease)
  B. Lack of contact of intraluminal fluid with absorptive surface
    1. Intestinal resection or bypass
    2. Enteroenteric fistulas (Crohn's disease)
  C. Deletion or inhibition of active ion absorption (congenital chloridorrhea)
II. Increased fluid secretion
  A. Passive secretion: increased hydrostatic pressure (obstruction of lymphatic drainage)
  B. Active secretion
    1. Secretory agent associated with activation of adenylate cyclase–cyclic AMP system
      a. Vasoactive intestinal peptide (watery diarrhea, hypokalemia, hypochlorhydria syndrome)
      b. Dihydroxy bile acids (acting on colon)
      c. Bacterial enterotoxins (*Vibrio cholerae* enterotoxin and *E. coli* heat-labile enterotoxin)
    2. Secretory agents associated with other intracellular second messengers
      a. Laxatives (bisacodyl, phenolphthalein, ricinoleic acid)
      b. Glucagon, substance P
      c. Toxins (staphylotoxin, *Clostridium perfringens* toxin, *E. coli* heat-stable enterotoxin, *Aeromonas* spp., *Plesiomonas* spp.)
    3. Villous adenoma (possible secretagogue)
III. Motor disturbances
  A. Irritable bowel syndrome
  B. Diabetic enteropathy
  C. Visceral scleroderma (results in bacterial overgrowth)
  D. Carcinoid syndrome
IV. Mucosal injury (multiple mechanisms involved)
  A. Bacterial (shigella, invasive *E. coli*)
  B. Inflammatory bowel disease (Crohn's disease, ulcerative colitis, collagenous and lymphocyte colitis)
  C. Ischemic bowel disease

Physical Examination. The physical examination is important as a basis for both diagnostic and therapeutic decisions. The state of hydration should be determined by assessing tissue turgor and by checking for orthostasis. A rectal examination and stool examination for blood and inflammatory cells should be part of the physical examination. There may be nonspecific extraintestinal manifestations of inflammatory bowel disease, for example, the presence of perianal disease in Crohn's disease.

Diagnostic Tests. The history and physical examination not only may suggest the diagnosis, but also enables the physician to approach diagnostic testing in an organized fashion. Fig. 339-1 outlines a diagnostic approach to patients with acute diarrhea. Most acute diarrheal attacks are self-limited and are probably viral in nature. Viral gastroenteritis is not accompanied by bloody diarrhea or inflammatory cells in the stool.

Fluid resuscitation is the mainstay of therapy, and electrolytes should be corrected. Antidiarrheal agents should be avoided in the presence of fever or bloody diarrhea. If the diarrheal illness is severe or is accompanied by the presence of fecal blood or inflammatory cells, further diagnostic studies are indicated. The patient should be referred to a gastroenterologist for flexible sigmoidoscopy, which allows for direct examination of the rectosigmoid mucosa. Findings of friability and ulcerations, although abnormal, are nonspecific features that can be noted in inflammatory or infectious causes of diarrhea. The presence of pseudomembranes suggests the diagnosis of *C. difficile* colitis.

Chronic Diarrhea

Chronic diarrhea is defined as recurrent diarrhea or diarrhea of greater than 3 weeks' duration. In general, chronic diarrhea is due to inflammatory processes, secretory conditions, or malabsorptive processes.

History. Inflammatory bowel disease should be considered in a young person with chronic diarrhea. Patients with ulcerative colitis tend to have bloody diarrhea, tenesmus, and urgency. Crohn's disease more often is associated with diarrhea, weight loss, and abdominal pain. Perianal disease is more common in patients with Crohn's disease. Extraintestinal manifestations, such as arthritis or skin lesions, may be present in both ulcerative colitis and Crohn's disease.

Drug ingestion is a common cause of chronic diarrhea. Drug-related causes of diarrhea may be evident from the patient's history of medication ingestion, for example, excessive ingestion of magnesium-containing antacids. Surreptitious use of laxatives should be considered in cases of chronic diarrhea of unclear cause.

Systemic illnesses associated with diarrhea are often evident from the history. Chronic diarrhea is common in patients with AIDS and is often multifactorial in nature. Disorders such as diabetes are usually known by the patient. Others, such as scleroderma, may become evident when the patient is examined. Patients with carcinoid syndrome may have a history of flushing, or explosive diarrhea. In the absence of metastatic liver disease, diarrhea in patients with carcinoid tumors may be related to partial small bowel obstruction resulting from the dense desmoplastic reaction that these tumors may induce locally. Hyperthyroidism may present as diarrhea, and the patient may give a history of heat intolerance, irritability, or weight loss despite a good appetite.

Infectious agents may also cause chronic diarrhea and should be suspected in a patient with an appropriate travel history or with a history of eating foods that harbor parasites and that may not be adequately cooked. Giardiasis should be suspected in patients who have traveled to endemic areas, who are taking immunosuppressants, or who are male homosexuals. Bacterial proliferation in the small intestine, which causes malabsorption and diarrhea, should be suspected in patients who have a predisposition to gastrointestinal stasis, such as occurs (1) after vagotomy, with or without partial gastrectomy; (2) after intestinal surgery, with the formation of blind loops; (3) in scleroderma; and (4) in diabetes. The exact nature of any previous surgery is an important part of the patient's history.

Malabsorption syndromes should be suspected in patients who lose weight despite a good appetite. In some patients, diarrhea improves

in etiology. However, acute infectious diarrhea, especially in underdeveloped nations, can be fatal.

In patients with acute diarrhea, a history of recent travel, contacts with patients with diarrhea, and ingestion of suspect foods should be sought. The type of food eaten may indicate the cause of the illness. Bacteria, including *Aeromonas* and *Plesiomonas* spp., have been implicated as foodborne and waterborne enteropathogens. *Bacillus cereus* has been associated with refried rice. *Giardia lamblia* should be considered in individuals in day care settings. Bloody diarrhea, suggesting mucosal invasion, may be due to *Shigella flexneri*, *Campylobacter jejuni*, or enteropathogenic *E. coli*. Microscopic or, less typically, gross blood, may occur after antibiotic use with the development of pseudomembranous colitis, caused by overgrowth of *Clostridium difficile*. Idiopathic inflammatory bowel disease may present as acute diarrhea, and the patient may be extremely ill (Box 339-1).

Medications can induce diarrhea. Potassium or theophylline elixirs containing sorbitol may cause diarrhea. Enteral feeds may also diarrhea as a result of their hypertonicity. Chemotherapeutic agents—including doxorubicin, methotrexate, and 5-fluorouracil—are associated with diarrhea.

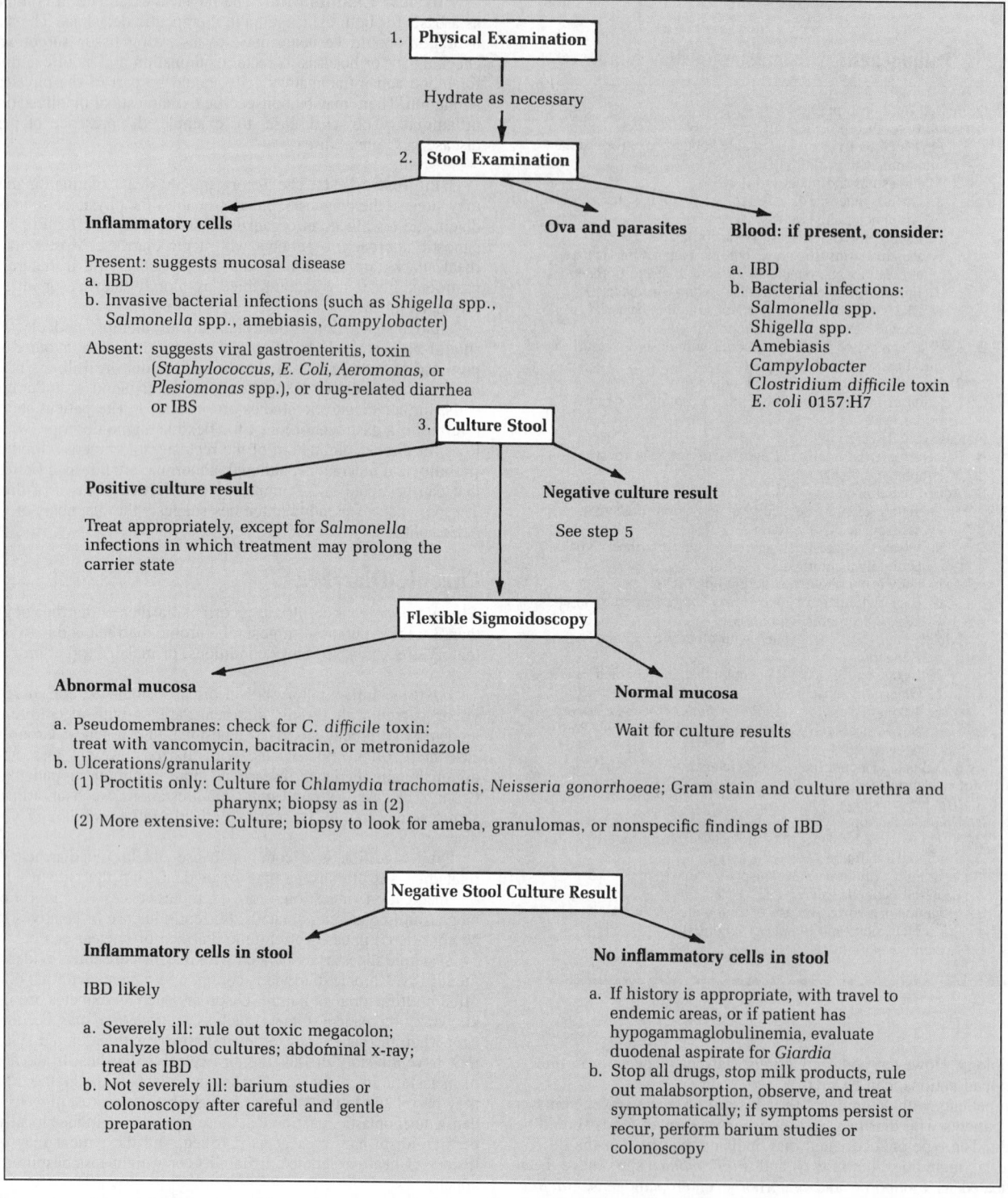

FIGURE 339-1   Diagnostic steps in the assessment of acute diarrhea. *IBD*, Inflammatory bowel disease; *IBS*, irritable bowel syndrome.

if they alter their diet in particular ways. Lactase deficiency is the most common cause of osmotic diarrhea. A history of chronic ethanol ingestion, recurrent attacks of pancreatitis, or surgical removal of the pancreas suggests pancreatic enzyme deficiency. A history of Crohn's disease or of surgical resection of the distal small bowel suggests bile salt depletion. Malabsorption syndromes usually present as large-volume, nonbloody diarrhea. The stool may be described by the patient as greasy, foul smelling, or floating, suggesting steatorrhea.

Many diseases that produce malabsorption have extraintestinal manifestations, such as arthritis in Whipple's disease. Secretory diarrheas are more difficult to diagnose by history alone; the diagnosis is best established by demonstrating the excretion of large volumes of stool in the absence of oral intake.

Irritable bowel syndrome usually occurs in the younger patient, is chronic, is often exacerbated by stress, and is not associated with blood in the stool or weight loss. Lymphocytic ("microscopic") and

✔ *WHEN TO REFER*

Patients with chronic diarrhea of unclear etiology, those with bloody stools or associated fever, and patients with inflammatory bowel disease should be referred to the gastroenterologist for further diagnostic evaluation or treatment. In addition, patients with uncontrollable, difficult-to-treat conditions and those with moderate to severe symptoms should be referred to the subspecialist.

collagenous colitis occur primarily in middle-aged women and cause chronic watery diarrhea. The colon usually appears normal, but histologic abnormalities including subepithelial collagen deposition and inflammation are present.

Physical Examination. The physical examination in patients with chronic diarrhea is important in assessing the degree of hydration and in suggesting associated systemic illness. For example, there may be resting tachycardia in hyperthyroidism, pulmonary stenosis murmur or tricuspid regurgitation murmur in carcinoid syndrome, and evidence of autonomic neuropathy or peripheral neuropathy in diabetes. Scleroderma may be diagnosed if the characteristic facies and skin change of the hands are present. There may be evidence of nutritional deficiencies in patients with chronic diarrhea associated with malabsorption. In Crohn's disease there may be abdominal tenderness or fullness, suggesting an inflammatory mass or evidence of perianal disease.

Diagnostic Tests. Diagnostic evaluation of the patient with chronic diarrhea is guided by the history and physical examination. It is important to determine whether there is an inflammatory component to the diarrhea by stool examination and/or flexible sigmoidoscopy. A detailed, stepwise diagnostic approach to a patient with chronic diarrhea is important. It should be first determined if the diarrhea is associated with inflammation of the mucosa and whether the cause is infectious or noninfectious. If no inflammation is demonstrable, an attempt is made to determine whether the diarrhea originates in the small or the large intestine. Large-volume diarrhea is more characteristic of a small bowel source and small-volume diarrhea is more suggestive of a colonic cause.

Therapy should be tailored to the underlying cause of the diarrhea. A therapeutic trial of dietary manipulation (e.g., a lactose-free diet) may be considered in a stable patient before more invasive diagnostic studies are pursued. Patients with inflammatory bowel disease may respond to acetylsalicylic acid (ASA) products or steroids. Cyclosporine, azathioprine, or 6-mercaptopurine have also been used. Patients with bacterial overgrowth often respond to antibiotic therapy. Tetracycline, ampicillin, ciprofloxacin, and metronidazole are the more common antibiotics used. Patients with pancreatic insufficiency will have decreased diarrhea with pancreatic replacement enzymes given with each meal, along with institution of a low-fat diet.

Constipation

Pathogenesis. Constipation is caused by a disorder of movement of material though the colon and/or rectum. Bowel function can be affected by structural abnormalities, metabolic disorders, neurologic abnormalities, or disorders of muscular function or motility disturbances. Medications frequently are associated with constipation (Box 339-2).

History. Important points in the history are the onset and duration of constipation and the presence of associated symptoms. Acute onset of constipation is suggestive of an organic etiology. Intestinal obstruction results in a decrease or cessation of bowel movements, abdominal distention, and crampy abdominal pain. Vomiting may occur. An ileus may also cause constipation and abdominal distention. However, vomiting often occurs early as a result of gastric and small intestinal hypomotility, and pain is less common.

A long history of constipation, especially if associated with ab-

---

BOX 339-2
Pathogenesis of constipation

I. Decreased fecal water content
  A. Dehydration
  B. Decreased oral intake
  C. Decreased bulk intake
II. Obstruction to flow
  A. Ileal
    1. Constipation by prevention of normal passage of intraluminal contents
    2. Presents with signs and symptoms of small bowel obstruction
  B. Colonic
    1. Extraluminal (diverticular abscess, adhesions, distended urinary bladder, mesenteric tumor, etc.)
    2. Intramural (intramural hematoma, etc.)
    3. Intraluminal (carcinoma, polyp, intussusception, etc.)
  C. Anal
    1. Extraluminal (fibrosis, etc.)
    2. Intraluminal (tumors, etc.)
III. Decreased or altered motility
  A. Generalized (may present as acute ileus)
    1. Drugs (opiates)
    2. Hypothyroidism and other metabolic disorders
    3. Intestinal pseudoobstruction
    4. Scleroderma, progressive systemic sclerosis
    5. Diabetic enteropathy
    6. Spinal cord injury (lumbosacral cord, paraplegia)
    7. Bed rest
  B. Colonic: irritable bowel syndrome
IV. Altered defecation reflex
  A. Hirschsprung's disease (short segment in adults)
  B. Secondary to painful rectal or anal lesions
  C. Other causes of idiopathic constipation associated with abnormal anal manometric findings
  D. Psychiatric illness

---

dominal pain and bloating is suggestive of irritable bowel syndrome. If the onset of constipation was early in infancy, congenital causes including Hirschsprung's disease should be considered. The onset of constipation in a middle-aged or older patient should always lead the physician to suspect the presence of colonic carcinoma. Associated symptoms may suggest systemic illnesses such as diabetes, scleroderma, and myxedema. A long history of obstructive symptoms and laparotomies should lead the physician to suspect intestinal pseudoobstruction.

Physical Examination. The physical examination may enable the physician to determine whether the patient has acute ileus or acute anatomic obstruction. Ileus is usually accompanied by a quiet, often distended abdomen, with stool present in the rectum. Organic obstruction is usually associated with abdominal distention, initially with high-pitched bowel sounds or rushes on auscultation, and often an empty ampulla on rectal examination. With time, the abnormal bowel sounds of acute obstruction may disappear.

On physical examination, findings of an underlying systemic disease such as scleroderma or myxedema should be sought. A careful neurologic examination should be performed. Rectal examination may demonstrate the presence of perianal disease. An empty ampulla, in the absence of enema administration, is noted in short-segment Hirschsprung's disease. The presence of blood on rectal exam suggests a mucosal lesion.

Diagnostic Approach. The diagnostic approach is directed by findings on the history and physical examination. Acute onset of absolute constipation (i.e., absence of passage of flatus or feces) suggests either complete bowel obstruction or an ileus. The patient should undergo plain upright abdominal radiography, which may show air-fluid levels. In complete obstruction there may be proximal distended loops of bowel and absent distal intraluminal air. In ileus there is usu-

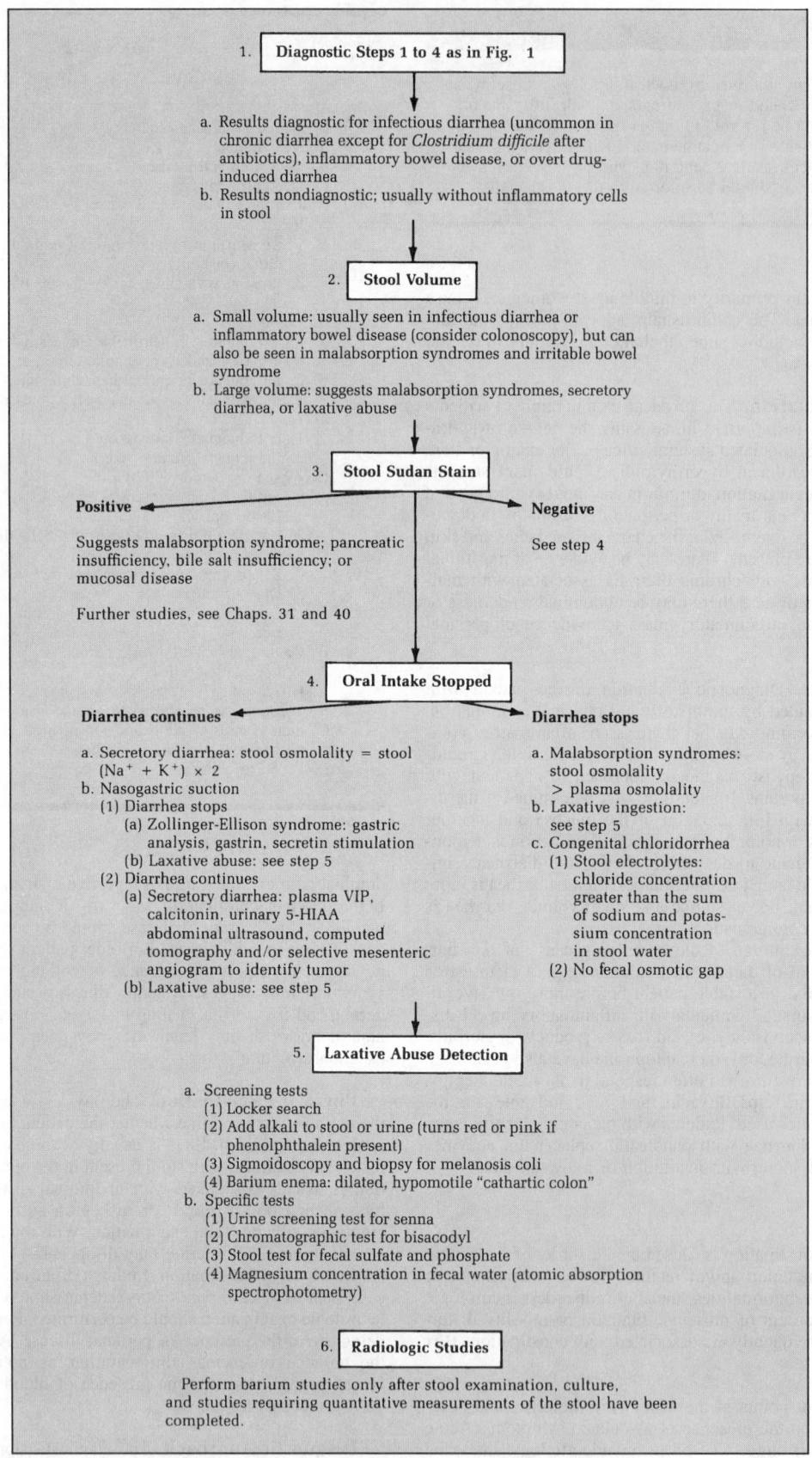

FIGURE 339-2   Diagnostic approach to the patient with chronic diarrhea. *VIP*, Vasoactive intestinal polypeptide; *5-HIAA*, 5-hydroxyindoleacetic acid.

BOX 339-3

Approach to the patient with chronic constipation

I. Systemic disease
   A. Often suggested by physical examination or by history
   B. Helpful laboratory tests include: electrolytes, BUN, tests of thyroid function, calcium, blood sugar
II. History of
   A. Bed rest
   B. Spinal cord lesion
   C. Autonomic neuropathy
   D. Peripheral neuropathy
III. Drug history: stop all potentially constipating drugs
IV. Assessment of gastrointestinal tract
   A. Rectal examination
      1. Tight sphincter, empty ampulla (Hirschsprung's disease)
      2. Anal and perianal disease (thrombosed hemorrhoid, fissure, fistulas, or abscess)
         a. Treat and observe
         b. Rule out associated Crohn's disease if perianal disease is present
      3. Blood in stool: proceed to flexible sigmoidoscopy and barium studies or colonoscopy
   B. Flexible sigmoidoscopy
      1. Normal mucosa: proceed to barium enema
      2. Abnormal: carcinoma, polyp, etc.: proceed with colonoscopy
   C. Barium studies or colonoscopy to rule out
      1. Obstructing lesion (carcinoma, polyp, diverticular mass)
      2. Stricture (neoplasm, inflammatory bowel disease, ischemia, radiation)
      3. Short-segment Hirschsprung's disease
      4. Small intestinal series if barium enema or colonoscopy normal to evaluate for small intestinal obstruction
   D. If cause of either an obstructing mass or stricture is not clear, perform colonoscopy for visual identification and biopsy
   E. If there is evidence of Hirschsprung's disease or if continued severe idiopathic constipation poorly responsive to medical therapy, perform anal manometry
   F. If there is no evidence of anal manometry abnormalities and no response to medical management, consider physiologic studies of colonic motility

---

ally air throughout the small and large intestines. The metabolic causes of constipation (i.e., electrolytes, calcium, blood urea nitrogen [BUN], thyroid tests) should be evaluated. The bowel should be decompressed in either case with a nasogastric tube. In the case of obstruction, further evaluation can be accomplished by either barium or endoscopic examination. If these procedures are unremarkable, a small bowel study may be appropriate (Box 339-3).

Physiologic Studies. If structural studies are unrevealing, studies of anal and colonic function should be considered. Anal manometry is useful for evaluating patients with anorectal dysfunction. Normally, rectal distention induces internal anal sphincter relaxation and reflex contraction of the external anal sphincter. In Hirschsprung's disease, or aganglionosis of segments of the colon, internal sphincter reflex relaxation is absent. Anal manometry is also helpful in evaluating sensation, compliance, and sphincter responses.

Colonic transit studies using radiopaque markers are helpful in assessing the extent and severity of colonic dysfunction. Patients with colonic inertia have delayed passage of the markers, which are scattered throughout the colon. In contrast, patients with rectoanal dysfunction have persistence of markers in the rectal region. Radioscintigraphy has also been used to evaluate colonic transit. At some centers, defecography is available for the detection of intussusception, rectocele, or pelvic floor abnormalities.

Management. In patients with idiopathic constipation, dietary management is often possible. Plenty of caffeine-free and alcohol-free fluids are important in management in patients with constipa-

✔ WHEN TO REFER

Patients with severe constipation, or those who do not respond to dietary manipulation and simple pharmacologic intervention, should be referred to a gastroenterologist. The gastroenterologist can also help guide the diagnostic evaluation of the patient with severe symptoms, including performing and interpreting the anal manometry.

tion. An increase of fiber in the diet to 25 to 40 g/day will increase stool weight and frequency. The institution of fiber should be slow and gradual to reduce the sensation of gas and bloating. Bulk-forming agents, taken with plenty of water, can be used in long-term management of patients with constipation. Saline agents, including those containing magnesium, phosphate, or citrate, act osmotically and are especially useful in the short-term management of constipation. Hyperosmotic agents (e.g., lactulose) and lubricants, (e.g., mineral oil) are useful agents in patients with chronic constipation. Stimulant agents should be avoided in chronic constipation because they can potentially cause damage to the bowel and electrolyte abnormalities.

IRRITABLE BOWEL SYNDROME

Irritable bowel syndrome (IBS) is an intestinal motility disorder of unknown cause. It is characterized by its symptom complex and by the lack of organic pathologic condition. The symptom complex includes abdominal pain, bloating, and alterations in bowel habits, with diarrhea and/or constipation. The symptoms are generally intermittent, chronic, or recurrent.

Incidence

IBS is one of the most frequently diagnosed disorders of the gastrointestinal tract and one of the most frequent conditions encountered by practicing physicians (40% to 70% of referrals to gastroenterologists). Surveys indicate that 14% to 22% of the general population experience symptoms suggestive of IBS.

Pathophysiology

A variety of psychosocial problems have been described in patients with IBS. Patients with IBS more often have abnormal personality patterns, including hypochondriasis, depression, and hysteria, and have abnormal illness attitudes. IBS patients overall, tend to have less adequate coping skills and greater physician-seeking behavior. An abuse history, either sexual or physical, should be sought in IBS patients with severe or refractory disease.

Motility alterations occur in patients with IBS. Intestinal smooth muscle cells have an inherent property of cyclic membrane depolarization and repolarization. The rate of cyclic depolarization, or the slow wave rate, determines the maximum frequency of contractions. In humans, there are two major slow wave frequencies in the colon, 3 and 6 cycles per minute, with 6 cycle per minute frequency accounting for 90% of recorded activity. In contrast, patients with IBS have 3 cycles per minute activity composing 40% of slow wave activity. Patients with IBS also have greater contractile activity in response to meal ingestion, cholecystokinin administration, or stress compared to normal patients. Abnormal irregular contractions may also occur in the small intestine in patients with IBS and may correlate with symptoms.

Patients with IBS appear to have heightened sensation to visceral stimulation. Balloon distension throughout the gastrointestinal tract causes pain at lower thresholds than in normal controls. Rectal hypersensitivity to balloon distension may prove to be a useful marker of IBS. Potentially, visceral afferents or the central processing of visceral information may be altered in patients with functional bowel disease.

✔ WHEN TO REFER

The majority of patients with irritable bowel syndrome can be evaluated and treated by the general medical physician. Patients with recalcitrant or severe symptoms may be referred to the gastroenterologist. Consultation to the specialist should be considered for those patients who do not respond to the usual dietary and behavioral changes. Associated psychiatric disorders should be considered and referral to a psychiatrist or psychologist may be helpful.

Clinical Presentation

Patients with irritable bowel syndrome present with chronic abdominal pain and altered bowel habits, which may be predominantly constipation or diarrhea or alternating diarrhea and constipation. There is a female predominance. Abdominal pain is often food- or stress-related, and the pain may be altered with defecation. The most common location for pain is the left lower quadrant. Associated symptoms of distention, bloating, and a feeling of incomplete evacuation are common. Patients often note mucus in the stools and looser stools with pain onset.

Diagnostic Studies

Diagnosis of IBS remains a process of exclusion, and major diseases to be ruled out include colonic neoplasms, diverticulosis, infectious causes of diarrhea, and inflammatory bowel disease. A typical history remains constant for years and might be that of a young women with a history of left lower quadrant pain with alternating constipation and diarrhea. Symptoms of IBS are not associated with weight loss or fever.

Patients with suspected IBS should have their symptoms assessed with a careful history (including dietary information) and physical examination. A focused screen for organic disease may include a blood count, sedimentation rate, fecal occult blood examination, stool studies for ova and parasites, and a flexible sigmoidoscopy with or without barium enema or colonoscopy. Further evaluation should be tailored to the individual patient.

Management

The key to the management of a patient with IBS is a good patient-physician relationship. Emotional support is vital, and the patient must be reassured that the physician does not think the symptoms are imaginary and that there is no life-threatening underlying illness. Stress management programs are useful for some patients.

The patient's diet should be reviewed and an association with symptoms be sought. Foods containing lactose, sorbitol, caffeine, fats, and legumes may contribute to symptoms in some patients. The management of constipation is essentially the addition of bulk to the diet in the form of fiber (such as bran) or bulk additives (such as psyllium seed). Evidence that bran is effective varies. It is important for patient tolerance that small, gradual increases of fiber be used.

Prescription medication may be considered in patients with persistent and moderate to severe symptoms who do not response to reassurance, education, diet manipulation, fiber, and development of coping skills. Medications should also be directed to the individual's symptoms. Anticholinergics, despite the lack of proven clinical efficacy, may be tried in patients in whom pain or constipation is problematic. Low doses of antidepressants may be useful in patients with continued pain. Prokinetic agents have been used in a subset of patients with constipation-predominant symptoms. Hormonal manipulation may benefit some female patients. Patients with diarrhea-predominant symptoms may respond to loperamide (Imodium). Research is ongoing for a potential clinical role of 5-hydroxytryptamine type 3 receptor antagonists and type 4 receptor agonists.

Prognosis

IBS is a chronic problem, with remissions and exacerbations. Patients should be advised of this and assured that the disease will not alter their life expectancy. Patients with severe symptoms of irritable bowel syndrome who do not respond to standard therapy may benefit from a referral to the gastroenterologist. In addition, patients with atypical signs or symptoms should undergo further evaluation by a subspecialist.

BIBLIOGRAPHY

Camilleri M, Thompson G, Fleshman JW, Pemberton JH: Clinical management of intractable constipation, *Ann Intern Med* 121:520-528, 1995.

Chopra S, Trier J: Diarrhea and malabsorption. In Chopra S, May RJ, editors: *Pathophysiology of gastrointestinal diseases,* Boston, 1989, Little, Brown.

Devroede G: Constipation. In Sleisenger MH, Fordtran JS, editors: *Gastrointestinal disease: pathophysiology, diagnosis and management,* ed 4, Philadelphia, 1989, WB Saunders.

Donowitz M, Kokke FT, Saidi R: Evaluation of patients with chronic diarrhea, *N Engl J Med* 332:725-729, 1995.

Drossman DA et al: Psychosocial factors in the irritable bowel syndrome, *Gastroenterology* 95:701, 1988.

Drossman DA, Talley NJ, Leserman J et al: Sexual and physical abuse and gastrointestinal illness, *Ann Intern Med* 123:782-794, 1995.

Guerrant RL, Bobak DA: Bacterial and protozoal gastroenteritis, *N Eng J Med* 325:327-340, 1991.

Kellow JE, Phillips SF: Altered small bowel motility in irritable bowel syndrome is correlated with symptoms, *Gastroenterology* 92:1885, 1987.

Keutch GT, Donowitz M: Pathophysiologic mechanisms of diarrheal diseases: diverse aetiologies and common mechanisms, *Scand J Gastroenterol Suppl* 84:33, 1983.

Lennard-Jones JE: Clinical management of constipation, *Pharmacology* 47:216-223, 1993.

Martelli H et al: Mechanisms of idiopathic constipation: outlet obstruction, *Gastroenterology* 75:623, 1978.

Mayer EA, Gebart GF: Basic and clinical aspects of visceral hyperalgesia, *Gastroenterology* 107:271-293, 1994.

McKee CP, Quigley EMM: Intestinal motility in irritable bowel syndrome: is IBS a motility disorder? *Dig Dis Sci* 38:1761-1762, 1993.

Mertz H, Naliboff B, Munakata J, Niazi N: Altered rectal perception is a biological marker of patients with irritable bowel syndrome, *Gastroenterology* 109:40-52, 1995.

Read NW, Timms JM: Defecation and the pathophysiology of constipation, *Clin Gastroenterol* 15:937, 1986.

Thompson WG, Creed F, Drossman DA et al: Functional bowel disease and functional abdominal pain, *Gastroenterology* 5:75-91, 1992.

CHAPTER

340 Diseases of Small Bowel Absorption

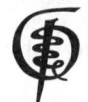

Michael R. Charlton and Edward V. Loftus, Jr.

The primary function of the small intestine is to efficiently extract nutrients from consumed foods. This is accomplished through a complex series of processes throughout the length of the small bowel. The healthy small intestine is elegantly adapted to this role through variations in gross anatomy, cellular structure and function, innervation, and hormonal production and responsiveness. The small intestine is generally a robust organ; however, each of the adaptive features necessary for the overall extraction of nutrients may be altered by disease. It is essential to possess an understanding of the physiology of normal small intestinal function to readily diagnose and manage the diseases that affect it. The extraction of nutrients requires both digestion and absorption. Although this section will focus on diseases of small intestinal absorption, a brief overview of the pertinent physiology is provided.

Digestion

Digestion is the process by which larger, more complex nutrients are broken down into smaller molecules that can be absorbed. Digestion is initiated in the mouth, through mastication and the mixing of saliva with food. The contribution of salivary enzymes to digestion is minimal. The great majority of digestion occurs in the stomach, through the hydrolytic actions of pepsin and hydrochloric acid; and in the proximal small bowel, through the actions of the pancreatic enzymes, chiefly trypsin, lipase, and amylase. As a result of digestion, the enterocyte is provided with monosaccharides, amino acids, peptides, fatty acids, and triglycerides. These nutrients are amenable to absorption by the small intestine. Although elemental diets, which do not require digestion, are now available, all other diets require some degree of digestion to occur for absorption to take place.

Absorption

Once digestion has taken place, the efficient absorption of nutrients requires luminal contents to be in intimate proximity with enterocytes. The small intestine has undergone a high degree of structural adaptation to maximize its surface area. Endoscopic examination of normal small bowel mucosal surface reveals intricate permanent folding of the mucosal surface, with the formation of plicae conniventes. Low power microscopic examination of a small intestinal fold will demonstrate that the mucosal epithelial surface is organized into villi. Higher power examination reveals that the luminal edge of the cells that make up the small intestinal villi are further organized into microvilli, referred to as the brush border (Fig. 340-1). There are approximately 2×10^8 microvilli/cm^2 of small intestinal luminal surface. This basic anatomic organization is constant throughout the length of the duodenum, jejunum, and ileum. The combined effect of mucosal folding, villi, and microvilli formation is a >600-fold increase in the surface area of the small intestine compared to the surface area of a simple cylinder of the same length. The total surface area of the small intestine is greater than 200m^2 and provides a large reserve of absorptive and secretory capacity. Once absorbed, nutrients enter the systemic circulation via the portal vein and liver or via lymphatics and the thoracic duct.

Clinical Features of Malabsorption

It has been said that we see only what we look for. This is particularly pertinent in the history and examination of patients with small bowel malabsorption. A detailed history and physical examination are cornerstones of the diagnosis and treatment of diseases of small intestinal malabsorption and will facilitate the development of the safest and least expensive evaluation for a given patient. Familiarity with the protean clinical manifestations of the malabsorption syndromes will aid the clinician in actively seeking evidence of generalized and specific nutrient deficiencies (Table 340-1). The presence or absence of a particular manifestation will vary tremendously with the underlying cause and severity of small intestinal malabsorption.

Intestinal Manifestations. Although the severity of symptoms may vary, some degree of diarrhea, flatulence, abdominal pain, and weight loss are almost ubiquitous. Stool frequency is usually increased in response to a combination of increased colonic delivery of fat, carbohydrate, fluid, and electrolytes, as well as the stimulatory effects of unabsorbed bile and hydroxy fatty acids on colonic secretion and motility. In cases of small bowel malabsorption in which stool frequency is not increased, stool volume will be. Patients with malabsorption often, although far from always, complain of pale, greasy, malodorous stools that are difficult to flush. Those patients who do not describe the classic steatorrheal stool usually have milder degrees of malabsorption but nonetheless have quantitative steatorrhea. Blood in the stool is atypical but may be found in patients who have underlying Crohn's disease or, rarely, ampullary carcinoma.

Increased flatulence is a common complaint of patients with malabsorption and is produced by the bacterial fermentation of dietary carbohydrates. In addition to producing flatulence, the excessive intestinal gas production contributes to the abdominal distention and discomfort that are so common in diseases of small intestinal malabsorption. Abdominal pain may be a prominent symptom in patients

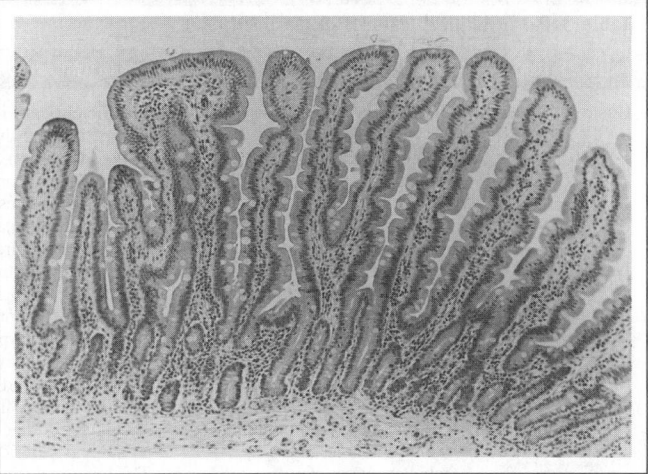

A

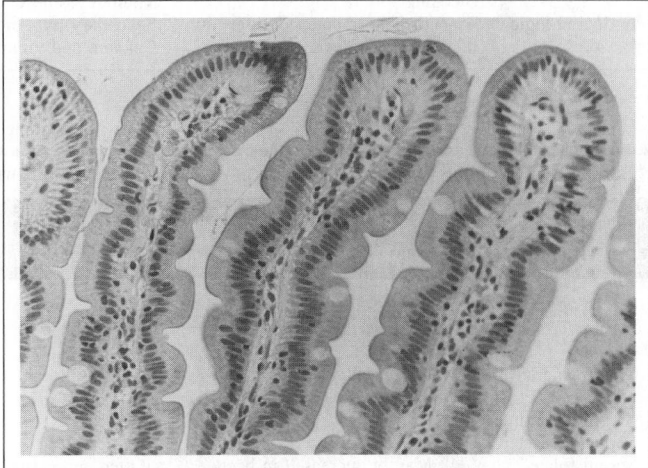

B

FIGURE 340-1 Normal jejunal mucosa. **A,** The normal villus to crypt ratio ranges from 4 : 1 to 6 : 1. Mononuclear inflammatory cells (predominantly plasma cells and lymphocytes) are evenly distributed throughout the lamina propria. Hematoxylin and eosin, medium power (180×). **B,** The epithelium is characterized by a dark, refractile outer "brush border" of microvilli, scattered goblet cells, and occasional intraepithelial lymphocytes. Hematoxylin and eosin, high power (400×).

Photomicrograph courtesy L.J. Burgart, M.D.

with Crohn's disease, chronic pancreatitis, pancreatic cancer, and adynamic ileus.

Weight loss is a common complaint in patients with established malabsorption and can be profound. Some patients are able to compensate for the increased fecal loss of nutrients by increasing their food intake. This should be readily apparent from the history.

Extraintestinal Manifestations. Every organ and tissue of the body can be affected by malabsorption (Table 340-1). Often it is one of the extraintestinal manifestations that cause a patient with malabsorption to first seek medical attention. Common extraintestinal manifestations are lassitude and skin changes, including ecchymoses and edema. Lassitude is often contributed to by associated anemia. Anemia is a prevalent finding and may be multifactorial. Many extraintestinal manifestations, such as night blindness, amenorrhea, impotence, and muscle cramps are noted only on direct questioning. Careful examination for the presence of peripheral neuropathy should be carried out in all patients in whom malabsorption is suspected.

Table 340-1 Clinical features of malabsorption

ORGAN/SYSTEM	SYMPTOM/SIGN	PATHOPHYSIOLOGY
Gastrointestinal	Weight loss	Insufficient calories secondary to malabsorption of fats, protein, and carbohydrate; diminished appetite, and dysgeusia from zinc deficiency
	Abdominal pain	Bowel distention, inflammation of serosa or peritoneum by underlying disease
	Diarrhea	Nutrient malabsorption (especially fats), decreased absorption and increased secretion of fluids and electrolytes (multifactorial, small and large intestine involved)
	Flatus	Bacterial fermentation of unabsorbed carbohydrates
	Glossitis, stomatitis, cheilosis	Deficiencies of iron, B_{12}, riboflavin, niacin, folate, and other micronutrients
Dermatologic	Purpura	Deficiency of vitamins C and K
	Dermatitis, follicular hyperkeratosis	Deficiencies of zinc, vitamin A, niacin, pyridoxine, and essential fatty acids
	Hyperpigmentism	Secondary hypopituitarism, adrenal insufficiency
	Edema	Protein malabsorption and protein-losing enteropathy resulting in decreased oncotic pressure, thiamine deficiency
Musculoskeletal	Bone pain, pathologic fractures	Osteomalacia and osteoporosis (multifactorial, including vitamin D and calcium malabsorption)
	Tetany	Calcium, magnesium, and vitamin D deficiency
Neurologic	Night blindness, xeropthalmia	Vitamin A deficiency
	Peripheral neuropathy	Vitamin B_{12} deficiency
	Cerebellar signs	Thiamine and vitamin E deficiency
Hematologic	Anemia	Macrocytic: folate and vitamin B_{12} deficiency
		Microcytic: iron and pyridoxine deficiency
	Bleeding	Vitamin K and C deficiency
Endocrinologic	Amenorrhea, impotence, infertility	Secondary hypopituitarism
	Increased PTH level	Calcium and vitamin D deficiency resulting in secondary hyperparathyroidism

Table 340-2 Useful tests in the evaluation of small bowel malabsorption

TEST	TYPICAL RESULTS — IMPAIRED INTALUMINAL DIGESTION	TYPICAL RESULTS — MUCOSAL DISEASE	COMMENTS
Screening tests			
Serum carotene	Decreased	Decreased	Good screening test when normal intake has been documented; poor sensitivity
Serum calcium	Decreased	Decreased	May need to correct values for hypoalbuminemia; poor sensitivity
Serum albumin	Normal or decreased	Decreased	Poor sensitivity
Serum cholesterol	Decreased	Decreased	Poor sensitivity
Serum folate	May be increased in bacterial overgrowth	Often decreased	Poor sensitivity; folate produced by small intestinal bacteria
Serum iron	Normal	Decreased in proximal small bowel disease	Poor sensitivity and specificity
Qualitative fecal fat	Fat globules	Fat globules	Sensitive screening test, may be false positive if mineral or castor oil ingested
Quantitative fecal fat	Increased	Increased	Sensitive but difficult, unpleasant, and expensive
Specific tests			
Vitamin B_{12}	Decreased in bacterial overgrowth and pancreatic insufficiency	Decreased in extensive ileal involvement	Requires normal renal function; all stages of Schilling test normal in proton pump inhibitor–related vitamin B_{12} deficiency
D-xylose absorption	Normal except in bacterial overgrowth	Decreased unless localized ileal disease	Requires normal renal function and gastric emptying; good discriminating test
Bentiromide	Decreased in pancreatic insufficiency	Normal	Simple; highly specific; requires normal renal function; excellent confirmatory test of pancreatic exocrine insufficiency
Secretin	Decreased in pancreatic insufficiency	Normal	Highly sensitive and specific when carried out correctly but difficult and expensive; rarely performed
Small bowel biopsy	Normal except in severe bacterial overgrowth	May be diagnositic (e.g., Celiac sprue)	Expensive but safe and simple; has potential to yield precise diagnosis; cost-effective when used appropriately
Lactulose breath	Increased H_2 excretion in 70% of pateints with bacterial overgrowth	Normal	Requires normal gastric emptying, detects lactase deficiency; simple test but has relatively poor sensitivity and specificity

Laboratory Findings

The diagnosis of small bowel malabsorption is usually suspected after a detailed history and physical examination. The clinician should initially seek to confirm or disprove his or her suspicion and then to identify the precise cause of small bowel malabsorption with the aid of the many diagnostic tools at their disposal (Table 340-2).

A practical algorithm for the investigation of suspected small bowel malabsorption is provided in Fig. 340-2. Once a history and

physical examination have raised the possibility of small bowel malabsorption, some routine blood tests should be obtained. The initial blood tests of choice should include a complete blood cell count, with prothrombin time and assays of serum levels of calcium, albumin, iron, carotene, and cholesterol. Vitamin B_{12} and folate levels are often added. None of these tests are particularly sensitive or specific for malabsorption. Examination of the stool, including the Sudan III stain for fat globules, is an excellent screening test for malabsorp-

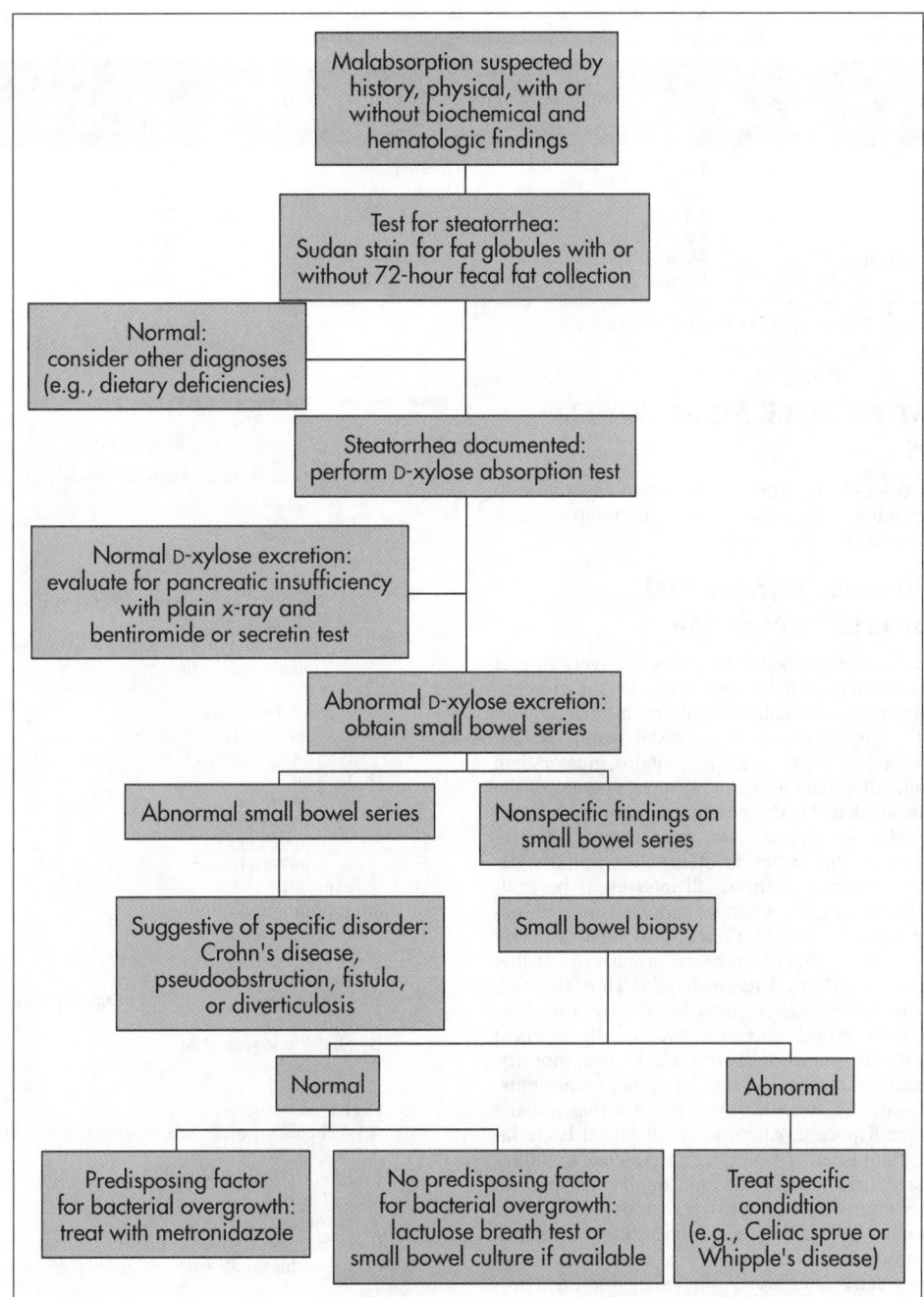

FIGURE 340-2   Diagnostic algorithm for the evaluation of small bowel malabsorption.

tion. Because the 72-hour fecal fat collection is expensive, unpleasant, and frequently carried out incorrectly, it can be obviated in the setting of a positive fecal Sudan III stain.

An abnormally low B_{12} level can be of great utility when followed up with a multi-stage Schilling test (Table 340-3). The increasingly frequent use of proton pump inhibitors, such as omeprazole and lansoprazole, has been shown to result in diminished dietary B_{12} absorption through impaired acidic release of dietary protein–bound B_{12}. The absorption of free B_{12}, as is administered in stage I of the Schilling test, will be normal in this setting.

Once small bowel malabsorption has been shown to be likely through these screening tests, the initial challenge is to distinguish between impaired intraluminal digestion, mucosal disease, and impaired lymphatic obstruction. Because the great majority of cases of small bowel malabsorption are due to either impaired intraluminal di-

gestion or mucosal disease, the first tests to be administered should facilitate distinguishing between these two entities. Measurement of the absorption and subsequent urinary excretion of D-xylose will distinguish between pancreatic and nonpancreatic causes. D-xylose is a five-carbon sugar that does not require pancreatic enzymes for absorption. Absorption is thus usually normal in exocrine pancreatic insufficiency and impaired in mucosal diseases. An abnormal (low) D-xylose excretion test should be followed up with a radiographic examination of the upper gastrointestinal tract. When the D-xylose and small bowel series have failed to indicate a cause of small bowel malabsorption, a small bowel biopsy is usually necessary. When applied sequentially, these three tests will yield a diagnosis in the great majority of cases. It should be noted that the D-xylose excretion test is not accurate in patients with impaired renal function or ascites, or in patients taking nonsteroidal antiinflammatory drugs (NSAIDs).

Table 340-3　Interpretation of the Schilling test

	STAGE I (^{57}CO-LABELED B$_{12}$)	STAGE II (^{57}CO-LABELED B$_{12}$ PLUS INTRINSIC FACTOR)	STAGE III (^{57}CO-LABELED B$_{12}$ PLUS PANCREATIC ENZYMES)	STAGE IV (^{57}CO-LABELED B$_{12}$ METRONIDAZOLE)
Pernicious anemia	Low	Normal	Low	Low
Pancreatic insufficiency	Low	Low	Normal	Low
Bacterial overgrowth	Low	Low	Low	Normal
Ileal dysfunction	Low	Low	Low	Low
Hypochlorhydria or achlorhydria	Normal	Normal	Normal	Normal
Dietary deficiency	Normal	Normal	Normal	Normal

"Low" or "normal" refers to the 24-hour urinary excretion of ^{57}Co-labeled B$_{12}$.

DISORDERS THAT PRODUCE SMALL BOWEL MALABSORPTION

It is easiest to consider diseases that affect small bowel absorption in terms of their pathophysiology: those that impair intraluminal digestion and those that impair mucosal absorption.

Disorders That Produce Intraluminal Maldigestion: Bacterial Overgrowth

Etiologic Factors. The healthy small bowel is relatively free of microorganisms. Fluid collected from the normal duodenum will contain on average $0-10^4$ organisms/ml, jejunum and proximal ileum will contain less than $0-10^5$ organisms/ml, and the distal ileum 10^3-10^9 organisms/ml. Colonic luminal fluid typically contains greater than 10^9 viable organisms/ml. Although the relatively sterile nature of the small intestine is contributed to by the combined antimicrobial effects of gastric acid production, mucus, bile, rapid enterocyte turnover, the ileocecal valve, and the secretion of IgA, the primary defense against bacterial overgrowth of the small intestine is peristalsis. This is supported by the fact that when bacterial overgrowth occurs, the flora making up the overgrowth are those that typically colonize the colon and not those that colonize the oropharynx or that are cultured from normal small bowel luminal fluid. Thus although impairment of any of the defense mechanisms listed may contribute to its development, small bowel bacterial overgrowth is most frequently associated with conditions of altered small bowel motility. Effective peristalsis requires integrity of small intestinal neuromuscular physiology and anatomic structure. Any process that impairs normal peristalsis can predispose a patient to small bowel bacterial overgrowth. Similarly, diminished IgA production, pancreaticobiliary secretion, and mucus or gastric acid production can all predispose to small bowel bacterial overgrowth. Box 340-1 provides a list of the clinical conditions that most frequently produce bacterial overgrowth. Although gastric acid production is often listed as a major factor in the maintenance of the relative sterility of the small intestine, prospective study of patients taking proton pump inhibitors for at least six months have failed to show an increase in small bowel bacterial overgrowth related to these agents.

Pathophysiologic Findings. Bacterial overgrowth can result in the malabsorption of fats, carbohydrates, and micronutrients. Mucosal damage—with subtotal villous atrophy, lamina proprial inflammation, and mucosal ulcerations—can result in generalized malabsorption but is not usually a prominent factor. More specific mechanisms bring about the malabsorption of fats, carbohydrates, and micronutrients.

Although the mechanism of carbohydrate malabsorption will vary with the dominant proliferating microorganism, bacterial overgrowth is frequently associated with diminished activity of the brush border disaccharidases. Disaccharidases are reduced through the action of anaerobic bacterial glycosidases and proteinases.

Fat is both maldigested and malabsorbed in small bowel bacterial overgrowth. Maldigestion occurs chiefly as a result of bacterial hydrolysis of conjugated bile salts, with concomitant impairment of pancreatic lipase activity. Deconjugated bile acids are more lipid soluble than conjugated bile acids and are thus absorbed in the proximal small bowel; selective absorption of conjugated bile acids occurs in the dis-

---

BOX 340-1
Causes of small bowel bacterial overgrowth

I. Structural lesions
　A. Small bowel diverticulosis
　B. Surgical
　　1. Afferent loop stasis post-Billroth II or Poly A partial gastrectomy
　　2. Side-to-side or side-to-end anastomosis
　　3. Continent ileostomy
　C. Strictures
　　1. Crohn's disease
　　2. Following radiation enteritis
　　3. Vascular disease
　D. Fistulas
　　1. Gastrocolic
　　2. Gastroileal
　　3. Jejunocolic
　　4. Jejunoileal
　E. Adhesions
　　1. Postoperative
　　2. Postinflammatory
II. Neuromuscular
　A. Postoperative adynamic ileus
　B. Drug-related (e.g., phenothiazines, opiates)
　C. Scleroderma
　D. Diabetic gastroparesis
　E. Amyloidosis
　F. Postvagotomy
III. Decreased gastric acid production
　A. Atrophic gastritis with or without pernicious anemia
　B. Postvagotomy with or without gastric resection
　C. Proton pump or high-dose H$_2$ receptor antagonist treatment
IV. Miscellaneous
　A. Portal enteropathy, cirrhosis
　B. Hypogammaglobulinemia or agammaglobulinemia
　C. Idiopathic (most frequent in the elderly)

---

tal ileum. The absorption of deconjugated bile acids in the proximal small bowel results in bile acid deficiency in the distal jejunum and ileum.

Vitamin B$_{12}$ (both free and bound to intrinsic factor) is utilized by luminal bacteria, which also produce inactive analogues of B$_{12}$. Vitamin B$_{12}$ deficiency may ensue and is regarded as one of the hallmarks of long-standing bacterial overgrowth. Bacterial fermentation of substrates results in the production of folate, which may subsequently be absorbed in abnormally large amounts. As a result, serum folate levels may actually be increased in small bowel bacterial overgrowth. Other water soluble vitamins are only rarely deficient in patients with bacterial overgrowth.

Fat-soluble vitamins—A, D and E—are occasionally lowered in patients with small bowel bacterial overgrowth due to impaired micelle formation and deconjugation of bile acids. In contrast, vitamin K levels are often normal or elevated due to bacterial production of this micronutrient. Coagulopathy is thus not a typical feature of bacterial overgrowth.

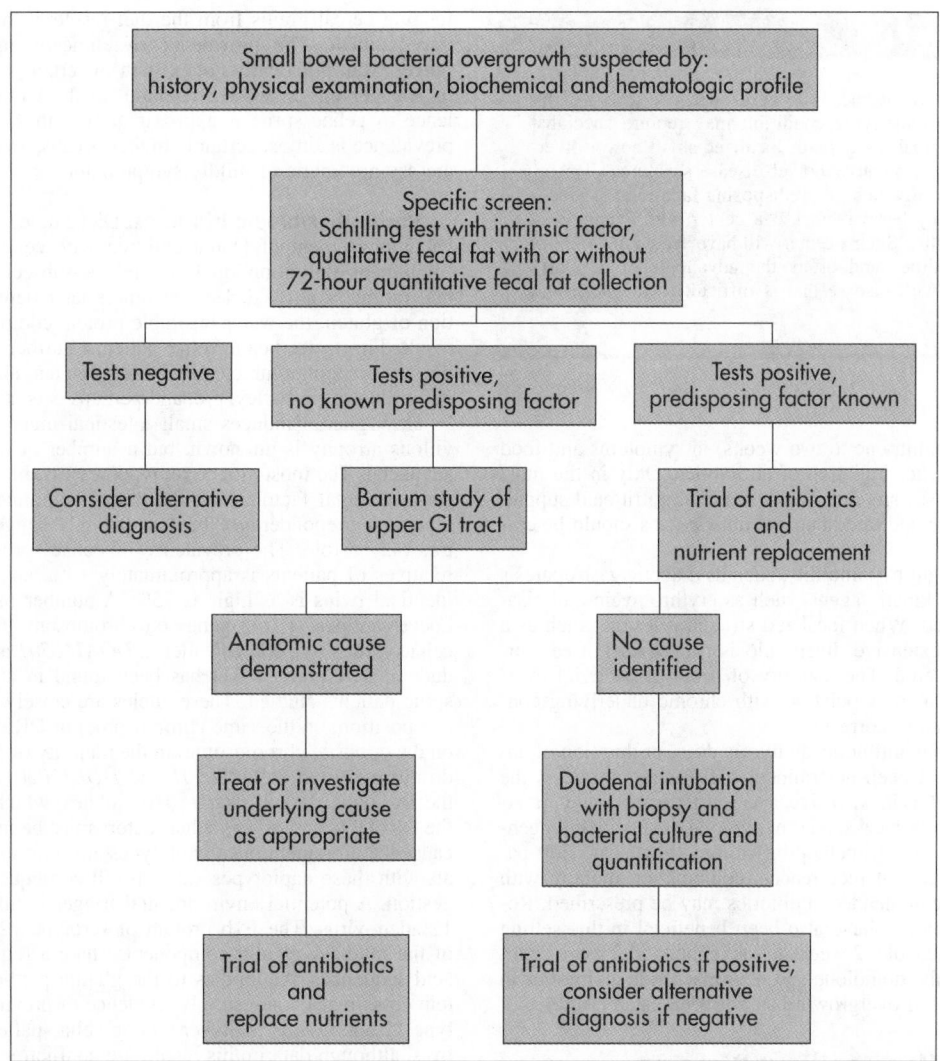

FIGURE 340-3   Algorithm for the management of suspected small bowel bacterial overgrowth. Qualitative fecal fat test may be carried out using stool microscopy and Sudan III stain. *3d,* three day.

Clinical Features and Diagnosis. Review of the pathogenesis of bacterial overgrowth will reveal that this condition is associated with maldigestion, malabsorption, and a potentially diverse set of micronutrient deficiencies. The symptoms of bacterial overgrowth may thus vary widely. Most patients will experience some degree of diarrhea, flatus, abdominal pain, and weight loss. Many patients will have symptoms related to the underlying cause of bacterial overgrowth, such as Crohn's disease, diabetes, scleroderma, or amyloidosis. In the case of strictures and adhesions, symptoms of the underlying condition may be indistinguishable from symptoms of small bowel bacterial overgrowth. It is important to bear in mind that the predisposing condition may have been present for years before the onset of the symptoms and signs of small bowel bacterial overgrowth.

Because of the high frequency of micronutrient deficiencies in the setting of bacterial overgrowth, systemic symptoms related to micronutrient deficiencies may be prominent. Common extraintestinal manifestations include megaloblastic anemia, arthritis, dermatitis, nephritis, and steatohepatitis. Bacterial antigen/antibody immune complex deposition may play a role in the development of joint, skin, and kidney lesions. Clinical symptoms and signs related to deficiencies of any of the listed micronutrients may also be apparent, such as glossitis and ecchymoses (see Table 340-1).

Because many of the predisposing conditions can cause symptoms that overlap with those of small bowel bacterial overgrowth, this diagnosis is easy to miss. Small bowel bacterial overgrowth should be considered in all patients who develop prolonged, unexplained diarrhea (particularly with features of steatorrhea), weight loss or macrocytic anemia. A practical algorithm for the diagnosis of small bowel-bacterial overgrowth is provided in Fig. 340-3. Much has been written about lactulose, glucose, ^{14}C-cholyglycine, and ^{14}C-xylose breath tests. With the possible exception of the lactulose-hydrogen breath test, these tests are not widely available and have poor sensitivity and specificity; they are rarely used in clinical practice. In patients who are known to have a predisposing factor and who present with suggestive symptoms (and/or signs), the combined presence of neutral fat globules in a stool sample stained with Sudan red and an abnormal Schilling test that fails to correct with intrinsic factor allows the presumptive diagnosis of small bowel bacterial overgrowth. Barium imaging of the upper GI tract is imperative for all patients in whom screening tests are positive in the absence of a known predisposing factor. Duodenal/jejunal intubation should be reserved for cases in which the diagnosis remains in doubt. Quantitative culture of jejunal fluid is a sensitive and specific test for small bowel bacterial overgrowth but is technically very difficult and should be performed at referral centers.

Management. Treatment of small bowel bacterial overgrowth comprises three elements: (1) restoration of adequate nutrition, (2) treatment of the underlying condition, and (3) antibiotic therapy.

In mild to moderate cases of small bowel bacterial overgrowth,

✔ *WHEN TO REFER*

Although the treatment of bacterial overgrowth per se is usually straightforward, the underlying condition may require specialist evaluation (e.g., surgical resection of localized small bowel diverticular disease or inflammatory bowel disease strictures). Recurrent cases and cases in which no predisposing factor can be identified should probably be evaluated at a center with expertise in gastrointestinal motility. Such a center will have access to the more unusual testing facilities and offers the advantage of regularly evaluating patients with disease that is difficult to diagnose and treat.

rapid improvement (within one to two weeks) in symptoms and food tolerance takes place after initiation of antibiotics. Only in the most severe or refractory cases are enteral or parenteral nutritional supplements needed. Documented micronutrient deficiencies should be corrected appropriately.

In cases related to gut hypomotility, such as diabetic gastroparesis or adynamic ileus, prokinetic agents such as erythromycin and cisapride may be employed. When localized structural lesions such as a focal stricture or nonextensive diverticulosis can be identified, surgery should be considered. The majority of cases of bacterial overgrowth, however, occur in association with chronic underlying conditions that are not readily corrected.

Although the optimal antibiotic, antibiotic dose, or duration of antibiotic course have not been determined, oral metronidazole is the most widely prescribed, is inexpensive, and is usually effective. Treatment should be for 2 to 4 weeks. Alternative oral agents include gentamicin, tetracycline, and trimethoprim-sulfamethoxazole. For patients who develop frequent recurrences, combination therapy with two or three of the recommended antibiotics may be prescribed. Rotating courses of antibiotics have also been beneficial in this setting (e.g., 2 weeks metronidazole; 2 weeks tetracycline; and 2 weeks gentamicin). The role of the quinolone and new macrolide antibiotics in the treatment of bacterial overgrowth has not been established.

Pancreatic and Hepatobiliary Diseases

The delivery of bile and pancreatic secretions into the lumen of the small bowel is essential for normal digestion and absorption (Chapter 326). Fortunately, humans are blessed with a large reserve of pancreatic exocrine capacity. Malabsorption does not usually occur until at least 90% of pancreatic exocrine function is lost. The most common cause of pancreatic exocrine insufficiency is chronic pancreatitis. Other conditions that may result in pancreatic insufficiency include tumors of the pancreas and ampulla and cystic fibrosis. These diseases are all reviewed in detail in Chapter 366.

Cirrhotic-stage liver disease, particularly the cholestatic forms such as primary biliary cirrhosis and primary sclerosing cholangitis, have a surprisingly high prevalence, >30%, of malabsorption secondary to reduced production and intraluminal delivery of bile salts. Furthermore, an association between primary biliary cirrhosis and celiac sprue has been reported. Descriptions of the clinical manifestations of these diseases are described in detail elsewhere in this book, but it should be noted that patients with cholestatic liver disease have impaired vitamin D and calcium metabolism and often develop prominent osteoporosis.

Tests of mucosal structure and function are usually normal in pancreatic and hepatobiliary causes of malabsorption.

DISORDERS OF MUCOSAL ABSORPTION
Celiac Sprue

Celiac sprue is a chronic inflammatory disorder of the small intestine resulting from the ingestion of certain substances found in cereal grains such as wheat, barley, rye, and perhaps oats. The inflammation produces villous atrophy, usually most prominent in the proximal small bowel, and results in malabsorption. Withdrawal of the of-

fending cereal grains from the diet results in histologic and clinical improvement. The prevalence of clinically apparent celiac sprue ranges from practically nonexistent in certain Third World areas to 1 in 300 persons in western Ireland. In the United States, the prevalence of celiac sprue is approximately 1 in 4500 persons. The true prevalence is almost certainly higher because many people with sprue are asymptomatic or mildly symptomatic.

Pathophysiologic Findings. Dicke noted the paradoxical clinical improvement of Dutch children with celiac disease during the "Winter of Starvation" in 1944 and the subsequent relapse when cereal rations improved. He and others later demonstrated that ingestion of gluten, the water-insoluble protein component of wheat flour, resulted in steatorrhea in celiac patients. Further work implicated gliadin, the alcohol-soluble component of gluten, along with corresponding prolamins in barley, rye, and perhaps oats, as the offending agent.

How gliadin induces small intestinal mucosal inflammation and villous atrophy is unknown, but a number of hypotheses have been advanced. The most attractive hypothesis is that genetic and possibly environmental factors alter the normal immune response to dietary gluten. A preponderance of data strongly suggests that genetic factors play a role. The prevalence of celiac sprue among first-degree relatives of patients is approximately 10%, and concordance among identical twins is as high as 75%. A number of class II human leukocyte antigen (HLA) genes on chromosome 6 are associated with celiac sprue. Two HLA-D alleles, *DQA1*0501* and *DQB1*0201,* produce a DQ2 antigen that has been found in at least 95% of celiac sprue patients studied. These alleles are closely linked to either DR3 (*cis* position, on the same chromosome) or DR5/DR7 (*trans* position, on the opposite chromosome) in the majority of patients. Patients who do not carry the *DQA1*0501* and *DQB1*0201* alleles tend to carry the *DQA1*0301* and *DQB1*0302* alleles, which are associated with the DR4DQ8 haplotype. Other factors must be involved, however, because the aforementioned haplotypes are common, and most individuals with these haplotypes suffer no ill consequences from gluten ingestion. A potential environmental trigger is infection with serotype 12 adenovirus. The E1b protein of serotype 12 adenovirus and one of the major α-gliadin components share a region of similar amino acid sequences. Antibodies to the gliadin peptide and the viral protein cross-react. Interestingly, evidence of previous exposure to serotype 12 adenovirus is higher among celiac patients than among controls, although data in this regard are conflicting. Thus viral infection might induce gluten sensitization in the genetically susceptible patient, but further studies are needed.

The inflammatory lesion in celiac sprue is likely a result of cell-mediated immune mechanisms. Class II HLA antigen expression is increased on intestinal epithelial cells and mononuclear cells. Intraepithelial lymphocyte density is increased, and exposure to gluten results in further increases in density. Gluten exposure also results in increased cytokine expression by lymphocytes.

The histologic lesion is variable in severity and extent (Fig. 340-4). In asymptomatic or mild illness the lesion may involve only the proximal small intestine. The lesion decreases in severity distally, probably a reflection of decreased distal contact with toxic gluten. The most characteristic finding is villous atrophy, either total (flat mucosa) or subtotal (broad, short villi). Overall, the mucosal thickness is normal and the crypts are elongated. Epithelial cells and their microvilli are shortened and irregular. In addition to increased intraepithelial lymphocytes, there are increased numbers of mononuclear cells and neutrophils in the lamina propria.

Malabsorption results from a decrease in both the quantity and the absorptive capacity of the mucosal surface. Other factors contributing to symptoms include excessive fluid secretion by damaged epithelium resulting in increased stool volume, loss of brush-border enzymes resulting in carbohydrate intolerance, and impaired release of enteric hormones such as cholecystokinin resulting in exocrine pancreatic insufficiency.

Clinical Features and Laboratory Findings. The spectrum of clinical presentation is quite broad and depends on the severity of the mucosal lesion. The spectrum ranges from isolated iron-deficiency or folate-deficiency anemia or unexplained osteopenia to full-blown malabsorption and malnutrition with dehydration and electrolyte ab-

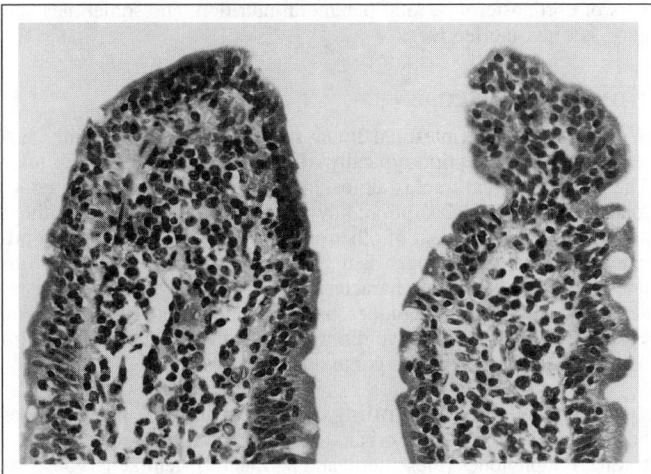

A

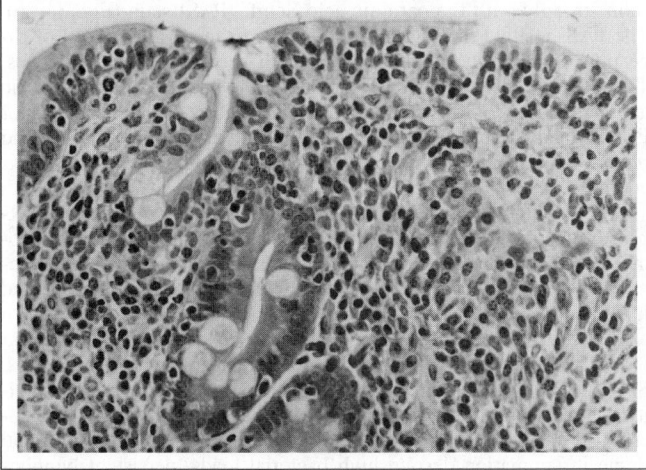

B

FIGURE 340-4 Celiac sprue at various degrees of severity. **A,** Mild. There is a significant degree of intraepithelial lymphocytosis despite the lack of mucosal flattening. Normally there are 20 to 40 lymphocytes per 100 epithelial cells. Hematoxylin and eosin, medium power (220×). **B,** Severe. Mucosal flattening of the small bowel due to celiac disease is always associated with marked intraepithelial lymphocytosis. Lamina propria mononuclear inflammation is also increased. Hematoxylin and eosin, high power (400×).

Photomicrograph courtesy L.J. Burgart, M.D.

normalities. Children with celiac disease present with diarrhea, abdominal distention, and failure to gain weight, typically after weaning as cereals are introduced into the diet. Symptoms may disappear during adolescence but often recur during adulthood. Adults with sprue may present with few or no gastrointestinal symptoms but with consequences of malabsorption such as anemia, osteopenia, peripheral neuropathy, or proximal myopathy. Celiac sprue has been associated with a number of autoimmune diseases including dermatitis herpetiformis, insulin-dependent diabetes mellitus, IgA deficiency, autoimmune thyroid disease, and polymyositis; gastrointestinal symptoms in these patients should be evaluated for sprue. Associations between celiac sprue and the idiopathic inflammatory bowel diseases (chronic ulcerative colitis, Crohn's disease, collagenous colitis, and lymphocytic colitis) have been described; therefore the diagnosis of sprue should be considered in such patients with "refractory" symptoms.

The association with dermatitis herpetiformis merits further attention. At least 90% of patients with this highly specific, pruritic papulovesicular eruption are found to have a small bowel lesion indistinguishable from sprue, even in the absence of malabsorption.

Conversely, approximately 10% of celiac sprue patients have dermatitis herpetiformis. The skin lesion usually improves with a gluten-free diet, but medical therapy directed toward the skin lesion (e.g., dapsone) has no effect on the intestinal abnormality.

The laboratory abnormalities also vary depending on the extent and severity of disease. In mild cases, iron deficiency may be the only abnormality; it results from a combination of decreased iron absorption and occult gastrointestinal bleeding. As severity increases, there is a greater likelihood of detecting classic abnormalities of malabsorption such as hypocalcemia, hypomagnesemia, hypoalbuminemia, and hypoprothrombinemia. Quantitative fecal fat is increased in all but the mildest of cases, and D-xylose absorption should be abnormal in these mild cases. Barium contrast examination of the small bowel reveals dilation, excess fluid, and segmentation of barium in moderate to severe enteropathy. However, these findings are not specific for celiac sprue, and the examination findings may be normal in mild illness.

Peroral biopsy of the small intestine remains critical in making a firm diagnosis. Endoscopic biopsy of the distal duodenum has largely replaced the Crosby capsule or Rubin tube. To make a definitive diagnosis of celiac sprue, three criteria should be met: (1) evidence of malabsorption (fecal fat or D-xylose), (2) small bowel biopsy showing subtotal or total villous atrophy with increased intraepithelial lymphocytes, and (3) clinical and histologic improvement after withdrawal of dietary gluten. Empiric withdrawal of gluten for idiopathic diarrhea is not recommended.

A number of noninvasive serologic tests to substantiate the diagnosis of celiac sprue are now clinically available, but no clear consensus on their role has been reached. Serum antigliadin IgA antibodies are highly sensitive but not as specific. The sensitivity and specificity of antiendomysial IgA antibodies approach 100%. Moreover, the antiendomysial antibodies tend to disappear after treatment with a gluten-free diet, so patient compliance can be measured. Unfortunately, these antibodies remain negative in patients with concomitant IgA deficiency. Because treatment of celiac sprue results in a permanent and dramatic change in life-style, a definitive diagnosis with small bowel biopsy must be recommended at this time. The greatest usefulness of serologic tests appears to be screening first-degree relatives of probands. Those relatives with positive serologic findings should undergo small bowel biopsy. Screening of the general population with serologic tests is not recommended.

Differential Diagnosis. The differential diagnosis based on clinical symptoms is quite broad because the symptoms are nonspecific and the spectrum of clinical presentation is wide. The symptoms of irritable bowel syndrome, perhaps the most common gastrointestinal disorder in the United States, are identical to those associated with a mild or moderate case of celiac sprue. Although the lesion found on small bowel biopsy is characteristic, it is not specific for celiac sprue. Similar histologic findings occur in infants with cow's milk sensitivity and in older children and adults with severe tropical sprue, eosinophilic enteritis, Zollinger-Ellison syndrome, radiation enteritis, and intestinal lymphoma.

Management. A gluten-free diet should be instituted after a firm diagnosis has been established. Wheat, barley, and rye should be definitely avoided. The toxicity of oats in sprue remains controversial, and this may be a reflection of the low concentration of the putative offending agent in oats. A consultation with a dietitian is quite helpful, because many processed foods contain wheat products. Rice- and corn-based recipes are nontoxic. Patients should be encouraged to contact one of the national support organizations for specific information, including gluten-free recipes.

Most patients improve symptomatically within weeks of beginning a gluten-free diet, but the histologic lesion may take months or even years to resolve. A repeat small bowel biopsy several months after institution of therapy is recommended. Vitamin and mineral deficiencies should be treated initially with supplementation, but typically the deficiencies are reversed rapidly as small bowel absorption normalizes. Although adolescents may tolerate gluten to a variable extent, they should be encouraged to maintain a strict gluten-free diet, especially since the relationship between dietary compliance and long-term complications such as lymphoma or adenocarcinoma is unclear.

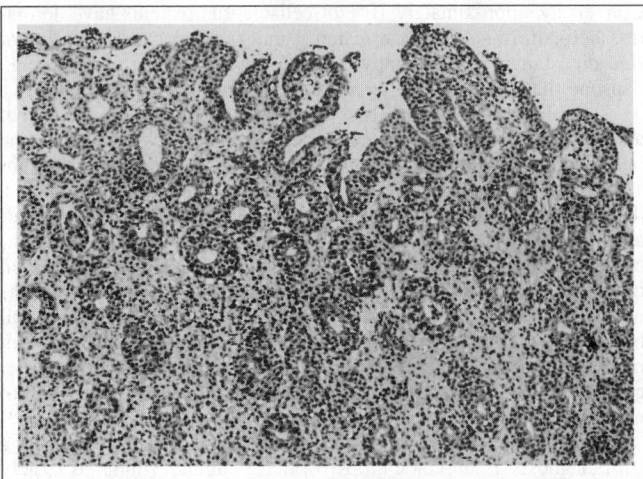

FIGURE 340-5 Enteropathy-associated T-cell lymphoma arising in sprue with marked infiltration of glandular epithelium by atypical lymphocytes. Hematoxylin and eosin, medium power (220×).

Photomicrograph courtesy L.J. Burgart, M.D.

Unclassified, Refractory, and Collagenous Sprue, and Nongranulomatous Ulcerative Jejunoileitis

A small group of patients with clinical and histologic features characteristic of celiac sprue do not respond to a strict gluten-free diet. By definition they do not have celiac sprue; rather, they have unclassified sprue. Occasional celiac sprue patients who were initially responsive to a gluten-free diet will become symptomatic again despite careful exclusion of dietary gluten, and hence have refractory sprue. These syndromes are ill-defined and somewhat heterogeneous from the standpoint of etiology and treatment. Occasional patients respond to withdrawal of other dietary items such as soybeans, chicken, tuna, or eggs. Other patients are found to have an associated microscopic or lymphocytic colitis. Still others have an underlying enteropathy-associated T-cell lymphoma, which on histologic examination can mimic sprue in its early stages. Initial treatment of unclassified and refractory sprue consists of oral corticosteroids, which can induce a remission in approximately 50% of patients. Azathioprine or cyclosporine may be beneficial in selected cases. A trial of total parenteral nutrition with careful stepwise reintroduction of dietary items may be helpful in identifying an offending non-gluten substance. A lack of response to these measures heralds a poor prognosis. Early referral of refractory patients to tertiary medical centers is recommended.

Some patients who fail to respond to, or relapse despite, a gluten-free diet are found to have a thick band of collagen in the lamina propria beneath the basement membrane of the intestinal epithelial cells. Whether such patients with collagenous sprue represent a separate disease entity is unclear, especially since some celiac sprue patients with similar histologic findings are gluten-responsive. An association with collagenous colitis has been described. Gluten-refractory patients should be treated with corticosteroids and/or immunosuppressive agents. In general, response to therapy and prognosis are poor.

Nongranulomatous ulcerative jejunoileitis (nongranulomatous chronic idiopathic enterocolitis) is another chronic inflammatory disease of the small bowel resulting in malabsorption. Its relationship to celiac sprue, unclassified sprue and enteropathy-associated T-cell lymphoma is unclear, and this likely reflects the grouping of several disorders under the same syndrome. Patients are typically middle-aged and present with abdominal pain, diarrhea, malabsorption, and gastrointestinal bleeding. A history of celiac sprue may or may not be present. Grossly there is extensive ulceration in the distal duodenum, jejunum, and sometimes ileum. The lesion can be indistinguishable on histologic examination from that of celiac sprue. The lesion appears to represent an early form of enteropathy-associated T-cell lymphoma in some patients (Fig. 340-5), so biopsy material should be carefully examined for evidence of neoplasia. Treatment, which consists of corticosteroids, total parenteral nutrition, and sometimes surgery, is often ineffective.

Whipple's Disease

Whipple's disease (intestinal lipodystrophy) is a rare, chronic, systemic bacterial infection typically affecting middle-aged white men. The gastrointestinal tract is almost always involved, and many symptoms arise from malabsorption; however, systemic symptoms or those arising from involvement of other organ systems sometimes predominate. The putative pathogen is a gram-positive bacillus that remains uncultured but has been characterized through polymerase chain reaction (PCR)-based techniques as an actinomycete-like organism. Formerly a fatal, progressive disease, it is quite responsive to antibiotics, although relapses are common.

Pathophysiologic Findings. The "Whipple's bacillus" has been located in numerous organs including small intestine, large intestine, lymph nodes (mesenteric and peripheral), central nervous system, eye, pericardium, endocardium, liver, lung, synovium, and skin. Small bowel biopsy typically shows flat or shortened villi with dilated lacteals, and the lamina propria is packed with macrophages that stain strongly with the periodic acid-Schiff (PAS) stain (Fig. 340-6). The PAS-positive material represents bacilli in various stages of digestion. In addition, there are free bacilli between the macrophages. The electron micrographic appearance of the bacillus is very specific and can be used to substantiate the diagnosis in the absence of PCR. Malabsorption results from a loss of absorptive surface, and protein-losing enteropathy due to mesenteric lymphatic obstruction is common.

The bacillus remains uncultured despite numerous attempts. PCR-based techniques were recently used to recover and identify ribosomal RNA from diseased duodenal tissue and lymph nodes. Phylogenetically the RNA appears most closely related to actinomycetes, and it has been named *Trophyrema whippeli*. Similar techniques have been used to recover *T. whippeli* RNA from peripheral blood and ocular tissue in patients with histologically normal small bowel biopsies. Several pieces of circumstantial evidence suggest that an abnormality of the host immune system is an important cofactor in pathogenesis: the rarity of disease, the lack of secondary infection, minimal tissue inflammation despite high bacterial loads, persistent lymphocytopenia, and diminished cutaneous delayed hypersensitivity. The HLA-B27 antigen is present more frequently than would be expected by chance.

Clinical and Laboratory Features and Diagnosis. Although signs and symptoms related to malabsorption and protein-losing enteropathy are frequent, the manifestations are often protean. Diarrhea and weight loss are often prominent, as is edema. Other symptoms depend on the degree of extraintestinal involvement. Approximately two thirds of patients have arthralgias or a nondestructive arthritis affecting the large joints. Joint symptoms may precede gastrointestinal symptoms by years. Fever, lymphadenopathy, pleuritis, pericarditis, cardiac murmurs, uveitis, and hyperpigmentation can also be features. CNS symptoms may include dementia; ophthalmoplegia; myoclonus; hypothalamic symptoms of disordered sleep, hunger, or thirst; ataxia; and the rare but pathognomonic oculomasticatory myorhythmia. Rarely patients present with prominent neurologic symptoms and little or no gastrointestinal involvement.

The diagnosis has been traditionally based on biopsy of involved tissue, usually from the duodenum or jejunum. Although the histologic lesion in the small bowel is specific, it can be patchy, and rarely the small bowel is uninvolved. If routine histologic findings are equivocal, electron microscopy of involved tissue reveals characteristic changes. PCR-based assays of blood and involved tissues may one day replace small bowel biopsy as the diagnostic test of choice, but more data regarding test specificity are required.

Differential Diagnosis. When gastrointestinal symptoms predominate, Whipple's disease can be confused with other malabsorptive disorders, but the small bowel histologic findings are quite specific, with one exception. Patients with acquired immunodeficiency syndrome (AIDS) who present with diarrhea may have a similar small intestinal lesion in that the PAS stain is strongly positive, but these

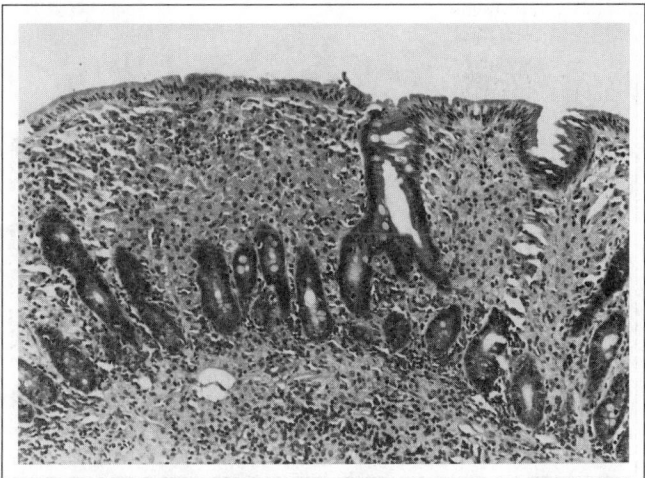

A

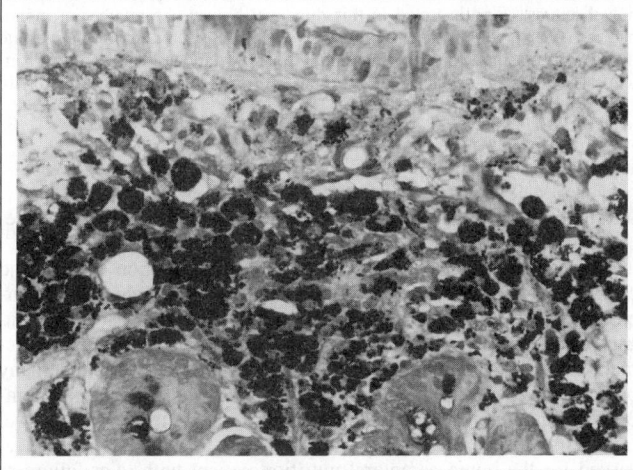

B

FIGURE 340-6 Whipple's disease. **A,** Characteristic foamy histiocytes within the lamina propria and resultant loss of villous architecture. Hematoxylin and eosin, medium power (200×). **B,** The individual bacilli show intense positive staining with PAS, which is resistant to diastase digestion. PAS and diastase, high power (480×).

Photomicrograph courtesy L.J. Burgart, M.D.

patients almost always have *Mycobacterium avium-intracellulare* infection. An acid-fast stain will differentiate the two conditions. Gastric and rectal biopsies should not be relied on to make a diagnosis of Whipple's disease because macrophages in these regions may normally stain for PAS.

Patients with predominantly extraintestinal symptoms can be difficult to diagnose. Whipple's disease should be considered in patients with fever of unknown origin, especially if lymphadenopathy and arthralgias are present; "sarcoidosis" that does not respond to conventional treatment; and unexplained neurologic symptoms, especially dementia, ophthalmoplegia, and myoclonus.

Management. The clinical response to antibiotics is usually quite gratifying. Gastrointestinal symptoms improve within days to weeks. The histologic abnormalities can take months or even years to resolve, although electron microscopy often demonstrates absence of viable bacilli. Clinical relapses have occurred in about one third of patients, especially those treated initially with tetracycline. CNS relapses may be antibiotic-resistant and fatal. Double-strength trimethoprim-sulfamethoxazole (TMP-SMX) twice daily for 1 year is the treatment of choice because it has excellent CNS penetration. For ill, hospitalized patients, a 2-week course of parenteral penicillin and streptomycin in addition to TMP-SMX is recommended. Short-

term vitamin and mineral supplementation may be required. For sulfa-allergic patients, chloramphenicol or cefixime is appropriate. Whether small bowel biopsies should be performed after completion of treatment to document eradication is controversial; certainly, a biopsy should be obtained when a clinical relapse is suspected. The use of PCR as a test-of-cure appears promising.

Tropical Sprue

Tropical sprue is a poorly understood disorder of small bowel absorption that occurs among residents of certain tropical areas, especially the Indian subcontinent, southeast Asia, and the Caribbean. The illness is endemic in these areas, both among natives and expatriates, although epidemics following outbreaks of acute diarrhea have occurred. Visitors have been known to develop the illness within weeks after a visit to the tropics, but it more typically occurs in expatriates who have lived in the tropics for at least 1 year. Expatriates may develop the illness months or even years after returning to temperate climes.

Pathophysiologic Features. The illness may be mediated by colonization of the small bowel with various toxigenic strains of coliform bacteria; however, bacteria are not uniformly cultured from the small bowel of tropical sprue patients, and viral infection may also be involved. Most but not all expatriates report an acute episode of diarrhea before the onset of illness. The mechanism by which coliforms or viruses persistently colonize the small bowel is unclear. In contradistinction to small bowel bacterial overgrowth, intraluminal concentrations of anaerobic bacteria are not elevated; thus malabsorption cannot be explained by deconjugation of bile salts. The offending agents are thought to elucidate cytotoxins or secretagogues, resulting in injury to the small intestinal epithelium. Since many patients improve with folate or vitamin B_{12} supplementation alone, malnutrition may somehow contribute to pathogenesis; however, well-nourished nonnative residents are susceptible to disease.

Small bowel biopsy typically shows broadened, shortened villi; elongated crypts; acute and chronic inflammation in the lamina propria; and lymphocytic infiltration of the epithelium. Small intestinal absorption is globally impaired, with net secretion of water and electrolytes, and diminished fat, carbohydrate and peptide absorption.

Clinical and Laboratory Features and Diagnosis. The illness frequently follows an episode of acute diarrhea and is characterized by steatorrhea, anorexia, abdominal pain and bloating, and weight loss. If the illness is unrecognized or untreated, nutritional deficiencies result in anemia, glossitis, stomatitis, and, rarely, neurologic complications of vitamin B_{12} deficiency.

Laboratory tests reveal megaloblastic anemia, folate and/or vitamin B_{12} deficiency, and impaired D-xylose, fat and vitamin B_{12} absorption. Small bowel biopsy usually reveals the changes noted, although rarely the injury can be so severe as to mimic celiac sprue, with total villous atrophy.

Management. Treatment consists of folic acid, 5 mg daily, and tetracycline, 250 mg four times daily. The response to therapy is often quite rapid, especially if the patient has returned to temperate climes, but the occasional patient will require therapy for up to 6 months. Nutritional supplements such as vitamin B_{12}, fat-soluble vitamins, and iron may be required as well. Recurrence is a possibility if the patient remains a resident of the tropics.

Radiation Enteropathy

Injury to the small bowel following radiation therapy to the pelvis, retroperitoneum, or mesentery is common. Acute histologic injury occurs in up to 90% of patients receiving 3000 cGy of radiotherapy, but clinical disease is typically mild and self-limited. Chronic radiation enteropathy presents months to years after completion of radiotherapy. Once thought to be an unusual complication, in some series up to 90% of patients receiving abdominal or pelvic irradiation demonstrate alterations in bowel habit or malabsorption. Chronic injury arises from an irreversible progressive obliterative endarteritis of the submucosa. The resulting ischemia can lead to mucosal ulceration, intestinal fibrosis, strictures, and fistulas.

The malabsorption is frequently multifactorial. Causes include bile salt malabsorption secondary to ileal involvement; small bowel bacterial overgrowth due to strictures, fistulas, and alterations in motility; intestinal lymphangiectasia due to lymphatic obstruction; and lactose intolerance due to brush border injury.

Although the overall diagnosis is straightforward when the history of radiotherapy is obtained, specific tests such as absorption of D-xylose or vitamin B_{12}, fecal fat collection, and barium examination of the small bowel may help delineate the exact nature of malabsorption. Treatment of mild disease consists of antidiarrheals, antispasmodics, cholestyramine, and a lactose-free diet. In moderate cases, a low-fat diet, oral antibiotics, or low-residue enteral feedings are employed. Severe cases may require total parenteral nutrition along with complete bowel rest. Surgery may be required for resection of high-grade strictures or persistent fistulas, but it is fraught with complications such as inadvertent enterotomies in a surgical field dense with adhesions, or poor anastomotic healing in the remaining diseased bowel.

Short Bowel Syndrome

Short bowel syndrome encompasses the clinical consequences of extensive intestinal resection, including diarrhea, fluid and electrolyte abnormalities, and malabsorption. In adults, Crohn's disease, intestinal infarction due to vascular insult, trauma, and radiation enteropathy are the most frequent conditions leading to extensive resection. In children, intestinal atresia, volvulus, or necrotizing enterocolitis may result in wide resection.

The type and severity of malabsorption depend on the extent and site of bowel resection. Removal of up to 50% of the small bowel is generally well tolerated from the standpoint of maintaining nutritional requirements. Proximal resection results in malabsorption of iron, calcium, and folate, whereas distal resections lead to vitamin B_{12} and bile salt malabsorption. In general, resection of the jejunum is better tolerated than ileal resection, because ileal mucosa is more adaptable. Limited resections (i.e., less than 100 cm) of terminal ileum may lead to cholerrheic or bile salt–induced diarrhea, which may respond to cholestyramine. However, wider resection results in more severe bile salt malabsorption for which increased hepatic synthesis of bile salts cannot compensate, and cholestyramine may actually worsen steatorrhea. Resection of the ileocecal valve results in faster intestinal transit and small bowel bacterial overgrowth, with its attendant effects on bile salts and vitamin B_{12}. The quality of the remaining intestinal mucosa affects severity, so patients with residual Crohn's disease or radiation enteropathy do more poorly. Patients with colon remaining are prone to oxalate hyperabsorption because the calcium that normally binds to oxalate in the intestinal lumen complexes instead with luminal fatty acids. Such patients are at risk for nephrolithiasis.

Treatment immediately following extensive resection consists of total parenteral nutrition, with careful replacement of fluid, electrolytes, vitamins, and minerals and antisecretory therapy with H_2 blockers or proton pump inhibitors to combat the gastric hypersecretion that usually occurs transiently. Elemental or semi-elemental enteral feeds should be introduced early (but slowly) so as to stimulate adaptation of the remaining intestinal mucosa. These enteral formulas should be diluted to reduce hyperosmolarity. Intraluminal administration of glutamine, the major fuel source for enterocytes, may further enhance intestinal adaptation.

Once evidence of ongoing adaptation has occurred, food may be gradually reintroduced. In patients with remaining colon, fat intake must be limited to minimize hydroxy-fatty acid–induced colonic diarrhea and to limit oxalate hyperabsorption. Such patients also require a low-oxalate diet. Fat and oxalate intake are less of an issue in patients with small intestinal ostomies; however, these patients may need to limit intake of high-osmolarity liquids. Lactose-free diets may help control diarrhea and bloating in patients with or without remaining colon. Medium-chain triglycerides (MCTs) are hydrolyzed, solubilized, and absorbed quite easily and may be a useful dietary supplement. Even when weight and overall nutritional parameters have stabilized, specific vitamin and mineral deficiencies may require ongoing supplementation. Vitamin B_{12}, fat-soluble vitamins, calcium, magnesium, iron, and zinc are the most common deficiencies seen.

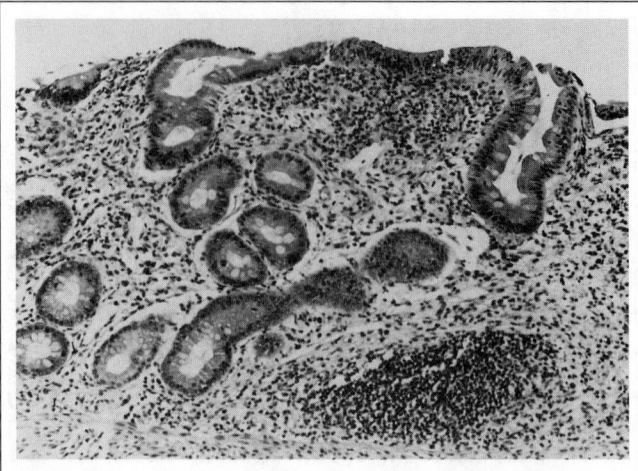

FIGURE 340-7 Hypogammaglobulinemia and related immunodeficiency states often show absence of plasma cells in the lamina propria of the small bowel mucosa. As illustrated in this duodenal biopsy, the number of mononuclear cells (predominantly lymphocytes) may be essentially normal despite the lack of plasma cells. The immunodeficiency state can lead to enteric infections, in this case causing a superficial neutrophilic infiltrate. Hematoxylin and eosin, medium power (180×).

Photomicrograph courtesy L.J. Burgart, M.D.

Intermittent treatment with antibiotics to combat small bowel bacterial overgrowth may be required.

A small subset of patients cannot avoid malnutrition or fluid and electrolyte abnormalities on oral intake and therefore require total parenteral nutrition indefinitely. Multidisciplinary home parenteral nutrition programs have refined the techniques of vascular access placement and care, patient education, and overnight infusion, so that many patients lead full, productive lives. However, infections and thrombotic complications remain a problem for some patients. Small bowel transplantation is an evolving technique that at present should be reserved for the home parenteral nutrition patient with liver failure or with no remaining vascular access.

Hypogammaglobulinemia

Diarrhea and malabsorption are seen in almost two thirds of patients with common variable hypogammaglobulinemia, one of the most common acquired defects of immunity. Infection with *Giardia lamblia* in these patients is common and results in mucosal inflammation and steatorrhea. Other disorders associated with common variable hypogammaglobulinemia include celiac sprue, unclassified or refractory sprue, selective IgA deficiency, pernicious anemia, small bowel bacterial overgrowth, Crohn's disease, and infectious gastroenteritis (both bacterial and viral pathogens).

The diagnosis should be suspected in patients with diarrhea, recurrent respiratory tract infections, recurrent and severe giardiasis, and diarrhea associated with prominent lymphoid nodular hyperplasia. Stool studies for bacterial pathogens, ova, and parasites may point to a specific cause. Duodenal aspirates for parasites and bacterial culture should be obtained. A low vitamin B_{12} level suggests bacterial overgrowth or Crohn's disease. Small bowel biopsy characteristically shows absence of plasma cells in the lamina propria (Fig. 340-7), but may also show evidence of giardiasis or a sprue-like condition.

Therapy is targeted toward the specific abnormality, such as metronidazole for giardiasis, antibiotics for bacterial overgrowth, or a gluten-free diet for celiac sprue. Patients who do not improve on a gluten-free diet despite the finding of villous atrophy on biopsy may benefit from corticosteroids or gamma globulin.

Eosinophilic Gastroenteritis

Eosinophilic gastroenteritis is a rare, idiopathic disorder of the gut characterized by eosinophilic infiltration of various gut wall layers

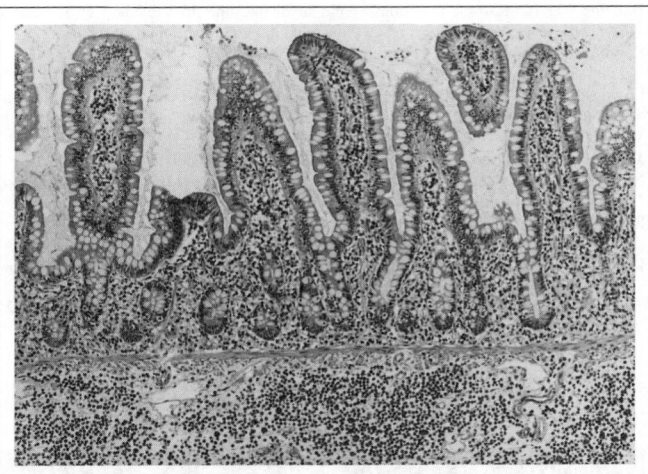

FIGURE 340-8 Eosinophilic enteritis is characterized by dense eosinophilic leukocyte infiltrates with no other histologic or clinical explanation (e.g., parasitic infection). The numerous inflammatory cells present in the submucosa are essentially all eosinophils. Although it can cause mucosal damage, it can also largely spare the mucosa as shown here. This feature may lead to false-negative mucosal endoscopic biopsies. Hematoxylin and eosin, medium power (180×).

Photomicrograph courtesy L.J. Burgart, M.D.

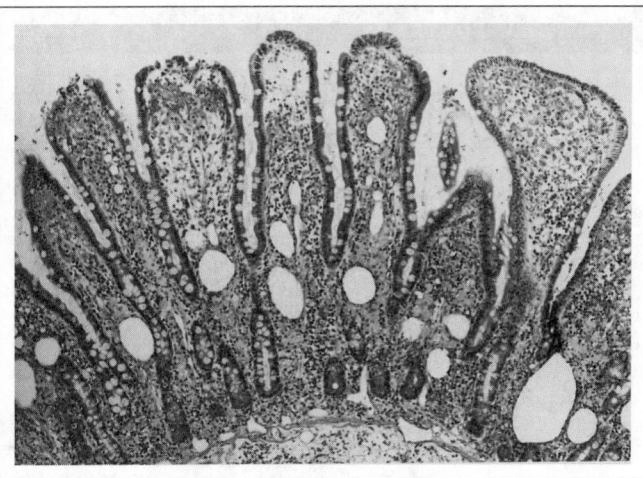

FIGURE 340-9 Intestinal lymphangiectasia, in this case secondary to Whipple's disease. The lymph channel dilation demonstrates the rich lymphatic network within the small bowel mucosa. Lymphangiectasia can result from mass effect or infection, or as a primary idiopathic process. Hematoxylin and eosin, medium power (180×).

Photomicrograph courtesy L.J. Burgart, M.D.

and peripheral eosinophilia. A personal or family history of atopy cannot be elicited in a substantial fraction of patients. Occasionally a history of symptoms precipitated by a specific foodstuff can be obtained, so food allergy may play a role; however, elemental or elimination diets benefit only a few patients.

Clinical features depend on the site and layer of gut wall involved. When eosinophilic infiltration is predominantly mucosal and submucosal, diarrhea, weight loss, abdominal pain, and malabsorption are the usual presenting symptoms. In addition to the usual laboratory features of malabsorption, there may be Charcot-Leyden crystals detected in the stool. Barium examination may demonstrate mucosal thickening of the stomach or small bowel. Biopsy of the small bowel demonstrates patchy infiltration of the mucosa and/or submucosa with numerous eosinophils (Fig. 340-8).

When the muscular layer of the gut is predominantly involved, symptoms are usually obstructive in nature. Barium examination reveals narrowing in the gastric antrum or small bowel, which can also mimic malignant disease. Since the eosinophilic infiltration is deep, endoscopic biopsies may be misleadingly normal, and a full-thickness biopsy may be required. Rarely, the serosal layer of the gut is primarily involved, and eosinophilic ascites is the presenting feature.

Treatment usually consists of a short course of oral corticosteroids, and response to therapy is usually dramatic. Efforts to exclude other illness such as hypereosinophilic syndrome, polyarteritis nodosa, and parasitic infestations should be made before starting corticosteroid therapy. Over the long term, disease activity will wax and wane, and repeat courses of steroids may be required. The occasional patient with a clear-cut history of symptoms triggered by food will benefit from an elemental or elimination diet.

Intestinal Lymphangiectasia

Lymphangiectasia is characterized by dilated lacteals due to intestinal, mesenteric, or more proximal lymphatic obstruction. When the dilated lacteals rupture, lymphocytes and protein-rich lymph exude into the intestinal lumen, resulting in lymphocytopenia and a protein-losing enteropathy. Lymphatic obstruction also leads to poor absorption of fat and fat-soluble vitamins. Intestinal lymphangiectasia may be a primary congenital malformation of the lymphatics or may occur secondary to another condition such as lymphoma, carcinoma, retroperitoneal fibrosis, sarcoidosis, tuberculosis, Whipple's disease, and constrictive pericarditis.

In primary intestinal lymphangiectasia, symptoms often appear in

infancy. Steatorrhea, growth failure, lymphocytopenia, and hypoalbuminemia suggest the diagnosis. Asymmetric lymphedema of the extremities is common. Secondary lymphangiectasia should be suspected in patients with underlying neoplasm or infection who develop steatorrhea, hypoalbuminemia, and weight loss. Small bowel biopsy reveals dilated lacteals and widened villi due to edema (Fig. 340-9). Computed tomography of the abdomen or echocardiography may be helpful in detecting the underlying abnormality in secondary lymphangiectasia.

Treatment should first be directed toward the underlying cause. For congenital disease, or for refractory secondary cases, MCT supplements should be substituted for long-chain triglycerides in the diet. MCTs are absorbed via the portal system rather than the lymphatics, thereby improving fat absorption and decreasing lymph flow. This may result in decreased protein loss and improvement of hypoalbuminemia.

Abetalipoproteinemia

Abetalipoproteinemia is a rare genetic disorder characterized by fat malabsorption, acanthocytosis of erythrocytes, and low plasma lipid levels. A defect in assembly of apolipoprotein B–containing lipoproteins results in failure to assemble and secrete chylomicrons and very-low-density lipoproteins. Mucosal absorption of lipids is normal but secretion is limited; thus small bowel biopsy reveals lipid-filled intestinal epithelial cells.

The disorder presents in infancy with steatorrhea, acanthocytosis, and neurologic sequelae of fat-soluble vitamin deficiencies such as ataxia, nystagmus, sensory loss, and retinopathy. Treatment consists of fat restriction, MCT supplements, and fat-soluble vitamin supplements.

Variants of abetalipoproteinemia, such as chylomicron retention disease (Anderson's disease) and normotriglyceridemic abetalipoproteinemia, represent selective abnormalities of lipoprotein B secretion. In these disorders, acanthocytosis is absent and plasma lipid levels are normal, but steatorrhea and neurologic abnormalities are present. Treatment is similar to that of classic abetalipoproteinemia.

Carbohydrate Intolerance

The absorption of carbohydrates requires hydrolysis of disaccharides to monosaccharides by enzymes located on the brush border of enterocytes. Carbohydrate intolerance results from primary deficiency of a specific disaccharidase or global deficiency secondary to a diffuse mucosal process.

✔ *WHEN TO REFER*

To establish the presence of small bowel malabsorption does not require specialist referral. Once small bowel malabsorption has been confirmed in a patient, however, a gastroenterologist will have much to offer in further diagnosis and management. Many of the investigations that may be required for the evaluation of malabsorption, especially the invasive ones, are best performed by a specialist. Furthermore, because the recommended therapies for some of the causes of malabsorption continue to evolve rapidly (e.g., for bacterial overgrowth), and the treatment of other causes may involve the use and titration of immunosuppressive agents, the advise of a specialist with regular experience in managing the causes of small bowel malabsorption can be invaluable. Consultation with a gastroenterlogist once small bowel malabsorption has been established would be the optimal course.

Adult lactase deficiency is the most common cause of carbohydrate intolerance, occurring in more than half the world's adult population. The prevalence of lactase deficiency with delayed onset is 5% to 15% in northern Europeans but is much higher in other populations, approaching 100% in Asians. In fact, a physiologic decline in lactase activity after weaning appears to be the norm.

Symptoms include abdominal distention, bloating, abdominal cramping, flatulence, and diarrhea following ingestion of milk. The amount of lactose required to produce symptoms varies considerably. Concomitant irritable bowel syndrome may result in symptoms of milk intolerance at lower amounts of ingestion.

The diagnosis is suspected when a history of milk intolerance is obtained, especially when the patient is from an ethnic group with a high prevalence of lactase deficiency. The diagnosis can be confirmed with the lactose tolerance test, when the ingestion of 50 g of lactose produces symptoms and there is a blunting of the normal 20 mg/dl increase in blood glucose. However, alterations in gastric motility and glucose metabolism lower the diagnostic accuracy of the test. The lactose hydrogen breath test, in which breath hydrogen is measured after ingestion of 50 g of lactose, is more sensitive and specific, but it may be affected by abnormalities in intestinal motility and colonic bacteria.

Treatment consists primarily of reduction of lactose in the diet. Complete withdrawal is rarely necessary. Lactase enzymes in capsule or tablet form can be taken with lactose-containing foods and beverages to avoid symptoms.

Congenital deficiencies of disaccharidases are rare but important causes of carbohydrate intolerance. Congenital lactase deficiency becomes manifest early in infancy as severe diarrhea after the introduction of breast milk or lactose-containing formulas and responds to withdrawal of lactose. Sucrase-isomaltase deficiency occurs in up to 10% of Native Alaskans and presents as diarrhea and weight loss shortly after weaning. Diagnosis is made by the oral sucrose tolerance test or sucrose hydrogen breath test, and a sucrose-free diet results in improvement. Congenital glucose-galactose malabsorption results from a defect in intestinal transport of glucose and galactose. Severe diarrhea begins shortly after birth. Treatment consists of fructose-based formulas and dietary exclusion of glucose and galactose.

The most common example of secondary carbohydrate intolerance is lactose intolerance following infectious gastroenteritis or before institution of treatment for celiac sprue. Treatment is directed toward the primary process, with gradual reintroduction of lactose.

BIBLIOGRAPHY

Brasitus TA, Sitrin MD: Short bowel syndrome. In Yamada T et al, editors: *Textbook of gastroenterology,* ed 2, Philadelphia, 1995, JB Lippincott, p. 1680.
Dicke WK: Coeliac disease: investigation of the harmful effects of certain types of cereal on patients with coeliac disease. Thesis, University of Utrecht, The Netherlands, 1950 (in Dutch).

Dobbins WO III: Chronic infections of the small intestine. In Yamada T et al, editors: *Textbook of gastroenterology,* ed 2, Philadelphia, 1995, JB Lippincott, p. 1630.
Kagnoff MF: Celiac disease. In Yamada T et al, editors: *Textbook of gastroenterology,* ed 2, Philadelphia, 1995, JB Lippincott, p. 1643.
Lloyd ML, Olsen WA: Disorders of epithelial transport in the small intestine. In Yamada T et al, editors: *Textbook of gastroenterology,* ed 2, Philadelphia, 1995, JB Lippincott, p. 1661.
Malagelada JR: Lactose intolerance, *N Engl J Med* 333:53, 1995.
Nostrant TT et al: Radiation injury. In Yamada T et al, editors: *Textbook of gastroenterology,* ed 2, Philadelphia, 1995, JB Lippincott, p. 2524.
Ramzan NN et al: Diagnosis and monitoring of Whipple's disease by polymerase chain reaction, *Ann Intern Med* 126:520-527, 1997.
Relman DA et al: Identification of the uncultured bacillus of Whipple's disease, *N Engl J Med* 327:293, 1992.
Talley NJ et al: Eosinophilic gastroenteritis: a clinicopathologic study of patients with disease of the mucosae, muscle layer and subserosal tissues, *Gut* 31:54, 1990.

CHAPTER

341   Idiopathic Inflammatory Bowel Disease

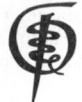

Stephen B. Hanauer

The term *inflammatory bowel disease* (IBD) encompasses a spectrum of infectious and noninfectious disorders of the gastrointestinal tract but refers primarily to two idiopathic syndromes: ulcerative colitis and Crohn's disease. *Ulcerative colitis* is manifest by a diffuse, continuous pattern of superficial inflammation limited to the colonic mucosa, always involving the rectum and extending proximal to an upper margin that varies between individuals. The pattern of ulcerative colitis is defined by the extent of disease: ulcerative proctitis is confined to the rectum, proctosigmoiditis to the sigmoid colon, left-sided colitis to the splenic flexure, or extensive (pan-)colitis involving the colon proximal to the splenic flexure. *Backwash ileitis* refers to minor involvement of the terminal ileum that may occur in the setting of extensive colitis. In contrast, the inflammatory process in *Crohn's disease* is focal, often transmural, and may affect any portion of the alimentary canal. Older synonyms for Crohn's disease include descriptive terms such as *terminal ileitis, granulomatous* or *regional enteritis,* or *colitis.* Presently Crohn's disease can be categorized by the site of macroscopic disease as *gastroduodenitis, jejunoileitis, ileitis, ileocolitis,* or *colitis.* Although Crohn's disease and ulcerative colitis represent an overlapping clinical spectrum, they will be discussed separately.

ETIOLOGIC FACTORS

The cause of IBD remains unknown. Although infectious agents have been implicated, particularly in Crohn's disease, in which atypical mycobacteria or measles viral antigen have been identified in a small minority of patients, Koch's postulates remain unfulfilled. Likewise, various immunologic phenomena have been described (e.g., variations in cytokine profiles or lymphocyte subpopulations), but a primary (predisposing) immunologic abnormality has yet to be elucidated. Currently, research into the etiology is focusing on genetic factors—a tenfold increased risk of disease has been recognized in first-degree relatives of patients. In addition, there is an increased concordance of disease type (including location and pattern of inflammation and complications) in maternal compared with paternal twins. The mode of inheritance is unclear, however, and is probably different for ulcerative colitis and Crohn's disease, with a strong likelihood of multiple genes being involved. Most investigators speculate that the diseases are related to the interaction of genetic susceptibility with as yet undiscovered environmental factors. Potential triggers may include normal intestinal constituents or a metabolic product of the gut microflora. To date, the only epidemilogic difference, aside from the family pattern of disease,

The authors thank Lawrence J. Burgart, M.D., for graciously providing all of the photomicrographs for this chapter.

between ulcerative colitis and Crohn's disease is exposure to cigarette smoking. Cigarette smoking has a protective effect against ulcerative colitis but is recognized to have a negative impact on Crohn's disease. It is uncommon for smokers to develop ulcerative colitis while they are still smoking, whereas smokers with Crohn's disease are more refractory to medical management and have a greater likelihood of developing recurrence after surgery. As yet, no specific dietary factor or psychologic profile has been found to predispose to the development of IBD.

INCIDENCE AND EPIDEMIOLOGY

The incidence and prevalence of IBD vary widely throughout the world but, as with other "autoimmune" disorders, there is a correlation between improved sanitation and the prevalence of IBD. These diseases are more common in the United States and Europe than in Asia or the tropics, where there is a high incidence of infectious diarrhea. In the United States and Europe, most studies indicate a range of 5 to 15 new cases per 100,000 population per year. The estimated prevalence approximates 100 cases per 100,000 population. Although the incidence of ulcerative colitis has stabilized in developed countries, the incidence of Crohn's disease appears to have increased. Furthermore, as IBD begins to appear in developing countries, the incidence of ulcerative colitis consistently occurs about one decade before the rise of Crohn's disease. This seems to be a true pattern rather than merely an increased awareness of the conditions. IBD affects both sexes equally. The peak age at onset is in the second to fourth decades, but new cases in infants and octogenarians also occur. Other interesting observations of unclear significance include an increased occurrence of IBD among Jews, at least in North America, and a greater incidence in whites than in non-white races. However, as stated, there is an increasing incidence and prevalence in developing countries corresponding to "Westernization" of diet and life-style.

CROHN'S DISEASE
Clinical Features

Crohn's disease can affect any portion of the gastrointestinal tract from the mouth to the anus. The pattern of intestinal involvement can be classified by the anatomic location and the pattern of gross inflammatory features. Most commonly the ileocecal (ileocolitis) region is involved (45%), followed in frequency by ileitis (30%) and colitis (15%). Less commonly the upper gastroduodenal regions are involved or the disease affects most of the small bowel (jejunoileitis). Aphthous ulcerations are common in patients, as are perianal manifestations of external skin tags (mistaken for hemorrhoids) and perianal abscesses of fistulae.

The classic pathologic features are focal, asymmetric, and transmural inflammation. Microscopic changes often are present in normal appearing mucosa at distant sites from macroscopically involved intestine. More than one area may be affected while the intervening bowel appears grossly normal, giving rise to so-called skip areas. Other typical gross findings are a thickened intestinal wall, mucosal fissuring, fistulas, inflammatory masses, and benign strictures. A "cobblestone" appearance results from normal or edematous mucosa that is transsected by communicating deep fissures and linear ulcerations. The pattern of inflammation can further categorize individuals or families with similar manifestations of inflammation alone (inflammatory subtype), strictures (fibrostenosing subtype) or inflammatory mass and fistula (fistulizing subtype). There is a consistency within individuals; recurrences after intestinal resection tend to be of the same inflammatory pattern.

The histologic lesions of Crohn's disease evolve from aphthous ulceration: lymphoid aggregation underneath M cells associated with erosions of the overlying mucosa. The microscopic ulcerations can extend in a variety of sizes and shapes: in a superficial pattern, producing linear ulcerations; through the mucosa and submucosa, producing transmural inflammation and fissures; or through the serosa into an adjacent structure, producing a fistula. The submucosa is edematous and contains nodular aggregates and dense infiltrates of lymphocytes and plasma cells. There may be lymphatic inflammation and secondary intestinal lymphangiectasia. Fibrosis may be ex-

tensive and may cause luminal narrowing, leading to bowel obstruction. Even the mesentery may be edematous and thickened, with mesenteric fat wrapping around the bowel. Mesenteric lymph nodes become hyperplastic and are densely packed with chronic inflammatory cells.

Another characteristic feature of Crohn's disease is the formation of noncaseating, sarcoidlike granulomas (Color Plate X-4). These are present in as many as 30% to 40% of conventionally examined, resected intestinal specimens and may also be found in areas that appear normal grossly and in the mesenteric lymph nodes. Although the presence of granulomas is extremely helpful in making the diagnosis of Crohn's disease, their absence does not rule out this diagnosis; they are far less commonly identified from typical mucosal biopsy specimens.

Clinical and Laboratory Findings

The clinical features of Crohn's disease depend on the site and severity of inflammation along the gastrointestinal tract. Common clinical features of Crohn's disease include diarrhea, abdominal pain, fever, and weight loss. Extraintestinal symptoms may precede abdominal complaints, especially in children in whom abnormalities of growth or sexual maturation, arthritis, or fevers of undetermined origin are common. Due to the protean manifestations and potential extraintestinal presentations, a delay in diagnosis is common.

Diarrhea is common with Crohn's disease and may have several possible causes. Inflammation of the small or large intestine leads to exudation of blood and protein as well as secretion of fluid and electrolytes. Depending on the location and extent of small bowel inflammation, there may be malabsorption of carbohydrates (e.g., lactose), fat, water- or fat-soluble vitamins, or vitamin B_{12}. Disease of the terminal ileum may cause malabsorption of bile salts, leading to ion and water secretion by the colon (so-called cholorrheic enteropathy). After resection of more than 100 cm of distal ileum, greater degrees of bile salt loss may occur, resulting in a greatly diminished total bile salt pool and producing steatorrhea caused by impaired intraluminal micelle formation. Small bowel strictures can cause stasis, producing malabsorption that results from bacterial overgrowth. Colon or rectal involvement may lead to diarrhea secondary to reduced colonic water resorption and accompanied by tenesmus and hematochezia. Occasionally, a submucosal vessel is eroded, leading to massive bleeding in Crohn's disease; this may be a presenting feature.

Abdominal pain is more common in Crohn's disease than in ulcerative colitis because of the transmural nature of intestinal inflammation and the location of pain receptors of the gut in the serosa and peritoneum. Nociceptors are not present in the mucosa. The location of pain is most often in the right lower quadrant, but it may be anywhere, reflecting the site of transmural involvement. If there is partial small bowel obstruction, the pain is often colicky and is aggravated by eating. A constant pain associated with spiking fever and leukocytosis should arouse suspicion of abscess formation. However, low-grade fever and malaise are common and may occur solely on the basis of bowel inflammation.

Perirectal disease, including abscess, fistulas, and anal fissures, may be a prominent feature of Crohn's disease (Color Plate X-5). Such conditions may precede or occur concomitantly with intestinal disease and should alert the clinician to search for evidence of Crohn's disease elsewhere in the bowel. Perirectal abscesses emanate from inflamed anal canal crypts and may occur in the absence of rectal or colonic disease.

Multiple nutritional deficiencies may be caused by poor dietary intake, malabsorption, and increased catabolism caused by inflammation. Weight loss and malnutrition may be dramatic, producing extreme cachexia. Females often become amenorrheic. In children, growth retardation and delayed sexual maturation are usually related to subtle avoidance of food and can be corrected by treatment of inflammation and restoration of nutritional requirements for growth.

A complete physical examination is often revealing of subtle manifestations of Crohn's disease. Evidence of weight loss and malnutrition should be sought. Patients are often febrile, with pale conjunctivae. Examination of the abdomen may reveal abdominal tenderness, palpable loops of thickened, inflamed bowel, or mass (typically in the right lower quadrant) caused by edematous, adherent loops of bowel or a chronic, walled-off abscess. Evidence of perirectal disease and extraintestinal manifestations of Crohn's disease must be carefully sought.

Laboratory findings are nonspecific. A complete blood cell count may show anemia, which is often multifactorial. Iron deficiency may be due to chronic blood loss or to iron malabsorption in the proximal small bowel. Persistent intestinal inflammation may contribute to the anemia of chronic disease. Macrocytic anemia may develop if terminal ileal disease or bacterial overgrowth leads to vitamin B_{12} malabsorption. Rarely, medications may produce anemia. For example, sulfasalazine may induce folate deficiency or cause hemolysis. The total leukocyte count and erythrocyte sedimentation rate are often elevated but do not always correlate with disease activity. Absolute lymphopenia may be especially associated with small bowel disease as well as malnutrition. Marked thrombocytosis may be related to inflammation or iron deficiency. Fluid and electrolyte imbalance is common in patients with diarrhea and/or malabsorption. Malabsorption of fat-soluble vitamins may lead to low serum carotene levels (vitamin A), hypocalcemia (vitamin D), or prolonged prothrombin times (vitamin K). Decreased protein intake and absorption, combined with increased catabolism and protein exudation into the gut, result in low plasma protein and albumin values and trace metal deficiencies (e.g., zinc).

Diagnosis

There is no single clinical feature or laboratory test that is diagnostic of Crohn's disease. Furthermore, no endoscopic, radiographic, or histologic feature is pathognomonic. Hence an index of suspicion must be present in the broad clinical spectrum for the possibility of Crohn's disease. The age of the patient and presenting symptom complex determine the context of the case and the differential diagnosis. In younger individuals presenting with abdominal pain, acute appendicitis, mesenteric adenitis, or ileitis due to *Yersinia* infection should be considered. In older individuals with a similar presentation of abdominal pain and fever and localized tenderness, diverticulitis, ischemic bowel disease, colon cancer, or lymphoma can mimic Crohn's disease. In patients presenting with diarrhea, fecal leukocytes should be sought and, if present, infectious etiologies such as amebiasis or bacterial enterocolitis due to pathogens including *Salmonella, Shigella, Campylobacter,* or *Clostridium difficile* should be ruled out with appropriate cultures or toxin assay. In patients with more insidious onset of abdominal pain and diarrhea, irritable bowel syndrome is excluded by the presence of weight loss, nocturnal symptoms, anemia, hematochezia, occult blood in the stool, or the presence of fecal leukocytes.

Most often, for a patient presenting with chronic diarrhea and abdominal pain, stools should be examined for ova and parasites and cultured for bacterial pathogens. Flexible sigmoidoscopy should be performed to search for distal colonic inflammation, recognizing that the rectum may be normal (spared) with typical aphthous (Color Plate X-6, *A*) or linear (Color Plate X-6, *B*) ulcerations present in the sigmoid colon, proximal colon, or terminal ileum. If fecal leukocytes are present or there is evidence of rectal bleeding or microscopic blood, the proximal colon and distal ileum need to be evaluated. This generally begins with colonoscopy, which allows accurate assessment of inflammation as well as the option of tissue sampling. At times, the colonoscopic examination may be curtailed due to stricture formation. Contrast radiography can substitute for colonoscopy and is often useful if endoscopic procedures are incomplete due to stricture formation; it is the most sensitive means to detect fistula tracts. The most common radiographic findings are mucosal nodules that cause a cobblestone appearance (Fig. 341-1), multiple ulcers, fissures, and strictures. Fistula tracts, either within the intestinal wall or between loops of bowel, may be identified. Patients who are acutely ill should have a plain abdominal radiograph in conjunction with a careful limited examination of the distal colon (flexible sigmoidoscopy), without prior catharsis to lessen the risk of toxic megacolon or perforation. In the acute setting, a computed tomography (CT) scan of the abdomen can help rule out an abscess, define an inflammatory mass of adhered bowel loops, and assess focal thickening of small or large bowel.

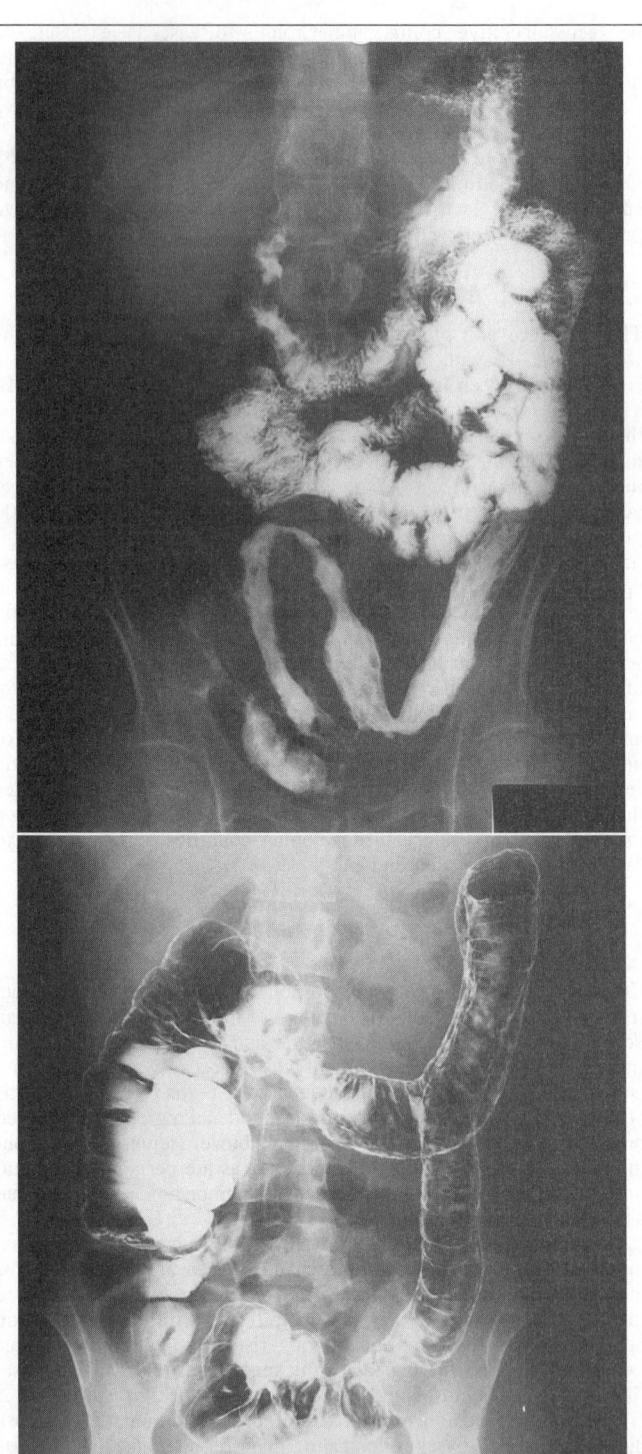

FIGURE 341-1 Radiograph features of Crohn's disease. **A,** Small bowel follow-through radiograph of Crohn's disease. Normal proximal small intestine with long inflamed ileal segment demonstrating cobblestone appearance with pseudodiverticula and separation of adjacent loops of bowel. **B,** Air-contrast radiograph of colon showing multiple smooth-surfaced, ovoid, and elongated mucosal cobblestones, with relatively mild involvement of the rectum.

Suspected small bowel disease (diarrhea, weight loss, abdominal pain) remains the domain of the barium contrast small bowel examination. Edema and thickening of the bowel wall may lead to separation of the loops and a "string sign," classically seen as a manifestation of severe luminal narrowing in the terminal ileum. An inflammatory mass or abscess may cause displacement of bowel loops and extrinsic compression of the bowel wall. Suspected abscesses may be further defined on CT scans or ultrasound. Labeled leukocyte scans with indium-111 or technetium-99 are used in some centers to localize suspected intestinal inflammation or suspected abscess.

Occasionally, the disease is diagnosed when a patient with suspected acute appendicitis undergoes laparotomy. The appendix looks normal, but the terminal ileum and its mesentery are inflamed. This form of acute terminal ileitis must be distinguished from a self-limited *Yersinia enterocolitica* infection by culture and serologic findings. If the cecum is grossly normal, the appendix may be safely removed to lessen confusion in the event of recurrent abdominal pain, but the terminal ileum should not be resected in the absence of other complications such as abscess.

Management

Because of the great variation in the clinical course of Crohn's disease, general recommendations applicable for individual patients are difficult to provide. Nevertheless, guidelines have been prepared by the American College of Gastroenterology that depend on the location and severity of Crohn's disease as well as the many potential complications. Although controlled trials are useful, the heterogeneous presentations and complications of Crohn's disease still leave many gaps in the "evidence base" for long-term management. Clinical trials have been hampered by the absence of gold-standard criteria for response, necessitating the use of nonspecific clinical indices or subjective determinations of clinical response. These endpoints have been achieved by a considerable proportion of placebo-treated patients, requiring careful interpretation of genuine therapeutic response. Nevertheless, the goals of therapy in Crohn's disease are to induce and then sustain clinical remissions or elimination of specific complications without inducing long-term side effects related to therapy.

Medical Therapy

General Therapy. When embarking on a therapeutic plan, the location of the disease, severity of symptoms, and complications are important for defining both antiinflammatory and symptomatic treatment. The impact on the short- and long-term quality of life is increasingly emphasized for this and other chronic diseases. The impact on the family and the psychologic sequelae for the patient must be kept in mind. Although there are no predisposing pychologic profiles for patients with Crohn's disease, both the disease and its therapies can have emotional and social consequences. General support for the patient's mental health, physical well-being, and nutritional status need to be maintained.

Nutrition. The importance of nutritional support cannot be overemphasized. While dietary factors have not been implicated in disease causation, dietary adjustments and nutritional assessment are essential to minimize symptoms and prevent complications. Both an elemental diet and total parenteral nutrition with bowel rest have been demonstrated to reduce the inflammatory sequelae of Crohn's disease, although these approaches are usually reserved for special circumstances because of difficulty with compliance and high cost. In some children or adolescent patients at specific risk for growth retardation due to malnutrition or corticosteroid side effects, these approaches are sometimes necessary. Most patients should be allowed to choose foods that are palatable, but dietary advise should be provided to minimize symptoms while providing adequate calories, protein, minerals, and vitamins for general health maintenance. Patients with diarrhea should be instructed on dietary factors that exacerbate symptoms such as undigested carbohydrates or fats in patients with ileal disease or resection. Milk products should be proscribed only in patients with true lactose intolerance. Location of disease predicts nu-

tritional sequelae. Supplementation of calcium, iron, magnesium, zinc, and water-soluble vitamins may be necessary when the proximal small bowel is diseased, whereas patients with ileal disease or resection may be deficient in fat-soluble vitamins and Vitamin B_{12}. Patients treated with corticosteroids require supplementation of calcium and possibly vitamin D to prevent osteoporosis. Iron stores should be maintained in patients with malabsorption or chronic bleeding and may require parenteral replacement if oral therapy is not sufficient or is poorly tolerated.

Antidiarrheal Measures. Treatment of diarrhea should be directed primarily at the underlying inflammatory process. Diphenoxylate, loperamide, and anticholinergics may provide symptomatic relief for patients with mild disease but should be avoided in the setting of severe colonic disease lest toxic dilation of the colon ensue. Because extensive (>100 cm) ileal disease or resection may lead to bile salt deficiency with steatorrhea, a low-fat diet will reduce fecal output. Conversely, for patients with diarrhea after short ileal resections, bile-salt malabsorption leads to increased colonic secretion. In this setting, adding an anion-exchange resin such as cholestyramine, which binds unabsorbed bile salts, will prevent diarrhea.

Antiinflammatory Agents. Several classes of antiinflammatory agents have had demonstrable benefits in controlled trials in Crohn's disease. These include the aminosalicylates, antibiotics, corticosteroids, and immunomodulators.

Sulfasalazine is the prototype aminosalicylate now recognized as a delivery system for mesalamine (5-aminosalicylic acid). In divided doses up to 4 to 6 g/day, sulfasalazine has been an effective drug for mild to moderate Crohn's disease, particularly for ileocolonic or colonic involvement. Sulfasalazine has been less effective for patients with purely small bowel disease. The activity of sulfasalazine in the distal bowel is explained by its metabolism by colonic flora to sulfapyridine and 5-aminosalicylic acid, the latter being the therapeutic moiety. Oral formulations of mesalamine have recently been used for both mild to moderately active Crohn's disease and to prolong remission after medical or surgical therapy. Mesalamine is effective in a dose-dependent manner. Divided doses up to 5 g/day have been used without evidence of the dose-related side effects observed with sulfasalazine.

Prednisone is an effective drug for moderately to severely ill patients. The daily dosage may be adjusted according to disease severity, with a maximum of 1 mg/kg of body weight. High-dose intravenous methylprednisolone therapy may be indicated in extremely ill patients on a bowel rest program. If rectal Crohn's disease is present, rectal administration of a steroid enema, suppository, or foam up to twice daily may be helpful. Although systemically administered steroids are certainly useful, serious side effects such as diabetes, hypertension, cataracts, and osteoporosis often limit long-term therapy. Alternate-day steroid therapy has been useful in children. The combination of an aminosalicylate and prednisone does not appear to be more effective than steroids alone, nor is there a long-term steroid-sparing effect. Steroids are used to treat acute disease but should not be used long term. There is no dosage that has been demonstrated to be safe and effective for long-term use to prevent relapse. Approximately 75% of patients requiring steroids to achieve benefits will require additional treatment after 1 year, and up to 40% may become steroid dependent.

Recently, newer glucocorticoid formulations have been developed for enteric delivery. Budesonide is a more potent antiinflammatory agent than prednisone and is rapidly metabolized by the liver. In a pH-dependent oral formulation, budesonide, 9 mg/day, has had palliative benefits comparable to those of prednisone, 40 mg/day for ileocolonic Crohn's disease without the severity of typical steroid-related side effects produced by prednisone. Long-term treatment at lower doses has not been beneficial.

A dilemma is presented by the Crohn's disease patient with fever, leukocytosis, and a palpable abdominal mass. It is usually best to treat such patients initially with intravenous antibiotics (e.g., metronidazole and an aminoglycoside or fluoroquinone, or a second- or third-generation cephalosporin) rather than with high-dose corticosteroids, which may produce septic complications.

Metronidazole appears to be an effective alternate drug in Crohn's disease; it is particularly useful for patients with ileocolonic or colonic involvement. For such patients, its efficacy is generally equivalent to that of sulfasalazine. Metronidazole also may be valuable in the management of perineal Crohn's disease. The dosage is 10-20 mg/kg/day, but beneficial effects may not be apparent before 4 to 6 weeks. Peripheral neuropathy, producing paresthesias that may persist after metronidazole is discontinued, is a common side effect.

Immunosuppressive Agents. Azathioprine and its metabolite 6-mercaptopurine (6-MP) have emerged in recent years as being clearly beneficial in Crohn's disease. Although not first-line agents, they are valuable in the treatment of refractory disease, problematic perianal disease, and fistulas. They also provide a steroid-sparing effect. Doses of up to 2.5 mg/kg body weight for azathioprine and 1.5 mg/kg for 6-MP have been safe and well tolerated with careful monitoring for bone marrow suppression (2%) and pancreatitis (3%). It may require 3 to 6 months for these agents to provide steroid-sparing or palliative benefits, and the duration of therapy is controversial; it appears that these drugs have long-term benefits lasting at least 3 to 4 years. Development of lymphoma is rare.

Methotrexate administered at 25 mg/week subcutaneously has also been demonstrated to provide steroid-sparing benefits for active Crohn's disease. Supplementation with folic acid, 1 mg/day, is recommended to minimize side effects, and both complete blood cell counts and liver enzymes require monitoring. Oral dosing has not been as efficacious, and the duration of benefits for treatment have not been defined.

High-dose intravenous cyclosporin has shown promise in refractory Crohn's disease and for healing Crohn's fistulae with a rapid onset of action. However, lower doses or oral therapy has not been beneficial, requiring the use of cyclosporine as a "bridge" to alternative long-term immune modulation with azathioprine or 6-MP. The narrow therapeutic margin for this combination has made the use of cyclosporine controversial; it is usually reserved for tertiary centers with transplantation experience.

Maintenance of Remission. Remission in Crohn's disease implies the resolution of inflammatory symptoms and systemic sequelae. Corticosteroids have not been demonstrated to maintain remissions in Crohn's disease and should be gradually tapered according to the rapidity of the therapeutic response. There are, however, steroid-responsive patients who repeatedly relapse after the usual drug withdrawal sequence. In this subgroup, drug administration may have to be tapered very slowly (no more than 2.5-5.0 mg each 14 days). In patients who redevelop symptoms, azathioprine or 6-MP may be used to extend the period of remission.

Patients who respond to an aminosalicylate or antibiotic without the need for corticosteroids should be continued on the same medication indefinitely, unless side effects occur or the disease relapses. Mesalamine has also been effective in reducing the clinical relapse rate in a proportion of patients after intestinal resection.

Surgical Therapy for Complications of Crohn's Disease

Operative treatment is indicated in Crohn's disease after failure of medical therapy or for complications. Surgery should not constitute primary therapy because there is an inevitable recurrence of Crohn's disease after intestinal resection. The incidence of disease recurrence is high, approaching 100% in patients with small intestinal involvement with long-term follow-up. The need for re-operation occurs in about 40% of patients by 15 years and is somewhat higher for ileo-colonic disease. Cigarette smoking increases both the likelihood of relapse and the need for subsequent surgery. Approximately 70% of patients with Crohn's disease ultimately require some form of surgery for this condition and usually see dramatic improvement in well-being and quality of life when resections are limited to actively inflamed segments. Most recently, stricturoplasty without resection has been beneficial for the resolution of obstructive symptoms without the need for extensive resections and concern regarding short-bowel syndrome. To procrastinate unduly while the patient is exposed to

uncontrollable disease sequelae and drug side effects is a disservice to the patient.

The complications of Crohn's disease and therefore the indications for surgery vary with the location of the involvement. Obstruction is one of the most common problems and occurs mainly with ileal or ileocolonic disease. A short trial of intestinal decompression, parenterally administered steroids, and transient bowel rest may be helpful. If this fails, surgical therapy should involve resection of the minimal amount of bowel necessary.

Abscess formation often is a sequela of luminal narrowing and/or transmural involvement and thus is associated mostly with ileal and ileocolonic involvement. Although antibiotic therapy should be instituted, it rarely is sufficient, and surgery is often required when a true abscess, rather than just matted loops of inflamed bowel, is present. A computed tomography (CT) scan or ultrasonogram can help locate and define the abscess. Guided percutaneous catheter drainage of abdominal abscesses has been successful in controlling the septic process and may suffice as a singular measure but, more typically, is useful in allowing an elective resection without the need for temporary diversion (stoma).

Fistula formation may occur with or without distal luminal obstruction. Fistulas require surgery only if they are symptomatic or if enough bowel is bypassed to cause severe malnutrition or other deleterious effects. Enteroenteric, enterocolonic, and enterovisicular fistulae are common, as are rectovaginal fistulae in women. Many fistula are asymptomatic or, as with many perianal fistula, can be controlled with medical therapy. Perianal abscesses should be incised and drained initially; this eventuates in perianal fistula with drainage that is often minimized with antibiotics or immune modulators. An aggressive surgical approach in which the surgeon attempts to remove all local disease may result in a draining, slow-healing perineal wound.

Less common complications include free perforation, massive hemorrhage, multiple small bowel strictures with bacterial overgrowth, carcinoma, and obstructive uropathy. The latter may occur in the absence of an abnormality identified by urinalysis if an inflamed intestinal mass compresses the right ureter, a situation common enough to make abdominal ultrasound an indicated part of the evaluation in most patients with ileocolonic disease.

Patients with colonic Crohn's disease may require surgery because of the disease's intractability to medical management, the development of toxic dilation of the colon, or the development of dysplasia or carcinoma. If the rectum remains grossly normal, a colectomy with ileorectal anastomosis may be considered. In the absence of ileal disease, a total colectomy and ileostomy is often curative for Crohn's disease confined to the colon. Although ileostomy dysfunction occurs somewhat more frequently in Crohn's disease patients than in ulcerative colitis patients who require proctocolectomy, the difference between dysfunction in the two groups is not great. In any event, the risk of subsequent small bowel problems should not be a deterrent when the physician is faced with the necessity of performing total colectomy. However, continent ileostomies or ileoanal anastomoses are contraindicated in patients with documented Crohn's disease.

ULCERATIVE COLITIS
Pathologic Findings

The key features of ulcerative colitis are a diffuse, continuous, superficial inflammation of the colon always involving the rectum and extending to a proximal cutoff to normal that varies between individuals. In acute ulcerative colitis, colonic mucosal—and on occasion submucosal—findings include diffuse vascular congestion, edema, hemorrhage, distorted crypt architecture, and cellular infiltration with plasma cells, lymphocytes, neutrophils, and eosinophils. Neutrophils invading into the colonic crypts are termed "crypt abscesses," which lead to microscopic ulceration and eventual crypt architectural distortion (Color Plate X-7, *B*), a hallmark of chronic inflammatory bowel disease. Goblet cells are usually depleted of mucus.

A common problem is the need to distinguish acute ulcerative colitis from acute colitis of infectious cause (*Salmonella, Shigella, Campylobacter, E. coli 0157:H7*, and amebae). Although there are no pathognomonic features, the finding of distorted crypt architecture and the presence not only of neutrophils but also of increased numbers of plasma cells and lymphocytes in the lamina propria is highly suggestive of ulcerative colitis. Crypt abscesses, which may also be seen in Crohn's disease and in the infectious colitides, are common and consist of accumulations of neutrophils, eosinophils, and cellular debris (Color Plate X-7, *A*). The muscularis mucosae may be hypertrophic, but rarely in ulcerative colitis does the inflammatory reaction invade below the muscularis mucosae.

In *chronic ulcerative colitis,* inflammation, edema, muscular hypertrophy, and deposition of fibrous tissue and fat may cause thickening, contraction, narrowing, and shortening—a "lead pipe" appearance. Inflammatory polyps (pseudopolyps) are common and represent mucosal remnants or accumulations of granulation tissue with or without overlying colonic epithelial cells. Mucosal bridges may result from mucosal undermining or from the attachment of the free ends of inflammatory polyps to adjacent mucosa. Injury and healing proceed concurrently, so that different areas in the bowel may simultaneously manifest all stages of reaction from acute inflammation to epithelial regeneration. The mucosa rarely becomes histologically normal, despite the remission of symptoms and the disappearance of endoscopically and radiologically apparent abnormalities. Thus biopsies of the rectal mucosa during remissions may reveal persistent foci of chronic inflammatory cells and evidence of mucosal atrophy and crypt architectural distortion (e.g., a loss of parallelism, branching, and decreased numbers of rectal glands) (Color Plate X-7, *C*).

Clinical and Laboratory Findings

The symptoms of ulcerative colitis are determined by the extent and severity of colonic inflammation. Patients with disease limited to the rectum (ulcerative proctitis) often present with constipation of stools but with frequent passage of blood or mucus. The more proximal the extent of colitis, the greater the tendency for diarrhea (and hematochezia) to predominate. Tenesmus and rectal urgency are typical in patients with active rectal inflammation. In acute severe disease, the patient often is febrile with 5 to 30 watery, bloody stools per day; dehydration; and anemia. Massive hemorrhage is rare because of the superficial nature of the mucosal inflammation in ulcerative colitis. However, depletion of iron stores, documented best in IBD by determining serum ferritin, and iron deficiency anemia are common. In more severe disease hypoalbuminemia due to protein exudation from the inflamed bowel can lead to edema and, rarely, hypercoagulability due to loss of anticoagulation factors. More often, the presentation and onset of ulcerative colitis is more insidious and mild, with one to four stools per day, minimal gross bleeding, and perhaps only vague abdominal discomfort. Associated symptoms include flatulence, rectal tenesmus, malaise, fatigue, anorexia, and loss of weight. Occasionally flares of colitis may be associated with constipation, perhaps as a result of inflammation-induced colonic dysmotility. Extracolonic complications (discussed later) involving the liver, skin, eyes, or joints may precede or accompany the colonic manifestations. In most patients, ulcerative colitis is chronic, with exacerbations and remissions.

The physical examination may not reveal an abnormality in patients with mild or distal colitis, but fever, tachycardia, pallor, and wasting are common in patients with extensive or more severe disease. The abdominal examination is usually benign with normal bowel sounds. Evidence of abdominal tenderness or rebound signify transmural inflammation and more severe or fulminant disease. Abdominal distension and diminished bowel sounds represent colonic dilation, one of the severe complications of ulcerative colitis. Despite the tendency toward chronic diarrhea, the perianal and rectal examination is most often normal aside from occasional perianal erythema. Significant hemorrhoids, skin tags, fissures, or abscess suggest Crohn's disease.

Laboratory findings include anemia due to iron deficiency or chronic disease. Sulfasalazine therapy rarely produces deficiency of folic acid or hemolysis. Serum ferritin is the most sensitive and specific test to assess the presence of iron stores in IBD since chronic disease and nutritional deficiencies can influence both serum iron and iron binding capacity. The leukocyte count and erythrocyte sedimentation rate may be elevated, especially in the presence of complications, and thrombocytosis may indicate disease activity (or iron deficiency). Prolonged diarrhea may lead to depressed serum levels of potassium, chloride, sodium, and magnesium; diarrhea may also re-

sult in metabolic acidosis. Low serum albumin levels may result from extensive protein loss into the gastrointestinal tract. Although there is no pathognomonic serologic marker for ulcerative colitis, the presence of antineutrophil cytoplasmic antibodies with a perinuclear immunofluorenscent pattern is present in between 60% and 80% of patients.

Diagnosis

Chapter 339 describes the differential approach to acute and chronic diarrhea syndromes and outlines the specific conditions that may affect the colon and need to be ruled out in establishing a diagnosis of ulcerative colitis (e.g., acute, self-limited bacterial colitis; *C. difficile* infection; amebiasis; ischemia; or radiation colitis).

Flexible sigmoidoscopy (proctosigmoidoscopy) is the most valuable diagnostic procedure in ulcerative colitis. The mucosal appearance of diffuse and continuous mucosal changes ranges in severity from mild hyperemia, fine granularity, petechiae, and minimal pinpoint bleeding (friability) to moderate or severe abnormalities such as mucopurulent exudate, frank ulceration, and spontaneous bleeding (Color Plate X-8, *B*). In ulcerative proctitis or left-sided colitis there is a distinct change to normal appearing mucosa at the margin of disease. Biopsies are usually nonspecific but demonstrate diffuse and superficial microscopic changes of crypt abscesses and crypt architectural distortion (Color Plate X-7). Biopsies may aid in the differentiation between acute self-limited colitis, *C. difficile* infection, and Crohn's colitis. Colonoscopy may be useful in demonstrating the extent of mucosal involvement in selected cases; in documenting Crohn's colitis, which may not involve the rectosigmoid; and in excluding colonic carcinoma in selected patients. However, colonoscopy is hazardous in patients with active acute disease because it may produce perforation or precipitate toxic megacolon. In patients presenting with severe disease or abdominal tenderness, a careful proctoscopic or flexible sigmoidoscopic examination in conjunction with a plain abdominal radiograph will demonstrate the presence of colitis and exclude toxic megacolon. The abdominal radiograph can also delineate the proximal extent of colitis by virtue of absent fecal material in the inflamed segments and lumenal air outlining edematous, ahaustral colon.

For the most part, contrast abdominal radiographs have been supplanted by endoscopic examinations, which allow a more critical review of the mucosa and histologic sampling for confirmation of the diagnosis. Air contrast barium enema examination should not be performed in patients with severely active colitis but can demonstrate fine mucosal serrations, a feathery outline, or well-circumscribed craters (Fig. 341-2). Other common findings include diminished or absent haustrations, straightening, narrowing, shortening, an irregular mosaic pattern produced by mucosal edema, diminished distensibility, spasm, and an increase in the retrorectal soft tissue space. The terminal ileum, although often normal, may in the presence of contiguous colonic involvement show similar superficial mucosal ulceration or irregularity ("backwash ileitis") with a lumen of increased or normal caliber, in contrast to the narrowing seen in Crohn's disease (Table 341-1). Partial or complete reversibility of the radiographic findings can occur in patients with ulcerative colitis in remission.

Strictures and inflammatory pseudopolyps may be difficult to differentiate from benign or malignant neoplasms without the aid of colonoscopy and biopsy. Benign strictures of the colon are found in 5% to 10% of patients with ulcerative colitis, are related to hypertrophy of the muscularis mucosae, and are reversible with healing. In contrast, the strictures seen in Crohn's disease are due to fibrosis and are permanent features. Strictures of ulcerative colitis are seldom multiple and, when irreversible with healing of colitis, usually indicate the presence of neoplasia.

Management

Therapeutic approaches in ulcerative colitis begin with an assessment of the extent and severity of colitis and also depend on a patient's response to prior interventions. Treatment is aimed at inducing and then maintaining remission of the inflammatory process while treating symptoms related to the abnormal motility and sensitivity of the colon due to acute or chronic inflammation. Therapy should encom-

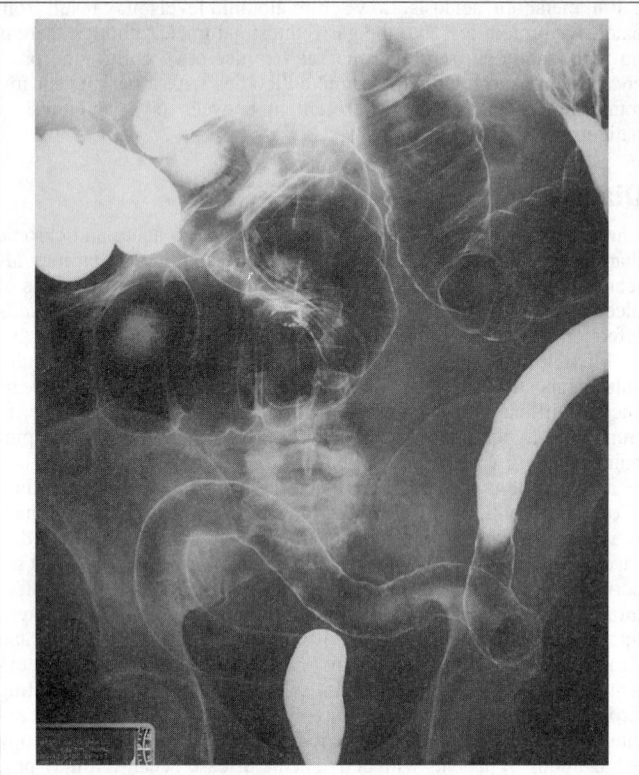

FIGURE 341-2 Radiography of ulcerative colitis. Air-contrast radiograph of the colon showing diffuse, continuous superficial inflammation, diminished haustrations, and numerous inflammatory polyps.

pass a broad program, emphasizing adequate nutrition and emotional support from the family, physician, and ancillary medical support staff. Diet in mild or quiescent disease is often unrestricted. If there is a question of lactose intolerance, dairy products should be avoided. In severe colitis, parenteral nutrition may be necessary for short periods but does not improve the natural history of the disease.

The goals of medical therapy in ulcerative colitis are to induce and maintain remission. Remission is defined as "the resolution of inflammatory symptoms (rectal bleeding, diarrhea, urgency, tenesmus) and regeneration of an intact colonic mucosa without ulceration, granularity, or significant friability." Maintenance of remission pertains to the prevention of relapse (recurrence of inflammatory symptoms and acute mucosal inflammation). Many patients with ulcerative colitis continue with mild symptoms of irritable bowel syndrome (e.g., abdominal cramps, loose bowel movements, bloating) which are distinguished from inflammatory symptoms by nocturnal bowel movements, the absence of bleeding, and evidence of a healed mucosa at sigmoidoscopy.

The cornerstone of drug therapy in mild to moderate cases of ulcerative colitis and for maintenance of remission has been the aminosalicylates. Sulfasalazine is the benchmark agent and is effective with a dose-response between 2 and 6 g/day for both active disease and maintaining remission. Sulfasalazine is cleaved by colonic bacteria into its two components: sulfapyridine and 5-aminosalicylic acid (5-ASA, mesalamine). The therapeutic properties of sulfasalazine are due to 5-ASA, whereas most of the side effects including intolerance (nausea, anorexia, headache) and hypersensitivity (rash, arthritis, pancreatitis) are ascribed to the sulfapyridine moiety. To obviate the disadvantages of sulfapyridine, new oral formulations providing delivery systems of 5-ASA have been developed that prevent the proximal intestinal absorption of 5-ASA to allow distal delivery to inflamed sites along the intestinal tract. 5-ASA appears to have topical (mucosal) antiinflammatory properties and is inactivated to acetylated 5-ASA after absorption. A dimer of 5-ASA (olsalazine) that is likewise cleaved by colonic bacteria, freeing the active 5-ASA, is also available. In addition, mesalamine suppositories are available for treatment of ulcerative proctitis and mesalamine enemas for disease distal to the splenic flexure. All forms of 5-ASA have proved beneficial in treating mild to moderately active disease and in maintaining remission. Although the newer preparations are better tolerated, they are no more effective but considerably more costly than sulfasalazine.

Corticosteroids are indicated to treat moderate to severe disease either as initial therapy or as an alternative when aminosalicylate therapy is not effective. Oral prednisone (40-60 mg/day), parenteral hydrocortisone (300-400 mg/day) or methylprednisolone (40-60 mg/day) may be used depending on the clinical severity. For proctitis or left-sided colitis, corticosteroid enemas may be given, but 20% to 80% of the dose may be absorbed, leading to systemic side effects. Newer, rapidly metabolized steroid enema preparations that do not have this effect (e.g., budesonide) are under development. Corticosteroids in any form are of no value in prolonging remission. Recently intravenous cyclosporine has been effective on a short-term basis for treating severely ill patients who have failed to improve with intravenous steroids. The ultimate benefits of cyclosporine remain controversial because of the narrow therapeutic window and the ultimate curability of ulcerative colitis with surgery. The immunosuppressive agents azathioprine and 6-MP have long-term steroid-sparing effects but are reserved for patients whose remissions are not maintained despite optimal dosing with aminosalicylate maintenance therapy.

Colectomy (removal of the entire colonic mucosa) is curative in ulcerative colitis since the disease never involves the small bowel. Even backwash ileitis resolves with colectomy. Surgery is indicated in ulcerative colitis in the setting of uncontrolled hemorrhage, free perforation, toxic megacolon, or evidence of dysplasia or carcinoma. Most frequently, however, colectomies are performed due to intractability: either failure to wean off of chronic steroid use or failure to improve despite an intensive inpatient regimen of intravenous corticosteroids.

The standard operation to cure ulcerative colitis is a proctocolectomy and ileostomy. However, in the past decade the ability to perform a colectomy and mucosal proctectomy with preservation of the distal colonic musculature and anal sphincter has allowed ileo-anal anastamoses with either a J-shaped or S-shaped ileal reservoir to replace the necessity of an external appliance for most patients with confirmed ulcerative colitis. This is now the preferred procedure in younger patients whose quality of life after surgery is excellent, with an average of 4-6 controlled, non-urgent bowel movements daily. The ileal reservoir occasionally becomes inflamed (pouchitis) in a similar superficial pattern as with ulcerative colitis, but the inflammation and resulting diarrhea, urgency, and extraintestinal symptoms resolve with antimicrobial therapy (e.g., metronidazole).

Prognosis

Prognosis for the initial attack of ulcerative colitis is affected by the severity and extent of the disease and by the age and physical condition of the patient. For example, the onset of ulcerative colitis in elderly or postpartum patients often is associated with a more stormy course. Factors associated with poorer long-term prognoses are extensive colonic involvement, associated liver disease (primary sclerosing cholangitis), severe initial attack, and onset either in childhood or after the age of 60 years. However, it is impossible to extrapolate general risk data to individual patients such that even the most severely ill patient may experience remarkable long-term recovery and maintenance of normal quality of life. For patients without liver disease, the life expectancy after the initial attack is similar to that of the general population. Exacerbations may be precipitated by cessation of cigarette smoking, intercurrent infections, use of oral antibiotics, menstruation, and, occasionally stress; although day-to-day life stresses have not been implicated in disease exacerbation. Nonsteroidal antiinflammatory drugs (NSAIDs) have a deleterious impact on ulcerative colitis and have been associated with disease initiation and exacerbations.

Unless the patient is currently ill, the disease is not a contraindication to becoming pregnant, and most pregnant patients with preexisting ulcerative colitis go on to a full-term normal delivery. Drug therapy (corticosteroids, aminosalicylates) does not appear to affect

Table 341-1   Clinical differentiation of ulcerative colitis and Crohn's disease

FINDINGS	ULCERATIVE COLITIS	CROHN'S DISEASE
Epidemiologic		
Cigarette smoking	Nonsmoker	Smoker
Serologic		
pANCA	Positive	Negative
Clinical		
Rectal bleeding	Present in most patients	Present in 50% of patients
Abdominal pain	Mild, rarely severe	Often present
Abdominal mass	Absent	Often present
Perianal lesions	Absent	Fissures, fistula, abscess, or "elephant-ear" tags common
Clubbing of fingers	Absent	Occasional
Endoscopic/radiographic		
Distribution	Diffuse, continuous, superficial, always involving rectum	Focal, asymmetric, with rectum spared in 50%
Mucosal detail	Granular, with pinpoint ulceration; pseudopolyps after healing	Aphthous or linear ulcers, cobblestone appearance
Small bowel	Patulous ileocecal valve with "backwash ileitis"	Strictured ileocecal valve, narrowed, ulcerated terminal ileum
Internal fistulae	Absent	Common: enteroenteric, rectovaginal, enterovesicular, enterocutaneous

fetal development. Although the pregnancy per se may not affect the course of the bowel disease, relapses occur in 25% to 50% of patients, especially during the first trimester and puerperium.

DIFFERENTIATION OF ULCERATIVE COLITIS AND CROHN'S COLITIS

Differentiating between ulcerative colitis and Crohn's colitis is important from therapeutic and prognostic standpoints. Ulcerative colitis is cured by colectomy, with excellent quality of life after an ileostomy or ileal pull-through. Conversely, Crohn's disease typically recurs after a resection, although proctocolectomy and ileostomy often "cures" Crohn's disease confined to the colon. The sphincter-saving ileal pouch operations are usually not performed for Crohn's disease because of complications within the pouch (e.g., recurrent disease, stricture or fistula formation). On the other hand, in patients with Crohn's disease of the colon, the medical options are somewhat greater, including use of antibiotics, which are ineffective in ulcerative colitis. The risk of colon cancer has been well clarified for ulcerative colitis related to the extent and duration of disease. The same two factors are probably related to the risk of cancer in Crohn's disease, although the focal nature of Crohn's and the inability to survey the entire colon due to stricturing make generalized recommendations for surveillance more controversial.

There is substantial overlap between ulcerative colitis and Crohn's disease with respect to epidemiologic factors, clinical manifestations, physical and laboratory findings, complications, and medical treatment. In approximately 20% of patients the distinction between ulcerative colitis and Crohn's disease confined to the colon is uncertain, leading to the classification of indeterminate colitis. In some patients the pattern may change over time or with therapy, usually from ulcerative colitis to Crohn's disease due to complications of perirectal disease, focal strictures, or a patchy distribution. Two recently identified clinical clues are smoking history and pANCA status. Since cigarette smoking prevents the development of ulcerative colitis, the presence of colitis in a smoker is more often Crohn's disease. On the other hand, pANCA-positive patients more often have ulcerative colitis or a pattern of Crohn's disease that resembles the course of ulcerative colitis. Table 341-1 summarizes the clinical and radiologic features by which ulcerative colitis and Crohn's colitis may be distinguished.

ADDITIONAL CONSIDERATIONS
Extraintestinal Manifestations

Extraintestinal features are common and may be the dominant or presenting manifestations of IBD. A useful classification relates these systemic problems to the major site of bowel involvement: (1) a "colitis-related" group, in which the severity of the extraintestinal disorder is more likely to vary directly with the activity of the bowel disease; (2) a group of disorders related to small bowel dysfunction; and (3) miscellaneous, nonspecific complications.

Of the colitis-related problems, seronegative arthritis or arthralgia is the most common (15% to 40%). The peripheral large joints (knees, ankles, wrists) are usually affected. The distribution is usually pauciarticular, asymmetric, and non-deforming. Peripheral joint manifestations either herald an attack or occur with colitis activity and respond to treatment of the bowel inflammation. In contrast, central arthritis (ankylosing spondylitis or sacroiliitis) is associated with the histocompatibility antigen HLA-B27, presents "out of synch" with the IBD activity, and progresses even after a curative colectomy in ulcerative colitis. Skin manifestations affect about 15% of patients with IBD and are principally seen as pyoderma gangrenosum (Color Plate X-9) and erythema nodosum. Similar to the peripheral arthritis, these complications usually parallel the course of the bowel disease. Oral aphthous ulcers (Color Plate X-10) are common in Crohn's disease and occasionally progress to more typical linear Crohn's ulcers. Significant eye complications, occurring in about 5% of IBD patients, include conjunctivitis, episcleritis, and uveitis. Uveitis is another HLA-B27–associated complication that follows a course independent from the intestinal inflammation.

The second group of disorders is more closely related to small bowel dysfunction. For example, there is an increased incidence of gallstones in Crohn's disease as a result of bile salt malabsorption from terminal ileal disease or resection. Nephrolithiasis may result from diarrhea and low urinary volume predisposing to uric acid stones or increased oxalate absorption from the colon in the presence of steatorrhea, producing hyperoxaluria and calcium oxalate stones. Hydronephrosis may result from ureteral obstruction by an inflammatory mass, usually at the ileocecal junction.

Metabolic bone disease is common in IBD and may be multifactorial, related to a combination of dietary exclusions (e.g., avoidance of milk), malabsorption of calcium or vitamin D in Crohn's disease of the small bowel, or long-term corticosteroid use. Adequate calcium intake of 1500 mg/day should be encouraged in all patients treated with steroids, and patients with extensive ileal Crohn's disease should be monitored for vitamin D deficiency. Corticosteroid use should be kept to a minimum to prevent accelerated osteoporosis. Hypertrophic osteoarthropathy ("clubbing") is occasionally noted with Crohn's disease.

Hepatic complications occur in approximately 5% of patients with IBD. The most common findings are a mild elevation in biliary and transaminase enzymes with hepatic steatosis due to nutritional deficiency or drug therapy including corticosteroids. A more specific complication related to IBD is primary sclerosing cholangitis (PSC), which runs a spectrum. At one end are asymptomatic mild elevations of alkaline phosphatase and gamma glutamyl transpeptidase. The associated hepatic pathology is a portal triaditis or pericholangitis, which are asymptomatic and usually not progressive. At the other end of the spectrum of PSC is a progressive inflammation of the intrahepatic and extrahepatic biliary tree that leads to a secondary biliary cirrhosis. The latter usually manifests with an elevated bilirubin level and transaminase values more than twice normal. Patients may present with jaundice, hepatosplenomegaly, or an episode of cholangitis. Cholangiocarcinoma is a rare complication of IBD and primary sclerosing cholangitis that may be difficult to distinguish from the benign biliary strictures of PSC. Other forms of chronic hepatitis may need to be excluded. In view of the spectrum of hepatic abnormalities associated with IBD, visualization of the biliary tree via ERCP or transhepatic cholangiography, as well as liver biopsy, may be indicated.

As a result of the acute phase inflammatory mediators released in IBD, hypercoagulability may manifest as thrombophlebitis. Rarely, loss of anticoagulant factors may occur in conjunction with protein-losing enterocolopathies. Secondary amyloidosis occasionally is a late manifestation of Crohn's disease.

Toxic Dilation of the Colon

Toxic dilation of the colon (toxic megacolon) is one of the few medical emergencies in IBD. Although it is much more common in ulcerative colitis, it can also complicate Crohn's colitis. Toxic megacolon is usually seen during exacerbations of chronic IBD but may be part of the initial episode in patients having an acute fulminating course. As with any presentation of acute colitis, it is crucial to exclude the infectious and other causes of colonic inflammation cited earlier. On clinical examination the patient appears severely ill, with fever, leukocytosis, abdominal distention, direct and even rebound abdominal tenderness, and diminished bowel sounds. Concomitant severe hemorrhage is also present in about one third of such patients. Plain radiographs of the abdomen show a dilated, ahaustral colon and a diameter in the transverse colon exceeding 6 cm (Fig. 341-3). On pathologic examination, the colon is characterized by mucosal denudation, necrotizing transmural inflammation, vasculitis, and thinning of the wall such that its consistency may approach that of wet tissue paper. The risk of imminent perforation is obvious. Precipitating factors may include use of opiates or anticholinergics, hypokalemia, and barium enema or colonoscopic examinations performed in the presence of very active disease. Toxic megacolon should be managed jointly by a medical and a surgical team. If perforation or peritonitis is not evident, a short period (48 to 72 hours) of intensive parenteral therapy, including high-dose intravenous administration of corticosteroids and broad-spectrum antibiotics, is usually indicated. Patients who do not respond with improvement in abdominal pain, distention, fever, and leukocytosis within 24 hours should be taken for emergent colectomy. Once colonic perforation occurs, mortality is a significant risk. Although some patients with colonic dilation who experience remission with medical management have relatively mild, easily controllable disease over the long term, up to 50% of patients who develop this complication ultimately require total proctocolectomy.

Bowel Cancer

The risk of colonic adenocarcinoma is clearly increased in patients with ulcerative colitis. Despite a 15-fold relative risk for patients with ulcerative colitis compared to the general population, only 3% to 4% of patients ultimately develop colon cancer. The risk factors for cancer in ulcerative colitis include the length of colon involved, the duration of colitis, and the presence of sclerosing cholangitis. The incidence of cancer begins to increase after 10 years of disease, increasing by about 1% per year and reaching an absolute risk of 30% after 35 years of disease. The risk is somewhat higher when the onset of disease occurs before 15 years of age. These data apply only to patients with pancolitis; those with disease confined to the rectum have little, if any, increase in risk of cancer. An intermediate risk exists for those with an intermediate extent of disease, but the limits of involvement cannot be adequately assessed in patients who have not under-

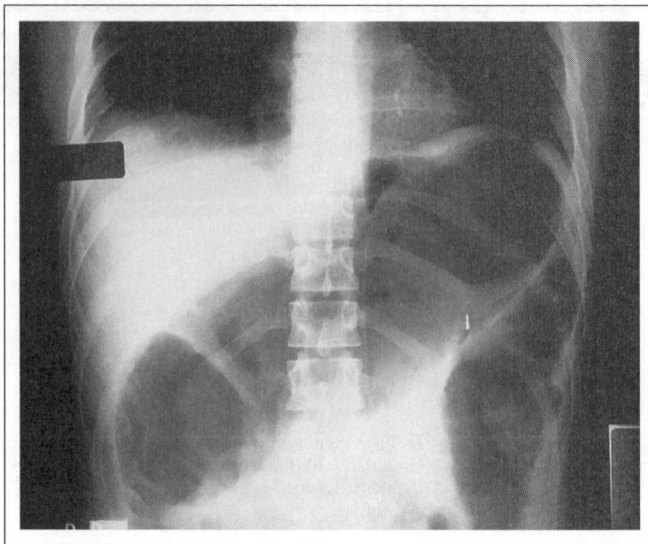

FIGURE 341-3 Plain abdominal radiograph of toxic megacolon. Dilated, ahaustral colon with thumb printing of colonic mucosa most prominent along the transverse colon.

gone complete colonoscopy. Because most colonic cancers appear in patients with quiescent ulcerative colitis, severity of disease is not considered to be a contributing factor.

Epithelial dysplasia is a precursor to carcinomas in ulcerative colitis. Compared to the general population in whom adenomatous polyps can be visualized, many dysplastic foci are present in flat, normal-appearing mucosa, although nodular or plaque-like lesions, or even adenomatous polyps may be identified. Dysplasia is a neoplastic condition that may be the superficial portion of an underlying carcinoma in ulcerative colitis. Dysplasia is often multifocal and associated with carcinomas distant from the herald lesion. Therefore colonoscopic surveillance with biopsies along the length of the colon are necessary for patients with longstanding (greater than 10 years) ulcerative colitis. Barium enemas are not sufficiently sensitive for surveillance in ulcerative colitis. Colitis cancers are often multicentric, occur more commonly beyond the reach of the sigmoidoscope, and may not produce clear-cut symptoms before the neoplasm is advanced. The prognosis is the same for cancers in ulcerative colitis when assessed according to stage and histology.

The preceding factors make cancer surveillance a difficult and important task. Patients with ulcerative colitis for more than 8 to 10 years should be entered into a colonoscopic surveillance program. This entails interval examinations of the entire colonic mucosa. Multiple random biopsies should be obtained from flat mucosa as well as from nodular or polypoid lesions. The presence of multiple postinflammatory polyps (pseudopolyps) may make surveillance impossible due to the inability to discriminate grossly between inflammatory and potentially neoplastic lesions. Standardization of the histologic criteria for the different degrees of dysplasia and recent worldwide studies defining the specificity and sensitivity of dysplasia have improved the usefulness of this diagnostic and prognostic modality. The presence of dysplasia confirmed by an expert pathologist is indication for colectomy due to the significant risk of synchronous cancer. Indeterminate interpretations of dysplasia due to active inflammation and regenerative atypia require careful reexamination after the colitis has been treated. Alternative precancer markers are greatly needed to improve the diagnostic and predictive accuracy of histologic dysplasia. Serial carcinoembryonic antigen determinations are of no predictive value.

Carcinoma also occurs more commonly in patients with longstanding Crohn's disease than in the general population, although not nearly to the degree noted in patients with ulcerative pancolitis. The vigilant surveillance procedures for colonic carcinoma described have yet to be applied systematically to patients with Crohn's colitis. Lym-

✔ WHEN TO REFER

The initial diagnosis of ulcerative colitis or Crohn's disease is often made by a primary care physician. Patients with mild or moderate symptoms of ulcerative colitis who respond to an aminosalicylate or topical corticosteroid should be placed on a maintenance medical program to prevent relapse. Those who remain well should be referred after 8 to 10 years for colonoscopic surveillance. Patients with moderate to severe symptoms should be referred to a gastroenterologist, and any hospitalized patient should be evaluated by a specialist. Patients with ulcerative colitis should not be maintained on corticosteroids, and steroid-dependent patients should also be evaluated by a specialist. Due to the spectrum of Crohn's disease and the multiple nutritional and systemic complications, most patients should be referred to a gastroenterologist for long-term management decisions. Certainly any patient who cannot be weaned from corticosteroids or one with long-standing disease deserves evaluation by a specialist.

phomas also have been seen more commonly in patients with IBD than in the general population, but the overall risk remains extremely low.

BIBLIOGRAPHY

Hanauer SB: Inflammatory bowel disease, *N Engl J Med* 334:841-848, 1996.
Hanauer SB, Meyers S: Practice guidelines—management of Crohn's disease in adults, *Am J Gastroenterol* 92(4):559-566, 1997.
Kornbluth A, Sachar DB: Practice guidelines—ulcerative colitis practice guidelines in adults, *Am J Gastroenterol* 92(2):204-211, 1997.
Kirsner JB, Shorter RG: *Inflammatory bowel disease,* ed 4, Philadelphia, Williams & Wilkins.

CHAPTER

342 Intestinal Obstruction and Peritonitis

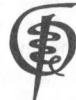

T. Edward Bynum

INTESTINAL OBSTRUCTION

Mechanical obstruction can occur at any site along the alimentary tract. In this chapter the discussion is confined to obstruction of the small and large intestines, a complication that is often associated with intraperitoneal adhesions from previous abdominal surgery, colonic carcinoma, fecal impaction (especially in the elderly), Crohn's disease, or diverticulitis. The intestine can be partially or completely obstructed by an extrinsic, intramural, or mucosal lesion that causes concentric or eccentric narrowing, ultimately leading to a severely reduced or obliterated lumen. Other ways the bowel can be obstructed are by volvulus or kinking of a loop, an intussusception, or a foreign body. See Box 342-1 for classification and differential diagnosis of intestinal obstruction.

Pathophysiology

Whatever the cause or mechanism of obstruction, the pathophysiology is similar. Initially, intestinal motor activity increases both above and below the site of obstruction. There is increased intestinal secretion by the intestine proximal to the obstruction to a degree that secretion often exceeds absorption. This leads to distention that, when combined with the increased motor activity, is clinically expressed as severe cramping abdominal pain, often recurring in waves. At this time, bowel sounds are hyperactive and high-pitched

---

BOX 342-1
Classification and differential diagnosis of intestinal obstruction

I. Paralytic ileus
II. Concentric narrowing
  A. Crohn's disease (benign or malignant stricture)
  B. Neoplasm (lymphoma, adenocarcinoma, other)
  C. Diverticulitis
  D. Resolved ischemic enteritis
III. Kinking of a loop
  A. Postoperative adhesions
  B. Incarcerated hernia
IV. Twisting of a loop
  A. Cecal volvulus
  B. Sigmoid volvulus
  C. Midgut volvulus
V. Intussusception
  A. Spontaneous
  B. Secondary to polyp or mass
VI. Foreign body
  A. Ingested
  B. Gallstone
VII. Pseudoobstruction

---

peristaltic rushes are often heard. The increased motor activity distal to the site of obstruction may lead to defecation, which does not relieve the pain. Later, bowel motor activity diminishes. During this phase, pain becomes more persistent, less severe, and less episodic, and bowel sounds may be normal or, more characteristically, continuous, and high-pitched. Still later, bowel motor activity ceases entirely; the bowel proximal to the site of obstruction becomes dilated, with characteristic air-fluid levels that are seen on upright plain radiographs of the abdomen. Bowel sounds are often absent. This last phase has been called *obstructive ileus* (as opposed to *paralytic ileus*). If the site of obstruction is at or distal to the ascending colon, the cecum can become greatly dilated; when its transverse diameter exceeds 12 to 14 cm, there is danger of cecal perforation.

If obstruction is caused by a volvulus or strangulated loop of bowel, impairment of the blood supply can lead to ischemic necrosis and possible perforation. In some instances, strangulation is heralded by fever and leukocytosis.

History

A patient who has obstruction usually gives a history of rather sudden onset of abdominal pain, the characteristics of which were described earlier, that may be accompanied by nausea, vomiting, and abdominal distention. After the patient has had obstruction of the jejunum or beyond for some time, usually several hours or longer, the emesis may become brownish and feculent, especially if the obstruction is located distal to the mid–small intestine. Initially the patient may have one or two urgent bowel movements, occasionally diarrhea, but then ceases to pass stool. One should inquire about previous abdominal surgery, recent (but less acute) changes in customary bowel habit, blood in the stool, family history of cancer or polyps, or previous symptoms or diagnosis of Crohn's disease.

Physical Examination

If physical examination is performed early in the course, there may be few, if any, abnormal findings. Late in the course the abdomen appears distended, with generally increased tympany to percussion, generalized tenderness, and often abnormal bowel sounds as previously described. If perforation complicates obstruction, there may be initial relief of pain. Pain subsequently returns, accompanied by rebound tenderness and fever as peritonitis develops fully. Rectal examination may reveal impacted stool or a mass.

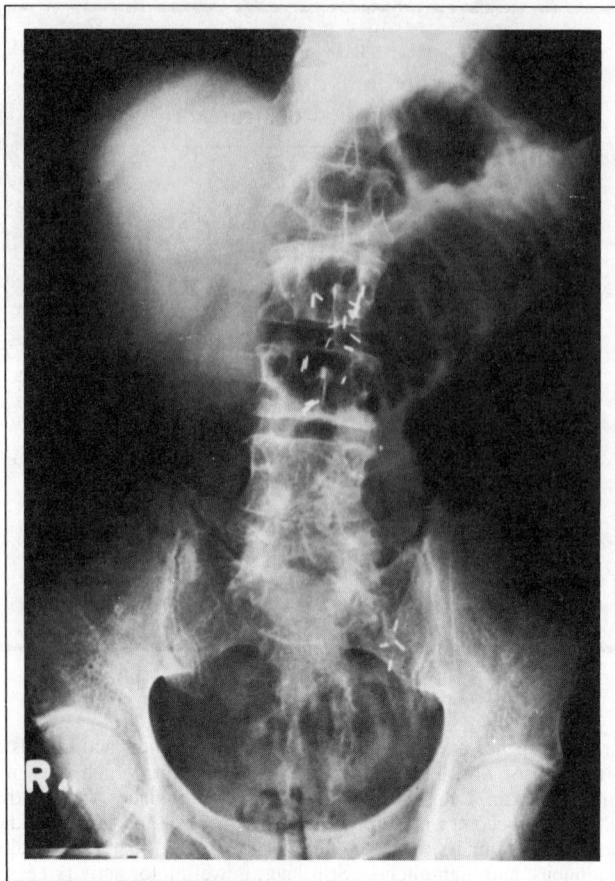

FIGURE 342-1 Plain radiograph of abdomen showing dilated loops of small bowel. The patient had obstruction in the proximal ileum. The clips indicate previous abdominal surgery.

Laboratory Tests

Laboratory tests are rarely helpful in the diagnosis of intestinal obstruction. Careful examination should be performed for inguinal, femoral, or mesenteric hernias. A rising white blood cell count may herald the development of strangulation, but strangulation may be present in the absence of leukocytosis, and leukocytosis may be due to other events not directly related to intestinal obstruction. Most other laboratory tests relate to specific diseases that can cause obstruction or to more general assessment of the patient's health, particularly with regard to the ability to tolerate surgical intervention. Electrolyte derangements and fluid depletion occur in prolonged obstruction consequent to sequestration of fluid and electrolytes in the bowel lumen or to severe emesis. Amylase release from ischemic bowel can lead to a false diagnosis of pancreatitis. Lipase level is usually normal. Acidosis with lactate is an ominous sign of intestinal infarction.

Radiographic Studies

Plain radiographs of the abdomen (KUB) show dilated loops of bowel (Fig. 342-1), often with air-fluid levels in upright views. The radiographs can reveal these changes, for example, in a patient who has abdominal pain, before abdominal distention and hypertympany are present on physical examination. Sometimes a sharp termination of dilated small bowel or colon can suggest a mechanical obstruction, whereas dilation from duodenum to anus is more likely caused by nonspecific (paralytic) ileus. Volvulus of the large bowel has a characteristic inverted "U" loop of bowel. Upright radiographs of the abdomen or of the chest should be obtained also, to look for free air under the diaphragm suggestive of perforation (see Fig. 335-2).

Barium should never be given orally when intestinal obstruction might be present unless obstruction in the large intestine has been unequivocally excluded. If the obstruction is not very low in the rectum (by rectal examination), the next study is a gentle barium enema. This might safely reveal the obstructing lesion if it is in the colon or effectively exclude the colon as the site of obstruction and direct subsequent medical (or surgical) attention to the small bowel, which can then be studied radiographically with contrast media. Barium enema can be used therapeutically to reduce a volvulus or intussusception. Computed tomography or sonography (ultrasound) of the abdomen is not particularly helpful in this clinical situation.

Endoscopy

Upper endoscopy and colonoscopy should not be performed if mechanical intestinal obstruction is suspected; these procedures require the introduction of air into the bowel to allow a field of view, which would further distend the bowel and possibly precipitate perforation. The exception is sigmoid volvulus, in which an experienced colonoscopist can often reduce the volvulus and relieve the obstruction.

Therapy

General therapy for intestinal obstruction is nasogastric intubation and intravenous administration of fluids, electrolytes, and glucose. Some advocate use of a long intestinal tube (such as the Miller-Abbott tube), but studies have demonstrated that nasogastric tube drainage results in decompression comparable to that achieved with longer tubes, and with less trouble.

Patients with upper small bowel obstruction sometimes vomit large quantities of fluid. If this emesis is largely gastric juice, alkalosis and significant hypokalemia can result. If it is mostly upper intestinal and pancreatic secretions, the patient may become acidotic from loss of bicarbonate. Obviously, intravenous fluid and electrolyte replacement must be tailored to the individual patient's deficiencies and requirements. If the site of obstruction is the lower small bowel or colon, vomiting is usually minor and the volume of emesis low. Nevertheless, the patient can have major contraction of intravascular volume caused by sequestration ("third spacing") of remarkably large volumes of fluid in the dilated and secreting bowel.

Because of the danger of strangulation, with consequent ischemic necrosis, it is generally wise to consider surgery early in intestinal obstruction, particularly if there is evidence suggesting obstruction produced by adhesions, volvulus, or an incarcerated hernia and if the patient is a reasonable surgical candidate. In many instances in which obstruction is due to concentric narrowing such as in Crohn's disease, intestinal lymphoma, or acute diverticulitis, medical therapy that is specific for the underlying disease may be sufficiently successful that obstruction is relieved without need for surgery.

Differential Diagnosis

Patients with nonobstructive paralytic ileus frequently have clinical and radiographic findings that are indistinguishable from those of mechanical obstruction of the intestine in its middle or late phase. In ileus, bowel sounds are characteristically absent (but the same may be true very late in the course of mechanical obstruction). Paralytic ileus occurs in peritonitis (of any cause), pneumonia, hypokalemia, sepsis, head trauma, severe general trauma, anticholinergic or opiate drug overdose, pulmonary embolus, myocardial infarction, shock, toxic megacolon, pancreatitis, and myxedema and after many types of surgery, especially if general anesthesia is used. Mechanical obstruction caused by concentric narrowing occurs in Crohn's disease; neoplasms (lymphoma, adenocarcinoma, sarcoma, etc.); and acute or chronic diverticulitis. Obstruction resulting from fecal impaction is especially common in the elderly. Kinking of a loop of bowel results from intraabdominal adhesions (most commonly caused by previous abdominal surgery, even if performed decades prior to the onset of obstruction) and to incarceration of bowel in a hernia. Twisting of the bowel causes obstruction in midgut, cecal, or sigmoid volvulus. Intussusception (the invagination of proximal bowel into the lumen of immediately distal bowel) is often a spontaneous event in young children but is almost always associated with a leading intraluminal mass (such as a polyp or other local nonconcentric neoplasm) in adults. Foreign bodies only rarely cause intestinal obstruction; if

---

BOX 342-2

Classification of intestinal pseudoobstruction

I. "Primary" (idiopathic intestinal pseudo-obstruction)
  A. Hollow visceral myopathy
    1. Familial
    2. Sporadic
  B. Neuropathic
    1. Abnormal myenteric plexus
    2. Normal myenteric plexus
II. Secondary
  A. Scleroderma
  B. Myxedema
  C. Amyloidosis
  D. Muscular dystrophy
  E. Hypokalemia
  F. Chronic renal failure
  G. Diabetes mellitus
  H. Drug toxicity caused by
    1. Anticholinergics
    2. Opiate narcotics
III. Ogilvie's syndrome

---

something gets past the pylorus, it usually makes it all the way through. The distal ileum is the one region where an ingested foreign body or large gallstone may become stuck. Obstruction caused by a gallstone impacted in the lumen of the distal small bowel is (somewhat confusingly) referred to as *gallstone ileus* (Chapter 364). The classic, if rather rare, findings that are seen on an abdominal radiograph indicating gallstone ileus are dilated loops of small bowel with air-fluid levels and air in the biliary tree, and rarely a calcified stone.

INTESTINAL PSEUDOOBSTRUCTION

Intestinal pseudoobstruction is a blanket term used to describe an array of intestinal motor disorders that are characterized by hypomotility, often with dilation of various portions of bowel. In the strictest sense the term refers to a clinical syndrome in which the patient experiences abdominal pain, dilated loops of intestine (often with air-fluid levels), and diarrhea or constipation, all of which suggest obstruction—but no true mechanical obstruction exists. In the loosest sense the term is a general classification under which the more specific diseases that may be responsible for the clinical presentation mentioned previously are included. This latter classification includes situations in which the clinical symptoms do not suggest obstruction but in which the findings on plain radiographic examination resemble mechanical obstruction or ileus and situations in which there are other clinical manifestations (such as diarrhea or malabsorption caused by bacterial overgrowth) related to bowel hypomotility.

Intestinal pseudoobstruction can be secondary to various disorders—such as scleroderma, amyloidosis, myxedema, muscular dystrophy, chronic renal failure, and hypokalemia—or can result from excessive drug therapy with anticholinergic agents or opiate narcotics (Box 342-2). This condition overlaps with paralytic ileus. Idiopathic intestinal pseudoobstruction includes sporadic and familial hollow visceral myopathy and a nonmyopathic disease in which the problem seems to reside in the autonomic innervation of the intestine.

Acute pseudoobstruction of the colon characterized by massive colonic dilation in the absence of mechanical obstruction in severely ill debilitated patients is commonly termed *Ogilvie's syndrome*. Predisposing conditions include recent surgery, neurologic disorders, serious infections, cardiorespiratory insufficiency, and metabolic disturbances, often coupled with the use of drugs that perturb colonic motility (anticholinergics or narcotics).

Pathophysiology

Hypomotility and dilatation of bowel loops occur because the smooth muscle of the muscularis propria is incapable of contracting in normal fashion and is even incapable of maintaining tone. Hypomotility

and dilation are caused by intrinsic disease in the muscle fibers themselves (hollow visceral myopathy, muscular dystrophy); by impaired muscle metabolism (myxedema, hypokalemia); by infiltration of the muscle by some abnormal material (scleroderma, amyloidosis, myxedema); or by impaired autonomic neural regulation of smooth muscle function (neuropathic idiopathic intestinal pseudoobstruction, anticholinergic toxicity).

Diagnosis

Surgery should be avoided in intestinal pseudoobstruction. Patients who have symptoms or signs of intestinal obstruction or ileus may have pseudoobstruction and should be evaluated for possible underlying disorders, especially those that can be readily corrected, such as drug toxicity, hypokalemia, and myxedema. If esophageal motility is also abnormal, consider scleroderma, amyloidosis, or idiopathic intestinal pseudoobstruction. The diagnosis of idiopathic intestinal pseudoobstruction becomes one of exclusion of those diseases that cause secondary pseudoobstruction. Because of the more common occurrence of pain, hollow visceral myopathy more often requires exploratory surgery to exclude mechanical obstruction and, in some cases, to resect or bypass segments of bowel in an attempt to improve nutrition or control symptoms. The definitive diagnosis of hollow visceral myopathy (and of the abnormal myenteric plexus forms of idiopathic intestinal pseudoobstruction) is a tissue diagnosis and requires careful evaluation of the histologic abnormalities of resected intestine.

Treatment

The therapy of some forms of secondary intestinal pseudoobstruction such as renal failure and drug toxicity involves treatment of the underlying disorder. For other disorders—such as scleroderma, amyloidosis, and muscular dystrophy—there is no successful therapy for the primary disease that can be expected to reverse or ameliorate the pseudoobstruction. There is no effective therapy that is specific for idiopathic intestinal pseudoobstruction. Consequently, for those forms of pseudoobstruction that are not readily amenable to cure, management consists of treating the complications. If the patient has bacterial overgrowth caused by intestinal stasis, manifested as diarrhea or malabsorption, recurrent cycles of broad-spectrum antibiotics can be successful, as in the treatment of other intestinal stasis syndromes (Chapter 340). Metoclopramide (Reglan), cisapride (Propulsid), and erythromycin have the pharmacologic potential to increase propulsive intestinal motility in pseudoobstruction and are worth a therapeutic trial in these patients. Overall effectiveness has not been great. Metoclopramide is limited by dystonic reactions and other central nervous system side effects. Obviously, anticholinergics and narcotics are contraindicated. Careful colonoscopic decompression, often in conjunction with a decompression tube, has been useful in Ogilvie's syndrome.

If nutrition is impaired, oral administration of liquid, low-residue, complete nutrition preparations may achieve, and assist in maintaining, adequate nutrition. A rare patient may require long-term total parenteral nutrition.

As mentioned previously, surgical therapy is occasionally attempted to bypass severely dilated loops in an effort to improve oral nutrition and perhaps to relieve pain, but its effectiveness varies greatly from patient to patient.

PERITONITIS

Inflammation of the peritoneum can be classified as acute or chronic, or as infectious, chemical, or idiopathic, depending on the type of etiologic event that has resulted in peritonitis. Innervation of the peritoneum is rich in sensory receptors for pain. Therefore a patient may be able to indicate the specific site of local peritonitis, such as that caused by contact with an adjacent inflamed intraabdominal organ.

The approach to the patient with acute peritonitis is described in Chapter 335. In patients with chronic peritonitis or forms of peritonitis that are rare or of obscure cause, important points from the history might be previous systemic disease or infection, type and timing of the onset of the symptoms, ethnic origin, and family history. On physical examination, tenderness, often with rebound tenderness, is characteristic for acute peritonitis. Patients with chronic peritonitis have little or no rebound tenderness. Paralytic ileus occurs frequently in acute peritonitis, so the absence of bowel sounds on auscultation of the abdomen is a common finding.

Plain radiographs of the abdomen may appear unremarkable, may suggest ascites, or may show free air if peritonitis is secondary to perforation of a hollow organ. An upright radiograph of the chest should be obtained in an effort to demonstrate free air under the diaphragm (Fig. 335-2).

Acute peritonitis commonly shows peripheral blood leukocytosis, but other blood tests are not likely to reveal an abnormality, except in patients with spontaneous bacterial peritonitis associated with cirrhosis and therefore abnormal liver test findings.

If ascites is present, diagnostic paracentesis is essential. The fluid in acute or chronic peritonitis is an exudate. The gross appearance of fluid obtained may help in the diagnosis. It may be purulent, feculent, hemorrhagic, or heavily bile stained. Fluid should be analyzed for cell count and differential, Gram stain, cultures (including those for tuberculous and anaerobic organisms), albumin (with simultaneous serum albumin), and amylase level.

After initial assessment and sometimes before all laboratory results are available, the physician must determine whether the patient has acute peritonitis related to a condition that requires early surgical intervention. If surgery is not indicated, further studies may be appropriate. One procedure that should be considered is peritoneoscopy, which can be done with local anesthesia with minimal risk and may make laparotomy unnecessary. Furthermore, it is the best method for obtaining biopsy specimens of the peritoneum. If chronic peritonitis seems to be present, percutaneous needle biopsy of the peritoneum (with needle and technique similar to that used for pleural biopsy) is an adequate method for obtaining a tissue specimen. Sixty to seventy-five percent of patients with tuberculous peritonitis have caseating granulomas that can be seen in specimens obtained by percutaneous needle biopsy (Chapter 367).

Differential Diagnosis

Infectious peritonitis can be caused by a wide array of organisms. If peritonitis results from rupture of a colonic diverticulum, cecal perforation secondary to colonic obstruction, toxic megacolon, ruptured appendix, or other type of colonic perforation, colonic organisms such as *Escherichia coli* or *Bacteroides* spp. may predominate. If a patient has preexisting ascites from whatever cause, but especially from cirrhosis, spontaneous bacterial peritonitis may occur (Chapter 354). The infecting organism may be *E. coli* or other coliforms, but because this infection is blood-borne, pneumococcal peritonitis is common, especially during winter months, when pneumonia is common. Tuberculous peritonitis is frequently an indolent infection, and correct diagnosis requires that it be suspected in patients who are at high risk for tuberculosis, such as HIV-positive patients. Tuberculosis and malignancy of the peritoneum are the most common causes of exudative ascites in patients without underlying liver disease. Gonococcal peritonitis occurs occasionally after massive gonococcemia. Chemical peritonitis occurs when the inflammation of the peritoneum is due primarily to the caustic effect of some substance rather than to infection by an organism. Offending substances are gastric acid, pancreatic fluid, bile, and starch. Miscellaneous or idiopathic peritonitis occurs in familial Mediterranean fever and in diseases associated with vasculitis such as systemic lupus erythematosus and polyarteritis nodosa. Specific therapy for the various causes of peritonitis is discussed in the various chapters that deal with those diseases.

BIBLIOGRAPHY

Abbasi AA et al: Myxedema ileus, *JAMA* 234:181, 1975.
Achem SR et al: Neuronal dysplasia and chronic intestinal pseudoobstruction, *Gastroenterology* 92:805, 1987.
Anuras S: Intestinal pseudoobstruction syndrome, *Annu Rev Med* 39:1, 1988.
Borhanmanesh F et al: Tuberculous peritonitis, *Ann Intern Med* 76:567, 1972.
Bynum TE: Disorders of bowel motility. In Eastwood GL, editor: *Core textbook of gastroenterology,* Philadelphia, 1989, JB Lippincott.
Endoscopic decompression for acute colonic pseudoobstruction, *Gastrointest Endosc* 44:144, 1996.

Fabri PJ, Rosemurgy A: Reoperation for small intestinal obstruction, *Surg Clin North Am* 71:131, 1991.
Maddaus MA et al: The biology of peritonitis and implications for treatment, *Surg Clin North Am* 68:431, 1988.
Richards WO, Williams LF Jr: Obstruction of the large and small intestine, *Surg Clin North Am* 68:355, 1988.
Stranghellini V et al: Chronic idiopathic intestinal pseudoobstruction, *Gut* 28:5, 1987.
Strodel WE, Brothers T: Colonoscopic decompression of pseudoobstruction and volvulus, *Surg Clin North Am* 69:1327, 1989.
Wilcox CM, Dismukes WE: Spontaneous bacterial peritonitis, *Medicine* 66:447, 1987.

CHAPTER

343 Tumors of the Small and Large Intestines

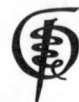

Charles J. Lightdale

MALIGNANT TUMORS OF THE SMALL INTESTINE
Relevant Physiology and Pathophysiology

That malignant tumors of the small intestine are quite uncommon is surprising considering the much higher frequency of malignancies originating in the large intestine and stomach. Liquidity of its contents, low bacterial population, rapid transit, rapid cell turnover, local immune responses, and active detoxifying enzyme systems, alone or in combination, have been suggested as contributing to the infrequency of small intestinal malignant tumors.

There are about 2000 new cases of small bowel cancer per year in the United States. The majority are adenocarcinomas. The disease is rare before age 30, when incidence gradually begins to rise steadily, peaking in the sixth decade. There is a slight preponderance of incidence in males, but no marked social differential. The incidence of small bowel cancer in different geographic regions seems to parallel the incidence of colonic carcinoma. In the Middle East the incidence of primary small intestinal lymphoma appears to exceed the incidence of other small intestinal malignancies.

Adenocarcinomas arise from the crypts of the mucosa of the small intestine. They develop most commonly in the proximal small bowel and least commonly toward the ileum. Clustering of duodenal adenocarcinomas in the periampullary region has implicated bile in the pathophysiology of these neoplasms. Histologically, adenocarcinomas of the small intestine most often resemble colonic rather than gastric adenocarcinomas. Metastases to local lymphatics are common; hematogenous spread and peritoneal seeding also occur.

Lymphomas originate in lymphoid cells within and beneath the mucosa of the small intestine and are more common in the distal small intestine. Hodgkin's disease is the least common primary lymphoid malignancy of the small bowel. Small bowel lymphomas are often multifocal and may infiltrate beneath the mucosa over a wide area.

The "Mediterranean lymphoma" prevalent in the Middle East appears to be a distinctive pathologic entity. The small intestinal lesion is usually diffuse, and the cells that characterize this neoplasm often have features of plasma cells, histiocytes, and atypical lymphocytes. Mediterranean lymphoma *(immunoproliferative small intestine disease)* affects the duodenum and proximal jejunum more commonly than the ileum. It may be associated with the production of an abnormal circulating immunoglobulin A (IgA) that contains only alpha chains (alpha chain disease), although not all diffuse mucosal lymphomas of the small intestine produce this immunoglobulin.

The smooth muscle layer of the muscularis externa of the small intestine may give rise to *leiomyosarcomas.* These are slightly more common in the proximal than in the distal small intestine. They metastasize by hematogenous spread to liver and lung and only rarely to regional lymph nodes.

Premalignant States and Risk Factors

Several conditions and diseases are associated with an increased incidence of small bowel adenocarcinoma or lymphoma.

Regional Enteritis (Crohn's Disease). Adenocarcinoma of the small bowel occurs more often in patients with regional enteritis than in age-matched controls and affects the ileum more often than the proximal bowel. Patients who have had segments of intestine bypassed surgically may be at higher risk.

Inherited Polyposis Syndromes. Several inherited intestinal polyposis syndromes are associated with an increased incidence of small intestinal adenocarcinoma. In familial adenomatous polyposis and Gardner's syndrome, adenomas and adenocarcinomas of the duodenum occur with increased frequency, particularly in the periampullary region (Chapter 365). Small intestinal (especially duodenal) adenocarcinoma has been reported in patients with Peutz-Jeghers syndrome, although the incidence is not high.

Celiac Sprue. An increased incidence of malignancy, especially lymphoma of the small intestine, has been reported in patients with celiac sprue. These lymphomas, derived from intestinal T cells, occur most frequently in the proximal small intestine. The association of celiac sprue with lymphoma has been questioned, because a diffuse intestinal lymphoma can also cause malabsorption, but evidence for this association is increasing. One study indicates that strict adherence to a gluten-free diet decreases the incidence of lymphoma. For further discussion see Chapter 340.

Immune Deficiency States. An increased incidence of lymphoma of the small intestine has been suggested in hereditary syndromes of decreased humoral or cellular immunity and also in acquired immunodeficiency. The latter group includes patients with acquired immunodeficiency syndrome (Chapter 346) and those treated with intensive radiation, chemotherapy, and immunosuppressives.

Laboratory and Other Diagnostic Tests

Patients with small intestinal tumors may be anemic and have occult blood in their stools. They may be hypoalbuminemic as a result of protein loss from the tumor and obstruction of lymphatics, especially patients with lymphomas that may infiltrate the mesentery. Malabsorption may produce excess fat in the stool, abnormal Schilling and D-xylose test results, prolonged prothrombin time, and low serum calcium and magnesium concentrations (Chapter 331).

Most malignant tumors of the small intestine can be detected in carefully performed barium contrast studies. A common error in evaluating patients with abdominal symptoms is to perform only a barium enema and upper gastrointestinal series. These examinations usually demonstrate only the most proximal and distal small bowel loops; therefore a small intestinal series should be performed. The detection of small lesions in the small intestine by barium radiographic study requires a skilled, interested, and attentive radiologist. The use of enteroclysis, or small bowel enema, can provide increased accuracy. In this more invasive technique, barium is instilled directly into the intestine by passage of a tube through the nose or mouth.

Duodenal tumors may be detected and biopsy specimens obtained by upper gastrointestinal endoscopy. Modern fiberscopes may reach the third portion of the duodenum, and longer enteroscopes have been developed. Most of the jejunum can be examined with "push"-type

---

✔ *WHEN TO REFER*

If the diagnosis of a small bowel tumor is made by radiologic examination, referral for gastrointestinal endoscopy may be appropriate for confirmation and histologic analysis. Most patients require surgical resection, but oncology referral may be appropriate as well for additional treatment of malignant small bowel neoplasms, most notably small bowel lymphoma.

---

enteroscopes that allow biopsy, and even the ileum can be seen using "sonde" enteroscopes, which rely on peristalsis for passage but have no biopsy capability. Tumors of the terminal ileum may be revealed in some patients if the ileocecal valve is passed with a colonoscope. Peroral biopsy via tubes passed under fluoroscopic control may obtain a biopsy specimen of small bowel malignancy, particularly in diffuse or multifocal lymphoma. Frequently the diagnosis of small bowel malignancy is made by the surgeon at the time of laparotomy, by palpation, and by biopsy.

Differential Diagnosis

Any of the small intestinal malignancies may ulcerate and bleed into the bowel lumen. Blood loss is generally not massive and may be occult. Leiomyosarcomas may be particularly vascular and may be a cause of gross bleeding with melena or grossly bloody stools. Tumors proximal to the ligament of Treitz occasionally cause hematemesis if they bleed rapidly.

Small bowel malignancies may narrow the intestinal lumen, creating partial obstruction that may cause cramping abdominal pain accompanied by loud peristaltic rushes and abdominal distention. Small bowel adenocarcinomas tend to create a ringlike constriction similar to that created by colonic adenocarcinomas. Small bowel tumors may also act as a lead point for an intussusception, producing intermittent obstruction. Higher grades of obstruction cause backing up of bowel contents, with nausea and vomiting; the vomiting may be feculent if the obstruction is in the distal small intestine and associated with stasis (Chapter 342).

Weight loss may be a prominent feature of small bowel malignancies. Malignant tumors in the abdomen frequently cause anorexia and decreased caloric intake. Abdominal pain caused by partial bowel obstruction may be exacerbated by food intake, contributing to anorexia. Bacterial overgrowth in the obstructed small intestine may be a cause of malabsorption, producing steatorrhea and weight loss (Chapter 340). Malabsorption is common with diffusely infiltrating small intestinal lymphomas.

Small bowel malignancies can, on occasion, cause acute abdominal catastrophes such as perforation, massive hemorrhage, or acute intestinal obstruction.

Management

Surgery is usually the first-line therapeutic modality for small bowel malignancy. A localized neoplasm is resected widely to ensure that resection margins are free of tumor. In the case of adenocarcinoma, surgery is the only possibility for cure; recurrences are more likely if the cancer has penetrated the serosa and invaded regional lymph nodes. Chemotherapy and radiation therapy can provide temporary palliation in a few patients with unresectable disease.

Radiation therapy and chemotherapy are important modalities for small bowel lymphomas as primary treatment and as adjuvant therapy after surgical resection. Perforation of the gastrointestinal tract caused by rapid lysis of lymphomatous areas has been described after radiation therapy or chemotherapy. Thus surgical resection with curative intent is widely held as preferable. Involvement of local lymph nodes is generally an indication for postoperative irradiation or chemotherapy. In widespread, unresectable disease, chemotherapy is indicated. Leiomyosarcomas are best treated with surgery. They are radioresistant, and chemotherapy has been largely ineffective.

CARCINOID TUMORS
Relevant Physiology and Pathophysiology

Carcinoid tumors are an interesting group of neoplasms that have their origin in the endocrine argentaffin cells in the small intestinal mucosa (argentaffinomas). They are found incidentally in 0.50% to 0.75% of autopsies. Carcinoid tumors occur frequently in the ileum, where argentaffin cells are more abundant, and 20% of these tumors are multifocal. Histologic criteria do not help the physician to distinguish benign from malignant carcinoid tumors. The tumors are invariably small. About 80% of tumors more than 2 cm in diameter metastasize; those less than 1 cm are almost always benign. Metastases are to local lymph nodes, liver, lung, and bone. Carcinoid tumors may induce a reactive fibrosis in the bowel mesentery, sometimes creating an angulated intestinal segment. Even malignant and metastatic carcinoid tumors are indolent. More than 50% of patients with unresectable local metastases survive 5 years, as do about 30% of those with liver metastases. About 10% of individuals with liver metastases survive more than 10 years.

Laboratory and Other Diagnostic Tests

The biochemical marker for the carcinoid syndrome is increased urinary excretion of 5-hydroxyindoleacetic acid (5-HIAA). More than 30 mg of 5-HIAA is usually excreted in 24 hours by patients with carcinoid syndrome. Less striking increases in urinary 5-HIAA may be found in some patients with malabsorption such as occurs in celiac disease and bacterial overgrowth syndromes. Blood serotonin and 5-hydroxytryptophan levels can now be determined; the latter is helpful if gastric carcinoid is suspected. When urinary 5-HIAA excretion is being tested, patients should avoid drugs that may produce false-positive test results, most notably glyceryl guaiacolate, phenothiazines, and methenamine mandelate. Foods rich in serotonin should also be avoided. These include pineapples, bananas, avocados, and walnuts.

Carcinoid tumors may secrete a variety of other hormones, including insulin, adrenocorticotropic hormone, melanocyte-stimulating hormone, gastrin, and glucagon. The endocrine cells from which carcinoid tumors originate are part of the amine content, precursor uptake, and decarboxylation (APUD) family. Foregut carcinoid tumors have also been associated with pluriglandular adenomatoses (e.g., pituitary, adrenal, and parathyroid tumors) and with pancreatic gastrinomas.

Differential Diagnosis

Carcinoid tumors of the small bowel seldom ulcerate and bleed and are usually too small to cause obstruction. They may, however, produce transient intussusceptions and cause cramping abdominal pain and diarrhea. These symptoms may be long standing and intermittent, suggesting irritable bowel syndrome or Crohn's disease.

In about one third of patients with liver metastases, carcinoid syndrome, which occurs rarely with only nodal metastases, develops. *Carcinoid syndrome* is characterized primarily by episodes of flushing and diarrhea. The flush may produce a cyanotic appearance, and if attacks are prolonged, facial edema and telangiectasis may develop. The mediator of the carcinoid flush is unknown. Kallikrein, bradykinin, other kinin peptides, substance P, prostaglandins, serotonin, and histamine have been implicated. The flush has been precipitated by ingestion of a meal and by administration of ethanol, calcium, epinephrine, isoproterenol, and pentagastrin. The diarrhea and cramps in this syndrome appear to be related to the production of serotonin (5-hydroxytryptamine).

Bronchial spasm is often part of carcinoid syndrome, and wheezing may become a prominent feature. Right-sided heart lesions, particularly pulmonary and tricuspid valvular fibrosis, may develop with associated murmurs of pulmonary stenosis and tricuspid insufficiency. Right-sided congestive heart failure may produce further hepatomegaly, ascites, pulmonary congestion, and edema.

Diarrhea in carcinoid syndrome is usually watery, episodic, and associated with abdominal cramping and loud borborygmi. Gastric carcinoids that tend to produce more 5-hydroxytryptophan than serotonin and that also may produce histamine usually are not associated with diarrhea.

Most patients with carcinoid syndrome have liver metastases, which are usually evident on physical examination and liver scans. Carcinoid tumors with nodal metastases that produce the syndrome may cause a palpable abdominal mass. Ovarian carcinoid tumors are usually detected by abdominal or pelvic examination, and bronchial carcinoid tumors by chest radiography.

Management

Carcinoid tumors of the small bowel should be surgically resected. If metastatic disease is present, the approach remains the same as in other bowel malignancies. In patients with the carcinoid syndrome all treatment must be carefully monitored and controlled to prevent

✔ WHEN TO REFER

Carcinoid tumors that appear to be resectable should be referred to an appropriate surgical specialist. Oncology referral should be obtained for patients with rapidly progressive metastatic carcinoid.

precipitating a carcinoid crisis. Chemotherapy has had some benefit in unresectable disease, but treatment efforts, in general, should be tempered by the usually indolent growth of these tumors. A variety of antiserotonin agents, antihistamines, antiadrenergics, antiprostaglandins, and steroids have been helpful in the carcinoid syndrome, but benefits must be weighed against side effects. Intravenous somatostatin has been used to ameliorate acute symptoms, and subcutaneous somatostatin analogs have become important agents for successful long-term control.

BENIGN TUMORS OF THE SMALL INTESTINE

Most benign small intestinal tumors cause no symptoms and are incidentally found during radiographic or endoscopic examination, surgery, or autopsy.

Adenomas may be polypoid or sessile, similar to their colonic counterparts. The potential for malignant change, however, appears to be less for small intestinal than for colonic adenomas. Isolated adenomas may bleed intermittently, but because they are usually small and soft, they rarely cause obstruction. Most occur in the upper small bowel, and in some cases an experienced endoscopist can remove them via cautery snare.

Leiomyomas, benign smooth muscle tumors, sometimes occur throughout the small intestine. They may have a rich blood supply and ulcerate and bleed profusely. They may also obstruct the lumen. Usually they produce a smooth filling defect, which can be seen on barium radiograph, as they grow beneath the bowel mucosa. Sometimes leiomyomas ulcerate, producing an umbilicated so-called target lesion, seen on barium radiographic examination as a mass with a central ulceration. Leiomyomas should generally be removed surgically if they cause symptoms.

Neurofibromas may arise as isolated lesions or as part of von Recklinghausen's disease, in which multiple tumors are often present. Neurofibromas tend to grow outward into the serosa and may become large, causing the intestine to twist around them and become obstructed.

Hamartomas are benign growths that may contain all the cellular elements of the small bowel mucosa. Peutz-Jeghers syndrome is characterized by multiple hamartomatous polyps in the gastrointestinal tract. The polyps seem to increase in number as the patient grows older and may bleed, cause obstruction, or cause intussusception. If surgery is required for these complications, it is generally recommended that the length of resected bowel be kept to a minimum.

Duodenal glands (Brunner's glands) are submucosal and mucosal mucus-secreting glands that are most prominent in the duodenal bulb but may extend into the jejunum. Adenomas that develop in this tissue may form polypoid and even pedunculated tumors. A single adenoma may be associated with chronic gastric hyperacidity, but diffuse hyperplasia of Brunner's glands is more common. Duodenal gland adenomas may sometimes contain adipose tissue, in which case they are considered hamartomatous. Duodenal gland adenomas only rarely cause symptoms. Endoscopic observation and biopsy confirmation are usually all that is required for diagnosis; a pedunculated lesion can be removed endoscopically by cautery snare.

MALIGNANT TUMORS OF THE LARGE INTESTINE
Relevant Physiology and Pathophysiology

Epidemiology and Incidence. A striking feature of colonic cancer is its geographic variation in incidence. The disease seems to occur primarily in industrialized Western countries. In the United States, about 134,000 new cases of colorectal cancer were diagnosed in 1996. Studies of migrant populations have shown fascinating changes in the incidence of colonic carcinoma. For example, in Japan the incidence of colonic cancer is increasing but remains relatively low. In Japanese families who have emigrated to the United States, however, within one generation colonic cancer occurs at a rate similar to that in the general American population.

Carcinogenesis and Its Inhibition. Diets high in fat and refined carbohydrate and low in plant fiber, more typical in the industrialized West, have been implicated in higher colonic cancer rates. There is some data to suggest that low-dose aspirin and other nonsteroidal antiinflammatory drugs may decrease colon cancer risk. At least 20 different classes of chemicals, some of which occur naturally in food (e.g., calcium), seem to have a protective effect against colon cancer in laboratory models.

Although the effects of environment continue to be studied and debated, genetic susceptibility to colonic cancer has become better defined. In certain groups hereditary colonic cancer risk has been clearly established. In the hereditary polyposis syndromes, particularly in familial adenomatous polyposis and in Gardner's syndrome, the risk is very high. These diseases, accounting for about 1% of colorectal cancer cases, are inherited as autosomal dominants with high penetrance. Familial polyposis coli is characterized by the growth of numerous adenomatous polyps in the colon, most markedly in the distal colon. The polyps frequently begin in childhood and increase in number with the patient's age. The colon may become carpeted with adenomas. Gardner's syndrome is characterized by multiple soft tissue tumors, fibromas, and osteomas, as well as colonic adenomas. In every patient with familial polyposis coli or Gardner's syndrome a colonic carcinoma will develop, with risk increasing as the patient becomes older. Other syndromes involving colonic polyposis and increased cancer risk include Turcot's syndrome, in which patients may have gliomas and medulloblastomas, and Oldfield's syndrome, in which patients have multiple sebaceous cysts. In the Peutz-Jeghers syndrome, characterized by abnormal pigmentation of the skin and mucous membranes and gastrointestinal hamartomas, there is a small increased risk of colonic adenocarcinoma.

Families have been identified with a marked hereditary increased risk of colonic carcinoma without florid polyposis, which has been called *hereditary nonpolyposis colorectal cancer* (HNPCC). HNPCC accounts for about 5% of new colorectal cancer cases. Two groups have been recognized. In Lynch syndrome I, cancers occur at an earlier age on average than sporadic colon cancers and are site specific to the colon. In Lynch syndrome II, patients have an additional susceptibility to other forms of cancer, particularly of the endometrium and ovaries. These syndromes are dominantly inherited and are characterized by the occurrence of small "flat adenomas" in the ascending colon. The "Amsterdam criteria" set the strictest standard for diagnosis of HNPCC: (1) three or more relatives with colorectal cancer; (2) at least one a first-degree relative of the other two; (3) diagnosis in one or more relatives before age 50; and (4) colorectal cancer involving at least two generations.

The actual gene responsible for familial adenomatous polyposis and variants including Gardner's syndrome and Turcot's syndrome has been identified on the long arm of chromosome 5 and sequenced (APC gene). In HNPCC, mutations in four genes on chromosomes 2, 3, and 7 are associated with 70% to 80% of cases.

Premalignant States. Patients with adenomatous polyps, especially villous adenomas, are considered at higher risk for colonic cancer. Evidence is mounting that there is a common sequence from adenoma to carcinoma. Invasive cancer has frequently been found in adenomatous tissue. Adenomas in patients with familial polyposis are similar to those in patients with single polyps. Several cases have been reported in which patients refused surgery for polyps that were subsequently observed over a period of years to become malignant. About one third of operative specimens from patients with colonic cancer also contain one or more adenomas.

A prior adenoma or colorectal cancer puts an individual at higher risk for subsequent colorectal neoplasia. On the other hand, colon adenomas are common, occurring in about 25% of patients over 50 years and increasing with age. Few adenomas progress to cancer, with an estimated incidence of only 2.5 polyps per 1000 per year. Progression from normal mucosa to adenoma seems related to a series of genetic abnormalities acquired after birth. Further abnormalities in both oncogenes and tumor suppressor genes result in further degen-

Table 343-1 Relationship of the Dukes' staging classification and TNM staging proposed by the American Joint Committee on Cancer and the International Union Against Cancer

	AJCC/UICC			
	T*	N†	M‡	DUKES
Stage 0	Tis	N0	M0	
Stage I	{ T1	N0	M0 }	A
	{ T2	N0	M0 }	
Stage II	{ T3	N0	M0 }	B
	{ T4	N0	M0 }	
Stage III	{ Any T	N1	M0 }	C
	{ Any T	N2, N3	M0 }	
Stage IV	Any T	Any N	M1	

*T = depth of cancer invasion: Tis, carcinoma in situ; T1, invasion of submucosa; T2, invasion of muscularis propria; T3, invasion to the subserosa; T4, invasion of visceral peritoneum, other organs, or structures.
†N = lymph node metastases: N0, no lymph node metastases; N1, metastases to one to three pericolic lymph nodes; N2, metastases to four or more pericolic nodes; N3, metastases to nodes along a named vascular trunk.
‡M = metastatic disease: M0, no distant metastasis; M1, any distant metastasis.

eration to carcinoma. A diminutive polyp takes an estimated average of 10 years to develop into an invasive carcinoma. About 75% of new cases of colorectal cancer occur in individuals with no known predisposing factors.

With increasing size, polyps tend to show increasing villous change and increasing dysplasia. An exception are some small colorectal flat adenomas reported most often from Japan, which seem to develop dysplasia and carcinoma in spite of their small size. Precancerous dysplastic changes have been described in the colonic mucosa of patients with long-standing ulcerative colitis and Crohn's disease, who have an increased risk of colonic cancer (Chapter 341).

In patients with colonic adenomas and carcinomas the zone of cell proliferation at the base of the colonic crypts has been shown to expand upward. Cells continue to show evidence of deoxyribonucleic acid (DNA) synthesis and other evidence of immature cellular structure and function at the mucosal surface. Such changes have also been found in patients with inflammatory bowel disease.

The incidence of colonic carcinoma is nearly the same in men and women, although incidence of rectal cancer is slightly higher in men and overall incidence is slightly higher in women. Colonic cancer before age 40 is uncommon and suggests possible familial disease. The mean age at diagnosis is about 65 years.

The location of cancers in the colon appears to be changing. Two decades ago about two thirds of colon cancers were reported to occur in the distal 25 cm of the rectosigmoid. More recently this proportion has decreased to one half or less of colonic cancers.

Most colonic adenocarcinomas form hard, nodular areas that grow irregularly. They may be polypoid and fungate and ulcerate, producing exophytic, bulky masses, or they may infiltrate around the bowel lumen, causing the classic "napkin-ring" lesion. Histologically, colonic cancers may vary from well-differentiated cells that appear normal (grade I) to highly anaplastic cells (grade IV) and may contain a variable amount of mucin. Colonic cancers, which produce intracellular mucin (signet-ring type), tend to be particularly aggressive. The pathologic staging of colonic cancer is based on depth of invasion and absence or presence of lymph node or distant metastases. The Dukes' staging system is most widely used, but there is increasing acceptance of the TNM (tumor, node, metastasis) system proposed by the American Joint Committee on Cancer (AJCC) and the International Union Against Cancer (UICC) (Table 343-1).

Only about 1% of colon malignancies are not adenocarcinomas. The most common of these are the lymphomas, primarily the diffuse histiocytic type. More common in immunosuppressed patients, such as those with HIV disease, these usually occur in either the cecal or the rectal areas. If polypoid, lymphomas may be impossible to distinguish grossly from adenocarcinomas. They may also infiltrate diffusely, producing a nodular, thickened bowel wall with ulcerations. Although less common, sarcomas may occur in the wall of the colon and resemble in behavior those found in the stomach and small intestine (Chapter 338).

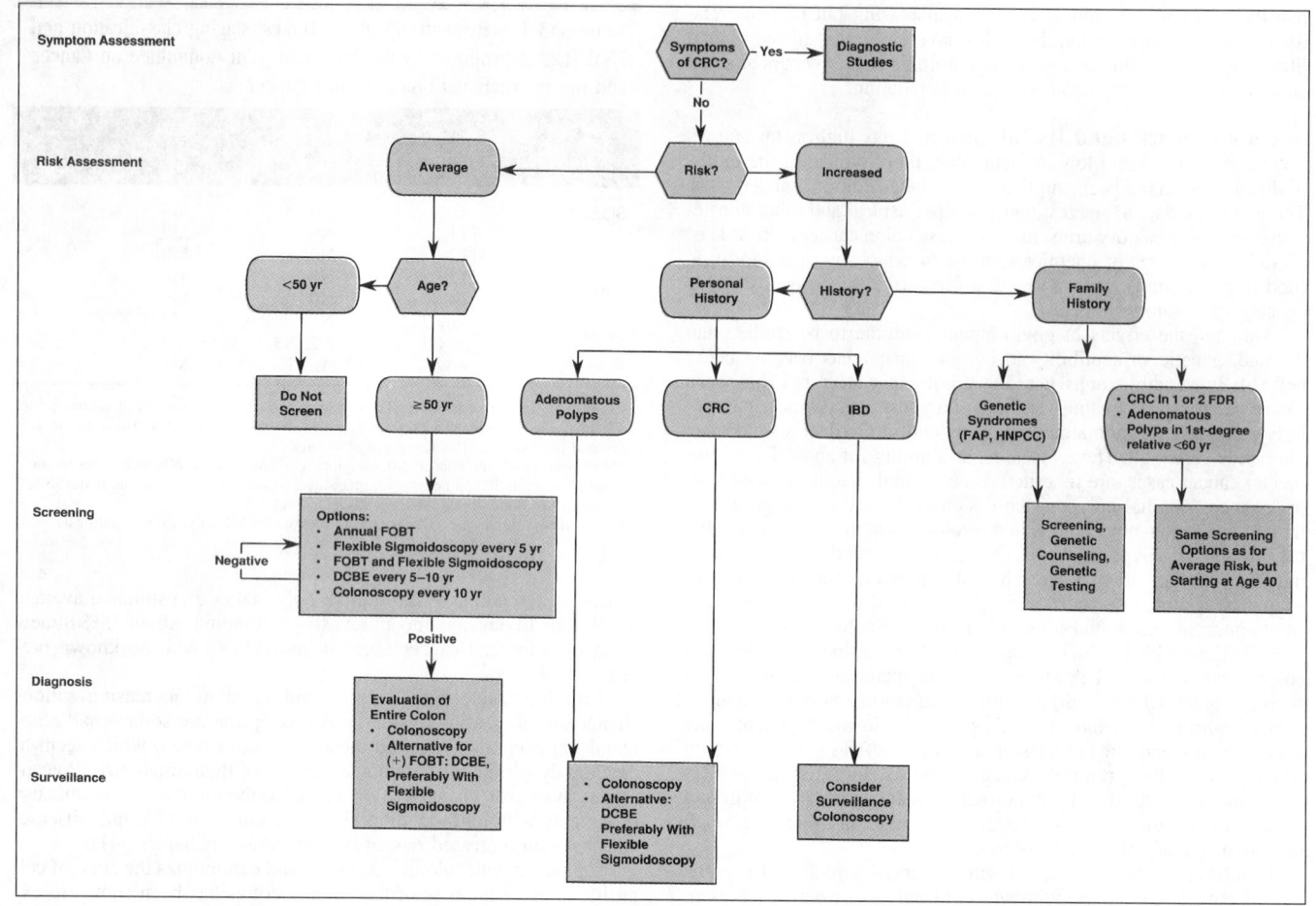

FIGURE 343-1   Algorithm of guidelines for screening approaches in patients at average risk and increased risk for the development of colorectal cancer, designed for prevention and early detection of the disease. *CRC*, Colorectal cancer; *IBD*, inflammatory bowel disease; *FOBT*, fecal occult blood test; *DCBE*, double contrast barium enema; *FAP*, familial adenomatous polyposis; *HNPCC*, hereditary nonpolyposis colorectal cancer; *FDR*, first-degree relatives.

From Winawer SJ, Fletcher RH, Miller L et al: *Gastroenterology* 112:594, 1997.

Laboratory and Other Diagnostic Tests

Laboratory findings that suggest the presence of colonic neoplasm include hypoalbuminemia, iron deficiency anemia, and occult blood in the stool. Elevated alkaline phosphatase concentration suggests colonic cancer metastatic to liver or bone. In liver metastases, bilirubin concentration remains normal until late in the course, and transaminase levels are usually normal or only slightly elevated.

Radiography and endoscopy are the primary means of establishing the diagnosis of large bowel cancer. Radiologists can detect fine mucosal details and small lesions with the air-contrast barium enema technique. It is a useful procedure for the identification of small polypoid lesions, although colonoscopy seems to be more sensitive.

Colonoscopy is used instead of barium enema or to confirm the presence of possibly cancerous lesions seen on barium enema and to document their nature by biopsy. With this information, appropriate therapy can be carried out with more assurance. Flexible sigmoidoscopes, essentially short colonoscopes, can be used with similar purpose for rectosigmoid lesions. For the most part, however, a full colon examination is preferred. Synchronous colonic carcinomas that are not evident on barium enema examination can be detected by colonoscopy; they occur in 1% to 5% of patients with colonic carcinoma. In addition, up to 40% to 50% of patients have synchronous adenomatous polyps.

Digital examination of the rectum may reveal a mass lesion. The digital rectal examination is an important part of the complete physical examination for many reasons and generally should not be omitted without reason. Abdominal mass lesions may be palpable at times. If there is metastatic spread to the liver, hepatomegaly may be noted, and the liver may feel hard and nodular and be slightly tender. Peritoneal metastases may cause ascites.

Endoscopic ultrasonography has been used to stage colorectal cancer, particularly rectal cancer. Locoregional staging with endoscopic ultrasound (EUS) for depth of tumor invasion and regional lymph node metastases has proved more accurate than pelvic computed tomography (CT) for rectal cancer staging. CT is still the best modality for the evaluation of distant metastases, such as to the liver.

Screening for Colorectal Cancer

The rationale for this approach is based on evidence that reduction in colorectal cancer mortality can be achieved through detection and surgical removal of early stage cancer, and by the removal of adenomatous polyps. Widely endorsed guidelines for colorectal cancer screening have been developed based on the division of the population into average risk and increased risk groups (Fig. 343-1). Those at increased risk include patients with first-degree relatives (parents, siblings, children) who have had colorectal cancer or adenomatous polyps, with a family history of familial adenomatous polyposis (FAP) or HNPCC, or with a personal history of adenomas or colorectal cancer. The screening tests used include fecal occult blood tests, flexible sigmoidoscopy, barium enema, and colonoscopy at varying onsets and intervals depending on the assessment of risk.

Genetic testing of populations for the APC gene is not feasible, since many different mutations of the gene have been found in different families. It is useful to screen family members within an affected kindred, but the significance of a negative test is uncertain. Similarly, the genetic mutations related to HNPCC are not useful in population screening but may have value in genetic identification within families at risk.

There has been recent interest in searching for mutated oncogenes in fecal DNA as a screening test for colonic neoplasia. Improved fecal occult blood tests are also under development, as is "virtual colonoscopy," an examination of the colon from images obtained during helical CT scanning. These tests have promise but have not reached a point of proven clinical utility.

The serum immunoassay for carcinoembryonic antigen (CEA) was developed to provide a means of early detection of colonic cancer. However, it is too insensitive and nonspecific to be a useful screening test. CEA concentration may also be elevated with other cancers and with benign conditions such as inflammatory bowel disease, alcoholic liver disease, and pancreatitis. The test is most useful in assessing the results of surgery. If CEA concentration is elevated preoperatively and falls to normal after curative resection, a second rise is a good indication of recurrence and may develop long before the cancer can be detected clinically. Surgical "second look" procedures have been advocated in this circumstance, but their value remains to be proved. Also, when initially high, CEA concentration has been used to gauge patient response to chemotherapy for metastatic disease.

Differential Diagnosis

The presenting symptoms vary according to the location of the neoplasm in the colon. Cancers that occur in the more voluminous and distensible cecum and right colon, where bowel contents are liquid, usually do not cause obstruction. These cancers tend to grow to large size and ulcerate, producing a gradual chronic blood loss. In some cases enough hemoglobin is lost to produce melena. Passage of reddish maroon stool sometimes occurs, indicating the diagnosis.

Large cecal masses may involve the ileocecal valve and produce apparent small bowel obstruction. Sometimes tumors of the ascending colon partially block the lumen. If the ileocecal valve is competent, the cecum becomes painfully dilated with gas and air, creating a tender right lower quadrant mass. Patients may massage this area and find relief as they force the trapped gas past the obstruction.

Cancers in the left colon, where the lumen is narrower and less distensible and the fecal stream is solid, commonly obstruct. This causes constipation and cramping abdominal pain. Sometimes a paradoxical diarrhea develops as some colonic contents are forced past a partially obstructing cancer. Bleeding from left-sided lesions may be bright red but is generally not massive. Patients with rectal cancers in particular tend to have bright red bleeding as well as tenesmus and small-caliber stools. Colonic cancers that advance to the stage at which they invade through the bowel wall may perforate it, leading to peritonitis. Anorexia and weight loss are common in advanced colonic cancer. Anorexia is intensified by partially obstructing lesions that may cause cramping abdominal pain associated with meals.

Colonic cancers may metastasize via lymphatic or hematogenous routes or both. Metastases to regional lymph glands, with intraabdominal spread, are most common. Metastases to the liver are frequently found. Lung and bone are other sites of metastatic spread.

Several conditions must be differentiated from colonic cancer. Diverticulitis may cause an inflammatory mass and obstruction that may resemble cancer, particularly in the sigmoid colon. Barium enema may sometimes be insufficient to distinguishing between a perforated diverticulum and a perforated carcinoma. Colonoscopy with biopsy is valuable for distinguishing these disorders from one another once the infectious process has been controlled but can be difficult if muscle hypertrophy, spasm, and mucosal edema are present.

In patients with ulcerative colitis, inflammatory strictures may be difficult to distinguish from malignant strictures. Again, the colonoscope is not always able to pass through the narrowed area. Frequently, however, a stricture has a component of muscle spasm, and such areas may be evaluated although they appear on barium enema examination to be too narrow for the colonoscope to pass. A cytology brush may be passed through the narrowed area, enabling the physician to detect malignant cells. Biopsy specimens from the proximal end of the stricture may not reveal a carcinoma present in the midportion or distal end. If any doubt exists, the stricture should be considered malignant until proved otherwise.

Benign-appearing polypoid lesions of the colon must be differentiated from carcinoma if they are larger than 7 mm in diameter. Simple biopsy of polyps may be misleading because a cancerous area may be missed as a result of sampling error. Cytologic specimens from polyps are not useful in practice because they do not permit differentiation of invasive carcinoma from the presence of atypical surface cells. Thus the best way to evaluate a polyp is to remove all of it by cautery snare. If a polypoid cancer with an involved margin is removed, resection of the involved segment of bowel and mesentery is usually indicated. Polyps 7 mm or smaller are not usually malignant and may be removed by fulguration ("hot") biopsy. In this technique the polyp is destroyed by electrocoagulation while a biopsy specimen is obtained.

Management

The only known curative treatment for colonic adenocarcinoma is surgical resection. The prognosis for recurrence after resection depends on the degree of bowel wall invasion by the cancer and the presence of lymph node or distant metastases. If resection is adequate, in the Dukes' A group only 5% to 10% of patients will have recurrent cancer in contrast to 20% to 30% in the Dukes' B group and to 50% in the Dukes' C group with cancer in the colon and 70% with cancer in the rectum.

The incidence and mortality of colorectal cancer has slightly decreased in the United States during the past decade. These observed declines may be due to better diets, removal of premalignant polyps, earlier diagnosis, and improved therapy in varying degrees and contributions.

Cancers in the right colon and left colon require right and left hemicolectomy, respectively. A wide margin should be taken with adequate resection of the mesentery and lymph nodes. Lesions in the rectosigmoid more than 6 to 8 cm from the anal verge may be treated by anterior resection, whereas sizeable cancers below this level require combined abdominal-perineal resection with colostomy. Small low rectal cancers may sometimes be curatively removed by wide local excision. Full-thickness excision, with perirectal lymph nodes if possible, is preferable to electrofulguration for local treatment because it allows pathologic analysis. In unresectable rectal cancer, electrocautery or laser treatment or stent insertion may provide palliation, sometimes precluding the need for colostomy. Resection of colon cancer using laparoscopic "minimally invasive" technique has proved feasible on a trial basis but requires additional follow-up studies.

Irradiation before surgery has been used in treating advanced rectal cancer. An unresectable lesion occasionally becomes resectable after treatment with 2000 to 3000 rad. Some physicians have advocated the routine use of preoperative radiotherapy for rectal lesions, but the results of studies have been conflicting. Postoperative irradiation for patients with rectal cancer at risk for residual disease has been advocated, and some radiation therapists advise a "sandwich" technique combining preoperative and postoperative treatment. In patients with advanced colorectal cancer, after resection of all gross disease, adjuvant therapy with a combination of 5-fluorouracil and levamisole has shown a significantly higher survival rate than in control subjects.

In patients with unresectable colonic cancer, both radiation therapy and chemotherapy have been widely used. Irradiation is usually employed for palliation and shrinkage of tumor masses in the pelvis. Chemotherapy remains unsatisfactory and experimental. 5-Fluorouracil has been the most widely used single agent; only about 15% to 20% of patients respond, most temporarily. Combination chemotherapy and modulation of 5-fluorouracil metabolism has not yet provided a noteworthy advance in colonic carcinoma treatment, although multiple-drug trials are in progress. A combination of radiation therapy and chemotherapy may have some increased benefit over either modality alone.

Infusions of 5-fluorouracil into the hepatic artery or portal vein, or both, have occasionally decreased hepatic metastases when systemic chemotherapy has failed. Patients with liver metastases have been treated with hepatic artery infusion via an implanted pump. A

✔ *WHEN TO REFER*

Patients at average risk for colorectal cancer can be screened successfully in the primary care setting. Patients with increased risk of colorectal cancer (those with first-degree relatives who have colorectal cancer or adenomas, a family history of familial adenomatous polyposis or hereditary nonpolyposis colorectal cancer, a personal history of colorectal cancer or adenomas, or long-standing inflammatory bowel disease) usually require more intensive screening, often involving periodic referral for colonoscopy. Colorectal adenomas should be removed at colonoscopy whenever possible. Patients with advanced colorectal cancer require expertise involving endoscopy, surgery, and oncologic treatment and should be referred to appropriate specialists as needed.

clear advantage over systemic treatment has not been demonstrated. A 5-year survival rate of about 20% has been reported in groups of patients who underwent surgical resection of localized liver metastases.

The judicious use of analgesics, sedatives, antidepressants, blood products, and nutritional supplements by a sympathetic physician can do much to enhance the quality of life for patients with metastatic colonic cancer.

BENIGN TUMORS OF THE LARGE INTESTINE

Adenomas of the colon constitute the great majority of polypoid lesions. The World Health Organization (WHO) has classified adenomas as (1) tubular, (2) villous, and (3) tubulovillous. Adenomas may be sessile, with a broad base, or have a large, thin pedicle containing fibrous tissue, blood vessels, and lymphatics. Polyps occur with greatest frequency in areas of the world where colonic cancer is common.

Most adenomas cause no symptoms. Bleeding from an adenoma may occur, more commonly with left-sided polyps. Bleeding usually is noted with bowel movements and is not profuse. Abdominal cramps may occur with large polyps. Intussusception of the large bowel from a benign adenoma is rare. Large villous adenomas may secrete copious amounts of potassium-rich mucus and cause diarrhea and hypokalemia when located in the distal large bowel.

It is estimated that 2% to 5% of single adenomas and 30% of villous adenomas become malignant, particularly if greater than 2 cm in diameter. Removing these benign tumors has been advocated as a means of preventing colonic cancer. Data from the National Polyp Study indicate that removal of all colonic adenomas at colonoscopy markedly decreases the expected incidence of colon cancer. However, whether removal of diminutive polyps (<0.3 cm) is essential remains controversial. After removal of all adenomas, surveillance colonoscopy at 3-year intervals seems adequate for most patients; adenomas that are found subsequently are usually small and tubular.

In familial polyposis coli and Gardner's syndrome, total proctocolectomy is recommended. In younger patients a subtotal colectomy with ileorectal anastomosis is sometimes performed, with endoscopic surveillance of the remaining rectum and fulguration of polyps at least twice yearly. However, because cancers have developed in the rectal segment, a great responsibility is placed on the physician when a proctocolectomy is not done. Ileoanal anastomosis is an option to avoid ileostomy if the rectum is removed.

Hyperplastic polyps should be differentiated from adenomas. They are characteristically small (often only 2 to 3 mm) mucosal excrescences that are usually smooth and sessile, although occasionally they have a short stalk. They appear most often in the rectosigmoid and seem unrelated to colonic neoplasia.

Juvenile polyps, usually pedunculated hamartomas, may be seen in adults as well as children. They may ulcerate and bleed or cause obstruction. With time they self-amputate spontaneously, but juvenile polyps that cause symptoms should be removed. Although there is no evidence that juvenile polyps undergo malignant change, the incidence of cancer of the colon appears to be higher in patients and family members of patients who have had juvenile polyps.

Carcinoid tumors may occur in the colon and especially the rec-

tum. As with carcinoid tumors in the small intestine, only tumors greater than 2 cm in size tend to metastasize. Carcinoid syndrome does not occur in patients with metastatic rectal carcinoid tumors.

Leiomyomas may occur in the colon but are much less common there than in the small bowel and stomach. *Lipomas* are the second most common benign colonic tumors. They are usually submucosal, and more than half are near the ileocecal valve. Lipomas may cause intussusception but are usually asymptomatic. They have a characteristic low-density appearance on CT scan. At colonoscopy they are seen to have a yellowish color and a soft, springy consistency and can be easily indented with a biopsy forceps, producing a "cushion" or "pillow" sign. Lipomas are usually sessile and, if asymptomatic, should be left alone.

BIBLIOGRAPHY

Basson MD, Ahlman H, Wangberg B, Modlin IM: Biology and management of the midgut carcinoid, *Am J Surg* 165:288, 1993.
DiSario JA, Burt RW, Vargas H et al: Small bowel cancer: epidemiological and clinical characteristics from a population-based registry, *Am J Gastroenterol* 89:699, 1994.
Fearon ER, Vogelstein B: A genetic model for colorectal tumorogenesis, *Cell* 61:759, 1990.
Harris AG, Redfern JS: Octreotide treatment of carcinoid syndrome: analysis of published dose-titration data, *Aliment Pharmacol Ther* 9:387, 1995.
Moertel BC et al: Levamisole and fluorouracil for adjuvant therapy of resected colon carcinoma, *N Engl J Med* 322:352, 1990.
Rex DK, Rahmani EY, Haseman JH et al: Relative sensitivity of colonoscopy and barium enema for detection of colorectal cancer in clinical practice, *Gastroenterology* 112:17, 1997.
Rustgi AK: Hereditary gastrointestinal polyposis and nonpolyposis syndromes, *N Engl J Med* 31:1694, 1994.
Steele G Jr: Accomplishment and promise in the understanding and treatment of colorectal cancer, *Lancet* 342:1092, 1993.
Winawer SJ, Fletcher RH, Miller L et al: Colorectal cancer screening: clinical guidelines and rationale, *Gastroenterology* 112:594, 1997.

CHAPTER

344 Vascular Diseases of the Intestine

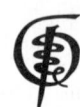

T. Edward Bynum

Mesenteric vascular disease is caused by the physical occlusion of a blood vessel (occlusive mesenteric vascular disease) *or* by low-flow states in which either the vessels are normal or the luminal compromise is insufficient to impair significantly the flow of blood to the tissues (nonocclusive, or "hemodynamic," mesenteric vascular disease). Major-vessel occlusion can result from an embolus (e.g., from the left atrium, mitral valve, arterial thrombus elsewhere, paradoxical embolism) or from thrombus formation. An arterial thrombus usually forms on an atheromatous plaque or spontaneously, as may occur in young women who are taking birth control pills. Rarely, other events cause major artery occlusion (e.g., surgical accidents, abdominal trauma, or encroachment by a malignant neoplasm). Small-vessel occlusion at the level of the arterioles is associated with systemic diseases such as thrombotic thrombocytopenic purpura, disseminated intravascular coagulation, polyarteritis nodosa, and systemic lupus erythematosus.

Nonocclusive mesenteric vascular disease is more common than occlusive mesenteric vascular disease and occurs in such low-flow and mesenteric vasoconstrictive states as severe congestive heart failure, aortic stenosis, shock (hemorrhagic, septic, cardiac), and cardiac arrhythmias and in concert with the use of vasoconstrictive drugs.

The incidence of mesenteric vascular disease is not known. Because of preterminal hypotension and rapid, postmortem autolysis of intestinal mucosa, the incidence figures obtained from autopsy series are overestimates. In the last 10 years the incidence, especially that of nonocclusive disease, appears to be declining. Perhaps this decline is due to better recognition of the pathophysiologic characteristics of shock and of mesenteric vascular disease, less use of vasoconstrictive drugs, better drugs for support of cardiovascular function, and better methods that assist respiration and maintain oxygenation.

PATHOPHYSIOLOGY

Ischemia or infarction of the intestine results when the bloodstream fails to carry oxygen and other nutrients in quantities sufficient for intestinal metabolic needs. This situation is obvious when a major artery supplying the intestine becomes completely occluded by an embolus or thrombus. The situation is less obvious, although more common, when there is no physical occlusion in the supplying vessels, as occurs in nonocclusive mesenteric ischemia and infarction. Nonocclusive mesenteric vascular disease is associated with a general threat to blood circulation such as hypovolemia (absolute or relative), hypotension, or shock. When effective circulating blood volume decreases, there is progressive vasoconstriction of mesenteric arterial vasculature, which shunts blood away from the splanchnic circulation into the general circulation. Teleologically, the less vital gastrointestinal tract is "sacrificed" in order to "protect" or "save" the more vital brain, heart, lungs, and kidneys. If vasoconstriction is combined with impaired cardiac output, severely depleted intravascular volume, or moderately compromised vascular channels, then a critical point may be reached at which the supply of oxygen falls below the minimum needed, and ischemia supervenes. If ischemia is severe or prolonged, infarction eventuates.

Intestinal villi are anatomically constructed so that the vessels within the villi can allow "countercurrent" exchange of oxygen. As a result, the villus tips are relatively hypoxemic even at full blood flow, so if there is a decline in intestinal blood flow, oxygen supply to the tips may rapidly become inadequate.

Fortunately, the gastrointestinal tract has a blood supply that is rich in collateral vessels, which provides considerable protection against occlusive vascular disease, especially when the occlusion develops slowly or involves the largest branches of the aorta. Chronic intestinal ischemia does not occur unless at least two of the three major mesenteric vessels (celiac axis, superior mesenteric artery, inferior mesenteric artery) are *completely* occluded. Unfortunately, this rich system of collaterals does not protect the gastrointestinal tract against nonocclusive vascular disease.

Infarction of the small intestine is associated with a high mortality, and the efficacy of therapy is low. Infarction of the colon is much more benign: the mortality is low and the colon frequently heals without residual complications.

PATHOLOGY

The earliest tissue changes in mesenteric ischemia are necrosis of villus tips in the small bowel and necrosis of the superficial epithelium in the colon. If the ischemic insult is more severe, deeper portions of the mucosa show hemorrhagic necrosis. Severe intestinal infarction is manifested by hemorrhagic necrosis of all layers of the bowel wall.

If blood flow is reinstituted, tissue injury becomes worse initially. Reperfusion actually increases cell necrosis because the reavailability of oxygen leads to the creation of toxic free radicals. However, the earliest lesion is fully reversible. Lesions of intermediate severity ulcerate or slough large areas of mucosa, after which repair takes place with ultimate reepithelialization but often with fibrous scarring and possible stricture formation. Very severe acute lesions may be associated with massive bleeding or perforation or lead to irreversible shock and death (especially as a consequence of small bowel infarction).

CLINICAL PRESENTATION

Patients with mesenteric ischemia have abdominal pain that is cramping, generalized or periumbilical, and often severe. In early stages the pain is not associated with any abnormalities evident on examination of the abdomen. Early in the course of intestinal ischemia a patient's pain is "out of proportion" to any other physical findings, particularly in small bowel ischemia. Colonic ischemia may be heralded by rectal bleeding as well as by abdominal pain. Therefore timely diagnosis of mesenteric vascular disease requires a high index of suspicion. Objective physical findings in the abdomen, particularly peritoneal signs, are a relatively late manifestation of bowel infarc-

tion, and at such a stage often little can be done to reverse the process or rescue the bowel.

Occlusive mesenteric vascular disease should be suspected in patients with known cardiac disease, particularly if they have mitral valve disease, marked left atrial enlargement, or atrial fibrillation. In patients with severe generalized atherosclerotic and arteriosclerotic vascular disease, the major mesenteric arteries may gradually and progressively become occluded until there is chronic ischemia of the intestine. When this situation is manifested by abdominal pain following the ingestion of food, it is termed *abdominal angina*. In rare instances, patients may have mild to moderate malabsorption secondary to severe chronic mesenteric ischemia. However, most patients lose weight because of "cardiac cachexia" or because they stop eating to prevent pain.

The possibility of small-vessel occlusive disease is suggested by the presence of known multisystem disease (collagen-vascular or "autoimmune" disease) or in situations in which disseminated intravascular coagulation might occur.

Nonocclusive mesenteric vascular disease occurs with congestive heart failure, cardiac arrhythmias, hypotension, or shock. Sympathomimetic drugs and digitalis glycosides are potent vasoconstrictors of the mesenteric vasculature. Fortunately, adrenergic drugs are no longer widely used, and digitalis only has significant splanchnic vasoconstrictive action if it is administered parenterally. However, nonocclusive intestinal infarction may occur with digitalis toxicity. When ischemia and infarction occur in the distal small bowel or in the colon, the patient may have bloody diarrhea or bright red blood from the rectum.

The laboratory offers little to aid in the specific diagnosis of mesenteric vascular disease. With intestinal infarction, moderate to severe leukocytosis is common. Serum amylase and alkaline phosphatase concentrations can be mildly to moderately elevated, because these enzymes are present in the intestinal epithelium.

DIAGNOSIS

It is very difficult to make the diagnosis of mesenteric ischemia or infarction with absolute certainty short of surgery or autopsy. Early diagnosis is mandatory and depends on the physician's high index of suspicion combined with an awareness of the clinical contexts in which the disease occurs. Mesenteric arteriography is helpful in documenting and locating a vascular occlusion. On the other hand, arteriograms may show radiographic evidence of vasoconstriction, or the arteries may appear entirely normal; either appearance is compatible with nonocclusive intestinal ischemia with or without infarction. If the arteriographic findings are compatible with nonocclusive disease, the catheter can be left in place for possible administration of a vasodilator drug intraarterially.

In less urgent clinical situations, barium contrast radiographs of the alimentary tract are often made to evaluate abdominal pain. "Thumbprinting" (indentation of the barium column caused by submucosal hemorrhage and edema) is characteristic of mesenteric vascular disease (Fig. 344-1) but also occurs in uremia, thrombocytopenia, Crohn's disease, and *Escherichia coli* O157:H7 colitis and after blunt trauma to the abdomen. Fibrous strictures may form in the colon after recovery from acute ischemia (Fig. 344-2).

TREATMENT

If the small bowel becomes acutely ischemic but does not progress to infarction, and if good blood flow can be reestablished, the lesion is usually reversible and there are no clinical sequelae. Infarction of the small bowel is not reversible, and the outcome is usually death or surgical resection. Therefore chronic strictures of the small bowel produced by ischemia are extremely rare. If occlusive disease is documented by angiography or if there is clinical evidence of infarction, surgery is indicated. Prompt embolectomy or bypass of the obstructed vessel may prevent infarction. If infarction has already occurred, all of the infarcted bowel must be resected. If the patient subsequently recovers but has had so much bowel resected that nutrition cannot be maintained by oral alimentation, parenteral alimentation must be established and often maintained indefinitely. When nonocclusive disease is suspected or known to be present, general support and measures designed to correct or alleviate such possible underlying prob-

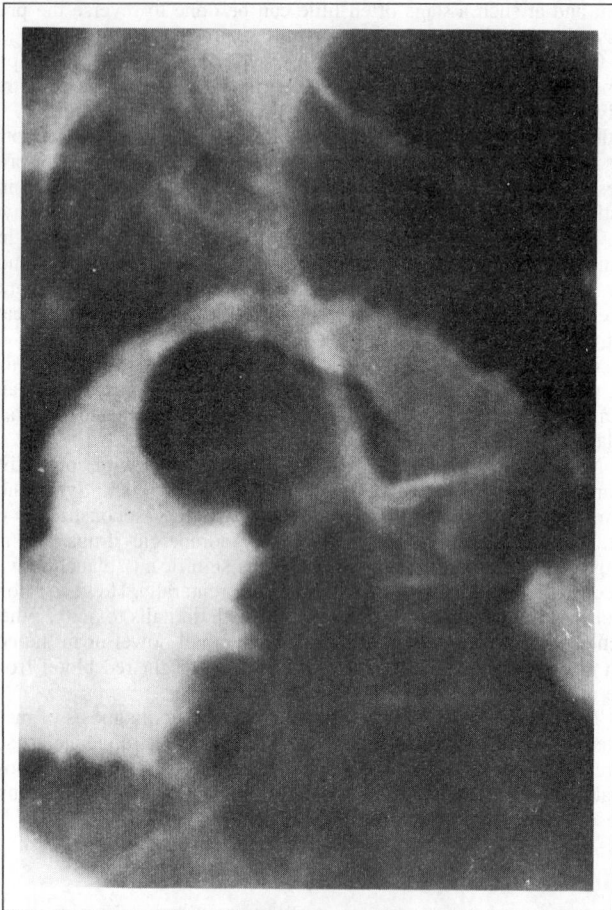

FIGURE 344-1 Spot film of barium enema in a patient with ischemic colitis, showing a large "thumbprint" and mucosal irregularity with spicules of barium at the margins of the barium column, indicating ulcerations.

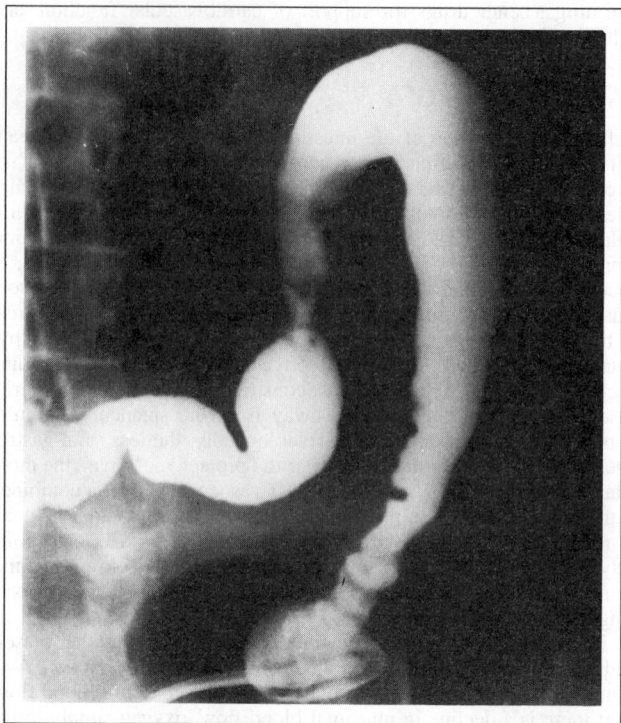

FIGURE 344-2 Spot film of barium enema, showing a smooth, tapered stricture of the sigmoid colon in a patient who had an episode of ischemic colitis 15 months previously.

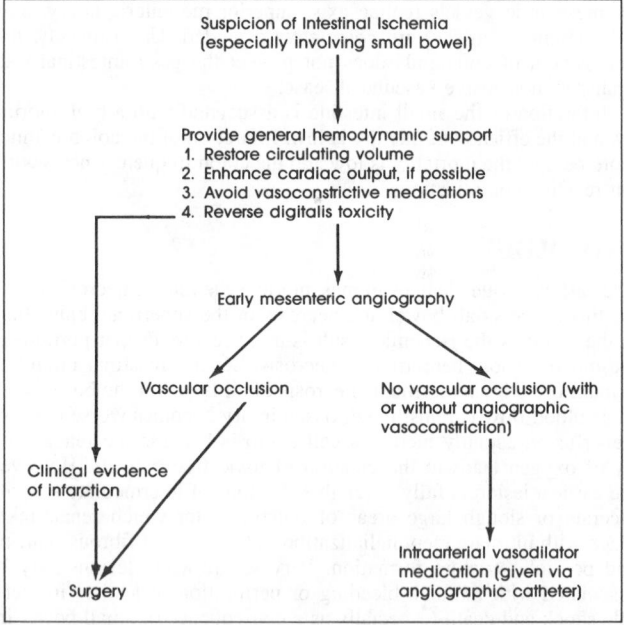

FIGURE 344-3 Suggested evaluation and therapy of mesenteric ischemia.

lems as hypovolemia, heart failure, or digitalis toxicity are crucial to restore circulating volume and enhance cardiac output. The goal is to restore perfusion of the intestine, reverse ischemia and tissue hypoxia, and prevent infarction. The diagnostic approach outlined in Fig. 344-3 is aggressive. However, mortality in patients with small bowel infarction is very high, and arteriography is quite safe when performed by experienced radiologists. Vasodilator drugs such as papaverine, glucagon, and the vasodilator prostaglandins can effectively increase mesenteric blood flow when administered intraarterially via a catheter placed during mesenteric arteriography. Vasodilator therapy is generally safe if general circulating volume has been restored and is maintained.

In the colon acute ischemia is frequently reversible, and extensive bowel wall infarction (with resultant toxic dilation or perforation) is rare. For the less than 15% of patients who have moderate ischemia of the colon that is not reversible, the outcome is a fibrous stricture (see Fig. 344-2). If the patient with a postischemic stricture of the colon has significant obstructive symptoms, the stricture must be dilated endoscopically or surgically resected. However, if symptoms are minimal, or if the stricture is discovered on a barium enema made for other indications, it may be left alone; many cases have shown gradual improvement or disappearance of the stricture over 6 to 12 months.

MESENTERIC VENOUS THROMBOSIS

There is no doubt that abdominal pain, intestinal ischemia, and perhaps intestinal infarction can result from thrombotic occlusion of mesenteric veins. Individual cases have been well documented in young women taking birth control pills and in other patients with hyperco-

aguable states. However, the overall incidence of this problem or its proportion of all cases of mesenteric vascular disease is difficult to determine. The reason for the difficulty is as follows: mesenteric venous thrombosis, particularly of the small branches draining the intestine, sometimes occurs as a result of ischemia (or infarction) caused by failure of perfusion because of either occlusion of the arterial supply or nonocclusive reduction in arterial blood flow. Therefore, if a patient actually has ischemia or infarction produced by nonocclusive disease, and thrombosis of mesenteric veins occurs secondarily, there has been a tendency to attribute the ischemia or infarction to the tangibly identified occlusion-thrombosis (i.e., that occurring in the mesenteric veins). Mesenteric vein thrombosis can be either the result of intestinal ischemia or infarction or the cause of it.

The largest vein draining the intestines is the portal vein. Complete occlusion of the portal vein is well known: portal vein thrombosis. The consequences of portal vein thrombosis are portal hypertension, esophageal varices, bleeding from varices, splenomegaly, and hypersplenism. Intestinal ischemia, intestinal infarction, malabsorption, or any measurable intestinal dysfunction does not result from portal vein thrombosis.

If mesenteric vein thrombosis is associated with infarction of the intestine, treatment is as outlined for infarction with prompt surgery after initial stabilization. Birth control pills should be discontinued if a woman is using that medication. If a hypercoaguable state is present, the treatment is that of the underlying disease and administration of anticoagulants.

BIBLIOGRAPHY

Bynum TE et al: The pathophysiology of nonocclusive intestinal ischemia. In Shepherd AP, Granger DN, editors: *Physiology of the intestinal circulation,* New York, 1984, Raven Press.

Bynum TE, Jacobson ED: Nonocclusive intestinal ischemia, *Arch Intern Med* 139:281, 1979.

Cooke M, Sande MA: Diagnosis and outcome of bowel infarction on an acute medical service, *Am J Med* 75:984, 1983.

Gandhi SK et al: Ischemic colitis, *Dis Colon Rectum* 39:88, 1996.

Geelkerken RH et al: Chronic mesenteric vascular syndrome, *Arch Surg* 126:1101, 1991.

Grendell JH, Ockner RK: Mesenteric venous thrombosis, *Gastroenterology* 82:358, 1982.

Kaleya RN et al: Aggressive approach to acute mesenteric ischemia, *Surg Clin North Am* 72:157, 1992.

Levine JS, Jacobson ED: Intestinal ischemic disorders, *Dig Dis Sci* 13:3, 1995.

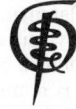

CHAPTER

345 Diverticular and Other Intestinal Diseases

Michael D. Apstein

Diverticula, either congenital or acquired, can arise in any portion of the gastrointestinal tract; they frequently cause no symptoms. For example, in 15% of the general population, one to three diverticula are present in the second portion of the duodenum. Although periampullary diverticula are associated with an increased risk of pigment gallstones, the diverticula themselves rarely cause symptoms. In the rare instances when congenital diverticula involve the colon, they are found in the cecum.

MECKEL'S DIVERTICULUM

Meckel's diverticulum is the most frequent congenital anomaly of the gastrointestinal tract, occurring in approximately 2% of the population. The diverticulum, most often located in the ileum within 100 cm of the ileocecal valve, is frequently lined with heterotrophic mucosa. The nature of the lining determines the clinical presentation. Melena, hematochezia, or pain reminiscent of acute appendicitis are the most common presentations in patients whose diverticulum is lined with acid-secreting gastric mucosa because of acid-induced ulceration of adjacent small bowel mucosa. In patients with non–acid-secreting mucosa in the diverticulum, intermittent small bowel obstruction caused by either intussusception or internal herniation secondary to a mesodiverticular band can occur. Although the majority of patients who become symptomatic do so by age 2, a Meckel's diverticulum should be considered in any young adult with melena, hematochezia, or small bowel obstruction. Scintigraphy with technetium-99 (^{99m}Tc)-pertechnetate (Meckel's scan) enhanced with

pentagastrin and a histamine 2 (H_2) blocker is the diagnostic test of choice in patients with a suspected Meckel's diverticulum and right lower quadrant pain or bleeding. Small bowel enteroclysis to visualize the diverticulum directly is the test of choice for patients with intermittent small bowel obstruction. Treatment of a patient with a symptomatic Meckel's diverticulum is surgical excision.

MULTIPLE JEJUNAL DIVERTICULOSIS

Multiple jejunal diverticulosis is an acquired disease that usually manifests itself in adulthood. Some patients probably have a variant of progressive systemic sclerosis limited to the gastrointestinal tract or an idiopathic visceral myopathy or neuropathy. The smooth muscle or myenteric plexus abnormality, in turn, produces localized wall weakness and/or uncoordinated motor activity resulting in formation of diverticula.

Only 10% to 40% of patients with multiple jejunal diverticulosis are symptomatic. Their symptoms are usually those of chronic intestinal pseudoobstruction (Chapter 342). The associated abnormal small intestinal motility and stasis within the diverticular lumens can result in bacterial overgrowth and malabsorption (Chapter 340). Additionally, there are isolated reports of inflammation, bleeding, or perforation of the diverticula.

Treatment is directed toward the underlying pathophysiologic process caused by the diverticula. Antibiotics are useful if bacterial overgrowth is present. Surgical resection of the involved diverticulum is the treatment of choice for perforation or uncontrollable bleeding but is of no use for chronic symptoms of intestinal pseudoobstruction.

COLONIC DIVERTICULAR DISEASE
Prevalence and Epidemiology

Prevalence rates of colonic diverticulosis vary tremendously depending on geographic area. For example, diverticulosis is so common in Western society that it almost could be considered a normal part of aging; 50% of individuals have colonic diverticula by age 70. However, diverticulosis is rare in Africa and other less industrialized parts of the world. This geographic variation in prevalence, the dramatic increase in prevalence in Western countries since 1900, and the appearance of the disease in Japanese immigrants to the West supports an environmental cause.

Many investigators believe dietary habits of a given population influence the prevalence of diverticulosis in that population. Diets low in fiber and other bulk and high in meat and refined carbohydrates have been implicated in the formation of colonic diverticula. The following statements offer support for this hypothesis: (1) vegetarians have a lower prevalence of diverticulosis than age-matched nonvegetarian control subjects; (2) the increase in prevalence in Western society has paralleled the increased dietary consumption of refined carbohydrate; (3) case-controlled studies have shown that patients with diverticula consume less dietary fiber than patients without diverticula. However, a true cause and effect relationship has yet to be established.

Pathology

A colonic diverticulum is a herniation of mucosa and submucosa through or between fibers of the major muscle layer (muscularis propria). Colonic diverticula may involve all portions of the colon (Fig. 345-1). They form at the site where the vasa recta (intramural branches of the marginal artery) penetrate the circular muscle (Fig. 345-2). As a result, the lumen of the diverticulum is separated from the vasa recta and peritoneum by only a few millimeters of mucosa and submucosa.

Diverticulitis results from a microperforation of the diverticular mucosa, submucosa, and adjacent serosa into the surrounding pericolic fat. Thus diverticulitis is primarily a pericolitis, not a true colitis; there is only localized involvement of the mucosa without extensive or diffuse mucositis. The pericolic infection ranges from a well-contained microabscess to one large enough to form an intraabdominal mass. Recurrent bouts of acute diverticulitis may lead to scarring, fibrosis, and stricture of the involved region.

Bleeding from colonic diverticula is caused by rupture of the un-

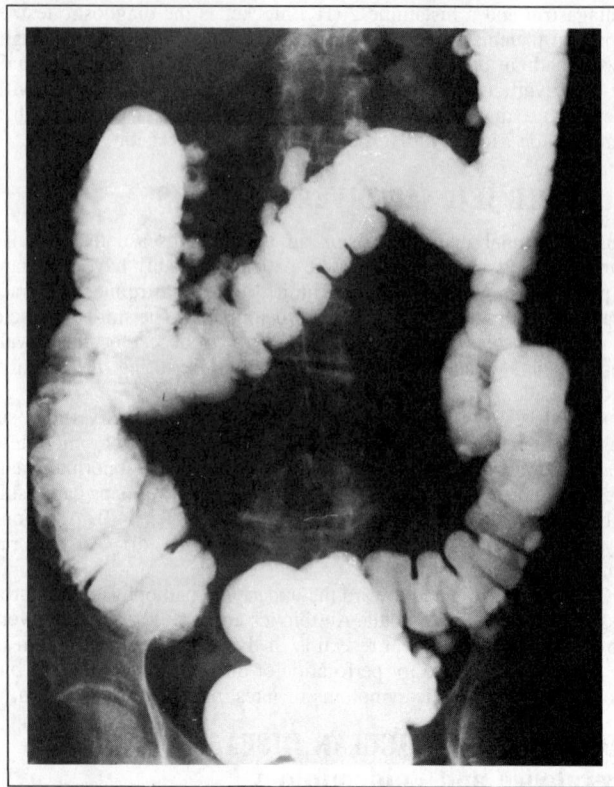

FIGURE 345-1   Single-column barium enema radiograph showing numerous diverticula of the colon.

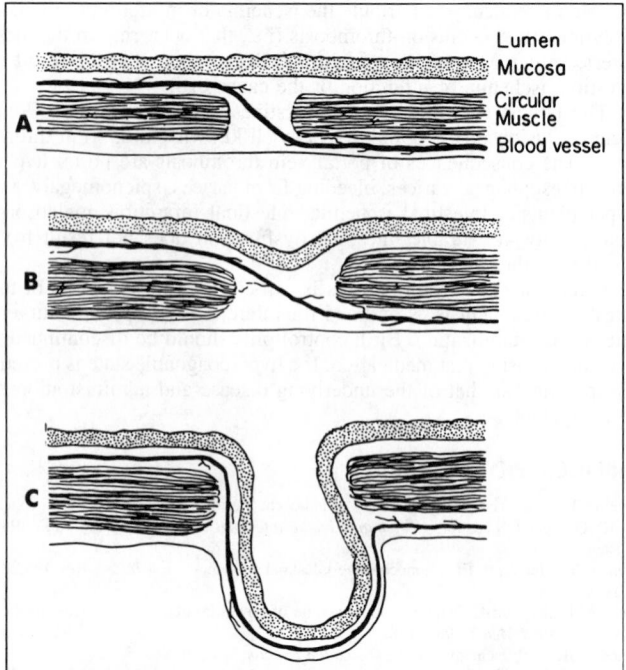

FIGURE 345-2   Structural dynamics of diverticular formation and vascular relationships. **A,** The long branch of the vas rectum artery penetrates the colonic wall through a connective tissue gap in the circular muscle. **B,** Early mucosal protrusion widens the connective tissue gap. **C,** With transmural extension of the diverticulum, the vas rectum is displaced over it. As a result, the lumen of the diverticulum is separated from the vas rectum by only a thin layer of mucosa and submucosa.

Modified from Meyers MA et al: *Gastroenterology* 71:577, 1976.

derlying vas rectum. Data suggest that injurious factors in the diverticular lumen produce eccentric damage to the underlying artery. Progressive weakness of the arterial wall results in rupture into the lumen of the diverticulum (Fig. 345-3).

Pathogenesis

Diverticula develop when intraluminal pressure exceeds the focal resistance of the colonic muscular layer, allowing the mucosa and submucosa to herniate. Studies examining the role of increased intraluminal pressure have given conflicting results. Some have implicated exaggerated, nonsynchronous contractions (spasms) in the sigmoid in response to food or drugs that stimulate contraction of the colonic smooth muscle. Segmentation and localized occlusion of short segments of the sigmoid occur, producing high intraluminal pressures in these localized occluded areas of the sigmoid colon. These investigators point to the 50% of patients with colonic diverticula who have marked thickening of the muscularis propria as evidence of spasm-induced muscle hypertrophy. However, others have not found an association between abnormal colonic motility and the presence of diverticulosis. In these studies there is a correlation between colonic motility and pain, but not diverticulosis. In fact, most patients with diverticulosis have normal colonic motility patterns. Whether diverticulosis is part of the spectrum of irritable bowel disease is also controversial.

Clinical Presentation and Diagnosis

The overwhelming majority of patients with diverticulosis never have symptoms. Symptoms result from the complications of diverticulosis: microperforation and diverticulitis or arterial rupture. Whether "painful diverticulosis" without a microperforation exists as a distinct entity or is just a manifestation of the irritable bowel syndrome is controversial. The clinical presentation of diverticulitis varies and depends on the extent of the perforation. Most commonly, the patient has a walled-off microabscess and experiences abdominal pain, fe-

ver, a change in bowel frequency (either constipation or diarrhea), and mild left lower quadrant tenderness and/or mass. Frequently, there is tenderness on rectal examination toward the area of inflammation. Laboratory tests usually reveal polymorphonuclear leukocytosis and an elevated sedimentation rate. Plain radiographs of the abdomen generally reveal normal results. This combination of findings is reminiscent of acute appendicitis; an older person who has "left-sided appendicitis" usually has diverticulitis.

Many patients with diverticulosis who experience cramping abdominal pain and irregular bowel movements have the irritable bowel syndrome and not diverticulitis. Diverticulitis should not be diagnosed in the absence of fever; tenderness; and, in most instances, leukocytosis. When diverticulitis is suspected in a patient with constipation, the administration of vigorous cathartics is contraindicated because of the risk of extending a microperforation. Occasionally patients present with an "acute abdomen" caused by peritonitis if the abscess has not been contained.

Rarely patients, especially men, present with pneumaturia or recurrent urinary tract infections from a colovesical fistula (Fig. 345-4). Since the uterus lies between the colon and bladder, women can present with a fecal discharge from the vagina.

An abdominal pelvic computed tomographic (CT) scan with oral contrast, the best method for confirming the diagnosis, is indicated when the clinical setting or course is atypical. It is safer than a barium enema and has the advantage of detecting other conditions that may mimic diverticulitis.

The differential diagnosis of acute diverticulitis includes localized Crohn's disease, colonic ischemia, a perforated colon cancer, pyelonephritis, ectopic pregnancy, salpingitis, or ovarian disease.

Colonoscopy is contraindicated early in the course of acute diverticulitis because of the risk of extending the microperforation. However, once the patient has been treated and is stable, a barium enema, flexible sigmoidoscopy, or colonoscopy to exclude a perforated colon cancer is imperative.

Bleeding from a diverticulum characteristically involves sudden

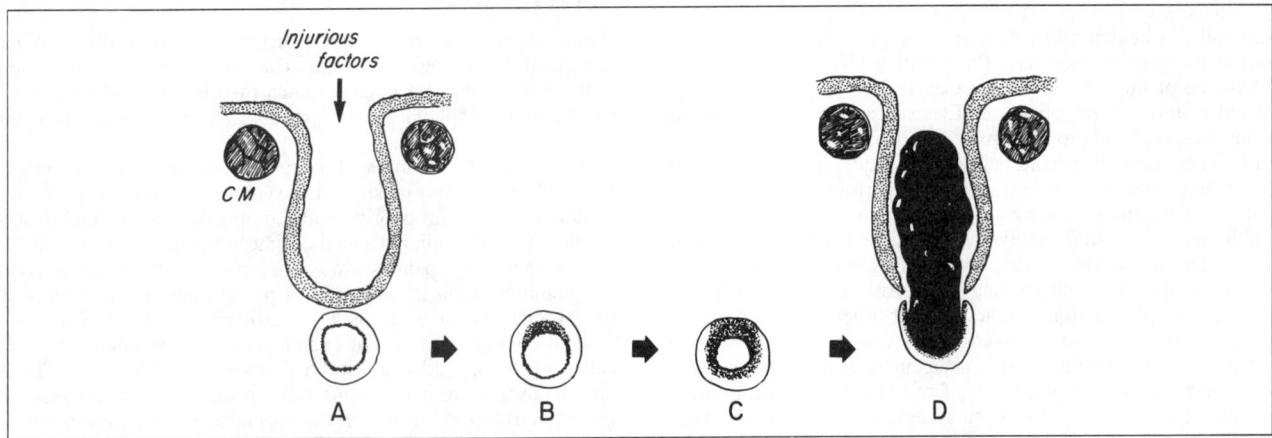

FIGURE 345-3   Proposed pathogenesis of diverticular bleeding. **A,** A cross-section through a diverticulum that has protruded between bands of circular muscle. Note the close apposition of the vas rectum artery to the dome of the diverticulum. Injurious factors in the lumen of the diverticulum cause initial damage to the vas rectum. **B,** Eccentric intimal thickening of the vas rectum vessel follows. **C,** Concentric intimal thickening with luminal accentuation occurs. **D,** Eccentric, acute rupture of the vas rectum into the lumen of the diverticulum. *CM,* Circular muscle.
Modified from Meyers MA et al: *Gastroenterology* 71:577, 1976.

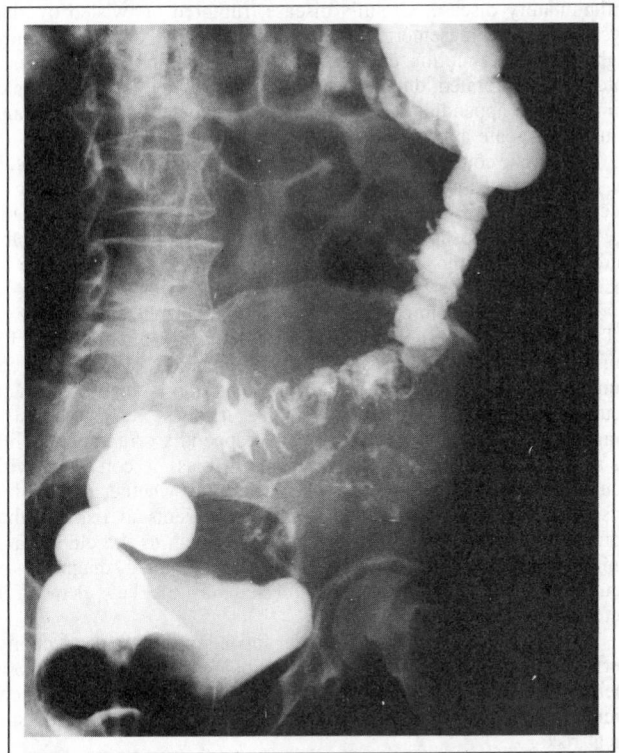

FIGURE 345-4   Barium enema radiograph in a patient with diverticulitis, showing a fistula from the sigmoid colon to the bladder. (The bladder is filled with barium, seen to the right of the rectum and rectosigmoid junction.)

passing of bright red or dark red blood from the rectum. It is almost always painless or, at most, associated with mild cramping. Occasionally, blood loss may be massive, leading to hemorrhagic shock or even death. Fortunately, most instances are self-limited, and bleeding ceases before the patient's life is endangered (and often before a precise diagnosis is made). Because the bleeding from a diverticulum results from the acute rupture of an artery, patients almost never experience occult gastrointestinal blood loss. Occult blood in the stool should be attributed to diverticula only when all other possible causes

(especially carcinoma of the cecum) have been confidently excluded. Diverticular bleeding occurs only very rarely in association with acute diverticulitis.

Sigmoidoscopy should be done promptly in the evaluation of patients who are thought to be bleeding from a colonic diverticulum to exclude another source of bleeding in the rectum or rectosigmoid. If sigmoidoscopy reveals that blood is coming from a location higher in the colon and if the patient continues to bleed briskly, the next diagnostic procedure should be a technetium-labeled red blood cell bleeding scan or a mesenteric arteriogram (Chapters 332 and 328). Colonoscopy is difficult during active lower gastrointestinal bleeding from any source; patients usually have not had a bowel-cleansing preparation, and blood mixed with even a small amount of feces cannot be removed adequately during colonoscopy to obtain a thorough examination. Furthermore, the risk of perforation is higher in the presence of diverticula. On the other hand, a 2- to 4-hour lavage with an osmotically balanced solution, such as GoLytely, administered orally facilitates localization of the bleeding site during colonoscopy in patients with acute colonic bleeding. Other diagnoses that need to be considered in the patient with brisk hematochezia are angiodysplasia (arteriovenous malformations) and, more rarely, colonic cancer or a massively bleeding lesion in the upper gastrointestinal tract. Angiodysplasia, small ectatic vascular lesions of the intestinal (frequently colonic) mucosa and submucosa, can be diagnosed with mesenteric angiography or with colonoscopy. Colonoscopy is more sensitive once the patient has stopped bleeding and the colon can be prepared adequately.

Treatment

Diets high in fiber have been recommended for patients with diverticulosis. Although these diets are probably beneficial in the irritable bowel syndrome, there is no conclusive evidence that any dietary changes will reduce the incidence of complications of diverticulosis or prevent formation of additional diverticula.

Some patients with mild diverticulitis can be treated as outpatients with a clear liquid diet and oral antibiotics such as ampicillin or tetracycline, 500 mg q6h. Addition of metronidazole to the regimen provides broader coverage for anaerobic bacteria. More symptomatic patients require hospitalization and bowel rest (nothing by mouth; intravenously administered fluid, electrolytes, and glucose; and nasogastric intubation if the patient has vomiting or an ileus) in addition to antibiotics. The choice of antibiotics for the hospitalized patient depends on the severity of the illness. Choices include intravenous ampicillin alone or, for more severely ill patients, combined with an aminoglycoside and clindamycin or metronidazole. Immediate surgery is necessary if generalized peritonitis is present. If medical therapy fails, as evidenced by a nonresolving or enlarging inflammatory mass, surgery is necessary. Preoperative CT-guided percutaneous drainage of the mass (abscess) may reduce the need for colostomy and a "three-stage" operation. Elective surgery is indicated for recurrent attacks; fistula formation; or, rarely, inability to exclude carcinoma. Since acute diverticulitis in patients under age 40 has a poor natural history, elective colonic surgery should be performed after a single episode. Partial colonic obstruction can occur during acute diverticulitis, although it frequently resolves during medical treatment. Months or years after an episode of acute diverticulitis, however, chronic obstruction may develop from scarring and fibrosis and may require surgery or endoscopic dilation to relieve the obstruction.

Bleeding from a colonic diverticulum ceases spontaneously in most patients. Therefore the early management of diverticular bleeding is supportive, with replacement of red blood cells and intravascular volume as indicated. If bleeding continues, selective intraarterial infusion of vasopressin (0.2 to 0.4 unit/min) into the artery supplying the bleeding site (as determined by angiography) stops the bleeding in more than 80% of patients. Intravenous vasopressin has no role in the treatment of diverticular bleeding. There are anecdotal reports of a barium enema's stopping diverticular hemorrhage. However, the success of this "therapy" is probably no greater than the rate at which diverticula stop bleeding spontaneously. Furthermore, the presence of barium in the colon interferes with angiographic localization of the site of bleeding. If diverticular bleeding persists despite intraarterial infusion of vasopressin, resection of the involved segment of colon is necessary. Twenty percent of patients who have had diverticular bleeding bleed again, whereas 50% rebleed if they have already bled twice. Therefore elective surgery is indicated for recurrent diverticular bleeding if the site can be localized with certainty. "Blind" hemicolectomy (right or left) is not prudent in patients with recurrent lower gastrointestinal bleeding in whom no specific site of blood loss has been identified.

AGANGLIONIC MEGACOLON

Megacolon is characterized by massive colonic dilation and constipation. It can be either congenital or acquired. In congenital megacolon (Hirschsprung's disease), the distal rectum lacks submucosal (Meissner's) and myenteric (Auerbach's) plexuses. The embryonic migration of ganglion cells to form these plexuses may be interrupted by intestinal ischemia secondary to structurally abnormal arteries or by an abnormal extracellular matrix microenvironment. The aganglionic segment may extend proximally for a variable distance from the distal rectum. Normal motor activity in this segment is lacking; the aganglionic segment is permanently contracted. As a consequence, the more proximal colon dilates secondary to the distal functional obstruction. In contrast, in acquired megacolon—which may be associated with Parkinson's disease, scleroderma, intestinal pseudoobstruction, Chagas' disease, amyloidosis, and drug-induced or idiopathic constipation—the entire rectum and colon are usually dilated.

Hirschsprung's disease, more common in males than in females, occurs approximately once in 5000 births. Although the clinical presentation occurs most often in infants, the diagnosis of Hirschsprung's disease should be considered in any adolescent or young adult with a history of severe, often lifelong, constipation. Patients frequently complain of abdominal distention and inability to pass flatus. They may have symptoms of large bowel obstruction with crampy abdominal pain, nausea, and vomiting. Digital examination reveals no stool in the rectum, but occasionally, on withdrawal of the examining finger or at sigmoidoscopy, a mass of stool is evacuated. A barium enema demonstrating distal narrowing and proximal dilation, most often at the level of the rectosigmoid, is characteristic. A lateral view frequently shows the transition zone best. Usually, definitive diagnosis can be made by rectal manometry (Chapter 339) and by suction biopsy that retrieves mucosa and submucosa, but a full-thickness rectal biopsy under general anesthesia may be necessary.

Surgery is the only treatment for Hirschsprung's disease. A temporary colostomy to relieve the functional obstruction may be indicated in some patients. However, several definitive procedures overcome the obstructing effect of the aganglionic segment yet preserve continence with minimal morbidity.

APPENDICITIS

Acute appendicitis most often occurs in adolescence and early adulthood, but no age is exempt. The cause is not known, although obstruction of the appendiceal lumen by a fecalith or hyperplasia of submucosal lymphoid tissue probably is a factor in promoting infection.

Clinically, the hallmark of acute appendicitis is the patient's history and progression of signs and symptoms. Classically, acute appendicitis starts with poorly localized epigastric or periumbilical abdominal pain that migrates to the right lower quadrant over the next 4 to 6 hours. The pain is always associated with anorexia. Nausea and vomiting occur in only 50% of patients and, in those, only after the pain has begun. There is no specific change in bowel habits.

The findings on physical examination vary depending on the location of the appendix and interval since the onset of pain. Tenderness is always present at some time in the course of an attack and corresponds to the location of the appendix: the right lower quadrant most frequently but also the right upper quadrant or flank in the case of a retrocecal appendix. The patient's temperature may be normal or mildly elevated. Fever above 101°F suggests a perforated appendix or alternative diagnosis.

Laboratory data are not diagnostic. The white blood cell count is usually but not invariably elevated. Values above 20,000 cells per cubic centimeter are rare and are consistent with a perforated appendix or another disease process.

Several other diseases may mimic symptoms and/or physical findings of acute appendicitis. The most common among these are pelvic inflammatory disease, Crohn's disease, ruptured or twisted ovarian cyst, and acute mesenteric adenitis. Occasionally, tubal pregnancy, right-sided diverticulitis, enteritis secondary to *Yersinia enterocolitica* infection, perforated duodenal ulcer, or acute pyelonephritis may mimic acute appendicitis. In addition, a perforated cecal carcinoma can mimic acute appendicitis in older individuals.

The classic course of acute appendicitis—epigastric pain that localizes to the right lower quadrant followed by nausea and vomiting—occurs in only 50% to 60% of individuals. Elderly patients and patients receiving immunosuppressive therapy may have blunted symptoms and physical findings, often delaying the diagnosis and leading to an increased rate of rupture with attendant increased mortality.

If the clinical picture is not clear, abdominal ultrasonography or CT scanning may be helpful. Ultrasonography is particularly useful during pregnancy and in children. Visualization of an enlarged, noncompressible appendix on ultrasonography is consistent with acute appendicitis; failure to visualize it does not exclude the diagnosis. On CT scanning an abnormal appendix or an appendolith in association with a right lower quadrant mass is consistent with acute appendicitis. CT scanning can determine whether perforation has occurred and is especially helpful in patients at risk for that complication or with atypical presentations, such as the elderly and immunosuppressed. Despite advances in radiologic diagnosis of acute appendicitis, clinical judgment remains the key element in determining therapy.

The accepted treatment for acute appendicitis is appendectomy, performed as soon as the diagnosis is apparent. Systemic antibiotic therapy has been effective in a number of patients with acute appendicitis but should be reserved for those who are unusually poor surgical risks.

Overlooked or delayed diagnosis of acute appendicitis can result in perforation of the appendix with subsequent increased immediate morbidity and mortality. Furthermore, the risk of subsequent tubal infertility increases sharply in women with a history of a perforated appendix. Very rarely does acute appendicitis resolve spontaneously without surgery or antibiotic therapy. Chronic appendicitis or recurrent acute appendicitis probably exists but must be extremely rare. Such a diagnosis should not be marshaled to account for chronic abdominal pain.

HEMORRHOIDS

Hemorrhoids are varicose veins of the anus and rectum. Most patients with hemorrhoids have no obvious predisposing factor. There is a familial tendency and an increased incidence in patients with irritable bowel syndrome who are constipated. Hemorrhoids develop frequently during pregnancy because the enlarging uterus obstructs veins that drain blood from the rectal area. In patients with portal hypertension, hemorrhoids (or dilated rectal veins that are clinically indistinguishable from hemorrhoids) are common, because this venous system participates in decompressing portal pressure.

In many patients, hemorrhoids are observed incidentally at the time of rectal, sigmoidoscopic, or colonoscopic examination and cause no symptoms. The major symptoms of hemorrhoids are bleeding, pain, itching, or rectal prolapse. Bleeding is usually painless. A patient may notice red blood on the toilet tissue or on the surface of formed stool; there may be dripping of blood into the water of the toilet bowl; or the patient's underclothing may become soiled with blood. Persistent, brisk bleeding is rare. Likewise, anemia resulting from hemorrhoidal bleeding is unusual and should prompt a more thorough investigation. Occult bleeding should not be attributed to hemorrhoids. Before any rectal bleeding can be attributed to hemorrhoids, sigmoidoscopy and a barium enema or colonoscopy should be performed to exclude other, more serious abnormalities. Pain is caused by thrombosis of a hemorrhoid. Itching represents low-order stimulation of pain fibers that occurs when a hemorrhoid becomes thrombosed. Itching may also be caused by fecal soiling, which can occur if the hemorrhoids causes mild sphincter incontinence in patients with loose stools.

Medical management of hemorrhoids requires treatment of any underlying condition. If a patient is constipated, a high-bulk diet and a hydrophilic substance such as psyllium seed mucilloid should be prescribed. Twice-daily sitz baths followed by insertion of an anesthetic hydrocortisone suppository are helpful. Patients should be advised to defecate when the urge is first experienced, avoid straining during defecation, and limit the amount of time spent sitting on a toilet. Although its effectiveness has not been evaluated objectively, witch hazel solution applied locally to the anus may reduce hemorrhoidal bleeding.

Indications for surgery are persistent bleeding and painful thrombosis not responding to medical therapy. A variety of surgical methods are used, including excision hemorrhoidectomy, rubber band ligation, cryosurgery, injection of sclerosing solutions, and extreme dilation of the anus. The rate of hemorrhoid recurrence is high after any method of surgical therapy.

SOLITARY ULCER SYNDROME

A single, usually large ulcer (often several centimeters in diameter) of unknown cause may occur in the cecum or in the midrectum. Solitary rectal ulcers have a high association with rectal prolapse and may be related to ischemia of a portion of the rectal mucosa produced by kinking or compression of the vasculature during prolapse.

Paradoxically, patients with solitary rectal ulcers rarely report rectal prolapse, possibly because they fail to notice the prolapse or because they are embarrassed to seek medical help. The usual presentation is rectal bleeding or, rarely, rectal pain. Because the ulcer is often large, with irregular edematous margins caused by granulation tissue, the lesion is often mistaken for carcinoma of the rectum after digital examination and/or sigmoidoscopy.

In patients with solitary rectal ulcers associated with rectal prolapse, the prolapse should be corrected surgically. Asymptomatic solitary rectal ulcers can be remarkably refractory, even to treatment with local adrenocorticosteroids. A stool softener and bulk agent (such as psyllium seed mucilloid) should be prescribed.

The patient with solitary cecal ulcer usually experiences lower gastrointestinal bleeding; very rarely, a cecal ulcer may be the source of colonic perforation. Entities to be excluded include Crohn's disease, carcinoma, or bleeding from some other site such as angiodysplasia or a diverticulum. Solitary cecal ulcers that cause symptoms require surgical resection.

ANAL FISSURE AND FISTULA

Stretching of the anal orifice during passage of a large, hard stool can tear the cutaneous-mucous membrane junction, resulting in a fissure. Anal inflammation secondary to any cause, such as herpes simplex type I or II, syphilis, or lymphogranuloma venereum, also facilitates formation of a fissure. On occasion, a fissure may bleed moderately. If it extends into a hemorrhoid, bleeding may become profuse. Most

> ✔ **WHEN TO REFER**
>
> Patients with acute abdominal pain or gastrointestinal bleeding benefit from early consultation with a surgeon, gastroenterologist, or both, depending on the situation. In addition, cases in which patients have significant comorbid disease, atypical presentation, and/or delayed response to treatment should be discussed with a radiologist to determine the ideal diagnostic studies and potential for either temporary or definitive interventional endoscopic or radiologic treatment.

commonly, a patient with anal fissure complains of pain, particularly during defecation, with well-localized anal tenderness. The initial treatment is stool softeners (such as psyllium seed mucilloid) and sitz baths. If pain is severe, astringent-anesthetic solutions, ointments, or salves containing a local anesthetic may be added. Local corticosteroids can be used if infection can be excluded. If not associated with underlying inflammatory disease such as Crohn's disease or infection, fissures usually heal rapidly when the stools are softened.

Fistulas at or near the anus (rectal fistula, perineal fistula, or perianal fistula) are distressingly common complications of Crohn's disease and may be the first manifestation of that disease (Chapter 341). When perianal fistulas occur in Crohn's disease, there may not be obvious involvement of the rectal mucosa; the principal focus may be in the distant bowel such as the terminal ileum. Short of local penetrating trauma, it is difficult to envision a cause for perianal fistula other than Crohn's disease. A perianal abscess can precede development of a perianal fistula. Patients with a perianal fistula have local pain, tenderness, swelling, and discharge of mucus, pus, or feces. The patient may have fecal incontinence if the fistula is severe and extends from rectal mucosa (and lumen) to perianal skin, bypassing the sphincter. If Crohn's disease is present, local surgery of the fistula may be followed by failure to heal and by further tissue breakdown. Therefore it is prudent to exclude conscientiously the possibility of otherwise occult or subclinical Crohn's disease before any local surgery is undertaken. Even then, better initial management might be prescription of antibiotics and stool softeners; local methylprednisolone injection; or, if the fistula is severe, bowel rest.

BIBLIOGRAPHY

Almy TP, Howell DA: Diverticular disease of the colon, *N Engl J Med* 302:324, 1980.

Barnes PRH et al: Hirschsprung's disease and idiopathic megacolon in adults and adolescents, *Gut* 27:534, 1986.

Birbaum BA, Balthazar EJ: CT of appendicitis and diverticulitis, *Radiol Clin North Am* 32:885-898, 1994.

Brian JE Jr, Stair JM: Noncolonic diverticular disease, *Surg Gynecol Obstet* 161:189, 1985.

Cho KC et al: Sigmoid diverticulitis: diagnostic role of CT comparison with barium enema studies, *Radiology* 176:111, 1990.

Ford MJ et al: Clinical spectrum of "solitary ulcer" of the rectum, *Gastroenterology* 84:1533, 1983.

Hughes LE et al: Local depot methylprednisolone injection for painful anal Crohn's disease, *Gastroenterology* 94:709, 1988.

Konvolinka CW: Acute diverticulitis under age forty, *Am J Surg* 167:562-565, 1994.

Krishnamurthy S et al: Jejunal diverticulosis: a heterogeneous disorder caused by a variety of abnormalities of smooth muscle or myenteric plexus, *Gastroenterology* 85:538, 1983.

Matsagas MI, Faturos N, Koulouras B, Giannoukas AD: Incidence, complications, and management of Meckel's diverticulum, *Arch Surg* 130:143-146, 1995.

Meyers MA et al: Pathogenesis of bleeding colonic diverticulosis, *Gastroenterology* 71:577, 1976.

Mueller PR et al: Sigmoid diverticular abscesses: percutaneous drainage as an adjunct to surgical resection in 24 cases, *Radiology* 164:321, 1987.

Parikh DH et al: Abnormalities in the distribution of laminin and collagen type IV in Hirschsprung's disease, *Gastroenterology* 102:1236, 1992.

Puylaert JBCM et al: A prospective study of ultrasonography in the diagnosis of appendicitis, *N Engl J Med* 317:666, 1987.

Stabile BE, Puccio E, van Sonnenberg E, Neff CC: Preoperative percutaneous drainage of diverticular abscesses, *Am J Surg* 159:99-105, 1990.

Taguchi T, Tanaka K, Ikeda K: Fibromuscular dysplasia of arteries in Hirschsprung's disease, *Gastroenterology* 88:1099, 1985.

Turgeon DK, Barnett JL: Meckel's diverticulum, *Am J Gastroenterol* 85:777, 1990.

Welch CE, Athanasoulis CA, Galdabini JJ: Hemorrhage from the large bowel with special reference to angiodysplasia and diverticular disease, *World J Surg* 2:73, 1978.

346 Gastrointestinal Manifestations of HIV Infection and AIDS

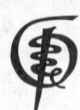

Donald P. Kotler

Gastrointestinal (GI) dysfunction is common in people infected with the human immunodeficiency virus type 1 (HIV-1), especially those with the acquired immunodeficiency syndrome (AIDS). The GI tract and other mucous membranes have an inherent vulnerability to enteric pathogens, produced by the absence of a strong physical barrier. The GI tract also is in intimate contact with a multitude of potential pathogens in the external (luminal) environment. The defense of the GI tract includes an immune system that is homologous to, but distinct from, systemic immunity. Nonimmunologic factors also contribute to the defense of the GI tract. Deficiencies in either immunologic or nonimmunologic defenses leads to a series of disease complications. The aim of this chapter is to codify the effects of AIDS on the GI tract. Diagnosis and management are organized into a series of clinical syndromes.

The topic of mucosal immunity is reviewed in detail elsewhere. Mucosal immunity in individuals infected with the human immunodeficiency virus type 1, the etiologic agent of AIDS, has not been studied thoroughly, though there is ample clinical evidence and some confirmatory experimental evidence of mucosal immune deficiency. Several studies have demonstrated cellular reservoirs for human immunodeficiency virus (HIV) in the GI tract. The evidence includes HIV deoxyribonucleic acid (DNA) and ribonucleic acid (RNA) by polymerase chain reaction and by in situ hybridization, and HIV protein antigens by immunohistochemical staining and enzyme-linked immunosorbent assay (ELISA). In vitro infection of intestinal epithelial cell lines by HIV has been accomplished. Animal studies indicate that intestinal cells are reservoirs for retroviruses. Significant associations among HIV expression in intestinal mucosa, clinical symptoms, and histopathologic alterations have been found.

GENERAL PRINCIPLES OF EVALUATION AND TREATMENT

A wide variety of GI complications may develop in HIV-infected individuals (Box 346-1). Proper clinical management requires an appreciation of the different disease presentations in this group. The specific pathogens producing disease in AIDS patients are different from those that usually affect immunocompetent individuals. A striking difference between HIV-infected and noninfected patients is the frequent coexistence of multiple enteric complications in AIDS patients. In most other circumstances, patients usually have a single disease entity, no matter how many or varied the symptoms: the so-called law of parsimony, or Occam's razor. The implication is that investigations should be thorough and not necessarily stop once a single pathogen is found. Clinical presentation and clinical course may be different in HIV-positive and HIV-negative individuals. The disease complications of AIDS are notable for their chronicity and, at present, susceptibility to suppression but resistance to cure. For this reason most treatments must be given chronically.

However, HIV-infected individuals also are subject to common illnesses, such as appendicitis. In either case, the pathologic features usually match the clinical symptoms and physical findings, so the inductive reasoning on which clinical diagnostics is based can be applied to gastrointestinal problems associated with HIV infection. It is important to remember that the clinical-pathologic correlations and the pathophysiologic mechanisms involved in disease expression are the same in HIV infection as in other diseases, and that they reflect the fundamental biology of the body's response to illness and injury.

BOX 346-1
Gastrointestinal pathogens in AIDS patients

Parasites
Cryptosporidium parvum
Enterocytozoon bieneusi
Encephalitozoon intestinalis
Isospora belli
Giardia lamblia
Entamoeba histolytica
*Blastocystis hominis**
Strongyloides stercoralis
Pneumocystis carinii

Bacteria
Salmonella spp.
Shigella spp.
Campylobacter spp.
Helicobacter pylori
Mycobacterium tuberculosis
Mycobacterium avium-intracellulare
Enteroadherent *Escherichia coli*
Clostridium difficile

Viruses
Human immunodeficiency virus*
Cytomegalovirus
Herpes simplex virus
Adenovirus
Epstein-Barr virus*
Human papillomavirus
Hepatitis B virus
Hepatitis C virus
Hepatitis D virus

Fungi
Candida albicans
Torulopsis glabrata
Coccidioides imitis
Cryptococcus neoformans
Histoplasma capsulatum

*Uncertain pathogenic potential.

CLINICAL SYNDROMES

The gastrointestinal complications of HIV infection and AIDS can be grouped into a series of clinical syndromes. These include disorders of food intake, dyspepsia, diarrhea, anorectal diseases, malignancies, gastrointestinal hemorrhage, diseases requiring surgery, hepatobiliary diseases, and pancreatic diseases.

Disorders of Food Intake

Oral candidiasis is the most commonly encountered complication in HIV-infected individuals. The most common species is *Candida albicans,* which is part of the normal enteric flora. The presenting symptoms are sore throat and, if there is concomitant esophageal involvement, odynophagia, as well as substernal discomfort. Esophageal disease may be asymptomatic. Food intake may be decreased, and increased sensitivity of the oral mucosa to foods may be noted. Erosions and plaques on the gingiva, palate, hypopharynx, and esophagus are seen. Bronchial, gastric, and intestinal mucosae are not involved grossly or microscopically. In most cases the diagnosis can be suggested by visual examination and confirmed by a response to treatment. Culture, biopsy, or brush cytologic evaluation may be confirmatory.

Oral candidiasis can be successfully treated with topical or systemic agents; esophageal candidiasis requires systemically active agents. Topical therapies include nystatin and clotrimazole troches

(Mycelex). Ketoconazole (Nizoral) and fluconazole (Diflucan) are effective systemic agents. Presumptive treatment of esophageal candidiasis, with more intensive evaluation limited to treatment failures, has been shown to be a cost-effective and safe management design. The infection is resistant to oral therapy in a small percentage of cases and must then be treated with intravenous amphotericin B. Few clinicians prescribe primary prophylaxis against candidiasis. Most clinicians maintain patients on secondary prophylaxis, though its advantage has not been shown objectively.

Oral hairy leukoplakia is a whitish, verrucous excrescence that occurs along the sides of the tongue. Epstein-Barr virus has been found in the lesions by molecular hybridization studies as well as by electron microscopic examinations. There are few symptoms. Acyclovir or ganciclovir therapy leads to resolution of the lesions.

Painful ulcers or ulcerating neoplasms of the oral cavity, hypopharynx, or esophagus may cause significant impairment of food intake. Small aphthous ulcers in the oral cavity are common and may resolve spontaneously or after administration of topical steroids. Thalidomide has been shown to be effective in refractory cases.

Some esophageal ulcers are infectious in etiology, and intracellular herpes simplex virus or cytomegalovirus inclusion bodies can be detected. Other esophageal ulcers are seen in which no etiologic agent can be identified. The presence of HIV in esophageal ulcers has been demonstrated, but its role in ulcer formation and progression is unknown. The ulcers are atypical in their large size and in the extensive undermining of the mucosa. The symptoms are refractory to antigastric secretory therapy and may respond poorly to opiates. Progressive malnutrition is the usual result in untreated cases. Corticosteroid therapy has been shown to produce symptomatic relief, weight gain, and ulcer healing in a substantial proportion of patients. Despite the potential hazards of steroid therapy, clinical experience has demonstrated that the treatment can be administered with relative safety. Thalidomide therapy also is effective in producing symptomatic relief and allowing healing to take place.

Neoplasms, such as Kaposi's sarcoma or lymphoma, may affect food intake by interfering with mastication or swallowing or by producing esophageal obstruction. These lesions may respond to a variety of therapies.

In many cases, food intake is diminished in the absence of pathologic lesions. The causes are diverse but fall into several general categories: focal or diffuse organic neurologic lesions, altered release of cytokines caused by systemic illnesses, anorexia as an indirect effect of malabsorption, alterations in taste, nausea, and psychologic or psychosocial factors.

Dyspepsia

Nausea and dyspepsia are very common symptoms in AIDS but rarely dominate the clinical picture. These symptoms may be due to a variety of pathologic processes. The stomach may be involved by disseminated infections such as those caused by cytomegalovirus (CMV), *Mycobacterium avium-intracellulare* (MAI), and fungi; or tumors such as Kaposi's sarcoma, lymphoma, or adenocarcinoma. Symptomatic gastritis caused by *Helicobacter pylori* has been described but appears not to be common, possibly because of frequent antibiotic usage in AIDS patients. Some medications, such as nonsteroidal antiinflammatory agents, promote gastric ulceration and produce dyspepsia. On the other hand, symptomatic peptic ulcer disease is uncommon in AIDS patients, possibly because of decreased gastric acid secretion. Dyspepsia is due to a low-grade pancreatitis in some patients and may precede the development of biliary tract disease (see later discussion).

The clinical symptoms are nonspecific. The presence of weight loss or fever implies a serious complication such as a systemic infection or ulcerating tumor. Treatment of dyspepsia depends on its cause. *Helicobacter pylori* in a symptomatic HIV-infected individual is treated in a manner similar to that for any other symptomatic patients. Diagnosis of CMV or MAI infection is an indication for antiinfective therapy. Widespread or ulcerating Kaposi's sarcoma is an indication for systemic chemotherapy, as is the presence of lymphoma.

Diarrhea and Wasting

Diarrhea and weight loss are very common problems in AIDS patients, occurring in up to three quarters during the disease course. The pathogenic mechanisms underlying diarrhea are multifactorial and related to the specific etiologic mechanism. Generally, symptoms can be attributed to either small intestinal injury and malabsorption or colitis. Although early studies reported large numbers of patients with unexplained diarrhea, an infectious agent can be found in the majority of AIDS patients if a comprehensive evaluation is performed. Conversely, a minority of HIV-infected individuals without AIDS who complain of diarrhea have an identifiable etiologic agent.

The clinical differentiation of malabsorptive from colitic disease is important in order to focus the diagnostic evaluation, though the possibility of multiple coexisting problems must be remembered. An algorithmic approach is shown in Fig. 346-1.

Parasites. *Cryptosporidium* spp. are the most widely recognized enteric pathogens in patients with AIDS. The infection has a worldwide distribution and is responsible for 5% to 10% of cases of severe diarrhea in American AIDS patients. The parasite may infect immunocompetent individuals who have a self-limited illness. Cryptosporidiosis has been implicated in traveler's diarrhea and in outbreaks of diarrheal disease in day care centers. On the other hand, cryptosporidiosis usually is chronic and protracted in AIDS patients. Spontaneous remissions occasionally occur and may be related to a relatively high number of CD4+ lymphocytes or temporal rise in CD4+ lymphocyte counts. The infection may spread to the biliary system, pancreas and gallbladder, and other areas.

Cryptosporidiosis can be diagnosed by special examination of stool specimens (Chapter 279) or intestinal biopsy specimens (Fig. 346-2). Therapeutic options for cryptosporidiosis are limited. Several antiparasitic agents are undergoing clinical trials. Treatment of diarrhea caused by cryptosporidiosis may be difficult. Diet modification may help in patients with mild disase. Hydrophilic bulking agents generally are not helpful. Opiates such as diphenoxylate, paregoric, or tincture of opium may be effective, though the amount required sometimes causes excessive sedation, and escalating doses may be required. Therapy with a somatostatin analog may be successful. Parenteral fluids may be required to maintain a normal state of hydration, and parenteral feedings may be required to maintain nutritional status.

Microsporidia have recently been recognized as a common cause of diarrhea in AIDS patients and may account for up to one quarter of cases of idiopathic diarrhea and progressive wasting. Two species producing intestinal disease have been identified. The majority of infections are caused by *Enterocytozoon bieneusi,* which is localized to the superficial epithelium. In most cases the diagnosis requires electron microscopy of intestinal biopsy specimens for confirmation (Fig. 346-2), though microsporidial spores have been identified in stool specimens and intestinal aspirates. The second species, *Encephalitozoon intestinalis,* can be distinguished ultrastructurally from *E. bieneusi.* In addition, the parasite may produce disseminated disease; organisms have been found in the kidney, liver, gallbladder, brain, and other sites.

Clinically, microsporidiosis resembles cryptosporidiosis and other diffuse small intestinal mucosal diseases; diarrhea is the major manifestation. Albendazole has demonstrated efficacy in *E. intestinalis* infections, but is less effective in *E. bieneusi* infections. Nutritional therapy is based on diet modification to decrease the fat and lactose content. Elemental diets, semielemental diets and parenteral nutrition have been used successfully in some patients.

Isospora belli has been reported frequently in AIDS patients from Haiti and West Africa, though fewer cases have been seen in northern climates. The symptoms are similar to those of cryptosporidiosis. Oocysts may be scarce in stool specimens (Color Plate VIII-1) and organisms rare in biopsy specimens (Fig. 346-2), so the diagnosis is more easily overlooked than is cryptosporidiosis. Successful disease suppression has been reported with trimethoprim sulfamethoxathole or pyrimethamine at various dosages but does not occur in every patient. Diarrhea often recurs on discontinuation of therapy so that chronic therapy with trimethoprim sulfamethoxathole, trimethoprim alone, or pyrimethamine and folinic acid is necessary.

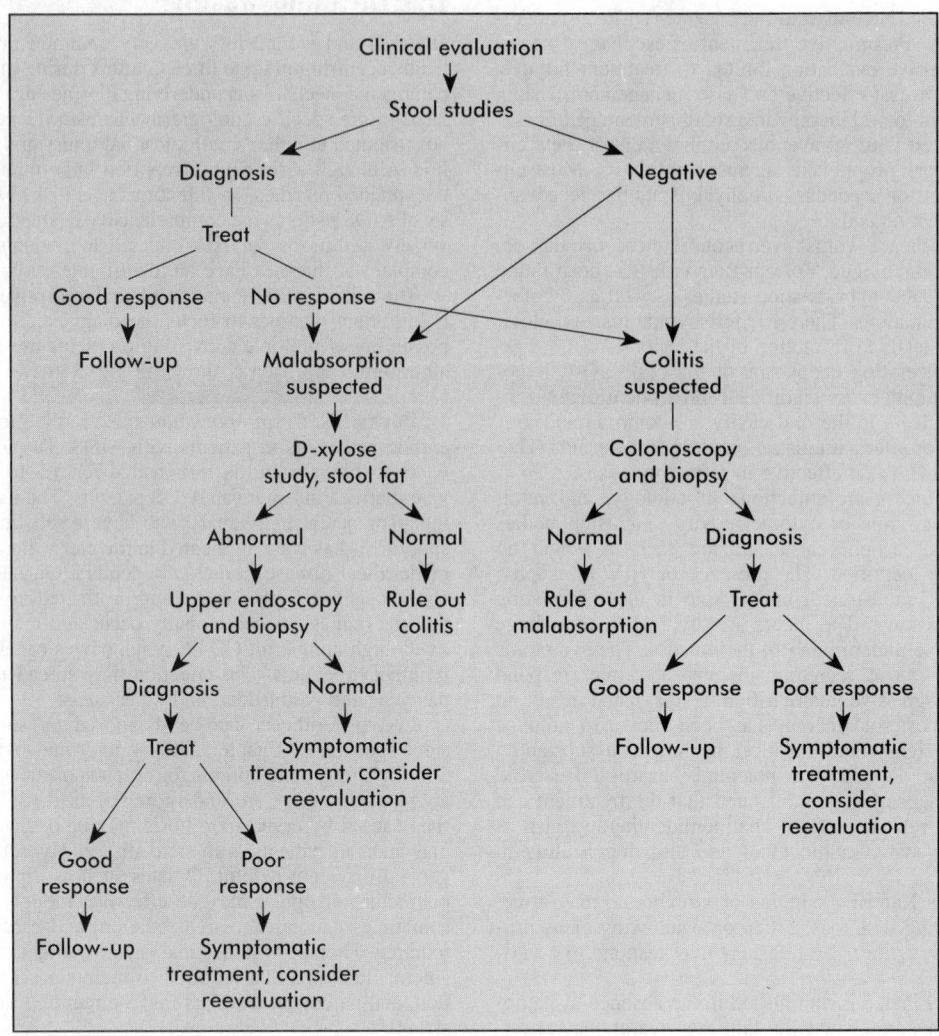

FIGURE 346-1   An approach to the evaluation of diarrhea and wasting in AIDS patients.

Giardiasis (Fig. 346-2) is not a common cause of acute diarrhea in AIDS. Drug therapy with quinacrine or metronidazole is indicated if cysts or trophozoites are found, though suspicion of other causes should be high. Like giardiasis, amebiasis is not a common cause of severe illness in HIV-infected patients. In the majority of cases, *Entamoeba histolytica* appears to act as a commensal organism. Although metronidazole therapy should be prescribed, the possibility of coexisting pathogens should be considered strongly. Other parasites have been reported, including *Strongyloides stercoralis,* which may produce a hyperinfection syndrome. *Blastocystis hominis,* which is considered by some but not by others to be an enteric pathogen, has been found in many HIV-seropositive people with diarrhea. Diarrhea may continue despite eradication of the organism.

Viruses. Disseminated cytomegalovirus infection is a progressive disease and contributes significantly to morbidity and mortality. CMV has been implicated in many GI syndromes and may infect any organ of the digestive system, but the most common presentation is CMV colitis. Patients complain of diarrhea, weight loss, and persistent fevers. In advanced cases the diarrhea may become bloody. Development of severe abdominal pain may signal intestinal infarction or perforation.

The diagnosis of CMV infection is made by histologic examination of tissue biopsy specimens. The key histopathologic feature is the characteristic intracellular inclusion. When inclusions are rare or atypical, immunohistologic or in situ hybridization techniques developed for clinical use may be helpful. Other available diagnostic techniques, such as viral culture and blood serologic analysis, generally are less useful.

Several agents are capable of inhibiting CMV replication. The most widely studied is ganciclovir. Clinical benefit from ganciclovir therapy in patients with serious CMV infection includes clinical stabilization, weight gain, and prolonged survival. Ganciclovir is administered intravenously using an induction regimen followed by maintenance therapy, given through a chronic indwelling catheter. The drug has hematologic toxicity and may produce neutropenia. Foscarnet is an antiviral agent with activity against HIV as well as CMV. Evidence of clinical benefit has been reported. Like ganciclovir, foscarnet must be given by intravenous infusion.

Adenoviruses are occasionally isolated from rectal swabs or biopsy specimens from AIDS patients with diarrhea and a stable or deteriorating course. Electron microscopic studies have demonstrated cytoplasmic inclusion bodies containing adenovirus in superficial epithelial cells.

The potential role of HIV as an enteric pathogen is incompletely defined. A prospective study of HIV-infected subjects with abdominal complaints demonstrated significant correlations among altered bowel habits, altered histologic features, biochemical evidence of intestinal injury, and evidence of HIV production, which were independent of enteric pathogens. Mucosal contents of HIV RNA and p24 antigen are higher in HIV-infected individuals without AIDS than in AIDS patients. In a companion study, tissue content of inflammatory cells varied with HIV disease progression and was highest in a subgroup of non-AIDS patients. Disproportionate depletion of CD4+

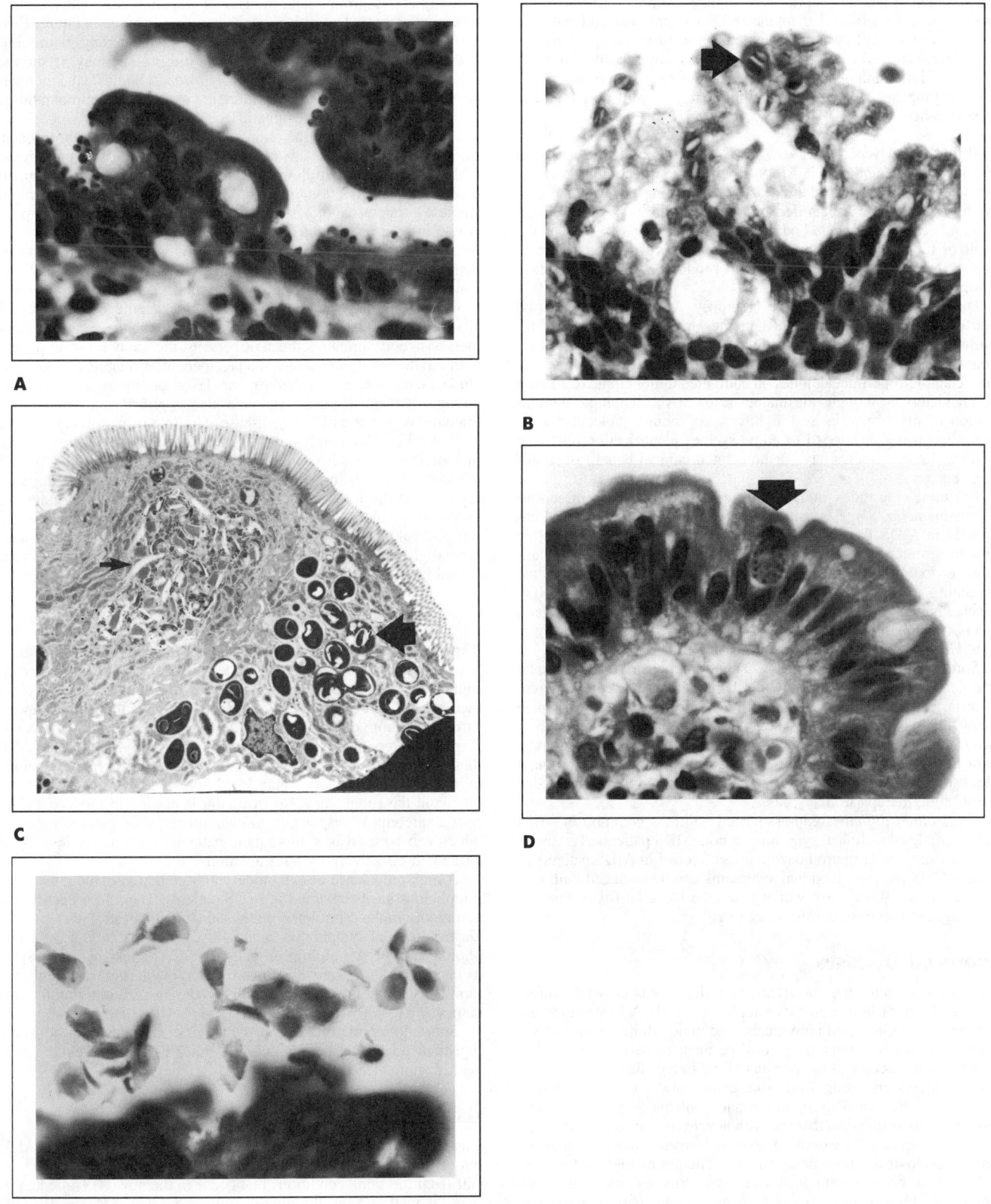

FIGURE 346-2   **A,** Cryptosporidial organisms located at the epithelial brush border in the jejunum (original magnification ×400). **B,** Developing microsporidial organisms in sloughing cells at the jejunal villus tip *(arrow)* (original magnification ×400). **C,** Transmission electron microscopic photograph demonstrating developing organisms in one cell *(small arrow)* and mature spores in an adjacent cell *(large arrow)* (×8000). **D,** Microgametocyte of *Isospora belli (arrow)* in a jejunal epithelial cell (original magnification ×400). **E,** Trophozoites of *Giardia lamblia* adjacent to jejunal epithelium (original magnification 400×).

lymphocytes in lamina propria were found. Lymphoid activation associated with generalized cytokine mRNA expression and mucosal inflammatory changes was documented. These results suggest that inflammation and HIV expression in mucosa are related. An HIV-associated inflammatory bowel disease could be an important factor in the pathogenesis of the immune deficiency as well as a factor in disease transmission.

Bacteria. *Mycobacterium avium-intracellulare* has been seen with increasing frequency in AIDS patients. The infection usually occurs late in the course of the disease in the setting of fever and progressive wasting. It is acquired orally or, possibly, by aerosol, and disseminates widely in the body. The intestinal lesion of MAI is the result of mucosal and submucosal infiltration with infected macrophages that block lymphatic flow and produce an exudative enteropathy.

Diagnosis is made by culture or biopsy. Acid-fast bacilli can be seen on stool examination, and their presence suggests possible intestinal involvement with MAI. Mucosal abnormalities on barium radiographs or thickening of the intestinal wall plus enlargement of mesenteric and retroperitoneal nodes on computed tomographic (CT) scan are characteristic though not diagnostic of MAI. Histologic demonstration of mycobacteria is straightforward, though molecular techniques are being developed to allow species identification on tissue sections. Recent studies have demonstrated clinical benefit of multidrug regimens.

Bacterial enteritides in HIV-infected persons include infections with *Salmonella, Shigella,* and *Campylobacter* species. Bacterial enteritides in AIDS frequently have a chronic, relapsing course, often with bacteremia. The diagnosis is straightforward with routine evaluation. Blood cultures as well as stool studies should be part of the evaluation of suspected infectious diarrhea with fever in an HIV-infected patient. Patients respond to antibiotic therapy with parenteral agents, though the incidence of disease recurrence after therapy is high. Chronic antibiotic administration may be needed.

Some patients with severe CD4+ lymphocyte depletion and chronic diarrhea have been shown to harbor infections with adherent bacteria, usually *E. coli.* The infection is identical to those seen in young infants, especially in the developing world. The infection is localized to the distal small intestine in the right colon in most cases. Clinically, the disease resembles ileal dysfunction, with predominant effects of malabsorbed bile acids and fat. The infection has responded to antibiotic therapy in many cases.

Clostridium difficile toxin-associated colitis is common in AIDS and resembles the clinical syndrome in non-AIDS patients. Treatment with vancomycin or metronidazole is as effective in AIDS patients as in non-AIDS patients. Residual symptoms can be managed with oral cholestyramine (Questran), which binds the bacterial toxin. Surveillance against recurrent colitis is necessary.

Anorectal Diseases

The anorectal region may be affected by ulcers, masses, warts, infections, and hemorrhoids. Herpes simplex virus (HSV) infections are common in HIV-infected individuals. The major clinical syndrome in AIDS is a slowly spreading, painful perineal or perianal ulcer. The primary lesion occurs at the pectinate line. Large, shallow, spreading perianal ulcers are recognized more commonly. The diagnosis may be indicated by visual examination and confirmed by viral culture. Most patients respond to therapy with acyclovir. Parenteral acyclovir therapy is required for extensive lesions. Herpes simplex virus resistant to acyclovir has been demonstrated. The use of foscarnet or ganciclovir may bring resolution. Cytomegalovirus also can cause anorectal ulcerations. Ganciclovir or foscarnet therapy may be associated with clinical resolution.

A variety of classic venereal diseases can produce anorectal ulcerations. Diagnosis and therapy of *Neisseria gonorrhea* proctitis is similar in AIDS and non-AIDS patients. Syphilis may have an atypical presentation in HIV-infected subjects, and serologic diagnosis is affected by the presence of immunodeficiency. Dark-field examination or immunohistologic studies of clinical specimens may be needed to identify the spirochete (Color Plate VIII-2). Prolonged intravenous antibiotic therapy is required. *Chlamydia trachomatis* is prevalent in

sexually active groups, and the risk of infection rises with the level of sexual activity. Definitive diagnosis is made by cell culture. Usual therapy is oral tetracycline or doxycycline. Therapy with either trimethoprim-sulfamethoxazole or sulfa drugs alone may be successful. Rectal spirochetosis has been recognized in homosexual men with or without HIV infections. The infection usually is asymptomatic and an incidental finding on evaluation.

Idiopathic ulcers of the anorectal region, similar to those occurring in the esophagus, are seen in AIDS patients. The presence of CMV, HSV, human papillomavirus (HPV), acid-fast bacilli, fungi, and other bacterial infections must be excluded by culture or histologic studies. Intralesional or systemic corticosteroids produce a prompt decrease in pain but have a variable effect on healing.

The incidence of anogenital neoplasms is increased in AIDS patients as it is in other immunosuppressed individuals. Kaposi's sarcoma and lymphoma are the most common neoplasms. Epidermoid cancers, including squamous cell and cloacagenic cancer, occur in anal skin and rectal glands, respectively. Although these cancers rarely metastasize in immunocompetent persons, they may do so in patients with AIDS. For these lesions, management after diagnostic biopsy includes excision, chemotherapy, or laser photocoagulation. Laser therapy of rectal Kaposi's sarcoma also is effective and may cause dramatic regression of bulky disease. The role of papillomavirus, the etiologic agent of condyloma acuminata (common venereal warts), in anorectal cancers is unclear. Specific serotypes of papillomaviruses are suspected as being cofactors for carcinogenesis in the anogenital region, and the incidence of squamous cell cancer of the anus was known to be increased in homosexual men before the recognition of AIDS. Leukoplakia of the anal canal, which is considered by some a premalignant lesion, is a common finding in HIV-infected homosexual men.

Malignancies

Kaposi's sarcoma in AIDS is histopathologically indistinguishable from classic Kaposi's sarcoma, endemic forms of Kaposi's sarcoma found in Africa, and the form that occurs during immunosuppressive therapy. Visceral involvement in AIDS patients with Kaposi's sarcoma is more common than in non–HIV-infected individuals with Kaposi's sarcoma. Visceral involvement may be asymptomatic. The diagnosis is made by visual inspection and confirmed by biopsy, though endoscopic biopsy may yield false-negative results if the tumor is in the submucosa. No treatment is needed in most cases. Kaposi's sarcoma is responsive to chemotherapy or radiation therapy, which can be used in symptomatic patients. Obstructive lesions can be treated effectively by laser ablation.

A high prevalence of extranodal, high-grade, non-Hodgkins B-cell lymphomas has been noted in AIDS patients. The tumor occurs most commonly in the central nervous system and the gastrointestinal tract. Gastrointestinal lymphomas in AIDS, especially the Burkitt's lymphoma subtype, are biologically aggressive. The lesions may respond to chemotherapy, using combination therapies. There are few long-term survivors, however, because of the underlying immunodeficiency.

Sporadic reports of AIDS patients with carcinomas in the gastrointestinal tract have been published, but a higher incidence has not been documented convincingly.

Gastrointestinal Hemorrhage

Gastrointestinal hemorrhage is not a common consequence of AIDS, but serious or life-threatening bleeding does occur. Bleeding may result from the same conditions that occur in the non–HIV-infected patient, as well as from the tumors and ulcers seen in AIDS. Episodes of massive arterial hemorrhage have occurred in patients with acute or chronic intestinal ulcers or rapidly progressive Kaposi's sarcoma.

The basic concepts of diagnosis and treatment are the same in HIV-infected and noninfected individuals (Chapter 332). Bleeding lesions may be visualized by endoscopy, and bleeding may be controlled locally. Angiographic localization of obscure lesions and pharmacologic control may be successful. If bleeding is related to a discrete ulcer, surgical excision may be indicated; surgery is less appropriate for patients with widespread disease. Proper management of bleeding neoplasms involves effective local control followed by systemic chemotherapy.

Complications Requiring Surgery

Disease complications requiring consideration of emergency surgical intervention occur in patients with AIDS. Perforated viscus occurs in AIDS, but the cause may more often be a solitary ulcer, CMV infection, or tumor rather than peptic ulcer disease or diverticulitis, which are the usual causes in patients without AIDS. Malignant obstruction usually is due to Kaposi's sarcoma or lymphoma rather than adenocarcinoma. Kaposi's sarcoma or lymphoma also may cause an intussusception. Some patients with clinical peritonitis have had, at laparotomy, only mild fibrinous exudate without obvious perforation.

Though the physical findings of the acute abdominal condition are not significantly affected by the presence of AIDS, the laboratory evaluation differs markedly from that expected. Elevated leukocyte counts with immature forms in the circulation may not be present, especially if there is preexisting leukopenia or prior treatment with myelosuppressive drugs. Isotopic imaging studies such as an indium-labeled white blood cell study or gallium scan may yield false-negative results in the presence of severe leukopenia. Imaging studies such as CT scan with luminal contrast may be particularly valuable in detecting extraluminal collections of pus or fluid.

Although the indications for surgery are the same in AIDS patients and non–HIV-infected patients, the expected outcomes may differ. One can anticipate the possibility of unusual pathogens, prolonged recovery times, and impaired wound healing in AIDS patients. The incidence of postoperative complications and mortality was high in several series but was due to the seriousness of the underlying disease complications. Complete recovery after major abdominal surgery is possible in AIDS patients and may be followed by prolonged survival. Laparoscopic surgery has been used successfully in cases of chronic cholecystitis.

Hepatobiliary Diseases

Three distinct clinical syndromes have been recognized: diffuse hepatocellular injury, granulomatous hepatitis, and sclerosing cholangitis. Many other patients with abnormal liver chemical findings have macrovesicular or microvesicular fatty infiltration or other nonspecific changes.

Diffuse hepatitis is most commonly a result of drug toxicity or hepatitis C or hepatitis D infection. Hepatitis B infection is clinically mild in most AIDS patients. Granulomatous hepatitis in AIDS patients is related to mycobacterial, fungal, or protozoal diseases or to drug toxicity. Fever and constitutional symptoms are prominent. Liver chemical test results demonstrate progressive elevations in the levels of alkaline phosphatase and γ-glutamyl transpeptidase. Liver biopsy reveals poorly formed granulomas. Special stains can presumptively identify the causative organism. Peliosis hepatis has been described in AIDS patients and is associated with infection by a *Rickettsia*-like organism. A syndrome of sclerosing cholangitis has been frequently recognized in AIDS patients and resembles the non-AIDS variety. The pathogenesis is unknown, although *Cryptosporidium* spp., microsporidia, and CMV inclusions have been observed in the biliary tract epithelium of some patients. Endoscopic retrograde examination demonstrates areas of narrowing and dilation of the intrahepatic and/or extrahepatic ducts with mucosal ulceration. Endoscopic papillotomy, dilation, or stent placement may give short-term relief. In long-term cases, progressive jaundice and liver failure may develop.

Pancreatic Diseases

Pancreatic disease in AIDS has received little attention and may not be recognized before postmortem examination. The pancreas may be affected by systemic diseases such as CMV, MAI, fungi, Kaposi's sarcoma, or lymphoma. Drug-induced pancreatitis is the most commonly recognized form. Hyperlipidemic pancreatitis has been observed. There are no reports of chronic pancreatitis as a specific complication of HIV infection. Pancreatic insufficiency is an uncommon cause of fat malabsorption in AIDS patients.

BIBLIOGRAPHY

Adal KA, Cockrell CJ, Petri WA: Cat scratch disease, bacillary angiomatosis, and other infections due to *Rochalimaea*, *N Engl J Med* 330:1509, 1994.

Benhamou Y, Caumes E, Gerosa Y et al: AIDS-related cholangiopathy: critical analysis of a prospective series of 26 patients, *Dig Dis Sci* 38:1113, 1993.

Cappell MS: Hepatobiliary manifestations of the acquired immune deficiency syndrome, *Am J Gastroenterol* 86:1, 1991.

Cappell MS, Geller AJ: The high mortality of gastrointestinal bleeding in HIV-seropositive patients: a multivariate analysis of risk factors and warning signs of mortality in 50 consecutive patients, *Am J Gastroenterol* 87:815, 1992.

Clayton F, Cronin WJ, Reka S et al: Rectal mucosal histopathology in HIV infection varies with disease stage and HIV protein content, *Gastroenterology* 103:919, 1992.

Dieterich DT, Kotler DP, Busch D et al: Ganciclovir treatment of cytomegalovirus colitis in AIDS: a randomized, double-blind, placebo-controlled multicenter trial, *J Infect Dis* 167:278, 1992.

Fox CH, Kotler DP, Tierney AR et al: Detection of HIV-1 RNA in intestinal lamina propria of patients with AIDS and gastrointestinal disease, *J Infect Dis* 159:467, 1989.

Knowles DM et al: Lymphoid neoplasia associated with the acquired immunodeficiency syndrome: the New York University Medical Center experience with 105 patients (1981-1986), *Ann Intern Med* 108:744, 1988.

Kotler DP: Gastrointestinal manifestations of HIV infection and AIDS. In Devita V, Hellman S, Rosenberg SA, editors: *AIDS: etiology, diagnosis, treatment and prevention*, ed 4, Philadelphia, 1997, JB Lippincott.

Kotler DP, Giang TT, Thiim M et al: Chronic bacterial enteropathy in patients with AIDS, *J Infect Dis* 171:552, 1995.

Kotler DP, Orenstein JM: Prevalence of intestinal microsporidiosis in HIV-infected individuals referred for gastroenterological evaluation, *Am J Gastroenterol* 89:1998, 1994.

Kotler DP, Reka S, Chow K, Orenstein JM: Effects of enteric parasitoses and HIV infection upon small intestinal structure and function in patients with AIDS, *J Clin Gastroenterol* 16:10, 1993.

Laine L, Dretler RH, Conteas CN et al: Fluconazole compared with ketoconazole for the treatment of candida esophagitis in AIDS, *Ann Intern Med* 117:655, 1992.

Orenstein JM: Microsporidiosis in the acquired immunodeficiency syndrome, *J Parasitol* 77:843, 1991.

Scannell KA: Surgery and human immunodeficiency virus disease, *J Acquir Immune Defic Syndr Hum Retroviral* 2:43, 1989.

Soave R, Johnson WD Jr: *Cryptosporidium* and *Isospora belli* infections, *J Infect Dis* 157:225, 1988.

Wilcox CM, Diehl DL, Cello JP et al: Cytomegalovirus esophagitis in patients with AIDS: a clinical, endoscopic, and pathologic correlation, *Ann Intern Med* 113:589, 1991.

Wilcox CM, Schwartz DA: A pilot study of oral corticosteroid therapy for idiopathic esophageal ulcerations associated with human immunodeficiency virus infection, *Am J Med* 93:131, 1992.

Young LS et al: Mycobacterial infections in AIDS patients, with an emphasis on the *Mycobacterium avium* complex, *Rev Infect Dis* 8:1024, 1986.

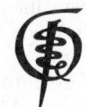

CHAPTER

347 Nutrition and Internal Medicine

Elliot Weser and Eleanor A. Young

Nutrition plays an important role in the quality of life and in the prevention and treatment of disease. Many of the currently known nutrients are essential for life. Thus nutrition influences virtually every area of medicine.

Data from animal experiments indicate that the control of food intake by the central nervous system represents a basic integrative physiologic system. The existence of a "feeding center" in the lateral area of the hypothalamus and "satiety center" in the ventromedial nucleus of the hypothalamus is well established. Stimulation of the satiety center results in inhibiting food-eating behavior; ablation of the ventromedial nucleus (satiety center) results in hyperphagia. Numerous other reflexes associated with food intake are integrated and coordinated by these centers, resulting in a complex but basic system that regulates feedback control of nutrient intake. In addition, some enteric hormones are known to play a role in a gut-neural axis, which also affects eating behavior. Overriding this system in humans are cortical functions, such as psychologic influences, which add to the complexity of this regulation. Nevertheless, increased caloric consumption and obesity have been associated with hypothalamic injury or disease as well as frontal lobotomy and bilateral frontal cortical lesions, suggesting that this basic control system does operate in humans. Although the findings of recent studies have indicated that specific genes may predispose to clinical obesity, the exact mechanisms by which they relate to the aforementioned processes remain unclear.

A complex array of metabolic, biochemical, and hormonal alterations occur within the host in response to systemic infection. These responses have nutritional consequences that vary in relation to the severity and duration of the illness. Both acute and chronic infections may deplete the body stores of nutrients and precipitate nutritional deficiency. This deficiency may result in greater susceptibility to secondary or superimposed infections as well as a general decrease in the ability to withstand the stress of disease. Additionally, severe protein-calorie malnutrition leads to impairment of nonspecific host defense mechanisms and specific forms of immune responsiveness, especially in hospitalized or ambulatory patients who have failed to maintain an adequate nutrient intake either as a result of disease or as a consequence of therapy (cytotoxic drugs, radiation, hemodialysis, etc.).

A close relationship also exists between nutrient intake and the gastrointestinal tract. Structural and functional changes within the small bowel may be produced by deficiencies in nutrient intake. Gastrointestinal disease may modify the digestion, absorption, and metabolism of nutrients and lead to secondary nutritional deficiencies (Chapter 326).

The liver is important in the utilization and storage of many nutrients. Abnormalities in the metabolism of protein, carbohydrates, fats, vitamins, and minerals often occur in liver disease and may have a significant impact on nutritional status. In time, this may affect the liver's ability to cope with further injury and contribute to the clinical complications of liver disease.

Epidemiologic studies suggest that 30% to 50% of all human cancers may be related to nutritional factors that contribute to colon, prostate, and breast cancer. The complexity of such relationships precludes an understanding of precise mechanisms at this time. On the other hand, a great deal of clinical experience is available for documenting the profound nutritional effects induced by cancer and the various modalities of therapy. Malnutrition may result from anorexia, impaired food intake (e.g., obstruction, nausea, reduced taste acuity, malabsorption, protein-losing enteropathy, and disturbances of electrolyte and fluid balance. Radiation therapy, surgery, and chemotherapy used in neoplastic diseases frequently predispose the patient to nutritional problems precipitated by reduced taste acuity, dysphagia, bowel damage caused by radiation, direct toxic effect of drugs on the gastrointestinal tract, or resection of some portion of the gastrointestinal tract. Nutritional support therefore must be an essential component in the overall treatment plan for patients with cancer. This requires frequent assessment of the nutritional status of the patient, selection of appropriate nutritional therapy, and competent delivery of such support. Nutritional status, tumor growth, and antitumor treatment are interrelated, and the physician must have sufficient expertise to provide optimum medical management for cancer patients.

Nutritional status may be significantly compromised by chronic renal disease. Defective conversion of vitamin D_3 to 1,25-dihydroxycholecalciferol may cause decreased calcium and phosphorus absorption from the intestine, uremic osteodystrophy, and enhanced calcium reabsorption by the kidney. Renal disease may also affect the ability of the kidney to synthesize and catabolize certain hormones and amino acids; to degrade peptides and small proteins (e.g., insulin, glucagon, parathyroid hormone); and to produce or utilize certain amino acids (e.g., serine, alanine). Malnutrition can significantly affect renal function (e.g., glomerular filtration rate is decreased, as is the ability to concentrate and acidify urine). Thus nutritional therapy is an important consideration in the management of patients with renal disease. Hemodialysis or peritoneal dialysis may reduce the adverse effects of chronic renal insufficiency on nutritional status. However, inadequate protein and calorie intake may still contribute to malnutrition in patients undergoing dialysis. During dialysis, there are losses of free amino acids, peptides, bound amino acids, glucose, and water-soluble vitamins. Even in patients on maintenance dialysis therapy, body tissue wasting may continue as a result of catabolic effects related to complicating disease, endocrine disorders, blood loss, poor dietary intake, emotional depression, and anorexia.

Regulatory mechanisms of hormone action may alter metabolism and influence the distribution and utilization of nutrients within the body. Inappropriate hormonal secretion in some disease states may have profound nutritional consequences. Examples include diabetes mellitus; hypoglycemia; parathyroid-induced disorders of calcium, phosphorus, and magnesium metabolism; renal osteodystrophy; myxedema; and hyperthyroidism. Maturity-onset diabetes mellitus, the most common of the endocrine disorders, is frequently associated with obesity, elevated blood glucose and serum triglyceride levels, increased incorporation of triglycerides into prebetalipoproteins, elevated insulin levels, hypertension, and an accelerated rate of development of atherosclerosis. Restriction of calories to achieve and maintain desirable weight causes prompt reduction in serum insulin, blood glucose, and plasma triglyceride levels. Weight reduction or salt restriction may significantly improve hypertension in both diabetic and nondiabetic patients.

The nervous system tends to be more resistant to the effects of malnutrition than other body systems, and clinical manifestations occur only with an extreme degree and duration of nutrient depletion. Nutritional diseases of the nervous system are related to conditions of chronic stress, psychiatric disease, infection, hemodialysis, and alcoholism. Thiamine deficiency may lead to Wernicke's encephalopathy and Korsakoff's syndrome or to polyneuropathy. Deficiencies of niacin, pyridoxine (vitamin B_6), folate, and vitamin B_{12} may also lead to peripheral or central nervous system manifestations.

Anemia is probably the most common expression of nutritional deficiency in human beings. A deficiency of iron leading to hypochromic, microcytic anemia is widely recognized as the most important cause of anemia in the world. Depletion of body stores of folate or vitamin B_{12} leads to megaloblastic anemia. Anemia as a result of copper, vitamin E, and vitamin B_6 deficiencies has also been well described.

It is clear from these examples that nutritional deficiencies or excesses may be associated with a variety of diseases seen in the practice of clinical medicine. Malnutrition may precipitate or complicate existing disease states or be the end result of a disease process. The importance of nutrition requires that the physician be knowledgeable about its role in health and disease.

MALNUTRITION

Nutrition in health or disease is never an isolated phenomenon but is influenced by numerous interrelated factors. Nutrition is the provision of adequate calories and essential nutrients to maintain health. In contrast, malnutrition refers to a state of bad or poor nutritional status. Although malnutrition is frequently considered strictly within the context of undernutrition, it is important that a broader view be taken in the practice of internal medicine.

One or a combination of several diseases may produce malnutrition. However, social, economic, psychologic, cultural, religious, and even political influences should be considered in the overall assessment of malnutrition. The five major factors contributing to malnutrition are undernutrition, overnutrition, imbalance of nutrients, increased nutrient requirements, and malabsorption.

Undernutrition

Undernutrition may result from inadequate intake of food or a deficiency of one or more specific nutrients.

Inadequate Intake of Food. Inadequate food intake may lead to a state of malnutrition depending on (1) the degree or severity of reduced food intake, (2) the duration of reduced food intake, (3) whether reduced food intake occurs during critical periods of rapid growth (infancy, adolescence, pregnancy), (4) the baseline body stores of nutrients, and (5) the presence of other factors such as fever, infection, immune status, and stress.

Primary chronic protein-calorie malnutrition is the predominant nutritional problem worldwide. In recent years, significant progress has been made in preventing malnutrition in many areas, yet malnutrition remains a critical factor in disease prevention and health promotion in half of the countries of the world. The prevalence of protein-calorie malnutrition is directly related to inadequate food supply for the populations at greatest risk. Worldwide, 1.3 billion people

Table 347-1   Comparative characteristics of kwashiorkor and marasmus

KWASHIORKOR	MARASMUS	MARASMIC KWASHIORKOR
Edema; enlarged liver caused by fat accumulation; hair: dry, brittle, easily pluckable; skin: scaly, hyperpigmented, erythematous	Obvious starved appearance; hair: sparse, thin, dry; skin: thin, dry, wrinkled	Combined clinical characteristics of kwashiorkor and marasmus Major features: (1) Edema of kwashiorkor with or without skin lesions (2) Muscle wasting and decreased subcutaneous fat of marasmus
Adequate fat reserves and muscle mass over short periods of adequate caloric but low protein intake	Severe fat and muscle wasting over prolonged periods of reduced caloric intake	
Depressed cellular immune functions	Diminished skinfold thickness: <3 mm	Biochemical features of kwashiorkor and marasmus are seen. Alterations of severe protein deficiency usually predominate
Reduced wound-healing capacity	Height/weight ratio: $<80\%$ of standard	
Increased susceptibility to infection	Midarm circumference: <15 cm	
Lymphopenia: <1500 cells/mm^3	Serum albumin level: >2.8 g/dl	
Serum albumin level: <2.8 g/dl	Normal to low	
Serum transferrin level: 150 mg/dl		

are too poor to afford enough food to keep themselves fully productive. Hunger is on the increase in many places, notably in Africa, Middle East, and Latin America.

Although protein-calorie malnutrition is much less prevalent in the United States, it does exist. The documentation of widespread malnutrition in the United States during the 1960s called forth development and expansion of federal food and nutrition programs to end hunger. A great deal of progress toward this goal was achieved. However, currently the challenge of malnutrition is again a critical problem as a result of increased growth of the number of persons living below the poverty line, cutbacks of many federally subsidized nutrition programs, and growing numbers of persons seeking emergency food assistance. Substantive reports document evidence that there is a significant increase in hunger and malnutrition in the United States. At present, approximately 20 to 30 million people in the United States face hunger. Hunger is more widespread now than it was 10 or 15 years ago. Every fifth child lives below the poverty line.

Documented protein-calorie malnutrition among hospitalized patients in the United States has been shown to range from 40% to 70%. These reports suggest that for hospitalized patients there are inadequate nutritional support, little or no attempt to reverse malnutrition, lack of concern and knowledge regarding nutritional status, and lack of clearly defined institutional goals regarding nutritional assessment.

Reduced total food intake is considered by many investigators as one of the major causes of weight loss leading to undernutrition in patients after total gastrectomy. After partial gastrectomy, approximately one half of patients lose weight and do not again achieve their ideal body weight. Reduced food intake may lead to malnutrition after small bowel resection and after jejunoileal or gastric bypass or volume reduction in markedly obese patients. Anorexia, loss of appetite, reduced food intake, and subsequent progressive tissue wasting are characteristically observed in patients with cancer.

Patients with anorexia nervosa experience significant weight loss and have an intractable negative attitude toward eating and weight gain that overrides hunger, admonitions, reassurance, and threats. Self-induced starvation results in cachexia, severe metabolic defects, and, if unchecked, death (Chapter 334).

Other groups of patients at high risk for development of protein-calorie malnutrition are those with chronic alcoholism, renal disease, or draining abscesses, wounds, or fistulas and those receiving intravenous glucose support alone, with no oral intake.

Regardless of the cause of protein-calorie malnutrition, special attention should be given to nutrition in patients who are grossly underweight (weight/height ratio below 80% of standard) or who have recently lost 10% or more of their usual body weight.

Protein-calorie malnutrition should be further diagnosed as either marasmus (simple starvation) or kwashiorkor (acute visceral attrition). Table 347-1 indicates the comparative characteristics of kwashiorkor and marasmus. These two distinct forms of protein-calorie malnutrition differ in cause, pathophysiologic characteristics, symptom complex, and treatment requirements. For these reasons, differential di-

agnosis should be carefully made so that an appropriate nutritional support plan can be initiated.

Combined kwashiorkor and marasmus occurs when a chronically undernourished patient becomes acutely ill or stressed. This usually leads to a serious, life-threatening situation in which vigorous nutritional therapy is critical.

Overnutrition

Overnutrition is an excess intake of total calories or of a specific nutrient and represents another example of malnutrition.

Excessive Intake of Calories. Excessive intake of calories leads to obesity, a pathologic condition characterized by an accumulation of excess body fat. Obesity is the most prevalent form of malnutrition in the United States, afflicting approximately 40 to 80 million persons. Obesity alters a number of metabolic variables and may complicate diseases encountered in clinical medicine.

Excessive Intake of a Single Nutrient. Excessive intake of a single nutrient may produce an adverse effect, leading to malnutrition. Most vitamins and minerals are needed in only trace amounts. Usual therapeutic doses of water-soluble vitamins are normally excreted without ill effects. However, megavitamin therapy with pharmacologic doses of water-soluble vitamins may have toxic side effects. The fat-soluble vitamins are even more likely to be toxic.

Excess intake of minerals is much more likely to have a toxic effect than excess intake of vitamins. Hypermagnesemia has been reported in patients with renal insufficiency who are taking magnesium-containing drugs (e.g., antacids). High blood concentrations of magnesium (8 mEq/L) lead to central nervous system depression, profound paralysis of the skeletal muscles, and respiratory distress.

Iron overload causing hemachromatosis and fluoride excess producing fluorosis are discussed in the sections on excess intake of minerals (Chapters 358 and 316).

Malnutrition produced by excess intake of trace metals is well documented. Excess iodide may lead to an inhibition of thyroid hormone synthesis, hypothyroidism, and iodide goiter. Acute copper intoxication in human beings causes nausea, vomiting, epigastric pain, diarrhea, headache, dizziness, and weakness. In severe cases, copper toxicity may lead to tachycardia, hypertension, coma, jaundice, hemolytic anemia, hemoglobinuria, uremia, and death. Toxic reactions generated by excess intake of manganese, cobalt, selenium, and cadmium have also been reported.

Imbalance of Nutrients

Imbalance of nutrients may produce malnutrition. A protein's quality and biologic value are determined largely by the amino acids it contains. Low levels of essential amino acids or disproportionate ratios of amino acids alter the biologic value of a protein. Therefore, in a diet limited largely to protein of vegetable origin, protein intake has to be greater than in a diet that includes protein of animal origin, because the amino acid ratio in animal proteins is more beneficial than that in vegetable proteins.

Heating a protein food in the presence of carbohydrate (Maillard reaction) produces an amino acid—carbohydrate complex that is not digested by human beings, with preferential binding of the essential amino acid lysine. This binding may result in an 80% loss of lysine, altering the amino acid ratio and decreasing the quality of protein present. This concept finds practical application in the processing of oral liquid formulas and solutions for total parenteral nutrition.

Folate therapy in a patient without adequate reserves of vitamin B_{12} can result in rapidly progressive subacute combined degeneration of the spinal cord, with neurologic deficits that may be irreversible.

Abnormalities of amino acid metabolism and urea formation are involved in the pathogenesis of hepatic encephalopathy (Chapter 354). The present therapy for hepatic encephalopathy produces a negative nitrogen balance, because it is based on decreasing the production of ammonia by reducing protein intake. In recent efforts to maintain nitrogen balance, a special mixture of amino acids has been used to normalize the amino acid pattern found in encephalopathy, and the keto analogs of amino acids have been used to offset hyperammonemia and negative nitrogen balance.

Many nutritional factors can increase urinary calcium, including increased vitamin D, magnesium, sodium, and vitamin A. Consumption of acids, ketogenic diets, and diets with a low calcium/phosphorus ratio cause hypercalciuria. Recent studies demonstrate that increased intake of dietary protein causes increased urinary excretion.

Nutrient imbalances other than deficiencies of iron, folate, or vitamin B_{12} have been shown to influence hematopoiesis. Anemia is often present in protein-calorie malnutrition and is thought to be due to an insufficient production of erythropoietin. Anemia characterized by neutropenia has been documented in copper deficiency. Vitamin B_6–responsive sideroblastic anemia is likely due to a defect in heme synthesis, although the exact location of the enzymatic block is not known. The hematologic effects of vitamin E deficiency in human beings have been debated. Hemolytic anemia has been clearly documented in premature babies maintained on tocopherol-deficient, high–polyunsaturated fat formulas. It is suggested that in the absence of adequate vitamin E, polyunsaturated fats in the erythrocyte membrane structure are peroxidized.

Increased Nutrient Requirements

Increased nutrient requirements may lead to malnutrition unless intake of the specific nutrients required is similarly increased.

Fever and infection increase the need for nutrients. All infections result in aberrations of nutritional balance, with most notable effects on protein and nitrogen balance. Not only does the infectious agent block utilization of nutrients as an integral part of its attack on the host, but the host exhibits a series of metabolic reactions to infection that are detrimental to nutrition. Host defense responses include the synthesis of phagocytes and leukocytes, the production of immunoglobulins, and the synthesis of a variety of nonspecific proteins associated with the reaction to infection. Thus there are both increased losses of and increased requirements for nutrients, particularly protein, during infection.

Major injury, burns, undue stress, and fractures all increase the need for nutrients. For example, a severely burned patient may require about 6000 to 9000 kcal per day to maintain energy balance. In severe burns, weight loss during the recovery period may be 30% to 40% of the patient's preburn weight. Protein requirements may range from 3.2 to 3.9 g per kilogram of body weight (early catabolic phase) to 2.0 to 2.5 g per kilogram of body weight (early anabolic phase). Requirements for water and electrolytes are also elevated.

Nutrient requirements may also be increased by exposure to heat and to cold and by living at high altitudes. Athletes have increased demand for calories, but there is no evidence that protein, mineral, or vitamin needs are greater than in healthy nonathletes. Energy expenditure in the developmentally disabled patient or in the orthopedically handicapped patient may be increased or decreased, and caloric needs must be adjusted accordingly to prevent malnutrition.

Malabsorption of Nutrients

Failure to absorb one or more dietary nutrients as a result of inadequate digestion or intestinal mucosal transport often produces severe malnutrition. Malabsorption may involve not only carbohydrates, fats, and proteins, but also water, electrolytes, calcium, magnesium, trace minerals, water-soluble and fat-soluble vitamins, and drugs (Chapter 340). By appropriate management of patients with malabsorption, malnutrition may be prevented.

OBESITY

Recent National Health and Nutrition Examination (NHANES) studies of obesity in the United States included a sample of 8260 adults 20 years of age or older. Overall, approximately one third (33.4%) of all adults in the United States were estimated to be overweight and had a mean body mass index (BMI) of 26.3. These results indicate a striking increase of 8% in the prevalence of obesity in the United States over the past decade.

Although body weight that exceeds ideal standards as determined by age, sex, and height may be accounted for by greater bone or muscle mass, the majority of individuals who weigh more than 20% over their calculated ideal weight have excessive adipose mass. It is likely that the increase in regular exercise among various age-groups in the population will significantly alter the incidence of obesity.

Although reduced longevity may not be associated with mild obesity, it is associated with extreme obesity. Increased susceptibility to cardiovascular disease (particularly hypertension), diabetes, pulmonary dysfunction, and gallstones is more often noted in the obese. Perhaps underemphasized are the psychologic, social, cultural, and occupational problems experienced by these patients (particularly in extreme obesity). The generally accepted increased risks of complications associated with anesthesia and major surgical procedures are additional considerations for the patient and physician. Obesity may affect the management of many disease states and requires attention in the total approach to the patient.

Causes

Various attempts have been made to classify obesity. An etiologic classification suggests four causes: (1) genetic transmission, (2) hypothalamic injury, (3) endocrine disorders, and (4) energy intake in excess of energy output.

Among experimental animals, several strains of mice with genetically inherited forms of obesity have been identified. Genetic causes of obesity in human beings are less clearly defined. However, recent human genetic variation in the β_3-adrenergic receptor associated with an increased capacity to gain weight has been reported. Recent reports of positional cloning of the mouse gene and its human homolog, as well as the more recent isolation of human ob complementary DNA (cDNA) clone will likely lead to a clearer understanding of human obesity as well as more effective ways to manage and prevent obesity.

Human population studies also strongly suggest the existence of genetic factors in obesity. Studies have shown that when both parents are of desirable weight, <10% of their children are obese. However, when one parent is obese, 50% of the children are obese, and when both parents are obese, over 80% of the children are obese. Correlations of parent-child weights comparing natural children with adopted children show significantly higher body weight correlations of natural parent–child weights. Studies of adopted children indicate that, relative to body weight, thin children tend to resemble their natural parents rather than their foster parents. Identical twins reared apart show higher weight correlations than do fraternal twins or fraternal siblings.

Lesions of the hypothalamus induced by electrolytic, surgical, or chemical means can produce obesity in experimental animals, depending on the extent and location of the injury. There is an alteration of the set point at which body weight can be regulated, and excess weight gain is hypertrophic, caused mainly by enlargement of adipose cells with little change in the number of fat cells. There is clear evidence that injury to the hypothalamus can also produce obesity in human beings. Patients with obesity produced by hypothalamic injury are rare (about 100 such cases reported in the medical literature), and in such patients most hypothalamic injuries have been due to malignant tumors, inflammatory lesions, or trauma to the head.

The most striking form of obesity produced by endocrine abnormalities is seen in patients with Cushing's syndrome, insulinomas, or hyperinsulinemia associated with maturity-onset diabetes.

Obesity of specific hypothalamic or endocrine origin is thought to account for <2% of all obesity. The overwhelming cause of obesity for most people is energy intake in excess of energy output, and a number of contributing factors are associated with this imbalance.

Restricted physical activity is a major cause of human obesity. Studies have demonstrated that obese persons are relatively inactive; however, there is no evidence that the obese are less active because of their obesity or that they are obese because they are less physically active. In either case, the effects of exercise on weight loss are clear. When energy expenditure is increased without a corresponding increase in food intake, body weight decreases. If food intake increases proportionately to exercise, body weight does not alter. With low levels of exercise, body weight and food intake tend to be higher than with moderate to high levels of exercise. Thus there is strong support for some form of physical activity as part of weight-reduction programs.

Subtle biochemical mechanisms may be operative in the development of obesity. An interlocking system of chemical reactions may lead to a futile cycle of thermogenesis. In this system the thermal dissipation of food energy is much less marked in the obese than in the lean person. Thus, in the obese person, more food energy is shunted into the body stores of fat than is dissipated as body heat. Occasionally an obese person may consume approximately the same amount of calories as a lean person, yet remain obese. Recent studies have demonstrated that people differ with regard to energy requirements, ability to synthesize and dispose of fat, capacity to store fat, and appetite.

Socioeconomic factors may also contribute to obesity. Obesity has been shown to be 7 to 12 times more prevalent in lower socioeconomic population groups than in upper socioeconomic groups. Occupation, education, income, self image, susceptibility to mass media influence, residential environment, and ethnic and cultural norms are all factors that may affect body weight.

Obese persons may be relatively insensitive to the internal hunger-satiety cues and excessively sensitive to the external cues of appearance, variety, aroma, and taste of foods. The obese person tends to overeat for nonphysiologic reasons, for when the external cues are removed, the obese person spontaneously decreases food intake and loses weight. The underlying mechanisms that trigger the "on" or "off" signals related to these cues require further study.

Frequency of food intake is another factor that may lead to energy intake in excess of energy expenditure. Controlled metabolic studies in human beings have demonstrated that when food intake is held both quantitatively and qualitatively constant, meal feeding (administration of total daily calories in a large meal rather than in small, frequent meals) is associated with increased lipogenesis, body fat, and cholesterol and insulin output and with decreased glucose tolerance.

Adipose cellularity may also be a significant factor leading to excess body fat. Studies of hyperplastic obesity (overweight condition related to an excessive number of fat cells) and hypertrophic obesity (overweight condition related to a normal number of fat cells of excessive size) have shown that (1) the number of fat cells can increase at any age; (2) once fat cells are made, they cannot be decreased in number by weight reduction; (3) the ability to attain normal body weight in relation to height is decreased in a person with an excess number of fat cells; and (4) when obese subjects lose and subsequently regain weight, the rate of weight gain is more rapid in subjects with hyperplastic obesity.

Dietary Approaches

Caloric restriction and exercise are complementary approaches to weight reduction. A negative energy balance can be achieved by (1) decreasing caloric intake (approximately 3500 kcal equals 1 lb body fat) while keeping expenditure constant; (2) increasing caloric expenditure while keeping caloric intake constant; or (3) decreasing caloric intake and simultaneously increasing energy expenditure.

Although these thermodynamic facts are easy to understand, prac-

---

BOX 347-1
Guideline for weight-reduction diets

1. Decide on rate of weight loss to be achieved. For most patients a 1- to 2-lb weight loss per week is satisfactory.
2. Decrease caloric intake; 1 lb body fat = 3500 kcal.
3. Increase energy expenditure.
4. The percentage of calories should be 12% to 14% protein, <30% fat (with low saturated fat), and 50% to 60% carbohydrate (with very low sucrose).
5. Provide for adequate intake of vitamins, minerals, and water. Supplementation may be needed when calories are restricted to less than 1000 kcal.
6. Provide for adequate and ongoing counseling and reinforcement aimed at behavior modification.
7. Salt restriction may decrease the tendency toward excessive fluid retention and may be effective in the prevention or reduction of hypertension.

---

tical and realistic approaches to weight reduction are difficult for most obese patients and are strongly influenced by lifestyle, attitudes, knowledge, and understanding of the health-related risks of obesity, and a multitude of other biologic and social factors. Studies show that 15% to 20% of obese subjects are able to achieve a 20-lb weight loss by dietary means, but only 5% can achieve a weight loss greater than 40 lb. The percentage of patients who can maintain weight loss is substantially smaller.

Patients least likely to achieve weight reduction by dietary means (1) are morbidly obese, (2) have been obese since childhood or adolescence, (3) expect quick and dramatic results, (4) place the burden of success on the physician or on some special dietary manipulation, and (5) fail to realize that obesity is a serious disorder that is associated with significantly increased health problems.

There is no magic, miraculous, painless diet for weight reduction. The continual promulgation of new and faddish weight-reduction diets attests to this fact. The $39 billion diet industry (diet books, weight-reducing clinics, exercise equipment, diet pills, etc.) in the United States is considered by many to constitute a gigantic fraud on the American public. Most popular weight-reduction diets (Dr. Atkins', Dr. Stillman's, Pritikin, Scarsdale, Last Chance, Air Force, Mayo, Drinking Man's) have not been tested in controlled long-term studies, thus making scientific appraisal difficult. No matter which diet is selected, certain general guidelines should be followed (Box 347-1).

Total fasting may be appropriate for patients with refractory obesity or for those who must reduce body weight quickly for medical reasons. Fasting should occur only with adequate medical supervision. The extent and rate of weight loss are directly proportional to initial weight, with greatest and most rapid losses occurring in the heaviest subjects. Men usually lose weight more rapidly, predictably, and linearly than women. Initial rapid weight loss is accounted for predominantly by decrease in body water level; a 2- to 11-lb weight loss may occur in the first 24 hours of fasting. Weight loss produced by decrease in body water level subsequently diminishes. Hunger is experienced by fasting patients for the first 2 to 4 days only, although many patients continue to be preoccupied with food. Prolonged fasting is accompanied by a number of physiologic and metabolic changes that should be continually monitored, including decreased body water level; electrolyte shifts produced by increased urinary loss of sodium, potassium, calcium, and magnesium; decreased volume of plasma and extracellular fluid; postural hypotension; continued negative nitrogen balance with loss of lean body mass; ketonemia; ketonuria; mild metabolic acidosis; hyperuricemia; hypoglycemia (40 to 50 mg/dl); decrease in serum cholesterol level; depletion of water-soluble vitamins (if not supplemented); and reduction in body fat stores.

With a semistarvation diet (400 to 600 kcal/day), some of the consequences of total fasting are ameliorated. Large losses of lean body mass can be prevented if 40 to 60 g protein is consumed, and this is one of the major advantages of partial over total fasting.

Short-term fasting interspersed with days of reduced caloric intake (fasting 1 or 2 days/week) may be an efficient approach to weight reduction. This approach has produced little adverse psychologic or physiologic stress; however, it should be based on a realistic weight-reduction plan.

A low-calorie (400 kcal) diet consisting of liquid protein hydrolysates, synthetic amino acids, or solid protein food has become popular over the past 10 years. This approach is based on the premise that complete elimination of carbohydrate from the diet enhances ketosis, eliminates hunger, improves compliance, and spares body protein. This approach is currently considered experimental, and the efficacy and potential risks have not been established. In some 50 patients who died while on protein-sparing diets, acute cardiac arrhythmia was suggested as the most common cause of death. Protein-sparing diets have not been shown to elicit greater patient compliance, and greater long-term acceptance remains unproved. Furthermore, weight loss on a hypocaloric pure-protein diet has not been found to be superior to that on a hypocaloric mixed diet.

Many popular diets are based on some alteration of the major energy components. Regardless of the claims made by proponents of such diets, well-controlled metabolic studies demonstrate that the most important single factor in weight loss is reduction of total caloric intake. On a long-term basis, the rate of weight loss is similar regardless of the ratio of carbohydrate, fat, and protein in the diet if total caloric intake is less than caloric expenditure. In patients on low-carbohydrate diets, initial weight loss is more rapid than in patients on carbohydrate-containing diets, but this initial weight loss is due mainly to loss of water.

Numerous one-food diets (egg diet, grapefruit diet, banana diet, etc.) have been in vogue for many years; however, compliance with such regimens is short-lived. In addition, no one food contains all of the essential nutrients, and the utilization of any one food for extended periods of time results in nutritional deficiencies.

A lecithin–kelp–vitamin B_6–cider vinegar diet continues to be widely published, although a well-controlled metabolic study indicated no advantage in weight reduction when use of capsules containing these ingredients was compared with use of a placebo.

Weight Watchers, TOPS (Take Off Pounds Sensibly), and other group approaches have been somewhat more successful than diet alone. These diet programs apply behavior-modification techniques and place emphasis on changes in lifestyle.

Exercise

A regular plan of exercise is an essential component of every weight-reduction program. Consideration should be given to the specifics of an exercise plan, including the type, duration, place, and time of exercise to be accomplished on a day-to-day basis. In order to enhance and encourage compliance, an evaluation of the exercise program should be included as a component of the medical assessment of the patient's progress. Elderly or physically disabled patients may benefit from assistance from a physical therapist regarding appropriate kinds of exercise. Aerobic expenditure of energy (e.g., walking briskly, running, swimming, bicycling) at a relatively constant but low level may have optimum effects on the cardiovascular system. Increased pulse rate and cardiac output should be reached and sustained for at least 15 minutes to achieve the greatest benefits from exercise.

Other Approaches to Weight Reduction

Other approaches include behavior modification, self-management training, external reinforcement, psychotherapy, psychiatric analysis, hypnosis, acupuncture, and ear lobe stapling. Most of these therapies have focused on helping patients achieve dietary self-control through understanding and modification of the conditions that affect their eating behavior. Recent reviews of studies using these methodologies indicate that they have greatly contributed to our understanding of the complexities of obesity. Most studies report changes that are clinically small, are variable, and usually cease at termination of formal therapy. Support for the effectiveness of these methods of therapy to produce long-term weight loss or behavioral change in the obese patient is yet to be demonstrated.

Numerous commercial gimmicks for weight loss such as sauna baths, body wraps, sweat suits, and vibrators have no known advantage in weight reduction and may precipitate adverse medical complications. These therapies are an economic fraud in addition to being ineffective in weight reduction.

Medical Management

Although caloric restriction and increased energy expenditure are the basic treatment for obesity, the judicious use of amphetamines or other derivatives of phenylethylamine, particularly in the beginning phase of weight reduction, may be helpful. By stimulating the satiety center in the hypothalamus, amphetamines are thought to suppress appetite and inhibit intake. They are useful in patients with clear patterns of satiety and hunger. If the dose and timing of medication are correct, the patient may experience significant weight loss early in the diet and gain a sense of accomplishment as well as encouragement. In addition to suppressing appetite (and food intake), amphetamines stimulate the central nervous system, and patients may experience increased activity levels, which also contribute to weight reduction. Because these drugs have adrenergic effects on the heart and may cause serious arrhythmias, they should be used with caution in patients with heart disease, severe hypertension, hypothyroidism, glaucoma, agitated states, and history of previous drug abuse. An exception is fenfluramine, which has side effects of drowsiness, depression, and diarrhea, necessitating caution in its use in patients with depression or those taking central nervous system (CNS) depressants. Tolerance to amphetamines develops in approximately 4 to 6 weeks, and once tolerance develops they no longer adequately suppress the desire for food intake. Therefore amphetamines' usefulness is short-lived, and they are best used in patients with recent onset of obesity. In a patient already receiving dietary and behavioral treatment, amphetamines may increase weight reduction by only an additional 10%.

Numerous agents for weight reduction have become available as over-the-counter substances. These agents include phenylpropanolamine, benzocaine, bulk agents, spirulina, and a variety of food substances. Phenylpropanolamine is an active ingredient in many commercial products and is related chemically and pharmacologically to the phenylethylamines, although the side effects are generally milder. Nevertheless, the same precautions should be exercised in their use. The long-term effectiveness of these over-the-counter compounds is controversial and not medically proved.

Unless a patient has proven hypothyroidism, thyroid derivatives should not be used to produce weight loss. Dosages sufficient to cause weight reduction are likely to produce clinical hyperthyroidism. The use of human chorionic gonadotropin injections has also been advocated as a means of producing weight loss. Controlled studies have clearly shown that reduction in weight occurs only when this agent is used as an adjunct to caloric restriction. Resultant weight loss is completely accounted for by the ingestion of fewer calories.

Surgical Therapy

Recent studies of obesity in the United States demonstrate an overall 8% increase in the prevalence of severe obesity. In these persons, who are commonly referred to as the morbidly obese, the death rate may be up to 12 times that in a nonobese matched population. Only 10% or less of extremely obese persons who do manage to lose significant amounts of weight (50% to 60% of initial body weight) by rigid dietary regimens are able to maintain weight loss for more than a few years. For these reasons, surgical approaches have been designed to decrease the ability to ingest food or to reduce its absorption significantly. Currently, there is still much debate about the overall medical usefulness, ethics, and research assessment of these procedures.

Lipectomy and wiring of the jaw have not proved adequate or effective on a long-term basis. Most experience has been acquired with the jejunoileal bypass, which essentially creates a short gut and results in impaired absorption. In most cases, significant weight loss results, usually about 40% of initial weight. Some regain the weight after 3 years. Two major factors influencing loss of weight are degree of malabsorption, which is related to the length of unresected bowel and extent of adaptive changes; and reduction in caloric intake. The latter may occur as a result of unpleasant intestinal symptoms precipitated by food intake and/or an altered taste acuity or desire to eat.

Numerous complications have been associated with the jejunoileal bypass (apart from the high surgical and anesthetic risks) for extremely obese individuals. These complications include oxalate stones and renal disease, liver necrosis and failure, malnutrition and intractable diarrhea, severe electrolyte imbalances, immune-complex arthritis, osteomalacia, proctitis and hemorrhoids, vitamin deficiencies, nausea and vomiting, intestinal pseudoobstruction, and neuromyopathy. Because of the high incidence of these complications, jejunoileal bypass has largely been abandoned.

In recent years, gastric reduction surgery has replaced jejunoileal bypass as the preferred operation for morbid obesity. These procedures essentially create a gastric pouch that, because of its small size, limits the amount of food that can be eaten at any one time. Satisfactory weight loss appears to be well maintained in most patients. Although the metabolic complications associated with the jejunoileal bypass are not prevalent after these gastric procedures, they may result in complications, including bile reflux gastritis, staple dehiscence, anastomotic leaks, stenosis or ulceration, perforation of the gastric pouch, dumping syndrome, and failure to lose weight by patients who succeed in overcoming the limitations imposed by the gastric pouch. For some, malnutrition may also result from inadequate nutrient intake, too-rapid weight loss, and noncompliance in taking appropriate vitamin-mineral supplements. Nutrients most frequently reported to be deficient in patients with gastric reduction are thiamine, folate, vitamin B_{12}, vitamin A, and iron.

All surgical treatment for morbid obesity is palliative and not designed to treat the basic defect. Although genetic factors may predispose to obesity, an essential issue concerning treatment outcome relates to behavioral and epidemiologic factors. The NHANES studies that report an increased prevalence of obesity in the United States may be influenced by one or a combination of the following:

1. Use of cross-sectional studies of a "representative sample" of the United States population.
2. There have been no prospective studies in the same population sample that reflect changes over time.
3. Influence of population migration.
4. Variation in mortality rates over time.
5. Failure of estimates to show the proportion of individuals who became overweight, remained overweight, or lost weight, but, rather, only the net effect of changes in weight.

Other considerations contributing to obesity in the United States include the following:

1. High alcohol intake representing 5% to 7% of overall calorie intake.
2. Plentiful and very palatable foods high in sugar and fat.
3. Drive-by pick-up foods usually deep-fat fried and available at convenient stop-and-go stores.
4. Decrease in energy expenditure via exercise or active sports.
5. Increase in passive leisure time entertainment (e.g., TV, computer games).
6. Overall sedentary lifestyle.
7. Decrease in smoking leading to increased taste and smell perceptions, resulting in increased calorie intake.
8. Cultural factors that tend to increase negative or positive attitudes toward obesity.

VITAMINS

Vitamins play an important role in health maintenance and in specific treatment of a variety of diseases. The initial awareness of vitamins resulted from identification of a group of vitamin-deficiency diseases (i.e., pellagra, beriberi, rickets, and scurvy), now essentially eliminated in the United States but still present in underdeveloped countries. Vitamins are biologically active organic compounds that are essential for normal growth, development, and health and that cannot be synthesized by the body. They must be obtained from exogenous sources, mainly dietary, and transported via the circulation in very low concentrations to a target organ. The vitamins may be separated into two groups, depending on their absorptive media. Vitamins A, D, E, and K are fat-soluble and therefore intimately associated with lipid absorption. The nine water-soluble vitamins are thiamine

Table 347-2   Biochemical function of vitamins

VITAMIN	BIOCHEMICAL ACTION
A	Stabilization of cell membranes
	Formation of visual pigments
	Synthesis of mucopolysaccharides
D	Increased intestinal calcium and phosphorus absorption
	Initiation of calcification of bone and activation of alkaline phosphatase
	Help in maintenance of serum calcium and phosphorus
K	Catalysis of synthesis of factors VII, VIII, IX, and X
	Cofactor in oxidative phosphorylation
E	Biologic antioxidant
	Protection of unsaturated fatty acid membranes
Thiamine (B_1)	Coenzyme in thiamine pyrophosphate
	Catalysis of decarboxylation of pyruvic acid and α-ketoglutaric acid
Riboflavin (B_2)	Coenzyme in flavoprotein enzyme system
Niacin	Coenzyme in nicotinamide dinucleotide
	Codehydrogenase for metabolism of alcohol, lactate, α-hydroxybutyrate
Pyridoxine (B_6)	Coenzyme in pyridoxal phosphate
	Activity in transamination, decarboxylation, deamination, desulfuration
Folic acid	Coenzyme in pyrimidine metabolism
	Transfer of single carbon units
Cyanocobalamin (B_{12})	Coenzyme in hydroxocobalamin
	Methyl biosynthesis, transmethylation, nucleic acid synthesis
	Activation of folic acid coenzymes
Ascorbic acid (C)	Antioxidant-reducing substance
	Hydroxylation of proline, tryptophan
	Iron reduction, absorption
Biotin	Coenzyme for carbon dioxide fixation (carboxylation)
Panthothenic acid	Conversion to coenzyme A

(vitamin B_1), riboflavin (vitamin B_2), niacin, pyridoxine (vitamin B_6), folic acid, cyanocobalamin (vitamin B_{12}), ascorbic acid (vitamin C), pantothenic acid, and biotin. Four of the water-soluble vitamins are absorbed by active transport (thiamine, folic acid, ascorbic acid, and vitamin B_{12}) and the remaining five by passive diffusion through intestinal mucosa. The biochemical actions of the vitamins are listed in Table 347-2.

Vitamin-Deficiency Diseases

Vitamin A Deficiency. Vitamin A deficiency from dietary causes is rare in North America and Western Europe, but represents an important cause of blindness in Southeast Asia, parts of Africa, and Central and South America. In these areas, the deficiency usually results from general malnutrition (often associated with kwashiorkor) in infants and young children. In the United States, vitamin A deficiency in adults is likely to be secondary to severe malabsorption (steatorrhea of diverse origin) or a restricted diet such as in anorexia nervosa. Low serum vitamin A levels are found in abetalipoproteinemia. Recent nutrition surveys in the United States indicate significantly lower serum retinol levels in certain ethnic populations (e.g., Mexican-Americans in the Southwest).

The earliest symptoms of vitamin A deficiency are night blindness and xerosis (drying) of the conjunctivae. Xerophthalmia, or extreme dryness of the conjunctivae, may be associated with xerosis conjunctivae (Bitôt's spots) in the sclera, which are foamy, triangular white patches on the outer and inner sides of the cornea, consisting of shed corneal epithelium. The tarsal glands along the margin of the eyelid may enlarge and resemble a string of beads. Untreated, xerosis of the cornea, with photophobia, keratomalacia, corneal perforation, collapse of the iris, and lens extrusion, may occur. Abnormal keratinization of skin epithelium also occurs and may lead to folliculosis, follicular hyperkeratosis, and phrynoderma ("toad skin"). An early symptom is dry, rough, and pruritic skin.

In general, vitamin A deficiency responds rapidly to vitamin A–replacement therapy. If the eye lesions have progressed to the severe destructive stage, little can be done to restore vision. Mild cases of night blindness show rapid improvement (after the equivalent of 1000 units of vitamin A (as the vitamin itself or as fish liver oil). Keratomalacia, xerophthalmia, and advanced skin changes may require doses in excess of 100,000 units daily for several months.

Vitamin D Deficiency. In the United States, vitamin D deficiency in infants and children has become a rare disease largely because of the enrichment of cows' milk with vitamin D and sufficient exposure to sunlight. As a result, deficient mineralization of growing bones leading to growth retardation and rickets is uncommon. Vitamin D deficiency in adults is usually related to intestinal malabsorption or altered vitamin D metabolism as seen in chronic hepatic and renal diseases.

Osteomalacia—with bone pain, widespread demineralization of bone, and microfractures or compression fractures—may be a presenting feature. Often, hypocalcemia is present and may cause tetany.

Treatment of vitamin D deficiency and osteomalacia in the presence of malabsorption may require doses of vitamin D in excess of 50,000 units daily. In addition, 15 g of calcium gluconate or lactate daily may also be necessary. Acute tetany requires immediate treatment with intravenously administered calcium gluconate, usually given as 10 to 20 ml of a 10% solution.

Vitamin K Deficiency. It is unlikely that vitamin K deficiency occurs solely as a result of inadequate dietary intake. Amounts adequate to meet daily requirements are supplied not only from the diet but also from synthesis of vitamin K by intestinal bacteria. Inadequate absorption of vitamin K may occur in biliary obstruction and all other steatorrheic disorders, presumably because of its excretion with unabsorbed fat. Prolonged administration of antibiotics, particularly in children, may produce a deficiency that is probably related to altered or suppressed intestinal bacterial flora.

Hemorrhage is the clinical manifestation of vitamin K deficiency, which is usually indicated by decreased prothrombin activity in the blood not associated with concomitant liver disease. The hypoprothrombinemia is readily corrected by administration of vitamin K orally, 2 to 5 mg daily. Synthetic, water-soluble preparations are equally effective and particularly useful when bile duct obstruction or steatorrhea is present.

Vitamin E Deficiency. Although vitamin E is essential in human nutrition, no clearly established deficiency syndrome has been consistently reported, although there is evidence that vitamin E replacement prevents the neurologic and visual complications that develop in patients with abetalipoproteinemia (Chapter 340). It has been suggested that vitamin E deficiency in premature and low-birth-weight infants causes hemolytic anemia and peripheral edema. There is no convincing evidence that vitamin E has any beneficial effects on the human reproductive system, habitual abortion, or in the treatment of myoneurogenic diseases. It also remains unsettled whether vitamin E is beneficial in the treatment of cardiac disease. Vitamin E does contribute an antioxidant role important in cancer prevention.

Thiamine (Vitamin B$_1$) Deficiency. Thiamine deficiency occurs in countries where polished rice is the staple dietary cereal or in instances of deprivation associated with dietary habits (food faddism, weight-reducing diets, anorexia nervosa, etc.). In the United States, thiamine deficiency is most commonly associated with chronic alcoholism. Partial deficiency coupled with increased requirements (rapid growth, pregnancy, lactation, hyperthyroidism, gastrointestinal disease, etc.) may also lead to clinical manifestations. In these instances, multiple deficiencies often occur together, particularly those of thiamine, riboflavin, and niacin.

Clinical manifestations of thiamine deficiency are related to the degree and duration of the deficit. Milder states of deprivation produce polyneuritis or dry beriberi. Greater degrees of thiamine deficiency cause beriberi; heart disease; and, in severe cases, Wernicke's encephalopathy and Korsakoff's syndrome. In severely depleted alcoholic patients, glucose infusion without added thiamine may precipitate Wernicke's encephalopathy or cause an early form of the disease to progress rapidly. In general, B vitamins should be added with glucose solutions in all cases, even though this complication is not due primarily to vitamin deficiency.

The early symptoms of thiamine deficiency may be nonspecific and undiagnosed. Intellectual impairment, emotional disturbances, reduced strength, weight loss, fatigue, difficulty walking long distances, insomnia, headache, and muscle tenderness may occur. The progression of impairment is variable, leading to dry, wet, or acute beriberi. Dry and wet beriberi are probably different manifestations of polyneuritis, although the pathogenesis of the edema is not clear. Early in the dry form, the patient may experience paresthesia, numbness, and muscle pain, leading to a slow and deliberate gait. Tendon reflexes may be exaggerated and later decrease or disappear. Muscle weakness may ensue, particularly in the lower extremities and torso. Ultimately, foot or wrist drop occurs, as does aphonia, which indicates paralysis of laryngeal muscles.

The wet form of beriberi is associated with peripheral edema and serous effusions. Although cardiac abnormalities are common at some stage of beriberi, edema may occur in the absence of heart disease. Certainly, heart failure with cardiac enlargement, tachycardia, cyanosis, and late pulmonary edema causes edematous fluid accumulation.

Acute, fulminant beriberi heart disease is typically accompanied by severe dyspnea, pronounced palpitations, and intense precordial chest pain. Heart failure of beriberi has been characterized as a high-output type during the earlier stages of the disease. If untreated, beriberi heart disease runs a progressive course, resulting in death usually within 1 year.

Wernicke's encephalopathy is characterized by altered mentation, eye muscle paralysis, weakness, and ataxic gait. Nystagmus is invariably present, as is paralysis of conjugate gaze. After treatment is begun with thiamine, Korsakoff's syndrome may become apparent. Memory of recent events is impaired and often associated with marked confabulation. There may be amnesia with regard to events during past months or years. Untreated Wernicke's encephalopathy results in high mortality; early treatment may effect complete recovery. Some features of Korsakoff's syndrome may not disappear, however.

The diagnosis of thiamine deficiency can be substantiated by measuring 24-hour urinary thiamine excretion. Values from 0 to 15 μ/24 hr have been found in beriberi. The usual dosage for adults with mild beriberi is 10 mg thiamine taken orally three times daily. In severe cases and in Wernicke's encephalopathy, 25 mg thiamine should be given intravenously, immediately and then two times per day. Patients with acute beriberi heart disease should receive higher doses (about 100 mg) along with other treatment for heart disease.

Riboflavin (Vitamin B$_2$) Deficiency. Riboflavin deficiency is found in all parts of the world, including the United States. Inadequate dietary intake is the principal cause, although intestinal malabsorption or poor utilization in patients with cirrhosis of the liver may also produce the deficiency.

The principal manifestations are cheilosis, angular stomatitis, seborrheic dermatitis, and glossitis. Photophobia, lacrimation, and itching of the eyes may also occur. Fissures may extend out from the angles of the lips onto the cheek or into the mouth in severe cases, and scars may remain after treatment and healing. Erythematous skin lesions of the scrotum and vulva may develop, with scaling and desquamation. The tongue may be deeply fissured and have a purple appearance. There also may be superficial vascularization of the cornea, ultimately producing punctate opacification and ulceration. Conjunctivitis and iritis may accompany the corneal lesions.

The diagnosis should be suspected from the history and clinical findings and can be confirmed if there is decreased 24-hour urinary excretion of riboflavin. Normal values are usually greater than 1000 μ/24 hr. Values less than 50 μ/24 hr are diagnostic of riboflavin deficiency.

In adults, administration of 2 to 5 mg riboflavin three times daily for several weeks usually results in rapid healing of the lesions. Some of the ocular symptoms may be relieved if vitamin A is given before riboflavin therapy, and even greater resolution results with riboflavin. Adequate dietary intake of milk, liver, meat, eggs, and some green leafy vegetables prevents recurrence.

Niacin Deficiency. Niacin is a generic name for both nicotinic acid and nicotinamide, both biologically active and equivalent vitamins. The most prevalent cause of niacin deficiency (pellagra) in the United States is inadequate intake caused by chronic alcoholism. Often, increased requirements associated with physical labor or exposure to the sun may contribute to the clinical presentation. In areas of the world where corn is the staple, cereal pellagra is common among the poor. Corn is low in tryptophan, which is the amino acid precursor of niacin and also contains niacin in a bound and unusable form (niacytin). Niacin deficiency may also occur in patients with malignant carcinoid tumors, because a large amount of tryptophan is converted to 5-hydroxytryptamine (serotonin) instead of niacin. Isoniazid therapy has also been associated with niacin deficiency, presumably because of induced pyridoxine deficiency, which decreases the conversion of tryptophan to niacin.

Pellagra is characterized by dermatitis, diarrhea, inflammation of the mucous membranes, and mental symptoms. Early symptoms that may precede skin changes include anorexia, weight loss, mild digestive complaints, lassitude, irritability, depression, memory loss, anxiety, and confusion. Initially, dermatitis resembles ordinary sunburn, affecting particularly the parts of the body exposed to the sun. The affected skin may then become increasingly pigmented and clearly demarcated from uninvolved areas. Areas of irritation and trauma such as axillae, perineum, genitalia, elbows, and knees may also become involved. In chronic pellagra the skin assumes a thickened, hyperkeratinized, deeply pigmented appearance.

Acute pellagra causes a sore, red, and swollen tongue, with painful swallowing. Inflammatory changes may occur throughout the entire gastrointestinal tract, producing heartburn, abdominal pain, severe diarrhea, and rectal pain. Achlorhydria is common. Other mucous membranes are affected, causing urethritis and vaginitis. Mental changes may progress to include severe confusion, disorientation, delusions, mania, delirium, hallucinations, dementia, and psychotic states. Death occurs within 4 or 5 years if pellagra is not treated.

The diagnosis is confirmed by demonstration of a decrease in the urinary excretion of niacin metabolites, usually 3 mg/24 hr. Niacin should be given orally, because intestinal absorption is slower, and blood concentrations remain elevated for longer periods. The usual dose is approximately 50 mg niacin or nicotinamide, 10 times daily. In severe cases, parenteral nicotinamide therapy may be advisable for several days, 100 mg per day.

Pyridoxine (Vitamin B$_6$) Deficiency. Pyridoxine deficiency from inadequate intake is rare in the United States and generally occurs only with other vitamin B deficiencies. In some patients receiving isoniazid, a potent pyridoxine antagonist, pyridoxine deficiency may develop, particularly if they are slow acetylators of the drug.

The principal manifestation of pyridoxine deficiency is peripheral neuritis, which may be particularly severe in alcoholic patients. Pyridoxine-responsive anemia is one of the pyridoxine-dependent syndromes (Chapter 90). Treatment of pyridoxine deficiency is administration of 10 to 150 mg pyridoxine daily. In patients receiving isoniazid, neuritis may be prevented (or treated) with dosages of 50 to 100 mg pyridoxine daily.

Measurements of urinary vitamin B$_6$ and urinary 4-pyridoxic acid are useful in diagnosing deficiency. Excretion of less than 100 mg vitamin B$_6$ or 1.0 mg 5-pyridoxic acid should lead the physician to suspect pyridoxine deficiency. Tryptophan loading will also result in increased excretion of xanthurenic acid in the urine, because pyridoxine is a cofactor in normal tryptophan metabolism. In pyridoxine deficiency, the usual tryptophan metabolic pathway is blocked, and intermediates are converted into xanthurenic and kynurenic acids that are excreted in increased amounts into the urine.

Folic Acid and Vitamin B$_{12}$ Deficiency. Deficiencies of folic acid and vitamin B$_{12}$ are relatively common and result from inadequate dietary intake, or are secondary to gastrointestinal disease or increased metabolic requirements. Clinical manifestations and treatment of these deficiency states are described in Chapter 87.

Ascorbic Acid (Vitamin C) Deficiency. In adults, scurvy-producing ascorbic acid deficiency is seldom seen today. When it occurs, it does so primarily as a result of food faddism, chronic alcoholism, or psychiatric disorders. Scurvy usually develops after 4 to 7 months of vitamin C deprivation.

Nonspecific symptoms may be noted before any physical changes occur and include lassitude, irritability, weight loss, and aching pains in muscles and joints. Perifollicular hyperkeratotic papules may form on the buttocks, thighs, and legs, with fragmentation, coiling, and embedding of hairs in follicles. Petechiae occur around the hair follicles and may be most prominent on the legs. Hemorrhage appears in the skin, muscles, and gums, with progressive edema. These lesions may ulcerate, and scars from previous trauma may also break down. The gums become swollen, boggy, friable, hemorrhagic, and eventually infected, sometimes to the point of gangrene. Hemorrhage into tissues may produce hemarthroses, mucous membrane bleeding, gastrointestinal and genitourinary blood loss, nosebleed, and retinal and cerebral hemorrhages. Early in scurvy, radiographic examination may show interruption of the lamina dura, which, as gum tissue progressively deteriorates, leads to tooth loss. Anemia may develop because of chronic blood loss or impaired folic acid utilization.

By the time scurvy is clinically apparent, the plasma levels of vitamin C are usually zero. Although not readily available, the vitamin C content of white blood cells falls below 2 mg/100 g just before scurvy develops. Treatment with ascorbic acid produces rapid recovery. The usual dosage of 100 mg five to six times daily can be reduced to 100 mg three times daily after 4 or 5 days but should be continued until complete healing is apparent.

Biotin Deficiency. It is doubtful that biotin deficiency can result solely from inadequate intake, because biotin is produced by intestinal bacteria. The rare deficiency described in adults has been associated with large consumption of raw eggs for a period of several months. Raw eggs contain avidin, which binds biotin and prevents its absorption.

The clinical picture is characterized by nonpruritic dermatitis, lassitude, somnolence, depression, muscle pains, and hyperesthesia. Later, anorexia, nausea, anemia, and hypercholesterolemia appear. All manifestations disappear within 2 to 5 days after parenteral treatment with biotin, approximately 200 μ daily.

Pantothenic Acid Deficiency. Pantothenic acid is so widely available from food sources that a deficiency state is extremely rare. Experimentally produced pantothenic acid deficiency causes fatigue, malaise, sleep disturbances, personality changes, numbness, paresthesia, and muscle cramps. In association with malnutrition, hyperhidrosis, burning feet, painful toes, and a flat-footed gait have been described.

The diagnosis should be suspected whenever malnutrition and coexistent vitamin deficiencies exist, particularly beriberi, pellagra, and ariboflavinosis. Treatment with 20 to 40 mg calcium pantothenate per day intramuscularly should produce complete recovery; paresthesia may be the last symptom to disappear.

Vitamin-Dependent Metabolic Defects. A variety of rare diseases are characterized by a specific metabolic defect, usually an enzyme deficiency, in which the normal dietary vitamin content is not sufficient to prevent clinical manifestations. In patients with these metabolic defects, large doses of the specific vitamin may be effective in overcoming the metabolic block. Some vitamin-dependent metabolic diseases are listed in Table 347-3.

Therapeutic Use of Vitamins

A healthy adult consuming a wide variety of foods will ingest an adequate supply of vitamins to meet normal body requirements. Whenever dietary intake is curtailed for extended periods of time, supplemental vitamin therapy to prevent deficiency states seems justified. Curtailment of dietary vitamin intake is commonly associated with eating patterns in old age, debilitating illnesses, food faddism, food restriction for weight reduction, chronic alcoholism, anorexia nervosa, drug-nutrient antagonism, and insufficient supplementation during prolonged intravenous nutrition or long-term hemodialysis. A strict but carefully selected vegetarian diet can supply all the vitamins except vitamin B$_{12}$. This vitamin is found only in foods of animal origin and therefore needs to be ingested as a supplement.

Table 347-3 Vitamin-dependent metabolic diseases

DISEASE	BIOCHEMICAL DEFECT	VITAMIN
Hyperalaninemia and hyperpyruvic acidemia	Pyruvate decarboxylase	Thiamine
Maple syrup urine disease	Decarboxylation of ketoacid analogus of branched-chain amino acid	Thiamine
Thiamine-responsive lactic acidosis	Hepatic pyruvate decarboxylase	Thiamine
Hartnup disease	Tryptophan and neutral amino acid active transport system	Niacin
Cystathioninuria	Cystathionase	Pyridoxine
Xanthurenic aciduria	Binding of pyridoxal phosphate to kynureninase	Pyridoxine
Homocystinuira	Cystathionine synthase	Pyridoxine and vitamin B_{12}
Vitamin B_6-dependent infantile convulsions	Defect in glutamic acid decarboxylase	Pyridoxine
Vitamin B_6-responsive anemia	Defect in α-aminolevulinic acid synthetase	Pyridoxine
Folic acid malabsorption	Folic acid active transport system	Folic acid
Formiminotransferase deficiency	Formiminotransferase	Folic acid
Methylmalonic aciduria	Formation of coenzyme B_{12}	Vitamin B_{12}
Beta-methylcrotonylglycinuria	β-Methylcrotonyl-CoA carboxylase	Biotin

Table 347-4 Megadoses and toxicity of selected vitamins

VITAMIN	TOXIC LEVELS
Vitamin A	>25,000 IU/day ingested chronically
	>660,000 IU ingested acutely (adults)
	>330,000 IU ingested acutely (children)
Vitamin E	>2200 IU/day
Vitamin D	>10,000 IU/day ingested chronically
Nicotinic acid	>3 g/day
Pyridoxine	>2-6 g/day
Ascorbic acid	>2-4 g/day

Vitamin therapy may also be necessary in conditions associated with decreased absorption or increased need or utilization such as malabsorption, pregnancy, hyperthyroidism, carcinoid syndrome, or excessive urinary loss. Long-term use of certain drugs also increases the need for a specific vitamin (e.g., isoniazid and methyldopapyridoxine).

Megavitamin Therapy. Apart from megadoses of specific vitamins required in the treatment of rare vitamin-dependent metabolic disorders, there is little reason for administration of large doses of vitamins. Such doses can cause vitamin toxicity, a serious clinical problem. Megadoses and toxicity of selected vitamins are listed in Table 347-4. Toxicity may be modulated by the biochemical form of the vitamin consumed, the dosage taken, and whether consumption was acute or chronic.

Hypervitaminosis A. In adults, chronic hypervitaminosis A may produce fatigue; weakness; anorexia; irritability; vomiting; lethargy; loss of body hair; brittle nails; constipation; dry, scaly, rough skin; peripheral edema; and mouth fissures. In addition, hepatosplenomegaly (with significant liver damage and cirrhosis), cortical bone thickening, and increased intracranial pressure have been reported. Serum concentration of vitamin A is usually above 100 μ per deciliter. With cessation of vitamin intake, clinical symptoms rapidly improve, with gradual resolution of the cortical bone changes. Recent reports confirm that the use during pregnancy of the vitamin A analog *13-cis-retinoic acid* for skin disorders may cause serious birth defects.

Vitamin D Intoxication. Excessive doses of vitamin D, taken for several weeks, may produce polyuria, polydipsia, lethargy, nausea, vomiting, constipation, and hypertension. Increased intestinal absorption of calcium, hypercalcemia, and hypercalciuria lead to calcium deposition in the kidney and progressive renal insufficiency. Coma may result from hypercalcemia or hypertensive encephalopathy.

Ascorbic Acid Toxicity. Many claims have been made for the use of large daily doses of vitamin C, particularly for the prevention and treatment of the common cold and, more recently, for cancer. In numerous clinical trials, however, no significant benefits from vitamin C megadoses have been substantiated. There appear to be no significant toxic effects of megadoses of this vitamin in normal persons.

However, abortion, fetal deformity, false-positive test results for glycosuria, augmentation of warfarin anticoagulation, high-altitude hypoxia, enhancement of uricosuria and oxalate renal stones, and increased hemolysis in glucose-6-phosphate dehydrogenase deficiency have all been reported as special side effects.

Niacin Toxicity. The use of megadoses of niacin and some other vitamins in the treatment of schizophrenia has been publicized and referred to as orthomolecular psychiatry. There has been no clinical substantiation of the efficacy of such therapy, but it is known that toxic reactions may occur with large doses of niacin. These reactions include skin flushing, pruritus, hyperuricemia, hyperglycemia, postural hypotension, macular edema with loss of vision, and abnormal liver function test results.

Vitamin E Toxicity. Although many claims have been made for the use of megadoses of vitamin E, the results of clinical trials indicate that tocopherols may be of benefit in intermittent claudication. Vitamin E ingestion of more than 1200 IU per day has been reported to prolong prothrombin time, producing a "conditioned vitamin K deficiency."

Pyridoxine Toxicity. Previously, megadoses of water-soluble B-complex vitamins were considered relatively harmless, because it was assumed that they were rapidly excreted from the body. Recent reports of the toxic effect of megadoses of pyridoxine (2 to 6 g/day, or 1000 to 2700 times the recommended daily allowance [RDA]) confirm that even water-soluble vitamins can be toxic and have direct adverse effects. The pathogenesis of the peripheral neuropathologic effect observed is not yet known with certainty.

MINERALS

About 4% of human body weight is composed of inorganic elements or minerals, and 17 of these are considered to be essential for life. As shown in Table 347-5, these minerals are conveniently subdivided into macrominerals (i.e., those needed in the diet at levels of 100 mg per day or more) and microminerals, or trace elements (needed in amounts less than 100 mg per day). The trace elements constitute less than 0.1% of the total body weight.

All inorganic minerals are derived from seawater, the earth's crust, and the biosphere. In fact, the mineral composition of the human body is very similar to that of the earth and the sea. Biologists and chemists have long been fascinated by the way evolution has selected certain elements as the building stones of living organisms, including humans, and virtually ignored others.

In recent years there has been a remarkable escalation of research into the role of the inorganic minerals in nutritional and biochemical processes that take place both in health and in disease. Seven macrominerals are known to be essential for human life: calcium, phosphorus, sodium, potassium, chlorine, magnesium, and sulfur. The essential microminerals are iron, copper, cobalt, zinc, manganese, iodine, molybdenum, selenium, fluoride, and chromium (Table 347-5). Above a defined level of intake, any one of these minerals is toxic. On the other hand, a deficiency of any one of these nutrients results

Table 347-5 Minerals in medicine

MINERAL	ABSORPTION (%)	MECHANISM OF ACTION/FUNCTION
Macrominerals		
Calcium	20-30	Formation of bones, teeth
		Regulation of excitable tissues (striated, cardiac, and smooth muscles; nerves)
		Activation of some enzymes
		Blood clotting
Phosphorus	50-60	Mineralization of bones, teeth
		Component of DNA, RNA
		Regulation of acid-base balance
		Component of phosphorylated vitamins (thiamine, niacin, riboflavin, pyridoxine) and ATP
		Component of phospholipids
Sodium	≈100	Regulation of pH, osmotic pressure, water balance
		Conductivity or excitability of nerves, muscles
		Active transport of glucose, amino acids
Potassium	≈100	Regulation of osmotic pressure, acid-base balance
		Activation of number of intracellular enzymes
		Regulation of nerve and muscle excitability
Chlorine	≈100	Regulation of osmotic pressure, acid-base balance, water balance
		Component of gastric juice
Magnesium	35-40	Component of several enzyme systems involving ATP
		Maintenance of electrical potential in nerves and muscle membranes
Sulfur		Component of methionine, cysteine, cystine
		Component of vitamins: thiamine, pantothenic acid, biotin
		Component of insulin, glutathione, taurocholic acid
		Provides high-energy sulfur bonds (—SH)
Microminerals or trace elements		
Iron	5-15	Structural component of hemoglobin, myoglobin, cytochrome, and other enzymes
Copper	30-60	Cross-linking of elastin
		Required for mobilization of iron
		Component of ceruloplasmin
		Component of many enzymes (cytochrome C oxidase, tyrosinase, dopamine β-hydroxylase)
Cobalt	80-95	Component of vitamin B_{12}
Zinc	10-40	Component of over 80 metalloenzymes (carbonic anhydrase, carboxypeptidases A and B, alkaline phosphatase, alcohol dehydrogenase)
		Wound healing
		Metabolism of nucleic acids (thymidine kinase)
Manganese	10-40	Formation of mucopolysaccharides
		Activation of many enzymes
Iodine	≈100	Constituent of thyroxine, triiodothyronine
Molybdenum	40-100	Structural component of xanthine oxidase, aldehyde oxidase
Selenium	35-85	Active component of glutathione peroxidase
Fluoride	75-90	Structural component of calcium hydroxyapatite of bones and teeth
Chromium	10-25	Component of glucose tolerance factor

in malnutrition. The minerals may share certain characteristics of biologic importance, frequently related to their proximity in the periodic table, substituting one element for another in specific reactions. Interactions among minerals may be antagonistic, with one element that inhibits the metabolic action of another. Interactions may also be additive or synergistic, causing an effect greater than either element alone. Many factors may influence the metabolism of minerals: stress; nutritional status; disease states; patterns of exposure; or excess, deficiency, or imbalance of minerals.

The functions of the minerals vary in biologic expression from the whole organism to the isolated subcellular organelle. The mechanisms of action are equally diverse: structural components of enzymes and vitamins; active components in the synthesis of amino acids, deoxyribonucleic acid (DNA), and ribonucleic acid (RNA); catalysts in enzyme reactions through substrate binding, activation of enzyme-substrate complexes, or formation of metalloenzymes; and regulation of intracellular heme concentration, membrane transport, nerve conduction, muscle contraction, osmotic pressure, water, and acid-base balance.

Mineral Deficiencies

There are numerous examples of deficiency states related to inadequate intake of minerals; however, only selected examples are given here to emphasize the importance of this concept.

Iron Deficiency Anemia (see Chapter 86). Iron deficiency anemia is probably the most prevalent nutritional deficiency that af-

fects human beings. It is estimated that iron deficiency anemia may be present in approximately 50% of the population in some parts of the world. In the United States, prevalence figures indicate that approximately 20% of infants and children, 10% to 50% of women 15 to 45 years of age, and 15% to 58% of pregnant women are iron-deficient. Inadequate iron intake is one of the major reasons for iron deficiency anemia. The average American diet contains about 6 mg iron per 1000 cal consumed. With a 2000-cal intake, one would ingest about 12 mg iron. This amount (12 mg) does not afford a sufficient margin of safety above the average physiologic requirement to cover variation among all individuals in the general population. A specific, concerted effort must be made to select iron-rich foods to meet requirements, or iron supplements may be needed by high-risk groups (e.g., infants, pregnant women). Increased menstrual bleeding and hemorrhage from the alimentary tract are the most common causes of iron deficiency.

Zinc Deficiency. The trace metal zinc is closely associated with a variety of more than 80 zinc-containing proteins and enzymes. Zinc is essential for the catalytic functions and the structure of key enzymes that play a central role in metabolism, including alcohol dehydrogenase, alkaline phosphatase, carboxypeptidase, and carbonic anhydrase. Zinc deficiency has been reported in a variety of clinical circumstances, including acute inflammatory stress; some specific malignancies (e.g., leukemia); chronic infections (e.g., pneumonia, bronchitis); alcoholism; liver disease (e.g., cirrhosis); chronic renal disease; rheumatoid arthritis; inflammatory bowel disease; hemolytic anemias; and malabsorption syndromes. Zinc deficiency may also result from administration of zinc-chelating drugs (e.g., penicillamine), or total parenteral nutrition (TPN) without adequate zinc given in the solution. Acrodermatitis enteropathica was the first inherited zinc-deficiency disorder reported in human beings, and small amounts of zinc completely reverse all pathologic lesions and clinical manifestations. Other manifestations of zinc deficiency include poor wound healing, growth retardation, hypogonadism, impaired immune function, mental disturbances, diarrhea, altered taste and smell, and reduced night vision.

Mineral Deficiencies Associated With TPN. There has been increased awareness of deficiency states that may be precipitated by lack of a single mineral in the solutions used for TPN, including zinc, copper, selenium, and molybdenum. Mineral deficiencies occur with frequency in patients on TPN. The most common cause of trace mineral deficiency in such patients is the failure to provide a sufficient amount of each mineral to meet both losses from previous or ongoing illnesses or injury plus the normal maintenance requirements.

Mineral Deficiencies Associated With Digestive Disease. Abnormal conditions of the digestive tract may predispose to depletion of minerals, especially zinc. A deficiency of this mineral may occur as a result of geophagia; celiac diseases; short bowel syndrome; diarrheal fluid loss; ileostomy fluid loss; enterocolic, pancreaticocutaneous, or pancreaticocolic fistula; pancreatic insufficiency; and cystic fibrosis. Copper deficiency is less frequent than zinc deficiency and causes anemia, leukopenia, and neutropenia. Chromium deficiency is rare and occurs only in chronic TPN administration, usually manifested by an increase in glucose intolerance and peripheral neuropathy. Magnesium deficiency may be manifested by muscle cramps and sometimes tetany. Selenium deficiency after years of TPN usually is associated with myopathy or cardiomyopathy.

Excess Intake of Minerals

Excess intake of any one of the essential minerals may also lead to toxicity and malnutrition. In fact, excess mineral intake is more likely to have a toxic effect than excess vitamin intake because the upper and lower physiologic tolerances are within a narrower range.

Hypermagnesemia. Hypermagnesemia has been reported in patients with renal insufficiency who are taking magnesium-containing drugs (e.g., antacids). High blood concentrations of magnesium (8 mEq/liter) lead to central depression, profound paralysis of the skeletal muscles, and respiratory distress.

Iron Toxicity. Iron overload can result from enhanced absorption, parenteral infusion, or a combination of these two factors and produce hemochromatosis. Prolonged intake of medicinal iron by patients who no longer need it may also lead to iron overload. Because iron preparations in the United States are widely advertised, available without prescription, and consumed in large quantities, one should consider the possibility of iron overload in appropriate clinical situations.

Trace Mineral Toxicity. Malnutrition caused by excess trace metals is well documented. Excess iodide may lead to an inhibition of thyroid hormone synthesis, hypothyroidism, and iodide goiter. Acute copper intoxication in human beings causes nausea, vomiting, epigastric pain, diarrhea, headache, dizziness, and weakness. In severe cases, copper toxicity may lead to tachycardia, hypertension, coma, jaundice, hemolytic anemia, hemoglobinuria, uremia, and death. Toxic reactions of excess intake of manganese, cobalt, selenium, and cadmium have also been reported. Fluoride excess has been studied extensively as a result of fortification of the public water supply of countries all over the world to decrease the prevalence of dental caries. It is well established that excess fluoride intake during the developmental period of the teeth leads to dental fluorosis but may also promote stabilization of newly synthesized bone matrix and inhibit bone resorption.

Mineral Toxicity Related to Food Contamination. The toxic potential of trace metals in foods and beverages should not be overlooked. Excess contamination of foods and beverages with lead, mercury, cobalt, and cadmium has been reported and in some instances has led to toxicity and death.

Table 347-6 Some drug-nutrient interactions

DRUG	NUTRIENTS	MECHANISM
Antacids	Iron, phosphates	Malabsorption, binding
Tetracyclines	Iron (antacids)	Chelation
	Calcium	Calcium binding in bones
Cholestyramine	Triglycerides, calcium, fat-soluble vitamins	Malabsorption, bile-acid sequestration
5-Fluorouracil	Protein	Malabsorption, reduced peptidases
Metformin	Vitamin B$_{12}$	Malabsorption, mucosal damage
Colchicine		
Para-aminosalicylic acid		
Ethanol	Folate	Uncertain
	Magnesium	Possible malabsorption; increase in stool
	Zinc	Increased urinary loss
	Vitamin B$_6$	Reduced conversion to pyridoxal phosphate
Methyldopa	Vitamin B$_6$	Metabolic antagonism
Isoniazid	Vitamin B$_6$, tryptophan	Competition for active enzyme site
	Niacin	
Penicillamine	Vitamin B$_6$	Increased urinary loss
Diphenylhydantoin	Folate	Uncertain
Primidone		
Methotrexate	Folate	Direct antagonism: competition for active enzyme site
Pyrimethamine		
Triaminopteride		
Trimethoprim		
Coumadin	Vitamin K	Decreased synthesis
Barbiturates		Induction of warfarin inactivation
Oxyphenbutazone		Enhancement of warfarin action (displacement of albumin binding)
Oral contraceptives	Vitamin B$_6$	Altered metabolism
	Tryptophan	Increased protein binding
	Folate	Reduction in red cell levels

DRUG-NUTRIENT INTERACTION

Drugs may interfere with the effect or utilization of nutrients in many ways. In some instances, drug-nutrient interaction is an intentional effect. More often, drug-nutrient interaction impairs nutrient use and is undesirable. Drugs may decrease nutrient absorption; increase urinary excretion; directly compete with or antagonize nutrient action; displace the nutrient from a carrier protein; and interfere with the synthesis of an enzyme, coenzyme, or carrier essential for the metabolism of the nutrient. Some hormones may also alter nutrient metabolism, particularly those in oral contraceptives. Finally, substances present as components of a drug may produce alterations in nutrient status. Examples of drug-nutrient interactions are described in Table 347-6.

NUTRITIONAL ASSESSMENT

Advanced states of malnutrition may be recognized easily on visual inspection. Physical examination may reveal specific changes associated with malnutrition. However, a planned procedure of nutritional assessment enables the clinician to detect the presence of less obvious malnutrition. Nutritional assessment provides an objective char-

acterization of nutritional status and should be a routine aspect of the clinical evaluation of every hospitalized patient.

No single assessment tool can adequately characterize nutritional status; thus a profile of tests and measurements should be used. Several assessment plans have been published. The four assessment parameters most useful in determining nutritional status are anthropometric, laboratory, clinical, and dietary. A list of the helpful anthropometric and laboratory parameters is shown in Table 347-7. Muscle or lean body mass may be estimated by determining the creatinine/height index. This index, which has proved to be particularly useful in assessing nutritional status, can be determined from comparison with the desirable weights and normal urinary creatinine excretion for given heights shown in Tables 347-8 and 347-9, respectively.

Calorie and Nutrient Requirements

The patient's diet is designed to provide adequate calories and essential nutrients. Caloric needs are best estimated as follows:
1. The basal metabolic rate is determined by first using a height-weight nomogram to obtain body surface area (Fig. 347-1). The

---

Table 347-7   Nutritional assessment

MEASUREMENT	ASSESSMENT
A. Anthropometric measurements	
1. Weight (kg)	Body weight status
2. Height (cm)	Desirable weight of adults (see Table 347-8)
3. Weight/height ratio	Body weight status
4. % Ideal body weight = $\dfrac{\text{actual weight}}{\text{ideal body weight}} \times 100$	
5. % Usual body weight = $\dfrac{\text{actual weight}}{\text{usual weight}} \times 100$	
6. % Weight change = $\dfrac{\text{usual weight} - \text{actual weight}}{\text{usual weight}} \times 100$	
7. Arm circumference (cm)	
8. % Standard arm circumference = $\dfrac{\text{actual arm circumference}}{\text{standard arm circumference}} \times 100$	Body weight status

9. Triceps skinfold (mm)	Body fatness
	    Men: 8-23 mm
	    Women: 10-30 mm

10. % Standard triceps skinfold = $\dfrac{\text{actual triceps skinfold}}{\text{standard triceps skinfold}} \times 100$	
11. Arm muscle circumference (mm) = arm circumference (mm) − 0.314 × triceps skinfold (mm)	Lean muscle mass Midarm muscle circumference (120-140 mm)
12. % Standard arm muscle circumference = $\dfrac{\text{actual arm muscle circumference}}{\text{standard arm muscle circumference}} \times 100$	
B. Laboratory measurements	
1. Total iron-binding capacity (TIBC)(µg/dl)	Labile or visceral protein status Protein-calorie malnutrition
2. Serum transferrin = (0.8 × TIBC) − 43, mg/dl	Visceral protein status Protein-calorie malnutrition
3. Serum albumin (g/dl)	Visceral protein status Protein-calorie malnutrition
4. White blood cell count (WBC/mm³)	
5. Total lymphocyte count = $\dfrac{\text{percent lymphocytes} \times \text{WBC}}{100}$	Immune function
6. 24-hr urinary creatinine (mg)	Ideal urinary creatinine values (see Table 347-9)
7. Creatinine height index = $\dfrac{\text{actual urinary creatinine}}{\text{ideal urinary creatinine}} \times 100$	Muscle or lean body mass
8. 24-hr urinary nitrogen (g)	Body protein status
9. Nitrogen balance = $\dfrac{\text{protein intake}}{6.25}$ − (urinary urea nitrogen + 4)	Body protein status
10. Basal energy expenditure	Used to derive total caloric needs

11. Complete blood count (CBC)	Anemia:
	    Normocytic
	    Microcytic
	    Macrocytic

12. Skin tests
    Purified protein derivative (PPD)
    Candida spp.
    Dinitrochlorobenzene (DNCB)
	Immune function

Table 347-8   1983 Metropolitan Life Insurance Company height and weight table

| MEN* | | | | | WOMEN† | | | | |
| HEIGHT | | SMALL FRAME | MEDIUM FRAME | LARGE FRAME | HEIGHT | | SMALL FRAME | MEDIUM FRAME | LARGE FRAME |
FEET	INCHES				FEET	INCHES			
5	2	128-134	131-141	138-150	4	10	102-111	109-121	118-131
5	3	130-136	133-143	140-153	4	11	103-113	111-123	120-134
5	4	132-138	135-145	142-156	5	0	104-115	113-126	122-137
5	5	134-140	137-148	144-160	5	1	106-118	115-129	125-140
5	6	136-142	139-151	146-164	5	2	108-121	118-132	128-143
5	7	138-145	142-154	149-168	5	3	111-124	121-135	131-147
5	8	140-148	145-157	152-172	5	4	114-127	124-138	134-151
5	9	142-151	148-160	155-176	5	5	117-130	127-141	137-155
5	10	144-154	151-163	158-180	5	6	120-133	130-144	140-159
5	11	146-157	154-166	161-184	5	7	123-136	133-147	143-163
6	0	149-160	157-170	164-188	5	8	126-139	136-150	146-167
6	1	152-164	160-174	168-192	5	9	129-142	139-153	149-170
6	2	155-168	164-178	172-197	5	10	132-145	142-156	152-173
6	3	158-172	167-182	176-202	5	11	135-148	145-159	155-176
6	4	162-176	171-187	181-207	6	0	138-151	148-162	158-179

*Weights at ages 25 to 59 based on lowest mortality. Weight in pounds according to frame (in indoor clothing weighing 5 lb, shoes with 1 in heels).
†Weights at ages 25 to 59 based on lowest mortality. Weight in pounds according to frame (in indoor clothing weighing 3 lb, shoes with 1 in heels).

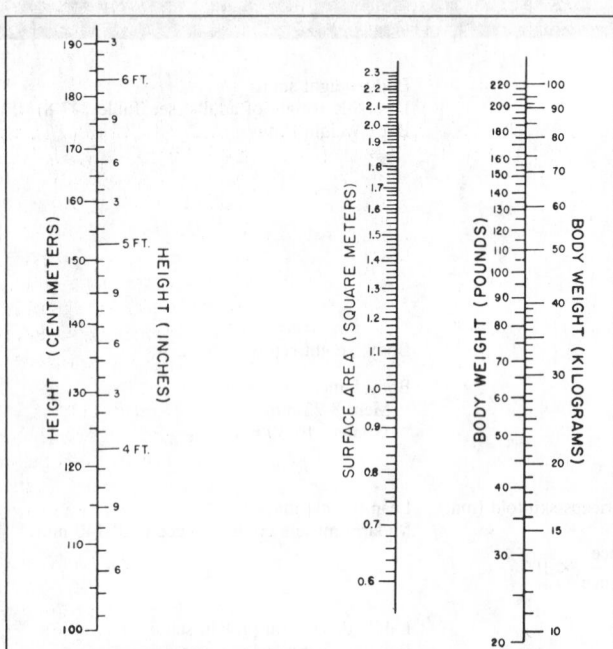

FIGURE 347-1   Nomogram for determining body surface area from height and weight. To determine body surface area from height *(left)* and weight *(right)*, these points are connected with a straight-edge and surface area is read from the middle scale.

From Wilmore DW: *The metabolic management of the critically ill,* New York, 1977, Plenum Medical.

metabolic rate for a given age and sex shown in Table 347-10 is then multiplied by the body surface area to provide the basal metabolic rate. This calculation can be made easily by use of the nomograph in Fig. 347-2.

2. The energy required for the patient's activity level is estimated from Table 347-11. This is then added to the basal metabolic rate to obtain total daily caloric needs.

3. The patient's daily caloric requirements depend on whether weight reduction, maintenance, or weight gain is needed. Hypocaloric, nitrogen-containing diets usually provide 400 to 1800 kcal per day, which is about 1000 kcal below estimated metabolic rate. Maintenance diets provide calories sufficient to meet estimated energy

needs. Hypercaloric diets generally provide 1000 kcal per day in excess of estimated needs. Patients with severe disease such as infection, sepsis, or cancer may require caloric intake significantly above daily metabolic rate to make up for existing defects or increased maintenance requirements.

4. The patient's nitrogen requirements can be determined from the nomograph shown in Fig. 347-3. Although healthy individuals maintain nitrogen balance with a nitrogen/total calorie ratio of 1 : 350, seriously ill patients benefit from a ratio of 1 : 150 because of their compromised protein status.

5. The appropriate route of feeding (oral, enteral, or parenteral) is determined from the patient's clinical condition. Route of intake usually influences selection of the diet's components.

6. Essential nutrients—including vitamins, minerals, and essential fatty acids—must be provided. The RDA (Tables 347-12 to 347-14) may serve as a guide, but special nutrient needs may require adjustment of daily doses above or below the RDA.

7. Reassessment is necessary at frequent intervals to ensure the success of nutritional support and determine changing requirements.

NUTRITIONAL MANAGEMENT

Nutritional management is an essential part of therapy for specific disorders and is an important adjunct in the treatment of many diseases. The incidence of protein-calorie malnutrition may range from 25% to 50% in hospitalized medical and surgical patients. Awareness of this important problem has grown, but practitioners of internal medicine still do not give it sufficient attention. Physicians' failure to record and use data (height, weight, weight history, dietary history, etc.); failure to assign specific responsibility for nutritional assessment and treatment; tendency to overlook patients' nutritional needs while obtaining numerous diagnostic studies; and failure to provide nutritional support before malnutrition is overt have all contributed to nutritional problems. Nutrient and calorie requirements are dramatically influenced by disease or injury and can be strikingly increased in critically ill patients.

Total Parenteral Nutrition

Indications. It is now possible to provide partial or complete nutrition by intravenous infusion of nutrient solutions. If gastrointestinal absorption and delivery of nutrients are inadequate, impossible for prolonged periods of time, or contraindicated, nourishment should be provided parenterally. Specific conditions in which parenteral feeding is indicated include mechanical bowel obstruction; postoperative ileus; acute inflammatory bowel disease; acute pancreatitis; short gut syndrome; proximal intestinal fistulas; severe burns; cancer cachexia

Table 347-9 Ideal urinary creatinine values

| | MEN* | | | WOMEN† | |
| HEIGHT | | IDEAL CREATININE | HEIGHT | | IDEAL CREATININE |
(in)	(cm)	(mg)	(in)	(cm)	(mg)
62	157.5	1288	58	147.3	830
63	160.0	1325	59	149.9	851
64	162.6	1359	60	152.4	875
65	165.1	1386	61	154.9	900
66	167.6	1426	62	157.5	925
67	170.2	1467	63	160.0	949
68	172.7	1513	64	162.6	977
69	175.3	1555	65	165.1	1006
70	177.8	1596	66	167.6	1044
71	180.3	1642	67	170.2	1076
72	182.9	1691	68	172.7	1109
73	185.4	1739	69	175.3	1141
74	188.0	1785	70	177.8	1174
75	190.5	1831	71	180.3	1206
76	193.0	1891	72	182.9	1240

From Margen S, Caan B, editors: *The Medical Clinics of North America symposium on applied nutrition in clinical medicine,* Philadelphia, 1979, WB Saunders.
*Creatinine coefficient (men) = 23 mg/kg of ideal body weight.
†Creatinine coefficient (women) = 18 mg/kg of ideal body weight.

Table 347-10 Metabolic rate

| | kcal/m²/h | |
AGES (YEARS)	MEN	WOMEN
18	40.0	35.9
19	39.2	35.5
20	38.6	35.3
25	37.5	35.2
30	36.8	35.1
35	36.5	35.0
40	36.3	34.9
45	36.2	34.5
50	35.8	33.9
55	35.4	33.3
60	34.9	32.7
65	34.4	32.2
70	33.8	31.7
75 and over	33.2	31.3

Modified from Fleisch A: *Helv Med Acta* 18:23, 1951.

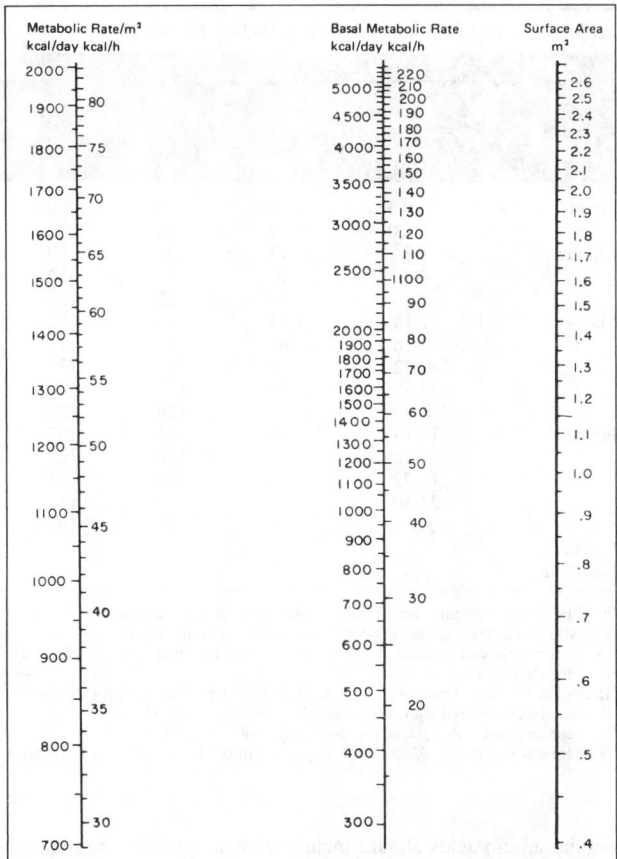

FIGURE 347-2 Prediction of daily metabolic requirements per square meter of body surface *(right)* for age and sex *(left)* (see Table 347-10). These points are connected with a straight-edge, and the predicted daily or hourly requirements are read from the middle scale.

From Wilmore DW: *The metabolic management of the critically ill,* New York, 1977, Plenum Medical

Table 347-11 Approximate energy output

TYPE OF WORK	CALORIES ADDED TO BASAL RATES (kcal/day)
Sedentary	400-800
Light work (professionals and businesspersons)	800-1200
Moderate work (mechanical)	1200-1800
Heavy work (laborers and athletes)	1800-4500

Modified from Wilmore DW: *The metabolic management of the critically ill,* New York, 1977, Plenum.

and adjunctive therapy; chronic debility; anorexia nervosa; and, occasionally, acute renal failure and hepatic or cardiac decompensation.

Nutrient Solutions. The two most important sources of calories are carbohydrates and fats. Infusion of 100 to 250 g glucose daily prevents ketosis and decreases catabolism of protein. Hypertonic solutions of glucose in final concentrations of 20% to 30% have been the major source of calories in solutions used for TPN. These solutions require the use of a central venous catheter to prevent the complications of thrombophlebitis. The availability of fat emulsions has added to the capability of supplying adequate energy needs parenterally. One major advantage of fat emulsions is that they supply 9 kcal per gram, more than twice the kilocalories supplied by a gram of glucose. In addition, fat emulsions are isotonic and may be administered through a peripheral vein. In combination with glucose and amino acids, fat emulsions administered by peripheral vein infusion can meet the total nutritional requirements of some patients with limited metabolic needs. In patients receiving prolonged TPN, essential fatty acid deficiency may be prevented by fat emulsion. Fat emulsions contain either soybean or cottonseed oil and consist mainly of oleic or linoleic fatty acid. One preparation currently used widely in the United States is a 10% soybean oil emulsion with an egg yolk stabilizer.

Nitrogen for parenteral solutions consists of either protein hydrolysates or mixtures of crystalline amino acids. Both types have been used successfully, but crystalline amino acids are preferred because it is possible to alter the solution to meet more appropriately the metabolic requirements of patients with specific organic diseases (e.g., renal disease, hepatic insufficiency). These requirements depend on physiologic conditions and increase as protein catabolism increases. In general, it is necessary to infuse between 80 and 160 g protein equivalent per 24 hours to ensure positive nitrogen balance. For nitrogen to be usable for tissue synthesis (instead of energy), the calorie/nitrogen ratio should be about 150 to 250 cal to 1 g nitrogen. In most TPN protocols, calorie/nitrogen ratio is 150:1. It is important to provide appropriate amounts of essential and nonessential amino acids in these mixtures, usually in a ratio of about 1.0:1.5. The non-

Table 347-12 Recommended daily dietary allowances[a]

		WEIGHT		HEIGHT			FAT-SOLUBLE VITAMINS		
	AGE (YEARS)	(kg)	(lb)	(cm)	(in)	PROTEIN (g)	VITAMIN A (µg R.E.)[b]	VITAMIN D (µg)[c]	VITAMIN E (mg α-T.E.)[d]
Infants	0.0-0.5	6	13	60	24	kg × 2.2	420	10	3
	0.5-1.0	9	20	71	28	kg × 2.0	400	10	4
Children	1-3	13	29	90	35	23	400	10	5
	4-6	20	44	112	44	30	500	10	6
	7-10	28	62	132	52	34	700	10	7
Males	11-14	45	99	157	62	45	1000	10	8
	15-18	66	145	176	69	56	1000	10	10
	19-22	70	154	177	70	56	1000	7.5	10
	23-50	70	154	178	70	56	1000	5	10
	51+	70	154	178	70	56	1000	5	10
Females	11-14	46	101	157	62	46	800	10	8
	15-18	55	120	163	64	46	800	10	8
	19-22	55	120	163	64	44	800	7.5	8
	23-50	55	120	163	64	44	800	5	8
	51+	55	120	163	64	44	800	5	8
Pregnant						+30	+200	+5	+2
Lactating						+20	+400	+5	+3

From Food and Nutrition Board, National Academy of Sciences–National Research Council: Recommended dietary allowances, ed 10, Washington, D.C., 1989.
[a]The allowances are intended to provide for individual variations among most normal persons as they live in the United States under usual environmental stresses. Diets should be based on a variety of common foods in order to provide other nutrients for which human requirements have been less well defined. See Table 347-14 for heights, weights, and recommended intake.
[b]Retinol equivalents. One retinol equivalent = 1 µg retinol or 6 µg β-carotene.
[c]As cholecalciferol. Ten µg cholecalciferol = 400 IU vitamin D.
[d]α-Tocopherol equivalents. One mg d-α-tocopherol = 1 α-T.E.
[e]N.E. (niacin equivalent) is equal to 1 mg of niacin or 60 mg of dietary tryptophan.

essential amino acids should include alanine, proline, arginine, glutamic acid, and histidine.

Sufficient electrolytes, vitamins, and minerals must be added to parenteral solutions to meet the needs of the patient. Additions may vary, depending on previous existing deficits, maintenance requirements (including daily losses), and deficiencies that may develop during prolonged therapy. For every 1000 cal infused, approximately 10 mEq sodium and chloride, 20 mEq potassium and phosphate, 8 mEq magnesium, and 5 mEq calcium is required just for metabolic utilization of nutrients in the solution. To these amounts should be added the daily basal losses of sodium, potassium, and chloride, so that the minimum daily requirement for common electrolytes is met. Cobalt, zinc, copper, manganese, and fluoride are required trace elements that must also be added to the solutions, although the precise daily requirements remain uncertain. Many hospital pharmacies compound a solution containing these trace minerals. The addition of water- and fat-soluble vitamins completes the basic solution. Usually, one ampul of a multiple vitamin preparation per day meets the daily recommended allowances, with the exception of those for folic acid, vitamin K, vitamin B$_{12}$, and iron. For maintenance, these compounds may be supplemented with parenteral injections at appropriate intervals. In some cases, insulin must be added to the solution to facilitate adequate utilization of the glucose present and to prevent hyperglycemia. A standard formula for basic parenteral nutrition administered through a central venous catheter is shown in Table 347-15. Variations in amounts of amino acids and sodium may be made to suit the needs of patients with renal, cardiac, and hepatic disease. Some incompatibilities or insolubilities are associated with these solutions. Addition of bicarbonate can form precipitates or cause inactivation of calcium, insulin, vitamin B complex, and vitamin C. If bicarbonate is required, it is usually given as the acetate salt of sodium or potassium. Exceeding the limits of calcium concentration may precipitate phosphate and sulfate salts. It is customary to begin total parenteral infusion at a rate of 10 dl per 24 hours and gradually increase the amount (by 10 dl) daily until estimated volume and calorie requirements are met.

Complications. Careful attention must be paid to preventing, detecting, and treating the many potential complications of TPN. Bacterial and fungal sepsis are major complications. Sepsis is usually associated with catheter placement, growth of organisms along the cutaneous-vascular route, and contamination of the closed system. Meticulous care must be taken of the insertion site, tubing, and filters, and a well-defined procedure must be established for documenting and treating infection. The central venous catheter should be used only for TPN: administration of "piggyback" medications, blood withdrawal, central venous pressure determination, and administration of other fluids or blood by this route should be prohibited. Mechanical malfunction of the central venous catheter also poses a risk for the patient. Embolism may occur with manipulation of the catheter or its connections, and thrombosis of the great veins may become a clinical problem if this produces emboli or sepsis. For these reasons, patients receiving TPN are best cared for by a team that includes the physician, a specially trained nurse, and a nutritionist.

The patient's metabolism must be monitored daily and alterations corrected immediately. Metabolic alterations include hyperosmolar nonketotic hyperglycemia (with or without coma) and severe hypoglycemia, particularly if there is sudden cessation of administration of the concentrated glucose solution. Hyperchloremic metabolic acidosis may develop from excessive chloride and monohydrochloride present in crystalline amino acid solutions. When protein hydrolysates are used as the source of nitrogen, sensitivity reactions and hyperammonemia may result. Prerenal azotemia may result from an excessive total dose or rate of infusion of the protein hydrolysate or amino acid solution.

Essential fatty acid deficiency can be prevented with biweekly infusion of a fat emulsion via a peripheral vein. Hypocalcemia and hypophosphatemia may result from inadequate administration of calcium and phosphate. Hypercalcemia may occur from excessive calcium and vitamin D administration. Other metabolic hazards include hypokalemia and hyperkalemia, hypomagnesemia and hypermagnesemia, deficiencies of chromium and other trace metals, anemia, bleeding, hypervitaminosis A, cholestasis, and the frequent occurrence of abnormal liver enzyme levels. Ten types of nutrient deficiencies during TPN have been described: phosphate, essential fatty acid, copper, zinc, chromium, folic acid, selenium, vitamin A, biotin, and molybdenum. Under certain circumstances of TPN, especially when associated with chronic disease states, some nonessential nutrients may

Table 347-12—cont'd

	WATER-SOLUBLE VITAMINS						MINERALS					
VITAMIN C (mg)	THIAMINE (mg)	RIBO-FLAVIN (mg)	NIACIN (mg N.E.)[E]	VITAMIN B_6 (mg)	FOLACIN[F] (μg)	VITAMIN B_{12} (μg)	CALCIUM (mg)	PHOS-PHORUS (mg)	MAGNESIUM (mg)	IRON (mg)	ZINC (mg)	IODINE (μg)
35	0.3	0.4	6	0.3	30	0.5[g]	360	240	50	10	3	40
35	0.5	0.6	8	0.6	45	1.5	540	360	70	15	5	50
45	0.7	0.8	9	0.9	100	2.0	800	800	150	15	10	70
45	0.9	1.0	11	1.3	200	2.5	800	800	200	10	10	90
45	1.2	1.4	16	1.6	300	3.0	800	800	250	10	10	120
50	1.4	1.6	18	1.8	400	3.0	1200	1200	350	18	15	150
60	1.4	1.7	18	2.0	400	3.0	1200	1200	400	18	15	150
60	1.5	1.7	19	2.2	400	3.0	800	800	350	10	15	150
60	1.4	1.6	18	2.2	400	3.0	800	800	350	10	15	150
60	1.2	1.4	16	2.2	400	3.0	800	800	350	10	15	150
50	1.1	1.3	15	1.8	400	3.0	1200	1200	300	18	15	150
60	1.1	1.3	14	2.0	400	3.0	1200	1200	300	18	15	150
60	1.1	1.3	14	2.0	400	3.0	800	800	300	18	15	150
60	1.0	1.2	13	2.0	400	3.0	800	800	300	18	15	150
60	1.0	1.2	13	2.0	400	3.0	800	800	300	10	15	150
+20	+0.4	+0.3	+2	+0.6	+400	+1.0	+400	+400	+150	h	+5	+25
+40	+0.5	+0.5	+5	+0.5	+100	+1.0	+400	+400	+150	h	+10	+50

[f]The folacin allowances refer to dietary sources as determined by *Lactobacillus casei* assay after treatment with enzymes ("conjugases") to make polyglutamyl forms of the vitamin available to the test organism.

[g]The RDA for vitamin B_{12} in infants is based on average concentration of the vitamin in human milk. The allowances after weaning are based on energy intake (as recommended by the American Academy of Pediatrics) and consideration of other factors such as intestinal absorption.

[h]The increased requirement during pregnancy cannot be met by the iron content of habitual American diets nor by the existing iron stores of many women; therefore, the use of 30-60 mg of supplemental iron is recommended. Iron needs during lactation are not substantially different from those of nonpregnant women, but continued supplementation of the mother for 2-3 months after parturition is advisable in order to replenish stores depleted by pregnancy.

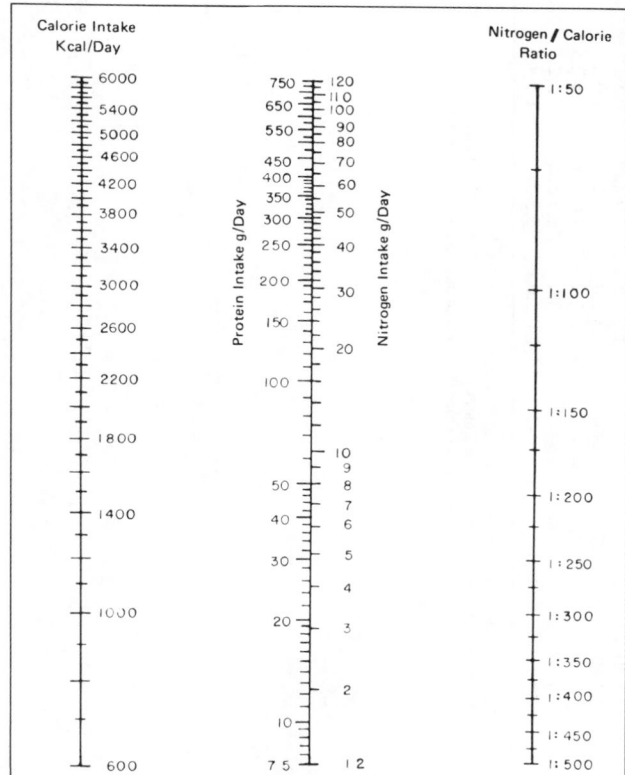

FIGURE 347-3   Nomogram for determining daily nitrogen requirements. Daily calorie requirements are located on the left scale, and a straight-edge is used to connect this point with the point on the right scale that indicates the desired nitrogen/calorie ratio (1:150 for most patients). Nitrogen intake is read from the right side of the center scale.

From Wilmore DW: *The metabolic management of the critically ill*, New York, 1977, Plenum Medical.

become limiting or deficient. Five such substances that require vigilance are tyrosine, cysteine, taurine, choline, and carnitine.

Peripheral Total Parenteral Nutrition

The objective of peripheral parenteral nutrition is to provide nutrition intravenously without inserting a central venous catheter. Peripheral infusion of amino acids, dextrose, and fat emulsion usually cannot provide adequate nonprotein calories to produce a positive nitrogen balance in adult patients under medical stress. Supplemental oral intake of these substances is necessary. Contraindications for peripheral parenteral nutrition include abnormalities in fat transport, uncontrolled diabetes mellitus (without insulin), liver disease, thrombocytopenia and/or coagulopathy, and severe chronic obstructive pulmonary disease. Basal requirements are usually met by infusing 1.5 liters of a 5% dextrose, 4.25% amino acid solution, and 1.0 to 1.5 liters of a 10% fat emulsion daily. Appropriate electrolytes are also added to meet daily requirements. Additional calories can be provided only by increasing the volume of the dilute dextrose solution, thus limiting the amount of calories that can be added.

Defined-Formula Diets and Other Supplements

Special low-residue, liquid-formula diets composed of all nutrients known to be required by human beings have been developed over the past decade. These defined-formula diets ("elemental" or "chemically defined" diets) are being extensively used in clinical medicine for patients who are unable to eat solid foods but who have a partially or totally intact and functioning gastrointestinal tract. Specialized defined-formula diets are thought to be readily and almost completely absorbed in the upper small intestine. They facilitate minimum delivery of residue to the lower bowel and are free of lactose. If oral intake of food is contraindicated, maintenance of adequate nutrition by a defined-formula diet may be an alternative to parenteral feeding. If the gastrointestinal tract is functioning, defined-formula diets have decided advantages over parenteral nutrition, because entry of nutrients into the gut stimulates maintenance of structure and function of the mucosa. Patients who may benefit from defined-formula diets are those with cancer, severe and persistent anorexia,

Table 347-13   Recommended dietary allowances: estimated safe and adequate daily dietary intakes of selected vitamins and minerals*

Category	AGE (YEARS)	VITAMINS			TRACE ELEMENTS†						ELECTROLYTES		
		VITAMIN K (µg)	BIOTIN (µg)	PANTOTHENIC ACID (mg)	COPPER (mg)	MANGANESE (mg)	FLUORIDE (mg)	CHROMIUM (mg)	SELENIUM (mg)	MOLYBDENUM (mg)	SODIUM (mg)	POTASSIUM (mg)	CHLORIDE (mg)
Infants	0-0.5	12	35	2	0.5-0.7	0.5-0.7	0.1-0.5	0.01-0.04	0.01-0.04	0.03-0.06	115-350	350-925	275-700
	0.5-1.0	10-20	50	3	0.7-1.0	0.7-1.0	0.2-1.0	0.02-0.06	0.02-0.06	0.04-0.08	250-750	425-1275	400-1200
Children	1-3	15-30	65	3	1.0-1.5	1.0-1.5	0.5-1.5	0.02-0.08	0.05-0.10	325-975	550-1650	550-1500	
	4-6	20-40	85	3-4	1.5-2.0	1.5-2.0	1.0-2.5	0.03-0.12	0.03-0.12	0.06-0.15	450-1350	775-2325	700-2100
	7-10	30-60	120	4-5	2.0-2.5	2.0-3.0	1.5-2.5	0.05-0.20	0.05-0.20	0.1-0.3	600-1800	1000-3000	925-2775
Adolescents	11+	50-100	100-200	4-7	2.0-3.0	2.5-5.0	1.5-2.5	0.05-0.20	0.05-0.20	0.15-0.50	900-2700	1525-4575	1400-4200
Adults		70-140	100-200	4-7	2.0-3.0	2.5-5.0	1.5-4.0	0.05-0.20	0.05-0.20	0.15-0.50	1100-3300	1875-5625	1700-5100

From Food and Nutrition Board, National Academy of Sciences–National Research Council, Washington, 1989.

*Because there is less information on which to base allowances, these figures are not given in Table 347-12 and are provided here in the form of ranges of recommended intakes.

†Because the toxic levels for many trace elements may be only several times the usual intake, the upper levels for the trace elements given in this table should not be habitually exceeded.

Table 347-14   Mean heights and weights and recommended energy intake; recommended dietary allowances*

CATEGORY	AGE (YEARS)	WEIGHT (kg)	WEIGHT (lb)	HEIGHT (cm)	HEIGHT (in)	ENERGY NEEDS (WITH RANGE) (kcal)	(MJ)
Males	11-14	45	99	157	62	2700 (2000-3700)	11.3
	15-18	66	145	176	69	2800 (2100-3900)	11.8
	19-22	70	154	177	70	2900 (2500-3300)	12.2
	23-50	70	154	178	70	2700 (2300-3100)	11.3
	51-75	70	154	178	70	2400 (2000-2800)	10.1
	76+	70	154	178	70	2050 (1650-2450)	8.6
Females	11-14	46	101	157	62	2200 (1500-3000)	9.2
	15-18	55	120	163	64	2100 (1200-3000)	8.8
	19-22	55	120	163	64	2100 (1700-2500)	8.8
	23-50	55	120	163	64	2000 (1600-2400)	8.4
	51-75	55	120	163	64	1800 (1400-2200)	7.6
	76+	55	120	163	64	1600 (1200-2000)	6.7
Pregnant						+300	
Lactating						+500	

From Food and Nutrition Board, National Academy of Sciences–National Research Council, Washington, 1989.
*The data in this table have been assembled with desirable weights for adults given in Table 347-12 for the mean heights of men (70 inches) and women (64 inches) between the ages of 18 and 34 years as surveyed in the U.S. population (HEW/NCHS data).
The energy allowances for the young adults are for men and women doing light work. The allowances for the two older groups represent mean energy needs over these age spans, allowing for a 2% decrease in basal (resting) metabolic rate per decade and a reduction in activity of 200 kcal/day for men and women between 51 and 75 years, 500 kcal for men over 75 years, and 400 kcal for women over 75. The customary range of daily energy output is shown for adults in parentheses and is based on a variation in energy needs of ±400 kcal at any one age, emphasizing the wide range of energy intake appropriate for any group of people.
Energy allowances for children through age 18 are based on median energy intakes of children of these ages followed in longitudinal growth studies. The values in parentheses are 10th and 90th percentiles of energy intake, to indicate the range of energy consumption among children of these ages.

Table 347-15   Standard formulation for total parenteral nutrition*

EACH 1000 ml CONTAINS:
    TOTAL CALORIES: 1000
    AMINO ACIDS: (4.25%, 180 cal) 42.5 g
    DEXTROSE: (25%, 850 cal) 250 g
    NITROGEN: 6.25 g
    VITAMINS: B complex (1 ml) and ascorbic acid equivalent (550 mg) every day; multivitamins (B group, A, D, E) (3.5 ml) and ascorbic
        acid equivalent (800 mg) once weekly
    OSMOLARITY: 1900 mOsm

FORMULA TYPE	K	NA	MG AS SULFATE	CA	P (mM)	P (mg)	CL	ACETATE	INSULIN (UNITS)
Standard	12	21	8	4.5	13.4	415	8	25	0
With added sodium	12	51	8	4.5	13.4	415	24	43	0
With added insulin	12	21	8	4.5	13.4	415	8	25	15
With added sodium and insulin	12	51	8	4.5	13.4	415	24	43	15
With added potassium	40	21	8	4.5	17.3	536	16	43	0
With added potassium and sodium	40	51	8	4.5	17.3	536	32	53	0
With added potassium and insulin	40	21	8	4.5	17.3	536	16	43	15
With added potassium, sodium, and insulin	40	51	8	4.5	17.3	536	32	53	15

*Values expressed in milliequivalents unless otherwise noted.

fistulas, severe malabsorption, coma, or impairment of swallowing mechanisms.

If the patient is unable to swallow, greatest tolerance is achieved if the liquid formula is delivered by continuous drip. Delivery may be by nasogastric or nasoduodenal tube or by gastrostomy or jejunostomy. Soft tubes made of silicone or polyurethane compounds are most acceptable. Care should be taken to follow recommended procedures for easy insertion and accurate placement of the feeding catheter.

Because all defined-formula diets are hyperosmolar, they are best tolerated if the concentration and rate of delivery are increased slowly. Accurate intake and output records must be kept, and the patient should be carefully monitored. Mechanical complications (e.g., aspiration, tracheoesophageal fistulas) and metabolic complications (e.g., hyperosmolar, hyperglycemic, nonketotic dehydration; fluid overload; nausea; vomiting; diarrhea) may occur and must be treated.

There are some contraindications for the use of defined-formula diets. Metabolic problems in patients with renal or hepatic disease may be exacerbated by the levels of protein, sodium, potassium phos-

phate, or magnesium present in the formula. Patients receiving corticosteroid treatment may not tolerate the amount of sodium in specific formulas. Patients with hypercalcemia may not tolerate the concentration of calcium.

The nutrient composition of defined-formula diets varies widely. This should be taken into consideration in the selection of a diet for an individual patient. Liquid formulas other than defined-formula diets may be effective for selected patients. These formulas may be used to supplement regular food intake, to increase the intake of one or more nutrients, or to provide the combination and proportion of nutrients most beneficial for the patient. Supplements should be selected for specific reasons, and their use carefully monitored by the physician.

BIBLIOGRAPHY

Beckmann D: Hunger: transforming the politics of hunger, Silver Springs, Md, 1993, Bread for the World Institute.
Bouchard C: Heredity and the path to overweight and obesity, *Med Sci Sports Exerc* 23(3):285-291, 1991.

Brown ML, editor: *Present knowledge in nutrition*, Washington DC, 1990, International Life Sciences Institute–Nutrition Foundation.

Brownell KD, Fairburn CG, editors: *Eating disorders and obesity*, New York, 1995, Guilford.

Byers T, Perry G: Dietary carotenes, vitamin C, and vitamin E as protective antioxidants in human cancers, *Annu Rev Nutr* 12:139-159, 1992.

Clement K, Vaisse C, Manning B St. J et al: Genetic variation in the β₃-adrenergic receptor and an increased capacity to gain weight in patients with morbid obesity, *N Engl J Med* 333:352-354, 1995.

Hennekens CH, editor: *Health promotion and disease prevention: the role of antioxidant vitamins 97* (suppl 3A-1S–3A-28S), 1994.

Himes JH, editor: *Anthropometric assessment of nutritional status*, New York, 1991, Wiley-Liss.

Hoehn RA, Huber R, Hennessey P: Feeding people—half of overcoming hunger: the U.S. feeding movement—fertile ground for an anti-hunger movement. In Cohen MJ, editor: *Hunger, 1994: transforming the politics of hunger*, Silver Springs, Md, 1993, Bread for the World Institute.

Kinney JM, Tucker HN, editors: *Energy metabolism: tissue determinants and cellular corollaries*, New York, 1992, Raven.

Kucamarski RJ, Flegal KM, Campbell SM, Johnson CL: Increasing prevalence of overweight among US adults: the national health and nutrition examination surveys, 1960 to 1991, *JAMA* 272:205-211, 1994.

Linder MD, editor: *Nutritional biochemistry and metabolism with clinical applications*, ed 2, New York, 1991, Elsevier.

Masuzaki H, Ogawa Y, Isse N et al: Human obese gene expression: adipocyte-specific expression and regional differences in adipose tissue, *Diabetes* 44:855-858, 1995.

McArdle WD, Katch FI, Katch VL: *Exercise physiology: energy, nutrition and human physiology*, ed 3, Philadelphia, 1991, Lea & Febiger.

Panetta LE: Congressional reports, *Health and Medicine* 2(3):18-19, 1984.

Rombeau JL, Caldwell MD, editors: *Clinical nutrition: enteral and tube feeding*, ed 2, Philadelphia, 1991, WB Saunders.

Shils ME, Olson JA, Shike M, editors: *Modern nutrition in health and disease*, ed 8, vol 1, vol 2, Philadelphia, 1994, Lea & Febiger.

Subcommittee on the Tenth Edition of the Recommended Dietary Allowances, Food and Nutrition Board: *recommended dietary allowances*, ed 10, Washington DC, 1989, National Research Council, National Academy of Sciences.

Van Itallie TB, Simopoulos AP, editors: *Obesity: new directions in assessment and management*, Philadelphia, 1995, Charles Press.

Zhang Y, Proenca R, Maffei M et al: Positional cloning of the mouse obese gene and its human homologue, *Nature* 372:425-432, 1994.

LIVER, BILIARY TREE, AND PANCREAS

I PHYSIOLOGIC, BIOCHEMICAL, AND IMMUNOLOGIC PRINCIPLES

348 Hepatic Metabolism

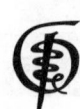

Seymour M. Sabesin

To consider the metabolic functions of the liver requires substantial discussion of the major biochemical processes in the body, particularly those that concern nutrient metabolism. The liver subserves central functions in the synthesis of proteins, carbohydrates, and lipids and is involved in many anabolic and catabolic reactions that regulate energy homeostasis in the fed and fasting states. Box 348-1 provides an overview of the major metabolic functions of the liver and lists some specialized functions such as the storage of certain metals and vitamins. Only a few hepatic functions are discussed in detail in this chapter. Other functions of the liver are considered in other chapters and will be referred to in the text.

The liver is important in certain processes in addition to macromolecular synthesis; these include (1) energy production; i.e., the use of carbohydrates, proteins, and fats for aerobic respiration in hepatic mitochondria (tricarboxylic acid cycle); (2) the metabolism and detoxification of drugs, vitamins, and hormones; (3) ammonia metabolism, leading to ureagenesis; and (4) maintenance of blood glucose levels and ketogenesis.

It is appropriate to consider briefly the major anabolic and catabolic functions of the liver. Liver disease may be associated with derangements in these functions, although marked impairment does not occur unless there has been a substantial loss of hepatic parenchymal tissue. A detailed analysis of all the metabolic functions of the liver comprises a major aspect of biochemistry; the objective here is to highlight the most important functions emphasizing processes that are most important physiologically and that are deranged readily in liver disease.

AMINO ACID AND PROTEIN METABOLISM

The liver is the major site of plasma protein synthesis. The liver synthesizes and then secretes into the plasma a variety of proteins, several of which subserve very specific functions (coagulation factors, transport proteins, etc.) (Box 348-1). In addition to synthesizing export proteins, the liver synthesizes the structural proteins and enzymes required for the maintenance of hepatocellular function. About 50% of hepatic protein synthesis is synthesis of proteins for export. The 12 g of albumin synthesized daily represents 25% of total hepatic protein synthesis in human beings.

Total body protein in an average 70-kg adult is approximately 12 kg. In a steady state, protein turnover reflects the synthesis and degradation of equal amounts of protein. Total body protein turnover is 200 to 300 g/day. When dietary supply is normal, liver and muscle use amino acids released by local protein degradation for up to 50% of their synthetic requirements. With dietary protein restriction this figure may be increased to 90%. Thus the amino acid pool available for protein synthesis is derived from the degradation of about 250 g of body protein plus variable amounts of dietary protein. Total body protein turnover also includes endogenous secretion of enzyme proteins, exfoliated cellular protein, and protein exuded into the gastrointestinal lumen. In the intestinal lumen all of these proteins mix with amino acids of dietary origin and undergo a similar digestive-absorptive process. Amino acids entering the portal vein originate from about 90 g of dietary protein, 50 g of exfoliated cellular protein, 16 g of secreted enzyme protein, and 2 g of exuded plasma protein.

The overall protein turnover rate is relatively stable, even with protein deprivation, reflecting compensatory changes in liver and muscle. With continued deprivation of exogenous amino acids, the mass of hepatic tissue protein decreases and the absolute rate of synthesis falls. In this way, the amino acid supply regulates the synthesis of proteins secreted by the liver into the plasma.

Most amino acids entering the liver via the portal vein are catabolized to urea in the Krebs-Henseleit cycle. The remainder are either utilized directly for protein synthesis (of either intracellular or plasma proteins), converted to special compounds (e.g., glutathione), or released into the blood as free amino acids. In the liver during a 12-hour absorptive period (12 noon to 12 midnight), 57% of incoming nitrogen is converted to urea, 6% is used for plasma protein synthesis, 14% is used for endogenous hepatic protein synthesis, and 23% is secreted into the circulation as free amino acids. During the nonabsorptive (fasting) period, the influx of amino acids in the portal blood is about one sixth of the absorptive level and is derived mostly from secreted and exfoliated protein. Plasma protein synthesis continues at the same rate as before, but amino acid release ceases and ureagenesis decreases by about two thirds. During fasting, hepatic tis-

---

BOX 348-1

Hepatic functions

I. Protein synthesis
  A. Albumin
  B. Blood coagulation proteins
    1. Fibrinogen (factor I)
    2. Prothrombin (factor II)
    3. Factors V, VII, IX, X
  C. Synthesis of other proteins
    1. Haptoglobin
    2. Ceruloplasmin
    3. Transferrin
    4. Alpha and beta globulins
    5. Complement factors
    6. Hormone transport proteins (e.g., sex steroid-binding globulins)
  D. Glycoprotein synthesis
  E. Synthesis of structural proteins and intracellular enzymes
II. Lipid synthesis
  A. Triglyceride
  B. Cholesterol
  C. Phospholipids
  D. Lipoproteins (very-low and very-high-density)
  E. Bile acids
III. Metabolic functions
  A. Biochemical oxidations
  B. Carbohydrate metabolism
    1. Glycogenesis
    2. Glycogenolysis
    3. Gluconeogenesis
    4. Glucose clearance from blood
    5. Lactate clearance from blood
    6. Nonglucose hexose metabolism (e.g., fructose and galactose)

  C. Amino acid metabolism for protein, carbohydrate, and lipid synthesis
  D. Free fatty acid metabolism
  E. Ketogenesis
  F. Ureagenesis
  G. Bilirubin metabolism: conjugation and excretion of bilirubin
  H. Lipoprotein uptake and catabolism (e.g., chylomicron remnants, LDL)
  I. Hormone metabolism
    1. Insulin
    2. Glucagon
    3. Growth hormone
    4. Glucocorticoids
    5. Catecholamines
    6. Thyroxine
    7. Sex steroid hormones
  J. Conjugation, solubilization, and deamination of drugs
IV. Specialized functions
  A. Bilirubin and bile salt secretion
  B. Reticuloendothelial functions
    1. Phagocytosis
    2. Processing of antigens (bacterial, viral, dietary) absorbed from the intestine
  C. Receptor-mediated uptake and endocytosis of many ligands (e.g., LDL)
  D. Storage functions
    1. Fat-soluble vitamins (A, D, K)
    2. Vitamin B_{12}
    3. Metals (iron, copper)
  E. Maintenance of plasma volume and electrolyte concentrations

---

sue protein goes into a catabolic phase and, together with alanine (released from muscle), contributes to ureagenesis and gluconeogenesis. All of these metabolic changes are mediated by enzymes concerned with synthesis of nonessential amino acids, transamination, ureagenesis, and gluconeogenesis.

Turnover of plasma amino acids is rapid. The total plasma pool of amino acids is about one two-hundredths the size of the influx. The tissue amino acid pool is about half the size of the absorbed amino acid load. It is composed mostly of glutamic acid, glutamine, alanine, and glycine, indicating that the turnover of plasma amino acids is associated with rapid transamination as well as utilization for protein synthesis. The liver is selective in its uptake of amino acids. For example, the branched-chain amino acids valine, isoleucine, and leucine are metabolized predominantly by muscle.

Albumin Synthesis

Albumin is synthesized exclusively in the liver at a rate in adults of 150 to 200 mg/kg/day. The half-life of albumin is 17 to 20 days but may be reduced with excessive losses from the body, as in protein-losing gastroenteropathy (Chapter 340) and massive proteinuria (Chapter 105). Albumin synthesis begins by association of messenger RNA with free ribosomal subunits in the hepatocyte cytosol. It is formed as a precursor molecule called *preproalbumin*. Portions of this molecule are subsequently removed within the hepatocyte, forming the final product, albumin, which is secreted from the cell. At the subcellular level, the time course for the assembly, intracellular transport, and secretion of albumin has been investigated by use of radioactively labeled amino acid precursors. The labeled amino acid is incorporated into the growing albumin chain within 1 minute. Sequentially, the radiolabeled albumin has its highest specific activity in the rough endoplasmic reticulum within 3 minutes, in the smooth endoplasmic reticulum within 6 minutes, and in the Golgi apparatus at 15

to 20 minutes. From the Golgi complex, the albumin molecules are packaged into secretory vesicles that migrate through the cytosol and fuse with the basolateral plasma membrane, thereby discharging the albumin into the perisinusoidal space of Disse.

About 0.3 to 0.4 mg of newly synthesized albumin per gram of liver tissue is present within hepatocytes. At a constant rate of synthesis and release, this quantity of albumin would turn over three times an hour; however, such a rate is two or three times greater than the normal synthetic rate of 150 to 200 mg/kg/day. Thus albumin synthesis and secretion operate at about one third of capacity.

Factors that regulate albumin synthesis are nutrition, hormonal balance, and osmotic pressure. Nutritional status is the prime factor, as albumin synthesis is very sensitive to the available supply of amino acids, particularly tryptophan. The livers of fasting animals produce less than half the amount of albumin that is synthesized by those of fed animals. The factors regulating albumin degradation are less well known. No organ has been implicated directly in albumin degradation. Fractional rates of albumin degradation are related directly to the albumin mass, serum albumin level, and dietary protein intake. When protein intake is limited, there is a low fractional rate of degradation.

Osmotic regulation of albumin synthesis is precise. The liver responds to reductions in extravascular osmotic pressure by increasing the rate of albumin synthesis. This effect is modulated by the osmotic pressure in the hepatic interstitial volume, only about one tenth of which is available for albumin distribution.

Hormones also influence hepatic protein metabolism, in part through their influences on nutrient metabolism. Examples of effects of hormones on hepatic protein synthesis include the anabolic effect of insulin on tissue and export protein synthesis and its anticatabolic effect on tissue protein degradation. Corticosteroids, growth hormone, and thyroid hormone stimulate albumin synthesis, whereas glucagon has an antianabolic effect on tissue and secretory proteins.

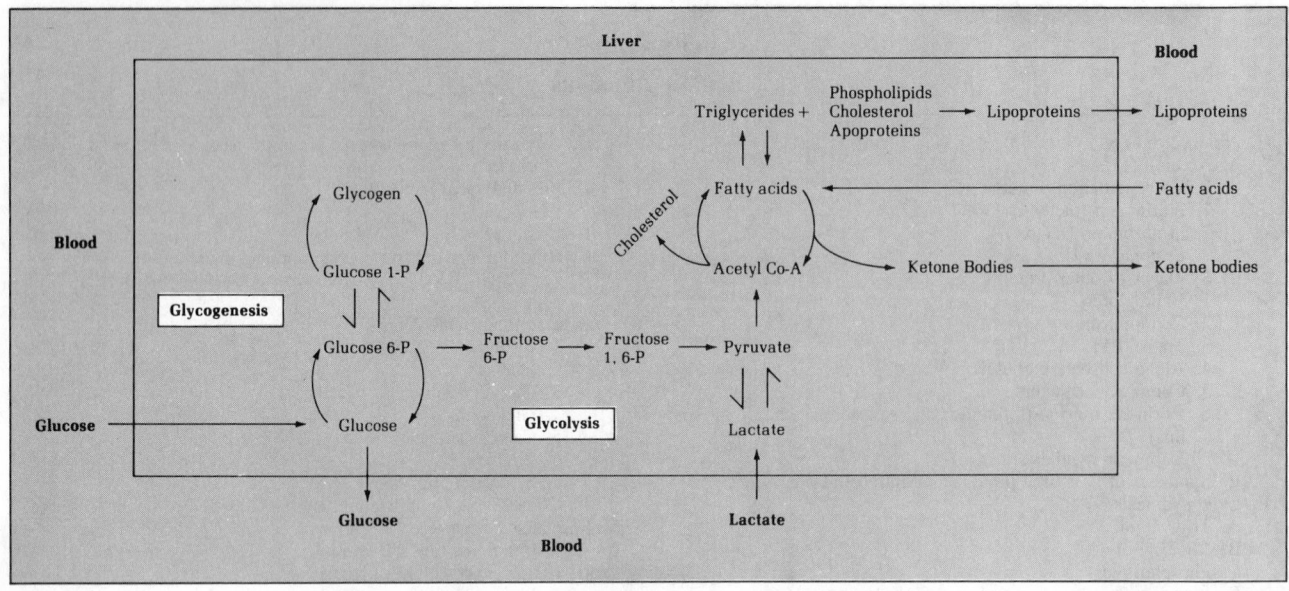

FIGURE 348-1   Simplified scheme of carbohydrate and lipid metabolism in the liver.

Ureagenesis

The formation of urea from ammonia is a unique hepatic function providing means by which the product of tissue and dietary nitrogen catabolism can be eliminated. Ureagenesis occurs in the Krebs-Henseleit cycle, which utilizes the four specific amino acids ornithine, citrulline, arginine, and aspartic acid to transform ammonia into urea. Urea is excreted primarily by the kidneys but also by the gastrointestinal tract (25%).

HEPATIC FORMATION OF SPECIALIZED PROTEINS
Coagulation Factors (see Chapter 84)

The liver is the site of synthesis of many blood-clotting factors (see Box 348-1). Factors II (prothrombin), VII, IX, and X are vitamin K responsive, and thus their synthesis is decreased if intestinal absorption of vitamin K is impaired. The half-life of several coagulation factors is quite short, varying from 4 hours for factor VII to 3 to 5 days for prothrombin. Prothrombin is synthesized as an inactive precursor whose conversion to an active coagulation protein requires vitamin K. The reduced form of vitamin K functions in the activation of an enzyme that removes gamma-carboxyglutamic acid from the precursor molecule. This reaction permits the conversion of prothrombin to thrombin, a process that requires factors V and X.

The liver synthesizes and degrades fibrinolytic factors and clears activated clotting factors from the circulation. Fibrinogen has a relatively constant fractional degradation rate, irrespective of plasma concentration. Alterations in fibrinogen synthesis may occur in liver disease, possibly due to the formation of functionally abnormal fibrinogens with reduced clotting ability.

Transferrin

Transferrin, the iron-binding protein, is synthesized principally but not exclusively in the liver. Its synthesis may be increased in iron deficiency states. Transferrin synthesis is predominant in determining the plasma transferrin concentration.

Ceruloplasmin

Ceruloplasmin, important for copper transport and homeostasis, is synthesized in the liver. Plasma ceruloplasmin levels are decreased in Wilson's disease (Chapter 359).

Alpha₁ Antitrypsin

Alpha$_1$ antitrypsin is synthesized by the liver, a process that is stimulated by acute stress. It is a serine protease inhibitor that may function to inactivate proteases released from intracellular sites. Alpha$_1$ antitrypsin is responsible for about 90% of the protease activity in plasma, but this is reduced to about 15% in patients with a hereditary defect in hepatic alpha-1 antitrypsin synthesis (Chapter 359).

Alpha-Fetoprotein

Alpha-fetoprotein is a normal secretory product of human fetal liver. Normally not present in plasma, its appearance in association with hepatocellular carcinomas (Chapter 362) is thought to reflect the derepression of fetal genomes. Alpha-fetoprotein may be associated with hepatic regeneration, as it has been reported in plasma after viral or toxic hepatitis and massive hepatic necrosis.

Ferritin

Ferritin is the principal form of available stored iron. Serum ferritin originates in part as a hepatic secretory protein. Serum ferritin concentration correlates well with total body iron stores. Thus it provides a good screening test for iron overload or deficiency. Serum ferritin may also be elevated in association with acute liver injury or ongoing chronic active hepatocellular necrosis. The function of circulating ferritin is not known, but knowledge of its role in tissue as a storage protein for iron is well established.

LIVER AND LIPID METABOLISM

The liver is involved in many aspects of lipid synthesis and metabolism (Fig. 348-1). It is a major site of triglyceride, cholesterol, and phospholipid synthesis. Cholesterol and phospholipids are used in part as constituents of hepatocyte membranes. In association with triglycerides they are also assembled into certain classes of lipoproteins that are then secreted into the circulation. Cholesterol is also used for bile acid synthesis, a process confined to the liver (Chapter 349).

Cholesterol synthesis is derived from acetate via its conversion to beta-hydroxy-beta-methylglutaryl-CoA (HMG-CoA). Regulation of the activity of the enzyme HMG-CoA reductase that controls this step is quite complex, depending in part on the hepatic uptake of cholesterol from dietary sources in chylomicron remnants. The regulation of the body cholesterol pool, which is relatively constant, is determined by a balance between synthesis and loss in the gastrointestinal tract and from desquamating cutaneous cells. Factors that regulate hepatic cholesterol synthesis include dietary cholesterol absorption, bile acid homeostasis, and the uptake of cholesterol from lipoproteins during their catabolism.

Fatty Acid Uptake and Utilization (see also Chapter 306)

Fatty acids liberated from adipose tissue are carried in the bloodstream bound to albumin. Approximately one third of the circulating fatty acids are removed by the liver, one third by skeletal muscle, and the rest by other tissues, especially myocardium. Hepatic triglyceride formation or accumulation is greatly affected by the rate at which fatty acids are presented to the liver. Fatty acids released from adipose tissue have a short half-life in the plasma: about 2 min. The liver can extract 30% of circulating free fatty acids in a single cycle.

After hepatic uptake, fatty acids may be oxidized or used for ketone body formation or for triglyceride and phospholipid synthesis (Fig. 348-1). Quantitatively, most of the fatty acids reaching the liver are resecreted into the bloodstream as triglycerides in the form of very-low-density lipoproteins (VLDL). After uptake of exogenously or endogenously derived fatty acids, hepatic triglyceride esterification occurs rapidly. Thus within 2 minutes after injection of radiolabeled fatty acids, most fatty acids recovered from the liver are already esterified. Esterification is closely linked to hepatic oxidative phosphorylation and is dependent on a ready supply of alpha-glycerophosphate, the precursor of glycerol supplied almost exclusively from glucose, and the availability of fatty acyl CoA. Glucose and insulin are extremely important in the regulation of hepatic triglyceride formation. Insulin regulates the activity of glucokinase that is essential for glucose phosphorylation, increases fatty acid synthesis from glucose, and promotes hepatic triglyceride secretion.

During fasting or when metabolic demands are great, fatty acids are used for ketone body formation. Fatty acid oxidation is important in removing excess lipid from the liver so that accumulation does not ordinarily occur. Fatty acids incorporated into phospholipids are stored in the formed membrane lipids or in the exchangeable phospholipid pools.

The rate of hepatic triglyceride synthesis is usually regulated by approximately equal hepatic secretion of triglyceride, but acute stresses such as mobilization of fatty acids from adipose tissue or a rapid and prolonged increase in dietary chylomicron triglyceride can result in increased hepatic triglyceride synthesis. The liver may respond to an increased fatty acid influx by increasing the rate of lipoprotein and ketone body formation, but the extent to which the activity of these pathways can increase is limited. If the rate at which fatty acids are brought to the liver exceeds the ability of the liver to metabolize and/or resecrete the fatty acids into the circulation as lipoproteins, storage of fat within the hepatocytes will ensue.

Lipoprotein Biosynthesis

The lipoproteins in fasting plasma are the metabolic products of newly synthesized (nascent) lipoproteins secreted by the liver or intestine. The liver contributes in many ways to the synthesis and metabolism of the plasma lipoproteins. Thus the liver synthesizes the major lipids and apoproteins of the plasma lipoproteins and secretes VLDL and high-density lipoproteins (HDL). VLDL and HDL are secreted as nascent particles whose lipid and apoprotein compositions are altered drastically in the plasma as a result of enzymatic transformations and exchange of lipids and apoproteins among various lipoprotein classes. These transformations, which are intrinsic to lipoprotein metabolism, are also dependent on other hepatic functions such as the synthesis of apoproteins C-II and A-I, which are the activators of lipoprotein lipase (LPL) and lecithin-cholesterol acyltransferase (LCAT), respectively. These enzymes are essential for the initiation of the lipoprotein metabolic pathways, as LPL is involved in the lipolysis of triglyceride-rich lipoproteins (chylomicrons and VLDL), and LCAT is responsible, in human beings, for all plasma cholesterol esterification. The liver is involved also in the uptake and degradation of chylomicron remnants, HDL, and LDL.

Significant advances have been made in lipoprotein metabolism

in the past few years, with particular relevance to the role of the liver.

Bile Acid Synthesis (see Chapter 349)

CARBOHYDRATE METABOLISM

The liver is essential for the regulation of carbohydrate metabolism, as it receives directly from the portal circulation most of the ingested carbohydrates and then, by hormonal regulation, controls the concentration of blood glucose in the fed and fasting states. The most important function of the liver in carbohydrate metabolism is its role in constantly regulating blood glucose levels, thereby providing a predictable supply of glucose for energy needs in tissues throughout the body (Fig. 348-1).

The metabolic actions of the liver with regard to carbohydrate metabolism and the maintenance of blood glucose levels are closely related to the liver's role in lipid (Fig. 348-1) and protein metabolism and to the fact that key hormones regulating carbohydrate homeostasis act mainly on the liver. These key hormones include insulin, glucagon, growth hormone, glucocorticoids, catecholamines, and thyroxine, all of which, except catecholamines, are catabolized by the liver. The liver's major role in carbohydrate metabolism can be subdivided into (1) functions that produce glucose, (2) functions that result in glucose storage as glycogen, and (3) the metabolism of hexoses and sugars other than glucose that are also derived from dietary sources. Processes involved in the maintenance of blood glucose concentration include (1) uptake and storage of glucose in the form of glycogen (glycogenesis), (2) conversion of stored glycogen into glucose (glycogenolysis), and (3) formation of glucose from noncarbohydrate sources (gluconeogenesis).

The main carbohydrates in the human diet are sucrose, fructose, lactose, and starch. Enzymatic hydrolysis of these substances yields glucose and fructose and smaller quantities of galactose. There is little fluctuation of blood glucose concentrations even after ingestion of large amounts of glucose. Glucose is disposed of rapidly and in large quantities, primarily by the liver. The importance of the liver in taking up a dietary glucose load is related not only to the anatomic location of the liver but also to the liver's sensitivity to insulin. Glucose disposal is autoregulated by glucose and insulin. Glucagon has short-term effects on glycogen breakdown but has a more sustained stimulatory effect on gluconeogenesis. Glucagon levels fall after glucose ingestion, and its effects are overcome by insulin. In contrast, glucocorticoids present in excess amounts can counteract the effects of insulin on glucose disposal in the liver. After its rapid diffusion into the liver, glucose is rapidly phosphorylated to glucose 6-phosphate by glucokinase. Most of the glucose is stored as glycogen. Glycolysis, from either glucose or glycogen, is relatively inactive in the liver, and less than 10% of glucose is disposed of by glycolysis. Glucose is also metabolized by the hexose monophosphate shunt.

The ingestion of glucose after fasting causes a rise in blood glucose levels and a concomitant release of insulin, which facilitates glucose uptake into cells. Approximately 60% of an oral glucose load is taken up by the liver and utilized for glycogen synthesis, triglyceride formation and, in small amounts, for glycolysis (Fig. 348-1). About 25% of the glucose is used by the brain and by non-insulin-dependent tissues as an energy source. During fasting, the liver maintains glucose homeostasis by glycogenolysis and gluconeogenesis. These two processes occur in response to decreased blood insulin levels and corresponding increases in glucagon concentration. The liver's capacity for glycogen storage is limited, about 70 g. With fasting, hepatic glycogen stores are depleted after 1 day; however, glucose consumption continues at a constant rate, stimulating hepatic gluconeogenesis.

The liver is the major site of gluconeogenesis, which utilizes three types of nonsugar precursors: glycogenic amino acids, lactate, and glycerol phosphate. The pathways leading to gluconeogenesis include the transamination of glycogenic amino acids. The alpha-ketoacids formed by transamination enter the gluconeogenic pathway either directly (pyruvate, oxaloacetate derived from alanine, and aspartate) or after further metabolic conversions (alpha-ketoglutarate from glutamate). Glycogenic amino acids are used for gluconeogenesis when dietary protein is high and there is insufficient dietary carbohydrate. This process is stimulated by glucocorticoid hormones. When oxygen consumption is insufficient to keep up with glucose utilization, as with vigorous muscular exercise, lactate produced in muscle is used for gluconeogenesis. The pathway leading to glucose formation from lactate involves first the oxidation of lactate to pyruvate and then entrance of pyruvate into the pathway, leading to glucose formation from glucose 6-phosphate. Glucose production from lactate can exceed 60 μmol/g liver/hr; however, this is very energy-demanding, consuming a considerable fraction of nucleotide triphosphates.

Lipid metabolism is important for glucose homeostasis, as the availability of glycerol phosphate for gluconeogenesis is derived from triglyceride and phospholipid metabolism. Triglyceride hydrolysis causes the release of free glycerol. The liver then converts glycerol to glycerol phosphate at the expense of adenosine triphosphate (ATP). In contrast, phospholipid hydrolysis leads directly to glycerol phosphate formation. Subsequently, glycerol phosphate is oxidized to dihydroxyacetone phosphate. When dietary carbohydrate is insufficient to maintain glucose homeostasis but fat intake is high, gluconeogenesis from the glycerol phosphate pathway takes place and the free fatty acids, released by triglyceride hydrolysis, are utilized for ketone body formation.

In short-term starvation the central nervous system (CNS) and peripheral nerves require glucose, whereas other tissues can use fatty acids and ketone bodies as energy substrates. The liver is essential to maintaining blood glucose levels, for it contains the enzyme glucose 6-phosphatase, which is necessary for the formation of glucose in the hepatocytes.

Lactate is the most important substance in gluconeogenesis, providing about 20% of total glucose after an overnight fast. More than 50% of the lactate is derived from glycogenolysis in extrahepatic tissues, principally muscle. Because muscle glycogen is derived from liver glucose, the utilization of lactate for gluconeogenesis does not represent a net increase in glucose synthesis. Gluconeogenesis from amino acids amounts to only about 6% to 12% of total glucose production after an overnight fast, but this percentage increases considerably if fasting continues. The principal amino acid for gluconeogenesis is alanine. Alanine is formed in peripheral tissues by transamination of pyruvate, but alanine is also synthesized from other amino acids. The regulation of gluconeogenesis is also sensitive to substrate availability; net glucose production increases with increasing precursor supply.

Most of the changes that occur in fasting can be attributed to alterations in the levels of circulating hormones that are superimposed on endogenous regulatory mechanisms. For example, as blood glucose concentrations fall, insulin secretion decreases and there are reciprocal elevations of glucagon secretion and increases in the concentrations of glucocorticoids, growth hormone, and catecholamines. The effects of glucocorticoids on peripheral tissues result in a release of alanine into the circulation, followed by an increased extraction of alanine by the liver, a process regulated by glucagon. The decrease in insulin lessens insulin's normal constraint on gluconeogenesis, which increases. At the same time glycogenolysis increases, due in part to lack of inhibition by glucose and insulin. With prolonged fasting there is an increase in adipose tissue lipolysis. This increase results in a marked increase in the uptake of free fatty acids by the liver, which results in increased ketone body formation, providing an alternative source of fuel for peripheral tissues and eventually for the CNS.

Metabolism of Other Hexoses

Fructose is an important caloric source. It is taken up and metabolized by the liver, where it is phosphorylated rapidly to fructose 1-phosphate. The latter enters the glycolytic/gluconeogenic pathway. Normally, about 70% of a fructose load appears as lactate, with the rest converted to glycogen. Galactose and other hexoses are also metabolized by the liver and are converted mostly to glucose or glycogen.

Ketogenesis

Ketone body formation, a process that occurs exclusively in the liver, is another essential hepatic function. Ketone bodies provide an energy source utilized by all tissues during starvation, and they are the only effective source of energy (other than glucose) for the CNS. The ketone bodies acetoacetate and beta-hydroxybutyrate are formed in the hepatocyte mitochondria from free fatty acids. This complex sequence of metabolic events depends in part on decreased insulin availability secondary to fasting or starvation. With insulin deficiency there is activation of lipolysis in peripheral adipose tissue, causing mobilization of free fatty acids. The rate of hepatic fatty acid oxidation is controlled by the activity of the carnitine acyltransferase system of enzymes that transports fatty acids into the mitochondria. During feeding, malonyl CoA, a potent inhibitor of carnitine acyltransferase I, prevents the transport of fatty acids into the mitochondria. This inhibition is removed during fasting by glucagon, which acts to lower the malonyl CoA concentration and increase the carnitine content of the liver. These changes enhance the capacity for fatty acid oxidation, and thus ketogenesis is activated. The rate of ketone body production is determined by the rate of delivery of free fatty acids from the periphery.

DETOXIFICATION

A major biochemical function of the liver is the detoxification and metabolism of drugs, vitamins, and hormones. The liver has a large capacity to modify exogenous and endogenous substances. Some compounds are metabolically converted to relatively inactive forms (e.g., steroid hormones), whereas others become more biologically active (e.g., vitamin D). Of prime importance in maintaining homeostasis and protecting the body against ingested toxins is the ability of the liver to metabolize and detoxify a wide variety of absorbed substances that reach it directly in the portal blood. Hepatic drug metabolism and drug-induced liver disease are considered in detail in Chapter 355.

HORMONE METABOLISM

The liver is involved in the metabolism of many hormones by virtue of its role in hormone biotransformation, inactivation, and excretion. In addition, many hormones exert direct effects on hepatic metabolic processes. Examples of the latter include the previously described effects of insulin, glucagon, and glucocorticoids on carbohydrate metabolism. The liver is particularly involved in steroid hormone metabolism. Steroid hormones are taken up from the circulation by the liver and then metabolized by hepatic enzymes, leading to their hydroxylation, oxidation, etc. The steroid hormones directly influence many of the liver's biochemical and physiologic functions. It is impossible to discuss all of the influences of hormones on the liver, because in some respects they encompass virtually all of its metabolic and physiologic functions. Therefore only examples of some key hormonal influences will be discussed.

The phagocytic function of the hepatic reticuloendothelial system is influenced directly by various steroid hormones. Estrogens stimulate phagocytosis, whereas glucocorticoids suppress reticuloendothelial function as assessed by the experimental inhibition of the clearance of infused particulate matter.

Insulin, glucocorticoids, estrogens, testosterone, thyroid hormone, and growth hormone are anabolic, increasing hepatic RNA synthesis and the rate of incorporation of amino acids into proteins. Hormones influence hepatic metabolism by regulating the synthesis of key enzymes involved in intermediary metabolism. There is considerable evidence that estrogens and progestins influence the plasma concentration of many proteins, presumably reflecting hormonal effects on hepatic synthesis, transport, and perhaps catabolism. Alteration in plasma concentration of certain proteins during pregnancy is an example of the physiologic regulation by hormones of hepatic protein production. Steroid hormones can induce key enzymes involved in porphyrin-heme synthesis, and by this means are important in the regulation of porphyrin and heme metabolism. The liver synthesizes special sex steroid-binding proteins and other globulins such as cortisol and thyroid-binding globulin (Chapter 282).

Hormones influence hepatic drug and chemical metabolism by their hormonal effects on hepatic enzymes involved in oxidative biotransformation and in drug conjugation. Sex hormones are particularly important in this regard, as evidenced by their effects on the oxidative capacity of the liver for certain drugs. Estrogens depress the rate of bile flow, and synthetic estrogens and progestins similarly depress the hepatic excretory capacity. The ability of the liver to excrete organic anions is compromised in pregnancy. Studies in pregnant women have demonstrated decreased capacity for the excretion of bilirubin and sulfobromophthalein sodium. The clinical counterpart of these hormonal effects is cholestasis, which sometimes occurs in pregnancy or after the use of oral contraceptives (Chapter 353). Steroid-induced cholestasis may also involve inhibitory effects on bilirubin conjugation, depressed bile salt synthesis, and other factors as yet poorly explained. The effects of liver injury on sex steroid biotransformation are discussed in Chapter 354.

BIBLIOGRAPHY

Ampola MG: The urea cycle: enzymes and defects. In Arias IM et al, editors: *The liver: biology and pathobiology,* New York, 1994, Raven Press.

Carr JM: Hemostatic disorders in liver disease. In Schiff L, Schiff ER, editors: *Diseases of the liver,* Philadelphia, 1993, JB Lippincott.

Cooper AD, Ellsworth JL: Lipoprotein metabolism. In Zakim D, Boyer TD, editors: *Hepatology,* Philadelphia, 1996, WB Saunders.

Cooper AJL: Role of the liver in amino acid metabolism. In Zakim D, Boyer TD, editors: *Hepatology,* Philadelphia, 1996, WB Saunders.

Donohue TM Jr., et al: Plasma protein metabolism. In Zakim D, Boyer TD, editors: *Hepatology,* Philadelphia, 1996, WB Saunders.

Glickman RM, Sabesin SM: Lipoprotein metabolism. In Arias IM et al, editors: *The liver: biology and pathobiology,* New York, 1994, Raven Press.

Havel RJ: Structure and metabolism of lipoproteins. In Scriver CR et al, editors: *The metabolic basis of inherited disease,* New York, 1995, McGraw-Hill.

Hellerstein K, Munro HN: Interaction of liver, muscle and adipose tissue in the regulation of metabolism in response to nutritional and other factors. In Arias IM, et al, editors: *The liver: biology and pathobiology,* New York, 1994, Raven Press.

Seifter S and England S: Energy metabolism. In Arias I et al, editors: *The liver: biology and pathobiology,* New York, 1994, Raven Press.

Vessey DA: Metabolism of xenobiotics by the liver. In Zakim D, Boyer TD, editors: *Hepatology,* Philadelphia, 1996, WB Saunders.

Vlahcevic ZR et al: Hepatic cholesterol metabolism. In Arias IM et al, editors: *The liver: biology and pathobiology,* New York, 1994, Raven Press.

Zakim D: Metabolism of glucose and fatty acids by the liver. In Zakim D, Boyer TD, editors: *Hepatology,* Philadelphia, 1996, WB Saunders.

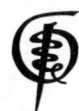

349 Bile Production and Secretion

James M. Crawford and Martin C. Carey

Bile is the "exocrine" secretion of the liver. Its solute composition is distinct, consisting principally of three kinds of lipids and a group of bile pigments in an aqueous electrolyte solution. The lipids of bile possess differing degrees of water solubility but are effectively solubilized by their physical-chemical interactions, enabling their transport in bile and delivery to the intestine. Hepatic secretion of bile facilitates the elimination of endogenous poorly water-soluble substances such as cholesterol; in the intestine, bile promotes the absorption of dietary lipids. This chapter highlights the mechanisms of bile formation and focuses on its unique solute composition and properties.

COMPOSITION

The concentration by weight of solutes in bile varies, depending on the extent of water secretion and reabsorption at different anatomic sites in the biliary system. Average solute concentrations are 3% (g/dl) in the hepatic ducts and 10% in the gallbladder. The solute composition of bile is shown in Fig. 349-1. Two thirds of the total solute mass is composed of bile salts, a family of closely related detergent-like molecules. The phospholipids of bile are less than a quarter of the mass and consist mostly (95%) of lecithin (phosphatidylcholine); the sterols are almost exclusively unesterified cholesterol. The bile pigment is bilirubin, which is conjugated predominantly with glucu-

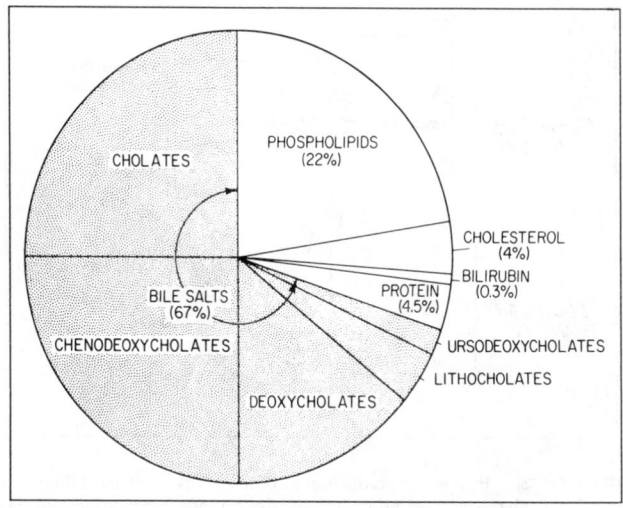

FIGURE 349-1 Typical solute composition of human gallbladder bile by weight percentage.

ronic acid. Present also are all the electrolytes found in plasma; low concentrations of glutathione; and a variety of proteins of diverse origin, including plasma apolipoproteins, albumin, and secretory IgA; liver lysosomal and plasma membrane enzymes; and high-molecular-weight glycoproteins, most of which are secreted as gallbladder mucins. In addition, bile contains trace amounts of heme, porphyrins, amino acids, vitamins, hormones, and many metals. Bile contains no glucose because of a high hepatic threshold for its secretion, and avid reabsorption in the biliary ductules. Hepatic bile contains a relatively high concentration of bicarbonate and maintains a pH of 7.0 to 8.0. Gallbladder secretion of protons and possibly reabsorption of bicarbonate give gallbladder bile a pH of 6.2 to 7.4.

BILE WATER PRODUCTION

In human beings the volume of bile produced each day varies from 500 to 1200 ml. Bile water production is an entirely passive process that occurs in response to active secretion of a number of solutes and is mediated both by hepatocytes and bile duct epithelial cells (Fig. 349-2). Hepatocellular water secretion, referred to as *canalicular*, follows osmotic gradients established primarily by the secretion of organic anions, particularly bile salts, with a much smaller contribution from glutathione. Sodium ions enter by a paracellular route through the "tight" junctions; water enters primarily via diffusion through the hepatocyte. Secretion of HCO_3^- across the canalicular membrane, mediated by a Cl^-/HCO_3^- exchanger, also promotes bile flow.

In human beings, about 80% of water secretion is canalicular in origin, most of which is bile salt–dependent. Thus with native bile salts, which aggregate within the proximal biliary tree to form polymolecular aggregates called *micelles* (from the New Latin *micella,* a grain), water secretion is less than with other secreted organic anions that do not aggregate extensively at canalicular concentrations.

The remainder of water secretion comes from the epithelial-ductular cells lining the intrahepatic and extrahepatic biliary tree. The gastrointestinal hormone *secretin* stimulates bile duct water secretion by binding to its basolateral receptor and increasing intracellular cyclic adenosine monophosphate (cAMP), which activates the apical membrane cystic fibrosis transmembrane conductance regulator (CFTR). The properties of this chloride secretory system are shared with many other epithelia, including the respiratory tree, small and large intestine, and pancreas, but secretin receptors are found on bile and pancreatic ductular cells only. Hydrophilic bile salts such as ursodeoxycholic acid can stimulate Cl^- secretion via Ca^{2+}-mediated mechanisms. Enhanced Cl^- secretion has several consequences: depolarization of the cell results in cellular HCO_3^- entry via the basolateral Na^+/HCO_3^- symport; luminal Cl^- and cellular HCO_3^- are exchanged by the apical membrane Cl^-/HCO_3^- exchanger; and Na^+ reaches the lumen by a paracellular route, thereby generating a

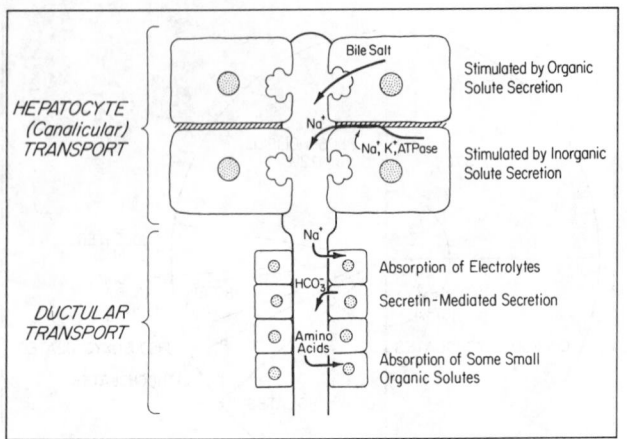

FIGURE 349-2 Bile water production at different levels of the biliary system. Canalicular water secretion follows the osmotic gradients established principally by secretion of bile salts, and, to a lesser extent, of glutathione and inorganic electrolytes (principally chloride, with operation of a chloride/HCO_3^- exchanger to produce a $NaHCO_3$-rich secretion). Ductular water secretion is mediated in large part by chloride entry into bile by the secretin-stimulated cystic fibrosis transmembrane conductance regulator (CFTR), followed by chloride/HCO_3^- exchange. In both hepatocytes and bile duct epithelial cells the basolateral Na^+, K^+-ATPase, and K^+ conductance channel act to maintain a high extracellular Na^+ concentration.

$NaHCO_3$-rich secretion. As with the hepatocyte, transcellular water movement follows the osmotic gradient. Unlike in the hepatocyte, apical membrane water channels have been identified in bile duct epithelial cells and may participate in water secretion.

Resorption of water occurs along the entire length of the bile duct system, but chiefly in the gallbladder secondary to electrolyte absorption and, to some extent, to the absorption of small organic solutes such as amino acids.

BILE LIPIDS
Bile Salts and the Enterohepatic Circulation

Bile salts* are synthesized from cholesterol, and have sharply defined hydrophobic (nonpolar) and hydrophilic (polar) surfaces. They are soluble amphiphilic molecules that possess detergent-like properties. In excess of their maximum monomeric concentrations, bile salt molecules self-associate via their hydrophobic portions to form small water-soluble micelles, incorporating a lesser number of molecules than is typical for detergents. The solute concentration at which these micelles form is just above the maximum monomeric solubility (1 to 3 mM), which is defined as the *critical micellar concentration*.

As part of the enterohepatic circulation that cycles bile salts from the liver to the gut and back to the liver again, bile salts are subject to structural transformations by both hepatocytes and gut bacteria. The changeable portion of the bile salt molecule is the polar surface (Fig. 349-3), resulting in significant variability in the amphiphilic properties of these molecules. For example, a bile salt with three hydroxyl groups (cholate) is completely water-soluble and readily forms micelles, whereas a bile salt with one hydroxyl group (lithocholate) is water-insoluble and cannot form micelles. In the liver the carboxyl side chain is conjugated to the amino acids taurine or glycine via an amide linkage, and much less commonly a sulfate or glucuronyl group is esterified to the hydroxyl group in the 3-carbon position. All of these conjugating groups can be removed by colonic bacterial

---

*The terms *bile salt* and *bile acid* are used interchangeably in this chapter. It should be recognized, however, that the salt (ionized) form of these molecules, which is found in bile and small intestine, is more polar and more water-soluble than the acid (protonated) form and thus is of greater physiologic importance. The sparingly soluble protonated bile acids are, in health, principally found only in the colon and in portal venous blood, but are converted completely to the salt form by conjugation during a single passage through the liver.

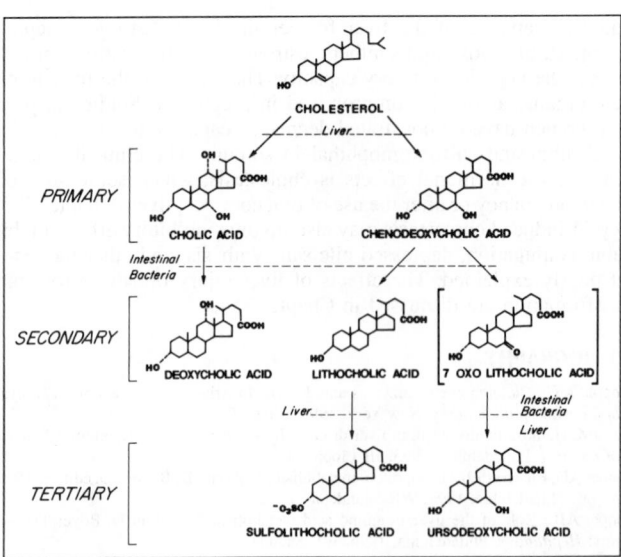

FIGURE 349-3 Major bile acids in human beings. The primary bile acids are synthesized from cholesterol in the liver. Subsequent bacterial (and/or hepatic) modifications result in secondary and tertiary bile acids. (Some authorities eschew the "tertiary" nomenclature and group all bacterially modified bile acids as "secondary" irrespective of subsequent bacterial or hepatic metabolism.) Normally, 7-oxolithocholic acid is a trace constituent of bile.

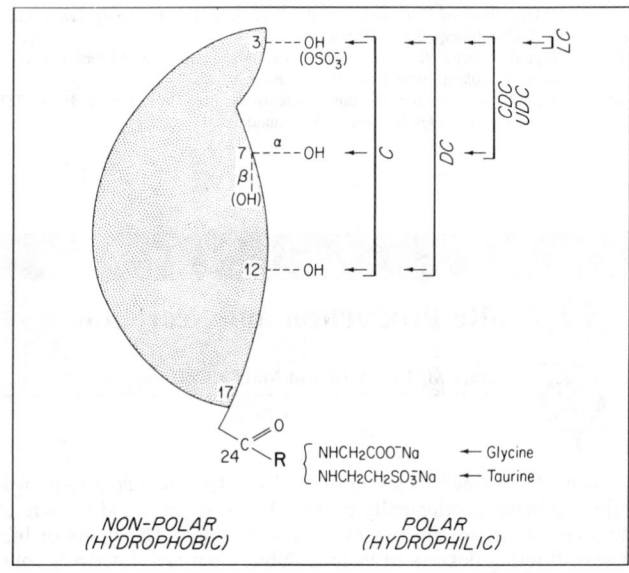

FIGURE 349-4 Amphiphilic structure of common human bile salts. Arrows indicate position and number of polar substituents. *C*, Cholates; *DC*, deoxycholates; *CDC*, chenodeoxycholates; *UDC*, ursodeoxycholates; *LC*, lithocholates; *R*, physiologic glycine or taurine conjugates found in bile and proximal small intestine. R is replaced by an OH group when bile salts are deconjugated in the colon. In UDC the C-7 OH group is equatorial ("β"); for all other common bile salts the C-7 OH group is perpendicular or axial ("α"). In LC the C-3 OH group is predominantly sulfated.

enzymes. Bile salts therefore must be viewed as a family of molecules whose physical-chemical properties are in a constant state of flux, as a result of important biochemical alterations by bacterial and hepatocellular enzymes and by the variable H^+ ion concentrations in the gastrointestinal tract, all of which change their aqueous solubilities.

Cholic and chenodeoxycholic acids (Fig. 349-4) are termed *primary bile acids* because they are synthesized de novo from unesterified cholesterol in hepatocytes. *Secondary bile acids* are formed by removal or dehydrogenation of the 7α-hydroxyl moiety on primary bile salts by anaerobic intestinal bacteria; *tertiary bile acids* result from hepatic or bacterial modifications of secondary bile acids.

Cholic and chenodeoxycholic acids are the end-products of an extensive series of enzymatic reactions beginning with microsomal 7α-hydroxylation of cholesterol. This reaction is rate limiting and is regulated by the magnitude of bile salt return to the liver in the portal venous blood. Subsequent synthetic steps involve additional hydroxylation to the steroid nucleus (principally by microsomal 12α-hydroxylase), hydroxylation of the 27-carbon in the mitochondria (sterol 27-hydroxylase), and cleavage of the branched aliphatic side chain of the parent cholesterol molecule by β-oxidation to form a 24-carbon carboxylated bile acid in peroxisomes. Hydroxylation of cholesterol in the C-27 position is also believed to play an important but as yet unquantified role in bile acid synthesis. Plasma lipoproteins ferry 27-hydroxycholesterol as a fatty acid ester generated in peripheral tissues to the liver, where it can be converted to chenodeoxycholic acid after 7α-hydroxylation by a hepatic enzyme different from that which 7α-hydroxylates cholesterol.

As the predominant organic solutes in bile, bile salts must be completely water-soluble under all pathophysiologic conditions. The hepatic conjugation reaction is a two-step process involving a microsomal enzyme (bile acid:CoA ligase) followed by a cytosolic enzyme (bile acid–S–CoA:glycine/taurine *N*-acyltransferase). Conjugation with taurine or glycine (see Fig. 349-3) lowers the pK_a value of the ionizable group—modestly in the case of glycine (which has a carboxyl group), and markedly in the case of taurine (which has a sulfonate group). The solubility of conjugated bile salts is thereby increased over that of the respective unconjugated bile acid for any physiologic bile salt concentration, calcium concentration, and pH.

In human beings the normal pattern of conjugation results in a glycine/taurine conjugated bile salt ratio of approximately 3:1. When excessive demands are placed on conjugation, the ratio can increase to 10:1 or even 20:1. This might occur when enhanced hepatic bile salt synthesis from cholesterol occurs in the setting of intestinal bile salt malabsorption, or when unconjugated ursodeoxycholic acid is given in pharmacologic doses for chronic liver disease or cholesterol gallstones. An additional specialized form of conjugation occurs for the highly insoluble secondary bile salt lithocholate. In human beings a small amount of this bile salt (about 20% of that generated by intestinal bacteria) is absorbed each day by the large intestine and is returned to the liver, where it is rendered water-soluble for biliary secretion by side-chain conjugation with glycine or taurine and, in 80% of the molecules, by sulfation at its single hydroxyl group (see Figs. 349-3 and 349-4).

In humans, three uncommon microsomal pathways involving glycosidic linkages of both conjugated and nonconjugated bile acids have been identified: hydroxyl or side-chain carboxylic glucuronidation, hydroxyl glucosidation, and hydroxyl *N*-acetylglucosaminidation. In cholestasis when bile flow is impaired, both sulfation and these specialized forms of glycosidation are induced, facilitating the elimination of all common bile acids in urine.

Deoxycholic and lithocholic acids, the physiologically important secondary bile acids (see Fig. 349-4), are formed in the distal small intestine and colon by the action of strictly anaerobic bacteria. Although bacterial enzymatic dehydroxylations and epimerizations result in the production of a large number of other molecular species, only these and 7-oxolithocholic acid are reabsorbed into the portal circulation and have a continuing biologic life. The majority of bacterially transformed bile salts are sparingly water-soluble, poorly characterized derivatives that are excreted directly in the feces or, if absorbed, in the urine.

The enterohepatic circulation of bile salts is a highly efficient conserving system (Fig. 349-5). After delivery to the gut, 95% to 98% of the bile salts are reabsorbed by the small intestine (chiefly in the ileum), returned to the liver via the portal vein, effectively taken up by hepatocytes, and resecreted into bile. Consequently, peripheral blood bile acid concentrations are extremely low (<5 μM), and urinary excretion is trivial in healthy persons. Because the bile salt secretion rate into bile over the period of a day is appreciably larger than the size of the bile salt pool, it is clear that each bile salt molecule must recirculate a number of times each day.

The small portion of secreted bile salts that is lost by fecal excretion is balanced by hepatic bile salt synthesis, thereby maintaining a

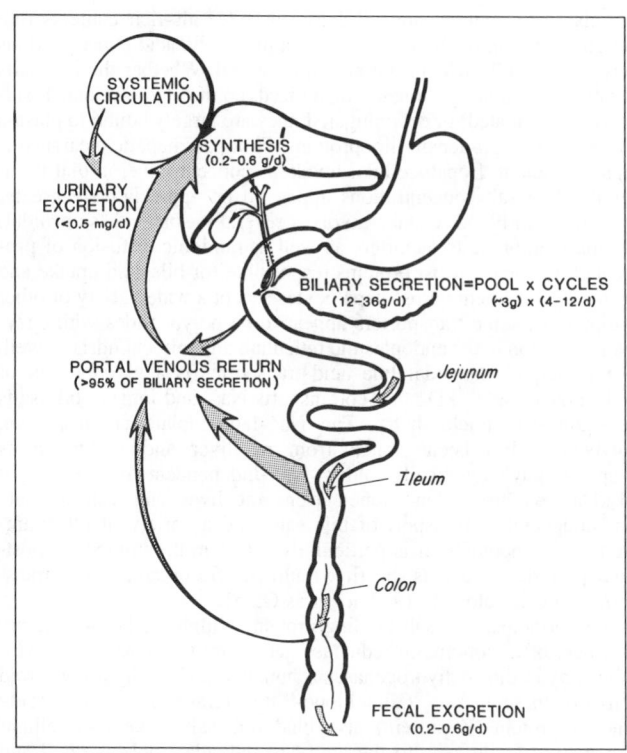

FIGURE 349-5   Enterohepatic circulation of bile salts in normal human beings. Arrows indicate bile salt movement within the biliary tree, intestine, portal venous system, and liver with a small "spill-over" into the systemic circulation. Fecal excretion is physiologically important since it must be balanced by catabolism of the same mass of cholesterol intrahepatically to replace the lost bile salts.

constant bile salt secretory rate. However, short-term variability in bile salt secretion rates arises from several sources: (1) gallbladder sequestration of a large fraction of the bile salt pool during periods of fasting (such as during sleep); (2) variable intestinal transit time, which is responsible for the rate of delivery of bile salts to sites of absorption; and (3) preferential absorption of bile salts of varying polarities at different levels of the intestinal tract. Specifically, dihydroxylated glycine-conjugated bile salts are moderately lipid-soluble, so they diffuse passively across the mucosa of the proximal intestine, and this accounts for a significant portion of their absorption. These relatively hydrophobic glycine-conjugated bile salts thus recirculate most rapidly, whereas taurine conjugates, which are always charged and therefore highly hydrophilic, are absorbed almost exclusively by active transport in the distal ileum, and recirculate more slowly. The mammalian ileal bile salt transporter is Na$^+$-dependent and Na$^+$-saturable, with a high affinity for a broad spectrum of bile salts containing a single fully dissociated anionic side chain. The functional Na$^+$–bile acid transporter in the rabbit ileum is composed of four integral 93-kDa and four peripheral 14-kDa subunits. The rabbit, human, and hamster transporters have now been cloned, and an identical apical polypeptide is present in the proximal tubules of the kidney. The renal transporter apparently serves as a backup mechanism to conserve monovalent bile salts in blood that have been filtered by the glomeruli.

Certain less stringent anaerobic intestinal bacteria enzymatically hydrolyze the peptide bond of conjugated bile salts to liberate "free" bile salts, a process called *deconjugation*. These free bile salts are readily protonated at quasineutral intestinal pH to form bile acids, which are absorbed by passive diffusion at all levels of the intestine. Because intestinal bacteria are confined primarily to the distal ileum and colon in healthy persons, unconjugated bile acids predominate in these portions of the gut and recirculate most slowly.

Most hepatic uptake and secretion of bile salts are Na$^+$-dependent and ATP-driven processes, respectively. When the gallbladder is stimulated to contract and discharge its bile salt–rich contents into the gut lumen in the hours following a meal, bile acid concentrations may approach 75 μM in portal venous blood. Whether the bile salts in portal blood are protonated or ionized, conjugated (amidated, sulfated, glycosidated) or deconjugated, they are largely bound to plasma albumin and high-density lipoproteins. First-pass hepatic clearance is highly efficient. Hepatocellular uptake is concentrative, in that intracellular bile salt concentrations appear to be appreciatively greater than in portal blood. Uptake involves several basolateral (sinusoidal) plasma membrane transporters as well as nonionic diffusion of protonated bile acids. Most proteins responsible for bile acid uptake and vectorial movement across hepatocytes accept a wide variety of other compounds; some transporters appear to be polypeptides with enzymatic function in the endoplasmic reticulum and mitochondria as well. The principal sinusoidal bile acid transporter is a glycoprotein of molecular mass 49-kDa that cotransports Na^+ and ionized bile salts in equimolar stoichiometry. The Na^+-taurocholate cotransporting polypeptide has been cloned from rat liver and is known as Ntcp. A phylogenetically older, Na^+-independent transporter of 54-kDa has also been cloned from rat liver and can mediate Na^+-independent transport of bile salts and a variety of other amphiphilic compounds. It is particularly active in the immediate postnatal period. Since it is the first multispecific organic anion–transporting protein cloned, it is known as Oatp1.

The principal bile salt binding proteins within the hepatocyte are members of a monomeric reductase gene family, consisting of cytosolic dihydrodiol dehydrogenase in humans, and 3α-hydroxysteroid dehydrogenase in rats. Glutathione-S-transferase and a fatty acid–binding protein (Z protein) also bind bile salts. The transcellular movement of bile salts to the apical (canalicular) pole is rapid and appears to be mediated by diffusion through the cytosol while bound to these soluble proteins. The unbound fraction of bile salts interacts reversibly with the membranes of intracellular organelles, including the Golgi apparatus, mitochondria, and endoplasmic reticulum; the latter interaction appears to stimulate biliary phospholipid movement to the canalicular membrane.

Bile salts are transported from the hepatocellular cytosol across the canalicular membrane into canalicular spaces against a chemical gradient of about 500-fold. Although it is certain that energy from ATP hydrolysis plays the major role, several candidate canalicular polypeptides each with a relative molecular mass (M_r) of about 100 kDa have been identified on the rat canalicular membrane. Although the negative intracellular electrical potential of about 30 to 40 mV can account for some of the driving force for bile salt secretion, a role for electrogenic transport remains controversial since a potential driven bile salt uptake system has also been identified in microsomes (endoplasmic reticulum), which invariably contaminate canalicular membrane preparations. A second, less specific ATP-driven transport system, the canalicular multifunctional organic anion transporter (cMOAT), has been cloned. This transporter mediates primary active secretion of a wide variety of divalent organic anions, including sulfated and glucuronidated bile salts and bilirubin glucuronides. Several stimuli—including enhanced transcellular flux of bile salts, cellular alkalinization, osmotic swelling, and possibly membrane potential—stimulate the insertion of transport proteins into the canalicular membrane. This occurs via microtubule-dependent delivery of protein-containing vesicles to the canalicular membrane from the basolateral membrane and intracellular sites, constituting a fundamental mechanism for regulation of transport capacity of the canalicular membrane for bile salts and other ions.

BILE LECITHIN SECRETION

Lecithin (phosphatidylcholine), the second most prevalent biliary solute, is also an amphiphilic molecule with two long-chain fatty acids composing its nonpolar hydrophobic portion and phosphorylcholine composing its polar hydrophilic portion. Unlike bile salts, however, lecithin molecules possess no true water solubility. Instead, pure lecithin forms bilayer membranes of lipid molecules interleaved with water and can incorporate substantial amounts of unesterified cholesterol, which is also water-insoluble. These self-aggregates are called *liquid crystals* and are prototypical of the unilamellar membranes of living cells.

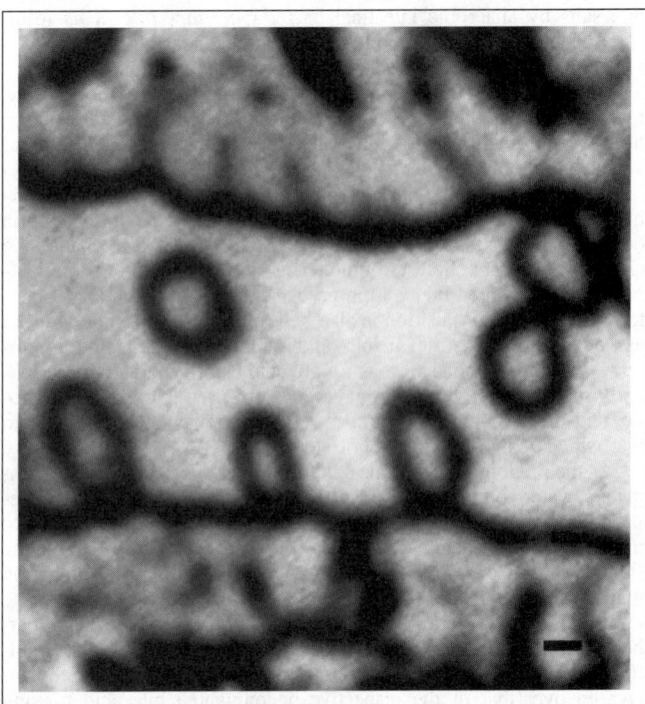

FIGURE 349-6 Electron micrograph of biliary vesicle formation and secretion on the exoplasmic face of the canalicular membrane. It is believed that biliary-type lecithin molecules are synthesized in the endoplasmic reticulum, released by bile salts, and delivered to the canalicular membrane via binding to cytosolic phosphatidylcholine transfer protein (PC-TP). Transmembrane translocation ("flipping") from the inner to the outer hemileaflet of the canalicular membrane most likely occurs via an mdr2-encoded P-glycoprotein (encoded by *MDR3* in humans). Bile salts probably aid lecithin secretion by inducing vesiculation of lecithin microdomains on the outer hemileaflet of the canalicular membrane. The electron spectroscopic image was taken of rat liver cryofixed in situ and shows that most vesicles are adherent to the luminal aspect of the canalicular membrane. The bar represents 500 Å.

Several principles are operative with regard to lecithin secretion. First, although bile lecithins are derived from hepatocytes, the pattern of molecular species (with predominantly palmitic acid in the C-1 position and linoleic or oleic acids in the C-2 position) is distinct, being less hydrophobic in character than the overall lecithin pattern found in hepatocyte membranes. Second, bile lecithins do not originate from lecithins internalized from circulating lipoproteins, including gut-derived chylomicra or, in the short term, from de novo synthesis within the hepatocyte. Third, bile salt secretion is required for elution of lecithin molecules into bile. Lecithin secretion increases in a curvilinear manner with increasing bile salt secretion over a wide range, plateauing at high rates of bile salt output.

Recent evidence suggests that acylglycerides within the endoplasmic reticulum, including triglycerides, are the major source for synthesis of biliary-type lecithin molecules. Subselection of these molecules intracellularly is most likely accomplished by a specific cytosolic phosphatidylcholine transfer protein (PC-TP), and their removal from the endoplasmic reticulum membrane can be activated by submicellar cytosolic concentrations of bile salts. PC-TP transports lecithin molecules in a 1:1 complex and is hypothesized to deposit them in the inner hemileaflet of the canalicular domain of the plasma membrane. A specific phospholipid transmembrane translocator then "flips" the lecithin molecules to the outer hemileaflet, where they form microdomains. The absence of lecithin in bile of mice lacking the P-glycoprotein encoded by the *mdr2* gene strongly implicates this protein as the "flippase" (the equivalent P-glycoprotein in humans is encoded by *MDR3*). Ionized bile salts, continuously secreted into the canalicular lumen, partition into these microdomains, and since they cannot "flip" back to the inner hemileaflet, they build up a critical pressure within these lecithin microdomains, resulting in selective ve-

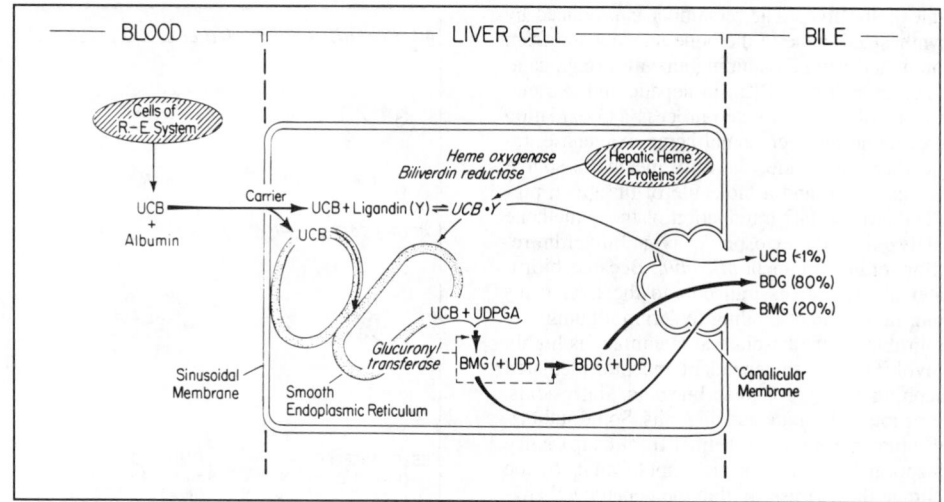

FIGURE 349-7 Metabolic determinants of biliary cholesterol secretion. The rate-limiting enzymes are 3-hydroxy-3-methylglutaryl CoA reductase (cholesterol [Ch] synthesis), acyl-CoA cholesterol acyltransferase (cholesteryl ester [ChE] synthesis), cholesteryl ester hydrolase (ChE hydrolysis), and cholesterol 7-hydroxylase (bile salt synthesis). The major lipoproteins, LDL as well as VLDL remnants, and chylomicron remnants are internalized by hepatocytes after binding to basolateral apolipoprotein B/E, hepatic lipase, and LRP receptors; HDL cholesterol and cholesteryl esters also transfer to the hepatocyte without internalization of HDL via docking with the sinusoidal SR-BI receptor.

siculation of the outer hemileaflet. *Unilamellar vesicles* (from the Latin *vesicula,* a small bladder) of 600 to 800 Å diameter are thereby formed on the outer face of the canalicular membrane and can be visualized by cryofixation techniques (Fig. 349-6). Because of the detergent action of the high bile salt concentrations present in the proximal biliary tree, these vesicles dissolve progressively into micelles.

BILE CHOLESTEROL SECRETION

As individual molecules, unesterified cholesterol is insoluble in water. Self-aggregates of cholesterol molecules precipitate as *cholesterol monohydrate crystals,* the major components of most gallstones. In the hepatocyte, cholesterol is solubilized by membrane phospholipids and, despite its synthesis in the endoplasmic reticulum, is found predominantly (80%) in the plasma membrane. Biliary cholesterol is derived principally from the cholesterol in the surface coat and within the lipid core of plasma lipoproteins. Cholesterol stored as esterified cholesterol and cholesterol that is newly synthesized by the liver make far smaller contributions to biliary cholesterol secretion. Cholesterol appears to arrive at the canalicular membrane independent of biliary lecithin molecules. Possible mechanisms for its delivery include (1) release from lysosomal hydrolysis of lipoprotein cholesteryl esters, followed by cytosolic trafficking via binding to sterol carrier protein–2 (SCP-2); (2) intracellular trafficking in "sterol-rich" vesicles; and (3) diffusion of free cholesterol from the surface coat of extracellular lipoproteins to the hepatocyte basolateral plasma membrane, followed by lateral diffusion to the canalicular domain. Because cholesterol readily "flip-flops" across membrane bilayers, it can distribute widely throughout both leaflets of cell membranes. It has been estimated that, in the healthy human, approximately 1% of hepatocellular free cholesterol is secreted into bile every hour.

As with lecithin, the relation of cholesterol secretion to bile salt secretion is curvilinear and plateaus at high bile salt secretion rates. However, the plateau for cholesterol secretion rate is considerably lower than that for lecithin, leading to wide variability in the relative secretion rates of bile salts, lecithin, and cholesterol under different physiologic conditions and among different individuals. It is not known whether cholesterol is released from the canalicular membrane in association with newly formed lecithin vesicles, or whether it is released so indirectly, being first extracted by luminal bile salts or by other, as yet unidentified, transporters.

The physiologic determinants of biliary cholesterol secretion (Fig. 349-7) are as follows:

1. The endocytosed lipoprotein cholesterol (from low-density lipoproteins and chylomicron remnants), which is dependent on sinusoidal expression of apolipoprotein B/E-receptor, hepatic lipase, and LDL-related protein (LRP) receptor activities.
2. The transferance to the hepatocyte of free and esterified cholesterol resulting mainly from transient docking of "circulating" or "plasma" high-density lipoproteins to a sinusoidal scavenger receptor known as SR-BI.
3. Hepatic cholesterol synthesis, catalyzed by the rate-limiting enzyme 3-hydroxy-3-methylglutaryl CoA reductase (HMG CoA reductase).
4. The disposition of cholesterol within the liver, which proceeds along four pathways:
   A. Esterification of free cholesterol to cholesteryl ester (catalyzed by acyl-CoA cholesterol acyltransferase, ACAT) during formation of very-low-density lipoprotein (VLDL), a process that is accelerated by increased triglyceride formation.
   B. Hydrolysis of cholesteryl esters by neutral (nonlysosomal) cholesteryl ester hydrolase (CEH).
   C. Conversion of free cholesterol to bile acids (catalyzed by cholesterol 7α-hydroxylase and stimulated principally by intestinal bile acid loss).
   D. Availability of solubilizing lipids within the canalicular lumen (i.e., bile salts and lecithins).

Over prolonged periods, biliary cholesterol secretion in humans can be increased by either increases in dietary cholesterol (via hepatic chylomicron remnant uptake), or increased return of peripheral tissue cholesterol in lipoproteins to the liver (as during rapid weight loss in obese patients). In the latter instance, fasting may also reduce the enterohepatic cycling of bile salts, producing in predisposed individuals a marked increase in the cholesterol/bile salt ratio in bile, and a resultant increased risk for cholesterol gallstone formation. Lastly, biliary cholesterol secretion may be increased during drug therapy for hypercholesterolemia.

BILIRUBIN PRODUCTION AND SECRETION

Bilirubin is the major end-product of the catabolism of heme. (For further discussion of bilirubin production and secretion, see Chapter 353.) Its production rate is about 350 mg/day, and it is derived principally (80%) from senescent red cell hemoglobin in the reticuloendothelial cells of the spleen and liver. The remainder is produced by destruction of newly synthesized heme in the bone marrow and from the turnover of myoglobin, and heme-containing enzymes (e.g., catalase) and coenzymes (e.g., cytochrome P_{450}) in hepatic and extrahepatic tissues. Bilirubin formation is a two-step process: (1) oxidation of the α-carbon bridge of heme by microsomal heme oxygenase, releasing a molecule of carbon monoxide (the only metabolic source of the gas in human beings), iron, and a molecule of the green pigment, biliverdin; and (2) the quantitative reduction of the γ-methene bridge of biliverdin, catalyzed by the cytosolic enzyme biliverdin reductase to form the yellow-orange pigment *bilirubin*. Because bilirubin is insoluble in water at pH 7.4, its transport to the liver takes place in plasma via tight, noncovalent binding to serum albumin.

Hepatic uptake of bilirubin by the basolateral membrane is highly efficient. The process involves a Na^+-independent, receptor-mediated uptake used also by unconjugated hydrophobic bile acids, fatty acids, and many drugs, but not by ionized conjugated bile salts. Some authorities believe that the bilirubin transporter is distinct from Oatp1 since it is inhibitable by cyclosporin A. Albumin itself is not taken up by the liver but appears to facilitate the process. Within the hepatocyte's cytosol, bilirubin is bound first to an acceptor protein, historically called *ligandin* (or protein Y), but now known to be glutathione-S-transferase. Binding to cytosolic fatty acid binding protein also occurs. It has been postulated that bilirubin transfers rapidly between intracellular membranes in vivo, and that binding proteins such as ligandin slow this process by retarding the rates of cytosolic diffusion.

Bilirubin is a substrate for uridine diphosphate glucuronosyltransferase (UGT) located in the endoplasmic reticulum, which couples β-D-glucuronic acid (or, less commonly, β-D-glucose or β-D-xylose) in ester linkage to one or both propionic acid side chains of bilirubin. The resulting conjugates are all water-soluble and are excreted rapidly in bile via the cMOAT system (see earlier discussion). Although transport via cMOAT is shared with many other organic dianions, lithocholate 3-sulfate and 3-O-glucuronide are the major utilizers of this transportor in health because of the enterohepatic circulation of the monohydroxy bile acids. Normally, the diconjugates (bilirubin diglucuronide with traces of bilirubin monoglucoside-monoglucuronide or monoxyloside-monoglucuronide diesters) predominate in bile (80%). The monoconjugates (bilirubin monoglucuronide with traces of monoglucoside or monoxyloside) constitute the remainder, and unconjugated bilirubin constitutes less than 1% of total bile pigments.

Bilirubin conjugates are waste products with no certain physiologic function, although they may act as antioxidants in liver and bile. In the adult, bilirubin conjugates are not reabsorbed from the intestine. However, the intraluminal bacterial flora of the colon deconjugate bilirubin and reduce the unconjugated form to a number of colorless urobilinogens. Urobilinogens are absorbed in part by passive diffusion from the colon cycle enterohepatically in the portal vein, and, after uptake into the hepatocytes (95%), are excreted in bile or in the urine (5%).

ASSEMBLY AND STRUCTURE OF BILE

Each of the major bile lipids contain large hydrophobic portions (steroid nucleus for bile salts and cholesterol, acyl hydrocarbon chains for lecithin) and relatively small polar functions (hydroxyl, carboxyl groups, or similar). Accordingly, these amphiphilic molecules form true (monomeric) solutions only when very dilute (Fig. 349-8). Above the limit of their monomeric concentrations, bile salts form micelles, lecithin molecules form stacked bilayer liquid crystals, and cholesterol molecules form *cholesterol monohydrate crystals.* When lecithin liquid crystals are dilute, especially in the presence of a submicellar bile salt concentration, the liquid crystals spontaneously form *vesicles.* Closed spherical structures of average 600 to 800 Å diameter are observed in freshly secreted canalicular bile by light scattering.

In hepatic and gallbladder biles, luminal concentrations of bile salts are well above their critical micellar concentrations, and their micelles have large capacities and solubilize lecithin and cholesterol molecules, leading to micellar dissolution of the secreted vesicles. The solubilization process is not a simple transition but proceeds via another liquid crystalline structure, a rod-shaped particle that is a fragment of a hexagonal liquid crystalline phase. With typical biliary compositions (see Fig. 349-1), the mixed micelles are not of uniform size, composition, or structure but are composed of two distinct species:

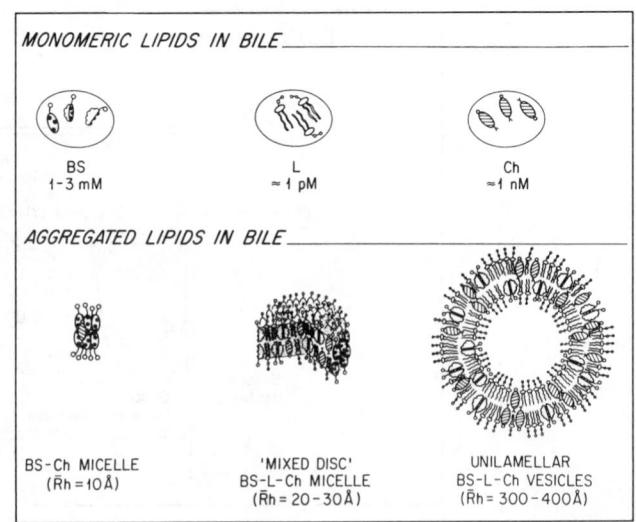

FIGURE 349-8 Schematic models of the major biliary lipid molecules with depictions of the average sizes and structures of the mixed micelles and unilamellar vesicles found in human bile. *BS,* Bile salt; *L,* lecithin; *Ch,* cholesterol; *Rh* mean hydrodynamic radius; *Å,* angstroms (10^{-10} m). Monomeric solubilities are given in SI units.

(1) bile salt–cholesterol micelles ("simple" mixed micelles), in which cholesterol is simply apposed to bile salt molecules; and (2) larger bile salt–lecithin–cholesterol micelles, in which a loosely organized fragment of a lecithin bilayer or rod is saturated with cholesterol and enveloped on its perimeter by bile salt molecules (Fig. 349-8). Cholesterol is about five times more soluble in mixed than in simple micelles because it interdigitates between the liquid hydrocarbon chains of the lecithin molecules.

All mammalian biles contain small unilamellar vesicles of lecithin-cholesterol and bile salt molecules that are about 10 times larger than the mixed micelles. These vesicles are found principally in hepatic bile but undergo continual transformation by bile salts into unsaturated mixed micelles during passage down the biliary tree. When bile salt micelles become saturated with cholesterol (a common occurrence in human hepatic and gallbladder bile), the biliary vesicles persist and become enriched in cholesterol by virtue of losing lecithin but not cholesterol molecules to bile salt micelles. In dilute human hepatic bile these vesicles are relatively stable and may be responsible for carrying up to 80% of the total biliary cholesterol content. Because of micellar solubilization in concentrated gallbladder bile, however, vesicles carry much less total cholesterol. The vesicles often become unstable and crystallize their cholesterol, setting the stage for cholesterol crystallization and gallstone formation.

In pure solution, bilirubin conjugates self-associate at concentrations in the 1- to 2-μM range to form dimers and, at higher concentrations, larger aggregates *(multimers).* Bilirubin multimers have no capacity to solubilize lecithin or cholesterol molecules. However, in the presence of both simple and mixed bile salt micelles, most of the conjugated bilirubin molecules in bile become strongly attached to the external hydrophilic parts, forming mixed aggregates of bile salts and bilirubin conjugates. As a consequence, bilirubin conjugates have little or no osmotic activity in bile. The small quantities of unconjugated bilirubin in bile may be preferentially associated with the hydrophobic interiors of biliary micelles and unilamellar vesicles.

PERTURBATIONS OF BILE PRODUCTION AND SECRETION
Obstructed Secretory Apparatus

The secretion of biliary lipids may fail as a result of functional or mechanical obstruction of the bile secretory apparatus. Obstruction can occur at any anatomic site in the biliary tree from liver cell to duodenum. Under these conditions the canalicular transport systems for bile salts and other ions redistribute partially to the basolateral plasma membrane. Moreover, the basolateral Na^+-dependent bile salt transporter is markedly down-regulated, potentially reducing the toxicity to hepatocytes of retained bile salts. Biliary lipids are shunted into the systemic circulation, leading to high levels of serum bile salt bound to albumin and all plasma lipoprotein classes; hyperbilirubinemia (jaundice); bilirubinuria; and the appearance of lipoprotein X, an abnormal, low-density lipoprotein containing biliary lecithin and unesterified cholesterol as unilamellar vesicles. In bile and blood, secondary bile salts disappear, and hepatic enzymes are induced to further hydroxylate, to sulfate, and glycosidate the primary bile salts, facilitating their renal clearance and urinary excretion. High levels of bile salts and perhaps other organic anions that are ordinarily secreted in bile and retained in blood and skin may induce severe pruritus.

Defective Bile Salt Synthesis

The bile salt pool may be reduced as a result of a congenital monoenzymatic defect or secondary to defective homeostatic mechanisms that are not fully understood. In these cases, hepatic bile salt synthesis is usually inappropriately low in the face of smaller than normal amounts of bile salt that are being recycled to the liver within the enterohepatic circulation. This is the situation in some nonobese cholesterol gallstone patients and in the normal newborn. In adults the shrunken bile salt pool may lead to a decrease in bile salt secretion rates, cholesterol-supersaturated or calcium (hydrogen) bilirubinate–supersaturated bile, and a propensity for gallstone formation.

Contaminated Small Bowel

In the contaminated small bowel syndrome, bile salt–metabolizing anaerobic bacteria colonize the jejunum, deconjugate and dehydroxylate bile salts, and result in the formation of sparingly soluble unconjugated deoxycholic and lithocholic acids in the small intestine. Only rarely do these hydrophobic bile acids precipitate intraluminally to form bile acid–fatty acid stones (enteroliths). More commonly the bile acids are absorbed by passive diffusion to enter portal venous blood and thereby short-circuit the enterohepatic circulation. Because intraluminal bile salt micelle formation is compromised, and unconjugated bile acids and anaerobic bacteria may injure the mucosa of the small intestine, malabsorption results (Chapter 340).

Increased Fecal Bile Salt Loss

Compensated Loss. Small bowel disease that is not extensive and involves the ileum (or the administration of certain drugs that bind intraluminally to bile salt) can lead to increased bile salt loss in the feces. In these instances, fecal loss is sufficiently small so that the liver can compensate with increased de novo synthesis from cholesterol to maintain the content of bile salts in the proximal small intestine above their critical micellar concentrations. However, the high flux of bile salt through the colon leads to secretory diarrhea and apparently promotes enterohepatic cycling of unconjugated bilirubin.

Decompensated Loss. The causes of decompensated fecal bile salt loss are often the same as those of a compensated loss but are more extensive and result in more severe clinical disease. In this situation, de novo synthesis of bile salt cannot keep pace with fecal loss, and a marked fall in the bile salt secretory rate results. This diminution in secretory rate leads to cholesterol-supersaturated or calcium (hydrogen) bilirubinate–supersaturated bile with the risk of gallstone formation; fat malabsorption; both bile salt– and fatty acid–induced secretory diarrhea; and increased oxalate absorption, hyperoxaluria, and an increased incidence of calcium oxalate kidney stones.

BIBLIOGRAPHY

Boyer JL: Bile duct epithelium: frontiers in transport physiology, *Am J Physiol* 270:G1-G5, 1996.

Carey MC, Duane WC: Enterohepatic circulation. In Arias IM, Boyer JL, Fausto N et al, editors: *The liver: biology and pathobiology*, New York, 1994, Raven Press, pp. 719-767.

Carey MC, LaMont JT: Cholesterol gallstone formation: 1. physical-chemistry of bile and biliary lipid secretion, *Prog Liver Dis* 10:139-163, 1992.

Cohen DE, Leonard MR and Carey MC: In vitro evidence that phospholipid secretion into bile may be coordinated intracellularly by the combined actions of bile salts and the specific phosphatidylcholine transfer protein of liver, *Biochemistry* 33:9975-9980, 1994.

Crawford JM: The role of vesicle-mediated transport pathways in hepatocellular bile secretion, *Sem Liver Dis* 16(1):16:169-189, 1996.

Crawford JM, Möckel G-M, Crawford AR et al: Imaging biliary lipid secretion in the rat: ultrastructural evidence for vesiculation of the hepatocyte canalicular membrane, *J Lipid Res* 36:2147-2163, 1995.

Green RM, Crawford JM: Hepatocellular cholestasis: pathobiology and histological outcome, *Semin Liver Dis* 15:372-389, 1995.

LaMont JT, Carey MC: Cholesterol gallstone formation: 2. pathobiology and pathomechanics, *Prog Liver Dis* 10:165-191, 1992.

Meier PJ: Molecular mechanisms of hepatic bile salt transport from sinusoidal blood to bile, *Am J Physiol* 269:G801-G812, 1995.

Möckel G, Gorti S, Tandon RK et al: Microscope laser light scattering spectroscopy of vesicles within canaliculi of rat hepatocyte couplets, *Am J Physiol* 269:G73-G84, 1995.

Noé B, Schleiss F, Wettstein M et al: Regulation of taurocholate excretion by a hypoosmolarity activated signal transduction pathway in rat liver, *Gastroenterology* 110:858-865, 1996.

Oude Elferink RPJ, Tytgat GNJ, Groen AK: The role of mdr2 P-glycoprotein in hepatobiliary lipid transport, *FASEB J* 11:19-28, 1997.

Smit JJM, Schinkel AH, Oude Elferink RPJ et al: Homozygous disruption of the murine mdr2 P-glycoprotein gene leads to a complete absence of phospholipid from bile and to liver disease, *Cell* 75:400-462, 1993.

Verkade HJ, Vonk RJ, Kuipers F: New insights into the mechanism of bile acid–induced biliary lipid secretion, *Hepatology* 21:1174-1189, 1995.

CHAPTER

350 Pancreatic Secretion

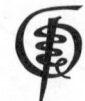

Laurence J. Miller

COMPOSITION, LOCATION, EMBRYOLOGIC DERIVATION, AND ORGANIZATION OF THE PANCREAS

The human pancreas is composed of distinct yet integrated exocrine and endocrine components, which are critical for the regulated assimilation of a meal, contributing toward its digestion and metabolism. It represents a finely lobulated, elongated solid organ, lying in the retroperitoneum at the level of the first lumbar vertebra, with its head in the duodenal sweep and its body and tail extending toward the hilum of the spleen. A clinically important uncinate process, representing a location for pancreatic carcinoma with a particularly poor prognosis, extends from the head of the gland posterior to the superior mesenteric vessels. Most of this organ serves an exocrine function to synthesize, secrete, and transport a large number of digestive enzymes in an electrolyte-rich alkaline milieu into the lumen of the duodenum. About one percent of the mass of the pancreas represents endocrine islets, which are scattered among the exocrine tissue. These are the site of synthesis and secretion of insulin, glucagon, and somatostatin. These two components, while physically distinct, are connected by an intrapancreatic islet-acinar portal circulation that provides a unique environment for the portion of the exocrine lobule affected. This has been the focus of intense investigation toward interactions between the endocrine and exocrine pancreas.

The pancreas develops from ventral and dorsal buds of endodermal cells, arising from the region of the caudal foregut that develops into the proximal duodenum (Fig. 350-1). As the duodenal sweep develops by rotating clockwise, the ventral bud moves to fuse with the dorsal bud. The ventral pancreatic bud develops into the uncinate process and the inferior portion of the mature pancreatic head, while the larger dorsal bud contributes the remainder of the gland. As these structures fuse, so do their component ductular elements, with the main pancreatic duct formed by the ductular component of the ventral bud and that of the distal portion of the dorsal bud. The proximal

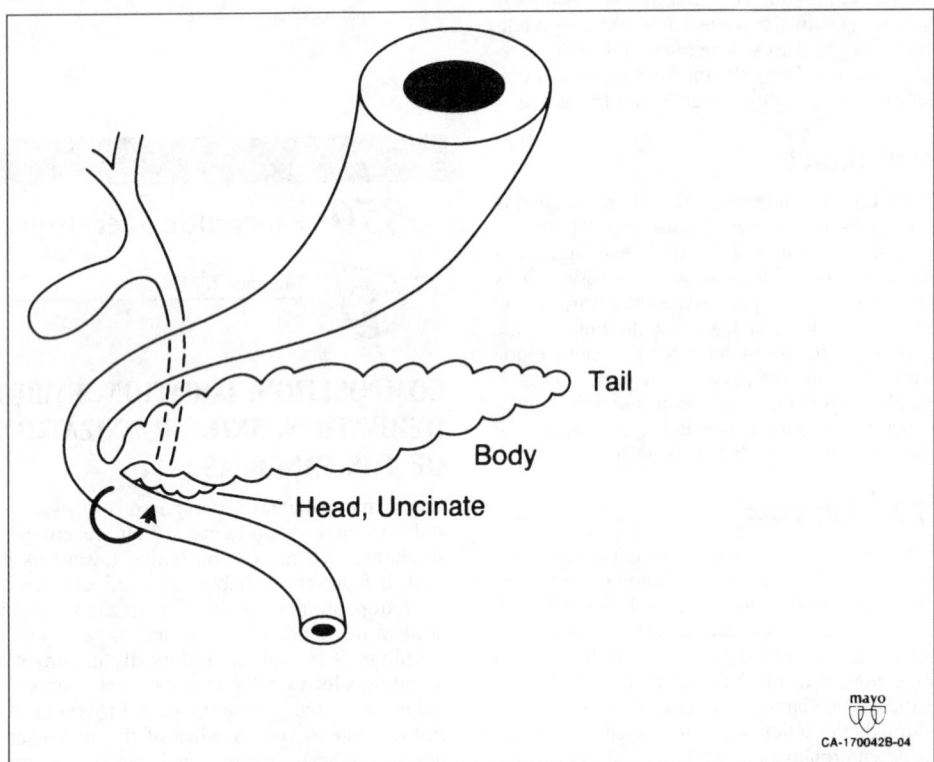

FIGURE 350-1   Pancreatic development. Shown are representations of the morphogenesis of the mature pancreas from dorsal and ventral buds of the primitive foregut. A critical rotation event occurs at the time of development of the duodenal sweep in which the pancreatic buds and their early ductular precursors fuse.

Continued.

region of the dorsal bud often persists as an accessory duct, contributing to the clinical entity of pancreas divisum.

The pancreatic parenchyma is derived from a common pool of endodermal precursor cells, which initially form a tubular network. These become primitive ductular structures. Acinar cells develop from clusters of cells at the distal ends of these structures, while islets develop from cells that migrate out of and between them. As the adult pancreas undergoes morphogenesis, the exocrine acinar cells organize into grape-like clusters (acini), which are organized into lobules by a hierarchy of structures that carry the secreted enzymes. Enzymesleave the apical pole of the acinar cells, at the level of the centroacinar cells, then move through intralobular or intercalated ducts, and into the in-

terlobular ducts. These traverse the loose connective tissue between the lobules in association with blood and lymphatic vessels and neural structures. The interlobular ducts coalesce to form the main pancreatic duct (Wirsung's duct) and the accessory duct (Santorini's duct), which drain into the duodenum.

The arterial supply of the pancreas comes from the celiac and superior mesenteric arteries, with the former giving rise to the pancreaticoduodenal and splenic arteries and the latter giving rise to the inferior pancreaticoduodenal artery. The veins travel adjacent to the arterial supply and drain into the portal vein either directly or indirectly via the splenic vein. The lymphatic drainage moves predominantly into the celiac nodes. A rich neural supply includes sympathetic, para-

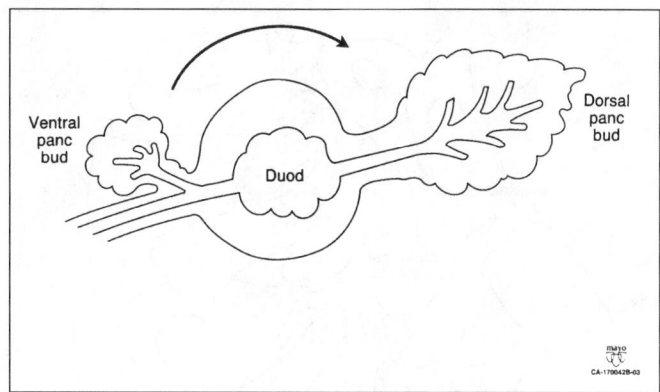

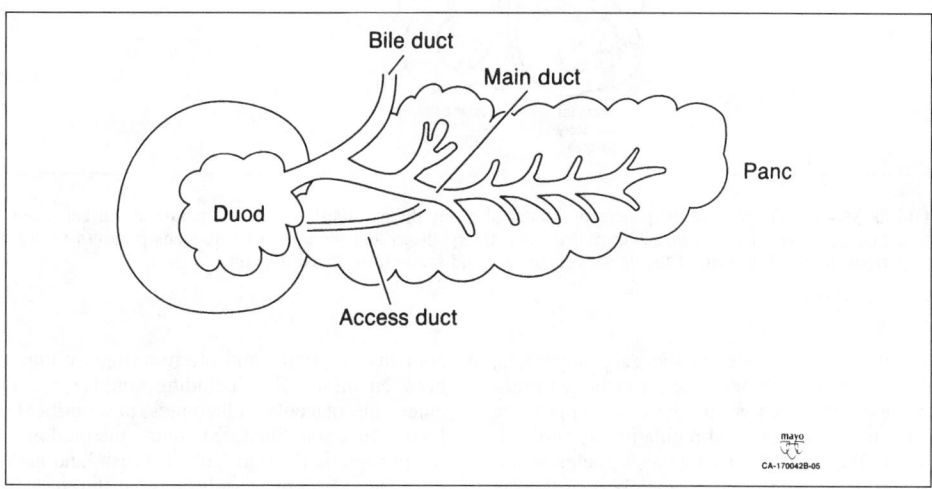

FIGURE 350-1, cont'd For legend see opposite page.

sympathetic, and peptidergic structures. The vagus gives rise to the preganglionic parasympathetic fibers, which largely traverse the celiac ganglion and terminate within intrinsic pancreatic ganglia. These give rise to fibers that terminate adjacent to the acinar cell clusters. Sympathetic fibers arising from the fifth through ninth thoracic ganglia lead to the celiac and superior mesenteric ganglia, where they give rise to postganglionic fibers that predominantly innervate the intrapancreatic vasculature. Pancreatic peptidergic fibers containing vasoactive intestinal polypeptide, peptide histidine isoleucine, calcitonin gene-related peptide, neuropeptide Y, substance P, gastrin-releasing peptide, enkephalin, and galanin have also been described.

In addition to understanding the venous and lymphatic drainage of the pancreas, knowledge of peripancreatic structures is important in the evaluation of the operability of malignancies arising within this organ. Posterior to the adult pancreas lies the inferior vena cava, superior mesenteric vessels, portal vein, celiac plexus, the crura of the diaphragm, and the left kidney. The common bile duct is often imbedded in the substance of the head of the pancreas as it courses toward the duodenum. The splenic artery runs along its upper border. Anterior to the pancreas is the lesser sac and the posterior gastric wall. Pancreatic neoplasms often reach substantial size and affect these associated structures before becoming clinically apparent, markedly reducing the ability to successfully treat these lesions.

CELLULAR ANATOMY, CELL BIOLOGY, AND PHYSIOLOGY OF THE EXOCRINE PANCREAS

Two types of cells are key in understanding pancreatic exocrine secretion: the acinar cell and the duct cell. Both are polarized epithelial cells, but each has its own specific role for its specialized secretory function and each has its own complement of receptors on its surface to enssure appropriate regulation and integration of its digestive functions. The acinar cell is the site of synthesis and regulated secretion

of the digestive enzymes, including proteases such as trypsin, chymotrypsin, carboxypeptidases A and B, and elastase, lipases, amylase, and ribonuclease. Normally, the proteases are secreted in inactive forms that become activated on entering the duodenum, where enterokinase converts trypsinogen to trypsin, which then activates the other enzymes in rapid succession. One of the postulated mechanisms for the initiation of pancreatitis is the premature activation of these proteases while still within the acinar cell. The mechanism for this and an effective way to block it are still not clear. The ductular tree provides a structural architecture for the acinar cells, conveys the secretory products of the acinar cells to the duodenum, and has an intrinsic secretory function for bicarbonate and electrolytes. It has been implicated in the pathogenesis of the pancreatic manifestations of cystic fibrosis and some forms of pancreatitis, and it is the likely origin of the vast majority of pancreatic carcinomas.

Acinar Cells

The acinar cell is the classic cellular model in which the biosynthetic and secretory cascade of events was initially described by Palade and his colleagues. The basal region of this pyramidal cell contains the nucleus and a well-developed biosynthetic machinery for the synthesis of proteins for export (Fig. 350-2). This includes an extensive network of rough endoplasmic reticulum and a prominent golgi apparatus, with scattered mitochondria to provide the needed energy. The apical portion of these cells is packed with maturing condensing vacuoles and mature zymogen granules, which are clustered adjacent to the microvillar membrane. Protein synthesis is initiated at the level of the membrane-bound ribosomes of the rough endoplasmic reticulum at the time of arrival of the messenger RNA that had been transcribed in the nucleus. The polypeptide chain cotranslationally traverses the microsomal membrane into the cisternal space. Posttranslational modifications begin there and proceed in an orderly man-

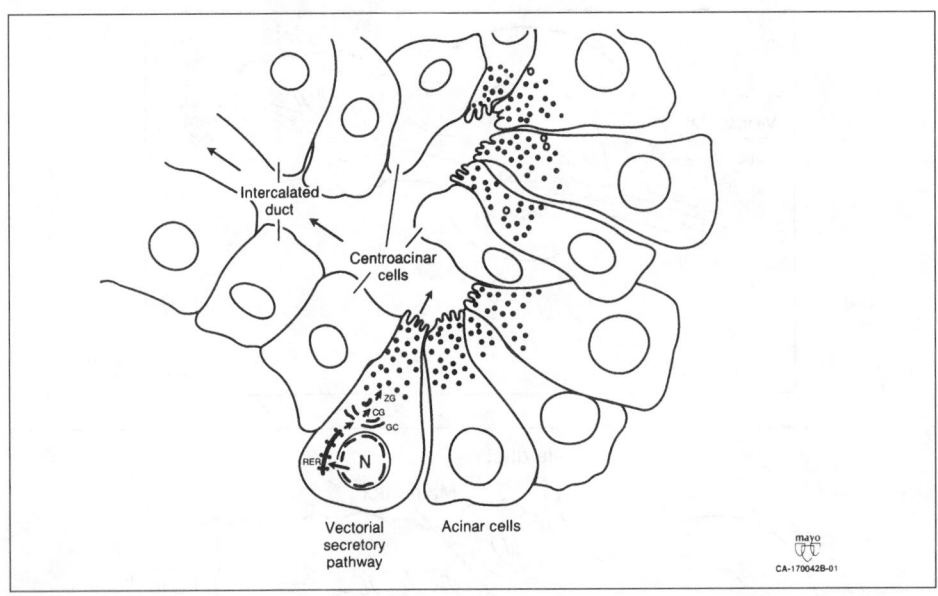

FIGURE 350-2 Diagram of the pancreatic lobule, showing the relationship between mature acinar cells, centroacinar cells, and the proximal intercalated duct. Biosynthesis and secretion of zymogens progress vectorially, from the basal domain of the acinar cell toward and through its apical domain.

ner as the protein moves through the stacks of the golgi apparatus, into condensing vacuoles, and ultimately into mature zymogen granules. The movement of these organelles within the cell seems to be dependent on a microtubular architecture and regulation by molecular motors such as kinesin. The process of exocytosis seems to involve small guanine nucleotide-binding proteins (members of the rab family), as well as synaptotagmins and synaptophysins. Ultimately, the membrane of the zymogen granule fuses with the apical plasmalemma and the contents are released into the lumen of the origin of the ductular tree, surrounded by centroacinar cells and the first ductular elements. The acinar cell must then recover the extensive new membrane from its apical domain by endocytosis, thereby recycling it for reuse in the active process of biosynthesis.

Key secretagogue receptors such as those for cholecystokinin have been localized to the basolateral plasmalemma of the pancreatic acinar cells. Thus stimulation by hormones and neurotransmitters comes from the location of the vascular supply and neural structures, and receptor occupation initiates well-defined cascades of biochemical events that terminate in apical exocytosis. The most relevant stimulus-activation cascades described to date include two groups of cascades of events initiated at guanine nucleotide-binding protein– (G protein)-bound receptors. In one, receptor occupation with agonists such as cholecystokinin and acetylcholine leads to the activation of phospholipase C, leading to the generation of inositol 1,4,5-trisphosphate and diacylglycerol, and the ultimate increase in intracellular calcium and activation of a number of key protein kinases. In the second, receptor occupation with agonists such as vasoactive intestinal polypeptide and secretin leads to the activation of adenylate cyclase with the generation of cyclic AMP (cAMP) and the activation of protein kinase A. Both cascades are capable of interaction and potentiation of the effects of the other cascade on secretion. Much recent evidence also links some of these events with regulation of other cellular activities such as growth.

Duct Cells

The duct cell is a cuboidal cell that is also polarized structurally and functionally, while having a structure quite distinct from that of the acinar cell. The endoplasmic reticulum, golgi complex, and secretory vesicles are much more sparse, and the mitochondria are much more prominent in these cells. This correlates with minimal protein synthetic function and substantial energy requirements to maintain its fluid and electrolyte secretory gradients. The apical plasmalemma contains microvilli and often a single cilium. Junctional complexes between these cells, including zonulae occludentes, zonulae adherentes, and macculae adherentes, are a critical component of their effective function. Scattered among the predominant ductular cell along the pancreatic duct are goblet, brush, and endocrine cells.

Although there are substantial differences in the secretagogue profile for duct cells from different species, all seem to respond to secretin by secreting a bicarbonate-rich fluid. There is a reciprocal relationship between the concentrations of bicarbonate and chloride (which are dependent on flow rate) due to an exchange mechanism between these anions. While bicarbonate concentration rises with increased flow rates, the fluid remains isotonic with plasma. There are few data characterizing potential heterogeneity among duct cells or identifying quantitative or qualitative differences in cells lining different size ducts along the ductular tree.

As noted previously, secretin seems to be a universal secretagogue for pancreatic duct cells of all species studied. Catecholamines and dopamine have both stimulatory and inhibitory effects on ducts of different species although they have no apparent effect on the human duct. Agents that may stimulate ductular secretion in some species include neurotensin, gastrin-releasing peptide, peptide histidine isoleucine, substance P, and enkephalin. Inhibitory agents include somatostatin, pancreatic polypeptide, peptide tyrosine tyrosine, glucagon, vasopressin, and calcitonin gene-related peptide. The physiologic roles of any of these potential transmitters is unclear.

Secretin stimulates the duct cell by binding to a G protein–coupled receptor that initiates the same cascade of events described for the acinar cell. This includes activation of adenylate cyclase. Of particular interest, this hormone and other agonists acting via receptors structurally related to it stimulate dual signalling pathways. In addition to the major activation of adenylate cyclase, they also stimulate the increase in intracellular calcium. Interactions between these two pathways clearly occur, and in a concentration-dependent manner. This is an active area of ongoing investigation.

Bicarbonate secretion by pancreatic duct cells seems to occur in two stages. The first involves active transport of bicarbonate across the basolateral plasmalemma, whereas the second involves passive diffusion down its electrochemical gradient across the apical plasmalemma. The vast majority of bicarbonate secreted into pancreatic juice comes from plasma, with only 7% coming from ductular metabolism. There is a requirement for sodium and potassium, consistent with a role for sodium-potassium-ATPase. Sodium/hydrogen exchangers, chloride/bicarbonate exchangers, and carbonic anhydrase also appear

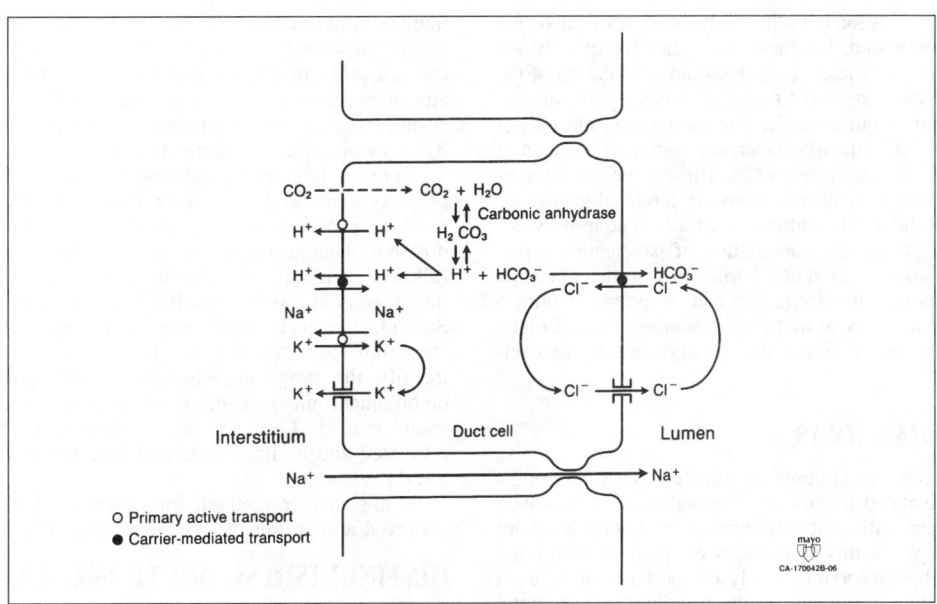

FIGURE 350-3   Proposed transport events through and around the pancreatic duct cell.

BOX 350-1
Neurohormonal regulation of pancreatic secretion

Stimulants and potentiators

Acetylcholine
Cholecystokinin
Secretin
Vasoactive intestinal polypeptide
Gastrin-releasing peptide
Calcitonin gene-related peptide
Peptide histidine isoleucine
Neurotensin
Substance P
Enkephalin
Motilin
Insulin
Epithelial growth factor

Inhibitors

Somatostatin
Pancreatic polypeptide
Peptide tyrosine tyrosine
Glucagon
Vasopressin

---

to have roles (Fig. 350-3). Of particular interest, in addition to the events which are postulated to occur within and through the duct cell, paracellular events are important as well. This provides a low-electrical-resistance, cation-selective path for sodium to cross the epithelial barrier. Molecular models for the function of this epithelium are still evolving.

INTEGRATED PANCREATIC SECRETORY PHYSIOLOGY

Pancreatic exocrine secretion is controlled by both hormonal and neural mechanisms (Box 350-1). Cholecystokinin (pancreozymin) was the first recognized hormonal stimulant of pancreatic secretion and the focus of extensive studies of secretory control in acinar cells, but the pendulum is swinging toward believing that the major stimulant role of pancreatic secretion in man is neuronal. Cholecystokinin is still a physiologic regulator of that activity, but it appears to be act-

ing at the cholecystokinin-A receptors that are present on neurons rather than those present directly on acinar cells of this species.

Vagal stimulation and cholecystokinin elicit flow of pancreatic juice rich in enzymes and low in bicarbonate. Vasoactive intestinal polypeptide and secretin elicit flow rich in bicarbonate and relatively poor in enzymes. Sympathetic stimulation inhibits secretion, likely via an effect on pancreatic blood flow.

Human pancreatic exocrine secretion is minimal during fasting, although it exhibits some cyclic activity with an increase that correlates with phase III of the migrating motor complex reaching the duodenum. This recurs at 60- to 90-minute intervals and represents only approximately 10% of the peak output observed in response to a meal. Ingestion of a meal at any time interrupts this cycle and changes the pattern of pancreatic output to that of the fed state. Like gastric secretion, pancreatic secretion can be stimulated by cephalic, gastric, and intestinal phases of digestion. During the earlier two phases, vagal influences are predominant. When nutrients enter the small intestine, hormonal mechanisms (including hormonally stimulated neural mechanisms) of stimulating the exocrine pancreas become prominent. The most stimulatory components of the meal include the lipid and protein, with carbohydrate only minimally stimulatory in an experimental setting. Both fatty acids and amino acids are known to stimulate cholecystokinin secretion from its site of synthesis in duodenal and jejunal I cells. The entry of acid into the duodenum is a potent stimulant of secretin secretion, which is likely the physiologic stimulant of ductular secretion. The coordinated stimulation of acinar cell and ductular secretion help to ensure adequate clearance of the enzymes and components that may have a tendency to form plugs or calculi in the ductular tree. These integrated processes appear to be defective in patients with cystic fibrosis or alcoholic pancreatitis.

There is a substantial "reserve capacity" of pancreatic enzymes secreted, with the amount entering the duodenum after a meal far in excess of that necessary for normal digestion. Maldigestion of fat and protein occurs only in severe pancreatic insufficiency in which lipase and trypsin output are reduced by greater than 90%. Although this is helpful when attempting to replace these enzymes with oral supplementation, their acid sensitivity interferes with delivery of active enzymes. Also, it is difficult to achieve the appropriate coordinated delivery of enzymes with nutrients when supplementing with exogenous enzymes.

MEASURING PANCREATIC SECRETION

Accurate measurement of human pancreatic enzyme secretion requires duodenal intubation and direct collection of secretions. There are simpler indirect methods such as the analysis of stool fat or the hydrolysis of a test compound, but these are indicative of only severe pancreatic exocrine insufficiency. Endoscopic cannulation of the pancreatic duct is the only method to directly collect pure, uncontaminated pancreatic juice, but it carries substantial risk and cannot be justified as a method to quantify pancreatic secretion. Instead, a marker-dilution method is usually employed. This can be used to correct for dilution by gastric contents and even for duodenal-gastric reflux. Under carefully validated conditions, such a technique provides highly sensitive and reproducible quantitation of pancreatic output. The typical test utilizes the infusion of a hormonal secretagogue such as cholecystokinin. Additional information can be provided with a slightly more complex analysis of output in response to a test meal, in which the phases of digestion and their integration are also relevant.

DIFFERENTIAL DIAGNOSIS

Increased pancreatic secretion is observed in a few clinical settings. Of interest, there are isolated reports of increased basal secretion in patients with acute pancreatitis, but antisecretory treatments have not been an effective therapy for this problem. Some patients with renal insufficiency also are hypersecretors, likely on the basis of reduced renal clearance of peptide hormones known to stimulate pancreatic secretion. While pancreatic enzymes and bicarbonate secretion are typically reduced in chronic pancreatitis, output of calcium and lactoferrin may be increased in that setting, possibly contributing toward calculus formation.

Reduced pancreatic exocrine secretion is the more common clinical concern. This may occur as a result of intrinsic pancreatic disease or extrapancreatic factors. The latter may include any process that interferes with the ability of ingested nutrients to release cholecystokinin, such as a gastric emptying disorder or a nonpancreatic maldigestive process like celiac disease or primary biliary cirrhosis. It may also represent extrapancreatic obstruction or any luminal condition that inactivates pancreatic enzymes, such as the hyperacidity of Zollinger-Ellison Syndrome. Intrapancreatic causes include chronic pancreatitis and intrapancreatic obstructive processes, of which pancreatic carcinoma is most concerning.

BIBLIOGRAPHY

Argent BE et al: The pancreatic duct cell, *Pancreas* 7:403-409, 1992.
Githens S: Pancreatic duct cell cultures, *Annu Rev Physiol* 56:419-443, 1994.
Go VLW et al, editors: *The pancreas: biology, pathobiology, and diseases*, ed 2, New York, 1993, Raven Press.
Singer MV, Ziegler R, Rohr G, editors: *Gastrointestinal tract and endocrine system*, Boston, 1995, Kluwer Academic.

This work was partially supported by grants from the National Institutes of Health, DK32878 and DK46577.

DIAGNOSTIC PROCEDURES AND TESTS

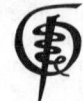

CHAPTER

351 Evaluation of Hepatobiliary Diseases

Albert J. Czaja

The evaluation of patients with hepatobiliary disease must be practical and achieveable by conventionally available resources. The immediate goals are to establish an accurate diagnosis and to institute an effective treatment strategy. The long-term objectives are to an-

ticipate consequences of the disease and its management and to modify treatment accordingly. By maintaining a systematic approach to each problem and by utilizing diagnostic tools to their maximal advantage, these objectives can be met in the majority of instances. A successful clinical evaluation must reflect a composite analysis that balances multiple complementary investigations.

Clinical, laboratory, radiologic, and histologic studies must be properly sequenced to navigate through the decision tree. Each study must contribute in a hierarchical fashion to resolution of the next problem. Diagnostic resources must be mustered to achieve the following. First, the duration of the disorder must be determined and the disease must be classified as an acute or chronic process. Second, the pattern of liver injury must be assessed and the "hepatitic" and "cholestatic" features must be counterbalanced to identify the prevailing character. Third, potential causes for the predominant injury pattern must be evaluated and the severity of the insult graded. Last, the aggressiveness of the disease must be estimated and its immediate and long-term outcome decided (Table 351-1).

In this chapter, methods for answering these critical questions are reviewed and promising new approaches to each problem discussed.

DISTINGUISHING ACUTE FROM CHRONIC DISEASE

The International Association for the Study of Liver (IASL) and the World Health Organization (WHO) have defined chronicity as continuous disease activity for at least 6 months. Diseases of lesser duration are categorized as acute, potentially self-limited disorders. This distinction is important since the diagnoses, treatment strategies, and outcomes are different in each instance. Patients with acute onset disease usually have hepatocellular injury attributable to an infection (virus, fungus, bacteria), drug, toxin (especially alcohol), or hemodynamic instability (hypotension, hypoxia, right heart failure). Choledocholithiasis may have a presentation similar to those of certain chronic liver diseases, especially autoimmune hepatitis, that have subclinical, indolent courses leading to an acute or even fulminant decompensation (Table 351-2). Patients with chronic liver disease commonly have viral (hepatitis B or hepatitis C virus infection), genetic (Wilson's disease, α-1 antitrypsin deficiency or hemochromatosis), immunologic (autoimmune hepatitis, primary biliary cirrhosis, primary sclerosing cholangitis), toxic (alcohol, methotrexate, various drugs), or metabolic (obesity, diabetes, malnutrition) bases for their findings (see Table 351-2). The suddenness of the presentation is determined mainly by clinical history, but the physical findings and laboratory tests must support this history. An acute onset does not necessarily indicate a recently acquired disease.

Physical findings that indicate chronic disease are muscle wasting, feminization in men, finger clubbing, spider nevi, palmar erythema, prominent abdominal wall venous pattern, and ascites. Sensitivity is variable depending on the presence or absence of cirrhosis, and the absence of one or more of the changes does not preclude advanced chronic liver disease. Indeed, 25% of patients with autoimmune hepatitis who present acutely have no features of chronicity.

The principal laboratory tests that indicate disease duration are the serum albumin level and prothrombin time (see Table 351-1). Alterations in these studies reflect changes in hepatic synthesis and differences in the serum half-life of albumin and the individual clotting factors that affect the prothrombin time. The serum gamma globulin level is also a useful indirect index of chronicity. Gamma globulin is not synthesized by the liver, but its serum level varies with the duration and severity of the inflammatory process.

Serum Albumin Level

Albumin is synthesized exclusively in the liver and 10 to 15 grams are produced each day. As a product of the liver, albumin is an important measure of hepatic synthetic function. The serum concentration is a static determination that reflects the rates of synthesis and degradation as well as the volume of distribution. A low serum albumin level connotes impaired hepatic synthesis due to hepatocyte injury or loss, increased urinary and/or enteric losses

Table 351-1 Diagnostic problems and evaluation strategies

DIAGNOSTIC PROBLEM	PARAMETERS	DEFINITIONS	EVALUATIONS
Disease duration	Acute vs. chronic	Acute: disease activity <6 months Chronic: disease activity ≥6 months or autoimmune hepatitis	Serum albumin Prothrombin time Serum γ-globulin Immunoglobulins Liver biopsy Hematology group
Pattern of injury	Hepatitic vs. cholestatic	Hepatitic: serum aminotransferase predominates Cholestatic: serum alkaline phosphatase predominates	AST, ALT, alkaline phosphatase and isoenzymes γ-glutamyl transferase 5′ nucleotidase
Establishing the diagnosis	Viral, drug, toxic, ischemic, hypoxic, inherited, immunologic, obstructive, or infiltrative	Demonstration of disease-specific markers and/or histologic findings	Serologic viral assays (A, B, and C), ceruloplasmin, iron and saturation, ferritin, α-1 phenotype SMA, ANA, anti-LKM1, AMA Ultrasonography, CT scan, MRI scan, or ERCP Arteriography, hepatic venography, PTC Liver biopsy
Disease severity and prognosis	Mild, moderate, or severe	No established definitions	Serum albumin Prothrombin time Pseudocholinesterase Bilirubin, ammonia Alpha fetoprotein Liver biopsy

AST, Aspartate aminotransferase; *ALT,* alanine aminotransferase; *SMA,* smooth muscle antibodies; *ANA,* antinuclear antibodies; *CT,* computed tomography; *MRI,* magnetic resonance imaging; *ERCP,* endoscopic retrograde cholangiopancreatography; *PTC,* percutaneous transhepatic cholangiography.

from conditions such as nephrotic syndrome or enteropathy, and/or extravascular distribution in ascites and edema fluid. The half-life of albumin in serum is 20 days, so marked abnormalities are typically absent in patients with acute liver disease unless loss or redistribution occurs. The liver can double its capacity to synthesize albumin, and the serum level can reflect this compensatory action. As a consequence, a normal serum albumin level can be falsely reassuring about the absence of liver disease. The rate of albumin synthesis is modulated by nutritional status, plasma colloid oncotic pressure, and inflammatory mediators (interleukin 1, tumor necrosis factor), and these factors must also be considered in the interpretation of a serum concentration. Poor nutrition predisposes to low serum albumin levels, which may exist before and despite the liver disease; high-colloid osmotic pressure downregulates albumin gene expression in rats and human hepatoma cells and can reduce albumin synthesis; and cytokines released during a chronic inflammatory reaction can inhibit albumin production.

Prothrombin Time

The prothrombin time assesses coagulation factors I (fibrinogen), II (prothrombin),V, VII, and X. These factors are products of the liver and important indices of hepatic synthetic function. Because the half-life of each factor in serum is short (from 6 hours for factor VII to 6 days for factor I), the prothrombin time can change rapidly as a result of liver injury. The abnormality itself connotes only the severity of liver damage, but in concert with a normal serum albumin level it provides a priori evidence of an acute liver disease. All the factors assessed by the prothrombin time, with the exception of factor V, are vitamin K dependent. Deficiencies in this vitamin due to fat malabsorption, the use of broad-spectrum antibiotics, or the administration of vitamin K antagonists (coumarin-like drugs, moxalactam) can perturb the test and confound its interpretation. As a consequence, all patients with a disturbance of prothrombin time warrant supplementation with vitamin K (10 mg intramuscularly) and a follow-up test after 24 hours. Correction of the abnormality indicates a vitamin K deficiency rather than a hepatocellular injury. Fixed or worsening abnormalities of prothrombin time have prognostic importance in acute liver failure and in chronic liver diseases whose prognosis is projected by scoring systems. Since factor V is not vitamin K dependent, it is a direct measure of hepatic synthetic function and disease severity. Its direct assessment, however, is commonly supplanted by the prothrombin time.

Table 351-2 Differential diagnosis

HEPATITIC PATTERN	CHOLESTATIC PATTERN
Acute	
Viral hepatitis	Drug or alcohol toxicity
Drug toxicity	Hepatitis A or C
Ischemic or hypoxic injury	Biliary obstruction (stone, pancreatitis)
Toxin exposure	Metabolic dysfunction (sepsis, hyperthy-
Exacerbated chronic hepatitis	roidism, hypercatabolic state, trauma)
Acute choledocholithiasis	Granulomatous hepatitis
	Primary or metastatic tumor
Chronic	Protracted hepatitis A
Viral hepatitis	Drug or alcohol toxicity
Drug toxicity	Biliary obstruction (stone, stricture,
Wilson's disease	tumor, chronic pancreatitis)
Hemochromatosis	Primary biliary cirrhosis
α-1 Antitrypsin deficiency	Primary sclerosing cholangitis
Autoimmune hepatitis	Autoimmune cholangitis
	Granulomatous hepatitis
	Cholangiocarcinoma
	Primary or metastatic tumor

Serum Gamma Globulin Level

Gamma globulin is produced by B lymphocytes, and its serum level can be enhanced by any process that persistently presents antigen to these immunocytes. Hypergammaglobulinemia does not have specificity for chronic liver disease, but in the clinical context of liver dysfunction, it connotes active liver inflammation, increased and persistent antigen presentation, excessive antibody production, and chronicity. The serum level in such patients is a function of the severity and duration of the inflammatory process.

Hypergammaglobulinemia may also have an etiologic connotation if the typically diffuse polyclonal gamma globulin response has a dominant isotype. Elevation mainly of immunoglobulin G supports the diagnosis of autoimmune hepatitis; a predominant increase in the concentration of immunoglobulin M is consistent with a chronic cholestatic disease such as primary biliary cirrhosis; and a high serum level of immunoglobulin A suggests chronic alcoholic liver disease. Conversely, a normal or low level of immunoglobulin A suggests a form of autoimmune hepatitis characterized by antibodies to liver/kidney microsome type 1 in serum (type 2 autoimmune hepatitis) or an intrinsic immunoglobulin A deficiency.

The antibodies that constitute the hypergammaglobulinemia of chronic liver disease are typically heterogeneous and nonpathogenic. Antibodies to bacteria (*Escherichia coli, Salmonella* sp., *Bacteroides* sp.) and viruses (measles, rubella, cytomegalovirus) have been described. This diverse humoral response may reflect the inability of the damaged liver to sequester exogenous antigens normally because of portal systemic shunting of blood and/or loss of Kupffer cell function. The hypergammglobulinemia may also harbor diagnostically useful antibodies, including those of autoimmune hepatitis (antinuclear antibodies, smooth muscle antibodies, and antibodies to liver/kidney microsome type 1), primary biliary cirrhosis (antimitochondrial antibodies), and chronic viral hepatitis (antibodies to hepatitis B and C viruses).

Hypergammaglobulinemia commonly accompanies active cirrhosis, but it is not a surrogate marker of cirrhosis. Depending on etiology, as many as 35% of patients with severe hepatocellular inflammation and no cirrhosis will have elevated serum gamma globulin levels. The levels of serum gamma globulin are typically higher in patients with cirrhosis than in those without cirrhosis, but individual serum values are not discriminatory.

The serum gamma globulin level should be assessed by protein electrophoresis in all patients in whom there is uncertainty about the acute or chronic nature of the disease. In this regard, its determination complements the results of the serum albumin level and prothrombin time. The gamma globulin level should also be determined to grade inflammatory activity and explore etiologic possibilities.

Liver Biopsy Examination

In most instances, the clinical history, physical examination, and analysis of the serum albumin level, prothrombin time, and serum gamma globulin concentration are sufficient to render a confident designation of acute or chronic liver disease. The liver biopsy procedure should not be done simply to assess the duration of illness; it is rarely helpful in patients with acute hepatitis. Exceptions include the rare individual with a presumed acute exacerbation of a previously chronic subclinical disease, the patient with a presumed infectious agent that may be detected in liver tissue, or the pregnant individual with a presumed acute fatty change that may warrant specific therapeutic interventions.

Ancillary Tests

Determinations of hemoglobulin level, leukocyte count, and platelet count can also reflect the nature and chronicity of the disease. A pancytopenia may be a consequence of hypersplenism or disseminated intravascular coagulation accompanying cirrhosis. Anemia can reflect bleeding, malnutrition, or hemolysis due to cirrhosis and portal hypertension, whereas an isolated thrombocytopenia may be an early sign of chronic liver disease and an evolving hypersplenism.

DETERMINING PATTERNS OF LIVER INJURY

Aspartate and alanine aminotransferase, alkaline phosphatase, gamma glutamyltransferase, and 5′ nucleotidase are intrahepatic enzymes whose abnormal concentration in serum reflects injury to liver cells and bile canaliculi. In patients with acute or chronic liver disease, the predominant enzyme abnormality permits classification of the injury pattern as hepatitic or cholestatic (see Table 351-1).

A hepatitic injury connotes damage to liver cells with necrosis or loss of surface membrane integrity ("cell leak") and it is manifested mainly by abnormalities in the serum alanine and aspartate aminotransferase levels. Direct hepatotoxins (drugs, chemicals, alcohol), acute or chronic viral infections (hepatitis A, B, and C viruses), hypoxia, ischemia (shock, heart failure), genetic or herditary disorders (Wilson's disease, hemochromatosis, α-1 antitrypsin deficiency), and self-perpetuating immunologic conditions (autoimmune hepatitis) are examples of hepatitic processes (see Table 351-2).

A cholestatic injury is manifested by abnormalities of the serum alkaline phosphatase, gamma glutamyltransferase, and/or 5′ nucleotidase levels. Extrahepatic biliary obstruction (choledocholithiasis, am-

pullary stenosis or neoplasm, enlargement of the pancreatic head due to pancreatitis or tumor, and stricture or neoplasm of the bile ducts), intrahepatic bile duct injury and/or loss (drugs, acute hepatitis A, chronic hepatitis C, primary biliary cirrhosis, autoimmune cholangitis, and primary sclerosing cholangitis), and infiltrative disorders (granulomatous hepatitis, sarcoidosis, and primary or metastatic malignancy) are examples of cholestatic processes (see Table 351-2).

Rarely are hepatitic or cholestatic patterns pure, and typically there are mixed enzyme abnormalities that require individual interpretation. The magnitude of elevation above the upper limit of normal must be determined for each of the pertinent laboratory indices and the principal derangement decided. Predominant abnormalities in the serum aminotransferase levels justify the designation of hepatitic injury, whereas predominant changes in the serum alkaline phosphatase, gamma glutamyltransferase, and/or 5′ nucleotidase levels support the designation of cholestatic injury. Proper characterization of the injury pattern is essential for the correct differential diagnosis and evaluation strategy (see Table 351-1).

Hyperbilirubinemia can occur with hepatitic and cholestatic processes and it does not by itself compel characterization. It typically reflects the composite functions of hepatic uptake, processing, and excretion; and its level is influenced by bilirubin load (hemolysis, shortened red blood cell survival) and the adequacy of alternate routes of excretion (renal function).

Serum Aminotransferase Level

Aspartate and alanine aminotransferases are enzymes within the cytosol of the hepatocyte that modulate the production of oxaloacetic acid, pyruvate, and glutamate. Their presence in serum in healthy individuals reflects normal liver cell turnover. Both enzymes are present in high concentration within the hepatocyte, and the release of only 1% of the hepatic pool of aspartate aminotransferase theoretically doubles the normal amount in serum. Blood levels of either enzyme, therefore, are extremely sensitive to liver cell injury.

Thirty-nine percent of the aspartate aminotransferase in liver cells is distributed in mitochondria, and its abnormal release in serum can signal mitochondrial injury. Alcohol is a mitochondrial toxin; this action may account for the observation that in alcoholic liver disease the serum aspartate aminotransferase level is commonly higher than the alanine aminotransferase level. Mitochondrial-derived aspartate aminotransferase can be measured in serum, but its lack of diagnostic specificity has limited its clinical application.

Individual serum aminotransferase levels do not correlate closely with the extent of liver cell necrosis, but ranges of enzyme abnormality have diagnostic value. The levels are rarely elevated above 500 IU/L (8.3 μKat/L) in obstructive jaundice and above 300 IU/L (5 μKat/L) in alcoholic liver disease. Levels above 1000 IU/L (16.6 μKat/L) indicate severe hepatocellular injury and a limited differential diagnosis. Acute virus infection, hepatocellular ischemia, or toxic injury are the principal considerations; spontaneous passage of a common bile duct stone or exacerbation of a subclinical chronic liver disease such as autoimmune hepatitis are infrequent alternative possibilities (see Table 351-2). Sustained elevation of the enzyme abnormality to 1000 IU/L (16.6 μKat/L) or higher also has a prognostic implication. In untreated patients with autoimmune hepatitis, an abnormality of this degree is associated with a 50% mortality within 3 years. Enzyme levels of up to 300 IU/L (5 μKat/L) are nonspecific and in these patients, the ratio of aspartate aminotransferase elevation to alanine aminotransferase elevation may influence the differential diagnosis. A ratio of greater than 2 supports the diagnosis of alcoholic liver disease, whereas a ratio of <1 suggests an acute hepatocellular injury, especially of viral or toxic cause.

Although neither aminotransferase has diagnostic specificity, the alanine type does have an almost exclusive liver origin. In contrast, aspartate aminotransferase is also found in heart, muscle, kidney, brain, pancreas, and erythrocytes. The tissue origin of a serum aspartate aminotransferase elevation cannot be determined by isoenzyme, and the hepatic origin of the abnormality must be deduced from the serum alanine aminotransferase level. As a consequence, measurement of the serum aspartate aminotransferase level in a patient with liver disease should always be accompanied by a simultaneous measurement of the alanine aminotransferase level.

It is important to note that the serum aspartate aminotransferase level can be markedly abnormal for months or years in individuals without disease of the liver or elsewhere. The enzyme can exist in blood as a macroenzyme by forming complexes with immunoglobulins A and G. The resultant large molecule may then persist in the circulation because of an inability to enter cells responsible for its catabolism. A macroenzyme can be suspected by the findings of normal serum alanine aminotransferase and creatine kinase levels in an otherwise healthy person. Confirmation of its presence requires testing of blood by exclusion chromatography, electrophoresis, and activation assays with pyridotal 5-phosphate.

Serum Alkaline Phosphatase Level

Cholestasis is most commonly assessed by the serum alkaline phosphatase level. This enzyme is in the canalicular membranes of hepatocytes and its synthesis is stimulated by obstruction, increased intraductal pressure and elevated tissue bile acid concentrations. Enzyme elevations, however, are not liver-specific, and alkaline phosphatase is also found in osteoblasts, placenta, and intestine. Isoenzyme determinations are available to define the tissue of origin and other laboratory indices of cholestasis, especially the serum gamma glutamyltransferase level, can confirm a liver source. Such confirmation is essential before embarking on other studies.

Normal values of serum alkaline phosphatase are age and sex dependent. In adolescent men (age 18 years), the upper limit of normal for alkaline phosphatase is 92% higher than the value for older men (age $\geq$19 years). In adolescent women of comparable age (age 17-23 years), the upper limit of normal is lower than that for similarly aged men but higher than that for older premenopausal women. After menopause (age 65 years), the normal range for women is higher than that for similarly aged men and premenopausal adult women. Age- and sex-related differences in the enzyme concentration undoubtedly reflect differences in bone mass and metabolism.

The serum alkaline phosphatase level is increased in at least 81% of patients with hepatocellular injury. Consequently, an abnormality alone is insufficient to define a cholestatic process. In chronic hepatitis, a greater than twofold elevation of serum alkaline phosphatase level above normal occurs in only 33% and a greater than fourfold increase occurs in only 10%. The greater the derangement in the alkaline phosphatase concentration the more prominent and clinically important is the cholestatic component. Enzyme elevations greater than fourfold the upper limit of normal are unusual in hepatitic processes and they justify a cholestatic designation (see Table 351-1).

A predominant cholestatic pattern suggests acute or chronic disease of the bile ducts at a microscopic and/or macroscopic level. Infiltrative disorders of the liver, however, must also be considered. Primary and metastatic tumors, granulomatous disorders, collagen vascular diseases with vasculitis, and drug toxicities must always be included in the differential diagnosis of a serum alkaline phosphatase abnormality, especially if the finding is isolated. Presumably the infiltrative process induces enzyme production by obstructing canaliculi (see Table 351-2).

Serum Gamma Glutamyltransferase Level

Gamma glutamyltransferase is present in the smooth endoplasmic reticulum and the canalicular plasma membrane of hepatocytes as well as the luminal membrane of biliary epithelial cells. Its activity can be induced by a variety of medications, especially dilantin and phenobarbital, and the serum level is commonly high in patients who consume excessive alcohol. Abnormalities attributable to enzyme induction may not be associated with intrinsic liver disease.

Biliary obstructive disease and focal infiltrative disorders elevate the enzyme level in serum and abnormalities of the serum gamma glutamyltransferase concentration have the same implications of cholestasis and/or infiltration as those of the serum alkaline phosphatase level (see Tables 351-1 and 351-2). Importantly, the presence and magnitude of the enzyme elevation may exceed that anticipated based on the clinical findings, suggesting that the test is nonspecific and/or overly sensitive to unimportant subclinical events.

The etiologic nonspecificity of the gamma glutamyltransferase elevation probably reflects the diverse distribution of the enzyme within the hepatocyte. Determination of the serum level should be done mainly in the context of an abnormal serum alkaline phosphatase level to support the likelihood of hepatic disease and a cholestatic disorder. The kidney, pancreas, and brain also contain gamma glutamyltransferase, but it is unclear if diseases of these organs produce clinically important or distinctive patterns of enzyme abnormality.

Serum 5' Nucleotidase Level

5' nucleotidase is found exclusively in the bile canalicular membranes of the liver, and it is a highly specific marker of cholestasis. The enzyme is tightly adherent to the canalicular membrane and can be solubilized only by exposure to bile acids within the biliary tree. Consequently, abnormal serum levels confidently reflect obstruction to bile flow at microscopic and/or macroscopic levels.

Serum elevations of 5' nucleotidase correlate closely with those of gamma glutamyltransferase, but the enzyme is not subject to induction by drugs or alcohol. Comparisons between serum levels of 5' nucleotidase, alkaline phosphatase, and gamma glutamyltransferase in patients with cancer have indicated that 5' nucleotidase has a higher predictive value for metastatic liver disease (86%) and lower false-positive rate (7%) than the other tests. In contrast, the serum gamma glutamyltransferase determination has a lower frequency of false-negative results (3%) but a higher frequency of false-positive results (35%). Accordingly, the 5' nucleotidase test is preferred in the evaluation of metastatic liver disease.

As a marker of extrahepatic biliary obstruction or intrinsic liver disease, the serum 5' nucleotidase level is less sensitive than the serum alkaline phosphatase level. Consequently, the serum alkaline phosphatase determination has supplanted the 5' nucleotidase assay as a screening test for these disorders. As a secondary test, however, determination of the 5' nucleotidase level adds specificity to the other findings.

Serum Leucine Aminopeptidase Level

Leucine aminopeptidase is found in almost all human tissues, but high activity is localized to the biliary epithelium. Like 5' nucleotidase, it is specific for cholestasis and it is as sensitive to obstructive, infiltrative, and space-occupying lesions of the liver. Unlike the serum alkaline phosphatase level, the leucine aminopeptidase level is not affected by bone disease; pregnancy is the only nonhepatic condition in which it is perturbed. As yet, measurement of the leucine aminopeptidase level has not been found to have special attributes that have recommended its general use.

Serum Bile Acid Level

Bile acids appear in serum because they have escaped the enterohepatic circulation (portal-systemic shunting) and/or hepatocytes have been unable to efficiently remove them from the portal circulation (diminished hepatic clearance). They are made by hepatocytes, excreted into bile by hepatocytes, metabolized by intestinal bacteria, absorbed by the terminal ileum, and recirculated to the liver via the portal vein. Consequently, there are many perturbations of a hepatitic or cholestatic nature that can affect their concentration in serum. Abnormalities lack diagnostic specificity, and determinations of the conjugated bile acid levels have not acquired widespread clinical application. Inactive cirrhosis in patients with normal liver tests may be detected by an elevated value that reflects subclinical portosystemic shunting. Elevation during pregnancy may be an early indication of intrahepatic cholestasis, and normal levels in patients with hyperbilirubinemia implicate a nonhepatic hemolytic disorder or Gilbert's syndrome. Since the conjugated serum bile acid level reflects the integrity of multiple interrelated physiologic events, the absence of an abnormality may be more useful clinically than detection of a disturbance. Postprandial assessments are as valuable as fasting levels.

MAKING THE DIAGNOSIS

Classification of the liver disease as an acute hepatitic, acute cholestatic, chronic hepatitic or chronic cholestatic process focuses the diagnostic evaluation and directs the testing sequence (see Tables 351-1 and 351-2). Assessment of an acute disorder typically includes serologic assays for viral markers; tests for chronic diseases that have an acute or fulminant presentation; serum levels of implicated drugs; and ultrasonography to identify changes suggestive of cirrhosis, fatty infiltration, mass or abscess formation, occlusion of hepatic, portal, or splenic veins, and biliary obstruction (see Table 351-2). Evaluation of a chronic disorder includes similar tests but focuses mainly on studies to exclude chronic viral infection, genetic or hereditary diseases, immunologic disorders, and infiltrative processes, and it may more commonly require liver biopsy examination. Chronic exposure to hepatotoxins and chronic biliary obstruction are other important diagnostic considerations in this category (see Table 351-2).

Viral Markers

Viruses can cause acute or chronic liver disease, and agents such as hepatitis A virus and hepatitis C virus can produce a cholestatic disorder. Viral infection, therefore, must be excluded in all patients regardless of the duration of illness or the pattern of liver injury. Hepatitis A, B, and C viruses are each capable of producing an acute illness, but only hepatitis B virus and hepatitis C virus induce a chronic viremia and long-term inflammatory reaction. Hepatitis A infection can produce a prolonged clinical illness ($\geq$6 months), but it is self-limited and without chronic consequence. In those few patients with chronic illness, especially in those who have an acute onset of symptoms and persistent cholestatic hepatitis, the test for hepatitis A virus infection (immunoglobulin M antibody positivity) can be diagnostic.

Multiple other viruses can produce acute hepatitis. Many have diagnostic assays and should be considered in the proper clinical context. The Epstein-Barr virus is a herpes virus that can produce an acute sporadic hepatitis that is characterized by pharyngitis, rash, lymphadenopathy, leukocytosis, and atypical lymphocytes on peripheral smear. Cytomegalovirus may produce a similar clinical syndrome and should be sought mainly in patients with immunocompromise. Hepatitis D (delta) virus has a single-stranded RNA core and a coat that consists of hepatitis B virus surface antigen. Consequently, it requires the hepatitis B virus for expression. Its diagnosis should be considered in patients with hepatitis B infection whose condition deteriorates. Hepatitis D virus is directly cytopathic to the liver and usually worsens the B disease. Coincidental acute infections with the B and D viruses are usually self-limited, whereas delta infections superimposed on chronic hepatitis B typically result in a severe, rapidly progressive disorder. Hepatitis E is a single-stranded RNA virus (calicivirus) that is transmitted by fecal-oral mechanisms akin to those of hepatitis A. It produces a self-limited infection, usually in epidemics, but among pregnant women it can be deadly. Hepatitis E infection is rare in Western countries but should be assessed for in patients from developing countries (Pakistan, India, Nepal, Russia, Somalia, Sudan, Algeria, and Mexico) who have sporadic or epidemic acute hepatitis.

The screening assays for viral infection in patients with acute hepatitic disease include those for immunoglobulin M antibody to hepatitis A virus, hepatitis B surface antigen, antibody to hepatitis B core antigen, and antibody to hepatitis C virus. Seropositivity for antibody to hepatitis B core antigen justifies a supplemental test to determine the presence of immunoglobulin M antibody to hepatitis B core antigen. The immunoglobulin M isotype typically predominates in serum for at least 6 months after an acute hepatitis B infection and it is a priori evidence of acute hepatitis B. Antibodies to delta virus should be sought in those patients who have hepatitis B virus infection to exclude a concidental acute infection with hepatitis D or a hepatitis D infection that is superimposed on a preexistent but subclinical chronic hepatitis B infection. Since antibodies to hepatitis C virus may develop late in the acute clinical illness, seronegativity early in the disease does not preclude infection. A succession of determinations throughout the clinical illness and into convalescence is necessary to fully discount the diagnosis. As an alternative, testing for hepatitis C virus RNA in blood by polymerase chain reaction assay secures the diagnosis even in the earliest stages of illness. The strong clinical suspicion of a viral infection in the absence of markers for the typical agents warrants additional tests for viruses such as Epstein-Barr virus and cytomegalovirus. Nonviral infections, including bacterial, parasitic, and rickettsial sources, may also require evaluation.

The screening tests for viral infection in patients with chronic hepatitic disease include the same studies for hepatitis B and C virus infection used in the evaluation of acute disease. The findings, however, are frequently supplemented to determine replicative activity, coexistent infections, and diagnostic specificity. Patients with hepatitis B surface antigen and antibody to hepatitis B core antigen must be assessed for hepatitis B e antigen (HBeAg), antibody to HBeAg, antibody to delta virus, and hepatitis B virus DNA in serum. The presence of HBeAg connotes active viral replication and increased infectivity. These findings can be substantiated by detection of hepatitis B virus DNA in serum. Such patients have active viremia and are candidates for antiviral therapy. Patients with active disease, absence of HBeAg, and hepatitis B virus DNA in serum have active B viremia and probable infection with a mutant (precore variant) of the hepatitis B virus. These patients are also candidates for antiviral therapy although they may be less responsive. Patients with antibody to hepatitis B core antigen, antibody to HBeAg, and absence of hepatitis B virus DNA in serum have a serologic profile that indicates a nonreplicative stage of infection. If these individuals have active clinical disease, a superimposed viral or toxic insult must be sought. Patients with antibodies to hepatitis C virus must have the specificity of the antibodies confirmed against recombinant hepatitis C virus-encoded antigens before the diagnosis is secure. The recombinant immunoblot assay (RIBA) is used for this purpose. A nonreactive RIBA indicates a false-positive result. Typically, false positivity is associated with a hypergammaglobulinemia that interferes with the immunoassay for antibodies to hepatitis C virus. False-positive test results and indeterminate RIBA reactions can be further assayed by seeking hepatitis C virus RNA in serum.

Viral infections are uncommon causes of acute cholestatic or chronic cholestatic diseases, but their potential relevance must not be overlooked. Hepatitis A virus can produce acute and slowly resolving cholestatic hepatitis, hepatitis C virus can variably damage bile ducts and produce the histologic changes of cholestasis, and hepatitis B virus can produce the syndrome of fibrosing cholestatic hepatitis in the setting of liver transplantation and rapid deterioration of the graft. Diagnosis is possible in each instance through application of conventional serologic assays.

Hereditary Markers

Wilson's disease, genetic hemochromatosis, and α-1 antitrypsin deficiency are the principal hereditary diseases of the liver; they mainly produce a chronic hepatitic syndrome (see Table 351-2). Determinations of the serum ceruloplasmin, iron, and α-1 antitrypsin levels screen for the diagnoses and additional tests, including liver biopsy examination, establish the condition.

Wilson's disease may have an acute fulminant hepatitic presentation or it may resemble chronic hepatitis. The onset of illness is typically between the ages of 6 years and 40 years, but the diagnosis has been made in older adults. Initial screening involves determination of the serum ceruloplasmin level. Ceruloplasmin is abnormally reduced in patients with the disease, and its concentration is strikingly decreased in the homozygous condition. Since ceruloplasmin is an acute phase reactant, its serum concentration may be increased in acute inflammatory diseases, chronic cholestatic conditions, and estrogen therapy. Consequently, a low value may be elevated into the normal range in rare cases of Wilson's disease (5%). To exclude this possibility, additional tests must be performed in patients with borderline values. Slit-lamp examination of the eyes for Kayser-Fleischer rings, measurement of urinary copper excretion, and liver biopsy assessment with quantitation of hepatic copper content may be required to clarify the situation. In patients with a fulminant presentation, the best laboratory indication of Wilson's disease is an increased serum copper concentration. The serum ceruloplasmin level may be low because of diminished hepatic synthetic function in patients with non-wilsonian fulminant hepatitis; urinary copper excretion may be nonspecifically increased in such patients; and liver biopsy assessment may be too hazardous to perform unless a transjugular approach is used. The presence of intravascular hemolysis and Kayser-Fleischer rings are other important aspects of the diagnosis in the fulminant setting.

Genetic hemochromatosis is suggested by an increased serum iron concentration and transferrin saturation. The range of abnormality in the transferrin saturation is broad, and the diagnosis of homozygous disease cannot be discounted in patients with only mild abnormalities (transferrin saturations, 55% to 70%). Virtually all homozygous patients have an increased serum ferritin level, and the combination of high transferrin saturation and ferritin level justify liver biopsy examination. The hepatocytic distribution of iron within the liver distinguishes genetic hemochromatosis from secondary conditions such as chronic hemolysis and transfusional overload in which iron is deposited mainly in Kupffer cells. The hepatic iron content can be determined in freshly obtained liver tissue or in paraffin blocks by atomic absorption spectrophotometry. Iron concentrations within the liver increase progressively with age in patients with genetic hemochromatosis and the interpretation of the hepatic iron concentration is facilitated by adjusting for age. This adjustment constitutes the hepatic iron index. The index should be calculated in each patient not only to define the presence of genetic hemochromatosis but also to distinguish a heterozygous from a homozygous condition. The hepatic iron index is determined by dividing the hepatic iron content in μmoles/g dry weight by the patient's age. If the hepatic iron level is given as μg/g dry weight, the value must be divided by 55.8 to convert to μmoles before dividing by age. The normal hepatic iron index is 0 to <1; the value for heterozygous disease is from 1 to 2 (rarely above 1.5); and the value for homozygous disease is >1.9. Unfortunately, hepatocellular necrosis can release iron and ferritin from intrahepatic stores and transiently increase the serum levels. Among patients with chronic viral hepatitis, 36% have elevated serum iron levels and 30% of male patients have abnormal serum ferritin levels. Serum aspartate aminotransferase concentrations correlate closely with the serum ferritin concentrations in such patients. Failure of the serum iron abnormalities to resolve with improvement in the indices of liver inflammation justifies liver tissue examination and performance of the appropriate hepatic iron studies.

Alpha-1 antitypsin deficiency can induce liver disease in infants and adults. In children, the disorder can produce a profound cholestatic disease that resembles mechanical obstruction, and it is associated with bile duct hypoplasia. Other infants may have histologic changes of giant cell hepatitis and hepatitic patterns of injury (neonatal hepatitis). Early deaths are unusual; it is in late childhood and early adolescence that the disease is frequently complicated by cirrhosis and liver failure. In adults, the disease produces a chronic hepatitic syndrome which is manifested as mild serum aminotransferase abnormalities and features of cirrhosis. The adult disease is probably different than the childhood disease as there is little historical data to link the two as a continuum. The diagnosis is made by demonstrating the presence of the deficiency phenotype (ZZ) in serum. The ZZ phenotype is associated with a low serum level of α-1 antitrypsin, and this low concentration is a surrogate marker for the disease. Serum levels, however, can fluctuate in response to concurrent inflammation, malignancy, estrogen therapy, and pregnancy. Accordingly, the α-1 antitrypsin level may be normal in some cases of partial deficiency, or extraneously increased levels may obscure distinctions between the heterozygous and homozygous states in others. The ZZ deficiency phenotype is found in 1% of patients with chronic liver disease and its frequency increases to 7% in patients younger than 20 years old. This percentage is higher than that found in normal subjects and it suggests that the ZZ phenotype does predispose to chronic liver disease in young adults. Partial deficiency phenotypes (MZ, MS, SS, and SZ) are found in 5% of patients with chronic liver disease and 6% of individuals with normal liver function. The similar frequencies of partial deficiency between patients and controls have suggested that in patients with chronic liver disease partial α-1 antitrypsin deficiency is coincidental and nonpathogenic. This concept is still debated. Liver biopsy assessment in patients with chronic liver disease and the ZZ phenotype discloses diastase-resistant PAS globules in 60%, whereas antibody-specifc immunofluorescence against the inclusion material is positive in 100%. In contrast, only 41% of patients with partial deficiency have diagnostic histologic findings by PAS staining after diastase digestion or by antibody-specific immunofluorescence. The intensity and the extent of the inclusions do not correlate closely with the histologic evidence of liver cell injury. Importantly, patients with hepatocellular cancer may have α-1 antitrypsin inclusions and the frequency of hepatocellular cancer is high in adults with ZZ deficiency and cirrhosis.

Immunologic Markers

The immunoserologic markers that are essential for the evaluation of chronic hepatitic or chronic cholestatic processes of an immunologic nature are antinuclear antibodies (ANAs), smooth muscle antibodies (SMAs), antibodies to liver/kidney microsome type 1 (anti-LKM1), and antimitochondrial antibodies (AMAs) (see Table 351-1). Additional assays of limited clinical availability detect antibodies to actin (anti-actin) and to the E2 subunits of the pyruvate dehydrogenase complex (anti-PDH-E2). The presence or absence of these various antibodies in the proper clinical setting can support the diagnosis of autoimmune hepatitis, primary biliary cirrhosis, or autoimmune cholangitis.

Autoimmune hepatitis is a chronic hepatitic disease that is characterized by the presence of at least periportal hepatitis (piecemeal necrosis or interface hepatitis) on histologic examination, hypergammaglobulinemia, and seropositivity for ANAs and/or SMAs, or anti-LKM1. Antinuclear antibodies and/or SMAs define type 1 autoimmune hepatitis, which is the most common form of the disease. Antibodies to LKM1 characterize type 2 autoimmune hepatitis, which affects mainly children (ages 2 years to 14 years) in Western Europe. Seropositivity for ANAs and/or SMAs is mutually exclusive of seropositivity for anti-LKM1 (4% overlap in adults), and the different autoantibody species define distinct clinical syndromes. Unfortunately, none of the autoantibodies is disease specific or pathogenic. Antinuclear antibodies occur in drug-induced chronic liver disease, chronic viral hepatitis, primary biliary cirrhosis, primary sclerosing cholangitis, autoimmune cholangitis, and nonalcoholic steatohepatitis. Similarly, SMAs are found in infectious mononucleosis; cytomegalovirus infection; multiple malignancies, including lymphoma, hypernephroma, and carcinoma; drug-related liver toxicities; chronic viral hepatitis; and primary biliary cirrhosis. Antibodies to LKM1 occur uncommonly in general but they have been described in chronic hepatitis C and in patients infected with herpes simplex type 1. The diagnosis of autoimmune hepatitis remains one of exclusion and it is not established solely by the demonstration of liver-related autoantibodies.

Antibodies to actin have a higher specificity for autoimmune hepatitis than SMA, but they are less sensitive to the diagnosis and are not generally available. Their presence, however, identifies patients who have a poorer prognosis after corticosteroid treatment. Shortcomings in diagnostic sensitivity and availability may be overlooked if this marker has prognostic advantages. Efforts to enhance the diagnostic specificity of ANAs by demanding only homogeneous patterns of indirect immunofluorescence on Hep-2 cell lines have only reduced diagnostic sensitivity. Only 34% of patients with autoimmune hepatitis have homogenous patterns of ANAs by indirect immunofluorescence, and these individuals have clinical syndromes similar to those with heterogeneous patterns. Perhaps the most important determinant of specificity for ANAs and SMAs is titer level. Titers of ≥1:80 are required for the definite diagnosis of autoimmune hepatitis, and titers ≥1:320 are rare in chronic viral hepatitis.

Primary biliary cirrhosis (nonsuppurative destructive cholangitis) is a chronic cholestatic syndrome that is characterized by bile duct injury and/or loss on histologic examination, and AMAs in serum. The reactivity to mitochondrial antigens by indirect immunofluorescence on murine kidney and stomach is very specific for the diagnosis if it is present in high titer (≥1:160). Low titers have less diagnostic specificity, and 20% of patients with autoimmune hepatitis have weak AMA positivity. These mitochondrial antibodies commonly have a low frequency of reactivity against the trypsin-sensitive antigen on the inner mitochondrial membrane that is specific for primary biliary cirrhosis. In addition, no more than 8% of patients with autoimmune hepatitis have anti-PDH-E2, which are the antibodies against the autoantigen of primary biliary cirrhosis. Consequently, the interpretation of AMA seropositivity may be flawed if titers are low and the serologic findings are not married closely to the clinical setting. The staining pattern on the distal tubule of the murine kidney can be exuberant, and the immunoreaction can be confused with the staining pattern on the proximal tubule that characterizes reactivity to LKM1. Difficulties in distinguishing AMAs from anti-LKM1 and vice versa can be eliminated by testing for anti-PDH-E2. Currently, tests for the antibodies specific for primary biliary cirrhosis are not generally available.

Autoimmune cholangitis is a chronic inflammation of the liver with mixed hepatic and cholestatic features. It is characterized by

ANAs and/or SMAs in serum and histologic evidence of bile duct injury. The disease has been variously designated as AMA-negative primary biliary cirrhosis or a variant of autoimmune hepatitis, but it is probably a separate entity. Invariably, ANAs are present and by definition AMAs are absent. Recent studies suggest that autoimmune cholangitis may have its own serologic identity as antibodies to carbonic anhydrase distinguish it from autoimmune hepatitis and primary biliary cirrhosis. Further studies are necessary to establish this relationship and justify the clinical application of an assay that is now reserved for investigational use.

Imaging Studies

Ultrasonography (US), computed tomography (CT), and endoscopic retrograde cholangiopancreatography (ERCP) are the imaging studies that are used most commonly in the evaluation of acute and chronic liver disease. Magnetic resonance imaging (MRI), visceral angiography, hepatic venography, percutaneous transhepatic cholangiography (PTC), and technetium radionuclide scans are performed in highly selected instances and usually after the other imaging tests. Each examination contributes nuances to the diagnosis, and they are all complementary. Individual studies must be chosen because of their potential value and not in accordance with a presumed hierarchal order. They are used to assess the configuration and size of the liver; the homogeneity of the hepatic parenchyma; the nature and extent of infiltrative processes; features of extrahepatic biliary obstruction; patency of hepatic, portal, and splenic veins; and the presence of ascites, lymphadenopathy, extrahepatic mass, and splenomegaly. Liver tissue samples, fluid specimens, and extrahepatic tissue samples can be obtained by needle aspiration under scan guidance and therapeutic interventions such as drainage, decompression, stone removal, and stenting can be performed. The resectability of a hepatic lesion can be evaluated, and anatomic features that impact on an individual's candidacy for liver transplantation can also be assessed.

Ultrasonography of the hepatobiliary tract evaluates the size and shape of the liver, hepatic parenchyma, gallbladder, intrahepatic and extrahepatic bile ducts, hepatic venous vasculature, perihepatic lymph nodes, spleen, and contiguous abdominal cavity. Distortion of the liver shape, reduction in size, and prominence of the caudate lobe suggest the presence of cirrhosis and a chronic hepatitic or cholestatic process. Hyperechogenicity of the parenchyma, especially in reference to the right kidney and spleen, and obscuration of the hepatic vasculature indicate a diffuse fatty infiltration. Coarsening of the hepatic echotexture connotes a diffuse parenchymal disease, whereas dilation of the intrahepatic and/or extrahepatic bile ducts implicates a biliary obstruction. Further evaluation of the distal common bile duct, pancreatic head, and its duct may define the cause. Focal intrahepatic lesions not only can be seen but the cystic or solid nature of the process can be determined. If characteristic sonographic features are present, a diagnosis such as cavernous hemangioma or focal fatty infiltrate can be rendered with accuracy. Hepatic vein thrombosis (Budd-Chiari syndrome), portal vein occlusion (cavernous transformation, tumor invasion, pancreatitis, and pylephlebitis), or splenic vein obstruction (gastric varices) can be assessed and other features of portal hypertension, including collateralization of intrabdominal blood vessels, ascites formation, and recanalization of the umbilical vein, can be documented. Failure of ultrasonography to demonstrate biliary obstruction does not exclude its existence; the clinical situation may mandate other biliary studies such as ERCP or transhepatic cholangiography. Marginally dilated extrahepatic ducts due to mechanical obstruction, diffusely strictured bile ducts associated with primary sclerosing cholangitis and/or cholangiocarcinoma, and lesions in the small intrahepatic ducts (cholangiocarcinoma, stones, and Caroli's disease) may be missed with this procedure.

Computed tomography provides different, but not necessarily better, information than ultrasonography, and both tests are frequently performed in the same patient. They are used mainly to evaluate the nature of an acute or chronic cholestatic (infiltrative) process. Rapid scanners produce sharper images of intraabdominal lesions than ultrasound, and the procedure is not compromised by large body habitus, abdominal gas, or bone interfaces. Its major use is in the identification of masses within the liver or abdomen; dynamic CT scans with intravenous contrast can provide diagnostic images. Cavernous hemangiomas are common lesions of the liver and they can be reliably distinguished from malignancies by a characteristic peripheral enhancement during rapid sequence contrast infusion followed by central filling. The administration of intravenous contrast dye also allows determination of the size and patency of the portal and hepatic veins, and CT is useful in the evaluation of Budd-Chiari syndrome and in the assessment of tumor resectability. Oral barium sulfate is commonly given in conjuction with the intravenous contrast dyes to better delineate space-occupying lesions and facilitates evaluation of tumor invasion. Marked attenuation of the liver signal by CT scan suggests steatohepatitis, and dilated intrahepatic and/or extrahepatic bile ducts connote a biliary obstruction whose location and cause is frequently delineated by examination of the biliary tree and pancreas. CT-guided biopsies can provide an objective basis for the visual impression.

Endoscopic retrograde cholangiopancreatography is a procedure that can extend the findings of ultrasonography and/or CT scan to a diagnostic conclusion. It also has a therapeutic potential. The presence of dilated intrahepatic and/or extrahepatic bile ducts, indeterminate mass at the head of the pancreas, dilated pancreatic duct, obscure right upper quadrant pain, and unexplained acute or chronic cholestatic laboratory findings justify its performance. It is the preferred procedure to evaluate unexplained cholestasis in the presence of nondilated bile ducts. In such cases, it may disclose characteristic changes of primary sclerosing cholangitis and/or cholangiocarcinoma, a focal proximal biliary obstruction (tumor, stone, or stricture), or a previously undetected dilated biliary tree due to stone, tumor, pancreatitis, or obstructing ampulla. The procedure permits direct visualization (and biopsy) of the ampulla for tumor or stenosis, delineation of the biliary and pancreatic ducts, removal of obstructing biliary stones and debris, brush cytology and biopsies of intraductal lesions, dilation and stenting of strictures, measurement of sphincteric pressures, assessment of biliary tract emptying, palliation of obstucting unresectable distal pancreatic or biliary malignancies, and sphincterotomy for improvement of bile duct drainage. There is an 8% frequency of complications, which include abdominal pain, infection, and pancreatitis. Intravenous antibiotics that are excreted into the biliary tree should be given immediately before the procedure if a mechanical biliary obstruction is anticipated.

Magnetic resonance imaging is one of several studies that can be selected to clarify uncertainties found with ultrasonography and/or CT scan. Its major advantages are the detection and characterization of small hepatic nodules and the visualization of abdominal blood vessels. The minimum detectable size for focal lesions within the liver is 1.5 cm, and 98% of hepatic masses $\geq$2 cm in diameter are visualized by MRI. Its sensitivity (64% versus 51%) and specificity (99% versus 94%) for liver metastases are greater than those for CT scan, but the resolution of small ($\leq$1 cm) lesions remains its pitfall. Nodular malignant tumors are better characterized by MRI than CT scan because of MRI's ability to detect tumor septae, pseudocapsule, and neovasculature. It also has a 90% accuracy in diagnosing cavernous hemangiomas, and it can frequently detect the central scar of focal nodular hyperplasia. The nature of nontumorous lesions such as cysts, abscesses, and focal fat are evaluated well by this technique, and portal vein thromboses, vascular invasion by tumor, and the etiology of Budd-Chiari syndrome can commonly be defined. Diffuse accumulations of fat, copper, and iron within the hepatic parenchyma can also be assessed by MRI, and it has greater sensitivity for these accumulations at low concentration than do other imaging modalities. MRI, however, does not provide quantitative information or a reliable method of studying changes in parenchymal concentration with time or therapy. The use of paramagnetic contrast agents enhances the sensitivity and specificity of the technique. Gadolinium diethylenetriamine pentaacetic acid accentuates normal liver tissue and enhances detection of focal nodules. When complexed with albumin, it remains in the intravascular space and delineates the vasculature. Some lesions are more crisply defined by CT scan than by MRI, and the technique should not be regarded as the final arbiter. Equivocal results are still common after an MRI examination, especially in the cirrhotic patient with regenerative or malignant nodules within the liver.

Arteriography is used mainly to evaluate portal hypertension, define the resectability of a focal intrahepatic lesion, assess the vascular anatomy before liver transplantation, design an effective central or distal shunt, deliver chemotherapy to an unresectable neoplasm, or embolize a malignant lesion, symptomatic arteriovenous shunt, or bleeding vessel. Its utility as a diagnostic tool has been largely supplanted by US, CT scan, and MRI. In contrast, hepatic venography remains a diagnostically important vascular study that should be used to evaluate unexplained ascites and rapid-onset hepatomegaly. The diagnosis of hepatic outflow obstruction can be made quickly, safely, and confidently using this procedure.

Radionuclide scans have also been largely replaced by ultrasonsography, CT scan, and MRI. Rarely, they may be necessary to characterize a cavernous hemangioma, implicate a focal nodular hyperplasia, or confirm a Budd-Chiari syndrome. A radiolabeled red blood cell scan can establish the presence of a cavernous hemangioma if other tests are equivocal. Similarly, a technetium sulfur colloid scan can indicate a focal nodular hyperplasia by filling out a discrete defect on CT scan, or it can implicate the Budd-Chiari syndrome by demonstrating a prominent caudate lobe on a background of decreased hepatic uptake. Other more powerful tools, however, portray the processes more completely.

Percutaneous transhepatic cholangiography is reserved for those patients with mechanical large bile duct obstruction in whom ERCP is unsuccessful in either establishing the diagnosis or bypassing the obstruction. Lesions at the bifurcation of the hepatic bile ducts or in the hepatic ducts themselves may not be accessible by ERCP. These lesions can often be reached by the transhepatic route. The lesion can be sampled and the dilated ducts can be drained internally by passage of a stent beyond the obstruction or externally by placement of a percutaneous drain. Dominant benign intraductal strictures can be dilated; stones can be removed; and malignant intraductal lesions can be palliated. Bleeding, sepsis, and bile peritonitis are serious but uncommon complications (1%), and parenteral antibiotic therapy should be administered before the procedure.

Liver Tissue Examination

The liver tissue examination should corroborate the clinical impression and establish the diagnosis. It should follow the appropriate laboratory assessments, and imaging studies and the histologic findings should not be unanticipated. All diseases of the liver have pathologic definitions and consequently a complete diagnosis requires this assessment. Rarely, however, is a liver tissue examination of value in the differential diagnosis of acute hepatitis or in extrahepatic biliary obstruction. In these circumstances, the biopsy procedure is justified only if an exacerbated chronic liver disease is expected; the specimen is likely to have the characteristic microvesicular fat droplets of Reye's syndrome or acute fatty liver of pregnancy; or the obstruction is due to primary sclerosing cholangitis. In each instance, the histologic findings may impact on immediate therapy.

Recent studies have confirmed that the percutaneous needle liver biopsy technique is safe and that it can be used successfully in the outpatient setting under well-monitored circumstances. Ultrasonographic guidance of the biopsy needle, however, improves the likelihood of harvesting diagnostic tissue and it reduces the low frequency of complications even further. Consequently, ultrasound guidance is now the preferred technique for liver biopsy.

Bleeding and abdominal pain, which may radiate to the right shoulder, are the most common complications of the procedure. Gallbladder puncture, bile peritonitis, and hematobilia are other rare consequences. The risk of clinically significant bleeding cannot be eliminated, so it is important to select patients for the procedure who have a low risk of hemorrhage. Salicylates should be avoided for at least 7 days before biopsy; abnormalities of prothrombin time should be treated with vitamin K, the hemoglobulin level should be at least 8 g/dl, the prothrombin time should not exceed control by more than 3 seconds (international normalized ratio <1.7), and platelet counts should be at least 50 x10⁹/L. Coagulation defects in excess of these guidelines should be corrected before biopsy by transfusion of packed red blood cells, platelets, and/or fresh frozen plasma. Patients at increased risk for hemorrhage (those with severe coagulopathy) should have a hemoglobin level of at least 10 g/dl with transfusion if necessary. Liver biopsy can be performed by the transjugular approach in patients with uncorrectable coagulopathy. With this method, the liver puncture is made from within the vasculature.

Cirrhosis is variably sampled by needle biopsy, and in chronic hepatitis multiple samples from different regions of the same liver at the same time show consistent features of cirrhosis in only 33% of instances. Cirrhosis, therefore, can be greatly underestimated by needle biopsy especially in a macronodular liver. Perhaps more importantly intraobserver consistency in diagnosing cirrhosis in the same biopsy specimen reviewed at different times is no greater than 78%. Consequently, patients may be wrongly diagnosed as having cirrhosis or not in 22% of instances. The application of rigid histologic criteria for cirrhosis is essential to minimize this error. Accordingly, the diagnosis of histologic cirrhosis requires a complete regenerative nodule with fibrosis. Specificity for the diagnosis is more important than sensitivity.

Laparoscopy and guided needle biopsy of the liver are probably more accurate methods of diagnosing cirrhosis than the closed technique. However, the interobserver and intraobserver error in the visual diagnosis of cirrhosis is unmeasured and the ability of laparoscopists to distinguish early cirrhosis from no cirrhosis and multilobular collapse and regeneration from established cirrhosis is uncertain. Fortunately, it is usually not critical in diagnosis and management to distinguish cirrhosis, and there are a phlethora of other less subjective tests by which to measure hepatic function and assess compensation. Perhaps the greatest value of laparoscopy currently is in the evaluation of ascites of unknown origin. Peritoneal and mesenteric surfaces can be inspected and granulomatous and lymphoproliferative disorders can be excluded.

Amino-Terminal Procollagen III Level

Procollagens are synthesized intracellularly and they have extension peptides at the amino and carboxy ends. The amino-terminal peptide is precursor specific and is cleaved and released into the circulation as procollagen is converted to collagen. The concentration of amino-terminal peptide in serum, therefore, is a reflection of collagen formation. Unfortunately, serum levels of the peptide correlate poorly with histologic and morphometric analyses of hepatic fibrosis and cirrhosis. Discrepancies probably relate to nonhepatic fibrogenesis (inflammatory diseases elsewhere in the body) and failure of the assay to account for collagen degradation. The net amount of fibrosis in the liver reflects the balance between collagen deposition and disappearance, and the assay for amino-terminal peptide measures only one aspect of this dynamic interaction. Hepatic inflammation stimulates reparative as well as cytolytic processes, and these actions increase collagen turnover. In chronic hepatitis, the procollagen III peptide level correlates with the standard laboratory tests of liver inflammation. Consequently, the major clinical value of the test is to provide additional reassurance about the presence or absence of such activity.

Serum Hyaluronic Acid Level

Hyaluronic acid is a polysaccharide that is synthetized by mesenchymal cells. It is an important component of the intercellular matrix of the liver and its level is increased in fibrosis. Clearance from plasma depends on the hepatic sinusoidal endothelial cells, and an elevated serum level reflects increased synthesis (fibrogenesis) and/or impaired clearance (decreased hepatic endothelial cell function or sinusoidal perfusion). Serum levels discriminate between the presence and absence of cirrhosis better than those for the amino-terminal procollagen III peptide, and abnormalities probably result from changes in sinusoidal endothelial cell function as a result of fibrosis. Measurements of the serum hyaluronic acid level are not yet part of the conventional battery of diagnostic tests.

ESTIMATIONS OF SEVERITY AND PROGNOSIS

The severity of an acute or chronic liver disease is reflected in its clinical manifestations and the tests of liver function and inflammation (Table 351-3). Patients with hepatic encephalopathy, renal insufficiency, ascites, and/or muscle wasting have poor hepatic function and a dismal immediate prognosis regardless of etiology. Patients with autoimmune hepatitis who have laboratory changes that indicate severe inflammation also have a poor prognosis, and failure of these patients to respond to corticosteroid therapy underscores the aggressiveness of their disease. In such patients, serum aspartate aminotrans-

Table 351-3   Prognostic indices

HEPATITIC PATTERN	CHOLESTATIC PATTERN
Acute	
Prothrombin time >50 seconds	Rising bilirubin and/or alkaline
Serum bilirubin >300 μmol/l	phosphatase and falling AST
Age <10 years and >40 years	Prolonged prothrombin time un-
≥7 Days from jaundice to coma	corrected by vitamin K
Renal insufficiency	Renal insufficiency
Persistent abnormalities >12	Hepatic encephalopathy
weeks	Muscle wasting
	Hepatic encephalopathy
Chronic	Renal insufficiency
Multilobular necrosis	Fixed hypoalbuminemia and hy-
Failure to improve elevated biliru-	poprothrombinemia
bin level after 2 weeks of corti-	Intractable ascites
costeroids if autoimmune	Gastrointestinal bleeding
hepatitis	Malignant infiltration
Muscle wasting	Child-Pugh class C
Hepatic encephalopathy	Mathematical models for primary
Renal insufficiency	biliary cirrhosis and primary
Fixed hypoalbuminemia and hy-	sclerosing cholangitis
poprothrombinemia	
Intractable ascites	
Gastrointestinal bleeding	
Child-Pugh class C	

ferase levels ten-fold or more of normal or five-fold or more of normal in conjunction with a hypergammaglobulinemia of at least twice normal are associated with a mortality of 50% within 3 years. The presence of bridging necrosis or mulilobular necrosis on histologic examination identifies individuals with an 82% frequency of cirrhosis and a mortality of 45% within 5 years. Laboratory tests of hepatic synthetic function (prothrombin time, serum albumin, and pseudocholinesterase levels), detoxification function (serum bilirubin and blood ammonia levels), and regenerative activity (alpha-fetoprotein level) are generic indices of disease severity. Combinations of abnormalities in different diseases have individual prognostic significance and these have been integrated into mathematical models that project outcome, as in primary biliary cirrhosis and primary sclerosing cholangitis; or as clinical constellations that connote severity, as in the Child-Pugh classification (Table 351-4). Quantitative liver function tests that reflect functioning hepatic mass and hepatic blood flow supplement these determinations, but their full potential as indices of prognosis has not been realized.

Hepatic Synthetic Function

The most practical and useful tests of hepatic synthetic function are the prothrombin time and the serum albumin level (see Table 351-3). The serum pseudocholinesterase level can supplement determinations of the serum albumin level if in the latter instance, the serum concentration has been altered by intravenous infusions.

In fulminant viral hepatitis, a prothrombin time >50 seconds (control, ≤15 seconds) is associated with a poor outcome as are a serum bilirubin level >300 μmol/l, age 10 years or older than 40 years, and an interval of at least 7 days between the onset of jaundice and the appearance of hepatic encephalopathy (see Table 351-3).

In chronic liver disease, the prothrombin time and serum albumin level are included in the formulation of the Child-Pugh classification. This classification continues to be the most practical and useful means of grading the severity of cirrhosis, and it should be calculated in each patient. Points are given for the presence or absence of ascites, degree of abnormality in prothrombin time, serum bilirubin level, serum albumin concentration, and the presence or absence of hepatic encephalopathy (see Table 351-4). The composite score determines the severity and this grade defines immediate mortality and the risk of hepatic complications.

In mathematical models of prognosis, the importance of the serum albumin level and prothromin time has also been recognized. When combined with the serum bilirubin level, patient's age, presence or absence of edema, and need for diuretic therapy, these indices accurately project survival by Cox Proportional Hazards Regres-

sion in patients with primary biliary cirrhosis (see Table 351-4). The combination of serum bilirubin level, patient's age, splenomegaly, and histologic stage project survival by a similar mathematical model in primary sclerosing cholangitis (see Table 351-4). These models are useful in the timing of liver transplantation, and they also provide a surrogate control group for the evaluation of new drugs.

Detoxification Function

Bilirubin is derived from the catabolism of heme proteins; its presence in serum reflects the rate of heme breakdown and the adequacy of hepatic uptake, conjugation, and canalicular excretion. Abnormal serum levels reflect perturbations at one or more of these steps. Serum levels can also be affected by renal function since a small but significant proportion of the bilirubin load is excreted by the kidneys. Determinations of the serum bilirubin level, therefore, are not direct measurements of hepatic excretory function. Insights into excretory activity are possible, however, if the conjugated (water-soluble) fraction of bilirubin is considered separately.

Conjugated or water-soluble bilirubin reflects hepatic processing. The pigment is delivered to the hepatocyte as a fat soluble byproduct of porphyrin metabolism. The unconjugated substrate can enter liver cells but cannot be excreted into bile by the canaliculus. Conjugation involves alteration of the molecule by direct hepatic action and incorporation of one or two glucuronic acids. Glucuronidation renders the bilirubin molecule polar and excretable in bile and urine. Abnormal elevation of the conjugated bilirubin fraction indicates an excretory block at the canaliculus or at any level in the biliary tree. Typically, the conjugated bilirubin fraction is increased in combination with the unconjugated fraction in any severe hepatocellular or cholestatic injury. The associated abnormalities in the serum aminotransferase, alkaline phosphatase, gamma glutamyltransferase, and/or 5' nucleotidase levels determine the hepatitic or cholestatic nature of the disease. Metabolic disturbances including sepsis, hyperthyroidism, hypotension, and anoxia commonly interfere with the energy-dependent step of canalicular excretion and can provoke a marked conjugated hyperbilirubinemia, especially after surgery, trauma, and burns (see Table 351-3). Inherited defects in bilirubin excretion as in the Dubin-Johnson syndrome or Rotor syndrome are characterized by conjugated hyperbilirubinemia, as are hepatocellular conditions due to drug, virus, or alcohol and diseases that mechanically obstruct bile ducts (see Table 351-3). A third of conjugated bilirubin is covalently bound to albumin as a "delta fraction." This fraction becomes more prominent with the duration of hyperbilirubinemia; it has a serum half-life that approximates that of albumin (15 days). The delta fraction is not excreted in urine and can result in slow resolution of the hyperbilirubinemia and a lingering concern about the adequacy of convalescence. The bilirubin level and its behavior over time reflect prognosis in primary biliary cirrhosis and in some acute and chronic liver diseases. A rising serum bilirubin concentration and a falling serum aminotransferase level indicate a poor prognosis in acute viral hepatitis. Similarly, failure of the bilirubin level to improve after 2 weeks of corticosteroid therapy denotes liver failure and imminent death from autoimmune hepatitis (see Table 351-3).

Ammonia is detoxified by the liver, and determinations of the blood ammonia level have been used as crude estimates of hepatic detoxification function. Ammonia is derived mainly from the diet and is present in food or is a consequence of dietary protein degradation by colonic bacteria. Other sources include small intestinal digestion of dietary protein, metabolism of endogenous glutamine by the small intestine, and the colonic breakdown of endogenous urea (25% to 30% of urea normally passes into the colon). Detoxification occurs in the liver, where ammonia is converted to urea, and in the skeletal muscle and brain, where it is combined with glutamic acid to form glutamine. Failure of the liver to detoxify ammonia because of decreased hepatic mass and/or shunting of portal blood around the liver raises the blood ammonia level. Since the blood ammonia concentration can be affected by blood flow, diet, and muscle mass, it is not a reliable measure of liver cell function and should not be used as such. Its major clinical value is to assess the nature of mental changes in patients who may have hepatic encephalopathy or in individuals who may have an inherited urea cycle defect. Since the skeletal muscle is a larger site for ammonia metabolism than the brain, the blood ammonia levels in patients with chronic encephalopathy are determined

Table 351-4   Quantitation of prognosis

| PROGNOSTIC VARIABLES | CHILD-PUGH SCORE* POINTS | | | MAYO PBC MODEL† | MAYO PSC MODEL‡ |
	1	2	3		
Bilirubin (mg/dl)	>1.1-2.0	>2.0-3.0	>3.0	X	X
Albumin (g/dl)		2.8-3.5	<2.8	X	
Prothrombin time (seconds above control)	1-3	4-6	>6	X (seconds)	
Encephalopathy		Grade 1-2	Grade 3-4		
Ascites		Mild	Moderate		
Age (years)				X	X
Edema (± diuretics)				X	
Splenomegaly					X
Histologic stage					X

*Child-Pugh classes: A, score 1-6; B, score 7-9; C, score 10-15.
†Mayo mathematical survival model for primary biliary cirrhosis (PBC): R (risk) = 0.871 log$_e$ (bilirubin) + −2.53 log$_e$ (albumin) + 0.039 (age) + 2.38 log$_e$ (prothrombin time) + 0.859 (edema).
‡Mayo mathematical survival model for primary sclerosing cholangitis (PSC): R (risk) = 0.535 log$_e$ (bilirubin) + 0.486 (histologic stage) + 0.041 (age) + 0.705 (splenomegaly).

mainly by muscle mass. Consequently, isolated blood ammonia levels correlate poorly with the level of encephalopathy. Serial determinations in the same patient correlate more closely with clinical change, and the sensitivity of the blood determination for hepatic encephalopathy can be increased if arterial levels are measured.

Hepatic Regenerative Activity

There are no clinical tests that reliably and safely assess hepatic regenerative activity. Alpha-fetoprotein is produced by fetal human liver cells, regenerating normal hepatocytes, malignant hepatocytes, and neoplastic embryonal cells of the gonads. Patients with fulminant hepatitis can produce alpha-fetoprotein, and this production can be measured in serum as a possible reflection of hepatocytic regenerative activity. The serum changes, however, correlate mainly with the duration of survival rather than actual survival, and the test does not have prognostic value. Similarly, 35% of patients with severe autoimmune hepatitis have abnormal serum alpha-fetoprotein levels at presentation; these findings do not distinguish the patients by outcome. Levels return to normal after corticosteroid therapy and resolution of the inflammatory process. Currently, determinations of the serum alpha-fetoprotein level should be used mainly for the assessment of patients with possible hepatocellular carcinoma.

Regenerative activity has been recognized and quantitated in patients with fulminant hepatitis by morphometric analysis of liver tissue. The quantitative result has been correlated with prognosis, and the assessment may have predictive value. Unfortunately, the procedure involves tissue sampling in critically ill patients with coagulopathy, and it is still uncertain if the prediction of outcome is better than that made by conventional tests. Histologic assessments in patients with advanced chronic liver disease can also identify hepatocytic regeneration. Without quantitation and correlation with outcome, however, these observations have no clinical importance.

Quantitative Liver Function Tests

Quantitative liver function tests have the potential to assess hepatocyte mass, project prognosis, and evaluate responses to therapy. Ideally, they would facilitate the selection of patients for hepatic resection, other major surgery, or liver transplantation. All such tests are based on the premise that hepatic clearance of a substance relates directly to hepatic blood flow and its hepatic extraction fraction. Substances that have a high first-pass clearance by the liver (extraction fraction ≈ 1.0) estimate hepatic blood flow, whereas substances with low hepatic clearance measure the functioning hepatic mass. Quantitative liver function tests have long been part of the diagnostic armamentarium, but they have not been generally available and they have failed to supplant conventional assays.

The galactose elimination test assesses the activity of the cytosolic enzyme, galactokinase. This activity correlates with hepatic weight and hepatocyte mass. The test, therefore, does quantitate hepatocyte function and has predicted survival in cirrhosis, fulminant hepatic failure, and primary biliary cirrhosis. Galactose, however, is excreted in urine; it is metabolized outside the liver; its catabolism is impaired by alcohol consumption; and its elimination decreases with age. These factors influence the interpretation and standardization of the test.

The monoethylglycinexylidide (MEGX) test measures the production of MEGX within 15 minutes after intravenous administration of lignocaine. The test assesses microsomal P450 function (CYP IIIA4), and it quantitates hepatic functional impairment. The activity of CYP IIIA4, however, fluctuates by ten-fold in healthy individuals, and test results are frequently variable. Indeed, the test has been unable to distinguish mild from severe disease on a consistent basis.

The aminopyrine breath test measures the microsomal demethylation of ^{13}C or ^{14}C methyl groups on aminopyrine. The formaldehyde that is produced is oxidized to $^{13}CO_2$ or $^{14}CO_2$, which is then exhaled at a rate that presumably reflects the functional microsomal mass. The rate-limiting demethylation step is catalyzed by several P450, and the test results reflect global microsomal activity (total hepatic P450 content), hepatic N-demethylase activity, and the surface area of the hepatic smooth endoplasmic reticulum. Unfortunately, the formation and excretion of CO_2 depend on many biochemical reactions that can affect the test results, and these interactions have hindered standardization of the test. In addition, results are affected by drugs that induce P450 function (barbiturates), tissue hypoxia (congestive heart failure), renal dialysis, and advancing age.

The hepatic metabolism of caffeine can be measured by plasma clearance, breath test, saliva clearance, or fasting serum level. Caffeine demethylation is mediated by a particular P450 isoenzyme (CAP1A2), which is not induced by drugs. It is affected by smoking, however, and this sensitivity can impair the value of the test as a probe of microsomal function. Caffeine metabolism does decrease with loss of hepatic mass, and test results do correlate with those of other quantitative liver tests. Findings, however, have not been assigned a prognostic significance or a superiority over those from other conventional studies.

The antipyrine clearance test measures the disappearance of a low-extraction drug that is metabolized by the cytochrome P450 system. The rate of disappearance of antipyrine does not depend on hepatic blood flow or drug dose, and clearance reflects the global P450 function of the liver. Since concentrations of antipyrine are similar in serum and saliva, the disappearance of the drug can be monitored in saliva samples collected 24 and 48 hours after a single oral dose. The rate of antipyrine metabolism is affected by cimetidine, estrogens, and anti-seizure medications, and side effects include allergic reactions (especially in those with known allergies to phenylbutazone or sulfinpyrazone) and hemolysis in those with glucose-6-phosphate dehydrogenase deficiency. Antipyrine clearance is decreased in patients with portal hypertension and ascites, and this reduction may reflect changes in liver function and/or the volume of drug distribution. The test does reflect survival in fulminant hepatic failure, disease activity in chronic hepatitis, and graft function after liver transplantation. Further studies must demonstrate its unique contributions to diagnosis and management.

Hepatic mitochondrial function has been measured in the rat by a breath test that quantitatively reflects the decarboxylation of ketoisocaproic acid. [13]C- and ^{14}C-ketoisocaproic breath tests have been used for the same purpose in humans, and preliminary studies indicate that they are able to distinguish alcoholic from nonalcoholic liver disease. Since mitochondrial function is impaired in many liver diseases, a test to quantitate this dysfunction would have broad clinical value, especially if it could discriminate levels of impairment and identify diseases that are characterized by mitochondrial injury (alcohol-related diseases and primary biliary cirrhosis). Further investigations are necessary before its introduction into the clinical arena.

SUMMARY

An accurate diagnosis can be obtained in most instances if patients with liver disease are evaluated in a systematic fashion. Clinical history, physical findings, laboratory tests, imaging studies, and liver tissue examination permit classification of such patients into categories that reflect disease duration, hepatitic or cholestatic nature, etiologic basis, and severity. By using the appropriate tests at each level of inquiry, the testing sequences can be logical, complementary, and cost effective. Novel assays, especially those that promise to quantitate liver function, will improve and replace current technologies. Diagnostic accuracy, however, will continue to depend on the physician.

BIBLIOGRAPHY

Bodily KO, Fitz JG: Approach to the patient with suspected liver disease. In Grendell JH, McQuaid KR, Friedman SL, editors: *Current diagnosis and treatment in gastroenterology,* Stamford, 1996, Appleton & Lange, p. 461.

Czaja AJ: Acute hepatitis. In Snape W Jr, editor: *Consultations in gastroenterology,* Philadelphia, 1995, WB Saunders, p. 659.

Czaja AJ: Autoantibodies, *Baillere's clinical gastroenterology* 9:723, 1995.

Czaja AJ: Chronic hepatitis. In Shearmann DJC, Finlayson NDC, Camilleri M, Carter DC, editors: *Diseases of the gastrointestinal tract and liver,* London, 1997, Churchill Livingstone, pp. 887-913.

Czaja AJ: Hepatomegaly. In Taylor RB, editor: *Difficult diagnosis 2,* Philadelphia, 1992, WB Saunders, p. 195.

Czaja AJ: Serologic markers of hepatitis A and B in acute and chronic liver disease, *Mayo Clin Proc* 54:721, 1979.

Czaja AJ, Wolf AM, Baggenstoss AH: Laboratory assessment of severe chronic active liver disease during and after corticosteroid therapy: correlation of serum aminotransferase and gamma globulin levels with histologic features, *Gastroenterology* 80:687, 1981.

Czaja AJ,Wolf AM, Baggenstoss AH: Clinical assessment of cirrhosis in severe chronic active liver disease: specificity and sensitivity of physical and laboratory findings, *Mayo Clin Proc* 55:360, 1980.

Davis GL et al: Prognostic and therapeutic implications of extreme serum aminotransferase elevation in chronic active hepatitis, *Mayo Clin Proc* 57:303, 1982.

McCullough AJ: Laboratory assessment of liver function and inflammatory activity in chronic active hepatitis. In Czaja AJ, Dickson ER, editors: *Chronic active hepatitis. the Mayo Clinic experience,* New York, 1986, Marcel Dekker, p. 205.

Reichen J, Widmer T, Cotting J: Accurate prediction of death by serial determination of galactose elimination capacity in primary biliary cirrhosis: a comparison with the Mayo model, *Hepatology* 14:504, 1991.

Renner EL: Liver function tests, *Baillere's clinical gastroenterology* 9:661, 1995.

Williams SJ, Farrell GC: Antipyrine clearance reflects spontaneous and interferon-induced changes in activity of chronic active hepatitis B, *Hepatology* 10:192, 1989.

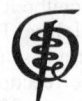

CHAPTER

352 Evaluation of Pancreatic Diseases

C.S. Pitchumoni

Measurements of pancreatic enzymes in serum and urine provide important information regarding assessment of pancreatic disease. They are simple to perform but are somewhat insensitive. The more sensitive pancreatic function tests are time-consuming and technically difficult, and they are not easily available in clinical practice except in

major university centers that are specializing in pancreatic disorders. The pancreatic imaging techniques have markedly improved recently and are now readily available in most hospitals. In general, the imaging studies are limited by their cost and poor sensitivity in early chronic pancreatitis.

SIMPLE PANCREATIC FUNCTION TESTS
Serum Amylase

Total serum amylase estimation has been used since 1929 and still is the mainstay in the diagnosis of acute pancreatitis. Two major sources of amylase exist in humans: the pancreas and salivary glands. Smaller amounts of salivary type amylases are produced by the lungs and fallopian tubes. Total serum amylase thus consists of two isoenzymes, salivary (S type) and pancreatic (P type). In clinical practice, total serum amylase activity is the one that is most often used in the diagnosis of acute pancreatitis in view of its low cost, easy availability, and a good sensitivity. The sensitivity of amylase in the diagnosis of acute pancreatitis depends upon the cut-off value taken for the upper limit of normal. A threefold elevation of amylase level, although it may slightly decrease the sensitivity, correlates well with a diagnosis of acute pancreatitis. Amylase levels have no prognostic value. However, levels tend to vary depending on the cause of pancreatitis. In gallstone-induced pancreatitis the levels are extremely high, whereas in alcohol-induced pancreatitis the levels are only mildly elevated. In hyperlipidemic pancreatitis the serum amylase level may not be appreciably elevated in nearly 50% of patients. The normal levels are the result of an amylase inhibitor in the serum of patients with hyperlipidemia, and serial dilutions overcome this impediment. Macroamylasemia is a condition seen in 1% to 2% of healthy population, where the amylase molecule is bound to an abnormal protein in the form of the IgA, IgG, or IgM to produce a larger molecular complex of nearly 150,000 daltons, which cannot be filtered into the urine. The condition is easily diagnosed by finding a normal or low urinary amylase in the presence of a high serum amylase level.

Although theoretically estimating pancreas-specific P isoamylase activity in the serum is a preferred method of diagnosis of acute pancreatitis, it has not been borne out in clinical practice. Estimation of P amylase is only marginally more sensitive and specific than total amylase levels when used in the diagnosis of acute pancreatitis.

Serum Lipase

Sources of lipase other than the pancreas are the stomach, tongue, and liver. However, lipase in the serum is exclusively pancreatic in origin. Technologic improvements in the estimation of lipase have made lipase assays useful in the diagnosis of acute pancreatitis. The newer techniques are faster and more reliable, and they compare favorably with amylase assays. In alcoholic pancreatitis, compared to the modest elevations of amylase levels noted, the levels of lipase are as high as five times normal. Another advantage of lipase estimation is that the levels of lipase remain elevated for a longer period of time than amylase. In contrast to common belief, lipase elevation is not specific for acute pancreatitis. Mild to moderate elevations (less than three times normal) are seen in a number of nonpancreatic conditions with abdominal pain, like ruptured aortic aneurysm, cholelithiasis, choledocholithiasis, and small bowel obstruction, and they are considered nonspecific for the diagnosis of acute pancreatitis.

Other Serum Markers

Other serum enzymes currently being evaluated in the diagnosis of pancreatic diseases include trypsin, elastase 1, polymorphonuclear (PMN) elastase, phospholipase A2, and ribonuclease (Rnase). Of these, trypsin appears to have a high sensitivity in detecting acute pancreatitis. The technique of trypsin assay is time consuming, and mild elevations are nonspecific for pancreatitis. Elastase 1, which tends to remain elevated for a long period of time, has no superiority over amylase estimation. Phospholipase A2 is produced by the acinar cells as an inactive proenzyme (proPLA2), which is converted to active form by trypsin. Very high levels of PLA2 are noted in severe acute pancreatitis. Serum Rnase as a marker of pancreatic necrosis is controversial.

PMN elastase is being studied as an early indicator of severity of acute pancreatitis. PMN elastase is produced by neutrophils, which participate in pancreatic injury by release of lysosomal proteases, mainly elastase. Polymorphonuclear elastase and C-reactive protein estimations, when performed during the first and second day of the disease, help to predict the severity with a high specificity and sensitivity. Values of PMN elastase >200 mg/ml and C-reactive protein >300 mg/l are seen only in severe acute pancreatitis. Human pancreas-specific protein (PASP) subsequently identified as pancreatic procarboxy peptidase B (PCB) has been recently characterized as a serum marker for pancreatitis. Early observations suggest that the elevations of PASP in the serum parallel the course of amylase and lipase initially, but stay high for a greater number of days. The test is new and has yet to be standardized.

Urinary Amylase and Lipase

Estimation of urinary amylase was once popular. The size of an amylase molecule is roughly 50,000 daltons, the critical size for passage through the glomerulus, but glomerular filtration of amylase is unpredictable. However, in acute pancreatitis the urinary clearance of amylase is twofold to fourfold. A number of conditions influence urinary amylase clearance, so urinary amylase levels are poor indicators of acute pancreatitis. Amylase/creatinine clearance ratio was originally proposed to diagnose acute pancreatitis. This test has been dropped from the list of diagnostic tests for acute pancreatitis, since experience has shown that it is neither sensitive nor specific for the diagnosis. Therefore, no further discussion of the test is warranted here.

Pancreatic lipase has a molecular weight of 48,000 daltons. The filtered lipase is reabsorbed in the tubules so that little or no lipase is found in the urine of normal individuals. Urinary lipase estimation has no place in the diagnosis of acute pancreatitis.

Complex Pancreatic Function Tests

In the natural history of chronic pancreatitis, progressive and permanent impairment of pancreatic secretion of bicarbonate and enzymes (exocrine secretions) as well as insulin and glucagon (endocrine secretion) occurs. In alcohol-induced chronic pancreatitis the onset of insufficiency is earlier and often quite severe. Malabsorption of fat does not occur until enzyme secretion is less than 10% of normal values, which does not occur until 5 to 10 years after the onset of alcohol-induced pancreatitis, or 20 to 25 years after the onset of idiopathic pancreatitis.

Exocrine pancreatic function can be measured directly or indirectly (Box 352-1). By duodenal aspirate we can measure the bicarbonate, amylase, lipase, and trypsin secretion directly, and evidence of pancreatic disease can be assessed long before the consequence of such enzyme and bicarbonate deficiency manifests as steatorrhea, creatorrhea, or carbohydrate malabsorption.

Pancreatic function tests in the diagnosis of chronic pancreatitis are indicated only when the diagnosis of pancreatic disease remains a possibility despite negative or inconclusive imaging studies (plain film of abdomen, ultrasound, computed tomography [CT] scan, and endoscopic retrograde cholangiopancreatography [ERCP]). These tests are traditionally classified as either noninvasive or tubeless tests, or invasive or tube tests (tests involving duodenal drainage).

A popular tubeless test is the Bentiromide (NBT-PABA) test, which depends on the intraduodenal hydrolysis by chymotrypsin of a synthetic peptide (bentiromide) bound to p-aminobenzoic acid (PABA). The liberated PABA is absorbed, conjugated in the liver, and eliminated in urine. The concentration of conjugated PABA excreted in the urine is a measure of pancreatic secretion of chymotrypsin. The test is positive only in those with marked insufficiency. In diseases of malabsorption due to other causes, as well as liver or kidney disease, the test is falsely positive. Many medications (sufonamides, sulfonylureas, laxatives, diuretics, and pancreatic enzymes) interfere with the test. An advantage of this simple test is that it helps to determine the indication for oral enzyme therapy. The pancreolauryl test is not available in the United States. The digestion of the di-xodeoic ester of fluorescein by pancreatic lipase is tested after oral administration of fluorescein-dilaurate. The test has a low sensitivity in the

---

BOX 352-1
Tests of pancreatic function

I. Tests of Exocrine Pancreatic Function
  A. Direct Pancreatic Function Tests
    1. Secretin stimulation test
    2. Combined secretin and CCK stimulation test
  B. Indirect pancreatic function test
    1. Lundh test meal stimulation
  C. Serum tests
    1. Amylase-isoamylase estimation
    2. Immunoreactive trypsin assay
  D. Stool tests
    1. Pancreatic elastase
    2. Chymotrypsin assay
    3. Staining of fat
    4. 72-Hour stool fat estimation
  E. Absorption tests
    1. Bentiromide (NBT-PABA test)
    2. Pancreolauryl test
    3. ^{131}I-labeled triolein test
    4. ^{131}I-labeled triolein and oleic acid test
  F. Miscellaneous tests
    1. Amino acid consumption test
    2. Schilling/dual labeled test
II. Tests for Endocrine Pancreatic function
  A. Glucose tolerance test
  B. Hemoglobin A1C
  C. Serum insulin/PP assays

---

diagnosis of early pancreatitis. Fecal chymotrypsin assay, performed in random stool samples, is simple and helpful in following patients already diagnosed having chronic pancreatitis, but has low sensitivity in diagnosing new-onset mild to moderate chronic pancreatitis. Another test that is being evaluated is the amino acid consumption test. Patients with chronic pancreatitis demonstrate less of a decrement in plasma amino acid concentration than healthy individuals following intravenous (IV) administration of secretin and CCK or cerluein. The fall in amino acid is a measure of amino acid incorporation into newly synthesized pancreatic enzymes. Stool fat estimation is not a test to diagnose chronic pancreatitis but only to establish and grade severity of steatorrhea. Other tests such as Triolein breath test, dual labelled Schilling test, and starch absorption test have very little use in the diagnosis of chronic pancreatitis.

The secretin-cholecystokinin stimulation test, a tube test that enjoyed wide popularity before the advent of modern imaging studies, is often quoted as the gold-standard. In the various modifications of this test (different doses and stimulants) gastroduodenal intubation is needed to collect duodenal samples. Bicarbonate level, amylase activity, and volume of duodenal samples are measured. As a functional test, the secretin-CCK test is the most sensitive test for detection of mild to moderate chronic pancreatitis if the test is performed carefully. The test is currently available only in some referral centers.

RADIOLOGICAL STUDIES

Pancreatic radiology has evolved considerably in the last three decades with the advent of abdominal sonography, CT scan of the abdomen, and magnetic resonance imaging. Endoscopic retrograde cholangiopancreaticography is the single most important development in pancreatic imaging, since it clearly delineates the ductal and even ductular morphology and provides an opportunity for therapeutic procedures. Conventional radiographs of the chest and abdomen continue to be important in the initial evaluation of the patient with suspected pancreatic disease. Newer modalities for scanning of certain islet cell tumors using octreotide scanning and intraoperative and endoscopic ultrasound appear to offer data not available through CT or MRI of the abdomen. The role of angiography has decreased with the increasing use of CT, and currently mostly limited to evaluation of nonspecific focal masses (ductal carcinoma vs. islet cell tumors).

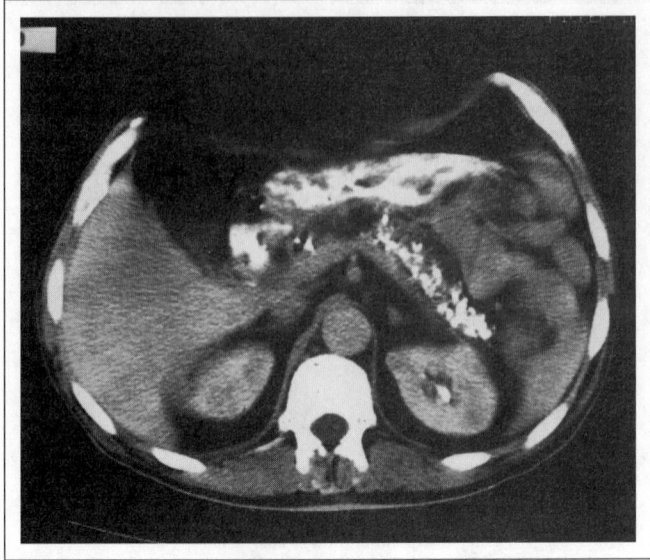

FIGURE 352-1   CT Scan of abdomen showing diffuse calculi and a small cyst.

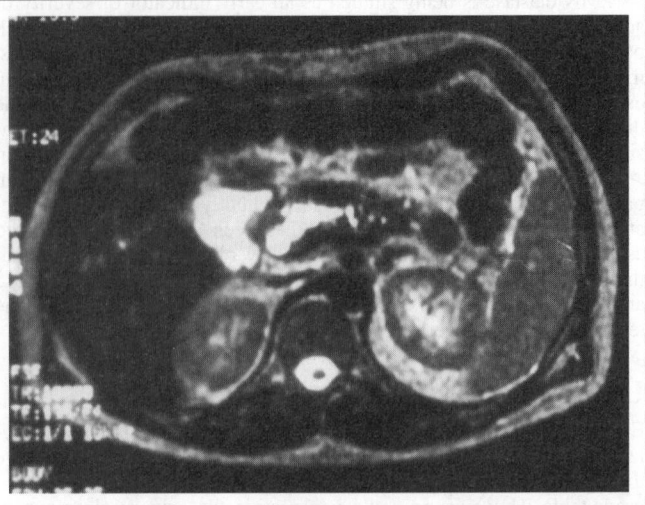

FIGURE 352-2   Magnetic resonance cholangiopancreaticography. 36-year-old alcoholic male with multiple episodes of chronic pancreatitis and obstructive jaundice. Note the dilated pancreatic duct in the region of head and the beaded appearance of the duct in the body and tail.

Plain radiography of the abdomen has the advantage of being readily available, inexpensive, and noninvasive. Pancreatic calculi are a marker of chronic pancreatitis. The calculi are often distributed through the main pancreatic duct, the bigger ones being close to the head of the pancreas. Pancreatic calculi in hereditary and tropical pancreatitis are larger than in alcoholic pancreatitis. Although presence of pancreatic calculi is highly specific for chronic pancreatitis, the sensitivity is poor since radio opaque calculi are not often seen in early stages of the disease.

Barium studies reveal findings that are mostly due to the pressure effects of pancreatic disease on the gastrointestinal tract and not of much help in the diagnosis. Deformities of the duodenum, widening of the duodenal loop, depression of the duodenogastric junction, mucosal fold alterations, and enlargement of the retrogastric space are indirect indicators of a possible pancreatic enlargement and fibrosis.

Ultrasonography

Ultrasonography of the abdomen is a noninvasive, safe, and relatively inexpensive procedure that has acquired its place as an important modality for pancreatic imaging. The disadvantage is that it is technician dependent, and obesity and bowel gas preclude adequate examination. In patients with acute pancreatitis it helps to evaluate gallstone disease and the size of common bile duct, in addition to providing valuable information on the pancreatic morphology. In acute pancreatitis the echo texture of the pancreas diminishes as a reflection of increased fluid content, and the gland is diffusely enlarged. Focal fluid collections, localized effusions in and around the pancreas, and pseudocysts are diagnosed with ultrasound. In chronic pancreatitis fibrosis and fatty infiltration produce a nonhomogenous echo texture. A dilated main pancreatic duct and pancreatic calculi can be identified. Adenocarcinoma of the pancreas appears as a hypoechoic focal mass.

Computed Tomography

Computed tomography has become a useful technique to diagnose and assess the severity of acute pancreatitis. Dynamic scanning after intravenous contrast has become the well-accepted procedure of choice in the evaluation of patients with acute pancreatitis. The ideal time to perform a CT scan in a patient with acute pancreatitis is on the third or fourth day, unless there are other reasons to evaluate the abdomen by CT initially (Chapter 366). In edematous pancreatitis the gland in one third to two thirds of cases appears diffusely enlarged, whereas with more severe forms of pancreatitis the borders of the

gland become indistinct and appear enlarged, and fluid collections appear. These fluid collections are not well outlined and are differentiated from pseudocysts that have a well-defined capsule. Pancreatic necrosis, infected or sterile, appears as low density areas within the inflamed mass. Presence of gas bubbles within the pancreas is seen only in 20% to 40% of abscesses. The best and most reliable method to diagnose infected pancreatic necrosis in aspiration and culture of material obtained by fine needle aspiration of the necrotic area under CT guidance.

The role of CT in chronic pancreatitis is to look for pancreatic ductal dilation, parenchymal atrophy, calculi, inflammatory and neoplastic masses, pseudocysts, and bile duct dilation. (Fig. 352-1) CT of the abdomen is an indispensable early diagnostic tool in the evaluation of a patient suspected of having carcinoma of the pancreas.

Endoscopic retrograde cholangiopancreatography has become the gold standard in the diagnosis of chronic pancreatitis. Although a normal pancreatogram does not always rule out chronic pancreatitis, in nearly 90% to 95% of patients the changes are diagnostic. In early chronic pancreatitis even if the main duct may be normal, the side branches may show sacculation. In more advanced disease the main duct is abnormal showing dilation, stricture, ("chain of lake" appearance) and intraductal filling defects. ERCP also helps to evaluate biliary strictures that complicate chronic pancreatitis, abrupt obstruction of the pancreatic duct (suggestive of carcinoma of the pancreas), and some cystic lesions communicating with ducts.

Magnetic Resonance Imaging

Magnetic resonance imaging has limited use in the evaluation of patients with acute or chronic pancreatitis. Although in the evaluation of patients with pancreatic cancer MRI has no significant advantage over CT, it plays a very useful role in the diagnosis of islet cell tumors and cystic neoplasms of the pancreas. Magnetic resonance cholangiopancreatography (MRCP) is a recent diagnostic tool that uses three-dimensional data sets for projection images, as well as arbitrary cross-sectional images of the pancreatic ducts (Fig. 352-2). Because MRCP is noninvasive, it might limit indications for diagnostic ERCP.

Endoscopic Ultrasonography

Endoscopic ultrasonography (EUS) permits the placement of the transducer into the duodenum or stomach under endoscopic guidance, to carry out scanning of the pancreas. The role of EUS in acute pancreatitis is not well studied. In detecting small pancreatic

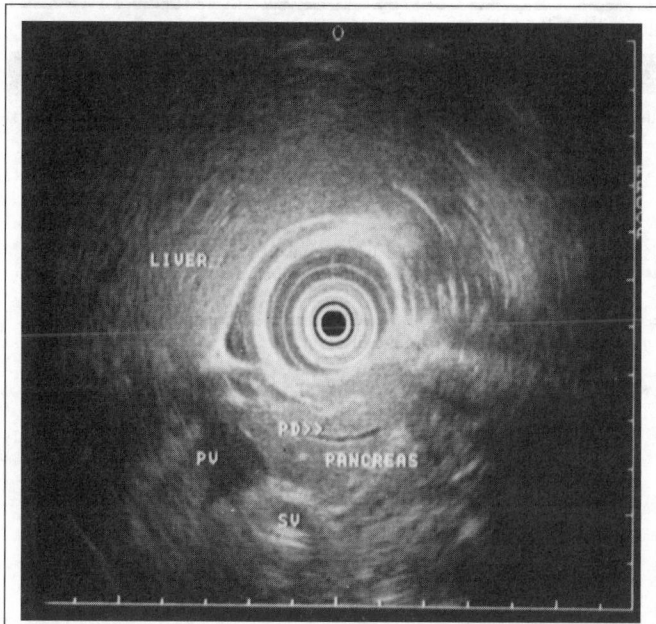

FIGURE 352-3 Endoscopic ultrasound demonstrating the pancreas and the main pancreatic duct *(PD) PV,* Portal vein; *SV,* splenic vein.

masses EUS appears to be superior to abdominal ultrasound and CT scan (Fig. 352-3).

Angiography

With the advent of less invasive and more sensitive studies such as EUS, CT, MRI, and ERCP to evaluate pancreatic lesions, the need for angiography is quite limited, since it is invasive and requires an experienced radiologist. Difficulties in interpretation of the very subtle changes of inflammation that mimic neoplasm make the procedure less attractive. A small group of patients with gastrointestinal bleeding due to erosion of an intrapancreatic blood vessel may require angiography for localization of the site of bleeding and therapy. A major valid indication for performance of a pancreatic angiogram today is in the localization of a small insulinoma.

BIBLIOGRAPHY

Bank S, Chow KW: Diagnostic tests in chronic pancreatitis, *Gastroenterologist* 2:224-232, 1994.

Banks PA, Gerzof SG, Lansevin RE et al: CT guided aspiration of suspected pancreatic infection, *Intl J Pancreatol* 18:265-270, 1995.

Boyd EJ, Wormsley KG: The assessment of chronic pancreatitis. In Burns GP, Bank S, editors: *Disorders of the pancreas: current issues in diagnosis and management,* New York, 1992, McGraw-Hill, pp. 283-314.

Freeny PC: Incremental dynamic bolus computed tomography of acute pancreatitis, *Intl Jl Pancreatol* 13:147-158, 1993.

Gumaste V: Diagnostic tests for acute pancreatitis, *Gastroenterologist* 2:119-130, 1994.

Printz H, Siegmund H, Woyte C et al: Human pancreas-specific protein (procarboxypeptidase B): a valuable marker in pancreatitis? *Pancreas* 10:222-230, 1995.

Schmid SW, Uhl W, Steinle A et al: Human pancreas-specific protein: a diagnostic and prognostic marker in acute pancreatitis and pancreas transplantation, *Int J Pancreatol* 19:165-170, 1996.

III CLINICAL SYNDROMES AND SPECIFIC DISEASE ENTITIES

CHAPTER

353 Jaundice and Disorders of Bilirubin Metabolism

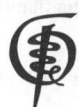

J. Donald Ostrow, Ronald P. J. Oude Elferink, and Piter J. Bosma

Jaundice, or icterus, is the yellowish discoloration of the skin, sclerae, and mucous membranes caused by retention of bilirubin and/or its conjugates. Carotene and lycopene may also cause yellowing of the skin but not the sclerae.

Jaundice may be the first or sole manifestation of disease. It is most easily seen in the normally white sclerae but is more difficult to detect in artificial or dim light and in blacks. Because jaundice is not usually detectable on clinical examination until total serum bilirubin levels are increased at least threefold to fourfold above normal, an elevation of this laboratory value on a blood chemistry screen is often the first indication of an abnormality in bilirubin metabolism.

PHYSIOLOGY: NORMAL BILIRUBIN METABOLISM

Bilirubin is a yellow, tetrapyrrolic pigment that is the major product of heme catabolism. As a result of internal hydrogen bonding of all the polar groups in unconjugated bilirubin, the pK'_a values of its two carboxyl groups are both above 7.0, and its interactions with water are limited, rendering it poorly water-soluble. Like other poorly water-soluble organic compounds, bilirubin is transported in the plasma bound to albumin, which limits its renal excretion. Bilirubin is cleared mainly by hepatocytes, which convert the pigment to a variety of water-soluble conjugates *(conjugated bilirubin),* principally the diglucuronides and monoglucuronides. This biotransformation is necessary for the excretion of bilirubin, and only traces of *unconjugated bilirubin* appear in the bile. Under normal conditions, conjugated bilirubins are efficiently excreted in bile, so that more than 96% of the bilirubin in normal plasma is unconjugated. The excreted conjugated bilirubin then traverses the biliary tree to the intestine, where bacterial flora metabolize the pigments to a variety of products that are eliminated, predominantly in the stool, along with varied proportions of unchanged bilirubin.

Bilirubin metabolism can be divided into 10 successive steps (Table 353-1, Figs. 353-1 and 353-2). The uptake, storage, conjugation, and secretion steps all apparently involve specific carriers or enzymes whose activity may be altered selectively by competitive or noncompetitive inhibition, induction, or genetic mutation. Disorders of the liver or biliary tree often preferentially involve one or more of these 10 steps, forming the basis for the classification and diagnosis of jaundice.

INDIVIDUAL STEPS IN BILIRUBIN METABOLISM
Bilirubin Formation

All bilirubin is derived from hemes and heme proteins (Fig. 353-3). Of the 3.8 ± 0.6 mg/kg of bilirubin produced per day, 75% to 80% derives from hemoglobin released during destruction of senescent red blood cells in the reticuloendothelial system. The remainder originates from nonhemoglobin heme proteins in the liver and from accelerated destruction in the marrow, spleen, and liver of immature or defectively formed red cells (ineffective erythropoiesis).

Regardless of the source, the normal pathways of heme catabolism involve its degradation by microsomal heme oxygenases I and

Table 353-1 Specific steps in bilirubin metabolism and related abnormalities that affect them

STEPS*	ABNORMALITIES

1. Formation of UCB† by catabolism of heme, mainly in reticuloendothelial cells	Overproduction of UCB:
	    Hemolysis (many Gilbert's)
	    Ineffective erythropoiesis

2. Delivery of UCB in the circulation, mainly via the portal vein, bound to plasma albumin	Right-sided congestive heart failure Portosystemic shunts: Cirrhosis or surgery
3. Uptake of UCB across the basolateral membrane into the hepatocyte, after dissociation from albumin	Competitive inhibition of UCB uptake by drugs Gilbert's syndrome possible bilitranslocase deficiency Fasting, hypothyroidism
4. Storage of UCB in the hepatocyte cytosol, bound to ligandin (limits regurgitation to plasma)	Competitive inhibition of UCB storage by drugs Rotor's syndrome (storage disease) Fever

5. Conjugation of UCB by microsomal B-UGT to form CB (mostly glucuronides)	Genetic deficiency of B-UGT1
	    Crigler-Najjar syndromes I and II (Arias' syndrome)
	    Gilbert's syndrome
	 Inhibition of conjugation by drugs, progestogens, fasting

6. Secretion of UCB into canalicular bile, mainly via ATP-dependent cMOAT	Specific cMOAT deficiency (Dubin-Johnson syndrome)
	 Rotor's syndrome (storage disease)
	 Hepatocellular jaundice: alcoholic, toxic, or viral hepatitis; cirrhosis
	 Canalicular cholestasis resulting from:
	    Estrogens, anabolic steroids, drugs, endotoxins (sepsis)
	    Total parenteral nutrition
	    Postoperative cholestasis
	    Benign recurrent cholestasis
	    Progressive familial intrahepatic cholestasis
	    Neonatal hepatitis

7. Flow of CB in bile down the biliary tree to the duodenum	Ductal cholestasis:
	    Intrahepatic cholestasis:
	       Primary biliary cirrhosis
	       Sclerosing cholangitis
	       Tumors, granulomas
	       Caroli's syndrome
	       Cystic fibrosis
	       Ductal plate malformations
	    Extrahepatic biliary obstruction:
	       Tumors, strictures, stones
	       Biliary atresia

8. Intestinal transit of CB and catabolism by gut flora to UCB and urobilinogens	Ileus, bacterial overgrowth Absence of anaerobic gut flora: Neonates, antibiotic therapy
9. Enterohepatic recirculation via portal venous blood to the liver (restart step 3)	Portosystemic shunting Acute cholecystitis Cholascos
10. Elimination in the feces	Obstipation

*Steps 1-6, 8, and 9 are immature in neonates.
†Normally, steps 5 or 6 may be rate-limiting.
UCB, Unconjugated bilirubin; *B-UGT*, biliribin uridine diphosphate glucuronosyltransferase; *CB*, conjugated bilirubins; *cMOAT*, canalicular multispecific organic anion transporter.

II to form carbon monoxide and biliverdin. Biliverdin is in turn converted to bilirubin by an enzyme in the cytosol, biliverdin reductase (Fig. 353-3). The heme oxygenase step is rate limiting. Both enzymes use NADPH as cofactor and are especially abundant in the hepatocytes, renal tubular epithelium, and reticuloendothelial cells.

Delivery of Bilirubin

Unconjugated bilirubin passes into the plasma, where it is almost completely bound to two sites on plasma albumin, with dissociation constants of 2×10^{-8} and 2×10^{-7} M, respectively. Albumin, 4 g/dl, has the capacity to bind up to 85 mg of bilirubin per deciliter; consequently, a large fraction of unbound, unconjugated bilirubin rarely occurs clinically except in the neonate, in whom the binding capacity and affinity of fetal albumin for bilirubin are less than in the adult. Conjugated bilirubin is also over 99% bound to albumin, though with less affinity than unconjugated bilirubin. The circulating conjugated bilirubin that is not bound can filter at the glomerulus, leading to bilirubinuria in patients with diseases that cause retention of conjugated bilirubin. Normally, most of the bilirubin formed comes from the spleen to the liver via the portal venous blood.

Hepatic Uptake and Storage (Clearance)

In the liver, unbound bilirubin and its albumin complex freely cross the porous sinusoidal endothelium to reach the liver cell surface in the space of Disse, where the unbound bilirubin is transported rapidly into the liver cell. Cellular uptake of bilirubin occurs by Na^+-independent, facilitated diffusion processes, mediated by at least two transporter proteins in the sinusoidal membrane of the hepatocyte: organic anion–transporting polypeptide (80 kDa) and bilitranslocase (37 kDa). Evidence is inconclusive for the transport function of two 55kDa basolateral membrane proteins that bind bilirubin and other organic anions (bilirubin-BSP–binding protein and organic anion–binding polypeptide). In the cytosol, unconjugated bilirubin is stored temporarily by binding to two groups of organic anion–binding proteins, which limits the passive reflux of bilirubin back into the plasma. Ligandin, the major bilirubin-binding protein, is the same as glutathione-S-transferase B. It is noteworthy that the basolateral uptake and cytosolic binding of conjugated bile salts are mediated by transport proteins different from those for bilirubin.

In the steady state the subsequent conjugation and active biliary secretion of bilirubin serve to maintain the gradient of unbound unconjugated bilirubin from the blood to the liver cell. The net clearance of bilirubin from plasma, which is determined by the difference

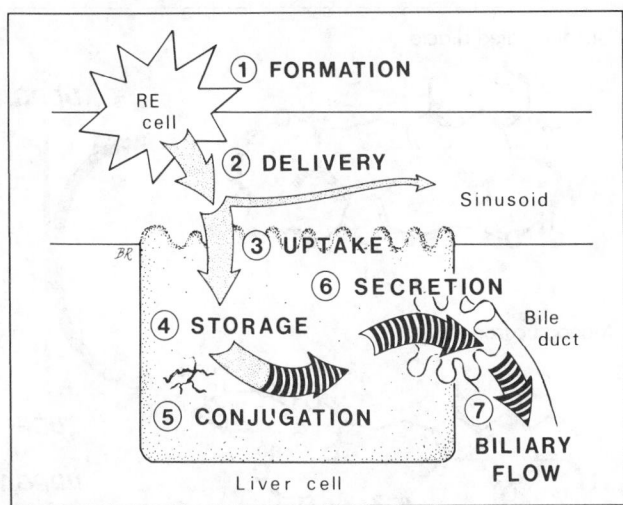

FIGURE 353-1 Normal hepatic bilirubin transport showing sequence of the seven steps from formation in the reticuloendothelial *(RE)* cell to flow in the biliary tree. *Stippled arrows,* unconjugated bilirubin; *striped arrows,* conjugated bilirubin; *squiggly figure,* endoplasmic reticulum.

Modified from Ostrow JD et al: *Unit I, Hepatic excretory function: undergraduate teaching project, American Gastroenterological Association,* Baltimore, 1975, Milner-Fenwick, slide 26.

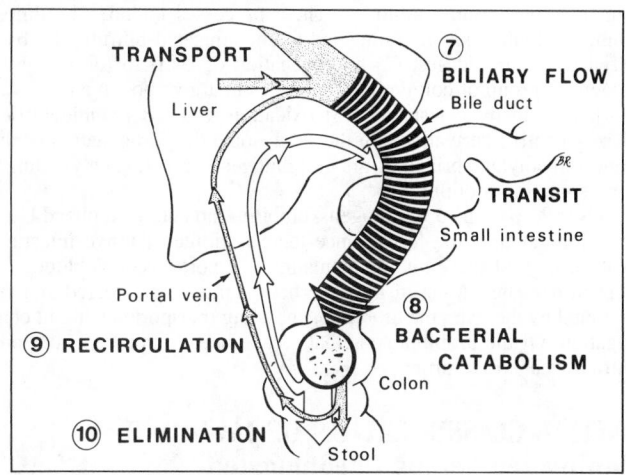

FIGURE 353-2 The enterohepatic circulation of bile pigments (symbols as in Fig. 353-1; *clear arrows,* urobilinogens).

Modified from Ostrow JD et al: *Unit I, Hepatic excretory function: undergraduate teaching project, American Gastroenterological Association,* Baltimore, 1975, Milner-Fenwick, slide 22.

between the rates of uptake and reflux, is normally 0.68 ± 0.14 ml/kg per minute, or 5.4% ± 1.4% of the bilirubin load, regardless of load. Various other organic anions, but not conjugated bile salts, share affinities for both the uptake carriers and ligandin. These compounds include rifampicin, sulfobromophthalein (BSP), indocyanine green (ICG), iopanoic acid, and the iminodiacetic acid (IDA) derivatives used for hepatobiliary scintiscanning.

Conjugation of Bilirubin

In the microsomes, unconjugated bilirubin (UCB) is converted to water-soluble conjugates by covalent coupling, mainly with glucuronic acid (Fig. 353-4), but also with glucose, xylose, and possibly sulfate. Each sugar is first activated by enzymatic formation of a high energy bond with uridine diphosphate and then transferred to bilirubin by a specific bilirubin-UDP glucuronosyltransferase (UGT1A or B-UGT1). Either one or both of the carboxyethyl side chains of UCB may be thus coupled, yielding monoconjugates and diconjugates, respectively. The diglucuronide normally accounts for over 85% of the bilirubin conjugates in the bile of adult humans, whereas the monoconjugate predominates in newborns. The proportions of monoglucuronide and nonglucuronide conjugates increase in various hepatobiliary diseases.

Secretion of Conjugated Bilirubin Into the Bile

After intracellular transfer of bilirubin conjugates to the canalicular membrane by poorly defined processes, bilirubin conjugates are secreted into the bile by an active, energy-dependent, Na^+-independent process, mediated by a 190-kDa transporter in the canalicular membrane. This canalicular multispecific organic anion transporter (cMOAT) is shared by many other organic dianions but not by conjugated bile salts, which are secreted by another ATP-dependent transporter. Though canalicular secretion of organic anions is aided by the electrical gradient produced by the −35-mV negative intracellular potential generated by the Na^+/K^+-ATPase in the basolateral membrane of the hepatocyte, canalicular secretion via cMOAT is powered primarily by hydrolysis of ATP. The energy dependence of all these transport processes renders them susceptible to impairment during hypoxia, shock, and severe circulatory stasis. The less than 1% of the total bilirubin in normal bile that is unconjugated derives mainly from hydrolysis of secreted conjugates and is a key factor in the formation of pigment (calcium-bilirubin) gallstones.

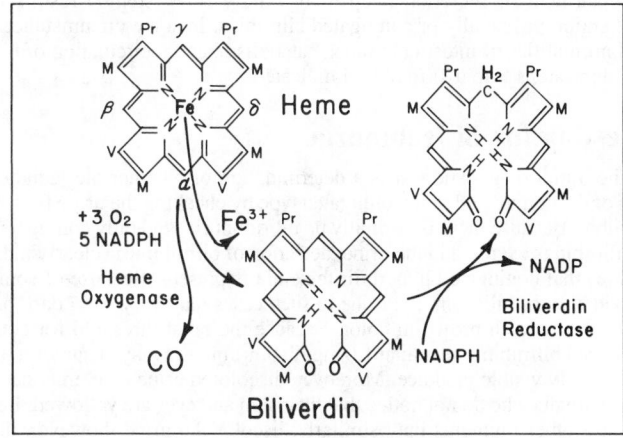

FIGURE 353-3. The formation of bilirubin from heme by the sequential action of the enzymes heme oxygenase and biliverdin reductase. *M,* Methyl; *V,* vinyl; *Pr,* propionic acid side chains.

Modified from Ostrow JD et al: *Unit I, Hepatic excretory function: undergraduate teaching project, American Gastroenterological Association,* Baltimore, 1975, Milner-Fenwick, slide 60.

Flow of Bilirubin Down the Biliary Tree

Bilirubin conjugates, in large part bound to biliary mixed micelles, pass with the bile successively from the canaliculi through the bile ductules, the interacinar (portal) bile ducts, intrahepatic ducts of progressively increasing caliber, and the extrahepatic bile ducts. Between meals the bile and bilirubin are stored mainly in the gallbladder, where conjugated bilirubin undergoes limited hydrolysis to unconjugated bilirubin, some of which may be absorbed. With feeding, much of the stored bile is emptied into the duodenum.

Intestinal Catabolism, Recirculation, and Elimination of Bile Pigments

In the small intestine, conjugated bilirubins are poorly absorbed but are partly hydrolyzed to unconjugated bilirubin by β-glucuronidases from the enterocytes (see Fig. 353-2). The intestinal catabolism of bile pigments, however, is mediated mainly by anaerobic ileocolonic flora, except in the germ-free intestine of neonates or patients receiving broad-spectrum antibiotics. These processes include (1) almost complete hydrolysis of conjugated to unconjugated bilirubin by bacterial β-glucuronidases; (2) hydrogenation of UCB to form urobilinogens, a group of colorless tetrapyrroles that give positive results to Ehrlich's aldehyde test; and (3) oxidation of UCB to unidentified diazo-negative derivatives. In the stool, some dehydrogenation of the central methylene bridge of the urobilinogens occurs, each yielding a corresponding urobilin.

Over 90% of the urobilinogens, urobilins, and unmetabolized UCB are eliminated in the feces, since there is limited passive intestinal reabsorption of these bile pigments into the portal venous blood, except in neonates. Most of the absorbed pigments are cleared and re-excreted by the liver, the urobilinogens being transported without conjugation. Of the urobilinogens that escape hepatic uptake, about one third appear in the urine.

INITIAL CLASSIFICATION OF JAUNDICE
Conjugated Versus Unconjugated Hyperbilirubinemia

Jaundice may be classified into two broad groups according to the predominant form of bilirubin, conjugated or unconjugated, that is retained in the plasma and tissues (Table 353-2). Unconjugated hyperbilirubinemia is caused by abnormalities in all steps up to and including the conjugation of bilirubin (steps 1 through 5). By contrast, impairment of secretion (step 6) or biliary flow (step 7) results in retention principally of conjugated bilirubins. In some circumstances, abnormalities of intestinal transit, catabolism, and recirculation of bilirubin (steps 8 to 10) may be implicated.

Testing for Bilirubinuria

The initial diagnostic test is a determination of whether the jaundice is of the conjugated or unconjugated type by checking the urine for bilirubin. Because there is normally no bilirubinuria, and only conjugated bilirubin is excreted in the urine, detection of bilirubinuria clearly indicates that conjugated hyperbilirubinemia is present. Because of some oxidation of bilirubin, the urine in such cases may vary from dark orange to reddish brown in color. Because the renal threshold for conjugated bilirubin is less than 1.0 mg/dl, bilirubinuria may occur without clinically visible jaundice. Moreover, discolored urine is often noticed by patients who do not notice that their skin and eyes are yellowed. Because other pigments may similarly discolor the urine, however, the presence of bilirubinuria must be confirmed chemically (Chapter 351).

Fractional Diazo Reaction of Serum

The simple test for bilirubinuria usually is sufficient to determine whether jaundice is of the conjugated or unconjugated type. This distinction, however, can be confirmed using the fractional diazo (van den Bergh's) reaction of serum bilirubin with a diazotized aromatic amine (Chapter 351).

Normally the total bilirubin concentration should not exceed 1.0 mg/dl (17 μM), with less than 0.2 mg/dl (3.5 μM) reacting directly. In pure unconjugated hyperbilirubinemia, no more than 15% of the total serum bilirubin may give a direct diazo reaction. In both situations the direct reaction is not caused by conjugated bilirubin but by endogenous accelerators of the diazo coupling of UCB or by other diazo-reactive substances.

In conjugated hyperbilirubinemia, more than 30%, and usually more than 50%, of the total serum bilirubin is direct reacting; there is also a significant indirect-reacting fraction, mainly as a result of unconjugated bilirubin formed by hydrolysis of the retained conjugates by tissue β-glucuronidases. The direct-reacting fraction consists not only of diconjugates and monoconjugates but also may contain up to 80% δ-bilirubin (BilAlb), a covalent amide conjugate of bilirubin to albumin. δ-bilirubin forms in any chronic conjugated hyperbilirubinemia by nonenzymatic transesterification of the acylbilirubin from glucuronic acid to —NH groups on albumin.

At total bilirubin concentrations below 3 mg/dl the inaccuracies of the direct diazo reaction render it desirable to use a new rapid,

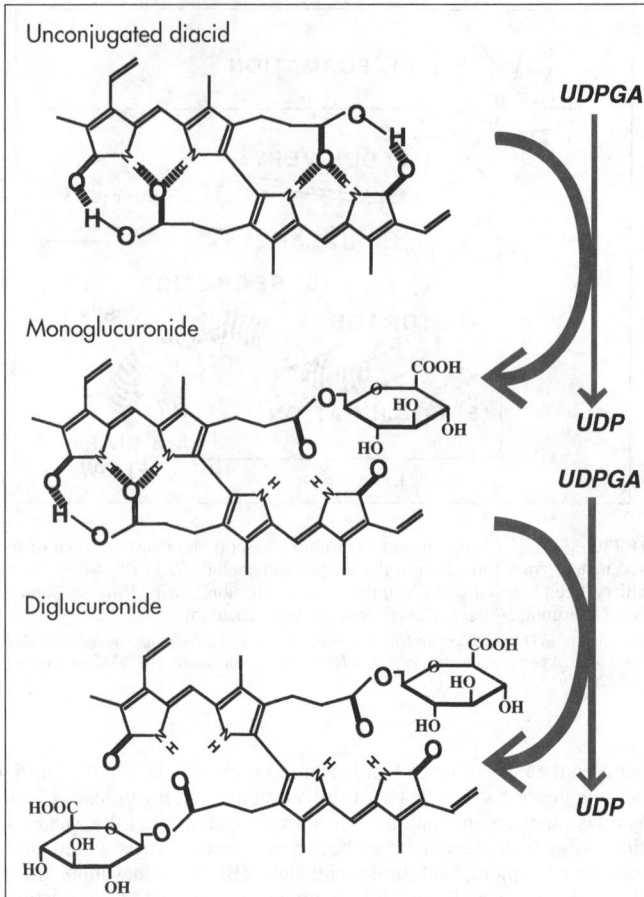

FIGURE 353-4   Structures of unconjugated bilirubin diacid and its monoglucuronide and diglucuronide conjugates. The serial action of a single microsomal enzyme, B-UGT1, transesterifies glucuronic acid (GA), glucose, or xylose from the activated UDP-sugar (e.g., UDPGA) to —COOH groups of one or both propionic acid side chains of bilirubin. Coupling of the polar, bulky, sugar moiety(s) to the —COOH group(s), which may also sterically hinder formation of the internal hydrogen bonds of bilirubin, renders the conjugates water-soluble and excretable into bile.

Modified from Ostrow JD, Berk PD: *Unit XXI, Hepatic transport and jaundice: undergraduate teaching project, American Gastroenterological Association,* Baltimore, 1989, Milner-Fenwick, slide 59.

simple, sensitive multilayer film method or HPLC to measure bilirubin glucuronides and δ-bilirubin; their increase in serum is diagnostic of hepatobiliary dysfunction, even when total serum bilirubin level is normal. At total bilirubin concentrations above 3 mg/dl, measurement of the direct and indirect diazo fractions suffices for the clinical distinction of conjugated from unconjugated hyperbilirubinemia.

PATHOPHYSIOLOGY AND CLASSIFICATION OF UNCONJUGATED HYPERBILIRUBINEMIA

Unconjugated hyperbilirubinemia (Fig. 353-5) is characterized by retention exclusively of unconjugated bilirubin in the serum, without bilirubinuria, as a result of insufficient hepatic clearance and/or conjugation of the load of the UCB produced each day. Unconjugated hyperbilirubinemia may be subclassified according to the step or steps in bilirubin metabolism that are deranged (see Table 353-1). The most common causes are (1) overproduction of unconjugated bilirubin caused by disorders of red blood cells; (2) impaired delivery of unconjugated bilirubin caused by circulatory disturbances involving the liver; and (3) functional or hereditary defects in uptake, storage, or conjugation of bilirubin. Immaturity of most steps of bilirubin me-

Table 353-2 Unconjugated versus conjugated hyperbilirubinemia

FINDING	UNCONJUGATED HYPERBILIRUBINEMIA	CONJUGATED HYPERBILIRUBINEMIA
Retained bilirubin	UCB	CB and UCB
Bilirubin in urine	No	Yes
Diazo reaction (direct/total)	<15%	>30% (usually >50%)
Abnormal steps	1-5 (Fig. 353-5)	6 or 7 (Fig. 353-6)
Usual causes	Hematologic, circulatory, or functional hepatic disorders	Hepatocellular or biliary tract disease
Compensatory mechanism	Catabolism of UCB to polar derivatives	Renal excretion of CB

CB, Conjugated bilirubin; *UCB,* unconjugated bilirubin.

tabolism produces a multifactorial, usually mild, temporary, unconjugated hyperbilirubinemia in virtually all neonates. This so-called physiologic jaundice of the newborn is much influenced by the high rates of production and intestinal reabsorption of UCB in neonates, and the partial starvation of suboptimal breast-feeding. It is usually more marked in premature or Asian infants and may be severe in newborns with complicating diseases, especially hemolytic disease caused by fetal-maternal Rh or ABO antigen incompatibility.

If serum UCB levels exceed 15 mg/dl, as in Crigler-Najjar I syndrome and some premature infants, unbound UCB may deposit in the central nervous system, causing neurologic dysfunction (bilirubin encephalopathy), which may be permanent or fatal (kernicterus). The underlying hematologic, circulatory, or functional disorders may also be serious in themselves. By contrast, the primary hepatic disorders are seldom life threatening per se, except in patients with endogenous portosystemic shunting because of cirrhosis. Therefore invasive diagnostic studies of the liver, including biopsy, are rarely indicated in patients with pure unconjugated hyperbilirubinemia.

Overproduction Jaundice

Excessive formation of bilirubin resulting from accelerated heme catabolism is a very common cause of unconjugated hyperbilirubinemia and often complicates and augments jaundice caused by other defects, such as Gilbert's syndrome. Because the hepatic component of bilirubin formation constitutes a small fraction of normal heme turnover and can increase no more than fivefold, it is rarely itself a cause of clinical jaundice. Consequently, overproduction jaundice is usually due to an erythroid disorder, and the exact diagnosis rests mainly on hematologic studies.

Decreased Delivery of Bilirubin

Decreased delivery of bilirubin to the liver cells caused by impairment of the hepatic circulation is the most common form of unconjugated jaundice. The delivery of other organic anion cholephiles is impaired also. This form of jaundice is most often due to right-sided congestive heart failure and clears as the heart failure is controlled. Another major cause is portosystemic shunting, caused by either cirrhosis or surgical anastomosis, which diverts the unconjugated bilirubin formed in the spleen directly into the systemic circulation.

Diminished Hepatic Clearance (Uptake and Storage)

Diminished hepatic uptake and/or storage of UCB may be acquired or hereditary. Acquired defects are often due to drugs, such as rifampicin, that competitively inhibit uptake and/or storage of UCB by binding to the same transporter and/or storage proteins, respectively. The jaundice usually resolves within 3 days after the offending drug is discontinued. Hypothyroidism may impair hepatic uptake of UCB, although it also increases ligandin levels. Febrile illnesses may cause retention of UCB, primarily because of decreased hepatic storage capacity and increased reflux of organic anions back into plasma.

Impaired clearance of UCB and related organic anions, but not of conjugated bile salts, is found in most patients with the hereditary disorder of conjugation, Gilbert's syndrome (see later discussion). Severe impairment of the storage of UCB and other organic anions is

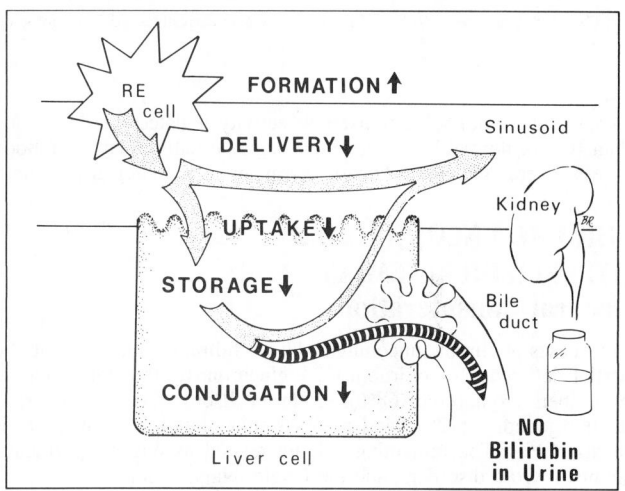

FIGURE 353-5 Abnormal bilirubin transport in unconjugated hyperbilirubinemia: steps that may be deranged (symbols as in Fig. 353-1). There is no bilirubinuria.

Modified from Ostrow JD et al: *Unit I, Hepatic excretory function: undergraduate teaching project, American Gastroenterological Association,* Baltimore, 1975, Milner-Fenwick, slide 27.

characteristic of Rotor's syndrome, but the associated decrease in canalicular secretion of conjugated bilirubins produces a predominantly conjugated hyperbilirubinemia.

Impaired Conjugation of Bilirubin

Bilirubin-UDP glucuronosyltransferase activity in liver is normal or increased in most hepatobiliary diseases. Exceptions are some patients with chronic persistent hepatitis, severe end-stage cirrhosis, acute hepatic failure, or Wilson's disease. Thus aside from impaired conjugation seen in neonates and patients with hyperthyroidism or caused by novobiocin or progestational steroids, most disorders of bilirubin conjugation are hereditary.

Gilbert's syndrome, the most common hereditary defect of bilirubin conjugation, is characterized by a chronic, mild, fluctuating unconjugated hyperbilirubinemia. This is caused by a frequently occurring mutation in the promotor region upstream of exon UGT1A–encoding bilirubin-UGT. Homozygosity for this mutation leads to an 80% decrease in the expression and activity of B-UGT1. When combined with overproduction and/or impaired clearance of bilirubin, unconjugated hyperbilirubinemia occurs. Bilirubin production and clearance are further (reversibly) altered during fasting and stress, often unmasking subclinical cases or augmenting the severity of visible jaundice.

The Crigler-Najjar syndromes are two more severe, rare, hereditary, recessive deficiencies of B-UGT1. In type I, there is no detectable bilirubin-UDP glucuronosyl transferase activity in the liver, and in several patients glucuronide conjugation of many phenolic substrates is impaired also. Jaundice is severe from the neonatal period, and kernicterus is the rule if the patients are untreated. In type II

Table 353-3 Disorders of bilirubin conjugation

	FINDINGS	CRIGLER-NAJJAR (type II (Arias)	GILBERT'S SYNDROME
Bilirubin-UDP glucuronosyltransferase (B-UGT1)	Undetectable	<10% of normal	20%-50% of normal
Organic anion kinetics (ICG, IDAs, BSP)	Normal	Normal	Clearance decreased in many patients
Bilirubin production rate	Usually normal	Usually normal	Increased in >50%
Serum bilirubin levels: range (mean) (mg/dl)	18-50 (27)	6-22 (13)	1-7 (3)
Bilirubins in bile	Trace UCB only	Mono-CB only	Mono-CB 30%-76%
Inheritance (autosomal)	Autosomal recessive	Autosomal recessive	Recessive plus other defects
Mutation in B-UGT1	Coding region	Coding region	Promotor (TATAA box)
Usual age of onset	1-3 days	1 day-10 years	10-30 years
Kernicterus	Usual if untreated	Occasionally	Never
Response to phenobarbital	None	Positive	Positive

ICG, Indocyanine green; _IDAs_, ^{99m}Tc–iodoacetic acid derivatives; _BSP_, sulfobromophthalein; _UCB_, unconjugated bilirubin; _CB_, conjugated bilirubins.

(Arias' syndrome) some transferase activity is detectable but at less than 10% of normal levels. Jaundice begins usually in late childhood, is less severe, and seldom causes kernicterus (see later discussion).

CHRONIC UNCONJUGATED HYPERBILIRUBINEMIAS
General Considerations

Most cases of chronic unconjugated hyperbilirubinemia are related to partial deficiency of bilirubin-UDP glucuronosyl transferase caused by Gilbert's syndrome (68%), erythroid disorders causing overproduction jaundice (12%), and portosystemic shunting because of cirrhosis (12%). The remaining 8% are related to surgical portocaval shunts, thyroid disorders, and the Crigler-Najjar syndromes.

Overproduction Jaundice

Etiology. Accelerated catabolism of heme to bilirubin, usually related to erythroid disorders, may be subclassified according to the source of the increased heme catabolism. _Hemolytic jaundice_ is due to accelerated destruction of circulating erythrocytes, for example, in sickle cell disease, hereditary spherocytosis, polycythemia vera, and acquired hemolytic anemias (e.g., with sepsis, autoimmune mechanisms, hypersplenism, or intracardiac valve prostheses). In _ineffective erythropoiesis_ the major source of added bilirubin is premature destruction of defective red cells in the marrow, liver, or spleen (e.g., in megaloblastic anemias, thalassemia, lead poisoning, and congenital erythropoietic porphyria). A mild hemolytic component may be present also. In the rare familial "shunt hyperbilirubinemia," rapid turnover of hepatic hemes is the primary defect, but dyserythropoiesis contributes also. Porphyria cutanea tarda and erythropoietic protoporphyria are also associated with accelerated turnover of hepatic hemes.

Pathophysiology and Clinical Features. In the steady state the rates of production and removal of UCB are equal and proportional to its concentration in the plasma. Thus increased production and delivery of UCB to the liver must result in an elevation of its concentration in the plasma. Because, with a normal liver, each threefold increase in bilirubin production results in a rise in serum UCB concentration of approximately 1.0 mg/dl, uncomplicated overproduction of UCB seldom elevates serum bilirubin concentrations above the level of 3.0 to 4.0 mg/dl that is necessary for jaundice to be clinically visible.

All forms of overproduction jaundice are accompanied by erythroid hyperplasia of the bone marrow and enhanced marrow uptake of ^{59}Fe from the circulation. The increased load of heme induces heme oxygenase in the liver and kidneys, resulting in augmented formation of bilirubin that is accommodated by enhanced uptake, conjugation, and excretion of bilirubin by the liver. The larger load of conjugated bilirubin presented to the intestinal bacteria results in greater output of urobilinogens in the feces. The increased bilirubin concentration in bile predisposes to formation of black pigment gallstones. Occasionally, significant retention of conjugated bilirubin may occur also if hemolysis is massive or if bilirubin secretion is diminished because of concomitant hepatobiliary disease.

Diagnosis and Treatment. Usually the presence of overproduction jaundice is revealed by findings of splenomegaly, anemia, or an abnormal peripheral blood smear. In some cases with compensated hemolysis these tests are normal, and hemolysis is suggested by reticulocytosis or a disproportionate elevation of lactic dehydrogenase compared with transaminases in the serum. More specific diagnosis then rests on other hematologic studies, discussed fully in Chapter 72. A serum UCB concentration in excess of that predicted for the rate of bilirubin production (assessed from ^{51}Cr–red cell survival) is evidence of an associated defect in clearance or conjugation of unconjugated bilirubin. Treatment is the therapy indicated for the underlying hematologic disorder.

Defects in Bilirubin Conjugation

Investigators have long been puzzled by the variable patterns and severity of defective conjugation of xenobiotics and bilirubin (Table 353-3) observed among subjects with bilirubin-UDP glucuronosyltransferase deficiency. These old observations have been explained by recent molecular biologic studies, which reveal that the UGT1 gene that encodes bilirubin-UGT1 also encodes the transferases that form glucuronides of phenolic substrates. By alternative splicing, at least 10 different UGT isozymes are encoded by the UGT1 gene. All members of this UGT1 family contain the constant region, encoded by four exons at the downstream region of this gene. This constant region includes the UDPGA-binding site and the endoplasmatic retention signal. Mutations in the constant region will affect all isozymes encoded by the UGT1 gene and impair conjugation of phenols as well as bilirubin. The upstream half of the gene contains exons that code for the unique binding sites for each subgroup of substrates; mRNA encoded by one of these exons is alternatively spliced onto mRNA from the constant region during gene transcription, yielding an individual mRNA for the transferase for each class of substrates. A mutation in one of these variable exons impairs the activity only of the transferase for the relevant substrates. The UGT2 family of UDP-glucuronosyltransferases for steroids and bile salts are encoded by other genes, explaining why those substrates are conjugated normally by subjects with deficiency of B-UGT1.

Because conjugation of bilirubin is essential to its excretion in bile, deficient conjugation must be compensated by alternate routes for catabolism of unconjugated bilirubin. Studies in Crigler-Najjar I patients and the comparable animal model, the Gunn rat, reveal two major pathways: (1) oxidation of bilirubin by microsomal cytochromes P_{450} IA1 and IA2 to form polar (probably hydroxyl) derivatives that can be excreted in bile without conjugation, and (2) diffusion of bilirubin directly across the intestinal wall with conversion to urobilinogens by intestinal bacteria. The relative importance of these two pathways and their function in patients with less severe defects in bilirubin conjugation are not known.

Gilbert's Syndrome

Etiology. This syndrome of benign, mild, chronic unconjugated hyperbilirubinemia (1 to 7 mg/dl) is related to a 50% to 80% decrease in the activity of hepatic bilirubin-UDP glucuronosyltransferase combined with impaired clearance and/or overproduction of bilirubin (Table 353-3). Gilbert's syndrome is caused by a homozygous elongation of the TATA box present in the promoter region of exon UGT1A, which encodes bilirubin UGT1. The TATA box is important for initiation of transcription; transcription factors bind to this promoter element. The abnormal allele contains a $(TA)_7TAA$ box, instead of the normal $(TA)_6TAA$ sequence, which results in a 70% to 80% decrease in the expression of B-UGT1.

Prevalence. The frequency of the allele with the elongated TATA box is estimated to be about 40%; thus up to 16% of the normal population is homozygous for the abnormal B-UGT promoter. As a result, 3% to 7% of men and 0.6% to 2.0% of women in asymptomatic populations have total serum bilirubin concentrations above 1.2 mg/dl without an increase in conjugated bilirubin. Among relatives of Gilbert's probands, 27% to 55% of siblings and 16% to 28% of parents also have mild unconjugated hyperbilirubinemia.

Pathophysiology. A 50% to 80% decrease in bilirubin conjugation is seldom sufficient by itself to produce hyperbilirubinemia and cannot in any case account for the increased serum bilirubin level seen in patients with Gilbert's syndrome. Thus male subjects who are homozygous for the Gilbert's allele have mean serum bilirubin levels of only 1.0 mg/dl, compared to 0.6 mg/dl in normal males. An associated disorder of bilirubin production and/or clearance must therefore be present for phenotypic expression of jaundice. Up to half the subjects have hemolysis, with UCB concentrations in the plasma in excess of the values predicted from the rates of bilirubin formation as estimated from the red blood cell life span. Kinetic studies, using low doses of BSP, suggest that most patients with Gilbert's syndrome also have defective clearance of all the organic anions that share the same transporter(s) as UCB. The relative contribution to total bilirubin uptake differs among the basolateral membrane organic anion transporters, one or more of which might be defective in a given patient. These contributing factors, which can explain the variable penetrance of the autosomal recessive conjugation defect, must be quite frequent to explain the high frequency of clinically apparent Gilbert's syndrome.

Pathology. Except for decreased rough endoplasmic reticulum, hypertrophy of the smooth endoplasmic reticulum, and mild parenchymal iron deposition in patients with associated erythroid disorders, the liver is structurally normal in patients with Gilbert's syndrome.

Clinical Features. Serum bilirubin concentrations are usually below the clinically detectable level of 3 to 4 mg/dl, and many subjects intermittently achieve normal values. Episodic increases in serum unconjugated bilirubin concentration occur with fasting, exertional or thermal stress, heavy alcohol intake, infections, or acute hemolysis, often unmasking previously subclinical jaundice. Hyperthyroidism, which impairs hepatic conjugation of bilirubin, also can aggravate jaundice from underlying Gilbert's syndrome.

The initial diagnosis is usually made in the second or third decade of life, when an elevated plasma UCB concentration is discovered during investigation of unrelated conditions. Hepatic size is usually normal, but splenomegaly may be present in patients with associated erythroid disorders. Except for hyperbilirubinemia, liver function tests are almost always normal. Serum bile acid concentrations are characteristically normal. As evidence of associated erythroid disorders, ^{51}Cr–red cell survival is decreased in 50% to 60% of patients, and over 80% show impaired incorporation of ^{59}Fe into circulating erythrocytes.

Crigler-Najjar Syndrome II (Arias' Syndrome)

This rare syndrome (see Table 353-3) of moderate, chronic unconjugated hyperbilirubinemia results from a decrease in the activity of bilirubin-UDP glucuronosyltransferase to less than 10% of normal.

The syndrome is inherited as an autosomal recessive defect in the coding region of B-UGT1. Heterozygotes show normal serum bilirubin levels except when they also carry the allele for Gilbert's syndrome (compound heterozygotes). Conjugation of other aglycones (e.g., menthol and aminophenols) may be deficient also, depending on the site of the mutation. Hepatic transport of other organic anions is unaffected. Jaundice may appear initially in late childhood as often as in infancy. Because serum bilirubin levels usually are 10 to 19 mg/dl (range can be 6 to 22 mg/dl), kernicterus seldom develops. Bilirubin in the bile is virtually all monoglucuronide.

Crigler-Najjar Syndrome I

This rare syndrome (Table 353-3), marked by severe unconjugated hyperbilirubinemia, is inherited as an autosomal recessive trait. No hepatic bilirubin-UDP glucuronosyltransferase activity is detectable, and the bile contains only traces of unconjugated bilirubin and nonglucuronide monoconjugates of bilirubin. Depending on the site of the mutation, it can be associated with severe but incomplete deficiency of glucuronide conjugation of salicylates, menthol, nitrophenols, and aminophenols, but conjugation of steroid hormones and bile salts is usually normal. Heterozygous parents and siblings have normal serum bilirubin concentrations but exhibit a 50% decrease in their capacity to conjugate and excrete loads of unconjugated bilirubin and often impairment in glucuronide conjugation of other aglycones.

Hepatic histologic condition and ultrastructure are normal. Jaundice in patients with Crigler-Najjar syndrome I is almost always manifested initially 1 to 3 days after birth, and serum unconjugated bilirubin concentrations plateau in excess of 20 mg/dl. Severe bilirubin encephalopathy is almost inevitable, causing severe mental retardation, dysarthria, ataxia, spasticity, and usually death in infancy or early childhood. Diagnosis and treatment are discussed in the following sections.

Diagnosis of Hereditary Unconjugated Hyperbilirubinemia

Routine Examinations. Once the presence of unconjugated hyperbilirubinemia is established, causes of reversible, acquired unconjugated hyperbilirubinemia, such as fever and right-sided heart failure, should be sought by history, physical examination, and routine laboratory tests. If acquired conditions are not evident, or if the jaundice does not resolve with appropriate therapy, one of the familial, functional disorders should be suspected. These syndromes can usually be distinguished by the patient's age at the onset of jaundice, the degree of elevation and variability of the serum bilirubin concentration, the presence or absence of kernicterus, and a history of jaundice in parents or siblings (see Table 353-3). Patients may not be aware of jaundice in their relatives, so it is essential to assess serum bilirubin levels in other family members.

Serum Bile Acid Levels. Serum bile acid levels are normal in all functional unconjugated hyperbilirubinemias; this is the noninvasive test of choice to exclude organic hepatobiliary diseases and/or portosystemic shunts.

Examination of the Bile. Determination of the proportion of unconjugated bilirubin, monoglucuronide, and diglucuronide in duodenal bile by either high-pressure liquid chromatography or analysis of azopigments is of further assistance in making the differential diagnosis (see Table 353-3) Patients with Gilbert's syndrome usually have at least 30% monoglucuronide in the bile, compared with less than 15% in most normal subjects. Patients with Crigler-Najjar syndrome type II have almost exclusively monoglucuronides in the bile. Patients with Crigler-Najjar syndrome type I show no glucuronide conjugates in the bile.

Effect of Fasting on Serum Bilirubin. In all the syndromes associated with decreased hepatic bilirubin-UDP glucuronosyltransferase activity, more than 90% of males, but only 40% to 50% of females, whose caloric intake is limited to less than 400 kcal daily for 24 to 48 hours will have an increase in plasma unconjugated bilirubin concentration to at least twice baseline values. By contrast, normal subjects and patients with unrelated hemolysis or liver diseases usually have less than a 50% increase in serum bilirubin levels during fasting. The hyperbilirubinemia reverses within 6 hours of refeeding. The mechanisms are believed to involve (1) mobilization during lipolysis of unconjugated bilirubin stored in depot fats; (2) impaired hepatocellular uptake of bilirubin; (3) decreased ligandin concentrations; (4) decreased substrate for uridine diphosphoglucose dehydrogenase, thus decreasing the supply of UDPGA for bilirubin conjugation; and (5) absorption of unconjugated bilirubin from the stagnant intestine. These phenomena assist in understanding the fluctuating severity of jaundice in patients with Gilbert's syndrome, but the fasting effect is too variable to be useful diagnostically.

Response to Phenobarbital. Differentiation of complete from partial conjugation defects can be confirmed by administration of phenobarbital in dosages of 2 to 5 mg/kg per day. Phenobarbital induces all the normal steps in hepatic bilirubin metabolism. Patients with Crigler-Najjar II or Gilbert's syndromes respond with a decline in serum bilirubin concentrations over 1 to 2 weeks to 30% to 50% of pretherapy values. In contrast, patients with Crigler-Najjar syndrome type I do not respond.

Percutaneous Liver Biopsy. Percutaneous liver biopsy is seldom necessary in the assessment of unconjugated hyperbilirubinemia, except when fatty liver, malignancy, or cirrhosis is suspected. Assay of decreased bilirubin-UDP glucuronosyltransferase activity is unnecessary and is a difficult, exacting procedure that often yields misleading results in inexpert hands.

Genetic Analysis and Prenatal Diagnosis. The UGT1 gene that encodes bilirubin-UGT1 and several other UGT1 isozymes has been isolated and characterized. Using specific oligonucleotides, this gene can be amplified by the polymerase chain reaction from genomic DNA, which can be isolated from leukocytes, fibroblasts, or, in case of a prenatal diagnosis, chorion cells. Subsequently, mutations causing B-UGT1 deficiency are identified by sequencing the amplified DNA. Thus genetic analysis does not require a percutaneous liver biopsy. To be sure that a prenatal diagnosis can be made in time, it is essential that the mutations present in the parents have been identified. Synthesis of a mutated bilirubin-UGT in tissue culture can be used to determine the residual activity of the mutated enzyme. This procedure has been used in making the differential diagnosis between type I and type II Crigler-Najjar patients. It is, however, a toilsome and expensive method.

Treatment of Unconjugated Hyperbilirubinemia

Amelioration of jaundice depends mainly on treatment of the underlying hematologic, circulatory, metabolic, or hepatic disorder. Jaundice itself is not harmful except in some neonates and in Crigler-Najjar I patients, in whom severe unconjugated hyperbilirubinemia may produce kernicterus. Phototherapy with blue light is the preferred treatment in young Crigler-Najjar I subjects and in neonatal jaundice. It acts by converting unconjugated bilirubin to geometric photoisomers that can be excreted in bile and urine without conjugation. The cosmetic embarrassment of milder chronic jaundice may be alleviated with high-dosage, long-term phenobarbital therapy. Such treatment is ineffective if any of the steps in bilirubin metabolism and transport are completely defective, as occurs in Crigler-Najjar syndrome type I. In such patients, induction of alternate pathways with the nontoxic indole-3-carbinol found in cruciferous vegetables is a potential new therapy. In neonates, frequent feeding of breast milk or formula minimizes fasting and limits the intestinal reabsorption of UCB. A newly accepted therapy in newborns is parenteral administration of tin protoporphyrin IX, a potent competitive inhibitor of heme oxygenase and thus of bilirubin synthesis. Treatments effective in animal models, but not established clinically, include removal of bilirubin by extracorporeal plasma perfusion through albumin-agarose and reverse-phase columns or columns of immobilized bilirubin oxidase; and oral administration of cholestyramine, charcoal, agar, or calcium phosphate to trap bilirubin in the intestine, interrupting its enterohepatic circulation. When severely jaundiced subjects respond in-

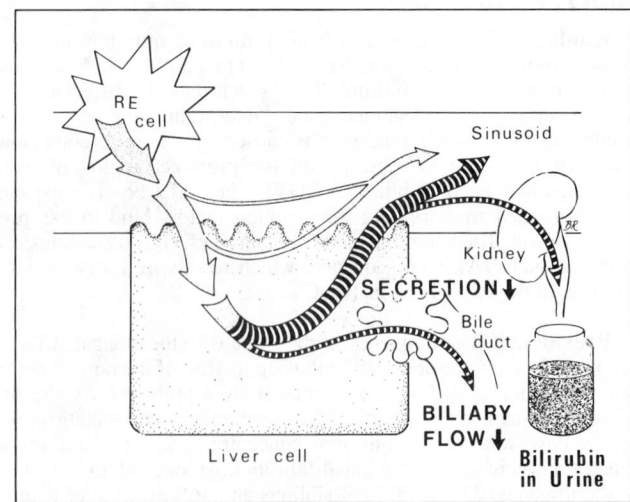

FIGURE 353-6 Abnormal bilirubin transport in conjugated hyperbilirubinemia; steps that may be deranged (symbols as in Fig. 353-1). Bilirubinuria is present. Regurgitation of bilirubin conjugates may occur via leaky tight junctions of bile canaliculi and/or ductules (not shown) as well as through the hepatocyte.

Modified from Ostrow JD et al: *Unit I, Hepatic excretory function: undergraduate teaching project, American Gastroenterological Association,* Baltimore, 1975, Milner-Fenwick, slide 28.

sufficiently to the usual therapies, neonates are treated by exchange transfusion to physically remove UCB, and Crigler-Najjar I subjects undergo liver transplantation.

PATHOPHYSIOLOGY AND CLASSIFICATION OF CONJUGATED HYPERBILIRUBINEMIA

Conjugated hyperbilirubinemia (Fig. 353-6) is characterized by retention principally of conjugated bilirubin in the serum. There is also significant elevation of the concentration of unconjugated bilirubin, in part because of hydrolysis of retained conjugated bilirubin by tissue β-glucuronidases, as well as contributions from associated hemolysis and/or impairment of delivery, uptake, and storage of unconjugated bilirubin.

All forms of conjugated hyperbilirubinemia involve a partial or complete deficiency in the canalicular secretion or biliary flow of conjugated bilirubins. ICG, cholephilic dyes, and IDA derivatives, which use the same transport system as conjugated bilirubin, are also excreted poorly. The retained conjugated bilirubins regurgitate through the hepatocytes into the lymph in the space of Disse and from there to the plasma. The small fraction of retained conjugated bilirubins that is not bound to plasma albumin filters at the glomerulus, producing the bilirubinuria which is diagnostic of conjugated hyperbilirubinemia. Renal excretion also constitutes the major alternate pathway for removal of conjugated bilirubin and other organic anions in the face of reduced hepatobiliary excretion.

With remission of hepatitis or relief of biliary obstruction, the urinary excretion of conjugated bilirubin terminates well before the serum level of "direct" bilirubin returns to normal. This occurs because δ-bilirubin is not excreted by the liver or kidneys and has the 14-day half-life of the albumin moiety; thus it persists in the plasma after the bilirubin glucuronides have been cleared within 3 to 4 days.

In contrast to unconjugated hyperbilirubinemia, jaundice with bilirubinuria almost always results from significant hepatobiliary disease, which may be classified further according to whether canalicular secretion or biliary flow is primarily impaired. Selective defects in canalicular secretion of bilirubin conjugates are characteristic of hereditary conjugated hyperbilirubinemias and common in hepatocellular diseases, whereas generalized defects in canalicular secretion or biliary flow produce the syndrome of cholestasis. Combined defects are often present, causing problems in differential diagnosis.

All forms of cholestasis may be distinguished from hepatocellular defects by the generalized retention of all components of bile and the consequences of marked retention of bile salts. These include decreased hepatic synthesis of cholesterol, inhibition of hepatic catabolism of cholesterol to bile salts, and hypercholesterolemia. Retained bile salts induce increased hepatic synthesis of alkaline phosphatase in the face of decreased hepatic excretion of this enzyme; this leads to elevation of alkaline phosphatase concentration in the serum, which is typically more marked in most forms of cholestasis. It is believed that toxic effects of retained hydrophobic bile salts cause the secondary hepatocellular injury that develops with prolonged cholestasis, and that the improvement in liver function, seen when the hydrophilic ursodeoxycholic acid is administered to such patients, may be due to replacement of the toxic bile salts with nontoxic ursodeoxycholate. Though both these concepts are controversial, most patients with chronic cholestasis are treated nowadays with oral ursodeoxycholic acid.

Step 6 Defects: Diminished Canalicular Secretion of Conjugated Bilirubins

The purest form of impaired secretion of conjugated bilirubin is the Dubin-Johnson syndrome, which results from an autosomal recessive defect in the cMOAT. In another uncommon hereditary disorder, Rotor's syndrome, impairment of canalicular transport of organic anions is less severe, but there is evidence of increased reflux of the conjugates from liver to plasma, so that the exact locus of the defect remains an enigma. Rifampicin may compete with bilirubin conjugates for secretion by cMOAT. In these conditions, canalicular morphology and secretion of bile salts are usually normal.

Preferential impairment of canalicular secretion of conjugated bilirubins, usually with limited impairment of bile acid secretion, is typical of the *hepatocellular diseases,* hepatitis and cirrhosis, most often caused by alcohol, drugs, toxins, or hepatitis viruses. These diseases often also affect the delivery, uptake, and storage of organic anions, causing associated increases in plasma concentrations of unconjugated bilirubin and bile salts.

More generalized damage to the canalicular membrane, usually evidenced by distortion and loss of microvilli in dilated canaliculi plugged with inspissated bile, results in impaired secretion of all components of bile, including bile salts and lipids, as well as bilirubin and other organic anion cholephiles. Such *canalicular cholestasis,* not involving larger biliary channels, is the most common form of intrahepatic cholestasis, and it sometimes complicates hepatocellular diseases. The canalicular tight junctions may become abnormally permeable, allowing bile constituents to regurgitate into the intercellular extensions of the space of Disse, and from there to the plasma.

Canalicular cholestasis is most often caused by drugs (e.g., cyclosporin A), steroid hormones, (e.g., estrogens), or by sepsis, and by total parenteral nutrition, but it may also occur in acute viral or alcoholic hepatitis. Drug-induced cholestasis usually occurs unpredictably in a few patients; may have many of the characteristics of an immunogenic reaction; and is usually associated with some degree of inflammation and hepatocellular necrosis, causing associated increases in serum transaminase levels (hepatocanalicular cholestasis). Drugs most often implicated include phenothiazines, diazepoxides, sulfonylureas, and antithyroid preparations such as methimazole.

Normal pregnancy or the administration of synthetic estrogens, 19-norprogestogens (19-nortestosterone derivatives), or 17-α-alkyl anabolic steroids impairs maximum hepatic secretory capacity for organic anion cholephiles in almost all subjects but unpredictably engenders a full-blown cholestatic syndrome in a small proportion of patients. Mild to severe canalicular cholestasis may occur after long, difficult surgical procedures with multiple blood transfusions. A similar syndrome sometimes occurs during lobar pneumonia, severe infections with endotoxemia and/or septicemia, total parenteral nutrition, and sickle cell anemia crises. Two rare hereditary syndromes, benign recurrent intrahepatic cholestasis and progressive familial intrahepatic cholestasis, are discussed in detail later. The former is characterized by intermittent prolonged episodes of pruritus, jaundice, and morphologic evidence of cholestasis, which revert to normal during remissions.

Step 7 Defects: Impaired Biliary Flow and Permeability

If any portion of the biliary tree, from the ductules to the sphincter of Oddi, becomes blocked or abnormally permeable, flow of bile is retarded, and excretion of all components of bile is decreased. Such *ductal cholestasis* may be classified primarily according to the locus of the damage to the biliary passages and secondarily according to the causative lesion or etiologic agent. Ductal cholestasis secondarily produces morphologic and functional changes in the canaliculi similar to those seen in canalicular cholestasis. Hepatocellular necrosis, periportal inflammation, and dilation of larger ducts may be variably associated, according to etiology, but are often minimal despite laboratory evidence of severe cholestasis.

Cholestasis Caused by Damage to the Interlobular Bile Ducts. Lesions of the ducts in the portal triads occur in primary biliary cirrhosis, in the sclerosing pericholangitis that accompanies inflammatory bowel disease, in about 20% of patients with postnecrotic cirrhosis, in patients on total parenteral nutrition, and in congenital intrahepatic biliary atresia. In biliary atresia and sclerosing pericholangitis the larger intrahepatic and extrahepatic bile ducts are usually affected also. Intrahepatic biliary atresia may sometimes be caused by accumulation of unusual, toxic bile salts resulting from hereditary defects in bile acid synthesis.

Pericholangitis, with associated canalicular cholestasis, occurs in almost 40% of patients who are on total parenteral nutrition for more than 4 to 6 weeks. Most of these patients have thick, dark bile and biliary sludge, and about one fourth develop calcium bilirubinate gallstones. The lesions are believed to be due to a combination of infrequent gallbladder emptying; accumulation of the toxic bile salt lithocholate in the biliary tree and liver; and bacterial overgrowth caused by stagnant intestinal motility, which results in translocation of bacteria and endotoxin into the circulation. Frequent administration of cholecystokinin to stimulate gallbladder and gut motility, and therapy with ursodeoxycholic acid and metronidazole, have been proposed as preventive measures.

Lesions of Interlobular and Larger Intrahepatic Bile Ducts. These ducts probably are the major site of blockage with multifocal lesions of the liver, which include granulomas, lymphomas, metastatic tumors, and primary hepatocellular carcinomas. These lesions often cause striking elevation of the serum alkaline phosphatase concentration, with little or no hyperbilirubinemia until late in the disease. Less common lesions involving the larger intrahepatic radicles include sclerosing cholangitis, intraductal papillomatosis, intraductal lithiasis, and the varied permutations and combinations of congenital biliary ectasias (Caroli's disease) and cystic disease (congenital hepatic fibrosis). The latter two diseases characteristically present as recurrent episodes of acute cholangitis, sometimes unaccompanied by jaundice.

Extrahepatic Cholestasis. Extrahepatic cholestasis is most often caused by focal lesions, especially carcinomas of the bile ducts, gallbladder, pancreas, or ampulla of Vater. Other common causes include choledocholithiasis, acute cholecystitis, and strictures of the common or hepatic ducts as a result of inadvertent injury during surgery. Less frequent causes are primary sclerosing cholangitis, fibrosis or edema of the head of the pancreas as a result of chronic or acute pancreatitis, congenital choledochal cysts, pancreatic pseudocysts, and benign polypoid epithelial tumors of the bile ducts. Extrahepatic obstructive lesions are usually remediable surgically or by endoscopic manipulation but lead to progressive liver damage and secondary biliary cirrhosis if untreated. In contrast, intrahepatic forms of cholestasis usually are treated medically.

Abnormalities of the Enterohepatic Circulation of Bile Pigments (Steps 8 to 10)

Some abnormalities simulate cholestasis as a result of increased recirculation of bile pigments and other components of bile. Cholascos (leakage of bile into the peritoneal cavity) results in jaundice due to result of the absorption of conjugated and unconjugated bilirubin, as

Table 353-4 Hepatocellular versus cholestatic jaundice

CLINICAL FINDING OR LABORATORY TEST	HEPATOCELLULAR JAUNDICE	CHOLESTATIC JAUNDICE CANALICULAR	CHOLESTATIC JAUNDICE DUCTAL
Pruritis	Uncommon	>75% of patients	> 75% of patients
Steatorrhea (insufficient micelles)	Uncommon	Common	Common
Serum bilirubin levels	Increased	Usually increased	Usually increased*
Serum bile acid levels	Increased	Increased	Usually very high
Serum alkaline phosphatase levels	Usually <3× normal	Usually >3× normal†	Usually >3× normal, often >10× normal
Serum cholesterol levels	Decreased or normal	Increased	Increased
Serum aminotransferases‡	Elevated, may be >1000 IU	Usually <300 IU, but may be >300 IU	Mildly elevated, seldom >300 IU
Prothrombin time and response to parenteral Vitamin K therapy	Usually increased; unresponsive to K	Sometimes increased; responds to K	

*Patients with hepatic metastases or granulomas, or chronic partial biliary obstruction, often have marked elevations of serum alkaline phosphatase with little or no increase in bilirubin levels.

†Alkaline phosphatase levels are often <3× normal in canalicular cholestasis caused by estrogens, anabolic steroids, endotoxins, or postoperative state.

‡Includes serum glutamic pyruvic transaminase (SGPT, alanine aminotransferase, ALT) and serum glutamic-oxalacetic transaminase (SGOT, aspartate aminotransferase, AST)

well as alkaline phosphatase and bile salts, across the peritoneal membrane. In acute cholangitis or cholecystitis, bacterial deconjugation of conjugated bilirubin and increased permeability of the gallbladder epithelium lead to increased absorption of bilirubins, and other bile components, from the gallbladder. Increased enterohepatic circulation of unconjugated bilirubin may occur with extensive ileal disease or resection.

DIFFERENTIAL DIAGNOSIS OF CONJUGATED HYPERBILIRUBINEMIA
Distinction of Hepatocellular from Cholestatic Jaundice

Once the presence of conjugated hyperbilirubinemia has been established, the next steps in differential diagnosis are (1) to determine whether jaundice is hepatocellular or cholestatic (see Table 353-4), and (2) to determine the level of the block to biliary flow if cholestasis is present (Chapter 351).

Itching, especially on the palms and soles, is virtually diagnostic of cholestasis but occurs in only 75% of cases. Recent data suggests that increased levels of endogenous opioids may be the cause of the itching. In those who do not itch, the presence of cholestasis may be surmised from an elevation of the serum alkaline phosphatase level more than threefold above normal, increased serum cholesterol level, absence of marked elevations of serum transaminases, and response of an abnormal prothrombin time to vitamin K. Steatorrhea may result from insufficient biliary excretion of bile salts into the intestine.

It may not be easy to distinguish cholestatic from hepatocellular jaundice for several reasons:
1. Some agents that typically cause hepatocellular disease (e.g., alcohol and hepatitis viruses) sometimes also affect bile canaliculi; drugs that characteristically cause intrahepatic cholestasis (e.g., chlorpromazine) may also damage hepatocytes.
2. Prolonged cholestasis, especially extrahepatic obstruction, secondarily damages the liver cells, possibly as a result of the toxic effects of retained bile salts.
3. All forms of cholestasis and hepatocellular disease, if prolonged, may lead to cirrhosis and portal hypertension.

The criteria in Table 353-4 are not infallible. For example, serum alkaline phosphatase values less than three times normal are common in patients with cholestasis caused by infections or estrogens, and occur in 15% of all patients with extrahepatic biliary obstruction. Alkaline phosphatase levels, moreover, may be increased as a result of bone or kidney disease, or pregnancy; thus the hepatic origin of the enzyme elevation may need verification by determination of serum 5′-nucleotidase, which is hepatospecific though less sensitive. Serum transaminase and lactic dehydrogenase activities may be markedly elevated in patients with primary or metastatic hepatic cancer, or when cholangitis complicates biliary obstruction.

Determination of the Site of Blockage in Cholestasis

Routine liver function tests are of absolutely no assistance in locating the site of a cholestatic lesion because all forms of cholestasis produce similar clinical, histologic, and biochemical abnormalities. Nonetheless, a careful history and physical examination, plus routine blood chemistry tests, can appropriately classify cholestatic jaundice in 85% to 90% of patients.

Clues from the history or physical examination that suggest a diagnosis of intrahepatic cholestasis include (1) age less than 40 years (viral and drug hepatitis are most common in this age-group); (2) liver span of more than 15 cm on percussion, especially if the liver is tender (this sign most often indicates alcoholic liver disease or malignancy but may be seen also in patients with primary biliary cirrhosis and sclerosing cholangitis); (3) drug addiction or homosexuality (high risk of transmission of hepatitis); and (4) history of alcoholism, or recent treatment with drugs or hormones known to cause jaundice, especially estrogens. Moreover, a decreased serum cholesterol concentration in the presence of an otherwise typical cholestatic syndrome should strongly suggest viral or alcoholic hepatitis as the cause.

Findings that favor a diagnosis of extrahepatic obstruction include (1) age greater than 60 years (in males in this age group, the obstruction is usually due to malignancy); (2) acholic (pale) stools persisting for more than 2 weeks; (3) colicky right upper quadrant pain and/or shaking chills compatible with choledocholithiasis and cholangitis; (4) severe jaundice without systemic symptoms (hepatocellular diseases with severe jaundice are almost always associated with systemic symptoms); and (5) a palpable (Courvoisier) gallbladder, an almost infallible sign of common bile duct obstruction, usually malignant.

When classification of cholestasis is difficult, upper abdominal ultrasonography is advised, followed by computerized tomographic (CT) scans if the sonogram is unsatisfactory. If intrahepatic cholestasis is suspected clinically and ultrasonography reveals no dilated ducts, liver biopsy is often helpful in establishing the etiology. If extrahepatic obstruction seems most likely clinically and noninvasive imaging reveals dilated ducts, endoscopic transduodenal cholangiopancreatography can be used to visualize, and even relieve, the obstructing lesion(s). In many centers this stepwise application of procedures has become routine in all patients with cholestasis.

In the neonate with cholestasis, hepatobiliary scintiscanning using ^{99m}Tc-labeled IDA derivatives is very useful to distinguish between biliary atresia and intrahepatic cholestases; appearance of the isotope in the duodenum essentially excludes extrahepatic atresia. In addition, because both neonatal hepatitis and metabolic defects (e.g., galactosemia, α-1 antitrypsin deficiency) often cause neonatal cholestasis, liver biopsy is frequently helpful.

Table 353-5   Dubin-Johnson and Rotor's syndromes

FINDING	DUBIN-JOHNSON SYNDROME	ROTOR'S SYNDROME
Hereditary defect	Autosomal recessive; absent cMOAT activity*	Dual defect of storage and biliary secretion
Serum total bilirubin (mg/dl):	1.8-9.9 in 90% of cases	2.7-7.9 in 90% of cases
Direct/total (mean)	60%	60%
Organic anion kinetics:		
Secretory maximum	<20% of normal	Mean 50% of normal
Storage capacity	Normal	<20% of normal
Late rise in conjugates in serum	>90% of cases	Never observed
Total urinary coproporphyrins:	Normal	Markedly increased
Ratio of isomer I to isomers I+III	>80%	<65%
Pigment in hepatocyte lysosomes	Almost always present	Never present
Gallbladder visualized on cholecystography	<25% of cases	Almost always
Gastrointestinal symptoms	>75% of cases	Seldom present
Hepatomegaly	>50% of cases	Rare
Usual age of onset	10-40 years	<20 years

*cMOAT, Canalicular multispecific anion transporter. A similar genetic defect is present in the analogous animal models (TR⁻, GY, and Eisai strains of rats).

BENIGN CHRONIC CONJUGATED HYPERBILIRUBINEMIAS
Dubin-Johnson Syndrome

Etiology. Patients with Dubin-Johnson syndrome (Table 353-5) and the TR⁻, GY, and Eisai strains of jaundiced rats with the analogous syndrome suffer from a hereditary autosomal recessive deficiency of the cMOAT protein that actively secretes organic anions, other than conjugated bile salts, into the canaliculus.

Incidence. Dubin-Johnson syndrome is found in about 1 of 1300 Sephardic Jews. The incidence in Western populations is probably lower. Males are affected twice as often as females.

Pathophysiology. Analyses of plasma disappearance curves—after intravenous administration of bilirubin, BSP, ICG, ¹³¹I–rose bengal, and iodipamide—indicate that the uptake and storage of these compounds are normal, but their maximum rate of secretion into bile is less than 10% of normal. The relatively normal initial plasma disappearance is followed in more than 90% of patients by a secondary rise in plasma concentration at 90 to 120 minutes as a result of reflux of unexcreted conjugates back into the plasma. This reflux occurs because the conjugated compounds are less well bound to cytoplasmic storage proteins than are the parent unconjugated substances. Kinetics, serum concentration, and biliary excretion of amidated bile salts are normal, but there is impaired secretion of ursodeoxycholic acid and bile acid 3-0-sulfates and glucuronides.

There is a high frequency of consanguinity, and about one third of tested siblings (but none of the parents) of children of Dubin-Johnson syndrome probands show increased serum conjugated bilirubin concentrations and a delayed rise in plasma BSP conjugates. Patients with Dubin-Johnson syndrome also exhibit a markedly increased coproporphyrin I/coproporphyrin III ratio in their urine, though total urinary coproporphyrin excretion is normal. This phenomenon apparently results from differential impairment of the biliary excretion of the two isomers. Heterozygous relatives have normal serum bilirubin and BSP test results but show an intermediate increase in the urinary coproporphyrin I/coproporphyrin III ratio.

Pathology. The liver is grossly black because of accumulation of a granular, melanin-like pigment in the lysosomes of perivenular hepatocytes. Liver histologic conditions and ultrastructure are otherwise usually normal.

Clinical Features. Jaundice is usually insidious in onset and begins in the second to fourth decades of life in 75% of patients. Serum bilirubin concentrations are less than 10 mg/dl in over 90% of patients, with an average of 60% direct-reacting bilirubin and a high proportion of δ-bilirubin. Bilirubin concentrations increase twofold to threefold during pregnancy, estrogen therapy, infections, trauma, or surgical procedures, often unmasking clinically latent jaundice.

Among patients with Dubin-Johnson syndrome, for unexplained reasons, the prothrombin time is prolonged in two thirds; factor VII is deficient in 40%; half have a palpably enlarged liver that is often tender; and three fourths have associated upper abdominal discomfort, nausea, or vomiting. These symptoms may mistakenly suggest a diagnosis of choledocholithiasis, especially since reduced secretion of iopanoic acid results in failure to visualize the gallbladder on oral cholecystography in 75% of patients. Dubin-Johnson syndrome, however, is readily distinguished by the absence of itching, the rarity of acholic stools, and minimal or no elevation of serum alkaline phosphatase and transaminases.

Diagnosis and Treatment. The family history should suggest a hereditary disorder. Cholestasis is excluded if serum bile acid levels are normal, and biliary tract disease can be excluded by ultrasonography or ⁹⁹ᵐTc DISIDA scintiscanning (with delayed films). The diagnosis may be confirmed by the typical increase in the coproporphyrin I/coproporphyrin III isomer ratio in the urine, with normal total coproporphyrin levels. Liver biopsy is rarely needed and may be misleading, since some patients lack the pigment. No treatment is known or necessary.

Rotor's Syndrome and Hepatic Storage Disease

These two related syndromes (see Table 353-5) are inherited in an autosomal recessive pattern. The chronic, predominantly conjugated hyperbilirubinemia results from a dual defect in transport of organic anions other than bile salts: severe impairment of storage and a mean 50% decrease in biliary secretion.

Incidence. These syndromes are rare. Most reported cases have been in Hispanic families. The sexes are almost equally affected.

Pathophysiology. In contrast to the Dubin-Johnson syndrome, the earlier portions of the plasma disappearance curves of unconjugated bilirubin, BSP, ICG, and iodipamide are markedly delayed because of reduction of storage capacity to less than 20% of normal. The reduced ligandin level, in the only patient thus tested, requires confirmation. Biliary secretory maximum is decreased also, to about one-half of normal values, and presumably accounts for the retention of bilirubin conjugates, but no late rise in plasma BSP conjugates is seen. The coexistence with Dubin-Johnson syndrome in some families and the 50% decrease in secretory capacity suggest that the secretory impairment in Rotor's syndrome might be due to one defective allele for cMOAT. Kinetic models that incorporate these dual transport defects reproduce the plasma disappearance curves obtained with BSP.

As in the Dubin-Johnson syndrome, the ratio of coproporphyrins I to III in the urine is elevated; in contrast, total urinary coproporphyrin is greatly increased as a result of an average 20-fold increase in the output of isomer I and a mean fourfold increase in the output of isomer III. Heterozygotes show intermediate increases in the ratio of coproporphyrin I to III in the urine, with a twofold to threefold increase in excretion of isomer I, as well as intermediate impairment of the clearance, storage, and biliary secretory maximum of BSP.

Pathology. Hepatic histologic findings are usually normal, and there is no pigment.

Clinical Features. Chronic, fluctuating jaundice usually develops in childhood or adolescence, with serum bilirubin concentrations usually in the range of 3 to 8 mg/dl; an average of 60% of serum bilirubin is direct-reacting. Unlike in Dubin-Johnson syndrome, the oral cholecystographic findings are normal, there is no hepatic enlargement, abdominal discomfort is rarely present, and jaundice is not aggravated by pregnancy. Serum bile acid concentrations are normal. Compared to Rotor's syndrome, hepatic storage disease causes more severe impairment of BSP storage capacity, and oral cholecystographic visualization of the gallbladder is delayed.

Diagnosis and Treatment. The same diagnostic considerations apply as described for Dubin-Johnson syndrome, but the differences in BSP secretory maximum and storage capacity, and the high total urinary coproporphyrin levels, are distinctive. No treatment is known or indicated.

FAMILIAL CHOLESTATIC SYNDROMES
Estrogen-Related Cholestasis

Etiology. Although estrogens impair the secretory maximum for BSP in all subjects, a small proportion of women develop marked retention of bile salts and severe pruritus on prolonged exposure to high levels of estrogens. Such exposure may result from ingestion of oral contraceptive pills or from pregnancy. Twenty percent of affected patients also develop conjugated hyperbilirubinemia. Progestational steroids potentiate the effect of estrogens by inhibiting their conjugation and detoxification. Occurrence of the syndrome in about 15% of mothers and sisters of probands favors a hereditary predisposition, but the genetic defect is not yet known.

Incidence. In most countries, estrogen-related cholestasis occurs in less than 0.5% of women during pregnancy and/or oral contraceptive use. The incidence in Sweden, however, is about 2%; in Chile it is about 10% among predominantly white probands and 28% among Araucanian Indians.

Pathophysiology. Increased levels of endogenous opioids may account for the pruritus. As in most steroid-related cholestasis, alkaline phosphatase levels are rarely more than three times normal except in patients with jaundice. Estrogen metabolism in these patients is normal except for the decreased conversion of 16-hydroxy estrones to estriols that is seen with cholestasis of any cause. The reasons for the sensitivity to estrogens and the irregular occurrence of the syndrome among the different pregnancies of a given patient are not known. Estrogen administration uniformly reproduces the syndrome in affected women, and the natural syndrome reverses spontaneously after parturition.

Pathology. During episodes of estrogen-related cholestasis, 80% of patients show the typical canalicular lesions of bile plugs, dilation, and loss of microvilli. There is no evidence of liver cell degeneration or necrosis, inflammation, or fibrosis. Histologic features revert to normal after remission.

Clinical Features. In women with estrogen-related cholestasis, pruritus usually begins without systemic prodromal symptoms, usually during the eighth or ninth month of gestation or within a few days of the start of estrogen therapy. If jaundice occurs, it usually develops 1 to 2 weeks later. Total serum bilirubin levels are rarely greater than 5 mg/dl; at least 50% of bilirubin is direct reacting. Serum transaminase levels are often elevated in the range of 100 to 200

units, and serum cholesterol is generally above 300 mg/dl, but serum alkaline phosphatase levels seldom exceed three times normal values. The liver and spleen are rarely enlarged. Though the syndrome is benign for the mothers, the infant is at increased risk from premature delivery or stillbirth. For unclear reasons, more than 50% of the patients, their mothers, and their sisters develop cholesterol gallstones.

Diagnosis. The family history and the relation of symptoms to pregnancy and/or oral contraceptive use should suggest estrogen-related cholestasis. The mild elevations of bilirubin, transaminases, and alkaline phosphatases and the absence of hepatomegaly, abdominal pain, fever, and systemic symptoms help to exclude choledocholithiasis, viral hepatitis, and the fearsome acute fatty liver of pregnancy. Abdominal ultrasonography can exclude biliary obstruction. Radiologic examinations and radioisotopic cholangiography are contraindicated in pregnancy.

Treatment. Termination of pregnancy or of oral contraceptive therapy invariably relieves the symptoms within hours to days. Cholestyramine may control itching; the effectiveness of phenobarbital and phototherapy has not been studied systematically. S-adenosylmethionine, 800 mg daily intravenously, reputedly reverses the syndrome in less than 1 week, but this is disputed. Controlled trials are underway to determine the effectiveness of opioid antagonists and of ursodeoxycholic acid against the pruritis.

Recurrent and Progressive Familial Cholestasis

Benign recurrent intrahepatic cholestasis (BRIC), a rare, autosomal recessive syndrome, causes recurrent prolonged episodes of severe cholestatic jaundice, usually unrelated to estrogen therapy or pregnancy. Males are affected almost twice as often as females. Keto and ring-unsaturated bile salts appear during attacks, but their etiologic role is doubtful. Genetic linkage analysis has localized the mutation to chromosome 18q21.2-3, the same region as the mutation in Byler's disease (see later discussion). Both diseases appear to involve primary genetic defects in the canalicular bile salt transporter.

In BRIC, retention of bile salts and itching dominate the attacks, associated with severe jaundice and systemic symptoms but little increase in serum cholesterol levels. Anorexia, combined with steatorrhea from decreased excretion of bile salts into the intestine, may cause weight loss during episodes. In addition to the typical lesions of canalicular cholestasis, there are also significant portal inflammatory infiltrates and hepatocellular lesions. Attacks usually begin in childhood or adolescence (before the age of 2 years in one third of patients) and often occur with regularity. Attacks typically begin with a prodrome of fatigue, malaise, and anorexia. Itching then begins, followed in 2 to 4 weeks by painless jaundice without fever. The liver is usually enlarged and is occasionally tender. Bilirubin concentrations usually plateau at 10 to 20 mg/dl. Transaminases may be elevated twofold to threefold. Attacks generally clear without sequelae in 1 to 4 months. Between episodes, liver function test results and histological features are normal. Diagnosis rests on the history of recurrent episodes of severe cholestasis from childhood and the limited abnormalities (other than marked bilirubinemia) revealed in liver function tests. Biliary obstruction can be excluded by ultrasonographic and radiologic visualization of the biliary tree. Prednisolone or ursodeoxycholic therapy may shorten attacks in some patients. Fat-soluble vitamin supplements should be given to patients with steatorrhea, and oral and parenteral hyperalimentaion may help to minimize weight loss. Treatment of itching is discussed earlier.

Byler's disease, a form of progressive familial intrahepatic cholestasis (PFIC), is a rare, autosomal recessive disorder, characterized by a severe defect in bile salt secretion. This results in hepatic fibrosis and failure, but minimal ductular proliferation, and serum γ-glutamyl transpeptidase (γ-GGT) values are normal. Another form of PFIC, with normal serum γ-GGT values, is caused by severe congenital defects in bile salt synthesis. A third form of PFIC is due to homozygous mutations in the MDR-3 canalicular flippase for lecithin. As in the comparable MDR-2 knockout mouse model, these patients have high γ-GGT values and show severe inflammation, fibrosis, and ductular proliferation and metaplasia in the liver. This is caused by the absence of biliary lecithins that normally protect the biliary epithelium from the toxic effects of secreted bile salts. PFIC may respond for a while to long-term ursodeoxycholic acid therapy, but liver transplantation is ultimately necessary.

POSTOPERATIVE CHOLESTASIS AND CHOLESTASIS RELATED TO SEVERE INFECTIONS

Mild or severe intrahepatic cholestasis may occur after long and difficult operations with multiple blood transfusions. The severe, less-common form develops in 3 to 4 days and peaks 9 to 18 days postoperatively. It results from a combination of (1) a large bilirubin load from transfusion of many units of blood plus internal bleeding, (2) impaired hepatic transport of bilirubin resulting from hypotension and anoxia, and (3) acute renal failure, with impairment of the urinary route for excretion of conjugated bilirubin. These patients may have conjugated hyperbilirubinemia of 20 to 40 mg/dl but serum alkaline phosphatase levels only three to five times normal. Centrilobular congestion and hemorrhagic necrosis with associated erythrophagocytosis are found at autopsy. The less severe form develops 1 to 2 days after prolonged surgery involving usually less than nine units of blood; shock, internal hemorrhage, and renal failure are absent. Serum bilirubin concentration is usually less than 10 mg/dl. Alkaline phosphatase levels are normal in 50% of patients and less than three times normal in the remainder. Histologic examination reveals the canalicular dilation and bile plugs typical of intrahepatic cholestasis. The syndrome resolves in 2 to 4 weeks unless additional complications supervene. Mild transaminase elevations exclude halothane or viral hepatitis, and the mild elevations of alkaline phosphatase in relation to bilirubin levels render extrahepatic obstruction unlikely. Treatment is directed at the underlying complications.

Similar syndromes occur with lobar pneumonia and severe infections, especially if accompanied by toxemia and/or septicemia. Though endotoxin does produce cholestasis experimentally, its role in the human syndrome is not established. The more severe picture occurs only with septicemic shock. The usual, milder syndrome does not affect the prognosis of the patient, and its histologic features are similar to those of mild postoperative cholestasis with, in addition, necrosis of periportal hepatocytes and dilation, plugging, and epithelial damage to the cholangioles.

BIBLIOGRAPHY

Berk PD and Noyer C, editors: Bilirubin metabolism and the hereditary hyperbilirubinemias, *Semin Liver Dis* 14:321-394, 1994.

Feuer G, and Di Fonzo CJ: Intrahepatic cholestasis: a review of biochemical-pathological mechanisms, *Drug Metabol Drug Interact* 10:1-161, 1992.

Frank BB et al: Clinical evaluation of jaundice: a guideline of the Patient Care Committee of the American Gastroenterological Association, *JAMA* 262:3031-3034, 1989.

Gartner LM: Neonatal jaundice, *Pediatr Rev* 15:422-432, 1994.

Lester R, editor: The pathogenesis of cholestasis: past and future trends, *Semin Liver Dis* 13:219-315, 1993.

Mews C, Sinatra FR: Cholestasis in infancy, *Pediatr Rev* 15:233-240, 1994.

Muraca M, Fevery J, Blanckaert N: Analytical aspects and clinical interpretation of serum bilirubins, *Semin Liver Dis* 8:137-149, 1988.

Okolicsanyi L, Nassuato G, Strazzabosco M: Familial hyperbilirubinemias: clinical aspects. In Tavoloni N, Berk PD, editors: *Hepatic transport and bile secretion: physiology and pathophysiology,* New York, 1993, Raven Press, pp. 649-664.

Ostrow JD: Therapeutic amelioration of jaundice: old and new strategies (editorial), *Hepatology* 8:683-689, 1988.

Ostrow JD, editor: *Bile pigments and jaundice: molecular, metabolic, and medical aspects,* New York, 1986, Marcel Dekker.

Ostrow JD, Mukerjee P, Tiribelli C: Structure and binding of unconjugated bilirubin: relevance for physiological and pathophysiological function, *J Lipid Res* 35:1715-1737, 1994.

Oude Elferink RPJ et al: Hepatobiliary secretion of organic compounds; molecular mechanisms of membrane transport, *Biochim Biophys Acta* 1421:215-268, 1995.

Quigley EM et al.: Hepatobiliary complications of total parenteral nutrition, *Gastroenterology* 104:286-301, 1993.

Reyes H: The spectrum of liver and gastrointestinal disease seen in cholestasis of prenancy, *Gastroenterol Clin North Am* 21:905-921, 1992.

Scheiman JM, Moseley RH: Cholestasis, *Compr Ther* 20:28-35, 1994.

Shah HA, Spivak W: Neonatal cholestasis: new approaches to diagnosis, evaluation, and therapy, *Pediatr Clin North Am* 41:943-966, 1994.

Sieg A et al: Subfractionation of serum bilirubins by alkaline methanolysis and thin layer chromatography: an aid in the differential diagnosis of icteric diseases, *J Hepatol* 11:159-164, 1990.

354 Principal Complications of Liver Failure

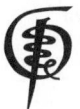

Steven Schenker and Anastacio M. Hoyumpa

The liver is a vital organ that has numerous anabolic (synthetic), catabolic (detoxifying), and storage functions. It also serves as a conduit by which portal blood enters the superior vena cava. Therefore liver failure may result in many derangements of normal body processes such as synthesis of protein; formation of glucose; detoxication of ammonia, various hormones, and drugs; storage of glycogen and certain vitamins; and maintenance of normal splanchnic blood flow. Many of these derangements are covered elsewhere in this book (Chapters 348 and 356); this discussion concerns only the following major manifestations of liver failure: hepatic encephalopathy, ascites, portal hypertension, the hepatorenal syndrome, hepatopulmonary syndrome, and endocrine disturbances.

HEPATIC ENCEPHALOPATHY
Clinical Features

Hepatic encephalopathy is a neuropsychiatric syndrome seen in some patients with liver failure. The disorder may be secondary to acute or chronic parenchymal liver disease, the latter frequently accompanied by spontaneous or surgically induced portosystemic shunting of blood. Rarely, encephalopathy may occur in children with congenital disorders of urea cycle enzymes and in patients with other types of hepatic dysfunction. The features common to all forms of hepatic encephalopathy are alterations of mental state, neurologic abnormalities, the presence of parenchymal liver disease, and, usually, certain characteristic but nonspecific laboratory findings. These clinical features are summarized in Table 354-1.

Hepatic encephalopathy can be considered as a spectrum of disorders. In acute liver failure, as seen in patients with fulminant viral or toxic hepatitis (i.e., due to acetaminophen or halothane) or with acute fatty liver of pregnancy, there are usually no obvious precipitants of encephalopathy. The course is explosive, with delirium, convulsions, and often cerebral edema and decerebrate rigidity. In about 80% of instances, the disorder is fatal.

By contrast, patients with chronic liver disease develop a more indolent type of neuropsychiatric disturbance, often called *portosystemic encephalopathy*. This disorder is often precipitated by specific events such as gastrointestinal hemorrhage, azotemia, or infection. The usual precipitating causes and their presumed mechanisms are shown in Table 354-2. Diagnosis of portosystemic encephalopathy depends on the identification of typical clinical features, the exclusion of other causes of encephalopathy, and, at times, on a therapeutic trial.

As can be seen in Table 354-1, an abnormal mental state is the *sine qua non* of all types of hepatic encephalopathy. The mental abnormality may consist only of slight alterations in judgment and other intellectual processes, nonspecific personality changes, and inappropriate behavior. Motor skills (i.e., driving) may be especially impaired and can be assessed by psychomotor testing. A graphic or semiquantitative assessment of intellectual performance also can be obtained by following the patient's handwriting, by asking the patient to do simple manual construction such as reproducing a five-pointed star, or by administering a numbers-connection (Reitan Trailmaking) test in which the patient connects sequential numbers by lines during a timed interval. The score is the time in seconds necessary to complete the task. Rapid, inexpensive, simple, and accurate, the numbers-connection test is more sensitive than the star construction test and handier than the electroencephalogram or the use of event-related (visual, auditory, somatosensory) evoked potentials. With more severe portosystemic encephalopathy, progressive inversion of sleep pattern, staring, apathy, drowsiness, and eventually deep coma may occur. Hy-

Table 354-1   Stages of hepatic encephalopathy

STAGE	SYMPTOMS	SIGNS	EEG
Prodrome	Loss of affect, euphoria, depression, apathy, inappropriate behavior, altered sleep pattern	Asterixis ±, constructional apraxia, writing difficulty	±
Impending coma	Confusion, disorientation, drowsiness	Asterixis, fetor hepaticus	++
Light coma	Marked confusion, arousable from sleep, response to stimuli	Asterixis, fetor hepaticus, rigidity of limbs, hyperflexia, clonus, extensor response, grasping and sucking reflexes	+++
Deep coma	Unconsciousness, no response to stimuli	Fetor hepaticus, no muscle tone, flaccid limbs, depressed reflexes	++++

±, May or may not be present; +, abnormal finding showing decreased electrical activity. Separation into various stages is not necessarily sharp, and EEG changes may not always correlate with the severity of coma. Hypothermia may be seen in the early stages, and hyperventilation at any state, of encephalopathy.

Table 354-2   Precipitating causes of portosystemic encephalopathy

CAUSE	PRESUMED MECHANISM	THERAPEUTIC IMPLICATION
Azotemia (spontaneous or diuretic-induced)	Increased enterohepatic circulation of urea nitrogen, with increased ammonia production Direct sedative effect of uremia Diuretic-induced hypokalemic alkalosis, increased renal vein ammonia output, resulting in enhanced transfer of ammonia across blood-brain barrier Excessive diuresis, leading to hypovolemia, prerenal azotemia, decreased perfusion of vital organs Separate role of hypokalemia in cerebral function	Avoidance of excessive diuresis Avoidance of potentially nephrotoxic agents (e.g., aminoglycosides)
Sedatives, tranquilizers, analgesics	Direct depressant effect on brain Hypoxia from depression of respiratory center	Cautious use of these drugs if unavoidable, with careful monitoring of response and adjustment of dosage; ideally, select agent metabolized normally in presence of liver disease, with short half-life, inactive metabolites, and no enhanced effect on the site of action (cerebral sensitivity)
Gastrointestinal bleeding	Substrate for increased production of ammonia and other nitrogenous toxins; 1 dl blood = 15-20 g protein Hypovolemia, shock, and hypoxia that compromise hepatic, cerebral, renal function, the latter leading to increased activity of the enterohepatic urea nitrogen cycle and increased ammonia production Contribution of ammonia in stored blood	Prophylactic use of lactulose and evacuation of blood from the intestine in bleeding, noncomatose patients with liver disease; avoid gastrointestinal irritants (alcohol, NSAIDs); measures needed to treat cough to minimize variceal bleeding from increased portal pressure during coughing or straining
Metabolic alkalosis	Diffusion of un-ionized ammonia across blood-brain barrier (see above)	K^+ replacement; in severe, unresponsive cases IV infusion of dilute HCl (1.5 dl 1 N HCl/1 L H_2O), 0.5-2.0 L/24 h
Excess dietary protein	Substrate for ammonia and other nitrogenous toxin production	Curtailment of dietary proteins, especially containing aromatic and sulfated amino acids and those with high ammonia-generating potential
Infection	Increased tissue catabolism, leading to more endogenous nitrogen load and increased ammonia production Dehydration and prerenal azotemia Hypoxia and/or hyperthermia that potentiates ammonia toxicity	Search for infection and early use of appropriate antibiotics
Constipation	Increased production and absorption of ammonia and other toxic nitrogen derivatives due to increased contact time between bacteria and nitrogenous substances Straining at stool that increases portal pressure, with subsequent variceal bleeding	Prophylactic use of stool softeners and laxatives

Modified from Hoyumpa AM et al: Hepatic encephalopathy, *Gastroenterology* 76:184-195, 1979.
NSAIDs, Nonsteroidal antiinflammatory drugs.

perventilation and hypothermia may be seen before the onset of coma. In about 50% of patients with portosystemic encephalopathy, fetor hepaticus may be detected. This is a sweetish, musty odor of the breath believed to be caused by exhaled mercaptans, products of impaired hepatic metabolism of the sulfur-containing amino acid methionine.

The most characteristic neurologic sign of hepatic encephalopathy is a flapping tremor of the hands called *asterixis.* It is best seen with the arms outstretched, wrists hyperextended, and fingers separated. The flap is maximum with sustained posture, is usually bilateral but asynchronous, and is frequently preceded by a lateral tremor of the fingers. Asterixis, which can also be detected as unsustained clonus in the feet, in tightly closed eyelids, pursed lips, or protruded

tongue, is thought to be due to improper integration of peripheral afferent information to the brainstem reticular formation. Asterixis is not specific for hepatic encephalopathy, however, because it occurs also in patients with uremia, pulmonary insufficiency, sedative overdose, and other metabolic neurologic derangements.

The other neurologic signs in classic hepatic encephalopathy are also believed to be caused by a metabolic rather than a structural brain disturbance. They are usually transient, changing (i.e., not localized), and potentially rapidly reversible. Thus early in portosystemic encephalopathy the patient may experience hyperreflexia, varying plantar extensor response, and spasticity. Later, with severe encephalopathy, depression of deep tendon reflexes is more common. In portosystemic encephalopathy, convulsions and decerebrate rigidity are rare. In some patients with portosystemic encephalopathy, two neurologic syndromes have been recognized. The first is called *hepatocerebral degeneration,* or pseudo-Wilsonian hepatic encephalopathy, as the neurologic signs resemble those of hepatolenticular degeneration. Prominent features include impairment of intellectual function, dysarthria, cerebellar ataxia, tremor, and athetoid movements. In contrast to Wilson's disease, however, there are no abnormalities of copper metabolism. The second syndrome, *spastic paraparesis,* consists of spasticity of the lower extremities, increased deep tendon reflexes, and extensor plantar responses. These motor disturbances are generally unaccompanied by sensory deficits or changes in cerebrospinal fluid pressure, protein concentration, or cell count. Unlike the more typical portosystemic encephalopathy, which responds to therapy in about 80% of instances, these less common neurologic syndromes are usually marked by slow, progressive deterioration, although improvement has been reported in a few patients treated with bromocriptine, a dopamine agonist, and occasionally with hepatic transplantation, which may result in normalization of the gait, disappearance of tremor, and marked improvement in mental function.

A number of abnormal laboratory findings are associated with hepatic encephalopathy. Changes in liver tests reflect an underlying hepatic disorder (Chapter 351). These tests do not, however, correlate with the presence or absence of hepatic encephalopathy, except for the prolonged prothrombin time in acute liver failure. Patients with hepatic encephalopathy, especially that secondary to chronic liver disease, also frequently show evidence of respiratory alkalosis due to hyperventilation and may have hypokalemic metabolic alkalosis due to diuretic overuse. Rarely, hypoglycemia is seen with fulminant liver failure. Abnormalities in nitrogen metabolism are characteristic. Arterial ammonia concentration is increased in about 90% of patients with hepatic encephalopathy. The arterial ammonia level, however, does not reflect well the degree of coma, probably because the assay is not fastidious enough, only single measurements are obtained, blood ammonia may not equate with brain ammonia, ammonia is not the sole "toxin" causing hepatic encephalopathy, and the clinical manifestations may lag behind the ammonia elevation by as long as 24 hours. Serial measurements of ammonia may be more helpful in following the clinical course of hepatic encephalopathy in individual patients. Spinal fluid glutamine, which reflects brain ammonia metabolism, and is usually increased, has greater stability than ammonia but requires a spinal tap. Glutamine measurements may be very helpful in distinguishing portosystemic encephalopathy from nonhepatic coma. Except for these findings, the cerebrospinal fluid in most patients with hepatic encephalopathy is usually normal. Occasionally, the spinal fluid protein concentration is elevated, in which case other causes of coma must be sought. The spinal fluid pressure may be elevated in patients with cerebral edema. Finally, patients with hepatic encephalopathy usually have an abnormal serum amino acid profile. Patients with coma due to acute liver failure have markedly elevated levels of all amino acids, and the levels tend to correlate with the degree of hepatic necrosis. On the other hand, patients with portosystemic encephalopathy exhibit an increase in aromatic amino acids and methionine, whereas branched-chain amino acid levels are depressed. Short- and long-chain fatty acid levels are likewise elevated in the blood.

Electroencephalograms in patients with hepatic encephalopathy show characteristic but nonspecific changes. These changes consist of slowing of cerebral electrical activity and high-voltage waves, starting bifrontally and progressing posteriorly. Focal abnormalities are not seen in uncomplicated hepatic encephalopathy. Similar changes in the electroencephalogram are seen in patients with other metabolic encephalopathies (e.g., uremia, drug intoxication).

Diagnosis of hepatic encephalopathy is based on the presence of typical clinical features (see Table 354-1) and the exclusion of other causes of altered mental state. Imaging techniques (computed tomography [CT] or magnetic resonance imaging [MRI]) may be helpful in excluding disorders, such as subdural or intracerebral bleeding, that can cause coma in a patient with liver disease. In fulminant hepatic failure, these techniques may show cerebral edema, but this finding is not as sensitive as abnormal pupillary changes. Papilledema is usually a late finding. In portosystemic encephalopathy, the CT scan and MRI may show frontal cortical atrophy, which may be associated with subclinical encephalopathy. In patients with cirrhosis, the MRI may

also show increased signal in the basal ganglia. This MRI finding may correlate with serum bilirubin and manganese levels but not with encephalopathy. The diagnosis of hepatic encephalopathy is often supported by the characteristic laboratory findings mentioned earlier, but these are not specific (i.e., elevated ammonia concentration may be due to liver disease, whereas the coma may have a different cause) and are not essential for the diagnosis. At times, a trial of therapy is helpful in making a diagnosis of portosystemic encephalopathy and should be used, provided other causes of coma continue to be sought.

Pathogenesis

The pathogenesis of hepatic encephalopathy is incompletely understood, and the mechanism or mechanisms that cause coma accompanying acute and chronic liver failure (and even different types of portosystemic encephalopathy) may differ. Despite these reservations, certain unifying concepts about the pathogenesis of hepatic encephalopathy have emerged.

First, hepatic encephalopathy seems usually to be a metabolic and neurophysiologic disorder often not accompanied by structural lesions in the brain. Thus it is potentially fully reversible, except in some patients with hepatocerebral degeneration and spastic paraparesis whose dysfunction may be progressive and who may have evidence of necrosis in the basal ganglia and demyelination in the spinal cord, respectively. In other patients with hepatic encephalopathy, the brain is either free of lesions or demonstrates astroglial proliferation and hypertrophy and/or cerebral edema, which, because of their inconsistency, are felt to be consequences rather than causes of hepatic encephalopathy. It is not known what precise anatomic sites in the brain are affected by hepatic encephalopathy, although it has been suggested that maintenance of consciousness depends on normal function of the reticular activating system in the brainstem and the modifying influence of the cortex. Presumably, therefore, these sites are affected. There is some evidence for selective sensitivity of the brainstem to the toxic effects of ammonia.

Second, hepatic encephalopathy may be a multifactorial problem. It may be caused by a synergistic interaction at the cerebral level of various "toxins" such as excess ammonia, short- and long-chain fatty acids, and possibly by mercaptans, an abnormal amino acid and neurotransmitter balance or by lack of some undefined vital protective substance(s). Various insults and physiologic derangements such as azotemia, infection, and hypokalemic alkalosis may summate with putative toxins to precipitate hepatic encephalopathy (see Table 354-2). It should be noted that the abnormal ratio of branched chain amino acid to aromatic amino acid does not necessarily correlate with the presence of encephalopathy. In patients taking sedatives, decreased drug metabolism with subsequent drug accumulation, increased penetration of the drug into the brain due to decreased drug binding to plasma proteins, and enhanced cerebral receptor sensitivity to the drug together may lead to increased susceptibility to encephalopathy. The relative importance of toxins, physiologic derangements, and cerebral susceptibility may vary with the type of liver disease and among patients.

Third, although the precise molecular basis of hepatic encephalopathy is uncertain, the mechanisms to be considered include altered energy metabolism, a derangement of the neuronal membranes, altered synaptic transmission resulting from an imbalance in cerebral neurotransmitters, or some combination of these. The possible mechanisms by which the various accumulated toxins may induce hepatic encephalopathy are diverse and are listed in Table 354-3. None of these toxins, however, has been unequivocally proven to be the cause of hepatic encephalopathy, although excess ammonia is clearly the leading candidate. The roles of mercaptans, fatty acids, and false neurotransmitters have been seriously questioned recently. An imbalance of excitatory and inhibitory amino acid neurotransmitters may also contribute to encephalopathy and currently seems the best explanation for hepatic coma. This imbalance may consist of decreased excitatory neurotransmitters (glutamate and aspartate) as a result of neuronal glutamate uptake and possibly increased gamma aminobutyrate (GABA) tone, an inhibitory effect. The latter does not appear to be due to greater influx of GABA into the brain (as originally proposed), but rather to the presence of a benzodiazepine-like substance that modulates the GABA receptor. This receptor (part of a supramolecu-

Table 354-3   Putative toxins and their mechanisms of action

TOXIN	POSSIBLE MECHANISM(S) OF ACTION*
Ammonia†	Direct effects on postsynaptic neuronal membrane
	Alteration of cytoplasmic/mitochondrial NADH/NAD ratio and malate-aspartate shuttle
	Decreased excitatory neurotransmission with impaired neuronal/astrocytic traffic
	Disturbance in energy metabolism
Mercaptan‡	Derangement of neuronal membrane activity via interference with $(Na^+ + K^+)$-ATPase activity
	Impairment of ammonia detoxication
Fatty acids‡	Impairment of ammonia detoxication
	Direct effects on neuronal/synaptic membranes
	Competition for intravascular binding of putative toxins
Various amino acids	Derangement of normal neurotransmitter status of brain (possibly false neurotransmitters)
	Generation of ammonia
	Generation of mercaptans
Other substances	Benzodiazepine-like GABA-ergicinhibitors

*Primary vs. secondary functional effects not defined.
†May especially affect glial function. Regional (i.e., brainstem) sensitivity may be present.
‡Possible contributing toxins.
Modified from Hoyumpa AM et al: Hepatic encephalopathy, *Gastroenterology* 76:184, 1979.

lar complex that also binds benzodiazepines and barbiturates) may also explain, at least partly, the enhanced cerebral sensitivity of patients with chronic liver disease to such sedatives. One major problem has been the inability to dissociate the causal from the casual neurochemical derangements; it is also difficult to establish valid experimental animal models of hepatic encephalopathy.

Therapy

The management of patients with portosystemic encephalopathy involves the following.
1. Treatment of the underlying hepatic disease, if possible
2. Identification and removal of factors that may have precipitated the encephalopathy
3. Reduction of the formation and influx of nitrogenous toxins into the brain by
   a. Alteration, reduction, or elimination of dietary protein
   b. Use of lactulose, antibiotics, or both
   c. Intestinal cleansing
   In addition, supportive care is provided to establish adequate caloric intake and to treat the complications of liver failure (e.g., hypoglycemia, gastrointestinal bleeding, and electrolyte abnormalities). Similar therapy is suitable for patients with coma due to acute liver failure, although its scientific basis and benefit for this group of patients are not as well documented.
   Identification of precipitating causes of portosystemic encephalopathy (see Table 354-2) and their treatment frequently result in clinical recovery. Often, the same factor induces recurrent portosystemic encephalopathy in the same patient. Development of spontaneous portosystemic encephalopathy, without a precipitating event or evident worsening of liver function, is uncommon and warrants reevaluation of the initial diagnosis.
   The major way to diminish the impact of nitrogenous toxins on patients with portosystemic encephalopathy is to reduce or eliminate dietary protein. The degree of protein restriction depends on the severity of the mental change. Patients with chronic liver disease require protein for hepatic regeneration; therefore complete withdrawal of dietary protein should be as brief as possible. Usually, with improvement of mental state, gradual increments of 10 to 20 g protein per day every 3 to 5 days are added and are adjusted to the clinical

response. In addition to restriction of the quantity of ingested protein, changes in the quality of protein may be beneficial. Vegetable protein may be tolerated better than animal protein, probably because (1) the greater amount of fiber promotes increased incorporation of, and subsequent elimination of, nitrogen in fecal bacteria that ultimately results in lowering blood ammonia and (2) it has a laxative effect. Another approach has been the use of amino acid mixtures high in branched-chain amino acids and low in methionine and aromatic acids. This approach is based on the observation that patients with portosystemic encephalopathy usually have low serum branched-chain and high aromatic amino acids, which may promote greater entry of aromatic amino acids into the brain and formation therein of false (weak) neurotransmitters. Thus the rationale is to normalize the serum amino acid profile of these patients with portosystemic encephalopathy in the hope of improving the presumed altered cerebral neurotransmitter states (see Table 354-3) and possibly of enhancing the metabolism of ammonia by muscle. The benefit of amino acid mixtures in the treatment of portosystemic encephalopathy is doubtful and controversial. Other recent studies have suggested that nitrogen-free ketoanalogs of essential amino acids may provide the carbon skeleton for complete amino acids and be aminated with endogenous nitrogen in patients. Further validating studies are needed before they can become part of routine management.
   Another standard therapeutic approach to portosystemic encephalopathy involves the use of lactulose, antibiotics, or both. Lactulose (a synthetic galactosidofructose), is given orally in doses of 60 to 120 ml per day in equally divided amounts so as to promote two to three soft stools daily with a pH of about 5.5. Low doses are given at first to determine patient tolerance and avoid diarrhea. Lactulose can also be given as an enema, 3 dl of lactulose syrup added to 7 dl of water. The drug, which is essentially not absorbed, (1) is broken down by gut bacteria to organic acids that lower colonic pH, thereby reducing the absorption of un-ionized ammonia and favoring the growth of low ammonia-producing bacteria, (2) serves as substrate for bacteria in utilizing ammonia, (3) promotes incorporation of fecal nitrogen by fecal bacteria, and (4) induces a more rapid evacuation of nitrogenous toxins from the bowel. Lactulose has few side effects, but gastric intolerance can occur, and large doses may produce osmotic diarrhea and occasional hypernatremia. Lactitol, a second-generation disaccharide in powder form, acts more promptly and has been shown to be as effective as lactulose but produces less diarrhea and flatulence. In populations with a high prevalence of lactase deficiency, lactose may be tried as an inexpensive substitute for lactulose. Recently, sodium benzoate, which combines with ammonia and is excreted as hippurate, reduces blood ammonia and has been used therapeutically with clinical benefit; however, in mice, sodium benzoate (50 times the human dose) produces a paradoxical increase in ammonia.
   Of the antibiotics, neomycin used to be widely employed but is now sparingly used. It is given in doses of 2 to 4 g per day orally or as a 1% enema. Oral treatment seems more reliable, except in the presence of ileus. The optimal dosage is not known, and the beneficial effect is presumed to be due to partial inactivation of bacteria that generate nitrogenous toxins from protein and urea. About 1% to 3% of neomycin may be absorbed from the upper and lower bowel. The drug may induce diarrhea by exerting a direct toxic effect on the gut mucosa or by altering the bacterial flora, although diarrhea usually occurs with higher dosages. Absorbed neomycin is excreted by the kidneys, and in patients with renal failure prolonged use of the drug may lead to its accumulation and to ototoxicity and nephrotoxicity. Metronidazole (250 mg QID) is another useful antibiotic, but it may produce peripheral neuropathy and central nervous system abnormalities, including convulsive seizures, especially with prolonged use.
   Either neomycin or lactulose may be used to treat patients with portosystemic encephalopathy, although lactulose is preferred in the presence of renal or hearing impairment and for prolonged therapy. Theoretically, neomycin might decrease the effectiveness of concomitant lactulose use by depressing the bacterial flora of the gut, but there is evidence that in some patients treatment with both drugs may be more effective than treatment with either drug alone. Moreover, efficient lactulose fermenters like *Lactobacillus acidophilus* and *Clostridium perfringens* are resistant to neomycin. If both neomycin and

lactulose are to be used, it would be prudent to check the stool pH and ascertain that addition of neomycin did not prevent the lactulose-induced decrease in stool pH, possibly obviating a beneficial effect of lactulose. A lactulose-metronidazole combination is probably undesirable because of metronidazole's activity against anaerobes. Bowel cleansing is an important adjunct for removing nitrogenous products from the bowel.

Rifaximin, a poorly absorbed antibiotic related to rifamycin, has been shown to be as effective as lactulose in the treatment of portal systemic encephalopathy when given at a dose of 1200 mg/day, but it has not yet been approved for use in the United States. The antibiotic is active against aerobic and anaerobic bacteria; combination lactulose-rifaximin regimen has not been evaluated.

Degradation of endogenous protein should be prevented by provision of at least 1600 cal/day in the form of glucose. Adequate vitamins should also be supplied, as patients with chronic liver disease often have deficiencies of these nutrients. Electrolyte abnormalities, especially hypokalemic alkalosis, require appropriate treatment. Severe resistant metabolic alkalosis, which causes increased generation of un-ionized ammonia and its passage into the more acid milieu of the brain, may require administration of arginine hydrochloride or diluted hydrochloric acid. There is no good therapy for respiratory alkalosis.

The treatment of encephalopathy due to fulminant hepatic failure poses an even greater challenge. For the most part, management consists of intensive supportive care, with close monitoring of vital functions and laboratory parameters, to allow prompt management of sepsis and cardiac, respiratory, gastrointestinal, renal, and other life-threatening complications. The apparent better survival rates in recent years, in fact, may be due to improved intensive care methods rather than to any specific treatment. In patients with fulminant hepatic failure, hypoglycemia must be looked for early and treated with glucose. These patients also often have a very prolonged prothrombin time and bleed easily. The incidence of gastrointestinal bleeding might be reduced by the prophylactic use of H_2-receptor antagonists, but these agents, especially in the elderly and those with concomitant renal failure and liver disease, may also cause mental obtundation. Infusion of fresh-frozen plasma may be beneficial, especially if bleeding is evident, but its effect is partial and transient and such therapy may lead to sodium and fluid overload and enhance consumptive coagulopathy. Heparin therapy for the consumptive coagulopathy that may accompany acute liver failure has not been helpful and may be risky. In acute liver failure, cerebral edema is a major cause of death. The precise pathogenesis of cerebral edema is still unclear. Altered permeability and inhibition of neuronal ($Na^+ + K^+$)-ATPase and osmolar changes due to ammonia metabolism have been cited as playing possible roles. Optimum therapy is uncertain. Initial encouraging results have been reported with mannitol.

There is no good evidence that corticosteroids, levodopa, or measures that provide temporary biologic support (e.g., exchange transfusions, absorbents) prolong the lives of patients with coma resistant to other measures, although improvement in the level of consciousness has been reported in some studies. Temporary liver assist measures are being studied. These include studies with cultured hepatocytes such as human hepatoblastoma cell liver or primary pig hepatocytes. Hepatic transplantation has been shown to improve the survival rate of patients with fulminant or subacute hepatic failure and is discussed in detail in Chapter 363. Other more novel approaches including the transplantation of hepatocytes rather than the whole or part of the liver, as well as the use of livers from nonhumans, are still highly experimental. The possibility that antagonists of benzodiazepine-like inhibitors will be effective therapy, at least temporarily, at the cerebral GABA receptor level is interesting and requires further study.

ASCITES
Clinical Picture

The ease and accuracy with which ascites is detected depend on the amount of fluid accumulated and the examiner's experience. Small amounts (1 liter or less) may be missed by physical examination.

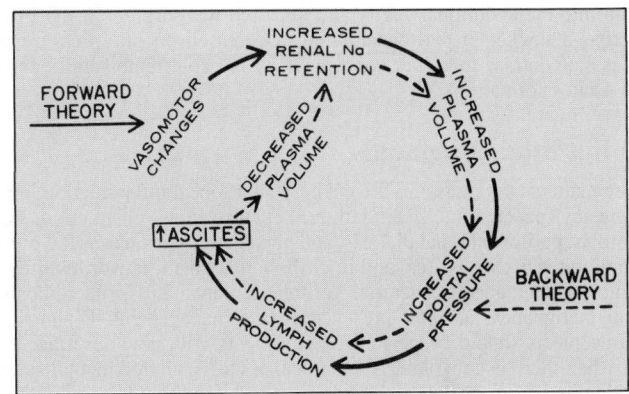

FIGURE 354-1 Theories of ascites formation. According to the backward theory of ascites formation, the basic defect is portal hypertension; increased physical force drives fluid into the abdominal cavity, eventually lowering the effective plasma volume and causing increased (compensatory) renal sodium reabsorption. Because a decreased effective plasma volume is a prominent feature, this proposed mechanism is also known as the *underfill theory.* When lymphatic drainage is overwhelmed, ascites ensues. According to the forward *(overflow)* theory of ascites formation, excessive renal sodium retention precedes the development of ascites. Hemodynamic changes induced by vasomotor alterations induce renal salt conservation. These hemodynamic changes consist of increased arteriovenous shunts, decreased peripheral resistance, decreased renal cortical blood flow, and eventual enhanced renal sodium reabsorption. Increase in sodium reabsorption leads to increase in total body sodium, increase in body and plasma volume, rise in portal pressure, and eventual ascites when lymphatic drainage does not keep up with fluid retention. From Galambos JT: Cirrhosis, *Major Probl Intern Med* 7:1, 1979.

Larger quantities may be perceived as abdominal distention, and initially as shifting dullness and then as a fluid wave on physical examination. As little as 200 ml may be detected as a puddle sign. Ascites may be seen radiologically as a diffuse haziness (ground-glass appearance) with separation of bowel loops. One hundred fifty milliliters or less can be appreciated ultrasonographically or by CT.

Pathogenesis

The accumulation of fluid in the peritoneal cavity of patients with cirrhosis results from an interaction of a number of factors. Those of principal importance are increased portal pressure and increased renal sodium reabsorption. Increased portal pressure, which is due principally to interference with portal flow in the cirrhotic liver and to increased total splanchnic plasma volume, disturbs the principle (Starling's hypothesis) that governs the normal interchange of fluid between the vascular compartment and tissue space and localizes the accumulation of fluid to the peritoneal cavity. The mechanism of increased reabsorption of sodium by the kidneys is uncertain but may be secondary to a decrease in "effective" plasma volume or more likely to hormonally mediated changes in sodium reabsorption in response to decreased perfusion of the renal cortex. Both portal hypertension and greater reabsorption of sodium are operative and interrelated in most patients with ascites, but there is debate as to which is the primary event. These interrelationships are shown schematically in Fig. 354-1 and are discussed in detail in Chapter 113. More recently, peripheral arterial vasodilation with subsequent sodium and water retention has been proposed as the initiating basis of ascites and as a unifying concept.

Also important in the development of ascites is an imbalance in the formation and removal of hepatic and gut lymph. When lymphatic drainage fails to compensate for increased lymph leakage, mainly due to elevated hepatic sinusoidal pressure, ascites develops. The fluid that leaves the hepatic sinusoids and seeps from the liver early in cirrhosis is generally rich in protein, while fluid escaping from the intestine later is low in protein because the intestinal capillaries are less permeable to protein than the hepatic sinusoids. Other nonrenal factors that contribute to ascites formation may include leakage of albumin into the abdominal cavity and impaired reabsorption of the fluid across a thickened peritoneal lining. Decreased oncotic pressure in plasma, contrary to earlier concepts, may not contribute significantly to ascites formation.

Differential Diagnosis

The main causes of ascites are cirrhosis, peritoneal inflammation, malignancy, pancreatitis, heart failure, hepatic venous obstruction, nephrosis, peritoneal renal dialysis, and myxedema. Cirrhosis is the most common cause of ascites, and in cirrhotic patients it is worthwhile to rule out spontaneous bacterial peritonitis, pancreatitis, tuberculosis, and malignancy, as their presence affects management. Diagnostic paracentesis should be performed in patients with new-onset ascites or when there is unexplained fever, leukocytosis, altered mental state, abdominal pain, or deterioration of general condition. Coagulopathy is not a contraindication, and many believe that prophylactic fresh-frozen plasma need not be administered. At times ultrasonographically guided paracentesis is necessary to best localize the fluid. The fluid should be routinely examined with regard to protein and albumin concentration, cell count and type, and amylase and cytology, and it should be cultured. An ascitic fluid/serum protein ratio of less than 0.5 suggests uncomplicated cirrhosis, whereas a larger ratio is more consistent with infection, cancer, or pancreatitis. There is substantial overlap, however, and high ascitic fluid protein may be seen in as many as 25% of cirrhotic patients with uncomplicated ascites. Such a condition may also be seen during effective diuresis. A low-protein ascites is reported in 30% of patients with malignant ascites. Thus the total ascitic protein should be interpreted carefully.

The serum-ascites albumin concentration gradient, a measure of oncotic pressure gradient that indicates the presence or absence of portal hypertension, provides better discrimination between the ascites of cirrhosis and that of malignancy. A gradient of >1.1 favors cirrhosis and portal hypertension, whereas a lower value favors a noncirrhotic etiology such as a malignancy. The mean number of polymorphonuclear neutrophils in the uninfected ascites is 60/mm^3. Neutrophil counts of >250 mm^3 (total white blood cell count × % of neutrophils ÷ 100) indicate peritonitis. Predominantly mononuclear fluid is suggestive of chronic infection such as tuberculosis. An elevated serum lactic dehydrogenase level (>400 units) in ascites or an ascitic fluid/serum lactic dehydrogenase ratio of more than 6.0 suggests the presence of malignancy. The presence of blood in the ascitic fluid also suggests malignancy, which may be confirmed by a positive cytologic examination, although atypical mesothelial cells may yield false-positive interpretations. Pancreatitic ascites typically has a high specific gravity, a high protein concentration, increased numbers of polymorphonuclear leukocytes, and, almost invariably, an elevated amylase concentration. Increased triglycerides in ascitic fluid indicate chylous ascites and suggest the presence of lymphatic disruption due to tumor, infection, or trauma. Rarely, chylous ascites is seen in uncomplicated cirrhosis. Debris and high cell counts may produce a cloudy fluid (pseudochylous ascites).

Complications

Many complications of ascites result directly from increased intra-abdominal pressure and thus are proportional to the volume and rate of accumulation of the fluid. Complications include anorexia, vomiting, reflux esophagitis, dyspnea, ventral hernia, and leakage of ascitic fluid into the chest and along other tissue planes (e.g., into the scrotum). In addition, the increased pressure may contribute to esophageal variceal bleeding.

A common complication of ascites is the development of spontaneous bacterial peritonitis. It occurs in 10% to 27% of patients with alcoholic cirrhosis, but may be seen in other forms of liver disease as well. The full-blown clinical picture consists of an abrupt onset of fever, chills, abdominal pain with rebound tenderness, absent bowel sounds, and leukocytosis. However, more commonly, the patient may have only unexplained fever, hypothermia, hypotension, abdominal discomfort, encephalopathy, or unexplained deterioration, or may be asymptomatic. Diagnostic paracentesis as well as cultures of the ascitic fluid and blood should be obtained. In most instances, only a

single organism is recovered, usually *Escherichia coli*, but a number of other bacteria have also been implicated. Three fourths are enteric organisms. In 70% of patients with acute bacterial infection, the blood culture is also positive. Anaerobic infection is rare. For optimal results, 10 ml of ascitic fluid should be inoculated into a blood culture bottle at the bedside. The sensitivity of this method is 93%. In contrast, if the usual method of inoculating 1 ml of fluid into agar plates or meat broth is used, the sensitivity is only 43%. Spontaneous bacterial peritonitis may be difficult to distinguish from peritonitis due to intestinal perforation in a patient with ascites. Favoring the latter are the following ascitic fluid features: protein >1.0 g/dl, glucose <50 mg/dl, lactic dehydrogenase >225 IU, and recovery of multiple microorganisms on culture.

Many factors are involved in the pathogenesis of spontaneous bacterial peritonitis, including impaired ability of the hepatic reticuloendothelial system to filter enteric bacteria, decreased antimicrobial activity of the ascitic fluid because of low complement levels, and loss of opsonins and phagocytic activity of neutrophils. Spontaneous bacterial peritonitis is probably acquired by hematogenous spread of microorganisms from foci of infection elsewhere (urinary tract, skin), or bacteremia secondary to invasive procedures. Low ascitic fluid protein (i.e., low opsonins) predisposes cirrhotic patients to spontaneous bacterial peritonitis.

There are two variants of spontaneous bacterial peritonitis: culture-negative neutrocytic ascites, in which the ascitic fluid neutrophil count exceeds 250/mm^3, and bacterascites, in which the ascitic fluid culture is positive but the neutrophil count is normal. These variants are otherwise similar clinically to the typical case and occur in the same clinical setting. They are managed as the main type.

Treatment of spontaneous bacterial peritonitis with a broad-spectrum antibiotic (cefotaxime) should be started promptly if the diagnosis is strongly suspected because of the high mortality, which may be as high as 78%. The usual dose of cefotaxime is 2 grams every 6 hours given intravenously, but recently 2 grams every 12 hours has been shown to be satisfactory also. Narrower spectrum antibiotics can be substituted when the sensitivity results are obtained. Aminoglycosides in conjunction with ampicillin are no longer advocated because of the potential for nephrotoxicity. The optimal duration of antibiotic treatment is not known; most clinicians treat for 7 to 10 days, but as short a period as 4 days has been satisfactory. Follow-up paracentesis at 48 hours may be helpful in that a fall in the ascitic fluid white count implies response to therapy, but it is usually not necessary unless the patient did not respond favorably. Patients who have an increased ascitic fluid neutrophil count but a negative culture should be treated similarly. An associated positive blood culture requires a longer course of antibiotics. Antibiotic therapy for spontaneous bacterial peritonitis is generally successful, but the probability of recurrence is high, particularly in patients who have an ascitic fluid protein of ≤1 g/dl, serum bilirubin > 4 mg/dl, and prothrombin time ≤45% of normal. In patients likely to have a recurrence, prophylactic oral nonabsorbable antibiotics or norfloxacin (400 mg/day) may be of benefit. Selective sterilization of the gut is usually accomplished within the first month. Ciprofloxacin 750 mg by mouth once a week for 6 months as well as trimothoprin-sulfamethoxazole double strength tablet daily 5 times a week have also been shown to significantly reduce the recurrence of spontaneous bacterial peritonitis.

Treatment

Because ascites is a complication of liver failure, management should start with attempts to improve hepatic function. Treatment for liver failure depends on the nature of the dysfunction and should include abstinence from alcohol, provision of nutrients for hepatic regeneration, and treatment with penicillamine for Wilson's disease or with corticosteroids for autoimmune chronic active hepatitis. In many instances, such therapy or spontaneous hepatic healing results in a decrease in ascites. It is also important to establish that ascites is not due to, or complicated by, another process; such verification is best accomplished by diagnostic paracentesis of 50 to 200 ml of fluid (see previous discussion). Measurements of baseline serum and urinary sodium concentrations are useful in deciding on further therapy of as-

Table 354-4 Suggested stepwise treatment of ascites

THERAPY	DOSAGE
Sodium restriction*	0.5-2.0 g/day
Bed rest	—
Spironolactone	50-600 mg/day
Furosemide† (or other loop diuretic) large volume paracentesis‡	40-400 mg/day
Peritoneovenous (LeVeen) shunt‡ or TIPS‡	—

Usual procedure is to start with sodium restriction (often with low dosages of spironolactone) and gradually increase spironolactone dosage, eventually adding furosemide if ascites is refractory. Incidence of side effects increases with intensity of diuretic use.
*With substantially reduced serum sodium levels (see text), water restriction may become necessary.
†If used alone, supplemental potassium is usually required.
‡See text.

cites. When urinary sodium is high (>10 mEq/L), the patient is likely to respond well to therapy. Moderate periods of bed rest and initial restriction of dietary sodium intake to 500 mg/day may cause significant diuresis in such patients. Rest should not preclude physical activity that is adequate to prevent muscle atrophy, and the diet should not be so restrictive as to result in inadequate intake of nutrients. In addition, patients with cirrhosis, particularly those with ascites, should not receive nonsteroidal antiinflammatory drugs as they may adversely affect renal plasma flow, glomerular filtration, and sodium excretion by reducing prostaglandin synthesis through cyclooxygenase inhibition (see discussion of hepatorenal syndrome).

If diuretics are required, it is wise to follow certain general principles. The maximum rate of peritoneal fluid reabsorption is only about 9 dl/day or less. Peripheral edema is mobilized more rapidly than ascites and tends to serve as a safety valve for fluid loss. Diuresis should not exceed 1 to 2 lb/day in the presence of edema and about 0.3 to 0.5 lb/day in the absence of edema. Otherwise, excessive diuresis may result in loss of plasma volume, with eventual azotemia, hyponatremia, hypokalemia, and encephalopathy. Thus the rate of diuresis, serum electrolyte concentration, and renal and mental function must be followed carefully, and the diuretic dosage adjusted according to response. Caution is particularly important when dry weight is approached and/or when larger doses of diuretics are needed to obtain a response.

When diuretics are used, it is reasonable to begin with spironolactone (Aldactone), 50 to 200 mg/day. This drug is an inhibitor of aldosterone-mediated distal tubular sodium reabsorption, and an effective dosage can be roughly titrated to urinary sodium excretion and overall diuretic response. Frequently, 200 mg/day is adequate, but if urinary sodium remains below 10 mEq/L and diuresis does not ensue, dosages of up to 300 to 600 mg/day may be used with success. The urinary sodium/potassium ratio may be helpful in adjusting the dose. Patients with a ratio of more than 1.0 are likely to respond to small doses (100 to 200 mg/day), whereas those with a lower ratio tend to need larger doses of spironolactone and to require loop diuretics. Spironolactone works slowly; diuresis begins in 3 to 4 days. This diuretic is not generally toxic, although gynecomastia in males, lactation in females, and hyperkalemia may be side effects.

Thiazides interfere with sodium reabsorption primarily in distal tubules. Both furosemide and ethacrynic acid impair sodium reabsorption in the loop of Henle. These drugs, which waste potassium, ideally should be used in conjunction with spironolactone, which conserves potassium. They should be administered intermittently and in the lowest effective dose so as to minimize the incidence of azotemia and electrolyte abnormalities. Some general and specific recommendations for diuretic therapy are shown in Table 354-4. In general, the higher the dose and the more potent the diuretic needed to obtain an effective response, the more severe the liver disease and the higher the complication rate from the drug. Diuretics should be stopped with the appearance of azotemia, encephalopathy, or electrolyte disturbances. Because the more potent loop diuretics may precipitate hypokalemic alkalosis, potassium supplements may be

needed. Cirrhotic patients with ascites may also have significant hyponatremia, especially after treatment with diuretics. Although hyponatremia may rarely result from sodium loss via diarrhea or excessive diuresis, it is usually due to overhydration induced by impaired generation of free water in the distal nephron. Dilutional hyponatremia requires water restriction to the equivalent of insensible loss (500 to 700 ml) plus urine output. Rarely, sodium intake may be increased cautiously if neurologic signs are evident but intravenous hypertonic sodium chloride should be avoided as it may cause pulmonary edema.

There are instances when ascites is so tense as to cause great discomfort, respiratory distress, formation and rupture of umbilical hernia, negative effects on cardiovascular function, and perhaps variceal bleeding. Therapeutic paracentesis is indicated to relieve these symptoms or to treat ascites that is refractory to the usual medical management. Serial large-volume paracentesis (4 to 6 L) with close monitoring of vital signs can be carried out safely. Large-volume paracentesis has been advocated also in patients who do not have tense ascites to relieve the ascites more quickly and to shorten the hospital stay, but the ascites often recurs unless subsequent control by diuretics and sodium restriction can be achieved. Most, but not all clinicians, advocate concomitant use of intravenous albumin with large volume paracentesis (40 g for each 5 liters removed) or equivalent and less expensive dextran to minimize any significant hemodynamic changes or deterioration of renal function. The role of paracenteses in lowering serum and ascitic complement and possible enhancement of spontaneous peritonitis requires further study.

Other measures have been tried to treat refractory ascites. In selected patients with good liver function, lowering of portal pressure with a side-to-side shunt has been used with some success. More recently, success has been reported with radiologically guided percutaneous placement of an intrahepatic shunt between portal and hepatic veins to lower portal pressure. This procedure is sometimes referred to as TIPS (transjugular intrahepatic portolsystemic shunt). The pertinent features of this procedure are summarized in Table 354-5. Another procedure involves the reinfusion of ascitic fluid by a peritoneovenous (LeVeen) shunt. A one-way, pressure-activated valve interposed in a tube connecting the peritoneal cavity and the superior vena cava is implanted. This shunt allows ascitic fluid to flow into the systemic circulation when a positive pressure gradient is generated between the peritoneal and venous systems. Although resistant ascites may respond to peritoneovenous shunt placement, the response is usually transient, and this treatment carries a significant incidence of serious complications. These include consumptive coagulopathy, pulmonary edema, infection, shunt occlusion, and precipitation of variceal bleeding. The procedure is clearly contraindicated in patients with peritoneal sepsis, severe coagulation abnormalities, heart failure, a history of variceal bleeding, and acute, severe liver disease. There is no evidence that this procedure improves with the use of serial paracentesis or prolongs life.

PORTAL HYPERTENSION
Clinical Features

Portal hypertension results from obstruction of portal blood flow due to extrahepatic or intrahepatic lesions. It is manifested by splenomegaly, ascites, and formation of collateral veins seen as prominent vessels in the anterior abdominal wall. Collateral vessels also develop at the esophagogastric junction due to dilation of the esophageal venous plexuses (esophageal varices) or of short gastric veins (gastric varices). Portal hypertension may be asymptomatic or may lead to variceal bleeding, hypersplenism, or ascites. Portal hypertension is a common complication of chronic liver disease, but it may rarely be seen also during acute hepatic decompensation in alcoholic or viral hepatitis. When it occurs in acute liver failure, portal hypertension may resolve as hepatic function improves. The clinical manifestations of portal hypertension may be the only overt evidence of chronic liver disease if hepatic fibrosis and cirrhosis are present without active hepatitis, or it may be accompanied by other signs of liver failure. In virtually all patients with clinically significant portal hypertension due to liver disease, careful clinical examination and laboratory tests reveal some hepatic abnormality.

Table 354-5 Transjugular intrahepatic portalsystemic shunt

Acceptable indications

Recurrent bleeding from esophageal varices not responsive to medical or endoscopic sclerotherapy or banding

Bleeding from gastric or intestinal varices not accessible to endoscopic sclerotherapy or banding

Bleeding from severe portal hypertensive gastropathy

Variceal bleeding in a patient awaiting a liver transplant

Potential (but still not fully accepted) indications

Refractory ascites

Budd-Chiari syndrome

Hepatorenal syndrome

Hepatopulmonary syndrome

Refractory hepatic hydrothorax

Not indicated

Initial variceal bleed

Prophylaxis for variceal bleed

Contraindications

Absolute

Severe right heart failure

Polycystic liver disease

Severe hepatic failure

Relative

Active intrahepatic or systemic infection

Severe portalsystemic encephalopathy poorly controlled by medical therapy

Complications

Acute: hemoperitoneum hemobilia, hepatic ischemia, cardiac puncture, pulmonary, edema, septicemia; migration of stent, hematoma, hypotension, arrhythmia, reaction to contrast material

Chronic: portal or splenic vein thrombosis, hemolysis, shunt stenosis, encephalopathy, worsening of liver functions

Table 354-6 Grades of liver disease severity (Child-Pugh classification)

CLINICAL AND BIOCHEMICAL PARAMETER	SCORES (POINTS) FOR INCREASING ABNORMALITY		
	1	2	3
Encephalopathy	None	1, 2	3, 4
Ascites	Absent	Slight	Moderate
Bilirubin (mg/dl)	1-2	2-3	>3
Albumin (g/dl)	>3.5	2.8-3.5	<2.8
Prothrombin time(s) prolonged	1-4	4-6	>6
For primary biliary cirrhosis			
Bilirubin (mg/dl)	1-4	4-10	>10

Class A = 5-6 points; class B = 7-9 points; class C = 10-15 points.

Variceal Hemorrhage

Bleeding from gastroesophageal varices is the most important complication of portal hypertension. Among patients with cirrhosis and esophageal varices 25% to 30% can be expected to present with this complication within 1 year of the detection of the varices. The presence of varices is best diagnosed by gastrointestinal endoscopy, which also reveals whether the varices are the site of bleeding. Barium swallow and arteriography are less sensitive or desirable methods of diagnosis. Sometimes CT detects esophageal varices or other intraperitoneal venous collaterals. Occasionally, varices are also present in the peritoneal cavity and other parts of the bowel, for example, small intestine, colonic, or rectum. Bleeding, however, usually is from the gastroesophageal area.

The precise mechanism of why varices bleed is still not completely clear, but variceal bleeding primarily reflects portal hypertension. Bleeding is usually seen when the portal pressure is >12 mm Hg. Aside from increased intravascular pressure, however, vessel wall thickness, radius, and transmural pressure (difference between intraluminal varix pressure and esophageal luminal pressure) play significant roles. Acid reflux is not believed to contribute significantly to the bleeding. Portal pressure can be measured by percutaneous hepatic or splenic manometry, via catheterization of the umbilical or portal veins or by determining the net wedge hepatic vein pressure (wedge pressure minus free hepatic vein pressure).

Factors that have been found to predict bleeding include severity of the liver disease Child-Pugh Class C (see Table 354-6), large varices, and the presence of microtelangiectatic changes vessels (red blebs, red wales, cherry red spots, bulges). Other possible harbingers of variceal bleeding are large spider nevi (>15 mm), and blue varices.

Demonstration of bleeding gastroesophageal varices requires further elucidation of the cause of the varices. Most commonly, they are due to chronic parenchymal liver disease with postsinusoidal and sinusoidal obstruction of the portal blood flow into the liver secondary to portal fibrosis and regenerating cirrhotic nodules. Sometimes, bleeding gastroesophageal varices may be due to postsinusoidal obstruction from hepatic vein thrombosis, venoocclusive disease, or to intrahepatic presinusoidal compression from sarcoidosis or schistosomiasis. These forms of portal hypertension can be confirmed by morphologic examination of liver tissue obtained by percutaneous or laparoscopic liver biopsy, by measurement of net wedge hepatic vein pressure, or by other techniques for determining postsinusoidal and sinusoidal pressure. It is essential to establish that the varices are not due solely to extrahepatic (presinusoidal) vascular obstruction caused by thrombosis, cavernomatous transformation of the portal vein, or by occlusion of the splenic vein due to pancreatitis, pseudocyst, or pancreatic carcinoma. The extrahepatic cause of the portal hypertension can be established by angiography, by finding a normal net wedge hepatic vein pressure, and by normal hepatic histology. Gastric varices alone without associated esophageal varices suggest a segmental portal hypertension secondary to splenic vein obstruction. It is essential to recognize this condition because it is curable by splenectomy. Rarely, portal hypertension may be due to increased portal volume caused by splenic arteriovenous malformations, or it may have no apparent explanation. Portal hypertension may also contribute to development of congestive gastropathy, a common cause of gastric bleeding in these patients. Congestive colopathy also has been described.

Treatment

The management of bleeding varices is best accomplished by a multidisciplinary team approach involving a gastroenterologist, a radiologist, and a surgeon, and consists of the initial evaluation and stabilization of the patient's hemodynamic state. With a large-bore tube, the stomach is lavaged with normal saline solution. Although this procedure may not stop the bleeding, the evacuation of blood clots permits better endoscopic inspection of the upper gastrointestinal tract, decreases the risk of portosystemic encephalopathy, and provides some idea as to whether the bleeding has stopped. Blood loss is replaced to maintain a systolic blood pressure of at least 90-100 mm Hg, and hemoglobin and hematocrit levels at 8 g/dl and 30% to 32% or more. Because the patient is often deficient in clotting factors, fresh frozen plasma is required, and platelets are given if thrombocytopenia is severe (<30,000/mm^3). Once the patient becomes hemodynamically stable, diagnostic evaluation is carried out to determine the nature and site of bleeding. It should be remembered that in a cirrhotic patient bleeding may be due to disorders other than varices, such as Mallory-Weiss tear; peptic ulcer; esophagitis, gastritis, or duodenitis; and portal hypertensive gastropathy. The precise diagnosis is best established by endoscopy. If bleeding is too profuse to permit endoscopy, then angiography may be used not only to locate the site of bleeding but also to define the vascular anatomy for possible surgery. To reduce or prevent portosystemic encephalopathy from the presence of blood in the gut, lactulose is given to promote evacuation of the bowels.

The second phase in the management of variceal bleeding consists of stopping the bleeding by pharmacologic, endoscopic, radiologic, surgical, or mechanical means.

Pharmacologic Agents

Intravenous vasopressin has been the traditional drug used in the management of acute variceal hemorrhage. One method is to administer 0.4 IU/min for 12 hours followed by decrements of 0.1 IU/min every12 hours for a total of 24-36 hours. Another way is to use up to 0.9 IU/min (if necessary) but only for 2 to 4 hours and then if ineffective, change to another form of treatment. The third option is to use lower doses, 0.2 IU/min for 48 hours for maximum benefit and to reduce the risks of toxicity (bradycardia, ischemia in various organs like the heart, intestines, and others because of intense vasoconstriction). The addition of nitroglycerin given transdermally, sublingually, or intravenously reduces the risk of vasopressin toxicity and enhances its efficacy. The intravenous route is preferred as it provides a more stable or consistent blood level. The initial dose of mitroglycerin is 40 μg/min, with increases of 40 μg/min every 15 minutes to a maximum of 400 μg/min. The systolic blood pressure is maintained no lower than 100 mm Hg, with dose adjustments when needed. Vasopressin analogues, such as glypressin and terlipressin, are less toxic but are not generally available in the United States.

More recently, somatostatin, or its longer acting analogue octreotide, has gained popularity and is becoming the agent of choice chiefly because, according to the majority of controlled trials, it is safer with only minor side effects, and it is at least as effective, if not more so, than either vasopressin alone or the vasopressin-nitroglycerin combination. Somatostatin is a 14-amino acid peptide that reduces splanchnic blood flow and wedged hepatic venous pressure. Its half-life is only 2 to 3 minutes. Because of its relative safety, it can be used in patients at risk for variceal bleeding even before the diagnosis is established. Slowing of the variceal bleeding permits a better endoscopic examination. The dose of somatastatin is an initial bolus of 250 μg. At the same time an infusion of 250 μg/h is started and continued for up to 5 days if needed. Octreotide, with a half-life of 90 minutes, is effective up to 8 hours. It is generally given as a continuous intravenous infusion of 25-50 μg/hr for 48 hours.

Endoscopic Procedures

Esophageal varices can be obliterated by injecting a sclerosant either intravariceally or paravariceally. This procedure has the potential of controlling acute variceal bleeding in 70% after one injection and in 80% to 90% after two sessions. Several subsequent courses at 2 to 4 weekly intervals may be necessary. However, bleeding from gastric varices or from distal gastrointestinal sites is generally not amenable to sclerotherapy. Rebleeding after sclerotherapy may occur; in many it is due to esophageal ulceration. Other complications of sclerotherapy include acute ones such as fever, chest pain, aspiration pneumonia, adult respiratory distress syndrome, perforation, mediastinitis, bacteremia, anaphylaxis, pneumoperitoneum, pneumatosis intestinalis, acute renal failure, intramural esophageal hematoma. The chronic complications include stricture, thrombosis of the portal vein or mesenteric vein, and prosthetic endocarditis. With the obliteration of esophageal varices, portal hypertensive gastropathy, which can bleed, may develop or worsen.

Ligation or banding of varices can also be accomplished endoscopically and is an effective alternative to sclerotherapy. Indeed, it is as effective as sclerotherapy with fewer complications and possibly better survival rates than the latter. In some centers this is the preferred procedure.

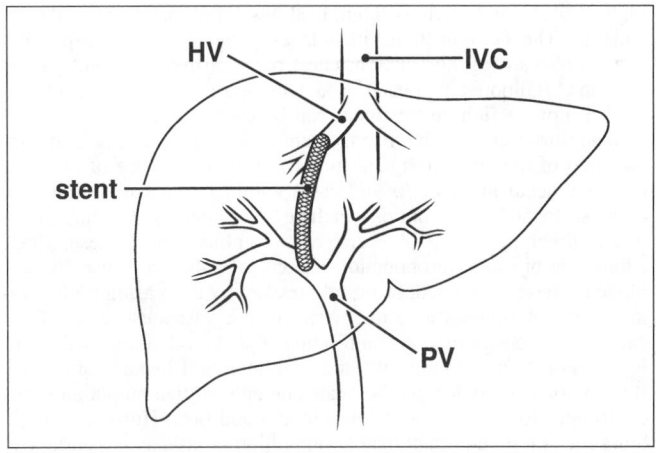

FIGURE 354-2   Algorithm for the management of bleeding varices.

Radiologic Methods

Interventional radiologists can now decompress portal hypertension by transjugular intrahepatic shunts (TIPS). A catheter is introduced into the jugular vein, then passed to the middle hepatic vein and into the right branch of the portal vein and splenic vein. The needle tract is dilated with a balloon, and an expandable stent is put in place in such a way that a communication or shunt is created between the hepatic and portal veins (Fig. 354-2). The indications, contraindications, and complications of this intrahepatic portosystemic shunt are summarized in Table 354-5.

Embolization of the coronary veins is another method that radiologists can offer to stop variceal bleeding.

Surgery

The usual surgical procedure in the management of variceal bleeding is the creation of a shunt between the inferior vena cava and the portal vein, either as an end-to-side or side-to-side anastomosis. Portacaval shunt is employed either as an emergency procedure or as an elective procedure to prevent recurrent bleeding. It is not advocated as a prophylactic measure in patients who have not previously bled. Portal decompression can be accomplished also by distal or proximal splenorenal or mesocaval shunt. These shunts have a significantly lower incidence of postoperative portosystemic encephalopathy but higher risks of shunt occlusion with subsequent recurrent variceal bleeding. The incidence of encephalopathy (20% to 30%) in patients with surgical extrahepatic portacaval shunt is comparable to those with transjugular intrahepatic shunt.

In patients who are not acceptable candidates for surgical shunts or are not responsive to medical therapy, devascularization procedures may offer alternative options. The Sugiura procedure is a two-step operation consisting of transthoracic esophageal devascularization and transection, and then transabdominal paraesophageal devascularization with splenectomy. Sugiura and colleagues report a rebleeding incidence of 2% and mortality of <5%. In other hands, however, mortality is as high as 55%, with rebleeding of 37% among survivors. A simpler procedure consists of esophageal transsection using mechanical stapling. Rebleeding in up to 55% of patients and survival of 45% have been observed.

Mechanical Compression of Varices

This is accomplished by balloon tamponade, in which balloons in the lower esophagus and stomach are inflated with air and the tube pulled taut against the gastric cardia, thus compressing the esophageal and/or gastric varices. To minimize aspiration, endotracheal intubation is done concurrently. In experienced hands active bleeding can be controlled in up to 90% of patients, but rebleeding is high (70%), and serious complications may occur in 15% of patients. The complications include esophageal rupture, aspiration pneumonia, airway obstruction, chest pains, arrhythmia, and gastric erosions. Balloon tamponade is a temporizing measure employed until a more definitive treatment can be carried out.

The third phase in the management of bleeding varices is the application of measures designed to prevent the recurrence of bleeding that may occur in about 70% of cases within 1 year with a mortality of close to 50%. The options include sclerotherapy, banding (ligation), surgery, TIPS, β-blockers, or a combination of these. Beta-adrenergic blockers (propranolol, nadolol) are the drugs usually employed. These agents reduce portal pressure by decreasing portal collateral blood flow as a result of splanchnic vasoconstriction. They cause vasoconstriction by inhibiting the vasodilating action of β2-adrenoreceptors in the splanchnic circulation. Blockade of cardiac β1-adrenoreceptors lowers the heart rate and cardiac output and thus contributes to the decreased splanchnic blood flow. However, the β1 blockade is less important than β2 inhibition in influencing portal hypertension, so that atenolol and other cardioselective β-blockers are less effective in the management of portal hypertension. The oral dose employed is adjusted in such a way as to achieve a reduction of the resting pulse rate by 25%, a change that may be associated with a 25% decrease in hepatic venous pressure and a reduction of the hepatic venous pressure gradient to <12 mm Hg. Clinical trials show a decrease of approximately 50% in the incidence of initial bleeding in patients with compensated liver disease, but survival is not improved. In a given patient it is difficult to predict the response of the portal pressure to β blockade. However, Doppler measurement of blood flow in the femoral artery, which, like the splanchnic circulation, has β2-adrenoreceptors, has been suggested as a useful noninvasive tool to select patients for therapy and to follow them.

Algorithm

Figure 354-3 shows step-by-step management of bleeding varices. Those patients who also have other manifestations of hepatic decompensation (e.g., ascites, coagulopathy, encephalopathy) should be considered for liver transplant provided they are not active alcoholics or have any contraindications such as infection or significant impairment of cardiac or pulmonary functions.

Hypersplenism

Obstruction to portal flow may cause hypersplenism, with increased destruction of all or some of the blood elements. These hematologic abnormalities are usually not severe and as a rule do not produce clinical problems or require therapy.

In the presence of a depressed platelet count, bleeding time is a good index of adequacy of hemostasis. It is important to rule out other causes of anemia, thrombocytopenia, and leukopenia (i.e., bone marrow suppression by drugs). Portal decompression by either surgery or TIPS may alleviate the manifestations of hypersplenism, but it is not uniformly effective.

HEPATORENAL SYNDROME
Clinical Picture

The development of unexplained progressive renal failure in a patient with liver disease should suggest the possibility of hepatorenal syndrome. This disorder is characterized by azotemia, usually oliguria, a concentrated urine with a urine/plasma osmolality ratio greater than 1.0, and a urinary sodium concentration of less than 10 mEq/L (often only 1 to 2 mEq/L). The urine is generally acid and may contain small amounts of protein, hyaline and granular casts, and a few erythrocytes. The syndrome usually appears in patients with decompensated cirrhosis and ascites, sometimes spontaneously but usually after forced diuresis, uncontrolled diarrhea, gastrointestinal hemorrhage, or other insults. Hepatorenal syndrome may also develop less commonly in acute liver failure due to alcoholism or viral or toxic hepatitis. This syndrome must be differentiated from other types of renal failure that may accompany liver diseases, including renal failure from exposure to toxins such as carbon tetrachloride or acetaminophen, leptospirosis or other infections, acute tubular necrosis due to hypotension from

gastrointestinal bleeding or aminoglycoside ingestion, and obstructive uropathy. In patients with acute tubular necrosis, the urine has low, fixed specific gravity; urinary sodium excretion is usually high; and there may be a characteristic sediment (Chapter 109). The other entities require a careful history, examination, and culture of the urine and at times a radiographic evaluation for diagnosis. It should be appreciated that patients with cirrhosis may have subtle renal dysfunction not reflected by the serum creatinine. The latter may be falsely low due to large plasma volume and decreased muscle mass. The physician should be sure that the renal failure in cirrhosis is not due to simple volume depletion from diarrhea, excessive diuresis, or leakage of ascitic fluid. Renal failure in some patients who respond to fluid repletion is mistakenly diagnosed as hepatorenal syndrome. This illustrates the prevailing confusion concerning the pathogenesis of hepatorenal syndrome, which may be a spectrum of functional renal failures, the early manifestations of which are reversible with fluid replacement. Until the pathogenesis of this syndrome is elucidated, the term *hepatorenal syndrome* should apply only to renal failure occurring in patients with liver disease whose renal dysfunction is unresponsive to short-term intravenous fluid repletion and in whom other known causes of renal failure are excluded.

Pathogenesis

The exact pathogenesis of hepatorenal syndrome is unclear. It is generally agreed that it is a functional disorder of the kidneys caused primarily by liver disease. This agreement is based on the observations that (1) there are no important morphologic changes in the kidneys, (2) the kidneys regain normal function when implanted in a recipient without liver disease, and (3) renal function improves when liver disease abates or if a healthy liver is implanted in the patient. Most evidence suggests that the primary abnormality in the kidneys is altered renal blood flow. Causes postulated have included changes in "effective" blood volume and increased sympathetic tone, possibly due to accumulation of false neurotransmitters at nerve endings, and increased peripheral as well as renal arteriovenous shunting, possibly due to accumulation and alteration of the normal balance of humoral agents such as prostaglandins, vasoactive peptides, and kinins. At present, the relative roles of these possible mechanisms (which are not mutually exclusive) are uncertain, although the concept of an altered humoral milieu is popular. Recent studies in rats suggest the presence of a hepatorenal reflex. Glutamine infusion into the mesenteric vein, but not to the jugular or femoral vein, induces hepatocyte swelling and decreased renal function. Renal or hepatic denervation abolishes these adverse effects on renal function. Glucagon infusion into the mesenteric vein, but not into the jugular vein, prevents the renal effects of glutamine infusion; these findings suggest the existence of a substance, possibly released from the liver, that is capable of regulating renal function by way of the hepatorenal innervations. The hepatorenal reflex, according to one theory, may be involved in establishing the initial retention of sodium and water in patients with cirrhosis. It may be that this syndrome reflects a continuum or spectrum of disorders, with a somewhat different mechanism for each type of dysfunction. A more likely possibility is that the hepatorenal syndrome starts with subclinical renal dysfunction due to decreased and/or unstable perfusion of the kidneys in many patients with severe liver disease, and that this is augmented in some patients by further liver failure and in most by various precipitants such as gastrointestinal hemorrhage.

Prognosis and Treatment

The prognosis of hepatorenal syndrome is very poor, indicating the lack of established, effective therapy. Defined rigorously (creatinine over 2.5 mg/dl), it is likely that mortality associated with this syndrome is 90% or more. The only favorable prognostic feature in one series of 30 patients was a urine volume of over 5 dl/24 hr.

Management of hepatorenal syndrome consists first of the exclusion of other, more treatable causes of renal failure such as infection, obstruction, or acute tubular damage. Another key approach is to identify, remove, or treat any factors known to precipitate renal failure in patients with severe liver disease; that is, diuretics should not be ad-

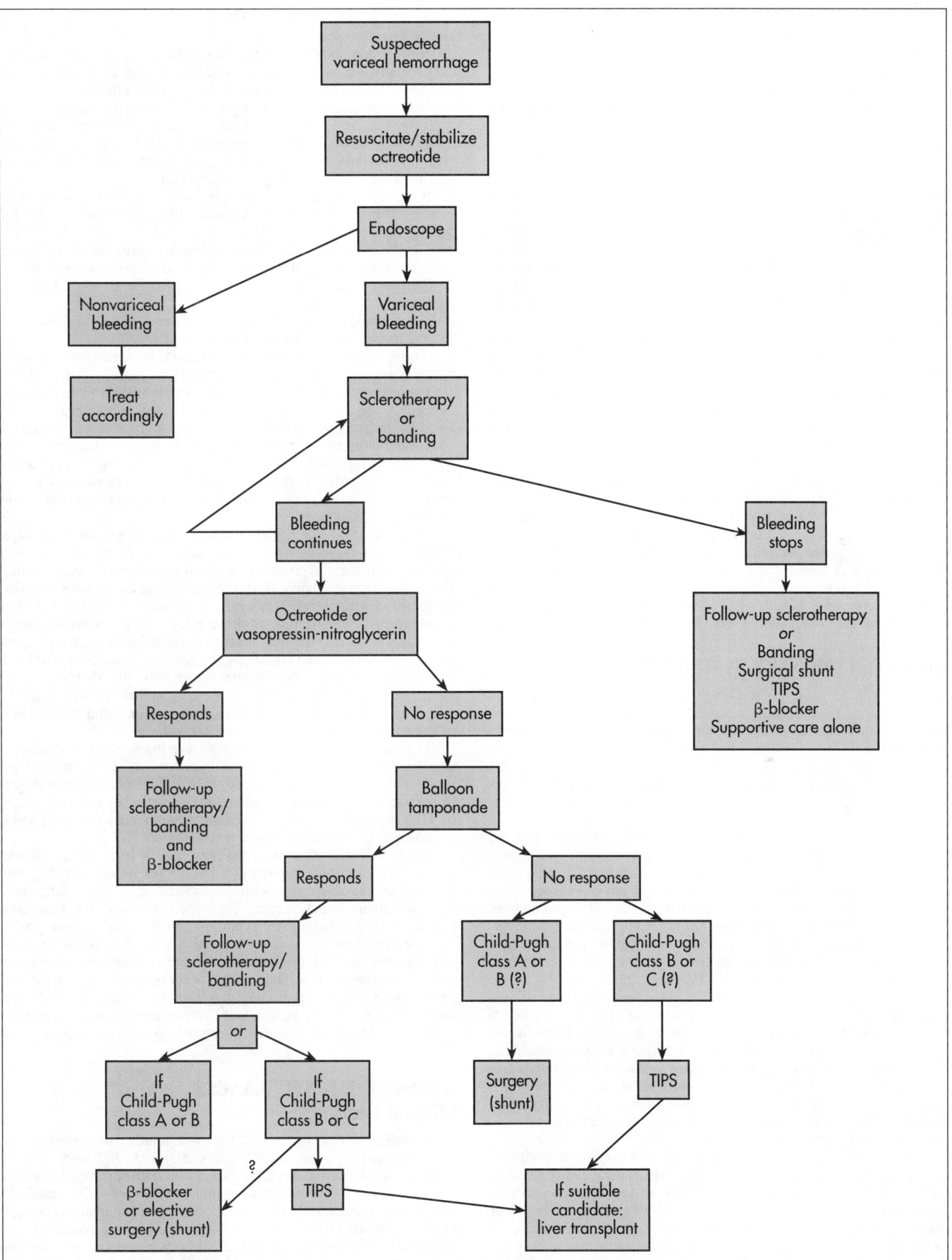

FIGURE 354-3 Algorithm for the management of bleeding varices. Practice may vary according to local resources, personnel, expertise, and preference. Where hepatic transplant is available, candidates may undergo TIPS placement sooner especially if sclerotherapy or banding for esophageal varices fails (gastric varices are generally not readily amenable to these procedures). Those who are not transplant candidates may benefit from portacaval shunt (side-to-side if ascites is present) to stop active bleeding or from distal splenorenal shunt if the patient is not actively bleeding and without ascites.

ministered, blood volume lost via hemorrhage or dehydration should be replaced, electrolyte problems should be corrected, and sepsis should be treated. As mentioned earlier, nonsteroidal antiinflammatory agents should not be administered to patients with severe liver disease, as there is evidence that these inhibitors of prostaglandin synthesis may precipitate renal failure, because prostaglandins help to maintain effective renal blood flow. All patients with apparent hepatorenal syndrome should undergo a short trial of fluid replacement with albumin, plasma, or saline to increase plasma volume in those few patients in whom a decrease in plasma volume (total or effective) is present but inapparent. Administration of fluid must be monitored carefully (preferably by central venous pressure measurements) to document adequate volume replacement and to reduce the risk of precipitating heart failure or variceal hemorrhage with excessive fluid administration. Fluid should be discontinued if there is no clear diuretic response.

Numerous agents have been tried in the treatment of hepatorenal syndrome. Most have been used on the premise that this disorder is due to renal vasoconstriction. Unfortunately, no consistent benefit has been observed in these trials, in which phentolamine, acetylcholine, papaverine, aminophylline, metaraminol, phenoxybenzamine hydrochloride (Dibenzyline), prostaglandin E$_1$, and dopamine have been used. In most trials, only a few patients were studied.

In patients with potentially reversible liver disease, renal failure may be transiently controlled with dialysis to allow the liver to heal with the hope that renal function will benefit.

There are a few reports of recovery from hepatorenal syndrome after portacaval shunt and orthotopic liver transplantation, but these are drastic measures inapplicable to most patients with this disorder. Perhaps TIPS (see earlier discussion) might be of benefit in patients who are not candidates for hepatic transplantation. The LeVeen shunt has been reported to benefit some of these patients. However, overall results from controlled studies have not been encouraging.

HEPATOPULMONARY SYNDROME

Patients with advanced liver disease may develop dyspnea even in the absence of obvious pulmonary disorder or congestive heart failure. They may have cyanosis and clubbing as a consequence of arterial hypoxemia. The Pao$_2$ on room air is frequently in the 60-70 mm Hg range but may be below 50 mm Hg. Characteristically patients develop more dyspnea and oxygen desaturation on standing or sitting (platysmia and orthodeoxia) and improve on assuming a recumbent position.

The precise mechanisms of the arterial hypoxemia are still not fully understood, but apart from decreased lung volume due to mechanical factors (elevation of the diaphragm because of ascites, basal atelectasis, and hydrothorax), there may be less obvious causes. Left-to-right shunting of blood may be present due to either intrapulmonary shunting through microscopic arteriovenous fistula or extrapulmonary venous interconnections. Lesions resembling the spider nevi commonly seen in the face, chest, and upper extremities of cirrhotic patients may be seen also in the lungs and pleura. Spider nevi on the skin may correlate with the presence of left-to-right shunt, digital clubbing, and cyanosis. A right-to-left shunting of blood may be facilitated also by the presence of anastomosis of periesophageal veins with mediastinal, pleuropericardial, and azygous veins. Connections between mediastinal venous plexus and bronchial or pulmonary veins may also occur; sometimes such communications may be large enough to allow emboli to pass and cause pulmonary embolism. Significant left-to-right shunting is likely to develop when the portal pressure exceeds the pulmonary pressure.

Hypoxemia in patients with advanced liver disease may also be related to ventilation/perfusion mismatch. Mechanical compression of distal airways by engorged bronchial blood vessels secondary to azygous venous hypertension may lead to airway trapping in the lower lung fields and decreased ventilation/perfusion ratio. In addition, inappropriate microvascular dilation may contribute to the ventilation/perfusion mismatch. The mechanism of the pulmonary vasodilation is not clear. One possibility is that there is a relative accumulation of vasodilator compounds that are not properly metabolized and cleared by the sick liver. The identity of such compounds has not been established. One possible candidate recently suggested is nitric oxide, an endothelium-derived vasodilator. Others propose the lack of vasocon-

stricting compounds or decreased sensitivity of the pulmonary vessels. Finally, the mechanical factors of diaphragm elevation, atelectasis, and effusion can clearly lead to impaired ventilation.

Pulmonary diffusion capacity may be reduced in about 20% of patients with cirrhosis. It is associated with a considerable thickening of the walls of the vessels in the lower lobes. It is further presumed that only erythrocytes immediately close to the capillary membrane are involved with alveolar gas equilibration.

Portal hypertension appears to play an important role in the pathogenesis of hepatopulmonary syndrome. This is suggested by the following observations.
1. Significant oxygen desaturation almost always occurs in the patient with esophageal varices, which reflect portal hypertension
2. Oxygen desaturation can be seen in patients with portal hypertension due to nonhepatic causes
3. Desaturation also occurs in posttransplant rejection in which there is a transient portal hypertension
4. Oxygen saturation improves when portal hypertension is relieved by placement of a transjugular intrahepatic portalsystemic shunt

These functional abnormalities are potentially reversible, and the concept of *hepatopulmonary syndrome* is now recognized. It is defined as the presence of hypoxemia (Pao$_2$ < 70 mm Hg) associated with intrapulmonary dilation and shunting and ventilation/perfusion inequality in a patient with liver disease. The presence of shunting is established with contrast enhanced echocardiography, by technetium-99 (^{99}Tc) macroaggregated albumin lung scanning or by pulmonary angiography.

With the advent of hepatic transplantation, recognition of hepatopulmonary syndrome has become important. In the past the presence of significant hypoxemia has been regarded as a contraindication to hepatic transplantation due to underlying functional rather than anatomic abnormalities. However, the hypoxemia with reversal of cyanosis and clubbing may improve after hepatic transplantation in much the same manner that functional renal impairment in hepatic failure can be improved after hepatic transplantation. Untreated hepatopulmonary syndrome is associated with a mortality of 40% 2.5 years after the onset of dyspnia. Thus it is important that the functional nature of the pulmonary abnormalities be determined and their relation to the hepatic disorder be better understood.

The treatment of hepatopulmonary syndrome should be directed at correcting the underlying portal hypertension. In the case of patients with end-stage liver disease, hepatic transplantation is needed to reverse the pulmonary failure. As mentioned earlier, the placement of TIPS has also been shown to improve pulmonary functions and is a useful bridge to eventual liver transplant.

Some patients with hypoxemia may benefit from the use of supplental oxygen (100% inspired O$_2$), but the response is variable. Pulmonary angiography is useful in evaluating patients with poor response to supplental oxygen. There are two types of angiographic patterns in hepatopulmonary syndrome: diffuse spidery abnormality is more prevalent and is associated with a good response to 100% inspired oxygen. The less common finding is the demonstration of discrete arteriovenous formations that occur predominantly in the lung bases. Patients with this finding may respond less well to 100% inspired oxygen and may be also less likely to improve with liver transplantation. More clinical experience is needed to confirm these impressions.

ENDOCRINE DISTURBANCES
Clinical Features

In patients with chronic hepatic failure, a number of endocrine disturbances may be observed (Chapters 292, 293, 300, and 301), including raised fasting levels of plasma growth hormone, abnormal glucose tolerance despite normal or high insulin levels, decreased thyroxine values, increased aldosterone, cushingoid features, and changes in sex hormones. Of these, the most dramatic are the prominent manifestations of hypogonadism that affect both sexes and overt feminization in males. In females, gonadal failure is characterized by atrophy of the uterus and breasts. There may be loss of libido, and, in females of childbearing age, menstrual periods are erratic, excessive, diminished, or absent altogether. As a result, these women may be unable to conceive. In postmenopausal women, hypogonadism may have little clinical consequence. Gonadal failure in males is manifested by gross and histologic evidence of testicular atrophy (50% to 75%) associated with impotence (79%) and, in those capable of ejaculation, with a marked decrease in sperm counts. Moreover, males with cirrhosis have decreased body hair (47%), slower beard growth, a smaller prostate, and decreased incidence of benign prostatic hypertrophy. Histologically, the testes of men with alcoholic liver disease have reduced germinal epithelium and moderate peritubular fibrosis, but the Leydig cells may be normal. In addition, males with cirrhosis assume several feminine physical characteristics, most often gynecomastia (14% to 52%), which may be unilateral initially, but which eventually becomes bilateral. Occasionally, patients with fibrolamellar carcinoma of the liver, a distinct variant of hepatocellular carcinoma, may develop gynecomastia as the presenting symptom. Other, less dramatic signs of feminization include a female body habitus and escutcheon (64%), cutaneous vascular spider nevi (74%), and palmar erythema (51%).

Presumed Mechanisms

There is a paucity of studies on the sex hormone changes in females. However, raised estrogen levels and impaired conversion of progesterone to pregnanediol have been noted in some females with cirrhosis. The precise mechanism of gonadal failure in females is still unclear. In contrast, more studies have been carried out to determine the mechanisms responsible for both hypogonadism and the overt feminization in male patients with cirrhosis. Therefore subsequent discussion will be confined mainly to hormonal changes observed in males.

The observation that in males with cirrhosis the urinary excretion of estrogens increases while that of testosterone decreases led to the theory that gynecomastia and the other endocrine features of cirrhosis were caused by an accumulation of estrogen due to impaired estrogen degradation by the liver. However, the clearance of estrogens in male cirrhotic patients may be normal; thus the matter is complex. Moreover, the available data are sometimes conflicting, perhaps because of differences in the methods of measuring the pertinent hormones and because of variations in the patient populations studied. Nevertheless, certain general remarks are warranted.

Androgen Formation and Regulation. Testosterone is converted by a series of biochemical steps from cholesterol, which may be synthesized de novo in the Leydig cells of the testes or extracted from the plasma pool. Only about 25 μg of testosterone is stored in normal testes, and to provide the average 6 mg secreted into the plasma in healthy young males, the total hormone content turns over approximately 200 times daily. Testosterone is transported in plasma, bound largely to a specific carrier protein (sex-hormone–binding globulin) and to albumin. Only 1% to 3% of testosterone remains free or unbound to plasma proteins, but it is this free fraction that is capable of combining with receptors to exert the biologic activity of the hormone. In the peripheral tissues, testosterone is converted to two active metabolites. Under the action of alpha$_5$-reductase, it is reduced to dihydrotestosterone, which possesses actions necessary for sexual differentiation and virilization. In addition, testosterone may be aromatized to estradiol. An estrogenic compound, estrone, which may be further converted to estriol, can also be derived from androstenedione, a testosterone precursor secreted principally from the adrenals. Primary liver cancer is capable of aromatizing androgens to estrogenic compounds, and this process may explain the feminization in patients with fibrolamellar carcinoma of the liver. Small amounts of dihydrotestosterone and estradiol may be derived directly from the testes and indirectly from the adrenal gland. Regulation of testosterone secretion is exerted largely by luteinizing hormone (LH) and to some extent by follicle-stimulating hormone (FSH), both from the pituitary. Testosterone in turn exerts a feedback influence on the pituitary to modulate the sensitivity of the gland to the LH-releasing hormone (LHRH) from the hypothalamus.

Hypogonadism. In male cirrhotic patients, the total testosterone concentrations in the plasma are significantly reduced. This hypotestosteronemia is associated with a marked increase in the sex-hormone–binding globulin. Consequently, the unbound testosterone fraction also falls. The low level of testosterone is due mainly to its diminished production by the testes. Despite an associated decrease

in metabolic clearance, and notwithstanding peripheral conversion from androstenedione, which can provide up to 15% of the testosterone, normal plasma testosterone levels are not maintained. Plasma dihydrotestosterone is also low in cirrhosis.

That plasma androgen levels are low in cirrhosis appears to be accepted. The question then arises as to whether these low levels result from a local gonadal lesion or from a central hypothalamic-pituitary impairment. Some data suggest a double defect. The presence of low testosterone levels despite elevated LH and FSH concentrations in one third of patients suggests hyporesponsiveness of the testes to the stimulation of these gonadotropins. Furthermore, the rise of testosterone levels after the administration of human chorionic gonadotropin is less in cirrhotic patients than in healthy controls. This finding indicates a reduced Leydig cell reserve and suggests a gonadal defect. On the other hand, the presence of normal amounts of LH and FSH in two thirds of patients despite low testosterone levels implies a subnormal hypothalamic-pituitary response. Such a central defect, believed by some to play the more important role, is confirmed by the failure of cirrhotic patients to exhibit an adequate increase in LH and FSH secretion after the administration of clomiphene, a drug that interacts with estrogen-receptor sites to prevent the normal feedback inhibition of estrogens on the secretion of LH- and FSH-releasing hormones. The defect is further localized to the hypothalamus, as indicated by the either normal or supranormal pituitary response to the gonadotropin-releasing hormone in cirrhotic patients. The basis for the hypothalamic defect is not clear.

Feminization. The three principal estrogens found in the plasma of normal males are estrone, estradiol, and estriol. Of these, the most biologically potent is estradiol. Like testosterone, it is bound in the plasma to the sex-hormone–binding globulin and to albumin. Whereas the affinity of the sex-hormone–binding globulin is greater for testosterone than for estradiol, albumin has a greater affinity for estradiol than for testosterone. As a result, alterations in the sex-hormone–binding globulin may lead to greater changes in the level of unbound testosterone than in that of unbound estradiol. The effect of changes in plasma albumin concentrations on levels of unbound testosterone and estradiol is still to be determined.

Although the biochemical basis for hypogonadism in chronic hepatic failure is fairly well established, the mechanism for feminization remains controversial. While there may be a positive initial correlation between elevated estradiol level and the presence of spider nevi, palmar erythema, or gynecomastia in patients with cirrhosis, follow-up observations reveal that spider nevi and palmar erythema may appear and disappear without obvious correlation with clinical or hormonal status. Moreover, there are no simple correlations between the severity of the disease on one hand and plasma estradiol concentration or gynecomastia on the other, or between the degree of liver disease and testicular volume or plasma testosterone levels.

Results of plasma estradiol measurements in cirrhotic male patients are variable, ranging from normal to increased. Mean values, however, are significantly higher in cirrhotic patients than in controls. In addition, estrone levels may be elevated in cirrhotic male patients, with higher levels present in those with than in those without gynecomastia, perhaps as a result of increased estrone formation from androstenedione. The clinical significance of estrone elevation is unclear, as its biologic activity is weak. Nevertheless, these data provide some basis for the concept cited earlier that features of feminization are related to the accumulation of estrogen, at least in some patients with cirrhosis. The elevation of plasma estradiol is not easily explained, however, and estradiol levels in cirrhotic patients are not always high. The critical factor in feminization may be not the absolute level of estradiol but rather the level of free estradiol in relation to the unbound fraction of testosterone. The net result of a raised estrogen/testosterone ratio or free estradiol/free testosterone ratio is a tendency to feminization. When these ratios were compared in cirrhotic patients with and without gynecomastia, however, significant differences were found in some but not in other studies. This finding suggests that factors other than sex hormone levels or ratios may be important. These factors remain obscure. There is no correlation between estrogen receptor content or circulating hormone.

It has also been postulated that prolactin may be involved in the development of gynecomastia. Increased numbers of prolactin-secreting cells have been noted in patients dying of cirrhosis. Plasma

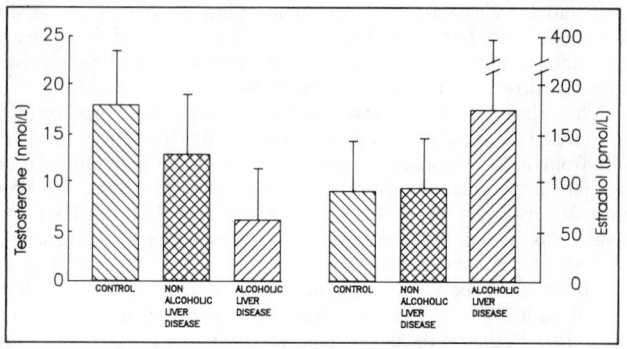

FIGURE 354-4   Testosterone and estradiol levels in patients with comparable nonalcoholic and alcoholic liver disease. Statistical comparison reveals that the testosterone levels of both groups of patients are significantly lower than controls and that those with alcoholic liver disease have lower values than those with nonalcoholic liver disease; estradiol levels are higher in patients with alcoholic liver disease than in two other groups in which values are similar. Thus liver disease causes changes in sex hormones, and these changes are made worse by alcohol.

Data from Bannister P et al: *Q J Med* 63:305, 1987.

prolactin levels are increased, with higher values in patients with gynecomastia than in those without it. Despite increased prolactin levels, galactorrhea is generally absent in cirrhotic males, with or without gynecomastia, raising questions regarding the clinical significance of such prolactin elevations. It has been proposed, however, that prolactin may potentiate the effect of estrogen by inducing or activating hepatic or other end-organ receptors for estrogens, thus contributing to the development of gynecomastia and enhancing the responsiveness of these receptors to estrogen action.

Malnutrition and Alcohol. Many aspects of the relationship between the endocrine features and the hormonal abnormalities of cirrhosis remain obscure, and it is possible that other important factors are involved. At least two factors, malnutrition and alcoholism, are frequently associated with cirrhosis. Loss of libido, testicular atrophy, and suppression of gonadotropin and testosterone may be observed in malnutrition. Gynecomastia may be seen on refeeding, perhaps related to a rise in gonadotropin and estrogen secretion during recovery.

The role of alcohol consumption has been extensively investigated. Many of the endocrine abnormalities of chronic liver disease are noted in patients with alcoholic cirrhosis, but similar physical signs and hormonal changes may also be seen in patients with nonalcoholic cirrhosis. Unlike patients with alcoholic cirrhosis, however, males with viral liver disease of comparable histologic and biochemical derangements may have normal testosterone levels and show little evidence of gonadal failure. In addition, the responses to clomiphene or LHRH factor may be normal in nonalcoholic patients. There is also ample evidence that short-term alcohol consumption by nonalcoholic subjects fed an adequate diet leads to decreased testosterone levels without changes in LH levels. These findings suggest both an impairment of central hypothalamic-pituitary function and a local gonadal defect. Moreover, the metabolic clearance of testosterone in these subjects is increased, possibly related to enhanced A-ring reductase activity and decreased plasma-binding capacity. More prolonged consumption of alcohol by these subjects is followed by a fall in LH. Thus alcohol itself may induce hormonal effects and perhaps even augment the influence of liver disease. Fig. 354-4 clearly illustrates this phenomenon. Finally, zinc deficiency, which may be seen in patients with alcoholic liver disease, may contribute to hypogonadism, probably by inducing Leydig cell failure.

Drugs. Gynecomastia related to drug use should be mentioned because one drug, spironolactone (Aldactone), is commonly used in the management of patients with cirrhosis. Spironolactone and cimetidine appear to be inhibitors of testosterone synthesis, and both may suppress, in a competitive manner, the binding of dihydrotestosterone to its receptors. Other drugs that may induce gynecomastia include digitalis, marijuana, heroin, busulfan, ethionamide, methyldopa, tricyclic antidepressants, calcium-channel blockers, acetylcholine esterase inhibitors, penicillamine, and omeprazole. In patients with gynecomastia, occult Leydig cell tumor of the testes should be ruled out.

BIBLIOGRAPHY

Arroyo V et al: Definition and diagnostic criteria of refractory ascites and hepatorenal syndrome in cirrhosis, *Hepatology* 23:164-176, 1996.

Bannister P et al: Sex hormone changes in chronic liver disease: a matched study of alcoholic vs. non-alcoholic liver disease, *Q J Med* (new series) 63:305, 1987.

Cavanaugh J, Niewoehner CB, Nuttall FQ: Gynecomastia and cirrhosis of the liver, *Arch Intern Med* 150:563-565, 1990.

Cello DP et al: Endoscopic sclerotherapy versus portacaval shunt in patients with severe cirrhosis and variceal hemorrhage, *N Engl J Med* 311:1589, 1984.

Conn HO et al: Propranolol in the prevention of the first hemorrhage from esophagogastric varices: a multicenter, randomized clinical trial, *Hepatology* 13:902-912, 1991.

De Franchis R et al: Prophylactic sclerotherapy in high-risk cirrhotics selected by endoscopic criteria, *Gastroenterology* 101:1087-1093, 1991.

Epstein M: Renal complications of liver disease, *Clin Symp* 37(5):31, 1985.

Galvaô-Tales A et al: Gonadal consequences of alcohol abuse: lessons from the liver, *Hepatology* 6:135, 1985.

Gines P et al: Paracentesis with intravenous infusion of albumin as compared with peritoneovenous shunting in cirrhosis with refractory ascites, *N Engl J Med* 325:829-835, 1991.

Gines P et al: Norfloxacine prevents spontaneous bacterial peritonitis recurrence in cirrhosis: results of a double-blind, placebo-controlled trial, *Hepatology* 12:716-724, 1990.

Herrera JL: Current medical management of cirrhotic ascites, *Am J Med Sci* 302:31-37, 1991.

Hoefs JC, Jonas GM: Diagnostic paracentesis. In Stollerman GH et al, editors: *Advances in internal medicine,* vol 37, St Louis, 1992, Mosby.

Hoyumpa AM, Jr, Schenker S: Perspective in hepatic encephalopathy, *J Lab Clin Med* 100:477, 1982.

Krowka, MJ: Hepatopulmonary syndrome versus portopulmonary hypertension: distinctions and dilemmas, *Hepatology* 25:1282-1284, 1997.

Kleber G et al: Prediction of variceal hemorrhage in cirrhosis: a prospective follow-up study, *Gastroenterology* 100:1332-1337, 1991.

Maruyama Y et al: Mechanism of feminization in male patients with nonalcoholic liver cirrhosis: role of sex hormone-binding globulin, *Gastroenterol Jpn* 26:435-439, 1991.

Pinto PC et al: Large-volume paracentesis in non-edematous patients with tense ascites: its effect on intravascular volume, *Hepatology* 8:207, 1988.

Prova Study Group: Prophylaxis of first hemorrhage from esophageal varices by sclerotherapy, propranolol or both in cirrhotic patients: a randomized multicenter trial, *Hepatology* 14:1016-1024, 1991.

Runyon BA: Spontaneous bacterial peritonitis: an explosion of information, *Hepatology* 8:171, 1988.

Runyon BA, Canawati HN, and Akriviadis EA: Optimization of ascitic fluid culture technique, *Gastroenterology* 95:1351-1355, 1988.

Schreir RW et al: Peripheral arterial vasodilation: determinant of functional spectrum of cirrhosis, *Semin Liver Dis* 14:14-22, 1994.

Teres J et al: Sclerotherapy vs. distal splenorenal shunt in the elective treatment of variceal hemorrhage: a randomized controlled trial, *Hepatology* 7:430, 1987.

CHAPTER

355   Acute and Chronic Viral Hepatitis

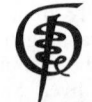

Rakesh Vinayek and Jorge Rakela

ACUTE VIRAL HEPATITIS

Viral hepatitis has been recognized as a clinical entity since antiquity. The hepatic diseases caused by various viruses share the common feature of inflammation of the liver, or hepatitis. Advances in virology, pathology, and more recently, molecular biology, have led to a surge of progress in the understanding of viral hepatitis. During the past three decades, five distinct hepatitis viruses have been discovered. Among those viruses, hepatitis B, D, and C viruses are transmitted parenterally, whereas hepatitis A and E viruses are transmitted enterally. Two new viral agents causing hepatitis in humans have recently been described by two independent teams of investigators. These include an agent called hepatitis GB virus C and hepatitis G virus (HGV). Further characterization has shown that they are identical viruses. An agent tentatively designated hepatitis F virus was described as a new enterically transmitted virus, but this was not substantiated.

The five hepatitis viruses, A through E, account for virtually all human viral hepatitis. Nonetheless, a small percentage of patients with typical signs and symptoms of acute viral hepatitis (<5% in the United States) who do not have serologic evidence of infection with any of the viruses may be infected with an unidentified hepatitis agent. These patients may be classified as having non-AE hepatitis.

A number of other viruses, however, may also produce hepatitis, including the herpes viruses (Epstein-Barr, cytomegalovirus, herpes simplex, and varicella-zoster), yellow fever virus, rubella virus, coxsackie virus, and adenovirus. Other exotic viruses (e.g., Marburg, Ebola, and Lassa) may also involve the liver as part of their systemic involvement.

Hepatitis A Virus

Hepatitis A virus (HAV) infection is distributed globally and it is also the most common form of hepatitis worldwide. The disease pattern and prevalence differ and correlate with the hygienic and sanitary conditions of a given geographic region. In developing countries with poor personal hygiene and sanitary standards, the prevalence of antibodies to HAV often exceeds 96%, with most persons infected as young children, at an age when HAV infection is often asymptomatic. This is in contrast with countries with high standards of sanitation and hygiene, in which antibodies to HAV can be found in the serum of 50% to 60% of the population older than 50 years of age, but in only 5% to 10% of those younger than 20 years of age. Paradoxically, because transmission in these areas often occurs in older age-groups, HAV infection is frequently symptomatic and more serious. Although there are no gender or race differences in susceptibility to infection, in developed countries the disease tends to be more common in specific risk groups, such as travelers to endemic areas, children and staff of day-care centers, individuals confined to custodial institutions or military barracks, homosexual men, and intravenous drug abusers. In the United States, hepatitis A has occurred in large nationwide epidemics approximately every 10 years, with the last increase in cases in 1989. The highest disease rates are in children ages 5 to 14 years. Community-wide outbreaks, with children often playing an important role in disease transmission, account for a large number of cases. The risk factors among cases reported to Centers for Disease Control and Prevention (CDC) include household or sexual contact with a patient with hepatitis (~24%), homosexual activity with a spread of virus through oral-anal contact (~11%), close contact with young children in day-care centers (~18%), recent international travel to endemic areas (6%), and intravenous drug abuse (~20%). Many persons (~40%) with antibodies to HAV do not identify risk factors; their source of infection may be other infected humans who are asymptomatic.

The hepatitis A virus is a small, single-stranded RNA virus belonging to the enterovirus group of the Picornavirus family, which also includes poliovirus, rhinoviruses, cocksackieviruses, and echoviruses. Four distinct genotypes have been recovered from infected humans, but these genotypes appear to be closely related antigenically, that is, all four genotypes belong to a single serotype. As with other enteroviruses, infection occurs via the alimentary tract, and primary replication probably occurs there as well. The incubation period is 2 to 6 weeks, and during this period, the virus infects the liver, is secreted into the bile, and is excreted in feces. High concentrations of HAV (10^8 viral particles/ml) are found in stool specimens from infected subjects; feces from these subjects are the primary source of HAV. Oral ingestion of HAV is the major route of transmission. HAV is detected in saliva and serum, but other than infected feces, only serum has been implicated in the transmission of the disease. In adults, viral concentrations in feces are highest during the late incubation period and fecal HAV excretion persists for less than 1 week after the onset of jaundice, but more recent observations using sensitive diagnostic assays such as polymerase chain reaction (PCR) have demonstrated that this excretion can extend for months after resolution of the illness.

HAV has also been detected during disease relapse as long as 2 months after onset of illness, and in infants born prematurely, HAV-RNA has been detected intermittently by PCR in stool specimens as long as 6 months after infection. Liver damage is probably not due to direct cytopathic effect of the virus but rather results from cell-mediated immune destruction of infected hepatocytes.

Person-to-person contact is the most common mode of HAV transmission; it is demonstrated by high rates of infection among household contacts of patients with hepatitis A and among children in day-care centers. Foodborne outbreaks also occur mainly through uncooked foods, foods touched by human hands after cooking, foods contaminated before wholesale distribution, and from ingestion of a variety of shellfish harvested from sewage-contaminated areas. Travel to developing countries in which HAV infection is endemic is also a risk factor for hepatitis A, and many cases of travel-related hepatitis occur in travelers with "standard" tourist itineraries and accommodations.

The onset of hepatitis is characteristically abrupt. Early symptoms include malaise, fatigue, nausea, vomiting, right upper quadrant discomfort, and fever, which may be impressive in early stages. The clinical signs, if present at all, are dark urine, light clay-colored stools, and scleral icterus that may appear during the first few days of illness. Diarrhea occurs in about one half of all infected children but is uncommon in adults. However, hepatitis A frequently causes minimal or no clinical symptoms at all.

The most striking laboratory findings include elevations of serum aminotransferase activities and serum bilirubin level. These enzyme activities may be minimally elevated or, in severe cases, may be elevated 100 times the upper limit of normal or more. Elevation of serum aminotransferases activity usually precedes a rise in serum bilirubin level. Other laboratory findings involve nonspecific elevations of acute phase reactants, immunoglobulins, and the erythrocyte sedimentation rate.

The entire acute illness may last one to several weeks, with complete resolutions of symptoms and abnormal serum chemistries; typically the aminotransferases begin to resolve before the serum bilirubin. Rarely, abnormal serum ALT levels may persist after the bilirubin level has returned to normal. Hepatitis A infection is not associated with chronic hepatitis, and a chronic carrier state has not been proven to exist. Hepatitis A in adults is usually an illness of extended convalescence. Fulminant hepatitis with a fatal outcome or requiring liver transplantation occurs almost exclusively in individuals above the age of 50. Severe manifestations of hepatitis A infections are more likely in individuals with underlying alcoholic liver disease or with chronic hepatitis due to other viral agents. Other infrequent clinical manifestations of hepatitis include cholestatic hepatitis A and relapsing hepatitis A. Patients with cholestatic hepatitis A have persistent jaundice and itching and laboratory evidence of intrahepatic cholestasis in the absence of substantial evidence of hepatocellular disease. Despite jaundice and itching, these patients feel quite well and do not appear to be infectious and do not seem to replicate large amounts of viral particles. Patients with relapsing hepatitis A experience a second discrete rise in serum aminotranferase activities after resolution of the initial bout of hepatitis, usually 2 to 3 months after the initial presentation. This second bout may be associated with fecal viral excretion. The prognosis for such cases is uniformly excellent, and symptoms and signs subside with complete resolution of clinical and chemical evidence of hepatitis A.

The diagnosis of hepatitis A is made by the demonstration of IgM antibodies against hepatitis A viral antigen (IgM anti-HAV). IgM anti-HAV is present in 99% of individuals at the time of their initial presentation. IgM anti-HAV usually peaks within the first month of illness and falls to undetectable levels within 6 to 12 months. This is superseded by the development of IgG antibodies against HAV antigen (IgG anti-HAV), which provides lifelong immunity against further infection with hepatitis A. The finding of IgG anti-HAV, but not IgM anti-HAV, in a patient with acute hepatitis indicates that the patient was previously exposed to hepatitis A but does not indicate current infection with hepatitis A virus.

Hepatitis B

Epidemiology. Hepatitis B virus (HBV) is a major cause of acute and chronic hepatitis, cirrhosis, and hepatocellular carcinoma (HCC). In the United States, an estimated 1 million to 1.25 million people have chronic HBV infection, with approximately 300 million chronic carriers worldwide. These persons are the major reservoir of HBV;

they are responsible for much of the cirrhosis worldwide and are also being implicated in 60% to 90% of HCC. An estimated 15% to 25% of persons with chronic HBV infection die prematurely of cirrhosis or HCC.

The prevalence of HBV infection varies greatly throughout the world. In areas of low endemicity (United States, Canada, Western Europe), less than 1% of adults are chronic carriers and less than 10% show evidence of prior HBV exposure, whereas in areas of high endemicity (Africa, Asia, and the Orient), 2% to 15% of adults are chronic carriers and 30% to 100% have markers of prior HBV infections. More than 75% of the world population lives in areas of intermediate to high endemicity. In the United States, adults and adolescents account for the majority of reported cases of HBV. Although a substantial number of children become infected in well-defined settings, more than 90% of these cases remain asymptomatic. During the past decade, an estimated 200,000 to 300,000 HBV infections occurred annually in the United States. The incidence of acute hepatitis B reached a peak in 1985 but by 1991 had declined by 40%. This decline was mainly a result of changes in disease transmission patterns, not because of hepatitis B vaccine use. The highest prevalence of HBV infection is found among persons born in areas of high HBV endemicity and their descendants, intravenous drug users, homosexual men, household contacts and sexual partners of HBV carriers, heterosexuals with multiple partners, hemodialysis patients, oncology and hemophilia patients receiving blood and blood products, institutionalized individuals including mentally retarded patients and prisoners, and health care personnel with occupational exposure to blood or blood products.

The risk of developing chronic HBV infection and the severity of acute illness varies inversely with the age at which infection is acquired. This factor accounts for the high carrier rate in areas of high endemicity, where exposure to HBV occurs at an early age. In such countries, chronicity develops among 90% of infants exposed at birth by vertical transmission from their mothers, and 25% to 50% of children between the ages of 1 and 5 years are exposed by horizontal transmission through open cuts, other skin lesions, or biting. In contrast, in areas of low endemicity, transmission is primarily by sexual or parenteral exposure (intravenous drug abuse), and only 6% to 10% of those acquiring HBV after the age of 6 years become chronic carriers. Individuals with an altered immune status, including dialysis patients and those on immunosuppressive drugs, are more likely to become chronic carriers.

The incubation period of HBV infection ranges from 45 to 160 days (average 120 days). It is transmitted primarily by percutaneous and mucous membrane exposure to infected body fluids. Hepatitis B surface antigen (HBsAg) has been detected in a wide variety of body fluids including saliva, serum, vaginal secretions, tears, breast milk, sweat, and urine, but only serum, saliva, and semen have been demonstrated to be infectious. Hepatitis Be antigen (HBeAg) positivity in serum correlates with the presence of whole virions containing HBVDNA. The risk of perinatal transmission is greatest to infants born to women with HBeAg-positive status and ranges 70% to 90% compared to 10% to 60% among infants born to mothers negative for HBeAg. The chronic infection is about 90% in the former group and 40% to 70% in the latter.

Transmission of HBV from persons with acute or chronic hepatitis B to their sexual partners is also an important source of infection; however, most people with chronic HBV infection are not aware that they are infected. These silent carriers are the most likely source of infection for persons with multiple sexual partners.

An important feature of the epidemiology of hepatitis B in the United States is that 30% to 40% of patients are not associated with an identifiable risk factor, which places them out of reach of immunization strategies that target only high-risk groups. The mode of transmission in these cases in not clear, but most likely it involves intimate contact with an unsuspected carrier. Most of those without known risk factors belong to minority populations with low socioeconomic status.

Hepatitis B is an efficient infectious agent. Approximately 10% of persons suffering an accidental needle stick from an HBV carrier develop hepatitis. Among health care personnel, 20% to 30% have evidence of prior HBV infection, compared with less than 10% of the general population.

Structure. HBV is a 42 nm diameter DNA virus. The outer coat is made of complex lipoprotein, the hepatitis B surface antigen (HBsAg). Excess coat protein circulates in the plasma as 22 nm diameter spherical and tubular aggregates that were identified by Blumberg as Australian Antigen in 1965. The virus contains a central hexagonal core consisting of a core antigen (HBcAg); a specific DNA polymerase; and circular, partially double stranded DNA (HBVDNA). The viral genome is 3.2 kb in size and is among the smallest of all known viruses.

Serologic Diagnosis of Hepatitis B. The diagnosis of HBV infection is more complex than HAV infection, primarily because of the presence of three different viral antigens: HBsAg, HBcAg, and HBeAg. These antigens result in the production of three different antibodies; hepatitis B surface antibody (anti-HBs), hepatitis B core antibody (anti-HBc) and hepatitis Be antibody (anti-HBe). In addition, the ability of HBV to persist as chronic infection leads to intricate serologic profiles.

Even though a variety of serologic tests are available for hepatitis B, the standard test for diagnosis of acute hepatitis B is the detection of IgM anti-HBc in serum by commercially available assays. The finding of HBsAg in serum from a patient with acute hepatitis B strongly suggests HBV as the causative agent, but the diagnosis must be confirmed with a positive IgM anti-HBc because of the possibility of underlying chronic HBV carrier state with a superimposed bout of non-B hepatitis. HBsAg is the first detectable evidence of infection with hepatitis B, appearing in serum within 3 to 6 weeks of exposure and up to 1 to 2 months before the onset of clinical disease. Its level begins to decline with onset of icterus and becomes undetectable during convalescence, sometimes disappearing before other laboratory tests (including serum bilirubin and aminotransferase levels) normalize but at other times not until several weeks after other test results have normalized. In a small percentage of patients with clinical hepatitis, HBsAg is undetectable at the time of initial presentation and anti-HBs has not yet developed. This interval between disappearance of HBsAg and development of anti-HBs was known as the "window period" that has been virtually eliminated with the availability of IgM anti-HBc and assays for direct detection of HBV-DNA. As the acute infection subsides, the level of IgM anti-HBc declines and is progressively replaced by IgG anti-HBc. Clearance of HBsAg generally indicates resolution of infection, and the development of anti-HBs provides immunity to future infection with hepatitis B. As a general rule, anti-HBs develops after HBsAg is no longer detectable. In a small proportion of patients (about 5%), anti-HBs is never detectable despite a successful resolution of acute hepatitis. However, in most individuals anti-HBV remains detectable for life.

HBeAg is detectable at the onset of illness and usually disappears after the serum alanine aminotransferase (ALT) level peaks. The detection of HBeAg suggests actively replicating and infectious virus in the blood, although infection can occur even after the development of (anti-HBe). The best marker of a patient's relative infectiousness is the presence of circulating viral DNA (HBV DNA).

Molecular Diagnosis of Hepatitis B. Application of molecular biological techniques and elucidation of genomic sequences of the individual hepatitis viruses have led to the development and clinical applicability of molecular diagnostic techniques that have rapidly become the standards against which serologic tests are compared. In comparison with immunoassays for viral peptide antigens or host antiviral antibodies, molecular diagnostic assays for viral nucleic acids offer several advantages. First, they provide direct evidence of replicative viral infection, which is especially important for evaluation of the natural history of infection, the hepatic and extrahepatic sites of replication, and response to antiviral therapies. Second, they are sensitive and specific regardless of the patient's immune response. Third, they are capable of detecting early infection, even before the onset of biochemical or clinical evidence of hepatocellular necrosis. In contrast, several weeks are often required for production of detectable titers of antiviral antibodies during acute viral hepatitis. Thus a serologic test may give false-negative results. Among molecular diagnostic techniques, slot blot or dot blot hybridization detects HBV DNA with a sensitivity of 10-500 pg/ml. The liquid hybridization column method is even more sensitive, detecting 1.6 pg/ml. Another new quantitative molecular technique, called *branched DNA assay* (bDNA), is even more sensitive than slot blot or dot blot hybridization and at least as sensitive as liquid hybridization. The technique involves capturing of viral DNA by virus-specific probes, followed by hybridization to branched DNA molecules, which are in turn detected by an enzyme-chemiluminescent substrate system. Recently, with the development of polymerase chain reaction (PCR) technique, several reports have demonstrated that PCR is more sensitive than hybridization, with a defection limit of approximately 10 to 50 genomes equivalent/ml.

Outcome of Hepatitis B Infection. In 90% to 95% of patients infected with HBV, there is complete resolution of symptoms and clearance of the virus; however, 0.1% to 1.0% of the patients develop fulminant hepatitis within several weeks of the onset of illness and 5% to 10% become chronic carriers. It is estimated that on an annual basis only 1% to 2% of chronic HBsAg carriers clear the virus and become HBsAg negative. When HBsAg persists in an individual without abnormal serum ALT levels or other indications of overt liver disease, the person is considered to be a "healthy" carrier. Anti-HBc is present in almost every case of chronic carrier state. Anti-HBs is absent in 60% to 80% but detectable in the remainder of the cases. In established chronic HBV infection, HBeAg tends to disappear in about 50% of patients over time, and anti-HBe becomes detectable. Often, a brief episode of significant elevation of serum ALT levels precedes seroconversion from HBeAg to anti-HBe. When HBeAg disappears, HBV replication ceases and serum ALT levels tend to normalize. These changes signal that the virus has entered a nonreplicative phase.

Asymptomatic carriers with normal serum aminotransferase levels usually do not progress to more serious forms of chronic liver disease, although these patients are at increased risk for developing hepatocellular carcinoma. Chronic carriers with or without symptoms may show mild, nonspecific changes or features of chronic hepatitis or even cirrhosis.

In the past, differences in the severity of HBV-induced liver disease have been attributed to differences in the host immune response. Recently, mutations in the HBV genome have been found that may have an influence on the course of liver disease. Several mutations have been described, the most common being a transition from G to A at nucleotide 1896 in the precore region, resulting in a stop codon and thus preventing HBeAg production. These mutations have been associated with immune escape phenomena and possibly more severe disease and resistance to alpha interferon therapy. Precore mutants have been found in patients with fulminant hepatitis in Israel, Southern Mediterranean, and Japan, but they appear to be rare in United States and France. Recently, mutations in the core promoter, with or without precore mutations, have been reported in patients with fulminant hepatic failure from Japan. Cluster mutations in the core gene associated with precore mutations have also been associated with progressive liver disease. Another subset of patients with chronic HBV infection are HBV-DNA positive but have no detectable HBsAg in the blood. Failure to detect HBsAg could be due to infection with a strain with mutation of "s" gene or due to very low levels of viremia. Recently, infection with HBV with "s" gene mutations have been implicated in posttransfusion hepatitis, chronic liver disease, and hepatocellular carcinoma. However, the role of HBV variants in the pathogenesis of liver disease is far from clear, and many of them are likely to be the result rather than the cause of particular host-virus interplay.

Hepatitis C Virus

Epidemiology. Hepatitis C virus (HCV) is the primary etiologic agent of parenterally transmitted non-A, non-B hepatitis and is also a major cause of acute and chronic hepatitis and cirrhosis worldwide. This virus is a 50-60 nm RNA virus and has a genome related to flaviviruses and pestiviruses. In the United States, the estimated incidence of acute hepatitis C remained stable through much of the 1980s but declined by more than 50% between 1989 and 1991. After correcting for underreporting and asymptomatic infections, the CDC estimates that an average of 150,000 HCV infections occurred annually during the last decade. Eighty percent to 90% of all posttransfu-

sion non-A, non-B hepatitis (NANBH) and 50% to 70% of sporadic community-acquired cases are positive for HCV antibody (anti-HCV). Virtually all people with acute HCV infection become chronically infected, and more than 60% of them develop chronic liver disease with persistent elevated serum aminotransferase levels regardless of the source of infection. Of those with chronic infection, chronic hepatitis or cirrhosis have been found in the majority of the cases within several years after the onset of their hepatitis. HCV also may be a major contributing cause of hepatocellular carcinoma. A strong association between the presence of anti-HCV and hepatocellular carcinoma has been demonstrated in several case-controlled studies.

The prevalence of anti-HCV is highly variable in the U.S. population. Results from the National Health and Nutrition Examination Survey (NHANES III) showed that the prevalence of HCV in the general United States population is 1.4%, which corresponds to 3.5 million anti-HCV persons nationwide. The highest rates are found among illicit intravenous drug users and hemophiliacs (20%), whereas somewhat lower rates are found among persons with high-risk sexual behaviors or sexual or household exposure to carriers (1% to 10%), as well as among health care workers (1% to 2%). The lowest rates of anti-HCV are found among volunteer blood donors (0.5% to 1%). Interpretation of the results of the enzyme immunoassays that screened for anti-HCV is limited by several factors.

1. These assays do not detect anti-HCV in 4% to 5% of the population infected with HCV
2. These assays do not distinguish between acute, chronic, or past infection
3. In the acute phase of hepatitis C, there may be a prolonged interval between onset of illness and seroconversion (window period)
4. In populations with a low prevalence of infection, the rate of false positivity for anti-HCV is usually high

The incubation period for hepatitis C following transfusion or accidental needle stick exposure has been reported to average 6 to 7 weeks. In contrast to HBV, HCV circulates at low titers in infected serum; no methods are available to measure infectivity, and the inconsistent reports of detection of HCV RNA in body fluids other than serum and plasma may reflect different titers of viruses in the infected people sampled.

The most efficient transmission of HCV is associated with direct percutaneous exposure, such as through transfusion of blood or blood products or transplantation of organs from infectious donors and sharing of contaminated needles among intravenous drug users. Health care workers experiencing needle stick injuries and dentists practicing oral surgery are also at risk for acquiring HCV infection. The incidence of HCV infection among health care workers with a needle stick exposure to blood from anti-HCV–positive source is found to be less than 10% when both anti-HCV testing and PCR are used to detect HCV infection. There is an annual attack rate of 2% to 6% in the hemophiliacs and 3% to 6% in hemodialysis patients (1% in hemodialysis staff). The greatest number of cases in the United States occur in illicit intravenous drug users, who make up 20% to 45% of all cases of hepatitis C. The risk of sexual and perinatal transmission remains controversial but appears to be very low. Several reports described no evidence of virus in the semen samples by PCR analysis from anti-HCV–positive patients. It clearly occurs at much lower frequency than in HBV infection probably because of lower circulatory concentrations of the virus. The number of cases among people without a specific source for their HCV infection continues to account for a substantial amount of disease. Low socioeconomic level is associated with a large proportion of those patients, with more than half reporting some type of high-risk behavior or contact, including history of imprisonment, one or more sexually transmitted diseases, or a history of illicit intravenous drug use.

Diagnostic Techniques for Hepatitis C. The identification of HCV was due in great part to the successful cloning of the virus and the development of anti-HCV–specific assays. First-generation enzyme-linked immunosorbent assay (ELISA) was directed at detecting antibody to a single epitope that had been cloned as a fusion protein (5-1-1). This test had poor sensitivity, delayed appearance of anti-HCV after acute infection, and high frequency of false-positive results. This problem was partially overcome by development of supplementary recombinant immunoblot assay-1 (RIBA-I) (Chiron Corp., Emeryville, Ca). To further improve the sensitivity and specificity, second- and third-generation ELISAs and RIBAs were devised through modifications of previously used antigens and the incorporation of an increasing number of new HCV antigens in each succeeding assay. These assays have shown that up to 60% of positive anti-HCV results in volunteer blood donors are false positive. Third-generation immunoassays currently under evaluation include the same HCV antigens as the second-generation assay and also an additional antigen corresponding to the NS5 region of HCV. This assay encompasses 60% of the amino acids encoded by the HCV genome and is expected to allow broader anti-HCV detection, significantly increasing our ability to diagnose HCV infection. RIBA-II assay includes the two HCV recombinant antigens, C100-3 and 5-1-1 of RIBA-I, and two additional antigens, C33C and C-22-3, and it is approved as a supplemental test for the diagnosis of HCV infection. The Matrix HCV dot blot immunoassay (Abbott Laboratories, Chicago, Illinois) employs C100, C33C, and core-derived HCV antigens. Comparison of RIBA II and the Matrix tests has shown a high degree of concordance, suggesting a similar capability to detect anti-HCV.

Molecular Diagnostic Assay for Hepatitis C. Since the initial cloning of HCV genomic sequences in 1989, molecular cloning has resulted in the production of recombinant HCV antigens in sufficient quantities for immunoassays. Because anti-HCV becomes detectable between 13 and 32 weeks after inoculation of chimpanzees with HCV, and HCVRNA is detectable by PCR as early as day 3, HCV RNA testing is superior to anti-HCV in diagnostic testing for early HCV infection. PCR for HCV RNA was first reported in 1990, with oligonucleotide primers from NS4 region of HCV genome. A nested PCR technique was subsequently developed to enhance sensitivity. However, conventional 30- to 40-cycle PCR using primers from 5'-untranslated region of HCV genome (5'UTR) achieves sensitivity comparable to that of nested PCR, simplifying the protocol and greatly decreasing labor intensity as well as decreasing the risk of false postivity. HCV RNA detection has been widely applied in the study and clinical management of chronic hepatitis C. The recently developed signal amplification technique for the detection and quantitation of virus, called branched DNA assay (bDNA), has been shown to have good correlation with PCR and noted to be easier to perform and less prone to contamination. The detection limit of the bDNA assay is 3.5×10^5 genome equivalent/ml. Riboprobe slot hybridization studies using both the sense and antisense riboprobes are excellent alternatives to PCR and have the potential advantages of being quantitative and without major risks of false positive results.

Hepatitis D Virus

The delta agent or hepatitis delta virus was first described by Rizzetto in 1977 and is a unique 35-37 nm defective RNA virus that requires the helper function of HBV or other hepadnaviruses to replicate. Hepatitis D virus (HDV) is found only in patients with HBV infection, and its outer coat is composed of HBsAg. Because HDV is only transmitted as a coinfection with HBV or as superinfection in a person already infected with HBV, the modes of transmission of HDV are similar to those of HBV with percutaneous exposure and sexual transmission. Perinatal HDV transmission is extremely rare. The global prevalence of HDV infection also corresponds to the prevalence of HBV infection, with some distinct features. Most countries with low endemicity of chronic HBV infection have low prevalence of HDV infection among HBV-infected persons. Among countries that are highly endemic for HBV infection, the prevalence of HDV infection can vary greatly. Regions with moderate to high HDV prevalence include Italy, Spain, Turkey, Egypt, and the Amazon basin in South America. In Asia and Africa, HBV infection is highly prevalent, but they have relatively low prevalence of HDV infection.

The assessment of prevalence rates of HDV infection from selected groups of patients in the United States with acute hepatitis B infection reveals that HDV accounts for 7500 infections annually. The prevalence of HDV infection among HBsAg-positive patients is low in the general population as represented by blood donors (1.4% to 8%) and highest in those with repeated percutaneous exposures such as intravenous drug users (20% to 53%) and hemophiliacs (48%

to 80%). Intermediate rates of HDV infection are found in HBsAg carriers with less intense or inapparent parenteral exposures, such as residents of institutions for the mentally handicapped (0% to 30%). Infection with HDV is virtually absent from populations with high rates of HBV infection resulting from transmission during infancy and childhood, including Native Alaskans.

HDV infection often results in severe acute hepatitis or rapidly progressive chronic liver disease. Acute HDV infection is often fulminant, and most patients with chronic hepatitis D have active disease with progression to cirrhosis and hepatic failure in a high proportion of cases. Because of the dependence of HDV on HBV, transmission can occur either as coinfection with HBV or by superinfection of an HBV carrier. A third type of transmission is recognized in the liver transplant setting where reinfection of a new donor organ occurs without the apparent support of HBV replication; this situation remains to be defined. Coinfection results in a pattern of acute B and D disease, which is usually transient and self-limiting but may also result in fulminant hepatic failure. Superinfection usually results in clinically severe disease indicated by sudden exacerbation in a chronic carrier of HBV.

The diagnosis of HDV infection relies mainly on assays for antibody to HDV antigen (HDAg). The diagnosis of acute hepatitis D is made by the detection of IgM antibodies or rising titers of IgG antibodies against HDAg (anti-HDV). High levels of anti-HDV correspond to ongoing HDV replication and chronic hepatitis D; accordingly, anti-HDV titers of >1:1000 help to distinguish chronic hepatitis D from past HDV infection. HDV infection can also be directly diagnosed by detecting HDAg by ELISA, RIA, and immunoblot methods. However, HDAg appears only transiently in serum during acute infection although it tends to persist in hepatocytes in chronic infection. Direct assays for serum HDV RNA are highly specific and sensitive and include hybridization assays using a variety of formats with either DNA- or RNA-specific probes or PCR that are capable of detecting 10 to 100 copies of the genome/ml in the infected serum.

Hepatitis E Virus

More than 50% cases of acute hepatitis in developing countries are caused by hepatitis E virus (HEV). HEV is an RNA virus related to the caliciviruses; it measures 27 to 32 nm in diameter. The most frequent mode of transmission of epidemic HEV is through fecally contaminated drinking water. Hepatitis E occurs most frequently in epidemics involving several thousand cases in developing countries of the Indian subcontinent, Asia, and Africa. Reports from the Indian subcontinent estimate that approximately 2 million adult cases of sporadic NANBH occur annually. The first extensively studied outbreak of waterborne hepatitis was reported from Delhi, India in 1956. Similar outbreaks have been reported from China, Burma, Indo-China, Algeria, Ghana, Ethiopia, Ivory Coast, and republic of Kirgizstan, with a higher fatality rate among females and the highest among pregnant women.

The mean incubation period for hepatitis E virus infection is 6 weeks (range, 2 to 9 weeks), and the clinical disease is self-limiting, similar to hepatitis A except for severity. Subclinical infection is known to occur in children and adults. Mortality is 1% to 2% in the general population. Sporadic cases of enterically transmitted hepatitis E also occur and may be the major cause of hepatitis E in areas of the world where it is endemic. Enteric hepatitis E appears to be self-limited with no chronic carrier state or long-term sequelae. Isolated cases have been reported in the United States in persons returning from areas endemic for HEV.

Clinical hepatitis E occurs in two phases: the prodromal phase, which is preicteric and is usually characterized by fever and nausea, and the icteric phase, which is characterized by icterus and dark urine. General symptoms include abdominal pain, anorexia, asthenia, diarrhea, fever, nausea, vomiting, pruritus, and hepatosplenomegaly. Although not a usual feature, fulminant hepatic failure has been associated with HEV.

Two types of histopathologic changes were observed in studies from the patients during the outbreaks in Delhi in 1956-1957, in Kashmir in 1978-1979, and in Ghana in 1962-1963. A cholestatic or "obstructive" type was found in a majority of cases, and a "standard" type with more typical features of acute viral hepatitis was observed in less than half the cases. The cholestatic type was characterized by bile stasis in canaliculi and gland-like transformation of parenchyma cells.

Laboratory diagnosis of HEV infection includes serologic identification of anti-HEV antibodies, immune electron microscopic identification of HEV particles in stools and serum, and PCR.

Hepatitis G Virus

It has become increasingly evident that there are patients with acute or chronic NANBH who are not infected with HCV, and there remains a risk of postransfusion hepatitis in recipients of blood that test negative for anti-HCV, HBsAg, or anti-HBc. These patients also have no evidence of infection with HDV or HEV. Recently, three new viral agents causing hepatitis have been described. These viruses have been cloned and turned out to be novel RNA viruses of the Flaviviridae family and were designated hepatitis GB virus A (HGBV-A), hepatitis GB virus B (HGBV-B) and hepatitis GB virus C (HGBV-C). HGBV-A and HGBV-B are tamarin viruses; HBGV-C is a human virus. The sequences of HGV and HGBV-C are more than 95% homologous, and the two are considered to be closely related strains of the same virus. The clinical implications of the identification of these agents remain largely unresolved. The agents are known to be parenterally transmitted and have been found in blood recipients, intravenous drug abusers, patients on hemodialysis, and hemophiliacs. In the United States, these viruses have been found in 1% to 2% of volunteer blood donors; thus they are more prevalent in the general population than HCV. No data are available on sexual or perinatal spread. Detection depends on the measurement of HGV-RNA by PCR.

Prospective studies have shown that the majority of HGV-infected transfusion recipients and dialysis patients have no biochemical evidence of liver disease. Only a small number of patients with community-acquired HGV infection have severe disease. In all cases of unexplained hepatitis, HGV has been found in approximately 10% of cases of acute hepatitis and in 5% cases of chronic hepatitis. Recently, HGV has been found in 25% of the patients with HCV infection before and after liver transplantation. The coinfection with HGV was not associated with more severe liver disease or graft rejection.

Non-A–Non-B–Non-C Hepatitis

Sensitive and specific assays are now available for all five forms of viral hepatitis (A through E). Nevertheless, 5% to 20% of cases of acute and chronic hepatitis are cryptogenic in that they cannot be attributed to any of the known forms of viral hepatitis and do not appear to be due to toxic, metabolic, or genetic conditions. The acute hepatitis is mild and self-limited, without any sequelae. Some cases are associated with parenteral exposure. In 20% to 30% of cases, chronic hepatitis is progressive and leads to end-stage liver disease. Transplantation for cryptogenic cirrhosis is generally not followed by recurrence of hepatitis in the graft. The major cause of fulminant hepatic failure in the United States is acute hepatitis of unknown cause. The prognosis is poor, and epidemiologic features rarely suggest a transmissible disease. Most cases of postransfusion hepatitis have been shown to be due to HCV. Nevertheless, a small proportion (10% to 20%) defies serologic categorization. The cases of hepatitis associated with aplastic anemia are often not attributable to a known cause of viral hepatitis. The hepatitis may be severe and fulminant, self-limited, or chronic. Molecular and state of the art techniques are critically needed to elucidate the cause of hepatitis in these cases.

Treatment of Acute Viral Hepatitis

General Measures. Acute viral hepatitis is in general a self-limited disease, with complete resolution of signs and symptoms and reversal of liver abnormalities in most cases. To date, no specific treatment is available, and major emphasis is placed on symptomatic and supportive measures and on the prevention of transmission. Most patients do not require hospitalization and can be managed appropriately at home. However, since the course of illness in a given patient is unpredictable, it is prudent to treat all attacks as potentially serious and use simple measures such as bed rest with activity as dictated by

the patient's own sense of malaise and fatigue. All potentially hepatotoxic agents and alcoholic beverages should be discontinued. Traditionally, a low-fat, high-carbohydrate diet has been recommended as it has been proved to be the most appetizing to the anorexic patient. Apart from this, no benefit accrues from the rigid insistence on low-fat diet. Hospitalization is indicated in patients with severe vomiting that precludes adequate oral intake; initial presenting features of ascites, edema, or hepatic encephalopathy; underlying chronic liver disease; coexistent serious medical condition; malnutrition; advanced age; laboratory findings of serum bilirubin >20 mg/dl; prolonged prothrombin time; low serum albumin; hypoglycemia; therapy with hepatotoxic or immunosuppressive agents; and pregnancy.

During the most severe phase of the illness, anorexia and nausea may be so severe that oral intake of any kind is minimal. In such instances, attention to fluid balance is important and it may be necessary to encourage the intake of small amount of fluids at frequent intervals along with the judicious use of antiemetics. As the patient's symptoms decrease and appetite improves, intake can be liberalized. Ambulation and activity can be increased as symptoms and laboratory test results improve. The decision to return to employment or school must take into consideration the patient's symptoms, the strenuousness of the work, and the potential for the transmission of the disease. In general, transmission is quite unlikely after the initial 2 to 3 weeks of illness with hepatitis A infection, whereas spread of hepatitis B or C ordinarily requires direct person-to-person contact. There is no convincing evidence to justify the use of corticosteroids in acute viral hepatitis, and they do not accelerate the rate of healing or alter the degree of liver necrosis. The steroids "whitewash" improves the morale of both the patient and physician but probably has little effect on the healing of the liver. Moreover, it may increase the risk of chronic infection in patients with acute hepatitis B.

Specific Measures. At present, there is no specific effective treatment for acute viral hepatitis but a number of features of acute viral hepatitis make antiviral therapy an attractive and viable option. First, acute viral hepatitis may be severe, with clinical symptoms lasting for several weeks and poorly tolerated in a substantial proportion of adult and elderly patients. Second, a small number of patients may develop fulminant hepatic failure (FHF). Finally a significant percentage of patients with hepatitis B, C, and D may go on to develop chronic hepatitis. Thus antiviral therapy could shorten the course of illness, ameliorate symptoms, accelerate recovery, and prevent FHF, chronicity, cirrhosis, and hepatocellular carcinoma. This therapeutic approach has not been evaluated so far.

Virtually all patients with hepatitis A recover completely and without any clinical sequalae. Only a very small proportion of adult patients experience relapsing episodes, and FHF occurs in 0.1% to 0.3% of hospitalized cases. Of the several agents that have been found to inhibit HAV replication in vitro, ribavirin (Virazole), a guanosine analog, is the only one tried in two randomized clinical trials and in dosages of 400-800 mg/day for 10 to 14 days. It was able to normalize liver function tests in patients with symptomatic hepatitis, although differences between the control and treated groups were not dramatic and there was no significant morbidity or mortality in the control group. Preliminary studies have also shown some usefulness of alpha-interferon in patients with severe and fulminant hepatitis A, although none was a randomized controlled trial.

Ninety-five percent of cases of acute hepatitis B have a self-limited course, and only 5% of patients develop chronic hepatitis; among those ill enough to be hospitalized, 1% may die from FHF. The success of alfa-interferon in treating chronic hepatitis B led to several clinical trials using this agent in acute and fulminant hepatitis B in an attempt to modify the severity and duration of symptoms and to induce recovery, but they failed to demonstrate any benefit from therapy. Foscarnet (trisodium phosphonoformate) has been used in a recent trial in a small group of patients with fulminant hepatitis B patients and has given somewhat encouraging results; further evaluation in randomized controlled trials is awaited. Despite the relatively large number of cases of FHF associated with HDV infection and the aggressive nature of hepatitis D, no controlled trials with interferon have been reported with HDV infection; in one pilot study alfa-interferon was found to have little effect on the course of acute or fulminant hepatitis D.

The high chronicity rate with hepatitis C infection and the knowledge that interferon was effective in a proportion of patients with chronic hepatitis C prompted several clinical trials of interferon in the acute phase of the infection with the aim of preventing chronicity. Common to all four prospective trials (three with alfa-interferon and one with beta-interferon) was the excellent tolerance and rapid normalization of aminotransferase levels in most treated patients. The response rate as defined by normalization of serum aminotransferase levels and the clearance of HCV RNA was better and sustained, and the relapse rate was lower with large total doses of interferon with prolonged treatment. These findings suggest that there may be a role for interferon therapy in a patient with newly diagnosed acute hepatitis C. This therapeutic approach needs further evaluation.

Patients developing fulminant or subfulminant hepatic failure in the context of acute viral hepatitis have a mortality rate close to 70%. In viral FHF, the causative agent has a considerable impact on outcome, with hepatitis A having the best outcome (50% survival rate), followed by hepatitis D (45%) and hepatitis B (23%), while NANBH has the worst prognosis (10% survival rate). Optimal care of the patients with FHF should be provided in an intensive care setting with special attention to complications that may prevent patients from undergoing liver transplantation, such as bleeding, sepsis, cerebral edema, renal failure, and respiratory failure. The role of antiviral therapy in FHF is speculative, and experience with the use of foscarnet for fulminant hepatitis B is limited and needs further trials. The results of orthotopic liver transplantation in FHF have improved remarkably over recent years, with a reported 1 year survival of 60% to 80%. Recently, the critical shortage of organs has spurred intensive exploration of the feasibility of developing liver assist devices to provide temporary support to patients with acute liver failure while they await transplantation. One such bioartificial liver assist device that is currently being evaluated passes a patient's blood through a column where purified hepatocytes may help remove toxins from the patients' blood. This device may help stabilize critically ill patients so that they may become clinically eligible for liver transplantation or the liver may regenerate and transplantation may no longer be required.

Prevention

Hepatitis A: General Measures. Since HAV is spread via the fecal-oral route—primarily by person-to-person transmission, including transmission by handling food and drinking water—and potentially by fomites, the same general sanitary and hygienic measures used to prevent transmission of any enteric illness should be used to control the spread of hepatitis A. To prevent household spread from an infected person, direct body contact should be limited to that necessary for care; attendants should wear gloves, and careful handwashing practices, including before food preparation and handling, are important. Food utensils, clothing, linen, needles, and excreta of infected patients should be handled separately and carefully, also by gloved attendants. The virus is readily inactivated by boiling or by exposure to formalin, chlorine, or ultraviolet radiation. In the hospital setting, strict isolation is usually not required for cooperative and informed patients with hepatitis A. In the home, similar measures should be implemented to the extent possible. During community outbreaks, insurance of safe drinking water and proper disposal of sewage can reduce the attack rate of HAV. In addition, all commercial food handlers should use good handwashing practices and personal hygiene to prevent food-borne outbreaks from occurring. Outbreaks of hepatitis A have been associated with ingestion of raw and undercooked shellfish; careful checking for contamination is essential.

Immunoprophylaxis

Immune globulin. Immune globulin (IG) has been shown to be safe and effective in preventing HAV infection in both preexposure and postexposure setup. The efficacy of IG prophylaxis following exposure to hepatitis A has been demonstrated to be between 80% and 90% if given within 10 to 14 days of exposure. Preexposure prophylaxis with IG has been shown to be efficacious in protecting against hepatitis A in individuals who are at high risk of exposure to HAV such as travelers, volunteers, and soldiers going to endemic areas. IG is prepared by the Cohn-Ondey cold ethanol fraction of human plasma

technique and contains predominantly IgG, with a trace amount of IgM, IgA, and other proteins. Donors for licensed IG preparation are screened for HBsAg, anti-HBc, anti-HCV, and anti-HIV in the United States and most countries. Since the institution of universal blood product screening, no episodes of transmission of HIV, HBV, or NANB has been reported except 112 possible cases of acute HCV in recipients of intravenous IG, as reported by the CDC.

The dose of IG for postexposure prophylaxis is 0.02ml/kg body weight, up to a maximum of 2 ml, although 5 ml has been advocated. Before the availability of hepatitis A vaccine, the preexposure dose of IG recommended for travelers to areas where hepatitis A is endemic was 0.02 ml/kg, which confers protection for 2 to 3 months; a dose of 0.06 ml/kg was used for persons traveling to an endemic area for a protracted period and appeared to be protective for up to 6 months. Before availability and licensing of hepatitis A vaccine in the United States, household and sexual contacts of persons with hepatitis A, children and staff at a day-care center with a reported case of hepatitis A, clients and staff for the developmentally disabled during the outbreak of hepatitis A, and food handlers and other workers in a restaurant where outbreak of hepatitis was reported were given IG. IG was not recommended for playmates at school, workplace contacts of index cases, or health care workers who cared for a patient with hepatitis A since the risk of transmissions was low.

Hepatitis A vaccine. Inactivated and recombinant HAV vaccines have been developed, and human trials with whole virus inactivated HAV vaccines have shown that the immunogenicity of these vaccines, when two or three doses are administered, approaches 100%. Adverse effects are minor, and controlled trials have shown a protective efficacy of 94% to 100%. An inactivated hepatitis virus vaccine prepared from an HAV strain, HM175 (Havrix) has recently been approved by the Food and Drug Administration. Complete (100%) seroconversion occurs after a series consisting of a primary dose and a second booster shot 6 to 12 months later. The standard dose of hepatitis A vaccine for adults contains 1440 ELISA units (United States) or 720 ELISA units (outside the United States) in 1 ml of solution. The lower concentration requires a three-dose series at 0, 1, and 12 months, and also achieves 100% seroconversion (defined as $\geq$20 mIU/ml). The worldwide pediatric formulation has a concentration of 360 ELISA units/ml; three doses are recommended at 0-1, and 6-12 month timing schedule. Coadministration of IG and hepatitis A vaccine lowers antibody levels to 50% compared with vaccine alone.

Groups recommended to receive hepatitis A vaccine include travelers to areas endemic for hepatitis A, military personnel, and special population such as Native Americans and Native Alaskans. Other groups that are potential candidates include day-care center students and workers, residents of institutions for the developmentally disabled, intravenous drug users, food handlers, homosexual males, persons with chronic liver disease, and sewage workers. Hepatitis A vaccine also may be very effective in controlling protracted community outbreaks of hepatitis A. Personal contact in a known case of hepatitis A forms the largest definable source of HAV transmission. IG remains the preferred method of prophylaxis; however, active immunoprophylaxis in the postexposure setting with the hepatitis A vaccine needs to be compared to IG immunization in clinical trials. Since 60% of persons acquiring Hepatitis A do not fit one of the high-risk groups, universal immunization may be needed to control the disease. Universal vaccination is certainly a desirable long-term goal, but questions about long-term immunity, feasibility of incorporating hepatitis A into routine vaccination schedules, and cost effectiveness of this approach must be answered. Hopefully, in coming years, the HAV vaccine will become important in preventing morbidity and mortality due to hepatitis A and will eventually lead to the eradication of this ubiquitous viral illness.

Hepatitis B: General Measures. Although HBV is not transmitted via the fecal-oral route, due consideration should be given to the general hygienic measures outlined for hepatitis A in both home and hospital. Sexual transmission is the main route of transmission among adults, but in the health care environment, transmission is possible via direct contact with the patient or needlestick exposure. Thus in the home, children are far less likely than the spouse to acquire hepatitis B from an acutely infected adult. In the hospital, strict isolation may not be necessary if excreta, needles, and other medical supplies and personal utensils are carefully handled and disposed.

Immunoprohylaxis

Immune globulins. Passive immunization with hepatitis B immune globulin with a high antibody titer is effective for passive immunization against hepatitis B when given prophylactically or within hours of exposure in accordance with established guidelines. If hepatitis vaccine is available, it should always be given with the HBIG. At present, its use is recommended for sexual partners of patients with acute hepatitis B within 2 weeks of contact, infants born to HBsAg-positive and/or HBeAg-positive mothers, inoculation of material known to be contaminated with HBV such as inadvertent puncture of a health professional by a needle from an HBsAg positive patient, accidental transfusion, or a splash of HBsAg positive blood or blood products into the eye or skin wound. The rationale for the use of HBIG depends on two essential components: there must be documentation of HBsAg in the material the person has been exposed to (requires identification of the source and appropriate serologic confirmation) and the exposed person must actually be at risk. If at the time of exposure the person is already positive for HBsAg (infected) or anti-HBs (i.e., immune, if the s/n value for radioimmunoassay exceeds 10), nothing will be gained by giving HBIG. Ideally, therefore, the serologic status of both "donor" and "recipient" should be evaluated before administering HBIG. The dose of HBIG for adults is 0.06 ml/kg, and the dose for children is 0.5 ml; these should be given as soon as possible combined with the first dose of vaccine.

Hepatitis B vaccine. The introduction in 1982 of a safe and effective hepatitis B vaccine from the plasma of hepatitis B carriers was a promising advance in an effort to control HBV infection. Despite its exhaustive inactivation process and its excellent safety and efficacy profiles, this first-generation vaccine met with limited acceptance because of unfounded fears about its safety. The 1987 introduction of a second-generation hepatitis B vaccine derived from recombinant yeasts containing the gene for hepatitis B surface antigen (HBsAg), the "s" gene, helped to allay these fears about the source and safety of the original plasma-derived vaccine. Two recombinant vaccines are available for routine use in the United States and are indistinguishable in immunogenicity from the plasma-derived vaccines. The vaccine is administered in three 20 μg doses—initially and at 1 month and 6 months later—and usually elicits production of anti-HBs in the recipient. Using the intramuscular route is important, and deltoid injection is more likely effective than gluteal administration. The vaccine is safe, but caution is recommended by the manufacturer for use in pregnant women. Booster doses of the vaccine are not recommended routinely, and the duration of protection probably is on the order of 5 years as indicated by anti-HBs titer of s/n >10 by RIA. Good responders have peak anti-HBs ≥100 IU/L and usually have long-term immunity; nonresponders have peak anti-HBs ≤10 IU/L and lack of protection.

The vaccine was initially recommended for use in high-risk groups and individuals. These include health care professionals (such as surgeons, dentists, and hospital and laboratory staff who come in contact with blood), dialysis patients and hemophiliacs, certain residents and staff of custodial care institutions, intravenous drug users, heterosexual and household contacts of HBsAg carriers, sexually active and promiscuous male homosexuals, babies born to HBsAg mothers, travelers to high-risk areas, and Native Alaskans. Because targeting high-risk groups has not been successful, the U.S. Public Health service has now recommended universal vaccination in childhood.

In immunocompetent adults, nonresponsiveness to hepatitis B vaccine has been reported to increase with such variables as age, obesity, smoking, male gender, improper site of vaccination (buttocks), and vaccination with commercial vaccine containing 10 μg of HBsAg proteins rather than that containing 20 μg of HBsAg. A small proportion of the population lacks an immune response to HBsAg and is genetically incapable of responding to hepatitis B vaccine. In immunocompromised persons, global immunosuppression rather than a specific genetic defect is the dominant factor that accounts for vaccine nonresponsiveness. In these populations, a more rational strategy for overcoming vaccine responsiveness is the combination of immune response modifiers with vaccine, such as

interleukin-2 and gamma interferon; preliminary reports of such use in hemodialysis patients are promising. Escape mutants of HBV have been found in vaccinated babies born to HBsAg-positive mothers; these mutants are not neutralized by vaccine-induced anti-HBs, and HBV infection occurs despite vaccination. The impact of such escape mutants on the success of hepatitis B vaccination remains to be determined. In the future, hepatitis vaccination may be achieved with synthetic peptides, anti-idiotypic antibodies, antireceptor vaccines, stimulation of T-cell responses to HBV proteins, adjuvant HBV proteins, live recombinant vaccines, and HBsAg expressed in transgenic plants. Some of these approaches may be cost competitive and drive down the price of the hepatitis B vaccine program.

Hepatitis D

There is no established method for active or passive immunization. Since HDV infection requires simultaneous or antecedent HBV infection, prevention of HBV protects against HDV.

Hepatitis C and NANBH

A problem largely confined to hepatitis C at present is that of posttransfusion hepatitis. The single most effective means of reducing the incidence of this disorder has been the exclusion of contaminated blood from commercial sources. There is a correlation between both elevated aminotransferase activity and anti-HBc positivity and the probability of posttransfusion hepatitis in a recipient; exclusion of such units is currently advised.

However, rejection of such blood products in certain areas of the world can cause a serious reduction in the blood donor pool without having a significant impact on the incidence of posttransfusion hepatitis. At the present time, hepatitis C is best prevented by the use of an all-volunteer blood donor population, reduction of blood use to essential need, use of autotransfusion whenever possible, and the careful screening of all blood products for the presence of anti-HCV. The possible role of preexposure (i.e., pretransfusion) use of IgG in the prevention of this disorder remains unclear, and at present IgG is not officially recommended for this purpose. At present, no HCV vaccine is on the horizon and there remains a dire need for an effective HCV vaccine to prevent HCV infection and its sequalae.

Hepatitis E

Hepatitis E prevention requires improved public sanitation. Passive protection by immune-serum globulin collected from the patients during the acute phase of the illness may be effective, but the data are sparse; more data are required before recommendations can be made. No vaccine is available as yet.

CHRONIC HEPATITIS

Chronic hepatitis is not a single disease but rather a syndrome that encompasses a constellation of clinical entities of diverse etiology, pathogenesis, histopathology, and clinical manifestations. In most cases, it is characterized by varying degrees of hepatocellular necrosis and inflammation that have evolved for at least 6 months. The necroinflammatory lesions are represented by focal areas of parenchymal necrosis and dropout, larger lobular areas of confluent necrosis with or without bridging, and periportal or piecemeal necrosis ("interphase hepatitis"). In its more severe forms, this inflammatory and necrotic process may lead to collapse of stromal elements, distortion of lobular architecture, and a reparative process consisting of fibrosis and nodular regeneration. For the lack of better definition of chronicity, chronic hepatitis is still defined as continuing necroinflammatory and fibrosing reaction in the liver without improvement for at least 6 months. In clinical practice, the continuous elevation of serum transaminases for greater than 6 months provides a simple operational definition. However, it must be stressed that in many cases, particularly in autoimmune hepatitis, the diagnosis can be made and therapy begun before such a time.

Chronic hepatitis was originally classified into two types: chronic persistent hepatitis (CPH), a milder category of disease that was be-

---

BOX 355-1
Etiology of chronic hepatitis

Chronic viral hepatitis
Hepatitis B
Hepatitis B with superimposed hepatitis D
Hepatitis C
Non A-E
Rubella, cytomegalus

Inborn errors of metabolism
Wilson's disease
Alpha-1-antitrypsin deficiency

Drugs and toxins
Methyldopa, isoniazid, nitrofurantoin, phenytoin, amiodarone, pro-
    phylthiouracil, sulfonamides, aspirin, acetaminophen, alcohol, dan-
    trolene, oxyphenisatin

Miscellaneous
Primary biliary cirrhosis
Primary sclerosing cholangitis
Autoimmune hepatitis

Cryptogenic

---

lieved not evolve to cirrhosis, and chronic active hepatitis (CAH), a more severe disease that could lead to cirrhosis. This proved to be an oversimplification of the problem, and a new term, *chronic lobular hepatitis,* was introduced. Unfortunately, this classification has often been misinterpreted as aiming at differentiation between separate disorders rather that just different grades of severity. Since the publication of the initial classification 25 years ago, there has been remarkable progress in understanding of chronic hepatitis, including recognition of various causes: viral hepatitis B, C, D, and NANBNC; several forms of autoimmune and inherited disorders; and adverse drug reactions. Better insight into the etiologic factors and pathogenesis of chronic hepatitis has also brought about a shift of emphasis in the classification from purely histologic features to a combination of histologic, clinical, and serologic factors. The revised classification incorporates many advances in the etiopathogenesis of this syndrome and is primarily based on the etiology because of the substantial differences in the clinical course, prognosis, and therapy of various etiologic categories. Each disease category needs to be further graded and staged in terms of histologic details, and whenever appropriate, these histologic details need to be objectively defined and assessed using well-characterized and standardized semiquantitative grading systems.

Etiologic Classification

Chronic hepatitis may be caused by chronic infection with HBV, HCV, or HDV; non–A-E hepatitis viruses; drugs and toxins; inborn errors of metabolism such as Wilson's disease and alpha-1-antitrypsin deficiency; autoimmune hepatitis; hemochromatosis; primary biliary cirrhosis; primary sclerosing cholangitis; and alcoholic liver disease (Box 355-1). In addition, a small percentage of patients (10% to 25%) remains whose chronic hepatitis is of unknown cause or is cryptogenic and poses a major diagnostic and therapeutic challenge. The proportion of patients with chronic hepatitis of each of these etiologic forms varies considerably from place to place, depending on the frequency of viral infection, ethnic background of the population, and prevalence of high-risk behaviors.

Clinical Assessment

Patients with chronic hepatitis can be classified clinically as having symptomatic or asymptomatic disease. The symptoms are often mild, somewhat nonspecific, and often overlooked; a small proportion of patients may be incapacitated by progressive liver failure and complications of portal hypertension. The most common symptoms of

chronic hepatitis are malaise and fatigue. It is usually intermittent, somewhat unpredictable, and worse at the end of the day. Less common symptoms are anorexia, nausea, weight loss, muscle and joint aches, arthritis, and abdominal pain. Other typical symptoms of liver disease such as jaundice and dark urine are rare except during severe exacerbations of chronic hepatitis or in patients with end-stage liver disease.

Laboratory tests are the most frequently used means of monitoring and grading severity of chronic hepatitis. Serum alanine or serum aspartate aminotransferase (ALT or AST) levels are increased in almost all cases with chronic hepatitis; however, at any given time, they may not correlate well with the histopathologic findings or long-term prognosis. An increase in ALT or AST measured over prolonged periods may reflect severity and has prognostic value, although normal ALT or AST values do not always reflect inactive disease. The severity of liver disease can be categorized on the basis of the degree of ALT increases: mild being less than three times higher (or <100U/L), moderate three to ten times higher (or 100 to 400 U/L) and severe more than 10 times higher (or >400U/L) than normal. However, ALT may be nearly normal with end-stage liver disease. Levels of other serum enzymes such as alkaline phosphatase and gamma-glutamyl transpeptidase are usually normal or minimally increased except during severe exacerbations or when cirrhosis is present. Similarly, serum bilirubin and albumin levels and prothrombin time are generally normal unless the disease is severe or advanced.

Histologic Grading. Despite recent advances in chemistry, virology, serology, and molecular biology techniques, liver biopsy remains an essential tool in the diagnosis and management of patients with chronic hepatitis. The usefulness of liver biopsy is not only in the establishment of diagnosis but also in grading of severity, staging or disease progression, detection and exclusion of other lesions, and evaluation of therapy. Grading also differs from staging in that it can change in either direction, whereas the stages of lesion are usually, though not invariably, progressive. Grading and staging are mainly carried out by means of conventional histologic stains: hematoxylin and eosin stain for general assessment and a connective tissue preparation for the assessment of fibrosis and structural alterations. Liver biopsy also provides opportunity to screen for diseases such as hemochromatosis, Wilson's disease, and alpha-1-antitrypsin deficiency with appropriate staining methods or quantitation of metals in tissue (e.g., iron, copper). In addition, immunohistochemical staining is helpful for detection of viral antigens in hepatocytes, and in situ hybridization and tissue PCR are being used increasingly for detection of viral nucleic acids in hepatocytes.

Histologic Features. Hepatitis, whether acute or chronic, is characterized by a combination of inflammatory cell infiltration and various forms of hepatocellular degeneration and necrosis. In most forms of chronic hepatitis, there is a prominent portal inflammatory reaction, consisting mainly of mononuclear cells, especially lymphocytes, macrophages, plasma cells, and sometimes eosinophils. There are also variable necrosis and inflammation involving hepatocytes that may be spotty, involving single cells or a group of cells adjacent to the portal tracts. Confluent necrosis denotes death of many adjacent hepatocytes and is called *bridging necrosis* when it links vascular structures. Although bridging necrosis can occur as a part of an otherwise uncomplicated and self-limited acute hepatitis, it may reflect a more severe injury that has a propensity to lead to progressive deterioration over a period of weeks to months ("subacute hepatic necrosis") or to cirrhosis. Paradoxically, among survivors of the most extreme form of acute liver injury, massive hepatic necrosis, chronic progressive liver disease is uncommon. *Piecemeal necrosis* is the death of hepatocytes at the interface between parenchyma and the inflamed connective tissue of a portal tract or fibrous septum. Individual hepatocytes may undergo different forms of damage, ranging from swelling (ballooning degeneration) to shrinkage (acidophilic change) and the formation of acidophilic or Councilman's bodies. In chronic hepatitis B, hepatocytes with ground glass appearance are seen, and these cells are stained with orcein or Victoria blue, or more specifically, by immunohistochemical methods with antiserum to HBsAg. In chronic hepatitis C, the hepatic lobules often exhibit microvesicular or macrovesicular steatosis, and portal tracts contain aggregates

Table 355-1 Components of the hepatitis activity index

COMPONENT	RANGE OF SCORES
Periportal necrosis with or without bridging necrosis	0-10
Interlobular degeneration and focal necrosis	0-4
Portal inflammation	0-4
Fibrosis	0-4

Table 355-2 Correlation between semiquantitative grading and verbal grades or diagnosis

HAI	BRIEF DESCRIPTION	POSSIBLE DIAGNOSIS IN OLD NOMENCLATURE
1-3	Minimal chronic hepatitis	Nonspecific reactive hepatitis, CLH, CPH
4-8	Mild chronic hepatitis	Severe CLH, CPH, mild CAH
9-12	Moderate chronic hepatitis	Moderate CAH
13-18	Severe chronic hepatitis	Severe CAH with bridging necrosis

HAI, Hepatitis activity index; *CLH*, chronic lobular hepatitis; *CPH*, chronic persistent hepatitis; *CAH*, chronic active hepatitis.

of lymphocytes, sometimes in follicular form, with formation of germinal centers with infiltration of small and medium sized bile ducts by lymphocytes. In chronic hepatitis D, no specific histologic features are seen, but necroinflammatory activity is often severe. The precise pattern and location of inflammation and hepatocellular damage vary from patient to patient and, to some extent, according to the cause of hepatitis.

Grading of Chronic Hepatitis Activity. In chronic hepatitis, grading is a measure of the severity of necroinflammatory process. The old categories of CPH, CAH, and chronic lobular hepatitis essentially represented a system of grading rather than staging. In recent years, semiquantitative grading or the assignment of numerical scores to different grades has become an important requirement for evaluation of various treatment modalities for chronic hepatitis. Several grading systems have been described, and the most widely used is the hepatitis activity index (HAI), also known as Knodell score. This consists of four separate scores for different components of the lesion (Table 355-1). It is important to note that only the first three categories represent grading, whereas the fourth is the method of staging. With the HAI or any other semiquantitative scoring systems, grades of necroinflammatory activity can be very approximately equated with grades or diagnoses as illustrated in Table 355-2.

The stage of chronic hepatitis is related to its time course and has significant prognostic and therapeutic implications. Its histologic evaluation is based on the extent of fibrosis and development of cirrhosis. Connective tissue stains are essential for staging. Several scoring systems have been proposed to evaluate the amount of fibrosis in chronic hepatitis as illustrated in Table 355-3; the differences between these scoring systems are not significant, and scores may be readily converted to verbal description for diagnostic purposes. Therefore, on the basis of guidelines and considerations discussed previously, the final diagnosis of chronic hepatitis should be based on three features: etiology, grade, and stage of the disease (e.g., chronic hepatitis B or C with moderate activity and moderate fibrosis).

In the following section, chronic hepatitis due to viral and autoimmune etiologies will be discussed in detail.

Chronic Hepatitis B

Chronic hepatitis B is a serious liver disorder that may result in cirrhosis, hepatocellular carcinoma, and death. It affects approximately 5% of the world population and is the ninth leading cause of death worldwide, placing it far ahead of acquired immunodeficiency syndrome in

both frequency and survival statistics. Approximately 5% to 10% of the adult patients with acute hepatitis B become chronic carriers, and most of them are asymptomatic and show minimal nonspecific changes on liver biopsy. Approximately 3% to 6% of cases develop progressive disease that progresses to chronic hepatitis and eventually cirrhosis. The degree of clinical and biochemical abnormalities does not necessarily correlate with the severity of histologic derangement, and liver biopsy is always required to determine the cause and prognosis, as well as to determine therapeutic options. Overall, chronic hepatitis B, with or without superimposed hepatitis D infection, represents approximately 20% of cases of chronic hepatitis.

Clinical Manifestations and Diagnosis. Typically, the patient comes to the clinician with general symptoms, physical signs, or abnormal serum biochemical tests. Only about 30% to 40% of patients with chronic hepatitis B offer antecedent history of acute viral hepatitis. Typically, the patient presents with vague symptoms of malaise, fatigue, and anorexia, which may be present for months before the patient seeks help. Many patients, particularly older patients, will already have cirrhosis at the time of initial presentation. Symptoms and physical signs may range from anorexia and fatigue to abdominal pain, amenorrhea, ascites, jaundice, arthralgia, hepatosplenomegaly, bleeding varices, and hepatic encephalopathy. Abnormal biochemical tests include elevated serum aminotransferases that may fluctuate from twofold to twentyfold above normal, variable increase of bilirubin and alkaline phosphatase, and increased gamma globulin. HBsAg is virtually always positive, as is anti-HBc.

An apparently stable patient with chronic liver disease may have clinical relapse, marked by increasing fatigue and rise in serum aminotransferase levels. Biochemical flare-ups precede seroconversion from a serum HBeAg-positive state, indicating active viral replication, to an HBeAg negativity, and later on, serum anti-HBe positivity. Seroconversion may be spontaneous in 10% to 15% of patients per annum, or it may follow antiviral therapy. Liver biopsy shows an exacerbation of hepatitis that ultimately subsides, and serum aminotransferase values fall. Subsequently, serum HBV-DNA usually becomes negative when anti-HBe has become positive. Spontaneous reactivation from an HBeAg negative to an HBeAg positive state has also been described. The liver disease becomes more active, and the picture is that of acute viral hepatitis that may be fatal. Reactivation may be marked serologically simply by finding a positive IgM anti-HBc; this is useful in making the diagnosis from a superimposed A, C, or D infection. Reactivation can follow cancer chemotherapy, organ transplantation, or use of immunosuppressive agents.

Treatment. The majority of the patients with chronic hepatitis B lead normal lives. Bed rest is not helpful, and no diet restriction is advocated. Alcohol consumption should be avoided. The patient must be counseled concerning personal infectivity, more so if he or she is HBeAg positive and/or HBV-DNA positive. Close family and sexual contacts should be screened for HBV infection and, if negative, hepatitis vaccination should be offered.

Needle biopsy is essential before the treatment is contemplated. Clearance of hepatocytes containing replicating or integrated nonreplicating HBV-DNA is necessary for effective treatment. This can be achieved with antiviral drugs, although the effects may not persist. Early treatment before extensive HBV-DNA integration is established might lead to complete eradication of the virus.

At present, alpha-interferon is the most extensively studied and effective treatment and the only approved antiviral agent for the treatment of chronic hepatitis B in the United States. More than 20 different subtypes of alfa-interferon have been identified, with the most biologically important being alpha-2. In a recently reported meta-analysis, all the randomized controlled trials analyzed showed that recombinant alpha-interferon-2b was beneficial. Based on these studies, the recommended treatment is 5 million units daily or 10 million units three times a week for 12 to 24 weeks. Response rate in most clinical trials is defined as suppression of HBV replication (loss of HBeAg and serum HBV DNA) and improvement in liver disease (normalization of ALT levels and reduction in histologic activity) and is approximately 35% to 40%. Overall, loss of HBsAg and viral replication markers occurred 6% and 20% more often in interferon-treated patients than in control subjects. Factors that are associated with fa-

Table 355-3   Scoring systems for staging of chronic hepatitis

SCORE	DESCRIPTION	KNODELL	SCIOT AND DESMET	SCHEUER
0	No fibrosis	No fibrosis	None	None
1	Mild fibrosis	Fibrous portal expansion	Periportal fibrous expansion	Enlarged fibrotic portal tracks
2	Moderate fibrosis		Portal-portal septa ($\geq$1 septum)	Periportal or portal-portal septa but intact architecture
3	Severe fibrosis	Bridging fibrosis (portal-portal or portal central linkage)	Portal-central septa ($\geq$1 septum)	Fibrosis with architectural distortion but no obvious cirrhosis
4	Cirrhosis	Cirrhosis	Cirrhosis	Probable or definite cirrhosis

vorable response to interferon therapy include high pretreatment serum ALT level, low pretreatment serum HBV DNA level, adult acquired HBV infection, active liver histology, female sex, HDV antibody and HIV antibody negative status, and heterosexual preference. Asian patients and children with active liver disease respond similarly to white adults. Most anti-HBe positive patients have inactive liver disease with no evidence of active HBV replication, and in most patients with cirrhosis, HBV replication is usually quiescent; interferon is of no benefit in these patients. Clinical trials have shown that gamma-interferon is less effective and more toxic than alpha-interferon. Most of the side effects of interferon are dose related and can be alleviated by dose reduction. Side effects include initial flu-like illness, fatigue, anorexia, nausea, weight loss, hair loss, emotional lability and depression, bone marrow suppression, induction of autoantibodies and enhancement of autoimmune disease, hypothyroidism, and less commonly, hyperthyroidism. Interferon should not be used in patients with a history of suicidal tendency, active psychiatric illness, autoimmune diseases, severe neutropenia or thrombocytopenia, concurrent severe systemic disorders, or decompensated cirrhosis. It is recommended that the patients have complete blood cell counts at the end of weeks 1 and 2 of therapy and monthly thereafter during treatment. The dose should be reduced or treatment discontinued depending on the magnitude of side effects, including the degree of thrombocytopenia and neutropenia.

Unfortunately, the majority of patients with chronic hepatitis B do not respond to the currently recommended interferon regimens. Various forms of combination therapy using immunomodulatory and antiviral agents have been studied or are currently under study in the hope of achieving additive or synergistic effects to interferon. The best hope for those who do not respond to interferon lies in the use of HBV DNA inhibitors such as nucleoside analogs (e.g., lamivudine, famciclovir) alone or combination with interferon. Lamivudine is an orally administered nucleoside analog that, in initial pilot studies, has been shown to be well tolerated and effective in inhibiting HBV replication. Studies on longer courses of lamivudine are ongoing, and preliminary results appear to be promising. Other antiviral agents such as adenine/arabinoside (ARA-A) and its monophosphate (ARA-AMP) are effective in inhibiting HBV replication, but their use is limited by the need for intramuscular administration and their neurotoxicity. Thymosin, an antiviral agent with an immunomodulatory effect, appeared promising in the pilot study but failed to confirm the initial optimism in a randomized controlled trial. The combination of interleukin-2 (IL-2) with alpha-interferon offers no additional antiviral but more adverse effects. Pilot studies showed that prednisone priming followed by interferon therapy could be more effective than alpha-interferon alone, but this was not confirmed by a randomized controlled trial. Although a small subset of patients with low ALT levels (<100 IU/L) may benefit, this remains to be confirmed. Prednisone priming has no role as a primary therapy; its role in nonresponders and in patients who relapse after previous response has not been conclusively evaluated.

Orthotopic liver transplantation (OLT) has become an established treatment for end-stage liver disease, and the survival rate of patients receiving OLT has improved remarkably over the past decade. However, the survival rates after OLT for chronic hepatitis B (HBV) infection have been less satisfactory because of HBV reinfection in the liver allograft, which evolves more rapidly than in the native liver, responds poorly to alpha-interferon treatment, and commonly leads to allograft failure in periods as short as 1 to 2 years. A particular lethal syndrome of recurrent HBV infection is that of *fibrosing cholestatic hepatitis* (FCH), which is characterized by unique clinical and histologic changes, is associated with marked cholestasis and hypoprothrombinemia, and is more likely to occur in patients with active pretransplant HBV replication than in those without. Low levels of pretransplantation viral replication (absence of HBV DNA and HBeAg) and HDV superinfection amid long-term immunoprophylaxis are associated with decreased recurrence and improved survival. In summary, the threat of recurrent infection and death from liver failure is ever present in patients undergoing OLT for chronic HBV infection; identification of pretransplant predictors of posttransplant outcome will aid in selection of patients more likely to benefit from OLT.

Chronic Hepatitis C

HCV is probably more important than HBV as a world-wide cause of chronic liver disease and cirrhosis. With the availability of more reliable assays for HCV, this infection is emerging as an extremely common and insidiously progressive disease that may result in chronic hepatitis, cirrhosis, and HCC. Chronic liver disease can follow blood transfusion or blood product–related acute disease, and 50% to 75% of patients with acute hepatitis C will develop chronic hepatitis while 20% will proceed to cirrhosis, usually after many years; this figure may approach 50% or more with long-term follow-up. The progression applies to symptomatic, asymptomatic, and non-icteric acute attacks. Factors believed to influence the rate of progression include the age at exposure, duration of infection, and degree of damage at the initial liver biopsy. The prospect of progressive liver injury over approximately 10 years has been shown to be greater in patients with moderately severe to severe chronic hepatitis than with mild chronic hepatitis. More than 90% of such patients go on to develop HCC. Many patients give no history of a previous blood transfusion or drug abuse, and the route of infection in these sporadic cases is unknown. Although posttransfusion hepatitis C affects men and women equally, 75% of those developing chronic hepatitis in one study were men.

Clinical Manifestations and Diagnosis. The most frequent complaint is fatigue, although patients may be completely symptom free. The most characteristic feature is fluctuating serum aminotransferases extending over many months or years. Similar to chronic hepatitis B, serum autoantibodies, hypergammaglobulinemia, and stigmata of chronic liver disease are rare, although positive tests for antinuclear antibodies may be present in some cases. Chronic HCV infection appears to be strongly associated with several extrahepatic conditions, including cryoglobulinemia, membranoproliferative glomerulonephritis, and porphyria cutanea tarda. The association with Mooren corneal ulcers and autoimmune thyroditis is suggested, but more data are needed to confirm this. The data for the association between HCV infection, Sjogren's syndrome, and lichen planus and idiopathic pulmonary fibrosis remain weak.

The diagnosis of chronic HCV is established by detecting anti-HCV and HCV RNA by methods described earlier in the chapter.

Treatment. As in chronic HBV infection, the majority of the patients lead normal lives. No diet restriction is advocated, and alcohol consumption should be strongly discouraged. Liver biopsy is essential before any therapeutic effort is undertaken. Therapeutic efforts toward controlling chronic HCV are justified by the insidiously progressive course of the disease, the risk of the development of cirrhosis or hepatic failure and the lack of spontaneous remission of the disease or clearance of the virus. The natural history and response to treatment are probably influenced by multiple factors including, but not limited to, viral genotype, level of viral replication, and histology. The desirable goal of treatment is eradication of HCV, but chronic suppression of HCV replication would be expected to have similar beneficial effects on the disease.

Currently, recombinant alpha-interferon 2b is the only approved treatment for chronic hepatitis C in the United States. Interferon therapy is currently indicated for all patients with chronic hepatitis C, with the exception of those patients with pronounced cytopenia, autoimmune disease including untreated thyroid disease, hepatic decompensation, and severe psychiatric conditions.

Standard initial therapy is recombinant interferon alfa-2b at a dose of three million units administered subcutaneously three times per week for 6 months. This regimen is effective in initially controlling the biochemical, histologic, and virologic activity of infection in 40% to 50% of treated patients. Approximately half the patients will not respond to interferon using a standard regimen. About 20% of these patients will respond if treated with five million units three times a week. It has been recently reported that hepatic iron content may correlate with response to interferon and that phlebotomy-induced iron deficiency may facilitate interferon action in patients who failed to initially respond to interferon. This observation needs to be confirmed in randomized controlled trials. In general, response to treatment is greatest in those patients without advanced inflammation and cirrhosis, with low levels of HCV RNA, and with non-1b genotype. HIV and HCV coinfected patients appear to respond no differently to interferon than do patients not infected with HIV, and interferon treatment should be considered in HIV-coinfected patients before onset of manifestations of immunodeficiency. About 60% to 90% of hemophiliacs have serologic evidence of HCV, and interferon treatment is as effective in this patient population as in others. In the case of cryoglobulinemia associated with HCV infection, cryoglobulin levels and associated disease improve or disappear in half of treated patients and the rest may require treatment with immunosuppressive agents including prednisone, cytoxan, and/or plasmapheresis.

Almost all responders (normal ALT levels) lose HCV RNA, detectable by PCR by the end of therapy. However, relapse occurs in 50% to 70% of patients after the end of the initial course and is associated with return of detectable HCV RNA. Unfortunately, the best way to treat relapse is not clear, although almost all patients will respond again when retreated. At this point, it is not clear whether repeated 6-month courses, a titrated long-term maintenance regimen, or fixed-dose treatment will benefit the patient.

While interferon treatment is quite effective, there is no doubt that it is far from optimal. Ongoing clinical trials will hopefully find better markers of response in order to fine tune treatment dosage and duration. Treatment options other than interferon are limited. Ribavirin, a broad-spectrum oral nucleoside analogue, has beneficial effects on serum aminotransferase levels in patients with chronic hepatitis C, but these effects are not accompanied by changes in serum HCV RNA levels, and biochemical changes are not sustained when ribavirin therapy is discontinued. Ursodeoxycholic acids, NSAIDs, and N-acetylcysteine have been proposed as adjunctive treatment to interferon, but experience with these agents is limited. New classes of therapeutic agents such as proteinase inhibitors, antisense oligonucleotides, and therapeutic vaccines may eventually be tested in clinical trials in the near future.

OLT is an established treatment for end-stage liver disease with HCV. Similar to HBV, HCV infection has a high frequency of recurrence in patients who receive transplants because of chronic hepatitis C. Patient and graft survival have been found to be low at 1 and 3 years when compared with a nonviral control group. The current tests for anti-HCV antibodies may underestimate the incidence of transmission and the prevalence of HCV infection among immunosuppressed organ recipients; hence RT-PCR should be routinely used in these patients to detect recurrent HCV. Interferon therapy can result in transient normalization of serum ALT levels and fall in HCV RNA. However, the greatest concern about the use of interferon in post–liver transplant has been the possibility of inducing allograft rejec-

tion, although, at times, there is a great deal of histologic overlap between recurrent hepatitis and changes of rejection.

Chronic Hepatitis D

Chronicity after HDV and HBV coinfection occurs in no more than 10% of patients. However, an acute delta hepatitis almost always becomes chronic following superinfection, presumably because chronic HBV infection is already established. The natural history of chronic HDV infection seems to be bimodal. In 10% to 15% of patients, liver failure develops within a few months to a few years. In the remainder, the disease runs an asymptomatic course that may last many years. The first pattern is typical in drug addicts, who have the highest levels of HBV and HDV replication. In these cases, progression to cirrhosis usually follows the classic histologic patterns of liver inflammation and bridging necrosis. Patients with chronic delta hepatitis tend to have severe or advanced liver disease on liver biopsy. Patients with cirrhosis related to HDV infection tend to be younger than those with cirrhosis from hepatitis B, suggesting that delta hepatitis has a more rapidly progressive course. In the United States, many patients with chronic delta hepatitis are found to have cirrhosis at first presentation. Although chronic HBV infection is a well-recognized risk factor for HCC, a similar association has not been clearly demonstrated for chronic HDV infection. Alpha-interferon is the only agent so far found to have a beneficial effect in chronic delta hepatitis. Even so, the relapse rate is very high unless HBsAg is cleared from the serum. Patients with decompensated cirrhosis due to chronic delta hepatitis are good candidates for OLT as recurrent HBV hepatitis is less frequent in these patients than among those with HBV infection alone.

Autoimmune Hepatitis

Autoimmune hepatitis is an unresolving inflammation of the liver that is characterized by periportal hepatitis on histologic examination and autoantibodies in the serum. First described by Waldenstrom in 1950 and Kunkel in 1951, the disease was thought to occur primarily in young women and demonstrated many autoimmune characteristics, including a positive lupus erythematosus (LE) cell phenomenon. It is now recognized that the disease occurs in all ages and both sexes. There are no pathognomonic features of the disease, and the diagnosis requires the exclusion of genetic disorders such as Wilson's disease, hemochromatosis, and alpha-1-antitrypsin deficiency; drug-related hepatitis (alpha-methyldopa, nitrofurantoin, propylthiouracil); and viral infection (chronic hepatitis B and C viral infections).

Etiologic Factors. The etiology is unknown, although immunologic changes are conspicuous and serum gamma globulin levels are markedly elevated. The autoantibodies associated with autoimmune hepatitis are neither pathogenic nor disease specific. Their presence supports the diagnosis but does not establish the diagnosis nor diminish the need for exclusion of other diseases with similar findings. In addition, patients with clinical, biochemical, and histologic features of autoimmune hepatitis may lack immunoserologic markers. These patients may have autoimmune hepatitis associated with an unconventional autoantibody, or they may be seronegative for conventional markers at the time of testing. The coexistence of autoantibodies and anti-HCV (their presence confirmed by recombinant immunoblot assays) and HCV RNA in sera of some patients with chronic hepatitis has raised the possibility of a viral cause in some patients.

Three subtypes of autoimmune hepatitis have been proposed based on distinct immunoserologic markers.

Type 1 Autoimmune Hepatitis. This so called classic or lupoid variety is the most common form of autoimmune hepatitis in the United States, constituting at least 80% of cases in adults. It is characterized by the presence of smooth muscle antibodies (SMA) and/or antinuclear antibodies (ANA); hypergammaglobulinemia; concurrent immunologic disorders; human leukocyte antigen (HLA) positivity for A1, B8, DR3, or DR4; and responsiveness to corticosteroids.

Typically, type 1 autoimmune hepatitis predominantly affects women, usually 15 to 40 years of age. An acute onset of illness occurs in one third of the patients, and these patients may be misdiagnosed as having acute viral hepatitis. A small proportion of these patients may have other immunologic disorders such as thyroiditis or Grave's disease, ulcerative colitis, or rheumatoid arthritis. The presence of ulcerative colitis may suggest the diagnosis of primary sclerosing cholangitis (PSC); cholangiography is required in all such patients because PSC may resemble autoimmune hepatitis or coexist with it. Genetic predisposition strongly influences disease expression and behavior in type 1 autoimmune hepatitis.

Patients with HLA-B8 are relatively younger than their counterparts with other phenotypes and have a greater degree of inflammatory activity on presentation. In addition, patients with HLA-B8 and HLA-A1 commonly relapse after corticosteroid therapy. Corticosteroid therapy fails commonly in individuals with HLA-DR3 phenotype, and these patients frequently require liver transplantation. In contrast, patients with the HLA-DR4 phenotype are older, have higher serum titer of ANA, have concomitant nonhepatic immunologic disease, and respond more commonly to corticosteroids. Unfortunately, the target antigen for type 1 autoimmune hepatitis is unknown and none of the autoantibodies associated with this disease are pathogenic.

Type 2 Autoimmune Hepatitis.

Type 2 autoimmune hepatitis is characterized by the presence of antibodies to liver/kidney microsomal type 1 (anti-LKM1) and absence of ANA and SMA in serum. Patients with type 2 disease are predominantly young children, but adults may be affected. In the United States the diagnosis is unusual among adults, occurring in only 4% of the patients with autoimmune hepatitis. Concurrent nonhepatic immunologic disorders are more common than in type 1, and patients may have vitiligo, autoimmune thyroiditis, type 1 insulin-dependent diabetes, autoimmune hemolytic anemia, idiopathic thrombocytopenic purpura, pernicious anemia, rheumatoid arthritis, and ulcerative colitis. Hypergammaglobulinemia is less pronounced than type 1, and organ-specific autoantibodies, including antithyroid antibodies, anti-islets of Langerhans antibodies, and anti-parietal cell antibodies, are common (30%). Type 2 disease may progress more rapidly to cirrhosis than type 1 disease. Unlike type 1, the target autoantigen of type 2 disease has been identified: cytochrome mono-oxygenase, P450IID6, which is recognized by anti-LKM1. Antibodies to P450IID6 characterize patients with type 2 autoimmune hepatitis. HCV infection has been closely associated with this condition in some parts of the world, and as many as 80% to 90% of patients with anti-LKM1 are seropositive for anti-HCV; a majority of these patients have true HCV infection. This observation has justified a proposal to subdivide type 2 autoimmune hepatitis into type 2a and 2b. Patients with type 2a are younger and more commonly women, lack anti-HCV, have higher titers of anti-LKM1, and are frequently positive for antibodies to P450IID6. In contrast, patients with type 2b have typical features of chronic viral infection with seropositivity for anti-HCV and infrequently anti-P450IID6 positivity.

Type 3 Autoimmune Hepatitis. Type 3 autoimmune hepatitis is characterized by the presence of antibodies to soluble liver antigen (anti-SLA). Patients with type 3 have many features of type 1 disease. They are mostly women of all age-groups, and they lack ANA, LKM1, and thyroid antibodies but are commonly seropositive for SMA, AMA, and antibodies to liver membrane antigen. This type has not yet been linked to HCV infection.

Treatment

Prospective, randomized, controlled trials have shown beneficial effects of steroids alone or in combination with low doses of azathioprine. Remission is induced in approximately 70% of patients within 2 years, with improvement in symptoms, laboratory abnormalities, and inflammatory changes seen on liver biopsy. An initial daily dose of 60 mg of prednisone or 30 mg prednisone combined with 50 mg of azathioprine is effective, tapered gradually over several weeks to months to a daily maintenance dose of 20 mg of prednisone or 10 mg of prednisone plus 50 mg of azathioprine. If a favorable response is not observed within 2 to 3 months, treatment should be discontinued. Patients receiving treatment should be examined and their liver

function tests monitored periodically, and liver biopsies may need to be repeated at intervals of 6 months to 1 year depending on circumstances. Most significantly ill patients with autoimmune hepatitis require continued immunosuppression. In a stable patient in whom serum aminotransferases return to a level less than twice normal and liver biopsy shows subsidence of the inflammatory and necrotic changes, an attempt should be made to gradually taper the treatment. Relapse after withdrawal of immunosuppression occurs in 50% of patients during the first 6 months and 70% during the first 36 months.

Immunosuppression does not prevent progression to cirrhosis: 40% of treated patients develop cirrhosis within 10 years. The HLA haplotype B8, DR3 is associated with earlier age of onset, increased inflammation, more frequent relapses, and greater requirement for OLT. Limited data is available regarding the efficacy of other potent immunosuppressive agents such as cyclosporine and tacrolimus. Extrahepatic malignancies develop in 5% of patients immunosuppressed for at least 42 months, with mean time to development of malignancy being 9.7 years and the relative risk being 1.4 compared to age- and sex-matched controls.

OLT is an established treatment for end-stage liver disease related to autoimmune hepatitis. The success rate of OLT for patients with autoimmune hepatitis is similar to that achieved in other adult diseases. Recurrence of autoimmune hepatitis after liver transplantation seems to be extremely infrequent.

BIBLIOGRAPHY

Alter MJ, Mast EE: The epidemiology of viral hepatitis in the United States, *Gastroenterol Clin North Am* 23:437, 1994.

Bader TF: Hepatitis A vaccine, *Am J Gastroenterol* 91(2):217, 1996.

Bloom BS: A reappraisal of hepatitis B virus vaccination strategies using cost effectiveness analysis, *Ann Intern Med* 118:298, 1993.

Centers for Disease Control: Protection against viral hepatitis: recommendation of the Immunization Practices Advisory Committee (ACIP), *MMWR* 39:1, 1990.

Czaja AJ: Autoimmune hepatitis: evolving concepts and treatment strategies, *Dig Dis Sci* 40:435, 1995.

Davis GL et al: Treatment of chronic hepatitis C with recombinant interferon alpha: a multicenter randomized controlled trial, *N Engl J Med* 321:1501, 1989.

Desmet VJ et al: Classification of chronic hepatitis: diagnosis, grading and staging, *Hepatology* 19(6):1513, 1994.

Fried MW: Therapy of chronoc viral hepatitis, *Med Clin North Am* 80(5):957, 1996.

Hollinger FB et al, editors: *Viral hepatitis,* ed 2, New York, 1991, Raven Press.

Hoofnagle JH: Therapy of acute and chronic viral hepatitis, *Adv Intern Med* 39:241, 1994.

Hoofnagle JH, Peters M, Mullen KD et al: Randomized controlled trial of recombinant human alpha interferon in patients with chronic hepatitis B, *Gastroenterology* 95:1318, 1988.

Johnson PJ et al: Meeting report: International Autoimmune Hepatitis Group, *Hepatology* 18(4):998, 1993.

Knodell RG et al: Formulation and application of a numerical scoring system for assessing histological activity in asymptomatic chronic active hepatitis, *Hepatology* 1(5):431, 1981.

Lee WM: Acute liver failure, *N Engl J Med* 329(25):1862, 1993.

Linnen J et al: Molecular cloning and disease association of hepatitis G virus: a transfusion-transmissible agent, *Science* 271:505, 1996.

Sjogren MH: Serologic diagnosis of viral hepatitis, *Med Clin North Am* 80(5):929, 1996.

Winkur PL, Stapleton JT: Immunoglobulin prophlaxis for hepatitis A, *Clin Infect Dis* 14:580, 1992.

CHAPTER

356 Drug- and Toxin-Induced Liver Disease

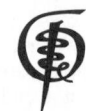

Hyman J. Zimmerman

A large number of chemical and biologic agents can induce hepatic injury (Box 356-1). Some hepatotoxins are plant or fungal products; some are minerals; and many are products, by-products, or wastes of the chemical and pharmaceutical industries.

Exposure to toxic agents can occur in domestic, occupational, or clinical settings. Some natural toxins—such as the peptides of

Amanita phalloides and related poisonous mushrooms, the pyrrolizidine alkaloids, and the toxin of the cycad nut—are taken as food or as folk medicine in ignorance of their toxicity. Other natural toxins (e.g., aflatoxin) are ingested because climatic conditions favor their presence as unsuspected contaminants of food. Synthetic hepatotoxins also may be ingested as accidental contaminants of food. Domestic exposure to hepatotoxins includes accidental or suicidal ingestion or inhalation of known toxins (e.g., carbon tetrachloride [CCl$_4$]) or of large overdoses of medicinal agents (e.g., acetaminophen).

Occupational exposure to hepatotoxic agents has led to hepatic injury in the past; however, improved industrial hygiene seems to have reduced the incidence. Pollution of the environment by toxic industrial by-products and wastes is of great concern, but the magnitude of the hepatotoxic threat remains to be defined.

Drug-induced hepatic injury is the facet of hepatotoxicity of most relevance to clinicians. A large number of medicinal agents can produce liver damage. The importance of drug-induced hepatic injury rests on both its frequency and its character. Although reactions to drugs account for fewer than 10% of all cases of apparent hepatitis, they assume more importance with advancing age, accounting for as many as 50% of cases of apparent hepatitis in patients older than 50 years. Furthermore, drug-induced hepatic injury plays a prominent role in the causation of massive hepatic necrosis, accounting for about 25% of cases. The importance of drug toxicity as a cause of fatal hepatic necrosis stems from the gravity of the hepatocellular type of drug-induced injury.

Of increasing concern, but only vaguely substantiated, is the risk of acquiring chronic hepatic disease, particularly neoplasms, from prolonged occupational exposure to toxic chemicals. Of validated concern is the risk of chronic disease from ingestion of mycotoxins and other natural hepatotoxins. Aflatoxins are a documented cause of hepatocellular carcinoma and a suspected cause of cirrhosis in some parts of the world, and pyrrolizidine alkaloids can cause venoocclusive disease and cirrhosis. Drugs also can lead to chronic hepatic disease.

SUSCEPTIBILITY OF THE LIVER TO CHEMICAL INJURY

The great susceptibility of the liver to damage by chemical agents is presumably a consequence of its primary role in the disposition of foreign substances. The position of the liver as portal to the tissues for ingested agents and the concentration of xenobiotics in the liver may contribute to its special vulnerability. The role of the liver in the metabolic conversions of foreign compounds is even more relevant to its susceptibility.

Biotransformation of foreign compounds has been traditionally considered detoxifying. Such reactions, however, can also convert nontoxic agents to potentially toxic products. It has become clear that formation of reactive, toxic, and metabolic intermediates within the hepatocyte accounts for the injury it sustains from many toxic chemicals and drugs.

Most of the biotransformations are catalyzed by the drug-metabolizing enzyme system called the *mixed function oxidase* (MFO) or *cytochrome P-450*. This enzyme consists of a number of isozymes (isoforms), each of which has special catalyzing properties for different substrates.

Modification of the ability to metabolize foreign chemicals results from exposure to a number of compounds. Administration of phenobarbital and exposure to insecticides and many other agents enhance the ability of the liver to metabolize a large number of compounds. This phenomenon, which involves an increase in the amount and activity of cytochrome P-450, has been called *induction*. Accordingly, induction enhances the hepatotoxicity of agents that are converted to toxic products by the isoform of cytochrome P-450 that has been induced.

Among the agents that enhance the ability to metabolize foreign compounds and thereby increase the hepatotoxic effects of a number of toxic chemicals is ethanol. The increased susceptibility of alcoholics to hepatic injury from carbon tetrachloride, acetaminophen, or isoniazid seems attributable, at least in part, to the enhancement of conversion of these agents to their toxic metabolites by the alcohol induction of the isoform of cytochrome P-450 that is involved in the

metabolism of these compounds. Conversely, inhibition of conversion of toxic agents to their active metabolic products by agents that inhibit the P-450 may decrease the toxic effects of the drug. Cimetidine, for example, inhibits the P-450, thus decreasing the hepatotoxic effects of acetaminophen for experimental animals. (Effectiveness of cimetidine in poisoning in humans remains to be demonstrated.)

CLASSIFICATION OF HEPATOTOXIC AGENTS

Two main categories of agents produce hepatic injury: predictable (intrinsic) hepatotoxins and nonpredictable (idiosyncratic) hepatotoxins. Idiosyncratic hepatotoxins produce hepatic injury only in unusually susceptible persons. The distinguishing characteristics of each type are listed in Table 356-1.

The division of hepatotoxic effects into intrinsic or idiosyncratic types is oversimplified. A spectrum of toxic potential exists, ranging from that of agents (e.g., phosphorus) that damage the liver of almost all members of a variety of species to drugs (e.g., penicillin) that hardly ever produce hepatic injury. The relative roles of host susceptibility and intrinsic toxicity of an agent might be portrayed as the two axes of a graph (Fig. 356-1).

Intrinsic Hepatotoxins

There are two main types of intrinsic hepatotoxins: direct and indirect. Direct hepatotoxins destroy hepatocytes by direct physicochemical attack, that is, peroxidation and denaturation of proteins or other destructive alteration of cell membranes. Indirect hepatotoxins divert or competitively inhibit essential metabolites, react selectively with and distort molecules essential for cell integrity, or in other ways interfere with specific metabolic or secretory functions of the hepatocyte. The effect of either type may be mediated by an active metabolite of the agent or by the native molecule.

Intrinsic hepatotoxins are either cytotoxic or cholestatic. Cytotoxic hepatotoxins produce steatosis, necrosis, or both. Steatosis results from interference with synthesis of apoprotein, assembly of the lipoprotein complex required for transport of lipid from the liver, mitochondrial oxidation of fatty acids, or other defects in lipid metabolism.

BOX 356-1

Types of hepatotoxic agents

I. Inorganic agents
  A. Metals and metalloids (antimony, arsenic, beryllium, cadmium, copper, iron, lead, manganese, phosphorus, thallium)
  B. Hydrazine derivatives
  C. Iodides
II. Organic agents
  A. Natural agents
    1. Plant toxins (albitocin, cycasin, amanitin, icterogenin, indospicine, lantana, ngaione, nutmeg, phalloidin, pyrrolizidines, safrol, tannic acid)
    2. Mycotoxins (aflatoxins, cyclochlorotine, ethanol, luteoskyrin, ochratoxin, rubratoxins, sterigmatocystins, griseofulvin, sporidesmin, tetracycline, and other antibiotics)
  B. Synthetic agents
    1. Nonmedicinal agents
      a. Haloalkanes and haloolefins
      b. Nitroalkanes
      c. Haloaromatic compounds
      d. Nitroaromatic compounds
      e. Organic amines
      f. Azo compounds
      g. Phenol and derivatives
      h. Various other organic compounds
    2. Medicinal agents (more than 300 drugs used for treatment and diagnosis)

Agents listed in this box vary considerably in their potential for causing hepatic injury.

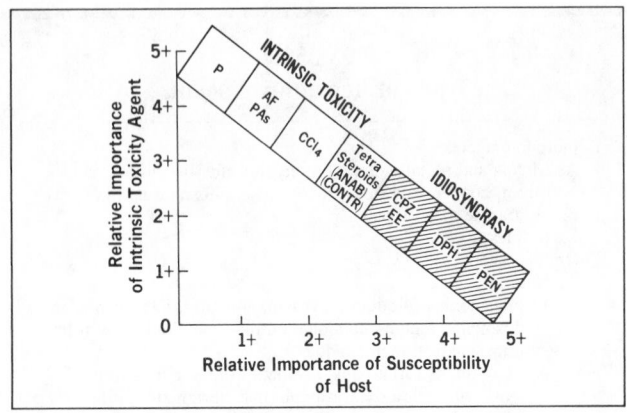

FIGURE 356-1 Interplay between intrinsic toxicity of chemical agent and susceptibility of exposed persons in the production of hepatic injury. Interplay can be expressed as dichotomy or as spectrum. *P,* Phosphorus; *AF,* aflatoxin; *PAs,* pyrrolizidine alkaloids; *CPZ,* chlorpromazine; *EE,* erythromycin estolate; *DPH,* diphenylhydantoin (phenytoin).

From Zimmerman HJ: Hepatotoxicity: adverse effects of drugs and other chemicals on the liver, New York, 1978, Appleton-Century-Crofts, p. 95.

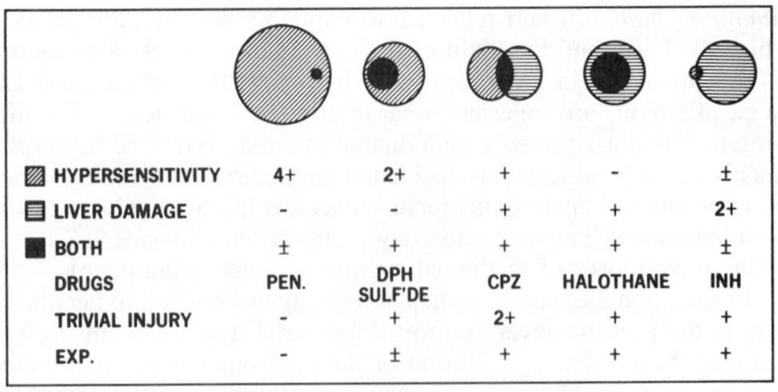

▨ HYPERSENSITIVITY	4+	2+	+	−	±
▤ LIVER DAMAGE	−	−	+	+	2+
▪ BOTH	±	+	+	+	±
DRUGS	PEN.	DPH SULF'DE	CPZ	HALOTHANE	INH
TRIVIAL INJURY	−	+	2+	+	+
EXP.	−	±	+	+	+

FIGURE 356-2 Relation between hypersensitivity and hepatic injury. Note that drugs such as penicillin *(PEN),* despite a marked tendency to produce hypersensitivity reactions, very rarely lead to liver damage and then only in association with hypersensitivity. Other drugs, such as phenytoin *(DPH)* and sulfonamides *(SULF'DE),* which are also prone to cause hypersensitivity, are much more likely to cause hepatic injury in association with hypersensitivity. A third group of drugs, represented by chlorpromazine *(CPZ)* and halothane, may produce liver damage with or without hypersensitivity, and a fourth group, represented by isoniaziod *(INH),* produces hepatic injury usually unaccompanied by hypersensitivity. All these drugs except penicillin produce a significant incidence of trivial injury in human beings and can produce injury in experimental animal models *(EXP.).*

From Zimmerman HJ: Drug hepatotoxicity: spectrum of clinical lesions. In Davis M, Tredger JM, Williams R, editors: Drug reactions and the liver, London, 1981, Pittman, p. 43.

Table 356-1 Features that distinguish intrinsic hepatotoxins from those that produce hepatic injury as idiosyncratic reactions

	CHARACTERISTICS			
BASIS FOR HEPATIC INJURY	**EXPERIMENTAL REPRODUCIBILITY**	**DOSE DEPENDENCE**	**INCIDENCE IN HUMAN BEINGS**	**LATENT PERIOD**
Intrinsic hepatotoxicity* (true, predictable hepatotoxic agents)	Yes†	Yes	High‡	Often short and relatively uniform
Idiosyncratic reaction* (unpredictable hepatotoxic agents)	No§	No§	Low	Often long and quite variable

*Terms preferred by this author. Terms in parentheses are those used by other authors.
†May apply only to some species.
‡Depends on dosage.
§If due to metabolic idiosyncrasy, may be reproducible experimentally in specially manipulated animal models.

Necrosis results from obscure mechanisms, presumably selective lesions of the membranes of the hepatocyte. Cholestatic hepatotoxins produce selective interference with mechanisms or structures involved in the excretion of bile or uptake of its constituents from the blood.

Idiosyncratic Hepatic Injury

Hepatic injury that occurs unpredictably in a small proportion of recipients of some drugs is an expression of a special susceptibility of the patient rather than of intrinsic toxicity of the agent. Idiosyncratic hepatic injury appears to be a manifestation of hypersensitivity or of aberrant metabolism of the drug.

The liver injury may be attributed to hypersensitivity if it is accompanied by clinical signs (fever, rash, eosinophilia) and histologic hallmarks (eosinophilic or granulomatous inflammation in the liver) of hypersensitivity. These characteristics, especially when supported by a prompt recurrence of the syndrome after a challenge dose, permit the inference that the hepatic injury is caused by a drug allergy and that the drug or a metabolite has acted as a hapten. This form of injury usually develops after a "sensitization" period of 1 to 5 weeks.

Lack of hypersensitivity and failure to evoke prompt recurrence of the hepatic injury with one or two challenge doses of the suspected drug suggest an alternative mechanism for the liver damage, presumably the production of hepatotoxic metabolites. This form of injury appears after widely variable latent periods ranging from weeks to months. For a number of drugs, evidence is strong that metabolic idiosyncrasy accounts for the injury they produce. Isoniazid, valproic acid, perhexiline maleate, and amiodarone produce hepatic injury that

seems clearly ascribable to toxic metabolites that are produced to a greater degree by patients who develop hepatic injury than by those who remain uninjured.

Metabolic idiosyncrasy may also be the mechanism by which hypersensitivity develops. Phenytoin leads to injury that appears to be classically hypersensitivity provoked. The apparent hapten is a reactive metabolite (the arene oxide) of phenytoin that accumulates in patients who have an inborn defective ability to convert the arene oxide to a nonreactive metabolite.

Even among agents that produce hypersensitivity reactions there are several categories of association of hypersensitivity with hepatic injury (Fig. 356-2). Some drugs (e.g., phenytoin) produce hepatic injury only in association with systemic features of an allergic response. Others (e.g., chlorpromazine) produce hepatic injury that may or may not be accompanied by systemic features suggestive of drug allergy. Still other drugs that lead to generalized hypersensitivity (penicillin) do not necessarily cause hepatic injury. These observations, the high incidence of mild hepatic dysfunction among recipients of some drugs (e.g., chlorpromazine), and the toxic effects of these drugs in experimental animal models have led to the hypothesis that hypersensitivity leads to overt hepatic disease if the causative drug also has some intrinsic hepatotoxic potential.

Mechanisms of injury are classified in Table 356-2. Toxins encountered in the home or workplace are intrinsic, direct, or indirect. Medicinal agents have been included in each of the classifications, although known potent intrinsic hepatotoxins such as CCl_4 and chloroform are no longer in clinical use. Some intrinsic hepatotoxins, however, are still used in clinical medicine. Some, such as acetamin-

Table 356-2 Classification of hepatotoxic agents and major characteristics of each group

CLASS OF AGENT	INCIDENCE	EXPERIMENTAL REPRODUCTION	DOSE DEPENDENCY	MECHANISM	HISTOLOGIC LESION	EXAMPLE
Intrinsic toxicity Direct	High	Yes	Yes	Direct physicochemical distortion and destruction by peroxidation and related effects	Necrosis	
Cytotoxic Cholestatic Indirect Cytotoxic	High	Yes	Yes	Interference with specific metabolic pathways leading to structural injury by covalent binding or other metabolic distortion	Hepatocytes Ducts Necrosis or steatosis	CCl$_4$ Paraquat Acetaminophen Tetracyclines
Cholestatic	High	Yes	Yes	Interference with excretory pathways leading to cholestasis	Bile casts	Anabolic steroids (C-17 alkylated)
Host idiosyncrasy Immunologic (hypersensitivity)	Low	No	No	Drug allergy	Necrosis or cholestasis	Phenytoin Chlorpromazine Erythromycins
Metabolic	Low	No	No	Production of hepatotoxic metabolites	Necrosis or cholestasis	Isoniazid Valproic acid Benoxaproten

Table 356-3 Histologic types of acute toxic hepatic injury and associated biochemical and clinical aspects

HISTOLOGIC LESIONS	BIOCHEMICAL ABNORMALITIES OF SERUM*			CLINICAL ASPECTS	EXAMPLES
	AMINOTRANSFERASES (AST AND ALT)	ALKALINE PHOSPHATASE	CHOLESTEROL		
Cytotoxic Necrosis					
Zonal	↑ (10-500×)	↑ (1-2×)	N, ↓	Hepatic and renal failure	CCl$_4$, MSH, ACM, HALO
Diffuse	↑ (10-200×)	↑ (1-2×)	N, ↓	Severe hepatitis-like disease	INH, methyldopa, HALO
Steatosis	↑ (5-20×)	↑ (1-2×)	↓	Resembles fatty liver of pregnancy and Reye's syndrome	Tetracycline, aspirin†
Cholestatic					
With pericholangitis (hepatocanalicular)	↑ (1-10×)	↑ (3-10X)	↑	Resembles obstructive jaundice	CPZ, EE
Without pericholangitis (canalicular)	↑ (1-5×)	↑ (1-3×)	N, ↑	Resembles obstructive jaundice	Anabolic and contraceptive steroids
Mixed (mixture of cytotoxic and cholestatic)	↑ (10-100×)	↑ (1-10×)	N, ↑	May resemble hepatitis or obstructive jaundice	PBZ, PAS, sulfonamides, DPH

*Degree of abnormality indicated as times increase. N, normal; N, ↑ or ↓, normal or slightly abnormal.
†Aspirin in therapeutic doses may contribute to development of Reye's syndrome in children exposed to influenza A, varicella, or other viral illness. A similar lesion is produced by poisonous overdose of aspirin.
ACM, Acetaminophen; *CPZ,* chlorpromazine; *DPH,* phenytoin; *EE,* erythromycin estolate; *HALO,* halothane; *INH,* isoniazid; *MSH,* poisonous mushrooms; *PAS,* para-aminosalicylate; *PBZ,* phenylbutazone.

ophen, are usually hepatotoxic only in large overdoses or in patients whose susceptibility is enhanced by other factors (e.g., alcohol). Others lead to cytotoxic injury (e.g., tetracycline and oncotherapeutic agents) or cholestatic injury (anabolic and contraceptive steroids) even at doses in the therapeutic range.

CLINICAL ASPECTS OF CHEMICAL HEPATIC INJURY

Chemical hepatic injury has a broad range of clinical manifestations. It may occur as an unexpected idiosyncratic reaction to a therapeutic drug dosage or as the expected consequence of an agent's intrinsic toxicity. Hepatic injury may be acute or chronic. Liver disease may be the only clinical manifestation of the chemical's adverse effect, or it may be accompanied by evident injury to other organs or by systemic manifestations. Liver disease may develop within several days after ingestion of a toxic dose of a known hepatotoxin, after 1 to 5 weeks of taking a drug whose hepatic injury involves hypersensitiv-

ity, or after weeks to many months of taking a drug that causes injury as a result of metabolic idiosyncrasy.

Acute Hepatic Injury

Acute toxic hepatic injury may be (1) mainly cytolytic, involving overt damage to hepatocytes; (2) cholestatic, involving mainly arrested bile flow; or (3) mixed, that is, with prominent cytotoxic and cholestatic features (Table 356-3). Most intrinsic toxins produce mainly cytotoxic injury; only a few produce injury that is mainly cholestatic. Some drugs that produce idiosyncratic hepatic damage produce mainly cholestatic injury; others produce cytotoxic injury; and some produce either or a mixed form of injury.

Cytolytic injury includes necrosis, steatosis, or both. There are two types of cholestatic injury. One is accompanied by portal inflammation and evident, although slight, hepatocyte injury. This type is called *sensitivity,* or *hepatocanalicular, cholestasis.* The second type is accompanied by little inflammation and even less hepatocyte injury and

Table 356-4 Systemic manifestations that may be associated with drug hepatotoxicity

MANIFESTATIONS	DRUGS
Allergic reactions	
Fever, rash, eosinophilia	Para-aminosalicylate, anticonvulsants
Pseudomononucleosis	Oxyphenisatin
Lymph node hyperplasia	
Lymphocytosis	
Autoantibodies	
LE factor	
Hemolytic anemia	Methyldopa
Bone marrow injury	Phenylbutazone, anticonvulsants
Renal injury	Sulindac, methoxyflurane
Gastrointestinal ulcer, pancreatitis	Phenylbutazone, tetracycline

is called *steroid-induced,* or *canalicular, cholestasis.* The hepatocanalicular type is exemplified by chlorpromazine jaundice and the canalicular type by anabolic or contraceptive steroid jaundice.

Clinical and biochemical features of toxic hepatic injury mirror the morphologic features. Hepatic necrosis leads to hepatocellular jaundice and a syndrome resembling that of viral hepatitis. Values for serum aspartate aminotransferase (AST) and serum alanine aminotransferase (ALT) are often very high (Table 356-3)—10 to 200 times the upper limit of normal (ULN) or even higher—and values for alkaline phosphatase are usually modestly increased (less than three times the ULN). The chief clinical manifestations are fatigue, anorexia, and nausea. Severe cases of toxic hepatic injury are manifested by deep jaundice, and hemorrhagic phenomena, coma, and death may develop. Indeed, the most important aspect of drug-induced hepatocellular jaundice is its tendency to result in fulminant hepatic failure. Mortality has ranged from 10% to 50%. Survival of the acute phase usually leads to complete recovery.

Acute steatosis, such as that caused by parenterally administered tetracycline or overdoses of aspirin, leads to clinical and biochemical features resembling those of the acute fatty liver of pregnancy and of Reye's syndrome, which it also mimics histologically. (In these conditions the steatosis is microvesicular, in contrast to the macrovesicular steatosis of alcoholic fatty liver.) Jaundice is usually relatively slight. Aminotransferase levels are usually somewhat lower than those in patients with hepatic necrosis (less than 20 times the ULN). The illness, however, is serious.

Cholestatic injury resembles extrahepatic obstructive jaundice. Jaundice and pruritus are the main clinical manifestations. Aminotransferase levels are only modestly elevated (usually less than eight times the ULN). There are biochemical counterparts to the two morphologic types of cholestasis. In the hepatocanalicular type, alkaline phosphatase levels are usually elevated to more than three times the ULN and cholesterol levels are elevated; in the canalicular type the values for alkaline phosphatase and cholesterol are normal or slightly elevated. Cholestatic injury, with a case mortality of less than 1%, has a far better prognosis than cytotoxic injury. In rare instances, however, cholestatic jaundice may fail to resolve and evolves into a syndrome resembling primary biliary cirrhosis ("the vanishing bile duct syndrome").

The clinical syndrome of chemical hepatic injury may indicate liver disease alone or with systemic manifestations and evidence of injury to other organs (Table 356-4). Fever, rash, and eosinophilia are characteristic of reactions caused by some drugs, and in some instances these features are accompanied by lymph node enlargement, lymphocytosis, and "atypical" circulating lymphocytes, leading to a syndrome that resembles infectious mononucleosis and serum sickness ("pseudomononucleosis"). Bone marrow, lung, and skin may be involved in systemic reactions. Renal injury may be a component of generalized hypersensitivity caused by some drugs (e.g., phenytoin, sulfonamides) or the result of the nephrotoxic effect of a metabolite of a drug (e.g., methoxyflurane). Renal injury is particularly prominent in poisoning by CCl_4, phosphorus, and poisonous mushrooms.

Chronic Liver Damage

Chemical hepatic injury can also lead to chronic lesions. These lesions include chronic active hepatitis, steatosis, phospholipidosis, granulomatous disease, several vascular lesions, several forms of cirrhosis, noncirrhotic portal hypertension, and several types of hepatic tumors (Table 356-5). Chronic active hepatitis has occurred as a reaction to oxyphenisatin, methyldopa, nitrofurantoin, sulfonamides, propylthiouracil, clometacine, papaverine, and other drugs. The syndrome resembles the autoimmune type of chronic active hepatitis. Several drugs that lead to phospholipidosis also lead to hyaline degeneration of the alcoholic hyaline type (Mallory's body). Amiodarone and perhexiline maleate have been incriminated in the production of a lesion that includes Mallory's bodies and cirrhosis.

HEPATOTOXIC REACTIONS AND CIRCUMSTANCES OF EXPOSURE

A host of agents with hepatotoxic potential have been used in the munitions, rocketry, plastics, paint, cosmetic, pharmaceutical, and other chemical industries. Nevertheless, overt acute hepatic injury is a rare consequence of occupational exposure to toxic chemicals and is more likely to be acquired in the home (Table 356-6). The risk of chronic subtle injury continues to be a concern, but there are scant data to support this. The toxicity of several of these agents warrants description in more detail.

Carbon Tetrachloride Poisoning

Instances of CCl_4 intoxication are now rare. Most victims are alcoholics because alcoholism enhances susceptibility by increasing transformation of CCl_4 to a toxic metabolite and leads to increased carelessness with its use. Inhalation or accidental ingestion has been the mode of exposure.

The clinical syndrome consists of hepatic failure accompanied by renal failure. Minutes to hours after exposure, there are usually neurologic and gastrointestinal manifestations and a variable degree of vascular collapse. There may then be a period of abatement, followed by the appearance of hepatic injury within 2 to 4 days of exposure. The current mortality appears to be considerably lower than the 25% previously noted, presumably because of the improved outlook provided by treatment of the renal failure with hemodialysis. Early treatment with acetylcysteine and hyperbaric oxygen has been proposed to have benefit.

Laboratory findings include neutrophilic leukocytosis, anemia, and azotemia. The urinary sediment reflects the acute tubular necrosis. Serum values of aminotransferases can reach astronomic levels—up to 700 times the normal.

Mushroom and Phosphorus Poisoning

A clinical syndrome somewhat similar to that seen with CCl_4 poisoning results from poisoning by the hepatotoxic mushroom *A. phalloides* and related species. The mortality, however, is about 25%. The patient presents with severe diarrhea, which is followed by a period of ameliorated symptoms and subsequently by severe hepatic and renal failure. In the liver, there is steatosis and centrilobular necrosis. The mortality is about 25%. A prothrombin concentration less than 10% of normal is strongly predictive of a fatal outcome, whereas a value above 40% of normal is predictive of survival.

Phosphorus poisoning is characterized by severe gastrointestinal symptoms and shock and by phosphorescence and garliclike odor of excreta and vomit. It leads to fulminant hepatic and renal failure, with a mortality also in excess of 50%. The liver shows mainly steatosis, at first at the periphery of the lobule and then throughout. Necrosis may be present and is also predominantly peripheral.

Acetaminophen Poisoning

This mild analgesic has virtually no side effects when administered in the usual therapeutic doses. It produces severe centrilobular hepatic necrosis if large doses are ingested, usually in suicide attempts. Necrosis is produced by an active metabolite that binds covalently to tissue macromolecules. The small amounts of active metabolite nor-

Table 356-5 Chronic hepatic disease caused by drugs

LESION OR SYNDROME	CAUSATIVE AGENTS
Cytotoxic	
Chronic necroinflammatory disease (chronic active hepatitis)	Oxyphenisatin, iproniazid isoniazid, methyldopa, sulfonamides, nitrofurantoin, dantrolene, propylthiouracil
Subacute hepatic necrosis	Drugs listed above for chronic inflammatory disease, occupational toxins (e.g., TNT)
Steatosis	Ethanol, methotrexate antineoplastic agents, valproate, glucocorticoids
Phospholipidosis* and pseudoalcoholic disease†	Coralgil‡ perhexiline maleate amiodarone
Cholestatic	
Chronic intrahepatic cholestasis	Chlorpromazine, and several other phenothiazines, several tricyclic antidepressants, ajmaline; organ arsenical, tolbutamide thiobendazole, etc.
Sclerosing cholangitis	Floxuridine
Cirrhosis	
Micronodular	Ethanol, methotrexate inorganic arsenical
Macronodular	Ethanol, methotrexate inorganic arsenical (also agents listed above for chronic inflammatory disease)
"Primary biliary"	See chronic intrahepatic cholestasis
Congestive "cirrhosis"	Oral contraceptive steroids, thioguanine, pyrrolizidine alkaloids, urethan (x-ray)
Vascular lesions	
Peliosis hepatis and/or marked sinusoidal dilatation	Anabolic and contraceptive steroids, phalloidin, oxazepam, azathioprine
Hepatic vein thrombosis	Contraceptive steroids
Veno-occlusive disease	Pyrrolizidine alkaloids, urethan, thioguanine, and other antineoplastic drugs, radiation injury
Neoplasm	
Adenoma	Anabolic and contraceptive steroids
Carcinoma	
Hepatocellular	Anabolic and contraceptive steroids, Thorotrast
Cholangiocellular	
Angiosarcoma	Vinyl chloride, Thorotrast, inorganic arsenicals
Other	
Hepatoportal sclerosis	Vinyl chloride, inorganic arsenicals
Centrilobular fibrosis	Vitamin A excess, methyldopa
Granulomas	Allupurinol, hydralazine, penicillin, phenylbutazone, quinidine, sulfonamides, sulfonylureas, and many other drugs

*Accumulation of phospholipids in lysosomes, with ultimate development of cirrhosis.
†Hyaline degeneration (Mallory's bodies) resembling alcoholic liver disease. This lesion can lead to cirrhosis.
‡Trade name for 4,4′-diethylaminoethoxyhexesterol dihydrochloride (a drug formerly used in Japan to treat arteriosclerotic heart disease).

Table 356-6 Known or potential* domestic hepatotoxic agents

AGENT	EXPOSURE	LESION
Chlorinated hydrocarbons	Careless use; accidental; solvent sniffing	Centrilobular necrosis, steatosis
Phosphorus (yellow)	Suicidal or accidental	Steatosis, periportal necrosis
Toxic chemicals as inadvertent contaminants of food		
4′,4-Diaminodiphenylmethane	Contaminant of flour ("Epping jaundice")	Cholestatic jaundice
Hexachlorobenzene	Fungistatic added to wheat	Steatosis, necrosis, toxic porphyria
Chlorinated biphenyls	Contaminant of rice (Japan)	Steatosis, necrosis
Toxic foods of plant origin		
A. phalloides and related species	Ingested as food in ignorance of toxicity	Centrilobular necrosis, steatosis
Cycad nut	Ingested as food in ignorance of toxicity	Necrosis, steatosis, cirrhosis, hepatocellular carcinoma
Senecio, Heliotropium, and Crotalaria spp. and other plants that contain pyrrolizidine alkaloids	Ingested as additive to foods, as medicinal decoction, or as abortifacient	Centrilobular necrosis, veno-occlusive disease, congestive cirrhosis, steatosis
Nutmeg	Ingested as abortifacient	Steatosis, midzonal necrosis
Ngaione	Potential food toxin	
Mycotoxins*		
Aflatoxins (Aspergillus flavus and related species)	Present mainly in legumes and other foods of vegetable origin when climatic conditions permit	Steatosis, necrosis, cirrhosis, hepatocellular carcinoma
Ochratoxin		
Luteoskyrin		
Other mycotoxins		

*Evidence for hepatotoxicity mainly epidemiologic and experimental.

mally formed from a therapeutic dose are readily detoxified by reacting with glutathione. Hepatic necrosis occurs only when the amount of active metabolite produced exceeds the binding capacity of glutathione. This occurs when the drug dose is large and especially in association with factors that increase the fraction of drug converted to an active metabolite (alcoholism, inducing drugs, stress, fasting) or that decrease the availability of glutathione. Doses have exceeded 15 g in about 80% of suicide cases.

Acetaminophen also has been reported to produce hepatic injury as a therapeutic mishap. This effect has involved mainly alcoholics in whom severe hepatic injury develops because they have taken large therapeutic doses or in whom susceptibility to acetaminophen injury is enhanced by the induction of cytochrome P-450 or by depletion of glutathione secondary to the alcoholism and fasting. Instances of non-alcoholic individuals in whom hepatic injury develops secondary to therapeutic doses of the drug or who have enhanced susceptibility also have been reported. A number of infants who have sustained hepatic injury from presumably excessive doses administered as antipyretics have also been reported.

Clinical Features. The clinical course of acetaminophen poisoning consists of three phases. The first, which comes within hours of intake, consists of acute gastrointestinal symptoms. The second phase, which continues for approximately 2 days, is characterized by abatement of symptoms. During this apparent subsidence, biochemical evidence of hepatic injury appears. Oliguria is usual. The third phase, that of overt hepatic damage, becomes clinically apparent 3 to 5 days after ingestion, with the appearance of jaundice. Renal failure may occur.

Biochemical Changes. AST and ALT values are very high, reaching levels up to 1000 times normal, but the bilirubin level is often only modestly elevated. Clotting abnormalities may be severe, and the one-stage prothrombin time is a useful prognostic indicator.

Histologic Changes. The liver shows centrilobular (zone 3) necrosis and sinusoidal congestion. The kidney may show tubular necrosis.

Prognosis and Treatment. Hepatic failure, as evidenced by hemorrhagic phenomena and hepatic encephalopathy, has occurred in as many as third of patients who develop jaundice. Many have died. The prognosis of an overdose of acetaminophen seems to correlate with blood levels of drug between 4 and 15 hours after ingestion. Early treatment with agents that replete glutathione has been effective in reducing the severity of hepatic injury. Indeed, acetylcysteine given within 16 hours of ingestion appears to prevent significant injury. Almost all patients so treated have survived. If it is administered after a longer interval, acetylcysteine seems to have questionable benefit.

Hepatic Injury Induced By Other Medicinal Agents (Table 356-7)

Halothane. Halothane can cause serious hepatic disease. Despite a very low incidence of overt injury (estimated to be 1 in 2500 exposed), its severity (20% to 50% case mortality in recognized toxicity) and widespread use make it an important cause of hepatic failure. The incidence is somewhat greater in females, is enhanced by obesity, and is low in children. Approximately 75% of patients in reported cases had prior exposure to the anesthetic. Many of the patients who developed jaundice had had fever after previous exposure. Onset of the syndrome is abrupt, usually with fever, and occurs a few days after exposure. Patients with fatal cases develop deepening jaundice, hemorrhagic phenomena, and coma. Aminotransferase levels are very high, leukocytosis is frequently present, and eosinophilia occurs in more than 40% of patients. The mechanism appears to involve both hypersensitivity and a toxic metabolite. The centrilobular (zone 3) necrosis observed in many cases supports the likelihood that a hepatotoxic metabolite of halothane contributes to the injury.

Enflurane. This closely related anesthetic also has been reported to produce similar hepatic injury, although apparently the incidence is even lower. The lesser degree of biotransformation of enflurane appears to account for the lower incidence of injury. Isoflurane, also a related compound, has produced hardly any instances of hepatic injury. At this writing only two reported patients exposed to the drug have had injury that was convincingly attributed to isoflurane. Sevoflurane and desflurane have yet to be reported as causes of hepatic injury.

Methoxyflurane. Methoxyflurane has led to similar instances of hepatic necrosis. It can also produce renal injury.

Chlorpromazine. Chlorpromazine, a phenothiazine widely used to treat psychosis and as a tranquilizer, can lead to hepatocanalicular jaundice in about 0.5% of recipients. A number of other phenothiazines produce similar injury. The mechanism for chlorpromazine-induced injury appears to involve both mild intrinsic toxicity and hypersensitivity (see description of idiosyncratic injury).

Phenytoin. Phenytoin and related anticonvulsants produce hepatocellular injury accompanied by sufficient evidence of cholestasis to warrant categorizing the lesion as a mixed hepatocellular injury. It is accompanied by prominent features of hypersensitivity and leads to a syndrome resembling serum sickness. Several other anticonvulsants have been incriminated in the production of hepatic injury. Carbamazepine has led to instances of hepatic injury either resembling those produced by phenytoin or with marked cholestasis. It also leads to granulomatous lesions of the liver. Another anticonvulsant, valproate, has led to a number of instances of fatal hepatic disease characterized by microvesicular steatosis and necrosis. Encephalopathy and increased blood ammonia levels may precede other evidence of hepatic injury. The mechanism appears to be metabolic idiosyncrasy.

Drugs Used to Treat Rheumatic and Other Musculoskeletal Diseases. All of the many nonsteroidal antiinflammatory drugs (NSAIDs) have been incriminated in the production of hepatic injury, although there are variations in potential for producing liver disease, in the mechanism for its production, and in the type of injury produced. Some agents produce hepatic injury accompanied by prominent hallmarks of hypersensitivity, whereas others appear to produce the injury as the result of a metabolic idiosyncrasy. Some NSAIDs produce hepatocellular injury, and others sometimes cause cholestatic jaundice. One recently abandoned agent (benoxaprofen) led to severe cholestasis and renal failure. Other drugs used in rheumatic disease (penicillamine, gold compounds) produce rare instances of idiosyncratic liver damage (usually cholestasis). The increasing use of methotrexate to treat rheumatoid arthritis has been expected to produce cases of steatosis and cirrhosis. The low dose used, however, has produced little evidence of hepatic injury. Salicylates have only recently been found to cause hepatic injury, despite almost a century of extensive clinical use. The injury, anicteric hepatocellular damage associated with high aminotransferase levels, occurs when blood levels are high (>15 mg/dl). An important observation is the association of Reye's syndrome (Chapter 358) with aspirin use. Although this incrimination of aspirin has been debated, it seems convincing and attributable to the conjoint adverse effects of the drug and viral infection. Poisonous overdoses of aspirin can lead to similar hepatic injury.

Alkylated Anabolic Steroids and Oral Contraceptives. These agents are indirect cholestatic hepatotoxins. They lead to hepatic dysfunction and canalicular jaundice. The adverse effect is dose related, and the incidence of jaundice is low at ordinary dosages. Contraceptive steroids have produced jaundice in a very small proportion of the millions of patients who have taken them. The higher incidence in patients with a personal or family history of jaundice of pregnancy and the clustering of cases in Chile and Scandinavia demonstrate that genetic susceptibility is relevant (Chapter 353).

Chronic lesions that can be induced by contraceptive and anabolic steroids include hepatic adenoma, peliosis hepatis, and carcinoma. The development of the Budd-Chiari syndrome in patients taking oral contraceptives seems to be attributable to the known thrombogenic effects of the estrogenic component (Chapter 360).

Isoniazid, Rifampin, and Amoxicillin. Isoniazid leads to hepatocellular jaundice in about 1% of recipients. The incidence is age related. It approaches 3% in patients over 50 but is rare below the age of 20. Susceptibility appears to be enhanced by alcoholism. The inference that acetylator status affects susceptibility is controversial. The injury is apparently caused by toxic metabolites of isoniazid. Clinical features resemble those of severe acute viral hepatitis. Values for AST and ALT are often in the thousands. The mortality for icteric patients exceeds 10%.

Minor elevations (below 200 units) of AST and ALT appear in 10% to 20% of patients during the first 2 months of isoniazid therapy

Table 356-7   Types of acute hepatic injury caused by drugs in various therapeutic categories

	CYTOTOXIC (HEPATOCELLULAR) AND MIXED[2]	CHOLESTATIC AND MIXED[2]	SOME CYTOTOXIC AND SOME CHOLESTATIC[3]
Anesthetics*	Enflurane Fluroxene Halothane Isoflurane?[10] Methoxyflurane		
Neuropsychotropics	Amineptine Clozapine Cocaine Famoxitine Hydrazides (all) Maprotiline Metopimazine Methylphenidate Molindone Tranylcypromine Tricyclics (most) Zimelidine	Chlorpromazine (and other phenothiazines) Haloperidol Trimipramine Benzodiazepines	Chlordiazepoxide Diazepam Mianserin Trazodone Tricyclics (some)
Anticonvulsants	Phenytoin Progabide Valproate[5] Felbamate		Carbamazepine Phenobarbital
Analgesic, antiinflammatory, anti–muscle spasm, antigout agents	Acetaminophen Chlorzoxazone Clomatacine Dantroline Diclofenac Fenclozic acid Glafenine Ibuprofen Indomethacin Salicylates Pirprofen Tolmetin Zoxazolamine	Benoxaprofen Diflunisal Penicillamine Propoxyphene	Allopurinol[4] Gold compounds Naproxen Phenylbutazone[4] Piroxicam Sulindac
Hormonal derivatives and drugs used in endocrine disease	Acetohexamide Carbutamide Cyclofenil Glipizide Metahexamide Propylthiouracil[4] Tamoxifen Diethylstibestrol	Carbimazole Chlorpropamide[4] Tolazemide[4] Tolbutamide[4] Methimazole Methylthiouracil Anabolic and contraceptive steroids Danazol	Thiouracil
Antimicrobials	Amodiaquine Amphotericin B Antimonials Clindamycin Hycanthone Hydroxystilbamidine Didanosine Ketoconazole Mebendazole Mepacrine Metronidazole P-Aminosalicylate Rifampin Sulfonamides[4] Sulfones Tetracyclines[5] Prothionamide	Amoxicillin-clavulanate Erythromycin[7] Griseofulvin Thiabendazole Menelamine Cloxacillin Zidovudine Dicloxacillin Floxacillin	Cephalosporins Chloramphenicol Clarithromycin Nitrofurantoin[4] Penicillin[8] Sulfamethoxazole-trimethoprim Sulfadoxine-pyrimethamine Idoxyuridine Zidovudine Ampicillin Oxacillin

1. Hepatic injury produced by volatile anesthetic agents is always cytotoxic.
2. Mixed forms of injury are categorized according to the predominant injury as cytotoxic or cholestatic.
3. Refers to agents that are inconsistent in the form of injury produced with some instances having been cholestatic and others cytotoxic.
4. Can cause granulomas.
5. Microvesicular steatosis. Valproate injury also includes necrosis in some cases.
6. Macrovesicular steatosis.
7. E-estolate, E-ethylsuccinate, E-proprionate, E-stearate.
8. Semisynthetic penicillins and penicillin.
9. Some of these agents alone or as combinations lead to veno-occlusive disease.
10. Two credible cases reported. Sevoflurane and desflurane were each incriminated in one case.
11. Also leads to phospholipidosis.
12. Can lead to changes resembling alcoholic liver disease (alcoholic hyaline).
13. Responsible for "toxic oil" epidemic in Spain.
14. Responsible for "Epping jaundice."

Continued.

Table 356-7   Types of acute hepatic injury caused by drugs in various therapeutic categories—cont'd

	CYTOTOXIC (HEPATOCELLULAR) AND MIXED[2]	CHOLESTATIC AND MIXED[2]	SOME CYTOTOXIC AND SOME CHOLESTATIC[3]
Cardiovascular drugs	Amiodarone[5,11,12] Aprindin Benziodarone Diltiazem Methyldopa Mexiletine Hydralazines[4] Nicotinic acid Nifedipine[12] Papaverine Perhexiline[5,11,12] Procainamide Pyridinol carbamate Quinidine[4] Suloctidil Ticrynafen Tocainamide Labetolol Lisinopril	Ajmaline Captopril Chlorthalidone Coumadin Phenindone Prajmaline Propafenone Thiazides Verapamil[4]	Amrinone Disopyramide Enalapril
Antineoplastic[9]	Asparaginase[5,6] Cis-platinum[5] Cyclophosphamide Dacarbazine Diethylstibestrol (DES)[12] Doxorubicin Etoposide Fluorouracil Indicine-N-oxide Methotrexate[6] N-Methyl-formamide[5] Mithramycin 6-Mercaptopurine Nitrosoureas Tamoxifen Thioguanine[7] Vincristine Flutamide	Aminoglutethamide Busulfan Floxuridine	Azathioprine
Miscellaneous	Disulfiram Iodide ion Oxyphenisatin Phenazopyridine Salizopyridine Tannic acid Vitamin A Para-aminobenzoic acid (PABA)	Propoxyphene Rapeseed oil–aniline[13] Methylene dianiline[14]	Cimetidine Ranitidine Etretinate

and may subside despite continued administration of the drug. Perhaps this curious phenomenon represents metabolic adjustment with decreased production of toxic metabolites. Nevertheless, periodic measurement of aminotransferase levels, with withdrawal of the drug when values exceed three times the ULN, would probably serve to prevent serious hepatic injury. Administration of rifampin has been alleged to potentiate the ability of isoniazid to produce liver damage. Alone, rifampin leads to rare instances of hepatocellular jaundice. Presumably unrelated is the ability of rifampin to produce unconjugated hyperbilirubinemia. The drug apparently competes with other substances for excretion into bile or uptake from sinusoidal blood.

Amoxicillin in combination with the β-lactamase inhibitor *clavulanic acid* has recently drawn attention as a cause of hepatic injury. The combination (trade name, Augmentin) has led to a number of instances of cholestatic jaundice.

Methyldopa. Methyldopa leads to hepatocellular jaundice in less than 1% of recipients. Aminotransferase levels are high, and serum alkaline phosphatase values are modestly elevated. The liver shows diffuse degeneration and necrosis. Death from hepatic failure has occurred in about 10% of reported cases. The mechanism of injury probably involves both hypersensitivity and toxic metabolites. A lesion resembling chronic, active hepatitis has also been observed in recipients of methyldopa.

Methotrexate. Methotrexate has been in clinical use for 40 years. There have been many reports that it causes fatty liver and cirrhosis, especially in patients who have received it as long-term treatment for psoriasis. The development of chronic liver disease appears to depend on total dose; duration of therapy; and, particularly, the interval between doses. Significant liver disease seems far more likely to develop in patients who receive doses more frequently than once per week than in those who take the drug less frequently. Alcohol intake enhances susceptibility to methotrexate-associated hepatic injury. Unfortunately, the development of the histologic lesion is not reliably reflected in abnormal liver function test results or serum enzyme values. The mechanism for the production of the lesion is unclear, but it seems probable that methotrexate is an intrinsic hepatotoxin of the indirect type, with low potency and insidious effect.

Herbal Remedies and Other Plant Toxins

A number of herbal drugs employed as folk medicine, nontraditional and unconventional remedies, health aids, and nutritional supplements have led to instances of hepatic injury (Table 356-8). These plant products tend to produce hepatocellular or mixed injury. Several of them lead to veno-occlusive disease. Several are known toxins with a dose-related hepatotoxic effect (pyrrolizidine alkaloids, pennyroyal

Table 356-8 Herbal products that can lead to hepatic injury

HERBAL PRODUCT	SOURCE	ACTIVE INGREDIENT	OSTENSIBLE EFFECT	HEPATIC INJURY
Comfrey	*Syphytum* spp.	PAs	Nutritional supplement	VOD
Gordolobo yerba tea	*Senecio* spp.	PAs	Health aid	VOD
Mate tea	Ilex	PAs	Health aid	VOD
Chinese herb preparations				
Medicinal tea	*Compositae* spp.	?PAs*	Medicinal	VOD
"Chinese herbs"	"Fu-san-chi"	?Glycerrhyza	Medicinal	Hepatitis
Jin Bu Auan	*Lycopodium serratum*	?Levotetrahydropalmitine	Anodyne; hypnotic	"Hepatitis"; also micro-vesicular steatosis
Germander	*Tencrium* spp. *Chainaedrys* spp.	Furanoneo-clerodane	Weight loss	Necrosis, zone 3
Chaparral leaf	*Larria tridanta; Larria diva-riatae* ("creosote bush"; "greasewood")	Nordihydroguaiaretic (NDGA) acid	Medicinal	Necrosis, zone 3
Mistletoe (plus other herbs)			Health aid	"Chronic hepatitis"
Margosa oil	*Azadirachta indica*	Pulegone		Microvesicular steatosis
Pennyroyal oil	*Labiatae* spp.	Pulegone Isonpulegone	Abortifacient Also medicinal	Necrosis, microvesicular steatosis

*The contents of this preparation are not clear. The entity is suggested in view of the character of the injury.
PA, Pyrrolizidine alkaloid; *VOD*, veno-occlusive disease.

and margosa oils); others appear to reflect idiosyncratic response of the involved individuals.

DIAGNOSIS

Recognition that hepatic disease is caused by drugs or other chemicals is most often based on circumstantial evidence. A history of exposure should be sought in every patient with hepatic disease. If such a history exists, its relevance should be judged according to the character of the hepatic disease and the known propensity of the agent for producing it.

A known toxin (e.g., CCl_4, acetaminophen) should be suspected as the cause of acute hepatocellular injury that progresses rapidly to hepatic failure, especially if hepatic failure is preceded by neurologic or gastrointestinal complaints, renal failure, and exposure to the toxin.

Drug-induced injury should be suspected as the cause of acute hepatic disease. If the hepatic injury is accompanied by fever and eosinophilia, the likelihood of drug-induced disease increases. Lack of these features, of course, does not exclude the diagnosis of drug-induced hepatic disease.

Distinction of drug-induced hepatocellular injury from viral hepatitis involves epidemiologic information; serologic studies to exclude hepatitis A, B, and C viruses; and a history that reveals exposure to a drug known to produce hepatocellular injury. Distinction of drug-induced cholestatic jaundice from extrahepatic obstructive jaundice may be difficult, and the special radiographic and sonographic techniques for distinction of intrahepatic cholestasis from extrahepatic obstruction may be needed (Chapter 348). The physician should strongly suspect that intrahepatic cholestasis is drug induced. If liver biopsy reveals cholestasis with an eosinophil-rich portal inflammation, the diagnosis of the hepatocanalicular type of drug-induced jaundice is probable. Cholestasis without portal inflammation may be of the canalicular type (see Table 356-3).

Disappearance of hepatic abnormality after withdrawal of an incriminated drug and recurrence of hepatic dysfunction or hyperbilirubinemia after a test dose of it support the diagnosis of drug-induced injury. Failure of the liver to develop abnormalities on readministration, however, does not preclude the diagnosis of drug-induced injury; in some patients with drug-induced jaundice the liver may fail to show a recurrence of hepatic dysfunction after a test dose. Furthermore, some drugs reproduce the hepatic injury only after weeks of readministration.

Recognition that chronic disease is the result of drug or other chemical injury is often more difficult. Awareness of the lesions that can be produced and of the agents that have been incriminated helps alert the physician to possible etiologic relationships. Reversal of lesions—for example, those of chronic active hepatitis—after withdrawal of a suspected drug offers a helpful clue.

TREATMENT

Treatment consists of removal of the causative agent and provision of supportive care. Early detection of drug-induced injury and withdrawal of the offending agent may prevent the development of more severe hepatic disease. Supportive treatment for patients with hepatocellular injury is similar to that for patients with acute viral hepatitis. Large dosages of glucocorticoids have been used to treat the hepatic failure of drug-induced acute hepatocellular disease, but the effectiveness of this treatment remains to be proved.

Supportive treatment for patients with hepatocanalicular injury involves alleviation of pruritus and, if the syndrome is prolonged, treatment of malabsorption. Cholestyramine may alleviate the itching, as may phenobarbital. Glucocorticoid therapy appears to be of little benefit in the drug-induced cholestatic syndrome. Ursodiol may be of benefit.

BIBLIOGRAPHY

American Academy of Pediatrics, Committee of Infectious Diseases: Aspirin and Reye's syndrome, *Pediatrics* 69:810, 1982.

Black M: Acetaminophen hepatotoxicity, *Annu Rev Med* 35:577, 1984.

Brechot C: *Primary liver cancer: etiological and progression factors,* Boca Raton, Fla, 1994, CRC Press.

Farber E, Fisher MM, editors: *Toxic injury of the liver,* New York, 1980, Dekker.

Farrell GS: *Drug-induced liver disease,* New York, 1994, Churchill Livingston.

Gram L, Bentsen KD: Hepatic toxicity of antiepileptic drugs: a review, *Acta Neurol Scand* 68(suppl 97):81, 1983.

Kaplowitz N, editor: Recent advances in drug metabolism and toxicity, *Semin Liver Dis* vol 10(4), New York, 1990, Thieme Medical Publishers.

Larrey D, Pageaux GP: Hepatotoxicity of herbal remedies and mushrooms, *Semin Liv Dis* 15:183, 1995.

Lewis JH, editor: Drug-induced liver disease, *Gastroenterol Clin North Am,* vol 24, December 1995.

Maddrey WC: Drug-related acute and chronic hepatitis, *Clin Gastroenterol* 9:213, 1980.

Mitchell JR et al: Metabolic activation: biochemical basis for many drug-induced liver injuries, *Prog Liver Dis* 5:259, 1976.

Pessayre D, Larrey D: Drug-induced hepatitis, *Baillieres Clin Gastroenterol* 2:385, 1988.

Powell PR, Jackson JM, Williams R: Hepatotoxicity to sodium valproate: a review, *Gut* 25:673, 1984.

Sharp JR, Ishak KG, Zimmerman HJ: Chronic active hepatitis and severe hepatic necrosis associated with nitrofurantoin, *Ann Intern Med* 92:14, 1980.

Stricker BH: *Drug-induced hepatic injury,* Amsterdam, 1992, Elsevier.

Zimmerman HJ: *Hepatotoxicity: adverse effects of drugs and other chemicals on the liver,* New York, 1978, Appleton-Century-Crofts.

Zimmerman HJ: Effects of alcohol on other hepatotoxins, *Alcohol Clin Exp Res* 10:3, 1986.

Zimmerman HJ, Maddrey WC: Toxic and drug-induced hepatitis. In Schiff L, Schiff ER, editors: *Diseases of the liver,* ed 7, Philadelphia, 1993, Lippincott.

Zimmerman HJ, Maddrey WC: Acetaminophen (Paracetamol) hepatotoxicity with regular intake of alcohol: analysis of instances of therapeutic misadventure, *Hepatology* 22:767-773, 1995.

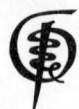

CHAPTER

357 Alcoholic Liver Diseases and Nonalcoholic Steatohepatitis

David W. Crabb and Mats Estonius

The medical and social effects of excess alcohol consumption comprise one of the largest groups of problems encountered by physicians. It is estimated that the prevalence of problem drinking (alcohol abuse and alcoholism) ranges from 7% to 10% of the adult population in the United States. Because of this high prevalence, alcohol abuse arises in the differential diagnosis of virtually all cases of hepatocellular disease and is the most common cause of serious liver disease in Western cultures. Unfortunately, diagnostic tests that help the physician determine cumulative alcohol consumption are unsatisfactory at present; moreover, heavy alcohol use is not sufficient to cause advanced liver injury, since only 20% of heavy drinkers will progress beyond the stage of alcoholic fatty liver. Thus liver disease in alcoholic patients is not always the result of alcohol and demands a thorough evaluation, especially for coexistent hepatitis virus infection. Liver disease in patients not thought to be alcoholic should still prompt an investigation into the patient's drinking history.

This chapter presents current concepts of alcohol-induced liver injury, differential diagnoses for the common presentations of liver disease in alcoholics, and the current knowledge about treatment for both the underlying alcoholism and the liver disease. Nonalcoholic steatohepatitis, which closely resembles alcoholic hepatitis histologically (although not clinically) is also discussed.

PATHOPHYSIOLOGY

The pathophysiology of alcoholic liver injury is complex and differs for the three different stages of disease.

Genetic Factors in Alcoholic Liver Disease

The risk of alcoholic liver injury is modified by genetic factors. The single largest study of genetic factors is the Veterans' Affairs (VA) twin panel that demonstrated a 26% concordance for alcoholism and a 16% concordance for cirrhosis among monozygotic twins. This was significantly higher than the 12% and 7% concordances among dizygotic twins. Approximately 50% of this concordance was estimated to be caused by genetic effects. To date, the exact identity of these factors has not been determined. Much attention has been paid to factors that modify rates of alcohol metabolism, which in part is responsible for its toxicity. This varies by at least three fold even within ethnic group and gender. The most well-understood differences between individuals that could alter metabolic rates are in the enzymes responsible for ethanol oxidation (Table 357-1).

Alcohol is first oxidized to acetaldehyde and then to acetate, as shown in Fig. 357-1. There are as many as eight genes for alcohol dehydrogenase (ADH), one gene for cytochrome P-4502E1 (CYP2E1), and perhaps eight for aldehyde dehydrogenases (ALDH). The *ADH2, ADH3, CYP2E1,* and *ALDH2* loci are polymorphic in humans and characteristics of these variants have been studied intensively in the last 5 years. In summary, high-activity *ADH2*2* genes are associated with mild flushing and are less common in alcoholics. A recent study suggested that Asians with *ADH2*2* who drink heavily may have higher risk for alcoholic liver disease than those without *ADH2*2*. Individuals with *ADH2*3* alleles have slightly faster rates of alcohol elimination, but the effect on risk for alcoholism has not been studied. The data on the association between a high-activity *CYP2E1* gene and liver disease are controversial. The *ALDH2* allele that encodes a subunit with a lysine for glutamate substitution is associated with the alcohol flush reaction, lower levels of drinking, and low frequency of alcoholism. However, in ALDH2-deficient individuals who drink heavily, there may be increased susceptibility to alcoholic hepatitis. Thus, in the case of *ADH2*2* and *ALDH2*2*, it is hypothesized that high rates of acetaldehyde production or low rates of acetaldehyde oxidation reduce the risk of alcoholism but might increase the risk of liver injury in those who drink heavily. Another important genetic factor in alcoholic liver injury is gender, possibly because of decreased first-pass metabolism of ethanol and increased alcohol metabolic rates in women. It bears emphasizing that additional factors must influence alcohol metabolic rates, and the basis for the wide variation in development of alcoholic liver injury remains largely unknown.

Effects of Alcohol Metabolism

There are many effects of the products of alcohol metabolism, reduced nicotinamide-adenine dinucleotide (NADH), and acetaldehyde. The large load of NADH generated in the cytosol and mitochondria results in inhibition of a number of NAD^+-dependent enzymes or shifts in their equilibrium toward the more reduced compound. Thus enzymes of β-oxidation are inhibited, blocking the oxidation of fatty acids. This is the major cause of the fatty liver, increased export of very low density lipoprotein (VLDL), and hypertriglyceridemia associated with alcohol use. Pyruvate is reduced to lactate, which impairs the liver's ability to synthesize glucose and can cause hypoglycemia in the fasted state. When alcohol consumption ceases after a long binge, free fatty acid levels are high and the rate of ketogenesis increases as fatty acid oxidation resumes, resulting in ketosis.

Acetaldehyde generated from ethanol is chemically reactive and has been implicated in a number of effects on hepatocytes. Acetaldehyde can modify liver proteins and deoxyribonucleic acid (DNA), forming neoantigens (protein-acetaldehyde adducts) that could be recognized by the immune system. Acetaldehyde also modifies tubulin and impairs endocytosis, secretion, and intracellular protein trafficking. Acetaldehyde has also be implicated in reducing cellular (espe-

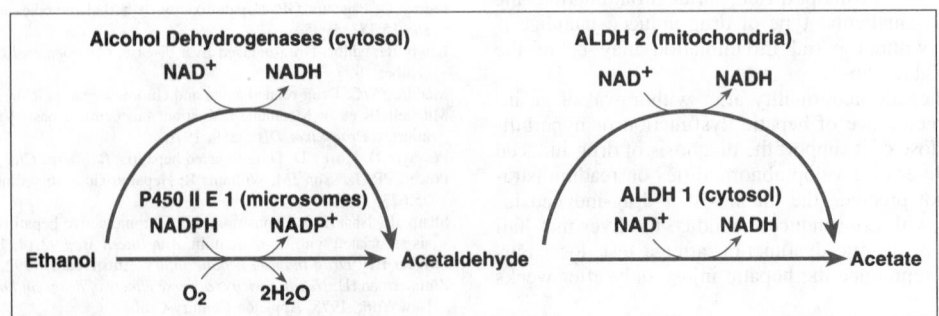

FIGURE 357-1 Alcohol metabolic pathway. Ethanol is sequentially oxidized to acetaldehyde by alcohol dehydrogenases or cytochrome P-450 IIE1 and then to acetate by aldehyde dehydrogenases (ALDH). NAD^+ and NADH are the oxidized and reduced forms of nicotinamide adenine dinucleotide, and $NADP^+$ and NADPH are the oxidized and reduced forms of nicotinamide adenine dinucleotide phosphate, respectively.

cially mitochondrial) glutathione (GSH) levels, rendering the liver more susceptible to oxidant stresses.

Nutritional Interactions with Ethanol

Although ethanol consumption alone can cause substantial liver injury in animal models, the nutritional status of the animal affects the degree of injury. Chronic administration of ethanol to baboons and mini-pigs, or to rats (by continuous gastric infusion, the Tsukamoto-French model), causes fatty liver, hepatic necrosis, and fibrosis. Some of the baboons progress to cirrhosis. This injury can be modified by dietary manipulations: cirrhosis is prevented by including polyunsaturated lecithin (specifically dilinoleoyl phosphatidylcholine) in the baboons' diet. The phosphatidylcholine appears to reverse the ethanol-induced reduction in phosphatidylethanolamine N-methyltransferase activity and thus maintains normal membrane composition. Paradoxically, the development of liver injury in the rat model requires high dietary polyunsaturated fat (corn or fish oil) and is prevented by substituting saturated fat. The deleterious effect of a diet high in polyunsaturated fat appears to result from these lipids' susceptibility to free radical attack and their ability to induce CYP2E1. Alcoholics are also commonly deficient in vitamin A, yet appear to be at increased risk of vitamin A toxicity because of microsomal enzyme induction. Deficiency in protein or vitamin E might exacerbate glutathione depletion and free radical toxicity.

Centrilobular Injury in Alcoholic Liver Disease

Mechanisms for alcoholic liver disease must account for the more severe injury in the centrilobular zone. Chronic alcohol use increases hepatic oxygen consumption to a greater extent than hepatic blood flow, resulting in relative hypoxia of the centrilobular zone of the liver. Part of this increased oxygen consumption may be caused by the induction of CYP2E1 activity. This enzyme is most active in the centrilobular zone of the liver, is induced by heavy alcohol use, and contributes to increased alcohol metabolism in drinkers. The enzyme can oxidize nearly 100 xenobiotics, including isoniazid and acetamin-

ophen, and contributes to the hepatotoxicity of these drugs. The enzyme also generates excessive oxygen radicals, and these may contribute to centrilobular liver injury. In the Tsukamoto-French model, inhibitors of CYP2E1 activity attentuated the liver injury caused by ethanol. The oxidant stress on the liver is also affected by the production of cytokines by activated Kupffer cells. Tumor necrosis factor (TNF) in particular can stimulate the production of oxygen radicals. Oxygen radical formation is enhanced by the presence of iron, which is commonly increased, by unknown mechanisms, in the livers of alcoholics. Chronic ethanol use also markedly reduces the mitochondrial glutathione pool, reducing the effectiveness of antioxidant defenses to remove toxic lipid peroxides.

Hepatic Fibrosis and Regeneration

The common mechanism for hepatic fibrosis is collagen synthesis by stimulated Ito cells. Chronic alcohol feeding stimulates the production of soluble factors (including transforming growth factor β-[TGFβ] and platelet-derived growth factor [PDGF]) by Kupffer cells that stimulate Ito cell proliferation and collagen formation. The Ito cells from animals on a high polyunsaturated fat diet were in turn more sensitive to these Kupffer cell–derived factors. The activated Ito cells may be further stimulated by acetaldehyde. Activation of both Kupffer and Ito cells may result from alcohol-induced increases in portal vein endotoxin. Inactivation of Kupffer cells with gadolinium chloride and reduction in the number of gram-negative organisms in the colon by adminstration of nonabsorbable antibiotics prevented the increase in alcohol metabolic rate, the increase in liver oxygen consumption, and the liver injury seen in the Tsukamoto-French model. Thus activation of these nonparenchymal liver cells may be central to the toxicity of ethanol. It is also interesting to speculate that activation of these cells by ethanol potentiates the fibrotic response to viral hepatitis, possibly accounting for the apparent synergistic effect of hepatitis C and heavy alcohol use. Coexistent infection with hepatitis C virus (HCV) is common in alcoholism, with as many as 40% of alcoholics with cirrhosis having HCV infection. Doubtless, many alcoholics with mildly abnormal transaminase levels who in the past were considered to have fatty liver in fact had HCV infection. Lastly, ethanol inhibits the ability of liver cells to regenerate by interfering with the necessary signal transduction pathways. These effects of ethanol on the liver are summarized in Box 357-1.

PATHOLOGY

Although it is believed that alcoholic liver disease progresses from the ubiquitous fatty liver through alcoholic hepatitis, and finally in some patients to cirrhosis, all three stages may coexist in a given patient. The fatty liver of alcoholism contains macrovesicular fat that is often more severe in the centrilobular zone (Fig. 357-2). Enlarged, abnormal megamitochondria may be present and reflect the effects of alcohol on this organelle. Although fatty liver is generally both benign and reversible, a large amount of fat may obscure more advanced features such as pericellular and perivenular fibrosis.

Alcoholic hepatitis is characterized by macrovesicular fat, infiltration of the liver with inflammatory cells (lymphocytes and especially polymorphonuclear leukocytes), and evidence of cell necrosis, such as ballooning hepatocytes or Mallory's hyaline (Fig. 357-3). Cirrhosis is of course characterized by liver fibrosis and regenerating nodules (Fig. 357-4). The central veins are often impossible to find as a result of lobular collapse and central fibrosis. Because cirrhosis

---

BOX 357-1
Mechanisms of liver injury caused by ethanol

Effects of ethanol
High NADH concentrations → inhibition of β-oxidation
Increased oxygen consumption → centrilobular hypoxia
Induction of CYP2E1 → generation of oxygen radicals, lipid peroxidation, increased sensitivity to drugs (acetaminophen)
Mitochondrial dysfunction
Inhibition of regeneration of injured liver cells
Inhibition of phosphatidylcholine synthesis
Sensititization of Kupffer and Ito cells (via endotoxin?)

Effects of acetaldehyde
Microtubular dysfunction → abnormal vesicular trafficking
Stimulation of collagen synthesis by Ito cells
Formation of acetaldehyde-protein adducts
Reduction in mitochondrial glutathione

NADH, Reduced nicotinamide-adenine dinucleotide.

Table 357-1 Enzyme systems that metabolize alcohol

ENZYME	LOCATION	KINETIC PROPERTIES	VARIANTS
Alcohol dehydrogenases (ADH)	Cytosol	Low Km for ethanol	High Vmax variants (β2 and β3) and high Km (β3) enzymes
Cytochrome P-4502E1	Microsomes	High Km (10 mM) for ethanol	High-activity variant for ethanol in promoter region of gene in Asians
Aldehyde dehydrogenases (ALDH)	Cytosol and mitochondria	Very low Km (μM) for acetaldehyde	Inactive variant common in Asians

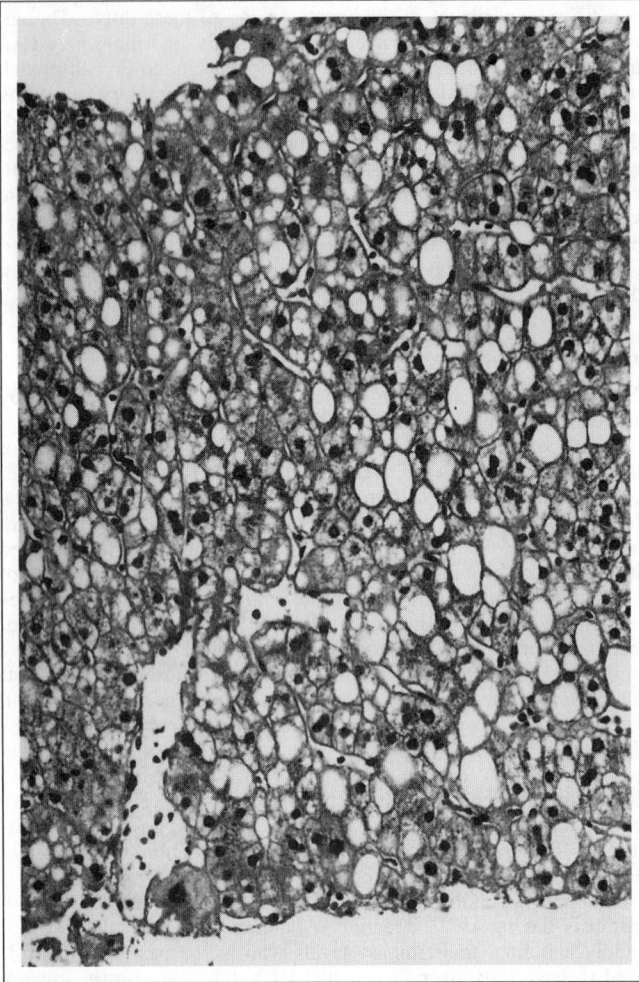

FIGURE 357-2 Alcoholic fatty liver. The hepatocytes are filled with large droplets of triglyceride, obscuring cellular detail and displacing the nuclei peripherally. The large amount of fat in the cells interferes with intrahepatic blood flow and contributes to the hypoxia of the centrilobular zone.

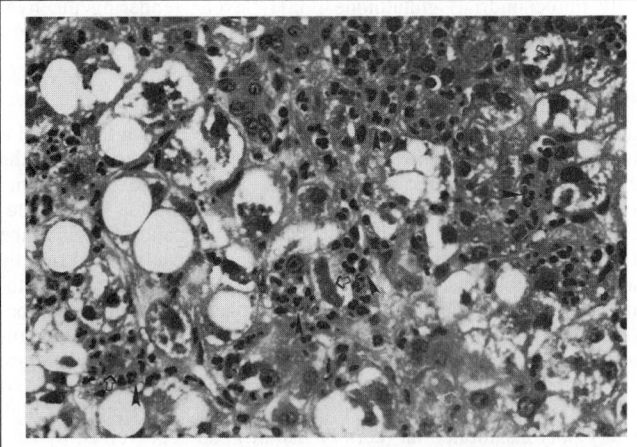

FIGURE 357-3 Alcoholic hepatitis. The liver typically contains macrovesicular fat *(left)* and demonstrates evidence of cell death (ballooning degeneration and the collapse of intermediate filaments to form Mallory's bodies, *open arrows*). In addition, the liver is infiltrated with acute (polymorphonuclear leukocytes, *closed arrow heads*) and chronic (lympohcytes) inflammatory cells. Pericellular fibrosis is present but difficult to discern without connective tissue stains.

may be the end stage of many different processes, the presence of features of alcoholic hepatitis or alcoholic fatty liver may help with the diagnosis. Less common pathologic variants of alcoholic liver disease include microvesicular steatosis and sclerosing hyaline necrosis (extensive inflammation of the pericentral zone with destruction of the the central veins). Patients with typical alcoholic hepatitis combined with features of chronic active hepatitis (expansion of portal tracts with lymphocytes, piecemeal necrosis of adjacent hepatocytes) often are infected with hepatitis B or C viruses.

CLINICAL PRESENTATION AND DIFFERENTIAL DIAGNOSIS
Alcoholic Fatty Liver

Alcoholic fatty liver usually is clinically silent. It may be recognized by the presence of hepatomegaly or by mild abnormalities of liver tests. Such abnormalities should prompt one to consider alcohol abuse if it has not previously been suspected. In alcoholic patients, other causes for liver injury, especially hepatitis C infection and acetaminophen toxicity, should be sought. On hepatic ultrasound, fatty liver appears as nonhomogenous echoes; on computed tomography (CT) scan, low attenuation of the liver suggests the presence of fat. However, neither of these imaging techniques can confidently make the diagnosis of fatty liver because of the many other causes of increased echogenicity of the liver and the frequent coexistence of fatty change

with more severe alcoholic liver disease. The differential diagnosis of fatty liver is shown in Table 357-2.

Alcoholic Hepatitis

Alcoholic hepatitis may also be clinically silent but is more likely than fatty liver to cause symptoms such as fatigue, right upper quadrant discomfort, nausea, or jaundice (Table 357-3). Although many physicians attempt to make the diagnosis of alcoholic hepatitis based merely on abnormal transaminases in an alcoholic patient, this cannot confidently be done without a liver biopsy. The liver is usually enlarged, and the patient may have stigmata of chronic parenchymal liver disease and of portal hypertension. In the more seriously ill patients, jaundice, fever, leukocytosis, ascites, and hepatic encephalopathy are generally present. The transaminases are elevated, often with a greater increase in the SGOT than the SGPT. Although a ratio of SGOT/SGPT over 2 is most common in alcoholic liver disease (occurring in about 70% of patients), it is sometimes seen in other liver diseases, and lower ratios are seen in alcoholic liver disease. The presence of fever, right upper abdominal pain, and leukocytosis will raise the possibility of acute biliary tract disease, necessitating, at the minimum, an ultrasound examination. In the patient without gallstones and no biliary duct dilation, the inflammatory signs and symptoms are attributed to the hepatic inflammation. However, intrahepatic ducts may not dilate in cirrhotic livers, even with obstruction.

Alcoholic Cirrhosis

Alcoholic cirrhosis is clinically indistiguishable from other forms of cirrhosis, except that certain physical examination features (such as parotid gland enlargement and testicular atrophy) are more often associated with alcoholic liver disease than with other causes of cirrhosis. Patients with well-compensated cirrhosis may only exhibit a mildly enlarged liver with minimal abnormalities of the blood liver tests. It is a common misconception that cirrhotic livers are usually small; in the case of actively drinking alcoholics, the cirrhotic liver is usually enlarged by the presence of fat and retained cellular proteins, as well as the increased amount of connective tissue. The frequency of various symptoms and physical examination findings in alcoholic cirrhosis is shown in Table 357-3.

Nonalcoholic Steatohepatitis

There exist patients with histologic liver disease indistiguishable from alcoholic hepatitis with or without cirrhosis, but who do not drink

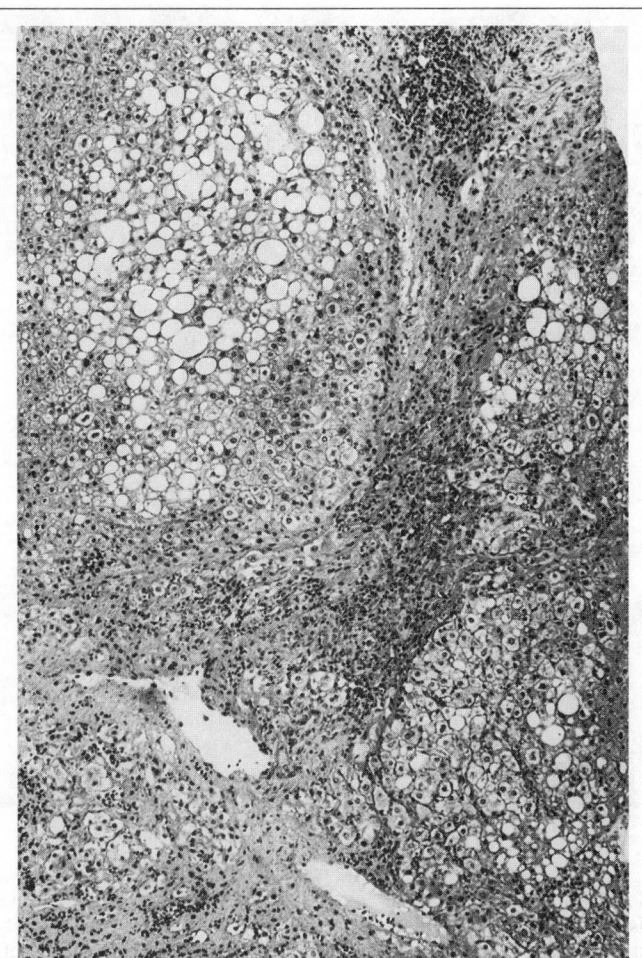

FIGURE 357-4 Alcoholic cirrhosis. The end stage of alcoholic liver injury is cirrhosis. The collagen content of the liver is increased in the form of fibrous bands extending from portal to portal tract or from portal to central vein (middle of photomicrograph), dividing the liver into small nodules. Lobular architecture is distorted, and the central veins may be difficult to identify within the regenerating nodule. If the patient is actively drinking, macrovesicular fat is common (as shown here), and alcoholic hepatitis may also be present.

Table 357-2 Differential diagnosis of fatty liver and steatohepatitis

Macrovesicular fat

Alcohol abuse
Obesity
Hepatitis C
Protein calorie malnutrition
Diabetes mellitus
Wilson's disease
Medications: amiodarone, glucocorticoids, estrogen, methotrexate

Microvesicular fat

Alcoholic foamy degeneration
Acute fatty liver of pregnancy
Reye's syndrome
Medications: tetracycline, valproic acid

Steatohepatitis

Alcohol abuse
Nonalcoholic steatohepatitis (NASH)
   Idiopathic
   Jejunoileal bypass and massive intestinal resection
   Wilson's disease
   Abetalipoproteinemia
   Diabetes mellitus
   Obesity
   Limb lipodystrophy
   Weber-Christian disease
   Parenteral nutrition
   Medications: methotrexate, amiodarone, corticosteroids, high-dose estrogen, nifedipine
      Historical interest: perhexiline maleate, diethylaminoethoxyhexestrol

Table 357-3 Signs and symptoms of alcoholic hepatitis and cirrhosis

	ALCOHOLIC HEPATITIS	CIRRHOSIS
Abdominal pain	50%	25%
Fever	20%-50%	5%-10%
Jaundice	30%-80%	20%
Encephalopathy	20%	—
Hepatomegaly	80%-95%	90%
Evidence of portal hypertension	40%-70%	20%-50%
Upper gastrointestinal bleeding	30%	25%
Stigmata of chronic liver disease	30%-60%	50%

These represent estimates summarized from several clinical series. The frequency of findings in cirrhosis refers to the early clinical features, that is, those present at the time of diagnosis.

heavily. This condition is termed *nonalcoholic steatohepatitis* (NASH). Some cases of cryptogenic cirrhosis may also have originated as NASH. The differential diagnosis of steatohepatitis includes the entities shown in Table 357-2. The most commonly associated entities include obesity, type II diabetes, and glucocorticosteroid use. More recent case series indicate that patients without these features may still have steatohepatitis, and several other drugs are also now implicated.

The pathophysiology of NASH is less well understood than that of alcoholic steatohepatitis. In fact, it is not established whether the fatty liver causes the inflammation or whether an inflammatory insult results in fatty liver, and thus it is best considered a syndrome. It is possible that induction of CYP2E1 is important in this disease, since obesity and ketone bodies (e.g., acetone) induce the enzyme. In addition, the steatohepatitis of jejunoileal bypass may be the result of high levels of portal venous endotoxin. Although HCV can cause fatty change in the liver, it is not a cause of NASH. Of the drugs that can cause NASH (see Table 357-2), some are only of historical interest, but amiodarone is important because of its wide use for cardiac arrhythmias. It causes phospholipidosis, with accumulation of phospholipid lamellae in lysosomes seen at the electron microscopic level. This has been attributed to inhibition of lysosomal phospholipases by amiodarone. It is difficult to discern a common pathophysiologic ba-

sis for these causes of NASH. Perhaps steatohepatitis is a stereotyped response to altered liver lipid metabolism of diverse causes.

The diagnosis of NASH requires a liver biopsy and exclusion of alcohol abuse, so the diagnosis is difficult to make with confidence. It is less likely to cause symptoms than alcoholic hepatitis, and fever, jaundice, ascites, or stigmata of portal hypertension are distinctly unusual. Patients affected typically have either hepatomegaly or abnormal liver tests without stigmata of liver disease. The elevated SGOT/SGPT ratio seen in alcoholic liver disease is not usually present in NASH, and albumin levels less than 3.5 g/dl, prolonged prothrombin times, and increased bilirubin or globulin levels are rare. The radiologic findings are those described for fatty liver and have the same limitations. Fever and leukocytosis are quite uncommon. Because the disorder causes few symptoms, it is common for the biopsy to show more serious liver lesions than anticipated.

Diagnosis of Alcoholism

Because the diagnosis of NASH requires exclusion of alcohol abuse and alcohol consumption is very common, this raises the question of

---

BOX 357-2
The CAGE questionaire

Have you felt you should **C**UT down on your drinking?
Have people **A**NNOYED you by criticizing your drinking?
Have you ever felt bad or **G**UILTY about your drinking?
Have you ever had a drink first thing in the morning to steady your nerves or to get rid of a hangover (**E**YE-OPENER)?

---

the threshold limits for alcoholic liver injury. For men, the safe limit is estimated to be about four drinks (40 g of ethanol) per day. For women, the threshold is lower, about two drinks per day. Thus consumption below these limits probably does not cause liver injury and would not explain the finding of steatohepatitis on the biopsy. The patient and family members should be questioned about quantity and frequency of drinking, as well as whether alcohol is interfering with social, school, family, or work activities. The CAGE test is a simple set of questions that effectively screens for alcohol abuse (Box 357-2). Positive answers to two or more questions suggests alcohol abuse, and additional attempts to establish drinking behavior are warranted. Unfortunately, there is no simple blood test to document alcohol consumption. The determination of the blood level of carbohydrate-deficient transferrin (CDT) is currently the best test for recent heavy alcohol use. The appearance of CDT results from inhibition by ethanol of 2,6-sialyl transferase in the liver. This enzyme adds terminal sialic acid residues to transferrin before it is secreted by the liver. The CDT test is currently not approved for routine clinical use in the United States.

Patient Management

Patients with alcoholic fatty liver may not need to have a liver biopsy performed. If other causes of mild liver test abnormalities are excluded (e.g., drug side effects are excluded; HCV and HBV serologic tests are negative; there are no abnormalities of copper and iron metabolism and no evidence [negative ANA and anti–smooth muscle antibody] of an autoimmune form of hepatitis), the patient's alcohol abuse can be addressed and the liver size and tests can be monitored. Although this approach does not exclude the possibility that there is early alcoholic hepatitis or even cirrhosis, it excludes other treatable diseases and focuses medical attention on keeping the patient sober, which itself promotes longevity.

When alcoholic hepatitis reaches medical attention, it is usually rather severe. These patients are universally malnourished, and one important part of their care is to ensure adequate caloric and protein intake. They generally tolerate protein (e.g., up to 1 g/kg/day) despite the propensity for encephalopathy. Trials of parenteral nutrition or supplementation with amino acids have suggested an improvement in liver function. Therefore good nutrition should be ensured by the oral route, by use of a feeding tube, or by parenteral nutrition. A number of studies have examined the usefulness of corticosteroids in alcoholic hepatitis. Metaanalysis of these trials has suggested that severely ill patients probably benefit. Often the diagnosis cannot be confirmed by biopsy because of coagulopathy (unless a transjugular approach is used). The degree of severity can be estimated from a severity index, developed by Maddrey's group, calculated as the bilirubin + (4.6 × the prolongation in prothrombin time). Scores over 32 indicate a high likelihood of dying from the attack of hepatitis and the need for intervention with steroids. Since clinical laboratories now report the prothrombin time as the INR, it is useful to recall that an INR of 1.7 is approximately the same degree of coagulopathy as a prothrombin time 4 seconds prolonged. An additional indicator of the need for treatment is hepatic encephalopathy not caused by gastrointestinal (GI) bleeding. Patients with GI bleeding, renal failure, or active infection should not be treated because of the risk that the steroids will worsen these problems. Patients are usually given 40 mg of prednisone per day for 30 days, with a rapid taper off the steroids. No other therapy is widely accepted at this time.

Alcoholic cirrhosis is not reversible, but cessation of drinking pro-

✔ **WHEN TO REFER**

The disorder underlying these conditions is alcoholism, a notoriously difficult condition to treat. Most primary care physicians will need to refer alcoholic patients to colleagues skilled in addiction medicine and encourage participation in support activities such as Alcoholics Anonymous. This is clearly required if transplantation is considered. There is a new medication now approved to help control alcohol craving, the opioid antagonist *naltrexone,* that should be used in conjunction with counseling or behavior modification techniques. Patients suspected to have only fatty liver can be managed with abstention from alcohol, serologic evaluation for other causes of liver disease, and follow-up of liver tests over time. Patients with more advanced forms of alcoholic liver disease and those needing a liver biopsy should be referred to a gastroenterologist or hepatologist. Patients with biopsy-proven cirrhosis or clinical findings of advanced liver disease should be considered for transplantation at an early stage. General criteria that will guide the primary care physician are that patients need to be younger than 65; have no significant other medical problems such as heart, renal, or pulmonary disease; not have diabetic complications; have patent hepatic veins and arteries and no evidence for hepatoma; be able to prove abstention with participation in therapy for alcoholism for a least 6 months; and have adequate social support systems. It is far better to refer a patient for evaluation who ultimately is found not be be an eligible candidate than to wait until the patient is quite ill with variceal bleeding, intractable ascites or encephalopathy, or infection, at which point it is unlikely that a liver can be found in time to help the patient. Currently, results of transplantation for alcoholic liver disease are among the best of any indication.

longs life and is an essential prerequisite to liver transplantation if that is contemplated. Two trials are currently underway that may modify the approach to these patients. Colchicine is being examined for its efficacy in cirrhosis (based on earlier long-term studies), and polyunsaturated lecithin is being tested for alcoholic fibrosis, based on studies done with alcohol-fed baboons. Until the results of these studies are known, cirrhotic patients need careful attention to general medical care and nutrition. To minimize protein malnutrition, protein restriction should be instituted only after other measures, such as lactulose, fail to control encephalopathy. In addition, some hepatologists choose to perform endoscopy these patients to assess the presence of varices and then treat with β-blockers if large varices are present. This has been shown to decrease the risk of the first variceal bleed. Patients with ascites should have the ascites fluid examined. Those with low protein levels (less than 1 g/dl) are at increased risk of spontaneous bacterial peritonitis (SBP) because of reduced opsonizing activity in the fluid. Recurrence of SBP can be reduced by prophylactic antibiotics (norfloxin or trimethoprim-sulfamethoxazole), which of course carries with it the risk of promoting bacterial antibiotic resistance.

One additional consideration needs to be emphasized for alcoholic patients. They are highly sensitive to the toxicity of acetaminophen because of the induction of the CYP2E1 enzyme system. Transaminase levels over 300 in alcoholics are rarely caused by alcoholic hepatitis or cirrhosis and, if over 1000, are very commonly caused by recent heavy use of acetaminophen-containing medications (without suicidal intent). Because the drug will have been taken several days before the elevated transaminases are detected, acetaminophen is usually not detected in the blood. These patients need to be warned not to take conventional doses of acetaminophen and to read labels of over-the-counter medications to prevent accidental overdose. Toxicity has been observed with dosages as low as 4 g per 24 hours (only eight extra-strength Tylenol).

There is no proven therapy for NASH aside from surgical revision of a jejunoileal bypass. It seems reasonable to encourage abstention from alcohol and achieving ideal body weight, with particular attention to restricting dietary fat. If the patient is diabetic, close glycemic control may be encouraged, since endogenous synthesis of triglycerides from glucose is a potential source of liver fat. Longitudinal studies have shown spontaneous resolution only rarely, and a minority of patients slowly progress from steatohepatitis to cirrhosis. Nonetheless, they still seem to have fewer problems with complications such as bleeding or ascites than do patients with alcoholic liver disease.

BIBLIOGRAPHY

Adachi Y et al: Inactivation of Kupffer cells prevents early alcohol-induced liver injury, *Hepatology* 20:453-60, 1994.

Bacon BR et al: Nonalcoholic steatohepatitis: an expanded clinical entity, *Gastroenterology* 107:1103-7, 1994.

Behrens U et al: Carbohydrate-deficient transferrin, a marker for chronic ethanol consumption in different ethnic populations: *Alc Clin Exp Res* 12:427-432, 1988.

Cohen JA, Kaplan MM: The SGOT/SGPT ratio: an indicator of alcoholic liver injury, *Dig Dis Sci* 24:835-840, 1979.

Crabb DW: The liver, *Rec Dev Alcohol* 11:207-231, 1993.

Crabb DW: Ethanol oxidizing enzymes: role in ethanol metabolism and alcoholism and alcoholic liver disease, *Prog Liver Dis* 13:151-172, 1995.

Diehl AM, Goodman Z, Ishak KG: Alcohol-like liver disease in nonalcoholics, *Gastroenterology* 95:1056-1062, 1988.

French SW et al: Effect of ethanol on cytochrome P450 (CYP2E1), lipid peroxidation, and serum protein adduct formation in relationship to liver pathology pathogenesis, *Exp Mol Pathol* 58:61-75, 1993.

Friedman SL: The cellular basis of hepatic fibrosis: mechanisms and treatment strategies, *N Engl J Med* 328:1828-1835, 1993.

Hrubec Z, Omenn GS: Evidence of genetic predisposition to alcoholic cirrhosis and psychosis: twin concordances for alcoholism and its biological endpoints by zygosity among male veterans, *Alcohol Clin Exp Res* 5:207-215, 1981.

Imperiale TF, McCullough AJ: Do corticosteroids reduce mortality from alcoholic hepatitis? a metaanalysis of the randomized trials, *Ann Intern Med* 113:299-307, 1990.

Lelbach WK: Cirrhosis in the alcoholic and its relation to the volume of alcohol abuse, *Ann NY Acad Sci* 285:85-105, 1975.

Lieber CS: Alcohol and the liver: 1994 update, *Gastroenterology* 106:1085-1105, 1994.

Lucey MR: Liver transplantation for the alcoholic patient, *Gastroenterol Clin North Am* 22:243-256, 1993.

Marsano L, McClain CJ: Nutrition and alcoholic liver disease, *JPEN* 15:337-344, 1991.

Mayfield D, McLeod G, Hull P: The CAGE questionnaire: validation of a new alcoholism screening instrument, *Am J Psych* 131:1121-1123, 1974.

Seeff LB et al: Acetaminophen toxicity in alcoholics, *Ann Intern Med* 104:399-404, 1986.

CHAPTER

358   Primary Biliary Cirrhosis, Primary Sclerosing Cholangitis, and Other Cholangiopathies

Adil E. Bharucha and Keith D. Lindor

INTRODUCTION

The cholangiopathies are a diverse group of hepatobiliary diseases in which cholangiocytes, or bile duct epithelial cells, are the primary target of pathologic processes. The cholangiopathies include immune-mediated, infectious, genetic or developmental, neoplastic, drug-induced, vascular, and idiopathic conditions.

The structure, function, and gene expression of cholangiocytes vary along the course of the biliary tree. The intrahepatic biliary ductal system is composed of ductules (<50 μm); interlobular ducts (50 to 100 μm); septal ducts (100 to 400 μm); and segmental ducts (400 to 500 μm). The intrahepatic ductal system drains into the extrahepatic ductal system, which ultimately empties into the duodenum. Because the peribiliary capillary plexus is derived exclusively from the hepatic artery, the intrahepatic biliary ductal system is particularly susceptible to ischemic damage.

Newer in vivo and in vitro experimental models have enhanced our understanding of cholangiocyte function. In general, cholangiocytes selectively proliferate in response to a variety of stimuli, participate in hormone-responsive bile formation, contain multiple transport proteins, communicate with each other, and are immunologically active. Cytokines (e.g., interferon-γ; interleukin-1, [IL-1]; interleukin-2 [IL-2]; and tumor necrosis factor–α (TNF-α) induce increased expression of class I major histocompatibility complex (MHC) and aberrant expression of class II MHC and adhesion mol-

ecules on cholangiocytes. Cytokines or cytotoxic T lymphocytes also activate fas, a surface receptor mediating apoptosis expressed by cholangiocytes. Lastly, cytokines induce the expression of adhesion molecules on arteriolar and portal venous endothelial cells. Adhesion molecules promote leukocyte adhesion and transendothelial migration into the portal tracts. These changes render cholangiocytes particularly susceptible to CD8 and CD4 helper T (Th1) cytotoxic T-lymphocyte destruction and confer antigen-presenting cell phenotype and function to cholangiocytes.

PRIMARY BILIARY CIRRHOSIS

Primary biliary cirrhosis (PBC), a chronic cholestatic liver disease of presumed autoimmune origin, is characterized by progressive, nonsuppurative, destructive cholangitis, fibrosis, and eventually cirrhosis with its attendant complications. In secondary biliary cirrhosis, longstanding extrahepatic bile duct obstruction ultimately results in clinical manifestations that are similar to PBC.

Epidemiology and Pathogenesis

PBC is an uncommon disease with an incidence of 5.8 to 15 cases per million per year and an estimated prevalence of 37 to 144 cases per million. The observed geographic differences in disease distribution are probably the result of differences in health care delivery systems rather than true variations in disease occurrence. About 95% of patients with PBC are women; the peak age of onset is between 30 and 65 years. The disease never occurs in childhood but has been reported in asymptomatic elderly individuals. Familial clustering is uncommon. Human leukocyte antigen (HLA) associations with PBC are weaker than those in autoimmune hepatitis or primary sclerosing cholangitis (PSC). In the United States and Europe, HLA DR8 confers a relative risk of PBC of only 2.0 to 3.3, and is present in 11% to 36% of patients. Except for DQB1*0402, which is in linkage disequilibrium with DR8, no DP or DQ associations have been found in whites.

Although the etiology of PBC is unknown, the duct destruction is believed to result from T cell–mediated inflammation. Arguments cited in favor of immune-mediated bile duct destruction include a cytotoxic T-lymphocytic portal infiltrate; several abnormalities in immunologic regulation; and an association with other autoimmune diseases, such as autoimmune thyroiditis, scleroderma, rheumatoid arthritis, and Sjögren's syndrome.

Ninety to ninety-five percent of white patients with PBC have antimitochondrial antibodies (AMAs). Conversely, AMAs are almost always absent in patients with mechanical bile duct obstruction. AMAs are also found in 10% to 30% of patients with autoimmune chronic active hepatitis and occasionally in patients with primary sclerosing cholangitis and drug-induced hepatitis. The anti-M2 antibody, directed against the E2 subunit of enzymes of the 2-oxoacid dehydrogenase complex located on the inner mitochondrial membrane, is the most specific AMA for PBC. Although AMAs inhibit enzyme function in vitro but not in vivo, the relationship between antibodies and ductal destruction is unclear. Nonsuppurative destructive cholangitis appears to be mediated by T cells rather than humoral immune mechanisms. Moreover, the absence of immunoglobulin on the basolateral membranes of biliary epithelial cells is evidence against antibody-mediated biliary epithelial destruction. Lastly, in patients with histologic features of PBC without antimitochondrial antibodies (so-called AMA-negative PBC, or autoimmune cholangitis), the age, gender predilection, disease duration, natural history and biochemical features are similar to those of AMA-positive PBC. Antinuclear (ANA) or anti–smooth muscle antibodies are found in 95% of patients with AMA-negative PBC.

Clinical Features, Natural History, and Associated Conditions

With the widespread use of screening laboratory tests, PBC may be diagnosed at a presymptomatic stage in patients with an elevated alkaline phosphatase of liver origin or with hypercholesterolemia. The serum antimitochondrial antibody is positive, and a liver biopsy, even in patients with minimally elevated alkaline phosphatase, is invariably abnormal and generally consistent with PBC.

The median duration of the presymptomatic phase is 7 years. The early symptoms of PBC, primarily pruritus and fatigue, begin insidiously. Pruritus may at first be localized, occur intermittently, and paradoxically resolve as the disease progresses. Consequences of cholestasis include jaundice, hyperpigmentation, hypercholesterolemia with xanthomas and xanthelasmas, and steatorrhoea with fat-soluble vitamin deficiency (vitamins A, D, E and K). In the United States, osteopenia associated with PBC is almost always caused by osteoporosis rather than osteomalacia. Although approximately 35% of patients with PBC have lumbar spine bone mineral densities below the fracture threshold, the true incidence of spontaneous fractures is not known. The accelerated bone loss in osteoporosis is caused by decreased bone formation rather than increased bone resorption. Ultimately, patients can develop cirrhosis and its complications, such as ascites, variceal bleeding, and encephalopathy. In addition to the autoimmune diseases associated with PBC, patients with PBC may have renal tubular acidosis, possibly related to excess renal copper deposition or an undefined immunologic process, usually asymptomatic pigment gallstones; pulmonary disease such as nodules, interstitial fibrosis, or interstitial giant cell granulomas; and an unexplained susceptibility to urinary tract infections in women.

Laboratory and Other Diagnostic Tests

A cholestatic biochemical pattern, indicated by a threefold to fourfold elevation in the alkaline phosphatase and γ-glutamyltranspeptidase, with normal or minimally elevated aminotransferases, is characteristic for the disease. The absolute values of serum alkaline phosphatase or aminotransferases are of no prognostic significance. Biochemical features of advanced disease are indicative of a poor prognosis and include a high serum bilirubin, low serum albumin, and a prolonged prothrombin time uncorrectable with vitamin K administration. Almost 80% of patients with PBC have hyperlipidemia, with different patterns in early and late disease. In the early stages the rise in serum high-density lipoproteins, some of which are abnormally large, exceeds that of low-density and very-low-density lipoproteins. Conversely, advanced disease is accompanied by markedly elevated low-density lipoproteins, low high-density lipoproteins, and the presence of lipoprotein X—an abnormal lipoprotein found in patients with chronic cholestasis. Patients with PBC do not have a higher risk for complications related to atherosclerotic disease despite extremely high serum cholesterol values. Reduced levels of lipoprotein (a) and the markedly elevated high-density lipoprotein levels during early disease may account for this phenomenon. Although hepatic copper concentrations are elevated in both Wilson's disease and PBC, the serum ceruloplasmin is characteristically elevated in PBC and the high copper level is a consequence rather than a cause of the liver disease.

A liver biopsy demonstrating the florid duct lesion, characterized by the formation of a poorly defined, noncaseating granuloma around, and segmental epithelial degeneration within, small and medium bile ducts is virtually diagnostic of PBC (Fig. 358-1). More frequently, a biopsy in early disease merely reveals ductopenia (defined as the absence of interlobular bile ducts in more than 50% of portal tracts), which may be consistent with either PBC or PSC. In this instance the presence of AMA confirms the diagnosis of PBC. If AMAs are absent, an endoscopic retrograde cholangiopancreatography (ERCP) is necessary to exclude PSC. Histologically, the disease progresses from stage 1 (portal inflammation only) through stages 2 (periportal inflammation, interface hepatitis, small duct proliferation) and 3 (bridging fibrosis) to culminate in stage 4 (cirrhosis).

Differential Diagnosis

Extrahepatic biliary obstruction caused by stones, strictures, or tumors can often be excluded by ultrasonography. Although the clinical, biochemical, and histologic features of hepatic and biliary sarcoidosis resemble PBC, sarcoidosis has a predilection for black males, is always accompanied by extrahepatic, usually pulmonary, manifestations of the disease, and serum AMAs are absent. In patients with drug-induced chronic cholestasis the onset is relatively acute and serum AMAs are absent. Although hepatitis and B and hepatitis C may cause biliary lesions indistinguishable from PBC, biliary granulomas and significant duct loss are unusual. Primary sclerosing cholangitis

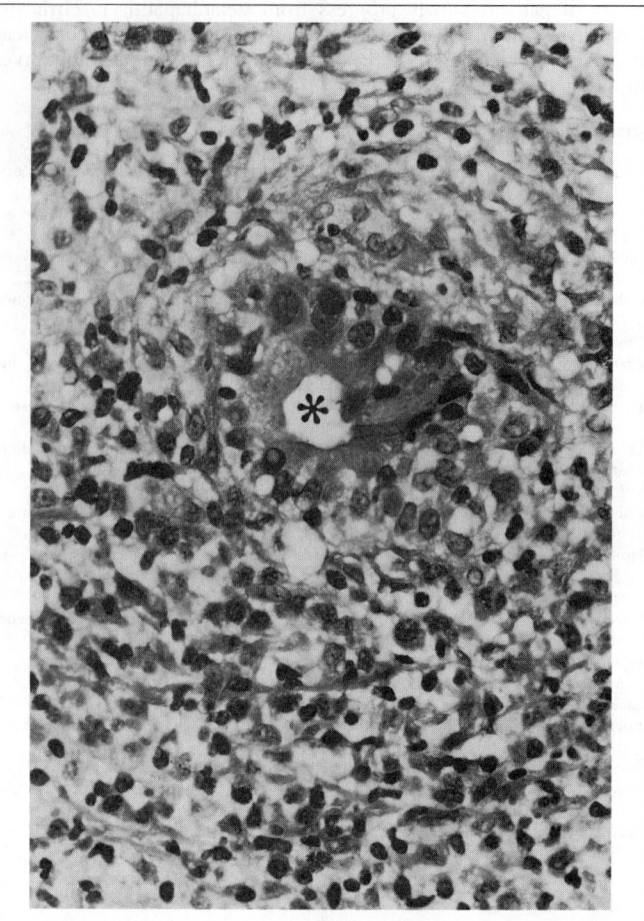

FIGURE 358-1   Needle biopsy specimen from 51-year-old woman with primary biliary cirrhosis. Florid, nonsuppurative, destructive cholangitis; the mixed inflammatory infiltrate obscures the duct outline. The lumen (*) is patent.

favors men with inflammatory bowel disease; serum AMAs are absent; and the cholangiographic findings (discussed later) are diagnostic. In contrast to patients with PBC, patients with autoimmune cholangitis are generally ANA-positive or smooth muscle antibody–positive (titer greater than 1:40) and AMA–negative with normal to borderline elevated serum IgM. Finally, we believe the term *idiopathic adult ductopenia* should be restricted to immunocompetent patients with cholestasis resulting from bile duct injury and loss with no identifiable cause, that is, absence of a history of ulcerative colitis, autoimmune disease, and implicable drug intake; no serum antibodies (ANA, anti–smooth-muscle antibody, AMA); and normal cholangiography.

Management

In contrast to immunosuppressive agents such as corticosteroids, cyclosporine, penicillamine, and methotrexate, ursodeoxycholic acid (UDCA) and colchicine are safe and well tolerated and improve biochemical parameters in PBC. In a study comparing UDCA alone and colchicine alone with placebo, the beneficial effects of UDCA on clinical, biochemical, and histologic findings were superior to those of colchicine. UDCA at a dose of 13 to 15 mg/kg produces a sustained improvement in serum bilirubin and liver enzymes in approximately 50% of patients with PBC; liver biochemistries normalize in approximately 20% of patients. Although patients with biochemically and histologically less severe disease and greater enrichment of biliary bile are more likely to respond to UDCA, patients with advanced PBC should not be excluded from receiving treatment with UDCA. The effects on symptoms and liver histology are difficult to interpret because clinical endpoints such as fatigue and pruritus are subjective

✔ *WHEN TO REFER*

Patients with PBC who do not demonstrate a response to UDCA should be referred to centers conducting trials evaluating newer drugs or combination therapies for PBC. Patients with advanced disease (stage 3 or 4) or indications for liver transplantation (serum bilirubin >8 mg/dl, recurrent variceal bleeding despite banding or sclerotherapy, diuretic-resistant ascites, hepatic encephalopathy, severe pruritus, fatigue, or osteoporosis) should be referred to a liver transplant center. Although the various survival models are useful in estimating survival, they do not take the patient's quality of life into consideration. For instance, patients with severe fatigue, pruritus, or metabolic bone disease may benefit from liver transplantation at an earlier stage of disease.

and influenced by placebo effect, and liver biopsies are subject to problems of sampling error. A combined analysis of data from 3 large multicenter randomized trials suggests that UDCA improved survival free of transplant (defined as time to transplant or death without transplant).

Orthotopic liver transplantation (OLT) is an effective and accepted therapeutic modality for patients with advanced PBC, with 1- and 5-year survivals of 80% to 90% and 60% to 70%, respectively. Clinical indications for liver transplantation include disabling fatigue, intractable pruritus, progressive malnutrition, refractory ascites with or without spontaneous bacterial peritonitis, recurrent or progressive hepatic encephalopathy, variceal bleeding not controlled with sclerotherapy or banding, hypoxemia secondary to the hepatopulmonary syndrome, and the hepatorenal syndrome. Deciding the optimal timing for transplantation is facilitated using survival models for PBC. Although patients with early disease are anticipated to have an excellent survival after transplantation, these patients will also have a reasonable quality of life for extended periods without liver transplantation. Conversely, liver transplantation has a high mortality and morbidity in patients who are bed bound or ventilator dependent or who develop either sepsis or the hepatorenal syndrome before liver transplantation.

Although both UDCA and the nonabsorbed resin *cholestyramine* relieve pruritus, the antihistamines are rarely helpful. Depending on the severity of pruritus, from 4 to 24 g of cholestyramine daily may be required, given in 4-g doses with meals. Pruritus refractory to UDCA and cholestyramine may respond to Rifampin in a dose of 300 mg twice daily.

Although controlled studies in PBC are lacking, the evidence in postmenopausal women and a retrospective study in PBC suggest that low-dose estrogens may slow the rate of bone loss without worsening cholestasis. Because hypercholesterolemia does not increase the risk for atherosclerotic vascular disease in PBC, no treatment is necessary. Lastly, patients with advanced liver disease and significant steatorrhoea may develop fat-soluble vitamin deficiencies. Vitamin D deficiency as evidenced by low serum 25 (OH) D2 levels is correctable with 50,000 IU of vitamin D given once a week. Vitamin A deficiency is uncommon, may present as night blindness, can be documented with low serum vitamin A levels, and is treated with 25,000 to 50,000 IU two to three times per week. Because excessive vitamin A replacement is associated with hepatotoxicity, serum levels should be repeated after several months of therapy. If the prothrombin time is prolonged, replacement with water-soluble vitamin K at 5 mg/day should be instituted, and continued if the prothrombin time improves. Vitamin E deficiency occurs rarely in PBC. Typically, vitamin E deficiency is associated with posterior column involvement, areflexia, loss of proprioception, or ataxia. However, the response to oral or parenteral vitamin E supplementation is poor.

PRIMARY SCLEROSING CHOLANGITIS

Primary sclerosing cholangitis (PSC)—which is characterized by progressive inflammation, destruction, and fibrosis of intrahepatic and extrahepatic bile ducts—predominantly afflicts young men with inflammatory bowel disease.

Epidemiology and Pathogenesis

Seventy percent of patients are men, 70% have coexistent inflammatory bowel disease, and the average age at diagnosis is 40 years. In contrast, only 2.5% to 7% of patients who present with ulcerative colitis will have or develop PSC. A recent increase in the incidence of PSC is probably attributable to an enhanced awareness of the disease; routine screening with biochemical liver tests, especially in patients with ulcerative colitis; and the widespread availability of ERCP. HLA haplotypes associated with PSC include HLA B8, DR3, and DR52a; the first two haplotypes are not increased in chronic ulcerative colitis. HLA DR3 and HLA DR2 are associated with high and low levels of tumor necrosis factor–α (TNF-α) production, respectively. In HLA DR3–negative patients, there is an independent association with HLA DR2. The HLA DR4 haplotype is underrepresented in PSC when compared with healthy controls, consequent to the increased frequency of the HLA DR2 and DR3 alleles. Patients with HLA DR4 may be prone to more rapid disease progression.

The pathogenesis of PSC is uncertain. Experimentally, cholangitis can be induced by immunizing rodents with syngeneic or allogeneic cholangiocytes. Further, adoptive transfer with splenic lymphocytes from cholangiocyte-immunized animals has been shown to induce cholangitis in naive rats. Patients with PSC, but not other cholestatic disorders, have a serum antibody directed against a shared epitope on biliary and colonic epithelial cells. Another hypothesis based on similarities between PSC and the hepatobiliary abnormalities in a genetically susceptible rat model with experimental small-bowel bacterial overgrowth suggests that absorption of bacterial cell-wall products, primarily peptidoglycan-polysaccharide (PG-PS), across a leaky intestinal membrane activates Kupffer's cells to produce cytokines, including TNF-α. These cytokines may cause hepatobiliary inflammation.

Clinical Features and Natural History

Most patients with PSC are asymptomatic or have minimal symptoms such as pruritus or fatigue at diagnosis. Only 10% to 15% of patients have bacterial cholangitis, as evidenced by episodes of fever and abdominal pain, with or without jaundice, at presentation. PSC generally runs a progressive course resulting in biliary fibrosis, cirrhosis with portal hypertension, and premature death from liver failure. Although the natural history of PSC is not as well understood as that of PBC, the median survival from diagnosis ranges from 9 to 11 years. Asymptomatic patients live longer than patients who were symptomatic at diagnosis. The new Mayo model for PSC contains five variables—namely, age, serum bilirubin, blood hemoglobin concentration, hepatic histologic stage, and splenomegaly—that can be used to estimate survival at any point in the disease course. A shortcoming is that the PSC model does not take into account the risk of developing a cholangiocarcinoma.

The specific complications of PSC are bacterial cholangitis, gallbladder and biliary stones, dominant bile duct strictures, and cholangiocarcinoma. Bacterial cholangitis occurs more frequently in patients who have had previous biliary surgery or developed a dominant biliary stricture. Patients with bacterial cholangitis may have only right upper quadrant pain; fever; or a sudden deterioration in liver biochemistries attributable to back pressure resulting from biliary strictures, debris, and/or stones. In addition to antibiotic coverage, patients with suspected bacterial cholangitis merit endoscopic removal of debris, cytologic brushing, and dilatation of strictures. Biliary operations have a limited role in PSC because they increase the risk of strictures and bacterial cholangitis and may compromise OLT. A selected group of noncirrhotic PSC patients with benign dominant extrahepatic strictures may benefit from biliary-enteric bypass. Long-term prophylactic antibiotic coverage with ciprofloxacin may be beneficial in preventing recurrent bouts of cholangitis. In patients with PSC, cholelithiasis and choledocholithiasis may be difficult to diagnose.

Cholangiocarcinoma, which occurs in 5% to 15% of patients with PSC, often presents as a clinical deterioration (recent weight loss, rapid increase in serum bilirubin); is associated with a poor prognosis; and, except in the setting of experimental protocols, generally precludes OLT. Abdominal ultrasound and computed tomography (CT) are insensitive in diagnosing early cholangiocarcinoma. Although ERCP frequently demonstrates a dominant stricture, the distinction between benign and malignant strictures is difficult. Tumor markers such as carcinoembryonic antigen (CEA) and carbohydrate antigen 19-9 (CA 19-9) may be of value in detecting cholangiocarcinoma in patients with PSC, although detecting tumors at a resectable stage is difficult.

Laboratory Diagnosis

Almost all patients have an elevated serum alkaline phosphatase level, usually greater than five times normal. Similarly, a majority display mild elevations in serum aminotransferases. Bilirubin levels may fluctuate but increase with disease progression. In early disease the serum albumin is normal unless patients have active inflammatory bowel disease. As in other cholestatic diseases, levels of urinary and serum copper and the serum ceruloplasmin level are increased.

Eighty percent of patients with PSC, with or without ulcerative colitis, have perinuclear antineutrophilic cytoplasmic antibodies (pANCA). The antigenic target for pANCA is unknown. pANCA are of limited value in distinguishing PSC from other causes of chronic liver disease, since they are also found in patients with autoimmune hepatitis, primary biliary cirrhosis, and chronic viral hepatitis. Hypergammaglobulinemia, increased IgM levels, antinuclear antibodies, and anti–smooth muscle antibodies are less frequent in PSC than in autoimmune chronic active hepatitis or primary biliary cirrhosis.

In the absence of extrahepatic obstruction or secondary sclerosing cholangitis, the cholangiographic findings of bile duct stricture with or without dilatation are the diagnostic hallmark of PSC (Fig. 358-2). Sclerosing cholangitis of secondary origin has been reported with choledocholithiasis or previous biliary tract surgery, floxuridine administration, acquired immunodeficiency syndrome, and histiocytosis. Rarely, conditions such as lymphoma, cholangiocarcinoma, hepatocellular carcinoma, amyloidosis, polycystic disease of the liver, intrahepatic thrombosis, and advanced cirrhosis may involve intrahepatic ducts and cause cholangiographic abnormalities that resemble PSC. "Small-duct PSC" refers to a small minority of inflammatory bowel disease patients with disease limited to the small intrahepatic ducts, identifiable on biopsy but not cholangiograms.

The commonest pathologic findings in PSC are periductal fibrosis and inflammation and bile duct proliferation alternating with ductal obliteration and ductopenia. The classic onion-skin lesion is virtually pathognomonic of PSC but is uncommonly seen (Fig. 358-3).

Differential Diagnosis

Differential diagnosis includes PBC, drug-induced cholestasis, idiopathic adulthood ductopenia, cholestatic alcoholic hepatitis, and cholestatic viral hepatitis. Other conditions with cholangiographic abnormalities that may mimic PSC include extrahepatic obstruction from stones; surgical strictures or tumors (cholangiocarcinoma, metastatic adenocarcinoma, lymphoma); hepatic arterial floxuridine infusion orchemoembolization; bile duct irradiation; and, increasingly, AIDS cholangiopathy.

Management

Drugs such as D-penicillamine, colchicine, azathioprine, methotrexate, cyclosporine, and corticosteroids do not benefit patients with PSC. Although uncontrolled studies suggest that ursodeoxycholic acid improves biochemical parameters in PSC, final recommendations must await the results of controlled trials. Endoscopic balloon dilatation and stenting may alleviate symptoms in patients with biliary strictures but do not influence the natural history of the disease. Liver transplantation is the treatment of choice for patients with advanced disease. The clinical indications for liver transplantation and the application of survival models are, in general, similar for PSC and PBC. One- and three-year survivals after liver transplantation for PSC are 85% and 75%, respectively.

VIRAL CHOLANGITIS

In adults, viral cholangitis occurs in two distinct settings. Chronic hepatitis C and, less frequently, hepatitis B may be associated with portal lymphocytic aggregates or intraepithelial lymphocytic infiltration, generally causing mild and focal damage of ducts 50 to 70 μm

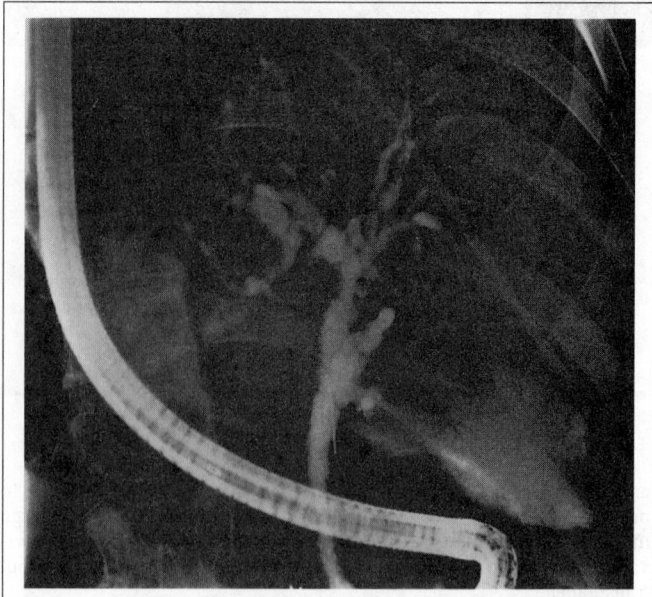

FIGURE 358-2 Retrograde cholangiogram showing typical features of primary sclerosing cholangitis (PSC). The intrahepatic and extrahepatic ducts are irregular and display multifocal strictures, dilatations, and outpouchings.

in diameter. In contrast to PBC, ductopenia and chronic cholestasis are extremely rare.

In AIDS, biliary disease is less common than hepatitis but is being recognized with increasing frequency. Pathologic and microbiologic examinations of multiple ampullary, duodenal, and biliary aspirates and biopsy specimens demonstrate another infectious organism—commonly cytomegalovirus (CMV), *Cryptosporidium* sp., *Mycobacterium avium,* or microsporidian—or a tumor such as Kaposi's sarcoma or lymphoma in as many as 70% of patients. Because some organisms such as *Cryptosporidium* spp. have not been proven to be cytopathic, the significance of isolating them is questionable. The human immunodeficiency virus (HIV) has not been localized to biliary epithelium. More than 85% of patients with AIDS cholangiopathy present with right upper quadrant pain. The remainder have fever, jaundice, and abnormal biochemical liver tests, notably alkaline phosphatase. The mean serum transaminase is usually less than 100 U/L and the serum bilirubin normal or mildly elevated. Although the abdominal ultrasound and CT scan frequently demonstrate abnormalities such as dilated intrahepatic or extrahepatic ducts, thickening of the bile duct wall, and distal tapering of the common bile duct, ERCP is necessary to make the diagnosis. Moreover, noninvasive studies are normal in nearly one third of patients with abnormal bile ducts at ERCP. More than 50% of patients with AIDS cholangiopathy have a combination of papillary stenosis and sclerosing cholangitis. The remainder have either papillary stenosis, sclerosing cholangitis, or a long extrahepatic duct stricture. A marked improvement in pain, but not biochemical parameters of liver function, has been noted after endoscopic sphincterotomy in patients with moderate to severe right upper quadrant pain and papillary stenosis. Other unproven treatments include balloon dilatation and/or stent placement for bile duct obstruction, chemotherapy for patients with Kaposi's sarcoma or lymphoma involving the bile duct, and ganciclovir for CMV.

DRUG-INDUCED AND TOXIC CHOLANGITIS

The bland cholestasis characteristic of oral contraceptives and anabolic steroids, as well as cholestasis with hepatitis caused by chlorpromazine and erythromycin, are discussed in other chapters; this section will focus on drug-induced cholestasis with bile duct injury and chronic cholestasis.

Drug-induced cholestasis with bile duct injury is unusual and characterized histologically by acute mixed-cell inflammatory destruction of the bile ductules (cholangiolitis) or bile ducts (cholangitis), occa-

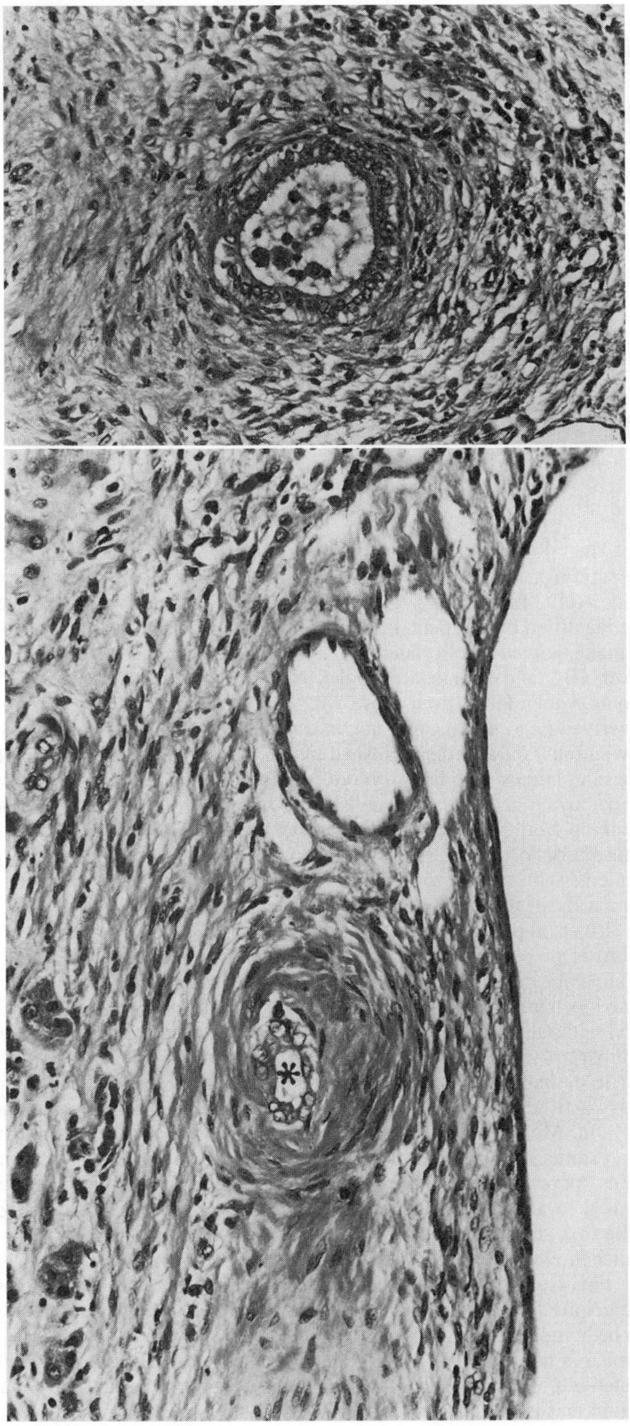

FIGURE 358-3   A, Fibrous cholangitis with concentric periductal fibrosis and mixed inflammatory infiltrates. Note cellular debris in lumen. **B,** Fibrous-obliterative cholangitis. The lumen(*) is markedly narrowed.

sionally accompanied by ductular proliferation. Ampicillin, barbiturates, carbamazepine, dextropropoxyphene, hydralazine, phenothiazines, phenytoin, and quinidine have been implicated in this pattern of injury. In 1965, toxic contamination by aromatic amines of flour used in baking bread was responsible for the outbreak of jaundice in Epping, England. Although patients usually present with jaundice and pruritus, other symptoms such as fever, abdominal pain, and tender hepatomegaly mimic extrahepatic bile duct obstruction. Because the histologic findings may be identical to those of biliary obstruction, an awareness of this entity may prevent unnecessary cholangiogra-

✔ WHEN TO REFER

Ideally, patients with PSC should be referred to a medical center for enrollment into therapeutic trials. Patients with complications such as new-onset jaundice or symptomatic deterioration in cholangitis should be referred to a specialist for consideration of endoscopic cholangiography. Patients with advanced disease should be referred to a liver transplantation center for evaluation.

phy or surgery. Although the outcome of drug-induced bile-duct injury is unknown, limited experience suggests that a few patients with severe cholangitis develop ductopenia.

Drug-induced chronic cholestasis is diagnosed when alterations in biochemical liver tests, primarily alkaline phosphatase or bilirubin, persist for 6 months or longer after the presumed offending agent is discontinued. Drug-induced chronic cholestasis in association with ductopenia, the vanishing duct syndrome, has been reported with the phenothiazines, tricyclic antidepressants, erythromycin, cotrimoxazole, tetracycline, and phenytoin. Fortunately, most patients with ductopenia recover completely or have biochemical cholestasis without jaundice. A few patients may have continuing jaundice or, rarely, develop biliary cirrhosis with portal hypertension.

ISCHEMIC CHOLANGITIS

Ischemic cholangitis is most frequently recognized to occur after liver transplantation and in patients who undergo hepatic arterial chemoembolization or receive infusions of floxuridine, an antineoplastic agent. Cholangiography reveals multiple, segmental, nonanastomotic strictures and dilatations. The management of ischemic cholangitis is similar to that for primary or secondary sclerosing cholangitis.

BIBLIOGRAPHY

Harnois DM, Lindor KD: Primary sclerosing cholangitis, *Dig Dis* (in press).
Hay E: Bone disease in cholestatic liver disease, *Gastroenterology* 108:276-283, 1995.
King PD, Blitzer BL: Drug-induced cholestasis: pathogenesis and clinical features, *Semin Liver Dis* 10:316-321, 1990.
Laurin JM, Lindor KD: Primary biliary cirrhosis, *Dig Dis* 12:331-350, 1994.
Lim AG, Jazrawi RP, Northfield TC: The ursodeoxycholic acid story in primary biliary cirrhosis, *Gut* 37:301-4, 1995.
Ludwig J et al: Chronic cholestasis in a young man, *Hepatology* 20:1351-1355, 1994.
Nakanuma Y et al: Pathology and immunopathology of primary biliary cirrhosis with emphasis on bile duct lesions: recent progress, *Semin Liver Dis* 15:313-328, 1995.
Roberts SK, LaRusso NF: Pathobiology of biliary epithelia, *Curr Opin Gastroenterol* 10:526-533, 1994.
Wiesner RH: Current concepts in primary sclerosing cholangitis, *Mayo Clin Proc* 69:969-982, 1994.

CHAPTER

359   Hemochromatosis, Wilson's Disease, and Other Genetic Liver Diseases Affecting the Adult

Kris V. Kowdley and Anthony S. Tavill

HEREDITARY HEMOCHROMATOSIS
Physiology and Pathophysiology

Hereditary hemochromatosis (HHC) is the most common genetic disease in white persons of Northern Hemisphere descent (Table 359-1). The disorder is inherited in an autosomal recessive pattern; the gene frequency is estimated to be approximately 1:20, and the frequency of homozygosity is reported to range from 1:250 to

Table 359-1 Genetic disorders leading to liver disease in the adult

DISEASE	ESTIMATED HETEROZYGOTE FREQUENCY	DIAGNOSTIC TESTS	EXTRAHEPATIC MANIFESTATIONS	TREATMENT
Hereditary hemochromatosis	1 in 8	Serum iron studies Hepatic iron concentration Hepatic iron index	Diabetes mellitus Congestive heart failure Arthritis Hypogonadism Hyperpigmentation	Phlebotomy Liver transplantation
Wilson's disease	1 in 90	Serum ceruloplasmin 24-hour urinary copper Hepatic copper concentration Slit-lamp exam for Kayser-Fleischer rings	Neuropsychiatric changes Kayser-Fleischer rings Renal tubular dysfunction Autonomic dysfunction Arthritis	D-Penicillamine Trientine Zinc salts Liver transplantation
α_1-Antitrypsin deficiency	1 in 23	α_1-antitrypsin level α_1-antitrypsin phenotype Liver biopsy for PAS-positive globules	Emphysema at early age	Liver transplantation Replacement α_1-antitrypsin therapy for lung disease

Modified from Tung B, Kowdley KV: Inherited liver diseases affecting the adult, *The Gastroenterologist* 4:245-261, 1996.

1:700. The pathophysiology of the disease is related to increased iron absorption in the proximal small intestine, leading to excessive iron deposition in the liver, heart, pancreas, skin, and joints, leading to end-organ damage.

Regulation of iron absorption in normal persons is at the level of the small intestine. In the presence of iron deficiency, decreased small-bowel mucosal ferritin expression and up-regulation of transferrin receptor expression are observed, leading to increased iron absorption. After iron repletion, mucosal ferritin stores increase and transferrin receptor expression is down-regulated, leading to a decrease in iron absorption. In persons with HHC this regulation is lost; despite increased iron stores, mucosal ferritin levels are low and transferrin receptor expression is high in the intestine, and excessive absorption of dietary iron is observed.

Hepatic iron deposition in HHC is localized primarily to the hepatocytes and biliary epithelial cells; iron-induced cytotoxicity leads to fibrosis, cirrhosis, liver failure, and hepatocellular carcinoma. Iron deposition in the heart results in a restrictive cardiomyopathy and congestive heart failure. Diabetes mellitus and joint disease related to pancreatic and articular iron deposition may also occur.

Genetics

The gene for HLA-linked HHC had previously been localized to the short arm of chromosome 6. A homozygous mutation in gene (HFE) that codes for an HLA class-I–like protein has been recently identified in more than 80% of homozygous HHC patients of Northern European descent. This mutation (C282Y) results in a cystine-to-tyrosine substitution at amino acid 282 of the HFE gene product. A second mutation (H63D), which results in a histidine-to-aspartic acid substitution at amino acid 63, has also been identified. Approximately 5% of patients who on phenotyping appeared to have HHC were compound heterozygotes (heterozygous for C282Y and H63D) in Feder's study. However, the clinical significance of the H63D mutation in HHC is unclear since this mutation is present in 7% of the general population.

Laboratory and Other Diagnostic Tests

Serum iron studies are generally the first diagnostic tests used to screen for HHC. These include serum iron and TIBC, which are used to calculate the percentage saturation (Fe/TIBC), and serum ferritin. Several large studies have examined the role of serum markers of iron status to screen for HHC. A fasting serum transferrin iron saturation ≥60% (in men) or ≥50% (in women) is sensitive in identifying asymptomatic persons with HHC. If the serum ferritin is also elevated, further evaluation is appropriate. Because both increased serum iron and decreased TIBC may be observed in advanced liver disease, these criteria may not be reliable in distinguishing HHC patients with established liver disease from patients with liver diseases from other causes.

The "gold standard" for the diagnosis of HHC is measurement of hepatic iron concentration (HIC) and calculation of the hepatic iron index (HIC [in μmol/g]/age [in years]). Homozygotes with HHC can be identified by a hepatic iron index ≥1.9, whereas heterozygotes and patients with alcoholic siderosis have a hepatic iron index ≤1.9. However, HIC and hepatic iron index cannot differentiate patients with homozygous HHC from those with certain forms of secondary iron overload (e.g., thalassemia major, transfusional iron overload). These two groups may be distinguished by the pattern of hepatic iron staining. In patients with homozygous HHC the iron is found primarily in hepatocytes and bile duct cells, with a decreasing gradient of iron staining from hepatocytes in the portal areas of the hepatic lobule to those around the central veins (zone 1 > zone 3 of Rappaport); in patients with certain forms of secondary iron overload, iron is found primarily in reticuloendothelial (Kupffer's) cells.

Liver biopsy is also essential for prognosis in HHC. Patients with fibrosis or cirrhosis have a significantly decreased life expectancy compared with those without established liver disease. Because routine biochemical tests cannot reliably differentiate between those with and without fibrosis, liver biopsy is needed for staging the degree of fibrosis.

In patients in whom the diagnosis is equivocal even after liver biopsy and hepatic iron measurement, quantitative phlebotomy can be helpful. Most homozygotes with symptomatic HHC have total body iron stores of more than 20 grams. Because each unit of blood contains approximately 250 mg of iron, the number of phlebotomies required to achieve iron deficiency can be used to calculate mobilizable iron stores. Patients who become iron deficient after only a few phlebotomies are unlikely to be homozygotes.

Finally, in first-degree relatives of HHC patients, HLA typing can be helpful. Those who share both HLA A and B haplotypes are likely to be homozygous and can be expected to develop iron overload. HLA typing is not useful for population screening or as a diagnostic test in putative probands, since it is frequently present in the normal population and is not always present in HHC homozygotes.

Diagnosis

This identification of putative HFE gene will likely have a significant impact on diagnostic testing for HHC. However, there remain many unanswered questions regarding genetic testing for HHC that preclude sole use of this test as a "gold standard" for diagnosis. First, the C282Y mutation may be insensitive for identifying patients with phenotypic evidence of HHC since it may be absent in 20% to 30% of apparent HHC patients. Second, some patients who appear phenotypically homozygous may not manifest iron overload. Therefore, most experts would agree that serum transferrin-iron saturation, ferritin levels, and liver biopsy should be used to diagnose HHC in index patients. Genotyping may be adequate for confirming the diagnosis of siblings of probands in the absence of abnormal LFTs or significant iron overload (i.e., serum ferritin <500 ng/ml). Liver biopsy

✔ *WHEN TO REFER*

Any patient with a confirmed elevation of serum transferrin iron saturation (≥60% in males, ≥50% in females) and elevated serum ferritin should be referred for evaluation of end-organ involvement and consideration of liver biopsy. Patients with elevated serum transferrin iron saturation but normal serum ferritin level may be followed with repeat determinations on a biannual basis and referred for further evaluation if serum ferritin becomes elevated. HLA-A and B identical first-degree relatives of probands should also be referred for evaluation of possible homozygosity for HHC. Genotyping may also have a role in screening family members of C282Y homozygous HHC patients.

remains important in current clinical practice for diagnosis of HHC and determination of whether cirrhosis is present.

Differential Diagnosis

The diagnosis of HHC can be straightforward in asymptomatic persons with elevated serum iron studies and characteristic liver biopsy findings. However, it is always important to exclude secondary causes for iron overload, such as increased red cell turnover associated with ineffective erythropoiesis, or transfusional iron overload. Furthermore, serum iron studies may falsely suggest HHC in patients with advanced liver disease, particularly when associated with excessive alcohol intake or chronic viral hepatitis. Measurement of HIC and calculation of hepatic iron index is crucial in this setting to confirm the diagnosis of homozygous HHC. Some African patients who chronically consume beer brewed in steel drums may develop a syndrome resembling homozygous HHC, although recent data suggest that a non–HLA-linked primary disorder of iron loading may be present in some African populations.

Management

The mainstay of management of iron reduction is phlebotomy. Iron reduction prior to the development of hepatic fibrosis may improve survival in HHC. Patients identified prior to the development of fibrosis who are compliant with phlebotomy can enjoy normal life expectancy, whereas survival is significantly diminished in those in whom fibrosis or cirrhosis has already occurred. The therapeutic goals are to reduce the serum transferrin-iron saturation to ≤15% and serum ferritin to ≤50 ng/ml. Phlebotomies are generally performed weekly or occasionally twice weekly early during treatment. Because many patients have >20 grams of body iron, initial iron reduction may take up to 1 to 2 years. Once patients have been iron depleted, periodic monitoring of serum ferritin and phlebotomy 3 to 5 times per year is adequate.

There is probably minimal benefit in limiting the intake of iron-rich foods such as red meat; however, patients should be advised to avoid iron supplements and to limit the intake of vitamin C, which can increase iron absorption to an even greater degree in HHC patients. Patients should also significantly curtail the intake of alcohol, which can increase iron absorption, as well as accelerate the development of hepatic fibrosis.

There are studies in European patients with HHC that suggest a higher prevalence of chronic viral hepatitis. Therefore it is probably advisable to screen HHC patients for chronic hepatitis, particularly if serum liver biochemical tests are elevated. Patients with established cirrhosis should be followed closely because of a significantly increased risk of hepatocellular carcinoma. The most common screening methods employ periodic hepatic ultrasonography and measurement of serum α-fetoprotein levels.

Liver transplantation for HHC-related end-stage liver disease is disappointing. One-year survival after liver transplantation for HHC is only around 50%; despite a high prevalence of primary liver cancer, increased mortality appears to be the result of sepsis and cardiac complications.

WILSON'S DISEASE
Physiology and Pathophysiology

Wilson's disease is characterized by a defect in copper transport, leading to toxic accumulation of copper in brain, liver, skin, kidney, and the skeletal system. The disease is inherited in an autosomal recessive pattern, and the gene has been localized to chromosome 13. The frequency of homozygosity is estimated to be 1:30,000, and for the asymptomatic heterozygous carrier state it is estimated to be 1:90. The clinical manifestations of the disease are caused by copper overload in various tissues.

Under normal circumstances, regulation of copper metabolism is maintained via biliary excretion, which is the major route of elimination of copper. The defect in the copper transport process across the biliary canaliculus results in failure of biliary copper excretion and accumulation of copper in hepatocytes and other tissues as hepatic storage capacity is saturated.

Hepatic manifestations of Wilson's disease are highly variable. Patients may present with asymptomatic hepatomegaly, acute fulminant hepatitis, chronic active hepatitis, or with evidence of cirrhosis and portal hypertension, or neurologic manifestations. The earliest pathologic finding in Wilson's disease is fatty change in parenchymal liver cells and glycogenated nuclei. Gradually there is progression to chronic hepatitis and cirrhosis.

Patients with Wilson's disease often have associated extrahepatic manifestations. Neurologic manifestations include motor abnormalities such as speech abnormalities, involuntary movements, ataxia, or spasticity; patients may also present with psychiatric symptoms and signs. A Coombs' test–negative hemolytic anemia may be present, often in patients with acute hepatitis. Renal tubular dysfunction caused by copper deposition in tubules can result in a distal renal tubular acidosis and excess urinary spillage of phosphate, urate, calcium, and bicarbonate. Renal osteodystrophy and stone formation may occur as a result of hypercalciuria.

Laboratory and Other Diagnostic Tests

The classic physical findings in Wilson's disease are Kayser-Fleischer rings. These are fine copper deposits in Descemet's membrane in the cornea visible by slit-lamp examination. Sunflower cataracts resulting from copper deposits in the anterior and posterior lens capsule may also occur. It is important to remember that Kayser-Fleischer rings may be seen in other liver disorders, such as primary biliary cirrhosis, in which copper excretion is impaired as a result of loss of bile ducts. The serum ceruloplasmin level is low (<20 mg/dl in as many as 95% of patients). Ceruloplasmin in the serum can act as an acute-phase reactant and therefore may occasionally be increased to approximately normal levels; however, elevated ceruloplasmin levels are not usually seen even under these circumstances in Wilson's disease. Furthermore, a minority of heterozygotes may have serum ceruloplasmin levels below 20 mg/dl, although this is observed only in 15% of patients. The "gold standard" is liver biopsy and measurement of hepatic copper concentration. Normal hepatic copper concentration is ≤50 μg/gram dry weight; patients with Wilson's disease generally have hepatic copper concentrations greater than 250 μg/gram. If there is question about the diagnosis or if liver biopsy cannot be performed, quantitative urinary copper excretion can be diagnostic. Normal urinary excretion of copper in 24 hours is less than 20 to 40 μg; patients with Wilson's disease have urinary copper levels ≥100 μg. Patients with Wilson's disease also have increased excretion of copper after oral D-penicillamine, whereas unaffected persons do not. Plasma copper levels are generally not performed in routine clinical practice for the diagnosis of Wilson's disease, although the free (non-ceruloplasmin) serum copper is increased and may be a helpful measurement in those homozygotes with normal ceruloplasmin levels.

Management

Drug therapy to chelate and mobilize excess body copper stores or limit copper absorption is the main form of treatment. Reduction or elimination of copper-rich foods such as liver, shellfish, nuts, and chocolate is reasonable but not adequate; lifelong therapy with copper-chelating agents is required. The two chelators available in clinical practice are D-penicillamine and triethyl tetramine (trien or trientene). These agents increase urinary excretion of free copper and result in net cupriuresis, improvement of symptoms, and reduction of hepatic and central nervous system (CNS) copper concentrations. The usual dosage of D-penicillamine is 1 to 2 grams a day four times daily. Pyridoxine, 25 mg daily, is also given to counteract D-penicillamine's antipyridoxine effects. Adverse reactions to D-penicillamine occur in as many as 20% of patients and include fever, rash, lymphadenopathy, and cytopenias. Lower initial doses may reduce allergic symptoms, and patients can often be desensitized to these reactions. More uncommon but potentially more serious are adverse effects such as nephrotic syndrome, myasthenia, or arthralgias. Patients who develop these complications can be treated with triethyl tetramine (trien), which is another copper-chelating agent currently approved by the FDA for treatment. Compliance with medical therapy may be a problem, particularly in younger patients, and must be emphasized. There are numerous reports of patients with liver failure and death caused by late noncompliance.

An additional therapy for Wilson's disease is elemental zinc. Orally administered zinc competes with copper for intestinal absorption and reduces copper stores by this mechanism. Dosages of 75 to 300 mg a day have been reported to improve neurologic symptoms and maintain remission in patients with Wilson's disease, but some authors have questioned the efficacy of zinc therapy. Zinc therapy may be most useful in asymptomatic patients with early disease or those who have already been copper depleted with a chelating agent.

Liver transplantation is an effective therapy for both fulminant and chronic liver failure caused by Wilson's disease. Because the genetic defect is expressed phenotypically in the liver, liver transplantation effectively cures the disease.

α_1-ANTITRYPSIN DEFICIENCY
Physiology and Pathophysiology

α_1-Antitrypsin (α_1-AT) deficiency, the leading cause of genetic liver disease in children, was first described in 1968 by Freier and co-workers. The disease can be a cause of chronic hepatitis, cirrhosis, and hepatocellular carcinoma in adults.

The gene for α_1-AT has been localized to q31 to q32.2 on chromosome 14. There are more than 100 alleles for the α_1-AT gene, which code for a variety of monomeric glycoproteins with varying amino acid sequences and carbohydrate side chains. These variants of α_1-AT are classified alphabetically according to phenotype (Pi) on the basis of electrophoretic migration pattern on agarose gels from low to high isoelectric points. Variants can be classified as "normal," "deficient," or "dysfunctional" based on the level and activity of α_1-AT. The most common normal variant is the M phenotype. The Z phenotype, which is the most common phenotype associated with significant liver disease, is characterized by a single lysine for glutamic acid amino acid substitution at position 342. The frequency of the homozygous form of this phenotype (PiZZ) is variably reported to range from 1:1600 to 1:8000.

The single amino acid substitution in the α_1-AT protein leads to defective folding and polymerization of the normally monomeric protein. It is believed that the polymeric α_1-AT cannot be properly exported from the intracellular production site through the Golgi apparatus. Liver injury in α_1-AT is believed to be a consequence of (1) intracellular accumulation of the α_1-AT protein in the rough endoscopic reticulum of hepatocytes, leading to chronic hepatitis; and (2) hepatocellular carcinoma. Therefore patients with the "null" phenotype, who have almost undetectable production of α_1-AT, are more prone to develop emphysema than liver disease, presumably because there is not enough α_1-AT produced to accumulate in the liver and lead to hepatic damage, whereas the deficiency of α_1-AT in extracellular fluids leads to unimpaired protease damage in extrahepatic sites.

The prevalence of clinically evident liver disease resulting from α_1-AT deficiency is not as high as would be expected based on the frequency of the PiZZ phenotype in the population. In a prospective study of 200,000 Swedish infants, 127 had the phenotype for homozygous deficiency of α_1-AT. However, only 22 of 127 showed signs of liver disease in infancy, 2 of whom died from liver disease. The re-

✔ **WHEN TO REFER**

The diagnosis of Wilson's disease should be entertained in any patient with chronic hepatitis of unknown etiology, particularly in patients younger than 40 years. Serum ceruloplasmin level should be obtained prior to referral, since this test may be strongly suggestive of the diagnosis in some cases. Similarly, any patient with unexplained neurologic or psychiatric symptoms and evidence of liver disease should be referred for evaluation and consideration of liver biopsy. Fresh liver tissue should be sent for quantitative hepatic copper concentration. It may be possible to retrospectively measure hepatic copper concentration from tissue fixed in formalin and embedded in paraffin. Slit-lamp examination for Kayser-Fleischer rings may be very helpful, particularly in patients with neurologic manifestations. Siblings of patients with Wilson's disease should be screened for the diagnosis and also referred for liver biopsy if appropriate.

mainder were followed at ages 16 and 18; none of the patients who survived developed overt evidence of liver disease. This study demonstrated that patients with homozygous α_1-AT deficiency generally have a good prognosis, and that development of clinically significant liver disease may depend on other genetic or environmental factors. In fact, it has been estimated that only 3% of children with α_1-AT deficiency require liver transplantation. Possible cofactors for development of overt liver disease include alcohol use, viral infection, and fever. One study has reported that adult patients with homozygous and heterozygous α_1-AT deficiency had an increased prevalence of hepatitis B and C infection. In patients with cirrhosis a significant proportion also had a history of alcohol abuse. Only 9% of patients with cirrhosis and 17% with chronic active hepatitis had no evidence of a second cause of liver disease. It has been proposed that degradation of the defective α_1-AT is impaired in patients with secondary liver diseases, leading to greater intrahepatic accumulation of the defective protein and possibly greater liver injury.

Laboratory and Other Diagnostic Tests

Three methods are available to establish the diagnosis of α_1-AT deficiency: measurement of serum α_1-AT level; α_1-AT phenotyping; and histologic assessment of liver tissue for α_1-AT. Serum α_1-AT levels are generally decreased, usually in the range of 15 to 200 mg/dl; the normal range is 150 to 350 mg/dl. Phenotyping of α_1-AT can be used to identify patients with α_1-AT deficiency; most patients with liver disease have the PiZZ phenotype, although multiple other phenotypes have been associated with liver disease. Biochemical liver tests and general histologic examinations are nonspecific for α_1-AT deficiency. However, special stains can be used to identify α_1-AT in the liver. The protein can be identified as diastase-resistant, periodic acid Schiff's reagent–positive, cytoplasmic globules in periportal hepatocytes. Confirmation by histochemical and immunocytochemical techniques is helpful. However, patients who are heterozygous for α_1-AT deficiency may also have evidence of α_1-AT globules on liver biopsy specimens; therefore liver biopsy findings alone may be inadequate for identifying homozygous α_1-AT deficiency.

Management

Replacement of α_1-AT is primarily useful for prevention of pulmonary damage. Intravenous infusions of α_1-AT can preserve alveolar levels of the antiprotease and possibly prevent lung damage. Replacement of the protein is not helpful in the management of liver disease. Currently, liver transplantation is the only therapeutic option for patients with end-stage liver disease. Long-term survival after liver transplantation for this indication is effective and corrects the underlying defect, since the defective α_1-AT is produced in the liver, and liver transplantation effectively replaces the α_1-AT genotype. It is hoped that, in the future, targeted gene therapy to the liver using a variety of viral and other vectors can replace the defective α_1-AT gene

✔ *WHEN TO REFER*

Any patient with evidence of chronic hepatitis and/or cirrhosis, particularly if the presentation is in adolescence or early adulthood, should be referred for evaluation and consideration of liver biopsy. It is appropriate to measure serum level of α_1-AT level as part of initial screening and perform α_1-AT phenotyping if a low level is detected.

✔ *WHEN TO REFER*

Patients with persistently abnormal liver tests of a cholestatic pattern in the setting of CF should be referred for evaluation, particularly if associated with evidence of extrahepatic obstruction (elevated serum bilirubin, dilated ducts on ultrasonography), in which case ERCP may be helpful to demonstrate the presence of biliary strictures. Liver biopsy may be helpful to demonstrate the presence of biliary cirrhosis.

with normal copies of the gene. Family members of patients with the disease should be screened for the presence of the PiZZ phenotype.

CYSTIC FIBROSIS
Physiology and Pathophysiology

Cystic fibrosis (CF) is an autosomal recessive disorder with a frequency of homozygosity of 1:2500 in whites. Defective salt and water transport across epithelial tissues in this disease can lead to damage to multiple organs, such as the pancreas, liver, and lungs. Liver disease may present in childhood or early adulthood and is usually characterized by cholestasis. Bile duct damage and biliary cirrhosis can occur, with development of extrahepatic bile duct strictures or damage to intrahepatic bile ducts. Decompensated liver disease and portal hypertension may result. The etiologic finding of liver failure is attributed to bile duct obstruction from inspissated mucus, leading to cholestasis, bile duct proliferation, and biliary cirrhosis. Secondary liver damage may be caused by the toxic effects of hydrophobic bile salts, which may accumulate in the liver after long-standing cholestasis, either from direct toxicity or from immune activation against damaged hepatocytes.

Laboratory and Other Diagnostic Tests

The diagnosis of CF-related liver disease should be suspected in patients who present with cholestatic liver enzyme abnormalities (elevated serum alkaline phosphatase, γ-glutamyl transpeptidase) in the setting of CF. Endoscopic retrograde cholangiopancreatography (ERCP) may be helpful to demonstrate extrahepatic bile duct obstruction and may be used to place biliary stents if dominant strictures are observed. Some have suggested that any child or young adult presenting with liver disease of unknown cause should be screened for CF. The classic diagnostic test for CF is the sweat test, which detects elevated chloride and sodium in the sweat of affected patients. Genotyping can also be performed to test probands, as well as family members. Liver biopsy may demonstrate focal or complete biliary cirrhosis, but there are no pathognomonic findings. There may be wide variability in the histologic lesion within the liver. Patients may also show signs of pancreatic insufficiency resulting from exocrine failure, and steatorrhea may be present, which is apparent on quantitative fecal fat testing.

Management

Bile acid therapy with ursodeoxycholic acid (UDCA) is beneficial in CF-related liver disease. UDCA is a water-soluble bile acid that decreases the lithogenicity of bile and promotes bile flow. These properties of UDCA may lead to improvement in serum liver biochemical tests in patients with biliary cirrhosis. UDCA may delay liver transplantation in patients with primary biliary cirrhosis, an autoimmune disease that has some similarity in its cholestatic features to CF-related liver disease.

Patients with portal hypertension and variceal bleeding have been treated with portosystemic shunts, either surgical or via a transjugular approach (TIPSS). Liver transplantation has been successfully performed in patients with advanced liver disease associated with CF, but patient selection is crucial. Patients are at higher risk of infectious complications and may do poorly if they have limited pulmonary reserve or pulmonary hypertension.

BIBLIOGRAPHY

Bassett ML, Halliday JW, Powell LW: Value of hepatic iron measurements in early hemochromatosis and determination of the critical iron level associated with fibrosis, *Hepatology* 6:24-29, 1986.

Colombo C et al: Ursodeoxycholic acid therapy in cystic fibrosis–associated liver disease: a dose-response study, *Hepatology* 16:924-929, 1992.

Edwards CQ, Kushner JP: Screening for hemochromatosis, *N Engl J Med* 328:1616-1620, 1993.

Gaskin KJ et al: Liver disease and common-bile-duct stenosis in cystic fibrosis, *N Engl J Med* 318:340-346, 1988.

Gordeuk V et al: Iron overload in Africa: interaction between a gene and dietary iron content, *N Engl J Med* 326:95-100, 1992.

Jazwinska EC et al: Localization of the hemochromatosis gene close to D6S105, *Am J Hum Genet* 53:347-352, 1993.

Kowdley KV et al: Primary liver cancer and survival in patients undergoing liver transplantation for hemochromatosis, *Liver Transplantation and Surgery* 1:237-241, 1995.

Kowdley KV, May EJ, Tavill AS: Inherited metabolic liver diseases, *Curr Opin Gastroenterology* 11:219-227, 1995.

Lugwig J: The liver biopsy diagnosis of Wilson's disease, *J Am J Clin Pathol* 102:443, 1994.

Niederau C et al: Survival and causes of death in cirrhotic and in noncirrhotic patients with primary hemochromatosis, *N Engl J Med* 313:1256-1262, 1985.

Perlmutter DH: Liver disease associated with 1-antitrypsin deficiency. In Ockner RK, Boyer J, editors: *Progress in liver disease,* vol 11, Philadelphia, 1993, Saunders, pp. 139-165.

Pietrangelo A et al: Regulation of transferrin, transferrin receptor, and ferritin genes in human duodenum, *Gastroenterology* 102:802, 1992.

Propst T et al: High prevalence of viral infection in adults with homozygous and heterozygous α_1-antitrypsin deficiency and chronic liver disease, *Ann Intern Med* 117:641-654, 1992.

Schienberg IH, Sternlieb I: Wilson's disease. In Smith LH, editor: *Major problems in internal medicine,* Philadelphia, 1984, Saunders, pp. 1-179.

Schoen RE, Sternlieb I: Clinical aspects of Wilson's disease, *Am J Gastroenterol* 85:1453-1457, 1990.

Sternlieb I: Perspectives on Wilson's disease, *Hepatology* 12:1234-1239, 1990.

Stremmel W et al: Wilson disease: clinical presentation, treatment, and survival, *Ann Intern Med* 115:720-726, 1991.

Sveger T: The natural history of liver disease in 1-AT deficient children, *Acta Paediatr Scand* 77:847-851, 1988.

Tavill AS: Hemochromatosis. In Schiff L, Schiff ER, editors: *Diseases of the liver,* Philadelphia, 1993, Lippincott.

Teckman JH, Perlmutter DH: Conceptual advances in pathogenesis and treatment of childhood metabolic liver disease, *Gastroenterology* 108:1263-1272, 1995.

Wu Y et al: A lag in intracellular degradation of mutant 1-antitrypsin correlates with liver disease phenotype in homozygous PIZZ 1-antitrypsin deficiency, *Proc Natl Acad Sci USA* 91:9014-9018, 1994.

Yarze JC, Martin P, Munoz SJ: Wilson's disease: current status, *Am J Med* 92:643-654, 1992.

CHAPTER

360 Hepatic Veno-Occlusive Diseases

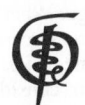

Stephen C. Hauser

Veno-occlusive diseases of the liver may involve either the portal venous system (*portal vein obstruction*) or the hepatic veins. Hepatic venous obstruction is subdivided on the basis of topographic and etiologic differences into the *Budd-Chiari syndrome,* which affects one or more of the major hepatic veins and/or the inferior vena cava, and *veno-occlusive disease,* which involves microscopic centrilobular and small sublobular veins within the liver.

BUDD-CHIARI SYNDROME

Budd-Chiari syndrome is the result of an occlusive process, usually thrombotic, involving one or more of the three major hepatic veins (right, middle, and left), with or without extension of thrombus into the inferior vena cava. Moreover, any condition involving the inferior vena cava itself at or above the entrance of the hepatic veins, such as a web or tumor, also can produce the Budd-Chiari syndrome. Although severe right-sided congestive heart failure and constrictive pericarditis may present with a clinical picture similar to that of Budd-Chiari syndrome, a careful physical examination that includes evaluation of the jugular venous pulse should clarify the diagnosis.

Excluding webs, which most often occur in patients from the Orient and South Africa, an underlying disorder can be identified in approximately 70% of patients with the Budd-Chiari syndrome. Nearly 20% of patients are women who have taken oral contraceptives, are pregnant, or have recently delivered a child. It is likely that the hypercoagulable state present in each of these conditions is responsible for the hepatic vein thrombosis. Another 20% of patients with Budd-Chiari syndrome are found to have hematologic conditions characterized by hypercoagulable states, including myeloproliferative syndromes (polycythemia rubra vera, paroxysmal nocturnal hemoglobinuria); deficiencies of antithrombotic factors (antithrombin III, protein C, protein S); and the presence of circulating antiphospholipid antibodies. Other conditions associated with the Budd-Chiari syndrome include trauma to the liver, infections (bacterial, amebic, or fungal abscess); malignant tumors (especially hepatoma); and other space-occupying lesions (adenomas, cysts). Many patients with so-called idiopathic Budd-Chiari syndrome eventually are found to have an occult myeloproliferative syndrome.

Budd-Chiari syndrome often presents as an insidious, chronic illness with nonspecific symptoms such as anorexia, nausea, vomiting, and generalized wasting. The three cardinal findings that suggest the diagnosis are *abdominal pain, hepatomegaly,* and *ascites.* The latter two findings eventually occur in nearly all cases. Some patients will develop splenomegaly, venous collaterals, and pedal edema. Large collaterals on the back suggest occlusion of the inferior vena cava. Symptoms and signs of cirrhosis are found in the late, preterminal stages of the disease. A few patients present with an acute illness mimicking fulminant hepatitis. In most cases, liver function test results are mildly elevated and are of little diagnostic value. The ascitic fluid may be either a transudate or an exudate. The serum-ascites albumin concentration gradient should be greater than 1.1 gm/dl. The usual natural history of untreated Budd-Chiari syndrome is one of gradual deterioration complicated by hepatic failure over a period of months to years. Given the nonspecific features of the illness, its insidious onset, and the lack of diagnostic value of standard laboratory tests, a high index of suspicion is prudent in patients with unexplained hepatomegaly, abdominal pain, and ascites.

Three noninvasive tests at present are useful in establishing the diagnosis of the Budd-Chiari syndrome: computer tomography (CT) with rapid intravenous contrast administration; real-time ultrasound with pulsed Doppler; and magnetic resonance imaging (MRI). MRI and ultrasound are the more useful of the noninvasive tests because they do not require intravenous contrast and are readily able to demonstrate the presence or absence of flow in the hepatic veins and inferior vena cava. A liver biopsy of an affected area will demonstrate typical findings, including centrilobular congestion, sinusoidal dilatation, and atrophy of hepatocytes. Hepatic venography and visceral angiography are important to localize the precise areas involved by the thrombotic process and may help to elucidate the etiology. Whether the inferior vena cava, portal vein, or other adjacent structures are involved is critical in considering possible surgical treatment. Referral of patients to an experienced hepatologist is prudent in consideration of the complex decisions required in the diagnosis and management of Budd-Chiari syndrome.

Treatment of Budd-Chiari syndrome depends on the anatomic location and extent of the thrombotic process, the etiology, the duration of the illness, and the presence or absence of cirrhosis. Predis-

posing conditions, such as polycythemia, should be treated, and oral contraceptives should be avoided. Antithrombotic treatment (heparin, warfarin, thrombolytic agents) is useful in only the few cases in which the diagnosis is made early in the course of the thrombotic process. Medical treatment of ascites or the performance of a LeVeen shunt may diminish the ascites but will not ameliorate the detrimental effects of hepatic venous obstruction on the liver. In the rare case of a membranous web, balloon membranotomy (angioplasty) or surgical resection or bypass may eliminate the obstruction. In many cases with centrilobular congestion on liver biopsy, the surgical creation of a portosystemic shunt to decompress the liver will greatly benefit the patient. If the inferior vena cava is involved, grafts can be constructed from the portal-mesenteric system to the right atrium. Transjugular intrahepatic portosystemic shunts (TIPS) have proven useful in the short term, but their propensity to thrombose limits their long-term effectiveness. Patients with advanced cirrhosis, hepatic encephalopathy, or coagulopathy are best managed by liver transplantation (Chapter 363).

VENO-OCCLUSIVE DISEASE

Veno-occlusive disease (VOD) is a nonthrombotic, fibrotic process that occludes and obliterates centrilobular and small sublobular veins in the liver. VOD occurs as a result of toxic injury secondary to pyrrolizidine plant alkaloids (i.e., herbal and "bush" teas derived from *Senecio, Crotolaria,* and *Heliotropium* genera); high-dose hepatic irradiation; and a number of chemotherapeutic and immunosuppressive agents (i.e., cyclophosphamide, cytosine arabinoside, azathioprine). VOD is most commonly a problem in patients given total body irradiation and/or high doses of cytotoxic agents in preparation for bone marrow transplantation. Hepatitis before transplantation, increasing age, and infection increase the risk for VOD, which overall is 20% to 50%. Much like Budd-Chiari syndrome, VOD presents clinically with abdominal pain, hepatomegaly, and ascites. Posttransplant VOD usually occurs 1 to 3 weeks after the graft. Weight gain may be an early sign of impending VOD. Eventually, most patients develop jaundice. Serum transaminase and alkaline phosphatase levels may be normal or greatly elevated. VOD in posttransplant patients often pursues a rapid downhill course, with mortality as high as 50%, although many patients appear to have a mild illness and recover completely. A liver biopsy often will confirm the clinical diagnosis, demonstrating centrilobular congestion and hepatocellular necrosis, as well as typical subendothelial fibrotic occlusion of central veins. Viral and fungal hepatitis, cholestatic hepatitis caused by drugs or parenteral nutrition, and unrecognized sepsis are the most important differential diagnoses to consider. Graft-versus-host disease usually occurs later. Unfortunately, no beneficial treatment has yet been found.

PORTAL VEIN OBSTRUCTION

Obstruction of the portal vein may occur at any point along its course, including small venous branches within the liver. Splenic and mesenteric veins also may be involved. In most cases of extrahepatic portal vein obstruction, collaterals bypass the occluded site, resulting in so-called cavernous transformation of the portal vein. Thrombosis of the extrahepatic portal vein may occur secondary to trauma (including surgical procedures in the upper abdomen), neoplasm, infection, inflammation, and thrombotic disorders. In neonates, umbilical sepsis may be a precipitating factor, although some cases may be congenital. Portal vein obstruction caused by cirrhosis (especially in the Orient) and occult myeloproliferative disorders are being recognized more frequently. Overall, the etiology of extrahepatic portal vein obstruction remains unknown in as many as half the cases. Noncirrhotic obstruction of small intrahepatic portal venous radicules may occur secondary to toxins such as arsenic, copper, vinyl chloride monomer, and cytotoxic drugs, or it may be idiopathic.

Acute obstruction of the portal vein may initially be accompanied by ascites, but this usually disappears or is minimal. Liver function test results in noncirrhotic patients usually remain normal. However, portal hypertension with varices, which may or may not bleed, is common. Children with varices may have bleeding episodes, especially around puberty, but the frequency of variceal hemorrhage often declines after puberty.

Angiography is crucial to identify the exact location and extent of the obstruction. Noninvasive tests such as real-time ultrasound with pulsed Doppler and magnetic resonance angiography also are useful. The presence of cirrhosis can be excluded by liver biopsy. Intrahepatic portal venous obstruction involving small venous radicules may be difficult to appreciate by angiography and in some cases even in percutaneous liver biopsy specimens. Treatment includes identification of the cause; endoscopic sclerotherapy or band ligation for bleeding varices; and, in those few patients who continue to bleed from varices despite endoscopic treatment, TIPS or shunt surgery. Hypersplenism with thrombocytopenia, anemia, or pain rarely requires surgery.

BIBLIOGRAPHY

Bearman SI: The syndrome of hepatic veno-occlusive disease after marrow transplantation, *Blood* 85:3005, 1995.

Blum U et al: Noncavernomatous portal vein thrombosis in hepatic cirrhosis: treatment with transjugular intrahepatic portosystemic shunt and local thrombolysis, *Radiology* 195:153, 1995.

Cohen J, Edelman RR, Chopra S: Portal vein thrombosis: a review, *Am J Med* 92:173, 1992.

Dilwari JB et al: Hepatic outflow obstruction (Budd-Chiari syndrome): experience with 177 patients and a review of the literature, *Medicine* 73:21, 1994.

Hauser SC, Gollan JL: Budd-Chiari syndrome. In Taylor MB et al, editors: *Gastrointestinal emergencies,* Baltimore, 1992, Williams & Wilkins.

McDonald GB et al: Veno-occlusive disease of the liver and multiorgan failure after bone marrow transplantation: a cohort study of 355 patients, *Ann Intern Med* 118:255, 1993.

Ringe B et al: What is the best surgery for Budd-Chiari syndrome: venous decompression or liver transplantation? A single-center experience with 50 patients, *Hepatology* 21:1337, 1995.

Shaked A et al: Portosystemic shunt versus orthotopic liver transplantation for the Budd-Chiari syndrome, *Surg Gynecol Obstet* 174:453, 1992.

Shill M, Henderson JM, Tavill AS: The Budd-Chiari syndrome revisited, *Gastroenterologist* 2:27, 1994.

Shulman HM, Hinterberger W: Hepatic veno-occlusive disease: liver toxicity syndrome after bone marrow transplantation, *Bone Marrow Transplant* 10:197, 1992.

CHAPTER

361   Liver Abscesses and Cysts

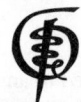   David R. Lichtenstein

LIVER ABSCESSES
Pyogenic Liver Abscess

Before the antibiotic era, pyogenic liver abscess was a disease of the young, most commonly occurring from embolization through the portal vein of bacteria originating in suppurative intraabdominal processes such as appendicitis or umbilical sepsis. Early recognition and treatment of these disorders have resulted in a decline in the incidence of pylephlebitis and subsequent liver abscess formation, so that pyogenic liver abscess is now seen predominantly in the middle-aged and elderly. Currently, the most common cause of liver abscess is biliary tract disease, usually biliary tract obstruction due to common bile duct stones or malignant disease (Box 361-1). Direct extension from contiguous sources, usually the gallbladder and adjacent viscera; necrotic tumor; direct trauma; systemic bacteremia with embolization through the hepatic artery; and unknown causes account for the remaining cases.

Pyogenic liver abscess is most often a chronic illness, with symptom onset preceding proper medical diagnosis by several weeks. Patients with pyogenic liver abscess most frequently present with nonspecific complaints of malaise, fever, and abdominal pain. The pattern of pain may vary from generalized abdominal pain to localized right upper quadrant discomfort. Right sided pulmonary symptoms with cough, pleuritic chest pain, right shoulder pain, and dyspnea may incorrectly suggest a primary pulmonary process. Physical findings related to pulmonary involvement may include crackles, friction rub,

and auscultatory evidence of effusion or consolidation in as many as 50% of patients. Symptoms of chronic illness such as weakness, fatigue, anorexia, and weight loss may occur in 25% to 75% of patients. Hepatomegaly, often with tenderness, is the most consistent physical sign. Laboratory tests are typically abnormal, with elevated leukocyte count, erythrocyte sedimentation rate, serum alkaline phosphatase, and aminotransferases. Jaundice occurs in advanced disease (large or multiple abscesses) or in cases associated with biliary tract obstruction.

Complications of pyogenic liver abscess are related to extension of the suppurative process. Extrahepatic extension with development of a subphrenic or subhepatic abscess occurs in up to 10% of cases. Abscesses may rarely extend into the pleural space, lung parenchyma, bronchi, pericardium, retroperitoneum, or intestine. Hemorrhage into the abscess and hemobilia are unusual complications. The development of diffuse abdominal pain, septic shock, and associated rise in liver function tests suggests the presence of a ruptured abscess.

At least half of liver abscesses are solitary, and more than two thirds are confined to the right lobe. Plain films of the chest and abdomen are abnormal in half of patients, revealing extraluminal gas, abnormal air-fluid levels, elevation of the right hemidiaphragm, right pleural effusion, or right lower lobe atelectasis. The majority of liver abscesses are identified by ultrasonography or computed tomography (CT) imaging. The typical ultrasonographic appearance is a hypoechoic or anechoic lesion with low level echoes often seen within the abscess corresponding to cellular debris. CT demonstrates a low-density mass. Ring enhancement may be seen corresponding to the rim of acute inflammatory reaction that surrounds the abscess. Necrotic tumors, hemorrhagic cysts, intrahepatic hematomas, or hepatic artery aneurysms may sometimes appear similar on imaging. Serologic tests are recommended in patients with liver abscess to exclude amebiasis. Needle aspirates of the abscess should undergo Gram stain and culture. Organisms are cultured from up to 90% of liver abscesses, and blood cultures are positive in up to 50%. Both blood and abscess cultures will be negative in fewer than 5% of patients. The predominant organisms cultured from pyogenic liver abscesses are enteric gram-negative aerobic rods, streptococci, and anaerobes.

The mortality of unrecognized or untreated pyogenic liver abscess approaches 100%. Mortality has been reduced to 10% to 15% owing to advances in antimicrobial therapy, earlier detection with newer imaging modalities, and development of noninvasive techniques for abscess drainage. Early imaging studies are necessary for diagnosis and localization of liver abscesses, assessment of extent of involvement, safe aspiration of abscess contents for culture, and drainage by indwelling catheter. Initial antibiotic coverage, while awaiting antibiotic sensitivities and ameba serologic findings, should include coverage for enteric gram-negative pathogens and anaerobes. This generally includes metronidazole in combination with an antipseudomonal

---

BOX 361-1

Pyogenic liver abscess: etiologic considerations and routes of infection

I. Biliary tract obstruction (40%)
   A. Benign (stone, stricture)
   B. Malignant
II. Hematogenous infection (10% to 20%)
   A. Infection via portal vein
      1. Diverticulitis
      2. Appendicitis
      3. Omphalitis
      4. Inflammatory disease of pancreas, spleen
   B. Infection via hepatic artery (bacteremia or septicemia from any cause)
III. Primary hepatic lesions (10%)
   A. Trauma (blunt abdominal trauma, penetrating liver injuries)
   B. Secondary bacterial infection of amebic abscess, cyst, or malignant lesion.
IV. Cryptogenic infection (20% to 40%)

penicillin, third-generation cephalosporin, or aminogylcoside. When cultures become available, antibiotic therapy should be adjusted accordingly. Recent studies have shown that appropriate antibiotics in combination with percutaneous needle or catheter drainage will effect a cure in a high percentage of patients. This modality of treatment is currently favored over surgical drainage in patients who do not require laparotomy for other reasons such as appendicitis. Occasionally antibiotic therapy alone will be appropriate, as in multiple small abscesses not amenable to drainage, or when a very favorable response to antibiotics occurs before the diagnosis of a pyogenic abscess has been established. The usual approach is to administer parenteral antibiotics for 10 to 14 days or until the patient becomes afebrile for several days, followed by a 6-week course of oral antibiotics. With this approach, a cure can be achieved in 75% of cases and an overall mortality of 10% to 15% should be expected. Mortality is adversely affected by the extent of liver involvement, the presence of multiple lesions because of poor accessibility of lesions to drainage, the presence of additional comorbid illnesses, and complications of abscess rupture or extension.

Amebic Liver Abscess

Although seven species of ameba may colonize the human colon, only *Entamoeba histolytica* is capable of tissue invasion and therefore able to cause hepatic abscess formation. Approximately 10% of the world population is infected with *E. Histolytica,* but only 10% of these patients develop clinical disease. Amebiasis occurs worldwide but is most prevalent in the tropics and subtropics, including Mexico, South America, Southeast Asia, and parts of western Africa. Most cases of amebic liver abscess seen in the United States have a history of residence or travel in these endemic areas. Other at-risk individuals include persons living in custodial institutions, homosexuals, and those with compromised immune systems.

The cysts of *E. hystolytica* pass through the gastrointestinal tract and change into trophozoites in the colon, where they invade the mucosa and are carried to the liver via the portal venous circulation. Symptoms and physical signs of amebic abscess are nonspecific and may suggest the presence of pyogenic liver abscess, although amebic abscess tends to be a more acute illness. Symptoms are typically present for less than 2 weeks at the time of diagnosis, but occasionally *E. histolytica* infection may take on an indolent clinical course, presenting as a fever of unknown origin. Intestinal infection is present in only 10% to 20% of cases, and most of these are carriers without invasive colonic disease. Abdominal pain is often well-localized to the right upper quadrant, and fever is nearly universal but may be intermittent. The pain is often pleuritic and referred to the right shoulder. Chills and night sweats are occasionally prominent. The constellation of symptoms is not specific and can be seen with pyogenic liver abscess, necrotic hepatic tumors, or infected hepatic cysts. Intercostal point tenderness is common. As in pyogenic abscess, pulmonary symptoms may be prominent. As many as 20% of amebic abscesses may not be recognized until they rupture or directly extend into adjacent structures. Abscesses may extend through the diaphragm, most commonly resulting in pleural effusion, empyema, or hepatobronchial fistula, and inferior extension may be seen into the peritoneal cavity, retroperitoneum, or adjacent viscera such as the stomach, duodenum, gallbladder, kidney, or pancreas. Bacterial superinfection, usually with enteric organisms, can occur spontaneously or after a drainage procedure, and carries a poor prognosis. Extension of lesions from the left lobe of the liver, though less commonly seen, is a serious and sometimes fatal complication. Such an occurrence may result in pericardial effusion, empyema, acute tamponade, or fibrinous constrictive pericarditis.

Laboratory tests are less dramatically abnormal than in pyogenic liver abscess. Anemia, leukocytosis without eosinophilia, and hypoalbuminemia are common. Alkaline phosphatase, LDH, and transaminase levels are increased in 70% to 80% but are more than twofold elevated in only about one third of patients. The bilirubin level is elevated in 50% of patients, but values exceeding 10 mg/dl are unusual and should suggest pyogenic abscess. In the absence of serologic confirmation or diagnostic aspiration, caution should be exercised in interpreting the therapeutic response to metronidazole or chloroquine. Metronidazole is effective against many anaerobes, and

chloroquine is an antipyretic; hence patients with pyogenic liver abscess or other intraabdominal infections may respond favorably to these antimicrobials. Diagnostic serologic tests to confirm amebic infection include complement fixation, indirect fluorescence antibody, gel diffusion precipitin, and indirect hemagglutination tests. These tests are positive in more than 90% of patients with proven amebic liver abscess; however, seropositivity is not specific to hepatic abscess, as it also occurs with active or prior invasive intestinal disease. In general, seropositivity in a patient with radiographic and clinical evidence of a hepatic abscess should be considered presumptive evidence for amebic abscess. Fixed preparations of aspirates and staining usually demonstrate the organisms, and culture using Robinson's medium is highly sensitive. In cases of diagnostic uncertainty, aspiration of the lesion under imaging guidance may be helpful. The presence of a thick red-brown fluid "anchovy paste" suggests amebic abscess, whereas foul-smelling contents with a positive Gram stain or culture confirm pyogenic liver abscess.

Hepatic imaging tests show that amebic abscess is most commonly (80%) located in the high anterior right lobe of the liver. Abscesses are typically solitary (85%) and vary in size from a few millimeters to several centimeters. Ultrasonography, computed tomography, and magnetic resonance imaging are comparably effective in the detection of amebic liver abscess; however, a distinction between an amebic and pyogenic abscess cannot be made accurately on radiographic findings alone.

Therapy with metronidazole, 750 mg three times daily for 10 days, is considered the treatment of choice. Follow-up treatment with the intestinal amebicide diiodohydroxyquin, 650 mg three times daily for 20 days, is sometimes recommended. Alternatively, dehydroemetine or emetine followed in sequence by chloroquine and diiodohydroxyquin is an accepted treatment regimen. Defervescence occurs rapidly, and 90% of patients are afebrile after a week of appropriate treatment. The time required for imaging tests to normalize ranges from 2 weeks to a year, depending on the initial size of the abscess. Therapeutic needle aspiration does not routinely facilitate resolution of the uncomplicated abscess and is rarely required. However, large lesions and those located in the left lobe should be considered for aspiration and drainage, since they pose a more immediate threat of rupture. Aspiration may also be helpful in resolving contiguous extension with pleural or pericardial collections, when the initial diagnosis is insecure, or when patients fail to improve in response to appropriate therapy.

HEPATIC CYSTS

Widespread application of hepatic imaging studies have led to an increased recognition of cystic diseases of the liver. Hepatic cysts may be classified into congenital or acquired (Box 361-2). Congenital cysts include solitary cysts, polycystic liver disease, and choledochal cysts, whereas acquired cysts are the result of trauma, inflammatory condi-

---

BOX 361-2
Classification of hepatic cysts

I. Congenital hepatic cysts
  A. Parenchymal cysts
    1. Solitary cyst
    2. Polycystic disease
  B. Ductal cysts
    1. Localized dilatation
    2. Multiple cystic dilatations of intrahepatic ducts (Caroli's disease)
II. Acquired hepatic cysts
  A. Inflammatory cysts
    1. Retention cyst
    2. Echinococcal cyst
  B. Neoplastic cyst
  C. Peliosis hepatis

tions, focal hepatic infarction, cystic neoplasms, and fluid collections such as biloma or hematoma.

Solitary Cysts

Solitary liver cysts are defined as cysts unassociated with systemic disease. The cysts may be solitary or multilocular and therefore would be more accurately termed simple, idiopathic, or sporadic hepatic cysts. The location, size, and appearance are quite variable. They may be intrahepatic or pedunculated, and range in size from a few millimeters to several centimeters in diameter. In adults, predominantly women are affected and the right lobe of the liver is most commonly involved. The origins of these cysts are unknown but are presumed to be congenital.

The cystic lesions are often incidental findings at the time of diagnostic imaging, laparotomy, or autopsy. Symptoms of epigastric fullness or pain, early satiety, nausea, and vomiting are uncommon and are related to compressive effects on hepatic parenchyma or adjacent structures. Complications of rupture, hemorrhage, biliary tract obstruction, and secondary infection of such cysts are extremely rare. CT scan typically reveals a hypodense nonenhancing homogeneous mass. Confusion can be caused by lesions with higher density related to hemorrhage, and in addition, solid tumors may occasionally have low attenuation numbers and appear cystic. For these reasons, ultrasonography is a more reliable means of confirming the cystic nature of the lesion and is considered the most useful radiographic study.

Treatment of solitary cysts is usually unnecessary, with invasive measures reserved for symptoms or complications. Surgical therapy depends on several factors and generally involves excision or cyst marsupialization. Ultrasonographically guided percutaneous aspiration of cyst fluid and injection of ethanol, minocycline, or hypertonic saline is an alternative to surgical therapy and will usually achieve a cure with one treatment session.

Polycystic Liver Disease

Polycystic liver disease is a disorder in which normal hepatic parenchyma is replaced by cystic lesions that appear to arise from clusters of small intrahepatic ducts that failed to involute during embryologic development. Although of biliary ductal origin, these cysts do not communicate directly with the biliary ductal system. Polycystic liver disease has an autosomal dominant pattern of inheritance with virtually complete penetrance and varying phenotypic expression. It is associated with multiple renal cysts in 50% of cases, and in some patients, multiple cysts can be found in other organs such as the pancreas, spleen, lung, and ovary. Conversely, liver cysts are found in a variable percentage of patients with polycystic kidney disease, ranging form 30% to 50%. The prevalence and number of hepatic cysts increases with age, female gender, and increased severity of renal impairment.

The majority of patients with polycystic liver disease are asymptomatic. However, patients may have symptoms from cyst compression of the extrahepatic biliary tree or abdominal pain resulting from stretching of the liver capsule or compression of adjacent viscera. Complications of hepatic cysts are unusual and include rupture, hemorrhage, secondary infection, biliary obstruction, portal hypertension, and rare malignant transformation. The most common cause of death in patients with both renal and hepatic cysts is kidney failure. Survival in the absence of associated renal disease is normal. Liver function test results are generally normal as hepatic parenchymal volume is preserved in spite of massive cystic involvement of the liver.

Treatment is generally not required, but a small subset of patients becomes incapacitated by massive liver enlargement and associated symptoms. Percutaneous aspiration of cyst fluid under ultrasonic guidance only temporarily alleviates symptoms; fluid usually reaccumulates. Ethanol sclerotherapy may delay recurrence, but experience with this treatment modality remains limited. Posttherapy alteration in cyst size and number is difficult to assess radiographically because the space formerly occupied by the collapsed cysts may be replaced by expansion of adjoining cysts. Surgical therapy involves fenestration techniques to unroof multiple cysts, resection of large cysts or groups of cysts, or resection of one or more hepatic lobes. Combined liver and kidney transplantation has been rarely performed in patients with renal failure and associated massive hepatic polycystic disease.

Echinococcal Cyst

Echinococcal disease in humans results from infection with the two species of cestodes, *Echinococcus granulosus* and *Echinococcus multilocularis.* The most common form is caused by *E. granulosus,* as a localized cystic disease known as hydatid cyst or echinococcal abscess. It is found most frequently in the liver (70%) or lung (25%) and less commonly in muscle, bone, kidney, and spleen.

Humans, along with other mammals such as sheep and cattle, act as intermediate hosts in the life cycle of *E. granulosus* by ingesting food or water contaminated by feces of the definitive hosts, usually dogs, wolves, or foxes. The ova are resistant to drying and may remain viable for weeks after being passed. On ingestion by the intermediate host, the external shell of the egg is digested by gastric acid, releasing the embryo into the upper bowel, with penetration into the intestinal mucosa to gain access to the portal circulation or lymphatic system until it becomes lodged in a capillary bed, usually within the liver or lung, where it develops into a mature cyst. The life cycle is completed when the definitive host eats contaminated offal.

The majority of patients with echinococcosis have resided in regions of the world where sheep are plentiful, including the Mediterranean, South America, France, Australia, South Africa, or other sheep and cattle farming areas. In the United States, Great Britain, and northern Europe, the disease is rare, appearing in travelers or immigrants from endemic areas.

Signs and symptoms are dependent on the size and location of the lesion. In the liver, the hydatid cyst of *E. granulosus* is usually solitary, is located in the right lobe, and causes no symptoms. Most commonly patients present with an abdominal mass noted incidentally on physical examination or abdominal imaging studies. The history may be remote since the lesions are extremely slow growing. Complications include secondary bacterial infection, allergic manifestations (anaphylactic shock and urticaria), and rupture (intrabiliary, intraperitoneal, and transdiaphragmatic). In rare cases, large cysts may compress or rupture directly into bile ducts, gallbladder, or blood vessels, causing jaundice, cholangitis, cholecystitis, or portal hypertension. Cysts may infrequently rupture upward into the pleural or pericardial spaces, lung parenchyma, or bronchi, or downward into the stomach, duodenum, colon, right kidney, or peritoneum. In contrast to the hydatid cyst of *E. granulosus,* which grows slowly and compresses adjacent host tissue, *E. multilocularis* is more virulent. It is characterized by a germinal membrane that permits formation of new cysts on its outer surface. The developing scolices invade adjacent tissue as an infiltrative process, and, on occasion, extend into blood vessels and metastasize to distant sites, where they resemble malignant mass lesions. The prognosis of this form is grave if the disease is extensive.

Eosinophilia is observed in 25% to 35% of cases but is more common in cases of cyst rupture. Echinococcal cysts may be identified using various imaging studies, but serologic tests are required for specific diagnosis. Indirect hemagglutination and complement-fixation tests are positive in 90% of patients with hepatic involvement and are useful confirmatory tests. Plain radiographs of the abdomen may reveal a rim of calcification as noted in up to 50% of patients, but this finding lacks specificity. Characteristically, the cysts have an inhomogeneous sonographic pattern with internal echoes corresponding to a disrupted endocyst, septation, debris, and daughter cysts. Otherwise, the lesions are sharply demarcated and appear as simple cysts in nearly half of cases. Liver biopsy is contraindicated.

Surgery is considered the most effective therapeutic approach, but it carries the risks of operative morbidity and spillage of fluid from the cysts, which can lead to anaphylaxis, dissemination of infection, and subsequent recurrence of cysts. Modern surgical management by omentoplasty, cystectomy, and partial hepatectomy have been found to be superior to marsupialization in reducing such complications. Small cysts should be excised, whereas large cysts should be extracted in a controlled environment through a cryogenic cone to minimize the risk of cyst spillage. Enucleation should be followed by instillation of a scolicidal agent, either silver nitrate or hypertonic saline solution, into the residual cystic cavity. Surgical morbidity approaches 5% to 10%, and mortality is less than 5%. Percutaneous aspiration of the cyst has been traditionally viewed as an absolute contraindication; however, in recent years, this view has been challenged. Percutaneous needle puncture and aspiration of hydatid cysts under ultrasound guidance when combined with a scolicidal agent may prove suitable for patients who refuse surgery or are poor operative candidates. Drug therapy with the anthelminthic benzimidazole derivative, albendazole, reduces the viability of protoscolices and cysts, and its hepatic metabolite, albendazole sulfoxide, is active against the larval cestodes. The administration of albendazole before surgery has been advocated in order to minimize the likelihood of recurrent disease. Drug therapy is also indicated to prevent secondary dissemination after the spontaneous or operative rupture of cysts. Albendazole may also be considered with inoperable or widespread disease, and for patients with other comorbid medical conditions who are unsuitable candidates for surgery.

Choledochal Cyst

Choledochal cyst is a disease manifest by dilation of the common bile duct in various anatomic patterns. The pathogenesis is unknown, but the current theory supports a congenital weakness of the bile duct wall combined with some degree of distal duct obstruction. Reflux of pancreatic juices caused by an anomalous junction of the pancreatic duct and common bile duct may contribute to cyst formation. Histologic findings show that the cyst wall consists of fibrous tissue and usually lacks epithelium or smooth muscle. The clinical manifestations of choledochal cysts vary considerably. The classic triad of pain, right upper quadrant mass, and jaundice occurs in less than 40% of patients. Epigastric pain is the most common symptom. Cholangitis, liver abscess, pancreatitis, portal venous thrombosis, and secondary biliary cirrhosis are less frequent manifestations. Diagnosis is confirmed by cholangiography. Treatment should consist of surgical drainage and, whenever possible, complete excision because of the high risk that carcinoma may develop in the biliary tree.

Peliosis Hepatis

Peliosis hepatis is characterized by the presence of blood-filled cystic spaces in the liver. A causal relationship exists to treatment with oral contraceptives and anabolic steroids. Bacillary peliosis hepatis secondary to *Bartonella henselae* has been reported in HIV-infected individuals and produces a similar lesion. Most patients are asymptomatic, and liver involvement is heralded by abnormal liver function tests or hepatomegaly. Progressive hepatic failure with impaired synthetic function may dominate the clinical picture. Fatalities have occurred after spontaneous rupture of a subcapsular cyst with exsanguinating intraperitoneal hemorrhage. Hepatic scintigraphy reveals hepatosplenomegaly with either patchy uptake of colloid in the liver or discrete filling defects. Percutaneous liver biopsy is often diagnostic but is potentially hazardous because of the vascular nature of the lesions. Discontinuation of the offending medication or treatment for the infecting agent in bacillary angiomatosis may result in variable regression of the peliotic lesions.

BIBLIOGRAPHY

Acunas B et al: Purely cystic hydatid disease of the liver: treatment with percutaneous aspiration and injection of hypertonic saline, *Radiology* 182:541, 1992.

Barnes PF et al: A comparison of amebic and pyogenic abscess of the liver, *Medicine* 66:472, 1987.

Behrns KE et al: Surgical management of hepatic hydatid disease, *Mayo Clin Proc* 66:1193, 1991.

Filice C et al: A new therapeutic approach for hydatid liver cysts: aspiration and alcohol injection under sonographic guidance, *Gastroenterology* 98:1366, 1990.

Gibney EJ: Amebic liver abscess, *Br J Surg* 77:843, 1990.

Hagiwara H et al: Successful treatment of a hepatic cyst by one-shot instillation of minocycline chloride, *Gastroenterology* 103:675, 1992.

Halvorsen RA et al: The variable CT appearance of hepatic abscesses, *Am J Roentgenol* 141:941, 1984.

Khuroo MS et al: Percutaneous drainage versus albendazole therapy in hepatic hydatosis: a prospective, randomized study, *Gastroenterology* 104:1452, 1993.

McDonald MI et al: Single and multiple pyogenic liver abscesses: natural history, diagnosis and treatment with emphasis on percutaneous drainage, *Medicine (Baltimore)* 63:291, 1984.

Milutinovic J et al: Liver cysts in patients with autosomal dominant polycystic kidney disease, *Am J Med* 68:741, 1980.

Perkocha LA et al: Clinical and pathological features of bacillary peliosis hepatitis in association with human immunodeficiency virus infection, *N Engl J Med* 323:1581, 1990.

Que F et al: Liver resection and cyst fenestration in the treatment of severe polycystic liver disease, *Gastroenterology* 108:487, 1995.

Seeto RK et al: Pyogenic liver abscess: changes in etiology, management, and outcome, *Medicine* 75:99, 1996.

CHAPTER

362 Hepatic Tumors

Gregory J. Gores

PRIMARY CARCINOMA OF THE LIVER
Hepatocellular Carcinoma

Incidence and Etiology. Hepatocellular carcinoma (HCC) is one of the most common cancers worldwide. The incidence varies widely, with a relatively low incidence in the United States of 4 per 100,000 up to an incidence of 113 per 100,000 in Mozambique. HCC is an aggressive cancer often leading to death within 6 months of diagnosis in symptomatic individuals. Thus the incidence and prevalence of this cancer worldwide are nearly identical. The geographic variation of HCC coincides with the prevalence of hepatitis B infection and high aflatoxin exposure, providing epidemiologic evidence linking these agents to its development. The peak incidence in the United States is in the fifth and sixth decades of life but is lower in high-incidence areas. HCC occurs predominantly in men, with a male/female ratio of approximately 3:1.

HCC is unique among human cancers in that the etiology in most instances is well understood. This cancer occurs predominantly in patients with cirrhosis and viral hepatitis. The most common causes of cirrhosis associated with HCC include hepatitis B, hepatitis B plus delta virus coinfection, hepatitis C, alcohol, α_1-antitrypsin deficiency, hemochromatosis, hereditary tyrosinemia, and cryptogenic cirrhosis. The risk for developing HCC with cirrhosis resulting from hepatitis C needs to be emphasized, since hepatitis C is extremely prevalent (0.5% to 1.5% of the population); and hepatitis C has replaced hepatitis B as the leading cause of HCC in many areas of the world. In men older than 40 years with cirrhosis from these causes, the overall incidence of HCC is 3% per year. These risk factors are additive; for example, the cumulative risk for the development of HCC in patients with alcoholic-induced cirrhosis who are hepatitis C antibody–positive may be as high as 81% over 10 years. Use of exogenous androgenic steroids has also been associated with HCC. Finally, HCC is more common in those areas of the world where intake of aflatoxin B_1 (a mutagen causing guanine-to-thymine transversions and guanine-to-adenine transitions) is high.

In contrast to the etiologic associations, the molecular events initiating HCC are obscure. Chronic hepatic necroinflammatory activity with cirrhosis is thought to provide a rich substrate for the development of HCC as a result of the mutagenic environment of inflammation, cellular injury, and hepatocellular regeneration. In addition to causing inflammation and cirrhosis, hepatitis B, a DNA virus, is thought to promote carcinogenesis by one of two mechanisms: (1) deregulation of cellular growth control genes by integration of viral DNA into the host genome; and (2) deregulation of cellular growth control genes by the viral-derived X protein, which functions as a transcription factor for both host and viral DNA. How hepatitis C, an RNA virus, promotes carcinogenesis remains unclear. Mutations of the tumor suppressor gene, p53, is common in many hepatocellular carcinomas. A hotspot guanine-to-thymine mutation at codon 249 of p53 is frequently identified in HCC from southern Africa and China, where aflatoxin B_1 exposure is high, implicating aflatoxin B_1 as a hepatic carcinogen. Although multiple other mutations and loss of heterozygosity of several chromosomes have been identified in HCC, none are found consistently, and the molecular events necessary for the initiation, promotion, and propagation of HCC remain unclear.

Clinical Features and Diagnosis. Patients with HCC may present with: (1) decompensation of their cirrhosis; (2) systemic or local symptoms referable to the cancer; (3) paraneoplastic manifestations; (4) symptoms resulting from metastases; and (5) a liver mass lesion identified incidentally on a radiographic procedure. Liver decompensation is a relatively common presentation of HCC and must be considered in anyone who presents with sudden and rapid decompensation of their liver disease. Symptoms of liver decompensation include ascites, variceal bleeding, jaundice, and unexplained severe fatigue with rapid muscle wasting and weight loss. Like any neoplastic condition, advanced HCC is frequently associated with anorexia, early satiety, malaise, weakness, nausea, vomiting, and weight loss. Local symptoms caused by the tumor mass are also common in advanced HCC. In particular, a self-limited, single episode of right upper quadrant abdominal pain resembling biliary colic is a common presenting symptom. The pain results either from an abrupt extension of the tumor through the liver capsule or limited hemorrhage and necrosis within the tumor. A variety of other local complications have been reported in advanced HCC, including chronic abdominal pain, an abdominal mass, hemoperitoneum from rupture of the tumor, hepatic vein obstruction leading to the Budd-Chiari syndrome, inferior vena cava obstruction with peripheral edema, shoulder pain and pleural effusions from diaphragmatic extension of the tumor, and jaundice or hemobilia caused by invasion of the tumor into bile ducts. Paraneoplastic manifestations are rare and include fever, leukocytosis, hypercalcemia, erythrocytosis, hypoglycemia, hypercholesterolemia, porphyria cutanea tarda, and hypertrophic pulmonary osteoarthropathy. Occasionally patients present with symptoms referable to metastatic disease. HCC may metastasize to bone, lung, skin, pituitary, spleen, and other sites. Tumor emboli may cause pulmonary arterial hypertension and respiratory compromise. Finally, the finding of an asymptomatic HCC is becoming increasingly more common as patients undergo radiographic imaging procedures of the liver to evaluate their known liver disease.

The physical findings observed in HCC depend on the stage of disease. Firm and/or tender hepatomegaly, a palpable liver mass, a liver bruit, a friction rub over the liver, jaundice, ascites, peripheral edema, and splenomegaly may be observed in HCC. However, the physical examination is frequently unrevealing in many patients with HCC in the United States, except for those physical findings commonly observed in cirrhosis.

Liver-derived serum biochemistries (alanine aminotransferase, aspartate aminotransferase, alkaline phosphatase, γ-glutamyl traspeptidase, and bilirubin) are frequently elevated in patients with HCC because of the underlying live disease. In patients in whom the elevations of liver-derived biochemistries are principally caused by the tumor mass, the alkaline phosphatase and γ-glutamyl transpeptidase may be disproportionately elevated in relation to the other liver tests. The serum ferritin may be elevated as a result of production and secretion of acidic isoferritins by the HCC.

Two tumor markers are used to diagnose HCC: (1) the serum α-fetoprotein (AFP), which is elevated in 60% to 80% of patients with HCC; and (2) the plasma des-γ-carboxyprothrombin (DCP), which is elevated in 50% to 80% of patients with HCC. The serum AFP determination is universally available, whereas the DCP determination is not widely performed. The AFP is a serum glycoprotein synthesized by embryonic liver cells, fetal yolk sac cells, regenerating liver, and HCC, and, occasionally, by other gastrointestinal and lung cancers, germ cell malignancies, and in some families without associated pathologic conditions. The serum AFP increases in the second and third trimesters of pregnancy. Patients with active acute and chronic hepatitis—especially patients with hepatitis B undergoing a seroconversion from HBeAg (+) and anti–HBeAg (−) status to HBeAg (−) and anti–HBeAg (+) status—also frequently have

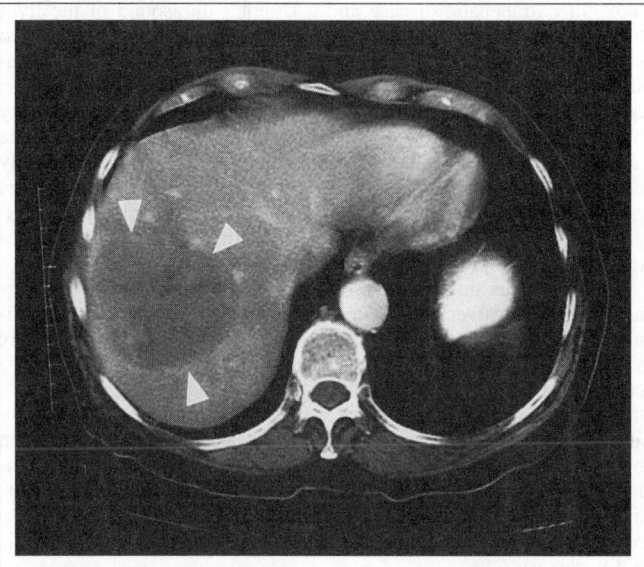

FIGURE 362-1   A computed tomography scan of a hepatocellular carcinoma in the right lobe of the liver *(arrow).*

elevated serum AFP concentrations in the absence of an HCC. Thus the AFP must be carefully assessed in the context of which it is measured. An AFP value greater than 400 ng/ml in chronic hepatitis B in the absence of a HBeAg seroconversion is strongly suggestive of an underlying HCC, as is a rapid and continuous rise of the serum AFP. In patients with non—hepatitis B related chronic liver disease, a serum AFP consistently greater than 200 ng/ml is worrisome for HCC. With a known liver mass, cirrhosis, and minimal hepatic necroinflammatory activity, an elevated serum AFP of any value is virtually diagnostic of HCC. Although elevated serum AFP values in chronic liver disease may be caused by active hepatic inflammation alone, careful imaging studies must be performed to exclude HCC, and these patients are an extremely high-risk group for the subsequent development of HCC (6- to 13-fold greater than patients with cirrhosis without an elevated serum AFP value). DCP is a form of prothrombin that is deficient in γ-carboxyglutamic acid residues, rendering the molecule inactive as a prothrombin. The plasma DCP is elevated in patients on Coumadin or with vitamin K deficiency, HCC, viral hepatitis, cirrhosis, and metastatic cancer. Multiple assays have been developed to measure this protein in plasma and, therefore, normal values vary from assay to assay. The DCP and AFP tests are complementary and increase the sensitivity for detecting HCC to approximately 85%.

A multitude of imaging modalities are available to image and stage HCC, including Doppler ultrasonography, spiral computed tomography (CT); magnetic resonance imaging (MRI); angiography; CT arterial portography (a rapid sequence CT scan performed in combination with angiography); Lipiodol angiography followed by CT scanning 2 weeks later; and laparoscopy. The following questions need to be addressed when staging HCC. What is the size, number, and location of the lesion(s)? Is vascular invasion present? What is the relationship of the tumor to the hepatic veins? Is there underlying cirrhosis? Is there extrahepatic disease? CT remains the best technique for determining if extrahepatic metastases have occurred, whereas Doppler ultrasound and MRI are excellent for determining if vascular invasion is present. All of the imaging modalities are useful for determining size, location, and multicentricity of the tumor. It should be noted, however, that the cirrhotic liver is difficult to image because: (1) portal hypertension and portosystemic shunting alter contrast enhancement of the liver; (2) macroregenerative nodules (MRN) present in the cirrhotic liver mimic small tumors; and (3) HCC in the cirrhotic liver may grow as an infiltrative tumor in the absence of a discrete mass. In patients without cirrhosis an abdominal CT scan and chest roentgenogram to look for extrahepatic disease and a Doppler ultrasound of the liver to determine if vascular invasion has occurred usually suffice to stage most patients with HCC (Fig. 362-1). In cirrhosis the sensitivity of ultrasound, CT, and angiography for detecting HCC is only 80%, 87%, and 90%, respectively. Thus multiple, complementary imaging studies are frequently necessary in patients with cirrhosis. The use of Lipiodol may be helpful in imaging HCC. Lipiodol is an oily compound that when injected into the hepatic arterial circulation is preferentially retained by HCC. A CT scan 2 weeks after a Lipiodol angiogram demonstrates a HCC with high contrast resulting from the retention of the Lipiodol within the tumor.

Percutaneous fine needle biopsy of the liver can be used to diagnose HCC. However, several caveats must be recognized by the clinician before having this procedure performed. First, HCCs are highly vascular, increasing the risk for hemorrhage. Second, the pathologist cannot distinguish between low-grade HCC and a benign lesion on the material usually obtained by a fine needle biopsy. Third, highly anaplastic HCCs are frequently interpreted as metastatic cancers, even by experienced pathologists. Fourth, the biopsy may promote vascular invasion and peritoneal seeding by the cancer. Finally, the information obtained by the biopsy should alter therapy. If the lesion is to be resected based on clinical circumstances, a preoperative biopsy is not necessary.

✔ *WHEN TO REFER*

The only definitive therapy for HCC is surgery. Surgical excision is largely restricted to those patients with no extrahepatic disease, unicentric disease limited to one lobe of liver, no vascular invasion, and no cirrhosis, or in cirrhotic patients with superb hepatic function and no portal hypertension. Despite these restrictive criteria, results following surgical resection are suboptimal, with 5-year survival rates of 20% to 30%. In the cirrhotic liver with HCC the remaining liver can be considered a premalignant organ in evolution to cancer. Because of this concept, many favor orthotopic liver transplantation (OLT) for patients with HCCs, especially HCCs smaller than 5 cm with no vascular invasion and less than three nodules in the liver. OLT also alleviates the problem of the underlying cirrhosis. Four-year survival rates with OLT for patients with selected HCC are 50% and are higher if preoperative chemoembolization is employed. If resection or OLT is not feasible, percutaneous ethanol injection, cyrosurgery, and chemoembolization can be considered. For patients with advanced intrahepatic or extrahepatic disease, therapy is frequently limited to supportive care, since there is no proven chemotherapy for HCC. In patients with advanced disease the average survival is only 6 months.

Management of HCC is complex, requiring the services of a multidisciplinary team experienced in hepatobiliary neoplasia. Indeed, consultations by a hepatologist, radiologist, hepatobiliary surgeon, transplant team, pathologist, and medical oncologist are usually necessary for the full evaluation of these patients. Thus all patients with HCC should be referred to an academic medical center experienced in the care of these patients.

Fibrolamellar Hepatocellular Carcinoma

Incidence and Etiology. Fibrolamellar hepatocellular carcinoma (FL-HCC) is an unusual variant of hepatocellular carcinoma characterized by unique histologic features. The histologic features include deeply eosinophilic malignant cells interspersed between laminated strands of collagen. FL-HCC accounts for 7% of all hepatocellular carcinomas in the Western world. This cancer does not have a gender predilection and occurs predominantly in patients younger than 40 years (90%). Cirrhosis, viral hepatitis, alcohol use, or a history of contraceptive pill use are unusual in FL-HCC.

Clinical Features and Diagnosis. The clinical presentation usually involves pain, fatigue, weight loss, nausea, fever, and a liver mass. Paraneoplastic syndromes such as erythrocytosis, hypercalce-

mia, and hypoglycemia are unusual. The serum alkaline phosphatase is usually elevated, whereas the serum transaminases are only modestly elevated. Unlike in HCC, the serum α-fetoprotein is usually normal in FL-HCC. The serum vitamin B_{12} level has been reported to be elevated in this cancer. FL-HCC often presents as a single, large mass on imaging studies of the liver, with no unique diagnostic features.

✔ *WHEN TO REFER*

These cancers are thought to be slow-growing cancers that metastasize late in their development. Thus FL-HCC is more often resectable (50% to 80%) on presentation than HCC. The 5-year survival in patients following hepatic resection is 56%. If the cancer is not amenable to resection as a result of anatomic considerations, liver transplantation is indicated. Survival following liver transplantation for FL-HCC is favorable (60% at 2 years). Those patients who have FL-HCC not amenable to resection or transplantation appear to have progressed to a more virulent stage of the tumor, and the median survival is only 13 months. As in usual HCC, therapy for patients with advanced cancer is largely supportive. All patients with FL-HCC should be referred to centers with multidisciplinary expertise in hepatobiliary neoplasia.

Intrahepatic Cholangiocarcinoma

Incidence and Etiology. Intrahepatic cholangiocarcinoma (ICC) is an adenocarcinoma arising from intrahepatic bile ducts. It is the second most common primary malignancy arising within the liver, accounting for approximately 10% to 20% of primary hepatic malignancies. Because ICC is an adenocarcinoma, it is frequently misdiagnosed as metastatic adenocarcinoma of unknown primary. Unfortunately, the misdiagnosis of ICC as metastatic adenocarcinoma frequently precludes appropriate attempts to surgically excise the cancer. Patients with primary sclerosing cholangitis, inflammatory bowel disease, Caroli's disease, chronic cholangitis with hepatic lithiasis, clonorchis sinesis infections, and a history of Thorotrast exposure are at risk for the development of ICC. Although ICC also occurs in patients with cirrhosis, it does so less frequently than hepatocellular carcinoma.

Clinical Features and Diagnosis. The mean age at presentation is 55 years. There is no gender predilection for this cancer. Abdominal pain or discomfort, malaise, weight loss, fatigue, nausea, anorexia, and fever are the primary presenting symptoms. Jaundice is unusual as a presenting symptom, unlike in extrahepatic bile duct cancer, which usually presents with jaundice. Liver-derived serum bio-

---

✔ *WHEN TO REFER*

Surgical excision is indicated in those patients without extrahepatic disease without vascular invasion and in those patients whose disease permits an anatomic resection without compromising hepatic function. The median survival in patients undergoing a curative resection is 3 years, with occasional long-term survivors. Results with orthotopic liver transplantation (OLT) for ICC are dismal, with virtual 100% recurrence in all patients; most transplant centers have abandoned OLT for ICC. Unfortunately, 80% of patients have lymph node metastasis, widespread hepatic involvement, or vascular invasion at the time of presentation; the median survival in these patients is only 5 months. There is no proven chemotherapy. The roles of chemoembolization, cryosurgery, and percutaneous ethanol injection have not been adequately evaluated. In patients with suspected or proven ICC, referral to a competent hepatobiliary surgeon is indicated to determine if the disease is potentially resectable.

chemistries are frequently elevated, especially the serum alkaline phosphatase. Unlike in hepatocellular carcinoma, the serum carcinoembryonic antigen (CEA) and CA 19-9 values are frequently elevated, whereas the α-fetoprotein (AFP) is normal. Indeed, in a patient with a unicentric liver mass, an elevated serum CEA, and a normal AFP, the diagnosis of ICC is highly likely. Patients may have firm and/or tender hepatomegaly or a palpable liver mass on physical examination. Patients with advanced and usually terminal disease can develop ascites, jaundice, splenomegaly and gastrointestinal bleeding.

Hepatic Epithelioid Hemangioendothelioma

Incidence and Etiology. Hepatic epithelioid hemangioendothelioma (HEHE) is a term used to designate a rare primary liver tumor composed of epithelioid, dendritic, and spindle-shaped cells with a very prominent fibroid stroma. Because the cells are positive for factor VIII, they are thought to arise from endothelial cells. HEHE may be associated with exposure to vinyl chloride; however, the cause in most cases is unclear.

Clinical Features and Diagnosis. This tumor is slightly more common in women and usually presents between the third and fifth decades of life. HEHE is an indolent, low-grade cancer that causes virtually no symptoms until the tumor is advanced. Furthermore, this vascular-derived tumor frequently invades vessels, promoting early intrahepatic and pulmonary metastases. Thus most patients present with advanced multicentric hepatic disease and symptoms of abdominal pain, abdominal fullness or distention, and weight loss. The serum alkaline phosphatase is elevated, with modest elevations of the transaminases. The α-fetoprotein and carcinoembryonic antigen levels are normal. Hepatomegaly is common on physical examination. Jaundice, ascites, and splenomegaly can occur but are rare. Imaging studies are nonspecific and reveal solid, nonhomogenous space-occupying liver masses. Usually, numerous lesions are present resembling diffuse hepatic metastases. A biopsy is necessary to make the diagnosis.

> ✔ *WHEN TO REFER*
>
> Management of HEHE is confounded by the highly variable natural history. For example, some patients die within 2 years of diagnosis, but survival for as long as 28 years following diagnosis without therapy has been reported. Occasionally, asymptomatic patients with early unicentric disease are identified; these patients should have their cancers resected. Most patients have extensive multicentric disease, however, precluding surgical extirpation of the disease. Liver transplantation should be considered in patients without extrahepatic disease who are not amenable to hepatic resection. Five-year survival may approach 76% in patients with extensive hepatic HEHE following liver transplantation. However, given the often extended survival of these patients without therapy, it is difficult to determine if survival is influenced by therapy. There is no accepted chemotherapy. All patients with HEHE should be referred to a major academic medical center with experience in hepatobiliary neoplasia and with an experienced liver transplant program.

BENIGN NEOPLASMS
Cavernous Hemangioma

Incidence and Etiology. Cavernous hemangiomas are extremely common and are present in 7% of adults in autopsy studies. A female predilection has been noted for this benign tumor. Cavernous hemangiomas are usually single but may be multicentric in as many as 30% of patients. They are composed of an extensive network of various-sized vascular spaces. The vascular spaces are lined by endothelial cells and are separated by fibrous stroma. Thrombosis, scarring, and calcifications may be present in large hemangiomas. The etiology is unclear.

Clinical Features and Diagnosis. Cavernous hemangiomas are usually asymptomatic and are identified incidentally on imaging studies of the liver performed for evaluation of abdominal pain and/or elevated serum-derived liver biochemical tests. Small lesions are asymptomatic and right upper quadrant pain should not be attributed to a small cavernous hemangioma. Growth of cavernous hemangiomas is rare, although occasional patients may present with massive lesions, the so-called *giant hemangiomas*. Giant cavernous hemangiomas may cause pain, abdominal distention, jaundice, the Budd-Chiari syndrome, and, rarely, hemorrhage. A Kasabach-Merritt syndrome with thrombocytopenia, hypofibrinogenemia, and increased fibrinogen degradation products has been described, with large hemangiomas replacing most of the liver. Malignant transformation does not occur. In the usual clinical situation the goal of the clinician is to not mistake a cavernous hemangioma for a more serious lesion. Fortunately, imaging studies of these lesions are usually diagnostic, allowing the clinician to dismiss the lesion as a health concern. On ultrasonography, cavernous hemangiomas are well-circumscribed, homogeneously hyperechoic lesions with smooth margins (Fig. 362-2). The differential hyperechoic lesions include small hepatocellular carcinomas, focal fat, angiolipomas, and metastases from neuroendocrine tumors and mucin-producing or highly vascular adenocarcinomas. In the patient with cirrhosis at risk for the development of hepatocellular carcinoma or a known primary malignancy, further radiographic studies are warranted to confirm the diagnosis of a suspected cavernous hemangioma. Technetium-99m–labeled (^{99m}Tc-labeled) red blood cell scintigraphy, dynamic bolus CT, and MRI are useful in confirming the diagnosis of a cavernous hemangioma. The diagnosis can be made with a high degree of specificity (100%) and sensitivity (80%) using ^{99m}Tc-labeled red blood cell scintigraphy. Cavernous heman-

> ✔ *WHEN TO REFER*
>
> The vast majority of patients with cavernous hemangioma can be reassured. In patients with large cavernous hemangiomas a repeat imaging study is suggested in 1 to 2 years to ensure no change. The rare patient with a symptomatic giant hemangioma may require surgical resection or, under extreme circumstances, even liver transplantation. Most patients with a cavernous hemangioma do not require a referral if the diagnosis is secure.

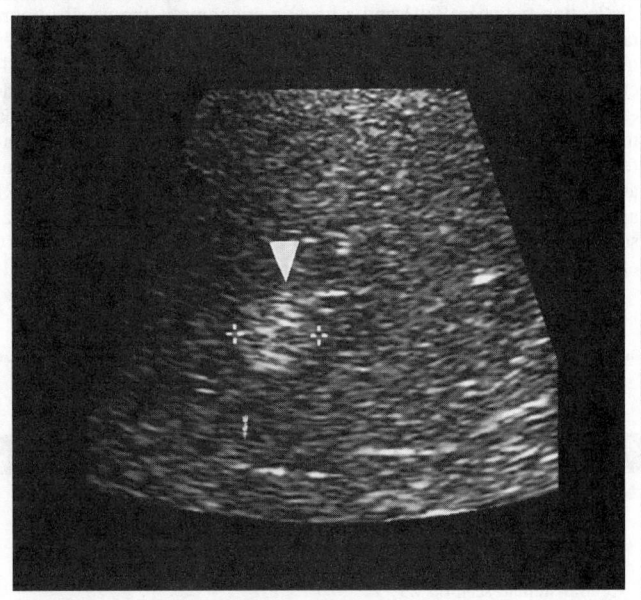

FIGURE 362-2   An ultrasound of a well-circumscribed, hyperechoic cavernous hemangioma of the liver *(arrow)*.

giomas demonstrate reduced perfusion on early images and a high concentration of the isotope within the lesion on late images (1 hour). This mismatch between early and late scintigraphic images is highly diagnostic of a cavernous hemangioma. Peripheral enhancement followed by delayed opacification of tumor is the classic CT appearance of a cavernous hemangioma. Cavernous hemangiomas are sharply demarcated, hyperintense lesions on T2-weighted spin echo MRI scans. Biopsies of these lesions should be avoided if possible because of the risk of hemorrhage. However, in patients with radiographic-indeterminate lesions caused by extensive thrombosis, necrosis, and scarring of the lesion or in patients with a known extrahepatic primary tumor in whom the diagnosis of a metastases would change therapy, a "skinny" needle biopsy can be performed safely by experienced radiologists. Because of the scarring, the biopsy may be relatively acellular, with occasional vascular elements. This relatively "dry aspirate" is diagnostic and should not prompt another biopsy.

Focal Nodular Hyperplasia

Incidence and Etiology. Focal nodular hyperplasia (FNH) is thought to occur by a reaction of the liver to an intrahepatic arterial malformation. The reaction consists of a proliferation of hepatocytes separated by fibrous septa. The arterial malformation is associated with a vascular stellate scar of connective tissue, as well as bile ductules. The presence of benign hepatic parenchyma with bile ductules in septal fibrosis is the diagnostic histologic feature. Although FNH occurs predominantly in women of childbearing age, it is not related to oral contraceptive use. However, estrogens and pregnancy may stimulate the growth, but the response is unpredictable. In patients found to have an incidental mass of the liver on imaging studies, 11% are FNHs. FNH may be multiple (10%) and may be associated with cavernous hemangiomas (22%), rarely with fibrolamellar hepatocellular carcinoma and occasionally with arterial venous malformations elsewhere in the body. A patient with progressive, multiple, and recurrent FNH following surgical resection has been described.

Clinical Features and Diagnosis. Most patients with FNH are asymptomatic. Occasional patients with large lesions may have abdominal discomfort or an abdominal mass. The physical examination is usually normal, as are liver-derived serum biochemical studies. The α-fetoprotein level is normal. The major decision when presented with a young women with a primary liver mass in the absence of underlying liver disease is whether the lesion is a cavernous hemangioma, FNH, a hepatic adenoma, or a fibrolamellar hepatocarcinoma. The distinction between FNH and a hepatic adenoma is the usual important clinical diagnostic dilemma (Table 362-I). Whereas FNH does not rupture or have the risk for malignant transformation, hepatic adenomas do. Thus FNH lesions can be observed, whereas hepatic adenomas should be resected. Fortunately, the diagnosis of FNH can be made by radiologic imaging studies in 70% of cases. The classic features on CT include hyperintense or isointense contrast enhancement and the presence of an avascular central scar. The diagnostic MRI appearance is isointensity on T1- and T2-weighted images, a central scar that is hyperintense on T2, and a homogenous signal intensity except for the central scar (Fig. 362-3). Technetium-99m sulfur colloid scintigraphy demonstrates hyperintense or isointense uptake by 50% to 60% of FNH as a result of the presence of Kupffer's cells; uptake of this colloid seldom occurs in hepatic adenomas, which are usually devoid of Kupffer's cells. Uptake of labeled iminodiacetic acid derivatives used in biliary tract scintigraphy also occur by the biliary elements of FNH, but the specificity of this observation is unclear.

✔ WHEN TO REFER

If the diagnosis of FNH is classic by radiographic imaging studies and the patient is asymptomatic with normal liver-derived serum biochemical studies, no medical or surgical intervention is warranted. Oral contraceptives should be discontinued to prevent potential further growth of the lesion. Symptomatic large lesions can be resected. If the diagnosis is uncertain and a hepatic adenoma still remains a diagnostic possibility, either the lesion should be resected or a large biopsy specimen should be obtained. Classic FNH does not require referral. However, if the lesion is not a classic FNH by radiographic imaging studies, referral to an academic medical center is warranted.

Hepatic Adenomas

Incidence and Etiology. Hepatic adenomas (HAs) are benign tumors composed of hepatocytes without bile ductules, fibrous septa, portal tracts, or central veins. These tumors occur predominantly in young women, and a strong association with oral contraceptives has been described, especially the older preparations with high-dose mestranol. Indeed, the incidence of HA in 1970 has been estimated to be 3 per 100,000 in long-term users of oral contraceptives. HAs also occur in patients with glycogen storage type IA disease and patients taking methandrostenolone and methyl testosterone; they are also a familiar condition associated with diabetes mellitus.

Clinical Features and Diagnosis. Most patients with HAs are women of childbearing age. The tumors are often identified as incidental liver masses. However, HAs have a propensity to rupture, presenting with intrahepatic hemorrhage or hemoperitoneum and shock. Limited intrahepatic hemorrhage causes pain. Large tumors may

Table 362-1 Focal nodular hyperplasia (FNH) vs. hepatic adenoma (HA)

	FNH	HA
Young women	+	+
Estrogen-stimulated growth	±	+
Rupture	−	+
Malignant transformation	−	+
Central stellate scan on CT or MRI	+	−
Increased or normal uptake on scintigraphy	+	−
Bile ducts in fibrous septa	+	−

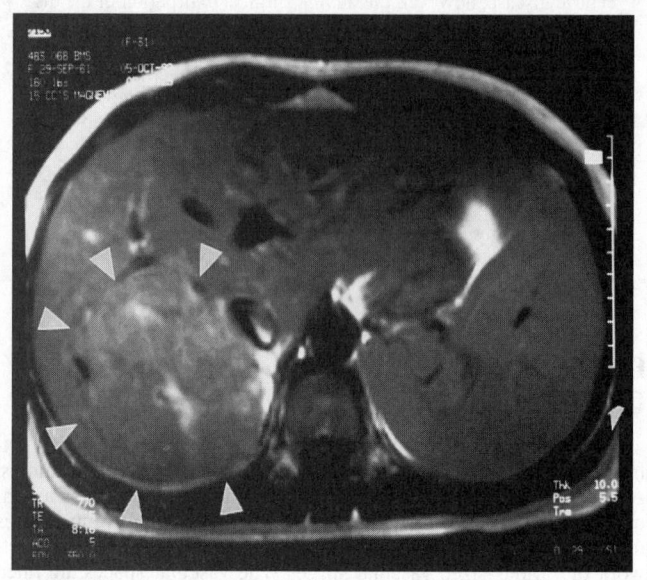

FIGURE 362-3 A T2-weighted MRI scan of a right, posterior lobe focal nodular hyperplasia. Note the hyperintense central scar in an otherwise homogenous isointense mass *(arrow)*.

cause abdominal discomfort. Rarely, night sweats and diarrhea are present. Hepatomegaly or a palpable mass may be present on examination, but commonly no abnormalities are observed. Aside from a mild elevation of the serum alkaline phosphatase, the liver-derived serum biochemistries and the α-fetoprotein are normal. Radiographic imaging studies are nonspecific, and the lesions cannot be differentiated from hepatocellular carcinoma by ultrasound, CT, or MRI. However, if intratumoral hemorrhage is present, the diagnosis of HA is favored. HAs are usually single but may be multiple, especially in patients with glycogen storage disease.

✔ WHEN TO REFER

Hepatic adenomas have been observed to decrease in size following withdrawal of oral contraceptives, but this is an infrequent occurrence. Moreover, growth despite withdrawal of oral contraceptive occurs, and adenomas have been observed with foci of malignancy and to dedifferentiate into hepatocellular cancer. Therefore most experienced hepatologists and hepatobiliary surgeons favor resection of HAs because of the risk of rupture and associated malignancy. In patients with glycogen storage disease and multiple, nonresectable HAs, liver transplantation should be performed because of the high rate of malignant degeneration of HA in this disease. All patients with HAs should be referred to a multidisciplinary team consisting of an experienced hepatologist and hepatobiliary surgeon.

BIBLIOGRAPHY

Bennett WF, Bova JG: Review of hepatic imaging and a problem-oriented approach to liver masses, *Hepatology* 12:761, 1990.

Cherqui D et al: Management of focal nodular hyperplasia and hepatocellar adenoma in young women: a series of 41 patients with clinical, radiological, and pathological correlations, *Hepatology* 22:1674-1681.

Farges O, Dadafkeh S, Bismuth H: Cavernous hemangiomas of the liver: are there any indications for resection? *World J Surgery* 19:19, 1995.

Gores GJ: Liver transplantation for malignant disease, *Gastroenterol Clin North Am* 16:627, 1987.

Kelleher MB et al: Epitheloid hemangioendothelioma of the liver: clinicopathological correlation of 10 patients treated with orthotopic liver transplantation, *Am J Surg Pathol* 13:399, 1989.

Okuda K: Hepatocellular carcinoma: recent progress, *Hepatology* 15:948, 1992.

Ruffin MT: Fibrolamellar hepatoma, *Am J Gastroenterol* 85:577, 1990.

Sadowski D et al: Progressive type of focal nodular hyperplasia characterized by multiple tumors and recurrence, *Hepatology* 21:970, 1995.

Schlinkert RT et al: Intrahepatic cholangiocarcinoma: clinical aspects, pathology, and treatment, *HPB Surg* 5:95, 1992.

Yamaguchi M et al: Prevalence of hepatocellular carcinoma in patients with alcoholic cirrhosis and prior exposure to hepatitis C, *Am J Gastroenterol* 88:39, 1993.

signaled the beginning of a new era. Encouraged by these results, a National Institute of Health Consensus Conference in 1983 concluded that liver transplantation had become a proven therapeutic modality and was no longer an experimental procedure. This far-reaching recommendation resulted in a rapid proliferation of transplant centers, since insurance companies and Medicare could no longer deny payment based on the premise that transplantation was experimental. In 1996 there were approximately 120 centers performing liver transplants in the United States. In busy centers, one can expect survival rates ranging from 60% to 90%, depending on the disease process and the recipient's clinical status before surgery. The debate has now shifted to donor availability, proper selection of recipients, timing of the transplant, and the place of transplantation in the overall scheme of financing health care. One should be reminded that the raison d'être for transplantation must include not only saving lives, but also restoring quality of life. Properly selected, the majority of patients should expect an improved and productive life after transplantation.

PATIENT SELECTION

As a general guideline, all patients with end-stage liver disease with an estimated life expectancy of 1 year or less should be considered as potential candidates for liver transplantation. The evaluation process is designed to answer specific questions surrounding the patient's candidacy (Box 363-1). Specific questions unique to a specific disease process must be satisfied, but overall the evaluation process is designed to uncover potential conditions that would preclude a successful transplant. Because the field of transplantation has matured, one can responsibly recommend transplantation earlier in the disease process, before complications ensue that lessen the chance for a favorable outcome.

INDICATIONS FOR TRANSPLANTATION

Specific diseases for which transplantation in the adult is indicated are listed in Box 363-2. Liver transplantation has been performed for almost all chronic end-stage liver diseases, selected congenital metabolic diseases, and fulminant hepatic failure. However, transplantation is more debatable in neoplastic and nonneoplastic disease where the disease present in the native liver can predictably be expected to recur. Long-term survival after transplantation in patients with cancer of the liver and biliary tree has been disappointing. This is particularly true for primary carcinoma of the bile ducts. Improved survival awaits development of effective modalities of adjuvant chemotherapy. These patients ideally should be transplanted only as part of an experimental protocol. In the past, transplantation of end-stage hepatitis B has resulted in recurrence of hepatitis in the graft, with dismal graft and patient survival. As a result, most centers in the United States considered chronic hepatitis B a contraindication to

CHAPTER

363 Liver Transplantation

Michael F. Sorrell and Jeremiah P. Donovan

The rapid evolution of liver transplantation has revolutionized the field of liver disease. The responsible physician is now obligated to consider the possibility of liver transplantation when confronted with a patient suffering from end-stage liver disease, for which an effective medical therapy is not available. After Starzl in Denver and Calne in Cambridge established the technical feasibility of liver transplantation, further progress was stymied by the lack of effective immunosuppression necessary for long-term survival. Survival after transplantation in the mid-1960s until 1980 never exceeded 25% to 30%. The emergence of cyclosporine A in 1980, with the concomitant dramatic increase in survival rates to between 60% and 80%,

---

BOX 363-1
Evaluation process

- What is the patient's diagnosis and how well is it established?
- What complications does the patient have, and what complications is the patient at risk of developing?
- How have the liver disease and its complications affected the patient's quality of life?
- Do any contraindications to transplantation exist?
- Does the patient have any concomitant disease process that would complicate transplantation?
- Will the patient be compliant with therapy after the transplant, and does he or she have the necessary psychosocial support structures to undergo the stresses associated with transplantation?
- Is the patient an adequate operative risk?
- Is there adequate financial support for the transplant?
- How soon should a transplant be considered to best optimize the patient's survival and quality of life?

BOX 363-2
Indications for liver transplantation in adults

I. Irreversible advanced chronic liver disease
  A. Predominantly cholestatic liver disease
    1. Primary biliary cirrhosis
    2. Primary sclerosing cholangitis
    3. Secondary biliary cirrhosis
    4. Alagille's syndrome
    5. Drug-induced biliary cirrhosis and cholestasis
    6. Caroli's syndrome
  B. Predominantly hepatocellular liver disease
    1. Chronic viral hepatitis
      a. Hepatitis B
      b. Hepatitis B with hepatitis D
      c. Hepatitis C
    2. Drug-induced liver disease
    3. Cryptogenic cirrhosis
    4. Autoimmune chronic active hepatitis with cirrhosis
    5. Alcoholic liver disease
    6. Wilson's disease
    7. Congenital hepatic fibrosis
  C. Vascular diseases that lead to hepatic dysfunction or portal hypertension or both
    1. Budd-Chiari syndrome
    2. Veno-occlusive disease
II. Hepatic malignancies not resectable without hepatic replacement but confined to the liver (hepatocellular carcinoma)
III. Fulminant hepatic failure
  A. Viral hepatitis (A, B, B+, D)
  B. Wilson's disease
  C. Drug- or toxin-induced hepatic failure
IV. Inherited metabolic disorders
  A. Hemophilia A
  B. Homozygous familial hypercholesterolemia
  C. Primary hyperoxaluria type I
  D. Others

BOX 363-3
Contraindications for liver transplantation

Absolute contraindications
- Active sepsis outside the biliary tract
- HIV-positive
- Extrahepatic malignancy
- Advanced cardiovascular disease
- Severe hypoxemia
- Active alcoholism
- Severe neurologic deficits

Relative contraindications
- Advanced age
- Biliary sepsis
- Extensive portal or mesenteric thrombosis
- Grade IV coma

---

transplantation. Utilizing high-dose intravenous hepatitis B immune globulin at the time of transplantation and long-term after transplantation, excellent graft and patient survival have recently been reported in both France and the United States. Unfortunately, intravenous hepatitis B immune globulin is not commercially available in the United States; therefore patients requiring intravenous hepatitis B immune globulin must be given immune globulin formulated for intramuscular use. A nucleoside analogue, lamivudine, has been to shown to inhibit replication of the hepatitis B virus and is being tested in trials designed to prevent recurrence of hepatitis B after liver transplantation. Fulminant liver failure secondary to hepatitis B infection does not exhibit the same proclivity for reinfection and chronicity. Satisfactory results can be expected when such patients are transplanted. It is important to recognize other comorbid conditions related to the underlying liver disease but not life-threatening by themselves, that may provide the impetus for early transplantation. Illustrative conditions would include severe osteopenic bone disease, intractable pruritus, and encephalopathy not responsive to medical therapy. Quality of life has become a more and more important factor in timing the transplant.

CONTRAINDICATIONS

As transplantation science has developed and experience has accumulated, the number of contraindications have decreased. These contraindications are outlined in Box 363-3. Many of the original contraindications were related to technical problems such as portal or mesenteric vein thrombosis or extensive right upper quadrant surgery that made the performance of the transplant hazardous. Advances in surgical technique have largely obviated such problems in experienced centers. With accumulated experience, age has become less of a factor. Survival rates approaching 90% have been obtained in low-risk patients over the age of 60 years. It has become clear that in-

creased survival rates are directly related to the condition of the patient at the time of transplantation. Shaw et al. demonstrated that when patients are stratified according to low-, intermediate-, and high-risk groups, actuarial survival rates of only 44.5% in 22 high-risk patients—compared with 85% and 90.5% for 27 intermediate-risk and 52 low-risk patients, respectively—were obtained.

SPECIFIC INDICATIONS IN THE ADULT
Alcoholic Cirrhosis

Perhaps no single indication for liver transplantation has caused so much controversy as transplantation in the alcoholic. Much of the debate has centered around the questions of potential recidivism in the recipient, as well as the concerns surrounding the use of a scarce resource in a patient with a "self-inflicted" disease. What is clear, however, is that survival after transplantation of the alcoholic parallels that of the nonalcoholic recipient. Recidivism rates of 11% to 12% at 1 year and 39% at 3 years after transplantation have been reported. However, these recidivism rates include any reported drinking episode. Destructive drinking—resulting in lack of treatment compliance, graft loss, or drunk driving—is much less common. There remain no absolute guidelines that predict return to drinking, but the best indicator of continuing sobriety is a period of at least 6 months of sobriety before transplantation. According to United Network Organ Sharing (UNOS) data, alcoholic liver disease is one of the two most frequent indications for transplantation in the United States.

Primary Biliary Cirrhosis

Historically, patients with primary biliary cirrhosis have been considered excellent candidates for transplantation. One- and five-year survival rates of 90% and 70%, respectively, have been reported. Timing of the operation has been difficult because of the indolent and fluctuating course inherent in the disease. Predictive models based on selected laboratory and clinical features have been proposed to aid in the decision-making process. Common indications for transplantation include variceal hemorrhage, recurrent encephalopathy, overwhelming fatigue, intractable pruritus, and hepatic osteodystrophy. Recurrence of primary biliary cirrhosis after successful liver transplantation has been reported by several different groups. This concept is not accepted by all, since the histologic appearance of recurrent disease and graft rejection is so similar that the distinction between recurrent primary biliary cirrhosis and rejection after liver biopsy is difficult at best.

Primary Sclerosing Cholangitis

In the majority of patients, primary sclerosing cholangitis occurs in association with ulcerative colitis. Rarely the inflammatory bowel disease will precede the duct lesion. Indications for transplantation are similar to those listed in regard to primary biliary cirrhosis. Predictive models to aid in the timing of transplantation have been proposed but are not yet of accepted clinical utility. One must be vigilant for the development of cholangiocarcinoma in these patients. In several series, cholangiocarcinoma was detected in 12% to 15% of patients for whom transplantation was considered.

Postnecrotic Cirrhosis

The etiologic agents responsible for the development of postnecrotic or cryptogenic cirrhosis include hepatitis C and B plus delta, as well as autoimmune hepatitis. A scattering of cases are caused by drugs such as methotrexate. In most transplant centers, hepatitis C–induced cirrhosis is the most frequent indication for transplantation. Recurrence of hepatitis C viremia after transplantation is universal, and recurrence of the hepatitis is frequent, but the subsequent course is often indolent. Management is often troublesome because of difficulty in distinguishing between recurrent hepatitis C and other causes of postoperative changes in liver function tests, such as rejection and biliary tract problems. Severe recurrent liver injury resulting from recurrent hepatitis C does occur and may require retransplantation. The initial results of retransplantation for hepatitis C have been rather poor. This may in part be the result of delaying the decision to retransplant until the patient is no longer an optimum candidate for transplantation. Further longitudinal experience with hepatitis C–transplanted patients will be necessary before accurate assessment of long-term outcomes can be estimated. Interferon is being used in various treatment protocols in the perioperative and postoperative period in an attempt to prevent or treat recurrent hepatitis C. At present, no antiviral therapy has proven effective in the patient with recurrent hepatitis C after liver transplantation. The presence of large numbers of patients with recurrent hepatitis C after transplantation will be one of the major challenges confronting the transplant community in the immediate future. Fewer patients with autoimmune cirrhosis have been transplanted, probably because of more effective treatment of the autoimmune process and the relative infrequency of the disease. There have been several reported cases of recurrent autoimmune hepatitis after transplantation.

Budd-Chiari Syndrome

The decision to transplant the patient with Budd-Chiari syndrome can be very difficult. Some patients can be treated with anticoagulation alone, whereas portosystemic shunting may be appropriate in others with less advanced disease. One must remember that what is possible is not obligatory. However, if the disease process is long-standing and cirrhosis is present, transplantation is the most feasible option. Outcome is excellent, although long-term anticoagulation is usually necessary.

Fulminant Hepatitis

Complex and difficult decisions surround the care of the patient with acute liver failure. In many instances, transplantation remains the best and often the only option in the desperately ill patient. The natural history of the well-characterized patient with fulminant failure and grade III to IV encephalopathy is such that one can predict with a certain degree of confidence mortality rates that will exceed 80%. In these instances, transplantation can be life saving. Improved survival has been associated with the employment of intracranial pressure–monitoring devices, as well as better selection and perioperative management of these unfortunate patients.

PEDIATRIC TRANSPLANTATION

The most common cause for transplantation in children is biliary atresia. In the well-prepared child, 1-year survival rates exceed 85%. It is generally felt that, if at all feasible, a Kasai (portoenterostomy) procedure should be done before liver transplantation. If successful, this will allow the child sufficient time to grow, thereby increasing the opportunity for obtaining a donor liver. Other indications for transplantation include α_1-antitrypsin deficiency, Wilson's disease unable to profit from chelation therapy, and any number of congenital and metabolic diseases. The major challenge remains the scarcity of do-

nor livers for the small child. Surgeons have responded to this problem in extremely innovative ways. The techniques of segmental and split liver grafts, plus the growing utilization of living related donors, have allowed for earlier and more optimum timing of transplantation.

THE DONOR LIVER

No discussion of liver transplantation would be complete without consideration of the donor liver. Donors are matched with recipients primarily by blood type and body size. The application of sophisticated tissue typing has not been found to be of clinical utility in the liver recipient as opposed to the kidney recipient. The improved survival in transplantation, with the subsequent proliferation of centers, has placed enormous demands on the donor pool. At present, more than 4000 liver transplants are performed each year in the United States. It is variously estimated that, at any one time, more than 40,000 potential recipients could benefit from liver transplantation. With the realization that the liver ages very little and atherosclerotic vascular disease is unusual in the hepatic artery, the age limits for donation have been raised upward to where, in limited series, donor livers in the 70-to-90 age range are being harvested. The problem is particularly acute in children, as discussed earlier. Unfortunately, the use of reduced-size grafts in children has accentuated the shortage in adults. The encouragement of organ donation is everyone's responsibility.

POSTOPERATIVE COURSE

Any number of medical and surgical complications can occur in the postoperative period. The most catastrophic event is primary graft failure immediately following transplantation. Known as *primary nonfunction*, it happens in approximately 3% of cases and requires immediate retransplantation. Hepatic artery thrombosis as the result of technical problems occurs most frequently in children, as opposed to adults, and may require retransplantation. Thrombosis of the hepatic artery may present under various guises, including rapidly increasing transaminases, high bilirubin level, bile duct strictures, or unexplained sepsis. Because the liver has a limited repertoire of response to injury, the transplant team must always confirm its clinical impression by carefully selected diagnostic testing. When graft dysfunction develops after the transplant, to err in diagnosis or treatment can be disastrous.

Rejection

At least one episode of acute rejection can be expected in approximately 70% of the patients undergoing transplantation. Acute rejection often occurs within the fifth to fourteenth postoperative day. When suspected, the diagnosis should be confirmed by percutaneous liver biopsy, since many other causes of graft dysfunction can mimic rejection. Standard immunosuppressive therapy of rejection includes additional steroids, plus the use of intravenous anti–T-cell monoclonal and polyclonal antibodies when indicated. In recalcitrant cases of acute rejection, switching to an alternate immunosuppressive drug may prove useful. An increasing number of drugs to treat newer rejection are in the investigational stage. The ideal immunosuppressive drug would prevent rejection without toxic side effects and without an increased susceptibility to infections.

Chronic rejection is clinically manifested by progressive, relentless cholestasis and histologically characterized by lymphocytic infiltration of the portal triads, arteriopathy, and disappearance of the interlobular bile ducts. It is estimated that chronic rejection develops in approximately 10% to 15% of transplants. It is not unusual for the patient to present with chronic rejection without previous evidence of acute rejection. Increased immunosuppression rarely will stay the course of documented chronic rejection. Retransplantation is often necessary.

Infection

In the postoperative period, infection is the predominant cause of mortality and morbidity. Cytomegalovirus (CMV) infection, either primary or reactivation, is present in 20% to 30% of patients. The most fearsome complication is that of systemic fungal infection, wherein mortality rates can exceed 90%. Bacterial infections account for more than 90% of clinically important infections after the patient has returned home. The risk of infection is markedly increased in patients with difficult, prolonged operations; an increased number of reoperations; and postoperative renal failure, and in those who require increased immunosuppression for control of rejection.

Other Considerations

Some impairment of renal function secondary to cyclosporine or FK 506 nephrotoxicity is a nearly constant feature in the posttransplant patient. On occasion the renal disease may become so severe that dialysis or renal transplantation is required. The development of malignancies, primarily lymphoproliferative in nature, are thought to be viral in origin and related to immunosuppressive therapy. Some tumors will respond to reduction in immunosuppression and the concomitant use of acyclovir. Chemotherapy has not proven useful in the majority of instances.

BIBLIOGRAPHY

Bismuth H, Sherlock DJ: Portasystemic shunting versus liver transplantation for Budd-Chiari syndrome, *Ann Surg* 214:581, 1991.

Klion FM et al: Prediction of survival of patients with primary biliary cirrhosis: examination of the Mayo Clinic model on a group of patients with known endpoint, *Gastroenterology* 102:310-313, 1992.

Lucey MR et al: Selection for and outcome of liver transplantation in alcoholic liver disease, *Gastroenterology* 102:1736-1741, 1992.

Maddrey WC, Sorrell MF: *Transplantation of the liver,* ed 2, Norwalk, Conn, 1995, Appleton & Lange.

National Institutes of Health Consensus Development Conference Statement: Liver Transplantation, June 20-23, 1983, *Hepatology* (suppl):107S-110S, 1983.

Samuel D et al: Liver transplantation in European patients with the hepatitis B surface antigen, *N Engl J Med* 329:1842-1847, 1993.

Shaw BW et al: Stratifying the causes of death in liver transplant recipients, *Arch Surg* 124:895-900, 1989.

Starzl TE, Demetris AJ, Van Thiel D: Liver transplantation, *N Engl J Med* 321:1014-1022,1092-1099, 1989.

Stieber AC et al: The surgical implications of the posttransplant lymphoproliferative disorders, *Transplant Proc* 23:1477-1479, 1991.

Whittington PF, Balistreri WF: Liver transplantation in pediatrics: indications, contraindications, and pretransplant management, *J Pediatr* 118:169-177, 1991.

Wright TL, Pereira B: Liver transplantation for chronic viral hepatitis, *Liver Transplantation and Surg* 1:30-42, 1995.

CHAPTER

364   Biliary Tract Stones and Associated Diseases

Michael D. Apstein

Gallstones are extremely common throughout the Western world. In the United States, 15% of the population, 35 million individuals, are estimated to have gallstones. Every year in the United States, 1 million patients are newly diagnosed with gallstones; half undergo cholecystectomy at an estimated annual cost of $6 billion. Despite new insights into the pathophysiology of gallstone disease, the key issues for physicians remain which patients should be treated and the roles of laparoscopic cholecystectomy and medical dissolution with oral bile acids. Biliary sludge has been recognized as a pathologic state capable of causing some, if not all, of the symptoms and complications of gallstones. Preventing gallstones with ursodiol in patients undergoing rapid weight loss is now approved by the Food and Drug Administration (FDA). Contact solvent dissolution and extracorporeal shock wave lithotripsy remain experimental and have limited applicability.

BILIARY TRACT STONES
Classification and Composition

Cholesterol stones and pigment (calcium [hydrogen] bilirubinate) stones are the two major categories of gallstones. Pigment stones are subdivided trivially as "brown" or "black." Black pigment stones are the more common pigment stones in Western populations and form principally under sterile conditions in the gallbladder. Brown pigment stones usually form de novo in infected, partially or intermittently obstructed bile ducts of patients following cholecystectomy. In Asians, brown pigment stones also form frequently in the intrahepatic bile ducts (hepatolithiasis) and also may involve the gallbladder.

The principal component of cholesterol stones is crystalline cholesterol monohydrate, usually greater than 70% by weight. Pigment stones are composed mostly of noncrystalline calcium (hydrogen) bilirubinate ("brown"), or polymer pigments ("black") derived from calcium (hydrogen) bilirubinate. Brown stones contain up to 30% cholesterol monohydrate, whereas black stones frequently contain none and only rarely as much as 10% cholesterol.

Both cholesterol and pigment stones always contain inorganic calcium salts. In the cholesterol and black pigment stones these salts are predominantly one polymorph (distinct crystalline form) of calcium carbonate or calcium phosphate. If stones contain sufficient amounts of crystalline calcium carbonates and phosphates, they are radiopaque. Calcium fatty acid soaps are typically found in brown pigment stones and render them radiolucent (Table 364-1). These stones also contain dead bacteria and their secretions.

Another component invariably present in gallbladder and bile duct stones is a poorly characterized glycoprotein mixture, previously called *unmeasured residue,* that represents mucus and other biliary proteins. Mucin glycoproteins pigmented with bilirubinate salts are found at the nuclei of all gallstones. Bile acids, free fatty acids, phospholipids, heavy metals, gas, and water are present in only trace amounts.

Because only cholesterol stones can be treated with nonsurgical therapies, identifying stone type by characteristics on plain abdominal x-ray films has practical importance even though it is imprecise and is now superseded by computed tomography (CT) scanning. Eighty percent of radiolucent gallstones and almost 100% with rim or central calcification are cholesterol stones; the remainder are brown pigment stones. Most diffusely calcified stones (70%) are black pigment stones. Overall, about 15% of gallstones are radiopaque on abdominal radiographs.

In addition to their chemical complexity, gallstones are physically heterogeneous. In appearance, cholesterol stones vary from yellow white to dark brown. If solitary (10%), they are usually round or mulberry shaped (Plate X-5). If multiple (90%), they are usually faceted and smooth (Plate X-6). Sizes range from less than 0.5 mm (gallsand) to 4 cm for solitary cholesterol gallstones. The cut surface demonstrates that the aggregated cholesterol monohydrate crystals have their long axes oriented radially to the nucleus. Mucin glycoproteins can be demonstrated in the nucleus and as a prosthesis dispersed throughout the stone. Solitary cholesterol stones always display pigmented centers composed of calcium (hydrogen) bilirubinate (Plate X-7). In the majority of cholesterol stones, discontinuous rings of calcium (hydrogen) bilirubinate, calcium salts, and amorphous material laminate the structure.

Black pigment stones almost always occur in multiples and are small (<5 to 10 mm), irregular in shape, often spiculated, and dark (usually black) (Plate X-8). Brown pigment stones are usually smooth, earthy to yellow in color, and often molded to the shape of the bile ducts. The content of mucin glycoproteins and other proteins in brown pigment stones is higher than that of cholesterol stones.

Pathophysiology

Gallstone formation, whether cholesterol or pigment, follows a logical pathophysiologic sequence: (1) bile becomes supersaturated with the insoluble solute, for example, cholesterol or calcium (hydrogen) bilirubinate (the chemical stage); (2) if supersaturation is extreme, homogeneous (spontaneous) nucleation may occur; if supersaturation is modest, the biliary tree, especially the gallbladder, must produce an

Table 364-1   Classification of gallstones

	CHOLESTEROL	POLYMER CALCIUM (HYDROGEN) BILIRUBINATE ("BLACK") PIGMENT	CALCIUM (HYDROGEN) BILIRUBINATE ("BROWN") PIGMENT
Primary location	Gallbladder	Gallbladder	90% biliary tree 10% gallbladder*
Number	Solitary (~10%) Multiple (90%)	Multiple	Solitary or multiple
Size	Up to 4 cm	2 to 5 mm	2 to 20 mm
Appearance	White-yellow-brown	Shiny black	Earthy brown
Hardness	Hard	Hard	Soft
Clinical associations	Hypersecretion of biliary cholesterol	Increased bilirubin secretion and bile salt deficiency	Anaerobic biliary infection and biliary obstruction
Cholesterol content	>70%	0%-10%	<30%
Calcium salts	Calcium carbonate or phosphate	Calcium phosphate carbonate and calcium (hydrogen) bilirubinate	Calcium (fatty acid) soaps, calcium (hydrogen) bilirubinate
Radiodensity	Lucent or rim calcification	70% opaque	Lucent

*Most likely secondary to prior episodes of healed, acute cholecystitis.

agent to induce nucleation (heterogeneous) and precipitation (the physical stage); and finally (3) stasis is required for the precipitates to agglomerate and grow to form macroscopic stones (the growth stage).

Cholesterol Stones

Patients with cholesterol gallstones typically have three pathophysiologic defects: supersaturation of bile with cholesterol, accelerated cholesterol nucleation, and sluggish gallbladder motility. However, recent studies suggest that a genetically mediated hypersecretion of cholesterol from the liver is the fundamental defect and the other pathophysiologic events are secondary.

Cholesterol Supersaturation. Cholesterol and bile salt secretions into bile are the body's major excretory routes for cholesterol. Cholesterol is insoluble in water but is solubilized in bile by the other biliary lipids (i.e., the detergent-like bile salts and the phospholipid lecithin) to form macromolecular, water-soluble complexes called *mixed micelles* and small unilamellar vesicles of lecithin and cholesterol (Chapter 349).

By plotting the relative molar compositions of bile salts, lecithin, and cholesterol in gallbladder and hepatic bile as a single point on triangular coordinates (Fig. 364-1), one can define the compositions in which the cholesterol is solubilized in mixed micelles or in the mixed micelles plus unilamellar vesicles. When plotted in this fashion, hepatic bile from both normal subjects and gallstone patients is "supersaturated" with cholesterol with respect to the solubilizing capacity of the micellar phase. However, a dilute bile system is extremely stable because the excess cholesterol is solubilized by metastable unilamellar vesicles, forming a two-phase (micellar and vesicular) system. Gallbladder bile from all cholesterol stone patients and approximately 50% of controls is also "supersaturated" with cholesterol with respect to the micellar phase. Bile from normal human beings contains relatively less cholesterol than that from gallstone patients. In gallstone subjects the higher relative contents of cholesterol are solubilized in supersaturated micelles and unilamellar vesicles. In concentrated gallbladder biles the vesicles become unstable and rapidly nucleate solid cholesterol crystals.

A relative excess of cholesterol molecules compared with molecules of the solubilizing lipids, bile salts, and lecithin must be present in bile before cholesterol gallstones can form. In this setting, cholesterol molecules can nucleate, crystallize, and precipitate from solution. In humans this imbalance between cholesterol and bile salts plus lecithin (lithogenic bile) is caused by hypersecretion of biliary cholesterol, hyposecretion of biliary bile salts, or both. A deficiency of biliary lecithin has not been identified.

Nucleation. Cholesterol precipitates (nucleates) from bile as the unilamellar vesicles that carry excess cholesterol fuse and become unstable when concentrated in the gallbladder (Fig. 364-1). The control of nucleation by pronucleating and antinucleating factors is critical

because most humans have supersaturated bile for hours during the day (fasting) yet do not form gallstones. A number of normal lipid and protein components of bile have been identified as pronucleating and antinucleating agents, but it is not known which ones are clinically relevant in normal and gallstone-forming biles. Gallbladder bile of persons with cholesterol stones precipitates cholesterol crystals about five times faster than do control gallbladder biles for the same degree of cholesterol supersaturation. Stimulation of the gallbladder mucosa by lithogenic bile induces hypersecretion of mucin glycoproteins. It is believed that mucin gel in the gallbladder lumen may be important in inducing nucleation. In fact, in lithogenic animal models, abnormal bile stimulates gallbladder mucin synthesis and secretion, whereas drugs that inhibit mucin production can prevent gallstones despite the persistence of supersaturated bile.

Gallbladder Dysmotility. Impaired gallbladder motility with increased gallbladder fasting and residual volumes (stasis) is an important primary defect predisposing to cholesterol gallstone formation. Animals fed a lithogenic diet demonstrate decreased gallbladder smooth muscle contractility and increased gallbladder fasting and residual volumes before gallstones develop. Furthermore, human gallbladder muscle contractility is reduced in patients with cholesterol gallstones compared to those with pigment stones. In cholesterol stone disease, gallbladder stasis allows cholesterol crystals to be entrapped by mucin glycoproteins, remain within the gallbladder, aggregate, and grow into macroscopic stones. Further, impaired gallbladder motor function is present in about 70% of gallstone patients consistent with the predominance of cholesterol stones.

Pigment Stones

Black pigment stones. Pathogenesis of black pigment gallstones is related to an increased biliary concentration of unconjugated bilirubin and ionized calcium, decreased biliary bile salt levels, and possibly gallbladder stasis. Both hepatic and gallbladder biles of black pigment stone patients without biliary infection or hemolytic states are supersaturated with calcium (hydrogen) bilirubinate and perhaps with calcium carbonate. The pigment supersaturation may result from (1) a defect in or overloading of hepatic conjugation with increased production of bilirubin monoglucuronides, (2) increased endogenous β-glucuronidase activity within the biliary tree, or (3) a deficiency of bile salt–lecithin solubilizers. Biliary ionized calcium then forms a high-affinity salt bond with two molecules of the acid species of unconjugated bilirubin, which precipitates and grows to form stones. Normally, bile salts both solubilize unconjugated bilirubin and bind ionized calcium. Consequently, decreased biliary bile salt levels strongly promote pigment stone formation by rendering more unconjugated bilirubin and free ionized calcium available for coprecipitation.

Very little is known about the nucleation or growth stage of black pigment stones, but it is likely that bilirubin and bile salt concentrations, biliary pH, calcium concentration, and gallbladder mucin glycoproteins play complementary roles. No work has been carried out on

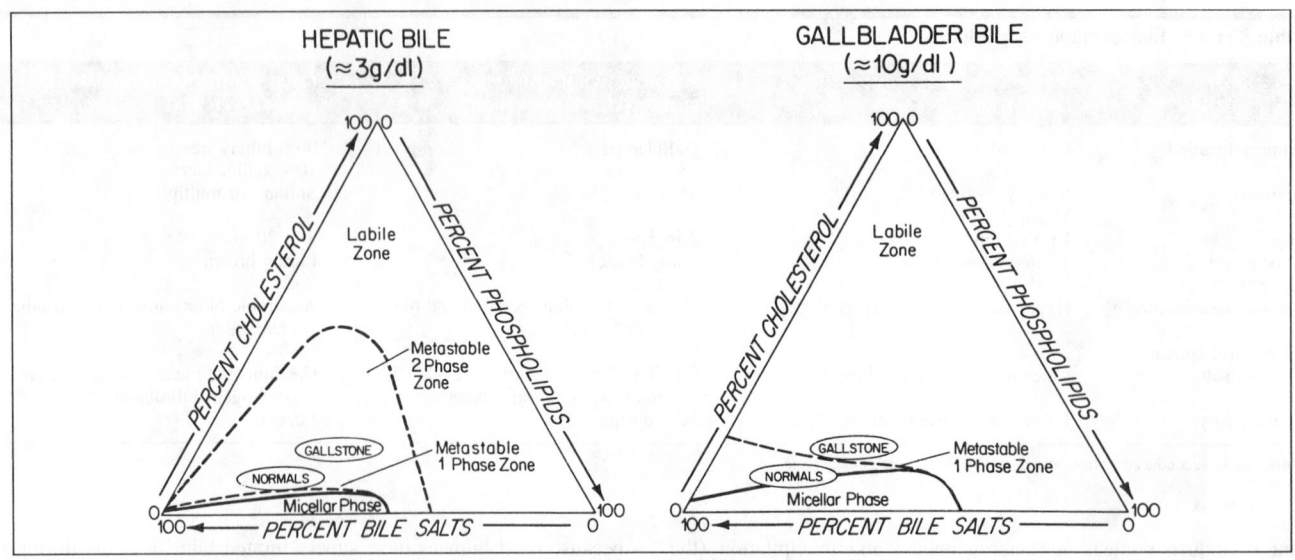

FIGURE 364-1   Relative lipid compositions of hepatic and gallbladder bile in normal subjects and in patients with cholesterol gallstones. In the micellar phase, bile is unsaturated with cholesterol; in the one-phase metastable zones, micelles are supersaturated with cholesterol but do not nucleate readily. In the two-phase metastable zone, unilamellar vesicles cooperate with supersaturated micelles to solubilize cholesterol. Outside these zones, bile nucleates spontaneously.

Table 364-2   Frequency of gallstone occurrence in selected groups and countries (autopsy series)

VERY COMMON (10%-70%)	COMMON (10%-30%)	INTERMEDIATE (<10%)	RARE (0%-1%)
United States (Indians)	United States (whites)	United States (blacks)	East Africa
South America (Indians)	Denmark	Japan (urban population)	West Africa
Ecuador	Norway	Thailand	New Guinea
Bolivia	United Kingdom	Northern India	Rural Japan
Chile	Italy	Canada (urban Eskimos)	Canada (rural Eskimos)
Mexico	New Zealand	China	Egypt
Canada (Indians)	Zimbabwe (whites)	Norway	Southern India
Sweden	Canada (whites)	Greece	
Czechoslovakia	Australia	Uzbekistan	
Germany	Finland	Indonesia	
	Japan	South Africa (Bantu)	
	South Africa (whites)		
	Russia		
	Ukraine		

Modified from Shaffer EA, Small DM: *Curr Probl Surg* 13:1, 1976; after Lowenfels AB, *Gut* 21:1090, 1980, and Brett M, Barker DJP: *Int J Epidemiol* 5:335, 1976; Carey MC, O'Donovan MA: Gallstone disease: current concepts in the epidemiology, pathogenesis and management. In *Harrison's principles of internal medicine* (Update V), New York, 1984, McGraw-Hill.

the polymerization of bile pigments. Because such stones occur predominantly in the gallbladder and always in noninfected bile, it is virtually certain that they form and grow by mechanisms chemically and physically distinct from those giving rise to brown pigment stones.

Brown pigment stones. Bacterial invasion is a prerequisite of brown pigment stone formation in both intrahepatic and extrahepatic bile ducts. Biliary tract infection results in high β-glucuronidase, conjugated bile salt hydrolase, and phospholipase A_1 activities in bile. The microbial β-glucuronidase, in contrast to the biliary tree enzyme, deconjugates bilirubin conjugates extremely rapidly at biliary pH and, as a result, the solubility of calcium (hydrogen) bilirubinate in bile is greatly exceeded. The conjugated bile salt hydrolase deconjugates bile salts and the phospholipase A_1 cleaves biliary lecithin, resulting in the formation of calcium bile salts and calcium soaps, respectively. Because of the limited capacity of human bile to solubilize any calcium salt and to maintain it in a metastable supersaturated solution, pigment stones can form in both intrahepatic and extrahepatic ducts. The appreciable cholesterol content in these stones results from depletion of the cholesterol solubilizers (bile salts and lecithin) by bacterial enzymatic hydrolysis.

Epidemiology

There is tremendous geographic variation in the prevalence as well as in the predominant type of gallstones (Table 364-2). Gallstones are much rarer in underdeveloped countries than in Western societies. In the West, 70% to 80% of gallstones are cholesterol, whereas pigment gallstones constitute the majority in rural areas of Japan, in other Asian countries, and in certain parts of Latin America.

The prevalence of cholesterol and pigment gallstones has changed dramatically in parts of the Orient during this century. After World War II, gallstones were rare and usually of the pigment variety in Japan and China. Since 1950 the prevalence of cholesterol gallstones has increased markedly in these countries, and the prevalence of pigment gallstones has fallen.

With the advent of ultrasonography, numerous studies have determined the true prevalence rates of gallstones in ambulatory, healthy populations. The pivotal study was carried out in the town of Sirimone, Italy, in the early 1980s, when males and females of all ages, 70% of the population, underwent abdominal ultrasonography. The prevalence of gallstones in women was shown to increase linearly with age from 2.9% in the 18- to 29-year-old group to 27% in the

BOX 364-1
Putative risk factors for gallstones

Cholesterol gallstones
Female gender
Parity
Obesity
Rapid weight loss
Advancing age
Family history
American Indian heritage
Gallbladder stasis syndromes
Medication: fibrates, estrogens, anabolic steroids, octreotide
Hypertriglyceridemia and low HDL cholesterol
Inborn errors of bile salt synthesis
Spinal cord injury

Pigment gallstones
Hemolytic disorders
Hepatic cirrhosis
Advancing age
Ileal disease, resection, bypass
Stasis syndromes (TPN, postvagotomy)
Chronic hypercalcemia
Advanced AIDS
Biliary infection

50- to 65-year-old group. Prevalence in men was half that in women. Other ultrasonographic studies of Western populations—Great Britain, Denmark, Germany, and Russia—confirm that gallstones are very common, with considerable intercontinental variation, Germany having the highest prevalence rates in Europe. In the United States, rigorous studies of randomly selected samples of whites are lacking, but, as is well known, certain U.S. and Canadian Indian tribes (Pima, Navajo, Chippewa, and MicMac) have epidemic rates of gallstones. Hispanic populations have a higher prevalence of gallstones than do U.S. whites.

PUTATIVE RISK FACTORS FOR GALLSTONE FORMATION

Putative risk factors for gallstones are listed in Box 364-1 and are summarized here.

Cholesterol Gallstones

For cholesterol gallstone disease, the putative risk factors probably modulate the underlying genetic predisposition.

Gender. Women have twice the risk as men of developing cholesterol gallstones because estrogen increases biliary cholesterol secretion. Before puberty this risk is negligible, and beyond menopause the increased risk disappears.

Parity. Pregnancy is an independent risk factor for cholesterol gallstones. The risk increases with increasing parity, especially with more than two children. During pregnancy, elevated estrogen and progesterone levels increase biliary cholesterol secretion. Elevated progesterone levels also inhibit gallbladder contractility. Forty percent of women develop "biliary sludge" in their gallbladder, a prestone condition, during pregnancy. Moreover, 12% of women form their first stones during pregnancy.

Obesity. Obesity is strongly associated with increased gallstone prevalence. The risk is proportional to the increase in total body fat. Obese people synthesize more cholesterol in both hepatic and nonhepatic tissues, transport it to the liver, and secrete more of it into bile, leading to bile that is often greatly supersaturated with cholesterol. Biliary cholesterol saturation reverts to normal after obese subjects achieve ideal body weight.

Rapid Weight Loss. Obese patients undergoing rapid weight loss (1% to 2% of body weight, or approximately 1 to 2 kg/week), either by very low caloric dieting or gastric stapling, have a 25% to 40% chance of developing gallstones within 4 months. During rapid weight loss, biliary cholesterol saturation increases acutely as cholesterol is mobilized from adipose tissue and skin and secreted into bile.

Advancing Age. Some but not all studies have demonstrated that biliary cholesterol saturation increases with advancing age as biliary cholesterol secretion increases and biliary bile salt synthesis decreases.

American Indians. Prevalence rates of gallstones among male and female Pima Indians are among the highest in the world: approximately 70% to 80% of men and women over 55 years of age have gallstones. In contrast to the low frequency of symptoms in whites or Pima men, 40% to 50% of Pima women over 35 years of age have symptoms or complications of gallstones.

Medications. Hypolipidemic drugs (clofibrate, gemfibrozil) that lower serum cholesterol by increasing biliary cholesterol secretion increase the risk of cholesterol gallstones by twofold to threefold. Sequestration of bile salts by drugs (cholestyramine, colestipol) does not result in an increased risk of gallstones because the liver compensates by increasing synthesis of bile salts to maintain normal bile salt secretion. Competitive inhibitors of 3-hydroxy-3-methylglutaryl coenzyme A (HMGCoA) reductase (lovastatin, simvastatin, pravastatin) *decrease* biliary cholesterol saturation. Estrogen therapy is associated with an increased risk of developing cholesterol gallstones in both men and women. Oral contraceptive steroids increase biliary cholesterol secretion and saturation but do not affect gallbladder motility.

Serum Lipids. An *inverse* correlation exists between high-density lipoprotein (HDL) cholesterol and gallstone prevalence. In contrast, there is a very strong *positive* correlation between plasma triglyceride concentrations, especially when combined with low HDL-cholesterol levels, and gallstone prevalence.

Diet. Increased intake of calories, refined carbohydrate (e.g., sucrose), cholesterol, and saturated fats have all been postulated to cause cholesterol gallstones. Patients with cholesterol gallstones secrete a greater fraction of dietary cholesterol into bile than do normal subjects. A diet high in bran has been reported to decrease biliary cholesterol saturation and potentially prevent stones. However, there is no conclusive evidence, with the exceptions of obesity and weight loss, that dietary habits influence cholesterol gallstone formation.

Spinal Cord Injury. Patients with spinal cord injury have a 10% incidence of forming gallstones within the first year after injury. This high risk, which is 20 times normal, is believed to be secondary to abnormal gallbladder motility and probably biliary hypersecretion of cholesterol from the progressive reduction in body mass.

Primary Biliary Cirrhosis. Patients with primary biliary cirrhosis have an increased prevalence of gallstones. Stone analysis has not been performed, but the elevated cholesterol saturation of bile in these patients suggest that they form cholesterol stones. The underlying pathophysiologic defects are not known.

Diabetes Mellitus. Despite obesity and increased total body cholesterol synthesis and decreased gallbladder motility seen in patients with diabetes, diabetes mellitus itself does not appear to be an independent risk factor for cholesterol gallstone disease. Studies describing such a correlation have failed to control for ethnic origin (e.g., American Indian), obesity, and hypertriglyceridemia.

Pigment Gallstones

Chronic Hemolysis. Inherited hemolytic anemias, sickle cell disease, spherocytosis, thalassemia, chronic hemolysis associated with artificial heart valves, and malaria dramatically increase the risk of pigment stone formation because of increased biliary secretion of total bilirubin conjugates, especially bilirubin monoglucuronide, at the expense of the bilirubin diglucuronides. The monoglucuronide is more easily hydrolyzed to unconjugated bilirubin in sterile bile than bilirubin diglucuronide, the predominant conjugate in healthy individuals.

Alcoholic Cirrhosis. Patients with alcoholic cirrhosis have an increased prevalence of pigment gallstones, which is positively correlated with age and severity of liver disease. Thirty percent to 60% of alcoholic cirrhotics have gallstones, almost half of which are black pigment stones. The precise pathophysiologic defects have not been identified, but subclinical hemolysis, defective bilirubin conjugation, alcohol-induced biliary secretion of unconjugated bilirubin into bile, and defective bile salt synthesis associated with liver disease have all been suggested.

Age. Increasing age is a risk factor for both hemolytic and nonhemolytic pigment gallstone formation in high-risk patients as well as the general population without any obvious risk factor for pigment stones. In fact, gallstones that recur after several cycles of successful gallstone dissolution appear to be age-related pigment stones.

Ileal Disease, Resection, and Bypass. Patients with ileal dysfunction have a strikingly increased risk for developing gallstones. Gallstones develop in approximately 30% to 50% of patients with ileal Crohn's disease; the risk correlates positively with the extent and duration of ileal dysfunction. Although ileal disease or resection leads to cholesterol supersaturation and cholesterol stone formation in some patients, careful studies now show that most patients with ileal dysfunction form black pigment, not cholesterol stones.

Biliary Infection. In the Orient, brown pigment stones are frequently found in the intrahepatic bile ducts and are always associated with infection by colonic organisms (usually *Escherichia coli*) or parasitic infestation (*Clonorchis sinensis, Ascaris lumbricoides,* or other helminths). In Western patients, intraductal stones developing after cholecystectomy are invariably associated with bile stasis, biliary tree infection, and/or retained suture material. Diverticula near the ampulla of Vater are associated with pigment gallstones in the bile ducts, presumably because the colonized diverticulum alters ampullary muscular tone and allows the biliary tract to become repeatedly infected with anaerobic bacteria.

Gallbladder Stasis. Impaired gallbladder emptying is an essential early defect in both cholesterol and pigment gallstone formation. In cholesterol stone disease, gallbladder stasis occurs in women during pregnancy and in patients with somatostatinoma or those receiving octreotide therapy, low fat–hypocaloric diets, and with spinal cord injury. Furthermore, increased fasting and residual gallbladder volumes have been demonstrated in the majority (70%) of white patients with gallstones.

For pigment stone disease, TPN is a powerful risk factor for gallstone formation. In one study, 100% of patients on TPN for longer than 6 weeks develop "biliary sludge" in their gallbladder. Routine ultrasonographic screening of adults on TPN for a mean of 23 months demonstrated that stones developed in 25% without and 39% with ileal disease. Gallstones form during TPN because of decreased gallbladder motility from lack of meal-stimulated cholecystokinin (CCK) release, resulting in increased fasting and residual volumes. The daily intravenous administration of CCK-octapeptide (via the existing central venous catheter) in patients receiving TPN corrects the motility defect and prevents stone formation. A similar, though less severe, defect occurs after vagotomy and is associated with a threefold to fivefold increased risk of gallstone formation. Stone composition in patients after vagotomy has not been determined.

DIAGNOSTIC TESTS FOR BILIARY TRACT STONES

Calcified stones are visualized as radiopaque shadows in the right upper quadrant in supine, upright, and lateral abdominal radiographs. Because 85% of stones are radiolucent, they are visualized only with an oral cholecystogram or by abdominal ultrasonography (see later). If radiopaque gallstones are seen elsewhere in the gut

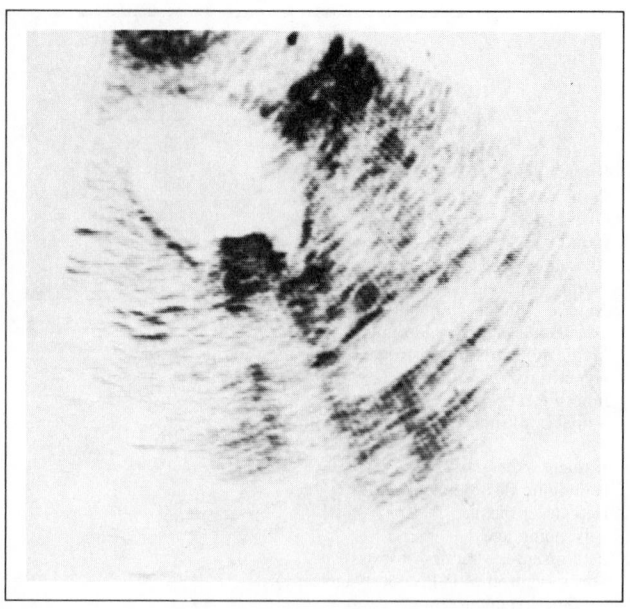

FIGURE 364-2   Ultrasonogram demonstrating a large gallstone in a dilated gallbladder. Note acoustic shadowing.

and/or air is present in the biliary tree, a spontaneous cholecystoenteric fistula should be suspected. If these patients have symptoms of intestinal obstruction, with air-fluid levels and dilated loops of small bowel, gallstone ileus is the most likely diagnosis. Air within the biliary system can also be seen in patients with an incompetent sphincter of Oddi, penetration of a chronic duodenal ulcer, or cholangitis with gas-forming organisms. In free perforation of the gallbladder, both gallstones and air may be seen free in the peritoneal cavity.

The time-honored radiologic examination of the gallbladder, oral cholecystography (OCG), has been replaced by ultrasonography because it is safer and more accurate.

Abdominal real-time ultrasonography reveals gallbladder stones as small as 3 mm in 95% to 97% of patients. The diagnosis of gallstones with the use of ultrasonography is certain when (1) the stone is within the gallbladder, (2) the stone is mobile, and (3) it casts an acoustic shadow (Fig. 364-2). By this means, a solitary gallstone can be differentiated from the less common adenomyoma of the gallbladder. Because x-rays are not involved and because radiocontrast agents occasionally induce toxic or allergic reactions, we believe that ultrasonography should be the initial examination of choice for stones in the gallbladder and biliary tree in both acute and nonacute situations.

Occasionally, ultrasonography gives false-negative results. If the clinical suspicion remains high, examination of the bile for crystals can be helpful (see later discussion).

The ultrasonographic examination, but not oral cholecystography, can detect "biliary sludge," multiple weak echoes without acoustic shadowing in the dependent part of the gallbladder. Biliary sludge is a mixture of mucin glycoproteins and microprecipitates of calcium (hydrogen) bilirubinate, liquid crystals of bile lipids, solid cholesterol monohydrate crystals, and microspheroliths of crystalline calcium carbonate or phosphate. Biliary sludge can form during prolonged fasting in debilitated hospitalized patients, during TPN, in the postoperative period, in patients with extrahepatic biliary obstruction, and in 40% of women during the last trimester of pregnancy.

Ultrasonographic examination may also demonstrate intraductal stones and/or dilatation of the intrahepatic or extrahepatic ductal systems. Although false-positive results are considered rare, the impression that the duct is normal may be in error in about 15% of cases. Obstruction may not correlate with dilatation of intrahepatic ducts because cirrhosis or cholangitis may have caused scarring, thereby preventing ductal dilatation. Furthermore, small stones in a greatly dilated duct are easily missed.

For radionuclide scanning, a ^{99m}Tc-labeled iminodiacetic acid derivative (usually DISIDA) is injected intravenously. The isotope is efficiently extracted by the liver and secreted into the biliary tree even when serum bilirubin levels are 10 to 20 mg/dl. Surface counting of the gamma emission from the radionuclide source outlines the biliary tree, including the gallbladder, and demonstrates flow into the duodenum. Cholescintigraphy effectively excludes acute cholecystitis if the gallbladder is demonstrated. If the gallbladder is not visualized but the radionuclide scan demonstrates patency of the biliary tree and free flow into the duodenum, the diagnosis of cholecystitis is very likely in the appropriate clinical setting.

Endoscopic retrograde cholangiopancreatography (ERCP) permits visualization of the biliary tree by retrograde injection of radiographic contrast material directly into the common duct after cannulation at the ampulla via a flexible fiberoptic duodenoscope (Chapter 328). ERCP is the diagnostic procedure of choice for evaluating the bile ducts. It also allows visualization of the periampullary region of the duodenum and the pancreatic duct. Most important, therapeutic maneuvers—such as stone extraction, sphincterotomy, stent placement—can be performed via this approach (Chapter 328).

Transhepatic cholangiography is now reserved for patients whose bile ducts cannot be visualized by ERCP. Major complications are rare but include hemorrhage, cholangitis, and bile peritonitis.

Duodenal drainage can be useful in searching for occult gallstone disease when the patient's symptoms are typical but results of the other tests are negative or equivocal. A sample of gallbladder bile is obtained via a duodenal tube after the patient is given a substance (preferably cholecystokinin octapeptide) intravenously that contracts the gallbladder. The bile samples and the centrifuged sediments should be examined with a polarizing microscope. The presence of flat, rhombohedral birefringent plates with notched corners and angles of approximately 79 and 101 degrees is diagnostic of cholesterol monohydrate crystals (Plate X-9). These crystals are never observed in normal bile. Calcium bilirubinate forms amorphous, birefringent, golden-yellow precipitates (Plate X-9) and, when present, suggests pigment or pigmented cholesterol stones. Rounded "cart-wheel" birefringent crystals that are not compressible are pathognomonic for inorganic calcium, especially carbonate salts. They are often present with calcified cholesterol or black pigment gallstones. Birefringent liquid crystals of cholesterol esters and methyl sterol esters in bile are observed only with cholesterolosis of the gallbladder. The microscopic identification of these precipitates in bile requires considerable skill and experience. When found in association with a suggestive clinical history, crystals or precipitates indicate the presence of biliary tract stones or cholesterolosis. False-positive tests, however, have been reported in patients with hepatic and non–stone-related pancreatic diseases.

NATURAL HISTORY OF ASYMPTOMATIC VERSUS SYMPTOMATIC GALLSTONES

Asymptomatic (silent) gallstones are detected during routine screening or diagnostic evaluation of chest or abdominal pain with a more obvious etiology. Recent epidemiologic evidence from large well-designed ultrasonographic screening studies in various parts of the world suggests that up to 80% of whites with "silent" stones have never experienced biliary pain or complications. Ultrasonographic screening of a young population (2 to 18 years) with sickle cell anemia has demonstrated that, although the prevalence of black pigment gallstones increases from approximately 10% in the 2- to 4-year-old age group to over 40% in the 15- to 18-year-old age group, only 22% of those with gallstones or sludge have biliary symptoms.

Data from typical Western populations suggest that the truly asymptomatic gallstone patient runs a relatively benign course, with only a 15% cumulative chance of developing symptoms over a 15-year period. In contrast, the mildly symptomatic patient (i.e., biliary pain not requiring hospitalization and no disruption of lifestyle) has a less benign course. These patients have a 20% chance of developing symptoms and complications over a 5-year period. Patients who are initially hospitalized for biliary pain have a greater than 50% chance of developing recurrent symptoms or complications over the next 20 years.

Gallstones may occasionally disappear. In about 7% of patients with multiple gallstones, but in less than 1% of patients with solitary cholesterol stones, the stones disappear spontaneously over a 10-year follow-up period, presumably via common bile duct migration into the duodenum. Spontaneous dissolution of stones is very rare.

Because of the benign course of patients with asymptomatic gallstones, the consensus of internists and surgeons is for expectant management only. A recent decision analysis demonstrated that prophylactic cholecystectomy for men with asymptomatic gallstones resulted in a *loss* of from 4 to 18 days of life expectancy depending on age. We advise these patients that they have a 10% to 30% chance of becoming symptomatic over the next 20 years, and they should be reevaluated only if symptoms occur.

Prophylactic cholecystectomy should be considered for several groups of patients with asymptomatic gallstones. One group is patients whose occupations require that they live for prolonged time periods in areas deficient in adequate medical facilities. In the past, because patients with diabetes who developed acute cholecystitis were thought to have a mortality rate as high as 15%, prophylactic cholecystectomies were recommended. Other associated conditions, such as cardiovascular disease, are responsible for this increased mortality. Nonetheless, patients with diabetes are disproportionately represented in series of deaths from gallstone disease. Despite a decision analysis concluding that prophylactic cholecystectomy in patients with diabetes shortened life span by 2 to 8 months regardless of patient age, the issue remains unsettled. We believe that the presence of diabetes per se is not an indication for prophylactic cholecystectomy. Because patients with nonfunctioning gallbladders have a worse long-term course, however, we recommend prophylactic cholecystectomy for a diabetic with a nonvisualizing gallbladder by radionuclide scanning. Gallbladder carcinoma is etiologically associated with gallstones and/or lithogenic bile, but its incidence in whites is very low (Chapter 365). Therefore prophylactic cholecystectomy to prevent gallbladder carcinoma in asymptomatic patients with stones is not recommended, except in two subgroups who have a fourfold to sevenfold increased risk: (1) American Indian women, and (2) patients with solitary stones that exceed 3.0 cm in diameter. Dissolution therapy with ursodiol (see later) would be inappropriate in these settings, since the gallstones themselves may not necessarily be the causative or even the promoting factor.

Four rare conditions require cholecystectomy even in the absence of gallstones because of the proven risk of gallbladder cancer: (1) gallbladder with a calcified wall ("porcelain" gallbladder); (2) gallbladder polyps >12 mm in absence of hyperplastic cholesterolosis in the remainder of the gallbladder; (3) anomalous pancreaticobiliary ductal junction; and (4) chronic *Salmonella typhosa* carriers.

The natural history of biliary sludge is variable. In many patients, biliary sludge in the gallbladder is innocuous and disappears soon after pregnancy or oral refeeding of the fasting patient. In others, however, biliary sludge may cause biliary pain, acute cholecystitis, or pancreatitis. The evolution of biliary sludge to gallstones has been documented during TPN and rapid weight loss and after pregnancy and spinal cord injury and supports the concept that biliary sludge represents an early but still reversible stage of gallstone formation.

BILIARY "COLIC"

The traditional designation for biliary pain, *biliary colic,* is a misnomer. The pain usually becomes severe within a few minutes of onset and is constant (i.e., does not wax and wane like that of intestinal colic). The pain is most commonly located in either the epigastrium or the right upper quadrant at the time of onset. Occasionally (<5% of patients) pain is felt in other parts of the abdomen or chest. Simultaneously referred pain in the scapular area or the posterior chest wall is common, as are nausea and vomiting, which often occur within 30 minutes of the onset of pain. Pain is usually intense for 1 to 4 hours and then resolves slowly, leaving the patient with a vague residual ache or soreness. As with renal "colic," the patient may have great difficulty lying still.

The timing of biliary colic is unpredictable, but the patient with known gallstones often associates its onset with the ingestion of a large or rich meal. Attacks may occur only once; every few years; or, in rare patients, daily. Patients with frequent episodes of pain should expect that pattern to continue in the future. It is believed that biliary pain is caused (1) by gallbladder contraction during transient cystic duct obstruction by a gallstone, or (2) by common duct contraction during passage of a stone. Because pain is as common in patients with large solitary stones as in patients with multiple stones, it may also be related to stones in the infundibulum of the gallbladder or even to viscous mucus obstructing the neck of the gallbladder. Resolution occurs once the stone drops back into the fundus of the gallbladder or migrates out of the common duct into the duodenum. Fatty food intolerance, belching, postprandial bloating, "flatulent dyspepsia," heartburn, regurgitation, or painless nausea and vomiting do not correlate at all with the presence of gallstones, are more likely to have other causes, and are rarely relieved permanently by cholecystectomy.

Physical examination of a patient during an attack of biliary pain is usually normal or reveals only mild right upper quadrant tenderness. Fever or leukocytosis is absent; if they are present, acute cholecystitis should seriously be suspected. Serum bilirubin, alkaline phosphatase, amylase, and transaminases should be normal when the stone obstructs the cystic duct but may be elevated if the stone has migrated into and obstructs the common bile duct.

Diagnosis

Ultrasonography is the test of choice for the diagnosis of gallstones or biliary sludge in the acute setting. For patients with symptoms highly suggestive of gallstones and repeatedly negative ultrasonography, microscopy of an aliquot of bile obtained by duodenal drainage to look for crystals or precipitates may provide the only clue that gallstone disease is present (Plate X-9).

Other common causes of abdominal pain should be considered in the differential diagnosis of biliary pain, including peptic ulcer disease, lobar pneumonia, alcoholic hepatitis, pancreatitis, and radicular pain caused by spinal lesions. Just as biliary colic may occasionally (~5% of patients) be felt only in the precordium, angina pectoris may cause pain in the abdomen, usually a subxiphoid location, and may be associated with nausea, heartburn, and regurgitation. A common cause for recurrent nonspecific dyspeptic symptoms, including abdominal pain, is the irritable colon syndrome; but the pain is usually located in the left upper or lower quadrant, and bowel habits are usually abnormal. Other forms of abdominal pain—such as that of renal colic, intestinal colic, and pain that occurs in the early phase of acute appendicitis—are usually readily distinguishable from biliary pain by their location and character.

Treatment

Patients with more than one attack of biliary pain should be treated definitively to prevent (1) future attacks of biliary pain; and (2) the complications of gallstones, including acute cholecystitis, cholangitis, and pancreatitis.

Cholecystectomy. Cholecystectomy is the treatment of choice for the majority of patients with biliary pain from gallstones. The operation relieves symptoms in more than 85% of individuals. In the vast majority of the others, cholecystectomy fails because the operation is performed for inappropriate symptoms. Elective, traditional (open) cholecystectomy is very safe. Mortality is related to age, sex, preexisting medical conditions, and nature of the operation (emergency for complications or elective).

The National Halothane Study of 27,600 cholecystectomies performed in the early 1960s revealed that operative mortality for elective procedures in women in moderately good health ranged from 0.05% below the age of 50 to 0.3% at age 70. Severe concomitant disease increased operative mortality to 1.3% and 1.7%, respectively. In all categories, men had roughly twice the operative mortality, probably because of a higher prevalence of "silent" cardiovascular disease. Operative mortality doubled with emergency operations and quadrupled when the common bile duct was explored. The most serious morbidity was due to bile duct injury, occurring in 0.2% of patients. Recent surveys in the 1980s suggest that overall U.S. mortality and morbidity is <1% and <5%, respectively.

Laparoscopic cholecystectomy has almost replaced open cholecystectomy, with more than 90% of elective operations being performed via this approach. However, no large randomized studies have compared the safety of the two approaches. Clear advantages of laparoscopic cholecystectomy include (1) far smaller scars; (2) reduced hospital stay (1 to 2 vs. 5 to 6 days); and (3) earlier return to normal activities (7 vs. 40 to 60 days). There is a higher rate of bile duct injury (0.8%) during laparoscopic than during traditional cholecystectomy but less overall morbidity. A bile duct injury and biliary leak should be suspected in patients who do not make a prompt recovery following laparoscopic cholecystectomy. Cholescintigraphy is an effective noninvasive technique for discovering a bile leak and should be performed as soon as one is suspected. Many leaks will seal after endoscopic sphincterotomy with stent placement to allow the unrestricted flow of bile into the duodenum.

Cholecystectomy causes no digestive sequelae other than postprandial diarrhea or softer bowel movements in about 1% of patients. There is no malabsorption of fat and no special diet is ever indicated. Earlier epidemiologic evidence suggested that cholecystectomy doubles the risk of developing right-sided colonic cancer; however, recent studies deny this association. For the minority of patients who continue to experience abdominal discomfort after cholecystectomy, the term *postcholecystectomy syndrome* has been used. This is an unfortunate term, since it implies that symptoms occur only as a consequence of the operation. Many patients with this label, however, simply have persisting preoperative discomfort and/or pain. Thus the clinician must distinguish between postoperative complications such as bile duct injury, adhesions, or retained stones, and misdiagnosed preoperative diseases such as irritable bowel syndrome, neoplasms, peptic ulcers, and pancreatitis.

Medical Dissolution Therapy. The naturally occurring bile acid *ursodeoxycholic acid* (ursodiol, Actigall) dissolves cholesterol gallstones by decreasing biliary cholesterol secretion and desaturating bile. Cholesterol molecules from the surfaces of gallstones are redissolved in newly desaturated micellar or vesicular solution.

Treatment with ursodiol is appropriate for mildly symptomatic patients with small, noncalcified cholesterol gallbladder stones. Additionally, selected patients who refuse or who are poor surgical candidates may be treated with ursodiol. Treatment with ursodiol is limited critically by the character and sizes of stones and severity of symptoms. The major disadvantages are that gallstones dissolve slowly (1 mm in diameter per month) and will recur in 50% of patients within 5 years of successful dissolution.

Before initiating ursodiol treatment, stone size, number, and calcium content must be determined by ultrasonography and abdominal flat plate. Small (<10 mm), noncalcified stones can be treated with 8 mg/kg of ursodiol administered in divided doses in the morning and at bedtime. Reassessment of stone size by ultrasonography after 6 months of therapy is the only specific follow-up required. Therapy should be discontinued if the patient shows lack of dissolution at follow-up. Ursodiol should be continued for 3 months after complete stone dissolution has been confirmed by ultrasonography. Frequent attacks of biliary pain occur rarely during dissolution therapy, and surgery may be required.

After complete dissolution, patients should be reevaluated for recurrent gallstones only if biliary tract symptoms recur. Surveillance ultrasonography is not recommended. Maintenance therapy with either low-dose ursodiol, or a low-cholesterol, high-fiber diet, may prevent gallstone recurrence, but conclusive evidence is lacking. Ursodiol is remarkably free of side effects and, unlike its predecessor, chenodiol, does not cause hepatic injury, diarrhea, or elevation of serum cholesterol. Patients should be advised, however, that the drug is expensive and that a second course of therapy for symptomatic recurrence may be required.

Lithotripsy. Extracorporeal shock wave lithotripsy (ESWL) is still investigational. It should be used only in conjunction with ursodiol treatment to accelerate dissolution of cholesterol stones. The focusing of shock waves onto gallstones causes fragmentation, transforming a large stone into myriads of small stones and fragments, which then either migrate into the duodenum without obstruction or dissolve more rapidly in ursodiol-induced unsaturated bile. Mildly symptomatic patients with a single lucent 1- to 2-cm stone in a functioning gallbladder are the best candidates for combination ESWL and ursodiol therapy. They have an 80% to 90% chance of complete stone and fragment dissolution after ESWL and 1 year of ursodiol therapy. ESWL has limited overall applicability, since only 10% to 15% of gallstone patients will have a solitary noncalcified stone. Severe side effects of ESWL are uncommon and are related to transient obstruction of the cystic or common bile ducts, resulting in acute cholecystitis or pancreatitis in 3% and 1%, respectively, usually within 48 hours of ESWL. Moreover, biliary pain occurs in 30% to 70% of patients during the first 3 months after lithotripsy.

Contact Solvent Dissolution. Methyl tert-butyl ether (MTBE) is being evaluated for direct contact dissolution of gallbladder stones. It is a powerful cholesterol solvent that, when repeatedly instilled into the gallbladder via a percutaneous transhepatic catheter, dissolves cholesterol stones in 2 to 8 hours. In skilled hands, complications and side effects appear to be few and principally involve biliary leakage on withdrawal of the catheter. Because both inorganic and organic calcium salts and mucin glycoproteins of stones are insoluble in MTBE, many patients are left with biliary sludge containing calcium salts at the end of therapy. MTBE is still investigational, and its use is confined to a small number of skilled centers. This therapy should be reserved for patients who are very symptomatic but not amenable to ursodiol treatment or surgery.

Specific Treatment Recommendations. Patients with biliary pain should be treated in the following ways:

1. Young (<50 years of age) patients with *recurrent* attacks of biliary pain who are otherwise in good health should undergo elective cholecystectomy, since the operative risk is small (<0.1%). Fifty percent of these patients will continue to have attacks of pain or will develop complications of their gallstones during the next 20 years if not treated. They will have significantly higher operative risks at that time. Oral dissolution therapy with ursodiol has little role in healthy, young symptomatic patients.
2. Patients with diabetes should undergo elective cholecystectomy after only *one* episode of biliary pain before they develop complications of gallstones. These patients have an increased operative mortality for complications of gallstones, but not for elective cholecystectomy.
3. The management of nondiabetic patients after a single episode of biliary pain is controversial. In young, otherwise healthy patients, cholecystectomy is reasonable. An expectant watch-and-wait approach to observe the frequency of attacks and to confirm that they are due to gallstones is equally reasonable. Patients with small, radiolucent stones—especially if they developed during weight loss, recent pregnancy, or use of medications—would be ideal candidates for ursodiol therapy during the period of observation. In older patients, concomitant medical problems that increase operative mortality and reduce life expectancy make the treatment decision more difficult. They physician must balance the risks of deferring treatment and possibly performing emergent rather than elective surgery against the chance that the patient will remain asymptomatic and die from other causes.
4. Patients who refuse surgery can be treated only with expectant management or, possibly, medical therapy.

Prevention of Gallstones

Patients receiving TPN for longer than 3 months not only invariably develop biliary sludge in their gallbladders, but also have more complications than would be expected in conventional populations with cholelithiasis. Therefore prophylactic medical therapy with daily administration of intravenous cholecystokinin-octapeptide (CCK-OP)—which prevents gallbladder stasis, sludge, and gallstone formation—is indicated.

Standard ursodiol (8 to 10 mg/kg/day) administration during the period of rapid weight loss prevents stone formation. Whether there is sufficient risk of gallstone formation in patients undergoing

more moderate weight loss to justify ursodiol prophylaxis is unknown.

COMPLICATIONS OF GALLSTONES
Cholecystitis

Ninety-five percent of episodes of acute inflammation of the gallbladder are associated with obstruction of the cystic duct by a gallstone. Stone impaction, chemical inflammation, and superimposed bacterial infection occur in sequence. Early in the course of acute cholecystitis, the bile may be sterile (50%), but within a few days bacteria can be cultured from the bile of nearly all patients. Bacterial infection is responsible for all the serious sequelae of acute cholecystitis, particularly empyema and perforation. Acalculous cholecystitis, which accounts for approximately 5% of cases, most often occurs in the severely ill and is associated with trauma, operative procedures, extensive burns, immobility, and prolonged fasting. Although the etiology is unknown, it is probably caused by occlusion of the cystic duct with biliary sludge. Less commonly, acalculous cholecystitis is related to parasitic infestation of the gallbladder (*Clonorchis sinensis, Ascaris lumbricoides, Fasciola hepatica);* diabetes mellitus; torsion of the gallbladder; and vasculitis. The outcome for patients with acalculous cholecystitis is generally worse than for patients with gallstone cholecystitis, since perforation, empyema, and gangrene of the gallbladder often complicate the clinical picture in a patient already in a perilous medical state.

Pathology. The pathologic changes in the gallbladder during the evolution of acute cholecystitis reflect the duration of cystic duct obstruction and superimposed bacterial inflammation. The earliest pathologic findings are erythema and edema with a fibrinosuppurative exudate. Histologically, there is subserosal edema, hemorrhage, and inflammatory infiltration, which progress to mucosal ulcerations within a few days. In rapid sequence, mural gangrene and abscess formation may ensue. If the acute process resolves, collagen deposits appear in about 1 to 2 weeks. Eventually the gallbladder becomes contracted and scarred around the enclosed gallstones, and a thick, pale wall forms. Because this lesion represents the healed stage of acute cholecystitis, it is not correct to label the condition *chronic cholecystitis.*

Empyema, by definition, indicates that the gallbladder is filled with pus, and results from suppurative cholecystitis. Its development often heralds gangrene of the gallbladder and/or perforation, which occurs most often at the fundus. When perforation occurs elsewhere, it is often the result of direct erosion by an impacted stone at the infundibulum. Because the greater omentum may become adherent to an acutely inflamed gallbladder, perforation may result in a pericholecystic abscess. If the inflamed gallbladder becomes adherent to an adjacent hollow viscus (usually the duodenum), a cholecystoenteric fistula may result. More commonly, perforation leads to free spillage of bile into the peritoneal cavity and bile peritonitis. Rarely, following chronic obstruction of the cystic duct, hydrops (mucocele) of the gallbladder develops.

Clinical Findings. The patient with acute cholecystitis experiences initial symptoms typical of biliary colic. Because 80% of patients have previously experienced biliary colic, they may believe that this abdominal pain is caused by a repeat attack; however, the symptoms do not abate with time. As inflammation progresses, the pain becomes more severe and becomes localized in the right upper quadrant. Referred pain may radiate to the middle of the back, to the right infrascapular area, or to the right shoulder. As in biliary colic, the patient is often restless; but in contrast to biliary colic, the intensity of the pain in acute cholecystitis is affected by movement, including respiration. The severity of pain varies from patient to patient; in some—particularly those with diabetes, the aged, and patients receiving corticosteroids—pain may be minimal or absent.

Anorexia, nausea, and occasionally vomiting begin soon after the onset of acute cholecystitis. Fever is usually low-grade (99.5° to 101.3° F, 37.5° to 38.5° C); in the elderly, fever may be the only clinical sign of acute cholecystitis. High fever and chills suggest a septic complication. In acute cholecystitis unassociated with choledocholithiasis, mild jaundice may develop as a result of edema of the nearby common bile duct and diffusion of bilirubin across the inflamed gallbladder mucosa. Nonetheless, hyperbilirubinemia of any magnitude in this setting should raise the possibility of choledocholithiasis.

In uncomplicated acute cholecystitis, bowel sounds may be diminished, and tenderness in the right upper quadrant of the abdomen or epigastrium is striking; palpation of the right upper quadrant may sharply aggravate pain and produce transient inspiratory arrest (Murphy's sign). A distended, tender gallbladder may be palpable in one third of patients, which suggests a first episode, since repeated attacks result in a scarred, nondistensible gallbladder. In the majority of patients, acute cholecystitis subsides spontaneously. Improvement is often noticeable within the first day or two, and the signs and symptoms gradually disappear in 1 to 4 days. If symptoms persist longer or increase in severity, the potential for perforation, gangrene, empyema, cholangitis, and septic shock requires prompt surgical therapy.

Laboratory Findings and Diagnostic Tests. During acute cholecystitis the leukocyte count is usually mildly elevated to 10,000 to 15,000 per milliliter but may be higher. Serum transaminases and alkaline phosphatase may rise to two to four times normal, and bilirubin to 4 mg/dl. Dramatic hyperbilirubinemia and alkaline phosphatase elevations strongly suggest choledocholithiasis. Serum amylase may be elevated if stones pass through the common bile duct, with or without associated pancreatitis, or if vomiting is severe. Supine and upright abdominal films may demonstrate gallstones, an enlarged gallbladder, or air in the biliary system or peritoneal cavity. Ultrasonographic examination is the quickest, simplest, and most reliable method of determining the presence or absence of stones. Lack of visualization of the gallbladder with opacification of the common bile duct by ^{99m}Tc DISIDA cholescintigraphy strongly suggests the diagnosis in the proper clinical setting.

Differential Diagnosis. In most patients the presence of right upper quadrant abdominal pain and tenderness, nausea, vomiting, and mild fever permits an accurate clinical diagnosis. Myocardial infarction or angina pectoris may mimic acute cholecystitis. An electrocardiogram may enable the physician to differentiate between these conditions, but T-wave inversions in the inferior leads may be associated with acute cholecystitis. The symptoms of pancreatitis may resemble cholecystitis, but the patient with pancreatitis usually has more intense nausea and vomiting, with epigastric and periumbilical pain penetrating through to the back. Serum or urinary amylase concentrations may be increased in both conditions. Lipemic serum and hypocalcemia also suggest pancreatitis, but cholecystitis and pancreatitis occasionally occur simultaneously. Acute appendicitis may mimic cholecystitis, but pain in appendicitis is usually localized to the right lower quadrant. Acute alcoholic hepatitis may cause diagnostic confusion, especially if incidental calcified gallstones are present. A history of recent alcohol abuse, more diffuse nonspecific abdominal symptoms, marked hepatomegaly, and other physical and laboratory findings of chronic liver disease may help to distinguish between these two entities. Finally, both pyelonephritis and pneumonia can present with abdominal pain and simulate acute cholecystitis, so urinalysis and chest roentgenograms should be obtained in all patients.

Treatment. In the majority of patients with cholecystitis, as with recurrent biliary colic, the treatment of choice is early surgery. Early surgery reduces the hazards of an emergency operation for worsening disease; the chances of missing a complication such as empyema or silent perforation; and the aggravation of preexisting cardiac, pulmonary, or renal disease. Work absenteeism and the expenses associated with hospitalization for interval cholecystectomy (approximately 6 weeks) can also be greatly reduced. If patients are good surgical risks, a brief period of conservative therapy may be necessary for stabilization before cholecystectomy. In most cases, cholecystectomy can be scheduled as a routine procedure within 48 hours of hospitalization. The patient should receive intravenous fluid replacement to counter dehydration from vomiting and fasting, nasogastric suction to diminish hormonal stimuli to the biliary tree, sufficient analgesia to combat pain, and a third-generation cephalosporin. If sepsis or other complications supervene, a third-generation cephalosporin and an aminoglycoside should be administered intravenously, and the risks

of surgery relative to the risks of continued delay must be assessed promptly. When emergency decompression becomes necessary, cholecystotomy, with evacuation of stones and pus followed by catheter drainage, may be the initial treatment of choice in such patients. Cholecystotomy is less risky than cholecystectomy and allows the acute infection to subside. Definitive surgery, however, is required 6 to 8 weeks later to remove the gallbladder to prevent a chronic mucous fistula and recurrent stone formation. Exploration of the common bile duct may also be necessary at the time of cholecystectomy if an intraoperative cholangiogram reveals ductal stones.

The natural history of patients with an episode of acute cholecystitis who do not undergo cholecystectomy is poor. Recurrences of biliary colic and complications are common, occurring in 50% of patients within 5 years.

Complications. The common complications of acute cholecystitis are empyema and perforation. Free perforation into the abdominal cavity may occur early in the course of cholecystitis and is associated with a high (approximately 30%) mortality rate, since it is often missed until bile peritonitis ensues. More often, perforation is localized by omental adhesions, producing a pericholecystic abscess, evident as a tender mass in the subhepatic region. Perforation into another hollow viscus (duodenum, colon, stomach, in that order) with fistula formation is less common. Many cholecystoenteric fistulas are discovered incidentally, as the acute perforation drains the gallbladder, relieving symptoms. However, cholecystocolonic fistulas may cause secretory diarrhea, fat malabsorption from diversion of bile, and profound bacterial contamination resulting in ascending cholangitis. A large gallstone ejected through a cholecystoduodenal fistula may obstruct the small intestine, causing gallstone ileus. Gallstone ileus should be suspected in the elderly and in patients with diabetes who present with acute, subacute, or intermittent small-bowel obstruction. Abdominal roentgenograms are typical of those seen in bowel obstruction and, in addition, reveal air in the biliary tree; in some cases a large, radiopaque gallstone may be evident in the right lower quadrant. The obstructing gallstones should be removed through an enterostomy. Cholecystectomy with repair of the fistula should be performed only if the patient subsequently has symptoms of biliary disease. Because of delay in making the diagnosis, the mortality of patients with gallstone ileus can be as high as 10% to 20%.

Choledocholithiasis

In Western countries the vast majority of common duct stones have migrated from the gallbladder; consequently, most common duct stones are cholesterol stones. In patients younger than 60 years the prevalence of common duct stones in association with gallbladder stones is about 8% to 15%. This prevalence increases to nearly 50% in patients aged 80 years and older. These data suggest that the longer stones are present in the gallbladder, the greater the likelihood they will migrate into the common bile duct. Nevertheless, most ductal stones are first discovered during exploration or intraoperative cholangiography at the time of cholecystectomy. Even after surgical exploration and removal of common duct stones, however, one or more stones, usually cholesterol, are left behind in 1% to 10% of patients. Stones that form in the duct (primary duct stones) are nearly always "brown" pigment stones. In the Western world, they are usually associated with cholangitis, which is often subclinical and caused by organisms producing β-glucuronidase and other enzymes capable of hydrolyzing bile salts and lecithin (e.g., *E. coli*). Bile stasis caused by ductal obstruction contributes to their formation. Pigment stones in the ductal systems (often in the intrahepatic radicles) of Eastern patients with intact gallbladders is not uncommon, but this finding is rare in Western patients (see Table 364-1), except in those with sclerosing cholangitis. In the Orient, parasitic infestation, with accompanying bacterial infection, appears to be a major cause of choledocholithiasis.

Clinical Findings. The natural history of choledocholithiasis is relatively benign in 50% of patients. Ten percent of patients with gallbladder stones pass them "silently" into the common duct and out into the intestines. In others, ductal stones are found incidentally during diagnostic evaluation or surgical exploration in patients with gallbladder stones. The natural history of stones that remain in the common bile duct is unpredictable, and patients may present with (1) cholangitis, (2) intermittent or persistent obstructive jaundice with or without pain, (3) acute pancreatitis, and (4) biliary pain without other complications. Long-standing common bile duct obstruction with or without intermittent painless jaundice may lead to secondary biliary cirrhosis.

Patients with ascending nonsuppurative cholangitis may present with jaundice, biliary colic, and fever (Charcot's intermittent fever). The cholangitis is often transient or intermittent because most stones only partially obstruct the common bile duct. In a typical attack a chill usually precedes fever and is followed by jaundice and dark urine from conjugated bilirubinuria. The pain is indistinguishable from that of classic biliary colic caused by gallbladder stones. Pain may be referred to the subxiphoid region, upper back, or shoulder and may be confused with that of pancreatitis, coronary disease, radicular neuritis, or lobar pneumonia. Usually, fever is moderate (100.4° to 102.2° F, 38° to 39° C), and pain and tenderness are localized to the right subcostal region. Symptoms usually subside within 24 to 48 hours with or without antibiotic administration, presumably because the stone is dislodged into a more capacious part of the common duct or is passed into the duodenum. The transient although often recurrent symptoms may not interfere with the patient's normal activities, so many patients first present after several weeks of mild recurrent fever. Most patients with jaundice resulting from choledocholithiasis do not have a palpable gallbladder because recurrent attacks of acute cholecystitis have left them with shrunken and fibrotic gallbladders. In contrast, patients who have a malignant process involving the distal biliary tree and who have not previously had cholecystitis usually have dilated and therefore potentially palpable gallbladders (Courvoisier's law).

In acute suppurative cholangitis, ductal obstruction is usually complete, cholangitis is unremitting, and ductal contents are purulent. Mental confusion, lethargy, and bacteremic shock are common accompanying features and overshadow those of cholestasis. Fortunately, this form of acute cholangitis is rare. Because the overwhelming infection advances rapidly, emergency biliary drainage is essential. If delays occur, the patient may die from generalized sepsis and shock within a few hours, or inflammation may spread, giving rise to pericholangitis and multiple hepatic abscesses. The usual prognosis for neglected suppurative cholangitis, even with antibiotic treatment, is extremely poor.

Laboratory Findings and Diagnostic Tests. In choledocholithiasis with or without cholangitis, the severity of jaundice varies, but serum bilirubin concentration is rarely greater than 15 mg/dl. Alkaline phosphatase, 5'-nucleotidase, and leucine aminopeptidase levels are substantially elevated, often paralleling serum bilirubin elevation. Hepatic transaminases are usually only mildly elevated to two or three times the upper limits of normal, but values as high as those reached in acute hepatitis are seen rarely, especially when there is associated ascending cholangitis. The leukocyte count is elevated to about 12,000 to 15,000 per milliliter but may be much higher in suppurative cholangitis. Blood cultures are usually positive in patients with suppurative cholangitis. With suspected persistent cholangitis, diagnostic procedures should be few, so that biliary tract drainage is not unduly delayed. In particular, if the patient is septic, with unequivocal signs and symptoms of suppurative cholangitis, prompt biliary tract decompression by endoscopic retrograde drainage and the administration of broad-spectrum antibiotics are desirable before definitive surgery. This approach has significantly reduced the mortality of acute suppurative cholangitis.

In contrast, if the patient is clearly not septic and is stable, with or without evident obstructive jaundice, the investigation can proceed at a more measured pace. Ultrasonographic examination may show a dilated common bile duct with or without a stone. Its sensitivity is low (~25%), however, because cholangitis can occur without ductal dilatation. Furthermore, stones in the common duct are far more difficult to visualize by ultrasonography than are stones in the gallbladder. CT is useful only if ultrasonography is technically inadequate or a pancreatic neoplasm is suspected as causing the obstruction. Magnetic resonance cholangiography (MRC) shows promise as a noninvasive method to identify stones, but ERCP remains the definitive

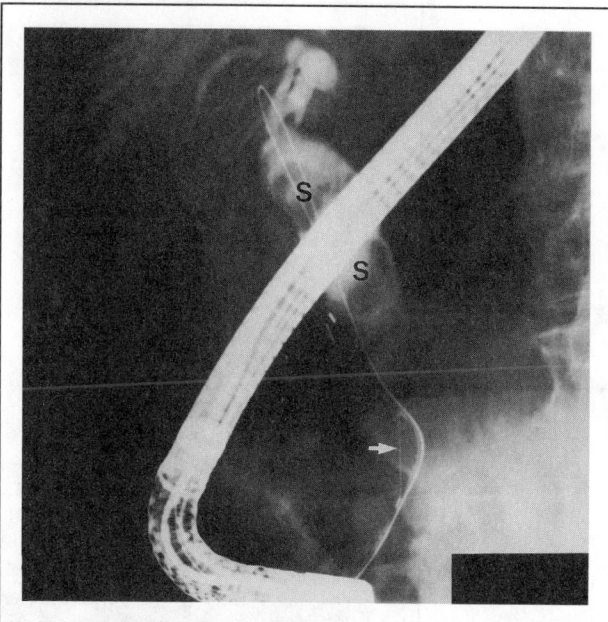

FIGURE 364-3   ERCP. The endoscope is positioned in the duodenum. Contrast material has been introduced retrograde into the common bile duct. Radiolucent gallstones are demonstrated in the common bile duct. A sphincterotome is shown extending from the endoscope in preparation for a sphincterotomy at the site of the sphincter *(arrow)*.
Courtesy of Dr. David Carr-Locke, Boston.

diagnostic test. If this test fails to demonstrate stones or duct dilatation, the stones have passed into the duodenum or the original diagnosis was in error.

Differential Diagnosis. Differentiation between choledocholithiasis, benign biliary stricture, and periampullary and biliary neoplasms can, as a rule, be made with ERCP. In neoplastic biliary obstruction, jaundice is relatively painless, and ascending cholangitis is rare. The most important group of conditions that must be excluded are those that cause intrahepatic cholestasis, in which surgery is contraindicated. These conditions include drug-induced cholestasis, alcoholic hepatitis, viral hepatitis, and complications of pregnancy.

Therapy. Rehydration with intravenously administered fluids is often required, and broad-spectrum antibiotic treatment should be initiated promptly if there is evidence of cholangitis. Endoscopic sphincterotomy and drainage of the biliary tree is not only relatively safe and effective but also, in many, the only procedure that need be performed. For other patients, however, surgical exploration should be performed once the patient's condition is stable. The operative approach to definitive biliary decompression will depend on the nature of the ductal obstruction, as well as the presence or absence of the gallbladder. Before definitive surgery, the anatomy of the biliary tree and the nature of the ductal obstruction should be delineated by direct cholangiography, usually by ERCP. Patients with common bile duct stones and an intact gallbladder who are good operative candidates should undergo ERCP, sphincterotomy, and endoscopic removal of common duct stones, followed promptly (1 to 2 days) by laparoscopic cholecystectomy.

Patients who are poor operative risks can be treated with sphincterotomy with removal of the common duct stone. With this treatment, they have only a 10% risk of developing subsequent cholecystitis of cholangitis. Patients with retained stones or newly formed stones after cholecystectomy should be treated by endoscopic sphincterotomy and stone extraction (Fig. 364-3). Even in those patients with a postoperative T-tube, an endoscopic sphincterotomy rather than an attempt at Dormia basket retrieval via the T-tube is preferable. The latter necessitates an 8- to 12-week wait for a fibrous tract to develop. Cholangitis or other complications could occur during this

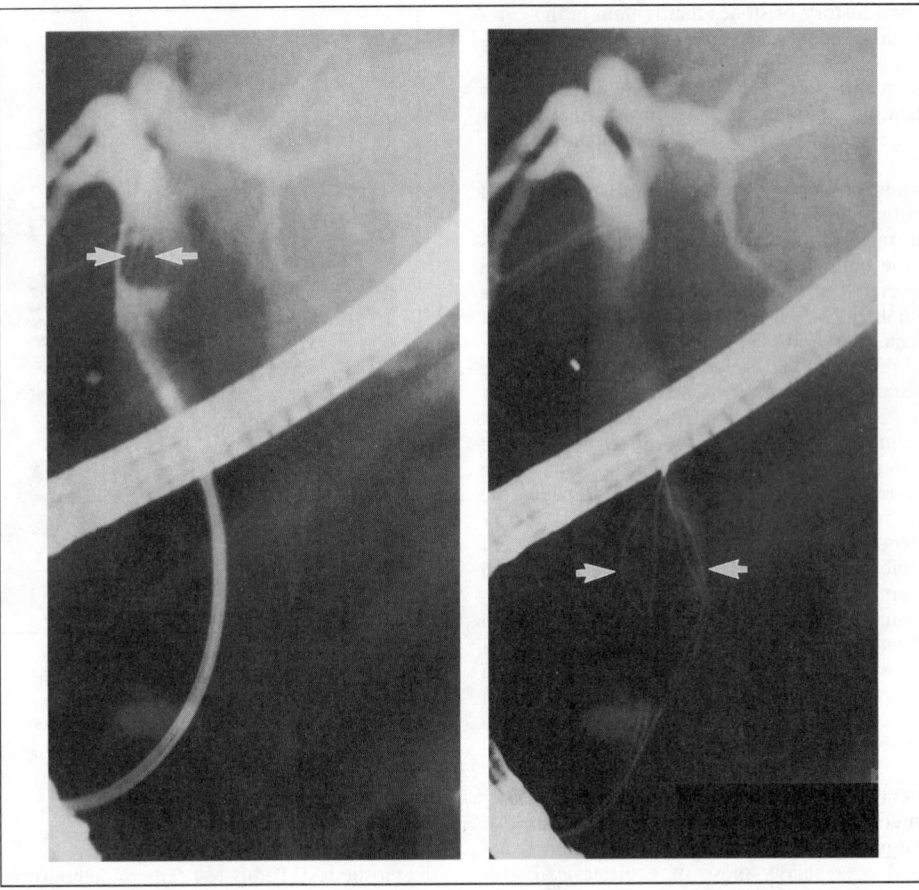

FIGURE 364-4   An endoscopic sphincterotomy has been performed after visualization of the common bile duct via ERCP. Common bile duct stones are crushed and removed with the aid of a mechanical lithotriptor directed *(arrows)* into the common bile duct.
Courtesy of Dr. David Carr-Locke, Boston.

period. Endoscopic sphincterotomy is safe and effective, with a mortality rate of ~1% and a success rate of >85%. Relative contraindications include stones greater than 2 cm, bile duct stricture proximal to the ampulla, an ampulla situated in a duodenal diverticulum, and significant coagulopathy. ESWL (still investigational) to fragment large stones in the common bile duct, coupled with endoscopic sphincterotomy, will allow removal of almost all retained stones (Fig. 364-4). Surgical removal and exploration of the common bile duct should be considered as a last resort but should be performed promptly if endoscopic sphincterotomy fails in a patient with an infected or obstructed biliary tree.

Attempted dissolution of retained common duct stones with T-tube infusion of cholesterol solvents—such as MTBE, monooctanoin (Capmul), or cholate—is neither safe nor effective. Complete extraction of intrahepatic stones at ERCP may be technically impossible, especially in the brown pigment stone hepatolithiasis syndrome, in which proximal ductal strictures and cisternal dilatation are commonly present. Such patients may require choledochoduodenostomy or even hepatic lobectomy to ensure stone removal and adequate drainage of the intrahepatic biliary tree.

Gallstone Pancreatitis

Gallstones or biliary sludge migrating from the gallbladder through the common bile duct and into the duodenum can cause pancreatitis. The pathogenesis appears related to temporary impaction of a gallstone or biliary sludge in the common channel of the pancreatic and biliary ducts; the semipatent common channel allows activated pancreatic enzymes, bile, and lipid digestive products to reflux into the pancreas.

Although an acute attack of gallstone pancreatitis is indistinguishable from an episode of acute pancreatitis from any other cause, it carries a high (10%) mortality. However, gallstone pancreatitis, unlike alcoholic pancreatitis, rarely results in chronic pancreatitis or pancreatic insufficiency, even after recurrent attacks.

The diagnosis of gallstone pancreatitis is based on the finding of stones or sludge in the gallbladder or biliary tree in the presence of acute pancreatitis. The detection of gallstones by manual sieving or ultrasonographic examination of the feces is also diagnostic in the correct clinical setting. Furthermore, two thirds of patients with idiopathic pancreatitis have biliary precipitates found in samples of bile obtained by duodenal drainage and hence can be diagnosed as having gallstone pancreatitis. Therefore the search for these precipitates should be made before classifying the pancreatitis as idiopathic.

The immediate medical treatment of acute gallstone pancreatitis is the same as that for acute pancreatitis of any other etiology (Chapter 363). If the patient fails to improve within 24 to 48 hours, emergency ERCP and sphincterotomy are indicated to remove the impacted stone. An elective cholecystectomy and common bile duct exploration are recommended as soon as the patient recovers from an acute attack. If cholecystectomy is delayed, 25% of patients will experience another attack of potentially fatal acute pancreatitis within 30 days and 50% within 11 months. If biliary sludge alone is the cause, medical dissolution treatment with ursodiol is an acceptable alternative because it prevents recurrent attacks.

Cholesterolosis

This pathologic change in the gallbladder and cystic duct wall consists of submucosal macrophages filled with cholesterol esters and

✔ *WHEN TO REFER*

Acutely ill patients with gallstones may need urgent surgical or endoscopic intervention and would benefit from early consultation with a surgeon and gastroenterologist. In addition, even patients who are not acutely ill with gallstones but whose liver function tests are abnormal are likely to have a complication of gallstones that will require consultation with a gastroenterologist trained in biliary endoscopy and/or a surgeon. Similarly, patients with symptoms highly suggestive of gallstones but negative imaging studies may benefit from duodenal intubation and examination of bile for cholesterol or bilirubin crystals. Most troublesome are patients with gallstones but with symptoms of other abdominal disease such as irritable bowel. In this setting a second opinion from a gastroenterologist can help reassure the patient and direct further evaluation and therapy.

smaller amounts of free cholesterol, triglycerides, fatty acids, and methyl sterols. The condition is extremely common, being found in as many as 40% of gallbladders removed for uncomplicated gallstones, and is often the sole lesion at autopsy. The yellow pigmentation produced by cholesterol and methyl sterol esters on the red mucosal background produces an appearance similar to that of a ripe strawberry (strawberry gallbladder). The etiology is unknown but appears to be secondary to enhanced transfer and esterification of lipids, particularly cholesterol, into the mucosa from bile. Grossly, the deposits are usually flat but may be raised and polypoid. If present as the sole gallbladder lesion, cholesterolosis usually causes no symptoms, although ill-defined episodic abdominal discomfort, which is probably unrelated, may occur. Abdominal ultrasonography may be diagnostic if mucosal excrescences that do not move with change of position are present. The diagnosis may be made if duodenal drainage is performed, followed by polarizing microscopy of the bile to look for birefringent liquid crystalline droplets composed of cholesterol esters. Relief of symptoms after cholecystectomy has been reported.

BIBLIOGRAPHY

Angelico M, DeSantis A, Capocaccia L: Biliary sludge: a critical update, *J Clin Gastroenterol* 12:656-662, 1990.

Apstein MD, Carey MC: Pathogenesis of cholesterol gallstones: a parsimonious hypothesis, *Eur J Clin Invest* 26:343-352, 1996.

Broomfield PH et al: Effects of ursodeoxycholic acid and aspirin on the formation of lithogenic bile and gallstones during loss of weight, *N Engl J Med* 319:1567-1572, 1988.

Cahalane MJ, Neubrand MW, Carey MC: Physical-chemical pathogenesis of pigment gallstones, *Semin Liver Dis* 8:317-328, 1988.

Carey MC, LaMont JT: Cholesterol gallstone formation. 1. Physical chemistry of bile and biliary lipid secretion, *Prog Liver Dis* 10:139-163, 1992.

Friedman GD, Raviola CA, Fireman B: Prognosis of gallstones with mild or no symptoms: 25 years of follow-up in a health maintenance organization, *J Clin Epidemiol* 42:127-136, 1989.

Friedman LS et al: Management of asymptomatic gallstones in the diabetic patient: a decision analysis, *Ann Intern Med* 109:913-919, 1988.

Gracie WA, Ransohoff DF: The natural history of silent gallstones: the innocent gallstone is not a myth, *N Engl J Med* 307:798-800, 1982.

Hofman AF: Primary and secondary prevention of gallstone disease: implications for patient management and research priorities, *Am J Surg* 165:541-548, 1993.

LaMont JT, Carey MC: Cholesterol gallstone formation. 2. Pathobiology and pathomechanics, *Prog Liver Dis* 10:165-191, 1992.

Lee SP, Maher K, Nicolls JF: Origin and fate of biliary sludge, *Gastroenterology* 94:170-176, 1988.

Leuschner U et al: Gallstone dissolution with methyl tert-butyl ether in 120 patients, *Dig Dis Sci* 36:193-199, 1992.

Marks AJ et al: The sequence of biliary events preceding the formation of gallstones in humans, *Gastroenterology* 103:566-570, 1992.

May GR, Shaffer EH: Should elective endoscopic sphincterotomy replace cholecystectomy for the treatment of high-risk patients with gallstone pancreatitis? (editorial), *J Clin Gastroenterol* 13:125-128, 1991.

Ransohoff DF et al: Prophylactic cholecystectomy or expectant management for silent gallstones, *Ann Intern Med* 99:199-204, 1983.

Ransohoff DF et al: Outcome of acute cholecystitis in patients with diabetes mellitus, *Ann Intern Med* 106:829-832, 1987.

Ros E et al: Occult microlithiasis in "idiopathic" acute pancreatitis: prevention of relapses by cholecystectomy or ursodeoxycholic acid therapy, *Gastroenterology* 101:1701-1709, 1991.

Sackmann M et al: The Munich gallbladder lithotripsy study: results of the first 5 years with 711 patients, *Ann Intern Med* 114:290-296, 1991.

Schoenfield LJ et al: The effect of ursodiol on the efficacy and safety of extracorporeal shock-wave lithotripsy of gallstones: the Dornier National Biliary Lithotripsy Study, *N Engl J Med* 323:1239-1245, 1990.

Southern Surgeons Club: A prospective analysis of 1518 laparoscopic cholecystectomies, *N Engl J Med* 324:1073-1078, 1991.

CHAPTER

365 Other Diseases of the Gallbladder and Biliary Tree

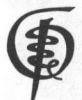

Stephen C. Hauser

A variety of diseases less common than cholelithiasis and choledocholithiasis that involve the gallbladder and biliary tree are discussed in this chapter. Patients with these disorders, like those with gallstone-related disease, may present with jaundice (sclerosing cholangitis, carcinoma of the bile ducts, benign stricture of the extrahepatic bile ducts, choledochal cyst, Caroli's disease); abdominal pain (carcinoma of the biliary tree, choledochal cyst, hemobilia, biliary dyskinesia); or fever (sclerosing cholangitis, Caroli's disease). Sclerosing cholangitis (PSC) is discussed in Chapter 358.

CARCINOMA OF THE BILE DUCTS

Primary adenocarcinoma of the bile ducts, or *cholangiocarcinoma,* accounts for the vast majority of tumors arising from the biliary ductal system. Anatomically, cholangiocarcinoma may originate in the intrahepatic bile ducts; in the hilar region where the hepatic ducts merge to form the common hepatic duct; or in the extrahepatic biliary tree, including the cystic duct and common bile duct. Intrahepatic bile duct carcinoma (peripheral cholangiocarcinoma) arises from very small bile ducts and is a rapidly growing tumor. Some carcinomas in this location consist of bile ductular as well as hepatocyte elements. Hilar cholangiocarcinoma, arising at or near the bifurcation of the common hepatic duct, is referred to as a Klatskin or bifurcation tumor (Fig. 365-1).

Cholangiocarcinoma is most common in the sixth decade and occurs with equal frequency in men and women. In persons from the Far East, chronic infestation with certain liver flukes, such as *Clonorchis sinensis* and *Opisthorchis viverrini,* has been associated with an increased incidence of cholangiocarcinoma, particularly the intrahepatic variety. The etiologic mechanism of this association is not known, but adenomatous proliferation of the ductular epithelium has been observed in the presence of these parasites. Interestingly, infestation with other flukes—including *Schistosoma mansoni, S. japonicum,* and *Fasciola hepatica*—has not been associated with cholangiocarcinoma. Other reported risk factors include chronic inflammatory bowel disease (usually ulcerative colitis, less often Crohn's colitis); PSC; administration of anabolic steroids and thorium dioxide (Thorotrast); chronic biliary typhoid infections; familial polyposis coli; cancer family syndrome; and congenital cystic disorders of the biliary tree (choledochal cyst and Caroli's disease). Workers in the automotive, aeronautic, and rubber industries also have a higher incidence of cholangiocarcinoma, presumably because of exposure to environmental toxic substances.

Patients with cholangiocarcinoma often present with symptoms of duct obstruction such as pruritus and jaundice, which may be intermittent early in the disease. Cholangitis is unusual, but anorexia, fatigue, abdominal pain, weight loss, and fever are common. Jaundice and hepatomegaly may be found on physical examination, and an enlarged gallbladder may occur with cholangiocarcinomas located below the common hepatic duct. Laboratory tests usually demonstrate

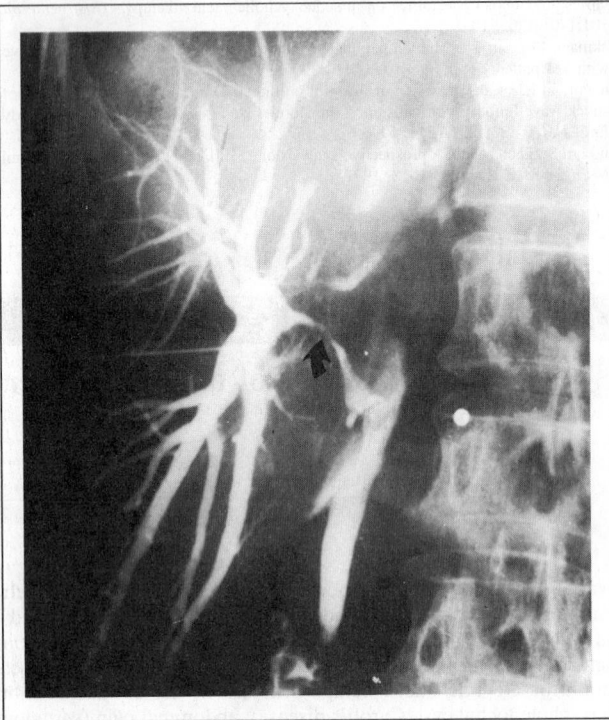

FIGURE 365-1 Klatskin-type cholangiocarcinoma, involving the common hepatic duct *(arrow)*, high in the porta hepatis close to the bifurcation, as demonstrated by percutaneous transhepatic cholangiogram. (The "skinny" needle is shown as a thin straight line of contrast material coming in from the left side of the cholangiogram.)

cholestasis, with an elevated serum alkaline phosphatase level in most cases.

Noninvasive tests—including ultrasound, computed tomography (CT), and magnetic resonance imaging (MRI)—may demonstrate dilated intrahepatic bile ducts proximal to the tumor, invasion of the adjacent liver parenchyma, and intraabdominal lymph node involvement. However, noninvasive tests may not identify the tumor itself, and radiographic visualization of the biliary tree is crucial to define the exact location and extent of the tumor. This is particularly important with Klatskin tumors, which can be difficult to find at surgery in patients in whom the tumor is not localized preoperatively. Either percutaneous transhepatic cholangiography or endoscopic retrograde cholangiography can be used. It is important to visualize the entire biliary tree to avoid overlooking a small focal tumor. Cytologic examination of material obtained by brushings, collecting bile, or fine-needle aspiration of the tumor site is diagnostic in about 50% of cases.

Most cholangiocarcinomas are unresectable, particularly when located at or above the hilus. Angiography and surgical exploration are required in selected patients to determine resectability. Palliative decompression of the obstructed biliary tree is useful. At present, this can be accomplished without surgical resection or bypass in many patients either by percutaneous transhepatic decompression, with placement of an endoprosthesis draining bile either externally or internally into the duodenum, or by endoscopic biliary decompression with nasobiliary or endoprosthetic stenting. Results with internal drainage are superior to those with external drainage. Radiotherapy can be useful for palliation in certain patients, whereas chemotherapy remains strictly investigational. Because many cholangiocarcinomas are slow growing, relief of biliary tract obstruction may prolong survival in some patients.

CARCINOMA OF THE AMPULLA OF VATER

Tumors in the vicinity of the ampulla of Vater may arise from the mucosa of the ampulla itself, the pancreatic duct, the distal common bile duct, or the duodenum. Nearly all of these tumors are adenocar-

cinomas. Noninvasive tests such as CT and invasive tests including endoscopic retrograde cholangiopancreatography and percutaneous transhepatic cholangiography are necessary to clarify the origin of adenocarcinomas in this region. This fact is important because patients with carcinoma of the ampulla of Vater—compared with other pancreatic, biliary tract, or small intestinal carcinomas—have a high 5-year survival rate (30% to 60%) after surgical resection of the pancreatic head and duodenum with pancreaticojejunostomy (Whipple's operation). Patients with familial polyposis coli, cancer family syndrome, and von Recklinghausen's disease are at increased risk for adenocarcinoma of the ampulla of Vater.

CARCINOMA OF THE GALLBLADDER

Nearly 5000 cases of gallbladder carcinoma are diagnosed in the United States annually. Over 80% of these are adenocarcinomas; the remainder are squamous cell and anaplastic carcinomas. The average age at presentation is 65, with a 2:1 female-male ratio. As many as 90% of gallbladder carcinoma patients also have gallstones, but the exact role of these stones, if any, in the etiology of gallbladder carcinoma is unclear. Because gallstones are so common and gallbladder carcinoma is so uncommon, the operative mortality of prophylactic cholecystectomy in the general population would be far higher than the number of deaths from gallbladder cancers that would be prevented. Specific groups of patients have been identified, however, in which prophylactic cholecystectomy is indicated. If left alone, about 50% of patients with porcelain gallbladders with patchy calcification of the gallbladder wall will develop gallbladder cancer. Chronic *Salmonella typhosa* carriers, women of American Indian heritage with gallstones, and patients with solitary gallstones larger than 3.0 cm in diameter are also at high risk of developing gallbladder cancer and should strongly be considered for prophylactic cholecystectomy.

The clinical presentation of gallbladder cancer is nonspecific and includes weight loss, pain, anorexia, nausea, and vomiting. A palpable mass, jaundice, fever, and chills also may occur. Laboratory findings also are nonspecific and include leukocytosis, anemia, and elevated serum alkaline phosphatase levels. Unfortunately, the tumor is usually silent until spread has occurred, and the diagnosis is rarely made when the tumor is still resectable. In fact, less than 20% of cases are diagnosed preoperatively. Ultrasound, CT, and MRI may demonstrate a mass as well as invasion of the liver. Survival beyond 1 year is uncommon. Occasionally, gallbladder carcinoma is found incidentally in gallbladders removed from patients with cholecystitis. If these have not yet penetrated the muscularis, they may be cured by surgery. Radiotherapy and chemotherapy are not effective in gallbladder cancer.

BENIGN STRICTURE OF EXTRAHEPATIC BILE DUCTS

Benign strictures of the extrahepatic bile ducts nearly always follow bile duct injury, most often as a result of surgery on either the ducts or the gallbladder, including minimally invasive surgery such as laparoscopic cholecystectomy. Inadvertent ligation of the extrahepatic bile duct may produce a symptomatic stricture in the immediate postoperative period, whereas more subtle injury may not produce symptoms until several years later. Depending on the degree of obstruction, the patient may be asymptomatic or have jaundice or may present with ascending cholangitis. Laboratory tests generally show evidence of cholestasis in symptomatic strictures with elevation of serum alkaline phosphatase and/or bilirubin levels. Ultrasound or CT may show dilated bile ducts proximal to the stricture. Chronic partial obstruction of the biliary tree may ultimately produce secondary biliary cirrhosis and portal hypertension. Percutaneous transhepatic cholangiography and endoscopic retrograde cholangiography are necessary to define the exact location of the stricture(s). In some instances it may be impossible to exclude cholangiocarcinoma. To further complicate the picture, brown pigment gallstones can form secondary to stasis, proximal to the stricture, and precipitate obstruction (Chapter 364). Depending on the clinical circumstances, surgical bypass or repair of the strictured duct by a skilled and experienced surgeon or balloon dilatation and/or stenting of the stricture may be required. Long strictures of the distal common bile duct may develop in alcoholic patients with chronic pancreatitis as a result of external compression of the duct by fibrosis and inflammation in the head of the pancreas. These patients require frequent cholangiographic evaluation as well as liver biopsies to determine when a biliary-enteric bypass procedure is indicated. If not corrected, partial biliary obstruction in this setting can result in secondary biliary cirrhosis within several months.

HEMOBILIA

Patients who bleed into the biliary tract often present with biliary colic, jaundice, and melena or hematemesis. The formation of clots within the biliary tree may cause jaundice. Hemobilia most often results from blunt or penetrating trauma to the abdomen. Transhepatic cholangiography, liver biopsy, biliary tract malignancy, gallstones, parasites, aneurysms, and varices of the biliary tree may be complicated by hemobilia. In certain patients, the bleeding may not stop spontaneously, and either surgical intervention or therapeutic angiographic embolization may be required.

HYPERPLASTIC CHOLECYSTOSIS

Hyperplastic cholecystosis refers to a loosely defined group of disorders affecting the gallbladder that includes adenomyomatosis, gallbladder polyps, and phrygian cap. *Adenomyomatosis* is defined as a generalized or segmental hyperplasia of the gallbladder epithelium. When localized, it may assume the shape of a polyp, which can be visualized by ultrasonography or cholecystography. In the absence of gallstones it is unlikely that adenomatosis produces symptoms. The same can be said for gallbladder polyps, most of which are cholesterol polyps, not true neoplasms. It is unknown if the phrygian cap deformity is congenital or acquired. For most patients with hyperplastic cholecystosis, therapy is not necessary, especially if the lesion is small (<10 mm) and does not change over time. However, if patients are symptomatic or have coexistent cholelithiasis or thickening of the gallbladder wall on ultrasound, or if the lesion increases in size, cholecystectomy is indicated.

BILIARY DYSKINESIA

A variety of dysmotility disorders of the biliary tract have been proposed to account for chronic abdominal pain that may resemble biliary colic in patients without gallstones. *Hyperkinesia* of the gallbladder is defined as excessive or abnormal contractility of the gallbladder after stimulation, such as after eating or after the administration of cholecystokinin. Gallbladder emptying can be studied by radionuclide scintigraphy with cholecystokinin octapeptide injection. Cholecystectomy may benefit selected patients. *Dyskinesia* refers to altered tonus of the sphincter of Oddi (usually increased pressure), disturbance in the coordination of contraction of the biliary ducts, and/or reduction in the speed of emptying of the biliary tree. Increased biliary ductal pressure secondary to diminished bile flow through the sphincter of Oddi may cause pain, transiently elevated results of liver function tests, dilatation of the ductal system, and delayed drainage of contrast after endoscopic retrograde cholangiography. Abnormal manometric pressure measurements of the sphincter of Oddi confirm the diagnosis, but it can be difficult to exclude organic papillary stenosis in some of these patients. Although endoscopic or surgical sphincterotomy may help selected patients with biliary dyskinesia, many patients with chronic abdominal pain syndromes suggestive of biliary dyskinesia probably suffer from the much more common irritable bowel syndrome. Hence objective findings such as manometric abnormalities or abnormal liver function test results are helpful in identifying patients who may benefit from surgery. Finally, it should be remembered that the presence of cholelithiasis and choledocholithiasis must be carefully excluded.

DEVELOPMENTAL ANOMALIES

Congenital abnormalities in the development of the biliary tract almost always present early in life. However, choledochal cysts and Caroli's disease, two conditions characterized by congenital dilatation of bile ducts, may become evident during adulthood. Choledochal

cysts may present as a right upper quadrant mass, with pain and jaundice. Ultrasound, CT, radionuclide scintigraphy, and cholangiography all can be useful in making the diagnosis. Because of the age-related increase in the incidence of carcinoma complicating choledochal cysts (up to 10% to 20%), surgical removal of the cyst and biliary reconstruction are recommended if possible. Caroli's disease is characterized by multiple areas of cystic dilatation involving the intrahepatic and, in some instances, the extrahepatic bile ducts. In some patients, only the bile ducts of certain segments or a single lobe of the liver are affected. Congenital hepatic fibrosis may also be present (Chapter 359). Fever, pain, jaundice, cholangitis, and secondary intrahepatic choledocholithiasis and abscess formation may occur periodically in patients with Caroli's disease. Cholangiography as well as ultrasound and CT can establish the diagnosis. Surgical drainage of the affected biliary radicles, partial hepatectomy in patients with localized disease, ursodeoxycholic acid administration, extracorporeal shock wave lithotripsy, and perhaps liver transplantation may benefit selected patients.

BIBLIOGRAPHY

Hogan WJ, Geenan JE, Dodds WJ: Dysmotility disturbances of the biliary tract: classification, diagnosis and treatment, *Semin Liver Dis* 7:302, 1987.
Levin B: Diagnosis and medical management of malignant disorders of the biliary tract, *Semin Liver Dis* 7:328, 1987.
May GR, Bender CE, Williams HJ: Radiologic approaches to the treatment of benign and malignant biliary tract disease, *Semin Liver Dis* 7:334, 1987.
Nagorney DM, McIlrath DC, Adson MA: Choledochal cysts in adults: clinical management, *Surgery* 96:656, 1984.
Nagorney DM, McPherson GAD: Carcinoma of the gallbladder and extrahepatic bile ducts, *Semin Oncol* 15:106, 1988.
Slivka A, Carr-Locke D: Therapeutic biliary endoscopy, *Endoscopy* 24:100, 1992.

CHAPTER

366   Pancreatic Diseases

C.S. Pitchumoni

ACUTE PANCREATITIS

Acute pancreatitis is an inflammatory condition of the pancreas, characterized clinically by moderate to severe epigastric pain and a broad spectrum of pathologic and clinical findings. The disease may remain localized to the region of the pancreas or may spread to involve remote organs and thereby manifest as multisystem disease. In contrast to chronic pancreatitis, there are no irreversible sequelae such as diabetes, steatorrhea, or pancreatic calculi. Factors that determine whether an episode of acute pancreatitis will be edematous (interstitial) or the severe necrotic form associated with serious complications are not clear. Terminology frequently used in the literature to describe the disease entity is found in Box 366-1.

Etiologic Factors. Alcoholism and biliary tract disease account for 90% of all cases of acute pancreatitis. It is generally accepted that biliary disease causes histologic and clinical acute pancreatitis, whereas the episodes of acute pancreatitis in chronic alcoholics mostly occur superimposed on some chronic damage.

In alcoholic pancreatitis, the first episode of clinical pancreatitis occurs after 15 to 20 years of heavy drinking and before the age of 35 to 40 years. Men are affected more often than women. A number of other etiologic factors that rarely cause acute pancreatitis are presented in Box 366-2. Many medications have been suspected, but the few that are clearly demonstrated to cause acute pancreatitis include immunosuppressive medications (6-mercaptopurine and azathioprine), sulfonamides, oral 5-aminosalicylic acid, metronidazole, tetracyclines, nitrofurantoin, valproic acid, corticosteroids, thiazide diuretics, furosemide, estrogens, methyldopa, pentamidine, and antiretroviral agents such as didanosine. Patients with type I, IV, and V (according to the Fredrickson classification) hyperlipidemia with serum

---

BOX 366-1
Acute pancreatitis terminology

Severe acute pancreatitis: associated with organ failure and/or local complications such as necrosis abscess, or pseudocyst
Mild acute pancreatitis: uneventful recovery occurs within 3 to 5 days; no organ dysfunction
Acute fluid collections: no defined wall; occurs in severe disease
Acute pseudocyst: collection of pancreatic juice enclosed by a wall of fibrous/granulation tissue
Pancreatic necrosis
  Sterile: diffuse or focal area or areas of nonviable parenchyma
  Infected: diagnosed by fine needle aspiration
Pancreatic abscess: circumscribed intraabdominal collection of pus in the pancreatic region

Modified from Bradley E: *Arch Surg* 128:586-590, 1993.

BOX 366-2
Etiologic factors of acute pancreatitis

Common
Alcohol
Biliary
Idiopathic

Occasional
Hyperlipidemia
Hypercalcemia
Post-ERCP
Medications*
Postoperative
Trauma

Rare
Hereditary pancreatitis
Vasculitis
Pancreas divisum
Penetrating peptic ulcer
Sphincter of Oddi dysfunction
Infections: mumps, coxsackie B, mycoplasma, ascariasis
Exposure to organophosphorus
Scorpion bite (Trinidad)
Post–renal transplant
Cardiopulmonary bypass surgery
Pancreatic cancer
Chronic renal failure

*Medications causing acute pancreatitis: *Definite:* azathioprine, thiazides, sulfonamide, furosemide, estrogens, tetracycline, valproic acid, pentamidine, dideoxyinosine. *Probable:* acetaminophen, ethacrynic acid, procainamide, erythromycin, L-aspariginase, metronidazole, chorthalidone, steroids.
ERCP, Endoscopic retrograde cholangiopancreatography

---

triglyceride levels in excess of 1000 mg/dl may develop recurrent episodes of acute pancreatitis.

Idiopathic pancreatitis describes attacks of pancreatitis for which no cause can be found. Some of these cases, on careful investigation of aspirated bile for crystals, have been secondary to microcalculi that eluded detection by ultrasonography or endoscopic retrograde cholangiopancreatography (ERCP).

Pathologic Factors and Pathophysiology. The pathologic findings range from microscopic interstitial edema and fat necrosis of the parenchyma to macroscopic areas of pancreatic and peripancreatic necrosis and hemorrhage. The areas of pancreatic necrosis may be sterile ("phlegmon") or infected (infected pancreatic necrosis). The presence and extent of necrosis are variable and are associated with the severity of disease.

Trypsin, phospholipase A2, elastase, and lipase have been proposed to play major roles in the auto-digestion of the pancreatic acinar cell that is characteristic of the disease. Active trypsin normally is formed from its inactive precursor trypsinogen only after contact with the duodenal mucosal enzyme enterokinase. The mechanism of activation of trypsinogen to trypsin within the acinar cell that initiates cellular injury has been studied in experimental animals. The initial abnormality is blockage of the secretion of pancreatic enzymes, leading to accumulation of zymogen granules within the cells. The next step is co-localization of zymogens with lysosomal enzymes within large vacuoles, which results in activation of trypsinogen to trypsin by cathepsin B (a lysosomal hydrolase). Increased fragility of lysosomes in pancreatic acinar cells has been observed in experimental pancreatitis. Activated trypsin subsequently activates other proteases and phospholipase A2, which cause intracellular injury. Extravasation of activated pancreatic juice into the parenchyma further aggravates the tissue injury in and around the pancreas. Biliary tract stone induced pancreatitis is observed to be initiated as a result of passage of stones into or through the terminal biliopancreatic ductal system. The sequence of events by which the passage of a stone causes pancreatitis is debatable. Presumably the impacted stone at the ampulla and the associated edema cause intraductal hypertension as a result of pancreatic ductal obstruction, and damages the ductal barrier, leading to co-localization of digestive zymogens and lysosomal enzymes.

Clinical Manifestations. Symptoms of acute pancreatitis vary considerably, from mild epigastric pain with no associated features to excruciating pain mimicking perforated peptic ulcer or mesenteric infarction.

Abdominal pain is moderate to severe and is usually localized to the epigastrium alone or to the epigastrium and left or right upper quadrant. The onset is often acute, reaching maximal intensity in 10 to 15 minutes. Pain is steady and boreing, with very little fluctuation in intensity. In nearly half of the cases, pain radiates straight through to the back and lasts for many hours. The typical pancreatic pain is relieved to some extent by lying on one side with the knees flexed or sitting forward with the knees flexed against the chest. However, many patients with severe acute pancreatitis do not get much pain relief with such maneuvers. The time interval between an alcoholic binge and the onset of abdominal pain varies but is usually many hours. In biliary pancreatitis symptoms appear soon after a meal. Nausea and vomiting develop shortly after the onset of pain, and vomiting does not offer any relief of pain. Severe acute pancreatitis in the absence of pain is extremely rare.

Patients with mild pancreatitis may not have any findings on abdominal examination except mild tenderness on deep palpation of the epigastrium. However, patients with more severe forms of pancreatitis look acutely ill and move restlessly in bed to assume a position that offers comfort. Low-grade fever, hypotension, and tachycardia are notable in severe pancreatitis. Orthostatic hypotension indicates hypovolemia as a result of vomiting or fluid loss in the retroperitoneal space. Initial examination of the abdomen typically reveals tenderness, distention, and hypoactive or, less often, absent bowel sounds. Abdominal rigidity is rare. A palpable mass is unusual but may occur a week after the onset of the disease. This may represent an inflammatory mass, infected necrosis, or a pseudocyst.

Examination of the chest may reveal limitation of diaphragmatic excursion, dullness to percussion over the bases of the lungs, and decreased breath sounds. Extreme shortness of breath indicates large pleural effusions, atelectasis, associated pneumonia, congestive heart failure, or adult respiratory distress syndrome. Rare clinical findings include scleral icterus, subcutaneous fat necrosis (predominantly over the extremities, buttocks, and trunk), hepatomegaly (in alcoholics), lipemia retinalis, and the presence of eruptive xanthomas (hyperlipidemic conditions). Other rare signs of severe pancreatitis associated with hemorrhage include ecchymotic discoloration of the flanks (Grey Turner's sign) or periumbilical region (Cullen's sign). Presence of high fever indicates cholangitis, massive pancreatic necrosis, or infection of a necrotic area.

Diagnosis. Every patient with moderate to severe abdominal pain of short duration (hours to days) is suspected to have pancreatitis. A detailed history, physical examination, and demonstration of elevated

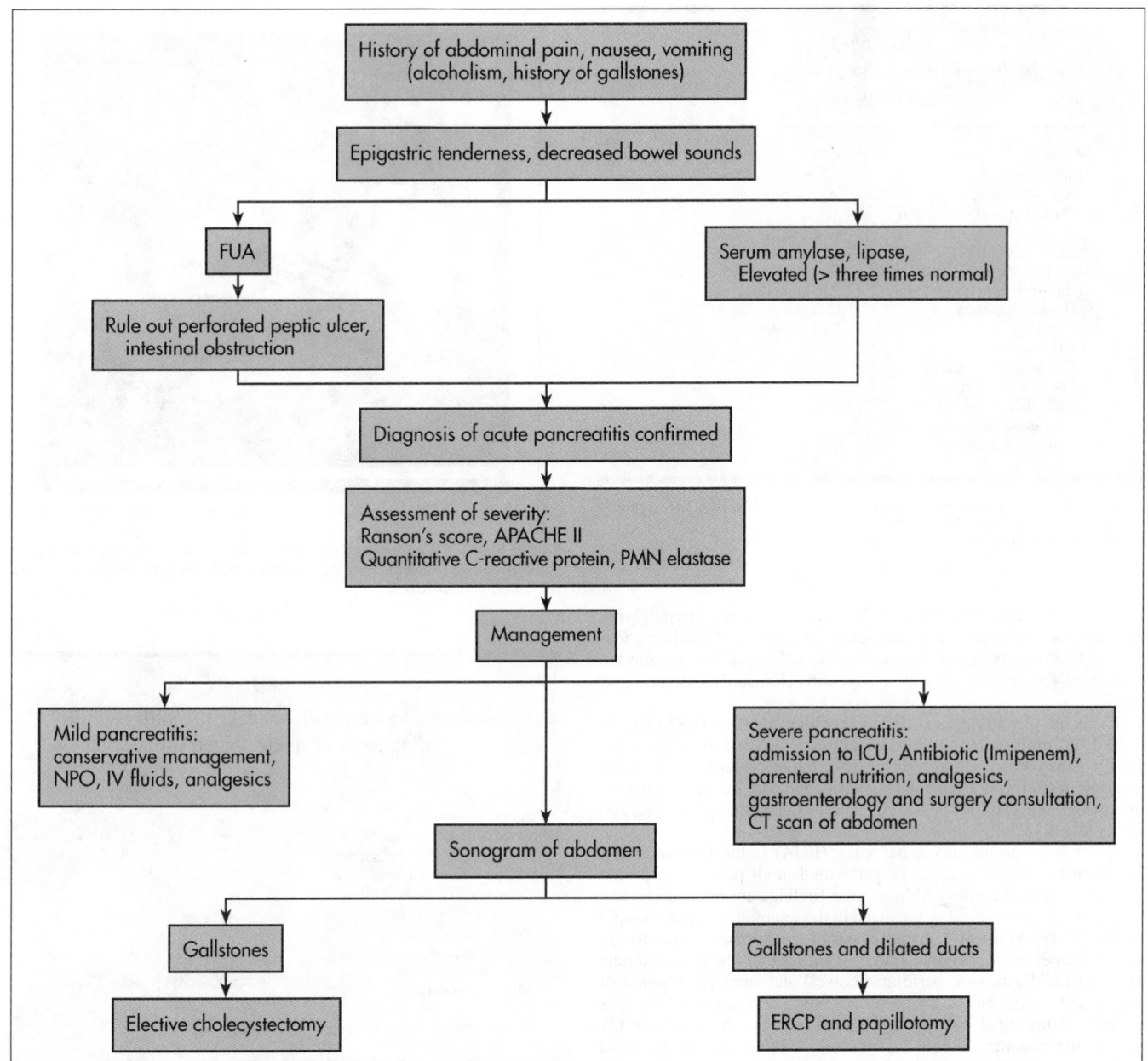

FIGURE 366-1   Assessment and management of acute pancreatitis.

serum amylase levels enable the physician to make a clinical diagnosis. In every patient suspected to have acute pancreatitis the three important questions to ask are (1) Is the hyperamylasemia due to pancreatitis or other diseases? (2) How severe is the episode? and (3) What is the etiologic factor for the episode of acute pancreatitis? (Fig. 366-1).

Determination of serum amylase level is the most important step in the diagnosis. In acute pancreatitis, hyperamylasemia is detectable shortly after the onset of symptoms, and the levels return to normal within 1 to 4 days. Prolonged hyperamylasemia suggests continuing necrosis of the pancreas, a complication such as pseudocyst or abscess, or pancreatic cancer. The degree of serum amylase elevation does not indicate severity of the disease. Hyperamylasemia may be seen in a number of conditions associated with abdominal pain, including biliary tract disease, intestinal obstruction, a perforated viscus, strangulation (of a bowel loop), dissecting aortic aneurysm, ectopic pregnancy, and strangulated ovarian cyst. Other conditions associated with hyperamylasemia include diabetic ketoacidosis, salivary disease, chronic renal failure, and certain nonpancreatic tumors that

seldom cause diagnostic difficulties. An amylase level elevation of three times normal is more likely related to acute pancreatitis than other causes of hyperamylasemia. Similarly, an elevated amylase that returns to normal with resolution of symptoms is strong evidence in favor of acute pancreatitis. The higher the amylase level, the more likely the pancreas is the source. An exception to this is that amylase levels may not be very elevated in those with hyprelipidemic pancreatitis. Although the cause of pancreatitis cannot be determined with certainty based on the degree of elevation of amylase, the levels are considerably higher in gallstone pancreatitis than in alcoholic pancreatitis. Urinary amylase values and urine amylase/creatinine clearance ratio studies are not reliable in the diagnosis of acute pancreatitis.

Serum lipase assays are more specific than amylase levels, since the pancreas is responsible for almost all of the lipase in the serum. Serum levels of pancreatic isoamylase, trypsin, and elastase have no additional value in the diagnosis of acute pancreatitis. The serum amylase levels usually return to normal by the fourth or fifth day, but lipase may not return to normal until the sixth or seventh day.

BOX 366-3

Representative prognostic scoring systems in acute pancreatitis*

Ranson	Glasgow
Admission	
Age >55 years	Age >50 years
WBC >16,000 cells/mm³	WBC >15,000
Glucose >200 mg/dl	Glucose >180 mg/dl
LDH >350 IU/L	BUN >45 mg/dl
AST >250 IU/L	PO_2 <60 mm Hg
Initial 48 hours	Albumin <3.2 g/dl
Hematocrit decrease	Calcium <8 mg/dl
>10%	LDH >600 IU/L
BUN increase >5 mg/dl	
Calcium <8 mg/dl	
PO_2 <60 mm Hg	
Base deficit >4 mEq/L	
Estimated fluid sequestra-	
tion >6 liters	

Modified from Ranson JAC et al: *Surg Gynecol Obstet* 143:209, 1976, and Neoptolemos VP et al: *Lancet* 2:979, 1988.

*Presence of three or more factors indicates poor prognosis.

Other laboratory abnormalities such as leukocytosis, hyperglycemia, increase in alanine aminotransferase, bilirubin and alkaline phosphatase levels, hypoxemia, hypocalcemia, and hypoalbuminemia are markers of the severity of acute pancreatitis (Ranson's criteria) (Box 366-3).

The acute physiology and chronic health evaluation II, (APACHE II) and the multiple organ system failure (MOSF) scores are more sensitive than Ranson's criteria in determining severity. The newer serologic tests for assessment of severity include elevated polymorphonuclear cell elastase (>200 mg/L) and C-reactive protein (>120 mg/L) levels.

A flat and upright abdominal x-ray (FUA) is the first and most important radiologic study to be performed in all patients suspected to have acute pancreatitis. Although the findings are nonspecific and include ileus, generalized or localized in the jejunum ("sentinel loop") or colon ("colon cut-off"), displacement of the stomach or duodenum and gallstones are occasional findings. Initial FUA helps to exclude air under the diaphragm (perforated bowel) and other conditions that mimic acute pancreatitis but need early surgical assessment such as findings of intestinal obstruction. If doubt exists, an immediate CT scan of the abdomen should be obtained. Radiographs of the chest may reveal elevation of the diaphragm, atelectasis, pneumonitis, pulmonary edema, and left-sided pleural effusion.

Initial ultrasonography of the abdomen will help to identify stones in the gallbladder or a dilated common bile duct with an impacted stone in addition to helping to assess the morphologic condition of the pancreas. CT scan need not be done routinely in all patients. Indications for CT scan include Ranson's score greater than three, refractory hypoxemia, hypotension, leucocytosis, fever, tender abdominal mass, hemodynamic deterioration, and evidence of hemorrhage (Cullen's or Grey Turner's sign). Features of acute pancreatitis include enlarged indistinct margins of the gland, alterations in enhancement patterns, fluid accumulations, and thickening of adjacent fascial planes. When the microcirculation of the edematous pancreas is intact, the pancreatic parenchyma is uniformly enhanced following intravenous (IV) contrast given by bolus technique, and contrast-enhanced CT (CECT) scan indicates interstitial pancreatitis (Fig. 366-2). If enhancement is patchy and large areas do not enhance at all, the process shows necrotizing pancreatitis. CT findings help not only in diagnosing pancreatitis but also in assessing the severity of the inflammatory process. Grade A or minimal edematous pancreatitis is indicated by normal pancreas, grade B by enlargement, grade C by peripancreatic inflammation, grade D by a single fluid collection, and grade E by multiple fluid collection (Balthazar criteria).

Determination of the etiologic factor is needed for appropriate

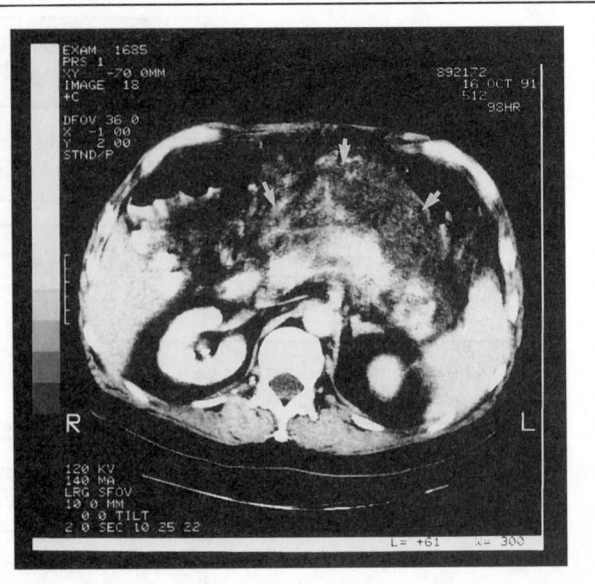

FIGURE 366-2   Computed tomography scan of pancreas in patient with acute pancreatitis. Note edema and inflammatory infiltration of peripancreatic and mesenteric fat *(arrows)*.

BOX 366-4

Diseases to be considered in the differential diagnosis of acute pancreatitis

Acute cholecystitis
Peptic ulcer disease
Intestinal obstruction
Acute gynecologic disorder
Mesenteric vascular disease
Appendicitis, diverticulitis
Abdominal aneurysm
Renal colic
Splenic rupture
Abdominal abscess
Myocardial infarction
Porphyria
Familial Mediterranean fever

management. Factors that predict biliary tract disease caused by pancreatitis include age over 50, female sex, amylase elevation of more than 4000 IU/ml, AST elevation of more than 100 U/L, and alkaline phosphatase of more than 300 IU/L. Alcoholic origin is more common in men with a long history of chronic alcoholism; the first episode is usually before age 40 years, and the degree of serum enzyme elevation is very modest. The lipase activity in alcoholic pancreatitis is usually high relative to the low amylase levels.

Differential Diagnosis. Abdominal pain associated with elevated amylase levels may occur in a number of conditions (Box 366-4). Acute cholecystitis with or without associated pancreatitis, perforated or a penetrating (posterior) peptic ulcer, intestinal obstruction or strangulation, ectopic pregnancy, and ruptured ovarian cyst are the most common entities to be excluded. In the majority of cases a detailed history and a thorough physical examination combined with judicious use of radiologic studies will clarify the diagnosis. Contrast-enhanced CT scan has reduced the need for exploratory laparotomy.

Management. The management of uncomplicated acute pancreatitis is essentially supportive, and the great majority of patients with mild pancreatitis can be managed on the regular hospital floor. While providing pain relief with parenteral analgesics, it is important to keep the pancreas at rest, maintain fluid and electrolyte balance, monitor hemodynamic and respiratory status, and provide close observation. Nasogastric tube aspiration of the stomach is needed only in moderate to severe acute pancreatitis to keep the stomach empty, to prevent aspiration in patients with vomiting, and to prevent gastric hydrochloric acid from entering the duodenum, thereby stimulating the pancreas. Oral intake of food is to be discontinued until pain disappears totally and amylase levels return to normal. Enteral feedings, when restarted, should initially be with liquids for the first 24 hours, then advanced as tolerated to a soft diet over the next 3 days. Peripheral parenteral nutrition (PPN) or total parenteral nutrition (TPN) may be needed for those who will be without food for a week or more.

Pain relief is provided by intramuscular injections of meperidine, 50-75 mg, given every 4 to 6 hours. Antibiotic therapy should be given to patients with severe acute pancreatitis, particularly to those with signs and symptoms of cholangitis. Infectious complications are the leading causes of death in acute pancreatitis. Ampicillin has low diffusion capacity in pancreatic tissue and should not be the antibiotic of choice. The antibiotics with good diffusion capacity are imipenem, ofloxacin, metronidazole, and mezlocillin; recent studies have shown that all patients with severe biliary pancreatitis benefit by antibiotic therapy. Those with necrotizing pancreatitis (diagnosed by CT) who receive imipenem 500, mg IV, every 12 hours for 2 weeks have a reduced incidence of septic complications. Severe acute pancreatitis is best treated in an intensive care unit, and an early surgical consult is advisable for closer surveillance. In order to provide appropriate fluid replacement, monitoring by Swan-Ganz catheter is desirable.

Peritoneal lavage in the management of severe acute pancreatitis has not shown any convincing benefit. Early ERCP and papillotomy should be the treatment of choice for those with severe acute pancreatitis and cholangitis. There is a definite role for surgery in acute pancreatitis with infected pancreatic necrosis, and the diagnosis is established by dynamic contrast-enhanced CT examination and CT-guided fine needle aspiration of the necrotic area, with smear for Gram staining and culture. Necrosectomy, placement of a large-caliber drain in the abscess cavity, and continuous irrigation with saline solution are recommended. The role of surgery in noninfected necrosis is debatable. Surgery is indicated in the treatment of pseudocysts that are larger than 5 cm in diameter, increasing in size, present for more than 6 weeks, are infected, or are symptomatic.

Complications of Acute Pancreatitis

Acute pancreatitis is a multisystem disease. The degree of inflammation and autodigestion of the pancreas determines the release of proteolytic enzymes, lipase, kinins, and peptides into the surrounding tissue and circulation.

The important local complications include sterile pancreatic necrosis, infected pancreatic necrosis, acute pancreatic pseudocyst, and pancreatic abscess (Boxes 366-1 and 366-5). Presence of fever, tachycardia, or CT findings do not help to distinguish infected from sterile necrosis. The role of fine needle aspiration in the differential diagnosis is well established. There is debate with regard to the need for surgery. Necrosectomy is perhaps indicated for those with early indicators of organ failure.

There is no debate with regard to the need for antibiotic therapy and surgery in those with infected pancreatic necrosis and pancreatic abscess.

A pancreatic pseudocyst that is less than 5 cm in size tends to disappear without surgical therapy. The cysts that usually require treatment are those which are more than 5 cm in diameter, have been present for more than 6 weeks, associated with severe pain, and show evidence of rapid expansion. Pseudocysts can be drained percutaneously, endoscopically, or surgically, depending on the number, size, and location of the cysts and the availability of expertise in the institution.

The systemic complications include hypocalcemia, hyperglycemia, hypoalbumenia, hyperlipidemia, and coagulation abnormalities. The four most important systemic complications that indicate organ system failure are shock (defined as systolic blood pressure of <80 mm Hg for at least 15 minutes), respiratory (P_{O_2} <60 mm Hg requiring oxygen therapy for >24 hours); renal (serum creatinine level

---

BOX 366-5
Complications of acute pancreatitis

Pancreatic

Necrosis: sterile vs. infected
Pseudocyst: infection, rupture, hemorrhage, abscess

Local nonpancreatic

Colonic infarction: lower gastrointestinal bleeding
Pancreatic ascites: high protein–high amylase ascites
Contiguous involvement: gastrointestinal bleeding, thrombosis of splenic vein, bowel infarction
Obstructive jaundice

Systemic

Pulmonary: hypoxia, pleural effusion, acute respiratory distress syndrome
Cardiac: shock, pericardial effusion, electrocardiogram changes, arrhythmias
Hematologic: disseminated intravascular coagulation, thrombotic thrombocytopenic purpura
Renal: azotemia, oliguria, myoglobinuria
Metabolic: hypocalcemia, hyperglycemia, acidosis, hypoalbuminemia
Central nervous system: psychosis, Puertscher's retinopathy
Peripheral: rhabdomyolysis, fat necrosis, bone necrosis, arthritis

---

>1.4 mg/dl during the hospitalization), and a sepsis-like picture (temperature >38.5° C and white blood cell count >20,000/mm³).

Hypocalcemia (<8.0 mg/dl) correlates strongly with a poor prognosis. The pathogenesis is attributed to massive calcium soap formation in areas of fat necrosis, hypoalbuminemia, and formation of calcium-free fatty acid complexes. Frank tetany is rare in view of near-normal levels of ionized calcium despite the fall in total calcium. During episodes of severe acute pancreatitis, transient hyperglycemia and glycosuria may occur. Diabetes in acute pancreatitis generally does not need any specific treatment. Hyperlipidemia, as a consequence of acute pancreatitis, seldom elevates the triglyceride levels above 500 mg/dl. Clinically significant coagulation abnormalities occur in severe acute pancreatitis. Disseminated intravascular coagulation (DIC), characterized by increased fibrin degradation products, thrombocytopenia, decreased level of factor VII, and increased levels of factors V and VIII and fibrinogen, occurs in severe acute pancreatitis. The mechanism of coagulation abnormalities is attributed to active circulating trypsin. Shock is attributed to hypovolemia, hemodynamic changes, and a possible myocardial depressant factor. The most serious respiratory complication is the adult respiratory distress syndrome (ARDS). Clinical features include severe dyspnea and extreme hypoxemia refractory to a high inspired oxygen concentration. Phospholipase A has been implicated in causing injury to the pulmonary capillary endothelium. Management of ARDS includes avoidance of fluid overload, prompt endotracheal intubation, positive end-expiratory pressure ventilation when necessary, and hemodynamic and nutritional support. Hypovolemia occurs in severe acute pancreatitis and is attributed to increased capillary permeability and sequestration of fluid in the retroperitoneal space. Thrombotic thrombocytopenic purpura (TTP) characterized by the classic pentad of symptoms (fever, microangiopathic hemolytic anemia, neurologic changes, thrombocytopenia, and acute renal failure) is a rare complication. Rhabdomyolysis when it occurs is usually associated with multiple organ system failure.

Acute pancreatitis may be associated with areas of fat necrosis in the subcutaneous tissue and bone marrow. Tender, raised, indurated nodules that may suppurate are localized to the pretibial soft tissues, the buttocks, thighs, upper arms, and trunk. Polyarthritis involving the metatarsal, interphalangeal, wrist, knee, and ankle joints frequently accompanies subcutaneous fat necrosis. Medullary bone involvement (painless) in long bones is incidentally detected on radiographs.

In uncomplicated mild interstitial pancreatitis the mortality is about 1% to 2%. When acute pancreatitis is complicated by respira-

✔ *WHEN TO REFER*

A great majority of patients with acute pancreatitis present no problem in diagnosis or management and recover with 2 to 3 days of fasting, adequate hydration, and analgesia. In contrast, nearly 20% of patients present with one or more major local or systemic complications requiring urgent care in an intensive care unit. The decision whether to admit a patient to a unit can be determined by the score system defined by Ranson or others, by the APACHE II system, or by assessing the circulating concentrations of C-reactive protein. In a small number of patients with hyperamylasemia and abdominal pain, the diagnosis may be in doubt or the patient may not show the expected signs of recovery in 2 to 3 days. In all these instances a prompt consultation from a gastroenterologist and a surgeon is warranted. In severe acute pancreatitis of biliary origin with cholangitis, sphincterotomy and stone extraction is indicated and a gastroenterologist with experience in endoscopic sphincterotomy is to be consulted. Fever, leucytosis, and persistent abdominal pain may indicate pancreatic necrosis, either infected or sterile. A radiologist's help is needed to do fine needle aspiration of a necrotic region seen on CT scan of abdomen to diagnose infected pancreatic necrosis, which is an indication for surgery. Thus a severe case of complicated pancreatitis is to be managed by a team of physicians including a gastroenterologist, a surgeon, and a radiologist.

tory failure, shock, renal failure, or a sepsis-like picture, the mortality is about 30% or higher.

CHRONIC PANCREATITIS

Chronic pancreatitis is defined as a disease that is characterized clinically by recurrent or persistent abdominal pain. Steatorrhea and/or diabetes are late manifestations of the disease. Morphologic features of the disease are irreversible destruction and permanent loss of exocrine parenchyma that may be either focal, segmental, or diffuse. In early stages it is impossible to differentiate an exacerbation of chronic pancreatitis from acute pancreatitis. In acute pancreatitis there is clinical and biologic restitution of the pancreas if the cause for pancreatitis was eliminated, and the pancreas is structurally and functionally normal between episodes.

Etiologic Factors. In the affluent nations, alcoholism is the leading cause of chronic pancreatitis, whereas in many developing nations a nonalcoholic type of calculous pancreatitis of undetermined origin (tropical, nutritional, Afro-Asian pancreatitis) may be the most common type. Other types of chronic pancreatitis include idiopathic varieties, hereditary pancreatitis, obstructive pancreatitis, and a miscellaneous group. Table 366-1 summarizes the major clinical features of the types.

With the increase in alcohol consumption in the Western nations, a parallel rise in the incidence of chronic pancreatitis has been observed. In the United States nearly 75 percent of cases of chronic pancreatitis are due to chronic alcoholism. Cigarette smoking appears to increase the predisposition for alcoholic pancreatitis. The hospitalization rates for chronic pancreatitis per 100,000 population are greater than three times higher for blacks than for white men (20.7 vs. 5.7), with the native Indians (Pima) having the lowest predisposition to the disease. The relatively low hospitalization rates for Native Americans with chronic pancreatitis are surprising given the high prevalence of gallstones and alcoholism among them. Overall, chronic pancreatitis is less frequent than acute pancreatitis, the ratio being 1:1.5 to 1:17 depending on the population group studied.

Pathologic Findings and Pathophysiology. Macroscopically the pancreas may appear enlarged in early stages (early stages of the disease), but in materials obtained at autopsy (late stages of the disease) the gland is often atrophic and may be adherent to adjacent structures. The gland feels nodular and gritty to touch over areas of calculi and cystic over dilated ducts and pseudocysts. Microscopic

features of the pancreas reveal patchy and focal involvement. (Fig. 366-3). The earliest changes are in acinar cells, which undergo atrophy and the zymogen granules within them decrease or disappear. Within a diseased pancreas are found areas where the pancreas is almost normal or shows only minimal changes, but in other parts the exocrine cells may be entirely replaced by loose areolar tissue or dense collagen. The ductal system shows an apparent increase of ductules. Uniform narrowing (long strictures) or short segment strictures and proximal dilations may be seen in the main pancreatic duct. Squamous and goblet cell metaplasia are notable. Intraductal calculi are usually seen in late cases. Stones in the pancreas may become bigger or smaller or may even disappear with progression of disease. Disappearance of pancreatic calculi ("vanishing pancreatic calcifications") is not to be considered a sign of malignancy as indicated in some previous reports. The nerves appear hypertrophied and prominent and may demonstrate accumulation of inflammatory cells in the perineural regions. The islet cells show atrophy in some areas, while surprisingly, in other areas, they may appear well preserved, and show hypertrophy (nesidioblastosis).

Pathogenesis. The pathogenesis of chronic pancreatitis is not well understood. The following discussion covers proposed hypotheses pertaining to alcohol-induced chronic pancreatitis (Box 366-6).

Unfavorable ductal flow. Sarles and co-workers, based on a number of elegant studies, have concluded that the pathophysiologic events begin as protein plug formation that gets calcified with calcium carbonate crystals, resulting in the formation of intraductal stones. In chronic alcoholics, the viscosity of pancreatic juice increases as a result of increased enzymatic as well as well as nonenzymatic (e.g., lactoferrin) proteins. An inherited or acquired deficiency of a special protein, with properties to prevent crystallization of calcium carbonate from a supersaturated solution (lithostathine, formerly known as pancreatic stone protein [PSP]), is reported to be the primary factor in the pathogenesis of chronic calculous pancreatitis.

Early acinar cell injury. Many believe that acinar cells are injured first, similar to liver cell injury in the alcoholic, and pancreatic secretory changes follow morphologic alterations. Fibrosis, ductular abnormalities, and stone formation are secondary to acinar cell injury. A number of factors such as metabolites of alcohol, unopposed free radical injury, increased fragility of organelles, lysosomal hypertrophy, and co-localization of lysosomal enzymes and zymogens participate in acinar cell injury and determine the severity of attack. Observations support acinar cell injury as the earliest event. There is an emergence of thought that chronic pancreatitis of the alcoholic is indeed only a late manifestation of recurrent acute pancreatitis (necrosis-fibrosis sequence of Kloppel) as a result of an ongoing acinar cell injury.

Clinical Features

Recurrent abdominal pain. Pain is the dominant symptom in nearly 85% of patients with chronic pancreatitis and the most common reason for patients to seek medical attention. It can be quite debilitating and intractable, with disruption of life-style often leading to functional incapacity, drug and alcohol addiction, a poor quality of life, and even suicidal tendencies. Painless chronic pancreatitis is diagnosed by detection of pancreatic calculi accidentally in flat plate or CT scan of the abdomen performed for unrelated diseases or in the workup of steatorrhea.

The characteristic features of pain in chronic pancreatitis are as follows. Steady, boreing and agonizing pain in the epigastrium or sometimes in the left upper quadrant, with radiation directly to the back between T12 and L2 vertebrae or to left shoulder is typical. Pain may be postprandial, associated with nausea and persistent vomiting that does not relieve the pain. Although drinking alcohol exacerbates pain, the pain may occur even during periods of abstinence with no identifiable cause. The pain may worsen with advancing disease but may decrease or even totally disappear with the onset of exocrine insufficiency ("burned out" pancreas). Pancreatic pain appears to be multifactorial in pathogenesis, explaining why pain relief does not always occur with medical, endoscopic, or surgical treatment. Ductal hypertension is the predominant mechanism, but ongoing acinar injury and structural changes of the nerves (hypertrophy, lack of nerve

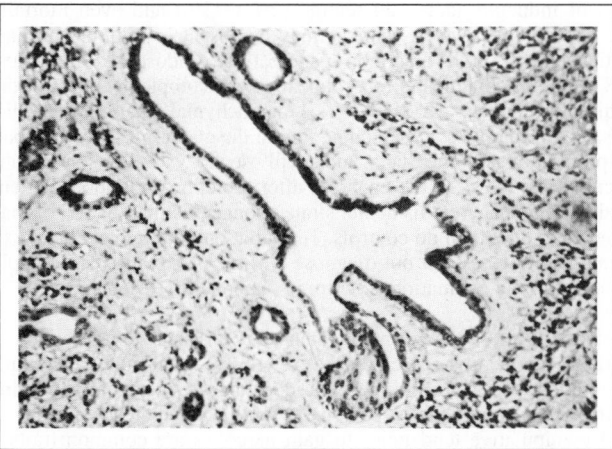

FIGURE 366-3   Chronic calcific alcoholic pancreatitis revealing dilation of large duct and surrounding fibrous tissues.

BOX 366-6
Pathogenetic hypotheses of alcoholic pancreatitis

Small duct hypotheses (unfavorable secretory changes)
   Increased viscosity
   Decreased lithostathine (pancreatic stone protein)
Early acinar cell injury
   Toxic metabolites
   Free radical injury
      Hyperstimulation of leukocytes
      Lysosomal hyperactivity
   "Necrosis-fibrosis" sequence
Big duct hypotheses (evidence weak)
   Biliary pancreatic reflux
   Sphincter of Oddi obstruction
   Duodenopancreatic reflux
   Increased ductal permeability

Table 366-1   Chronic pancreatitis: types, clinical features, and associated features

TYPE	CLINICAL FEATURES	ASSOCIATED FEATURES
Alcoholic	Mean age at onset 30-35 years Alcoholism for >15 years, >80 g/day	Painful episodes followed by calculi (9 yrs), later steatorrhea (13 yrs), diabetes (20 yrs)
Tropical	Afro-Asian countries Affects poor children and young adults Episodes of abdominal pain	Early onset of diabetes and calculi Diabetes and calculi in nearly 100% High incidence of pancreatic cancer
Hereditary	Caucasians Autosomal dominant Abdominal pain in childhood	Calculi later in life Pancreatic cancer at a young age

Idiopathic	Two types:
	   Early onset: painful, calculi, steatorrhea
	   Late onset (senile): painless
	Pancreatic calculi are an incidental finding
		Diabetes 2-3 decades later

Obstructive	Calculi rare, markedly dilated ducts Relieved by surgery	Secondary to ampullary obstruction
Pancreatitis divisum	Obstruction to the pancreatic juice at the lesser papilla	Congenital abnormality
Miscellaneous	Hyperlipidemia Hyperparathyroidism Celiac disease Billroth II gastrectomy Alpha-I antitrypsin deficiency Autoimmune	

sheaths, perineural inflammatory cells) also seem to play a role in the pathogenesis.

Malabsorption. In the natural history of chronic pancreatitis, steatorrhea occurs usually only after 10 years after of the onset of the disease and does not occur until the enzyme secretion is reduced to less than 10% of normal. Lipolytic activity decreases much faster than tryptic activity, explaining why steatorrhea occurs sooner and is more severe than azotorrhea. The stools may be bulky and formed, as opposed to the frank watery diarrhea seen in malabsorptive disorders secondary to small intestinal causes. Passage of oil droplets in the stool is often reported in chronic pancreatitis. Fecal weight tends to be lower and the fat content of the stool greater (more than 20 g/24 hours) in patients with pancreatic insufficiency than in patients with steatorrhea from other causes. Although overt vitamin B_{12} malabsorption is extremely rare, an abnormal Schilling test is often seen. Dietary vitamin B_{12} that is bound to salivary R protein is cleaved by pancreatic enzymes, transferring cobalamin to intrinsic factor.

Pancreatic diabetes. Although glucose intolerance is common early in the course of chronic pancreatitis, clinical diabetes occurs only relatively late in the disease in nearly 30% of patients with alcoholic pancreatitis. Pancreatic diabetes may be the presenting symptom as in patients with painless pancreatitis. The diabetic syndrome secondary to pancreatic disease is an example of acquired beta and alpha cell insufficiency associated with insulin resistance. In general,

pancreatic diabetes is mild and ketoacidosis is rare. Recent observations indicate that the risk and characteristics of retinopathy in alcoholic pancreatitis are similar to those with non–insulin-dependent diabetes mellitus (NIDDM). Neuropathy is common, probably because of the additive effect of alcohol abuse and malnutrition. The most dramatic manifestation of pancreatic diabetes is the frequent and profound hypoglycemic episodes, which may be fatal if not managed promptly.

Diagnosis. Chronic pancreatitis is to be considered in all patients with unexplained abdominal pain. Very few patients present with the classic triad of pancreatic calculi, diabetes mellitus, and steatorrhea. In the large majority of patients the diagnosis is suspected because of a history of abdominal pain characteristic of pancreatitis in origin, along with a longstanding history of alcoholism. Physical findings in alcoholic pancreatitis are nonspecific and include signs of chronic alcoholism, epigastric tenderness, and occasional associated hepatomegaly. A number of tests are available to confirm the diagnosis (Chapter 352).

In the early stages of chronic pancreatitis, during acute exacerbations, serum amylase and lipase values are moderately elevated, but the tests are of no use between acute exacerbations and in those with more advanced disease. Making a diagnosis of chronic pancreatitis solely based on mild elevations of serum amylase is not justifiable.

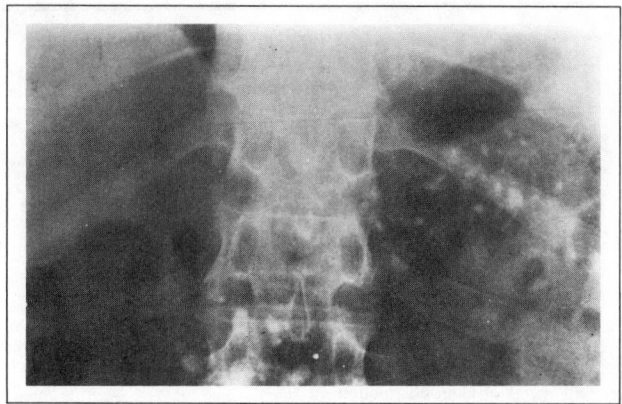

FIGURE 366-4   Flat abdominal x-ray film. Diffuse pancreatic calcification is visible.

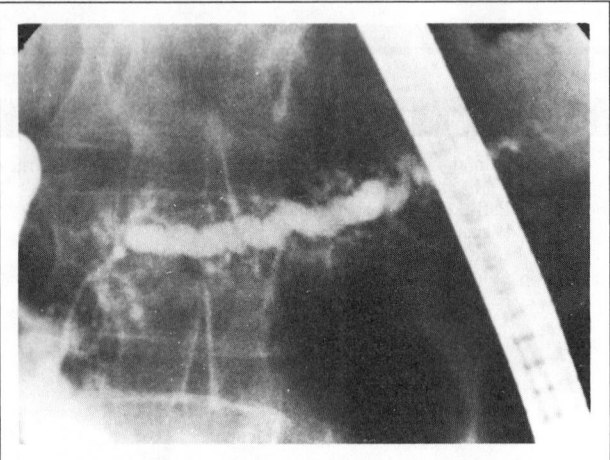

FIGURE 366-5   Endoscopic retrograde cholangiopancreatogram in a patient with advanced chronic pancreatitis, showing a diffusely dilated and tortuous main pancreatic duct.

In evaluating patients with atypical abdominal pain, one should remember the prevalence of macroamylasemia in the general population, which is about 5%. The high-molecular-weight amylase is not cleared in the urine, and there may be a persistent twofold to threefold elevation of the enzyme in the serum while the amylase levels are low in the urine.

Plain film of the abdomen including a chest film is the first radiologic study in all patients with initial or subsequent episodes of suspected chronic pancreatitis, to detect pancreatic calculi, and to exclude other intraabdominal causes of pain. The presence of pancreatic calculi is almost definite evidence for chronic pancreatitis (Fig. 366-4). In those with no pancreatic calculi, the two diagnostic modalities used to assess the many morphologic abnormalities of the pancreas are abdominal ultrasound and CT scan of the abdomen. The size of the pancreas, presence or absence of cysts, irregularities and size of ducts, parenchymal heterogeneity, presence or absence of calculi, and extrapancreatic complications such as common bile duct obstruction and dilation are detectable. Ultrasound has limited usefulness in obese patients and in those with increased bowel gas and thus CT is generally preferred. There are no data to demonstrate that magnetic resonance imaging is superior to CT scanning. ERCP is the new gold standard in the diagnosis of chronic pancreatitis (almost replacing the secretin CCK secretory test, which has become unpopular in view of its difficulty to be performed accurately). ERCP findings are highly sensitive (70% to 90%) and specific (90% to 100%) (Fig. 366-5). Dilation of side branches, stricture and dilations of main duct obstructions, and intraductular filling defects are diagnostic findings. The limitations of ERCP are its high cost, the associated complica-

tion of inducing acute pancreatitis (2% to 3%) and even mortality (0.1% to 0.2%). Ductal changes may be absent or minimal in many patients with mild alcoholic pancreatitis. Endoscopic ultrasound (EUS), a new diagnostic tool, appears to be complementary to other radiologic studies. EUS identifies parenchymal changes including cystic abnormalities, hyperechoic foci in the gland, presence of stones or protein plugs in the ducts, and small pseudocysts. The sonographic secretin test is US of the pancreas after secretin stimulation. Patients with chronic pancreatitis demonstrate a longer lasting dilation of main pancreatic duct than do controls. Tests that only help to evaluate exocrine insufficiency but not diagnose chronic pancreatitis are complementary in the evaluation of chronic pancreatitis (Chapter 352).

Management.   The management of an acute exacerbation of chronic pancreatitis is exactly the same as that of acute pancreatitis. Continued use of alcohol, narcotic dependence, recurrent abdominal pain, erratic eating habits, personality problems, aggressive behavior, and manipulative tendencies to gain narcotics are common traits in many patients. There is a need for a multidisciplinary team approach with an internist as the gatekeeper to coordinate, and a gastroenterologist, a psychiatrist, an experienced pancreatic surgeon, a social worker, and a diabetologist as consultants. The importance of abstinence from alcohol use cannot be overemphasized, since pain relief is usually higher and deterioration of pancreatic function is slower in abstinent patients. In this regard the help of a psychiatrist and an alcohol rehabilitation program are recommended. The diet should be small and low in fat (30%), to minimize the stimulation of pancreas. It should be nutritious, adequate in calories, high in protein (25% of calories), and moderate in carbohydrate (45%). In the management of pain, the first step is to try nonopioid analgesics, such as acetaminophen, salicylates, and NSAIDs, with or without antidepressants. Most patients, however, need opioid analgesics for symptomatic relief, and the initial doses should be low and the drug administered less frequently. Low-potency drugs such as Darvocet U100 or small doses of codeine derivatives with acetaminophen are the drugs of choice. A controversial form of therapy is treatment of pain with high doses of oral pancreatic enzymes.

It is speculated that extremely low levels of intraduodenal protease levels in chronic pancreatitis stimulate pancreatic enzyme secretion and increase intraductular pressure proximal to strictures. The converse will be that adequate amounts of proteases should decrease pancreatic secretion and intraduct pressure. In order to effect feedback inhibition of pancreatic secretion and offer pain relief, it is important to administer very large doses of a commercially available non–enteric coated pancreatic enzyme preparation with a high concentration of proteases. However, the best clinical response is seen only in a small group of female patients with idiopathic pancreatitis and normal fecal fat excretion, and is not of much use in patients with alcoholic pancreatitis.

Currently other forms of therapy are undergoing clinical trials. Octreotide acetate, a synthetic analog of somatostatin, when given subcutaneously is rapidly absorbed and inhibits pancreatic enzyme release and offers pain relief. The results are not consistent. Endoscopic therapies are frequently being used before surgical options are considered. The underlying principle of all endoscopic therapies is that the sole or the most important mechanism of pain in chronic pancreatitis is impaired outflow of pancreatic secretion as a result of strictures or calculi in the main pancreatic duct. The forms of endoscopic procedures currently available include (1) sphincterotomy, (2) internal drainage of pancreatic cysts, (3) extraction of stones from the pancreatic duct, (4) ductal ablation by glues, (5) guide-wire–catheter dilation of strictures, and (6) placement of pancreatic stents. Celiac plexus block using alcohol or phenol as neurolytic agents is not only technically difficult, but the relief of pain is often transient, sometimes lasting only a few days. Pancreatic surgery is aimed at drainage of the gland (pancreaticojejunostomy, or Puestow's procedure), resecting part of the gland, or total pancreatectomy. Resective procedures are associated with worsening of malabsorption and precipitation of diabetes.

Management of pancreatic insufficiency is with manipulation of diet and addition of supplementary oral enzymes. Substitution of dietary fat with medium-chain triglycerides (MCT) (fatty acids 8 to 10 carbon atoms in length) may be indicated temporarily to provide calories to relieve steatorrhea and promote weight gain. Medium-chain

---

BOX 366-7
Pancreatic enzyme therapy

Indication: steatorrhea, abdominal pain
Contraindication: allergy to pork protein
Side effects: hyperuricosuria (high doses in CF), impairment of folate absorption, impairment of iron absorption, colonic stricture (high doses)
For steatorrhea: enteric coated capsules
For pain: high-dose non–enteric coated tablets

BOX 366-8
Complications of chronic pancreatitis

Extrahepatic biliary obstruction (from fibrosis of the head of the pancreas, pressure from a pseudocyst)
  Asymptomatic alkaline phosphatase elevation
  Jaundice
  Second biliary cirrhosis, cholangitis
Pancreatic ascites/pleural effusion (from leakage of pancreatic juice into retroperitoneum, mediastinum, or pleural space)
  Elevated amylase and albumin in ascites, pleural fluid
Gastrointestinal bleeding (esophageal/gastric varices from splenic vein thrombosis)
  Bleeding esophageal varices
Metastatic fat necrosis (as a result of increased lipolytic activity in circulation)
  Subcutaneous fat necrosis
  Intramedullary fat necrosis
  Polyarthritis
Cirrhosis in alcoholic pancreatitis
  Prevalence varies (1% to 33%)
Cancers
  Extrapancreatic cancers: tongue, larynx, bronchus, colon, rectum, liver, skin, lip, bladder
  Pancreatic cancer

✔ *WHEN TO REFER*

Referral of a patient with suspected chronic pancreatitis to a subspecialist is needed for establishing when routine studies such as FUA, abdominal ultrasound, or CT scan of abdomen fail to reveal an abnormality. ERCP is required to diagnose chronic pancreatitis and to obtain valid data on the morphology of the pancreatic and biliary duct; thus a gastroenterologist with experience in the procedure is to be consulted. Once the diagnosis is established, a number of problems are to be addressed. Management of pain, associated alcoholism, and drug dependency necessitates consultations from a psychiatrist, a surgeon, and a therapeutic endoscopist. Abstinence from alcohol use and narcotic dependency cannot be achieved in most patients without the help of a drug or alcohol rehabilitation program. Recurrent and severe pain is quite frustrating to the patient as well as to the physician. The decision to do a pancreatic stent placement endoscopically is to be made only after a firm diagnosis of chronic pancreatitis is made. Only a few patients with isolated proximal stricture respond to this form of therapy, and the procedure is invasive, expensive, and associated with complications. If surgery is indicated, the choice of surgery (drainage vs. resection), choice of the patient for the surgery (patient compliance), and choice of the surgeon (only an experienced pancreatic surgeon) are important factors that influence the outcome. It is not often difficult to manage diabetes secondary to chronic pancreatitis, but a few cases with recurrent hypoglycemia may require help from an endocrinologist and a dietitian. A number of patients are diagnosed as having chronic pancreatitis with little evidence and are subjected to papillotomy and repeated stent placements; the primary care physician and the gastroenterologist should not fall into this trap.

---

triglycerides are better absorbed than the usual dietary fats (long-chain triglycerides) even in the presence of only very small amounts of lipase and in the absence of bile salts. The definitive therapy for the management of exocrine insufficiency is supplementation with commercially available pancreatic enzymes. Several factors are to be pointed out concerning the scientific basis of enzyme therapy (Box 366-7). It is necessary to administer up to fivefold to tenfold more lipase than what is normally required in the duodenum. To deliver such high concentrations requires taking a large number of tablets, up to eight with each meal; because of the high cost and other factors, decreased patient compliance is seen. Enteric coated microspheres (in contrast to the non–enteric coated preparation that is preferred in the management of pain) are more effective, cheaper, and better tolerated. The management of pancreatic diabetes requires caution. Hypoglycemia is the most common cause of death in diabetics secondary to chronic pancreatitis, and patients must be educated to recognize its early symptoms and to initiate prompt self-management. In administering insulin therapy, the golden rule is to err on the side of underinsulinization and not to target normoglycemia.

Complications (Box 366-8)

Obstructive jaundice in chronic pancreatitis, as a result of common bile duct (CBD) stenosis, is a frequent complication. The distal common bile duct that traverses the head of the pancreas is involved in acute exacerbations of chronic pancreatitis as a result of fibrosis of the head of the pancreas or by compression from a pseudocyst. Ultrasonography, percutaneous transhepatic cholangiography, and ERCP delineate the stricture and proximal dilation of the CBD and intrahepatic biliary radicles. Appropriate antibiotic therapy and decompres-

sion of the biliary tract by choledochoenterostomy avoid complications such as acute cholangitis and secondary biliary cirrhosis.

Fibrosis of the head of the pancreas may also involve the adjacent antrum of the stomach or duodenum, causing epigastric pain, postprandial fullness, nausea, and vomiting, mimicking pancreatic carcinoma. Diagnosis is established by upper gastrointestinal series and esophagogastroduodenoscopy. Surgical treatment may be needed to relieve obstruction.

Pancreatic pseudocysts are collections of pancreatic juice surrounded by a nonepithelial fibrous wall of granulation tissue. The indications for treatment of pseudocysts are discussed in the section on acute pancreatitis. Pancreatic ascites is caused by leakage of pancreatic juice as a result of a ruptured duct or pseudocyst. A pancreaticopleural fistula is the cause of pleural effusions. The diagnosis of pancreatic ascites and pleural effusion is made by demonstration of high amylase and protein in the aspirated fluid. Thrombosis of the splenic vein, splenic artery aneurysm, or pseudoaneurysm are complications of chronic pancreatitis. The splenic vein and portal vein may also be compressed by a pseudocyst or occluded by fibrosis from adjacent inflammation. A segmental form of portal hypertension characterized by gastric varices develops, and life-threatening variceal bleeding may occur. Splenectomy is curative. Unilateral or bilateral pleural effusion is often the result of a leaking pseudocyst or pleuropancreatic fistula, which can be demonstrated by ERCP and managed conservatively.

Prognosis. Chronic pancreatitis is a progressive disease with loss of exocrine and endocrine function. The effects of abstinence from alcohol on progression of the disease are not clear. The typical patient with alcoholic pancreatitis returns to the emergency room more and more frequently with pain that becomes constant, requiring round-the-clock doses of narcotics. Many become drug dependent and develop drug-seeking behavior. Some patients may reach the stage of "burned out" pancreas, when pain may totally disappear but steatorrhea and diabetes become prominent features. The adverse prognostic factors include continued alcoholism, cigarette smoking, IDDM, associated liver disease, and advancing age. Extrapancreatic and pancreatic malignancies might complicate chronic pancreatitis. Death is often as a result of upper gastrointestinal bleeding, hypoglycemia, or infections, or by suicide.

Table 366-2   Major presenting features of pancreatic cancer

	HEAD (%)	BODY AND TAIL (%)
Weight loss	92	100
Jaundice	82	7
Pain	72	87
Anorexia	64	33

Data from Howard JM, Jordan CL, Jr: *Curr Publ Cancer* 2:1, 1977.

EXOCRINE PANCREATIC TUMORS (TABLE 366-2)

Pancreatic adenocarcinoma is one of the most difficult and discouraging problems in clinical medicine. It is a highly lethal disease with a mortality rate well in excess of 95%. The disease is nearly always diagnosed at a relatively late stage because its signs and symptoms are often nonspecific and occur only after the disease has sufficiently advanced. The 5-year survival rate with adenocarcinoma of the pancreas in the United States is 1.3%, and the median survival is 4.1 months. Carcinoma of the ampulla of Vater, which represents 4% to 10% of patients with peripancreatic carcinoma, has a different clinical course and the 5-year survival rate is about 36%. Cystic neoplasms of the pancreas are extremely rare, more common in women (72%), and often misdiagnosed as pseudocysts. The overall prognosis of cystadenocarcinoma is very favorable, with a 75% cure rate with early diagnosis and surgery.

Epidemiology. Carcinoma of the exocrine pancreas is now the tenth most common cause of cancer, the second most common cancer of the gastrointestinal tract, and the fourth leading cause of cancer-related deaths in men (after lung, prostate, and colorectal cancers) and the fifth in women (after lung, breast, colorectal, and ovarian cancers). Approximately 25,000 new cases occur per year. Peak incidence of pancreatic cancer is in the seventh to eight decades. There is an increased incidence in males, and in blacks in general. Pancreatic cancer is primarily a disease of the developed world.

Risk Factors. Cigarette smoking has been strongly linked to pancreatic cancer. The onset of pancreatic cancer in smokers is 10 years before nonsmokers, and the relative risk compared to nonsmokers is nearly double. Occupational exposure to many industrial toxins (benzidine, beta-naphthylamine derivatives, metal dusts, coal tar derivatives) increases the risk. There also appears to be a good correlation between the mortality from pancreatic cancer and fat content in the diet. All forms of chronic pancreatitis, particularly hereditary pancreatitis and tropical pancreatitis, predispose to pancreatic cancer. There is a slight increase in the incidence of pancreatic cancer in those with longstanding diabetes. There are no conclusive data to associate drinking of coffee with the development of pancreatic cancer.

Pathologic Findings. Benign tumors of the pancreas are rare and are usually cystic. Seventy percent of carcinomas originate in the head of the gland, with the remainder being diffuse or situated in the body or tail. It is important to differentiate periampullary cancers arising from the duodenum or common bile duct and the rare cystadenocarcinoma from pancreatic carcinomas, as these lesions have a better prognosis and should be treated with aggressive surgery.

Approximately 90% of nonendocrine carcinomas develop from ductular epithelium and 1% from acinar cells; the remainder comprise a heterogenous group of unusual histologic types. Ductal adenocarcinoma occurs predominantly in the head of the gland (60% to 70%). Papillary, tubular, or acinar arrays of malignant cells with varying degrees of cellular differentiation are seen on microscopic examination. Ductal epithelium at a distance from the cancer often exhibits papillary hyperplasia, and carcinoma in situ occurs in up to 20% of cases. Acute or chronic pancreatitis may exist distal to an obstructing cancer, but calcification is rare. Spread occurs by direct extension, with early neural and lymph node invasion. Visceral metastases are most common in liver and peritoneum. The pancreas can also be the site of secondary metastatic deposits, most commonly from breast or lung cancer, or melanoma.

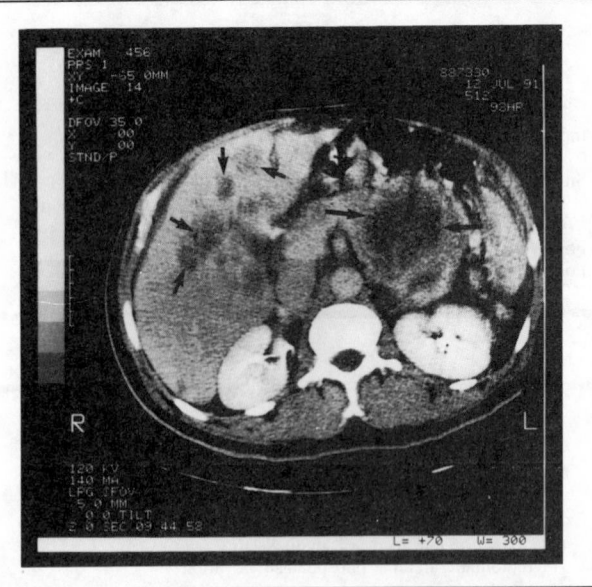

FIGURE 366-6   Computed tomography scan in a patient with carcinoma of the tail of the pancreas. Necrotic pancreatic mass *(long arrow)* and hepatic metastases *(short arrows)* are evident.

Clinical Features. Presenting symptoms and signs depend on the location and extent of the lesion (Table 366-2), but nonspecific and vague complaints such as depression or anxiety are the earliest features in half of patients. The classic triad of abdominal pain, weight loss, and obstructive jaundice indicates a cancer situated in the head of the gland that is usually advanced and incurable. A palpably enlarged, nontender gallbladder in a jaundiced patient without biliary colic usually signifies malignant obstruction of the terminal bile duct (Courvoisier's law) and is seen in 30% of patients with carcinoma of the head of the pancreas. Steatorrhea and severe weight loss may occur with proximal lesions. Cancer located in the pancreas body or tail may cause splenic vein obstruction, portal hypertension, and gastrointestinal bleeding. Otherwise, symptoms are similar no matter what the location of the tumor.

Abdominal pain is persistent, often postprandial and nocturnal, and is located in the upper abdomen. Weight loss is dramatic, progressive, and associated with aversion to food. Pruritus, ascites, hepatosplenomegaly, and constipation are other common features. Diabetes is observed in 50% of patients and may precede or follow other symptoms. Two thirds of patients with cancer of the head of the pancreas have light-colored stools. Physical findings are variable but include jaundice, epigastric tenderness, and the presence of an abdominal mass or palpable gallbladder. Migratory thrombophlebitis and palpable subcutaneous fat nodules with polyarthralgias and prominent epigastric bruits due to compression of splanchnic vessels are unusual but striking manifestations. Pancreatic cancers may be associated with the ectopic production of hormones, resulting in hypoglycemia or hypercalcemia and Cushing's and carcinoid syndromes.

Diagnosis and Staging. Most pancreatic tumors are unresectable when the patient is first seen, explaining the poor survival rate. There is no satisfactory screening test for asymptomatic patients. Many serologic markers have been investigated; the most extensively studied is CA19-9. The marker is nonspecific, but the level correlates with tumor volume; its only use is for observing patients after surgical resection. The available diagnostic techniques include noninvasive tests such as abdominal ultrasound, CT scan (Fig. 366-6), and MRI. Dynamic contrast-enhanced CT scan is more useful than US since it offers useful information on hepatic metastases and shows contiguous organ invasion and/or vascular involvement, predicting resectability. CT scanning has more than 90% sensitivity in the detection of pancreatic carcinoma. Magnetic resonance imaging is not superior to CT scan. ERCP (Fig. 366-7) is falling out of favor for the diagnosis of cancer of the pancreas. However, there is the advantage

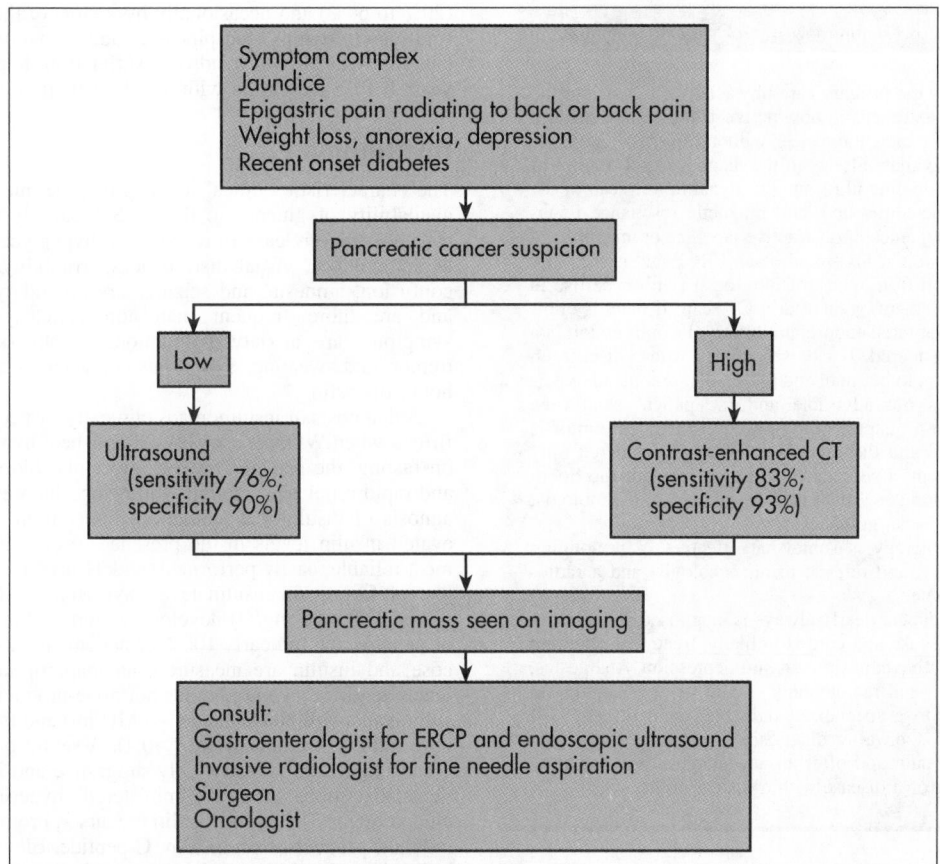

FIGURE 366-7   Algorithm for pancreatic cancer. MRI and EUS may detect small tumors missed by CT scan, although experience is limited. CT scan is recommended by some authors for all patients with suspected pancreatic cancer.

of obtaining pure pancreatic juice for cytologic study. If the tumor is in the head of the pancreas, contiguous involvement of both pancreatic and bile ducts may produce the "double duct" sign, indicating obstruction of both ducts. Otherwise, solitary irregular pancreatic ductal stenosis, abrupt occlusion of the main duct, and pooling of the contrast in irregular pockets indicate cancer. However, all these diagnostic techniques fail to detect tumors less than 2 cm in diameter. EUS is superior to abdominal US or CT scanning in diagnosing tumors less than 2 cm in diameter. The procedure is relatively new, and it may be difficult to differentiate focal chronic pancreatitis from tumors. Percutaneous fine needle biopsy is indicated only for inoperable cases before palliative therapy. The technique may possibly result in spread of tumor and should not be used for the definitive diagnosis of small resectable lesions. Pancreatic function tests are not useful in view of their low sensitivity and specificity.

Differential Diagnosis. Chronic alcoholic pancreatitis is sometimes difficult to distinguish from carcinoma, and accurate diagnosis may require invasive tests or laparotomy. Patients with mesenteric vascular disease (abdominal angina) and rarely those with retroperitoneal lymphomas may also present with abdominal pain and weight loss. In jaundiced patients, cancer must be differentiated from cholestatic liver disease, common bile duct stones, and ampullary or bile duct carcinoma. Pruritus and jaundice occur early in the course of ampullary carcinoma along with anemia and guaiac-positive stools. Endoscopic examination offers an opportunity to biopsy ampullary tumors.

Treatment and Prognosis. Despite many technical advances in the diagnostic and surgical approaches to patients with pancreatic cancer, no significant gains in long-term survival have been achieved. Treatment is palliative in the majority of cases. The Whipple resection (pancreaticoduodenectomy) for periampullary malignancies re-

mains the procedure of choice. A Whipple procedure, although seldom curative for cancer of the pancreas, can cure up to 30% of patients with carcinoma of the ampulla of Vater or the distal common bile duct. Palliative surgery for jaundice and gastric outlet obstruction is effective and indicated for those with a life expectancy of several months. Biliary decompression can be achieved less invasively either by percutaneous transhepatic drainage or endoscopically. The endoscopic approach in placing a biliary stent is preferable, since it avoids an external drainage tube and offers the same result as the percutaneous approach. Technical difficulties might preclude the procedure in some patients. Chemotherapy as a single modality plays only a palliative role. Combined chemotherapy (5-fluorouracil) and high-dose radiation therapy may help relieve pain but does not alleviate biliary or intestinal obstruction. Other chemotherapeutic agents of some use include mitomycin-C, anthracyclines (doxorubicin, epirubicin), ifosfamide, and nitrosoureas. Several combinations of single agents have been tried, and the two most widely used regimens have been 5FU, doxyrubicin, and mitomycin C (FAM) and streptozoticin, mitomycin, and 5FU (SMF).

Radiotherapy along with 5FU or SMF improves survival compared with radiation therapy or chemotherapy alone. The metabolic complications of diabetes and malabsorption, whether caused by malabsorption or by surgical resection, can be effectively managed with insulin and pancreatic enzyme supplementation. The most exciting new agent available for pancreatic cancer is the flourine substituted cytarabine analog gemcitabine. Gemcitabine is of interest not only because it produces partial antitumor responses, but also because it appears to improve quality of life by reducing the requirements for pain medication and maintaining performance status.

The primary care physician has the major role for offering palliative therapy in order to maximize comfort, physical, emotional, and interpersonal functioning. Since pain is one of the foremost symptoms, a systematic and sympathetic approach is required. Analgesics

✔ *WHEN TO REFER*

The difficult task for the primary care physician is to consider the multiple causes for extrahepatic obstructive jaundice and make a clinical diagnosis of pancreatic cancer without much delay. A variety of studies are available today in the diagnosis and staging of pancreatic cancer, including ultrasound or dynamic CT scan of the abdomen, endoscopic ultrasound, and magnetic resonance imaging. A patient with evidence of obstructive jaundice or unexplained epigastric pain and weight loss requires an ERCP and it is proper to seek a consultation from a gastroenterologist (with expertise in ERCP and stent placement) soon after a CT scan. If there is clinical evidence of cholangitis, endoscopic biliary decompression is a procedure to be considered. For those patients whose disease on CT evaluation appears to be small and resectable, preoperative percutaneous biopsy is not advisable and the patient should be promptly referred to an experienced surgeon. But if the tumor is deemed unresectable and the candidate is being considered only for palliative treatment, a percutaneous biopsy is needed to document the diagnosis and the patient is to be referred to a radiologist for biopsy under CT scan guidance.

Adjuvant chemotherapy appears to be somewhat effective in prolonging survival after surgery, and referral to an oncologist and a radiotherapist is appropriate.

Since pancreatic cancer nearly always is diagnosed at relatively late stages of the disease and cure is unlikely, treatment planning should include palliative care for pain and depression. Analgesics, celiac plexus blocks, and radiotherapy should be considered, and appropriate referral to a specialized pain management center, if available, is needed soon after diagnosis. The aim is to provide significant relief of pain and offer an acceptable level of quality of life in the setting of a disease with a dismal prognosis.

(nonopioid and opioid) are to be administered on a regular basis. Opioid analgesics are the central component to pain management. Patients should be placed on around-the-clock maintenance doses of medications. External beam radiation therapy and celiac plexus block may be needed in addition.

When it is clear that nothing can be done to influence the course of the disease, hospice care should be considered. Hospice services focus on comfort care, pain control, and emotional support for the patient and family.

ENDOCRINE TUMORS OF THE PANCREAS

Pancreatic endocrine tumors are exceedingly rare. These tumors share the property of staining for a variety of peptide hormones by immunocytochemistry and can be classified as functional or nonfunctional. Functional tumors produce distinct hormones and clinical syndromes; this category includes insulinoma, gastrinoma (Zollinger-Ellison syndrome), glucagonoma, VIPoma, GRFoma, and somatostatinoma. Some of these tumors may produce more than one hormone, causing a confusing clinical picture. Pancreatic polypeptide secreting tumor (PPoma) is a nonfunctioning tumor. The majority of nonfunctioning tumors occur sporadically in the fourth or fifth decade of life.

The major clinical features of some of these tumors are shown in Table 366-3. The overall prevalence of functional pancreatic tumors is approximately ten per million population, although autopsy materials show a much higher prevalence.

The origin of these tumors is not clear, but it was originally proposed that they were part of the diffuse neuroendocrine system. The islet cells belong to a family of endocrine and neuronal cells that constitute the so-called APUD (amine precursor uptake and decarboxylation) system, sharing certain cytochemical properties.

Pancreatic endocrine tumors may occur with an autosomal dominant inheritance as part of the multiple endocrine neoplasia type I (MEN-1) syndrome. These tumors are often multiple, have no sex preference, present in early adulthood, and manifest with other endocrinopathies. The MEN-1 syndrome is mostly characterized by parathyroid hyperplasia (in more than 90% of cases) and pituitary tumors

(20% to 60%) and occasionally by tumors of the adrenal cortex, thyroid gland, thymus, and pineal gland. An overwhelming majority of patients with MEN-1 syndrome suffer from hyperparathyroidism for years before presenting with a pancreatic tumor.

Insulinoma

The characteristic clinical features may be due to either insufficient availability of glucose to the CNS (neuroglycopenia) or excessive catecholamine release in response to hypoglycemia. Symptoms such as somnolence, visual disturbances, irritability, abnormal behavior, confusion, amnesia, and seizures are secondary to neuroglycopenia and are more frequent than adrenergic symptoms. Adrenergic symptoms are anxiety, palpitations, weakness, fatigue, headache, tremor, and sweating. Symptoms characteristically occur after many hours of fasting.

A diagnosis of insulinoma is clinically suspected although not confirmed when Whipple's triad is established: hypoglycemic symptoms on fasting, the presence of hypoglycemia (blood sugar <50 gm/dl), and rapid relief of symptoms following glucose ingestion. A firm diagnosis of insulinoma requires demonstration of inappropriately elevated insulin levels in the presence of clinical hypoglycemia. The most reliable, easily performed, widely used test is to observe the effect of fasting on insulin level. Symptomatic hypoglycemia (blood glucose of <50 mg/dl) develops within 24 hours of fasting in 75% of patients and in nearly 100% of patients in 72 hours. Levels of glucose and insulin are measured; an inappropriately elevated insulin level identifies an autonomous hormone-producing tumor. Plasma insulin levels will be elevated (>5 MU/ml) and the plasma insulin/glucose ratio will be abnormal (>0.4). A serum proinsulin/insulin ratio greater than 0.25 is also highly suggestive and is seen in 90% of patients. Factitious or "self administered" hyperinsulinism can be excluded by measuring the insulin precursor, proinsulin, and/or the degradation product of proinsulin, C-peptide. Elevation of either one is indicative of endogenous hyperinsulinism.

Provocative tests using tolbutamide, glucagon, amino acid arginine, and leucine are currently not advocated and are even considered dangerous.

CT scan is useful in localizing the site of the tumor. The recently introduced indium-labeled octreotide scan appears to be useful in defining occult insulinomas with somatostatin receptors (about 60%). Selective arteriography with or without digital substraction is a sensitive method. Percutaneous transhepatic portal venous sampling of hormone concentrations helps to localize the site(s) of hormone production. Intraoperative and endoscopic ultrasonography have the highest sensitivity in the diagnosis of this and other pancreatic tumors. Experience with MRI for the detection of insulinomas is limited, but MRI with dynamic gadolinium enhancement and fat suppression is reported to be a promising tool. Diazoxide suppresses insulin release, and an oral dose of 100 to 150 mg every 8 hours is effective in keeping the blood glucose at normal levels.

Administration of a long-acting somatostatin analog (Octreotide) has been successful in the treatment of insulinomas. Octreotide reduces plasma concentrations of many circulating peptides. By decreasing plasma concentrations of multiple peptide hormones (including insulin, gastrin, and glucagon), this agent may provide symptomatic relief. Surgery is the treatment of choice.

Gastrinoma

The pathophysiology, chemical features, and treatment of gastrinoma are discussed in detail in Chapter 336.

Glucagonoma

Glucagonomas usually occur in middle age or in the elderly. The typical features of glucagonoma syndrome include a specific form of dermatitis (necrolytic migratory erythema) that starts in the groin and migrates to the thighs, buttocks, perineum, and distal extremities. The initial erythematous areas later become raised, with vesicopustules and bullae. The blisters rupture, forming crusts, followed by healing with hyperpigmentation. Hypoaminoacidemia (alamine, glycine, and serine), glucose intolerance, weight loss, and anemia are important

Table 366-3   Neuroendocrine tumors of the pancreas

	INSULINOMA	GASTRINOMA	VIPOMA	GLUCAGONOMA	SOMATOSTATINOMA
Hormone	Insulin	Gastrin	VIP	Glucagon	Somatostatin
Size	Small	Small, solitary	Large	Large	Large
Malignant potential	Small (10%)	High (60%-80%)	High (60%-90%)	High (60%-90%)	High (60%-90%)

Clinical presentation	Neuroglycopenia:
	  Headache, lightheadedness, confusion, irrational behavior
	Hypoglycemic symptoms:
	  Tremor, sweating, palpitation, hyperphagia (catecholamine excess)
		Abdominal pain (peptic ulcer disease)
		Gastroesophageal reflux disease
		Diarrhea
			Large volume, watery diarrhea (secretory); stool isotonic; persists on fasting
			Hypokalemia
			Achlorhydria
				Migratory necrolytic erythema
				Glucose intolerance
				Weight loss
				Anemia
				Glossitis
					Diabetes (mild)
					Gallbladder disease
					Weight loss
					Diarrhea
					Steatorrhea
					Hypochlorhydria

Tumor location	>95% head, body, tail	<50% head	>90% tail	100% body, tail	50% head

✔ *WHEN TO REFER*

Islet cell tumors are extremely rare, and the diagnosis is seldom suspected early in the natural history of the clinical syndromes when the symptoms are not typical and mimic other disorders. However, because of their secretory products, these tumors produce characteristic pathophysiologic disturbances that become obvious at least some years after the onset of the syndrome. A common approach to all these neuroendocrine tumors is to establish the diagnosis, search for MEN-I syndrome, control the symptoms, localize the tumor, and finally, decide whether surgical therapy is appropriate. With the exception of those with advanced metastatic disease or MEN-I syndrome, an aggressive surgical approach is indicated for all patients. The primary care physician's major role is limited to providing symptomatic treatment, performing imaging studies, instituting nutritional support, and preventing complication. Diazoxide for insulinoma, and octreotide for glucagonoma and VIPoma are effective in controlling the metabolic consequences and symptoms of hormonal excess. Insulinoma being the most common islet cell tumor, the primary care physician should suspect the syndrome in the presence of neuroglycopenic symptoms (episodes of lightheadedness, confusion, visual disturbances, irrational behavior, seizures, and coma) and other adrenergic symptoms due to hypoglycemia. An endocrinologist's help in further evaluation is required, to chart out appropriate metabolic and diagnostic imaging studies. Other endocrine tumors of the islets occur less frequently and are most often identified on routine imaging studies, which leads to appropriate consultations. Most of these tumors, in view of their infrequency, are better referred to special centers with expertise for definitive management.

clinical manifestations. Depression, altered bowel habits, and life-threatening venous thrombosis are other features.

The diagnosis is suspected because of the characteristic skin rash or a pancreatic mass detected on CT scan in a patient with weight loss and diabetes. The diagnosis is confirmed by demonstrating serum glucagon levels above 1000 pg/ml (normal is <150 pg/ml). Serum glucagon level is moderately elevated (<500 pg/ml) in a number of conditions including renal failure hepatic failure, diabetic ketoacidosis, acromegaly, severe burns, and acute pancreatitis. However, these conditions do not cause confusion in the diagnosis of glucagonoma.

Tumor localization is fairly easy with most imaging techniques because most tumors are large (5 to 10 cm). CT scan, ultrasonography, and selective angiography confirm the diagnosis.

The principles of management are control of the symptoms, correction of hyperglycemia, and restoration of nutritional status while surgical therapy is being contemplated. Octreotide treatment (100 to 400 mg/day) improves symptoms of weight loss, abdominal pain, and diarrhea. Correction of anemia may require blood transfusions. Par-

enteral nutrition assists in restoring nutritional status and in healing the dermatitis. Nearly two thirds of patients have liver metastases at the time of diagnosis and are not candidates for surgery. Debulking of the tumor may offer benefit to some patients. Chemotherpy with various agents, including streptozotocin, 5-fluorouracil, and doxorubicin given in combination is suggested for patients with widely metastatic disease.

VIPoma

Patients with VIPoma (watery diarrhea–hypokalemia-achlorhydria [WDHA] syndrome) have large volume (70% of patients having more than 3 L of stool per day) secretory diarrhea, which causes hypokalemia, dehydration, and acidosis. The syndrome (also called Verner-Morrison syndrome) results from autonomous, unregulated secretion by a neuroendocrine tumor. The stool output does not decrease on fasting, and there is no osmotic gap in the stool. Other rare clinical features include a characteristic erythematous rash, weight loss, flushing (20%), hypercalcemia (without hyperparathyroidism), and non–anion gap acidosis. Profound hypokalemia (<2.5 mmol/L) is a frequent manifestation. Hypochorhydria is probably due to an inhibitory action on gastric acid secretion.

The diagnosis is established by demonstration of secretory diarrhea (stool osmolar gap 290 mOsm − 2 × (Na$^+$ + K$^+$) = <50), elevated VIP levels (normal levels are <170 pg/ml). Diagnosis is often made on surgical exploration after other causes of chronic secretory diarrhea, especially laxative and diuretic abuse, have been excluded. The principles of management include replenishment of fluid and electrolytes to correct dehydration, hypokalemia, and acidosis. A number of drugs are reported to control diarrhea, including prednisone, clonidine, indomethacin, phenothiazine, and lithium. Currently, Octreotide is the therapeutic agent of choice to control diarrhea. The dosage varies; some patients respond to a low dose of 50 to 100 mg three times a day and others need up to 1200 mg/day. Long-term treatment with octreotide may be needed in those with unresectable or metastatic VIPomas.

GRFoma

GRFoma is a rare cause of acromegaly, indistinguishable from that caused by pituitary adenoma. Growth hormone–releasing factor from the pancreatic adenoma stimulates the production of growth hormone from the pituitary. The clinical suspicion is aroused when a patient known to have a neuroendocrine tumor develops acromegaly. Increased plasma levels of GRF greater than 300 pg/ml confirm the diagnosis.

Somatostatinoma

Mild diabetes mellitus, gallbladder disease, weight loss, diarrhea, steatorrhea, and hypochlorhydria are the clinical features. The diagnosis is made by CT scan of abdomen, demonstration of elevated somatostatin level, and by immunohistochemistry of pancreatic tissue.

Nearly 50% of patients have other endocrinopathies, including MEN-I and MEN-II.

Somatostatinoma is often a diagnosed by accident in patients with large pancreatic tumors detected by imaging studies. Elevated somatostatin levels are late to manifest. The diagnosis is established by immunochemical identification of the resected tumor showing an increased number of D cells. Octreotide is contraindicated since the product of the tumor is somatostatin.

CYSTIC FIBROSIS

Cystic fibrosis (CF), an inborn error of metabolism, is the most common lethal genetic disease in the caucasian population of North America, Europe, and Australia, affecting between 1 in 2000 and 1 in 3000 live births. In the African-American population the prevalence is estimated to be exceedingly rare (about 1/17,000). This autosomal recessive disease affects males and females equally, and monozygotic twins have 100% concordance. It has been recently discovered that CF is caused by mutations of the cystic fibrosis transmembrane regulator (CFTR) gene, which is expressed in most epithelial cells. This gene is located on the long arm of chromosome 7, which encodes a protein of 1480 aminoacids. The discovery of CFTR gene, along with its role in the regulation of transmembrane channel chloride transport by cyclic AMP, has profoundly advanced our understanding of the pathophysiology of the disease, ion transport in secretory epithelia, and more importantly has established the feasibility of gene therapy for this disease. As many as 60% of patients with CF can expect to survive into adulthood and many into their thirties.

Current understanding of the pathophysiology of this multisystem disease indicates that epithelial cells from CF patients have reduced Cl-permeability, which impairs fluid and electrolyte secretion, resulting in luminal dehydration. Increased viscosity of exocrine secretions and increased electrolyte concentration in sweat and saliva are characteristic of CF. Abnormalities in exocrine secretion occur not only in sweat ducts but also in pancreatic, intestinal, and airway epithelia. Protein hyperconcentration in mucus increases viscosity and causes inspissation of secretions. Eosinophilic concretions are formed, which block the secretion from pancreatic acinar cells, intestinal glands, intrahepatic bile ducts, and the prostate. The disease thus affects the lungs, sinuses, pancreas, gastrointestinal tract, hepatobiliary system, sweat glands, and reproductive tract. Recurrent pulmonary infections and the eventual development of chronic pulmonary disease account for much of the morbidity. The airways become chronically colonized with antibiotic-resistant bacteria. Bronchitis, bronchiectasis, and fibrosis are the result. The majority of patients die of pulmonary disease.

Gastrointestinal manifestations of the disease occur in more than 80% of patients at the time of diagnosis. The earliest manifestation is meconium ileus that occurs in 15% of infants within 1 to 2 days after birth. Signs and symptoms of intestinal obstruction occur. Impaction of the small bowel is caused by inspissated meconium as a result of reduced water content.

Manifestations of exocrine pancreatic insufficiency become apparent by the age of 2 years, and nearly 90% of patients present with exocrine pancreatic insufficiency, which is essentially because of blockage of ductules by precipitated pancreatic secretions. Acinar disruption and autodigestion of the pancreas follow. A profound reduction in pancreatic bicarbonate secretion is a functional abnormality. Abnormalities of the pancreatic duct include dilation, strictures, and intraductal radiolucent and radiopaque calculi.

Failure to gain weight despite excellent appetite, as well as watery, bulky, greasy stools, become evident very early as a result of exocrine insufficiency. Steatorrhea leads to deficiencies of fat-soluble vitamins and hemorrhagic complications from vitamin K deficiency. Protein malabsorption leads to hypoproteinemia and edema. Recurrent acute pancreatitis is a rare manifestation. As the life expectancy of CF patients has improved, patients are noted to have an increased incidence of diabetes as a result of insulinopenia.

Rectal prolapse occurs in nearly 20% of children with CF. Older children may develop intestinal obstruction due to a poorly digested inspissated bolus of food material ("meconium ileus equivalent"). Liver diseasae is a complication in nearly 5% of patients and is caused by viscous, inspissated bile that interferes with bile flow. Neonatal

jaundice, fatty liver, cholestasis, sclerosing cholangitis, cirrhosis, portal hypertension, and gallstone disease are the consequences.

Diagnosis of CF is suspected in children with pancreatic insufficiency. A carefully performed quantitative electrolyte analysis of sweat collected using pilocarpine iontophoresis confirms the diagnosis. A sweat sodium or chloride level higher than 60 mmol/L is positive for CF (sensitivity 98% to 99%). Ultrasound of the pancreas is nonspecific but shows an irregularly enlarged pancreatic gland.

Management of cystic fibrosis is complex, and a multidisciplinary approach is needed. The quality in life of CF patients is determined by socioeconomic, nutritional, and environmental factors as well as the ready availability of adequate medical care. Treatment of psychosocial aspects is important. Besides prevention and treatment of respiratory infections, the most important aspect is appropriate nutritional support. In addition to maldigestion and malabsorption, the increased demand made by chronic respiratory infections creates a need for calorie intake of up to 130% to 150% of the recommended dietary allowance (RDA). Dietary fats should not be restricted in patients with CF, and fats should provide 40% to 50% of daily energy needs. Pancreatic enzyme supplementation is the mainstay of treatment, and enteric coated microspheres are more effective than enteric-coated tablets. Adjuvant therapy with H_2 receptor antagonists or a proton-pump inhibitor may be useful. Glucose polymers (Polycose) and medium-chain triglycerides (MCTs) are recommended to improve calorie intake. Fat-soluble vitamin supplementation is required to correct nutritional deficiencies. Providing vegetable oils in the diet prevents deficiency of essential fatty acids.

A disturbing side effect of consuming pancreatic enzyme supplements in large doses as needed in the management of CF is "fibrosing colonopathy," which causes strictures in the colon.

Ursodeoxycholic acid (UCDA) has shown beneficial effects in the treatment of cholestatic liver disease in CF.

An important development in the understanding of CF is the detection of CFTR, which has opened up the potential for gene therapy.

CONGENITAL ANOMALIES

Ectopic endocrine and/or exocrine pancreatic tissue is a common developmental anomaly that is rarely of clinical significance. The gastric antrum and proximal duodenum are the usual sites affected, but ectopia may also occur in the remainder of the small bowel, Meckel's diverticula, bile ducts, gallbladder, and the splenic hilum.

Annular pancreas results from an incomplete embryologic migration of the ventral pancreas, which instead encircles the second portion of the duodenum. Duodenal obstruction in the neonate is the usual presenting feature, but bile duct obstruction, pancreatitis, and duodenal ulcer may also occur. A smooth, symmetric constriction of the postbulbar duodenum with proximal dilation is the characteristic radiologic feature, and surgical bypass is the treatment of choice. Preoperative confirmation is possible with endoscopic pancreatography.

Pancreas divisum results when the ventral and dorsal portions of the pancreatic ductal system fail to fuse. Drainage of pancreatic secretions into the duodenum then occurs primarily through the accessory papilla. This very common congenital defect (3% to 7% of the population) is discovered more often in patients undergoing endoscopic retrograde cholangiopancreatography for documented attacks of acute pancreatitis than in those subjects having the test performed for evaluation of biliary disease or chronic unexplained abdominal pain. Stenosis of the minor duct or accessory papilla is the proposed pathogenetic mechanism. Surgical transduodenal sphincteroplasty or endoscopic sphincterotomy of the accessory papilla is variably successful in preventing recurrent attacks of pancreatitis and should probably by considered only when other potential causes have been excluded and when radiologic evidence of minor duct dilation is observed. In the occasional patient with irreversible chronic pancreatitis and pancreas divisum, sphincteroplasty has not been beneficial.

PANCREATIC TRAUMA

Traumatic injuries of the pancreas can occur after blunt or penetrating trauma or as a consequence of surgery. Penetrating abdominal wounds (e.g., gunshot and stab wounds) may lead to early lacerations, contusions, or hematomas of the gland or to the late complication of abscess, pseudocyst, or fistula. Associated major vascular and

✔ *WHEN TO REFER*

Cystic fibrosis is predominantly a disease of the pediatric population. However, some patients escape an early diagnosis because of atypical presentations or milder forms of the disease and grow to adolescence. Although the sweat electrolyte test is diagnostic, ideally the test should be performed in centers with experience. It is recommended that those with suspected or diagnosed CF be referred to one of the regional cystic fibrosis centers with diagnostic and therapeutic expertise. Patients with psychosocial problems, nutritional deficiencies, pancreatic insufficiency, or respiratory infections may need consultations with appropriate specialists. However, the primary care physician maintains a pivotal role in the management of the patient.

---

visceral injuries are common and result in 20% mortality for pancreatic trauma. Elevated amylase levels in serum or paracentesis fluid are diagnostic, and early surgery with external drainage or pancreatic resection is usually required. Blunt abdominal trauma less commonly results in pancreatic damage, but steering-wheel compression injuries are responsible for the uncommon entity of pancreatic transsection. When it occurs, postoperative acute pancreatitis usually follows biliary or gastric surgery; it is difficult to diagnose and results in a high mortality rate.

BIBLIOGRAPHY

N, Pitchumoni CS: Acute pancreatitis: a multisystem disease, *Gastroenterologist* 1:115-128, 1993.

Ahlgren JD: Epidemiology and risk factors in pancreatic cancer, *Semin Oncol* 23:241-250, 1996.

Ammann RW, Heitz PU, Kloppel G: Course of alcoholic chronic pancreatitis: a prospective clinicomorphological long-term study, *Gastroenterology* 111:224-231, 1996.

Banks P: Practice guidelines in acute pancreatitis, *Am J Gastroenterol* 92:377-386, 1997.

Balthazar EJ, Freeny PC, VanSonnenberg E: Imaging and intervention in acute pancreatitis, *Radiology* 193:297-306, 1994.

Bradley EL III: A clinically based classification system for acute pancreatitis, *Arch Surg* 128:586-590, 1993.

Folisch UR, Nitsche R, Ludtke R et al: Early ERCP and papillotomy compared with conservative treatment for acute biliary pancreatitis, *N Engl J Med* 336:237-242, 1997.

Go VLW, Everhart JE: Pancreatitis. In Everhart JE: Digestive diseases in the United States: epidemiology and impact, NIH pub. no. 94-1447, 1994, U.S. Department of Health and Human Services, National Institutes of Health, pp. 693-712.

Howard TJ, Wielske EA, Mogovero G et al: Classification and treatment of local septic complications of acute pancreatitis, *Am J Surg* 170:44-50, 1995.

Layer P, Yamamoto H, Kalthoff L et al: The different courses of early and late onset of idiopathic and alcoholic chronic pancreatitis, *Gastroenterology* 107:1481-1487, 1994.

Lee SP et al: Biliary sludge as a cause of acute pancreatitis, *N Engl J Med* 326:589, 1992.

Lerch M, Saluya A, Runzi M et al: Luminal endocytosis and intracellular targeting of acinar cells during early biliary pancreatitis, *J Clin Invest* 95:2222-2231, 1995.

Metz C, Jensen RT: Endocrine tumors of the pancreas. In Haurich WB, Berk JE, editors: *Bockus gastroenterology*, ed 5, Philadelphia, 1995, WB Saunders, pp. 3002-3034.

Schnall SF, MacDonald JS: Chemotherapy of adenocarcinoma of the pancreas, *Semin Oncol* 23:220-228, 1996.

Steer M, Waxman I, Freedman S: Chronic pancreatitis, *N Engl J Med* 332:1482-1490, 1995.

Steinberg W, Tenner S: Acute pancreatitis, *N Engl J Med* 330:1198-1210, 1995.

Taylor WF, Everhart JE: Pancreatic cancer. In Everhart JE: Digestive diseases in the United States: epidemiology and impact, NIH pub. no. 94-1447, U.S. Department of Health and Human Services, National Institutes of Health, 1994, pp. 249-270.

Tizzano EF, Buchwald M: Expression and organ damage in cystic fibrosis, *Ann Intern Med* 123:305-308, 1995.

Toskes PP: Medical management of chronic pancreatitis, *Scand J Gastroenterol* 208:74-80, 1995.

367 Diseases of the Peritoneum, Mesentery, and Omentum

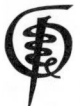

James M. McGill

INTRODUCTION

Diseases of the peritoneum are obscure and generally present with vague abdominal symptoms. These illnesses are often smoldering but at times are precipitous and life threatening. Because of the absence of a unique constellation of symptoms and discrete areas of the abdomen that are affected, peritoneal disorders are frequently "stumbled upon" rather than specifically sought after. An aid in the diagnosis of peritoneal disorders is to consider them in the differential diagnosis for numerous abdominal symptoms.

The peritoneum is a single-layered cellular membrane that lines the peritoneal cavity and forms two discrete layers: the visceral peritoneum and the parietal peritoneum. The visceral peritoneum covers the intraperitoneal organs (stomach, jejunum, transverse colon, liver, and spleen) and the anterior aspect of retroperitoneal organs (duodenum, right and left colon, pancreas, kidneys, and adrenal glands). The parietal peritoneum covers the peritoneal cavity, including the pelvis and inferior surface of the diaphragm. In males the parietal peritoneum is a sealed space, but in females it is open to the external environment via the fallopian tubes. In general, the peritoneum functions as a membrane for bidirectional diffusion of water and solutes and provides a lubricated surface over which the intraabdominal organs easily glide within the abdominal space.

The blood supply to the peritoneum is mainly through the splanchnic blood vessels, with a small contribution from the intercostal, lumbar, and iliac arteries. Important clinical differences exist regarding afferent nervous innervation of the peritoneal surfaces. Transmitted through the autonomic nervous system, noxious stimulation of the visceral peritoneum is perceived as diffuse, dull pain. In contrast, noxious stimulation of the parietal peritoneum, innervated by both visceral and somatic nerves, results in sharp, localized pain, often with rebound tenderness.

The mesentery is formed by the confluence of the peritoneal layers and serves to attach organs to the posterior portion of the abdominal wall. Important elements of the mesentery are sandwiched between these layers and include blood vessels, lymphatics, and lymph nodes.

Like the mesentery, the omentum is a specialized layering of peritoneum. In contrast to the posterior position of the mesentery, the omentum is an anterior structure that joins the stomach inferiorly to the transverse colon and laterally to the liver. Like the mesentery, the omentum holds a large number of blood vessels and lymphatics and appears to be a reservoir for infection-fighting macrophages.

Diseases originating in these tissues are uncommon; most often these peritoneal structures are "innocent bystanders." Frequently, peritoneal innervation serves as a sentinel for injury or inflammation in a surrounding organ. Occasionally disease originating from the peritoneal structures develops and is mistaken for that of an adjacent organ with a better appreciated clinical presentation (e.g., appendix, gallbladder). Perhaps the most important concept is that one must think about peritoneal disorders in the differential diagnosis of abdominal symptoms. The commonest signs and symptoms of peritoneal, mesenteric, and omental diseases are similar to those of other abdominal disorders, and they are summarized for the more common processes in Table 367-1.

DISEASES OF THE PERITONEUM
Infectious Peritonitis

Bacteria, fungi, and parasites have all been identified as causes for peritonitis. Pathogens enter the peritoneal space transmurally (bowel infection, not requiring perforation), through direct extension (fallopian tube, peritoneal catheter), or through the vascular or lymphatic

Table 367-1   Common signs and symptoms of peritoneal, mesenteric, and omental diseases

DISEASE	ABDOMINAL PAIN	ASCITES	FEVER	NAUSEA/ VOMITING	WEIGHT LOSS	MASS EFFECT	DIARRHEA	IRON DEFICIENCY	URETERAL OBSTRUCTION
Infectious peritonitis	+	+	+	+	−	−	±	−	−
Neoplasms	±	±	±	±	+	−	−	±	−
Cysts	+	−	−	±	−	+	−	−	−
Bleeding	+	−	±	+	−	±	±	−	−
Castleman's disease	±	−	−	−	±	+	−	+	−
Retractile mesenteritis	+	±	−	+	±	+	±	−	−
Mesenteric panniculitis	+	−	±	+	±	+	−	−	−
Retroperitoneal fibrosis	+	−	−	±	±	−	−	−	+
Adhesions/internal hernias	+	−	−	±	−	−	−	−	−
Abscess	+	±	+	±	±	±	±	−	−
Pseudomyxoma peritonei	±	−	−	−	±	+	−	−	−
Bile/duodenal/pancreatic/ lymph fluid or urine collection	+	−	±	±	−	−	±	−	−
Omental torsion	+	−	±	+	−	+	±	−	−
Recurrent polyserositis	+	−	+	±	±	−	−	−	−

+, Typically present; −, typically absent; ±, presence or absence is not characteristic.

systems. In clinical practice, infectious peritonitis is typically found in the following circumstances:

- Primary or spontaneous bacterial peritonitis (SBP)
- Secondary bacterial peritonitis
- Continuous ambulatory peritoneal dialysis–related peritonitis
- Sexually transmitted disease–related peritonitis (Fitz-Hugh-Curtis syndrome)
- Peritonitis in immunocompromised patients

In general, patients with any form of infectious peritonitis present with similar complaints of abdominal pain, distention, and fever. One surmises the probable cause based on the patient's history.

Spontaneous or Primary Bacterial Peritonitis

Spontaneous bacterial peritonitis occurs in patients with ascites caused by cirrhosis of the liver or nephrotic syndrome. It may also occur in patients with systemic lupus erythematosus receiving corticosteroids (see Chapter 357 for detailed discussion).

The clinical features, differential diagnosis, and approach to patients in acute (secondary) bacterial peritonitis are described in Chapters 335 and 342.

Continuous Ambulatory Peritoneal Dialysis-Related Peritonitis

Continuous ambulatory peritoneal dialysis (CAPD) is an increasingly common method of dialysis in patients with end-stage renal disease. The most common complication of this dialysis method is peritonitis. Although noninfectious causes can occur (e.g., foreign-body reaction to the catheter), infectious causes are far more common. Characteristically, a single organism (usually a gram-positive coccus) is identified, which most commonly infects through direct extension via the dialysis catheter. This may occur either by unsterile handling of the catheter or through dialysis solutions. Other methods of contamination are possible but less likely. Fungal infections have also been reported (most commonly, *Candida* infection). The presence of anaerobic or mixed flora suggests possible secondary peritonitis. Antimicrobial drugs, remedial instruction regarding sterile technique, and occasionally removal of the catheter with conversion to hemodialysis are treatment options.

Sexually Transmitted Disease–Related Peritonitis (Fitz-Hugh-Curtis Syndrome)

These disorders, predominantly seen in young women, result from intraperitoneal infection by either *Neisseria gonorrhoeae* or *Chlamydia trachomatis*. The patient typically complains of severe abdominal pain and fever. Peritoneal signs, often localized to the right upper quadrant, are found on examination. These symptoms, along with mi-

nor abnormalities in liver tests, raise suspicions of acute cholecystitis. Although noninvasive testing has not been found to be definitive for this disorder, ultrasound and computed tomography (CT) findings have been reported. The presence of normal biliary imaging along with the presence of adnexal tenderness and demonstration of gonococci (Gram stain) or chlamydia (immunoassay or DNA hybridization assay) and a positive culture of cervical mucus help to focus on perihepatitis as the diagnosis. In advanced stages of peritonitis, laparoscopy reveals perihepatitis with classic "violin string" adhesions between the parietal peritoneum and anterior surface of the liver. Therapeutic benefit may result if these adhesions are transected during laparoscopic examination. Appropriate antimicrobial therapy can lead to rapid resolution of symptoms.

Peritonitis in Immunocompromised Patients

Although tuberculosis, fungi, and parasites can infect the peritoneum in immunocompetent hosts (see CAPD-related peritonitis), in the United States the majority of patients are immunocompromised. Tuberculous peritonitis typically results from hematogenous or lymphangitic spread from another body site. (See Chapters 342 and 273.)

Fungal peritonitis can occur as a complication of bowel perforation and CAPD and is usually caused by *Candida albicans*. *Torulopsis glabrata*, *Histoplasma capsulatum*, *Coccidioides immitis*, and *Cryptococcus neoformans* may rarely cause peritonitis. Parasitic infestation is uncommon but may result from peritoneal infection with *Schistosoma mansoni*, *Enterobius vermicularis*, and *Ascaris lumbricoides*. *Strongyloides stercoralis* and *Entamoeba histolytica* can cause more fulminant peritonitis. Treatment is geared toward eradication of the causative organism.

Other Forms of Peritonitis

Granulomatous Peritonitis. Granulomatous peritonitis is a mixed group of infectious and noninfectious causes of peritonitis that results in granuloma formation. In addition to mycobacterial, fungal, and parasitic infections, a variety of noninfectious disorders can evoke a granulomatous inflammatory response in the peritoneum. These disorders include Crohn's disease, sarcoidosis, *C. immitis* infection, ruptured cystic teratomas, and adenocarcinomas. Lubricants from surgical gloves (e.g., cornstarch, talc) or cellulose fibers from surgical supplies may also initiate granulomatous peritonitis.

Aseptic (Chemical) Peritonitis. Chemical peritonitis usually develops as a complication of surgery or trauma resulting in a leak of bile, urine, or chyle. Initially, these episodes are sterile, but their presence promotes the growth of bacteria, resulting in septic peritonitis. Bile peritonitis is the most common cause. Bile peritonitis following rupture of an inflamed gallbladder, leakage around T-tubes,

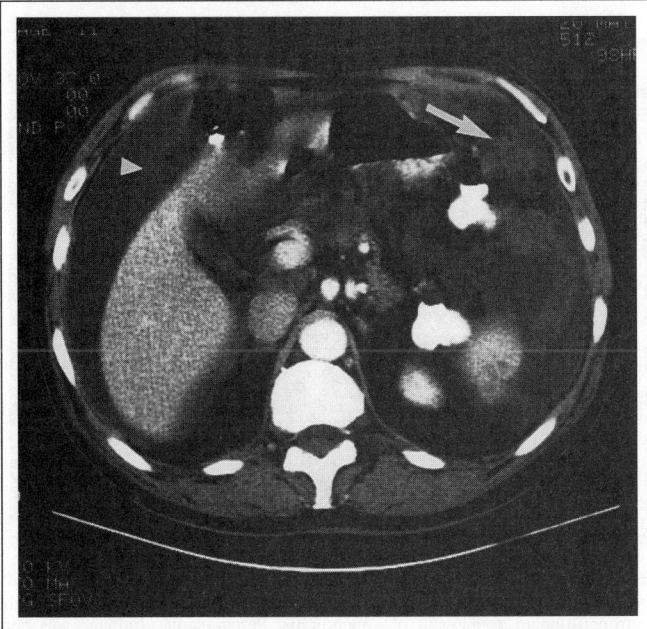

FIGURE 367-1 Peritoneal metastases. There is marked omental thickening in the left upper quadrant *(arrow)* and ascites *(arrow heads)* in this 68-year-old male patient with peritoneal metastatic disease from an unknown primary adenocarcinoma.

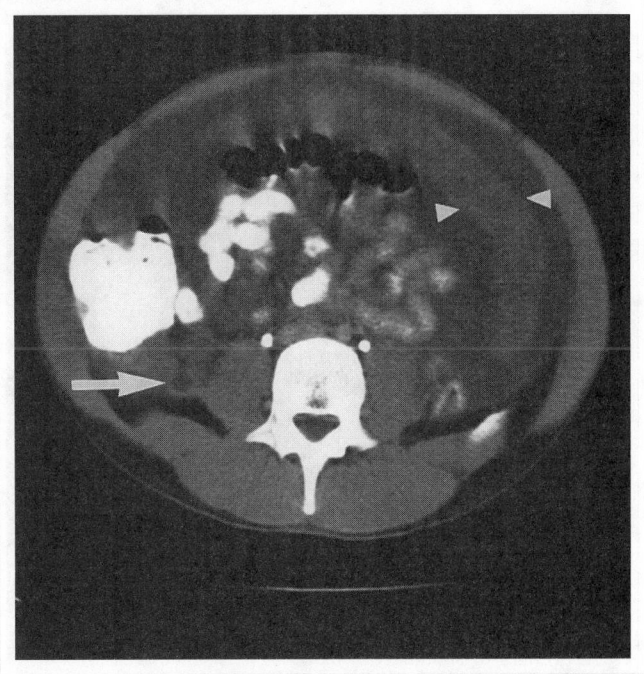

FIGURE 367-2 Pseudomyxoma peritonei. High-density gelatinous ascites and omental thickening *(arrow heads)* are present in this 38-year-old man who presented with abdominal distention. The cause of the pseudomyxoma peritonei is the low-density mucocele in the appendix *(arrow).*

and other procedural mishaps including percutaneous needle biopsy of the liver, is heralded by the rapid development of usually intense abdominal pain and often results in shock. Leakage of uninfected bile, as may occur consequent to abdominal trauma, often produces slowly progressive ascites with minimal abdominal pain. Depending on the situation, diagnosis is typically made by serial testing, first with hepatobiliary scintigraphy, which if positive is followed up with endoscopic retrograde cholangiography. The treatment of bile peritonitis consists of appropriate fluid and electrolyte replacement, broad-spectrum antibiotic therapy, and urgent gastroenterology and surgical consultation.

In the setting of gastrointestinal perforation, in addition to body fluids, barium sulfate may spill into the abdominal cavity during diagnostic radiographic evaluation. This is best avoided by using water-soluble contrast in patients suspected of having a perforated viscus.

Inflammatory Peritonitis. Although peritonitis can develop in patients who suffer from collagen vascular diseases (e.g., lupus) where serositis is one of the manifestations of their disease, it is reported to occur very rarely. Treatment is directed at the underlying disorder.

Recurrent polyserositis (familial Mediterranean fever) is an inherited disorder of unknown etiology characterized by recurrent, transient episodes of fever, peritonitis, and either arthritis or pleuritis. Recurrent polyserositis affects primarily persons of southern European and Middle Eastern ancestry. Colchicine has been shown to effectively prevent attacks and reduce complications such as amyloidosis.

Peritoneal Tumors

Metastatic lesions are the most common tumor of the peritoneum and typically present with ascites. Ascitic fluid cytologic examination is the usual means of diagnosis, though typically with low sensitivities. Carcinomas are more common than either lymphomas or sarcomas. Most commonly, adenocarcinomas from ovary, stomach, colon, breast, pancreas, or lung are involved (Fig. 367-1). Modest palliation may be achieved by repeated paracentesis, transperitoneal instillation of chemotherapeutic agents, or peritoneovenous shunting. In general, treatment is usually disappointing

and patient survival is brief. However, patients with malignant ascites resulting from ovarian carcinoma, breast cancer, and lymphoma may have a better prognosis, with appropriate treatment directed at the underlying malignancy.

Pseudomyxoma peritonei is a mucinous tumor affecting the peritoneum that has a natural history significantly different from other metastatic lesions (Fig. 367-2). This rare condition is characterized by the presence of gelatinous viscid material in the peritoneal cavity. The major causes are mucoceles of the appendix and mucinous cystadenocarcinomas of the ovary, pancreas, or appendix. Increasing abdominal girth in a patient who is otherwise well is frequent. An abdomen distended with what appears to be fluid that does not shift may suggest the diagnosis. The correct diagnosis can be readily made at laparoscopy. Removal of the gelatinous material along with the primary tumor and omentum should be attempted at laparotomy; instillation of a chemotherapeutic agent may be beneficial. Surgery may be curative and has a 5-year survival rate of approximately 50%.

Primary Tumors of the Peritoneum

Peritoneal mesothelioma is a rare tumor of the peritoneum associated with occupational exposure to asbestos in about 65% of patients. The development of peritoneal mesotheliomas has also been linked to exposure to thorium dioxide (Thorotrast). Exposure to asbestos need not be of long duration, but often the latent period between exposure and development of the tumor is 30 to 40 years. Approximately 65% of mesotheliomas arise from the pleura, 25% from the peritoneum, and 10% from the pericardium. Men are affected more frequently than women, and the highest prevalence is in the sixth decade. The most frequent initial symptom is abdominal pain. Severe weight loss and ascites (occasionally very viscid) are almost universal features. Many patients have clubbing and respiratory signs associated with asbestosis. Diagnosis is established most often at the time of laparotomy or autopsy. Although the histologic features of peritoneal mesothelioma are quite variable and not necessarily specific, the tumor has distinctive ultrastructural features that are often extremely helpful in making a specific diagnosis. The course is virulent; there is no effective therapy, and most patients die 1 to 2 years after diagnosis.

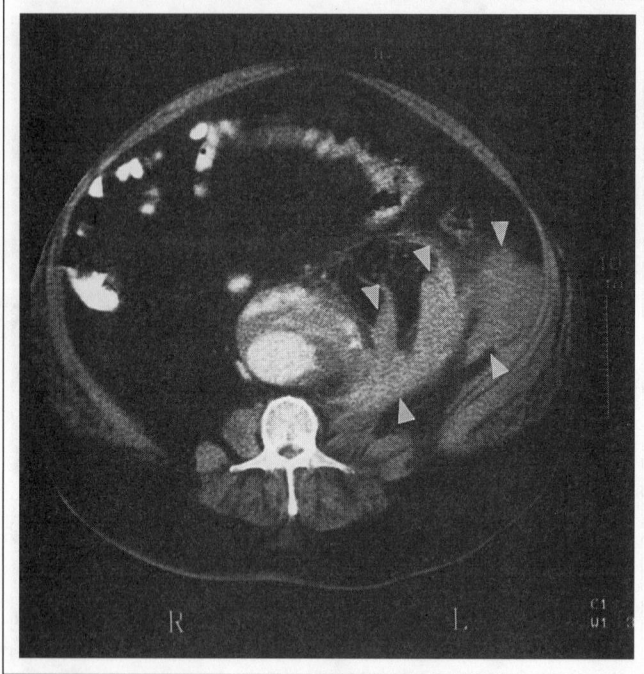

FIGURE 367-3 Retroperitoneal hemorrhage. High-density fluid representing hemorrhage *(arrow heads)* is present in the retroperitoneum and left paracolic gutter from a large, leaking abdominal aortic aneurysm.

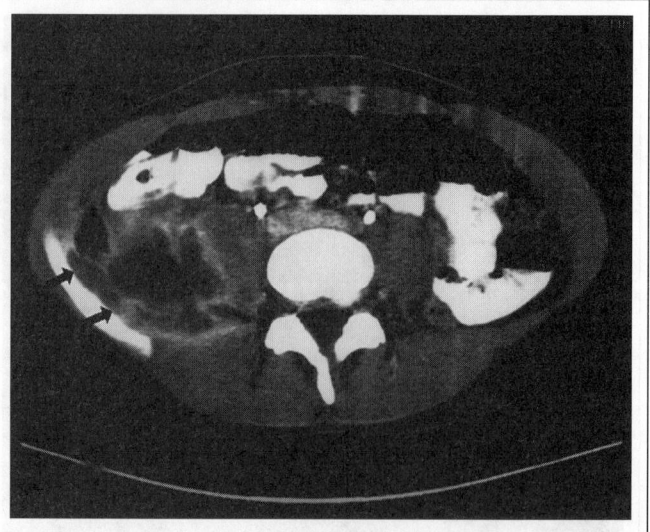

FIGURE 367-4 Retroperitoneal abscess. A large, septated fluid collection *(arrows)* with an enhancing rim of inflammatory tissue is present in the right retroperitoneum as a result of appendicitis. Percutaneous drainage was performed to treat the abscess before subsequent appendectomy.

DISEASES OF THE RETROPERITONEUM
Retroperitoneal Hemorrhage

Although retroperitoneal bleeds may be minor events, often they are severe and rapidly evolving. Typically the patient will experience pain, of variable severity, in the abdomen, back, flank, groin, or hips and present with hypovolemia and anemia (e.g., pallor, tachycardia, weakness) without an apparent bleeding site. Dominant clinical circumstances that favor development of retroperitoneal hemorrhage are trauma to the abdominal, lumbar, or pelvic regions; coagulation disorders (including therapeutic anticoagulation); and arterial or venous cannulation for angiographic catheterization or placement of central lines. Abdominal CT scanning is the preferred method of detection (Fig. 367-3). Treatment is supportive and includes correction of coagulation defects. Vascular surgical consultation for possible exploration and repair is prudent; it is mandatory when the bleed is a consequence of penetrating trauma.

Retroperitoneal Abscess

Abscesses in the retroperitoneum are typically an extension of gastrointestinal infection or inflammation (Crohn's disease, diverticulitis, appendicitis, perforation, pancreatitis) or renal or ureteral infection. Typically the illness is slowly progressive, having symptoms of fever; chills; night sweats; malaise; abdominal, flank, or back pain; nausea; vomiting; anorexia; weight loss; and general debility. Contrasted CT scan is the optimal means of diagnosis (Fig. 367-4). Antimicrobial therapy usually combined with drainage (percutaneous or surgical) is the current method of treatment.

Retroperitoneal Fibrosis

This entity is characterized by a well-delineated fibrous plaque centered around the sacral promontory, frequently enveloping the bifurcation of the aorta and extending laterally to the ureters and iliac vessels. Less commonly, the fibrotic process involves the kidneys, urinary bladder, duodenum, descending colon, spleen, pancreas, ovaries, and mesenteric blood vessels. Retroperitoneal fibrosis may occur in conjunction with other fibrotic processes such as mediastinal fibro-

sis, mesenteric fibrosis, sclerosing cholangitis, orbital pseudotumor, Dupuytren's contracture, Riedel's disease, and Peyronie's disease. Seventy percent of patients are in the fifth to seventh decade of life, and there is a 2:1 male predominance.

The cause of retroperitoneal fibrosis is unknown in two thirds of patients. In a recent review, methysergide was responsible for approximately 12% of all cases. In 8% of cases the process was associated with a malignant neoplasm, notably reticulum-cell sarcoma, lymphosarcoma, Hodgkin's disease, and carcinoid tumors. A clinical picture simulating retroperitoneal fibrosis has been described in patients with abdominal aortic aneurysms (perianeurysmal fibrosis). Retroperitoneal injury resulting from any mechanism is capable of inciting retroperitoneal fibrosis.

Poorly localized abdominal or back pain is the most frequent presenting symptom. Other presenting symptoms are constitutional: anorexia, malaise, nausea, fever, and weight loss. Anuria is the sole manifestation in 10% of patients. Other symptoms include lower extremity edema, intermittent claudication, jaundice, gastrointestinal bleeding, and toxic megacolon.

A rectal or abdominal mass is palpable in 15% of patients. Anemia and elevation of the erythrocyte sedimentation rate and blood urea nitrogen are common findings. Although the inferior vena cava is often encased by the fibrous tissue, signs of obstruction are rare. Most deaths result from renal failure or an underlying malignant process. The diagnosis may be suggested by contrast urography: the classic triad consists of bilateral ureteral narrowing at the level of the fifth lumbar vertebra; medial deviation of the ureters; and dilatation of the ureter, calyces, and pelvis. Although computed tomography (Fig. 367-5) and magnetic resonance imaging (MRI) may disclose characteristic abnormalities, exploratory laparotomy is necessary to establish the correct diagnosis and permit ureterolysis.

Corticosteroid therapy has been used as an adjunct to surgical measures or as primary therapy in patients in whom all studies are consistent with the diagnosis of idiopathic retroperitoneal fibrosis and in whom the operative risks appear prohibitive. Methotrexate and tamoxifen have also been reported to be beneficial. The long-term outlook is good, with the cumulative mortality being around 10%.

Retroperitoneal Tumors

Tumors arising in the retroperitoneum (not including those of specific organs, e.g., kidney, adrenal glands, pancreas) are unusual and can be expected to arise from connective tissue (including fat), the nerves and vessels that run through it, or residual urogenital tissues.

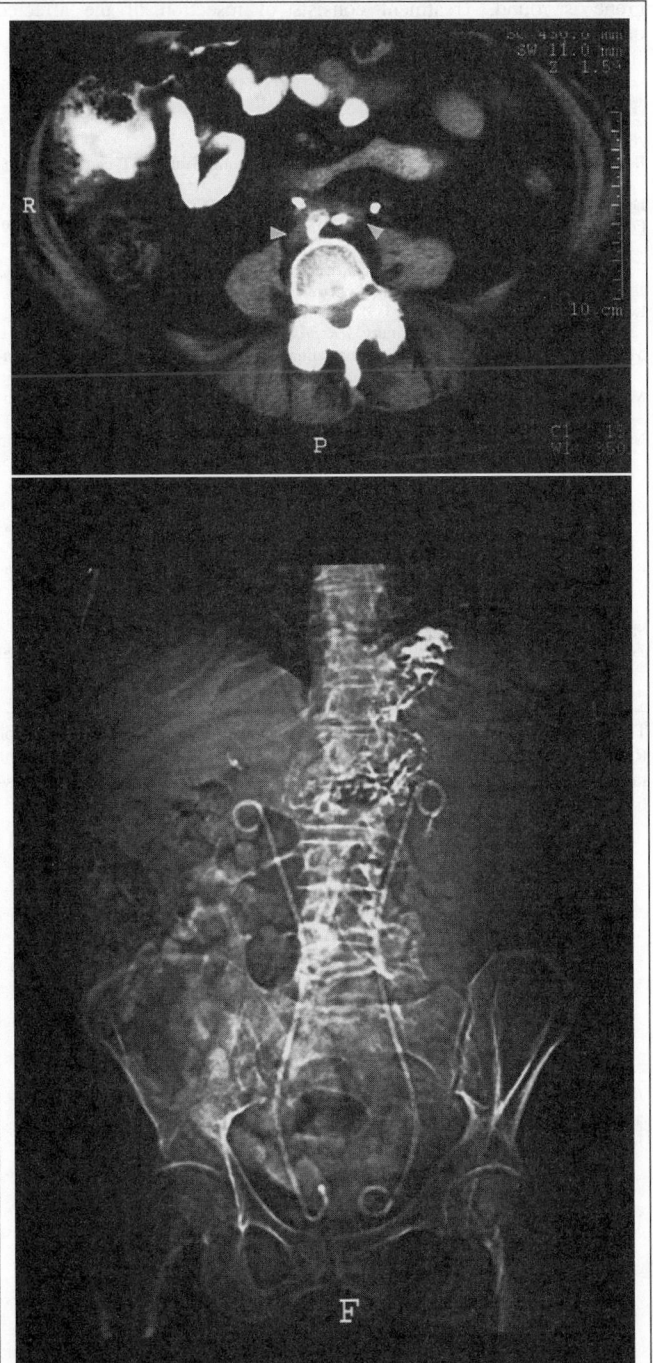

FIGURE 367-5 Retroperitoneal fibrosis. **A,** Fibrotic soft tissue *(arrow heads)* surrounds the calcified aorta in this 70-year-old woman who presented with renal failure. Bilateral ureteral stents are in place. **B,** The CT scout film demonstrates the medial deviation of the ureters caused by the retroperitoneal fibrosis.

Tumors are often asymptomatic or symptoms are mild and nonspecific. Precipitous pain may herald sudden hemorrhage into or around the tumor (see earlier discussion of retroperitoneal bleeding). Obstruction of the veins or lymphatic channels of the lower extremities may result in edema of the lower extremities. CT scan is the best method to diagnose retroperitoneal disease including tumors; the role of MRI scanning remains unsettled but will likely play an adjunctive role in determining the composition (fat or vascular) of retroperitoneal lesions. Except for lymphoma, surgical resection is the treatment, and this may be difficult or impossible depending on the size of the tumor or its particular involvement of adjacent structures. Oncologic consultation should be sought.

DISEASES OF THE MESENTERY
Inflammatory Disorders of the Mesentery

Although there are many terms used to describe them, inflammatory diseases of the mesentery are typically categorized as either mesenteric panniculitis or retractile mesenteritis, each at an end of the spectrum of what may be the same disease.

Mesenteric panniculitis (also called *mesenteric lipodystrophy)* is a disorder in which excessive fat accumulates in the mesentery, forming fat masses that subsequently degenerate and initiate inflammatory changes, resulting in fibrotic lesions. Patients are typically at least middle-age and are more often men. About 60% of patients have abdominal pain, nausea, vomiting, weight loss, and low-grade fever. The remaining 40% are incidentally discovered to have an abdominal mass at the time of physical examination or laparotomy. Radiographic examination often reveals separation of small-bowel loops, with kinking or angulation; CT findings include a low-density mass. If the fibrosis is more dense and accompanied by retraction of the mesentery, the disorder is considered retractile mesenteritis. At this point, patients may have small-bowel obstruction and intestinal lymphatic obstruction, producing protein-losing enteropathy, steatorrhea, and ascites. In general, the prognosis for mesenteric panniculitis is good. Some patients may have spontaneous regression; others may need limited surgery to bypass obstructed intestinal segments. In case reports, corticosteroids, azathioprine, and cyclophosphamide have been reported to be effective.

Mesenteric Fibromatosis

Mesenteric tumors or mesenteric desmoids are benign but locally invasive fibrous masses typically having dense central collagen. They are most frequently found in patients with familial polyposis disorders; 10% to 18% of patients with Gardner's syndrome will develop them. Although usually asymptomatic, the fibrous proliferation may cause obstructive symptoms. If large enough, the mass may be noted on physical examination and visualized by either ultrasound or CT scans. Therapeutic options are uncertain but typically involve surgical resection if possible. Medical treatment has been mostly anecdotal.

Mesenteric Hernia

A mesenteric hernia is an intraperitoneal herniation of a loop of bowel through a mesenteric defect. Most often the defect is single, 2 to 3 cm in diameter, and located in the mesentery of the small bowel. Mesenteric (internal) hernias account for 1% to 2% of intestinal obstruction in collected series of patients with intestinal obstruction. Patients may have a history of chronic intermittent abdominal distress. Complications include acute intestinal obstruction, volvulus, and gangrene of the bowel. A correct diagnosis is seldom made preoperatively, and mesenteric hernias can be missed at surgery. Treatment is surgical and consists of reduction of incarcerated bowel, repair of the defect, and resection of any nonviable bowel.

Mesenteric Cysts

These rare lesions develop most often in the second decade of life. They present as smooth, painless masses that can be made to move freely at right angles to the line of attachment of the mesentery. Large cysts may mimic ascites. Rupture, hemorrhage, or infection occurs rarely. Surgical excision is the preferred treatment.

Mesenteric Tumors

Mesenteric tumors may be benign (fibromas, lipomas, myomas) or malignant (lymphomas, sarcomas). Physical signs are similar to those mentioned for mesenteric cysts, with the exception that the tumor mass is often solid. Most are locally invasive, and cure is effected by excision. Metastatic tumors are significantly more common than primary tumors of the mesentery, characteristically involving the regional lymph nodes. Presentation depends on which adjacent organs are being affected by the tumor and the extent to which there is a fibrotic reaction with accompanying visceral obstruction or compression.

Mesenteric Giant Lymph Node Hyperplasia (Castleman's Disease)

Giant lymph node hyperplasia usually takes place in the chest, but it may occur in the abdomen, more commonly presenting as a mass in young women. It may present either as localized disease in the abdomen or abdominal involvement of multicentric disease, either as adenopathy or hepatosplenomegaly. The localized form is associated with iron deficiency anemia, has an excellent prognosis, and is cured with surgical resection. Treatment of the multicentric form has not yet been optimized and carries a poor prognosis.

DISEASES OF THE OMENTUM

The greater omentum has been called the "abdominal policeman," since it often limits the spread of intraperitoneal infections. Cysts and tumors of the omentum are similar in presentation to their mesenteric counterparts. By far the most dramatic disorder involving the omentum is torsion, which occurs predominantly in middle-age, obese men. As expected, the most common symptom is abdominal pain that is usually acute at onset. At times, this pain localizes to the right lower quadrant and, along with symptoms of nausea and vomiting, may present like appendicitis. Because it presents as an acute condition in the abdomen, patients are typically diagnosed surgically, where a hemorrhagic omental mass and possibly gan-

grene is found. Treatment consists of resection of the affected omentum.

BIBLIOGRAPHY

Amis ES: Retroperitoneal fibrosis, *AJR* 157:321, 1991.
Beauchamp RD: Diseases of the mesentery and omentum. In Yamada T, editor: *Textbook of gastroenterology,* Philadelphia, 1995, Lippincott.
Durst AL et al: Mesenteric panniculitis, *Surgery* 81:203, 1977.
Feliciano DV: Management of traumatic retroperitoneal hematoma, *Ann Surg* 211:109, 1990.
Fernandez RN, Daly JM: Pseudomyxoma peritonei, *Arch Surg* 115:409, 1980.
Janin Y, Stone AM, Wise L: Mesenteric hernia, *Surg Gynecol Obstet* 150:747, 1980.
Lopez-Zeno JA, Keith LG, Berger GS: The Fitz-Hugh-Curtis syndrome revisited: changing perspectives after half a century, *J Reprod Med* 30:567, 1985.
Marshall JB: Tuberculosis of the gastrointestinal tract and peritoneum, *Am J Gastroenterol* 88:989, 1993.
Morgenstern L, Berci G, Pasternak EH: Bile leakage after biliary tract surgery: a laparoscopic perspective, *Surg Endosc* 7:432, 1993.
Nance FC: Diseases of the peritoneum, retroperitoneum, mesentery, and omentum. In Haubrich WS, Schaffner F, Berk JE, editors: *Gastroenterology,* Philadelphia, 1995, Saunders.
Ruben RA, Chopra S: Bile peritonitis after liver biopsy: nonsurgical management of a patient with an acute abdomen: a case report with review of the literature, *Am J Gastroenterol* 82:265, 1987.
Runyon BA: Surgical peritonitis and other diseases of the peritoneum, mesentery, omentum, and diaphragm. In Sleisenger MH, Fordtran JS, editors: *Gastrointestinal Disease,* Philadelphia, 1993, Saunders.
Shahidi H, Myers JL, Kvale PA: Castleman's disease, *Mayo Clin Proc* 70:969, 1995.
Zemer D et al: Colchicine in the prevention and treatment of the amyloidosis of familial Mediterranean fever, *N Engl J Med* 314:1001, 1986.

The author wishes to thank Dr. Michael G. Khamis, Assistant Professor of Radiology, for his thoughtful review of the chapter and his contribution of radiographs. This work was supported in part by a Glaxo Institute for Digestive Health Basic Research Award.

PART ELEVEN

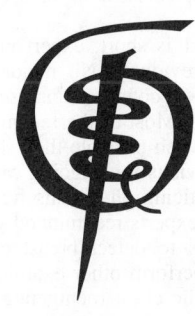

Special Topics in Internal Medicine

368 Periodic Health Examination

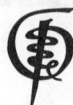

Suzanne W. Fletcher

The periodic health examination is a set of four clinical tasks carried out on asymptomatic persons: taking parts of a history, doing portions of a physical examination, ordering certain laboratory tests, and performing simple preventive maneuvers such as counseling patients and providing immunizations and chemoprevention. These tasks are undertaken to promote health and prevent disease or to find disease early in its course so that it can be treated before adverse health outcomes occur.

Over the past two decades the periodic health examination has evolved from the yearly physical examination, a general and untargeted checkup, to a lifetime program of "health protection packages." Certain history items, physical examinations, laboratory tests, immunizations, chemoprevention prescriptions, and counseling procedures are performed based on the age, sex, and risk category of each patient.

When physicians perform periodic health examinations, they usually do so in the context of ongoing care of their patients. Such a practice is called *case finding,* and it implies that the person initiating the examination has assumed the responsibility of following up any abnormality found. If the clinician is not committed to investigation of abnormal results, the examination should not be performed in the first place. Patients undergoing case finding in internal medicine practices frequently are not well and often have many symptoms. Case finding is that part of the examination directed toward medical conditions for which the patient is asymptomatic. For example, a physician practices case finding when he or she performs a periodic clinical breast examination on a patient who is without breast symptoms but who is being seen for diabetes and angina.

Routine physical examinations are among the 20 most frequent reasons for visits to internists' offices in all subspecialties except oncology and nephrology. Internists care for an age-group of patients for whom periodic health examinations are recommended with greater frequency than for any other group except pregnant women and very young children.

RECOMMENDATIONS

Several groups have made recommendations for the minimal set of tasks that should be included in periodic health examinations. Figure 368-1 is a summary of recent recommendations for adults made by major groups.

In the history, health behaviors regarding cigarette smoking, alcohol, diet, contraceptives, and seat belt use should be assessed, and appropriate counseling should be given when necessary. Some groups also suggest checking for other health-related behavior, as noted in Fig. 368-1.

Periodic physical examination recommendations are highly targeted and include examinations for obesity, hypertension, and visual and hearing loss, and for breast, cervical, and colorectal cancers. Recommended laboratory tests are aimed at breast, cervical, and colorectal cancers as well as hypercholesterolemia. Appropriate immunizations are recommended, as are chemoprophylaxis with folic acid for women of childbearing age and hormone replacement therapy for appropriate postmenopausal women.

The physician's role in counseling patients about healthful behaviors is growing. Smoking cessation is more likely to be successful with counseling. For control of hypercholesterolemia, the first step is dietary change; appropriately trained physicians can help patients learn better eating habits. Physician counseling increases seat belt use, as well as contraceptive use to prevent unplanned pregnancies, and it decreases alcohol use among problem drinkers. Other healthful behaviors also can be encouraged by physicians (Fig. 368-1), but the effectiveness of physician counseling in changing these behaviors has not yet been established.

Examination of Fig. 368-1 shows that recommended procedures and frequencies vary according to patients' ages. For example, carcinoma in situ of the cervix is more common in younger than in older women, and therefore most groups suggest more frequent Papanicolaou smears in young women. Breast cancer, on the other hand, becomes more common as a woman grows older, and recommendations regarding the search for breast cancer reflect this fact. For most women patients, this means that physicians should shift case-finding emphasis from cervical to breast cancer as the woman grows older.

The list of tasks in Fig. 368-1 is short; expert groups currently recommend fewer items than previously. No major group recommends routine complete blood cell counts, urinalyses, chest roentgenograms, or electrocardiograms. Most of the recommended procedures are also inexpensive, and when possible they should be incorporated into regularly scheduled visits for ongoing care.

Studies have shown that practicing physicians frequently do not perform some examinations that experts recommend with a high degree of consensus, such as tests to detect breast cancer in older women. Meanwhile, they often perform other examinations that are not recommended, such as periodic chest roentgenograms and electrocardiograms. Periodic health examinations should start with the items listed in Fig. 368-1.

Even when physicians are committed to periodic health examinations, it is not easy to incorporate the performance of indicated examinations into the ongoing care of patients being seen for established diseases. For example, it is difficult to remember that a given patient being seen for hypertension is also due for a breast examination, mammography, and a stool guaiac test. Prompting systems can help. Many practices include in each patient's medical record a flow sheet similar to that in Fig. 368-1; whenever a patient visits the practice, the flow sheet is consulted to see if any procedures are indicated. Computer prompting has also been used to help remind physicians to perform periodic tests.

UNDERLYING SCIENTIFIC PRINCIPLES

When physicians undertake periodic health examinations on asymptomatic patients, a decision must be made about which medical problems or diseases should be sought or prevented. This principle sounds straightforward, but often it is not. Thus a urinalysis—frequently ordered in routine examinations of young, asymptomatic, nonpregnant adults (but not recommended by any of the expert groups represented in Fig. 368-1)—might be used to search for any number of medical problems, including diabetes, asymptomatic urinary tract infections, and renal calculi. Before a urinalysis is performed, it is necessary to decide which, if any, of these conditions is worth screening for.

Three criteria have been developed for deciding whether a medical condition should be sought during a periodic health examination. In order of importance, these criteria are (1) the effectiveness of prevention or early treatment for the medical condition, (2) the severity of the condition, and (3) the quality of the proposed screening procedure. A good screening procedure should be sensitive, specific, simple, inexpensive, safe, and acceptable to patients and physicians.

The three criteria are fulfilled better for some conditions than for others, and judgment is involved in reaching decisions. As a result, some recommended procedures listed in Fig. 368-1 are made with much more certainty, scientific evidence, and consensus among various groups than other recommendations. Also, the correct frequency of repeat examinations undergoes constant modification as more information becomes available.

Physicians who examine their patients for unrecognized disease rarely find the disease. Even "common" diseases are uncommon; for breast cancer, several hundred women must be examined for each case of cancer found. Furthermore, because of low prevalence of disease in asymptomatic individuals, even very accurate tests with good sensitivities and specificities produce many false-positive results. Most abnormalities uncovered during periodic health examinations are not caused by the medical condition being sought. Targeting specific examinations according to a person's age, sex, and risk status helps to increase the prevalence of disease among those examined before the

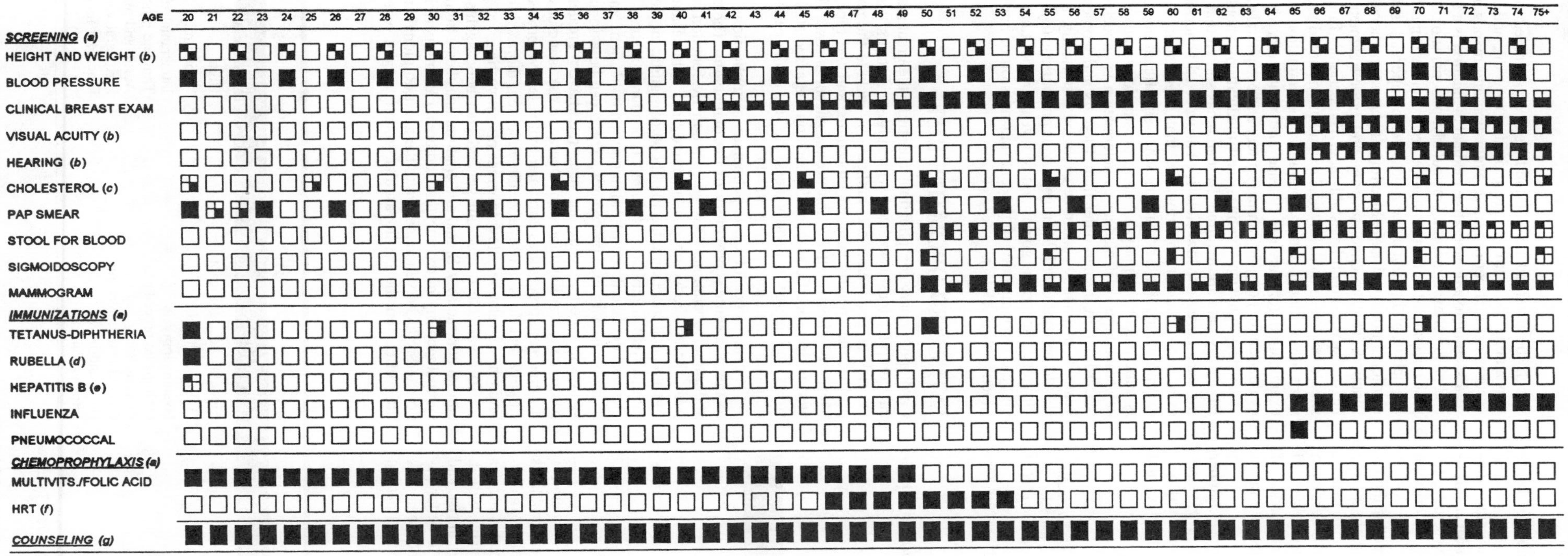

USPSTF - US Preventive Service Task Force
CTFPHE - Canadian Task Force on the Periodic Health Examination
ACP - American College of Physicians
AAFP - American Academy of Family Physicians

USPSTF	CTFPHE
ACP	AAFP

(*a*) Only clear recommendations in favor of the activity are included. (*a* and *b* recommendations by USPSTF and CTFPHE). Frequency of screening not clearly stated. Recommendations frequently differ for high risk groups.

(*b*) ACP has not considered these tests. USPSTF and CTFPHE recommend screening frequency be left to physician discretion.

(*c*) ACP and USPSTF recommend beginning in men at age 35 and women, age 45. They note that the frequency of cholesterol testing should depend on prior results and other risk factors. Those with lower risk factors may be screened less often.

(*d*) Screening women of child bearing age by seriologic testing or history of vaccination, followed by vaccination of susceptible women. Alternatively, all women in this age group could be offered vaccination without screening.

(*e*) Recommended routinely for young adults not previously immunized.

(*f*) May be discussed at later age if not previously discussed.

(*g*) All groups recommend regular counseling of appropriate patients for tobacco cessation, dietary fat/cholesterol, dietary fruits and vegetables, contraceptive use to prevent unintended pregnancy, use of seat belts, and problem alcohol drinking. No definite interval is specified. In addition, they note that the following activities reduce risk, but that the evidence is inadequate to determine whether physician counseling is effective in changing behavior:
- set hot water heater to <120-130 degrees
- fall prevention in older people
- regular physical activity
- motorcycle helmets
- smoke detector
- safe storage or removal of firearms
- sexually transmitted disease protection
- regular dental visits
- floss and brush teeth

FIGURE 368-1 Preventive care guidelines of expert groups for asymptomatic nonpregnant adults at average risk.

Data from U.S. Preventive Services Task Force: Guide to clinical preventive services, ed 2, Baltimore, 1996, Williams & Wilkins, and Medical Practice Committee, American College of Physicians: Periodic health examination: a guide for designing individualized preventive health care in the asymptomatic patient, *Ann Intern Med* 95:729, 1981.

examination is done, thereby cutting down on the number of false-positive test results.

The number of false-positive test results is also related to the number of examinations a physician carries out on a patient. Most physicians do not perform only one or two tests on patients presenting for checkups. Many order several dozen tests, which is easy to do with modern technology and automated blood tests.

A laboratory test result is usually defined as "abnormal" if the result falls outside the range covered by 95% of test results in a large group of people. This means that the more tests a physician orders, the greater the risk of a false-positive test. If the physician orders even 5 tests, 23% of healthy people will have an abnormal result; with 20 tests, 64%; and with 100 tests, over 99%. The resultant burden of financial, medical, and psychological costs among patients with false-positive test results may be large.

Physicians can guard against this problem by keeping the number of tests they perform to a minimum and by making sure they search only for medical conditions meeting the three criteria outlined earlier. Such strategies maximize the benefits and minimize the risks and costs of periodic health examinations.

BIBLIOGRAPHY

American Academy of Family Physicians: *Age charts for periodic health examination,* Kansas City, Mo, 1994, American Academy of Family Physicians (Reprint 510).
Canadian Task Force on the Periodic Health Examination: *Canadian guide to clinical preventive health care,* Ottawa, 1994, Canada Communications Group.
Eddy DM, editor: *Common screening tests,* Philadelphia, 1991, American College of Physicians.
Fletcher RH, Fletcher SW, Wagner EH: Prevention. In *Clinical epidemiology: the essentials,* ed 3, Baltimore, 1996, Williams & Wilkins.
Sox HC: Preventive health services in adults, *N Engl J Med* 330:1589, 1994.
U.S. Preventive Services Task Force: *Guide to clinical preventive services,* ed 2, Baltimore, 1996, Williams & Wilkins.

CHAPTER

369   Preoperative Evaluation

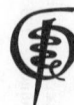

Jane Appleby, C. Jeffrey Griffin, and Valerie A. Lawrence

The goal of preoperative medical evaluation is to decrease operative morbidity and mortality by identifying and treating medical problems that contribute to perioperative risk. Medical complications of surgery have become relatively uncommon, so research in this area is difficult and many clinical issues have not been rigorously studied. However, identifying medical illnesses that increase surgical risk and defining potential complications presumably contribute to better patient management and improve outcome. Assessing the additional risk imposed by underlying illnesses can help the physician and patient weigh the potential benefits and risks of a procedure. Communication among the primary care provider, surgeon, and anesthesiologist ensures optimal perioperative evaluation and management.

Essential to a preoperative medical evaluation is a thorough history and physical examination. Particularly, patients should be asked about past responses to anesthesia and surgery, current medications, smoking habits, and recent acute illness. Also important is a past history of cardiopulmonary disease, bleeding diathesis, and hepatic or renal dysfunction. The presence, severity, and prior treatment of preexisting heart disease should be established. The patient's functional capacity should be determined. Physical examination should include an assessment of nutritional status, a pulmonary examination, a cardiovascular examination for valvular disease and ventricular dysfunction, plus evaluation for possible coronary artery and peripheral vascular disease.

History, physical findings, and medications should dictate what laboratory data are required. Research has shown that routine screening tests have very low yield for unsuspected abnormal findings and even less yield for abnormalities that affect surgical outcome. The exceptions include a hematocrit when significant operative blood loss is anticipated; a urinalysis before prosthetic, vascular, or neurosurgical procedures or if bladder catheterization is expected; and an electrocardiogram in men older than 40 years and women older than 55 years. If pregnancy cannot be excluded historically, a pregnancy test should be considered. Routine barrier precautions (eye covers, double gloving, impervious gowns and footwear), rather than routine screening, are recommended to prevent transmission of human immunodeficiency virus (HIV).

ESTIMATED OPERATIVE RISK

Cardiopulmonary complications constitute the great majority of medical complications associated with surgery. Factors that contribute to the risk of perioperative complications include the patient's clinical profile, the specific surgical procedure, and the type of anesthesia. Mortality directly attributable to anesthesia is low. The risk associated with a specific surgery depends on the associated hemodynamic stress, the degree of invasiveness, the risk to the patient, and the anticipated blood loss (Table 369-1).

The incidence of cardiopulmonary complications is also related to the procedure's proximity to the diaphragm. Thoracic and upper abdominal operations cause diaphragm dysfunction and inspiratory pain, thereby reducing postoperative tidal volume and cough effectiveness and increasing the likelihood of significant atelectasis, pneumonia, and ventilatory failure. Procedures lasting over 2 hours increase the likelihood of pulmonary complications and deep venous thrombosis. Vascular procedures, which can be associated with wide swings in blood pressure and heart rate, have a greater risk of perioperative myocardial infarction. Operative risk is increased 2 to 5 times for emergent procedures compared with elective procedures. Elective surgery that does not involve the abdomen, thorax, blood vessels, or brain has a relatively low inherent operative risk.

To a variable degree, all general anesthetic agents depress myocardial contractility. Spinal and epidural anesthesia produce prolonged sympathectomy in the anesthetized area, causing peripheral vasodilation and reduced venous return to the heart. Regional anesthetics have little effect on the cardiovascular system except when absorbed in

Table 369-1   Risk associated with surgical procedures

RISK	LOW (<1%)*	MODERATE (<5%)	HIGH (>5%)
Invasiveness	Minimal to moderate	Moderate to significant	High
Blood loss	<500 ml	500 to 1500 ml	>1500 ml
Examples	Cataract extraction	Hysterectomy	Intracranial surgery
	Cytoscopy	Orthopedic procedures	Thoracic procedures
	Laparoscopy	Prostatectomy	Aortic and major vascular
	Arthroscopy	Carotid endarterectomy	Peripheral vascular
	Inguinal hernia	Head and neck	Emergent major procedures
		Intraperitoneal	

*Percentages indicate the combined incidence of cardiac death and myocardial infarction.

large quantities. General, spinal, and epidural anesthesia are thought to carry an equal risk of myocardial infarction and cardiac death. Regional anesthesia is usually well tolerated regardless of the patient's clinical status.

The Dripps–American Society of Anesthesiology (ASA) classification of physical status was developed over 30 years ago for estimating perioperative mortality resulting from systemic disease. Postoperative mortality increases progressively with increasing ASA class: class I, healthy; class II, mild systemic disease; class III, severe systemic disease; class IV, incapacitating systemic disease that is a constant threat to life; and class V, moribund and not expected to survive 24 hours with or without operation. Disadvantages of the ASA classification system are that it is a subjective, relatively poorly defined classification system and that patients with many different types of illnesses undergoing surgical procedures with different overall complication rates are combined, exaggerating the operative risk in some and minimizing the risk in others. A further disadvantage is that the ASA classification does not specifically predict cardiopulmonary complications, which are the major source of surgical risk.

SYSTEMIC RISK FACTORS
Cardiovascular Risk Factors

Identification and Management of Cardiovascular Risk. The management of patients at risk for cardiac complications associated with elective noncardiac surgery depends on the patient's clinical risk profile and functional capacity, the urgency of the procedure, and the inherent risk of the planned surgery. In general, tests should be obtained only if they will alter management. Intervention is rarely indicated to lower the risk of surgery unless it would be advised independently of the anticipated procedure. Indications for preoperative angiography in patients with known or suspected coronary artery disease are similar to those for patients who are not being evaluated for surgery. Angiography may be helpful in patients who are candidates for revascularization and who have unstable angina, angina unresponsive to medical therapy, a high-risk noninvasive test, or a nondiagnostic or equivocal noninvasive test in a high-risk patient undergoing a high-risk procedure.

Clinical Risk Profile. Clinical markers that assist in the identification of patients at risk for perioperative myocardial infarction (MI) and cardiac death have been derived from several large prospective studies. Clinical findings associated with a high risk of perioperative cardiac events include unstable coronary syndromes (recent myocardial infarction, unstable or severe angina); severe valvular disease; significant arrhythmia (high-grade AV block, symptomatic ventricular arrhythmias in the presence of underlying heart disease, supraventricular arrhythmias with uncontrolled rate); and decompensated congestive heart failure. Stable angina, known coronary artery disease, compensated congestive heart failure, and diabetes mellitus are associated with moderate risk of perioperative cardiac events. Advanced age, electrocardiographic abnormalities, controlled arrhythmias, poor medical status, and evidence of systemic atherosclerosis indicate a low-risk profile. The presence of risk factors for coronary artery disease with a normal electrocardiograph and good functional status is associated with negligible operative risk. (Clinical predictors of perioperative cardiac risk are shown in Table 369-2).

Older landmark studies indicate the risk of reinfarction in patients who have surgery after a recent MI is approximately 30% in the first 3 months. In the next 4 to 6 months the risk of reinfarction is 11% to 16%. After 6 months the reinfarction rate declines 4% to 6%. Actual rates may be lower with today's technology and management. Patients who have had a recent myocardial infarction require risk stratification before elective surgery. If there is no indication of myocardium at risk by exercise stress testing, the likelihood of reinfarction after noncardiac surgery is low. Although there are no well-designed trials to guide the management of these patients, current recommendations are to wait at least 4 to 6 weeks after MI to perform elective surgery.

Functional Capacity. After the patient's clinical risk profile is determined, the next step in preoperative risk assessment is to determine the patient's functional capacity. Functional capacity is best expressed in metabolic equivalent levels (METs). The MET correlates with oxygen consumption. Functional capacity is excellent if greater than 7 METs can be achieved, moderate if 4 to 7 METs is achieved, and poor if less than 4 METs is achieved. The risk of perioperative cardiovascular complications is increased in patients who are unable to exercise to a level of 4 METs. Table 369-3 illustrates the Canadian Cardiovascular Society (CCS) functional classification scheme. Specific activities and associated METs correlating with each class are also indicated. If the patient's functional capacity is uncertain based on available history and clinical information, an exercise treadmill test may provide a more objective assessment.

Management. Once the patient's clinical risk profile, functional status, and the risk associated with the planned surgery have been determined, a stepwise approach (as recommended in recent practice guidelines published by the American Heart Association and the American College of Cardiology) can be used to determine the need for preoperative testing. This approach is shown in Fig. 369-1. All patients should have existing medical conditions optimally treated before surgery. If surgery is urgent or emergent, postoperative risk stratification may be more appropriate. Preoperative testing is not usually indicated in patients with a history of coronary revascularization within the 5 years before surgery who have no recurrence of symptoms or signs of myocardial ischemia. Similarly, an appropriate cardiac evaluation in the past 2 years indicating that the patient is low

Table 369-2   Clinical predictors of perioperative cardiovascular risk

NEGLIGIBLE RISK CLINICAL PROFILE	LOW-RISK CLINICAL PROFILE (1% TO 2%)	MODERATE RISK CLINICAL PROFILE (2% TO 5%)	HIGH-RISK CLINICAL PROFILE (>5%)
Normal ECG	Age >75	Stable angina	Recent MI‡
No CAD risks	Rhythm not sinus (i.e., AFIB)	CCS class 1 or 2 angina	Unstable angina
Age <75	>5 PVCs	Known CAD	CCS class 3 or 4 angina
	Low functional capacity*	Compensated CHF	Severe valvular disease
	Evidence of atherosclerosis	Diabetes mellitus	Significant arrhythmia§
	• CVA/TIA		Decompensated CHF
	• Prior vascular surgery		
	• Claudication		
	• Bruits on examination		
	Abnormal ECG†		

*Canadian Cardiovascular Society (CCS) class 3 or 4.
†Left ventricular hypertrophy, left bundle branch block, ST abnormalities.
‡Recent MI is defined as greater than 7 days but less than 30 days.
§High-grade AV block, symptomatic ventricular arrhythmia with underlying heart disease, supraventricular arrhythmia with uncontrolled rate.
Percentages in parentheses indicate the risk of cardiac complications (myocardial infarction, congestive heart failure, and cardiac death).
AFIB, Atrial fibrillation; *CAD,* coronary artery disease; *CCS,* Canadian Cardiovascular Society; *CHF,* congestive heart failure; *CVA,* cerebrovascular accident; *ECG,* electrocardiogram; *MI,* myocardial infarction; *TIA,* transient ischemic attack; *PVC,* premature ventricular contraction.

Table 369-3 Estimation of functional capacity of patients with cardiovascular disease

CLASS	CCS*	SPECIFIC ACTIVITY†
1	Angina with strenuous, rapid, or prolonged work.	Carry 24 lb up 8 steps, carry 80 lb, jog or walk 5 miles per hour. (7 METs)
2	Angina with walking more than two blocks or more than one flight of stairs.	Garden, rake, dance or walk at 4 mph on level ground. (5 METs)
3	Angina walking one or two blocks or one flight of stairs.	Shower, mop, walk 2.5 mph, push power mower. (2 METS)
4	Angina at rest or with any activity.	Can do none of the above or symptoms at rest.

*Canadian Cardiovascular Society (CCS) scale reported in *Circulation* 54:522, 1975.
.†Specific activity scale reported in *Circulation* 64:1227, 1981.

risk does not need to be repeated unless there are new symptoms that suggest myocardial ischemia. If the patient is not a candidate for revascularization, noninvasive testing to establish the diagnosis of severe coronary artery disease may not be indicated.

Patients who have a low-risk clinical profile with a good functional status (>4 METs) can usually proceed to surgery without preoperative testing. Patients with a low-risk clinical profile and a poor functional status (<4 METs) and patients with a moderate-risk clinical profile and good functional status will usually tolerate surgery that carries a low or intermediate risk of complications. However, this same group of patients may benefit from noninvasive evaluation before high-risk surgery. Patients with a moderate-risk clinical profile and poor functional status may also benefit from noninvasive testing before surgery. Elective surgery should be delayed or canceled in patients who have a high-risk clinical profile. Alternatively, coronary angiography, if indicated, should be performed preoperatively.

Noninvasive Testing. Exercise treadmill stress testing with and without nuclear imaging, dobutamine stress echocardiography, and intravenous dipyridamole myocardial perfusion imaging are the most commonly used preoperative noninvasive tests. Exercise testing is useful in ambulatory patients without significant electrocardiographic abnormalities. In the presence of left bundle branch block, left ventricular hypertrophy with strain, atrial fibrillation, or digoxin effect, exercise testing with myocardial perfusion imaging or exercise echocardiography should be considered. Dobutamine stress echocardiography or intravenous dipyridamole myocardial perfusion imaging are indicated if patients are not ambulatory or are unable to achieve an adequate workload using standard exercise testing.

Vascular Surgery. The evaluation of patients who require vascular surgery is particularly challenging. Because significant exercise limitation associated with claudication or other manifestations of peripheral vascular disease is often present, symptoms of myocardial ischemia may not be present even in patients with severe coronary artery disease.

In addition, patients with peripheral vascular disease have a high prevalence of coronary artery disease. Although routine preoperative screening using noninvasive testing is not indicated before vascular surgery, many patients will have a moderate-risk clinical profile and a poor functional capacity. Current recommendations are to perform noninvasive testing in this clinical setting.

If surgery is performed without preoperative noninvasive testing, close attention to optimal medical management, treatment with antianginal medications, communication with the anesthesiologist and surgeon, and vigilant postoperative surveillance for cardiac events are mandatory for this subset of patients. Because death in individuals with peripheral vascular disease is often related to coronary artery disease, coronary revascularization may improve long-term outcome. Thus reassessment of the need for coronary angiography after the patient has recovered from vascular surgery is imperative. Postoperative functional status may improve enough so that the symptoms of myocardial ischemia appear.

Noninvasive testing with dipyridamole thallium or dobutamine stress echocardiography in individuals with an intermediate clinical risk profile helps define the risk of cardiac complications associated with vascular procedures. The negative predictive value of a normal myocardial perfusion scan ranges from 95% to 100%. The risk of perioperative cardiac events in the presence of a fixed defect is higher than with a normal scan but is significantly lower than the risk of cardiac events noted if redistribution is present on the preoperative scan. Patients with fixed defects noted on preoperative perfusion imaging should have their medical regimen optimized and should be monitored for cardiac events in the postoperative period. Patients who have a reversible defect noted on preoperative dipyridamole thallium stress testing may have a high risk of perioperative cardiac events. The negative predictive value of a normal dobutamine echocardiogram ranges from 93% to 100%. The presence of new wall motion abnormalities at a low infusion rate of dobutamine indicates myocardium at risk. Management of patients with reversible defects on myocardial perfusion studies or new wall motion abnormalities on dobutamine echo is controversial. Equally acceptable alternatives include angiography and revascularization if indicated independent of surgery; treatment with maximal medical therapy and repeat noninvasive testing reserving angiography for those with persistent high-risk results; or optimizing the preoperative medication regimen (including β-blockers and nitrates) combined with postoperative monitoring for ischemia.

Perioperative Surveillance. Most postoperative myocardial infarctions occur within the first 48 hours of surgery; are rarely associated with chest pain; have a high mortality (30% to 50%); and are associated with reduced long-term survival. Surveillance for cardiac events with postoperative electrocardiograms, cardiac enzymes, and continuous electrocardiographic monitoring is indicated in selected patients. Patients with known or suspected coronary artery disease or patients who undergo procedures associated with a high risk of cardiac events should have an electrocardiogram immediately after surgery and on the first two postoperative days. Cardiac enzymes should be sent in patients who have electrocardiographic changes suggestive of ischemia or with clinical findings of pulmonary edema, unexplained tachycardia, hypotension, or hemodynamic instability. An electrocardiogram should be obtained for patients with a low or moderate clinical risk profile who demonstrate signs or symptoms suggestive of myocardial ischemia in the postoperative period. Prolonged postoperative ST-segment changes observed on ambulatory electrocardiographic monitors correlate highly with postoperative cardiac events. Unfortunately, this technology is limited by the delay in obtaining results and requires further research before common use.

The use of pulmonary artery catheters to reduce mortality and morbidity in the perioperative period has been advocated but not rigorously studied. Recent randomized trials comparing pulmonary artery catheters and central venous monitoring have not shown differences in perioperative myocardial infarction or cardiac death. In general, pulmonary artery catheters are recommended in patients who are at risk for major hemodynamic disturbances with surgery or who have a fixed cardiac output (e.g., severe valvular disease or left ventricular dysfunction).

Heart failure. The operative risk associated with congestive heart failure depends on the degree of left ventricular dysfunction. Patients with New York Heart Association (NYHA) functional class I or II symptoms and no jugular venous pressure elevation are not at a significantly higher risk of perioperative MI or pulmonary edema than asymptomatic patients. Perioperative management should include optimal medical therapy and careful management of fluids, electrolytes, and hematocrit. Patients with NYHA class III or IV heart failure, jugular venous pressure elevation, or a third heart sound (S_3) or resting left ventricular ejection fraction of less than 35% are at high risk of cardiac complications. Elective surgery should be delayed until heart failure is adequately controlled. Perioperative hemodynamic monitoring with a pulmonary artery catheter has not been carefully evaluated with controlled studies but may be beneficial.

Arrhythmias. Relevant factors in the incidence and severity of perioperative arrhythmias include underlying ischemic heart disease or left ventricular dysfunction, preoperative history of arrhythmias, depth of anesthesia, presence of aortic stenosis, postoperative infec-

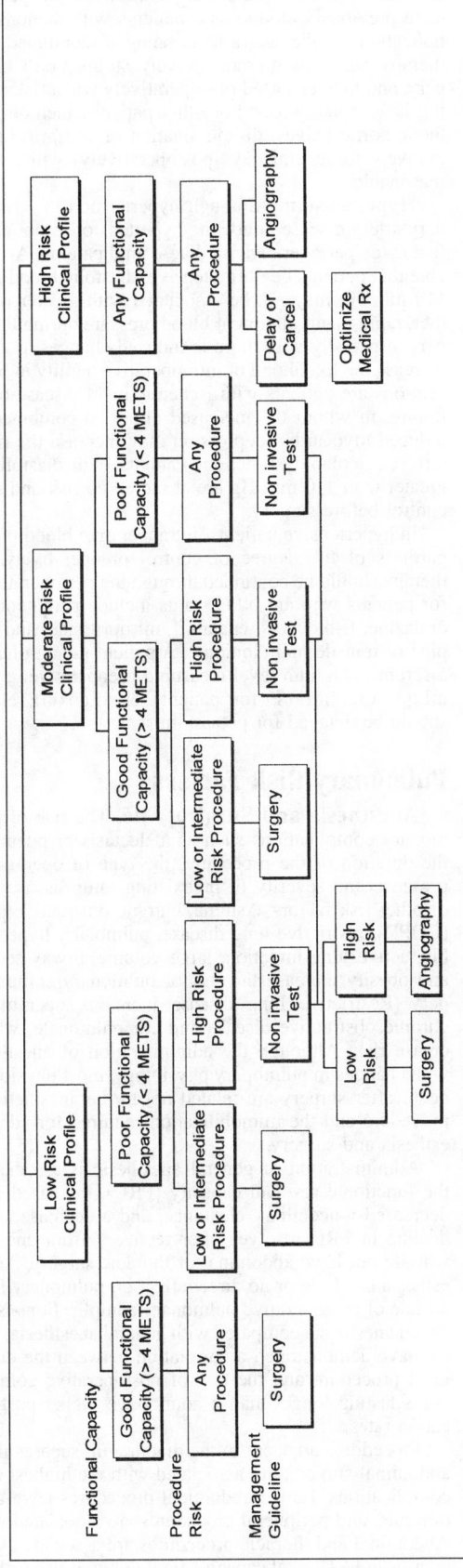

FIGURE 369-1   Management guidelines for patients at risk for perioperative cardiac complications.
Modified from ACC/AHA Task Force guidelines for perioperative cardiovascular evaluation for noncardiac surgery, *JACC*, 27(4): 910-948, 1996.

Notes:

- All patients must have medical conditions optimally treated prior to surgery.
- If functional status is uncertain evaluate by exercise treadmill testing.
- Coronary angiography and coronary revascularization is recommended in situations in which it would be advised independent of the anticipated surgery.
- Asymptomatic patients who have had coronary revascularization in the 5 years prior to presurgical evaluation usually do not require additional preoperative testing.
- Adequate cardiac evaluation in the 2 years prior to presurgical evaluation does not need to be repeated in patients without symptoms of myocardial ischemia or an interim change in clinical status.
- Risk factor reduction and risk stratification should be done after recovery from surgery in patients who do not have preoperative testing.

tion, hypoxia, hypokalemia, hypomagnesemia, use of digoxin, anemia, and increased levels of circulating catecholamines. Supraventricular tachycardia including atrial fibrillation occurs in about 4% of all surgical patients and should prompt evaluation for congestive heart failure, myocardial infarction, pericarditis, pulmonary embolism, infection, hypoxia, acidosis, hypokalemia, or aggravating drugs such as bronchodilators or epinephrine.

Symptomatic or hemodynamically significant arrhythmias require preoperative initiation of therapy. Cardioversion is not recommended until the underlying cause of the arrhythmia is identified and reversed. Postoperative bradyarrhythmias are usually caused by electrolyte disturbance, hypoxemia, or ischemia. Patients on chronic antiarrhythmic therapy should receive their usual oral dose the morning of surgery and as soon as possible after the operation. Patients taking quinidine may have prolonged neuromuscular blockade after exposure to neuromuscular blockers, so their respiratory status should be followed closely.

Conduction abnormalities. The presence of cardiac conduction disturbance requires careful evaluation for underlying cardiopulmonary disease, drug toxicity, or metabolic abnormality. Left or right bundle branch block or right bundle branch block plus left anterior hemiblock does not indicate a significant risk of perioperative second- or third-degree heart block. Asymptomatic patients with bifascicular block should have continuous intraoperative ECG monitoring but usually do not require a prophylactic temporary pacemaker. Symptoms of high-grade atrioventricular block or sinus node failure should be evaluated and treated before elective surgery.

The presence of a permanent pacemaker does not increase surgical mortality. Permanent pacemakers may need to be checked before surgery to verify normal function. Discharge of pacing impulses from demand pacemakers may be inhibited by electrocautery. Ground connections for cautery should be placed as far away from the pacemaker and heart as possible. If pacemaker inhibition still occurs, the pacemaker should be set in a fixed-rate mode.

Valvular heart disease. The indications for evaluation and treatment of valvular heart disease are identical in the operative and nonoperative setting. Valvular heart disease reduces the patient's ability to meet perioperative demands for increased cardiac output; increases the risk of bacterial endocarditis; and, in patients with prosthetic valves, may require modification of chronic anticoagulation. In general, mildly symptomatic patients (NYHA class I or II) tolerate surgery well, except those with aortic stenosis. For noncardiac surgery, hemodynamically important aortic stenosis increases perioperative mortality to about 13%, primarily from arrhythmias and pulmonary edema, compared with about 2% for other valvular disease. Patients with severe symptomatic aortic stenosis require valve replacement or rarely percutaneous valvuloplasty (if not a candidate for replacement) before elective, noncardiac operations with general, epidural, or spinal anesthesia.

Mitral stenosis increases the risk of perioperative atrial fibrillation. Preoperative administration of digoxin or β-blockers may slow the ventricular rate if atrial fibrillation occurs. Tachycardia increases the risk of postoperative congestive heart failure in patients with mitral stenosis because of reduced diastolic filling. Patients with severe mitral stenosis should have balloon valvuloplasty or valve repair before elective noncardiac surgery. For mitral and aortic regurgitation, risk of noncardiac surgery depends on the degree of left ventricular volume overload and decompensation. Well-compensated lesions are associated with minimally increased risk. Patients with moderate to severe regurgitation should have invasive hemodynamic monitoring and cautious afterload reduction if surgery cannot be delayed. Patients with moderate to severe aortic regurgitation are extremely sensitive to bradycardia and vasodilation. Valve replacement should be considered in patients with functional class III or IV valvular disease.

Patients with valvular heart disease undergoing procedures that produce transient bacteremia are at risk for bacterial endocarditis. Clean operations—such as orthopedic, ophthalmologic, and plastic surgical procedures—do not require antibiotics to prevent endocarditis. Antibiotic prophylaxis should be given to patients with disease of their native valves; hypertrophic cardiomyopathy; atrial septal defect (primum only); most congenital cardiac malformations; prosthetic valves; and with a history of previous bacterial endocarditis. For patients with mitral valve prolapse, prophylaxis is not recommended without documented regurgitant flow.

Perioperative management of patients on chronic anticoagulant therapy depends on the indication. Patients who should have minimal interruption of anticoagulation include those with mechanical prosthetic valves in the mitral position, dialysis patients whose shunts have previously clotted, and patients with demonstrated risk of embolization. While warfarin is being discontinued, full-dose heparin therapy can be used preoperatively, stopped 6 to 12 hours before surgery, and then restarted postoperatively when risk of surgical rebleeding is acceptably low. For other patients, including those with prosthetic aortic valves, discontinuation of warfarin (3 or 4 days preoperatively to several days postoperatively) without heparinization is reasonable.

Hypertension. Although hypertension is a risk factor for coronary artery disease, moderate hypertension is not an independent risk factor for perioperative cardiac complications. Although it is preferable that patients be normotensive, diastolic blood pressures less than 110 mm Hg may not be associated with greater operative risk. Further, rapid manipulation of blood pressure during the week before surgery, especially with diuretic-induced changes in volume status, may increase the likelihood of intraoperative lability in blood pressure. Exceptions are patients with ischemic heart disease or congestive heart failure, in whom the increased afterload combined with anesthetic-induced myocardial depression may increase the risk of ischemia or left ventricular dysfunction. Patients with diastolic blood pressures greater than 110 mm Hg are at increased risk and should have better control before surgery.

In hypertensive patients, intraoperative blood pressure is labile regardless of the degree of control preoperatively. Antihypertensive therapy should be continued through the perioperative period. Options for patients who are NPO status include parenteral methyldopa, hydralazine, β-blockers, enalapril, nitroprusside, and sublingual nifedipine or transdermal clonidine. A patient taking diuretics should have a serum potassium level measured preoperatively; if it is less than 3 mEq/L (3.5 mEq/L for patients on digoxin), elective procedures should be delayed for potassium repletion.

Pulmonary Risk Factors

Anesthesia and Surgical Site. The risk of postoperative pulmonary complications such as atelectasis or pneumonia depends on the duration of the procedure, the type of operation performed, the presence and severity of preexisting lung disease, and the presence of other risk factors. Asthma, chronic obstructive pulmonary disease (COPD), restrictive lung disease, pulmonary hypertension, hypercarbia, active lung infection, large volume airway secretions, smoking, and obesity increase the risk of pulmonary complications after surgery. Restrictive lung disease increases operative risk less than chronic obstructive disease and cor pulmonale, which markedly increase risk. Although the administration of anesthetic is associated with changes in pulmonary physiology, most physiologic changes that occur after surgery are related not to the anesthetic agent but to the procedure and the immobilization required for administration of anesthesia and surgery.

Administration of general anesthesic is associated with a fall in the functional residual capacity (FRC), increased airway secretions, decreased mucociliary clearance, and a decreased cough reflex. The decline in FRC resolves after recovery from anesthesia in patients who do not have abdominal or thoracic surgery. Although spinal anesthesia has little or no direct effect on pulmonary function, the overall rate of postoperative pulmonary complications is no different with spinal anesthesia compared with general anesthesia. A number of studies have demonstrated a correlation between the duration of the surgical procedure and the rate of postoperative complications. Procedures lasting longer than 2 hours have higher postoperative complication rates.

Procedures adjacent to the diaphragm, such as thoracic and upper abdominal surgery, are associated with the highest risk of pulmonary complications. Lower abdominal procedures have a lower complication rate, and peripheral procedures are associated with the least risk. Abdominal and thoracic procedures are associated with persistent decreases in FRC, vital capacity, tidal volume, residual volume, and sigh frequency. The decreases in these parameters are secondary, in part, to the supine position required for surgery and prolonged immobility that occurs in the perioperative period. Postoperative pain, narcotic medications, and diaphragmatic dysfunction that occurs after these procedures also contribute to these physiologic changes. Narcotic medications decrease cough and sigh frequency. As the FRC, or lung volume remaining at the end of a normal exhalation, declines and approaches the volume at which dependent airways collapse (closing volume), the collapse of alveoli leads to microatelectasis and macroatelectasis. Areas of atelectasis cause ventilation/perfusion mismatch and decreased arterial oxygenation. Patients with abnormalities that are associated with elevated closing volumes or depression of FRC are more likely to develop postoperative atelectasis and hypoxemia. Patients with asthma and chronic obstructive pulmonary disease (COPD) are likely to have elevated closing volumes. Obesity, neuromuscular disorders, skeletal abnormalities, and restrictive lung diseases are associated with depressed FRC.

Aspiration of gastric contents occurs in 7% to 16% of patients undergoing general anesthesia. Nasogastric tubes; autonomic dysfunction (e.g., diabetes); drugs that relax the lower esophageal sphincter; pregnancy; and emergency operations increase the risk of aspiration. Neutralization of gastric acid with H2-receptor blocking agents or antacids reduces the morbidity of aspiration. Aspiration of food or other particulate matter increases the morbidity of aspiration; at-risk patients should therefore be maintained without food by mouth until the risk of aspiration diminishes.

Nearly one half of patients undergoing abdominal procedures develop small pleural effusions within 3 days of operation. The effusion usually occurs on the side of surgery and resolves within 3 to 4 days.

Infection. Acute upper and lower respiratory tract infections increase the risk of postoperative atelectasis and pneumonia. Elective procedures should be delayed until acute infections have resolved.

Asthma. Poorly controlled asthmatic patients have an increased incidence of postoperative pulmonary complications. Patients with asthma may have increased airway obstruction during the perioperative period, partly related to the irritant effect of dehumidified, highly oxygenated inspired air, increased airway secretions, aspiration, administration of mast cell degranulating drugs, or spinal anesthesia above T6. High spinal anesthesia (above T6) may result in the blockade of bronchial efferent sympathetic input, leading to unopposed bronchial vagal stimulation and bronchospasm. Preoperative preparation should focus on the optimization of the patient's pulmonary function, as judged by an objective measurement of air flow, and by physical examination. Forced expiratory volume in one second (FEV_1), or peak expiratory flow rate, should be at or near baseline. Ideally, wheezing should be absent at induction. Patients with asthma who are at baseline can be maintained on their usual medication regimen through the operative period. There is evidence, however, to suggest that treatment with a 3- to 7-day course of systemic oral corticosteroids combined with perioperative IV hydrocortisone reduces the incidence of postoperative bronchospasm. Patients with bronchospasm preoperatively may also benefit from a course of corticosteroids along with more intensive therapy with inhaled β-adrenergic agonists and antibiotic treatment of bacterial respiratory infections. Several studies have demonstrated a low rate of steroid-related complications (e.g., adrenocortical insufficiency, postoperative infection, delayed wound healing) in asthmatic patients treated perioperatively with corticosteroids.

Chronic Obstructive Pulmonary Disease. Operative risk depends on the extent of underlying functional pulmonary impairment and the type of procedure. Unfortunately, pulmonary function tests and arterial blood gas analysis only approximately correlate with the likelihood of pulmonary complications. Maximum voluntary ventilation, FEV_1, and $Paco_2$ are the more reliable predictors of outcome. Roughly, risk of pulmonary complications is low when FEV_1 is greater than 2.0 liters, moderate for FEV_1 of 1.0 to 2.0 liters, and high with FEV_1 less than 1.0 liter. Hypercarbia, more than hypoxemia, identifies patients who may be difficult to wean from mechanical ventilation.

No single spirometric test accurately predicts complications. Further, critical appraisal of the evidence about spirometry's predictive value indicates that it is a poor screening test. Rather than being obtained routinely, preoperative spirometry should be used to define clinically apparent lung disease that has not been previously characterized, to determine if there is a bronchodilator response, when hypercarbia is suspected, or to assess other factors important to clinical decisions. Patients should not be denied potentially high-benefit surgery on the basis of marginal pulmonary function alone. With very careful management, many such patients can do well. Lung resection is a special situation, and risk assessment requires more sophisticated tests and the guidance of pulmonary specialists.

Prophylaxis of Pulmonary Complications. Ceasing cigarette smoking is recommended, but airway secretions may actually increase in the first few days after cessation. The necessary period of abstinence to reduce complications is not clear but appears to be about 2 months. For reversible airway disease, aerosolized bronchodilators and corticosteroids should be the primary therapy. If the patient has a purulent cough, antibiotics in the week before surgery may be helpful. Postoperatively, lung expansion maneuvers have been demonstrated to reduce complication rates. The maneuvers include deep breathing techniques, in which the patient takes 5 sequential deep breaths, holding each breath for 5 seconds and repeating the sequence every hour. Incentive spirometers can facilitate deep breathing techniques by documenting inhaled volume. Lung expansion maneuvers should be continued for 3 to 4 days after surgery. Continuous positive airway pressure (CPAP) is also effective in improving FRC postoperatively and may be particularly useful in high-risk patients who are unable or unwilling to perform voluntary lung expansion maneuvers.

Prevention of Thromboembolism. Clinical risk factors for postoperative deep venous thrombosis (DVT) are shown in Box 369-1.

Certain general surgical procedures, including abdominal or pelvic cancer surgery and prostatectomy, and certain orthopedic surgeries, including total knee and hip replacement surgery and hip fracture repair surgery, are associated with a very high risk of DVT. In any individual patient, risk factors may be multiple and are cumulative. For those patients at low risk for postoperative DVT (uncomplicated surgery of less than 30 minutes duration in patients younger than 40 years with no clinical risk factors), no specific preventive measures are necessary other than encouraging early ambulation. However, graduated compression elastic stockings may also be useful in this group of patients. For moderate risk patients (older than 40 years with no other clinical risk factors, undergoing major general surgical procedure of greater than 30 minutes duration), subcutaneous, low-dose, unfractionated heparin (LDUH) at 5000 units 2 hours before surgery followed by 5000 units every 12 hours or intermittent pneumatic compression (IPC), applied during the operation if possible, is recommended. For high-risk patients (older than 40 years with additional clinical risk factors, undergoing major general surgical procedures of greater than 30 minutes duration), subcutaneous LDUH (every 8 hours) or subcutaneous, fixed-dose, low-molecular-weight heparin (LMWH), beginning immediately postprocedure is recommended. Intermittent pneumatic compression is an alternative choice for prophylaxis in patients at risk for wound complication. For very-high-risk general surgery (patients with multiple DVT risk factors undergoing high-risk procedures such as prostatectomy or abdominal or pelvic cancer surgery), either (1) LDUH or LMWH used in combination with IPC, or (2) low-intensity warfarin (target INR, 2.0 to 3.0) is an effective prevention strategy.

There are several orthopedic and neurosurgical procedures associated with a very high risk of proximal DVT and pulmonary embolus that deserve special mention. All patients undergoing major orthopedic surgery of the lower limb (hip or knee replacement or repair of a hip fracture) should receive some form of prophylaxis. For elective hip replacement surgery, low-intensity warfarin, twice-daily subcutaneous LMWH, and adjusted subcutaneous LDUH (maintaining partial thromboplastin time [PTT] in the upper range of normal) are effective prophylactic regimens. For patients undergoing hip fracture surgery, low-intensity warfarin or LMWH is effective; either regimen should be started preoperatively, as soon as the patient is clinically stable. For both hip replacement and hip fracture surgery, combining

---

BOX 369-1

**Clinical risk factors for postoperative
venous thromboembolism**

Venous stasis
  Venous insufficiency
  Congestive heart failure
  Obesity
Age greater than 40 years
Prolonged immobilization
Paralysis
Hypercoagulable states
  Antithrombin III deficiency
  Protein C resistance or deficiency
  Protein S deficiency
  Plasminogen and plasminogen activation abnormalities
  Antiphospholipid antibodies
  Lupus inhibitor
  Hyperviscosity syndromes
  Myeloproliferative disorders
  Nephrotic syndrome
Previous deep venous thrombosis (DVT)
Cancer
Pregnancy
Myocardial infarction
Stroke
High-dose estrogen use
Fractures
  Pelvic
  Hip
  Leg
Multiple trauma
Spinal cord injury
Type of surgery
  Major general surgery (>30 to 60 min)
Orthopedic surgery
  Hip fracture repair
  Hip arthroplasty
  Knee arthroplasty
Prostatectomy

IPC with anticoagulant-based regimen may provide additional benefit. For total knee replacement surgery, postoperative LMWH or IPC is effective and should be continued postoperatively for at least 7 to 10 days regardless of hospital length of stay; the two in combination may be of benefit in patients with multiple clinical risk factors. For patients undergoing elective intracranial neurosurgery, IPC with or without elastic stockings is recommended. LDUH is an acceptable alternative therapy and, in combination with IPC, may be more effective than IPC or LDUH alone. Recommendations for prevention of venous thromboembolism are summarized in Table 369-4.

Prophylaxis with either LDUH or LMWH appears to be associated with no significant increase in the rate of major perioperative bleeding, although wound hematomas are more frequent. When anticoagulant therapy is contraindicated, intermittent pneumatic compression with or without graduated compression elastic stockings is generally effective. Intermittent pneumatic compression stockings should not be used in patients with significant lower extremity peripheral vascular disease or if there is a possibility of deep venous thrombosis in the lower limb. Placement of an inferior vena cava filter may also be considered in very-high-risk patients.

Hematologic Risk Factors

Most patients with mild to moderate anemia (hemoglobin level of 8 gm/dl to 10 gm/dl) without cardiac or pulmonary disease do not require transfusion before major surgery unless significant blood loss (more than 500 ml) is expected. Patients with significant cardiopulmonary disease affecting cardiac output and/or oxygen saturation (e.g., chronic obstructive pulmonary disease, congestive heart failure) should, in general, have a hemoglobin level greater than 10 gm/dl at

the time of surgery. Likewise, patients undergoing procedures in which blood loss is expected to be greater than 500 ml (e.g., aortobifemoral bypass, abdominal aortic aneurysm repair, internal fixation of a hip fracture) should have a hemoglobin greater than 10 gm/dl at the time of surgery. The benefits of homologous red cell transfusion (improved oxygen delivery to tissues and organs) must be weighed against the risks, including the transmission of infection and the occurrence of transfusion reactions.

A platelet count greater than 50,000/μl is adequate for patients undergoing most surgical procedures, although platelet counts greater than 100,000/μl are preferable for cardiac and central nervous system procedures. Minor surgery not involving the airway or blood vessels is usually safe with 30,000 platelets per microliter. Patients with dysfunctional platelets, regardless of the total count, may have a higher incidence of perioperative hemostatic complications. Ticlopidine and aspirin should be avoided for 1 to 2 weeks before noncardiac surgery. Other nonsteroidal antiinflammatory drugs that inhibit platelet function can be stopped 1 to 2 days before surgery.

Endocrine Risk Factors

The stress of anesthesia and surgery increases insulin and corticosteroid requirements. Diabetic patients have a higher incidence of postoperative wound and genitourinary infections, which may increase insulin requirements. Conversely, surgical resolution of infection, sepsis, and shock reduces postoperative insulin requirements.

Perioperative insulin requirements depend on the degree of glucose control and type of therapy before surgery. Oral hypoglycemic agents should be discontinued the day of surgery. In patients whose fasting serum glucose values are below 200 mg per deciliter, perioperative insulin is generally not required. Insulin-dependent diabetics and non–insulin-dependent diabetics with poor control need perioperative insulin. Several regimens are effective: (1) half the usual morning dose of insulin before surgery; (2) one third the usual daily dose of insulin before surgery and one third after; or (3) continuous infusion of 8 to 10 units of regular insulin in 5% glucose solution. Patients receiving supplemental insulin should have intravenous glucose until oral intake is adequate. Postoperatively, serum glucose should be checked regularly to guide insulin dosage.

Inability to meet perioperative requirements for corticosteroids may lead to adrenal crisis. Patients receiving adrenal-suppressing doses of steroids for a period of 1 week or more during the previous year, those currently taking corticosteroids, or those with a suspect pituitary-adrenal axis should receive supplemental corticosteroids perioperatively. If time allows, cortrosyn stimulation testing can be performed before surgery to determine adrenal function and the need for perioperative steroid administration. In cases of maximum stress, adequate replacement is hydrocortisone 100 mg intravenously or intramuscularly at midnight before surgery, the morning of surgery, and then every 6 to 8 hours for 24 hours or until postoperative complications resolve. Replacement should then be tapered over several days.

Hypothyroidism increases sensitivity to sedative and anesthetic agents and impairs ventricular function, ability to excrete a free water load, and ventilatory response to $PaCO_2$. However, available evidence suggests that mild to moderate hypothyroidism usually does not significantly increase surgical risk. When feasible, it is probably prudent to delay elective operations until replacement therapy is adequate. An important exception may be patients with angina undergoing coronary artery bypass surgery; risk of ischemia may increase with full thyroid replacement. Close attention should be paid to postoperative respiratory and volume status and serum sodium concentration.

Hyperthyroid patients undergoing surgery are at increased risk of thyroid storm. Elective operations should be delayed until the patient is euthyroid. For emergent or urgent operations, propranolol usually controls cardiovascular manifestations of hyperthyroidism and prevents thyroid storm.

Gastrointestinal and Hepatic Risk Factors

Anesthetic agents generally reduce blood flow to the liver and enhance the risk of surgery in patients with liver disease. Morbidity usually results from postoperative gastrointestinal bleeding, hepatic en-

Table 369-4 Perioperative prevention of venous thromboembolism (VTE)

	LOW RISK	MODERATE RISK	HIGH RISK	VERY HIGH RISK— GENERAL SURGERY	VERY HIGH RISK—ORTHOPEDIC SURGERY
Procedure	Minor surgery (<30 minutes) or ambulatory surgery	Major surgery (30 to 60 minutes)	Major surgery (>30 to 60 minutes)	Major surgery (>30 to 60 minutes)	Major surgery (>30 to 60 minutes)
Patient	<40 years old No clinical risk factors	>40 years old No clinical risk factors	>40 years old Additional risk factors or MI	>40 years old Risk factor of prior VTE, malignancy, CVA, or spinal cord injury	>40 years old Planned hip fracture repair, total hip or total knee arthroplasty
Recommendations	Early ambulation	LDUH (5000 U sq 2 hours preoperatively and q 12 hours postoperatively) **or** Graded compression elastic stockings **or** IPC	LDUH (5000 U sq q 8 hours) **or** LMWH **or** IPC	LDUH or LMWH **and** IPC	*Total hip and hip fracture:* LMWH **or** Low-intensity oral anticoagulation (INR 2.0 to 3.0 started preoperatively or immediately postoperatively). May consider IPC as adjuvant therapy. *Total knee* LMWH **or** IPC

CVA, Cerebrovascular accident; *IPC,* intermittent pneumatic compression; *INR,* international normalized ratio; *LDUH,* low-dose unfractionated heparin; *LMWH,* low-molecular-weight heparin; *MI,* myocardial infarction.

cephalopathy, acute renal failure, and infection. The operative mortality associated with acute liver disease is difficult to separate from the prognosis of the disease itself. Acute viral hepatitis, for example, has a 9% overall operative mortality, whereas 85% of patients with acute fulminant hepatic failure die after surgery. Alcoholic hepatitis also increases operative risk. Acute hepatitis is a relative contraindication to surgery, but the degree of risk is not well quantitated. The usual recommendation is to delay elective procedures until liver function tests have remained normal for 1 month.

Most data about operative risk of chronic liver disease come from patients undergoing portosystemic shunting procedures. Serum bilirubin greater than 10 mg per deciliter, albumin less than 3 g per deciliter, prothrombin time greater than 4 seconds above control, poorly controlled ascites, encephalopathy, and poor nutritional status are associated with increased risk of operative complications and death.

Perioperative management of patients with liver disease includes meticulous attention to fluids, electrolytes, and the dosage of hepatically metabolized drugs, plus preoperative lactulose or neomycin to decrease risk of encephalopathy in those with poor prognostic indicators or history of encephalopathy. Hypoglycemia and hypokalemia are more likely with nasogastric suctioning and decreased oral intake.

Peptic ulcer disease, gastritis, and reflux esophagitis can be exacerbated by stress of surgery and nasogastric tubes. The incidence of upper gastrointestinal bleeding can be reduced with H_2-receptor antagonists or hourly administration of antacids. Preoperative parenteral hyperalimentation should be considered for patients with malnutrition (e.g., inflammatory bowel disease, malabsorption syndrome) to improve wound healing and reduce postoperative infection, but the large Veterans Affairs Cooperative Trial did not find it to be effective in reducing complications in all patients.

Renal Risk Factors

Patients undergoing surgery generally have a small risk (about 1%) of developing acute renal failure (ARF) during the operative or postoperative period. However, the mortality associated with perioperative ARF is high, ranging from 10% in patients with isolated renal failure to greater than 90% in patients with multiorgan system failure. Surgery and anesthesia induce hemodynamic and hormonal changes that alter effective renal perfusion, which in turn may predispose patients to renal injury. Patients undergoing surgery may also be exposed to nephrotoxic agents such as radiocontrast material, nephrotoxic drugs, or high levels of myoglobin, increasing their risk for ARF. Finally, patients are at increased risk during the perioperative period of developing ARF from postrenal obstruction, resulting from either bladder dysfunction (e.g., following the administration of anticholinergic agents) or, less commonly, bilateral ureteral obstruction. Patients with prostate enlargement or neuropathy that affects bladder function are particularly predisposed to obstructive uropathy with anticholinergic medications. Bilateral ureteral obstruction may be caused by traumatic retroperitoneal hematoma, increased intraabdominal pressure, or inadvertent surgical ureteral ligation.

The most common cause of ARF in the surgical setting is acute tubular necrosis (ATN). Prolonged intraoperative hypotension is the strongest predictor of ARF after general surgical procedures. Contrast nephropathy may occur after vascular surgery because of the necessity for preoperative angiography and the high prevalence of elderly patients with chronic renal insufficiency who undergo vascular procedures. Contrast nephropathy is uncommon in patients with normal renal function but occurs in as many as 50% of patients with both diabetes and chronic renal insufficiency. The evaluation of ARF is the same in the operative and nonoperative setting.

Patients at high risk for perioperative ARF include those with underlying chronic renal insufficiency; prerenal states (including congestive heart failure, the nephrotic syndrome, and cirrhosis); and jaundice, as well as the elderly. Patients with the nephrotic syndrome are more susceptible to infection and vascular thrombosis, in addition to being at risk for ARF. Diabetes has been associated with an increased incidence of postoperative ARF in some studies. Operative procedures associated with a higher risk of ARF include aortic surgeries, coronary artery bypass graft surgery, and valve replacement surgery.

Patients at risk for perioperative acute renal failure should be managed with particular attention to maintenance of renal perfusion and euvolemia, as well as careful use or avoidance of agents that can cause toxic or obstructive nephropathies. Patients with mild to moderate chronic renal impairment generally have no increased operative morbidity provided that volume depletion and nephrotoxic drugs are avoided or drug dosage is appropriately modified and potassium administration is monitored. A timed creatinine clearance should be obtained before surgery in elderly patients so that the glomerular filtration rate (GFR) can be accurately estimated. Medication doses can then be appropriately adjusted for the GFR. Patients undergoing high-risk surgeries require increased vigilance regarding volume status; patients undergoing aortic or cardiac surgery may benefit from invasive hemodynamic monitoring to maintain optimal cardiac output and volume status. These patients also benefit from minimization of suprarenal cross-clamping and cardiopulmonary bypass times.

Patients with severe renal failure on chronic dialysis have only a 2% to 4% mortality for major elective surgery, but operative morbidity approaches 60%. The primary causes of death in these patients are sepsis and cardiac arrhythmias or dysfunction. Incidence of hyperkalemia, shunt or fistula thrombosis, pneumonia, wound infection, postoperative hypoventilation, pulmonary edema, and bleeding complications is increased. Maintaining serum potassium below 5 mEq per liter, replenishing bicarbonate stores, and controlling hypertension appear to reduce surgical risk. Dialysis within 24 hours of surgery is generally safe and may reduce the postoperative rise in serum potassium. A hematocrit of 20% to 30% is usually well tolerated. If transfusion is required, washed cells should be considered because of reduced potassium load.

BIBLIOGRAPHY

ACC/AHA Task Force: Guidelines for electrocardiography: A report of the American College of Cardiology/American Heart Association Task Force on Assessment of Diagnostic and Therapeutic Cardiac Procedures (Committee on Electrocardiography), *JACC* 19:473-481, 1992.

ACC/AHA Task Force: Guidelines for perioperative cardiovascular evaluation for noncardiac surgery, *JACC* 27(4):910-948, 1996.

Appleby J, Lawrence VA: Anesthesia: a review for the internist, *JGIM* 9:635-647, 1994.

Ashton CM et al: The incidence of perioperative myocardial infarction in men undergoing noncardiac surgery, *Ann Intern Med* 118:504-510, 1993.

Calandri C, Rand JH: Preoperative evaluation of hematologic status, *Mt Sinai J Med* 58(1):41-47, 1991.

Charlson ME et al: Surveillance for postoperative myocardial infarction after noncardiac operations, *Surgery, Gynecology, and Obstetrics* 167:407-414, 1988.

Clagett CP et al: Prevention of venous thromboembolism, *Chest* 108:312S-314S, 1995.

Hayden SP et al: Postoperative pulmonary complications: risk assessment, prevention, and treatment, *Cleve Clin J Med* 62(6):401-407, 1995.

Kabalin CS et al: Low complication rate of corticosteroid-treated asthmatics undergoing surgical procedures, *Arch Intern Med* 155:1379-1384, 1995.

Kellerman PS: Perioperative care of the renal patient, *Arch Intern Med* 154:1674-1688, 1994.

Klein JT, Rosen MJ: Preoperative evaluation of pulmonary status, *Mt Sinai J Med* 58:37-40, 1991.

Lawrence VA, Page CP, Harris GD: Preoperative spirometry before abdominal operations: a critical appraisal of its predictive value, *Arch Intern Med* 149:280-285, 1989.

Levine MN et al: Prevention of deep vein thrombosis after elective hip surgery: a randomized trial comparing low-molecular-weight heparin with standard unfractionated heparin, *Ann Intern Med* 114:545-551, 1991.

Lubin MF, Walker HD, Smith RB, editors: *Medical management of the surgical patient*, ed 3, Philadelphia, 1995, Lippincott.

MacPherson DS, Snow R, Lofgren RR: Preoperative screening: value of previous tests, *Ann Intern Med* 113:969-973, 1990.

Mangano DT, Goldman L: Preoperative assessment of patients with known or suspected coronary artery disease, *N Engl J Med* 333:1750-1756, 1995.

Mason JJ et al: The role of coronary angiography and coronary revscularization before noncardiac vascular surgery, *JAMA* 273(24):1919-1925, 1995.

Merli GJ, Weitz HH, editors: *Medical management of the surgical patient*, Philadelphia, 1992, Saunders.

Office of Medical Applications of Research, National Institutes of Health: Perioperative red blood cell transfusion, *JAMA* 260(18):2700-2703, 1988.

Veterans Affairs Total Parenteral Nutrition Cooperative Study Group: Perioperative total parenteral nutrition in surgical patients, *N Engl J Med* 325:525-532, 1991.

Zibrak JD et al: Indications for preoperative pulmonary function testing, *Ann Intern Med* 112:763-771, 1990.

Zibrak JD, O'Donnell CR: Indications for preoperative pulmonary function testing, *Clin Chest Med* 14:227-236, 1993.

CHAPTER

370 Prevention and Control of Injuries

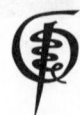

Arthur L. Kellerman

Throughout history, physicians have focused their efforts on diagnosis and treatment of disease. At least as many lives can be saved through prevention. Child and adult immunization, smoking cessation, promotion of healthy lifestyles, and screening for treatable conditions have contributed to a dramatic decline in deaths from many communicable and noncommunicable diseases. Comparable benefits can be achieved by preventing deaths from injury as well.

Injuries are the fourth leading cause of death in the United States. In contrast to heart disease, cancer, and stroke, which generally afflict older individuals, injuries disproportionately strike children and young adults. As a result, injuries account for more years of potential life lost before age 65 than all causes of cancer and all causes of heart disease *combined*. Each year, one out of every four Americans is injured seriously enough to require medical attention. Annual lifetime costs of injury (direct and indirect) are estimated to exceed $265 billion.

Injuries aren't "accidents." Epidemiologic research has demonstrated that injuries, like diseases, affect identifiable high-risk groups, follow an often predictable chain of events, and are therefore preventable. When an injury occurs, optimal provision of emergency care can save lives that would otherwise be lost. Rehabilitation can reduce the incidence of long-term disability. The combination of these strategies—prevention, acute care, and rehabilitation—has come to be termed *injury control*.

Energy is the etiologic agent of injury. Every time someone drives a car, hammers a nail, or irons a shirt, energy is harnessed to accomplish a task. As long as the demands of the task are exceeded by our capacity for control, work can be accomplished at little or no risk. If, however, the demands of the task momentarily exceed an individual's capacity (for example, a car hits a patch of ice) or an individual's capacity to control falls below the demands of the task (as a result of distraction, boredom, fatigue, or intoxication), an uncontrolled release of energy may occur.

If this energy is transferred to the victim, or *host*, at a rate or amount that exceeds the body's ability to tolerate it without damage, an injury will occur. In most cases, energy is transferred through an inanimate object, or *vehicle*. Examples include a speeding car, a hot iron, or a bullet. The severity of an injury and the consequences that follow can also be influenced by the *environment* in which it occurs. A crash into a concrete bridge pier is more devastating than a crash into an energy-absorbing barrier.

William Haddon was the first to apply the public health concepts of agent, host, vehicle, and environment to analyze and prevent injuries. His work formed the scientific basis for the field of injury control. Haddon also identified ten generic strategies to prevent or control injuries by breaking the chain of causation at various points (Box 370-1). Use of this list to identify the best strategy (or combination of strategies) to prevent or control a particular type of injury is known as *options analysis*.

Before Haddon's landmark work, injury prevention was confined to "safety training." Little effort was expended on correcting hazardous products or environments. In the 1950s, millions of federal highway dollars were spent on ineffective efforts to fix "the nut behind the wheel." Little progress was made until regulatory efforts were shifted towards improving motor vehicle design (e.g., safety belts, energy-absorbing interiors) and building safer roads (e.g., divided highway lanes, breakaway light poles).

Public education became more effective as well. Instead of promoting vague and complex concepts such as "drive safely," educators began to promote simple, concrete acts, such as "buckle up for safety." Over the next 30 years the collective impact of these efforts led to a marked reduction in the rate of death from motor vehicle crashes (Table 370-1).

Table 370-1 Haddon matrix (interventions to control motor vehicle–related injuries)

	PHASE		
FACTOR	**PREEVENT**	**EVENT**	**POSTEVENT**
Host	Driver education Alcohol and drug avoidance Fatigue avoidance Impaired vision or hearing correction	Physical conditioning Osteoporosis treatment	First aid training
Vehicle	Antilock brakes Motor vehicle inspection	Tempered glass Safety belts Air bags	Flame-retardant fabric Puncture-resistant gas tanks
Environment	Divided highways Pedestrian overpasses Speed limits	Breakaway poles Impact-absorbing barriers	Emergency number: 911 Trauma care systems Regional rehabilitation centers

---

BOX 370-1
Options analysis for injury prevention and control

1. Prevent creation of the hazard
2. Reduce the amount of hazard
3. Prevent the release of a hazard that already exists
4. Modify the rate or distribution of the release of the hazard from its source
5. Separate, by time or space, the hazard from that which is to be protected
6. Physically separate the hazard from that which is to be protected by barriers
7. Modify surfaces and basic structures to minimize injury
8. Make that which is to be protected more resistant to damage
9. Begin to counter damage already done
10. Stabilize, repair, and rehabilitate the injured person

Modified from Haddon W: The changing approach to the epidemiology, prevention, and amelioration of trauma: the transition to approaches etiologically rather than descriptively based, *Am J Pub Health* 58:1431, 1968.

PROMOTING INJURY CONTROL

Efforts to prevent injuries can be grouped into two broad categories. *Active countermeasures* require the conscious cooperation of individuals to be effective. Examples include use of manual safety belts, motorcycle helmets, and child safety seats. *Passive countermeasures* work automatically, without the conscious cooperation of the user. Examples include automatic safety belts, air bags, sprinkler systems, and the "kill switch" on many lawn mowers. Because passive countermeasures exert their protective effects at all times, they are generally more effective than active countermeasures. Manual safety belts decrease the risk of death or serious injury in a frontal collision by 45% to 55%, but they must be buckled to be effective. Air bags deploy virtually 100% of the time.

EDUCATION

Although the array of interventions to prevent injuries is broader than it once was, education remains the foundation of many injury prevention programs. Public education programs (such as driver education, child-pedestrian training, and bicycle rodeos) are popular and relatively easy to implement. Most rely on the premise that people change their behavior when they realize that doing so can reduce their risk of injury.

Unfortunately, education is not a particularly effective way to achieve sustained behavior change in populations. An evaluation of a $78 million federal "alcohol safety action program" showed that it failed to reduce alcohol-related fatalities in the target population. In another evaluation the impact of saturation advertising to promote use of safety belts was studied in a city served by two cable television systems. One system aired more than 1000 high-quality promotional spots. The other aired none. No difference was noted in subsequent rates of safety belt use among subscribers to either system.

Others have achieved more encouraging results. A comprehensive bicycle helmet promotion program increased rates of helmet use among children in Seattle, Washington. Education about fire safety coupled with distribution of smoke detectors led to a sharp decrease in residential fire deaths in Oklahoma City, Oklahoma.

The impact of public education is blunted by *attenuation of effect*. No matter how powerful a safety message may be, some people never encounter it. Some who see or hear the message actively reject it. Among those who believe the message, some are not sufficiently motivated to change their behavior. Among those who are, some fail to follow the message consistently or lapse back into old habits. Young males (the group at highest risk for serious injury) are particularly resistant to behavioral change.

Despite these limitations, education remains a key element of efforts to prevent injuries. Doctor-patient communication has been shown to be an important motivator for behavior change, and this can be used to promote appropriate injury prevention behaviors, such as use of helmets and safety belts. Education is also necessary to build support for more intrusive measures, such as safety legislation and product safety regulations.

ENFORCEMENT

When education is not enough to change behavior, compliance can be enhanced by adding the force of law. The impact of "mandatory use" laws can be impressive. Child safety seat legislation in Michigan reduced serious injuries to child occupants of motor vehicles by 25%. Imposition of a national 55-mph speed limit saved between 2000 and 4000 lives each year it was in effect. Raising the minimum age to purchase alcoholic beverages in 26 states decreased fatal nighttime crashes by an average of 13%.

Safety legislation can be strengthened by public education and effective law enforcement. In Elmira, New York, publicity and enforcement of the state's mandatory safety belt law increased rates of use from 49% to 77%. When belt use decreased 4 months later, a reminder campaign boosted rates to 80%.

Mandatory use laws are effective, but they are difficult to enact. Voters generally support measures to limit the dangerous actions of others (such as drunk-driving laws) but they are less willing to support laws that limit their own actions. Some consider any kind of safety legislation an infringement of "personal freedom."

Political backlash can lead to repeal of effective laws. Despite overwhelming evidence that motorcycle helmets save lives, 26 states repealed their mandatory motorcycle helmet laws when federal incentives were relaxed in 1976. Crash fatality rates in these states promptly increased an average of 40%. Arguments about personal freedom are offset by the realization that the victim is not the only one who suffers loss from a serious or fatal injury. In the final analysis, everyone bears the social and financial cost of preventable injuries.

ENGINEERING

When feasible, building a safer product or modifying a dangerous environment is usually the best option of all. Engineering safer products and environments can be costly, but it is often quite effective. It is generally simpler to design a safer product or roadway than to teach millions of people how to safely use a dangerous one.

For example, consider the problem of deaths and injuries from residential fires. Many occur when a smoldering cigarette is left on bedding or upholstery. Young children and the elderly face the highest risk of death because of their impaired mobility. Education about the dangers of smoking in bed has little impact. Installing a smoke detector, on the other hand, can cut household risk of death in half. Unfortunately, many people fail to check their smoke detector regularly to keep it in working order. Finally, large numbers of residential fires could be prevented if cigarette manufacturers modified their product to reduce its potential to start fires. This option is technically feasible, but it is opposed by the tobacco industry.

When manufacturers resist making needed changes to their products, it is sometimes possible to compel them to make changes through regulatory action. Many changes in automobile design have occurred as a result of federal regulations. Unfortunately, product safety laws are difficult to enact. Opponents argue that it raises the price of products and makes it difficult for manufacturers to compete. When legislative efforts fail, product liability lawsuits may be the only way to force an industry to modify a particularly hazardous product.

PRACTICING INJURY CONTROL

Physicians do not need training in epidemiology or public health to practice injury control. Many countermeasures can be promoted at the bedside or in an office setting (Box 370-2). Highly effective programs can be designed and implemented at the local level.

BOX 370-2

Physician counseling for injury prevention and control: adolescents and adults

---

Adolescents **should be periodically advised to**
1. Use safety belts every time you drive or ride in a motor vehicle*
2. Don't drink when driving a motorized vehicle or boating*
3. Wear a helmet every time you ride a bike or motorcycle, roller skate, or use in-line skates*

Adults **should be periodically advised to**
1. Use safety belts when operating or riding in a motor vehicle*
2. Don't drink when driving a motorized vehicle or boating*
3. Avoid alcohol when using motorized tools or a firearm†
4. Wear a safety helmet while riding a bicycle or motorcycle, or while skating†
5. Wear a mouth guard when playing a contact sport†
6. Install and maintain smoke detectors in your residence†
7. Keep any firearms stored in a locked container; store ammunition separately†
8. Be aware of safety rules and any hazards at your work site†

Older adults and caregivers **should be periodically advised to**
1. Inspect the home for adequate lighting†
2. Remove or correct tripping hazards, such as loose rugs, extension cords, and slick floor surfaces†
3. Install handrails and traction strips in stairways and bathtubs†
4. Reduce home water heater temperature to 120° F†
5. Encourage older adults without medical contraindications to exercise†

Modified from Department of Health & Human Services, Public Health Service, Office of Disease Prevention & Health Promotion: *Clinician's handbook of preventive services: put prevention into practice,* Washington, DC, 1994, U.S. Government Printing Office.
*Required in most states.
†Voluntary.

Step One: Define the Problem

Various sources of information can be used to define the scope of injuries in a community. Each has advantages and disadvantages. Vital statistics can reveal leading causes of injury-related death, but they do not provide information about nonfatal injuries. Hospital records and trauma registries contain useful information about serious nonfatal injuries, but neither source provides population-based data.

Injuries that are treated on an outpatient basis are often dismissed as minor, but they can result in significant long-term disability. This is particularly true for head, back, and hand injuries. Patients who visit a hospital emergency department with injury may be at increased risk for recurrent injury, especially if the index visit was precipitated by alcohol, drug use, or violence. Efforts to identify and intervene in such cases are justified.

Many hospitals assign an international classification of disease (ICD) "E-code" (external cause of injury code) to document the cause of every injury-related hospitalization. E-coding can substantially enhance community-based injury surveillance. Several states mandate E-coding of all hospital admissions, but only two code emergency department visits. Some injuries are easier to classify than others. Studies have shown, for example, that many victims of domestic violence are reluctant or afraid to report the true nature of their injuries.

Step Two: Identify Causes and Risk Factors

Once a particular type of injury has been identified as a priority, further research may be needed to identify factors that increase or decrease a victim's risk of injury. It is particularly important to determine *who* is being injured, *what* kind of injuries are involved, *when* they occur, *where* they occur, and, most important, *why* they occur.

Step Three: Develop and Test Interventions

Once a problem has been identified and its associated risk factors are understood, a variety of countermeasures can be considered. Options analysis (see earlier discussion and Box 370-1) is useful at this step. Careful attention must be given to the characteristics of the target population, the feasibility of the countermeasure, its acceptability to the target population, and its cost. If it is unclear which of several strategies is best, small-scale pilot programs may be useful to assess their impact. The most promising one can then be selected for full-scale implementation.

Most successful programs establish benchmarks and use them to measure their progress toward explicitly stated goals. For example, a program to prevent deaths and injuries from residential fires could measure program *structure* (e.g., number of staff hired or cooperative agreements signed), *process* (number of pamphlets distributed, home visits made, and smoke detectors installed), and *outcome* (number or rate of fire deaths, number or rate of hospital admissions resulting from burns and/or smoke inhalation).

Step Four: Implement Effective Interventions and Document Impact

If a program works, its effectiveness should be documented. Several years ago, researchers at the Harborview Injury Prevention and Research Center determined that bicycle riders who were injured in crashes were much less likely to sustain a serious head injury if they were wearing a helmet at the time of their crash. This observation sparked a nationwide effort to promote bicycle helmets. It also encouraged a small but growing number of states to enact mandatory bicycle helmet laws for children.

THE ROLE OF THE PHYSICIAN IN INJURY CONTROL

Physicians can save lives, reduce disability, and decrease health care costs by incorporating injury control into their daily practice. This can be accomplished in any of four ways.

Patient Education

Efforts to prevent and control injuries need not be implemented on a grand scale. In many age-groups the risk of death from injury is at least as great as the risk of death from disease. Injury prevention education should be incorporated into routine clinical practice (Box 370-2).

Emergency department and office visits for treatment of minor injuries are "teachable moments" that are ideal for promoting the value of injury prevention. In addition to treating the wound, the physician should identify and correct any factors that contributed to the injury. For example, an adult who has sustained a minor injury in a low-velocity motor vehicle crash should get a stern lecture about wearing his safety belt. An elderly woman who has fallen should be given instructions on how she might reduce her risk of falls in the future.

Data Collection and Program Evaluation

Prevention of illness and injury will become increasingly important in the future. As the principal focus of care shifts from the inpatient to the outpatient setting, data will be needed to monitor system performance, identify high-risk groups, and evaluate the impact of programs.

Research

Much can be learned from community-based epidemiologic research. High priority should be placed on studies of drug- and alcohol-impaired driving, firearm-related injuries, domestic violence, residential fires, drowning, and falls in the elderly. A portion of the funds for any intervention should be set aside for program evaluation. This is the only way to determine what works and what doesn't.

Advocacy

Physicians can accomplish a great deal by participating in the legislative process. Doctors make credible witnesses, and their testimony can positively influence local officials, state legislators, and federal officials. A pediatrician in Tennessee helped his state enact the nation's first child safety seat law. Joining forces with community-based organizations and other health care professionals is usually more effective than working alone. Physician leadership can play a key role in bringing groups together.

BIBLIOGRAPHY

Baker SP et al: *Injury fact book,* ed 2, New York, 1992, Oxford University Press.
Committee on Trauma Research: *Injury in America: a continuing public health problem,* Washington, DC, 1985, National Academy Press.
Department of Health and Human Services, Public Health Service, Office of Disease Prevention and Health Promotion: *Clinician's handbook of preventive services: put prevention into practice,* Washington, DC, 1994, U.S. Government Printing Office.
Haddon W: Advances in the epidemiology of injuries as a basis for public policy, *Public Health Rep* 95:411-421, 1980.
National Committee for Injury Prevention and Control: Injury prevention: meeting the challenge, *Am J Prev Med* (suppl), New York, 1989, Oxford University Press.
Rice DP et al: *Cost of injury in the United States: a report of Congress,* San Francisco, 1989, Institute for Health and Aging, University of California and Injury Prevention Center, Johns Hopkins University.
Rivasa FP, Grossman DC, Cummings P: Injury Prevention, *N Engl J Med* 337:543-548, 613-618, 1997.
Rosenberg M, Fenley MA: *Violence in America: a public health approach,* New York, 1991, Oxford University Press.
Waller J: *Injury control: a guide to the causes and prevention of trauma,* Lexington, Mass, 1985, Lexington Books.

CHAPTER

371 Women's Health

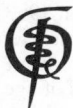

Jeane Ann Grisso, Michelle Berlin, Margo J. Krasnoff, and Anne W. Moulton

The heightened interest in women's health over the past decade has resulted in a number of efforts to improve the provision of health care services to women. In spite of promising developments in clinical care, the knowledge base underlying health care for women remains comparatively weak. Knowledge gaps in women's health are particularly striking for those women at highest risk of ill health: members of racial and ethnic minorities, elderly women, and those living in poverty. A number of national initiatives have begun to address the knowledge gap, including the creation of the Office on Women's Health within the Office of the Secretary for Health and Human Services, the Office of Research on Women's Health at the National Institutes of Health, and other women's health offices and programs at the Centers for Disease Control and Prevention, the Food and Drug Administration, and the Agency for Health Care Policy and Research and the Health Resources and Services Administration. As a result, the number of studies including women subjects has increased substantially, as have efforts to promote research on women's health issues. However, efforts to describe and promote women's health have tended to focus on diseases that are unique to or more prevalent in women, rather than on conditions that account for the greatest burden of mortality and morbidity in women.

OVERVIEW OF WOMEN'S HEALTH

As important as the medical aspects of pregnancy are (Chapter 372), the major causes of death and morbidity for women are not related to diseases that are reproductive in nature or that are unique to women. For example, the leading causes of death among women are similar to those among men. In addition, women in the United States constitute diverse populations whose health status varies greatly. Mortality rates are greater for black women compared with white women for every leading cause of death (Table 371-1). Black women are twice as likely to die from stroke, three times as likely to die from compli-

Table 371-1 Age-adjusted death rates for leading causes of death in U.S. women in 1993

CAUSE OF DEATH	WHITE WOMEN	BLACK WOMEN
All causes	367.7	578.8
Diseases of heart	99.2	165.3
Lung cancer	27.6	27.3
Injuries (unintentional, homicide, suicide)	24.2	35.6
Cerebrovascular diseases	22.7	39.9
Breast cancer	21.2	27.1
Chronic obstructive pulmonary diseases	17.8	12.2
Colorectal cancer	10.5	15.2
Pneumonia and influenza	10.4	13.5
Diabetes mellitus	10.0	26.9
Chronic liver disease and cirrhosis	4.6	6.6
Nephritis, nephrotic syndrome, and nephrosis	3.2	9.2
Septicemia	3.2	7.8
Human immunodeficiency virus infection	1.9	17.3

From the Centers for Disease Control and Prevention, National Center for Health Statistics: *Vital statistics rates in the United States, 1940-1960,* DHEW Pub. No. (PHS) 1677, Public Health Service, Washington, DC, 1968, U.S. Government Printing Office; *Vital statistics of the United States, vol 2, mortality, part A, for data years 1960-1993,* Washington, DC, Public Health Service. Data computed by the Division of Health and Utilization Analysis from data compiled by the Division of Vital Statistics. Death Rates per 100,000 virulent female population in that racial group.

cations of diabetes, and ten times as likely to die from complications of acquired immunodeficiency syndrome (AIDS).

The rates of illness and causes of death also vary by age. Among women 25 to 44 years of age, injuries (including unintentional, homicide, and suicide) are the leading cause of death. The homicide rate for women in this age-group reached a record high in 1993 and was five times greater among black women than among white women. For women ages 45 to 64 the leading causes of death are heart disease, lung cancer, and breast cancer. For women 65 years of age and older, heart disease constitutes 37% of all deaths, followed by lung cancer, chronic obstructive pulmonary disease, and stroke.

Demographic and economic shifts in the United States have had major effects on the health of American women. For example, 72% of persons 85 years of age and older are women, and the number of persons in this age-group is expected to double by the year 2020. Women make up 75% of residents in nursing homes, and the majority of community-dwelling elderly women live alone. Poverty is another major cause of illness and disability among women. Poverty has increased dramatically, especially among women of color. A major cause is change in the structure of the family. In 1950, 90% of children were born to married couples. In the 1990s, about 50% of children are born to single mothers, the majority of whom live in poverty. Overall, working women still earn 30% less than men, and they tend to have jobs that are demanding and highly stressful and over which they exercise little control. Moreover, women are still the primary child rearers, housekeepers, and caregivers of elderly parents; 14 million women in the United States have no medical insurance.

Another problem primarily affecting women in the United States is the fragmentation of primary care, since a woman often sees two different specialists for primary care, an internist and a gynecologist. Women may be less satisfied with their health care than men are. A recent survey showed that 40% of women had changed physicians because of dissatisfaction, 17% reported that their symptoms had been "trivialized" by a physician, and 30% reported being "talked down to" by a physician.

Four aspects of women's health are of particular importance to internists. Violence against women is a major public health problem that is unrecognized, particularly among internists. Internists should be competent in counseling and prescribing contraception in the context of their routine practices. Menopause is a normal life transition for women that is both biologic and social, with important health consequences. Finally, cardiovascular disease is the leading cause of death in women, and knowledge in recent years has greatly expanded regarding the unique characteristics of heart disease in women.

VIOLENCE AGAINST WOMEN

Violence against women was not discussed for many years in the medical community; in the last two decades there has been significant research to determine the prevalence and the medical consequences of this problem. Medical practitioners treating adult women will see primarily victims of domestic violence (also known as *intimate partner abuse* or *battering*) and patients who have experienced sexual and/or physical abuse while children. One of the most commonly accepted definitions of domestic violence is acts of physical violence perpetrated against women by current or former intimate partners, whether spousal or cohabiting. Using this definition, at least 30% of women in the general population have experienced some domestic violence, and 9% of women in the general population have experienced severe abuse. These acts carry a high likelihood of physical injury and include kicking, biting, hitting, choking, beating, threatening with a knife or gun, or using a knife or gun.

Domestic Violence

Domestic violence includes not only physical injury, but also behaviors used by one partner to maintain power and control over the other. These behaviors include threats and intimidation, progressive social isolation, emotional and psychologic torment leading to low self-esteem, sexual abuse, economic control, and threatening to harm a woman's children. Domestic violence can be found in heterosexual, as well as in male and female homosexual, relationships.

The ability to screen, recognize, and treat the manifestations of

---

> ### BOX 371-1
> ### Interviewing strategies for domestic violence
>
> - Are you in a relationship in which you have been physically hurt or threatened by your partner?
> - Are you in a relationship in which you felt you were treated badly? In what ways?
> - Has your partner ever destroyed things that you cared about?
> - Has your partner ever threatened or abused your children?
> - Has your partner ever forced you to have sex when you didn't want to? Does he ever force you to engage in sex that makes you feel uncomfortable?
> - We all fight at home. What happens when you and your partner fight or disagree?
> - Do you ever feel afraid of your partner?
> - Has your partner ever prevented you from leaving the house, seeing friends, getting a job, or continuing your education?
> - You mentioned that your partner uses drugs/alcohol. How does he act when he is drinking or on drugs? Is he ever verbally or physically abusive?
> - Do you have guns in your home? Has your partner ever threatened to use them when he was angry?

From Flitcraft A et al: *Diagnostic and treatment guidelines on domestic violence,* Chicago, 1992, American Medical Association.

---

domestic violence has been advocated as a core competency for those who care for women. Multiple studies of primary care and specialty practices have demonstrated that the prevalence of domestic violence among patients reflects that of the general population. McCauley and colleagues surveyed 1952 female community-based primary care patients in Baltimore through an anonymous waiting room questionnaire. One of every twenty women had experienced domestic violence in the last year; one of every five had experienced violence as an adult; and one of every three women had experienced violence as either a child or an adult. As widespread as the prevalence of violence is in this sample, it likely underrepresents the magnitude of the problem because of the strict definition of abuse used (physical violence or coerced sexual activities, excluding solely verbal abuse) and the use of a written questionnaire compared to a personal interview.

Three demographic features were most associated with abuse: age less than 36 years, separated or divorced status, and insurance coverage by medical assistance or no insurance. Compared to the patients who were not currently being abused, those currently abused experienced more physical symptoms and higher levels of depression, anxiety, and somatization. They were more likely to have been abusing alcohol or street drugs, to have lower levels of self-esteem, to have higher numbers of prior suicide attempts, and to have used an emergency department in the last 6 months. Physicians should screen female patients about domestic violence, in particular, with women presenting with multiple somatic symptoms or emotional distress. In addition, abuse must be considered in any woman who presents with an injury. The major clues with injuries are that the woman's explanation of how the injury occurred does not seem plausible, and that there has been a delay in seeking medical care. Because 23% of pregnant women experience domestic violence, all women who present for prenatal care should be screened for domestic violence. When a health care provider identifies domestic violence, inquiry about sexual assault should be undertaken as well.

Box 371-1 lists general recommendations concerning how to inquire about abuse. If a patient discloses abuse, physicians should include this in their documentation, determine the seriousness of this problem, and emphasize the need to link the patient with community resources that can address safety, advocacy, and support. Because the most dangerous time for a battered woman is when she decides to leave her abuser, the patient needs to develop an individualized safety plan. A skilled social worker or battered women's advocate can assist. Legal requirements vary; physicians should be aware of the state laws and the services available in their communities.

BOX 371-2
Factors suggesting a history of abuse

Psychologic issues
Difficulties in establishing trust
Difficulties in maintaining control
Helplessness and dependency
Feelings of shame and guilt

Medical disorders
Chronic pain
Severe constipation (especially pelvic-floor dyssynergia)
Eating disorders (bulimia nervosa, anorexia nervosa)
Unexplained vomiting
Sexual dysfunction

Psychiatric disorders
Somatoform disorders (somatization, conversion, hypochondriasis)
Dissociation disorders, including multiple-personality disorder
Posttraumatic stress disorder
Severe depression and panic disorder

Illness-related behaviors
Disability disproportionate to the clinical data
Attempts to validate disease and denial that psychologic factors may play a role
Placement of responsibility for health care with physician
Avoidance of health-promoting behaviors
Difficulty with procedures (rectal or vaginal examination, endoscopy)
Borderline behaviors (intense attachments, difficulty in dealing with uncertainties, demanding behaviors)

Unwanted outcomes
Multiple diagnostic procedures, treatments, and surgeries
Substance abuse (alcohol, medications, illegal drugs)
Disability and litigation seeking
Frequent and excessive use of health care services

Modified from Drossman DA et al: Sexual and physical abuse and gastrointestinal illness: review and recommendations, *Ann Intern Med* 123:782-794, 1995.

Child Sexual Abuse

In the Baltimore primary care survey, 22% of the women indicated that they had been physically or sexually abused before 18 years of age. Child sexual abuse can vary significantly in the frequency and severity of the sexual activity. It most commonly involves multiple sexual contacts that escalate over time. The onset of incest is usually before puberty, with an average duration of 4 years. Health care providers who care for adults can reasonably expect to treat survivors of childhood abuse whose symptoms may be related directly to their abuse. Those who have studied the consequences of abuse in female children have noted gastrointestinal and genitourinary symptoms among the most prominent physical manifestations following the assault. Common relationships between the abuse history and physical and psychologic conditions are listed in Box 371-2.

In contrast to domestic violence, for which routine screening has been advocated, inquiry about childhood abuse has been advised when the clinical data are suggestive and when the information will enhance the patient's outcome. The great majority of patients who have disclosed childhood abuse to their physicians have indicated that the opportunity to discuss the events was beneficial or at least not harmful. For some, however, breaking the silence can be highly stressful and anxiety provoking. If the patient discloses abuse, the physician can refer her (or him) to a qualified mental health professional for further psychologic assessment and therapy. When the patient denies a history of abuse but the nonverbal response is incongruous, the physician should continue to offer nonjudgmental support.

Once a history of abuse has been revealed, the physician should recognize that, for many survivors, issues of control over their bodies are very important. Examinations and procedures should be explained in detail. Routine parts of the physical examination, such as

Table 371-2   First-year failure rates of contraceptive methods, United States

Method	PERCENTAGE OF WOMEN WITH PREGNANCY IN FIRST YEAR OF USE	
	TYPICAL USE	**PERFECT USE**
Method		
No method	85	85
Withdrawal	19	4
Periodic abstinence	20	1-9
Topical agents		
Spermicides	21	6
Sponge	18-36	9-26
Barrier methods		
Condom		
Female	21	5
Male	12	3
Diaphragm with spermicide	18	6
IUDs		
Progesterone T	2	1.5
Copper T 380A	0.8	0.6
Hormonal agents		
Depo-Provera	0.3	0.3
Norplant	0.09	0.09
Birth control pills	3	
Progesterone only	—	0.5
Combination	—	0.1
Sterilization		
Female	0.4	0.4
Male	0.15	0.1

Modified from Hatcher RA et al: *Contraceptive technology reference #27*, New York, 1994, Irvington Publishers, Inc., pp. 113-114.

examination of the breasts and pelvic and rectal examinations might be particularly stressful for the patient, particularly if these were parts of the body involved in the abuse. Allowing the patient to control the pace of the examination sometimes helps to reduce fear. Mild sedation and collaboration with her psychotherapist may be required for the patient to undergo more invasive procedures such as a breast biopsy or colposcopy. Though it is beyond the scope of this chapter, physicians should be familiar with the symptoms of posttraumatic stress disorder in those who have survived childhood abuse, as well as those who are currently in an abusive relationship.

CONTRACEPTION

In the 1990 data collected by the National Center for Health Statistics, 59% of the 58 million reproductive-aged women (defined as ages 15 to 44) in the United States used a contraceptive method. Thus approximately 35 million U.S. women utilize contraception. The most popular forms of contraception employed by U.S. women are female sterilization (18%), birth control pill (17%), male condom (11%), and male sterilization (8%), followed by diaphragm (1.7%) and intrauterine device (IUD) (0.8%). The uses and failure rates of these methods are reviewed in Table 371-2.

Surgical Sterilization

Surgical sterilization remains the most popular method of permanent contraception. Female sterilization is effected by ligation or mechanical occlusion of the fallopian tubes; it can be performed during hospitalization for childbirth or as an outpatient procedure. The major benefits of this method are its relative safety, reliability, permanence, and lack of dependence on partner compliance. The major risks are that a surgical procedure is required, it must be considered permanent (i.e., it is not reliably reversible), and it provides no protection against sexually transmitted diseases. Vasectomy is an appropriate alternative for many couples. This procedure is simply and rapidly performed and is very effective and permanent. Although some concern has been raised about the possibility of an increased rate of prostate cancer among men who have undergone vasectomy, the data remain conflicting, with insufficient information available to recommend against this procedure.

Hormonal Contraception

Several types of hormonal contraception exist. The most common type of oral contraceptive is the combination pill, containing both estrogen and progesterone derivatives. Its major mechanism of action is the prevention of ovulation, with concomitant changes in the endometrial lining that discourage implantation. Although the pill is convenient, reversible, and reliable, it does not protect against sexually transmitted diseases (STDs), including human immunodeficiency virus (HIV).

Questions concerning safety and side effects have rendered "the pill" one of the most thoroughly studied medications ever devised. Early concerns centered around cardiovascular events among women taking the pill (i.e., thromboembolic events, myocardial infarction). However, with the current "low-dose" pills (containing generally 35 μg or less of estrogen), the risks of thromboembolic and cardiovascular events are low. A recurrent concern has been a possible association between the pill and breast cancer. An extensive reanalysis of the majority of the worldwide data indicates that women currently taking the pill, and for up to 10 years after stopping the pill, have a slight but real increased risk of having breast cancer detected (1.24 versus 1.07). However, for women who ceased taking the pill 10 or more years previously, no excess risk of breast cancer is found. Those cancers found among women who had taken the pill were more likely to be localized than those found among women who had never taken the pill. The overall message is that pill use does not appear to confer long-term risks of breast cancer. The Cancer and Steroid Hormone Study (CASH study) confirmed that the pill decreases the risk of endometrial and ovarian cancer, especially among women of low parity who are at highest risk of both forms of carcinomas, and that this decreased risk persisted long after pill use stopped. Pill use also decreases the risk of severe pelvic inflammatory disease, reduces dysmenorrhea, and decreases menstrual blood loss. Some pill-users note increased mood changes, including depression, whereas others do not. The previously noted increase of hepatocellular adenoma is much reduced with the current low-dose formulations.

Progesterone-only contraceptives exist in three forms in the United States: oral "mini-pill," injectable Depo-Provera, and implantable Norplant (a progesterone-containing IUD is discussed later). All three are thought to inhibit ovulation and alter cervical mucus such that sperm are inhibited. Although all three forms provide good contraceptive efficacy, each has particular advantages and disadvantages concerning administration and ease of reversibility. Norplant, for example, is excellent for women who have difficulty remembering to take pills daily or have difficulty returning for injections periodically; although it is quickly reversible, removal of the implants is occasionally difficult. Women using Depo-Provera are more likely to develop amenorrhea than Norplant users; although Depo-Provera does not require surgical insertion, the injections need to be repeated approximately every 12 weeks and reversal of contraception may take 6 months. And, like the combination pill, these agents do not provide protection against STDs.

Intrauterine Device

The intrauterine device is quite effective and, in the right patients, is quite safe. Although its mechanism of action remains indeterminate, it is a good choice for monogamous, parous women desiring a long-acting and reversible form of contraception. It does not provide protection against STDs acquired with sexual activity (in addition, a transient increased risk of pelvic inflammatory disease [PID] at the time of insertion may occur as a result of the insertion process and may increase dysmenorrhea among some patients).

Barrier Contraception

Barrier methods of contraception, including condoms (both male and female) and the diaphragm, offer protection against STDs as well as contraception. Condoms remain a very popular form of contraception and, particularly with respect to HIV, are effective in preventing the acquisition of STDs. The diaphragm, when correctly used with an appropriate spermicidal agent, provides excellent protection against STDs. A difficulty with these methods is the need to utilize them correctly each time and every time intercourse occurs. With male condoms, for example, true breakage does not occur frequently with vaginal intercourse, but slippage (i.e., the condom slipping partially or completely from the penis) can occur.

Topical Agents

Topical agents have an important role in providing protection against STDs as well as contraception. Contraceptive foams, jellies, and suppositories, as well as the contraceptive sponge, have the advantages of easy availability and portability. As with the barrier methods, topical agents must be used with each episode of intercourse. Nonoxynol 9, the active ingredient in these contraceptives, is an effective agent against STDs including HIV; however, some individuals develop irritation or allergy with frequent use.

MENOPAUSE
Epidemiology

Life expectancy for women is gradually increasing and is now estimated to be approximately 78 years. Thus, for most women, up to one third of their total life span occurs after menopause. The average age at menopause is approximately 51, although the range is about 42 to 58. The only consistently identified predictor of age at menopause is smoking history: women who smoke undergo menopause an average of 2 years earlier than nonsmokers.

Physiology

Menopause is traditionally defined as a permanent cessation of menses for 12 months and a follicle-stimulating hormone (FSH) level >40 mIU/ml. The hormonal changes leading up to menopause occur over a 5- to 10-year period and are referred to as the perimenopausal transition. They include changes in ovarian sex steroid biosynthesis and pituitary gonadotropin secretion. After menopause the only functioning component of the postmenopausal ovary is the stroma, the site of androgen production. Although testosterone levels do not change after menopause, androstenedione levels decrease by approximately 50%. The postmenopausal ovary appears to make little or no estrogen, and circulating estrogen in postmenopausal women is derived primarily from peripheral conversion of androstenedione and testosterone to estrone.

Clinical Presentation

The earliest clinical finding during the perimenopausal transition for most women is a decrease in cycle length. Although they initially experience short cycles (mean cycle length, 23 days), they may also have long, anovulatory cycles that are interspersed with the shorter cycle. The most common symptom of menopause is the vasomotor flush. Approximately 75% of women going through natural menopause experience flushes, and as many as 90% of women who have surgical menopause have them, but limited data suggest that there may be significant cultural variation. The hot flush describes the subjective feeling of warmth that precedes any physiologically measurable change and is characterized by visible redness of the chest, neck, and face, usually followed by sweating in the same distribution. Nocturnal hot flushes are more common than daytime hot flushes and have been associated with disturbances in sleep patterns. Many perimenopausal and postmenopausal women experience insomnia-related symptoms that can result in fatigue, irritability, and, in some cases, depression. Estrogen treatment of these symptomatic women results in improved sleep latency and an increased percentage of rapid eye movement (REM) sleep. Hot flushes are treated very successfully by hormone replacement therapy. Other treatment alternatives include clonidine at 0.1 mg twice daily, medroxyprogesterone acetate at 10 mg daily, and β-blockers. A variety of nonpharmacologic methods for minimizing hot flashes (often suggested by patients) include avoidance of factors known to precipitate hot flashes: stress, hot weather, warm rooms, hot drinks, alcohol, caffeine, and spicy foods. Paced respirations, deep breathing, and other biofeedback relaxation techniques have also been helpful.

Genitourinary atrophy occurs 3 to 5 years after the cessation of menses. The vagina and outer third of the urethra are estrogen-responsive tissues, and many patients experience vaginal dryness, dyspareunia, and urinary symptoms secondary to estrogen withdrawal. Most of the genitourinary symptoms respond to hormone replacement therapy (HRT). Women who are not otherwise receiving hormone replacement therapy usually respond well to vaginal estrogen. Other modalities of treatment include vaginal lubrication with over-the-counter products.

Preventive Issues

In addition to the symptoms associated with menopause, there are two chronic conditions that are affected by menopause: osteoporosis and ischemic heart disease, which must be factored into decisions about HRT. An increased risk of osteoporosis is related to an accelerated decrease in bone mass in the years following menopause. There is no abrupt change in cardiovascular risk as a woman goes through menopause, but her risk starts to climb substantially in the 10 to 15 years after menopause. Substantially more women die of heart disease than of breast cancer.

Approach to the Woman at Menopause

Although most of the existing literature on menopause focuses on the use of hormone replacement therapy, there are other important issues to consider in the treatment of postmenopausal women. Menopause offers a convenient time for examining health maintenance and preventive measures in women who may not have previously seen an internist. The changes in cholesterol occur with declining estrogen levels, and cholesterol screening should probably be conducted annually. Usually a nonfasting high-density lipoprotein (HDL) and total cholesterol level is acceptable. Counseling about calcium intake of 1000 to 1500 mg of calcium daily and regular weight-bearing exercise is particularly important for women at midlife for prevention of osteoporosis. A review of cancer-screening guidelines for women ages 50 and above is helpful, including mammography, Pap smears, and screening for colorectal cancer.

A discussion of hormone replacement therapy should be initiated with every menopausal woman, with the knowledge that most of the studies to date are observational and have been performed primarily using white women. The two most popular regimens include cyclic estrogen with progestin and combined continuous estrogen and progestin. The cyclic regimen consists of 0.625 mg of conjugated estrogen and 5 mg of medroxyprogesterone acetate on days 1 through 12 of the month. The continuous regimen, which is much more suitable for older women who have an atrophic endometrial lining, consists of daily use of 0.625 mg per day of conjugated estrogen and 2.5 mg per day of medroxyprogesterone acetate. The latter regimen can be associated with unpredictable vaginal bleeding in women 6 to 12 months after initiation of therapy, whereas women on the cyclic regimen will experience normal periods for several years. The nationally funded Women's Health Initiative, a randomized double-blind placebo-controlled trial of HRT looking at cardiovascular disease end-points as well as breast cancer and colon cancer, is not expected to yield data for 10 to 15 years. For women who have had a hysterectomy or who have heart disease or a strong family history of heart disease, HRT is probably indicated. Contraindications to hormonal therapy include known or suspected breast or uterine cancer, active liver disease, or active thrombophlebitis or thromboembolic disorders. Relative contraindications include chronic hepatic dysfunction and a strong family history of breast cancer.

CORONARY DISEASE RISK FACTORS, AND DIAGNOSIS

Coronary artery disease (CAD) is the number one cause of death in women above the age of 40. There are approximately 250,000 coronary deaths per year in women (of which 100,000 are premature). Compared to those for white women, rates of CAD are higher in black women and lower in Hispanic and Asian women. There is increasing evidence that CAD is different in women with respect to the role of risk factors, clinical presentation, and diagnosis.

Risk Factors

Traditional cardiac risk factors do have predictive value in women, but the magnitude of the effect of these risk factors is different for women than for men. There are also unique risk factors and, thus, preventive strategies for women. Diabetes is probably the most important risk factor because it essentially eliminates any female advantage over men for the development of CAD. Hypertension is an important CAD risk factor in women because it is so prevalent, occurring in 20% of white women and 40% of black women. It is particularly prevalent in women as they age, occurring in more than 60% of white women and more than 75% of black women over the age of 65. Most of the literature on serum lipids has been done on males. However, pooled data on women suggest that for women younger than 65, there is an increased CAD risk associated with elevated total and low-density lipoprotein (LDL) cholesterol and low HDL cholesterol. For women older than 65, only low HDL cholesterol is associated with increased risk for coronary heart disease (CHD). Data in minority women are less conclusive. Smoking remains an important risk factor for CAD in women and probably the most important risk factor for CAD in premenopausal women. Obesity is a risk factor for CAD in women but not in men, and this risk persists even after controlling for associated risk factors such as hypertension, diabetes, and elevated cholesterol. Higher rates of CAD are observed in upper-body or truncal obesity versus lower-body or hip distribution ("apple" versus "pear" configuration). Family history of CAD is an independent risk factor for CAD in women, with a similar effect regardless of whether the affected parent is male or female. Information on the current lower-dose oral contraceptive pills suggest they are not associated with an increased CAD risk.

The slower progression of atherosclerosis for women than for men has been attributed to the beneficial effects of estrogen through several mechanisms. Only 25% to 50% of the beneficial effect of estrogen is actually mediated through improvement in serum lipids. Other postulated mechanisms include estrogen's activity on estrogen receptors in endothelial and smooth muscle cells to reduce the impact on endothelial functions, as well as clotting at those sites. For natural menopause the risk of heart disease increases slowly with the decline of serum estrogen levels. In contrast, both early menopause and early surgical menopause are associated with an increased risk of CAD. There have been more than 20 epidemiologic studies on the use of hormone replacement therapy (in most cases, estrogen alone) and the risk of developing CAD, and the majority have shown a risk reduction of about 50%. The long-term effect of the addition of progesterone (which is essential for a woman who still has a uterus) is less clear. The recent short-term *prospective estrogen and progesterone intervention trial* (PEPI trial) suggests that current hormone replacement therapy regimens (HRT) that include progesterone only partially diminish the beneficial effects of estrogen on lipids.

Finally, there are psychosocial factors that appear to have an impact on the development of CAD in women (even after controlling for other cardiac risk factors), including lower educational level, lower socioeconomic status, type of occupation (especially those that involve high levels of responsibility with little control), multiple social roles, loss of social support, suppressed anger, and depression.

Differences in Clinical Manifestations of CAD in Women

Chest pain is more common in women than in men, and, except in older women, nonischemic causes of chest pain predominate, including variant (vasospastic) and microvascular angina, several gastrointestinal causes, musculoskeletal disease, and psychiatric disease. Of note, chest pain can be a manifestation of the perimenopausal transition, especially in association with palpitations. Overall, the relationship between the type of presenting chest pain and the prevalence of angiographically significant disease is not as strong in women as it is in men. The prevalence of coronary artery disease in men with typical exertional angina is over 80%, in contrast to a prevalence of 58% in women with exertional angina.

Women with CAD are more likely to present with angina than myocardial infarction as their first manifestation of the disease. They are also more likely to have anginal symptoms associated with mental stress, sleep, and rest, in contrast to males, whose symptoms are more likely to be associated with exertion. Women also have more symptoms in addition to chest pain, such as nausea, vomiting, dyspnea, fatigue, and radiation of the pain to the neck and shoulders.

Differences in Evaluation of CAD in Women

It is useful to stratify women into three categories of risk based on risk factors and the quality of the presenting chest pain when considering the appropriate diagnostic procedure (exercise versus pharmacologic stress, echocardiography versus nuclear imaging, etc.) for the additional evaluation of CAD. In women whose likelihood of disease is less than 20% (e.g., young women without risk factors and atypical pain), exercise stress testing is more likely to yield a false-positive result than a true-positive result; all cardiac testing should be avoided and other sources of chest pain should be explored. In women of moderate risk (risk between 20% and 80%) the decision depends on several variables, including the patient's resting electrocardiogram, capacity for exercise, risk factors, and comorbidities. In women of high risk (>80%), most clinicians would favor direct referral to cardiac catheterization.

IMPLICATIONS

A recent report on women and medicine issued by the Council on Graduate Medical Education concludes that physicians have not been well prepared to meet the challenges of women's health. The report recommends that fundamental changes be instituted in the way physicians are educated and health care is delivered. Physicians, particularly internists, can serve a key role in improving health care for women by implementing multidisciplinary approaches, improving patient-provider communication, obtaining skills in office-based gynecology, and learning effective and culturally competent ways to respond to the needs of economically and socially diverse groups of women. Although there has been a rapid rise in awareness of women's health, there remain major gaps in knowledge. Ultimately, the goal of health care professionals is to achieve such progress in approaches and understanding that "women's health" will no longer need to be a separate concern.

BIBLIOGRAPHY

Alpert EJ: Violence in intimate relationships and the practicing internist: new "disease" or new agenda? *Ann Intern Med* 123:774-771, 1995.

Centers for Disease Control and Prevention, National Center for Health Statistics: *Vital statistics rates in the United States, 1940-1960,* Grove RD, Hetzel AM: DHEW Pub. No (PHS) 1677. Public Health Service, Washington, DC, 1968, U.S. Government Printing Office; *Vital statistics of the United States, vol 2, mortality, part A, for data years 1960-93,* Washington, DC, 1995, Public Health Service. Data computed by the Division of Health and Utilization Analysis from data compiled by the Division of Vital Statistics.

Collaborative Group on Hormonal Factors in Breast Cancer: Breast cancer and hormonal contraceptives: collaborative reanalysis of individual data on 53,497 women with breast cancer and 100,239 women without breast cancer from 54 epidemiologic studies, *Lancet* 347:12713-12727, 1996.

Drossman DA et al: Sexual and physical abuse and gastrointestinal illness: review and recommendations, *Ann Intern Med* 123:782-794, 1995.

Flitcraft A et al: *Diagnostic and treatment guidelines on domestic violence,* Chicago, 1992, American Medical Association.

Grady D et al: Hormone therapy to prevent disease and prolong life in postmenopausal women, *Ann Intern Med* 117:1016-1037, 1992.

Greendale GA: The menopause: health implications and clinical management, *J Am Geriatr Soc* 41:426-436, 1993.

Kawachi I, Colditz GA, Hankinson S: Long-term benefits and risks of alternative methods of fertility control in the United States, *Contraception* 50:1-16, 1994.

Peterson LS: *Contraceptive use in the United States, 1982-90: advance data from vital statistics; no 260,* Hyattsville, Md, 1995, National Center for Health Statistics.

U.S. Department of Health and Human Services; Public Health Service Health Resources and Services Administration: *Council on Graduate Medical Education fifth report: Women and medicine; physician education in women's health; women in the physician workforce,* July 1995, pub no HRSA-P-DM-95-1.

372 Medical Disorders During Pregnancy

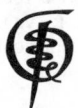

Andrea J. Singer

Although relatively few medical disorders can prevent pregnancy, virtually the entire spectrum of disease can complicate it. This chapter highlights some of the most frequently encountered medical disorders during pregnancy. Others are discussed elsewhere in this text. In each case the unique interaction of medical disease and pregnancy is emphasized. Recommendations for treatment reflect the understanding that management of serious medical disorders frequently requires the use of medications potentially harmful to the fetus. Yet many untreated medical diseases are detrimental to the fetus and jeopardize the health of the mother as well.

ENDOCRINE DISORDERS
Diabetes Mellitus, Type I

Beginning in early gestation, glucose and various gluconeogenic amino acids reach the fetus against a concentration gradient by facilitated diffusion. Since maternal loss of glucose and gluconeogenic substrate to the fetus conspires to cause maternal hypoglycemia, it is often necessary to reduce the total daily insulin dosage during the first trimester.

At approximately 24 weeks' gestation, the so-called diabetogenic stress of pregnancy begins. At this time, basal insulin levels are higher than normal nongravid levels, and eating produces a twofold to threefold greater outpouring of insulin. Increased plasma insulin is opposed by diminished responsiveness to insulin in the periphery. This insulin resistance is thought to result, at least in part, from the contraregulatory hormones—such as human placental lactogen, prolactin, and cortisol—produced by the placenta. Thus in the second half of gestation, insulin requirements predictably increase in women with type I diabetes. In addition, gestational diabetes is most likely to begin at this time.

Major congenital anomalies remain the leading cause of death among infants of diabetic mothers. In insulin-dependent diabetes mellitus (IDDM) pregnancies, poor preconception diabetic control, duration of diabetes of greater than 10 years, and the presence of diabetic vasculopathy have been identified as risk factors for a major congenital anomaly. An IDDM pregnancy carries an especially high risk for neural tube anomalies (19.5 per 1000 versus 2 per 1000 for nondiabetic pregnancies). In addition, there is a fivefold increase in cardiac abnormalities, which include ventricular septal defects, transposition of the great vessels, and coarctation of the aorta. Renal anomalies, including agenesis and ureteral duplication, and gastrointestinal anomalies, such as duodenal atresia and anorectal atresia, are also more common. Prenatal diagnosis of fetal anomalies is aided by tests for potential risk (maternal glycosylated hemoglobin levels); maternal serum α-fetoprotein estimation for neural tube defects; and a fetal anatomic survey by ultrasound at 18 to 20 weeks gestation.

Most, if not all, of the aforementioned anomalies are formed early in gestation, by 8 weeks after the last menstrual period. Furthermore, the teratogenic potential of hyperglycemia has been established by animal and human studies. It is therefore mandatory to initiate diabetes education and optimal blood glucose control before conception to prevent major congenital malformations. A useful marker for this

Table 372-1   O'Sullivan criteria for detecting gestational diabetes (100-g oral glucose tolerance test)

INTERVAL	WHOLE BLOOD* (MG/DL)	PLASMA* (MG/DL)
Fasting	90	105
1 hour	165	190
2 hours	145	165
3 hours	125	145

*Values represent two standard deviations above the mean.

treatment goal is the near normalization of maternal glycosylated hemoglobin concentration before attempting conception. Good metabolic control before conception also reduces the risk of spontaneous abortion to no greater than that of nondiabetic women.

Excessive fetal growth, or macrosomia (birth weight greater than 4500 g), has been the hallmark of a diabetic pregnancy. This altered fetal growth can be explained in part by the fact that maternal hyperglycemia leads to fetal hyperglycemia as glucose passes through the placenta by facilitated diffusion. The fetal response is one of increased insulin production, and insulin is the most important growth hormone in the fetus. Improved maternal glycemic control helps to reduce the incidence of macrosomia, but it does not eliminate it. Other factors may predispose or contribute to fetal macrosomia, including maternal weight, maternal weight gain during pregnancy, parity, and genetic factors.

Gestational Diabetes

Gestational diabetes is defined as carbohydrate intolerance of variable severity with onset during the present pregnancy. The definition applies regardless of whether insulin is used for treatment or the condition persists after pregnancy, but it does not exclude the possibility that glucose intolerance may have antedated the pregnancy.

The American College of Obstetricians and Gynecologists recommends that screening for gestational diabetes be done for women with one or more risk factors, including maternal age of 30 years or greater, family history of diabetes, previous macrosomic infant, previous stillbirth, previous malformed infant, obesity, hypertension, or glycosuria. The American Diabetes Association and the Centers for Disease Control and Prevention recommend screening all pregnant women between the twenty-fourth and twenty-eighth gestational week with a 50-g oral glucose challenge. A plasma glucose value of 140 mg per deciliter or greater 1 hour after a 50-g oral glucose dose indicates the need for a full diagnostic glucose tolerance test. It does not, by itself, establish the diagnosis. Diagnosis is based on results of the 100-g oral glucose tolerance test, interpreted according to the diagnostic criteria of O'Sullivan and Mahan (Table 372-1).

All patients with gestational diabetes are at significant risk for fetal macrosomia with consequent birth trauma, as well as other neonatal complications, including hypoglycemia, hypocalcemia, and hyperbilirubinemia.

All women with gestational diabetes should receive appropriate nutritional and exercise counseling. If dietary management does not consistently maintain the fasting blood glucose concentration below 105 mg per deciliter or the 2 hour postprandial glucose concentration below 120 mg per deciliter, insulin therapy should be initiated. Oral hypoglycemic agents are contraindicated during pregnancy. If insulin is prescribed, human preparations are preferred to minimize antigenicity.

Women who had gestational diabetes should be evaluated at the first postpartum visit by a 2-hour, 75-g glucose tolerance test to detect overt diabetes.

Thyroid Disease

Several special considerations of thyroid dysfunction during pregnancy should be kept in mind. First, signs and symptoms of disordered thyroid function may be mimicked by pregnancy itself. Second, increases in thyroid-binding proteins during pregnancy alter standard thyroid function tests. Third, placental transfer of most thyroid hormones is minimal. Finally, most antithyroid drugs freely cross the placenta and are potentially active in the fetal thyroid.

Profound hypothyroidism is often associated with impaired fertility and is uncommon during pregnancy. On the other hand, mild hypothyroidism is a frequent concomitant illness during pregnancy. Therapy consists of full thyroid hormone replacement. When replacement is adequate, thyroid-stimulating hormone levels return to normal, but this may take up to 8 weeks for maximum effect. There is no evidence to suggest that replacement dosages of thyroid medication suppress fetal thyroid function.

Graves' disease is the major cause of thyrotoxicosis in women of childbearing age and thus in pregnancy. The clinical course of Graves' disease is known to vary during gestation. Thyrotoxicosis often improves during pregnancy and worsens postpartum.

Since radioactive iodide therapy is contraindicated during pregnancy, therapeutic options include antithyroid medications and surgery. Two important points require emphasis before specific treatment of hyperthyroidism is considered. First, mild hyperthyroidism appears to be well tolerated during pregnancy. Second, antithyroid drugs freely cross the placenta and are active against the fetal thyroid.

Both propylthiouracil (PTU) and methimazole have been used successfully during pregnancy. PTU crosses the placenta only about one fourth as well as methimazole and is preferred for use during pregnancy. Propranolol has been used during pregnancy to control severe adrenergic symptoms before antithyroid medications have had sufficient time to take effect. Propranolol does not block production of thyroid hormone. Surgery should be reserved for patients with hypersensitivity to antithyroid drugs, for poorly compliant patients, and for the occasional patient in whom reasonable dosages of antithyroid drugs have been ineffective. Patients with Graves' disease who have undergone thyroidectomy may still have high concentrations of thyroid-stimulating immunoglobulin; consequently, their offspring are vulnerable to neonatal thyrotoxicosis.

Hyperparathyroidism

Primary hyperparathyroidism does not appear to impair fertility, but it is known to result in a high rate of fetal complications such as spontaneous abortions, stillbirths, and neonatal tetany. Maternal hyperparathyroidism causes maternal hypercalcemia, which in turn facilitates increased placental calcium transport. High fetal calcium concentrations suppress the fetal parathyroid so that after delivery the neonate is functionally hypoparathyroid. Deprived of its maternal source of calcium, the neonate becomes vulnerable to tetany in the immediate postpartum period.

Medical therapy for hyperparathyroidism during pregnancy is appropriate only for a short period. Surgical exploration of the neck is the recommended treatment for a pregnant patient with rising serum calcium concentration, worsening symptoms, or hyperparathyroid crisis unresponsive to medical therapy. Many authors believe that the high incidence of maternal and neonatal complications associated with hyperparathyroidism makes surgery the treatment of choice even if the disease is mild. Surgery should ideally be performed during the second trimester.

Pituitary Adenomas

Prolactin-secreting adenomas account for approximately 30% of all pituitary adenomas. Fewer than 7% of patients with intrasellar microadenomas (size less than 10 mm) manifest clinical evidence of tumor expansion during pregnancy. On the other hand, macroadenomas (size greater than 10 mm) are associated with a 17% incidence of complications during pregnancy. Symptoms of headache, visual disturbance, and nausea are the most common. These symptoms tend to occur most frequently during the first trimester and can be mistaken for symptoms of pregnancy.

For patients with microadenomas treated with bromocriptine to achieve pregnancy, the drug should be discontinued as soon as pregnancy is diagnosed. It is generally accepted that periodic measurement of serum prolactin levels are of minimal benefit during pregnancy, since serum prolactin levels do not always rise with pregnancy-induced tumor enlargement. Because of the low incidence of microadenoma growth during pregnancy, it is not necessary to perform routine visual field testing. Routine clinical evaluation with particular attention to symptoms of headache and visual disturbances constitutes prudent follow-up. For patients with known microadenomas who become symptomatic, immediate computed tomography (CT) scanning or magnetic resonance imaging (MRI) is indicated.

For women with macroadenomas confined to the sella, the risk of enlargement during pregnancy is small. For women with larger macroadenomas that have suprasellar extension, there is a 15% to 35% risk of clinically significant tumor enlargement during pregnancy. Patients with suprasellar extension of their tumors should consider transsphenoidal tumor resection before conception. Unfortunately, tumor growth during gestation cannot be predicted by prepregnancy tumor size or serum prolactin concentration. Patients at highest risk include those with neurologic or visual symptoms before pregnancy.

All patients with macroadenomas should have monthly neurologic examinations and visual field tests. As with microadenomas, periodic serum prolactin levels are not helpful. CT scanning or MRI should be performed when tumor growth is clinically suspected. Bromocriptine can be used during pregnancy to decrease tumor size rapidly. In previously symptomatic patients with suprasellar extension, continuation of bromocriptine throughout pregnancy is prudent, since sudden reexpansion of the tumor has been reported. Surgery is rarely necessary.

There is no evidence that breast-feeding causes tumor enlargement. Nevertheless, patients with macroadenomas should be followed closely for symptoms or signs of tumor expansion during breast-feeding.

RENAL DISORDERS

Pregnancy is associated with a variety of anatomic and functional changes of the kidneys and lower urinary tract. Caliceal, pelvic, and ureteral dilatation occurs during the first trimester and persists throughout gestation up to 12 weeks postpartum. Hydronephrosis and hydroureter have direct clinical consequences because urinary stasis contributes to the propensity to develop pyelonephritis in women with asymptomatic bacteriuria.

The most significant alteration in renal function during pregnancy is a progressive increase in the glomerular filtration rate, which begins as early as 2 weeks' gestation. Creatinine and urea production do not increase during pregnancy. Therefore a serum concentration of creatinine and urea considered normal for a nonpregnant woman may be elevated in the gravida and should be investigated.

Acute renal failure during pregnancy most often results from severe preeclampsia or eclampsia. Management of acute renal failure during pregnancy is essentially the same as that for nonpregnant patients (see Chapter 109). Particular attention should be given to fluid and electrolyte balance and adequate nutrition.

Many women with chronic renal disease have diminished fertility. Nevertheless, some patients with moderately severe disease and some who have received renal transplants do conceive. The major determinants of pregnancy outcome in women with chronic renal disease are the presence of hypertension and the severity of pregestational renal insufficiency. The severity of renal insufficiency has a direct effect on the outcome of pregnancy. Pregnancies in women with a pregestational serum creatinine concentration greater than 1.5 mg per deciliter or a creatinine clearance less than 70 to 80 ml per minute are associated with an increase in perinatal mortality and the onset or worsening of hypertension.

HYPERTENSIVE DISORDERS

Hypertension is among the most commonly seen medical disorders of pregnancy. Up to 30% of pregnancies are complicated by hypertension, about half being chronic essential hypertension. Preeclampsia occurs in 5% to 10% of pregnant women. Arterial blood pressure greater than 140 mm Hg systolic and 90 mm Hg diastolic or a rise in blood pressure more than 30 mm Hg systolic and 15 mm Hg diastolic over baseline warrant a diagnosis of hypertension. A useful classification of hypertensive disorders of pregnancy is presented in Box 372-1.

Preeclampsia and Eclampsia

Diagnosis. Preeclampsia is a multiorgan disease unique to pregnancy. The condition is characterized by the development of elevated

---

> ### BOX 372-1
> ### Classification of hypertensive disorders of pregnancy
>
> 1. Preeclampsia, eclampsia
> 2. Chronic hypertension (140/90 mm Hg)
> 3. Chronic hypertension with superimposed preeclampsia or eclampsia
> 4. Late or transient hypertension

> ### BOX 372-2
> ### Signs and symptoms of severe preeclampsia
>
> 1. Blood pressure 160 mm Hg systolic or 110 mm Hg diastolic
> 2. Proteinuria >5 g per 24 hours or 3+ or 4+ proteinuria as determined by dipstick
> 3. Oliguria <400 ml per 24 hours
> 4. Epigastric or right upper quadrant pain
> 5. Abnormal coagulation tests (thrombocytopenia, prolonged partial thromboplastin time (PTT) or prothrombin time (PT), hypofibrinogenemia)
> 6. Elevated liver enzymes
> 7. Pulmonary edema
> 8. Persistent headache, visual disturbance, lethargy, clonus, or other signs of significant central nervous system (CNS) irritability

---

blood pressure, proteinuria, and generalized edema. The condition may also be recognized by visual changes, headache, hyperreflexia, fundoscopic changes, and the presence of hyperuricemia. Eclampsia is the presence of generalized seizures or coma in a patient with preeclampsia. Preeclampsia usually occurs after 20 weeks' gestation and before the seventh postpartum day. The vast majority of women who develop preeclampsia are nulliparous and frequently at the extremes of their childbearing years. Other identified risk factors for preeclampsia include family history of preeclampsia, history of preeclampsia in a previous pregnancy, multiple gestation, and hydatidiform mole. Chronic hypertension and underlying vascular disease increase the likelihood that superimposed preeclampsia will develop. Pregnant women with diastolic blood pressure consistently greater than 75 mm Hg in the second trimester or greater than 85 mm Hg in the third trimester should be observed closely for signs of preeclampsia.

It is clinically useful to separate preeclampsia into mild and severe disease. In most cases the development of severe preeclampsia requires delivery, regardless of gestational age. Box 372-2 lists criteria frequently used to indicate severe disease if any are present. Even in mild disease, careful frequent evaluation is necessary because of the possibility of rapid deterioration and the development of eclampsia. Nearly 25% of eclamptics experience their first seizure with "mild" disease.

A subset of severe preeclamptic patients develop hemolysis (H), elevated liver enzymes (EL), and low platelets (LP), or the "HELLP syndrome." The majority of cases occur between the twenty-seventh and thirty-sixth week of gestation, but approximately one third occur postpartum, with peak laboratory abnormalities on the day or two following delivery. Presenting symptoms in women with the HELLP syndrome include right upper quadrant or epigastric pain, malaise, nausea or vomiting, and headache. Physical examination may reveal right upper quadrant tenderness, edema, and weight gain, but hypertension and proteinuria may be absent. Maternal mortality is about 1% to 3% in tertiary care settings, but rates as high as 25% have been reported in community hospitals. Complications of the HELLP syndrome include disseminated intravascular coagulation, abruptio placenta, acute renal failure, and pulmonary edema.

Pathophysiology. Systemic alteration in vascular endothelial function leading to reduced organ perfusion appears to be the basic pathologic mechanism in preeclampsia. This abnormality is the result of a cascade of events that begins with an abnormal immunologic reaction to placental implantation that prevents trophoblastic invasion of the uterine spiral arteries. The arteries reach only about 40% of the diameter achieved in normal pregnancy, and the placenta, in turn, becomes chronically hypoperfused. This hypoperfusion leads to the elaboration of toxic mediators, which may then cause endothelial dysfunction. The end result is hypoperfusion of vital organs and activation of the clotting cascade.

Management. Early detection, close surveillance, and timely delivery are the requirements for the management of preeclampsia. Delivery is the ultimate cure, and although always appropriate for the mother, it may not be best for the fetus.

Although some experts advocate hospital admission for all preeclamptic patients, reliable women with mild disease who are remote from term may safely be managed as outpatients. Bed rest is a traditional management strategy for hypertension in pregnancy and is generally employed. Although bed rest does help control blood pressure, it does not change maternal or fetal outcome. Neither sodium nor fluid restriction is indicated. Weekly evaluation of kidney, liver, and coagulation function is important. Weekly or twice-weekly antepartum fetal surveillance is required to ensure adequate placental function. Serial ultrasound evaluation of fetal growth is also used. Evidence of significant intrauterine growth retardation is an indication for delivery. If maternal and fetal conditions are stable, delivery near term or with biochemical evidence of fetal lung maturity before 37 weeks is advisable.

Severe preeclampsia or eclampsia requires delivery. Patients should be treated with magnesium sulfate, 4 to 8 grams, given intravenously over 10 to 20 minutes until normal or diminished deep tendon reflexes are achieved. Continuous intravenous administration of magnesium sulfate, 2 to 3 grams per hour, is usually required to maintain diminished reflexes and serum magnesium levels in the therapeutic range of 6 to 8 mEq per liter. Respiratory depression can occur rapidly with intravenous infusion and may be reversed by slow intravenous administration of 10 ml of 10% calcium gluconate. Respiratory depression may be aggravated by concurrent use of narcotics or benzodiazepines. Oliguria decreases magnesium excretion, increasing the possibility of respiratory depression. Magnesium sulfate treatment should continue for at least 24 hours postpartum.

Arterial blood pressure of 180/110 mm Hg or higher requires treatment. Hydralazine is most often effective when administered in an intravenous bolus of 5 mg. Boluses may be repeated every 15 to 30 minutes if diastolic blood pressure remains at 110 mm Hg, up to a cumulative dose of 20 mg. Diastolic blood pressures below 90 mm Hg are undesirable because of the negative impact on uterine and placental blood flow. If blood pressure control is not achieved, labetalol, 20 mg intravenous bolus, or nifedipine, 10 mg orally, may be necessary to lower diastolic blood pressure.

Recurrence of seizures in a preeclamptic patient requires administration of 10 mg of diazepam, followed by loading and maintenance infusions of magnesium sulfate as outlined earlier. Experience with phenytoin in preeclamptic seizures has been limited.

Vaginal delivery is usually possible once the patient with severe preeclampsia is stabilized. Prostaglandin cervical ripening and oxytocin induction can be used to achieve delivery even in patients with an unfavorable cervix. With rare exceptions, attempts at vaginal delivery should be made in most patients with severe preeclampsia or eclampsia. The majority of patients spontaneously begin diuresis within 24 to 36 hours after delivery. Swan-Ganz catheterization and hemodynamic monitoring are rarely required postpartum unless severe oliguria is encountered. Total fluid intake should be maintained at 2000 to 2500 ml per 24 hours.

Most preeclamptic primigravidas become normotensive shortly after delivery, although elevated blood pressure can persist in a minority of patients for up to 6 weeks. Hypertension that persists 12 weeks postpartum should be considered chronic and should be appropriately evaluated.

Chronic Hypertension

Diagnosis. Without documentation of elevated blood pressure before pregnancy, chronic hypertension can only be presumed. The vast majority of patients who present with elevated blood pressure before the twentieth week of gestation, however, have chronic hypertension. Signs of long-standing hypertension in the retina or other organ systems strongly suggest the diagnosis. Women with chronic hypertension are at high risk of developing superimposed preeclampsia manifest by worsening hypertension, diffuse edema, or proteinuria. In patients with severe labile hypertension, a search for underlying vascular, renal, or endocrine causes should be considered.

Management. Complicating cardiac, renal, neurologic, and retinal disease must be excluded in all women with chronic hypertension, ideally before pregnancy. Medications should be reviewed and, if necessary, changed appropriate for pregnancy. Use of low-dose aspirin at 60 to 80 mg/day has been advocated by some to decrease the likelihood of superimposed preeclampsia. Patients with mild hypertension *not* receiving medication are generally treated conservatively during pregnancy, with mild sodium restriction, increased bed rest, and daily home blood pressure measurements. Smoking must be eliminated. If blood pressure exceeds 140/100 mm Hg, oral antihypertensive medication is usually administered using the fewest number and safest drugs necessary to maintain diastolic blood pressure near 90 mm Hg. Lowering diastolic blood pressure consistently below 90 mm Hg is not desirable because uterine blood flow may be reduced and fetal growth impaired.

Methyldopa is currently the drug of choice in the United States for treating significant chronic hypertension during pregnancy. Hydralazine has also been used extensively, with no evidence of fetal compromise. Use of β-adrenergic blocking agents during pregnancy was originally condemned, particularly with respect to their effect on uteroplacental hemodynamics. Infrequent neonatal side effects include mild bradycardia and hypoglycemia. A number of prospective series using labetalol for treatment of chronic hypertension support its safety during pregnancy. The use of diuretics in pregnancy continues to be controversial. As long as maternal electrolytes remain normal, no detrimental effects have been observed in the fetus or neonate when diuretics have been initiated *before* pregnancy. Given the other alternatives available for treatment of hypertension during pregnancy, it is inadvisable to initiate diuretics during gestation except in the circumstance of cardiac decompensation. Although oral nifedipine can be an effective agent in the control of acute hypertension during pregnancy, there is little experience with long-term administration of calcium-blocking drugs during pregnancy. Therefore its widespread use to treat chronic hypertension throughout gestation awaits additional study. Angiotensin-converting enzyme (ACE) inhibitors have been associated with impairment of fetal growth, severe oligohydramnios, anatomic abnormalities, renal failure, and death in up to 20% of neonates when used in the second and third trimester. Women in their childbearing years treated for chronic hypertension should not be treated with ACE inhibitors unless adequate contraception can be ensured.

Maternal and Fetal Effects. Women with chronic hypertension during pregnancy are at risk for superimposed preeclampsia and abruptio placenta and for developing fetal intrauterine growth retardation. Development of these sequelae is more likely in women with long-standing severe hypertension and in those with preexisting cardiac or renal involvement, or in those with diastolic pressures greater than 110 mm Hg during the first trimester. Early documentation of fetal age is mandatory, with monthly ultrasound evaluation of growth and development in the second half of pregnancy. Weekly antepartum fetal evaluation is mandatory during the last 6 to 8 weeks of pregnancy, or earlier if poor fetal growth is noted. In circumstances of significant fetal growth retardation or suspicious antepartum fetal testing, delivery is indicated regardless of gestational age.

Late or Transient Hypertension

Hypertension without proteinuria or abnormal edema that develops late in gestation or in the puerperium is referred to as *late* or *transient hypertension*. Blood pressure normalizes by the tenth postpartum day. Often it may be difficult to differentiate transient hypertension from early preeclampsia. Almost half of the women with transient hypertension in pregnancy subsequently develop long-standing chronic hypertension.

CARDIOVASCULAR DISORDERS

Normal pregnancy is accompanied by changes in blood volume, heart rate, blood pressure, cardiac output, and ventilation. Cardiac output begins to rise during the first trimester, peaks at an approximate 40% increase by 20 to 24 weeks, then declines during the last 8 weeks of gestation. The increase in cardiac output during early pregnancy is primarily caused by an increase in stroke volume. As pregnancy advances, heart rate increases, whereas stroke volume falls to nonpregnant levels.

Immediately after delivery, with relief of compression on the inferior vena cava, cardiac output may increase as much as 10% to 20%. Following this transitory rise in cardiac output, values fall progressively to baseline levels. Nonpregnant levels are reached by the end of the second postpartum week. During the initial postpartum period, relative bradycardia is common.

Atrial premature contractions, ectopic atrial tachycardia, and paroxysmal supraventricular tachycardia (PSVT) may be recognized for the first time during pregnancy or may increase in frequency and severity during pregnancy in previously diagnosed patients. Similarly, the awareness of ventricular tachycardia may also increase during pregnancy. Potential reasons for these occurrences include increased myocardial irritability as a consequence of increased blood volume; increased sinus heart rate, which may cause altered myocardial refractoriness and altered reentry patterns; and increased cardiac excitability and numbers of α-adrenergic receptors secondary to increased estrogen levels. Regardless of the mechanism, the treatment of arrhythmias during pregnancy is complicated by concerns for fetal well-being, and therefore depends on the maternal hemodynamic response and severity of symptoms. Nonpharmacologic therapy is strongly preferred and includes observation, rest, recumbency, and reassurance. Vagal maneuvers may aid in both diagnosis and treatment, and esophageal pacing can be quite effective. Although almost all of the antiarrhythmic agents are labeled FDA pregnancy risk category C (i.e., risk cannot be ruled out), most of these drugs are well tolerated by mother and fetus and can be used if deemed necessary. The use of phenytoin is contraindicated because of the risk of teratogenesis, and amiodarone and bretylium should be reserved for life-threatening situations. Temporary and permanent pacing have been used during pregnancy safely, as has direct current cardioversion.

Most patients with valvular heart disease can successfully complete pregnancy. If necessary, there is ample experience with valvular surgery during pregnancy. Yet it is extremely important that women with known valvular heart disease be evaluated before pregnancy and that, if necessary, corrective surgery be performed before conception.

Mitral stenosis is by far the most common rheumatic valvular lesion encountered in pregnant women. Increased heart rate, blood volume, and transmitral flow are all associated with normal pregnancy and tend to exacerbate the severity of mitral stenosis. Mitral regurgitation generally poses little threat during pregnancy except in severe cases, when volume overload can produce congestive heart failure. Mild aortic stenosis is usually well tolerated. Cardiac catheterization is indicated during pregnancy when aortic stenosis is associated with left ventricular failure, syncope, or angina. Aortic regurgitation is often ameliorated during pregnancy because there is a reduction in total peripheral resistance.

Primary or secondary pulmonary hypertension, Eisenmenger's syndrome, and cardiomyopathy with persistent left ventricular failure all pose an unacceptably high risk of maternal mortality. Women with these conditions should not become pregnant, and those who do conceive should be encouraged to terminate pregnancy in the first trimester.

Marfan's syndrome is associated with aortic dissection and myxomatous degeneration of the aortic and mitral valves. Historically, these patients have been advised to avoid pregnancy. More recent reports, however, suggest a favorable outcome for women with Marfan's syndrome who lack significant cardiovascular involvement.

THROMBOEMBOLIC DISORDERS (CHAPTER 63)

Thromboembolic disease is the leading cause of nonobstetric postpartum maternal mortality. In the United States, one half of all thromboembolic events in women younger than 40 years are related to pregnancy. The risk of deep vein thrombophlebitis (DVT) during pregnancy has been reported to be five times higher than in nonpregnant individuals and is probably even higher in the immediate postpartum period. The risk of pregnancy-associated thromboembolism is further increased in patients with prior DVT or pulmonary embolism (PE), advanced maternal age, multiparity, prolonged bed rest, varicose veins, or obesity, as well as those with a variety of inherited or acquired coagulation disorders. Postpartum risks are increased by cesarean delivery (a fourfold to tenfold increase over vaginal delivery).

The diagnosis of deep vein thrombophlebitis or pulmonary embolism may be suspected clinically but usually requires radiographic confirmation. Noninvasive methods include high-resolution compression ultrasonography coupled with color Doppler imaging and impedance plethosmography to assess for DVT, as well as ^{99}Tc ventilation-perfusion lung scan to assess for PE. Given the 15% to 40% mortality of untreated maternal PE, if results of noninvasive testing are not definitive or if therapy will be altered by an invasive diagnostic procedure (such as pulmonary angiogram), the benefits of the procedure outweigh the risks to mother and fetus. The only examination contraindicated during pregnancy is ^{125}I-fibrinogen scanning, because the dose of radiation to the fetal thyroid is clinically significant.

Initial treatment of acute venous thrombosis and pulmonary embolism requires intravenous heparin given in a high dosage sufficient to prolong the activated partial thromboplastin time (PTT) 1.5 to 2.5 times the control value. The heparin requirements to treat acute venous thrombosis seem to be greater during pregnancy than in the nonpregnant state. In addition, failure to reach adequate anticoagulation in the first 24 hours of treatment greatly increases the risk of recurrent thrombosis. Therefore an initial intravenous bolus of 7500 to 10,000 units is administered, followed by a continuous infusion of heparin at 15 to 20 U/kg/hr. Intravenous treatment is usually continued for 5 to 10 days to allow for organization and firm attachment of the thrombus to the vessel wall. The patient then begins self-injected, adjusted high-dose subcutaneous heparin every 8 to 12 hours. The dose is determined by dividing the 24-hour intravenous required dose into two to three subcutaneous injections daily. The goal again is to maintain the midinterval PTT at 1.5 to 2.5 times the control value. Alternatively, continuous infusion of heparin can be arranged for the patient. Anticoagulation is continued throughout pregnancy and for approximately 3 months postpartum. Though heparin is the anticoagulant of choice during pregnancy, heparin-induced thrombocytopenia and osteoporosis are important adverse effects that must be watched.

There are insufficient data to conclude which regimen provides the safest maximal protection against recurrent antepartum thrombosis. Antepartum thromboembolism prophylaxis should be considered, however, in pregnant women with a prior history of DVT or PE; women with antithrombin III, protein C, or protein S deficiency; and women with the antiphospholipid antibody syndrome.

Unlike heparin, warfarin freely crosses the placenta. Use of warfarin during the first trimester has been associated with a variety of neonatal malformations, including nasal hypoplasia, frontal bossing, and short stature with stippled epiphyses. Use during the second and third trimesters has been associated with central nervous system abnormalities and fetal and placental hemorrhage resulting in fetal death. Warfarin should be avoided throughout pregnancy, and patients already taking warfarin and desiring to conceive should be switched to heparin before conception.

Low-molecular-weight heparin may afford some advantages during pregnancy because of its long half-life, which may allow for once-daily dosing. It has been used in a small number of pregnant women who have had adverse reactions to heparin, and it does not appear to cross into fetal circulation. There are limited data, however, and its use cannot be recommended at this time.

Heparin appears to be safe for use during lactation because it does not enter breast milk. Warfarin also appears to be safe in women who breastfeed their infants. Small studies have found little or no warfarin activity in breast milk or infant's plasma.

ASTHMA (CHAPTER 188)

Asthma is one of the most common illnesses and the most common obstructive pulmonary disease encountered during pregnancy. Asthma may occur for the first time during pregnancy. Approximately one third of pregnant women with asthma improve, one third remain the same, and one third get worse. Regardless of their clinical status, pregnant women with asthma need effective pharmacologic and nonpharmacologic treatment to ensure their health and the health of their infants. Uncontrolled asthma can produce serious fetal and maternal complications; therefore aggressive management of the asthmatic pregnant patient is always indicated. Maternal complications in women with uncontrolled asthma include preeclampsia, gestational hypertension, hyperemesis gravidarum, vaginal hemorrhage, and preterm labor. Fetal complications include intrauterine growth retardation, preterm birth, low birth weight, increased perinatal mortality, and neonatal hypoxia.

Management of asthma is altered very little by pregnancy. As in the nonpregnant patient, effective management comprises four integral components: (1) objective measures for monitoring maternal lung function and fetal well-being; (2) avoidance and control of asthma triggers, including treating associated conditions such as sinusitis, rhinitis, and gastroesophageal reflux; (3) pharmacologic therapy; and (4) patient education.

Considerable experience with the use of methylxanthines during pregnancy has been accumulated. There has been no evidence of teratogenicity or fetal injury. The dosage does not usually need to be altered, but it is advisable to measure serum concentrations to ensure a therapeutic response and minimize side effects.

Adrenergic agents are effective bronchodilators used alone or in conjunction with methylxanthines. There has been extensive clinical experience with these drugs during pregnancy, with few reports of adverse effects. Administration of adrenergic medication by inhalation provides the most rapid relief of acute asthma with the fewest side effects. Older oral preparations containing phenobarbital should be avoided throughout pregnancy.

Cromolyn sodium prevents release of histamine and is useful for prophylaxis against acute asthma. It has no bronchodilating activity and is not useful for treatment of acute attacks. Cromolyn appears to have no maternal or fetal toxicity.

Acute bronchospasm unresponsive to bronchodilator therapy often improves with the antiinflammatory effect of corticosteroids. Oral, inhaled, and intravenous corticosteroids are all considered safe for use during pregnancy. Inhaled corticosteroids such as beclomethasone may allow a reduction in the dosage of oral preparations or the frequency of use of β-sympathomimetic inhalers.

HEPATIC DISORDERS

The most common cause of jaundice in pregnant women in the United States is viral hepatitis. With the exception of hepatitis E infection, the clinical course and histologic findings of hepatitis A, B, C, and delta hepatitis do not differ between well-nourished pregnant women and nonpregnant individuals.

Acute Hepatitis A

Pregnant women with hepatitis A generally do not transmit the infection to their offspring. Presumably, the risk of transmission is limited by the brief viremic period and the lack of fecal contamination during delivery. Management does not differ from that of nonpregnant patients. In uncomplicated cases there is no rational basis for restricting protein intake or providing excessive quantities of carbohydrate. Effective prophylaxis against hepatitis A can be achieved with immune globulin and should be offered to pregnant women with household or sexual contacts who have acute hepatitis A.

Acute Hepatitis B

Infection with the hepatitis B virus (HBV) is a major cause of acute and chronic hepatitis, cirrhosis, and primary hepatocellular carcinoma throughout the world. Although pregnancy does not affect the course of hepatitis B and hepatitis B does not appear to affect the pregnancy adversely, concern centers around the vertical transmission of this virus from mother to child, which occurs at the time of birth. Certain features appear to determine the likelihood and rate of perinatal transmission of HBV, including the period in pregnancy during which in-

fection occurs, the mother's infectivity as measured by her HB_eAg status, and the mother's racial and geographic background. Women who have acute hepatitis B during the first or second trimester rarely transmit the infection to their neonates and only do so if they become HB_sAg carriers. On the other hand, women who contract the infection during the third trimester or near the time of delivery have a very high probability of transmitting the virus to their offspring. Mothers positive for both HB_sAg and HB_eAg infect more than 80% of untreated infants. Transmission by asymptomatic mothers is much higher in Asian countries (30% to 70%) than it is in the United States (5% to 20%) and most Western countries.

The most common outcome of infection in the newborn is persistent antigenemia, and up to 90% become HBV carriers. Some ultimately develop chronic active hepatitis, cirrhosis, and primary hepatocellular carcinoma. In addition, female carriers may subsequently perpetuate the cycle of perinatal transmission when they become pregnant. Because of the high prevalence of infection with hepatitis B virus, routine screening for Hb_sAg is recommended for all pregnant women. All infants of mothers who have active or chronic hepatitis should receive hepatitis B immune globulin during the first 12 hours after birth. They should then be immunized with hepatitis B vaccine during the first week of life, 1 month later, and again at approximately 6 months of age, a practice that is now standard for all infants.

Hepatitis C

Infection with hepatitis C (HCV) is a serious health problem. Despite the relatively benign nature of the acute infection, there is a high frequency of progression to chronic hepatitis (up to 50%), cirrhosis (20% to 25%), and hepatocellular carcinoma. Vertical transmission of HCV may occur but seems to be far less common than that for HBV. Coinfection with human immunodeficiency virus (HIV) in the mother may enhance transmission of HCV to the neonate.

Delta Hepatitis and Hepatitis E

Delta hepatitis (HDV) is caused by a defective RNA virus that is dependent on HBV for replication. Infection with HDV can occur as coinfection, which requires acquisition of HBV and HDV at the same time, or as superinfection with HDV in a chronic carrier of HBV. Perinatal transmission of HDV is very rare. Delta infection in the neonate can only occur if HDV is transmitted along with HBV; HBV carriers superinfected with HDV are usually anti-HB_e–positive and therefore are much less likely to transmit HBV to their offspring.

Hepatitis E is a serious disease in pregnant women and is responsible for a high frequency of fatal, fulminant hepatitis in up to 20% of cases.

Intrahepatic Cholestasis of Pregnancy

Intrahepatic cholestasis of pregnancy (ICP) results from failure of the liver to excrete bile acids appropriately. Although the cause has not been clearly delineated, hormonal and genetic factors are suspected. ICP is more common in women with a family history of the disease and in women who have had cholestasis while taking oral contraceptives. The disorder also tends to recur in subsequent pregnancies.

Despite the fact that the disease is usually referred to as benign, an increased incidence of preterm labor, stillbirths, fetal distress, and meconium staining has been reported with ICP. Affected women should therefore be treated at centers capable of caring for premature infants. Increased postpartum bleeding may result from decreased absorption of vitamin K.

ICP typically occurs during the third trimester and is characterized by generalized pruritus, which may be severe and is often worse at night. Twenty percent to 60% of women may subsequently develop jaundice. Laboratory data reveal elevated serum bilirubin concentration, but usually below 6 mg per deciliter. Liver tests reflect cholestasis without significant evidence of hepatocellular injury.

Symptomatic relief of pruritus may be achieved with the bile salt–binding resin cholestyramine. Patients should be followed closely for signs of preterm labor and fetal well-being. Prophylactic vitamin K should be administered to prevent increased bleeding.

Acute Cholecystitis

Despite the cholestatic effect of estrogen and impaired gallbladder emptying, there is no proved increased incidence of acute cholecystitis or common duct obstruction during gestation. Cholecystectomy is performed in 1 per 1000 to 3000 pregnancies. Clinical presentation generally does not differ from that in nonpregnant individuals. During late gestation, however, cholecystitis can be confused with the right upper quadrant pain that often accompanies preeclampsia. Acute appendicitis during pregnancy may also present with right upper quadrant pain. The presence of gallstones can usually be established with ultrasonography.

Initial management, even when pancreatitis is present, should be conservative. Surgery should be reserved for cases in which there is suspicion of perforation, failure to respond to medical therapy within 4 to 5 days, persistent obstructive jaundice, or repeated attacks of biliary colic, and for patients in whom other acute surgical abdominal diseases (e.g., acute appendicitis) cannot be ruled out.

Acute Fatty Liver of Pregnancy

Acute fatty liver of pregnancy (AFLP) is a relatively uncommon disease of unknown cause. In the past, maternal and fetal mortality rates had been reported to be as high as 85%. At present, early detection, rapid delivery following diagnosis, and aggressive supportive care have reduced maternal and fetal mortality to less than 20%.

The obstetric history of a patient with AFLP parallels preeclampsia. The disease presents during the third trimester, with the mean gestational age at onset of 36 weeks. The incidence of AFLP is highest in primiparas and women with multiple gestations.

Initial manifestations are sudden but nonspecific. Nausea, vomiting, and abdominal pain are the most common presenting complaints. Jaundice often follows these nonspecific symptoms. If untreated, the disease typically progresses to hepatic failure, disseminated intravascular coagulation, renal failure, gastrointestinal or uterine bleeding, pancreatitis, seizures, coma, and/or death.

Transaminases are typically elevated in the range of 300 to 500 units. Levels above 1000 units suggest fulminant hepatitis. Serum bilirubin may be normal early in the course of AFLP, but it rises if pregnancy is not terminated. Hematologic abnormalities include leukocytosis, microangiopathic hemolytic anemia, and thrombocytopenia. Hypoglycemia is common and may be profound. Liver biopsy is usually diagnostic and characterized by the accumulation of microvesicular fat within hepatocytes, but may not be appropriate to perform in the presence of significant coagulopathy.

AFLP is managed by immediate delivery and intensive medical support. Despite appropriate care, the patient's condition may deteriorate further postpartum. Survivors have no long-term sequelae and liver histologic condition returns to normal. Liver transplantation has been successful in women with fulminant hepatic failure whose condition did not improve. In subsequent pregnancies, AFLP does not appear to recur.

DIGESTIVE TRACT DISORDERS
Hyperemesis Gravidarum

Hyperemesis gravidarum is a condition of pregnant women in which intractable vomiting early in gestation causes dehydration, electrolyte disturbances, and/or nutritional deficiencies with accompanying weight loss. Also known as the "pernicious vomiting of pregnancy," hyperemesis gravidarum occurs in approximately 3.5 per 1000 pregnancies. Hyperemesis gravidarum is more common in primigravidas; younger women, especially those less than 20 years of age; women with less than 12 years of education; obese women; and nonsmokers. Multiple gestations and the presence of trophoblastic disease also appear to predispose to this disorder. Though generally a self-limited condition, the natural history of hyperemesis gravidarum is one of slow recovery with frequent relapses. Fluid, electrolyte, and nutritional derangements can lead to renal and hepatic dysfunction. Other associated disturbances include neurologic abnormalities, retinal hemorrhage, Mallory-Weiss tear, and acid aspiration syndrome.

The treatment of hyperemesis gravidarum is generally supportive and includes reassurance, small frequent meals, restricting the amount of fat and indigestible material in meals, and encouraging intake of carbohydrates. For severe or refractory cases, parenteral hyperalimentation may be required. The most effective way to judge recovery is not only by cessation of vomiting and correction of fluid and electrolyte abnormalities, but also by weight stabilization and weight gain.

Inflammatory Bowel Disease

Both ulcerative colitis and Crohn's disease have a predilection for young adults, with peak occurrence between the second and fourth decade of life. It is therefore not at all uncommon to encounter a woman with inflammatory bowel disease (IBD) who is pregnant or who wishes to become pregnant. The issues of particular interest to both the patient with IBD and her physician are the ability to conceive, the influence of IBD on pregnancy, the influence of pregnancy on the underlying bowel disease, and the effect of therapy on the fetus.

Fertility. Ulcerative colitis appears to have little effect on fertility. Crohn's disease, however, has been associated with decreased fertility rates. Though reported fertility rates vary by study, most agree that conception among women with Crohn's disease generally occurs during periods of disease remission. In addition, surgical removal of diseased bowel has been associated with restoration of normal fertility, with postoperative rates of conception approximating those of the population at large. Other factors that contribute to diminished fertility in Crohn's disease include adnexal involvement by the chronic inflammatory process resulting in tubal occlusion, decreased libido associated with the systemic illness, nutritional deficiencies, and the presence of perineal disease, which may result in a physical or psychologic impediment to intercourse.

Influence of IBD on Pregnancy. In general, ulcerative colitis and Crohn's disease do not have a detrimental effect on the outcome of pregnancy. The incidence of live births, congenital anomalies, spontaneous abortions, and stillbirths is similar to that in pregnancies without associated IBD. Exceptions to these optimistic findings indicate that the risk of spontaneous abortion and prematurity may be greater in women whose disease is active at the time of conception than in those who conceive when their disease is quiescent. Women with IBD who experience severe exacerbations during pregnancy and those in whom Crohn's disease develops for the first time during gestation may also have increased fetal risk.

Previous bowel resection or proctocolectomy with ileostomy does not affect the course of pregnancy. The mode of delivery should be based on obstetric indications. Displacement, enlargement, and prolapse of the ileal stoma can occur, however.

Influence of Pregnancy on IBD. The effect of pregnancy on IBD is variable and appears to be related to disease activity at the time of conception. Of patients whose IBD is quiescent at the onset of pregnancy, approximately 75% remain free of symptoms throughout gestation. If relapse does occur, it usually does so during the first trimester in both ulcerative colitis and Crohn's disease. In the less common situation in which pregnancy occurs in the presence of active disease, the prognosis is less favorable. Approximately 70% of these women show no improvement in their disease or become worse as gestation progresses. Although many reports suggest that women who manifest the onset of IBD during pregnancy have the highest risk of serious problems, more recent clinical data do not unanimously reflect this experience. When IBD does first arise during pregnancy, it is most likely to do so in the first or second trimester. Disease behavior during one pregnancy is not predictive of behavior during subsequent pregnancies.

Treatment. The management of IBD differs little during pregnancy. Maintenance therapy with sulfasalazine can be continued throughout pregnancy in women who have taken it before conception. The drug may also be initiated to treat exacerbations. There is no evidence that the medication should be discontinued near the time of delivery, nor that use during breast-feeding harms the newborn. If necessary, corticosteroids may be used to manage IBD during pregnancy and lactation. In general, patients on chronic corticosteroid therapy are given increased doses for labor and delivery. Metronidazole and the immunosuppressives 6-mercaptopurine and azathioprine should be avoided during pregnancy because of possible teratogenic effects of these agents.

RHEUMATIC DISORDERS
Systemic Lupus Erythematosus

Many reports have suggested that the frequency of exacerbations of systemic lupus erythematosus (SLE) is increased during pregnancy and the postpartum period. There are no convincing data, however, to support this concern. The natural history of the disease is variable, and older series were reported before the effective use of corticosteroids or immunosuppressives. The risk of exacerbations does seem to be minimized in patients who are in complete clinical remission at the time of conception.

A number of factors play a role in the increased frequency of fetal loss, prematurity, and intrauterine growth retardation that occur in SLE. These factors include maternal hypertension and renal disease, namely, proteinuria and decreased creatinine clearance, prior history of fetal death, and the presence of antiphospholipid antibodies. Though initially felt to be directly correlated, lupus activity itself has not been shown to independently affect pregnancy outcome. It has been observed that there is a relationship between fetal heart block and maternal SLE. It appears that maternal anti-Ro (SS-A) or anti-La (SS-B) antibody crosses the placenta and may directly damage fetal cardiac tissue. Only 1% to 5% of the children from mothers with anti-Ro (SS-A) or anti-La (SS-B) antibody develop neonatal lupus, characterized by transient photosensitive skin rash, permanent congenital complete heart block, or both. The absence of these antibodies in maternal serum suggests that a child is unlikely to be affected. The occurrence and severity of neonatal lupus are unrelated to maternal disease activity.

Many patients with SLE demonstrate spontaneous remission and do not require treatment. However, flares do occur. The diagnosis of flare in the gravid patient can be difficult because, in pregnancy, common symptoms suggestive of lupus flare—such as arthralgia, palmar and facial erythema, and proteinuria—often have causes unrelated to SLE. More reliable indicators of active disease during pregnancy include increasing levels of anti-DNA antibody, alternative pathway hypocomplementemia, true arthritis, aphthous ulcers, and lymphadenopathy. Serious flares involving the kidneys or central nervous system reduce fetal survival and pose a serious threat to maternal well-being. These patients require treatment, and corticosteroids are the mainstay of therapy. Treatment should not be deferred because of pregnancy. The management of antiphospholipid antibody syndrome in pregnancy without active SLE includes a regimen of heparin and low-dose aspirin. Some studies advocate the use of prednisone, but this remains controversial.

Rheumatoid Arthritis

Most reports indicate that pregnancy has a favorable effect on the clinical course of rheumatoid arthritis. Up to 75% of patients experience a significant remission. Furthermore, remission during one pregnancy often indicates that a similar remission may be experienced in a subsequent pregnancy.

Whenever possible, every effort should be made to control arthritic symptoms with adequate rest; physical and occupational therapy; local heat; and, if necessary, intraarticular corticosteroid injections. Gold, antimalarials, nonsteroidal antiinflammatory drugs, and cytotoxic agents should be avoided during pregnancy. Acetaminophen and low-dose corticosteroids can be used if needed.

All women with rheumatoid arthritis should be evaluated for significant cervical spine disease, especially subluxation, before delivery. It is advisable to restart antirheumatic therapy shortly after parturition because the disease will flare in the majority of patients within 6 to 9 months postpartum.

HEMATOLOGIC DISORDERS
Anemia

Because plasma volume increases more than red cell volume, the hematocrit during pregnancy can be expected to fall to as low as 35% by the beginning of the third trimester. Generally, a hemoglobin value of less than 11 g per deciliter defines anemia during pregnancy.

Pure macrocytic anemia in pregnancy, with the presence of hypersegmented neutrophils, usually represents folate deficiency. Pernicious anemia is extremely rare during pregnancy. Anemia secondary to folate deficiency is frequently combined with iron deficiency and requires oral iron in addition to 1 mg of folic acid daily.

In nonmacrocytic anemia, a low serum ferritin concentration is diagnostic of deficient iron stores. Reticulocytosis can be demonstrated within 2 weeks of oral iron supplementation. Parenteral iron administration is rarely necessary.

Hemoglobinopathy or thalassemia should be suspected in patients who have a previous history of anemia, African or Mediterranean ancestry, and a normal serum ferritin concentration. Hemoglobin electrophoresis is necessary to establish the diagnosis.

The most frequently encountered hemoglobinopathies involve abnormal hemoglobins S and C and β-thalassemia, either isolated or in combination. Sickle cell trait (HbAS) is common but comparatively benign. Conversely, sickle cell disease (HbSS) and hemoglobin SC disease (HbSC) are frequently complicated by preeclampsia, infection, painful crises, and increased perinatal loss.

Bleeding Disorders

Approximately 7% of healthy pregnant women have mild to moderate thrombocytopenia (platelet count 80 to 150×10^9 per liter). Neither these women nor their offspring manifest abnormal bleeding. This condition has been designated incidental thrombocytopenia of pregnancy and requires no treatment.

Idiopathic Thrombocytopenic Purpura. Idiopathic thrombocytopenic purpura (ITP) is a common autoimmune disorder in which patients form antiplatelet autoantibodies against platelet-specific antigens. The condition frequently affects young women; consequently, one can anticipate that many patients with ITP will become pregnant while their illness is active. The major concern during pregnancy is whether infants born to mothers with ITP are at risk of serious bleeding during delivery and whether they can be identified before delivery.

Unfortunately, it has been determined that there is no relationship between maternal platelet count and the infant's platelet count. Similarly, measurement of platelet-associated IgG on maternal platelets does not predict neonatal thrombocytopenia. In a prospective series of more than 7000 women, Burrows found that severe thrombocytopenia at the time of delivery occurs in less than 5% of infants. Moreover, Burrows found that one of the best predictors of severe neonatal thrombocytopenia is a previously affected infant. Thus the type of delivery should be decided solely on obstetric indications. After delivery a fetal cord platelet count should be obtained immediately and the infant's platelet count followed carefully over the next week. Maternal indications for treatment of thrombocytopenia should not differ from those for nonpregnant individuals.

Disseminated Intravascular Coagulation. Disseminated intravascular coagulation (DIC) is associated with a number of complications of pregnancy. Abruptio placenta, amniotic fluid embolus, severe preeclampsia, retained dead fetus, sepsis, and second-trimester abortion can all be associated with DIC. Treatment of the underlying disease, including delivery, is the mainstay of therapy.

Von Willebrand's Disease. Von Willebrand's disease encompasses a group of inherited disorders of platelet function and factor VIII activity. Transfusions of cryoprecipitate or specific clotting factors are necessary if measured factor VIII activity falls below 50% during labor. Patients with type I von Willebrand's disease may also respond favorably to treatment with desmopressin.

INFECTIOUS DISEASES
Sexually Transmitted Diseases

Gonorrhea and Chlamydia. Infection with *Neisseria gonorrhoeae* and/or *Chlamydia trachomatis* may have a deleterious effect on both mother and fetus, including preterm delivery, premature rupture of membranes, chorioamnionitis, and postpartum infection. Because of these consequences and the fact that the majority of gonorrheal and chlamydial infections are asymptomatic during pregnancy, routine endocervical culture is indicated in high-risk populations. Primary treatment of gonorrhea infections during pregnancy is ceftriaxone administered intramuscularly at 125 mg once or spectinomycin in penicillin-allergic patients. Alternatives to the tetracyclines and quinolones that are used for the treatment of chlamydial infection but are contraindicated during pregnancy include erythromycin and amoxicillin.

Bacterial Vaginosis. Bacterial vaginosis is a common syndrome in which the normal, lactobacillus-predominant vaginal flora is replaced with multiple organisms, including *Gardnerella vaginalis, Mycoplasma hominis,* and anaerobic bacteria. It is one of the most common genital infections found during pregnancy, with between 12% and 22% of gravid women affected. Bacterial vaginosis has been associated with preterm delivery, premature rupture of membranes, chorioamnionitis, and postpartum infection. A recent study confirms the association between bacterial vaginosis and the preterm delivery of low-birth-weight infants. Though screening and treatment of bacterial vaginosis during pregnancy may significantly reduce the risk of preterm birth in the general population, further prospective, randomized clinical trials are needed to help establish practice guidelines for the treatment of this syndrome in all pregnant women. Currently, screening is generally advocated for women at high risk for delivering a premature infant.

Syphilis. Because of its detrimental fetal and maternal effects, including congenital disease, syphilis must be treated as soon as the diagnosis is confirmed by specific serologic tests. Nonspecific serologic tests (Venereal Disease Research Laboratory [VDRL], rapid plasma reagin [RPR]) should be performed monthly after treatment. Rising titers indicate inadequate therapy.

Herpes Simplex. The incidence of neonatal herpes simplex virus (HSV), which includes central nervous system infection leading to mental retardation and sometimes death, appears to be increasing as genital herpes becomes more common. Exposure of the infant to HSV can often be prevented by cesarean delivery if maternal genital herpes lesions are recognized at the onset of labor. Unfortunately, most neonatal HSV infections result from asymptomatic maternal shedding of HSV, as indicated by the fact that only one third of the mothers of infants with neonatal herpes have signs of HSV infections.

Recently, the Infectious Disease Society for Obstetrics-Gynecology has endorsed the following recommendations for women with a history of genital herpes.

A. In women with a history of genital herpes, but without lesions:
  1. Weekly prenatal cultures should be abandoned because there is poor predictive value for identifying the patient who will be shedding virus at the time of delivery.
  2. In the absence of genital herpetic lesions, vaginal delivery should be expected (unless other indications for cesarean delivery are present).
  3. To identify potentially exposed neonates, a culture for herpes virus may be obtained from either the mother on the day of delivery or from the neonate.
  4. Isolation is not necessary for the mother.
  5. It is recognized that, with such a policy, there is a small risk (approximately 1 per 1000) of neonatal infection.
B. In women with herpetic lesions of the genital tract when either labor or membrane rupture occurs:
  1. Cesarean delivery can reduce the risk of neonatal herpes virus infection.
  2. Ideally, cesarean delivery should be performed before or within 4 to 6 hours of membrane rupture, but it may be of benefit in preventing neonatal herpes regardless of duration of membrane rupture.
C. In women with genital herpetic lesions at or near term, but before labor or membrane rupture, cultures collected at 3- to 5-day intervals may be performed to ensure the absence of virus at the time of birth and to increase the likelihood of vaginal delivery.

Viral Infections

Cytomegalovirus. Cytomegalovirus (CMV) is the most common congenital viral disease in the United States. From 0.2% to 2.2% of all infants acquire infection during the perinatal period. The consequences of this infection can be devastating and include deafness, neurologic complications, developmental learning disabilities, multiple physical defects, and stillbirth. Infant mortality may be as high as 20% to 30% in primary CMV infections.

Unfortunately, the presence or absence of seroreactivity does not correlate with the presence or absence of the virus on body surfaces or in body secretions. Accurate diagnosis must be established by isolation of the virus from such sites as urine and endocervical secretions. Because there is no satisfactory therapy available for CMV infections in either adults or newborns, it is ideal for women who are pregnant or are contemplating pregnancy and are known to be seronegative to avoid exposure to CMV from such obvious sources as day-care centers and renal dialysis units.

Varicella-Zoster. Despite the fact that varicella infections are among the most common communicable diseases in the general population, they are relatively infrequent during pregnancy because most women have been infected with chickenpox as children.

Transmission of the virus to the fetus during the first 20 weeks of gestation has been reported to result in a clinical syndrome of intrauterine growth retardation, hypoplasia of the extremities, cutaneous scars, cortical atrophy, microcephaly, cataracts, chorioretinitis, microophthalmia, and psychomotor retardation. The exact risk of this congenital syndrome is unknown but is probably less than 1% to 2%.

A more common problem has been maternal varicella in the peripartum period, producing neonatal chickenpox. If a mother develops varicella within 4 days before delivery or 2 days after, there is a 25% chance that the newborn will become infected. During this interval the newborn acquires the virus but is delivered before the mother has produced a varicella-specific antibody response capable of crossing the placenta and protecting the fetus. Such infants may have as high as 30% mortality. When more than 5 days have elapsed between the onset of maternal rash and delivery, sufficient delay has occurred for a maternal antibody response to develop and the fetus is passively immunized, thus ameliorating the severity of the disease. If parturition occurs during the 7-day period of risk for disseminated neonatal infection, newborns should be passively immunized using varicella-zoster immune globulin.

Rubella. Rubella infection during the first trimester can lead to congenital rubella syndrome in greater than 80% of fetuses. Congenital rubella syndrome is characterized by intrauterine growth retardation, prematurity, increased risk for spontaneous abortion, and stillbirth, as well as severe neurologic, ophthalmologic, and cardiac complications. An estimated 10% to 15% of young adults remain susceptible to rubella, and limited outbreaks continue to be reported, particularly in universities and hospitals. Every effort should be made to vaccinate all nonpregnant young women unless there is proof of immunity or a specific contraindication to the vaccine. Because of the theoretic risk to the fetus, women should be counseled not to become pregnant for 3 months after vaccination.

If a pregnant woman is inadvertently vaccinated or becomes pregnant within 3 months of vaccination, she should be counseled about the theoretic risks of congenital rubella syndrome. She should be reassured, however, that a Centers for Disease Control prospective study of susceptible pregnant women who received rubella vaccine within 3 months of conception and who carried their pregnancies to term showed a negligible risk of rubella syndrome.

Parvovirus. Infection with parvovirus B_{19} produces a common childhood illness called *erythema infectiosum* or *fifth disease*. This disease is characterized by fever and a lacy macular rash often described as a "slapped cheek" appearance. Because of its affinity for erythroid cells, parvovirus is a common cause of transient aplastic crisis in children and adults. Parvovirus does cross the human placenta and may lead to severe, life-threatening anemia and nonimmune hydrops in the fetus if maternal infection is acquired during pregnancy. The greatest risk to the fetus occurs during the first 20 weeks of gestation, a period that corresponds to the major development of erythroid precursors. The risk of congenital malformation appears negligible. Nonimmune hydrops in the fetus after maternal infection appears to occur in 5% to 10% of cases. Serial ultrasound evaluation of the at-risk fetus is recommended after documented maternal infection. Intrauterine red cell transfusions for the fetus may be necessary to avoid fetal death secondary to anemia.

Acquired Immunodeficiency Syndrome (AIDS). A woman may learn of her human immunodeficiency virus (HIV) status from prenatal screening. Initial assessment of the pregnant HIV-infected patient should not differ from that of a nonpregnant individual and therefore may consist of obtaining complete blood counts and antibody titers to toxoplasmosis and cytomegalovirus; tuberculosis skin testing; determination of hepatitis B surface antigen, VDRL, and cryptococcal antigen status; cervical cultures for gonorrhea and chlamydia; and administration of Pneumovax. Viral load and CD4 counts should be checked periodically to determine whether or not the patient is a candidate for antiretroviral therapy or *Pneumocystis carinii* pneumonia prophylaxis.

HIV may be transmitted from infected women to their offspring by three possible routes: to the fetus in utero through the maternal circulation, to the infant during labor and delivery by inoculation or ingestion of blood and other infected fluids, and to the infant shortly after birth through infected breast milk. Based on currently available information, there is approximately a 25% to 35% rate of perinatal transmission. All women known to be infected with HIV should receive detailed counseling.

Toxoplasmosis

Toxoplasma gondii infection is a protozoan infection to which most adults have antibody protection. When immunocompetent adults do become infected, they are usually asymptomatic or experience only mild constitutional symptoms and lymphadenopathy. Primary infection during pregnancy, however, can have serious consequences for the fetus, including seizures, hydrocephaly, microcephaly, jaundice, chorioretinitis, increased risk of prematurity, and low birth weight. The most severe cases of congenital toxoplasmosis are seen in fetuses infected early in gestation. There can be a 60% reduction in the rate of complications if treatment is instituted. When primary infection is recognized after 14 weeks' gestation, treatment with pyrimethamine and sulfadiazine along with leucovorin should be started. The safety of these medications before 14 weeks' gestation has not been demonstrated. Prevention remains the goal, and pregnant women should be instructed to avoid potential sources of exposure, such as undercooked meat and cat feces.

Urinary Tract Infections

Pregnant women are predisposed to infections of the urinary tract because of dilation of the ureters and collecting systems, smooth muscle relaxation caused by increased progesterone concentrations, and glycosuria.

Between 5% and 10% of pregnant women have asymptomatic bacteriuria. If untreated, up to 40% of these women suffer acute pyelonephritis during pregnancy or the puerperium. Acute pyelonephritis is more severe in pregnant women and is associated with maternal complications as well as increased preterm labor and low birth weight. Screening urine cultures in all women during early gestation, with appropriate treatment and follow-up, minimizes the occurrence of significant infection during the third trimester. Patients with treated bacteriuria or a history of frequent urinary tract infections may need to be screened more frequently. Treatment of asymptomatic bacteriuria can be accomplished with ampicillin or nitrofurantoin. Quinolones are contraindicated. A 7- to 10-day course of antibiotics is used; short course (1- to 3-day) regimens should be avoided. Pyelonephritis should be aggressively managed with hospitalization, rehydration, and intravenous antibiotic therapy based on in vitro sensitivities. Table 372-2 lists some common antibiotics and special considerations for their use during pregnancy.

Table 372-2   Antibiotic use during pregnancy

ANTIBIOTIC	SPECIAL CONSIDERATIONS DURING PREGNANCY
Penicillin G	Safe in nonallergic patients; dosage requirements increased during pregnancy
Ampicillin	Dosage requirements increased during pregnancy; can lower urinary estriols; unconjugated serum estriol unaffected
Amoxicillin	Same as ampicillin
Cephalosporins	Dosage requirements increased during pregnancy; some cross-sensitivity in penicillin-allergic patients; may affect urinary estriols; no effect on unconjugated serum estriol
Erythromycin	Generally safe; placental transfer is erratic, but the fetal liver concentrates the drug
Tetracycline	Abnormal fetal teeth and bone development; increased risk of maternal liver and pancreatic disease; contraindicated in pregnancy
Chloramphenicol	May cause "gray baby syndrome"; avoid in pregnancy
Clindamycin	Fetal effects are unknown; may rarely cause pseudomembranous colitis in the mother
Vancomycin	Potential fetal ototoxicity; should be reserved for life-threatening infections in patients allergic to penicillin
Metronidazole	Mutagenic and carcinogenic in animals; may be necessary to use for symptomatic parasitic infections during second and third trimesters
Nitrofurantoin	Generally safe but has been rarely associated with hemolytic anemia in the newborn; few systemic effects
Quinolones	Contraindicated in pregnancy
Sulfonamides	Competes with bilirubin for albumin binding; should not be used in last trimester to avoid neonatal kernicterus
Trimethoprim	Folic acid antagonist; should be avoided during pregnancy unless no alternative available

Aminoglycosides
  Amikacin
  Gentamicin
  Kanamycin
  Streptomycin
  Tobramycin
	Possible fetal and maternal ototoxicity and renal toxicity; maternal serum levels should be monitored closely but are usually in low range because of rapid renal clearance

NEUROLOGIC DISORDERS
Seizures

Approximately 50% of women with epilepsy have no change in the frequency of their seizures during pregnancy, 40% to 45% have more frequent seizures, and 5% to 10% have fewer.

All patients treated with anticonvulsants who desire pregnancy should be carefully evaluated regarding the accuracy of the diagnosis of epilepsy and the continuing need for anticonvulsant therapy. In patients who have been seizure-free for 2 years or more, preconception anticonvulsant drug withdrawal may be considered. The major anticonvulsant drugs—phenytoin, phenobarbital, valproic acid, and carbamezapine—are teratogenic. The incidence of fetal malformations is correlated with the number of medications taken and with dosage. Patients should be advised, however, that the risk of poor fetal outcome is also high for women who experience grand mal seizures during pregnancy.

To maintain therapeutic concentrations of phenytoin and phenobarbital throughout pregnancy, it is usually necessary to increase the dosage as gestation advances. Patients receiving anticonvulsants should have serum drug concentrations measured at least monthly. Adequate folate supplementation must be provided. Dosages of anticonvulsants need to be decreased within 1 week after delivery to avoid toxicity. Breast-feeding is not absolutely contraindicated, but infants must be closely monitored for side effects from the medications.

Multiple Sclerosis

The effect of pregnancy on the course of multiple sclerosis has been variable. Several studies have demonstrated that the number and severity of relapses diminish during pregnancy, particularly during the third trimester. In the past it has been suggested that exacerbations should be anticipated after delivery. More recent reports have not substantiated this concern.

Acute attacks are best managed with bed rest. The use of corticosteroids for severe attacks is advocated by some neurologists, but the efficacy of steroids for multiple sclerosis remains controversial.

BIBLIOGRAPHY

Barbour LA, Pickard J: Controversies in thromboembolic disease during pregnancy: a critical review, *Obstet Gynecol* 86:621, 1995.

Bishnoi A, Sachmechi I: Thyroid disease during pregnancy, *Am Fam Physician* 53:215, 1996.

Boumpas DT et al: Systemic lupus erythematosus: emerging concepts, *Ann Intern Med* 123:42, 1995.

Garner P: Type I diabetes mellitus and pregnancy, *Lancet* 346:157, 1995.

Hillier SL et al: Association between bacterial vaginosis and preterm delivery of a low-birth-weight infant, *N Engl J Med* 333:1737, 1995.

Jackson P, Bash DM: Management of the uncomplicated pregnant diabetic client in the ambulatory setting, *Nurse Pract* 19:64, 1994.

Knox TA, Olans LB: Liver disease in pregnancy, *N Engl J Med* 335:569, 1996.

Lee SH et al: Effects of pregnancy on first onset and symptoms of paroxysmal supraventricular tachycardia, *Am J Cardiol* 76:675, 1995.

Maccato M: Herpes in pregnancy, *Clin Obstet Gynecol* 36:869, 1993.

Mestman JH, Goodwin TM, Montoro MM: Thyroid disorders of pregnancy, *Endocrinol Metabol Clin North Am* 24:41, 1995.

Mishra L, Seeff LB: Viral hepatitis, A through E, complicating pregnancy, *Gastroenterol Clin North Am* 21:873, 1992.

Page RL: Treatment of arrhythmias during pregnancy, *Am Heart J* 130:871, 1995.

Petri M: Systemic lupus erythematosus and pregnancy, *Rheum Dis Clin North Am* 20:87, 1994.

Report of the Working Group on Asthma and Pregnancy Executive Summary: *Management of asthma during pregnancy,* NIH Pub. No. 93-3279A, 1993.

Sibai BM: Treatment of hypertension in pregnant women, *N Engl J Med* 335:257, 1996.

Sturridge F, de Swiet M, Letsky E: The use of low molecular weight heparin for thromboprophylaxis in pregnancy, *Br J Obstet Gynaecol* 101:69, 1994.

Usta IM et al: Acute fatty liver of pregnancy: an experience in the diagnosis and management of fourteen cases, *Am J Obstet Gynecol* 171:1342, 1994.

Wendel PJ, Wendel GD: Sexually transmitted diseases in pregnancy, *Semin Perinatol* 17:443, 1993.

Zamorski MA, Green LA: Preeclampsia and hypertensive disorders of pregnancy, *Am Fam Physician* 53(5):1595, 1996.

CHAPTER

373 Gerontology and Geriatric Medicine

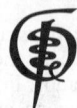

Michael S. Katz and Meghan B. Gerety

It's no art to grow old;
It is art to endure it.
Johann Wolfgang von Goethe

Elderly people are subject to deteriorating function, diverse diseases, and environmental challenges that potentiate the development of frailty and the inability to live independently. Geriatric medicine, defined as the medical care of elderly persons, is characterized by the comprehensive assessment and management of the older patient with chronic disability and multiple medical and social problems. The goal of geriatric medicine is generally to optimize function in the elderly patient with debilitating conditions. To accomplish this goal, the physician must combine medical expertise with a knowledge of gerontology (the study of aging) and a recognition that numerous clinical disciplines in addition to internal medicine (e.g., clinical pharmacol-

ogy, psychiatry, neurology, rehabilitation medicine, nursing) are essential to comprehensive management of the elderly patient.

GERONTOLOGY
Demography and Epidemiology

The elderly population of the United States has grown dramatically over the twentieth century and is projected to expand further during the early decades of the next century. The number of persons ages 65 and older increased from 4% of the population in 1900 to 12% in 1990. With the aging of the "baby boom" generation born after World War II, the 65-and-older age-group is anticipated to account for 17% of the population by the year 2020; by 2040, 21% of all persons living in the United States will be 65 or older. The growth of the older population reflects improvements in public health, socioeconomic conditions, and medical care that have resulted in decreased mortality rates of all age-groups, including elderly persons. Since 1900, life expectancy estimates at birth and at age 65 have increased, respectively, by 25 years and 5 years; currently, life expectancy averages 75 years at birth and 82 years at age 65. The 85-and-older age-group is the most rapidly growing segment of the U.S. population, and it is expected that more than 100,000 centenarians will be living by the year 2000.

The aging of the population during the twentieth century has heightened the demand for comprehensive health services to increased numbers of older persons susceptible to chronic illness and disability. Although persons 65 and older represent 12% of the population, this group accounts for more than one third of U.S. health care expenditures. Older people undergo more frequent and more prolonged hospitalizations and visit physicians more often than younger individuals. Eighty-five percent of people over 65 have at least one chronic illness, and 30% have three or more chronic diseases. One half of community-dwelling persons 65 and older report symptoms of arthritis. Other commonly reported conditions, in order of decreasing prevalence, include hypertension, decreased hearing, heart disease, and visual impairment. Older individuals with chronic illness are subject to functional impairment and eventual loss of the ability to live independently. Most noninstitutionalized persons over 65 maintain adequate basic function, as assessed by personal care activities (basic activities of daily living [basic ADLs], see later discussion). However, one quarter of this population has difficulty performing activities required for independent living (instrumental ADLs). The proportion of older persons institutionalized in nursing homes increases dramatically with age, rising from 1% of those 65 to 74, to 6% of those 75 to 84, to 22% of the 85-and-older age-group. Current projections indicate that 43% of persons over age 60 will live in nursing homes for some period during their lives.

The three leading causes of mortality in elderly persons, accounting for three quarters of all deaths in those 65 and older, are cardiovascular disease (predominantly coronary artery disease), malignant neoplasms (most often of the lung, breast, prostate, and colon), and cerebrovascular disease. Since 1968, mortality rates from coronary artery disease have decreased in all age-groups, including those over 65. This decrease is thought to result from risk factor reduction associated with control of hypertension, cessation of cigarette smoking, and decreased cholesterol intake. Over the same time period, cancer mortality in elderly persons has increased, probably as a reflection of the decline in mortality from coronary artery disease.

Although disease and disability are common at advanced age, it remains unclear whether the continued growth of the older population into the next century will lead by necessity to increased numbers of debilitated elderly persons requiring extensive medical and social support. Some investigators have argued that disease prevention and health promotion measures might be developed to promote a "compression of morbidity"—that is, to delay (or even eliminate) the onset of chronic illness and disability in people surviving to advanced age. The concept of limiting disease morbidity before death has been extended to age-related decrements in function of individuals without disease. Physiologic functioning is highly variable among older individuals, even though aging populations without discernible disease on the average are characterized by physiologic decline. Thus "normal" aging occurring in the absence of disease has been classified into two categories: *usual,* in which aging is accompanied by typical nonpathologic losses of physiologic function, and *successful,* in which physiologic decline during aging is minimal or even absent. Physiologic losses during usual aging have been attributed to the modifying effects of extrinsic variables (e.g., diet, exercise, psychosocial factors) on basic aging processes. Various extrinsic variables are known to be risk factors for specific diseases common in elderly persons (e.g., coronary artery disease risk factors). Accordingly, the gerontologic literature emphasizes the need for future research into strategies by which modifications of life-style and environment might reduce morbidity and maintain vitality in increasing numbers of older people.

Biology of Aging

Theories of Aging. Aging can be defined in biologic terms as those processes occurring during the postmaturational life span that progressively decrease the ability of an organism to adapt to environmental change and increase the likelihood of dying. The cellular and organismal mechanisms underlying aging are unknown, although it is generally agreed that aging is likely to be due to more than one primary process. For descriptive purposes, theories of aging can be classified into two broad categories, according to which aging is attributed to either (1) genetically programmed processes or (2) accumulation of damage to critical cellular or tissue constituents. These two classes of theories, like many individual theories of aging, are not mutually exclusive.

Genetic theories. Considerable evidence points to a genetic basis for aging. Perhaps the strongest evidence in this regard is the finding that maximum life span is species-specific and varies markedly among different species. Compelling evidence for genetic control of life span has also been provided by studies in which selective breeding of *Drosophila melanogaster* and the nematode *Caenorhabditis elegans* has been used to produce populations with increased longevity. The existence in humans of genetic progeroid syndromes (e.g., Werner's syndrome, Hutchinson-Gilford syndrome) characterized by premature occurrence of the aging phenotype further supports a role for genetics in aging. In addition, familial studies of longevity have demonstrated greater similarity between monozygotic twins than between dizygotic twins and nontwin siblings.

Current efforts to delineate the genetic determinants of aging draw on classic evolutionary theory as well as modern molecular biology. It has been suggested that aging evolved as a selected trait conferring advantage to the reproductively fit members of a species by eliminating old individuals in competition for the same resources. Support for this view is limited because animals in the wild do not usually survive to old age. Under these circumstances, aging would not be expected to provide added advantage to younger individuals. Alternative theories postulating genetic control of aging do not presuppose that aging is a selected trait of evolutionary value. For example, aging has been hypothesized to result from the expression of genes that exhibit "antagonistic pleiotropy"—that is, have opposite effects on fitness characteristics. In this case, genes selected for early reproductive fitness might also result in decreased fitness and aging later in life. Aging could also be caused by destructive genes expressed only late in the life span, after the period of reproductive fitness; such genes would presumably not be subject to strong negative selection and would thereby be maintained in a species despite their negative effects. Studies to identify specific genes that regulate aging have been conducted in lower organisms such as *C. elegans* and the budding yeast *Saccharomyces cerevisiae*. Mutation of a single gene called *age-1* has been found to lengthen life in *C. elegans,* whereas controlled expression of the viral oncogene *v-Ha-ras* in *S. cerevisiae* prolongs the life span of this organism. The relevance of these findings to the genetic control of aging in higher organisms, including humans, is unknown.

Damage theories. Prominent theories advocating the involvement of accumulated damage in aging processes are related conceptually to the long-standing view that metabolic rate is an important determinant of aging. According to this view the metabolism of fuels necessary to sustain life has deleterious effects on the organism that may cause aging. Over the past century an inverse relationship between metabolic rate and life span has been observed repeatedly, though not invariably, in mammalian species as well as invertebrates.

However, more recent studies comparing a large number and variety of animal species call the relationship between metabolic rate and aging into question. For example, birds, which have a relatively long life span, have very high metabolic rates. In addition, food restriction of rodents is well known to increase life span and retard processes attributable to aging but has no effect on metabolic rate per unit lean mass. Thus, although not all available data support a metabolic rate hypothesis of aging, a number of theories suggest possible mechanisms by which essential metabolism might create damage and thereby hasten aging processes.

Free radical theory. The free radical theory of aging, first proposed in the 1950s and currently under increasing scrutiny, postulates a major role for oxidative metabolism in causing cumulative damage. Highly reactive oxygen species, such as the superoxide and hydroxyl free radicals and also the hydrogen peroxide molecule, are generated in the course of normal oxidative metabolism. These intermediates are thought to cause damage and eventual aging through reactions with nucleic acid, protein, and lipid components of cells. Protective enzymes (e.g., superoxide dismutase, catalase) eliminate toxic oxygen intermediates, and, in some instances, transcription of the genes encoding these antioxidant enzymes declines with age. To some extent, therefore, the proposition that free radical damage causes aging is representative of theories invoking a genetic basis for aging.

Over the past decade a great deal of evidence has been obtained in support of the free radical theory of aging. For example, many types of free radical damage (e.g., lipid peroxidation, protein oxidation, oxidation of DNA) have been found to increase with increasing age in both invertebrate and mammalian animal models. Moreover, food restriction has consistently been shown to reduce the levels of free radical damage in tissues of rodents. Using transgenic techniques, investigators are now studying the effect of overexpressing antioxidant enzymes on aging. Recent studies with *D. melanogaster* show that flies overexpressing both superoxide dismutase and catalase have less free radical damage and longer life spans, which is the strongest evidence to date in support of the free radical theory of aging.

Glycation theory. A prominent theory relating fuel utilization to damage and aging holds that toxic effects of glucose may mediate aging processes. Glucose and other reducing sugars undergo nonenzymatic glycation reactions with proteins and nucleic acids to generate glycoadducts termed *advanced glycosylation end-products* (AGEs). It has been proposed that AGEs cause aging by cross-linking or otherwise modifying biologic molecules involved in critical physiologic processes. The glycation theory is especially provocative because recent studies demonstrating prevention of AGE formation by aminoguanidine suggest potential interventions to retard aging processes.

Somatic mutation theory. The somatic mutation theory of aging originated in 1959 when it was hypothesized that the accumulation of DNA damage in somatic cells was a basic mechanism in the aging process. It was proposed that the accumulation of DNA damage eventually resulted in the inactivation of genes and death of the cells. Over the ensuing years support for this theory of aging has waxed and waned; however, it has become increasingly apparent over the past decade that many steps in DNA metabolism are altered with age in a variety of tissues and animal models. In addition, many of the age-related alterations in DNA metabolism are retarded by food restriction. For example, tissues from food-restricted rodents show increased DNA repair activity and reduced levels of DNA damage and mutations. Studies of Werner's syndrome, a genetic disease with many clinical findings suggestive of accelerated aging, indicate that this disease may be associated with defects in DNA metabolism. Although no deficit in DNA repair has been observed in patients with Werner's syndrome, cells from these patients show an increased mutation frequency. Recently the gene product responsible for Werner's syndrome has been identified as a mutated, putative DNA helicase, an enzyme normally involved in DNA functions (e.g., replication, repair) requiring DNA unwinding. This observation is consistent with the hypothesis that Werner's syndrome patients age prematurely because of an accelerated accumulation of DNA damage and/or mutations with age.

Cellular aging. A distinctive approach to the study of aging has been to use human cells in tissue culture to investigate a cellular basis for aging. This line of research began 35 years ago with the observation that normal human fibroblasts grown in culture exhibit a limited number of population doublings. The doubling capacity of cultured fibroblasts was found to be inversely related to the age of the donor and directly related to maximum life span among different species. Findings such as these have led some to contend that aging in vivo is expressed in culture and that aging is an intrinsic characteristic of cells proliferating in vitro. However, others have cautioned against using cultured cells as a model of aging because the relevance of replicative potential in vitro to aging processes in vivo is yet to be established.

Physiologic Changes. It is generally agreed that human aging is accompanied by physiologic deterioration. However, studies of the effects of aging on physiologic function are subject to several limitations. First, the physiologic consequences of aging are often difficult to distinguish from the superimposed effects of diseases and life-style changes common in elderly persons. Second, physiologic decline is highly variable among elderly persons and also among different organ systems of any given individual. As noted earlier, individual variation may be attributable to factors extrinsic to the primary aging processes. Third, most studies of age differences in physiologic function have been cross-sectional in design. Such studies may fail to identify important cohort effects and secular trends. Despite the limitations of cross-sectional data, longitudinal studies in general confirm a decline in physiologic function with advancing age. Finally, because functional losses during aging reflect diminished homeostatic control mechanisms, age changes in physiologic systems are usually maximal under conditions of stress and may not be demonstrable at rest.

The following sections summarize examples of major physiologic changes observed during human aging.

Body composition and homeostatic regulation. Changes in body composition include a decline in lean body mass (primarily as a result of decreased muscle mass) with a proportionate increase in body fat. These changes are important determinants of physiologic function and therapeutic intervention in elderly persons. For example, reduced muscle mass is thought to account in large part for the decline in maximum oxygen consumption during exercise (VO_{2max}) demonstrable with increasing age. In addition, increases in body fat may increase the volume of distribution of lipophilic drugs and prolong their pharmacologic actions. Of note, changes in body composition in elderly persons are probably caused not only by primary aging processes but also by extrinsic factors such as physical inactivity and altered dietary intake. Age changes in homeostatic controls include impaired baroreflex sensitivity, which may predispose older persons to orthostatic hypotension, and diminished thermoregulation, which increases susceptibility to hypothermia and heatstroke.

Cardiovascular function. Numerous studies have been conducted to evaluate functional changes of the cardiovascular system during aging. A well-established observation is that the pattern of left ventricular filling shifts with age. In older individuals early diastolic filling is reduced, and there is increased reliance on atrial contraction to maintain adequate left ventricular filling. Although the precise mechanism of this age-related change remains under investigation, the consensus view is that with aging the heart becomes less compliant and requires higher pressures for the same degree of filling. Reduced compliance (increased stiffness) of the heart may be due to increases in connective tissue as well as to the presence of ventricular hypertrophy, which is known to be more prevalent in older age groups. The hypertrophy, in turn, may result from age-associated decreases in arterial compliance that increase impedance to ventricular ejection. Increases in arterial stiffness with age are multifactorial in origin; causes include hypertension, increased collagen deposition in the arterial tree, calcification, and underlying atherosclerosis. The net result of the increased ventricular stiffness, as reflected by altered filling pattern, is that older persons may develop signs and symptoms of pulmonary congestion (rales, dyspnea on exertion) in the absence of systolic dysfunction. Discerning the presence of diastolic dysfunction in older patients is important because the management of these patients differs from management of those with traditional heart failure. In older patients with diastolic dysfunction, augmentation of contractile strength with drugs such as digoxin serves no purpose and may indeed be harmful. Gentle diuresis and aggressive control of coexistent hypertension are the most useful therapies for this type of patient.

β-adrenergic responsiveness of the heart is also known to decline with advancing age. During vigorous exercise, heart rate increases to a lesser extent in older persons than in younger individuals. This age-related change has been attributed to diminished β-adrenergic modulation of heart rate during exercise. An age-associated increase in plasma catecholamine (norepinephrine) has been documented at rest and during exercise, but the relationship between this finding and decreased β-adrenergic responsiveness with age has not been clarified.

Pulmonary function. Pulmonary function declines with advancing age. Elastic recoil of the lung decreases during aging, possibly from loss of alveolar attachments to parenchymal elastic fibers. Decreased lung elasticity contributes to age-related increases in functional residual capacity (resting volume of the lungs after a normal expiration) and residual volume (volume remaining after maximum expiration). Loss of elastic recoil, which results in early collapse of peripheral airways during forced expiration, may also account in part for age-associated decreases in forced vital capacity (total volume forcibly exhaled after full inspiration) and the volume forcibly exhaled in 1 second (FEV_1). In addition, decreasing elasticity with age progressively increases the closing volume (lung volume at which peripheral airways collapse) to the extent that, in some elderly individuals, airway closure may occur during normal respiration. Arterial oxygen tension (PaO_2) declines with age, largely as a result of a ventilation-perfusion imbalance created by airway collapse in well-perfused areas of the lung. Diminished ventilatory responses to hypoxia and hypercapnia are also demonstrable in elderly persons and are thought to reflect decreased chemoreceptor function.

Renal function. Age-related decrements have been observed in kidney function and the regulation of electrolyte and fluid balance. Anatomic changes of the aging kidney include a gradual decline in mass (especially prominent in the renal cortex), a decrease in the total number of glomeruli, and increased glomerulosclerosis. Glomerular filtration rate, as assessed by creatinine clearance, falls progressively with increasing age. However, the decline in creatinine clearance with age is highly variable; some individuals evaluated longitudinally over many years exhibit no age-related decrease in creatinine clearance. The ability of the kidney to decrease urinary sodium excretion in response to sodium restriction is impaired in older individuals. This defect in sodium conservation may be due, at least in part, to an age-related decline in renin and aldosterone levels documented under basal and stimulated conditions. Several factors contribute to age changes in the regulation of extracellular fluid volume. Vasopressin (antidiuretic hormone) release in response to hypertonic saline infusion is *greater* in older individuals than in younger subjects, reflecting an age-related increase in sensitivity of hypothalamic osmoreceptors. Despite this increase in vasopressin release, kidney responsiveness to vasopressin falls with age, resulting in impaired urinary concentrating ability after water deprivation. In addition, thirst and drinking responses to water deprivation are decreased in elderly individuals. The urinary concentrating defect and reduced thirst in elderly persons increase the risk of dehydration during illness.

Endocrine function. Considerable attention in the endocrine literature has been focused on age changes in glucose metabolism. Glucose tolerance decreases during aging. In healthy aging adults, plasma glucose measured 2 hours after an oral glucose load increases by about 9 mg/dl per decade; fasting plasma glucose increases by 1 mg/dl per decade. The impairment of glucose tolerance at advanced ages is independent of obesity and physical inactivity, which are common accompaniments of aging and can themselves contribute to glucose intolerance. The primary cause of decreased glucose tolerance during aging is insulin resistance in peripheral tissues, especially muscle. Numerous studies have shown that insulin binding to cell receptors does not change with age, and thus a postreceptor abnormality is thought to account for the age-related defect in insulin action. Although insulin secretion may also be impaired with age, circulating insulin levels are not diminished in older individuals, probably because of an age-related decline in insulin clearance. Decreased glucose tolerance during aging does not generally result in glucose levels in the diabetic range. However, as postulated by the glycation theory of aging, modest elevations in glucose over time could influence the development of physiologic deterioration or age-associated disease. In this regard, fasting plasma glucose and glycosylated hemoglobin are highly correlated in nondiabetic subjects over a wide age range. Some epidemiologic data suggest that glucose elevations even within the nondiabetic range increase the risk of cardiovascular disease. It remains controversial whether the predictive value of glucose is independent of established cardiovascular risk factors such as insulin, which may be elevated in elderly individuals with insulin resistance.

Another endocrine variable of potential importance during aging is the growth hormone–insulin-like growth factor 1 (IGF-1) axis. Pituitary secretion of growth hormone declines with increasing age. Many of the anabolic effects of growth hormone are mediated by IGF-1, which is produced by the liver and other tissues in response to growth hormone. As with growth hormone secretion, circulating IGF-1 levels decrease with age. Body composition changes in elderly persons (i.e., reduced lean body mass, increased body fat) resemble those found in nonelderly individuals with growth hormone deficiency. These findings have led to the hypothesis that age-related changes in body composition are due, at least in part, to decreased growth hormone secretion. In support of this hypothesis, studies have demonstrated that growth hormone administration to healthy elderly men with low IGF-1 levels increases lean body mass and decreases fat mass. Clinical trials of growth hormone administration are currently being extended to frail elderly populations subject to malnutrition and other catabolic conditions.

Immune function. Depressed function of the immune system with aging may predispose elderly persons to infectious diseases and malignancy. An age-related decline in cell-mediated immunity is characterized by decreased proliferation of T lymphocytes in response to mitogenic stimulation. Impaired T-cell proliferation with age may be due to defective intracellular transduction of mitogenic signals. In addition, interleukin-2 (IL-2) synthesis and IL-2 receptor expression, which are required for T-cell proliferation, are both decreased with age. Interestingly, only a portion of the T-lymphocyte population undergoes functional decline; the mechanisms underlying this heterogeneity of the lymphocyte pool are yet to be identified. Thymic involution and loss of thymic hormones are thought to play a role in decreased T-cell function during aging. Age changes in humoral immunity include increased production of autoantibodies, including antiidiotypic antibodies, and decreased antibody responses to foreign antigens. These changes may reflect age-related alterations in T-cell regulation of B-cell function.

GERIATRIC MEDICINE
Special Considerations in the Approach to the Geriatric Patient

Atypical Presentation of Illness. It has been claimed that physiologic changes with aging cause an alteration of host-disease response in older persons. The level of evidence for increased frequency of "atypical" illness presentation in elders is weak, since most reports are case series or case control studies from teaching hospitals and academic referral clinics. The contributions of disease burden and disability, both independent of age, are usually not explored. Although it is inappropriate to reach a conclusion that age systematically changes host-disease response, age and other factors may indeed affect signs and symptoms of illness in some elders.

Factors that interact to influence the responses of older persons to illness include age-associated changes in physiologic functions (host factors), the burden of comorbid disease (disease factors), and treatments for disease (treatment factors). Accurate ascertainment of illness is made difficult by host factors such as hearing and visual impairment, memory loss, and aphasia. Other important host factors include alterations in perception of pain and other symptoms, and the occasional absence of signs or symptoms typically noted in younger individuals (e.g., fever in infectious illness such as pneumonia). Disease-disease interactions are also common in older persons. Acute illness in one system may stress the already reduced reserve capacity of another, producing unrelated signs and symptoms that distract diagnostic efforts away from the correct etiologic condition. For example, urosepsis may present as delirium in a person with impaired cognitive function. Illnesses may also mask one another; for example, activity limitation by osteoarthritis may obscure symptoms of coronary artery disease. Finally, treatment for one illness may unmask a previously undiagnosed pathologic condition. For example, urinary

outlet obstruction may become symptomatic for the first time when a pharmacologic agent with anticholinergic properties provokes urinary retention.

Because host, disease, and treatment factors that may alter manifestations of disease are so common in elders, physicians may wish to change their approach to diagnosis in these persons. Even when signs and symptoms appear straightforward, an evaluation to uncover occult contributing disease may be appropriate. Certain nonspecific syndromes should be regarded as sentinel events requiring thorough investigation. These syndromes include failure to thrive, acute change in appetite, decline in self-care capacity, onset of falls, immobility ("taking to bed"), change in intellectual function, and new incontinence.

Functional Status Assessment. The effects of age, disease, and environment all interact and express themselves through a final common pathway—functional status. *Functional status* is a term used to describe the capacity of an individual to function in multiple domains (physical, mental, social, emotional) and at multiple levels (organ function, function of the person as a whole, function of the person in society). Care of the older person should focus not only on optimizing health but also on improving or maintaining function. Formal assessment of functional status serves four primary purposes. First, assessment may reveal previously undetected medical or psychiatric diagnoses that warrant evaluation or treatment. Second, functional status assessment provides the context within which goals of therapy and intensity of diagnostic evaluation may most appropriately be set. Third, repetition of functional assessment may be used to gauge the impact of therapy. Finally, identification of functional deficits predicts need for social and environmental interventions. Thus any evaluation of an older or chronically ill patient should be accompanied by an assessment of functional status.

A substantial body of literature published over the last decade has advocated an interdisciplinary approach to geriatric functional assessment. The team approach may include primary care physicians, nurses, social workers, psychologists or psychiatrists, pharmacists, and nutritionists in the care of a single patient. However, an interdisciplinary approach may be impractical for many physicians' practices. For this reason a stratified approach to the evaluation of the older patient is preferred, one that progresses in intensity and complexity as illness and functional disability increase. Three patient categories determine the assessment strategy: (1) apparently healthy elderly persons, (2) frail elderly persons (i.e., functionally impaired or medically ill community-dwelling elderly patients), and (3) institutionalized or severely impaired elderly patients.

Assessment across these patient categories may be performed with instruments (Table 373-1) consisting of standardized questions or semistructured interviews that can be incorporated into the review of systems. The instruments shown in Table 373-1 were chosen to allow a functional status assessment to be conducted in the office or nursing home, where a physician and nurse may be the sole members of the interdisciplinary team. Although performing additional assessments for frailer persons increases the time required for evaluation, it also increases diagnostic yield. Time commitment of the physician to functional status assessment can be minimized by using self-report questionnaires completed by the patient or caregiver while in the waiting room or administered by an office assistant.

Physical function can be assessed most simply with basic and instrumental activities of daily living (ADLs). Basic ADLs are personal care activities including bathing, dressing, grooming, toileting, continence, transfers (bed-to-chair, chair-to-toilet), and ambulation. Dependence in personal care activities indicates the need for personal assistance in the home unless a return to independence can be achieved. Instrumental ADLs are the tasks necessary to maintain an independent household. They include ability to take medications, manage finances, telephone, shop, keep house, prepare meals, and use transportation. Dependence in these tasks indicates the need for social services rather than personal assistance.

Brief instruments are also available to screen for cognitive impairment, gait and balance abnormalities, incontinence, depressive symptoms, and social support requirements (Table 373-1). Social function is ideally evaluated by a social worker with an intake interview that details the patient's financial resources, social supports, and prefer-

Table 373-1 Geriatric assessment instruments

DOMAIN	EXAMPLE	PATIENT CATEGORY	ASSESSOR	TIME REQUIRED (MINUTES)
Functional status				
General functioning	Medical Outcomes Study SF-36	HE	Questionnaire, MD or assistant	10
Basic ADLs	Katz ADLs, Lawton PSMS	FE, IE	Questionnaire, MD or assistant	<5
Instrumental ADLs	Lawton IADLs, OARS ADLs	HE, FE, IE	Questionnaire, MD or assistant	<5
Cognition	MMSE, SPMSQ	FE, IE	Interviewer administered	10
Gait and balance	Performance-oriented mobility assessment	FE, IE	MD or other health professional	5-10
Incontinence	Structured history	HE, FE, IE	MD or assistant	<5
Depression	Geriatric Depression Scale	HE, FE, IE	Questionnaire, MD or assistant	<5
Social support	OARS Social Support Questionnaire	FE, IE	Questionnaire, MD or assistant	10-15

ADLs, Activities of daily living; *PSMS,* Personal Self-Maintenance Scale; *OARS,* Older Americans Research and Service Center; *MMSE,* Mini-Mental State Exam; *SPMSQ,* Short Portable Mental Status Questionnaire; *FE,* frail elderly; *IE,* institutionalized or severely impaired elderly; *HE,* healthy elderly; *MD,* physician
Modified with permission from Chiodo L, Gerety MB: Medical evaluation of the geriatric patient. In Katz MS, editor: *Geriatric medicine,* New York, 1991, Churchill Livingstone.

ences for social intervention. Environmental assessment is ideally accomplished during a home visit, including a thorough inventory detailing sanitary conditions, safety, and accessibility. If a home visit is not feasible, a home access and safety questionnaire completed in the physician's office can substitute. The Occupational Safety and Health Administration (OSHA) publishes a comprehensive checklist to be used by consumers in assessing the home.

Geriatric Clinical Pharmacology. Although only 12% of the population is older than 65, this group accounts for more than 30% of all medication consumption in the United States. Multiple drug use is costly and confers significant clinical risk. Epidemiologic evidence has implicated adverse drug reactions as causal factors in as many as 10% of hospital admissions. Strong associations exist between specific drug classes and common disabling conditions in elderly patients. Neuroleptics, long-acting benzodiazepines, and other psychoactive drugs have been implicated as risk factors for falls and hip fracture. Cognitive impairment, depression, incontinence, gastrointestinal bleeding, and renal insufficiency have also been linked to drug toxicity.

The role of age as a determinant of drug response is controversial. Many studies have convincingly demonstrated that older persons are at greater risk than younger persons for adverse drug events. This association holds across hospital and community settings. Age per se, however, probably confers minimal risk. If disease burden and number of medications are held constant, the association between age and adverse reactions weakens. In fact, marked heterogeneity exists among aged individuals in pharmacokinetic and pharmacodynamic responses to drugs. It is likely that many interacting factors contribute to variation in drug response and increased susceptibility to adverse drug events. These factors include cumulative burden of chronic (and often progressive) illness, intermittent acute illnesses, number of medications, physician prescribing behavior, and patient compliance.

Age-related changes in pharmacokinetic and pharmacodynamic responses to drugs are outlined in Table 373-2. Renal and hepatic functions are often significantly reduced by age and age-associated disease. Adjustments of drug dosage or dosing interval are often required to compensate. Creatinine clearance may be estimated using the Cockcroft equation:

$$\text{Creatinine clearance} = \frac{(140 - \text{Age[yr]}) \times \text{Weight (kg)}}{72 \times \text{Serum creatinine (mg/dl)}} \quad \textbf{(EQ. 1)}$$
$$\text{(multiply by 0.85 for females)}$$

For patients with creatinine clearance less than 50 ml/min, dosage and/or dosing intervals should be adjusted for all drugs that are cleared by the kidney and have a narrow therapeutic index. Most clinicians already adjust doses for aminoglycosides, but care must also be taken with many antibiotics, especially ticarcillin, Timentin (ticarcillin and clavulanate), cephalosporins, imipenem, and ciprofloxacin. Other drugs requiring dose adjustment in elderly patients include digoxin, allopurinol, lithium, amantadine, and H_2 blockers. More comprehensive information about dosage adjustments can be found in other sources. Hepatic function cannot be easily estimated. Dos-

Table 373-2 Pharmacokinetic and pharmacodynamic changes with aging

PHYSIOLOGIC CHANGE	PHARMACOLOGIC EFFECT
Gastrointestinal	
↓ Gastric motility	Negligible
↓ Gastric pH	Negligible
Body composition	
↓ Lean body mass	Water-soluble drugs ↑ Serum concentration, ↓Vd, ↓t½
↑ Total body fat	Lipid-soluble drugs ↓ Serum concentration, ↑ Vd, ↑ t½
↓ Albumin	Highly (>90%) protein-bound drugs ↑ Free (active)/bound drug
Metabolism	
↓ Phase I reactions (e.g., oxidation)	Oxidatively metabolized drugs →↓ Metabolism, ↓ clearance, ↑ t½
→ Phase II reactions (e.g., glucuronidation)	No effects
↓ Hepatic blood flow	Drugs with flow-dependent metabolism ↓ Clearance, ↑ t½
Renal function	
↓ Creatinine clerance	Renally excreted drugs ↓ Clearance, ↑ t½
Target organ	
↓ Cellular mass (e.g., brain)	CNS-active drugs ↑ Drug effect
↓ Receptor function β-Adrenergic response	β-Adrenergic drugs ↓ Effect of β₁-active drugs →↓ Effect of β₂-active drugs
↓ Baroreceptor response	Drugs with orthostatic potential ↑ Orthostasis ↓ Heart rate, ↓ blood pressure compensation

↑, Increase; ↓, decrease; →, no change; *Vd,* volume of distribution; t½, half-life.
From Gerety MB et al: Adverse drug reactions and altered clinical pharmacology in the elderly: a guide for modification of prescribing. In Katz MS, editor: *Geriatric medicine,* New York, 1991, Churchill Livingstone.

age adjustments should be made for hepatically metabolized drugs under conditions of altered hepatic blood flow or function. These conditions include congestive heart failure, primary liver diseases, and β-adrenergic blockade.

Pharmacodynamic properties of drugs may be altered in elders because of smaller target organ mass or reduced cellular function. This is particularly true of drugs with primary or secondary CNS effects.

Initial doses of CNS-active drugs should be approximately one half of the usual starting adult dose. Slow titration to the desired therapeutic end-point is preferred.

The physician's prescribing behavior should reflect age-associated changes in drug response. Each patient's drug regimen must be carefully tailored, regularly reviewed, and periodically adjusted. A mounting body of evidence suggests that it is both safe and beneficial to discontinue medications with no apparent indication, even if they have been prescribed for long periods of time. The best strategy is to discontinue agents one at a time, carefully monitoring for recurrence of the original indication or changes in effectiveness of concomitantly prescribed medications.

Nutrition. Physiologic changes occurring with age often interact with socioeconomic factors and chronic disease to produce poor nutrition status in elderly persons. The U.S. National Health, Examination, and Nutrition Survey indicates that older persons often consume as few as 1000 Kcal/day. As many as 60% of hospitalized patients and 50% to 70% of institutionalized persons may suffer from mild to moderate malnutrition. Coexisting diseases often make traditional markers of malnutrition, such as serum albumin, difficult to interpret. Nevertheless, these markers continue to have clear-cut associations with treatment outcomes. Clinical and biochemical markers such as weight loss, low body weight, and low serum albumin are strongly associated with prolonged hospital stays, poor outcome from surgery, and mortality.

Numerous factors contribute to inadequate nutrition. Socioeconomic factors include lack of education about appropriate nutrients, inadequate economic resources, and social isolation. Neuropsychologic diseases such as depression and dementia may result in reduced appetite. Functional disability and immobility make it difficult to use transportation, acquire groceries, and prepare food. Age-associated physiologic changes in thirst, taste, and smell may also reduce food consumption. Dental dysfunction and periodontal disease, common in elders, may be important factors in poor nutritional intake in elderly patients.

Assessment of nutritional status in younger persons often involves anthropometric measurements, serum albumin and transferrin levels, total lymphocyte counts, and cell-mediated immune responses to dermal antigen injections. In elderly persons many of these nutritional variables are subject to age- and disease-associated changes. A simple, clinically oriented evaluation of nutritional status may be useful. A nutritionally focused history should elicit changes in weight (significant if >10% weight loss occurs over 6 months or 5% over 1 month) and determine whether weight is stable or still declining. Changes in eating habits or the presence of symptoms that interfere with food intake or digestion should be noted. The physical examination should focus on underlying causes of weight loss as well as signs of malnutrition (cachexia, interosseous wasting, loss of muscle mass) or nutrient deficiency (angular cheilitis or glossitis). Oral examination should include inspection of teeth, gums, fit of dentures, and oropharyngeal lesions that may interfere with mastication or oral intake.

The American Society for Parenteral and Enteral Nutrition has published guidelines suggesting threshold criteria for nutritional intervention. Supplemental feeding is recommended for persons with obvious malnutrition or borderline nutritional status whenever a prolonged (5- to 7-day) period of hypocaloric intake is anticipated. If nutritional status is uncertain, daily calorie counts should be obtained and supplemental feedings instituted if caloric intake is inadequate. An adequate trial of supplemental oral feeding should be attempted before tube feeding or parenteral nutrition is instituted.

Sensory Impairment. Hearing and vision impairments are common chronic conditions that limit communication and isolate aged individuals. From a diagnostic perspective, these impairments make it more difficult to obtain a history and evaluate an individual appropriately. Although other specialists may be necessary to rehabilitate sensory impairment, internists must be able to screen for impairment and refer for appropriate management.

Hearing impairment. Clinically significant hearing loss affects about one in three individuals 65 years of age or older, and one half of all persons between 75 and 79. The most common pattern of hearing loss in elderly persons is termed *presbycusis* and is characterized by bilateral high-frequency sensorineural loss. The etiology of presbycusis is undetermined.

Most speech occurs at frequencies from 1000 to 3000 Hz. No universally accepted audiometric definition of hearing loss exists, but an average loss of more than 25 decibels (dB) at 500, 1000, or 2000 Hz is recognized by most audiologists as evidence for significant hearing impairment. Clinicians can evaluate hearing quickly, reliably, and inexpensively with self-report or physical diagnostic tests. The Hearing Handicap Inventory for the Elderly–Screening (HHIE-S) is a 10-item questionnaire with scores predictive of hearing loss and successful rehabilitation. A hand-held otoscope with a built-in audiometer produces a standard screening signal at a known distance. An audiometer signal of 40 dB at 1000 and 2000 Hz can be used to detect hearing loss with a sensitivity of 94%.

To facilitate communication during the clinical interview, the physician should speak clearly and slowly and be positioned in front of the patient so that lip reading may be used to facilitate speech interpretation. Assistive listening devices (ALDs, pocket amplifiers) can enhance understanding, relieve the strain of listening, and reduce the need for shouting.

Hearing-impaired patients with recognized handicap should be referred to an audiologist for full audiometry and the appropriate prescription of a hearing aid. In clinical trials, hearing aids have been demonstrated to improve communication function, reduce depressive symptoms, and improve cognitive performance. For patients who cannot afford hearing aids, ALDs provide a less expensive means of general amplification.

Visual impairment. Visual impairment affects 1 in 6 persons ages 75 to 84 and 1 in 4 persons age 85 and older. Total blindness is operationally defined as a visual acuity of 20/200 or worse in the better eye; although only 1% of persons older than 65 meet this definition, they account for the majority of blind persons in the United States. Many impairments, such as loss of accommodation of the lens or corneal abnormalities, can be managed by appropriate refraction with glasses or contact lenses. However, a variety of other conditions (macular degeneration, cataracts, diabetic retinopathy, glaucoma) lead to blindness and require ophthalmologic care and vision rehabilitation.

Visual loss leads directly to loss of independence in instrumental and basic ADLs, decreased physical activity, and symptoms of depression. The greatest threat posed by visual impairment to a functionally independent aged individual is the loss of driving privileges. Most states require a best corrected visual acuity of 20/40 to operate an automobile. Visual loss also increases the risk of falls and injury.

The internist should screen for visual impairment and, with appropriate referral, take steps to overcome its impact. Near and far vision may be screened effectively using a variety of visual acuity charts with Snellen letters (or symbols if the patient is illiterate or cognitively impaired). Ophthalmoscopy may identify cataracts or retinal changes of diabetes and macular degeneration. Because the prevalence of visual impairment is so high in the elderly population, age >65 may be used as an independent criterion for referral to an ophthalmologist if an eye examination has not been performed in the previous 2 years.

Hazards of Bed Rest. Although a time-honored treatment for many illnesses, imposition of bed rest is now understood to pose significant physiologic and psychologic hazards. The physiologic effects of immobility were originally described in young healthy adult males as part of the space program. Because of marginal reserve in physiologic systems affected by immobilization, elderly persons are particularly prone to adverse effects of bed rest. Almost all the adverse consequences of immobility are preventable with simple, practical maneuvers.

The physiologic consequences of bed rest are global. After less than 2 days, blood volume decreases, cardiac output declines, and pulmonary volumes decrease. Urinary concentrating ability decreases, and calcium and nitrogen losses often exceed intake. Appetite decreases and bowel motility slows. Constipation or overflow fecal incontinence may occur. Decreased muscular strength, decreased endurance, and muscle atrophy also occur. Collagen fibers in tendinous and joint capsular structures begin to realign themselves along lines of stress into contractures after only 96 hours. Skin breakdown may begin to occur over bony prominences. Tissue pressure that exceeds capillary pressure for more than 2 hours may produce histologic findings of early tissue necrosis. Addition of shear forces (sliding downward in bed), heat, and humidity may hasten the formation of pressure ulcers. Stasis in the lower extremities and the pelvic venous system increases the risk of deep vein thrombosis. Arterial and venous responses to the upright position are diminished, with resultant postural hypotension. Both peripheral and central nervous system functions are altered. Emotional lability, decreased concentration, poor short-term memory, and diminished intellectual functioning are seen after prolonged immobility.

The effects of bed rest may be prevented or ameliorated using simple precautionary measures and rehabilitation techniques. Assumption of the upright (seated, standing, or weight-bearing) posture for a few minutes several times a day minimizes fluid, electrolyte, and calcium losses and helps retain vascular tone and baroreflex action. Passive range of motion exercises—that is, moving joints through full range of motion only once per day—may prevent contractures. A few submaximal contractions of major muscle groups minimize loss of strength. Special attention should be paid to muscle groups important for bed mobility, transfers, and ambulation. These muscle groups include hip and knee flexors and extensors and trunk musculature. The most effective exercises for these muscle groups in patients who must experience periods of immobility are functional activities, including supine-to-sit, sit-to-supine, transfer from bed to chair and chair to bed, sit-to-stand, and ambulation. Frequent changes of position and time out of bed will also prevent pressure ulcer formation. Routine orders for hospitalized elderly patients should include being out of bed for all meals and ambulation at least daily. Nurses and physicians should encourage patients to perform these activities with minimal to no assistance.

The hazards of bed rest are so great that bed rest should be prescribed only when no other alternative exists. Physicians, nurses, and rehabilitation therapists often unwittingly conspire to produce complications of bed rest in the interest of "patient safety," despite the obvious risks of immobility.

Geriatric Syndromes

Many of the problems affecting aged individuals should be viewed as syndromes, that is, collections of signs and symptoms with a number of potential causes. Only now are the causes and effective treatments of these conditions beginning to be understood.

Dementia. Dementia (Chapter 142) is a syndrome of global intellectual deterioration. The fourth edition of the American Psychiatric Association's *Diagnostic and Statistical Manual of Mental Disorders (DSM-IV)* defines the clinical features that serve as diagnostic criteria for the dementia syndrome. Dementia is characterized by a chronic loss of previously established intellectual ability that interferes with occupational and social function. Memory impairment is essential to the diagnosis and must be accompanied by at least one other deficit in cognitive areas such as language, perception, visuoconstructive function, calculation, abstract thinking, judgment, and executive function. Personality change may also occur, but level of consciousness is maintained. Global cognitive impairment distinguishes the dementia syndrome from the decline in recent memory that often accompanies advanced age ("benign senescent forgetfulness"). Moreover, progressive deterioration with normal attention and alertness differentiate the dementia syndrome from acute confusional states such as delirium.

Alzheimer's disease (Chapter 142) accounts for more than one half of all cases of dementia. The prevalence of Alzheimer's disease may be greater than previously suspected. In a community-based study the prevalence rates for probable Alzheimer's disease were 10% of those over the age of 65 and 47% of those older than 85. A widely used set of criteria for the clinical diagnosis of *probable* Alzheimer's disease has been proposed by a work group of the U.S. Department of Health and Human Services Task Force on Alzheimer's disease. The diagnosis requires that dementia be established by clinical examination, formal mental status tests (e.g., Mini–Mental State Examination, Blessed Dementia Scale), and neuropsychologic testing. Other disorders (see following discussion) that could account for progressive in-

tellectual decline must be absent. The diagnosis of *definite* Alzheimer's disease requires histopathologic evidence (neuritic plaques, neurofibrillary tangles) rarely obtained premortem.

Dementing disorders other than Alzheimer's disease are discussed in Chapter 142. In autopsy series, 10% to 20% of cases of dementia have been attributed to multiple cerebral infarcts (*multiinfarct* or *vascular dementia*), with an equal number of cases caused by multiinfarct dementia coexisting with Alzheimer's disease. A much lower prevalence (1% to 4%) of multiinfarct dementia has been described in geriatric outpatients presenting with suspected dementia, although this population may exclude patients referred for neurologic rather than geriatric evaluation. Characteristics suggesting vascular dementia include abrupt onset, history of strokes, focal neurologic findings, stepwise deterioration, and history or presence of hypertension.

Much has been written about treatable causes of *reversible* dementia, in contrast to *irreversible* disorders such as Alzheimer's disease and multiinfarct dementia. Medication toxicity, metabolic disorders such as hypothyroidism, and depression are considered the most common causes of reversible dementia. Cognitive impairment accompanying depression is sometimes called *pseudodementia*. In general, geriatric outpatients with reversible dementia have shorter duration of symptoms, are less demented, and use more prescription drugs than those with irreversible dementia.

Between 10% and 20% of dementias have been classified as "reversible" on the basis of their association with common treatable conditions that may affect mentation. Treatment of these associated conditions usually results in only modest, transient improvement of cognitive function. It is especially important to recognize that even in patients with "irreversible" dementia, cognitive improvement may follow treatment of coexisting medical disorders. Some treatable conditions such as hearing impairment can produce social isolation and other findings mistakenly attributed to cognitive impairment. These concerns have led some to question the practical significance of the term *reversible dementia* and to emphasize instead the treatment of comorbid conditions that contribute to overall loss of function in the demented patient.

In addition to a history and physical examination, neuropsychologic testing may be required to meet the diagnostic criteria for probable Alzheimer's disease. Initial laboratory evaluation with complete blood cell count, blood chemistries (including electrolytes, glucose, creatinine, and calcium), and thyrotropin testing is recommended to identify treatable abnormalities contributing to "reversible" dementia or other dysfunction in the demented patient. Neuroimaging, either by computed tomography (CT) or magnetic resonance imaging (MRI), is probably not applicable to every dementia work-up and is recommended especially for patients with recent onset of symptoms, atypical presentation, rapid deterioration, unexplained focal neurologic findings, history of head injury, and manifestations of normal-pressure hydrocephalus (i.e., incontinence or gait disturbance). Neuroimaging may also be useful to reassure patients and caregivers. Positron emission tomography (PET) and single-photon emission computed tomography (SPECT) have demonstrated reduced metabolic activity in the temporal and parietal region of patients with Alzheimer's disease. However, the clinical utility of these newer imaging techniques in the diagnostic evaluation of dementia remains to be determined.

Management of the demented patient is directed at (1) treating reversible conditions that exacerbate functional decline and (2) reducing behavioral disturbances through environmental modification or, if necessary, pharmacologic therapy. Education of the patient's caregiver(s) is also an essential aspect of a comprehensive therapeutic plan. Instruction on the nature of the patient's illness and the availability of community respite services can improve patient care as well as reduce caregiver burden and thereby enhance quality of life for the caregiver.

Currently, no effective medical treatments exist for the irreversible dementias. The cholinergic hypothesis of Alzheimer's disease has led to recent clinical trials of the cholinesterase inhibitors *tacrine* (tetrahydroaminoacridine, THA) and *donepezil* as potential therapeutic agents. Clinical trials in multiple sites suggest that some Alzheimer's disease patients treated with cholinesterose inhibitors respond over the short term with clinically meaningful improvement of cognitive

Table 373-3 Frequently used drugs for treatment of depression in elderly patients

| DRUG CLASS | MAJOR SIDE EFFECTS | | | | DRUG INTERACTION POTENTIAL | USUAL GERIATRIC DOSAGES |
	ANTICHOLINERGIC	SEDATION	AGITATION	CARDIOVASCULAR		
Tricyclics						
Desipramine	+	+	−	+ +	High	25-100 mg daily (PM)
Nortriptyline	+ +	+ +	−	+ +	High	25-100 mg daily (PM)
Heterocyclics						
Trazodone	−	+ + +	−	+ +	Moderate	50-200 mg* daily (PM)
Bupropion	−	±	+	+	Low	50-100 mg bid-tid†
Serotonergics						
Fluoxetine	−	−	+ +	+	Low	10-20 mg daily (AM)
Sertraline	±	±	±	±	Low	50-150 mg daily (AM)
Paroxetine	−	±	−	−	Moderate	10-40 mg‡ daily (AM or PM)
Monoamine oxidase inhibitor						
Phenelzine	+ +	+ +	−	+ + +	High	15-30 mg tid
Other						
Venlafaxine	±	±	+	±	Moderate	25-100 mg bid

*Dosages sufficiently high for antidepressant action are commonly associated with sedation.
†Dosages above 450 mg daily are associated with increased risk of seizures.
‡Nonlinear metabolism may cause unpredictably high serum levels within therapeutic dosage range.

function. However, drug toxicity with tacrine is substantial, and long-term efficacy or either agent is unproved.

Depression. Depressive disorders are common among elderly persons, particularly women. Over a lifetime, cumulative risk of experiencing a depressive disorder is higher for women (20% to 25%) than for men (7% to 12%). Point prevalence rates for major depression in community-dwelling elderly women (4% to 9%) are twice as high as in older men (2% to 4%). Illness, not gender, is the most striking risk factor for depression. If medical treatment setting is used as a proxy for illness burden, point prevalence of depression increases from 9% to 15% of elderly patients seen in primary care practices to 15% to 25% of patients in geriatric clinics and 33% to 45% of elders in hospitals and nursing homes. Although depression is common in treatment settings for elders, epidemiologic research suggests that depressive disorders are *not* more common in elderly than in younger persons.

Despite its prevalence, depression remains an underdiagnosed and undertreated disorder in elderly persons. Primary care physicians, including geriatricians, often do not uncover symptoms in a typical medical encounter. Patients, families, and physicians may interpret low mood, anhedonia, and somatic symptoms of depression as part of aging or chronic illness. Discovery of depression is aided by routine use of depression screening questionnaires (see Table 373-1). Sixty percent to 70% of persons with positive screening tests meet DSM-IV criteria for major depression.

Drugs appear to have no advantage over psychotherapy, and response rates may be improved when both types of therapy are combined. Results of treatment trials in older individuals parallel results in younger populations. It is important to note that among patients with a first episode of major depression, long-term prognosis may be better for older persons than for younger persons. Benefits of treatment for elderly patients with significant comorbid illnesses or functional disability are unknown, since most trials of antidepressant therapy have not included these patients. Potential benefits of therapy are substantial, however, and it is recommended that frail and chronically ill persons should not be denied treatment.

Both doses and dosing intervals of drugs commonly used for the treatment of depression may need to be modified for older persons. In some cases, dose reductions and longer dosing intervals are necessitated by reduced drug clearance (prolonged half-life) related to decreased renal or hepatic function. More commonly, however, modification of doses may be required because of enhanced pharmacodynamic effects of antidepressant agents in older persons. Table 373-3 displays commonly administered antidepressant agents, their principal side effects, and suggested doses for elders.

Falls. Falls are a common and significant public health problem. In general, falls occur when intrinsic compensatory mechanisms cannot overcome a postural stress. Falls are defined as events that result in a person inadvertently coming to rest on the ground or at a lower level. Definitions of accidental falls usually exclude those resulting from loss of consciousness (syncope), sudden paralysis (stroke), or seizure.

Approximately one third of community-dwelling persons over 65 years of age fall each year. Fall rates increase with illness and functional disability. In the nursing home, one half of residents fall at least once annually, with fall rates of 1.6 to 2.4 per person year. Across all settings, one of six falls results in injury, usually of soft tissue. One in twenty falls results in a fracture (commonly wrist, ribs, and hip), and approximately 1% of falls result in hospitalization. Importantly, injury is the sixth leading cause of death in persons over 65, and many injuries are fall related. Injuries, however, are not the only consequence of falls. When persons who have fallen are interviewed, 50% express fear of falling and 30% report reduced activities. Reduced physical function, decreased physical activity, loss of confidence, and fall-related anxiety are all associated with falls. Without evaluation and/or treatment, falls can subtly reduce quality of life and limit social participation.

Evaluation of falls should focus on identification of modifiable risk factors. Risk factors can be classified as intrinsic (within the patient) or extrinsic (outside the patient). Although some risk factors are related to age, the majority are related to age-associated disease. Epidemiologic studies show that the number of fall risk factors is highly correlated with the likelihood of falling and benefit from fall interventions. Two-year fall incidence is <5% for persons with only one risk factor, but rises to almost 80% for persons with more than four risk factors. When applied to relatively healthy community dwellers, fall interventions reduce the number of falls and the proportion of persons falling by approximately 10% over a year of follow-up. In contrast, similar interventions delivered to persons with multiple fall risk factors reduce falls by almost one third.

Intrinsic risk factors. Important intrinsic risk factors include impairments of physical function, neurologic disorders, sensory deficits, and postural hypotension. Significant and modifiable aspects of physical function important to falls include strength, balance, gait, and sensory function. With age, strength declines, postural sway increases, gait becomes slower and less fluid, and vision and hearing become

---

BOX 373-1
Items in a performance-oriented assessment of mobility

Balance measures

Sitting balance (leaning versus steady)
Ability to rise from chair (number of attempts, assisted versus unassisted)
Immediate standing balance (first 5 seconds)
Standing balance (wide based, narrow based, or assisted)
Sternal nudge (steady, staggers, or falls)
Standing balance, eyes closed (steady versus unsteady)
360-degree turn (continuous versus discontinuous steps)
Sitting down (safe, smooth motion versus unsafe or unsmooth motion)

Gait Measures

Gait initiation (hesitation versus no hesitation)
Step length and height (foot clears floor and passes stance foot)
Step symmetry (right and left steps appear equal)
Step continuity
Gait path (straight versus marked deviation)
Trunk (straight versus flexed)
Walk stance (narrow based versus broad based)

---

more impaired. Reduced strength, poor balance, and slow gait speed impair the recovery of equilibrium following postural stress and are associated with falls; these impairments also limit compensatory strategies to avoid falls. Over the last decade, useful, standardized performance-based measures to evaluate gait, balance, and strength have been validated. These tools can both identify deficits and suggest modes of treatment.

One available validated clinical tool is the Performance-Oriented Mobility Assessment (POMA) (Box 373-1). Much of this rapid (<2 minutes) evaluation can be accomplished while watching the patient rise from a waiting room chair and walk to the examination room. Deficits identified during mobility assessment may form the basis of a diagnostic and therapeutic plan. For instance, multiple attempts to rise from a chair may indicate weakness of the hip flexors and extensors, which may be remediable with strength training. Asymmetric step length may provoke a search for asymmetric lower extremity weakness or hip osteoarthritis treatable with assistive devices or analgesics.

Neurologic problems such as cerebellar and vestibular dysfunction, residua from strokes, and dementia may contribute to fall risk. Parkinsonism increases the risk of falling ten-fold. Proprioceptive problems should prompt screening for vitamin B_{12} deficiency and cervical spondylosis. Musculoskeletal disorders such as rheumatoid arthritis, osteoarthritis, foot problems (bunions, hammer toes), and primary muscle disorders impair mobility and increase the risk of falling. Postural hypotension, most likely to occur during the postprandial period, contributes to falls. Lastly, vision and hearing impairments are each independently associated with falls. Successful multifactorial fall interventions include optimal management of underlying disease, correction of sensory impairments, and rehabilitation of physical function.

Extrinsic risk factors. In contrast to intrinsic factors that increase the risk of falling, extrinsic factors may be more readily manageable. Poorly fitting shoes providing little support or inadequate traction should be replaced by low-heeled shoes with firm, nonskid soles. Long, loose garments may also cause tripping and should be avoided.

Most falls occur in and around the home. Structured home safety checks should be included in all fall evaluations. In randomized trials, one half of community elders have preferred to use home safety checklists rather than having a professional home assessment. However, in cases of a questionable home environment, home safety assessments should be performed by family, case managers, or a rehabilitation therapist. Particular attention should be paid to walking surfaces. Slick floors and surfaces (especially in bathrooms), loose rugs,

and obstacles (low pieces of furniture, electric cords) may all predispose to falls and injuries. Poor lighting, especially on stairwells, may lead to a fall. Examples of remedial actions include installation of tub rails, nonslip strips, and tub chairs in bathrooms. Removal of obstacles and placement of nonslip rugs make walking surfaces safer. Adequate lighting, handrails, appropriately sized step rises, and maintenance of steps in good repair make stairways safer. Although interventions focused only on the environment have not been shown to be effective in reducing falls, successful multifactoral interventions always include home assessment and modification.

Both number and type of medications are associated with fall risk and with hip fracture. All classes of psychotropic drugs (phenothiazines, butyrophenones, benzodiazepines, antidepressants), especially those with long half-lives and active metabolites, have been shown to increase the risk of hip fracture twofold. A faller's drug regimen should be carefully scrutinized and the use of these agents minimized or eliminated. The evidence that antihypertensives predispose patients to falls and injuries is less compelling, but these agents may increase fall risk by causing postural hypotension. Alcohol is clearly a risk factor for falls and injuries in younger adults, but evidence that alcohol consumption is a contributor to falling in aged individuals is lacking. Persons who use multiple drugs are at increased risk of falling irrespective of the class of agents. Medications should be reviewed to document need, find the lowest effective dosage, and reduce the total number of medicines taken.

Appropriate fall management depends on the results of the evaluation and the combination of identified risk factors (Fig. 373-1). Interventions to reduce fall risk are most effective when therapies are specific to identified risk factors. Single-factor interventions—such as exercise, medication change, or environmental alterations—may individually be of benefit but are more powerful when combined. Some factors (e.g., a dim light bulb in a stairwell) are easier to correct than others. Management of disease contributing to falls should be optimized. Suspect medications should be reduced or eliminated. Sensory impairments should be appropriately rehabilitated. Neuromuscular, gait, and balance deficits may often be improved through supervised physical therapy or exercise programs. Exercise modalities demonstrated to reduce falls include lower extremity strength training, physical therapy, and balance training. Physical therapy is also useful to teach safer performance of common physical maneuvers, such as transfer techniques or rising slowly from chair or bed. Patients at high risk should establish methods to seek assistance when a fall occurs. Although caregivers are the primary source of help, elders who live alone may need a remote alert system, such as a call button worn around the neck and connected to a central emergency notification system.

Urinary Incontinence. Urinary incontinence is a common problem, increasing in prevalence with age, functional disability, cognitive impairment, and burden of disease. From 1% to 10% of all community-dwelling elderly persons over the age of 65 report some degree of incontinence. Approximately 15% to 25% of all hospitalized persons and more than one half of nursing home residents have episodes of incontinence. Only one third to one half of affected persons seek medical treatment for incontinence, even though treatment may be beneficial.

The continence mechanism relies on simultaneous and integrated actions of many physiologic systems. Continence is maintained by a balance between pressure within the bladder *(expulsive forces)* and the bladder outlet *(retentive forces)*. In normal individuals, accumulation of urine in the bladder occurs isotonically—that is, without a rise in bladder pressure. β-Adrenergic stimulation relaxes the bladder detrusor musculature during filling. α-Adrenergic stimulation maintains tonic contraction of the bladder neck and the intrinsic urinary sphincter. When a critical volume-pressure threshold is reached, the first desire to void is perceived and may be heightened by an accompanying involuntary detrusor contraction. In response to the urge to void, healthy individuals voluntarily suppress bladder contractions (reducing expulsive pressure) and contract pelvic floor musculature (increasing retentive pressure) until voiding is possible. Voiding is initiated by cholinergic stimulation of detrusor contraction, together with relaxation of the bladder neck, external sphincter, and pelvic floor musculature.

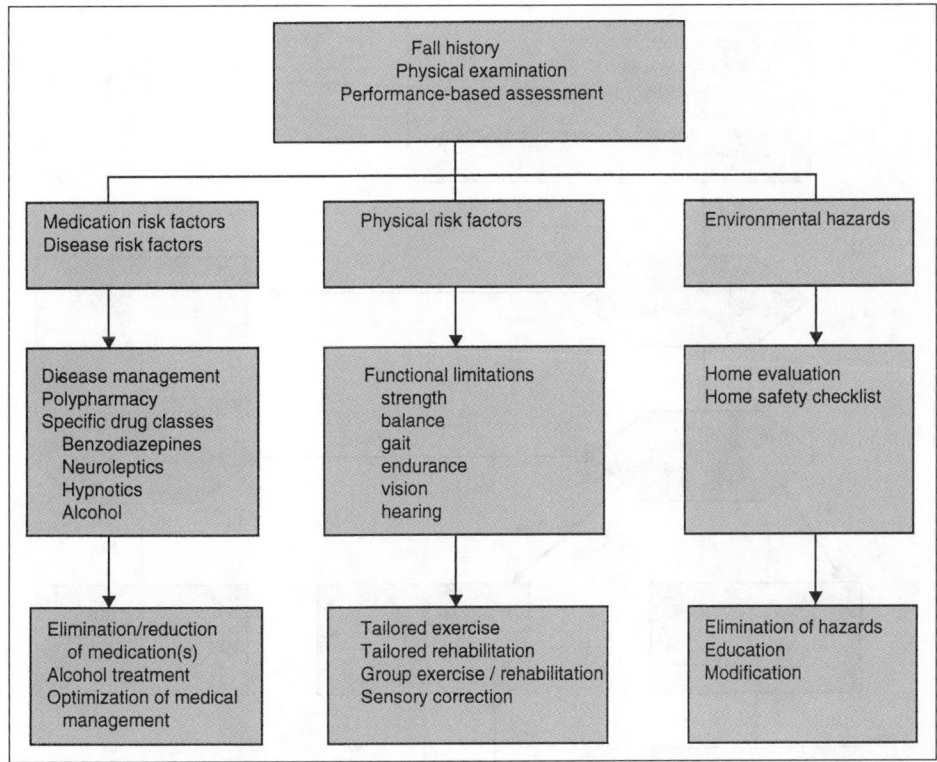

FIGURE 373-1   Fall evaluation and management strategy.

Cross-sectional studies of older persons have suggested changes in micturition physiology with age and disease. Bladder filling may not be isotonic because detrusor compliance decreases with age. Urge to void and involuntary detrusor contractions may occur at smaller bladder volumes. Older individuals are less able to suppress involuntary detrusor contractions, with a corresponding decrease in ability to postpone voiding. Bladder outlet pressure is less affected by age than by disease. Prostatism and urethral stricture may increase bladder outlet pressure. In contrast, postmenopausal or multiparous women may have reduced outlet resistance. Patterns of fluid excretion also change with aging. Although younger individuals excrete most fluid intake during the day, excretion may occur primarily at night in persons of advanced age. Nocturia, a relatively reliable sign of prostatism in younger men, may be less reliable in older men.

Incontinence may be acute or chronic. Chronic urinary incontinence is commonly classified into one of several syndromes: urge, stress, functional, and overflow incontinence. These syndromes have characteristic symptoms, urodynamic profiles, and potential etiologies, but may overlap in as many as one third of incontinent persons (*mixed incontinence*).

Urge incontinence is loss of moderate amounts of urine associated with a strong desire to void. Urinary loss is the result of an involuntary bladder contraction that overcomes outlet resistance. Postvoid residual urine volume usually does not exceed 200 ml. Nocturnal episodes of incontinence are common. Although the most common causes of urge incontinence are neurologic (e.g., stroke, dementing disorders, upper motor neuron disease), this syndrome often occurs in neurologically normal individuals, especially men with prostatism.

Urodynamic evaluation of the patient with urge incontinence reveals frequent involuntary bladder contractions, many associated with a strong desire to void. However, the amplitude (strength) of bladder contractions varies widely. Indeed, some persons have weak contractions, a condition known as *detrusor hyperactivity with impaired bladder contractility* (DHIC). Instead of complete bladder emptying, individuals with DHIC may void small amounts of urine and have a high postvoid residual volume. This syndrome has been described in

elderly, predominantly female nursing home residents. Its importance and prevalence in a general population are uncertain.

Stress incontinence is the involuntary loss of urine with maneuvers that increase intraabdominal pressure. Patients describe loss of small to moderate amounts of urine with actions such as coughing, laughing, and sneezing. Few of these episodes are accompanied by a strong urge to urinate, and nocturnal incontinence is uncommon. In women, this condition is typically associated with multiparity, gynecologic surgeries, or menopausal atrophic urethritis. Males usually experience stress incontinence as a result of intrinsic sphincter damage during prostatectomy. Urodynamic studies of persons with pure stress incontinence demonstrate detrusor pressure higher than urethral pressure when the patient voluntarily increases intraabdominal pressure. Postvoid residual volume is usually normal.

Functional incontinence, observed in persons with impaired mobility and/or cognition, is apparently unrelated to neuromuscular disorders of the continence mechanism. Although urodynamic studies may be normal, persons with functional incontinence may be unable to reach the toilet or fail to respond appropriately to the urge to urinate. Although this syndrome is a diagnosis of exclusion, it may be the leading cause of incontinence in hospitalized and institutionalized patients.

Overflow incontinence is characterized by involuntary loss of small to moderate amounts of urine, an overdistended bladder, and a high postvoid residual volume. Patients may have almost constant dribbling or intermittent loss of small amounts of urine. This syndrome is most often secondary to chronic, severe outlet obstruction, such as prostatism and urinary stricture. In individuals with only moderate outlet obstruction or relatively weak detrusor contractions, overflow incontinence may be precipitated by drugs that decrease detrusor contractile strength (anticholinergics, smooth muscle relaxants) or increase outlet pressure (α-adrenergic agonists). New onset of mechanical obstruction (fecal impaction) or acute changes in mental status may also precipitate urinary retention and overflow incontinence.

Not all individuals with urinary incontinence need evaluation or treatment. Some persons experience relatively little distress or inconvenience, with infrequent or small-volume incontinent episodes.

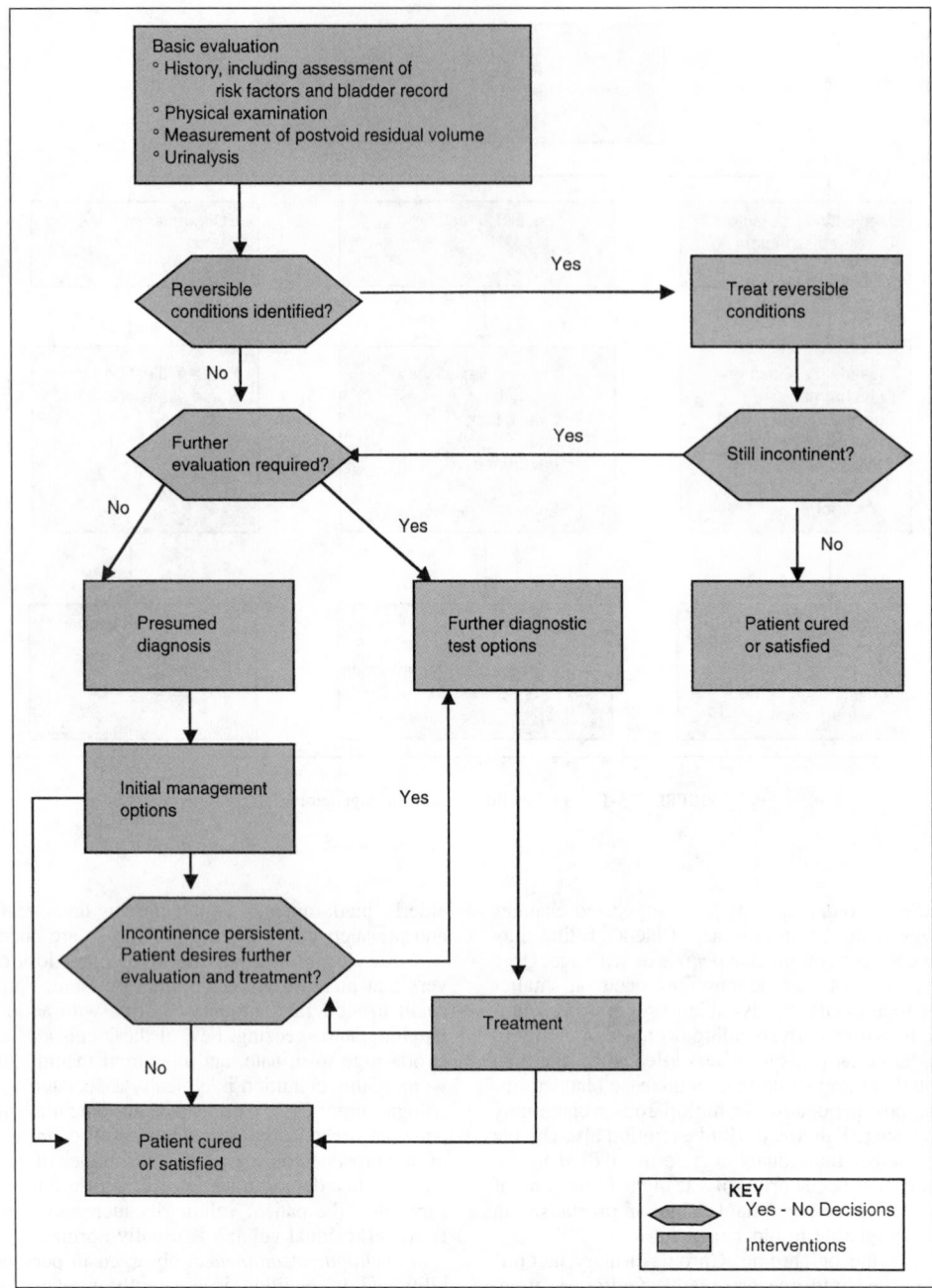

FIGURE 373-2   Evaluation and management of urinary incontinence in primary care.
From AHCPR pub no 96-0682, Rockville, Md, 1996, U.S. Department of Health and Human Services.

Medical evaluation should focus on confirming the presence of the disorder, identifying individuals for whom more extensive evaluation may be required, and finding reversible contributing factors or transient causes. An evaluation and management algorithm proposed by the Agency for Health Care Policy and Research in its Clinical Practice Guidelines is presented in Figure 373-2. Causes of transient incontinence that should be addressed first include acute changes in mental status, urinary tract infection, atrophic urethritis, stool impaction, and medications (diuretics, caffeine, agents with anticholinergic properties, and any that affect alertness). A history of prior gynecologic and urologic conditions or surgical procedures should be elicited. Associated symptoms such as dysuria, nocturia, hematuria, hesitancy, or change in bowel habits should be determined.

The physical examination should focus on abdominal, pelvic, and rectal findings, including masses, prostatic enlargement, fecal impaction, atrophic urethritis, vaginitis, cystocele, rectocele, or uterine pro-

lapse. Neurologic examination should evaluate general mental status, focal neurologic deficits, autonomic neuropathy, and spinal cord reflexes (bulbocavernosus reflex, perianal wink). Evaluation of the lower urinary tract should include measurement of postvoid residual volume, and may include maneuvers to detect stress incontinence. All individuals discovered to have a large postvoid residual volume (>200 ml) should undergo evaluation for urinary tract obstruction and detrusor function, followed by appropriate treatment.

Laboratory evaluation should focus on detection of secondary causes of urinary incontinence, including urinary tract infection, malignancies, and metabolic abnormalities (hyperglycemia, hypokalemia, hypercalcemia) that increase urinary flow.

Several nonpharmacologic therapeutic measures apply across the syndromes of stress, urge, and functional incontinence. These include scheduled toileting, bladder retraining, pelvic floor exercises, and improved toilet access. *Scheduled toileting,* at intervals determined by the frequency of incontinent episodes, maintains a small volume of urine in the bladder, reducing the likelihood of incontinent episodes. *Bladder retraining* is the only therapy that prolongs the interval between perception of the urge to void and onset of incontinence. Retraining is also useful to reduce the frequency of stress incontinent episodes. When combined, scheduled toileting and bladder retraining can decrease both stress and urge incontinent episodes by 50% to 75%.

Originally conceived as a treatment for stress incontinence, *pelvic floor exercises* are also beneficial for urge incontinence. Known as *Kegel's exercises,* repeated contractions of the pubococcygeus muscle increase bladder outlet resistance. Contractions should be sustained for up to 10 seconds, followed by an equal period of relaxation. Sets of 10 to 30 contractions should be repeated several times daily. Effects may be noted within several weeks, but the exercises must be continued indefinitely, because cessation is likely to be followed by recurrence of incontinence.

Drug therapy is a useful adjunct to behavioral modalities in the management of incontinence. When behavioral and pharmacologic treatments are used simultaneously in motivated individuals without severe cognitive impairment, incontinent episodes may be reduced by as much as 75%. In general, pharmacotherapy is not recommended for individuals with functional incontinence. However, an empiric trial of drug therapy may be warranted if behavioral measures fail and patient or caregiver stress is intolerable.

Many drugs have been tried for urge incontinence, but only a few have been demonstrated to be efficacious. Oxybutynin, the most commonly used agent, is a smooth muscle relaxant with anticholinergic properties. This drug reduces detrusor pressure and increases bladder capacity, but may cause urinary retention in patients with high postvoid residual volumes. Because it may cause confusion, oxybutynin should be used with great caution in cognitively impaired persons. For urge incontinence associated with prostatism, the α-adrenergic blocking agents terazosin and prazosin relax prostatic smooth muscle, increase urinary flow, and may reduce episodes of incontinence. 5α-Reductase inhibitors (e.g., finasteride) have shown promise in shrinking prostate volume and increasing urinary flow rates but appear not to be effective in men with only moderately enlarged prostatic volume.

Stress incontinence may be treated with α-adrenergic agents (tricyclic antidepressants, phenylpropanolamine), which produce mild increases in bladder outlet pressure. Estrogen replacement therapy (topical or systemic) may increase bladder outlet pressure by treating postmenopausal urethral atrophy. Persons with intractable stress incontinence may greatly benefit from surgical intervention (bladder suspension or artificial sphincter placement).

BIBLIOGRAPHY

Abrams WB et al, editors: *The Merck manual of geriatrics,* ed 2, Whitehouse Station, 1995, Merck & Co, Inc.

Branch LG, Horowitz A, Carr C: The implications for everyday life of incident self-reported visual decline among people over age 65 living in the community, *Gerontologist* 329:359-365, 1989.

Depression Guideline Panel: *Depression in primary care, vol 1, Detection and diagnosis,* Rockville, Md, 1993, AHCPR pub no 93-0550, Agency for Health Care Policy and Research, Public Health Service, U.S. Department of Health and Human Services.

Depression Guideline Panel: *Depression in primary care, vol 2, Treatment of major depression,* Rockville, Md, 1993, AHCPR pub no 93-0551, Agency for Health Care Policy and Research, Public Health Service, U.S. Department of Health and Human Services.

Felson DT et al: Impaired vision and hip fracture: the Framingham Study, *J Am Geriatr Soc* 37:495-500, 1989.

Finch CE: *Longevity, senescence, and the genome,* Chicago, 1990, University of Chicago Press.

Gurwitz JH, Avorn J: The ambiguous relation between aging and adverse drug reactions, *Ann Intern Med* 114:956-966, 1991.

Harper CM, Lyles YM: Physiology and complications of bedrest, *J Am Geriatr Soc* 36:1047-1054, 1988.

Hazzard RH et al, editors: *Principles of geriatric medicine and gerontology,* ed 3, St Louis, 1994, McGraw-Hill.

Katz MS, editor: *Geriatric medicine,* New York, 1991, Churchill Livingstone.

Lepor H et al: The efficacy of terazosin, finasteride, or both in benign prostatic hyperplasia, *N Engl J Med* 335:533-539, 1996.

Masoro EJ: Biology of aging: facts, thoughts, and experimental approaches, *Lab Invest* 65:500-510, 1991.

Masoro EJ, editor: *Handbook of physiology, section 11: aging,* New York, 1995, Oxford University Press.

McDowell I: *Measuring health: a guide to rating scales and questionnaires,* New York, 1996, Oxford University Press.

Mulrow CD, Lichtenstein MJ: Screening for hearing impairment in the elderly: rationale and strategy, *J Gen Intern Med* 6:249-258, 1991.

National Institutes of Health: Geriatric assessment methods for clinical decision making, *J Am Geriatr Soc* 35:1071-1078, 1987.

Orr WC, Sohal RS: Extension of life-span by overexpression of superoxide dismutase and catalase in *Drosophila melanogaster, Science* 263:1128-1130, 1994.

Ouslander JG et al: Predictors of successful prompted voiding among incontinent nursing home residents, *JAMA* 273:1366-1370, 1995.

Province MA et al: The effects of exercise on falls in elderly patients: a preplanned meta-analysis of the FICSIT trials, *JAMA* 273:1341-1347, 1995.

Sullivan DH et al: Impact of nutrition status on morbidity and mortality in a select population of geriatric rehabilitation patients, *Am J Clin Nutr* 51:749-758, 1990.

Tinetti ME et al: A multifactorial intervention to reduce the risk of falling among elderly people living in the community, *N Engl J Med* 331:821-827, 1994.

Tinetti ME, Speechley M: Prevention of falls among the elderly, *N Engl J Med* 320:1055-1059, 1989.

Urinary Incontinence Guideline Panel: *Urinary incontinence in adults: clinical practice guidelines,* Rockville, Md, 1996, AHCPR pub no 96-0682, Agency for Health Care Policy and Research, Public Health Service, U.S. Department of Health and Human Services.

Ware JE Jr, Sherbourne CD: The MOS 36-item Short-Form Health Survey (SF-36), *Med Care* 30:473-483, 1992.

Ware JE Jr et al: *SF-36 health survey: manual and interpretation guide,* Boston, 1993, Health Institute, New England Medical Center.

Yu C-N et al: Positional cloning of the Werner's syndrome gene, *Science* 272:258-262, 1996.

CHAPTER

374   Substance Abuse

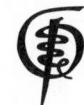

Booker T. Bush

Epidemiology

The use of alcohol and other substances is quite common in the United States. The rate of problematic use or dependence on alcohol and other substances varies according to the reporting criteria. Up to 8% of Americans report dependence on alcohol, 2% amphetamine abuse or dependence, 0.3% cocaine abuse, and slightly fewer than 1% reported dependence or abuse of opioids. In medical and surgical practice the prevalence of these problems is much higher, with rates ranging from 20% to 40% of patients, depending on the institutional setting.

Substance abuse causes increased morbidity, disability, and fiscal costs to society. Alcohol abuse has long been a factor known to cause death as a result of motor vehicle accidents and other forms of trauma, as well as disability caused by hepatic, cardiac, neurologic, neoplastic, and pancreatic disease. More recently, research has linked the abuse of alcohol and other substances with domestic violence and other psychiatric conditions. Nicotine, an addictive agent found in tobacco, prompts chronic use of tobacco, a major risk factor for the development of cardiovascular, peripheral vascular, neoplastic, pulmonary, and cerebrovascular disease. Cocaine may induce vascular spasm and hemorrhage, causing cardiac damage and CNS ischemia; depression and fatigue follow discontinuation of the drug. Intravenous narcotic addiction carries the risks of human immunodeficiency virus (HIV) infection, recurrent infection, hepatitis, or death from overdose. Although medical complications of substance abuse are substantial, the economic and social costs are greater, with lost productivity in the workplace, instability in social relationships, and loss of self-esteem.

Diagnostic Criteria

Health care providers should screen all patients for substance abuse. At minimum, a careful history should include quantity and frequency of use of alcohol, tobacco, and other substances. A cluster of cogni-

BOX 374-1

Criteria for substance dependence

A maladaptive pattern of substance use leading to significant impairment or distress as manifested by three or more of the following:

1. *Tolerance.* A need for increased amounts of the substance to achieve intoxication or desired effect; markedly diminished effect with continued use of the same amount of the substance.
2. *Withdrawal.* The characteristic withdrawal syndrome for the substance; the same or a closely related substance is taken to relieve or avoid withdrawal symptoms.
3. The substance is often taken in larger amounts than intended.
4. There is a persistent desire to cut down or control substance use.
5. A great deal of time is spent obtaining the substance, using the substance, or recovering from its effects.
6. Important social, occupational, or recreational activities are given up or reduced because of the substance use.
7. The substance use is continued despite knowledge of having a persistent or recurrent physical or psychological problem that is likely to have been caused or exacerbated by the substance.

BOX 374-2

Criteria for substance abuse

A maladaptive pattern of substance use leading to clinically significant impairment or distress as manifested by one or more of the following:

1. Recurrent substance abuse, resulting in failure to fulfill major role obligations at work, school, or home.
2. Recurrent substance use in situations in which it is physically hazardous (e.g., driving).
3. Recurrent substance-related legal problems.
4. Continued substance use despite having persistent or recurrent social or interpersonal problems caused or exacerbated by the effects of the substance.

BOX 374-3

Substance abuse history

Family history of alcohol abuse
Inventory of all medications and substances
Quantity and frequency of alcohol use
History of previous treatment
Medical complications from alcohol abuse, including withdrawal
Social and occupational complications related to substance abuse
Psychiatric diagnoses (depression, anxiety, bipolar disorder)

tient, usually through information learned from the history and physical examination. If the patient agrees that the behavior is a problem, he or she enters the next stage, *contemplation.* The patient may see the problem but feels ambivalent about whether the benefits from changing will outweigh the discomfort from ceasing the behavior. Substance abuse continues at this stage because, at least in the short term, the patient feels better with the substance than without the substance. Patients in the contemplation stage need assistance from their physicians to see that behavioral change will indeed benefit them. It is useful to guide the patient to see that the risks associated with substance abuse usually outweigh the benefits. Once patients have decided to change, they enter a stage called *preparation.* They set a target date, prepare to stop the old behavior, and replace it with new behaviors. When the change is made, the patient has entered the *action* phase. Ongoing support and monitoring by the physician can be very helpful during this time.

Relapse is a common behavior, especially with regard to addiction. Patients may relapse from the action phase to a contemplative or even precontemplative stage, and then they need to again weigh the pros and cons of taking action. The provider strategy should include feedback about the patient's behavior while substance-free, to help remind the patient of the substantial benefits of the behavioral change.

ALCOHOL ABUSE AND DEPENDENCE

Alcoholism is a common problem. As many as 20% of patients seen in an ambulatory setting meet the criteria for alcohol abuse or dependence. The disease can have a high morbidity with social and economic dysfunction, as well as a high mortality because of the increased risk of death from motor vehicle accidents and trauma, cirrhosis, cardiomyopathy, and dementia. Despite these factors, it is a treatable disorder.

When taking the history, clinicians should note quantity and frequency of use of alcohol. Women who drink more than three drinks on a single occasion or more than seven drinks per week and men who drink more than four drinks on a single occasion or more than fourteen drinks per week should be assessed for potential problems. The CAGE questionnaire (Have you ever **Cut** down on your drinking? Does anyone **Annoy** you about your drinking? Do you feel **Guilty** about your alcohol use? Do you use alcohol as an **Eye-opener?**) is an excellent tool for screening for alcohol-related problems. The Michigan Alcoholism Screening Test (MAST) is a diagnostic questionnaire of alcohol dependence and abuse for patients who have concerns about alcohol use. In patients who offer positive answers to screening questions or report large quantities of alcohol intake, a complete assessment should include the elements in Box 374-3. Specific information regarding the impact of alcohol use on relationships and other activities of daily living is important, especially in the early stages of alcohol abuse, when physical problems may not yet be an issue. The history and physical examination should assess the items in Boxes 374-3 and 374-4.

Although some patients may present with acute intoxication or medical complications related to substance use, many show no symptoms or signs at all. The symptoms of alcohol abuse include sleep disturbance, peptic symptoms, poor concentration, short-term memory deficits, and irritability. Some patients will present to the physician

tive, behavioral, social, and physiologic symptoms signify substance abuse or dependence when use continues. Repeated self-administration of the substance may result in tolerance, withdrawal, and compulsive drug-taking behaviors. Dysfunction or disability commonly occurs first in close interpersonal relationships, then progresses to financial, occupational, and, later, physical problems.

One predisposing factor for addiction is a positive family history of substance abuse. Although a clear association exists between substance abuse and psychiatric conditions such as posttraumatic stress disorder, depression, and bipolar disorder, these disorders are not clearly causative of its development. The DSM-IV criteria for substance dependence and abuse are defined in Boxes 374-1 and 374-2.

General Approach to Treatment

The general approach to intervention is similar for various substances. When the clinician recognizes an addictive disorder, the next step is to assess the patient's motivation to change the behavior. Instead of simply asking a patient to change, the clinician should intervene in a manner appropriate to the patient's readiness. In a series of smoking cessation studies, Prochaska discovered and described the stages that individuals evolve through as they change behaviors. These stages, along with models of how to approach each with treatment, summarized are as follows.

The first stage is *pre-contemplation.* In this stage the problematic behavior is evident to many observers but not the patient. Asking patients who are unaware of their behavior to change that behavior is usually not helpful. The appropriate intervention is to *educate* the pa-

---

BOX 374-4

Physical examination

Elevated blood pressure
Anxiety, tremulousness
Rosacea, rhinophyma, telangiectasias
Obstructive lung disease
Tachycardia, heart failure
Hepatosplenomegaly
Peripheral neuropathy
Evidence of trauma or domestic violence

BOX 374-6

Signs and symptoms of alcohol withdrawal

Anxiety
Sleeping problems
Agitation
Tremors
Tachycardia
Diaphoresis
Elevated blood pressure
Visual and auditory hallucinations

BOX 374-5

**Laboratory evaluation for the patient
with substance abuse**

Complete blood cell count with indices
Blood urea nitrogen (BUN), creatinine
Liver transaminases, alkaline phosphatase, γ-glutamyl transpeptidase
Serum albumin, total protein
Calcium, magnesium
Uric acid
Toxicologic screen (urine and serum)

---

with medical conditions that are a direct result of alcohol use, such as alcoholic hepatitis and cirrhosis, pancreatitis, congestive heart failure caused by alcoholic cardiomyopathy, or peripheral neuropathy. Other patients may come to medical attention for an issue such as unstable angina and then have their treatment complicated by the appearance of an alcohol withdrawal syndrome. The approach to the management of an individual depends on the clinical presentation and the patient's motivation to change the behavior.

The physical examination should seek evidence of damage related to substance use. Chronic alcohol use elevates blood pressure and may be a cause of difficult-to-control hypertension. Alcohol withdrawal causes increased anxiety and tremor with tachycardia. Because of alcohol's effects on androgens, acne and rosacea are common skin findings with its abuse. Alcohol abuse may cause hepatic inflammation and is a common cause of a "stocking-glove" neuropathy similar to that seen with diabetes mellitus. Ecchymoses, fractures, and other evidence of falls or inflicted trauma are also common.

When a patient reports heavy alcohol intake or there are physical findings suggesting an alcohol abuse–related disorder, it is important to perform a careful laboratory evaluation to screen for additional alcohol-related disorders, as outlined in Box 374-5. Because the sensitivity of these tests can be quite low, normal laboratory results do not exclude a substance use disorder. As a bone marrow suppressant, alcohol can cause a macrocytic anemia or even pancytopenia. Macrocytosis in the absence of vitamin B_{12}, folate deficiency, or hemolysis should prompt a more thorough alcohol use history. When people use alcohol as a major nutritional source, the blood urea nitrogen may become abnormally low, reflecting poor protein intake. Alcohol may cause hepatitis, leading to an elevation in liver transaminase levels, and, in the setting of cirrhosis, the albumin frequently falls, whereas the total protein level remains normal or even elevated. When a patient uses a substance metabolized by the hepatic P_{450} system (e.g., alcohol, benzodiazepines, nicotine, or many therapeutic drugs), the γ-glutamyl transpeptidase (GGT) elevates. Alcohol use elevates high-density lipoprotein (HDL) cholesterol (which is likely the reason for its beneficial effect in reducing cardiovascular risk). Magnesium diuresis from alcohol may result in hypomagnesemia with resultant cardiac arrhythmias. If hypomagnesemia persists, PTH will fail to function, and hypocalcemia may occur.

Alcohol Withdrawal

The symptoms and signs of alcohol withdrawal (Box 374-6) occur after reduction or cessation of alcohol intake. Their severity correlates with the dosage and duration of alcohol use. Symptoms may occur because of the withdrawal syndrome itself or because of an intercurrent acute illness that prompts cessation of alcohol use. When increased anxiety, confusion, nausea, vomiting, tremulousness, and other symptoms occur, it is critical to identify them as alcohol withdrawal so that appropriate therapy may begin.

Management of severe alcohol withdrawal involves the use of cross-tolerant medications such as benzodiazepines or barbiturates. For simple alcohol withdrawal, benzodiazepines are the mainstay of therapy. In patients withdrawing from multiple sedative medications, barbiturates are a treatment option. The choice of benzodiazepine depends on the presence or absence of liver disease or the age of the patient. If concern regarding hepatic metabolism exists, a short-acting benzodiazepine, such as lorazepam or oxazepam, may be used, whereas, for a patient with normal hepatic metabolism, long-acting medications, such as chlordiazepoxide or diazepam, are preferable.

Three regimens now exist for treatment of alcohol withdrawal: fixed-schedule dosing, "front-loading" therapy, and symptom-triggered therapy. A randomized clinical trial comparing symptom-triggered therapy with fixed-schedule dosing showed that those treated according to symptoms required much less medication for successful detoxification than those on a fixed schedule. Many addiction treatment specialists, however, now prefer front-loading therapy, in which the patient is administered an "intoxicating" amount of benzodiazepine and then receives a tapered dose (Table 374-1) to ensure that the patient receives adequate medication to prevent worsening of the withdrawal syndrome. When patients are also being treated for an intercurrent medical problem, such as pneumonia in a patient with chronic obstructive pulmonary disease (COPD), it may be difficult to use high-dose benzodiazepines for treatment of withdrawal, since undue sedation may result. In this case a symptom-triggered regimen may be more useful.

Another syndrome of alcohol withdrawal is delirium tremens, in which classic signs and symptoms occur along with confusion (delirium). For individuals who develop delirium tremens, mortality can be as high as 6% to 10%. Therapy, including the use of parenteral benzodiazepines, should occur in a carefully monitored environment, since a high morbidity is associated with the syndrome, as well as risks inherent to high-dose sedation. The most commonly used regimen is diazepam administered intravenously in doses of 10 to 20 mg every 30 minutes until symptoms are controlled. In delirium tremens it is not unusual to require doses of 80 to 140 mg of diazepam to calm the patient. In the setting of end-stage liver disease, a short-acting benzodiazepine such as lorazepam may be preferable.

Seizures may both precede and complicate alcohol withdrawal. These seizures are usually grand mal, rather than focal or recurrent. In the setting of status epilepticus and alcohol withdrawal, the clinician should assume that a primary seizure disorder exists separate from the withdrawal. Adequate dosing of benzodiazepines usually serves to prevent alcohol withdrawal seizures, rather than initiation of anticonvulsant therapy. For patients with a history of a primary

Table 374-1 Pharmacologic treatment of alcohol withdrawal

	STANDARD REGIMEN	HEPATIC SYNTHETIC DYSFUNCTION OR NEED FOR PARENTERAL DOSING
Fixed-schedule dosing	Diazepam 20 mg orally q6h on day 1, 10 mg q6h on day 2, 5 mg q6h on day 3	Lorazepam 1-2 mg IM or orally q4h with taper over 3 day.
Front-loading therapy	Diazepam 20 mg orally q2h until sedated	Lorazepam 1-2 mg IM or orally every 2 hours until symptoms resolve
Symptom-triggered therapy	Diazepam 20 mg orally q1-2h while the patient has symptoms	Lorazepam 1-2 mg IM or orally every 2 hours while needed

seizure disorder, anticonvulsant therapy should continue during alcohol withdrawal treatment.

Long-Term Treatment

Treatment for alcohol abuse may be as simple as advice that leads to a behavioral change, or as complex as an alcohol detoxification program followed by inpatient rehabilitation. Recommendations should be based on specific needs of patients.

Twelve-step programs such as Alcoholics Anonymous (AA) have a long history of success with treating alcoholism. These programs offer patients support, behavioral therapy, and education about alcohol's risks. Participation in such programs provides patients with the opportunity to change their social systems to allow abstinence from alcohol. Clinicians may wish to consult their local AA chapters to "match" their patients with groups.

Patients who require detoxification may receive treatment either on an ambulatory or inpatient basis. Those with a stable home and work situation who are neither medically unstable nor suicidal may do well in an ambulatory program. Medically or psychiatrically unstable patients, or those who have failed ambulatory detoxification, should receive inpatient treatment, preferably within an addictions treatment program offering appropriate rehabilitation services.

If patients relapse after detoxification, prolonged rehabilitation may be appropriate, either in an inpatient or a day treatment setting. These programs both detoxify patients and offer more psychologic support, including 12-step programs, family meetings, and, on occasion, further psychiatric care.

Pharmacologic therapy for alcohol abuse has seen rapid growth. Disulfiram (Antabuse), which inhibits alcohol metabolism and thus causes increased blood levels of acetaldehyde, prevents alcohol use by causing nausea and vomiting upon alcohol ingestion. Through its interaction with μ-receptors in the brain, naltrexone (ReVia) decreases the euphoria that accompanies alcohol use. This medication has reduced the frequency of relapse of alcohol use in dependent patients. Research has also shown that it decreases the amount of alcohol that patients in treatment programs ingest. Benzodiazepines play an important role in detoxification. Their role in maintaining sobriety, however, is unclear, except in the management of a primary anxiety disorder. Serotonin reuptake inhibitors have also proven to be important adjunctive therapy in patients with primary depressive disorders abstaining from alcohol use.

The clinician has an important role in following the patient during treatment, offering continued assessment of the patient's physical status as well as ongoing support.

TOBACCO USE AND NICOTINE ADDICTION

Although using tobacco is not commonly regarded as substance abuse in the same sense as alcohol abuse and dependence, it should be. Tobacco is the only commonly used substance that, even in moderation, will likely produce disease and death. The 435,000 U.S. deaths per year attributable to tobacco exceed all other preventable causes combined.

Intervention and Management

Many people quit smoking successfully on their own. Because of the surgeon general's warnings and extensive public health educational efforts, most smokers are already aware that tobacco is dangerous to their health. Many smokers report that they have tried to quit at least once. Although 95% of smokers quit tobacco use independently of any formal program, such success occurs only after a number of attempts to stop. The physician must encourage and reassure patients that relapse is common in nicotine addiction, but success is possible. Clinicians must not only screen patients for tobacco use and recommend stopping, but also continue to raise the issue of tobacco use with their patients in subsequent contacts, offering different strategies for cessation.

When patients choose to discontinue tobacco use, they may develop a characteristic nicotine withdrawal syndrome that includes craving, irritability, anxiety, anger, restlessness, increased appetite, and weight gain. The use of nicotine replacement, via nicotine gum or continuous-release nicotine patches, may alleviate these symptoms. Detoxification programs are most effective when combined with counseling and ongoing contact with a clinician.

Nicotine-replacement therapy can delay withdrawal symptoms until psychologic and behavioral issues resolve. The patient should agree to stop cigarette use totally upon initiation of nicotine-replacement therapy. If the patient begins to smoke again, nicotine-replacement therapy must end. Counseling and written materials about proper use should always accompany nicotine-replacement therapy. Nicotine replacement is contraindicated during pregnancy, breast feeding, angina, and in patients with arrhythmias. In patients with dental problems or temporomandibular joint dysfunction, nicotine gum is contraindicated.

Although nicotine-replacement therapy is now available without a prescription, many patients benefit from a medically modeled plan of care. Nicotine patches are available in 21 mg, 14 mg, and 7 mg doses. For a patient who uses a pack or more per day, a standard replacement regimen is as follows: a 21 mg patch daily for 4 to 6 weeks, a 14 mg patch for 4 weeks, followed by a 7 mg patch for 4 weeks. Some patients may need a slower program, which can last for as long as 6 months, whereas other patients require therapy for only 6 weeks. Ongoing follow-up of the treatment regimen—along with continued advice from a physician or a 12-step program (Smokers Anonymous) regarding new behaviors, exercise, and avoidance of smoking cues—are helpful for treatment success.

COCAINE ADDICTION

Cocaine-related biomedical and psychosocial problems remain a major public health problem in the United States. The 1993 National Household Survey on Drug Abuse estimated that 4.5 million Americans used cocaine in 1992 and 1.3 million persons reported monthly use. There were 30,900 cocaine-related visits to emergency departments over a 3-month period in 1992, most of which were for cardiovascular, cerebrovascular, and gastrointestinal problems induced by the drug.

Symptoms of Use

Cocaine, a stimulant with potent vasoconstrictor properties, causes an intense euphoria and alertness combined with a sense of confidence, heightened sexual feelings, and indifference to concerns or cares. As the cocaine effect wears off, these subjective feelings are followed by despondency and dejection. Cocaine is similar to other drugs that cause euphoric and dysphoric mood swings. It may be used orally, intranasally, or by intravenous injection or inhalation of the freebase form or "crack" cocaine. Mood enhancement heightens when the route of administration allows for rapid rise of serum cocaine levels. Intravenous and crack cocaine use offer rapid rise in levels, whereas intranasal inhalation prompts a less intense high. Cocaine has a very short half-life of 60 minutes, and its plasma metabolites are excreted in the urine.

Toxic effects related to cocaine use include not only cardiovascular and cerebrovascular ischemic events, but also reproductive dysfunction, hepatic necrosis, and pulmonary disease. Disorders of sleep, anxiety, mood, and delirium and psychotic disorders are also common.

Cocaine intoxication produces feeling of euphoria and heightened awareness. In large doses, highly distressing paranoid states may occur. Habitual cocaine use has profound effects on the dopaminergic and neuroadrenergic modulation of central nervous system function. Animal studies suggest that dopaminergic pathways serve as important mediators of cocaine's reinforcing properties. Dopamine depletion causes symptoms of depression and fatigue, and likely causes the "crash" that patients experience as they discontinue cocaine.

Management of Abuse

Patients in acute cocaine withdrawal experience agitation followed by severe depression, with tremors, muscle aches, and excessive sleep. The depression usually clears in a few days. Antidepressant therapy may aggravate cardiac arrhythmias associated with acute cocaine intoxication. Although a specific treatment does not exist, careful reassurance and support are important because these patients may be at high risk for suicide.

The long-term management of chronic cocaine abuse and psychologic dependence is similar to the treatment for other substance abuse disorders. This includes a goal of abstinence from all drugs, including alcohol, and relapse prevention through self-help groups such as Cocaine Anonymous, other 12-step programs, and psychotherapy. Because dopamine depletion causes profound depressive symptoms that may persist, many experimental protocols use antidepressant medications to maintain abstinence. Studies have shown that bromocriptine and other dopaminergic agents can increase the time that addicted individuals remain in treatment. Longer term studies of these, however, have not shown improved treatment success. Research at present looks towards blocking cocaine and dopamine receptors, as well as cocaine vaccines, as possible forms of therapy.

NARCOTIC ADDICTION
Effects of Use

Of the opioids, morphine, heroin, codeine, oxycodone, and meperidine are the most commonly abused. Because of its lipid solubility, heroin crosses the blood-brain barrier more quickly than other opioids, causing more intense euphoria and sedation. All opioids are quickly metabolized and excreted in the urine. Opioid overdose causes respiratory depression, bradycardia, coma, and death. Overdose may occur when opioids are combined with other drugs such as cocaine ("speedballs") and alcohol. Since the potency of heroin can vary, an unsuspecting user may die from the usual dose of drug.

Many complications occur because of the intravenous mode of delivery. Along with frequent staphylococcal infections from nonsterile technique, the risk of HIV infection and hepatitis B and C infections as a result of sharing needles are major problems. Even patients who avoid intravenously using opioids develop other complications inherent to addiction. Their lives become focused on obtaining the drug, frequently disrupting their relationships, social interactions, and ability to remain employed.

Treatment of Opiate Abuse

Opiate overdose may occur when patients obtain more drug effect than anticipated. Such patients develop pinpoint pupils, somnolence, coma, bradycardia, and respiratory depression. These signs and symptoms are reversible by administering a narcotic antagonist such as naloxone. If a patient overdoses on a long-acting opioid such as methadone, prolonged therapy with a narcotic antagonist is necessary.

Although opiate withdrawal is not life threatening, patients can become extremely dysphoric. Heroin withdrawal begins 12 to 14 hours after use, peaks at 36 to 48 hours, and has a total duration of 7 to 10 days. Because of its longer half-life, methadone withdrawal begins 24 to 48 hours after the last dose, with peak symptoms occurring 6 days later. The duration of acute withdrawal may last as long as 2 weeks. Craving and drug-seeking behavior occur first. In medical settings, patients exhibit many behaviors to obtain opiates to relieve these symptoms. The craving is followed by a "crawling" sensation in the skin, diaphoresis, and rhinorrhea. Anxiety, fear, and sleep disturbance accompany the other withdrawal symptoms. Musculoskeletal pain in the back, joints, and abdomen, along with nausea and diarrhea, soon follow. Physical examination shows agitation, diaphoresis, increased lacrimation, piloerection, and dilated pupils. Tachycardia, tachypnea, and hypertension may appear, but these are less intense than seen in alcohol or sedative withdrawal. Fever, seizures, hallucinations, and delirium do not occur with opioid withdrawal and, when present, suggest either polydrug withdrawal or an associated medical illness.

During the patient's hospital stay, methadone may be offered to relieve symptoms of withdrawal. If the patient was on a methadone maintenance program before hospital admission, the same dose should be offered. If the patient is withdrawing from heroin, an initial dose of 20 mg of methadone should be given after documenting evidence of withdrawal. It is unusual for a heroin-addicted patient to need more than 40 mg of methadone per day. It is illegal in the United States for physicians to prescribe methadone for maintenance or detoxification outside of inpatient settings, so this therapy can only be offered during brief hospitalizations.

If methadone therapy is not an option, clonidine can also be useful for opiate detoxification because of its α_2-adrenergic blockade. Clonidine is very effective for treating drug craving, sweating, piloerection, anxiety, and agitation. It may not be effective for insomnia, muscle cramps, and gastrointestinal symptoms. A standard protocol is to administer 0.2 mg of clonidine three times a day for up to 3 weeks. Lower dosages are indicated in patients who develop hypotension.

After detoxification, patients frequently benefit from ongoing participation in 12-step programs such as Narcotics Anonymous and Alcoholics Anonymous, or addictions-oriented psychotherapy. Many patients, however, will require long-term therapy, such as methadone maintenance, to abstain from heroin or other narcotic abuse. Participation in such programs may continue for years before withdrawal from methadone therapy occurs. There is also a role for naltrexone (narcotic antagonist) therapy in highly motivated patients who choose not to use methadone. These treatment decisions should occur within an addictions treatment program, with ongoing participation by the medical provider.

BIBLIOGRAPHY

Bush B et al: Screening for alcohol abuse using the CAGE questionnaire, *Am J Med* 82:231-235, 1987.

Mendelson JH, Mello NK: Management of cocaine abuse and dependence, *N Engl J Med* 334:905-972, 1996.

Prochaska JO, DiClemente CC, Norcross JC: In search of how people change: applications to addictive behaviors, *Am Psychol* 47:1102-1114, 1992.

Saitz R: Recognition and management of occult alcohol withdrawal, *Hosp Pract* 30:49-58, 1995.

Saitz R et al: Individualized treatment for alcohol withdrawal: a randomized double-blind controlled trial, *JAMA* 272:519-523, 1994.

375 Chronic Fatigue Syndrome

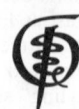

Daniel J. Clauw

Chronic fatigue is very common, affecting approximately 20% of the general population. Usually there is an identifiable medical or psychiatric cause for this fatigue. Sometimes, however, severe fatigue is not attributable to other causes and is accompanied by other symptoms, such as pain in multiple areas of the body and difficulties with sleep and memory. This symptom complex has been termed the *chronic fatigue syndrome* (CFS). Although this term has been adopted recently, this constellation of symptoms has been described for centuries in the medical literature. Many previous terms used to describe this condition, such as chronic Epstein-Barr virus (EBV) syndrome and chronic candidiasis, were attempts to link the symptom complex to an underlying pathophysiologic process. The generic term now used to describe this illness reflects the fact that the cause of CFS is unclear at present.

Although there has been substantial progress in defining the clinical features of CFS, it is difficult to consider this a discrete entity. Most individuals who fulfill criteria for CFS also satisfy criteria for one or more systemic conditions (e.g., fibromyalgia, somatoform disorders) and/or localized entities (e.g., irritable bowel syndrome, migraine and tension headaches, and premenstrual syndrome). In fact, there is increasing evidence that CFS falls within a spectrum of conditions that may share common inciting and aggravating factors, clinical symptoms, and underlying pathophysiologic mechanisms. It is easier to understand CFS when the aggregate data on this and related disorders are combined, so this chapter will emphasize findings that have been consistently noted in CFS, as well as in these "allied conditions."

DEFINITION

In 1994 the Centers for Disease Control and Prevention (CDC) convened an International Chronic Fatigue Syndrome Study Group to reformulate criteria for this illness. The definition that resulted from this conference is included in Fig. 375-1. There were several reasons for a new definition, including the fact that some objective findings required in previous criteria (e.g., pharyngitis, lymphadenopathy) are actually uncommon in CFS. More commonly, the patient with CFS experiences a sore throat rather than inflammation of the pharynx, and tender nodes rather than enlargement of the lymph nodes. In the new CFS definition, five of the eight minor criteria are pain based, reinforcing the fact that diffuse pain is common in this condition, which accounts for the significant overlap between CFS and fibromyalgia.

EPIDEMIOLOGY

Although CFS has commonly been described as occurring in clusters, most individuals do not develop this illness as part of an epidemic. In fact, the notion that CFS usually occurs after an infection is not supported by recent studies, which demonstrate that "pseudo-epidemics" of this illness may occur because of a high background rate of unrecognized cases in the population, and that common infective episodes seen in primary care only rarely lead to chronic fatigue. As of 1996, there were no true population-based studies published that used the 1994 CDC definition to estimate the point prevalence of CFS. The studies that were available either employed methodologies that might underestimate the true prevalence of CFS (e.g., cases were selected from clinic-based samples) or used older, more restrictive CFS criteria. It is likely that the point prevalence of CFS is of the same order of magnitude as fibromyalgia, which affects approximately 2% of the population. Women are affected much more often than men, although the precise ratio is unclear. Many case series have suggested that this disorder occurs more frequently in affluent white individuals, but this finding is likely more reflective of an increased access to health care by these individuals than a true difference in susceptibility.

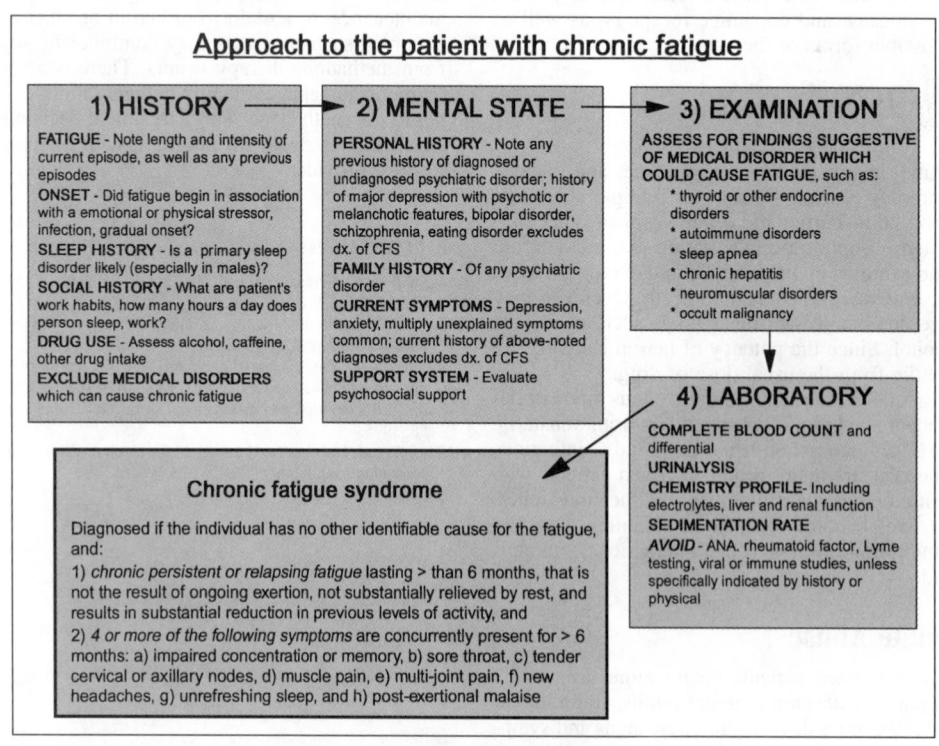

FIGURE 375-1 A suggested approach to the evaluation of the individual with chronic fatigue. The CFS definition noted is the 1994 Centers for Disease Control and Prevention (CDC) definition.

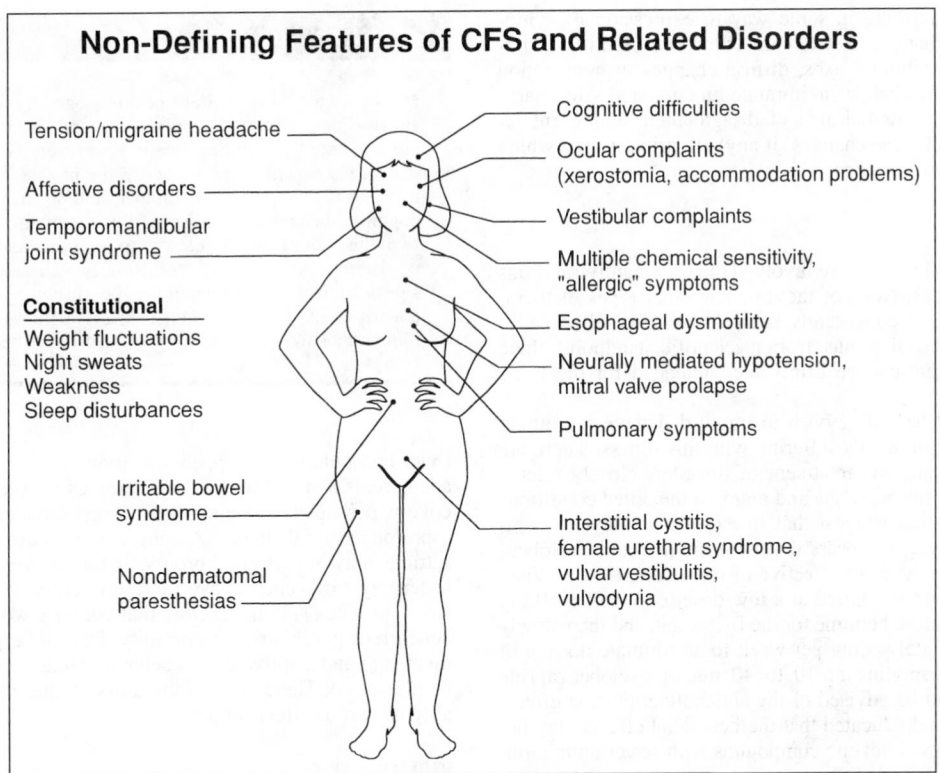

Non-Defining Features of CFS and Related Disorders

Tension/migraine headache

Affective disorders

Temporomandibular joint syndrome

Constitutional
Weight fluctuations
Night sweats
Weakness
Sleep disturbances

Irritable bowel syndrome

Nondermatomal paresthesias

Cognitive difficulties

Ocular complaints (xerostomia, accommodation problems)

Vestibular complaints

Multiple chemical sensitivity, "allergic" symptoms

Esophageal dysmotility

Neurally mediated hypotension, mitral valve prolapse

Pulmonary symptoms

Interstitial cystitis, female urethral syndrome, vulvar vestibulitis, vulvodynia

FIGURE 375-2 Nondefining clinical features of chronic fatigue syndrome and related disorders.

CLINICAL FEATURES

Although the seminal clinical features of CFS are included in the CDC criteria (see Fig. 375-1), there are clearly many other symptoms that occur commonly in this disorder and in related systemic conditions such as fibromyalgia (Fig. 375-2). These associated symptoms and allied conditions will not be discussed in detail, but they probably are mediated by many of the same pathophysiologic mechanisms that are responsible for CFS (e.g., central disturbances in pain processing, autonomic and neuroendocrine dysfunction, psychologic factors).

The relationship between affective disorders and CFS is important, since many individuals with this illness will have evidence of psychiatric comorbidity; some physicians even view CFS as primarily a psychiatric disease. The current CDC case definition for CFS excludes individuals with a past or current history of a major depressive disorder with psychotic or melancholic features, bipolar disorders, schizophrenia, delusional disorders, dementia, and anorexia nervosa or bulimia. Despite these exclusions, a significant number of CFS patients (perhaps 50%) will meet criteria for other psychologic conditions, such as somatoform disorder, less severe forms of depression, and anxiety disorders.

There are several reasons for this: (1) the diagnostic features of these psychiatric disorders overlap significantly with those of CFS (e.g., fatigue, sleep disturbance, "physiologically unexplained" symptoms), (2) many individuals develop anxiety or depression because of this or any other chronic illnesses, and (3) there may be common pathophysiologic mechanisms responsible for both CFS and some psychiatric disorders (e.g., abnormalities in the hypothalamic-pituitary axes, imbalances of central neurotransmitter levels). Most patients with CFS do not have features of major depression such as anhedonia (loss of interest in normal activities) and suicidal ideations and will often have prompt resolution of psychiatric features if their CFS symptoms are controlled.

LABORATORY AND OTHER OBJECTIVE ABNORMALITIES

There is no specific diagnostic test for CFS, and many individuals with this entity will have completely normal results from laboratory studies. It is important to recognize, however, that there are several common laboratory tests that are abnormal in a significant percentage of CFS patients, including tests of serum antinuclear antibodies (ANA), IgG levels, immune complexes, alkaline phosphatase, cholesterol, and triglycerides. There are also many other laboratory abnormalities that are commonly seen in this condition, including elevations in titers to several ubiquitous viruses (e.g., EBV, human herpesvirus-6 [HHV-6]) and low natural killer cell number and function. Although these mild abnormalities in immune function have not generally been shown to correlate with clinical status, and most of these same immune aberrations are noted in a variety of chronic stressful situations (e.g., spouses of Alzheimer's patients, prisoners of war, students taking final exams), there is still debate about whether any of these abnormalities contribute to symptomatology. Although these and other tests (e.g., SPECT brain scans, quantitative electroencephalogram [EEG]) are frequently abnormal in this disorder, this testing should be reserved for research settings, since at present there is no known diagnostic or prognostic value.

SUSPECTED PATHOGENIC MECHANISMS

The cause of CFS remains unclear, and, given the heterogeneity of this disorder, it is unlikely that there will be a single cause identified. There are limited data to suggest that there may be a familial or genetic predisposition to develop CFS, fibromyalgia, and other allied conditions. There is much better evidence to suggest that this symptom complex can either begin indolently or be triggered by a variety of stressors, including immune stimuli (e.g., infections), physical trauma, and emotional stress. The same stressors that can initiate CFS can also frequently lead to exacerbations of disease. Once this cascade of symptoms begins, there are a variety of abnormalities identified that may all contribute in some way to expression of symptoms, including disturbances in autonomic function, blunting of numerous hypothalamic pituitary axes, diffuse changes in nociception (pain tolerance), and the changes in immune function and viral markers noted earlier. The principal area of disagreement at present revolves around which of these changes (if any) are primary, and which are secondary (i.e., epiphenomena).

TREATMENT

Most therapeutic trials in CFS have involved the use of antiviral drugs or immune interventions. None of these or any other types of therapeutic interventions have consistently been shown to be effective in controlled randomized trials. Thus, from a scientific standpoint, there are no interventions that can be firmly recommended for the treatment of CFS.

However, it would be a disservice to imply that there is nothing that can be done for individuals suffering with this illness. There are reasonable data regarding the treatment of disorders closely related to CFS—for example, fibromyalgia and many of the allied conditions noted in Fig. 375-2—that suggest that low doses of tricyclic compounds can be effective. It appears that amitriptyline and cyclobenzaprine may be among the most effective of these compounds. When used, these drugs should be started at a low dose (e.g., half a 10-mg tablet) several hours before bedtime for the first week, and then slowly escalated by approximately 5 mg per week to an ultimate dosage of 30 to 70 mg of amitriptyline or 10 to 40 mg of cyclobenzaprine nightly. Patients should be advised of the anticholinergic side effects of these medications and educated that the beneficial effects may not occur for several weeks. Tricyclic compounds with fewer anticholinergic side effects may be substituted if amitriptyline and cyclobenzaprine are not tolerated, but these alternative drugs are typically not as effective. Serotonin reuptake inhibitors (e.g., fluoxetine, sertraline, paroxetine) can also be used; these agents might work better when used in combination with a nightly dose of a tricyclic compound than when used alone.

Anecdotal experience suggests that many other agents may be effective for relief of certain symptoms or features of CFS. Drugs such as trazodone or zolpidem can be helpful for insomnia and may be preferable to other hypnotics because these agents do not impair stage III and IV sleep. Low doses of nonsteroidal antiinflammatory drugs or tramadol may be helpful adjuncts as analgesics and are generally preferable to the use of narcotics, if possible. Newer classes of antidepressants (e.g., bupropion for fatigue or in those who gain weight with tricyclics) may be helpful in certain instances; again, these drugs may be more effective if combined with a low dose of a tricyclic compound. There is a subset of individuals with CFS and related disorders who have autonomic dysfunction, which may be demonstrable with provocative maneuvers such as tilt-table testing. These individuals may benefit from high-salt diets, low doses of fludrocortisone (given with potassium supplements), low doses of β-blockers, or disopyramide. A host of nutritional supplements have been touted as beneficial in this condition, although only one (intramuscular magnesium) has been shown to be effective in a placebo-controlled trial, and only a few others (e.g., melatonin, DHEA) have a sound theoretical basis for use.

Nonpharmacologic therapy is important in this disorder. Patient education is vital, and can sometimes be augmented by local and national patient support groups. Low-impact aerobic exercise may be extremely beneficial in some patients. For this therapy to be tolerated, the patient typically must begin at a very low level (e.g., 3 to 5 minutes per day) and increase slowly over several months. Significant lifestyle adjustments are sometimes necessary to minimize symptoms, and many patients with this disorder eventually end up with some form of disability. Psychotherapy may be helpful in some individuals, and cognitive-behavioral programs that combine clinical, psychologic, and physical aspects of therapy may also be useful.

PROGNOSIS

It is difficult to assess the prognosis and natural history of CFS because of the differences between patients seen in primary and tertiary care centers, as well as lack of uniformity in measures of disease ac-

✔ **WHEN TO REFER**

Most patients with CFS are best managed by a primary care physician. For patients who do not respond to the simple treatments already noted, it can be of benefit to assemble an informal multidisciplinary team to help manage the patient. This may consist of a physical therapist, psychologist, and/or an individual skilled in cognitive-behavioral therapy. If this treatment approach is ineffective, the patient can be referred to an individual or center with expertise in treating this illness. Referring these patients to multiple subspecialists should generally be discouraged, since this frequently leads to fragmented care and a focus on specific symptoms rather than the overall health of the patient.

tivity and outcome. It appears as though a significant percentage of adolescents and children who develop CFS experience a complete recovery, perhaps because many of these individuals are suffering from a prolonged viral illness. Among adults, those seen in primary care settings may have a good prognosis for recovery, whereas those seen in tertiary care centers have more refractory disease and thus have a worse prognosis. Other factors that confer a worse prognosis include concurrent psychiatric comorbidity, lack of response to initial treatment, and maladaptive illness behaviors (e.g., "victimization," learned helplessness). There are no laboratory studies that have been predictably shown to affect prognosis.

BIBLIOGRAPHY

Bates DW et al: Clinical laboratory test findings in patients with chronic fatigue syndrome, *Arch Int Med* 155:97-103, 1995.

Clauw DJ: Fibromyalgia: more than just a musculoskeletal disease, *Am Fam Phys* 52:843-851, 1995.

Fukuda K et al: Chronic fatigue syndrome: a comprehensive approach to its definition and study, *Ann Int Med* 121:953-959, 1994.

Gatti G et al: Psychoemotional, cognitive, chronoendocrine, and immune responses to a survival performance in an African desert, *Ann N Y Acad Sci* 251-256, 1994.

Krupp L, Mendelson W, Friedman R: An overview of chronic fatigue syndrome, *J Clin Psychiatry* 52(10):403-410, 1991.

Wilson A et al: Science and speculation: the treatment of chronic fatigue syndrome, *Am J Med* 96:544-550, 1994 (abstract).

CHAPTER

376 Common Eye Problems

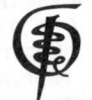

William G. Tsiaras and Ananth V. Mudgill

The eye and its visual pathways can be affected by a myriad of systemic ailments. There are also numerous ocular diseases that can adversely affect patients' physical and emotional status. The ability to perform direct ophthalmoscopy allows the physician to view the retina and its vasculature, the optic nerve, and the pigmented uveal tissues. All these structures can manifest the effects of systemic diseases, making eye evaluation an important part of the physical examination. Ocular manifestations of neurologic disorders, including eye movement disorders, are covered in Chapter 195. The purpose of this chapter is to discuss several of the more common ophthalmologic conditions that affect patients, particularly the elderly.

VISUAL LOSS

Loss of vision can be transient or of longer duration. Transient vision loss is that lasting less than 24 hours; it is usually caused by ocular manifestations of a neurologic or vascular process (see Chapter 195). Binocular vision loss lasting a few seconds is referred to as *visual*

Table 376-1   Differential diagnosis of vision loss lasting more than 24 hours

AMBLYOPIA	STRABISMIC, ANISOMETROPIC
Anterior segment	Corneal disease (edema, dystrophy, infection, leukoma); cataract; hyphema; uveitis
Vitreous	Opacities such as blood, inflammation, asteroid hyalosis
Retina and choroid	Macular degenerations and dystrophies; infectious and inflammatory chorioretinitis or retinochoroiditis; retinal detachment; vascular occlusive disease; toxic and traumatic retinopathies; tumors
Optic nerve	Glaucoma and other optic neuropathies such as hereditary, vascular, traumatic, inflammatory, toxic, or nutritional; tumors (glioma, schwannoma, meningioma)
Visual pathway (nonphysiologic)	Vascular, neoplastic, inflammatory, infectious, degenerative

obscurations. These obscurations can be the result of increased intracranial pressure (ICP) being transmitted to the optic discs, resulting in papilledema. Conditions such as subarachnoid or intracerebral hemorrhage, benign intracranial hypertension (Chapter 309), or central nervous system (CNS) tumors that result in increased ICP can cause visual obscurations.

Transient visual loss lasting from several seconds to several minutes is typical of vascular insufficiency, such as with amaurosis fugax or vertebrobasilar artery insufficiency. Patients with vertebrobasilar insufficiency may initially have transient bilateral visual disturbances and pronounced oculomotor deficits. Patients with carotid insufficiency usually present with monocular or binocular symptoms lasting several minutes. These visual symptoms may be associated with other lateralizing neurologic symptoms.

Visual loss lasting more than 24 hours encompasses a broader differential, as listed in Table 376-1. Important components of the history include the presence of pain; acuteness of onset; and coexisting systemic diseases such as hypertension, diabetes, hypercholesterolemia, or cardiac disease. Retinal artery occlusions and ischemic optic neuropathies that can cause sudden and painless visual loss are discussed in Chapter 195.

THE AGING EYE

The physiologic and pathologic changes associated with aging are diverse. This section discusses several common conditions that affect the general population and are associated with aging: presbyopia, cataracts, glaucoma, macular degeneration, and retinal vascular diseases.

Presbyopia

Presbyopia in the broadest sense refers to progressive loss of the eye's accommodative ability secondary to the natural hardening of the crystalline lens. The lens is most malleable during childhood and the early adult years, and it progressively loses its ability to change shape with age. Adolescents generally have 10 to 16 diopters of accommodation. Adults at age 40 have 4 to 8 diopters of accommodation, and after age 50 this decreases to less that 2 diopters of accommodation. Presbyopia is readily correctable with reading glasses, and it is considered a normal aging phenomenon rather than a disease process.

Cataracts

Cataracts are lens opacities of the crystalline lens. Characteristically, acquired age-related cataracts produce painless and gradual loss of vision. The prevalence of cataracts is 50% in people between ages 65 and 74. This increases to 70% in those over the age of 75. In the initial stages of typical age-related cataract formation, near vision may paradoxically improve, although distant vision is blurred. This "second sight" may allow the patient to read without glasses; the phenomenon of second sight is due to myopia induced by increased convexity of the aging lens.

Glaucoma

Glaucoma is a broad term encompassing a heterogeneous group of disorders affecting all age groups and linked by the common triad of increased intraocular pressure, cupping and atrophy of the optic nerve head, and visual field loss. The major types of glaucoma are primary open angle glaucoma, angle closure (primary and secondary) glaucoma, congenital glaucoma, and secondary glaucoma.

Primary open angle glaucoma (POAG) is the most common form of glaucoma in the United States, comprising about 60% to 70% of all adult cases. The disease occurs primarily in patients over 50 years of age but can develop in younger patients. The risk of POAG increases with each decade of life to nearly 15% incidence in the population over age 80. It is the leading cause of legal blindness in African-American patients and the third leading cause of legal blindness among whites. (Legal blindness is defined as vision less than or equal to 20/200 in the best eye with correction, or a visual field no greater than 20 degrees in its widest diameter.) Close relatives of patients with glaucoma have a five to six times greater risk of glaucoma. Additional risk factors for POAG include African-American race, diabetes, cardiovascular disease, elevated intraocular pressure, and myopia.

POAG is insidious in onset and slowly progressive. Pain is not characteristic. Central vision is spared until late in the disease process, and therefore significant visual loss from glaucoma can occur without symptoms. Diagnosis consists of measuring the intraocular pressure, examining the optic disc, and testing the visual fields. The normal range of intraocular pressure is 10 to 21 mm Hg. Nearly 50% of patients with glaucoma have initial intraocular pressures less than 21 mm Hg. These patients may have undetected intermittent pressure elevations as a result of diurnal variations in the intraocular pressure. Furthermore, intraocular pressure elevation alone is not diagnostic; some patients tolerate elevated intraocular pressures (ocular hypertension) without vision loss, whereas others may be more susceptible and exhibit glaucomatous damage with pressures in the normal range. Hence the management of a patient with glaucoma requires close long-term follow-up, consisting of visual field testing and optic nerve evaluation.

Primary open angle glaucoma is caused by a relative obstruction to aqueous humor outflow from the trabecular meshwork. Medical treatment therefore includes agents that reduce the production of aqueous humor or facilitate nontrabecular aqueous outflow through the uveoscleral pathway. Six classes of drugs are available for the treatment of glaucoma: adrenergic agonists, β-adrenergic blocking agents, parasympathomimetic agents, carbonic anhydrase inhibitors, hyperosmotic agents, and prostaglandin analogs (Table 376-2).

Other forms of glaucoma seen in adults are less common, including secondary open angle glaucomas and primary and secondary angle closure glaucomas. Secondary open angle glaucomas are due to an identifiable cause for the obstruction of aqueous outflow, without direct apposition of the iris to the trabecular meshwork. Examples include intraocular inflammation, intraocular tumors, trauma with leakage of lens material, pseudoexfoliation, and pigmentary glaucoma. Angle closure glaucomas involve iris apposition to the trabecular meshwork, blocking the drainage of aqueous humor. The cause is usually pupillary block in primary angle closure glaucoma and inflammation in secondary angle closure glaucoma.

Age-Related Macular Degeneration

In the United States, age-related macular degeneration (AMD) is the leading cause of irreversible visual impairment and blindness in patients over 50 years of age. The course of normal senescence results in a number of changes in the macula that culminate in a reduction in the number of photoreceptors, a reduction in the number of melanin granules in the retinal pigment epithelium (RPE), and an increase in the amount of waste products within the RPE. Bruch's membrane, ordinarily an elastic membrane, also becomes laden with debris that is deposited from the overlying RPE. This results in progressive mineralization, loss of elasticity, and increased fragility of Bruch's mem-

Table 376-2 Commonly used glaucoma medications

CLASS	AGENTS	EFFECT	SIDE EFFECTS
Parasympathomimetics	*Cholinergics:* Pilocarpine Carbachol	Improves aqueous outflow	Miosis, poor night vision, myopia, brow ache, angle closure, retinal tear/detachment
	Anticholinesterase: Demecarium bromide Echothiophate iodide	Improves aqueous outflow	Miosis, iris pigment cysts, myopia, cataract, retinal detachment/tear, angle closure, abdominal cramps, delayed recovery from succinylcholine
Adrenergic agonists	*Nonselective:* Epinephrine Dipivefrin	Improves aqueous outflow	Irritation, contact blepharitis, blurred vision, cystoid macular edema in aphakia, tachycardia, hypertension, angina
	Selective a-2: Apraclonidine (primarily used after laser surgery)	Reduces aqueous secretion	Topical irritation, vasovagal attack
β-Adrenergic blocking agents	*Nonselective:* Timolol Carteolol Metipranolol Levobunolol	Reduces aqueous secretion	Blurring, follicular conjunctivitis, congestive heart failure, hypotension, gastrointestinal upset, bronchospasm, impotence
	Selective: Betaxolol	Reduces aqueous secretion	Same as above except fewer pulmonary side effects
Carbonic anhydrase inhibitors (CAI)	Acetazolamide, Methazolamide, Dichlorphenamide Dorzolamide (topical)	Reduces aqueous secretion	Malaise, paresthesias, nausea, anorexia, renal stones, hypokalemia, acidosis, aplastic anemia, agranulocytosis, thrombocytopenia, loss of libido, acute respiratory failure
Prostaglandin analog	Latanoprost	Improves uveoscleral outflow	Conjunctival irritation, iris pigmentation
Hyperosmotic agents (intravenous)	Glycerol Isosorbide Mannitol Urea	Reduces vitreous volume	Congestive heart failure, headache, subdural hemorrhage (urea), hypertension, diabetic ketoacidosis (glycerol)

All of these medications are topical except the hyperosmotic agents and carbonic anhydrase inhibitors, of which only dorzolamide is topical.

brane. Recognized risk factors for the development of visual loss from AMD include increasing age, hyperopia, light iris color, family history, and cigarette smoking.

Although most patients with AMD manifest only drusen (small yellow-white lesions under the RPE, Color Plate XI-1) or RPE atrophy, approximately 90% of patients who suffer severe visual loss from AMD do so because of the development of choroidal neovascularization (CNV). This involves a break in Bruch's membrane through which neovascular vessels from the choroid invade the sub-RPE space. Intraretinal or subretinal hemorrhaging or lipid exudation often follows, causing elevation and displacement of the photoreceptors in the macula (Color Plate XI-2).

Patients with CNV often note metamorphopsia (distortion of objects), central or paracentral scotomas, or sudden and nonspecific changes in central vision. Successful treatment of exudative AMD (CNV) depends on early recognition. In cases of extrafoveal CNV it is important to make the diagnosis before the central hemorrhage and exudate involves the fovea. Fluorescein angiography is indicated at the earliest possible opportunity to confirm the diagnosis.

There is no known effective medical treatment or prevention for macular degeneration. However, certain presentations of neovascular AMD may be amenable to laser therapy. The possible role of nutritional supplementation with specific vitamins, minerals, or antioxidants needs further study. Standard current therapy uses laser surgery.

RETINAL VASCULAR DISEASE

Retinal vascular diseases, particularly atherosclerotic and arteriolosclerotic vascular occlusive diseases, are common infirmities of the aging eye, and they are reflective of systemic vasculopathic processes. Evaluation of the retinal circulation offers an excellent opportunity to assess the vascular status of the patient in general.

Hypertensive Retinopathy

The term *hypertensive eye disease* encompasses a myriad of hypertension-induced changes that occur in the retinal arterioles, reti-

nal parenchyma, choroid, and optic nerve. Acute hypertensive retinopathy includes the following ophthalmoscopically visible changes:

1. Diffuse arteriolar narrowing from vasoconstriction occurs with reduction of the arteriolar-to-venule lumen diameter ratio (normally, 2:3). In the acute setting this is reversible. Vasoconstriction is an autoregulatory phenomenon caused by stimulation of the vascular tone of the muscular retinal arteries.

2. Hemorrhages resulting from hypertension most commonly appear in either a dot-blot pattern or a flame shape by ophthalmoscopy (Color Plate XI-3). The difference in appearance is due to the topographic location of the blood within the retina. Flame-shaped hemorrhages are most commonly located in the nerve fiber layer, which is the layer closest to the vitreous cavity, where the nerve fibers travel to the optic nerve following an arcuate course similar to that of the larger blood vessels. Hence the flame-shaped hemorrhages usually parallel the vascular system. Deeper hemorrhages appear rounder and blotlike because the blood is forced together between the more vertically oriented deeper retinal tissues. Blot hemorrhages are less common and suggest a more severe hypertensive state. Neither type of hemorrhage is specific to hypertension. Both may be seen in a variety of vascular disruptive diseases, such as diabetes.

3. Cotton wool patches represent infarcts of the nerve fiber layer, a finding that also is not specific to hypertension (Color Plate XI-4). On ophthalmoscopic examination these appear as blurred, grayish white areas with feathery amorphous edges. They are more commonly located within the major vascular arcades or close to the optic nerve, where the nerve fiber layer is thickest. The clinical appearance of the cotton wool spot is due to closure of the capillary circulation, resulting in swelling of the nerve fibers and proliferation of their organelles.

4. Hard exudates are another finding related to hypertensive vascular damage to end arterioles or capillaries, resulting in plasma leakage into the deeper retina. As the plasma fluid subsequently begins to resolve, the residual lipid material remaining in the extravascular retinal tissue becomes hard exudate. In hyperten-

sion this exudate can be deposited in the perifoveal area of the macula in a stellate pattern referred to as a *macular star* (Color Plate XI-5). This pattern is due to the topography of the macula, where Henle's layer (the outer plexiform layer) is radially and obliquely oriented. Neither the macular star nor other retinal hard exudates are specific to hypertensive retinopathy, but when these changes are attributed to hypertension, they are indicative of more serious disease.

5. Microaneurysms may also occur as part of hypertensive retinopathy, especially around cotton wool spots. These dilatations of the vascular lumen can lead to retinal edema. Microaneurysms are most commonly found in diabetics and next most frequently seen in hypertensive retinopathy.

6. Acute hypertension—such as in patients with preeclampsia, eclampsia, pheochromocytoma, or accelerated hypertension—can also result in hypertensive choroidopathy. Zones of nonperfusion of the choriocapillares may occur initially, as determined by fluorescein angiography. Focal detachments of the overlying RPE may also occur, rarely leading to retinal detachment.

7. Either acute or chronic hypertension can result in hypertensive optic neuropathy. Patients may manifest flame-shaped hemorrhages at or near the optic disc, blurring of disc margins, congestion of the retinal veins, and florid disc edema, which may be confluent with edema and exudate in the macula (macular star). Disc edema is an essential finding with malignant hypertension (Color Plate XI-6).

Chronic hypertensive changes lead to arteriolosclerosis of the retinal vessels. These changes include the following:

1. Luminal narrowing with reduction of the arteriole-to-venule lumen diameter ratio (normally 2:3). This is due to thickening of the vessel wall from arteriolosclerosis.

2. Light reflex changes are also seen and are the result of progressive arteriolosclerosis. Mild arteriolar light reflex changes manifest as a broader and duller appearance to the arterioles. With moderate sclerosis the arterioles assume a burnished copper appearance ("copper wire"). Further sclerosis results in "silver wiring," in which the arteriole is so thick that the blood column can no longer be visualized (Color Plate XI-6).

3. Arteriovenous branching abnormalities are changes that are seen at arteriovenous crossings. Arteriovenous nicking (Gunn's sign) occurs as the thickened artery compresses the vein at the crossing point, where the two vessels share a common adventitial sheath. Because the common adventitial sheath acts as a nondistensible annulus, the walls of the more compliant vein are believed to become compressed when the overlying arteriole undergoes sclerosis and thickening (Color Plate XI-3). Continued compression can result in a vein occlusion.

4. Vascular occlusive complications include branch retinal artery occlusion, central retinal artery occlusion, branch retinal vein occlusion, and central retinal vein occlusion. Ischemia secondary to vascular occlusion may result in neovascularization of the retina, vitreous hemorrhage, and tractional retinal detachment.

Diabetic Retinopathy

Diabetic retinopathy can appear similar to hypertensive eye disease. Unlike hypertensive retinopathy, however, diabetic retinopathy is the leading cause of blindness in the United States for individuals between 20 and 64 years of age. This blindness usually is the result of nonresolving vitreous hemorrhage, tractional retinal detachment, or diabetic macular edema. Since diabetic retinopathy can be asymptomatic in its most treatable stages, it is crucial for physicians to facilitate early diagnosis through regularly scheduled ocular examinations.

Diabetic retinopathy is a highly specific vascular complication of both type I and type II diabetes mellitus. Within the diabetic population the prevalence of all types of retinopathy increases with age and the duration of diabetes. It is rare to find diabetic retinopathy in children less than 10 years of age regardless of the duration of diabetes. After 20 years of diabetic disease, nearly all patients with insulin-dependent diabetes mellitus and more that 60% of patients with non-insulin-dependent diabetes mellitus have some degree of retinopathy.

The pathogenesis of diabetic microvascular disease is unknown.

Hyperglycemia is believed to result in glycosylation of tissue proteins, leading to vascular endothelial damage. The ultrastructural vascular changes include basement membrane thickening and loss of pericytes, resulting in decreased caliber of the capillary lumen and a breakdown of the blood-retinal barrier. Eventually the microcirculation may become focally occluded, resulting in the angiographic sign of capillary nonperfusion, which causes retinal ischemia. Early in the course of diabetic retinopathy, autoregulation of the retinal vasculature may be impaired, which can further potentiate retinal damage and ischemia. The pathogenesis of neovascularization remains unclear, although observations implicate substances released from ischemic retina that stimulate new vessel formation.

The specific retinal lesions found in diabetic retinopathy include those already described under hypertensive retinopathy: microaneurysms, intraretinal hemorrhages (dot-blot and flame shaped), cotton wool spots, and hard exudates (Color Plates XI-3, XI-7, XI-8, and XI-9). Other important findings are intraretinal microvascular abnormalities (IRMAs), venous caliber abnormalities, diabetic macular edema, and proliferative changes consisting of neovascularization within the retinal circulation.

Intraretinal microvascular abnormalities represent either new vessel growth within the retina or, more likely, preexisting vessels with endothelial cell proliferation that become shunts through areas of nonperfusion (Color Plate XI-7). Multiple IRMAs represent a severe stage of nonproliferative retinopathy and indicate that frank neovascularization is likely.

Venous caliber abnormalities are another indicator of severe retinal hypoxia. The most common presentation of this is venous beading (Color Plate XI-7). Adjacent to the veins are often large areas of nonperfusion showing venous beading.

Proliferative retinopathy is marked by proliferating endothelial cell tubules and fibrous tissue, where the extraretinal fibrovascular proliferation extends beyond the plane of the retina into the vitreous chamber. It is contraction of either these fibrovascular bands or the vitreous body to which they are attached that results in pulling on the retina, leading to retinal detachment or retinal breaks. Rupture of the fragile neovascular vessels results in vitreous hemorrhage (Color Plate XI-8).

Diabetic macular edema is another common cause of visual morbidity, since retinal edema either directly involves or threatens the center of the macula as a result of abnormal vascular permeability in diabetic retinopathy. The diagnosis of macular edema is best made by assessing for retinal thickening with slit-lamp biomicroscopy, which allows binocular visualization.

The ophthalmoscopic retinal findings are used to stratify diabetic retinopathy into various stages of disease activity. In the broadest sense, diabetic retinopathy is classified as nonproliferative diabetic retinopathy (NPDR) or proliferative diabetic retinopathy (PDR). The distinction between the two is that PDR includes the intraretinal findings of NPDR with the addition of neovascularization, which leads to complications such as vitreous hemorrhage and retinal detachment. Diabetic macular edema can be present at any stage of diabetic retinopathy.

Four important national collaborative and randomized clinical studies have formed the basis of clinical management of patients with diabetic retinopathy. The Diabetic Retinopathy Study (DRS) demonstrated a 50% or greater reduction in the rates of severe visual loss (SVL) in eyes treated with panretinal photocoagulation. The Early Treatment Diabetic Retinopathy Study (ETDRS) showed that there was no benefit for panretinal photocoagulation in eyes with mild or moderate NPDR as defined by strict criteria. This study also showed a 50% or greater reduction in the rates of moderate visual loss in eyes treated with laser for clinically significant macular edema. Aspirin therapy was also evaluated in the ETDRS and was found to be of no ocular benefit, but it caused no increased risk of vitreous hemorrhage. The Diabetic Retinopathy Vitrectomy Study showed that for patients with type 1 diabetes who have severe vitreous hemorrhage, early vitrectomy (within 6 months versus at 1 year) was beneficial. There was no such benefit for type 2 or mixed patients. The Diabetes Control and Complications Trial demonstrated that intensive insulin therapy can delay the onset and slow the progression of diabetic retinopathy, nephropathy, and neuropathy in patients with type 1 disease.

It is important to emphasize that additional health and medical issues can also influence the development and progression of diabetic

BOX 376-1

Systemic differential diagnosis of branch and central retinal arterial occlusive disease

Embolus
    Calcific from cardiac valves
    Cholesterol from carotid arteries
    Platelet-fibrin from large vessel arteriosclerosis
Trauma
Sickle cell disease
Oral contraceptives
Coagulation disorders
Mitral valve prolapse
Vasculitis
Connective tissue disorders, including giant cell arteritis
Cardiac myxoma
Migraine
Endocarditis

BOX 376-2

Systemic differential diagnosis of branch and central retinal venoocclusive disease

Systemic arterial hypertension
Diabetes mellitus
Drugs (oral contraceptives, diuretics)
Blood dyscrasias (polycythemia vera)
Dysproteinemias
Vasculitis
Migraine
Hypercoagulable state (including malignancy)

retinopathy. These issues include pregnancy, chronic hyperglycemia, hypertension, renal disease, and hyperlipidemia. All patients with diabetes mellitus should have an annual dilated eye exam to evaluate for diabetic retinopathy. Patients with diabetic retinopathy are then followed more closely depending on the activity of the retinopathy.

Retinal Venoocclusive Disease

Occlusive diseases of the major retinal vessels are usually related to or caused by collateral systemic ailments, as listed in Boxes 376-1 and 376-2. Retinal arterial occlusive disease is discussed in the context of neurologic disorders in Chapter 195. This section discusses the etiology and management of retinal venous occlusive disease.

Venoocclusive diseases are among the most common retinal vascular diseases seen by ophthalmologists. Retinal vein occlusions are broadly divided anatomically into branch and central retinal vein occlusions.

Branch retinal vein occlusions (BRVOs) are lesions that most commonly occur at an arteriovenous crossing point (Color Plate XI-9). The fundus findings typically consist of flame-shaped and blot hemorrhages, retinal edema, and often cotton-wool spots in the sector of retina drained by the affected vein. The supratemporal quadrant of the fundus is most commonly affected. Occlusions of the nasal retina may never become clinically manifest, since the area of distribution is usually asymptomatic. The total area of retina involved depends on the size and location of the involved vein. In general, the closer the point of occlusion is to the optic nerve, the greater is the extent of the affected retina and the more serious are the sequelae.

The visual prognosis after a branch retinal vein occlusion is most related to the extent of capillary damage within the macula and to the level of retinal ischemia. Fluorescein angiography is useful in assessing the extent and location of capillary nonperfusion. In the acute

setting after a BRVO, vision can be reduced from macular edema, retinal hemorrhage, or perifoveal capillary occlusion, which results in foveal ischemia. In the chronic setting, permanent visual loss from BRVO is often the sequela of one or more of the following: macular ischemia, cystoid macular edema, exudative macular edema, pigmentary macular disturbance, or retinal fibrosis. Despite these potential complications, the overall prognosis following BRVO remains good: 50% to 60% of untreated patients maintain visual acuities of 20/40 or better after 1 year.

In 1984 the Branch Retinal Vein Occlusion Study (BRVOS) reported that macular argon laser photocoagulation improved the visual outcome in eyes where there was no perifoveal capillary nonperfusion and where macular edema alone was responsible for reduced vision in the range from 20/40 to 20/200. Because spontaneous remission may occur, treatment should be delayed for 3 months.

Central retinal vein occlusion (CRVO) is an entity that is well recognized by most clinicians because of its dramatic and distinctive "blood and thunder" appearance (Color Plate XI-10). In its classic presentation there is marked dilatation and tortuousity of the retinal veins and extensive superficial and deep retinal hemorrhages and cotton wool spots in all quadrants. Edema of both the retina and optic nerve are also seen, which contributes to the painless blurring or loss of vision that patients report.

Central retinal vein occlusions are broadly divided into two categories: (1) ischemic, and (2) nonischemic or venous stasis retinopathy, which produces less significant clinical symptoms. In several large series two thirds of CRVOs were found to be nonischemic.

The management of patient with CRVO begins with treatment of associated medical conditions. The common ocular complications include macular edema, hemorrhage, and neovascularization. As with other retinal diseases the proliferation of new blood vessels is a complication of retinal ischemia. With CRVOs, neovascularization may take place on the optic disc, on the retina, and even more anteriorly on the iris (rubeosis iridis) and around the trabecular meshwork of the angle. Unlike the other ischemic eye diseases, CRVO involves anterior neovascularization more commonly than neovascularization of the optic disc or retina. Iris and angle neovascularization are the most feared complications, since they may result in fulminant neovascular glaucoma by occluding the trabecular meshwork, leading to pain and blindness. This frequently occurs around 3 months after the occlusive event and is often referred to as *90-day glaucoma*. Among ischemic eyes, rubeosis iridis with or without glaucoma occurs in 45% to 80% of cases. In nonischemic eyes the incidence of rubeosis is reported to be less than 5%. In 1995 the Central Vein Occlusion Study Group (CVOSG) reported that laser treatment for macular edema caused by CRVO was of no benefit in improving visual acuity.

OPHTHALMIC MANIFESTATIONS OF AIDS

Eye disease is an important cause of morbidity in patients with the acquired immunodeficiency syndrome (AIDS). Visual morbidity can be severe, and blindness has been suggested as a leading cause of suicide in patients with AIDS. In more than 70% of patients with AIDS, ocular manifestations of the disease develop at some time during the course of the illness, and 90% of patients have ocular disease at autopsy. Ocular manifestations can involve virtually any eye structure, as seen in Box 376-3.

Common Infectious Manifestations of AIDS—Anterior Segment

Molluscum contagiosum is a skin infection caused by a DNA virus of the Poxviridae group. The typical lesion is a pearly white, dome-shaped, umbilicated 3- to 5-mm nodule on the eyelid or eyelid margin. When the lid margin is involved, conjunctivitis is commonly seen, since virus particles also infect the conjunctiva. Unlike normal hosts, in whom the infection is self-limited and fewer than 10 lesions are present at any one time, the patient with AIDS has lesions that are larger, more numerous, and difficult to eradicate.

Herpes zoster ophthalmicus (HZO), caused by the varicella-zoster virus, may be the first manifestation of a human immunodeficiency virus (HIV) infection, and HIV should be suspected if HZO is seen in an individual under age 40. Clinically, the illness is characterized

BOX 376-3
Ocular manifestations of acquired immunodeficiency syndrome

Eyelids
Molluscum contagiosum
Kaposi's sarcoma

Cornea/conjunctiva
Keratoconjunctivitis sicca
Bacterial/fungal ulcerative keratitis
Herpes simplex
Herpes zoster ophthalmicus
Conjunctival microvasculopathy
Kaposi's sarcoma

Retina, choroid, and vitreous
Microvasculopathy
Endophthalmitis
Cytomegalovirus retinitis
Acute retinal necrosis
Syphilis
Toxoplasmosis
Pneumocystis choroidopathy
Cryptococcosis
Mycobacterial infection
Intraocular lymphoma
Candidiasis
Histoplasmosis

Drugs associated with ocular toxicity
Rifabutin
Didanosine

Neuroophthalmic
Disc edema
Primary or secondary optic neuropathy
Cranial nerve palsies

Orbital
Lymphoma
Infection
Pseudotumor

CMV retinitis is the most common intraocular infection associated with HIV and accounts for most of the severe visual loss in these patients. The prevalence may be as high as 40% in some patient populations, and 40% of those affected may lose central vision in both eyes by the time of death. This tends to be a late manifestation of the disease, with patients having AIDS for many months before CMV retinitis develops. The CD4 count is usually less than 0.10×10^9/L, and more often less than 0.05×10^9/L.

Symptoms of CMV retinitis depend on its initial location. Peripheral lesions may not be symptomatic, or the patient may complain of floaters or loss of peripheral vision. More posterior lesions, which involve the macula, are readily symptomatic and may result in paracentral or central scotomas. The diagnosis of CMV retinitis is made by careful examination of the dilated fundus. Three general patterns of CMV retinitis have been described: hemorrhagic, brush fire, and granular. The classic form of CMV retinitis is the hemorrhagic type, which has been termed "crumbled cheese and ketchup" or "pizza pie" (Color Plate XI-11). Histopathologic studies of postmortem eyes show extensive areas of full-thickness retinal and retinal pigment epithelial necrosis. The differential diagnosis includes cotton-wool spots, toxoplasmosis, *Candida* infection, syphilis, herpes simplex retinitis, and herpes zoster retinitis.

Two drugs are currently approved in the United States for the treatment of CMV retinitis: ganciclovir and foscarnet. Ganciclovir (Cytovene, DHPG [dihydroxy propoxymethyl guanine]) is an antiviral acyclic nucleoside analog of acyclovir that derives its pharmacologic activity from its structural similarity to guanosine. Because of its similarity to guanosine, it is phosphorylated by cells infected with CMV and thus inhibits viral DNA polymerase and viral proliferation. Foscarnet (trisodium phosphonoformate hexahydrate), a pyrophosphate analog, is an inhibitor of DNA polymerase and reverse transcriptase, making it effective against the herpes class of viruses and providing activity against HIV. Patients who are treated with ganciclovir require close monitoring of blood cell counts because of reversible myelosuppression, resulting in neutropenia and thrombocytopenia. Patients treated with foscarnet require close monitoring of renal function and electrolytes because of nephrotoxic side effects, which are usually reversible. CMV retinitis recurrence is common during maintenance therapy, occurring in up to 85% of patients. Lifelong maintenance treatment is necessary to slow the progression of retinitis.

To obviate systemic toxicity from anti-CMV therapy, local therapy can be administered into the eye with intravitreal injections of foscarnet or ganciclovir. Because of the short half-life of these drugs in the vitreous, patients require one or two injections per week. Complications of the intravitreal injections include endophthalmitis and retinal detachment. Sustained-release ganciclovir implant therapy is another local therapeutic strategy that allows several months between ocular treatment. Some suggest that intraocular treatment can be supplemented with oral treatment to avoid parenteral therapy.

Toxoplasmic a infection is second only to CMV infection as the cause of retinitis in the AIDS patient. Toxoplasmic retinitis in the AIDS patient appears to occur from newly acquired primary infection or from dissemination to the retina from latent extraocular sites. More than half of patients with AIDS and toxoplasmic retinitis have associated encephalitis, and therefore AIDS patients with newly diagnosed toxoplasmic retinitis should undergo computed tomography of the brain with contrast media to rule out toxoplasmic encephalitis. On ocular examination a granulomatous anterior uveitis and vitreitis is commonly seen.

by a vesicular rash in the distribution of the ophthalmic branch of the trigeminal nerve and may be associated with blepharitis, keratitis, conjunctivitis, and uveitis. The HIV patient often has a prolonged and severe course. HZO should be treated with systemic acyclovir (10 mg/kg every 8 hours intravenously or 600 to 800 mg by mouth five times per day), and the patient should be followed closely for evidence of disseminated infection. Topical steroids for uveitis should be administered only under the close supervision of an ophthalmologist, because steroid use places the patient at high risk for superinfections and glaucoma. After the acute episode the patient needs to be followed closely by an ophthalmologist, since relapses are common. Varicella-zoster virus may also involve the retina, as discussed later in the section on acute retinal necrosis.

Common Infectious Manifestations of AIDS—Posterior Segment

The HIV virus has been shown to infect retinal tissue, including the capillary endothelium and neuroretinal cells. The infection of capillary endothelial cells and the associated deposition of immune complexes may play a role in the formation of cotton-wool spots commonly seen in patients with AIDS. Other etiologic possibilities of cotton-wool spots include disseminated intravascular coagulopathy or hematologic sludging resulting from increased red blood cell aggregation and blood viscosity. Regardless of etiology, the compromised endothelial cells may then allow cytomegalovirus (CMV)-infected monocytes to pass into the retina, leading to CMV retinitis.

Common Noninfectious Manifestations of AIDS

Kaposi's sarcoma (KS) is a multifocal, malignant sarcoma characterized by vascular tumors of the skin, oral mucosa, and internal organs. KS occurs in approximately 10% of patients with AIDS, and 20% of patients with AIDS-related KS have ophthalmic involvement. The eyelids, conjunctiva, and orbit can become involved, and this may be the initial manifestation of AIDS. Subconjunctival hemorrhages are in the differential diagnosis and are caused by the thrombocytopenia that is often seen in HIV-infected patients. In any case of nonresolving subconjunctival hemorrhage the diagnosis of KS should be considered. With KS infiltration of the orbit, proptosis, ptosis, eyelid edema, and diplopia from ocular nerve palsies may occur. The various forms of treatment include excision, chemotherapy, cryotherapy, and radiation therapy, which may provide palliative relief but are not curative. Recurrences are common.

Keratoconjunctivitis sicca is a dry eye condition that is well known to occur in Sjögren's syndrome, which is associated with autoimmune diseases such as rheumatoid arthritis. Keratoconjunctivitis sicca is seen in 10% to 15% of HIV-infected patients. Salivary gland biopsies reveal intense lymphocyte infiltration of glandular parenchyma. This condition is usually well managed with routine topical lubricant therapy, such as artificial tears.

Burkitt's lymphoma has also been associated with AIDS. This is a diffuse non-Hodgkin's lymphoma that may involve the eyelids, orbit, and leptomeningeal tissue. When involving the orbital structures, patients may present with a nontender anterior orbital mass, ptosis, eyelid edema, subconjunctival hemorrhage, or diplopia from ocular nerve palsies.

Patients with AIDS often complain vaguely of blurred vision and photophobia. The pathophysiologic mechanisms for these complaints are not fully understood. Complaints of darkening vision may be a result of primary HIV-related optic neuropathy. Complaints of night blindness may be related to malabsorption of vitamin A. Difficulties of accommodation and progression of myopia may be related to the multiple medications and multiple medical problems common in these patients; these issues are readily managed with appropriate refraction. Any patient with AIDS and visual complaints, such as floaters or new-onset blurred vision, should be readily referred for ophthalmic consultation to rule out opportunistic infection.

BIBLIOGRAPHY

Albert D et al: AIDS and its ophthalmic manifestations. In McMullen WW, D'amico DJ, editors: *Principles and practice of ophthalmology,* vol 5, Philadelphia, 1994, WB Saunders.

Albert D et al: Retina manifestations of AIDS: diagnosis and treatment. In Albert D, Jakobiec F, editors: *Principles and practice of ophthalmology,* vol 2, Philadelphia, 1994, WB Saunders.

American Academy of Ophthalmology: *Basic and clinical science course: lens and cataract—section 11,* section I and II, San Francisco, 1994, American Academy of Ophthalmology.

American Academy of Ophthalmology: *Basic and clinical science course: glaucoma—section 10,* San Francisco, 1996, American Academy of Ophthalmology.

American Academy of Ophthalmology: *Basic and clinical science course: retina,* San Francisco, 1996, American Academy of Ophthalmology.

Bressler NM, Bressler SB, Gragoudas ES: Age-related macular degeneration: drusen and geographic atrophy. In Albert D, Jakobiec F, editors: *Principles and practice of ophthalmology,* vol 2, Philadelphia, 1994, WB Saunders.

Culbertson WW: Infections of the retina in AIDS, *Int Ophthalmol Clin* 29:108-118, 1989.

Jabs DA, Green WR, Fox R, et al: Ocular manifestations of the acquired immune deficiency syndrome, *Ophthalmology* 96(7):1092-1099, 1989.

Tasman W, Jaeger EA, editors: *Duane's biomedical foundations of clinical ophthalmology,* vol 3, Philadelphia, 1995, JB Lippincott.

Whitcup SM: Ocular manifestations of AIDS, *JAMA* 275(2):142-144, 1996.

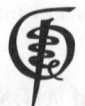

CHAPTER

377 Common Ear, Nose, and Throat Problems

Earl H. Harley

EMERGENCIES AND URGENT CONDITIONS
Supraglottitis (Epiglottitis)

Supraglottitis can be insidious in adults, beginning with severe sore throat and progressing to odynophagia and fever. Stridor and airway embarrassment are late findings in adults. There may be a paucity of physical findings in the oropharynx, especially in those who have had tonsillectomy. Radiographic examination often reveals an enlarged epiglottis and the typical "thumbprint sign." However, this sign is variable and its absence does not rule out supraglottitis. Flexible laryngoscopy with a fiberoptic scope (often performed in the emergency department) will reveal the typical pattern of swelling and inflammation in the supraglottic structures. These patients should be admitted to the hospital and observed closely for progression of airway symptoms. Antibiotic treatment should be directed initially against *Haemophilus influenzae* type b while culture results are pending.

Peritonsillar Abscess (Quinsy)

Peritonsillar abscess (PTA) is a complication of acute tonsillitis often caused by *Streptococcus pyogenes* (group A β-hemolytic streptococcus). In most instances, PTA occurs in the superior pole of the tonsil and often presents with deviation of the uvula to the opposite side. Peritonsillar abscess usually occurs in young adults but may occur at any age. Patients typically develop a sore throat with progressive symptoms of difficulty swallowing, "hot potato speech," trismus, and drooling. Earache on the side of the abscess is a common symptom. Drainage of the abscess and antibiotic therapy are the main treatments. Needle aspiration successfully accomplishes this drainage in 70% to 80% of the cases. Occasionally otolaryngologists will perform an incision and drainage (I&D) procedure. Quinsy tonsillectomy, removal of the tonsil during the acute phase of the disease, has many proponents but is usually reserved for patients who fail to respond to needle aspiration and/or I&D and continue to have severe symptoms.

Angioedema

Angioedema may present with life-threatening swelling in the oropharynx and larynx. The most common identifiable etiologic factor is the use of angiotensin-converting enzyme inhibitors. The swelling typically occurs after the first several doses of medication.

Often there is marked swelling of the lips, tongue, and mucosa, including the uvula and facial structures. These patients are at risk for airway obstruction, but usually the swelling remains limited to the lips and tongue. Although treatment with antihistamine drugs is usually sufficient, patients may require endotracheal intubation and observation in the intensive care unit. Supplemental oxygen, subcutaneous epinephrine, and an antihistamine should be given. Corticosteroids may be used, but they will not have an immediate effect. The swelling resolves over a period of 24 to 48 hours.

Facial Nerve Paralysis

If a specific cause of the facial paralysis is not determined, this entity is referred to as *Bell's palsy.* Bell's palsy is treated with corticosteroids. Because of a suspected viral etiology, antiviral agents such as acyclovir may be considered. If there is complete paralysis of the nerve, electrical testing should be performed. If at least 10% of the fibers are still intact, the nerve has a good chance of recovery. If less than 10% of the nerve fibers are intact, surgical decompression of the facial nerve can be considered but is rarely necessary.

In other forms of facial nerve paralysis, management is dependent on etiology. For example, traumatic injury to the facial nerve may require decompression or repair of the injured segments. Regardless of the cause of the facial nerve paralysis, care of the eye and cornea are of paramount concern to prevent exposure keratitis.

Acute Airway Obstruction

The following is a partial list of conditions that may acutely compromise the airway: angioedema, severe tonsillitis (especially mononucleosis tonsillitis), deep neck infections, blunt facial trauma, blunt neck trauma, supraglottitis, caustic ingestions, and tumors. One should always remember to use the simplest intervention possible. Often insertion of a nasal airway is all that is needed to correct the problem. Sometimes endotracheal intubation is necessary. Emergency or bedside tracheotomies are only rarely done. In the true emergency situation when a surgical airway is required, a cricothyrotomy is a much safer procedure.

EAR DISORDERS

Otalgia

Otalgia may be due to an otologic or a nonotologic disorder. Areas outside of the ear produce otalgia, which is chiefly mediated by branches of the fifth, seventh, or ninth cranial nerves. In the absence of physical findings referable to the ear, one must investigate adjacent structures.

Musculoskeletal disorders such as temporomandibular joint (TMJ) dysfunction or myofascial disorder affecting the sternocleidomastoid muscle may cause ear discomfort. Otalgia may be of a dental etiology. Pharyngeal infections such as severe tonsillopharyngitis or peritonsillar abscess may refer pain to the ear. Occult cancers of the tonsil, base of tongue, and pyriform sinuses are notorious in their propensity to refer pain to the ear via the tympanic branch of the glossopharyngeal nerve.

Tinnitus

Tinnitus may be associated with hearing loss. Persistent tinnitus should be investigated with an audiogram because this may be an early symptom of a tumor. In Ménière's disease, tinnitus may be a low pitch roar. Tinnitus may be pulsatile secondary to a vascular abnormality, such as a glomus tumor. Certain medications, such as aspirin and quinine, also produce tinnitus (see discussion of vertigo).

Otorrhea

Otorrhea is frequently associated with otitis externa. Another common cause is drainage secondary to a cholesteatoma, especially chronic ear drainage that does not respond to antibiotics and ototopical therapy. A rare cause of otorrhea is a cerebrospinal fluid fistula, which usually occurs after trauma such as a basal skull or temporal bone fracture, but it may be spontaneous.

Vertigo

Vertigo should be distinguished from dizziness and lightheadedness. The latter symptoms are often secondary to metabolic or cardiac disorders, whereas vertigo is of an otologic or neurologic origin. The most common cause of vertigo is viral labyrinthitis or vestibular neuronitis. Ménière's disease, benign positional vertigo, migraine syndrome, multiple sclerosis, syphilis, and acoustic neuroma are other causes.

Evaluation of vertigo dictates a thorough history, including medications and toxic exposures, and physical examination, including a neurologic assessment. An audiogram and electronystagmogram are often necessary in pinpointing the exact nature of the vertigo. Serum glucose, lipids, and thyroid function tests may be useful. Serologic tests for syphilis should be obtained in some patients to rule out a luetic cause of the vertigo. Magnetic resonance imaging (MRI) of the temporal bone is the most widely employed imaging study because it allows evaluation for acoustic neuroma or other cerebropontine angle tumors and multiple sclerosis.

Ménière's disease is a common cause of vertigo. Ménière's disease is endolymphatic hydrops, characterized by fullness in the ear(s), episodic vertigo, and hearing loss. It is usually unilateral, but it may progress to become bilateral. Most patients can be treated conservatively with a low-salt diet, low-dose diuretics, and labyrinthine sedatives such as meclizine. Occasionally, low-dose benzodiazepines are useful. Only 15% to 20% of patients with Ménière's disease require surgical intervention. Surgery is indicated for severe disabling disease or to arrest the progression of the disease, especially hearing loss. Endolymphatic shunting and vestibular nerve sections are used to stabilize patients with Ménière's disease whose hearing has not deteriorated. If the hearing has already decreased significantly, a labyrinthectomy can be employed. Streptomycin is used for a so-called medical labyrinthectomy for patients with severe bilateral Ménière's disease who have normal hearing; streptomycin will destroy the labyrinth while preserving hearing.

Otitis Externa (OE)

Acute otitis externa is characterized by pain, swelling, and drainage from the affected ear and tenderness on manipulation of the auricle or the tragus and a watery or a mucopurulent drainage. Swelling of the canal is variable.

Initial therapy is usually empirical. Unless the host is immunocompromised, culture and sensitivity is reserved for recalcitrant infections, which may be caused by *Pseudomonas* species.

Gentle cleansing of the ear canal is a very important part of treatment. The infection is usually localized, and acidic drops or ototopical antibiotics usually suffice. Because the edema is so marked in some cases, the canal is completely occluded and it is impossible to instill otic drops. In these instances an ear wick is advisable. The pain accompanying OE is often severe enough to require narcotics for relief.

Swimmer's ear is form of OE; it can be prevented with the prophylactic use of 2% acetic acid and 70% alcohol solution after swimming.

Chronic OE causes itching and dry skin. Eczema and seborrhea contribute to chronic OE. The application of baby oil or steroid preparations can be beneficial.

Fungal OE, or otomycosis, is occasionally encountered. *Aspergillus* species are the most frequent offending organisms. These saprophytic infections usually occur in conjunction with underlying bacterial infections. The ear should be cleansed and ototopical drops applied. Antifungal agents such as clotrimazole may be useful for difficult infections.

Middle Ear Disorders

Eustachian tube dysfunction produces otalgia by creating negative pressure in the middle ear because of poor ventilation. Often, allergic diathesis is the underlying cause of this dysfunction. Nasal steroids are often used to reduce local edema and improve tubal function. Valsalva's maneuver can be useful in improving middle ear function.

Acute suppurative otitis media may occur with upper respiratory tract infections and with allergic symptoms. Secretory otitis occurs mainly in allergic diseases. Of note are chronic middle ear effusions, which may be the presenting symptoms in a patient with a nasopharyngeal mass such as nasopharyngeal carcinoma. Also, human immunodeficiency virus–acquired immunodeficiency syndrome (HIV-AIDS) produces hyperplasia of tissue in Waldeyer's ring, which obstructs the eustachian tube. A middle ear effusion may be the first clinical symptom of HIV-AIDS.

If an infection does not respond readily to appropriate antibiotics to cover the usual bacteria, *Streptococcus pneumoniae and Haemophilus influenzae,* tympanocentesis can be both diagnostic and therapeutic.

Perforation of the tympanic membrane may result from acute or chronic ear infections or from trauma. Most acute perforations heal completely without intervention. Nonhealing perforations may be patched or may require surgical repair.

Chronic otitis media may develop into cholesteatoma (keratoma). Cholesteatoma occurs when squamous epithelium develops in the middle ear and mastoid. It may present with pain, otorrhea, and hearing loss. Occasionally the drainage takes on a bloody appearance. Vertigo and facial nerve weakness are less common symptoms associated with cholesteatoma. Retraction of the epitympanic (pars flaccida) portion of the tympanic membrane may be the earliest physical finding. Eventually the patient develops a perforation in the pars flaccida. Granulation tissue and aural polyps may also be seen. A cholesteatoma is treated surgically with a tympanomastoidectomy.

There are several other notable complications of otitis media. These include acute mastoiditis, lateral sinus thrombosis, facial nerve palsy, labyrinthitis, extradural abscess, subdural abscess, brain abscess, and otitic hydrocephalus. Treatments for these complications range from myringotomy to mastoidectomy to craniotomy.

Hearing Loss

Normal hearing ranges from 0 dB to 20 dB. Persons with hearing thresholds greater than 20 dB are considered to have a hearing loss.

Hearing losses are divided into three categories: conductive, sensorineural, and mixed. Hearing can be estimated with the use of tuning forks. It is customary practice to use the 512-Hz tuning fork for this purpose. Weber's test and the Rinne test have the most practical application as hearing screens. Weber's test is performed in the midline: forehead, occiput, central maxillary teeth, or alveolus. Weber's test is normal when the sound is perceived in the midline or is equally distinct in either ear. When there is a conductive hearing loss, Weber's test lateralizes to the affected ear. When there is a sensorineural hearing loss, Weber's test lateralizes to unaffected ear. The Rinne test must be used in conjunction with Weber's test. The Rinne test measures air-versus-bone conduction. Air conduction is normally twice as long as bone conduction. If there is a significant conductive hearing loss, the results will be reversed and bone conduction will be greater than air. In a sensorineural hearing loss, air conduction continues to be greater than bone in both ears.

Conductive hearing losses are caused by such problems as cerumen occlusion in the ear canal, fluid in the middle ear, chronic otitis media with or without cholesteatoma, tympanic membrane perforation, ossicular erosion, otosclerosis, and tumors of the external or middle ear. These types of losses are often amenable to medical or surgical intervention. Sensorineural hearing losses whereby there is damage to hair cells and nerves in the inner ear can be caused by such varied etiologic factors as acoustic trauma, presbycusis, acoustic neuroma, ototoxic drugs, autoimmune disease, idiopathic sudden sensorineural hearing loss, perilymphatic fistula, and infectious agents such as syphilis.

Idiopathic sudden sensorineural hearing loss is an acute onset of decreased hearing thresholds greater than 30 dB that occurs in less than 3 days. There are several possible causes. These include viral, vascular, and autoimmune causes. A short course of corticosteroids may be useful in sudden sensorineural hearing loss. To be effective, the steroid should be given as soon after the onset as possible.

NOSE AND SINUS DISORDERS
Rhinitis

The most common cause of chronic rhinitis is allergy. The symptoms are often seasonal, but they may be perennial if the patient is allergic to dust, household pets, or foods. This condition is often confused with vasomotor rhinitis, which may represent a non–IgE-mediated allergy. A total IgE level and nasal smear for eosinophils may help to distinguish the two entities. The mainstay of therapy for either is inhaled nasal steroids, with which there is typically a delayed onset of action from several days to a week. In addition to decongestants, antihistamines are often useful. Topical decongestants such as phenylephrine used for periods of 2 to 3 days are helpful before the onset of action of steroids. Care must be exercised because of the development of rhinitis medicamentosa. Recent experience with ipratropium in treating various forms of rhinitis, including allergic and acute rhinitis, is encouraging. For severely allergic patients, immunotherapy is often indicated.

There are several other notable causes of rhinitis. These include the rhinitis associated with pregnancy, medications, and metabolic disorders. A most bothersome form of rhinitis is secondary to abuse of over-the-counter nasal sprays. Such ill-advised usage leads to rhinitis medicamentosa, a constant state of vasodilation. Treatment involves abrupt discontinuance of the spray with systemic decongestants and inhaled nasal steroids to help the patient through the difficult phase of withdrawing from the nasal sprays.

Nasal Obstruction

Nasal polyps are often seen in allergic patients. A short course of systemic steroids can be useful in treating these patients. Immunotherapy and often polypectomy may also be part of the treatment. Other causes of nasal polyps include cystic fibrosis and inverting papilloma, a potentially premalignant lesion that should be completely surgically excised.

Nasal septal deviation is a common cause of nasal obstruction. The deviation may be posttraumatic, but often it is not. If the patient complains of symptomatic nasal obstruction, a septoplasty or nasal reconstruction may be indicated.

Epistaxis

Eighty percent to ninety percent of epistaxis, at least in children, occurs in the anterior part of the nose in an area known as Kiesselbach's plexus. The remaining 10% to 20% of epistaxis is posterior and usually occurs in older adults with atherosclerosis and hypertension. Bleeding disorders may present as epistaxis.

Anterior epistaxis is usually easily treated with local pressure and occasionally with silver nitrate cauterization. Rarely, anterior nasal packing is required. Patients are advised to keep the mucous membranes supple with either saline solution or petroleum jelly.

Patients with posterior epistaxis may require hospitalization for control of their hypertension, and they may require posterior nasal packing for several days. Posterior nasal packing, however, is a procedure involving some risks. There are several reports of hypoxia, hypotension, and death in these sometimes fragile patients. The mechanism is arguably secondary to a "nasopulmonary" reflex. Patients with posterior nasal packs, especially the elderly, with underlying cardiovascular disease, should be admitted for observation and monitored closely.

Nasal Fracture

The diagnosis of nasal fracture is based on history of injury and physical findings of ecchymosis, tenderness, and deformity. Radiographic studies may be of little value. Although reduction of the nasal fracture can safely be delayed until the edema subsides in 5 to 10 days, it is imperative to consider a septal hematoma as soon after the injury as possible. The hallmark of a septal hematoma is increasing nasal obstruction following blunt nasal trauma. This hematoma must be promptly drained in order to avoid a septal abscess and subsequent deformity of the nose secondary to destruction of septal cartilage.

Sinusitis

The maxillary and ethmoid sinuses are the most common sinuses to be involved. The final common pathway for all sinusitis is obstruction, edema with occlusion of the sinus ostia, and subsequent infection. Viral upper respiratory tract infections or underlying allergic phenomena are the most common reasons for recurrent acute sinusitis. Other common predisposing factors are nasal septal deviation, nasal polyps, irritation from cigarette smoke, and barotrauma. Persons with HIV-AIDS; cystic fibrosis; or ciliary disorders, such as in Kartagener's syndrome, also suffer frequent sinus infections.

Purulent nasal drainage, headaches, facial pain, pressure on bending over, anosmia, and cough are common symptoms of acute sinusitis. Purulent nasal discharge and cough are sensitive but not very specific symptoms of sinus infection. On the other hand, maxillary toothache is a highly specific.

In patients with reactive airway disease, bronchospasm may be precipitated by a sinus infection. This may be caused by aspiration of purulent secretions, enhanced vagal stimulation in the infected sinus, excessive drying of the lower airway because of nasal obstruction, or production of cytokines and bronchoconstrictive mediators in the infected sinus. Control of sinus disease can have a beneficial effect on the lower airway.

Transillumination of the frontal and maxillary sinuses may be of some benefit in elucidating the diagnosis. Normal transmission of light may eliminate consideration of sinusitis, whereas opaque transillumination helps to diagnose sinusitis. Dull transillumination is less helpful in making a diagnosis.

Imaging studies can be performed, but they may not be necessary in all cases of acute sinusitis when the history and physical findings are typical. The most useful studies are plain radiographs and computed tomography (CT). Ultrasound has been advocated by some, but it has not proved to be very reliable.

The most common bacteria in acute sinusitis are *Streptococcus pneumoniae* and *Haemophilus influenzae*. Occasionally *Staphylococcus aureus* invades the sinus cavity. As the disease becomes more chronic, anaerobic organisms can be seen. Fungal sinusitis also occurs, and *Aspergillus* species can infect otherwise healthy patients. In diabetic and immunocompromised patients, *Mucor* species can be involved.

The major treatment goals in the management of sinusitis are reduction of edema, facilitation of drainage, and control of infection. Saline nasal irrigations and decongestants promote reduction of mucosal edema and opening of the sinus ostia. Decongestants may be given topically or systemically. Antihistamines alone or in combination with decongestants cause drying but may be used judiciously in selected allergic patients. Mucoevacuants such as guaifenesin are also useful in sinusitis.

Amoxicillin is considered to be the first line antibiotic of choice. Other suitable antibiotics include trimethoprim-sulfamethoxazole. If patients do not respond clinically to these drugs, cephalosporins and newer macrolides may be necessary. If a β-lactamase organism is suspected, amoxicillin with clavulanic acid is efficacious. Unsuitable antibiotics in the treatment of acute sinusitis include tetracycline (because of resistant pneumococcus); penicillin; erythromycin; and cephalexin (because of resistant *H. influenzae*).

In rare instances of acute sinusitis the patient does not respond readily to treatment. In these cases a maxillary sinus puncture can be performed in the office by the otolaryngologist. The sinus is usually punctured via the inferior meatus or the canine fossa under a topical and/or locally injected anesthesia. Trephination may be necessary for unresolving acute frontal sinusitis. Chronic sinusitis is considered to be an infection that persists to some degree for at least 3 months. Patients with chronic sinusitis may suffer frequent exacerbations of infection. Inhaled nasal steroids have proved to be beneficial as maintenance therapy in chronic sinusitis. Systemic steroids are often used when allergic polyposis and allergic fungal sinusitis are a component of the disease process. Definitive management of chronic sinusitis may include surgical intervention.

There are several serious and potentially fatal complications of sinusitis. These complications can be divided into sinus, orbital, and central nervous system (CNS). The most notable sinus complication is a mucocele or mucopyocele. The most common type of mucocele or mucopyocele is the frontoethmoid variety. A mucocele is an expanding cyst that may erode through bone into adjacent structures. These are slow-growing destructive lesions that must be removed. These are not to be confused with mucus retention cysts, which are not erosive and rarely require removal.

Orbital extension of sinusitis is usually secondary to ethmoiditis. The lamina papyracea is a very thin bone that divides the ethmoid sinus from the orbit. Chandler has classified orbital complications into five stages: periorbital cellulitis (preseptal), orbital cellulitis, subperiosteal orbital abscess, orbital abscess, and cavernous thrombosis. Intravenous antibiotics may suffice in the early stages. However, surgery is usually required in the advanced stages.

The CNS complications of sinusitis usually arise in the frontal sinuses and less often the sphenoid sinuses. Meningitis, epidural abscess, subdural abscess, and brain abscess are all potential complications.

ORAL, PHARYNGEAL, AND LARYNGEAL DISORDERS
Oral Cavity

Common problems of the oral cavity include aphthous ulcers and herpetic stomatitis. There are no good treatments for aphthous ulcers, but rinsing with solutions containing antibiotics such as erythromycin may be beneficial. Recurrent herpetic lesions are best managed symptomatically. Acyclovir or similar antiviral agents should be reserved for more severe cases.

Leukoplakia is a white lesion of the oral cavity, often simply representing hyperkeratosis. The incidence of malignant transformation is less than 10%. If the lesion is not removed, one must follow the patient closely. Erythroplakia is a red lesion of the oral cavity and is more likely to be malignant or premalignant.

Tonsillopharyngitis

Viral tonsillopharyngitis is the most common cause of throat infection. Group A β-hemolytic strep (GABHS) infection is also common. Other organisms such as mycoplasma and chlamydia infect the throat. Infectious mononucleosis tonsillitis may be severe and cause great difficulty with swallowing and occasionally with breathing.

Tonsillectomy is indicated for patients who suffer recurrent tonsillopharyngitis, especially GABHS. In general, four to five episodes of tonsillitis per year meets the threshold for tonsillectomy. Also, a recurrent peritonsillar abscess or suspected tumors are indications for tonsillectomy.

Snoring

Loud snoring may indicate airway obstruction. The snoring may be secondary to septal deviation, nasal allergy, nasal polyps, redundant soft palate, or large tonsils.

Although initial therapy should include assistance in sleeping prone, patients may benefit from surgery, particularly if airway obstruction is associated with sleep apnea. Uvulopharyngopalatoplasty (UPPP) and laser-assisted uvulopalatoplasty (LAUP) have been used with variable success. Septoplasty, geniohyoid advancement, or tongue reduction may be required. Tracheotomy is reserved for patients with severe obstruction with hypoxia and hypercapnia who do not respond to continuuous positive airway pressure (CPAP) and/or less aggressive surgery such as UPPP.

Hoarseness

Acute laryngitis may be of viral etiology. The treatment should consist of voice rest, fluids, and humidification. If the patient has a lower airway–induced cough, it should be treated to decrease the irritation to the larynx. In singers and other professionals who rely on their voices, a short course of systemic steroids may be beneficial.

Hoarseness lasting more than 2 to 3 weeks should be referred to the otolaryngologist to rule out a laryngeal tumor. If the chronic hoarseness is secondary to vocal misuse and resultant vocal cord nodules, a referral for speech therapy should be part of the management. Inhaled steroids may have some benefit in chronic laryngitis.

Hoarseness may also be secondary to vocal cord paralysis. Vocal cord paralysis may be secondary to a viral disease or to other infectious disorders such as Lyme disease. Also, it may be the presenting sign of mediastinal adenopathy from metastatic lung cancer. Blunt trauma also may cause vocal cord paralysis. If a specific treatable etiology is not identified, the patient should be referred to speech pathology for vocal exercises. The patient may be a candidate for surgery to improve vocal function or improve the airway if the paralysis is bilateral.

Recurrent respiratory papillomatosis (RRP) causes hoarseness and occasionally airway obstruction. Adults may have the more aggressive juvenile form or the less aggressive adult-onset form. Laser excision is the preferred treatment for RRP. Interferon has been successfully used in difficult cases. Methotrexate and retinoic acid have also been employed for recalcitrant disease that does not respond to more conventional therapy.

NECK DISORDERS
Deep Neck Infections

Infections of the dental area, tonsils, and pharynx are common sources of infection extending into the fascial planes of the neck and producing a deep neck infection. The presenting symptoms of deep neck infections include odynophagia, dysphagia, drooling, trismus, and poor oral intake. Airway occlusion is a potential problem from the expanding suppuration and associated edema. Because fascial planes of the neck communicate with the mediastinum, infections in the neck may result in mediastinitis.

Adenopathy

Cervical adenopathy is often secondary to acute viral or bacterial sources. Also, infectious mononucleosis as well as mycobacterial and fungal disease are causes of inflammatory cervical nodes. Antibiotics may be given empirically. If the patient does not respond, a work-up may be performed. A fine needle aspiration, chest roentgenogram, and skin tests for tuberculosis and fungal diseases should be done. An excisional biopsy may be necessary in rare instances.

In middle-aged or elderly adults, persistent cervical adenopathy is of greater concern because of the possibility of metastatic cancer from regional or remote organs. In about 85% of cases the malignancy is a squamous cancer from a head and neck site. The other 15% of malignancies are lymphoma, sarcoma, or metastasis from regions outside of the head and neck. Cancers originating in the head and neck areas usually metastasize to the anterior or posterior triangles of the neck. When the nodal mass is in the supraclavicular area, the cancer is most likely from a site below the clavicle. A right supraclavicular node may originate from the lung or breast, whereas a left supraclavicular node is often from the gastrointestinal tract (Virchow's node).

Benign Neck Cysts

Thyroglossal duct cysts, branchial cleft cysts, and dermoid cysts are common cystic lesions. Other types of benign cysts occur in the neck. These include thymic cysts, parathyroid cysts, and thyroid cysts.

Thyroglossal duct cysts occur in the midline. The tract begins at the foramen cecum of the tongue, and the cyst presents at the level of the hyoid bone in the midline. These cysts are often asymptomatic but may eventually become infected and fistulize. Surgery is definitive treatment.

Branchial cleft anomalies occur in the lateral part of the neck. These anomalies present as cysts, sinuses, or fistulae. The most common type of branchial cleft anomaly is found along the anterior border of the sternocleidomastoid muscle and has an internal opening in the tonsillar fossa. They sometimes become symptomatic in association with an upper respiratory tract infection. Surgical excision is the treatment of choice.

Acute Inflammation of Salivary Glands

The event may be precipitated by a stone (sialolithiasis). About 80% of salivary stones are radiopaque. Thus they may be visualized on roentgenograms of the area involved. The submandibular gland is the most common gland infected, and the parotid gland is the second most common gland infected. *Staphylococcus aureus* is almost always the responsible bacterial organism. Treatment consists of hydration, sialogogues such as hard candy, and antistaphylococcal antibiotics such as oxacillin or cephalexin.

Cystic lesions of the parotid gland occur frequently in HIV-AIDS. These cysts are often bilateral and are treated by needle aspiration, repeatedly if necessary. Occasionally, sclerosing agents can be injected into the cyst cavity after aspiration. Surgical excision of the cysts is rarely indicated.

Head and Neck Cancer

Most malignancies of the head and neck are squamous cell cancers (SCC), excluding thyroid, parathyroid, and parotid cancers; lymphoma; and sarcoma. Typically patients with SCC of the head and neck have histories of heavy alcohol and tobacco use. The presenting symptoms may be a unilateral earache, dysphagia and/or odynophagia, hoarseness, or neck mass. Radiation is the usual treatment in early stages. In advanced stages, multimodality treatment is usually required for a successful outcome.

CHAPTER

378 Drug Interactions and Adverse Effects

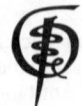

David A. Flockhart

The unpredictability of adverse drug reactions and the substantial morbidity they cause are not subjects of debate. Each year in the United States, approximately two billion prescriptions are filled, and time constraints placed on both physicians and pharmacists have made it increasingly difficult for either to counsel patients thoroughly about the possibility of adverse reactions to medications that are intended to have therapeutic benefit.

Side effects are strictly defined as effects of a drug that are beyond those intended for therapeutic benefit, and they encompass both adverse effects and beneficial ones, such as the improvement in prostatic symptoms experienced by men treated with α_1-adrenergic blocking agents for hypertension. In fact, the vast majority of patients report that they have experienced an adverse side effect of some drug. Even if these side effects might appear innocuous to health professionals (e.g., the drowsiness associated with some antihistamines, or the fungal vaginitis or diarrhea frequently associated with antibiotic use), they can be of great concern to patients. For physicians the importance of familiarity with adverse effects and of counseling patients about them is emphasized by the fact that inappropriate prescribing of medications is cited as the second most common cause of malpractice suits.

Although the Food and Drug Administration has an aggressive program called Medwatch to encourage health care professionals to use forms contained in every copy of the *Physicians' Desk Reference* to report adverse events caused by drugs, most experts agree that more than 90% of these events go unreported. The medical consequences of these events are substantial. In a recent study conducted at the Harvard teaching hospitals, 6.5% of inpatients experienced a confirmed injury brought about by drugs, and a further 5.5% were the potential victims of mistakes that could have caused harm. There is particular cause for concern in the burgeoning aged population, for whom 3% to 11% of hospital admissions may be due to unintended consequences of drug-related therapy.

Among these adverse effects of pharmaceuticals, drug interactions appear to account for 5% to 10% of reported events. For example, cardiac arrests resulting from the coprescription of antihistamines such as terfenadine (Seldane) and astemizole (Hismanal) with erythromycin or ketoconazole alerted many physicians and researchers to the potential importance of drug interactions. Indeed, the effectiveness of medical communication about life-threatening coprescriptions has been challenged by the observation that terfenadine continued to be coprescribed with erythromycin 4 years after the interaction was reported, and that more than 30% of pharmacists failed to note such coprescriptions and warn patients. Drug interactions are an increasing concern as the number of available prescription medications for a variety of disorders increases, and as the number of different prescriptions taken by individual patients, particularly the elderly, increases.

Although we generally think of drug interactions in a negative light, it is also important to note that they may be used to therapeutic benefit. For example, ketoconazole has been used to decrease the metabolism of cyclosporine and thus reduce the required dose and the costs associated with cyclosporine therapy. A similar strategy has been employed with ketoconazole to slow the metabolism of methadone.

MECHANISMS OF DRUG INTERACTIONS

A drug interaction with a particular medicine may be caused by either a change in the concentration of that medicine (a pharmacokinetic effect) or a change in the drug's effect. Although it is often possible for health care professionals to predict a pharmacodynamic interaction if the clinical effect of the drug is known (e.g., verapamil and metoprolol both slow heart rate), it is not as easy to recognize the possibility of a pharmacokinetic interaction. It is possible to simplify a search for possible sites of interaction by following a medication through the body.

First, interactions can occur as a result of coprecipitation of chemicals that are not compatible in intravenous solutions, before any medication enters the body. A good example is the interaction between gentamicin and cefoxitin. These drugs coprecipitate if mixed in high concentrations, resulting in complete loss of any drug effect and, often, the loss of the intravenous access. The simple way to avoid these interactions is to avoid infusing these medications simultaneously if possible, especially via the same intravenous line either by "piggybacking" or through the same central line. Hospital pharmacies and intensive care units have detailed listings of such incompatibilities available.

Second, drugs can interact in the stomach, where insoluble complexes may be formed between cations such as calcium or aluminium

Table 378-1 Characteristics of Human Cytochrome P_{450} Isoforms Relevant to Drug Metabolism

ISOFORM	CHARACTERISTICS
CYP1A2	Activity increased in smokers
CYP2C9	Absent in 1% of whites
CYP2C19	Absent in 15%-20% of Asians and 2%-5% of whites
CYP2D6	Absent in 7% of whites
CYP2E1	Activity increased by alcohol
CYP3A4	Wide range of activity in liver and GI tract

(in milk, cheese, antacids, or sucralfate) or iron and drugs such as tetracycline, digoxin, or fluoroquinolone antibiotics. Resins such as cholestyramine and kaolin-pectin may decrease the absorption of thyroid hormones or warfarin by a similar mechanism. The acid environment in the stomach is itself important to the solubility, and therefore to the absorption of some drugs (e.g., ketoconazole), and so it is important to realize that the potent proton pump inhibitors now available (omeprazole, lansoprazole and pantoprazole) are also potent inhibitors of ketoconazole absorption. Prokinetic drugs—such as metoclopramide, cisapride and erythromycin—can not only affect the extent of the aforementioned interactions, but also speed the absorption of drugs in the small intestine. Conversely, drugs that slow gastric emptying via anticholinergic or other mechanisms may slow the absorption of any drug.

Interactions may occur in the gastrointestinal (GI) system beyond the stomach. A number of drugs, notably digoxin, are degraded by commensal bacteria in the small and large bowel, and the use of antibiotics may not only result in diarrhea, but also in an increase in absorption as a result of decreased intestinal degradation.

Third, and probably most important, the pharmacokinetics of drugs that are metabolized in the liver or in the intestinal mucosa can be powerfully altered by drugs that induce or inhibit metabolism. Metabolism usually results in the conversion of a drug to a form that is more easily eliminated, either directly or after further processing via the conjugation reactions with glucuronides, glutathione, or acetyl moieties that are referred to as *phase 2 metabolism.* Inhibition of metabolism may slow elimination of the parent drug, particularly if metabolism is very active, or if there is a large "first-pass" effect. This effect involves metabolism during the first pass of the drug through the intestinal-hepatic "wall" of metabolic enzymes that is positioned strategically to protect us against plant toxins. Within this diverse, powerful, and adaptable system of defense, the group of enzymes referred to as cytochrome P_{450} play a dominant, and often rate-limiting role.

Cytochrome P_{450}-Based Interactions

Over the past 20 years it has become clear that the human cytochrome P_{450} system involves a large number of enzymes with distinct characteristics. The nomenclature of these enzymes is unfortunately genetically based, and it is not possible to infer anything about functional similarity of cytochrome P_{450} isoforms that have similar nomenclatures. For example, the drug specificity and the regulation of the cytochrome isoforms called 2C9 and 2C19 are very different, whereas both CYP1A2 and CYP2D6 are involved in the metabolism of imipramine.

Although more than 20 cytochrome P_{450} isoforms have been identified in human liver and intestine, only a few of these are importantly involved in drug metabolism. The distinctive characteristics of six of the most clinically relevant isoforms are summarized in Table 378-1.

It is notable that the only cytochrome P_{450} isoform induced by tobacco is CYP1A2, and that this is the primary isoform responsible for the metabolism of theophylline. One would expect that other drugs, such as imipramine, that have cytochrome P_{450} 1A2 as a dominant metabolic route, would be affected by smoking in the same way that we know theophylline is, and that drugs that decrease theophylline metabolism, such as ciprofloxacin and fluvoxamine, would also decrease imipramine metabolism.

Similarly, it is notable that CYP2C9, CYP2D6, and CYP2C19 exhibit genetic polymorphism. This has important clinical consequences. For example, poor metabolizers of CYP2C9 are likely to have a longer half-life for *S*-warfarin, the active enantiomer of this racemic drug. As a result, one might expect those individuals to take longer to reach steady state, and that greater plasma concentrations and drug effects will be seen in this group. Similarly, the large number of poor metabolizers of CYP2C19 in the Asian population are more likely to experience prolonged sedation as the result of persistent high concentrations of diazepam after routine dosing. Lastly, it is important that poor metabolizers may not make an active metabolite that contributes significantly to a drug's effect.

An example of an important clinical consequence of the absence of metabolism of a drug is the case of codeine. The analgesic, sedative, and pupillary effects of codeine are largely brought about by the active metabolites morphine and morphine glucuronide. As a result, individuals who cannot carry out the cytochrome P_{450} 2D6–mediated conversion of codeine to morphine experience notably lower opiate effects. Patients taking codeine and fluoxetine who report little analgesic effect of the opiate are likely not malingerers, but people in whom no morphine results from codeine administration.

The effects of alcohol on cytochrome P_{450} 2E1 are important because they result in an increased synthesis of the hepatotoxic metabolite of acetaminophen *N-acetyl paraquinone,* and this may in part explain the sensitivity of regular consumers of alcohol to acetaminophen-induced hepatic injury. Significant amounts of cytochrome P_{450} 3A in the intestine contribute to the metabolism of drugs, such as cyclosporine, that demonstrate a large first-pass effect. The great variability in activity of this isoform contributes to the difficulty in predicting cyclosporine pharmacokinetics in a given patient.

Understanding the principal cytochrome P_{450} isoform(s) involved in a drug's metabolism can help anticipate which other drugs might inhibit or increase a drug's metabolism. Table 378-2 summarizes clinically important drugs that are metabolized by cytochrome P_{450} isoforms and describes commonly prescribed inhibitors and inducers of each isoform. One can use this table to identify likely pharmacologic inducers and inhibitors of an individual drug of concern.

For example, this table can be used to predict the slowing of imipramine metabolism by inhibitors of theophylline metabolism, such as the serotonin reuptake inhibitor fluvoxamine, and that smokers would experience faster metabolism of imipramine. Although this approach cannot predict the quantitative changes that occur in an individual patient, it does provide a means to focus upon likely interactions.

As a result of the metabolism of *S*-warfarin by cytochrome P_{450} 2C9, fluconazole or isoniazid inhibits *S*-warfarin's metabolism. Such interactions with warfarin have the potential to be fatal and should be carefully monitored. Among substrates of cytochrome P_{450} 2C9, phenytoin is a special case. It is metabolized primarily by the cytochrome P_{450} isoforms 2C9 and 2C19. Therefore potent inhibitors of cytochrome P_{450} 2C9, such as fluconazole or ticlopidine, may have pronounced inhibitory effects on phenytoin disposition in poor metabolizers who do not have cytochrome P_{450} 2C19 activity. The doses of phenytoin in routine therapeutic use easily saturate these metabolic routes; as a result the drug exhibits nonlinear pharmacokinetics that may result in dramatic increases in concentration when a small increase in dose occurs. These may be particularly pronounced in genetically poor metabolizers of either cytochrome P_{450} 2C9 or cytochrome P_{450} 2C19.

Another example is the effect of fluoxetine, paroxetine, and quinidine in decreasing the metabolism and thus increasing the half-life of desipramine, clomipramine, or amitriptylline. One would expect that patients who experience little analgesia with codeine might be poor metabolizers of cytochrome P_{450} 2D6 and might experience adverse effects as a result of prolonged high concentrations of thioridazine, haloperidol, or most of the prescribed β-blockers (excluding atenolol, which undergoes purely renal elimination).

In the case of drugs metabolized by cytochrome P_{450} 2E1, isoniazid predisposes to acetaminophen toxicity by the same mechanism that alcohol does: increased activity of the enzyme. Disulfiram (Antabuse) slows both acetaminophen and chlorzoxazone (Parafon Forte, Paraflex) metabolism.

The sedative hypnotic *triazolam* is metabolized by CYP3A, and rifampin, which induces its metabolism, renders the drug ineffective, whereas ketoconazole decreases metabolism, resulting in prolonged

Table 378-2 Commonly used drugs that are substrates, inhibitors, and inducers of human cytochrome P_{450} isoforms

1A2	2C19	2C9	2D6	2E1	3A4
Substrates					
Theophylline	Phenytoin	S-Warfarin	Codeine	Acetaminophen	Alprazolam
					Triazolam
Imipramine	Diazepam	Phenytoin	Amitriptyline	Chlorzoxazone	Cyclosporine
			Desipramine		
Propranolol	Imipramine	Tamoxifen	Imipramine	Ethanol	FK-506
	Clomipramine				
Clozapine	Amitriptyline	Tolbutamide	Metoprolol		Terfenadine
			Timolol		Astemizole
	Propranolol	Diclofenac	Carvedilol		Cisapride
		Ibuprofen			Indinavir
	Lansoprazole	Naproxen	Ondansetron		Ritonavir
	Omeprazole				Saquinavir
	Pantoprazole	Losartan	Propafenone		Diltiazem
					Felodipine
			Haloperidol		Nifedipine
			Risperidone		Lovastatin
Inhibitors					
Cimetidine	Fluoxetine	Fluconazole	Amiodarone	Disulfiram	Erythromycin
Ciprofloxacin	Omeprazole	Isoniazid	Fluoxetine		Clarithromycin
Fluvoxamine	Ticlopidine		Paroxetine		Itraconazole
Ofloxacin			Quinidine		Ketoconazole
			Ticlopidine		Cimetidine
					Indinavir
Inducers					
Tobacco	Barbiturates	Rifampin		Ethanol	Rifampin
	Carbamazepine	Prednisone		Isoniazid	Phenytoin
	Norethindrone				Carbamazepine
	Rifampin				Glucocorticoids
					Barbiturates

sedation in affected patients. Other short-acting benzodiazepines such as midazolam and alprazolam, nonsedating antihistamines such as terfenadine and astemizole, and other drugs such as cyclosporine or FK-506 that have cytochrome P_{450} 3A as their dominant metabolic route are affected in the same way by rifampin or ketoconazole.

Some drugs do not have a single dominant route of metabolism. For example, propranolol is metabolized by at least three different cytochrome P_{450} isoforms: CYP1A2, CYP2C19, and CYP2D6. As a result, large changes in any one of these enzymes have little effect on propranolol pharmacokinetics, and it is only when multiple pathways are affected (e.g., in cirrhosis) that clinically relevant changes result.

Interactions Caused by Protein Binding

Only drug that is not bound to protein can exert a pharmacologic effect. Thus many have thought that the displacement of bound drug from binding sites on albumin or α_1-acid glycoprotein may result in increased efficacy or toxicity. In fact, this is nearly always a transient and clinically insignificant phenomenon, because any change in the free concentration of a drug is followed by rapid redistribution and an adjustment in clearance by metabolism, secretion, or renal filtration that quickly results in a new equilibrium. Consequently, protein displacement is likely to be clinically important only if a drug has a small volume of distribution, rapid onset of action, and a narrow therapeutic index. Many of the interactions previously attributed to protein displacement were likely a result of a simultaneous decrease in clearance by inhibition of metabolism or renal secretion.

Renal Interactions

Nearly all renal interactions that occur between the water-soluble drugs eliminated by the kidney occur as the result of competition for the renal tubular transport system. They become clinically important only when a significant proportion of renal elimination occurs via secretion as opposed to glomerular filtration. This interaction can be used for therapeutic benefit, as it is when probenicid is used to block the tubular secretion of penicillin in order to achieve enhanced therapeutic effect. Predictably, it can also have adverse consequences, as when trimethoprim or cimetidine blocks the renal clearance of amantadine, leading to sedation, or when salicylates reduce methotrexate elimination, resulting in hematologic toxicity.

Pharmacodynamic Interactions

Pharmacodynamic interactions are simple to anticipate if one is aware of the mechanism responsible for a drug's effect. One might anticipate that dopamine antagonists such as haloperidol or other antipsychotic agents will decrease the effect of L-DOPA or dopamine itself via competition at dopamine receptors. Similarly, it is not surprising that β-antagonists blunt the effects of albuterol or salmeterol and significantly complicate the treatment of asthma with these drugs, or of congestive heart failure with dopamine and dobutamine. Other examples of understood direct receptor–based interactions include the antagonism of clonidine's antihypertensive effect by tricyclic antidepressant via α_2-blockade in the brain, and increased anticholinergic effects brought about by combining any of the antihistamines, antinauseants, neuroleptics, or antidepressants known to share with atropine the ability to block cholinergic receptors.

Pharmacodynamic interactions may be the result of independent mechanisms that result in a similar effect. For example, a loop diuretic may (via potassium depletion) worsen electrocardiac QT prolongation brought about by quinidine or thioridazine. Likewise, dangerous hyperkalemia may result from the coprescription of a potassium-sparing diuretic with an angiotensin-converting enzyme inhibitor or angiotensin receptor blocker.

PRINCIPLES OF MANAGEMENT

How does one keep track of or anticipate unwanted drug interactions? A high index of suspicion is appropriate when any two drugs are prescribed, and it is very important to recall that patients may keep pharmaceuticals long after the original prescription, so that any new drug prescribed should be considered a possible interactor wth others the patient may have been prescribed in the past. Perhaps the most important principle for any health care professional in this regard is that of the personal formulary: know well the drugs you use. If the drug is highly metabolized in the liver, it may help to identify the principal enzyme involved. Know the potential interactions and side effects and have an organized system to evaluate any novel drug for its admission onto your formulary.

Drug interactions that occur with agents that have a narrow therapeutic index have a greater potential to cause harm than do drugs whose therapeutic index is wide. Similar problems are more likely to occur when the drug interaction involves a compound that demonstrates nonlinear pharmacokinetics (wherein dose is not proportional to serum concentration when metabolism becomes saturated), such as phenytoin. Physicians should familiarize themselves with these drugs and, if one is prescribed, take extra care to monitor the patient's medication regimen and response to therapy.

The following are principles that may help physicians approach the problem of drug-drug interactions at the clinical level. They are offered to assist the physician in minimizing the likelihood of prescribing drug combinations that have the potential to precipitate unwanted drug effects.

Identify Patient Risk Factors

In older patients the influence of age on the absorption, distribution, metabolism, and excretion of drugs must be considered a major risk factor. In addition, patients who have impaired renal or hepatic function and disorders such as achlorhydria, diabetes, or cardiovascular disease are at greater risk for undesirable drug interactions. Patients who smoke, use alcohol, or who have dietary deficiencies handle drugs differently, and they should be identified as higher-risk patients.

Take a Thorough Drug History and Maintain Complete Medication Records

A complete and up-to-date record of both prescription and nonprescription drugs must be taken, maintained, and utilized. Many avoidable interactions have occurred because the prescribing physician was unaware of medications prescribed by another physician or because the patient used nonprescription medications that were not documented in the patient's records. Patients may be confused when a drug is dispensed in both its brand and generic names, thus leading some patients to believe they are different drugs that should both be taken. Studies show that at least 30% of all elderly patients receive drugs from more than one prescriber. Nearly all pharmacies maintain computerized medication profiles for their patients. Physicians should recommend that patients obtain all of their prescription and nonprescription medications from one pharmacy and make sure that this pharmacy maintains and uses these records in filling prescriptions. The pharmacist may be in the best position to detect potential drug-related problems and to inform the prescriber(s) regarding severity of the situation.

Be Knowledgeable About the Actions of the Drugs Being Prescribed

Physicians should be familiar with the primary and secondary pharmacologic properties of the drugs they prescribe. Drug-drug interactions are likely to be clinically significant if they lead to substantial changes in drug pharmacokinetics or pharmacodynamics, or if they involve agents that have a narrow therapeutic-toxic ratio. It is helpful to know whether the prescribed drugs are metabolized by the cytochrome P_{450} systems in the liver, as is the case with warfarin, quinidine, phenytoin, or cyclosporine, or whether the drugs are excreted unchanged primarily by the kidney. It is also helpful to be familiar with the drugs that have the potential to interfere with the hepatic metabolism of other drugs such as cimetidine and the barbiturates.

Consider Therapeutic Alternatives

Many documented drug interactions are not absolute contraindications, and two interacting drugs may continue to be coprescribed if the patient is properly monitored and dosage adjustment is made to compensate for the altered response. However, in situations in which another agent with similar therapeutic properties and less risk of interaction is available, it should be considered for use.

Avoid Complex Therapeutic Regimens Whenever Possible

The likelihood of drug interactions increases as the number of drugs taken increases. Whenever a new drug is added to the patient's therapeutic regimen, the physician should review the medication profile to determine whether another drug can be discontinued. An important principle is that the best way to treat an adverse effect of one drug is *not* to add another. In addition, the use of medications or dosage regimens that permit less frequent administration may help avoid interactions that result from an alteration of absorption. Dosing schedules should be designed to be as simple as possible to maximize compliance.

Educate the Patient

Too often patients know very little about their illnesses, let alone the benefits and problems that may result from their drug therapy. It has been well documented that patients who understand this information are more likely to be compliant with their medications and are more likely to identify drug-induced side effects. Patients should be encouraged to be aggressive health care consumers, to ask questions about their medications, and to report any unusual or unexpected responses.

Monitor Therapy

All patients should be closely monitored not only for the risk of drug-induced problems occurring from drug interactions, but also for noncompliance and for adverse effects occurring from the use of individual agents. A low index of suspicion on the part of the prescriber has been cited as one reason why drug interactions are not commonly documented in clinical practice. New symptoms should be suspected as being drug-related until that possibility is excluded. In particular, symptoms in the elderly such as drowsiness, confusion, insomnia, forgetfulness, or irritability are often attributed to the aging process when, in fact, they may be the result of a drug interaction and can be prevented through dosage adjustment or change in the therapeutic regimen. The identification of drug-induced illnesses should be a common occurrence in a physician's daily practice.

Individualize Therapy

It is well recognized that patients' responses to the same drug can vary widely. With many agents it is difficult to predict drug response when a drug is used alone; the challenge is much greater when drugs are used in combination.

Identify and Utilize Proper Resources for Information

It is impossible for prescribing physicians to keep current with the entire range of information dealing with drug interactions. The personal formulary is an important means of staying up to date on specific medications that a physician prescribes, but it is also necessary to have a reference source available. In addition to the commonly used *United States Pharmacopeia Drug Index* and *Physicians Desk Reference,* several useful references are now available in computer CD-ROM format. These are useful as a source of *possible* drug interactions and of those that have been reported, but they cannot substitute for a physician's judgment in ascertaining the likelihood of a given interaction in a specific patient. Many patients use these sources extensively, and at least one such reference source should be easily available to all practitioners. It is also highly recommended that health care professionals utilize the expertise of a clinical pharmacologist or pharmacist who is knowledgeable in the area of drug interactions; these individuals can provide excellent consultation and information to the physician and patient alike.

BIBLIOGRAPHY

Bajpai M et al: Role of S-mephenytoin hydroxylase in the metabolism of phenytoin, *Pharm Res* 11:S348, 1994.

Bates DW et al: Incidence of adverse drug events and potential adverse drug events: implications for prevention: ADE Prevention Study Group, *JAMA* 274:29-34, 1995.

Beard K: Adverse drug reactions as a cause of hospital admissions in the aged, *Drugs Aging* 2:298-325, 1992.

Black DJ et al: A metabolically based drug interaction between fluconazole and warfarin: in vivo studies, *Drug Metab Dispo* 24:422-428, 1996.

Cadle RM et al: Fluconazole-induced symptomatic phenytoin toxicity, *Ann Pharmacother* 28:191-194, 1994.

Flockhart DA: Drug interactions and the cytochrome P_{450} system: the role of cytochrome P_{450} 2C19, *Clin Pharmacokinet* 29:45-52, 1995.

Ketter TA et al: The emerging role of cytochrome P_{450} in psychopharmacology, *J Clin Psychopharm* 15:387-398, 1995.

May DG: Genetic differences in drug disposition, *J Clin Pharmacol* 34:881-897, 1994.

Peck CC, Temple R, Collins JM: Understanding consequences of concurrent therapies, *JAMA* 269:1550-1552, 1993.

Woosley RL et al: Mechanism of cardiotoxicity of terfenadine, *JAMA* 269:403-409, 1993.

Wright JM: Drug interactions. In Melmon KL et al, editors: *Clinical pharmacology*, New York, 1992, McGraw-Hill, pp. 1012-1021.

APPENDIX

ADULT IMMUNIZATION OVERVIEW*

Vaccines and toxoids recommended for adults, by age groups,
United States

AGE		VACCINE/TOXOID					
	Influenza	Pneumococcal	Measles	Mumps	Rubella	Varicella	Td[1]
18-24			X	X	X	X	X
25-64			X[2]	X	X[3]	X	X
65+	X	X				X	X

[1]Td = Tetanus and diphtheria toxoids, adsorbed (for adult use), which is a combined preparation containing <2 flocculation units of diphtheria toxoid.
[2]One dose for all persons born in 1957 or later, two doses for health care workers, college students, travelers born in 1957 or later.
[3]Those born after 1956.

Influenza Vaccine (7/16/97)

Indications:
a. Adults 65 years of age and older.
b. Adults of any age with chronic cardiovascular or pulmonary disorders, including asthma.
c. Residents of nursing homes or other facilities for patients with chronic medical conditions.
d. Adults with chronic metabolic diseases (including diabetes), renal dysfunction, anemia, immunosuppressive or immunodeficiency disorders, which required regular medical follow-up or hospitalization in the past year.
e. Groups, including household members and care givers, who can transmit influenza to persons at high risk.
Dose: 0.5 ml intramuscular (IM) each fall.
Contraindications: Anaphylactic allergy to eggs.

Tetanus and Diphtheria Toxoids Combined (Td) (7/16/97)

Indications: All adults.
Dose: 0.5 intramuscular (IM). Two doses 4-6 weeks apart, third dose 6-12 months after the second. No need to repeat doses if the schedule is interrupted.
Contraindications: Neurologic or severe hypersensitivity reaction to prior dose.
Wound Management:
Patients with three or more previous tetanus toxoid doses:
a. Give Td for clean, minor wounds only if more than 10 years since last dose.
b. For other wounds, give Td if over 5 years since last dose.
Patients with less than 3 or unknown number of prior tetanus toxoid doses:
a. Give Td for clean, minor wounds.
b. Give Td and TG (tetanus immune globulin) for other wounds.

Pneumococcal Vaccine (7/16/97)

Indications:
a. Adults 65 years of age and older.
b. Adults of any age with significant chronic cardiovascular or pulmonary disorders, including asthma.
c. Adults of any age with splenic dysfunction, asplenia, Hodgkin's disease, multiple myeloma, cirrhosis, alcoholism, renal failure, CSF leaks, immunosuppressive conditions.
d. Persons with functional or anatomic asplenia, transplant patients, patients with chronic kidney disease, immunosuppressed or immunodefi-

cient persons, and others at highest risk of fatal infection 5 years after prior dose.
Dose: 0.5 ml intramuscular (IM) or subcutaneous (SC).
Contraindications: Allergy to vaccine components or to thimerosol; people who have ITP.
Comments: If elective splenectomy or immunosuppressive therapy is planned, give vaccine 2 weeks ahead, if possible.

Measles and Mumps Vaccines† (7/16/97)

Indications:
Primary Schedule
a. Adults born after 1956 without written documentation of immunization on or after the first birthday.
b. Health care personnel born since 1956 who are at risk of exposure to patients with measles should have documentation of two doses of vaccine on or after the first birthday or of measles seropositivity.
c. HIV-infected persons.
d. Travelers to foreign countries.
e. Persons entering college.
Dose: 0.5 ml subcutaneous (SC). At least one dose on or after first birthday. (Two doses if in college, in health care profession or traveling to a foreign country, with second dose at least 1 month after the first).
Contraindications:
a. Immunosuppressive therapy or immunodeficiency including HIV-infected persons with severe immunosuppression.
b. Anaphylactic allergy to eggs or neomycin.
c. Pregnancy.
d. Immune globulin preparation or blood/blood product received in preceding 3-11 months.
†These vaccines can be given in the combined form measles-mumps-rubella (MMR). Persons already immune to one or more components can still receive MMR.

Rubella Vaccine‡ (7/16/97)

Indications:
Primary Schedule
a. Adults (especially women) without written documentation of immunization on or after the first birthday or of seropositivity.
b. Male and female health care personnel who are at risk of exposure to patients with rubella and who may have contact with pregnant patients should have at least one dose of vaccine on or after the first birthday.
Dose: 0.5 ml subcutaneous (SC).
Contraindications:
a. Immunosuppressive therapy or immunodeficiency including HIV-infected persons with severe immunosuppression.
b. Pregnancy.
c. Immune globulin preparation or blood/blood product received in preceding 3-11 months.
Women should avoid pregnancy for 3 months after immunization.
‡These vaccines can be given in the combined form measles-mumps-rubella (MMR). Persons already immune to one or more components can still receive MMR.

Hepatitis A Vaccine (7/16/97)

Indications:
a. Persons traveling to or working in countries with high or intermediate endemicity of infection.
b. Men who have sex with men.
c. Drug users.
d. Persons who work with HAV-infected primates or with HAV in a research laboratory setting.
e. Persons with chronic liver disease.
f. Persons with clotting factor disorders.
g. Foodhandlers, where health authorities or private employers determine vaccination to be cost effective.
HAVRIX: Adults 18 years of age and older: Two doses, separated by 6-12 months.

---

*Adapted from the recommendations of the Advisory Committee on Immunization Practices (ACIP), 7/16/97. Foreign travel and less commonly used vaccines such as typhoid, rabies, and meningococcal are not included.
Data from Centers for Disease Control and Prevention: http://www.cdc.gov/nip/adult.htm

VAQTA: Adults 17 years of age and older: Two doses, separated by 6 months.

Dose: 1.0 ml intramuscular (IM).

Contraindications: A history of hypersensitivity to alum or the preservative 2-phenoxyethanol. The safety of hepatitis A vaccine during pregnancy has not been determined, though the theoretical risk to the developing fetus is expected to be low. The risk of vaccination should be weighed against the risk of hepatitis A in women who may be at high risk of exposure to HAV.

Hepatitis B Vaccine (7/16/97)

Indications:

a. Persons with occupational risk of exposure to blood or blood-contaminated body fluids.

b. Clients and staff of institutions for the developmentally disabled.

c. Hemodialysis patients.

d. Recipients of clotting-factor concentrates.

e. Household contacts and sex partners of HBV carriers.

f. Adoptees from countries where HBV infection is endemic.

g. Certain international travelers.

h. Injecting drug users.

i. Sexually active homosexual and bisexual men.

j. Sexually active heterosexual men and women with multiple sex partners or recent episode of a sexually transmitted disease.

k. Inmates of long-term correctional facilities.

l. All adolescents 11-12 years of age.

Three doses: first two 1 month apart, third dose 6 months after first.

No need to start series over if schedule interrupted. Can start series with one manufacturer's vaccine and finish with another.

Dose (Adult): 1.0 ml intramuscular (IM).

Booster: Need unclear. None presently recommended.

Contraindications: Anaphylactic allergy to yeast.

a. Persons with serologic markers of prior or continuing hepatitis B infection (carriage) do not need immunization.

b. For hemodialysis patients and other immunodeficient or immunosuppressed patients, vaccine dosage is doubled or special preparation is used.

c. Pregnant women should be sero-screened for HbsAg, and if positive, their infants should be given postexposure prophylaxis.

d. Postexposure prophylaxis: consult ACIP recommendations, local health department, or the immunization program.

Poliovirus Vaccine (IPV and OPV) (7/16/97)

IPV—Inactivated vaccine
OPV—Oral (live) vaccine

Indications:

Primary Schedule

a. Health care workers and laboratory workers who may be in close contact with patients excreting wild poliovirus or who handle specimens from such patients.

b. Members of community with current disease caused by wild polio viruses.

c. Travelers to developing countries.

Dose: 0.5 ml subcutaneous (SC).

Unimmunized adults: IPV—two doses at 4-8 week intervals, third dose 6-12 months after second (can be as soon as 2 months).

Partially immunized adults: Complete primary series with vaccine. IPV schedule shown above. OPV schedule is two doses 6-8 weeks apart and third dose 6-12 months after second (can be given as early as 6-8 weeks after second if need urgently). No need to repeat doses if schedule is interrupted.

Booster: OPV—none. IPV—need unclear, possibly one dose every 5 years.

Contraindications:

IPV

a. Pregnancy

b. Anaphylactic allergy to neomycin or streptomycin.

OPV

a. Vaccine recipient or household contact is immunodeficient or immunosuppressed (including HIV infection).

b. Pregnancy is relative contraindication; OPV may be used if immediate protection is needed.

c. Anaphylactic allergy to neomycin or streptomycin.

In episode of potential exposure to wild poliovirus, adults who had only three doses of OPV previously may be given one more dose.

Varicella Vaccine (7/16/97)

Indications:

a. Adults of any age without a reliable history of varicella disease or vaccination, or who are seronegative for varicella.

b. All susceptible health care workers.

c. Susceptible family contacts of immunocompromised persons.

d. Susceptible persons in the following groups who are at high risk for exposure:

• Persons who live or work in environments in which transmission of VZV is likely (e.g., teachers of young children, day care employees) or can occur (e.g., college students, military personnel)

• Nonpregnant women of childbearing age

• International travelers

Two doses separated by 4-8 weeks. If more than 8 weeks elapse following the first dose, the second dose can be administered without restarting the schedule.

Dose: 0.5 ml subcutaneous (SC).

Contraindications:

a. Anaphylactic allergy to gelatin or neomycin.

b. Immunosuppressive therapy or immunodeficiency (including HIV infection).

c. Family history of congenital or hereditary immunodeficiency in first-degree relatives, unless the immune competence of the potential vaccine recipient has been clinically substantiated or verified by a laboratory.

d. Pregnancy.

e. Immune globulin preparation or blood/blood product received in preceding 5 months.

Women should be asked if they are pregnant before receiving varicella vaccine, and are advised to avoid pregnancy for 1 month following each dose of vaccine.

INDEX

A

A-band, 39
A-I Milano apolipoprotein, 1897
A wave
  atrial septal defect, 281
  hypertrophic cardiomyopathy, 266
  jugular venous pulse, 66, 69
  mitral regurgitation, 250-251
  primary pulmonary hypertension, 294
  pulmonic stenosis, 288
  tricuspid stenosis, 255
AA amyloidosis, 1283
Abdomen
  aortic aneurysm, 300
  arteriography, 2033-2034
  heart failure, 165
  imaging studies
    gallstones, 2224
    Hodgkin's disease, 694
    pancreatic disease, 2145-2147
    ultrasound, 2033
  intestinal obstruction, 2077-2079
    abdominal pain, 2032
    colon cancer, 2085
    cystic fibrosis, 2246
    Meckel's diverticulum, 2089
    mesenteric hernia, 2251
    radiography, 2032
    small intestinal malignancies, 2081
  intraabdominal catastrophe, 1476
  intraabdominal disease, 1396-1402
    actinomycosis, 1665
    anaerobic bacteria, 1617-1618
    clostridial, 1575
    diagnosis, 1399-1400
    enterococcal infection, 1562
    gram-negative bacteremia, 1446
    intraperitoneal abscess, 1398
    lymphadenopathy, 598-599
    pancreatic abscess, 366, 1399
    pleural effusion, 508
    primary intraperitoneal infection, 1396
    retroperitoneal abscess, 1398
    secondary intraperitoneal infection,
      1396-1398
    splenic abscess, 1398-1399
    treatment, 1400-1402
  peritonitis, 2079-2080, 2247-2249
    abdominal evaluation, 2032
    acquired immunodeficiency syndrome, 1476
    anaerobic bacteria, 1617
    bile, 2249
    candidal, 1661
    dialysis-related, 791
    paralytic ileus, 2078
    primary, 1396
    systemic lupus erythematosus, 1214
  radionuclide studies
    intraabdominal abscess, 1400
    intraabdominal infection, 1399
Abdominal angina, 2087
Abdominal aorta, 299
  aneurysm, 300, 2250
  infection, 1398
Abdominal bruit, 321
Abdominal distention
  celiac disease, 2063
  intestinal obstruction, 2077

Abdominal distention—cont'd
  lactase deficiency, 2068
  ulcerative colitis, 2073
Abdominal film
  abdominal pain, 2032
  acute pancreatitis, 2236
  chronic pancreatitis, 2240
  intestinal diseases, 2007
  intestinal obstruction, 2078
  pancreatic disease, 2146
  pyogenic liver abscess, 2209
Abdominal mass
  abdominal aortic aneurysm, 300
  Castleman's disease, 2252
  focal nodular hyperplasia, 2216
  hypertrophic pyloric stenosis, 2044
  renal cell carcinoma, 898
  retroperitoneal fibrosis, 2250
Abdominal pain, 2030-2035
  abscess
    amebic, 2210
    pyogenic liver, 2209
    splenic, 1399
  acute cholecystitis, 2227
  acute intermittent porphyria, 1926
  amebiasis, 1682
  autosomal dominant polycystic kidney disease,
    873
  Budd-Chiari syndrome, 2208
  cancer
    carcinoid tumor of small bowel, 2082
    colon, 2085
    gastric, 2046
    intrahepatic cholangiocarcinoma, 2214
    pancreatic, 2242
    peritoneal mesothelioma, 2249
    pheochromocytoma, 1829
    renal cell carcinoma, 898
  cirrhosis, 2197
  classification, causes, and pathophysiology,
    2030-2031
  Crohn's disease, 2069
  diverticulosis, 2090
  eosinophilic enteritis, 2067
  epidemic pleurodynia, 1489
  gallbladder, 2233
  gallstones, 2225-2226
  giant peristaltic contractions, 1979-1980
  hepatitis
    alcoholic, 2197
    chronic, 2180
  human immunodeficiency virus, 1476
  intestinal obstruction, 2077
  irritable bowel syndrome, 2056
  laboratory tests, 2032
  lactase deficiency, 2068
  Lassa fever, 1510
  liver biopsy complication, 2141
  malabsorption, 2057
  mesenteric ischemia, 2087
  mesenteric panniculitis, 2251
  pancreatitis
    acute, 2234
    chronic, 2238
  patient evaluation, 2031-2032
  peritoneal mesenteric and omental diseases,
    2248
  peritonitis, 1397-1398
  post ischemic colon, 2088

Abdominal pain—cont'd
  postcoarctation syndrome, 287
  radiography, 2032-2033
  Rocky Mountain spotted fever, 1543
  Salmonella, 1599
  shigellosis, 1602-1603
  systemic lupus erythematosus, 1215
  systemic sclerosis, 1229
  thrombotic thrombocytopenic purpura, 615
  toxic megacolon, 2076
  tropical sprue, 2065
Abdominal skin reflex, 964
Abducens nerve palsy, 1062
Aberrant right subclavian artery, 291
Abetalipoproteinemia, 1897
  malabsorption, 2067
  vitamin A deficiency, 2105
  vitamin E deficiency, 2106
Ablative procedures
  prostate cancer, 719
  rotational ablation device, 118-119
  sudden death survivors, 190
  ventricular tachycardia, 140
Abnormal, defined, 6
Abnormal eye movements, 1062-1063
Abnormal hematocrit, 586-590
ABO compatibility testing, 573
Abortion
  chromosome abnormality, 1728
  inflammatory bowel disease, 2278
  lupus inhibitor, 629
  relapsing fever, 1645
  sickle cell disease, 659
Abortive poliomyelitis, 1487
Abscess
  amebiasis, 1682
  bacterial prostatitis, 1462
  brain, 1413-1416
    Acanthamoeba, 1684
    acquired immunodeficiency syndrome,
      1414
    acute meningitis, 1407
    amebic, 1682
    anaerobic bacteria, 1617
    antibiotic therapy, 1415-1416
    Bacteroides, 1414
    sinusitis, 2309
    supratentorial, 1416
  clostridial, 1575
  compromised host, 1388
  Crohn's disease, 2069, 2072
  echinococcal, 2111-2212
  epidural, 1013
    computed tomography, 920
    intracranial, 1418
    sinusitis, 2309
    spinal, 1418-1419
  facial pain, 962
  fever of unknown origin, 1376
  intraperitoneal, 1398
  liver, 2209-2210
  lung
    anaerobic bacteria, 1617
    nephritis associated with, 844
  nontuberculous mycobacterial infection,
    1639
  osteomyelitis, 1433
  pancreatic, 366, 1399
  peritonsillar, 1393, 1617, 2306

2317

Abscess—cont'd
  renal
    imaging studies, 754-755
    nephritis associated with visceral abscess,
      844
  retroperitoneal, 1398, 2250
  septal, 2308
  spinal, 1418
  splenic, 1398-1399
  subdural, 2309
  subphrenic, 508
  surgical drainage, 1621
  tuboovarian
    anaerobic bacteria, 1618
    clostridial, 1575
  ulcerative colitis, 2072, 2073, Plate X-5
  urinary tract infection, 1456
  visceral, 844
Absence seizure, 979
Absidia, 1659
Absolute lymphocytosis, 592
Absorption
  cholesterol, 1884
  intestinal, 1985-1989, 2057
  iron, 641
  magnesium, 1939, 1940
  malabsorption, 2056-2068
    abetalipoproteinemia, 2067
    bacterial overgrowth, 2060-2062
    carbohydrate intolerance, 2067-2068
    carbohydrates, 1987
    celiac sprue, 2062-2063
    chronic diarrhea, 2051-2052
    chronic pancreatitis, 2145, 2239
    clinical features, 2057-2058
    congenital glucose-galactose, 878
    Crohn's disease, 270, 2069
    cystic fibrosis, 2246
    digestion process, 2056-2057
    eosinophilic enteritis, 2067
    eosinophilic gastroenteritis, 2066-2067
    hypogammaglobulinemia, 2066
    intestinal lymphangiectasia, 2067
    laboratory findings, 2058-2060
    magnesium, 1940
    multiple jejunal diverticulosis, 2089
    negative phosphate balance, 1935
    pancreatic and hepatobiliary diseases, 2062
    radiation enteropathy, 2065-2066
    serum electrolytes, 2005
    short bowel syndrome, 2066
    small intestinal tumors, 2081
    stool examination, 2006
    tests for, 2006-2007
    tropical sprue, 2065
    vitamin B_{12} deficiency, 648
    vitamin K deficiency, 607, 626
    weight loss, 1749
    Whipple's disease, 2064-2065
Abulia, 1032
Abuse
  child, 2269
  elderly, 4
  substance, 2293-2297
    alcohol, 2294-2296
    candidiasis, 1661
    cellulitis, 1420
    cocaine, 2296-2297
    hepatitis A virus infection, 2173
    hepatitis B virus infection, 2174
    impotence, 1761
    infective endocarditis, 226, 229-230
    mood disorders, 1036
    narcotics, 2297
    personality disorders, 1039
    renal disease, 853
    tetanus risk, 1572
    tobacco, 2296
    tricuspid regurgitation, 256
    weight loss, 1749
  ABVD regimen, 694-695

Academic detailing, 25
Acalculous cholecystitis, 2227
Acanthamoeba, 1683-1684
Acanthocyte, 662, 667
Acanthocytosis, 2067
Acanthosis, 1302, 2016
Acanthosis nigricans, 1316, Plate VII-17
  congenital total lipodystrophy, 1900
  diabetic patient, 1323
  gastric cancer, 2046
  insulin resistance, 1862
  lipodystrophy, 1901
Acanthosis palmaris, 1319
Acarbose, 1858
Accelerated acute rejection of kidney, 794
Accelerated atherosclerosis in nephrotic
    syndrome, 766
Accelerated atrioventricular junctional rhythm,
    144
Accelerated idioventricular rhythm, 149, 150,
    223
Accelerated junctional rhythm, 144
Accelerated transplant coronary artery disease,
    341
Accessory pathway, 90
Accessory pathway reentry tachycardia, 134,
    142-143, 145
Accupril; *see* Quinapril
Acebutolol
  hypertension, 325
  properties, 203
Acetaldehyde, 2194-2195
Acetaminophen, 1259-1260
  analgesic-associated nephropathy, 870-871,
    890
  chronic pancreatitis, 2240
  glucose-6-phosphate dehydrogenase
    deficiency, 664
  hepatic injury, 2191
  human cytochrome P450 isoforms, 2312
  influenza, 1492
  interference with oral anticoagulants, 636
  osteoarthritis, 1268
  poisoning, 2188-2190
Acetanilid, 663
Acetate
  cholesterol metabolism, 1884
  total parenteral nutrition formula, 2117
Acetazolamide
  cystine stones, 804
  glaucoma, 2302
  inhibitor of carbonic anhydrase, 835
  normotensive renal potassium wasting, 828
Acetoacetate, 2122
  cholesterol metabolism, 1884
Acetoacetic acid, 743, 834
Acetohexamide
  diabetes mellitus, 1858
  hepatic injury, 2191
Acetohydroxamic acid, 804
Acetone, 743
Acetophenetidin, 664
Acetyl coenzyme A
  carbohydrate metabolism, 1851
  effects of fasting, 1852-1853
Acetylcholine, 56, 930
  parietal cell receptors, 1981, 1983
  peripheral chemoreceptor signal, 353
  peristalsis, 1977
  potassium channel, 59
  vasoactive effects on pulmonary circulation,
    363
Acetylcholine receptor antibody, 1157
Acetylcysteine, 2190
Acetylsalicylic acid
  acute erosive gastritis, 2041
  adult Still's disease, 1243
  analgesic-associated nephropathy, 870-871
  angina, 205, 207
  arterial thromboembolism, 639
  atrial fibrillation, 148, 640, 1088

Acetylsalicylic acid—cont'd
  decreased colon cancer risk, 2083
  glucose-6-phosphate dehydrogenase
    deficiency, 664
  hepatic injury, 2190
  increased frequency of bleeding, 605
  induction of anaphylaxis, 1193
  influenza, 1492
  interference with oral anticoagulants, 636
  ischemic heart disease, 200
  myocardial infarction, 212, 217
  non-Q wave myocardial infarction, 218
  pericardial heart disease, 278
  platelet aggregation studies, 570
  platelet cyclooxygenase and, 611
  during pregnancy, 2275
  prosthetic heart valve, 258, 640
  pulmonary parenchymal reactions, 476
  pulmonary toxicity, 479
  restenosis, 124
  rheumatic diseases, 1258
  rheumatic fever, 1257
  rheumatoid arthritis, 1207
  subacute thyroiditis, 1812
  superficial thrombophlebitis, 311
  thrombotic stroke, 1004
  unstable angina, 639
Achalasia, 2001, 2021-2022
Achievement tests, 903
Achilles tendinitis, 1197-1198, 1238
Achlorhydria
  acid secretory values, 2003
  pellagra, 2107
  Schilling test, 2060
Acid
  excretion in chronic renal failure, 779
  production, 834
  renal excretion, 739-741
Acid-base balance, 836-841
  chronic renal failure, 779
  hypocalcemia, 1930
  internal potassium balance, 825
  metabolic acidosis, 836-839
    acute renal failure, 772
    chronic renal failure, 779, 786
    glucose-6-phosphate dehydrogenase
      deficiency, 1881
    gram-negative bacteremia, 1449
    hyperkalemia, 832-833
    internal potassium balance, 825
    normotensive renal potassium wasting, 828
    obstructive uropathy, 886
    potassium and, 838-839
    respiratory compensation, 834
  metabolic alkalosis, 839-841
    changes in arterial pH, 353
    consequence of vomiting, 2028
    hepatic encephalopathy, 2163
    hypertensive renal potassium wasting, 828
    hypokalemia, 827, 829-830
    normotensive renal potassium wasting, 828
    portosystemic encephalopathy, 2160
    renal excretion of potassium, 741
  patient evaluation, 840, 841
  physiology, 834-836
  potassium balance disorders, 825-834
    external potassium balance, 825, 826
    hyperkalemia, 830-833
    hypokalemia, 826-830
    internal potassium balance, 825-826
  regulation by lung, 351
  renal acidification, 739-741
  renal response, respiratory acidosis
    acute respiratory failure, 412, 414, 416
    chronic obstructive pulmonary disease with
      acute respiratory failure, 417
    hyperkalemia, 831
    hyperphosphatemia, 1938
    mechanical ventilation, 416
    renal response, 835-836

Acid-base balance—cont'd
  respiratory alkalosis
    carbon dioxide partial pressure, 834
    gram-negative bacteremia, 1449
    hypokalemia, 827
    hypophosphatemia, 1936
    renal excretion of potassium, 741
    renal response, 835
  sodium balance disorders, 816-825
    cirrhosis, 818-820
    congestive heart failure, 817-818
    edematous states, 816-817
    extrarenal sodium depletion, 823
    idiopathic edema, 821
    nephrotic syndrome, 820-821
    salt-wasting states, 823
    sodium depletion of renal origin, 823-825
    use of diuretics, 821-823
  water balance disorders, 805-816
    hypernatremia, 813-816
    hyponatremia, 809-813
    principles of osmoregulation, 805-809
Acid-base nomogram, 836
Acid ceramidase deficiency, 1918
Acid-fast stain, 1371
  acute meningitis, 1408
  leprosy, 1650
  Mycobacterium avium complex, Plate VIII-36
  nocardiosis, 1665
Acid-hydrolase enzymes, 536
Acid lipase deficiency, 1919
Acid reflux, 2001
Acidemia
  blood pH, 834
  internal potassium balance, 825
  isovaleric, 1908
  precapillary pulmonary hypertension, 295
  propionic, 1908
Acidification, urinary, 739-741, 747
Acidosis, 834
  chronic renal failure, 779
  Fanconi's syndrome, 882
  galactosemia, 1883
  hypercalciuria, 798
  hyperventilation, 355
  hypocalcemia, 1930
  lactic
    anion gap acidosis, 836
    diabetes mellitus, 1866-1867
    gram-negative sepsis, 1450, 1452
    use of nucleoside analog, 1451
  metabolic, 836-839
    acute renal failure, 772
    chronic renal failure, 779, 786
    glucose-6-phosphate dehydrogenase
      deficiency, 1881
    gram-negative bacteremia, 1449
    hyperkalemia, 832-833
    internal potassium balance, 825
    normotensive renal potassium wasting, 828
    obstructive uropathy, 886
    potassium and, 838-839
    respiratory compensation, 834
  osteomalacia, 1953
  renal bone disease, 1961
  renal tubular
    Fanconi's syndrome, 882
    hypercalciuria, 798
    osteomalacia with, 1954, 1955
    renal magnesium wasting, 1940
    tests of renal acidification, 747
  respiratory
    acute respiratory failure, 412, 414, 416
    chronic obstructive pulmonary disease with
      acute respiratory failure, 417
    hyperkalemia, 831
    hyperphosphatemia, 1938
    mechanical ventilation, 416
    renal response, 835-836
  serum calcium, 1744
  VIPoma, 2245

Aciduria
  argininosuccinic, 1907
  methylmalonic, 1908
Acinar cell, 2131-2132
  injury in chronic pancreatitis, 2238
  pancreatic tumor, 2242
Acinetobacter
  antibiotic selection, 1347
  normal flora, 1368
Acinus, 360
  emphysema, 439
Acne, 1304-1306
  drug-induced, 1313, 1315
  folliculitis, 1420
  prolactin-secreting pituitary adenoma, 1786
Acne conglobata, 1305
Acne rosacea, 1305
Acne vulgaris, 1304-1306
Acoustic neuroma, 1070
  brainstem auditory evoked potential, 911
  neurofibromatosis, 1921
Acquired hepatocerebral degeneration, 1102
Acquired ichthyosis, 1316
Acquired immunodeficiency syndrome,
      1470-1479, 1533-1534
  acute meningitis, 1407
  adenopathy, 599
  aplastic anemia, 672
  autoimmune hemolytic anemia, 669
  biliary disease, 2202
  brain abscess, 1414
  carcinogenesis, 548
  cardiovascular involvement, 333
  clinical stages, 1471-1472
  clinical syndromes, 1474-1479
  cryptococcosis, 1667
  cryptosporidiosis, 1679
  cutaneous manifestations, 1325-1329
  cyclosporiasis, 1680
  cytomegalovirus infection, 1528
  dementia, 987, 1478
  diagnosis, 1472
  ecthyma, 1420
  epidemiology, 1470-1471
  esophageal ulcerations, 2020
  etiology and pathophysiology, 1470
  evaluation and management, 1472-1474
  fever and rash, 1381
  fever of unknown origin, 1377
  flow cytometry, 1152
  folliculitis, 1420
  gastrointestinal manifestations, 2094-2099
  generalized lymphadenopathy, 599
  gram-negative bacteremia, 1446
  hemophilia, 622
  histoplasmosis, 1655
  hypogonadism, 1843
  isosporiasis, 1680
  meningitis, 1404, 1409
  microsporidiosis, 1680
  nephropathy, 853
  neutropenia, 593
  nocardiosis, 1666
  nontuberculous mycobacterial infection, 1638,
      1639
  nosocomial infection, 1361
  ophthalmic manifestations, 2304-2306
  pericardial effusion, 272
  Pneumocystis carinii pneumonia, 1692-1696
  during pregnancy, 2281
  prevention, 1479
  primary sclerosing cholangitis, 2202
  prognosis and treatment goals, 1479
  prostatic infections, 1463
  retrovirus, 1533-1534
  Salmonella, 1601-1602
  septic arthritis, 1254, 1255
  shigellosis, 1603
  spinal infection, 1013
  syphilis, 1640, 1641
  T-cell function, 1343

Acquired immunodeficiency syndrome—cont'd
  thrombocytopenia, 605
  toxoplasmosis, 1677
  transfusion-associated, 575
  transfusion-transmitted, 575
  tuberculosis, 1626
  weakness, 1754
  weight loss, 1750
Acquired immunodeficiency syndrome-related
      complex, 1472
Acquired inhibitors of blood coagulation,
      628-630
Acquired lipoatrophic diabetes, 1903
Acquired partial lipodystrophy, 1902
Acquired renal cystic disease, 788, 874-875
Acral lentiginous melanoma, 1299
Acridine orange stain, 1371
Acrocyanosis, 310, 669-670
Acrodermatitis enteropathica, 2110
Acrokeratosis paraneoplastica, 1317, 1318
Acromegaloidism, 1782
Acromegaly, 1769, 1782-1785
  amenorrhea, 1759
  arthropathy, 1246-1247
  clinical manifestations, 1782, 1784
  diagnosis, 1782-1783
  general appearance, 63
  hyperphosphatemia, 1938
  insulin resistance, 1862
  therapy, 1783-1784
  weakness, 1754
Acromioclavicular joint, 1164
Acrylamide, 1020
ACTH; *see* Adrenocorticotropic hormone
Actin antibody, 2139
Actin filament, 39
Actinic keratoses, 1297
Actinobacillus, 230
Actinomyces, 1664-1665
  actinomycetoma, 1660
  normal flora, 1368
  pleural effusion, 507
Action myoclonus, 996
Action potential, 36, 37-38, 1976
  Purkinje fiber, 132
Activated partial thromboplastin time
  to monitor heparin dosage, 633
  venous thromboembolism, 632
Activated plasminogen streptokinase activator
      complex, 213
Activation gate, 37-38
Activation-induced cell death, 1144
Activator calcium, 39
Active countermeasures, 2265
Active transport, 1986
Activin, 1835
Activities of daily living, 2285
  chronic obstructive pulmonary disease, 445
Activity
  after cardiac transplantation, 343
  aortic regurgitation, 241
  during bed rest, 2288
  cardiovascular response, 49
  chronic fatigue syndrome, 2300
  chronic obstructive pulmonary disease, 445
  coronary blood flow, 194
  effect on vasopressin release, 1791
  heart failure, 164
  hypertension management, 324
  increased bone mass in postmenopausal
      women, 1947
  increased potassium loss from cells, 831
  intermittent claudication, 308-309
  ischemic heart disease, 200
  neutrophilia, 590
  obesity, 2103, 2104
  palpitations, 130
  pulmonary rehabilitation, 435-436
  rheumatoid arthritis, 1206-1207
  rhinitis therapy, 1182
  silent myocardial ischemia, 194

Activity—cont'd
  skeletal muscle blood flow, 46
  walk through angina, 195
Activity front, 1979
Acute bacterial prostatitis, 1462
Acute confusional state, 1031
Acute disseminated encephalomyelitis, 1010
Acute fatty liver of pregnancy, 2278
Acute febrile neutrophilic dermatosis, 1318-1319
Acute hemorrhagic conjunctivitis, 1490
Acute hemorrhagic leukoencephalopathy, 1010
Acute hepatic encephalopathy, 1079-1080
Acute infectious lymphocytosis, 592
Acute inflammatory demyelinating
        polyradiculoneuropathy, 1018
Acute intermittent porphyria, 1926
Acute interstitial nephritis, 868, 889-890
Acute interstitial pneumonia, 448, 452
Acute intoxication, 1080
Acute ischemia, 978
Acute lymphoblastic leukemia, 682-683, Plate
        IV-5
  abnormal lymphocytes in peripheral blood,
        595
  curability with chemotherapy, 552
  lymphosarcoma cell leukemia *versus*, 594
  molecular diagnostics, 562
Acute monocytic leukemia, 591
Acute myelogenous leukemia, 689-690, 691
  aberrant hematopoietic cellular proliferation
        and maturation, 534
  chromosomal abnormalities, 544
  curability with chemotherapy, 552
  eosinophil abnormalities, 680-681
  molecular diagnostics, 562
  myelofibrosis, 677
  potassium wasting, 828
  second malignancy, 586
  sideroblastic anemia, 645
Acute myeloid leukemia 1 core binding factor
        beta, 545
Acute myelomonocytic leukemia, 680-681
Acute nephritic syndrome, 763-764
Acute nonlymphocytic leukemia, 689
Acute occlusive arterial disease, 307-308
Acute phase response, 1130
Acute rejection
  after liver transplantation, 2219
  lung, 520-522
  renal transplantation, 794
Acute renal failure, 768-776
  acute interstitial nephritis, 889-890
  cancer with, 775
  clinical course, complications, and prognosis,
        772-773
  diagnosis, 770-772
  essential mixed cryoglobulinemia, 857
  etiology, 768-769
  following bone marrow transplantation,
        775-776
  hemolytic-uremic syndrome, 858
  hyperphosphatemia, 1938
  liver disease with, 774-775
  management, 773-774
  obstructive uropathy, 885
  operative risk, 2263-2264
  pathophysiology, 769
  postoperative cholestasis, 2159
  during pregnancy, 775, 2274
  pulmonary-renal syndrome, 775
  radiocontrast nephropathy, 775
  renal allograft, 775
  rhabdomyolysis, 775
  Rocky Mountain spotted fever, 1543
Acute respiratory distress syndrome
  acquired immunodeficiency syndrome, 1475
  acute lung injury, 371-372
  acute pancreatitis, 2237
  with acute respiratory failure, 418
  gram-negative bacteremia, 1449
  mixed venous oxygen saturation, 393

Acute respiratory distress syndrome—cont'd
  multiple organ dysfunction syndrome, 421-423
  pathogenesis, 1341
  pressure-controlled ventilation, 419
  pulmonary edema, 168, 424, 425
  streptococcal toxic shock syndrome, 1558
  transfusion-associated lung injury, 1480
Acute respiratory failure, 412-420
  adult respiratory distress syndrome with, 418
  artificial airway, 416-417
  chronic obstructive pulmonary disease with,
        417-418, 446
  classification, 413, 414
  diagnosis, 413-414
  mechanical ventilation, 397, 416, 418-420
  oxygenation measures, 415-416
  pathophysiology, 412-413
  principles of management, 414, 415
  respiratory acidosis, 416
  tuberculosis, 1628
  without lung disease, 418
Acute toxic exposure, 473
Acute tubular necrosis
  acute renal failure, 769-770
  anti-neutrophil cytoplasmic antibodies-positive
        crescentic glomerulonephritis, 847
  clinical course complications and prognosis,
        772-773
  diagnosis, 771
  liver disease, 774-775
  operative risk, 2263
  prophylaxis, 773
Acute viral hepatitis
  hepatitis A virus, 2173
  hepatitis B virus, 2173-2175
  hepatitis C virus, 2175-2176
  hepatitis delta virus, 2176
  hepatitis E virus, 2176-2177
  hepatitis G virus, 2177
  non-A–non-B, 2177
  prevention, 2178-2179
  treatment, 2177-2178
Acute visceral attrition, 2101
Acyanotic tetralogy, 289
Acyclovir
  effects on kidney, 869
  facial nerve paralysis, 2306
  herpesvirus infections, 1526
    after marrow transplantation, 578-579
    esophagitis, 2020
    herpes simplex virus, 1524-1525
    herpes zoster ophthalmicus, 2305
    varicella and zoster, 1527
  prophylactic
    compromised host, 1390
    lung transplantation, 518
Acyl-coarctation of aorta cholesterol
        acyltransferase, 2127
Acylglycerides, 2126
Adalat; *see* Nifedipine
ADC; *see* Acquired immunodeficiency
        syndrome-related complex
Addison's disease, 1823-1824
  adrenocortical antibodies, 1157
  autoantibodies, 1155
  cutaneous manifestations, 1322-1323
  hypercalcemia, 1928
  hyperkalemia, 831
  hyperpigmentation of gums, Plate VII-14
  infertility and oligospermia, 1846
  lymphocytosis, 593
  weight loss, 1749
Adductor reflex, 964
Adenine, 50
Adenine/arabinoside, 2182
Adenine phosphoribosyltransferase, 1269
Adeno-associated virus, 1503
Adenocarcinoma
  ampulla of Vater, 2232
  Barrett's epithelium, 2018
  breast, 707

Adenocarcinoma—cont'd
  colonic, 2076-2077
  endometrium, 713-714
  esophageal, 2023-2024
  gallbladder, 2232
  gastric, 2039, 2045-2050
  intrahepatic cholangiocarcinoma, 2214
  lung, 487, 725
  pancreatic, 2242
  prostate, 717-720
  small bowel, 2080
  unknown primary site, 730, 732
Adenohypophysis, 1773-1788
  anatomy, 1773-1774
  Cushing's disease, 1786-1787
  empty sella syndrome, 1787
  gonadotropin-secreting pituitary tumor, 1787
  growth hormone-secreting pituitary tumor,
        1782-1785
  hyperprolactinemia, 1785-1786
  hypopituitarism, 1776-1777
  hypothalamic-pituitary adrenal system, 1774
  hypothalamic-pituitary axis, 1773-1774
  hypothalamic-pituitary gonadal system,
        1774-1775
  hypothalamic-pituitary growth hormone
        system, 1775
  hypothalamic-pituitary prolactin system,
        1775-1776, 1777
  hypothalamic-pituitary thyroid system, 1774
  pituitary apoplexy, 1777-1781
  pituitary tumor, 1781-1782
  thyroid-stimulating hormone-secreting tumor,
        1787
Adenoid cystic carcinoma, 491
Adenoma
  adrenal, 1820, 1822
  aldosterone-secreting, 1823
  bronchial, 491-492
  colon, 2086
  hepatic, 2216-2217
  pancreatic, 1876
  parathyroid, 1965
  pituitary, 1781-1782
    gonadotropin-secreting, 1787
    growth hormone-secreting, 1782-1785
    impotence, 1762
    during pregnancy, 2273-2274
    thyroid-stimulating hormone-secreting,
        1787, 1807
  renal, 753, 899
  small bowel, 2082
  thyroid, 1813-1814
Adenoma sebaceum, 1922
Adenomatous polyp
  gastric, 2046
  risk for colon cancer, 2083
Adenomyomatosis, 2233
Adenopathy
  adenovirus infection, 1503
  cervical, 1385
  hilar
    brucellosis, 1606
    computed tomography, 386
    tuberculosis, 1628
  infectious mononucleosis, 1529
  inguinal, 1444
  non-Hodgkin's lymphoma, 697
  scarlet fever, 1421
  syphilis, 1640
Adenosine, 139, 1140, 1141
  atrial flutter, 144
  atrioventricular nodal reentrant tachycardia,
        141-142, 144, 145
  dipyridamole stress scintigraphy, 103-104
  response of arrhythmias, 134, 135
  sustained ventricular tachycardia and wide
        QRS complex tachycardia, 150
  uncommon types of sustained ventricular
        tachycardia, 153

Adenosine—cont'd
  vasoactive effects on pulmonary circulation, 363
  Wolff-Parkinson-White syndrome, 142
Adenosine deaminase deficiency, 1177
Adenosine diphosphate
  hyperuricemia, 1270
  platelet aggregation, 536
  platelet function disorders, 612
  platelet release reaction, 611
Adenosine receptor, 59
Adenosine thallium scintigraphy, 198-199
Adenosine triphosphatase
  heart failure, 159-160
  inhibition by digitalis, 173
Adenosine triphosphate
  bile salt transport, 2126
  carbohydrate metabolism, 1851
  cardiac contraction, 39
  cystic fibrosis transmembrane conductance regulator, 480
  depletion in hypophosphatemia, 1936
  hereditary fructose intolerance, 1880
  hormone action, 1711
  hyperuricemia, 1270
  muscle testing, 1025
  peristalsis, 1977
  potassium channel inhibition, 59
  secretion of conjugated bilirubin into bile, 2149
  shock, 176, 178
  thyroid hormone formation, 1798
  vasoactive effects on pulmonary circulation, 363
Adenovirus, 1503-1504
  acquired immunodeficiency syndrome, 2096
  compromised host, 1388
  culture, 1369
  pericarditis, 272
  pharyngitis, 1393
  respiratory tract infection, 1390
Adenovirus vector, 1732
Adenylate cyclase
  activation, 1711, 2132
  cellular modulation of contractility, 41
  signal transduction, 58
  thyroid hormone formation and metabolism, 1797
ADH; *see* Antidiuretic hormone
Adhesion
  cell-to-cell, 370
  platelet, 611
    platelet-endothelial cell adhesion molecule-1, 370
    subendothelium, 536
Adhesion molecule, 370, 372
Adhesive capsulitis, 1197
Adhesive proteins, 536
Adipose cellularity, 2103
Adipose tissue
  adrenergic responses, 1828
  free fatty acid mobilization from, 1853
  lipodystrophies, 1899-1903
  obesity, 1751
  triglyceride storage, 1884
Adjunctive therapy, 554
  anaerobic infection, 1621
  bacterial meningitis, 1412-1413
  breast cancer, 709
  cryptococcosis, 1669-1670
  myocardial infarction, 215-218
Adjustment disorder with depressed mood, 1036
Adjustment sleep disorder, 944
Adolescent
  anorexia nervosa, 1749, 1769-1770, 2030
    criteria, 2028
    hypogonadism, 1842
    protein calorie malnutrition, 2101
  atrial septal defect, 280
  bulimia nervosa, 2028

Adolescent—cont'd
  growth and development disorders, 1766-1773
    breast growth abnormalities, 1770
    constitutional delay of pubertal growth, 1768
    Crohn's disease, 1768
    evaluation of pubertal growth, 1770-1772
    familial tall stature, 1769
    growth hormone deficiency, 1769
    hypothyroidism, 1768-1769
    idiopathic short stature, 1769
    Klinefelter's syndrome, 1769
    puberty, 1766-1768
    therapy, 1772
    Turner's syndrome, 1769
    weight abnormalities, 1769-1770
  juvenile cystinosis, 1910
  juvenile nephronophthisis, 875, 892
  juvenile-onset diabetes mellitus, 1854
  juvenile osteoporosis, 1945
  juvenile polyps, 2086
  juvenile rheumatoid arthritis, 273
  thyrotoxicosis, 1808
ADP; *see* Adenosine diphosphate
Adrenal adenoma, 1822
Adrenal cancer, 1822
  aldosterone-secreting adenoma, 1823
  computed tomography, 1734
  Cushing's syndrome, 1820
Adrenal cortex, 1817-1826
  aldosterone, 1741
    aldosterone-producing adenoma, 321
    cirrhosis, 819
    excess, 1822-1823
    hyperkalemia, 832
    hypertension, 321
    hypertensive renal potassium wasting, 828
    hypoaldosteronism, 824, 1824
    hypomagnesemia, 1941
    secretion, 1818
    sodium balance, 738
  androgens, 1741
  congenital adrenal hyperplasia, 1824-1825
  cortisol
    Addison's disease, 1824
    congenital adrenal hyperplasia, 1825
    Cushing's syndrome, 1820-1821
    feedback inhibition tests, 1736
    glucose production, 1874, 1875
    hypercortisolism, 1820
    hypoglycemia, 1877
    integrated fuel homeostasis, 1853
    plasma, 1740
    secretion, 1818
    urinary free, 1741
  Cushing's syndrome, 1819-1822
    amenorrhea, 1759
    arthropathy, 1247
    cutaneous manifestations, 1323
    dexamethasone suppression test, 1737
    endocrine paraneoplastic syndromes, 583
    general appearance, 63
    hypertension, 321-322
    hypokalemia, 829
    insulin resistance, 1862
    mediastinal mass, 513
    medullary thyroid carcinoma, 1816
    obesity, 2103
    plasma cortisol levels, 1740
    screening tests, 1826
    weakness, 1754
  glucocorticoids, 1740-1741
    calcium homeostasis, 1720
    deficiency, 838
    effects on potassium transport, 741
    enhancement of cognitive function, 1076
    gluconeogenesis, 2122
    human cytochrome P450 isoforms, 2312
    overproduction in Cushing's syndrome, 1819-1820
    vasopressin inhibition, 1791

Adrenal cortex—cont'd
  hormone synthesis and secretion, 1817-1819
  hypofunction, 1823-1824
  mass, 1825-1826
  mineralocorticoids, 1741-1742
    deficiency, 824
    effects on potassium transport, 741
    excess, 840, 1822-1823
    renal hydrogen ion secretion, 741
    sodium-retaining action, 738
Adrenal gland
  disease
    arthropathy, 1247
    cutaneous manifestations, 1322-1323
    dementia, 987
    gynecomastia, 1765
    hypothalamic-pituitary adrenal system, 1774
    structure and function, 1817
Adrenal hyperplasia
  congenital, 1824-1825
  hirsutism, 1755
  hyperkalemia, 831
  hypertensive renal potassium wasting, 828
Adrenal insufficiency, 1823-1824
  acquired immunodeficiency syndrome, 1475
  hypoglycemia, 1876
  lymphocytosis, 592
  sepsis *versus,* 1451
  sodium depletion, 824
Adrenal mass, 1825-1826
  hypertension, 321
Adrenal medulla, 1826-1831
  catecholamines, 1826-1827; *see also*
      Catecholamines
    agents interfering with assays, 1740
    biosynthesis and metabolism, 1826-1827
    compensatory mechanisms, 159
    degradation, 1714
    hypertension, 316
    integrated fuel homeostasis, 1853
    internal potassium balance, 825
    measurement, 938
    neurogenic pulmonary edema, 1099
    plasma, 1740
    synthesis, 1710
    transient hypokalemia, 826
    uncommon types of sustained ventricular tachycardia, 153
    urinary, 1740
    vasoactive effects on pulmonary circulation, 363
  hormones, 1739-1740
  hyperfunction, 1828
  hypofunction, 1827-1828
  pheochromocytoma, 1828-1831
    autonomic hyperactivity, 935
    hypercalcemia, 1928
    hypertension, 322
    insulin resistance, 1862
    neurofibromatosis, 1921
    weight loss, 1749
Adrenalectomy
  adrenal medulla hypofunction following, 1827
  Cushing's syndrome, 1821
Adrenergic-dependent torsades de pointes, 152-153
Adrenergic receptors, 931, 1827
  cardiac function, 56-58
Adrenocortical antibody, 1157
Adrenocorticosteroids; *see also* Corticosteroids
  biosynthesis, 1817, 1818
  myasthenia gravis, 1022
  regulation of secretion, 1817-1819
  rheumatoid arthritis, 1207
  systemic lupus erythematosus, 1216-1217
Adrenocorticotropic hormone, 1774
  Addison's disease, 1823-1824
  Cushing's syndrome, 1737, 1820, 1821-1822
  deficiency, 1777, 1823-1824
  dexamethasone suppression test, 1736-1737
  ectopic secretion, 1735

Adrenocorticotropic hormone—cont'd
  gout, 1274
  hirsutism, 1756
  hypopituitarism treatment, 1779-1780
  increase after nausea induction, 2025
  regulation of adrenocortical secretion,
      1817-1819
  stimulation tests, 1741
Adrenogenital syndrome, 828
Adrenomedullin, 1826
Adriamycin; *see* Doxorubicin
Adson's maneuver, 306
Adult hypergonadotropic hypogonadism, 1844,
    1845
Adult hypogonadotropic hypogonadism, 1844,
    1845
Adult hypophosphatasia, 1954
Adult lactase deficiency, 2068
Adult-onset diabetes mellitus, 1854
Adult Still's disease, 1243
Adult T-cell leukemia, 1532
Advance directive, 12-13
Advanced glycosylation end-products, 2283
Advanced Maillard products, 861
Advanced sleep phase syndrome, 945
Adventitial reticular cell, 531
Adventitious lung sounds, 402
Advocacy, injury control, 2267
Adynamic bone disease, 1961, 1962
Adynamic ileus, 1977
  pseudomembranous colitis with, 1570
Adynamic renal bone disease, 1963
Aerobic bacteria
  antibiotic selection, 1347
  compromised host, 1388
  Corynebacterium, 1347, 1565-1567
    erythrasma, 1422
    normal flora, 1368
  Legionella pneumophila, 1621-1625
    acute interstitial nephritis, 889, 890
    nosocomial infection, 1363
  Listeria monocytogenes, 1576-1578
    after heart transplantation, 1090
    fever, 1387
    meningitis, 1403, 1478
  Neisseria gonorrhoeae, 1581-1585
    beta-lactamases, 1345
    diarrhea, 1476
    immunoglobulin A, 1337
    peritonitis, 1396, 2248
    septic arthritis, 1251
    urethritis, 1455
  Neisseria meningitidis, 1339, 1578-1581
    immunoglobulin A, 1337
    meningitis, 1402-1403
    normal microflora, 1368, 1615
    synergistic nonclostridial anaerobic
        myonecrosis, 1424
  Aeromonas, 1593
    compromised host, 1388
    diarrhea, 1427, 2051
Aerosol face mask, 428-429
Aerosol medications, 430-431
  asthma, 1189-1190
Affective disorders, 2299
Affinity maturation, 1111, 1125
Afibrinogenemia, 625
Aflatoxin
  carcinogenesis, 548
  hepatocellular carcinoma, 2185, 2212
African trypanosomiasis, 1687-1689
Afterdepolarization, 132
Afterload, 42
  aortic regurgitation, 240
  cardiogenic shock, 176
  heart failure, 158-159
  nitroglycerin effect, 126
Agammaglobulinemia, 1490
Aganglionic megacolon, 2092
Age
  alveolar-arterial oxygen difference, 351
  antibacterial selection, 1346

Age—cont'd
  antihypertensive agent choices, 326
  asthma, 1192
  atrial fibrillation, 146
  bacterial meningitis, 1403
  bone loss, 1946
  bone mineral content, 1715
  contraindication to transplantation, 792
  dementia, 985
  depressive disorders, 1036
  domestic violence, 2268
  gallstone risk factor, 2223, 2224
  glomerulonephritis, 842
  Haemophilus influenzae infections, 1586
  headache syndromes, 960
  heart failure, 157, 158
  hepatitis A virus infection, 2173
  hepatitis B virus infection, 2174
  hypertension, 312
  idiopathic nephrotic syndrome, 850
  lymphadenopathy, 597
  metabolic rate, 2113
  nosocomial infection, 1361
  obstructive uropathy, 884
  osteoarthritis, 1264
  ovarian cancer, 716
  parvovirus B19 infection, 1513
  prostate cancer, 717
  recommended daily dietary allowances, 2114
  rickets, 1949
  risk of stroke, 1001
  serum alkaline phosphatase level, 2137
  testicular function, 1839-1840
Age-related macular degeneration, 2301-2302
Agglutination reactions, 1373
Agglutination test, 1371-1372
  bacterial meningitis, 1408
  brucellosis, 1606
  Treponema pallidum, 1642
  tularemia, 1608
  venous thromboembolism, 632
Aging
  biology, 2283-2285
  changes in osmoregulatory system, 1789
  eye problems, 2301-2302
  hormones and, 1076-1077
  osteoarthritis risk, 1264
  peripheral vascular disease, 305
  voiding dysfunction, 1065-1066
Agnogenic myeloid metaplasia, 677
Agraphia, 978
AICD; *see* Automatic implantable cardioverter
    defibrillator
AIDP; *see* Acute inflammatory demyelinating
    polyradiculoneuropathy
AIDS; *see* Acquired immunodeficiency
    syndrome
Air conditioner lung, 460
Air-entrainment mask, 429
Air exchange, 366, 367
Air pollution, 438
Air space enlargement, 439
Air space flooding, 424
Air travel, 447
AIRE study, 172
Airway
  comatose patient, 950
  cystic fibrosis, 480
  head trauma, 1044
  hyperreactivity
    asthma, 1185-1186
    chronic obstructive pulmonary disease, 439
  interstitial lung disease, 450
  obstruction
    acute, 2306
    anaphylaxis, 1193
    angioedema, 2306
    asthma, 1188
    chronic obstructive pulmonary disease, 438
    exercise tests, 379
    heart failure *versus,* 168

Airway—cont'd
  obstruction—cont'd
    maximal expiratory and inspiratory
        flow-volume curve, 377
    sarcoidosis, 458
    sleep-induced, 527-528
    snoring, 2309
    spirometry, 377
  occupational disease, 471-473
  sinusitis, 2308
  upper airway resistance syndrome, 526-527,
      943
Airway resistance, 347
  Cheyne-Stokes respiration, 354
  upper airway resistance syndrome, 943
  ventilated patient, 399
Ajmaline, 2192
Akathisia, 1042
Akinetic mutism, 977, 1032
Akinetic/rigid syndrome, 992
Akinetic seizure, 954, 979
AL amyloidosis, 1282-1283
Alanine
  gluconeogenesis, 2122
  related diseases, 1904
Alanine aminotransferase
  acetaminophen poisoning, 2190
  acute pancreatitis, 2236
  chronic hepatitis, 2180
  hepatic injury, 2136, 2188
  hepatitis A infection, 2173
  hepatitis B infection, 2175
Albendazole
  echinococcal cyst, 2212
  Enterocytozoon bieneusi, 1474
  intestinal helminths, 1697, 1698
  microsporidiosis, 1679, 1681
  Strongyloides stercoralis, 1699
  tissue nematode infection, 1700
  whipworm, 1696
  Wuchereria bancrofti, 1699
Albright's hereditary osteodystrophy, 1932
Albumin
  albuminuria
    diabetic nephropathy, 859, 1870
    galactosemia, 1883
  within alpha-granules, 536
  bilirubin, 2147
  in bronchoalveolar lavage fluid, 367
  fatty acid transport, 2121
  grades of liver disease severity, 2166
  hepatic synthesis, 2119
  hepatic uptake of bilirubin, 2128
  hypoalbuminemia, 765
    acute pancreatitis, 2237
    amebic liver abscess, 2210
    anion gap acidosis, 836
    intestinal disease, 2005
    intestinal lymphangiectasia, 2067
    nephrotic syndrome, 765
    serum magnesium, 1942
    transudative pleural effusion, 507
  plasma
    nephrotic syndrome, 765
    unconjugated bilirubin, 2148
  proteinuria, 743, 760
  serum
    adult respiratory distress syndrome, 421
    heart failure, 166
    hypercalcemia, 1929
    kwashiorkor, 2101
    liver disease, 2134-2135
    nephrotic syndrome, 765
    nutritional assessment, 2111
    peritonitis, 2080
    primary biliary cirrhosis, 2200
    primary sclerosing cholangitis, 2202
    small bowel malabsorption, 2058
  total serum calcium, 1744
Albuminuria
  diabetic nephropathy, 859, 1870
  galactosemia, 1883

Albuterol
  hyperkalemia, 833
  pertussis, 1613
Alcohol
  alcohol-tobacco amblyopia, 1081
  arrhythmia, 133
  atrial fibrillation, 146
  bleeding time, 612
  cancer risk, 550
  carcinogenesis, 548
  cytochrome P450 2E1, 2311
  dilated cardiomyopathy, 265
  effects on lipoproteins, 1890
  esophageal cancer, 2023
  hypertension, 318, 319, 324
  inhibition of folate metabolism, 647
  interference with oral anticoagulants, 636
  medical interview of usage, 3-4
  metabolic disorders, 1080-1081
  metabolism, 2194-2195
  mood disorders, 1036
  myopathy, 1030
  nausea and vomiting, 2026
  neuropathy, 1019
  personality disorders, 1039
  risk of falls, 2290
  sideroblastic anemia, 645
  sleep disorders, 945
  withdrawal, 2295-2296
    seizure, 982
    sympathetic nervous system overactivity, 934-935
Alcohol dehydrogenases, 2194, 2195
Alcohol-dependent sleep disorder, 945
Alcohol-tobacco amblyopia, 1081
Alcoholic fatty liver, 2196, 2197
Alcoholic hepatitis, 2196, 2197
  acute cholecystitis *versus*, 2228
  operative risk, 2263
Alcoholic ketoacidosis, 743
Alcoholic ketosis, 1865
Alcoholic liver disease, 2194-2199
  canalicular cholestasis, 2155
  cirrhosis, 2196
  hepatitis, 2196, 2197
    acute cholecystitis *versus*, 2228
    hepatitis A infection, 2173
    operative risk, 2263
  liver transplantation, 2218
  risk of gallstone formation, 2224
  serum aminotransferase levels, 2136
Alcoholic pancreatitis, 2144
Alcoholics Anonymous, 2296
Alcoholism, 2294-2296
  acute meningitis, 1407
  acute pancreatitis, 2233
  alcoholic ketosis, 1865
  carbon tetrachloride poisoning, 2188
  chronic pancreatitis, 2238
  cirrhosis, 2172
  diagnosis, 2197-2198
  hypomagnesemia, 1941
  hypophosphatemia, 1936
  niacin deficiency, 2107
  porphyria cutanea tarda, 1927
  thiamine deficiency, 2106
  weight loss, 1749
Aldactazide; *see* Spironolactone
Aldehyde dehydrogenases, 2194, 2195
Aldolase, 1025
Aldolase B, 1880
Aldomet; *see* Methyldopa
Aldosterone
  excess, 1822-1823
  hyperaldosteronism
    cirrhosis, 819
    hypertensive renal potassium wasting, 828
    hypomagnesemia, 1941
  hyperkalemia, 832
  hypertension, 321

Aldosterone—cont'd
  hypoaldosteronism
    hyporeninemic, 1824
    sodium depletion, 824
  plasma, 1741
    aldosterone-producing adenoma, 321
    hypertension, 321
  potassium, 825
  secretion, 1818
  sodium balance, 738
  sodium retention in cirrhosis, 819
Alendronate
  osteoporosis, 1948
  Paget's disease, 1957
Alexia, 978
Alfa-interferon
  chronic myelogenous leukemia, 687
  hepatitis C infection, 2178
  polycythemia vera, 689
Algodystrophy, 1247
Alimentary tract
  adrenergic responses, 1828
  antirheumatic drug toxicity, 1261
  beta-blockers, 202
  calcium absorption, 1717
  diabetic autonomic neuropathy, 1872-1873
  diverticular disease
    diverticulitis, 2085
    diverticulosis, 1996, 2060
    esophageal, 2020-2021
    gastric, 2044
    intestinal, 2089-2092
  drug interactions, 2311
  endoscopy, 1993-1998
  esophageal disease, 2014-2024
    achalasia, 2021-2022
    benign tumors, 2023
    cancer, 2023-2024
    chemical and physical injury, 2018-2019
    esophageal spasm, 2022-2023
    esophageal webs, rings, and diverticula, 2020-2021
    evaluation, 1998-2002
    gastroesophageal reflux, 2014-2018
    infectious esophagitis, 2019-2020
    weight loss, 1749
  features of malabsorption, 2058
  febrile compromised patient, 1388
  gastric secretion, 1980-1985
  gastritis, 2041-2044
    atrophic, 2045
    Helicobacter pylori, 1592-1593
    operative risk, 2263
  gastroenteritis, 1425-1432
    bacterial agents, 1425-1427
    coronavirus, 1502
    diagnosis, 1430-1431
    diarrhea, 1429-1430
    eosinophilic, 2066-2067
    immunoglobulin A nephropathy, 845
    parasitic agents, 1428-1429
    pathophysiology, 1425
    prophylaxis for traveler's diarrhea, 1432
    rotavirus and Norwalk-like virus, 1519-1522
    Salmonella, 1599
    Staphylococcus aureus, 1548-1549
    treatment, 1431-1432
    Vibrio parahaemolyticus, 1596-1597
    viral agents, 1427-1428
  gastrointestinal bleeding, 2008-2014
    acquired immunodeficiency syndrome, 2098-2099
    alcoholic hepatitis and cirrhosis, 2197
    antacids and antisecretory agents, 2013
    Campylobacter jejuni, 1591
    chronic renal failure, 783, 784
    colon cancer, 2085
    colonoscopy, 1996
    cutaneous manifestations, 1320
    diagnostic and therapeutic studies, 2011-2013
    esophageal varices, 2013-2014
    fulminant hepatic failure, 2163

Alimentary tract—cont'd
  gastrointestinal bleeding—cont'd
    gastric cancer, 2046
    initial management, 2010-2011
    portosystemic encephalopathy, 2160
    small intestinal malignancies, 2081
    technetium 99m studies, 2004
    upper gastrointestinal endoscopy, 1994
  inflammatory bowel disease, 2068-2077
    arthropathy, 1245-1246
    chronic diarrhea, 2051
    colonoscopy, 1996
    Crohn's disease, 2069-2072
    cutaneous findings, 1321
    differentiation of ulcerative colitis and Crohn's disease, 2075
    etiology, 2068-2069
    extraintestinal manifestations, 2075-2076
    fever and rash, 1385
    incidence and epidemiology, 2069
    increased risk of cancer, 548, 2076-2077
    portal triad lesions, 2155
    during pregnancy, 2278-2279
    primary sclerosing cholangitis, 2201
    secondary hyperoxaluria, 799, 804
    stool examination, 2006
    toxic megacolon, 2076
    ulcerative colitis, 2072-2075
  intestinal absorption, 1985-1989
    cholesterol, 1884
    magnesium, 1939, 1940
  intestinal immunity, 1989-1993
  intestinal obstruction, 2077-2079
    abdominal pain, 2032
    colon cancer, 2085
    cystic fibrosis, 2246
    Meckel's diverticulum, 2089
    radiography, 2032
    small intestinal malignancies, 2081
  intestinal vascular disease, 2086-2089
    iron absorption from, 641
  irritable bowel syndrome, 2055-2056
    abdominal pain, 2035
    celiac sprue *versus,* 2063
    colonic dysmotility, 2007
    diarrhea, 2052
  Kaposi's sarcoma, 1330
  malabsorption, 2056-2068
    abetalipoproteinemia, 2067
    bacterial overgrowth, 2060-2062
    carbohydrate intolerance, 2067-2068
    carbohydrates, 1987
    celiac sprue, 2062-2063
    chronic diarrhea, 2051-2052
    chronic pancreatitis, 2145, 2239
    clinical features, 2057-2058
    congenital glucose-galactose, 878
    Crohn's disease, 270, 2069
    cystic fibrosis, 2246
    digestion process, 2056-2057
    eosinophilic enteritis, 2067
    eosinophilic gastroenteritis, 2066-2067
    hypogammaglobulinemia, 2066
    intestinal lymphangiectasia, 2067
    laboratory findings, 2058-2060
    magnesium, 1940
    multiple jejunal diverticulosis, 2089
    negative phosphate balance, 1935
    pancreatic and hepatobiliary diseases, 2062
    radiation enteropathy, 2065-2066
    serum electrolytes, 2005
    short bowel syndrome, 2066
    small intestinal tumors, 2081
    stool examination, 2006
    tests for, 2006-2007
    tropical sprue, 2065
    vitamin B_{12} deficiency, 648
    vitamin K deficiency, 607, 626
    weight loss, 1749
    Whipple's disease, 2064-2065
  manifestations of acquired immunodeficiency syndrome, 2094-2099

Alimentary tract—cont'd
motor function, 1976-1980
neurogastroenterology, 1100-1102
operative risks, 2262-2263
origin of sodium loss, 823
peptic ulcer disease, 2035-2041
acid secretory values, 2003
Helicobacter pylori, 1592-1593
operative risk, 2263
peritonitis, 2079-2080, 2247-2249
abdominal evaluation, 2032
acquired immunodeficiency syndrome, 1476
anaerobic bacteria, 1617
candidal, 1661
dialysis-related, 791
paralytic ileus, 2078
primary, 1396
systemic lupus erythematosus, 1214
polyarteritis nodosa, 1220
primary hyperparathyroidism, 1966
prophylaxis in compromised host, 1390
relationship with nutrient intake, 2100
spinal cord injury, 1050
stomach cancer, 2045-2050
systemic lupus erythematosus, 1215
systemic sclerosis, 1229-1230, 1232
toxicity of chemotherapeutic agents, 584-585
toxicity of nonsteroidal antiinflammatory
drugs, 1258-1259
Alkalemia
blood pH, 834
internal potassium balance, 825
Alkali, 2043
Alkaline phosphatase
acute cholecystitis, 2228
acute pancreatitis, 2236
amebic liver abscess, 2210
bone and mineral disorders, 1744-1745
choledocholithiasis, 2229
hepatitic injury, 2136
hepatocellular *versus* cholestatic jaundice,
2156
human immunodeficiency virus infection,
1473
hypophosphatasia, 1954
lipodystrophy, 1901
liver disease, 2137
osteomalacia, 1949
Paget's disease, 1956
postoperative cholestasis, 2159
primary biliary cirrhosis, 2200
primary sclerosing cholangitis, 2202
renal bone disease, 1964
Alkaline tide, 742
Alkalinization
bile salt transport, 2126
cast nephropathy, 865
Alkalosis, 834
hypocalcemia, 1930
hypokalemia, 827
metabolic, 839-841
changes in arterial pH, 353
consequence of vomiting, 2028
hypertensive renal potassium wasting, 828
hypokalemia, 827, 829-830
normotensive renal potassium wasting, 828
renal excretion of potassium, 741
respiratory
carbon dioxide partial pressure, 834
gram-negative bacteremia, 1449
hypokalemia, 827
hypophosphatemia, 1936
renal excretion of potassium, 741
renal response, 835
serum calcium, 1744
Alkaptonuria, 1170, 1280-1282, 1910
Alkeran; *see* Melphalan
Alkylating agents
carcinogenesis, 548
chronic lymphocytic leukemia, 685
effects on kidney, 869

Alkylating agents—cont'd
essential thrombocythemia, 688
minimal change disease, 851
pulmonary parenchymal reactions, 476
rheumatic disease, 1262
ALL; *see* Acute lymphoblastic leukemia
All-trans retinoic acid
acne vulgaris, 1305
acute myelogenous leukemia, 690
cancer treatment, 555
pulmonary parenchymal reactions, 476
pulmonary toxicity, 478
Allele, 1721
autosomal recessive inheritance pattern, 1725
human leukocyte antigen, 1115-1118
Allele specific oligonucleotide, 1724
Allelic exclusion, 1110, 1125
Allelic loss, 546
Allen test, 305
Allergen
allergic contact dermatitis, 1303
rhinitis, 1182
Allergic asthma, 1139
Allergic bronchopulmonary aspergillosis, 483
Allergic contact dermatitis, 1303
Allergic granulomatosis, 465-467, 1220
Allergic reaction
antirheumatic drug toxicity, 1261
chronic rhinitis, 2308
contact dermatitis, 1303
insulin, 1861
otitis media, 2307
penicillin, 1346
streptokinase, 637-638
transfusion, 574-575
Allergic rhinitis, 1181, 1183
Allergic tubulointerstitial nephritis, 832
Allergic vasculitis, 465-467
Allograft rejection
heart, 339-341
hematopoietic stem cell, 578
kidney, 793-794
liver, 2219
lung, 520-524
Alloimmune thrombocytopenic purpura, 616
Alloimmunization
platelet transfusion, 573
sickle cell disease, 659
Allopurinol
hepatic injury, 2191
leishmaniasis, 1686
multiple myeloma, 702
tophaceous gout, 1275
uric acid stones, 804
Alopecia
drug-induced, 1313
heparin-associated, 635
lupus erythematosus, 1291
syphilis, 1641
vitamin D-dependent rickets, type II, 1953
Alpha-1,4-glucosidase deficiency, 1881
Alpha-actin protein, 59
Alpha-actinin, 59
Alpha-adrenergic antagonists
angina, 205
chronic pernio, 310
hypertension, 325, 326
hypertensive emergency, 328
impotence, 1764
neurogenic pulmonary edema, 1099
pheochromocytoma, 1831
Raynaud's phenomenon, 310
reflex sympathetic dystrophy, 311
Alpha-adrenergic receptors, 1827
7-Alpha-dydroxylation of cholesterol, 1884
Alpha-dystroglycan, 1027
Alpha-fetoprotein
hepatic formation, 2120
hepatocellular carcinoma, 2143, 2213
testicular cancer, 720
Alpha-glucosidase inhibitors, 1858

Alpha-granule, 536
Alpha-heavy-chain disease, 704
Alpha-interferon
chronic hepatitis B, 2181-2182
fulminant hepatitis A, 2177
multiple myeloma, 702
Alpha-interferon 2b, 2183
Alpha-ketoacids, 2121
Alpha-mannosidosis, 1916
Alpha-receptors, 56-58
Alpha-satellite deoxyribonucleic acid, 561, 562
Alpha-syntrophin, 1027
Alpha-thalassemia, 656
Alpha-tropomyosin, 61
Alpha-tubulin, 59
Alpha$_1$-adrenergic blockers
hypertension, 325
urge incontinence, 2293
Alpha$_1$-antitrypsin
absorption of vitamin B$_{12}$, 2007
deficiency, 2206-2207
chronic hepatitis, 2180
hepatocellular carcinoma, 2212
hereditary markers, 2139
liver transplantation, 2219
hepatic formation, 2120
venous thromboembolism, 632
Alpha$_1$-globulin, 565
Alpha$_1$-protease inhibitor deficiency, 439-440
Alpha$_2$-adrenergic agonists
chronic hypertension during pregnancy, 2275
drug-induced immune hemolytic anemia, 670
drug-nutrient interactions, 2110
hepatic injury, 2192
hepatocellular jaundice, 2192
hot flashes, 2271
hypertension, 325
interference with catecholamine assays, 1740
opiate detoxification, 2297
pheochromocytoma, 322, 1830
spasticity after spinal cord injury, 1051
testing for growth hormone reserve, 1775
Alpha$_2$ antiplasmin, 618
Alpha$_2$-antiplasmin, 538, 540
Alpha$_2$ macroglobulins
rheumatoid arthritis, 1202
shock states, 176
Alpha$_2$ plasmin inhibitor deficiency, 625
Alphavirus, 1514-1519
Alport's syndrome, 794, 876-877
Alprazolam
anxiety disorders, 1035
human cytochrome P450 isoforms, 2312
Altace; *see* Ramipril
Altered state of consciousness
abnormal respiratory rhythms, 1097-1098
coma, 947
epilepsy, 981
Alternative complement pathway, 1135
activation, 1338
bacteremia, 1448
inherited defects, 1179-1180, 1339
meningitis, 1404
Alternative mRNA splicing, 51
Altitude insomnia, 944
Alu sites, 1723
Aluminum toxicity
dialysis encephalopathy, 785, 1106
renal bone disease, 1961
rickets and osteomalacia in renal disease,
1953
Alveolar amyloidosis, 452
Alveolar-arterial oxygen difference, 351-352
Alveolar arterial oxygen tension gradient, 500
Alveolar epithelium, 348, 371
Alveolar gas, 348
Alveolar hemorrhage, 454-455
Alveolar hyperventilation, 378
Alveolar hypoventilation, 412-413
Alveolar hypoxia, 295

Alveolar macrophage, 367-369, 1127
  hypersensitivity pneumonitis, 462
  interstitial lung disease, 450
  lung injury, 370, 372
  lung repair, 374
  sarcoidosis, 457
  silicosis, 475
  sputum examination, 380-381
  tuberculosis, 1627
Alveolar pressure, 362
Alveolar ventilation, 348
Alveolitis
  asbestosis, 474
  interstitial lung diseases, 448
  sarcoidosis, 457, 459
Alveolocapillary membrane, 346
Alveolus
  defense mechanisms, 366, 367
  diffuse alveolar damage, 448
  effects of lung inflation, 362
  hypersensitivity pneumonitis, 460
  normal recovery from injury, 374
  pulmonary edema, 424
  wall components, 370-371
Alzheimer's disease, 985-987
  dementia, 2288
  electroencephalography, 907, 910
  localized amyloidosis, 1285
Alzheimer's Disease Assessment Scale, 904
Amadori product, 861
Amantadine
  disordered thinking, 1041
  influenza, 1492
  Parkinson's disease, 992
Amaurosis fugax, 1057-1058
Amblyopia ex anopia, 1062
Ambulatory blood pressure monitoring, 312, 313
Ambulatory electrocardiography
  aortic stenosis, 238
  arrhythmias, 134, 135
  ischemic heart disease, 197, 198
  mitral valve prolapse, 254
  myocarditis, 263
  sudden death survivor, 189-190
  sustained monomorphic ventricular
    tachycardia, 151
  tetralogy of Fallot, 289
Amebiasis, 1681-1683
  acquired immunodeficiency syndrome, 2096
  liver abscess, 2210
  meningitis, 1409
  pleural effusion, 507
  traveler, 1465-1466
Ameboma, 1682
Amenorrhea, 1757-1760
  anorexia nervosa, 1769
  hirsutism, 1756
  hypothalamic, 1837
  malabsorption, 2057
  prolactin-secreting pituitary adenoma, 1786
American Diabetes Association diet, 1857
American Heart Association
  guidelines for coronary angioplasty, 124
  recommended diet, 1893
American trypanosomiasis, 1689-1690
Amikacin, 1356
  bacterial meningitis, 1411
  dosage, 1349
  effects on kidney, 868
  enterococci resistance, 1561
  mycobacterial disease, 1631
  use during pregnancy, 2281
Amiloride
  heart failure, 170
  hyperkalemia, 832
  hypertension, 325
  nephrogenic diabetes insipidus, 884
  stone formation reduction, 803
Amine precursor uptake and decarboxylation
  system, 2244
Amineptine, 2191

Amines, 1708
Amino acid-carbohydrate complex, 2102
Amino acid consumption test, 2145
Amino acid disorders
  metabolic, 1903-1911
    branched-chain amino acids, 1907-1908
    histidinemia, 1906
    hyperphenylalaninemia, 1904-1905
    lysine disorders, 1907
    sulfur-containing amino acids, 1908-1909
    tyrosinemia, 1905-1906
    urea cycle defects, 1906-1907
  storage, 1909-1910
  transport, 1910-1911
Amino acids
  absorption, 1988
  apoproteins, 1885
  cholecystokinin stimulation, 2133
  functions of minerals, 2109
  glucose homeostasis during fasting, 1852
  glycogenic, 2121-2122
  hepatic encephalopathy, 2161, 2162
  hepatic metabolism, 2118-2120
  hyperdibasic aminoaciduria, 1910
  mutations in leprechaunism, 1900
  for parenteral solutions, 2113-2114
  protein metabolism, 1851-1852
Amino-terminal procollagen III, 2141
Amino-terminal variable domain, 1122
Aminoaciduria, 879
  dicarboxylic, 879-880
  Fanconi's syndrome, 882
  galactosemia, 1883
  neutral, 879
Aminoglutethimide
  breast cancer, 710, 711
  Cushing's disease, 1786-1787
  ectopic adrenocorticotropic hormone secretion,
    1822
  hepatic injury, 2192
Aminoglycoside-modifying enzymes, 1345
Aminoglycosides, 1355-1356
  antibacterial mechanisms, 1345
  antimicrobial mechanisms, 1344
  auditory effects, 972
  bacterial meningitis, 1411
  bacterial pneumonia after lung transplantation,
    517
  brucellosis, 1605
  cholesterol-absorption blockade, 1890-1891
  cystic fibrosis, 482
  dosage, 1349
  drug-induced lysosomopathies, 1919
  effect on vestibular function, 972
  effects on kidney, 868
  enterococci resistance, 1561
  glucose-6-phosphate dehydrogenase
    deficiency, 664
  gram-negative sepsis, 1452
  hepatic encephalopathy, 2162-2163
  infective endocarditis, 231, 232
  Meniere's disease, 2307
  mycobacterial disease, 1631
  plague, 1610
  respiratory exacerbations in cystic fibrosis, 483
  septic arthritis, 1253
  tularemia, 1608
  use during pregnancy, 2281
Aminoglycosidic aminocyclitols, 1355-1356
Aminoguanidine, 861
Aminolevulinic acid dehydrase deficiency, 1927
Aminophylline
  anaphylaxis, 1194
  asthma, 1190
  dipyridamole stress scintigraphy, 103
Aminopyrine breath test, 2143
4-Aminoquinolines, 1208
Aminorex, 477
Aminosalicylates
  Crohn's disease, 2071
  mycobacterial disease, 1631

Aminosalicylates—cont'd
  during pregnancy, 2278
  pulmonary toxicity, 479
  rheumatic disease, 1260, 1261-1262
  rheumatoid arthritis, 1208
  ulcerative colitis, 2074
5-Aminosalicylic acid
  Crohn's disease, 2071
  ulcerative colitis, 2074
Aminotransferases
  alcoholic hepatitis, 2196
  chronic hepatitis, 2180
  chronic hepatitis B, 2181
  chronic hepatitis C, 2182
  hepatitis A, 2173
  hepatitis B, 2175
  hepatocellular *versus* cholestatic jaundice,
    2156
  liver disease, 2136-2137
Amiodarone, 138
  angina, 205
  atrioventricular reciprocating tachycardia, 143
  heart failure, 174
  hepatic injury, 2192
  human cytochrome P450 isoforms, 2312
  hypertrophic obstructive cardiomyopathy, 269
  interference with oral anticoagulants, 636
  pulmonary parenchymal reactions, 476
  pulmonary toxicity, 478
  uncommon types of sustained ventricular
    tachycardia, 153
Amiodiaquine, 2191
Amitriptyline, 1037
  chronic fatigue syndrome, 2300
  human cytochrome P450 isoforms, 2312
  prophylaxis of migraine, 962
AML; *see* Acute myelogenous leukemia
Amlodipine
  heart failure, 174
  hypertension, 325
  interaction with cyclosporin, 793
  properties, 204
Ammonia
  acid-base homeostasis, 835
  acute toxic exposure, 473
  decreased synthesis, 838
  hepatic detoxification function, 2142
  hepatic encephalopathy, 1080, 2161, 2162
  hyperammonemia, 1907
  urea cycle, 1906
Ammonium
  renal acidification, 740
  urinary, 747
  urinary crystals, 746
  urine pH, 742
Ammonium chloride loading test, 747
Amnesia, 985
Amnesic syndrome, 1031-1032
Amniocentesis, 619
Amoxapine, 1037
Amoxicillin, 1352
  chlamydial infection, 1537
  dosage, 1350
  Helicobacter pylori, 1593
  hepatic injury, 2190-2192
  infective endocarditis prophylaxis, 234
  Lyme disease, 1254, 1647
  peptic ulcer disease, 2040
  sinusitis, 1183, 2309
  typhoid fever, 1601
  use during pregnancy, 2281
Amoxicillin-clavulanate
  Haemophilus ducreyi, 1589
  hepatic injury, 2191
  Pasteurella, 1609
  sinusitis, 1395
Amphetamines
  arrhythmia, 133
  interference with catecholamine assays, 1740
  narcolepsy, 943
  treatment for obesity, 2104

Amphotericin B, 1653
  amebic meningoencephalitis, 1684
  aspergillosis, 1659
  candidal infection, 1663, 1664
  coccidioidomycosis, 1254, 1474, 1657
  cryptococcosis, 1669
  effects on kidney, 869
  esophageal candidiasis, 2020
  febrile neutropenic patient, 1389
  hepatic injury, 2191
  histoplasmosis, 1474, 1655
  leishmaniasis, 1686
  lung transplantation
    aspergillosis, 520
    candidiasis, 519
    prophylaxis, 518
  meningitis
    acquired immunodeficiency syndrome
      patient, 1478
    bacterial, 1410, 1411
    cryptococcal, 1474
  zygomycosis, 1659
Ampicillin, 1352
  bacterial meningitis, 1411
  chronic obstructive pulmonary disease, 444
  diverticulosis, 2091
  dosage, 1350
  drug-induced bile duct injury, 2203
  enterococci resistance, 1561
  Haemophilus ducreyi, 1589
  Haemophilus influenzae, 1410, 1588
  hepatic injury, 2191
  infective endocarditis, 232
  intraabdominal infection, 1401
  sinusitis, 1183
  typhoid fever, 1601
Ampicillin-sulbactam
  activity against major anaerobes, 1620
  osteomyelitis, 1436
  peritonitis, 1402
Amplification assay, 1372-1373
Ampulla of Vater carcinoma, 2232
Amputation
  diabetes mellitus, 1872
  osteomyelitis, 1436
Amrinone
  dilated cardiomyopathy, 264
  hepatic injury, 2192
  shock, 182
Amygdala, 1075
Amylase
  abdominal pain, 2032
  acute pancreatitis, 2144, 2235
  hyperamylasemia, 2235
  intestinal obstruction, 2078
  macroamylasemia, 2144
  pancreatic disease, 2144
  peritonitis, 2080
  urinary, 2145
Amylase/creatinine clearance ratio, 2145
Amylo-1,6-glucosidase deficiency, 1882
Amyloid, 863
Amyloidosis, 1282-1285
  AL type, 863, 865
  alveolar, 452
  cutaneous manifestations, 1316-1317
  familial Mediterranean fever, 877
  Fanconi's syndrome, 882
  hyperkalemia, 832
  intestinal pseudoobstruction, 2079
  multiple myeloma, 701
  nephrotic syndrome, 767
  rheumatoid arthritis, 1205
Amylopectin, 1987
Amylopectinosis, 1882
Amylose, 1987
Amyotrophic lateral sclerosis, 1015
  referral, 1021
  respiratory failure, 1097
Anabolic steroids
  hepatic injury, 2190, 2191
  interference with oral anticoagulants, 636

Anaerobic bacteria
  antibiotic selection, 1348
  Bacteroides, 1613-1621
    bacteremia and endocarditis, 1618
    brain abscess, 1414
    central nervous system infections, 1617
    classification and characteristics, 1613-1614
    diagnosis, 1618-1619
    gram-negative bacteremia, 1446
    head and neck infections, 1616-1617
    intraabdominal infections, 1617-1618
    necrotic skin and soft tissue infections, 1618
    normal flora, 1368
    obstetric and gynecologic infections, 1618
    pathophysiology, 1614-1616
    pleuropulmonary infections, 1617
    prevention, 1621
    therapy, 1619-1621
  bile salt secretion, 2125
  Clostridium, 1567-1576
    bacteremia, 1576
    cellulitis, 1422
    food-borne, 1568-1570
    gas gangrene, 1422-1423
    gastrointestinal tract, 1567-1568
    hemolytic anemia, 667
    myonecrosis, 1574-1576
    neurologic syndromes, 1570-1572
    tetanus, 1572-1574
  compromised host, 1388
  enterococci, 1560-1564
    nosocomial infections, 1362
    resistance to vancomycin, 1346
  Haemophilus influenzae, 1585-1590
    acquired immunodeficiency syndrome, 1329
    antibiotic selection, 1347
    chronic bronchitis, 443
    clinical diseases, 1586-1589
    cystic fibrosis airway infection, 480
    epidemiology, 1586
    epiglottitis, 1393
    erysipelas, 1420
    meningitis, 1402-1403
    osteomyelitis, 1433
    respiratory tract infection, 1390
    septic arthritis, 1251
    sickle cell disease, 658
    sinusitis, 1183
    subdural empyema, 1417
  normal flora, 1368, 1614, 1615
  sinusitis, 1394
Anagrelide, 688
Anal fissure, 2069, 2093, Plate X-5
Anal manometry, 2055
Anal reflex, 964
Analgesics, 1259
  acute pancreatitis, 2237
  acute stone passage, 803
  cause of end-stage renal failure, 890
  chronic pancreatitis, 2240
  cystic fibrosis, 482
  gastrointestinal endoscopy, 1994
  gouty arthritis, 1274
  hepatic injury, 2191
  human cytochrome P450 isoforms, 2312
  interference with oral anticoagulants, 636
  low back pain, 967
  migraine, 961
  multiple myeloma, 702
  nephrotoxicity, 870-871
  nonopioid, 1259-1260
    acute erosive gastritis, 2041
    adult Still's disease, 1243
    analgesic-associated nephropathy, 870-871, 890
    angina, 205, 207
    arterial thromboembolism, 639
    atrial fibrillation, 148, 640, 1088
    chronic pancreatitis, 2240
    cystic fibrosis, 482
    decreased colon cancer risk, 2083

Analgesics—cont'd
  nonopioid—cont'd
    glucose-6-phosphate dehydrogenase
      deficiency, 664
    gouty arthritis, 1274
    hepatic injury, 2190, 2191
    human cytochrome P450 isoforms, 2312
    increased frequency of bleeding, 605
    induction of anaphylaxis, 1193
    influenza, 1492
    interference with oral anticoagulants, 636
    ischemic heart disease, 200
    myocardial infarction, 212, 217
    non-Q wave myocardial infarction, 218
    osteoarthritis, 1268
    pericardial heart disease, 278
    platelet aggregation studies, 570
    platelet cyclooxygenase and, 611
    poisoning, 2188-2190
    during pregnancy, 2275
    prosthetic heart valve, 258, 640
    pulmonary parenchymal reactions, 476
    pulmonary toxicity, 479
    restenosis, 124
    rheumatic diseases, 1258
    rheumatic fever, 1257
    rheumatoid arthritis, 1207
    subacute thyroiditis, 1812
    superficial thrombophlebitis, 311
    thrombotic stroke, 1004
    unstable angina, 639
  opioid
    abdominal pain, 2032
    abuse, 2297
    acute intermittent porphyria, 1926
    acute pancreatitis, 2237
    acute stone passage, 803
    cancer pain, 580, 581
    cough, 408, 409
    cytochrome P450 2D6-mediated conversion,
      2311
    effect on vasopressin release, 1791
    human cytochrome P450 isoforms, 2312
    myocardial infarction, 212, 216
    pulmonary edema, 169
    pulmonary toxicity, 479
    restless legs syndrome, 944
    sedation during gastrointestinal endoscopy,
      1994
    status migrainosus, 962
  pancreatic cancer, 2243-2244
  pericardial heart disease, 278
  portosystemic encephalopathy, 2160
  rheumatic diseases, 1259-1260
  rheumatoid arthritis, 1207
  sickle cell disease, 658
Anaphylactoid purpura, 857
Anaphylactoid reaction, 637, 1193
Anaphylatoxin, 1338
Anaphylatoxin inactivator, 1135
Anaphylaxis, 1193-1195
  epinephrine, 182
  intravenous iron dextran, 644
  transfusion, 574-575
Anaplastic astrocytoma, 1069
Anaplastic large cell lymphoma, 697
Anaplastic thyroid carcinoma, 1815-1816
Anasarca, 747
Anatomic and physiologic barriers to infection,
  1335
Anatomic substrates
  balance, 971-972
  neuroendocrine regulation, 1075
Ancrod, 635
Ancylostoma duodenale, 1698
Anderson-Fabry disease, 878
Anderson's disease, 1882, 2067
Androgens, 1741
  amenorrhea, 1759
  aplastic anemia, 674
  breast cancer, 710
  calcium homeostasis, 1720

Androgens—cont'd
  hereditary angioedema, 1180
  hirsutism, 1755-1757
  hypogonadotropic syndromes, 1841-1843
  hypopituitarism treatment, 1780
  liver failure, 2171
  metabolism, 1838-1839
  myelofibrosis, 677
  prostate cancer, 719
  puberty, 1767
Androstanediol glucuronide, 1742
Androstenedione, 1742, 1817
Anemia
  acute myelogenous leukemia, 689
  acute renal failure, 773
  amebic liver abscess, 2210
  aplastic, 671-674, 675
    failure of hematopoiesis, 533
    hematopoietic stem cell transplantation, 576
    hepatitis associated with, 2177
    nosocomial infection, 1361
  celiac sprue, 2062
  chest pain, 128
  chronic disease, 642-643
  chronic myelogenous leukemia, 686
  chronic renal failure, 783
  congenital erythropoietic porphyria, 1925
  Crohn's disease, 2070
  disseminated tuberculosis, 1635
  Fanconi's, 672
  gastric cancer, 2046
  giant-cell arteritis, 304
  glucagonoma, 2244
  Goodpasture's syndrome, 847
  hematopoietic abnormalities, 534
  hemolytic, 661-671
    acquired, 666-668
    congenital erythropoietic porphyria, 1925
    dietary factors, 2102
    drug-induced, 670
    hereditary, 662-666
    homozygous beta thalassemia, 654
    hypophosphatemia, 1936
    immune, 668-670
    Mycoplasma pneumoniae pneumonia, 1539-1540
    patient evaluation, 661-662
    risk of pigment stone formation, 2223-2224
    splenomegaly, 601
    thrombotic thrombocytopenic purpura, 615
  high-output failure, 160
  hypersplenism, 601
  infective endocarditis, 228
  intestinal disease, 2005
  iron deficiency, 642-645, 2109
    celiac sprue, 2062
    folate deficiency, 650
    Goodpasture's syndrome, 847
    hookworm infection, 1698
    intestinal disease, 2005
    peritoneal mesenteric and omental diseases, 2248
    during pregnancy, 2279
    splenomegaly, 601
    ulcerative colitis, 2073
    upper gastrointestinal endoscopy, 1994
  low hematocrit, 586
  macroglobulinemia, 704
  malabsorption, 2057
  malaria, 1673
  megaloblastic, 646-650
  multiple myeloma, 701
  myelodysplastic syndrome, 676
  myelofibrosis, 677
  neurologic aspects, 1103
  non-Hodgkin's lymphoma, 697
  nutritional deficiency, 2100
  operative risk, 2262
  osteopetrosis, 1958
  overproduction jaundice, 2152
  oxygen transport, 350

Anemia—cont'd
  pernicious
    autoantibodies, 1155
    dementia, 987
    dizziness, 972
    gastric antibodies, 1157
    gastric cancer, 2045
    hypokalemia, 827
    Lambert-Eaton myasthenic syndrome with, 1024
    neurologic aspects, 1103
    during pregnancy, 2279
    Schilling test, 2060
    type A gastritis, 2042
    vitamin B_{12} deficiency, 650
  during pregnancy, 2279
  primary hyperparathyroidism, 1966
  prosthetic heart valve, 258
  protein-calorie malnutrition, 2102
  protoporphyria, 1926
  red blood cell mass, 586
  renal cell carcinoma, 898
  sickle cell, 656-660, Plate IV-4
    acute meningitis, 1407
    arthropathy, 1246
    hypergonadotropic hypogonadism, 1843
    neurologic aspects, 1103
    renal manifestations, 891
    thrombosis, 609
  sideroblastic, 645-646
  Sjögren syndrome, 1210
  systemic lupus erythematosus, 1215
  ulcerative colitis, 2073
  Waldenström macroglobulinemia, 704
Anesthesia
  cardiopulmonary complications, 2256-2257
  hepatic injury, 2190, 2191
  nephrotoxicity, 871
  pulmonary risk factors, 2260-2261
Aneuploidy, 1727-1728
Aneurysm
  angiography, 927
  aortic, 299-300
    aortic ejection sounds, 74
    aortitis, 302
  candidal, 1663
  carotid artery, 1762
  computed tomography, 106
  coronary sinus, 291
  hemorrhagic stroke, 997-998
  involvement in polycystic kidney disease, 872
  left ventricular, 221
  Marfan syndrome, 299, 1289
  mediastinal mass, 513
  peripheral arterial, 309
  syphilitic, 1641
Angelman's syndrome, 1729
Angina, 194-196
  abdominal, 2087
  antihypertensive agent choices, 326
  continuous ambulatory electrocardiographic recording, 94
  coronary arteriography, 199-200
  coronary artery bypass graft, 206-207
  heart failure, 167
  hypertrophic obstructive cardiomyopathy, 266
  macrovascular disease, 1868
  myocardial revascularization, 205-206
  nitroglycerin and nitrates, 201, 202
  percutaneous transluminal coronary angioplasty *versus* coronary artery bypass graft, 118
  pharmacologic stress testing, 104
  systemic lupus erythematosus, 1215
Angina at rest, 126
Angina pectoris, 125-126, 195-196
  acute cholecystitis *versus,* 2228
  aortic regurgitation, 241
  aortic stenosis, 236
  mitral stenosis, 245
  pulmonic stenosis, 288
  thyroid hormone therapy-induced, 1810

Angiocentric immunoproliferative disorders, 1225
Angiodysplasia, 624
Angioedema
  drug-induced, 1315-1316
  emergency management, 2306
  losartan-induced, 327
Angiofibroma, 1922
Angiofollicular lymph node hyperplasia, 599
Angiography, 111, 112
  after valve replacement, 259
  aortic regurgitation, 242
  Budd-Chiari syndrome, 2208
  cerebral, 925-926, 927
    coma, 950
    epilepsy, 982
  cholangiocarcinoma, 2232
  hepatocellular carcinoma, 2213
  intestinal bleeding, 2007
  mitral stenosis, 248
  mitral valve prolapse, 254
  portal venous obstruction, 2209
  precapillary pulmonary hypertension, 296
  preoperative, 2257
  pulmonary, 388-389
    hepatopulmonary syndrome, 2170
    primary pulmonary hypertension, 294-295
    pulmonary thromboembolism, 502
  pulmonic stenosis, 288
  radionuclide, 104-105
  renal, 751
    chronic renal failure, 782
    renal mass, 752
    renovascular disease, 755
    renovascular hypertension, 321
  stroke, 1003
  tetralogy of Fallot, 289
  variceal bleeding, 2167
  ventricular septal defect, 284
Angioimmunoblastic lymphadenopathy, 599, 1247-1248
Angiokeratoma corporis diffusum, 878
Angiolupoid plaque, 1324
Angiomatosis, bacillary
  acquired immunodeficiency syndrome, 1474, 1477
  typical lesion, Plate VIII-40
Angiomyolipoma, 753, 899
Angiopeptin, 124
Angioplasty, 116-125
  approach to specific lesions, 120-121
  background, 116-117
  Budd-Chiari syndrome, 2208
  complications, 122
  devices, 117-120, 121
  myocardial infarction, 121-122, 214-215
  myocardial revascularization, 205-206
  pathophysiology, 116
  primary, 122, 123, 124
  randomized trials, 117, 118
  referral, 124
  rescue, 122
  restenosis, 122-124
  shock, 183
Angiosarcoma
  cardiac, 330
  drug-induced, 2189
  immunohistochemistry, 731
  incidence, 329
Angiostrongylus cantonensis, 1700, 1702
Angiostrongylus costaricensis, 1700, 1702
Angiotensin-converting enzyme, 459, 1818
Angiotensin-converting enzyme inhibitor renography, 894
Angiotensin-converting enzyme inhibitors, 832, 861-862
  chronic interstitial nephritis, 893
  congestive heart failure, 818
  congestive heart failure-associated hyponatremia, 818
  cost-utility analysis, 16
  cystinuria, 804-805

Angiotensin-converting enzyme inhibitors—cont'd
  development of chronic cough, 407
  diabetic nephropathy, 862
  diastolic heart failure, 168
  dilated cardiomyopathy, 264
  effects on sodium currents, 59
  focal glomerular sclerosis, 852
  heart failure, 160, 169-172
  hypertension, 324, 325, 327
  hypertensive emergency, 328
  hypotonic hyponatremic syndromes, 812
  induction of angioedema, 2306
  induction of cough, 477
  microvascular disease in diabetic patient, 1870
  myocardial infarction, 217
  during pregnancy, 2275
  prevention or delay of end-stage renal disease,
       782
  proteinuria, 760
  pulmonary toxicity, 479
  renovascular hypertension, 896
  restenosis, 124
  sudden death survivors, 190
  systemic sclerosis, 1232-1233
  typical medical regimen six months after
       transplantation, 343
Angiotensin I, 1818
Angiotensin II
  cardiac growth and hypertrophy, 55
  heart failure, 160, 161, 162, 817
  regulation of adrenocortical secretion,
       1817-1819
  renal acid excretion, 740
  vasoactive effects on pulmonary circulation,
       363
  vasopressin secretion, 1790
Angiotensinogen, 1818
Angle closure glaucoma, 2301
Angular cheilitis, 1311
Angular stomatitis, 2106
Anhidrosis, 935
Anhydrides, 472
Aniline dye, 548, 868
Animal dander, 1183
Animal-transmitted infection
  balantidiasis, 1690-1691
  brucellosis, 1604-1607
  echinococcosis, 2111
  histoplasmosis, 1654
  Lyme disease, 1646
  Pasteurella, 1609
  rabies, 1505-1508
  travel-related, 1465
  tularemia, 1607-1609
Anion gap, 838, 864
Anion gap acidosis, 836-837
Anions in body water compartments, 736
Anisakis, 1700, 1702
Ankle
  arthrography, 1164
  periarticular problems, 1197-1198
  rheumatoid arthritis, 1203
Ankle jerk, 964
Ankle systolic pressure, 305
Ankylosing hyperostosis of Forestier, 1168, 1170
Ankylosing spondylitis, 1238-1239
  aortitis, 302, 303
  calcium pyrophosphate dihydrate deposition
       disease *versus,* 1279
  colitis-related, 2075
  hypoventilation, 356
  interstitial lung disease, 453-454
  neurologic manifestations, 1095
  osteophytosis, 1170, 1171
  sacroiliac joint abnormalities, 1173
Ann Arbor staging of Hodgkin's disease, 694
Annular pancreas, 2246
Anomia, 975
Anomic aphasia, 976
Anorchia, 1843
Anorectal manometry, 2008

Anorexia, 2029-2030
  acute cholecystitis, 2227
  acute hyponatremia, 811
  acute viral hepatitis, 2177
  adrenal insufficiency, 1876
  appendicitis, 2092
  ascites, 2164
  benign recurrent intrahepatic cholestasis, 2158
  chronic hepatitis, 2180, 2181
  chronic renal failure, 781, 784, 786
  colon cancer, 2085
  intrahepatic cholangiocarcinoma, 2214
  neurohormonal regulation, 1077
  peritonitis, 1398
  primary hyperparathyroidism, 1967
  pyogenic liver abscess, 2209
  sarcoidosis, 458
  small intestinal malignancies, 2081
  tropical sprue, 2065
  ulcerative colitis, 2073
Anorexia nervosa, 1749, 2030
  adolescent, 1769-1770
  criteria, 2028
  hypogonadism, 1842
  protein calorie malnutrition, 2101
Anosmia, 1182
Anosodiaphoria, 1033
Anosognosia, 1033
Anserine bursitis, 1197
Antacids
  drug-nutrient interactions, 2110
  gastrointestinal bleeding, 2013
  interference with oral anticoagulants, 636
  negative phosphate balance, 1935
  typical medical regimen six months after
       transplantation, 343
Antagonistic pleiotropy, 2283
Anterior cerebral artery occlusion, 1005
Anterior circulation large-vessel occlusive
       disease, 1004-1005
Anterior cord syndrome, 1048
Anterior epistaxis, 2308
Anterior horn cell disease, 916-917
Anterior ischemic optic neuropathy, 1058-1059
Anterior lead, 83
Anterior mediastinal tumor, 512-513
Anterior nasal diphtheria, 1566
Anterior pituitary, 1773-1788
  anatomy, 1773-1774
  Cushing's disease, 1786-1787
  Cushing's syndrome, 1819-1822
    amenorrhea, 1759
    arthropathy, 1247
    cutaneous manifestations, 1323
    dexamethasone suppression test, 1737
    endocrine paraneoplastic syndromes, 583
    general appearance, 63
    hypertension, 321-322
    hypokalemia, 829
    insulin resistance, 1862
    mediastinal mass, 513
    medullary thyroid carcinoma, 1816
    obesity, 2103
    plasma cortisol levels, 1740
    screening tests, 1826
    weakness, 1754
  empty sella syndrome, 1787
  gonadotropin-secreting pituitary tumor, 1787
  growth hormone-secreting pituitary tumor,
       1782-1785
  hyperprolactinemia, 1785-1786
  hypopituitarism, 1776-1777, 1779-1781
  hypothalamic-pituitary adrenal system, 1774
  hypothalamic-pituitary axis, 1773-1774
  hypothalamic-pituitary gonadal system,
       1774-1775
  hypothalamic-pituitary growth hormone
       system, 1775
  hypothalamic-pituitary prolactin system,
       1775-1776, 1777
  hypothalamic-pituitary thyroid system, 1774

Anterior pituitary—cont'd
  pituitary apoplexy, 1777-1781
  pituitary tumor, 1781-1782
  thyroid-stimulating hormone-secreting tumor,
       1787
Anterior spinal artery myelopathy, 1012
Anthracyclines
  cardiotoxicity, 584
  pancreatic cancer, 2243
Anthralin, 1301
Anthrax, 1423
Anthropometric measurements, 2111
Anti-idiotypic networks, 1114
Anti-idiotypic response, 1114
Anti-Ro antibody, 1291
Anti-topoisomerase, 1231
Antiandrogen therapy, 1305
Antianginal agents
  achalasia, 2022
  angina, 196, 201, 202, 203
  angina pectoris, 126, 127
  aortic regurgitation, 243
  arrhythmias, 138
  atrial fibrillation, 147, 223
  autonomic dysreflexia, 1049
  chronic hypertension during pregnancy, 2275
  glaucoma, 2302
  heart failure, 170, 173-174, 818
  hepatic injury, 2192
  human cytochrome P450 isoforms, 2312
  hypertension, 325, 327
  hypertensive emergency, 328
  hypertrophic obstructive cardiomyopathy, 269
  interaction with cyclosporin, 793
  interference with catecholamine assays, 1740
  ischemic heart disease, 200-201, 202
  mitral stenosis, 248
  multifocal atrial tachycardia, 144
  myocardial infarction, 212, 216, 218
  non-Q wave myocardial infarction, 218
  primary pulmonary hypertension, 295
  properties, 204
  prophylaxis of migraine, 962
  pulmonary edema, 169
  Raynaud's phenomenon, 310, 1227
  typical medical regimen six months after
       transplantation, 343
  variceal bleeding, 2167
Antianxiety agents, 1037
  alcohol withdrawal, 1080, 2295
  anxiety disorders, 1035
  cancer pain, 580
  delirium tremens, 2295, 2296
  depression in elderly patient, 2289
  disordered thinking, 1041
  hepatic injury, 2191
  human cytochrome P450 isoforms, 2312
  interference with oral anticoagulants, 636
  muscle spasm in tetanus, 1573
  for nausea and vomiting, 2027
  preeclampsia, 2275
  prophylaxis of migraine, 962
  sedation during gastrointestinal endoscopy,
       1994
  spasticity, 997
    after spinal cord injury, 1051
  status epilepticus, 982, 983
Antiarrhythmics, 134-139
  angina, 203, 205, 207
  aortic regurgitation, 243
  arrhythmia, 138
  arrhythmias, 138
  atrial fibrillation, 147, 223
  atrial flutter, 144, 146
  atrioventricular reciprocating tachycardia, 143
  before cardiac transplantation, 336
  cluster headache prophylaxis, 962
  constrictive pericarditis, 279
  dilated cardiomyopathy, 264
  drug-induced bile duct injury, 2203
  effects of magnesium deficiency, 1942

Antiarrhythmics—cont'd
effects on sodium currents, 59
glucose-6-phosphate dehydrogenase
deficiency, 664
heart failure, 170, 173, 174
hepatic injury, 2192
human cytochrome P450 isoforms, 2312
hypertension, 325
hypertensive emergency, 328
hypertrophic obstructive cardiomyopathy, 269
interaction with calcium channel blockers, 204
interaction with cyclosporin, 793
interference with catecholamine assays, 1740
interference with oral anticoagulants, 636
malaria, 1674-1675
multifocal atrial tachycardia, 144
myocardial infarction, 217
pharmacokinetics, 137
premature ventricular contractions, 149
properties, 203, 204
prophylaxis of migraine, 962
pulmonary parenchymal reactions, 476
pulmonary toxicity, 478
sudden death survivor, 189-191
sustained ventricular tachycardia and wide
QRS complex tachycardia, 150
uncommon types of sustained ventricular
tachycardia, 153
ventricular tachyarrhythmia, 223, 224
Wolff-Parkinson-White syndrome, 142
Antiasthmatics
asthma, 1190, 1191, 1192
Cheyne-Stokes respiration, 354
chronic obstructive pulmonary disease, 434,
444
with acute respiratory failure, 417
human cytochrome P450 isoforms, 2312
hyperkalemia, 833
pertussis, 1613
during pregnancy, 2277
rhinitis, 1182, 1183
Antibacterial agents; *see* Antibiotics
Antibiotics, 1343-1361
acne vulgaris, 1305
actinomycosis, 1665
activity against major anaerobes, 1620
acute epiglottitis, 1393
acute infectious exacerbations of chronic
obstructive pulmonary disease, 434
acute otitis media, 1395
acute pancreatitis, 2237
allergy, 1194
amebiasis, 1683
amebic liver abscess, 2210
aminoglycosidic aminocyclitols, 1355-1356
anaerobic bacteria, 1619-1620
antimicrobial combinations, 1360
antimicrobial mechanisms, 1344
aplastic anemia, 672
asthma, 1191
babesiosis, 1676
bacillary angiomatosis, 1474
bacterial meningitis, 1410-1412
bacterial overgrowth, 2062
bacterial peritonitis, 1400-1402
bacterial pneumonia after lung transplantation,
517
bacterial prostatitis, 1463
bacterial vaginosis, 1443
bactericidal effect, 1344
balantidiasis, 1691
beta-lactams, 1355
brain abscess, 1415-1416
brucellosis, 1605, 1606
Campylobacter enteritis, 1592
campylobacteriosis, 1432
cellulitis, 1420
cephalosporins, 1352-1355
chlamydial infection, 1537
choice of appropriate agent, 1346-1351
choledocholithiasis, 2229

Antibiotics—cont'd
cholera, 1596
chronic obstructive pulmonary disease, 444
with respiratory failure, 418
clostridial infection, 1576
Clostridium difficile colitis, 1569, 1570
coagulase-negative staphylococcal infection,
1552
compromised host, 1388
Crohn's disease, 2072
cystic fibrosis, 482
dermal infection, 1424
dermatitis-aggravating *Staphylococcus aureus*
infection, 1303
Dientamoeba fragilis, 1691
diphtheria, 1567
diverticulosis, 2091-2092
dosage, 1349, 1350
drug-induced bile duct injury, 2203
drug-nutrient interactions, 2110
effect on vestibular function, 972
effects on kidney, 868
endocarditis, 231
enterococci resistance, 1561
erysipelas, 1420
erythrasma, 1422
erythromycin and clindamycin, 1357
evaluation of response, 1360
Fanconi's syndrome induction, 882
furuncle, 1421
generation of alkalosis, 840
giardiasis, 1685
glucose-6-phosphate dehydrogenase
deficiency, 664
gonorrhea, 1584, 1585
gram-negative bacteremia, 1452, 1453
gram-negative sepsis, 1452
Haemophilus ducreyi, 1589
Haemophilus influenzae, 1588
Helicobacter pylori, 1593
hepatic encephalopathy, 2162
hepatic injury, 2190-2192
human cytochrome P450 isoforms, 2312
iliac crest biopsy, 1747
induction of acute interstitial nephritis, 889
infectious eczematoid dermatitis, 1304
infective endocarditis, 230-233
infective endocarditis prophylaxis, 234
interaction with cyclosporin, 793
interference with oral anticoagulants, 636
intestinal pseudoobstruction, 2079
intraabdominal infection, 1401
Legionella pneumophila, 1624
leptospirosis, 1645
liver abscess, 2209-2210
Lyme disease, 1254, 1647-1648
macrolides, 1357-1358
measurement of bone formation, 1949
mechanism of resistance, 1345
mechanisms of antimicrobial action,
1343-1345
mechanisms of antimicrobial resistance,
1345-1346
meningococcal disease, 1580
metronidazole, 1358-1359
mycobacterial disease, 1631
Mycoplasma hominis infection, 1541
Mycoplasma pneumoniae pneumonia, 1540
non-group A streptococcal infection,
1563-1564
nonvenereal treponematosis, 1644
osteomyelitis, 1435, 1436
Pasteurella, 1609
penicillins, 1351-1352
peptic ulcer disease, 2040
peritonitis, 1402
pertussis, 1613
pill esophagitis, 2019
plague, 1610
platelet dysfunction caused by, 612
Pneumocystis carinii pneumonia, 1694

Antibiotics—cont'd
polymyxins, 1358
portosystemic encephalopathy, 2162
prophylaxis for traveler's diarrhea, 1432
prophylaxis in lung transplantation, 518
prosthetic valve endocarditis, 230-233
pulmonary parenchymal reactions, 476
quinolone antibiotics, 1359
reaction with antiarrhythmics, 136-137
relapsing fever, 1646
renal effects, 868-869
resistance of *Staphylococcus aureus,* 1345
respiratory exacerbations in cystic fibrosis,
483
rheumatic fever, 1258
rhinitis, 1183
rickettsial infection, 1545
septic arthritis, 1253
shigellosis, 1603
sinusitis, 1183, 1395, 2309
spinal epidural abscess, 1418
spontaneous bacterial peritonitis, 2164
staphylococcal infection, 1551
Staphylococcus epidermidis, 1552
streptococcal pharyngitis, 1393
streptococcal resistance, 1559-1560
structural formula, 1351
subdural empyema, 1418
sulfonamides and trimethoprim, 1358
syphilis, 1643
tetanus, 1574
tetracyclines and chloramphenicol, 1356-1357
toxoplasmosis, 1474, 1678
trichomoniasis, 1441, 1443, 1691
tropical sprue, 2065
tularemia, 1608
typhoid fever, 1432, 1601
urethritis, 1441
urinary tract antiseptics, 1359-1360
use during pregnancy, 2281
vancomycin, 1358
vitamin K deficiency, 626
Whipple's disease, 2065
wound botulism, 1572
Yersinia enterocolitica, 1605
Antibodies to liver/kidney microsome type 1
autoimmune hepatitis, 2184
hepatobiliary disease, 2139
Antibody, 1110, 1121-1126
acute nephritic syndrome, 764
adrenocortical, 1157
anti-Ro, 1291
anticardiolipin, 629, 1160
anticentromere, 1293
antiepithelial cell, 1218
antierythrocyte, 668
antiglomerular basement membrane, 842, 843
disease, 454
rapidly progressive glomerulonephritis,
846-849
antiidiotype, 1146
antiinsulin, 1861-1862
antilymphocyte
for recurrent rejection, 341
renal transplantation, 792
antimitochondrial
hepatobiliary disease, 2139
primary biliary cirrhosis, 2139, 2199
antineutrophil, 847-849, 1160
acute glomerulonephritis, 771
crescentic glomerulonephritis, 847
Kawasaki's disease, 1219
primary sclerosing cholangitis, 2202
vasculitis, 1218-1219
Wegener's granulomatosis, 858, 1219, 1223
antinuclear, 1158-1160
hepatobiliary disease, 2139
primary biliary cirrhosis, 2199
progressive systemic sclerosis, 1159-1160
Raynaud's phenomenon, 1227
Sjögren syndrome, 1209, 1210-1211

Antibody—cont'd
  antinuclear—cont'd
    systemic lupus erythematosus, 1212, 1216
    systemic sclerosis, 1231
    type 1 autoimmune hepatitis, 2183
  antiphospholipid
    syndrome, 1093, 1292
    venous thrombosis, 311
  antiplatelet, 558
  antithyroglobulin, 1738-1739
  antithyroid, 1801
  antithyroid peroxidase, 1738-1739
  antitreponemal, 1642
  autoantibody, 1155-1160
    Addison's disease, 1155
    autoimmune hemolytic anemia, 1155
    autoimmune hepatitis, 2183
    bullous pemphigoid, 1155
    chronic active hepatitis, 1155
    diffuse toxic goiter, 1155
    drug-induced immune hemolytic anemia,
      670
    enzyme-linked immunosorbent assay, 1156
    Goodpasture's syndrome, 1155
    Graves' disease, 1155
    Hashimoto's thyroiditis, 1155
    idiopathic thrombocytopenic purpura, 1155
    immune complex formation, 842
    immunofluorescence, 1156
    inflammatory myopathies, 1235, 1236-1237
    interpretation of serum tests, 1156-1157
    Lambert-Eaton myasthenic syndrome, 1075
    myasthenia gravis, 1155
    myoclonus, 1075
    neurologic paraneoplastic syndromes, 1075
    opsoclonus, 1075
    pemphigus vulgaris, 1155
    pernicious anemia, 1155
    polymyositis, 1143, 1155
    primary antiphospholipid antibody
      syndrome, 1155
    primary biliary cirrhosis, 1155
    retinal degeneration, 1075
    rheumatoid arthritis, 1155
    rheumatoid factor, 1160-1161
    Sjögren syndrome, 1155
    systemic lupus erythematosus, 1155
    systemic sclerosis, 1231
    vasculitis, 1155
    vitiligo, 1155
    Wegener's granulomatosis, 468
  autoimmune disease laboratory tests, 1156
  autoimmune hypoparathyroidism, 1931
  B-cell response, 1110
  barrier to infection, 1335
  Campylobacter, 1590
  cardiac muscle, 1157
  cardiolipin, 629
  centromere/kinetochore, 1159
  Cryptococcus neoformans, 1667
  cytoskeletal, 1158
  deficiency syndromes, 1175-1176
  deoxyribonucleic acid, 1158-1159
  Donath-Landsteiner
    autoimmune hemolytic anemia, 668
    paroxysmal cold hemoglobinuria, 670
  enzyme-linked immunosorbent assay, 1372
  fluorescent treponemal antibody-absorption
    test, 1642
  gamma globulin, 1020, 1021
  gastric, 1157
  gene rearrangement, 1125-1126
  genetics, 1121-1126
  glomerular diseases, 841-843
  Goodpasture's syndrome, 847
  hemophilia A, 620
  hepatobiliary disease, 2139-2140
  histone, 1159
  Hu, 1158
  human immunodeficiency virus, 1533
  human T-cell leukemia virus type 1, 1532

Antibody—cont'd
  hypergammaglobulinemia of chronic liver
    disease, 2136
  hypersensitivity pneumonitis, 461
  immediate hypersensitivity, 1139
  immunoassay, 1733-1734
  immunoglobulin A, 1110, 1122-1123
    within alpha-granules, 536
    barrier to infection, 1335
    biclonal gammopathy, 705
    Bordetella pertussis, 1612-1613
    in bronchoalveolar lavage fluid, 367
    Campylobacter infection, 1590-1591
    deficiency, 1176, 1991-1993
    influenza antibody, 1487
    liver disease, 2135-2136
    Mediterranean lymphoma, 2080
    nephropathy, 845, 877
    nephrotic syndrome, 765
    pemphigus, 1295
    Peyer's patch B-cells, 1990
    plasma cells in lamina propria, 1990
    properties and distribution, 1336
    secretory, 1990-1993
    small bowel secretion, 2060
    systemic lupus erythematosus, 1216
  immunoglobulin D, 1110, 1123, 1336
  immunoglobulin E, 1110, 1123
    anaphylaxis, 1193
    asthma, 1188
    in bronchoalveolar lavage fluid, 367
    Churg-Strauss syndrome, 465
    drug eruption, 1313
    food allergy, 1993
    immediate-type hypersensitivity reaction,
      1139
    in vitro assay, 1154
    intestinal immunity, 1990-1991
    occupational asthma, 471
    parasite-induced eosinophilia, 1705
    properties and distribution, 1336
  immunoglobulin G, 1110, 1122
    within alpha-granules, 536
    barrier to infection, 1335
    biclonal gammopathy, 705
    Bordetella pertussis, 1612-1613
    in bronchoalveolar lavage fluid, 367
    brucellosis, 1606
    Campylobacter infection, 1590
    Coccidioides immitis, 1657
    Graves' disease, 1805
    Haemophilus influenzae infection, 1587
    immune thrombocytopenic purpura, 616
    Lyme disease, 1646-1647
    membranoproliferative glomerulonephritis,
      854
    membranous nephropathy, 853
    myasthenia gravis, 1021
    nephrotic syndrome, 765
    parvovirus B19 infection, 1514
    properties and distribution, 1336
    respiratory defense, 366
    rheumatoid arthritis, 1201
    rheumatoid factors, 1160
    schematic diagram, 1122
    thyroid-stimulating hormone receptor
      antibody, 1801
    toxoplasmosis, 1678
    transient hypogammaglobulinemia of
      infancy, 1176
    warm-reacting antibody hemolytic anemia,
      668-669
  immunoglobulin M, 1110, 1122
    barrier to infection, 1335
    biclonal gammopathy, 705
    Bordetella pertussis, 1612-1613
    in bronchoalveolar lavage fluid, 367
    brucellosis, 1606
    Campylobacter infection, 1590
    Coccidioides immitis, 1657
    cold agglutinin disease, 669-670

Antibody—cont'd
  immunoglobulin M—cont'd
    cytomegalovirus, 1528
    hepatitis A, 2173
    hyper-immunoglobulin M syndrome, 1176,
      1343
    Lyme disease, 1646
    nephrotic syndrome, 765
    parvovirus B19 infection, 1513
    properties and distribution, 1336-1337
    rheumatoid arthritis, 1201
    rheumatoid factor, 1160-1161
    systemic lupus erythematosus, 1216
    toxoplasmosis, 1678
    Waldenström macroglobulinemia, 703-704,
      865
  immunology, 1121-1126
  indirect immunofluorescence assays,
    1373-1374
  influenza, 1487
  insulin resistance, 1861
  islet cell, 1158
  Lyme disease, 1646-1647
  mechanisms contributing to diversity,
    1124-1125
  mitochondrial, 1157
  monoclonal, 565
    cancer treatment, 555
    cardiac transplantation, 1090
    evaluation of cellular immune function,
      1151
    gram-negative infection, 1454
    gram-negative sepsis, 1453
    multiple myeloma, 701
    renal transplantation, 792
  mouse monoclonal antihuman T lymphocyte,
    523
  myasthenia gravis, 1020, 1021, 1022
  Mycoplasma pneumoniae, 1540
  myelin, 1158
  pancreatic islet cell, 1158
  parainfluenza, 1495
  paraneoplastic syndromes, 1158
  pemphigoid, 1295
  phospholipids, 1160
  precipitating, 461
  properties and distribution, 1336-1337
  rabies, 1506
  radioimmunoassays and enzyme
    immunoassays, 1374
  reticulin, 1157-1158
  Sjögren syndrome, 1209, 1210-1211
  skin, 1158
  smooth muscle, 1157, 2200
    hepatobiliary disease, 2139
    type 1 autoimmune hepatitis, 2183
  striated-muscle, 1157
  structure, 1122-1123
  subacute cutaneous lupus erythematosus, 1291
  thyroglobulin, 1157
  thyroid, 1157
    Hashimoto's thyroiditis, 1811
    hypothyroidism, 1809
  thyroid-stimulating hormone receptor, 1801
  toxoplasmosis, 1678
  tubulointerstitial renal disease, 889
  type A gastritis, 2042
  vasculitis, 1218-1219
  warm, 668
  Western blotting, 52
  Yo, 1158
Antibody-dependent cellular cytotoxicity, 1153
Antibody genes, 1123-1126
Anticardiolipin antibody, 1160
  lupus inhibitor, 629
Anticardiolipin lupus anticoagulant, 1292
Anticentromere antibody, 1293
Anticholinergic agents
  asthma, 1191, 1192
  chronic obstructive pulmonary disease, 444
    with acute respiratory failure, 417

Anticholinergic agents—cont'd
dystonia, 995
irritable bowel syndrome, 2056
multiple sclerosis, 1010
rhinitis, 1183
vasodepressor syncope, 956
Anticholinesterase, 2302
Anticholinesterase agents
Lambert-Eaton myasthenic syndrome, 1024
myasthenia gravis, 1022
Anticipation, 1726
Anticipatory vomiting, 582
Anticoagulation therapy
acute aortic obstruction, 304
after myocardial infarction, 639
angina, 205, 207
arterial thromboembolism, 639
atrial fibrillation, 147-148, 640, 1088
Budd-Chiari syndrome, 2219
during cardiac catheterization, 108
coronary stenting, 120
deep vein thrombosis, 311, 504
dilated cardiomyopathy, 264
disseminated intravascular coagulation, 628
drug-induced immune thrombocytopenia, 615-616
fulminant hepatic failure, 2163
heart failure, 174-175
human cytochrome P450 isoforms, 2312
hyperkalemia, 832
hypertrophic obstructive cardiomyopathy, 269
left ventricular thrombus, 221
mast cell, 1142
mitral stenosis, 248
myocardial infarction, 212, 217
non-Q wave myocardial infarction, 218
during pregnancy, 2276
primary pulmonary hypertension, 295
prosthetic heart valve, 258, 640
prothrombin time, 571
pulmonary thromboembolism, 503
recurrent embolism, 641
reocclusion of infarct-related vessel, 214
restenosis, 124
thrombotic stroke, 1004
unstable angina, 639
venous thromboembolism, 311, 632-638
Anticonvulsants, 982-984
antidepressant effects, 479
anxiety disorders, 1035
brain tumor, 1072
cluster headache prophylaxis, 962
diabetes insipidus, 1797
drug-induced bile duct injury, 2203
euthyroid hypothyroxinemia, 1804
glucose-6-phosphate dehydrogenase deficiency, 664
hepatic injury, 2186, 2190, 2191
human cytochrome P450 isoforms, 2312
induction of osteomalacia, 1953
interaction with cyclosporin, 793
interference with oral anticoagulants, 636
during pregnancy, 2281
prophylaxis of migraine, 962
pulmonary hypersensitivity reactions, 479
pulmonary parenchymal reactions, 476
pulmonary toxicity, 479
restless legs syndrome, 944
serum bilirubin levels, 2154
spasticity after spinal cord injury, 1051
status epilepticus, 983
supratentorial brain abscess, 1416
vasopressin inhibition, 1791
Antidepressants, 1037
anxiety disorders, 1035
cancer pain, 580
chronic fatigue syndrome, 2300
cocaine intoxication, 2297
depression in elderly patient, 2289
human cytochrome P450 isoforms, 2312
interference with oral anticoagulants, 636

Antidepressants—cont'd
irritable bowel syndrome, 2056
prophylaxis of migraine, 962
Antidiabetic agents
diabetes insipidus, 1796
diabetes mellitus, 1858
hepatic injury, 2191
human cytochrome P450 isoforms, 2312
Antidiarrheals
Crohn's disease, 2071
diarrhea, 1431-1432
irritable bowel syndrome, 2056
Antidiuretic hormone
aging and, 2284
biochemistry, 1788-1789
congestive heart failure, 817
deficiency, 1777
diabetes insipidus, 883, 1793-1795
diverticular bleeding, 2092
gastrointestinal bleeding, 2012-2013
heart failure, 160, 161
hypopituitarism treatment, 1781
increase after nausea induction, 2025
nephrogenic diabetes insipidus, 883
physiology, 1789-1793
pituitary stimulation tests, 1736
plasma, 1737-1738
variceal bleeding, 2167
vasoactive effects on pulmonary circulation, 363
water balance, 739
Antidote
heparin, 635
oral anticoagulants, 637
thrombolytic therapy, 638
Antidromic atrioventricular reciprocating tachycardia, 144
Antidromic tachycardia, 142
Antiemetics, 962
Antiepileptics, 982-984
anticonvulsant-induced osteomalacia, 1953
antidepressant effects, 479
diabetes insipidus, 1797
drug-induced bile duct injury, 2203
euthyroid hypothyroxinemia, 1804
glucose-6-phosphate dehydrogenase deficiency, 664
hepatic injury, 2186, 2190, 2191
human cytochrome P450 isoforms, 2312
interaction with cyclosporin, 793
interference with oral anticoagulants, 636
during pregnancy, 2281
pulmonary hypersensitivity reactions, 479
pulmonary parenchymal reactions, 476
pulmonary toxicity, 479
serum bilirubin levels, 2154
status epilepticus, 983
supratentorial brain abscess, 1416
vasopressin inhibition, 1791
Antiepiligrin cicatricial pemphigoid, 1296
Antiepithelial cell antibody, 1218
Antierythrocyte antibody, 668
Antiestrogens
breast cancer, 710
endometrial cancer, 714
fibrocystic breast disease, 1850
medication-induced hypercalcemia, 1928
Antifreeze, 866
Antifungal agents, 1652-1654
amebic meningoencephalitis, 1684
aspergillosis, 1659
candidal infection, 1663, 1664
after lung transplantation, 519
esophageal, 2020
vulvovaginal, 1442
coccidioidomycosis, 1254, 1474, 1657
cryptococcosis, 1669
Cushing's disease, 1786
ectopic adrenocorticotropic hormone secretion, 1821-1822
effects on kidney, 869

Antifungal agents—cont'd
febrile neutropenic patient, 1389
hepatic injury, 2191
histoplasmosis, 1474, 1655
human cytochrome P450 isoforms, 2312
interaction with cyclosporin, 793
interference with oral anticoagulants, 636
leishmaniasis, 1686
lung transplantation
aspergillosis, 520
candidiasis, 519
prophylaxis, 518
meningitis
acquired immunodeficiency syndrome patient, 1478
bacterial, 1411
cryptococcal, 1474
otomycosis, 2307
paracoccidioidomycosis, 1657
pityriasis versicolor, 1309-1310
renal effects, 869
superficial fungal infections, 1309
therapeutic drug interactions, 2310
tinea unguium, 1311
trichomoniasis, 1443
typical medical regimen six months after transplantation, 343
zygomycosis, 1659
Antigen, 1111-1112
activation of mast cells and basophils, 1140
autoantigen, 1142
basic immunology, 1174-1175
binding, 1110-1111
CA125, 716
carbohydrate antigen 19-9, 2202
carcinoembryonic
cholangiocarcinoma, 2202
colon cancer, 2085
gastric cancer, 2047
intrahepatic cholangiocarcinoma, 2215
competitive binding assays, 1372
cryptococcal, 1477-1478
CTLA-4, 1145
development of rash, 1380-1381
epithelial membrane, 731
extractable nuclear, 1159
factor VIII procoagulant, 618
Giardia lamblia, 1685
hepatitis A, 2173
hepatitis B e, 2138, 2174
human leukocyte, 1115-1121
celiac disease, 2062
epidermolysis bullosa acquista, 1296
genetics, 1115-1118
Hodgkin's disease, 691
Lyme disease, 1254
primary biliary cirrhosis, 2199, 2201
psoriasis, 1300
role in disease, 1120-1121
sarcoidosis, 457
tissue distribution, structure, and function, 1118-1120
typing, 1120
human lymphocyte, 1111
hypersensitivity pneumonitis, 460
hypersensitivity vasculitis, 1221
immediate-type hypersensitivity reaction, 1139
immunologic memory, 1108
Jo-1, 1159
K, 1456
Langerhans' cell granulomatosis, 463
leukocyte common, 731
lymphocyte activation, 1114
microbial, 1336
pemphigus vulgaris, 1293
polysaccharide, 1446
processing, 1111-1112
HLA molecules, 1119-1120
presentation to lymphocyte, 596
proliferating cell nuclear, 1159
prostate-specific, 553, 717

Antigen—cont'd
  radioimmunoassays and enzyme
    immunoassays, 1374
  scl-70, 1159
  skin tests, 1153
  smooth-muscle, 1157
  SS-A/Ro, 1159
  SS-B/La, 1159
  subepithelial immune complex deposits, 842
  superantigen, 1127
    bacterial, 1112
    streptococcal, 1555
    systemic tolerance, 1143
  systemic lupus erythematosus, 1142-1143
  thyroid microsomal, 1157
  von Willebrand's factor, 618
Antigen challenge, 379, 462
Antigen-presenting cell, 368, 1111-1112, 1126
Antigen receptor, 1127
Antigen-receptor homology motif 1, 1174, 1175
Antigen-recognition activation motif, 1174, 1175
Antigenic drift, 1484
Antigenic shift, 1484
Antiglobulin test, 587
Antiglomerular basement membrane antibody,
    842, 843, 846-849
Antiglomerular basement membrane antibody
    disease, 454
Antiglomerular basement membrane
    glomerulonephritis, 847
Antigout agents
  alcoholic hepatitis, 2198
  calcium pyrophosphate dihydrate deposition
    disease, 1278
  drug-nutrient interactions, 2110
  familial Mediterranean fever, 877, 1243
  glucose-6-phosphate dehydrogenase
    deficiency, 664
  gouty arthritis, 1274-1275
  hepatic injury, 2191
  leishmaniasis, 1686
  multiple myeloma, 702
  pericardial heart disease, 278
  pericarditis, 221
  primary biliary cirrhosis, 2200
  pulmonary parenchymal reactions, 476
  reactive amyloidosis, 1283
  tophaceous gout, 1275
  uric acid stones, 804
Antihelmintics
  echinococcal cyst, 2212
  Enterocytozoon bieneusi, 1474
  intestinal helminths, 1697, 1698
  microsporidiosis, 1679, 1681
  Strongyloides stercoralis, 1699
  tissue nematode infection, 1700
  whipworm, 1696
  Wuchereria bancrofti, 1699
Antihistamines
  anaphylaxis, 1194
  angioedema, 2306
  antiemesis, 2027, 2028
  asthma, 1191
  chronic rhinitis, 2308
  dermatomyositis, 1292
  glucose-6-phosphate dehydrogenase
    deficiency, 664
  human cytochrome P450 isoforms, 2312
  rhinitis, 1182
  sinusitis, 2309
Antihypertensives, 324, 325
  aortic regurgitation, 243
  autonomic dysreflexia, 1049
  bleeding varices, 2168
  chronic hypertension during pregnancy, 2275
  cystinuria, 804-805
  diabetic nephropathy, 861, 862
  diabetic retinopathy, 861
  dilated cardiomyopathy, 264
  drug-induced bile duct injury, 2203
  drug-induced immune hemolytic anemia, 670
  drug-nutrient interactions, 2110

Antihypertensives—cont'd
  elderly patient, 327
  glaucoma, 2302
  heart failure, 170, 172, 173-174, 818
  hepatic injury, 2192
  hepatocellular jaundice, 2192
  hot flashes, 2271
  human cytochrome P450 isoforms, 2312
  hypertension, 325, 327
  hypertensive emergency, 328
  increased intracranial pressure, 1084
  interaction with nonsteroidal antiinflammatory
    drugs, 322
  interference with catecholamine assays, 1740
  interference with oral anticoagulants, 636
  myocardial infarction, 217
  opiate detoxification, 2297
  pheochromocytoma, 322, 1830
  preeclampsia, 2275
  properties, 203
  pulmonary toxicity, 479
  renovascular hypertension, 896
  spasticity after spinal cord injury, 1051
  testing for growth hormone reserve, 1775
  typical medical regimen six months after
    transplantation, 343
  urge incontinence, 2293
Antihyperuricemic therapy, 1274
Antiidiotype antibody, 1146
Antiinfective therapy, 1343-1361; *see also*
    Antibiotics
  aminoglycosidic aminocyclitols, 1355-1356
  antimicrobial combinations, 1360
  beta-lactams, 1355
  cephalosporins, 1352-1355
  choice of appropriate agent, 1346-1351
  compromised host, 1388
  erythromycin and clindamycin, 1357
  evaluation of response, 1360
  macrolides, 1357-1358
  mechanisms of antimicrobial action,
    1343-1345
  mechanisms of antimicrobial resistance,
    1345-1346
  metronidazole, 1358-1359
  penicillins, 1351-1352
  polymyxins, 1358
  quinolone antibiotics, 1359
  sulfonamides and trimethoprim, 1358
  tetracyclines and chloramphenicol, 1356-1357
  urinary tract antiseptics, 1359-1360
  vancomycin, 1358
Antiinflammatory drugs
  Crohn's disease, 2071
  gout, 1274
  nonsteroidal
    ankylosing spondylitis, 1239
    asthma induction, 1187
    cancer pain, 580
    chronic fatigue syndrome, 2300
    decreased colon cancer risk, 2083
    fever of unknown origin, 1380
    focal glomerular sclerosis, 852
    gastric ulcer induction, 2036, 2037
    gouty arthritis, 1274
    hepatic injury, 2190
    induction of acute interstitial nephritis, 889
    induction of bronchospasm, 477
    inhibition of platelet cyclooxygenase, 611
    interaction with antihypertensives, 322
    low back pain, 966
    neck pain, 971
    nephrotoxicity, 853, 870-871
    osteoarthritis, 1267-1268
    pericardial heart disease, 278
    pericarditis, 221
    pulmonary parenchymal reactions, 476
    pulmonary toxicity, 479
    rheumatic diseases, 1258-1259
    rheumatoid arthritis, 1207
    systemic lupus erythematosus, 1216
  sarcoidosis, 459

Antiinsulin antibody, 1861-1862
Antilymphoblast globin, 1090
Antilymphocyte antibody
  for recurrent rejection, 341
  renal transplantation, 792
Antimalarial agents
  rheumatic disease, 1261
  rheumatoid arthritis, 1208
  systemic lupus erythematosus, 1217
Antimanic agents
  associated goiter, 1809
  cluster headache prophylaxis, 962
  dilated cardiomyopathy, 265
  disordered thinking, 1041
  mania, 1038
  medication-induced hypercalcemia, 1928
  role in Ebstein's anomaly, 280, 289
Antimetabolites, 869
Antimicrobial combinations, 1360
Antimicrobial resistance, 1345-1346
  chemotherapeutic drugs, 554
  enterococci, 1346, 1561
  Neisseria gonorrhoeae, 1582
  Neisseria meningitidis, 1579, 1582
  nosocomial infection, 1363
  Salmonella typhi, 1601
  staphylococci, 1345
  streptococci, 1559-1560
  tumor response to drug treatment, 552
Antimicrobial susceptibility testing, 1346
  anaerobic bacteria, 1619-1621
  tuberculosis, 1632
Antimicrobial therapy, 1343-1361; *see also*
    Antibiotics
  aminoglycosidic aminocyclitols, 1355-1356
  antimicrobial combinations, 1360
  bacterial meningitis, 1410-1412
  beta-lactams, 1355
  brucellosis, 1606-1607
  cephalosporins, 1352-1355
  choice of appropriate agent, 1346-1351
  clostridial infection, 1576
  compromised host, 1388-1389
  erythromycin and clindamycin, 1357
  evaluation of response, 1360
  gram-negative bacteremia, 1452, 1453
  Haemophilus influenzae, 1588
  Helicobacter pylori, 1593
  hepatic injury, 2191
  infective endocarditis, 230-233
  liver abscess, 2209-2210
  macrolides, 1357-1358
  mechanisms of antimicrobial action, 1343-1345
  mechanisms of antimicrobial resistance,
    1345-1346
  metronidazole, 1358-1359
  penicillins, 1351-1352
  polymyxins, 1358
  prosthetic valve endocarditis, 230-233
  pulmonary parenchymal reactions, 476
  quinolone antibiotics, 1359
  sulfonamides and trimethoprim, 1358
  tetracyclines and chloramphenicol, 1356-1357
  typhoid fever, 1601
  urinary tract antiseptics, 1359-1360
  urinary tract infection, 1459
  vancomycin, 1358
  Yersinia enterocolitica, 1611
Antimitochondrial antibody
  hepatobiliary disease, 2139
  primary biliary cirrhosis, 2199
Antimonials, 2191
Antimony, 867
Antineoplastic agents
  breast cancer, 710
  effects on kidney, 869
  gastric cancer, 2048
  hepatic injury, 2192
  pancreatic cancer, 2243
  pulmonary parenchymal reactions, 476
  pulmonary toxicity, 478
  renal effects, 869-870

Antineutrophil cytoplasmic antibody, 847-849, 1160
  acute glomerulonephritis, 771
  vasculitis, 1218-1219
  Wegener's granulomatosis, 858, 1223
Antinuclear antibody, 1158-1160
  hepatobiliary disease, 2139
  primary biliary cirrhosis, 2199
  Raynaud's phenomenon, 1227
  Sjögren syndrome, 1209, 1210-1211
  systemic lupus erythematosus, 1212, 1216
  systemic sclerosis, 1231
  type 1 autoimmune hepatitis, 2183
Antiparkinsonian agents, 992
  acromegaly, 1784-1785
  cocaine intoxication, 2297
  fibrocystic breast disease, 1850
  gonadotropin-secreting pituitary tumor, 1787
  hepatic encephalopathy, 2161
  hyperprolactinemia, 1786
  interaction with cyclosporin, 793
  Parkinson's disease, 991, 992
  prolactinoma, 1759
  restless legs syndrome, 944
  schizophrenia, 1042
  use during pregnancy, 2274
Antiperistaltic contractions, 1977
Antiphospholipid antibody
  syndrome, 1093, 1292
  venous thrombosis, 311
Antiplatelet agents
  arterial thromboembolism, 639
  coronary stenting, 120
Antiplatelet antibody, 558
Antiprotozoal agents
  African trypanosomiasis, 1689
  leishmaniasis, 1686
  Pneumocystis carinii pneumonia, 1694, 1695
  renal effects, 869
  secretion clearance and lung expansion, 430
Antipsychotics
  disordered thinking, 1041
  drug-induced lysosomopathies, 1919
  hepatic injury, 2186, 2190, 2191
  human cytochrome P450 isoforms, 2312
  interference with catecholamine assays, 1740
  for nausea and vomiting, 2027
  pituitary stimulation tests, 1736
  schizophrenia, 1042
  status migrainosus, 962
  vasopressin inhibition, 1791
Antipyrine clearance test, 2143-2144
Antiretroviral therapy, 1473
Antirheumatic drugs, 1258-1263
  analgesics, 1259-1260
  disease-modifying antirheumatic drugs, 1260-1262
  glucocorticoids, 1262-1263
  nonsteroidal antiinflammatory drugs, 1258-1259
Antisecretory agents
  gastroesophageal reflux, 2018
  gastrointestinal bleeding, 2013
Antiseptics, urinary tract, 1359-1360
  antibacterial mechanism, 1345
  enterococcal infection, 1563
  hemolysis in glucose-6-phosphate dehydrogenase deficiency, 663
  hepatic injury, 2191
  interference with catecholamine assays, 1740
  pulmonary parenchymal reactions, 476
  pulmonary toxicity, 478
  use during pregnancy, 2281
Antiserum, gram-negative sepsis, 1453
Antispastics, 997, 1055
  hepatic injury, 2191
  multiple sclerosis, 1009
  spasticity after spinal cord injury, 1051
Antistreptolysin O titer, 1555
  acute glomerulonephritis, 771
  rheumatic fever, 1257
Antithrombin assay, 572

Antithrombin III, 538, 539
  disseminated intravascular coagulation, 628
  gram-negative infection, 1454
  inactivation of coagulation factors, 539
  inhibition of fibrin formation, 535
  shock states, 176
  thrombosis, 609
  venous thromboembolism, 631
Antithrombosis therapy
  activation of plasminogen to plasmin, 540
  angina, 205
  angioplasty after, 121-122
  atrial fibrillation, 640
  cardiac catheterization in ischemic heart disease, 113
  cost-utility analysis, 16
  deep venous thrombosis, 311
  myocardial infarction, 212-214
  primary angioplasty *versus,* 122, 123
  pulmonary embolism, 503
  shock, 182-183, 184, 185
  venous thromboembolism, 632, 637
Antithymocyte globulin
  aplastic anemia, 672, 674
  OKT3-induced meningitis, 1090
Antithyroglobulin antibody, 1738-1739
Antithyroid antibody, 1801
Antithyroid peroxidase antibody, 1738-1739
Antitoxin
  botulinum, 1571
  diphtheria, 1567
  gas gangrene, 1576
  tetanus, 1573
Antituberculosis agents, 1630-1633
  acquired immunodeficiency syndrome, 1473, 1474
  antimicrobial mechanisms, 1344
  bacterial meningitis, 1411
  brucellosis, 1605, 1606
  drug-nutrient interactions, 2110
  effects on kidney, 868
  glucose-6-phosphate dehydrogenase deficiency, 664
  Haemophilus influenzae, 1589
  hepatic injury, 2190-2192
  human cytochrome P450 isoforms, 2312
  infective endocarditis, 231, 232
  interaction with cyclosporin, 793
  interference with oral anticoagulants, 636
  leprosy, 1651
  meningococcal disease, 1580
  mycobacterial disease, 1631
  prevention of tuberculosis, 1637
  prophylaxis in lung transplantation, 518
  silicosis with positive tuberculin reaction, 475
  Staphylococcus epidermidis, 1552
Antitumor antibiotics
  effects on kidney, 869
  pulmonary toxicity, 584
Antitussive drugs, 408
Antiulcer agents
  gastroesophageal reflux, 2018
  hepatic injury, 2192
  human cytochrome P450 isoforms, 2312
  interference with oral anticoagulants, 636
  peptic ulcer disease, 2040
  reaction with antiarrhythmics, 135-136
  typical medical regimen six months after transplantation, 343
Antiviral agents
  acquired immunodeficiency syndrome, 1474
  chronic hepatitis B, 2182
  disordered thinking, 1041
  facial nerve paralysis, 2306
  hepatic injury, 2191
  herpes zoster ophthalmicus, 2305
  herpesvirus infections, 1526
    after marrow transplantation, 578-579
    esophagitis, 2020
    herpes simplex virus, 1524-1525
  influenza, 1492
  Parkinson's disease, 992

Antiviral agents—cont'd
  prophylactic
    compromised host, 1390
    lung transplantation, 518
  renal effects, 869
  varicella and zoster, 1527
Anton's syndrome, 1033
Antral gastritis, 2042
Antrum
  chronic gastritis, 2042
  movement of food, 1978
  stomach, 1981
Anuria
  acute tubular necrosis, 772
  obstructive uropathy, 886
  retroperitoneal fibrosis, 2250
Anus
  fissure and fistula, 2093
  hemorrhoids, 2092-2093
  manifestations of acquired immunodeficiency syndrome, 2098
Anxiety, 1034-1035
  autonomic overactivity, 934
  chest pain, 129
  chronic fatigue syndrome, 2299
  dyspnea, 432, 437
  hyperventilation, 355
  hypoglycemia, 1875
  hypoglycemic coma, 1867
  palpitations, 130, 131
  pancreatic cancer, 2242
  pheochromocytoma, 1829
  thyrotoxicosis, 1804
Anxiolytics, 1037
  alcohol withdrawal, 1080, 2295
  anxiety disorders, 1035
  cancer pain, 580
  delirium tremens, 2295, 2296
  depression in elderly patient, 2289
  disordered thinking, 1041
  hepatic injury, 2191
  human cytochrome P450 isoforms, 2312
  interference with oral anticoagulants, 636
  muscle spasm in tetanus, 1573
  for nausea and vomiting, 2027
  preeclampsia, 2275
  prophylaxis of migraine, 962
  sedation during gastrointestinal endoscopy, 1994
  spasticity, 997
    after spinal cord injury, 1051
  status epilepticus, 982, 983
Aorta
  aberrant right subclavian artery, 291
  angiography, 111
  coarctation, 286-287
  diseases, 299-304
    aortic aneurysm, 299-300
    aortitis, 302-303
    atherosclerosis, 299
    dissection of aorta, 300-302, 303
    Marfan syndrome, 299
    mycotic aneurysm, 299, 300
    occlusive disease, 304
    syphilis, 303
  hemodynamic data, 110
  magnetic resonance imaging, 389
  Takayasu's arteritis, 1224
  trauma, 304
  traumatic rupture, 333
Aortic aneurysm, 299-300
  aortic ejection sounds, 74
  aortitis, 302
Aortic arch, 299
Aortic baroreceptors, 162
Aortic dissection
  aortic regurgitation, 244
  chest pain, 128
  transesophageal echocardiography, 97
Aortic ejection sounds, 74
Aortic isthmus, 299
Aortic pressure, 299

Aortic regurgitation, 239-245
  ankylosing spondylitis, 303
  aortic dissection, 300
  aortic ejection sounds, 74
  Austin Flint murmur, 79
  bicuspid aortic valve, 287
  cardiac auscultation, 68
  cardiac catheterization, 113-114
  chest pain, 128
  differential diagnosis, 180
  dissection of aorta, 301
  Doppler image, Plate II-3
  Marfan syndrome, 299
  pandiastolic murmur, 79-80
  during pregnancy, 2276
  pulsus bisferiens, 65
  rheumatic fever, 1256
  Takayasu's arteritis, 311
  ventricular septal defect with, 285
Aortic root angiography, 113, 114
Aortic stenosis, 235-239
  angina, 127
  aortitis, 302
  cardiac auscultation, 68
  cardiac catheterization, 113
  congenital, 287
  differential diagnosis, 180
  mesenteric vascular disease, 2086
  murmur, 79-80
  pandiastolic murmur, 79-80
  pulsus bisferiens, 65
  second heart sound, 72
Aortic valve area, 111
Aortic valve disease
  bicuspid aortic valve, 287
  passive pulmonary hypertension, 298
Aortic valvular ejection sounds, 74
Aortitis, 302-303
Aorto-enteric fistula, 2010
Aortography
  acute aortic obstruction, 304
  coarctation of aorta, 286
  coronary arteriovenous fistula, 292
  dissection of aorta, 301, 302
  patent ductus arteriosus, 286
  peripheral arterial aneurysm, 309
  ventricular septal defect with aortic
      regurgitation, 285
Aortopulmonary septal defect, 286
APC tumor suppressor, 547
Apex phonocardiogram, 69, 70
Aphasia, 975-977
Aphasic agraphia, 978
Aphasic alexia, 978
Aphemia, 977
Apheresis, 574
Aphonia, 977
Aphthous ulcer, 2309
  Crohn's disease, 2069, Plate X-6, Plate X-10
  human immunodeficiency virus, 2095
Apical approach in echocardiography, 95
Apical impulse
  coarctation of aorta, 286
  ischemic heart disease, 197
Apical lead, 83
Apical movements, 67
Aplasia
  bone marrow
    acute myelogenous leukemia, 690
    megakaryocytic hypoplasia, 614
  pure red blood cell, 674-675
  pure white blood cell, 675
Aplastic anemia, 671-674, 675
  failure of hematopoiesis, 533
  hematopoietic stem cell transplantation, 576
  hepatitis associated with, 2177
  nosocomial infection, 1361
Aplastic crisis, 657
  hereditary spherocytosis, 664
  parvovirus B19 infection, 1513

Apnea, 524-525
  Cheyne-Stokes respiration, 354
  posthyperventilation, 1097
  sleep apnea syndrome, 354-355
  testing for brain death, 951
Apneustic breathing, 1098
Apocrine glands, 933
Apolipoprotein A, 1285, 1897
Apolipoprotein B, 1897
Apolipoprotein C, 1898
Apolipoprotein E, 1897-1898
Apolipoproteins, 1885
  atherosclerosis, 60
  nephrotic syndrome, 766
  synthesis abnormalities, 1897
Apomorphine
  effect on vasopressin release, 1791
  pituitary stimulation tests, 1736
Apoplexy, pituitary, 1777-1781
Apoproteins, 1885
Apoptosis, 1112
  autoimmunity and, 1144-1145
  role of protooncogene products, 542-543
Appendectomy, 2092
Appendicitis, 2092
  acute cholecystitis *versus,* 2228
  omental torsion *versus,* 2252
Appendicular skeleton, 1164-1169
Appetite
  anorexia, 2029
  Cushing's syndrome, 1820
  thyrotoxicosis, 1804
Apraclonidine, 2302
Apraxia of gait, 973
Apraxia of gaze, 1033
Apraxic agraphia, 978
Apresoline; *see* Hydralazine
Aprindin, 2192
Aprosodia, 1033
Aprosody, 977
Aptitude tests, 903
Aquaporin-2, 808
Arachidonic acid
  inflammatory response, 1448
  nonsteroidal antiinflammatory drugs and, 1258
  oxidation products, 1140
Arbovirus, 1465, 1514-1519
Arbutamine stress testing, 104
ARC; *see* Acquired immunodeficiency
          syndrome-related complex
Arcanobacterium haemolyticum, 1566
ARDS; *see* Acute respiratory distress syndrome
Area-counts technique, 104
Areflexic bladder, 1050
Arenavirus, 1508-1511
Arfonad; *see* Trimethaphan
Argentaffinoma, 2081
Argentinian hemorrhagic fever, 1511
Arginase, 1906
Arginine
  hyperargininemia, 1907
  pituitary stimulation tests, 1736
  related diseases, 1904
  testing for growth hormone reserve, 1775
Arginine hydrochloride, 831
Arginine vasopressin
  control of, 808
  heart failure, 162
  osmoregulatory system, 807
  renal response, 808-809
  renal retention of acquired water, 806
Argininosuccinate lyase, 1906
Argininosuccinate synthetase, 1906
Argininosuccinic aciduria, 1907
Arginisuccinic acid, 1904
Argyria, 1313
Arias' syndrome, 2152, 2153
Arimidex, 710, 711
Arm circumference, 2111
Arm muscle circumference, 2111
Aromatase inhibitors, 710, 711

Aromatic amino acids, 1981
Arousal disorders, 945-946
Arrhythmia, 131-156
  abnormal jugular venous pulse, 66
  accelerated idioventricular rhythm, 149, 150,
      223
  antiarrhythmics, 134-139
    angina, 203, 205, 207
    aortic regurgitation, 243
    arrhythmia, 138
    arrhythmias, 138
    atrial fibrillation, 147, 223
    atrial flutter, 144, 146
    atrioventricular reciprocating tachycardia,
        143
    before cardiac transplantation, 336
    cluster headache prophylaxis, 962
    constrictive pericarditis, 279
    dilated cardiomyopathy, 264
    drug-induced bile duct injury, 2203
    effects of magnesium deficiency, 1942
    effects on sodium currents, 59
    glucose-6-phosphate dehydrogenase
        deficiency, 664
    heart failure, 170, 173, 174
    hepatic injury, 2192
    human cytochrome P450 isoforms, 2312
    hypertension, 325
    hypertensive emergency, 328
    hypertrophic obstructive cardiomyopathy,
        269
    interaction with calcium channel blockers,
        204
    interaction with cyclosporin, 793
    interference with catecholamine assays,
        1740
    interference with oral anticoagulants, 636
    malaria, 1674-1675
    multifocal atrial tachycardia, 144
    myocardial infarction, 217
    pharmacokinetics, 137
    premature ventricular contractions, 149
    properties, 203, 204
    prophylaxis of migraine, 962
    pulmonary parenchymal reactions, 476
    pulmonary toxicity, 478
    sudden death survivor, 189-191
    sustained ventricular tachycardia and wide
        QRS complex tachycardia, 150
    uncommon types of sustained ventricular
        tachycardia, 153
    ventricular tachyarrhythmia, 223, 224
    Wolff-Parkinson-White syndrome, 142
  atrial tachycardia
    ectopic, 143-144, 146
    multifocal, 144, 146
    response to carotid sinus massage or
        intravenous adenosine, 134
  bradycardia, 153-156
    calcium channel blocker-induced, 205
    hypothyroidism, 334, 1809
    Legionnaire's disease, 1623
    myocardial infarction, 222
    postinfarction, 223
    sinus, 153-154, 155
    torsades de pointes, 151-152
  during cardiac catheterization, 108
  cardiogenic syncope, 954
  continuous ambulatory electrocardiographic
      recording, 94
  dilated cardiomyopathy, 264
  hypertrophic obstructive cardiomyopathy, 266,
      269
  hypokalemia, 829
  intraventricular conduction abnormalities, 156
  magnesium deficiency, 1942
  mitral valve prolapse, 254
  myocardial abnormalities in neurologic
      disease, 1087
  myocardial contusion, 332
  neurologic aspects, 1088

Arrhythmia—cont'd
  nonpharmacologic therapy, 139-140
  operative risk, 2258-2260
  palpitation *versus,* 130-131
  pathophysiology, 131-134
  pharmacologic therapy, 134-139
  during pregnancy, 2276
  sinus tachycardia, 141
    dilated cardiomyopathy, 264
    increased automaticity, 132
    myocardial infarction, 223
    palpitations, 130
    response to carotid sinus massage or
        intravenous adenosine, 134
    restrictive cardiomyopathy, 270-271
  supraventricular tachycardia, 141-148
    accelerated atrioventricular junctional
        rhythm, 144
    atrial fibrillation, 146-148
    atrial flutter, 144-146
    atrioventricular nodal reentrant tachycardia,
        141-142, 144, 145
    ectopic atrial tachycardia, 143-144, 146
    mitral valve prolapse, 254
    multifocal atrial tachycardia, 144, 146
    palpitations, 130
    premature atrial contractions, 141
    sinus tachycardia, 141
    supraventricular tachyarrhythmias, 141, 142,
        143
    Wolff-Parkinson-White syndrome, 142-143,
        145
  tachycardia
    acute mitral regurgitation, 252
    acute pancreatitis, 2234
    aortic regurgitation, 244
    atrioventricular nodal reentrant, 134,
        141-142, 144, 145
    atrioventricular reciprocating, 142-143, 145
    gas gangrene, 1423, 1575
    hypoglycemia, 1875
    hypoglycemic coma, 1867
    mitral valve prolapse, 254
    murmur, 76
    myocarditis, 262
    pacemaker-mediated, 139
    pulmonary thromboembolism, 500
    thyrotoxicosis, 1804
  tachycardia-bradycardia syndrome, 154, 155,
        954
  ventricular, 148-153
    accelerated idioventricular rhythm, 149, 150
    automatic implantable cardioverter
        defibrillator, 140
    cardiogenic syncope, 954
    complication of pulmonary artery
        catheterization, 395
    fibrillation, 153
    hypertrophic obstructive cardiomyopathy,
        269
    mitral valve prolapse, 254
    myocardial infarction, 180, 223
    nonsustained ventricular tachycardia, 149
    palpitations, 130
    polymorphic, 151-153
    polymorphic ventricular tachycardia,
        151-153
    premature ventricular contractions, 148-149
    response to carotid sinus massage or
        intravenous adenosine, 134
    sudden death, 187
    sustained monomorphic ventricular
        tachycardia, 150-151
    sustained ventricular tachycardia with wide
        QRS complex tachycardia, 149-150,
        151
Arsenic, 867
  basal cell carcinoma, 1297
  carcinogenesis, 548
  sensorimotor neuropathy, 1020
  sideroblastic anemia, 645

Arsenic hydride, 668
Arsine, 867
Arsine hydride, 668
Arterial blood gases
  acid-base imbalances, 840
  acquired immunodeficiency syndrome, 1477
  acute respiratory failure, 412
  asthma, 1189
  chronic obstructive pulmonary disease, 442
  effect of ventilation, 353
  effects of oxygen breathing, 352
  mechanical ventilation, 397
  Pneumocystis carinii pneumonia, 1694
  primary pulmonary hypertension, 294
  pulmonary artery catheterization, 391
  pulmonary edema, 425
  pulmonary thromboembolism, 501
Arterial carbon dioxide tension, 349-350
  acute respiratory failure, 412
  Cheyne-Stokes breathing, 354
  chronic obstructive pulmonary disease, 446
  before lung resection, 497
  ventilatory control studies, 378
Arterial diameter, 46
Arterial hypertension; *see* Hypertension
Arterial occlusion
  basilar, 973
  continuous murmur, 81
  embolectomy, 307-308
  reocclusion of infarct-related vessel, 214
  retinal artery, 1058
Arterial pulses, 64-65, 66, 67
Arterial supply
  adrenal gland, 1817
  anterior pituitary, 1773
  pancreas, 2130
  peritoneum, 2247
  posterior pituitary, 1788
  respiratory muscle endurance and fatigue, 358
Arterial thromboembolism, 638-641, 766
Arteriography
  abdominal, 2033-2034
  brain tumor, 1068
  chronic occlusive arterial disease, 308
  coronary, 111
    aortic stenosis, 287
    cardiac catheterization with, 108, 109
    congenital abnormalities of coronary
        arteries, 291
    congenital coronary arteriovenous fistula,
        292
    heart failure, 167
    ischemic heart disease, 113
    mitral regurgitation, 251
    mitral stenosis, 248
    mitral valve prolapse, 254
    myocardial ischemia, 199-200
    sudden cardiac survivor, 188
    transplant donor, 339
    ventricular septal defect, 284
  gastrointestinal bleeding, 2012
  hepatic, 2140-2141
  insulinoma, 2244
  mesenteric, 2087
  before parathyroid surgery, 1970
  renal
    renal artery stenosis, 895
    renal cell carcinoma, 898
    renal mass, 752
  temporal arteritis, 311
Arteriolosclerosis, 2303
Arteriosclerosis, 64
Arteriovenous fistula
  continuous murmur, 81
  pulmonary, 499
  pulmonary angiogram, 388
Arteriovenous malformation
  dural, 928
  hemorrhagic stroke, 998
Arteriovenous nicking in hypertension, Plate
        XI-3

Arteriovenous oxygen difference
  hemodynamic data, 110
  pulmonary artery catheterization, 391
Arteriovenous shunt, 2014
Arteritis
  giant cell, 304, 311, 959, 1223-1224
    anterior ischemic optic neuropathy, 1059
    fever of unknown origin, 1378
    glucocorticoid protocol, 1263
    neurologic manifestations, 1092
  polyarteritis nodosa, 334, 856, 1219-1220
    crescentic glomerulonephritis, 848
    diffuse immune-complex vasculitis, 454
    glucocorticoid protocol, 1263
    microscopic, 1220-1221
    neurologic manifestations, 1092, 1095
  Takayasu's, 311, 470-471, 1224
    aortic obstruction and inflammation,
        303-304
    neurologic manifestations, 1092, 1095
  temporal, 311, 959, 1223-1224
    anterior ischemic optic neuropathy, 1059
    glucocorticoid protocol, 1263
    neurologic manifestations, 1092
Arthralgia
  colitis-related, 2075
  endocarditis, 227
  Lassa fever, 1510
  mixed cryoglobulinemia, 1249
  myxoma, 330
  parvovirus B19 infection, 1513
  rubella, 1501
  Whipple's disease, 2064
Arthritis
  acute meningitis, 1407
  antirheumatic drugs, 1258-1263
    analgesics, 1259-1260
    disease-modifying antirheumatic drugs,
        1260-1262
    glucocorticoids, 1262-1263
    nonsteroidal antiinflammatory drugs,
        1258-1259
  calcium oxalate arthropathy, 1280
  calcium pyrophosphate dihydrate deposition
        disease, 1276-1279
  chest discomfort, 129
  chronic hepatitis, 2180
  coccidioidomycosis, 1656-1657
  colitis-related, 2075
  endocarditis, 227
  enteropathic, 1242
  evaluation of joint complaints, 1198-1200
  gouty, 1271-1272
    joint space narrowing, 1166
    osseous erosions, 1167-1168
    soft tissue swelling, 1165
  imaging evaluation, 1164-1174
    advanced methods, 1173
    appendicular skeleton, 1164-1169
    axial skeleton, 1169-1171, 1172
    foot, 1172
    hand, 1171-1172
    hip, 1173
    knee, 1172-1173
    sacroiliac joint, 1172, 1173
    techniques and modalities, 1064
    wrist, 1172
  infectious, 1250-1256
  Lyme disease, 1647
  Milwaukee shoulder/knee syndrome,
        1279-1280
  mumps complication, 1496
  osteoarthritis, 1199, 1264-1268
    glucocorticoid protocol, 1263
    hand, 1171
    joint space narrowing, 1166, 1167
    knee, 1172-1173
    wrist, 1172
  Paget's disease, 1957
  parvovirus B19 infection, 1513

Arthritis—cont'd
polyarthritis, 1198, 1199-1200, 1245
acute pancreatitis, 2237
septic, 1250-1251
systemic lupus erythematosus, 1214
systemic sclerosis, 1229
Yersinia enterocolitica, 1611
pseudorheumatoid, 1279
psoriatic, 1240-1242
reactive, 1239-1240
relapsing polychondritis, 1243
rheumatic fever, 1256
rheumatoid, 1200-1209
aortitis, 303
atlantoaxial subluxation, 1171, 1172
autoantibodies, 1155
cardiac involvement, 334
course and prognosis, 1205-1206
diagnosis, 1206
differential diagnosis, 1206
extraarticular manifestations, 1202, 1203-1205
glucocorticoid protocol, 1263
gold salt-induced pulmonary disease, 478
interstitial lung disease, 453
intervertebral disk space narrowing, 1169-1170
laboratory findings, 1205
lymphocytosis of large granular lymphocytes, 679
management, 1206-1209
neurologic manifestations, 1093-1095
pericarditis, 272-273
pleural effusion, 508
radiologic findings, 1205
soft tissue swelling, 1165
synovial effusion, 1163
septic, 1250-1251
Haemophilus influenzae, 1588
Neisseria meningitidis, 1579
reactive arthritis *versus,* 1240
Staphylococcus aureus, 1549
Whipple's disease, 2064
Yersinia enterocolitica, 1611
Arthrocentesis, 1161
Arthrography
evaluation of arthritis, 1164
rheumatoid arthritis, 1203
Arthropathy
adult Still's disease, 1243
Behçet disease, 1243
calcium oxalate, 1280
coagulation disorders, 1246
endocrine diseases, 1246-1247
familial Mediterranean fever, 1242-1244
foreign body synovitis, 1244
hyperlipoproteinemia, 1245
inflammatory bowel disease, 1245-1246
intermittent hydroarthrosis, 1244
malignancy, 1247-1248
Milwaukee shoulder/knee syndrome, 1279-1280
multicentric reticulohistiocytosis, 1245
neurologic disorders, 1247
osteonecrosis, 1244
palindromic rheumatism, 1243-1244
panniculitis, 1245
pigmented villonodular synovitis, 1244-1245
relapsing polychondritis, 1243
relapsing seronegative symmetric synovitis with pitting edema, 1243
sarcoidosis, 1245
sickle cell disease, 1246
Whipple's disease, 1246
Arthropod-borne infection
Lyme disease, 1646
viral, 1514-1519
Arthus's reaction, 1138
Articular cartilage
calcium pyrophosphate dihydrate crystals, 1277

Articular cartilage—cont'd
osteoarthritis, 1265
rheumatoid arthritis, 1201-1202
urate crystals, 1271
Artificial airway, 416-417
Artificial kidney, 789
Artificial tears, 1211-1212
Aryl hydrocarbon hydroxylase, 486
Asbestos, 473-474
carcinogenesis, 548
mesothelioma, 510, 2249
pleural effusion, 508
Asbestosis, 474
Ascaris lumbricoides, 1698
brown pigment stones, 2224
peritonitis, 2248
Ascending aorta, 111, 299
Aschoff body, 1256
Aschoff nodule, 235, 245
Ascites
alcoholic hepatitis, 2198
Budd-Chiari syndrome, 2208
cancer
gastric, 2046
hepatocellular carcinoma, 2213
pancreatic, 2242
chronic pancreatitis, 2241
cirrhosis, 818
constrictive pericarditis, 277
creatinine clearance, 747
galactosemia, 1883
gastrointestinal tuberculosis, 1636
grades of liver disease severity, 2166
heart failure, 165
hereditary fructose intolerance, 1880
laparoscopy, 2141
liver failure, 2163-2165
peritoneal mesenteric and omental diseases, 2248
peritonitis, 2080
portal hypertension, 2165
primary biliary cirrhosis, 2200
pseudomyxoma peritonei, 2249
uremic serositis, 784
varicose veins, 311
Ascorbic acid
beta-thalassemia, 656
biochemical function, 2105
cystinosis, 1910
deficiency, 2107
glucose-6-phosphate dehydrogenase deficiency, 664
megadoses and toxicity, 2108
recommended daily dietary allowances, 2115
ASD; *see* Atrial septal defect
Aseptic meningitis, 1409, 1488
Aseptic peritonitis, 2248-2249
Ash leaf spots, 1922
Asherman's syndrome, 1760
Ashman phenomenon, 147
Asparaginase
effects on kidney, 870
hepatic injury, 2192
Asparagine, 1904
Aspartate aminotransferase
acetaminophen poisoning, 2190
acute pancreatitis, 2236
chronic hepatitis, 2180
hepatitic injury, 2136
myocardial infarction, 211
toxic hepatic injury, 2188
Aspartic acid, 1904
Aspartylglycosaminuria, 1917
Aspergillus, 1658-1659
azole antifungals, 1654
bronchiectasis, 484
compromised host, 1388
fever, 1387
hypersensitivity pneumonitis, 460
meningitis, 1404
normal flora, 1368

Aspergillus—cont'd
otomycosis, 2307
posttransplant infection
heart, 1090
lung, 520
serodiagnosis, 1653
sinusitis, 2308
Asphyxia
obstructive sleep apnea, 525
sleep-disordered breathing events, 524
Aspiration, 1998-1999
abnormal swallowing, 1998
achalasia, 2022
amebic liver abscess, 2210
esophageal disease, 1998-1999
synovial fluid, 1161
transtracheal, 385
upper gastrointestinal endoscopy, 1995
vomiting consequence, 2028
Aspiration pneumonia, Plate VIII-7
Aspirin
acute erosive gastritis, 2041
adult Still's disease, 1243
analgesic-associated nephropathy, 870-871
angina, 205, 207
arterial thromboembolism, 639
atrial fibrillation, 148, 640, 1088
decreased colon cancer risk, 2083
glucose-6-phosphate dehydrogenase deficiency, 664
hepatic injury, 2190
increased frequency of bleeding, 605
induction of anaphylaxis, 1193
influenza, 1492
interference with oral anticoagulants, 636
ischemic heart disease, 200
myocardial infarction, 212, 217
non-Q wave myocardial infarction, 218
pericardial heart disease, 278
platelet aggregation studies, 570
platelet cyclooxygenase and, 611
during pregnancy, 2275
prosthetic heart valve, 258, 640
pulmonary parenchymal reactions, 476
pulmonary toxicity, 479
restenosis, 124
rheumatic diseases, 1258
rheumatic fever, 1257
rheumatoid arthritis, 1207
subacute thyroiditis, 1812
superficial thrombophlebitis, 311
thrombotic stroke, 1004
unstable angina, 639
Aspirin idiosyncrasy, 1181
Asplenic patient, 602
Assay
amplification, 1372-1373
catecholamines, 938
Clostridium difficile toxin, 1431
coagulation factor, 571
competitive binding, 1372
complement, 1339
fixation, 1373
presence of immune complex, 1149
total hemolytic, 1147-1148
enzyme immunoassay, 1372
adenovirus, 1504
infectious disease, 1373-1374
Legionella pneumophila, 1623
Norwalk virus, 1522
rotavirus, 1521
enzyme-linked immunosorbent assay
Bordetella pertussis, 1612-1613
Borrelia burgdorferi, 1647
brucellosis, 1606
Cryptococcus neoformans, 1668
detection of autoantibodies, 1156
Helicobacter pylori, 1592-1593
hepatitis C, 2175-2176
human immunodeficiency virus infection, 1472

Assay—cont'd
  enzyme-linked immunosorbent assay—cont'd
    Lassa fever virus, 1510
    measles, 1499
    mumps, 1497
    septic arthritis, 1252
    serum total thyroxine and triiodothyronine
      levels, 1800
    toxoplasmosis, 1678
    venous thromboembolism, 632
  immune complex, 1149
  immunofluorescence, 1152, 1371, 1373-1374
    Alport's syndrome, 877
    babesiosis, 1676
    Borrelia burgdorferi, 1647
    detection of autoantibodies, 1156
    focal glomerular sclerosis, 852
    glomerulonephritis, 842
    human immunodeficiency virus, 1472
    idiopathic nephrotic syndrome, 850
    immune complex detection, 1149
    infectious disease, 1373-1374
    Legionella pneumophila, 1623
    mumps, 1497
    poststreptococcal glomerulonephritis,
      843-844
    rapidly progressive glomerulonephritis,
      848
    Rocky Mountain spotted fever, 1544
    toxoplasmosis, 1678
  immunometric, 1734
  lipopolysaccharide, 1450
  lymphocyte cytotoxicity, 1152
  monocyte-macrophage, 1153
  parathyroid hormone, 1968-1969
  radioimmunoassay, 1372
    albumin excretion, 761
    brucellosis, 1606
    detection of autoantibodies, 1156
    infectious disease, 1373-1374
    microalbuminuria, 743
    paper disk, 1154
    parathyroid hormone, 1745-1746
    principles, 1733-1734
    thyroid hormone, 1738
  recombinant immunoblot, 2138
  ribonuclease protection, 53-54
  ristocetin-cofactor, 569-570
  stem cell, 531
Assessment of Treatment with Lisinopril and
  Survival, 171
Assist/control ventilation, 397
Asteatotic dermatitis, 1303
Astemizole
  human cytochrome P450 isoforms, 2312
  rhinitis, 1182
Asterixis, 2160
Asteroid body, 1324
Asthma, 1185-1193
  Churg-Strauss syndrome, 465
  clinical manifestations, 1187-1188
  cough, 406
  diagnosis and differential diagnosis, 1189
  epidemiology and pathology, 1185
  heart failure *versus,* 168
  laboratory findings, 1188-1189
  management, 1189-1192
  occupational, 471-472, 473
  operative risk, 2261
  pathophysiology, 1185-1187
  patterns of pulmonary function abnormalities,
    379
  physical findings, 403
  during pregnancy, 2276-2277
  prognosis, 1192-1193
  pulmonary rehabilitation, 432-437
  sputum expectoration, 408
  wheezing, 404
Astrocytoma, 925, 1069
Asymmetric apical hypertrophy, 265

Asymptomatic illness
  bacteriuria, 1461
  brucellosis, 1605
  gallstones, 2225
Atabrine; *see* Quinacrine
Ataxia
  acute ethanol intoxication, 1080
  cerebrotendinous xanthomatosis, 1898
  complication of chemotherapy, 1072
  Crigler-Najjar syndrome, 2153
  Friedreich's, 1088
  megaloblastic anemia, 648
  multiple sclerosis, 1055
Ataxia-telangiectasia, 549
  autosomal recessive immunodeficiency, 1178
  cutaneous changes and malignancy, 1319
Ataxic breathing, 1098
Ataxic dysarthria, 977
Atelectasis
  physical findings, 403
  pulmonary embolism, 501, 632
  secretion clearance and lung expansion,
    429-430
Atenolol
  elderly patient, 327
  hypertension, 325
  interference with oral anticoagulants, 636
  properties, 203
ATG; *see* Antithymocyte globulin
Atheroembolism, 308
  abdominal aortic aneurysm, 309
  renal, 897
Atherosclerosis
  abdominal aortic aneurysm, 300
  aortic disease, 299
  apolipoproteins, 60
  cardiac catheterization, 107
  cerebrotendinous xanthomatosis, 1898
  chronic occlusive arterial disease, 308
  disorder in apolipoprotein A metabolism, 1897
  femoral pulses, 64
  interventional cardiac catheterization, 116-125
    approach to specific lesions, 120-121
    background, 116-117
    complications, 122
    coronary angioplasty for acute myocardial
      infarction, 121-122
    devices, 117-120, 121
    pathophysiology, 116
    primary coronary angioplasty, 122
    randomized trials, 117, 118
    referral, 124
    rescue coronary angioplasty, 122
    restenosis, 122-124
  ischemic heart disease, 192, 193
  ischemic stroke, 998-1000
  lipoproteins, 60, 1888-1889
  peripheral arterial aneurysm, 309
  peripheral artery disease, 305
  renal artery stenosis, 894
  renovascular disease, 755
  rheumatoid arthritis, 334
  thrombus formation, 638
Atherosclerotic plaque, 195, 1888
Atherosclerotic renovascular disease, 896
Athetoid movements, 2161
Athlete's foot, 1308
Athyreotic cretinism, 1809
Atlantoaxial subluxation, 1171, 1172
ATLAS survival trial, 171
ATN; *see* Acute tubular necrosis
Atonia, 942
Atopic dermatitis, 1302-1303
Atorvastatin, 1891
Atovaquone, 1694
ATP; *see* Adenosine triphosphate
Atresia
  biliary
    liver transplantation, 2219
    portal triad lesions, 2155
  tricuspid, 291

Atrial depolarization, 83-84
Atrial enlargement, 88
Atrial fibrillation, 146-148
  anticoagulant therapy, 639-640
  atrioventricular reciprocating tachycardia, 142
  calcium channel blockers, 138
  constrictive pericarditis, 277
  diastolic filling murmur, 78
  flecainide, 138
  mitral regurgitation, 251
  mitral stenosis, 245, 246
  myocardial infarction, 223
  neurologic aspects, 1088
  occlusive mesenteric vascular disease, 2087
  palpitations, 130
  risk of stroke, 1001
  SPAF study, 134
  thyrotoxicosis, 1804
  tricuspid regurgitation, 256
Atrial flutter, 144-146
  calcium channel blockers, 138
  flecainide, 138
  palpitations, 130
  response to carotid sinus massage or
    intravenous adenosine, 134
Atrial gallop, 74
Atrial myxoma, 78, 330
Atrial natriuretic peptide, 55
  heart failure, 160, 161, 162, 166
  hypertension, 317-318
  sodium balance, 738
  sodium retention in cirrhosis, 819-820
Atrial premature beats
  myocardial infarction, 223
  during pregnancy, 2276
Atrial septal defect, 280-282
  atrial fibrillation, 146
  Ebstein's anomaly, 289
  precapillary pulmonary hypertension, 296-297
Atrial tachycardia
  palpitations, 130
  response to carotid sinus massage or
    intravenous adenosine, 134
Atrioventricular block, 153-156
  atrial fibrillation, 148
  during cardiac catheterization, 108
  cardiogenic syncope, 954
  myocardial infarction, 222-223
  myocarditis, 263
  pacemaker, 139
  palpitations, 130
  paroxysmal atrial tachycardia, 143
  rheumatic fever, 1257
  right ventricular infarction, 220
  supraventricular tachyarrhythmias, 141
Atrioventricular canal defect, 282-283
Atrioventricular fistula, 160
Atrioventricular nodal artery, 132
Atrioventricular nodal reentrant tachycardia,
    141-142, 144, 145
  myocardial infarction, 223
  response to carotid sinus massage or
    intravenous adenosine, 134
Atrioventricular node, 131-132
  accelerated atrioventricular junctional rhythm,
    144
  accessory pathways, 90
  automatic implantable cardioverter
    defibrillator, 140
  cardiac cycle, 36
  conduction disturbance in myocardial
    infarction, 222
  reentrant circuit, 133
Atrioventricular reciprocating tachycardia,
    142-143, 145
Atrioventricular valve
  diastolic murmur, 78-79, 80
  opening snap, 74-75
  restrictive cardiomyopathy, 270
Atromid-S; *see* Clofibrate
Atrophic gastritis, 2045

Atrophic vaginitis, dysuria, 763
Atrophy
  chronic aortic obstruction, 304
  chronic atrophic gastritis, 2042
  diabetic dermopathy, 1873
  gastric, 1983, 2042
  genitourinary, 2271
  gyrate, 1909
  multiple system, 935, 1098
  olivopontocerebellar, 935, 992-993
  retinal gyrate, 1909
  rheumatoid arthritis, 1204
  Sudeck's, 1247
Attenuation artifact, 101
Attenuation of effect, 2265
Atypical hyperplasia, 600
Atypical lymphocyte, 595
Atypical lymphoreticular granulomatous
        vasculitis, 470
Audiogram, 974
AUDIT questions, 4
Auditory hallucination, 1041
Auer rod, 594, 689, 690, Plate IV-6
Augmentation therapy
  alpha₁-protease inhibitor deficiency, 441
  bronchiolitis obliterans syndrome, 523-524
Aura, 957, 979-980
Aural polyp, 2307
Auranofin
  rheumatic disease, 1260, 1261
  rheumatoid arthritis, 1208
Auscultation
  cardiac, 68-71
  evaluation of respiratory disease, 402, 403
  prosthetic heart valve, 259
  pulmonic regurgitation, 257
  subclavian artery, 306
Auspitz's sign, 1300
Austin Flint murmur, 78-80, 241
Autoantibody, 1155-1160
  Addison's disease, 1155
  autoimmune hemolytic anemia, 1155
  autoimmune hepatitis, 2183
  bullous pemphigoid, 1155
  chronic active hepatitis, 1155
  diffuse toxic goiter, 1155
  drug-induced immune hemolytic anemia, 670
  enzyme-linked immunosorbent assay, 1156
  Goodpasture's syndrome, 1155
  Graves' disease, 1155
  Hashimoto's thyroiditis, 1155
  idiopathic thrombocytopenic purpura, 1155
  immune complex formation, 842
  immunofluorescence, 1156
  inflammatory myopathies, 1235, 1236-1237
  interpretation of serum tests, 1156-1157
  laboratory tests for serum antibodies in
        autoimmune disease, 1156
  myasthenia gravis, 1155
  neurologic paraneoplastic syndromes, 1075
  pemphigus vulgaris, 1155
  pernicious anemia, 1155
  polymyositis, 1143, 1155
  primary antiphospholipid antibody syndrome,
        1155
  primary biliary cirrhosis, 1155
  rheumatoid arthritis, 1155
  rheumatoid factor, 1160-1161
  Sjögren syndrome, 1155
  systemic lupus erythematosus, 1155
  systemic sclerosis, 1231
  vasculitis, 1155
  vitiligo, 1155
  Wegener's granulomatosis, 468
Autoantigen, 1142
Autocrine secretion, 487
Autocrine stimulation, 544
Autograft, 261
Autoimmune disease
  abnormality in normal self-tolerance, 1142-1147
  Addison's disease, 1823-1824

Autoimmune disease—cont'd
  celiac sprue, 2063
  cholangitis, 2139-2140
  chronic aortic regurgitation, 239
  fever of unknown origin, 1376, 1377-1378
  Graves' disease
    antithyroid antibodies, 1801
    autoantibodies, 1155
    during pregnancy, 2273
    thyroid scan, 1802
    thyrotoxicosis, 1804, 1805-1807
    weakness, 1754
  hemolytic anemia, 668, 1155
  hepatitis, 2183-2184
    immunoserologic markers, 2139
    serum aminotransferase levels, 2136
  hypergonadotropic hypogonadism, 1843
  hypoparathyroidism, 1931
  immune complexes, 1138, 1149
  infertility and oligospermia, 1846
  insulin resistance, 1862
  laboratory tests for serum antibodies, 1156
  Lambert-Eaton myasthenic syndrome, 1023
  lymphocytic hypophysitis, 1776
  lymphoproliferative syndrome, 1128
  multiple sclerosis, 1008
  myasthenia gravis, 1020-1023
    abnormal eye movements, 1063
    autoantibodies, 1155
    cardiac abnormalities, 1087
    peripheral neuropathy *versus,* 1014
    respiratory failure, 1097
    weakness, 1754
  neurologic aspects, 1091-1095
  pemphigus vulgaris, 1293-1294
  self/nonself discrimination, 1109
  silent thyroiditis, 1807, 1812
  Sjögren syndrome, 1209-1212
    anti-Ro antibody, 1291
    autoantibodies, 1155
    Fanconi's syndrome, 882
    inflammatory myopathies, 1236
    interstitial lung disease, 453
    neurologic manifestations, 1095
    renal involvement, 891
    systemic sclerosis, 1230
  thrombocytopenic purpura, 616-617
  thyroiditis, 1811
Autoimmunity, 1142-1147, 1261
Autologous blood transfusion, 572-573
Autologous stem cell transplantation, 577
Automated blood cell analysis, 555-556
Automated reagin test, 1642
Automatic atrial tachycardia, 143
Automatic behavior in narcolepsy, 942
Automatic implantable cardioverter defibrillator,
        139-140
  sustained monomorphic ventricular
        tachycardia, 151
  ventricular fibrillation, 153
Automaticity, 132
Automatism, 979
Autonomic dysreflexia
  bladder-emptying dysfunction, 1066
  spinal cord injury, 1049
Autonomic failure, 935-936
  diabetic autonomic neuropathy, 1872-1873
  mitral valve prolapse, 254
  orthostatic hypotension, 953
Autonomic fibers, 1011
Autonomic nervous system, 930-938
  autonomic failure, 935-936
  autonomic overactivity, 934-935
  bladder control, 933, 935
  cardiovascular reflexes, 936-938
  cardiovascular regulation, 931-932
  chronic renal failure, 784
  genital function, 933-934
  local autonomic disorders, 936, 937
  neuroanatomy, 930, 931, 932
  neurochemistry, 930-931, 933

Autonomic nervous system—cont'd
  pupil physiology, 932-933, 934
  sweating, 933
  testing, 936
  vomiting, 2025
Autonomic overactivity, 934-935
Autoradiography, 52
Autoreactivity, 1146
Autoregulation
  blood flow, 46-47
  cerebral bacterial meningitis, 1405
  cerebral blood flow, 952
  relationship with intracranial pressure, 1082
Autosomal dominant inheritance, 1726
Autosomal dominant polycystic kidney disease,
        872-874
Autosomal recessive inheritance, 1725-1726
Autosomal recessive polycystic kidney disease,
        874
Autosomal recessive severe combined
        immunodeficiency resulting from
        JAK3 deficiency, 1177
Autosome, 1727
Auxotyping system, 1581
Avascular necrosis, 1214
Avidin, 2107
Axial skeleton, 1169-1171, 1172
Axillary artery hyperabduction maneuver, 306
Axillary dissection, 709
Axillary nerve mononeuropathy, 1017
Axillary node
  lymphadenopathy, 597-598
  metastasis, 732
Axillary temperature, 1375
Axis deviation, 85
Axonopathy, 1019
5-Azacytidine, 656
Azathioprine
  autoimmune hepatitis, 2184
  hepatic injury, 2192
  interstitial lung disease, 451
  lung transplantation, 516
  myasthenia gravis, 1022-1023
  prevention and therapy of rejection, 340-341
  renal transplantation, 792
  rheumatic disease, 1260, 1262
  typical medical regimen six months after
        transplantation, 343
  ulcerative colitis, 2074
Azithromycin, 1357-1358
  chlamydial infection, 1537
  dosage, 1349
  Mycobacterium avium-intracellulare complex,
        1474
  Mycoplasma pneumoniae pneumonia, 1540
  urethritis, 1441
Azlocillin, 1350
Azole antifungals, 1653-1654
  candidiasis, 1663
  coccidioidomycosis, 1254
  cryptococcosis, 1669
Azoospermia, 1845-1846
Azotemia
  analgesic nephropathy, 890
  hepatic encephalopathy, 2159
  hepatorenal syndrome, 2168
  infective endocarditis, 228
  leptospirosis, 1645
  metformin-induced, 1858
  portosystemic encephalopathy, 2160
  volume depletion on diuretics, 169
AZT; *see* Zidovudine
Aztreonam, 1355
  dosage, 1350
  gram-negative sepsis, 1452

B

B cell, 1108, 1109
  antibody response, 1110
  assay, 1153

B cell—cont'd
  basic immunology, 1174-1175
  chronic lymphocytic leukemia, 684-685
  differentiation, 1113
  gamma globulin production, 2135
  human immunodeficiency virus infection,
    1470
  lamina propria, 1990, 1991
  lymphoid follicles, 596
  non-Hodgkin's lymphoma, 697
  Peyer's patches, 1989
  primary disorders, 1343
  pulmonary, 368
  systemic lupus erythematosus, 1213
  tolerance, 1143, 1144
B cell antigen receptor, 1174
B cell lymphoma
  chromosomal abnormalities, 544
  gastric, 2038
  molecular diagnostics, 563
B cell receptor, 1123
B-mode ultrasound
  proximal venous thrombosis, 502
  stroke, 1003
Babesiosis, 1675-1676
  hemolytic anemia, 667
  peripheral blood smear, 557
  transfusion-transmitted, 575, 576
Baby boom generation, 2282
Bacillary angiomatosis
  acquired immunodeficiency syndrome, 1474,
    1477
  typical lesion, Plate VIII-40
Bacillary peliosis hepatis, 2212
Bacille Calmette-Guérin, 1637-1638
Bacillus anthracis, 1347
Bacillus cereus, 1430
Bacillus subtilis, 2043
Bacitracin, 1569, 1570
Back pain, 963-971
  abdominal aortic aneurysm, 300
  brucellosis, 1605
  endocarditis, 227
  esophageal cancer, 2024
  gastric cancer, 2046
  low back pain, 963-968
  neck, 968-971
  neuronal disease, 1017
  Paget's disease, 1955
  pancreatic abscess, 1399
  retroperitoneal abscess, 1398
  retroperitoneal fibrosis, 2250
  spinal epidural abscess, 1418
  vertebral compression fracture, 1945
  vertebral osteomyelitis, 1433
Background retinopathy, 1870
Backwash ileitis, 2068
Baclofen
  multiple sclerosis, 1009
  spasticity, 997, 1055
  spinal cord injury, 1051
Bacterascites, 2164
Bacteremia, 1445-1455
  after stem cell transplantation, 578
  anaerobic bacteria, 1618
  Campylobacter, 1590
  clinical manifestations, 1449-1450
  clostridial, 1576
  compromised host, 1388
  diagnosis, 1450-1451
  enterococcal, 1562
  epidemiology, 1445-1446
  erysipelas, 1420
  Haemophilus influenzae, 1586, 1587
  infective endocarditis, 228
  laboratory findings, 1450
  meningitis, 1404
  microbiology, 1446
  nosocomial, 1364, 1480
  pathogenesis, 1446-1447
  pathophysiology, 1447-1448

Bacteremia—cont'd
  prevention, 1453-1454
  Salmonella, 1600
  serum bactericidal activity, 1339
  shigellosis, 1603
  staphylococcal, 1550
  streptococcal toxic shock, 1421
  therapy, 1451-1453
Bacterial infection
  acquired immunodeficiency syndrome,
    1328-1329, 1474, 2098
    cutaneous, 1477
    streptococcal, 1328-1329
  acute cholecystitis, 2227
  acute pharyngitis, 1392
  after liver transplantation, 2220
  Bacteroides, 1613-1621
    antibiotic selection, 1348
    bacteremia and endocarditis, 1618
    brain abscess, 1414
    central nervous system infections, 1617
    classification and characteristics, 1613-1614
    diagnosis, 1618-1619
    gram-negative bacteremia, 1446
    head and neck infections, 1616-1617
    intraabdominal infections, 1617-1618
    necrotic skin and soft tissue infections,
      1618
    normal flora, 1368
    obstetric and gynecologic infections, 1618
    pathophysiology, 1614-1616
    pleuropulmonary infections, 1617
    prevention, 1621
    therapy, 1619-1621
    virulence factors, 1615-1616
  Bordetella pertussis, 1611-1613
  brown pigment stones formation, 2222, 2224
  brucellosis, 1604-1607
  Campylobacter, 1590-1593
  cell wall synthesis, 1343
  chlamydial, 1534-1538
  chronic bronchitis, 443
  clostridial, 1567-1576
    bacteremia, 1576
    food-borne, 1568-1570
    gastrointestinal tract, 1567-1568
    myonecrosis, 1574-1576
    neurologic syndromes, 1570-1572
    tetanus, 1572-1574
  Corynebacterium diphtheriae, 1565-1567
  culture, 1367-1369
  cystic fibrosis, 480
  diarrhea, 1425-1427, 2051
  differential diagnosis of fever and rash, 1384
  empyema, 507
  endocarditis, 225-235
    acute meningitis, 1407
    anaerobic bacteria, 1618
    antimicrobial therapy, 230-233
    aortic regurgitation, 244
    aspergillosis, 1658
    bicuspid aortic valve, 287
    brain abscess, 1414
    Brucella, 1606
    brucellosis, 1606
    candidiasis, 1664
    clinical syndrome, 227-228
    coagulase-negative staphylococci,
      1550-1551
    differential diagnosis, 229
    drug user, 229-230
    endocardial cushion defect, 283
    enterococcal, 1562
    fever of unknown origin, 1376-1377
    Haemophilus influenzae, 1586
    hypertrophic obstructive cardiomyopathy,
      269
    laboratory findings, 228-229
    mitral regurgitation, 250
    mitral valve prolapse, 255
    mycotic aneurysm, 299

Bacterial infection—cont'd
  endocarditis—cont'd
    nephritis with, 844
    neurologic aspects, 1089-1090, 1409
    pathophysiology, 225-227
    prophylaxis, 233, 234-235
    prosthetic heart valve, 230, 258-259, 261
    Q fever, 1545
    referral, 233-234
    rheumatic fever, 1256
    Staphylococcus aureus, 1550
    ventricular septal defect, 283
    weight loss, 1750
  enterococcal, 1560-1564
    antibiotic selection, 1347
    normal flora, 1368
    nosocomial infections, 1362
    resistance to vancomycin, 1346
  esophageal, 2019-2020
  fever of unknown origin, 1376
  gram-negative bacteremia, 1445-1455
    clinical manifestations, 1449-1450
    diagnosis, 1450-1451
    epidemiology, 1445-1446
    laboratory findings, 1450
    microbiology, 1446
    pathogenesis, 1446-1447
    pathophysiology, 1447-1448
    prevention, 1453-1454
    therapy, 1451-1453
  Haemophilus, 1585-1590, Plate VIII-5
    acquired immunodeficiency syndrome, 1329
    antibiotic selection, 1347
    bacterial meningitis, 1402-1403
    beta-lactamases, 1345
    cellulitis, Plate VIII-26
    chronic bronchitis, 443
    clinical diseases, 1586-1589
    complement deficiency, 1339
    cystic fibrosis airway infection, 480
    epidemiology, 1586
    epiglottitis, 1393
    erysipelas, 1420
    Gram stain, Plate VIII-8
    immunoglobulin A, 1337
    osteomyelitis, 1433
    pericarditis, 272
    phagocytosis defects, 1341
    respiratory tract infection, 1390
    septic arthritis, 1251
    sickle cell anemia, 658
    sinusitis, 1183, 1394, 2308
    subdural empyema, 1417
  immune complexes, 1149
  labyrinthitis, 972
  Legionella pneumophila, 1621-1625
  leprosy, 1648-1651
  Listeria monocytogenes, 1576-1578
  meningitis
    clinical manifestations, 1406, 1407
    differential diagnosis, 1408-1409
    enterococcal, 1562
    epidemiology and etiology, 1402-1403
    laboratory investigation, 1406-1408
    Neisseria meningitidis, 1578-1579
    pathogenesis and pathophysiology,
      1404-1406
    treatment, 1409-1413
    tuberculous, 1636
  mycoplasmal, 1538-1541
  nasopharyngitis-sinusitis, 1183
  Neisseria gonorrhoeae, 1581-1585
    beta-lactamases, 1345
    diarrhea, 1476
    immunoglobulin A, 1337
    peritonitis, 1396, 2248
    septic arthritis, 1251
    urethritis, 1455
  Neisseria meningitidis, 1339, 1578-1581
    immunoglobulin A, 1337
    meningitis, 1402-1403

Bacterial infection—cont'd
non-group A streptococcal, 1563-1564
nosocomial, 1362
Pasteurella, 1609
pericarditis, 272
peritonitis, 2247-2248
posttransplant
cardiac, 341
lung, 517-518
renal, 794
respiratory tract, 1390-1396
Salmonella, 1598-1602
seizure, 980
Shigella, 1602-1604
spirochetes, 1640-1648
Borrelia, 1645-1648
leptospires, 1644-1645
Treponema pallidum, 1640-1644
splenic dysfunction, 1338
staphylococcal, 1546-1553
acquired immunodeficiency syndrome,
1328-1329
antibiotic selection, 1347
antimicrobial resistance, 1345
bacterial meningitis, 1403
brain abscess, 1414
cellulitis, 1420
characteristics, 1547
coagulase-negative, 1550-1551
cystic fibrosis airway infection, 480
dermatitis with, 1303
empyema, 507
epidemiology, 1547-1548
erysipelas, 1420
furuncles and carbuncles, 1421
impetigo, 1419
infective endocarditis, 226
lung recipient, 517
nosocomial infections, 1362
osteomyelitis, 1433
pancreatic abscess, 1399
pathophysiology, 1548
polyarticular septic arthritis, 1251
prevention, 1553
respiratory tract infection, 1390
scalded-skin syndrome, 1384, 1421
septic arthritis, 1251
toxic shock syndrome, 1421-1422
treatment, 1551-1553
urinary tract infection, 1457
streptococcal, 1553-1560
acquired immunodeficiency syndrome,
1328-1329, 1477
acute interstitial nephritis, 890
antibiotic selection, 1347
bacterial meningitis, 1402-1403
brain abscess, 1414
cell structure and extracellular products,
1554-1556
chronic bronchitis, 443
empyema, 507
endocarditis, 226
epidemiology, 1553-1554
impetigo, 1419
lung recipient, 517
mitral stenosis, 248
osteomyelitis, 1433
pharyngitis, 1391-1392, 1556
poststreptococcal glomerulonephritis, 843,
1559
primary peritonitis, 1396
respiratory tract, 1390
rheumatic fever, 1256, 1558-1559
scarlet fever, 1556
sickle cell disease, 658
sinusitis, 1183
soft-tissue infection, 1556-1557
spinal epidural abscess, 1418
toxic shock-like syndrome, 1384
toxic shock syndrome, 1421, 1557-1558
treatment, 1559-1560

Bacterial infection—cont'd
tuberculosis, 1625-1638
acquired immunodeficiency syndrome,
1472, 1473, 1474
after lung transplantation, 520
characteristics of *Mycobacterium
tuberculosis,* 1625-1626
chemotherapy, 1630-1633
clinical spectrum, 1628
dysuria, 762
empyema, 507
epidemiology, 1626-1627
extrapulmonary, 1633-1637
fever of unknown origin, 1376
hypercalcemia, 1928
joint disease, 1254
pathogenesis, 1627
pericarditis, 272
prevention, 1637-1638
prostate, 1463
public health considerations, 1638
pulmonary, 1628-1630
renal dysfunction, 892-893
silicosis-related, 475
skeletal, 1437
weight loss, 1750
tularemia, 1607-1609
urinary tract, 1455-1464
clinical symptoms and diagnosis, 1458-1459
epidemiology, 1457-1458
management, 1459-1462
microbiology, 1457
pathogenesis, 1455-1456
pathology, 1456-1457
prevention, 1462
prostatitis, 1462-1463
vaginosis, 762, 1443, 2280
Vibrio, 1593-1598
Whipple's disease, 2064-2065
Yersinia, 1609-1611
Bacterial overgrowth
malabsorption, 2060-2062
multiple jejunal diverticulosis, 2089
Schilling test, 2060
small intestinal malignancies, 2081
Bacterial superantigens, 1112
Bacterial synergy, 1616
Bacteriologic index, 1649
Bacteriuria, 1457
catheter-associated, 1480
management, 1459
Bacteroides, 1613-1621
antibiotic selection, 1348
bacteremia and endocarditis, 1618
brain abscess, 1414
central nervous system infections, 1617
classification and characteristics, 1613-1614
diagnosis, 1618-1619
gram-negative bacteremia, 1446
head and neck infections, 1616-1617
intraabdominal infections, 1617-1618
necrotic skin and soft tissue infections, 1618
normal flora, 1368
obstetric and gynecologic infections, 1618
pathophysiology, 1614-1616
pleuropulmonary infections, 1617
prevention, 1621
susceptibility to empiric antimicrobial therapy,
1400
therapy, 1619-1621
virulence factors, 1615-1616
Bagassosis, 460
Baker's cyst, 1203
BAL; *see* Bronchoalveolar lavage
Balance, anatomic substrate, 971-972
Balanitis
candidal, 1442, 1662
dysuria, 763
Balantidiasis, 1690-1691
Balkan endemic nephropathy, 893

Balloon angioplasty
chronic total occlusions, 120
complications, 122
stent *versus,* 119-120
Takayasu's arteritis, 311
Balloon atrial septostomy, 290, 291
Balloon-expandable stent implantation with
balloon angioplasty, 119
Balloon flotation catheter, 108
Balloon tamponade, 2013, 2167-2168
Balloon valvuloplasty, 288
Balthazar criteria, 2236
Bamboo spine, 1170
Band neutrophil, 532
Banding, esophageal varices, 2167
Barbiturates
alcohol withdrawal, 2295
drug-induced bile duct injury, 2203
drug-nutrient interactions, 2110
human cytochrome P450 isoforms, 2312
increased intracranial pressure, 1084
interference with oral anticoagulants, 636
BARI trial, 117
Barium poisoning, 827
Barium studies
acute abdominal pain, 2032-2033
colonoscopy after, 1996
constipation, 2055
diverticulitis, 2091
esophageal cancer, 2024
esophageal disease, 1999-2000
gastroduodenal diseases, 2002
gastrointestinal bleeding, 2013
intestinal diseases, 2007
intestinal obstruction, 2078
ischemic colitis, 2088
mesenteric ischemia, 2087
progressive systemic sclerosis, 2023
small bowel bacterial overgrowth, 2061
small intestinal tumors, 2081
Baroreceptor reflex, 931
Baroreceptors
aortic, 162, 299
blood pressure, 931, 932
carotid, 162
heart failure, 162, 164
vasopressin release, 808
Baroregulatory system, 1790
Barotrauma
mechanical ventilation, 397
multiple organ dysfunction syndrome
complication, 422-423
Barr body, 1727, 1743
Barrel chest, 402
Barrett's esophagus, 2000, 2016, 2017-2018
cancer surveillance, 1995
esophageal cancer, 2023
increased risk of cancer, 548
Barrier contraception, 2270
Bartholinitis, 1444, 1536
Bartholin's glands
exam for sexually transmitted disease, 1439
gonococcal infection, 1583
Bartonellosis
acquired immunodeficiency syndrome, 1329
hemolytic anemia, 667
Bart's hemoglobin, 656
Bartter's syndrome
generation of alkalosis, 839-840
renal magnesium wasting, 1940
renal potassium wasting, 828
Basal acid output, 2003
Basal body temperature, 1743
Basal cell carcinoma, 1297, Plate VII-5
Basal cell nevus syndrome, 1319
Basal energy expenditure, 2111
Basal metabolic rate, 2111-2112, 2113
cancer, 1749-1750
lipodystrophy, 1901
Basal tests, 1732
Base production, 834

Basedow's disease, 1805-1807
Basic calcium phosphate crystal arthropathy, 1279-1280
Basic calcium phosphate crystals, 1162-1163
Basidiobolomycosis, 1660
Basilar artery occlusion, 973, 1005
Basophil, 1109, 1342
  abnormalities, 680-681
  hemolytic anemia, 662
  immediate hypersensitivity, 1139-1140
Basophilia, 591, 680-681
Basophilic leukemia, 1983
Basophilic normoblast, 531mPlate IV-3
Bassen-Kornzweig disease, 1101
Battering, 2268
Bauer-Kirby method, 1346
Bayes' theorem, 93
Bazex's syndrome, 1317, 1318
BCL-2 protooncogene, 542-543, 1126
  non-Hodgkin's lymphoma, 697
BCNU; *see* Bischlorethylinitrosourea
BCR protooncogene, 543
Becker muscular dystrophy, 62
Beclomethasone
  during pregnancy, 2277
  rhinitis, 1182
Bed rest
  ascites, 2165
  chronic venous insufficiency, 312
  common cold, 1392
  dilated cardiomyopathy, 264
  diphtheria, 1567
  hazards, 2287-2288
  preeclampsia, 2275
  rheumatoid arthritis, 1206-1207
  streptococcal pharyngitis, 1393
Bee sting, 668
Beef tapeworm, 1696
Beer-drinker's potomania, 811
Behavior
  epilepsy, 984
  hormonal milieu, 1076
Behavior modification, 2104
Behavioral neurology, 1030-1034
Behçet disease, 469
  arthropathy, 1243
  genital ulcerations, 1444
  pulmonary vasculitis, 454
Bejel, 1644
Belching, 2015
Bellini duct carcinoma, 899
Bell's palsy, 1017, 2306
Benazepril, 325
Bence Jones protein
  multiple myeloma, 862
  screening tests, 567
Bence Jones proteinuria
  serum protein electrophoresis, 565
  streptococcal superantigen method, 743
  Waldenström macroglobulinemia, 865
Beneficence, 10
Beneficence-in-trust, 10
BENESTENT trial, 119, 124
Benign adolescent gynecomastia, 1770, 1772
Benign breast disease, 1846-1850
Benign chronic conjugated hyperbilirubinemia, 2157-2158
Benign cystinosis, 1910
Benign familial hypercalcemia, 1969
Benign focal amyotrophy, 1015
Benign intracranial hypertension, 1070
Benign lymphocytic angiitis and granulomatosis, 469
Benign monoclonal gammopathy, 705-706
Benign mucous membrane pemphigoid, 1296
Benign neck cyst, 2310
Benign paroxysmal positional vertigo, 972
Benign pleural disease, 474

Benign prostatic hyperplasia, 717
  bladder-emptying dysfunction, 1066
  clinical guideline, 20
  hematuria, 757
Benign recurrent intrahepatic cholestasis, 2158
Benign stricture of extrahepatic bile ducts, 2232-2233
Benign tumor
  breast, 708
  bronchial adenoma, 491-492
  cardiac, 329
  cavernous hemangioma, 2215-2216
  colon, 2086
  esophageal, 2023
  gastric, 2050
  small bowel, 2082
  thyroid, 1813-1814
Benoxaprofen, 2190, 2191
Bentiromide, 2058, 2145
Benzathine penicillin
  rheumatic fever, 1258
  streptococcal pharyngitis, 1393
  syphilis, 1643
Benzene, 672
Benziodarone, 2192
Benzodiazepines
  alcohol withdrawal, 2295
  Alzheimer's disease, 986
  anxiety disorders, 1035
  delirium tremens, 2295, 2296
  disordered thinking, 1041
  ethanol withdrawal, 1080
  hepatic injury, 2191
  human cytochrome P450 isoforms, 2312
  hypnotic-dependent sleep disorders, 944
  multiple sclerosis, 1009
  muscle spasm in tetanus, 1573
  for nausea and vomiting, 2027
  preeclampsia, 2275
  sedation during gastrointestinal endoscopy, 1994
  spasticity, 997
  spinal cord injury, 1051
  status epilepticus, 982, 983
Benzols, 548
Benzonatate, 409
Benzoquinone acetic acid, 1280-1281
Benzoyl peroxide, 1305
Benztropine
  disordered thinking, 1041
  Parkinson's disease, 992
  status migrainosus, 962
Benzylpenicillin, 1351-1352
  bacterial peritonitis, 1400
  dosage, 1350
  endocarditis, 231
  resistance of *Staphylococcus aureus,* 1345
  rheumatic fever, 1258
  septic arthritis, 1253
  use during pregnancy, 2281
Bepridil
  angina, 203
  arrhythmias, 138
  properties, 204
Berger's disease, 877
Beriberi, 265, 2106
  cardiomyopathy, 262
  high-output failure, 160
Bernard-Soulier syndrome, 536, 603, 611
Bernstein test, 2017
Berry aneurysm, 997
Beryllium disease, 475
BEST survival trial, 171
Beta 1-syntrophin, 1027
Beta-adrenergic agonists
  asthma, 1190
  chronic obstructive pulmonary disease, 417, 444
  cystic fibrosis, 482
  hyperkalemia, 833
  pertussis, 1613
  pulmonary toxicity, 479

Beta-adrenergic receptor, 1827
Beta-adrenergic receptor kinase, 57-58
Beta-alanine, 1904
Beta arrestin, 57
Beta-blocker Evaluation Survival Trial, 171
Beta-blockers
  acute intermittent porphyria, 1926
  arrhythmias, 138
  atrial fibrillation, 147, 148
  atrial flutter, 146
  bleeding varices, 2168
  cost-utility analysis, 16
  diastolic heart failure, 168
  dilated cardiomyopathy, 264
  dissection of aorta, 301
  elderly patient, 327
  glaucoma, 2302
  Graves' disease, 1806-1807
  heart failure, 160, 174
  high thyroxine levels, 1803
  human cytochrome P450 isoforms, 2312
  hypertension, 324, 325, 327
  hypertensive emergency, 328
  hypertrophic obstructive cardiomyopathy, 269
  induction of bronchospasm, 477
  interaction with calcium channel blockers, 204
  interference with oral anticoagulants, 636
  mitral stenosis, 248
  mitral valve prolapse, 255
  multifocal atrial tachycardia, 144
  myocardial infarction, 216
  myocardial ischemia, 201-203
  non-Q wave myocardial infarction, 218
  palpitations, 131
  during pregnancy, 2273
  properties, 203
  prophylaxis of migraine, 962
  sudden death survivors, 190
  tetralogy of Fallot, 289
  thyrotoxic storm, 1808
  uncommon types of sustained ventricular tachycardia, 153
  variceal bleeding, 2013-2014
  Wolff-Parkinson-White syndrome, 142
Beta-carotene, 1926
Beta-dystroglycan, 1027
Beta-endorphin
  effect on vasopressin release, 1791
  increase after nausea induction, 2025
Beta-galactocerebrosidase deficiency, 1918
Beta-galactosidase deficiency, 1919
Beta-glucocerebrosidase deficiency, 1918
Beta-hydroxybutrate, 2122
Beta-hydroxybutyric acid, 743, 834
Beta-interferon
  hepatitis C infection, 2178
  multiple sclerosis, 1010
  renal cell carcinoma, 898
Beta-lactam antibiotics, 1355
  cephalosporins, 1352-1355
    activity against major anaerobes, 1620
    acute epiglottitis, 1393
    bacterial meningitis, 1411
    coagulase-negative staphylococcal infection, 1552
    dosage, 1349
    effects on kidney, 868
    gonorrhea, 1584, 1585
    gram-negative sepsis, 1452
    Haemophilus ducreyi, 1589
    Haemophilus influenzae, 1588
    hepatic injury, 2191
    induction of acute interstitial nephritis, 889
    infective endocarditis, 231, 232
    intraabdominal infection, 1401
    Lyme disease, 1647-1648
    meningococcal disease, 1580
    peritonitis, 1402
    prophylaxis in lung transplantation, 518
    respiratory exacerbations in cystic fibrosis, 483

Beta-lactam antibiotics—cont'd
cephalosporins—cont'd
septic arthritis, 1253
sinusitis, 1395
spinal epidural abscess, 1418
spontaneous bacterial peritonitis, 2164
subdural empyema, 1418
syphilis, 1643
typhoid fever, 1601
use during pregnancy, 2281
effects on kidney, 868
enterococci resistance, 1561, 1562
Haemophilus influenzae, 1588
Helicobacter pylori, 1593
induction of acute interstitial nephritis, 889
penicillin, 1351-1352
actinomycosis, 1665
activity against major anaerobes, 1620
acute pancreatitis, 2237
allergy, 1194
anaerobic bacteria, 1619-1620
bacterial meningitis, 1410, 1411
bactericidal effect, 1344
brain abscess, 1416
chlamydial infection, 1537
chronic obstructive pulmonary disease, 444
clostridial infection, 1576
coagulase-negative staphylococcal infection, 1552
dermatitis-aggravating *Staphylococcus aureus* infection, 1303
diphtheria, 1567
diverticulosis, 2091
dosage, 1350
drug-induced bile duct injury, 2203
effects on kidney, 868
enterococci resistance, 1561
erysipelas, 1420
Haemophilus ducreyi, 1589
Haemophilus influenzae, 1588
Helicobacter pylori, 1593
hepatic injury, 2190-2192
infectious eczematoid dermatitis, 1304
infective endocarditis, 231, 232, 234
interference with oral anticoagulants, 636
intraabdominal infection, 1401
Lyme disease, 1254, 1647
meningococcal disease, 1580
non-group A streptococcal infection, 1563-1564
nonvenereal treponematosis, 1644
osteomyelitis, 1436
Pasteurella, 1609
peptic ulcer disease, 2040
peritonitis, 1402
relapsing fever, 1646
respiratory exacerbations in cystic fibrosis, 483
rheumatic fever, 1258
septic arthritis, 1253
sinusitis, 1183, 1395, 2309
staphylococcal scalded-skin syndrome, 1421
staphylococcal infection, 1551
streptococcal pharyngitis, 1393
streptococcal resistance, 1559-1560
structural formula, 1351
subdural empyema, 1418
syphilis, 1643
tetanus, 1574
typhoid fever, 1601
use during pregnancy, 2281
wound botulism, 1572
Beta-lactamases
alteration or inactivation, 1345
head and neck infections, 1617
intraabdominal abscess, 1400
Beta-myosin heavy chain, 59
Beta-receptor, 45, 56-58
Beta-sitosterol, 1891
Beta streptococci, 1347

Beta-subunit human chorionic gonadotropin, 1742
Beta-thalassemia, 576, 652-656, Plate IV-4
Beta thromboglobulin, 638
Beta-tubulin, 59
Beta$_2$-microglobulin, 1111
Beta$_2$-microglobulin amyloidosis, 1284
Betapace; *see* Sotalol
Betaseron, 1010
Betaxolol
glaucoma, 2302
hypertension, 325
properties, 203
Betazole hydrochloride, 2003
Bethanechol, 2018
Bethesda unit, 620
Bezafibrate, 1892
Bezoar, 2044
Bicarbonate, 834
acid-base balance, 835-836
bile, 2123
body water compartments, 736
chronic renal failure, 779
cystine stones, 804
Fanconi's syndrome, 882
intestinal absorption, 1988
metabolic acidosis, 839
pancreatic duct cells, 2132-2133
regulation by lung, 351
renal acidification, 740-741, 747
respiratory acidosis, 416
secretion into gastric mucus, 1984
Bicarbonate-carbon dioxide buffer system, 834
Biceps femoris reflex, 964
Biceps jerk, 964
Bicipital tendinitis, 1196-1197
Biclonal gammopathy, 566, 705
Bicuspid aortic valve, 235, 287
Bicycle ergometer, 93
Bifascicular block, 156
Bifid arterial pulse, 266
Bifidobacterium, 1368
Biguanides, 1857
Bilateral acoustic neurofibromatosis, 1922
Bile, 2123-2129
acute gastritis, 2041
assembly and structure, 2128
bile lipids, 2124-2126
bile water production, 2123-2124
bilirubin production and secretion, 2127-2128
cholesterol excretion, 1884
cholesterol gallstones, 2221
cholesterol secretion, 2127
composition, 2123
concentration of antimicrobial agents, 1351
conjugated bilirubins, 2147
defective bile salt synthesis, 2129
increased fecal bile salt loss, 2129
intestinal absorption of lipids, 1986
lecithin secretion, 2126-2127
obstructed secretory apparatus, 2128-2129
role in digestion, 1980
secretion of conjugated bilirubin into, 2149
in vomitus, 2028
Bile acid coarctation of aorta ligase, 2125
Bile acid S-coarctation of aorta glycine/taurine N-acyltransferase, 2125
Bile acid sequestrants, 1890, 1894
Bile acids
cholesterol, 1884
defective synthesis, 1898
hepatocellular *versus* cholestatic jaundice, 2156
liver disease, 2137
malabsorption, 2060
unconjugated hyperbilirubinemia, 2153
vitamin D absorption, 1951
Bile ducts
carcinoma, 2231-2232
lesions, 2155

Bile ducts—cont'd
obstruction
cholestasis, 2156
cystic fibrosis, 2207
primary biliary cirrhosis, 2199
resorption of water, 2124
stricture, 2201, 2202, 2232-2233
Bile peritonitis, 2249
Bile pigments
abnormal enterohepatic circulation, 2155-2156
intestinal catabolism, recirculation, and elimination, 2149-2150
Bile salt binding proteins, 2126
Bile salts, 2123
benign recurrent intrahepatic cholestasis, 2158
black pigment stones, 2221-2222
cholesterol gallstones, 2221
cystic fibrosis, 2207
defective synthesis, 2129
enterohepatic circulation, 2124-2126
fat maldigestion and malabsorption, 2005
gastric refluxate, 2015
increased fecal bile salt loss, 2129
intestinal absorption of lipids, 1986-1987
Bilharziasis, 1702-1703
Biliary atresia
liver transplantation, 2219
portal triad lesions, 2155
Biliary cirrhosis
systemic lupus erythematosus, 1215
systemic sclerosis, 1230
Biliary colic, 2225-2227
acute cholecystitis, 2227
hemobilia, 2233
Biliary disease
acquired immunodeficiency syndrome, 2098-2099
acute pancreatitis, 2233
benign stricture of extrahepatic bile ducts, 2232-2233
biliary dyskinesia, 2233
bilirubin metabolism disorders, 2147-2159
classification, 2150, 2151
conjugated hyperbilirubinemia, 2154-2156
Dubin-Johnson syndrome, 2157
familial cholestatic syndromes, 2158-2159
normal bilirubin metabolism, 2147-2150
postoperative cholestasis, 2159
Rotor's syndrome and hepatic storage disease, 2157-2158
unconjugated hyperbilirubinemia, 2150-2154
carcinoma of ampulla of Vater, 2232
carcinoma of bile ducts, 2231-2232
conjugated hyperbilirubinemia, 2154
developmental anomalies, 2233
drug-induced and toxic cholangitis, 2202-2203
evaluation, 2134-2144
distinguishing acute from chronic disease, 2134-2136
estimations of severity and prognosis, 2141-2144
hereditary markers, 2138-2139
imaging studies, 2140-2141
immunologic markers, 2139-2140
liver biopsy, 2141
patterns of liver injury, 2136-2137
viral markers, 2138
fever of unknown origin, 1376
gallbladder cancer, 2232
hemobilia, 2233
hyperplastic cholecystosis, 2233
impaired lipid ingestion, 1987
ischemic cholangitis, 2203
liver abscess, 2209
malabsorption, 2062
osteomalacia, 1951-1952
primary biliary cirrhosis, 2199-2201
antimitochondrial antibodies, 2139
autoantibodies, 1155
gallstone risk factor, 2223

Biliary disease—cont'd
  primary biliary cirrhosis—cont'd
    liver transplantation, 2218
    malabsorption, 2062
    mitochondrial antibodies, 1157
  primary sclerosing cholangitis, 2201-2202, 2203
    extrahepatic cholestasis, 2155
    inflammatory bowel disease, 2075-2076
    liver transplantation, 2218-2219
    malabsorption, 2062
  viral cholangitis, 2202
Biliary dyskinesia, 2233
Biliary obstruction
  cholestasis, 2156
  conjugated hyperbilirubinemia, 2154
  cystic fibrosis, 2207
  primary biliary cirrhosis, 2199
  serum alkaline phosphatase level, 2137
Biliary sludge, 2220
  gallstone pancreatitis, 2230
  pericholangitis, 2155
  ultrasonographic examination, 2224
Biliary stent in pancreatic cancer, 2243
Biliary tract stones, 2220-2231
  asymptomatic *versus* symptomatic, 2225
  biliary colic, 2225-2227
  brown pigment stones formation, 2222
  cholecystitis, 2227-2228
  choledocholithiasis, 2228-2230
  cholesterol stones, 2221, 2222
  cholesterolosis, 2230-2231
  classification and composition, 2220, 2221
  Crohn's disease, 2075
  defective bile salt synthesis, 2129
  diagnostic tests, 2224-2225
  epidemiology, 2222-2223
  gallstone pancreatitis, 2230
  hereditary spherocytosis, 665-666
  pathophysiology, 2220-2221
  pigment stones, 2221-2222
  during pregnancy, 2278
  risk factors, 2223-2224
  sickle cell disease, 657, 659
Bilirubin, 2123
  acute cholecystitis, 2228
  acute pancreatitis, 2236
  black pigment stones, 2221-2222
  conjugated hyperbilirubinemia
    benign chronic, 2157-2158
    differential diagnosis, 2156
    pathophysiology and classification, 2154-2156
  conjugation, 2149, 2150
  delivery, 2148
  formation, 2147-2148, 2149
  grades of liver disease severity, 2166
  hepatic excretory function, 2142
  hepatic uptake and storage, 2148-2149
  hereditary spherocytosis, 665-666
  hyperbilirubinemia
    conjugated *versus* unconjugated, 2150, 2151
    hepatic function, 2136
    hereditary fructose intolerance, 1880
    sickle cell disease, 657
  impaired conjugation, 2151-2152
  intestinal catabolism, recirculation, and elimination of bile pigments, 2149-2150
  laboratory testing, 744
  metabolic disorders, 2147-2159
    classification, 2150, 2151
    conjugated hyperbilirubinemia, 2154-2156
    Dubin-Johnson syndrome, 2157
    familial cholestatic syndromes, 2158-2159
    normal bilirubin metabolism, 2147-2150
    postoperative cholestasis, 2159
    Rotor's syndrome and hepatic storage disease, 2157-2158
    unconjugated hyperbilirubinemia, 2150-2154

Bilirubin—cont'd
  multimers, 2128
  production and secretion, 2127-2128
  serum
    acquired immunodeficiency syndrome cholangiopathy, 2202
    adult respiratory distress syndrome, 421
    Dubin-Johnson and Rotor's syndromes, 2157
    estrogen-related cholestasis, 2158
    Gilbert's syndrome, 2153
    hepatitis A virus, 2173
    hepatocellular *versus* cholestatic jaundice, 2156
    primary biliary cirrhosis, 2200
    unconjugated hyperbilirubinemia
      chronic, 2152-2154
      diagnosis, 2153-2154
      pathophysiology, 2150-2152
      treatment, 2154
Bilirubin-BSP-binding protein, 2148
Bilirubin conjugates, 2128
Bilirubin diglucuronides, 2224
Bilirubin monoglucuronide, 2224
Bilirubin-UDP glucuronosyltransferase, 2149, 2151, 2152
Bilirubinuria, 2150
Biliverdin, 2128, 2148
Biliverdin reductase, 2148, 2149
Bilobed neutrophil, Plate IV-6
Binocular vision loss, 2300-2301
Bioartificial liver assist device, 2178
Biochemical markers
  bone and mineral disorders, 1746-1747
  carcinoid syndrome, 2082
  osteoporosis, 1947
Bioethics, 9-13
Biofeedback
  Raynaud's phenomenon, 310, 1227
  stroke patient, 1055
Biologic enzymes, 472
Biologic markers
  breast cancer, 708
  lung cancer, 490
  medullary thyroid carcinoma, 1816
  testicular cancer, 720
Biologic response modifiers, 555
Biologic valves, 260
Biomedical futility, 12
Biopsy
  achalasia, 2022
  Barrett's esophagus, 2018
  bone, 1747, 1949
  bone marrow
    aplastic anemia, 672, 673
    hairy cell leukemia, 684
    Hodgkin's disease, 694
    lymphoma, 698
    non-Hodgkin's lymphoma, 698
  Campylobacter jejuni infection, 1591
  cancer
    breast, 708
    cervical, 715
    gastric, 2046
    head and neck, 724
    Hodgkin's disease, 691, 692
    lung, 490
    melanoma, 1299
    prostate, 718
    small bowel, 2081
    squamous cell carcinoma, 1298
    thyroid, 1816
    of unknown primary site, 730
  candidal infection, 1663
  cardiac transplant rejection, 339-340
  dilated cardiomyopathy, 263
  endometrial, 713
  endomyocardial, 108
  esophageal, 2000
  fever and rash, 1385
  fever of unknown origin, 1380

Biopsy—cont'd
  gastric, 2002
  iliac crest, 1747, Plate IX-5
  intestinal disorders, 2007
  liver, 2136, 2141
    cholestasis, 2156
    chronic hepatitis, 2180
    hepatic epithelioid hemangioendothelioma, 2215
    hepatocellular carcinoma, 2214
    hereditary hemochromatosis, 2204
    peliosis hepatis, 2212
    portal hypertension, 2166
    primary biliary cirrhosis, 2199
    protoporphyria, 1926
    unconjugated hyperbilirubinemia, 2153
  lung, 382-384
    bleomycin-induced pulmonary diseases, 477
    bronchial adenoma, 491-492
    bronchiolitis obliterans syndrome, 522
    bronchoscopy-guided, 383-384
    hypersensitivity pneumonitis, 461
    interstitial lung disease, 451
    Langerhans' cell granulomatosis, 464
    lung cancer, 490
    open, 385-386
    pleural disease, 506
    solitary pulmonary nodule, 494
  lymph node, 600
    acquired immunodeficiency syndrome, 1476
    Hodgkin's disease, 691, 692
    Mycobacterium avium complex, Plate VIII-36
  malignant pleural effusion, 508
  mediastinal mass, 512
  melanoma, 1299
  mucosal
    Helicobacter pylori, 2003
    small intestine, 2008
  muscle, 1235
  myelofibrosis, 677
  myocarditis, 263
  pleural, 382-383
    granuloma, 382
    pleural disease, 506
  renal, 748
    diabetic glomerulopathy, 860
    focal glomerular sclerosis, 852
    hematuria, 748
    isolated proteinuria, 761
    membranoproliferative glomerulonephritis, 854
    minimal change disease, 851
    nephrotic syndrome, 767
    polyarteritis nodosa, 856
    rapidly progressive glomerulonephritis, 848
    systemic lupus erythematosus, 1215
    Wegener's granulomatosis, 858
  salivary gland, 1211
  sarcoidosis, 459
  small bowel
    adenocarcinoma, 2081
    celiac sprue, 2063
    eosinophilic enteritis, 2067
    tropical sprue, 2065
  squamous cell carcinoma, 1298
  temporal arteritis, 311
  temporal artery, 1223, 1224
  thyroid, 1802
  toxoplasmosis, 1678
  transbronchial
    acute lung allograft rejection, 521
    cytomegalovirus pneumonia in lung allograft, 518
    cytomegalovirus pneumonitis, Plate VIII-37
    through fiberoptic bronchoscope, 384
  transthoracic, 385
    mediastinal mass, 512
    solitary pulmonary nodule, 494
  vertebral osteomyelitis, 1435
Wegener's granulomatosis, 467

Biotin
  biochemical function, 2105
  deficiency, 2107
  propionic acidemia, 1908
  recommended daily dietary allowances, 2116
Biotinidase deficiency, 1908, 1909
Bipedal lymphangiography
  Hodgkin's disease, 694
  testicular cancer, 720-721
Bipolar disorder, 946, 1035, 1036, 1038
Birbeck granules, 463
Bird breeder's lung, 460
Birds
  causing occupational asthma, 472
  Chlamydia psittaci, 1535
Birth, changes in fetal circulation, 280
Bischlorethylinitrosourea, 584
Bismuth
  acute renal failure, 867
  diarrhea, 1431-1432
  Helicobacter pylori, 1593
  traveler's diarrhea, 1467
Bisoprolol
  hypertension, 325
  properties, 203
Bisphosphonates
  hypercalcemia, 1929, 1974
  induction of osteomalacia, 1953
  osteoporosis, 1948
  Paget's disease, 1957
  primary hyperparathyroidism, 1971
Bite cell
  glucose-6-phosphate dehydrogenase
    deficiency, 664
  hemolytic anemia, 662
Bite wound, rabies, 1505
Bitot's spots, 2105
Biventricular assist device, 185, 186
Björk-Shiley spherical occluder, 259, 260
Black death, 1609-1610
Black fever, 1687
Black pigment stones, 2220, 2221-2222, Plate
    X-14
Black sputum, 475
Blackfly, 1699-1701
Blackhead, 1305
Blackwater fever, 667, 1673
Bladder
  adenovirus infection, 1504
  autonomic control, 933, 935
  autonomic failure, 935
  cancer, 550
  dysfunction in diabetes mellitus, 1873
  emptying, 1065, 1066
  interstitial cystitis, 763
  intravenous pyelogram, 749
  multiple sclerosis, 1055
  neurology, 1065-1067
  renal imaging studies, 756
  retraining, 2293
  spinal cord injury, 1050
  stroke patient, 1054
  urodynamic testing, 938
  voiding dysfunction, 1065-1066
Bladder neck obstruction, 768
Bladder outlet obstruction, 771
Blalock-Taussig procedure, 289
Blast crisis, 687
Blastocystis hominis, 1476, 1691, 2096
Blastomyces dermatidis, 1657
Blastomycosis, 1657
  bone infection, 1437
  joint disease, 1255
  serodiagnosis, 1653
  skin lesion, Plate VIII-48
Blebs, 509
Bleeding, 978, 2041-2044
  acute hemorrhagic conjunctivitis, 1490
  acute hypertensive retinopathy, 2302
  anal fissure, 2093
  colon cancer, 2085

Bleeding—cont'd
  from colonic diverticulum, 2089-2090, 2091,
    2092
  complication of thrombolytic therapy, 637
  diabetic retinopathy, 2303
  epistaxis, 2308
  erosive esophagitis, 2017
  essential thrombocythemia, 688
  gastric cancer, 2046
  gastrointestinal, 2008-2014
    acquired immunodeficiency syndrome,
      2098-2099
    antacids and antisecretory agents, 2013
    Campylobacter jejuni, 1591
    chronic renal failure, 783, 784
    colonoscopy, 1996
    cutaneous manifestations, 1320
    diagnostic and therapeutic studies, 2011-2013
    esophageal varices, 2013-2014
    initial management, 2010-2011
  hemobilia, 2233
  hemophilia A, 619
  hemorrhoids, 2093
  heparin-induced, 634-635
  intracranial
    complication of systemic cancer, 1071
    computed tomography, 919
    endocardial hemorrhage with, 1087
    factor XIII deficiency, 624
    hemophilic patient, 620
    hemorrhagic stroke, 997, 998
  liver biopsy complication, 2141
  macroglobulinemia, 704
  Mallory-Weiss syndrome, 2028
  Meckel's diverticulum, 2090-2091
  myocardial contusion, 332
  peptic ulcer, 2037, 2039-2040
  platelet function disorders, 612
  prosthetic heart valve, 261
  pulmonary hemorrhage syndromes, 454-455
  pyogenic liver abscess, 2209
  relationship to platelet count, 612
  retinal vein occlusion, Plate XI-9
  retroperitoneal, 2250
  scurvy, 2107
  side effect of oral anticoagulant therapy, 636
  subarachnoid, 960, 1043
  variceal
    hepatocellular carcinoma, 2213
    portal hypertension, 2165-2168, 2166
    portal vein obstruction, 2208
    primary biliary cirrhosis, 2200
  vitamin K deficiency, 2106
  vitreous, Plate XI-8
Bleeding diathesis, 1001
Bleeding disorders, 602-610
  coagulation dysfunction, 606-608
  increased risk for thrombosis, 608-609
  multiple hemostatic defects, 608
  plasma coagulation, 570-571
  platelets and
    blood vessels, 602-605
    platelet function, 568-570
  during pregnancy, 2279
  preoperative assessment, 609-610
  pseudothrombocytopenia, 610
  relapsing fever, 1645
  risk in multiple myeloma, 700
  screening tests, 571-572
Bleeding time, 569
  nonsteroidal antiinflammatory drugs and, 1259
  platelet function disorders, 612
Bleomycin
  effects on kidney, 869
  Hodgkin's disease, 694-695
  hypersensitivity, 460
  non-Hodgkin's lymphoma, 699
  pulmonary parenchymal reactions, 476
  pulmonary toxicity, 477-478, 584
  testicular cancer, 721
Blepharitis, 1211

Blindness
  amaurosis fugax, 1057-1058
  Behçet disease, 1243
  candidal endophthalmitis, 1662
  central retinal vein occlusions, 2304
  diabetic retinopathy, 2303
  giant-cell arteritis, 304, 311
  glaucoma, 2301
  human immunodeficiency virus, 1478
  onchocerciasis, 1701
  vitamin A deficiency, 2105
Blink reflex, 917, 1066
Blister
  bullous impetigo, 1419
  bullous pemphigoid, 1295-1296
  necrotizing fasciitis, 1422
Blister cell, Plate IV-4
  glucose-6-phosphate dehydrogenase
    deficiency, 664
  hemolytic anemia, 662
Bloating
  lactase deficiency, 2068
  tropical sprue, 2065
Blocadren; *see* Timolol
Blood
  abetalipoproteinemia, 1897
    malabsorption, 2067
    vitamin A deficiency, 2105
    vitamin E deficiency, 2106
  acidemia
    blood pH, 834
    internal potassium balance, 825
    isovaleric, 1908
    precapillary pulmonary hypertension, 295
    propionic, 1908
  agammaglobulinemia, 1175, 1490
  alkalemia
    blood pH, 834
    internal potassium balance, 825
  automated blood cell analysis, 555-556
  benign chronic conjugated hyperbilirubinemia,
    2157-2158
  Bruton's agammaglobulinemia, 1175
  chromosome analysis, 1727
  citrullinemia, 1907
  congenital afibrinogenemia, 625
  congenital dysfibrinogenemia, 625
  conjugated hyperbilirubinemia, 2154-2156
    benign chronic, 2157-2158
    differential diagnosis, 2156
    pathophysiology and classification,
      2154-2156
  cryoglobulinemia, 1222, 1248-1250
  dysbetalipoproteinemia, 60, 1898
  dyslipoproteinemia, 60
  dysproteinemia, 700-706
    heavy-chain diseases, 704
    monoclonal gammopathy of undetermined
      significance, 705-706
    multiple myeloma, 700-703
    platelet dysfunction, 611-612
    renal manifestations, 862-866
    Waldenström macroglobulinemia, 703-704
  essential mixed cryoglobulinemia, 857
  euthyroid hyperthyroxinemia, 1803, 1804
  euthyroid hypothyroxinemia, 1804
  familial dysalbuminemic hyperthyroxinemia,
    1803
  familial dysbetalipoproteinemia, 1898
  fibrinolysis, 539-540
  flow cytometry analysis, 558-559, 1151-1152
  hemostasis, 534-540
    bleeding disorders, 602-610
    plasma coagulation, 570-571
    platelet function disorders, 610-613
    platelets and platelet function, 535-537,
      568-570
    screening tests for thrombotic disorders,
      571-572
    secondary, 537-539
    thrombocytopenia, 613-617

Blood—cont'd
  hereditary tyrosinemia, 2212
  histidinemia, 1906
  hormone transport, 1713
  hyperammonemia, 1907
  hyperargininemia, 1907
  hyperbilirubinemia
    conjugated *versus* unconjugated, 2150, 2151
    hepatic function, 2136
    hereditary fructose intolerance, 1880
    sickle cell disease, 657
  hypergammaglobulinemia, 1233, 2136
    chronic liver disease, 2136
    human immunodeficiency virus infection, 1470
    liver inflammation, 2135-2136
    myxoma, 330
  hypergastrinemia, 2002, 2003
  hyperinsulinemia, 319
  hyperlipoproteinemia, 1245, 1892
  hyperlysinemia, 1907
  hyperphenylalaninemia, 1904-1905
  hyperprolactinemia, 1785-1786
    basal pituitary hormone measurement, 1737
    milk discharge, 1848
    testicular dysfunction, 1841
  hyperproteinemia, 806
  hyperthyroxinemia, 1803, 1804
  hypoalbuminemia, 765
    acute pancreatitis, 2237
    amebic liver abscess, 2210
    anion gap acidosis, 836
    intestinal disease, 2005
    intestinal lymphangiectasia, 2067
    nephrotic syndrome, 765
    serum magnesium, 1942
    transudative pleural effusion, 507
  hypoalphalipoproteinemia, 1896, 1898
  hypobetalipoproteinemia, 1897
  hypogammaglobulinemia
    Crohn's disease, 2066
    multiple myeloma, 864
    serum protein electrophoresis, 565-566
  hypoprothrombinemia, 1104, 2106
  hypothyroxinemia, 1804
  immunohistochemistry, 558-559
  kerotic hyperglycinemia, 1908
  lipoproteinemia, 60
  macroglobulinemia, 704
  measurement of hormone concentrations, 1733
  metabolic disorders
    conjugated hyperbilirubinemia, 2154-2156
    unconjugated hyperbilirubinemia, 2150-2154
  methemoglobinemia, 351, 660
    angina, 201
    oxidant hemolysis, 667
  mixed cryoglobulinemia, 1249
  molecular and cellular biology of hematopoiesis, 530-534
  peripheral
    abnormal nucleated cells in, 594-596
    megaloblastic anemia, 648
    smear, 556-557
    source of hematopoietic cells, 577
  source of DNA, 51
  specimens, 1367
  tyrosinemia, 1905-1906
  unconjugated hyperbilirubinemia, 2150-2154
    chronic, 2152-2154
    conjugated *versus,* 2150, 2151
    diagnosis, 2153-2154
    pathophysiology, 2150-2152
    treatment, 2154
  in vomitus, 2028
  Waldenström macroglobulinemia, 703-704
    bleeding problems, 612
    immunoelectrophoresis, 566-567
    plasmacytoid lymphocytes, 595
    renal involvement, 865-866
Blood ammonia, 2142

Blood-brain barrier, 1404-1405
Blood casts, 745
Blood cell count
  abnormal, 590-596
    nucleated cells in peripheral blood, 594-596
    quantitative alterations in normal nucleated cells, 590-594
  asthma, 1188
  fever of unknown origin, 1379
  flow cytometry analysis, 1151-1152
  gastrointestinal bleeding, 2011
  heart failure, 166
  hemolytic anemia, 661
  impotence, 1763
  nutritional assessment, 2111
Blood coagulation disorders, 617-630
  acquired inhibitors of blood coagulation, 628-630
  disseminated intravascular coagulation, 627-628
  factor deficiencies, 624
  fibrinogen abnormalities, 625
  hemophilia A, 617-622
  hemophilia B, 622
  liver disease, 626-627
  protease inhibitors deficiencies, 625
  vitamin K deficiency, 625-626
  von Willebrand's disease, 622-624
Blood culture
  bacteremia, 1450
  choledocholithiasis, 2229
  diarrhea, 1431
  fever and rash, 1385
  fever of unknown origin, 1379
  fungal infection, 1652
  Haemophilus influenzae, 1588
  illness in returned traveler, 1469
  infective endocarditis, 228
  Legionella pneumophila, 1623
  liver abscess, 2209
  meningitis, 1406
  Neisseria meningitidis, 1580
  osteomyelitis, 1434
  splenic abscess, 1398-1399
Blood flow
  autoregulation, 46-47
  cerebral
    bacterial meningitis, 1405
    brain resuscitation, 1085
    increased intracranial pressure, 1081
    syncope, 952
  control of coagulation, 539
  coronary
    angina pectoris, 126
    calcium channel blockers, 203-204
    determinants, 193-195
    echocardiography, 97-100
    heart failure, 161-162, 164
    hypertension, 316
    positron emission tomography, 106
  pulmonary, 360-364
    atrial septal defect, 282
    pulmonary hypertension, 293, 363
    pulmonic stenosis, 288
    tetralogy of Fallot, 288
    total anomalous pulmonary venous connection, 291
    tricuspid atresia, 291
  renal
    congestive heart failure, 817
    hepatorenal syndrome, 2168
    hypokalemia, 829
    obstructive uropathy, 884-885
    prerenal azotemia, 768, 769
  sodium transport, 738
Blood folate, 649
Blood gases
  acid-base imbalances, 840
  acquired immunodeficiency syndrome, 1477
  acute respiratory failure, 412
  asthma, 1189

Blood gases—cont'd
  chronic obstructive pulmonary disease, 442
  effect of ventilation, 353
  effects of oxygen breathing, 352
  mechanical ventilation, 397
  Pneumocystis carinii pneumonia, 1694
  primary pulmonary hypertension, 294
  pulmonary artery catheterization, 391
  pulmonary edema, 425
  pulmonary thromboembolism, 501
Blood glucose
  insulin release, 1714
  insulinoma, 2244
  metabolic actions of liver, 2121
  metabolic encephalopathy, 1079
  Somogyi phenomenon, 1861
Blood loss
  bleeding varices, 2166
  gastrointestinal bleeding, 2010
  iron deficiency, 642
Blood oxygen level-dependent imaging, 922
Blood pH, 834
Blood pigments, 744
Blood pressure; *see also* Hypertension
  baroreceptor impulses, 931, 932
  cardiac output, 316
  coronary artery disease, 200
  effects of reduction on coronary heart disease, 322
  exercise test, 379
  extracellular fluid volume contraction, 824
  heart failure, 173
  during hemodialysis, 790
  hypertension, 312-329
    acute glomerulonephritis, 771
    aldosterone excess, 1822
    antirheumatic drug toxicity, 1261
    aortic aneurysm, 299
    aortic ejection sounds, 74
    aortic stenosis, 236-237
    arteriovenous nicking, Plate XI-3
    atherosclerosis risk, 192
    atrial fibrillation, 146
    autonomic overactivity, 934
    autosomal dominant polycystic kidney disease, 873
    chronic renal failure, 781, 783
    coronary artery disease, 200
    coronary artery disease in women, 2271
    cyclosporin A-associated, 870
    diabetic glomerulopathy, 860
    diagnostic tests, 329
    differential diagnosis, 320-322
    dissection of aorta, 301
    environmental mechanisms, 319
    essential mixed cryoglobulinemia, 857
    exertional angina, 127
    focal glomerular sclerosis, 852
    frequency, 312-314
    headache, 960
    hemorrhagic stroke, 998
    hyperkalemia, 833
    hypertensive retinopathy, 2302-2303
    hypothyroidism, 1809
    increased intracellular sodium and calcium, 317-318
    increased intracranial pressure, 1084
    increased peripheral resistance, 314-319
    increased sodium intake, 318-319
    management, 322-329
    membranoproliferative glomerulonephritis, 854
    microvascular disease in diabetic patient, 1870
    mitral stenosis, 245
    natural history, 319-322
    neurofibromatosis, 1921
    obstructive sleep apnea and, 526
    operative risk, 2260
    peripheral arterial aneurysm, 309
    peripheral vascular disease, 305

Blood pressure—cont'd
  hypertension—cont'd
    pheochromocytoma, 1828, 1829-1830
    poststreptococcal glomerulonephritis, 844
    during pregnancy, 2275
    primary hyperparathyroidism, 1966-1967
    proteinuria, 760
    referral, 329
    renal cell carcinoma, 898
    renal sodium retention, 86
        316-317, 318
    renal transplant recipient, 795
    risk of stroke, 1001
    stress, 316
    types, 314, 315
  Hypertension Detection and Follow-up
        Program, 312
  hypotension, 175
    acute pancreatitis, 2234
    adrenal insufficiency, 1823
    after cardiac transplantation, 335
    after stroke, 1007
    calcium channel blocker-induced, 205
    cardiac tamponade, 275
    cardiogenic shock, 175-187; *see also*
        Cardiogenic shock
    comatose patient, 950
    dissection of aorta, 301
    gram-negative bacteremia, 1449
    heart failure, 173
    hypermagnesemia, 1943
    hypovolemic hypernatremia, 816
    Lassa fever, 1510
    penetrating injury to heart, 332
    rabies, 1506
    right ventricular infarction, 178
    thrombolytic agents, 213
    vasopressin release, 1792
  influence on vasopressin, 1789-1790
  measurement, 64
  pheochromocytoma, 1831
  portal hypertension
    alcoholic hepatitis and cirrhosis, 2197
    ascites formation, 2163
    autosomal recessive polycystic kidney
        disease, 874
    cystic fibrosis, 2207
    hepatopulmonary syndrome, 2170
    liver failure, 2165-2168
    splenomegaly, 601
  precautions in measurement, 312-313, 314
  preeclampsia, 2274
  preventive care guidelines, 2255
  pulmonary hypertension, 293-299
    acquired immunodeficiency syndrome, 333
    cardiac catheterization, 108
    cardiac transplantation, 338
    chronic obstructive pulmonary disease,
        446-447
    continuous-wave Doppler echocardiography,
        99
    cor triatriatum, 291
    drug-induced, 477
    exertional angina, 127
    Graham Steell murmur, 80
    interstitial lung disease, 452
    mitral regurgitation, 250
    mitral stenosis, 245, 248
    neurogenic pulmonary edema, 1099
    obesity, 334
    passive, 297-298
    pathophysiology, 363-364
    precapillary, 293-297
    primary and secondary causes, 497-499
    reactive, 298
    systemic sclerosis, 1230
    Takayasu's arteritis, 470
  relationship with intracranial pressure, 1082
  renovascular hypertension, 321, 829, 893-896
  response to standing, 937

Blood pressure—cont'd
  syncope, 952
  Valsalva's maneuver, 937
Blood products
  hepatitis B virus infection, 2174
  human immunodeficiency virus transmission,
        1471
Blood smear, 556-557
  abnormal red blood cell indices in nonanemic
        patient, 588
  acute nephritic syndrome, 764
  babesiosis, 557
  cold agglutinin disease, 670
  iron deficiency, 643
  left shift on, 591
  malaria, 1674
  multiple myeloma, 701
  neutropenia, 593
  overproduction jaundice, 2152
  thrombocytopenia, 613
Blood supply
  adrenal gland, 1817
  anterior pituitary, 1773
  pancreas, 2130
  peritoneum, 2247
  posterior pituitary, 1788
  respiratory muscle endurance and fatigue, 358
Blood tests
  abdominal pain, 2032
  flow cytometry analysis, 1151-1152
  gastrointestinal bleeding, 2011
  heart failure, 166
  hemolytic anemia, 661
  hypertension, 318
  impotence, 1763
  meningitis, 1406
  nutritional assessment, 2111
  small bowel malabsorption, 2058
Blood transfusion, 572-576
  adverse effects, 564-576
  bleeding ulcer, 2039-2040
  cold agglutinin disease, 670
  fever after, 1480
  gastrointestinal bleeding, 2010
  granulocyte, 573-574
  hepatitis C virus, 2175
  human immunodeficiency virus transmission,
        1471
  myelofibrosis, 677
  plasma, 573
  platelets, 573
  postoperative cholestasis, 2159
  whole blood and red cell, 572-573
Blood urea nitrogen
  dialysis disequilibrium syndrome, 1105
  gastrointestinal bleeding, 2011
  glomerular filtration rate, 747
  syndrome of inappropriate antidiuretic
        hormone, 489
  uremic syndrome, 776
Blood vessels; *see also* Cardiovascular system
  aberrant right subclavian artery, 291
  adrenergic responses, 1828
  aneurysm
    angiography, 927
    aortic, 74, 299-300, 302
    candidal, 1663
    carotid artery, 1762
    computed tomography, 106
    coronary sinus, 291
    hemorrhagic stroke, 997-998
    Marfan syndrome, 299, 1289
    syphilitic, 1641
  angioplasty, 116-125
    approach to specific lesions, 120-121
    background, 116-117
    Budd-Chiari syndrome, 2208
    complications, 122
    devices, 117-120, 121
    myocardial infarction, 121-122, 214-215

Blood vessels—cont'd
  angioplasty—cont'd
    myocardial revascularization, 205-206
    pathophysiology, 116
    primary, 122, 123, 124
    randomized trials, 117, 118
    referral, 124
    rescue, 122
    restenosis, 122-124
    shock, 183
  angiosarcoma
    cardiac, 330
    drug-induced, 2189
    immunohistochemistry, 731
    incidence, 329
  aortic disorders, 299-304
    aortic aneurysm, 299-300
    aortitis, 302-303
    atherosclerosis, 299
    dissection of aorta, 300-302, 303
    Marfan syndrome, 299
    mycotic aneurysm, 299, 300
    occlusive disease, 304
    syphilis, 303
  auscultation, 306
  bleeding disorders, 602-605
  heart failure, 161-162, 164
  hemostasis, 535-537
  lipoprotein levels, 60
  peripheral vascular disease, 304-312
    anticoagulant therapy, 641
    arteritis, 311
    occlusive peripheral arterial disease,
        307-309
    peripheral arterial aneurysm, 309
    peripheral arteries, 305-307
    peripheral veins, 311-312
    vasospastic disorders, 309-311
  polyangiitis, 1221
  polyarteritis nodosa, 334, 856, 1219-1220
    crescentic glomerulonephritis, 848
    diffuse immune-complex vasculitis, 454
    glucocorticoid protocol, 1263
    microscopic, 1220-1221
    neurologic manifestations, 1092, 1095
  subclavian artery aneurysm, 309
Blood volume
  hypertension, 316
  influence on vasopressin, 1789-1790
  nephrotic syndrome, 820
  peritonitis, 1398
Bloom's syndrome, 549
Blot hemorrhage, 2302
Blue rubber bleb nevus syndrome, 1320
Blunt trauma
  abdominal arteriography, 2033
  cardiac, 332
  pancreas, 2246-2247
  thromboangiitis obliterans, 308
  traumatic pericardial disease, 273
Blurred vision
  cataracts, 2301
  human immunodeficiency virus-infected
        patients, 2306
  hypoglycemia, 1875
Boarding-school amenorrhea, 1757
BOAT trial, 124
Body composition, 2284
Body fat
  aging and, 2284
  obesity, 1750-1753
  puberty, 1768
Body fluids, 736-737
Body louse
  relapsing fever, 1645-1658
  typhus fever, 1544
Body mass index, 1751
Body plethysmography, 378
Body surface area, 2112
Body surface leads, 82-83

Body temperature, 1375; *see also* Fever
  effect on vasopressin release, 1791
  hyperthermia, 1375, 1936
  hypothermia
    bacteremia, 1449
    electrocardiographic abnormalities, 89, 90
    hypokalemia, 827
    myxedema coma, 1810
    peritonitis, 1398
Body water
  cellular and extracellular compartments, 806
  compartmentalization, 736
  influence on vasopressin, 1789, 1792
Boerhaave's syndrome, 2019, 2028
Boil, 1421
Bolivian hemorrhagic fever, 1511
Bolus escape, 2000
Bolus impaction, 2019
Bombesin, 487
Bone
  aluminum accumulation in, 1961
  biochemical markers of resorption and
        formation, 1746-1747
  biopsy, 1949
  erosion in arthritis, 1167-1168
  formation, 1949, 1971, 1972
  graft in osteomyelitis, 1435-1436
  histomorphometry, 1747
  homeostasis, 1714-1721
    calcium metabolism, 1717-1720
    cellular physiology, 1716
    effects of hormones, 1720
    functions of skeleton, 1714-1715
    matrix formation and calcification, 1716
    natural history of skeleton, 1715-1716
    stress and coupling, 1716
  loss in primary biliary cirrhosis, 2200
  magnesium concentration, 1939, 1940
  measurement of mineral content, 1747
  mineralization, 1961
  mucopolysaccharidosis, 1912
  osteogenesis imperfecta, 1287
  osteomyelitis, 1433-1437
  outgrowths, 1170, 1171
  potassium, 825
  remodeling, 1715-1716
  resorption
    biochemical markers, 1746-1747
    effects of parathyroid hormone, 1718
    lytic metastases, 1971, 1972
    osteopetrosis, 1958
    primary hyperparathyroidism, 1966
    systemic sclerosis, 1229
  sclerosis, 1168
  skeletal metastases, 1971-1974
  solitary plasmacytoma, 703
  turnover, 1715-1716
  X-linked hypophosphatemic rickets, 880
Bone densitometry, 1947
Bone density
  arthritis, 1165
  osteomalacia, 1949-1950
  osteoporosis, 1944
  postmenopausal women with primary
        hyperthyroidism, 1970
  primary hyperparathyroidism, 1966
Bone disease
  actinomycosis, 1665
  brucellosis, 1605-1606
  chronic renal failure, 785-786
  diagnostic approach, 1744-1748
  fibrous dysplasia, 1960-1961
  hyperparathyroidism, 1965-1971
    arthropathy, 1246
    calcium pyrophosphate dihydrate deposition
        disease, 1279
    chronic renal failure, 785
    diagnosis, 1967-1969
    humoral hypercalcemia of malignancy
        versus, 1973-1974

Bone disease—cont'd
  hyperparathyroidism—cont'd
    hypermagnesemia, 1943
    kidney stone formation, 798
    mixed uremic osteodystrophy, 1963
    osteomalacia, 1950
    pathology and etiology, 1965-1966
    during pregnancy, 2273
    prevalence, 1965, 1966
    renal osteodystrophy, 1961
    renal transplant recipient, 795
    renal wasting of phosphate, 1935
    symptoms and signs, 1966-1967
    treatment, 1969-1971
  nephrotic syndrome, 767
  nontuberculous mycobacterial infection,
        1639
  osteomalacia, 1949-1955
    after parathyroidectomy, 1965
    bone biopsy, 1747
    chronic hypophosphatemia, 1936
    chronic renal failure, 785
    proximal renal tubular acidosis, 837
    renal osteodystrophy, 1961
    vitamin D deficiency, 2106
    vitamin D metabolism, 1719
    X-linked hypophosphatemic rickets, 880
  osteopetrosis, 1958-1959
  osteoporosis, 1944-1949
    bone biopsy, 1747
    brucellosis, 1606
    calcitonin therapy, 1719
    glucocorticoid-induced, 1263
    heparin, 635
    menopause, 2271
    multiple myeloma, 864
    reduction in bone density, 1165
    rheumatoid arthritis, 1205
  Paget's disease, 1955-1958
  renal osteodystrophy, 1961-1965
  Staphylococcus aureus, 1549
  syphilis, 1641
  tuberculosis, 1634, 1635
Bone Gla protein, 1716
Bone marrow
  acute lymphoblastic leukemia, 682-683
  analysis of marrow cells, 557-558
  erythroid precursors, Plate IV-3
  exit of blood cells from, 533-534
  failure in osteopetrosis, 1958
  hairy cell leukemia, 683-684
  Hodgkin's disease, 693
  iron in, Plate IV-9
  myelofibrosis, 676-677
    acute myelogenous leukemia, 677
    megakaryocytic hypoplasia, 614
    neutrophilic leukocytosis, 591
    polycythemia vera, 688
  myelopoiesis, 532, 593
  myeloproliferative disorders, 685-691
    acute myelogenous leukemia, 689-690, 691
    bleeding and thrombosis, 611
    chronic, 686
    essential thrombocytopenia, 687-688
    immature granulocytes, 594
    myelodysplastic syndromes, 690-691
    myelogenous leukemia, 686-687
    neutrophilic leukocytosis, 591
    polycythemia vera, 688
  myelosuppression
    monocytosis, 591
    stem cell transplantation, 577-578
  normal, Plate IV-1
  overproduction jaundice, 2152
  plasma cell, Plate IV-8
  ringed sideroblast, Plate IV-11
  source of hematopoietic cells, 577
  toxicity of chloramphenicol, 1356
  vitamin B_{12} deficiency, Plate IV-7

Bone marrow aplasia
  acute myelogenous leukemia, 690
  megakaryocytic hypoplasia, 614
Bone marrow examination
  aplastic anemia, 672, 673
  aspirate smear, 557-558
  hairy cell leukemia, 684
  Hodgkin's disease, 694
  human immunodeficiency virus infection,
        1473
  iron deficiency anemia, 643
  megaloblastic anemia, 648
  neutropenia, 593
  non-Hodgkin's lymphoma, 698
  small cell lung cancer, 726
Bone marrow failure, 671-677
  aplasias of single cell lineages, 674-675
  aplastic anemia, 671-674, 675
  myelodysplasia, 675-676
  myelofibrosis, 676-677
  thrombocytopenia, 605
Bone marrow fibrosis, 686
Bone marrow hypoplasia, 573
Bone marrow precursor cell, 530
Bone marrow transplantation
  acute lymphoblastic leukemia, 683
  acute myelogenous leukemia, 690
  acute renal failure following, 775-776
  aplastic anemia, 674
  beta-thalassemia, 656
  chronic myelogenous leukemia, 687
  lysosomal storage disease, 1920
  multiple myeloma, 702, 865
  myelodysplastic syndrome, 676
  neurologic complications, 1104-1105
  osteopetrosis, 1959
  sickle cell disease, 660
  Wiskott-Aldrich syndrome, 1178
Bone mass, 1716
  osteoporosis, 1944
  puberty, 1768
Bone membrane, 1716
Bone morphogenetic proteins, 1720
Bone pain
  after renal transplantation, 795
  hyperparathyroid bone disease, 1963
  hypophosphatemia, 1936
  leukemia, 1247
  malignant involvement in skeleton, 1972
  multiple myeloma, 700, 864
  osteomalacia, 1949
  primary hyperparathyroidism, 1966
  vitamin D deficiency, 2106
Bone scan
  ankylosing spondylitis, 1238-1239
  osteomalacia, 1950
  osteomyelitis, 1434
  Paget's disease, 1956
  prostate cancer, 718
  small cell lung cancer, 726
Bone volume, 1716
BOOP; *see* Bronchiolitis obliterans-organizing
        pneumonia
Borborygmi, 2032
Borderline high hematocrit, 590
Borderline hypertension, 314
Borderline low hematocrit, 588
Bordetella pertussis, 1611-1613
  antibiotic selection, 1347
  persistent cough, 407
Bornholm disease, 1489
Borrelia burgdorferi, 1646-1648
  identification, 1251
  Lyme disease, 1254
Borrelia recurrentis, 1645-1646
Boston diagnostic aphasia examination, 903
Botulinum toxin
  focal dystonia, 996
  spasticity after spinal cord injury, 1052
Botulism, 1570-1572, 1754

Bouchard's node, 1199, 1266
Boutonneuse fever, 1545
Boutonniere deformity, 1203
Bovine deoxyribonuclease, 482
Bovine thrombin, 1146
Bowel sounds, 2032, 2077
Bowel wall infarction, 2088
Bowen's disease, 1297
BPH; *see* Benign prostatic hyperplasia
Brachial artery blood pressure, 64
Brachial plexus injury, 1055
Brachial pressure, 305-307
Brachyesophagus, 2018
Bradycardia, 153-156
  calcium channel blocker-induced, 205
  hypothyroidism, 334, 1809
  Legionnaire's disease, 1623
  myocardial infarction, 222
  postinfarction, 223
  sinus, 153-154, 155
  torsades de pointes, 151-152
Bradykinesia, 989
Bradykinin
  effect on vasopressin release, 1791
  lung filtration, 346
  shock, 176
  vasoactive effects on pulmonary circulation,
    363
Bradyzoite, 1676
Brain
  ammonia metabolism, 2142-2143
  cerebral angiography, 925-926, 927
  cerebrovascular disease, 997-1007
    amnesic syndrome, 1032
    atrial fibrillation, 146
    clinical separation of stroke subtypes,
      1000-1002
    depression, 1036
    dizziness, 973
    embolism, 1006
    hemorrhagic stroke, 997-998, 1006
    hypertension, 314, 315, 322-323
    ischemic stroke, 998-1000
    laboratory diagnosis, 1002-1004
    parkinsonism, 993
    prevention, complications, and
      rehabilitation, 1006-1007, 1054-1055
    sickle cell disease, 659
    thrombotic stroke, 1004-1006
  computed tomography, 917-918, 919, 920
  control of ventilation, 353
  electroencephalography, 905-908
  emetic center, 581
  encephalitis
    acquired immunodeficiency syndrome, 1477
    herpes, 1524
    measles, 1498
    mumps, 1496
    parkinsonism, 993
    picornavirus infection, 1487
    poliomyelitis, 1488
    viral, 1488
  glucose requirements, 1874
  hepatic encephalopathy, 2161
  herniation, 905, 1044
  magnetic resonance imaging, 912-924
  metabolic encephalopathy, 1078-1079
  metastasis in small cell lung cancer, 489
  mucopolysaccharidosis, 1912
  rabies, 1505
  syphilis, 1641
  target for circulating hormones, 1076
Brain abscess, 1413-1416
  Acanthamoeba, 1684
  acute meningitis, 1407
  amebic, 1682
  anaerobic bacteria, 1617
  sinusitis, 2309
Brain death, 1083
  criteria, 951
  transplant donor, 338-339

Brain disease
  acute confusional state, 1031
  amnesic syndrome, 1032
  bladder-emptying dysfunction, 1066
  emotional expression disorders, 1033-1034
  frontal lobe syndrome, 1032-1033
Brain injury, 1043-1045
  dementia, 988
  endocardial hemorrhage, 1087
  frontal lobe syndrome, 1032
  increased intracranial pressure, 1084
  rehabilitation, 1055-1056
  seizure, 980
Brain natriuretic peptide, 738
Brain resuscitation, 1085
Brain scan, 926-929
Brain stem
  diseases causing dizziness, 973
  regulation of gastric acid secretion, 1981
Brain tumor
  computed tomography, 920
  dementia, 988
  depression, 1037
  headache, 960
  magnetic resonance imaging, 923
  neurooncology, 1067-1070
  seizure, 980
  tuberous sclerosis, 1922
Brainstem auditory evoked potentials,
    911-912
Branch retinal vein occlusions, 2304
Branched-chain amino acids, 1907-1908
Branched deoxyribonucleic acid assay
  hepatitis B infection, 2175
  hepatitis C infection, 2176
  human immunodeficiency virus infection
    diagnosis, 1472
Branchial cleft cyst, 2310
Branching enzyme deficiency, 1882
Brandt-Daroff exercises, 972
Branhamella, 1368
Branham's sign, 81
Brazilian purpuric fever, 1589
Break point cluster region gene, 563
Breast
  adolescent growth abnormalities, 1770
  anatomy and physiology, 1846-1849
  benign disease, 1846-1850
  gynecomastia, 1764-1766
  preventive care guidelines, 2255
  proliferative lesions, 1850
Breast cancer, 706-713
  axillary nodal metastases, 732
  curability with chemotherapy, 552
  hypercalcemia of malignancy, 1973
  incidence and death rates, 550
  neoplastic pericarditis, 272
  oral contraceptives and, 2270
  pulmonary metastases, 493
  risks in benign breast lesions, 1846,
    1847-1848, 1849
  screening, 25, 552
  second malignancy, 586
  supraclavicular lymphadenopathy, 598
Breast-feeding
  human immunodeficiency virus transmission,
    1471
  oxytocin action, 1792
Breath sounds
  chronic obstructive pulmonary disease, 442
  interstitial lung disease, 450
  pleural disease, 505
Breath urea test, 2003
Breathing
  abnormalities of control, 352-357
  asthma, 1188
  neural control, 358
  sleep-disordered, 943-944
Breathing retraining, 436
Breathing techniques, 482

Breathlessness, 404, 405
  acute lung allograft rejection, 521
  acute pancreatitis, 2234
  acute pericarditis, 273
  aortic stenosis, 236
  asthma, 1187
  atrial septal defect, 281
  behavioral control of breathing, 356-357
  bronchiolitis obliterans syndrome, 522
  cardiac tamponade, 275
  chronic obstructive pulmonary disease, 442
  complete transposition of great arteries, 290
  dilated cardiomyopathy, 263
  exercise testing, 379
  heart failure, 163
  human immunodeficiency virus, 1477
  hypersensitivity pneumonitis, 461
  hypertrophic obstructive cardiomyopathy, 266
  idiopathic pulmonary fibrosis, 453
  interstitial lung disease, 450
  ischemic heart disease, 196-197
  Langerhans' cell granulomatosis, 464
  lung cancer, 488
  lymphomatoid granulomatosis, 470
  malignant mesothelioma, 510
  mediastinal abnormality, 511
  mitral regurgitation, 250
  mitral stenosis, 246
  pleural disease, 505
  pneumothorax, 509
  precapillary pulmonary hypertension, 293
  psychologic considerations, 432
  pulmonary edema, 168
  pulmonary function tests, 375
  pulmonary hypertension, 498
  pulmonary thromboembolism, 500
  pulmonary veno-occlusive disease, 298
  respiratory muscle failure, 359
  right atrial myxoma, 330
  sarcoidosis, 458
  spontaneous pneumomediastinum, 514
  systemic lupus erythematosus, 1215
  systemic sclerosis, 1230
  Wegener's granulomatosis, 468
Breslow thickness, 1299
Bretylium, 1740
Brevibloc; *see* Esmolol
Bridging necrosis, 2180
Brief Cognitive Rating Scale, 904
Brief reactive psychosis, 1041
Brill-Zinsser disease, 1544
Brim sign, 1956
British antilewisite
  arsenic poisoning, 867
  rheumatoid arthritis, 1208
Broad-spectrum antibiotics, 1356
Broca's aphasia, 976
Bromocriptine
  acromegaly, 1784-1785
  cocaine intoxication, 2297
  fibrocystic breast disease, 1850
  gonadotropin-secreting pituitary tumor, 1787
  hepatic encephalopathy, 2161
  hyperprolactinemia, 1786
  interaction with cyclosporin, 793
  Parkinson's disease, 991, 992
  prolactinoma, 1759
  use during pregnancy, 2274
Bronchial adenoma, 491-492
Bronchial allergen challenge, 1154
Bronchial artery angiogram, 388-389
Bronchial challenge testing, 379, 1188
Bronchial constriction, 348
Bronchiectasis, 483-485
  cough, 406
  cystic fibrosis, 480
  double lung allograft, 515
  dyspnea, 404
  high-resolution computed tomography, 387
  sputum expectoration, 408
Bronchiolar diseases, 455

Bronchiole, 1828
Bronchiolitis
    chronic obstructive pulmonary disease, 439
    cystic fibrosis, 480
    desquamative interstitial pneumonia, 449
    follicular bronchitis/bronchiolitis, 455
    Langerhans' cell granulomatosis, 463
Bronchiolitis obliterans, 517, 522-524, 1503
Bronchiolitis obliterans-organizing pneumonia,
        448, 452-453
Bronchioloalveolar carcinoma, 487
Bronchitis
    asthma *versus,* 1189
    chronic
        API deficiency, 440
        defined, 437-438
        hemoptysis, 411
        pathogenesis, 442
        pathology, 439
        patterns of pulmonary function
                abnormalities, 379
    cough, 406
    follicular bronchitis/bronchiolitis, 455
    parainfluenza, 1494
    physical findings, 403
    sputum expectoration, 408
Bronchoalveolar lavage, 383, 384
    acute lung allograft rejection, 521
    cytomegalovirus pneumonia in lung allograft,
            518
    interstitial lung disease, 451
    Pneumocystis carinii, 1694
    reimplantation response, 517
    sarcoidosis, 459
Bronchoconstriction
    asthma, 1187
    pulmonary edema, 424
    wheezing, 404
Bronchodilators, 377-378
    asthma, 1189-1190
    chronic obstructive pulmonary disease, 417,
            443-444
    cough, 408
    cystic fibrosis, 482
    hyperkalemia, 833
    pertussis, 1613
    during pregnancy, 2277
    pulmonary rehabilitation, 434
    stimulant-dependent sleep disorder, 945
Bronchogenic cyst, 513
Bronchopleural fistula
    chronic obstructive pulmonary disease, 447
    tuberculous empyema, 507
Bronchoprovocation inhalation tests, 379
Bronchoscopy, 383-384
    acquired immunodeficiency syndrome, 1477
    diagnosis and staging of lung cancer, 489-490
    hemoptysis, 411
    lung cancer, 726
Bronchospasm, 2082
    asthma, 1187, 1188
    beta-adrenergic blocker-induced, 202
    dobutamine stress imaging, 104
    drug-induced, 476, 477
    mitomycin toxicity, 478
    sinusitis, 2308
    wheezing with, 404
Brown pigment stones, 2220, 2221, 2222
Brown-Séquard syndrome, 1012, 1048
Brown tumor, 1966
Brucellosis, 1604-1607
    antibiotic selection, 1347
    fever of unknown origin, 1377
    weight loss, 1750
Bruch's membrane, 2301-2302
Brudzinski's sign, 1406
Brugia malayi, 1699
Bruising, 602, 603
    acute lymphoblastic leukemia, 682
    aplastic anemia, 672
    Churg-Strauss syndrome, 466

Bruising—cont'd
    differential diagnosis of fever and rash, 1384
    Ehlers-Danlos syndromes, 1288
    gram-negative bacteremia, 1449
    Henoch-Schönlein purpura, 1222
    idiopathic myelofibrosis, 677
    immune thrombocytopenic, 1472
    mixed cryoglobulinemia, 1249
    posttransfusion, 616
    Rocky Mountain spotted fever, Plate VIII-18
    Wegener's granulomatosis, 468
Bruit
    auscultation of subclavian artery, 306
    chronic aortic obstruction, 304
    renovascular hypertension, 321
    Takayasu's arteritis, 303
Brunner's glands, 2082
Brush border, 2057
Brushing, esophageal, 2000
Bruton's agammaglobulinemia, 1175
Bruxism, 946
btk/tec family, 1175
Bubonic plague, 1610
Buccal smear, 1743
Buclizine hydrochloride, 2027
Budd-Chiari syndrome, 2208
    imaging studies, 2140
    liver transplantation, 2219
    oral contraceptives, 2190
Budesonide
    Crohn's disease, 2071
    rhinitis, 1182
Buerger's disease, 308
Buffers, 834
Bulbar poliomyelitis, 1488
Bulbocavernous reflex, 964, 1051
Bulimia
    criteria, 2028
    neurohormonal regulation, 1077
Bulla
    chronic obstructive pulmonary disease, 447
    diabetic patient, 1323
    emphysema, 439
    fixed drug eruption, 1315
    idiopathic thrombocytopenic purpura, Plate
            IV-10
    Langerhans' cell granulomatosis, 465
    porphyria cutanea tarda, 1927
    staphylococcal scalded-skin syndrome, 1421
    sun-induced, 1307
Bullous diseases, 1158, 1293-1297
Bullous impetigo, 1419
Bullous pemphigoid, 1155, 1295-1296
Bullous systemic lupus erythematosus, 1296
Bumetanide
    cause of renal potassium wasting and
            alkalosis, 828
    heart failure, 170
    hyperkalemia, 833
    interference with oral anticoagulants, 636
Bundle branch block, 86
    aortic stenosis, 237
    Ebstein's anomaly, 290
    electrocardiography, 87, 88
    endocardial cushion defect, 283
    exercise imaging, 104
    intraventricular conduction abnormalities, 156
    myocardial infarction, 88, 223
    myocarditis, 263
    thrombolytic therapy, 214
Bundle branch reentry ventricular tachycardia, 153
Bundle of His, 132
    accelerated atrioventricular junctional rhythm,
            144
    accessory pathways, 90
    arrhythmia, 134
    cardiac cycle, 36
    conduction disturbance in myocardial
            infarction, 222
    electrical impulse, 84
    intraventricular conduction abnormalities, 156

Bunyavirus, 1514-1519
Bupropion, 1037
    chronic fatigue syndrome, 2300
    depression in elderly patients, 2289
Burkholderia cepacia, 480
Burkitt's lymphoma, 695
    chromosomal translocation, 544
    hypophosphatemia, 1936
    ocular involvement, 2306
Burn
    gram-negative bacteremia, 1446
    hypophosphatemia, 1936
    increased nutrient requirements, 2102
    intravascular hemolysis, 668
    lye, 2019
    nosocomial infection, 1361
Bursitis, 1196
Burst-forming unit-erythroid, 531
Burst-forming unit-megakaryocyte, 532
Buspirone, 1035
Busulfan
    chronic myelogenous leukemia, 687
    hepatic injury, 2192
    hepatic toxicity, 585
    myelofibrosis, 677
    pulmonary parenchymal reactions, 476
    pulmonary toxicity, 478, 584
Butterfly rash, 1213, 1214
Buttock cell, 594
Buttressing, 1168
Butyrophenones, 582
BVAD; *see* Biventricular assist device
Byler's disease, 2158-2159
Bypass
    cardiopulmonary
        heart-lung allograft, 515
        nosocomial infection, 1480
        postperfusion syndrome, 668
        transient thrombocytopenia, 614
    coronary artery
        cardiogenic shock, 185
        cost-utility analysis, 16
        internal mammary artery, 206
        ischemic heart disease, 206-207
        patient on dialysis, 783
        percutaneous transluminal coronary
                angioplasty *versus,* 117, 118
        triiodothyronine levels following, 1811
    gastric, 1753, 1876
    ischemic bowel, 2087
    jejunoileal, 2104-2105
    Takayasu's arteritis, 311
Bypass Angioplasty Revascularization
        Investigation, 117
Byssinosis, 460
Bystander effect, 1142

C

C-CAT trial, 124
^{14}C-cholyglycine absorption test, 2007
C-fos protein, 50-51, 55
C-jun protein, 50-51, 55
C-ketoisocaproic breath test, 2144
C-kit ligand, 1128
C-kit ligand stem cell factor, 532
C-MOPP regimen, 699
C-Mpl ligand, 532
C-myc protooncogene, 55, 1126
C-peptide, 1744, 1877
C-reactive protein
    acute meningitis, 1408
    brain abscess, 1415
    diagnosis of pancreatic disease, 2145
    osteomyelitis, 1434
    rheumatic fever, 1257
C region, 1111
C-terminal assay, 1745
^{14}C-triolein breath test, 2006-2007
C type of natriuretic peptide, 738
C-urea breath test, 2037

C wave
  cardiac cycle, 71
  jugular venous pulse, 65
C-xylose breath test, 2061
C1
  activation, 1133, 1134
  deficiency, 1179
C1-alpha-hydroxylase, 1961
C1-esterase inhibitor, 1454
C1 inhibitor, 1135
  deficiency, 1148, 1180
C1s, 1133
C2, 1133
  deficiency, 1179
C3, 1338
  activation, 1134, 1135
  antigenic assay, 1147-1148
  deficiency, 1179, 1339
  partial lipodystrophy, 1902
C3 convertase, 1133
C3 nephritic factor, 1148, 1180
  membranoproliferative glomerulonephritis, 854
  partial lipodystrophy, 1902
C3a, 1448
C3bBb, 1338
C4, 1133
  antigenic assay, 1147-1148
  deficiency, 1179
C4-binding protein, 1135
C4b2b complex, 1135
C5, 1135
C5a, 1136
  bacteremia, 1448
C9, 1137
C282Y mutation, 2204
CA125 antigen, 716
Cachectin, 1750
Cachexia
  diabetic neuropathic, 1749
  oculopharyngeal dystrophy, 1028
  retroperitoneal abscess, 1398
Cadherins, 1293
Cadmium
  carcinogenesis, 548
  chronic tubulointerstitial nephritis, 891
  renal toxicity, 867
Café-au-lait spot, 1920
Caffeine
  arrhythmia, 133
  demethylation, 2143
  fibrocystic breast disease, 1849, 1850
  premature ventricular contractions, 149
  stimulant-dependent sleep disorder, 945
CAGE questionnaire, 3, 4, 2198, 2294
Calan; *see* Verapamil
Calcific retinal embolus, 1057, 1058
Calcific tendinitis, 1168, 1196
Calcification
  bicuspid aortic valve, 287
  bone formation, 1949
  bone matrix, 1716
  constrictive pericarditis, 277
  gastrointestinal brucellosis, 1606
  hyperparathyroid bone disease, 1963
  intervertebral disk, 1170-1171
  intraarticular and periarticular, 1169
  medullary sponge kidney, 875
  mitral stenosis, 245
  nontoxic goiter, 1812
  pineal, 1083
  pleural, 510
  pseudohypoparathyroidism, 1932
  silicosis, 475
  solitary pulmonary nodule, 493
  systemic sclerosis, 1228-1229
  valve replacement surgery, 257
Calcimimetics, 1971
Calcinosis, 1232
Calcitonin
  bone and mineral disorders, 1746
  calcium stimulation tests, 1739

Calcitonin—cont'd
  medullary thyroid carcinoma, 1732, 1816,
    2005
  osteoporosis, 1948
  Paget's disease, 1956-1957
  reflex sympathetic dystrophy syndrome, 1247
  role in calcium metabolism, 1718-1719
  uremia, 786
Calcitonin gene-related peptide, 1718, 1982
Calcitonin receptor, 1719
Calcitriol
  osteoporosis, 1948
  renal bone disease, 1964
  renal osteodystrophy, 1961
  rickets, 881
  X-linked hypophosphatemic rickets, 880
Calcium
  abnormalities of impulse formation, 132
  aortic stenosis, 237
  body water compartments, 736
  chronic renal failure, 779
  drug-nutrient interactions, 2110
  functions, 2109
  heart failure, 160
  hypercalcemia, 1927-1930
    acute renal failure, 773
    calcitonin therapy, 1719
    causes and differential diagnosis, 1927-1928
    chronic nephrocalcinosis, 891
    clinical features, 1928-1929
    congenital aortic stenosis, 287
    1,25-dihydrotachysterol, 1954
    efforts of ionized calcium on cell metabolic
      processes, 1717
    electrocardiographic abnormalities, 89, 90
    endocrine paraneoplastic syndromes, 583
    interstitial lung disease, 452
    kidney stone formation, 798
    lung cancer, 489
    malignancy, 1972-1974
    medication-induced, 1928
    multiple myeloma, 700, 702, 864
    nonparathyroid endocrine disorders, 1928
    Paget's disease, 1956
    predominant hyperparathyroid bone disease,
      1964
    primary hyperparathyroidism, 1965, 1966,
      1967
    renal cell carcinoma, 898
    renal magnesium wasting, 1940-1941
    sarcoidosis, 458
    steroid suppression test, 1746
    treatment, 1929-1930
    urinary cyclic adenosine monophosphate,
      1746
    vitamin D toxicity, 1928
  hypercalciuria
    dietary factors, 2102
    hypophosphatemia, 1936
    hypophosphatemic rickets, 1952-1953
    mechanisms, 797-798
    sarcoidosis, 458
    urine calcium, 1744
  hyperkalemia therapy, 833
  hyperphosphatemia, 1938
  hypertension, 317-318
  hypocalcemia, 1930-1934
    acute pancreatitis, 2237
    acute renal failure, 773
    after massive transfusion, 2011
    chronic renal failure, 779, 785-786
    clinical features, 1932-1933
    differential diagnosis, 1931-1932
    efforts of ionized calcium on cell metabolic
      processes, 1717
    electrocardiographic abnormalities, 89, 90
    ethylene glycol poisoning, 866
    hyperphosphatemia, 1938
    hypomagnesemia, 1942
    nephrotic syndrome, 767
    osteomalacia, 1949

Calcium—cont'd
  hypocalcemia—cont'd
    relative hypoparathyroidism, 1932
    treatment, 1933-1934
    vitamin D deficiency, 2106
  hypocalciuria, 1942
  intestinal absorption, 1988-1989
  mediation of hormone action, 1711-1712
  metabolism, 1717-1720
  osteoporosis, 1947
  parenteral solutions, 2114
  platelet aggregation, 536
  recommended daily dietary allowances, 2115
  secondary hyperparathyroidism, 881
  serum
    bone and mineral disorders, 1744
    hypercalcemia, 1929
    hypercalcemia of malignancy, 1974
    hypocalcemia, 1930
    osteomalacia, 1949
    primary hyperparathyroidism, 1967
    small bowel malabsorption, 2058
  smooth muscle contraction, 1976
  storage in bone, 1715
  supplements in rickets or osteomalacia, 1954
  total parenteral nutrition formula, 2117
  urine
    bone and mineral disorders, 1744
    crystals, 746
    hypercalciuria, 1744
    primary hyperparathyroidism, 1968
Calcium acetate, 785
Calcium-activated calmodulin kinase, 41
Calcium ATPase of plasma membrane, 58
Calcium ATPase of sarcoplasmic reticulum, 58
Calcium carbonate
  chronic pancreatitis, 2238
  hyperphosphatemia, 774
  hypocalcemia, 1934
  renal bone disease, 1964
  renal osteodystrophy, 785
  urinary crystals, 746
Calcium carbonate-apatite stone, 799
Calcium channel, 58-59
  abnormalities of impulse formation, 132
  cardiac conduction, 38
  cellular modulation of contractility, 40
Calcium channel blockers
  achalasia, 2022
  angina, 203
  aortic regurgitation, 243
  arrhythmias, 138
  asthma, 1191
  autonomic dysreflexia, 1049
  chronic hypertension during pregnancy, 2275
  diabetic nephropathy, 862
  diastolic heart failure, 168
  heart failure, 174
  human cytochrome P450 isoforms, 2312
  hypertension, 324, 325, 327
  hypertrophic obstructive cardiomyopathy, 269
  interaction with cyclosporin, 793
  ischemic heart disease, 203-205
  myocardial infarction, 216-217
  prevention or delay of end-stage renal disease,
    782
  primary pulmonary hypertension, 295
  properties, 204
  prophylaxis of migraine, 962
  Raynaud's phenomenon, 310, 1227
  renovascular hypertension, 896
Calcium chloride
  after massive transfusion, 2011
  hypermagnesemia, 1943
Calcium citrate, 1934
Calcium-containing stone, 797-799, 803-804
Calcium fatty acid soaps, 2220
Calcium gluconate
  hyperkalemia, 833
  hypermagnesemia, 1943
  vitamin D deficiency, 2106

Calcium oxalate
  arthropathy, 1280
  ethylene glycol poisoning, 866
  urinary crystals, 746
Calcium oxalate dihydrate crystals, 801
Calcium oxalate monohydrate crystals, 801
Calcium oxalate stones
  increased fecal bile salt loss, 2129
  obstructive uropathy, 885
Calcium phosphate crystals, 801
Calcium pyrophosphate dihydrate crystals, 1162
Calcium pyrophosphate dihydrate deposition
        disease, 1276-1279
  cyst formation, 1168
  hand, 1171
  intraarticular and periarticular calcification,
        1168
  osteoarthritis, 1267
  septic arthritis *versus,* 1252
  wrist, 1172
Calcium-regulating hormones, 1946-1947
Calcium salts, 2220
Calcium sensor, 1718
Calculus
  biliary tract stones, 2220-2231
    asymptomatic *versus* symptomatic, 2225
    biliary colic, 2225-2227
    cholecystitis, 2227-2228
    choledocholithiasis, 2228-2230
    cholesterol stones, 2221, 2222
    cholesterolosis, 2230-2231
    classification and composition, 2220, 2221
    Crohn's disease, 2075
    defective bile salt synthesis, 2129
    diagnostic tests, 2224-2225
    epidemiology, 2222-2223
    gallstone pancreatitis, 2230
    hereditary spherocytosis, 665-666
    pathophysiology, 2220-2221
    pigment stones, 2221-2222
    during pregnancy, 2278
    risk factors, 2223-2224
    sickle cell disease, 657, 659
  bilirubin, 665-666
  cystine, 1910
  pancreatic, 2238, 2239, 2240
  renal, 796-805
    autosomal dominant polycystic kidney
        disease, 873
    calcium-containing stones, 797-799
    cystine stones, 799-800
    differential diagnosis, 800
    laboratory and diagnostic testing, 800, 801,
        802
    management, 803-805
    medullary sponge kidney, 875
    obstructive uropathy, 885
    physiology and pathophysiology, 797
    spinal cord injured patient, 1050
    struvite stones, 799
    uric acid stones, 799
    urine calcium, 1744
California encephalitis, 1515, 1517
Callosal apraxia, 976
Calmodulin, 55, 1711-1712, 1717
Caloric intake
  diabetes mellitus, 1856-1857
  effects on lipoproteins, 1890
  elderly, 2287
  excessive, 2101
  obesity, 1752-1753
  renal insufficiency in diabetic patient, 1870
Caloric test, 948
Calorie requirements, 2111-2112
CaM-K; *see* Calcium-activated calmodulin
        kinase
cAMP; *see* Cyclic adenosine monophosphate
Campylobacter, 1590-1593
  acquired immunodeficiency syndrome, 1476
  compromised host, 1388
  gay bowel syndrome, 1429

Campylobacter coli, 1590
Campylobacter fetus, 1590
Campylobacter jejuni, 1590, 1591-1592
  antibiotic selection, 1347
  Bruton's agammaglobulinemia, 1175
  diarrhea, 1426-1427
Canadian Cardiovascular Society
  classification of angina pectoris, 127
  Functional Classification Scheme, 2257
Canalicular cholestasis, 2155, 2188
Canalicular multifunctional organic anion
        transporter, 2126
Canalicular multispecific organic anion
        transporter, 2149
Canalicular water secretion, 2123, 2124
Cancellous bone, 1714-1715, 1963
Cancer
  acquired immunodeficiency
        syndrome-associated, 1329
  acute meningitis, 1407
  acute renal failure with, 775
  adrenal, 1822
    aldosterone-secreting adenoma, 1823
    computed tomography, 1734
    Cushing's syndrome, 1820
  ampulla of Vater, 2232, 2242
  bile ducts, 2231-2232
  bladder, 550
  bowel, 2076-2077
  breast, 706-713
    axillary nodal metastases, 732
    curability with chemotherapy, 552
    hypercalcemia of malignancy, 1973
    incidence and death rates, 550
    neoplastic pericarditis, 272
    oral contraceptives and, 2270
    pulmonary metastases, 493
    risks in benign breast lesions, 1846,
        1847-1848, 1849
    screening, 25, 552
    second malignancy, 586
    supraclavicular lymphadenopathy, 598
  cervical, 714-715
  chemotherapy, 554-555
  chronic abdominal pain, 2035
  colon, 2082-2086
    allelic loss, 546
    Campylobacter jejuni infection *versus,* 1591
    colonoscopy, 1996
    curability with chemotherapy, 552
    hereditary nonpolyposis, 549
    incidence and death rates, 550
    physiology and pathophysiology, 2082-2083
    risk in ulcerative colitis, 2075
    screening, 552-553
  complications, 579-586
    nausea and vomiting, 581-582
    neutropenia and fever, 582
    pain, 580-581
    paraneoplastic syndromes, 582-583
    radiation therapy, 585
    secondary malignancies, 585-586
    therapy, 583-586
  curability, 551-552
  cutaneous manifestations, 1316-1320
  diagnosis and staging, 550-551
  disseminated intravascular coagulation, 628
  elderly, 2282
  endometrial, 713-714
  epidemiology, 550
  esophageal, 2023-2024
  exposure to chemical agents, 868
  gallbladder, 2232
  genetics, 540-549
    environmental agents, 548-549
    genetic stability and tumor formation, 549
    multistep genetic pathway to tumor
        formation, 547-548
    oncogenes, 541-545
    tumor suppressor genes, 545-547
  head and neck, 722-724

Cancer—cont'd
  hematopoietic stem cell transplantation,
        576-577
  Hodgkin's disease, 691-695
    acquired ichthyosis, 1316
    chemotactic defects, 1340
    curability with chemotherapy, 552
    fever of unknown origin, 1377
    infertility, 585
    internal lymphadenopathy, 598
    molecular diagnostics, 563-564
    secondary malignancies, 585-586
    stomach involvement, 2049
    thyroid gland failure, 1809
  hypercalcemia of malignancy, 1972-1974
  immunosuppression-related, 795
  leukemia, 685-691
    abnormal lymphocytes in peripheral blood,
        595
    acute lymphoblastic, 682-683
    acute myelogenous leukemia, 689-690, 691
    arthropathy, 1247
    cardiac metastasis, 331
    chromosomal abnormalities, 544
    chronic, 686
    curability with chemotherapy, 552
    essential thrombocythemia, 687-688
    fever of unknown origin, 1377
    hematopoietic stem cell transplantation,
        576-577
    incidence and death rates, 550
    lymphoid, 682-685
    lysozymuria, 760
    mast cell, 681
    megakaryocytic hypoplasia, 614
    molecular diagnostics, 562-563
    myelodysplastic syndrome, 676
    myelodysplastic syndromes, 690-691
    myelogenous leukemia, 686-687
    myeloproliferative disorders, 685-691
    neoplastic pericarditis, 272
    nosocomial infection, 1361
    plasma cell, 703
    platelet abnormalities, 611
    polycythemia vera, 688
    second malignancy, 586
    splenomegaly, 601
  lung, 486-492, 724-729
    asbestos-related, 474
    bronchial adenoma, 491-492
    clinical presentation, 487-488
    diagnosis and staging, 489-490
    ectopic production of adrenocorticotropic
        hormone, 1820
    genetic predisposition, 486
    hamartoma, 492
    hemoptysis, 411
    hypertrophic osteoarthropathy, 1247
    incidence and death rates, 550
    magnetic resonance imaging, 389
    malignant effusion, 508
    metastasis, 489, 492
    molecular biology, 487
    neoplastic pericarditis, 272
    nervous system metastasis, 489
    oat cell carcinoma, 1024
    occupational exposure, 476
    papilloma, 492
    paraneoplastic syndromes, 488-489
    pathology, 487
    prevention, 491
    pulmonary metastasis, 492
    screening, 490
    solitary pulmonary nodule, 493-497
    staging, 725-726
    treatment, 490-491
  metastases
    breast cancer, 707, 710-711
    carcinoid tumors, 2082
    colon cancer, 2085
    complications, 1070-1073, 1074

Cancer—cont'd
  metastases—cont'd
    cutaneous, 1316
    esophageal cancer, 2024
    gastric cancer, 2046
    hepatocellular carcinoma, 2213
    involving heart, 330-332
    lung cancer, 489, 492, 726
    megakaryocytic hypoplasia, 614
    neoplastic pericarditis, 272
    pancreatic tumor, 2242
    peritoneal tumors, 2249
    prostate cancer, 718
    renal cell carcinoma, 898
    skeletal, 1971-1974
    solitary pulmonary nodule, 494
    testicular cancer, 720
  molecular diagnostics, 559-564
    clonality, 559
    DNA analysis, 559-561
    fluorescence in situ hybridization, 561, 562
    leukemia, 562-563
    lymphoma, 563-564
  multiple myeloma, 700-703
    anion gap acidosis, 836
    bleeding problems, 612
    monoclonal gammopathy of undetermined significance, 705
    nephrotic syndrome, 767
    plasmacytoid lymphocytes, 595
    streptococcal superantigen method, 743
  neurologic complications, 1070-1074
  neurooncology, 1067-1074
  neutrophilia, 590
  non-Hodgkin's lymphoma, 695-700
    bone marrow biopsy section, 558
    heart involvement, 331
    molecular diagnostics, 563
  nutritional factors, 2100
  ovarian, 715-716
    curability with chemotherapy, 552
    peritoneal carcinomatosis, 732
    thyrotoxicosis, 1807
  pancreatic, incidence and death rates, 550
  prevention, 550
  prostate, 717-720
    elevated prostate specific antigen, 732
    incidence and death rates, 550
    obstructive uropathy, 885
    osteoblastic bone formation, 1971
    pulmonary metastases, 493
    screening, 553
  radiation therapy, 553-554
  radionuclide angiography, 105
  renal cell carcinoma, 898-899
    incidence and death rates, 550
  risk of stroke, 1001
  screening, 552-553
  stomach, 2045-2050, Plate X-3
    adenocarcinoma, 2039, 2045-2050
    carcinoid, 2082
    peptic ulcer disease *versus,* 2038
  surgical treatment, 553
  testicular, 720-722
    curability with chemotherapy, 552
    gynecomastia, 1764, 1765
    impotence, 1762
  thyroid, 1814-1817
    Hashimoto's thyroiditis, 1811
    pulmonary metastases, 493
    serum calcitonin, 1746
    thyroid biopsy, 1802
  unknown primary site, 729-733
  upper gastrointestinal endoscopic surveillance, 1995
  vitamin E, 2106
  weight loss, 1749-1750
Cancer and steroid hormone study, 2270
Cancer-associated myositis, 1236

Candida, 1310-1312, 1660-1664
  acquired immunodeficiency syndrome, 1328, 1476, 2094
  after renal transplantation, 794
  compromised host, 1388
  continuous ambulatory peritoneal dialysis-related peritonitis, 2248
  diabetic patient, 1323
  drug-induced infection, 1313
  endocarditis, 226
  esophageal infection, 2019-2020
  fever, 1383, 1387
  gastric infection, 2043
  genital lesions, 1444
  lung transplantation, 517, 518, 519-520
  meningitis, 1404, 1409
  normal flora, 1368
  odynophagia, 1998
  peritonitis, 1397
  rash, 1383
  serodiagnosis, 1653
  Sjögren syndrome, 1212
  urinary tract infection, 1457
  vaginitis, 762
  vulvovaginal infection, 1442
Candidemia, 1662
Cannon wave, 66
Cannula
  hospital-acquired bloodstream infection, 1364
  oxygen administration, 445
  pancreatic secretion measurement, 2134
  peripheral artery, 390
CAPD; *see* Continuous ambulatory peritoneal dialysis
Capillary blood gas, 349
Capillary endothelium, 348, 371
Capillary exchange, 47-48
Capillary hydrostatic pressure
  microvascular fluid exchange, 346
  shock, 177
Capillary perfusion, 349
Capillary permeability, 424
Capillary pressure, 168, 424
Capillary wedge pressure, 183, 361, 362
Capitation, 32-33
Caplan's syndrome, 475, 1204
Capnography, 396, 431
Capoten; *see* Captopril
Capreomycin, 1631
Capsaicin
  cancer pain, 580
  osteoarthritis, 1268
Capsid, 1483
Capsomer, 1483
Capsule
  bacterial, 1446
  streptococcal, 1554
Captopril, 1741-1742
  cystinuria, 804-805
  diabetic nephropathy, 862
  dilated cardiomyopathy, 264
  heart failure, 170, 172
  hepatic injury, 2192
  hypertension, 325
  myocardial infarction, 217
  pulmonary toxicity, 479
  renovascular hypertension, 321
Capture beat, 150
Carbacephems, 1349
Carbachol, 2302
Carbamazepine, 983
  diabetes insipidus, 1797
  drug-induced bile duct injury, 2203
  hepatic injury, 2190, 2191
  human cytochrome P450 isoforms, 2312
  interaction with cyclosporin, 793
  interference with oral anticoagulants, 636
  pulmonary hypersensitivity reactions, 479
  pulmonary parenchymal reactions, 476
  vasopressin inhibition, 1791
Carbamoylphosphate synthetase, 1906, 1907

Carbapenems
  dosage, 1349
  effects on kidney, 868
Carbenicillin, 1350, 1352
Carbidopa-levodopa, 944
Carbimazole, 2191
Carbohydrate antigen 19-9, cholangiocarcinoma, 2202
Carbohydrate-deficient transferrin test, 2198
Carbohydrates
  chronic renal failure, 786
  effects on cholesterol, 1890
  ground substance, 1289-1290
  hepatic metabolism, 2121-2122
  heritable disorders of metabolism, 1879-1883
    galactosemia, 1882-1883
    glycogen storage diseases, 1880-1882
    nondiabetic melliturias, 1879-1880
  hydrogen breath test, 2006
  intestinal absorption, 1987
  intolerance, 197
  leprechaunism, 1900
  malabsorption, 2060, 2067-2068
  metabolism, 1851
Carbolfuchsin stain, 1371
Carbon-11 acetate, 106
Carbon dioxide
  hypercapnia
    acute respiratory failure, 412
    chronic obstructive pulmonary disease, 442
    hypoventilation and, 356
    mechanical ventilation, 397
    obstructive lung disease, 356
    during sleep, 354
    vasopressin secretion, 1790-1791
    ventilatory response to hypoxia, 353
  hypocapnia, 355-356
    hyperventilation-induced, 525
    pulmonary edema, 425
    to reduce increased intracranial pressure, 1084
  vasoactive effects on pulmonary circulation, 363
  ventilatory response to, 353
Carbon dioxide angiography, 895
Carbon dioxide dissociation curve, 348, 349
Carbon dioxide partial pressure
  asthma, 1189
  Cheyne-Stokes breathing, 354
  medullary chemoreceptors, 353
  obstructive lung disease, 357
  primary pulmonary hypertension, 294
  regulation of, 834
  renal hydrogen ion secretion, 741
  ventilatory control studies, 378
Carbon disulfide, 1020
Carbon monoxide
  oxygen transport disorders, 350
  poisoning, 993
  single-breath diffusing capacity, 378
Carbon monoxide diffusing capacity
  bleomycin-induced pulmonary diseases, 477
  chronic obstructive pulmonary disease, 442
  hypersensitivity pneumonitis, 461
  interstitial lung disease, 450
Carbon tetrachloride, 866
  aplastic anemia, 672
  poisoning, 2188
Carbonate, 1715
Carbonic acid, 834
Carbonic anhydrase
  bicarbonate, 835
  deficiency in osteopetrosis, 1958
  renal acid excretion, 740
Carbonic anhydrase inhibitors, 835
  cystine stones, 804
  glaucoma, 2302
  normotensive renal potassium wasting, 828
Carboxyhemoglobin, 443
Carboxyterminal constant domain, 1122
Carbuncle, 1421, 1456

Carbutamide, 2191
Carcinoembryonic antigen
  cholangiocarcinoma, 2202
  colon cancer, 2085
  gastric cancer, 2047
  intrahepatic cholangiocarcinoma, 2215
Carcinoid, 2082
  bronchial, 491-492
  chronic diarrhea, 2051
  colon, 2086
  gastric, 2050
  intestinal, 2081-2082
  medullary thyroid carcinoma, 1816
  niacin deficiency, 2107
  renal, 899
  weight loss, 1749
Carcinoma
  adenocarcinoma
    ampulla of Vater, 2232
    breast, 707
    cancer of unknown primary site, 732
    chemotherapy, 732
    colonic, 2076-2077
    endometrium, 713-714
    esophageal, 2018, 2023-2024
    gallbladder, 2232
    gastric, 2039, 2045-2050
    intrahepatic cholangiocarcinoma, 2214
    lung, 487, 725
    pancreatic, 2242
    prostate, 717-720
    small bowel, 2080, 2081
    of unknown primary site, 730
  adenoid cystic, 491
  adrenal, 1822
    aldosterone-secreting adenoma, 1823
    computed tomography, 1734
    Cushing's syndrome, 1820
  basal cell, 1297, Plate VII-5
  Bellini duct, 899
  bile ducts, 2231-2232
  bladder, 550
  breast, 706-713
    axillary nodal metastases, 732
    curability with chemotherapy, 552
    hypercalcemia of malignancy, 1973
    incidence and death rates, 550
    neoplastic pericarditis, 272
    oral contraceptives and, 2270
    pulmonary metastases, 493
    risks in benign breast lesions, 1846,
      1847-1848, 1849
    screening, 25, 552
    second malignancy, 586
    supraclavicular lymphadenopathy, 598
  bronchioloalveolar, 487
  cervix, 714-715
  cholangiocarcinoma, 2231-2232
    inflammatory bowel disease, 2076
    intrahepatic, 2214-2215
    primary sclerosing cholangitis, 2201-2202
  choriocarcinoma, 493
  collecting duct, 899
  colon, 2082-2086
    allelic loss, 546
    Campylobacter jejuni infection *versus,* 1591
    colonoscopy, 1996
    curability with chemotherapy, 552
    hereditary nonpolyposis, 549
    incidence and death rates, 550
    physiology and pathophysiology, 2082-2083
    risk in ulcerative colitis, 2075
    screening, 552-553
  Crohn's disease
    colonic carcinoma, 2076
    small bowel adenocarcinoma, 2081
  endometrial, 713-714
  esophageal, 2023-2024
  gallbladder, 2232
  gastric, 2046, 2047
  germ cell tumor, 732

Carcinoma—cont'd
  head and neck, 732
  hepatocellular, 2212-2214
    aflatoxin, 2185, 2212
    allelic loss, 546
    alpha-fetoprotein, 2143, 2213
    chronic hepatitis B, 2181
    drug-induced, 2189
    fibrolamellar, 2214
    hepatitis B virus, 2173
    hepatitis C virus, 2175
    liver biopsy, 2214
    porphyria cutanea tarda, 1927
  Hürthle cell, 1815
  liver
    fibrolamellar hepatocellular carcinoma,
      2214
    hepatocellular carcinoma, 2212-2214
    intrahepatic cholangiocarcinoma, 2214-2215
  lung, 486-492, 724-729
    asbestos-related, 474
    bronchial adenoma, 491-492
    clinical presentation, 487-488
    diagnosis and staging, 489-490
    ectopic production of adrenocorticotropic
      hormone, 1820
    epidermoid, 487
    genetic predisposition, 486
    hamartoma, 492
    hemoptysis, 411
    hypertrophic osteoarthropathy, 1247
    incidence and death rates, 550
    magnetic resonance imaging, 389
    malignant effusion, 508
    molecular biology, 487
    neoplastic pericarditis, 272
    nervous system metastasis, 489
    oat cell, 1024
    occupational exposure, 476
    papilloma, 492
    paraneoplastic syndromes, 488-489
    pathology, 487
    prevention, 491
    pulmonary metastasis, 492
    screening, 490
    small cell, 487, 488, 726-729
    solitary pulmonary nodule, 493-497
    staging, 725-726
    treatment, 490-491
  lymphoma *versus,* 731
  ovarian, 732
    curability with chemotherapy, 552
  ovary, 715-716
    curability with chemotherapy, 552
    peritoneal carcinomatosis, 732
    thyrotoxicosis, 1807
  pancreatic, 550
  papillary
    renal, 899
    thyroid, 1815
  parathyroid, 1965-1966
  prostate, 717-720
    elevated prostate specific antigen, 732
    incidence and death rates, 550
    obstructive uropathy, 885
    osteoblastic bone formation, 1971
    pulmonary metastases, 493
    screening, 553
  renal cell, 898-899
    abdominal mass, 898
    anemia, 898
    computed tomography, 751-752
    incidence and death rates, 550
    renal arteriography, 898
  small cell
    lung, 487, 488, 726-729
    renal, 899
  squamous cell, 1297-1298, Plate VII-5
    acquired immunodeficiency
      syndrome-associated, 1329
    biopsy, 1298

Carcinoma—cont'd
  squamous cell—cont'd
    cancer of unknown primary site, 732
    cervical lymph nodes, 732
    lung, 487
    tongue, Plate IV-14
    of unknown primary site, 730
    upper aerodigestive tract, 722-724
  stomach, 2038, 2045-2050, Plate X-3
  testicular, 720-722
    gynecomastia, 1764, 1765
    impotence, 1762
  thyroid, 1814-1817
    anaplastic, 1815-1816
    biologic markers, 1816
    Hashimoto's thyroiditis, 1811
    pulmonary metastases, 493
    serum calcitonin, 1746
    thyroid biopsy, 1802
  ulcerative colitis, 2076
  verrucous, 723
Carcinoma in situ
  breast, 1847
  cause of renal magnesium wasting, 1940
Cardene; *see* Nicardipine
Cardiac arrest
  electroencephalography, 908
  neurologic aspects, 1088-1089
Cardiac arrhythmia, 131-156
  abnormal jugular venous pulse, 66
  accelerated idioventricular rhythm, 149, 150,
    223
  antiarrhythmics, 134-139
    angina, 203, 205, 207
    aortic regurgitation, 243
    arrhythmia, 138
    arrhythmias, 138
    atrial fibrillation, 147, 223
    atrial flutter, 144, 146
    atrioventricular reciprocating tachycardia, 143
    before cardiac transplantation, 336
    cluster headache prophylaxis, 962
    constrictive pericarditis, 279
    dilated cardiomyopathy, 264
    drug-induced bile duct injury, 2203
    effects of magnesium deficiency, 1942
    effects on sodium currents, 59
    glucose-6-phosphate dehydrogenase
      deficiency, 664
    heart failure, 170, 173, 174
    hepatic injury, 2192
    human cytochrome P450 isoforms, 2312
    hypertension, 325
    hypertensive emergency, 328
    hypertrophic obstructive cardiomyopathy, 269
    interaction with calcium channel blockers,
      204
    interaction with cyclosporin, 793
    interference with catecholamine assays, 1740
    interference with oral anticoagulants, 636
    malaria, 1674-1675
    multifocal atrial tachycardia, 144
    myocardial infarction, 217
    pharmacokinetics, 137
    premature ventricular contractions, 149
    properties, 203, 204
    prophylaxis of migraine, 962
    pulmonary parenchymal reactions, 476
    pulmonary toxicity, 478
    sudden death survivor, 189-191
    sustained ventricular tachycardia and wide
      QRS complex tachycardia, 150
    uncommon types of sustained ventricular
      tachycardia, 153
    ventricular tachyarrhythmia, 223, 224
    Wolff-Parkinson-White syndrome, 142
  atrial tachycardia
    ectopic, 143-144, 146
    multifocal, 144, 146
    response to carotid sinus massage or
      intravenous adenosine, 134

Cardiac arrhythmia—cont'd
  bradycardia, 153-156
    calcium channel blocker-induced, 205
    hypothyroidism, 334, 1809
    Legionnaire's disease, 1623
    myocardial infarction, 222
    postinfarction, 223
    sinus, 153-154, 155
    torsades de pointes, 151-152
  during cardiac catheterization, 108
  cardiogenic syncope, 954
  continuous ambulatory electrocardiographic
      recording, 94
  dilated cardiomyopathy, 264
  hypertrophic obstructive cardiomyopathy, 266,
      269
  hypokalemia, 829
  intraventricular conduction abnormalities, 156
  magnesium deficiency, 1942
  mitral valve prolapse, 254
  myocardial abnormalities in neurologic
      disease, 1087
  myocardial contusion, 332
  neurologic aspects, 1088
  nonpharmacologic therapy, 139-140
  operative risk, 2258-2260
  palpitation *versus,* 130-131
  pathophysiology, 131-134
  pharmacologic therapy, 134-139
  during pregnancy, 2276
  sinus tachycardia, 141
    dilated cardiomyopathy, 264
    increased automaticity, 132
    myocardial infarction, 223
    palpitations, 130
    response to carotid sinus massage or
        intravenous adenosine, 134
    restrictive cardiomyopathy, 270-271
  supraventricular tachycardia, 141-148
    accelerated atrioventricular junctional
        rhythm, 144
    atrial fibrillation, 146-148
    atrial flutter, 144-146
    atrioventricular nodal reentrant tachycardia,
        141-142, 144, 145
    ectopic atrial tachycardia, 143-144, 146
    mitral valve prolapse, 254
    multifocal atrial tachycardia, 144, 146
    palpitations, 130
    premature atrial contractions, 141
    sinus tachycardia, 141
    supraventricular tachyarrhythmias, 141, 142,
        143
    Wolff-Parkinson-White syndrome, 142-143,
        145
  tachycardia
    acute mitral regurgitation, 252
    acute pancreatitis, 2234
    aortic regurgitation, 244
    atrioventricular nodal reentrant, 134,
        141-142, 144, 145
    atrioventricular reciprocating, 142-143, 145
    gas gangrene, 1423, 1575
    hypoglycemia, 1875
    hypoglycemic coma, 1867
    mitral valve prolapse, 254
    murmur, 76
    myocarditis, 262
    pacemaker-mediated, 139
    pulmonary thromboembolism, 500
    thyrotoxicosis, 1804
  tachycardia-bradycardia syndrome, 154, 155,
      954
  ventricular, 148-153
    accelerated idioventricular rhythm, 149, 150
    automatic implantable cardioverter
        defibrillator, 140
    cardiogenic syncope, 954
    complication of pulmonary artery
        catheterization, 395
    fibrillation, 153

Cardiac arrhythmia—cont'd
  ventricular—cont'd
    hypertrophic obstructive cardiomyopathy,
        269
    mitral valve prolapse, 254
    myocardial infarction, 180, 223
    nonsustained ventricular tachycardia, 149
    palpitations, 130
    polymorphic, 151-153
    polymorphic ventricular tachycardia,
        151-153
    premature ventricular contractions, 148-149
    response to carotid sinus massage or
        intravenous adenosine, 134
    sudden death, 187
    sustained monomorphic ventricular
        tachycardia, 150-151
    sustained ventricular tachycardia with wide
        QRS complex tachycardia, 149-150,
        151
Cardiac Arrhythmia Suppression Trial, 134,
    190-191
Cardiac calcium adenosine triphosphatase, 55
Cardiac catheterization, 107-116
  angiography, 111, 112
  aortic regurgitation, 113-114, 242
  aortic stenosis, 113, 238
  atrial septal defect, 282
  cardiac output, 109-110
  cardiomyopathies, 115-116
  chronic constrictive pericarditis, 116
  circulatory shunts and resistances, 110-111
  coarctation of aorta, 286-287, 287
  complete transposition of great arteries, 290
  constrictive pericarditis, 277-278, 279
  dilated cardiomyopathy, 264
  Ebstein's anomaly of tricuspid valve, 290
  echocardiography, 100
  endocardial cushion defect, 283
  heart failure, 167
  hypertrophic cardiomyopathy, 268
  indications, 107-108
  interventional, 116-125
    approach to specific lesions, 120-121
    background, 116-117
    complications, 122
    coronary angioplasty for acute myocardial
        infarction, 121-122
    devices, 117-120, 121
    pathophysiology, 116
    primary coronary angioplasty, 122
    randomized trials, 117, 118
    referral, 124
    rescue coronary angioplasty, 122
    restenosis, 122-124
  ischemic heart disease, 113
  left ventricular function, 111-113
  mitral regurgitation, 114, 115, 251
  mitral stenosis, 114-115, 248
  mitral valve prolapse, 254
  patent ductus arteriosus, 286
  precapillary pulmonary hypertension, 296, 297
  pressure management, 108-109, 110
  primary pulmonary hypertension, 294
  pulmonic regurgitation, 257
  risks, 108, 109
  shock, 184
  sudden cardiac survivor, 188
  techniques, 108
  tetralogy of Fallot, 289
  tricuspid regurgitation, 256
  tricuspid stenosis, 256
Cardiac conduction system, 81
Cardiac contraction, 37-41
Cardiac cycle, 36-37, 71-72
  electrocardiography, 81-82
Cardiac function, 36-47
  after heart transplantation, 342-343
  cardiac cycle, 36-37
  cardiac output and systemic hemodynamics,
      46-47

Cardiac function—cont'd
  cellular basis of cardiac contraction, 37-41
  diastolic function, 43-46
  structure and function of ventricle, 41-42
  systolic function, 42-43
Cardiac gating, 389
Cardiac imaging, 212
Cardiac index, 110
  effects of pharmacologic interventions, 183
  hemodynamic data, 110
  pulmonary artery catheterization, 181, 391
Cardiac muscle antibodies, 1157
Cardiac neurosis, 131
Cardiac noninvasive techniques, 91-107
  chest radiography, 91, 92
  computed tomography, 106
  continuous ambulatory electrocardiographic
      recording, 94
  echocardiography, 94-100
  exercise electrocardiographic testing, 91-94
  gamma camera imaging agents, 105
  ischemic heart disease, 198-199
  magnetic resonance imaging, 106-107
  myocardial perfusion imaging, 101-104
  positron emission tomography, 105-106
  radionuclide angiography, 104-105
  sudden cardiac death survivor, 188
Cardiac output, 46-47
  acute respiratory failure, 414
  after cardiac transplantation, 342
  aortic regurgitation, 241
  aortic stenosis, 236
  blood pressure, 316
  cardiac catheterization, 109-110
  cardiogenic shock, 176
  cardiogenic syncope, 954
  changes during pregnancy, 2276
  congestive heart failure, 817
  dilated cardiomyopathy, 263
  exercise stress testing, 91
  heart failure, 159
  lung filtering and, 346
  mitral stenosis, 245
  mixed venous oxygen saturation, 393
  oxygen transport, 350
  pheochromocytoma, 1829
  positive end-expiratory pressure depression,
      398, 415
  pulmonary hypertension, 364
  pulmonary vascular resistance, 361
  shock, 176
  thermodilution, 392-393
  tricuspid stenosis, 255
  weakness, 1755
Cardiac sarcoidosis, 458
Cardiac surgery
  aortic stenosis, 287
  atrial fibrillation after, 146
  atrial septal defect, 282
  coarctation of aorta, 287
  common aortopulmonary trunk, 290
  hypertrophic cardiomyopathy, 270
  patent ductus arteriosus, 286
  pericardial effusion following, 274
  sternal osteomyelitis after, 1551
  tetralogy of Fallot, 289
  triiodothyronine levels following, 1811
Cardiac tamponade, 275-276
  after valve replacement, 259
  chronic renal failure, 784
  management, 278
  metabolic pericarditis, 273
  pulsus paradoxus, 65
Cardiac transplantation, 335-344
  dilated cardiomyopathy, 264-265
  evaluation and medical therapy of heart
      failure, 335-336
  function after, 342-343
  future directions, 343-344
  neurologic aspects, 1090-1091
  pericardial effusion following, 274

Cardiac transplantation—cont'd
  referral for, 335
  rejection and immunosuppression, 339-342
  selection, 336-339
Cardiac tumor, 329-332
Cardiogenic shock, 175-187
  clinical presentation, 177-180
  clinical trials, 184, 185
  coronary angioplasty, 183
  coronary artery bypass graft, 185
  differential diagnosis, 175, 176
  evaluation and treatment, 180, 181
  hemodynamic alterations, 176, 177
  mechanical intervention, 184, 185-186
  myocardial function, 176
  myocardial infarction, 218-219
  pharmacologic therapy, 181-182
  reperfusion therapy, 182-183
  serum lactate and anaerobic metabolism, 176,
    178
Cardiogenic syncope, 954
Cardiolipin antibody, 629
Cardiomegaly
  atrial septal defect, 281
  coarctation of aorta, 286
  dilated cardiomyopathy, 264
  heart failure, 165
  patent ductus arteriosus, 285
  Pompe's disease, 1881
Cardiomyopathy, 262-271
  accelerated idioventricular rhythm, 149
  acquired immunodeficiency syndrome, 333
  atrial fibrillation, 146
  cardiac catheterization, 115-116
  Chagas's disease, 1690
  contractile and cytoskeletal proteins, 59-60
  dilated, 263-265
    acquired immunodeficiency syndrome, 333
    cardiac catheterization, 115
    molecular biology, 61-62
    radionuclide angiography, 104
    transplant candidate, 335
  echocardiography, 100
  hypertrophic, 265-270
    cardiac catheterization, 115-116
    chest pain, 128
    molecular biology, 61-62
    pulsus bisferiens, 65
    restriction fragment length polymorphism,
      54-55
    sudden cardiac death, 187
  metabolic myopathy, 1086-1087
  molecular biology, 60-62
  myocarditis, 262-263
  radionuclide angiography, 104
  restrictive, 270-271
  sarcoidosis, 458
  uremic, 784
Cardiopulmonary arrest, 907, 908
Cardiopulmonary bypass
  heart-lung allograft, 515
  nosocomial infection, 1480
  postperfusion syndrome, 668
  transient thrombocytopenia, 614
Cardiopulmonary resuscitation, 12
Cardiotoxicity
  amiodarone, 138
  chemotherapeutic agents, 584
  digitalis, 138
Cardiovascular reflexes, 936-938
Cardiovascular system
  aging and, 2284
  autonomic physiology, 931-932
  candidal infection, 1663
  computed tomography, 106
  molecular biology, 49-63
    adrenergic receptors and G proteins, 56-58
    cardiac growth and hypertrophy, 55-56, 57
    cardiomyopathies, 60-62
    contractile and cytoskeletal proteins, 59-60
    DNA cloning, 52-53

Cardiovascular system—cont'd
  molecular biology—cont'd
    DNA code, 49-50
    DNA libraries, 54
    electrophoresis, 51-52
    gene expression and regulation, 50-51
    gene transfer, 55
    ion channels, 58-59
    isolation and digestion of DNA, 51
    lipoproteins, apolipoproteins, and
      atherosclerosis, 60
    polymerase chain reaction, 55, 56
    recombinant techniques, 51
    restriction fragment length polymorphism,
      54-55
    RNA analysis, 53-54
    sequencing, 54
    Southern, Northern, Western, and
      Southwestern blotting, 52
  operative risks, 2257-2260
  physical examination, 63-81
    arterial pulses, 64-65, 66, 67
    auscultation, 68-71
    blood pressure measurement, 64
    cardiac cycle, 71-72
    general appearance, 63-64
    heart murmurs, 75-81
    heart sounds, 72-75, 76
    inspection and palpation, 67-68, 70, 71
    jugular venous pulse, 65-67, 68, 69
  physiology, 36-49
    capillary exchange, 47-48
    cardiac cycle, 36-37
    cardiac output and systemic hemodynamics,
      46-47
    cellular basis of cardiac contraction, 37-41
    coronary circulation, 48-49
    diastolic function, 43-46
    response to dynamic exercise, 49
    structure and function of ventricle, 41-42
    systolic function, 42-43
  spinal cord injury, 1049
  sudden cardiac death, 187-191
  trauma, 332-333
Cardioversion
  arrhythmias, 139
  atrial fibrillation, 147-148, 223
  atrial flutter, 145
  mitral stenosis, 248
Carditis
  Lyme disease, 1648
  rheumatic fever, 1256-1257
Cardizem; *see* Diltiazem
Cardura; *see* Doxazosin
Carmustine
  multiple myeloma, 702
  nephrotoxicity, 891
  pulmonary disease induction, 478
  pulmonary parenchymal reactions, 476
Carnitine acyltransferase, 2122
Caroli's disease, 2233
Carotene, 2058
Carotid artery
  aneurysm, 1762
  atherosclerotic lesions, 998
  extracranial carotid angiography, 927
  occlusive disease, 1004-1005, 1089
Carotid baroreceptors, 162
Carotid digital subtraction angiography, 928
Carotid insufficiency, 2301
Carotid pulse, 64, 66, 286
Carotid sinus massage, 134
Carotid sinus syncope, 956
Carotid ultrasonography, 929
Carpal spasm, 1933
Carpal tunnel syndrome, 1017
  beta₂-microglobulin amyloidosis, 1284
  hypothyroidism, 1809
  nerve conduction studies, 915-916
  uremic patient, 1105
Carpentier-Edwards aortic prosthesis, 260

Carrier
  hemophilia A, 619
  hemophilia B, 622
  hepatitis B, 2174, 2175
  Neisseria gonorrhoeae, 1582
  Salmonella, 1599-1600
  Staphylococcus aureus, 1552-1553
  Streptococcus pyogenes, 1556
  typhoid fever, 1601
  X-linked hypophosphatemic rickets, 880
Carrier proteins, 1713
Carteolol
  glaucoma, 2302
  hypertension, 325
  properties, 203
Cartilage
  alkaptonuria, 1281
  calcium pyrophosphate dihydrate crystals,
    1277
  proteoglycans, 1289
  relapsing polychondritis, 1243
Cartrol; *see* Carteolol
Carvallo's sign
  Ebstein's anomaly of tricuspid valve, 290
  tricuspid regurgitation, 256
Carvedilol
  dilated cardiomyopathy, 264
  heart failure, 174
  human cytochrome P450 isoforms, 2312
  hypertension, 325, 327
Case finding, 2254
Casein hydrolysate, 1953
Cast nephropathy, 863
CAST study; *see* Cardiac Arrhythmia
    Suppression Trial
Castleman's disease, 599, 1295, 2252
Casts
  acute nephritic syndrome, 764
  acute pyelonephritis, 1456
  acute renal failure, 771
  poststreptococcal glomerulonephritis, 844
  pyelonephritis, 1458
  urinalysis, 745, 746
  Wegener's granulomatosis, 1223
Catabolism of bile pigments, 2149-2150
Catalase, 2283
Catamenial pneumothorax, 509
Cataplexy, 942-943
Catapres; *see* Clonidine
Cataract, 2301
  diabetes mellitus, 1871
  galactosemia, 1883
Catch-22 syndrome, 1729
Catechol-O-methyltransferase, 930, 1826, 1827
Catecholamines
  agents interfering with assays, 1740
  biosynthesis and metabolism, 1710, 1826-1827
  compensatory mechanisms, 159
  degradation, 1714
  dopamine
    acute tubular necrosis, 773-774
    biosynthesis, 1826
    cocaine intoxication, 2297
    dilated cardiomyopathy, 264
    gram-negative bacteremia, 1451
    heart failure, 173, 174
    mediator of emetic reflex, 2026
    multiple organ dysfunction syndrome, 422
    myocardial infarction, 218
    Parkinson's disease, 990-991
    prolactin inhibition, 1775
    shock, 180
  epinephrine, 56, 930
    anaphylaxis, 1193-1194
    angioedema, 2306
    asthma, 1190
    biosynthesis and metabolism, 1826-1827
    effects on potassium transport, 741
    glaucoma, 2302
    glucose production, 1874, 1875
    hypertension, 316

Catecholamines—cont'd
  epinephrine—cont'd
    normal plasma levels, 1827
    shock, 180-181
  integrated fuel homeostasis, 1853
  internal potassium balance, 825
  measurement, 938
  neurogenic pulmonary edema, 1099
  norepinephrine, 56, 930
    biosynthesis and metabolism, 1826-1827
    cardiac growth and hypertrophy, 55
    heart failure, 159, 160, 161, 166, 818
    hypertension, 316
    lung filtration, 346
    normal plasma levels, 1827
    shock, 180
    sodium retention, 819
    vasopressin inhibition, 1791
  plasma, 1740
  transient hypokalemia, 826
  uncommon types of sustained ventricular
    tachycardia, 153
  urinary, 1740
  vasoactive effects on pulmonary circulation,
    363
Cathepsin, 373
Catheter
  balloon flotation, 108
  directional atherectomy, 117-118
  hospital-acquired bloodstream infection, 1364
  protected brush, 384-385
  pulmonary artery balloon, 169
  Swan-Ganz, 383, 390-395
    adult respiratory distress syndrome, 421
    heart failure, 167
  transluminal extraction, 118, 121
Catheter ablation
  sudden death survivors, 190
  ventricular tachycardia, 140
Catheter-associated infection
  bacteremia, 1364
  candidal, 1663
  gram-negative bacteremia, 1446
  multiple organ dysfunction syndrome, 423
  Staphylococcus epidermidis, 1551
  urinary tract, 1462
Catheter balloon commissurotomy, 249
Catheter balloon valvuloplasty, 239
Catheter-tipped transducer, 100
Catheterization
  cardiac, 107-116
    angiography, 111, 112
    aortic regurgitation, 113-114, 242
    aortic stenosis, 113, 238
    approach to specific lesions, 120-121
    atrial septal defect, 282
    background, 116-117
    cardiac output, 109-110
    cardiomyopathies, 115-116
    chronic constrictive pericarditis, 116
    circulatory shunts and resistances, 110-111
    coarctation of aorta, 286-287
    complete transposition of great arteries, 290
    complications, 122
    constrictive pericarditis, 277-278, 279
    coronary angioplasty for acute myocardial
      infarction, 121-122
    devices, 117-120, 121
    dilated cardiomyopathy, 264
    Ebstein's anomaly of tricuspid valve, 290
    echocardiography, 100
    endocardial cushion defect, 283
    heart failure, 167
    hypertrophic cardiomyopathy, 268
    indications, 107-108
    ischemic heart disease, 113
    left ventricular function, 111-113
    mitral regurgitation, 114, 115, 251
    mitral stenosis, 114-115, 248
    mitral valve prolapse, 254
    patent ductus arteriosus, 286

Catheterization—cont'd
  cardiac—cont'd
    pathophysiology, 116
    precapillary pulmonary hypertension, 296,
      297
    pressure management, 108-109, 110
    primary coronary angioplasty, 122
    primary pulmonary hypertension, 294
    pulmonic regurgitation, 257
    randomized trials, 117, 118
    referral, 124
    rescue coronary angioplasty, 122
    restenosis, 122-124
    risks, 108, 109
    shock, 184
    sudden cardiac survivor, 188
    techniques, 108
    tetralogy of Fallot, 289
    tricuspid regurgitation, 256
    tricuspid stenosis, 256
  pulmonary artery, 390-395
    gram-negative bacteremia, 1451
    right ventricular infarction, 220
    sepsis, 1450
    shock, 181
  urinary, 1462
Cation, 736
Cation pump enzymes, 58
Cauda equina syndrome, 1048
Caustic esophageal stricture, 2019
CAVEAT I trial, 124
Caveolar-vesicle junctions, 1672
Cavernous hemangioma, 614, 2215-2216
Cavernous sinus, 1773
Cavernous thrombosis, 2309
CD3ε deficiency, 1177
CD3γ deficiency, 1177
CD4 molecule, 1113, 1533
CD4 receptor, 1470
CD4+ T-cell, 1114
  adult T-cell leukemia, 1532
  human immunodeficiency virus infection,
    1470, 1472-1473
  hypersensitivity pneumonitis, 461-462
  inflammatory myopathies, 1234
  Pneumocystis carinii, 1693
  respiratory, 367, 368
  sarcoidosis, 456, 457
CD4+ thymocyte, 1112, 1113
CD8 deficiency, 1177-1178
CD8 molecule, 1113, 1127
CD8+ T-cell, 1114, 1127
  Graves' disease, 1805
  human immunodeficiency virus infection, 1533
  hypersensitivity pneumonitis, 461, 462
  inflammatory myopathies, 1234
  intraepithelial, 1990
  multiple myeloma, 701
  respiratory, 367, 368
  sarcoidosis, 456
CD8+ thymocyte, 1112, 1113
CD28, 1113
CD40L, 1113
CD59, 1135
  deficiency, 1180
CD80, 1113
CD86, 1113
Cecal ulcer, 2093
Cefazolin
  activity against major anaerobes, 1620
  infective endocarditis, 231
  septic arthritis, 1253
Cefixime, 1354, 1584
Cefmetazole, 1354
Cefoperazone, 1354, 1620
Cefotaxime, 1354
  activity against major anaerobes, 1620
  acute epiglottitis, 1393
  bacterial meningitis, 1411
  Haemophilus influenzae, 1410, 1588
  spontaneous bacterial peritonitis, 2164

Cefotetan, 1354, 1620
Cefoxitin, 1354
  activity against major anaerobes, 1620
  intraabdominal infection, 1401
Cefpodoxime, 1354
Cefprozil, 1354
Ceftazidime, 1354
  activity against major anaerobes, 1620
  bacterial meningitis, 1411
  prophylaxis in lung transplantation, 518
  Pseudomonas aeruginosa, 1410
  respiratory exacerbations in cystic fibrosis,
    483
Ceftibuten, 1354
Ceftizoxime, 1354
  activity against major anaerobes, 1620
  gonorrhea, 1585
Ceftriaxone, 1354
  activity against major anaerobes, 1620
  bacterial meningitis, 1411
  gonorrhea, 1584, 1585
  Haemophilus ducreyi, 1589
  Haemophilus influenzae, 1410, 1588
  infective endocarditis, 231, 232
  Lyme disease, 1647-1648
  meningococcal disease, 1580
  septic arthritis, 1253
  syphilis, 1643
  typhoid fever, 1601
Cefuroxime, 1354
  acute epiglottitis, 1393
  sinusitis, 1395
Celiac disease, 1991
Celiac sprue
  incidence of malignancy, 2081
  malabsorption, 2062-2063
Celiprolol, 203
Cell
  abnormalities in myocardial failure, 159-160
  growth and differentiation, 541
  radiation-induced death, 585
Cell adhesion molecule, 370
Cell cycle
  regulation, 542
  relevance to cancer treatment, 551
Cell-mediated immunity, 1126-1132
  amebiasis, 1682
  barrier to infection, 1335
  celiac disease, 2062
  cellular constituents, 1127-1128
  coccidioidomycosis, 1656
  Cryptococcus neoformans, 1667
  cytokines and immunoregulation, 1128-1132
  delayed-type hypersensitivity, 1132
  derangements, 1132
  evaluation, 1150-1153, 1175
  histoplasmosis, 1654
  leprosy, 1650
  mononuclear phagocyte system, 1342
  myasthenia gravis, 1021
  Pneumocystis carinii pneumonia, 1693
  Rocky Mountain spotted fever, 1543
Cell membrane
  bacterial, 1344
  linoleic acid, 1884
  red blood cell defects, 664-666
Cell surface molecule, 1151
Cell surface receptor, 370, 1710-1711
Cell-to-cell adhesion, 370
Cell volume, 805
Cell wall
  bacterial, 1343-1344
  gram-negative microorganism, 1447
  Streptococcus pyogenes, 1555
Cellular aging, 2283-2284
Cellular biology
  bone, 1716
  hematopoiesis, 530-534
Cellulitis, 1420
  acute meningitis, 1407
  clostridial, 1422, 1575

Cellulitis—cont'd
  erysipelas, 1420
  Haemophilus influenzae, 1586, 1588, Plate
    VIII-26
  nonclostridial crepitant, 1422
  Streptococcus pyogenes, 1556
Central alveolar hypoventilation syndrome, 943
Central apnea, 354-355
Central cord syndrome, 1012, 1047-1048
Central diabetes insipidus, 815
Central inhibitors, 325, 326
Central nervous system
  acquired immunodeficiency syndrome, 1477
  acute intermittent porphyria, 1926
  acute meningitis, 1402
  acute respiratory failure, 413-414
  alimentary motor function, 1977-1978
  antirheumatic drug toxicity, 1261
  chronic renal failure, 784
  cocaine intoxication, 2297
  coccidioidomycosis, 1656
  control of food intake, 2099
  cryptococcosis, 1667-1668
  features of malabsorption, 2058
  glucose requirements, 1874
  hormonal regulation, 1075-1078
  Krabbe's disease, 1918
  lung cancer, 726
  lymphoma, 1069, 1477
  malignant lymphoma, 697
  measles complications, 1498
  mumps, 1496
  neurofibromatosis, 1920
  peripheral nervous system *versus,* 1014
  primary angiitis, 1225
  regulation of gastric acid secretion, 1981
  syphilis, 1641
  toxoplasmosis, 1677
  Whipple's disease, 2064
Central nervous system hypersomnolence, 943
Central nervous system infection
  actinomycosis, 1665
  anaerobic bacteria, 1617
  brain abscess, 1413-1416
  brucellosis, 1606
  cryptococcosis, 1669
  depression, 1037
  febrile compromised patient, 1387
  intracranial epidural abscess, 1418
  intracranial subdural empyema, 1416-1418
  meningitis, 1402-1413
    clinical manifestations, 1406, 1407
    differential diagnosis, 1408-1409
    epidemiology and etiology, 1402-1404
    fever, 1385, 1387
    headache, 960
    laboratory investigation, 1406-1408
    OKT3-induced, 1090
    pathogenesis and pathophysiology,
      1404-1406
    prognosis, 1413
    rash, 1385
    respiratory alkalosis, 355
    treatment, 1409-1413
  Naegleria fowleri, 1684
  spinal epidural abscess, 1418-1419
  tuberculosis, 1636
Central neurogenic hyperventilation, 1097
Central pontine myelinolysis, 813, 1080
Central retinal artery occlusion, 1058
Central retinal vein occlusion, 2304, Plate XI-10
Central sleep apnea, 528, 943
Central tentorial herniation syndrome, 1044
Central venous pressure, 65-68
Centrifugal lipodystrophy, 1903
Centrilobular emphysema, 439
Centrilobular injury in alcoholic liver disease,
  2195
Centroacinar emphysema, 439
Centromere/kinetochore antibody, 1159

Cephalexin
  dermatitis-aggravating *Staphylococcus aureus*
    infection, 1303
  infectious eczematoid dermatitis, 1304
Cephalic tetanus, 1573
Cephalometric measurements, 355
Cephalosporins, 1352-1355
  activity against major anaerobes, 1620
  acute epiglottitis, 1393
  bacterial meningitis, 1411
  coagulase-negative staphylococcal infection,
    1552
  dosage, 1349
  effects on kidney, 868
  gonorrhea, 1584, 1585
  gram-negative sepsis, 1452
  Haemophilus ducreyi, 1589
  Haemophilus influenzae, 1588
  hepatic injury, 2191
  induction of acute interstitial nephritis, 889
  infective endocarditis, 231, 232
  intraabdominal infection, 1401
  Lyme disease, 1647-1648
  meningococcal disease, 1580
  peritonitis, 1402
  prophylaxis in lung transplantation, 518
  respiratory exacerbations in cystic fibrosis,
    483
  septic arthritis, 1253
  sinusitis, 1395
  spinal epidural abscess, 1418
  spontaneous bacterial peritonitis, 2164
  Streptococcus pneumoniae meningitis, 1410
  subdural empyema, 1418
  syphilis, 1643
  typhoid fever, 1601
  use during pregnancy, 2281
Cephalothin, 1354
Cephalothoracic progressive lipodystrophy,
  1902
Cephapirin, 1354
Cephradine, 1354
Ceramide trihexoside lipidosis, 1918-1919
Ceramides, 1917
Cerebellar ataxia
  complication of chemotherapy, 1072
  hepatic encephalopathy, 2161
  multiple sclerosis, 1055
Cerebellar infarction, 973
Cerebral aneurysm, 1089
Cerebral angiography, 925-926, 927
  coma, 950
  epilepsy, 982
Cerebral blood flow
  bacterial meningitis, 1405
  brain resuscitation, 1085
  increased intracranial pressure, 1081
  syncope, 952
Cerebral cortex
  diseases causing dizziness, 973
  epileptic hyperactivity, 978-979
Cerebral edema
  acute hyponatremia, 811
  bacterial meningitis, 1405
  hepatic encephalopathy, 2161
Cerebral embolism, 955, 1006
Cerebral hemorrhage, 609
Cerebral infarction
  endocarditis, 1089
  magnetic resonance imaging, 922
  vascular dementia, 988-989
Cerebral malaria, 1674
Cerebral perfusion pressure, 1081
  head trauma, 1043
  increased intracranial pressure, 1081-1082
Cerebral T-wave, 1087
Cerebritis, 1549-1550
Cerebrospinal fluid
  culture
    coccidioidomycosis, 1657
    Haemophilus influenzae, 1588

Cerebrospinal fluid—cont'd
  examination, 904-905
    central nervous system tuberculosis, 1636
    cryptococcosis, 1668
    meningitis, 1407-1408
    multiple sclerosis, 1009
    Neisseria meningitidis, 1580
    pituitary apoplexy, 1779
    rabies, 1506
    Rocky Mountain spotted fever, 1544
    spinal lesion, 1012
    syphilis, 1641, 1642
    toxoplasmosis, 1677
  fistula, 2307
  hormone transport, 1713
  hydrocephalus
    brain tumor, 1067
    dementia, 988
    Maroteaux-Launy syndrome, 1915
    posttraumatic, 1045
    radionuclide cisternography, 926
  leak in head trauma, 1044
  meningitis, 1404-1405
  papilledema, 1060
  pleocytosis, 1496
  shunt infection, 1551
Cerebrotendinous xanthomatosis, 1898
Cerebrovascular accident, 997-1007
  amnesic syndrome, 1032
  atrial fibrillation, 146
  during cardiac catheterization, 108
  clinical separation of stroke subtypes, 1000-1002
  depression, 1036
  dizziness, 973
  embolism, 1006
  hemorrhagic, 997-998, 1006
  hypertension, 314, 315, 322-323
  ischemic, 998-1000
  laboratory diagnosis, 1002-1004
  parkinsonism, 993
  prevention, complications, and rehabilitation,
    1006-1007, 1054-1055
  respiratory rhythm abnormalities, 1098
  sickle cell disease, 659
  systemic lupus erythematosus, 1093
  thrombotic, 1004-1006
Cerebrovascular disease, 997-1007
  amnesic syndrome, 1032
  anticoagulant therapy, 640
  antihypertensive agent choices, 326
  atrial fibrillation, 146
  clinical separation of stroke subtypes,
    1000-1002
  depression, 1036
  dizziness, 973
  elderly, 2282
  embolism, 1006
  hemorrhagic, 997-998, 1006
  hemorrhagic stroke, 997-998, 1006
  hypertension, 322-323
  hypertension risk factors, 314, 315
  ischemic, 998-1000
  ischemic stroke, 998-1000
  laboratory diagnosis, 1002-1004
  parkinsonism, 993
  prevention, complications, and rehabilitation,
    1006-1007
  rehabilitation, 1054-1055
  respiratory rhythm abnormalities, 1098
  sickle cell disease, 659
  syncope *versus,* 954, 955
  systemic lupus erythematosus, 1093
  thrombotic, 1004-1006
Ceruloplasmin
  hepatic formation, 2120
  primary biliary cirrhosis, 2200
  primary sclerosing cholangitis, 2202
  Wilson's disease, 2138, 2205
Cervical adenopathy, 2309-2310
  fever and rash, 1385
  infectious mononucleosis, 1529

Cervical cord astrocytoma, 925
Cervical esophagus, 1978
Cervical lymph nodes
  cancer, 724
  containing squamous cell carcinoma, 732
  esophageal cancer, 2024
  lymphadenopathy, 597
  toxoplasmosis, 1677
Cervical pain, 968-971, 1392-1393
  herpangina, 1488-1489
  Lassa fever, 1510
  Mycoplasma pneumoniae pneumonia, 1539
  rheumatic fever, 1256
  scarlet fever, 1421
  spontaneous pneumomediastinum, 514
  subacute thyroiditis, 1811
Cervical spine
  atlantoaxial subluxation, 1171, 1172
  computed tomography, 920
  magnetic resonance imaging, 925
  radiculopathy, 1015-1016
  spinal epidural abscess, 1418
  spondylosis, 925, 1012-1013
  syndromes, 969
  trauma, 1048-1049
Cervical venous hum, 81
Cervical web, 2020
Cervicitis, 1441-1442, 1618
Cervix
  cancer, 714-715
  cervicitis, 1441-1442, 1618
  dysplasia, 714
  exam for sexually transmitted disease, 1439
  normal microflora, 1615
Cestode
  intestinal, 1696-1697
  tissue, 1704-1705
Ceta-carboxyl glutamic acid, 625
Cetirizine, 1182
Chagas' disease, 1689-1690
  esophageal achalasia, 2021
  gastrointestinal motility, 1978
  transfusion-transmitted, 575, 576
Chagoma, 1690
Chalk bone disease, 1958
Chancre, 1640, Plate VIII-34
Chancroid, 1444
  Haemophilus ducreyi, 1589
  traveler's disease, 1466
Chaotic atrial rhythm, 144, 146
Chaparral leaf, 2193
Charcot-Bouchard microaneurysm, 998
Charcot-Leyden crystals
  asthma, 1185
  sputum examination, 380
Charcot-Marie-Tooth dystrophy, 1754
Charcot's arthropathy, 1246
Charcot's intermittent fever, 2229
Charcot's joint, 1247, 1871-1872
Chédiak-Higashi syndrome, 1919
  chemotactic defects, 1340
  granule abnormalities, 1341
Cheese worker's lung, 460
Cheilosis, 2106
Chelation therapy
  acute lead nephropathy, 867
  beta-thalassemia, 655-656
  iron overload, 646
  Wilson's disease, 1102, 2205-2206
Chemical carcinogens, 548
Chemical exposure
  aplastic anemia, 672
  carcinogenesis, 868
  esophageal injury, 2018-2019
  hemoglobinuria, 867-868
  hemolytic anemia, 667
  hepatic injury, 2187-2193
    acetaminophen poisoning, 2188-2190
    carbon tetrachloride poisoning, 2188
    clinical aspects, 2187-2188

Chemical exposure—cont'd
  hepatic injury—cont'd
    medicinal agents, 2190-2192
    mushroom and phosphorus poisoning, 2188
  occupational asthma, 472
Chemical-induced nephropathy, 866-871
Chemical peritonitis, 2248-2249
Chemical worker's lung, 460
Chemiluminescence immunoassay, 1734
Chemoattractants, 450
Chemokines, 1127, 1129, 1130
  acquired immunodeficiency syndrome, 1533
  vascular cell production, 371
Chemoprevention, 550
  endocarditis, 233, 234-235
  Haemophilus influenzae, 1589
  influenza, 1493
  plague, 1610
  Pneumocystis carinii pneumonia, 1695
  tuberculosis, 1637
Chemoreceptor
  carbon dioxide partial pressure, 353
  chemoreceptor trigger zone, 2026
  modulation of ventricular function, 45
  pericardial, 271
  peripheral chemoreceptor signal, 353
  response to hypoxia, 353
  ventilation, 352-353
Chemoreceptor trigger zone, 2026
Chemotactic mediators, 1140-1142
Chemotaxis, 1340-1341
Chemotherapeutic agents
  induction of impotence, 1762
  pulmonary toxicity, 478
  toxicity, 584-585
Chemotherapy
  acute interstitial nephritis, 889
  acute lymphoblastic leukemia, 683
  adenocarcinoma, 732
  adrenal cancer, 1822
  amyloidosis, 865
  brain tumor, 1069
  breast cancer, 709, 711-712
  carcinoid tumor of small bowel, 2082
  cervical cancer, 715
  chronic myelogenous leukemia, 687
  colon cancer, 2085
  endometrial cancer, 714
  gastric cancer, 2048
  herpesvirus infections, 1526
  Hodgkin's disease, 694-695
  induction of hypocalcemia, 1932
  leprosy, 1651
  lung cancer, 727, 729
  metastatic cancer, 1073-1074
  multiple myeloma, 702
  myelodysplastic syndrome, 676
  nausea and vomiting, 581-582
  neurologic complications, 1072
  non-Hodgkin's lymphoma, 698-699
  ovarian cancer, 716
  pancreatic cancer, 2243
  polycythemia vera, 688
  principles, 554-555
  prostate cancer, 720
  small intestinal malignancies, 2081
  testicular cancer, 721
  thyroid lymphoma, 1816
  toxicity, 579
  tuberculosis, 1630-1633
Chenodeoxycholic acid, 1884, 1898, 2124-2125
Chest
  chronic obstructive pulmonary disease, 442
  inspection and palpation, 67-68, 70, 71
  magnetic resonance imaging, 389-390
Chest compression, 332
Chest pain, 125-129
  angina, 196
  anxiety, 1034
  coronary artery disease in women, 2271-2272
  coronary sinus aneurysm, 291

Chest pain—cont'd
  cryptococcosis, 1668
  dissection of aorta, 301
  epidemic pleurodynia, 1489
  esophageal origin, 1999
  exercise thallium-201 imaging, 101
  gastroesophageal reflux, 128
  hypertrophic obstructive cardiomyopathy, 266
  Lassa fever, 1510
  lung cancer, 488
  lung disease, 408-410
  lymphomatoid granulomatosis, 470
  malignant mesothelioma, 510
  mediastinal abnormality, 511
  mitral stenosis, 245, 246
  mitral valve prolapse, 254, 255
  myocardial infarction, 209-210
  myopericarditis, 1489
  pharmacologic stress testing, 104
  pheochromocytoma, 1829
  pleuritic pain *versus,* 505
  pneumothorax, 509
  primary pulmonary hypertension, 294
  pulmonary embolism, 500
  spontaneous pneumomediastinum, 514
  thallium-201 imaging, 101
  thoracic aortic aneurysm, 300
  thyroid hormone therapy-induced, 1810
  tuberculosis, 1628
  Wegener's granulomatosis, 468
Chest pain center, 129
Chest physiotherapy
  cystic fibrosis, 482
  secretion clearance and lung expansion, 430
Chest radiography, 386
  acquired immunodeficiency syndrome, 1477
  acute pericarditis, 273-274
  acute respiratory failure, 414
  alpha$_1$-protease inhibitor deficiency, 440
  amiodarone-induced pulmonary disease, 478
  aortic regurgitation, 241, 242
  aortic stenosis, 237, 238, 287
  asthma, 1189
  atrial septal defect, 281
  bronchiectasis, 484
  chronic obstructive pulmonary disease, 442
  Churg-Strauss syndrome, 466
  coarctation of aorta, 286
  complete transposition of great arteries, 290
  congenital abnormalities of coronary arteries, 292
  congenital coronary arteriovenous fistula, 292
  cor pulmonale, 498
  cystic fibrosis, 481
  dissection of aorta, 301
  Ebstein's anomaly of tricuspid valve, 290
  endocardial cushion defect, 282
  evaluation of respiratory disease, 403-404
  fever of unknown origin, 1379
  giant bullae, 447
  heart, 91, 92
  heart failure, 165
  hemoptysis, 411
  Hodgkin's disease, 694
  hypertrophic cardiomyopathy, 267
  hypothyroidism, 1810
  idiopathic pulmonary fibrosis, 453
  interstitial lung disease, 451
  ischemic heart disease, 197
  Legionnaire's disease, 1623
  lymphomatoid granulomatosis, 470
  mitral regurgitation, 251, 253
  mitral stenosis, 247
  mitral valve prolapse, 254
  myocardial infarction, 212
  patent ductus arteriosus, 285
  pericardial effusion, 274
  Pneumocystis carinii pneumonia, 1693
  primary pulmonary hypertension, 294
  pulmonary edema, 425
  pulmonary thromboembolism, 501

Chest radiography—cont'd
  pulmonic regurgitation, 257
  pulmonic stenosis, 288
  sarcoidosis, 458
  solitary pulmonary nodule, 493-494, 495
  sudden cardiac survivor, 188
  tetralogy of Fallot, 289
  total anomalous pulmonary venous connection, 291
  tricuspid regurgitation, 256
  tricuspid stenosis, 255
  ventricular septal defect, 284
  Wegener's granulomatosis, 468
Chest syndrome, 658
Chest wall
  causes of respiratory muscle weakness, 359
  compliance, 347
  computed tomography, 387
  inspection and palpation, 67-68, 70, 71
  mechanoreceptors, 353
  pain, 410
  projection of lungs on, 403
Chest wall syndrome, 410
Cheyne-Stokes respiration, 353-354, 1097-1098
CHF-STAT survival trial, 171
Chiasmal disease, 1060
Chicken plucker's lung, 460
Chickenpox, 1525-1527, 2280
Chief cell, 1981, 1982
Chief cell receptor, 1984
Chief complaint, 2
Child, 616
  alpha₁-antitrypsin deficiency, 2206
  atrial septal defect, 281
  automatic atrial tachycardia, 143
  autosomal recessive polycystic kidney disease, 874
  bacterial meningitis, 1403
  bacteriuria, 1457
  bullous impetigo, 1419
  chronic bullous disease, 1296
  congenital heart disease, 280-292
    aberrant right subclavian artery, 291
    aortic stenosis, 287
    aortopulmonary septal defect, 286
    atrial septal defect, 280-282
    bicuspid aortic valve, 287
    coarctation of aorta, 286-287
    complete transposition of great arteries, 290
    congenitally corrected transposition of great arteries, 290
    cor triatriatum, 291
    coronary artery abnormalities, 291-292
    coronary sinus aneurysm, 291
    disturbances of conduction, 292
    Ebstein's anomaly of tricuspid valve, 289-290
    endocardial cushion defect, 282-283
    etiology, 280
    fetal circulation and changes associated with birth, 280
    infective endocarditis, 225, 226
    malposition of heart, 291
    partial transposition of pulmonary veins, 282
    patent ductus arteriosus, 285-286
    pericardial, 273, 291-292
    tetralogy of Fallot, 288-289
    total anomalous pulmonary venous connection, 290-291
    tricuspid atresia, 291
    truncus arteriosus, 290
    valvular pulmonic stenosis with intact ventricular septum, 288
    ventricular septal defect, 283-285
  cretinism, 1809
  cryptosporidiosis, 1679
  epidemic pleurodynia, 1489
  gonorrhea, 1583-1584
  hand-foot-mouth syndrome, 1489
  hepatitis A virus, 2173

Child—cont'd
  hypertension, 328
  hypoglycemia, 1876
  hypophosphatasia, 1954
  idiopathic nephrotic syndrome, 850
  infectious pericarditis, 272
  juvenile cystinosis, 1910
  juvenile nephronophthisis, 875, 892
  juvenile-onset diabetes mellitus, 1854
  juvenile osteoporosis, 1945
  juvenile polyps, 2086
  juvenile rheumatoid arthritis, 273
  liver transplantation, 2219
  minimal change disease, 851
  neurofibromatosis, 1921
  Niemann-Pick disease, 1918
  osteomyelitis, 1433
  patent ductus arteriosus, 285
  pertussis, 1611
  pulmonic stenosis, 288
  radiation-induced thyroid carcinoma, 1816-1817
  recommended daily dietary allowances, 2114-2115, 2116
  safety seat legislation, 2265
  septic arthritis, 1252
  sexual abuse, 2269
  shigellosis, 1602
  staphylococcal scalded-skin syndrome, 1421
  toxoplasmosis, 1677
  type 2 autoimmune hepatitis, 2184
  whipworm infestation, 1696
Child-Pugh classification, 2142, 2143, 2166
Childhood-onset insomnia, 942
Chills
  amebic liver abscess, 2210
  babesiosis, 1676
  bacteremia, 1449
  bacterial meningitis, 1406
  bacterial prostatitis, 1462
  erysipelas, 1420
  hypersensitivity pneumonitis, 461
  infectious mononucleosis, 1529
  influenza, 1490
  lymphogranuloma venereum, 1535
  malaria, 1673
  Mycoplasma pneumoniae pneumonia, 1539
  transfusion reaction, 574
  tularemia, 1607
  urinary tract infection, 1458
Chinese herbs
  hepatic injury, 2193
  nephropathy, 893
Chinese liver fluke, 1703
CHIP-28 pores, 808
Chlamydia epididymitis, 1444
Chlamydia pneumoniae, 407, 1534, 1535
Chlamydia psittaci, 1377, 1534, 1535
Chlamydia trachomatis, 1534-1538
  culture, 1370
  diarrhea, 1476
  dysuria, 762, 763
  Giemsa stain, Plate VIII-11
  gonorrhea with, 1584
  nongonococcal urethritis, 1440
  peritonitis, 2248
  during pregnancy, 2279-2280
  primary peritonitis, 1396
  reactive arthritis, 1240
  traveler's disease, 1466
  urethritis, 1455
Chloral hydrate, 636
Chlorambucil
  amyloidosis, 1283
  breast cancer, 710
  chronic lymphocytic leukemia, 685
  minimal change disease, 851
  non-Hodgkin's lymphoma, 698
  pulmonary parenchymal reactions, 476
  rheumatic disease, 1260, 1262
  Waldenström macroglobulinemia, 704

Chloramphenicol, 1356-1357
  activity against major anaerobes, 1620
  acute epiglottitis, 1393
  antimicrobial mechanisms, 1344
  aplastic anemia, 672
  bacterial meningitis, 1411
  cholera, 1596
  enterococci resistance, 1561
  glucose-6-phosphate dehydrogenase deficiency, 664
  Haemophilus influenzae, 1588
  hepatic injury, 2191
  intraabdominal infection, 1401
  mechanism of resistance, 1345
  relapsing fever, 1646
  rickettsial infection, 1545
  typhoid fever, 1601
  use during pregnancy, 2281
  Yersinia enterocolitica, 1605
Chlordane, 867
Chlordiazepoxide
  alcohol withdrawal, 2295
  hepatic injury, 2191
  interference with oral anticoagulants, 636
Chloride
  body water compartments, 736
  hyperchloremic metabolic acidosis, 779, 837, 2114
  intestinal absorption, 1988
  parenteral solutions, 2114
  primary hyperparathyroidism, 1974
  recommended daily dietary allowances, 2116
  secretory system, 2123-2124
  total parenteral nutrition formula, 2117
Chloridorrhea, 839
Chlorine, 2109
2-Chlorodeoxyadenosine
  hairy cell leukemia, 684
  Waldenström macroglobulinemia, 704
Chloroform, 866
Chloroguanidine, 664
Chloroquine
  amebiasis, 1683
  amebic liver abscess, 2210
  drug-induced lysosomopathies, 1919
  glucose-6-phosphate dehydrogenase deficiency, 664
  malaria, 1465, 1467, 1674
  porphyria cutanea tarda, 1927
  rheumatic disease, 1261
  rheumatoid arthritis, 1208
  systemic lupus erythematosus, 1217
Chlorozotocin, 476
Chlorpromazine
  drug-induced lysosomopathies, 1919
  hepatic injury, 2186, 2190, 2191
  interference with catecholamine assays, 1740
  for nausea and vomiting, 2027
  pituitary stimulation tests, 1736
Chlorpropamide
  diabetes insipidus, 1796
  diabetes mellitus, 1858
  hepatic injury, 2191
Chlorthalidone
  elderly patient, 327
  heart failure, 170
  hepatic injury, 2192
  hypertension, 325
Chlorzoxazone
  hepatic injury, 2191
  human cytochrome P450 isoforms, 2312
Cholangiocarcinoma, 2231-2232
  inflammatory bowel disease, 2076
  intrahepatic, 2214-2215
  primary sclerosing cholangitis, 2201-2202
Cholangiocyte, 2199
Cholangiography, 1997
  Caroli's disease, 2233
  choledochal cyst, 2212
  ischemic cholangitis, 2203

Cholangitis
autoimmune, 2139-2140
choledochal cyst, 2212
clostridial, 1575
common bile duct obstruction, 2229
drug-induced, 2202-2203
fever of unknown origin, 1376
ischemic, 2203
primary biliary cirrhosis, 2199
primary sclerosing cholangitis, 2201
Cholascos, 2155-2156
Cholate, 2124
Cholcystokinin-octapeptide, 2227
Cholecalciferol, 1710
Cholecystectomy, 2226
cholecystitis, 2228
choledocholithiasis, 2229
gallbladder cancer, 2232
hereditary spherocytosis, 665
during pregnancy, 2278
prophylactic, 2225
Cholecystitis
gallstones, 2227-2228
Haemophilus influenzae, 1588
during pregnancy, 2278
Cholecystoenteric fistula, 2228
Cholecystokinin
absorption of protein, 1987
amino acid consumption test, 2145
chronic pancreatitis, 2240
chronic renal failure, 784
intestinal absorption of lipids, 1986
pancreatic acinar cells, 2132
pancreatic exocrine secretion, 2133
pepsinogen secretion, 1984
pericholangitis, 2155
role in digestion, 1980
Cholecystosis, 2233
Choledochal cyst, 2155, 2212, 2233
Choledocholithiasis
extrahepatic cholestasis, 2155
gallstones, 2228-2230
primary sclerosing cholangitis, 2202
Cholelithiasis, 483
Cholera, 1593-1598
acute diarrhea, 1425-1426
risk to travelers, 1464
sodium depletion, 823
Cholescintigraphy
bile leak, 2226
gallstones, 2225
Cholestanol, 1898
Cholestasis
benign strictures of extrahepatic bile ducts,
2232
determination of blockage site, 2156
drug-induced, 2203
estrogen-related, 2158
during pregnancy, 2277
secondary hepatocellular injury, 2155
serum alkaline phosphatase level, 2137
steroid-induced, 2123
Cholestatic hepatotoxins, 2186, 2187
Cholestatic injury, 2188
Cholestatic jaundice, 2156
Cholesteatoma, 2307
Cholesterol
adrenal steroid biosynthesis, 1817
atherosclerosis, 1888-1889
bile, 2127
effects of diet, 1890
estrogen-related cholestasis, 2158
foam cell formation, 60
hepatocellular *versus* cholestatic jaundice,
2156
hydroxy-methyl-glutaryl coenzyme A
reductase inhibitors, 1891
hypercholesterolemia, 1892-1894
familial, 60
periodic health examination, 2254
hyperlipidemia, 1892-1894

Cholesterol—cont'd
hypoalphalipoproteinemia, 1896, 1898
lipid absorption, 1987
metabolism, 1883-1884
population distribution, 1893
preventive care guidelines, 2255
small bowel malabsorption, 2058
steroid hormones, 1709
synthesis in liver, 1885, 2120-2121
synthesis of bile salts, 2124
uremic patient, 786
Cholesterol 7α-hydroxylase, 2127
Cholesterol-absorption blockers, 1890-1891
Cholesterol and Recurrent Events study, 1891
Cholesterol crystals, 1163, 2127, 2128
embolism, 999, 1057
light microscopy, Plate X-15
Cholesterol esters
cholesterolosis, 2230-2231
high density lipoproteins, 1887
lipid absorption, 1987
lipoproteins, 1885
storage disease, 1898
Cholesterol-lowering agents, 1891
bile acid blockade, 1890
Clostridium difficile colitis, 1569, 1570
drug-nutrient interactions, 2110
gallstone risk factor, 2223
hyperoxaluria, 804
lipoprotein lipase potentiation, 1892
primary biliary cirrhosis, 2201
protoporphyria, 1926
restenosis, 124
secondary hypertriglyceridemia, 1895
Cholesterol stones, 2221, 2222, 2223
Cholesterolosis, 2230-2231
Cholesteryl ester hydrolase, 2127
Cholesteryl ester storage disease, 1919
Cholestyramine
bile acid blockade, 1890
Clostridium difficile colitis, 1569, 1570
drug-nutrient interactions, 2110
hyperoxaluria, 804
interference with oral anticoagulants, 636
primary biliary cirrhosis, 2201
protoporphyria, 1926
Cholic acid, 1884, 2124-2125
Cholinergic agents
glaucoma, 2302
induction of bronchospasm, 477
pepsinogen secretion, 1984
Cholinergic crisis, 1022
Cholinesterase inhibitors, 2288
Cholorrheic enteropathy, 2069
Chondritis, 410
Chondroblast, 1716
Chondrocalcinosis, 1169, 1276
Chondrocyte
calcium pyrophosphate dihydrate deposition
disease, 1276
osteoarthritis, 1265
Chondroitin 4-sulfate, 1142
Chondromalacia patellae, 1266
CHOP regimen
gamma heavy-chain disease, 704
non-Hodgkin's lymphoma, 699-700
Chordal rupture, 252
Chorea
rheumatic fever, 1257
systemic lupus erythematosus, 1093
Choreic movements, 994
Choriocarcinoma
curability with chemotherapy, 552
pulmonary metastases, 493
Chorionic gonadotropin, 1742
Chorionic villus sampling, 619
Chorioretinitis, 1678
Choroidal neovascularization, 2302
Christmas disease, 622
Chromaffin cell, 1817, 1828

Chromium
carcinogenesis, 548
deficiency, 2110
functions, 2109
recommended daily dietary allowances, 2116
Chromium-51-labeled autologous platelets, 614
Chromium scan, 2004
Chromoblastomycosis, 1659-1660
Chromosomal abnormalities, 1727-1729
acute lymphoblastic leukemia, 682
acute myelogenous leukemia, 689
cancer, 487, 544
hypertrophic cardiomyopathy, 265
lysosomal storage disease, 1912
myelodysplastic syndrome, 676
Chromosomal analysis, 1743
Chromosomal mapping, 60-61
Chromosome, 1727, 1728
DNA code, 49
interstitial microdeletion, Plate IX-1
Chronic acquired hepatocerebral degeneration,
1080
Chronic active hepatitis, 1155, 2180
Chronic atrophic gastritis, 2042
Chronic bacterial prostatitis, 1462-1463
Chronic bronchitis, 472-473
API deficiency, 440
defined, 437-438
hemoptysis, 411
pathogenesis, 442
pathology, 439
patterns of pulmonary function abnormalities,
379
Chronic daily headache, 962
Chronic effusive pericarditis, 274
Chronic ethanol toxicity, 1081
Chronic fatigue syndrome, 1375, 2298-2300
Chronic granulomatous disease, 1341
Chronic granulomatous prostatitis, 1463
Chronic hepatitis, 2179-2184
autoimmune, 2183-2184
clinical assessment, 2180-2181
etiologic classification, 2180
hepatitis B virus, 2181-2182
hepatitis C virus, 2182-2183
hepatitis D virus, 2183
treatment, 2184
Chronic idiopathic neutropenia, 679
Chronic idiopathic neutrophilia, 590
Chronic inflammatory demyelinating
polyradiculoneuropathy, 1018
Chronic inflammatory disease, 1160
Chronic interstitial pneumonia–not otherwise
specified, 449
Chronic lobular hepatitis, 2180
Chronic lymphocytic leukemia, 684-685, Plate
IV-5
abnormal lymphocytes in peripheral blood,
595
lymphocytosis, 592
lymphosarcoma cell leukemia *versus,* 594
molecular diagnostics, 563
Chronic lymphocytic thyroiditis, 1811
Chronic mucocutaneous candidiasis, 1311-1312,
1662
Chronic myelocytic leukemia, Plate IV-6
Chronic myelogenous leukemia, 686-687
chromosomal abnormalities, 544
molecular diagnostics, 562-563
myelofibrosis *versus,* 677
neutrophilic leukocytosis, 591
translocation, 560
Chronic myelomonocytic leukemia, 676
Chronic nonbacterial prostatitis, 1463
Chronic obstructive pulmonary disease, 437-447
acute respiratory failure, 413-414
with acute respiratory failure, 417-418
airflow obstruction, 438
alpha₁-protease inhibitor deficiency, 439-440
clinical features, 442
complications, 445-447

Chronic obstructive pulmonary disease—cont'd
  cough syncope, 953
  definition, 437-438
  diagnosis, 443
  dyspnea, 404
  epidemiology, 438-439
  heart failure *versus,* 168
  hypercapnia, 356
  laboratory findings, 442-443
  lung transplantation, 445
  occupational, 473
  operative risk, 2261
  pathogenesis, 441-442
  pathology, 439
  physical appearance, 63
  physical examination, 442
  precapillary pulmonary hypertension,
      295-296
  prognosis and course, 447
  pulmonary rehabilitation, 432-437
  secondary polycythemia, 588
  sleep studies with monitoring of oxygen
      saturation, 380
  treatment, 443-445
  weight loss, 1750
Chronic occlusive arterial disease, 307, 308-309
Chronic pain
  abdominal, 2030
  depression, 1037
Chronic pancreatitis, 2242
Chronic paroxysmal hemicrania, 947
Chronic pernio, 310
Chronic persistent hepatitis, 2179-2180
Chronic pyelonephritis, 1456
Chronic rejection
  after liver transplantation, 2219
  lung, 522-524
  renal transplantation, 794
Chronic renal failure, 776-796
  abnormal platelet function, 605
  cardiopulmonary complications, 783-784
  clinical presentation and diagnosis, 780-782
  conservative treatment, 787
  dialysis, 789-791
  diminished fertility, 2274
  endocrine function abnormalities, 786-787
  etiology and incidence, 777
  gastrointestinal tract disturbances, 784
  hematologic disorders, 783
  hyperkalemia, 832
  hypertension, 783
  hypogonadism, 1843
  immunologic and infectious complications,
      784-785
  neuromuscular abnormalities, 784
  nutritional and metabolic alterations, 786
  osmolol gap, 806
  pathophysiology, 777-780
  prevention or delay of end-stage renal disease,
      782-783
  renal osteodystrophy, hyperphosphatemia,
      hypocalcemia, and bone and joint
      disease, 785-786
  renal replacement therapy, 788
  renal salt-washing, 824
  renal transplantation, 791-796
Chronic renal insufficiency, 776
Chronic superficial gastritis, 2042
Chronic tardive dyskinesia, 995
Chronic tophaceous gout, 1272, 1275
Chronic tubulointerstitial nephropathy, 890-892
Chronic vegetative state, 977
Chronic venous insufficiency, 311-312
Chronobiology, 940
Chuputti flour, 1951
Churg-Strauss syndrome, 453, 465-467, 1220
Chvostek's sign, 1932
Chyle, 509
Chylomicron, 60, 1885, 1888, 1987
  abetalipoproteinemia, 1897
  familial deficiency of lipoprotein lipase, 1898

Chylomicron—cont'd
  obesity, 1752
  retention disease, 2067
Chylomicron remnants, 1885, 1888-1889
Chylothorax, 382, 509
Chylous ascites, 2164
Chymotrypsin, 373
Cicatricial pemphigoid, 1296
Cidofovir, 1526
Cierny and Mader classification of osteomyelitis,
    1436
Cimetidine
  gastroesophageal reflux, 2018
  hepatic injury, 2192
  human cytochrome P450 isoforms, 2312
  induction of acute interstitial nephritis, 889
  interference with oral anticoagulants, 636
  peptic ulcer disease, 2040
  reaction with antiarrhythmics, 135-136
Cineangiography, 269
Cingulate gyrus, 1075
Ciprofloxacin, 1359
  bacterial pneumonia after lung transplantation,
      517
  Campylobacter enteritis, 1592
  dosage, 1350
  effects on kidney, 868
  enterococci resistance, 1561
  Haemophilus ducreyi, 1589
  human cytochrome P450 isoforms, 2312
  interference with oral anticoagulants, 636
  mycobacterial disease, 1631
  Pasteurella, 1609
  prophylaxis for traveler's diarrhea, 1432
  respiratory exacerbations in cystic fibrosis,
      483
  shigellosis, 1603
  spontaneous bacterial peritonitis, 2164
  typhoid fever, 1432, 1601
Ciprostene, 124
Circadian rhythm sleep disorders, 945
Circadian rhythms, 940, 1733
Circulating immune complexes, 1138
  endocarditis, 227
  Lyme disease, 1647
  measurement, 1148-1149
Circulating leukocyte
  abnormalities of phagocytes, eosinophils, and
      basophils, 678-681
  decreased volume, 593-594
  increased volume, 590-593
Circulating lymphoma cell, 594
Circulatory shock, 175-187, 180
  clinical presentation, 177-180
  clinical trials, 184, 185
  coronary angioplasty, 183
  coronary artery bypass graft, 185
  differential diagnosis, 175, 176
  evaluation and treatment, 180, 181
  hemodynamic alterations, 176, 177
  mechanical intervention, 184, 185-186
  myocardial function, 176
  myocardial infarction, 218-219
  pharmacologic therapy, 181-182
  reperfusion therapy, 182-183
  serum lactate and anaerobic metabolism, 176,
      178
Circulatory shunts and resistances, 110-111
Circulatory syncope, 952-954
Circumlocutions, 975, 976
Cirrhosis
  Anderson's disease, 1882
  ascites, 2163, 2164
  autoimmune hepatitis, 2184
  Budd-Chiari syndrome, 2208
  chemotactic defects, 1340
  chronic hepatitis B, 2181
  chronic hepatitis C, 2182
  coagulation disorder, 607
  constrictive pericarditis *versus,* 277
  cystic fibrosis, 483

Cirrhosis—cont'd
  decreased delivery of bilirubin to liver,
      2151
  drug-induced, 2189
  edema, 816
  gonadal failure, 2171
  gynecomastia, 1765
  hepatitis B virus, 2173-2174
  hepatitis C virus, 2175
  hepatocellular carcinoma, 2212
  hypergammaglobulinemia, 2136
  hypersplenism, 614
  hypogonadism, 1843
  impairment of canalicular secretion of
      conjugated bilirubins, 2155
  impotence, 1761
  liver biopsy, 2141
  liver fibrosis, 2195-2196
  porphyria cutanea tarda, 1927
  portal triad lesions, 2155
  portal vein obstruction, 2208
  primary biliary cirrhosis, 2199
  primary peritonitis, 1396
  risk of gallstone formation, 2224
  sodium balance dysfunction, 818-820
  splenomegaly, 601
  transudative pleural effusion, 507
  Wilson's disease, 2205
Cis-retinoic acid, 550
Cisapride
  diabetic gastroparesis, 1873
  gastroesophageal reflux, 2018
  human cytochrome P450 isoforms, 2312
  intestinal pseudoobstruction, 2079
Cisplatin
  cervical cancer, 715
  chemotherapy-induced nausea and vomiting,
      581
  effects on kidney, 869
  endometrial cancer, 714
  esophageal cancer, 2024
  hepatic injury, 2192
  lung cancer, 728, 729
  nephrotoxicity, 584, 891
  testicular cancer, 721
Cisternography, 926-929
Citrate, 799
Citrate anticoagulant, 570
Citric acid, 797, 799
Citrulline, 1904
Citrullinemia, 1907
Cladosporium, 1660
Clam shell procedure, 516
Clara cell, 366, 371
Clarithromycin, 1357-1358
  dosage, 1350
  Helicobacter pylori, 1593
  hepatic injury, 2191
  human cytochrome P450 isoforms, 2312
  Mycobacterium avium-intracellulare, 1474
  Mycoplasma pneumoniae pneumonia, 1540
  peptic ulcer disease, 2040
Clasp-knife phenomenon, 997
Classic angina, 194
Classic esophageal spasm, 2022
Classical pathway, 1133-1135
  activation, 1338
  bacteremia, 1448
  deficiencies of early components, 1179
Clathrin, 1886
Claudication, 1001
Clearance, 746
  amylase/creatinine clearance ratio, 2145
  antiarrhythmic drugs, 136-137
  antipyrine, 2143-2144
  bilirubin, 2147, 2148-2149
  creatinine, 746-747, 2286
  free-water, 739, 748
  low-density lipoproteins, 1890-1891
  osmolar, 748

Clearance—cont'd
secretion, 429-430
chronic obstructive pulmonary disease, 444
cystic fibrosis, 482
pulmonary rehabilitation, 436
vasopressin, 1791
Click, 75, 76
congenital aortic stenosis, 287
mitral valve prolapse, 254
Climacteric, male, 1844
Clindamycin, 1357
acne vulgaris, 1305
activity against major anaerobes, 1620
antimicrobial mechanisms, 1344
babesiosis, 1676
dosage, 1350
hepatic injury, 2191
infective endocarditis prophylaxis, 234
intraabdominal infection, 1401
osteomyelitis, 1436
pill esophagitis, 2019
Pneumocystis carinii pneumonia, 1694
prophylaxis in lung transplantation, 518
toxoplasmosis, 1474, 1678
use during pregnancy, 2281
Clinical bioethics, 9-13
Clinical Dementia Rating Scale, 904
Clinical practice guidelines, 23-26
methods of quality improvement, 19-20
Clinical risk profile, 2257
Clinitest, 743
CLL; *see* Chronic lymphocytic leukemia
Clofazimine, 1651
Clofibrate
diabetes insipidus, 1796-1797
gallstone risk factor, 2223
interference with catecholamine assays, 1740
interference with oral anticoagulants, 636
lipoprotein lipase potentiation, 1892
Clomatacine, 2191
Clomiphene, 1736, 1841, 1842
Clomipramine, 1037
cataplexy, 943
human cytochrome P450 isoforms, 2312
Clonal specificity, 1108
Clonal succession model, 530
Clonality, 559
Clonazepam, 983
anxiety disorders, 1035
restless legs syndrome, 944
spasticity after spinal cord injury, 1051
Clonic seizure, 979
Clonidine
hot flashes, 2271
hypertension, 325
interference with catecholamine assays, 1740
opiate detoxification, 2297
pheochromocytoma, 322, 1830
spasticity after spinal cord injury, 1051
suppression, 1740
testing for growth hormone reserve, 1775
Cloning
deoxyribonucleic acid, 52-53
positional, 1724
Clonorchis sinensis, 1703, 2231
Clostridium, 1567-1576
bacteremia, 1576
cellulitis, 1422
food-borne, 1568-1570
gastrointestinal tract, 1567-1568
myonecrosis, 1574-1576
neurologic syndromes, 1570-1572
normal flora, 1368
tetanus, 1572-1574
Clostridium botulinum, 1570-1572
Clostridium difficile, 1568-1570
acquired immunodeficiency syndrome, 2098
compromised host, 1388
stool examination, 2006
ulcerative colitis *versus,* 2073

Clostridium perfringens, 1567
antibiotic selection, 1348
bacteremia, 1576
diarrhea, 1430
food poisoning, 1568
gas gangrene, 1422-1423
hemolytic anemia, 667
infectious gastritis, 2043
intraabdominal infection, 1397
myonecrosis, 1574-1576
neomycin resistance, 2162
Clostridium ramosum, 1574-1576
Clostridium septicum, 1423
Clostridium tetani, 1572-1574
Clot stability test, 571
Clotrimazole
esophageal candidiasis, 2020
otomycosis, 2307
trichomoniasis, 1443
typical medical regimen six months after
transplantation, 343
Clotting factors
assay, 571
congenital deficiency, 624
hepatic formation, 2120
Cloxacillin
dosage, 1350
hepatic injury, 2191
Clozapine
hepatic injury, 2191
human cytochrome P450 isoforms, 2312
Parkinson's disease, 992
schizophrenia, 1042
CLR, 1133
Clubbing
atrial septal defect, 281
Crohn's disease, 2075
hepatopulmonary syndrome, 2170
hypertrophic osteoarthropathy, 1247
infective endocarditis, 228
interstitial lung disease, 450
tetralogy of Fallot, 289
Clue cell, 1443
Cluster headache, 959
sleep-related, 947
treatment, 962
Cluster of differentiation, 1113, 1151
CMF regimen, 709
CMFVP regimen, 711-712
CMV; *see* Cytomegalovirus
Coagulase-negative staphylococci, 1547,
1550-1551
endocarditis, 226
Staphylococcus epidermidis, 1546
antibiotic selection, 1347
bacterial meningitis, 1403
epidemiology, 1548
nosocomial infections, 1362, 1551-1552
prosthetic valve endocarditis, 1550-1551
septic arthritis, 1251
therapy, 1552
Coagulation, 537-539
control mechanisms, 539
plasma, 570-571
Coagulation disorders, 606-608, 617-630
acquired inhibitors of blood coagulation,
628-630
arthropathy, 1246
disseminated intravascular coagulation,
627-628
factor deficiencies, 624
fibrinogen abnormalities, 625
hemophilia A, 617-622
hemophilia B, 622
liver disease, 626-627
nephrotic syndrome, 766
protease inhibitors deficiencies, 625
vitamin K deficiency, 625-626
von Willebrand's disease, 622-624

Coagulation factors
assay, 571
congenital deficiency, 624
hepatic formation, 2120
Coagulation inhibitors, 571, 608, 629
Coagulopathy
acute pancreatitis, 2237
chronic renal failure, 783
fulminant hepatic failure, 2163
gram-negative bacteremia, 1448
paraneoplastic dermatoses, 1317
primary pulmonary hypertension, 294
Coal tar psoriasis, 1301-1302
Coal worker's pneumoconiosis, 475
Coaptation, 884
Coarctation of aorta, 286-287
Cobalamin, 1080, 1989
Cobalt
functions, 2109
hard metal disease, 475-476
Cocaine, 2296-2297
arrhythmia, 133
hepatic injury, 2191
pupil response, 933
pupillometry, 938
Coccidioides immitis, 1655-1657
hazard to laboratory personnel, 1369
meningitis, 1409
peritonitis, 2248
respiratory infection, acquired
immunodeficiency syndrome, 1477
Coccidioidomycosis, 1655-1657, 1679-1680
acquired immunodeficiency syndrome, 1474
bone infection, 1437
joint disease, 1254
pleural effusion, 507
serodiagnosis, 1653
Cock-croft equation, 2286
Codeine
abuse, 2297
cancer pain, 581
cough, 408, 409
cytochrome P450 2D6-mediated conversion,
2311
human cytochrome P450 isoforms, 2312
pulmonary toxicity, 479
restless legs syndrome, 944
Codominant, 1724
Codon, 50
Cofactors of coagulation, 538
Cognition
impairment in elderly, 2288
thought disorders, 1041-1043
Cognitive failure dementia, 985-989
Coin lesion, 493
Colchicine
alcoholic hepatitis, 2198
calcium pyrophosphate dihydrate deposition
disease, 1278
drug-nutrient interactions, 2110
familial Mediterranean fever, 877, 1243
glucose-6-phosphate dehydrogenase
deficiency, 664
gouty arthritis, 1274-1275
pericardial heart disease, 278
pericarditis, 221
primary biliary cirrhosis, 2200
pulmonary parenchymal reactions, 476
reactive amyloidosis, 1283
Cold
common, 1180-1185, 1390-1392
cryoglobulinemia, 1248
increased nutrient requirements, 2102
Cold agglutinin disease, 669-670
Cold agglutinins, 1540
Cold core, 1523
Cold exposure
chest pain, 126
Raynaud's phenomenon, 1226-1227
Cold pressor test, 937

Colectomy
  Crohn's disease, 2072
  toxic megacolon, 2076
  ulcerative colitis, 2074
Colestipol, 1890
Colic
  biliary, 2225-2227
    acute cholecystitis, 2227
    hemobilia, 2233
  esophageal, 1999
  renal
    diagnostic algorithm, 754
    medullary sponge kidney, 875
Colipase, 1987
Colistimethate, 483
Colistin, 1350, 1358
Colitis
  acquired immunodeficiency syndrome, 1476
  Campylobacter jejuni, 1591-1592
  chronic gastrointestinal bleeding, 2014
  chronic renal failure, 784
  Clostridium difficile, 1568-1570
  Entamoeba histolytica, 1681
  fecal leukocytes, 1430, 1431
  pseudomembranous, 1568-1570, 1996
  ulcerative, 2072-2075
    Crohn's disease *versus*, 2075
    cutaneous findings, 1321
    diagnosis, 2073, 2074
    enteropathic arthropathy, 1245-1246
    histologic features, Plate X-5
    increased risk of cancer, 548
    management, 2073-2074
    pathologic findings, 2072-2073
    prognosis, 2074-2075
Collaborative self-management, 435
Collagen
  bone organic matrix, 1716
  cardiac, 41
  diabetic nephropathy, 861
  disorders of structure and metabolism,
    1286-1289
  hepatic fibrosis, 2195
  lung extracellular matrix, 371
  platelet adhesion to subendothelium, 536
  types and tissue distribution, 1286
  urinary excretion of pyridinium and
    deoxypyridinium crosslinks, 1745
Collagen vascular disease, 453-454
  alveolar hemorrhage with, 455
  fever of unknown origin, 1376, 1377-1378
  neurologic manifestations, 1092
Collateral circulation
  coarctation of aorta, 286
  nitroglycerin effects, 201
  portal hypertension, 2165
Collecting duct
  carcinoma, 899
  crystal attachment, 797
  renal concentrating and diluting mechanisms,
    739, 740
Collecting tubule, 835
Colles' fracture, 1945
Colloid droplets, 1797
Colon
  adenocarcinoma, 2076-2077
  balantidiasis, 1690-1691
  cancer, 2082-2086
    allelic loss, 546
    Campylobacter jejuni infection *versus*, 1591
    colonoscopy, 1996
    curability with chemotherapy, 552
    hereditary nonpolyposis, 549
    incidence and death rates, 550
    physiology and pathophysiology, 2082-2083
    risk in ulcerative colitis, 2075
    screening, 552-553
  colitis
    acquired immunodeficiency syndrome, 1476
    Campylobacter jejuni, 1591-1592

Colon—cont'd
  colitis—cont'd
    chronic gastrointestinal bleeding, 2014
    chronic renal failure, 784
    Clostridium difficile, 1568-1570
    Entamoeba histolytica, 1681
    fecal leukocytes, 1430, 1431
    Crohn's disease, 1996, 2069-2072
     Campylobacter jejuni infection *versus*, 1591
     chronic diarrhea, 2051
     clinical features, 2069
     Colonic carcinoma, 2076
     cutaneous findings, 1321
     delay in secondary sexual development,
      1768
     diagnosis, 2070-2071
     endoscopic photographs, Plate X-6
     fever of unknown origin, 1378
     fissured ulcer, Plate X-4
     granulomatous gastritis, 2043
     heteropathic arthropathy, 1245-1246
     hypogammaglobulinemia, 2066
     impotence, 1763
     laboratory findings, 2069-2070
     management, 2071-2072
     oral aphthous ulcer, Plate X-10
     perianal fistula, 2093
     perianal manifestations, Plate X-5
     pregnancy and, 2278
     risk of gallstone formation, 2224
     short bowel syndrome, 2066
     small bowel adenocarcinoma, 2081
     ulcerative colitis *versus*, 2075
    diverticular disease, 2089-2092
    evaluation, 2004-2008
    flexible sigmoidoscopy, 1995
    increased fecal bile salt loss, 2129
    infarction, 2087, 2088
    Kaposi's sarcoma, Plate VIII-39
    luminal fluid, 2060
    normal microflora, 1615
    polyp, 2073
    radiologic examination, 2007
    rigid proctoscopy, 1995
    role in digestion, 1980
    secondary intraperitoneal infection, 1396
    systemic sclerosis, 1230
    toxic dilation, 2076
    transit studies, 2055
    ulcerative colitis, 2072-2075
     chronic diarrhea, 2051
     colon cancer *versus*, 2085
     colonoscopy, 1996
     Crohn's disease *versus*, 2075
     cutaneous findings, 1321
     diagnosis, 2073, 2074
     endoscopic features, Plate X-8
     enteropathic arthropathy, 1245-1246
     heteropathic arthropathy, 1245-1246
     histologic features, Plate X-5
     increased risk of cancer, 548
     management, 2073-2074
     pathologic findings, 2072-2073
     pregnancy and, 2278
     primary sclerosing cholangitis, 2201
     prognosis, 2074-2075
Colonoscopy, 1996
  acute lower gastrointestinal bleeding, 2012
  colonic diverticulum, 2091
  constipation, 2055
  Crohn's disease, 2070
  diarrhea, 1476
  intestinal obstruction, 2078
Colony-forming unit-blast, 531
Colony-forming unit-bone marrow, aPlate IV-2
Colony-forming unit-erythroid, 531
Colony-forming unit-granulocyte, erythrocyte,
  macrophage, megakaryocyte, 531
Colony-forming unit-granulocyte macrophage,
  532

Colony-forming unit-megakaryocyte, 532
Colony-forming unit-spleen, 531
Colony-forming unit–granulocyte, 532
Colony-forming unit–macrophage, 532
Color of urine, 742
Color return, venous filling times and, 305
Color vision, 1057
Colorado tick fever, 1511-1512
Colovesical fistula, 2090
Colposcopy, 715
Coltivirus, 1511-1512
Coma, 947-950, 1081-1086
  acute hyponatremia, 811
  eclampsia, 2274
  electroencephalography, 907, 909
  hepatic encephalopathy, 2160
  hyperosmolar nonketotic, 1865-1866
  hypoglycemia, 1875
  Jolliffe's disease, 1101
  myxedema, 1810-1811
  rabies, 1505
  thrombotic thrombocytopenic purpura, 615
  toxic hepatic injury, 2188
Coma vigil, 1032
Combination therapy
  antimicrobial, 1360
  breast cancer, 709, 711-712
  myelodysplastic syndrome, 676
  non-small cell lung cancer, 727-728
Combined hyperlipedmias, 1895-1896
Combined tension-migraine headache, 958
Comedone, 1305
Comfrey, 2193
Commercial air travel, 447
Commissurotomy
  aortic stenosis, 239
  mitral stenosis, 248
  tricuspid stenosis, 256
Common aortopulmonary trunk, 290
Common atrioventricular canal defect, 282-283
Common bile duct, 2130
  choledochal cyst, 2212
Common cold, 1180-1185, 1390-1392
  coronavirus, 1502
  rhinovirus, 1487
Common duct stones, 2228-2230
Common faint, 952
Common variable immunodeficiency, 1176, 1343
  gastric cancer, 2046
Communication hydrocephalus, 926-929
Compartmentalization of body water, 736
Compatibility testing, 573
Compensated hemolytic anemia, 587
Compensatory mechanisms
  arrhythmia, 159
  shock, 177, 179
Competence, decision making capacity, 11-12
Competitive binding assays, 1372
Competitive protein binding, 1734
Complement, 1132-1138
  activation, 1110, 1133-1135
  assay, 1149
  barrier to infection, 1335
  deficiency, 1178-1180, 1338-1339
  effector functions, 1136-1137
  gram-negative bacteremia, 1448
  history and nomenclature, 1133
  hypocomplementemia, 1147, 1148
    acute nephritic syndrome, 764
    membranoproliferative glomerulonephritis,
     854
    partial lipodystrophy, 1902
  infectious diseases, 1338-1339
  lung injury, 374
  measurement, 1147-1150
  meningitis, 1404
  regulation, 1135-1136
  respiratory defense, 366
  synovial fluid, 1163
  systemic lupus erythematosus, 1216

Complement factor B, 766
Complement-fixation assay, 1373
Complement membrane proteins, 1133
Complement receptor, 1338
   deficiency, 1179-1180
Complement receptor 1, 1135
complement receptor type 1, 1136
Complement serum proteins, 1133
Complementary deoxyribonucleic acid libraries,
      54
Complete blood count
   flow cytometry analysis, 1151-1152
   gastrointestinal bleeding, 2011
   heart failure, 166
   hemolytic anemia, 661
   impotence, 1763
   nutritional assessment, 2111
Complete heart block, 180, 223
Complete thromboplastins, 570-571
Complete transposition of great arteries, 290
Complex carbohydrates, 1289-1290
Complex inheritance, 1726-1727
Complex partial seizure, 979
Compliance, 1081
   aortic, 299
   increased intracranial pressure, 1081
   pulmonary blood flow, 362
Compound motor action potential, 914
Comprehension
   neurologic examination, 902
   testing in aphasia, 975
Compression
   mediastinal mass, 511
   optic nerve, 1060
   spinal cord, 1011-1012, 1071
   variceal bleeding, 2167-2168
Compromised host
   cytomegalovirus, 1528
   fever, 1386-1390
   herpes simplex virus infection, 1524
   measles, 1498
   multiple organ dysfunction syndrome, 422
   nocardiosis, 1666
   nontuberculous mycobacterial infection, 1639
   peritonitis, 2248
   precautions before international travel,
         1468-1469
   Staphylococcus aureus, 1550
   Staphylococcus epidermidis, 1551
   zoster, 1527
Compulsive water drinking, 815
Computed tomographic angiography, 926
Computed tomography, 512
   abdominal, 2033
   acute maxillary sinusitis, 1394
   acute pancreatitis, 2236
   adrenal mass, 321
   aldosterone excess, 1823
   ankylosing spondylitis, 1239
   appendicitis, 2092
   benign strictures of extrahepatic bile ducts,
         2232
   brain abscess, 1414, 1415
   Budd-Chiari syndrome, 2208
   cancer
      brain tumor, 1067-1069
      cholangiocarcinoma, 2232
      gastric, 2046
      hepatocellular carcinoma, 2213
      lung, 489, 726
      non-Hodgkin's lymphoma, 698
      renal cell carcinoma, 898
      testicular, 720-721
   Caroli's disease, 2233
   cavernous hemangioma, 2216
   cholestasis, 2156
   chronic obstructive pulmonary disease, 442
   chronic pancreatitis, 2240
   coma, 949-950
   constrictive pericarditis, 277
   Crohn's disease, 2070

Computed tomography—cont'd
   dementia, 988
   electron beam, 106
   epilepsy, 981, 982
   evaluation of arthritis, 1164, 1173
   focal nodular hyperplasia, 2216
   gallstones, 2220
   giant bullae, 447
   gynecomastia, 1765
   head trauma, 1044
   heart, 106
   hematuria, 757
   hemoptysis, 411
   hepatic encephalopathy, 2161
   hepatobiliary tract, 2140
   hypothalamic-pituitary disease, 1734
   incidentaloma, 1830
   insulinoma, 1878, 2244
   intestinal disease, 2007
   intraabdominal abscess, 1400
   ischemic heart disease, 198
   lesions causing headache, 961
   low back pain, 966
   measurement of bone mineral density, 1748
   Meckel's diverticulum, 2090
   meningitis, 1406-1407
   multiple sclerosis, 1009
   myocardial infarction, 212
   neck pain, 969
   neurologic disorders, 917-918, 919, 920
   obstructive sleep apnea, 355
   osteomyelitis, 1434
   pancreatic, 2145
   pancreatic disease, 2146
   pancreatic tumor, 2242
   pelvis, 756
   peptic ulcer disease, 2037
   pericardial effusion, 275
   peripheral arterial aneurysm, 309
   pleural disease, 506
   posterior fossa, 974
   pulmonary, 386-387
   pyogenic liver abscess, 2209
   renal, 750
      abscess, 755
      autosomal dominant polycystic kidney
            disease, 873
      obstructive uropathy, 754, 886-887
      renal mass, 751-752
      upper urinary tract tumor, 899
   retroperitoneal abscess, 2250
   retroperitoneal fibrosis, 2251
   secondary polycythemia, 589-590
   septic arthritis, 1252
   simple cyst, 871-872
   sinusitis, 2308
   solitary pulmonary nodule, 495, 497
   spinal lesion, 1012
   stroke, 973, 1002-1003
   subdural empyema, 1417-1418
   Taenia solium, 1704
   thoracic aortic aneurysm, 300
   toxoplasmosis, 1477, 1478
   tuberous sclerosis, 1922
Computer-based medical record, 27-28
Concentration of solute, 806
Condom, 2270
Conducting airways, 365
Conduction aphasia, 976
Conduction disturbances, 131-156
   bradyarrhythmias and atrioventricular block,
         153-156
   congenital, 292
   congenital long Q-T syndrome, 62
   dilated cardiomyopathy, 264
   electrocardiography, 86-87
   intraventricular, 156
   myocardial infarction, 222-224
   nonpharmacologic therapy, 139-140
   operative risk, 2260
   pathophysiology, 131-134

Conduction disturbances—cont'd
   pharmacologic therapy, 134-139
   supraventricular tachycardia, 141-148
      accelerated atrioventricular junctional
            rhythm, 144
      atrial fibrillation, 146-148
      atrial flutter, 144-146
      atrioventricular nodal reentrant tachycardia,
            141-142, 144, 145
      ectopic atrial tachycardia, 143-144, 146
      multifocal atrial tachycardia, 144, 146
      premature atrial contractions, 141
      sinus tachycardia, 141
      supraventricular tachyarrhythmias, 141, 142,
            143
      Wolff-Parkinson-White syndrome, 142-143,
            145
   ventricular arrhythmias, 148-153
      accelerated idioventricular rhythm, 149, 150
      nonsustained ventricular tachycardia, 149
      polymorphic ventricular tachycardia,
            151-153
      premature ventricular contractions, 148-149
      sustained monomorphic ventricular
            tachycardia, 150-151
      sustained ventricular tachycardia with wide
            QRS complex tachycardia, 149-150,
            151
      ventricular fibrillation, 153
Conduction tissue, 36
Conduction velocity, 914-915
Conductive hearing loss, 2308
Condylomata lata, 1641
Conflict of interest, 12
Confrontation visual field testing, 1057
Confusion, 985
   acute confusional state, 1031
   acute hyponatremia, 811
   bacterial meningitis, 1406
   hepatic encephalopathy, 2160
   hypoglycemia, 1875
   hypoglycemic coma, 1867
   streptococcal toxic shock syndrome, 1557
Confusional arousals, 945
Congenital contractural arachnodactyly, 1289
Congenital coronary arteriovenous fistula, 292
Congenital disorders
   absence of pericardium, 273
   adrenal hyperplasia, 1824-1825
   cytomegalovirus, 1527-1528
   defective bile salt synthesis, 2129
   diabetic mother, 2272
   evaluation of respiratory disease, 402
   hematologic, 617-625
      factor deficiencies, 624
      Fanconi's anemia, 672
      fibrinogen abnormalities, 625
      hemophilia A, 617-622
      hemophilia B, 622
      protease inhibitors deficiencies, 625
      von Willebrand's disease, 622-624
   herpes simplex virus, 1524
   hypogonadism, 1840
   lactase deficiency, 2068
   malaria, 1672
   Meckel's diverticulum, 2089
   mediastinal cyst, 513
   obesity, 1751, 1752
   pancreatic, 2246
   rubella, 1501
   syphilis, 1641-1642
   toxoplasmosis, 1677
   varicella, 1527
   vitamin K deficiency, 626
Congenital end-plate acetylcholinesterase
      deficiency, 1023
Congenital erythropoietic porphyria, 1925
Congenital glucose-galactose malabsorption, 878
Congenital heart disease, 280-292
   aberrant right subclavian artery, 291
   aortic stenosis, 287

Congenital heart disease—cont'd
  aortic valve stenosis, 235
  aortopulmonary septal defect, 286
  atrial septal defect, 280-282
  bicuspid aortic valve, 287
  brain abscess, 1414
  cardiac catheterization, 108
  cardiogenic syncope, 954
  coarctation of aorta, 286-287
  complete transposition of great arteries, 290
  congenitally corrected transposition of great arteries, 290
  cor triatriatum, 291
  coronary artery abnormalities, 291-292
  coronary sinus aneurysm, 291
  disturbances of conduction, 292
  Ebstein's anomaly of tricuspid valve, 289-290
  echocardiography, 100
  endocardial cushion defect, 282-283
  etiology, 280
  fetal circulation and changes associated with birth, 280
  infective endocarditis, 225, 226
  malposition of heart, 291
  mitral regurgitation, 250
  partial transposition of pulmonary veins, 282
  patent ductus arteriosus, 285-286
  pericardial, 273, 291-292
  precapillary pulmonary hypertension, 296-297
  pulmonic regurgitation, 257
  pulmonic stenosis, 256
  tetralogy of Fallot, 288-289
  total anomalous pulmonary venous connection, 290-291
  tricuspid atresia, 291
  truncus arteriosus, 290
  valvular pulmonic stenosis with intact ventricular septum, 288
  ventricular septal defect, 283-285
Congenital long Q-T syndrome, 59, 61, 62
Congenital myasthenia, 1023
Congenital rubella syndrome, 2280
Congenital total lipodystrophy, 1900-1902
Congenitally corrected transposition of great arteries, 290
Congestive cardiomyopathy, 263-265
  molecular biology, 61-62
  pulmonary hypertension, 298
  transplant candidate, 335
Congestive heart failure, 156-175
  advanced renal disease, 784
  after stroke, 1007
  angiotensin-converting enzyme inhibitors, 169-172
  antiarrhythmic therapy, 174
  anticoagulation, 174-175
  antihypertensive agent choices, 326
  atrial fibrillation, 146
  beta-adrenergic blockers, 174
  calcium channel blockers, 174
  cardiac catheterization, 17, 108
  cardiac output, 159
  cellular abnormalities of myocardial failure, 159-160
  Cheyne-Stokes respiration, 353
  Churg-Strauss syndrome, 466
  clinical manifestations, 163-165
  compensatory mechanisms, 159
  complete transposition of great arteries, 290
  diabetes mellitus, 334
  diastolic heart failure, 167-168
  differential diagnosis, 168
  diuretics, 169, 170
  Ebstein's anomaly, 290
  edema, 816
  epidemiology and prognosis, 157-158
  high-output failure, 160
  infective endocarditis, 228
  inotropic agents, 172-173, 174
  laboratory and diagnostic testing, 165-167
  mesenteric vascular disease, 2086

Congestive heart failure—cont'd
  myocarditis, 262-263
  neuroendocrine activity, 160, 161, 162, 163
  neurohormonal hypothesis, 161
  operative risk, 2258
  pathogenesis, 158-159
  patient and family counseling, 167
  peripheral vascular and reflex control abnormalities, 161-162, 164
  Pompe's disease, 1881
  proteinuria, 760
  pulmonary edema, 168-169
  rabies, 1506
  radionuclide angiography, 104-105
  rheumatic fever, 1256
  sodium and water retention, 162-163
  sodium balance dysfunction, 817-818
  splenomegaly, 601
  syphilis, 1641
  thrombosis, 609
  transudative pleural effusion, 507
  vasodilators, 173-174
  ventricular septal defect, 284
  weight loss, 1750
Congestive Heart Failure Survival Trial of Antiarrhythmic Therapy, 171
Conidiobolomycosis, 1660
Conjugate eye movement disturbances, 1063-1065
Conjugated bilirubin, 2147
Conjugated bilirubin fraction, 2142
Conjugated hyperbilirubinemia
  benign chronic, 2157-2158
  differential diagnosis, 2156
  pathophysiology and classification, 2154-2156
  unconjugated *versus,* 2150, 2151
Conjunctiva, renal osteodystrophy, 1963
Conjunctivitis
  acute hemorrhagic, 1490
  adenovirus, 1504
  American trypanosomiasis, 1690
  Chlamydia trachomatis, 1536
  Kawasaki's disease, 1225
  keratoconjunctivitis sicca
    human immunodeficiency virus-infected patients, 2306
    Sjögren syndrome, 1209-1212
  measles, 1498
  staphylococcal toxic shock syndrome, 1421
  trachoma, 1535
  tularemia, 1608
Connecting peptide, 1744
Connective tissue disease
  associated myositis, 1236
  chronic aortic regurgitation, 239
  cutaneous manifestations, 1290-1293
  heritable and developmental, 1286-1290
  neurologic aspects, 1091-1095
  pericarditis, 272
  peripheral neuropathy, 1016
  pleural effusion, 508
  rheumatoid arthritis *versus,* 1206
  systemic sclerosis, 1228
Connective tissue mast cell, 1139
Conn's syndrome, 828
Consanguinity
  autosomal recessive inheritance pattern, 1725-1726
  leprechaunism, 1899
Conscious sedation, 1994
Consciousness
  abnormal respiratory rhythms, 1097-1098
  coma, 947
  epilepsy, 981
  hepatic encephalopathy, 2160
CONSENSUS survival trial, 171, 172
Consolidation of lung, 403
Constipation, 2053-2055
  autonomic failure, 935
  calcium channel blocker-induced, 205
  Chagas's disease, 1690

Constipation—cont'd
  chemotherapy-induced, 585
  colon cancer, 2085
  gastric cancer, 2046
  irritable bowel syndrome, 2056
  neurofibromatosis, 1921
  pancreatic cancer, 2242
  portosystemic encephalopathy, 2160
  systemic sclerosis, 1230
Constitutional delay, 1768, 1843
Constrictive pericarditis, 277-278
  cardiac catheterization, 116
  central venous pressure, 66-67
  heart failure *versus,* 168
  management, 278-279
  restrictive cardiomyopathy *versus,* 271
  transudative pleural effusion, 507
Consultant, medical genetic diagnosis, 1730
Consumptive coagulopathy, 627
Contact dermatitis, 1303-1304
Contact urticaria, 1304
Contaminated small bowel syndrome, 2129
Contiguous focus osteomyelitis, 1434, 1435-1436
Continuous ambulatory electrocardiographic recording, 94
Continuous ambulatory peritoneal dialysis, 790-791
  chronic renal failure, 788
  induction of peritonitis, 2248
Continuous arteriovenous hemofiltration, 791
Continuous loop recorder, 134
Continuous murmur, 80
Continuous positive airway pressure
  acute respiratory failure, 415-416, 418
  obstructive apnea, 355, 527-528
  precapillary pulmonary hypertension, 296
Continuous quality improvement, 18
Continuous-wave Doppler echocardiography, 98
Contraception, 2269-2270
  intrauterine device, 2270
    actinomycosis, 1665
    endometrial scarring, 1760
  oral contraceptives, 2270
    drug-nutrient interactions, 2110
    estrogen-related cholestasis, 2158
    fibrocystic breast disease, 1850
    hepatic vein thrombosis, 2208
    hirsutism, 1756-1757
    hypertension, 320
    migraine, 957
Contract, physician, 33
Contractile proteins, 59-60
Contractile system, 39-41
Contractility, 112
  cardiogenic shock, 176, 179
Contracting factors, 318
Contraction
  cardiac, 37-41
  respiratory muscles, 357-358
Contracture
  rheumatoid arthritis, 1203
  spinal cord injury, 1052
  systemic sclerosis, 1229
Contraregulatory mechanisms, 177, 179
Contrast media
  computed tomography, 386
  induction of anaphylaxis, 1193, 1194
  nephrotoxicity, 871
Contrast radiographic studies, 2032
Contrast venography, 502
Control of bone resorption and growth, 1716
Controlled mechanical ventilation, 397, 418-419
Contusion
  brain, 1043
  myocardial, 332
Conus medullaris syndrome, 1048
Convergence-retractory nystagmus, 1064
Conversion disorder, 1040
Converting enzyme inhibitors, 832

Convulsion
  hepatic encephalopathy, 2160
  uremia, 784
Cooley's anemia, 654
Coombs' test
  autoimmune hemolytic anemia, 669
  chronic lymphocytic leukemia, 685
  drug-induced immune hemolytic anemia, 670
  increased reticulocyte count, 587
Cooperative New Scandinavian Enalapril
    Survival Study, 171, 172
Cooperativity of hemoglobin, 652
COPD; *see* Chronic obstructive pulmonary
    disease
Copolymer I, 1010
Copper
  acute renal failure, 867
  deficiency, 2110
  functions, 2109
  primary sclerosing cholangitis, 2202
  recommended daily dietary allowances, 2116
  sideroblastic anemia, 645
  Wilson's disease, 1102, 2138, 2205
Copper wiring, Plate XI-4
Coproporphyrin, 1926-1927, 2157-2158
Coproporphyrinogen oxidase, 1923
Cor pulmonale, 442, 446-447, 498
Cor triatriatum, 291, 298
Cord blood screening, 660
Cordarone; *see* Amiodarone
Cordis stent, 120
Cordotomy, 581
Coreg; *see* Carvedilol
Corgard; *see* Nadolol
Cori cycle, 1750, 1852
Corkscrew esophagus, 2023
Cornea
  Acanthamoeba infection, 1684
  acute hemorrhagic conjunctivitis, 1490
  herpes keratitis, 1524
  Hurler's syndrome, 1912
Coronary angioplasty, 116-125
  for acute myocardial infarction, 121-122
  approach to specific lesions, 120-121
  background, 116-117
  complications, 122
  devices, 117-120, 121
  myocardial revascularization, 205-206
  pathophysiology, 116
  primary, 122, 123, 124
  randomized trials, 117, 118
  referral, 124
  rescue, 122
  restenosis, 122-124
  shock, 183
Coronary arteriography, 111
  aortic stenosis, 287
  cardiac catheterization with, 108, 109
  congenital abnormalities of coronary arteries,
    291
  congenital coronary arteriovenous fistula, 292
  heart failure, 167
  ischemic heart disease, 113
  mitral regurgitation, 251
  mitral stenosis, 248
  mitral valve prolapse, 254
  myocardial ischemia, 199-200
  sudden cardiac survivor, 188
  transplant donor, 339
  ventricular septal defect, 284
Coronary arteritis
  rheumatoid arthritis, 334
  systemic lupus erythematosus, 1215
Coronary artery
  arteriogram, 109
  congenital abnormalities, 291-292
  magnetic resonance imaging, 107
  penetrating injuries, 333
Coronary artery bypass graft
  cardiogenic shock, 185
  cost-utility analysis, 16

Coronary artery bypass graft—cont'd
  ischemic heart disease, 206-207
  patient on dialysis, 783
  percutaneous transluminal coronary
    angioplasty *versus*, 117, 118
  triiodothyronine levels following, 1811
Coronary artery disease, 264
  after cardiac transplantation, 341
  atrial fibrillation, 146
  cardiac catheterization, 107-108, 113
  chest pain, 127
  diabetes mellitus, 334, 1869
  echocardiography, 100
  elderly, 2282
  electron beam computed tomography, 106
  exercise stress testing, 93
  heart failure, 158, 167
  interventional cardiac catheterization, 116-125
    approach to specific lesions, 120-121
    background, 116-117
    complications, 122
    coronary angioplasty for acute myocardial
      infarction, 121-122
    devices, 117-120, 121
    pathophysiology, 116
    primary coronary angioplasty, 122
    randomized trials, 117, 118
    referral, 124
    rescue coronary angioplasty, 122
    restenosis, 122-124
  ischemic heart disease, 192, 193
  neurologic aspects, 1089
  preoperative evaluation, 2258
  radionuclide angiography, 105
  risk of stroke, 1001
  sudden cardiac death, 188
  technetium-99m sestamibi imaging, 102-103
  thallium-201 imaging, 101
  thyroid hormone replacement therapy
      complications, 1810
  transplant candidate, 335
  valve replacement surgery, 257-258
  women, 2271-2272
Coronary artery spasm, 194, 200
Coronary blood flow, 48-49
  angina pectoris, 126
  calcium channel blockers, 203-204
  determinants, 193-195
Coronary heart disease
  effects of blood pressure reduction, 322
  endogenous hypertriglyceridemia, 1895
  hydroxy-methyl-glutaryl conenzyme A
      reductase inhibitors, 1891
  hypercholesterolemia, 1892-1893
  hypertension, 314, 315
  lipoprotein lipase potentiation drugs, 1892
  plasma cholesterol, 1888
  systemic lupus erythematosus, 1215
  total cholesterol/HDL cholesterol ratio, 1897
Coronary perfusion pressure, 45-46
Coronary revascularization, 16
Coronary sinus, 292
Coronary sinus aneurysm, 291
Coronary vasospasm
  after revascularization surgery, 207
  amrinone, 182
  angioplasty-induced, 122
  coronary arteriography, 200
  myocardial infarction, 209
  variant angina, 194
Coronavirus, 1502-1503
  common cold, 1391
  pharyngitis, 1392
  respiratory tract infection, 1390
Corrigan pulse, 65, 241
Corrosive gastritis, 2043
Cortical anarthria, 977
Cortical-basal ganglionic degeneration, 992
Cortical bone, 1714-1715
Cortical function, 1078
Cortical mapping of brain function, 922

Cortical stuttering, 977
Cortical vein thrombosis, 928
Corticospinal tract, 1011
Corticosteroids
  acute interstitial nephritis, 889
  acute lung allograft rejection, 521
  anti-glomerular basement membrane antibody
      disease, 454
  antibody-mediated insulin resistance, 1861
  antiphospholipid syndrome, 1292
  asthma, 1190-1191, 1192
  autoimmune hepatitis, 2184
  biosynthesis, 1817, 1818
  brain abscess, 1416
  breast cancer, 709
  bronchiolitis obliterans syndrome, 523
  bullous pemphigoid, 1296
  chemotherapy-induced nausea and vomiting,
      582
  chronic lymphocytic leukemia, 685
  chronic obstructive pulmonary disease, 434,
      444
    with acute respiratory failure, 417-418
  Churg-Strauss syndrome, 467
  cluster headache prophylaxis, 962
  crescentic glomerulonephritis, 848
  Crohn's disease, 2071, 2072
  cutaneous complications of sarcoidosis, 1325
  cutaneous lesions in lupus erythematosus,
      1291-1292
  cystic fibrosis, 482
  dermatomyositis, 1292
  drug-induced thrombocytopenia, 615
  eosinophilic enteritis, 2067
  eosinophilic fasciitis, 1234
  Epstein-Barr virus infection, 1529
  fever of unknown origin, 1380
  giant-cell arteritis, 304
  Goodpasture's syndrome, 847
  gout, 1274
  gram-negative sepsis, 1453
  Hodgkin's disease, 694-695
  human cytochrome P450 isoforms, 2312
  hypersensitivity pneumonitis, 462
  immune hemolytic anemia, 669
  immune thrombocytopenic purpura, 616
  inflammatory myopathies, 1237
  interstitial lung disease, 451
  lung transplantation, 516
  lupus erythematosus, 1291
  minimal change disease, 851
  multiple myeloma, 702
  multiple sclerosis, 1010
  myasthenia gravis, 1022
  myelofibrosis, 677
  myelopathy, 1013
  myocarditis, 263
  for nausea and vomiting, 2027
  neurologic complications, 1072, 1090
  neutropenia, 679
  non-Hodgkin's lymphoma, 698-699
  optic neuritis, 1060
  osteoarthritis, 1268
  pemphigus vulgaris, 1294
  pericardial heart disease, 278
  perioperative requirements, 2262
  Pneumocystis carinii pneumonia, 1695
  during pregnancy, 2277
  prevention and therapy of rejection, 340
  psoriasis, 1301
  pulmonary edema, 427-428
  pulmonary rehabilitation, 434
  pulmonary tuberculosis, 1633
  reflex sympathetic dystrophy syndrome, 1247
  regulation of albumin synthesis, 2119
  regulation of secretion, 1817-1819
  relapsing polychondritis, 1243
  relapsing seronegative symmetric synovitis
      with pitting edema, 1243
  renal transplantation, 792
  retroperitoneal fibrosis, 2250

Corticosteroids—cont'd
rheumatic fever, 1257
rheumatoid arthritis, 1207-1208
rhinitis, 1182-1183
sarcoidosis, 459
systemic lupus erythematosus, 1216-1217
Takayasu's arteritis, 311
temporal arteritis, 959
tendinitis, 1198
thrombotic thrombocytopenic purpura, 615
tropical spastic paraparesis, 1533
tuberculous meningitis, 1412
tuberculous pericarditis, 1637
typhoid fever, 1601
typhus fever, 1546
typical medical regimen six months after
transplantation, 343
ulcerative colitis, 2074
Wegener's granulomatosis, 468, 1223
Corticotroph cell, 1773, 1774
Corticotropin-releasing factor, 1774
Corticotropin-releasing hormone, 1735
Cortisol
Addison's disease, 1824
congenital adrenal hyperplasia, 1825
Cushing's syndrome, 1820-1821
feedback inhibition tests, 1736
glucose production, 1874, 1875
hypercortisolism, 1820
hypoglycemia, 1877
integrated fuel homeostasis, 1853
plasma, 1740
secretion, 1818
urinary free, 1741
Cortisol-binding globulin, 1835
Cortisone
conversion from cortisol, 1819
rheumatoid arthritis, 1207
Cortrosyn stimulation test, 1774
Corynebacterium, 1565-1567
antibiotic selection, 1347
erythrasma, 1422
normal flora, 1368
Cosmid, 52
Cost-benefit analysis, 15
Cost-effectiveness analysis, 15-16
Cost-identification analysis, 16
Cost-utility analysis, 16
Costal chondritis, 410
Costoclavicular maneuver, 306
Costs and outcomes, 14-16
ethics and, 13
heart failure, 157, 158
Cosyntropin
aldosterone excess, 1823
congenital adrenal hyperplasia, 1825
Cotrimoxazole
interference with oral anticoagulants, 636
Pneumocystis carinii pneumonia, 519
Cotton wool patches, 2302
Cotton-wool spots, Plate XI-4
acquired immunodeficiency syndrome patient,
2305
retinal vein occlusion, Plate XI-9
Cough, 404-408, 409
acute lung allograft rejection, 521
acute pharyngitis, 1393
Ascaris lumbricoides, 1698
asthma, 1187
blastomycosis, 1657
bronchiectasis, 484
bronchiolitis obliterans syndrome, 522
chronic bronchitis, 437
common cold, 1391
croup, 1393
dilated cardiomyopathy, 263
drug-induced, 476, 477
hypersensitivity pneumonitis, 461
idiopathic pulmonary fibrosis, 453
influenza, 1490
interstitial lung disease, 450

Cough—cont'd
irritant receptors, 353
Langerhans' cell granulomatosis, 464
Lassa fever, 1510
lung cancer, 488
lymphomatoid granulomatosis, 470
malignant mesothelioma, 510
mediastinal abnormality, 511
Mycoplasma pneumoniae pneumonia, 1539
pertussis, 1611-1613
pleural disease, 505
Pneumocystis carinii pneumonia, 1694
secretion clearance and lung expansion, 429
sinusitis, 2308
systemic lupus erythematosus, 1215
tuberculosis, 1628
tularemia, 1608
typhoid fever, 1601
Wegener's granulomatosis, 468, 1222
Cough suppressants, 408
Cough syncope, 408, 953
Cough-variant asthma, 407
Coumadin
drug-nutrient interactions, 2110
hepatic injury, 2192
restenosis, 124
Coumarin
primary pulmonary hypertension, 295
vitamin K deficiency, 626
Coumarin derivatives, 295
Councilman's body, 2180
Counseling
genetic disorders, 1730-1731
heart failure, 167
human immunodeficiency virus diagnosis,
1472
medical interview, 2, 3
periodic health examination, 2254
Counterimmunoelectrophoresis, 1408
Coupling of bone formation to bone resorption,
1716
Courvoisier gallbladder, 2156
Courvoisier law, 2242
Cowden's syndrome, 1319
Cow's milk
Campylobacter jejuni infection, 1591
food allergy insomnia, 944
intolerance, 1993, 2068
Cox proportional hazards regression, 2142
Coxiella burnetti, 1543
Coxsackievirus
acute hemorrhagic conjunctivitis, 1490
compromised host, 1388
hand-foot-mouth syndrome, 1489
herpangina, 1488
myopericarditis, 1489-1490
pathogenesis, 1486
pericarditis, 272
pharyngitis, 1393
pleural effusion, 507
poliomyelitis, 1488
Cozaar; *see* Losartan
CPAP; *see* Continuous positive airway pressure
CPPD; *see* Calcium pyrophosphate dihydrate
deposition disease
Crack cocaine, 2297
Crackles
evaluation of respiratory disease, 402
interstitial lung disease, 450
Langerhans' cell granulomatosis, 464
pulmonary thromboembolism, 501
Cranial arteritis, 311
Cranial nerve palsy, 1017
Cranial nerves
diabetes mellitus, 1871
effects of pituitary tumor, 1781-1782
neurologic examination, 902
obstructive apnea, 355
Cranial neuralgia, 958
Cranial neuropathy, 1072
Craniotomy, 1069

Creatine kinase
evaluation of muscle disease, 1025
hypothyroidism, 1809
inflammatory myopathies, 1235
myocardial infarction, 211-212
Creatine phosphokinase, 1755
Creatinine, 746
hepatorenal syndrome, 2168
measurement of hormone concentration in
urine, 1733
prerenal azotemia, 770
serum, 746
adult respiratory distress syndrome, 421
crescentic glomerulonephritis, 848
heart failure, 166
increased during angiotensin-converting
enzyme inhibitor therapy, 896
multiple myeloma, 701
thrombotic thrombocytopenic purpura, 858
toxicity of nonsteroidal antiinflammatory
drugs, 870
uremic syndrome, 776
syndrome of inappropriate antidiuretic
hormone, 489
Creatinine clearance, 746-747, 2286
Creatinine height index, 2111
Creatinine index, 746
Cremasteric reflex, 964
Creola body
asthma, 1185
sputum examination, 380
Crepitus
gas gangrene, 1423
systemic sclerosis, 1229
Crescentic glomerulonephritis, 846-849
Crescents
glomerular disease, 764
glomerulonephritis, 842
CREST syndrome, 1228, 1293
Cretinism, 1809
Creutzfeldt-Jakob disease
dementia, 987-988
electroencephalography, 907
transfusion-transmitted, 575, 576
CRF; *see* Corticotropin-releasing factor
Cricoid achalasia syndrome, 2021
Cricopharyngeal spasm, 2015
Crigler-Najjar syndromes, 2151-2152, 2153
Critical care medicine; *see also* Pulmonary
disease
acute respiratory failure, 412-420
adult respiratory distress syndrome with,
418
artificial airway, 416-417
chronic obstructive pulmonary disease with,
417-418, 446
classification, 413, 414
diagnosis, 413-414
mechanical ventilation, 397, 416, 418-420
oxygenation measures, 415-416
pathophysiology, 412-413
principles of management, 414, 415
respiratory acidosis, 416
without lung disease, 418
breathing control abnormalities, 352-357
chest pain, 408-410
cough, 404-408, 409
dyspnea, 404, 405
expectoration, 408
hemoptysis, 410-411
intensive care monitoring, 390-396
end-tidal carbon dioxide, 396
peripheral artery catheterization, 390
pulmonary artery catheterization, 390-395
pulse oximetry, 396
transcutaneous oxygen and carbon dioxide,
396
laboratory and diagnostic tests
imaging methods, 386-390
invasive, 380-386
pulmonary function tests, 375-380

Critical care medicine—cont'd
 lung injury and repair, 370-375
 medical history, 401-402
 multiple organ dysfunction syndrome, 421-423
 physical examination, 402-404
 pulmonary blood flow, 360-364
 pulmonary edema, 423-428
  acute toxic, 473
  adult respiratory distress syndrome, 421
  drug-induced, 477
  hemoptysis, 410
  pneumothorax, 510
  pulmonary artery wedge pressure, 395
 pulmonary rehabilitation, 432-437
 respiratory muscle failure, 357-360
 respiratory pathophysiology, 346-352
  nonrespiratory functions of lung, 346-347
  oxygen transport disorders, 350-352
  respiratory function, 347-350
 respiratory therapy, 428-432
 respiratory tract host defense mechanisms,
  364-369
 wheezing, 404, 405
Critical-illness polyneuropathy, 1085, 1097
Critical micellar concentration, 2124
Critical pathway, 20-22, 28
Crixivan; *see* Indinavir
Crohn's disease, 1996, 2069-2072
 Campylobacter jejuni infection *versus,* 1591
 chronic diarrhea, 2051
 clinical features, 2069
 colonic carcinoma, 2076
 cutaneous findings, 1321
 delay in secondary sexual development,
  1768
 diagnosis, 2070-2071
 endoscopic photographs, Plate X-6
 fever of unknown origin, 1378
 fissured ulcer, Plate X-4
 granulomatous gastritis, 2043
 heteropathic arthropathy, 1245-1246
 hypogammaglobulinemia, 2066
 impotence, 1763
 laboratory findings, 2069-2070
 management, 2071-2072
 oral aphthous ulcer, Plate X-10
 perianal fistula, 2093
 perianal manifestations, Plate X-5
 pregnancy and, 2278
 risk of gallstone formation, 2224
 short bowel syndrome, 2066
 small bowel adenocarcinoma, 2081
 ulcerative colitis *versus,* 2075
Cromolyn sodium
 asthma, 1191, 1192
 during pregnancy, 2277
 rhinitis, 1182
Cross-bridge, 39
Cross-reactive immunologic material, 1925
Cross-reactive immunologic material negative
  mutation, 1925
Cross-reactive immunologic material positive
  mutation, 1925
Cross-reactivity, 1146
Crossed aphasia, 976-977
Crossmatching, 573
Croup, 1393-1394
Crude coal tar, 1301-1302
Crust
 bullous impetigo, 1419
 chickenpox, 1525
 ecthyma, 1420
 genital lesions, 1442
 impetigo, 1419
Cryocrit, 1250
Cryoglobulinemia, 1222, 1248-1250
Cryoglobulins, 705-706, 1222, 1248
 hepatitis C virus, 1138
 mixed essential cryoglobulinemia, 857
 presence of immune complex, 1149

Cryoprecipitate
 afibrinogenemia, 625
 hemophilia A, 621
 hemostatic defects in liver disease, 627
 platelet disorder, 613
 von Willebrand's disease, 624
Cryotherapy
 hemorrhoids, 2093
 squamous cell carcinoma, 1298
Crypt abscess in ulcerative colitis, 2072, 2073,
  Plate X-5
Cryptococcus, 1667-1670
 acquired immunodeficiency syndrome, 1329
 after heart transplantation, 1090
 Blastomyces dermatidis versus, 1657
 compromised host, 1388
 India ink preparation, Plate VIII-50
 meningitis, 1404
  acquired immunodeficiency syndrome, 1477
  fundoscopic view, Plate VIII-51
 normal flora, 1368
 peritonitis, 2248
 serodiagnosis, 1653
Cryptorchidism, 720
Cryptosporidium, 1679-1680
 acquired immunodeficiency syndrome, 1474,
  1476, 2095, 2097
 cholangitis, 2202
 compromised host, 1388
 diarrhea, 1428
 Kinyoun stain, Plate VIII-32
 oocyst, Plate VIII-33
 T-cell deficiencies, 1993
Crystal deposition disease, 1276
Crystal nucleation, 797
Crystalline cholesterol monohydrate, 2220
Crystalline zinc, 1859
Crystallization of uric acid, 1271
Crystalluria, 866
Crystals
 arthritis associated calcium-containing crystals,
  1276-1280
 synovial fluid, 1162
 urinalysis, 745-746
Crytococcemia, 1668
CT; *see* Computed tomography
CTLA-4 antigen, 1145
Cubital tunnel syndrome, 915-916
Cullen's sign, 2234
Culture
 acute maxillary sinusitis, 1394-1395
 acute meningitis, 1408
 anaerobic bacteria, 1619
 bacteremia, 1450
 Bordetella pertussis, 1612
 Borrelia burgdorferi, 1647
 brucellosis, 1606
 Campylobacter, 1591-1592
 Candida, 1661
 Clostridium difficile, 1569
 Coccidioides immitis, 1657
 cytomegalovirus, 1528
 diarrhea, 1431
 fever and rash, 1385
 fever of unknown origin, 1379
 fungal infection, 1652
 gonococcal infection, 1584
 Haemophilus influenzae, 1588
 Helicobacter pylori, 2003
 impetigo, 1419
 infective endocarditis, 228
 Legionella pneumophila, 1623
 liver abscess, 2209
 meningitis, 1406
 Mycobacterium tuberculosis, 1628
 Neisseria gonorrhoeae, 1439
 Neisseria meningitidis, 1580
 osteomyelitis, 1434
 poststreptococcal glomerulonephritis, 844
 splenic abscess, 1398-1399
 staphylococcal, 1548

Culture—cont'd
 tissue, 1369
 urinary tract infection, 762
 Vibrio cholerae, 1595
Culture-negative neurocytic ascites, 2164
Curability of cancer, 551-552
Curettage and electrodesiccation
 basal cell carcinoma, 1297
 squamous cell carcinoma, 1298
Curschmann's spirals, 380, 1185
Cushing disease, 1786-1787
Cushing response, 934
Cushing syndrome, 1819-1822
 amenorrhea, 1759
 arthropathy, 1247
 cutaneous manifestations, 1323
 dexamethasone suppression test, 1737
 endocrine paraneoplastic syndromes, 583
 general appearance, 63
 hypertension, 321-322
 hypokalemia, 829
 insulin resistance, 1862
 mediastinal mass, 513
 medullary thyroid carcinoma, 1816
 obesity, 2103
 plasma cortisol levels, 1740
 screening tests, 1826
 weakness, 1754
Cutaneous anergy, 1150-1151
Cutaneous candidiasis, 1310-1311, 1312
Cutaneous diphtheria, 1566
Cutaneous disorders, 1290-1332
 acne vulgaris, 1304-1306
 allergic granulomatosis, 1220
 anaphylaxis, 1193
 biopsy, 1298
 blastomycosis, Plate VIII-48
 bullous diseases, 1293-1297
 connective tissue disease, 1290-1293
 coumarin-induced necrosis, 636
 cutaneous anergy, 1150-1151
 cutis laxa, 1289
 dermatitis, 1302-1304
  herpetiformis, 1296-1297
  Pityrosporum, 1309-1310
 drug reactions, 1312-1316
 Ehlers-Danlos syndrome, 1287-1288
 endocrine disorders, 1322-1324
 eosinophilic fasciitis, 1233
 febrile compromised patient, 1388
 gastrointestinal disease, 1320-1322
 human immunodeficiency virus, 1325-1329,
  1477
 hypersensitivity vasculitis, 1221
 Kaposi's sarcoma, 1330-1331, Plate VIII-38
 lupus erythematosus, 1290-1292
 malignancy, 1297-1298
  cutaneous T-cell lymphoma, 1331-1332
  immunosuppression-related, 795
  internal, 1316-1320
  melanoma, 1298-1300
 meningococcemia, Plate VIII-21
 mycosis fungoides, 1331-1332
 photodermatoses, 1306-1307
 Pseudomonas aeruginosa, Plate VIII-23
 pseudoxanthoma elasticum, 1289
 psoriasis, 1300-1302
 sarcoidosis, 458, 1324-1325
 Sézary's syndrome, 1331-1332
 Sjögren syndrome, 1210
 sodium loss through, 823
 spinal cord injury, 1051
 sporotrichosis, Plate VIII-24
 superficial fungal infections, 1307-1312
  candidiasis, 1310-1312
  clinical presentation, 1308-1309
  dermatophyte infection, 1307-1308
  diagnostic procedures, 1309
  Pityrosporum infection, 1309-1310
 systemic lupus erythematosus, 1213-1214
Cutaneous larva migrans, 1700, 1702

Cutaneous T-cell lymphoma, 1331-1332
Cutis laxa, 1289, 1320
CVID; *see* Common variable immunodeficiency
Cvostek's sign, 1030
CVP regimen
  gamma heavy-chain disease, 704
  non-Hodgkin's lymphoma, 698-699
Cyanide, 1020
Cyanocobalamin, 649-650, 2105
  absorption test for malabsorption, 2007
  bacterial overgrowth, 2060
  biochemical function, 2105
  cellular metabolism, 647
  chronic gastritis, 2043
  deficiency, 1080, 1101, 2107
    bone marrow, Plate IV-7
    clinical presentation, 647-648
    intestinal disease, 2005
    metabolic myelopathy, 1013
    neurologic aspects, 1103
    thrombocytopenia, 605, 614
  diabetic polyneuropathy, 1871
  intestinal absorption, 1989
  megaloblastic anemia, 646-647, 649
  recommended daily dietary allowances, 2115
  small bowel malabsorption, 2058
Cyanosis
  atrial septal defect, 281
  cardiovascular examination, 63
  common aortopulmonary trunk, 290
  complete transposition of great arteries, 290
  Ebstein's anomaly of tricuspid valve, 290
  gram-negative bacteremia, 1449
  hepatopulmonary syndrome, 2170
  interstitial lung disease, 451
  mitral stenosis, 245
  patent ductus arteriosus, 285
  Pompe's disease, 1881
  Raynaud's phenomenon, 1226
  reflex sympathetic dystrophy, 310-311
  tetralogy of Fallot, 289
  total anomalous pulmonary venous connection, 291
  tricuspid atresia, 291
  venous thromboembolism, 631
Cyclic adenosine monophosphate, 57
  activation of adenyl cyclase, 1711
  alimentary tract motor function, 1976
  bile water production, 2123
  bone and mineral disorders, 1746
  cellular modulation of contractility, 41
  cystic fibrosis transmembrane conductance regulator, 480
  diarrhea, 2050
  fibrocystic breast changes, 1847
  glycogen storage diseases, 1880-1881
  histamine receptors on parietal cells, 1981
  hormone action, 1711
  nephrogenic diabetes insipidus, 883
  pancreatic acinar cell secretions, 2132
  parathyroid hormone mediator, 1718
  pepsinogen secretion, 1984, 1985
  thyroid hormone formation, 1798
Cyclic edema, 821
Cyclic guanosine monophosphate, 1712
  alimentary tract motor function, 1976
  ischemic heart disease, 201
Cyclic guanosine triphosphate, 1712
Cyclizine hydrochloride, 2027
Cyclobenzaprine, 2300
Cyclogenil, 2191
Cyclooxygenase
  aspirin-induced platelet release defect, 611
  nonsteroidal antiinflammatory drugs and, 1258-1259
Cyclopentanoperhydrophenanthrene nucleus, 1708, 1817
Cyclophosphamide
  acute interstitial nephritis, 889
  amyloidosis, 1283
  aplastic anemia, 674

Cyclophosphamide—cont'd
  breast cancer, 709, 710
  cardiotoxicity, 584
  Churg-Strauss syndrome, 467
  crescentic glomerulonephritis, 848
  dilated cardiomyopathy, 265
  effect on vasopressin release, 1791
  effects on kidney, 869
  focal glomerular sclerosis, 852
  Goodpasture's syndrome, 847
  graft-*versus*-host disease, 578
  hepatic injury, 2192
  hepatic toxicity, 585
  interstitial lung disease, 451
  lupus nephritis, 857
  microscopic polyarteritis nodosa, 1221
  minimal change disease, 851
  multiple myeloma, 702
  nephrotoxicity, 584
  non-Hodgkin's lymphoma, 698-699
  pulmonary parenchymal reactions, 476
  pulmonary toxicity, 478
  rheumatic disease, 1260, 1262
  toxicity, 579
  Wegener's granulomatosis, 468, 858
Cycloserine, 1343
  mycobacterial disease, 1631
  nocardiosis, 1666
Cyclospora, 1428-1429, 1680
Cyclosporin
  aplastic anemia, 675
  asthma, 1191
  cardiac transplantation, 1090
  Crohn's disease, 2072
  effects on kidney, 870
  graft-*versus*-host disease, 578
  human cytochrome P450 isoforms, 2312
  lung transplantation, 516
  nephrotoxicity, 891
  paraneoplastic pemphigus, 1295
  prevention and therapy of rejection, 340
  psoriasis, 1302
  renal transplantation, 793
  rheumatic disease, 1260, 1262
  typical medical regimen six months after transplantation, 343
  ulcerative colitis, 2074
Cylindrical bronchiectasis, 483
CYP2E1
  alcoholic hepatitis, 2198
  enzyme system, 2195, 2198
  nonalcoholic steatohepatitis, 2197
Cyproheptadine, 1786
Cyproterone, 1757
Cyst
  Baker's, 1203
  benign neck, 2310
  branchial cleft, 2310
  bronchogenic, 513
  choledochal, 2212, 2233
  echinococcal, 2211-2212
  Entamoeba histolytica, 1681, 2210, Plate VIII-52
  formation in arthritis, 1168, 1169
  Giardia lamblia, 1684, Plate VIII-53
  hepatic, 2210-2212
  mediastinal mass, 513
  mesenteric, 2251
  ovarian, 1837
    amenorrhea, 1759
    cancer *versus,* 716
    gonadotropic pulsations, 1836
    hirsutism, 1756
    insulin resistance, 1862
    21-hydroxylase deficiency, 1824
  pericardial, 273
  Pneumocystis carinii, 1693, Plate VII-10
  renal, 871-876
    acquired, 874-875
    dialysis complication, 788
    tubulointerstitial abnormalities, 892

Cyst—cont'd
  renal cell carcinoma, 898
  von Hippel-Lindau syndrome, 1923
Cystathionine, 1904
Cystathioninuria, 1909
Cystatin C, 1285
Cysteamine, 1910
Cysteine, 1904
Cystic bronchiectasis, 483-484
Cystic fibrosis, 479-483
  autosomal recessive inheritance pattern, 1725
  double lung allograft, 515
  nasal polyps, 2308
  pancreatic involvement, 2246
  sinopulmonary-infertility syndrome, 1845
Cystic fibrosis transmembrane conductance regulator, 480, 2123
Cystic fibrosis transmembrane regulator gene, 2246
Cystic medial necrosis, 1730
  aortic disease, 299
  fibrillin, 1289
  mitral regurgitation, 249
  mitral valve prolapse, 253
  during pregnancy, 2276
  tall stature, 1769
Cystic parathyroid adenomatosis, 1965
Cysticercosis, 1696, 1704-1705
Cystine
  cystinuria, 1910
  related diseases, 1904
Cystine stone, 799-800, 804-805
Cystinosis, 1919
  amino acid storage disorder, 1909-1910
  Fanconi's syndrome, 881
Cystinuria, 799-800, 1910
  management, 804
Cystitis, 1261, 1455
Cystometrogram, 938
Cystoscopy
  hematuria, 757
  interstitial cystitis, 763
  upper urinary tract tumor, 899
Cytapheresis, 574
Cytarabine, 699
Cytochrome P450
  alcohol metabolism, 2195
  biotransformation, 2185
  drug interactions, 2311-2312
  hepatic clearance of antiarrhythmic drugs, 136-137
  inhibition by cimetidine, 135-136
  quantitative liver function tests, 2143-2144
Cytogenetics
  aplastic anemia, 672
  cancer of unknown primary site, 731
  stem cell transplantation, 578
Cytokeratin, 731
Cytokines, 1110, 1128-1132
  activation of alveolar epithelial cells, 371
  anemia of chronic disease, 642-643
  asthma, 1186
  bacterial meningitis, 1405
  calcium homeostasis, 1720
  cancer treatment, 555
  cholangiocyte susceptibility, 2199
  as endogenous pyrogens, 1375
  heart failure, 161
  as hematopoietic growth factors, 532
  inflammatory response, 1448
  interstitial lung disease, 449, 450
  lung injury, 370, 372
  macrophage secretion, 368
  mast cell, 1142
  measurement, 1153
  multiple organ dysfunction syndrome, 421
  natural immunity and inflammation, 1129-1130
  regulation of hematopoiesis, 1128
  regulation of lymphoid growth and differentiation, 1130-1131
  release during hemodialysis, 790

Cytokines—cont'd
　respiratory defense, 366
　rheumatoid arthritis, 1202
　sarcoidosis, 457
　signal transduction, 1131-1132
　tubulointerstitial renal disease, 889
Cytology
　Barrett's esophagus, 2018
　Chlamydia trachomatis, 1536
　gastric biopsy, 2002
　gastric carcinoma, 2046
　pericardial effusion, 274
　synovial fluid, 1162, 1163
　upper urinary tract tumor, 899
Cytolytic therapy, 523
Cytomegalovirus, 1527-1529
　acquired immunodeficiency syndrome, 1328,
　　　2096
　acute hepatitis, 2138
　acute interstitial nephritis, 890
　after cardiac transplantation, 341-342
　after liver transplantation, 2219
　after lung transplantation, 518-519
　after stem cell transplantation, 579
　blindness, 1478
　cholangitis, 2202
　compromised host, 1388
　culture, 1369
　diarrhea, 1476
　esophageal infection, 2019-2020
　fever, 1475
　fever of unknown origin, 1377
　human immunodeficiency virus-associated
　　　dementia, 987
　immunocompromised patient, 1387
　odynophagia, 1998
　pneumonitis, Plate VIII-37
　during pregnancy, 2280
　renal transplantation, 785, 795
　retinitis, 2305
　retinochoroiditis, Plate VIII-41
　transfusion-associated, 575-576
Cytomegalovirus retinitis, Plate XI-11
Cytopenia
　hairy cell leukemia, 683
　splenectomy, 602
Cytoplasmic anti-neutrophil cytoplasmic
　　　antibodies
　vasculitis, 1218
　Wegener's granulomatosis, 1223
Cytoplasmic granule, 1339
Cytoplasmic membrane
　bacterial, 1344
　Streptococcus pyogenes, 1555
Cytoplasmic receptors, 1712-1713
Cytosine, 50
Cytosine arabinoside
　acute myelogenous leukemia, 690
　myelodysplastic syndrome, 676
　pulmonary toxicity, 478
Cytoskeletal antibody, 1158
Cytoskeletal proteins, 59-60
Cytosolic dihydrodiol dehydrogenase, 2126
Cytotoxic agents, 1844
　antiphospholipid syndrome, 1292
　breast cancer, 710
　crescentic glomerulonephritis, 848
　focal glomerular sclerosis, 852
　lupus nephritis, 857
　rheumatoid arthritis, 1209
Cytotoxic cerebral edema, 1405
Cytotoxic hepatotoxins, 2185-2186, 2187
Cytotoxic T-cell, 1114
　assay, 1152
　cell-mediated immunity, 1132

D

D cell, 1981, 1982
D-dimer
　unstable angina, 195
　venous thromboembolism, 632

D segment, 1111
D-xylose absorption, 2058
D-xylose excretion test, 2059
D4T; *see* Stavudine
Da Costa's syndrome, 131
Dacarbazine
　hepatic injury, 2192
　Hodgkin's disease, 694-695
Dacron graft, 300
Dactylitis, 1241
DAD; *see* Delayed afterdepolarization
DAG; *see* Diacylglycerol
Daily caloric requirements, 2112
Daily metabolic requirements, 2113
Damage theories of aging, 2283
Danaparoid sodium, 635
Danazol
　benign pubertal gynecomastia, 1772
　fibrocystic breast disease, 1849-1850
　hepatic injury, 2191
　hereditary angioedema, 1180
　immune hemolytic anemia, 669
　immune thrombocytopenic purpura, 617
　interaction with cyclosporin, 793
Dander, 1183
Dantrolene
　hepatic injury, 2191
　spasticity, 997
　spinal cord injury, 1051
Dapsone
　cutaneous lesions in lupus erythematosus,
　　　1292
　dermatitis herpetiformis, 1297
　leprosy, 1651
　Pneumocystis carinii pneumonia, 1473, 1474,
　　　1694, 1695
　prophylaxis in lung transplantation, 518
　relapsing polychondritis, 1243
Dark-field microscopy
　leptospirosis, 1645
　relapsing fever, 1645
　syphilis, 1642
　Treponema pallidum, Plate VIII-2
Data gathering
　injury control, 2267
　medical interview, 2, 3
Daunorubicin
　acute myelogenous leukemia, 690
　dilated cardiomyopathy, 265
Dawn phenomenon, 1861
Daytime bloaters, 2017
DDAVP; *see* Desmopressin
DDC; *see* Zalcitabine
DDD pacemaker, 139
DDI; *see* Didanosine
de Musset's sign, 241
Dead space, 348
Dead space volume, 348
Deafness, 2307-2308
　Alport's syndrome, 876
　central nervous system disease, 974
　elderly, 2287
　Lassa fever, 1510
　mumps complication, 1496
　neonatal cytomegalovirus, 1528
　otitis media, 1395
DeBakey classication of aortic dissection, 301
Debrancher enzyme deficiency, 1882
Debridement
　clostridial infection, 1576
　gas gangrene, 1423-1424
　necrotizing fasciitis, 1422
　osteomyelitis, 1435
　synergistic nonclostridial anaerobic
　　　myonecrosis, 1424
Debrisoquine, 486
Decay-accelerating factor, 1135, 1180
Decerebrate rigidity, 2160
Decision making
　patient capacity, 11-12
　threshold model, 9

Decongestants
　chronic rhinitis, 2308
　rhinitis, 1182
　sinusitis, 2309
　stimulant-dependent sleep disorder, 945
Deconjugation, 2125
Decortication, 296
Decubitus ulcer
　after stroke, 1007, 1054
　elderly, 22887
　spinal cord injury, 1051
Deep tendon reflexes
　hepatic encephalopathy, 2160
　hypermagnesemia, 1943
　spinal cord injury, 1051
Deep venous thrombosis, 311
　critical pathway, 21
　diagnosis, 502
　paraneoplastic dermatoses, 1317
　during pregnancy, 2276
　pulmonary embolism, 631
　risk factors for postoperative, 2261-2262
　spinal cord injury, 1049
　superficial thrombophlebitis, 638
Deerfly, 1701
Deerfly fever, 1607-1609
Defecation, 1980
Defecation syncope, 953
Defecography, 2055
Defeminization, 1755
Defense mechanisms, 1336-1343
　bacterial meningitis, 1404-1406
　candidiasis, 1661
　choice of antibiotics, 1351
　complement system, 1338-1339
　febrile neutropenic patient, 1389-1390
　gram-negative bacteremia, 1446-1447
　humoral immunity, 1336-1337
　patterns of infection in impaired patient, 1335
　phagocytic cells, 1339-1343
　respiratory tract, 364-369
　spleen, 1337-1338
　urinary tract infection, 1456
Deferoxamine
　iron overload, 646
　removal of aluminum from bone, 1964-1965
Defibrillation
　sudden cardiac death survivors, 190
　ventricular fibrillation, 153
Defined-formula diet, 2115-2117
Degeneration
　acquired hepatocerebral, 1102
　infective endocarditis, 225, 226
　joint disease, 1264-1268
　nucleus pulposus, 1169-1170
　peripheral vascular disease, 305
　polyarthritis, 1199
Deglutition, 1999-2000
Degos disease, 1320, 1321
Degranulation, 1340
Dehydration
　cholera, 1595
　dementia, 987
　diabetes insipidus, 1795
　diabetic ketoacidosis, 1863
　hematocrit, 824
　lactic acidosis, 1867
　nephrogenic diabetes insipidus, 883
　primary hyperparathyroidism, 1967
　red blood cell mass, 586
　VIPoma, 2245
7-Dehydrocholesterol, 1719
Dehydroemetine, 1683
Dehydroepiandrosterone
　biosynthesis, 1817
　migraine, 961-962
　plasma, 1741
　puberty, 1766
Dehydroepiandrosterone sulfate, 1741, 1766
5'-Deiodinase, 1802
Deiodination, 1799
Delavirdine, 1474

Delayed afterdepolarization, 132
Delayed allograft function, 793-794
Delayed gastric emptying, 1979
  anorexia nervosa, 2030
  diagnosis, 2003-2004
Delayed puberty, 1842
  hypogonadism, 1843
  treatment, 1844, 1845
Delayed response, occupational asthma, 471
Delayed sleep phase syndrome, 945
Delayed-type hypersensitivity, 1127
  allergic contact dermatitis, 1303
  cell-mediated immunity, 1132
  drug eruption, 1313
  in vivo assessment of cell-mediated immunity,
      1150-1151
Delirium, 1031
  bacterial meningitis, 1406
  bubonic plague, 1610
  disordered thinking, 1041
  gas gangrene, 1423
  megaloblastic anemia, 648
Delirium tremens, 985, 1080, 2295
Delta agent, 2176
Delta-amino-levulinic acid synthase, 1923
Delta fraction, 2142
Delta hepatitis, 2277
Delta sleep, 939
Delta wave, 90
Demecarium bromide, 2302
Demeclocycline
  iliac crest biopsy, 1747
  isovolemic hypotonic hyponatremia, 813
Dementia
  cognitive failure, 985-989
  dialysis, 908, 1105-1106
  disordered sleep, 946-947
  elderly, 2288-2289
  electroencephalography, 907, 910
  human immunodeficiency virus, 1478
  megaloblastic anemia, 648
  psychologic testing, 904
  Wernicke's encephalopathy, 1100-1102
dementia, 987
Demethylchlortetracycline, 1747
Demineralization, 1966
Demyelinating diseases, 1007-1011
  acute disseminated encephalomyelitis, 1010
  acute hemorrhagic leukoencephalopathy, 1010
  multiple sclerosis, 1007-1009
  progressive multifocal leukoencephalopathy,
      1010
  transverse myelitis, 1010
Demyelinating neuropathy, 1018
Demyelination
  motor conduction velocities, 915
  vitamin B_{12} deficiency, 648
Dendritic cell, 596
  cell-mediated immunity, 1128
  eosinophilic granuloma, 463
  self-tolerance and autoimmunity, 1146
Denervation, transplanted heart, 342
Dengue, 1465, 1515, 1516, 1517
Denial, maladaptive illness behavior, 1040
Dense granule, 536
Dense tubular system, 536
Densensitization, 1183
Densitometry, 1947
Dental procedures, infective endocarditis, 227,
      233
Dental sepsis, 1414
Dentinogenesis imperfecta, 1287
Dentition
  hypophosphatasia, 1954
  rickets, 1949
Deoxycholic acids, 2125
2-Deoxycoformycin, 684
11-Deoxycorticosteroid, 1741
Deoxypyridinium crosslinks, 1745
Deoxypyridinoline, 1745
Deoxyribonucleases, group A streptococci, 1555

Deoxyribonucleic acid, 49-50
  antibodies to, 1158-1159
  assay, 1472
  bacterial synthesis and replication, 1344
  cardiac growth and hypertrophy, 55-56, 57
  cloning, 52-53, 559
  electrophoresis, 51-52
  fluorescence in situ hybridization, 561, 562
  functions of minerals, 2109
  gene expression and regulation, 50-51
  gene transfer, 55
  human immunodeficiency virus infection, 1470
  hybridization, 52, 1841, Plate IX-1
  hypomethylation, 548
  inherent properties fundamental to
      recombinant techniques, 51
  isolation and digestion, 51
  mismatch repair system, 549
  nucleic acid-based tests, 1372-1373
  physical basis for inheritance, 1721
  polymerase chain reaction, 55, 56, 561
  radiation damage, 553
  restriction fragment length polymorphism,
      54-55
  ribonucleic acid analysis, 53-54
  sequencing, 54
  somatic mutation of aging, 2283
  Southern, Northern, Western, and
      Southwestern blotting, 52
  Southern blot analysis, 52, 560-561
Deoxyribonucleic acid-dependent ribonucleic
      acid polymerase, 1344
Deoxyribonucleic acid libraries, 54
Deoxyribonucleic acid ligase, 52
Deoxyribonucleic acid markers, 60-61
Deoxyribonucleic acid probe
  Chlamydia trachomatis, 1536
  hemophilia, 619
  Southern blot analysis, 52, 560
Deoxyribonucleic acid restriction enzyme, 54
Deoxyribonucleic acid virus
  adenovirus, 1503-1504
  hepatitis B virus, 2174
  herpesvirus, 1522-1530
    characteristics, 1522-1523
    cytomegalovirus, 1527-1529
    Epstein-Barr virus, 1529-1530
    herpes simplex virus, 1523-1525
    human herpesvirus 6, 1530
    human herpesvirus 8, 1530
    varicella zoster virus, 1525-1527
Deoxyribose sugar chain, 49
Depakote; *see* Valproate
Dependence, alcohol, 2294-2296
Depo-Provera, 2270
Depolarization, 82
  atrial, 83-84
  smooth muscle, 1976
  ventricular, 84
Depression, 1035-1038
  after stroke, 1007
  chronic abdominal pain, 2035
  chronic fatigue syndrome, 2299
  chronic heart failure, 169
  cognitive impairment, 2288
  dialysis patient, 787
  disordered thinking, 1041
  dyspnea and, 432, 437
  elderly, 2289
  impotence, 1760-1761
  irritable bowel syndrome, 2055
  menopause, 2270
  neurohormonal regulation, 1077
  pancreatic cancer, 2242
  Parkinson's disease, 992
  systemic lupus erythematosus, 1093
  weight loss, 1749
DeQuervain's tenosynovitis, 1197
DeQuervain's thyroiditis, 1807, 1811-1812
Dermatitis, 1302-1304
  biotin deficiency, 2107
  glucagonoma, 2244

Dermatitis—cont'd
  niacin deficiency, 2107
  Pityrosporum, 1309-1310
  stasis, 312
Dermatitis herpetiformis, 1296-1297, 2063, Plate
      VII-4
Dermatology, 1290-1332; *see also* Skin
  acne vulgaris, 1304-1306
  bullous diseases, 1293-1297
  cutaneous malignancies, 1297-1298
  cutaneous manifestations
    connective tissue disease, 1290-1293
    drug reactions, 1312-1316
    endocrine disorders, 1322-1324
    gastrointestinal disease, 1320-1322
    human immunodeficiency virus, 1325-1329
    internal malignancy, 1316-1320
    sarcoidosis, 1324-1325
  dermatitis, 1302-1304
    biotin deficiency, 2107
    glucagonoma, 2244
    herpetiformis, 1296-1297
    niacin deficiency, 2107
    Pityrosporum, 1309-1310
    stasis, 312
  Kaposi's sarcoma, 1330-1331
  melanoma, 1298-1300
  mycosis fungoides, 1331-1332
  photodermatoses, 1306-1307
  psoriasis, 1300-1302
  Sézary's syndrome, 1331-1332
  superficial fungal infections, 1307-1312
    candidiasis, 1310-1312
    clinical presentation, 1308-1309
    dermatophyte infection, 1307-1308
    diagnostic procedures, 1309
    Pityrosporum infection, 1309-1310
Dermatolysis, 1289
Dermatomyositis, 1200, 1234, 1235, 1292
  Gottron's papules, Plate VII-3
  heart disease, 1087
  neurologic manifestations, 1092
  paraneoplastic dermatoses, 1317, 1318
Dermatomyositis-polymyositis, 453
Dermatopathic lymphadenopathy, 599
Dermatophyte infection, 1307-1308
Dermatophytosis, 1328
Dermatoses, paraneoplastic, 1316-1319
Dermoid
  mediastinal, 513
  neck, 2310
Dermopathy, diabetic, 1873
Des-gamma-carboxyprothrombin, 2213
Descending aorta, 299
Desferrioxamine
  beta-thalassemia, 655-656
  osteomalacia in renal disease, 1953
Designated donation of blood, 573
Desipramine, 1037
  depression in elderly, 2289
  human cytochrome P450 isoforms, 2312
Desmin, 59
Desmogleins, 1293
Desmopressin
  diabetes insipidus, 1796
  hemophilia A, 621
  nephrogenic diabetes insipidus, 883
  structure, 1789
  uremia, 613
  von Willebrand's disease, 624
Desoxycorticosterone escape phenomenon, 738
Desquamation
  scarlet fever, 1421
  toxic shock syndrome, 1421, Plate VIII-20
Desquamative interstitial pneumonia, 449
Detergent worker's lung, 460
Detoxification, 2122, 2142-2143, 2296
Detrusor, 933, 1065, 1066
  hyperactivity with impaired bladder
      contractility, 2291
  hyperreflexia, 935
Detrusor-sphincter dyssynergia, 1050

Devascularization procedures, 2167
Developmental abnormalities, 1766-1773
  biliary tract, 2233
  breast growth abnormalities, 1770
  complete transposition of great arteries, 290
  connective tissue disease, 1286-1290
  constitutional delay of pubertal growth, 1768
  Crohn's disease, 1768
  evaluation of pubertal growth, 1770-1772
  familial tall stature, 1769
  Fanconi's syndrome, 882
  growth hormone deficiency, 1769, 1777
  hypothyroidism, 1768-1769
  idiopathic short stature, 1769
  intestinal lymphangiectasia, 2067
  juvenile nephronophthisis, 875
  Klinefelter's syndrome, 1769
  neurofibromatosis, 1921
  puberty, 1766-1768
  rickets, 881
  tetralogy of Fallot, 289
  therapy, 1772
  Turner's syndrome, 1769
  weight abnormalities, 1769-1770
Developmental arrest, 1757
Dexamethasone
  bacterial meningitis, 1412-1413
  brain abscess, 1416
  chemotherapy-induced nausea and vomiting,
    582
  Cushing's syndrome, 1821
  metastatic cancer, 1073
  multiple myeloma, 702
  for nausea and vomiting, 2027
  non-Hodgkin's lymphoma, 699
  suppression test, 1736-1737
Dexfenfluramine, 261
Dextro-transposition of great arteries, 290
Dextroamphetamine, 943, 1038
Dextrocardia, 91
Dextromethorphan, 408, 409
Dextropropoxyphene
  drug-induced bile duct injury, 2203
  interference with oral anticoagulants, 636
Dextroversion, 291
DHP receptor, 38
Di-isocyanates, 472
Diabetes Control and Complications Trial, 2303
Diabetes insipidus, 883-884, 1793-1795
Diabetes mellitus, 1850-1874
  acute meningitis, 1407
  atrial fibrillation, 146
  cardiovascular involvement, 333-334
    cardiac transplantation, 338
    coronary artery disease in women, 2271
    hypertension, 328
    ischemic heart disease, 200
  chemotactic defects, 1340
  chronic pancreatitis, 2239
  classification, 1853-1856
  complications, 1862-1874
    acute mononeuropathies, 1872
    alcoholic ketosis, 1865
    arthropathy, 1246
    autonomic dysfunction, 936, 1087,
      1872-1873
    chronic renal failure, 781, 786, 859
    dermopathy, 1873
    diabetic ketoacidosis, 1862-1865
    diabetic nephropathy, 859-862
    gallstones, 2223
    hyperosmolar nonketotic coma, 1865-1866
    hypoglycemic coma, 1867
    hyporeninemic hypoaldosteronism, 1824
    impotence, 1760, 1844
    lactic acidosis, 1866-1867
    localized amyloidosis, 1285
    macrovascular disease, 1868-1869
    microalbuminuria, 743
    microvascular disease, 1869-1870
    nephropathy, 1870

Diabetes mellitus—cont'd
  complications—cont'd
    neuromuscular disease, 1872
    neuropathy, 1871-1872
      during pregnancy, 1873-1874, 2272-2273
    retinopathy, 1870-1871, 2303-2304
    stroke, 1001
    weight loss, 1749
  cutaneous manifestations, 1323
  dysbetalipoproteinemia, 1898
  emptying of solid radiopaque markers, 2004
  hyperventilation, 355
  hypoglycemia, 1875
  management, 1856-1862
    antibiotic selection, 1348
    antihypertensive agent choices, 326
    dietary, 1856-1857
    insulin therapy, 1858-1862
    oral hypoglycemic agents, 1857-1858
  nutritional consequences, 2100
  operative risk, 2262
  pancreatic cancer, 2242
  physiology, 1851-1853
  Prader-Labhart-Willi syndrome, 1842
  prevention of coma, 1867-1868
  reflux esophagitis, 2023
  renal transplant recipient, 795
  secondary combined hyperlipidemia, 1896
  secondary hypertriglyceridemia, 1895
  somatostatinoma, 2245
Diabetic amyotrophy, 1017, 1872
Diabetic hyperglycemia, 831
Diabetic ketoacidosis, 1862-1865
  anion gap acidosis, 836
  effects on fetus, 1874
  hypokalemia, 829
  hypomagnesemia, 1941
  hypophosphatemia, 1935-1936, 1938
  ketone bodies, 743
Diabetic macular edema, 2303
Diabetic motor neuropathy, 1017
Diabetic nephropathy, 859-862, 1870
  microalbuminuria, 743, 761
  nephrotic syndrome, 767
Diabetic neuropathy, 1871-1872
Diabetic retinopathy, 1870-1871, 2303-2304
  exudative, Plate IX-3
  hemorrhagic, Plate IX-2
  microvascular abnormalities and venous
    beading, Plate XI-7
  neovascularization of optic nerve, Plate XI-8
  proliferative, Plate IX-4
Diabetic Retinopathy Study, 2303
Diabetic Retinopathy Vitrectomy Study, 2303
Diabetogenic stress of pregnancy, 2272
Diabinese; *see* Chlorpropamide
Diacylglycerol, 57, 542, 1712
Diagnosis-related groups, 27
Diagnostic testing; *see* Laboratory and diagnostic
    testing
Dialysate, 789
Dialysis
  acquired cystic disease, 874
  acute renal failure, 774
  aluminum intoxication, 1961
  bone and joint disease, 785-786
  chronic renal failure, 776, 789-791
  ethylene glycol poisoning, 866
  hemolytic-uremic syndrome, 858
  hyperkalemia, 774, 833
  hyperparathyroid bone disease, 1963
  hypovolemic hypernatremia, 816
  malnutrition, 2100
  operative risk, 2264
  urinary tract obstruction, 887
Dialysis-associated pericarditis, 273, 278
Dialysis dementia, 908, 1105-1106
Dialysis disequilibrium syndrome, 790, 1105
Dialyzer, 789
Diamond-Blackfan syndrome, 674-675
Diaper rash, 1661-1662

Diaphragm
  cardiac auscultation, 68
  contraceptive, 2270
  muscle contracture, 357-358
  paralysis, 359
Diaphragma sella, 1773
Diaphysis, 1716
Diarrhea, 1425-1432, 2050-2055
  acquired immunodeficiency syndrome,
    2095-2098
  acute, 2050-2051
  alpha heavy-chain disease, 704
  autonomic failure, 935
  bacterial agents, 1425-1427
  balantidiasis, 1691
  Campylobacter jejuni, 1591
  candidiasis, 1661
  carcinoid tumor of small bowel, 2082
  celiac disease, 2063
  chemotherapy-induced, 585
  cholera, 1594, 1595
  chronic, 2051-2053, 2054
  Clostridium difficile, 1568-1570
  Clostridium perfringens food poisoning, 1568
  colon cancer, 2085
  colonoscopy, 1996
  common variable immunodeficiency, 1991
  compromised host, 1388
  Crohn's disease, 2069
  cyclosporiasis, 1680
  diabetic, 1749, 1872
  diagnosis, 1430-1431
  Entamoeba histolytica, 1681
  eosinophilic enteritis, 2067
  fecal bile salt loss, 2129
  frequency, 1429-1430
  galactosemia, 1882
  generation of alkalosis, 839
  giant peristaltic contractions, 1979
  Giardia lamblia, 1337, 1684-1685
  hepatic adenoma, 2217
  hepatitis A virus infection, 2173
  human immunodeficiency virus infection,
    1476, 1533
  hyperchloremic metabolic acidosis, 837
  hypogammaglobulinemia, 2066
  infectious, 1101
  irritable bowel syndrome, 2056
  Isospora belli, 1680
  lactase deficiency, 2068
  Lassa fever, 1510
  malabsorption, 2057
  parasitic agents, 1428-1429
  pathogenesis, 2050
  pathophysiology, 1425
  pellagra, 2107
  peritoneal mesenteric and omental diseases,
    2248
  potassium depletion, 827-828
  Rocky Mountain spotted fever, 1543
  rotavirus and Norwalk-like virus, 1519-1522
  Salmonella, 1599
  shigellosis, 1602-1603
  short bowel syndrome, 2066
  sodium depletion, 823
  somatostatinoma, 2245
  thyrotoxicosis, 1805
  traveler's, 1432, 1464
  treatment, 1431-1432
  ulcerative colitis, 2073
  VIPoma, 2245
  viral agents, 1427-1428
  Whipple's disease, 2064
Diastole, 72
  filling sounds, 74
  flow velocities, Plate II-1
Diastolic filling murmur, 78-79, 80
Diastolic function, 43-46
Diastolic heart failure, 167-168, 180
Diastolic murmur, 78-79, 80
Diastolic pressure measurement, 64

Diastolic ventricular interaction, 45
Diazepam
    alcohol withdrawal, 1080, 2295
    delirium tremens, 2295, 2296
    hepatic injury, 2191
    human cytochrome P450 isoforms, 2312
    muscle spasm in tetanus, 1573
    for nausea and vomiting, 2027
    preeclampsia, 2275
    sedation during gastrointestinal endoscopy,
        1994
    spasticity, 997
    spinal cord injury, 1051
    status epilepticus, 982, 983
Diazoxide
    glucose-6-phosphate dehydrogenase
        deficiency, 1881
    hyperinsulinism, 1878
    hypertensive emergency, 328
DIC; *see* Disseminated intravascular coagulation
Dicarboxylic aminoaciduria, 879-880
Dichlorophenoxyacetic acid, 1020
Dichlorphenamide, 2302
Diclofenac, 1259
    hepatic injury, 2191
    human cytochrome P450 isoforms, 2312
    psoriatic arthritis, 1242
Dicloxacillin
    dermatitis-aggravating *Staphylococcus aureus*
        infection, 1303
    dosage, 1350
    hepatic injury, 2191
    infectious eczematoid dermatitis, 1304
    interference with oral anticoagulants, 636
    respiratory exacerbations in cystic fibrosis,
        483
Dicrotic pulse, 65
Didanosine
    acquired immunodeficiency syndrome, 1475
    hepatic injury, 2191
Didronel; *see* Etidronate
Diencephalic epilepsy, 934
Dientamoeba fragilis, 1691
Diet
    acute intermittent porphyria, 1926
    breast cancer, 706
    cancer risk, 550
    celiac disease, 2063
    chronic pancreatitis, 2240
    chronic renal failure, 786
    constipation, 2055
    defined-formula, 2115-2117
    diabetes mellitus, 1856-1857
    diarrhea, 1431
    diverticulosis, 2091
    effects on lipoprotein metabolism, 1889-1890
    endogenous hypertriglyceridemia, 1894-1895
    galactosemia, 1883
    gallstone risk factor, 2223
    gastroesophageal reflux, 2018
    gestational diabetes, 2273
    hemorrhoids, 2093
    hyperkalemia, 774
    hyperoxaluria, 804
    hypertension management, 324
    hyperuricemia, 1275
    hypophosphatemia, 1937
    irritable bowel syndrome, 2056
    kidney stone formation, 798
    lipodystrophy, 1902
    nephrotic syndrome, 765, 767
    obesity, 2103-2104
    phenylketonuria, 1905
    plasma renin activity, 1741
    recurrent stone disease, 803
    renal insufficiency in diabetic patient, 1870
    vitamin K deficiency, 626
Dietary fats, 1986
Dietary fiber, 2055
Dietary hyperlipidemia, 1892
Diethylcarbamazine, 1699, 1700, 1701

Diethylene glycol, 866
Diethylstilbestrol
    breast cancer, 710, 711
    carcinogenesis, 548
    hepatic injury, 2191, 2192
Difficulty initiating and maintaining sleep, 940
Diffuse alveolar damage, 448
Diffuse esophageal spasm, 2022, 2023
Diffuse fasciitis with eosinophilia, 1233-1234
Diffuse idiopathic skeletal hyperostosis, 1168,
        1170, 1246
Diffuse intravascular coagulation, 373
Diffuse osteomyelitis, 1436-1437
Diffuse proliferative lupus nephritis, 856
Diffuse toxic goiter
    antithyroid antibodies, 1801
    autoantibodies, 1155
    during pregnancy, 2273
    thyroid scan, 1802
    thyrotoxicosis, 1804, 1805-1807
    weakness, 1754
Diffusing capacity for carbon monoxide, 348
Diffusion limitation, 413
Diflunisal
    hepatic injury, 2191
    interference with oral anticoagulants, 636
DIG survival trial, 171
DiGeorge syndrome, 1178, 1342, 1931-1932
Digestion, 2056-2057
    gastric secretion, 1981
    pancreatic exocrine secretion, 2133
Digestive enzymes, 2129
Digital angiography, 111
Digital rectal examination, 717
Digital subtraction angiography, 925
Digitalis
    aortic regurgitation, 243
    arrhythmias, 138
    atrial flutter, 146
    dilated cardiomyopathy, 264
    electrocardiographic abnormalities, 90
    heart failure, 172-173
    interaction with calcium channel blockers, 204
    mitral regurgitation, 252
    mitral stenosis, 248
    shock, 182
    toxicity
        accelerated atrioventricular junctional
            rhythm, 144
        accelerated idioventricular rhythm, 149
        hyperkalemia, 831
        hypokalemia, 829
        nonocclusive intestinal infarction, 2087
    tricuspid regurgitation, 256
Digitalis Investigators Group, 171
Diglucuronides, 2147, 2150
Diglycine, 1988
Digoxin
    aortic regurgitation, 243
    arrhythmias, 138
    atrial fibrillation, 147
    before cardiac transplantation, 336
    constrictive pericarditis, 279
    effects of magnesium deficiency, 1942
    heart failure, 170, 173
    interaction with calcium channel blockers, 204
    Wolff-Parkinson-White syndrome, 142
Dihydropteridine reductase deficiency, 1905
Dihydropyridine
    angina, 203
    heart failure, 174
    hypertension, 325
Dihydropyridine receptor, 58
    hypokalemic periodic paralysis, 826
    potassium channel, 59
Dihydrotestosterone, 1742, 1766, 1839
Dihydroxyphenylalanine, 930
Dihydroxyphenylglycol, 930
1,25-Dihydroxyvitamin D, 1710, 1719
    hypercalcemia, 1928
    hypocalcemia, 1934

1,25-Dihydroxyvitamin D—cont'd
    hypoparathyroidism, 1931
    measurement, 1746
    osteomalacia, 1952, 1953, 1954
    osteopetrosis, 1959
    osteoporosis, 1947
    primary hyperparathyroidism, 1968
    rickets, 1954
Diiodohydroxyquin, 2210
Diiodotyrosine, 1710
Dilacor; *see* Diltiazem
Dilantin; *see* Phenytoin
Dilated cardiomyopathy, 263-265
    acquired immunodeficiency syndrome, 333
    cardiac catheterization, 115
    molecular biology, 61-62
    radionuclide angiography, 104
    transplant candidate, 335
Dilemma, 10
Diltiazem
    angina, 203
    arrhythmias, 138
    atrial fibrillation, 147, 223
    hepatic injury, 2192
    human cytochrome P450 isoforms, 2312
    hypertension, 325
    interaction with cyclosporin, 793
    mitral stenosis, 248
    multifocal atrial tachycardia, 144
    non-Q wave myocardial infarction, 218
    primary pulmonary hypertension, 295
    properties, 204
    typical medical regimen six months after
        transplantation, 343
Dimenhydrinate, 2027
Dimethylpropionitrile, 1020
Dimorphic fungi, 1654-1660
Dipetalonema perstans, 1701
Dipetalonema streptocera, 1701
Diphenhydramine
    glucose-6-phosphate dehydrogenase
        deficiency, 664
    for nausea and vomiting, 2027
Diphenylhydantoin
    drug-nutrient interactions, 2110
    inhibition of folate metabolism, 647
    pulmonary parenchymal reactions, 476
2,3-Diphosphoglycerate, 1934
Diphtheria, 1565-1567
    acute interstitial nephritis, 890
    skin signs and risk factors, 1423
    weakness, 1754
Diphtheroids, 1566
Diphyllobothrium latum, 1696-1697
Dipivefrin, 2302
Diploid, 1727
Diplopia, 1062
    hypoglycemic coma, 1867
    ocular Kaposi's sarcoma, 2305
    pituitary apoplexy, 1778
Dipstick test
    acute renal failure, 771
    hematuria, 757
    protein, 567
    proteinuria, 761
Dipyridamole-thallium scintigraphy, 103
    ischemic heart disease, 198-199
    preoperative, 2258
Direct-acting oral vasodilator therapy, 173-174
Direct antiglobulin test, 669
Direct detection techniques, 1370-1373
Direct immunofluorescence, 1371
    pemphigus vulgaris, 1293
    systemic lupus erythematosus, 1213
Direct medical costs, 14
Direct medical outcomes, 18
Directed donation of blood, 573
Directional atherectomy, 117-118
Dirofilaria immitis, 468-469, 1701
Dirofilariasis tenuis, 1701
Disaccharidases, 2068

Disaccharides, 1987
Discoid lupus, 1290-1291
Disease
  Addison's, 1823-1824
    adrenocortical antibodies, 1157
    autoantibodies, 1155
    cutaneous manifestations, 1322-1323
    hypercalcemia, 1928
    hyperkalemia, 831
    hyperpigmentation of gums, Plate VII-14
    infertility and oligospermia, 1846
    lymphocytosis, 593
    weight loss, 1749
  Alzheimer's, 985-987
    dementia, 2288
    electroencephalography, 907, 910
    localized amyloidosis, 1285
  Anderson-Fabry, 878
  Anderson's, 1882, 2067
  Basedow's, 1805-1807
  Bassen-Kornzweig, 1101
  Behçet, 469
    arthropathy, 1243
    genital ulcerations, 1444
    pulmonary vasculitis, 454
  Berger's, 877
  Bornholm, 1489
  Bowen's, 1297
  Brill-Zinsser, 1544
  Buerger's, 308
  Byler's, 2158-2159
  Caroli's, 2233
  Castleman's, 599, 1295, 2252
  Chagas,' 1689-1690
    esophageal achalasia, 2021
    gastrointestinal motility, 1978
    transfusion-transmitted, 575, 576
  Creutzfeldt-Jakob
    dementia, 987-988
    electroencephalography, 907
    transfusion-transmitted, 575, 576
  Crohn's, 1996, 2069-2072
    Campylobacter jejuni infection *versus,* 1591
    chronic diarrhea, 2051
    clinical features, 2069
    colonic carcinoma, 2076
    cutaneous findings, 1321
    delay in secondary sexual development, 1768
    diagnosis, 2070-2071
    endoscopic photographs, Plate X-6
    fever of unknown origin, 1378
    fissured ulcer, Plate X-4
    granulomatous gastritis, 2043
    heteropathic arthropathy, 1245-1246
    hypogammaglobulinemia, 2066
    impotence, 1763
    laboratory findings, 2069-2070
    management, 2071-2072
    oral aphthous ulcer, Plate X-10
    perianal fistula, 2093
    perianal manifestations, Plate X-5
    pregnancy and, 2278
    risk of gallstone formation, 2224
    short bowel syndrome, 2066
    small bowel adenocarcinoma, 2081
    ulcerative colitis *versus,* 2075
  Cushing's, 1786-1787
  Degos, 1320, 1321
  Engelmann's, 1959
  Fabry's, 1918-1919
  Fazio-Londe, 1015
  Gaucher's, 576, 1918
  Gierke's, 1881
  Graves,' 1805-1807
    antithyroid antibodies, 1801
    autoantibodies, 1155
    during pregnancy, 1808, 2273
    thyroid scan, 1802
    thyrotoxic storm, 1807-1808
    thyrotoxicosis, 1804, 1805-1807
    weakness, 1754

Disease—cont'd
  Günther's, 1925
  Hansen's, 1648-1651
  Hartnup, 879, 1910, 1911
  Hirschsprung's, 1980, 2053, 2092
  Hodgkin's, 691-695
    acquired ichthyosis, 1316
    chemotactic defects, 1340
    curability with chemotherapy, 552
    fever of unknown origin, 1377
    infertility, 585
    internal lymphadenopathy, 598
    molecular diagnostics, 563-564
    secondary malignancies, 585-586
    stomach involvement, 2049
    thyroid gland failure, 1809
  Huntington's, 994
  immune function, 1108-1109
  Jolliffe's, 1101
  Kahler's, 700-703
  Kawasaki's, 1225
    anti-neutrophil cytoplasmic antibodies, 1219
    exanthem, 1385
  Kimmelstiel-Wilson's, 1870
  Korsakoff's, 1100-1102
  Krabbe's, 1918
  Legionnaire's, 1623
  Letterer-Siew, 463
  Lyme, 1254, 1646-1648
    fever and rash, 1383
    hoarseness, 2309
    influence of season and geographic setting, 1381
    meningitis, 1409
    transfusion-transmitted, 575
  Marchiafava-Bignami, 1081
  McArdle's, 1025, 1029
  Menetrier's, 2043, 2049
  Ménière's, 972, 2307
  Milroy's, 1420
  Mondor's, 410
  Niemann-Pick, 943, 1918
  Osler-Weber-Rendu, 2014
  Paget's, 1955-1958
    breast, 707
    calcitonin therapy, 1719
    high-output failure, 160
    serum alkaline phosphatase, 1744
    urinary hydroxyproline, 1745
  Parkinson's, 989-992
    depression, 1036
    reflux esophagitis, 2023
    respiratory rhythm abnormalities, 1098
  Parry's, 1805-1807
  Peyronie's, 1761
  Pick's, 987
  Plummer's, 1807
  Pompe's, 1881
  Refsum's, 1754
  Reiter, 1200
  relationship to mood disorders, 1036
  relevance of murine defects, 1145
  role of human leukocyte antigen complex, 1120-1121
  Sandhoff, 1919
  Steinert, 62
  Still's, 1243
  systemic
    causing dementia, 987
    esophageal motility disorders produced by, 2023
    glomerular involvement, 855-859
    hypogonadotropic hypogonadism, 1842
  Tangier, 1897
  Tay-Sachs, 1919
  Thomsen's, 1028
  transfusion-transmitted, 575-576
    babesiosis, 1676
    human immunodeficiency virus transmission, 1471
    malaria, 1672-1673

Disease—cont'd
  triangular model, 1361
  van Buchem's, 1959
  von Hippel-Lindau, 1922-1923
  von Recklinghausen, 2050
  von Willebrand's, 611, 622-624
    factor VIII concentration, 604
    during pregnancy, 2279
  Werdig-Hoffman, 1015
  Whipple
    arthropathy, 1246
    dementia, 987
    enteropathic arthritis *versus,* 1242
    fever of unknown origin, 1378
    malabsorption, 2064-2065
    neurologic aspects, 1101
  Wilson's, 2205-2206
    chronic hepatitis, 2180
    hereditary markers, 2138
    irreversible portosystemic encephalopathy, 1102
    liver transplantation, 2219
    osteoarthritis, 1267
  Wolman, 1898, 1919
Disease-disease interactions, 2285
Disease management, 26
Disease-modifying antirheumatic drugs, 1207, 1208, 1260-1262
Disk-diffusion method, 1346
Disk herniation
  computed tomography, 920
  magnetic resonance imaging, 924
  myelogram, 926
Disopyramide, 137
  hepatic injury, 2192
  hypertrophic obstructive cardiomyopathy, 269
  vasodepressor syncope, 956
Disordered thinking, 1041-1043
Dissection of aorta, 300-302, 303
  aortic regurgitation, 244
  chest pain, 128
  transesophageal echocardiography, 97
Disseminated gonococcal infection, 1583
  fever and rash, 1382
  polyarticular septic arthritis, 1250-1251
  skin lesion, Plate VIII-22
Disseminated intravascular coagulation, 609, 627-628
  acute head injury, 1045
  acute pancreatitis, 2237
  chronic liver disease, 607
  complication of systemic cancer, 1071
  gram-negative bacteremia, 1450
  hemolytic anemia, 666
  liver disease, 627
  meningococcal disease, 1580
  neurologic aspects, 1104
  paraneoplastic dermatoses, 1317
  during pregnancy, 2279
  thrombotic thrombocytopenic purpura, 615
Disseminated tuberculosis, 1634-1635
Dissociated sensory loss, 1012
Dissociation curves, 348
Distal acinar emphysema, 439
Distal glycolytic enzyme deficiency, 1029
Distal interphalangeal joint
  osteoarthritis, 1266
  rheumatoid arthritis, 1202-1203
Distal latency, 914-915
Distal nephron, 741
Distal renal tubular acidosis, 828, 837-838
Disturbances of conduction, 292
Disulfiram, 2296
  hepatic injury, 2192
  human cytochrome P450 isoforms, 2312
  interference with catecholamine assays, 1740
  interference with oral anticoagulants, 636
Dithiothreitol, 1910
Diulo; *see* Metolazone

Diuresis
  osmotic, 824
  postobstructive, 887
  solute, 1793, 1794
Diuretics, 822
  acute tubular necrosis, 773-774
  aortic regurgitation, 243
  ascites, 2165
  cause of renal potassium wasting and
      alkalosis, 828
  chronic hypertension during pregnancy, 2275
  cirrhotic ascites, 822
  cirrhotic patient, 820
  congestive heart failure-associated
      hyponatremia, 818
  constrictive pericarditis, 279
  cystine stones, 804
  diabetes insipidus, 1797
  diabetic nephropathy, 862
  dyspnea, 163
  elderly patient, 327
  generation of alkalosis, 839
  glaucoma, 2302
  heart failure, 169, 170
  hirsutism, 1757
  hypercalcemia, 1929
  hyperkalemia, 832, 833
  hypertension, 324, 325, 326
  hyponatremia, 811
  increased intracranial pressure, 1084
  induction of gynecomastia, 2172
  inhibitor of carbonic anhydrase, 835
  interference with oral anticoagulants, 636
  isovolemic hypotonic hyponatremia, 813
  medication-induced hypercalcemia, 1928
  microvascular disease in diabetic patient, 1870
  mitral regurgitation, 252
  nephrogenic diabetes insipidus, 884
  nephrotic syndrome, 767, 821
  normotensive renal potassium wasting, 828
  potassium depletion, 828
  pulmonary edema, 168-169
  rhabdomyolysis, 775
  sodium balance disorders, 821-823
  stone formation reduction, 803
Diversity gene segment, 1124
Diverticulitis, 2085
Diverticulosis
  colonoscopy, 1996
  small bowel bacterial overgrowth, 2060
Diverticulum
  esophageal, 2020-2021
  gastric, 2044
  intestinal, 2089-2092
Dizziness, 972, 973
  hypertrophic cardiomyopathy, 266
  ischemic heart disease, 197
  Lassa fever, 1510
DM kinase, 62
DMARDS; *see* Disease-modifying antirheumatic
      drugs
DNA; *see* Deoxyribonucleic acid
Do not resuscitate order, 12
Dobrava virus, 1516
Dobutamine
  dilated cardiomyopathy, 264
  heart failure, 173, 174
  myocardial infarction, 218
  neurogenic pulmonary edema, 1099
  shock, 180
  stress perfusion scintigraphy, 199
Dobutamine stress echocardiography, 104
  ischemic heart disease, 199
  preoperative, 2258
Dog heartworm, 468
Dog tapeworm, 1705
Dohle's body, 594
Dolichostenomelia, 1289
Doll's eye response, 947-948
Domain, immunoglobulin, 1122
Domain subunit structure, 1110

Domestic violence, 4, 2268
Dominance, 1721, 1724
Dominant trait, 1721
Domperidone, 2027
Donath-Landsteiner antibody
  autoimmune hemolytic anemia, 668
  paroxysmal cold hemoglobinuria, 670
Donepezil, 986, 2288
Donor
  cardiac, 338-339
  hematopoietic stem cell, 577
  kidney, 791-792
  liver, 2219
  lung, 515-516
Donovanosis, 1444
Dopa, 1826
L-Dopa, 1775
Dopa decarboxylase, 1826
Dopamine
  acute tubular necrosis, 773-774
  biosynthesis, 1826
  cocaine intoxication, 2297
  dilated cardiomyopathy, 264
  gram-negative bacteremia, 1451
  heart failure, 173, 174
  mediator of emetic reflex, 2026
  multiple organ dysfunction syndrome, 422
  myocardial infarction, 218
  Parkinson's disease, 990-991
  prolactin inhibition, 1775
  shock, 180
Dopamine beta hydroxylase, 930
Dopamine-receptor blockers
  lipodystrophy, 1902
  vasopressin inhibition, 1791
Dopaminergic pathways, 1076
Doppler echocardiography
  aortic regurgitation, 242
  aortic stenosis, 238, 287
  atrial septal defect, 281-282
  cardiac tamponade, 276
  deep venous thrombosis, 311
  diastolic heart failure, 168
  dilated cardiomyopathy, 264
  Ebstein's anomaly, 290
  endocardial cushion defect, 283
  hypertrophic cardiomyopathy, 268, 269
  infective endocarditis, 229
  mitral regurgitation, 251, 253
  patent ductus arteriosus, 285-286
  primary pulmonary hypertension, 294
  pulmonic stenosis, 288
  total anomalous pulmonary venous connection,
      291
  tricuspid stenosis, 256
  ventricular septal defect, 284, 285
Doppler effect, 97
Doppler flow velocity profile, 45
Doppler ultrasound
  aortic regurgitation, 244
  hepatocellular carcinoma, 2213
Doppler waveform, 929
Dorolamide, 2302
Dorsal column, 1011
Dorsal rhizotomy, 581
Dosage compensation, 1727
Dot blot hybridization, 2174
Double duct sign, 2243
Double effect principle, 13
Double lung transplantation, 515
  cystic fibrosis, 483
  emphysema, 445
Double-positive thymocyte, 1113
Double product, 91, 126, 193
Down-beat nystagmus, 1064
Down regulation, 1712, 1718
Down syndrome
  Hashimoto's thyroiditis, 1811
  hypergonadotropic hypogonadism, 1843
  ostium primum defect, 282-283

Doxazosin
  chronic pernio, 310
  hypertension, 325
  Raynaud's phenomenon, 310
  reflex sympathetic dystrophy, 311
Doxepin, 1037
Doxorubicin
  anthracycline-induced cardiotoxicity, 584
  breast cancer, 709, 710, 712
  dilated cardiomyopathy, 265
  endometrial cancer, 714
  gastric cancer, 2048
  hepatic injury, 2192
  Hodgkin's disease, 694-695
  multiple myeloma, 702
  non-Hodgkin's lymphoma, 699
  pancreatic cancer, 2243
  toxicity, 105
Doxycycline
  bacillary angiomatosis, 1474
  brucellosis, 1605, 1606
  chlamydial infection, 1537
  cholera, 1596
  chronic obstructive pulmonary disease, 444
  dosage, 1350
  esophagitis, 2019
  gonorrhea, 1585
  leptospirosis, 1645
  Lyme disease, 1254, 1647
  malaria, 1467
  Mycoplasma hominis infection, 1541
  relapsing fever, 1646
  rickettsial infection, 1545
  syphilis, 1643
  urethritis, 1441
dP/dt; *see* Maximal rate of pressure rise
DPT vaccine, 1567, 1574
Dracunculus medinensis, 1700, 1701
Drainage
  duodenal
    cholesterolosis, 2231
    gallstone, 2225
  peritonitis, 1402
  peritonsillar abscess, 2306
Dressler's syndrome, 221-222
  pericarditis, 273
  pleural effusion, 508
DRGs; *see* Diagnosis-related groups
Dripps-American Society of Anesthesiology
      classification of physical status, 2257
Dronabinol, 2027
Drooling, 1999
Drop attack, 955
Droperidol, 2027
Drowning, 668
Drug abuse, 2293-2297
  alcoholism, 2294-2296
    acute meningitis, 1407
    acute pancreatitis, 2233
    alcoholic ketosis, 1865
    carbon tetrachloride poisoning, 2188
    chronic pancreatitis, 2238
    cirrhosis, 2172
    diagnosis, 2197-2198
    hypomagnesemia, 1941
    hypophosphatemia, 1936
    niacin deficiency, 2107
    porphyria cutanea tarda, 1927
    thiamine deficiency, 2106
    weight loss, 1749
  candidiasis, 1661
  cellulitis, 1420
  cocaine, 2296-2297
  hepatitis A virus infection, 2173
  hepatitis B virus infection, 2174
  impotence, 1761
  infective endocarditis, 226, 229-230
  mood disorders, 1036
  narcotics, 2297
  personality disorders, 1039
  renal disease, 853

Drug abuse—cont'd
  tetanus risk, 1572
  tobacco, 2296
  tricuspid regurgitation, 256
  weight loss, 1749
Drug allergy
  hepatic injury, 2186
  penicillins, 1352
Drug fever, 1378
Drug history
  arrhythmia, 133
  drug interaction management, 2313
Drug hypersensitivity reaction
  acquired immunodeficiency syndrome,
    1326-1327
  cutaneous manifestations, 1312-1316
  pleural effusion, 508
  primary pulmonary hypertension, 294
  tuberculosis, 1632
Drug-induced disorders
  acute confusional state, 1031
  acute pancreatitis, 2233
  adverse pulmonary reactions, 476-479
  arrhythmia, 133, 134-135
  bone marrow failure, 671-672
  canalicular cholestasis, 2155
  causing occupational asthma, 472
  cholangitis, 2202-2203
  chronic diarrhea, 2051
  delayed gastric emptying, 1979
  dyskinesia, 995
  Fanconi's syndrome, 882
  fever and rash, 1381
  generalized lymphadenopathy, 599
  goiter, 1809
  gynecomastia, 1765
  hemolytic anemia, 667-668, 670
  hypercalcemia, 1928
  hyperglycemia, 1855
  hypertension, 322
  hypoglycemia, 1875-1876
  immune thrombocytopenia, 615-616
  impotence, 1760, 1761
  incontinence, 2293
  intestinal pseudoobstruction, 2079
  liver disease, 2184-2193
    acetaminophen poisoning, 2188-2190
    acute hepatic injury, 2187-2188
    carbon tetrachloride poisoning, 2188
    chronic liver damage, 2188
    classification of hepatotoxic agents,
      2185-2187
    diagnosis, 2193
    herbal remedies and plant toxins, 2192-2193
    medications, 2190-2192
    mushroom and phosphorus poisoning, 2188
    susceptibility of liver to chemical injury,
      2185
    treatment, 2193
  lupus erythematosus, 1217-1218
    pericarditis, 273
    pleural effusion, 508
  lysosomopathies, 1919
  megakaryocytic hypoplasia, 614
  mood disorders, 1036
  myopathy, 1030
  nausea and vomiting, 2026-2027
  neutropenia, 679
  orthostatic hypotension with syncope, 953-954
  parkinsonism, 993
  pemphigus, 1294
  renal
    acute interstitial nephritis, 889
    chronic tubulointerstitial nephropathy, 890
    nephropathy, 866-871
    renal magnesium wasting, 1940
    tubulointerstitial disease, 888
  sensorimotor neuropathy, 1020
  vitamin K deficiency, 626
Drug-induced tolerance, 1143

Drug interactions, 2310-2314
  antiarrhythmic drugs, 137
  azole antifungals, 1654
  mechanisms, 2310-2312
  oral anticoagulants, 636-637
  principles of management, 2312-2313
Drug reactions
  anaphylaxis, 1194-1195
  neutropenia, 593
  nosocomial infection, 1480
Drug resistance
  chemotherapeutic drugs, 554
  enterococci, 1346
  Haemophilus influenzae, 1588
  isoniazid, 1632
  mechanisms of antimicrobial resistance,
    1345-1346
  Neisseria gonorrhoeae, 1582
  Neisseria meningitidis, 1579
  Salmonella typhi, 1601
  staphylococci, 1345
  streptococci, 1559-1560
  tumor response to drug treatment, 552
Drugs
  effect on vasopressin release, 1790, 1791
  effects of lipoproteins, 1890-1892
  effects on electrocardiography, 90
  esophageal injury, 2019
  fall risk, 2290
  geriatric clinical pharmacology, 2286-2287
  hepatic detoxification, 2122
  hepatotoxicity, 2184-2193
    acetaminophen poisoning, 2188-2190
    acute hepatic injury, 2187-2188
    carbon tetrachloride poisoning, 2188
    chronic liver damage, 2188
    classification of hepatotoxic agents,
      2185-2187
    diagnosis, 2193
    herbal remedies and plant toxins, 2192-2193
    medications, 2190-2192
    mushroom and phosphorus poisoning, 2188
    susceptibility of liver to chemical injury,
      2185
    treatment, 2193
  lipoprotein lipase potentiation, 1892
  lipoprotein synthesis inhibitors, 1891-1892
  neuroendocrinology, 1077
  overdose, 418
Drusen, Plate XI-1
Dry beriberi, 2106
Dry eye
  Sjögren syndrome *versus,* 1209-1212
  systemic sclerosis, 1230
Dry mouth
  Lambert-Eaton myasthenic syndrome, 1024
  Sjögren syndrome, 1209-1212
  systemic sclerosis, 1230
Dry-powder inhaler, 430, 431
DT vaccine, 1567
DTH; *see* Delayed-type hypersensitivity
Dual-beam photon absorptiometry, 1748
Dual-energy x-ray absorptiometry, 1748
Dual-isotope rest ^{2}01T1/exercise ^{9}9mTc
  sestamibi study, 102
Dubin-Johnson syndrome, 2142, 2155, 2157
Duchenne muscular dystrophy, 1026
  cardiomyopathy, 62
  myocardial dysfunction, 1086
Duck fever, 460
Duct cell, 2132-2133
Duct ectasia, 1846, 1848
Ductal carcinoma in situ, breast, 707
Ductal cholestasis, 2155
Ductal hyperplasia, 1846
Ductular obstruction in cystic fibrosis, 480
Ductular water secretion, 2123-2124
Ductus arteriosus, 280, 285
Ductus venosus, 280
Duffy blood group system, 1672
Dukes' staging classification, 2083

Duodenal drainage
  cholesterolosis, 2231
  gallstone, 2225
Duodenal gland adenoma, 2082
Duodenum
  absorption of iron, 1988
  alpha heavy-chain disease, 704
  ectopic pancreatic tissue, 2246
  endoscopic examination, 1994
  iron absorption, 1988
  movement of food, 1978
  secretin release, 1986
  ulcer, 2003
  visualization, 2002
Duplex scan, 929
Durable powers of attorney for health care,
  12-13
Dural arteriovenous malformation, 928
Dural rheumatoid nodule, 1094
Dural venous sinus thrombosis, 928
Duret hemorrhage, 1082-1083
Duroziez's sign, 65, 241
Dust, hypersensitivity pneumonitis, 460
Dutch hypothesis, 439
DVT; *see* Deep venous thrombosis
Dwarf tapeworm, 1697
Dyazide; *see* Dyrenium
DynaCare; *see* Isradipine
Dynamic compliance, 347
Dyrenium, 325
Dysarthria, 977
  Crigler-Najjar syndrome, 2153
  hepatic encephalopathy, 2161
Dysautonomia, 1087
Dysbetalipoproteinemia, 60, 1898
Dysentery
  causes, 1430
  Shigella, 1445
Dysfibrinogenemia, 625
Dysfibrinogens, 627
Dysgenesis
  gonadal, 1769, 1838
  reticular, 1177
Dysgenesis, reticular, 1177
Dyshidrotic hand dermatitis, 1304
Dyskinesia
  biliary, 2233
  drug-induced, 995
  gallbladder, 2233
Dyslipidemia, 326
Dyslipoproteinemia, 60
Dysmotility, gallbladder, 2221, 2224
Dysmyelination, 1007
Dysostoses, 1286
Dysostosis multiplex, 1912
Dyspepsia, 2039
  acquired immunodeficiency syndrome,
    2095
  upper gastrointestinal endoscopy, 1994
Dysphagia, 1998
  anaplastic thyroid carcinoma, 1815
  aortic dissection, 300
  deep neck infections, 2309
  erosive esophagitis, 2017
  esophageal cancer, 2024
  esophageal disease, 1998
  gastric cancer, 2046
  human immunodeficiency virus, 1476
  infectious esophagitis, 2020
  Lassa fever, 1510
  oropharyngeal, 1998
  Riedel's thyroiditis, 1812
  stroke patient, 1054
  systemic sclerosis, 1229
  upper gastrointestinal endoscopy, 1994
Dysplasia
  angiodysplasia, 624
  carcinoma in ulcerative colitis, 2076
  cervix, 714
  epithelial, 2076
  esophageal, 2018

Dysplasia—cont'd
  fibromuscular
    renovascular disease, 755-756
    renovascular hypertension, 893
  fibrous, 1960-1961
  hereditary onychoosteodysplasia, 877
  mammary, 708
  myelodysplasia, 611, 675-676
  osteochondrodysplasia, 1286
  progressive diaphyseal, 1959
  renal-retinal, 875
  right ventricular, 153
  skeletal, 1286-1290
Dysplastic nevus, 1298
Dyspnea, 404, 405
  acute lung allograft rejection, 521
  acute pancreatitis, 2234
  acute pericarditis, 273
  aortic dissection, 300
  aortic stenosis, 236
  ascites, 2164
  asthma, 1187
  atrial septal defect, 281
  behavioral control of breathing, 356-357
  bronchiolitis obliterans syndrome, 522
  cardiac tamponade, 275
  chronic obstructive pulmonary disease, 442
  complete transposition of great arteries, 290
  constrictive pericarditis, 277
  dilated cardiomyopathy, 263
  exercise testing, 379
  heart failure, 163
  hepatopulmonary syndrome, 2170
  human immunodeficiency virus, 1477
  hypersensitivity pneumonitis, 461
  hypertrophic obstructive cardiomyopathy, 266
  hypothyroidism, 334
  idiopathic pulmonary fibrosis, 453
  interstitial lung disease, 450
  ischemic heart disease, 196-197
  Langerhans' cell granulomatosis, 464
  lung cancer, 488
  lymphomatoid granulomatosis, 470
  malignant mesothelioma, 510
  mediastinal abnormality, 511
  mitral regurgitation, 250
  mitral stenosis, 246
  myopericarditis, 1489
  patent ductus arteriosus, 285
  pleural disease, 505
  pneumothorax, 509
  precapillary pulmonary hypertension, 293
  psychologic considerations, 432
  pulmonary edema, 168
  pulmonary function tests, 375
  pulmonary hypertension, 498
  pulmonary thromboembolism, 500
  pulmonary veno-occlusive disease, 298
  pulmonic stenosis, 288
  respiratory muscle failure, 359
  right atrial myxoma, 330
  sarcoidosis, 458
  spontaneous pneumomediastinum, 514
  systemic lupus erythematosus, 1215
  systemic sclerosis, 1230
  Wegener's granulomatosis, 468
Dysprosody, 976, 977
Dysproteinemia, 700-706
  heavy-chain diseases, 704
  monoclonal gammopathy of undetermined
    significance, 705-706
  multiple myeloma, 700-703
  platelet dysfunction, 611-612
  renal manifestations, 862-866
  Waldenström macroglobulinemia, 703-704
Dyssomnias, 940-945
Dyssynergia, 1065, 1066
Dysthyroid ophthalmopathy, 1063
Dystonia, 946, 995
Dystrophin, 51, 59-60, 62, 1026
Dystrophin-associated glycoproteins, 1027

Dystrophy
  facioscapulohumeral, 1027
  lipodystrophy, 1899-1903
    centrifugal, 1903
    congenital total, 1900-1902
    insulin resistance, 1861
    intestinal, 2064-2065
    leprechaunism, 1899-1900
    lipoatrophic diabetes, 1902-1903
    membranous lipodystrophy, 1903
    mesenteric, 1903, 2251
    partial, 1902, 1903
    renal involvement, 877-878
  muscular
    Becker, 62
    cardiac disease, 1086
    chromosomal mapping, 61
    Duchenne, 62, 1026, 1086
    dystrophin, 59-60
    Erb's, 1026-1027, 1028, 1086
    Fukuyama, 1028
    limb girdle, 1026-1027, 1028, 1086
    molecular biology, 61-62
    respiratory failure, 1097
    weakness, 1754
  mytonic, 1027-1028
  oculopharyngeal, 1028
  osteodystrophy
    Albright's hereditary, 1932
    chronic renal failure, 779, 780
    mixed uremic, 1963
  pseudo-Hurler, 1916
  renal osteodystrophy, 1961-1965
    calcium acetate, 785
    chronic renal failure, 785-786
    hyperparathyroidism, 1961
    hyperphosphatemia, 1938
Dysuria, 762-763
  bacterial prostatitis, 1462
  hematuria, 757
  Lassa fever, 1510
  urethritis, 1440
  urinary tract infection, 1458
  vulvovaginal candidiasis, 1442

E

E-coding, 2266
E-mail, 28
EAD; *see* Early afterdepolarization
Ear
  chronic tophaceous gout, 1272
  Haemophilus influenzae infection, 1587, 1588
  hearing handicap inventory for
    elderly-screening, 2287
  hearing loss, 2307-2308
    Alport's syndrome, 876
    central nervous system disease, 974
    elderly, 2287
    Lassa fever, 1510
    mumps complication, 1496
    neonatal cytomegalovirus, 1528
    otitis media, 1395
  hearing test, 2255
  middle ear disorders, 2307
  otalgia, 2307
  otitis externa, 2307
  otitis media, 1395
  otogenic subdural empyema, 1417
  otoneurology, 971-975
  otorrhea, 2307
  otosclerosis, 974
  tinnitus, 2307
  toxicity of chemotherapeutic agents, 585
  vertigo, 2307
  Wegener's granulomatosis, 468
Earache, 2307
  acute otitis media, 1395
  peritonsillar abscess, 2306
Early afterdepolarization, 132
Early repolarization, 89-90

Early Treatment Diabetic Retinopathy Study,
    2303
EAST trial, 117
Eastern equine encephalitis, 1515, 1517
Eaton-Lambert syndrome, 489
Ebstein's anomaly of tricuspid valve, 256,
    289-290
Eccentrocyte, 662, Plate IV-4
Eccrine glands, 933
Eccrine testing, 938
Echinococcal cyst, 2211-2212
Echinococcosis, 1466
Echinococcus granulosus, 507, 1705, 2111
Echinococcus multilocularis, 1705
Echinostomas ilocanum, 1698
Echocardiography, 94-100
  after valve replacement, 259
  aortic regurgitation, 241-242, 244
  aortic stenosis, 238, 287
  atrial septal defect, 281-282
  cardiac structure and function, 95-97
  cardiac tamponade, 276
  cardiac tumor, 331-332
  clinical indications, 100
  coarctation of aorta, 286
  common aortopulmonary trunk, 290
  constrictive pericarditis, 277
  cor pulmonale, 498
  dexfenfluramine and, 261
  diastolic function, 45
  diastolic heart failure, 168
  dilated cardiomyopathy, 264
  Ebstein's anomaly, 290
  endocardial cushion defect, 283
  fenfluramine and, 261
  fever of unknown origin, 1380
  flow velocities and direction, 97-100
  heart failure, 165-167
  hypertrophic cardiomyopathy, 267, 268, 269
  infective endocarditis, 229
  left-ventricular performance, 166
  mitral regurgitation, 251, 253
  mitral stenosis, 248
  mitral valve prolapse, 254
  myocardial infarction, 212
  myocardial ischemia, 199
  patent ductus arteriosus, 285-286
  penetrating injury to heart, 332
  pericardial effusion, 274-275
  precapillary pulmonary hypertension, 296
  primary pulmonary hypertension, 294
  pulmonary edema, 169
  pulmonic stenosis, 288
  restrictive cardiomyopathy, 271
  sudden cardiac survivor, 188, 189
  syncope, 956
  total anomalous pulmonary venous connection,
    291
  transplant donor, 339
  transplanted heart, 343
  tricuspid regurgitation, 256
  tricuspid stenosis, 256
  truncus arteriosus, 290
  ventricular septal defect, 284, 285
Echolalia, 976, 977
Echothiophate iodide, 2302
Echovirus
  exanthems, 1489
  pericarditis, 272
Eclampsia, 2274-2275
ECM; *see* Extracellular matrix
Economics
  cost-benefit analysis, 15
  cost-effectiveness analysis, 15-16
  cost-identification analysis, 16
  cost-utility analysis, 16
  costs and outcomes, 14-16
  infection control programs, 1365
  poverty of elderly women, 2268
Ecthyma, 1420

Ecthyma gangrenosum, Plate VIII-23
  gram-negative bacteremia, 1450
  Pseudomonas septicemia, 1382
  skin signs and risk factors, 1423
Ectopic adrenocorticotropic hormone syndrome,
      489
Ectopic atrial tachycardia, 143-144, 146, 2276
Ectopic coronary artery, 291
Ectopic secretion of human chorionic
      gonadotropin, 583
Eczema, 1302-1304
  drug-induced, 1313
  otitis externa, 2307
  sun-induced, 1307
Eczema craquelé, 1303
Edema
  acute aortic obstruction, 304
  acute glomerulonephritis, 771
  acute pancreatitis, 2234
  arthritis, 1164-1166
  cerebral
    acute hyponatremia, 811
    bacterial meningitis, 1405
    head trauma, 1044
    hepatic encephalopathy, 2161
  Churg-Strauss syndrome, 466
  constrictive pericarditis, 277
  dilated cardiomyopathy, 263
  eosinophilic fasciitis, 1233
  gastric outlet obstruction, 2040
  gastroesophageal reflux, 2015
  heart failure, 165
  hypernatremia, 815
  hyponatremia, 811-812
  kwashiorkor, 2101
  nephrotic syndrome, 765-766, 820-821
  optic disc, 2303, Plate XI-2
  osteomyelitis, 1433
  papilledema, 1060
    bacterial meningitis, 1406
    brain herniation after lumbar puncture,
        905
    cryptococcosis, 1669
    fundoscopic view, Plate VIII-51
    hepatic encephalopathy, 2161
    osteomalacia, 1949
    Rocky Mountain spotted fever, 1543
    subdural empyema, 1417
  paravertebral, 1171
  permeability, 346-347
  poststreptococcal glomerulonephritis, 844
  pulmonary, 423-428
    acute toxic, 473
    adult respiratory distress syndrome, 421
    aortic regurgitation, 244
    chronic renal failure, 783-784
    congenital aortic stenosis, 287
    dilated cardiomyopathy, 263
    drug-induced, 477
    heart failure, 165
    hemoptysis, 410
    hypertrophic obstructive cardiomyopathy,
        266
    malaria, 1673
    mitral stenosis, 247
    myocardial contusion, 332
    neurogenic, 1099-1100
    papillary muscle rupture, 219
    patent ductus arteriosus, 285
    pneumothorax, 510
    precapillary pulmonary hypertension, 293
    pulmonary artery wedge pressure, 395
    treatment, 168
    ventricular septal defect, 284
  rheumatoid arthritis, 1201, 1202
  right atrial myxoma, 330
  Rocky Mountain spotted fever, 1543
  scurvy, 2107
  sodium balance dysfunction, 816-817
  staphylococcal scalded-skin syndrome, 1421
  superior vena caval obstruction, 511

Edema—cont'd
  systemic sclerosis, 1228
  venous thromboembolism, 631
  Whipple's disease, 2064
Edinger-Westphal nucleus, 932-933
EDRF; *see* Endothelium-derived relaxing factor
EDTA; *see* Ethylenediamine tetraacetic acid
EEG; *see* Electroencephalography
Effective blood volume
  arginine vasopressin release, 810-811
  congestive heart failure, 817, 818
  edema, 816
  edematous cirrhotic patient, 819
  heart failure, 162
  nephrotic syndrome, 820
Effective osmols, 806
Effective plasma volume, 816
Effusion
  degenerative polyarthritis, 1199
  middle ear, 2307
  pericardial, 274-275
    acquired immunodeficiency syndrome, 333,
        1478
    acute pericarditis, 274
    cardiac metastasis, 332
    echocardiography, 100
    heart murmur, 76
    hypothyroidism, 1809
    management, 278
  pleural, 505
    asbestos exposure, 474
    chronic pancreatitis, 2241
    classification of, 506
    dilated cardiomyopathy, 263
    heart murmur, 76
    hypothyroidism, 1809
    lymphomatoid granulomatosis, 470
    malignant, 507-508
    physical findings, 403
    pyogenic liver abscess, 2209
    thoracentesis, 381
    ultrasound, 389
  rheumatoid arthritis, 1203
  synovial, 1162
Effusive-constrictive pericarditis, 278
Eflornithine, 1689
Ehlers-Danlos syndrome, 1287-1289, 1320
Ehrlichiosis, 1545
Ehrlich's aldehyde test, 2150
Eisenmenger's reaction
  atrial septal defect, 281
  patent ductus arteriosus, 285
  precapillary pulmonary hypertension, 296
  ventricular septal defect, 283, 284
Eisenmenger's syndrome, 515
Ejaculation, 934
Ejection click, 287
Ejection fraction, 42, 112
  aortic regurgitation, 241
  dilated cardiomyopathy, 264
  heart failure, 159
  prognosis of ischemic heart disease, 208
Ekbom syndrome, 1103
El Tor biotype *Vibrio cholerae,* 1594, 1595
Elastance, ventricular, 42-43
Elastase
  acute pancreatitis, 2234
  diagnosis of pancreatic diseases, 2144
  gram-negative bacilli, 1446
  lung damage, 373
Elastase-antielastase hypothesis of emphysema,
      441
Elastic recoil
  aging and, 2284
  restenosis, 122
Elastic stockings, 312
Elastic strings, 504
Elastic tissue disease, 1289
Elastin, 1289
  emphysema, 441
  lung extracellular matrix, 371

Elbow
  bursitis, 1197
  rheumatoid arthritis, 1203
Elderly, 2282-2293
  abuse, 4
  aortic stenosis, 236-237
  asymptomatic bacteriuria, 1461
  biology of aging, 2283-2285
  changes in osmoregulatory system, 1789
  chronic lymphocytic leukemia, 684
  dementia, 2288-2289
  demography and epidemiology, 2282-2283
  depression, 2289
  eye problems, 2300-2306
    age-related macular degeneration,
        2301-2302
    cataracts, 2301
    diabetic retinopathy, 2303-2304
    glaucoma, 2301, 2302
    hypertensive retinopathy, 2302-2303
    presbyopia, 2301
    visual loss, 2300-2301
  falls, 2289-2290, 2291
  health care expenditure, 14
  hematuria, 757
  hormones and, 1076-1077
  hyperkalemia, 832
  hypertension, 312, 327
  multiple myeloma, 700
  myelodysplasia, 676
  myocardial infarction, 210, 211
  osteoarthritis, 1264
  peripheral vascular disease, 305
  prolonged bleeding times, 569
  special considerations, 2285-2288
  thrombolytic therapy, 214
  urinary incontinence, 2290-2293
  voiding dysfunction, 1065-1066
Electrical activation of ventricle, 36-37
Electrical control activities, 1976
Electrical potentials, electrocardiogram, 82
Electrical response activity, 1976
Electrical stimulation, 967
Electrical substrate, 188, 189
Electrocardiographic stress testing, 91-94
Electrocardiography, 81-91
  acute pericarditis, 273, 274
  aortic regurgitation, 241
  aortic stenosis, 237, 287
  arrhythmia, 133-134, 135
  atrial fibrillation, 146-147
  atrial flutter, 144, 146
  atrial septal defect, 281, 282
  atrioventricular reciprocating tachycardia, 142,
      145
  cardiac electrical activity, 81-82
  cardiac tamponade, 276
  chamber enlargement and hypertrophy, 87-88
  coarctation of aorta, 286
  conduction abnormalities, 86-87
  congenitally corrected transposition of great
      arteries, 290
  constrictive pericarditis, 277
  cor pulmonale, 498
  dilated cardiomyopathy, 264
  dissection of aorta, 301
  drug and metabolic effects, 90
  early repolarization, 89-90
  endocardial cushion defect, 283
  heart failure, 166
  hepatic encephalopathy, 2161
  hypertension, 318
  hypertrophic cardiomyopathy, 267
  hypothyroidism, 1809-1810
  interpretation, 84-86
  ischemic heart disease, 88-89, 197-198
  lung cancer, 488
  mitral regurgitation, 251, 253
  mitral stenosis, 247
  mitral valve prolapse, 254

Electrocardiography—cont'd
  myocardial abnormalities in neurologic
      disease, 1087-1088
  myocardial infarction, 211
  myocarditis, 263
  P wave, 83-84
  palpitations, 130, 131
  pericarditis, 89
  precapillary pulmonary hypertension, 296
  preoperative medical evaluation, 2256
  primary pulmonary hypertension, 294
  pulmonary thromboembolism, 501
  pulmonic regurgitation, 257
  pulmonic stenosis, 288
  QRS complex, 84
  sick sinus syndrome, 154
  silent myocardial ischemia, 194
  ST segment, 84
  standard leads, 82-83
  sudden cardiac survivor, 188
  supraventricular tachyarrhythmias, 141, 142,
      143
  sustained ventricular tachycardia and wide
      QRS complex tachycardia, 150
  syncope, 956
  T wave, 84
  tetralogy of Fallot, 289
  tricuspid regurgitation, 256
  tricuspid stenosis, 256
  U wave, 84
  ventricular septal defect, 284
Electrocoagulation, 2011-2012
Electroconvulsive therapy, 1038
Electrode
  electrocardiographic, 82
  needle electromyography, 916
Electroencephalography, 905-908
  brain death, 1083
  coma, 950
  dementia, 988
  dialysis encephalopathy, 1105
  epilepsy, 981
  metabolic encephalopathy, 1079
  pseudoseizure attacks, 984
  sleep states, 939
  stroke, 1003
Electrolyte disorders
  acid-base balance disorders, 836-841
      metabolic acidosis, 836-839
      metabolic alkalosis, 839-841
      patient evaluation, 840, 841
  cholera, 1595
  diabetic ketoacidosis, 1864
  electrocardiographic abnormalities, 90
  hyperosmolar nonketotic coma, 1866
  intestinal disorders, 2005-2006
  multiple myeloma, 864
  polymorphic ventricular tachycardia, 152
  potassium balance, 825-834
      external potassium balance, 825, 826
      hyperkalemia, 830-833
      hypokalemia, 826-830
      internal potassium balance, 825-826
  renal tubular transport disorders, 878-884
      aminoaciduria, 879
      dicarboxylic aminoaciduria, 879-880
      Fanconi's syndrome, 881-882
      Hartnup disease, 879
      iminoglycinuria, 880
      nephrogenic diabetes insipidus, 883-884
      renal glycosuria, 878-879
      renal phosphate wasting syndromes, 880
      X-linked hypophosphatemic rickets,
          880-881
  sodium balance, 816-825
      cirrhosis, 818-820
      congestive heart failure, 817-818
      edematous states, 816-817
      extrarenal sodium depletion, 823
      idiopathic edema, 821
      nephrotic syndrome, 820-821

Electrolyte disorders—cont'd
  sodium balance—cont'd
      salt-wasting states, 823
      sodium depletion of renal origin, 823-825
      use of diuretics, 821-823
  water balance disorders, 805-816
      hypernatremia, 813-816
      hyponatremia, 809-813
      principles of osmoregulation, 805-809
  weakness, 1754
Electrolytes
  intestinal absorption, 1988
  loss during vomiting, 2028
  parenteral solutions, 2114
Electromechanical coupling, 1976
Electromyographic biofeedback, 1055
Electromyography, 814-917
  determination of weakness, 1755
  low back pain, 966
  muscle disease, 1025-1026
  myasthenia gravis, 1022
  neck pain, 969
  plexopathy, 1017
  respiratory muscle fatigue, 358
  sleep states, 939
  sphincter, 938
Electron beam computed tomography, 106
Electron microscopy
  Alport's syndrome, 876-877
  cancer of unknown primary site, 731
  focal glomerular sclerosis, 852
  glomerulonephritis, 842
  idiopathic nephrotic syndrome, 850
  minimal change disease, 849
  poststreptococcal glomerulonephritis, 843-844
  primary hyperparathyroidism, 1968
Electronic mail, 28
Electrophoresis, 567-568
  multiple myeloma, 701
  separation and identification of
      deoxyribonucleic acid, 51-52
  serum gamma globulin level, 2136
  serum protein, 565-566
Electrophysiologic studies
  arrhythmias, 134
  sick sinus syndrome, 154
  sudden death survivor, 188, 190
  syncope, 956
  ventricular fibrillation, 224
Elephantiasis nostras, 1423, Plate VIII-27
Elevation pallor, 305
11β-OH steroid dehydrogenase deficiency,
      828-829
ELISA; *see* Enzyme-linked immunosorbent
      assay
Elliptocyte, Plate IV-4
  hemolytic disease, 662
  hereditary elliptocytosis, 665, 666
Ellis van Creveld syndrome, 280
Elongation factor 2, 1446
Embolectomy
  embolic arterial occlusion, 307-308
  pulmonary thromboembolism, 503
Embolic arterial occlusion, 307
Embolism
  acute aortic obstruction, 304
  acute pulmonary hypertension, 297
  candidal, 1663
  cholesterol crystal, 1057
  fat, 658
  heart failure, 174-175
  infective endocarditis, 228
  ischemic stroke, 998-1000
  mitral stenosis, 246
  myxoma, 330
  primary pulmonary hypertension, 293
  prosthetic heart valve, 261
  pulmonary, 630-638
      acute pulmonary hypertension, 297
      atrial fibrillation, 146
      chest pain, 128

Embolism—cont'd
  pulmonary—cont'd
      deep venous thrombosis, 311
      echocardiography, 100
      embolectomy, 503
      heart failure *versus,* 168
      lung scan, 387-388
      nephrotic syndrome, 766
      nosocomial, 1480-1481
      during pregnancy, 2276
      pulmonary angiogram, 388
      pulmonary edema *versus,* 425
      sepsis *versus,* 1451
      wheezing, 1189
  renal artery, 896-897
  stroke, 1006
Embolization
  infective endocarditis, 226, 227
  myxoma, 330
  prosthetic valve problems, 258
  variceal bleeding, 2167
Embryology, pancreatic, 2129-2131
Emergency management, 2306-2310
  acute airway obstruction, 2306
  acute aortic obstruction, 304
  acute mitral regurgitation, 219
  angioedema, 2306
  aortic dissection, 300
  facial nerve paralysis, 2306
  head trauma, 1045
  neurologic problems, 1081-1086
  peritonsillar abscess, 2306
  supraglottitis, 2306
Emesis, 2025-2029
  acute cholecystitis, 2227
  acute pancreatitis, 2234
  appendicitis, 2092
  ascites, 2164
  autonomic failure, 935
  bacterial meningitis, 1406
  biliary colic, 2225
  bubonic plague, 1610
  chemotherapy-induced, 581-582
  chronic renal failure, 784
  galactosemia, 1882
  generation of alkalosis, 839
  hepatitis A virus, 2173
  hepatocellular carcinoma, 2213
  herpangina, 1488
  hyperemesis gravidarum, 2278
  hypertrophic pyloric stenosis, 2044
  intestinal obstruction, 2077, 2078
  Lassa fever, 1510
  mesenteric panniculitis, 2251
  normotensive renal potassium wasting, 828
  Norwalk virus, 1522
  pancreatic abscess, 1399
  peptic ulcer, 2037
  peritoneal mesenteric and omental diseases,
      2248
  peritonitis, 1398
  pheochromocytoma, 1829
  Rocky Mountain spotted fever, 1543
  rotavirus, 1521
  solitary liver cyst, 2111
  thrombotic thrombocytopenic purpura, 615
Emetic center, 581
Emetic reflex, 2025, 2026
Emory Angioplasty *vs.* Surgery Trial, 117
Emotion
  chest pain, 126, 129
  palpitations, 130
  physician-patient relationship, 2
Emotional expression disorders, 1033-1034
Emotional stress
  chronic fatigue syndrome, 2299
  effect on vasopressin release, 1791
  hypertension, 316
  hypogonadism, 1842
  increased catecholamines, 1828
  increased nutrient requirements, 2102

Emotional stress—cont'd
  irritable bowel syndrome, 2056
  long-term modulation of ventricular function,
    46
  neuroendocrinology, 1077
  neutrophilia, 590
  palpitations, 130
  skeletal growth, 1716
Emperipolesis, 680
Emphysema
  API deficiency, 440
  asthma *versus,* 1189
  defined, 438
  heart murmur, 76
  mediastinal, 513-514
  mediastinal crunch, 75
  pathogenesis, 441-442
  pathology, 439
  patterns of pulmonary function abnormalities,
    379
  physical findings, 403
  pulmonary hypertension, 498
  second heart sound, 73
Empiric treatment
  anaerobic infection, 1619-1621
  diarrhea, 1431-1432
  febrile compromised patient, 1388-1390
  infectious diseases, 1380
  purulent meningitis, 1411
Employee health, 1365
Empty sella syndrome, 1787
Emptying of radiopaque markers, 2004
Empyema, 507
  acalculous cholecystitis, 2227, 2228
  actinomycosis, 1665
  anaerobic bacteria, 1617
  clostridial, 1575
  computed tomography, 387
  intracranial subdural, 1416-1418
  tuberculous, 1634
Enalapril
  congestive heart failure, 818
  dilated cardiomyopathy, 264
  heart failure, 170
  hepatic injury, 2192
  hypertension, 325
  hypertensive emergency, 328
  myocardial infarction, 217
  typical medical regimen six months after
    transplantation, 343
Encephalitis
  acquired immunodeficiency syndrome, 1477
  herpes, 1524
  measles, 1498
  mumps, 1496
  parkinsonism, 993
  picornavirus infection, 1487
  poliomyelitis, 1488
  viral, 1488, 1516-1518
Encephalitozoon, 1680-1681, 2095
Encephalopathy
  alcoholic hepatitis and cirrhosis, 2197
  aluminum intoxication, 1964
  blood ammonia levels, 2143
  complication of chemotherapy, 1072
  Crigler-Najjar syndrome, 2153
  dialysis, 1105-1106
  grades of liver disease severity, 2166
  hepatic
    abnormalities of amino acid metabolism and
      urea formation, 2102
    liver failure, 2159-2163
  hypertensive crisis, 328
  hypophosphatemia, 1936
  hypoxic-ischemic, 950-951
  Lyme disease, 1647
  metabolic, 948-949, 1078-1080
  pancreatic, 1101
  primary biliary cirrhosis, 2200
  reversible portosystemic, 1102
  uremic, 784

Encephalopathy—cont'd
  Wernicke's, 1081
    amnesic syndrome, 1032
    thiamine deficiency, 1100-1102, 2106
End-diastolic volume, 112
End-plate acetylcholinesterase deficiency, 1023
End-stage renal disease, 776
  bone and joint disease, 785-786
  cardiopulmonary complications, 783-784
  chronic renal failure, 782-783
  diabetic nephropathy, 859
  dialysis, 789-791
  endocrine function abnormalities, 786-787
  etiology and incidence, 777
  gastrointestinal tract disturbances, 784
  glomerular diseases, 841-859
    acquired immunodeficiency syndrome
      nephropathy, 853
    adverse reaction to nonsteroidal
      antiinflammatory agents, 853
    focal glomerular sclerosis, 851-852
    glomerular involvement in systemic
      diseases, 855-859
    heroin nephropathy, 853
    immunoglobulin A nephropathy, 845
    loin pain-hematuria syndrome, 845-846
    mechanisms and consequences of immune
      glomerular injury, 841-843
    membranoproliferative glomerulonephritis,
      854-855
    membranous nephropathy, 853-854
    mesangial proliferative disease, 851
    minimal change disease, 849-851
    nephritis associated with visceral abscess,
      844
    postinfectious glomerulonephritis, 843-844
    rapidly progressive glomerulonephritis,
      846-849
    subacute bacterial endocarditis, 844
  hematologic disorders, 783
  hyperphosphatemia, 785-786
  hypertension, 320-321, 783
  hypocalcemia, 785-786
  immunologic and infectious complications,
    784-785
  membranoproliferative glomerulonephritis, 854
  membranous nephropathy, 854
  mixed uremic osteodystrophy, 1962
  neuromuscular abnormalities, 784
  nutritional and metabolic alterations, 786
  poststreptococcal glomerulonephritis, 844
  renal osteodystrophy, 785-786
  renal replacement therapy, 788
  renal transplantation, 791-796
  tubulointerstitial damage, 888
End-systolic pressure-volume relation, 42-43
End tidal carbon dioxide measurement, 431
End-tidal carbon dioxide monitoring, 396
Endarterectomy, 1004
Endarteritis, 1641
Endemic cretinism, 1809
Endemic diarrhea, 1429-1430
Endemic pemphigus foliaceus, 1294
Endobronchial biopsy, 491-492
Endobronchial obstruction
  coughing, 407-408
  lung cancer, 491
Endocardial cushion defect, 282-283
Endocarditis, 225-235
  acute meningitis, 1407
  anaerobic bacteria, 1618
  antimicrobial therapy, 230-233
  aortic regurgitation, 244
  aspergillosis, 1658
  bicuspid aortic valve, 287
  brucellosis, 1606
  candidiasis, 1664
  clinical syndrome, 227-228
  coagulase-negative staphylococci, 1550-1551
  differential diagnosis, 229
  drug user, 229-230

Endocarditis—cont'd
  endocardial cushion defect, 283
  enterococcal, 1562
  fever of unknown origin, 1376-1377
  Haemophilus influenzae, 1586
  hypertrophic obstructive cardiomyopathy, 269
  laboratory findings, 228-229
  mitral regurgitation, 250
  mitral valve prolapse, 255
  mycotic aneurysm, 299
  neurologic aspects, 1089-1090
  pathophysiology, 225-227
  prophylaxis, 233, 234-235
  prosthetic heart valve, 230, 258-259, 261
  Q fever, 1545
  referral, 233-234
  rheumatic fever, 1256
  Staphylococcus aureus, 1550
  ventricular septal defect, 283
Endocardium
  metastatic disease, 331
  restrictive cardiomyopathy, 270
Endochondral bone formation, 1716
Endocrine disorders
  adolescent growth and development,
    1766-1773
    breast growth abnormalities, 1770
    constitutional delay of pubertal growth,
      1768
    Crohn's disease, 1768
    evaluation of pubertal growth, 1770-1772
    familial tall stature, 1769
    growth hormone deficiency, 1769
    hypothyroidism, 1768-1769
    idiopathic short stature, 1769
    Klinefelter's syndrome, 1769
    puberty, 1766-1768
    therapy, 1772
    Turner's syndrome, 1769
    weight abnormalities, 1769-1770
  adrenal cortex, 1817-1826
    adrenal hypofunction, 1823-1824
    adrenal mass, 1825-1826
    congenital adrenal hyperplasia, 1824-1825
    Cushing's syndrome, 1819-1822
    hormone synthesis and secretion, 1817-1819
    hypofunction, 1823-1824
    mass, 1825-1826
    mineralocorticoid excess, 1822-1823
  adrenal medulla, 1826-1831
    hyperfunction, 1828
    hypofunction, 1827-1828
  altered libido, 1760-1764
  amenorrhea, 1757-1760
    anorexia nervosa, 1769
    hirsutism, 1756
    hypothalamic, 1837
    malabsorption, 2057
    prolactin-secreting pituitary adenoma, 1786
  arthropathy, 1246-1247
  benign disease of breast, 1846-1850
  chronic renal failure, 786-787
  cutaneous manifestations, 1322-1324
  diabetes mellitus, 1850-1874
    acute mononeuropathies, 1872
    alcoholic ketosis, 1865
    antibiotic selection, 1348
    antihypertensive agent choices, 326
    arthropathy, 1246
    autonomic dysfunction, 936, 1087,
      1872-1873
    cardiac transplantation, 338
    cardiovascular involvement, 333-334
    chronic pancreatitis, 2239
    chronic renal failure, 781, 786, 859
    classification, 1853-1856
    coronary artery disease in women, 2271
    cutaneous manifestations, 1323
    dermopathy, 1873
    diabetic ketoacidosis, 1862-1865
    diabetic nephropathy, 859-862

Endocrine disorders—cont'd
diabetes mellitus—cont'd
  dietary, 1856-1857
  emptying of solid radiopaque markers, 2004
  gallstones, 2223
  hyperosmolar nonketotic coma, 1865-1866
  hypertension, 328
  hyperventilation, 355
  hypoglycemia, 1875
  hypoglycemic coma, 1867
  hyporeninemic hypoaldosteronism, 1824
  impotence, 1760, 1844
  insulin therapy, 1858-1862
  ischemic heart disease, 200
  lactic acidosis, 1866-1867
  localized amyloidosis, 1285
  macrovascular disease, 1868-1869
  management, 1856-1862
  microalbuminuria, 743
  microvascular disease, 1869-1870
  nephropathy, 1870
  neuromuscular disease, 1872
  neuropathy, 1871-1872
  nutritional consequences, 2100
  operative risk, 2262
  oral hypoglycemic agents, 1857-1858
  pancreatic cancer, 2242
  physiology, 1851-1853
  Prader-Labhart-Willi syndrome, 1842
  during pregnancy, 1873-1874, 2272-2273
  prevention of coma, 1867-1868
  reflux esophagitis, 2023
  renal transplant recipient, 795
  retinopathy, 1870-1871
  somatostatinoma, 2245
  weight loss, 1749
gynecomastia, 1764-1766
  benign adolescent, 1770
  end-stage renal disease, 787
  impotence, 1763
  Klinefelter's syndrome, 1843
  liver disease, 1843
  prolactin-secreting pituitary adenoma, 1786
  small cell lung cancer, 489
heritable disorders of carbohydrate
  metabolism, 1879-1883
  galactosemia, 1882-1883
  glycogen storage diseases, 1880-1882
  nondiabetic mellyturias, 1879-1880
hirsutism, 1755-1757
  prolactin-secreting pituitary adenoma, 1786
  21-hydroxylase deficiency, 1824
hyperparathyroidism, 1965-1971
  arthropathy, 1246
  calcium pyrophosphate dihydrate deposition
    disease, 1279
  diagnosis, 1967-1969
  humoral hypercalcemia of malignancy
    versus, 1973-1974
  hypermagnesemia, 1943
  kidney stone formation, 798
  osteomalacia, 1950
  pathology and etiology, 1965-1966
  during pregnancy, 2273
  prevalence, 1965, 1966
  renal transplant recipient, 795
  renal wasting of phosphate, 1935
  symptoms and signs, 1966-1967
  treatment, 1969-1971
hypoglycemia, 1874-1879
  acute fatty liver of pregnancy, 2278
  adrenal medulla hypofunction, 1828
  amylo-1,6-glucosidase deficiency, 1882
  cholera, 1595
  chronic pancreatitis, 2241
  diagnosis, 1877-1878
  dizziness, 972
  effects on fetus, 1874
  endocrine paraneoplastic syndromes, 583
  epilepsy *versus,* 981

Endocrine disorders—cont'd
hypoglycemia—cont'd
  glucose-6-phosphate dehydrogenase
    deficiency, 1881
  gram-negative bacteremia, 1449
  growth hormone deficiency, 1777
  hereditary fructose intolerance, 1880
  hypoglycemic coma, 1867
  insulin-induced, 202, 826, 1735-1736
  insulinoma, 2244
  leprechaunism, 1900
  metabolic encephalopathy, 1079
  neurologic aspects, 1101
  pathophysiology, 1875-1876
  physiology, 1874-1875
  Somogyi phenomenon, 1861
  syncope *versus,* 954-955
  treatment, 1878
  vasopressin stimulation, 1790
hypokalemia, 829
hypothalamic, 1773-1788
  amenorrhea, 1757-1759
  Cushing's disease, 1786-1787
  empty sella syndrome, 1787
  gonadotropin-secreting pituitary tumor,
    1787
  growth hormone-secreting pituitary tumor,
    1782-1785
  hyperprolactinemia, 1785-1786
  hypopituitarism, 1776-1777
  obesity, 1751, 1752, 2102-2103
  pituitary apoplexy, 1777-1781
  pituitary tumor, 1781-1782
  thyroid-stimulating hormone-secreting
    tumor, 1787
impotence, 1760-1764
lipid and lipoprotein disorders, 1883-1898
  apoliprotein synthesis abnormalities,
    1897-1898
  atherosclerosis, 1888-1889
  dietary factors, 1889-1890
  effects of drugs, 1890-1892
  enzyme abnormalities, 1898
  hyperlipidemia, 1892-1896
  hypoalphalipoproteinemia, 1896
  lipid metabolism, 1883-1884
  lipoprotein metabolism, 1885-1888
lipodystrophies, 1899-1903
  centrifugal lipodystrophy, 1903
  congenital total lipodystrophy, 1900-1902
  insulin resistance, 1861
  intestinal, 2064-2065
  leprechaunism, 1899-1900
  lipoatrophic diabetes, 1902-1903
  membranous lipodystrophy, 1903
  mesenteric, 2251
  mesenteric lipodystrophy, 1903
  partial lipodystrophy, 1902, 1903
  renal involvement, 877-878
liver failure, 2170-2172
myopathy, 1030
nonparathyroid, 1928
obesity, 1750-1753
osteoarthritis, 1266-1267
ovarian, 1832-1838
  amenorrhea, 1759-1760
  hirsutism, 1755-1756
  laboratory and diagnostic testing, 1835-1836
pheochromocytoma, 1828-1831
  autonomic hyperactivity, 935
  hypercalcemia, 1928
  hypertension, 322
  neurofibromatosis, 1921
  weight loss, 1749
posterior pituitary, 1795-1797
  diabetes insipidus, 1793-1795
  testing, 1737-1738
during pregnancy, 2272-2274
testicular, 1838-1846
  androgen metabolism, 1838-1839
  assessment of clinical status, 1840

Endocrine disorders—cont'd
testicular—cont'd
  assessment of hormonal status, 1840-1841
  genetic analysis, 1841
  hypogonadotropic syndromes, 1841-1843
thyroid disease, 1797-1817
  acute psychiatric illness, 1803
  arthropathy, 1246
  benign neoplasms, 1813-1814
  cutaneous manifestations, 1322
  dementia, 987
  dysthyroid ophthalmopathy, 1063
  euthyroid hyperthyroxinemia, 1803, 1804
  euthyroid hypothyroxinemia, 1804
  euthyroid sick syndrome, 1802-1803
  goiter, 1812-1813
  hypothyroidism, 1808-1811
  imaging techniques, 1801-1802
  impotence, 1762
  invasive techniques, 1802
  laboratory tests, 1800-1801
  Lambert-Eaton myasthenic syndrome with,
    1024
  malignancy, 1814-1817
  mood disorders, 1036
  myasthenia gravis with, 1022
  during pregnancy, 2273
  thyroid gland anatomy, 1797, 1798
  thyroid hormone formation and metabolism,
    1797-1799
  thyroiditis, 1811-1813
  thyrotoxicosis, 1804-1808
  L-thyroxine therapy, 1803-1804
weakness, 1753-1755
weight loss, 1748-1759
Endocrine islets, 2129
Endocrine paraneoplastic syndromes, 583
Endocrine stomach, 1981
Endocrine system
aging and, 2284-2285
anterior pituitary, 1773-1788
  anatomy, 1773-1774
  hypothalamic-pituitary adrenal system, 1774
  hypothalamic-pituitary axis, 1773-1774
  hypothalamic-pituitary gonadal system,
    1774-1775
  hypothalamic-pituitary growth hormone
    system, 1775
  hypothalamic-pituitary prolactin system,
    1775-1776, 1777
  hypothalamic-pituitary thyroid system, 1774
bone and mineral homeostasis, 1714-1721
  calcium metabolism, 1717-1720
  cellular physiology, 1716
  effects of hormones, 1720
  functions of skeleton, 1714-1715
  matrix formation and calcification, 1716
  natural history of skeleton, 1715-1716
  stress and coupling, 1716
features of malabsorption, 2058
laboratory and diagnostic testing, 1732-1744
  adrenal medullary hormones, 1739-1740
  androgens, 1741
  female gonadal function, 1742-1743
  general principles, 1732-1735
  genetic studies, 1743
  glucocorticoids, 1740-1741
  hypothalamic-pituitary testing, 1735-1737
  male gonadal function, 1742
  mineralocorticoids, 1741-1742
  posterior pituitary testing, 1737-1738
  thyroid function tests, 1738-1739
operative risks, 2262
physiology, 1708-1714
  classes of hormones, 1708
  hormone secretion, 1713-1714
  hormone synthesis, 1708-1710
  mechanisms of hormone action, 1710-1713
posterior pituitary, 1788-1797
  anatomy, 1788
  biochemistry, 1788-1789

Endocrine system—cont'd
  posterior pituitary—cont'd
    diabetes insipidus, 1793-1795
    disorders, 1795-1797
    physiology, 1789-1793
    testing, 1737-1738
Endocytosis, 1797, 1986
Endogenous hypertriglyceridemia, 1894
Endogenous pyrogen, 1386
Endoglycosides, 1289
Endolimax nana, 1692
Endolymph, 972
Endolymphatic hydrops, 2307
Endometrial cancer, 713-714
Endometriosis, 1618
Endomyocardial biopsy, 108
  cardiac transplant rejection, 340
  myocarditis, 263
Endoperoxides, 1141
Endophthalmitis, 1662
Endorphin, 353
Endoscopic retrograde cholangiopancreatography,
    1997, 2140, 2145
  acquired immunodeficiency syndrome
      cholangiopathy, 2202
  acute pancreatitis, 2237
  benign strictures of extrahepatic bile ducts, 2232
  choledocholithiasis, 2229
  chronic pancreatitis, 2146, 2240
  cystic fibrosis, 2207
  gallstones, 2225
  pancreatic tumor, 2242-2243
Endoscopic sphincterotomy, 2230
Endoscopic ultrasound, 1997
  chronic pancreatitis, 2240
  esophageal cancer, 2024
  gastric carcinoma, 2046, 2047
  pancreatic cancer, 2243
  pancreatic disease, 2146-2147
Endoscopy, Plate X-6
  abdominal pain, 2034
  Barrett's esophagus, 2018
  bronchoscopy, 383-384
    acquired immunodeficiency syndrome, 1477
    hemoptysis, 411
    lung cancer, 489-490, 726
    sarcoidosis, 459
    solitary pulmonary nodule, 494
  chronic pancreatitis, 2240
  colonoscopy, 1996
    acute lower gastrointestinal bleeding, 2012
    colonic diverticulum, 2091
    constipation, 2055
    Crohn's disease, 2070
    diarrhea, 1476
    intestinal obstruction, 2078
  esophagogastroduodenoscopy, 1994
  esophagoscopy, 2000
    erosive esophagitis, 2017
    esophageal varices, 2167
    infectious esophagitis, 2020
  fever of unknown origin, 1379
  gastroduodenal diseases, 2002
  gastrointestinal, 1993-1998
  gastrointestinal bleeding, 2011
  gastroscopy, 2041
  intestinal disorders, 2007
  intestinal obstruction, 2078
  pancreatic secretion measurement, 2134
  peptic ulcer, 2037, 2039
  rhinopharyngeal, 1181
  sigmoidoscopy, 1995-1996
    balantidiasis, 1691
    colonic diverticulum, 2091
    constipation, 2055
    Crohn's disease, 2070
    diarrhea, 1476
    intestinal disease, 2007
    preventive care guidelines, 2255
    ulcerative colitis, 2073, Plate X-8
  stomach cancer, 2046

Endothelial-leukocyte adhesion molecule-1, 372
Endothelin
  heart failure, 160
  hypertension, 316, 319
  multiple organ dysfunction syndrome, 421
  vasoactive effects on pulmonary circulation,
    363
Endothelin-1, 1448
Endothelium
  capillary, 348, 371
  hypertension, 318
  injury in ischemic heart disease, 192
  modulation of arterial tone, 47
  pulmonary vasculitides, 453
Endothelium-derived hyperpolarizing factor, 48
Endothelium-derived relaxing factor
  atherosclerosis, 999
  hypertension, 316
  modulation of arterial tone, 48
Endotoxin, 1362-1363, 1446
  inflammatory response, 1448
  Neisseria meningitidis, 1579
Endotracheal intubation
  acute respiratory failure, 416-417
  angioedema, 2306
  mechanical ventilation, 399
  pulmonary edema, 425-426
Energy output, 2113
Enflurane, 2190, 2191
Engelmann's disease, 1959
Engineering controls, 1364-1365
Enhancer, 50, 51
Enoxicin, 636
ENR; *see* Eosinophilic nonallergic rhinitis
Entamoeba coli, 1692
Entamoeba hartmanni, 1692
Entamoeba histolytica, 1681-1683, Plate VIII-52
  acquired immunodeficiency syndrome, 1476
  diarrhea, 1428, 1476
  gay bowel syndrome, 1429
  liver abscess, 2210
  peritonitis, 2248
Enteral nutrition
  acute pancreatitis, 2237
  multiple organ dysfunction syndrome, 422
Enteric cyst, 513
Enteric fever, 1601
Enteric infection, 1425-1432
  bacterial agents, 1425-1427
  diagnosis, 1430-1431
  diarrhea, 1429-1430
  parasitic agents, 1428-1429
  pathophysiology, 1425
  prophylaxis for traveler's diarrhea, 1432
  traveler's risk, 1467, 1469
  treatment, 1431-1432
  viral agents, 1427-1428
Enteric nervous system, 1977, 1981
Enteric protein loss, 2007
Enteritis
  acquired immunodeficiency syndrome, 1476
  Campylobacter, 1591-1592
  fever of unknown origin, 1378
  regional, 2081
  Vibrio, 1596
Enteritis necroticans, 1568
Enterobacteriaceae
  antibiotic selection, 1347
  bacteremia, 1445
  brain abscess, 1414
  folliculitis, 1420
  normal flora, 1368
  Salmonella, 1598-1602
  Shigella, 1602-1604
  susceptibility to empiric antimicrobial therapy,
    1400
  synergistic nonclostridial anaerobic
    myonecrosis, 1424
  urinary tract infection, 1457
Enterobiasis, 1696
Enterobius vermicularis, 2248

Enterochromaffin-like cell, 1981-1982
Enteroclysis, 2007, 2081
Enterococci, 1560-1564
  antibiotic selection, 1347
  endocarditis, 226, 232
  normal flora, 1368
  nosocomial infections, 1362
  resistance to vancomycin, 1346
Enterocolitis
  Campylobacter jejuni, 1591-1592
  nongranulomatous chronic idiopathic, 2064
  Salmonella, 1599-1600
  Yersinia enterocolitica, 1611
Enterocyte, 2057
Enterocytozoon, 1680, 1681
Enterocytozoon bieneusi, 1474, 2095
Enterohepatic circulation, 2149
  bile pigment abnormalities, 2155-2156
  bile salts, 2124-2126
  relationship with low-density lipoprotein
    receptors, 1891
  vitamin D deficiency, 1951
Enteropathic arthritis, 1242
Enteropathic arthropathy, 1245-1246
Enteropathogenic *Escherichia coli,* 1426
Enteropathy, radiation, 2065-2066
Enteroscopy, 1995
Enterotoxigenic *Escherichia coli,* 1426
Enterotoxin
  cholera, 1594
  Clostridium perfringens, 1568
Enterotoxin F, 1362
Enterovirus
  acute hemorrhagic conjunctivitis, 1490
  culture, 1369
  epidemiology, 1484
  hand-foot-mouth syndrome, 1489
  hepatitis A virus, 2173
  pathogenesis, 1485, 1486
  poliomyelitis, 1488
  viral meningitis, 1403-1404
Entomophthoramycosis, 1660
Enuresis, 946
Environmental factors
  interstitial lung disease, 452
  lung cancer, 486
  nosocomial infection, 1363
  systemic lupus erythematosus, 1212
  tumor formation, 548-549
Environmental sleep disorder, 944
Enzymatic disorders
  hematopoietic stem cell transplantation, 576
  hemolytic anemia, 662-664
Enzyme immunoassay, 1372
  adenovirus, 1504
  infectious disease, 1373-1374
  Legionella pneumophila, 1623
  Norwalk virus, 1522
  rotavirus, 1521
Enzyme-linked immunosorbent assay
  Bordetella pertussis, 1612-1613
  Borrelia burgdorferi, 1647
  brucellosis, 1606
  Cryptococcus neoformans, 1668
  detection of autoantibodies, 1156
  Helicobacter pylori, 1592-1593
  hepatitis C, 2175-2176
  human immunodeficiency virus infection,
    1472
  Lassa fever virus, 1510
  measles, 1499
  mumps, 1497
  septic arthritis, 1252
  serum total thyroxine and triiodothyronine
    levels, 1800
  toxoplasmosis, 1678
  venous thromboembolism, 632
Enzyme therapy
  lysosomal storage disease, 1919
  treatment of inherited disorders, 1731

Enzymes
acid-hydrolase, 536
acyl-coarctation of aorta cholesterol
acyltransferase, 2127
adenine phosphoribosyltransferase, 1269
adenosine triphosphatase
heart failure, 159-160
inhibition by digitalis, 173
adenylate cyclase
activation, 1711, 2132
cellular modulation of contractility, 41
signal transduction, 58
thyroid hormone formation and metabolism,
1797
adrenal steroid biosynthesis, 1817
alanine aminotransferase
acetaminophen poisoning, 2190
acute pancreatitis, 2236
chronic hepatitis, 2180
hepatic injury, 2136, 2188
hepatitis A infection, 2173
hepatitis B infection, 2175
alcohol metabolism, 2195
aldolase, 1025
aldolase B, 1880
alkaline phosphatase
acute cholecystitis, 2228
acute pancreatitis, 2236
amebic liver abscess, 2210
bone and mineral disorders, 1744-1745
choledocholithiasis, 2229
hepatitic injury, 2136
hepatocellular *versus* cholestatic jaundice,
2156
human immunodeficiency virus infection,
1473
hypophosphatasia, 1954
lipodystrophy, 1901
liver disease, 2137
osteomalacia, 1949
Paget's disease, 1956
postoperative cholestasis, 2159
primary biliary cirrhosis, 2200
primary sclerosing cholangitis, 2202
renal bone disease, 1964
aminoglycoside-modifying, 1345
aminotransferases
alcoholic hepatitis, 2196
chronic hepatitis, 2180
chronic hepatitis B, 2181
chronic hepatitis C, 2182
hepatitis A, 2173
hepatitis B, 2175
hepatocellular *versus* cholestatic jaundice,
2156
liver disease, 2136-2137
amylase
abdominal pain, 2032
acute pancreatitis, 2144, 2235
hyperamylasemia, 2235
intestinal obstruction, 2078
macroamylasemia, 2144
pancreatic disease, 2144
peritonitis, 2080
urinary, 2145
anti-topoisomerase, 1231
anticholinesterase, 2302
arginase, 1906
argininosuccinate lyase, 1906
argininosuccinate synthetase, 1906
aryl hydrocarbon hydroxylase, 486
asparaginase
effects on kidney, 870
hepatic injury, 2192
aspartate aminotransferase
acetaminophen poisoning, 2190
acute pancreatitis, 2236
chronic hepatitis, 2180
hepatitic injury, 2136
myocardial infarction, 211
toxic hepatic injury, 2188

Enzymes—cont'd
beta-adrenergic receptor kinase, 57-58
bile acid coarctation of aorta ligase, 2125
bile acid S-coarctation of aorta glycine/taurine
N-acyltransferase, 2125
bilirubin-UDP glucuronosyltransferase, 2149,
2151, 2152
C1-alpha-hydroxylase, 1961
calcium-activated calmodulin kinase, 41
carbamoylphosphate synthetase, 1906, 1907
carbonic anhydrase
bicarbonate, 835
deficiency in osteopetrosis, 1958
renal acid excretion, 740
carnitine acyltransferase, 2122
catalase, 2283
catechol-O-methyltransferase, 930, 1826, 1827
cation pump, 58
cholesterol 7α-hydroxylase, 2127
cholesteryl ester hydrolase, 2127
congenital adrenal hyperplasia, 1824-1825
coproporphyrinogen oxidase, 1923
creatine kinase
evaluation of muscle disease, 1025
hypothyroidism, 1809
inflammatory myopathies, 1235
myocardial infarction, 211-212
creatine phosphokinase, 1755
delta-amino-levulinic acid synthase, 1923
deoxyribonucleic acid-dependent ribonucleic
acid polymerase, 1344
deoxyribonucleic acid ligase, 52
deoxyribonucleic acid restriction enzyme, 54
digestive, 2129
disaccharidases, 2068
dopa decarboxylase, 1826
dopamine beta hydroxylase, 930
elastase
acute pancreatitis, 2234
diagnosis of pancreatic diseases, 2144
gram-negative bacilli, 1446
lung damage, 373
pancreatic diseases, 2144
fructokinase, 1879
fructose 1-phosphate aldolase, 1880
functions of minerals, 2109
gamma glutamyltransferase, 2136, 2137
glucose phosphate isomerase, 663
glutathione-S-transferase, 2126, 2128,
2148-2149
gram-negative bacteria, 1447
guanylate cyclase, 1712
heme biosynthesis, 1923
heme oxygenase, 2149
herpes virus thymidine kinase, 555
hexokinase, 663
hypoxanthine-guanine
phosphoribosyltransferase, 1269
Janus kinases, 1131-1132
lactate dehydrogenase
amebic liver abscess, 2210
ascites, 2164
beta-thalassemia, 655
hemolytic anemia, 661
hereditary spherocytosis, 665
human immunodeficiency virus infection,
1473
myocardial infarction, 211
non-Hodgkin's lymphoma, 698
overproduction jaundice, 2152
prosthetic valve problems, 258
lecithin-cholesterol acetyltransferase, 60, 1898,
2121
leucine aminopeptidase, 2137
leukocyte esterase, 1458
lipase
abdominal pain, 2032
acute pancreatitis, 2234, 2235
gastric, 1986
intestinal obstruction, 2078
pancreatic disease, 2144

Enzymes—cont'd
lipoprotein metabolism, 1898, 2121
lysosomal, 1911
macroenzyme, 2137
malonyl-coenzyme A, 1851, 1863, 2122
mast cell, 1142
myophosphorylase deficiency, 1025, 1029
ornithine transcarbamoylase deficiency, 1907
pancreatic
assessment of pancreatic disease, 2144
chronic pancreatitis, 2240, 2241
cystic fibrosis, 2246
parietal cell hydrogen-potassium-ATPase,
1983, 1984
peptidases, 1988
phenylethanolamine N-methyltransferase,
1826, 1827
phosphoglycerate kinase, 663
polymorphonuclear elastase, 2144, 2145
porphobilinogen deaminase, 1926
propionyl-CoA carboxylase, 1908
prostatic acid phosphatase, 718
protein kinase
mitogen-activated, 541
myotonic muscular dystrophy, 62
protein kinase A
pancreatic acinar cell secretions, 2132
regulation, 57
protein kinase C, 1712
protoporphyrinogen oxidase, 1923
pyrimidine-5′ nucleotidase, 663
pyruvate dehydrogenase, 1851
pyruvate kinase
deficiency, 664
hemolytic anemia, 663
replication of DNA, 1721-1722
ribonuclease, 2144
ribonucleic acid polymerase, 50
serine proteases, 442
serine-threonine kinases, 542
11-β-Steroid dehydrogenase, 1819
sterol metabolism, 1898
synthesis in liver, 2118
Taq polymerase, 55
triose phosphate isomerase, 663
tyrosine aminotransferase deficiency,
1905-1906
urea cycle, 1906
urease
breath urea test, 2003
pyelonephritis, 1456
uridine diphosphate glucuronosyltransferase,
2128
uridine-glucose-galactose-1-phosphate-
uridylyltransferase, 1882-1883
urokinase
activation of plasminogen to plasmin, 540
deep venous thrombosis, 311
myocardial infarction, 213
pulmonary embolism, 503
venous thromboembolism, 637
uroporphyrinogen decarboxylase, 1923
vasopressinase, 808, 1791
virilization at puberty, 1844
Eosinophil, 1109, 1341-1342
abnormalities, 680-681
asthma, 1185, 1186
Churg-Strauss syndrome, 466-467
sputum examination, 380
Eosinophil chemotactic factors, 1140
Eosinophilia, 591, 680-681, 744
after international travel, 1469
asthma, 1188
causes, 1342
echinococcal cyst, 2111
eosinophilic enteritis, 2067
eosinophilic gastritis, 2043
intestinal disease, 2005
parasite-induced, 1705-1706
tropical pulmonary eosinophilia, 1701
tubulointerstitial disease, 888

Eosinophilia-myalgia syndrome, 681, 1234
Eosinophilic fasciitis, 1231, 1233-1234
Eosinophilic gastritis, 2043
Eosinophilic gastroenteritis, 2066-2067
Eosinophilic granuloma, 463-465
Eosinophilic granulomatous vasculitis, 465-467
Eosinophilic nonallergic rhinitis, 1181, 1183
Eosinophilic pneumonia, 455
Eosinophilic pneumonitis, 477
Ependymoma, 1070
Ephedrine, 1740
EPIC trial, 121, 124
Epidemic pleurodynia, 1489
Epidemiologic research, 2267
Epidermal growth factor, 1131, 1720
Epidermoid carcinoma, 487
Epidermolysis bullosa acquista, 1296
Epidermophyton, 1307-1308
Epididymitis, 1444
Epidural abscess, 1013
    intracranial, 1418
    sinusitis, 2309
    spinal, 1418-1419
Epidural block, 581
Epidural hematoma, 1043, 1044, 1045
Epigastric pain
    acute pancreatitis, 2233
    appendicitis, 2092
    choledochal cyst, 2212
    gastric cancer, 2046
    granulomatous gastritis, 2043
    peptic ulcer disease, 2039
Epigastric reflex, 964
Epiglottitis, 1393-1394
    emergency management, 2306
    Haemophilus influenzae, 1586, 1588
Epilepsy, 978-985
    anticonvulsant-induced osteomalacia, 1953
    clinical seizure patterns, 979-980
    diagnosis and laboratory evaluation, 980-982
    electroencephalography, 906-907
    etiology, 980
    pathophysiology, 978-979
    posttraumatic, 1045
    during pregnancy, 2281
    psychologic issues and behavior changes,
        984-985
    syncope *versus,* 954
    treatment, 982-984
Epileptogenic focus, 979
EPILOG study, 121
Epimastigote, 1688
Epinephrine, 56, 930
    anaphylaxis, 1193-1194
    angioedema, 2306
    asthma, 1190
    biosynthesis and metabolism, 1826-1827
    effects on potassium transport, 741
    glaucoma, 2302
    glucose production, 1874, 1875
    hypertension, 316
    normal plasma levels, 1827
    shock, 180-181
Epiphyseal plate, 1716
Epirubicin
    cardiotoxicity, 584
    pancreatic cancer, 2243
Episcleritis, 1204
Epistaxis, 286, 2308
Epitaxial nucleation, 797
Epithelial dysplasia, 2076
Epithelial hyperplasia of esophagus, 2016
Epithelial membrane antigen, 731
Epithelioid angiomatosis, 1423
Epithelioid granuloma, 456-457, 470
Epithelium
    airway, 365
    alveolar, 348, 371
    Barrett's esophagus, 2016
    bile water production, 2123
    interstitial lung disease, 450

Epitope, 1110
Epitrochlear nodes, 598
Epivir; *see* Lamivudine
Epoxy resin lung, 460
Epsilon-aminocaproic acid, 638
Epsilon-globin chain, 651
Epsilon heavy chain, 1123
Epstein-Barr virus, 1529-1530
    acquired immunodeficiency syndrome, 1328
    acute hepatitis, 2138
    acute interstitial nephritis, 889
    aplastic anemia, 672
    Burkitt's lymphoma, 695
    carcinogenesis, 548
    fever of unknown origin, 1377
    Hodgkin's disease, 691
    infectious mononucleosis, 1393
    pericarditis, 272
    posttransplant
        cardiac, 1090-1091
        lung, 519
        renal, 795
    Sjögren syndrome, 1210
Epstein syndrome, 603
Equilibrium radionuclide method, 104
Erb's muscular dystrophy, 1026-1027, 1028,
        1086
ERCP; *see* Endoscopic retrograde
        cholangiopancreatography
Ergocalciferol, 1719
Ergonovine, 200
Ergotamine tartrate, 961-962
Erosio interdigitalis blastomycetica, 1662
Erosive esophagitis, 2017
Erosive osteoarthritis, 1266
Eruptive xanthoma, Plate VII-18
Erysipelas, 1420, 1556, Plate VIII-25
Erysipeloid, 1423
Erythema
    genital lesions, 1442
    hand-foot-mouth syndrome, 1489
    insulin allergy, 1861
    rheumatoid arthritis, 1202
    scarlet fever, 1421
    staphylococcal scalded-skin syndrome, 1421
    streptococcal cellulitis, 1556
    systemic lupus erythematosus, 1213
Erythema gyratum repens, 1317, 1318
Erythema infectiosum, 1384
    parvovirus B19 infection, 1513
    during pregnancy, 2280
Erythema marginatum, 1384
    rheumatic fever, 1257, 1559
Erythema migrans, 1254, 1384, 1646
Erythema multiforme, 1384
    drug-induced, 1313
    paraneoplastic pemphigus, 1295
Erythema nodosum, 1245, Plate VII-12
    Behçet disease, 1243
    cutaneous findings, 1321
    drug-induced, 1313
    inflammatory bowel disease, 2075
Erythema nodosum leprosum, 1650
Erythematous maculopapular reaction,
        1306-1307
Erythrasma, 1422
Erythritol tetranitrate, 201, 202
Erythrocyte, 531, Plate IV-4
    abnormalities in intestinal disorders, 2005
    automated blood cell analysis, 555-556
    babesiosis, 1676
    chronic myeloproliferative disorders, 686
    Doppler effect, 97
    examination of peripheral blood smear,
        556-557
    flow cytometry, 558
    gas transfer, 348
    hemolytic anemia, 661-671
        acquired, 666-668
        drug-induced, 670
        hereditary, 662-666

Erythrocyte—cont'd
    hemolytic anemia—cont'd
        homozygous beta thalassemia, 654
        immune, 668-670
        patient evaluation, 661-662
        splenomegaly, 601
        thrombotic thrombocytopenic purpura, 615
    hemostatic defects in liver disease, 627
    life span, 642
    malaria, 1672
    megaloblastic anemia, 648
    membrane defects, 664-666
    nucleated, 595-596
    polycythemia
        Budd-Chiari syndrome, 2208
        high hematocrit, 588-590
        neutrophilic leukocytosis, 591
        RBC mass, 586
        tetralogy of Fallot, 289
    polycythemia vera, 688
    processing of immune complexes, 1137
    prosthetic heart valve, 258
    pure red blood cell aplasia, 674-675
    unconjugated hyperbilirubinemia, 2150
    urinalysis, 744
    venous thrombus, 631
Erythrocyte fragmentation syndromes, 666-667
Erythrocyte protoporphyrin, 643
Erythrocyte sedimentation rate
    acute pericarditis, 274
    ankylosing spondylitis, 1238
    brain abscess, 1415
    Churg-Strauss syndrome, 465
    giant-cell arteritis, 304
    headache, 961
    infective endocarditis, 228
    myxoma, 330
    osteomyelitis, 1434
    rheumatic fever, 1257
    rheumatoid arthritis, 1205
    spinal epidural abscess, 1418
    subdural empyema, 1417
Erythrocytosis, 443
Erythroderma
    drug-induced, 1314
    psoriasis, 1301
    toxic shock syndrome, 1383, 1421
Erythrohepatic porphyria, 1925-1926
Erythroid precursor, 530, Plate IV-3
Erythromycin, 1357-1358
    acne vulgaris, 1305
    antimicrobial mechanisms, 1344
    bacillary angiomatosis, 1474
    Campylobacter enteritis, 1592
    campylobacteriosis, 1432
    chlamydial infection, 1537
    diphtheria, 1567
    dosage, 1350
    effects on kidney, 868
    enterococci resistance, 1561
    erythrasma, 1422
    Haemophilus ducreyi, 1589
    Helicobacter pylori, 1593
    hepatic injury, 2191
    human cytochrome P450 isoforms, 2312
    infective endocarditis prophylaxis, 234
    interaction with cyclosporin, 793
    interference with oral anticoagulants, 636
    intestinal pseudoobstruction, 2079
    Legionella pneumophila, 1624
    Lyme disease, 1647
    Mycoplasma pneumoniae pneumonia, 1540
    pertussis, 1613
    reaction with antiarrhythmics, 136-137
    relapsing fever, 1646
    streptococcal resistance, 1559
    urethritis, 1441
    use during pregnancy, 2281
Erythrophagocytosis, 662
Erythroplakia, 722, 2309, Plate IV-13

Erythropoiesis, 531
  hemochromatosis, 646, 2205
  ineffective, 646, 2152
  iron-deficient, 644
  iron for, 642
  sideroblastic anemia, 645
Erythropoietic protoporphyria, 1306, 1925-1926, 2152
Erythropoietin, 532-533, 1129
  anemia therapy, 534
  dialysis, 790
  nephrotic syndrome, 765
  production of red blood cells, 586
  secondary polycythemia, 588
Escape beat, 132
Escape phenomenon, 1718
Escape rhythm, 132
Eschar, 1422
Escherichia coli
  antibiotic selection, 1347
  attachment mechanisms, 1446
  bacteremia, 1445
  bacterial meningitis, 1403
  brown pigment stones, 2224
  diarrhea, 1426
  empyema, 507
  nosocomial infections, 1362
  osteomyelitis, 1433
  primary peritonitis, 1396
  sickle cell disease, 658
  spinal epidural abscess, 1418
  spontaneous bacterial peritonitis, 2164
  susceptibility to empiric antimicrobial therapy, 1400
  synergistic nonclostridial anaerobic myonecrosis, 1424
  urinary tract infection, 1457
Esidrix; *see* Hydrochlorothiazide
Esmolol
  angina, 207
  arrhythmias, 138
  atrial fibrillation in myocardial infarction, 223
  hypertensive emergency, 328
  properties, 203
Esophageal colic, 1999
Esophageal dysphagia, 1998
Esophageal endoscopy, 2000
Esophageal manometry, 2000-2001, 2022
Esophageal pH, 2015
Esophageal pressure, 358
Esophageal ring, 2020
Esophageal spasm, 128, 2022-2023
Esophageal stretch, 1999
Esophageal varices
  portal hypertension, 2166
  treatment, 2013-2014
Esophageal web, 1999, 2020
Esophagitis, 2014
  acquired immunodeficiency syndrome, 1474
  heartburn *versus,* 1999
  reflux and regurgitation, 1998, Plate X-1
Esophagogastroduodenoscopy, 1994
Esophagoscopy, 2000
Esophagus, 2014-2024
  achalasia, 2021-2022
  benign tumors, 2023
  cancer, 2023-2024
  cardiac imaging, 95-97
  chemical and physical injury, 2018-2019
  endoscopic examination, 1994
  erosion, 2015-2016
  esophageal spasm, 2022-2023
  esophagitis, 2014
    acquired immunodeficiency syndrome, 1474
    heartburn *versus,* 1999
    reflux and regurgitation, 1998, Plate X-1
  evaluation, 1998-2002
  gastroesophageal reflux, 2014-2018
  infectious esophagitis, 2019-2020
  movement of food, 1978

Esophagus—cont'd
  rupture, 128
    pleural effusion, 508
    thoracentesis, 382
    traumatic pneumomediastinum, 514
  stricture, 1994, 1999-2000, 2018
  systemic sclerosis, 1229
  thrush, 1661
  ulcer, 2095
  webs, rings, and diverticula, 2020-2021
  weight loss, 1749
Espundia, 1687
ESRD; *see* End-stage renal disease
Essential fructosuria, 1879
Essential hypertension; *see* Hypertension
Essential light chain, 39
Essential mixed cryoglobulinemia, 857-858
Essential myoclonus, 996
Essential thrombocythemia, 557, 687-688
Essential tremor, 994
Esterification, 2121
Esterified cholesterol, 2127
Estimated operative risk, 2256-2257
Estradiol
  chronic hepatic failure, 2171
  evaluation of ovarian secretory capacity, 1742
  feedback effects, 1834
  gonadotropin secretion, 1714
  measurement, 1835
  normal levels, 1836
  osteoporotic fractures, 1948
  puberty, 1766
  testing for male gonadal function, 1742
  testosterone aromatization, 1839
Estriol, 2171
Estrogen
  breast cancer, 708, 709-710
  calcium homeostasis, 1720
  cholestasis, 2158
  cirrhosis patient, 2171
  decreased bone mass, 1946
  deficiency in menopause, 1833
  feedback inhibition tests, 1736
  gynecomastia, 1764
  hepatic metabolism, 2122-2123
  medication-induced hypercalcemia, 1928
  menopause, 2271
  porphyria cutanea tarda, 1927
  puberty, 1767
  thyroxine-binding globulin levels, 1803
Estrogen therapy
  acne vulgaris, 1305
  gallstone risk factor, 2223
  hypopituitarism, 1780-1781
  osteoporotic fractures, 1948
Estrone, 2171
Ethacrynic acid
  cause of renal potassium wasting and alkalosis, 828
  heart failure, 170
  hyperkalemia, 833
Ethambutol
  mycobacterial disease, 1631
  Mycobacterium avium-intracellulare complex, 1474
  tuberculosis, 1474
  tuberculous meningitis, 1412
Ethanol
  alcohol-tobacco amblyopia, 1081
  arrhythmia, 133
  atrial fibrillation, 146
  bleeding time, 612
  cancer risk, 550
  carcinogenesis, 548
  cytochrome P450 2E1, 2311
  dilated cardiomyopathy, 265
  drug-nutrient interactions, 2110
  effects on lipoproteins, 1890
  esophageal cancer, 2023
  human cytochrome P450 isoforms, 2312
  hypertension, 318, 319, 324

Ethanol—cont'd
  inhibition of folate metabolism, 647
  interference with catecholamine assays, 1740
  interference with oral anticoagulants, 636
  medical interview of usage, 3-4
  metabolic disorders, 1080-1081
  metabolism, 2194-2195
  mood disorders, 1036
  myopathy, 1030
  nausea and vomiting, 2026
  neuropathy, 1019
  nutritional interactions, 2195
  personality disorders, 1039
  risk of falls, 2290
  sideroblastic anemia, 645
  sleep disorders, 945
  withdrawal, 1080-1081, 2295-2296
    seizure, 982
    sympathetic nervous system overactivity, 934-935
Ethics, 9-13
Ethidium bromide stain, 51
Ethinyl estradiol, 710
Ethionamide
  leprosy, 1651
  mycobacterial disease, 1631
  tuberculous meningitis, 1412
Ethmoiditis, 2309
Ethmozine; *see* Moricizine
Ethopropazine, 992
Ethosuximide, 983
Ethyl alcohol, 866
Ethylene dichloride, 866
Ethylene glycol, 837, 866
Ethylene oxide, 1020
Ethylenediamine tetraacetic acid
  blood culture anticoagulant, 1373
  coagulation assays, 570
  lead mobilization test, 867
  thrombocytopenia, 613
Etidronate
  heterotopic ossification, 1051
  hypercalcemia, 1929, 1974
  Paget's disease, 1957
Etodolac, 1259
Etoposide
  hepatic injury, 2192
  lung cancer, 728
  non-Hodgkin's lymphoma, 699
  testicular cancer, 721
Etretinate
  hepatic injury, 2192
  psoriasis, 1301, 1302
Eubacterium, 1368
Euglobulin, 567
Eugonadotropic disorders, 1845
Eumycetoma, 1660
Eunuchoidism, hypogonadotropic, 1841-1842
Eustachian tube dysfunction, 2307
Euthyroid goiter, 1812-1813
Euthyroid hyperthyroxinemia, 1803, 1804
Euthyroid hypothyroxinemia, 1804
Euthyroid sick syndrome, 1801, 1802-1803
Evans's syndrome, 616
Event monitor, 94
Event recorder, 134
Evidence-based guidelines, 24
Evoked responses, 908-914, 1009
Ewart's sign, 274
Ewing's sarcoma, 731
Exanthem
  chickenpox, 1525
  Colorado tick fever, 1512
  dengue fever, 1465
  dermatomyositis, 1235
  differential diagnostic value, 1384-1385
  disseminated gonococcal infection, 1583
  drug-induced, 1313-1314
  fever with, 1380-1386
  glucagonoma, 2245
  graft-*versus*-host disease, 578

Exanthem—cont'd
Hartnup disease, 879, 1910, 1911
herpangina, 1488
hookworm, 1698
hypersensitivity vasculitis, 1221
Lassa fever, 1510
lymphomatoid granulomatosis, 470
meningococcal infection, 1406
meningococcemia, 1579
myxoma, 330
parvovirus B19 infection, 1513
photodermatosis, 1306-1307
relapsing fever, 1645
Rocky Mountain spotted fever, 1543
rubella, 1501
scarlet fever, 1421
syphilis, 1641
toxic shock syndrome, 1421
trimethoprim-sulfamethoxazole-induced, Plate
VII-13
typhoid fever, 1601
vasculitis, 1225
VIPoma, 2245
viral, 1489
Excess blasts, 676
Excess dietary protein, 2160
Excessive daytime sleepiness, 940, 942-943
Exchange lists, 1857
Excitation-contraction coupling system, 38-39
Excitation system, 37-38
Exclusive contract, 33
Exercise
after cardiac transplantation, 343
aortic regurgitation, 241
during bed rest, 2288
cardiovascular response, 49
chronic fatigue syndrome, 2300
chronic obstructive pulmonary disease, 445
coronary blood flow, 194
effect on vasopressin release, 1791
heart failure, 164
hypertension management, 324
increased bone mass in postmenopausal
women, 1947
increased potassium loss from cells, 831
increased skeletal muscle blood flow, 46
intermittent claudication, 308-309
ischemic heart disease, 200
neutrophilia, 590
obesity, 2104
palpitations, 130
pulmonary rehabilitation, 435-436
rheumatoid arthritis, 1206-1207
rhinitis therapy, 1182
silent myocardial ischemia, 194
Exercise-induced disorders
anaphylaxis, 1193
asthma, 1187
hypoxemia, 450
proteinuria, 760
Exercise testing, 91-94
aortic regurgitation, 242
aortic stenosis, 238
clinical applications, 93-94
heart failure, 166-167
ischemic heart disease, 197-198
mitral valve prolapse, 254
myocardial perfusion imaging with, 101
physiology, 91
preoperative, 2258
procedures, 93
pulmonary function, 379-380
risk stratification, 224
technical aspects, 93
Exertional angina, 194
Exfoliative dermatitis, 1314
Exocrine glands
pancreas, 2131-2133
Sjögren syndrome, 1210
Exocrine stomach, 1981
Exocytosis, 1713

Exon, 1708-1709, 1721
Exophthalmos, 1805-1806
Exotoxin
bullous impetigo, 1419
nosocomial infections, 1362
staphylococcal scalded-skin syndrome, 1421
Yersinia pestis, 1609-1610
Exotoxin A, 1362, 1446
Expectoration, 408
Experimental autoimmune myasthenia gravis,
1021
Experimental tolerance, 1143-1145
Expiration-inspiration ratio, 937
Explicit approach to developing guidelines, 24
Exploratory laparotomy, 2034
Exposure
chemical
acute toxic, 473
aplastic anemia, 672
asbestos, 474
cadmium, 891
carcinogenesis, 868
esophageal injury, 2018-2019
hemoglobinuria, 867-868
hemolytic anemia, 667
hepatic injury, 2187-2193
occupational asthma, 472
cold, 126
irritant contact dermatitis, 1303
occupational lung diseases, 471
radiation, 868, 892
Expressivity, 1721
Exserohilum, 1660
Extensor finger and hand jerk, 964
External dysuria, 762
External pulsatile ventricular assist device, 185,
186
Exteroceptive reflex, 964
Exton's test, 567
Extracellular fluid
arginine vasopressin, 808, 809
calcium in, 1717
interstitial and plasma components, 805
ionic composition, 736
potassium, 825
principles of osmoregulation, 805-806
Extracellular fluid volume, 816
aging and, 2284
hypernatremic states, 813-814
Extracellular matrix
diabetes mellitus, 860-861
lung, 371
proteoglycans, 1289
Extracellular pathogens, 1334
Extracorporeal shock wave lithotripsy, 803
common bile duct stones, 2230
gallstones, 2226-2227
Extractable nuclear antigens, 1159
Extrahepatic bile ducts, 2232-2233
Extrahepatic cholestasis, 2155
Extrahepatic ductal system, 2199
Extramedullary hematopoiesis, 1103
Extramedullary plasmacytoma, 703
Extraocular muscles
diabetic mononeuropathy, 1872
pituitary apoplexy, 1778
Extrapulmonary tuberculosis, 1633-1637
Extrarenal sodium depletion, 823
Extreme axis deviation, 85
Extreme lyonization, 619
Extrinsic allergic alveolitis, 460
Extrinsic coagulation pathway, 537
Extrinsic sleep disorders, 944-945
Exudate
acute hypertensive retinopathy, 2302-2303
acute pericarditis, 274
acute pharyngitis, 1393
bacterial meningitis, 1405
diabetic retinopathy, Plate IX-3
gastrointestinal tuberculosis, 1636
macular star, Plate XI-5

Exudate—cont'd
peritonitis, 2080
pleural disease, 507-508
pleural effusion, 506
pleural fluid classification, 382
Eye, 2300-2306
Acanthamoeba infection, 1684
acquired immunodeficiency syndrome,
2304-2306
acute hemorrhagic conjunctivitis, 1490
age-related macular degeneration, 2301-2302
candidal endophthalmitis, 1662
cataracts, 2301
diabetes mellitus, 1871
galactosemia, 1883
Chlamydia trachomatis, 1536
conjunctivitis
acute hemorrhagic, 1490
adenovirus, 1504
American trypanosomiasis, 1690
Chlamydia trachomatis, 1536
Kawasaki's disease, 1225
measles, 1498
staphylococcal toxic shock syndrome,
1421
trachoma, 1535
tularemia, 1608
diabetic retinopathy, 1870-1871, 2303-2304
exudative, Plate IX-3
hemorrhagic, Plate IX-2
microvascular abnormalities and venous
beading, Plate XI-7
neovascularization of optic nerve, Plate
XI-8
proliferative, Plate IX-4
Ehlers-Danlos syndromes, 1287, 1288
glaucoma, 2301, 2302
Graves' disease, 1805-1806
herpes keratitis, 1524
Hurler's syndrome, 1912
hypertensive retinopathy, 2302-2303
hypothyroidism, 1809
immunologically privileged site, 1145
keratoconjunctivitis sicca
human immunodeficiency virus-infected
patients, 2306
Sjögren syndrome, 1209-1212
Marfan syndrome, 1289
movements after cardiac arrest, 1088
neurofibromatosis, 1920-1921
neurologic disorders, 1056-1065
abnormalities of vision, 1056-1057
disturbances of conjugate eye movements,
1063-1065
eye movement abnormalities, 1062-1063
ocular vascular disease, 1057-1062
Niemann-Pick disease, 1918
Paget's disease, 1955
presbyopia, 2301
pseudoxanthoma elasticum, 1289
retinal venoocclusive disease, 2304
rheumatoid arthritis, 1204
riboflavin deficiency, 2106
sarcoidosis, 458
Sjögren syndrome, 1209-1212
syphilis, 1642
toxoplasmosis, 1677
trachoma, 1535-1536
tuberous sclerosis, 1922
tularemia, 1608
visual loss, 2300-2301
vitamin A deficiency, 2105-2106
Vittaforma infection, 1681
von Hippel-Lindau disease, 1922, 1923
Wegener's granulomatosis, 468
Eyeworm, 1700
Eysenck Personality Inventory, 903
Ezymes
tyrosine aminotransferase deficiency,
1905-1906

F

F-actin, 1027, 1157
F wave, 915, 916
¹8F,2-fluoro-2-deoxyglucose, 105-106
Fab fragment, 1110, 1122
Fabry's disease, 1918-1919
Face mask, intermittent positive-pressure
    breathing, 430
Facial flushing
  autonomic overactivity, 934
  calcium channel blocker-induced, 205
  carcinoid syndrome, 2082
  human immunodeficiency virus infection,
    1327
  mitral stenosis, 245
  VIPoma, 2245
Facial nerve paralysis, 2306
Facial pain, 962-963
Facies
  mucopolysaccharidosis, 1912
  pseudohypoparathyroidism, 1932, 1933
Facilitated diffusion, 1986
Facioscapulohumeral dystrophy, 1027, 1086
Factitious illness, 1040
  fever, 1375-1376
  gastrointestinal bleeding, 2014
  thyrotoxicosis, 1807
Factor deficiencies, 624
Factor H, 1135
  deficiency, 1180
Factor I, 537-539, 1135
  abnormalities, 625
  chronic renal failure, 783
  congenital disorders of blood coagulation, 618
  deficiency, 1180
  hereditary amyloidosis, 1285
  plasma, 571
  platelet aggregation, 611
  prothrombin time, 2135
  replacement for hypofibrinogenemia, 573
  serum protein electrophoresis, 565
  synthesis, 2120
Factor II, 538
  congenital disorders of blood coagulation, 618
  deficiency, 624
  hypoprothrombinemia, 1104, 2106
  prothrombin time, 2135
  synthesis, 2120
  vitamin K defects, 2005
Factor IX, 538
  assay, 606
  congenital disorders of blood coagulation, 618
  hemophilia B, 622
  sources, 621
  synthesis, 2120
  vitamin K defects, 2005
Factor IX concentrates, 622
Factor V, 538
  congenital disorders of blood coagulation, 618
  deficiency, 624
  mutant, 609
  prothrombin time, 2135
  shock states, 176
  venous thrombus, 631
Factor VII, 538
  congenital disorders of blood coagulation, 618
  deficiency, 624
  Dubin-Johnson syndrome, 2157
  prothrombin time, 2135
  shock states, 176
  synthesis, 2120
  vitamin K defects, 2005
Factor VIII, 538
  activities, 618
  assay, 606
  chronic renal failure, 783
  congenital disorders of blood coagulation, 618
  hemophilia A, 617-618
  molecular defects, 618-619
  sources, 621
  venous thromboembolism, 632

Factor VIII—cont'd
  von Willebrand factor and, 622
  von Willebrand's disease, 604
Factor VIII concentrate, 621
Factor VIII inhibitors, 628-629
Factor VIII procoagulant antigen, 618
Factor X, 538
  activation, 537
  congenital disorders of blood coagulation, 618
  deficiency, 624
  prothrombin time, 2135
  synthesis, 2120
  vitamin K defects, 2005
Factor Xa, 537
Factor XI, 538
  congenital disorders of blood coagulation, 618
  deficiency, 624
  sepsis syndrome, 1448
Factor XII
  congenital disorders of blood coagulation, 618
  deficiency, 624
  lung damage, 373
  sepsis syndrome, 1448
Factor XIII, 538
  congenital disorders of blood coagulation, 618
  deficiency, 624
Factor XIII zymogen, 539
Factor XIIIa, 539
Facultative anaerobic bacteria
  bacterial synergy, 1616
  enterococci, 1560-1564
    antibiotic selection, 1347
    normal flora, 1368
    nosocomial infections, 1362
    resistance to vancomycin, 1346
  Haemophilus, 1585-1590
    acquired immunodeficiency syndrome, 1329
    antibiotic selection, 1347
    bacterial meningitis, 1402-1403
    chronic bronchitis, 443
    clinical diseases, 1586-1589
    cystic fibrosis airway infection, 480
    epidemiology, 1586
    epiglottitis, 1393
    erysipelas, 1420
    normal flora, 1368
    osteomyelitis, 1433
    respiratory tract infection, 1390
    septic arthritis, 1251
    sickle cell disease, 658
    sinusitis, 1183
    subdural empyema, 1417
Failure of diagnosis, 2034
Faintness, 952-957
Falls, elderly, 2289-2290, 2291
False aneurysm, 333
False-negative results, 6, 7
False-positive results, 6, 7
Famiciclovir, 1526
Familial adenomatous polyposis, 1319, 2081
Familial autoimmune endocrine deficiency
    syndrome, 1846
Familial benign essential hematuria, 877
Familial cholestatic syndromes, 2158-2159
Familial combined hyperlipidemia, 60, 1896
Familial dysalbuminemic hyperthyroxinemia,
    1803
Familial dysbetalipoproteinemia, 1898
Familial hypercholesterolemia, 60, 1894
Familial hypertriglyceridemia, 1895
Familial hypertrophic cardiomyopathy, 61-62,
    265
Familial hypocalciuric hypercalcemia, 1928,
    1969
  hypermagnesemia, 1943
  urine calcium, 1744
Familial hypoparathyroidism, 1931
Familial idiopathic dilated cardiomyopathy,
    61-62
Familial iminoglycinuria, 1910-1911
Familial lipoatrophic diabetes, 1902-1903

Familial lipodystrophy, 1752
Familial Mediterranean fever
  abdominal pain, 2031
  arthropathy, 1242-1244
  fever of unknown origin, 1378
  peritonitis, 2249
  reactive amyloidosis, 1283
  renal involvement, 877
Familial nephrogenic diabetes insipidus, 883-884
Familial polyposis coli, 2083
Familial short stature, 1769
Familial tall stature, 1769
Family history
  arrhythmia, 133
  breast cancer, 706
  estrogen-related cholestasis, 2158
  psoriasis, 1300
  respiratory disease, 402
  substance abuse, 2294
Famotidine
  gastroesophageal reflux, 2018
  interference with oral anticoagulants, 636
Famoxitine, 2191
Fanconi's anemia, 549, 672
Fanconi's syndrome
  aminoaciduria, 879
  chronic lead nephropathy *versus,* 867
  multiple myeloma, 864
  proximal tubule abnormalities, 747
  proximal tubule defect, 837
  renal tubular transport defects, 881-882
Farber lipogranulomatosis, 1918
Farmer's lung, 460
Fas ligand, 1128, 1144
Fas protein, 1144-1145
Fascicular block, 86-87
Fasciculations, 916
Fasciitis
  clostridial, 1575
  eosinophilic, 1233-1234
  necrotizing, 1422
Fasciola hepatica, 1703-1704, 2231
Fasciolopsis buski, 1697-1698
Fasting
  effect on diarrhea, 2006
  effect on serum bilirubin, 2153-2154
  gluconeogenesis, 2122
  glucose homeostasis during, 1852
  obesity, 2103-2104
  pancreatic exocrine secretion, 2133
  serum gastrin levels, 2003
Fasting hyperglycemia, 1860
Fasting hypoglycemia, 1875, 1876, 1877, 1878
Fasting serum phosphate level, 1934
Fat
  cystic fibrosis diagnosis, 481-482
  dietary, 1986
  fecal, 2058
  malabsorption, 2060
  puberty, 1768
  urinary, 745, 746
Fat embolism, 658
Fat emulsion, 2113
Fat necrosis, 2234, 2237
Fat-soluble vitamins, 2060
Fatigue, 1753
  acute lung allograft rejection, 521
  acute lymphoblastic leukemia, 682
  aldosterone excess, 1822
  aplastic anemia, 672
  atrial septal defect, 281
  benign recurrent intrahepatic cholestasis, 2158
  cardiac tamponade, 275
  chronic fatigue syndrome, 2298-2300
  chronic hepatitis, 2180
  chronic hepatitis B, 2181
  chronic hepatitis C, 2182
  coarctation of aorta, 286
  constrictive pericarditis, 277
  diabetes insipidus, 1793
  giant-cell arteritis, 304

Fatigue—cont'd
 heart failure, 164
 hepatitis A virus, 2173
 hepatocellular carcinoma, 2213
 hypothyroidism, 334
 infectious mononucleosis, 1529
 insulin-dependent diabetes mellitus, 1854
 intrahepatic cholangiocarcinoma, 2214
 macroglobulinemia, 704
 mitral stenosis, 246
 mitral valve prolapse, 254
 multiple sclerosis, 1008
 myxoma, 330
 pheochromocytoma, 1829
 primary biliary cirrhosis, 2200
 primary sclerosing cholangitis, 2201
 prolactin-secreting pituitary adenoma, 1786
 pulmonic stenosis, 288
 pyogenic liver abscess, 2209
 sarcoidosis, 458
 ulcerative colitis, 2073
Fatty acids, 1883-1884
 cholecystokinin stimulation, 2133
 deficiency in total parenteral nutrition, 2113,
  2114
 hepatic encephalopathy, 2161, 2162
 metabolism
  during fasting, 1852-1853
  hepatic, 2121
  intestinal, 1987
  myocardial energy, 40
 synthesis, 1851
Faucial diphtheria, 1566
Fazio-Londe disease, 1015
Fc fragment, 1110, 1122
FDG; *see* ¹8F,2-fluoro-2-deoxyglucose
Febrile seizure, 982
Fecal chymotrypsin assay, 2145
Fecal incontinence
 anal fissure and fistula, 2093
 Hirshsprung's disease, 1980
Fecal leukocyte test, 1430-1431
Feces
 bile acid excretion, 2125
 bilirubin excretion, 2150
 hepatitis A virus, 2173
 increased fecal bile salt loss, 2129
Fed pattern, 1979
Fee-for-service, 30
Feedback, physician performance data, 21-22
Feedback regulation
 cortisol, 1817-1818
 gastrin secretion, 1982
 hormone secretion, 1714
 ovarian function, 1833, 1834-1835
Feeding center, 2099
Feeding disorders, 1077-1078
Feeding tube, 1995
Felbamate, 2191
Felodipine
 angina, 203
 human cytochrome P450 isoforms, 2312
 hypertension, 325
 interference with oral anticoagulants, 636
 properties, 204
Felty's syndrome
 neutropenia, 593, 679
 rheumatoid arthritis, 1205
 splenomegaly, 601
Female, 2267-2272
 breast cancer, 706-713
  axillary nodal metastases, 732
  hypercalcemia of malignancy, 1973
  screening, 25, 552
  second malignancy, 586
  supraclavicular lymphadenopathy, 598
 cervical cancer, 714-715
 cervicitis, 1441-1442
 Chlamydia trachomatis, 1536
 contraception, 2269-2270
 coronary artery disease, 2271-2272

Female—cont'd
 dysuria, 762-763
 endometrial cancer, 713-714
 examination for sexually transmitted disease,
  1439
 gonadal function testing, 1742-1743
 gonococcal infection, 1583
 height and weight table, 2112
 hypertension, 313
 mean heights and weights and recommended
  energy intake, 2117
 menopause, 2270-2271
 ovarian cancer, 715-716
  carcinoid tumor, 2082
  peritoneal carcinomatosis, 732
 pelvic inflammatory disease, 1583
 recommended daily dietary allowances,
  2114-2115, 2116
 secondary sexual development, 1771
 sterilization, 2269-2270
 violence against women, 2268-2269
Feminization
 chronic hepatic failure, 2171-2172
 Cushing's syndrome, 1820
Femoral artery aneurysm, 309
Femoral head osteonecrosis, 1244
Femoral nerve mononeuropathy, 1017
Femoral pulse, 64
Femorofemoral extracorporeal bypass, 185-186
Femur
 fracture, 1945
 Paget's disease, 1955, 1956
Fenclozic acid, 2191
Fenfluramine, 621, 1902, 2104
Fenofibrate, 1892
Fentanyl
 cancer pain, 581
 sedation during gastrointestinal endoscopy,
  1994
Ferric oxide dust, 476
Ferritin, 642
 hepatic formation, 2120
 hereditary hemochromatosis, 2139, 2204
 iron overload, 646
 iron status, 643
Ferrochelatase, 1923
Ferrous iron, 351
Ferrous sulfate, 644
Fertility
 antirheumatic drug toxicity, 1261
 chemotherapy, 585
 germinal cell dysfunction, 1844-1846
 gonococcal salpingitis, 1583
 hirsutism, 1755
 inflammatory bowel disease, 2278
 21-hydroxylase deficiency, 1824
FES; *see* Functional electrical stimulation
Fetal alcohol syndrome, 280
Fetal blood sampling, 619
Fetal circulation, 280
Fetor hepaticus, 2160
Fetus
 antibiotic toxicity, 1348
 blood sampling for hemophilia A, 619
 chronic hypertension during pregnancy, 2275
 diabetic mother, 2272
 fetal alcohol syndrome, 280
 Listeria monocytogenes infection, 1577
 maternal mumps, 1497
 oral anticoagulant administration, 636
 parvovirus B19 infection, 1513-1514
 syphilis, 1640
 viral infections, 2280-2281
Fever, 1375
 acute febrile neutrophilic dermatosis,
  1318-1319
 acute lung allograft rejection, 521
 acute pancreatitis, 2234
 adenovirus infection, 1503
 African trypanosomiasis, 1688
 after cardiac transplantation, 341

Fever—cont'd
 after international travel, 1469
 after stem cell transplantation, 578
 alcoholic hepatitis and cirrhosis, 2197
 babesiosis, 1676
 bacteremia, 1449
 bacterial meningitis, 1406
 bacterial prostatitis, 1462
 blastomycosis, 1657
 Boutonneuse fever, 1545
 brain abscess, 1414
 brucellosis, 1605
 bubonic plague, 1610
 cancer patient, 582
 Colorado tick fever, 1512
 common bile duct obstruction, 2229
 complication of thrombolytic therapy, 637
 compromised host, 1386-1390
 Crohn's disease, 2069
 dengue, 1465, 1516
 diphtheria, 1566
 diverticulosis, 2090
 enteric, 1601
 epidemic pleurodynia, 1489
 erysipelas, 1420
 hepatitis A virus, 2173
 Hodgkin's disease, 693
 hospitalized patient, 1479-1482
 human immunodeficiency virus, 1475
 hypersensitivity pneumonitis, 461
 hyperventilation, 355
 idiopathic pulmonary fibrosis, 453
 increased nutrient requirements, 2102
 infectious mononucleosis, 1529
 infective endocarditis, 227
 influenza, 1490
 interstitial lung disease, 450
 intestinal disease, 2005
 intrahepatic cholangiocarcinoma, 2214
 Lassa fever, 1510
 leptospirosis, 1644
 lymphangitis, 1420
 lymphogranuloma venereum, 1535
 malaria, 1464, 1673
 mesenteric panniculitis, 2251
 metal fume, 473
 Mycoplasma pneumoniae pneumonia, 1539
 myopericarditis, 1489
 myxoma, 330
 necrotizing fasciitis, 1422
 otitis media, 1395
 pathogenesis, 1386-1387
 peritoneal mesenteric and omental diseases, 2248
 peritonitis, 1398
 pharyngitis, 1393
 pleural disease, 505
 pyogenic liver abscess, 2209
 Q fever, 1545
 rash with, 1380-1386
 relapsing febrile nodular panniculitis, 1245
 rheumatic, 1256-1258
 Rocky Mountain spotted fever, 1543
 rotavirus, 1521
 Salmonella infection, 1599
 sarcoidosis, 458
 scarlet fever, 1421, 1556
 shigellosis, 1602-1603
 spinal epidural abscess, 1418
 splenic abscess, 1399
 staphylococcal scalded-skin syndrome, 1421
 staphylococcal toxic shock syndrome, 1421
 streptococcal toxic shock syndrome, 1557
 subdural empyema, 1417
 supraglotittis, 2306
 systematic inflammatory response syndrome,
  1445
 transfusion reaction, 574
 tularemia, 1607
 typhoid fever, 1600-1602
 urinary tract infection, 1458
 viral infection, 1487

Fever blister, 1523
Fever of unknown origin, 1375-1380
  vasculitis, 1225
  Whipple's disease, 2065
Fexofenadine, 1182
FGS; *see* Focal glomerular sclerosis
FHIT gene, 546
Fiber, constipation, 2055
Fiberoptic bronchoscopy, 383-384
  hemoptysis, 411
  lung cancer, 490
  sarcoidosis, 459
  solitary pulmonary nodule, 494
Fiberoptic reflectance oximetry, 393
Fibric acid, 1892
Fibric acid derivatives, 767
Fibrillation, 916
  atrial, 146-148
    anticoagulant therapy, 639-640
    atrioventricular reciprocating tachycardia, 142
    calcium channel blockers, 138
    constrictive pericarditis, 277
    diastolic filling murmur, 78
    flecainide, 138
    mitral regurgitation, 251
    mitral stenosis, 245, 246
    myocardial infarction, 223
    neurologic aspects, 1088
    occlusive mesenteric vascular disease, 2087
    palpitations, 130
    risk of stroke, 1001
    SPAF study, 134
    thyrotoxicosis, 1804
    tricuspid regurgitation, 256
  ventricular, 153
    during cardiac catheterization, 108
    hyperkalemia, 833
    myocardial infarction, 223-224
    potassium therapy, 830
Fibrillin, 1289
Fibrin
  formation, 537-539
  infective endocarditis, 225, 226
  lung repair, 375
  pulmonary fibrosis, 450
  unstable angina, 195
  venous thrombus, 631
Fibrin clotting time, 571
Fibrin degradation products
  fibrinolysis, 540
  pulmonary thromboembolism, 501
  screening test, 571
Fibrinogen, 537-539, 1135
  abnormalities, 625
  chronic renal failure, 783
  congenital disorders of blood coagulation, 618
  deficiency, 1180
  hereditary amyloidosis, 1285
  plasma, 571
  platelet aggregation, 611
  prothrombin time, 2135
  replacement for hypofibrinogenemia, 573
  serum protein electrophoresis, 565
  synthesis, 2120
  venous thromboembolism, 632
Fibrinogen concentration, 571
Fibrinoid degeneration, 999
Fibrinoid material, 1213
Fibrinolysis, 539-540
  disseminated intravascular coagulation, 609
  lung injury, 373-374
  screening test, 571
  thrombosis, 609
Fibrinopeptide A
  unstable angina, 195, 539
  venous thromboembolism, 632
Fibrinopeptide B, 539
Fibroadenoma, breast, 1846
Fibroblast
  alveolar interstitial space, 371
  chemotaxis, 375

Fibroblast—cont'd
  interstitial lung disease, 450
  low-density lipoprotein receptors, 1886
  Paget's disease, 1955
  rheumatoid arthritis, 1202
  scleroderma, 1228
  tubulointerstitial renal disease, 889
Fibroblast growth factor, 1131, 1720
Fibrocartilage, 1277-1278
Fibrocystic disease of breast, 1846
Fibrolamellar hepatocellular carcinoma, 2214
Fibroma
  cardiac, 330
  incidence, 329
  mesenteric, 2251
Fibromatosis, mesenteric, 2251
Fibromuscular dysplasia
  renovascular disease, 755-756
  renovascular hypertension, 893
Fibromyalgia, 1195-1196, 2298
Fibronectin
  erythroleukemic, 533
  lung repair, 375
  respiratory defense, 366
Fibrosarcoma, 329
Fibrosing cholestatic hepatitis, 2182
Fibrosing mediastinitis, 512
Fibrosis
  asbestosis, 474
  bicuspid aortic valve, 287
  chronic mediastinitis, 514
  chronic myeloproliferative disorders, 686
  chronic pancreatitis, 2241
  cirrhosis
    cystic fibrosis, 483
    liver fibrosis, 2195-2196
  cystic, 479-483
    acute pancreatitis, 2246
    airway disease, 480
    allergic bronchopulmonary aspergillosis, 483
    autosomal recessive inheritance pattern, 1725
    double lung allograft, 515
    intestinal obstruction, 2246
    malabsorption, 2246
    nasal polyps, 2308
    pancreatic involvement, 2246
    sinopulmonary-infertility syndrome, 1845
  hepatic, 2195
  hypersensitivity pneumonitis, 461
  idiopathic myelofibrosis purpura, 677
  inflammation-fibrosis hypothesis of emphysema, 441
  interstitial lung disease, 448, 450
  Langerhans' cell granulomatosis, 464
  lung repair, 374
  myelofibrosis, 676-677
    neutrophilic leukocytosis, 591
    polycythemia vera, 688
  pneumonitis with, 476-477
  primary biliary cirrhosis, 2199
  primary sclerosing cholangitis, 2201
  progressive massive, 475
  pulmonary
    asbestos-related, 473-474
    high-resolution computed tomography, 387
    idiopathic, 453
    systemic sclerosis, 1230
  retroperitoneal, 885, 2250, 2251
Fibrothorax, 296
Fibrous dysplasia, 1960-1961
Fibrous myopathy, 1229
Fick principle, 109
Field defect, 1848
Fifth disease, 1513
  during pregnancy, 2280
  septic arthritis, 1255
Filariasis, 1466, 1699
Filling pressure, 41-42
Filtering function of lung, 346

Fimbriae
  bacterial meningitis, 1404
  gram-negative bacteria, 1447
Finasteride
  prostate cancer, 718
  urge incontinence, 2293
Fine-needle aspiration
  lung cancer, 490
  thyroid, 1802, 1814
Finger
  acrocyanosis, 310
  herpetic whitlow, 1524
Finkelstein's test, 1197
First-generation cephalosporins, 1352
First heart sound, 72
  aortic regurgitation, 244
  atrial septal defect, 281
  hypertrophic cardiomyopathy, 266
  mitral regurgitation, 251
  mitral stenosis, 245
  myocarditis, 262
  pulmonic regurgitation, 257
First-pass effect, 2311
FIRST survival trial, 171
FISH; *see* Fluorescence in situ hybridization
Fish oil, 845, 1884
Fish tapeworm, 1696-1697
Fissure, anal, 2093, Plate X-5
Fistula
  anal, 2093
  aorto-enteric, 2010
  arteriovenous
    angiogram, 388
    continuous murmur, 81
    coronary, 292
    pulmonary, 499
  atrioventricular, 160
  bronchopleural
    chronic obstructive pulmonary disease, 447
    tuberculous empyema, 507
  cerebrospinal fluid, 2307
  cholecystoenteric, 2228
  colovesical, 2090
  Crohn's disease, 2069, 2070, 2072
  perianal, 2093
  perilymph, 973
  sinus of Valsalva, 291
  small bowel bacterial overgrowth, 2060
Fitz-Hugh-Curtis syndrome, 1583, 2248
Fixed drug eruption, 1314-1315
Flaccid dysarthria, 977
Flank pain
  kidney stones, 800
  obstructive uropathy, 885-886
  urinary tract infection, 1458
Flash pulmonary edema, 169, 177
Flatulence
  lactase deficiency, 2068
  malabsorption, 2057
  ulcerative colitis, 2073
Flatworm, 1696-1697
Flavivirus, 1514-1519
Flea, *Yersinia pestis*, 1610
Flecainide, 138
Flexible sigmoidoscopy, 1995-1996
  constipation, 2055
  Crohn's disease, 2070
  intestinal disease, 2007
  ulcerative colitis, 2073
Flexion contracture, 1203
Flexor finger jerk, 964
Flexural dermatitis, 1303
Flolan International Randomized Survival Trial, 171
Flow cytometry
  peripheral blood and bone marrow cells, 558-559
  peripheral blood leukocytes, 1151-1152
Flow velocity in echocardiography, 97-100
Floxacillin, 2191

Floxuridine
  effects on kidney, 869
  hepatic injury, 2192
Fluconazole, 1653, 1654
  candidiasis, 1663
    after lung transplantation, 519
    esophageal, 2020
    vulvovaginal, 1442
  coccidioidomycosis, 1254, 1474, 1657
  cryptococcosis, 1669
  effects on kidney, 869
  esophagitis, 1474
  funguria, 1462
  human cytochrome P450 isoforms, 2312
  inhibitor of cytochrome P450, 2311
  interaction with cyclosporin, 793
  interference with oral anticoagulants, 636
  meningitis
    acquired immunodeficiency syndrome, 1478
    bacterial, 1411
    cryptococcal, 1474
  prophylaxis in lung transplantation, 518
  sporotrichosis, 1658
Flucytosine, 1653, 1654
  cryptococcosis, 1669
  endocarditis, 232
  prophylaxis in lung transplantation, 518
Fludarabine
  chronic lymphocytic leukemia, 685
  Waldenström macroglobulinemia, 704
Fludrocortisone
  Addison's disease, 1824
  hyporeninemic hypoaldosteronism, 832
  hypotension, 1828
  vasodepressor syncope, 956
Fluency, testing in aphasia, 975
Fluid exchange, 346-347
Fluid management
  acute diarrhea, 2051
  acute renal failure, 773
  choledocholithiasis, 2229
  cholera, 1596
  diabetic ketoacidosis, 1864
  diarrhea, 1431
  hepatorenal syndrome, 2170
  hypercalcemia, 1929
  hypercalciuria, 798
  hyperosmolar nonketotic coma, 1866
  hyponatremia, 812
  pulmonary edema, 427
  rotavirus infection, 1521
  uric acid nephrolithiasis, 804
Fluid restriction
  compulsive water drinkers, 815
  hypotonic hyponatremic syndromes, 812-813
  serum osmolality, 806
  syndrome of inappropriate antidiuretic
    hormone, 489
Fluid retention
  after cardiac transplantation, 343
  aortic regurgitation, 241
  heart failure, 162-163
Fluke
  cholangiocarcinoma, 2231
  intestinal, 1697-1698
  tissue, 1702-1704
Flumazenil, 1080
Flunisolide, 1182
Fluorescein conjugated antihuman globulin, 1458
Fluorescence in situ hybridization, 561, 562,
  563, Plate IX-1
Fluorescent treponemal antibody-absorption test,
  1642
Fluoride
  excess ingestion, 1959
  functions, 2109
  induction of skeletal fluorinosis, 1953
  osteogenesis imperfecta, 1287
  recommended daily dietary allowances, 2116
5-Fluorocytosine, 1663
Fluorodeoxyuridine, 585

Fluoroquinolones, 1359
  acute pancreatitis, 2237
  antimicrobial mechanisms, 1344
  bacterial pneumonia after lung transplantation,
    517
  Campylobacter enteritis, 1592
  dosage, 1350
  effects on kidney, 868
  enterococcal infection, 1563
  enterococci resistance, 1561
  gonorrhea, 1584
  Haemophilus ducreyi, 1589
  human cytochrome P450 isoforms, 2312
  interference with oral anticoagulants, 636
  mycobacterial disease, 1631
  Mycoplasma pneumoniae pneumonia, 1540
  Pasteurella, 1609
  prophylaxis for traveler's diarrhea, 1432
  respiratory exacerbations in cystic fibrosis,
    483
  shigellosis, 1603
  spontaneous bacterial peritonitis, 2164
  traveler's diarrhea, 1432
  typhoid fever, 1432, 1601
  urethritis, 1441
  urinary tract infection, 1459-1461
Fluoroscopy
  after valve replacement, 259
  examination of deglutition, 1999-2000
  ischemic heart disease, 198
Fluorosis, 1959
5-Fluorouracil
  breast cancer, 709, 710
  colon cancer, 2085
  drug-nutrient interactions, 2110
  effects on kidney, 869
  endometrial cancer, 714
  esophageal cancer, 2024
  gastric cancer, 2048
  gastrointestinal toxicity, 585
  hepatic injury, 585, 2192
  pancreatic cancer, 2243
  squamous cell carcinoma, 1298
Fluoxetine, 1037
  chronic fatigue syndrome, 2300
  depression in elderly patients, 2289
  human cytochrome P450 isoforms, 2312
  interference with oral anticoagulants, 636
Fluoxymesterone
  adult hypergonadotropic hypogonadism, 1845
  breast cancer, 710
Fluphenazine, 1791
Fluroxene, 2191
Flushing
  autonomic overactivity, 934
  calcium channel blocker-induced, 205
  carcinoid syndrome, 2082
  human immunodeficiency virus infection,
    1327
  mitral stenosis, 245
  VIPoma, 2245
Flutamide
  hepatic injury, 2192
  prostate cancer, 719
Flutter, atrial, 134, 144-146
Fluvastatin, 1891
Fluvoxamine, 1037, 2312
Flying W pattern for pulmonary hypertension, 99
Foam cell formation, 60
Foamy macrophage, 462
Focal dystonia, 995-996
Focal emphysema, 439
Focal glomerular sclerosis, 849, 851-852
Focal nodular hyperplasia, 2216
Focal proliferative lupus nephritis, 856
Fogo selvagem, 1294
Folate
  cellular metabolism, 647
  deficiency
    alcoholic patient, 1081
    clinical presentation, 647-648

Folate—cont'd
  deficiency—cont'd
    intestinal disease, 2005
    neurologic aspects, 1103
    during pregnancy, 2279
    thrombocytopenia, 614
  drug-nutrient interactions, 2110
  hemostatic defects in liver disease, 627
  immune hemolytic anemia, 669
  intestinal absorption, 1989
  megaloblastic anemia, 647, 649
  recommended daily dietary allowances, 2115
Folic acid
  bacterial, 1344-1345
  biochemical function, 2105
  Crohn's disease, 2072
  deficiency, 605, 2107
  diabetic polyneuropathy, 1871
  folate deficiency treatment, 650
  pure red blood cell aplasia, 675
  sickle cell disease, 658
  tropical sprue, 2065
Folinic acid
  Pneumocystis carinii pneumonia, 1694
  prophylaxis in lung transplantation, 518
  toxoplasmosis, 1474, 1678
Folkow hypothesis of hypertension, 316
Follicle-stimulating hormone, 1775
  amenorrhea, 1757-1758
  cirrhosis, 2171
  constitutional delay of puberty, 1768
  estrogen feedback inhibition tests, 1736
  gonadotropin-secreting pituitary tumor, 1787
  gynecomastia, 1764, 1765
  hypogonadotropic eunuchoidism, 1841-1842
  impotence, 1763
  Klinefelter's syndrome, 1843
  laboratory and diagnostic testing, 1835, 1836
  neonatal, 1832
  normal levels, 1836
  ovarian feedback mechanisms, 1834-1835
  pituitary secretion, 1834
  polycystic ovarian disease, 1837
  puberty, 1766, 1767
  reproductive years, 1832-1833
  spermatogenesis, 1839
Follicular bronchitis/bronchiolitis, 455
Follicular dendritic cell, 1128
Follicular thyroid carcinoma, 1815
Folliculitis, 1420
  candidal, 1662
  hot tub, 1423, Plate VIII-28
  human immunodeficiency virus infection, 1326
  Pityrosporum, 1309-1310
Food
  cholecystokinin stimulation, 2133
  faddism, 1750
  gastric secretion stimulation, 1981
  heartburn, 1999
  interactions with oral anticoagulants, 636
  intolerance in esophageal disease, 1999
  mineral toxicity related to contamination, 2110
  movement through gut segments, 1978-1980
  pancreatic exocrine secretion, 2133
Food allergy insomnia, 944
Food-borne disease
  botulism, 1570-1571
  brucellosis, 1604
  Clostridium perfringens, 1568
  diarrhea, 1429, 1430
  hepatitis A virus, 2173
  Salmonella, 1599
  shigellosis, 1602
  Yersinia enterocolitica, 1611
Food intake
  disorders in acquired immunodeficiency
    syndrome, 2094-2095
  obesity, 1752, 2103
  overnutrition, 2101
  undernutrition, 2100-2101
  weight loss, 1748, 1749

Foot
  arthritis, 1172
  chronic pernio, 310
  damage in leprosy, 1650
  diabetes mellitus, 1872
  ischemic ulceration, 308
  osteomyelitis, 1434
  psoriatic arthritis, 1241
  rheumatoid arthritis, 1203
  tinea pedis, 1308
Foramen ovale, 280
Force-frequency relation, 40-41
Forced expiratory volume in 1 second
  aging and, 2284
  asthma, 1188-1189
  bronchiolitis obliterans syndrome, 522-523
  bronchoprovocation inhalation tests, 379
  chronic obstructive pulmonary disease, 442
  chronic simple silicosis, 474
  coal worker's pneumoconiosis, 475
  cystic fibrosis, 481
  giant bullae, 447
  hypersensitivity pneumonitis, 461
  inhaled bronchodilator studies, 377-378
  before lung resection, 497
  obstructive lung disease, 357
  operative risk, 2261
  spirometry, 376
  upper airway obstruction, 376
Forced expiratory volume in 1 second/forced
    vital capacity ratio, 376
Forced vital capacity
  aging and, 2284
  bronchoprovocation inhalation tests, 379
  cystic fibrosis, 481
  hypersensitivity pneumonitis, 461
  inhaled bronchodilator studies, 377-378
  spirometry, 376
Forchheimer spots, 1501
Foreign body
  cardiac, 333
  esophageal, 2019
  gastric, 2044
  synovitis, 1244
  tumor formation, 548
  upper gastrointestinal endoscopy, 1995
Formal consensus, 24
Formaldehyde
  aminopyrine breath test, 2143
  corrosive gastritis, 2043
Formula, defined-formula diet, 2115-2117
Fort Bragg fever, 1621
Foscarnet
  cytomegalovirus, 1529
    blindness, 1478
    retinitis, 2305
  effects on kidney, 869
  fulminant hepatitis B, 2177
  herpesvirus infections, 1526
  retinitis, 1474
Fosinopril
  heart failure, 170, 172
  hypertension, 325
  nephrotic syndrome, 767
Four-gland hyperplasia, 1965
Fournier's gangrene, 1424
Fourth heart sound, 73-74, 75
  aortic stenosis, 236
  hypertrophic cardiomyopathy, 266
  mitral regurgitation, 251
  myocardial infarction, 210
  myocarditis, 262
  pulmonic stenosis, 288
Fourth-nerve palsy, 1062
Fraction 1, 1609-1610
Fraction of inspired oxygen
  acute respiratory failure occurring with acute
    respiratory distress syndrome, 418
  aerosol face mask, 428-429
  hypoxemia caused by ventilation/perfusion
    mismatching, 413

Fraction of inspired oxygen—cont'd
  nasal prongs, 428
  oxygen toxicity, 415
Fractional diazo reaction of serum, 2150
Fractional excretion of phosphate, 1745
Fractional excretion of sodium, 747
  acute renal failure, 770
  chronic renal failure, 778
  syndrome of inappropriate antidiuretic
    hormone, 489
Fracture
  cough, 408
  falls, 2289
  increased nutrient requirements, 2102
  nose, 2308
  osteomalacia, 1949
  osteopetrosis, 1958
  osteoporosis, 1944
  pathologic, 864
    fibrous dysplasia, 1960
    multiple myeloma, 864
    Paget's disease, 1955
    primary hyperparathyroidism, 1966
  rib, 410
  skull, 1043, 1045
  spinal cord injury with, 1046
  vertebral crush, 1944-1945
Fragile site, 546
Fragile-X syndrome, 1726
Fragility fracture, 1944
Framingham Heart Study, 1888
  atrial fibrillation, 146
  heart failure, 158
  hypertension, 314
Francisella tularensis, 1607-1609
  antibiotic selection, 1347
  hazard to laboratory personnel, 1369
Frank-Starling mechanism, 159
Frank-Starling relation, 40, 41-42
Frankel classification system, 1047
Fraudelent fever, 1481
Freckles, 1920
Free bile salts, 2125
Free cortisol, 1818-1819
Free fatty acids, 1884, 1931
Free intraperitoneal air, 2032, 2033
Free-living amebae, 1683-1684
Free radical theory of aging, 2283
Free thyroid hormone concentration, 1738
Free thyroxine, 1801
Free thyroxine index, 1800
Free triiodothyronine, 1801
Free-water clearance, 748
Free-water reabsorption, 739
Frequency
  bacterial prostatitis, 1462
  diabetes insipidus, 1793
  urinary tract infection, 1458
Frequency and dysuria syndrome, 763
Fresh-frozen plasma, 573, 1339
  bleeding varices, 2166
  disseminated intravascular coagulation, 628
  factor XI deficiency, 624
  fulminant hepatic failure, 2163
  hemophilia A, 621
  hemophilia B, 622
  hemostatic defects in liver disease, 627
  vitamin K deficiency, 626
Freshwater drowning, 668
Friction rub, 75
  acute pericarditis, 273
  myocarditis, 262
  myopericarditis, 1490
Friedreich's ataxia, 1088
Frontal alexia, 978
Frontal lobe syndrome, 1032-1033
Frontal subdural empyema, 1417
Frontoethmoidal sinusitis, 1414
Frozen deglycerolized red blood cells, 572
Frozen shoulder, 1197
Fructokinase, 1879

Fructose
  absorption, 1987
  enzymatic hydrolysis, 2121
  hepatic metabolism, 2122
  intolerance, 1880
    Fanconi's syndrome, 882
    hypoglycemia, 1876
Fructose 1-phosphate aldolase, 1880
Fructosuria, 1879
FSH; *see* Follicle-stimulating hormone
Fucosidosis, 1916-1917
Fukuyama congenital muscular dystrophy, 1028
Fulminant hepatic failure
  acute viral hepatitis, 2177
  hepatic encephalopathy, 2163
Fulminant hepatitis
  alpha-fetoprotein, 2143
  hepatic encephalopathy, 2159
  hepatitis A infection, 2173
  liver transplantation, 2219
Functional assessment of cell-mediated
    immunity, 1152-1153
Functional capacity, 2257, 2258
Functional cardiovascular disease, 131
Functional dyspepsia, 2039
Functional electrical stimulation
  spinal cord injury, 1053
  stroke patient, 1055
Functional platelet release defects, 611
Functional prepubertal castrate syndrome, 1843
Functional residual capacity, 348
  administration of general anesthesia,
    2260-2261
  aging and, 2284
  chronic obstructive pulmonary disease, 442
Functional status assessment, 18-19, 2285-2286
Fundoplication, 2018
Fundus, 1981, 2041-2042
Fungal infection, 1651-1660
  acquired immunodeficiency syndrome, 1328,
    1329
  Actinomyces, 1664-1665
  Addison's disease, 1823
  after liver transplantation, 2219-2220
  antifungal therapy, 1652-1654
  arthritis, 1254-1255
  aspergillosis, 1658-1659
  blastomycosis, 1657
  candidiasis, 1660-1664
  chromoblastomycosis and mycetoma,
    1659-1660
  coccidioidomycosis, 1655-1657
  Cryptococcus neoformans, 1667-1670
  culture, 1370
  diagnosis, 1652, 1653
  differential diagnosis of fever and rash, 1384
  endocarditis, 226
  esophageal infection, 2019-2020
  fever, 1387
  fever of unknown origin, 1377
  histoplasmosis, 1654-1655
  infectious gastritis, 2043
  meningitis, 1404
  nocardiosis, 1665-1666
  nosocomial, 1362
  osteomyelitis, 1437
  paracoccidioidomycosis, 1657
  penicilliosis, 1658
  peritonitis, 2247-2248
  phaeohyphomycosis, 1660
  pleural effusion, 507
  posttransplant
    heart, 342
    kidney, 794
    lung, 519-520
    stem cell, 578
  prosthetic valve endocarditis, 230
  sporotrichosis, 1658
  superficial, 1307-1312
    candidiasis, 1310-1312
    clinical presentation, 1308-1309

Fungal infection—cont'd
  superficial—cont'd
    dermatophyte infection, 1307-1308
    diagnostic procedures, 1309
    Pityrosporum infection, 1309-1310
  uremic patient, 784
  urinary tract, 1462
  zygomycetes, 1659
Fungi
  dimorphic, 1654-1660
  normal flora, 1368
Furosemide
  acute tubular necrosis, 773
  ascites, 2165
  cause of renal potassium wasting and
    alkalosis, 828
  congestive heart failure-associated
    hyponatremia, 818
  heart failure, 169, 170
  hypercalcemia, 1929
  hyperkalemia, 833
  hypertension, 325
  induction of acute interstitial nephritis, 889
  isovolemic hypotonic hyponatremia, 813
  pulmonary edema, 169
Furuncle, 1421
Fusarium, 1659
Fusiform aneurysm, 299
Fusion beat, 149, 150
Fusobacterium, 1368

G

G-banded chromosome, Plate IX-1
G cell, 1981, 1982
G protein-linked 7-membrane spanning protein,
    1718
G proteins
  activation of adenyl cyclase, 1711
  adrenergic receptors, 1827
  cardiac function, 56-58
  cardiac sodium currents, 59
  fibrous dysplasia, 1960
  pancreatic acinar cells, 2132
  pancreatic duct cell secretions, 2132
  pepsinogen secretion, 1984, 1985
  signal transduction, 541
Gabapentin
  mania, 1038
  restless legs syndrome, 944
Gadolinium-135 dual-beam photon
    absorptiometry, 1748
Gag clause, 33
Gag reflex, 1999
Gait
  Alzheimer's disease, 986
  apraxia, 973
  brain tumor, 1067
  multiple sclerosis, 1055
  neurologic examination, 903
  osteomalacia, 1949
  syphilis, 1641
Galactitol, 1883
Galactokinase, 1882, 1883
Galactorrhea, 1786
Galactose
  absorption, 1987
  elimination test, 2143
  hepatic metabolism, 2122
Galactosemia, 1882-1883
  Fanconi's syndrome, 882
  reactive hypoglycemia, 1876
Galactosuria, 1879
Gallbladder
  benign stricture of extrahepatic bile ducts,
    2232-2233
  bile salt secretion rates, 2125
  biliary dyskinesia, 2233
  cancer, 2232
    carcinoma of ampulla of Vater, 2232
    carcinoma of bile ducts, 2231-2232

Gallbladder—cont'd
  cancer—cont'd
    extrahepatic cholestasis, 2155
    prophylactic cholecystectomy, 2225
  developmental anomalies, 2233
  Dubin-Johnson and Rotor's syndromes, 2157
  dysmotility, 2221, 2224
  gallstones, 2220-2231
    asymptomatic *versus* symptomatic, 2225
    biliary colic, 2225-2227
    cholecystitis, 2227-2228
    choledocholithiasis, 2228-2230
    cholesterol stones, 2221, 2222
    cholesterolosis, 2230-2231
    classification and composition, 2220, 2221
    Crohn's disease, 2075
    defective bile salt synthesis, 2129
    diagnostic tests, 2224-2225
    epidemiology, 2222-2223
    gallstone pancreatitis, 2230
    hereditary spherocytosis, 665-666
    pathophysiology, 2220-2221
    pigment stones, 2221-2222
    during pregnancy, 2278
    risk factors, 2223-2224
    sickle cell disease, 657, 659
  hemobilia, 2233
  hepatobiliary disease
    acquired immunodeficiency syndrome,
      2098-2099
    benign stricture of extrahepatic bile ducts,
      2232-2233
    biliary dyskinesia, 2233
    carcinoma of ampulla of Vater, 2232
    carcinoma of bile ducts, 2231-2232
    conjugated hyperbilirubinemia, 2154-2156
    developmental anomalies, 2233
    distinguishing acute from chronic disease,
      2134-2136
    drug-induced and toxic cholangitis,
      2202-2203
    Dubin-Johnson syndrome, 2157
    estimations of severity and prognosis,
      2141-2144
    familial cholestatic syndromes, 2158-2159
    fever of unknown origin, 1376
    gallbladder cancer, 2232
    hemobilia, 2233
    hereditary markers, 2138-2139
    hyperplastic cholecystosis, 2233
    imaging studies, 2140-2141
    immunologic markers, 2139-2140
    impaired lipid ingestion, 1987
    ischemic cholangitis, 2203
    liver biopsy, 2141
    malabsorption, 2062
    normal bilirubin metabolism, 2147-2150
    osteomalacia, 1951-1952
    patterns of liver injury, 2136-2137
    postoperative cholestasis, 2159
    primary biliary cirrhosis, 2199-2201
    primary sclerosing cholangitis, 2201-2202,
      2203
    Rotor's syndrome and hepatic storage
      disease, 2157-2158
    unconjugated hyperbilirubinemia, 2150-2154
    viral cholangitis, 2202
    viral markers, 2138
  hyperplastic cholecystosis, 2233
  movement of food, 1980
  somatostatinoma, 2245
Gallium nitrate, 1974
Gallium scan, 388
  acute pericarditis, 274
  amebiasis, 1683
  amiodarone-induced pulmonary disease, 478
  osteomyelitis, 1434
Gallop, 73, 75
  aortic regurgitation, 244
  dilated myocarditis, 263
  heart failure, 165

Gallstone ileus, 2079, 2228
Gallstone pancreatitis, 2230
Gallstones, 2220-2231, Plate X-11, Plate X-12
  asymptomatic *versus* symptomatic, 2225
  biliary colic, 2225-2227
  black pigment, Plate X-14
  calcium bilirubinate, Plate X-13
  cholecystitis, 2227-2228
  choledocholithiasis, 2228-2230
  cholesterol stones, 2221, 2222
  cholesterolosis, 2230-2231
  classification and composition, 2220, 2221
  Crohn's disease, 2075
  defective bile salt synthesis, 2129
  diagnostic tests, 2224-2225
  epidemiology, 2222-2223
  gallbladder carcinoma, 2232
  gallstone pancreatitis, 2230
  hereditary spherocytosis, 665-666
  liver abscess, 2209
  pathophysiology, 2220-2221
  pigment stones, 2221-2222
  during pregnancy, 2278
  primary sclerosing cholangitis, 2201
  risk factors, 2223-2224
  sickle cell disease, 657, 659
GALT; *see* Gut-associated lymphoid tissue
Galvanic skin reflex, 938
Gamma-aminobutyric acid
  effects of tetanus, 1573
  hepatic encephalopathy, 2161-2162
Gamma camera imaging agents, 105
Gamma delta T-cell, 1127
Gamma globulin
  hypergammaglobulinemia, 1233
    human immunodeficiency virus infection,
      1470
    liver inflammation, 2135-2136
    myxoma, 330
  hypogammaglobulinemia
    malabsorption, 2066
    multiple myeloma, 864
    serum protein electrophoresis, 565-566
Gamma globulin antibody, 1020, 1021
Gamma glutamyltransferase
  hepatitic injury, 2136
  liver disease, 2137
Gamma heavy-chain disease, 704
Gamma-interferon
  activation of macrophage, 369
  osteopetrosis, 1959
Gamma knife surgery, 1069
Ganciclovir
  cytomegalovirus, 1478
  herpes esophagitis, 2020
  herpesvirus infections, 1526
  prophylaxis in lung transplantation, 518
  retinitis, 1474, 2305
Ganglionectomy, 278
Ganglioneuroma, 1830
Gangliosidoses, 1919
Gangrene
  chronic aortic obstruction, 304
  gallbladder, 2227
  gas, 1422-1424
  group A streptococci, 1557
  mesenteric hernia, 2251
  progressive bacterial synergistic, 1425
  Raynaud's phenomenon, 1227
  Streptococcus pyogenes, Plate VIII-30
Gardnerella
  bacterial vaginosis, 762, 1443
  normal flora, 1368
  during pregnancy, 2280
Gardner's syndrome
  cutaneous changes and malignancy, 1319
  mesenteric fibromatosis, 2251
  risk for colonic cancer, 2083
  small bowel adenocarcinoma, 2081
Gas chromatography-mass spectrometry, 1904

Gas exchange, 347-350
  failure, 397
  microvascular fluid exchange, 346
  monitoring, 390-396
    peripheral artery catheterization, 390
    pulmonary artery catheterization, 390-395
    pulse oximetry, 396
    transcutaneous oxygen and carbon dioxide, 396
Gas gangrene, 1422-1424, 1575-1576
Gasoline vapors, 867
Gasserian ganglion syndrome, 1071
Gastrectomy
  reactive hypoglycemia following, 1876
  risk of gastric cancer, 2045
  undernutrition, 2101
Gastric acid, 1981-1983
  abnormalities of secretion, 1983-1984
  barrier to infection, 1335
  gastric cancer, 2046
  hypersecretory gastropathy, 2043
  measurement, 2002-2003
  regulation, 1981, 1982
  small bowel bacterial overgrowth, 2060
Gastric adenocarcinoma, 2039, 2045-2050
Gastric analysis, 2002-2003
  peptic ulcer, 2038
Gastric antibody, 1157
Gastric atrophy, 2042
Gastric bezoar, 1979, 2044
Gastric biopsy, 2002
Gastric bypass, 1753
  reactive hypoglycemia following, 1876
Gastric carcinoid, 2082
Gastric emptying, 1978-1979, 2003-2004
  anorexia nervosa, 2030
  gastroesophageal reflux, 2015
  gastroparesis, 2044
Gastric glands, 1981, 1982
Gastric inhibitory polypeptide, 784
Gastric isotopic scanning, 2004
Gastric lavage, 2010-2011
Gastric lipase, 1986
Gastric outlet obstruction, 2027, 2040
Gastric pits, 1981, 1982
Gastric polyp, 2045-2046
Gastric pressure, 358
Gastric reduction surgery, 2105
Gastric secretion, 1980-1985
  hypersecretory gastropathy, 2043
Gastric ulcer
  acid secretory values, 2003
  gastric biopsy and cytology, 2002
  upper gastrointestinal endoscopy, 1994
Gastric vagotomy, 2040-2041
Gastric varices, 2166
Gastrin
  calcitonin release, 1718
  chronic renal failure, 784
  enterochromaffin-like cells, 1981-1982
  gastric cancer, 2046
  hypergastrinemia, 2003
  pepsinogen secretion, 1984
  peptic ulcer, 2038
  serum, 2003
  tests, 1743
Gastrinoma, 2005
Gastritis, 2041-2044
  atrophic, 2045
  Helicobacter pylori, 1592-1593
  operative risk, 2263
Gastrocolic reflex, 1980
Gastroenteritis, 1425-1432
  bacterial agents, 1425-1427
  coronavirus infection, 1502
  diagnosis, 1430-1431
  diarrhea, 1429-1430
  eosinophilic, 2066-2067
  immunoglobulin A nephropathy, 845
  parasitic agents, 1428-1429
  pathophysiology, 1425

Gastroenteritis—cont'd
  prophylaxis for traveler's diarrhea, 1432
  rotavirus and Norwalk-like virus, 1519-1522
  Salmonella, 1599
  Staphylococcus aureus, 1548-1549
  treatment, 1431-1432
  Vibrio parahaemolyticus, 1596-1597
  viral agents, 1427-1428
Gastroesophageal reflux, 2014-2018
  development of chronic cough, 407
  pain, 128
  pH measurement, 2001
Gastroesophageal squamocolumnar junction, 2000
Gastrointestinal bleeding, 2008-2014
  acquired immunodeficiency syndrome, 2098-2099
  alcoholic hepatitis and cirrhosis, 2197
  antacids and antisecretory agents, 2013
  Campylobacter jejuni, 1591
  chronic renal failure, 783, 784
  colon cancer, 2085
  colonoscopy, 1996
  cutaneous manifestations, 1320
  diagnostic and therapeutic studies, 2011-2013
  esophageal varices, 2013-2014
  fulminant hepatic failure, 2163
  gastric cancer, 2046
  hepatic encephalopathy, 2159
  initial management, 2010-2011
  portosystemic encephalopathy, 2160
  small intestinal malignancies, 2081
  technetium 99m studies, 2004
  upper gastrointestinal endoscopy, 1994
Gastrointestinal disease
  adenovirus, 1504
  Blastocystis hominis, 1691
  brucellosis, 1606
  Campylobacter jejuni, 1591-1592
  chronic renal failure, 784
  clostridial infection, 1567-1568
  cutaneous manifestations, 1320-1322
  diverticular
    diverticulitis, 2085
    diverticulosis, 1996, 2060
    esophageal, 2020-2021
    gastric, 2044
    intestinal, 2089-2092
  esophageal, 2014-2024
    achalasia, 2021-2022
    benign tumors, 2023
    cancer, 2023-2024
    chemical and physical injury, 2018-2019
    esophageal spasm, 2022-2023
    esophageal webs, rings, and diverticula, 2020-2021
    evaluation, 1998-2002
    gastroesophageal reflux, 2014-2018
    infectious esophagitis, 2019-2020
    weight loss, 1749
  evaluation, 2004-2008
  gastric analysis, 2002-2003
  gastric biopsy and cytology, 2002
  gastric emptying, 2003-2004
  Helicobacter pylori, 1592-1593
    abnormalities of gastric acid secretion, 1984
    acquired immunodeficiency syndrome, 2095
    acute gastritis, 2041
    increased risk of cancer, 548
    monocytoid B lymphoma, 697
    peptic ulcer, 2035-2036
    risk of gastric cancer, 2045
    testing for, 2003
    type B gastritis, 2042-2043
  infection, 1425-1432
    bacterial agents, 1425-1427
    diagnosis, 1430-1431
    diarrhea, 1429-1430
    parasitic agents, 1428-1429
    pathophysiology, 1425
    prophylaxis for traveler's diarrhea, 1432

Gastrointestinal disease—cont'd
  infection—cont'd
    traveler's risk, 1467, 1469
    treatment, 1431-1432
    viral agents, 1427-1428
  inflammatory bowel disease, 2068-2077
    arthropathy, 1245-1246
    chronic diarrhea, 2051
    colonoscopy, 1996
    Crohn's disease, 2069-2072
    cutaneous findings, 1321
    differentiation of ulcerative colitis and Crohn's disease, 2075
    etiology, 2068-2069
    extraintestinal manifestations, 2075-2076
    fever and rash, 1385
    incidence and epidemiology, 2069
    increased risk of cancer, 548, 2076-2077
    portal triad lesions, 2155
    during pregnancy, 2278-2279
    primary sclerosing cholangitis, 2201
    secondary hyperoxaluria, 799, 804
    stool examination, 2006
    toxic megacolon, 2076
    ulcerative colitis, 2072-2075
  intestinal obstruction, 2077-2079
    abdominal pain, 2032
    colon cancer, 2085
    cystic fibrosis, 2246
    Meckel's diverticulum, 2089
    radiography, 2032
    small intestinal malignancies, 2081
  intestinal pseudoobstruction, 2079
  intestinal vascular disease, 2086-2089
  irritable bowel syndrome, 2055-2056
    abdominal pain, 2035
    celiac sprue *versus,* 2063
    colonic dysmotility, 2007
    diarrhea, 2052
  malabsorption, 2056-2068
    abetalipoproteinemia, 2067
    bacterial overgrowth, 2060-2062
    carbohydrate intolerance, 2067-2068
    carbohydrates, 1987
    celiac sprue, 2062-2063
    chronic diarrhea, 2051-2052
    chronic pancreatitis, 2145, 2239
    clinical features, 2057-2058
    congenital glucose-galactose, 878
    Crohn's disease, 270, 2069
    cystic fibrosis, 2246
    digestion process, 2056-2057
    eosinophilic enteritis, 2067
    eosinophilic gastroenteritis, 2066-2067
    hypogammaglobulinemia, 2066
    intestinal lymphangiectasia, 2067
    laboratory findings, 2058-2060
    magnesium, 1940
    multiple jejunal diverticulosis, 2089
    negative phosphate balance, 1935
    pancreatic and hepatobiliary diseases, 2062
    radiation enteropathy, 2065-2066
    serum electrolytes, 2005
    short bowel syndrome, 2066
    small intestinal tumors, 2081
    stool examination, 2006
    tests for, 2006-2007
    tropical sprue, 2065
    vitamin B_{12} deficiency, 648
    vitamin K deficiency, 607, 626
    weight loss, 1749
    Whipple's disease, 2064-2065
  mineral deficiencies, 2110
  noncardiac causes of chest pain, 128
  peptic ulcer disease, 2035-2041
    acid secretory values, 2003
    Helicobacter pylori, 1592-1593
    operative risk, 2263
  peritonitis, 2079-2080, 2247-2249
    abdominal evaluation, 2032
    acquired immunodeficiency syndrome, 1476

Gastrointestinal disease—cont'd
  peritonitis—cont'd
    anaerobic bacteria, 1617
    candidal, 1661
    dialysis-related, 791
    paralytic ileus, 2078
    primary, 1396
    systemic lupus erythematosus, 1214
  secondary nutritional deficiencies, 2100
  serum gastrin, 2003
  stomach cancer, 2045-2050
  tuberculous, 1636
  visualization of stomach and duodenum, 2002
  vitamin D deficiency, 1951-1952
  weight loss, 1749
  Yersinia enterocolitica, 1611
Gastrointestinal endoscopy, 1993-1998
Gastrointestinal peptides, 1077
Gastrointestinal system
  adrenergic responses, 1828
  antirheumatic drug toxicity, 1261
  beta-blockers, 202
  calcium absorption, 1717
  diabetic autonomic neuropathy, 1872-1873
  drug interactions, 2311
  effects of parathyroid hormone, 1718
  endoscopy, 1993-1998
  features of malabsorption, 2058
  febrile compromised patient, 1388
  gastric secretion, 1980-1985
  intestinal absorption, 1985-1989
    cholesterol, 1884
    magnesium, 1939, 1940
  intestinal immunity, 1989-1993
  iron absorption from, 641
  Kaposi's sarcoma, 1330
  manifestations of acquired immunodeficiency
    syndrome, 2094-2099
  neurogastroenterology, 1100-1102
  operative risks, 2262-2263
  origin of sodium loss, 823
  polyarteritis nodosa, 1220
  primary hyperparathyroidism, 1966
  prophylaxis in compromised host, 1390
  pulmonary metastases, 492
  relationship with nutrient intake, 2100
  sodium loss, 823
  spinal cord injury, 1050
  systemic lupus erythematosus, 1215
  systemic sclerosis, 1229-1230, 1232
  toxicity of chemotherapeutic agents, 584-585
  toxicity of nonsteroidal antiinflammatory
    drugs, 1258-1259
Gastrokinetic drugs, 2018
Gastroparesis, 2044
  autonomic failure, 935
  diabetic, 1872-1873
Gastroplasty, 1753
Gastroscopy, 2041
GATA-1, erythroid development, 651
Gated blood pool scintigraphy, 199
  aortic regurgitation, 242
  aortic stenosis, 238
  mitral regurgitation, 253
Gatekeeper, managed care, 32-33
Gaucher's disease, 576, 1918
Gay bowel syndrome, 1429, 1445
Gaze-evoked nystagmus, 1064
Gaze nystagmus, 973-974
Gelsolin, 1285
Gemcitabine, 2243
Gemfibrozil
  gallstone risk factor, 2223
  lipoprotein lipase potentiation, 1892
  secondary hypertriglyceridemia, 1895
Gender
  gallstone risk factor, 2223
  headache syndromes, 960
Gene
  DNA code, 49
  expression and regulation, 50-51

Gene products, 551
Gene rearrangement
  analysis, 560
  antibody, 1125-1126
Gene therapy
  cancer treatment, 555
  lysosomal storage disease, 1920
  treatment of inherited disorders, 1731-1732
Gene transcription, 50
  globin genes, 651, 652
  impairment in beta-thalassemia, 654
Gene transfer, 55
Generalized autonomic disorders, 934-936
Generalized lymphadenopathy, 599-600
Generalized seizure, 979
Generalized tonic-clonic convulsion, 979
Genetic code, 49-50
Genetic counseling, 1921
Genetic disorders, 1721-1732
  abetalipoproteinemia, 2067
  alpha₁ antitrypsin deficiency, 2206-2207
  amenorrhea, 1760
  azoospermia, 1845-1846
  choice of antimicrobials, 1346-1348
  chromosomal abnormalities, 1727-1729
  chronic tubulointerstitial nephropathy, 892
  counseling and prenatal diagnosis, 1730-1731
  cutaneous changes and malignancy, 1319
  diagnosis and management, 1729-1730, 1731
  fever of unknown origin, 1378
  hereditary hemochromatosis, 2203-2205
  hereditary tyrosinemia, 1905
  heritable disorders of carbohydrate
    metabolism, 1879-1883
    galactosemia, 1882-1883
    glycogen storage diseases, 1880-1882
    nondiabetic mellondurias, 1879-1880
  human chromosomes, 1727, 1728
  hyperlipidemia, 1892
  mechanisms of monogenic inheritance,
    1724-1726
  molecular genetics of human genome,
    1721-1724
  multifactorial inheritance, 1726-1727
  positional cloning, 1724
  treatment, 1731-1732
  Wilson's disease, 2205-2206
Genetic hypoparathyroidism, 1931
Genetic linkage analysis, 60-61
Genetic testing, 1730, 1731
  colon cancer, 2085
  endocrine, 1743
  hereditary hemochromatosis, 2204, 2205
  unconjugated hyperbilirubinemia, 2153
Genetic theories of aging, 2283
Genetics
  acute myelogenous leukemia, 689
  alcoholic liver disease, 2194, 2195
  Alport's syndrome, 876
  antibody, 1121-1126
  asthma, 1187
  autosomal dominant polycystic kidney disease,
    872
  autosomal recessive polycystic kidney disease,
    874
  cancer, 540-549
    breast, 706-707
    colon, 2083
    environmental agents, 548-549
    gastric, 2045
    genetic stability and tumor formation, 549
    lung, 486
    multistep genetic pathway to tumor
      formation, 547-548
    oncogenes, 541-545
    ovarian, 715-716
    relevance to cancer treatment, 551
    tumor suppressor genes, 545-547
  celiac disease, 2062
  Crigler-Najjar syndrome, 2153
  epilepsy, 980

Genetics—cont'd
  Gilbert's syndrome, 2153
  gout, 1271
  Graves' disease, 1805
  hematology
    fibrinogen abnormalities, 625
    hemoglobinopathies, 650-651
    hemophilia A, 619
  hereditary amyloidosis, 1284
  hereditary hemochromatosis, 2204
  human leukocyte antigen complex, 1115-1118
  hypercalciuria, 798
  hypertrophic cardiomyopathy, 265
  hypogonadotropic eunuchoidism, 1841-1842
  hypophosphatemic rickets, 1952
  inflammatory bowel disease, 2068
  inherited myopathies, 1028
  juvenile nephronophthisis and medullary
    cystic disease, 875
  molecular biology of cardiovascular system,
    49-63
    adrenergic receptors and G proteins, 56-58
    cardiac growth and hypertrophy, 55-56, 57
    cardiomyopathies, 60-62
    contractile and cytoskeletal proteins, 59-60
    DNA cloning, 52-53
    DNA code, 49-50
    DNA libraries, 54
    electrophoresis, 51-52
    gene expression and regulation, 50-51
    gene transfer, 55
    ion channels, 58-59
    isolation and digestion of DNA, 51
    lipoproteins, apolipoproteins, and
      atherosclerosis, 60
    polymerase chain reaction, 55, 56
    recombinant techniques, 51
    restriction fragment length polymorphism,
      54-55
    RNA analysis, 53-54
    sequencing, 54
    Southern, Northern, Western, and
      Southwestern blotting, 52
  neurofibromatosis, 1921
  obesity, 1751, 2102
  osteoarthritis risk, 1264
  osteoporosis, 1946
  polycystic liver disease, 2111
  psoriasis, 1300
  rheumatoid arthritis, 1201
  sickle cell disease, 657
  Sjögren syndrome, 1210
  systemic lupus erythematosus, 1212
  tuberous sclerosis, 1922
  vasopressin deficiency, 1795-1796
  von Hippel-Lindau disease, 1922
Geniohyoid advancement, 2309
Genital herpes, 1523-1524
Genital infection, *Mycoplasma hominis,*
  1540-1541
Genital lesions, sexually transmitted infection,
  1444
Genitourinary atrophy, 2271
Genitourinary tract
  anaerobic bacterial infection, 1618
  autonomic regulation, 933-934
  brucellosis, 1606
  diabetic autonomic neuropathy, 1873
  gram-negative bacteremia, 1446
  hematuria, 757
  normal flora, 1614
  spinal cord injury, 1050
  tuberculosis, 1634
Genodermatoses, 1319-1320
Genome, molecular genetics, 1721-1724
Genotype, 50
  cystic fibrosis, 481
  non-Hodgkin's lymphoma, 697
Gentamicin
  bacterial meningitis, 1411
  brucellosis, 1605

Gentamicin—cont'd
  dosage, 1349
  effect on vestibular function, 972
  effects on kidney, 868
  enterococci resistance, 1561
  infective endocarditis, 231, 232
  septic arthritis, 1253
  tularemia, 1608
  use during pregnancy, 2281
Geophagia, 827
Geriatric medicine, 2282-2293
  aortic stenosis, 236-237
  asymptomatic bacteriuria, 1461
  biology of aging, 2283-2285
  changes in osmoregulatory system, 1789
  chronic lymphocytic leukemia, 684
  dementia, 2288-2289
  demography and epidemiology, 2282-2283
  depression, 2289
  elder abuse, 4
  eye problems, 2300-2306
    age-related macular degeneration,
      2301-2302
    cataracts, 2301
    diabetic retinopathy, 2303-2304
    glaucoma, 2301, 2302
    hypertensive retinopathy, 2302-2303
    presbyopia, 2301
    visual loss, 2300-2301
  falls, 2289-2290, 2291
  health care expenditure, 14
  hematuria, 757
  hormones and, 1076-1077
  hyperkalemia, 832
  hypertension, 312, 327
  multiple myeloma, 700
  myelodysplasia, 676
  myocardial infarction, 210, 211
  osteoarthritis, 1264
  peripheral vascular disease, 305
  prolonged bleeding times, 569
  special considerations, 2285-2288
  thrombolytic therapy, 214
  urinary incontinence, 1065-1066, 2290-2293
Germ cell tumor
  cytogenetics, 731
  mediastinal, 513
  ovarian, 716
  pineal, 1070
  poorly differentiated carcinoma, 732
  testicular, 720
Germander, 2193
Germinal cell dysfunction, 1844-1846
Germinal center of lymphoid follicle, 597
Germinal epithelium, 1832
Germinoma, pineal, 1070
Gerontology, 2282-2285
Gerstmann's syndrome, 978
GESICA survival trial, 171
Gestational diabetes, 1856, 2273
Gestational iron deficiency, 642
GFR; *see* Glomerular filtration rate
GHRH; *see* Growth hormone-releasing hormone
Giant cavernous hemangioma, 614
Giant cell arteritis, 304, 311, 959, 1223-1224
  anterior ischemic optic neuropathy, 1059
  fever of unknown origin, 1378
  glucocorticoid protocol, 1263
  neurologic manifestations, 1092
Giant cell granulomatous vasculitis, 470-471
Giant cell interstitial pneumonia, 448
Giant cell thyroiditis, 1811-1812
Giant hemangioma, 2215
Giant molluscum, 1327
Giant peristaltic contraction, 1979
Giantism, 1769
Gianturco-Roubin stent, 119
Giardia lamblia, 1684-1685
  acquired immunodeficiency syndrome, 1476,
    2096
  compromised host, 1388

Giardia lamblia—cont'd
  diarrhea, 1428, 1429, 2051
  gay bowel syndrome, 1429
  hypogammaglobulinemia, 2066
  immunodeficiency syndromes, 1993
  trophozoite and cyst, Plate VIII-53
Gibbs-Donnan effect, 736, 805
Giemsa stain, 1371
  Borrelia, 1646
  Chagas' disease, 1690
  Chlamydia trachomatis, 1536, Plate VIII-11
  fever and rash, 1385
  Helicobacter pylori, 2003
  leishmaniasis, 1685, 1687, Plate VIII-12
  malaria, 1674
  plague, 1610
  Plasmodium falciparum, Plate VIII-14
  Plasmodium vivax, Plate VIII-15
  Pneumocystis carinii, 1693, Plate VIII-10
  Trypanosoma brucei rhodesiense, Plate
    VIII-16
  Trypanosoma cruzi, Plate VIII-17
Gierke's disease, 1881
Gilbert's syndrome, 2151, 2152, 2153
Gingiva
  anaerobic infection, 1617
  normal microflora, 1615
Gingivitis, 1617
GISSI III study, 172
Gitelman's syndrome, 828
Gla protein, 1716, 1747
Glafenine, 2191
Glandular stomach, 1981
Glanzmann's thrombasthenia, 536, 570, 611
Glasgow Coma scale, 1043
Glaucoma
  diabetes mellitus, 1871
  elderly, 2301, 2302
  nitrates, 201
Gleason grading system for prostate cancer, 717,
  718
Gleet, 1440
Glenohumeral joint, 1164
Gliadin, 2062
Glioblastoma multiforme, 1068, 1069
Glipizide
  diabetes mellitus, 1858
  hepatic injury, 2191
Glitter cell, 744
Global aphasia, 976
Globin gene, 650-651
Globulins, 760
Globus sensation, 1998
Glomerular basement membrane, 876
  nail-patella syndrome, 877
  proteinuria, 760
Glomerular capillary permeability, 760
Glomerular diseases, 841-859
  acquired immunodeficiency syndrome
    nephropathy, 853
  acute nephritic syndrome, 763
  adverse reaction to nonsteroidal
    antiinflammatory agents, 853
  Alport's syndrome, 876-877
  diabetic nephropathy, 859
  focal glomerular sclerosis, 851-852
  glomerular involvement in systemic diseases,
    855-859
  hematuria, 757
  heroin nephropathy, 853
  immunoglobulin A nephropathy, 845
  loin pain-hematuria syndrome, 845-846
  mechanisms and consequences of immune
    glomerular injury, 841-843
  membranoproliferative glomerulonephritis,
    854-855
  membranous nephropathy, 853-854
  mesangial proliferative disease, 851
  minimal change disease, 849-851
  nephritis associated with visceral abscess, 844
  postinfectious glomerulonephritis, 843-844

Glomerular diseases—cont'd
  rapidly progressive glomerulonephritis,
    846-849
  subacute bacterial endocarditis, 844
Glomerular filtration, 760
Glomerular filtration rate, 737-738, 746-747
  aging and, 2284
  chronic renal failure, 776, 777, 778
  congestive heart failure, 817
  diabetic nephropathy, 859
  hyperphosphatemia, 1938
  hypokalemia, 829
  nephrotic syndrome, 821
  obstructive uropathy, 885
  during pregnancy, 2274
  prerenal azotemia, 769
  tubulointerstitial disease, 888
Glomerular permeability
  acute renal failure, 769
  nephrotic syndrome, 765
Glomerular ultrafiltration, 737
Glomerulonephritis
  acute renal failure, 769
  Alport's syndrome, 876-877
  casts, 745
  chemotactic defects, 1340
  immune complexes, 1149
  immunoglobulin A nephropathy, 845
  infective endocarditis, 227
  loin pain-hematuria syndrome, 845-846
  membranoproliferative, 854-855
  microscopic polyarteritis nodosa, 1220-1221
  postinfectious, 843-845
  poststreptococcal, 1559
  posttransplantation, 794
  primary renal diseases, 841, 842
  rapidly progressive, 846-849
  Sjögren syndrome, 1210
  vasculitis, 1225
Glomerulosclerosis
  chronic renal failure, 778
  monoclonal light chain deposition disease, 863
  progressive glomerular diseases, 842
Glomerulus
  calcium reabsorption, 1718
  diabetic nephropathy, 859
Glossitis, 2106
Glossopharyngeal neuralgia, 953
Glottis, 404-406
Glucagon
  chronic renal failure, 784
  fasting hypoglycemia, 1878
  glucagonoma, 2245
  glucose production, 1874, 1875
  glycolysis, 1851
  hypoglycemic coma, 1867
  integrated fuel homeostasis, 1853
  regulation of albumin synthesis, 2119
Glucagonoma, 2244-2245
Glucocorticoids, 1740-1741
  anaphylaxis, 1194
  asthma, 1190-1191
  calcium homeostasis, 1720
  deficiency, 838
  dermatitis, 1303
  drug-induced acute hepatocellular disease,
    2193
  effects on potassium transport, 741
  enhancement of cognitive function, 1076
  gluconeogenesis, 2122
  hirsutism, 1756, 1757
  human cytochrome P450 isoforms, 2312
  hypopituitarism treatment, 1779-1780, 1781
  immune hemolytic anemia, 669
  metastatic cancer, 1073
  overproduction in Cushing's syndrome,
    1819-1820
  pure red blood cell aplasia, 674-675
  remediable aldosteronism, 828
  rheumatic diseases, 1262-1263
  sarcoidosis, 459

Glucocorticoids—cont'd
before surgery, 2262
vasopressin inhibition, 1791
Gluconeogenesis, 1851, 1852, 2121
Glucose
absorption, 1987
acute meningitis, 1408
blood
insulin release, 1714
insulinoma, 2244
metabolic actions of liver, 2121
metabolic encephalopathy, 1079
Somogyi phenomenon, 1861
cerebral requirements, 1874
conjugation of bilirubin, 2149
diabetes mellitus, 1855-1856
diabetic nephropathy, 860-861
fasting hypoglycemia, 1878
hepatic metabolism, 2121
homeostasis during fasting, 1852
hyperglycemia
acute pancreatitis, 2236, 2237
cataracts, 1871
diabetes mellitus, 1850
diabetic glomerulopathy, 860
diabetic ketoacidosis, 1863
diabetic mother, 2272-2273
diabetic retinopathy, 2303
drug-induced, 1855
glucagonoma, 2245
gram-negative bacteremia, 1449
hyperosmolar nonketotic coma, 1866
hypophosphatemia, 1935
lactic acidosis, 1867
potassium diffusion out of cells, 826
weakness, 1754
hyperkalemia, 833
hypoglycemia, 1874-1879
acute fatty liver of pregnancy, 2278
adrenal medulla hypofunction, 1828
amylo-1,6-glucosidase deficiency, 1882
cholera, 1595
chronic pancreatitis, 2241
diagnosis, 1877-1878
dizziness, 972
effects on fetus, 1874
endocrine paraneoplastic syndromes, 583
epilepsy *versus*, 981
fulminant hepatic failure, 2163
glucose-6-phosphate dehydrogenase
deficiency, 1881
gram-negative bacteremia, 1449
growth hormone deficiency, 1777
hereditary fructose intolerance, 1880
hypoglycemic coma, 1867
insulin-induced, 202, 826, 1735-1736
insulinoma, 2244
leprechaunism, 1900
metabolic encephalopathy, 1079
neurologic aspects, 1101
pathophysiology, 1875-1876
physiology, 1874-1875
Somogyi phenomenon, 1861
syncope *versus*, 954-955
treatment, 1878
vasopressin stimulation, 1790
hypoglycemic coma, 1867
hypoglycorrhachia
bacterial meningitis, 1407
spinal fluid examination, 904
hypophosphatemia, 1935, 1936
leprechaunism, 1900
lipodystrophy, 1901
metabolic encephalopathy, 1079
metabolic myopathy, 1028
myocardial energy metabolism, 40
plasma, 743
fasting hypoglycemia, 1877
hypoglycemia, 1875
regulation of hepatic triglyceride formation,
2121

Glucose—cont'd
renal glycosuria, 878-879
suppression of growth hormone, 1737
synovial fluid, 1163
urinary, 743
Glucose-6-phosphate dehydrogenase
deficiency, 1881
eccentrocytes, Plate IV-4
hemolytic anemia, 663-664
red blood cell enzyme defect, 588
hemolytic anemia, 663
malaria and, 1674
muscle phosphofructokinase deficiency, 1882
myeloproliferative disorders, 686
Glucose-galactose malabsorption, 2068
Glucose phosphate isomerase, 663
Glucose tolerance, 1855
acromegaly, 1783
aging and, 2284-2285
glucagonoma, 2244
Glucuronic acid, 2123, 2149
3-O-Glucuronide, 2128
Glutamate, 1076
Glutamic acid, 1904
Glutamic oxaloacetic transaminase
alcoholic hepatitis, 2196
hypothyroidism, 1809
Glutamic pyruvic transaminase, 2196
Glutamine
hepatic encephalopathy, 2161
related diseases, 1904
Glutathione-S-transferase, 2126, 2128,
2148-2149
Gluteal reflex, 964
Gluten, celiac disease, 2062
Gluten-sensitive enteropathy, 1296
Glutethimide derivatives
breast cancer, 710, 711
Cushing's disease, 1786-1787
ectopic adrenocorticotropic hormone secretion,
1822
hepatic injury, 2192
Glycation theory of aging, 2283
Glycerol
bacterial meningitis, 1413
glaucoma, 2302
Glycerol phosphate, 2122
Glyceryl guaiacolate, 1740
Glycine
bile acid conjugation, 2125
hyponatremia, 812
isovaleric acidemia, 1908
related diseases, 1904
Glycogen
storage in liver, 2121
synthesis, 1851
Glycogen storage diseases, 1880-1882
Glycogenic amino acids, 2121-2122
Glycols, 866
Glycolysis, 1851, 2121
Glycopeptides, 1561
Glycoprotein cell surface membrane receptors,
1710-1711
Glycoproteins
dystrophin-associated, 1027
lung extracellular matrix, 371
mucin, 2220
platelet membrane, 536
Glycosaminoglycans
lung extracellular matrix, 371
mucopolysaccharidosis, 1912
Glycosuria
acute pancreatitis, 2237
Fanconi's syndrome, 882
renal, 878-879
Glycylleucine, 1988
Gnathostoma spinigerum, 1700, 1702
GnRH; *see* Gonadotropin-releasing hormone
Goblet cell, 365
Goeckerman regimen, 1301-1302

Goiter
euthyroid, 1812-1813
euthyroid hyperthyroxinemia, 1803
Hashimoto's thyroiditis, 1811
substernal, 513
thyroid-stimulating hormone receptor
antibodies, 1801
thyrotoxicosis, 1804
Goitrous hypothyroidism, 1809
Gold compounds
acute renal failure, 867
aplastic anemia, 672
asthma, 1191
hepatic injury, 2191
pulmonary parenchymal reactions, 476
pulmonary toxicity, 478-479
rheumatic disease, 1260
rheumatoid arthritis, 1208
Goldie-Coldman hypothesis, 552
Golfer's elbow, 1197
Golgi apparatus, 1709
Gonadal dysgenesis, 1769, 1838
Gonadal steroids, 1076
Gonadal toxins, 1844
Gonadotroph cell, 1773, 1774
Gonadotropin-releasing hormone, 1774-1775
adult hypogonadotropic hypogonadism, 1845
amenorrhea, 1757-1759
constitutional delay of puberty, 1768
gonadotropin-secreting pituitary tumor, 1787
gynecomastia, 1763-1764
hypogonadotropic eunuchoidism, 1841-1842
hypothalamic amenorrhea, 1837
hypothalamic secretion, 1834
impotence, 1763
ovarian feedback mechanisms, 1834-1835
ovarian function, 1832, 1833-1834
puberty, 1766, 1767
testing, 1735
Gonadotropins, 1775
basal measurements, 1737
deficiency, 1777, 1841
constitutional delay, 1843
hypopituitarism treatment, 1780-1781
laboratory and diagnostic testing, 1835, 1836
ovarian, 1833-1835
Gonads
dysfunction in end-stage renal disease, 787
function testing, 1742-1743
hypergonadotropic disorders, 1845
hypogonadism
acromegaly, 1782
chronic hepatic failure, 2170-2171
evaluation of testicular function, 1840
gonadotropin deficiency, 1777
gynecomastia, 1764, 1765
impotence, 1761
Prader-Labhart-Willi syndrome, 1842
hypogonadotropic eunuchoidism, 1841-1842,
1843
hypogonadotropic hypogonadism, 1842,
1843-1844
hypothalamic-pituitary gonadal system,
1774-1775
Gonococcal infection
Neisseria gonorrhoeae, 1581-1585
beta-lactamases, 1345
complement deficiencies, 1179
diarrhea, 1476
immunoglobulin A, 1337
peritonitis, 2248
primary peritonitis, 1396
septic arthritis, 1251
urethritis, 1455
polyarticular septic arthritis, 1250-1251
skin lesion, Plate VIII-22
urethritis, 1440
Gonorrhea, 1581-1585
dysuria, 762, 763
during pregnancy, 2279-2280
urethritis, 1440

Goodpasture's syndrome, 454, 846-849
  acute glomerulonephritis with hemoptysis, 775
  autoantibodies, 1155
  immune complexes, 1138
Gordolobo yerba tea, 2193
Gordon's syndrome, 832
Gorlin formula, 111
Gorlin's syndrome, 1319
Gottron's papule, 1292, Plate VII-3
Gottron's sign, 1235
Gout, 1268-1276
  after renal transplantation, 795
  chronic renal failure, 785
  osteoarthritis, 1267
  primary hyperparathyroidism, 1966
  septic arthritis *versus*, 1252
  uric acid stones, 799
Gouty arthritis, 1271-1272
  joint space narrowing, 1166
  osseous erosions, 1167-1168
  soft tissue swelling, 1165
Gowers' maneuver, 1026
Graafian follicle, 1832
Graded compression elastic stockings, 504
Gradient-echo image formation, 919
Graft
  autograft, 261
  rejection
    heart, 339-341
    hematopoietic stem cell, 578
    kidney, 793-794
    liver, 2219
    lung, 520-524
  Staphylococcus epidermidis infection, 1551
  thoracic aortic aneurysm, 300
Graft coronary artery disease, 341
Graft-*versus*-host disease
  bone marrow transplantation, 1104
  hematopoietic stem cell transplantation, 578
  transfusion reaction, 575
Graham Steell murmur, 80
  mitral stenosis, 247
  pulmonic regurgitation, 257
Grain handler's lung, 460
Gram-negative bacilli
  antibiotic selection, 1347
  Legionella pneumophila, 1621-1625
  meningitis, 1403
  normal flora, 1614
  primary peritonitis, 1396
  Salmonella, 1598-1602
  septic arthritis, 1251
  Shigella, 1602-1604
  Vibrio, 1593-1598
  Yersinia, 1609-1611
Gram-negative bacteremia, 1445-1455
  anaerobic bacteria, 1618
  clinical manifestations, 1449-1450
  diagnosis, 1450-1451
  epidemiology, 1445-1446
  laboratory findings, 1450
  microbiology, 1446
  pathogenesis, 1446-1447
  pathophysiology, 1447-1448
  prevention, 1453-1454
  therapy, 1451-1453
Gram-negative cocci
  antibiotic selection, 1347
  Neisseria gonorrhoeae, 1581-1585
  normal flora, 1614
Gram-negative coccobacilli
  Bordetella pertussis, 1611-1613
  Brucella, 1604-1607
  Francisella tularensis, 1607-1609
  Haemophilus, 1585-1890
  Pasteurella, 1609
Gram-positive bacilli, 1565-1578
  clostridial infections, 1567-1576
    bacteremia, 1576
    food-borne, 1568-1570
    gastrointestinal tract, 1567-1568

Gram-positive bacilli—cont'd
  colstridial infections—cont'd
    myonecrosis, 1574-1576
    neurologic syndromes, 1570-1572
    tetanus, 1572-1574
  Corynebacterium diphtheriae, 1565-1567
  Listeria monocytogenes, 1576-1578
  normal flora, 1614
  Whipple's disease, 2064
Gram-positive cocci, Plate VIII-4
  antibiotic selection, 1347
  enterococci, 1560-1564
    antibiotic selection, 1347
    normal flora, 1368
    nosocomial infections, 1362
    resistance to vancomycin, 1346
  normal flora, 1614
  pneumonia, Plate VII-1
  Staphylococcus aureus, 1546
    acquired immunodeficiency syndrome,
      1328-1329
    antibiotic selection, 1347
    antimicrobial resistance, 1345
    brain abscess, 1414
    cellulitis, 1420
    cystic fibrosis airway infection, 480
    dermatitis with, 1303
    empyema, 507
    erysipelas, 1420
    furuncles and carbuncles, 1421
    impetigo, 1419
    infective endocarditis, 226
    lung recipient, 517
    nosocomial infections, 1362
    osteomyelitis, 1433
    pancreatic abscess, 1399
    polyarticular septic arthritis, 1251
    respiratory tract infection, 1390
    staphylococcal scalded-skin syndrome, 1421
    urinary tract infection, 1457
  Staphylococcus epidermidis, 1546
    antibiotic selection, 1347
    bacterial meningitis, 1403
    nosocomial infections, 1362
    septic arthritis, 1251
Gram stain, 1346, 1370, 1371
  actinomycosis, 1665
  anaerobic bacteria, 1619
  anaerobic pneumonia, Plate VII-1
  aspiration pneumonia, Plate VIII-7
  bacterial meningitis, 1407, 1408
  bullous impetigo, 1419
  chronic bronchitis, 443
  clostridial cellulitis, 1422
  fever and rash, 1385
  gas gangrene, 1423
  gonococcal infection, 1584
  gram-negative bacteremia, 1451
  Haemophilus influenzae, 1588
  impetigo, 1419
  infectious esophagitis, 2020
  infective endocarditis, 228
  Legionella pneumophila, 1622
  liver abscess, 2209
  lymphangitis, 1420
  meningococcal meningitis, Plate VIII-9
  necrotizing fasciitis, 1422
  plague, 1610
  pneumococcus, Plate VIII-3
  procedure, 1371
  rectal mucosa, 1439
  septic arthritis, 1251, 1252
  synovial fluid, 1163
  tularemia, 1608
  urethral discharge, 1440
Grand mal seizure, 979, 1215
Granisetron, 581, 2027
Granulation tissue, 1201-1202
Granule
  actinomycosis, 1664-1665
  neutrophil, 1339

Granulocyte, 594, Plate IV-6
Granulocyte colony stimulating factor, 532, 1129
  aplastic anemia, 674
  chemotherapy-induced neutropenia, 1339
  febrile neutropenic patient, 1389-1390
  neutropenia, 678
Granulocyte-macrophage colony stimulating
    factor, 532, 1128, 1129
  aplastic anemia, 674
  febrile neutropenic patient, 1389-1390
  neutropenia, 678
  neutrophil production, 1339
  rheumatoid arthritis, 1201
Granulocyte transfusion, 573-574, 674
Granulocytopenia
  after stem cell transplantation, 578
  gram-negative bacteremia, 1446
Granuloma
  Churg-Strauss syndrome, 467
  Crohn's disease, 2069
  eosinophilic, 463-465
  human immunodeficiency virus infection,
    1327
  hypersensitivity pneumonitis, 461
  megakaryocytic hypoplasia, 614
  pleural biopsy, 382
  primary biliary cirrhosis, 2200
  sarcoidosis, 456
  syphilis, 1641
Granuloma annulare, 1327
Granulomatosis infantisepticum, 1577
Granulomatous disease
  acute beryllium disease, 475
  fever of unknown origin, 1376, 1378
  gastritis, 2043
  hepatitis, 1378
  interstitial nephritis, 888, 892-893
  leprosy, 1648-1651
  lung, 456
  nephritis, 892-893
  pulmonary vasculitis, 465-471
  Wegener's granulomatosis, 467-468, 469,
    1222-1223
    acute nephritic syndrome, 764
    anti-neutrophil cytoplasmic antibodies, 1219
    crescentic glomerulonephritis, 848
    lung involvement, 453
    neurologic manifestations, 1092, 1095
    renal involvement, 858
Granulomatous peritonitis, 2248
Granulomatous thyroiditis, 1811-1812
Granulosa cell, 1832
Graves' disease, 1805-1807
  antithyroid antibodies, 1801
  autoantibodies, 1155
  during pregnancy, 1808, 2273
  thyroid scan, 1802
  thyrotoxic storm, 1807-1808
  thyrotoxicosis, 1804, 1805-1807
  weakness, 1754
Gray matter, 978-979
Great arteries, complete transposition, 290
Greenfield filter, 632
Grey Turner's sign, 2234
GRFoma, 2245
Griseofulvin
  hepatic injury, 2191
  interference with oral anticoagulants, 636
  tinea unguium, 1311
Gross national product, health care expenditure,
    14
Ground substance, 1289-1290
Group A streptococci, 1553-1560
  cell structure and extracellular products,
    1554-1556
  cellulitis, 1420
  ecthyma, 1420
  epidemiology, 1553-1554
  erysipelas, 1420
  lymphangitis, 1420
  pharyngitis, 1556

Group A streptococci—cont'd
 poststreptococcal glomerulonephritis, 1559
 primary peritonitis, 1396
 respiratory tract infection, 1390
 rheumatic fever, 1256, 1558-1559
 scarlet fever, 1421, 1556
 soft-tissue infection, 1556-1557
 toxic shock syndrome, 1557-1558
 treatment, 1559-1560
Group B streptococci, 1403, 1564
Group C and G *pyogenes*-like streptococci, 1564
Group Study of Heart Failure in Argentina, 171
Growth abnormalities, 1766-1773
 Anderson's disease, 1882
 breast growth abnormalities, 1770
 complete transposition of great arteries, 290
 constitutional delay of pubertal growth, 1768
 Crohn's disease, 1768
 evaluation of pubertal growth, 1770-1772
 familial tall stature, 1769
 Fanconi's syndrome, 882
 growth hormone deficiency, 1769, 1777
 hypothyroidism, 1768-1769
 idiopathic short stature, 1769
 intestinal lymphangiectasia, 2067
 juvenile nephronophthisis, 875
 Klinefelter's syndrome, 1769
 neurofibromatosis, 1921
 puberty, 1766-1768
 rickets, 881
 tetralogy of Fallot, 289
 therapy, 1772
 Turner's syndrome, 1769
 weight abnormalities, 1769-1770
Growth factors, 532-533, 1128
 Haemophilus influenzae, 1586
 lung cancer, 487
 lung repair, 370
 mobilization of hematopoietic stem and
  progenitor cells, 533
 as therapeutic agents, 534
Growth hormone, 1775
 acromegaloidism, 1782
 acromegaly, 1769, 1782-1785
  amenorrhea, 1759
  arthropathy, 1246-1247
  clinical manifestations, 1782, 1784
  diagnosis, 1782-1783
  general appearance, 63
  hyperphosphatemia, 1938
  insulin resistance, 1862
  therapy, 1783-1784
  weakness, 1754
 aging and, 2285
 calcium homeostasis, 1720
 deficiency, 1769, 1777
 glucose production, 1874, 1875
 glucose suppression of, 1737
 GRFoma, 2245
 hypersomatotropism, 1782
 hypopituitarism treatment, 1781
 hypothalamic-pituitary growth hormone
  system, 1775
 puberty, 1767
 regulation of albumin synthesis, 2119
 secretion during sleep, 940
Growth hormone neurosecretory dysfunction,
 1769
Growth hormone-releasing factor, 2245
Growth hormone-releasing hormone, 1775
 acromegaly, 1782
 deficiency, 1769
 puberty, 1767
Growth plate, 1716
GTP; *see* Guanosine triphosphate
Guaifenesin
 rhinitis, 1183
 sinusitis, 2309
Guanabenz, 325
Guanadrel, 325
Guanafacine, 325

Guanarito virus, 1509
Guanethidine
 hypertension, 325
 interference with catecholamine assays, 1740
Guanine, 50
Guanine nucleotide binding protein, 1932, 1934
 pepsinogen secretion, 1984, 1985
Guanosine diphosphate, 57, 541, 1711
Guanosine triphosphate
 cellular modulation of contractility, 41
 G proteins, 56-57, 1711
 signal transduction, 541
Guanylate cyclase, 1712
Guided needle biopsy, 2141
Guillain-Barré syndrome
 autonomic hyperactivity, 935
 blood pressure control, 1087
 botulism *versus,* 1571
 Campylobacter jejuni infection, 1591
 complication of influenza, 1491
 F wave, 916
 poliomyelitis *versus,* 1488
 respiratory failure, 1085-1086, 1097
 weakness, 1754
Guinea worm, 1700, 1701
Gumma, 1640
Gums, hyperpigmentation, Plate VII-14
Gunn's sign, 2303
Günther's disease, 1925
GUSTO trial, 213, 214
Gut-associated lymphoid tissue, 1989-1990, 1991
Guttate psoriasis, 1301
Gynecologic cancer, 713-717
 cervical, 714-715
 endometrial, 713-714
 ovarian, 715-716
Gynecomastia, 1764-1766
 benign adolescent, 1770
 chronic hepatic failure, 2171-2172
 end-stage renal disease, 787
 impotence, 1763
 Klinefelter's syndrome, 1843
 liver cancer, 2171
 liver disease, 1843
 prolactin-secreting pituitary adenoma, 1786
 small cell lung cancer, 489

H

H reflex, 915, 916
Haddon matrix, 2265
Haemophilus, 1585-1590
 normal flora, 1368
 prosthetic valve endocarditis, 230
Haemophilus aegyptius, 1589
Haemophilus aphrophilus, 1586, 1589
Haemophilus ducreyi, 1466, 1586, 1589
Haemophilus haemolyticus, 1586
Haemophilus influenzae, Plate VIII-5
 acquired immunodeficiency syndrome, 1329
 antibiotic selection, 1347
 bacterial meningitis, 1402-1403
 beta-lactamases, 1345
 cellulitis, Plate VIII-26
 chronic bronchitis, 443
 clinical diseases, 1586-1589
 complement deficiency, 1339
 cystic fibrosis airway infection, 480
 epidemiology, 1586
 epiglottitis, 1393
 erysipelas, 1420
 Gram stain, Plate VIII-8
 immunoglobulin A, 1337
 osteomyelitis, 1433
 pericarditis, 272
 phagocytosis defects, 1341
 respiratory tract infection, 1390
 septic arthritis, 1251
 sickle cell anemia, 658
 sinusitis, 1183, 1394, 2308
 subdural empyema, 1417

Haemophilus influenzae type b vaccine, 1588-1589
Haemophilus parainfluenzae, 1586, 1589
Haemophilus paraphrophilus, 1586, 1589
Hair
 adrenal insufficiency, 1823
 argininosuccinic aciduria, 1907
 hirsutism, 1755
 hypothyroidism, 1809
 lupus erythematosus, 1291
 tinea capitis, 1308
 trichomycosis axillaris, 1422
Hair follicle, 1755
 folliculitis, 1420
Hair loss
 drug-induced, 1313
 heparin-associated, 635
 lupus erythematosus, 1291
 syphilis, 1641
 vitamin D-dependent rickets, type II, 1953
Hairy cell, 595, Plate IV-5
Hairy cell leukemia, 683-684
 characteristic cells, 595
 molecular diagnostics, 563
 myelofibrosis *versus,* 677
 splenomegaly, 601
Hairy cell leukoplakia
 acquired immunodeficiency syndrome, 1328,
  1478
 oral, Plate VIII-42
Halazone, 1685
Hallucination, 1033
 auditory, 1041
 ethanol withdrawal, 1080
 narcolepsy, 942
 visual, 1061-1062
Haloperidol
 disordered thinking, 1041
 hepatic injury, 2191
 human cytochrome P450 isoforms, 2312
 for nausea and vomiting, 2027
 schizophrenia, 1042
 status migrainosus, 962
 vasopressin inhibition, 1791
Halothane, 2190, 2191
HAM; *see* Human T-cell leukemia
  virus-associated myelopathy
Hamartoma, 492, 2082
Hamilton's Depression Rating Scale, 903
Hamman-Rich syndrome, 452
Hamman's sign, 75, 514
Hand
 acrocyanosis, 310
 arthritis, 1171-1172
 candidal paronychia, 1662
 chronic occlusive arterial disease, 308
 damage in leprosy, 1650
 dermatitis, 1304
 diabetic neuromuscular disease, 1872
 hand-foot-mouth syndrome, 657, 1489
 Raynaud's phenomenon, 310
 tinea manus, 1308
Hand-foot-mouth syndrome, 1489
Hand-foot syndrome, 657
Hand-Schuller-Christian syndrome, 463
Handwashing, 1365
Hangout interval, 72
Hansen's disease, 1648-1651
Hantaan virus, 1515, 1516
Hantavirus, 1515, 1516
Haplotype, 650-651, 1117-1118, 1722
Haptoglobin, 661
Hard metal disease, 475-476
Hardy-Weinberg formula, 1725
Harkavy syndrome, 465-467
Hartnup disease, 879, 1910, 1911
Harvey's sign, 79
Hashimoto's thyroiditis, 1811
 antithyroid antibodies, 1801
 autoantibodies, 1155
 hypothyroidism, 1808, 1809
 thyroid lymphoma, 1816

Haustra, 1980
Haustral contraction, 1980
Haversian canal, 531
Havrix, 2178
Hawaii virus, 1522
Hawkins' sign, 1197
HBsAg, 2174
Head
    computed tomography, 917-918, 919, 920
    magnetic resonance imaging, 921
    radiation-induced thyroid carcinoma,
        1816-1817
Head and neck cancer, 722-724, 732
Head trauma, 1043-1045
    dementia, 988
    endocardial hemorrhage, 1087
    frontal lobe syndrome, 1032
    increased intracranial pressure, 1084
    seizure, 980
Headache, 957-962
    acute hyponatremia, 811
    acute pharyngitis, 1393
    aldosterone excess, 1822
    bacterial meningitis, 1406
    brain abscess, 1414
    brain tumor, 1067
    brucellosis, 1605
    bubonic plague, 1610
    calcium channel blocker-induced, 205
    central nervous system disease, 973
    coarctation of aorta, 286
    dengue fever, 1465
    diabetes insipidus, 1793
    effect of nitrate therapy, 201
    epidemic pleurodynia, 1489
    erysipelas, 1420
    evaluation, 960-961
    giant-cell arteritis, 304
    herpangina, 1488
    human immunodeficiency virus, 1477-1478
    hypoglycemic coma, 1867
    influenza, 1490
    Lassa fever, 1510
    lumbar puncture-induced, 905
    Lyme disease, 1647
    lymphocytic choriomeningitis virus, 1509
    lymphogranuloma venereum, 1535
    mechanisms, 957, 958
    meningococcemia, 1579
    Mycoplasma pneumoniae pneumonia, 1539
    neurofibromatosis, 1921
    neuronal disease, 1017
    osteomalacia, 1949
    pheochromocytoma, 322
    pituitary apoplexy, 1778
    pituitary tumor, 1781, 1786
    rheumatoid arthritis, 1203
    Rocky Mountain spotted fever, 1543
    scarlet fever, 1421, 1556
    sleep-related, 947
    stroke, 1001
    subdural empyema, 1417
    superior vena caval obstruction, 511
    systemic lupus erythematosus, 1093, 1215
    tetralogy of Fallot, 289
    treatment, 961-962
    types, 957-960
Health care delivery, 31
Health care expenditure, 14-16
Health care management, 26
Health maintenance organization, 30-31
Health Plan and Employer Data and
    Information Set, 19, 34
Health status instruments, 14
Healthy People 2000, 19
Hearing handicap inventory for
    elderly-screening, 2287
Hearing loss, 2307-2308
    Alport's syndrome, 876
    central nervous system disease, 974
    elderly, 2287

Hearing loss—cont'd
    Lassa fever, 1510
    mumps complication, 1496
    neonatal cytomegalovirus, 1528
    otitis media, 1395
Hearing test, 2255, 2308
Heart
    adrenergic responses, 1828
    aging and, 2284
    anaphylaxis, 1193
    arrhythmia, 131-156
        accelerated atrioventricular junctional
            rhythm, 144
        accelerated idioventricular rhythm, 149, 150
        atrial fibrillation, 146-148
        atrial flutter, 144-146
        atrioventricular nodal reentrant tachycardia,
            141-142, 144, 145
        bradyarrhythmias and atrioventricular block,
            153-156
        ectopic atrial tachycardia, 143-144, 146
        intraventricular conduction abnormalities,
            156
        multifocal atrial tachycardia, 144, 146
        nonpharmacologic therapy, 139-140
        nonsustained ventricular tachycardia, 149
        pathophysiology, 131-134
        pharmacologic therapy, 134-139
        polymorphic ventricular tachycardia,
            151-153
        premature atrial contractions, 141
        premature ventricular contractions, 148-149
        sinus tachycardia, 141
        supraventricular tachyarrhythmias, 141, 142,
            143
        sustained monomorphic ventricular
            tachycardia, 150-151
        sustained ventricular tachycardia with wide
            QRS complex tachycardia, 149-150,
            151
        ventricular fibrillation, 153
        Wolff-Parkinson-White syndrome, 142-143,
            145
    autonomic regulation, 931-932
    candidal infection, 1663
    cardiac catheterization, 107-116
        angiography, 111, 112
        aortic regurgitation, 113-114, 242
        aortic stenosis, 113, 238
        atrial septal defect, 282
        cardiac output, 109-110
        cardiomyopathies, 115-116
        chronic constrictive pericarditis, 116
        circulatory shunts and resistances, 110-111
        coarctation of aorta, 286-287
        complete transposition of great arteries, 290
        constrictive pericarditis, 277-278, 279
        dilated cardiomyopathy, 264
        Ebstein's anomaly of tricuspid valve, 290
        endocardial cushion defect, 283
        heart failure, 167
        hypertrophic cardiomyopathy, 268
        indications, 107-108
        interventional, 116-125
        ischemic heart disease, 113
        left ventricular function, 111-113
        mitral regurgitation, 114, 115, 251
        mitral stenosis, 114-115, 248
        mitral valve prolapse, 254
        patent ductus arteriosus, 286
        precapillary pulmonary hypertension, 296,
            297
        pressure management, 108-109, 110
        primary pulmonary hypertension, 294
        pulmonic regurgitation, 257
        risks, 108, 109
        shock, 184
        sudden cardiac survivor, 188
        techniques, 108
        tetralogy of Fallot, 289
        tricuspid regurgitation, 256

Heart—cont'd
    cardiac catheterization—cont'd
        tricuspid stenosis, 256
    cardiogenic shock, 175-187
        clinical presentation, 177-180
        clinical trials, 184, 185
        coronary angioplasty, 183
        coronary artery bypass graft, 185
        differential diagnosis, 175, 176
        evaluation and treatment, 180, 181
        hemodynamic alterations, 176, 177
        mechanical intervention, 184, 185-186
        myocardial function, 176
        pharmacologic therapy, 181-182
        reperfusion therapy, 182-183
        serum lactate and anaerobic metabolism,
            176, 178
    Chagas's disease, 1690
    changes during pregnancy, 2276
    chest pain, 125-129
    congestive heart failure, 156-175
        after valve replacement, 259
        angiotensin-converting enzyme inhibitors,
            169-172
        antiarrhythmic therapy, 174
        anticoagulation, 174-175
        beta-adrenergic blockers, 174
        calcium channel blockers, 174
        cardiac catheterization, 17
        cardiac output, 159
        cardiac transplantation, 335-336
        cellular abnormalities of myocardial failure,
            159-160
        clinical manifestations, 163-165
        compensatory mechanisms, 159
        diastolic heart failure, 167-168
        differential diagnosis, 168
        diuretics, 169, 170
        epidemiology and prognosis, 157-158
        high-output failure, 160
        inotropic agents, 172-173, 174
        laboratory and diagnostic testing, 165-167
        neuroendocrine activity, 160, 161, 162, 163
        neurohormonal hypothesis, 161
        pathogenesis, 158-159
        patient and family counseling, 167
        peripheral vascular and reflex control
            abnormalities, 161-162, 164
        pulmonary edema, 168-169, 423
        sodium and water retention, 162-163
        therapy before cardiac transplantation, 336
        vasodilators, 173-174
    diabetic autonomic neuropathy, 1873
    effects of hyperkalemia, 832
    effects of hypokalemia, 829
    effects of hypomagnesemia, 1942
    effects of spinal cord injury, 1049
    electrical activity, 81-82
    electrocardiography, 81-91
        acute pericarditis, 273, 274
        aortic regurgitation, 241
        aortic stenosis, 237, 287
        arrhythmia, 133-134, 135
        atrial flutter, 144, 146
        atrial septal defect, 281, 282
        atrioventricular reciprocating tachycardia,
            142, 145
        cardiac electrical activity, 81-82
        cardiac tamponade, 276
        chamber enlargement and hypertrophy,
            87-88
        coarctation of aorta, 286
        conduction abnormalities, 86-87
        congenitally corrected transposition of great
            arteries, 290
        constrictive pericarditis, 277
        cor pulmonale, 498
        dilated cardiomyopathy, 264
        dissection of aorta, 301
        drug and metabolic effects, 90
        early repolarization, 89-90

Heart—cont'd
  electrocardiography—cont'd
    endocardial cushion defect, 283
    heart failure, 166
    hypertrophic cardiomyopathy, 267
    interpretation, 84-86
    ischemic heart disease, 88-89, 197-198
    lung cancer, 488
    mitral regurgitation, 251, 253
    mitral stenosis, 247
    mitral valve prolapse, 254
    myocardial infarction, 211
    myocarditis, 263
    P wave, 83-84
    palpitations, 130, 131
    pericarditis, 89
    precapillary pulmonary hypertension, 296
    primary pulmonary hypertension, 294
    pulmonary thromboembolism, 501
    pulmonic regurgitation, 257
    pulmonic stenosis, 288
    QRS complex, 84
    ST segment, 84
    standard leads, 82-83
    sudden cardiac survivor, 188
    supraventricular tachyarrhythmias, 141, 142,
      143
    sustained ventricular tachycardia and wide
      QRS complex tachycardia, 150
    T wave, 84
    tetralogy of Fallot, 289
    tricuspid regurgitation, 256
    tricuspid stenosis, 256
    U wave, 84
    ventricular septal defect, 284
  hypotension
    after cardiac transplantation, 335
    calcium channel blocker-induced, 205
    dissection of aorta, 301
    heart failure, 173
    penetrating injury to heart, 332
  interventional cardiac catheterization, 116-125
    approach to specific lesions, 120-121
    background, 116-117
    complications, 122
    coronary angioplasty for acute myocardial
      infarction, 121-122
    devices, 117-120, 121
    pathophysiology, 116
    primary coronary angioplasty, 122
    randomized trials, 117, 118
    referral, 124
    rescue coronary angioplasty, 122
    restenosis, 122-124
  lipodystrophy, 1901
  lung cancer and, 488
  magnetic resonance imaging, 389-390
  malposition, 291
  manifestations of neurologic disease,
    1086-1088
  Marfan syndrome, 1289
  molecular biology, 49-63
    adrenergic receptors and G proteins, 56-58
    cardiac growth and hypertrophy, 55-56, 57
    cardiomyopathies, 60-62
    contractile and cytoskeletal proteins, 59-60
    DNA cloning, 52-53
    DNA code, 49-50
    DNA libraries, 54
    electrophoresis, 51-52
    gene expression and regulation, 50-51
    gene transfer, 55
    ion channels, 58-59
    isolation and digestion of DNA, 51
    lipoproteins, apolipoproteins, and
      atherosclerosis, 60
    polymerase chain reaction, 55, 56
    recombinant techniques, 51
    restriction fragment length polymorphism,
      54-55
    RNA analysis, 53-54

Heart—cont'd
  molecular biology—cont'd
    sequencing, 54
    Southern, Northern, Western, and
      Southwestern blotting, 52
  noninvasive cardiac testing, 91-107
    chest radiography, 91, 92
    computed tomography, 106
    continuous ambulatory electrocardiographic
      recording, 94
    echocardiography, 94-100
    exercise electrocardiographic testing, 91-94
    gamma camera imaging agents, 105
    ischemic heart disease, 198-199
    magnetic resonance imaging, 106-107
    myocardial perfusion imaging, 101-104
    positron emission tomography, 105-106
    radionuclide angiography, 104-105
    sudden cardiac death survivor, 188
  obstructive sleep apnea and, 526
  operative risks, 2257-2260
  palpitations, 130-131
  pericardial tuberculosis, 1636-1637
  physical examination, 63-81
    arterial pulses, 64-65, 66, 67
    auscultation, 68-71
    blood pressure measurement, 64
    cardiac cycle, 71-72
    general appearance, 63-64
    heart murmurs, 75-81
    heart sounds, 72-75, 76
    inspection and palpation, 67-68, 70, 71
    jugular venous pulse, 65-67, 68, 69
  physiology, 36-49
    capillary exchange, 47-48
    cardiac cycle, 36-37
    cardiac output and systemic hemodynamics,
      46-47
    cellular basis of cardiac contraction, 37-41
    coronary circulation, 48-49
    diastolic function, 43-46
    response to dynamic exercise, 49
    structure and function of ventricle, 41-42
    systolic function, 42-43
  polyarteritis nodosa, 1220
  rheumatic fever, 1256-1258
  rheumatoid arthritis, 1204
  sickle cell disease, 657
  sudden cardiac death, 187-191
    aortic stenosis, 236, 238-239
    congenital aortic stenosis, 287
    diabetic autonomic neuropathy, 1873
    Ebstein's anomaly, 290
    familial hypertrophic cardiomyopathy, 61
    hypertrophic cardiomyopathy, 270
    hypertrophic obstructive cardiomyopathy,
      269
    obesity, 1753
    pituitary apoplexy, 1778
    primary pulmonary hypertension, 294
    prosthetic valve problems, 258
    tetralogy of Fallot, 289
    ventricular fibrillation, 153
    Wolff-Parkinson-White syndrome, 142
  systemic lupus erythematosus, 1215
  systemic sclerosis, 1230, 1232
  toxicity of chemotherapeutic agents, 584
  transplantation, 335-344
    anomalous origin of left coronary artery,
      292
    evaluation and medical therapy of heart
      failure, 335-336
    function after, 342-343
    future directions, 343-344
    referral for, 335
    rejection and immunosuppression, 339-342
    selection, 336-339
    tumor, 329-332
Heart block, 153-156
  atrial fibrillation, 148
  during cardiac catheterization, 108

Heart block—cont'd
  cardiogenic syncope, 954
  hypermagnesemia, 1943
  myocardial infarction, 222-223
  myocarditis, 263
  neurologic aspects, 1088
  pacemaker, 139
  palpitations, 130
  paroxysmal atrial tachycardia, 143
  rheumatic fever, 1257
  right ventricular infarction, 220
  supraventricular tachyarrhythmias, 141
Heart disease
  aortic, 299-304
    aortic aneurysm, 299-300
    aortitis, 302-303
    atherosclerosis, 299
    dissection of aorta, 300-302, 303
    Marfan syndrome, 299
    mycotic aneurysm, 299, 300
    occlusive disease, 304
    syphilis, 303
  cardiac transplantation, 335-344
    dilated cardiomyopathy, 264-265
    evaluation and medical therapy of heart
      failure, 335-336
    function after, 342-343
    future directions, 343-344
    pericardial effusion following, 274
    referral for, 335
    rejection and immunosuppression, 339-342
    selection, 336-339
  cardiac tumor, 329-332
  cardiomyopathy, 262-271
    accelerated idioventricular rhythm, 149
    acquired immunodeficiency syndrome, 333
    atrial fibrillation, 146
    cardiac catheterization, 115-116
    Chagas's disease, 1690
    chest pain, 128
    contractile and cytoskeletal proteins, 59-60
    dilated, 263-265
    echocardiography, 100
    hypertrophic, 128, 187, 265-270
    metabolic myopathy, 1086-1087
    molecular biology, 60-62
    myocarditis, 262-263
    radionuclide angiography, 104
    restrictive, 270-271
    sarcoidosis, 458
    sudden cardiac death, 187
    uremic, 784
  chronic renal failure, 783-784
  congenital, 280-292
    aberrant right subclavian artery, 291
    aortic stenosis, 287
    aortopulmonary septal defect, 286
    atrial septal defect, 280-282
    bicuspid aortic valve, 287
    coarctation of aorta, 286-287
    complete transposition of great arteries, 290
    congenitally corrected transposition of great
      arteries, 290
    cor triatriatum, 291
    coronary artery abnormalities, 291-292
    coronary sinus aneurysm, 291
    disturbances of conduction, 292
    Ebstein's anomaly of tricuspid valve,
      289-290
    endocardial cushion defect, 282-283
    etiology, 280
    fetal circulation and changes associated
      with birth, 280
    malposition of heart, 291
    partial transposition of pulmonary veins,
      282
    patent ductus arteriosus, 285-286
    pericardial defects, 291-292
    precapillary pulmonary hypertension,
      296-297
    tetralogy of Fallot, 288-289

Heart disease—cont'd
  congenital—cont'd
    total anomalous pulmonary venous
        connection, 290-291
    tricuspid atresia, 291
    truncus arteriosus, 290
    valvular pulmonic stenosis with intact
        ventricular septum, 288
    ventricular septal defect, 283-285
  contractile and cytoskeletal proteins, 59-60
  cost-utility analysis, 16
  esophageal disease with, 1999
  hypertension, 312-329
    aortic aneurysm, 299
    aortic stenosis, 236-237
    atherosclerosis risk, 192
    coronary artery disease, 200
    diagnostic tests, 329
    differential diagnosis, 320-322
    dissection of aorta, 301
    environmental mechanisms, 319
    exertional angina, 127
    frequency, 312-314
    increased intracellular sodium and calcium,
        317-318
    increased peripheral resistance, 314-319
    increased sodium intake, 318-319
    management, 322-329
    mitral stenosis, 245
    natural history, 319-322
    obstructive sleep apnea and, 526
    peripheral arterial aneurysm, 309
    proteinuria, 760
    referral, 329
    renal sodium retention, 316-317, 318
    renovascular, 321
    risk factors, 314, 315
    stress, 316
    types, 314, 315
  infective endocarditis, 225-235
    acquired immunodeficiency syndrome, 333
    antimicrobial therapy, 230-233
    aortic regurgitation, 244
    aspergillosis, 1658
    brucellosis, 1606
    candidiasis, 1664
    clinical syndrome, 227-228
    coagulase-negative staphylococci,
        1550-1551
    differential diagnosis, 229
    drug user, 229-230
    fever and rash, 1383
    general appearance, 63
    Haemophilus influenzae, 1586
    laboratory findings, 228-229
    mitral regurgitation, 250
    pathophysiology, 225-227
    prophylaxis, 233, 234-235
    prosthetic heart valve, 230, 258-259
    referral, 233-234
    Staphylococcus aureus, 1550
  interstitial lung disease with, 452
  ischemic, 192-208
    antianginal therapy, 205
    beta-adrenergic blockers, 201-203
    calcium channel blockers, 203-205
    clinical manifestations, 195-197
    coronary angioplasty and revascularization,
        205-207
    electrocardiography, 88-89
    etiology, 192, 193
    laboratory studies, 197-200
    nitroglycerin and nitrates, 200-201, 202
    nuclear cardiology techniques, 101
    pathophysiology, 192-195
    physical examination, 197
    prognosis, 208
    radionuclide angiography, 105
    therapeutic approaches, 207-208
  lipoproteins and apolipoproteins, 60
  menopause, 2271

Heart disease—cont'd
  myocardial infarction, 209-225
    accelerated atrioventricular junctional
        rhythm, 144
    acute cholecystitis *versus,* 2228
    acute mitral regurgitation, 219, 220
    adjunctive therapy, 215-218
    angioplasty, 214-215
    angiotensin-converting enzyme inhibitors,
        172
    anomalous origin of left coronary artery,
        292
    anticoagulant therapy, 639
    aortic dissection, 300
    atrioventricular block, 156
    beta-blockers, 138
    during cardiac catheterization, 108
    cardiac imaging, 212
    cardiogenic shock, 176, 177
    chest pain, 127
    clinical presentation, 209-211
    complete heart block, 180
    congenital abnormalities of coronary
        arteries, 292
    coronary angioplasty, 121-122
    coronary artery bypass graft, 185
    during coronary artery bypass graft, 206
    echocardiography, 100
    electrical complications, 222-224
    electrocardiographic manifestations, 211
    electrocardiography, 88-89
    incidence, 209
    infarct expansion and left ventricular
        aneurysm, 221
    laboratory tests, 211-212
    left ventricular failure, 218-219
    left ventricular mural thrombosis, 638
    left ventricular thrombus, 221, 222
    macrovascular disease, 1868
    mechanical complications, 219
    mitral regurgitation, 250
    myocardial rupture, 219, 220
    neurologic aspects, 1089
    nuclear cardiology techniques, 101
    PAMI trial, 122
    pathophysiology, 209, 210
    percutaneous transluminal coronary
        angioplasty *versus* coronary artery
        bypass graft, 118
    pericarditis, 221-222
    pericarditis after, 273
    premature ventricular contractions, 149
    preoperative, 2257
    radionuclide angiography, 105
    rehabilitation and preventive cardiology,
        224
    right ventricular infarction, 220-221
    risk stratification, 224
    sepsis *versus,* 1451
    shock, 176, 177, 180
    stent, 119
    sustained monomorphic ventricular
        tachycardia, 151
    thrombolytic therapy, 212-214
    ventricular fibrillation, 153
    ventricular septal rupture, 219-220
    ventricular tachycardia, 180
    neurologic aspects, 1088-1090
    occlusive mesenteric vascular disease with,
        2087
  pericardial, 271-279
    acute pericarditis, 273-274
    after myocardial infarction, 221-222
    cardiac tamponade, 275-276
    chest pain, 128
    constrictive pericarditis, 277-278
    electrocardiography, 89
    etiology, 272-273
    management, 278-279
    pericardial effusion, 274-275
    referral, 279

Heart disease—cont'd
  pericardial—cont'd
    restrictive cardiomyopathy *versus,* 271
  peripheral vascular disease, 304-312
    anticoagulant therapy, 641
    arteritis, 311
    occlusive peripheral arterial disease,
        307-309
    peripheral arterial aneurysm, 309
    peripheral arteries, 305-307
    peripheral veins, 311-312
    vasospastic disorders, 309-311
  physical examination of cardiovascular
      system, 63-81
    arterial pulses, 64-65, 66, 67
    auscultation, 68-71
    blood pressure measurement, 64
    cardiac cycle, 71-72
    general appearance, 63-64
    heart murmurs, 75-81
    heart sounds, 72-75, 76
    inspection and palpation, 67-68, 70, 71
    jugular venous pulse, 65-67, 68, 69
  pregnancy and, 2276
  pulmonary hypertension, 293-299
    chronic obstructive pulmonary disease,
        446-447
    interstitial lung disease, 452
    passive, 297-298
    precapillary, 293-297
    primary and secondary causes, 497-499
    reactive, 298
  secondary polycythemia, 588-589
  sudden cardiac death, 187
  syphilis, 1641
  valvular, 235-262
    aortic regurgitation, 239-245
    aortic stenosis, 235-239
    mitral regurgitation, 249-253
    mitral stenosis, 245-249
    mitral valve prolapse, 253-255
    multivalvular, 257
    prosthetic valves, 257-261
    pulmonic regurgitation, 256-257
    pulmonic stenosis, 256
    tricuspid regurgitation, 256
    tricuspid stenosis, 255-256
Heart failure, 156-175
  advanced renal disease, 784
  after stroke, 1007
  after valve replacement, 259
  angiotensin-converting enzyme inhibitors,
      169-172
  antiarrhythmic therapy, 174
  anticoagulation, 174-175
  antihypertensive agent choices, 326
  atrial fibrillation, 146
  beta-adrenergic blockers, 174
  calcium channel blockers, 174
  cardiac catheterization, 17, 108
  cardiac output, 159
  cardiac transplantation, 335-336
  cellular abnormalities of myocardial failure,
      159-160
  Cheyne-Stokes respiration, 353
  Churg-Strauss syndrome, 466
  clinical manifestations, 163-165
  compensatory mechanisms, 159
  Congestive Heart Failure Survival Trial of
      Antiarrhythmic Therapy, 171
  coronary sinus aneurysm, 291
  diabetes mellitus, 334
  diastolic heart failure, 167-168
  differential diagnosis, 168
  diuretics, 169, 170
  edema, 816
  epidemiology and prognosis, 157-158
  high-output failure, 160
  infective endocarditis, 228
  inotropic agents, 172-173, 174
  laboratory and diagnostic testing, 165-167

Heart failure—cont'd
  mesenteric vascular disease, 2086
  myocarditis, 262-263
  neuroendocrine activity, 160, 161, 162, 163
  neurohormonal hypothesis, 161
  operative risk, 2258
  pathogenesis, 158-159
  patient and family counseling, 167
  peripheral vascular and reflex control
     abnormalities, 161-162, 164
  Pompe's disease, 1881
  proteinuria, 760
  pulmonary edema, 168-169, 423
  rabies, 1506
  radionuclide angiography, 104-105
  rheumatic fever, 1256-1257
  sodium and water retention, 162-163
  sodium balance dysfunction, 817-818
  splenomegaly, 601
  syphilis, 1641
  therapy before cardiac transplantation, 336
  thiamine deficiency, 2106
  thrombosis, 609
  transudative pleural effusion, 507
  vasodilators, 173-174
  ventricular septal defect, 284
  weight loss, 1750
Heart-lung transplantation, 515
Heart murmur, 75-81
  aortic regurgitation, 241
  aortic stenosis, 236, 287
  atrial septal defect, 281
  bicuspid aortic valve, 287
  cardiac auscultation, 70
  coarctation of aorta, 286
  congenital coronary arteriovenous fistula, 292
  dilated cardiomyopathy, 263-264
  Ebstein's anomaly of tricuspid valve, 290
  hypertrophic obstructive cardiomyopathy,
     266-267
  infective endocarditis, 227
  ischemic heart disease, 197
  left atrial myxoma, 330
  mitral regurgitation, 251
  mitral stenosis, 246-247
  mitral valve prolapse, 253, 254
  myocardial infarction, 210
  patent ductus arteriosus, 285
  pulmonic regurgitation, 257
  rheumatic fever, 1256
  sinus of Valsalva fistula, 291
  tetralogy of Fallot, 289
  tricuspid stenosis, 255
  ventricular septal defect, 283
Heart rate
  aging and, 2284
  changes during pregnancy, 2276
  exercise testing, 94, 379
  myocardial oxygen demand, 192-193
  palpitations, 130
  power spectral analysis, 937
  response to standing, 937
  short-term modulation of ventricular function,
     45-46
  systematic inflammatory response syndrome,
     1445
  Valsalva's maneuver, 937
Heart sounds, 67-68, 72-75, 76
  anginal attack, 196
  aortic regurgitation, 241, 244
  aortic stenosis, 236
  atrial septal defect, 281
  cardiac auscultation, 68-70
  chronic obstructive pulmonary disease, 442
  dilated cardiomyopathy, 263-264
  Ebstein's anomaly, 290
  heart failure, 165
  hypertrophic cardiomyopathy, 266-267
  ischemic heart disease, 197
  mitral regurgitation, 251
  mitral stenosis, 245

Heart sounds—cont'd
  mitral valve prolapse, 254
  myocardial infarction, 210
  myocarditis, 262
  primary pulmonary hypertension, 294
  pulmonic regurgitation, 257
  pulmonic stenosis, 288
  spontaneous pneumomediastinum, 514
Heartburn, 1999
  erosive esophagitis, 2017
  upper gastrointestinal endoscopy, 1994
Heat, reduced sperm production, 1846
Heavy chain
  human leukocyte antigen, 1111, 1118
  immunoglobulin, 1110
Heavy-chain diseases, 704
Heavy chain gene, 1124
Heavy chain locus, 1125
Heavy metals
  Fanconi's syndrome, 882
  hypoparathyroidism, 1931
  nephrotoxicity, 867, 891
Heberden's node, 1199
  osteoarthritis, 1266
  pseudoosteoarthritis, 1279
HEDIS; *see Health Plan and Employer Data
     and Information Set*
Heerfordt's syndrome, 459
Height, 2112
  preventive care guidelines, 2255
  puberty, 1767, 1770
  recommended daily dietary allowances, 2114,
     2117
Height and weight table, 2112
Heinz body, 557, 600, Plate IV-4
  beta-thalassemia, 654
  glucose-6-phosphate dehydrogenase
     deficiency, 664
Helicobacter pylori, 1592-1593
  abnormalities of gastric acid secretion, 1984
  acquired immunodeficiency syndrome, 2095
  carcinogenesis, 548
  gastric cancer risk, 2045
  gastritis, 2041, 2042-2043
  monocytoid B lymphoma, 697
  peptic ulcer, 2035-2036
  testing for, 2003
Helium dilution technique, 378
Helix-loop-helix proteins, 51
Heller's myotomy, 2022
HELLP syndrome, 615, 775, 2274
Helminth infection, 1696-1706
  brown pigment stones, 2224
  eosinophilia, 1705-1706
  intestinal worms, 1696-1698
  intestinal worms with tissue migratory phases,
     1698-1699
  tissue worms, 1699-1705
  travel-related, 1466
Helper T-cell, 1127
  differentiation, 1130-1131
  human immunodeficiency virus infection,
     1470
  oral tolerance, 1143
  respiratory, 367
  sarcoidosis, 1324
Hemangioendothelioma, 2215
Hemangioma
  cavernous, 2215-2216
  giant cavernous, 614
  incidence, 329
Hemangiopericytoma, 321
Hemarthrosis, 606, 619-620
Hematemesis
  gastric cancer, 2046
  gastrointestinal bleeding, 2010
  hemobilia, 2233
  infectious esophagitis, 2020
  peptic ulcer, 2037
  upper gastrointestinal endoscopy, 1994
Hematin, 1926

Hematochezia
  gastrointestinal bleeding, 2010
  Meckel's diverticulum, 2089
Hematocrit, 555
  abnormal, 586-590
  bleeding varices, 2166
  chronic myeloproliferative disorders, 686
  gastrointestinal bleeding, 2011
  hypertension, 318
  salt and water depletion, 824
Hematogenous osteomyelitis, 1433, 1435
Hematologic disease
  abnormal hematocrit, 586-590
  abnormal nucleated blood cell counts, 590-596
    nucleated cells in peripheral blood, 594-596
    quantitative alterations in normal nucleated
      cells, 590-594
  abnormalities of phagocytes, eosinophils, and
     basophils, 678-681
  anemia
    acute myelogenous leukemia, 689
    acute renal failure, 773
    amebic liver abscess, 2210
    celiac sprue, 2062
    chest pain, 128
    chronic disease, 642-643
    chronic myelogenous leukemia, 686
    chronic renal failure, 783
    congenital erythropoietic porphyria, 1925
    Crohn's disease, 2070
    disseminated tuberculosis, 1635
    Fanconi's, 672
    gastric cancer, 2046
    giant-cell arteritis, 304
    glucagonoma, 2244
    Goodpasture's syndrome, 847
    hematopoietic abnormalities, 534
    high-output failure, 160
    hypersplenism, 601
    infective endocarditis, 228
    intestinal disease, 2005
    low hematocrit, 586
    macroglobulinemia, 704
    malabsorption, 2057
    malaria, 1673
    megaloblastic, 646-650
    multiple myeloma, 701
    myelodysplastic syndrome, 676
    myelofibrosis, 677
    neurologic aspects, 1103
    non-Hodgkin's lymphoma, 697
    nutritional deficiency, 2100
    operative risk, 2262
    osteopetrosis, 1958
    overproduction jaundice, 2152
    oxygen transport, 350
    during pregnancy, 2279
    primary hyperparathyroidism, 1966
    prosthetic heart valve, 258
    protein-calorie malnutrition, 2102
    protoporphyria, 1926
    red blood cell mass, 586
    renal cell carcinoma, 898
    sideroblastic, 645-646
    Sjögren syndrome, 1210
    systemic lupus erythematosus, 1215
    ulcerative colitis, 2073
    Waldenström macroglobulinemia, 704
  anemia of chronic disease, 642-643
  aplastic anemia, 671-674, 675
    failure of hematopoiesis, 533
    hematopoietic stem cell transplantation, 576
    hepatitis associated with, 2177
    nosocomial infection, 1361
  arthropathy, 1246
  bleeding disorders, 602-610
    blood vessels, 602-605
    coagulation dysfunction, 606-608
    increased risk for thrombosis, 608-609
    multiple hemostatic defects, 608
    plasma coagulation, 570-571

Hematologic disease—cont'd
  bleeding disorders—cont'd
    platelet function, 568-570
    preoperative assessment, 609-610
    pseudothrombocytopenia, 610
    risk in multiple myeloma, 700
    screening tests, 571-572
  blood transfusion, 572-576
    adverse effects, 564-576
    cold agglutinin disease, 670
    granulocyte, 573-574
    myelofibrosis, 677
    plasma, 573
    platelets, 573
    whole blood and red cell, 572-573
  bone marrow failure, 671-677
    aplasias of single cell lineages, 674-675
    aplastic anemia, 671-674, 675
    myelodysplasia, 675-676
    myelofibrosis, 676-677
  chronic renal failure, 783
  chronic tubulointerstitial nephropathy, 891-892
  coagulation disorders, 617-630
    acquired inhibitors of blood coagulation,
        628-630
    disseminated intravascular coagulation,
        627-628
    factor deficiencies, 624
    fibrinogen abnormalities, 625
    hemophilia A, 617-622
    hemophilia B, 622
    liver disease, 626-627
    protease inhibitors deficiencies, 625
    vitamin K deficiency, 625-626
    von Willebrand's disease, 622-624
  deoxyribonucleic acid analysis, 561-564
  disseminated tuberculosis, 1635
  hemoglobinopathy, 350-351, 650-660
    arthropathy, 1246
    neurologic aspects, 1103
    during pregnancy, 2279
    prenatal diagnosis and screening, 660
    sickle cell disease, 656-660
    thalassemia, 652-656
  hemolytic anemia, 661-671
    acquired, 666-668
    congenital erythropoietic porphyria, 1925
    dietary factors, 2102
    drug-induced, 670
    hereditary, 662-666
    homozygous beta thalassemia, 654
    hypophosphatemia, 1936
    immune, 668-670
    Mycoplasma pneumoniae pneumonia,
        1539-1540
    patient evaluation, 661-662
    risk of pigment stone formation, 2223-2224
    splenomegaly, 601
    thrombotic thrombocytopenic purpura, 615
  iron deficiency anemia, 642-645, 2109
    celiac sprue, 2062
    folate deficiency, 650
    Goodpasture's syndrome, 847
    hookworm infection, 1698
    intestinal disease, 2005
    peritoneal mesenteric and omental diseases,
        2248
    during pregnancy, 2279
    splenomegaly, 601
    ulcerative colitis, 2073
    upper gastrointestinal endoscopy, 1994
  lymphadenopathy, 596-600
  megaloblastic anemia, 646-650, 827
  molecular and cellular biology of
        hematopoiesis, 530-534
  neurohematology, 1103-1105
  pernicious anemia
    autoantibodies, 1155
    dementia, 987
    dizziness, 972
    gastric antibodies, 1157

Hematologic disease—cont'd
  pernicious anemia—cont'd
    gastric cancer, 2045
    hypokalemia, 827
    Lambert-Eaton myasthenic syndrome with,
        1024
    neurologic aspects, 1103
    during pregnancy, 2279
    Schilling test, 2060
    type A gastritis, 2042
    vitamin B_{12} deficiency, 650
  during pregnancy, 2279
  sickle cell anemia, 656-660, Plate IV-4
    acute meningitis, 1407
    arthropathy, 1246
    hypergonadotropic hypogonadism, 1843
    neurologic aspects, 1103
    renal manifestations, 891
    thrombosis, 609
  sideroblastic anemia, 645-646
  splenectomy, 602
  splenomegaly, 600-602
  thrombocytopenia, 613-617
    acute myelogenous leukemia, 689
    cirrhosis, 627
    evaluation, 569
    gram-negative bacteremia, 1449, 1450
    hemolytic-uremic syndrome, 858
    hemorrhagic fever, 1511
    heparin-induced, 634-635
    hypersplenism, 601
    lymphocytic choriomeningitis virus,
        1509
    malaria, 1673
    neurologic aspects, 1104
    petechiae, 603
    during pregnancy, 2279
    pure amegakaryocytic thrombocytopenic
        purpura, 675
    vitamin B_{12} deficiency, 648
    Wiskott-Aldrich syndrome, 1178
  thrombosis, 630-641
    acute aortic obstruction, 304
    aortic aneurysm, 300
    arterial, 308, 638-641
    Behçet disease, 469
    bleeding disorders, 608-609
    dissection of aorta, 302
    essential thrombocythemia, 688
    hypertrophic obstructive cardiomyopathy,
        269
    lupus inhibitor, 629
    myocardial infarction, 209, 210, 221, 222
    nephrotic syndrome, 766
    peripheral arterial aneurysm, 309
    plasma coagulation, 570-571
    platelets and platelet function, 568-570
    polycythemia vera, 688
    primary pulmonary hypertension, 293
    prosthetic heart valve, 258
    pulmonary, 388, 499-504
    renal artery, 756
    screening tests, 571-572
    superficial thrombophlebitis, 638
    unstable angina, 195
    venous, 311, 630-638
Hematoma
  bleeding patient, 603
  head trauma, 1043-1045
  hemophilia, 606, 620
  purpura *versus,* 603
  septal, 2308
Hematopoiesis
  cytokine regulation, 1128
  molecular and cellular biology, 530-534
Hematopoietic cords, 531
Hematopoietic cytokine receptor superfamily,
    1128
Hematopoietic growth factors, 674
Hematopoietic regulatory molecules, 532-533

Hematopoietic stem cell, 530-531
  paroxysmal nocturnal hemoglobinuria, 668
  transplantation, 576-579
Hematoxylin and eosin preparation
  Negri body, Plate VIII-43
  peripheral lymph node hyperplasia, Plate
      VIII-35
Hematuria, 756-758
  acute nephritic syndrome, 763
  Alport's syndrome, 876
  autosomal dominant polycystic kidney disease,
      873
  bacterial prostatitis, 1462
  crescentic glomerulonephritis, 848
  focal glomerular sclerosis, 852
  Goodpasture's syndrome, 847
  in hemophilic patient, 620
  idiopathic nephrotic syndrome, 850
  immunoglobulin A nephropathy, 845
  kidney stones, 800
  loin pain-hematuria syndrome, 845-846
  obstructive uropathy, 886
  poststreptococcal glomerulonephritis, 844
  renal biopsy-induced, 748
  renal cell carcinoma, 898
  thrombotic thrombocytopenic purpura, 615,
      858
  upper urinary tract tumor, 899
  urinary tract infection, 1458
Heme
  absorption, 1988
  bile, 2123
  bilirubin, 2128, 2147-2148, 2149
  biosynthesis, 1923
  oxygen transport, 652
  reagent stick test, 744
Heme-heme interaction, 652
Heme oxygenase, 2149
Hemiacidrin, 804
Hemicraniectomy, 1084
Hemineglect, 1033
Hemispatial neglect, 1033
Hemobilia, 2209, 2233
Hemochromatosis, 646
  calcium pyrophosphate dihydrate deposition
      disease, 1279
  cardiomyopathy, 262
  chronic hepatitis, 2180
  hepatocellular carcinoma, 2212
  hereditary, 2203-2205
  hypogonadism, 1843
  impotence, 1761, 1762
  iron absorption, 1988
  osteoarthritis, 1267
Hemodialysis, 867
  acute renal failure, 774
  chronic renal failure, 789-790
  hepatitis C virus infection, 2175
  hypercalcemia, 1929
  hyperkalemia, 833
  hyperphosphatemia, 1939
  induction of beta$_2$-microglobulin amyloidosis,
      1284
  malnutrition, 2100
  neurologic complications, 1105-1106
  transient thrombocytopenia, 614
  urea cycle disorders, 1906
Hemodynamic monitoring, 390-396
  adult respiratory distress syndrome, 421
  aortic regurgitation, 243
  cardiac catheterization, 107-116
    angiography, 111, 112
    aortic regurgitation, 113-114
    aortic stenosis, 113
    cardiac output, 109-110
    cardiomyopathies, 115-116
    chronic constrictive pericarditis, 116
    circulatory shunts and resistances, 110-111
    indications, 107-108
    ischemic heart disease, 113
    left ventricular function, 111-113

Hemodynamic monitoring—cont'd
  cardiac catheterization—cont'd
    mitral regurgitation, 114, 115
    mitral stenosis, 114-115
    pressure management, 108-109, 110
    risks, 108, 109
    techniques, 108
  cardiac tamponade, 276
  constrictive pericarditis, 277-278, 279
  end-tidal carbon dioxide, 396
  heart failure, 167
  myocardial infarction, 218, 219
  peripheral artery catheterization, 390
  pulmonary artery catheterization, 390-395
  pulse oximetry, 396
  sepsis, 1450
  shock, 180
  transcutaneous oxygen and carbon dioxide, 396
Hemodynamic pulmonary edema, 168
Hemodynamics
  normal at rest, 110
  proteinuria, 760-761
Hemofiltration, 791
Hemoglobin, 555
  bleeding varices, 2166
  chronic liver disease, 2136
  gastrointestinal bleeding, 2011
  hemoglobinopathies, 350-351, 650-660
    arthropathy, 1246
    neurologic aspects, 1103
    during pregnancy, 2279
    prenatal diagnosis and screening, 660
    sickle cell disease, 656-660
    thalassemia, 652-656
  hemoglobinuria
    chemical exposure, 867-868
    hemolytic anemia, 661
    March, 666-667
    paroxysmal cold, 670
    paroxysmal nocturnal, 668
  insulin therapy in diabetes mellitus, 1859-1860
  iron, 642
  multiple myeloma, 701
  proteinuria, 760
  urinalysis, 744
Hemoglobin oxygen-carrying capacity, 110
Hemoglobin-oxygen dissociation curve, 652
Hemoglobinopathy, 350-351, 650-660
  arthropathy, 1246
  neurologic aspects, 1103
  during pregnancy, 2279
  prenatal diagnosis and screening, 660
  sickle cell disease, 656-660
  thalassemia, 652-656
Hemoglobinuria
  chemical exposure, 867-868
  hemolytic anemia, 661
  March, 666-667
  paroxysmal cold, 670
  paroxysmal nocturnal, 668
Hemolysins, 1446
Hemolysis
  babesiosis, 1676
  galactosemia, 1883
  hemolytic anemia, 661-671
    acquired, 666-668
    drug-induced, 670
    hereditary, 662-666
    homozygous beta thalassemia, 654
    immune, 668-670
    patient evaluation, 661-662
    splenomegaly, 601
    thrombotic thrombocytopenic purpura, 615
  hemophilia, 622
  hyperkalemia, 831
  hypophosphatemia, 1936
  malaria, 1673
  Mycoplasma pneumoniae pneumonia, 1539-1540
  preeclamptic patient, 2274

Hemolysis—cont'd
  prosthetic heart valve, 258
  risk of pigment stone formation, 2223-2224
  sickle cell disease, 657
Hemolytic anemia, 661-671
  acquired, 666-668
  congenital erythropoietic porphyria, 1925
  dietary factors, 2102
  drug-induced, 670
  hereditary, 662-666
  homozygous beta thalassemia, 654
  hypophosphatemia, 1936
  immune, 668-670
  Mycoplasma pneumoniae pneumonia, 1539-1540
  patient evaluation, 661-662
  risk of pigment stone formation, 2223-2224
  splenomegaly, 601
  thrombotic thrombocytopenic purpura, 615
Hemolytic jaundice, 2152
Hemolytic transfusion reaction, 574
Hemolytic-uremic syndrome, 615, 666, 858
Hemophagocytic syndrome, 680
Hemophilia
  arthropathy, 1246
  hepatitis C virus infection, 2175
  Ivy method bleeding time, 606
  partial thromboplastin time, 571
Hemophilia A, 617-622
Hemophilia B, 622
Hemopneumothorax, 510
Hemoptysis, 410-411
  anaplastic thyroid carcinoma, 1815
  anti-GBM antibody disease, 454
  bronchial artery angiogram, 388
  bronchiectasis, 484
  chronic obstructive pulmonary disease, 442
  cystic fibrosis, 482-483
  Goodpasture's syndrome, 847
  lung cancer, 488
  mitral stenosis, 246
  tuberculosis, 1628
  Wegener's granulomatosis, 468, 1222
Hemorrhage, 978, 2041-2044
  acute hemorrhagic conjunctivitis, 1490
  acute hypertensive retinopathy, 2302
  anal fissure, 2093
  colon cancer, 2085
  from colonic diverticulum, 2089-2090, 2091, 2092
  complication of thrombolytic therapy, 637
  diabetic retinopathy, 2303
  epistaxis, 2308
  erosive esophagitis, 2017
  essential thrombocythemia, 688
  gastric cancer, 2046
  gastrointestinal, 2008-2014
    acquired immunodeficiency syndrome, 2098-2099
    antacids and antisecretory agents, 2013
    Campylobacter jejuni, 1591
    chronic renal failure, 783, 784
    colonoscopy, 1996
    cutaneous manifestations, 1320
    diagnostic and therapeutic studies, 2011-2013
    esophageal varices, 2013-2014
    initial management, 2010-2011
  hemobilia, 2233
  hemophilia A, 619
  hemorrhoids, 2093
  heparin-induced, 634-635
  inherited deficiencies of protease inhibitors, 625
  intracranial
    complication of systemic cancer, 1071
    computed tomography, 919
    endocardial hemorrhage with, 1087
    factor XIII deficiency, 624
    hemophilic patient, 620
    hemorrhagic stroke, 997, 998

Hemorrhage—cont'd
  liver biopsy complication, 2141
  macroglobulinemia, 704
  Mallory-Weiss syndrome, 2028
  Meckel's diverticulum, 2090-2091
  myocardial contusion, 332
  peptic ulcer, 2037, 2039-2040
  platelet function disorders, 612
  prosthetic heart valve, 261
  pulmonary hemorrhage syndromes, 454-455
  pyogenic liver abscess, 2209
  relationship to platelet count, 612
  retinal vein occlusion, Plate XI-9
  retroperitoneal, 2250
  scurvy, 2107
  side effect of oral anticoagulant therapy, 636
  subarachnoid, 960, 1043
  variceal
    hepatocellular carcinoma, 2213
    portal hypertension, 2165-2168, 2166
    portal vein obstruction, 2208
    primary biliary cirrhosis, 2200
  vitamin K deficiency, 2106
  vitreous, Plate XI-8
Hemorrhagic bullae, Plate IV-10
Hemorrhagic cystitis, 1504
Hemorrhagic diathesis, 1103-1104
Hemorrhagic fever, 1465, 1511
  dengue, 1516, 1517
  hazard to laboratory personnel, 1369
Hemorrhagic stroke, 997-998, 1006
Hemorrhoidectomy, 2093
Hemorrhoids, 483, 2092-2093
Hemosiderin, 642
  erythrocyte fragmentation syndromes, 667
  hemolytic anemia, 661
Hemostasis, 534-540
  bleeding disorders, 602-610
    coagulation dysfunction, 606-608
    increased risk for thrombosis, 608-609
    multiple hemostatic defects, 608
    platelets and blood vessels, 602-605
    preoperative assessment, 609-610
    pseudothrombocytopenia, 610
  plasma coagulation, 570-571
  platelet function disorders, 610-613
  platelets and platelet function, 535-537, 568-570
  screening tests for thrombotic disorders, 571-572
  secondary, 537-539
  sepsis syndrome, 1448
  spinal cord injury, 1049
  thrombocytopenia, 613-617
Hemothorax, 508-509
Henderson-Hasselbalch equation, 834
Henle's loop
  calcium reabsorption, 1718
  magnesium reabsorption, 1939
  potassium transport, 741
  renal concentrating and diluting mechanisms, 739, 740
Henoch-Schönlein purpura, 454, 857, 1222
HEp-2 cell adherence assay, 1426, 1427
Heparin
  acute aortic obstruction, 304
  after myocardial infarction, 639
  angina, 205, 207
  during cardiac catheterization, 108
  deep venous thrombosis, 311
  disseminated intravascular coagulation, 628
  drug-induced immune thrombocytopenia, 615-616
  fulminant hepatic failure, 2163
  hyperkalemia, 832
  mast cell, 1142
  myocardial infarction, 212, 217
  non-Q wave myocardial infarction, 218
  during pregnancy, 2276
  pulmonary thromboembolism, 503
  recurrent embolism, 641

Heparin—cont'd
  reocclusion of infarct-related vessel, 214
  restenosis, 124
  unstable angina, 639
  venous thromboembolism, 311, 632, 633
Heparin cofactor II, 539
Heparinoid, 634
Hepatic adenoma, 2216-2217
Hepatic artery thrombosis, 2219
Hepatic encephalopathy
  abnormalities of amino acid metabolism and
      urea formation, 2102
  liver failure, 2159-2163
Hepatic epithelioid hemangioendothelioma, 2215
Hepatic fibrosis, 2195
Hepatic iron concentration, 2204
Hepatic iron index, 2139, 2204
Hepatic metabolism, 2118-2123
  amino acids and protein, 2118-2120
  carbohydrates, 2121-2122
  detoxification, 2122
  hormones, 2122-2123
  lipids, 2120-2121
Hepatic phosphorylase b kinase deficiency, 1882
Hepatic storage disease, 2157-2158
Hepatic triglyceride lipase, 1886
Hepatic vein
  drug-induced thrombosis, 2189
  transjugular intrahepatic shunt, 2167
  veno-occlusive disease, 585, 2207-2208
Hepatic venoocclusive disease, 585, 2207-2209
Hepatitis
  acquired immunodeficiency syndrome, 2099
  acute viral infection, 2172-2179
    hepatitis A virus, 2173
    hepatitis B virus, 2173-2175
    hepatitis C virus, 2175-2176
    hepatitis delta virus, 2176
    hepatitis E virus, 2176-2177
    hepatitis G virus, 2177
    non-A–non-B, 2177
    prevention, 2178-2179
    treatment, 2177-2178
  alcoholic, 2196, 2197, 2295
  chronic, 2179-2184
    autoimmune, 2183-2184
    clinical assessment, 2180-2181
    etiologic classification, 2180
    hepatitis B virus, 2181-2182
    hepatitis C virus, 2182-2183
    hepatitis D virus, 2183
    treatment, 2184
  chronic viral infection, 2179-2184
  coagulation disorder, 607
  conjugated hyperbilirubinemia, 2154
  dialysis-related, 790
  drug-induced hepatocellular injury *versus,*
      2193
  enteroviral, 1490
  fever of unknown origin, 1376
  hepatorenal syndrome, 2168
  impairment of canalicular secretion of
      conjugated bilirubins, 2155
  inflammatory bowel disease, 2076
  isoniazid-induced, 1637
  liver transplantation, 2219
  operative risk, 2263
  serum alkaline phosphatase level, 2137
  systemic lupus erythematosus, 1215
  transfusion-associated, 575
    hemophilic patient, 621
  travel-related, 1465
  Wilson's disease, 2205
Hepatitis A, 2138, 2173
  acute, 2173
  aplastic anemia, 672
  posttransfusion, 575
  during pregnancy, 2277
  prevention, 2178
  transfusion-transmitted, 575
  traveler, 1465

Hepatitis A vaccine, 1493, 2178
Hepatitis A viral antigen, 2173
Hepatitis activity index, 2181
Hepatitis B, 2138, 2173-2175
  acute, 2173-2175
  carcinogenesis, 548
  chronic, 2181-2182
  hepatocellular carcinoma, 2212
  immune complexes, 1137-1138
  polyarteritis nodosa, 1219
  during pregnancy, 2277
  prevention, 2178-2179
  primary biliary cirrhosis *versus,* 2200
  septic arthritis, 1255
  transfusion-associated, 575
  viral cholangitis, 2202
Hepatitis B e antigen, 2138, 2174
Hepatitis B immune globulin, 2218
Hepatitis B vaccine, 2179
  hemophilic patient, 621-622
  preventive care guidelines, 2255
Hepatitis C, 2138, 2175-2176
  acute, 2175-2176
  alcoholic, 2195
  chronic, 2182-2183
  hepatocellular carcinoma, 2212
  membranoproliferative glomerulonephritis, 854
  postnecrotic cirrhosis, 2219
  during pregnancy, 2277
  primary biliary cirrhosis *versus,* 2200
  transfusion-transmitted, 575
  viral cholangitis, 2202
Hepatitis D, 2138
  acute, 2176
  chronic, 2183
Hepatitis E, 2138, 2176-2177
  during pregnancy, 2277
  traveler, 1465
Hepatitis G, 2177
Hepatitis GB virus A, 2177
Hepatitis GB virus B, 2177
Hepatitis GB virus C, 2177
Hepatobiliary disease
  acquired immunodeficiency syndrome,
      2098-2099
  benign stricture of extrahepatic bile ducts,
      2232-2233
  biliary dyskinesia, 2233
  bilirubin metabolism disorders, 2147-2159
    classification, 2150, 2151
    conjugated hyperbilirubinemia, 2154-2156
    Dubin-Johnson syndrome, 2157
    familial cholestatic syndromes, 2158-2159
    normal bilirubin metabolism, 2147-2150
    postoperative cholestasis, 2159
    Rotor's syndrome and hepatic storage
        disease, 2157-2158
    unconjugated hyperbilirubinemia,
        2150-2154
  carcinoma of ampulla of Vater, 2232
  carcinoma of bile ducts, 2231-2232
  conjugated hyperbilirubinemia, 2154
  developmental anomalies, 2233
  drug-induced and toxic cholangitis, 2202-2203
  evaluation, 2134-2144
    distinguishing acute from chronic disease,
        2134-2136
    estimations of severity and prognosis,
        2141-2144
    hereditary markers, 2138-2139
    imaging studies, 2140-2141
    immunologic markers, 2139-2140
    liver biopsy, 2141
    patterns of liver injury, 2136-2137
    viral markers, 2138
  fever of unknown origin, 1376
  gallbladder cancer, 2232
  hemobilia, 2233
  hyperplastic cholecystosis, 2233
  impaired lipid ingestion, 1987
  ischemic cholangitis, 2203

Hepatobiliary disease—cont'd
  malabsorption, 2062
  osteomalacia, 1951-1952
  primary biliary cirrhosis, 2199-2201
    autoantibodies, 1155
    mitochondrial antibodies, 1157
  primary sclerosing cholangitis, 2201-2202,
      2203
  viral cholangitis, 2202
Hepatocanalicular cholestasis, 2187
Hepatocellular carcinoma, 2212-2214
  allelic loss, 546
  chronic hepatitis B, 2181
  drug-induced, 2189
  fibrolamellar, 2214
  hepatitis B virus, 2173
  hepatitis C virus, 2175
  porphyria cutanea tarda, 1927
Hepatocellular jaundice, 2156
Hepatocerebral degeneration, 1102, 2161
Hepatocyte
  albumin synthesis, 2119
  alcoholic fatty liver, 2196
  bile salts and, 2124
  bilirubin clearance, 2147
  direct hepatotoxins, 2185
  focal nodular hyperplasia, 2216
Hepatoerythropoietic porphyria, 1927
Hepatojugular reflux, 65
Hepatomegaly
  alcoholic fatty liver, 2196
  alcoholic hepatitis and cirrhosis, 2197
  amylo-1,6-glucosidase deficiency, 1882
  Budd-Chiari syndrome, 2208
  cholangiocarcinoma, 2231
  Dubin-Johnson and Rotor's syndromes, 2157
  galactosemia, 1882
  hepatic epithelioid hemangioendothelioma,
      2215
  idiopathic myelofibrosis, 677
  pyogenic liver abscess, 2209
Hepatopulmonary syndrome, 2170
Hepatorenal reflex, 2168
Hepatorenal syndrome, 775, 2168-2170
Hepatosplenomegaly
  brucellosis, 1606
  constrictive pericarditis, 277
  gangliosidoses, 1919
  heavy-chain disease, 704
  hereditary fructose intolerance, 1880
  melanoma, 1299
  mucopolysaccharidosis, 1912
  neonatal cytomegalovirus, 1528
  Niemann-Pick disease, 1918
  pancreatic cancer, 2242
  peliosis hepatis, 2212
  right atrial myxoma, 330
  tularemia, 1607
Hepatotoxicity
  chemotherapeutic agents, 585
  drugs and toxins, 2184-2193
    acetaminophen poisoning, 2188-2190
    acute hepatic injury, 2187-2188
    carbon tetrachloride poisoning, 2188
    chronic liver damage, 2188
    classification of hepatotoxic agents,
        2185-2187
    diagnosis, 2193
    herbal remedies and plant toxins, 2192-2193
    medications, 2190-2192
    mushroom and phosphorus poisoning, 2188
    susceptibility of liver to chemical injury,
        2185
    treatment, 2193
Herbal remedies, 2192-2193
Herbicides, 867
Hereditary amyloidosis, 1284-1285
Hereditary angioedema, 1180
Hereditary axonopathy, 1019
Hereditary coproporphyria, 1926-1927
Hereditary elliptocytosis, 665, 666

Hereditary fructose intolerance, 1880
Hereditary hemochromatosis, 646, 2203-2205
  hereditary markers, 2138-2139
Hereditary hemolytic anemia, 662-666
Hereditary hemorrhagic telangiectasia, 1321
Hereditary motor and sensory polyneuropathy,
  1018
Hereditary nonpolyposis colon cancer, 549, 2083
Hereditary onychoosteodysplasia, 877
Hereditary persistence of fetal hemoglobin, 654
Hereditary pyropoikilocytosis, 665, 666
Hereditary sideroblastic anemia, 645
Hereditary spherocytosis, 664-666, Plate IV-4
Hereditary stomatocytosis, 665, 666
Hereditary telangiectasia, 2014
Hereditary transport disorder, 828
Hereditary tyrosinemia, 2212
Hereditary xerocytosis, 666
Hering-Breuer reflex, 353
Hermansky-Pudlak syndrome, 611
Herniation
  ascites, 2164
  brain, 1044, 1082
  colonic diverticulum, 2089
  heart, 292
  hiatal, 2014, 2028
  intravertebral disk
    computed tomography, 920
    magnetic resonance imaging, 924
    myelogram, 926
  mesenteric, 2251
  tonsillar, 1044
Heroin
  abuse, 2297
  nephropathy, 853
  pulmonary parenchymal reactions, 476
  pulmonary toxicity, 479
Herpangina, 1393, 1487, 1488-1489
Herpes encephalitis, 1524
Herpes genitalis, 1444
Herpes gestationis, 1296
Herpes keratitis, 1524
Herpes simplex virus, 1523-1525
  acquired immunodeficiency syndrome, 1328,
    2098
  anal fissure and fistula, 2093
  cervicitis, 1442
  compromised host, 1388
  culture, 1369
  cutaneous lesion, 1477
  diarrhea, 1476
  encephalitis, 907, 1409
  esophageal infection, 2019-2020
  multinuclear giant cells, Plate VIII-13
  odynophagia, 1998
  pharyngitis, 1393
  posttransplant
    lung transplantation, 518, 519
    stem cell transplantation, 578-579
  during pregnancy, 2280
Herpes virus thymidine kinase, 555
Herpes zoster, 1527
  acquired immunodeficiency syndrome, 1328
  chest discomfort, 129
  cranial nerve palsy, 1017
  Hodgkin's disease, 693
  thoracolumbar radiculopathy, 1016
Herpes zoster ophthalmicus, 2304-2305
Herpesviruses, 1522-1530
  characteristics, 1522-1523
  cytomegalovirus, 1527-1529
    acquired immunodeficiency syndrome,
      1328, 2096
    acute hepatitis, 2138
    acute interstitial nephritis, 890
    after cardiac transplantation, 341-342
    after liver transplantation, 2219
    after lung transplantation, 518-519
    after stem cell transplantation, 579
    blindness, 1478
    cholangitis, 2202

Herpesviruses—cont'd
  cytomegalovirus—cont'd
    compromised host, 1388
    culture, 1369
    diarrhea, 1476
    esophageal infection, 2019-2020
    esophagitis, 2020
    fever, 1475
    fever of unknown origin, 1377
    human immunodeficiency virus-associated
      dementia, 987
    immunocompromised patient, 1387
    odynophagia, 1998
    pneumonitis, Plate VIII-37
    during pregnancy, 2280
    renal transplantation, 785, 795
    retinitis, 2305, Plate XI-11
    retinochoroiditis, Plate VIII-41
    transfusion-transmitted, 575-576
  Epstein-Barr virus, 1529-1530
    acquired immunodeficiency syndrome, 1328
    acute hepatitis, 2138
    acute interstitial nephritis, 889
    after cardiac transplantation, 1090-1091
    after lung transplantation, 519
    aplastic anemia, 672
    Burkitt's lymphoma, 695
    carcinogenesis, 548
    fever of unknown origin, 1377
    Hodgkin's disease, 691
    infectious mononucleosis, 1393
    pericarditis, 272
    renal transplant recipient, 795
    Sjögren syndrome, 1210
  esophageal infection, 2019-2020
  fever of unknown origin, 1377
  hemophagocytic syndrome, 680
  herpes simplex virus, 1523-1525
    acquired immunodeficiency syndrome,
      1328, 2098
    anal fissure and fistula, 2093
    cervicitis, 1442
    compromised host, 1388
    culture, 1369
    cutaneous lesion, 1477
    diarrhea, 1476
    encephalitis, 907, 1409
    esophageal infection, 2019-2020
    multinuclear giant cells, Plate VIII-13
    odynophagia, 1998
    pharyngitis, 1393
    posttransplant
      lung transplantation, 518, 519
      stem cell transplantation, 578-579
    during pregnancy, 2280
  human herpesvirus 6, 1530
  human herpesvirus 8, 1530
  renal transplant recipient, 795
  varicella-zoster virus, 1525-1527
    acquired immunodeficiency syndrome, 1328
    after stem cell transplantation, 579
    compromised host, 1388
    culture, 1369
    esophageal infection, 2019-2020
    pericarditis, 272
    during pregnancy, 2280
Herpetic stomatitis, 2309
Herpetic whitlow, 1524
Hertough's sign, 1322
Heterochromatic body, 1727
Heterogeneous nucleation, 797
Heteromorphisms, 1727
Heterophytes heterophytes, 1698
Heterotopic ossification, 1050-1051
Heterozygous beta-thalassemia, 654-656, Plate
  IV-4
Heterozygous thalassemia, 588
Hexacarbons, 1020
Hexokinase, 663
Hexose monophosphate shunt, 662-663, 2121
Hexoses, 1879, 2122

HG factor, 1296
Hiatal hernia, 2014
  Mallory-Weiss syndrome, 2028
Hibernating myocardium, 105
High-altitude pulmonary hypertension, 295
High-ceiling diuretics, 821-822
High-density lipoproteins, 1886, 1887-1888
  atherosclerosis, 1889
  atherosclerotic coronary artery disease, 192
  fatty acids and, 2121
  gallstone prevalence, 2223
  hypoalphalipoproteinemia, 1896, 1898
  ischemic heart disease, 192
  macrovascular disease, 1868
  nephrotic syndrome, 766
  population distribution, 1897
  primary biliary cirrhosis, 2200
  uremic patient, 786
High-frequency jet ventilator, 398
High-frequency oscillator, 398
High-frequency positive pressure ventilator, 398
High-frequency ventilation, 398
High hematocrit, 588-590
High-molecular-weight kininogen deficiency, 624
High-molecular-weight neutrophil chemotactic
  factor, 1140
High-output failure, 160
High oxygen affinity syndrome, 660
High-proliferative-potential colony forming cell,
  531
High resolution computed tomography, 484
High-resolution computed tomography
  hypersensitivity pneumonitis, 462
  interstitial lung disease, 451
  Langerhans' cell granulomatosis, 464
  pulmonary, 387
  sarcoidosis, 457
High-response inhibitors, 620
Hikojima serotype *Vibrio cholerae,* 1594
Hila, 386-387
Hilar adenopathy
  brucellosis, 1606
  computed tomography, 386
  tuberculosis, 1628
Hilar cholangiocarcinoma, 2231
Hinge region, 1122
Hip
  arthritis, 1173, 1203
  arthrography, 1164
  fracture, 2290
  total hip replacement, 504
  trochanteric bursitis, 1197
Hippocampus, 1075
Hippocratic oath, 10
Hirschsprung's disease, 1980, 2053, 2092
Hirsutism, 1755-1757
  prolactin-secreting pituitary adenoma, 1786
  21-hydroxylase deficiency, 1824
Hirudin
  heparin-induced thrombocytopenia, 635
  reocclusion of infarct-related vessel, 214
His bundle, 132
  accelerated atrioventricular junctional rhythm,
    144
  accessory pathways, 90
  arrhythmia, 134
  cardiac cycle, 36
  conduction disturbance in myocardial
    infarction, 222
  electrical impulse, 84
  intraventricular conduction abnormalities, 156
Histamine, 1140, 1141
  acid secretion stimulation, 1982
  effect on vasopressin release, 1791
  measurements, 1154
  pepsinogen secretion, 1984, 1985
  shock, 176
  stimulated acid output, 2003
  variant angina, 194
  vasoactive effects on pulmonary circulation,
    363

Histamine₁-antihistamines, 1182
Histamine₁ receptors, 1140
Histamine₂-receptor antagonists
    gastroesophageal reflux, 2018
    hepatic injury, 2192
    human cytochrome P450 isoforms, 2312
    interference with oral anticoagulants, 636
    peptic ulcer disease, 2040
    reaction with antiarrhythmics, 135-136
    typical medical regimen six months after
        transplantation, 343
Histamine₂ receptors, 1140, 1981
Histamine₃ receptors, 1982
Histidine, 1904
Histidine-alpha-deaminase, 1906
Histidinemia, 1906
Histiocyte, 2065
Histiocytic granuloma, 470
Histiocytosis, 463-465, 2202
Histologic grading of acute cellular rejection, 521
Histomorphometry, bone, 1747
Histone, 50
Histone antibody, 1159
Histoplasma capsulatum, 1654-1655
    mononuclear phagocytes, 1342
    peritonitis, 2248
Histoplasmosis, 1654-1655
    acquired immunodeficiency syndrome, 1474,
        1475, 1477
    pericarditis, 272
    serodiagnosis, 1653
History; *see* Patient history
Hives, 574
Hivid; *see* Zalcitabine
HMG CoA; *see* Hydroxy-methyl-glutaryl
        coenzyme A
HMO; *see* Health maintenance organization
Hoarseness, 2309
    acute laryngitis, 1393
    anaplastic thyroid carcinoma, 1815
    aortic dissection, 301
    esophageal cancer, 2024
    lung cancer, 488
    mediastinal abnormality, 511
    mediastinal mass, 512
    parainfluenza, 1495
Hodgkin's disease, 691-695
    acquired ichthyosis, 1316
    chemotactic defects, 1340
    curability with chemotherapy, 552
    fever of unknown origin, 1377
    infertility, 585
    internal lymphadenopathy, 598
    molecular diagnostics, 563-564
    secondary malignancies, 585-586
    stomach involvement, 2049
    thyroid gland failure, 1809
Hoesch test, 1926
Hole zones of collagen, 1716
Hollenhorst plaque, 1057
Hollow visceral myopathy, 2079
Holt-Oram syndrome, 280
Holter monitoring
    aortic stenosis, 238
    arrhythmias, 134, 135
    bradyarrhythmias and atrioventricular blocks,
        153
    ischemic heart disease, 197, 198
    mitral valve prolapse, 254
    myocarditis, 263
    sudden death survivor, 189-190
    sustained monomorphic ventricular
        tachycardia, 151
    tetralogy of Fallot, 289
Home management
    blood glucose monitoring, 1860
    diuretics in heart failure, 169
    oxygen therapy, 429
    pulmonary rehabilitation, 435
    ventilator-dependent patient with chronic
        obstructive pulmonary disease, 437

Homeostasis
    acid-base, 835-836
        chronic renal failure, 779
        cirrhosis, 818-820
        congestive heart failure, 817-818
        edematous states, 816-817
        external potassium balance, 825, 826
        extrarenal sodium depletion, 823
        hyperkalemia, 830-833
        hypernatremia, 813-816
        hypocalcemia, 1930
        hypokalemia, 826-830
        hyponatremia, 809-813
        idiopathic edema, 821
        internal potassium balance, 825-826
        metabolic acidosis, 836-839
        metabolic alkalosis, 839-841
        nephrotic syndrome, 820-821
        patient evaluation, 840, 841
        physiology, 834-836
        principles of osmoregulation, 805-809
        regulation by lung, 351
        renal acidification, 739-741
        salt-wasting states, 823
        sodium depletion of renal origin, 823-825
        use of diuretics, 821-823
    aging and, 2284
    bone and mineral, 1714-1721
        calcium metabolism, 1717-1720
        cellular physiology, 1716
        effects of hormones, 1720
        functions of skeleton, 1714-1715
        matrix formation and calcification, 1716
        natural history of skeleton, 1715-1716
        stress and coupling, 1716
    during fasting, 1852
    immune, 1114
    insulin regulation, 1853
Homocysteine, 649, 1904
Homocystinuria, 609, 1908-1909
Homogentisic acid, 1280, 1282, 1910
Homograft valve, 261
Homology units, 1122
Homonymous visual field defects, 1060-1062
Homosexual patient
    gay bowel syndrome, 1429
    gonococcal proctitis, 1583
    hepatitis A virus infection, 2173
    hepatitis B virus infection, 2174
    human immunodeficiency virus transmission,
        1471
Homozygous alpha₁-protease inhibitor
        deficiency, 440
Homozygous beta-thalassemia, 654, Plate IV-4
Honey, infant botulism, 1572
Honeycomb lung, 450
Honeymoon effect, 1861
Hookworm, 1698
Hoover's sign, 358, 402
Horizontal meridian, 1058
Hormonal ablation in prostate cancer, 719
Hormonal contraception, 2270
Hormonal derivatives, 2191
Hormonal factors, 1213
Hormonal therapy
    cancer, 554-555
        breast, 710-711
        endometrial, 714
    fibrocystic breast disease, 1849-1850
    menopause, 2271
Hormone receptors, 1710-1713
    breast cancer, 707
    regulation, 1712
    vasopressin, 1791
Hormone responsive elements, 1712-1713
Hormones, 1708-1714; *see also* Endocrine
        system
    adrenal medulla, 1826-1827
    bone and mineral homeostasis, 1714-1721
        calcium metabolism, 1717-1720
        cellular physiology, 1716

Hormones—cont'd
    bone and mineral homeostasis—cont'd
        effects of hormones, 1720
        functions of skeleton, 1714-1715
        matrix formation and calcification, 1716
        natural history of skeleton, 1715-1716
        stress and coupling, 1716
    carcinoid tumor secretion, 2082
    classes, 1708
    control of bone resorption and growth, 1716
    eating behavior, 2099
    gastrointestinal motility, 1978
    hepatic metabolism, 2122-2123
    hypothalamic-pituitary adrenal system, 1774
    hypothalamic-pituitary axis, 1773-1774
    hypothalamic-pituitary gonadal system,
        1774-1775
    hypothalamic-pituitary growth hormone
        system, 1775
    hypothalamic-pituitary prolactin system,
        1775-1776, 1777
    hypothalamic-pituitary thyroid system, 1774
    laboratory and diagnostic testing, 1732-1744
        adrenal medullary hormones, 1739-1740
        androgens, 1741
        female gonadal function, 1742-1743
        general principles, 1732-1735
        genetic studies, 1743
        glucocorticoids, 1740-1741
        hypothalamic-pituitary testing, 1735-1737
        male gonadal function, 1742
        mineralocorticoids, 1741-1742
        posterior pituitary testing, 1737-1738
        thyroid function tests, 1738-1739
    magnesium balance, 1941
    mechanisms of action, 1710-1713
    neurohypophyseal, 1077
    neurotransmitter regulation, 1076
    pancreatic exocrine secretion, 2133
    paraneoplastic syndromes, 582-583
    posterior pituitary, 1788-1789
    puberty, 1766-1767
    regulation of albumin synthesis, 2119
    regulation of central nervous system,
        1075-1078
    secretion, 1713-1714
    synthesis, 1708-1710
    testicular function, 1840-1841
    uremia, 786
Horner's syndrome, 932
    aortic dissection, 301
    lung cancer, 488
    mediastinal mass, 512
    radiation therapy-induced, 1073
Horse antihuman thymocyte globulin, 523
Horsefly, 1701
Hospice care, 2244
Hospital-acquired illness
    catheter-associated bacteremia, 1364
    fever, 1479-1482
Hospital epidemiologist, 1364
Hospital infection control, 1361-1366
Hospitalization
    acute pericarditis, 279
    acute viral hepatitis, 2177
    myocardial infarction, 218
Host defense mechanisms, 1336-1343
    bacterial meningitis, 1404-1406
    candidiasis, 1661
    choice of antibiotics, 1351
    complement system, 1338-1339
    febrile neutropenic patient, 1389-1390
    gram-negative bacteremia, 1446-1447
    humoral immunity, 1336-1337
    patterns of infection in impaired patient, 1335
    phagocytic cells, 1339-1343
    respiratory tract, 364-369
    spleen, 1337-1338
    urinary tract infection, 1456
Host-disease response, 2285

Host factors
  candidiasis, 1661
  choice of appropriate antimicrobial agents,
    1346-1351
  nosocomial infection, 1361-1362
  obligate anaerobic bacteria, 1614, 1615
Hot flush, 2270-2271
Hot tub folliculitis, 1420, 1423, Plate VIII-28
Hounsfield units, 386
Housekeeping gene, 49
Housemaid's knee, 1197
Howell-Evans syndrome, 1319
Howell-Jolly body, 600, 602, 654, Plate IV-4
HPFH; *see* Hereditary persistence of fetal
    hemoglobin
HSV; *see* Herpes simplex virus
Hu antibody, 1158
Hughes-Stovin syndrome, 469
Human chorionic gonadotropin, 1833
  adult hypogonadotropic hypogonadism, 1845
  gastric cancer, 2047
  gynecomastia, 1764
  impotence, 1763
  testicular cancer, 720
Human cyclic neutropenia, 679
Human diploid cell vaccine, 1506, 1507, 1508
Human genome, 1721-1724
Human granulocytic ehrlichiosis, 1545
Human herpesvirus 6, 1530
Human herpesvirus 8, 1530
Human immunodeficiency virus infection,
    1470-1479, 1533-1534
  acute meningitis, 1407
  adenopathy, 599
  aplastic anemia, 672
  autoimmune hemolytic anemia, 669
  biliary disease, 2202
  brain abscess, 1414
  carcinogenesis, 548
  cardiovascular involvement, 333
  clinical stages, 1471-1472
  clinical syndromes, 1474-1479
  cryptococcosis, 1667
  cryptosporidiosis, 1679
  cutaneous manifestations, 1325-1329
  cyclosporiasis, 1680
  cytomegalovirus infection, 1528
  dementia, 987, 1478
  diagnosis, 1472
  ecthyma, 1420
  epidemiology, 1470-1471
  esophageal ulcerations, 2020
  etiology and pathophysiology, 1470
  evaluation and management, 1472-1474
  fever and rash, 1381
  fever of unknown origin, 1377
  flow cytometry, 1152
  folliculitis, 1420
  gastrointestinal manifestations, 2094-2099
  generalized lymphadenopathy, 599
  gram-negative bacteremia, 1446
  hemophilia, 622
  histoplasmosis, 1655
  hypogonadism, 1843
  isosporiasis, 1680
  meningitis, 1404, 1409
  microsporidiosis, 1680
  nephropathy, 853
  neutropenia, 593
  nocardiosis, 1666
  nontuberculous mycobacterial infection, 1638,
    1639
  nosocomial infection, 1361
  ophthalmic manifestations, 2304-2306
  pericardial effusion, 272
  Pneumocystis carinii pneumonia, 1692-1696
  during pregnancy, 2281
  prevention, 1479
  primary sclerosing cholangitis, 2202
  prognosis and treatment goals, 1479
  prostatic infections, 1463

Human immunodeficiency virus infection—cont'd
  retrovirus, 1533-1534
  Salmonella, 1601-1602
  septic arthritis, 1254, 1255
  shigellosis, 1603
  spinal infection, 1013
  syphilis, 1640, 1641
  T-cell function, 1343
  thrombocytopenia, 605
  toxoplasmosis, 1677
  transfusion-transmitted, 575
  tuberculosis, 1626
  weakness, 1754
  weight loss, 1750
Human leukocyte antigen, 1115-1121
  celiac disease, 2062
  epidermolysis bullosa acquista, 1296
  genetics, 1115-1118
  Hodgkin's disease, 691
  Lyme disease, 1254
  primary biliary cirrhosis, 2199, 2201
  psoriasis, 1300
  role in disease, 1120-1121
  sarcoidosis, 457
  tissue distribution, structure, and function,
    1118-1120
  typing, 1120
Human leukocyte antigen-B27
  ankylosing spondylitis, 1238
  enteropathic arthritis, 1242
Human leukocyte antigen class I molecule,
    1118-1119
Human leukocyte antigen class II gene, 1120
Human leukocyte antigen class II molecule, 1119
Human leukocyte antigen typing, 1120
  hereditary hemochromatosis, 2204, 2205
  myasthenia gravis, 1020
Human lymphocyte antigen, 1111
Human monocytic ehrlichiosis, 1545
Human papillomavirus, 492
  carcinogenesis, 548
  cervical carcinoma, 549
Human rabies immunoglobulin, 1508
Human T-cell leukemia virus-associated
    myelopathy, 1532
Human T-cell leukemia virus type 1, 1531, 1532
  carcinogenesis, 548
  spinal infection, 1013
Human tetanus immunoglobulin, 1573
Humate-P, 624
Humidification, 429, 1180
Humidifier lung, 460
Humoral hypercalcemia of malignancy, 1972
Humoral immunity, 1336-1337
  aging and, 2285
  evaluation, 1175
  inflammatory myopathies, 1234
  spleen, 1337-1338
Hungry bone syndrome, 1936, 1940
Hunter's syndrome, 1912
Huntington's disease, 994
Hurler-Scheie syndrome, 1912
Hurler's syndrome, 1912
Hürthle cell carcinoma, 1815
Hutchinson's teeth, 1642
Hutchison's sign, 1299
Hyaline cast, 745
  acute renal failure, 771
  systemic lupus erythematosus, 1215
Hyaluronic acid, 2141
Hyaluronidase, 1555
Hycanthone, 2191
Hydatid cyst, 2111-2212
Hydatid disease, 507, 1705
Hydralazine
  aortic regurgitation, 243
  autonomic dysreflexia, 1049
  congestive heart failure, 818
  drug-induced bile duct injury, 2203
  heart failure, 170, 173-174
  hepatic injury, 2192

Hydralazine—cont'd
  hypertension, 325, 327
  hypertensive emergency, 328
  interference with catecholamine assays, 1740
  preeclampsia, 2275
Hydramnios, 883
Hydration
  acute diarrhea, 2051
  acute renal failure, 773
  choledocholithiasis, 2229
  cholera, 1596
  diabetic ketoacidosis, 1864
  diarrhea, 1431
  hepatorenal syndrome, 2170
  hypercalcemia, 1929
  hypercalciuria, 798
  hyperosmolar nonketotic coma, 1866
  hyponatremia, 812
  multiple myeloma, 702
  pulmonary edema, 427
  therapy of uric acid nephrolithiasis, 804
  urinary tract infection, 1459
Hydrazides, 2191
Hydrocarbons, 867
Hydrocephalus
  brain tumor, 1067
  dementia, 988
  Maroteaux-Lamy syndrome, 1915
  posttraumatic, 1045
  radionuclide cisternography, 926
Hydrochloric acid
  achlorhydria
    acid secretory values, 2003
    pellagra, 2107
    Schilling test, 2060
  acute erosive gastritis, 2041
  gastric refluxate, 2015
  hypochlorhydria
    Helicobacter pylori, 1984
    Schilling test, 2060
    somatostatinoma, 2245
Hydrochlorothiazide
  heart failure, 170
  hypertension, 325, 326
  pulmonary parenchymal reactions, 476
  pulmonary toxicity, 479
  stone formation reduction, 803
Hydrocodone, 581
Hydrocortisone
  dermatitis, 1303
  hirsutism, 1756
  hypopituitarism treatment, 1779-1780, 1781
  before surgery, 2262
Hydrodiuril; *see* Hydrochlorothiazide
Hydrogen bonds, 50
Hydrogen breath test, 2006
Hydrogen ions
  magnetic resonance imaging, 918-919
  renal acidification, 740
  secretion and excretion, 835
  vasoactive effects on pulmonary circulation,
    363
Hydrogen peroxide
  aging and, 2283
  lung damage, 373
Hydrolytic digestion, 1112
Hydrometer, 742
Hydromorphone, 581
Hydronephrosis, 884
  abdominal mass, 886
  renal imaging studies, 753-754
Hydroperoxyeicosatetraenoic acid, 1140
Hydrostatic pleural pressure, 505
Hydrostatic pressure
  alveolocapillary membrane, 346
  circulatory shock, 177
  pulmonary edema, 168
Hydrostatic pulmonary edema, 168
4-Hydroxy-debrisoquine, 486
Hydroxy-methyl-glutaryl coenzyme A, 1884,
    2120

Hydroxy-methyl-glutaryl coenzyme A reductase, 1884, 2120
Hydroxy-methyl-glutaryl coenzyme A reductase inhibitors, 1891
  coronary artery disease in diabetic patient, 1869
  hyperlipidemia, 200
Hydroxyamphetamine, 933, 938
Hydroxyapatite, 1716
Hydroxychloroquine
  cutaneous lesions in lupus erythematosus, 1292
  dermatomyositis, 1237, 1292
  rheumatic disease, 1260, 1261
  systemic lupus erythematosus, 1217
18-Hydroxycorticosterone, 1741
5-Hydroxyindoleacetic acid, 2082
Hydroxyl glucosidation, 2125
Hydroxyl N-acetylglucosaminidation, 2125
Hydroxyl radicals
  aging and, 2283
  lung damage, 373
11-Hydroxylase deficiency, 1824
17α-Hydroxylase deficiency, 1844
21-Hydroxylase deficiency, 1824
24-Hydroxylase system, 1719
1-Hydroxylation, 1719
Hydroxymethylbilane, 1923
17-Hydroxyprogesterone, 1741
Hydroxyproline, 1745
Hydroxystilbamidine, 2191
Hydroxyurea
  beta-thalassemia, 656
  chronic myelogenous leukemia, 687
  essential thrombocythemia, 688
  myelofibrosis, 677
  polycythemia vera, 688
  sickle cell disease, 659-660
25-Hydroxyvitamin D, 1719
  measurement, 1746
  rickets or osteomalacia, 1954
Hydroxyzine
  for nausea and vomiting, 2027
  rhinitis, 1182
Hygroton; *see* Chlorthalidone
Hylorel; *see* Guanadrel
Hymenolepis nana, 1696, 1697
Hymenoptera, 1194
Hyperabduction maneuver, 306
Hyperacute rejection
  renal transplantation, 793
  xenografts, 1138
Hyperaldosteronism
  cirrhosis, 819
  hypertensive renal potassium wasting, 828
  hypomagnesemia, 1941
Hyperammonemia, 1907
Hyperamylasemia, 2235
Hyperargininemia, 1907
Hyperbaric oxygen therapy, 1576
Hyperbilirubinemia
  conjugated
    benign chronic, 2157-2158
    differential diagnosis, 2156
    pathophysiology and classification, 2154-2156
    unconjugated *versus,* 2150, 2151
  hepatic function, 2136
  hereditary fructose intolerance, 1880
  sickle cell disease, 657
  unconjugated
    chronic, 2152-2154
    diagnosis, 2153-2154
    pathophysiology, 2150-2152
    treatment, 2154
Hypercalcemia, 1927-1930
  acute renal failure, 773
  calcitonin therapy, 1719
  causes and differential diagnosis, 1927-1928
  chronic nephrocalcinosis, 891
  clinical features, 1928-1929

Hypercalcemia—cont'd
  congenital aortic stenosis, 287
  1,25-dihydrotachysterol, 1954
  effects of ionized calcium on cell metabolic processes, 1717
  electrocardiographic abnormalities, 89, 90
  endocrine paraneoplastic syndromes, 583
  interstitial lung disease, 452
  kidney stone formation, 798
  lung cancer, 489
  malignancy, 1972-1974
  medication-induced, 1928
  multiple myeloma, 700, 702, 864
  nonparathyroid endocrine disorders, 1928
  Paget's disease, 1956
  predominant hyperparathyroid bone disease, 1964
  primary hyperparathyroidism, 1965, 1966, 1967
  renal cell carcinoma, 898
  renal magnesium wasting, 1940-1941
  sarcoidosis, 458
  steroid suppression test, 1746
  treatment, 1929-1930
  urinary cyclic adenosine monophosphate, 1746
  vitamin D toxicity, 1928
Hypercalciuria
  dietary factors, 2102
  hypophosphatemia, 1936
  hypophosphatemic rickets, 1952-1953
  mechanisms, 797-798
  sarcoidosis, 458
  urine calcium, 1744
Hypercaloric diet, 2112
Hypercapnia
  acute respiratory failure, 412
  chronic obstructive pulmonary disease, 442
  hypoventilation and, 356
  mechanical ventilation, 397
  obstructive lung disease, 356
  during sleep, 354
  vasopressin secretion, 1790-1791
  ventilatory response to hypoxia, 353
Hyperchloremic acidosis, 779
Hyperchloremic metabolic acidosis, 837, 2114
Hypercholesterolemia, 1892-1894
  familial, 60
  periodic health examination, 2254
Hypercoagulable states
  hepatic vein thrombosis, 2208
  inflammatory bowel disease, 2076
  neurologic aspects, 1104
  pulmonary embolism, 499
Hypercortisolism, 1820
Hyperdibasic aminoaciduria, 1910
Hyperemesis gravidarum, 2278
Hyperemia, Raynaud's phenomenon, 1226
Hyperfiltration
  diabetic glomerulopathy, 860
  glomerular damage, 842
Hyperfunction, adrenal medulla, 1828
Hypergammaglobulinemia, 1233
  human immunodeficiency virus infection, 1470
  liver inflammation, 2135-2136
  myxoma, 330
Hypergastrinemia, 2002, 2003
Hyperglycemia
  acute pancreatitis, 2236, 2237
  cataracts, 1871
  diabetes mellitus, 1850
  diabetic glomerulopathy, 860
  diabetic ketoacidosis, 1863
  diabetic mother, 2272-2273
  diabetic retinopathy, 2303
  drug-induced, 1855
  glucagonoma, 2245
  gram-negative bacteremia, 1449
  hyperosmolar nonketotic coma, 1866
  hypophosphatemia, 1935
  lactic acidosis, 1867

Hyperglycemia—cont'd
  potassium diffusion out of cells, 826
  weakness, 1754
Hypergonadotropic disorders, 1845
Hyperimmunoglobulin M syndrome, 1176, 1343
Hyperinfection syndrome, 1403
Hyperinsulinemia, 319
Hyperinsulinism, 1876, 1877, 1878
Hyperkalemia, 830-833
  acute renal failure, 772-773
  chronic renal failure, 777
  decreased ammonia synthesis, 838
  electrocardiographic changes, 89, 90, 772
  heart failure, 172
  mineralocorticoid deficiency, 1824
  supportive treatment, 774
  toxicity of nonsteroidal antiinflammatory drugs, 870
Hyperkalemic periodic paralysis, 831
Hyperkalemic renal tubular acidosis, 831
Hyperkeratotic lupus erythematosus, 1291
Hyperkinesia, 2233
Hyperkinetic dysarthria, 977
Hyperkinetic movement disorders, 993-997
Hyperkinetic pulmonary hypertension, 296
Hyperkinetic pulse, 64-65, 66
Hyperlipidemia, 1892-1896
  acute pancreatitis, 2233-2234, 2237
  amylo-1,6-glucosidase deficiency, 1882
  atherosclerotic coronary artery disease, 192
  combined, 1895-1896
  coronary artery disease, 200
  cutaneous manifestations, 1323-1324
  glucose-6-phosphate dehydrogenase deficiency, 1881
  hypercholesterolemia, 1892-1894
  hypertriglyceridemia, 1894-1895
  insulin resistance, 1862
  ischemic heart disease, 197
  lipodystrophy, 1901
  myocardial infarction, 210
  nephrotic syndrome, 766
  osmolal gap, 806
  risk of stroke, 1001
Hyperlipoproteinemia, 1245, 1892
Hyperlysinemia, 1907
Hypermagnesemia, 1943, 2101, 2110
  acute renal failure, 773
  hypocalcemia, 1931
Hypernatremia, 748, 813-816
Hypernephroma, 1377
Hyperosmolar nonketotic coma, 1865-1866
Hyperosmotic agents
  constipation, 2055
  glaucoma, 2302
Hyperostosis corticalis generalisata, 1959
Hyperoxaluria
  renal allograft dysfunction, 794
  stone formation, 799
  therapy, 804
Hyperparathyroid bone disease
  chronic renal failure, 785
  mixed uremic osteodystrophy, 1963
  renal osteodystrophy, 1961
Hyperparathyroidism, 1965-1971
  arthropathy, 1246
  calcium pyrophosphate dihydrate deposition disease, 1279
  diagnosis, 1967-1969
  humoral hypercalcemia of malignancy *versus,* 1973-1974
  hypermagnesemia, 1943
  kidney stone formation, 798
  osteomalacia, 1950
  pathology and etiology, 1965-1966
  during pregnancy, 2273
  prevalence, 1965, 1966
  renal transplant recipient, 795
  renal wasting of phosphate, 1935
  symptoms and signs, 1966-1967
  treatment, 1969-1971

Hyperphenylalaninemia, 1904-1905
Hyperphosphatemia, 1938-1939
  acute renal failure, 773
  chronic renal failure, 779, 785-786
  renal bone disease, 1964
  renal osteodystrophy, 1961
Hyperpigmentation
  Addison's disease, Plate VII-14
  adrenal disease, 1322-1323
  adrenal insufficiency, 1823
  neurofibromatosis, 1920
Hyperpipecolatemia, 1907
Hyperplasia
  adrenal
    congenital, 1824-1825
      hirsutism, 1755
      hyperkalemia, 831
      hypertensive renal potassium wasting, 828
    atypical, 600
  benign prostatic, 717
    bladder-emptying dysfunction, 1066
    clinical guideline, 20
    hematuria, 757
  ductal, 1846
  esophageal, 2016
  focal nodular, 2216
  four-gland, 1965
  hyperplastic cholecystosis, 2233
  hyperplastic gastric polyps, 2045, 2046
  hyperplastic obesity, 2103
  hyperplastic polyps, 2086
  lymph node
    angiofollicular, 599
    hematoxylin and eosin preparation, Plate
      VIII-35
    mesenteric, 2252
  reactive macrophage, 680
  squamous cell, 2016
  thymic, 1022
Hyperplastic cholecystosis, 2233
Hyperplastic gastric polyps, 2045, 2046
Hyperplastic obesity, 2103
Hyperplastic polyps, 2086
Hyperpolization, smooth muscle, 1976
Hyperprolactinemia, 1785
  basal pituitary hormone measurement, 1737
  milk discharge, 1848
  testicular dysfunction, 1841
Hyperprosody, 977
Hyperproteinemia, 806
Hyperreflexia, 2160
Hyperresponsive airway, 439
Hypersalivation, 1998-1999
Hypersecretory gastropathy, 2043
Hypersegmented neutrophil, Plate IV-6
Hypersensitivity
  antituberculosis agents, 1632
  chemotherapy agents, 585
  delayed-type, 1127
    allergic contact dermatitis, 1303
    cell-mediated immunity, 1132
    drug eruption, 1313
    in vivo assessment of cell-mediated
      immunity, 1150-1151
  esophageal, 2016-2017
  hepatic injury, 2186
  immediate, 1139-1142
    laboratory methods, 1153-1155
  stinging insect, 1194
Hypersensitivity pneumonitis, 460-463
  drug-induced, 477
  isocyanate-induced, 473
Hypersensitivity vasculitis, 1221-1222
Hypersomatotropism, 1782
Hypersplenism, 601-602
  hemolysis, 668
  neutropenia, 593
  portal hypertension, 2165-2168
  thrombocytopenia, 614
Hyperstat; *see* Diazoxide

Hypertension, 312-329
  acute glomerulonephritis, 771
  aldosterone excess, 1822
  antirheumatic drug toxicity, 1261
  aortic aneurysm, 299
  aortic ejection sounds, 74
  aortic stenosis, 236-237
  arteriovenous nicking, Plate XI-3
  atherosclerosis risk, 192
  atrial fibrillation, 146
  autonomic overactivity, 934
  autosomal dominant polycystic kidney disease,
    873
  chronic renal failure, 781, 783
  coronary artery disease, 200, 2271
  cyclosporin A-associated, 870
  diabetic glomerulopathy, 860
  diagnostic tests, 329
  differential diagnosis, 320-322
  dissection of aorta, 301
  environmental mechanisms, 319
  essential mixed cryoglobulinemia, 857
  exertional angina, 127
  focal glomerular sclerosis, 852
  frequency, 312-314
  glomerulonephritis, 842
  headache, 960
  hemorrhagic stroke, 998
  hyperkalemia, 833
  hypertensive retinopathy, 2302-2303
  hypothyroidism, 1809
  idiopathic nephrotic syndrome, 850
  increased intracellular sodium and calcium,
    317-318
  increased intracranial pressure, 1084
  increased peripheral resistance, 314-319
  increased sodium intake, 318-319
  management, 322-329
    child, 328
    drug therapy, 324, 325, 326-327
    elderly patient, 327
    guidelines, 324-326
    nondrug therapies, 323-324
    patient compliance, 328-329
    results of clinical trials, 322-323
  membranoproliferative glomerulonephritis, 854
  microvascular disease in diabetic patient, 1870
  mitral stenosis, 245
  natural history, 319-322
  neurofibromatosis, 1921
  obstructive sleep apnea and, 526
  operative risk, 2260
  peripheral arterial aneurysm, 309
  peripheral vascular disease, 305
  pheochromocytoma, 1828, 1829-1830
  portal
    alcoholic hepatitis and cirrhosis, 2197
    ascites formation, 2163
    autosomal recessive polycystic kidney
      disease, 874
    cystic fibrosis, 2207
    hepatopulmonary syndrome, 2170
    liver failure, 2165-2168
    splenomegaly, 601
  poststreptococcal glomerulonephritis, 844
  during pregnancy, 2275
  primary hyperparathyroidism, 1966-1967
  proteinuria, 760
  pulmonary, 293-299
    acquired immunodeficiency syndrome, 333
    cardiac catheterization, 108
    cardiac transplantation, 338
    chronic obstructive pulmonary disease,
      446-447
    continuous-wave Doppler echocardiography,
      99
    cor triatriatum, 291
    dexfenfluramine and, 261
    drug-induced, 477
    exertional angina, 127
    fenfluramine and, 261

Hypertension—cont'd
  pulmonary—cont'd
    Graham Steell murmur, 80
    interstitial lung disease, 452
    mitral regurgitation, 250
    mitral stenosis, 245, 248
    neurogenic pulmonary edema, 1099
    obesity, 334
    passive, 297-298
    pathophysiology, 363-364
    precapillary, 293-297
    primary and secondary causes, 497-499
    reactive, 298
    systemic sclerosis, 1230
    Takayasu's arteritis, 470
  referral, 329
  renal cell carcinoma, 898
  renal sodium retention, 316-317, 318
  renal transplant recipient, 795
  renovascular, 321, 829, 893-896
  risk of stroke, 1001
  stress, 316
  types, 314, 315
Hypertension Detection and Follow-up Program,
  312
Hypertensive choroidopathy, 2303
Hypertensive crisis, 328
Hypertensive optic neuropathy, 2303
Hypertensive retinopathy, 2302-2303
Hyperthecosis, 1759, 1837
Hyperthermia, 1375, 1936
Hyperthyroidism
  atrial fibrillation, 146
  cardiovascular involvement, 334
  gynecomastia, 1765
  hypercalcemia, 1928
  hypercalciuria, 798
  impotence, 1762
  nontoxic goiter, 1812
  operative risk, 2262
  physical appearance, 63
  during pregnancy, 2273
  proximal myopathy, 1030
  serum thyroid-stimulating hormone levels,
    1801
  thyroid scan, 1735, 1802
  thyrotoxicosis *versus,* 1804
  weakness, 1754
Hyperthyroxinemia, 1803, 1804
Hypertonic hyponatremia, 810
  clinical manifestations, 811
  treatment, 812, 813
Hypertonicity, 806
  arginine vasopressin release, 807
  potassium diffusion out of cells, 826
Hypertrichosis lanuginosa acquista, 1317, 1318
Hypertriglyceridemia, 1894-1895
  with elevated cholesterol levels, 1895-1896
  lack of apolipoprotein C, 1898
Hypertrophic cardiomyopathy, 265-270
  cardiac catheterization, 115-116
  chest pain, 128
  molecular biology, 61-62
  pulsus bisferiens, 65
  restriction fragment length polymorphism,
    54-55
  sudden cardiac death, 187
Hypertrophic lupus erythematosus, 1291
Hypertrophic obstructive cardiomyopathy, 265
Hypertrophic osteoarthropathy, 489, 1247
Hypertrophic pyloric stenosis, 2044
Hypertrophy
  contractile and cytoskeletal proteins, 59-60
  dilated cardiomyopathy, 263
  electrocardiography, 87-88
  hypertension, 316
  left ventricular
    anomalous origin of left coronary artery,
      292
    aortic regurgitation, 239-240
    aortic stenosis, 235, 236

Hypertrophy—cont'd
  left ventricular—cont'd
    electrocardiography, 87
    hypertrophic obstructive cardiomyopathy, 266
    mitral regurgitation, 250
    molecular biology, 55-56, 57
  right ventricular
    cor triatriatum, 291
    electrocardiography, 87-88
    pulmonic stenosis, 288
    reactive pulmonary hypertension, 298
    tetralogy of Fallot, 288
Hyperuricemia, 1268-1276
  acute renal failure, 773
  after renal transplantation, 795
  calcium pyrophosphate dihydrate deposition disease, 1277
  glucose-6-phosphate dehydrogenase deficiency, 1881
  multiple myeloma, 700, 702
  Paget's disease, 1956
Hyperuricosuria, 799
Hyperventilation, 349-350
  central neurogenic, 1097
  to enhance ventilatory endurance, 360
  hypocapnia and, 355-356
  obesity, 334
  obstructive sleep apnea, 525
  presyncope, 955
  to reduce increased intracranial pressure, 1084
  relationship of ventilation to perfusion, 349
Hyperventilation-induced hypocapnia, 525
Hyperviscosity
  neurologic aspects, 1104
  rheumatoid arthritis, 1205
  tetralogy of Fallot, 289
  Waldenström macroglobulinemia, 865-866
Hypervitaminosis A, 2108
Hypervolemic hypernatremia, 814
Hypnic jerks, 946
Hypnogogic hallucination, 942
Hypnotic-dependent sleep disorder, 944-945
Hypoalbuminemia
  acute pancreatitis, 2237
  amebic liver abscess, 2210
  anion gap acidosis, 836
  intestinal disease, 2005
  intestinal lymphangiectasia, 2067
  nephrotic syndrome, 765
  serum magnesium, 1942
  transudative pleural effusion, 507
Hypoaldosteronism
  hyporeninemic, 1824
  sodium depletion, 824
Hypoalphalipoproteinemia, 1896, 1898
Hypoaminoacidemia, 2244
Hypobetalipoproteinemia, 1897
Hypocalcemia, 1930-1934
  acute pancreatitis, 2237
  acute renal failure, 773
  after massive transfusion, 2011
  chronic renal failure, 779, 785-786
  clinical features, 1932-1933
  differential diagnosis, 1931-1932
  efforts of ionized calcium on cell metabolic processes, 1717
  electrocardiographic abnormalities, 89, 90
  ethylene glycol poisoning, 866
  hyperphosphatemia, 1938
  hypomagnesemia, 1942
  nephrotic syndrome, 767
  osteomalacia, 1949
  relative hypoparathyroidism, 1932
  treatment, 1933-1934
  vitamin D deficiency, 2106
Hypocalciuria, 1942
Hypocapnia, 355-356
  hyperventilation-induced, 525
  pulmonary edema, 425
  to reduced intracranial pressure, 1084

Hypochloremic hypokalemic metabolic alkalosis, 2028
Hypochlorhydria
  Helicobacter pylori, 1984
  Schilling test, 2060
  somatostatinoma, 2245
Hypochromia, 654
Hypochromic microcyte, 662
Hypocitraturia, 797, 799
Hypocomplementemia, 1147, 1148
  acute nephritic syndrome, 764
  membranoproliferative glomerulonephritis, 854
  partial lipodystrophy, 1902
Hypofunction
  adrenal cortex, 1823-1824
  adrenal medulla, 1827-1828
Hypogammaglobulinemia
  acute meningitis, 1407
  malabsorption, 2066
  multiple myeloma, 864
  serum protein electrophoresis, 565-566
Hypoglycemia, 1874-1879
  acute fatty liver of pregnancy, 2278
  adrenal medulla hypofunction, 1828
  amylo-1,6-glucosidase deficiency, 1882
  cholera, 1595
  chronic pancreatitis, 2241
  diagnosis, 1877-1878
  dizziness, 972
  effects on fetus, 1874
  endocrine paraneoplastic syndromes, 583
  epilepsy *versus,* 981
  fulminant hepatic failure, 2163
  glucose-6-phosphate dehydrogenase deficiency, 1881
  gram-negative bacteremia, 1449
  growth hormone deficiency, 1777
  hereditary fructose intolerance, 1880
  hypoglycemic coma, 1867
  insulin-induced, 202, 826, 1735-1736
  insulinoma, 2244
  leprechaunism, 1900
  metabolic encephalopathy, 1079
  neurologic aspects, 1101
  pathophysiology, 1875-1876
  physiology, 1874-1875
  Somogyi phenomenon, 1861
  syncope *versus,* 954-955
  treatment, 1878
  vasopressin stimulation, 1790
Hypoglycemic coma, 1867
Hypoglycorrhachia
  bacterial meningitis, 1407
  spinal fluid examination, 904
Hypogonadism
  acromegaly, 1782
  chronic hepatic failure, 2170-2171
  evaluation of testicular function, 1840
  gonadotropin deficiency, 1777
  gynecomastia, 1764, 1765
  impotence, 1761
  Prader-Labhart-Willi syndrome, 1842
Hypogonadotropic eunuchoidism, 1841-1842, 1843
Hypogonadotropic hypogonadism, 1842, 1843-1844
Hypokalemia, 826-830
  arrhythmia, 133
  chronic tubulointerstitial nephritis, 891
  consequences, 829-830
  diarrhea, 2005
  diuretic-induced, 326
  electrocardiographic abnormalities, 89, 90
  Fanconi's syndrome, 882
  hypomagnesemia, 1942
  with potassium depletion, 827
  treatment, 830
  VIPoma, 2245
  vomiting consequence, 2028
  without potassium depletion, 826-827

Hypokalemic periodic paralysis, 58, 826, 1029-1030
Hypokinetic dysarthria, 977
Hypokinetic pulse, 65, 66
Hypomagnesemia, 1939-1943
  acute renal failure, 773
  hypocalcemia, 1931
Hypomagnesuria, 797
Hypomania, 1036
Hypomethylation, 548
Hypomotility
  after spinal cord injury, 1050
  intestinal pseudoobstruction, 2079
  systemic sclerosis, 1229-1230
Hyponatremia, 809-813
  acute intermittent porphyria, 1926
  acute renal failure, 773
  after stroke, 1007
  cirrhotic patient with ascites, 2165
  congestive heart failure, 817-818
  disorders of urinary dilution, 748
  heart failure, 172
  hypokalemia and, 830
  Legionnaire's disease, 1623
  malaria, 1674
  meningitis, 1406
  metabolic encephalopathy, 1079
  Rocky Mountain spotted fever, 1544
Hypoparathyroidism
  dementia, 987
  hypocalcemia with, 1931-1932
  myopathy, 1030
  osteomalacia, 1952
  urinary cyclic adenosine monophosphate, 1746
Hypoperfusion
  ischemic stroke, 998-1000
  preeclampsia, 2275
  shock, 175, 177
Hypopharyngeal cancer, 723
Hypophonia, 977
Hypophosphatasia, 1854
Hypophosphatemia, 1935-1938
  cardiomyopathy, 262
  diabetic ketoacidosis, 1864-1865
  dilated cardiomyopathy, 265
  hemolysis associated with liver disease, 667
  hereditary fructose intolerance, 1880
  renal phosphate wasting, 880
  X-linked hypophosphatemic rickets, 880
Hypophosphatemic osteomalacia, 1952-1953
Hypophyseal-portal blood supply, 1773
Hypophysiotropic-releasing hormones, 1077
Hypopituitarism, 1776-1777, 1779-1781
Hypoplasia
  bone marrow, 573
  megakaryocytic, 614
  thymic, 1342
Hypopnea, 524-525
Hypoprosody, 977
Hypoprothrombinemia, 1104, 2106
Hyporeninemic hypoaldosteronism, 831-832, 1824
Hyposensitization, rhinitis, 1183
Hyposmia, 1182
Hypotension
  acute pancreatitis, 2234
  adrenal insufficiency, 1823
  after cardiac transplantation, 335
  after stroke, 1007
  calcium channel blocker-induced, 205
  cardiac tamponade, 275
  cardiogenic shock, 175-187
    clinical presentation, 177-180
    clinical trials, 184, 185
    coronary angioplasty, 183
    coronary artery bypass graft, 185
    differential diagnosis, 175, 176
    evaluation and treatment, 180, 181
    hemodynamic alterations, 176, 177
    mechanical intervention, 184, 185-186
    myocardial function, 176

Hypotension—cont'd
  cardiogenic shock—cont'd
    pharmacologic therapy, 181-182
    reperfusion therapy, 182-183
    serum lactate and anaerobic metabolism,
      176, 178
  comatose patient, 950
  dissection of aorta, 301
  gram-negative bacteremia, 1449
  heart failure, 173
  hypermagnesemia, 1943
  hypovolemic hypernatremia, 816
  Lassa fever, 1510
  orthostatic
    acute pancreatitis, 2234
    autonomic failure, 935
    causes, 1828
    diabetic autonomic neuropathy, 1873
    megaloblastic anemia, 648
    with syncope, 953-954
  penetrating injury to heart, 332
  rabies, 1506
  right ventricular infarction, 178
  staphylococcal toxic shock syndrome, 1421
  thrombolytic agents, 213
  vasopressin release, 1792
Hypothalamic amenorrhea, 1837
Hypothalamic disorders, 1773-1788
  amenorrhea, 1757-1759
  Cushing's disease, 1786-1787
  empty sella syndrome, 1787
  gonadotropin-secreting pituitary tumor, 1787
  growth hormone-secreting pituitary tumor,
    1782-1785
  hyperprolactinemia, 1785-1786
  hypopituitarism, 1776-1777
  obesity, 1751, 1752, 2102-2103
  pituitary apoplexy, 1777-1781
  pituitary tumor, 1781-1782
  thyroid-stimulating hormone-secreting tumor,
    1787
  tumor
    cachexia, 1749
    impotence, 1762
Hypothalamic-pituitary adrenal system, 1774
Hypothalamic-pituitary axis, 1773-1774
Hypothalamic-pituitary gonadal system,
  1774-1775
Hypothalamic-pituitary growth hormone system,
  1775
Hypothalamic-pituitary prolactin system,
  1775-1776, 1777
Hypothalamic-pituitary testing, 1735-1737
Hypothalamic-pituitary-testis axis, 1839, 1840
Hypothalamic-pituitary thyroid system, 1774
Hypothalamus
  anatomy, 1773-1774
  control of food intake, 2099
  dysfunction, 1776
  fever, 1375
  gonadotropin-releasing hormone secretion,
    1834
  hypothalamic-pituitary adrenal system, 1774
  hypothalamic-pituitary axis, 1773-1774
  hypothalamic-pituitary gonadal system,
    1774-1775
  hypothalamic-pituitary growth hormone
    system, 1775
  hypothalamic-pituitary prolactin system,
    1775-1776, 1777
  hypothalamic-pituitary testing, 1735-1737
  hypothalamic-pituitary thyroid system, 1774
  hypothalamus-pituitary-testis axis, 1839, 1840
  integration of autonomic function, 930
  neuroendocrine regulation, 1075
  puberty, 1766
  regulation of thyroid function, 1799
  sweating, 933
Hypothermia
  bacteremia, 1449
  electrocardiographic abnormalities, 89, 90

Hypothermia—cont'd
  hypokalemia, 827
  myxedema coma, 1810
  streptococcal toxic shock syndrome, 1557
Hypothyroidism, 1808-1811
  arthropathy, 1246
  calcium pyrophosphate dihydrate deposition
    disease, 1279
  cardiovascular involvement, 334
  cutaneous manifestations, 1322
  delay in secondary sexual development,
    1768-1769
  dizziness, 974
  hyperprolactinemia, 1785
  impaired hepatic uptake of bilirubin, 2151
  impotence, 1762
  mood disorders, 1036
  operative risk, 2262
  physical appearance, 63
  during pregnancy, 2273
  proximal myopathy, 1030
  serum thyroid-stimulating hormone levels,
    1801
  weakness, 1754
Hypothyroxinemia, 1804
Hypotonia, 1842
Hypotonic hyponatremia, 810-813
Hypotonicity, 806, 807-808
Hypoventilation, 349-350
  acute respiratory failure, 412-413
  hypercapnia and, 356
  neuropulmonology, 1096
  obstructive sleep apnea, 525
  precapillary pulmonary hypertension, 296
Hypovolemia
  acute pancreatitis, 2237
  after stroke, 1007
  mesenteric vascular disease, 2086
  Rocky Mountain spotted fever, 1543
  vasopressin release, 1792
Hypovolemic hypernatremia, 814
Hypovolemic shock, 176, 177
Hypoxanthine-guanine phosphoribosyltransferase,
  1269
Hypoxemia
  asthma, 1189
  causes, 349
  diffusion limitation, 413
  gram-negative bacteremia, 1449, 1450
  hepatopulmonary syndrome, 2170
  interstitial lung disease, 450
  Langerhans' cell granulomatosis, 464
  mechanical ventilation, 396-397
  prescription of oxygen, 429
  pulmonary edema, 425
  pulmonary hypertension, 498
  pulmonary thromboembolism, 500
  systemic lupus erythematosus, 1215
  ventilation-perfusion ratio mismatch, 413
Hypoxia
  chemoreceptor response to, 353
  chest pain, 128
  electroencephalography, 907, 908
  erythropoietin, 586
  retinal, 2303
  during sleep, 354
  vasopressin secretion, 1790-1791
Hypoxic-ischemic encephalopathy, 950-951
Hypoxic pulmonary vasoconstriction, 294, 363
Hypoxic vasoconstriction, 498
Hysterectomy, ovarian cancer, 716
Hysteria, 1040
Hysterical faint, 955
Hytrin; *see* Terazosin

I

I-band, 39
I cell disease, 1916
Iatrogenic pericardial disease, 273
IBS; *see* Irritable bowel syndrome

Ibuprofen, 1259
  cystic fibrosis, 482
  hepatic injury, 2191
  human cytochrome P450 isoforms, 2312
  interference with oral anticoagulants, 636
  pericardial heart disease, 278
ICD; *see* International Classification of Diseases
Icterus, 2147-2159
  alcoholic hepatitis and cirrhosis, 2197
  amebic liver abscess, 1682
  cholangiocarcinoma, 2231
  choledocholithiasis, 2229
  cholestatic hepatitis A, 2173
  chronic pancreatitis, 2241
  classification, 2150, 2151
  conjugated hyperbilirubinemia, 2154-2156
  Dubin-Johnson syndrome, 2157
  familial cholestatic syndromes, 2158-2159
  galactosemia, 1882
  gastric cancer, 2046
  hemobilia, 2233
  hepatocellular carcinoma, 2213
  hereditary fructose intolerance, 1880
  hereditary spherocytosis, 664
  idiopathic myelofibrosis, 677
  leptospirosis, 1645
  neonatal cytomegalovirus, 1528
  normal bilirubin metabolism, 2147-2150
  postoperative cholestasis, 2159
  during pregnancy, 2277
  pyogenic liver abscess, 2209
  Rotor's syndrome and hepatic storage disease,
    2157-2158
  toxic hepatic injury, 2188
  unconjugated hyperbilirubinemia, 2150-2154
Idarubicin, 584
Ideal body weight, 2111
Ideomotor apraxia, 976
Idiopathic adult ductopenia, 2200
Idiopathic cervical dystonia, 996
Idiopathic costochondritis, 129
Idiopathic edema, 821
Idiopathic granulomatosis, 1378
Idiopathic hypercalciuria, 798
Idiopathic hypereosinophilic syndrome, 681
Idiopathic hypersomnia, 943
Idiopathic hypertrophic subaortic stenosis, 265
Idiopathic insomnia, 942
Idiopathic interstitial pneumonia, 579
Idiopathic membranous nephropathy, 767
Idiopathic myelofibrosis, 677
Idiopathic nephrotic syndrome, 849-855
Idiopathic orthostatic hypotension, 936
Idiopathic osteoporosis, 1945
Idiopathic pancreatitis, 2234
Idiopathic pulmonary fibrosis, 387, 453
Idiopathic pulmonary hemosiderosis, 455
Idiopathic seminiferous tubular failure, 1845
Idiopathic short stature, 1769
Idiopathic sideroblastic anemia, 645
Idiopathic sudden sensorineural hearing loss,
  2308
Idiopathic thrombocytopenic purpura, 603-604
  autoantibodies, 1155
  petechiae and bullae, Plate IV-10
  during pregnancy, 2279
Idiosyncratic hepatic injury, 2186-2187
Idiotype, 1114
  autoreactivity, 1146
Idoxuridine, 1526, 2191
Iduronidase deficiency, 1912
Ifosphamide
  cardiotoxicity, 584
  pancreatic cancer, 2243
Ileal conduit, 837
Ileostomy
  Crohn's disease, 2072
  ulcerative colitis, 2074
Ileum
  bile salts reabsorption, 2125
  carcinoid tumors, 2081

Ileum—cont'd
  increased fecal bile salt loss, 2129
  Meckel's diverticulum, 2089
  Schilling test, 2060
Ileus
  abdominal pain, 2032
  chronic renal failure, 784
  constipation, 2053-2055
  gallstone, 2228
  postcoarctation syndrome, 287
  radiography, 2032
Iliac crest biopsy, 1747, Plate IX-5
Ilizarov external fixation method, 1436
Imaging studies
  abdominal
    Hodgkin's disease, 694
      pancreatic disease, 2145-2147
  amebic liver abscess, 2210
  anaerobic bacterial infection, 1619
  ankylosing spondylitis, 1239
  arthritis, 1164-1174
    advanced methods, 1173
    appendicular skeleton, 1164-1169
    axial skeleton, 1169-1171, 1172
    evaluation of arthritis, 1164, 1173
    foot, 1172
    hand, 1171-1172
    hip, 1173
    knee, 1172-1173
    sacroiliac joint, 1172, 1173
    septic arthritis, 1252
    techniques and modalities, 1064
    wrist, 1172
  cancer
    brain tumor, 1067-1069
    head and neck, 723-724
    hepatocellular carcinoma, 2213-2214
    lung, 726
    renal cell carcinoma, 898
    testicular, 720-721
    upper urinary tract tumor, 899
  cardiac, 106-107
    acute pericarditis, 273-274
    aortic regurgitation, 241, 242
    aortic stenosis, 237, 238, 287
    atrial septal defect, 281
    coarctation of aorta, 286
    common aortopulmonary trunk, 290
    complete transposition of great arteries, 290
    congenital abnormalities of coronary
      arteries, 292
    congenital coronary arteriovenous fistula,
      292
    constrictive pericarditis, 277, 278
    dissection of aorta, 301
    Ebstein's anomaly of tricuspid valve, 290
    endocardial cushion defect, 282
    heart failure, 165
    ischemic heart disease, 198
    mitral regurgitation, 251, 253
    mitral stenosis, 247
    mitral valve prolapse, 254
    myocardial infarction, 212
    patent ductus arteriosus, 285
    pericardial effusion, 274-275
    primary pulmonary hypertension, 294
    pulmonic regurgitation, 257
    pulmonic stenosis, 288
    sudden cardiac death survivor, 188
    tetralogy of Fallot, 289
    total anomalous pulmonary venous
      connection, 291
    tricuspid regurgitation, 256
    tricuspid stenosis, 255
    ventricular septal defect, 284
  cholestasis, 2156
  dementia, 2288
  diabetes insipidus, 1795
  echinococcal cyst, 2111
  endocrine, 1734-1735
  gynecomastia, 1765

Imaging studies—cont'd
  hemoptysis, 411
  hepatic encephalopathy, 2161
  incidentaloma, 1830
  inflammatory myopathies, 1235, 1236
  intestinal disease, 2007
  liver abscess, 2209
  liver disease, 2140-2141
  mediastinal mass, 512
  neck pain, 969
  neurologic
    brain tumor, 1067-1069
    head trauma, 1044
    neurologic disorders, 918-924
    stroke, 1002-1003
  non-Hodgkin's lymphoma, 698
  obstructive sleep apnea, 355
  pelvis, 756
  peptic ulcer, 2037
  peripheral arterial aneurysm, 309
  pulmonary, 386-390
    acute respiratory failure, 414
    amiodarone-induced pulmonary disease, 478
    bronchiectasis, 484
    chronic obstructive pulmonary disease, 442
    cor pulmonale, 498
    cystic fibrosis, 481
    evaluation of respiratory disease, 403-404
    idiopathic pulmonary fibrosis, 453
    interstitial lung disease, 451
    lung cancer, 489, 726
    pleural disease, 506
    pulmonary edema, 425
    pulmonary thromboembolism, 501-502
    solitary pulmonary nodule, 493-494, 495
  renal, 748-756
    acute inflammation, 754-755
    angiography, 751
    autosomal dominant polycystic kidney
      disease, 873
    computed tomography, 750
    hematuria, 757
    intravenous pyelography, 748-749
    lower urinary tract, 756
    magnetic resonance imaging, 750-751
    nuclear medicine, 750
    obstructive uropathy, 753-754, 886-887
    renal abscess, 755
    renal cell carcinoma, 898
    renal mass, 751-753
    renovascular disease, 755-756
    retrograde pyelography, 751
    simple cyst, 871-872
    ultrasonography, 749-750
  secondary polycythemia, 589-590
  sinusitis, 2308
  spinal lesion, 1012
  thyroid disease, 1801-1802
Imidazoles
  candidiasis, 1442, 1663
  tinea pedis, 1311
Imino carrier, 1988
Iminoglycinuria, 880
Imipenem, 1355
  activity against major anaerobes, 1620
  acute pancreatitis, 2237
  dosage, 1349
  enterococci resistance, 1561
  gram-negative sepsis, 1452
  peritonitis, 1402
Imipramine, 1037
  anxiety disorders, 1035
  human cytochrome P450 isoforms, 2312
Immature granulocyte, 594
Immediate hypersensitivity, 1139-1142,
    1153-1155
Immobility, physiologic consequences, 2287
Immune cell, 1109, 1152
Immune complexes, 1137-1138
  common tests, 1148
  drug-induced immune hemolytic anemia, 670

Immune complexes—cont'd
  glomerular diseases, 841-843
  infective endocarditis, 227
  leprosy, 1650
  measurement, 1148-1149
  membranoproliferative glomerulonephritis, 854
  mixed cryoglobulins, 1249
  pulmonary vasculitides, 453
  rapidly progressive glomerulonephritis, 846
  rheumatoid arthritis, 1201
  tubulointerstitial renal disease, 889
  vasculitis, 1218
Immune deposits, glomerular, 841-843
Immune exclusion, 1336
Immune hemolytic anemia, 668-670
Immune heparin-induced thrombocytopenia,
    634-635
Immune pericarditis, 272-273
Immune response, 1108-1115
  aging and, 2285
  antigens and antigen processing, 1111-1112
  cell-mediated immunity, 1126-1132
    cellular constituents, 1127-1128
    cytokines and immunoregulation, 1128-1132
    delayed-type hypersensitivity, 1132
    derangements, 1132
    evaluation, 1150-1153, 1175
    myasthenia gravis, 1021
  cellular components, 1109
  cervical cancer, 714
  chlamydial infection, 1535
  evaluation, 1175
  gram-negative bacteremia, 1452-1453, 1454
  gram-negative disease, 1446
  Haemophilus influenzae, 1586-1587
  humoral immunity, 1336-1337
  immunoglobulin superfamily, 1110-1111
  leprosy, 1649-1650
  lymphocyte differentiation and activation,
    1112-1114
  redundancy and multiplicity, 1336
  Salmonella, 1599
  self/nonself discrimination, 1108-1109
  silicosis, 475
  soluble factors, 1110
  T-cell subsets and immunoregulation, 1114
  tolerance and autoimmunity, 1142-1147
  tubulointerstitial disease, 888-889
Immune sera, 1138
Immune thrombocytopenia, 615-616
Immune thrombocytopenic purpura, 616-617,
    1472
Immunity
  cell-mediated, 1126-1132
    barrier to infection, 1335
    cellular constituents, 1127-1128
    cytokines and immunoregulation, 1128-1132
    delayed-type hypersensitivity, 1132
    derangements, 1132
    evaluation, 1150-1153, 1175
    mononuclear phagocyte system, 1342
    myasthenia gravis, 1021
  humoral, 1336-1337
    evaluation, 1175
    inflammatory myopathies, 1234
    spleen and, 1337-1338
  intestinal, 1989-1993
  malaria, 1673
Immunization
  preventive care guidelines, 2255
  before traveling, 1467-1468
  tuberculosis, 1637-1638
Immunoassay, 1733-1734
  matrix hepatitis C virus dot blot, 2176
  parathyroid hormone, 1968-1969
Immunoblotting, 567
Immunocompromised patient
  cytomegalovirus, 1528
  fever, 1386-1390
  herpes simplex virus infections, 1524
  measles, 1498

Immunocompromised patient—cont'd
multiple organ dysfunction syndrome, 422
nocardiosis, 1666
nontuberculous mycobacterial infection, 1639
peritonitis, 2248
precautions before international travel,
1468-1469
Staphylococcus aureus, 1550
Staphylococcus epidermidis, 1551
zoster, 1527
Immunodeficiency states
aplastic anemia, 672
chronic lymphocytic leukemia, 684
gastric cancer, 2046
hematopoietic stem cell transplantation, 576
increased incidence of lymphoma of small
intestine, 2081
intestinal disease, 2005
primary, 1174-1178
Immunodiffusion assay, 1373
Immunoelectrophoresis, 566-567, 568
Immunoenzyme techniques, 1371
Immunofixation, 566, 567
plasma cell dyscrasias, 864
urine, 568
Immunofluorescence, 1152, 1371
Alport's syndrome, 877
detection of autoantibodies, 1156
focal glomerular sclerosis, 852
glomerulonephritis, 842
human immunodeficiency virus, 1472
idiopathic nephrotic syndrome, 850
immune complex detection, 1149
Legionella pneumophila, 1623
mumps, 1497
poststreptococcal glomerulonephritis, 843-844
rapidly progressive glomerulonephritis, 848
Rocky Mountain spotted fever, 1544
Immunoglobulin A, 1110, 1122-1123
within alpha-granules, 536
barrier to infection, 1335
biclonal gammopathy, 705
Bordetella pertussis, 1612-1613
in bronchoalveolar lavage fluid, 367
Campylobacter infection, 1590-1591
deficiency, 1176, 1991-1993
influenza antibody, 1487
liver disease, 2135-2136
Mediterranean lymphoma, 2080
nephropathy, 845, 877
nephrotic syndrome, 765
pemphigus, 1295
Peyer's patch B-cells, 1990
plasma cells in lamina propria, 1990
properties and distribution, 1336
secretory, 1990-1993
small bowel secretion, 2060
systemic lupus erythematosus, 1216
Immunoglobulin amyloidosis, 1282-1283
Immunoglobulin D, 1110, 1123, 1336
Immunoglobulin E, 1110, 1123
anaphylaxis, 1193
asthma, 1188
in bronchoalveolar lavage fluid, 367
Churg-Strauss syndrome, 465
drug eruption, 1313
food allergy, 1993
immediate-type hypersensitivity reaction, 1139
in vitro assay, 1154
intestinal immunity, 1990-1991
occupational asthma, 471
parasite-induced eosinophilia, 1705
properties and distribution, 1336
Immunoglobulin enhancer sequence, 1123
Immunoglobulin G, 1110, 1122
within alpha-granules, 536
barrier to infection, 1335
biclonal gammopathy, 705
Bordetella pertussis, 1612-1613
in bronchoalveolar lavage fluid, 367
brucellosis, 1606

Immunoglobulin G—cont'd
Campylobacter infection, 1590
Coccidioides immitis, 1657
Graves' disease, 1805
Haemophilus influenzae infection, 1587
immune thrombocytopenic purpura, 616
Lyme disease, 1646-1647
membranoproliferative glomerulonephritis, 854
membranous nephropathy, 853
myasthenia gravis, 1021
nephrotic syndrome, 765
parvovirus B19 infection, 1514
properties and distribution, 1336
respiratory defense, 366
rheumatoid arthritis, 1201
rheumatoid factors, 1160
schematic diagram, 1122
thyroid-stimulating hormone receptor antibody,
1801
toxoplasmosis, 1678
transient hypogammaglobulinemia of infancy,
1176
warm-reacting antibody hemolytic anemia,
668-669
Immunoglobulin heavy chain deletions, 1176
Immunoglobulin M, 1110, 1122
barrier to infection, 1335
biclonal gammopathy, 705
Bordetella pertussis, 1612-1613
in bronchoalveolar lavage fluid, 367
brucellosis, 1606
Campylobacter infection, 1590
Coccidioides immitis, 1657
cold agglutinin disease, 669-670
cytomegalovirus, 1528
hepatitis A, 2173
hyper-immunoglobulin M syndrome, 1176,
1343
Lyme disease, 1646
nephrotic syndrome, 765
parvovirus B19 infection, 1513
properties and distribution, 1336-1337
rheumatoid arthritis, 1201
rheumatoid factor, 1160-1161
systemic lupus erythematosus, 1216
toxoplasmosis, 1678
Waldenström macroglobulinemia, 703-704,
865
Immunoglobulin superfamily, 1110-1111, 1174
Immunoglobulins, 1110
agammaglobulinemia, 1490
as B-cell receptors, 1123
basic immunology, 1174-1175
deficiencies, 1337
diversity, 1111
evaluation in serum and urine, 564
hepatitis A, 2178
hepatitis B, 2179
quantitation of, 567
respiratory defense mechanism, 367
rheumatoid arthritis, 1201
Southern blot analysis, 560
Immunohistochemistry, 1152
analysis of peripheral blood and bone marrow
cells, 559
cancer of unknown primary site, 730-731
characterization and classification of cancers,
730
detection of autoantibodies, 1156
Hodgkin's disease, 692-693
non-Hodgkin's lymphoma, 696
Immunologic barriers to infection, 1335
Immunologic disorders, 1174-1263
anaphylaxis, 1193-1195
antirheumatic drugs, 1258-1263
analgesics, 1259-1260
disease-modifying antirheumatic drugs,
1260-1262
glucocorticoids, 1262-1263
nonsteroidal antiinflammatory drugs,
1258-1259

Immunologic disorders—cont'd
arthropathy
adult Still's disease, 1243
Behçet disease, 1243
calcium oxalate, 1280
coagulation disorders, 1246
endocrine diseases, 1246-1247
familial Mediterranean fever, 1242-1244
foreign body synovitis, 1244
hyperlipoproteinemia, 1245
inflammatory bowel disease, 1245-1246
intermittent hydrarthrosis, 1244
malignancy, 1247-1248
Milwaukee shoulder/knee syndrome,
1279-1280
multicentric reticulohistiocytosis, 1245
neurologic disorders, 1247
osteonecrosis, 1244
palindromic rheumatism, 1243-1244
panniculitis, 1245
pigmented villonodular synovitis,
1244-1245
relapsing polychondritis, 1243
relapsing seronegative symmetric synovitis
with pitting edema, 1243
sarcoidosis, 1245
sickle cell disease, 1246
Whipple's disease, 1246
asthma, 1185-1193
clinical manifestations, 1187-1188
diagnosis and differential diagnosis, 1189
epidemiology and pathology, 1185
laboratory findings, 1188-1189
management, 1189-1192
pathophysiology, 1185-1187
prognosis, 1192-1193
chronic renal failure, 784-785
cryoglobulinemia, 1222, 1248-1250
diffuse fasciitis with eosinophilia, 1233-1234
evaluation of joint complaints, 1198-1200
Graves' disease, 1805-1807
antithyroid antibodies, 1801
autoantibodies, 1155
during pregnancy, 2273
thyroid scan, 1802
thyrotoxicosis, 1804
weakness, 1754
inflammatory myopathy, 1234-1237
inherited complement deficiencies, 1178-1180
joint infection, 1250-1256
lymphadenopathy, 597
pathogenetic processes, 1108
periarticular rheumatic complaints, 1195-1198
primary immunodeficiency disorders,
1174-1178
Raynaud's phenomenon, 310, 1226-1227
cryoglobulinemia, 1248
scleroderma, 1293
systemic sclerosis, 1229, 1232
transient monocular blindness, 1058
rheumatic fever, 1256-1258
rheumatoid arthritis, 1200-1209
aortitis, 303
atlantoaxial subluxation, 1171, 1172
cardiac involvement, 334
course and prognosis, 1205-1206
diagnosis, 1206
differential diagnosis, 1206
extraarticular manifestations, 1202,
1203-1205
glucocorticoid protocol, 1263
gold salt-induced pulmonary disease, 478
interstitial lung disease, 453
intervertebral disk space narrowing,
1169-1170
laboratory findings, 1205
lymphocytosis of large granular
lymphocytes, 679
management, 1206-1209
pericarditis, 272-273
pleural effusion, 508

Immunologic disorders—cont'd
  rheumatoid arthritis—cont'd
    radiologic findings, 1205
    soft tissue swelling, 1165
  rhinitis, 467, 1180-1185
  Sjögren syndrome, 1209-1212
    anti-Ro antibody, 1291
    Fanconi's syndrome, 882
    inflammatory myopathies, 1236
    interstitial lung disease, 453
    renal involvement, 891
    systemic sclerosis, 1230
  spondyloarthropathy, 1200, 1237-1242
  systemic lupus erythematosus, 1200,
      1212-1218
    alveolar hemorrhage with, 455
    bullous, 1296
    cardiac involvement, 334
    clinical features, 1213-1215
    cutaneous lesions, 1290
    diagnosis, 1216
    drug-induced lupus syndromes, 1217-1218
    etiology, 1212-1213
    incidence and prevalence, 1212
    interstitial lung disease, 453
    laboratory findings, 1215-1216
    neutropenia, 593
    pathogenesis, 1213
    pleural effusion, 508
    renal involvement, 856-857
    treatment, 1216-1217
  systemic sclerosis, 334, 1228-1233
  vasculitis, 1218-1226
    alveolar hemorrhage with, 454
    angiocentric immunoproliferative disorders,
        1225
    anti-neutrophil cytoplasmic
        antibodies-positive crescentic
        glomerulonephritis, 847-848
    Behçet disease, 1243
    Churg-Strauss syndrome, 1220
    classification, 1219
    clinical approach, 1225-1226
    giant cell arteritis, 1223-1224
    glomerular involvement, 855-859
    hypersensitivity vasculitis, 1221-1222
    hypokalemia, 829
    Kawasaki's disease, 1225
    leukocytoclastic, 1315
    microscopic polyarteritis nodosa, 1220-1221
    panniculitis, 1245
    pathogenesis, 1218-1219
    petechiae, 603
    polyangiitis, 1221
    polyarteritis nodosa, 1219-1220
    primary angiitis of central nervous system,
        1225
    pulmonary, 454, 465-471
    rheumatoid arthritis, 1203
    Sjögren syndrome, 1210
    systemic lupus erythematosus, 1213-1214
    systemic sclerosis, 1230
    Takayasu's arteritis, 1224
    Wegener's granulomatosis, 1222-1223
Immunologic memory, 1108
Immunologic privilege, 1145
Immunologic testing
  infectious disease, 1371-1372
  liver disease, 2139-2140
  for monoclonal proteins, 565
Immunologically mediated neutropenia, 679
Immunology
  antibody, 1121-1126
  autoantibodies, 1155-1160
  cell-mediated immunity, 1126-1132
    cellular constituents, 1127-1128
    cytokines and immunoregulation, 1128-1132
    delayed-type hypersensitivity, 1132
    derangements, 1132
  complement system, 1132-1138

Immunology—cont'd
  human leukocyte antigen complex, 1115-1121
    genetics, 1115-1118
    role in disease, 1120-1121
    tissue distribution, structure, and function,
        1118-1120
    typing, 1120
  immediate hypersensitivity, 1139-1142
  immune response, 1108-1115
    antigens and antigen processing, 1111-1112
    cellular components, 1109
    immunoglobulin superfamily, 1110-1111
    lymphocyte differentiation and activation,
        1112-1114
    self/nonself discrimination, 1108-1109
    soluble factors, 1110
    T-cell subsets and immunoregulation, 1114
  rheumatoid factor, 1160-1161
  synovial fluid analysis, 161-1163
  tolerance and autoimmunity, 1142-1147
Immunometric assay, 1734
Immunoperoxidase, 1544
Immunophenotyping, 558-559
Immunoproliferative disease
  angiocentric, 1225
  Mediterranean lymphoma, 2080
  vascular inflammatory diseases, 1219
Immunoprophylaxis
  compromised host, 1390
  hepatitis A, 2178
  hepatitis B, 2179
Immunoreactive parathyroid hormone, 1745-1746
Immunosuppression
  anemia
    aplastic, 674, 675
    immune hemolytic, 669
  Crohn's disease, 2072
  induction of malignant lymphoma, 695-696
  lupus nephritis, 857
  myasthenia gravis, 1022-1023
  myocarditis, 263
  pure red blood cell aplasia, 675
  purine nucleoside analogs, 684
  renal effects, 870
  rheumatoid arthritis, 1209
  risk of brain abscess, 1414
  systemic lupus erythematosus, 1217
  transfusion reaction, 575
  transplantation
    cardiac, 340-341
    lung, 516
    renal, 792-793
Immunotherapy
  asthma, 1191
  nasal polyps, 2308
  rhinitis, 1183
  testing for immunoglobulin E, 1154-1155
Impedance, heart failure, 158-159
Impedance plethysmography
  calf vein thrombosis, 633
  proximal venous thrombosis, 502
Impetigo, 1419
Impetigo contagiosa, 1556
Implantable cardioverter-defibrillator, 190
Impotence, 1760-1764
  autonomic dysfunction, 935
  diabetes mellitus, 1844
  diabetic autonomic neuropathy, 1873
  diuretic-induced, 326
  Lambert-Eaton myasthenic syndrome, 1024
  liver failure, 2171
Imprint, 1370, 1371
Imprinting, 1729
In situ melanoma, 1299
Inactivation gate, 37-38
Inadequate sleep hygiene, 944
Inborn errors of metabolism
  amino acids, 1904
  Fanconi's syndrome, 881
    aminoaciduria, 879
    chronic lead nephropathy *versus*, 867

Inborn errors of metabolism—cont'd
  Fanconi's syndrome—cont'd
    multiple myeloma, 864
    proximal tubule abnormalities, 747
    proximal tubule defect, 837
    renal tubular transport defects, 881-882
  fructosuria, 1879
  galactosemia, 1882-1883
  glucose-6-phosphate dehydrogenase
      deficiency, 1881
    eccentrocytes, Plate IV-4
    hemolytic anemia, 663-664
    red blood cell enzyme defect, 588
  porphyrias, 1923-1927
  vitamin D-dependent rickets, 1952
Incentive spirometry, 429-430
Incidentaloma, 1830
Inclusion body myositis, 1236
Inclusion conjunctivitis, 1536
Incompetent lower esophageal sphincter, 2015
Incomplete left bundle branch block, 87
Incomplete right bundle branch block, 87
Incompletely dominant, term, 1724
Incontinence, 1065-1066
  autonomic failure, 935
  fecal
    anal fissure and fistula, 2093
    Hirshsprung's disease, 1980
  urinary
    elderly, 2290-2293
    hyperosmolar nonketotic coma, 1866
    spinal epidural abscess, 1418
Increased intracranial pressure
  bacterial meningitis, 1405
  headache, 960
  medical treatment, 1084
  pathophysiology, 1081-1082
Incubating syphilis, 1640
IND; *see* Indinavir
Indapamide, 325
Indayl-carbenicillin, 1350
Indemnity-based insurance, 30
Independent assortment, 1721
Independent practice association, 30, 31
Inderal; *see* Propranolol
India ink preparation
  Cryptococcus neoformans, 1668, Plate VIII-50
  meningitis
    acquired immunodeficiency syndrome, 1477
    acute, 1408
Indicator-dilution method, 110
Indicine-N-oxide, 2192
Indigenous microflora, 1614, 1615
Indinavir
  acquired immunodeficiency syndrome, 1474
  human cytochrome P450 isoforms, 2312
Indirect costs of medical care, 14
Indirect immunofluorescence, 1373-1374
  babesiosis, 1676
  Borrelia burgdorferi, 1647
  detection of autoantibodies, 1156
  infectious disease, 1373-1374
  Legionella pneumophila, 1623
  toxoplasmosis, 1678
Indium-111 antimyosin Fab fragments, 105
Indium scan
  gastric, 2004
  osteomyelitis, 1434
Indole-3-carbinol, 2153
Indomethacin, 1259
  hepatic injury, 2191
  patent ductus arteriosus, 286
  pericardial heart disease, 278
Industrial bronchitis, 472-473
Indwelling catheter, risk of urinary tract
    infection, 1462
Ineffective erythropoiesis, 533, 646, 2152
Ineffective osmols, 805
Infant
  botulism, 1572
  Chlamydia trachomatis, 1536

Infant—cont'd
  congenital heart disease, 280-292
    aberrant right subclavian artery, 291
    aortic stenosis, 287
    aortic valve stenosis, 235
    aortopulmonary septal defect, 286
    atrial septal defect, 280-282
    bicuspid aortic valve, 287
    brain abscess, 1414
    cardiac catheterization, 108
    cardiogenic syncope, 954
    coarctation of aorta, 286-287
    complete transposition of great arteries, 290
    congenitally corrected transposition of great
      arteries, 290
    cor triatriatum, 291
    coronary artery abnormalities, 291-292
    coronary sinus aneurysm, 291
    disturbances of conduction, 292
    Ebstein's anomaly of tricuspid valve,
      289-290
    echocardiography, 100
    endocardial cushion defect, 282-283
    etiology, 280
    fetal circulation and changes associated
      with birth, 280
    infective endocarditis, 225, 226
    malposition of heart, 291
    mitral regurgitation, 250
    partial transposition of pulmonary veins,
      282
    patent ductus arteriosus, 285-286
    pericardial, 273, 291-292
    precapillary pulmonary hypertension,
      296-297
    pulmonic regurgitation, 257
    pulmonic stenosis, 256
    tetralogy of Fallot, 288-289
    total anomalous pulmonary venous
      connection, 290-291
    tricuspid atresia, 291
    truncus arteriosus, 290
    valvular pulmonic stenosis with intact
      ventricular septum, 288
    ventricular septal defect, 283-285
  cytomegalovirus, 1527
  galactosemia, 1882-1883
  gonorrhea, 1583-1584
  hepatitis B virus infection, 2174
  hyperinsulinism, 1876
  hypertrophic pyloric stenosis, 2044
  nephrogenic diabetes insipidus, 883
  Niemann-Pick disease, 1918
  osteomyelitis, 1433
  pertussis, 1611
  radiation-induced thyroid carcinoma,
    1816-1817
  recommended daily dietary allowances,
    2114-2115, 2116
  respiratory syncytial virus, 1499-1500
  toxoplasmosis, 1677
  transient hypogammaglobulinemia, 1176
Infantile hypophosphatasia, 1954
Infantile nephropathic cystinosis, 1909
Infarct expansion, 221
Infarction
  bowel wall, 2088
  cerebellar, 973
  cerebral
    endocarditis, 1089
    magnetic resonance imaging, 922
    vascular dementia, 988-989
  intestinal, 2087
  mesenteric venous thrombosis, 2088
  myocardial, 209-225
    acute mitral regurgitation, 219, 220
    adjunctive therapy, 215-218
    angioplasty, 214-215
    angiotensin-converting enzyme inhibitors,
      172
    anticoagulant therapy, 639

Infarction—cont'd
  myocardial—cont'd
    cardiac imaging, 212
    chest pain, 127
    clinical presentation, 209-211
    complete heart block, 180
    congenital abnormalities of coronary
      arteries, 292
    coronary angioplasty, 121-122
    coronary artery bypass graft, 185
    echocardiography, 100
    electrical complications, 222-224
    electrocardiography, 88-89, 211
    incidence, 209
    infarct expansion and left ventricular
      aneurysm, 221
    laboratory tests, 211-212
    left ventricular failure, 218-219
    left ventricular mural thrombosis, 638
    left ventricular thrombus, 221, 222
    mechanical complications, 219
    mitral regurgitation, 250
    myocardial rupture, 219, 220
    neurologic aspects, 1089
    pathophysiology, 209, 210
    pericarditis, 221-222, 273
    premature ventricular contractions, 149
    rehabilitation and preventive cardiology,
      224
    right ventricular infarction, 220-221
    risk stratification, 224
    sepsis *versus,* 1451
    shock, 176, 177, 180
    sustained monomorphic ventricular
      tachycardia, 151
    thrombolytic therapy, 212-214
    ventricular septal rupture, 219-220
    ventricular tachycardia, 180
  pituitary, 1777-1781
  pulmonary
    complication of pulmonary artery
      catheterization, 395
    pleural effusion, 508
    pulmonary embolism, 500, 502
  renal artery thrombosis, 897
  retinal, 1057-1058
Infection
  acute confusional state, 1031
  acute interstitial nephritis, 890
  acute renal failure, 773
  antibiotic selection, 1347, 1348-1349
  antirheumatic drug toxicity, 1261
  aplastic anemia, 674
  bacterial; *see* Bacterial infection
  within bullae, 447
  cancer patient, 582
  cholestasis related to, 2159
  chronic axonopathy, 1019
  chronic lymphocytic leukemia, 685
  chronic renal failure, 784-785
  complement deficiency, 1339
  deep neck, 2309
  disseminated intravascular coagulation, 628
  empyema, 507
  esophageal, 2019-2020
  fever of unknown origin, 1376
  gastrointestinal tract, 1425-1432
    bacterial agents, 1425-1427
    diagnosis, 1430-1431
    diarrhea, 1429-1430
    parasitic agents, 1428-1429
    pathophysiology, 1425
    prophylaxis for traveler's diarrhea, 1432
    traveler's risk, 1467, 1469
    treatment, 1431-1432
    viral agents, 1427-1428
  generalized adenopathy, 599
  hepatic encephalopathy, 2159
  hospital infection control, 1361-1366
  immune complexes, 1137-1138
  increased nutrient requirements, 2102

Infection—cont'd
  infectious gastritis, 2043
  interstitial lung disease, 452
  intraabdominal, 1396-1402
    diagnosis, 1399-1400
    intraperitoneal abscess, 1398
    pancreatic abscess, 1399
    primary intraperitoneal infection, 1396
    retroperitoneal abscess, 1398
    secondary intraperitoneal infection,
      1396-1398
    splenic abscess, 1398-1399
    treatment, 1400-1402
  joint, 1250-1256
  lymphadenopathy, 597
  multiple organ dysfunction syndrome, 422
  nausea and vomiting, 2026
  nephrotic syndrome, 766
  neutropenia, 593, 678
  neutrophilia, 590
  obstructive uropathy, 886
  operative risk, 2261
  osteomyelitis, 1433-1437
  portosystemic encephalopathy, 2160
  postsplenectomy, 602
  posttransplant
    cardiac, 335, 341-342
    hematopoietic stem cell transplantation,
      578-579
    liver, 2219-2220
    renal, 794-795
  during pulmonary rehabilitation, 434
  rheumatoid arthritis, 1205
  risk in multiple myeloma, 700
  sickle cell disease, 658
  skin and subcutaneous, 1419-1425
  sputum expectoration, 408
  traveler's, 1464-1470
    arboviral and animal-transmitted viral
      infections, 1465
    diarrhea, 1464
    evaluation of problems after international
      travel, 1469-1470
    helminth infections, 1466
    malaria, 1464-1465
    pretravel advice, 1466-1469
    protozoan infections, 1465-1466
    sexually transmitted disease, 1466
    typhoid, 1465
    viral hepatitis, 1465
  urinary tract, 1455-1464
    clinical symptoms and diagnosis, 1458-1459
    epidemiology, 1457-1458
    management, 1459-1462
    microbiology, 1457
    pathogenesis, 1455-1456
    pathology, 1456-1457
    prevention, 1462
    prostatitis, 1462-1463
  viral; *see* Viral infection
  weight loss, 1750
Infection control, 1361-1366
Infection control committee, 1364
Infection control staff, 1364
Infectious arthritis, 1250-1256
Infectious diarrhea, 1101
Infectious disease
  acquired immunodeficiency syndrome,
    1470-1479
    autoimmune hemolytic anemia, 669
    brain abscess, 1414
    cardiovascular involvement, 333
    clinical stages, 1471-1472
    clinical syndromes, 1474-1479
    cryptococcosis, 1667
    cryptosporidiosis, 1679
    cutaneous manifestations, 1325-1329
    cyclosporiasis, 1680
    cytomegalovirus infection, 1528
    dementia, 987
    diagnosis, 1472

Infectious disease—cont'd
  acquired immunodeficiency syndrome—cont'd
    ecthyma, 1420
    epidemiology, 1470-1471
    etiology and pathophysiology, 1470
    evaluation and management, 1472-1474
    flow cytometry, 1152
    folliculitis, 1420
    generalized lymphadenopathy, 599
    gram-negative bacteremia, 1446
    histoplasmosis, 1655
    isosporiasis, 1680
    meningitis, 1404
    microsporidiosis, 1680
    nephropathy, 853
    nocardiosis, 1666
    nontuberculous mycobacterial infection,
        1638, 1639
    nosocomial infection, 1361
    pericardial effusion, 272
    Pneumocystis carinii pneumonia, 1692-1696
    prevention, 1479
    prognosis and treatment goals, 1479
    prostatic infections, 1463
    retrovirus, 1533-1534
    Salmonella, 1601-1602
    septic arthritis, 1254, 1255
    shigellosis, 1603
    syphilis, 1640, 1641
    T-cell function, 1343
    toxoplasmosis, 1677
    tuberculosis, 1626
    weight loss, 1750
  antiinfective therapy, 1343-1361
    aminoglycosidic aminocyclitols, 1355-1356
    antimicrobial combinations, 1360
    beta-lactams, 1355
    cephalosporins, 1352-1355
    choice of appropriate agent, 1346-1351
    erythromycin and clindamycin, 1357
    evaluation of response, 1360
    macrolides, 1357-1358
    mechanisms of antimicrobial action,
        1343-1345
    mechanisms of antimicrobial resistance,
        1345-1346
    metronidazole, 1358-1359
    penicillins, 1351-1352
    polymyxins, 1358
    quinolone antibiotics, 1359
    sulfonamides and trimethoprim, 1358
    tetracyclines and chloramphenicol,
        1356-1357
    urinary tract antiseptics, 1359-1360
    vancomycin, 1358
  bacterial, 2064-2065
    acquired immunodeficiency syndrome, 2098
    acute pharyngitis, 1392
    Bacteroides, 1613-1621
    Bordetella pertussis, 1611-1613
    brucellosis, 1604-1607
    Campylobacter, 1590-1593
    cell wall synthesis, 1343
    chlamydial, 1534-1538
    chronic bronchitis, 443
    clostridial, 1567-1576
    Corynebacterium diphtheriae, 1565-1567
    culture, 1367-1369
    cystic fibrosis, 480
    diarrhea, 1425-1427
    differential diagnosis of fever and rash,
        1384
    empyema, 507
    endocarditis, 226
    enterococcal, 1560-1564
    fever of unknown origin, 1376
    furuncles and carbuncles, 1421
    Haemophilus, 1585-1590
    immune complexes, 1149
    impetigo, 1419
    labyrinthitis, 972

Infectious disease—cont'd
  bacterial—cont'd
    Legionella pneumophila, 1621-1625
    leprosy, 1648-1651
    leptospirosis, 1644-1645
    Listeria monocytogenes, 1576-1578
    lung recipient, 517
    Lyme disease, 1645-1648
    meningitis, 1402-1409
    mycoplasmal, 1538-1541
    nasopharyngitis-sinusitis, 1183
    Neisseria gonorrhoeae, 1581-1585
    Neisseria meningitidis, 1578-1581
    non-group A streptococcal, 1563-1564
    nosocomial, 1362
    osteomyelitis, 1433
    pancreatic abscess, 1399
    Pasteurella, 1609
    pericarditis, 272
    pharyngitis, 1391-1392, 1556
    poststreptococcal glomerulonephritis, 843,
        1559
    primary peritonitis, 1396
    respiratory tract, 1390-1396
    rheumatic fever, 1256, 1558-1559
    Salmonella, 1598-1602
    scalded-skin syndrome, 1384, 1421
    scarlet fever, 1556
    seizure, 980
    septic arthritis, 1251
    Shigella, 1602-1604
    sickle cell disease, 658
    sinusitis, 1183
    soft-tissue, 1556-1557
    spinal epidural abscess, 1418
    splenic dysfunction, 1338
    staphylococcal, 1546-1553
    streptococcal, 1553-1560
    syphilis, 1640-1644
    toxic shock-like syndrome, 1384
    toxic shock syndrome, 1421-1422,
        1557-1558
    tuberculosis, 1625-1638
    tularemia, 1607-1609
    urinary tract, 1455-1464
    vaginosis, 762, 1443
    Vibrio, 1593-1598
    Yersinia, 1609-1611
  basic principles, 1334-1336
  brain abscess, 1413-1416
  chlamydial, 1444, 1534-1538
    diarrhea, 1476
    dysuria, 762, 763
    fever of unknown origin, 1377
    gonorrhea with, 1584
    persistent cough, 407
    primary peritonitis, 1396
    reactive arthritis, 1240
    urethritis, 1440, 1455
  fever
    compromised host, 1386-1390
    hospitalized patient, 1479-1482
    rash with, 1380-1386
    of unknown origin, 1375-1380
  fungal, 1651-1660
    acquired immunodeficiency syndrome,
        1328, 1329
    Actinomyces, 1664-1665
    after stem cell transplantation, 578
    antifungal therapy, 1652-1654
    arthritis, 1254-1255
    aspergillosis, 1658-1659
    blastomycosis, 1657
    candidiasis, 1310-1312, 1660-1664
    chromoblastomycosis and mycetoma,
        1659-1660
    coccidioidomycosis, 1655-1657
    Cryptococcus neoformans, 1667-1670
    culture, 1370
    dermatophyte, 1307-1308
    diagnosis, 1652, 1653

Infectious disease—cont'd
  fungal—cont'd
    differential diagnosis of fever and rash,
        1384
    endocarditis, 226
    fever, 1387
    fever of unknown origin, 1377
    heart recipient, 342
    histoplasmosis, 1654-1655
    kidney recipient, 794
    lung recipient, 519-520
    meningitis, 1404
    nocardiosis, 1665-1666
    nosocomial, 1362
    osteomyelitis, 1437
    paracoccidioidomycosis, 1657
    penicilliosis, 1658
    phaeohyphomycosis, 1660
    Pityrosporum, 1309-1310
    pleural effusion, 507
    sporotrichosis, 1658
    uremic patient, 784
    urinary tract, 1462
    zygomycetes, 1659
  gastrointestinal tract infection, 1425-1432
    bacterial agents, 1425-1427
    diagnosis, 1430-1431
    diarrhea, 1429-1430
    parasitic agents, 1428-1429
    pathophysiology, 1425
    prophylaxis for traveler's diarrhea, 1432
    treatment, 1431-1432
    viral agents, 1427-1428
  gram-negative bacteremia, 1445-1455
    clinical manifestations, 1449-1450
    diagnosis, 1450-1451
    epidemiology, 1445-1446
    laboratory findings, 1450
    microbiology, 1446
    pathogenesis, 1446-1447
    pathophysiology, 1447-1448
    prevention, 1453-1454
    therapy, 1451-1453
  helminths, 1696-1706
    eosinophilia, 1705-1706
    intestinal worms, 1696-1698
    intestinal worms with tissue migratory
        phases, 1698-1699
    tissue worms, 1699-1705
    travel-related, 1466
  hemolytic anemia, 667
  hospital infection control, 1361-1366
  host defense, 1336-1343
    complement system, 1338-1339
    humoral immunity, 1336-1337
    phagocytic cells, 1339-1343
    spleen, 1337-1338
  immune complexes, 1149
  intraabdominal, 1396-1402
    anaerobic bacteria, 1617-1618
    clostridial, 1575
    diagnosis, 1399-1400
    enterococcal infection, 1562
    gram-negative bacteremia, 1446
    intraperitoneal abscess, 1398
    pancreatic abscess, 1399
    pleural effusion, 508
    primary intraperitoneal infection, 1396
    retroperitoneal abscess, 1398
    secondary intraperitoneal infection,
        1396-1398
    splenic abscess, 1398-1399
    treatment, 1400-1402
  intracranial epidural abscess, 1418
  intracranial subdural empyema, 1416-1418
  laboratory and diagnostic testing, 1366-1374
    bacteria culture, 1367-1369
    Chlamydiae, Rickettsiae, and Mycoplasmas,
        1370
    direct detection techniques, 1370-1373
    fungus culture, 1370

Infectious disease—cont'd
  laboratory and diagnostic testing—cont'd
    serology, 1373-1374
    skin testing, 1374
    test interpretation, 1366-1367
    virus culture, 1369-1370
  meningitis, 1402-1413
    acquired immunodeficiency syndrome,
        1477-1478
    aseptic, 1488
    brain abscess *versus,* 1414
    candidal, 1662-1663
    clinical manifestations, 1406, 1407
    coccidioidomycosis, 1657
    cryptococcal, 1474, 1667-1668
    differential diagnosis, 1408-1409
    enterococcal, 1562
    epidemiology and etiology, 1402-1404
    fever, 1385, 1387
    Haemophilus influenzae, 1586, 1587
    headache, 960
    laboratory investigation, 1406-1408
    leptospirosis, 1644
    OKT3-induced, 1090
    pathogenesis and pathophysiology,
        1404-1406
    prognosis, 1413
    rash, 1385
    respiratory alkalosis, 355
    Staphylococcus aureus, 1549-1550
    toxoplasmosis, 1677
    treatment, 1409-1413
    tuberculous, 1636
  mycoplasmal, 1538-1541
    cold agglutinin disease, 669, 670
    persistent cough, 407
    pleural effusion, 507
  osteomyelitis, 1433-1437
    anaerobic infection, 1617
    fever of unknown origin, 1377
    Haemophilus influenzae, 1588
    intervertebral disk space narrowing, 1169
    sickle cell disease, 658
    Staphylococcus aureus, 1549
    sternal, 1551
  parasitic
    acquired immunodeficiency syndrome,
        1474, 2095-2096
    coccidian, 1679-1680
    depression, 1037
    diarrhea, 1428-1429, 1431
    fever of unknown origin, 1377
    helminths, 1696-1706
    immune complexes, 1149
    neurologic aspects, 1101
    pleural effusion, 507
    rheumatoid factor, 1160
    transfusion-transmitted, 576
    travel-related, 1465-1466
  peripheral neuropathy, 1016
  Pneumocystis carinii, 1692-1696
    acquired immunodeficiency syndrome,
        1473, 1474, 1477, 1534
    after stem cell transplantation, 579
    lung transplantation, 518, 519
    RNA typing studies, 1652
    sputum examination, 380
  during pregnancy, 2279-2281
  protozoan, 1671-1692
    African trypanosomiasis, 1687-1689
    amebiasis, 1681-1683
    babesiosis, 1675-1676
    balantidiasis, 1690-1691
    Blastocystis hominis, 1691
    Chagas' disease, 1689-1690
    cryptosporidiosis, 1679-1680
    cyclosporiasis, 1680
    Dientamoeba fragilis, 1691
    giardiasis, 1684-1685
    isosporiasis, 1680
    leishmaniasis, 1685-1687

Infectious disease—cont'd
  protozoan—cont'd
    malaria, 1671-1675
    microsporidiosis, 1680-1681
    Naegleria and *Acanthamoeba,* 1683-1684
    nonpathogenic protozoa, 1692
    sarcocystosis, 1680
    toxoplasmosis, 1676-1679
    travel-related, 1465-1466
    trichomoniasis, 1691
  respiratory tract infection, 1390-1396
    acute interstitial pneumonia, 448, 452
    after stem cell transplantation, 579
    after stroke, 1007
    bronchiolitis obliterans-organizing
        pneumonia, 448, 452-453
    bronchoalveolar lavage, 384
    brucellosis, 1606
    cancer patient, 582
    chest pain, 129
    Chlamydia pneumoniae, 1535
    common cold, 1290-1392
    cystic fibrosis, 480
    desquamative interstitial pneumonia, 449
    eosinophilic pneumonia, 455
    febrile compromised patient, 1387-1388
    gram-negative bacteremia, 1446
    Haemophilus influenzae, 1586, 1588
    influenza with, 1486, 1491
    laryngitis, croup, and epiglottitis, 1393-1394
    lung recipient, 517-518
    lymphoid interstitial pneumonia, 449
    multiple organ dysfunction syndrome, 423
    Mycoplasma pneumoniae, 1538-1539
    Neisseria meningitidis, 1579
    nosocomial, 1480
    oculopharyngeal dystrophy, 1028
    otitis media, 1395
    pharyngitis, 1392-1393
    Pneumocystis carinii pneumonia, 380, 518,
        519, 1473, 1474, 1477
    pulmonary edema *versus,* 425
    risk in multiple myeloma, 700, 703
    sinusitis, 1394-1395
    sputum examination, 380
    Staphylococcus aureus, 1549
    usual interstitial pneumonia, 449
    varicella, 1527
  rickettsial, 1541-1546
    culture, 1370
    differential diagnosis of fever and rash,
        1384
    fever of unknown origin, 1377
  sexually transmitted, 1437-1445
    cervical cancer, 714
    cervicitis, 1441-1442
    Chlamydia trachomatis, 1535
    diagnosis, 1438-1439
    early diagnosis and treatment in human
        immunodeficiency virus prevention,
        1471
    epidemiology, 1437-1438
    gonorrhea, 1581-1585
    inguinal adenopathy, 1444
    miscellaneous syndromes, 1444-1445
    skin and mucous membrane lesions, 1444
    syphilis, 1640-1644
    traveler's risk, 1466
    urethritis, 1440-1441
    vulvovaginitis, 1441, 1442-1443
  skin and subcutaneous infections, 1419-1425
  spinal epidural abscess, 1418-1419
  spirochetes, 1640-1648
    Borrelia, 1645-1648
    leptospires, 1644-1645
    normal flora, 1614
    transfusion-transmitted, 576
    Treponema pallidum, 1640-1644
  travel-related, 1464-1470
    arboviral and animal-transmitted viral
        infections, 1465

Infectious disease—cont'd
  travel-related—cont'd
    diarrhea, 1464
    evaluation of problems after international
        travel, 1469-1470
    helminth infections, 1466
    malaria, 1464-1465
    pretravel advice, 1466-1469
    protozoan infections, 1465-1466
    sexually transmitted disease, 1466
    typhoid, 1465
    viral hepatitis, 1465
  urinary tract infection, 1455-1464
    clinical symptoms and diagnosis, 1458-1459
    epidemiology, 1457-1458
    management, 1459-1462
    microbiology, 1457
    pathogenesis, 1455-1456
    pathology, 1456-1457
    prevention, 1462
    prostatitis, 1462-1463
  viral
    activation of protooncogenes, 543
    acute pharyngitis, 1392
    adenovirus, 1503-1504
    after renal transplantation, 794-795
    aplastic anemia, 672
    arenavirus, 1508-1511
    cell-mediated immunity, 1132
    Colorado tick fever, 1511-1512
    common cold, 1390-1392
    coronavirus, 1502-1503
    culture, 1369-1370
    cytomegalovirus, 1527-1529
    diarrhea, 1427-1428
    differential diagnosis of fever and rash,
        1384
    Epstein-Barr virus, 1529-1530
    fever of unknown origin, 1377
    hand-foot-mouth syndrome, 1489
    hemophagocytic syndrome, 680
    hepatitis, 790, 1465, 1490
    herpangina, 1488-1489
    herpes simplex virus, 1523-1525
    Hodgkin's disease, 691
    human herpesvirus 6, 1530
    human herpesvirus 8, 1530
    immune complexes, 1149
    immunocompromised patient, 1387
    influenza, 1490-1491
    lymphonodular pharyngitis, 1489
    measles, 1497-1499
    meningitis, 1488
    mumps, 1495-1497
    myocarditis, 262
    myopericarditis, 1489-1490
    neurologic complications, 1491
    Norwalk-like virus, 1521-1522
    parainfluenza, 1494-1495
    paralytic poliomyelitis, 1487-1488
    paramyxovirus, 1494
    parvovirus, 1512-1514
    pericarditis, 272
    picornavirus and orthomyxovirus,
        1483-1494
    progressive multifocal leukoencephalopathy,
        1010
    pure red blood cell aplasia, 675
    rabies, 1505-1508
    respiratory syncytial virus, 1499-1500
    respiratory tract, 1390-1396
    retrovirus, 1531-1534
    rotavirus, 1520-1521
    rubella, 1500-1502
    septic arthritis, 1255
    Sjögren syndrome, 1210
    travel-related, 1465
    uremic patient, 784
    varicella zoster virus, 1525-1527
  weight loss, 1750
Infectious eczematoid dermatitis, 1304

Infectious gastritis, 2043
Infectious mononucleosis
　abnormal lymphocytes in peripheral blood, 595
　acute infectious lymphocytosis *versus*, 592
　adenopathy, 599
　cervical lymphadenopathy, 597
　cytomegalovirus, 1528
　Epstein-Barr virus, 1529
　inguinal adenopathy, 1444
Infectious pericarditis, 272
Infective endocarditis, 225-235
　acquired immunodeficiency syndrome, 333
　antimicrobial therapy, 230-233
　aortic regurgitation, 244
　aspergillosis, 1658
　brucellosis, 1606
　candidiasis, 1664
　clinical syndrome, 227-228
　coagulase-negative staphylococci, 1550-1551
　differential diagnosis, 229
　drug user, 229-230
　fever and rash, 1383
　general appearance, 63
　Haemophilus influenzae, 1586
　laboratory findings, 228-229
　mitral regurgitation, 250
　pathophysiology, 225-227
　prophylaxis, 233, 234-235
　prosthetic heart valve, 230, 258-259
　referral, 233-234
　Staphylococcus aureus, 1550
Inferior vena cava
　Budd-Chiari syndrome, 2208
　venous thromboembolism, 632
Inferior vena cava filter, 638
Infertility
　antirheumatic drug toxicity, 1261
　germinal cell dysfunction, 1844-1846
　gonococcal salpingitis, 1583
　hirsutism, 1755
　21-hydroxylase deficiency, 1824
Infiltrates
　acute lung allograft rejection, 521
　bronchiolitis obliterans syndrome, 522
　crescentic glomerulonephritis, 848
　Goodpasture's syndrome, 847
　hypersensitivity pneumonitis, 461
　Langerhans' cell granulomatosis, 464
　meningococcemia, 1579
　reimplantation response, 517
Infiltrating duct carcinoma, breast, 707
Infiltrative lung disease, 448
Inflammation
　acute cholecystitis, 2227
　American trypanosomiasis, 1690
　asthma, 1185-1187
　bacterial prostatitis, 1462
　celiac sprue, 2062
　chronic abdominal pain, 2035
　containment of infection, 1336
　cytokines, 1129-1130
　DeQuervain's thyroiditis, 1807
　dermatomyositis, 1292
　eczema, 1302
　eosinophilic fasciitis, 1233
　fibrocystic breast disease, 1848
　gastritis, 2041
　glomerulonephritis, 842
　gonococcal infection, 1582
　gouty arthritis, 1272
　hepatitis, 2180
　histoplasmosis, 1655
　intravascular catheter-induced, 1480
　lupus erythematosus, 1291
　mesenteric, 2251
　myelitis, 1011
　myocarditis, 262
　neutrophilia, 590-591
　osteoarthritis, 1265
　otitis media, 1395

Inflammation—cont'd
　peritonitis, 1398, 2079-2080
　plaque disruption, 195
　polyarthritis, 1199-1200
　primary biliary cirrhosis, 2199
　primary granulomatous pulmonary vasculitis, 465
　primary sclerosing cholangitis, 2201
　psoriasis, 1300-1302
　rate of albumin synthesis, 2135
　renal, 754-755
　rheumatic fever, 1256
　rheumatoid arthritis, 1201
　salivary gland, 2310
　subarachnoid space, 1405
　ulcerative colitis, 2073
　vascular, 1218-1226
　　alveolar hemorrhage with, 454
　　angiocentric immunoproliferative disorders, 1225
　　Churg-Strauss syndrome, 1220
　　classification, 1219
　　clinical approach, 1225-1226
　　giant cell arteritis, 1223-1224
　　glomerular involvement, 855-859
　　hypersensitivity vasculitis, 1221-1222
　　hypokalemia, 829
　　Kawasaki's disease, 1225
　　microscopic polyarteritis nodosa, 1220-1221
　　pathogenesis, 1218-1219
　　petechiae, 603
　　polyangiitis, 1221
　　polyarteritis nodosa, 1219-1220
　　primary angiitis of central nervous system, 1225
　　pulmonary, 454, 465-471
　　rheumatoid arthritis, 1203
　　Sjögren syndrome, 1210
　　systemic lupus erythematosus, 1213-1214
　　Takayasu's arteritis, 1224
　　Wegener's granulomatosis, 1222-1223
　vasculitis, 1218-1226
　　angiocentric immunoproliferative disorders, 1225
　　Churg-Strauss syndrome, 1220
　　classification, 1219
　　clinical approach, 1225-1226
　　giant cell arteritis, 1223-1224
　　hypersensitivity vasculitis, 1221-1222
　　Kawasaki's disease, 1225
　　microscopic polyarteritis nodosa, 1220-1221
　　pathogenesis, 1218-1219
　　polyangiitis, 1221
　　polyarteritis nodosa, 1219-1220
　　primary angiitis of central nervous system, 1225
　　Takayasu's arteritis, 1224
　　Wegener's granulomatosis, 1222-1223
Inflammation-fibrosis hypothesis of emphysema, 441
Inflammatory bowel disease, 2068-2077
　arthropathy, 1245-1246
　chronic diarrhea, 2051
　colonoscopy, 1996
　Crohn's disease, 2069-2072
　cutaneous findings, 1321
　differentiation of ulcerative colitis and Crohn's disease, 2075
　etiology, 2068-2069
　extraintestinal manifestations, 2075-2076
　fever and rash, 1385
　incidence and epidemiology, 2069
　increased risk of cancer, 548, 2076-2077
　portal triad lesions, 2155
　during pregnancy, 2278-2279
　primary sclerosing cholangitis, 2201
　secondary hyperoxaluria, 799, 804
　stool examination, 2006
　toxic megacolon, 2076
　ulcerative colitis, 2072-2075
Inflammatory carcinoma of breast, 707

Inflammatory cell
　lung injury, 372-373
　in stool, 2006
　tubulointerstitial disease, 888
Inflammatory mediators
　asthma, 1187
　gram-negative bacteremia, 1448
Inflammatory myopathy, 1234-1237
　glucocorticoid protocol, 1263
　weakness, 1754
Inflammatory pericarditis, 272-273
Inflammatory peritonitis, 2249
Influenza vaccine, 1493
　chronic obstructive pulmonary disease, 434
　cystic fibrosis, 482
　interference with oral anticoagulants, 636
　preventive care guidelines, 2255
　renal transplant recipient, 795
Influenza virus, 1483-1484
　acute febrile undifferentiated illness, 1487
　acute hemorrhagic conjunctivitis, 1490
　acute pharyngitis, 1392-1393
　aseptic meningitis, 1488
　characteristics, 1483
　chemoprophylaxis, 1493
　chronic meningoencephalitis, 1490
　classification, 1483-1485
　common cold, 1487
　culture, 1369
　diagnosis, 1492
　encephalitis, 1488
　epidemic pleurodynia, 1489
　epidemiology, 1484-1485
　exanthems, 1489
　hand-foot-mouth syndrome, 1489
　hepatitis, 1490
　herpangina, 1488-1489
　lymphonodular pharyngitis, 1489
　myopericarditis, 1489-1490
　neurologic complications, 1491
　paralytic poliomyelitis, 1487-1488
　pathogenesis, 1485-1487
　pericarditis, 272
　prevention, 1492-1493
　pulmonary complications, 1491
　treatment, 1492
　uncomplicated influenza, 1490-1491
Informal consensus, 23
Information technology, 25-26
Informed consent, 12
Infradian rhythm, 1719
Infrared absorption spectrophotometry, 396
Infundibular process, 1788
Infundibular stenosis, 289
Infundibulum, 1788
Inguinal adenopathy, 1444, 1640
Inguinal lymph nodes
　containing squamous cell carcinoma, 732
　lymphadenopathy, 598
Inguinal orchiectomy, 720, 721
Inhalants, 452
Inhaled bronchodilator studies, 377-378
Inhaler, 1190
Inherited complement deficiencies, 1178-1180
Inherited polyposis syndrome, 2081
Inhibin, 1767, 1839
Inhibin A, 1835
Inhibin B, 1835
Injury; *see* Trauma
Injury control, 2264
Inner ear, 972
Innervation
　alimentary tract, 1977-1978
　bladder, 933, 935
　genital system, 933-934
　lower urinary tract, 1065
　pancreas, 2130-2131
　peritoneal surfaces, 2247
　pupil, 932-933, 934
Innocent murmur, 77, 78
Inositol phosphate, 57

Inositol triphosphate, 1712
Inotropic agents
　acute tubular necrosis, 773-774
　aortic regurgitation, 243
　arrhythmias, 138
　atrial flutter, 146
　cocaine intoxication, 2297
　dilated cardiomyopathy, 264
　electrocardiographic abnormalities, 90
　gram-negative bacteremia, 1451
　heart failure, 172-173, 174
　interaction with calcium channel blockers, 204
　mitral regurgitation, 252
　mitral stenosis, 248
　multiple organ dysfunction syndrome, 422
　myocardial infarction, 218
　neurogenic pulmonary edema, 1099
　Parkinson's disease, 990-991
　prolactin inhibition, 1775
　shock, 180, 182
　stress perfusion scintigraphy, 199
　tricuspid regurgitation, 256
Insect
　anaphylaxis, 1194
　causing occupational asthma, 472
　ecthyma, 1420
　hemolysis, 668
Insecticides, 867
Insomnia, 940
　chronic fatigue syndrome, 2300
　lesions of anterior hypothalamus, 940
　menopause, 2270
　restless legs syndrome, 1103
Inspiration
　abdominal muscles and, 358
　alveolar gas and dead space, 348
Inspiratory muscles, 357
　chronic obstructive pulmonary disease, 418
　ventilatory pump, 347
Instructional hypothesis, 530
Insufficiency
　adrenal, 1823-1824
　　acquired immunodeficiency syndrome, 1475
　　hypoglycemia, 1876
　　lymphocytosis, 592
　　sepsis *versus,* 1451
　　sodium depletion, 824
　carotid, 2301
　pancreatic, 2133
　　cystic fibrosis, 2246
　　impaired lipid ingestion, 1987
　　Schilling test, 2060
　renal
　　Alport's syndrome, 876
　　antihypertensive agent choices, 326
　　chronic, 776
　　diabetic patient, 1870
　　familial Mediterranean fever, 877
　　hypoglycemia, 1876
　　multiple myeloma, 700
　　obstructive uropathy, 886
　venous, 311-312
　vertebrobasilar artery, 2301
Insufficient sleep syndrome, 944
Insulin
　aging and, 2284-2285
　calcium homeostasis, 1720
　chronic renal failure, 786
　diabetes mellitus, 1850
　dosage during first trimester, 2272
　feedback regulation, 1714
　glucose production, 1874
　hyperinsulinemia, 319
　hyperinsulinism, 1876, 1877, 1878
　hyperkalemia, 833
　hypertension, 316
　hypertonic hyponatremia, 812
　hypokalemia without potassium depletion, 826
　insulinoma, 2244
　integrated fuel homeostasis, 1853
　internal potassium balance, 825

Insulin—cont'd
　measurement, 1743
　myocardial energy metabolism, 40
　perioperative requirements, 2262
　prevention of hypoglycemia, 1875
　protein metabolism, 1851-1852
　regulation of hepatic triglyceride formation,
　　2121
　serum phosphate level, 1936
　testing for adrenocorticotropic hormone
　　reserve, 1774
　testing for growth hormone reserve, 1775
　total parenteral nutrition formula, 2117
　vasopressin stimulation, 1790
Insulin-dependent diabetes mellitus, 1853-1854
　autoantibodies, 1155
　diabetic mother, 2272
　diabetic nephropathy, 859
　weight loss, 1749
Insulin-induced hypoglycemia, 1735-1736
Insulin-like growth factor-1
　acromegaly, 1782, 1783
　aging and, 2285
　growth hormone stimulation, 1775
　normal age-related changes, 1737
　puberty, 1767
Insulin-like growth factor binding proteins, 1775
Insulin-like growth factor-II, 1876
Insulin-like growth factors
　calcium homeostasis, 1720
　osteoporosis, 1947
Insulin receptor, 1900
Insulin resistance, 1861-1862
　bacteremia in diabetic patient, 1450
　hirsutism, 1756
　leprechaunism, 1900
　lipodystrophy, 1901
　polycystic ovarian disease, 1837
　during pregnancy, 2272
Insulin therapy
　diabetes mellitus, 1858-1862
　diabetic glomerulopathy, 860, 861
　diabetic ketoacidosis, 1865
　hyperosmolar nonketotic coma, 1866
　hypoglycemic coma, 1868
　lactic acidosis, 1867
　during pregnancy, 1874
Insulinoma, 2244
　endocrine tests, 1743
　hyperinsulinism, 1876
　surgery, 1878
Intact nephron hypothesis, 777
Intangible costs, 14
Integrins, 370
Integumentary system, 1290-1332
　adrenergic responses, 1828
　allergic granulomatosis, 1220
　anaphylaxis, 1193
　barrier to infection, 1335
　biopsy, 1298
　candidal infection, 1661-1662
　coumarin-induced necrosis, 636
　cutaneous anergy, 1150-1151
　dermatitis, 1302-1304
　　biotin deficiency, 2107
　　glucagonoma, 2244
　　herpetiformis, 1296-1297
　　niacin deficiency, 2107
　　Pityrosporum, 1309-1310
　　stasis, 312
　drug reactions, 1312-1316
　endocrine disorders, 1322-1324
　features of malabsorption, 2058
　febrile compromised patient, 1388
　gastrointestinal disease, 1320-1322
　hypothyroidism, 1809
　infection, 1419-1425
　leishmaniasis, 1685-1687
　malignancy, 1297-1298
　　cutaneous T-cell lymphoma, 1331-1332
　　immunosuppression-related, 795

integumentary system—cont'd
　malignancy—cont'd
　　internal, 1316-1320
　　Kaposi's sarcoma, 1330-1331
　　melanoma, 1298-1300
　nails
　　candidal paronychia, 1662
　　nail-patella syndrome, 877
　　psoriasis, 1300, 1301
　　psoriatic nail disease, 1241
　　tinea unguium, 1308
　niacin deficiency, 2107
　normal flora, 1614, 1615
　nosocomial infection, 1480
　riboflavin deficiency, 2106
　skin lesions
　　acne vulgaris, 1304-1306
　　anaerobic bacterial infection, 1618
　　bejel, 1644
　　bullous diseases, 1293-1297
　　celiac sprue, 2063
　　chromoblastomycosis and mycetoma,
　　　1659-1660
　　clostridial infection, 1575-1576
　　coccidioidomycosis, 1656
　　connective tissue disease, 1290-1293
　　cutis laxa, 1289
　　diabetic dermopathy, 1873
　　Ehlers-Danlos syndrome, 1287-1288
　　eosinophilic fasciitis, 1233
　　Fabry's disease, 1918-1919
　　fibrous dysplasia, 1960
　　gram-negative bacteremia, 1449-1450
　　hand-foot-mouth syndrome, 1489
　　human immunodeficiency virus, 1325-1329
　　hypersensitivity vasculitis, 1221
　　impetigo contagiosa, 1556
　　leprosy, 1649, 1650
　　lupus erythematosus, 1290-1292
　　mycosis fungoides, 1331-1332
　　onchocerciasis, 1701
　　pellagra, 1101
　　photodermatoses, 1306-1307
　　pinta, 1644
　　porphyrias, 1925
　　pseudoxanthoma elasticum, 1289
　　psoriasis, 1300-1302
　　sarcoidosis, 458, 1324-1325
　　sexually transmitted infection, 1444
　　Sézary's syndrome, 1331-1332
　　Sjögren syndrome, 1210
　　sporotrichosis, 1658
　　syphilis, 1640-1641
　　tuberous sclerosis, 1922
　　tularemia, 1607-1608
　　yaws, 1644
　sodium loss through, 823
　spinal cord injury, 1051
　staphylococcal infection, 1549
　superficial fungal infections, 1307-1312
　　candidiasis, 1310-1312
　　clinical presentation, 1308-1309
　　dermatophyte infection, 1307-1308
　　diagnostic procedures, 1309
　　Pityrosporum infection, 1309-1310
　systemic sclerosis, 1228-1229
　thyrotoxicosis, 1804
　vitamin A deficiency, 2105
　vitamin D synthesis, 1719
Intensive care monitoring, 390-396
　end-tidal carbon dioxide, 396
　peripheral artery catheterization, 390
　pulmonary artery catheterization, 390-395
　pulse oximetry, 396
　transcutaneous oxygen and carbon dioxide,
　　396
Intensive care unit
　acute respiratory failure, 414
　multiple organ dysfunction, 423
Intention tremor, 994
Intercalated disk, 36

Intercellular adhesion molecule-1, 372
Intercellular immunoglobulin A vesicopustular
　　dermatosis, 1295
Interdigestive housekeepers, 1979
Interdigestive migrating motor complexes, 1979
Interdigitating dendritic cell, 1128
Interferon, 1129, 1130
　　effects on kidney, 870
　　hepatitis C infection, 2178
Interferon-alfa
　　chronic myelogenous leukemia, 687
　　hepatitis C infection, 2178
　　polycythemia vera, 689
Interferon-alpha
　　cancer treatment, 555
　　common cold, 1392
Interferon-beta, 421
Interferon-gamma, 1129
　　activation of macrophages, 1130-1131
　　calcium homeostasis, 1720
　　psoriasis, 1300
Interferon therapy
　　cancer treatment, 555
　　chronic hepatitis B, 2181-2182, 2183
　　chronic hepatitis C, 2183
　　fulminant hepatitis A, 2177
　　membranoproliferative glomerulonephritis, 854
　　multiple myeloma, 702
　　multiple sclerosis, 1010
　　osteopetrosis, 1959
Interleukin-1, 1128-1130
　　gram-negative bacteremia, 1447, 1448
　　multiple organ dysfunction syndrome, 421
　　pyelonephritis, 1456
　　pyrogenic actions, 1386
　　rheumatoid arthritis, 1201
　　sarcoidosis, 457
Interleukin-1α, 372
Interleukin-1 receptor antagonist, 1454
Interleukin-2, 1129
　　cancer treatment, 555
　　effects on kidney, 870
　　pulmonary toxicity, 478
　　renal cell carcinoma, 898
　　T-cell replication, 369
Interleukin-2 receptor, 1177
Interleukin-3, 1129
Interleukin-3/GM-CSF fusion, 532
Interleukin-4, 1129, 1131
Interleukin-5, 1129
Interleukin-6, 532, 1129, 1130
　　bacterial meningitis, 1405
　　multiple myeloma, 701
　　multiple organ dysfunction syndrome, 421
　　pyelonephritis, 1456
　　sepsis, 1448
Interleukin-7, 1129
Interleukin-8, 1129
　　bacterial meningitis, 1405
　　multiple organ dysfunction syndrome, 421
　　sepsis, 1448
Interleukin-9, 1129
Interleukin-10, 1129
　　bacterial meningitis, 1405
　　inhibitor of cell-mediated immunity, 1131
Interleukin-11, 532
Interleukin-12, 1129
Interleukin-13, 1129
Interleukin-14, 1131
Interleukin-15, 1129
Interleukin-16, 1131
Interleukin-17, 1131
Interleukins, 532, 1128, 1947
Intermediate-density lipoproteins, 1886
Intermittent arthropathy, 1242-1244
Intermittent claudication, 308-309, 641
Intermittent hydrarthrosis, 1244
Intermittent mandatory ventilation, 397-398,
　　418-419
Intermittent pneumatic compression, 504,
　　2261-2262

Intermittent positive pressure breathing, 430
Intermittent proteinuria, 761
Internal carotid artery siphon, 1004
Internal dysuria, 762
Internal mammary artery, coronary artery bypass
　　graft, 206
Internal nodes, 598-599
Internal sphincter, 933, 1065
International Classification of Diseases, 27
International classification of sleep disorders,
　　940, 941
International Headache Society, 957
International Normalized Ratio, 571, 635
International Sensitivity Index, 571
International 10-20 system of electrode
　　placement, 905
Internet-based medical information, 28-29
Internuclear ophthalmoplegia, 1008
Interphalangeal joint
　　multicentric reticulohistiocytosis, 1245
　　psoriatic arthritis, 1241
Interstitial cells of Cajal, 1976
Interstitial compartment, 424
Interstitial cystitis, 763
Interstitial edema, 1405
Interstitial fibrosis
　　diffusing capacity, 378
　　systemic sclerosis, 1230
　　tubulointerstitial disease, 888
Interstitial fluid, 736
Interstitial hereditary nephropathies, 876-878
Interstitial infiltrate, 403, 848
Interstitial lung disease, 448-456
　　clinical features, 450-451
　　clinicopathologic classification, 449
　　diagnosis and management, 451-452
　　dyspnea, 404
　　etiologic factors, 452
　　exercise tests, 379
　　imaging techniques, 451
　　lung pathology, 448-449
　　pathogenesis, 449-450
　　pathophysiology, 450
　　pulmonary hypertension, 498
　　unknown origin, 452-456
Interstitial nephritis, 769, 889-890
Interstitial space
　　cells of, 371
　　egress of fluid during shock, 176, 177
Interstitium, alveolocapillary membrane, 348
Intertrigo, candidal, 1310, 1311, 1662
Interventional cardiac catheterization, 116-125
　　approach to specific lesions, 120-121
　　background, 116-117
　　complications, 122
　　coronary angioplasty for acute myocardial
　　　　infarction, 121-122
　　devices, 117-120, 121
　　pathophysiology, 116
　　primary coronary angioplasty, 122
　　randomized trials, 117, 118
　　referral, 124
　　rescue coronary angioplasty, 122
　　restenosis, 122-124
Intervertebral disk
　　calcification, 1170-1171
　　disk space narrowing in arthritis, 1169-1170
　　herniation
　　　　computed tomography, 920
　　　　magnetic resonance imaging, 924
　　　　myelogram, 926
　　spondylosis deformans, 1266
Interview, 2, 3
Intestinal absorption, 1985-1989
　　cholesterol, 1884
　　magnesium, 1939, 1940
Intestinal disorders
　　aganglionic megacolon, 2092
　　amebiasis, 1682
　　anal fissure and fistula, 2093
　　appendicitis, 2092

Intestinal disorders—cont'd
　　candidiasis, 1661
　　colon cancer, 2082-2086
　　　　allelic loss, 546
　　　　Campylobacter jejuni infection *versus,* 1591
　　　　colonoscopy, 1996
　　　　curability with chemotherapy, 552
　　　　hereditary nonpolyposis, 549
　　　　incidence and death rates, 550
　　　　physiology and pathophysiology, 2082-2083
　　　　risk in ulcerative colitis, 2075
　　　　screening, 552-553
　　diverticular, 2089-2092
　　enteric infection, 1425-1432
　　　　bacterial agents, 1425-1427
　　　　diagnosis, 1430-1431
　　　　diarrhea, 1429-1430
　　　　parasitic agents, 1428-1429
　　　　pathophysiology, 1425
　　　　prophylaxis for traveler's diarrhea, 1432
　　　　treatment, 1431-1432
　　　　viral agents, 1427-1428
　　evaluation, 2004-2008
　　gastroenteritis, 1425-1432
　　　　bacterial agents, 1425-1427
　　　　coronavirus, 1502
　　　　coronavirus infection, 1502
　　　　diagnosis, 1430-1431
　　　　diarrhea, 1429-1430
　　　　eosinophilic, 2066-2067
　　　　immunoglobulin A nephropathy, 845
　　　　parasitic agents, 1428-1429
　　　　pathophysiology, 1425
　　　　prophylaxis for traveler's diarrhea, 1432
　　　　rotavirus and Norwalk-like virus, 1519-1522
　　　　Salmonella, 1599
　　　　Staphylococcus aureus, 1548-1549
　　　　treatment, 1431-1432
　　　　Vibrio parahaemolyticus, 1596-1597
　　　　viral agents, 1427-1428
　　hemorrhoids, 2092-2093
　　increased bile salt loss in feces, 2129
　　inflammatory bowel disease, 2068-2077
　　　　arthropathy, 1245-1246
　　　　chronic diarrhea, 2051
　　　　colonoscopy, 1996
　　　　Crohn's disease, 2069-2072
　　　　cutaneous findings, 1321
　　　　differentiation of ulcerative colitis and
　　　　　　Crohn's disease, 2075
　　　　etiology, 2068-2069
　　　　extraintestinal manifestations, 2075-2076
　　　　fever and rash, 1385
　　　　incidence and epidemiology, 2069
　　　　increased risk of cancer, 548, 2076-2077
　　　　portal triad lesions, 2155
　　　　during pregnancy, 2278-2279
　　　　primary sclerosing cholangitis, 2201
　　　　secondary hyperoxaluria, 799, 804
　　　　stool examination, 2006
　　　　toxic megacolon, 2076
　　　　ulcerative colitis, 2072-2075
　　malabsorption, 2056-2068
　　　　abetalipoproteinemia, 2067
　　　　bacterial overgrowth, 2060-2062
　　　　carbohydrate intolerance, 2067-2068
　　　　celiac sprue, 2062-2063
　　　　clinical features, 2057-2058
　　　　digestion process, 2056-2057
　　　　eosinophilic gastroenteritis, 2066-2067
　　　　hypogammaglobulinemia, 2066
　　　　intestinal lymphangiectasia, 2067
　　　　laboratory findings, 2058-2060
　　　　pancreatic and hepatobiliary diseases, 2062
　　　　radiation enteropathy, 2065-2066
　　　　short bowel syndrome, 2066
　　　　tropical sprue, 2065
　　　　Whipple's disease, 2064-2065
　　secondary hyperoxaluria, 799
　　small intestine tumor, 2080-2081
　　solitary ulcer syndrome, 2093

Intestinal disorders—cont'd
systemic sclerosis, 1229-1230
vascular disease, 2086-2089
Intestinal ileus, 829
Intestinal immunity, 1989-1993
Intestinal lipodystrophy, 2064-2065
Intestinal lymphangiectasia, 2067
Intestinal metaplasia, 2042
Intestinal motility
barrier to infection, 1335
evaluation, 2007-2008
intestinal pseudoobstruction, 2079
irritable bowel syndrome, 2055
Intestinal obstruction, 2077-2079
abdominal pain, 2032
colon cancer, 2085
constipation, 2053-2055
cystic fibrosis, 2246
Meckel's diverticulum, 2089
mesenteric hernia, 2251
radiography, 2032
small intestinal malignancies, 2081
Intestinal pseudoobstruction, 2079, 2089
Intestinal villus, 1991
Intestinal worms
cestodes, 1696-1697
nematodes, 1696
with tissue migratory phases, 1698-1699
Intestine
bile salt secretion rates, 2125
catabolism, recirculation, and elimination of
bile pigments, 2149-2150
dilated loops, 2032
normal flora, 1614, 1615
Intimate partner abuse, 2268
Intoxication
alcohol, 1080
aluminum, 1961, 1964
cocaine, 2297
salicylates, 355, 1451
vitamin D, 2108
Intraabdominal catastrophe, 1476
Intraabdominal disease, 1396-1402
anaerobic bacteria, 1617-1618
clostridial, 1575
diagnosis, 1399-1400
enterococcal infection, 1562
gram-negative bacteremia, 1446
intraperitoneal abscess, 1398
pancreatic abscess, 1399
pleural effusion, 508
primary intraperitoneal infection, 1396
retroperitoneal abscess, 1398
secondary intraperitoneal infection, 1396-1398
splenic abscess, 1398-1399
treatment, 1400-1402
Intraabdominal lymphadenopathy, 598-599
Intraabdominal pressure, 2164
Intraaortic balloon counterpulsation, 205
Intraaortic balloon pump
cardiogenic shock, 185
coarctation of aorta, 287
Intraarterial digital subtraction angiography, 895
Intraarticular bone ankylosis, 1166-1167
Intraarticular calcification, 1169
Intraarticular corticosteroids, 1207-1208
Intracavitary radiation in cervical cancer, 715
Intracellular fluid
calcium in, 1717
ionic composition, 736
magnesium, 1939, 1940
principles of osmoregulation, 805-806
Intracellular killing defects, 1341
Intracellular pathogens, 1334
Intracerebral hematoma, 1043, 1044, 1045
Intracranial epidural abscess, 1418
Intracranial hemorrhage
complication of systemic cancer, 1071
computed tomography, 919
endocardial hemorrhage with, 1087
factor XIII deficiency, 624

Intracranial hemorrhage—cont'd
hemophilic patient, 620
hemorrhagic stroke, 997, 998
Intracranial pressure
bacterial meningitis, 1405
head trauma, 1043, 1044
headache, 958
papilledema, 1060
pathophysiology, 1081-1082
visual obscurations, 2301
Intracranial subdural empyema, 1416-1418
Intradermal hemorrhage, Plate VIII-45
Intraepithelial lymphocyte, 1990
Intrahepatic bile duct carcinoma, 2231
Intrahepatic biliary ductal system, 2199
Intrahepatic cholangiocarcinoma, 2214-2215
Intrahepatic cholestasis of pregnancy, 2277
Intraluminal maldigestion, 2060-2062
Intraocular pressure, 2301
Intraoperative enteroscopy, 1995
Intraoperative radiation therapy, 2048
Intraperitoneal infection, 1396-1398
Intrarenal reflux, 892
Intraretinal microvascular abnormalities, 2303
Intraspinal bacterial infection, 1418-1419
Intrauterine device, 2270
actinomycosis, 1665
endometrial scarring, 1760
Intravascular catheter-induced inflammation,
1480
Intravenous fluids, 2078
Intravenous immunoglobulin
Bruton's agammaglobulinemia, 1175
immune hemolytic anemia, 669
immune thrombocytopenic purpura, 617
inflammatory myopathies, 1237
multiple myeloma, 703
myasthenia gravis, 1023
posttransfusion purpura, 616
Intravenous pyelography, 748-749
hematuria, 757
nephrotic syndrome, 766
obstructive uropathy, 753, 754
postrenal azotemia, 771
renal mass, 753
Intravenous urography
medullary sponge kidney, 875
renal cell carcinoma, 898
upper urinary tract tumor, 899
Intraventricular conduction abnormalities, 156
Intrinsic coagulation pathway, 537
Intrinsic hepatoxins, 2185-2186
Intrinsic renal disease
acute renal failure, 768-769
diagnosis, 771-772
management, 773
pathophysiology, 769
Intrinsic sleep disorders, 940-944
Intrinsic sympathomimetic activity, 327
Intron, 1708-1709, 1721
Intubation
acute respiratory failure, 416-417
angioedema, 2306
botulism, 1571
gastrointestinal bleeding, 2010
head trauma, 1044
intestinal obstruction, 2078
mechanical ventilation, 399
pulmonary edema, 425-426
Intussusception, 2078
Invasive diagnostic techniques
angiography, 111, 112
after valve replacement, 259
aortic regurgitation, 242
Budd-Chiari syndrome, 2208
cerebral, 925-926, 927
cholangiocarcinoma, 2232
hepatocellular carcinoma, 2213
intestinal bleeding, 2007
mitral stenosis, 248
mitral valve prolapse, 254

Invasive diagnostic techniques—cont'd
angiography—cont'd
portal venous obstruction, 2209
precapillary pulmonary hypertension, 296
preoperative, 2257
pulmonary, 294-295, 388-389, 2170
pulmonic stenosis, 288
radionuclide, 104-105
renal, 751, 752, 782
stroke, 1003
tetralogy of Fallot, 289
variceal bleeding, 2167
ventricular septal defect, 284
aortography
acute aortic obstruction, 304
coarctation of aorta, 286
coronary arteriovenous fistula, 292
dissection of aorta, 301, 302
patent ductus arteriosus, 286
peripheral arterial aneurysm, 309
ventricular septal defect with aortic
regurgitation, 285
bone biopsy, 1747, Plate IX-5
bone marrow examination
aplastic anemia, 672, 673
aspirate smear, 557-558
hairy cell leukemia, 684
Hodgkin's disease, 694
human immunodeficiency virus infection,
1473
iron deficiency anemia, 643
lymphoma, 558
megaloblastic anemia, 648
neutropenia, 593
non-Hodgkin's lymphoma, 698
small cell lung cancer, 726
cardiac catheterization, 107-116
angiography, 111, 112
aortic regurgitation, 113-114, 242
aortic stenosis, 113, 238
atrial septal defect, 282
cardiac output, 109-110
cardiomyopathies, 115-116
chronic constrictive pericarditis, 116
circulatory shunts and resistances, 110-111
coarctation of aorta, 286-287
complete transposition of great arteries, 290
constrictive pericarditis, 277-278, 279
dilated cardiomyopathy, 264
Ebstein's anomaly of tricuspid valve, 290
echocardiography, 100
endocardial cushion defect, 283
heart failure, 167
hypertrophic cardiomyopathy, 268
indications, 107-108
ischemic heart disease, 113
left ventricular function, 111-113
mitral regurgitation, 114, 115, 251
mitral stenosis, 114-115, 248
mitral valve prolapse, 254
patent ductus arteriosus, 286
precapillary pulmonary hypertension, 296,
297
pressure management, 108-109, 110
primary pulmonary hypertension, 294
pulmonic regurgitation, 257
risks, 108, 109
shock, 184
sudden cardiac survivor, 188
techniques, 108
tetralogy of Fallot, 289
tricuspid regurgitation, 256
tricuspid stenosis, 256
endoscopy, Plate X-6
abdominal pain, 2034
Barrett's esophagus, 2018
bronchoscopy, 383-384
chronic pancreatitis, 2240
colonoscopy, 1996
esophagogastroduodenoscopy, 1994
esophagoscopy, 2000

Invasive diagnostic techniques—cont'd
  endoscopy—cont'd
    fever of unknown origin, 1379
    gastroduodenal diseases, 2002
    gastrointestinal, 1993-1998
    gastrointestinal bleeding, 2011
    gastroscopy, 2041
    intestinal disorders, 2007
    intestinal obstruction, 2078
    pancreatic secretion measurement, 2134
    peptic ulcer, 2037, 2039
    rhinopharyngeal, 1181
    sigmoidoscopy, 1995-1996
    stomach cancer, 2046
    ulcerative colitis, 2073, Plate X-8
  liver biopsy, 2136, 2141
    acute fatty liver of pregnancy, 2278
    Budd-Chiari syndrome, 2208
    cholestasis, 2156
    chronic hepatitis, 2180
    fever of unknown origin, 1380
    hepatic epithelioid hemangioendothelioma, 2215
    hepatocellular carcinoma, 2214
    hereditary hemochromatosis, 2204
    peliosis hepatis, 2212
    portal hypertension, 2166
    primary biliary cirrhosis, 2199
    protoporphyria, 1926
    unconjugated hyperbilirubinemia, 2153
    veno-occlusive disease, 2208
    Wilson's disease, 2205
  lung biopsy, 382-384
    bleomycin-induced pulmonary diseases, 477
    bronchial adenoma, 491-492
    bronchiolitis obliterans syndrome, 522
    bronchoscopy-guided, 383-384
    hypersensitivity pneumonitis, 461
    interstitial lung disease, 451
    Langerhans' cell granulomatosis, 464
    lung cancer, 490
    open, 385-386
    pleural disease, 506
    solitary pulmonary nodule, 494
  lymph node biopsy, 600
    acquired immunodeficiency syndrome, 1476
    angioimmunoblastic lymphadenopathy, 1248
    Hodgkin's disease, 691, 692
    Mycobacterium avium complex, Plate VIII-36
  mucosal biopsy
    Helicobacter pylori, 2003
    small intestine, 2008
  muscle biopsy
    determination of weakness, 1755
    electromyography *versus,* 917
    inflammatory myopathies, 1235
  needle aspiration, 383, 384
    bone, 1747
    dilated cardiomyopathy, 263
    kidney, 748
    lymph node, 600
    necrotizing fasciitis, 1422
    peritonsillar abscess, 2306
    transthoracic, 385
    tuberculous pleurisy, 507
  pleural biopsy, 382-383
    granuloma, 382
    lung cancer, 490
    pleural disease, 506
  pulmonary, 380-386
    bronchoalveolar lavage, 384
    bronchoscopy and biopsy, 383-384
    mediastinoscopy and mediastinotomy, 385
    open lung biopsy, 385-386
    pleural biopsy, 382-383
    protected brush catheter, 384-385
    sputum examination, 380-381
    Swan-Ganz catheterization, 383
    thoracentesis, 381-382
    thoracoscopy, 385

Invasive diagnostic techniques—cont'd
  pulmonary—cont'd
    transthoracic needle aspiration, 385
    transtracheal aspiration, 385
  renal biopsy, 748
    chronic renal failure, 782
    diabetic glomerulopathy, 860
    focal glomerular sclerosis, 852
    hematuria, 748
    isolated proteinuria, 761
    membranoproliferative glomerulonephritis, 854
    minimal change disease, 851
    nephrotic syndrome, 767
    polyarteritis nodosa, 856
    rapidly progressive glomerulonephritis, 848
    renal atheroembolism, 897
    systemic lupus erythematosus, 1215
    Wegener's granulomatosis, 858
  small bowel biopsy
    adenocarcinoma, 2081
    celiac sprue, 2063
    eosinophilic enteritis, 2067
    small bowel malabsorption, 2058
    tropical sprue, 2065
    upper gastrointestinal endoscopy, 1995
  thyroid, 1802
  transbronchial biopsy
    acute lung allograft rejection, 521
    cytomegalovirus pneumonia in lung allograft, 518
    cytomegalovirus pneumonitis, Plate VIII-37
    through fiberoptic bronchoscope, 384
  transthoracic biopsy, 385
    mediastinal mass, 512
    solitary pulmonary nodule, 494
Inverse psoriasis, 1301
Inverse ratio ventilation, 398
  acute respiratory failure, 418-419
  multiple organ dysfunction, 423
Inversion, 1728
Invertebrate peptides, 1077
Inverting papilloma, 2308
Invirase; see Saquinavir
Involucrum, 1433
Iodamoeba bütschlii, 1692
Iodide
  excess intake, 2110
  Graves' disease, 1806
  hepatic injury, 2192
Iodinated glycerol
  rhinitis, 1183
  secretion clearance and lung expansion, 430
Iodine
  functions, 2109
  induction of thyrotoxicosis, 1807
  nontoxic goiter, 1812, 1813
  recommended daily dietary allowances, 2115
  thyroid hormone formation, 1797
Iodine-123 phenylpentadecanoic acid, 105
Iodine-123 radiolabeled metaiodobenzylguanidine, 1830
Iodine-125-fibrinogen leg scanning, 502
Iodine-125 single-beam photon absorptiometry, 1747
Iodine-131 thyroid scan, 1801-1802
Iodoquinol
  amebiasis, 1683
  balantidiasis, 1691
Iodothyronines, 1708
Ion channels, 58-59
Ionizing radiation, 553
  acute myelogenous leukemia, 689
  carcinogenesis, 548
  tumor formation, 548
IPA; *see* Independent practice association
IPF; *see* Idiopathic pulmonary fibrosis
IPPA; *see* Iodine-123 phenylpentadecanoic acid

Ipratropium bromide
  asthma, 1191, 1192
  chronic obstructive pulmonary disease, 417, 444
  rhinitis, 1183
Iron
  absorption, 641
  beta-thalassemia, 655-656
  drug-nutrient interactions, 2110
  functions, 2109
  hereditary hemochromatosis, 2139, 2204
  intestinal absorption, 1988
  normal bone marrow, Plate IV-9
  overload, 646, 2101, 2110
    transfusion reaction, 575
  porphyria cutanea tarda, 1927
  recommended daily dietary allowances, 2115
  small bowel malabsorption, 2058
  splenic storage, 600
  stores and mobilization, 642
  toxicity, 2110
Iron deficiency anemia, 642-645, 2109
  celiac sprue, 2062
  folate deficiency, 650
  Goodpasture's syndrome, 847
  hookworm infection, 1698
  intestinal disease, 2005
  microcytic hypochromic cells, Plate IV-4
  peritoneal mesenteric and omental diseases, 2248
  during pregnancy, 2279
  splenomegaly, 601
  ulcerative colitis, 2073
  upper gastrointestinal endoscopy, 1994
Iron dextran replacement, 644
Iron stain, 558
Irradiation gastritis, 2043-2044
Irregular breathing, 353-354
Irregular sleep-wake pattern, 945
Irreversible dementia, 2288
Irreversible portosystemic syndromes, 1102
Irreversibly sickled cells, 657
Irritable bowel syndrome, 2055-2056
  abdominal pain, 2035
  celiac sprue *versus,* 2063
  colonic dysmotility, 2007
  diarrhea, 2052
Irritant contact dermatitis, 1303
Irritant receptors, 353
ISA; *see* Intrinsic sympathomimetic activity
Ischemia
  anterior spinal artery, 1012
  chronic occlusive arterial disease, 308
  exercise stress testing, 93
  foot ulceration, 308
  intestinal, 2087
  myocardial, 192-208
    anomalous origin of left coronary artery, 292
    antianginal therapy, 205
    aortic dissection, 300
    beta-adrenergic blockers, 201-203
    calcium channel blockers, 203-205
    clinical manifestations, 195-197
    congenital abnormalities of coronary arteries, 291-292
    coronary angioplasty and revascularization, 205-207
    etiology, 192, 193
    during exercise, 91
    laboratory studies, 197-200
    myocardial infarction, 209
    nitroglycerin and nitrates, 200-201, 202
    pathophysiology, 192-195
    physical examination, 197
    prognosis, 208
    technetium-99m sestamibi imaging, 102-103
    therapeutic approaches, 207-208
  peripheral artery cannulation, 390
  peripheral artery disease, 305
  potassium channel, 59

Ischemic cardiomyopathy
  dilated cardiomyopathy, 264
  radionuclide angiography, 104
Ischemic cholangitis, 2203
Ischemic forearm lactate test, 1025
Ischemic heart disease, 192-208
  antianginal therapy, 205
  beta-adrenergic blockers, 201-203
  calcium channel blockers, 203-205
  cardiac catheterization, 113
  chest pain, 125
  clinical manifestations, 195-197
  coronary angioplasty and revascularization,
      205-207
  electrocardiography, 88-89
  etiology, 192, 193
  laboratory studies, 197-200
  neurologic aspects, 1089
  nitroglycerin and nitrates, 200-201, 202
  nuclear cardiology techniques, 101
  pathophysiology, 192-195
  physical examination, 197
  prognosis, 208
  pulmonary hypertension, 298
  radionuclide angiography, 105
  systemic lupus erythematosus, 1215
  therapeutic approaches, 207-208
Ischemic necrosis, 2078
Ischemic pneumonitis, 632
Ischemic stroke, 998-1000
ISIS IV study, 172, 217
Islet cell antibody, 1158
Ismelin; *see* Guanethidine
Isochromosome 12 in germ cell tumor, 732
Isocoproporphyrins, 1927
Isocyanates, 471
Isoflurane, 2191
Isoforms, 51
Isolated gonadotropin deficiency, 1843
Isolated growth hormone deficiency, 1176
Isolated levocardia, 291
Isolated proteinuria, 761
Isolated ultrafiltration, 791
Isolation, 1365
Isolation and identification
  bacteria, 1367-1369
  virus, 1370
Isolation of speech area, 976
Isoleucine
  disorders of branched-chain amino acid
      metabolism, 1908
  related diseases, 1904
Isometric exercise, 91
Isometric hand grip, 937
Isoniazid
  bacterial meningitis, 1411
  drug-nutrient interactions, 2110
  glucose-6-phosphate dehydrogenase
      deficiency, 664
  hepatic injury, 2190-2192
  human cytochrome P450 isoforms, 2312
  interference with oral anticoagulants, 636
  mycobacterial disease, 1631
  Mycobacterium tuberculosis meningitis, 1410
  prevention of tuberculosis, 1637
  prophylaxis in lung transplantation, 518
  silicosis with positive tuberculin reaction, 475
  tuberculosis, 1473, 1474
Isophane insulin, 1859, 1860-1861
Isoproterenol
  effect on vasopressin release, 1791
  hypoxemia, 363
  interference with catecholamine assays, 1740
  shock, 180
Isoptin; *see* Verapamil
Isosorbide, 2302
  achalasia, 2022
  angina, 201, 202
  congestive heart failure, 818
  heart failure, 170, 173-174

Isospora belli, 1680
  acquired immunodeficiency syndrome, 1474,
      1476, 2095
  compromised host, 1388
  mature oocyst, Plate VIII-1
  T-cell deficiencies, 1993
Isotonic exercise
  electrocardiographic stress testing, 91
  hypertension management, 324
Isotonic expansion of body fluid, 806
Isotonic hyponatremia, 810
  clinical manifestations, 811
  treatment, 812, 813
Isotonic saline, 1939
Isotope switching, 1176
Isotretinoin, 1305
Isotype, 1110, 1122
Isotype switching, 1110, 1124, 1125
Isovaleric acidemia, 1908
Isovolemic hypernatremia, 814-815
Isovolumic contraction, 37
Isovolumic relaxation, 37, 44
Isradipine
  hypertension, 325
  properties, 204
Itching
  benign recurrent intrahepatic cholestasis, 2158
  candidal vaginitis, 1661
  cholangiocarcinoma, 2231
  cholestatic hepatitis A, 2173
  conjugated hyperbilirubinemia, 2156
  estrogen-related cholestasis, 2158
  genital lesions, 1444
  hemorrhoids, 2093
  hepatocellular *versus* cholestatic jaundice,
      2156
  Hodgkin's disease, 693
  hookworm, 1698
  human immunodeficiency virus infection,
      1326
  otitis externa, 2307
  pancreatic cancer, 2242
  paraneoplastic dermatoses, 1317, 1318
  polycythemia vera, 688
  primary biliary cirrhosis, 2200
  primary sclerosing cholangitis, 2201
  protoporphyria, 1925
  transfusion reaction, 574
  vulvovaginal candidiasis, 1442
Ito cell, 2195
ITP; *see* Immune thrombocytopenic purpura
Itraconazole, 1653-1654
  aspergillosis, 1658
  blastomycosis, 1657
  coccidioidomycosis, 1254, 1474
  cryptococcosis, 1670
  esophagitis, 1474
  histoplasmosis, 1474, 1655
  human cytochrome P450 isoforms, 2312
  interaction with cyclosporin, 793
  interference with oral anticoagulants, 636
  paracoccidioidomycosis, 1657
  sporotrichosis, 1658
  tinea unguium, 1311
IUD; *see* Intrauterine device
Ivermectin
  onchocerciasis, 1701
  Strongyloides stercoralis, 1699
  tissue nematode infection, 1700
  Wuchereria bancrofti, 1699
Ivy method bleeding time, 606
Ixodes, 1254, 1646

J

J chain, 1990
J point, 84, 89
J receptor, 353
J segment, 1111
Jacksonian seizure, 979
JAK3 deficiency, 1177

Janeway lesion
  infective endocarditis, 228, 1383
  lupus erythematosus, 1291
Janus kinases, 1131-1132
Japanese encephalitis, 1465, 1515
Jarisch-Herxheimer reaction, 1642-1643
Jaundice, 2147-2159
  alcoholic hepatitis and cirrhosis, 2197
  amebic liver abscess, 1682
  cholangiocarcinoma, 2231
  choledocholithiasis, 2229
  cholestatic hepatitis A, 2173
  chronic pancreatitis, 2241
  classification, 2150, 2151
  conjugated hyperbilirubinemia, 2154-2156
  Dubin-Johnson syndrome, 2157
  familial cholestatic syndromes, 2158-2159
  galactosemia, 1882
  gastric cancer, 2046
  hemobilia, 2233
  hepatocellular carcinoma, 2213
  hereditary fructose intolerance, 1880
  hereditary spherocytosis, 664
  idiopathic myelofibrosis, 677
  leptospirosis, 1645
  neonatal cytomegalovirus, 1528
  normal bilirubin metabolism, 2147-2150
  postoperative cholestasis, 2159
  during pregnancy, 2277
  pyogenic liver abscess, 2209
  Rotor's syndrome and hepatic storage disease,
      2157-2158
  toxic hepatic injury, 2188
  unconjugated hyperbilirubinemia, 2150-2154
JCAHO; *see* Joint Commission on Accreditation
      of Healthcare Organizations
Jejunoileal bypass, 2104-2105
Jejunum, alpha heavy-chain disease, 704
Jerk nystagmus, 1064
Jervell and Lange-Nielsen syndrome, 62, 153
Jet lag, 945
Jin Bu Auan, 2193
Jitter, 917
Jo-1 antigen, 1159
Jock itch, 1308
Jodbasedow syndrome, 1804, 1807
Johnson & Johnson Interventional Systems stent,
      120
Joint
  contracture in spinal cord injury, 1052
  effusion, 1433
  evaluation of complaints, 1198-1200
  hematoma in hemophiliac, 619-620
  primary hyperparathyroidism, 1966
  space narrowing in arthritis, 1165-1166
Joint Commission on Accreditation of Healthcare
      Organizations, 17
Joint disease
  amyloidosis, 1282-1285
    AL type, 863, 865
    alveolar, 452
    cutaneous manifestations, 1316-1317
    familial Mediterranean fever, 877
    Fanconi's syndrome, 882
    hyperkalemia, 832
    multiple myeloma, 701
    nephrotic syndrome, 767
    rheumatoid arthritis, 1205
  arthropathy
    adult Still's disease, 1243
    Behçet disease, 1243
    coagulation disorders, 1246
    endocrine diseases, 1246-1247
    familial Mediterranean fever, 1242-1244
    foreign body synovitis, 1244
    hyperlipoproteinemia, 1245
    inflammatory bowel disease, 1245-1246
    intermittent hydrarthrosis, 1244
    malignancy, 1247-1248
    multicentric reticulohistiocytosis, 1245
    neurologic disorders, 1247

Joint disease—cont'd
  arthropathy—cont'd
    osteonecrosis, 1244
    palindromic rheumatism, 1243-1244
    panniculitis, 1245
    pigmented villonodular synovitis,
      1244-1245
    relapsing polychondritis, 1243
    relapsing seronegative symmetric synovitis
      with pitting edema, 1243
    sarcoidosis, 1245
    sickle cell disease, 1246
    Whipple's disease, 1246
  brucellosis, 1605-1606
  calcium pyrophosphate dihydrate deposition
    disease, 1276-1279
  chronic renal failure, 785-786
  connective tissue disease
    associated myositis, 1236
    cutaneous manifestations, 1290-1293
    heritable and developmental, 1286-1290
    peripheral neuropathy, 1016
    pleural effusion, 508
    rheumatoid arthritis *versus,* 1206
  evaluation of complaints, 1198-1200
  gout and hyperuricemia, 1268-1276
    acute renal failure, 773
    after renal transplantation, 795
    calcium pyrophosphate dihydrate deposition
      disease, 1277
    chronic renal failure, 785
    multiple myeloma, 702
    osteoarthritis, 1267
    uric acid stones, 799
  gouty arthritis, 1271-1272
    joint space narrowing, 1166
    osseous erosions, 1167-1168
    soft tissue swelling, 1165
  infections, 1250-1256
  intermittent hydrarthrosis, 1244
  ochronosis and alkaptonuria, 1280-1282
  osteoarthritis, 1199, 1264-1268
    glucocorticoid protocol, 1263
    hand, 1171
    joint space narrowing, 1166, 1167
    knee, 1172-1173
    wrist, 1172
  palindromic rheumatism, 1243-1244
  polyarthritis, 1245
    acute pancreatitis, 2237
    systemic lupus erythematosus, 1214
    systemic sclerosis, 1229
    Yersinia enterocolitica, 1611
  rheumatoid arthritis, 1200-1209
    course and prognosis, 1205-1206
    diagnosis, 1206
    differential diagnosis, 1206
    extraarticular manifestations, 1202,
      1203-1205
    laboratory findings, 1205
    management, 1206-1209
    radiologic findings, 1205
  Staphylococcus aureus, 1549
  synovial fluid analysis, 161-1163
  systemic lupus erythematosus, 1214
  systemic sclerosis, 1229
  tuberculosis, 1634, 1635
  Yersinia enterocolitica, 1611
Jolliffe's disease, 1101
Jones criteria for rheumatic fever, 1257
Jugular foramen syndrome, 1071
Jugular vein
  distention in right ventricular infarction, 178
  heart failure, 164
Jugular venous pulse, 65-67, 68, 69
  atrial septal defect, 281
  cardiac tamponade, 275
  mitral regurgitation, 250
  primary pulmonary hypertension, 294
  pulmonic stenosis, 288
  tricuspid regurgitation, 256

Junin virus, 1508-1509
Justice, 10
Juvenile cystinosis, 1910
Juvenile nephronophthisis, 875, 892
Juvenile-onset diabetes mellitus, 1854
Juvenile osteoporosis, 1945
Juvenile polyps, 2086
Juvenile rheumatoid arthritis, 273

K

K antigen, 1456
K cell, 491
K complex, 939
Kahler's disease, 700-703
Kala-azar, 1685, 1687
Kaliuresis, 831
Kallikrein, 373
Kallmann's syndrome, 1769, 1841-1842
Kanamycin, 1356
  auditory effects, 972
  dosage, 1349
  enterococci resistance, 1561
  mycobacterial disease, 1631
  use during pregnancy, 2281
Kaolin, 476
Kaposi's sarcoma, 1320-1321, 1329, 1533,
    2098
  acquired immunodeficiency syndrome,
    1477
  cholangitis, 2202
  colon lesion, Plate VIII-39
  cutaneous lesions, 1330-1331, Plate VIII-38
  heart involvement, 331
  human herpesvirus 8, 1530
  ophthalmic involvement, 2305
  oral involvement, 2095
Kappa chain deficiency, 1176
Kappa light chain, 1110
Kappa light chain locus, 1123, 1124
Karyotype, 1727
Karyotype analysis
  hemophilia A, 619
  Klinefelter's syndrome, 1843
  medical genetic diagnosis, 1730
  testicular, 1841
Kasabach-Merritt syndrome, 614, 2215
Kauffmann-White classification of *Salmonella,*
    1598
Kawasaki's disease, 1225
  anti-neutrophil cytoplasmic antibodies, 1219
  exanthem, 1385
Kayexalate; *see* Sodium polystyrene sulfonate
Kayser-Fleischer rings, 1102, 2138, 2205
Kearns-Sayre syndrome, 62, 1029, 1088
Kegel's exercise, 2293
Kenyan tick typhus, 1545
Keratinization, 1304
Keratinocyte, 1300
Keratitis
  Acanthamoeba, 1684
  facial nerve paralysis, 2306
  herpes, 1524
  syphilis, 1642
Keratoconjunctivitis sicca
  human immunodeficiency virus-infected
    patients, 2306
  Sjögren syndrome, 1209-1212
Keratoma, 2307
Kerion, 1308, 1309
Kerley B line
  heart failure, 165
  passive pulmonary hypertension, 297
  pulmonary edema, 425
Kerlone; *see* Betaxolol
Kernig's sign, 1406
Kerosene, 672
Kerotic hyperglycinemia, 1908
Ketanserin, 124
Keto acids, 1853

Ketoacidosis
  alcoholic, 743
  diabetic, 1862-1865
    anion gap acidosis, 836
    effects on fetus, 1874
    hypokalemia, 829
    hypomagnesemia, 1941
    hypophosphatemia, 1935-1936, 1938
    ketone bodies, 743
Ketoconazole, 1653-1654
  candidiasis, 1664
  Cushing's disease, 1786
  ectopic adrenocorticotropic hormone secretion,
    1821-1822
  effects on kidney, 869
  esophageal candidiasis, 2020
  hepatic injury, 2191
  human cytochrome P450 isoforms, 2312
  interaction with cyclosporin, 793
  interference with oral anticoagulants, 636
  leishmaniasis, 1686
  paracoccidioidomycosis, 1657
  pityriasis versicolor, 1309-1310
  therapeutic drug interactions, 2310
Ketogenesis, 1852-1853, 2122
Ketone body, 1853
  fatty acids and, 2121
  formation, 2122
  laboratory testing, 743
Ketoprofen, 636, 1259
Ketorolac, 1259
  cancer pain, 580
  interference with oral anticoagulants, 636
Ketosis, 1881
Ketosis-prone diabetes mellitus, 1854
Ketosis-resistant diabetes mellitus, 1854
17-Ketosteroid reductase deficiency, 1844
17-Ketosteroids, 1741
Ketotic hypoglycemia, 1876
Ketotifen, 1191
Kidney, 735-899
  acid-base balance disorders, 836-841
    metabolic acidosis, 836-839
    metabolic alkalosis, 839-841
    patient evaluation, 840, 841
  acute nephritic syndrome, 763-764
  acute renal failure, 768-776
    acute interstitial nephritis, 889-890
    cancer with, 775
    clinical course, complications, and
      prognosis, 772-773
    diagnosis, 770-772
    essential mixed cryoglobulinemia, 857
    etiology, 768-769
    following bone marrow transplantation,
      775-776
    hemolytic-uremic syndrome, 858
    liver disease with, 774-775
    management, 773-774
    obstructive uropathy, 885
    pathophysiology, 769
    pregnancy, 775
    pulmonary-renal syndrome, 775
    radiocontrast nephropathy, 775
    renal allograft, 775
    rhabdomyolysis, 775
  adrenergic responses, 1828
  aging and, 2284
  Anderson-Fabry disease, 878
  antibiotic toxicity, 1348
  antirheumatic drug toxicity, 1261
  brucellosis, 1606
  calcium reabsorption, 1718
  changes during pregnancy, 2274
  chronic renal failure, 776-796
    abnormal platelet function, 605
    cardiopulmonary complications, 783-784
    clinical presentation and diagnosis, 780-782
    conservative treatment, 787
    dialysis, 789-791
    endocrine function abnormalities, 786-787

Kidney—cont'd
 chronic renal failure—cont'd
  etiology and incidence, 777
  gastrointestinal tract disturbances, 784
  hematologic disorders, 783
  hyperkalemia, 832
  hypertension, 783
  immunologic and infectious complications, 784-785
  neuromuscular abnormalities, 784
  nutritional and metabolic alterations, 786
  osmolol gap, 806
  pathophysiology, 777-780
  prevention or delay of end-stage renal disease, 782-783
  renal osteodystrophy, hyperphosphatemia, hypocalcemia, and bone and joint disease, 785-786
  renal replacement therapy, 788
  renal salt-washing, 824
  renal transplantation, 791-796
 cystic disease, 871-876
 diabetic nephropathy, 859-862
  microalbuminuria, 743, 761
  nephrotic syndrome, 767
 drug- and chemical-induced nephropathy, 866-871
 drug interactions, 2312
 dysproteinemia, 862-866
 dysuria, 757, 762-763
 effects of heart failure, 162-163
 effects of hypokalemia, 829
 familial Mediterranean Fever, 877
 glomerular and interstitial hereditary nephropathies, 876-878
 glomerular diseases, 841-859
  acquired immunodeficiency syndrome nephropathy, 853
  acute nephritic syndrome, 763
  adverse reaction to nonsteroidal antiinflammatory agents, 853
  Alport's syndrome, 876-877
  diabetic nephropathy, 859
  focal glomerular sclerosis, 851-852
  glomerular involvement in systemic diseases, 855-859
  hematuria, 757
  heroin nephropathy, 853
  immunoglobulin A nephropathy, 845
  loin pain-hematuria syndrome, 845-846
  mechanisms and consequences of immune glomerular injury, 841-843
  membranoproliferative glomerulonephritis, 854-855
  membranous nephropathy, 853-854
  mesangial proliferative disease, 851
  minimal change disease, 849-851
  nephritis associated with visceral abscess, 844
  postinfectious glomerulonephritis, 843-844
  rapidly progressive glomerulonephritis, 846-849
  subacute bacterial endocarditis, 844
 hematuria, 756-758
  acute nephritic syndrome, 763
  Alport's syndrome, 876
  autosomal dominant polycystic kidney disease, 873
  crescentic glomerulonephritis, 848
  focal glomerular sclerosis, 852
  Goodpasture's syndrome, 847
  in hemophilic patient, 620
  immunoglobulin A nephropathy, 845
  kidney stones, 800
  loin pain-hematuria syndrome, 845-846
  obstructive uropathy, 886
  poststreptococcal glomerulonephritis, 844
  renal biopsy-induced, 748
  renal cell carcinoma, 898
  thrombotic thrombocytopenic purpura, 858
  upper urinary tract tumor, 899
 hepatorenal syndrome, 2168-2170

Kidney—cont'd
 imaging studies, 748-756
  acute inflammation, 754-755
  angiography, 751
  computed tomography, 750
  intravenous pyelography, 748-749
  lower urinary tract, 756
  magnetic resonance imaging, 750-751
  nuclear medicine, 750
  obstructive uropathy, 753-754
  renal mass, 751-753
  renovascular disease, 755-756
  retrograde pyelography, 751
  ultrasonography, 749-750
 laboratory and diagnostic tests
  acidification, 747
  biopsy, 748
  fractional excretion of sodium, 747
  glomerular filtration rate, 746-747
  microscopic examination of urine sediment, 744-746
  urinalysis, 742-744
  urinary concentration and dilution, 748
 leptospirosis, 1645
 lipodystrophy, 877-878, 1901
 nail-patella syndrome, 877
 nephrolithiasis, 796-805
  calcium-containing stones, 797-799
  cystine stones, 799-800
  differential diagnosis, 800
  laboratory and diagnostic testing, 800, 801, 802
  management, 803-805
  physiology and pathophysiology, 797
  struvite stones, 799
  uric acid stones, 799
 nephrotic syndrome, 765-768
  acquired immunodeficiency syndrome nephropathy, 853
  adverse reaction to nonsteroidal antiinflammatory agents, 853
  clinical manifestations and pathophysiology, 765-766
  complications, 766-767
  diagnosis and management, 767
  familial Mediterranean fever, 877
  Fanconi's syndrome, 882
  focal glomerular sclerosis, 851-852
  glycosuria, 879
  Henoch-Schönlein purpura, 857
  heroin nephropathy, 853
  hyponatremia, 812
  immunofixation, 568
  lipiduria, 745
  lipodystrophy, 877
  membranoproliferative glomerulonephritis, 854-855
  membranous nephropathy, 853-854
  mesangial proliferative disease, 851
  minimal change disease, 849-851
  sodium balance dysfunction, 820-821
  transudative pleural effusion, 507
 obstructive uropathy, 753-754, 884-887
 operative risks, 2263-2264
 physiology, 736-741
  composition of body fluids, 736-737
  glomerular ultrafiltration, 737
  potassium transport, 741
  renal acidification, 739-741
  sodium balance, 737-739
  water metabolism, 739, 740
 polyarteritis nodosa, 1219-1220
 potassium balance disorders, 825-834
  external potassium balance, 825, 826
  hyperkalemia, 830-833
  hypokalemia, 826-830
  internal potassium balance, 825-826
 potassium losses, 828-829
 proteinuria, 758-761
  acquired immunodeficiency syndrome patient, 853

Kidney—cont'd
 proteinuria—cont'd
  acute nephritic syndrome, 764
  Bence Jones, 863
  crescentic glomerulonephritis, 848
  diabetic glomerulopathy, 860
  familial Mediterranean fever, 877
  focal glomerular sclerosis, 852
  Goodpasture's syndrome, 847
  hematuria, 757
  immunoglobulin A nephropathy, 845
  isolated, 761
  laboratory testing, 743
  lipodystrophy, 877
  mechanisms, 759-761
  membranous nephropathy, 854
  minimal change disease, 851
  nephrotic syndrome, 765
  poststreptococcal glomerulonephritis, 844
  subepithelial immune complex deposits, 842
  systemic lupus erythematosus, 1215
  thrombotic thrombocytopenic purpura, 615
  Wegener's granulomatosis, 468
 pulmonary metastases, 493
 regulation of acid-base homeostasis, 835-836
 regulation of phosphate, 1935
 regulator of magnesium balance, 1939
 renal cell carcinoma, 898-899
  computed tomography, 751-752
  incidence and death rates, 550
 renal osteodystrophy, 1961-1965
 renal tuberculosis, 1634
 renal tubular transport disorders, 878-884
  aminoaciduria, 879
  dicarboxylic aminoaciduria, 879-880
  Fanconi's syndrome, 881-882
  Hartnup disease, 879
  iminoglycinuria, 880
  nephrogenic diabetes insipidus, 883-884
  renal glycosuria, 878-879
  renal phosphate wasting syndromes, 880
  X-linked hypophosphatemic rickets, 880-881
 renovascular disease, 893-897
  hypertension, 314
  renal failure, 782
  renal imaging studies, 755-756
 rheumatoid arthritis, 1204
 secondary polycythemia, 589-590
 sodium balance disorders, 816-825
  cirrhosis, 818-820
  congestive heart failure, 817-818
  edematous states, 816-817
  extrarenal sodium depletion, 823
  idiopathic edema, 821
  nephrotic syndrome, 820-821
  salt-wasting states, 823
  sodium depletion of renal origin, 823-825
  use of diuretics, 821-823
 sodium depletion, 823-825
 systemic lupus erythematosus, 1213, 1215
 systemic sclerosis, 1230, 1232-1233
 thin basement membrane nephropathy, 877
 toxicity of chemotherapeutic agents, 584
 transplantation
  allograft dysfunction, 793-794
  chronic renal failure, 791-796
  cytomegalovirus infection, 785
  focal glomerular sclerosis after, 852
  immunosuppression, 792-793
  kidney donor, 791-792
  membranous nephropathy, 854
  multiple myeloma, 865
  myeloma kidney, 703
  recipient, 792
 tubulointerstitial disease, 888-893
  hematuria, 757
  nephritis and uveitis syndrome, 890
 vasopressin clearance, 1791
 von Hippel-Lindau syndrome, 1923

Kidney—cont'd
  water balance disorders, 805-816
    hypernatremia, 813-816
    hyponatremia, 809-813
    principles of osmoregulation, 805-809
  Wegener's granulomatosis, 1222-1223
Kidney stones, 796-805
  autosomal dominant polycystic kidney disease,
    873
  calcium-containing stones, 797-799
  cystine stones, 799-800
  differential diagnosis, 800
  laboratory and diagnostic testing, 800, 801,
    802
  management, 803-805
  medullary sponge kidney, 875
  obstructive uropathy, 885
  physiology and pathophysiology, 797
  spinal cord injured patient, 1050
  struvite stones, 799
  uric acid stones, 799
  urine calcium, 1744
Kidneys, ureters, and bladder
  intestinal obstruction, 2078
  before intravenous pyelography, 748, 749
  obstructive uropathy, 886
  staghorn calculus, 755
Killip classification, 182, 183, 210, 211
Kimmelstiel-Wilson's disease, 859, 1870
Kinesin, 2132
Kininogen, 374
Kinyoun stain
  cryptosporidia, 1680, Plate VIII-32
  procedure, 1371
Klatskin tumor, 2231, 2232
Klebsiella, Plate VIII-6
  antibiotic selection, 1347
  bacteremia, 1445
  spinal epidural abscess, 1418
  susceptibility to empiric antimicrobial therapy,
    1400
  synergistic nonclostridial anaerobic
    myonecrosis, 1424
  urinary tract infection, 1457
Kleine-Levin syndrome, 943
Klinefelter's syndrome, 1729, 1769
  clinical features, 1844
  gynecomastia, 1764
  Hashimoto's thyroiditis, 1811
  hypergonadotropic hypogonadism, 1843
  impotence, 1762
Klonopin; *see* Clonazepam
Knee
  arthritis, 1172-1173
  arthrography, 1164
  bursitis, 1197
  calcium pyrophosphate dihydrate crystals,
    1277, 1278
  chondromalacia patellae, 1266
  pseudogout, 1279
  rheumatoid arthritis, 1203
Knee jerk, 964
Knodell score, 2181
Koate-HS, 624
Koebner's phenomenon, 1300
Koplick's spots, 1385
Korotkoff sounds
  aortic regurgitation, 241
  blood pressure measurement, 64
  pulsus paradoxus, 65
Korsakoff's psychosis, 1081
Korsakoff's syndrome
  amnesic syndrome, 1032
  thiamine deficiency, 2106
  Wernicke's encephalopathy, 1100-1102
Krabbe's disease, 1918
Krebs-Henseleit cycle, 2118, 2120
KS; *see* Kaposi's sarcoma
KUB; *see* Kidneys, ureters, and bladder
Kulchitsky's cell, 491

Kupffer cell, 1127
  hepatic fibrosis and regeneration, 2195
  primary biliary cirrhosis, 2201
Kussmaul respiration, 834
  diabetes mellitus, 355
  diabetic ketoacidosis, 1863
Kussmaul's sign
  cardiac tamponade, 275
  constrictive pericarditis, 277
  myocardial infarction, 210
  right ventricular infarction, 178, 220
Kveim test, 459, 1324
Kwashiorkor, 2101, 2105
Kyphoscoliosis
  hypoventilation, 356
  neurofibromatosis, 1921
  precapillary pulmonary hypertension, 296
Kyphosis
  mitral valve prolapse, 254
  vertebral crush fracture, 1945
Kytril; *see* Granisetron

L

Labeled macroaggregated albumin, 387
Labetalol
  chronic hypertension during pregnancy, 2275
  dissection of aorta, 301
  hepatic injury, 2192
  hypertension, 325
  hypertensive emergency, 328
  properties, 203
Labia
  exam for sexually transmitted disease, 1439
  trichomoniasis, 1443
Laboratory and diagnostic testing
  bone and mineral disorders, 1744-1748
    fibrous dysplasia, 1960
    hyperphosphatemia, 1938-1939
    hypophosphatemia, 1937
    osteomalacia, 1949
    osteoporosis, 1947
    renal bone disease, 1964
  chronic fatigue syndrome, 2299
  endocrine, 1732-1744
    adrenal medullary hormones, 1739-1740
    androgens, 1741
    diabetes insipidus, 1794-1795
    diabetes mellitus, 1855-1856
    diabetic ketoacidosis, 1863
    female gonadal function, 1742-1743
    general principles, 1732-1735
    genetic studies, 1743
    glucocorticoids, 1740-1741
    goiter, 1813
    gynecomastia, 1765-1766
    hirsutism, 1756
    hyperparathyroidism, 1968-1969
    hypoglycemia, 1877-1878
    hypothalamic-pituitary testing, 1735-1737
    hypothyroidism, 1809-1810
    impotence, 1763
    male gonadal function, 1742
    mineralocorticoids, 1741-1742
    ovarian disorders, 1835-1836
    pheochromocytoma, 1830
    posterior pituitary testing, 1737-1738
    thyroid disease, 1800-1801
    thyroid function tests, 1738-1739
  gastrointestinal
    abdominal pain, 2032
    colon cancer, 2084
    Crohn's disease, 2069-2070
    endoscopy, 1993-1998
    esophageal cancer, 2024
    esophageal disease, 1999-2000
    gastrointestinal bleeding, 2011-2013
    intestinal carcinoid, 2082
    intestinal obstruction, 2078
    malabsorption, 2058-2060
    peptic ulcer disease, 2036-2038

Laboratory and diagnostic testing—cont'd
  gastrointestinal—cont'd
    small intestine tumor, 2081
    stomach cancer, 2046-2047
    ulcerative colitis, 2073
  heart, 63-81, 91-116
    acute pericarditis, 274
    angiography, 111, 112
    aortic regurgitation, 113-114, 241-242
    aortic stenosis, 113, 237-238
    arterial pulses, 64-65, 66, 67
    auscultation, 68-71
    blood pressure measurement, 64
    cardiac cycle, 71-72
    cardiac output, 109-110
    cardiac tamponade, 276
    cardiomyopathies, 115-116
    chest radiography, 91, 92
    chronic constrictive pericarditis, 116
    circulatory shunts and resistances, 110-111
    computed tomography, 106
    constrictive pericarditis, 277, 278
    continuous ambulatory electrocardiographic
      recording, 94
    echocardiography, 94-100
    exercise electrocardiographic testing, 91-94
    gamma camera imaging agents, 105
    general appearance, 63-64
    heart failure, 165-167
    heart murmurs, 75-81
    heart sounds, 72-75, 76
    hypertension, 320
    hypertrophic cardiomyopathy, 267-269
    indications, 107-108
    inspection and palpation, 67-68, 70, 71
    ischemic heart disease, 113, 197-200
    jugular venous pulse, 65-67, 68, 69
    left ventricular function, 111-113
    magnetic resonance imaging, 106-107
    mitral regurgitation, 114, 115, 251
    mitral stenosis, 114-115, 248
    mitral valve prolapse, 254
    myocardial infarction, 211-212
    myocardial perfusion imaging, 101-104
    pericardial effusion, 274-275
    positron emission tomography, 105-106
    pressure management, 108-109, 110
    radionuclide angiography, 104-105
    risks, 108, 109
    techniques, 108
  hematology and cancer, 555-572
    acute lymphoblastic leukemia, 682-683
    acute myelogenous leukemia, 689-690
    aplastic anemia, 672, 673
    breast cancer, 708
    cervical cancer, 714-715
    chronic lymphocytic leukemia, 684-685
    clonality, 559
    DNA analysis, 559-561
    endometrial cancer, 713
    evaluation of peripheral blood and bone
      marrow cells, 555-559
    fluorescence in situ hybridization, 561, 562
    glucose-6-phosphate dehydrogenase
      deficiency, 663-664
    hairy cell leukemia, 683-684
    hematopoiesis, 530-534
    hereditary spherocytosis, 663-664
    leukemia, 562-563
    lung cancer, 487-488
    lymphoma, 563-564
    megaloblastic anemia, 648-649
    melanoma, 1299
    monoclonal proteins, 564-568
    multiple myeloma, 701
    myelodysplastic syndrome, 676
    myelofibrosis, 677
    ovarian cancer, 716
    plasma coagulation, 570-571
    platelets and platelet function, 568-570
    prostate cancer, 717-718

Laboratory and diagnostic testing—cont'd
  hematology and cancer—cont'd
    serum and urine monoclonal proteins,
      564-568
    sickle cell disease, 658
    testicular cancer, 720-721
    thalassemia, 654-655, 656
    thrombotic disorders, 571-572
    Waldenström macroglobulinemia, 704
  hepatic, 2137-2141
    alpha₁ antitrypsin deficiency, 2206
    hereditary hemochromatosis, 2204
    lipodystrophies, 1901
  hepatobiliary, 375-400
    biliary colic, 2226
    cholecystitis, 2228
    choledocholithiasis, 2229
    gallstones, 2224-2225
    primary biliary cirrhosis, 2200
    primary sclerosing cholangitis, 2202
    unconjugated hyperbilirubinemia,
      2153-2154
  imaging methods, 386-390
  immunologic
    asthma, 1188-1189
    autoantibodies, 1155-1160
    complement measurement, 1147-1150
    evaluation of cell-mediated immunity,
      1150-1153, 1175
    gout, 1273
    imaging evaluation of arthritis, 1164-1174
    immediate hypersensitivity, 1153-1155
    infectious arthritis, 1251-1252
    inflammatory myopathies, 1235
    rheumatoid factor, 1160-1161
    rhinitis, 1181-1182
    synovial fluid analysis, 1161-1163
    systemic lupus erythematosus, 1215-1216
  infectious disease, 1366-1374
    actinomycosis, 1665
    bacteria culture, 1367-1369
    botulism, 1571
    brain abscess, 1415, 1416
    candidiasis, 1663
    Chlamydiae, Rickettsiae, and Mycoplasmas,
      1370
    Clostridium difficile, 1569
    Clostridium perfringens, 1568
    diphtheria, 1566
    direct detection techniques, 1370-1373
    enteric infection, 1430-1431
    fever and rash, 1385-1386
    fever of unknown origin, 1379-1380
    fungus culture, 1370
    gram-negative bacteremia, 1450-1451
    intracranial subdural empyema, 1416-1418
    leprosy, 1650-1651
    leptospirosis, 1645
    listeriosis, 1577
    Lyme disease, 1647
    meningitis, 1406-1408
    osteomyelitis, 1434-1435
    relapsing fever, 1645-1646
    Rocky Mountain spotted fever, 1544
    serology, 1373-1374
    sexually transmitted, 1439
    shigellosis, 1603
    skin testing, 1374
    spinal epidural abscess, 1418
    streptococcal toxic shock syndrome, 1558
    syphilis, 1642, 1643
    test interpretation, 1366-1367
    tetanus, 1573
    tuberculosis, 1628
    virus culture, 1369-1370
  neurologic disorders, 917-930
    autonomic failure, 935-936
    autonomic overactivity, 934-935
    bladder control, 933, 935
    carotid ultrasonography, 929
    coma, 949-950

Laboratory and diagnostic testing—cont'd
  neurologic disorders—cont'd
    computed tomography, 917-918, 919, 920
    conventional radiography, 924-926
    electroencephalography, 905-908
    electromyography, 814-917
    evoked responses, 908-914
    genital function, 933-934
    head trauma, 1044
    history and examination, 902-903
    local autonomic disorders, 936, 937
    magnetic resonance imaging, 918-924
    multiple sclerosis, 1009
    myasthenia gravis, 1022
    principles, 5-9
    psychologic testing, 903-904
    pupil physiology, 932-933, 934
    radionuclide studies, 926-929
    spinal fluid examination, 904-905
    stroke, 1002-1004
    syncope, 955-956
  pancreatic
    acute pancreatitis, 2234-2236
    chronic pancreatitis, 2239-2240
    exocrine pancreatic tumor, 2242-2243
  pulmonary
    bronchoalveolar lavage, 384
    bronchoprovocation inhalation tests, 379
    bronchoscopy and biopsy, 383-384
    exercise tests, 379-380
    inhaled bronchodilator studies, 377-378
    intensive care monitoring, 390-396
    lung volume determination, 378
    mediastinoscopy and mediastinotomy, 385
    open lung biopsy, 385-386
    pleural biopsy, 382-383
    protected brush catheter, 384-385
    single-breath diffusing capacity, 378, 379
    sleep studies, 380
    spirometry, 376-377
    sputum examination, 380-381
    Swan-Ganz catheterization, 383
    thoracentesis, 381-382
    thoracoscopy, 385
    transthoracic needle aspiration, 385
    transtracheal aspiration, 385
    ventilatory control studies, 378-379
    Wilson's disease, 2205
  renal, 742-756
    acidification, 747
    acute inflammation, 754-755
    angiography, 751
    biopsy, 748
    computed tomography, 750
    fractional excretion of sodium, 747
    glomerular filtration rate, 746-747
    hematuria, 757
    intravenous pyelography, 748-749
    lower urinary tract, 756
    magnetic resonance imaging, 750-751
    microscopic examination of urine sediment,
      744-746
    multiple myeloma and plasma cell
      dyscrasias, 864
    nephrolithiasis, 800
    nuclear medicine, 750
    obstructive uropathy, 753-754
    proteinuria, 761
    renal mass, 751-753
    renovascular disease, 755-756
    retrograde pyelography, 751
    ultrasonography, 749-750
    urinalysis, 742-744
    urinary concentration and dilution, 748
Labyrinthectomy, 975
Labyrinthitis, 972
Laceration
  cardiac, 332
  Mallory-Weiss, 2019
LaCrosse encephalitis, 1515, 1517
Lactase deficiency, 2052

Lactate
  gluconeogenesis, 2122
  ischemic forearm lactate test, 1025
  shock, 176, 178
  vitamin D deficiency, 2106
Lactate dehydrogenase
  amebic liver abscess, 2210
  ascites, 2164
  beta thalassemia, 655
  hemolytic anemia, 661
  hereditary spherocytosis, 665
  human immunodeficiency virus infection, 1473
  myocardial infarction, 211
  non-Hodgkin's lymphoma, 698
  overproduction jaundice, 2152
  prosthetic valve problems, 258
Lactation
  antibiotic selection, 1348
  mean heights and weights and recommended
    energy intake, 2117
  recommended daily dietary allowances,
    2114-2115, 2116
Lactic acid, 834
Lactic acidosis
  anion gap acidosis, 836
  diabetes mellitus, 1866-1867
  gram-negative bacteremia, 1450
  gram-negative sepsis, 1452
  use of nucleoside analog, 1451
Lactitol, 2162
Lactobacillus acidophilus
  neomycin resistance, 2162
  normal flora, 1368
  vaginal, 1456
Lactoferrin, 367
Lactose
  enzymatic hydrolysis, 2121
  hydrogen breath test, 2068
  hydrolysis, 1987
  tolerance test, 2068
  urinary, 1880
Lactose-positive *Vibrio,* 1597
Lactotroph cell, 1773, 1774
Lactulose
  constipation, 2055
  hydrogen breath test, 2061
  portosystemic encephalopathy, 2162-2163
  small bowel malabsorption, 2058
Lacune, 999, 1001
Laennec's cirrhosis, 1378
Lambda light chain, 1110
Lambert-Eaton myasthenic syndrome, 1023-1024
  autoantibody, 1075
  peripheral neuropathy *versus,* 1014
Lamina papyracea, 2309
Lamina propria
  airway, 365
  chronic superficial gastritis, 2042
  esophageal, 2015
  lymphoid cell, 1990
  ulcerative colitis, Plate X-7
Laminectomy, 1419
Laminin 5, 1296
Lamivudine, 2218
  acquired immunodeficiency syndrome, 1474
  chronic hepatitis B, 2182
Landouzy-Dejerine dystrophy, 1027, 1086
Langerhans' cell, 1128
Langerhans' cell granulomatosis, 463-465
Langerhans' cell histiocytosis, 680
Language disorders, 975-978
Lanosterol, 1884
Lansoprazole
  gastroesophageal reflux, 2018
  human cytochrome P450 isoforms, 2312
Laparoscopy
  abdominal pain, 2034
  cholecystectomy, 2226
  cirrhosis, 2141
  fundoplication, 2018
  gastrointestinal, 1997-1998

Laparotomy, 2002
Laplace relation, 42
Large cell lung carcinoma, 487
Large cell lymphoma, 697, 698
Large granular lymphocyte, 592, 679, 1109, 1127
Large intestine; *see* Colon
Laryngeal ascent, 1999
Laryngeal nerve
    aortic dissection, 300
    thoracic aortic aneurysm, 300
Laryngitis, 1393-1394, 1494, 2309
Laryngospasm
    hypocalcemia, 1933
    sleep-related, 947
Larynx
    abnormal swallowing, 1998
    angioedema, 2306
    cancer, 723
    dysfunction in asthma, 1189
    hoarseness, 2309
    laryngitis, 1393-1394
    sleep-related laryngospasm, 947
Laser therapy
    angioplasty, 119
    macular degeneration, 2302
    photocoagulation, 2011-2012
    uvulopalatoplasty, 2309
    uvuloplasty, 528
Lasix; *see* Furosemide
Lassa fever, 1369, 1509-1511
Latanoprost, 2302
Late elective angioplasty, 215
Late potential, 134
Lateral lead, 83
Lateral medullary infarction, 1005
Lateral spinothalamic tract, 1011
Lateral tentorial herniation syndrome, 1044
Latex agglutination
    bacterial meningitis, 1408
    venous thromboembolism, 632
Latex allergy, 1193, 1304
Latex fixation test, 1161
Laurence-Moon-Biedl syndrome
    hypogonadism, 1842
    hypopituitarism, 1776
    obesity, 1752
Law and morality, 10
Law enforcement, 2265
Law of parsimony, 2094
Laxatives
    abuse
        hyperchloremic metabolic acidosis, 837
        stool examination, 2006
    constipation, 2055
    induction of hyperphosphatemia, 1939
    portosystemic encephalopathy, 2162-2163
Lead poisoning
    abdominal pain, 2031
    chronic tubulointerstitial nephritis, 891
    Fanconi's syndrome, 882
    nonoxidative hemolysis, 667-668
    renal toxicity, 867
    sensorimotor neuropathy, 1020
Lean body mass
    aging and, 2284
    puberty, 1768
Leber's hereditary optic neuropathy, 1029
Lechithin-cholesterol acetyltransferase, 60, 1898, 2121
Lecithin, 1883
    bile, 2126-2127
    cholesterol gallstones, 2221
    lipid absorption, 1987
Lecithin-kelp-vitamin B$_6$-cider vinegar diet, 2104
Left anterior fascicular block, 86-88
Left atrial depolarization, 83
Left atrium
    mitral regurgitation, 250
    mitral stenosis, 245, 247
    myxoma, 330
    radiographic views, 92

Left axis deviation, 85
Left bundle branch block, 86
    aortic stenosis, 237
    exercise imaging, 104
    intraventricular conduction abnormalities, 156
Left heart catheterization, 108
Left posterior fascicular block, 86-88
Left-shifted neutrophilia, 591
Left-sided heart failure, 180
Left-to-right shunt, 110, 393
    aortopulmonary septal defect, 286
    atrial septal defect, 280
    coronary arteriovenous fistula, 292
    endocardial cushion defect, 282
    hepatopulmonary syndrome, 2170
    pulmonary hypertension, 296
    tetralogy of Fallot, 288, 289
    total anomalous pulmonary venous connection, 290-291
    truncus arteriosus, 290
    ventricular septal defect, 283
Left ventricle
    angiography, 111
    hemodynamic data, 110
    hypertrophic cardiomyopathy, 265
    radiographic views, 92
Left ventricular aneurysm
    mitral regurgitation, 251
    myocardial infarction, 221
Left ventricular assist device, 186
Left ventricular dilation, 105
Left ventricular dysfunction
    angina pectoris, 127
    atrial fibrillation, 146
    automatic implantable cardioverter defibrillator, 140
    dicrotic pulse, 65
    heart failure, 157, 158
        echocardiography and radionuclide ventriculography, 166
        exercise testing, 166-167
    myocardial infarction, 210, 218-219
    nuclear cardiology techniques, 101
    passive pulmonary hypertension, 297-298
    prognosis of ischemic heart disease, 208
    pulmonary edema, 424
    pulsus alternans, 65
    shock, 177
    tricuspid regurgitation, 256
    wheezing, 1189
Left ventricular ejection fraction
    aortic regurgitation, 243-244
    mitral regurgitation, 250
    radionuclide angiogram, 104, 105
    technetium-99m sestamibi imaging, 102-103
Left ventricular ejection period, 71
Left ventricular end diastolic pressure, 394
Left ventricular end diastolic volume
    aortic regurgitation, 240
    relationship of pulmonary artery wedge pressure and, 394
Left ventricular filling, 275
Left ventricular function, 111-113, 157
Left ventricular hypertrophy
    anomalous origin of left coronary artery, 292
    aortic regurgitation, 239-240
    aortic stenosis, 235, 236
    electrocardiography, 87
    hypertrophic obstructive cardiomyopathy, 266
    mitral regurgitation, 250
Left ventricular outflow obstruction
    cardiogenic syncope, 954
    coarctation of aorta, 286
    hypertrophic cardiomyopathy, 265
    systolic ejection murmur, 77
Left ventricular stroke volume, 240-241
Left ventricular stroke work index, 391
Left ventricular systolic function
    aortic regurgitation, 242-243
    aortic stenosis, 236
    myocardial infarction, 212

Leg
    acute aortic obstruction, 304
    blood pressure measurement, 64
    ecthyma, 1420
    peripheral arterial aneurysm, 309
    peripheral vascular disease, 305-307
    varicose veins, 311
Leg pain
    retroperitoneal abscess, 1398
    venous thrombosis, 631
Legal blindness, 2301
Legionella micdadei, 1624
Legionella pneumophila, 1621-1625
    acute interstitial nephritis, 889, 890
    antibiotic selection, 1347
    nosocomial infection, 1363
Legionnaire's disease, 1623
Leiden mutation, 631
Leiomyoma
    colon, 2086
    esophageal, 2023
    small bowel, 2082
    stomach, 2049
Leiomyosarcoma
    small bowel, 2080
    stomach, 2049-2050
Leishmaniasis, 1685-1687
    Giemsa stain, Plate VIII-12
    traveler, 1466
Lens, presbyopia, 2301
Lente, 1859, 1860-1861
Lentigo maligna, 1299
Lepore hemoglobin, 654
Leprechaunism, 1899-1900
Lepromatous leprosy, 1640, 1649
Lepromin test, 1650
Leprosy, 1648-1651
Leptin, 1128, 1751
Leptocyte, 662
Leptospiral meningitis, 1409
Leptospires, 1644-1645
Leser Trélat, 1317, 1318
Letterer-Siew disease, 463
Leu-enkephalin, 363
Leucine
    disorders of branched-chain amino acid metabolism, 1908
    related diseases, 1904
Leucine aminopeptidase, 2137
Leucine zipper proteins, 50-51
Leucovorin, 1474
Leukemia, 682-691
    abnormal lymphocytes in peripheral blood, 595
    acute lymphoblastic, 682-683
    arthropathy, 1247
    cardiac metastasis, 331
    chromosomal abnormalities, 544
    curability with chemotherapy, 552
    fever of unknown origin, 1377
    hematopoietic stem cell transplantation, 576-577
    incidence and death rates, 550
    lymphoid, 682-685
    lysozymuria, 760
    mast cell, 681
    megakaryocytic hypoplasia, 614
    molecular diagnostics, 562-563
    myelodysplastic syndrome, 676
    myeloproliferative disorders, 685-691
        acute myelogenous leukemia, 689-690, 691
        chronic, 686
        essential thrombocythemia, 687-688
        myelodysplastic syndromes, 690-691
        myelogenous leukemia, 686-687
        polycythemia vera, 688
    neoplastic pericarditis, 272
    nosocomial infection, 1361
    plasma cell, 703
    platelet abnormalities, 611
    second malignancy, 586
    splenomegaly, 601

Leukemic blast, Plate IV-6
Leukemic reticuloendotheliosis, 683
Leukemoid reaction, 591
Leukocidin, 1362
Leukocyte
  abnormal blood cell count, 590-596
    nucleated cells in peripheral blood, 594-596
    quantitative alterations in normal nucleated
      cells, 590-594
  abnormalities of phagocytes, eosinophils, and
    basophils, 678-681
  acute lymphoblastic leukemia, 682-683
  automated blood cell analysis, 556
  chronic myelogenous leukemia, 687
  chronic myeloproliferative disorders, 686
  examination of peripheral blood smear, 557
  fecal, 2006
  immune system, 1109
  pure white blood cell aplasia, 675
  source of deoxyribonucleic acid, 51
  urinalysis, 744
  urinary, 744
Leukocyte adhesion deficiency, 1152, 1180
Leukocyte alkaline phosphatase
  chronic myelogenous leukemia, 687
  essential thrombocythemia, 688
Leukocyte collagenase, 373
Leukocyte common antigen, 731
Leukocyte count
  acute cholecystitis, 2228
  acute pericarditis, 274
  bacterial meningitis, 1407
  bacterial prostatitis, 1463
  choledocholithiasis, 2229
  chronic liver disease, 2136
  Colorado tick fever, 1512
  compromised host, 1388
  human immunodeficiency virus infection,
    1473
  mumps, 1497
  Mycoplasma pneumoniae pneumonia, 1539
  osteomyelitis, 1434
  primary peritonitis, 1399
  synovial fluid, 1162, 1163, 1164
  systematic inflammatory response syndrome,
    1445
Leukocyte differential count, 556
Leukocyte elastase, 373
Leukocyte esterase, 1458
Leukocyte-reduced red blood cell, 572
Leukocytoclastic vasculitis, 1315
Leukocytosis
  abdominal pain, 2032
  acute pancreatitis, 2236
  amebic liver abscess, 2210
  chronic myelogenous leukemia, 687
  gastrointestinal bleeding, 2011
  gram-negative bacteremia, 1449, 1450
  infective endocarditis, 228
  intestinal disease, 2005
  intraabdominal infection, 1399
  Legionnaire's disease, 1623
  lymphangitis, 1420
  Meckel's diverticulum, 2090
  meningitis, 1406
  myxoma, 330
  necrotizing fasciitis, 1422
  peritonitis, 2080
  polycythemia vera, 688
  release of cellular potassium, 831
  Rocky Mountain spotted fever, 1544
Leukocyturia, 742
Leukodystrophy, 1007, 1918
Leukoencephalopathy
  acute hemorrhagic, 1010
  bone marrow transplant recipient, 1104-1105
  progressive multifocal, 987, 1010
Leukoerythroblastosis, 591
Leukopenia
  Colorado tick fever, 1512
  gram-negative bacteremia, 1449, 1450

Leukopenia—cont'd
  hypersplenism, 601
  infective endocarditis, 228
  Lassa fever, 1510
  lymphocytic choriomeningitis virus, 1509
  measles, 1498, 1499
  systemic lupus erythematosus, 1215
  vitamin B_{12} deficiency, 648
Leukoplakia, 722, 2309
  hairy cell
    acquired immunodeficiency syndrome,
      1328, 1478
    oral, Plate VIII-42
  tongue, Plate IV-12
Leukotriene A_4, 1140
Leukotriene B_4, 1140, 1448
Leukotriene D_4, 1140
Leukotriene E_4, 1140
Leukotriene receptor antagonists, 1191
Leukotrienes
  asthma, 1187
  sepsis, 1448
  vasoactive effects on pulmonary circulation,
    363
Leuprolide, 719
Leustatin; *see* 2-Chlorodeoxyadenosine
Levatol; *see* Penbutolol
LeVeen shunt
  ascites, 2165
  hepatorenal syndrome, 2170
Level of consciousness
  abnormal respiratory rhythms, 1097-1098
  coma, 947
  epilepsy, 981
Levine's sign, 125
Levobunolol, 2302
Levodopa
  dystonia, 995
  glucose-6-phosphate dehydrogenase
    deficiency, 664
  interference with catecholamine assays, 1740
  Parkinson's disease, 991, 992
  pituitary stimulation tests, 1736
Levorphanol, 581
Lewis leads, 134
Leydig cell, 1838
  dysfunction in Klinefelter's syndrome, 1843
  male climacteric, 1844
Leydig tumor
  gynecomastia, 1764
  impotence, 1762
LH; *see* Luteinizing hormone
Lhermitte's phenomenon, 1008
Libido, 1760-1764
  chronic hepatic failure, 2170
  prolactin-secreting pituitary adenoma, 1786
Lichen myxedematosus, 705
Lichen planus-like eruption, 1315
Lichenification, 1302
Lichenoid eruption, 1315, 1327
Licorice
  metabolic alkalosis, 840
  mineralocorticoid excess, 321
  pseudohyperaldosteronism, 1819
Lid retraction, 1063
Liddle's syndrome, 828
Lidocaine, 137-138
  myocardial infarction, 217
  premature ventricular contractions, 149
  pulmonary parenchymal reactions, 476
  ventricular tachyarrhythmia, 223, 224
Life expectancy, 2282
Lifestyle
  celiac disease, 2063
  hypertension management, 323
  osteoporosis, 1947
Ligand, 1110
Ligand binding, 541, 543
Ligand-gated receptor, 1710
Ligandin, 2128, 2148-2149

Ligase chain reaction
  Chlamydia trachomatis, 1536
  Neisseria gonorrhoeae, 1584
Ligation of esophageal varices, 2013, 2167
Light chain
  immunoglobulin, 1110, 1122
  multiple myeloma, 862-863
  proteinuria, 760
  sarcomere, 39
Light chain deposition, 882
Light chain gene, 1123-1124
Light chain glomerulopathy, 863
Light microscopy
  analysis of crystals in synovial fluid, 1163
  cancer of unknown primary site, 730
  cholesterol monohydrate crystals, Plate X-15
  glomerulonephritis, 842
  idiopathic nephrotic syndrome, 850
  poststreptococcal glomerulonephritis, 843-844
  rapidly progressive glomerulonephritis, 848
Lightheadedness, 972
Lignin, 1951
Limb electrode, 82
Limb-girdle muscular dystrophy, 1026-1027,
  1028, 1086
Limit setting disorder, 944
Limulus lysate, 1408
Lincomycin, 1344
Linear growth during puberty, 1767
Linear immunoglobulin A bullous dermatosis,
  1296
Linear scleroderma, 1228
Link protein, 1289
Linkage, 1721
Linkage analysis, 1724
Linkage disequilibrium, 1117
Linked angina, 195, 196
Linoleic acid, 1883-1884, 1889
Linolenic acid, 1884
Lioresal; *see* Baclofen
Lipase
  abdominal pain, 2032
  acute pancreatitis, 2234, 2235
  gastric, 1986
  intestinal obstruction, 2078
  pancreatic disease, 2144
Lipectomy, 2104
Lipemia, 1901
Lipid A, 1362, 1446
Lipid A analogues, 1454
Lipid A endotoxin, 176
Lipid effusion, 509
Lipid-lowering agents
  myocardial infarction, 218
  nephrotic syndrome, 767
Lipid storage diseases, 1917-1919
  vasopressin deficiency, 1795
  weakness, 1754
Lipids
  atherosclerosis, 60
  bile, 2123, 2124-2126
  gallstone prevalence, 2223
  hepatic metabolism, 2120-2121
  hyperlipidemia, 1892-1896
    acute pancreatitis, 2233-2234, 2237
    amylo-1,6-glucosidase deficiency, 1882
    atherosclerotic coronary artery disease, 192
    combined, 1895-1896
    coronary artery disease, 200
    cutaneous manifestations, 1323-1324
    glucose-6-phosphate dehydrogenase
      deficiency, 1881
    hypercholesterolemia, 1892-1894
    hypertriglyceridemia, 1894-1895
    insulin resistance, 1862
    ischemic heart disease, 197
    lipodystrophy, 1901
    myocardial infarction, 210
    nephrotic syndrome, 766
    osmolal gap, 806
    risk of stroke, 1001

Lipids—cont'd
  intestinal absorption, 1986-1987
  metabolism, 1883-1884
    chronic renal failure, 786
    metabolic myopathy, 1028
    rare disorders, 1896-1898
  solubility of beta-blockers, 327
  storage diseases, 1917-1919
  transport by lipoproteins, 1885
Lipiduria, 765, 766
Lipiodol, 2214
Lipoatrophic diabetes mellitus, 1862, 1902-1903
Lipoatrophy, 1873
Lipodystrophy, 1899-1903
  centrifugal, 1903
  congenital total, 1900-1902
  insulin resistance, 1861
  intestinal, 2064-2065
  leprechaunism, 1899-1900
  lipoatrophic diabetes, 1902-1903
  membranous lipodystrophy, 1903
  mesenteric, 1903, 2251
  partial, 1902, 1903
  renal involvement, 877-878
Lipogenesis, 1851
Lipogranuloma of mesentery, 1903
Lipohyalinosis, 999
Lipohypertrophy, 1873
Lipoid dermatoarthritis, 1245
Lipoid nephrosis, 849-851
Lipoma
  cardiac, 330
  colon, 2086
  computed tomography, 387
  incidence, 329
  mesenteric, 2251
Lipomastia, 1764
Lipopolysaccharide
  anaerobic gram-negative bacteria, 1616
  cytokines and, 421
  gram-negative organism infection, 1447
  Shwartzman reaction, 1380
Lipopolysaccharide-neutralizing proteins, 1454
Lipoprotein lipase, 1885, 2121
  drug potentiation, 1892
  familial deficiency, 1898
Lipoprotein X, 1894, 2200
Lipoproteinemia, 60
Lipoproteins
  abetalipoproteinemia, 1897
    malabsorption, 2067
    vitamin A deficiency, 2105
    vitamin E deficiency, 2106
  atherosclerosis, 60, 1888-1889
  drugs inhibiting synthesis, 1891-1892
  effects of diet, 1889-1890
  effects of drugs, 1890-1892
  hepatic biosynthesis, 2121
  hyperlipoproteinemia, 1245, 1892
  hypoalphalipoproteinemia, 1896, 1898
  metabolism, 1885-1888
  nephrotic syndrome, 766
  plasma, 1886, 1889-1890
  rare disorders of lipid metabolism, 1896-1898
Liquid crystals, 2126
Liquid-formula diets, 2115-2117
Liquid hybridization column method, 2174
Liquid oxygen, 429, 435
Liquor carbonic detergents, 1302
Lisch nodule, 1920
Lisinopril
  heart failure, 170
  hepatic injury, 2192
  hypertension, 325
Listeria monocytogenes, 1576-1578
  after heart transplantation, 1090
  antibiotic selection, 1347
  compromised host, 1388
  fever, 1387
  meningitis, 1403, 1478

Lithium carbonate
  associated goiter, 1809
  cluster headache prophylaxis, 962
  dilated cardiomyopathy, 265
  disordered thinking, 1041
  mania, 1038
  medication-induced hypercalcemia, 1928
  role in Ebstein's anomaly, 280, 289
Lithocholate, 2124, 2125
Lithocholate 3-sulfate, 2128
Lithocholic acids, 2125
Lithostathine, 2238
Lithotripsy, 2226-2227
Livedo reticularis, 310
  antiphospholipid syndrome, 1292
  systemic lupus erythematosus, 1213
Liver
  abscess, 2209-2210
  adrenergic responses, 1828
  albumin synthesis, 2134
  alkaline phosphatase, 1745
  amebiasis, 1682
  antibiotic toxicity, 1348
  antirheumatic drug toxicity, 1261
  bile production and secretion, 2123-2129
    assembly and structure of bile, 2128
    bile cholesterol, 2127
    bile lecithin, 2126
    bile water production, 2123-2124
    bilirubin, 2127-2128
    composition of bile, 2123
    defective synthesis, 2129
    enterohepatic circulation, 2124-2126
    obstructed secretory apparatus, 2128-2129
  bilirubin uptake and clearance, 2148-2149
  cholesterol excretion, 1884
  cyst, 2210-2212
  drug interactions, 2311
  galactosemia, 1882
  gluconeogenesis, 1851, 1852
  heart failure, 165
  hepatic metabolism, 2118-2123
    amino acids and protein, 2118-2120
    carbohydrates, 2121-2122
    detoxification, 2122
    hormones, 2122-2123
    lipids, 2120-2121
  hepatobiliary disease
    acquired immunodeficiency syndrome, 2098-2099
    benign stricture of extrahepatic bile ducts, 2232-2233
    biliary dyskinesia, 2233
    carcinoma of ampulla of Vater, 2232
    carcinoma of bile ducts, 2231-2232
    conjugated hyperbilirubinemia, 2154-2156
    developmental anomalies, 2233
    distinguishing acute from chronic disease, 2134-2136
    drug-induced and toxic cholangitis, 2202-2203
    Dubin-Johnson syndrome, 2157
    estimations of severity and prognosis, 2141-2144
    familial cholestatic syndromes, 2158-2159
    fever of unknown origin, 1376
    gallbladder cancer, 2232
    hemobilia, 2233
    hereditary markers, 2138-2139
    hyperplastic cholecystosis, 2233
    imaging studies, 2140-2141
    immunologic markers, 2139-2140
    impaired lipid ingestion, 1987
    ischemic cholangitis, 2203
    liver biopsy, 2141
    malabsorption, 2062
    normal bilirubin metabolism, 2147-2150
    osteomalacia, 1951-1952
    patterns of liver injury, 2136-2137
    postoperative cholestasis, 2159
    primary biliary cirrhosis, 2199-2201

Liver—cont'd
  hepatobiliary disease—cont'd
    primary sclerosing cholangitis, 2201-2202, 2203
    Rotor's syndrome and hepatic storage disease, 2157-2158
    unconjugated hyperbilirubinemia, 2150-2154
    viral cholangitis, 2202
    viral markers, 2138
  hereditary fructose intolerance, 1880
  Hodgkin's disease, 693
  involvement in polycystic kidney disease, 872
  ketogenesis, 1852-1853
  operative risks, 2262-2263
  peliosis hepatis, 2212
  protoporphyria, 1926
  sarcoidosis, 458
  susceptibility to chemical injury, 2185
  synthesis of complement components, 1132
  toxicity of chemotherapeutic agents, 585
  vasopressin clearance, 1791
Liver biopsy, 2136, 2141
  acute fatty liver of pregnancy, 2278
  Budd-Chiari syndrome, 2208
  cholestasis, 2156
  chronic hepatitis, 2180
  fever of unknown origin, 1380
  hepatic epithelioid hemangioendothelioma, 2215
  hepatocellular carcinoma, 2214
  hereditary hemochromatosis, 2204
  peliosis hepatis, 2212
  portal hypertension, 2166
  primary biliary cirrhosis, 2199
  protoporphyria, 1926
  unconjugated hyperbilirubinemia, 2153
  veno-occlusive disease, 2208
  Wilson's disease, 2205
Liver cancer, 2212-2217
  carcinoid tumor metastases, 2082
  cavernous hemangioma, 2215-2216
  fibrolamellar hepatocellular carcinoma, 2214
  focal nodular hyperplasia, 2216
  hepatic adenoma, 2216-2217
  hepatic epithelioid hemangioendothelioma, 2215
  hepatocellular carcinoma, 2212-2214
  intrahepatic cholangiocarcinoma, 2214-2215
  metastases from colon, 2085-2086
Liver disease
  aberrations in tyrosine metabolism, 1906
  abscess, 2209-2210
  acute renal failure with, 774-775
  acute viral hepatitis
    hepatitis A virus, 2173
    hepatitis B virus, 2173-2175
    hepatitis C virus, 2175-2176
    hepatitis delta virus, 2176
    hepatitis E virus, 2176-2177
    hepatitis G virus, 2177
    non-A-non-B, 2177
    prevention, 2178-2179
    treatment, 2177-2178
  alcoholic, 2194-2199
  alpha$_1$ antitrypsin deficiency, 2206-2207
  chronic hepatitis, 2179-2184
    autoimmune, 2183-2184
    clinical assessment, 2180-2181
    etiologic classification, 2180
    hepatitis B virus, 2181-2182
    hepatitis C virus, 2182-2183
    hepatitis D virus, 2183
    treatment, 2184
  cyst, 2210-2212
  cystic fibrosis, 2246
  dementia, 987
  drug- and toxin-induced, 2184-2193
    acetaminophen poisoning, 2188-2190
    acute hepatic injury, 2187-2188
    carbon tetrachloride poisoning, 2188

Liver disease—cont'd
 drug- and toxin-induced—cont'd
  chronic liver damage, 2188
  classification of hepatoxic agents,
    2185-2187
  diagnosis, 2193
  herbal remedies and plant toxins, 2192-2193
  medications, 2190-2192
  mushroom and phosphorus poisoning, 2188
  susceptibility of liver to chemical injury,
    2185
  treatment, 2193
 electroencephalography, 907, 909
 evaluation, 2134-2144
  distinguishing acute from chronic disease,
    2134-2136
  estimations of severity and prognosis,
    2141-2144
  hereditary markers, 2138-2139
  imaging studies, 2140-2141
  immunologic markers, 2139-2140
  liver biopsy, 2141
  patterns of liver injury, 2136-2137
  viral markers, 2138
 hemolysis, 667
 hemophilia, 621
 hemostatic abnormalities, 607, 626-627
 hepatic venoocclusive disease, 2207-2209
 hepatitis
  acquired immunodeficiency syndrome, 2099
  alcoholic, 2196, 2197, 2295
  coagulation disorder, 607
  dialysis-related, 790
  enteroviral, 1490
  fever of unknown origin, 1376
  inflammatory bowel disease, 2076
  isoniazid-induced, 1637
  liver transplantation, 2219
  operative risk, 2263
  serum alkaline phosphatase level, 2137
  systemic lupus erythematosus, 1215
  transfusion-associated, 575, 621
  travel-related, 1465
  Wilson's disease, 2205
 hepatitis A, 2138, 2173
  acute, 2173
  aplastic anemia, 672
  posttransfusion, 575
  during pregnancy, 2277
  traveler, 1465
  vaccine, 1493
 hepatitis B, 2138, 2173-2175
  acute, 2173-2175
  chronic, 2181-2182
  immune complexes, 1137-1138
  polyarteritis nodosa, 1219
  during pregnancy, 2277
  septic arthritis, 1255
  transfusion-associated, 575
  vaccine, 621-622, 2255
 hepatitis C, 2138, 2175-2176
  acute, 2175-2176
  alcoholic, 2195
  chronic, 2182-2183
  membranoproliferative glomerulonephritis,
    854
  during pregnancy, 2277
 hepatitis D, 2138
  acute, 2176
  chronic, 2183
 hepatitis E, 2138, 2176-2177
  during pregnancy, 2277
  travel-related, 1465
 hepatitis G, 2177
 hereditary hemochromatosis, 2203-2205
 hypogonadism, 1843
 impact on nutritional status, 2100
 liver transplantation, 2217-2220
 neurohepatology, 1102-1103
 operative risk, 2262-2263
 osteomalacia, 1951-1952

Liver disease—cont'd
 porphyrias, 1925
 portal hypertension, 2165
 during pregnancy, 2277-2278
 vitamin D deficiency, 1951-1952
 Wilson's disease, 2205-2206
Liver enzymes, 2136-2137
 acetaminophen poisoning, 2190
 acute pancreatitis, 2236
 choledocholithiasis, 2229
 chronic hepatitis, 2180
 hepatic injury, 2136
 hepatitic injury, 2136
 hepatitis A virus, 2173
 hepatitis B infection, 2175
 hepatocellular *versus* cholestatic jaundice,
   2156
 myocardial infarction, 211
 preeclamptic patient, 2274
Liver failure, 2159-2172
 acute fatty liver of pregnancy, 2278
 Anderson's disease, 1882
 ascites, 2163-2165
 bleeding diathesis, 612
 Budd-Chiari syndrome, 2208
 endocrine disturbances, 2170-2172
 hepatic encephalopathy, 2159-2163
 hepatopulmonary syndrome, 2170
 hepatorenal syndrome, 2168-2170
 hyperventilation, 355
 leptospirosis, 1644
 liver transplantation, 2219
 peliosis hepatis, 2212
 portal hypertension, 2165-2168
 primary sclerosing cholangitis, 2201
 sarcoidosis, 458
Liver fluke, 1703-1704
Liver function tests
 Budd-Chiari syndrome, 2208
 fever of unknown origin, 1379
 gram-negative bacteremia, 1450
 hepatic encephalopathy, 2161
 hepatocellular carcinoma, 2213
 human immunodeficiency virus infection,
   1473
 lipodystrophy, 1901
 quantitative, 2143-2144
Liver scan, 2141
 amebiasis, 1683
 cavernous hemangioma, 2215-2216
 cholestasis, 2156
 focal nodular hyperplasia, 2216
Liver transplantation, 2217-2220
 alpha$_1$-antitrypsin deficiency, 2206
 autoimmune hepatitis, 2184
 chronic hepatitis B, 2182
 chronic hepatitis C, 2183
 glucose-6-phosphate dehydrogenase
   deficiency, 1881
 hepatic encephalopathy, 2163
 hepatic epithelioid hemangioendothelioma,
   2215
 hepatocellular carcinoma, 2214
 hepatopulmonary syndrome, 2170
 hereditary hemochromatosis, 2205
 neurologic effects, 1102
 primary biliary cirrhosis, 2201
 vancomycin resistant enterococcal infection,
   1562
 veno-occlusive disease following, 2208
 Wilson's disease, 2206
Living-related donor renal transplantation,
   791-792
Living will, 12-13
Loa loa, 1700, 1701
Lobar atelectasis, 482
Lobectomy
 lung cancer, 490
 non-small cell lung cancer, 726
 thyroid carcinoma, 1815
Lobomycosis, 1660

Local area network for hematopoiesis, 531
Local autonomic disorders, 936, 937
Local tolerance, 1145
Localized amyloidosis, 1285
Localized lipodystrophy, 1903
Localized osteomyelitis, 1436
Locked-in patient, 977
Lockjaw, 1573
Locus, 1721
Locus control region, 651
Loffler's syndrome, 455
Logarithm of odds of disequilibrium, 1724
Logorrhea, 975
Loin pain-hematuria syndrome, 845-846
Lomefloxacin, 1350, 1359
Lomustine, 476
Lone atrial fibrillation, 146
Long-acting thyroid stimulator, 1157
Long-acting thyroid stimulator protector, 1157
Long-axis views, 95, 96
Long bones
 fibrous dysplasia, 1960
 hematogenous osteomyelitis, 1433
 mechanism of bone formation, 1716
 osteopetrosis, 1958
 Paget's disease, 1955
Long Q-T syndrome, 62
Long-term bone marrow culture-initiating cell,
   531
Long-term oxygen therapy, 444-445
Long thoracic nerve mononeuropathy, 1017
Loniten; *see* Minoxidil
Loop diuretics, 822
 acute tubular necrosis, 773
 ascites, 2165
 cause of renal magnesium wasting, 1940
 cause of renal potassium wasting and
   alkalosis, 828
 congestive heart failure-associated
   hyponatremia, 818
 generation of alkalosis, 839
 heart failure, 169, 170
 hypercalcemia, 1929
 hyperkalemia, 833
 hypertension, 325
 interference with oral anticoagulants, 636
 isovolemic hypotonic hyponatremia, 813
 nephrotic syndrome, 767
 pulmonary edema, 169
Loop of Henle
 calcium reabsorption, 1718
 magnesium reabsorption, 1939
 potassium transport, 741
 renal concentrating and diluting mechanisms,
   739, 740
Looser's zone, 1950
Loperamide
 diarrhea, 1431-1432
 irritable bowel syndrome, 2056
Lopressor; *see* Metoprolol
Loracarbef, 1354
 dosage, 1349
 sinusitis, 1395
Loratadine, 1182
Lorazepam
 alcohol withdrawal, 2295
 anxiety disorders, 1035
 delirium tremens, 2295, 2296
 disordered thinking, 1041
 muscle spasm in tetanus, 1573
 for nausea and vomiting, 2027
 status epilepticus, 983
Losartan
 heart failure, 174
 human cytochrome P450 isoforms, 2312
 hypertension, 325, 327
Loss of energy, 1753
Loss of heterozygosity, 546
Lotensin; *see* Benazepril
Louis-Bar syndrome, 1319

Louse
  epidemic typhus, 1544
  relapsing fever, 1645-1658
Lovastatin, 1891
  gallstone risk factor, 2223
  human cytochrome P450 isoforms, 2312
  restenosis, 124
Low back pain, 963-968
  endocarditis, 227
Low-calorie diet, 2104
Low-density lipoprotein receptors
  fibroblast, 1886
  relationship with enterohepatic circulation,
    1891
Low-density lipoproteins, 1886-1887
  abetalipoproteinemia, 1897
  atherosclerosis, 60, 192, 1889
  drugs enhancing clearance, 1890-1891
  effects of carbohydrates, 1890
  hypoalphalipoproteinemia, 1896, 1898
  ischemic heart disease, 192
  nephrotic syndrome, 766
  uremic patient, 786
Low-dose unfractionated heparin, 2261-2262
Low hematocrit, 586-588
Low-molecular-weight heparin, 634
  deep venous thrombosis, 504, 2261-2262
  during pregnancy, 2276
  unstable angina, 639
Low-pressure volume receptors, 817
Low-turnover osteomalacia, 1961, 1962, 1963
Lower esophageal ring, Plate X-2
Lower esophageal sphincter
  achalasia, 2021-2022, 2022
  assessment, 2001
  defective relaxation, 1978
  gastroesophageal reflux disease, 2015
  Schatzki's rings, 2020
Lower extremity
  acute aortic obstruction, 304
  blood pressure measurement, 64
  ecthyma, 1420
  peripheral arterial aneurysm, 309
  peripheral vascular disease, 305-307
  varicose veins, 311
Lower-limb somatosensory evoked potential,
    913-914
Lower motor neuron deficit, 1015
Lower respiratory tract infection
  acute interstitial pneumonia, 448, 452
  after stroke, 1007
  bronchiolitis obliterans-organizing pneumonia,
    448, 452-453
  bronchoalveolar lavage, 384
  cancer patient, 582
  chest pain, 129
  Chlamydia pneumoniae, 1535
  cystic fibrosis, 480
  desquamative interstitial pneumonia, 449
  eosinophilic pneumonia, 455
  fever, 1387
  gram-negative bacteremia, 1446
  Haemophilus influenzae, 1586, 1588
  influenza with, 1486, 1491
  lymphoid interstitial pneumonia, 449
  Mycoplasma pneumoniae, 1538-1539
  Neisseria meningitidis, 1579
  nosocomial, 423, 1480
  oculopharyngeal dystrophy, 1028
  Pneumocystis carinii pneumonia, 1692-1696
    acquired immunodeficiency syndrome,
      1473, 1474, 1477
    lung transplantation, 518, 519
    sputum examination, 380
  posttransplant
    lung, 517-518
    stem cell, 579
  pulmonary edema *versus,* 425
  risk in multiple myeloma, 700, 703
  sputum examination, 380
  Staphylococcus aureus, 1549

Lower respiratory tract infection—cont'd
  usual interstitial pneumonia, 449
  varicella, 1527
Lower urinary tract
  neurology, 1065-1067
  renal imaging studies, 756
Lowe's syndrome, 882, 1911
Lozol; *see* Indapamide
Lucio phenomenon, 1650
Luft's syndrome, 1749
Lukes-Butler classification of Hodgkin's disease,
    693
Lumbar disk herniation, 963-964
Lumbar puncture, 904-905
  central nervous system tuberculosis, 1636
  dementia, 988
  determination of weakness, 1755
  febrile seizure, 982
  meningococcemia, 1580
  non-Hodgkin's lymphoma, 698
Lumbar spine
  ankylosing spondylitis, 1238-1239
  computed tomography, 920
  dual-beam photon absorptiometry, 1748
  magnetic resonance imaging, 924
  Paget's disease, 1955
  vertebral osteomyelitis, 1433
  weight bearing radiograph, 1164
Lumbar sympathectomy, 310
Lumbosacral nerve root disorders, 966
Lumbosacral radiculopathy, 1016
Luminal; *see* Phenobarbital
Lumpectomy, 709
Lung
  abscess, 1617
  adverse drug reactions, 476-479
  aging and, 2284
  antirheumatic drug toxicity, 1261
  breathing control abnormalities, 352-357
  complications of influenza, 1491
  heart failure, 165
  hepatopulmonary syndrome, 2170
  host defense mechanisms, 364-369
  imaging, 386-390
  intensive care monitoring, 390-396
    end-tidal carbon dioxide, 396
    peripheral artery catheterization, 390
    pulmonary artery catheterization, 390-395
    pulse oximetry, 396
    transcutaneous oxygen and carbon dioxide,
      396
  invasive diagnostic techniques, 380-386
    bronchoalveolar lavage, 384
    bronchoscopy and biopsy, 383-384
    mediastinoscopy and mediastinotomy, 385
    open lung biopsy, 385-386
    pleural biopsy, 382-383
    protected brush catheter, 384-385
    sputum examination, 380-381
    Swan-Ganz catheterization, 383
    thoracentesis, 381-382
    thoracoscopy, 385
    transthoracic needle aspiration, 385
    transtracheal aspiration, 385
  mechanisms of injury and repair, 370-375
  operative risks, 2260-2262
  pulmonary blood flow, 360-364
  pulmonary function tests, 375-380
    bronchoprovocation inhalation tests, 379
    exercise tests, 379-380
    inhaled bronchodilator studies, 377-378
    lung volume determination, 378
    single-breath diffusing capacity, 378, 379
    sleep studies, 380
    spirometry, 376-377
    ventilatory control studies, 378-379
  pulmonary rehabilitation, 432-437
  respiratory pathophysiology, 346-352
    nonrespiratory functions of lung, 346-347
    oxygen transport disorders, 350-352
    respiratory function, 347-350

Lung—cont'd
  respiratory therapy, 428-432
  rheumatoid arthritis, 1204
  systemic lupus erythematosus, 1215
  systemic sclerosis, 1230, 1232
  technetium-99m sestamibi uptake, 103
  toxicity of chemotherapeutic agents, 584
  transfusion-associated injury, 1480
  transfusion reaction, 574
  Waldenström macroglobulinemia, 704
  zones, 393
Lung biopsy
  bleomycin-induced pulmonary diseases, 477
  bronchiolitis obliterans syndrome, 522
  hypersensitivity pneumonitis, 461
  interstitial lung disease, 451
  Langerhans' cell granulomatosis, 464
  open, 385-386
Lung cancer, 486-492, 724-729
  asbestos-related, 474
  bronchial adenoma, 491-492
  clinical presentation, 487-488
  diagnosis and staging, 489-490
  ectopic production of adrenocorticotropic
    hormone, 1820
  genetic predisposition, 486
  hamartoma, 492
  hemoptysis, 411
  hypertrophic osteoarthropathy, 1247
  incidence and death rates, 550
  magnetic resonance imaging, 389
  malignant effusion, 508
  metastasis
    nervous system, 489
    pulmonary, 492
  molecular biology, 487
  neoplastic pericarditis, 272
  oat cell carcinoma of lung, 1024
  occupational exposure, 476
  papilloma, 492
  paraneoplastic syndromes, 488-489
  pathology, 487
  prevention, 491
  screening, 490
  solitary pulmonary nodule, 493-497
  staging, 725-726
  treatment, 490-491
Lung compliance, 347, 398
Lung disease
  acute respiratory failure, 412-420
    adult respiratory distress syndrome with, 418
    artificial airway, 416-417
    chronic obstructive pulmonary disease with,
      417-418, 446
    classification, 413, 414
    diagnosis, 413-414
    mechanical ventilation, 397, 416, 418-420
    oxygenation measures, 415-416
    pathophysiology, 412-413
    principles of management, 414, 415
    respiratory acidosis, 416
    without lung disease, 418
  adverse drug reactions, 476-479
  aspergillosis, 1658-1659
  asthma, 1185-1193
    Churg-Strauss syndrome, 465
    clinical manifestations, 1187-1188
    cough, 406
    diagnosis and differential diagnosis, 1189
    epidemiology and pathology, 1185
    laboratory findings, 1188-1189
    management, 1189-1192
    occupational, 471-472, 473
    pathophysiology, 1185-1187
    patterns of pulmonary function
      abnormalities, 379
    physical findings, 403
    prognosis, 1192-1193
    pulmonary rehabilitation, 432-437
    sputum expectoration, 408
    wheezing, 404

Lung disease—cont'd
  bronchiectasis, 483-485
  chest pain, 128-129, 408-410
  chronic obstructive pulmonary disease,
      437-447
    with acute respiratory failure, 413-414,
        417-418
    airflow obstruction, 438
    alpha$_1$-protease inhibitor deficiency,
        439-440
    clinical features, 442
    complications, 445-447
    definition, 437-438
    diagnosis, 443
    dyspnea, 404
    epidemiology, 438-439
    hypercapnia, 356
    laboratory findings, 442-443
    lung transplantation, 445
    occupational, 473
    pathogenesis, 441-442
    pathology, 439
    physical examination, 442
    prognosis and course, 447
    pulmonary rehabilitation, 432-437
    sleep studies with monitoring of oxygen
        saturation, 380
    treatment, 443-445
  cough, 404-408, 409
  cryptococcosis, 1667, 1668
  cystic fibrosis, 479-483
  diagnostic imaging, 386-390
  dysfunction of host defenses, 369
  dyspnea, 404, 405
  expectoration, 408
  heart failure *versus*, 168
  hemoptysis, 410-411
  high-resolution computed tomography, 387
  hypersensitivity pneumonitis, 460-463
  interstitial, 448-456
    clinical features, 450-451
    clinicopathologic classification, 449
    diagnosis and management, 451-452
    dyspnea, 404
    etiologic factors, 452
    exercise tests, 379
    imaging techniques, 451
    lung pathology, 448-449
    pathogenesis, 449-450
    pathophysiology, 450
    pulmonary hypertension, 498
    unknown origin, 452-456
  invasive diagnostic techniques, 380-386
    bronchoalveolar lavage, 384
    bronchoscopy and biopsy, 383-384
    mediastinoscopy and mediastinotomy, 385
    open lung biopsy, 385-386
    pleural biopsy, 382-383
    protected brush catheter, 384-385
    sputum examination, 380-381
    Swan-Ganz catheterization, 383
    thoracentesis, 381-382
    thoracoscopy, 385
    transthoracic needle aspiration, 385
    transtracheal aspiration, 385
  Langerhans' cell granulomatosis, 463-465
  mediastinal disease, 510-514
  medical history, 401-402
  multiple organ dysfunction syndrome,
      421-423
  neoplasms, 486-492; *see also* Lung cancer
  nocardiosis, 1666
  nontuberculous mycobacterial infection, 1639
  occupational, 471-476
  pertussis, 1611-1613
  physical examination, 402-404
  pleural, 505-510
  Pneumocystis carinii pneumonia, 1692-1696
  pneumonic plague, 1610
  primary granulomatous pulmonary vasculitis,
      465-471

Lung disease—cont'd
  pulmonary edema, 423-428
    acute toxic, 473
    adult respiratory distress syndrome, 421
    drug-induced, 477
    hemoptysis, 410
    pneumothorax, 510
    pulmonary artery wedge pressure, 395
  pulmonary hypertension
    cardiac transplantation, 338
    chronic obstructive pulmonary disease,
        446-447
    drug-induced, 477
    exertional angina, 127
    interstitial lung disease, 452
    pathophysiology, 363-364
    primary and secondary causes, 497-499
    Takayasu's arteritis, 470
  pulmonary rehabilitation, 431, 432-437
  pulmonary thromboembolism, 499-504
  pulmonary transplantation, 514-524
    allograft rejection, 520-524
    chronic obstructive pulmonary disease, 445
    complications, 516-520
    future trends, 524
    immunosuppression, 516
    indications, 514-515
    outcome, 516
    selection of donor and recipient, 515-516
  respiratory therapy, 428-432
  sarcoidosis, 456-459
  sleep-related, 524-528
  solitary pulmonary nodule, 493-497
  tuberculosis, 1628-1630
  tularemia, 1608
  wheezing, 404, 405
Lung expansion, 429-430
Lung fluke, 507, 1704
Lung scan, 387-388
  Behçet disease, 469
  primary pulmonary hypertension, 294
  pulmonary embolism, 297
  pulmonary thromboembolism, 501-502
Lung transplantation, 514-524
  allograft rejection, 520-524
  chronic obstructive pulmonary disease, 445
  complications, 516-520
  cystic fibrosis, 483
  future trends, 524
  immunosuppression, 516
  indications, 514-515
  interstitial lung disease, 452
  outcome, 516
  selection of donor and recipient, 515-516
Lung volume, 378
  aging and, 2284
  chronic obstructive pulmonary disease, 442
  diaphragm and, 358
  drug-induced pneumonitis, 477
  effects of lung inflation, 362
Lupron, 710
Lupus anticoagulant, 609
Lupus erythematosus, Plate VII-2
  cutaneous lesions, 1290-1292
  glucocorticoid protocol, 1263
Lupus hair, 1291
Lupus inhibitor, 629
Lupus nephritis
  hyperkalemia, 832
  nephrotic syndrome, 767
  tubulointerstitial involvement, 891
Lupus pernio, 458, 1324, Plate VII-21
Lupus pneumonitis, 1215
Lupus profundus, 1291
Luteinizing hormone, 1775
  alcoholic cirrhosis, 2172
  amenorrhea, 1757-1758
  cirrhosis, 2171
  constitutional delay of puberty, 1768
  estrogen feedback inhibition tests, 1736
  gonadotropin-secreting pituitary tumor, 1787

Luteinizing hormone—cont'd
  gynecomastia, 1764, 1765
  hypogonadotropic eunuchoidism, 1841-1842
  impotence, 1763
  Klinefelter's syndrome, 1843
  laboratory and diagnostic testing, 1835, 1836
  neonatal, 1832
  normal levels, 1836
  ovarian feedback mechanisms, 1834-1835
  pituitary secretion, 1834
  polycystic ovarian disease, 1837
  puberty, 1766, 1767
  reproductive years, 1832-1833
  testosterone stimulation, 1838
Lutembacher's syndrome, 245, 280
lycosphingolipid metabolism, 878
Lye
  carcinogenesis, 548
  corrosive gastritis, 2043
  esophageal injury, 2019
Lye stricture, 1999-2000
Lyme disease, 1254, 1646-1648
  fever and rash, 1383
  hoarseness, 2309
  influence of season and geographic setting,
      1381
  meningitis, 1409
  transfusion-transmitted, 575
Lymph node
  adenopathy, 513
    adenovirus infection, 1503
    cervical, 1385
    infectious mononucleosis, 1529
    inguinal, 1444
    non-Hodgkin's lymphoma, 697
    scarlet fever, 1421
    syphilis, 1640
  biopsy, 600
    acquired immunodeficiency syndrome, 1476
    angioimmunoblastic lymphadenopathy, 1248
    Hodgkin's disease, 691, 692
    Mycobacterium avium complex, Plate
        VIII-36
  breast cancer, 707
  hilar adenopathy
    brucellosis, 1606
    computed tomography, 386
    tuberculosis, 1628
  Hodgkin's disease, 691-695
    acquired ichthyosis, 1316
    chemotactic defects, 1340
    curability with chemotherapy, 552
    fever of unknown origin, 1377
    infertility, 585
    internal lymphadenopathy, 598
    molecular diagnostics, 563-564
    secondary malignancies, 585-586
    stomach involvement, 2049
    thyroid gland failure, 1809
  hyperplasia
    angiofollicular, 599
    hematoxylin and eosin preparation, Plate
        VIII-35
    mesenteric, 2252
  lymphangitis, 1420
  morphology, 1152
  non-Hodgkin's lymphoma, 695-700
    acquired immunodeficiency syndrome, 1329
    bone marrow biopsy section, 558
    Epstein-Barr virus, 1529
    heart involvement, 331
    molecular diagnostics, 563
    stomach involvement, 2049
  nontuberculous mycobacterial infection, 1639
  rheumatoid arthritis, 1205
  structure and function, 596-597
  tularemia, 1607-1608
Lymphadenitis
  elephantiasis nostra, 1420
  Toxoplasma gondii, 1677

Lymphadenopathy, 596-600
  angioimmunoblastic, 1247-1248
  brucellosis, 1606
  bubonic plague, 1610
  chronic lymphocytic leukemia, 684
  diphtheria, 1566
  heavy-chain disease, 704
  human immunodeficiency virus infection,
      1471-1472, 1476
  impetigo, 1419
  leishmaniasis, 1687
  Lyme disease, 1647
  lymphogranuloma venereum, 1535
  melanoma, 1299
  rheumatoid arthritis, 1205
  rubella, 1501
  sinus histiocytosis, 680
  syphilis, 1640
  systemic lupus erythematosus, 1215
  toxoplasmosis, 1677
  tularemia, 1607-1608
Lymphangiography
  Hodgkin's disease, 694
  testicular cancer, 720-721
Lymphangioleiomyomatosis, 455
Lymphangitis, 1420, 1557
Lymphatic filariasis, 1699, 1700
Lymphatic obstruction
  erysipelas, 1420
  intestinal lymphangiectasia, 2067
Lymphatic tuberculosis, 1633
Lymphatics
  barrier to infection, 1335
  hormone transport, 1713
  microvascular fluid exchange, 346
  pancreas, 2130
  pyelonephritis, 1456
  removal of protein from pleural space, 505
Lymphoblast, 594, 595
Lymphocyte, Plate IV-5
  airway, 365
  alcoholic liver disease, 2195
  apoptosis, 1144
  basic immunology, 1174-1175
  chronic lymphocytic leukemia, 684-685
  defects, 1342-1343
  differentiation and activation, 1112-1114
  hypersensitivity pneumonitis, 461
  immune system, 1109
  lamina propria, 1990, 1991
  malignant, 696
  migration, 1989-1990, 1991
  myasthenia gravis, 1022
  respiratory, 367-368
  rheumatoid arthritis, 1201
  sarcoidosis, 457
  source of DNA, 51
Lymphocyte cytotoxicity assays, 1152
Lymphocytic choriomeningitis virus, 1509
Lymphocytic granulomatous vasculitis, 469-470
Lymphocytic lymphoma, 595
Lymphocytopenia, 593-594
  intestinal lymphangiectasia, 2067
  systemic lupus erythematosus, 1215
Lymphocytosis, 592-593
  chronic lymphocytic leukemia, 685
  pertussis, 1612
Lymphoepithelioma, 723, 724
Lymphogranuloma venereum, 1444
  anal fissure and fistula, 2093
  Chlamydia trachomatis, 1535
  inguinal adenopathy, 1444
Lymphoid cell
  abnormal, 594-595
  cytokine regulation of growth and
      differentiation, 1130-1131
  lamina propria, 1990
  morphologic considerations, 592
  pathologic gene rearrangements, 1126
  Southern blot, 561
Lymphoid clonality, 558

Lymphoid follicle, 596-597
Lymphoid infiltrative disorders, 455
Lymphoid interstitial pneumonia, 449
Lymphoid leukemia, 682-685
Lymphoid organs, 1108
Lymphoid tissue, gut-associated, 1989-1990,
    1991
Lymphokine-activated killer cell, 519-520, 1127
Lymphokines, 1128
  human immunodeficiency virus infection,
      1470
  tuberculosis, 1627
Lymphoma
  abnormal lymphocytes in peripheral blood,
      595
  acquired immunodeficiency syndrome, 1329
    central nervous system, 1477
    non-Hodgkin's lymphoma, 1329
  after cardiac transplantation, 342
  anaplastic large cell, 697
  B-cell
    chromosomal abnormalities, 544
    gastric, 2038
    molecular diagnostics, 563
  bone marrow biopsy section, 558
  Burkitt's, 695
    chromosomal translocation, 544
    hypophosphatemia, 1936
    ocular involvement, 2306
  cardiac, 329
  cholangitis, 2202
  chylothorax, 509
  colon, 2083
  cytogenetics, 731
  fever of unknown origin, 1377
  Hodgkin's disease, 691-695
    acquired ichthyosis, 1316
    chemotactic defects, 1340
    curability with chemotherapy, 552
    fever of unknown origin, 1377
    infertility, 585
    internal lymphadenopathy, 598
    molecular diagnostics, 563-564
    secondary malignancies, 585-586
    stomach involvement, 2049
    thyroid gland failure, 1809
  immunosuppression-related, 795
  incidence and death rates, 550
  large cell, 697, 698
  lymphocytic, 595
  lymphosarcoma cell leukemia, 594
  mantle cell, 697
  marginal zone, 697
  mediastinal mass, 513
  Mediterranean, 2080
  mesenteric, 2251
  metastatic carcinoma *versus,* 731
  molecular diagnostics, 563-564
  monocytoid B, 697
  mucosa-associated lymphoid tissue, 697, 2038
  neoplastic pericarditis, 272
  non-Hodgkin's, 695-700
    acquired immunodeficiency syndrome, 1329
    bone marrow biopsy section, 558
    Epstein-Barr virus, 1529
    heart involvement, 331
    molecular diagnostics, 563
    stomach involvement, 2049
  poorly differentiated carcinoma, 732
  primary central nervous system, 920, 1069
  pseudolymphoma, 599, 2049
  small bowel, 2080
  stomach, 2049
  T cell, 682, 695
    chromosomal abnormalities, 544
    cutaneous, 1331-1332
    enteropathy-associated, 2064
    hypercalcemia of malignancy, 1973
    molecular diagnostics, 563
  thyroid, 1816
Lymphomatoid granulomatosis, 470

Lymphonodular pharyngitis, 1489
Lymphopenia
  human immunodeficiency virus infection,
      1473
  intestinal disease, 2005
  kwashiorkor, 2101
  myocardial infarction, 212
Lymphoproliferative disorders
  after prolonged immunosuppression, 1090
  angioimmunoblastic lymphadenopathy,
      1247-1248
  generalized lymphadenopathy, 599
Lymphosarcoma cell, 594, 595
Lymphosarcoma cell leukemia, 594, 684, Plate
      IV-5
Lymphotoxin, 1129, 1130
Lynch syndrome, 2083
Lysine
  cystinuria, 1910
  hyperlysinemia, 1907
  metabolic disorders, 1907
  related diseases, 1904
Lysis centrifugation method, 1367
Lysosomal acid lipase, 1898
Lysosomal enzymes, 1142, 1911, 2234
Lysosomal storage diseases, 1911-1920
  Chédiak-Higashi syndrome, 1919
  cystinosis, 1919
  drug-induced lysosomopathies, 1919
  general considerations, 1911-1912
  lipid storage diseases, 1917-1919
  lysosomal physiology, 1911
  mucolipidoses, 1915-1917
  mucopolysaccharidoses, 1912-1915
  treatment, 1919-1920
Lysosome, 536, 1911
  acute pancreatitis, 2234
  aminoglycoside toxicity, 868
  thyroid hormone transport, 1797
Lysozyme, 760
  bacterial meningitis, 1408
  hereditary amyloidosis, 1285
  neutrophil, 1339
Lysozymuria, 760
Lyspro analog, 1859

M

M-BACOD regimen, 699
M cell, 1989, 1990
M component
  amyloidosis, 1283
  plasma cell dyscrasias, 864
M-line, 39
M-mode echocardiography, 95
  aortic regurgitation, 242
  aortic stenosis, 238
  constrictive pericarditis, 277
  hypertrophic cardiomyopathy, 267
  mitral valve prolapse, 254
  pericardial effusion, 274-275
  tricuspid regurgitation, 256
M protein, 564, 1554-1555
  multiple myeloma, 700
Machine operator's lung, 460
Machupo virus, 1509
MACOP-B regimen, 699
Macroadenoma
  hyperprolactinemia, 1785-1786
  local neurologic effects, 1781-1782
  during pregnancy, 2273, 2274
Macroaggregated albumin, 387
Macroamylasemia, 2144
Macroangiopathic hemolytic anemia, 666-667
Macrocephaly, neurofibromatosis, 1921
Macrocytic anemia
  intestinal disease, 2005
  during pregnancy, 2279
Macrocytosis, Plate IV-4
Macroenzyme, 2137

Macroglobulinemia
  cryoglobulinemia, 1248
  immunofixation, 566
Macrolides, 1357-1358
  acne vulgaris, 1305
  antimicrobial mechanisms, 1344
  bacillary angiomatosis, 1474
  Campylobacter enteritis, 1592
  campylobacteriosis, 1432
  chlamydial infection, 1537
  diphtheria, 1567
  dosage, 1349, 1350
  effects on kidney, 868
  enterococci resistance, 1561
  erythrasma, 1422
  Haemophilus ducreyi, 1589
  Helicobacter pylori, 1593
  hepatic injury, 2191
  human cytochrome P450 isoforms, 2312
  infective endocarditis prophylaxis, 234
  interaction with cyclosporin, 793
  interference with oral anticoagulants, 636
  intestinal pseudoobstruction, 2079
  Legionella pneumophila, 1624
  Lyme disease, 1647
  Mycobacterium avium-intracellulare complex,
    1474
  Mycoplasma hominis infection, 1541
  Mycoplasma pneumoniae pneumonia, 1540
  peptic ulcer disease, 2040
  pertussis, 1613
  reaction with antiarrhythmics, 136-137
  relapsing fever, 1646
  streptococcal resistance, 1559
  urethritis, 1441
  use during pregnancy, 2281
Macrominerals, 2108
Macrophage, 1127-1128, 1342
  abnormalities, 680
  airway, 365
  alveolar, 367-369, 1127
    hypersensitivity pneumonitis, 462
    interstitial lung disease, 450
    lung injury, 370, 372
    lung repair, 374
    sarcoidosis, 457
    silicosis, 475
    sputum examination, 380-381
    tuberculosis, 1627
  asthma, 1186-1187
  cerebrospinal fluid, 1129
  desquamative interstitial pneumonia, 449
  interstitial lung disease, 450
  Langerhans' cell granulomatosis, 464
  low-density lipoprotein receptors, 1886-1887
  lung repair, 375
  pathogenesis of emphysema, 441
  reactive macrophage hyperplasia, 680
  respiratory defense, 366
  sarcoidosis, 457
  splenic, 600
  tuberculosis, 1627
Macrophage colony-stimulating factor, 532
Macropsia, 1033
Macrosomia, 2273
Macrovascular disease, 1868-1869
Macular degeneration, 2301-2302, Plate XI-1
Macular star, 2303, Plate XI-5
Macule
  chickenpox, 1525
  coal, 475
  differential diagnosis of fever and rash, 1384
  fever and rash, 1382
  leprosy, 1650
  neurofibromatosis, 1920
  photodermatosis, 1306-1307
  rubella, 1501
  systemic candidiasis, 1312
Madura foot, 1658

Magnesium, 1939-1944
  asthma, 1191
  body water compartments, 736
  chronic renal failure, 779
  depletion in hypokalemia, 828
  drug-nutrient interactions, 2110
  functions, 2109
  hypermagnesemia, 1943, 2101, 2110
    acute renal failure, 773
    hypocalcemia, 1931
  hypocalcemia, 1931
  hypomagnesemia, 1939-1943
    acute renal failure, 773
    hypocalcemia, 1931
  hypomagnesuria, 797
  normal metabolism, 1939, 1940
  recommended daily dietary allowances, 2115
  regulation of renal magnesium excretion, 1939
  retention after acute magnesium loading, 1942
  serum, 1942
  storage in bone, 1715
  total parenteral nutrition formula, 2117
Magnesium ammonium phosphate crystals, 799
Magnesium chloride, 1942
Magnesium gluconate, 1942
Magnesium oxide, 1942
Magnesium phosphate, 746
Magnesium sulfate
  hypomagnesemia, 1943
  myocardial infarction, 217
  preeclampsia, 2275
Magnetic resonance angiography, 107, 919
  brain, 925-926
  renovascular hypertension, 894-895
Magnetic resonance cholangiography, 2229
Magnetic resonance cholangiopancreatography,
    2146
Magnetic resonance imaging
  ankylosing spondylitis, 1239
  aortic stenosis, 287
  brain abscess, 1414, 1415
  brain tumor, 1067-1069
  Budd-Chiari syndrome, 2208
  cavernous hemangioma, 2216
  cholangiocarcinoma, 2232
  coma, 950
  common aortopulmonary trunk, 290
  constrictive pericarditis, 277, 278
  dementia, 988
  diabetes insipidus, 1795
  endocrine evaluation, 1735
  epilepsy, 981-982
  evaluation of arthritis, 1164, 1173
  focal nodular hyperplasia, 2216
  gynecomastia, 1765
  head, 1416
  heart, 106-107
  hepatic encephalopathy, 2161
  hepatobiliary tract, 2140
  hepatocellular carcinoma, 2213
  incidentaloma, 1830
  inflammatory myopathies, 1235, 1236
  insulinoma, 2244
  intraabdominal abscess, 1400
  lesions causing headache, 961
  low back pain, 966
  measurement of bone mineral density, 1748
  mediastinal mass, 512
  meningitis, 1406-1407
  multiple sclerosis, 1009, 1010
  myxoma, 330
  neck pain, 969
  neurologic disorders, 918-924
  osteomyelitis, 1434-1435
  pancreas, 2145
  pancreatic disease, 2146
  pancreatic tumor, 2242
  pericardial effusion, 275
  pituitary, 1782
  posterior fossa, 974

Magnetic resonance imaging—cont'd
  pulmonary, 389-390
  renal, 750-751
  renal cell carcinoma, 898
  renal mass, 752-753
  septic arthritis, 1252
  spinal epidural abscess, 1418
  spinal lesion, 1012
  stroke, 1003
  subdural empyema, 1417-1418
  tetralogy of Fallot, 289
  thoracic aortic aneurysm, 300
  total anomalous pulmonary venous connection,
    291
  toxoplasmosis infection, 1477, 1478
  truncus arteriosus, 290
  tuberous sclerosis, 1922
  ventricular septal defect, 284
  vertigo, 2307
Magnetic resonance spectroscopy, 922-924
Maillard reaction, 2102
Major depression, 1036, 2299
Major histocompatibility complex, 1115
  antigen binding, 1111, 1141
  T-cell recognition, 1174, 1175
Major histocompatibility complex class I
    molecule, 1127
Major histocompatibility complex class II
    molecule
  deficiency, 1177
  induction of organ-specific autoimmunity,
    1145-1146
Malabsorption, 2056-2068
  abetalipoproteinemia, 2067
  alpha heavy-chain disease, 704
  bacterial overgrowth, 2060-2062
  carbohydrates, 1987, 2067-2068
  celiac sprue, 2062-2063
  chronic diarrhea, 2051-2052
  chronic pancreatitis, 2145, 2239
  clinical features, 2057-2058
  congenital glucose-galactose, 878
  Crohn's disease, 270, 2069
  cystic fibrosis, 2246
  digestion process, 2056-2057
  eosinophilic enteritis, 2067
  eosinophilic gastroenteritis, 2066-2067
  hypogammaglobulinemia, 2066
  intestinal lymphangiectasia, 2067
  laboratory findings, 2058-2060
  magnesium, 1940
  multiple jejunal diverticulosis, 2089
  negative phosphate balance, 1935
  pancreatic and hepatobiliary diseases, 2062
  radiation enteropathy, 2065-2066
  serum electrolytes, 2005
  short bowel syndrome, 2066
  small intestinal tumor, 2081
  stool examination, 2006
  tests for, 2006-2007
  tropical sprue, 2065
  vitamin B_{12} deficiency, 648
  vitamin K deficiency, 607, 626
  weight loss, 1749
  Whipple's disease, 2064-2065
Maladaptive illness behavior, 1040
Maladie de Roger, 283
Malaise
  acute lung allograft rejection, 521
  bacterial prostatitis, 1462
  benign recurrent intrahepatic cholestasis, 2158
  chronic hepatitis, 2180
  common cold, 1391
  erysipelas, 1420
  hepatitis A, 2173
  hepatitis B, 2181
  influenza, 1490
  intrahepatic cholangiocarcinoma, 2214
  myopericarditis, 1489
  myxoma, 330

Malaise—cont'd
pyogenic liver abscess, 2209
retroperitoneal abscess, 1398
sarcoidosis, 458
scarlet fever, 1421
thrombotic thrombocytopenic purpura, 615
Malar flush, 245
Malaria, 1671-1675
fever of unknown origin, 1377
hemolytic anemia, 667
nephrotic syndrome, 767
peripheral blood smear, 557
Plasmodium falciparum, Plate VIII-14
Plasmodium vivax, Plate VIII-15
during pregnancy, 1468
transfusion-transmitted, 575, 576
travel-related, 1464-1465, 1467
Maldigestion
cystic fibrosis, 2246
pancreatic insufficiency, 2133
Male
breast cancer, 712-713
candidal balanitis, 1662
chancre, Plate VIII-34
Chlamydia trachomatis, 1536
climacteric, 1844
ejaculation, 934
genital examination for sexually transmitted
disease, 1438-1439
gonadal function testing, 1742
gonadotropin-secreting pituitary tumor, 1787
gynecomastia, 1764-1766
height and weight table, 2112
hypertension, 313
impotence, 1760-1764
autonomic dysfunction, 935
diabetes mellitus, 1844, 1873
diuretic-induced, 326
Lambert-Eaton myasthenic syndrome, 1024
liver failure, 2171
lymphogranuloma venereum, 1535
mean heights and weights and recommended
energy intake, 2117
prostate cancer, 717-720
elevated prostate specific antigen, 732
incidence and death rates, 550
obstructive uropathy, 885
osteoblastic bone formation, 1971
pulmonary metastases, 493
screening, 553
prostatectomy, 719
prostatic hypertrophy, 885
prostatitis, 1462-1463
recommended daily dietary allowances,
2114-2115, 2116
secondary sexual development, 1771
testicular cancer, 720-722
urethritis, 1440-1441
dysuria, 763
gonococcal, 1582
pellagra, 2107
Ureaplasma urealyticum, 1540-1541
Malformation
arteriovenous
dural, 928
hemorrhagic stroke, 998
vascular
angiography, 927
hemorrhagic stroke, 998
Malignancy; *see also* Cancer
acquired immunodeficiency
syndrome-associated, 1329, 2098
after cardiac transplantation, 342
antirheumatic drug toxicity, 1261
arthropathy, 1247-1248
bone metastases, 1971-1974
cancer of unknown primary tissue, 729-733
cardiac tumor, 329
cervical adenopathy, 2309-2310
chronic axonopathy, 1019

Malignancy—cont'd
colon, 2082-2086
complications, 579-586
nausea and vomiting, 581-582
neutropenia and fever, 582
pain, 580-581
paraneoplastic syndromes, 582-583
radiation therapy, 585
secondary malignancies, 585-586
therapy, 583-586
cutaneous, 1297-1298
cutaneous manifestations, 1316-1320
depression, 1037
esophageal, 2023-2024
fever of unknown origin, 1376
hypercalcemia, 1927, 1972-1974
immunosuppression-related, 795
insulin resistance, 1861
lymphadenopathy, 597, 599-600
molecular diagnostics, 559-564
clonality, 559
DNA analysis, 559-561
fluorescence in situ hybridization, 561, 562
leukemia, 562-563
lymphoma, 563-564
multiple myeloma, 700-703
neurofibromatosis, 1921
recurrent thromboembolic disease, 608-609
secondary, 585-586
small intestine, 2080-2081
splenomegaly, 601
sputum examination, 380
T-cell function, 1343
thyroid, 1814-1817
Malignant atrophic papulosis, 1320, 1321
Malignant effusion, 381-382
Malignant histiocytosis
fever of unknown origin, 1377
monocyte-macrophage abnormalities, 680
Malignant hypertension
hypokalemia, 829
optic nerve disc edema, Plate XI-2
Malignant hyperthermia, 1030
Malignant melanoma, 1298-1300
atypical mole, Plate VII-7
basal cell carcinoma *versus,* 1297
cardiac metastasis, 331
immunohistochemistry, 731
neoplastic pericarditis, 272
poorly differentiated carcinoma, 732
pulmonary metastases, 493
superficial spreading, Plate VII-8
Malignant mesothelioma, 510
asbestos exposure, 474
fasting hypoglycemia, 1876
high molecular weight keratins, 731
incidence, 329
intramyocardial, 330
peritoneal, 2249
pleural biopsy, 382-383
Malignant pleural effusion, 488, 507-508
Malignant transformation, 1108
Malingering, 1040
Mallory-Weiss syndrome, 2019, 2028
Mallory's body, 2188
Malnutrition
anorexia nervosa, 2030
chronic axonopathy, 1019
chronic obstructive pulmonary disease, 436, 445
chronic renal failure, 786
cirrhosis, 2172
excess mineral intake, 2110
nephrotic syndrome, 767
nosocomial infection, 1361
nutritional assessment, 2111
nutritional management, 2112-2117
vitamin A deficiency, 2105
Malonyl-coenzyme A, 1851, 1863, 2122
Malposition of heart, 291
Malt worker's lung, 460

Malta fever, 1604-1607
Mammary dysplasia, 708
Mammography, 552
breast cancer, 707
fibrocystic breast disease, 1849
preventive care guidelines, 2255
United States Preventive Services Task Force
guidelines, 25
Man-in-the-barrel syndrome, 951
Managed care, 29-34
Managed indemnity plan, 31
Manchester Comparative Reagent, 635
Manganese
functions, 2109
recommended daily dietary allowances, 2116
Mania, 1036, 1041
Manic-depressive disorder, 1035
Mannitol
acute tubular necrosis, 773
glaucoma, 2302
increased intracranial pressure, 1084
rhabdomyolysis, 775
Mannoheptulose, 1879-1880
Mannose 6-phosphate residue, 1911
Mannose-binding protein
activation of classical pathway, 1133
deficiency, 1179
Manometry
anorectal, 2008
esophageal, 2000-2001
Mansonella ozzardi, 1701
Mantle cell lymphoma, 697
Mantoux method, 1629
Maple bark stripper's lung, 460
Maple syrup urine disease, 1908
Maprotiline, 1037, 2191
Marble bone disease, 1958
Marble brain disease, 1958
March hemoglobinuria, 666-667
Marchiafava-Bignami disease, 1081
Marfan syndrome, 1730
aortic disease, 299
fibrillin, 1289
mitral regurgitation, 249
mitral valve prolapse, 253
during pregnancy, 2276
tall stature, 1769
Marginal zone lymphoma, 697
Margosa oil, 2193
Marijuana, 2028
Maroteaux-Lamy syndrome, 1915
Marsden, Hallett, and Fahn classification of
myoclonus, 996
Mass
abdominal
abdominal aortic aneurysm, 300
Castleman's disease, 2252
focal nodular hyperplasia, 2216
hypertrophic pyloric stenosis, 2044
renal cell carcinoma, 898
retroperitoneal fibrosis, 2250
adrenal, 1825-1826
breast cancer, 707-708
gastric biopsy and cytology, 2002
hepatocellular carcinoma, 2213
ovarian cancer, 716
renal, 749-751
retroperitoneal fibrosis, 2250
scrotal, 721
testicular cancer, 721
upper gastrointestinal endoscopy, 1994
Mass effect, 978
Mass median aerodynamic diameter, 430
Mass movement, 1980
Mass spectroscopy, 396
Mast cell, 1109
asthma, 1185, 1186
enzymes and proteoglycans, 1142
immediate hypersensitivity, 1139-1140
mastocytosis, 681

Mast cell leukemia, 681
Mastectomy, 709
Mastitis, 1848
Mastocytosis, 681
    gastric acid hypersecretion, 1983
    nasal, 1181
Mastoiditis
    anaerobic infection, 1617
    Haemophilus influenzae, 1588
    Wegener's granulomatosis, 468
Mate tea, 2193
Material Safety Data Sheets, 471
Matrix formation and calcification, 1716
Matrix hepatitis C virus dot blot immunoassay,
    2176
Matrix metalloproteinases, 1265
Mattis Dementia Rating Scale, 904
Maturity-onset diabetes mellitus, 1854
Maxik; *see* Trendolapril
Maxillary sinus puncture, 2309
Maxillary sinusitis, 1394-1395
Maximal expiratory flow-volume curve, 376,
    377
Maximal inspiratory airway pressure, 431
Maximal mid-expiratory flow
    chronic obstructive pulmonary disease, 473
    cystic fibrosis, 481
Maximal oxygen consumption, 166-167
Maximal rate of pressure rise, 43
Maximal voluntary ventilation, 379
Maximum acid output, 2003
Maximum oxygen uptake, 91
Maximum urine osmolality, 739
Maximum voluntary ventilation maneuver, 420
Maxzide; *see* Dyrenium
May-Hegglin anomaly, 603
Mazoplasia, 1848
Mazzotti test, 1701
MB isoenzyme of creatine kinase
    left ventricular aneurysm, 221
    myocardial infarction, 211-212
McArdle's disease, 1025, 1029
McCune-Albright syndrome, 1960
MCD; *see* Minimal change disease
McLeod's syndrome, 666
MCV; *see* Mean corpuscular volume
MDC survival trial, 171
Mean arterial pressure, 817
Mean cell hemoglobin, 555
Mean cell volume, 555, 556
    gastrointestinal bleeding, 2011
    hemolytic anemia, 661
Mean corpuscular volume
    beta-thalassemia, 654-655
    megaloblastic anemia, 648
    microcytosis, 643
Mean platelet volume, 556
Mean pulmonary artery pressure, 500
Means-Lerman scratch, 334
Measles, 1497-1499
    compromised host, 1388
    culture, 1369
Mebendazole
    Ascaris lumbricoides, 1698
    hepatic injury, 2191
    intestinal helminths, 1697
    pinworm infestation, 1696
    whipworm, 1696
Mechanical disorders
    chronic tubulointerstitial nephropathy, 892
    gastroesophageal reflux disease, 2015
    myocardial infarction, 219
Mechanical valve, 259-260
Mechanical ventilation, 396-400
    acute respiratory failure, 416, 418-419
        with chronic obstructive pulmonary disease,
            446
        weaning, 420
    chronic obstructive pulmonary disease, 417
    endotracheal intubation and tracheotomy, 399
    gram-negative sepsis, 1452

Mechanical ventilation—cont'd
    initiation, 396-397
    modes, 397-398
    monitoring ventilatory mechanics, 398-399
    pulmonary edema, 426-427
    respiratory acidosis, 416
    respiratory muscle failure, 359-360
    weaning, 399-400, 420
Mechanoreceptor
    modulation of ventricular function, 45
    pericardial, 271
    ventilation, 353
Mechanoreceptors
    chest wall, 353
    modulation of ventricular function, 45
    pericardial, 271
    ventilation, 353
Meckel's diverticulum, 2014, 2089
Meclizine, 2027
Meclofenamate, 852
Meconium ileus, 2246
Median eminence, 1788
Median nerve
    damage in leprosy, 1650
    mononeuropathy, 1017
    somatosensory evoked potential, 913
Mediastinal crunch, 75
Mediastinal disease, 510-514
Mediastinal pain, 505
Mediastinitis, 514
    deep neck infections, 2309
    fibrosing, 512
Mediastinoscopy, 385
    lung cancer, 726
    mediastinal mass, 512
Mediastinotomy, 385
Mediastinum, 510-511
    computed tomography, 386-387
    magnetic resonance imaging, 389
Mediator
    asthma, 1187
    emetic reflex, 2026
    endotoxin, 1448
    fever, 1386-1387
    gouty arthritis, 1271-1272
    gram-negative bacteremia, 1448
    immediate hypersensitivity, 1139, 1140-1142
    release, 1136
Medicaid, 31-32
Medical genetics, 1721-1732
    chromosomal abnormalities, 1727-1729
    counseling and prenatal diagnosis, 1730-1731
    diagnosis and management of inherited
        disorders, 1729-1730, 1731
    human chromosomes, 1727, 1728
    mechanisms of monogenic inheritance,
        1724-1726
    molecular genetics of human genome,
        1721-1724
    multifactorial inheritance, 1726-1727
    positional cloning, 1724
    treatment of genetic disorders, 1731-1732
Medical history; *see* Patient history
Medical informatics, 26-29
Medical interview, 2, 3
Medical practice, 1-34
    clinical bioethics, 9-13
    costs and outcomes, 14-16
    implementation of clinical practice guidelines,
        23-26
    managed care, 29-34
    medical informatics, 26-29
    physician-patient encounter, 2-5
    principles of diagnostic testing, 5-9
    quality of care, 16-22
Medical record
    computer-based, 27-28
    drug interactions, 2313
Medicare
    health care expenditure, 14
    managed care, 31-32

Medicare—cont'd
    reimbursement of long-term oxygen therapy,
        429
Mediterranean anemia, 654
Mediterranean fever, 1604-1607
Mediterranean lymphoma, 2080
Mediterranean spotted fever, 1545
Medium-chain triglycerides
    chronic pancreatitis, 2240-2241
    cystic fibrosis, 2246
MEDLINE, 29
Medroxyprogesterone
    hot flashes, 2271
    obstructive sleep apnea, 528
    osteoporotic fractures, 1948
    progesterone withdrawal test, 1742
Medtronic Hall valve, 260
Medulla oblongata, 2025
Medullary chemoreceptors, 353
Medullary cords, 596
Medullary cystic disease, 875, 892
Medullary hypertonicity, 808-809
Medullary osteomyelitis, 1436
Medullary sponge kidney, 875
Medullary thyroid carcinoma, 1732, 1816
Medulloblastoma, 1070
Medwatch, 2310
Mefloquine, 1467
Megacolon
    aganglionic, 2092
    Chagas's disease, 1690
    toxic, 1591
Megaesophagus, 1690
Megakaryocyte
    evaluation of thrombocytopenia, 569
    platelet development from, 535-536
Megakaryocytic hypoplasia, 614
Megakaryocytopoiesis, 532
Megaloblast, 646
Megaloblastic anemia, 646-650
    hypokalemia, 827
    macrocytosis, Plate IV-4
Megavitamin therapy, 2108
Megestrol acetate
    breast cancer, 710
    endometrial cancer, 714
Meig's syndrome, 508
Melanoma, 1298-1300
    atypical mole, Plate VII-7
    basal cell carcinoma *versus,* 1297
    cardiac metastasis, 331
    immunohistochemistry, 731
    neoplastic pericarditis, 272
    poorly differentiated carcinoma, 732
    superficial spreading, Plate VII-8
Melanoptysis, 475
Melarsoprol, 1689
MELAS syndrome, 1029
Melatonin, 1708
Melena
    gastric cancer, 2046
    gastrointestinal bleeding, 2010
    hemobilia, 2233
    infectious esophagitis, 2020
    Meckel's diverticulum, 2089
    peptic ulcer, 2037
    upper gastrointestinal endoscopy, 1994
Meleney's synergistic gangrene, 1425
Melphalan
    multiple myeloma, 702
    pulmonary parenchymal reactions, 476
Membrane attack complex, 1136-1137, 1179
Membrane cofactor protein, 1135
Membrane excitability disorders, 1026
Membrane exon, 1124
Membrane proteins, 1338
Membrane receptors, 1710-1711
Membranoproliferative glomerulonephritis,
    854-855
Membranous lipodystrophy, 1903
Membranous lupus nephritis, 856-857

Membranous nephropathy, 853-854, 1213
Memorial Sloan-Kettering staging system for
    non-seminomatous germ cell tumors,
    721
Memory B-cell, 1113
Memory cell, 1126
Memory impairment
    amnesic syndrome, 1031-1032
    chronic fatigue, 2298
    elderly, 2288
Memory testing, 902
Menadione, 625, 664
Menaphthone, 664
Menaquinone, 625
Menelamine, 2191
Menetrier's disease, 2043, 2049
Ménière's disease, 972, 2307
Meningeal carcinomatosis, 1071-1072
Meningeal inflammation, 958
Meningeal irritation, 960
Meningioma, 1069
Meningitis, 1402-1413
    acquired immunodeficiency syndrome,
        1477-1478
    aseptic, 1488
    brain abscess *versus,* 1414
    candidal, 1662-1663
    clinical manifestations, 1406, 1407
    coccidioidomycosis, 1657
    cryptococcal, 1667-1668
        acquired immunodeficiency syndrome, 1474
        fundoscopic view, Plate VIII-51
    differential diagnosis, 1408-1409
    enterococcal, 1562
    epidemiology and etiology, 1402-1404
    fever, 1385, 1387
    Haemophilus influenzae, 1586, 1587, Plate
        VIII-8
    headache, 960
    laboratory investigation, 1406-1408
    leptospirosis, 1644
    meningococcal, Plate VIII-9
    OKT3-induced, 1090
    pathogenesis and pathophysiology, 1404-1406
    picornavirus infection, 1487
    prognosis, 1413
    rash, 1385
    respiratory alkalosis, 355
    sinusitis, 2309
    Staphylococcus aureus, 1549-1550
    toxoplasmosis, 1677
    treatment, 1409-1413
    tuberculous, 1636
Meningococcal meningitis, 1403
    Gram stain, Plate VIII-9
    Neisseria meningitidis, 1578-1581
Meningococcemia, 1579-1580
    fever and rash, 1382
    skin lesion, Plate VIII-21
Meningoencephalitis
    adenovirus, 1504
    African trypanosomiasis, 1688
    agammaglobulinemia, 1490
    headache, 960
    Listeria, 1577
    Naegleria fowleri, 1683-1684
    Toxoplasma gondii, 1677
Meningovascular syphilis, 1641
Menopausal insomnia, 947
Menopause, 2270-2271
    erosive osteoarthritis, 1266
    osteoporosis, 1946, 1947
    ovarian function, 1833
Menorrhagia
    end-stage renal disease, 787
    von Willebrand's disease, 624
Menotropin, 1759
Menstrual-associated sleep disorder, 947
Menstruation
    acromegaly, 1782
    breast changes during, 1846

Menstruation—cont'd
    chronic hepatic failure, 2170
    end-stage renal disease, 787
Mental failure, 985
Mental illness
    anxiety, 1034-1035
    disordered sleep, 946
    maladaptive illness behavior, 1040
    mood disorders, 1035-1038
    personality disorders, 1039-1040
    somatization, 1040
    thought disorders, 1041-1043
Mental retardation
    alpha-mannosidosis, 1916
    Crigler-Najjar syndrome, 2153
    galactosemia, 1883
    mucopolysaccharidosis, 1912
    neonatal cytomegalovirus, 1528
    phenylketonuria, 1905
    Prader-Labhart-Willi syndrome, 1842
    total lipodystrophy, 1901
Mental status
    acute confusional state, 1031
    chronic fatigue, 2298
    gram-negative bacteremia, 1449
    hepatic encephalopathy, 2159
    impotence, 1760-1761
    metabolic encephalopathy, 1078
    neurologic examination, 902
    Parkinson's disease, 992
    psychometric tests, 903
    relapsing fever, 1645
Mepacrine, 2191
Meperidine
    abdominal pain, 2032
    abuse, 2297
    acute intermittent porphyria, 1926
    acute pancreatitis, 2237
    cancer pain, 580, 581
    sedation during gastrointestinal endoscopy, 1994
    status migrainosus, 962
Mercaptans, 2161, 2162
Mercaptoproprionylglycine, 804-805
6-Mercaptopurine
    Crohn's disease, 2072
    hepatic injury, 2192
    ulcerative colitis, 2074
Mercuric chloride, 867
Mercury
    acute renal failure, 867
    sensorimotor neuropathy, 1020
Merosin, 1027
MERRF syndrome, 996
Mesalamine
    Crohn's disease, 2071
    ulcerative colitis, 2074
Mesangial cell
    AL type of amyloidosis, 863
    diabetic nephropathy, 859
    membranoproliferative glomerulonephritis, 854
Mesangial deposits, 842, 843, 845
Mesangial lupus nephritis, 856
Mesangial nephritis, 1213, 1215
Mesangial proliferative disease, 851
Mesenteric arteriography, 2087
Mesenteric cyst, 2251
Mesenteric fibromatosis, 2251
Mesenteric giant lymph node hyperplasia, 2252
Mesenteric hernia, 2251
Mesenteric lipodystrophy, 1903, 2251
Mesenteric panniculitis, 2251
Mesenteric tumor, 2251-2252
Mesenteric vascular disease, 2086-2089
Mesenteric vein
    obstruction, 81, 2208
    thrombosis, 2088-2089
Mesentery, 2247
Mesocaval shunt, 2167
Mesothelioma
    asbestos-related, 474
    fasting hypoglycemia, 1876

Mesothelioma—cont'd
    high molecular weight keratins, 731
    incidence, 329
    intramyocardial, 330
    peritoneal, 2249
    pleural biopsy, 382-383
Messenger ribonucleic acid, 1721
    analysis, 53-54
    DNA code, 49, 50
    hormone synthesis, 1709
Metabolic acidosis, 836-839
    acute renal failure, 772
    chronic renal failure, 779, 786
    glucose-6-phosphate dehydrogenase
        deficiency, 1881
    gram-negative bacteremia, 1449
    hyperkalemia, 832-833
    internal potassium balance, 825
    normotensive renal potassium wasting, 828
    obstructive uropathy, 886
    potassium and, 838-839
    respiratory compensation, 834
Metabolic alkalosis, 839-841
    changes in arterial pH, 353
    consequence of vomiting, 2028
    hepatic encephalopathy, 2163
    hypertensive renal potassium wasting, 828
    hypokalemia, 827, 829-830
    normotensive renal potassium wasting, 828
    portosystemic encephalopathy, 2160
    renal excretion of potassium, 741
Metabolic bone disease
    Fanconi's syndrome, 882
    inflammatory bowel disease, 2075
    osteomalacia, 1949-1955
        after parathyroidectomy, 1965
        bone biopsy, 1747
        chronic hypophosphatemia, 1936
        chronic renal failure, 785
        proximal renal tubular acidosis, 837
        renal osteodystrophy, 1961
        vitamin D deficiency, 2106
        vitamin D metabolism, 1719
        X-linked hypophosphatemic rickets, 880
    osteopetrosis, 1958-1959
    osteoporosis, 1944-1949
        bone biopsy, 1747
        brucellosis, 1606
        calcitonin therapy, 1719
        glucocorticoid-induced, 1263
        heparin, 635
        menopause, 2271
        multiple myeloma, 864
        reduction in bone density, 1165
        rheumatoid arthritis, 1205
    Paget's disease, 1955-1958
Metabolic disorders, 1078-1081
    acute confusional state, 1031
    alcohol-related, 1080-1081
    amino acid metabolism disorders, 1903-1911
        branched-chain amino acids, 1907-1908
        histidinemia, 1906
        hyperphenylalaninemia, 1904-1905
        lysine disorders, 1907
        sulfur-containing amino acids, 1908-1909
        tyrosinemia, 1905-1906
        urea cycle defects, 1906-1907
    amino acid storage disorders, 1909-1910
    amino acid transport disorders, 1910-1911
    choice of antimicrobials, 1346-1348
    chronic abdominal pain, 2035
    chronic axonopathy, 1019
    chronic effects, 1080
    chronic renal failure, 786
    chronic tubulointerstitial nephropathy, 890-891
    diabetes mellitus complications, 1862-1874
        alcoholic ketosis, 1865
        diabetic ketoacidosis, 1862-1865
        diabetic nephropathy, 859-862
        gallstones, 2223
        hyperosmolar nonketotic coma, 1865-1866

Metabolic disorders—cont'd
  diabetes mellitus complications—cont'd
    hypoglycemic coma, 1867
    hyporeninemic hypoaldosteronism, 1824
    impotence, 1760, 1844
    lactic acidosis, 1866-1867
    weight loss, 1749
  disordered thinking, 1041
  effects on electrocardiogram, 90
  heritable disorders of carbohydrate
      metabolism, 1879-1883
    galactosemia, 1882-1883
    glycogen storage diseases, 1880-1882
    nondiabetic mellituarias, 1879-1880
  hypercalcemia, 1927-1930
    acute renal failure, 773
    calcitonin therapy, 1719
    causes and differential diagnosis, 1927-1928
    chronic nephrocalcinosis, 891
    clinical features, 1928-1929
    1,25-dihydrotachysterol, 1954
    efforts of ionized calcium on cell metabolic
        processes, 1717
    electrocardiographic abnormalities, 89, 90
    endocrine paraneoplastic syndromes, 583
    interstitial lung disease, 452
    kidney stone formation, 798
    lung cancer, 489
    malignancy, 1972-1974
    medication-induced, 1928
    multiple myeloma, 700, 702, 864
    nonparathyroid endocrine disorders, 1928
    Paget's disease, 1956
    predominant hyperparathyroid bone disease,
        1964
    primary hyperparathyroidism, 1965, 1966,
        1967
    renal cell carcinoma, 898
    renal magnesium wasting, 1940-1941
    sarcoidosis, 458
    steroid suppression test, 1746
    treatment, 1929-1930
    urinary cyclic adenosine monophosphate,
        1746
    vitamin D toxicity, 1928
  hypocalcemia, 1930-1934
    acute pancreatitis, 2237
    acute renal failure, 773
    after massive transfusion, 2011
    chronic renal failure, 779, 785-786
    clinical features, 1932-1933
    differential diagnosis, 1931-1932
    efforts of ionized calcium on cell metabolic
        processes, 1717
    electrocardiographic abnormalities, 89, 90
    ethylene glycol poisoning, 866
    hyperphosphatemia, 1938
    hypomagnesemia, 1942
    nephrotic syndrome, 767
    osteomalacia, 1949
    relative hypoparathyroidism, 1932
    treatment, 1933-1934
    vitamin D deficiency, 2106
  interference with detoxification function, 2142
  interstitial lung disease with, 452
  lipid and lipoprotein, 1883-1898
    apoliprotein synthesis abnormalities,
        1897-1898
    atherosclerosis, 1888-1889
    dietary factors, 1889-1890
    effects of drugs, 1890-1892
    enzyme abnormalities, 1898
    hyperlipidemia, 1892-1896
    hypoalphalipoproteinemia, 1896
    lipid metabolism, 1883-1884
    lipoprotein metabolism, 1885-1888
  lipodystrophies, 1899-1903
    centrifugal lipodystrophy, 1903
    congenital total lipodystrophy, 1900-1902
    leprechaunism, 1899-1900
    lipoatrophic diabetes, 1902-1903

Metabolic disorders—cont'd
  lipodystrophies—cont'd
    membranous lipodystrophy, 1903
    mesenteric lipodystrophy, 1903
    partial lipodystrophy, 1902, 1903
  lysosomal storage diseases, 1911-1920
    Chédiak-Higashi syndrome, 1919
    cystinosis, 1919
    drug-induced lysosomopathies, 1919
    general considerations, 1911-1912
    lipid storage diseases, 1917-1919
    lysosomal physiology, 1911
    mucolipidoses, 1915-1917
    mucopolysaccharidoses, 1912-1915
    treatment, 1919-1920
  magnesium, 1939-1944
    chronic renal failure, 779
    drug-nutrient interactions, 2110
    hypermagnesemia, 1943
    hypocalcemia, 1931
    hypomagnesemia, 1939-1943
  megaloblastic anemia, 648
  metabolic encephalopathy, 1078-1079
  multifocal atrial tachycardia, 144
  myelopathy, 1013
  osteoarthritis, 1266-1267
  peripheral neuropathy, 1016
  phakomatoses, 1920-1923
  phosphate, 1934-1939
    chronic renal failure, 779
    hyperphosphatemia, 1938-1939
    hypophosphatemia, 1935-1938
    hypophosphatemic rickets, 1952
    renal osteodystrophy, 785
    renal phosphate wasting syndromes, 880
    rickets, 881
  porphyrias, 1923-1927
  seizures, 980
  vitamin-dependent, 2107, 2108
Metabolic encephalopathy, 1078-1080
  coma, 948-949
  electroencephalography, 907-908
Metabolic equivalent, 2257, 2258
  cardiac rehabilitation, 224
  exercise stress testing, 91
Metabolic myopathy, 1028-1030, 1086-1087
Metabolic pericarditis, 273
Metabolic rate, 2113
  aging and, 2283
Metabolic testing, 1730
Metabolism
  bilirubin, 2147-2150
  bone and mineral homeostasis, 1714-1721
    calcium metabolism, 1717-1720
    cellular physiology, 1716
    effects of hormones, 1720
    functions of skeleton, 1714-1715
    matrix formation and calcification, 1716
    natural history of skeleton, 1715-1716
    stress and coupling, 1716
  calcium, 1717-1720
  catecholamines, 1826-1827
  hepatic, 2118-2123
    amino acids and protein, 2118-2120
    carbohydrates, 2121-2122
    detoxification, 2122
    hormones, 2122-2123
    lipids, 2120-2121
  lipids, 1883-1884, 1896-1898
  lipoproteins, 1885-1888
  role of lung, 346
  shock, 176, 178
  thyroid hormone, 1797-1799
  toxicity of chemotherapeutic agents, 584
  vitamin B$_{12}$ and folate, 647
Metachromatic leukodystrophy, 1918
Metagonimus yokogawai, 1698
Metahexamide, 2191
Metaiodobenzylguanidine, 105
  pheochromocytoma, 1830
  thyroid, 1735

Metal fume fever, 473
Metallothionein, 867
Metals causing occupational asthma, 472
Metamorphopsia, 1033, 2302
Metamyelocyte, 532
Metanephrine, 322, 1739
Metaplasia
  agnogenic myeloid, 677
  atrophic gastritis mucosa, 2042
  epithelial, 2016
  mucosal, 2000, 2016, 2017-2018
Metastases
  breast cancer, 707, 710-711
  carcinoid tumors, 2082
  colon cancer, 2085
  complications, 1070-1073, 1074
  cutaneous, 1316
  esophageal cancer, 2024
  gastric cancer, 2046
  hepatocellular carcinoma, 2213
  involving heart, 330-332
  lung cancer, 489, 492, 726
  megakaryocytic hypoplasia, 614
  neoplastic pericarditis, 272
  pancreatic tumor, 2242
  peritoneal tumor, 2249
  prostate cancer, 718
  renal cell carcinoma, 898
  skeletal, 1971-1974
  solitary pulmonary nodule, 494
  testicular cancer, 720
Metatarsophalangeal joint, 1203
Metered dose inhaler, 430-431
Metformin
  diabetes mellitus, 1857-1858
  drug-nutrient interactions, 2110
Methacholine, 933
Methacholine test, 379
Methadone, 2297
  cancer pain, 580, 581
  pulmonary parenchymal reactions, 476
  pulmonary toxicity, 479
Methamphetamine hydrochloride, 943
Methanol, 837
Methazolamide, 2302
Methemoglobinemia, 351, 660
  angina, 201
  oxidant hemolysis, 667
Methenamine, 1360
  antibacterial mechanism, 1345
  interference with catecholamine assays, 1740
Methicillin, 1352
  brain abscess, 1416
  dosage, 1350
Methicillin-resistant staphylococci, 1551
Methimazole
  Graves' disease, 1806
  hepatic injury, 2191
  during pregnancy, 2273
Methionine
  related diseases, 1904
  stone formation, 798
Methotrexate
  asthma, 1191
  breast cancer, 709, 710
  Crohn's disease, 2072
  dermatomyositis, 1292
  drug-induced hypersensitivity pneumonitis,
      477
  drug-nutrient interactions, 2110
  effects on kidney, 869
  graft-*versus*-host disease, 578
  hepatic injury, 585, 2192
  inflammatory myopathies, 1237
  inhibition of folate metabolism, 647
  nephrotoxicity, 584
  non-Hodgkin's lymphoma, 699
  psoriasis, 1302
  psoriatic arthritis, 1242
  pulmonary toxicity, 478
  retroperitoneal fibrosis, 2250

Methotrexate—cont'd
  rheumatic disease, 1260-1261
  rheumatoid arthritis, 1208-1209
  stomatitis, 584-585
3-Methoxy-4-hydroxyphenylglycol, 930
Methoxyflurane
  effects on kidney, 871
  hepatic injury, 2190, 2191
8-Methoxypsorlen, 1302
Methyl bromide, 1020
N-Methyl-formamide, 2192
Methyl tert-butyl ether, 2227
Methyldopa
  chronic hypertension during pregnancy, 2275
  drug-induced immune hemolytic anemia, 670
  drug-nutrient interactions, 2110
  hepatic injury, 2192
  hepatocellular jaundice, 2192
  hypertension, 325
  interference with catecholamine assays, 1740
Methylene blue
  hemolysis in glucose-6-phosphate
      dehydrogenase deficiency, 663
  infectious diseases, 1603
Methylene dianiline, 2192
Methylmalonic acid, 649
Methylmalonic aciduria, 1908
Methylparatyrosine, 1740
Methylphenidate
  depression, 1038
  hepatic injury, 2191
  interference with catecholamine assays, 1740
  narcolepsy, 943
Methylprednisolone
  acute lung allograft rejection, 521
  antiphospholipid syndrome, 1292
  asthma, 1192
  brain abscess, 1416
  bronchiolitis obliterans syndrome, 523
  chronic obstructive pulmonary disease with
      respiratory failure, 418
  crescentic glomerulonephritis, 848
  Crohn's disease, 2071
  cutaneous lesions in lupus erythematosus,
      1291-1292
  lung transplantation, 516
  multiple myeloma, 702
  multiple sclerosis, 1010
  myelopathy, 1013
  for nausea and vomiting, 2027
  optic neuritis, 1060
  prevention and therapy of rejection, 340
  rheumatic fever, 1257
  rheumatoid arthritis, 1207
  systemic lupus erythematosus, 1216-1217
  ulcerative colitis, 2074
Methyltestosterone, 1845
Methylthiouracil, 2191
Methylxanthines
  anaphylaxis, 1194
  asthma, 1190, 1192
  Cheyne-Stokes respiration, 354
  chronic obstructive pulmonary disease, 417,
      434, 444
  dipyridamole stress scintigraphy, 103
  human cytochrome P450 isoforms, 2312
  interference with catecholamine assays, 1740
  during pregnancy, 2277
Methysergide
  cluster headache prophylaxis, 962
  prophylaxis of migraine, 962
  retroperitoneal fibrosis, 2250
Metipranolol, 2302
Metoclopramide
  gastroesophageal reflux, 2018
  interaction with cyclosporin, 793
  intestinal pseudoobstruction, 2079
  morning sickness, 2029
  for nausea and vomiting, 2027
  pituitary stimulation tests, 1736
  status migrainosus, 962

Metolazone
  heart failure, 169, 170
  hypertension, 325
  nephrotic syndrome, 767
Metopimazine, 2191
Metoprolol
  human cytochrome P450 isoforms, 2312
  hypertension, 325
  interference with oral anticoagulants, 636
  properties, 203
Metoprolol in Dilated Cardiomyopathy study,
    171
Metronidazole, 1358-1359
  activity against major anaerobes, 1620
  acute pancreatitis, 2237
  amebiasis, 1683
  amebic liver abscess, 2210
  bacterial overgrowth, 2062
  bacterial vaginosis, 1443
  balantidiasis, 1691
  brain abscess, 1416
  Clostridium difficile colitis, 1569, 1570
  Crohn's disease, 2072
  dosage, 1350
  giardiasis, 1685
  hepatic encephalopathy, 2162
  hepatic injury, 2191
  interference with oral anticoagulants, 636
  intraabdominal infection, 1401
  liver abscess, 2209
  subdural empyema, 1418
  trichomoniasis, 1441, 1443, 1691
  use during pregnancy, 2281
Metyrapone
  Cushing's disease, 1786
  ectopic adrenocorticotropic hormone secretion,
      1822
  testing for adrenocorticotropic hormone
      reserve, 1774
  tests of feedback inhibition, 1736
Mevalonic acid, 1884
Mexiletine, 138, 2192
Mexitil; *see* Mexiletine
Mezlocillin, 1352
  activity against major anaerobes, 1620
  acute pancreatitis, 2237
  dosage, 1350
  enterococci resistance, 1561
MG; *see* Myasthenia gravis
Mianserin, 2191
MIBG; *see* Iodine-123 radiolabeled
      metaiodobenzylguanidine
Micelle, 2124
  flow of bilirubin down biliary tree, 2149
  lipid digestion, 1987
Miconazole, 636
Micro-satellite deoxyribonucleic acid, 1723
Microadenoma
  amenorrhea, 1759
  during pregnancy, 2273, 2274
  prolactin-secreting, 1785-1786
Microalbuminuria, 743, 761, 859-860
Microaneurysm, 2303
Microangiopathic hemolytic anemia, 666-667
Microcirculation, 47-48
Microcomedone, 1305
Microcytic anemia, 2005
Microcytosis, 643
  beta-thalassemia, 654, 655
  without iron deficiency, 588
Microdeletion on chromosome 22, 1729
Microfilaments, 536
Microflora, 1367, 1368
  bile salt secretion, 2125
  intestinal catabolism of bile pigments,
      2149-2150
  intraabdominal infection, 1397
  obligate anaerobic bacteria, 1614, 1615
Microglia, 1127
Microhemagglutination test, 1642
Microhematuria, 744

Microminerals, 2108
Microorganisms, 1334; *see also* Bacterial
      infection; Viral infection
  choice of appropriate antimicrobial agents,
      1346
  development of rash, 1380-1381
  hazardous to laboratory personnel, 1369
  laboratory testing, 1366-1374
    bacteria culture, 1367-1369
    Chlamydiae, Rickettsiae, and Mycoplasmas,
        1370
    direct detection techniques, 1370-1373
    fungus culture, 1370
    serology, 1373-1374
    skin testing, 1374
    test interpretation, 1366-1367
    virus culture, 1369-1370
  nosocomial infection, 1362-1363
  small bowel, 2060
Micropolyspora faeni, 461
Micropsia, 1033
Microsatellites, 549
Microscopic polyarteritis nodosa, 856,
    1220-1221
Microscopy, 843-844, 1370-1371
  acute renal failure, 771
  dark-field
    leptospirosis, 1645
    relapsing fever, 1645
    syphilis, 1642
    Treponema pallidum, Plate VIII-2
  electron
    Alport's syndrome, 876-877
    cancer of unknown primary site, 731
    focal glomerular sclerosis, 852
    glomerulonephritis, 842
    idiopathic nephrotic syndrome, 850
    minimal change disease, 849
    poststreptococcal glomerulonephritis,
        843-844
    primary hyperparathyroidism, 1968
  hematuria, 757
  light
    analysis of crystals in synovial fluid, 1163
    cancer of unknown primary site, 730
    cholesterol monohydrate crystals, Plate
        X-15
    glomerulonephritis, 842
    idiopathic nephrotic syndrome, 850
    poststreptococcal glomerulonephritis,
        843-844
    rapidly progressive glomerulonephritis, 848
  urine sediment, 744-746
Microsleeps, 942
Microspherocyte, 668, 669
Microsporida, 1680-1681
  acquired immunodeficiency syndrome, 1476,
      2095
  compromised host, 1388
Microsporum, 1307-1308
Microtubules, 59
Microvascular angina, 195
Microvascular disease, 1869-1870
Microvascular fluid exchange, 346-347
Microvillus, 2057
Microx; *see* Metolazone
Micturition, 933
Micturition center, 933
Micturition syncope, 953
Mid-systolic ejection murmur, 76
Mid-systolic nonejection sound, 76
Midazolam, 1994
Middle cerebral artery occlusion, 1004-1005
Middle ear
  acute otitis media, 1395
  disorders, 2307
Middle fossa syndrome, 1071
Middle mediastinal tumor, 513
Midesophageal diverticula, 2021
Midesophageal stricture, 2017
Mifepristone, 1787

Migraine, 957-959
  epilepsy *versus,* 981
  treatment, 961-962
  visual hallucinations, 1062
Mild aplastic anemia, 671
Miliary lesions in lung, 1635
Miliary tuberculosis, 1409
Milieu interieur, 1075
Milk intolerance, 1993, 2068
Milkman's syndrome, 1950
Miller's lung, 460
Milrinone
  dilated cardiomyopathy, 264
  heart failure, 173, 174
Milroy's disease, 1420
Milwaukee shoulder/knee syndrome, 1279-1280
Mineral dusts, 476
Mineralization of bone, 1716
  osteomalacia and rickets, 1953-1954
Mineralocorticoids, 1741-1742
  deficiency, 824
  effects on potassium transport, 741
  excess, 840, 1822-1823
  renal hydrogen ion secretion, 741
  sodium-retaining action, 738
Minerals, 2108-2110
  disorders, 1744-1748
  excess intake, 2101
  measurement of bone mineral content, 1747
  parenteral solutions, 2114
  physiology of bone and mineral homeostasis,
      1714-1721
    calcium metabolism, 1717-1720
    cellular physiology of bone, 1716
    effects of hormones, 1720
    functions of skeleton, 1714-1715
    matrix formation and calcification, 1716
    natural history of skeleton, 1715-1716
    stress and coupling, 1716
Mini-mental state examination, 904
Minimal change disease, 767, 849-851
Minimal lupus nephritis, 856
Minimum inhibitory concentration, 1346
Minimum urine osmolality, 739
Minipress; *see* Prazosin
Minnesota Multiphasic Personal Inventory, 903
Minocycline
  leprosy, 1651
  rheumatic disease, 1260, 1262
  urethritis, 1441
Minoxidil
  hypertension, 325, 327
  interference with catecholamine assays, 1740
Minute ventilation
  acute respiratory failure occurring with acute
      respiratory distress syndrome, 418
  exercise test, 379
  removal from mechanical ventilation and
      weaning, 420
MIP; *see* Managed indemnity plan
Mirror-image dextrocardia, 291
Missile wound to head, 1045
Mistletoe, 2193
Mite, 1183
Mithramycin
  effects on kidney, 869
  hepatic injury, 2192
Mitochondrial abnormalities, 1029
Mitochondrial antibody, 1157
Mitochondrial cardiomyopathy, 62
Mitogen, 1152
Mitogen-activated protein kinase, 541
Mitogenic factor, 1556
Mitogenic growth factors, 1202
Mitomycin
  breast cancer, 710
  effects on kidney, 869
  gastric cancer, 2048
  pancreatic cancer, 2243
  pulmonary parenchymal reactions, 476
  pulmonary toxicity, 478

Mitotane
  Cushing's disease, 1787
  Cushing's syndrome, 1821
Mitral valve
  hypertrophic cardiomyopathy, 265
  occlusive mesenteric vascular disease, 2087
  radiographic views, 92
Mitral valve area, 111
Mitral valve prolapse, 253-255
  acquired immunodeficiency syndrome, 333
  arrhythmia, 133
  atrial septal defect, 280, 281
  auscultatory findings, 75, 76
  chest pain, 128, 129
  infective endocarditis, 225, 226
  mitral regurgitation, 249
  palpitations, 131
  von Willebrand's disease, 624
Mitral valve regurgitation, 249-253
  atrial septal defect, 281
  cardiac catheterization, 114, 115
  dexfenfluramine and, 261
  diastolic heart failure, 167
  dicrotic pulse, 65
  differential diagnosis, 180
  Doppler image, Plate II-4
  fenfluramine and, 261
  hypertrophic cardiomyopathy, 265
  mitral valve prolapse, 253
  myocardial infarction, 219, 220
  nonejection systolic sounds, 75
  pansystolic murmur, 77
  during pregnancy, 2276
  restrictive cardiomyopathy, 271
  shock, 177
  weakness, 1755
Mitral valve stenosis, 245-249
  cardiac catheterization, 114-115
  diastolic filling murmur, 78, 80
  operative risk, 2260
  during pregnancy, 2276
  pulmonary hypertension, 298
  pulsed-Doppler echocardiography, 99
  weakness, 1755
Mixed acid-base disorders, 836
Mixed angina, 194
Mixed connective tissue disease
  interstitial lung disease, 453
  neurologic manifestations, 1092, 1095
Mixed cryoglobulins, 1249
Mixed function oxidase, 2185
Mixed lymphocyte reaction, 1152
  human leukocyte antigen typing, 1120
Mixed micelle, 2221
Mixed uremic osteodystrophy, 1961, 1962, 1963
Mixed venous hemoglobin saturation, 427
Mixed venous oxygen saturation, 393, 394
MMR vaccine, 1499
Mobility assessment, 2290
Mobitz type I block, 154, 155
Mobitz type II block, 154-155, 156
Modafinil, 943
Modified Bernoulli equation, 98-99
Modified Kinyoun stain, 1476
Modified mini-mental state examination, 904
Modified sham feeding, 2003
Moduretic; *see* Amiloride
Moexipril, 325
Mold, 1183
Mole, Plate VII-7
  basal cell carcinoma *versus,* 1297
  melanoma risk, 1298
Molecular biology
  cancer, 559-564
    clonality, 559
    DNA analysis, 559-561
    fluorescence in situ hybridization, 561, 562
    leukemia, 562-563
    lung cancer, 487-488
    lymphoma, 563-564

Molecular biology—cont'd
  cardiovascular system, 49-63
    adrenergic receptors and G proteins, 56-58
    cardiac growth and hypertrophy, 55-56, 57
    cardiomyopathies, 60-62
    contractile and cytoskeletal proteins, 59-60
    DNA cloning, 52-53
    DNA code, 49-50
    DNA libraries, 54
    electrophoresis, 51-52
    gene expression and regulation, 50-51
    gene transfer, 55
    ion channels, 58-59
    isolation and digestion of DNA, 51
    lipoproteins, apolipoproteins, and
        atherosclerosis, 60
    polymerase chain reaction, 55, 56
    recombinant techniques, 51
    restriction fragment length polymorphism,
        54-55
    RNA analysis, 53-54
    sequencing, 54
    Southern, Northern, Western, and
        Southwestern blotting, 52
  globin biosynthesis, 651-652, 653
  hematopoiesis, 530-534
Molecular genetics, 1721-1724
Molecular immunology, 1110-1111
Molecular mimicry, 1121, 1146
Molecular testing
  hepatitis B virus, 2174
  hepatitis C virus, 2175-2176
  medical genetic diagnosis, 1730
Molindone, 2191
Molluscum contagiosum
  acquired immunodeficiency syndrome, 1327
  ocular involvement, 2304
Molybdenum
  functions, 2109
  recommended daily dietary allowances, 2116
Mondor's disease, 410
Monitoring
  ambulatory blood pressure, 312, 313
  blood glucose, 1860
  drug interactions, 2313
  hemodynamic, 390-396
    adult respiratory distress syndrome, 421
    aortic regurgitation, 243
    cardiac catheterization, 107-116
    cardiac tamponade, 276
    constrictive pericarditis, 277-278, 279
    end-tidal carbon dioxide, 396
    heart failure, 167
    myocardial infarction, 218, 219
    peripheral artery catheterization, 390
    pulmonary artery catheterization, 390-395
    pulse oximetry, 396
    sepsis, 1450
    shock, 180
    transcutaneous oxygen and carbon dioxide,
        396
  Holter
    aortic stenosis, 238
    arrhythmias, 134, 135
    bradyarrhythmias and atrioventricular blocks,
        153
    ischemic heart disease, 197, 198
    mitral valve prolapse, 254
    myocarditis, 263
    sudden death survivor, 189-190
    sustained monomorphic ventricular
        tachycardia, 151
    tetralogy of Fallot, 289
  mechanical ventilation, 398-399
  respiratory, 431
  sleep studies, 380
Monoamine oxidase, 930, 1826, 1827
Monoamine oxidase inhibitors
  anxiety disorders, 1035
  depression, 1037
  interference with catecholamine assays, 1740

Monoarthropathy, 1244-1245
Monoarticular arthritis, 1198-1199
Monobactams
    dosage, 1350
    effects on kidney, 868
Monoclonal antibody
    cancer treatment, 555
    evaluation of cellular immune function, 1151
    gram-negative infection, 1454
    gram-negative sepsis, 1453
    multiple myeloma, 701
Monoclonal cryoproteins, 1249, 1250
Monoclonal gammopathy
    differential diagnosis, 565
    of undetermined significance, 705-706, 1104
Monoclonal light chain deposition disease,
        862-866
Monoclonal protein
    benign monoclonal gammopathy, 705-706
    multiple myeloma, 700, 701
    serum and urine, 564-568
Monocular diplopia, 1033
Monocyte, 1109
    abnormalities, 680
    lung injury, 370
    meningitis, 1404
    sarcoidosis, 457
Monocyte-macrophage assay, 1153
Monocyte-macrophage colony-stimulating factor,
        1128
    calcium homeostasis, 1720
    osteopetrosis, 1958
Monocytoid B lymphoma, 697
Monocytosis, 591, 680
Monodeiodination, 1799
Monoethylglycinexylidide, 2143
Monogenic inheritance, 1724-1726
Monoglucuronide, 2147, 2150, 2153
Monoglutamate, 1989
Monoiodotyrosine, 1710
Monokines, 1128
Mononeuropathy, 1017
    diabetic, 1872
    nerve conduction studies, 915
    uremic patient, 1105
Mononeuropathy multiplex, 1017
Mononuclear granulomatous vasculitis, 467-469
Mononuclear phagocyte, 1127-1128, 1342
Mononucleosis
    abnormal lymphocytes in peripheral blood,
        595
    acute infectious lymphocytosis *versus,* 592
    adenopathy, 599
    atypical lymphocytes, Plate IV-5
    cervical lymphadenopathy, 597
    cytomegalovirus, 1528
    Epstein-Barr virus, 1529
    inguinal adenopathy, 1444
Monopril; *see* Fosinopril
Monosaccharides, 1987
Monosodium urate crystal, 1162
Monosodium urate crystal deposition disease,
        1277
Monounsaturated fatty acids, 1889-1890
Mood assessment tests, 903
Mood disorders, 1035-1038
    disordered thinking, 1041
Mood-stabilizing drugs, 1038
Mooren corneal ulcer, 2182
MOP-BAP regimen, 694-695
MOPP-ABV regimen, 694-695
MOPP regimen
    compromised androgen production, 1844
    Hodgkin's disease, 694-695
Morality, law and, 10
Moraxella catarrhalis
    acute laryngitis, 1393
    chronic bronchitis, 443
    normal flora, 1368
    respiratory tract infection, 1390
    sinusitis, 1183, 1394

Morgans, 1721
Moricizine, 137, 636
Morning sickness, 2029
Morphea, 1228, 1231, 1293
Morphine
    abdominal pain, 2032
    abuse, 2297
    acute stone passage, 803
    cancer pain, 580, 581
    effect on vasopressin release, 1791
    myocardial infarction, 212, 216
    pulmonary edema, 169
Morphologic index, 1649
Morquio's syndrome, 1915
Mosaicism, 1727-1728
Mosquito vector
    arbovirus infection, 1514
    Dirofilaria immitis granulomatous vasculitis,
        468
    malaria, 1671-1675
    Wuchereria bancrofti, 1699
Motilin, 1978, 1979
Motility
    barrier to infection, 1335
    diarrhea, 2050
    esophageal, 2001
        achalasia, 2021-2022
        spasm, 2022-2023
    evaluation, 2007-2008
    hypomotility
        after spinal cord injury, 1050
        intestinal pseudoobstruction, 2079
        systemic sclerosis, 1229-1230
    intestinal
        barrier to infection, 1335
        evaluation, 2007-2008
        intestinal pseudoobstruction, 2079
        irritable bowel syndrome, 2055
Motion sickness, 2025
Motor control disorders, 989-997
    chorea
        non-Huntington, 994-995
        rheumatic fever, 1257
        Sydenham's, 994-995
        systemic lupus erythematosus, 1093
    disorders with increased tone, 997
    hyperkinetic movement disorders, 993-997
    Parkinson's disease, 989-992
        depression, 1036
        reflux esophagitis, 2023
        respiratory rhythm abnormalities, 1098
    secondary, 992-993
Motor function
    alimentary tract, 1976-1980
    impaired gallbladder, 2221
    neurologic examination, 902-903
Motor nerve conduction studies, 914
Motor paralytic bladder, 1066
Motor unit action potential, 916, 1025
Mouse monoclonal antihuman T lymphocyte
        antibody, 523
Mouth
    anaerobic infection, 1616-1617
    aphthous ulcer in Crohn's disease, Plate X-10
    cancer, 723
    common problems, 2309
    hand-foot-mouth syndrome, 1489
    movement of food, 1978
    oral candidiasis, 1476, 1661, 2094-2095
    physical examination, 1999
    psoriasis, 1300
    Sjögren syndrome, 1209-1212
Moxalactam, 1354, 1355
MRI; *see* Magnetic resonance imaging
MS; *see* Multiple sclerosis
Mu heavy-chain disease, 704
Mucin, 1984
Mucin glycoproteins, 2220
Mucocele, 2309
Mucociliary elevator, 1335
Mucocutaneous leishmaniasis, 1687

Mucocutaneous lymph node syndrome, 1385
Mucocutaneous telangiectasia, 63-64
Mucoevacuants, 1183
Mucolytic agents, 430
Mucopolysaccharidoses, 576, 1912-1915
Mucopyocele, 2309
Mucormycosis, 1868
Mucosa
    absorption disorders, 2062-2063
    adrenal insufficiency, 1823
    alimentary tract, 1976
    barrier to infection, 1335
    candidiasis, 1310
    colon
        colonic diverticulum, 2089
        Kaposi's sarcoma, Plate VIII-39
        ulcerative colitis, 2073
    Crohn's disease, 2069, Plate X-6
    esophageal, 2015
    extracellular fluid volume contraction, 824
    gastric cancer, 2046
    gastritis, 2041
    jejunal, 2057
    Meckel's diverticulum, 2090
    meningitis, 1404
    small intestinal, 1986
    squamous cell carcinoma of upper digestive
        tract, 722-724
    ulceration in chronic renal failure, 784
    vitamin B$_{12}$ deficiency, 648
Mucosa-associated lymphoid tissue, 2049
Mucosa-associated lymphoid tissue lymphoma,
        697, 2038
Mucosal airway cell, 365
Mucosal biopsy
    Helicobacter pylori, 2003
    small intestine, 2008
Mucosal mast cell, 1139
Mucosal metaplasia, 2000, 2016, 2017-2018
Mucous membrane
    fever and rash, 1385
    gonococcal infection, 1582
    hemorrhagic bullae, Plate IV-10
    jaundice, 2147
    pellagra, 2107
    pemphigus vulgaris, 1293
    sexually transmitted infection, 1444
    syphilis, 1640, 1641
    thrush, 1661
Mucus
    asthma, 1185
    expectoration, 408
    gastric, 1984
Muerto Canyon virus, 1515, 1517-1518
MUGA nuclear scan, 104
Muir-Torre syndrome, 1319
Mulibrey nanism, 277
Multicentric reticulohistiocytosis, 1245, 1317,
        1318
Multifactorial inheritance, 1726-1727
Multifactorial traits, 1721
Multifocal atrial tachycardia, 144, 146
Multiinfarct dementia, 2288
Multiple cerebral infarct, 988-989
Multiple end-organ endocrine deficiency
        syndrome, 1931
Multiple endocrine neoplasia
    medullary thyroid carcinoma, 1816
    pancreatic endocrine tumor, 2244
    pheochromocytoma, 1829
    primary hyperparathyroidism, 1968
    thyroid cancer, 1814, 2005
Multiple-gated acquisition study, 104
Multiple hamartoma syndrome, 1319
Multiple jejunal diverticulosis, 2089
Multiple myeloma, 700-703
    amyloidosis with, 1316-1317
    anion gap acidosis, 836
    bleeding problems, 612
    cryoglobulinemia, 1248
    Fanconi's syndrome, 882

Multiple myeloma—cont'd
  monoclonal gammopathy of undetermined
    significance, 705
  nephrotic syndrome, 767
  neurologic aspects, 1104
  plasmacytoid lymphocytes, 595
  renal involvement, 862-863, 891-892
  streptococcal superantigen method, 743
Multiple organ dysfunction syndrome
  acute pancreatitis, 2237
  adult respiratory distress syndrome, 421-423
  streptococcal toxic shock, 1421
Multiple reentrant wavelet mechanism, 146
Multiple Risk Factor Intervention Trial, 1888
Multiple sclerosis, 1007-1009
  brain magnetic resonance imaging, 921
  brainstem auditory evoked potential, 911-912
  depression, 1036
  neurorehabilitation, 1055
  pattern-reversal visual evoked response, 911
  during pregnancy, 2282
  transverse myelitis with, 1013
Multiple sleep latency test, 943
Multiple sulfatase deficiency, 1918
Multiple system atrophy, 935, 1098
Multiple tropic hormone deficiencies, 1841
Multivalvular heart disease, 257
Mumps, 1495-1497
  culture, 1369
  hypergonadotropic hypogonadism, 1843
  impotence, 1762
  pericarditis, 272
  septic arthritis, 1255
  subacute thyroiditis, 1811
Munchausen's syndrome-by-proxy, 2027
Murine plague, 1610
Murine typhus, 1544
Murmur, 75-81
  aortic regurgitation, 241
  aortic stenosis, 236, 287
  atrial septal defect, 281
  bicuspid aortic valve, 287
  cardiac auscultation, 70
  coarctation of aorta, 286
  congenital coronary arteriovenous fistula, 292
  dilated cardiomyopathy, 263-264
  Ebstein's anomaly of tricuspid valve, 290
  hypertrophic obstructive cardiomyopathy,
    266-267
  infective endocarditis, 227
  ischemic heart disease, 197
  left atrial myxoma, 330
  mitral regurgitation, 251
  mitral stenosis, 246-247
  mitral valve prolapse, 253, 254
  myocardial infarction, 210
  patent ductus arteriosus, 285
  pulmonic regurgitation, 257
  rheumatic fever, 1256
  sinus of Valsalva fistula, 291
  tetralogy of Fallot, 289
  tricuspid stenosis, 255
  ventricular septal defect, 283
Murray Valley encephalitis, 1515
Muscarinic receptors, 56
Muscle, 1024-1030
  biopsy
    determination of weakness, 1755
    electromyography *versus,* 917
    inflammatory myopathies, 1235
  electromyography, 1025-1026
  hyperkalemia, 832
  hypokalemia, 829
  hypomagnesemia, 1942
  laboratory evaluation, 1025
  lipid metabolism disorders, 1029
  magnesium in, 1939, 1940
  muscular dystrophy
    Becker, 62
    cardiac disease, 1086
    chromosomal mapping, 61

Muscle—cont'd
  muscular dystrophy—cont'd
    Duchenne, 62, 1026, 1086
    dystrophin, 59-60
    Erb's, 1026-1027, 1028, 1086
    facioscapulohumeral, 1027
    Fukuyama, 1028
    limb girdle, 1026-1027, 1028, 1086
    molecular biology, 61-62
    oculopharyngeal, 1028
    respiratory failure, 1097
    weakness, 1754
  myalgia
    acute pharyngitis, 1393
    bacterial meningitis, 1406
    brucellosis, 1605
    common cold, 1391
    giant-cell arteritis, 304
    herpangina, 1488
    hypersensitivity pneumonitis, 461
    influenza, 1490
    Lassa fever, 1510
    Lyme disease, 1647
    myxoma, 330
  myasthenia gravis, 1020-1023
    abnormal eye movements, 1063
    autoantibodies, 1155
    cardiac abnormalities, 1087
    peripheral neuropathy *versus,* 1014
    respiratory failure, 1097
    weakness, 1754
  myoclonic epilepsy and ragged red fibers,
    996, 1029
  myoclonic seizure, 979
  myoclonus, 996
    autoantibody, 1075
    nocturnal, 944
    ocular, 1064
  myopathy, 1024-1030
    chronic ethanol abuse, 1081
    complication of chemotherapy, 1072
    Duchenne muscular dystrophy, 1026
    electromyography, 1025-1026
    facioscapulohumeral dystrophy, 1027
    inflammatory, 1234-1237
    laboratory evaluation, 1025
    limb girdle muscular dystrophy, 1026-1027,
      1028
    metabolic, 1028-1030
    mytonic dystrophy, 1027-1028
    oculopharyngeal dystrophy, 1028
    pathology, 1026
    respiratory failure, 1097
    rheumatoid arthritis, 1094, 1204
    rickets, 1949
    weakness, 1754
  myositis
    complication of influenza, 1492
    rheumatoid arthritis, 1094
    streptococcal, 1557
    vasculitis, 1225
  pathology, 1026
  phosphofructokinase deficiency, 1882
  phosphorylase deficiency, 1882
  polymyalgia rheumatica
    glucocorticoid protocol, 1263
    neurologic manifestations, 1092
Muscle cramps
  hypokalemia, 829
  malabsorption, 2057
Muscle relaxants
  anaphylaxis, 1194
  asthma, 1190
  dipyridamole stress scintigraphy, 103
  neck pain, 971
  osteoarthritis, 1268
Muscle spasm
  headache associated with, 958
  peritonitis, 1398
  tetanus, 1573-1574
Muscle strength rating, 1025

Muscle wasting
  acquired immunodeficiency syndrome,
    2095-2098
  constrictive pericarditis, 277
  hepatocellular carcinoma, 2213
  marasmus, 2101
  muscle disease, 1025
  muscle phosphorylase deficiency, 1882
Muscle weakness, 1753-1755
  acute aortic obstruction, 304
  acute lymphoblastic leukemia, 682
  aldosterone excess, 1822
  aplastic anemia, 672
  differential diagnosis, 1754
  hyperkalemia, 832
  hypernatremia, 815
  hypokalemia, 829
  hypophosphatemia, 1936
  inflammatory myopathies, 1234
  Lambert-Eaton myasthenic syndrome,
    1023-1024
  macroglobulinemia, 704
  mitral valve prolapse, 254
  muscle disease, 1024
  muscle phosphorylase deficiency, 1882
  myasthenia gravis, 1022
  myocardial infarction, 209
  peripheral neuropathy *versus,* 1014-1015
  primary hyperparathyroidism, 1966
  primary pulmonary hypertension, 294
  rheumatoid arthritis, 1204
  rickets, 1949
  sarcoidosis, 458
  spinal epidural abscess, 1418
  systemic lupus erythematosus, 1214
  thiamine deficiency, 2106
  thrombotic thrombocytopenic purpura, 615
  thyrotoxicosis, 1805
  tropical spastic paraparesis, 1532
Muscular dystrophy
  Becker, 62
  cardiac disease, 1086
  chromosomal mapping, 61
  Duchenne, 62, 1026, 1086
  dystrophin, 59-60
  Erb's, 1026-1027, 1028, 1086
  Fukuyama, 1028
  limb girdle, 1026-1027, 1028, 1086
  molecular biology, 61-62
  respiratory failure, 1097
  weakness, 1754
Muscular subaortic stenosis, 265
Musculocutaneous nerve mononeuropathy, 1017
Musculoskeletal system
  actinomycosis, 1665
  biochemical markers of bone turnover, 1746
  brucellosis, 1605-1606
  chronic renal failure, 785-786
  congenital total lipodystrophy, 1900
  diagnostic approach, 1744-1748
  effects of hormones, 1720
  features of malabsorption, 2058
  fibrous dysplasia, 1960-1961
  functions, 1714-1715
  hyperparathyroidism, 1965-1971
    arthropathy, 1246
    calcium pyrophosphate dihydrate deposition
      disease, 1279
    chronic renal failure, 785
    diagnosis, 1967-1969
    humoral hypercalcemia of malignancy
      versus, 1973-1974
    hypermagnesemia, 1943
    kidney stone formation, 798
    mixed uremic osteodystrophy, 1963
    osteomalacia, 1950
    pathology and etiology, 1965-1966
    during pregnancy, 2273
    prevalence, 1965, 1966
    renal osteodystrophy, 1961
    renal transplant recipient, 795

Musculoskeletal system—cont'd
  hyperparathyroidism—cont'd
    renal wasting of phosphate, 1935
    symptoms and signs, 1966-1967
    treatment, 1969-1971
  imaging evaluation of arthritis, 1164-1171,
    1172
  metastatic disease, 1971-1974
  natural history, 1715-1716
  nephrotic syndrome, 767
  neurofibromatosis, 1921
  nontuberculous mycobacterial infection, 1639
  osteomalacia, 1949-1955
    after parathyroidectomy, 1965
    bone biopsy, 1747
    chronic hypophosphatemia, 1936
    chronic renal failure, 785
    proximal renal tubular acidosis, 837
    renal osteodystrophy, 1961
    vitamin D deficiency, 2106
    vitamin D metabolism, 1719
    X-linked hypophosphatemic rickets, 880
  osteopetrosis, 1958-1959
  osteoporosis, 1944-1949
    bone biopsy, 1747
    brucellosis, 1606
    calcitonin therapy, 1719
    glucocorticoid-induced, 1263
    heparin, 635
    menopause, 2271
    multiple myeloma, 864
    reduction in bone density, 1165
    rheumatoid arthritis, 1205
  Paget's disease, 1955-1958
  primary hyperparathyroidism, 1966
  renal osteodystrophy, 1961-1965
  skeletal tuberculosis, 1437, 1634, 1635
  spinal cord injury, 1050-1051
  Staphylococcus aureus, 1549
  syphilis, 1641
  systemic lupus erythematosus, 1214
  tuberculosis, 1634, 1635
Mushroom poisoning, 2188
Mushroom worker's lung, 460
Mutant factor V, 609
Mutism, 977, 1032
Myalgia
  acute pharyngitis, 1393
  bacterial meningitis, 1406
  brucellosis, 1605
  common cold, 1391
  giant-cell arteritis, 304
  herpangina, 1488
  hypersensitivity pneumonitis, 461
  influenza, 1490
  Lassa fever, 1510
  Lyme disease, 1647
  myxoma, 330
Myasthenia gravis, 1020-1023
  abnormal eye movements, 1063
  autoantibodies, 1155
  cardiac abnormalities, 1087
  peripheral neuropathy *versus,* 1014
  respiratory failure, 1097
  weakness, 1754
Myasthenic crisis, 1022
Myasthenic syndrome, 489
Myc gene
  Burkitt translocations, 544
  lung cancer, 487
  non-Hodgkin's lymphoma, 697
Mycetoma, 447, 1659-1660
Mycobacterial infection
  arthritis, 1254-1255
  compromised host, 1388
  nontuberculous infections, 1638-1639
  tuberculosis, 1625-1638
    acquired immunodeficiency syndrome,
      1472, 1473, 1474
    after lung transplantation, 520

Mycobacterial infection—cont'd
  tuberculosis—cont'd
    characteristics of *Mycobacterium
      tuberculosis,* 1625-1626
    chemotherapy, 1630-1633
    clinical spectrum, 1628
    dysuria, 762
    empyema, 507
    epidemiology, 1626-1627
    extrapulmonary, 1633-1637
    fever of unknown origin, 1376
    hypercalcemia, 1928
    joint disease, 1254
    pathogenesis, 1627
    pericarditis, 272
    prevention, 1637-1638
    prostate, 1463
    public health considerations, 1638
    pulmonary, 1628-1630
    renal dysfunction, 892-893
    silicosis-related, 475
    skeletal, 1437
    weight loss, 1750
Mycobacterium avium-intracellulare complex,
  1638-1639
  acid-fast stain, Plate VIII-36
  acquired immunodeficiency syndrome, 1329,
    1473-1474, 2098
Mycobacterium fortuitum, 1638
Mycobacterium haemophilum, 1329
Mycobacterium kansasii, 1638-1639
Mycobacterium leprae, 1648-1651
Mycobacterium marinum, 1423, Plate VIII-31
Mycobacterium scrofulaceum, 1638-1639
Mycobacterium tuberculosis, 1625-1638
  acquired immunodeficiency syndrome, 1472,
    1473, 1474, 1477
  after lung transplantation, 518, 520
  characteristics, 1625-1626
  chemotherapy, 1630-1633
  clinical spectrum, 1628
  dysuria, 762
  empyema, 507
  epidemiology, 1437
  extrapulmonary tuberculosis, 1633-1637
  fever of unknown origin, 1376
  hypercalcemia, 1928
  joint disease, 1254
  meningitis, 1478
  mononuclear phagocytes, 1342
  nosocomial infection, 1363
  pathogenesis, 1627
  pericarditis, 272
  prevention, 1637-1638
  primary peritonitis, 1396
  prostate, 1463
  public health considerations, 1638
  pulmonary tuberculosis, 1628-1630
  renal dysfunction, 892-893
  septic arthritis, 1251
  silicosis-related, 475
  skeletal tuberculosis, 1437
  weight loss, 1750
Mycophenolate mofetil
  bronchiolitis obliterans syndrome, 523
  lung transplantation, 516
  renal transplantation, 793
Mycoplasma, 1370, 1538-1541
  normal flora, 1368
Mycoplasma fermentans, 1541
Mycoplasma hominis, 2280
Mycoplasma penetrans, 1541
Mycoplasma pirum, 1541
Mycoplasma pneumoniae, 1538-1541
  cold agglutinin disease, 669, 670
  persistent cough, 407
  pleural effusion, 507
Mycoses, 1651-1660
  acquired immunodeficiency syndrome, 1328,
    1329
  Actinomyces, 1664-1665

Mycoses—cont'd
  antifungal therapy, 1652-1654
  arthritis, 1254-1255
  aspergillosis, 1658-1659
  blastomycosis, 1657
  candidiasis, 1310-1312, 1660-1664
    acquired immunodeficiency syndrome,
      1328, 1476, 2094
    after renal transplantation, 794
    compromised host, 1388
    continuous ambulatory peritoneal
      dialysis-related peritonitis, 2248
    diabetic patient, 1323
    drug-induced infection, 1313
    endocarditis, 226
    esophageal infection, 2019-2020
    fever, 1383, 1387
    gastric infection, 2043
    genital lesions, 1444
    lung transplantation, 517, 518, 519-520
    meningitis, 1404, 1409
    odynophagia, 1998
    peritonitis, 1397
    rash, 1383
    serodiagnosis, 1653
    Sjögren syndrome, 1212
    urinary tract infection, 1457
    vaginitis, 762
    vulvovaginal infection, 1442
  chromoblastomycosis and mycetoma,
    1659-1660
  coccidioidomycosis, 1655-1657
  Cryptococcus neoformans, 1667-1670
  culture, 1370
  diagnosis, 1652, 1653
  differential diagnosis of fever and rash, 1384
  endocarditis, 226
  fever, 1387
  fever of unknown origin, 1377
  histoplasmosis, 1654-1655
  meningitis, 1404
  nocardiosis, 1665-1666
  nosocomial, 1362
  osteomyelitis, 1437
  paracoccidioidomycosis, 1657
  penicilliosis, 1658
  phaeohyphomycosis, 1660
  pleural effusion, 507
  posttransplant
    heart, 342
    kidney, 794
    lung, 519-520
    stem cell, 578
  sporotrichosis, 1658
  superficial, 1307-1312
    candidiasis, 1310-1312
    clinical presentation, 1308-1309
    dermatophyte infection, 1307-1308
    diagnostic procedures, 1309
    Pityrosporum infection, 1309-1310
  uremic patient, 784
  urinary tract, 1462
  zygomycetes, 1659
Mycosis fungoides, 1331-1332
Mycotic aneurysm, 299, 300
Mydriasis, 932-933
Myelin antibody, 1158
Myelin body, 878
Myelitis, 1011
Myeloblast, 532
  acute myelogenous leukemia, 689, 690
  leukemic, Plate IV-6
Myelocyte, 532
Myelodysplasia, 611, 675-676
Myelodysplastic sideroblastic anemia, 645
Myelodysplastic syndromes, 675-676, 690-691
Myelofibrosis, 676-677
  acute myelogenous leukemia, 677
  megakaryocytic hypoplasia, 614
  neutrophilic leukocytosis, 591
  polycythemia vera, 688

Myelography, 924, 926, 1012
Myeloid leukemia, 559
Myeloid precursor, 530
Myeloma
  bone marrow plasma cell, Plate IV-8
  hypercalcemia of malignancy, 1973
  incidence and death rates, 550
  multiple, 700-703
    amyloidosis with, 1316-1317
    anion gap acidosis, 836
    bleeding problems, 612
    cryoglobulinemia, 1248
    Fanconi's syndrome, 882
    monoclonal gammopathy of undetermined
      significance, 705
    nephrotic syndrome, 767
    neurologic aspects, 1104
    plasmacytoid lymphocytes, 595
    renal involvement, 862-863, 891-892
    streptococcal superantigen method, 743
  multiple organ dysfunction syndrome *versus,*
    422
  osteosclerotic, 703
  serum calcium concentration, 1744
Myelomatosis, 700-703
Myelopathy, 1011-1014
  complication of chemotherapy, 1072
  human T-cell leukemia virus-associated, 1532
  tropical spastic paraparesis, 1532
Myeloperoxidase
  deficiency, 1341
  vasculitis, 1218
Myelopoiesis, 532, 593
Myeloproliferative disorders, 685-691
  acute myelogenous leukemia, 689-690, 691
  bleeding and thrombosis, 611
  chronic, 686
  essential thrombocytopenia, 687-688
  immature granulocytes, 594
  myelodysplastic syndromes, 690-691
  myelogenous leukemia, 686-687
  neutrophilic leukocytosis, 591
  polycythemia vera, 688
Myelosuppression
  monocytosis, 591
  stem cell transplantation, 577-578
Myo-D transcription factor, 51
Myoadenylate deaminase deficiency, 1029
Myocardial contractility, 111-113
  cardiogenic shock, 179
Myocardial contrast echocardiography, 100
Myocardial contusion, 332
Myocardial depressant substance, 1448
Myocardial infarction, 209-225
  accelerated atrioventricular junctional rhythm,
    144
  acute cholecystitis *versus,* 2228
  acute mitral regurgitation, 219, 220
  adjunctive therapy, 215-218
  angioplasty, 214-215
  angiotensin-converting enzyme inhibitors, 172
  anomalous origin of left coronary artery, 292
  anticoagulant therapy, 639
  aortic dissection, 300
  atrioventricular block, 156
  beta-blockers, 138
  during cardiac catheterization, 108
  cardiac imaging, 212
  cardiogenic shock, 176, 177
  chest pain, 127
  clinical presentation, 209-211
  complete heart block, 180
  congenital abnormalities of coronary arteries,
    292
  coronary angioplasty, 121-122
  during coronary artery bypass graft, 185, 206
  echocardiography, 100
  electrical complications, 222-224
  electrocardiography, 88-89, 211
  incidence, 209

Myocardial infarction—cont'd
  infarct expansion and left ventricular
    aneurysm, 221
  laboratory tests, 211-212
  left ventricular failure, 218-219
  left ventricular thrombus, 221, 222, 638
  macrovascular disease, 1868
  mechanical complications, 219
  mitral regurgitation, 250
  myocardial rupture, 219, 220
  neurologic aspects, 1089
  nuclear cardiology techniques, 101
  PAMI trial, 122
  pathophysiology, 209, 210
  percutaneous transluminal coronary
    angioplasty *versus* coronary artery
    bypass graft, 118
  pericarditis, 221-222, 273
  premature ventricular contractions, 149
  preoperative, 2257
  radionuclide angiography, 105
  rehabilitation and preventive cardiology, 224
  right ventricular infarction, 220-221
  risk stratification, 224
  sepsis *versus,* 1451
  shock, 176, 177, 180
  stent, 119
  sustained monomorphic ventricular
    tachycardia, 151
  thrombolytic therapy, 212-214
  ventricular fibrillation, 153
  ventricular septal rupture, 219-220
  ventricular tachycardia, 180
Myocardial ischemia, 192-208
  anomalous origin of left coronary artery, 292
  antianginal therapy, 205
  aortic dissection, 300
  beta-adrenergic blockers, 201-203
  calcium channel blockers, 203-205
  clinical manifestations, 195-197
  congenital abnormalities of coronary arteries,
    291-292
  coronary angioplasty and revascularization,
    205-207
  etiology, 192, 193
  during exercise, 91
  laboratory studies, 197-200
  myocardial infarction, 209
  nitroglycerin and nitrates, 200-201, 202
  pathophysiology, 192-195
  physical examination, 197
  prognosis, 208
  technetium-99m sestamibi imaging, 102-103
  therapeutic approaches, 207-208
Myocardial oxygen consumption, 48-49
  exercise stress testing, 91
Myocardial oxygen demand
  beta-adrenergic blockers, 201-202
  chest pain, 126
  ischemic heart disease-193, 192
  myocardial infarction, 212
Myocardial oxygen supply
  aortic stenosis, 236
  determinants, 193-195
Myocardial pain, 505
Myocardial perfusion imaging, 101-104
Myocardial perfusion scintigraphy
  ischemic heart disease, 198-199
  mitral valve prolapse, 254
Myocarditis, 262-263
  acquired immunodeficiency syndrome, 333
  diphtheria, 1566
  Neisseria meningitidis, 1579
Myocardium
  aortic regurgitation, 239
  cardiac cycle, 36
  coronary blood flow, 48
  metastatic disease, 331
  myocardial energy metabolism, 40
  myopericarditis, 1489-1490
  positron emission tomography, 105-106

Myocardium—cont'd
  revascularization, 205-206
  rupture, 177-178, 219, 220
  systemic lupus erythematosus, 1215
Myoclonic epilepsy and ragged red fibers, 996,
  1029
Myoclonic seizure, 979
Myoclonus, 996
  autoantibody, 1075
  ocular, 1064
Myocyte
  contraction, 36
  myocardial energy metabolism, 40
Myofibril, 38, 265
Myogenic tone, 47-48
Myoglobin
  myocardial infarction, 211
  proteinuria, 760
  urinalysis, 744
Myoglobinuria
  chemical exposure, 867-868
  toxic shock syndrome, 1421
Myoma, mesenteric, 2251
Myonecrosis, 1574-1576
Myopathy, 1024-1030
  chronic ethanol abuse, 1081
  complication of chemotherapy, 1072
  Duchenne muscular dystrophy, 1026
  electromyography, 1025-1026
  facioscapulohumeral dystrophy, 1027
  inflammatory, 1234-1237
  laboratory evaluation, 1025
  limb girdle muscular dystrophy, 1026-1027,
    1028
  metabolic, 1028-1030
  mytonic dystrophy, 1027-1028
  oculopharyngeal dystrophy, 1028
  pathology, 1026
  respiratory failure, 1097
  rheumatoid arthritis, 1094, 1204
  rickets, 1949
  weakness, 1754
Myopericarditis, 1489-1490
Myophosphorylase deficiency, 1025, 1029
Myoplasmic calcium spike, 38
Myosin, 39
Myosin-binding protein, 61
Myosin heavy chain, 59
Myosin heavy chain gene expression, 50
Myosin light chain, 59
Myositis
  complication of influenza, 1492
  rheumatoid arthritis, 1094
  streptococcal, 1557
  vasculitis, 1225
Myotonia congenita, 1028, 1086
Myotonic dystrophy, 1843
Myotonic muscular dystrophy, 1027-1028
  heart failure, 1086
  molecular biology, 62
Mysoline; *see* Primidone
Myxedema
  electrocardiographic abnormalities, 90
  general appearance, 63
  hypothyroidism, 1809
  hypoventilation, 356
  pericarditis with effusion, 273
Myxedema coma, 1810-1811
Myxoma, 329, 330
  diastolic murmur, 78
  fever of unknown origin, 1377
Myxomatous proliferation of mitral leaflet tissue,
  253
Myxovirus, 1390

N

N-acetyl paraquinone, 2311
N-acetylcysteine
  cystic fibrosis, 482
  secretion clearance and lung expansion, 430

N-acetylglucosamine, 1911
N-acetylglutamate, 1906
N-aspartyl-beta-glucosaminidase deficiency, 1917
N-nucleotide addition, 1111
N region, 1124
Nabilone, 2027
Nabumetone, 1259
NACI study, 122
NADH; *see* Reduced nicotinamide-adenine
    dinucleotide
Nadolol
    bleeding varices, 2168
    hypertension, 325
    properties, 203
Naegleria, 1683-1684
Nafcillin, 1352
    bacterial meningitis, 1411
    brain abscess, 1416
    coagulase-negative staphylococcal infection,
        1552
    dosage, 1350
    infective endocarditis, 231
    interference with oral anticoagulants, 636
    respiratory exacerbations in cystic fibrosis,
        483
    septic arthritis, 1253
    staphylococcal scalded-skin syndrome, 1421
    Staphylococcus aureus meningitis, 1410
    subdural empyema, 1418
Nail
    candidal paronychia, 1662
    nail-patella syndrome, 877
    psoriasis, 1300, 1301
    psoriatic nail disease, 1241
    tinea unguium, 1308
Nail-patella syndrome, 877
Nalidixic acid, 1359
    dosage, 1350
    hemolysis in glucose-6-phosphate
        dehydrogenase deficiency, 663
    interference with catecholamine assays, 1740
Naloxone
    comatose patient, 950
    gram-negative sepsis, 1453
    morphine reversal, 216
Naltrexone, 2296
Naphthalene, 663
Naproxen, 1259
    gouty arthritis, 1274
    hepatic injury, 2191
    human cytochrome P450 isoforms, 2312
    interference with oral anticoagulants, 636
Narcolepsy, 942-943, 981
Narcotic analgesics
    abdominal pain, 2032
    abuse, 2297
    acute intermittent porphyria, 1926
    acute pancreatitis, 2237
    acute stone passage, 803
    cancer pain, 580-581
    chronic pancreatitis, 2240
    cough, 409
    cytochrome P450 2D6-mediated conversion,
        2311
    effect on vasopressin release, 1791
    gastrointestinal motility, 1978
    human cytochrome P450 isoforms, 2312
    myocardial infarction, 212, 216
    pancreatic cancer, 2244
    pulmonary edema, 169
    pulmonary toxicity, 479
    restless legs syndrome, 944
    rheumatic disease, 1260
    sedation during gastrointestinal endoscopy,
        1994
    status migrainosus, 962
Nasal allergen challenge, 1154
Nasal congestion, 1181, 1391
Nasal continuous positive airway pressure,
    527-528

Nasal discharge
    common cold, 1391
    sinusitis, 1394, 2308
Nasal mastocytosis, 1181
Nasal mucosa, 1180-1185
Nasal obstruction, 2308
Nasal pack, 2308
Nasal polyp, 482, 1183, 2308
Nasal prongs, 415, 428
Nasal septal deviation, 2308
Nasal spray abuse, 2308
NASH; *see* Nonalcoholic steatohepatitis
Nasogastric intubation
    acute pancreatitis, 2237
    gastrointestinal bleeding, 2010
    intestinal obstruction, 2078
Nasogastric suctioning, 839
Nasopharyngitis-sinusitis, 1183
Nasopharynx
    bacterial meningitis, 1404
    cancer, 492, 723
    meningococcal infections, 1579
    nasopharyngitis-sinusitis, 1183
    Pasteurella, 1609
National Acute Spinal Cord Injury Study II,
    1048
National Committee on Quality Assurance, 19,
    33-34
National Health and Nutrition Examination
    Survey, 312
National neurofibromatosis foundation, 1922
National tuberous sclerosis association, 1922
Native valve endocarditis, 226, 230, 1550
Natriuretic hormone
    hypertension, 317-318
    sodium retention in cirrhosis, 819-820
Natriuretic peptides, 738
Natural immunity, 1129-1130
Natural killer cell, 1109
    cell-mediated immunity, 1127
    function assessment, 1152-1153
Nausea, 2025-2029
    acquired immunodeficiency syndrome, 2095
    acute cholecystitis, 2227
    acute hyponatremia, 811
    acute pancreatitis, 2234
    acute viral hepatitis, 2177
    appendicitis, 2092
    autonomic failure, 935
    biliary colic, 2225
    bubonic plague, 1610
    calcium channel blocker-induced, 205
    chemotherapy-induced, 581-582
    chronic hepatitis, 2180
    chronic renal failure, 784
    constrictive pericarditis, 277
    hepatitis A virus, 2173
    hepatocellular carcinoma, 2213
    intestinal obstruction, 2077
    intrahepatic cholangiocarcinoma, 2214
    mesenteric panniculitis, 2251
    myocardial infarction, 209
    Norwalk virus, 1522
    pancreatic abscess, 1399
    peptic ulcer, 2037
    peritoneal mesenteric and omental diseases,
        2248
    peritonitis, 1398
    pheochromocytoma, 1829
    Rocky Mountain spotted fever, 1543
    solitary liver cyst, 2111
    thrombotic thrombocytopenic purpura, 615
    vasopressin stimulation, 1790
NBTE; *see* Nonbacterial thrombotic endocarditis
Nebulin, 59
Nebulized medications, 430-431
Nebulizer, 431, 1189-1190
Necator americanus, 1698
Neck
    acute inflammation of salivary glands, 2316
    adenopathy, 2309-2310

Neck—cont'd
    benign cyst, 2310
    deep neck infections, 2309
    head and neck cancer, 722-724, 2316
        carcinoma of unknown origin, 732
        radiation-induced, 1816-1817
    hypoparathyroidism after surgery, 1931
Neck pain, 968-971, 1392-1393
    herpangina, 1488-1489
    Lassa fever, 1510
    Mycoplasma pneumoniae pneumonia, 1539
    rheumatic fever, 1256
    scarlet fever, 1421
    spontaneous pneumomediastinum, 514
    subacute thyroiditis, 1811
Necrobiosis lipoidica diabeticorum, 1323, Plate
    VII-16
Necrobiotic xanthogranuloma, 1317, 1318
Necrolytic migratory erythema, 1317, 1318
Necrosectomy, 2237
Necrosis
    acute pancreatitis, 2234
    acute toxic hepatic injury, 2187
    alcoholic liver disease, 2195
    avascular, 1214
    chronic hepatitis, 2179
    coumarin-induced, 636
    gastroesophageal reflux, 2015
    intestinal obstruction, 2078
    ischemic heart disease, 192
    mesenteric ischemia, 2087
    myocardial contusion, 332
    myocardial infarction, 209
Necrotizing eosinophilic granuloma, 466-467
Necrotizing fasciitis, 1422, 1557
Necrotizing lymphadenitis, 1378
Necrotizing sarcoid granulomatosis, 470
Necrotizing soft tissue infections, 1422-1425
Necrotizing vasculitis, 1219-1220
    leprosy, 1650
    postcoarctation syndrome, 287
Nedocromil, 1191, 1192
Needle aspiration, 383, 384
    bone, 1747
    dilated cardiomyopathy, 263
    kidney, 748
    lymph node, 600
    necrotizing fasciitis, 1422
    peritonsillar abscess, 2306
    transthoracic, 385
    tuberculous pleurisy, 507
Needle electromyography, 916-917
Needle pericardiocentesis, 278
Needle stick
    hepatitis B, 2174
    hepatitis C, 2175
Neer's sign, 1197
Nefazodone, 1037
Negative free water clearance, 739
Negative nitrogen balance, 786
Negative predictive value, 7-8
Negative selection, 1112, 1113
Negri body, 1505, Plate VIII-43
Neisseria gonorrhoeae, 1581-1585
    beta-lactamases, 1345
    complement deficiencies, 1179
    diarrhea, 1476
    immunoglobulin A, 1337
    peritonitis, 2248
    primary peritonitis, 1396
    septic arthritis, 1251
    urethritis, 1455
Neisseria meningitidis, 1339, 1578-1581
    immunoglobulin A, 1337
    meningitis, 1402-1403
NEL; *see* Nelfinavir
Nelfinavir, 1474
Nematode
    intestinal, 1696
    tissue, 1699-1702
    with tissue migratory phases, 1698-1699

Neoadjuvant chemotherapy, 554
Neointimal formation, 122
Neologisms, 975, 976
Neomycin, 1356
  auditory effects, 972
  cholesterol-absorption blocker, 1890-1891
  effects on kidney, 868
  hepatic encephalopathy, 2162-2163
Neonatal alloimmune thrombocytopenia, 616
Neonatal lupus, 2279
Neonatal osteomyelitis, 1433
Neoplasm
  adrenal, 1825-1826
  benign
    breast, 708
    bronchial adenoma, 491-492
    cardiac, 329
    cavernous hemangioma, 2215-2216
    colon, 2086
    esophageal, 2023
    gastric, 2050
    small bowel, 2082
    thyroid, 1813-1814
  brain
    computed tomography, 920
    dementia, 988
    depression, 1037
    headache, 960
    magnetic resonance imaging, 923
    neurooncology, 1067-1070
    seizure, 980
    tuberous sclerosis, 1922
  breast, 708
  bronchial adenoma, 491-492
  cardiac, 329-332
  colon, 2082-2086
  cytogenetics, 731
  esophageal, 2023-2024
  fever of unknown origin, 1377
  formation, 540-549
    environmental agents, 548-549
    genetic stability, 549
    multistep genetic pathway, 547-548
    oncogenes, 541-545
    tumor suppressor genes, 545-547
  gastric, 2045-2050
  hepatic, 2212-2217
  Hodgkin's disease, 691-695
  hypercalcemia of malignancy, 1972-1974
  lung, 486-492
  mediastinal, 512-513
  membranous nephropathy with, 854
  mesenteric, 2251-2252
  neurofibromatosis, 1920-1921
  non-Hodgkin's lymphoma, 695-700
  ovarian, 716, 1838
  pancreatic
    endocrine, 2244-2246
    exocrine, 2242-2244
    fasting hypoglycemia, 1876
    islet cell tumor, 1928
    pancreatic polypeptide secreting tumor, 2244
  peritoneal, 2249
  pheochromocytoma, 1828-1831
    autonomic hyperactivity, 935
    hypercalcemia, 1928
    hypertension, 322, 1829-1830
    neurofibromatosis, 1921
    weight loss, 1749
  pituitary, 1781-1782
    Cushing's disease, 1786-1787
    gonadotropin-secreting, 1787
    growth hormone-secreting, 1782-1786
    hyperprolactinemia, 1785
    thyroid-stimulating hormone-secreting, 1787
    vasopressin deficiency, 1795
  poorly differentiated carcinoma, 732
  radiation sensitivity of, 553
  renal cell carcinoma, 898-899
  renin-secreting, 321, 829

Neoplasm—cont'd
  response to drug treatment, 552
  retroperitoneal, 2250-2251
  small intestine, 2080-2081
  spinal, 1013
  testicular, 720
    gynecomastia, 1764, 1765
    impotence, 1762
  von Hippel-Lindau disease, 1922
  Wilms' tumor, 829, 899
    curability with chemotherapy, 552
    hypokalemia, 829
Neoplastic disease
  fever of unknown origin, 1377
  immune complexes, 1149
  interstitial lung disease, 452
  paraneoplastic pemphigus, 1295
  paraneoplastic syndromes, 582-583
    antibodies, 1158
    arthropathy, 1247
    dementia, 987
    dermatoses, 1316-1319
    lung cancer, 488-489
    myelopathy, 1013
  pericarditis, 272
Neovascularization
  central retinal vein occlusions, 2304
  diabetic retinopathy, 1870, Plate IX-4
  optic nerve, Plate XI-8
Nephelometric immunoassay, 1147
Nephrectomy, 898
Nephritic syndrome
  anti-neutrophil cytoplasmic antibodies-positive glomerulonephritis, 848
  essential mixed cryoglobulinemia, 857
  immunoglobulin A nephropathy, 845
  poststreptococcal glomerulonephritis, 844
  rapidly progressive glomerulonephritis, 846
Nephritis
  acute interstitial, 889-890
  alveolar hemorrhage, 454
  associated with visceral abscess, 844
  imaging studies, 754
  radiation, 868
  sporadic streptococcal pharyngitis, 844
  thrombocytopenia, 603
Nephrocalcin, 797
Nephrogenic diabetes insipidus, 815, 883-884, 1793, 1795
Nephrolithiasis, 796-805
  calcium-containing stones, 797-799
  Crohn's disease, 2075
  cystine stones, 799-800
  differential diagnosis, 800
  laboratory and diagnostic testing, 800, 801, 802
  management, 803-805
  physiology and pathophysiology, 797
  struvite stones, 799
  uric acid stones, 799
Nephron
  light chain nephrotoxicity, 863
  loss in chronic renal failure, 777-778
  potassium transport, 741
  renal concentrating and diluting mechanisms, 739
Nephropathy
  acquired immunodeficiency syndrome, 853
  analgesic, 890
  chronic tubulointerstitial, 890-892
  diabetic, 859-862, 1870
    microalbuminuria, 743, 761
    nephrotic syndrome, 767
  drug- and chemical-induced, 866-871
  glomerular and interstitial, 876-878
  hematuria, 757
  heroin, 853
  immunoglobulin A, 845
  membranous, 853-854
  pigment, 867-868
  thin basement membrane, 877
  urate, 1273

Nephrotic proteinuria, 764
Nephrotic syndrome, 765-768
  acquired immunodeficiency syndrome nephropathy, 853
  adverse reaction to nonsteroidal antiinflammatory agents, 853
  amyloidosis, 1282-1283
  clinical manifestations and pathophysiology, 765-766
  complications, 766-767
  diagnosis and management, 767
  familial Mediterranean fever, 877
  Fanconi's syndrome, 882
  focal glomerular sclerosis, 851-852
  glycosuria, 879
  Henoch-Schönlein purpura, 857
  heroin nephropathy, 853
  hypercholesterolemia, 1894
  hyponatremia, 812
  immunofixation, 568
  lipiduria, 745
  lipodystrophy, 877
  membranoproliferative glomerulonephritis, 854-855
  membranous nephropathy, 853-854
  mesangial proliferative disease, 851
  minimal change disease, 849-851
  operative risk, 2263
  primary peritonitis, 1396
  sodium balance dysfunction, 820-821
  transudative pleural effusion, 507
Nephrotomogram, 751
Nephrotoxicity, 866-871
  chemotherapeutic agents, 584
  cyclosporin A, 794
  diagnostic and therapeutic agents, 868-871
  environmental and occupational agents, 866-868
Nerve block, 581
Nerve compression, 700
Nerve conduction studies, 914-917
  low back pain, 966
  neck pain, 969
Nervous system
  acquired immunodeficiency syndrome, 1477
  acute intermittent porphyria, 1926
  acute meningitis, 1402
  acute respiratory failure, 413-414
  alimentary motor function, 1977-1978
  antirheumatic drug toxicity, 1261
  chronic renal failure, 784
  cocaine intoxication, 2297
  coccidioidomycosis, 1656
  complications of systemic cancer, 1070-1074
  control of food intake, 2099
  cryptococcosis, 1667-1668
  features of malabsorption, 2058
  glucose requirements, 1874
  hormonal regulation, 1075-1078
  infective endocarditis, 228
  Krabbe's disease, 1918
  lung cancer, 726
  lymphoma, 1477
  malignant lymphoma, 697
  measles complications, 1498
  metastatic lung cancer, 489
  mumps, 1496
  neurofibromatosis, 1920
  peripheral nervous system *versus,* 1014
  polyneuritis
    diphtheria, 1566
    thiamine deficiency, 2106
  polyneuropathy, 1017-1020
    critical-illness, 1085
    diabetes mellitus, 1871-1872
    nerve conduction studies, 915
  polyradiculopathy, 1017
  primary angiitis, 1225
  primary central nervous system lymphoma, 1069
  regulation of gastric acid secretion, 1981

Nervous system—cont'd
  respiratory muscle control, 358
  sarcoidosis, 458
  spinal cord injury, 1051-1052
  syphilis, 1641
  toxoplasmosis, 1677
  Whipple's disease, 2064
Nervous system infection
  actinomycosis, 1665
  anaerobic bacteria, 1617
  brain abscess, 1413-1416
  brucellosis, 1606
  cryptococcosis, 1669
  depression, 1037
  febrile compromised patient, 1387
  intracranial epidural abscess, 1418
  intracranial subdural empyema, 1416-1418
  meningitis, 1402-1413
    clinical manifestations, 1406, 1407
    differential diagnosis, 1408-1409
    epidemiology and etiology, 1402-1404
    fever, 1385, 1387
    headache, 960
    laboratory investigation, 1406-1408
    OKT3-induced, 1090
    pathogenesis and pathophysiology,
      1404-1406
    prognosis, 1413
    rash, 1385
    respiratory alkalosis, 355
    treatment, 1409-1413
  Naegleria fowleri, 1684
  spinal epidural abscess, 1418-1419
  tuberculosis, 1636
Netilmicin
  dosage, 1349
  effects on kidney, 868
  enterococci resistance, 1561
Neural tube defects
  diabetic mother, 2272
  maternal megaloblastic anemia, 647
Neuralgia
  glossopharyngeal, 953
  trigeminal, 962-963
Neurally mediated syncope, 952-954
Neuritic leprosy, 1650
Neuritis
  diphtheria, 1566
  optic, 1060
  pyridoxine deficiency, 2107
  rheumatoid arthritis, 1094
  traumatic intercostal, 410
Neuroanatomy, 930, 931, 932
Neuroarthropathy, 1168-1169
Neurocardiology, 1086-1091
Neurochemistry, 930-931, 933
Neurocirculatory asthenia, 131
Neuroendocrine secretion, 1076
Neuroendocrine system
  central nervous system involvement, 1075
  heart failure, 160, 161, 162, 163
Neuroendocrine tumor, pancreatic, 2245
Neuroendocrinology, 1075-1078
Neurofibroma, 547
  neurofibromatosis, 1920
  small bowel, 2082
Neurofibromatosis, 1726, 1920-1922
Neurofibromin, 1921
Neurogastroenterology, 1100-1102
Neurogenic bladder, 768
Neurogenic diabetes insipidus, 1793-1795
Neurogenic pulmonary edema, 1099-1100
Neurogenic respiratory failure, 1096-1097
Neurogenic shock, 176, 180
Neurogenic tumor, mediastinal, 513
Neuroglycopenia, 2244
Neurohematology, 1103-1105
Neurohepatology, 1102-1103
Neurohormonal hypothesis of heart failure, 161
Neurohumoral modulation of ventricular
      function, 45-46

Neurohypophyseal hormones, 1077
Neurohypophysis, 1788-1797
  anatomy, 1788
  biochemistry, 1788-1789
  diabetes insipidus, 1793-1795
  disorders, 1795-1797
  physiology, 1789-1793
  testing, 1737-1738
Neurokinin A, 353
Neuroleptics
  cancer pain, 580
  disordered thinking, 1041
  schizophrenia, 1042
Neurologic complications
  acute renal failure, 773
  brain abscess, 1414
  cerebrotendinous xanthomatosis, 1898
  chemotherapy, 1072
  coccidioidomycosis, 1657
  critical medical illness, 1085
  fall risk, 2290
  hepatic encephalopathy, 2160-2161
  hypothyroidism, 1809
  infective endocarditis, 228
  megaloblastic anemia, 647
  pituitary adenoma, 1781-1782
  polyarteritis nodosa, 1220
  porphyrias, 1925
  spinal epidural abscess, 1418
  stroke, 1001
  syphilis, 1641
  systemic cancer, 1070-1074
  thrombotic thrombocytopenic purpura, 615
Neurologic disorders
  abnormal swallowing, 1998
  anxiety, 1034-1035
  arthropathy, 1247
  back pain, 963-971
    low back pain, 963-968
    neck, 968-971
    neuronal disease, 1017
  botulism, 1570-1572
  brain death criteria, 951
  cognitive failure dementia, 985-989
  coma, 947-950, 1081-1086
    acute hyponatremia, 811
    electroencephalography, 907, 909
    Jolliffe's disease, 1101
  demyelinating diseases, 1007-1011
    acute disseminated encephalomyelitis, 1010
    acute hemorrhagic leukoencephalopathy,
      1010
    multiple sclerosis, 1007-1009
    progressive multifocal leukoencephalopathy,
      1010
    transverse myelitis, 1010
  epilepsy, 978-985
    clinical seizure patterns, 979-980
    diagnosis and laboratory evaluation,
      980-982
    electroencephalography, 906-907
    etiology, 980
    pathophysiology, 978-979
    posttraumatic, 1045
    psychologic issues and behavior changes,
      984-985
    syncope *versus*, 954
    treatment, 982-984
  facial pain, 962-963
  faintness, 952-957
  head trauma, 1043-1045
    dementia, 988
    endocardial hemorrhage, 1087
    frontal lobe syndrome, 1032
    increased intracranial pressure, 1084
    seizure, 980
  headache, 957-962
    acute hyponatremia, 811
    brain tumor, 1067
    calcium channel blocker-induced, 205
    central nervous system disease, 973

Neurologic disorders—cont'd
  headache—cont'd
    effect of nitrate therapy, 201
    evaluation, 960-961
    giant-cell arteritis, 304
    lumbar puncture-induced, 905
    mechanisms, 957, 958
    neuronal disease, 1017
    rheumatoid arthritis, 1203
    sleep-related, 947
    stroke, 1001
    superior vena caval obstruction, 511
    systemic lupus erythematosus, 1093, 1215
    treatment, 961-962
    types, 957-960
  hypoxic-ischemic encephalopathy, 950-951
  impotence, 1761
  laboratory and diagnostic testing
    electroencephalography, 905-908
    electromyography, 914-917
    evoked responses, 908-914
    history and examination, 902-903
    psychologic testing, 903-904
    spinal fluid examination, 904-905
  Lambert-Eaton myasthenic syndrome,
      1023-1024
  maladaptive illness behavior, 1040
  metabolic disorders, 1078-1081
  mood disorders, 1035-1038
  muscle disease, 1024-1030
    Duchenne muscular dystrophy, 1026
    electromyography, 1025-1026
    facioscapulohumeral dystrophy, 1027
    laboratory evaluation, 1025
    limb girdle muscular dystrophy, 1026-1027,
      1028
    metabolic myopathies, 1028-1030
    myotonic dystrophy, 1027-1028
    oculopharyngeal dystrophy, 1028
    pathology, 1026
  myasthenia gravis, 1020-1023
  myelopathy, 1011-1014
  neck pain, 968-971
  neuromuscular junction disease, 1020-1024
    congenital myasthenia, 1023
    Lambert-Eaton myasthenic syndrome,
      1023-1024
    myasthenia gravis, 1020-1023
    peripheral neuropathy *versus*, 1014-1015
  neurooncology, 1067-1074
    intracranial neoplasms, 1067-1070
    neurologic complications of systemic
      cancer, 1070-1074
  neuroradiologic studies, 917-930
    carotid ultrasonography, 929
    computed tomography, 917-918, 919, 920
    conventional radiography, 924-926
    magnetic resonance imaging, 918-924
    radionuclide studies, 926-929
  neurorehabilitation, 1053-1056
  ocular manifestations, 1056-1065
    abnormalities of vision, 1056-1057
    disturbances of conjugate eye movements,
      1063-1065
    eye movement abnormalities, 1062-1063
    ocular vascular disease, 1057-1062
  parkinsonism and movement disorders,
      989-997
    disordered sleep, 946-947
    disorders with increased tone, 997
    hyperkinetic movement disorders, 993-997
    Parkinson's disease, 989-992
    secondary, 992-993
  peripheral neuropathy, 1014-1020
    after stroke, 1007
    autonomic hyperactivity, 935
    chemotherapy-induced, 585
    chronic renal failure, 781, 784
    complication of chemotherapy, 1072
    differential diagnosis, 1014-1015
    electromyography, 1017

Neurologic disorders—cont'd
  peripheral neuropathy—cont'd
    headache, back pain, multiple cranial nerve
      palsies, and polyradiculopathy, 1017
    management, 1020
    polyneuropathy, 1017-1020
    progressive lower motor neuron deficit with
      or without upper motor neuron deficit,
      1015
    proximal pain in one limb, with sensory,
      motor, or reflex abnormalities,
      1015-1017
    rheumatoid arthritis, 1094
    vasculitis, 1225
  persistent vegetative state, 950-951
  personality disorders, 1039-1040
  during pregnancy, 2281-2282
  respiratory failure, 1085-1086
  sleep disorders, 939-947
    dyssomnias, 940-945
    medical and psychiatric disorders, 946-947
    parasomnias, 945-946
  somatization, 1040
  speech and language, 975-978
  spinal cord injury, 1045-1053
    classification, 1046-1047
    epidemiology, 1046
    mass reflex of autonomic overactivity, 934
    rehabilitation, 1052-1053
    respiratory failure, 1097
    subacute management, 1049-1052
    syndromes, 1047-1049
  stroke, 997-1007
    amnesic syndrome, 1032
    atrial fibrillation, 146
    clinical separation of stroke subtypes,
      1000-1002
    depression, 1036
    dizziness, 973
    embolism, 1006
    hemorrhagic, 997-998, 1006
    hypertension, 322-323
    hypertension risk factors, 314, 315
    ischemic, 998-1000
    laboratory diagnosis, 1002-1004
    parkinsonism, 993
    prevention, complications, and
      rehabilitation, 1006-1007
    rehabilitation, 1054-1055
    respiratory rhythm abnormalities, 1098
    sickle cell disease, 659
    systemic lupus erythematosus, 1093
    thrombotic, 1004-1006
  syncope, 952-957
  thought disorders, 1041-1043
Neurologic examination, 902-903
  botulism, 1571
  dementia, 988
  low back pain, 966
  stroke, 1001-1002
  urinary incontinence in elderly, 2292
  vertigo, 2307
Neurologic level of injury, 1046, 1053
Neurologic paraneoplastic syndromes, 1071,
  1073, 1074
Neurology
  behavioral, 1030-1034
  lower urinary tract, 1065-1067
  neurocardiology, 1086-1091
  neuroendocrinology, 1075-1078
  neurogastroenterology, 1100-1102
  neurohematology, 1103-1105
  neurohepatology, 1102-1103
  neuronephrology, 1105-1106
  neurooncology, 1067-1074
    intracranial neoplasms, 1067-1070
    neurologic complications of systemic
      cancer, 1070-1074
  neuropulmonology, 1095-1100
  neurorheumatology, 1091-1095
  otoneurology, 971-975

Neuroma
  acoustic, 1070
    brainstem auditory evoked potential, 911
    neurofibromatosis, 1921
  ganglioneuroma, 1830
Neuromuscular disorders
  acute respiratory failure without lung disease,
    418
  chronic renal failure, 784
  diabetic, 1872
  hyperkalemia, 832
  hypomagnesemia, 1942
  muscle disease, 1024-1030
    Duchenne muscular dystrophy, 1026
    electromyography, 1025-1026
    facioscapulohumeral dystrophy, 1027
    laboratory evaluation, 1025
    limb girdle muscular dystrophy, 1026-1027,
      1028
    metabolic myopathies, 1028-1030
    myotonic dystrophy, 1027-1028
    oculopharyngeal dystrophy, 1028
    pathology, 1026
  noncardiac causes of chest pain, 129
  pulmonary rehabilitation, 437
  respiratory muscle weakness, 359
Neuromuscular junction
  disorders, 1020-1024
    congenital myasthenia, 1023
    Lambert-Eaton myasthenic syndrome,
      1023-1024
    myasthenia gravis, 1020-1023
    peripheral neuropathy *versus,* 1014-1015
  electromyography, 917
Neuromyopathy, 489
Neuron
  injury in bacterial meningitis, 1405-1406
  intramural, 1978
  neurohypophysis, 1788
  upper motor neuron deficit, 1015
Neuronal transplantation, 1054
Neuronephrology, 1105-1106
Neuronitis, vestibular, 972
Neurooncology, 1067-1074
  intracranial neoplasms, 1067-1070
  neurologic complications of systemic cancer,
    1070-1074
Neuropathic bladder, 1066
Neuropathic joint disease, 1247
Neuropathy
  cardiac abnormalities, 1087
  complication of chemotherapy, 1072
  connective tissue disease, 1093
  diabetic, 1871-1872
  hypertensive optic, 2303
  Leber's hereditary optic neuropathy, 1029
  leprosy, 1649
  nerve conduction studies, 915
  optic, 1060
  pancreatic diabetes, 2239
  peripheral, 1014-1020
    chemotherapy-induced, 585
    chronic renal failure, 781, 784
    complication of chemotherapy, 1072
    differential diagnosis, 1014-1015
    electromyography, 1017
    headache, back pain, multiple cranial nerve
      palsies, and polyradiculopathy, 1017
    management, 1020
    polyneuropathy, 1017-1020
    progressive lower motor neuron deficit with
      or without upper motor neuron deficit,
      1015
    proximal pain in one limb, with sensory,
      motor, or reflex abnormalities,
      1015-1017
    vasculitis, 1225
  rheumatoid arthritis, 1204
  uremic, 1105
Neuropeptide Y, 934
Neuropeptides, 1075

Neurophysin, 808, 1788, 1792
Neuropsychiatric manifestations
  systemic lupus erythematosus, 1215
  vitamin B_{12} deficiency, 648
Neuropsychologic tests, 903
Neuropsychotropics, 2191
Neuropulmonology, 1095-1100
  abnormal respiratory rhythms in altered states
    of consciousness, 1097
  neurogenic respiratory failure, 1096-1097
  respiratory rhythm abnormalities in conscious
    patient, 1098-1099
Neuroradiologic studies, 917-930
  carotid ultrasonography, 929
  computed tomography, 917-918, 919, 920
  conventional radiography, 924-926
  magnetic resonance imaging, 918-924
  radionuclide studies, 926-929
Neurorehabilitation, 1053-1056
Neurorheumatology, 1091-1095
Neurosecretion, 1075
Neurosurgery, 984
Neurosyphilis, 1642
Neurotoxin, 1567
Neurotransmitters, 930-931
  chemoreceptor trigger zone, 2026
  emetic response, 581
  hepatic encephalopathy, 2161
  hormones as, 1076
  hormones *versus,* 1708
  influence on sleep, 940
  pain, 580
Neutral aminoaciduria, 879
Neutral protamine, 1859
Neutralization tests, 1373
Neutropenia, 593, 678-679
  acute myelogenous leukemia, 689
  aplastic anemia, 672
  cancer patient, 582
  candidiasis, 1661
  compromised host, 1388-1389
  cytotoxic drug-induced, 1340
  granulocyte transfusion, 573-574
  peripheral blood smear, 557
Neutrophil, 1339-1341, Plate IV-6
  abnormalities, 678-680
  asthma, 1186
  bacterial meningitis, 1405
  barrier to infection, 1335
  chronic bronchitis, 442
  gram-negative bacteremia, 1448
  Langerhans' cell granulomatosis, 464
  megaloblastic anemia, 648
  pathogenesis of emphysema, 441
  phagocytosis, 1109
  ulcerative colitis, 2072-2073
Neutrophil count, 1388
Neutrophilia, 557, 590-591, 678
Nevirapine, 1474
Nevus, Plate VII-7
  basal cell carcinoma *versus,* 1297
  melanoma risk, 1298
New flow across capillary, 737
New World hookworm, 1698
Newborn
  autosomal recessive polycystic kidney disease,
    874
  bacterial meningitis, 1403
  bullous impetigo, 1419
  Chlamydia trachomatis, 1536
  coxsackievirus myocarditis, 1490
  cytomegalovirus, 1527
  herpes simplex virus, 2280
  herpes simplex virus infection, 1524
  hypocalcemia, 1931-1932
  Listeria monocytogenes, 1577
  maternal hepatitis B, 2277
  maternal hyperparathyroidism, 2273
  myasthenia gravis, 1021
  myopericarditis, 1489-1490
  neonatal alloimmune thrombocytopenia, 616

Newborn—cont'd
neonatal hypocalcemia, 1968
neurofibromatosis, 1921
osteomyelitis, 1433
ovarian function, 1832
physiologic jaundice of, 2151
septic arthritis, 1252
staphylococcal scalded-skin syndrome, 1421
tetanus neonatorum, 1573
transient tyrosinemia of, 1905
varicella, 1527
vitamin K deficiency, 625-626
NF1 gene, 546-547, 1921
Niacin
biochemical function, 2105
deficiency, 987, 2107
drug-nutrient interactions, 2110
megadoses and toxicity, 2108
recommended daily dietary allowances,
2115
Nicardipine
angina, 203
hypertension, 325
hypertensive emergency, 328
interaction with cyclosporin, 793
properties, 204
Nickel, 548
Nicotinamide, 879, 2107
Nicotinamide adenine dinucleotide, 861
Nicotinamide adenine dinucleotide phosphate,
663
Nicotine
effect on vasopressin release, 1791
withdrawal syndrome, 2296
Nicotine patch, 2296
Nicotinic acid
deficiency, 1101, 2107
diabetes mellitus, 1869
hepatic injury, 2192
hypercholesterolemia, 1894
lipoprotein synthesis inhibition, 1891-1892
megadoses and toxicity, 2108
Niemann-Pick disease, 943, 1918
Nifedipine
achalasia, 2022
angina, 203
aortic regurgitation, 243
autonomic dysreflexia, 1049
chronic hypertension during pregnancy, 2275
hepatic injury, 2192
human cytochrome P450 isoforms, 2312
hypertension, 325, 327
hypertrophic obstructive cardiomyopathy, 269
interference with catecholamine assays, 1740
primary pulmonary hypertension, 295
properties, 204
prophylaxis of migraine, 962
Raynaud's phenomenon, 310, 1227
Night blindness
human immunodeficiency virus-infected
patients, 2306
vitamin A deficiency, 2105
Night burners, 2017
Night sweats
amebic liver abscess, 2210
hepatic adenoma, 2217
Hodgkin's disease, 693
Nightmares, 946
Nikolsky's sign, 1293
Nil disease, 849-851
Nimbus hemopump, 186
Nimodipine, 203
90-day glaucoma, 2304
Ninhydrin, 1904
Nipent; *see* 2-Deoxycoformycin
Nipride; *see* Nitroprusside
Niridazole
hemolysis in glucose-6-phosphate
dehydrogenase deficiency, 663
tissue nematode infection, 1700

Nisoldipine
angina, 203
hypertension, 325
properties, 204
Nitazoxamide, 1679
Nitrates
beta-adrenergic blockers with, 202
dilated cardiomyopathy, 264
gastric cancer, 2045
heart failure, 173-174
ischemic heart disease, 200-201, 202
myocardial infarction, 216
Nitrazepam, 636
Nitrazie paper, 742-743
Nitrendipine, 203, 204
Nitric oxide
bacterial meningitis, 1405
endotoxemia and cirrhosis, 820
erectile function, 934
hepatopulmonary syndrome, 2170
hypertension, 316, 319
lung injury, 373
modulation of arterial tone, 48
modulation of ventricular function, 45
peripheral chemoreceptor signal, 353
peristalsis, 1977
precapillary pulmonary hypertension, 296
pulmonary vasodilation, 363
sepsis, 1448
vasoactive effects on pulmonary circulation, 363
Nitric oxide products, 370
Nitric oxide synthase inhibitors, 1454
Nitrofurantoin, 1359-1360
dosage, 1350
enterococcal infection, 1563
hemolysis in glucose-6-phosphate
dehydrogenase deficiency, 663
hepatic injury, 2191
pulmonary parenchymal reactions, 476
pulmonary toxicity, 478
use during pregnancy, 2281
Nitrofurtimox, 1690
Nitrogen
chronic renal failure, 786
nutritional assessment, 2111
for parenteral solutions, 2113-2114
requirements, 2112, 2115
Nitrogen-containing diet, 2112
Nitrogen mustard, 694-695
Nitrogen washout-helium dilution technique, 378
Nitroglycerin
angina, 196
angina pectoris, 126, 127
hypertensive emergency, 328
interference with catecholamine assays, 1740
ischemic heart disease, 200-201, 202
myocardial infarction, 212, 216, 218
pulmonary edema, 169
variceal bleeding, 2167
Nitropress; *see* Nitroprusside
Nitroprusside
dilated cardiomyopathy, 264
heart failure, 173, 174
hypertensive emergency, 328
myocardial infarction, 218
pulmonary edema, 169
shock, 182
testing for diabetic ketoacidosis, 1863-1864
Nitrosamines, 2045
Nitrosureas
effects on kidney, 869
hepatic injury, 2192
pancreatic cancer, 2243
pulmonary parenchymal reactions, 476
pulmonary toxicity, 478, 584
Nizatidine
gastroesophageal reflux, 2018
interference with oral anticoagulants, 636
Nocardia, 1665-1666
compromised host, 1388
pleural effusion, 507

Nocturia
bacterial prostatitis, 1462
chronic renal failure, 778, 780
disorders of urinary concentration, 748
Nocturnal angina, 195, 196
Nocturnal eating (drinking) syndrome, 944
Nocturnal myoclonus, 944
Nocturnal paroxysmal dystonia, 946
Nodular diabetic glomerular sclerosis, 859
Nodular melanoma, 1299
Nodular sclerosis, 692
Nodule
acne vulgaris, 1305
asbestos exposure, 474
Aschoff, 235, 245
Churg-Strauss syndrome, 466
cutaneous manifestation of internal
malignancy, 1316
Ehlers-Danlos syndrome, 1287
Langerhans' cell granulomatosis, 464
lymphomatoid granulomatosis, 470
necrotizing sarcoid granulomatosis, 470
rheumatic fever, 1257, 1559
rheumatoid, 1094, 1203
solitary pulmonary, 493-497
splenic, 531
sporotrichosis, Plate VIII-24
superficial thrombophlebitis, 311
thyroid adenoma, 1814
toxic nodular goiter, 1807
trichomycosis axillaris, 1422
Wegener's granulomatosis, 468
Nomogram
acid-base, 836
daily nitrogen requirements, 2115
for determining body surface area, 2112
heparin, 633, 634
hypertension, 323
Non-A–non-B hepatitis, 575, 2177
Non-group A streptococci, 1563-1564
Non-Hodgkin's lymphoma, 695-700
acquired immunodeficiency syndrome, 1329
bone marrow biopsy section, 558
Epstein-Barr virus, 1529
heart involvement, 331
molecular diagnostics, 563
stomach involvement, 2049
Non-Huntington chorea, 994-995
Non-insulin–dependent diabetes mellitus, 1854
diabetic nephropathy, 859
obesity, 1752
secondary combined hyperlipidemia, 1896
secondary hypertriglyceridemia, 1895
Non-O1 *Vibrio cholerae,* 1596
Non-Q wave infarction, 89, 218
Non-rapid eye movement narcolepsy, 943
Non-rapid eye movement sleep, 939-940
Non-small cell lung cancer, 725-729
Nonagglutinable vibrios, 1593, 1596
Nonalcoholic steatohepatitis, 2196-2197
Nonallergic rhinitis, 1181
Nonbacterial thrombotic endocarditis, 1089
Noncardiogenic pulmonary edema, 477
Noncholera vibrios, 1593, 1596
Nonclostridial crepitant cellulitis, 1422
Nonconvulsive status epilepticus, 984
Nondiabetic melliturias, 1879-1880
Nondipper, 313
Nonejection systolic sounds, 75, 76
Nonendocrine paraneoplastic syndromes, 583
Nonenterococcal group D streptococci, 1564
Nonenzymatic glycation, 861
Nongonococcal urethritis, 1440
Nongranulomatous ulcerative jejunoileitis, 2064
Noninflammatory rhinitis, 1181
Noninvasive cardiac testing, 91-107
chest radiography, 91, 92
computed tomography, 106
continuous ambulatory electrocardiographic
recording, 94
echocardiography, 94-100

Noninvasive cardiac testing—cont'd
  exercise electrocardiographic testing, 91-94
  gamma camera imaging agents, 105
  ischemic heart disease, 198-199
  magnetic resonance imaging, 106-107
  myocardial perfusion imaging, 101-104
  positron emission tomography, 105-106
  radionuclide angiography, 104-105
  sudden cardiac death survivor, 188
Nonketotic hyperglycemia, 829
Nonketotic hyperglycinemia, 1909
Nonmaleficence, 10
Non–twenty-four hour sleep-wake syndrome, 945
Nonopioid analgesics, 1259-1260
  acute erosive gastritis, 2041
  adult Still's disease, 1243
  analgesic-associated nephropathy, 870-871, 890
  angina, 205, 207
  arterial thromboembolism, 639
  atrial fibrillation, 148, 640, 1088
  chronic pancreatitis, 2240
  cystic fibrosis, 482
  decreased colon cancer risk, 2083
  glucose-6-phosphate dehydrogenase deficiency, 664
  gouty arthritis, 1274
  hepatic injury, 2190, 2191
  human cytochrome P450 isoforms, 2312
  increased frequency of bleeding, 605
  induction of anaphylaxis, 1193
  influenza, 1492
  interference with oral anticoagulants, 636
  ischemic heart disease, 200
  myocardial infarction, 212, 217
  non-Q wave myocardial infarction, 218
  osteoarthritis, 1268
  pericardial heart disease, 278
  platelet aggregation studies, 570
  platelet cyclooxygenase and, 611
  poisoning, 2188-2190
  during pregnancy, 2275
  prosthetic heart valve, 258, 640
  pulmonary parenchymal reactions, 476
  pulmonary toxicity, 479
  restenosis, 124
  rheumatic diseases, 1258
  rheumatic fever, 1257
  rheumatoid arthritis, 1207
  subacute thyroiditis, 1812
  superficial thrombophlebitis, 311
  thrombotic stroke, 1004
  unstable angina, 639
Nonoxidative hemolysis, 667-668
Nonparathyroid endocrine disorders, 1928
Nonparoxysmal junctional tachycardia, 134
Nonpathogenic protozoa, 1692
Nonpenetrant, 1721
Nonperistaltic contraction, 1978
Nonproliferative diabetic retinopathy, 2303
Nonsecretory myeloma, 703
Nonsense mutation, 654
Nonsteroidal antiinflammatory drugs
  ankylosing spondylitis, 1239
  asthma induction, 1187
  cancer pain, 580
  chronic fatigue syndrome, 2300
  decreased colon cancer risk, 2083
  fever of unknown origin, 1380
  focal glomerular sclerosis, 852
  gastric ulcer induction, 2036, 2037
  gouty arthritis, 1274
  hepatic injury, 2190
  induction of acute interstitial nephritis, 889
  induction of bronchospasm, 477
  inhibition of platelet cyclooxygenase, 611
  interaction with antihypertensives, 322
  low back pain, 966
  neck pain, 971
  nephrotoxicity, 853, 870-871

Nonsteroidal antiinflammatory drugs—cont'd
  osteoarthritis, 1267-1268
  pericardial heart disease, 278
  pericarditis, 221
  pulmonary parenchymal reactions, 476
  pulmonary toxicity, 479
  rheumatic diseases, 1258-1259
  rheumatoid arthritis, 1207
  systemic lupus erythematosus, 1216
Nonsustained ventricular tachycardia, 149, 224
Nontoxic goiter, 1812-1813
Nontuberculous mycobacterial infections, 1638-1639
Nontyphoidal *Salmonella*, 1598-1600
Nonvenereal treponematosis, 1644
Noonan's syndrome, 1769, 1843
Noradrenergic pathways, 1076
Norepinephrine, 56, 930
  biosynthesis and metabolism, 1826-1827
  cardiac growth and hypertrophy, 55
  heart failure, 159, 160, 161, 166, 818
  hypertension, 316
  lung filtration, 346
  normal plasma levels, 1827
  shock, 180
  sodium retention, 819
  vasopressin inhibition, 1791
Norethandrolone, 674
Norethindrone, 2312
Norfloxacin, 1359
  dosage, 1350
  enterococcal infection, 1563
  prophylaxis for traveler's diarrhea, 1432
  shigellosis, 1603
  spontaneous bacterial peritonitis, 2164
Normal, defined, 6
Normal flora, 1367, 1368
  bile salt secretion, 2125
  intestinal catabolism of bile pigments, 2149-2150
  intraabdominal infection, 1397
  obligate anaerobic bacteria, 1614, 1615
Normal saline, 775
Normetanephrine, 930, 1739
Normocalcemic hyperparathyroidism, 1967-1968
Normodyne; *see* Labetalol
Norpace; *see* Disopyramide
Norplant, 2270
North American Symptomatic Carotid Endarterectomy Trial, 1058
Northern blot, 52
Nortriptyline, 1037
  anxiety disorders, 1035
  depression in elderly patients, 2289
  prophylaxis of migraine, 962
Norvasc; *see* Amlodipine
Norvir; *see* Ritonavir
Norwalk-like virus, 1521-1522
Norwalk virus, 1428, 1429, 1521-1522
Nose
  allergen challenge, 1154
  applied anatomy and physiology, 1180-1181
  cancer, 723
  epistaxis, 2308
  fracture, 2308
  lupus pernio, Plate VII-21
  mastocytosis, 1181
  nasal congestion, 1181, 1391
  nasal discharge
    common cold, 1391
    sinusitis, 1394, 2308
  nasal mucosa, 1180-1185
  obstruction, 2308
  packing, 2308
  polyp, 482, 1183, 2308
  rhinitis, 2308
  septal deviation, 2308
  sinusitis, 2308-2309
    acquired immunodeficiency syndrome, 1478
    after lung transplantation, 520
    anaerobic infection, 1617

Nose—cont'd
  sinusitis—cont'd
    antibiotic therapy, 1183
    complication of influenza, 1492
    cystic fibrosis, 482
    endotracheal tube infection, 416
    epidural abscesses and, 1418
    facial pain, 962
    Haemophilus influenzae, 1588
    nosocomial, 1480
    subdural empyema and, 1416-1417
    Wegener's granulomatosis, 467
Nosebleed, 2308
Nosema, 1680-1681
Nosocomial infection, 1361-1366
  Candida, 1660-1661, 1662
  enterococcal, 1561
  fever, 1479-1482
  gram-negative bacteremia, 1445
  meningitis, 1403
  pneumonia, 423
  staphylococcal, 1550
Notching, coarctation of aorta, 286
Novacor left ventricular assist system, 186
NSAIDS; *see* Nonsteroidal antiinflammatory drugs
NSG; *see* Necrotizing sarcoid granulomatosis
Ntcp polypeptide, 2126
Nuchal rigidity
  bacterial meningitis, 1406
  Lyme disease, 1647
  meningococcemia, 1579
Nuclear cardiology techniques, 100-106
  gamma camera imaging agents, 105
  myocardial perfusion imaging, 101-104
  positron emission tomography, 105-106
  radionuclide angiography, 104-105
Nuclear factor-beta, 372
Nuclear medicine
  obstructive uropathy, 754
  osteomalacia, 1949-1950
  renal, 750
Nuclear receptor, 1712-1713
Nucleated red blood cell, 595-596
Nucleic acid-based tests, 1372-1373
Nucleoside analogs, 704
5′-Nucleotidase
  choledocholithiasis, 2229
  hepatitic injury, 2136
  hepatocellular *versus* cholestatic jaundice, 2156
  liver disease, 2137
Nucleotide, 52
Nucleotide exchange factors, 541
Nucleus tractus solitarius, 46
Numbers-connection test, 2159
Nummular dermatitis, 1303
Nutcracker esophagus, 2022
Nutrients
  excessive intake of single nutrient, 2101
  imbalance, 2101-2102
  requirements, 2111-2112
Nutrition, 2099-2118
  drug-nutrient interactions, 2110, 2111
  elderly, 2287
  malnutrition, 2100-2102
  management, 2112-2117
  minerals, 2108-2110
  nutritional assessment, 2111-2112, 2113
  obesity, 2102-2105
  vitamins, 2105-2108
Nutritional assessment, 2111-2112, 2113
Nutritional disorders
  alcohol-related, 1081
  chronic renal failure, 786
  Crohn's disease, 2069
  vitamin D deficiency, 1951
Nutritional status
  elderly, 2287
  nosocomial infection, 1361
  rate of albumin synthesis, 2135

Nutritional status—cont'd
  regulation of albumin synthesis, 2119
  susceptibility or tolerance to noxious agents, 866
Nutritional support
  acute renal failure, 774
  acute respiratory failure, 420
  alcoholic hepatitis, 2198
  chronic obstructive pulmonary disease, 445
  cystic fibrosis, 2246
  to increase respiratory muscle strength, 360
  multiple organ dysfunction syndrome, 422
  pulmonary rehabilitation, 435, 436
NVP; *see* Nevirapine
Nystagmus, 973-974, 1064, 2106
Nystatin
  candidiasis, 1312, 2020
  thrush, 1663
  typical medical regimen six months after transplantation, 343

O

O polysaccharides, 1447
Oat cell carcinoma of lung, 1024
Oath of Hippocrates, 10
Oatpl polypeptide, 2126
Obesity, 1750-1753, 2102-2105
  adolescent, 1769-1770
  cardiovascular mortality and morbidity, 334
  causes, 2102-2103
  coronary artery disease in women, 2271
  creatinine clearance, 747
  diabetes mellitus, 1854
  diagnosis, 1751
  dietary approaches, 2103-2104
  differential diagnosis, 1752
  dysbetalipoproteinemia, 1898
  exercise, 2104
  gallstone risk factor, 2223
  heart murmur, 76
  hypertension, 319
  hypogonadism, 1842-1843
  insulin resistance, 1861, 1862
  ischemic heart disease, 200
  obstructive sleep apnea, 525
  osteoarthritis risk, 1264
  pathophysiology, 1751-1752
  Prader-Labhart-Willi syndrome, 1842
  second heart sound, 73
  treatment, 1752-1753
  varicose veins, 311
Obesity-hypoventilation syndrome, 354, 528
Obligate anaerobic bacteria
  Bacteroides, 1613-1621
    antibiotic selection, 1348
    bacteremia and endocarditis, 1618
    brain abscess, 1414
    central nervous system infections, 1617
    classification and characteristics, 1613-1614
    diagnosis, 1618-1619
    gram-negative bacteremia, 1446
    head and neck infections, 1616-1617
    intraabdominal infections, 1617-1618
    necrotic skin and soft tissue infections, 1618
    normal flora, 1368
    obstetric and gynecologic infections, 1618
    pathophysiology, 1614-1616
    pleuropulmonary infections, 1617
    prevention, 1621
    therapy, 1619-1621
  Mycobacterium leprae, 1648-1651
Observation, neurologic examination, 902
Obsessive-compulsive behavior, 996, 1032, 1039
Obstruction
  airway
    acute, 2306
    anaphylaxis, 1193
    angioedema, 2306
    asthma, 1188

obstruction—cont'd
  airway—cont'd
    chronic obstructive pulmonary disease, 438
    sarcoidosis, 458
    sleep-induced, 527-528
    snoring, 2309
    spirometry, 377
  aortic, 304
  bile duct
    cholestasis, 2156
    cystic fibrosis, 2207
    primary biliary cirrhosis, 2199
  biliary secretory apparatus, 2128-2129
  bladder
    bladder neck, 768
    bladder outlet, 771
    emptying dysfunction, 1066
  endobronchial
    coughing, 407-408
    lung cancer, 491
  gastric outlet, 2027, 2040
  hydrocephalus
    brain tumor, 1067
    dementia, 988
    Maroteaux-Launy syndrome, 1915
    posttraumatic, 1045
    radionuclide cisternography, 926
  intestinal, 2077-2079
    abdominal pain, 2032
    colon cancer, 2085
    cystic fibrosis, 2246
    Meckel's diverticulum, 2089
    radiography, 2032
    small intestinal malignancies, 2081
  left ventricular outflow
    cardiogenic syncope, 954
    coarctation of aorta, 286
    hypertrophic cardiomyopathy, 265
    systolic ejection murmur, 77
  lymphatic
    erysipelas, 1420
    intestinal lymphangiectasia, 2067
  nasal, 2308
  portal vein, 2208-2209
  renal, 884-887, 1457
    chronic renal failure, 781
    chronic tubulointerstitial disease, 892
    postrenal azotemia, 768
  right ventricular outflow
    abnormal jugular venous pulse, 66
    cardiogenic syncope, 954
    hypertrophic cardiomyopathy, 266
    systolic ejection murmur, 77
  splenic vein, 2208
  superior vena caval, 511-512
    abnormal jugular venous pulse, 66
    transudative pleural effusion, 507
  ureteral
    peritoneal mesenteric and omental diseases, 2248
    posttransplantation, 794
Obstructive airway disease
  exercise tests, 379
  heart failure *versus*, 168
  maximal expiratory and inspiratory flow-volume curve, 377
Obstructive ileus, 2077
Obstructive jaundice
  chronic pancreatitis, 2241
  serum aminotransferase levels, 2136
Obstructive sleep apnea, 354-355, 524-528, 943
Obstructive uropathy, 884-887
  renal imaging studies, 753-754
  urinary tract infection, 1457
Occam's razor, 2094
Occipital alexia, 978
Occipital condyle syndrome, 1071
Occlusion
  aortic, 304
  basilar artery, 973
  central retinal artery, 1058

Occlusion—cont'd
  hypertensive retinopathy, 2303
  mesenteric vascular disease, 2086
  retinal vein
    central, Plate XI-10
    cotton-wool spots, Plate XI-9
  vertebral artery, 1005
Occlusive peripheral arterial disease, 305-309, 310
Occult blood loss, 2017
Occult constrictive pericarditis, 278
Occupational exposure
  hepatotoxic agents, 2185
  pancreatic cancer, 2242
Occupational history, 401
Occupational lung disease, 471-476
  brucellosis, 1604
  chronic obstructive pulmonary disease, 439
  hypersensitivity pneumonitis, 462
  interstitial lung disease, 452
  lung cancer, 486
Occupational Safety and Health Administration, 471
Occupational therapy
  osteoarthritis, 1267
  pulmonary rehabilitation, 436
  spinal cord injury, 1052
  stroke patient, 1054
Ochronosis, 1170, 1280-1282
Octreotide
  acromegaly, 1785
  chronic pancreatitis, 2240
  glucagonoma, 2245
  hypoglycemia, 1878
  insulinoma, 2244
  variceal bleeding, 2167
  VIPoma, 2245
Ocular bobbing, 1064
Ocular disease, 2300-2306
  Acanthamoeba, 1684
  acquired immunodeficiency syndrome, 2304-2306
  age-related macular degeneration, 2301-2302
  candidal endophthalmitis, 1662
  cataracts, 2301
  Chlamydia trachomatis, 1536
  diabetic retinopathy, 1870-1871, 2303-2304
  Ehlers-Danlos syndromes, 1287, 1288
  glaucoma, 2301, 2302
  Graves' disease, 1805-1806
  herpes keratitis, 1524
  hypertensive retinopathy, 2302-2303
  hypothyroidism, 1809
  immunologically privileged site, 1145
  Marfan syndrome, 1289
  neurofibromatosis, 1920-1921
  neurologic disorders, 1056-1065
    abnormalities of vision, 1056-1057
    disturbances of conjugate eye movements, 1063-1065
    eye movement abnormalities, 1062-1063
    ocular vascular disease, 1057-1062
  Niemann-Pick disease, 1918
  Paget's disease, 1955
  presbyopia, 2301
  pseudoxanthoma elasticum, 1289
  retinal venoocclusive disease, 2304
  rheumatoid arthritis, 1204
  riboflavin deficiency, 2106
  sarcoidosis, 458
  Sjögren syndrome, 1209-1212
  syphilis, 1642
  toxoplasmosis, 1677
  trachoma, 1535-1536
  tuberous sclerosis, 1922
  tularemia, 1608
  visual loss, 2300-2301
  vitamin A deficiency, 2105-2106
  Vittaforma infection, 1681
  von Hippel-Lindau disease, 1922, 1923
  Wegener's granulomatosis, 468

Ocular flutter, 1064
Ocular motor nerve disorders, 1062-1063
Ocular myoclonus, 1064
Ocular sarcoidosis, 458
Ocular sympathetic pathways, 934
Oculogyric crisis, 1510
Oculomasticatory myorhythmia, 1101
Oculomotor nerve palsy, 1062-1063
Oculopharyngeal dystrophy, 1028
Oculosympathetic paralysis, 932
Odor
    bacterial vaginosis, 1443
    vomitus, 2028
Odynophagia, 1998
    deep neck infections, 2309
    esophageal disease, 1998
    infectious esophagitis, 2020
    supraglottitis, 2306
    upper gastrointestinal endoscopy, 1994
Ofloxacin, 1359
    acute pancreatitis, 2237
    dosage, 1350
    enterococcal infection, 1563
    gonorrhea, 1584
    human cytochrome P450 isoforms, 2312
    mycobacterial disease, 1631
    prophylaxis for traveler's diarrhea, 1432
    traveler's diarrhea, 1432
    typhoid fever, 1432
    urethritis, 1441
Ogilvie's syndrome, 2079
Ohm's law, 46
OKT3 monoclonal antibody
    cardiac transplantation, 1090
    renal transplantation, 792
Olanzapine, 1042
Old World hookworm, 1698
Oldfield's syndrome, 2083
Olecranon bursa, 1197
Oleic acid, 1883, 1889-1890
Olestra, 1891
Oligoarticular arthritis, 1198
Oligodendroglioma, 1068
Oligomenorrhea
    prolactin-secreting pituitary adenoma, 1786
    21-hydroxylase deficiency, 1824
Oligospermia, 1845
Oliguria
    acetaminophen poisoning, 2190
    acute tubular necrosis, 772
    anti-neutrophil cytoplasmic antibodies-positive
        glomerulonephritis, 848
    preeclampsia, 2274
    toxicity of nonsteroidal antiinflammatory
        drugs, 870
Olivopontocerebellar atrophy, 935, 992-993
Omega-3 fatty acids, 1884
    nephrotic syndrome, 767
    platelet release defects, 611
    restenosis, 124
Omentum, 2247, 2252
Omeprazole
    gastroesophageal reflux, 2018
    Helicobacter pylori, 1593
    human cytochrome P450 isoforms, 2312
    interference with oral anticoagulants, 636
    peptic ulcer disease, 2040
    prophylaxis for traveler's diarrhea, 1432
Onchocerca volvulus, 1699-1701
Oncocytoma, renal, 753, 899
Oncogene
    breast cancer, 707
    disruption during tumor formation, 543-545
    lung cancer, 487
    normal function, 541-543
    parathyroid neoplasia, 1966
Oncology; *see* Cancer
Oncotic pressure
    pulmonary edema, 168, 424
    shock, 177

Ondansetron, 581
    human cytochrome P450 isoforms, 2312
    for nausea and vomiting, 2027
Ondine's curse, 378, 1096-1097
Oocyst, 1676
    Cryptosporidium, Plate VIII-33
    Isospora belli, Plate VIII-1
Oocyte, 1832
Oophorectomy, 711
Oophoritis, 1496
Opa proteins, 1581
OPAD; *see* Occlusive peripheral arterial disease
Open angle glaucoma, 2301
Open biopsy
    cancer of unknown primary site, 730
    lung, 385-386
Opening snap, 74-75
    mitral stenosis, 247
Operability, 728
Operative risks, 2256-2264
    cardiovascular, 2257-2260
    endocrine, 2262
    estimated, 2256-2257
    gastrointestinal and hepatic, 2262-2263
    hematologic, 2262
    pulmonary, 2260-2262
    renal, 2263-2264
Ophthalmopathy, 2300-2306
    Acanthamoeba, 1684
    acquired immunodeficiency syndrome,
        2304-2306
    age-related macular degeneration, 2301-2302
    candidal endophthalmitis, 1662
    cataracts, 2301
    Chlamydia trachomatis, 1536
    diabetic retinopathy, 1870-1871, 2303-2304
    Ehlers-Danlos syndromes, 1287, 1288
    glaucoma, 2301, 2302
    Graves' disease, 1805-1806
    herpes keratitis, 1524
    hypertensive retinopathy, 2302-2303
    hypothyroidism, 1809
    immunologically privileged site, 1145
    Marfan syndrome, 1289
    neurofibromatosis, 1920-1921
    neurologic disorders, 1056-1065
        abnormalities of vision, 1056-1057
        disturbances of conjugate eye movements,
            1063-1065
        eye movement abnormalities, 1062-1063
        ocular vascular disease, 1057-1062
    Niemann-Pick disease, 1918
    Paget's disease, 1955
    presbyopia, 2301
    pseudoxanthoma elasticum, 1289
    retinal venoocclusive disease, 2304
    rheumatoid arthritis, 1204
    riboflavin deficiency, 2106
    sarcoidosis, 458
    Sjögren syndrome, 1209-1212
    syphilis, 1642
    toxoplasmosis, 1677
    trachoma, 1535-1536
    tuberous sclerosis, 1922
    tularemia, 1608
    visual loss, 2300-2301
    vitamin A deficiency, 2105-2106
    Vittaforma infection, 1681
    von Hippel-Lindau disease, 1922, 1923
    Wegener's granulomatosis, 468
Opiates
    addiction, 2297
    poisoning, 948
    pulmonary parenchymal reactions, 476
    pulmonary toxicity, 479
    vasopressin inhibition, 1791
Opinion leader, 25
Opioid analgesics
    abdominal pain, 2032
    abuse, 2297
    acute intermittent porphyria, 1926

Opioid analgesics—cont'd
    acute pancreatitis, 2237
    acute stone passage, 803
    cancer pain, 580, 581
    cough, 408, 409
    cytochrome P450 2D6-mediated conversion,
        2311
    effect on vasopressin release, 1791
    human cytochrome P450 isoforms, 2312
    myocardial infarction, 212, 216
    pulmonary edema, 169
    pulmonary toxicity, 479
    restless legs syndrome, 944
    sedation during gastrointestinal endoscopy,
        1994
    status migrainosus, 962
Opioid peptides, 1077
Opioids
    abuse, 2297
    cancer pain, 580-581
    chronic pancreatitis, 2240
    gastrointestinal motility, 1978
    pancreatic cancer, 2244
Opisthorchis felineus, 1704
Opisthorchis viverrini, 2231
Opisthorchis viverroni, 1704
Opportunistic infection
    acquired immunodeficiency syndrome,
        1327-1329, 1470, 1473-1474
    acute interstitial nephritis, 890
    after lung transplantation, 520
    after renal transplantation, 794
    bronchiectasis, 484
    neutropenia, 678
    nocardiosis, 1666
    odynophagia, 1998
    prophylaxis in compromised host, 1390
Opportunistic molds, 1652
Opsoclonus, 1064, 1075
Opsonins, 366
Opsonization, 1136, 1386
Optic disc, 1061
    anterior ischemic optic neuropathy, 1058-1059
    edema, 2303
Optic glioma, 1920-1921
Optic nerve
    anterior ischemic optic neuropathy, 1058-1059
    chemotherapy-induced damage, 1072
    edema, Plate XI-2
    glaucoma, 2301
    neovascularization, Plate XI-8
Optic neuritis, 1060
    multiple sclerosis, 1007-1008
    pattern-reversal visual evoked response, 911
Optic neuropathy, 1060
    anterior ischemic, 1058-1059
    chronic ethanol abuse, 1081
Optimal medical care, 23
Options analysis, 2264, 2265
Oral candidiasis, 1476, 2094-2095
Oral cavity
    anaerobic infection, 1616-1617
    aphthous ulcer in Crohn's disease, Plate X-10
    cancer, 723
    common problems, 2309
    hand-foot-mouth syndrome, 1489
    movement of food, 1978
    oral candidiasis, 1476, 1661, 2094-2095
    physical examination, 1999
    psoriasis, 1300
    Sjögren syndrome, 1209-1212
Oral cholecystography, 2224
Oral contraceptives, 2270
    drug-nutrient interactions, 2110
    estrogen-related cholestasis, 2158
    fibrocystic breast disease, 1850
    gallstone risk factor, 2223
    hepatic adenoma, 2216
    hepatic injury, 2190
    hepatic vein thrombosis, 2208
    hirsutism, 1756-1757

Oral contraceptives—cont'd
  hypertension, 320
  migraine, 957
Oral glucose tolerance test
  acromegaly, 1783
  gestational diabetes, 1856, 2273
Oral hairy cell leukoplakia, Plate VIII-42
Oral hairy leukoplakia
  acquired immunodeficiency syndrome,
    1328
  human immunodeficiency virus, 2095
Oral hypoglycemic agents, 1857-1858
Oral tolerance, 1143-1144, 1993
Orbit
  abscess, 2309
  cellulitis, 2309
  sinusitis, 2309
Orchiectomy
  prostate cancer, 719
  testicular cancer, 720
Orchitis
  impotence, 1762
  picornavirus infection, 1487
Orchitis-epididymitis, 1496
Organ-specific autoimmunity, 1145-1146
Organic acidemia, 1904
  disorders of branched-chain amino acids,
    1907-1908
  hyperammonemia, 1907
Organic hypogonadotropism, 1841
Organic solvents, 866-867
Organification, 1710
Organomegaly, 1911-1912
Organophosphate poisoning, 1754
Organophosphorus esters, 1020
Orientia tsutsugamushi, 1545
Orinase; *see* Tolbutamide
Ornithine
  cystinuria, 1910
  related diseases, 1904
  urea cycle, 1906
Ornithine transcarbamoylase deficiency, 1907
Orolabial herpes simplex virus-1 infection,
    1523
Oropharyngeal dysphagia, 1998
Oropharynx
  angioedema, 2306
  barium contrast examination, 1999
  cancer, 723
  movement of food, 1978
  normal flora, 1614, 1615
  supraglotittis, 2306
  tularemia, 1608
Orthochromatic normoblast, 531, Plate IV-3
Orthocolic reflex, 1980
Orthodromic accessory pathway, 142
Orthodromic atrioventricular reciprocating
    tachycardia, 144
Orthomyxovirus, 1483-1494
  acute febrile undifferentiated illness, 1487
  acute hemorrhagic conjunctivitis, 1490
  aseptic meningitis, 1488
  characteristics, 1483
  chemoprophylaxis, 1493
  chronic meningoencephalitis, 1490
  classification, 1483-1485
  common cold, 1487
  diagnosis, 1492
  encephalitis, 1488
  epidemic pleurodynia, 1489
  epidemiology, 1484-1485
  exanthems, 1489
  hand-foot-mouth syndrome, 1489
  hepatitis, 1490
  herpangina, 1488-1489
  influenza, 1490-1491
  lymphonodular pharyngitis, 1489
  myopericarditis, 1489-1490
  neurologic complications, 1491
  paralytic poliomyelitis, 1487-1488
  pathogenesis, 1485-1487

Orthomyxovirus—cont'd
  prevention, 1492-1493
  pulmonary complications, 1491
  treatment, 1492
Orthopedic surgery
  osteoarthritis, 1268
  rheumatoid arthritis, 1209
Orthophosphates, 1934
Orthopnea
  aortic regurgitation, 241
  dilated cardiomyopathy, 263
  heart failure, 163
  mitral regurgitation, 250
  mitral valve prolapse, 254
  precapillary pulmonary hypertension, 293
  pulmonary veno-occlusive disease, 298
Orthostatic hypotension
  acute pancreatitis, 2234
  autonomic failure, 935
  causes, 1828
  diabetic autonomic neuropathy, 1873
  megaloblastic anemia, 648
  with syncope, 953-954
Orthostatic proteinuria, 760-761
Orthovoltage machine, 553
OSA; *see* Obstructive sleep apnea
Oscillopsia, 1064
Osler node
  infective endocarditis, 227-228, 1383
  lupus erythematosus, 1291
Osler-Weber-Rendu syndrome, 2014
  cutaneous manifestations, 1321
  scleroderma, 1293
Osmolal gap, 806
Osmolality, 806
  plasma, 806
    capillary exchange, 47
    increased, 739
  serum, 806
    hyponatremia, 811
  urine, 742
    acute renal failure, 770
    chronic renal failure, 778
    nephrogenic diabetes insipidus, 883
    renal concentrating and diluting
      mechanisms, 739
    syndrome of inappropriate antidiuretic
      hormone, 489
Osmolar clearance, 748
Osmometer, 742
Osmoreceptor, 1790
Osmoregulation, 805-809, 1789
Osmotic demyelination syndrome, 1080
Osmotic diuresis, 824
Osmotic pressure
  influence on vasopressin, 1789
  regulation of albumin synthesis, 2119
Osmotic shock, 813
Osp-A vaccine, 1648
Ossification
  ankylosing spondylitis, 1239
  paravertebral, 1170
Osteitis fibrosa cystica, 1966, 1967
Osteoarthritis, 1199, 1264-1268
  glucocorticoid protocol, 1263
  hand, 1171
  joint space narrowing, 1166, 1167
  knee, 1172-1173
  osteoporosis with, 1945
  wrist, 1172
Osteoarthrosis, 1264-1268
Osteoblast, 1716
  alkaline phosphatase, 1744
  Paget's disease, 1955
  predominant hyperparathyroid bone disease,
    1962
Osteocalcin, 1716
  Paget's disease, 1956
  serum, 1747
Osteochondrodysplasia, 1286

Osteoclast, 1127, 1716
  1,25-dihydroxyvitamin D effects,
    1719-1720
  effects of calcitonin, 1718-1719
  osteopetrosis, 1958
  Paget's disease, 1955, 1956
  predominant hyperparathyroid bone disease,
    1962
Osteoclast-activating factor
  bone destruction, 1973
  calcium homeostasis, 1720
Osteocyte, 1716, 1962
Osteodystrophy
  Albright's hereditary, 1932
  chronic renal failure, 779, 780
  mixed uremic, 1963
  renal, 1961-1965
    calcium acetate, 785
    chronic renal failure, 785-786
    hyperparathyroidism, 1961
    hyperphosphatemia, 1938
Osteogenesis imperfecta, 1287
Osteogenic sarcoma, 552
Osteoid
  bone formation, 1949
  maturation, 1716
Osteomalacia, 1949-1955
  after parathyroidectomy, 1965
  bone biopsy, 1747
  chronic hypophosphatemia, 1936
  chronic renal failure, 785
  iliac crest biopsy, Plate IX-5
  proximal renal tubular acidosis, 837
  renal osteodystrophy, 1961
  vitamin D deficiency, 2106
  vitamin D metabolism, 1719
  X-linked hypophosphatemic rickets, 880
Osteomyelitis, 1433-1437
  anaerobic infection, 1617
  fever of unknown origin, 1377
  Haemophilus influenzae, 1588
  intervertebral disk space narrowing, 1169
  sickle cell disease, 658
  Staphylococcus aureus, 1549
  sternal, 1551
Osteonecrosis
  after renal transplantation, 795
  arthropathy, 1244
  joint space narrowing, 1166, 1167
  sickle cell disease, 659
  systemic lupus erythematosus, 1214
Osteopenia
  osteoporosis, 1944
  reduction in bone density, 1165
Osteopetrosis, 1958-1959
Osteophytosis, 1168, 1170, 1171
Osteoporosis, 1944-1949
  bone biopsy, 1747
  brucellosis, 1606
  calcitonin therapy, 1719
  glucocorticoid-induced, 1263
  heparin, 635
  menopause, 2271
  multiple myeloma, 864
  primary biliary cirrhosis, 2200
  reduction in bone density, 1165
  rheumatoid arthritis, 1205
Osteoporosis circumscripta, 1956
Osteoprogenitor cell, 1716
Osteosarcoma, 493
Osteosclerotic myeloma, 703
Ostium primum atrial septal defect, 282-283
Ostium secundum atrial septal defect, 280
Ostwald-100 viscometer, 567
O'Sullivan criteria for detecting gestational
    diabetes, 2273
Otalgia, 2307
Otitis
  epidural abscesses and, 1418
  Haemophilus influenzae, 1586, 1588
Otitis externa, 2307

Otitis media, 1395, 2307
  acute meningitis, 1407
  anaerobic infection, 1616-1617
  cerebral abscess and, 1413
  complication of influenza, 1492
Otogenic subdural empyema, 1417
Otomycosis, 2307
Otoneurology, 971-975
Otorrhea, 1407, 2307
Otosclerosis, 974
Ototopical antibiotics, 2307
Ototoxicity of chemotherapeutic agents, 585
Ouabain, 317-318
Ouchterlony immunodiffusion, 567
Outcomes research, 14-15
Ovary, 1832-1838
  amenorrhea, 1759-1760
  cancer, 715-716
    curability with chemotherapy, 552
    peritoneal carcinomatosis, 732
    thyrotoxicosis, 1807
  carcinoid tumor, 2082
  hirsutism, 1755-1756
  laboratory and diagnostic testing, 1835-1836
  modulation of gonadotropin secretion,
    1833-1835
  pathophysiologic disorders, 1836-1838
  physiology, 1832-1833
  ultrasound, 1734
Overfill theory of edema formation, 766
Overflow incontinence, 2291
Overflow proteinuria, 760
Overflow theory of ascites formation, 819, 2163
Overlap syndrome, 1221, 1228
Overnutrition, 2101
Overproduction jaundice, 2151, 2152
Oxacillin
  bacterial meningitis, 1411
  coagulase-negative staphylococcal infection,
    1552
  dosage, 1350
  hepatic injury, 2191
  septic arthritis, 1253
  Staphylococcus aureus meningitis, 1410
Oxalate
  ethylene glycol poisoning, 866
  hyperoxaluria
    renal allograft dysfunction, 794
    stone formation, 799
    therapy, 804
Oxalic acid, 891
Oxaloacetate, 1851
Oxamniquine, 1703
Oxaprozin, 1259
Oxazepam, 2295
Oxidants, 373
Oxidative burst, 1340
Oxidative hemolysis, 667
Oximetry, 431
7-Oxolithocholic acid, 2125
Oxybutynin
  bladder capacity increase, 1065
  multiple sclerosis, 1010
  urge incontinence, 2293
Oxycodone
  abuse, 2297
  cancer pain, 581
Oxygen, 379
Oxygen consumption
  cardiac output, 109-110
  chronic alcohol use, 2195
  determination, 109-110
  pulmonary artery catheterization, 391
  pulmonary edema, 427
Oxygen delivery
  effect of smoking, 589
  multiple organ dysfunction syndrome, 422
  pulmonary artery catheterization, 391
  pulmonary edema, 427
  respiratory care treatment modalities, 428-431
  shock, 176, 178

Oxygen dissociation curve, 348
Oxygen free radicals
  chronic ethanol use, 2195
  lung injury, 370
  theory of aging, 2283
Oxygen-hemoglobin affinity, 350
Oxygen-hemoglobin curve, 350
Oxygen-hemoglobin dissociation curve, 349, 412
Oxygen mask, 415
Oxygen partial pressure
  acquired immunodeficiency syndrome, 1477
  acute respiratory failure, 412
  aging and, 2284
  Cheyne-Stokes breathing, 354
  chronic obstructive pulmonary disease, 446
  effect on vasopressin release, 1791
  hepatopulmonary syndrome, 2170
  oxygen transport, 350
  primary pulmonary hypertension, 294
  pulmonary embolism, 500
  during sleep, 354
Oxygen therapy, 428-429
  acute respiratory failure, 415
  carbon dioxide retention with, 352
  chronic cor pulmonale, 447
  chronic obstructive pulmonary disease
    with acute respiratory failure, 417
    long-term, 444-445
  effects on blood gases, 352
  myocardial infarction, 216
  precapillary pulmonary hypertension, 296
  pulmonary edema, 169, 425-426
  pulmonary hypertension, 499
  pulmonary rehabilitation, 434-435
  pulmonary toxicity, 479
Oxygen toxicity
  management of acute respiratory failure, 415
  multiple organ dysfunction syndrome
    complication, 422
Oxygen transport, 350
  acid-base regulation by lung, 351
  alveolar-arterial oxygen difference, 351-352
  oxygen-hemoglobin curve, 350
  role of hemoglobin, 652
Oxygenation
  acute respiratory failure, 414, 415-416
  hypoxemia
    asthma, 1189
    causes, 349
    chemoreceptor response to, 353
    chest pain, 128
    diffusion limitation, 413
    electroencephalography, 907, 908
    erythropoietin, 586
    gram-negative bacteremia, 1449, 1450
    hepatopulmonary syndrome, 2170
    interstitial lung disease, 450
    Langerhans' cell granulomatosis, 464
    mechanical ventilation, 396-397
    prescription of oxygen, 429
    pulmonary edema, 425
    pulmonary hypertension, 498
    pulmonary thromboembolism, 500
    retinal, 2303
    during sleep, 354
    systemic lupus erythematosus, 1215
    vasopressin secretion, 1790-1791
    ventilation-perfusion ratio mismatch, 413
Oxymetholone, 674
Oxyntic cell, 1981, 1982
Oxyphenbutazone, 2110
Oxyphenisatin, 2192
Oxytocin
  biochemistry, 1788-1789
  physiology, 1789-1793

P

P-R interval, 85, 132
  aortic regurgitation, 241
  atrial septal defect, 281

P-R interval—cont'd
  atrioventricular conduction abnormalities, 154,
    155
  congenitally corrected transposition of great
    arteries, 290
  Ebstein's anomaly, 290
  ectopic atrial tachycardia, 143
  endocardial cushion defect, 283
  hypertrophic cardiomyopathy, 267
  hypokalemia, 829
  multifocal atrial tachycardia, 144
  Wolff-Parkinson-White syndrome, 142
P-R segment, 84
  acute pericarditis, 89, 273
P wave, 83-84
  accelerated atrioventricular junctional rhythm,
    144
  aortic stenosis, 237
  arrhythmia, 134
  atrioventricular conduction abnormalities, 154
  cardiac tamponade, 276
  Ebstein's anomaly, 290
  ectopic atrial tachycardia, 143
  effects of pacemaker, 90
  hyperkalemia, 832
  hypokalemia, 829
  left atrial abnormality, 88
  mitral regurgitation, 251
  mitral stenosis, 247
  premature atrial contractions, 141
  sinoatrial block, 153
  sinus bradycardia, 153
  sinus tachycardia, 141
  supraventricular tachyarrhythmias, 141
  tricuspid stenosis, 256
p21 gene, 547
p53 gene, 547
PABA; *see* Paraaminobenzoic acid
PAC; *see* Premature atrial contractions
Pacemaker
  arrhythmia, 139, 140
  atrial fibrillation, 148
  atrial flutter, 145-146
  atrioventricular block, 156
  bradyarrhythmias and atrioventricular blocks,
    153
  effects on electrocardiogram, 90
  extra cardiac sounds, 75
  hypertrophic obstructive cardiomyopathy, 269
  intraventricular conduction abnormalities, 156
  nosocomial infection, 1480
  sick sinus syndrome, 154
Pacemaker cell, 132
Pacemaker-mediated tachycardia, 139
Pacemaker syndrome, 139
Pacesetter potentials, 1976
Pachydermatoglyphy, 1319
Packed red blood cells, 572
  aplastic anemia, 673
  sickle cell disease, 659
Paclitaxel
  breast cancer, 710
  cardiotoxicity, 584
  lung cancer, 728
  multiple myeloma, 702
  ovarian cancer, 716
  prostate cancer, 720
Paget's disease, 1955-1958
  breast, 707
  calcitonin therapy, 1719
  high-output failure, 160
  serum alkaline phosphatase, 1744
  urinary hydroxyproline, 1745
Pain
  abdominal, 2030-2035
  acute aortic obstruction, 304
  acute cholecystitis, 2227
  acute occlusive arterial disease, 307
  acute pancreatitis, 2234
  acute pericarditis, 273
  acute pharyngitis, 1393

Pain—cont'd
  amebiasis, 1682
  anal fissure, 2093
  angina, 196
  anxiety, 1034
  aortic dissection, 128
  appendicitis, 2092
  autosomal dominant polycystic kidney disease, 873
  bacterial meningitis, 1406
  bacterial prostatitis, 1462
  biliary colic, 2225
  Bornholm disease, 1489
  brucellosis, 1605
  cancer, 580-581
    gastric, 2046
    lung, 488
    renal cell carcinoma, 898
    retroperitoneal tumor, 2251
  central retinal vein occlusions, 2304
  chest, 125-129
  chronic aortic obstruction, 304
  chronic fatigue, 2298
  chronic pancreatitis, 2238-2239
  Churg-Strauss syndrome, 465-466
  common bile duct obstruction, 2229
  common cold, 1391
  cryptococcosis, 1668
  dissection of aorta, 301
  dysuria, 762
  effect on vasopressin release, 1791
  epidemic pleurodynia, 1489
  esophageal, 1999
  esophageal spasm, 128
  Fabry's disease, 1918-1919
  facial, 962-963
  fibrocystic breast disease, 1848
  fibromyalgia, 1195
  fibrous dysplasia, 1960
  gas gangrene, 1423
  gastric lymphoma, 2049
  gastric volvulus, 2044
  gastroesophageal reflux, 128
  giant-cell arteritis, 304
  granulomatous gastritis, 2043
  hemorrhoids, 2093
  hepatocellular carcinoma, 2213
  herpangina, 1488
  Hodgkin's disease, 693
  human immunodeficiency virus, 1476
  hypersensitivity pneumonitis, 461
  hypertrophic obstructive cardiomyopathy, 266
  infectious esophagitis, 2020
  influenza, 1490
  irritable bowel syndrome, 2056
  kidney stones, 800
  Lassa fever, 1510
  lung disease, 408-410
  Lyme disease, 1647
  lymphomatoid granulomatosis, 470
  malignant involvement in skeleton, 1972
  malignant mesothelioma, 510
  Meckel's diverticulum, 2089
  mediastinal abnormality, 511
  medullary sponge kidney, 875
  mitral stenosis, 246
  mitral valve prolapse, 254
  multiple myeloma, 700
  myocardial infarction, 209-210
  myxoma, 330
  neck, 963-971
  nonsteroidal antiinflammatory drugs, 1259
  obstructive uropathy, 885-886
  omental torsion, 2252
  osteoarthritis, 1264-1268
  osteomalacia, 1949
  osteomyelitis, 1433
  otalgia, 2307
  otitis externa, 2307
  Paget's disease, 1955
  peptic ulcer disease, 2036-2037

Pain—cont'd
  pericardial, 128
  peritoneal, 2247
  pharmacologic stress testing, 104
  pheochromocytoma, 1829
  pleuritic pain *versus,* 505
  preeclampsia, 2274
  principle of double effect, 13
  retroperitoneal abscess, 1398
  retroperitoneal hemorrhage, 2250
  rheumatic fever, 1256
  rheumatoid arthritis, 1202
  shingles, 1527
  sickle cell disease, 657
  solitary liver cyst, 2111
  spontaneous pneumomediastinum, 514
  staphylococcal scalded-skin syndrome, 1421
  streptococcal toxic shock syndrome, 1557
  on swallowing, 1998
  systemic lupus erythematosus, 1214, 1215
  systemic sclerosis, 1229
  tetanus, 1573
  thoracic aortic aneurysm, 300
  urinary tract infection, 1458
  Wegener's granulomatosis, 468
Palate
  erythroplakia, Plate IV-13
  herpangina, 1488
  rubella, 1501
Palilalia, 977
Palindromic rheumatism, 1243-1244
Palliation
  cholangiocarcinoma, 2232
  esophageal cancer, 2024
  pancreatic cancer, 2243
  peritoneal tumors, 2249
Pallor
  acute lymphoblastic leukemia, 682
  acute occlusive arterial disease, 307
  elevation, 305
  idiopathic myelofibrosis, 677
  juvenile nephronophthisis, 875
  multiple myeloma, 701
  Raynaud's phenomenon, 1226
Palmaz-Schatz stent, 119, 120, 121
Palmitic acid, 1883
Palpation
  chest wall and bony thorax, 67-68, 70, 71
  evaluation of respiratory disease, 402
  thyroid, 1797
Palpitation, 130-131
  aortic regurgitation, 241
  dilated cardiomyopathy, 263
  hypertrophic obstructive cardiomyopathy, 266
  hypoglycemia, 1875
  ischemic heart disease, 197
  mitral regurgitation, 250
  mitral stenosis, 246
  mitral valve prolapse, 254
  pheochromocytoma, 322
  premature ventricular contractions, 149
  primary pulmonary hypertension, 294
Pamaquine, 663
PAMI trial, 122
Pamidronate
  hypercalcemia, 1929-1930, 1974
  Paget's disease, 1957
Panacinar emphysema, 439
Pancarditis, 1256
Pancellular hereditary persistence of fetal hemoglobin, 654
Pancreas
  abscess, 1399
  adrenergic responses, 1828
  calculi, 2238, 2239, 2240
  cellular anatomy, cell biology, and physiology, 2131-2133
  composition, location, embryologic derivation, and organization, 2129-2131
  computed tomography, 1734
  congenital anomalies, 2246

Pancreas—cont'd
  cystic fibrosis, 481-482, 483
  function tests, 2144-2145
  integrated pancreatic secretory physiology, 2133
  measurement of pancreatic secretion, 2133-2134
  pseudocyst
    acute pancreatitis, 2237
    chronic pancreatitis, 2241
  transplantation, 1101-1102
  trauma, 2246-2247
  von Hippel-Lindau syndrome, 1923
Pancreas divisum, 2246
Pancreas-specific protein, 2145
Pancreatic ascites, 2164
Pancreatic cancer
  endocrine tumor, 2244-2246
  exocrine tumor, 2242-2244
  extrahepatic cholestasis, 2155
  fasting hypoglycemia, 1876
  incidence and death rates, 550
  islet cell tumor, 1928
  pancreatic polypeptide secreting tumor, 2244
Pancreatic diabetes, 2239
Pancreatic disease, 2233-2247
  acquired immunodeficiency syndrome, 2098-2099
  congenital anomalies, 2246
  cystic fibrosis, 2246
  encephalopathy, 1101
  evaluation, 2144-2147
  malabsorption, 2062
  neurologic aspects, 1101
  osteomalacia, 1951-1952
  pancreatitis, 2233-2241
    activation of proteases within acinar cell, 2130
    acute, 2233-2238
    acute cholecystitis *versus,* 2228
    alcoholic ketosis, 1865
    chronic, 2238-2241
    chronic renal failure, 784
    endoscopic retrograde cholangiopancreatography, 1997
    exocrine pancreatic tumor, 2242
    extrahepatic cholestasis, 2155
    gallstone, 2230
    hypocalcemia, 1932
    hypomagnesemia, 1941
    intestinal obstruction *versus,* 2078
    lack of apolipoprotein C, 1898
    mumps complication, 1496
    pancreatic abscess, 1399
    panniculitis, 1245
    sepsis *versus,* 1451
  pleural effusion, 508
  reduced pancreatic exocrine secretion, 2134
  trauma-induced, 2246-2247
Pancreatic encephalopathy, 1101
Pancreatic enzymes
  assessment of pancreatic disease, 2144
  chronic pancreatitis, 2240, 2241
  cystic fibrosis, 2246
Pancreatic insufficiency
  cystic fibrosis, 2246
  impaired lipid ingestion, 1987
  Schilling test, 2060
Pancreatic islet cell antibody, 1158
Pancreatic lipase, 1987
Pancreatic stone protein, 2238
Pancreaticoduodenectomy, 2243
Pancreatitis, 2233-2241
  activation of proteases within acinar cell, 2130
  acute, 2233-2238
  acute cholecystitis *versus,* 2228
  alcoholic ketosis, 1865
  chronic, 2238-2241
  chronic renal failure, 784
  cystic fibrosis, 2246

Pancreatitis—cont'd
  endoscopic retrograde
      cholangiopancreatography, 1997
  exocrine pancreatic tumor, 2242
  extrahepatic cholestasis, 2155
  gallstone, 2230
  hypocalcemia, 1932
  hypomagnesemia, 1941
  intestinal obstruction *versus,* 2078
  lack of apolipoprotein C, 1898
  mumps complication, 1496
  pancreatic abscess, 1399
  panniculitis, 1245
  sepsis *versus,* 1451
Pancreatography, 1997
Pancreolauryl test, 2145
Pancreozymin, 2133
Pancytopenia
  aplastic anemia, 671
  hairy cell leukemia, 683
  megaloblastic anemia, 647
  myelodysplastic syndrome, 676
  neutropenia, 593
Pandiastolic aortic regurgitant murmur, 79-80
Panic attack, 355-356
Panic disorder
  anxiety, 1034
  chest pain, 128
Panniculitis, 1245
Pansystolic regurgitant murmur, 76, 77, 79
Pantoprazole, 2312
Pantothenic acid, 2116
  biochemical function, 2105
  deficiency, 2107
PAP; *see* Pulmonary alveolar proteinosis
Papanicolaou smear
  cervical cancer, 714-715
  preventive care guidelines, 2255
Papaverine
  hepatic injury, 2192
  impotence, 1764
Paper disk radioimmunoassay technique, 1154
Papillae, esophageal, 2015
Papillary carcinoma
  renal, 899
  thyroid, 1815
Papillary fibroelastoma
  cardiac, 330
  incidence, 329
Papillary muscle
  acute mitral regurgitation, 252
  rupture, 177, 219, 220
Papillary necrosis
  analgesic nephropathy, 890
  complications of acute pyelonephritis, 1456
  obstructive uropathy, 885
Papilledema, 1060
  bacterial meningitis, 1406
  brain herniation after lumbar puncture, 905
  cryptococcosis, 1669
  fundoscopic view, Plate VIII-51
  hepatic encephalopathy, 2161
  osteomalacia, 1949
  Rocky Mountain spotted fever, 1543
  subdural empyema, 1417
Papilloma
  breast, 1848
  inverting, 2308
  lung, 492
Papillomatosis
  breast, 1846, 1850
  recurrent respiratory, 2309
Papillomavirus
  carcinogenesis, 548
  cervical carcinoma, 549
Papillotomy, 2237
Pappenheimer body, 654, Plate IV-4
Paprika splitter's lung, 460
Papule
  acne vulgaris, 1305
  differential diagnosis of fever and rash, 1384

Papule—cont'd
  genital lesions, 1442
  Gottron's, Plate VII-3
  hand-foot-mouth syndrome, 1489
  human immunodeficiency virus, 1325
  rickettsialpox, 1545
  sarcoidosis, 1324, Plate VII-20
  systemic candidiasis, 1312
PAR; *see* Pulmonary arteriolar resistance
Para-aminobenzoate, 664
Para-aminosalicylic acid
  drug-nutrient interactions, 2110
  hepatic injury, 2191
Paraabducen nucleus, 1063
Paraaminobenzoic acid
  Bentiromide test, 2145
  folic acid metabolism, 1344
  hepatic injury, 2192
Paracarcinomatous neuropathy, 1020
Paracellular transport, 1988
Paracentesis
  abdominal pain, 2032
  ascites, 2164, 2165
  intraabdominal infection, 1399
  refractory ascites, 820
Paracicatricial emphysema, 439
Paracoccidioides brasiliensis, 1653, 1657
Paracrine function, 1708
Paracrine modulation of ventricular function, 45
Paradoxical emboli, 999
Paragonimus westermani, 507, 1704
Parainfluenza, 1494-1495
  common cold, 1391
  culture, 1369
Paralexia, 1033
Paralysis
  acute occlusive arterial disease, 307
  botulism, 1571
  diaphragmic, 359
  facial nerve, 2306
  gaze, 1033
  hyperkalemic periodic, 831
  hypokalemic, 1029-1030
  hypokalemic periodic, 826
  picornavirus infection, 1487
  rabies, 1506
Paralytic ileus, 1977, 2077
  intestinal obstruction *versus,* 2078
  peritonitis, 2080
Paralytic poliomyelitis, 1487-1488
Paramyotonia congenita, 1028
Paramyxovirus, 1390, 1494
Paranasal sinus cancer, 723
Paraneoplastic pemphigus, 1295
Paraneoplastic syndromes, 582-583
  antibodies, 1158
  arthropathy, 1247
  dementia, 987
  dermatoses, 1316-1319
  lung cancer, 488-489
  myelopathy, 1013
Paraprotein, 564
Paraproteinemia, 1104
Paraquat, 452, 867
Parasellar syndrome, 1071
Paraseptal emphysema, 439
Parasitic infection
  acquired immunodeficiency syndrome, 1474, 2095
  coccidian, 1679-1680
  depression, 1037
  diarrhea, 1428-1429, 1431
  fever of unknown origin, 1377
  helminths, 1696-1706
    eosinophilia, 1705-1706
    intestinal worms with tissue migratory phases, 1698-1699
    strictly intestinal worms, 1696-1698
    tissue worms, 1699-1705
    travel-related, 1466
  immune complexes, 1149

Parasitic infection—cont'd
  neurologic aspects, 1101
  peritonitis, 2247-2248
  pleural effusion, 507
  rheumatoid factor, 1160
  transfusion-transmitted, 576
  travel-related, 1465-1466
Parasomnias, 945-946
Parasternal approach in echocardiography, 95
Parasternal impulses, 67
Parasympathetic nervous system, 930
  alimentary motor function, 1977
  pupil innervation, 932
Parasympathomimetics
  asthma, 1191, 1192
  chronic obstructive pulmonary disease, 417, 444
  dystonia, 995
  glaucoma, 2302
  irritable bowel syndrome, 2056
  multiple sclerosis, 1010
  rhinitis, 1183
  vasodepressor syncope, 956
Parathion, 867
Parathyroid
  accumulation of aluminum in, 1961
  adenoma, 1965
  carcinoma, 1965-1966
  cyst, 2310
  osteoporosis, 1947
Parathyroid hormone, 1718, 1932, 1933
  assay, 1734
  calcium absorption in gut, 1717
  chronic renal failure, 777, 778
  hypercalcemia of malignancy, 1972
  hyperparathyroid bone disease
    chronic renal failure, 785
    mixed uremic osteodystrophy, 1963
    renal osteodystrophy, 1961
  hyperparathyroidism, 1965-1971
    arthropathy, 1246
    calcium pyrophosphate dihydrate deposition disease, 1279
    diagnosis, 1967-1969
    humoral hypercalcemia of malignancy *versus,* 1973-1974
    hypermagnesemia, 1943
    kidney stone formation, 798
    osteomalacia, 1950
    pathology and etiology, 1965-1966
    during pregnancy, 2273
    prevalence, 1965, 1966
    renal transplant recipient, 795
    renal wasting of phosphate, 1935
    symptoms and signs, 1966-1967
    treatment, 1969-1971
  hypoparathyroidism, 1931
    dementia, 987
    hypocalcemia with, 1931-1932
    myopathy, 1030
    osteomalacia, 1952
    urinary cyclic adenosine monophosphate, 1746
  intestinal magnesium absorption, 1939
  kidney stone formation, 798
  neurologic complications of uremia, 1105
  1-hydroxylation, 1719
  osteomalacia, 1949
  radioimmunoassay, 1745-1746
  regulator of urinary phosphate excretion, 1935
  role in calcium metabolism, 1718
Parathyroid hormone-related protein, 583
  calcium homeostasis, 1720
  syndrome of humoral hypercalcemia of malignancy, 1927
Parathyroidectomy, 1969-1970
  hypophosphatemia, 1936
  predominant hyperparathyroid bone disease, 1965
Paravertebral ossification, 1170
Paravertebral swelling, 1171

Paravertebral sympathetic chain and ganglia, 930
Parenchymal lung disease
  occupational, 473
  single lung allograft, 514
Parenchymal renal disease
  acute renal failure, 768-769
  diagnosis, 771-772
  pathophysiology, 769
Parenteral nutrition
  acute pancreatitis, 2237
  hypercalcemia after, 1928
  potassium depletion, 827
  short bowel syndrome, 2066
Paresthesia
  acute occlusive arterial disease, 307
  hypocalcemia, 1932
  hypothyroidism, 1809
  megaloblastic anemia, 648
Paretic dysarthria, 977
Parietal alexia, 978
Parietal cell
  acid secretion by, 1981
  regulation by enterochromaffin-like cells,
    1981-1982
Parietal cell hydrogen-potassium-ATPase, 1983,
  1984
Parietal cell receptors, 1981, 1983
Parietal pain, 2030
Parietal peritoneum, 2247
Parietal pleura, 505
Parkinsonian tremor, 994
Parkinsonism, 989-997
  disordered sleep, 946-947
  disorders with increased tone, 997
  fall risk, 2290
  hyperkinetic movement disorders, 993-997
  impotence, 1761
  Parkinson's disease, 989-992
  secondary, 992-993
Parkinson's disease, 989-992
  depression, 1036
  reflux esophagitis, 2023
  respiratory rhythm abnormalities, 1098
Parkinson's-plus syndromes, 992-993
Paromomycin
  amebiasis, 1683
  cryptosporidiosis, 1474, 1476
  giardiasis, 1685
Paronychia, candidal, 1310-1311, 1312, 1662
Parotid gland cyst, 2310
Parotitis
  acute meningitis, 1407
  chronic renal failure, 784
  facial pain, 962
  mumps, 1496
Paroxetine, 1037
  chronic fatigue syndrome, 2300
  depression in elderly patient, 2289
  human cytochrome P450 isoforms, 2312
Paroxysmal atrial tachycardia, 143-144, 146
Paroxysmal cold hemoglobinuria, 670
Paroxysmal nocturnal dyspnea, 163
Paroxysmal nocturnal hemoglobinuria, 668, 1148
Paroxysmal supraventricular tachycardia, 2276
Paroxysmal vertigo, 981
Parry's disease, 1805-1807
Pars flaccida, 2307
Pars nervosa, 1788
Partial anomalous pulmonary venous connection,
  282
Partial code, 12
Partial complex seizure, 954
Partial lipodystrophy, 1902, 1903
Partial nephrectomy, 898
Partial pressure of oxygen inspired, 348
Partial seizure, 979
Partial thromboplastin time, 570-571
  acquired coagulation inhibitors, 630
  disseminated intravascular coagulation, 609
  fibrinogen abnormalities, 625
  gastrointestinal bleeding, 2011

Partial thromboplastin time—cont'd
  hemophilia, 606
  hemophilia A, 618
  hemophilia B, 622
  hemostatic abnormalities in liver disease, 627
  vitamin K deficiency, 626
Partial thromboplastins, 571
Partial transposition of pulmonary veins, 282
Parvovirus, 1512-1514
  during pregnancy, 2280
  septic arthritis, 1255
Passive countermeasures, 2265
Passive diffusion, 1985-1986
Passive head-up tilt-testing, 956
Passive pressure-volume relation, 44-45
Passive pulmonary hypertension, 297-298
Passive smoking
  chronic obstructive pulmonary disease, 438
  lung cancer, 486
Passovoy, 618, 624
Pasteurella, 1347, 1609
Pastia's lines, 1421
Patella, chondromalacia patellae, 1266
Patent ductus arteriosus, 280, 285-286
  cardiac auscultation, 68
  complete transposition of great arteries, 290
  continuous murmur, 81
  precapillary pulmonary hypertension, 296
  pulmonary hypertension, 296
  pulmonic stenosis, 288
  tricuspid atresia, 291
Paternalism, 11
Pathogens
  laboratory and diagnostic testing, 1366-1374
    bacteria culture, 1367-1369
    Chlamydiae, Rickettsiae, and Mycoplasmas,
      1370
    direct detection techniques, 1370-1373
    fungus culture, 1370
    serology, 1373-1374
    skin testing, 1374
    test interpretation, 1366-1367
    virus culture, 1369-1370
  nosocomial, 1362
  sexually transmitted, 1438
Pathologic fracture
  fibrous dysplasia, 1960
  multiple myeloma, 864
  Paget's disease, 1955
  primary hyperparathyroidism, 1966
Patient autonomy, 10, 12
Patient compliance
  antihypertensive therapy, 328-329
  antituberculosis therapy, 1632
  continuous oxygen therapy, 435
  death after cardiac transplantation, 338
Patient education
  asthma, 1189
  clinical guidelines, 25
  diabetes mellitus, 1856
  drug interactions, 2313
  injury prevention, 2267
Patient history
  abdominal pain, 2031-2032
  abnormal swallowing, 1998
  abnormalities of vision, 1056
  acute pericarditis, 273
  anxiety, 1034
  aortic regurgitation, 241
  aortic stenosis, 236
  arrhythmia, 133
  asthma, 1187-1188
  bleeding patient, 603
  cardiac tamponade, 275-276
  chest pain, 127, 129
  chronic fatigue, 2298
  chronic obstructive pulmonary disease, 442
  chronic renal failure, 782
  constipation, 2053
  constrictive pericarditis, 277
  fever and rash, 1381

Patient history—cont'd
  fever of unknown origin, 1378
  gastrointestinal bleeding, 2010
  gynecomastia, 1764
  hirsutism, 1756
  human immunodeficiency virus infection,
    1472
  impotence, 1760-1761
  inflammatory myopathies, 1235
  inherited disease, 1730
  lung disease, 401-402
  mitral regurgitation, 250
  mitral stenosis, 246
  mitral valve prolapse, 254
  neurologic disorders, 902-903
  neurologic examination, 902
  nosocomial infection, 1482
  palpitations, 130
  pericardial effusion, 274
  personality disorders, 1039
  preoperative medical evaluation, 2256
  pulmonic regurgitation, 257
  rhinitis, 1181-1182
  sexually transmitted disease, 1438
  site of blockage in cholestasis, 2156
  sudden cardiac survivor, 188
  syncope, 955
  tricuspid regurgitation, 256
  tricuspid stenosis, 255
Patient positioning
  cardiac auscultation, 70-71
  jugular venous pulse, 65
  rigid proctoscopy, 1995
Patient preference assessment, 14-15
Patient satisfaction, 18-19
PATP; *see* Pure amegakaryocytic
          thrombocytopenic purpura
Pattern-reversal visual evoked potential, 910-911
Patterson-Kelly syndrome, 2020
Paul Bunnell test, 1529
PBC; *see* Primary biliary cirrhosis
PCOD; *see* Polycystic ovarian disease
PCR; *see* Polymerase chain reaction
PDA; *see* Patent ductus arteriosus
$P(A-a)O_2$; *see* Alveolar-arterial oxygen difference
Peak acid output, 2003
Peak exercise oxygen consumption, 337
Peak height velocity, 1767, 1768, 1770
Peak weight velocity, 1767, 1768, 1770
Peau d'orange, 1322, 1420
PEB regimen, 721
Pectus excavatum, 254
Pedal plantar flexion, 305
Pedigree, 1730
Peduncular hallucinosis, 1033
PEEP; *see* Positive end-expiratory pressure
Pel-Ebstein fever, 693
Pelger-Huët anomaly, 594, Plate IV-6
Peliosis hepatis, 2212
Pellagra
  Hartnup disease, 879
  neurologic aspects, 1101
  niacin deficiency, 2107
Pelvic examination
  abdominal pain, 2032
  cancer of unknown primary site, 731
Pelvic floor exercises, 2293
Pelvic infection
  actinomycosis, 1665
  amenorrhea, 1760
  anaerobic bacteria, 1618
  enterococcal, 1562
Pelvic inflammatory disease, 1583
Pelvis
  clostridial abscess, 1575
  erysipelas, 1420
  osteopetrosis, 1958
  Paget's disease, 1955, 1956
Pemoline, 943
Pemphigoid, 1295-1296
Pemphigoid gestationis, 1296

Pemphigus, 1293-1295
Pemphigus erythematosus, 1294
Pemphigus foliaceus, 1294
Pemphigus vulgaris, 1155, 1293-1294
Penbutolol, 325
Penetrance, autosomal dominant disorders, 1726
Penetrating aortic ulcer, 301
Penetrating artery disease, 1005-1006
Penetrating trauma
    aortic, 304
    cardiac, 332
    pancreas, 2246
    traumatic pericardial disease, 273
D-Penicillamine
    cystinuria, 804-805, 1910
    drug-nutrient interactions, 2110
    hepatic injury, 2191
    induction of myasthenia gravis, 1021
    induction of pemphigus, 1294
    pulmonary parenchymal reactions, 476
    pulmonary reactions, 477
    pulmonary toxicity, 479
    rheumatic disease, 1260, 1261
    rheumatoid arthritis, 1208
    systemic sclerosis, 1232
    Wilson's disease, 1102, 2206
Penicillin, 1351-1352
    actinomycosis, 1665
    activity against major anaerobes, 1620
    acute pancreatitis, 2237
    allergy, 1194
    anaerobic bacteria, 1619-1620
    bacterial meningitis, 1410, 1411
    bactericidal effect, 1344
    brain abscess, 1416
    bullous impetigo, 1419
    chlamydial infection, 1537
    chronic obstructive pulmonary disease, 444
    clostridial infection, 1576
    coagulase-negative staphylococcal infection,
        1552
    dermatitis-aggravating *Staphylococcus aureus*
        infection, 1303
    diphtheria, 1567
    diverticulosis, 2091
    dosage, 1350
    drug-induced bile duct injury, 2203
    effects on kidney, 868
    enterococci resistance, 1561
    erysipelas, 1420
    Haemophilus ducreyi, 1589
    Haemophilus influenzae, 1588
    Helicobacter pylori, 1593
    hepatic injury, 2190-2192
    infectious eczematoid dermatitis, 1304
    infective endocarditis, 231, 232
    infective endocarditis prophylaxis, 234
    interference with oral anticoagulants, 636
    intraabdominal infection, 1401
    Lyme disease, 1254, 1647
    meningococcal disease, 1580
    non-group A streptococcal infection,
        1563-1564
    nonvenereal treponematosis, 1644
    osteomyelitis, 1436
    Pasteurella, 1609
    peptic ulcer disease, 2040
    peritonitis, 1402
    relapsing fever, 1646
    respiratory exacerbations in cystic fibrosis,
        483
    rheumatic fever, 1258
    septic arthritis, 1253
    sinusitis, 1183, 1395, 2309
    staphylococcal infection, 1551
    staphylococcal scalded-skin syndrome, 1421
    streptococcal pharyngitis, 1393
    streptococcal resistance, 1559-1560
    Streptococcus pneumoniae meningitis, 1410
    structural formula, 1351
    subdural empyema, 1418

Penicillin—cont'd
    syphilis, 1643
    tetanus, 1574
    typhoid fever, 1601
    use during pregnancy, 2281
    wound botulism, 1572
Penicillin-binding proteins, 1344, 1555
Penicillin G, 1351-1352
    bacterial peritonitis, 1400
    dosage, 1350
    endocarditis, 231
    Neisseria meningitidis meningitis, 1410
    resistance of *Staphylococcus aureus*, 1345
    rheumatic fever, 1258
    septic arthritis, 1253
    use during pregnancy, 2281
Penicillin V
    dosage, 1350
    streptococcal pharyngitis, 1393
Penicilliosis, 1658
Penicillium, 1368, 1658
Penis
    autonomic control of erection, 933-934
    candidal balanitis, 1662
    chancre, Plate VIII-34
    exam for sexually transmitted disease,
        1438-1439
    impotence, 1760-1764
    lymphogranuloma venereum, 1535
Pennyroyal oil, 2193
Pentaerythritol tetranitrate, 201, 202
Pentagastrin, 1739
    provocative testing, 1746
    stimulated acid output, 2003
Pentamidine
    African trypanosomiasis, 1689
    effects on kidney, 869
    leishmaniasis, 1686
    Pneumocystis carinii pneumonia, 1694,
        1695
    secretion clearance and lung expansion, 430
Pentaquine, 663
Pentostam; *see* Sodium stibogluconate
Pentosuria, 1879
Pentoxifylline, 309
Pepsin, 1980, 1984
    gastric refluxate, 2015
Pepsinogen, 1984-1985
Peptic ulcer disease, 2035-2041
    acid secretory values, 2003
    Helicobacter pylori, 1592-1593
    operative risk, 2263
Peptidases, 1988
Peptide hormones, 1708-1709
Peptides, G cell stimulation, 1981
Peptidoglycan, 1343
Peptococcus, 1368
Peptones, 1981, 1984
Peptostreptococcus, 1368
Percent overweight, 1751
Perception disorders, 1033
    stroke patient, 1055
Percussion
    abdomen, 2032
    evaluation of respiratory disease, 402, 403
    pleural disease, 505
Percutaneous balloon pericardiotomy, 332
Percutaneous catheter drainage, 1402
Percutaneous endoscopic gastrostomy, 1995
Percutaneous needle biopsy
    diagnosis and staging of lung cancer,
        489-490
    iliac crest, 1747
    kidney, 748
    liver, 2141, 2154
    pleural, 382
Percutaneous transhepatic cholangiography,
        1997, 2141, 2232
Percutaneous transhepatic portal venous
        sampling, 2244

Percutaneous transluminal coronary angioplasty,
        108, 308, 309
    cost-utility analysis, 16
    myocardial infarction, 214-215
    randomized trials, 117, 118
    shock, 183, 185
Percutaneous transluminal renal angioplasty, 896
Perennial rhinitis, 1181
Perforation
    acute otitis media, 1395
    gallbladder, 2227, 2228
    intestinal obstruction, 2077
    peptic ulcer disease, 2039
    tympanic membrane, 2307
Performance-oriented mobility assessment, 2290
Perfusion, 349
    hypoxic pulmonary vasoconstriction, 363
    multiple organ dysfunction syndrome, 422
Perfusion imaging, 212
Perfusion lung scan, 387-388
    pulmonary thromboembolism, 501-502
Pergolide
    Parkinson's disease, 991, 992
    restless legs syndrome, 944
Perhexiline, 2192
Perianal fistula, 2093
Perianal ulcer
    acquired immunodeficiency syndrome, 2098
    Crohn's disease, Plate X-5
Periarteritis, 1092
Periarticular calcification, 1169
Periarticular osteoporosis, 1165
Periarticular rheumatic complaints, 1195-1198
Pericardial cyst, 273, 513
Pericardial defect, congenital, 291-292
Pericardial effusion, 274-275
    acquired immunodeficiency syndrome, 333, 1478
    acute pericarditis, 274
    cardiac metastasis, 332
    echocardiography, 100
    heart murmur, 76
    hypothyroidism, 1809
    management, 278
Pericardial fluid
    cardiac tamponade, 276
    constrictive pericarditis, 278
    pericardial effusion, 274
    tuberculous pericarditis, 1636
Pericardial friction rub, 75
    acute pericarditis, 273
    myocardial contusion, 332
Pericardial heart disease, 271-279
    abnormal jugular venous pulse, 66
    cardiac catheterization, 108
    cardiac tamponade, 275-276
    computed tomography, 106
    etiology, 272-273
    management, 278-279
    pericardial effusion, 274-275
    pericarditis
        acute, 273-274
        chest pain, 128
        constrictive, 277-278
        electrocardiography, 89
        myocardial infarction, 221-222
        restrictive cardiomyopathy *versus*, 271
    referral, 279
Pericardial knock, 74, 277
Pericardial pain, 273, 505
Pericardial pressure, 271-272, 275
Pericardial tamponade, 332
Pericardial tuberculosis, 1636-1637
Pericardial window, 278
Pericardiectomy, 278-279
Pericardiocentesis
    cardiac tamponade, 276
    penetrating injury to heart, 332
    pericardial heart disease, 278
Pericarditis
    acute, 273-274
    arrhythmia, 133

Pericarditis—cont'd
  atrial fibrillation, 146
  chest pain, 128
  chronic renal failure, 784
  constrictive, 277-278
    cardiac catheterization, 116
    central venous pressure, 66-67
    management, 278-279
    restrictive cardiomyopathy *versus,* 271
    transudative pleural effusion, 507
  electrocardiography, 89
  etiology, 272-273
  management, 278-279
  myocardial infarction, 221-222
  myocarditis, 262
  restrictive cardiomyopathy *versus,* 271
  rheumatic fever, 1257
  rheumatoid arthritis, 1204
  systemic lupus erythematosus, 1214
  systemic sclerosis, 1230
  tuberculous, 1636-1637
Pericardium, 271-272
  metastatic disease, 331
  myopericarditis, 1489-1490
  passive pressure-volume relationship, 44-45
  radiation injury, 273
Pericholangitis, 2155
Pericyte, 371
Perilymph fistula, 973
Perimeningeal infection, 1413-1419
Perimenstrual syndrome, 1077
Perinatal transmission of human
    immunodeficiency virus, 1471
Perinephritic hematoma, 748
Perinuclear antineutrophil cytoplasmic antibody
  primary sclerosing cholangitis, 2202
  vasculitis, 1218
Periodic acid-Schiff stain
  Cryptosporidium oocyst, Plate VIII-33
  Whipple's disease, 2064, 2065
Periodic alternating nystagmus, 1064
Periodic health examination, 2254-2256
Periodic hyperlysinemia, 1907
Periodic limb movement disorder, 944
Periodontal infection, 1617
Perioperative surveillance, 2258
Periorbital cellulitis, 2309, Plate VIII-26
Periostitis, 1200, 1241, 1641
Peripheral arterial aneurysm, 309
Peripheral arterial vasodilatation hypothesis,
    818-819
Peripheral artery catheterization, 390
Peripheral blood
  abnormal nucleated cells in, 594-596
  chromosome analysis, 1727
  megaloblastic anemia, 648
  source of hematopoietic cells, 577
Peripheral blood leukocyte, 1151-1152
Peripheral blood smear, 556-557
  abnormal red blood cell indices in nonanemic
      patient, 588
  acute nephritic syndrome, 764
  babesiosis, 557
  cold agglutinin disease, 670
  iron deficiency, 643
  left shift on, 591
  multiple myeloma, 701
  neutropenia, 593
  overproduction jaundice, 2152
  thrombocytopenia, 613
Peripheral blood stem cell transplantation,
    702
Peripheral cholangiocarcinoma, 2231
Peripheral circulation
  capillary exchange and microcirculatory
      control mechanisms, 47-48
  cardiac output and systemic hemodynamics,
      46-47
  coronary circulation, 48-49
Peripheral inhibitors, 325, 326

Peripheral leukocyte count
  spinal epidural abscess, 1418
  subdural empyema, 1417
Peripheral lymph node hyperplasia, Plate VIII-35
Peripheral nerve, 930
  injury in stroke patient, 1055
  relation of reflexes, 964
Peripheral nervous system
  bladder control, 933
  central nervous system *versus,* 1014
  detrusor muscle areflexia, 935
Peripheral neuritis, 2107
Peripheral neuropathy, 1014-1020
  acute intermittent porphyria, 1926
  after stroke, 1007
  autonomic hyperactivity, 935
  chemotherapy-induced, 585
  chronic renal failure, 781, 784
  complication of chemotherapy, 1072
  diabetes mellitus, 1871-1872
  differential diagnosis, 1014-1015
  electromyography, 1017
  headache, back pain, multiple cranial nerve
      palsies, and polyradiculopathy, 1017
  malabsorption, 2057
  management, 1020
  polyneuropathy, 1017-1020
  progressive lower motor neuron deficit with or
      without upper motor neuron deficit,
      1015
  proximal pain in one limb, with sensory,
      motor, or reflex abnormalities, 1015-1017
  rheumatoid arthritis, 1094
  vasculitis, 1225
Peripheral pulses, 64
Peripheral resistance, 316, 317, 318
Peripheral total parenteral nutrition, 2115
Peripheral vascular disease, 304-312
  anticoagulant therapy, 641
  arteritis, 311
  contraindication to renal transplantation, 792
  occlusive peripheral arterial disease, 307-309
  peripheral arterial aneurysm, 309
  peripheral arteries, 305-307
  peripheral veins, 311-312
  preoperative evaluation, 2258
  vasospastic disorders, 309-311
Peripheral vascular resistance
  cirrhosis, 818
  hypertension, 316
Peripheral vascular system
  heart failure, 161-162, 164
  systemic sclerosis, 1229
Perirectal disease, 2069
Perirectal pain, 1476
Peristalsis
  alimentary motor function, 1977
  assessment, 2000
  defense against bacterial overgrowth of small
      intestine, 2060
  gastroesophageal reflux disease, 2015
  hypertrophic pyloric stenosis, 2044
Peristaltic contractions, 1977
Peritoneal carcinomatosis, 732
Peritoneal dialysis
  acute renal failure, 774
  chronic renal failure, 790-791
  hypercalcemia, 1929
  malnutrition, 2100
Peritoneoscopy, 1997-1998
Peritoneovenous shunt, 822
Peritoneum, 2247
Peritonitis, 2079-2080, 2247-2249
  abdominal evaluation, 2032
  acquired immunodeficiency syndrome, 1476
  anaerobic bacteria, 1617
  candidal, 1661
  dialysis-related, 791
  paralytic ileus, 2078
  primary, 1396
  systemic lupus erythematosus, 1214

Peritonsillar abscess, 1393, 1617, 2306
Peritubular capillary forces, 738
Perlèche, 1311
Permanent pacing, 139
Permeability, antibiotic, 1345
Permeability edema, 346-347
Permissive hypercapnia, 397, 423
Pernicious anemia
  Addison's disease, 1823-1824
    adrenocortical antibodies, 1157
    autoantibodies, 1155
    cutaneous manifestations, 1322-1323
    hypercalcemia, 1928
    hyperkalemia, 831
    hyperpigmentation of gums, Plate VII-14
    infertility and oligospermia, 1846
    lymphocytosis, 593
    weight loss, 1749
  dementia, 987
  dizziness, 972
  gastric antibodies, 1157
  gastric cancer, 2045
  hypokalemia, 827
  Lambert-Eaton myasthenic syndrome with, 1024
  neurologic aspects, 1103
  during pregnancy, 2279
  Schilling test, 2060
  type A gastritis, 2042
  vitamin B_{12} deficiency, 650
Pernicious vomiting of pregnancy, 2278
Pernio, 310
Peroneal nerve
  damage in leprosy, 1650
  lower-limb somatosensory evoked potentials,
      914
  mononeuropathy, 1017
Peroneal palsy, 1017
Perphenazine, 2027
Perserverative speech disorders, 977
Persistent diarrhea, 1429-1430
Persistent hyperlysinemia, 1907
Persistent hyperphenylalaninemia, 1905
Persistent vegetative state, 950-951
Personality change in elderly, 2288
Personality disorders, 1039-1040, 1041
Personality tests, 903
Pertussis, 592, 1611-1613
PES; *see* Programmed electrical stimulation
Petechiae
  aplastic anemia, 672
  differential diagnosis of fever and rash, 1384
  gram-negative bacteremia, 1449
  idiopathic thrombocytopenic purpura, Plate
      IV-10
  infective endocarditis, 227
  intradermal hemorrhage of vasculitis, Plate
      VIII-45
  neonatal cytomegalovirus, 1528
  Rocky Mountain spotted fever, 1382, Plate
      VIII-18
  scurvy, 2107
  thrombocytopenia, 603
Petit mal seizure, 979
Peutz-Jeghers syndrome
  cutaneous changes and malignancy, 1319-1320
  gastric polyp, 2046
  risk for colonic cancer, 2083
  small bowel adenocarcinoma, 2081
Peyer's patches, 1989-1990, 1991
Peyronie's disease, 1761
pH
  bile, 2123
  chronic renal failure, 779
  esophageal, 2001
  indigenous microflora, 1614
  mucus gel, 1984
  oxygen-hemoglobin affinity, 350
  serum calcium, 1744
  stool, 2006
  urinary, 742-743
  vaginal discharge, 1439

Phaeohyphomycosis, 1660
Phage cloning systems, 52
Phagocyte, 1339-1343
    abnormalities, 678-681
    cell-mediated immunity, 1127-1128
    cell surface receptors, 1136
    immunologic defects, 1386
Phagocytosis
    barrier to infection, 1335
    calcium pyrophosphate dihydrate crystals,
        1277
    defects, 1341
    splenic role, 600
Phagosome, 1340
Phakomatoses, 1920-1923
Pharmacodynamics
    changes with aging, 2286
    drug interactions, 2312
Pharmacokinetics, 2286
Pharmacologic stress imaging, 103-104
Pharmacologic testing of autonomic nervous
        system, 938
Pharmacomechanical coupling, 1976
Pharyngitis, 1392-1393
    acute meningitis, 1407
    adenovirus infection, 1503
    gonococcal, 1583
    infectious mononucleosis, 1529
    Lassa fever, 1510
    lymphonodular, 1489
    parainfluenza, 1494
    picornavirus infection, 1487
    scarlet fever, 1421
    staphylococcal toxic shock syndrome, 1421
    Streptococcus pyogenes, 1556
Pharyngoconjunctival fever, 1393, 1503-1504
Pharynx
    abnormal swallowing, 1998
    diphtheria, 1566
    movement of food, 1978
    obstructive sleep apnea, 525
    sore throat, 1392-1393
        acute pharyngitis, 1392
        chronic fatigue, 2298
        common cold, 1391
        epidemic pleurodynia, 1489
        hand-foot-mouth syndrome, 1489
        herpangina, 1488-1489
        infectious mononucleosis, 1529
        influenza, 1490
        Lassa fever, 1510
        Mycoplasma pneumoniae pneumonia, 1539
        peritonsillar abscess, 2306
        rheumatic fever, 1256
        scarlet fever, 1421
        spontaneous pneumomediastinum, 514
        subacute thyroiditis, 1811
        supraglotittis, 2306
        tonsillopharyngitis, 2309
Phase 2 metabolism, 2311
Phenacetin, 870-871, 890
Phenazopyridine, 2192
Phenelzine, 1037
    anxiety disorders, 1035
    depression in elderly patients, 2289
Phenindione, 2192
Phenobarbital, 983
    anticonvulsant-induced osteomalacia, 1953
    hepatic injury, 2191
    interaction with cyclosporin, 793
    during pregnancy, 2281
    serum bilirubin levels, 2154
    status epilepticus, 983
Phenothiazines
    acute intermittent porphyria, 1926
    antiemesis, 2028
    chemotherapy-induced nausea and vomiting,
        582
    drug-induced bile duct injury, 2203
    marrow suppression, 679

Phenotype, 50, 1721
    alpha$_1$-antitrypsin deficiency, 2206
    somatic mutator, 549
Phenoxybenzamine, 1830, 1831
Phentermine, 261
Phentolamine
    hypertensive emergency, 328
    impotence, 1764
    neurogenic pulmonary edema, 1099
    pheochromocytoma, 1831
Phenylalanine
    alkaptonuria, 1280
    breast cancer, 710
    G cell stimulation, 1981
    hyperphenylalaninemia, 1904-1905
    phenylketonuria, 1905
    related diseases, 1904
Phenylalanine carrier, 1988
Phenylbutazone
    glucose-6-phosphate dehydrogenase
        deficiency, 664
    hepatic injury, 2191
    interference with oral anticoagulants, 636
Phenylephrine
    chronic rhinitis, 2308
    pupil response, 933
Phenylethanolamine N-methyltransferase, 1826,
        1827
Phenylethylamine, 2104
Phenylhydrazine, 663
Phenylketonuria, 1731, 1904-1905
Phenylpiperazine, 1037
Phenylpropanolamine, 2104, 2293
Phenytoin, 983
    anticonvulsant-induced osteomalacia, 1953
    drug-induced bile duct injury, 2203
    euthyroid hypothyroxinemia, 1804
    glucose-6-phosphate dehydrogenase
        deficiency, 664
    hepatic injury, 2186, 2190, 2191
    human cytochrome P450 isoforms, 2312
    interaction with cyclosporin, 793
    interference with oral anticoagulants, 636
    during pregnancy, 2281
    pulmonary hypersensitivity reactions, 479
    status epilepticus, 983
Pheochromocytoma, 1828-1831
    autonomic hyperactivity, 935
    hypercalcemia, 1928
    hypertension, 322
    insulin resistance, 1862
    neurofibromatosis, 1921
    weight loss, 2298
Phialophora, 1660
Philadelphia chromosome, 544, 545, 562, 686,
        1728
Phlebothrombosis, 1007
Phlebotomus fever virus, 1515
Phlebotomy
    hereditary hemochromatosis, 2204, 2205
    polycythemia vera, 590, 688
    tetralogy of Fallot, 289
    ventricular septal defect, 285
Phlegm, 408
Phlegmasia cerulea dolens, 631
Phonocardiography, 259
Phosphate, 1934-1939
    body water compartments, 736
    chronic renal failure, 779
    dilated myocarditis, 265
    hyperphosphatemia, 1938-1939
        acute renal failure, 773
        chronic renal failure, 779, 785-786
        renal bone disease, 1964
        renal osteodystrophy, 1961
    hypophosphatasia, 1854
    hypophosphatemia, 1935-1938
        cardiomyopathy, 262
        diabetic ketoacidosis, 1864-1865
        dilated cardiomyopathy, 265
        hemolysis associated with liver disease, 667

Phosphate—cont'd
    hypophosphatemia—cont'd
        hereditary fructose intolerance, 1880
        renal phosphate wasting, 880
        X-linked hypophosphatemic rickets, 880
    hypophosphatemic osteomalacia, 1952-1953
    hypophosphatemic rickets, 1952
    renal osteodystrophy, 785
    renal phosphate wasting syndromes, 880
    replacement in diabetic ketoacidosis, 1864
    rickets, 881
    serum, 1934
        bone and mineral disorders, 1745
        hypoparathyroidism, 1931
        primary hyperparathyroidism, 1968
        rickets, 881
        storage in bone, 1715
        titratable buffer, 835
        urine pH, 742
Phosphate binders, 1964
Phosphate salts, 1938
Phosphatidyl inositol, 542
Phosphatidylcholine, 2123, 2126-2127, 2195
Phosphatidylcholine transfer protein, 2126
Phosphatidylinositol, 1712
Phosphaturia, 1935
Phosphodiester bonds, 49
Phosphodiesterase inhibitors, 1454
Phosphofructokinase deficiency, 1029, 1882
Phosphoglycerate kinase, 663
Phospholamban, 41
Phospholipase A2
    acute pancreatitis, 2234
    diagnosis of pancreatic diseases, 2144
Phospholipase C
    activation, 57
    hormone function, 1712
    pepsinogen secretion, 1984, 1985
Phospholipids
    antibodies to, 1160
    bile, 2123
    lipoproteins, 1885
    metabolism, 1883-1884
    synthesis in liver, 2120
5-Phosphoribosyl-1-pyrophosphate, 1269
Phosphorus
    functions, 2109
    poisoning, 2188
    recommended daily dietary allowances, 2115
    renal osteodystrophy, 1961
    serum
        bone and mineral disorders, 1745
        primary hyperparathyroidism, 1968
    total parenteral nutrition formula, 2117
Photoallergens, 1307
Photodermatosis, 1306-1307
Photophobia
    acute hemorrhagic conjunctivitis, 1490
    human immunodeficiency virus-infected
        patients, 2306
Photosensitivity, 1306-1307
    drug-induced, 1315
    human immunodeficiency virus infection, 1327
    lupus erythematosus, 1291
    protoporphyria, 1926
Phototherapy
    dermatitis, 1303
    psoriasis, 1302
    unconjugated hyperbilirubinemia, 2153
Phototoxic agents, 1306
Phrygian cap, 2233
Physical activity
    after cardiac transplantation, 343
    aortic regurgitation, 241
    during bed rest, 2288
    cardiovascular response, 49
    chronic fatigue syndrome, 2300
    chronic obstructive pulmonary disease, 445
    coronary blood flow, 194
    effect on vasopressin release, 1791
    heart failure, 164

Physical activity—cont'd
  hypertension management, 324
  increased bone mass in postmenopausal
    women, 1947
  increased potassium loss from cells, 831
  increased skeletal muscle blood flow, 46
  intermittent claudication, 308-309
  ischemic heart disease, 200
  neutrophilia, 590
  obesity, 2103, 2104
  palpitations, 130
  pulmonary rehabilitation, 435-436
  rheumatoid arthritis, 1206-1207
  rhinitis therapy, 1182
  silent myocardial ischemia, 194
  skeletal muscle blood flow, 46
  walk through angina, 195
Physical examination, 5
  abdominal pain, 2032
  acute diarrhea, 2051
  acute pericarditis, 273
  alcoholism, 2295
  appendicitis, 2092
  arrhythmia, 133
  asthma, 1188
  bleeding patient, 603
  cancer of unknown primary site, 731
  cardiac tamponade, 275-276
  cardiovascular system, 63-81
    arterial pulses, 64-65, 66, 67
    auscultation, 68-71
    blood pressure measurement, 64
    cardiac cycle, 71-72
    general appearance, 63-64
    heart murmurs, 75-81
    heart sounds, 72-75, 76
    inspection and palpation, 67-68, 70, 71
    jugular venous pulse, 65-67, 68, 69
  chronic diarrhea, 2053
  chronic fatigue, 2298
  chronic obstructive pulmonary disease, 442
  chronic renal failure, 782
  constipation, 2053
  constitutional delay of puberty, 1768
  constrictive pericarditis, 277
  Crohn's disease, 2069-2070
  esophageal disease, 1999
  fever, 1387
  fever and rash, 1381
  fever of unknown origin, 1378-1379
  fibrocystic breast disease, 1848-1849
  gastric cancer, 2046
  gastrointestinal bleeding, 2010
  gynecomastia, 1764
  heart failure, 164-165
  hematuria, 757
  hirsutism, 1756
  impotence, 1761
  inflammatory myopathies, 1235
  intestinal disease, 2004-2005
  intestinal obstruction, 2077
  ischemic heart disease, 197
  low back pain, 966
  lung disease, 402-404
  myocardial infarction, 210
  nephrotic syndrome, 767
  neurologic disorders, 902-903
  nosocomial infection, 1482
  pericardial effusion, 274
  periodic health examination, 2254
  postrenal azotemia, 771
  preoperative medical evaluation, 2256
  prerenal azotemia, 770
  puberty, 1770
  reactive arthritis, 1240
  rhinitis, 1181-1182
  sexually transmitted disease, 1438-1439
  site of blockage in cholestasis, 2156
  syncope, 955-956
  vertigo, 2307
  weight loss, 1750

Physical therapy
  neck pain, 971
  osteoarthritis, 1267
  pulmonary rehabilitation, 436
  spinal cord injury, 1052
  stroke patient, 1054
  vestibular, 975
Physician, role in injury control, 2266-2267
Physician-patient encounter, 2-5
Physician performance data, 21-22
Physician profile, 33
Physicians Desk Reference, 2313
Physiologic consequences of aging, 2284-2285
Physiologic delayed puberty, 1843
Physiologic jaundice of newborn, 2151
Physiologic third heart sound, 73-74
Physiology
  autonomic nervous system, 931-934
  bone and mineral homeostasis, 1714-1721
    bone formation, 1949
    calcium metabolism, 1717-1720
    cellular physiology of bone, 1716
    effects of hormones, 1720
    functions of skeleton, 1714-1715
    matrix formation and calcification, 1716
    natural history of skeleton, 1715-1716
    stress and coupling, 1716
  breast, 1846-1849
  cardiovascular, 36-49
    capillary exchange, 47-48
    cardiac cycle, 36-37
    cardiac output and systemic hemodynamics,
      46-47
    cellular basis of cardiac contraction, 37-41
    coronary circulation, 48-49
    diastolic function, 43-46
    exercise stress testing, 91
    response to dynamic exercise, 49
    structure and function of ventricle, 41-42
    systolic function, 42-43
  endocrine, 1708-1714
    classes of hormones, 1708
    diabetes mellitus, 1851-1853
    hormone secretion, 1713-1714
    hormone synthesis, 1708-1710
    hypoglycemia, 1874-1875
    mechanisms of hormone action, 1710-1713
    ovary, 1832-1833
  gastrointestinal
    alimentary tract motor function, 1976-1980
    gastric secretion, 1980-1985
    intestinal absorption, 1985-1989
  hepatic, 2118-2123
    amino acids and protein metabolism,
      2118-2120
    bile production and secretion, 2123-2129
    carbohydrate metabolism, 2121-2122
    detoxification, 2122
    hormone metabolism, 2122-2123
    lipid metabolism, 2120-2121
  lysosomal, 1911
  nasal, 1180-1181
  neurologic, 939-940
  pancreatic, 2129-2134
  posterior pituitary, 1789-1793
  pulmonary, 346-375
    abnormalities of breathing control, 352-357
    mechanisms of lung injury and repair,
      370-375
    nonrespiratory functions of lung, 346-347
    oxygen transport disorders, 350-352
    pulmonary blood flow, 360-364
    respiratory function, 347-350
    respiratory muscles, 357-360
    respiratory tract host defense mechanisms,
      364-369
  renal, 736-741
    acid-base homeostasis, 834-836
    composition of body fluids, 736-737
    glomerular ultrafiltration, 737
    potassium transport, 741

Physiology—cont'd
  renal—cont'd
    renal acidification, 739-741
    sodium balance, 737-739
    water metabolism, 739, 740
Physiotherapy
  cystic fibrosis, 482
  secretion clearance and lung expansion, 430
Phytobezoar, 2044
Phytonadione, 625
Pica behavior, 1103
Pick's disease, 987
Pickwickian syndrome, 334, 354
Picornavirus, 1483-1494
  acute febrile undifferentiated illness, 1487
  acute hemorrhagic conjunctivitis, 1490
  aseptic meningitis, 1488
  characteristics, 1483
  chemoprophylaxis, 1493
  chronic meningoencephalitis, 1490
  classification, 1483-1485
  common cold, 1487
  diagnosis, 1492
  encephalitis, 1488
  epidemic pleurodynia, 1489
  epidemiology, 1484-1485
  exanthems, 1489
  hand-foot-mouth syndrome, 1489
  hepatitis, 1490
  hepatitis A virus, 2173
  herpangina, 1488-1489
  influenza, 1490-1491
  lymphonodular pharyngitis, 1489
  myopericarditis, 1489-1490
  neurologic complications, 1491
  paralytic poliomyelitis, 1487-1488
  pathogenesis, 1485-1487
  prevention, 1492-1493
  pulmonary complications, 1491
  treatment, 1492
Piecemeal necrosis, 2180
Pigbel, 1568
Pigment nephropathy, 867-868
Pigment stones, 2221-2224
Pigmentation
  Addison's disease, Plate VII-14
  adrenal disease, 1322-1323
  adrenal insufficiency, 1823
  alkaptonuria, 1281
  neurofibromatosis, 1920
Pigmented casts, 745
Pigmented villonodular synovitis
  arthropathy, 1244-1245
  soft tissue swelling, 1164, 1165
Pilocarpine
  glaucoma, 2302
  pupil response, 933
  pupillometry, 938
Pimozide, 1902
Pinch test, 1751
Pindolol
  hypertension, 325
  properties, 203
Pineal gland
  calcification, 1083
  neuroendocrine regulation, 1075
  tumor, 1069-1079
Pineoblastoma, 1069-1079
Pineocytoma, 1069-1079
Pink tetralogy, 289
Pinta, 1644
Pinworm, 1696
PIOPED; *see* Prospective Investigation of
        Pulmonary Embolism Diagnosis study
Pipecolic acid, 1904, 1907
Piperacillin, 1253
  activity against major anaerobes, 1620
  dosage, 1350
  enterococci resistance, 1561
  intraabdominal infection, 1401
  respiratory exacerbations in cystic fibrosis, 483

Piperazine, 1698
Piriformis syndrome, 965
Piroxicam, 1259
  hepatic injury, 2191
  interference with oral anticoagulants, 636
Pirprofen, 2191
Pitressin, 1794, 1796
Pitting and culling functions of spleen, 600
Pittsburgh pneumonia agent, 1621, 1624
Pituitary, 1773-1788
  amenorrhea, 1759
  anterior
    anatomy, 1773
    Cushing's disease, 1786-1787
    empty sella syndrome, 1787
    hyperprolactinemia, 1785-1786
    hypopituitarism, 1776-1777
    hypothalamic-pituitary adrenal system, 1774
    hypothalamic-pituitary axis, 1773-1774
    hypothalamic-pituitary gonadal system,
      1774-1775
    hypothalamic-pituitary growth hormone
      system, 1775
    hypothalamic-pituitary prolactin system,
      1775-1776, 1777
    hypothalamic-pituitary testing, 1735-1737
    hypothalamic-pituitary thyroid system, 1774
    pituitary apoplexy, 1777-1781
  gonadotropin secretion, 1834
  hypergonadotropic hypogonadism, 1843-1844
  hypothalamus-pituitary-testis axis, 1839, 1840
  posterior, 1788-1797
    anatomy, 1788
    biochemistry, 1788-1789
    diabetes insipidus, 1793-1795
    disorders, 1795-1797
    physiology, 1789-1793
    testing, 1737-1738
  thyroid-stimulating hormone secretion, 1799
Pituitary adenoma, 1781-1782
  gonadotropin-secreting, 1787
  growth hormone-secreting, 1782-1785
  impotence, 1762
  during pregnancy, 2273-2274
  thyroid-stimulating hormone-secreting, 1787,
    1807
  vasopressin deficiency, 1795
Pituitary apoplexy, 1777-1781
Pituitary hormones, 1077
  adrenocorticotropic hormone, 1774
    Addison's disease, 1823-1824
    Cushing's syndrome, 1737, 1820,
      1821-1822
    deficiency, 1777, 1823-1824
    gout, 1274
    hirsutism, 1756
    hypopituitarism treatment, 1779-1780
    increase after nausea induction, 2025
    regulation of adrenocortical secretion,
      1817-1819
    stimulation tests, 1741
  growth hormone, 1775
    acromegaly, 1782-1785
    aging and, 2285
    calcium homeostasis, 1720
    deficiency, 1769, 1777
    glucose production, 1874, 1875
    glucose suppression of, 1737
    hypersomatotropism, 1782
    hypopituitarism treatment, 1781
    hypothalamic-pituitary growth hormone
      system, 1775
    puberty, 1767
    regulation of albumin synthesis, 2119
    secretion during sleep, 940
  neurally-mediated release, 1714
  prolactin, 1776
    chronic hepatic failure, 2171-2172
    hyperprolactinemia, 1785-1786
    hypothalamic-pituitary prolactin system,
      1775-1776, 1777

Pituitary hormones—cont'd
  prolactin—cont'd
    puberty, 1767
    stimulation tests, 1736
Pituitary snuff-taker's lung, 460
Pityriasis versicolor, 1309-1310
Pityrosporum, 1309-1310
  acquired immunodeficiency syndrome, 1326,
    1328
  normal flora, 1368
PiZZ alpha₁-protease inhibitor deficiency, 440
PiZZ phenotype, 2206
PKU; *see* Phenylketonuria
Placenta, 636
Plague, 1423, 1609-1610
Plain film
  abdominal pain, 2032
  chronic pancreatitis, 2240
  echinococcal cyst, 2111
  evaluation of arthritis, 1164
  intestinal diseases, 2007
  intestinal obstruction, 2078
  pancreatic disease, 2146
  pyogenic liver abscess, 2209
Plant toxins, 2192-2193
Plantar response, 903
Plants causing occupational asthma, 472
Plaque
  asbestos exposure, 474
  atherosclerotic, 1888
  leprosy, 1650
  myocardial infarction, 209, 210
  psoriasis, 1300
  retroperitoneal fibrosis, 2250
  sarcoidosis, 1324
  thrush, 1661
  tinea capitis, 1308
  unstable angina, 195
Plasma
  acquired coagulation inhibitors, 630
  defect in thrombotic thrombocytopenic
    purpura, 615
  electrolyte content, 736
  hormone transport, 1733
Plasma albumin
  nephrotic syndrome, 765
  unconjugated bilirubin, 2148
Plasma aldosterone, 1741
  aldosterone-producing adenoma, 321
  hypertension, 321
Plasma bicarbonate, 779
Plasma catecholamines, 1740
Plasma cell
  airway, 365
  bone marrow, Plate IV-8
  chronic atrophic gastritis, 2042
  lamina propria, 1990, 1991
  pulmonary, 368
  synthesis of light chains, 863
Plasma cell dyscrasias, 862-863, 891-892
Plasma cell granulomatous vasculitis, 467-469
Plasma cell labeling index, 701
Plasma cell leukemia, 595, 703
Plasma cell myeloma, 700-703
Plasma cholesterol
  hyperlipidemia, 1892-1894
  population distribution, 1893
Plasma coagulation, 570-571
Plasma cortisol, 1740
Plasma creatinine concentration, 746, 747
Plasma dehydroepiandrosterone, 1741
Plasma exchange therapy, 574
  Goodpasture's syndrome, 847
  thrombotic thrombocytopenic purpura, 615,
    858
Plasma fibrinogen, 571, 783
Plasma gastrin, 784
Plasma glucose, 743
  fasting hypoglycemia, 1877
  hypoglycemia, 1875
Plasma growth hormone, 2245

Plasma insulin, 2244
Plasma lipids, 60
Plasma lipoproteins, 1886, 1889-1890
Plasma magnesium, 1939
Plasma norepinephrine
  congestive heart failure, 818
  heart failure, 166
Plasma oncotic pressure, 346
Plasma osmolality, 806
  capillary exchange, 47
  change in plasma vasopressin, 1789, 1790
  diabetes insipidus, 1794-1795
  increased, 739
Plasma proteins
  alpha-fetoprotein
    hepatic formation, 2120
    hepatocellular carcinoma, 2143, 2213
    testicular cancer, 720
  alpha₁-antitrypsin
    absorption of vitamin B₁₂, 2007
    hepatic formation, 2120
    venous thromboembolism, 632
  alpha₂ macroglobulins
    rheumatoid arthritis, 1202
    shock states, 176
  antithrombin III, 538, 539
    disseminated intravascular coagulation, 628
    gram-negative infection, 1454
    inhibition of fibrin formation, 535
    shock states, 176
    thrombosis, 609
  inactivation of coagulation factors, 539
  inhibition of fibrin formation, 535
  protein C, 538, 539
    assay, 572
    gram-negative infection, 1454
    inhibition of fibrin formation, 535
    thrombin formation, 537, 539
    thrombosis, 609
    thrombotic thrombocytopenic purpura, 614
    venous thrombus, 631
  proteinuria, 760
  synthesis in liver, 2118
  total serum calcium, 1744
  venous thromboembolism, 631
Plasma renin, 1741
  chronic renal failure, 783
  heart failure, 160, 161
  renal artery stenosis, 895
Plasma 17-hydroxyprogesterone, 1741
Plasma testosterone
  amenorrhea, 1759
  congenital adrenal hyperplasia, 1825
  hirsutism, 1756
Plasma transfusion, 573
Plasma triglycerides, 1892
Plasma urea nitrogen/creatinine ratio, 770
Plasma vasopressin, 883, 1737-1738
Plasma volume
  ascites, 818, 2163
  hepatorenal syndrome, 2170
  hypertonic dehydration, 824
  hypovolemia
    acute pancreatitis, 2237
    after stroke, 1007
    mesenteric vascular disease, 2086
    Rocky Mountain spotted fever, 1543
    vasopressin release, 1792
  sickle cell disease, 657
Plasma von Willebrand's factor, 569
Plasma water, 736
Plasmacytoid lymphocyte, 595, Plate IV-5
Plasmacytoma, 703
Plasmalemmal excitation system, 37-38
Plasmapheresis
  antiphospholipid syndrome, 1292
  cast nephropathy, 865
  myasthenia gravis, 1023
  plasma exchange therapy, 574
  thrombotic thrombocytopenic purpura, 615
  thyroid storm, 1808

Plasmapheresis—cont'd
  before transplantation, 341
  Waldenström macroglobulinemia, 865-866
Plasmid, 52, 53, 1582
Plasmid-mediated modification of target site, 1345-1346
Plasmid-profile analysis, 1547
Plasmin
  fibrinolysis, 539-540
  screening test for fibrinolysis, 571
Plasmin-plasminogen activator-inhibitor system, 373
Plasminogen, 538, 540
Plasminogen activator inhibitor
  congenital disorders of blood coagulation, 618
  deficiency, 625
Plasminogen activator inhibitor-1, 538, 540
Plasmodium falciparum, 1671-1675, Plate VIII-14
Plasmodium malariae, 1671
Plasmodium ovale, 1671
Plasmodium vivax, 1671, Plate VIII-15
Plateau waves, 1082
Platelet
  adhesion, 536, 611
  aggregation, 570, 611
    nitroglycerin and nitrates, 201
    secretion and, 536
    unstable angina, 195
  arterial thrombus, 638
  automated blood cell analysis, 556
  bleeding disorders, 602-605
  chronic myeloproliferative disorders, 686
  chronic renal failure, 783
  coagulant activity, 570
  decreased production causing thrombocytopenia, 614
  development from megakaryocyte, 535-536
  evaluation of hemostasis and thrombosis, 568-570
  examination of peripheral blood smear, 557
  function disorders, 610-613
  hypophosphatemia, 1936
  infective endocarditis, 225, 226
  Lassa fever, 1510
  lung injury, 374
  non–immune-mediated destruction, 614
  ristocetin-induced agglutination, 569
  structure and contents, 536
  thrombin generation, 537
Platelet activating factor, 1140, 1141
  bacterial meningitis, 1405
  gram-negative organism infection, 1447
  sepsis, 1448
  vasoactive effects on pulmonary circulation, 363
Platelet activating factor receptor antagonists, 1454
Platelet concentrates
  acquired coagulation inhibitors, 630
  hemostatic defects in liver disease, 627
Platelet count, 556
  chronic liver disease, 2136
  essential thrombocythemia, 688
  evaluation of hemostasis and thrombosis, 568-569
  gastrointestinal bleeding, 2011
  hemostatic disorders, 603
  iron deficiency, 644
  operative risk, 2262
  posttransfusion, 573
  posttransfusion purpura, 616
  relationship to bleeding time, 612
  streptococcal toxic shock syndrome, 1558
  thrombocytopenia, 613
Platelet-derived growth factor, 1131
  calcium homeostasis, 1720
  chronic alcoholism, 2195
  tubulointerstitial renal disease, 889
  venous ulceration, 312

Platelet-endothelial cell adhesion molecule-1, 370
Platelet factor 3 availability, 570
Platelet factor 4, 536, 638
Platelet-fibrinogen-platelet unit, 536
Platelet membrane glycoproteins, 536
Platelet transfusion, 573
  aplastic anemia, 673-674
  bleeding varices, 2166
  myelofibrosis, 677
Pleistophora, 1680
Plendil; see Felodipine
Plesiomonas, 1427, 1593, 2051
Pleura, 505
  computed tomography, 387
  thoracentesis, 381-382
Pleural biopsy, 382-383
  lung cancer, 490
  pleural disease, 506
Pleural calcification, 510
Pleural diseases, 505-510
Pleural effusion, 505
  asbestos exposure, 474
  chronic pancreatitis, 2241
  classification of, 506
  dilated cardiomyopathy, 263
  heart murmur, 76
  hypothyroidism, 1809
  lymphomatoid granulomatosis, 470
  malignant, 507-508
  physical findings, 403
  pyogenic liver abscess, 2209
  thoracentesis, 381
  ultrasound, 389
  uremic serositis, 784
Pleural fluid, 381, 505
Pleural friction rub, 410, 505-506
Pleural pain, 410
Pleural rub, 273
Pleural space, 505
  hemothorax, 508
  pneumothorax, 509
Pleural tuberculosis, 1633-1634
Pleural ultrasound, 506
Pleurisy, 410, 505
  rheumatoid arthritis, 1204
  tuberculous, 507
Pleuritic pain, 505
  myopericarditis, 1489
  pneumothorax, 509
  pulmonary embolism, 500
  tuberculosis, 1628
Pleuritis, 410
  systemic lupus erythematosus, 1214
  tuberculous, 1633-1634
  Wegener's granulomatosis, 1222
Pleuropneumonia-like organism, 1538
Pleuroscopy, 385
Plexiform lesion, 294
Plexopathy, 1016-1017, 1073
Plicamycin, 1974
Ploidy analysis, 559
Plucked chicken sign, 1321
Plummer-Vinson syndrome, 2020
Plummer's disease, 1807
Plummer's nails, 1322
Pluripotent hematopoietic stem cell, 530, Plate IV-2
PND; see Paroxysmal nocturnal dyspnea
Pneumococcal vaccine, 2255
Pneumococcus
  antibiotic selection, 1347
  Gram stain, Plate VIII-3
  meningitis, 1403
Pneumoconiosis, 475, 476
Pneumoconstriction, 500
Pneumocystis carinii, 1692-1696
  acquired immunodeficiency syndrome, 1473, 1474, 1477, 1534
  after stem cell transplantation, 579
  compromised host, 1388

Pneumocystis carinii—cont'd
  Giemsa stain, Plate VIII-10
  lung transplantation, 518, 519
  nodular thyroiditis, 1812
  RNA typing studies, 1652
  sputum examination, 380
Pneumocyte
  alveolar epithelium, 371
  shock states, 176
Pneumomediastinum, 513-514
Pneumonectomy, 490
Pneumonia
  actinomycosis, 1665
  acute cholecystitis *versus,* 2228
  acute interstitial, 448, 452
  acute meningitis, 1407
  adenovirus infection, 1503
  after stroke, 1007
  anaerobic bacteria, 1617
  aspiration, Plate VIII-7
  bronchiolitis obliterans-organizing, 448, 452-453
  bronchoalveolar lavage, 384
  cancer patient, 582
  chest pain, 129
  Chlamydia pneumoniae, 1535
  cholestasis, 2159
  cystic fibrosis, 480
  desquamative interstitial, 449
  eosinophilic, 455
  fever, 1387
  gram-negative bacteremia, 1446
  Gram stain, Plate VII-1
  Haemophilus influenzae, 1586
  influenza with, 1486, 1491
  Legionella pneumophila, 1622
  lymphoid interstitial, 449
  multiple organ dysfunction syndrome, 423
  Mycoplasma pneumoniae, 1538-1539
  Neisseria meningitidis, 1579
  nocardiosis, 1666
  nosocomial, 1480
  oculopharyngeal dystrophy, 1028
  Pneumocystis carinii, 1692-1696
    acquired immunodeficiency syndrome, 1473, 1474, 1477
    lung transplantation, 518, 519
    sputum examination, 380
  posttransplant
    lung, 517-518
    stem cell, 579
  pulmonary edema *versus,* 425
  risk in multiple myeloma, 700, 703
  sputum examination, 380
  Staphylococcus aureus, 1549
  tularemia, 1608
  usual interstitial, 449
  varicella, 1527
Pneumonic plague, 1610
Pneumonitis
  anaerobic bacteria, 1617
  Ascaris lumbricoides, 1698
  cytomegalovirus, Plate VIII-37
  with fibrosis, 476-477
  hypersensitivity, 460-463
    isocyanate-induced, 473
  radiation-induced, 411
Pneumoperitoneum, 1398
Pneumothorax, 509-510
  acquired immunodeficiency syndrome, 1477
  chronic obstructive pulmonary disease, 447
  cystic fibrosis, 482
  hemothorax with, 508
  Langerhans' cell granulomatosis, 464, 465
  lymphangioleiomyomatosis, 455
  physical findings, 403
  pulmonary edema *versus,* 425
  spontaneous, 128-129
  transthoracic needle aspiration, 385
POEMS syndrome, 703
Poikilocyte, 662

Poikiloderma, 1292
Point mutation, 1722, 1900
Point of service plan, 31
Poiseuille's equation, 46
Poisoning
  acetaminophen, 2188-2190
  barium, 827
  carbon monoxide, 993
  carbon tetrachloride, 2188
  interstitial lung disease, 452
  lead
    abdominal pain, 2031
    chronic tubulointerstitial nephritis, 891
    Fanconi's syndrome, 882
    nonoxidative hemolysis, 667-668
    renal toxicity, 867
    sensorimotor neuropathy, 1020
  medicinal agents, 2190-2192
  mushroom and phosphorus, 2188
Polio vaccine, 1492-1493
Poliomyelitis, 1487-1488
Poliovirus, 1486
Pollen, allergic rhinitis, 1183
Polyangiitis, 1221
Polyarteritis nodosa, 334, 856, 1219-1220
  crescentic glomerulonephritis, 848
  diffuse immune-complex vasculitis, 454
  glucocorticoid protocol, 1263
  microscopic, 1220-1221
  neurologic manifestations, 1092, 1095
Polyarthritis, 1198, 1199-1200, 1245
  acute pancreatitis, 2237
  septic, 1250-1251
  systemic lupus erythematosus, 1214
  systemic sclerosis, 1229
  Yersinia enterocolitica, 1611
Polychlorinated biphenyls, 1020
Polychromatic normoblast, 531, Plate IV-3
Polychromatophilia, Plate IV-4
Polyclonal gammopathies, 565
Polyclonal protein, 564-565
Polycyclic hydrocarbons, 2045
Polycystic liver disease, 2211
Polycystic ovarian disease, 1837
  amenorrhea, 1759
  gonadotropic pulsations, 1836
  hirsutism, 1756
  insulin resistance, 1862
  21-hydroxylase deficiency, 1824
Polycythemia
  Budd-Chiari syndrome, 2208
  high hematocrit, 588-590
  neutrophilic leukocytosis, 591
  red blood cell mass, 586
  tetralogy of Fallot, 289
Polycythemia vera, 588-590, 688-689
Polydipsia
  diabetes insipidus, 1793-1794
  diabetic ketoacidosis, 1863
  disorders of urinary concentration, 748
  hypokalemia, 829
  insulin-dependent diabetes mellitus, 1854
  juvenile nephronophthisis, 875
  nephrogenic diabetes insipidus, 883
  schizophrenia, 1796
Polygenic traits, 1721
Polyglutamate, 1989
Polyhydramnios, 883
Polyimmunoglobulin receptor, 1990
Polymerase chain reaction, 55, 56, 561,
    1723-1724
  adenovirus, 1504
  alpha-thalassemia, 656
  babesiosis, 1676
  Chlamydia trachomatis, 1536
  chronic hepatitis C, 2183
  chronic myelogenous leukemia, 563
  hepatitis A virus, 2173
  hepatitis B virus, 2175
  hepatitis C virus, 2176
  herpes simplex virus, 1524

Polymerase chain reaction—cont'd
  human immunodeficiency virus infection,
    1472
  human leukocyte antigen typing, 1120
  infectious esophagitis, 2020
  Lassa fever virus, 1510
  Mycobacterium tuberculosis, 1629
  Neisseria meningitidis, 1580
  non-Hodgkin's lymphoma, 563
  Norwalk virus, 1522
  nucleic acid-based tests, 1372
  parvovirus B19, 1514
  rabies, 1506
  septic arthritis, 1251
Polymorphic ventricular tachycardia, 151-153
Polymorphism, 1722
Polymorphonuclear elastase, 2144, 2145
Polymorphonuclear leukocyte, 1109
  gram-negative disease, 1446
  rheumatoid arthritis, 1205
Polymorphonuclear lymphocyte, 2195
Polymorphonuclear neutrophil
  gonorrhea, 1439
  lung injury, 372-373
  respiratory defense, 366
  tissue injury, 1341
Polymorphous light eruption, 1306
Polymyalgia rheumatica
  glucocorticoid protocol, 1263
  neurologic manifestations, 1092
Polymyositis, 1234
  autoantibodies, 1143, 1155
  heart disease, 1087
  neurologic manifestations, 1092
  weakness, 1754
Polymyxin B
  dosage, 1350
  gram-negative infection, 1454
Polymyxins, 1344, 1350, 1358
Polyneuritis
  diphtheria, 1566
  thiamine deficiency, 2106
Polyneuropathy, 1017-1020
  critical-illness, 1085
  diabetes mellitus, 1871-1872
  nerve conduction studies, 915
Polyol pathway, 861
Polyp
  aural, 2307
  bronchiolitis obliterans-organizing pneumonia,
    448
  colon
    colonoscopy, 1996
    evaluation, 2085
    ulcerative colitis, 2073
  gallbladder, 2233
  gastric, 2045-2046
  nasal, 1183, 2308
Polypharmacy, 2313
Polyploidization, 532
Polyploidy, 1727
Polyradiculopathy, 1017
Polyribosome, 1709
Polysomnography, 939
  arousal disorders, 946
  narcolepsy, 942
  obstructive sleep apnea, 526
Polyunsaturated fatty acids, 1883-1884, 1889
Polyuria
  after relief of obstruction, 887
  chronic renal failure, 778
  diabetes insipidus, 815, 1793-1794
  diabetic ketoacidosis, 1863
  disorders of urinary concentration, 748
  Fanconi's syndrome, 882
  hypercalcemia, 1929
  hypokalemia, 829
  insulin-dependent diabetes mellitus, 1854
  juvenile nephronophthisis, 875
  nephrogenic diabetes insipidus, 883, 884
  primary hyperparathyroidism, 1967

Pompe's disease, 1881
Pontiac fever, 1623
Pontine gaze center, 1063
Pontine paramedian reticular formation, 1063
Poorly differentiated adenocarcinoma, 732-733
Poorly differentiated carcinoma, 730, 732-733
Popliteal artery aneurysm, 309
Population health outcomes, 19
Porcine heterograft, 260
Pork tapeworm, 1696
Porphobilinogen, 1923
Porphobilinogen deaminase, 1926
Porphyria, 1923-1927, 2031
Porphyria cutanea tarda, 1307, 1927, Plate
    VII-10
  accelerated turnover of hepatic hemes, 2152
  human immunodeficiency virus infection,
    1327
Porphyromonas gingivalis, 1614
Portacaval shunt, 2167
Portal hypertension
  alcoholic hepatitis and cirrhosis, 2197
  ascites formation, 2163
  autosomal recessive polycystic kidney disease,
    874
  cystic fibrosis, 2207
  hepatopulmonary syndrome, 2170
  liver failure, 2165-2168
  splenomegaly, 601
Portal vein
  obstruction, 2208-2209
  thrombosis, 2089
  transjugular intrahepatic shunt, 2167
Porter-Silber chromogen, 1819, 1821
Portosystemic encephalopathy, 2159-2160
Portosystemic shunt, 2151
Positional cloning, 1724
Positioning
  cardiac auscultation, 70-71
  jugular venous pulse, 65
  rigid proctoscopy, 1995
Positive airway pressure, 430
Positive end-expiratory pressure, 398
  acute respiratory failure, 415-416, 418
  alveolar pressure, 363
  neurogenic pulmonary edema, 1099
  pulmonary artery wedge pressure, 394
  pulmonary edema, 426-427
Positive nitrogen balance, 786
Positive predictive value, 7-8
Positive sharp waves, 916
Positron emission tomography
  brain, 929
  coronary blood flow, 199
  cortical mapping of brain function, 922
  dementia, 2288
  heart, 105-106
  myocardial infarction, 212
  stroke, 1003
Postcapillary pulmonary hypertension, 497
Postcardiotomy syndrome, 273
Postcholecystectomy syndrome, 2226
Postcoarctation syndrome, 287
Postencephalitic parkinsonism, 993
Posterior alexia, 978
Posterior cerebral artery occlusion, 1005
Posterior circulation large artery occlusive
    disease, 1005
Posterior column syndrome, 1048
Posterior interosseous palsy, 1017
Posterior mediastinal tumor, 513
Posterior pituitary, 1788-1797
  anatomy, 1788
  biochemistry, 1788-1789
  diabetes insipidus, 1793-1795
  disorders, 1795-1797
  physiology, 1789-1793
  testing, 1737-1738
Posterior tibial nerve mononeuropathy, 1017
Posterior tibial reflex, 964
Posteroventral medial pallidotomy, 992

Postexposure prophylaxis in rabies, 1507, 1508
Postganglionic neuron, 930
Postgonococcal urethritis, 1440
Posthypercapnic alkalosis, 840
Posthyperventilation apnea, 1097
Postinfectious glomerulonephritis, 843-844
Postmyocardial infarction, 326
Postnasal drip, 407
Postnecrotic cirrhosis, 2219
Postobstructive diuresis, 887
Postoperative care
  liver transplantation, 2219
  minidose heparin therapy, 504
  prosthetic heart valve, 259
Postoperative cholestasis, 2159
Postoperative wound infection, 1363-1364
Postpartum factor VIII inhibitors, 629
Postperfusion syndrome, 259, 668
Postpericardiotomy syndrome, 259
Postpolio syndrome, 1015
Postprandial alkaline tide, 742
Postprandial angina, 194-195
Postprandial dyspepsia, 2016-2017
Postprandial hypoglycemia, 1877
Postrenal azotemia
  diagnosis, 771
  etiology, 768
  management, 773
  pathophysiology, 769
Postsplenectomy infection, 656, 1338
Poststreptococcal glomerulonephritis, 764, 843, 1559
Postsurgical hypoparathyroidism, 1931
Postsynaptic receptor agonists, 938
Posttranscriptional regulation, 51
Posttransfusion purpura, 616
Posttransplant lymphoproliferative disease
  cardiac transplantation, 1090
  lung transplantation, 519
  renal transplantation, 795
Posttraumatic hypersomnia, 943
Posttraumatic stress disorder
  head injury, 1045
  neuroendocrinology, 1077
Postural change
  autonomic regulation of cardiovascular response, 931-932
  plasma norepinephrine, 938
Postural drainage
  cystic fibrosis, 482
  secretion clearance and lung expansion, 430
Postural hypotension, 2290
Posture
  blood pressure measurement, 314
  gastroesophageal reflux, 2018
  idiopathic edema, 821
Potassium, 825-834
  abnormalities of impulse formation, 132
  aldosterone secretion modulation, 1818
  alimentary tract motor function, 1976
  body water compartments, 736
  excretion in chronic renal failure, 778-779
  external potassium balance, 825, 826
  functions, 2109
  hyperkalemia, 830-833
    acute renal failure, 772-773
    chronic renal failure, 777
    decreased ammonia synthesis, 838
    electrocardiographic abnormalities, 89, 90
    electrocardiographic changes, 772
    heart failure, 172
    mineralocorticoid deficiency, 1824
    supportive treatment, 774
    toxicity of nonsteroidal antiinflammatory drugs, 870
  hyperkalemic periodic paralysis, 831
  hyperkalemic renal tubular acidosis, 831
  hyperosmolar nonketotic coma, 1866
  hypertension, 319

Potassium—cont'd
  hypokalemia, 826-830
    arrhythmia, 133
    chronic tubulointerstitial nephritis, 891
    consequences, 829-830
    diarrhea, 2005
    diuretic-induced, 326
    electrocardiographic abnormalities, 89, 90
    Fanconi's syndrome, 882
    hypomagnesemia, 1942
    with potassium depletion, 827
    treatment, 830
    VIPoma, 2245
    vomiting consequence, 2028
    without potassium depletion, 826-827
  hypokalemic paralysis, 1029-1030
  hypokalemic periodic paralysis, 58, 826
  internal potassium balance, 825-826
  intestinal absorption, 1988
  metabolic acidosis and, 838-839
  parenteral solutions, 2114
  proton pump, 1983
  recommended daily dietary allowances, 2116
  renal hydrogen ion secretion, 741
  renal transport, 741
  replacement in diabetic ketoacidosis, 1864
  serum, 840
  total parenteral nutrition formula, 2117
  vasoactive effects on pulmonary circulation, 363
  wasting in distal renal tubular acidosis, 838
Potassium channel, 59
  cardiac conduction, 38
Potassium citrate, 803
Potassium hydroxide preparation
  blastomycosis, 1657
  candidiasis, 1439
  fungal culture, 1309, 1310
  infectious esophagitis, 2020
Potassium iodide, 1658
Potassium-losing diuretics, 822
Potassium phosphate
  hypophosphatemia, 1937
  stone formation reduction, 803-804
Potassium-sparing diuretics, 822
  ascites, 2165
  cirrhotic ascites, 822
  diuretic-induced hypokalemia, 832
  heart failure, 170
  hirsutism, 1757
  hyperkalemia, 832
  hypertension, 325
  hypomagnesemia, 1942-1943
  induction of gynecomastia, 2172
  nephrogenic diabetes insipidus, 884
  stone formation reduction, 803
Potts procedure, 289
Poverty, elderly women, 2268
Powassan encephalitis, 1514, 1515
Power spectral analysis, 937
PPD; *see* Purified protein derivative
PPO; *see* Preferred provider organization
Practice guidelines, 23
PRAD 1 protooncogene, 1966
Prader-Labhart-Willi syndrome, 1842
Prader orchidometer, 1771
Prader-Willi syndrome, 1729
  hypopituitarism, 1776
  obesity, 1752
PRAISE survival trial, 171
Prajmaline, 2192
Prausnitz-Kustner reaction, 1154
Pravastatin, 1891
  gallstone risk factor, 2223
  hyperlipidemia, 200
  nephrotic syndrome, 767
  typical medical regimen six months after transplantation, 343
Praxis, 902

Praziquantel
  intestinal helminths, 1697
  schistosomiasis, 1703
  Taenia solium, 1704-1705
Prazosin
  hypertension, 325
  urge incontinence, 2293
Pre-B receptor, 1125
Precapillary pulmonary hypertension, 293-297, 497
Precipitating antibody, 461
Precipitin reactions, 1373
PRECISE/MOCHA survival trial, 171
Precocious puberty, 1921
Precordial electrode, 82-83
Precordial movements, 67
Predictive value, 7-8, 1366
Prednisolone
  interstitial lung disease, 451
  tuberculous pericarditis, 1637
Prednisone
  acute interstitial nephritis, 889
  antibody-mediated insulin resistance, 1861
  asthma, 1192
  autoimmune hepatitis, 2184
  breast cancer, 709
  bronchiolitis obliterans syndrome, 523
  bullous pemphigoid, 1296
  chronic lymphocytic leukemia, 685
  chronic obstructive pulmonary disease, 434, 444
  Churg-Strauss syndrome, 467
  cluster headache prophylaxis, 962
  crescentic glomerulonephritis, 848
  Crohn's disease, 2071
  cutaneous lesions in lupus erythematosus, 1291
  cystic fibrosis, 482
  dermatomyositis, 1292
  drug-induced thrombocytopenia, 615
  eosinophilic fasciitis, 1234
  Epstein-Barr virus infection, 1529
  Goodpasture's syndrome, 847
  gout, 1274
  Hodgkin's disease, 694-695
  human cytochrome P450 isoforms, 2312
  hypersensitivity pneumonitis, 462
  immune hemolytic anemia, 669
  immune thrombocytopenic purpura, 616
  minimal change disease, 851
  multiple myeloma, 702
  myasthenia gravis, 1022
  non-Hodgkin's lymphoma, 698-699
  optic neuritis, 1060
  pemphigus vulgaris, 1294
  pericardial heart disease, 278
  Pneumocystis carinii pneumonia, 1695
  reflex sympathetic dystrophy syndrome, 1247
  relapsing seronegative symmetric synovitis with pitting edema, 1243
  rheumatic fever, 1257
  rheumatoid arthritis, 1207
  sarcoidosis, 459
  systemic lupus erythematosus, 1216-1217
  thrombotic thrombocytopenic purpura, 615
  transplantation
    lung, 516
    prevention and therapy of rejection, 340
    renal, 792
    typical medical regimen six months after, 343
  tropical spastic paraparesis, 1533
  tuberculous meningitis, 1412
  tuberculous pericarditis, 1637
  ulcerative colitis, 2074
  Wegener's granulomatosis, 468
Predominant hyperparathyroid bone disease, 1962-1963
Preeclampsia, 775, 2274-2275
Preexposure prophylaxis in rabies, 1507-1508
Preferred provider organization, 30, 31

Preganglionic neuron, 930
Pregnancy, 2272-2282
    acute renal failure, 775
    after renal transplantation, 796
    antibiotic selection, 1348
    arginine vasopressin release, 808
    asthma, 2276-2277
    atrial septal defect, 282
    bacteriuria during, 1457-1458
    cardiovascular disorders, 2276
    chronic hypertension, 2275
    diabetes mellitus during, 1873-1874
    dissection of aorta, 301
    endocrine disorders, 2272-2274
    estrogen-related cholestasis, 2158
    gallstone risk factor, 2223
    gestational diabetes, 1856
    gonorrhea during, 1583-1585
    hematologic disorders, 2279
    hepatic disorders, 2277-2278
    hyperemesis gravidarum, 2278
    immune thrombocytopenic purpura, 617
    infectious diseases, 2279-2281
    inflammatory bowel disease, 2278-2279
    listeriosis, 1577
    malaria during, 1674
    mean heights and weights and recommended
        energy intake, 2117
    measles during, 1498
    neurologic disorders, 2281-2282
    neutrophilia, 590
    oral anticoagulant administration during, 636
    parvovirus B19 infection during, 1513-1514
    pemphigoid gestationis, 1296
    precautions before international travel,
        1468-1469
    preeclampsia and eclampsia, 2274-2275
    primary hyperparathyroidism during, 1968
    recommended daily dietary allowances,
        2114-2115, 2116
    red blood cell mass, 586
    renal disorders, 2274
    rheumatic disorders, 2279
    rhinitis during, 1183-1185
    sickle cell disease, 659
    systemic lupus erythematosus during, 1217
    thromboembolic disorders, 2276
    thyrotoxicosis during, 1808
    toxoplasmosis during, 1677
    transient antidiuretic hormone resistance, 883
    ulcerative colitis during, 2074-2075
    vomiting, 2029
Pregnenolone, 1709
Prekallikrein deficiency, 624
Preleukemic syndromes, 645
Preload, 42
    cardiogenic shock, 176
    heart failure, 158
    relationship of pulmonary artery wedge
        pressure and, 394
Preload recruitable stroke work, 43
Premature atrial contractions, 141
Premature beat
    increase in blood pressure, 65, 67
    palpitations, 130
Premature ovarian failure, 1760, 1838
Premature ventricular contractions, 134, 148-149
Prematurity, inflammatory bowel disease, 2278
Premenstrual insomnia, 947
Prenatal diagnosis
    genetic disorders, 1730-1731
    hemophilia A, 619
    lysosomal storage disease, 1912
    thalassemia and hemoglobinopathies, 660
    unconjugated hyperbilirubinemia, 2153
Prenatal stress, 1076
Preoperative evaluation, 2256-2264
    bleeding disorders, 609-610
    cardiovascular risk factors, 2257-2260
    dipyridamole or adenosine stress imaging, 104
    endocrine risk factors, 2262

Preoperative evaluation—cont'd
    estimated operative risk, 2256-2257
    gastrointestinal and hepatic risk factors,
        2262-2263
    hematologic risk factors, 2262
    pulmonary risk factors, 2260-2262
    renal risk factors, 2263-2264
Prepatellar bursitis, 1197
Prepro-parathyroid hormone, 1718
Preproalbumin, 2119
Preprohormone, 1709
Prerenal azotemia
    chronic renal failure, 783
    diagnosis, 770-771
    etiology, 768
    hyperkalemia, 832
    hypovolemic hypernatremia, 816
    liver disease, 774
    management, 773
    pathophysiology, 769
    total parenteral nutrition, 2114
    volume depletion on diuretics, 169
Presbycusis, 2287
Presbyopia, 2301
Preservation injury in lung transplantation,
        516-517
Pressure controlled ventilation
    acute respiratory failure, 418-419
    multiple organ dysfunction, 423
Pressure half-time, 99
Pressure sore
    after stroke, 1007, 1054
    elderly, 22887
    spinal cord injury, 1051
Pressure support ventilation, 398
    acute respiratory distress syndrome, 418-419
    weaning, 400
Pressure transducer, 108
Pressure-volume area, 44
Presyncope, 266, 952
Presystolic gallop, 74
Pretibial myxedema, 1322, 1806
Prevotella, 1614
prima facie, 10
Primaquine
    hemolysis in glucose-6-phosphate
        dehydrogenase deficiency, 663
    malaria, 1674
    Pneumocystis carinii pneumonia, 1694
Primary aldosteronism, 321
Primary angiitis of central nervous system, 1225
Primary antiphospholipid antibody syndrome,
        1155
Primary bile acids, 2124
Primary biliary cirrhosis, 2199-2201
    antimitochondrial antibodies, 2139
    autoantibodies, 1155
    gallstone risk factor, 2223
    liver transplantation, 2218
    malabsorption, 2062
    mitochondrial antibodies, 1157
Primary care provider, 32
Primary central nervous system lymphoma, 1069
Primary combined hyperlipidemia, 1896
Primary coronary angioplasty, 122, 123, 124
Primary endogenous hypertriglyceridemia, 1895
Primary granulomatous pulmonary vasculitis,
        465-471
Primary hyperparathyroidism, 1965-1971
Primary hypodipsia, 815
Primary immunodeficiency disorders, 1174-1178
Primary open angle glaucoma, 2301
Primary peristalsis, 1978
Primary pulmonary hypertension, 293-295, 498,
        514
Primary sclerosing cholangitis, 2201-2202, 2203
    extrahepatic cholestasis, 2155
    inflammatory bowel disease, 2075-2076
    liver transplantation, 2218-2219
    malabsorption, 2062
Primary systemic amyloidosis, 1316-1317

Primer extension, 55
Primidone, 983, 2110
Primrose oil, 1850
Principlism, 10
Prinivil; *see* Lisinopril
Prinzmetal's angina, 192, 194
Pro-opiomelanocortin, 1774
Proadrenomedullin, 1826
Proarrhythmia, 134-135
Probenecid
    glucose-6-phosphate dehydrogenase
        deficiency, 664
    tophaceous gout, 1275
Probucol, 1891
Procainamide, 137
    glucose-6-phosphate dehydrogenase
        deficiency, 664
    hepatic injury, 2192
Procaine penicillin, 1643
Procalcitonin, 1718
Procan; *see* Procainamide
Procarbazine
    Hodgkin's disease, 694-695
    pulmonary parenchymal reactions, 476
    pulmonary toxicity, 478
Procardia; *see* Nifedipine
Prochlorperazine
    for nausea and vomiting, 2027
    status migrainosus, 962
Procollagens, 2141
Proctitis, 1444-1445
    acquired immunodeficiency syndrome, 1476,
        2098
    gonococcal, 1583
Proctocolectomy
    Crohn's disease, 2072
    toxic megacolon, 2076
    ulcerative colitis, 2074
Proctoscopy, 1995
Proctosigmoidoscopy
    acute lower gastrointestinal bleeding, 2012
    ulcerative colitis, 2073
Proenzymes of coagulation, 538
PROFILE survival trial, 171
Progabide, 2191
Progesterone
    breast cancer, 708
    effects on breast, 1846
    feedback effects, 1834
    hypopituitarism treatment, 1781
    measurement, 1835
    normal levels, 1836
    precapillary pulmonary hypertension, 296
    puberty, 1767
    reduction in arterial carbon dioxide tension,
        356
    testing for female gonadal function, 1742
    withdrawal test, 1742
Progesterone-only contraceptives, 2270
Progestins
    breast cancer, 710
    fibrocystic breast disease, 1850
    hepatic metabolism, 2122, 2123
Programmed cell death, 542-543, 1144
Programmed electrical stimulation, 151, 152
Progressive bacterial synergistic gangrene, 1425
Progressive bulbar palsy, 1015
Progressive diaphyseal dysplasia, 1959
Progressive external ophthalmoplegia, 1029
Progressive familial cholestasis, 2158-2159
Progressive generalized lymphadenopathy, 599
Progressive massive fibrosis, 475
Progressive multifocal leukoencephalopathy,
        1010
    human immunodeficiency virus-associated
        dementia, 987
    rheumatoid arthritis, 1094
Progressive myoclonus epilepsy, 996
Progressive pulmonary sarcoidosis, 458
Progressive supranuclear palsy, 992

Progressive systemic sclerosis, 1293
  antinuclear antibody, 1159-1160
  cardiac involvement, 334
  interstitial lung disease, 453
  multiple jejunal diverticulosis, 2089
  pulmonary hypertension, 296
  reflux esophagitis, 2023
Prolactin, 1776
  chronic hepatic failure, 2171-2172
  hyperprolactinemia, 1785-1786
    basal pituitary hormone measurement, 1737
    milk discharge, 1848
    testicular dysfunction, 1841
  hypothalamic-pituitary prolactin system,
    1775-1776, 1777
  pseudoseizure, 984
  puberty, 1767
  stimulation tests, 1736
Prolactin-inhibiting factor, 1775
Prolactin-secreting adenoma, 1785-1786
  amenorrhea, 1759
  impotence, 1763
  during pregnancy, 2273
Prolapse
  mitral valve, 253-255
    acquired immunodeficiency syndrome, 333
    arrhythmia, 133
    atrial septal defect, 280, 281
    auscultatory findings, 75, 76
    chest pain, 128, 129
    infective endocarditis, 225, 226
    mitral regurgitation, 249, 253
    palpitations, 131
    von Willebrand's disease, 624
  rectal
    cystic fibrosis, 483, 2246
    solitary rectal ulcers, 2093
Proliferating cell nuclear antigen, 1159
Proliferative diabetic retinopathy, 2303
Proline, 1904
Prolonged insertional activity, 916
Prolymphocyte, 595
Prolymphocytic leukemia
  abnormal lymphocytes in peripheral blood,
    595
  lymphosarcoma cell leukemia *versus,* 594
ProMACE-CytaBOM regimen, 699
Promethazine
  for nausea and vomiting, 2027
  status migrainosus, 962
  vasopressin inhibition, 1791
PROMISE survival trial, 171
Promoter, 50, 51, 651
Promyelocyte, 532
Pronator syndrome, 1017
Pronestyl; *see* Procainamide
Pronormoblast, 531, Plate IV-3
Proopiomelanocortin, 1708
Propafenone, 138
  hepatic injury, 2192
  human cytochrome P450 isoforms, 2312
  interference with oral anticoagulants, 636
Proparathyroid hormone, 1718
Properdin, 1133
Prophylactic cholecystectomy, 2225
Prophylaxis
  acute tubular necrosis, 773
  cerebral embolism, 1006
  cryptococcosis, 1670
  deep venous thrombosis, 311
  gram-negative infection, 1454
  Haemophilus influenzae, 1589
  infection after lung transplantation, 517, 518
  infective endocarditis, 233, 234-235
  Lassa fever, 1510
  meningococcal disease, 1580
  opportunistic infection, 1473-1474
  platelet transfusion, 573
  Pneumocystis carinii pneumonia, 1695
  pulmonary complications of surgery, 2261
  rabies, 1507-1508

Prophylaxis—cont'd
  reinfection of urinary tract, 1461
  sickle cell disease, 658
  staphylococcal infections, 1553
  traveler's diarrhea, 1432
Prophyrinogens, 1924
Propionibacterium acnes, 1304-1305, 1368
Propionic acidemia, 1908
Propionyl-CoA carboxylase, 1908
Propofol, 1573-1574
Propoxyphene
  hepatic injury, 2191, 2192
  pulmonary parenchymal reactions, 476
  pulmonary toxicity, 479
Propranolol
  acute intermittent porphyria, 1926
  arrhythmias, 138
  bleeding varices, 2168
  Graves' disease, 1806-1807
  high thyroxine levels, 1803
  human cytochrome P450 isoforms, 2312
  hypertension, 325
  hypertensive emergency, 328
  hypertrophic obstructive cardiomyopathy, 269
  interference with oral anticoagulants, 636
  palpitations, 131
  during pregnancy, 2273
  properties, 203
  prophylaxis of migraine, 962
  tetralogy of Fallot, 289
  thyrotoxic storm, 1808
  Wolff-Parkinson-White syndrome, 142
Propylene glycol, 866
Propylthiouracil
  Graves' disease, 1806
  hepatic injury, 2191
  during pregnancy, 2273
  thyroid storm, 1808
Prosody, 977
Prospect Hill virus, 1516
Prospective estrogen and progesterone
    intervention trial, 2271
Prospective Investigation of Pulmonary
    Embolism Diagnosis study, 502
Prospective Randomized Amlodipine Survival
    Evaluation, 171
Prospective Randomized Evaluation of
    Carvedilol on Symptoms and
    Exercise/Multicenter Oral Carvedilol
    Heart Failure Assessment, 171
Prospective Randomized Flosequinan Longevity
    Profile, 171
Prospective Randomized Milrinone Survival
    Evaluation, 171
Prostacyclin
  angina, 205
  primary pulmonary hypertension, 295
  shock, 176
  thrombotic thrombocytopenic purpura, 614
Prostaglandin analog, 2302
Prostaglandin D$_2$, 1140
Prostaglandin E$_1$
  hepatorenal syndrome, 2170
  impotence, 1764
  primary pulmonary hypertension, 295
  vasoactive effects on pulmonary circulation,
    363
Prostaglandin E$_2$
  gram-negative sepsis, 1448
  shock, 176
Prostaglandin-generating factor, 1141
Prostaglandin I$_2$, 1448
Prostaglandin synthetase inhibitors, 832, 884
Prostaglandins, 1141
  calcium homeostasis, 1720
  effect on vasopressin release, 1791
  fever, 1375
  heart failure, 160
  inflammatory response, 1448
  lung filtration, 346

Prostaglandins—cont'd
  nonsteroidal antiinflammatory drugs and,
    1258-1259
  osteoporosis, 1947
  pepsinogen secretion, 1984, 1985
  sepsis, 1448
  sodium retention, 819
  vasoactive effects on pulmonary circulation,
    363
Prostate
  cancer, 717-720
    elevated prostate specific antigen, 732
    incidence and death rates, 550
    obstructive uropathy, 885
    osteoblastic bone formation, 1971
    pulmonary metastases, 493
    screening, 553
  hypertrophy, 885
  prostatism, 326
  prostatitis, 1462-1463
Prostate-specific antigen, 553, 717
Prostatectomy, 719
Prostatic acid phosphatase, 718
Prostatic intraepithelial neoplasia, 717
Prostatism, 326
Prostatitis, 1461, 1462-1463
Prostatodynia, 1463
Prosthetic infection
  candidal, 1551
  nosocomial, 1480
  staphylococcal, 1551
Prosthetic valve, 257-261
  anticoagulant therapy, 640
  infective endocarditis, 230, 231-232,
    1550-1551
  transesophageal echocardiography, 97
Protamine sulfate, 635
Protamine zinc, 1859
Protease inhibitors
  acquired immunodeficiency syndrome, 1474
  deficiencies, 625
Proteases
  gram-negative bacilli, 1446
  lung injury, 373
  pancreatic, 2131
Protected brush catheter, 384-385
Protein
  acinar cell, 2131
  amino acid content and sequence, 50
  bacterial synthesis, 1344
  bile acid uptake, 2126
  body water compartments, 736
  in bronchoalveolar lavage fluid, 367
  deposition in amyloidosis, 1282
  drug-nutrient interactions, 2110
  effects of diet, 1890
  hepatic metabolism, 2118-2120
  hyperproteinemia, 806
  increased delivery, 760
  intestinal absorption, 1987-1988
  metabolism, 1851-1852
  recommended daily dietary allowances, 2114
  restriction
    chronic interstitial nephritis, 893
    chronic renal failure, 786, 787
    diabetic nephropathy, 862
    hepatic encephalopathy, 1080, 2162
    renal osteodystrophy, 785
    urea cycle disorders, 1906
Protein binding drug interactions, 2312
Protein C, 538, 539
  assay, 572
  gram-negative infection, 1454
  inactivation of coagulation factors, 539
  inhibition of fibrin formation, 535
  thrombin formation, 537, 539
  thrombosis, 609, 631
  thrombotic thrombocytopenic purpura, 614
Protein Ca, 537, 539
Protein-calorie malnutrition, 436, 2100-2101
Protein F, 1556

Protein kinase
  mitogen-activated, 541
  myotonic muscular dystrophy, 62
Protein kinase A
  pancreatic acinar cell secretions, 2132
  regulation, 57
Protein kinase C, 1712
Protein precipitation method, 761
Protein S, 538
  assay, 572
  thrombosis, 609
  venous thromboembolism, 631
Protein-sparing diet, 2104
Protein tyrosine kinases, 1127, 1175
Protein Y, 2128
Proteinases
  interstitial lung disease, 450
  rheumatoid arthritis, 1202
Proteinuria, 758-761
  acquired immunodeficiency syndrome patient, 853
  acute nephritic syndrome, 764
  amyloidosis, 1283
  Bence Jones, 863
  constrictive pericarditis, 277
  crescentic glomerulonephritis, 848
  diabetic glomerulopathy, 860
  familial Mediterranean fever, 877
  focal glomerular sclerosis, 852
  Goodpasture's syndrome, 847
  heavy-chain disease, 704
  hematuria, 757
  immunoglobulin A nephropathy, 845
  isolated, 761
  laboratory testing, 743
  Lassa fever, 1510
  lipodystrophy, 877
  mechanisms, 759-761
  membranous nephropathy, 853, 854
  minimal change disease, 851
  nephrotic syndrome, 765
  partial lipodystrophy, 1902
  poststreptococcal glomerulonephritis, 844
  preeclampsia, 2274
  subepithelial immune complex deposits, 842
  systemic lupus erythematosus, 1215
  thrombotic thrombocytopenic purpura, 615
  urinary tract infection, 1458
  Wegener's granulomatosis, 468
Proteoglycans, 1142, 1289
Proteus
  antibiotic selection, 1347
  bacteremia, 1445
  infectious gastritis, 2043
  spinal epidural abscess, 1418
  susceptibility to empiric antimicrobial therapy, 1400
  synergistic nonclostridial anaerobic myonecrosis, 1424
  urinary tract infection, 1457
Prothionamide, 2191
Prothrombin, 538
  congenital disorders of blood coagulation, 618
  deficiency, 624
  hypoprothrombinemia, 1104, 2106
  prothrombin time, 2135
  synthesis, 2120
  vitamin K defects, 2005, 2106
Prothrombin complex concentrates
  hemophilia B, 622
  vitamin K deficiency, 626
Prothrombin time, 571
  acquired coagulation inhibitors, 630
  adult respiratory distress syndrome, 421
  disseminated intravascular coagulation, 609
  fibrinogen abnormalities, 625
  gastrointestinal bleeding, 2011
  grades of liver disease severity, 2166
  hemophilia, 606
  hemostatic abnormalities in liver disease, 627

Prothrombin time—cont'd
  hepatocellular *versus* cholestatic jaundice, 2156
  liver disease, 2135
  platelet coagulant activity, 570
  primary biliary cirrhosis, 2200, 2201
  test of hepatic synthetic function, 2142, 2143
  vitamin K defects, 626, 2005
  warfarin monitoring, 635
Prothymocyte, 1112
Proton pump, 1983
Proton pump inhibitors, 2018, 2040
Protooncogene, 541
Protoporphyria, 1925-1926
Protoporphyrin, 1923
Protoporphyrinogen oxidase, 1923
Protozoan infection, 1671-1692
  African trypanosomiasis, 1687-1689
  amebiasis, 1681-1683
    acquired immunodeficiency syndrome, 2096
    liver abscess, 2210
    meningitis, 1409
    pleural effusion, 507
    traveler, 1465-1466
  babesiosis, 1675-1676
  balantidiasis, 1690-1691
  Blastocystis hominis, 1691
  Chagas' disease, 1689-1690
    esophageal achalasia, 2021
    gastrointestinal motility, 1978
    transfusion-transmitted, 575, 576
  cryptosporidiosis, 1679-1680
  cyclosporiasis, 1680
  Dientamoeba fragilis, 1691
  giardiasis, 1684-1685
  isosporiasis, 1680
  leishmaniasis, 1685-1687
  malaria, 1671-1675
    fever of unknown origin, 1377
    hemolytic anemia, 667
    nephrotic syndrome, 767
    peripheral blood smear, 557
    Plasmodium falciparum, Plate VIII-14
    Plasmodium vivax, Plate VIII-15
    during pregnancy, 1468
    transfusion-transmitted, 575, 576
    travel-related, 1464-1465, 1467
  microsporidiosis, 1680-1681
  Naegleria and *Acanthamoeba,* 1683-1684
  nonpathogenic protozoa, 1692
  during pregnancy, 2281
  sarcocystosis, 1680
  toxoplasmosis, 1676-1679
    acquired immunodeficiency syndrome, 1473, 1474, 1477, 1478
    brain abscess, 1414
    compromised host, 1388
    fever of unknown origin, 1377
    lung transplantation, 518, 520
    during pregnancy, 2281
    travel-related, 1465-1466
  trichomoniasis, 1442-1443, 1691
Protriptyline, 1037
  cataplexy, 943
  obstructive sleep apnea, 528
Provocative testing
  bronchial challenge, 379, 1188
  photodermatoses, 1307
Provoked seizure, 980
Proximal convoluted tubule, 1718
Proximal diabetic neuropathy, 1017
Proximal femoral fracture, 1945
Proximal interphalangeal joint, 1202
Proximal nephron, 741
Proximal renal tubular acidosis, 828, 837-838
Proximal tubular reabsorption, 738
Proximal tubule
  reabsorption of bicarbonate, 835
  renal cell carcinoma, 898
Proximal-vein thrombosis, 631
Prurigo, 1326

Pruritus
  benign recurrent intrahepatic cholestasis, 2158
  candidal vaginitis, 1661
  cholangiocarcinoma, 2231
  cholestatic hepatitis A, 2173
  conjugated hyperbilirubinemia, 2156
  estrogen-related cholestasis, 2158
  genital lesions, 1444
  hemorrhoids, 2093
  hepatocellular *versus* cholestatic jaundice, 2156
  Hodgkin's disease, 693
  hookworm, 1698
  human immunodeficiency virus infection, 1326
  otitis externa, 2307
  pancreatic cancer, 2242
  paraneoplastic dermatoses, 1317, 1318
  polycythemia vera, 688
  primary biliary cirrhosis, 2200
  primary sclerosing cholangitis, 2201
  protoporphyria, 1925
  transfusion reaction, 574
  vulvovaginal candidiasis, 1442
Prussian blue stain, 558
  iron in normal bone marrow, Plate IV-9
  ringed sideroblast, Plate IV-11
PSC; *see* Primary sclerosing cholangitis
PSC 833, 702
Pseudallescheria, 1659
Pseudo-Hurler dystrophy, 1916
Pseudo-von Willebrand's disease, 623
Pseudo-Wilsonian hepatic encephalopathy, 2161
Pseudoaneurysm, 178, 299
Pseudoarthrosis, 1921
Pseudobulbar affect, 1033
Pseudobulbar palsy, 1999
Pseudochylothorax, 509
Pseudochylous ascites, 2164
Pseudochylous effusion, 382
Pseudoclaudication, 308
Pseudocyst
  acute pancreatitis, 2237
  chronic pancreatitis, 2241
Pseudodementia, 2288
Pseudodysphagia, 1998
Pseudofracture in osteomalacia, 1950
Pseudogene, globin, 650-651
Pseudogout, 1278-1279
  primary hyperparathyroidism, 1966
  renal osteodystrophy, 1963
Pseudohyperaldosteronism, 1819
Pseudohyperkalemia, 831
Pseudohypoaldosteronism, 832
Pseudohypoglycemia, 1877
Pseudohyponatremia, 810, 812
Pseudohypoparathyroidism, 1932, 1933
  osteomalacia, 1952
  urinary cyclic adenosine monophosphate, 1746
Pseudolymphoma, 599, 2049
Pseudomacrocytosis, 588
Pseudomembranous colitis, 1568-1570, 1996
Pseudomonas
  bacteremia, 1445
  cystic fibrosis airway infection, 480
  empyema, 507
  folliculitis, 1420
  lung recipient, 517
  normal flora, 1368
  otitis externa, 2307
  prosthetic valve endocarditis, 230
  septicemia, 1382
  spinal epidural abscess, 1418
  urinary tract infection, 1457
Pseudomonas aeruginosa
  acquired immunodeficiency syndrome, 1329
  antibiotic selection, 1348
  antimicrobial combinations, 1360
  compromised host, 1388
  cutaneous lesion, Plate VIII-23
  diabetic patient, 1323
  susceptibility to empiric antimicrobial therapy, 1400

Pseudomyxoma peritonei, 2249
Pseudoneurotrophic joint, 1279
Pseudoobstruction, intestinal, 2079
Pseudoosteoarthritis, 1279
Pseudopolyp, ulcerative colitis, 2073, Plate X-8
Pseudopseudohypoparathyroidism, 1932
Pseudorheumatoid arthritis, 1279
Pseudosciatica, 965
Pseudosepsis, 1451
Pseudothrombocytopenia, 610, 613
Pseudotumor, hemophilia, 606
Pseudotumor cerebri, 1061, 1070
Pseudoxanthoma elasticum, 1289, 1321
Psittacosis, 1377, 1535
Psoriasis, 1300-1302, Plate VII-9
    human immunodeficiency virus infection,
        1325-1326
    intraarticular bone ankylosis, 1166-1167
Psoriatic arthritis, 1240-1242
Psychiatric disorders
    anorexia nervosa, 2030
    anxiety, 1034-1035
    chronic fatigue syndrome, 2299
    hypogonadism, 1842
    maladaptive illness behavior, 1040
    mood disorders, 1035-1038
    mutism, 977
    neurohormonal regulation, 1077
    palpitations, 131
    personality disorders, 1039-1040
    sleep disorders, 946-947
    somatization, 1040
    thought disorders, 1041-1043
    thyroid disease, 1803
    weight loss, 1749
Psychogenic abdominal pain, 2031, 2034-2035
Psychogenic coma, 949
Psychogenic spell, 981
Psychogenic vomiting, 2027
Psychologic factors
    amenorrhea, 1757-1758
    anorexia, 2029
    breast cancer, 712
    chest pain, 129
    impotence, 1760-1761
    irritable bowel syndrome, 2055
Psychologic support
    cancer pain, 581
    multiple sclerosis, 1009
    osteoarthritis, 1267
    pulmonary rehabilitation, 435-437
    spinal cord injury, 1052
Psychologic testing, 903-904
Psychomotor seizure, 979
Psychophysiologic insomnia, 940-942
Psychosis
    disordered thinking, 1041
    hypothyroidism, 1809
    systemic lupus erythematosus, 1093
Psychotherapy, 2300
Psyllium, 636
PT; *see* Prothrombin time
PTCA; *see* Percutaneous transluminal coronary
    angioplasty
Pteroylmonoglutamate, 1989
PTLD; *see* Posttransplant lymphoproliferative
    disease
PTT; *see* Partial thromboplastin time
Puberty, 1766-1767
    disorders of growth and development,
        1768-1770
    evaluation of growth and development,
        1770-1772
    growth during, 1767-1768
    gynecomastia, 1765
    impotence, 1761
    ovarian function, 1832
    testicular function, 1839-1840
Public education programs, 2265
Public health considerations in tuberculosis,
    1638

Pulmonary alveolar proteinosis, 455-456
Pulmonary angiography, 388-389
    hepatopulmonary syndrome, 2170
    primary pulmonary hypertension, 294-295
    pulmonary thromboembolism, 502
Pulmonary arterial resistance, 110
Pulmonary arteriolar resistance, 111
Pulmonary arteriovenous fistula, 499
Pulmonary artery, 360
    aneurysm, 469
    biventricular assist device, 185
    hemodynamic data, 110
    primary pulmonary hypertension, 294
    root ejection sounds, 74
    rupture, 395
    stenosis, 81
Pulmonary artery balloon catheter, 169
Pulmonary artery catheter, 390-395
    gram-negative bacteremia, 1451
    right ventricular infarction, 220
    sepsis, 1450
    shock, 181
Pulmonary artery diastolic pressure, 392
Pulmonary artery pressure
    normal at rest, 110
    pulmonary hypertension, 293, 363, 364, 498
    pulmonic regurgitation, 257
Pulmonary artery pressure-flow relationship, 361
Pulmonary artery wedge pressure, 391-392,
        393-394
    cardiac *versus* noncardiac edema, 425
    effects of pharmacologic interventions, 183
    mitral stenosis, 245
Pulmonary blood flow, 360-364
    atrial septal defect, 282
    pulmonary hypertension, 293, 363
    pulmonic stenosis, 288
    tetralogy of Fallot, 288
    total anomalous pulmonary venous connection,
        291
    tricuspid atresia, 291
Pulmonary capillary hydrostatic pressure,
        394-395
Pulmonary capillary wedge pressure
    gram-negative bacteremia, 1451
    heart failure, 173, 174
    hemodynamic data, 110
    pulmonary artery catheterization, 181
Pulmonary diagnostic imaging, 386-390
Pulmonary disease
    acute respiratory failure, 412-420
        adult respiratory distress syndrome with, 418
        artificial airway, 416-417
        chronic obstructive pulmonary disease with,
            417-418, 446
        classification, 413, 414
        diagnosis, 413-414
        mechanical ventilation, 397, 416, 418-420
        oxygenation measures, 415-416
        pathophysiology, 412-413
        principles of management, 414, 415
        respiratory acidosis, 416
        without lung disease, 418
    adverse drug reactions, 476-479
    asthma, 1185-1193
        Churg-Strauss syndrome, 465
        clinical manifestations, 1187-1188
        cough, 406
        diagnosis and differential diagnosis, 1189
        epidemiology and pathology, 1185
        laboratory findings, 1188-1189
        management, 1189-1192
        occupational, 471-472, 473
        pathophysiology, 1185-1187
        patterns of pulmonary function
            abnormalities, 379
        physical findings, 403
        prognosis, 1192-1193
        pulmonary rehabilitation, 432-437
        sputum expectoration, 408
        wheezing, 404

Pulmonary disease—cont'd
    bronchiectasis, 483-485
        cough, 406
        cystic fibrosis, 480
        double lung allograft, 515
        dyspnea, 404
        high-resolution computed tomography, 387
        sputum expectoration, 408
    chest pain, 128-129, 408-410
    chronic obstructive pulmonary disease, 437-447
        with acute respiratory failure, 413-414,
            417-418
        airflow obstruction, 438
        alpha$_1$-protease inhibitor deficiency,
            439-440
        clinical features, 442
        complications, 445-447
        definition, 437-438
        diagnosis, 443
        dyspnea, 404
        epidemiology, 438-439
        hypercapnia, 356
        laboratory findings, 442-443
        lung transplantation, 445
        occupational, 473
        pathogenesis, 441-442
        pathology, 439
        physical examination, 442
        prognosis and course, 447
        pulmonary rehabilitation, 432-437
        sleep studies with monitoring of oxygen
            saturation, 380
        treatment, 443-445
    cough, 404-408, 409
    cystic fibrosis, 479-483
    diagnostic imaging, 386-390
    dysfunction of host defenses, 369
    dyspnea, 404, 405
    expectoration, 408
    hemoptysis, 410-411
    high-resolution computed tomography, 387
    hypersensitivity pneumonitis, 460-463
    interstitial, 448-456
        clinical features, 450-451
        clinicopathologic classification, 449
        diagnosis and management, 451-452
        dyspnea, 404
        etiologic factors, 452
        exercise tests, 379
        imaging techniques, 451
        lung pathology, 448-449
        pathogenesis, 449-450
        pathophysiology, 450
        pulmonary hypertension, 498
        unknown origin, 452-456
    invasive diagnostic techniques, 380-386
        bronchoalveolar lavage, 384
        bronchoscopy and biopsy, 383-384
        mediastinoscopy and mediastinotomy, 385
        open lung biopsy, 385-386
        pleural biopsy, 382-383
        protected brush catheter, 384-385
        sputum examination, 380-381
        Swan-Ganz catheterization, 383
        thoracentesis, 381-382
        thoracoscopy, 385
        transthoracic needle aspiration, 385
        transtracheal aspiration, 385
    Langerhans' cell granulomatosis, 463-465
    mediastinal disease, 510-514
    medical history, 401-402
    multiple organ dysfunction syndrome, 421-423
    neoplasms, 486-492; *see also* Lung cancer
    occupational, 471-476
    physical examination, 402-404
    pleural, 505-510
    primary granulomatous pulmonary vasculitis,
        465-471
    pulmonary edema, 423-428
        acute toxic, 473
        adult respiratory distress syndrome, 421

Pulmonary disease—cont'd
  pulmonary edema—cont'd
    drug-induced, 477
    hemoptysis, 410
    pneumothorax, 510
    pulmonary artery wedge pressure, 395
  pulmonary hypertension
    cardiac transplantation, 338
    chronic obstructive pulmonary disease,
      446-447
    drug-induced, 477
    exertional angina, 127
    interstitial lung disease, 452
    pathophysiology, 363-364
    primary and secondary causes, 497-499
    Takayasu's arteritis, 470
  pulmonary rehabilitation, 431, 432-437
  pulmonary thromboembolism, 499-504
  pulmonary transplantation, 514-524
    allograft rejection, 520-524
    chronic obstructive pulmonary disease, 445
    complications, 516-520
    future trends, 524
    immunosuppression, 516
    indications, 514-515
    outcome, 516
    selection of donor and recipient, 515-516
  respiratory therapy, 428-432
  sarcoidosis, 456-459
  sleep-related, 524-528
  solitary pulmonary nodule, 493-497
  Waldenström macroglobulinemia, 704
  Wegener's granulomatosis, 1222
  wheezing, 404, 405
Pulmonary edema, 423-428
  acute toxic, 473
  adult respiratory distress syndrome, 421
  aortic regurgitation, 244
  chronic renal failure, 783-784
  congenital aortic stenosis, 287
  dilated cardiomyopathy, 263
  drug-induced, 477
  heart failure, 165
  hemoptysis, 410
  hypertrophic obstructive cardiomyopathy, 266
  malaria, 1673
  mitral stenosis, 247
  myocardial contusion, 332
  neurogenic, 1099-1100
  papillary muscle rupture, 219
  patent ductus arteriosus, 285
  pneumothorax, 510
  precapillary pulmonary hypertension, 293
  pulmonary artery wedge pressure, 395
  treatment, 168
  ventricular septal defect, 284
Pulmonary embolectomy, 503
Pulmonary embolism, 499-504, 630-638
  acute pulmonary hypertension, 297
  atrial fibrillation, 146
  chest pain, 128
  deep venous thrombosis, 311
  echocardiography, 100
  heart failure *versus,* 168
  lung scan, 387-388
  nephrotic syndrome, 766
  nosocomial, 1480-1481
  during pregnancy, 2276
  pulmonary angiogram, 388
  pulmonary edema *versus,* 425
  sepsis *versus,* 1451
  wheezing, 1189
Pulmonary fibrosis
  asbestos-related, 473-474
  asbestosis, 474
  systemic sclerosis, 1230
Pulmonary function tests, 375-380
  acquired immunodeficiency syndrome, 1477
  acute lung allograft rejection, 521
  asthma, 1188-1189
  bronchiolitis obliterans syndrome, 522

Pulmonary function tests—cont'd
  bronchoprovocation inhalation tests, 379
  chronic obstructive pulmonary disease,
    442-443
  drug-induced pneumonitis, 477
  exercise tests, 379-380
  hypersensitivity pneumonitis, 461
  inhaled bronchodilator studies, 377-378
  interstitial lung disease, 451
  Langerhans' cell granulomatosis, 464
  before lung resection, 497
  lung volume determination, 378
  precapillary pulmonary hypertension, 296
  single-breath diffusing capacity, 378, 379
  sleep studies, 380
  spirometry, 376-377
  ventilatory control studies, 378-379
  Wegener's granulomatosis, 1222
Pulmonary hemorrhage, 454-455
  Goodpasture's syndrome, 847
Pulmonary hypertension, 293-299
  acquired immunodeficiency syndrome, 333
  cardiac catheterization, 108
  cardiac transplantation, 338
  chronic obstructive pulmonary disease,
    446-447
  continuous-wave Doppler echocardiography,
    99
  cor triatriatum, 291
  dexfenfluramine and, 261
  drug-induced, 477
  exertional angina, 127
  fenfluramine and, 261
  Graham Steell murmur, 80
  interstitial lung disease, 452
  mitral regurgitation, 250
  mitral stenosis, 245, 248
  neurogenic pulmonary edema, 1099
  obesity, 334
  passive, 297-298
  pathophysiology, 363-364
  phentermine and, 261
  precapillary, 293-297
  primary and secondary causes, 497-499
  reactive, 298
  systemic sclerosis, 1230
  Takayasu's arteritis, 470
Pulmonary infarction
  complication of pulmonary artery
    catheterization, 395
  pleural effusion, 508
Pulmonary infiltrates
  acute lung allograft rejection, 521
  bronchiolitis obliterans syndrome, 522
  crescentic glomerulonephritis, 848
  eosinophilia, 1698, 1702
  Goodpasture's syndrome, 847
  hypersensitivity pneumonitis, 461
  Legionnaire's disease, 1623
  meningococcemia, 1579
  Pneumocystis carinii pneumonia, 1693
  reimplantation response, 517
Pulmonary nodule, solitary, 493-497
Pulmonary regurgitant murmur, 80
Pulmonary rehabilitation, 431, 432-437
  benefits, 432-433
  chronic obstructive pulmonary disease, 445
  exercise conditioning, 435-436
  follow-up care, 437
  medical intervention, 434-435
  nutritional evaluation and therapy, 435
  occupational therapy, 436
  physical therapy, 436
  program structure, 433-434
  psychosocial management, 435-437
  referral, 433
Pulmonary-renal syndrome, 775
Pulmonary sarcoidosis, 1245
Pulmonary shunt, 426
  pulmonary artery catheterization, 391
Pulmonary toilet, 516

Pulmonary toxicity, chemotherapeutic agents,
  584
Pulmonary transplantation, 514-524
  allograft rejection, 520-524
  chronic obstructive pulmonary disease, 445
  complications, 516-520
  future trends, 524
  immunosuppression, 516
  indications, 514-515
  outcome, 516
  selection of donor and recipient, 515-516
Pulmonary tuberculosis, 1628-1630
Pulmonary ultrasonography, 389
Pulmonary vascular disease, 454
  atrial septal defect, 280
  common aortopulmonary trunk, 290
  double lung allograft, 515
  primary granulomatous vasculitis, 465-471
  tetralogy of Fallot, 289
  ventricular septal defect, 283
Pulmonary vascular resistance, 361
  mitral stenosis, 245
  patent ductus arteriosus, 285
  pulmonary artery catheterization, 391
  pulmonary hypertension, 363
Pulmonary vein, 360
  partial transposition, 282
  stenosis, 298
  total anomalous pulmonary venous connection,
    290-291
Pulmonary veno-occlusive disease, 298
Pulmonary venous congestion, 91
Pulmonic regurgitation, 80, 256-257
Pulmonic stenosis, 256
  with intact ventricular septum, 288
  systolic murmur, 266
  tetralogy of Fallot, 288-289
Pulse
  acute occlusive arterial disease, 307
  aortic regurgitation, 241
  aortic stenosis, 236
  extracellular fluid volume contraction, 824
  heart failure, 165
  hypertrophic obstructive cardiomyopathy, 266
  jugular venous, 65-67, 68, 69
    atrial septal defect, 281
    cardiac tamponade, 275
    mitral regurgitation, 250
    primary pulmonary hypertension, 294
    pulmonic stenosis, 288
    tricuspid regurgitation, 256
  mitral stenosis, 246
  Quincke's, 241
Pulse oximetry, 378-379, 396
  adult respiratory distress syndrome, 421
  pulmonary edema, 425
Pulsed Doppler echocardiography, 98
Pulseless disease, 311, 470-471, 1224
  aortic obstruction and inflammation, 303-304
  neurologic manifestations, 1092, 1095
Pulsus alternans, 65, 67, 264
Pulsus bisferiens, 65
Pulsus paradoxus, 65, 67
  asthma, 1188
  cardiac tamponade, 275-276
  constrictive pericarditis, 277
Pulsus parvus et tardus pulse, 65
Pupil
  autonomic regulation, 932-933, 934
  brain death, 951, 1083
Pupillometry, 938
Pure agraphia, 978
Pure alexia, 978
Pure amegakaryocytic thrombocytopenic
  purpura, 675
Pure autonomic failure, 936
Pure red blood cell aplasia, 674-675
Pure sideroblastic anemia, 645
Pure white blood cell aplasia, 675
Pure word blindness, 978
Pure word mutism, 977

Purified protein derivative
    human immunodeficiency virus infection,
        1473
    Mycobacterium tuberculosis, 1629
Purine metabolism, 1269
Purine nucleoside analogs, 684
Purine nucleoside phosphorylase deficiency,
    1177
Purkinje fiber
    action potential, 132
    cardiac cycle, 36
Purpura, 602, 603
    Churg-Strauss syndrome, 466
    differential diagnosis of fever and rash, 1384
    gram-negative bacteremia, 1449
    Henoch-Schönlein purpura, 1222
    idiopathic myelofibrosis, 677
    immune thrombocytopenic, human
        immunodeficiency virus infection,
        1472
    mixed cryoglobulinemia, 1249
    posttransfusion, 616
    Rocky Mountain spotted fever, Plate VIII-18
    Wegener's granulomatosis, 468
Pursed-lip breathing, 402, 436
Pursuit eye movement, 1063
Push enteroscopy, 1995
Pustular psoriasis, 1301
Pustule
    acne vulgaris, 1305
    differential diagnosis of fever and rash, 1384
    disseminated gonococcal infection, 1382
    ecthyma, 1420
    impetigo, 1419
    systemic candidiasis, 1312
Puumala virus, 1516
PVC hypothesis, 134
Pyarthrosis, 1586, 1588
Pyelonephritis, 1455
    acute cholecystitis *versus,* 2228
    dysuria, 763
    imaging studies, 754-755
    during pregnancy, 2281
Pyknodysostosis, 1959
Pyloric stenosis, 2044
Pylorus, movement of food, 1978
Pyoderma, streptococcal, 1556
Pyoderma gangrenosum, 705, Plate X-9
    cutaneous findings, 1321-1322
Pyogenic liver abscess, 2209-2210
Pyopneumothorax, 510
Pyrazinamide
    mycobacterial disease, 1631
    tuberculosis, 1474
Pyridinium crosslinks, 1745
Pyridinol carbamate, 2192
Pyridinoline, 1745, 1947
Pyridostigmine, 1022
Pyridoxine
    biochemical function, 2105
    deficiency, 1101, 2107
    hyperoxaluria, 804
    megadoses and toxicity, 2108
    sideroblastic anemia, 645-646
    tuberculosis, 1474
    Wilson's disease, 2206
Pyridoxine-responsive anemia, 2107
Pyrimethamine
    brain abscess, 1416
    coccidian parasitic disease, 1679
    drug-nutrient interactions, 2110
    glucose-6-phosphate dehydrogenase
        deficiency, 664
    isosporiasis, 1680
    prophylaxis in lung transplantation, 518
    toxoplasmosis, 1474, 1477, 1678, 1679
Pyrimidine-5′ nucleotidase, 663
Pyrogenic exotoxins, group A streptococci,
    1555-1556
Pyrogens, 1375, 1386-1387
Pyrophosphate, 1276, 1277

Pyrophosphate analogs
    hypercalcemia, 1929
    primary hyperparathyroidism, 1971
Pyropoikilocytosis, 665, 666
Pyrosis, 1999
Pyruvate dehydrogenase, 1851
Pyruvate kinase
    deficiency, 664
    hemolytic anemia, 663
Pyuria
    with dysuria, 762
    reactive arthritis, 1240
    urinary tract infection, 1458

Q

Q fever, 1543, 1545
Q wave, 84
    congenitally corrected transposition of great
        arteries, 290
    constrictive pericarditis, 277
    hypertrophic cardiomyopathy, 267
    ischemic heart disease, 197
    myocardial infarction, 88
    tetralogy of Fallot, 289
Q wave myocardial infarction, 209, 218
QRS axis, 85
    atrial abnormality, 88
    endocardial cushion defect, 283
    pulmonary hypertension, 296
QRS complex, 84, 132
    accelerated atrioventricular junctional rhythm,
        144
    atrial fibrillation, 147
    atrial septal defect, 281
    atrioventricular block in myocardial infarction,
        223
    atrioventricular conduction abnormalities,
        153-154
    cardiac tamponade, 276
    conduction abnormalities, 86
    effects of pacemaker, 90
    hyperkalemia, 832
    hypokalemia, 829
    left ventricular hypertrophy, 87
    multifocal atrial tachycardia, 144
    premature ventricular contractions, 148
    sinoatrial block, 153
    sinus bradycardia, 153
    supraventricular tachyarrhythmias, 141, 142
    sustained ventricular tachycardia and wide
        QRS complex tachycardia, 149-150,
        151
    wide QRS complex tachycardia, 149-150, 151
    Wolff-Parkinson-White syndrome, 142
QRS duration, 85, 150
QRS interval, 833
QRS vector, 85, 148
QT interval, 85
    effects of quinidine, 137
    mitral valve prolapse, 254
    polymorphic ventricular tachycardia, 152
    proarrhythmia, 135
Quadruple-bolus testing, 1776, 1777
Qualitative fecal fat, 2058
Quality assurance, 17
Quality improvement, 17-18
    methods for, 19-22
    physician response, 22
Quality of care, 16-22
    managed care, 33-34
Quantitation of immunoglobulins, 567
Quantitative fecal fat, 2058
Quantitative liver function tests, 2143-2144
Quinacrine
    cutaneous lesions in lupus erythematosus,
        1292
    giardiasis, 1685
    rheumatic disease, 1261
    systemic lupus erythematosus, 1217

Quinapril
    heart failure, 170
    hypertension, 325
Quincke's pulse, 241
Quinidine, 137
    atrial fibrillation, 147
    atrial flutter, 144, 146
    drug-induced bile duct injury, 2203
    glucose-6-phosphate dehydrogenase
        deficiency, 664
    hepatic injury, 2192
    human cytochrome P450 isoforms, 2312
    interference with catecholamine assays, 1740
    interference with oral anticoagulants, 636
    malaria, 1674-1675
Quinine
    babesiosis, 1676
    drug-induced immune thrombocytopenia, 615
    glucose-6-phosphate dehydrogenase
        deficiency, 664
    interference with catecholamine assays, 1740
    malaria, 1465, 1674-1675
Quinolones, 1359
    acute pancreatitis, 2237
    bacterial pneumonia after lung transplantation,
        517
    Campylobacter enteritis, 1592
    dosage, 1350
    effects on kidney, 868
    enterococcal infection, 1563
    enterococci resistance, 1561
    gonorrhea, 1584
    Haemophilus ducreyi, 1589
    Helicobacter pylori, 1593
    human cytochrome P450 isoforms, 2312
    interference with oral anticoagulants, 636
    mycobacterial disease, 1631
    Mycoplasma hominis infection, 1541
    osteomyelitis, 1436
    Pasteurella, 1609
    prophylaxis in compromised host, 1390
    respiratory exacerbations in cystic fibrosis, 483
    shigellosis, 1603
    spontaneous bacterial peritonitis, 2164
    traveler's diarrhea, 1432
    typhoid fever, 1432, 1601
    urethritis, 1441
    use during pregnancy, 2281
Quinsy, 1393, 2306

R

R-prime wave, 84
R wave, 84
    atrial septal defect, 281
    cardioversion, 139
    chronic cor pulmonale, 445
    endocardial cushion defect, 283
    myocardial infarction, 88, 211
    sinus tachycardia, 141
    tetralogy of Fallot, 289
Rabbit brain thromboplastin, 639
Rabbit fever, 1607-1609
Rabbit ileal intestinal loop test, 1426, 1429
Rabies, 1505-1508, Plate VIII-43
Race
    chronic obstructive pulmonary disease, 438
    end-stage renal disease, 777
    glucose-6-phosphate dehydrogenase
        deficiency, 663
    heart failure, 157-158
    hypertension, 319
    osteoarthritis risk, 1264
    prostate cancer, 717
    risk of stroke, 1001
Radial immunodiffusion, 567
Radial nerve mononeuropathy, 1017
Radial reflex, 964
Radiation-induced disorders
    enteropathy, 2065-2066
    esophagitis, 2019

Radiation-induced disorders—cont'd
gastric, 2043
iatrogenic pericardial disease, 273
impotence, 1762
interstitial lung disease, 452
myelopathy, 1013
pneumonitis, 411
renal injury, 868, 892
Radiation sensitivity of tumor, 553
Radiation therapy
acromegaly, 1784
breast cancer, 709
cervical cancer, 715
colon cancer, 2085
complications, 585
endometrial cancer, 714
esophageal cancer, 2024
head and neck cancer, 724
Hodgkin's disease, 694
malignant pericardial effusions, 332
non-Hodgkin's lymphoma, 700
non-small cell lung cancer, 727, 728-729
pancreatic cancer, 2243
principles, 553-554
prostate cancer, 719
small intestinal malignancies, 2081
testicular cancer, 721
thyroid lymphoma, 1816
toxicity, 579
neurologic, 1072-1073
pulmonary, 479
Radical mastectomy, 709
Radical nephrectomy, 898
Radical prostatectomy, 719
Radiculopathy
complication of chemotherapy, 1072
needle electromyography, 917
Radioactive iodine scan, 1813
Radioallergosorbent test, 1154, 1304
Radiocontrast nephropathy, 775
Radioenzymatic conversion, 1734
Radiographic contrast media
induction of anaphylaxis, 1193, 1194
nephrotoxicity, 871
Radiography
abdominal pain, 2032-2033
achalasia, 2022
acute maxillary sinusitis, 1394
arthritis, 1164-1174
advanced methods, 1173
appendicular skeleton, 1164-1169
axial skeleton, 1169-1171, 1172
foot, 1172
hand, 1171-1172
hip, 1173
knee, 1172-1173
sacroiliac joint, 1172, 1173
techniques and modalities, 1064
wrist, 1172
chronic pancreatitis, 2240
diagnosis and staging of lung cancer, 489
echinococcal cyst, 2111
endocrine, 1734-1735
evaluation of arthritis, 1164
intestinal disorders, 2007
intestinal obstruction, 2078
intraabdominal infection, 1399
ischemic heart disease, 198
Legionnaire's disease, 1623
low back pain, 966
meningitis, 1406-1407
multiple myeloma, 701
neurologic disorders, 924-926
osteoarthritis, 1267
osteomalacia, 1949-1950
osteomyelitis, 1434
Paget's disease, 1956
pancreatic disease, 2145-2147
pleural effusion, 506
Pneumocystis carinii pneumonia, 1693
pyogenic liver abscess, 2209

Radiography—cont'd
renal bone disease, 1964
sinus, 1181-1182
spontaneous pneumomediastinum, 514
swallowing assessment, 2000
tuberculosis, 1628, 1629
ulcerative colitis, 2073, 2074
Radioimmunoassay, 1372
albumin excretion, 761
brucellosis, 1606
detection of autoantibodies, 1156
infectious disease, 1373-1374
microalbuminuria, 743
parathyroid hormone, 1745-1746
principles, 1733-1734
thyroid hormone, 1738
Radioiodine therapy, 1806
Radioisotope studies, 1734-1735
Radiology
brain abscess, 1415, 1416
head trauma, 1044
intracranial subdural empyema, 1416-1418
ischemic heart disease, 198
rheumatoid arthritis, 1205
spinal epidural abscess, 1418
stone passage, 800
Radionuclide angiography
cardiac function, 104-105
dilated cardiomyopathy, 264
Radionuclide cisternography, 926-929
Radionuclide-derived ejection fraction, 251
Radionuclide studies
acute lower gastrointestinal bleeding, 2012
bone
ankylosing spondylitis, 1238-1239
osteomalacia, 1950
osteomyelitis, 1434
Paget's disease, 1956
prostate cancer, 718
septic arthritis, 1252
small cell lung cancer, 726
brain, 926-929
fever of unknown origin, 1379-1380
gallium, 388
acute pericarditis, 274
amebiasis, 1683
amiodarone-induced pulmonary disease, 478
osteomyelitis, 1434
gallstones, 2225
gastric, 2004
hepatic, 2141
intraabdominal abscess, 1400
intraabdominal infection, 1399
liver, 2141
amebiasis, 1683
cavernous hemangioma, 2215-2216
cholestasis, 2156
focal nodular hyperplasia, 2216
lung, 387-388
primary pulmonary hypertension, 294
pulmonary embolism, 297, 387-388,
501-502
mitral valve prolapse, 254
neurologic disorders, 926-929
parathyroid tumor, 1970
proximal venous thrombosis, 502
renal, 750
hydronephrosis, 754
pediatric urinary tract infection, 1459
thyroid, 1801-1802
Graves' disease, 1802
hyperthyroidism, 1735, 1802
Radionuclide ventriculography
heart failure, 165-167
myocardial ischemia, 199
Radiopaque marker study, 2004
Radiotherapy; *see* Radiation therapy
RAG-1 gene, 1123
RAG-2 gene, 1123
Raji cell assay, 1149

Rales
dilated cardiomyopathy, 263
heart failure, 165
RALES survival trial, 171
Ramipril
heart failure, 172
hypertension, 325
Ramsay-Hunt syndrome, 1527
Randomized Aldactone Evaluation Study, 171
Ranitidine
gastroesophageal reflux, 2018
hepatic injury, 2192
interference with oral anticoagulants, 636
peptic ulcer disease, 2040
Ranson's criteria of acute pancreatitis, 2236
Rapamycin
effects on kidney, 870
renal transplantation, 793
Rapeseed oil, 1234, 1884, 2192
Rapid eye movement sleep, 939-940
narcolepsy, 942
parasomnias usually associated with, 946
Rapid eye movement sleep behavior disorder,
946
Rapid plasma reagin test, 1642
Rapidly progressive glomerulonephritis, 846-849
acute nephritic syndrome, 763
alveolar hemorrhage, 455
Rappaport classification, 696
ras gene, 541, 1175
lung, 487
mutation, 544
myelodysplastic syndrome, 676
Rash
chickenpox, 1525
Colorado tick fever, 1512
dengue fever, 1465
dermatomyositis, 1235
differential diagnostic value, 1384-1385
disseminated gonococcal infection, 1583
drug-induced, 1313-1314
fever with, 1380-1386
glucagonoma, 2245
graft-*versus*-host disease, 578
Hartnup disease, 879, 1910, 1911
hookworm, 1698
hypersensitivity vasculitis, 1221
Lassa fever, 1510
lymphomatoid granulomatosis, 470
meningococcal infection, 1406
meningococcemia, 1579
myxoma, 330
parvovirus B19 infection, 1513
photodermatosis, 1306-1307
relapsing fever, 1645
Rocky Mountain spotted fever, 1543
rubella, 1501
scarlet fever, 1421
syphilis, 1641
toxic shock syndrome, 1421
typhoid fever, 1601
vasculitis, 1225
VIPoma, 2245
Rat plague, 1610
Ratbite fever, 1377, 1381
Rate nephelometer, 567
Rate-pressure product, 91
Raynaud's phenomenon, 310, 1226-1227
cryoglobulinemia, 1248
myxoma, 330
scleroderma, 1293
systemic sclerosis, 1229, 1232
transient monocular blindness, 1058
Rb-1 gene, 546
Reactive amyloidosis, 1283
Reactive arthritis, 1239-1240
Reactive hypoglycemia, 1875, 1876
Reactive lymphocyte, 592
Reactive macrophage hyperplasia, 680
Reactive oxygen species, 1405
Reactive pulmonary hypertension, 298

Reagent stick test, 743, 744
Reagent strip test, 742, 743
Reagin, 1139
Reannealling, 52
Rebound headache, 961
Rebound tenderness, 1398, 2080
Receiver operating characteristic curve, 8-9
Receptive alexia, 978
Receptor
  adenosine, 59
  adrenergic, 931
    cardiac function, 56-58
    G proteins, 1827
  alpha-adrenergic, 56-58, 1827
  antigen, 1127
  B-cell, 1123
  B-cell antigen, 1174
  baroreceptors
    aortic, 162, 299
    blood pressure, 931, 932
    carotid, 162
    heart failure, 162, 164
    vasopressin release, 808
  beta-adrenergic, 45, 56-58, 1827
  calcitonin, 1719
  CD4, 1470
  cell surface, 370, 1710-1711
  chemoreceptors
    carbon dioxide partial pressure, 353
    chemoreceptor trigger zone, 2026
    modulation of ventricular function, 45
    pericardial, 271
    peripheral chemoreceptor signal, 353
    response to hypoxia, 353
    ventilation, 352-353
  chief cell, 1984
  complement, 1135, 1179-1180, 1338
  cytoplasmic, 1712-1713
  DHP, 38
  dihydropyridine, 58
    hypokalemic periodic paralysis, 826
    potassium channel, 59
  glycoprotein cell surface membrane,
    1710-1711
  hematopoietic cytokine, 1128
  histamine₁, 1140
  histamine₂, 1140, 1981
  histamine₃, 1982
  hormone, 1710-1713
    breast cancer, 707
    regulation, 1712
    vasopressin, 1791
  insulin, 1900
  interleukin-2, 1177
  irritant, 353
  J, 353
  ligand-gated, 1710
  low-density lipoprotein
    fibroblast, 1886
    relationship with enterohepatic circulation,
      1891
  low-pressure volume, 817
  mechanoreceptors
    chest wall, 353
    modulation of ventricular function, 45
    pericardial, 271
    ventilation, 353
  membrane, 1710-1711
  muscarinic, 56
  nuclear, 1712-1713
  osmoreceptor, 1790
  parietal cell, 1981, 1983
  polyimmunoglobulin, 1990
  pre-B, 1125
  ryanodine, 38, 58
  segment, 1710
  seven-transmembrane segment, 1710
  single transmembrane segment, 1710
  stretch, 45
  surface, 1710

Receptor—cont'd
  T cell, 1127, 1174
    antigen binding, 1111
    apoptosis and autoimmunity, 1144
    Southern blot analysis, 560
  thyroid-stimulating hormone, 1805
  tyrosine kinase, 541, 543
Receptor editing, 1113
Receptor mediated ion channels, 58
Recessive trait, 1721
Recessiveness, 1721, 1724
Recipient
  kidney, 792
  lung, 515-516
Reciprocal changes, 89
Recombinant human DNAase
  cystic fibrosis, 482
  secretion clearance and lung expansion, 430
Recombinant human erythropoietin, 676
Recombinant immunoblot assay, 2138, 2176
Recombinant tissue plasminogen activator
  pulmonary embolism, 503
  venous thromboembolism, 637
Recombination, 1721
Recruitment, 361
Rectal examination
  abdominal pain, 2032
  acute diarrhea, 2051
  cancer of unknown primary site, 731
  constipation, 2053, 2055
  prostate cancer, 717
Rectal prolapse
  cystic fibrosis, 483, 2246
  solitary rectal ulcers, 2093
Rectal temperature, 1375
Rectum
  bleeding in colonic ischemia, 2087
  carcinoid tumor, 2086
  defecation, 1980
  exam for sexually transmitted disease, 1439
  flexible sigmoidoscopy, 1995
  hemorrhoids, 2092-2093
  manifestations of acquired immunodeficiency
    syndrome, 2098
  ulcer, 2093
  ulcerative colitis, 2072-2075
Recurrent disease
  cervical cancer, 715
  familial cholestasis, 2158-2159
  gastric ulcer, 2003
  hypersomnia, 943
  nephrolithiasis, 800, 801, 802
  peptic ulcer disease, 2040
  polyserositis, 2249
  pulmonary edema, 169
  respiratory papillomatosis, 2309
  systemic embolism, 641
  urinary tract infection, 1455
Recurrent laryngeal nerve
  aortic dissection, 300
  thoracic aortic aneurysm, 300
Red blood cell, 531, Plate IV-4
  abnormalities in intestinal disorders, 2005
  automated blood cell analysis, 555-556
  babesiosis, 1676
  chronic myeloproliferative disorders, 686
  Doppler effect, 97
  examination of peripheral blood smear,
    556-557
  flow cytometry, 558
  gas transfer, 348
  hemolytic anemia, 661-671
    acquired, 666-668
    drug-induced, 670
    hereditary, 662-666
    homozygous beta thalassemia, 654
    immune, 668-670
    patient evaluation, 661-662
    splenomegaly, 601
    thrombotic thrombocytopenic purpura,
      615

Red blood cell—cont'd
  hemostatic defects in liver disease,
    627
  life span, 642
  malaria, 1672
  megaloblastic anemia, 648
  membrane defects, 664-666
  nucleated, 595-596
  polycythemia
    Budd-Chiari syndrome, 2208
    high hematocrit, 588-590
    neutrophilic leukocytosis, 591
    red blood cell mass, 586
    tetralogy of Fallot, 289
  polycythemia vera, 688
  processing of immune complexes, 1137
  prosthetic heart valve, 258
  pure red blood cell aplasia, 674-675
  unconjugated hyperbilirubinemia, 2150
  urinalysis, 744
  venous thrombus, 631
Red blood cell casts, 745
  crescentic glomerulonephritis, 848
  poststreptococcal glomerulonephritis, 844
Red blood cell distribution width, 555, 556
  beta-thalassemia, 654
  iron deficiency, 644
Red blood cell index, 556, 588
Red blood cell mass, 586
Red blood cell size, 555
Red cell transfusion, 572-573
Red eye syndrome, 1963
Red pulp, splenic, 600
Red thrombi, 638, 999
Reduced nicotinamide-adenine dinucleotide
  carbohydrate metabolism, 1851
  effects of alcohol metabolism, 2194
5α-Reductase deficiency, 1844
Reduplicative paramnesia, 1031
Reduviid bug, 1689-1690
Reed-Sternberg cell, 563-564, 692
Reentry, 132-133
  sudden death, 187-188
Refeeding phenomenon, 840
Referred pain, 2030-2031
  acute cholecystitis, 2227
  chest discomfort, 125
Reflex myoclonus, 996
Reflex-response interval variation, 936-937
Reflex sympathetic dystrophy, 310-311, 1055,
    1247
Reflex syncope, 953
Reflex tachycardia, 204
Reflexes
  deep tendon
    hepatic encephalopathy, 2160
    hypermagnesemia, 1943
    spinal cord injury, 1051
  neurologic examination, 903
  thiamine deficiency, 2106
Reflexive coughing, 404
Reflux, 1998-1999
  bile, 2041
Reflux esophagitis, 2014-2018, Plate X-1
  ascites, 2164
  chest pain, 128
  operative risk, 2263
Reflux nephropathy, 892
Refluxate, 2015
Refractory anemia, 676
Refsum's disease, 1754
Regeneration, hepatic, 2143
Regional anesthesia, cardiopulmonary
    complications, 2257
Regional enteritis, 2081
Regional lymphadenopathy, 597-599
Regitine; *see* Phentolamine
Regulatory light chain, 39
Regulatory proteins of coagulation, 538
Regulatory proteins of complement, 1135
Regurgitant volume, 111

Regurgitation
  achalasia, 2022
  aortic, 239-245
    ankylosing spondylitis, 303
    aortic dissection, 300
    aortic ejection sounds, 74
    Austin Flint murmur, 79
    bicuspid aortic valve, 287
    cardiac auscultation, 68
    cardiac catheterization, 113-114
    chest pain, 128
    dexfenfluramine and, 261
    differential diagnosis, 180
    dissection of aorta, 301
    fenfluramine and, 261
    Marfan syndrome, 299
    pandiastolic murmur, 79-80
    during pregnancy, 2276
    pulsus bisferiens, 65
    rheumatic fever, 1256
    Takayasu's arteritis, 311
    ventricular septal defect with, 285
  mitral, 249-253
    atrial septal defect, 281
    cardiac catheterization, 114, 115
    dexfenfluramine and, 261
    diastolic heart failure, 167
    dicrotic pulse, 65
    differential diagnosis, 180
    Doppler image, Plate II-4
    fenfluramine and, 261
    hypertrophic cardiomyopathy, 265
    myocardial infarction, 219, 220
    nonejection systolic sounds, 75
    pansystolic murmur, 77
    during pregnancy, 2276
    restrictive cardiomyopathy, 271
    shock, 177
    weakness, 1755
  pulmonic, 256-257
  tricuspid, 256
    abnormal jugular venous pulse, 66-67
    dilated cardiomyopathy, 264
    infective endocarditis, 229
    nonejection systolic sounds, 75
    pansystolic murmur, 77
    restrictive cardiomyopathy, 271
Rehabilitation
  after renal replacement therapy, 788
  alcohol abuse, 2296
  breast cancer, 712
  head and neck cancer, 724
  myocardial infarction, 224
  pulmonary, 431, 432-437
    benefits, 432-433
    chronic obstructive pulmonary disease, 445
    exercise conditioning, 435-436
    follow-up care, 437
    medical intervention, 434-435
    nutritional evaluation and therapy, 435
    occupational therapy, 436
    physical therapy, 436
    program structure, 433-434
    psychosocial management, 435-437
    referral, 433
  septic arthritis, 1254
  spinal cord injury, 1052-1053
  stroke, 1006-1007, 1054-1055
Rehabilitation engineering, 1052-1053
Rehydration
  acute diarrhea, 2051
  acute renal failure, 773
  choledocholithiasis, 2229
  cholera, 1596
  diabetic ketoacidosis, 1864
  diarrhea, 1431
  hepatorenal syndrome, 2170
  hypercalcemia, 1929
  hypercalciuria, 798
  hyperosmolar nonketotic coma, 1866
  hyponatremia, 812

Rehydration—cont'd
  pulmonary edema, 427
  rotavirus infection, 1521
  uric acid nephrolithiasis, 804
Reiger's anomaly, 1903
Reimbursement for patient care, 32-33
Reimplantation response, 516-517
Reinfection
  brucellosis, 1607
  Legionella, 1623
  urinary tract, 1455, 1461
Reitan trailmaking test, 2159
Reiter syndrome, 1200, 1239-1240
  dysuria, 763
  human immunodeficiency virus infection, 1326
  nongonococcal urethritis, 1441
  septic arthritis *versus,* 1252
  soft tissue swelling, 1165
Rejection
  heart, 339-341
  hematopoietic stem cell, 578
  kidney, 793-794, 891
  liver, 2219
  lung, 520-524
Relapsing fever, 1645-1648
Relapsing illness
  brucellosis, 1606-1607
  Clostridium difficile colitis, 1570
  coccidioidomycosis, 1657
  febrile nodular panniculitis, 1245
  fever of unknown origin, 1377
  polychondritis, 1243
  seronegative symmetric synovitis with pitting
    edema, 1243
  typhoid fever, 1601
  urinary tract infection, 1455, 1461
Relationship building, 2, 3
Relative hypoparathyroidism, 1932
Relative lymphocytosis, 592
Relative polycythemia, 588
Relative risk, 1120
Relative volume curve, 104, 105
Relaxation techniques
  hypertension management, 324
  psychophysiologic insomnia, 941-942
  pulmonary rehabilitation, 436
Remodeling, restenosis, 122
Renal abscess
  imaging studies, 754-755
  nephritis associated with visceral abscess, 844
Renal acidification, 739-741, 747
Renal acidosis, 837-838
Renal allograft, 775
Renal angiography
  chronic renal failure, 782
  renovascular hypertension, 321
Renal arteriography
  renal artery stenosis, 895
  renal cell carcinoma, 898
  renal mass, 752
Renal artery
  blood supply to adrenals, 1817
  renovascular hypertension, 894-895
Renal artery stenosis, 755, 756
  continuous murmur, 81
  neurofibromatosis, 1921
  renovascular hypertension, 893-894
Renal artery thrombosis, 896-897
Renal biopsy
  chronic renal failure, 782
  diabetic glomerulopathy, 860
  focal glomerular sclerosis, 852
  isolated proteinuria, 761
  membranoproliferative glomerulonephritis, 854
  minimal change disease, 851
  nephrotic syndrome, 767
  polyarteritis nodosa, 856
  rapidly progressive glomerulonephritis, 848
  renal atheroembolism, 897
  systemic lupus erythematosus, 1215
  Wegener's granulomatosis, 858

Renal blood flow
  congestive heart failure, 817
  hepatorenal syndrome, 2168
  hypokalemia, 829
  obstructive uropathy, 884-885
  prerenal azotemia, 768, 769
  sodium transport, 738
Renal bone disease, 1961-1965
Renal calculi, 796-805
  autosomal dominant polycystic kidney disease,
    873
  calcium-containing stones, 797-799
  cystine stones, 799-800
  differential diagnosis, 800
  laboratory and diagnostic testing, 800, 801,
    802
  management, 803-805
  medullary sponge kidney, 875
  obstructive uropathy, 885
  physiology and pathophysiology, 797
  spinal cord injured patient, 1050
  struvite stones, 799
  uric acid stones, 799
  urine calcium, 1744
Renal cell carcinoma, 898-899
  computed tomography, 751-752
  incidence and death rates, 550
Renal chromophobe carcinoma, 899
Renal colic
  diagnostic algorithm, 754
  medullary sponge kidney, 875
Renal disease, 735-899
  acid-base balance disorders, 836-841
    metabolic acidosis, 836-839
    metabolic alkalosis, 839-841
    patient evaluation, 840, 841
  acute nephritic syndrome, 763-764
  acute renal failure, 768-776
    acute interstitial nephritis, 889-890
    cancer with, 775
    clinical course, complications, and
      prognosis, 772-773
    diagnosis, 770-772
    essential mixed cryoglobulinemia, 857
    etiology, 768-769
    following bone marrow transplantation,
      775-776
    hemolytic-uremic syndrome, 858
    liver disease with, 774-775
    management, 773-774
    obstructive uropathy, 885
    pathophysiology, 769
    pregnancy, 775
    pulmonary-renal syndrome, 775
    radiocontrast nephropathy, 775
    renal allograft, 775
    rhabdomyolysis, 775
  Alport's syndrome, 876-877
  Anderson-Fabry disease, 878
  brucellosis, 1606
  chronic renal failure, 776-796
    abnormal platelet function, 605
    cardiopulmonary complications, 783-784
    clinical presentation and diagnosis, 780-782
    conservative treatment, 787
    dialysis, 789-791
    endocrine function abnormalities, 786-787
    etiology and incidence, 777
    gastrointestinal tract disturbances, 784
    hematologic disorders, 783
    hyperkalemia, 832
    hypertension, 783
    immunologic and infectious complications,
      784-785
    neuromuscular abnormalities, 784
    nutritional and metabolic alterations, 786
    osmolol gap, 806
    pathophysiology, 777-780
    prevention or delay of end-stage renal
      disease, 782-783

Renal disease—cont'd
  chronic renal failure—cont'd
    renal osteodystrophy, hyperphosphatemia,
      hypocalcemia, and bone and joint
      disease, 785-786
    renal replacement therapy, 788
    renal salt-washing, 824
    renal transplantation, 791-796
  complement depression, 1147-1148
  cystic, 871-876
  dementia, 987
  diabetic nephropathy, 859-862
    microalbuminuria, 743, 761
    nephrotic syndrome, 767
  drug- and chemical-induced nephropathy,
    866-871
  dysuria, 757, 762-763
  familial Mediterranean Fever, 877
  glomerular, 841-859
    acquired immunodeficiency syndrome
      nephropathy, 853
    acute nephritic syndrome, 763
    adverse reaction to nonsteroidal
      antiinflammatory agents, 853
    Alport's syndrome, 876-877
    diabetic nephropathy, 859
    focal glomerular sclerosis, 851-852
    glomerular involvement in systemic
      diseases, 855-859
    hematuria, 757
    heroin nephropathy, 853
    immunoglobulin A nephropathy, 845
    loin pain-hematuria syndrome, 845-846
    mechanisms and consequences of immune
      glomerular injury, 841-843
    membranoproliferative glomerulonephritis,
      854-855
    membranous nephropathy, 853-854
    mesangial proliferative disease, 851
    minimal change disease, 849-851
    nephritis associated with visceral abscess,
      844
    postinfectious glomerulonephritis, 843-844
    rapidly progressive glomerulonephritis,
      846-849
    subacute bacterial endocarditis, 844
  glomerular and interstitial hereditary
    nephropathies, 876-878
  gouty, 1273
  hematuria, 756-758
    acute nephritic syndrome, 763
    Alport's syndrome, 876
    autosomal dominant polycystic kidney
      disease, 873
    crescentic glomerulonephritis, 848
    focal glomerular sclerosis, 852
    Goodpasture's syndrome, 847
    in hemophilic patient, 620
    immunoglobulin A nephropathy, 845
    kidney stones, 800
    loin pain-hematuria syndrome, 845-846
    obstructive uropathy, 886
    poststreptococcal glomerulonephritis, 844
    renal biopsy-induced, 748
    renal cell carcinoma, 898
    thrombotic thrombocytopenic purpura, 858
    upper urinary tract tumor, 899
  hyperparathyroidism, 1966
  impact on nutritional status, 2100
  kidney transplantation
    allograft dysfunction, 793-794
    chronic renal failure, 791-796
    cytomegalovirus infection, 785
    focal glomerular sclerosis after, 852
    immunosuppression, 792-793
    kidney donor, 791-792
    membranous nephropathy, 854
    multiple myeloma, 865
    myeloma kidney, 703
    recipient, 792
  lipodystrophy, 877-878

Renal disease—cont'd
  metabolic acidosis, 836
  nail-patella syndrome, 877
  nephrolithiasis, 796-805
    calcium-containing stones, 797-799
    cystine stones, 799-800
    differential diagnosis, 800
    laboratory and diagnostic testing, 800, 801,
      802
    management, 803-805
    physiology and pathophysiology, 797
    struvite stones, 799
    uric acid stones, 799
  nephrotic syndrome, 765-768
    acquired immunodeficiency syndrome
      nephropathy, 853
    adverse reaction to nonsteroidal
      antiinflammatory agents, 853
    clinical manifestations and pathophysiology,
      765-766
    complications, 766-767
    diagnosis and management, 767
    familial Mediterranean fever, 877
    Fanconi's syndrome, 882
    focal glomerular sclerosis, 851-852
    glycosuria, 879
    Henoch-Schönlein purpura, 857
    heroin nephropathy, 853
    hyponatremia, 812
    immunofixation, 568
    lipiduria, 745
    lipodystrophy, 877
    membranoproliferative glomerulonephritis,
      854-855
    membranous nephropathy, 853-854
    mesangial proliferative disease, 851
    minimal change disease, 849-851
    sodium balance dysfunction, 820-821
    transudative pleural effusion, 507
  neuronephrology, 1105-1106
  obstructive uropathy, 753-754, 884-887
  osteomalacia and rickets, 1953
  potassium balance disorders, 825-834
    external potassium balance, 825, 826
    hyperkalemia, 830-833
    hypokalemia, 826-830
    internal potassium balance, 825-826
  potassium losses, 828-829
  during pregnancy, 2274
  proteinuria, 758-761
    acquired immunodeficiency syndrome
      patient, 853
    acute nephritic syndrome, 764
    Bence Jones, 863
    crescentic glomerulonephritis, 848
    diabetic glomerulopathy, 860
    familial Mediterranean fever, 877
    focal glomerular sclerosis, 852
    Goodpasture's syndrome, 847
    hematuria, 757
    immunoglobulin A nephropathy, 845
    isolated, 761
    laboratory testing, 743
    lipodystrophy, 877
    mechanisms, 759-761
    membranous nephropathy, 854
    minimal change disease, 851
    nephrotic syndrome, 765
    poststreptococcal glomerulonephritis, 844
    subepithelial immune complex deposits, 842
    systemic lupus erythematosus, 1215
    thrombotic thrombocytopenic purpura, 615
    Wegener's granulomatosis, 468
  renal cell carcinoma, 751-752, 898-899
  renal tubular transport disorders, 878-884
    aminoaciduria, 879
    dicarboxylic aminoaciduria, 879-880
    Fanconi's syndrome, 881-882
    Hartnup disease, 879
    iminoglycinuria, 880
    nephrogenic diabetes insipidus, 883-884

Renal disease—cont'd
  renal tubular transport disorders—cont'd
    renal glycosuria, 878-879
    renal phosphate wasting syndromes, 880
    X-linked hypophosphatemic rickets, 880-881
  renovascular, 893-897
  renovascular disease
    hypertension, 314
    renal failure, 782
    renal imaging studies, 755-756
  sodium balance disorders, 816-825
    cirrhosis, 818-820
    congestive heart failure, 817-818
    edematous states, 816-817
    extrarenal sodium depletion, 823
    idiopathic edema, 821
    nephrotic syndrome, 820-821
    salt-wasting states, 823
    sodium depletion of renal origin, 823-825
    use of diuretics, 821-823
  sodium depletion, 824
  thin basement membrane nephropathy, 877
  tubulointerstitial, 888-893
  tubulointerstitial disease
    hematuria, 757
    nephritis and uveitis syndrome, 890
  water balance disorders, 805-816
    hypernatremia, 813-816
    hyponatremia, 809-813
    principles of osmoregulation, 805-809
Renal failure
  acetaminophen poisoning, 2190
  acute, 768-776
    acute interstitial nephritis, 889-890
    cancer with, 775
    clinical course, complications, and
      prognosis, 772-773
    diagnosis, 770-772
    essential mixed cryoglobulinemia, 857
    etiology, 768-769
    following bone marrow transplantation,
      775-776
    hemolytic-uremic syndrome, 858
    liver disease with, 774-775
    management, 773-774
    obstructive uropathy, 885
    pathophysiology, 769
    pregnancy, 775
    pulmonary-renal syndrome, 775
    radiocontrast nephropathy, 775
    renal allograft, 775
    rhabdomyolysis, 775
  Anderson-Fabry disease, 878
  anti-GBM antibody disease, 454
  carbon tetrachloride poisoning, 2188
  chronic, 776-796
    abnormal platelet function, 605
    cardiopulmonary complications, 783-784
    clinical presentation and diagnosis, 780-782
    conservative treatment, 787
    dialysis, 789-791
    endocrine function abnormalities, 786-787
    etiology and incidence, 777
    gastrointestinal tract disturbances, 784
    hematologic disorders, 783
    hyperkalemia, 832
    hypertension, 783
    immunologic and infectious complications,
      784-785
    neuromuscular abnormalities, 784
    nutritional and metabolic alterations, 786
    osmol gap, 806
    pathophysiology, 777-780
    prevention or delay of end-stage renal
      disease, 782-783
    renal osteodystrophy, hyperphosphatemia,
      hypocalcemia, and bone and joint
      disease, 785-786
    renal replacement therapy, 788
    renal salt-washing, 824
    renal transplantation, 791-796

Renal failure—cont'd
  Churg-Strauss syndrome, 466
  crescentic glomerulonephritis, 848
  diabetes mellitus, 1876
  diabetic nephropathy, 859
  drug abuser, 853
  electroencephalography, 907
  focal glomerular sclerosis, 852
  gynecomastia, 1765
  hyperkalemia, 832
  hyperphosphatemia, 1938
  infantile nephropathic cystinosis, 1909
  intestinal pseudoobstruction, 2079
  liver disease, 2168
  malaria, 1673
  meningitis, 1406
  multiple myeloma, 864
  multiple organ dysfunction syndrome, 422
  neuronephrology, 1105-1106
  operative risk, 2263
  polyarteritis nodosa, 856
  streptococcal toxic shock syndrome, 1558
  thrombotic thrombocytopenic purpura, 615
Renal failure casts, 745
Renal failure index, 770
Renal function
  after liver transplantation, 2220
  aging and, 2284
  aminoglycoside toxicity, 868
  antibiotic toxicity, 1348
  diabetes insipidus, 1793-1794
  effects of hypokalemia, 829
  focal glomerular sclerosis, 852
  gram-negative bacteremia, 1450, 1451-1452
  immunoglobulin A nephropathy, 845
  lipodystrophy, 1901
  poststreptococcal glomerulonephritis, 844
  during pregnancy, 2274
Renal function tests, 746-748
  fractional excretion of sodium, 747
  glomerular filtration rate, 746-747
  renal acidification, 739-741
  urinary concentration and dilution, 748
Renal glycosuria, 878-879
Renal imaging studies, 748-756
  acute inflammation, 754-755
  angiography, 751
  computed tomography, 750
  intravenous pyelography, 748-749
  lower urinary tract, 756
  magnetic resonance imaging, 750-751
  nuclear medicine, 750
  obstructive uropathy, 753-754
  renal mass, 751-753
  renovascular disease, 755-756
  retrograde pyelography, 751
  ultrasonography, 749-750
Renal infarction, 897
Renal insufficiency
  Alport's syndrome, 876
  antihypertensive agent choices, 326
  diabetic patient, 1870
  familial Mediterranean fever, 877
  hypoglycemia, 1876
  multiple myeloma, 700
  obstructive uropathy, 886
Renal magnesium-wasting syndrome, 1940
Renal mass
  computed tomography, 750
  renal imaging studies, 751-753
  ultrasonography, 749-750
Renal osteodystrophy, 1961-1965
  chronic renal failure, 785-786
  hyperphosphatemia, 1938
Renal parenchymal disease
  hematuria, 757
  hypertension, 314, 320-321
Renal pelvic tumor, 899
Renal phosphate wasting, 880, 1935, 1952

Renal physiology, 736-741
  composition of body fluids, 736-737
  glomerular ultrafiltration, 737
  potassium transport, 741
  renal acidification, 739-741
  sodium balance, 737-739
  water metabolism, 739, 740
Renal potassium wasting, 828-829
Renal replacement therapy, 788
Renal-retinal dysplasia, 875
Renal scan
  hydronephrosis, 754
  pediatric urinary tract infection, 1459
Renal transplantation
  allograft dysfunction, 793-794
  chronic renal failure, 791-796
  cytomegalovirus infection, 785
  focal glomerular sclerosis after, 852
  immunosuppression, 792-793
  kidney donor, 791-792
  membranous nephropathy, 854
  multiple myeloma, 865
  myeloma kidney, 703
  neurologic complications, 1106
  recipient, 792
Renal tuberculosis, 1634
Renal tubular acidosis
  Fanconi's syndrome, 882
  hypercalciuria, 798
  osteomalacia with, 1954, 1955
  renal magnesium wasting, 1940
  tests of renal acidification, 747
Renal tubular transport disorders, 878-884
  aminoaciduria, 879
  dicarboxylic aminoaciduria, 879-880
  Fanconi's syndrome, 881-882
  Hartnup disease, 879
  iminoglycinuria, 880
  nephrogenic diabetes insipidus, 883-884
  renal glycosuria, 878-879
  renal phosphate wasting syndromes, 880
  X-linked hypophosphatemic rickets, 880-881
Renal tubule, 1718
Renal ultrasonography
  chronic renal failure, 782
  postrenal azotemia, 771
  renal cell carcinoma, 898
  tubulointerstitial disease, 888
Renal vein, 1817
Renal vein thrombosis
  acute renal failure, 769
  membranous nephropathy with, 854
  nephrotic syndrome, 766
Renin
  aldosterone secretion regulation, 1818
  heart failure, 160, 161
  hyperkalemia, 831-832
  hypertension, 319
  hypertensive renal potassium wasting, 828-829
Renin-angiotensin-aldosterone system, 817
  cardiac growth and hypertrophy, 55-56
  heart failure, 160, 162, 163
  renovascular hypertension, 893-894
Renin-secreting tumor
  hypertension, 321
  hypokalemia, 829
Renovascular disease, 893-897
  hypertension, 314
  renal failure, 782
  renal imaging studies, 755-756
Renovascular hypertension, 321, 829, 893-896
Reoperation, prosthetic heart valve, 258, 261
Repair mechanisms of lung, 374-375
Reperfusion therapy, 182-183
Repetition, testing for aphasia, 975
Repetitive nerve stimulation, 1024
Repetitive stimulation studies, 917
Repolarization, myocardial infarction, 88
Reporter gene, 54

Rescriptor; *see* Delavirdine
Rescue angioplasty, 215
Rescue coronary angioplasty, 122
RESCUE trial, 122
Research, injury control, 2267
Resectability, 728
Reserpine
  hypertension, 325, 327
  interference with catecholamine assays, 1740
Reservoir, 1363
Reset osmostat, 812, 815
Residual urinary volume, 938
Residual volume
  aging and, 2284
  interstitial lung disease, 450
  spirometry, 376
Residual volume/total lung capacity ratio
  cystic fibrosis, 481
  Langerhans' cell granulomatosis, 464
Resistance
  antimicrobial, 1345-1346
    chemotherapeutic drugs, 554
    enterococci, 1346, 1561
    mechanisms of antimicrobial resistance, 1345-1346
    Neisseria gonorrhoeae, 1582
    Neisseria meningitidis, 1579, 1582
    nosocomial infection, 1363
    staphylococci, 1345
    streptococci, 1559-1560
    tumor response to drug treatment, 552
  aortic, 299
  pulmonary blood flow, 361-362
Resistant ovary syndrome, 1760
Resorption of bone, 1716
Respiration
  adverse drug reactions, 476-479
  breathing control abnormalities, 352-357
  neural control, 358
  during normal sleep, 525
  pathophysiology, 346-352
    nonrespiratory functions of lung, 346-347
    oxygen transport disorders, 350-352
    respiratory function, 347-350
  respiratory muscles, 357-360
Respiratory acidosis
  acute respiratory failure, 412, 414, 416
  chronic obstructive pulmonary disease with
    acute respiratory failure, 417
  hyperkalemia, 831
  hyperphosphatemia, 1938
  mechanical ventilation, 416
  renal response, 835-836
Respiratory alkalosis
  carbon dioxide partial pressure, 834
  gram-negative bacteremia, 1449
  hypokalemia, 827
  hypophosphatemia, 1936
  renal excretion of potassium, 741
  renal response, 835
Respiratory alternans, 418
Respiratory cells, 367-369
Respiratory control system, 352
Respiratory disease
  acute respiratory failure, 412-420
    adult respiratory distress syndrome with, 418
    artificial airway, 416-417
    chronic obstructive pulmonary disease with, 417-418, 446
    classification, 413, 414
    diagnosis, 413-414
    mechanical ventilation, 397, 416, 418-420
    oxygenation measures, 415-416
    pathophysiology, 412-413
    principles of management, 414, 415
    respiratory acidosis, 416
    without lung disease, 418
  adenovirus, 1503-1504
  adverse drug reactions, 476-479

Respiratory disease—cont'd
asthma, 1185-1193
Churg-Strauss syndrome, 465
clinical manifestations, 1187-1188
cough, 406
diagnosis and differential diagnosis, 1189
epidemiology and pathology, 1185
laboratory findings, 1188-1189
management, 1189-1192
occupational, 471-472, 473
pathophysiology, 1185-1187
patterns of pulmonary function
abnormalities, 379
physical findings, 403
prognosis, 1192-1193
pulmonary rehabilitation, 432-437
sputum expectoration, 408
wheezing, 404
bronchiectasis, 483-485
chest pain, 128-129, 408-410
Chlamydia trachomatis, 1536
chronic obstructive pulmonary disease, 437-447
with acute respiratory failure, 413-414,
417-418
airflow obstruction, 438
alpha$_1$-protease inhibitor deficiency,
439-440
clinical features, 442
complications, 445-447
definition, 437-438
diagnosis, 443
dyspnea, 404
epidemiology, 438-439
hypercapnia, 356
laboratory findings, 442-443
lung transplantation, 445
occupational, 473
pathogenesis, 441-442
pathology, 439
physical examination, 442
prognosis and course, 447
pulmonary rehabilitation, 432-437
sleep studies with monitoring of oxygen
saturation, 380
treatment, 443-445
cough, 404-408, 409
cystic fibrosis, 479-483
diagnostic imaging, 386-390
dysfunction of host defenses, 369
dyspnea, 404, 405
expectoration, 408
hemoptysis, 410-411
high-resolution computed tomography, 387
hypersensitivity pneumonitis, 460-463
interstitial, 448-456
clinical features, 450-451
clinicopathologic classification, 449
diagnosis and management, 451-452
dyspnea, 404
etiologic factors, 452
exercise tests, 379
imaging techniques, 451
lung pathology, 448-449
pathogenesis, 449-450
pathophysiology, 450
pulmonary hypertension, 498
unknown origin, 452-456
invasive diagnostic techniques, 380-386
bronchoalveolar lavage, 384
bronchoscopy and biopsy, 383-384
mediastinoscopy and mediastinotomy, 385
open lung biopsy, 385-386
pleural biopsy, 382-383
protected brush catheter, 384-385
sputum examination, 380-381
Swan-Ganz catheterization, 383
thoracentesis, 381-382
thoracoscopy, 385
transthoracic needle aspiration, 385
transtracheal aspiration, 385

Respiratory disease—cont'd
Langerhans' cell granulomatosis, 463-465
mediastinal disease, 510-514
medical history, 401-402
multiple organ dysfunction syndrome, 421-423
neoplasms, 486-492; *see also* Lung cancer
occupational, 471-476
physical examination, 402-404
pleural, 505-510
primary granulomatous pulmonary vasculitis,
465-471
pulmonary edema, 423-428
acute toxic, 473
adult respiratory distress syndrome, 421
drug-induced, 477
hemoptysis, 410
pneumothorax, 510
pulmonary artery wedge pressure, 395
pulmonary hypertension
cardiac transplantation, 338
chronic obstructive pulmonary disease,
446-447
drug-induced, 477
exertional angina, 127
interstitial lung disease, 452
pathophysiology, 363-364
primary and secondary causes, 497-499
Takayasu's arteritis, 470
pulmonary rehabilitation, 431, 432-437
pulmonary thromboembolism, 499-504
pulmonary transplantation, 514-524
allograft rejection, 520-524
chronic obstructive pulmonary disease, 445
complications, 516-520
future trends, 524
immunosuppression, 516
indications, 514-515
outcome, 516
selection of donor and recipient, 515-516
renal compensation, 835-836
respiratory therapy, 428-432
sarcoidosis, 456-459
sleep-related, 524-528
solitary pulmonary nodule, 493-497
wheezing, 404, 405
Respiratory distress
anaplastic thyroid carcinoma, 1815
Riedel's thyroiditis, 1812
Respiratory failure, 359
botulism, 1571
diphtheria, 1566
Legionnaire's disease, 1623
neurogenic, 1096-1097
neurologic disease, 1085-1086
precapillary pulmonary hypertension, 295-296
Respiratory inductive plethysmography, 431
Respiratory lining secretions, 365
Respiratory monitoring, 431
Respiratory muscles, 357-360
chronic obstructive pulmonary disease with
respiratory failure, 418
drug-induced dysfunction, 477
failure in hypophosphatemia, 1936
ventilatory failure, 347
Respiratory paralysis, 1926
Respiratory rate
abnormalities in conscious patient, 1098-1099
altered states of consciousness, 1097-1098
autonomic overactivity, 934
carbon dioxide partial pressure, 834
volume-controlled ventilatory mode, 419
Respiratory syncytial virus, 1499-1500
common cold, 1391
culture, 1369
Respiratory therapy, 428-432
Respiratory tract infection, 1390-1396
after stroke, 1007
bronchoalveolar lavage, 384
brucellosis, 1606

Respiratory tract infection—cont'd
cancer patient, 582
chest pain, 129
common cold, 1290-1392
cystic fibrosis, 480
febrile compromised patient, 1387-1388
gram-negative bacteremia, 1446
Haemophilus influenzae, 1586, 1588
influenza with, 1486, 1491
laryngitis, croup, and epiglottitis, 1393-1394
Neisseria meningitidis, 1579
nosocomial, 423, 1480
oculopharyngeal dystrophy, 1028
otitis media, 1395
pharyngitis, 1392-1393
Pneumocystis carinii pneumonia
acquired immunodeficiency syndrome,
1473, 1474, 1477
lung transplantation, 518, 519
sputum examination, 380
pneumonia
acute interstitial, 448, 452
bronchiolitis obliterans-organizing
pneumonia, 448, 452-453
Chlamydia pneumoniae, 1535
desquamative interstitial, 449
eosinophilic, 455
lymphoid interstitial, 449
Mycoplasma pneumoniae, 1538-1539
usual interstitial, 449
posttransplant
lung, 517-518
stem cell, 579
pulmonary edema *versus,* 425
risk in multiple myeloma, 700, 703
sinusitis, 1394-1395
sputum examination, 380
Staphylococcus aureus, 1549
varicella, 1527
Rest
ascites, 2165
chronic venous insufficiency, 312
common cold, 1392
dilated cardiomyopathy, 264
diphtheria, 1567
hazards, 2287-2288
preeclampsia, 2275
rheumatoid arthritis, 1206-1207
streptococcal pharyngitis, 1393
Rest angina, 196
Restenosis
after coronary angioplasty, 205-206
Palmaz-Schatz stent, 119, 121
pathobiology, 122-124
unstable angina, 195
Resting membrane potential, 1976
Resting potential, 37
Restless legs syndrome, 784, 944, 1103
Restriction endonuclease enzymes, 51
Restriction endonuclease mapping, 656
Restriction endonucleases, 1822
Restriction fragment length polymorphism,
54-55, 1722-1723
stem cell transplantation, 578
Restrictive cardiomyopathy, 66, 270-271
Restrictive pericarditis, 277
RET protooncogene
medullary thyroid carcinoma, 1816
pheochromocytoma, 1829
Retching, 2026
Reticular dysgenesis, 1177
Reticulin antibody, 1157-1158
Reticulocyte, 531, Plate IV-4
Reticulocyte count
anemia, 586-587
beta thalassemia, 654
decreased, 587
increased, 587-588
Reticulocyte index, 556, 661, 669
Reticulocyte maturity index, 558

Reticulocytosis, 556-557, 670
Reticuloendothelial system
  hepatic bilirubin transport, 2148
  sarcoidosis, 458
Retina
  acquired immunodeficiency syndrome,
      2304-2306
  arterial embolism, 1057
  cherry-red spots
    gangliosidoses, 1919
    Niemann-Pick disease, 1918
  circulation, 1057
  degeneration, 1075
  detachment, 2303
  diabetic retinopathy, 1870-1871, 2303-2304
    exudative, Plate IX-3
    hemorrhagic, Plate IX-2
    microvascular abnormalities and venous
        beading, Plate XI-7
    neovascularization of optic nerve, Plate
        XI-8
    proliferative, Plate IX-4
  gyrate atrophy, 1909
  Paget's disease, 1955
  retinal artery occlusion, 1058
  retinal pigment epithelium, 2301-2302
  retinal vein occlusion
    central, Plate XI-10
    cotton-wool spots, Plate XI-9
  retinitis
    acquired immunodeficiency syndrome, 1474
    cytomegalovirus, Plate XI-11
    toxoplasmosis, 1677
  vascular disease, 2302-2304
Retinal artery occlusion, 1058
Retinal cherry-red spots
  gangliosidoses, 1919
  Niemann-Pick disease, 1918
Retinal gyrate atrophy, 1909
Retinal pigment epithelium, 2301-2302
Retinal vein occlusion
  central, Plate XI-10
  cotton-wool spots, Plate XI-9
Retinitis
  acquired immunodeficiency syndrome, 1474
  cytomegalovirus, Plate XI-11
  toxoplasmosis, 1677
Retinoblastoma, 546
Retinoblastoma susceptibility gene, 486
Retinochoroiditis, Plate VIII-41
Retinoic acid receptor gene, 545
Retinoids, 555
Retinopathy
  diabetic, 1870-1871, 2303-2304
    exudative, Plate IX-3
    hemorrhagic, Plate IX-2
    microvascular abnormalities and venous
        beading, Plate XI-7
    neovascularization of optic nerve, Plate
        XI-8
    proliferative, Plate IX-4
  hypertensive, 2302-2303
Retractile mesenteritis, 2251
Retransplantation, lung, 523
Retrocalcaneal bursitis, 1198
Retrochiasmic disease, 1060-1062
Retrograde pyelography, 751, 757
Retroperitoneal abscess, 1398, 2250
Retroperitoneal fibrosis, 885, 2250, 2251
Retroperitoneal hematoma, 620
Retroperitoneal hemorrhage, 637, 2250
Retroperitoneal lymph node dissection, 721
Retroperitoneal tumor, 1876, 2250-2251
Retrovir; *see* Zidovudine
Retrovirus, 1531-1534
  spinal infection, 1013
  transfusion-associated, 575
  tumorigenic, 541
  vector, 1732

Revascularization
  catheter-based, 205
  chronic occlusive arterial disease, 308
  coronary angioplasty, 124
  myocardial infarction, 218-219
  shock, 184
  unstable angina, 195
Reverse cholesterol transport, 1887
Reverse splitting of heart sound, 74
Reverse transcriptase, 50
Reverse transcriptase inhibitors, 1474
Reverse transcriptase polymerase chain reaction
  coronavirus, 1502
  respiratory syncytial virus, 1500
  rubella, 1501
Reversible dementia, 2288
Reversible portosystemic encephalopathy, 1102
Review of systems, 2
Reye's syndrome, 1491
RFLP; *see* Restriction fragment length
      polymorphism
Rh determination, 573
Rh factor mismatches, 1146
Rhabdomyolysis
  acute renal failure, 775
  binge drinking, 1081
  hyperphosphatemia, 1938
  hypokalemia, 829
  hypophosphatemia, 1936
Rhabdomyoma
  cardiac, 330
  incidence, 329
Rhabdomyosarcoma
  cardiac, 330
  immunohistochemistry, 731
  incidence, 329
Rheumatic disease
  complement assay, 1147
  during pregnancy, 2279
Rheumatic fever, 1256-1258, 1558-1559
  accelerated atrioventricular junctional rhythm,
      144
  fever of unknown origin, 1378
Rheumatic heart disease
  aortic stenosis, 235
  infective endocarditis, 225, 226
  mitral regurgitation, 249, 250
  mitral stenosis, 245
  during pregnancy, 2276
  tricuspid stenosis, 255
  valve replacement surgery, 257
Rheumatism, palindromic, 1243-1244
Rheumatoid aortic stenosis, 235
Rheumatoid arteritis, 1203
Rheumatoid arthritis, 1200-1209
  aortitis, 302, 303
  atlantoaxial subluxation, 1171, 1172
  autoantibodies, 1155
  cardiac involvement, 334
  course and prognosis, 1205-1206
  diagnosis, 1206
  differential diagnosis, 1206
  extraarticular manifestations, 1202,
      1203-1205
  glucocorticoid protocol, 1263
  gold salt-induced pulmonary disease, 478
  interstitial lung disease, 453
  intervertebral disk space narrowing,
      1169-1170
  laboratory findings, 1205
  lymphocytosis of large granular lymphocytes,
      679
  management, 1206-1209
  neurologic manifestations, 1093-1095
  pericarditis, 272-273
  pleural effusion, 508
  during pregnancy, 2279
  radiologic findings, 1205
  soft tissue swelling, 1165
  synovial effusion, 1163

Rheumatoid disease
  amyloidosis, 1282-1285
    AL type, 863, 865
    alveolar, 452
    cutaneous manifestations, 1316-1317
    familial Mediterranean fever, 877
    Fanconi's syndrome, 882
    hyperkalemia, 832
    multiple myeloma, 701
    nephrotic syndrome, 767
    rheumatoid arthritis, 1205
  antirheumatic drugs, 1258-1263
    analgesics, 1259-1260
    disease-modifying antirheumatic drugs,
        1260-1262
    glucocorticoids, 1262-1263
    nonsteroidal antiinflammatory drugs,
        1258-1259
  arthropathy
    adult Still's disease, 1243
    Behçet disease, 1243
    coagulation disorders, 1246
    endocrine diseases, 1246-1247
    familial Mediterranean fever, 1242-1244
    foreign body synovitis, 1244
    hyperlipoproteinemia, 1245
    inflammatory bowel disease, 1245-1246
    intermittent hydroarthrosis, 1244
    malignancy, 1247-1248
    multicentric reticulohistiocytosis, 1245
    neurologic disorders, 1247
    osteonecrosis, 1244
    palindromic rheumatism, 1243-1244
    panniculitis, 1245
    pigmented villonodular synovitis, 1244-1245
    relapsing polychondritis, 1243
    relapsing seronegative symmetric synovitis
        with pitting edema, 1243
    sarcoidosis, 1245
    sickle cell disease, 1246
    Whipple's disease, 1246
  calcium pyrophosphate dihydrate deposition
      disease, 1276-1279
  cardiovascular involvement, 334
  chronic renal failure, 785-786
  connective tissue disease
    associated myositis, 1236
    cutaneous manifestations, 1290-1293
    heritable and developmental, 1286-1290
    neurologic aspects, 1091-1095
    peripheral neuropathy, 1016
    pleural effusion, 508
    rheumatoid arthritis *versus,* 1206
    systemic sclerosis, 1228
  eosinophilic fasciitis, 1233-1234
  evaluation of joint complaints, 1198-1200
  gout and hyperuricemia, 1268-1276
    acute renal failure, 773
    after renal transplantation, 795
    calcium pyrophosphate dihydrate deposition
        disease, 1277
    chronic renal failure, 785
    multiple myeloma, 702
    osteoarthritis, 1267
    uric acid stones, 799
  gouty arthritis, 1271-1272
    joint space narrowing, 1166
    osseous erosions, 1167-1168
    soft tissue swelling, 1165
  imaging evaluation of arthritis, 1164-1174
    advanced methods, 1173
    appendicular skeleton, 1164-1169
    axial skeleton, 1169-1171, 1172
    foot, 1172
    hand, 1171-1172
    hip, 1173
    knee, 1172-1173
    sacroiliac joint, 1172, 1173
    techniques and modalities, 1064
    wrist, 1172

Rheumatoid disease—cont'd
  infections, 1250-1256
  inflammatory myopathies, 1234-1237
  intermittent hydroarthrosis, 1244
  joint infections, 1250-1256
  neurorheumatology, 1091-1095
  ochronosis and alkaptonuria, 1280-1282
  osteoarthritis, 1199, 1264-1268
    glucocorticoid protocol, 1263
    hand, 1171
    joint space narrowing, 1166, 1167
    knee, 1172-1173
    wrist, 1172
  palindromic rheumatism, 1243-1244
  periarticular rheumatic complaints, 1195-1198
  rheumatic fever, 1256-1258
  rheumatoid aortic stenosis, 235
  rheumatoid arteritis, 1203
  rheumatoid arthritis, 1200-1209
    aortitis, 303
    atlantoaxial subluxation, 1171, 1172
    autoantibodies, 1155
    cardiac involvement, 334
    course and prognosis, 1205-1206
    diagnosis, 1206
    differential diagnosis, 1206
    extraarticular manifestations, 1202,
      1203-1205
    glucocorticoid protocol, 1263
    gold salt-induced pulmonary disease, 478
    interstitial lung disease, 453
    intervertebral disk space narrowing,
      1169-1170
    laboratory findings, 1205
    lymphocytosis of large granular
      lymphocytes, 679
    management, 1206-1209
    neurologic manifestations, 1093-1095
    pericarditis, 272-273
    pleural effusion, 508
    during pregnancy, 2279
    radiologic findings, 1205
    soft tissue swelling, 1165
    synovial effusion, 1163
  rheumatoid factor, 1160
  spondyloarthropathies, 1237-1242
  synovial fluid analysis, 161-1163
  systemic lupus erythematosus, 1200,
    1212-1218
    alveolar hemorrhage with, 455
    autoantibodies, 1155
    bullous, 1296
    cardiac involvement, 334
    clinical features, 1213-1215
    complement assay, 1147
    cutaneous lesions, 1290
    diagnosis, 1216
    drug-induced lupus syndromes, 1217-1218
    etiology, 1212-1213
    fever of unknown origin, 1377
    incidence and prevalence, 1212
    interstitial lung disease, 453
    laboratory findings, 1215-1216
    multiple cerebral infarct, 989
    neurologic manifestations, 1092, 1093
    neutropenia, 593
    pathogenesis, 1213
    pleural effusion, 508
    during pregnancy, 2279
    renal involvement, 856-857
    self-antigens, 1142-1143
    synovial effusion, 1163
    treatment, 1216-1217
  systemic sclerosis, 1229
Rheumatoid effusion, 382
Rheumatoid factor, 1138, 1160-1161
  infective endocarditis, 228
  rheumatoid arthritis, 1205
  Sjögren syndrome, 1209, 1211
Rheumatoid nodule, 1203

Rheumatoid pneumoconiosis, 1204
Rhinitis, 1180-1185, 2308
  parainfluenza, 1494
  Wegener's granulomatosis, 467
Rhinitis medicamentosa, 2308
Rhinomanometry, 1182
Rhinopharyngeal endoscopy, 1181
Rhinoprobe, 1181
Rhinorrhea, 1181
  acute meningitis, 1407
  pertussis, 1612
Rhinosporidiosis, 1660
Rhinovirus
  common cold, 1391
  epidemiology, 1484
  pathogenesis, 1485-1486
  pharyngitis, 1392
  respiratory tract infection, 1390
Rhizomucor, 1659
Rhizopus, 1659
Rhodotorula, 1368
Rhonchus, 402
Rhythmic movement disorder, 946
Rhythmol; *see* Propafenone
Rib fracture, 410
Rib notching in coarctation of aorta, 286
Ribavirin
  chronic hepatitis C, 2183
  hepatitis A virus, 2177
  influenza, 1492
  Lassa fever, 1510
  parainfluenza, 1495
  respiratory syncytial virus, 1500
  secretion clearance and lung expansion, 430
Riboflavin
  biochemical function, 2105
  deficiency, 2106
  recommended daily dietary allowances, 2115
Ribonuclease, 2144
Ribonuclease protection assay, 53-54
Ribonucleic acid
  analysis, 53-54
  cDNA library, 54
  functions of minerals, 2109
  human immunodeficiency virus infection,
    1470
  northern blotting, 52
  viral, 1483
Ribonucleic acid polymerase, 50
Ribonucleic acid virus
  arenavirus, 1508-1511
  Colorado tick fever, 1511-1512
  coronavirus, 1502-1503
  hepatitis C virus, 2175
  hepatitis delta virus, 2176
  hepatitis E virus, 2176
  paramyxovirus, 1494
  picornavirus, 1483-1494
    acute febrile undifferentiated illness, 1487
    acute hemorrhagic conjunctivitis, 1490
    aseptic meningitis, 1488
    characteristics, 1483
    chemoprophylaxis, 1493
    chronic meningoencephalitis, 1490
    classification, 1483-1485
    common cold, 1487
    diagnosis, 1492
    encephalitis, 1488
    epidemic pleurodynia, 1489
    epidemiology, 1484-1485
    exanthems, 1489
    hand-foot-mouth syndrome, 1489
    hepatitis, 1490
    herpangina, 1488-1489
    influenza, 1490-1491
    lymphonodular pharyngitis, 1489
    myopericarditis, 1489-1490
    neurologic complications, 1491
    paralytic poliomyelitis, 1487-1488
    pathogenesis, 1485-1487

Ribonucleic acid virus—cont'd
  picornavirus—cont'd
    prevention, 1492-1493
    pulmonary complications, 1491
    treatment, 1492
  rabies, 1505-1508
  retrovirus, 1531-1532
  rotavirus, 1520
  rubella, 1500-1502
Riboprobe slot hybridization studies, 2176
Ribosome, 49
  bacterial, 1344
  hormone synthesis, 1709
Ribosome lamella complexes, 595
Ribozyme, 1721
Richter's syndrome, 685
Rickets, 1949-1950
  chronic hypophosphatemia, 1936
  nephrotic syndrome, 767
  proximal renal tubular acidosis, 837
  vitamin D metabolism, 1719
  X-linked hypophosphatemic, 880-881
Rickettsia prowazekii, 1544
Rickettsia typhi, 1544
Rickettsial infection, 1541-1546
  culture, 1370
  differential diagnosis of fever and rash, 1384
  fever of unknown origin, 1377
  Rocky Mountain spotted fever, 1541-1544
    fever and rash, 1382
    influence of season and geographic setting,
      1381
    purpura and petechiae, Plate VIII-18
    rickettsial invasion, Plate VIII-19
    sepsis *versus,* 1451
    vasculitis, Plate VIII-44
Rickettsialpox, 1545
Riedel's thyroiditis, 1809, 1812
Rifabutin, 1474
Rifampin
  antimicrobial mechanisms, 1344
  bacterial meningitis, 1411
  brucellosis, 1605, 1606
  effects on kidney, 868
  Haemophilus influenzae, 1589
  hepatic injury, 2190-2192
  human cytochrome P450 isoforms, 2312
  induction of acute interstitial nephritis, 889
  infective endocarditis, 231, 232
  interaction with cyclosporin, 793
  interference with oral anticoagulants, 636
  leprosy, 1651
  meningococcal disease, 1580
  mycobacterial disease, 1631
  Mycobacterium tuberculosis meningitis, 1410
  Staphylococcus epidermidis, 1552
  tuberculosis, 1474
Rifaximin, 2163
Rift valley fever, 1465
Right atrial depolarization, 83
Right atrial pressure
  normal at rest, 110
  pulmonary hypertension, 364
Right atrium
  biventricular assist device, 185
  coronary arteriovenous fistula, 292
  hemodynamic data, 110
  myxoma, 330
  radiographic views, 92
  total anomalous pulmonary venous connection,
    290-291
  tricuspid stenosis, 255
Right axis deviation, 85
Right bundle branch block
  aortic stenosis, 237
  Ebstein's anomaly, 290
  electrocardiography, 87, 88
  endocardial cushion defect, 283
  intraventricular conduction abnormalities, 156

Right heart catheterization, 108
  complications, 395
  systemic sclerosis, 1230
Right-sided heart failure
  abnormal jugular venous pulse, 66
  carcinoid syndrome, 2082
  cor pulmonale, 498
  pulmonary embolism, 632
  varicose veins, 311
Right-to-left shunt, 110-111, 283
  atrial septal defect, 280
  Ebstein's anomaly, 289, 290
  hepatopulmonary syndrome, 2170
  precapillary pulmonary hypertension, 296
  tetralogy of Fallot, 288
  total anomalous pulmonary venous connection,
    290-291
  ventricular septal defect, 284-285
Right ventricle
  coronary arteriovenous fistula, 292
  Ebstein's anomaly, 289
  hemodynamic data, 110
  primary pulmonary hypertension, 294
  radiographic views, 92
  tricuspid atresia, 291
Right ventricle pressure, 110
Right ventricular dysplasia, 153
Right ventricular hypertrophy
  cor triatriatum, 291
  electrocardiography, 87-88
  pulmonic stenosis, 288
  reactive pulmonary hypertension, 298
  tetralogy of Fallot, 288
Right ventricular infarction, 178-180, 220-221
Right ventricular outflow obstruction
  abnormal jugular venous pulse, 66
  cardiogenic syncope, 954
  hypertrophic cardiomyopathy, 266
  systolic ejection murmur, 77
Right ventricular stroke volume, 281
Right ventricular stroke work index, 391
Right ventricular systolic pressure
  constrictive pericarditis, 277-278
  pulmonary hypertension, 498-499
Rigid bronchoscopy, 383, 384
Rigid dysarthria, 977
Rigid endoscopy, 1181
Rigid proctoscopy, 1995
Rigidity
  hepatic encephalopathy, 2160
  Parkinson's disease, 989
Riley-Day syndrome, 1087
Rim sign, 754
Rimantadine, 1492
Ringed sideroblast, 645, 676, Plate IV-11
Rinne test, 2308
Risk stratification, 224
Risperidone, 1042
Ristocetin-cofactor assay, 569-570
Ristocetin-induced platelet aggregation, 622, 623
Risus sardonicus, 1573
RIT; *see* Ritonavir
Ritonavir
  acquired immunodeficiency syndrome, 1474
  human cytochrome P450 isoforms, 2312
Ritrodine, 479
River blindness, 1699-1701
RNA; *see* Ribonucleic acid
Robertsonian type translocation, 1728
ROC curve, 8-9
Rocky Mountain spotted fever, 1541-1544
  fever and rash, 1382
  influence of season and geographic setting,
    1381
  purpura and petechiae, Plate VIII-18
  rickettsial invasion, Plate VIII-19
  sepsis *versus*, 1451
Rodent handler's disease, 460
Romaña's sign, 1690
Romano-Ward syndrome, 62, 153
Romberg test, 903

Romhilt-Estes score, 87
Root ejection sounds, 74
Rorschach test, 903
Rose spots, 1601
Rostral ventral lateral medulla, 46
Rotational ablation device, 118-119
Rotator cuff tendinitis, 1196-1197
Rotavirus, 1520-1521
  antigen test, 1431
  compromised host, 1388
  diarrhea, 1427-1428
Roth spots, 228
Rotor's syndrome, 2142, 2157-2158
Rouleau formation, 704, Plate IV-4
Rounded atelectasis, 474
Roundworm
  intestinal, 1696
  tissue, 1699-1702
  with tissue migratory phases, 1698-1699
  travelers infection, 1466
RPGN; *see* Rapidly progressive
    glomerulonephritis
RR interval
  atrial fibrillation, 147
  atrioventricular conduction abnormalities, 154
RSV; *see* Respiratory syncytial virus
RU-486; *see* Mifepristone
Rubber band ligation, 2093
Rubella, 1500-1502
  congenital heart disease, 280
  culture, 1369
  during pregnancy, 2280
  pulmonic stenosis, 288
  septic arthritis, 1255
Rubella vaccine, 2255
Rubeola, 1385
Rubeosis iridis, 2304
Ruffled border, 1716
Rumination syndrome, 2027
Rupture
  aneurysm
    aortic, 300
    peripheral arterial, 309
  aortic, 304, 333
  chordal, 252
  esophageal, 128, 2019
    pleural effusion, 508
    thoracentesis, 382
    traumatic pneumomediastinum, 514
  myocardial, 177-178, 219, 220
  papillary muscle, 177, 219, 220
  pulmonary artery, 395
  ventricular septum, 219-220
Russian spring-summer encephalitis, 1514, 1515
Ryanodine receptor, 38, 58

S

S fimbriae, 1404
S-prime wave, 84
S-T segment, 84
  acute pericarditis, 89, 273, 274
  aortic regurgitation, 241, 244
  early repolarization, 89
  effect of digitalis, 90
  exercise stress testing, 93
  hypokalemia, 829
  ischemic heart disease, 197
  left ventricular hypertrophy, 87
  myocardial infarction, 88
  myocarditis, 263
  myopericarditis, 1490
  pulmonary hypertension, 296
  Q wave myocardial infarction, 211
  right ventricular infarction, 178
  silent myocardial ischemia, 194
  variant angina, 194
S wave, 84
  chronic cor pulmonale, 445
Sabia virus, 1509
Saccadic eye movement, 1063

Saccular aneurysm, 299
Sacroiliac joint
  ankylosing spondylitis, 1238-1239
  arthritis, 1172, 1173
Sacroiliitis
  brucellosis, 1606
  colitis-related, 2075
Saddle-nose deformity, 1222
SAFE questions for domestic violence, 4
Safety belts, 2265
Saint Jude valve, 259, 260
St. Louis encephalitis, 1515, 1517
Salicylates
  adult Still's disease, 1243
  anion gap acidosis, 836
  euthyroid hypothyroxinemia, 1804
  hepatic injury, 2190, 2191
  intoxication, 355, 1451
  pericarditis, 221
  rheumatic diseases, 1258
Saline infusion test, 1741
Saline irrigation, 1182
Saline load test, 2004
Salivary gland
  acute inflammation, 2310
  mumps, 1495-1497
  Sjögren syndrome, 1209-1212
Salivary stones, 2310
Salizopyridine, 2192
Salmeterol, 1190
Salmon calcitonin, 1719, 1956-1957
Salmonella, 1598-1602
  acquired immunodeficiency syndrome, 1472,
    1476
  antibiotic selection, 1348
  compromised host, 1388
  diarrhea, 1426, 1430
  gay bowel syndrome, 1429
  mycotic aortic aneurysm, 299
  neurologic aspects, 1101
  reactive arthritis, 1240
  sickle cell anemia, 658
Salmonella typhi, 1465
  gallbladder cancer, 2232
  vaccine, 1596
Salpingitis
  anaerobic bacteria, 1618
  Chlamydia trachomatis, 1536
  gonococcal, 1583
  Mycoplasma hominis, 1541
Salsalate, 1259
Salt intake
  ascites formation, 818
  chronic renal failure, 778
  extracellular fluid volume, 737
  heart failure, 169
  hypercalciuria, 798
  hypertension, 318-319
Salt restriction
  acute renal failure, 774
  ascites, 2165
  autosomal dominant polycystic kidney disease,
    873
  chronic renal failure, 787
  cirrhotic patient, 820
  hypertension, 324
  hypertension management, 324
  hypokalemia, 830
  kidney stones, 800
  nephrotic syndrome, 767
  thiazide treatment program, 803
Salt-wasting states, 823
Sand fly, 1685
Sandhoff disease, 1919
Sanfilippo's syndrome, 1914-1915
Sanger technique, 54
Santorini's duct, 2130
Saphenous vein, coronary artery bypass graft, 206
Saquinavir
  acquired immunodeficiency syndrome, 1474
  human cytochrome P450 isoforms, 2312

Sarcocystosis, 1680
Sarcoglycan proteins, 1027
Sarcoidosis, 456-459
  arthropathy, 1245
  chemotactic defects, 1340
  cutaneous manifestations, 1324-1325
  dyspnea, 404
  fever of unknown origin, 1378
  granulomatous gastritis, 2043
  papule, Plate VII-20
  renal dysfunction, 892
  steroid suppression test, 1746
Sarcoma
  cardiac, 330
  colon, 2083
  Ewing's, 731
  Kaposi's, 1320-1321, 1329, 1533, 2098, Plate
      VII-22
    acquired immunodeficiency syndrome, 1477
    cholangitis, 2202
    colon lesion, Plate VIII-39
    cutaneous lesions, Plate VIII-38
    cutaneous manifestations, 1330-1331
    heart involvement, 331
    ophthalmic involvement, 2305
    oral involvement, 2095
  mesenteric, 2251
  osteogenic, 552
  Paget's disease, 1956
  renal, 898
Sarcomere, 39
  cardiac, 59
Sarcoplasmic reticulum, 38
Sarcoplasmic reticulum calcium-pump proteins,
      38, 39, 40-41
Sarcotubular system, 38
Satellite bubo, 1640
Satiety center, 2099
Saturated fatty acids, 1889
Saturday-night palsy, 1017
SAVE trial, 172
SAVED trial, 120
Scabies, 1444
Scalded-skin syndrome, 1384, 1421, 1549, Plate
      VIII-29
Scalene maneuver, 306
Scalp, tinea capitis, 1308, 1309
Scan
  acute lower gastrointestinal bleeding, 2012
  bone
    ankylosing spondylitis, 1238-1239
    osteomalacia, 1950
    osteomyelitis, 1434
    Paget's disease, 1956
    prostate cancer, 718
    septic arthritis, 1252
    small cell lung cancer, 726
  brain, 926-929
  gallium, 388
    acute pericarditis, 274
    amebiasis, 1683
    amiodarone-induced pulmonary disease, 478
    osteomyelitis, 1434
  gallstones, 2225
  gastric, 2004
  intraabdominal abscess, 1400
  intraabdominal infection, 1399
  liver, 2141
    amebiasis, 1683
    cavernous hemangioma, 2215-2216
    cholestasis, 2156
    focal nodular hyperplasia, 2216
  lung, 387-388
    Behçet disease, 469
    primary pulmonary hypertension, 294
    pulmonary embolism, 297, 387-388,
        501-502
  mitral valve prolapse, 254
  neurologic disorders, 926-929
  parathyroid tumor, 1970
  proximal venous thrombosis, 502

Scan—cont'd
  renal, 750
    hydronephrosis, 754
    pediatric urinary tract infection, 1459
  thyroid, 1801-1802
    Graves' disease, 1802
    hyperthyroidism, 1735, 1802
  xenon, 387
Scandinavian Simvastatin Survival Study, 218,
      1891
Scapulohumeral reflex, 964
Scarlatina toxins, 1555-1556
Scarlet fever, 1421, 1556, 1557
Schatzki's rings, 2020
Schaumann body, 456, 1324
Scheduled toileting, 2292-2293
Scheie's syndrome, 1912
Schilling test, 2059, 2060
  absorption of vitamin B$_{12}$, 2007
  chronic pancreatitis, 2239
  small bowel bacterial overgrowth, 2061
  vitamin B$_{12}$ deficiency, 649
Schirmer's test, 1209
Schistocyte, Plate IV-4
  disseminated intravascular coagulation, 627
  hemolytic anemia, 587, 662, 666
Schistosoma haematobium, 548
Schistosoma japonicum, 1702-1703
  cholangiocarcinoma, 2231
  pulmonary hypertension, 297
Schistosoma mansoni, 1702-1703
  cholangiocarcinoma, 2231
  granulomatous vasculitis, 470
  peritonitis, 2248
  pulmonary hypertension, 297
Schizophrenia
  disordered thinking, 1041-1042
  polydipsia, 1796
Schmidt's syndrome, 1823-1824, 1838
Schmorl's node, 1266
Schüffner's dots, 1672, Plate VIII-15
Schwann cell, 1871
Schwann cell tumor, 973
SCI; *see* Spinal cord injury
Sciatic nerve mononeuropathy, 1017
Sciatica, 965
SCID; *see* Severe combined immunodeficiency
Scimitar sign, 91
Scimitar syndrome, 282
Scintigraphy
  bone
    ankylosing spondylitis, 1238-1239
    osteomalacia, 1950
    osteomyelitis, 1434
    Paget's disease, 1956
    prostate cancer, 718
    septic arthritis, 1252
    small cell lung cancer, 726
  intraabdominal abscess, 1400
  intraabdominal infection, 1399
  liver, 2141
    amebiasis, 1683
    cavernous hemangioma, 2215-2216
    cholestasis, 2156
    focal nodular hyperplasia, 2216
  lung, 387-388
    Behçet disease, 469
    primary pulmonary hypertension, 294
    pulmonary embolism, 297, 501-502
  mitral valve prolapse, 254
  neurologic disorders, 926-929
  parathyroid tumor, 1970
  renal, 750
    hydronephrosis, 754
    pediatric urinary tract infection, 1459
  thyroid, 1801-1802
Scl-70 antigen, 1159
Sclera, 2147
Scleritis, 1204
Sclerodactyly, 1293

Scleroderma, 1228-1233
  autoantibodies, 1155
  cutaneous manifestations, 1293
  delayed gastric emptying, 1979
  intestinal pseudoobstruction, 2079
  neurologic manifestations, 1092, 1095
  reflux esophagitis, 2023
Sclerosing adenoma, 1846
Sclerosing agents, 332
Sclerosing cholangitis, 2099
Sclerosing pericholangitis, 2155
Sclerosis
  amyotrophic lateral, 1015
    referral, 1021
    respiratory failure, 1097
  arteriolosclerosis, 2303
  arteriosclerosis, 64
  atherosclerosis
    abdominal aortic aneurysm, 300
    aortic disease, 299
    apolipoproteins, 60
    cardiac catheterization, 107
    cerebrotendinous xanthomatosis, 1898
    chronic occlusive arterial disease, 308
    disorder in apolipoprotein A metabolism,
        1897
    femoral pulses, 64
    ischemic heart disease, 192, 193
    ischemic stroke, 998-1000
    lipoproteins, 60, 1888-1889
    peripheral arterial aneurysm, 309
    peripheral artery disease, 305
    renal artery stenosis, 894
    renovascular disease, 755
    rheumatoid arthritis, 334
    thrombus formation, 638
  bone, 1168
  focal glomerular, 849, 851-852
  glomerulosclerosis
    chronic renal failure, 778
    monoclonal light chain deposition disease,
        863
    progressive glomerular diseases, 842
  multiple, 1007-1009
    brain magnetic resonance imaging, 921
    brainstem auditory evoked potential,
        911-912
    depression, 1036
    neurorehabilitation, 1055
    pattern-reversal visual evoked response,
        911
    during pregnancy, 2282
    transverse myelitis with, 1013
  nodular
    diabetic glomerular, 859
    Hodgkin's disease, 692
  otosclerosis, 974
  progressive systemic sclerosis, 1293
    antinuclear antibody, 1159-1160
    cardiac involvement, 334
    interstitial lung disease, 453
    multiple jejunal diverticulosis, 2089
    pulmonary hypertension, 296
    reflux esophagitis, 2023
  systemic, 1228-1233
    cardiac involvement, 334
    neurologic manifestations, 1092,
        1095
    reflux esophagitis, 2023
  tuberous, 1922
Sclerotherapy
  esophageal varices, 2167
  gastrointestinal bleeding, 2011-2012
  induction of pericarditis, 273
  polycystic liver disease, 2111
  varicose veins, 311
Scoliosis
  Marfan syndrome, 1289
  mitral valve prolapse, 254
  neurofibromatosis, 1921
Scopolamine, 2027

Screening
 cancer, 552-553
  breast, 25, 707
  colorectal, 2084-2085
  lung, 490
 coagulation inhibitors, 571
 cost-utility analysis, 16
 DNA and cDNA libraries, 54
 fibrinolysis, 571
 gestational diabetes, 2273
 hearing impairment in elderly, 2287
 monoclonal proteins, 567
 preventive care guidelines, 2255
 sexual problems, 4
 small bowel malabsorption, 2059
 substance abuse, 2293-2294
 thalassemia and hemoglobinopathies, 660
 thrombotic disease, 571-572
 transplant donor, 339
Scrotal mass, 722
Scrub typhus, 1545
Scurvy, 2107
Seafood, *Vibrio* gastroenteritis, 1593-1594
Seasonal allergic rhinoconjunctivitis, 1181
Seasonal rhinitis, 1181
Sebaceous follicle, 1304
Seborrhea, 2307
Seborrheic dermatitis
 human immunodeficiency virus infection,
  1326
 riboflavin deficiency, 2106
Sebum, 1305
Second-degree atrioventricular block, 222-223
Second-generation cephalosporins, 1352-1354
Second heart sound, 72-73, 74
 anginal attack, 196
 aortic regurgitation, 244
 aortic stenosis, 236
 atrial septal defect, 281
 hypertrophic cardiomyopathy, 266
 pulmonic stenosis, 288
Secondary bile acids, 2124-2125
Secondary combined hyperlipidemia, 1896
Secondary crystal growth, 797
Secondary diabetes mellitus, 1854-1855
Secondary hypertriglyceridemia, 1895
Secondary malignancy, 585-586
Secondary parkinsonism, 992-993
Secondary peristalsis, 1978
Secondary polycythemia, 588-590
Secondary sexual development, 1768, 1770-1772
Secretin
 bile duct water secretion, 2123
 intestinal absorption of lipids, 1986
 pancreatic duct cells, 2132
 pepsinogen secretion, 1984
 small bowel malabsorption, 2058
 stimulation test, 1743
Secretin-cholecystokinin stimulation test, 2145
Secretion clearance, 429-430
 chronic obstructive pulmonary disease, 444
 cystic fibrosis, 482
 pulmonary rehabilitation, 436
Secretomotor fibers in nose, 1181
Secretory component, 1110, 1122, 1990
 in alveolar fluid, 367
Secretory granule, 536
Secretory immunoglobulin A, 1122, 1990-1993
Secretory leucoprotease inhibitor, 442
Sectral; *see* Acebutolol
Sedatives
 human cytochrome P450 isoforms, 2312
 interference with oral anticoagulants, 636
 portosystemic encephalopathy, 2160
 sedation during gastrointestinal endoscopy,
  1994
Segment receptor, 1710
Segmental contraction, 1977, 1979
Segmental esophageal spasm, 2022
Segmental mastectomy, 709
Segmented neutrophil, 532

Segregation, 1721
Seizure
 acute confusional state, 1031
 after stroke, 1007
 alcohol withdrawal, 2295-2296
 amylo-1,6-glucosidase deficiency, 1882
 autonomic overactivity, 934
 bacterial meningitis, 1406
 brain abscess, 1414
 brain tumor, 1067
 eclampsia, 2274
 endocardial hemorrhage, 1087
 endocarditis, 1089
 epilepsy, 978-985
  clinical seizure patterns, 979-980
  diagnosis and laboratory evaluation, 980-982
  electroencephalography, 906-907
  etiology, 980
  pathophysiology, 978-979
  posttraumatic, 1045
  psychologic issues and behavior changes,
   984-985
  syncope *versus,* 954
  treatment, 982-984
 hereditary fructose intolerance, 1880
 human immunodeficiency virus, 1478
 hypoglycemia, 1875
 hypoglycemic coma, 1867
 during pregnancy, 2281-2282
 pseudobulbar affect, 1033-1034
 respiratory rhythm abnormalities, 1098
 shigellosis, 1603
 sleep-related, 947
 status epilepticus, 1085
 stroke, 1001
 subdural empyema, 1417
 syncope *versus,* 954
 systemic lupus erythematosus, 1093, 1215
 thrombotic thrombocytopenic purpura, 615
 tuberous sclerosis, 1922
 vitamin B_6 deficiency, 1101
 withdrawal, 1080
Selective arteriography, 2012-2013
Selective deficiency of immunoglobulin G
  subclasses, 1176
Selective estrogen receptor modulators, 1850
Selective immunoglobulin A deficiency, 1991,
  2046
Selegeline, 990, 992
Selenium
 functions, 2109
 fungal infection, 1311
 recommended daily dietary allowances, 2116
Self-induced emesis, 2027
Self/nonself discrimination, 1108-1109
Self recognition, 1108
Self-tolerance, 1142
Sella turca, 1773
Semen analysis, 1742
Semicircular canals, 971-972
Semilente, 1859
Semilunar valve, 78-79, 80
Semimembranosus and semitendinosus reflex,
  964
Seminiferous tubules, 1839, 1845
Seminoma
 mediastinal, 513
 testicular, 721
Semistarvation diet, 2103
Semustine, 869
Sengstaken-Blakemore tube, 2013
Senile purpura, 603
Sensitivity and specificity, 6-7, 1366
Sensitivity cholestasis, 2187
Sensorimotor neuropathy, 1020
Sensorineural hearing loss, 2308
Sensory alexia, 978
Sensory examination, 903
Sensory impairment
 diabetes mellitus, 1871-1872
 fall risk, 2290

Sensory nerve conduction studies, 915
Sentinel lymph node biopsy, 1299
Seoul virus, 1516
Sepsis, 1445-1455
 acute respiratory failure occurring with acute
  respiratory distress syndrome, 418
 canalicular cholestasis, 2155
 clinical manifestations, 1449-1450
 diagnosis, 1450-1451
 epidemiology, 1445-1446
 laboratory findings, 1450
 Listeria, 1577
 microbiology, 1446
 mixed venous oxygen saturation, 393
 multiple organ dysfunction syndrome, 421
 nosocomial fever, 1480
 pathogenesis, 1446-1447
 pathophysiology, 1447-1448
 postsplenectomy, 1338
 prevention, 1453-1454
 therapy, 1451-1453
 total parenteral nutrition, 2114
 transfusion reaction, 575
 Vibrio vulnificus, 1597
Septal abscess, 2308
Septal defect
 aortopulmonary, 286
 atrial, 280-282
  atrial fibrillation, 146
  Ebstein's anomaly, 289
  precapillary pulmonary hypertension,
   296-297
 ventricular, 283-285
  with aortic regurgitation, 285
  complete transposition of great arteries, 290
  differential diagnosis, 180
  murmur, 77, 79
  precapillary pulmonary hypertension, 296
  pulmonary hypertension, 296
  tetralogy of Fallot, 288-289
  tricuspid atresia, 291
Septal hematoma, 2308
Septal Q wave, 84
Septata intestinalis, 1474
Septi-chek system, 1369
Septic arthritis, 1250-1251
 Haemophilus influenzae, 1588
 Neisseria meningitidis, 1579
 reactive arthritis *versus,* 1240
Septic scarlet fever, 1556, 1557
Septic shock, 176, 1445
 cholestasis, 2159
 differential diagnosis, 180
 peritonitis, 1398
 pyogenic liver abscess, 2209
Septicemic plague, 1610
Septoplasty, 2309
Sequential estrogen-progesterone stimulation,
  1742-1743
Sequoiosis, 460
Serine, 1904
Serine proteases, 442
Serine-threonine kinases, 542
Serologic testing, 1372, 1373-1374
 acute nephritic syndrome, 764
 adenovirus, 1504
 agglutination reactions, 1373
 albumin excretion, 761
 amebiasis, 1683
 amebic liver abscess, 2210
 asthma, 1188
 babesiosis, 1676
 Bordetella pertussis, 1612-1613
 Borrelia burgdorferi, 1647
 brucellosis, 1606
 chlamydial infection, 1536-1537
 chronic renal failure, 782
 Coccidioides immitis, 1657
 complement-fixation assays, 1373
 cytomegalovirus, 1528
 detection of autoantibodies, 1156

Serologic testing—cont'd
echinococcal cyst, 2111
enzyme immunoassay, 1374
fever and rash, 1385
fever of unknown origin, 1379
fungal infection, 1652, 1653
Helicobacter pylori, 2037
histoplasmosis, 1655
indirect immunofluorescence assays, 1373-1374
infectious disease, 1373-1374
infective endocarditis, 228
Legionella pneumophila, 1623
leishmaniasis, 1687
leptospirosis, 1645
liver abscess, 2209
Lyme disease, 1647
microalbuminuria, 743
neutralization tests, 1373
Norwalk virus, 1522
parathyroid hormone, 1745-1746
parenchymal renal disease, 771
precipitin reactions, 1373
principles, 1733-1734
radioimmunoassays, 1374
rotavirus, 1521
syphilis, 1641, 1642, 1643
systemic lupus erythematosus, 857
systemic sclerosis, 1231
thyroid hormone, 1738
toxoplasmosis, 1678
Western blot assay, 1374
Serositis, 1214-1215
Serotonergic projections, 1076
Serotonin
emetic response, 581
lung filtration, 346
migraine, 959
variant angina, 194
vasoactive effects on pulmonary circulation, 363
Serotonin reuptake inhibitors, 1037
alcohol abuse, 2296
cataplexy, 943
chemotherapy-induced nausea and vomiting, 582
chronic fatigue syndrome, 2300
depression, 1037, 2289
human cytochrome P450 isoforms, 2312
interference with oral anticoagulants, 636
Serous labyrinthitis, 972
Serpasil; *see* Reserpine
Serratia
antibiotic selection, 1348
susceptibility to empiric antimicrobial therapy, 1400
Sertoli cell, 1839
dysfunction causing infertility, 1844-1846
Sertoli-cell–only syndrome, 1845
Sertoli-Leydig cell tumor, 1838
Sertraline, 1037
chronic fatigue syndrome, 2300
depression, 2289
Serum alanine aminotransferase
acetaminophen poisoning, 2190
acute pancreatitis, 2236
chronic hepatitis, 2180
hepatic injury, 2136, 2188
hepatitis A infection, 2173
hepatitis B infection, 2175
Serum albumin
adult respiratory distress syndrome, 421
heart failure, 166
hypercalcemia, 1929
kwashiorkor, 2101
liver disease, 2134-2135
nephrotic syndrome, 765
nutritional assessment, 2111
peritonitis, 2080
primary biliary cirrhosis, 2200
primary sclerosing cholangitis, 2202
small bowel malabsorption, 2058

Serum alkaline phosphatase
bone and mineral disorders, 1744-1745
hepatocellular *versus* cholestatic jaundice, 2156
liver disease, 2137
osteomalacia, 1949
Paget's disease, 1956
primary biliary cirrhosis, 2200
primary sclerosing cholangitis, 2202
renal bone disease, 1964
Serum aminotransferases
alcoholic hepatitis, 2196
alcoholic liver disease, 2136
chronic hepatitis, 2180
chronic hepatitis B, 2181
chronic hepatitis C, 2182
hepatitis A virus, 2173
hepatitis B, 2175
hepatocellular *versus* cholestatic jaundice, 2156
liver disease, 2136-2137
Serum amylase
abdominal pain, 2032
acute pancreatitis, 2235
pancreatic disease, 2144
Serum anion gap, 840
Serum-ascites albumin concentration gradient, 2164
Serum aspartate aminotransferase
acetaminophen poisoning, 2190
acute pancreatitis, 2236
chronic hepatitis, 2180
hepatitic injury, 2136
myocardial infarction, 211
toxic hepatic injury, 2188
Serum bile acids
hepatocellular *versus* cholestatic jaundice, 2156
liver disease, 2137
unconjugated hyperbilirubinemia, 2153
Serum bilirubin
acquired immunodeficiency syndrome cholangiopathy, 2202
adult respiratory distress syndrome, 421
Dubin-Johnson and Rotor's syndromes, 2157
estrogen-related cholestasis, 2158
Gilbert's syndrome, 2153
hepatitis A virus, 2173
hepatocellular *versus* cholestatic jaundice, 2156
primary biliary cirrhosis, 2200
Serum bone Gla protein, 1747
Serum calcitonin, 1746
Serum calcium
bone and mineral disorders, 1744
hypercalcemia, 1929
hypercalcemia of malignancy, 1974
hypocalcemia, 1930
osteomalacia, 1949
primary hyperparathyroidism, 1967
small bowel malabsorption, 2058
Serum carotene, 2058
Serum chloride, 1974
Serum cholesterol
estrogen-related cholestasis, 2158
hepatocellular *versus* cholestatic jaundice, 2156
small bowel malabsorption, 2058
Serum creatine kinase, 211
Serum creatinine, 746
adult respiratory distress syndrome, 421
crescentic glomerulonephritis, 848
heart failure, 166
increase during angiotensin-converting enzyme inhibitor therapy, 896
multiple myeloma, 701
thrombotic thrombocytopenic purpura, 858
toxicity of nonsteroidal antiinflammatory drugs, 870
uremic syndrome, 776
Serum cryptococcal antigen titer, 1477-1478

Serum ferritin
hereditary hemochromatosis, 2139, 2204
iron overload, 646
iron status, 643
Serum gamma globulin, 2135-2136
Serum gamma glutamyltransferase, 2137
Serum gastrin, 2003
Serum glucagon, 2245
Serum glucose, 1855-1856
Serum glutamic oxaloacetic transaminase
alcoholic hepatitis, 2196
hypothyroidism, 1809
infectious mononucleosis, 1529
Serum glutamic pyruvic transaminase
alcoholic hepatitis, 2196
infectious mononucleosis, 1529
Serum hyaluronic acid, 2141
Serum iron
hereditary hemochromatosis, 2204
iron deficiency anemia, 643
small bowel malabsorption, 2058
Serum lactate, 176, 178
Serum lactate dehydrogenase
ascites, 2164
human immunodeficiency virus infection, 1473
Serum leucine aminopeptidase, 2137
Serum lipase
abdominal pain, 2032
acute pancreatitis, 2235
pancreatic disease, 2144
Serum lipids, 2223
Serum magnesium, 1942
Serum markers, 2144-2145
Serum monoclonal proteins, 564-568
Serum osmolality, 806, 811
Serum osmolar gap, 840
Serum parathyroid hormone, 1964
Serum phosphate, 1934
bone and mineral disorders, 1745
hypoparathyroidism, 1931
primary hyperparathyroidism, 1968
rickets, 881
Serum potassium, 840
Serum prolactin, 984
Serum protein electrophoresis, 565
Serum proteins, 1163
Serum sodium, 1079
Serum testosterone, 1763
Serum thyroglobulin, 1739, 1801
Serum thyroid-stimul-ating hormone, 1801, 1802
Serum thyroxine
euthyroid hyperthyroxinemia, 1803, 1804
goiter, 1813
Graves' disease, 1806
hypothyroidism, 1809
Serum total carbon dioxide, 840
Serum total thyroxine, 1800
Serum total triiodothyronine, 1800
Serum transaminases
acute cholecystitis, 2228
alcoholic hepatitis, 2196
estrogen-related cholestasis, 2158
Serum transferrin
iron deficiency, 644
kwashiorkor, 2101
nutritional assessment, 2111
Serum triiodothyronine
goiter, 1813
Graves' disease, 1806
hypothyroidism, 1809
Serum viral ribonucleic acid, 1473
Serum viscometry, 567
Serum vitamin B_{12}, 649
Sestamibi imaging
coronary artery disease, 102-103
ischemic heart disease, 199
Seven-transmembrane segment receptor, 1710
Severe aplastic anemia, 671

Severe combined immunodeficiency, 1177-1178, 1343
  flow cytometry, 1152
  hematopoietic stem cell transplantation, 576
Severity adjustment systems, 18
Sex chromosome, 1727
Sex chromosome abnormalities, 1729
Sex steroids
  calcium homeostasis, 1720
  hepatic synthesis, 2122-2123
  laboratory and diagnostic testing, 1835
Sexual abuse, 2269
Sexual activity
  human immunodeficiency virus transmission, 1471
  reinfection of urinary tract, 1461
  risk of urinary tract infection, 1457
Sexual differentiation, 1077
Sexual function
  after spinal cord injury, 1050
  autonomic control, 933-934
  medical interview, 4-5
Sexually transmitted disease, 1437-1445
  cervical cancer, 714
  cervicitis, 1441-1442
  Chlamydia trachomatis, 1535
  diagnosis, 1438-1439
  early diagnosis and treatment in human immunodeficiency virus prevention, 1471
  epidemiology, 1437-1438
  gonorrhea, 1581-1585
    dysuria, 762, 763
    during pregnancy, 2279-2280
    urethritis, 1440
  hepatitis B virus infection, 2174
  hepatitis C virus infection, 2175
  inguinal adenopathy, 1444
  miscellaneous syndromes, 1444-1445
  peritonitis, 2248
  during pregnancy, 2279-2280
  skin and mucous membrane lesions, 1444
  syphilis, 1640-1644
    acquired immunodeficiency syndrome, 2098
    anal fissure and fistula, 2093
    aortic disease, 303
    aortitis, 302
    granulomatous gastritis, 2043
    meningitis verus, 1409
    neuroarthropathy, 1168
    palmar lesions, Plate VIII-47
    penile chancre, Plate VIII-34
    during pregnancy, 2280
    secondary, Plate VIII-46
    transfusion-transmitted, 575, 576
  traveler's risk, 1466
  Trichomonas vaginalis, 1691
  urethritis, 1440-1441
  vulvovaginitis, 1441, 1442-1443
Sézary cell, 595, Plate IV-5
Sézary syndrome, 1331-1332
Sham code, 12
Sharp wave, 906, 907
Shear stress, 48
Shellfish, *Vibrio* gastroenteritis, 1593-1594
Shift work sleep disorder, 945
Shiga bacillus, 1426
Shigella, 1602-1604
  acquired immunodeficiency syndrome, 1476
  antibiotic selection, 1348
  compromised host, 1388
  diarrhea, 1426, 1430
  dysentery, 1445
  gay bowel syndrome, 1429
  neurologic aspects, 1101
Shin spots, 1323
Shingles, 1328, 1527
Shipyard eye, 1504
Shock, 175-187
  acute pancreatitis, 2237
  aortic dissection, 300

Shock—cont'd
  candidemia, 1662
  cardiogenic, 175-187
    clinical presentation, 177-180
    clinical trials, 184, 185
    coronary angioplasty, 183
    coronary artery bypass graft, 185
    differential diagnosis, 175, 176
    evaluation and treatment, 180, 181
    hemodynamic alterations, 176, 177
    mechanical intervention, 184, 185-186
    myocardial function, 176
    myocardial infarction, 218-219
    pharmacologic therapy, 181-182
    reperfusion therapy, 182-183
    serum lactate and anaerobic metabolism, 176, 178
  dengue fever, 1516
  disseminated intravascular coagulation, 628
  gas gangrene, 1423
  gastric volvulus, 2044
  gram-negative bacteremia, 1449
  hypovolemic, 176, 177
  mesenteric vascular disease, 2086
  septic, 176, 1445
    differential diagnosis, 180
    peritonitis, 1398
  spinal, 1011-1012
    spinal cord injury, 1051
  streptococcal toxic shock syndrome, 1558
Shohl's solution, 804
Short-axis views, 95, 96
Short bowel syndrome, 2066
Short stature, 1769
  growth hormone deficiency, 1777
  neurofibromatosis, 1921
  Prader-Labhart-Willi syndrome, 1842
  pseudohypoparathyroidism, 1932, 1933
Short tandem repeat polymorphisms, 60-61
Shortness of breath, 404, 405
  acute lung allograft rejection, 521
  acute pancreatitis, 2234
  acute pericarditis, 273
  aortic dissection, 300
  aortic stenosis, 236
  ascites, 2164
  asthma, 1187
  atrial septal defect, 281
  behavioral control of breathing, 356-357
  bronchiolitis obliterans syndrome, 522
  cardiac tamponade, 275
  chronic obstructive pulmonary disease, 442
  complete transposition of great arteries, 290
  constrictive pericarditis, 277
  dilated cardiomyopathy, 263
  exercise testing, 379
  heart failure, 163
  hepatopulmonary syndrome, 2170
  human immunodeficiency virus, 1477
  hypersensitivity pneumonitis, 461
  hypertrophic obstructive cardiomyopathy, 266
  hypothyroidism, 334
  idiopathic pulmonary fibrosis, 453
  interstitial lung disease, 450
  ischemic heart disease, 196-197
  Langerhans' cell granulomatosis, 464
  lung cancer, 488
  lymphomatoid granulomatosis, 470
  malignant mesothelioma, 510
  mediastinal abnormality, 511
  mitral regurgitation, 250
  mitral stenosis, 246
  mitral valve prolapse, 254
  myopericarditis, 1489
  patent ductus arteriosus, 285
  pleural disease, 505
  pneumothorax, 509
  precapillary pulmonary hypertension, 293
  psychologic considerations, 432
  pulmonary edema, 168
  pulmonary function tests, 375

Shortness of breath—cont'd
  pulmonary hypertension, 498
  pulmonary thromboembolism, 500
  pulmonary veno-occlusive disease, 298
  pulmonic stenosis, 288
  respiratory muscle failure, 359
  right atrial myxoma, 330
  sarcoidosis, 458
  spontaneous pneumomediastinum, 514
  systemic lupus erythematosus, 1215
  systemic sclerosis, 1230
  Wegener's granulomatosis, 468
Shoulder
  adhesive capsulitis, 1197
  arthrography, 1164
  periarthritis, 1196-1197
Shoulder-hand syndrome, 1055, 1247
Shoulder-pad sign, 1165
Show code, 12
Shunt
  acute respiratory failure, 413
  arteriovenous, 2014
  blood flow measurements, 110-111
  Ebstein's anomaly of tricuspid valve, 290
  hexose monophosphate, 662-663, 2121
  left-to-right, 110, 393
    aortopulmonary septal defect, 286
    atrial septal defect, 280
    coronary arteriovenous fistula, 292
    endocardial cushion defect, 282
    hepatopulmonary syndrome, 2170
    pulmonary hypertension, 296
    tetralogy of Fallot, 288, 289
    total anomalous pulmonary venous connection, 290-291
    truncus arteriosus, 290
    ventricular septal defect, 283
  right-to-left, 110-111, 283
    atrial septal defect, 280
    Ebstein's anomaly, 289, 290
    precapillary pulmonary hypertension, 296
    tetralogy of Fallot, 288
    total anomalous pulmonary venous connection, 290-291
    ventricular septal defect, 284-285
  transjugular intrahepatic portosystemic, 2167
    ascites, 2165, 2166
    Budd-Chiari syndrome, 2208
    cirrhotic ascites, 822-823
    cystic fibrosis, 2207
    hepatopulmonary syndrome, 2170
    hepatorenal syndrome, 2170
Shunt hyperbilirubinemia, 2152
Shunt infection, 1551
Shwartzman reaction, 1380
Shy-Drager syndrome, 935, 992
Sialidosis, 1916
Sialitis, 1496
Sialolithiasis, 2310
Sick cell syndrome, 812
Sick sinus syndrome, 154, 1001
Sickle cell disease, 656-660, Plate IV-4
  acute meningitis, 1407
  arthropathy, 1246
  hypergonadotropic hypogonadism, 1843
  neurologic aspects, 1103
  renal manifestations, 891
  thrombosis, 609
Sickle cell trait, 657, 2279
Side-chain carboxylic glucuronidation, 2125
Side effects, 2310
Sideroblast, 645
Sideroblastic anemia, 645-646, Plate IV-11
Siderosis, 476
Sigmoid esophagus, 2000
Sigmoidoscopy
  balantidiasis, 1691
  colonic diverticulum, 2091
  diarrhea, 1476
  preventive care guidelines, 2255
Sign of Leser Trélat, 1317, 1318

Signal averaged electrocardiography, 134, 149
Signal recognition peptide, 1709
Signal transducers and activators of transcription, 1131
Signal transduction, 541, 543
  chief cell receptors, 1984
  cytokines, 1131-1132
  G proteins, 56-57
  parietal cell receptors, 1981, 1983
Silencers, 50, 51
Silent ischemia
  diabetes mellitus, 334
  diabetic autonomic neuropathy, 1873
Silent mutation, 1722
Silent myocardial ischemia, 194
  continuous ambulatory electrocardiographic recording, 94
  therapeutic approach, 208
Silent thyroiditis, 1807, 1812
Silicoproteinosis, 456
Silicosis, 474-475
Silver methenamine stain, 2020
Silver wiring, Plate XI-6
Simple cyst
  imaging and pathologic findings, 751
  renal, 871-872
Simple partial seizure, 979
Simvastatin, 1891
  gallstone risk factor, 2223
  hyperlipidemia, 200
  interference with oral anticoagulants, 636
  nephrotic syndrome, 767
Sin Nombre virus, 1516
Single-beam photon absorptiometry, 1747-1748
Single-breath diffusing capacity, 378, 379
Single-chain urokinase-type tissue plasminogen activator, 213
Single-fiber electromyography, 917
Single lung transplantation, 445, 514
Single nephron glomerular filtration rate, 777
Single photon emission computed tomography, 100-101
  brain, 929
  cardiac transplantation, 1090
  dementia, 2288
  stroke, 1003
Single-positive thymocyte, 1113
Single transmembrane segment receptor, 1710
Sinoatrial block, 153-154, 155
Sinoatrial node, 83, 131
Sinopulmonary-infertility syndrome, 1845
Sinorhinitis
  Churg-Strauss syndrome, 465
  Wegener's granulomatosis, 467
Sinus arrest, 153, 155
  rapid eye movement sleep-related, 946
Sinus bradycardia, 153-154, 155
  myocardial infarction, 222
Sinus histiocytosis, 680
Sinus node artery, 131
Sinus of Valsalva
  aneurysm, 81
  fistula, 291
  Marfan syndrome, 299
Sinus ostia, 2308
Sinus tachycardia, 141
  dilated cardiomyopathy, 264
  increased automaticity, 132
  myocardial infarction, 223
  palpitations, 130
  response to carotid sinus massage or intravenous adenosine, 134
  restrictive cardiomyopathy, 270-271
Sinuses
  disorders, 2308-2309
  radiography, 1181-1182
Sinusitis, 1394-1395, 2308-2309
  acquired immunodeficiency syndrome, 1478
  acute meningitis, 1407
  after lung transplantation, 520
  anaerobic infection, 1617

Sinusitis—cont'd
  antibiotic therapy, 1183
  complication of influenza, 1492
  cystic fibrosis, 482
  endotracheal tube infection, 416
  epidural abscess and, 1418
  facial pain, 962
  Haemophilus influenzae, 1588
  nosocomial, 1480
  subdural empyema and, 1416-1417
  Wegener's granulomatosis, 467
Sipple's syndrome, 1829
Sister Mary Joseph's nodule, 1316
Sitophobia, 2029
Situs inversus, 291
Sixth-nerve palsy, 1062
Sjögren syndrome, 1209-1212
  anti-Ro antibody, 1291
  autoantibodies, 1155
  Fanconi's syndrome, 882
  inflammatory myopathies, 1236
  interstitial lung disease, 453
  neurologic manifestations, 1095
  renal involvement, 891
  systemic sclerosis, 1230
Skeletal dysplasia, 1286-1290
Skeletal muscle
  ammonia metabolism, 2142-2143
  effects of fasting, 1852
  electrolyte content of intracellular water, 736
  hypokalemia, 829
  hypophosphatemia, 1936
  inflammatory myopathies, 1234-1237
  leptospirosis, 1645
  muscle phosphorylase deficiency, 1882
  polymyositis, 1234
    autoantibodies, 1143, 1155
    heart disease, 1087
    neurologic manifestations, 1092
    weakness, 1754
  Pompe's disease, 1881
  potassium, 825
  systemic sclerosis, 1229
Skeletal tuberculosis, 1437, 1634, 1635
Skeleton
  actinomycosis, 1665
  biochemical markers of bone turnover, 1746
  brucellosis, 1605-1606
  chronic renal failure, 785-786
  congenital total lipodystrophy, 1900
  diagnostic approach, 1744-1748
  effects of hormones, 1720
  fibrous dysplasia, 1960-1961
  functions, 1714-1715
  hyperparathyroidism, 1965-1971
    arthropathy, 1246
    calcium pyrophosphate dihydrate deposition disease, 1279
    chronic renal failure, 785
    diagnosis, 1967-1969
    humoral hypercalcemia of malignancy *versus,* 1973-1974
    hypermagnesemia, 1943
    kidney stone formation, 798
    mixed uremic osteodystrophy, 1963
    osteomalacia, 1950
    pathology and etiology, 1965-1966
    during pregnancy, 2273
    prevalence, 1965, 1966
    renal osteodystrophy, 1961
    renal transplant recipient, 795
    renal wasting of phosphate, 1935
    symptoms and signs, 1966-1967
    treatment, 1969-1971
  imaging evaluation of arthritis, 1164-1171, 1172
  metastatic disease, 1971-1974
  natural history, 1715-1716
  nephrotic syndrome, 767
  nontuberculous mycobacterial infection, 1639

Skeleton—cont'd
  osteomalacia, 1949-1955
    after parathyroidectomy, 1965
    bone biopsy, 1747
    chronic hypophosphatemia, 1936
    chronic renal failure, 785
    proximal renal tubular acidosis, 837
    renal osteodystrophy, 1961
    vitamin D deficiency, 2106
    vitamin D metabolism, 1719
    X-linked hypophosphatemic rickets, 880
  osteopetrosis, 1958-1959
  osteoporosis, 1944-1949
    bone biopsy, 1747
    brucellosis, 1606
    calcitonin therapy, 1719
    glucocorticoid-induced, 1263
    heparin, 635
    menopause, 2271
    multiple myeloma, 864
    reduction in bone density, 1165
    rheumatoid arthritis, 1205
  Paget's disease, 1955-1958
  primary hyperparathyroidism, 1966
  renal osteodystrophy, 1961-1965
  Staphylococcus aureus, 1549
  syphilis, 1641
  tuberculosis, 1634, 1635
Skew deviation, 1063
Skin, 1290-1332
  acanthosis nigricans, 1316, Plate VII-17
    congenital total lipodystrophy, 1900
    diabetic patient, 1323
    gastric cancer, 2046
    insulin resistance, 1862
    lipodystrophy, 1901
  acanthosis palmaris, 1319
  adrenergic responses, 1828
  allergic granulomatosis, 1220
  anaphylaxis, 1193
  barrier to infection, 1335
  biopsy, 1298
  candidal infection, 1661-1662
  coumarin-induced necrosis, 636
  cutaneous anergy, 1150-1151
  dermatitis, 1302-1304
    biotin deficiency, 2107
    glucagonoma, 2244
    herpetiformis, 1296-1297
    niacin deficiency, 2107
    Pityrosporum, 1309-1310
    stasis, 312
  drug reactions, 1312-1316
  endocrine disorders, 1322-1324
  extracellular fluid volume contraction, 824
  features of malabsorption, 2058
  febrile compromised patient, 1388
  gastrointestinal disease, 1320-1322
  hypothyroidism, 1809
  infection, 1419-1425
  jaundice, 2147
  leishmaniasis, 1685-1687
  livedo reticularis, 310
  malignancy, 1297-1298
    cutaneous T-cell lymphoma, 1331-1332
    immunosuppression-related, 795
    internal, 1316-1320
    Kaposi's sarcoma, 1330-1331
    melanoma, 1298-1300
  niacin deficiency, 2107
  normal flora, 1614, 1615
  nosocomial infection, 1480
  rash
    chickenpox, 1525
    Colorado tick fever, 1512
    dengue fever, 1465
    dermatomyositis, 1235
    differential diagnostic value, 1384-1385
    disseminated gonococcal infection, 1583
    drug-induced, 1313-1314
    fever with, 1380-1386

Skin—cont'd
  rash—cont'd
    glucagonoma, 2245
    graft-*versus*-host disease, 578
    Hartnup disease, 879, 1910, 1911
    hookworm, 1698
    hypersensitivity vasculitis, 1221
    Lassa fever, 1510
    lymphomatoid granulomatosis, 470
    meningococcal infection, 1406
    meningococcemia, 1579
    myxoma, 330
    parvovirus B19 infection, 1513
    photodermatosis, 1306-1307
    relapsing fever, 1645
    Rocky Mountain spotted fever, 1543
    rubella, 1501
    scarlet fever, 1421
    syphilis, 1641
    toxic shock syndrome, 1421
    typhoid fever, 1601
    vasculitis, 1225
    VIPoma, 2245
  riboflavin deficiency, 2106
  sodium loss through, 823
  spinal cord injury, 1051
  staphylococcal infection, 1549
  systemic sclerosis, 1228-1229
  thyrotoxicosis, 1804
  vitamin A deficiency, 2105
  vitamin D synthesis, 1719
Skin antibody, 1158
Skin bioelectric recordings, 938
Skin lesion
  acne vulgaris, 1304-1306
  anaerobic bacterial infection, 1618
  bejel, 1644
  blastomycosis, Plate VIII-48
  bullous diseases, 1293-1297
  bullous impetigo, 1419
  celiac sprue, 2063
  chromoblastomycosis and mycetoma,
    1659-1660
  clostridial infection, 1575-1576
  coccidioidomycosis, 1656
  connective tissue disease, 1290-1293
  cutis laxa, 1289
  diabetic dermopathy, 1873
  disseminated gonococcal infection, Plate
    VIII-22
  ecthyma, 1420
  Ehlers-Danlos syndrome, 1287-1288
  endocarditis, 227
  eosinophilic fasciitis, 1233
  Fabry's disease, 1918-1919
  fibrous dysplasia, 1960
  furuncles and carbuncles, 1421
  gram-negative bacteremia, 1449-1450
  hand-foot-mouth syndrome, 1489
  human immunodeficiency virus, 1325-1329
  hypersensitivity vasculitis, 1221
  impetigo contagiosa, 1556
  Kaposi's sarcoma, Plate VIII-38
  leprosy, 1649, 1650
  lupus erythematosus, 1290-1292
  lymphogranuloma venereum, 1535
  meningococcemia, Plate VIII-21
  mycosis fungoides, 1331-1332
  necrotizing fasciitis, 1422
  onchocerciasis, 1701
  pellagra, 1101
  photodermatoses, 1306-1307
  pinta, 1644
  porphyrias, 1925
  Pseudomonas aeruginosa, Plate VIII-23
  pseudoxanthoma elasticum, 1289
  psoriasis, 1300-1302, Plate VII-9
    human immunodeficiency virus infection,
      1325-1326
    intraarticular bone ankylosis, 1166-1167
  Rocky Mountain spotted fever, Plate VIII-18

Skin lesion—cont'd
  sarcoidosis, 458, 1324-1325
  sexually transmitted infection, 1444
  Sézary's syndrome, 1331-1332
  Sjögren syndrome, 1210
  sporotrichosis, 1658, Plate VIII-24
  staphylococcal scalded-skin syndrome, 1421
  superficial fungal infections, 1307-1312
    candidiasis, 1310-1312
    clinical presentation, 1308-1309
    dermatophyte infection, 1307-1308
    diagnostic procedures, 1309
    Pityrosporum infection, 1309-1310
  synergistic nonclostridial anaerobic
    myonecrosis, 1424
  syphilis, 1640-1641
  tuberous sclerosis, 1922
  tularemia, 1607-1608
  yaws, 1644
Skin test
  Coccidioides immitis, 1657
  evaluation of cellular immune response,
    1150
  immediate hypersensitivity, 1153-1154
  infectious disease, 1374
  meningitis, 1409
  nutritional assessment, 2111
  rhinitis, 1182
  skeletal tuberculosis, 1437
  solitary pulmonary nodule, 494
  tuberculin, 1629-1630
Skull
  barrier to infection, 1335
  fracture, 1043, 1045
    acute meningitis, 1407
  osteopetrosis, 1958
  Paget's disease, 1955, 1956
  radiograph, 924
SLE; *see* Systemic lupus erythematosus
Sleep
  breathing during, 354-355
  chronic fatigue, 2298
  disturbance in heart failure, 164
  hormone release during, 1713
  menopause, 2270
  normal, 525
  paroxysmal nocturnal dyspnea, 164
  physiology, 939-940
Sleep apnea, 354-355, 402
Sleep architecture, 939
Sleep bruxism, 946
Sleep-disordered breathing events, 524
Sleep disorders, 939-947
  chronic obstructive pulmonary disease,
    445-446
  chronic renal failure, 784
  dyssomnias, 940-945
  medical and psychiatric disorders, 946-947
  parasomnias, 945-946
  respiratory disorders, 524-528
Sleep efficiency, 939
Sleep enuresis, 946
Sleep history, 526
Sleep onset association disorder, 944
Sleep paralysis, 942, 946
Sleep-related epileptic seizure, 947
Sleep starts, 946
Sleep state misperception, 942
Sleep studies, 380
Sleep terrors, 946
Sleep-wake transition disorders, 946
Sleepwalking, 945-946
Slit diaphragms, 760
Slot blot, 2174
Slow-channel syndrome, 1023
Slow-reacting substance of anaphylaxis, 1140,
  1141
Slow ventricular tachycardia, 149
Slow wave, 906, 907, 1976
Slow wave sleep, 939
Small airways disease, 450

Small bowel biopsy
  celiac sprue, 2063
  eosinophilic enteritis, 2067
  small bowel malabsorption, 2058
  tropical sprue, 2065
  upper gastrointestinal endoscopy, 1995
Small bowel enema, 2081
Small cell lung cancer, 487, 726-729
  curability with chemotherapy, 552
  paraneoplastic syndromes, 488
Small cell renal carcinoma, 899
Small-fiber neuropathy, 1018
Small intestine
  absorption diseases, 2056-2068
    abetalipoproteinemia, 2067
    bacterial overgrowth, 2060-2062
    carbohydrate intolerance, 2067-2068
    celiac sprue, 2062-2063
    clinical features, 2057-2058
    digestion process, 2056-2057
    eosinophilic gastroenteritis, 2066-2067
    hypogammaglobulinemia, 2067
    intestinal lymphangiectasia, 2067
    laboratory findings, 2058-2060
    pancreatic and hepatobiliary diseases, 2062
    radiation enteropathy, 2065-2066
    short bowel syndrome, 2066
    tropical sprue, 2065
    Whipple's disease, 2064-2065
  bile salts reabsorption, 2125
  evaluation, 2004-2008
  infarction, 2087-2088
  intestinal obstruction, 2077-2079
  intestinal pseudoobstruction, 2079
  movement of food, 1979-1980
  normal microflora, 1615
  peritonitis, 2079-2080, 2247-2249
    abdominal evaluation, 2032
    acquired immunodeficiency syndrome, 1476
    anaerobic bacteria, 1617
    candidal, 1661
    dialysis-related, 791
    paralytic ileus, 2078
    primary, 1396
    systemic lupus erythematosus, 1214
  secondary intraperitoneal infection, 1396
  tumor, 2080-2081
Small lymphocyte, 594, 595
Small nuclear ribonuclear particles, 1159
Smear, 556-557, 1370, 1371
  blood
    abnormal red blood cell indices in
      nonanemic patient, 588
    acute nephritic syndrome, 764
    cold agglutinin disease, 670
    iron deficiency, 643
    left shift on, 591
    malaria, 1674
    multiple myeloma, 701
    neutropenia, 593
    overproduction jaundice, 2152
    thrombocytopenia, 613
  illness in returned traveler, 1469
  Tzanck, 1371
    herpes simplex virus, 1524
    herpesvirus infection, 1439
    impetigo, 1419
    molluscum contagiosum, 1327-1328
Smoke detector, 2266
Smokers Anonymous, 2296
Smoking
  alcohol-tobacco amblyopia, 1081
  alcoholic pancreatitis, 2238
  asthma, 1189
  cancer
    bladder, 868
    deaths, 550
    esophageal, 2023
    lung, 486, 725
    pancreatic, 2242

Smoking—cont'd
cancer—cont'd
squamous cell carcinoma of upper
aerodigestive tract, 722
chest pain, 126
chronic obstructive pulmonary disease, 438
chronic occlusive arterial disease, 308
coronary artery disease, 200
diabetic, 1869
in women, 2271
development of chronic cough, 407
evaluation of respiratory disease, 401-402
inflammatory bowel disease, 2069
Langerhans' cell granulomatosis, 463
polycythemia, 588, 589
premature ventricular contractions, 149
Smoking cessation
chronic obstructive pulmonary disease, 443
peripheral arterial disease, 308
prevention of lung cancer, 491
pulmonary rehabilitation, 434
Smoldering multiple myeloma, 701, 703
Smooth muscle
alimentary tract, 1976
alveolar interstitial space, 371
contraction, 1976
effects of vasopressin, 1791
vascular
modulation of arterial tone, 47
pulmonary vessels, 360
Smooth muscle antibody, 1157, 2200
hepatobiliary disease, 2139
primary biliary cirrhosis, 2200
type 1 autoimmune hepatitis, 2183
Smooth muscle-reactive mediators, 1140
Snail-borne fluke, 1698
Snake bite, 668
Sneddon's syndrome, 1292
Sneezing, common cold, 1391
Snoring, 2309
Socioeconomic factors
chronic obstructive pulmonary disease, 438
nutritional status in elderly, 2287
obesity, 2103
Sodium
aging and, 2284
aldosterone secretion modulation, 1818
bile water production, 2123
body water compartments, 736
diabetes insipidus, 1794-1795
extrarenal depletion, 823
functions, 2109
heart failure, 162-163, 169
hepatic uptake and secretion of bile salts, 2125
hypernatremia, 748, 813-816
hypertension, 316-319
hypertonic hyponatremia, 810
clinical manifestations, 811
treatment, 812, 813
hypervolemic hypernatremia, 814
hyponatremia, 809-813, 1079
acute intermittent porphyria, 1926
acute renal failure, 773
after stroke, 1007
cirrhotic patient with ascites, 2165
congestive heart failure, 817-818
disorders of urinary dilution, 748
heart failure, 172
hypokalemia and, 830
Legionnaire's disease, 1623
malaria, 1674
meningitis, 1406
metabolic encephalopathy, 1079
Rocky Mountain spotted fever, 1544
ileal bile salt transport, 2125
intestinal absorption, 1988
mineralocorticoid deficiency, 1824
parenteral solutions, 2114
reabsorption
ascites formation, 2163
glomerular filtration rate, 738

Sodium—cont'd
recommended daily dietary allowances, 2116
renal depletion, 823-825
replacement in diabetic ketoacidosis, 1864
secretion of conjugated bilirubin into bile,
2149
storage in bone, 1715
total parenteral nutrition formula, 2117
vasopressin stimulation, 1789
Sodium balance, 737-739
disorders, 816-825
cirrhosis, 818-820
congestive heart failure, 817-818
edematous states, 816-817
extrarenal sodium depletion, 823
idiopathic edema, 821
nephrotic syndrome, 820-821
salt-wasting states, 823
sodium depletion of renal origin, 823-825
use of diuretics, 821-823
fractional excretion of sodium, 747
Sodium benzoate, 2162
Sodium bicarbonate
acute renal failure, 774
cystine stones, 804
hyperkalemia therapy, 833
lactic acidosis, 1867
rhabdomyolysis, 775
Sodium bicarbonaturia, 2028
Sodium-calcium exchanger pump, 58
cardiac conduction, 38
cellular modulation of contractility, 40
Sodium channels, 59
Sodium chloride, 737
Sodium cromoglycate, 482
Sodium diatrizoate, 1740
Sodium fluoride, 1948
Sodium-glucose transporters, 878-879
Sodium intake
ascites formation, 818
chronic renal failure, 778
extracellular fluid volume, 737
heart failure, 169
hypercalciuria, 798
hypertension, 318-319
Sodium nitroprusside
dilated cardiomyopathy, 264
heart failure, 173, 174
hypertensive emergency, 328
myocardial infarction, 218
pulmonary edema, 169
shock, 182
testing for diabetic ketoacidosis, 1863-1864
Sodium polystyrene sulfonate, 774, 833
Sodium potassium-activated adenosine
triphosphatase, 58, 805
abnormalities of impulse formation, 132
cardiac contraction, 37-38
hypertension, 317-318
intestinal carbohydrate absorption, 1987
plasma potassium concentration, 825
secretion of conjugated bilirubin into bile, 2149
thyroid hormone formation and metabolism,
1797
water and iron absorption, 1988
Sodium restriction
acute renal failure, 774
ascites, 2165
autosomal dominant polycystic kidney disease,
873
chronic renal failure, 787
cirrhotic patient, 820
hypertension, 324
hypertension management, 324
hypokalemia, 830
kidney stones, 800
nephrotic syndrome, 767
thiazide treatment program, 803
Sodium retention
aortic regurgitation, 241
chronic renal failure, 778

Sodium retention—cont'd
congestive heart failure, 817
edema, 816
hypertension, 316-317, 318
toxicity of nonsteroidal antiinflammatory
drugs, 870
Sodium stibogluconate, 1687
Sodium-taurocholate cotransporting polypeptide,
2126
Soft palate
erythroplakia, Plate IV-13
herpangina, 1488
rubella, 1501
Soft tissue infection
anaerobic bacteria, 1618
enterococcal, 1562
necrotizing, 1422-1425
nontuberculous mycobacterial, 1639
nosocomial, 1480
Pasteurella, 1609
Streptococcus pyogenes, 1556-1557
Sokolow-Lyon criteria, 87
Solar urticaria, 1306-1307
Soldier's heart, 131
Solitary cyst
hepatic, 2211
renal, 871-872
Solitary myeloma, 703
Solitary plasmacytoma of bone, 703
Solitary pulmonary nodule, 493-497
computed tomography, 386
Dirofilaria immitis granulomatous vasculitis,
469
Solitary ulcer syndrome, 2093
Soluble mucin, 1984
Solute concentration, osmoregulation, 805-806
Solute diuresis, 1793, 1794
SOLVD; *see* Studies of Left Ventricular
Dysfunction
Solvent/detergent method of viral inactivation of
fresh frozen plasma, 573
Somatic mutation, 1111, 2283
Somatic mutator phenotype, 549
Somatic pain, 2030
Somatization, 1040
Somatomedin C, 1716, 1720
Somatosensory evoked responses, 912-914
low back pain, 966
neck pain, 969
Somatostatin
gastrin inhibition, 1982
tests, 1743
variceal bleeding, 2167
Somatostatin analog, 1785
Somatostatinoma, 2245-2246
Somatotroph cell, 1773, 1774
Somogyi phenomenon, 1861
Sonde enteroscopy, 1995
Sorbitol, 812, 861
Sore throat, 1392-1393
acute pharyngitis, 1392
chronic fatigue, 2298
common cold, 1391
epidemic pleurodynia, 1489
hand-foot-mouth syndrome, 1489
herpangina, 1488-1489
infectious mononucleosis, 1529
influenza, 1490
Lassa fever, 1510
Mycoplasma pneumoniae pneumonia, 1539
peritonsillar abscess, 2306
rheumatic fever, 1256
scarlet fever, 1421
spontaneous pneumomediastinum, 514
subacute thyroiditis, 1811
supraglotitis, 2306
Sotalol, 138
hypertrophic obstructive cardiomyopathy, 269
properties, 203
South African tick bite fever, 1545
Southeast Asian ovalocytosis, 666

Southern blot, 52, 560-561, 1722-1723
  non-Hodgkin's lymphoma, 696
Southwestern blot, 52
SP-40,40, 1135
SPAF study, 134
Spasm
  bronchospasm, 2082
    asthma, 1187, 1188
    beta-adrenergic blocker-induced, 202
    dobutamine stress imaging, 104
    drug-induced, 476, 477
    mitomycin toxicity, 478
    sinusitis, 2308
    wheezing with, 404
  carpal, 1933
  coronary
    after revascularization surgery, 207
    amrinone, 182
    angioplasty-induced, 122
    coronary arteriography, 200
    myocardial infarction, 209
    variant angina, 194
  cricopharyngeal, 2015
  esophageal, 2022-2023
  laryngospasm
    hypocalcemia, 1933
    sleep-related, 947
  muscle
    headache associated with, 958
    peritonitis, 1398
    tetanus, 1573-1574
Spasmodic torticollis, 996
Spastic contractions, 1977
Spastic dysarthria, 977
Spastic paraparesis, 2161
Spasticity, 997
  after spinal cord injury, 1051
  Crigler-Najjar syndrome, 2153
  hepatic encephalopathy, 2160, 2161
  neurorehabilitation, 1055
Specialized columnar epithelium, 2016
Specific gravity of urine, 742
Specificity, 6-7, 1734
Specimen collection and handling
  anaerobic culture, 1619
  bacteria, 1367
  complement assay, 1147
  virus, 1369-1370
Spectinomycin, 1356, 1585
Spectrin, 59, 664
Speech
  disorders, 975-978
  echolalia, 976, 977
  neurologic examination, 902
  therapy for stroke patient, 1054-1055
Sperm, semen analysis, 1742
Spermatogenesis, 1839
  chemotherapy, 585
  disorders affecting, 1844-1846
Spermatogonia, 1839
Sphenoid sinus, 1773
Sphenoidal sinusitis, 1414
Spherocyte
  anemia, 587
  hemolytic disease, 662
  hereditary spherocytosis, 664-666
Spherocytosis
  cold agglutinin disease, 670
  hereditary, 664-666
Sphincter, urodynamic testing, 938
Sphincter of Oddi
  ductal cholestasis, 2155
  gallbladder, 2233
  gallstones, 2224
  movement of food, 1980
Sphincterotomy
  choledocholithiasis, 2229
  gallbladder, 2233
Sphingolipids, 1917
Sphingomyelinase deficiency, 1918
Sphygmomanometer, 64

Spider bite, 668
Spike potentials, 1976
Spike wave, 906, 907
Spinal accessory nerve mononeuropathy, 1017
Spinal anesthesia, 2257
Spinal canal, 924
Spinal cord
  lower-limb somatosensory evoked potentials,
    914
  multiple myeloma, 700
  multiple sclerosis, 1008
  myelitis, 1011
  myelodysplasia, 611, 675-676, 690-691
  myelography, 924, 926, 1012
  myelopathy, 1011-1014
    complication of chemotherapy, 1072
    human T-cell leukemia virus-associated,
      1532
    tropical spastic paraparesis, 1532
  subacute combined degeneration, 1080
Spinal cord compression, 1011-1012, 1071
Spinal cord injury, 1045-1053
  classification, 1046-1047
  epidemiology, 1046
  gallstone risk factor, 2223
  mass reflex of autonomic overactivity, 934
  rehabilitation, 1052-1053
  respiratory failure, 1097
  subacute management, 1049-1052
  syndromes, 1047-1049
Spinal epidural abscess, 1418-1419
Spinal fluid examination, 904-905
Spinal meningitis, 1578
Spinal radiography, 966
Spinal root signs and symptoms, 1016
Spinal shock, 1011-1012
  spinal cord injury, 1051
Spinal tumor, 1013
Spine
  computed tomography, 918, 920
  lung cancer metastasis, 489
  osteomalacia, 1950
  osteomyelitis, 1169
  Paget's disease, 1955
  plain film, 924
  rheumatoid arthritis, 1202
  spondylosis deformans, 1266
Spinhaler, 431
Spirochetes, 1640-1648
  Borrelia, 1645-1648
    identification, 1251
    Lyme disease, 1254
  leptospires, 1644-1645
  normal flora, 1614
  syphilis, 1640-1644
    acquired immunodeficiency syndrome, 2098
    anal fissure and fistula, 2093
    aortic disease, 303
    aortitis, 302
    granulomatous gastritis, 2043
    meningitis verus, 1409
    neuroarthropathy, 1168
    palmar lesions, Plate VIII-47
    penile chancre, Plate VIII-34
    during pregnancy, 2280
    secondary, Plate VIII-46
    transfusion-transmitted, 575, 576
Spirometry, 376-377
  asthma, 1189
  incentive, 429-430
  oxygen consumption, 109-110
Spironolactone
  ascites, 822, 2165
  heart failure, 170
  hirsutism, 1757
  hyperkalemia, 832
  hypertension, 325
  induction of gynecomastia, 2172
Spleen
  abscess, 1398-1399
  brucellosis, 1606

Spleen—cont'd
  Hodgkin's disease, 693
  humoral immunity, 1337-1338
  hypersplenism, 601-602
    hemolysis, 668
    neutropenia, 593
    portal hypertension, 2165-2168
    thrombocytopenia, 614
  sickle cell disease, 657-658
  structure and function, 600
Splenectomy
  acute meningitis, 1407
  beta-thalassemia, 656
  gastric cancer, 2048
  hairy cell leukemia, 684
  hemolytic anemia, 667, 669
  hereditary spherocytosis, 665
  immune thrombocytopenic purpura, 616
  myelofibrosis, 677
  neutropenia, 679
  pyruvate kinase deficiency, 664
  risk of infection, 1338
Splenic artery, 2130
Splenic nodule, 531
Splenic vein
  obstruction, 2208
  transjugular intrahepatic shunt, 2167
Splenomegaly, 600-602
  amylo-1,6-glucosidase deficiency, 1882
  chronic myelogenous leukemia, 686-687
  hairy cell leukemia, 683
  hemolytic anemia, 661
  hereditary spherocytosis, 664
  idiopathic myelofibrosis, 677
  infective endocarditis, 228
  malaria, 667, 1673, 1674
  myelodysplastic syndrome, 676
  overproduction jaundice, 2152
  portal hypertension, 2165
  rheumatoid arthritis, 1205
  rubella, 1501
  thrombocytopenia, 614
Splinter hemorrhage, 228
Splitting of second heart sound, 72-73, 74
Spondylitis
  alkaptonuric, 1281
  ankylosing, 1238-1239
    aortitis, 303
    calcium pyrophosphate dihydrate deposition
      disease *versus,* 1279
    hypoventilation, 356
    interstitial lung disease, 453-454
    osteophytosis, 1170, 1171
    sacroiliac joint abnormalities, 1173
  brucellosis, 1606
  inflammatory bowel disease, 1246
Spondyloarthropathy, 1200, 1206, 1237-1242
Spondylosis, cervical, 925, 1012-1013
Spondylosis deformans, 1266
Spontaneous abortion
  chromosome abnormality, 1728
  inflammatory bowel disease, 2278
  lupus inhibitor, 629
  relapsing fever, 1645
  sickle cell disease, 659
Spontaneous bacterial peritonitis, 2164, 2198,
    2248
Spontaneous nystagmus, 973-974
Spontaneous pneumomediastinum, 513-514
Spontaneous pneumothorax, 128-129, 509
Spontaneous staphylococcal bacteremia, 1550
Spore-forming bacteria
  Clostridium, 1567-1576
    antibiotic selection, 1348
    bacteremia, 1576
    cellulitis, 1422
    food-borne, 1568-1570
    gas gangrene, 1422-1423
    gastrointestinal tract, 1567-1568
    hemolytic anemia, 667
    myonecrosis, 1574-1576

Spore-forming bacteria—cont'd
Clostridium—cont'd
neurologic syndromes, 1570-1572
normal flora, 1368
tetanus, 1572-1574
normal flora, 1614
Sporotrichosis, 1658
lymphangitic spread, Plate VIII-49
skin lesion, 1423, Plate VIII-24
Springwater cyst, 513
Spur cell anemia, 667
Spurious hyperkalemia, 830-831
Spurious hypokalemia, 826
Sputum examination, 380-381
acquired immunodeficiency syndrome, 1477
asthma, 1188
bronchiectasis, 484
chronic obstructive pulmonary disease, 443
diagnosis and staging of lung cancer, 489-490
Haemophilus influenzae, 1588
Legionnaire's disease, 1623
Mycobacterium tuberculosis, 1628
Pneumocystis carinii, 1694
solitary pulmonary nodule, 494
superior vena caval obstruction, 511
Sputum expectoration, 408
Squamous cell carcinoma, 1297-1298, Plate
VII-5
acquired immunodeficiency
syndrome-associated, 1329
esophageal, 2023-2024
head and neck, 2310
lung, 487
tongue, Plate IV-14
of unknown primary site, 730, 732
upper aerodigestive tract, 722-724
Squamous cell hyperplasia, 2016
Square root sign, 270
Src protooncogene, 1958
SS-A/Ro antigen, 1159
SS-B/La antigen, 1159
Stabilization
myocardial infarction, 212
shock, 180
Stable angina
coronary arteriography, 199-200
myocardial revascularization, 206
therapeutic approach, 207
Staghorn calculus, 755
Staging
breast cancer, 708-709
cervical cancer, 715
chronic hepatitis, 2180
endometrial cancer, 714
exocrine pancreatic tumor, 2242-2243
Hodgkin's disease, 694
lung cancer, 489-490, 725-726
melanoma, 1299
multiple myeloma, 701, 702
non-Hodgkin's lymphoma, 698
osteomyelitis, 1436-1437
ovarian cancer, 716
Stain, 1370, 1371
acid-fast, 1371
acute meningitis, 1408
leprosy, 1650
Mycobacterium avium complex, Plate
VIII-36
nocardiosis, 1665
acridine orange, 1371
carbolfuchsin, 1371
chromosome, 1727, 1728
ethidium bromide, 51
Giemsa, 1371
Borrelia, 1646
Chagas' disease, 1690
Chlamydia trachomatis, 1536, Plate VIII-11
fever and rash, 1385
Helicobacter pylori, 2003
leishmaniasis, 1685, 1687, Plate VIII-12
malaria, 1674

Stain—cont'd
Giemsa—cont'd
plague, 1610
Plasmodium falciparum, Plate VIII-14
Plasmodium vivax, Plate VIII-15
Pneumocystis carinii, 1693, Plate VIII-10
Trypanosoma brucei rhodesiense, Plate
VIII-16
Trypanosoma cruzi, Plate VIII-17
Gram, 1346, 1370, 1371
actinomycosis, 1665
anaerobic bacteria, 1619
anaerobic pneumonia, Plate VII-1
aspiration pneumonia, Plate VIII-7
bacterial meningitis, 1407, 1408
bullous impetigo, 1419
chronic bronchitis, 443
fever and rash, 1385
gas gangrene, 1423
gonococcal infection, 1584
gram-negative bacteremia, 1451
Haemophilus influenzae, 1588
impetigo, 1419
infectious esophagitis, 2020
infective endocarditis, 228
Legionella pneumophila, 1622
liver abscess, 2209
lymphangitis, 1420
meningococcal meningitis, Plate VIII-9
necrotizing fasciitis, 1422
plague, 1610
pneumococcus, Plate VIII-3
rectal mucosa, 1439
septic arthritis, 1251, 1252
synovial fluid, 1163
tularemia, 1608
urethral discharge, 1440
Kinyoun
cryptosporidia, 1476, 1680, Plate VIII-32
procedure, 1371
methylene blue, 1603
periodic acid-Schiff
Cryptosporidium oocyst, Plate VIII-33
pulmonary alveolar proteinosis, 455
Whipple's disease, 2064, 2065
Prussian blue, 558
iron in normal bone marrow, Plate IV-9
ringed sideroblast, Plate IV-11
septic arthritis, 1251-1252
silver methenamine, 2020
Sudan black, 481-482
trichome, *Entamoeba histolytica,* Plate VIII-52
Wright, 1371
CFU-GEMM, Plate IV-2
fever and rash, 1385
granulocyte, Plate IV-6
hemolytic anemia, 661, 662
leishmaniasis, 1687
lymphocyte, Plate IV-5
plague, 1610
Ziehl-Neelsen, 1371
cryptosporidiosis, 1680
Cryptosporidium oocyst, Plate VIII-33
Mycobacterium leprae, 1650-1651
septic arthritis, 1252
synovial fluid, 1163
Standard arm circumference, 2111
Standard arm muscle circumference, 2111
Standard triceps skinfold, 2111
Standards of Practice Committee of American
Sleep Disorders Association, 943
Standing position
heart rate response, 937
nonejection sounds, 76
Stanford classification of aortic dissection, 301
Staphylococcal coagglutination, 1408
Staphylococcal scalded-skin syndrome, 1384,
1421, 1549, Plate VIII-29
Staphylococcal toxic shock syndrome,
1421-1422, 1549

Staphylococcus, 1546-1553, Plate VIII-4
characteristics, 1547
coagulase-negative, 1550-1551
epidemiology, 1547-1548
fever and rash, 1382
mycotic aortic aneurysm, 299
normal flora, 1368
pathophysiology, 1548
pericarditis, 272
prevention, 1553
treatment, 1551-1553
urinary tract infection, 1457
Staphylococcus aureus, 1546
acquired immunodeficiency syndrome,
1328-1329
antibiotic selection, 1347
antimicrobial resistance, 1345
brain abscess, 1414
bullous impetigo, 1419
cellulitis, 1420
compromised host, 1388
cystic fibrosis airway infection, 480
dermatitis with, 1303
diseases produced by, 1548-1550
empyema, 507
endocarditis, 226
epidemiology, 1547-1548
erysipelas, 1420
folliculitis, 1420
food-borne diarrhea, 1430
furuncles and carbuncles, 1421
impetigo, 1419
infective endocarditis, 226
lung recipient, 517
lymphangitis, 1420
nosocomial infections, 1362
osteomyelitis, 1433
pancreatic abscess, 1399
polyarticular septic arthritis, 1251
respiratory tract infection, 1390
sialolithiasis, 2310
sinusitis, 1394, 2308
splenic abscess, 1398
staphylococcal scalded-skin syndrome, 1421
urinary tract infection, 1457
Staphylococcus epidermidis, 1546
antibiotic selection, 1347
bacterial meningitis, 1403
epidemiology, 1548
nosocomial infections, 1362
prosthetic valve endocarditis, 230, 1550-1551
septic arthritis, 1251
Starch, 1987
enzymatic hydrolysis, 2121
Starch granulomatous vasculitis, 470
Starling forces
ascites, 818
edema, 816
exchange of fluid between plasma and
interstitial compartments, 737
pulmonary edema, 168, 424
Starr-Edwards ball valve, 259-260
Starvation, 2101
hepatic ketogenesis, 1852-1853
hepatic maintenance of blood glucose levels,
2122
magnesium depletion, 1940
negative phosphate balance, 1935
Starvation ketosis, 743
Stasis
cholestasis
benign strictures of extrahepatic bile ducts,
2232
determination of blockage site, 2156
estrogen-related, 2158
during pregnancy, 2277
secondary hepatocellular injury, 2155
serum alkaline phosphatase level, 2137
steroid-induced, 2123
chronic venous insufficiency, 312
elderly, 2288

Stasis—cont'd
  gastric, 1979
  varicose veins, 311
STAT proteins, 1131
Static compliance, 347
  ventilated patient, 399
Statins, 1891
  gallstone risk factor, 2223
  hypercholesterolemia, 1894
  hyperlipidemia, 200
  interference with oral anticoagulants, 636
  myocardial infarction, 218
  nephrotic syndrome, 767
  secondary hypertriglyceridemia, 1895
  typical medical regimen six months after
    transplantation, 343
Stationary cycling, 436
Status epilepticus, 1085
Status migrainosus, 962
Stavudine, 1474
STD; *see* Sexually transmitted disease
Stearic acid, 1883
Steatohepatitis, 2196-2197
Steatorrhea
  alpha heavy-chain disease, 704
  chronic pancreatitis, 2239
  Crohn's disease, 2069
  diabetic, 1749
  hepatocellular *versus* cholestatic jaundice,
    2156
  intestinal lymphangiectasia, 2067
  malabsorption, 2057
  pancreatic cancer, 2242
  somatostatinoma, 2245
  stool examination, 2006
  tropical sprue, 2065
Steatosis, 2187
Steel mouse, 534
Steele-Richardson-Olszewski syndrome, 992
Steinert disease, 62
Stem cell, 530-531, Plate IV-2
  assay, 531
  neoplasms, 686-689
  transplantation, 576-579, 702
Stem cell factor, 1128, 1129
Stenosis
  aortic, 235-239, 287
    angina, 127
    aortitis, 302
    cardiac auscultation, 68
    cardiac catheterization, 113
    chronic, 304
    congenital, 287
    differential diagnosis, 180
    mesenteric vascular disease, 2086
    murmur, 79-80
    pandiastolic murmur, 79-80
    pulsus bisferiens, 65
    second heart sound, 72
  continuous-wave Doppler echocardiography,
    99
  mitral, 245-249
    cardiac catheterization, 114-115
    diastolic filling murmur, 78, 80
    operative risk, 2260
    during pregnancy, 2276
    pulmonary hypertension, 298
    pulsed-Doppler echocardiography, 99
    weakness, 1755
  pulmonary artery, 81
  pulmonic, 256
    with intact ventricular septum, 288
    systolic murmur, 266
  pyloric, 2044
  renal artery, 755, 756
    continuous murmur, 81
    neurofibromatosis, 1921
    renovascular hypertension, 893-894
  restenosis, 122-124
  single photon emission computed tomography,
    101

Stenosis—cont'd
  subclavian, 1005
  thallium-201 imaging, 101
  tricuspid, 78, 255-256, 1755
  valve orifice size, 111
Stensen's duct
  mumps, 1496
  Sjögren syndrome, 1209
Stent
  biliary, 2243
  coronary, 119-120
Stent Restenosis Study, 119
Stereotactic needle aspiration of brain abscess,
    1416
Stereotactic radiosurgery
  brain tumor, 1069
  neurologic complications, 1073
Stereotyped patterns, 981
Sterile pyuria, 744
Sterilization, surgical, 2269-2270
Sternal osteomyelitis, 1551
11-β-Steroid dehydrogenase, 1819
Steroid hormones
  degradation, 1714
  metabolism, 2122
  nuclear and cytoplasmic receptors, 1712
  synthesis, 1709-1710
Steroid-induced cholestasis, 2188
Steroid suppression test, 1746
Steroids
  acute interstitial nephritis, 889
  acute lung allograft rejection, 521
  anabolic
    hepatic injury, 2190, 2191
    interference with oral anticoagulants, 636
  antibody-mediated insulin resistance, 1861
  antiphospholipid syndrome, 1292
  asthma, 1192
  autoimmune hepatitis, 2184
  bacterial meningitis, 1412-1413
  brain abscess, 1416
  breast cancer, 709
  bronchiolitis obliterans syndrome, 523
  bullous pemphigoid, 1296
  cancer pain, 580
  chemotherapy-induced nausea and vomiting,
    582
  chronic lymphocytic leukemia, 685
  chronic obstructive pulmonary disease, 418,
    434, 444
  chronic rhinitis, 2308
  chronic sinusitis, 2309
  Churg-Strauss syndrome, 467
  cluster headache prophylaxis, 962
  crescentic glomerulonephritis, 848
  Crohn's disease, 2071
  Cushing's syndrome, 1821
  cutaneous lesions in lupus erythematosus,
    1291-1292
  cystic fibrosis, 482
  dermatitis, 1303
  dermatomyositis, 1292
  drug-induced thrombocytopenia, 615
  eosinophilic fasciitis, 1234
  Epstein-Barr virus infection, 1529
  focal glomerular sclerosis, 852
  Goodpasture's syndrome, 847
  gout, 1274
  hirsutism, 1756
  Hodgkin's disease, 694-695
  human cytochrome P450 isoforms, 2312
  hypersensitivity pneumonitis, 462
  hypopituitarism treatment, 1779-1780, 1781
  immune hemolytic anemia, 669
  immune thrombocytopenic purpura, 616
  interstitial lung disease, 451
  lung transplantation, 516
  lupus nephritis, 857
  metastatic cancer, 1073
  minimal change disease, 851
  multiple myeloma, 702

Steroids—cont'd
  multiple sclerosis, 1010
  myasthenia gravis, 1022
  myelopathy, 1013
  nasal polyp, 1183
  for nausea and vomiting, 2027
  non-Hodgkin's lymphoma, 698-699
  optic neuritis, 1060
  ovarian, 1832
  pemphigus vulgaris, 1294
  pericardial heart disease, 278
  Pneumocystis carinii pneumonia, 1695
  prevention and therapy of rejection, 340
  reflex sympathetic dystrophy syndrome, 1247
  relapsing seronegative symmetric synovitis
    with pitting edema, 1243
  renal transplantation, 792
  restenosis, 124
  rheumatic fever, 1257
  rheumatoid arthritis, 1207
  sarcoidosis, 459
  before surgery, 2262
  systemic lupus erythematosus, 1216-1217
  temporal arteritis, 311
  thrombotic thrombocytopenic purpura, 615
  toxoplasmosis, 1678
  tropical spastic paraparesis, 1533
  tuberculous meningitis, 1412
  tuberculous pericarditis, 1637
  typical medical regimen six months after
    transplantation, 343
  ulcerative colitis, 2074
  Wegener's granulomatosis, 468, 858
Sterol carrier protein-2, 2127
Sterols, 1719
Stevens-Johnson syndrome, 1313, Plate VII-11
  nongonococcal urethritis, 1441
  vesicular lesions, 1384
Stiff-man syndrome, 996
Stimulant-dependent sleep disorder, 945
Stimulated acid output, 2003
Stimulation tests, 1732
  adrenocorticotropic hormone, 1741
  testis, 1840-1841
  thyroid-stimulating hormone, 1739
Stimulus-control therapy, 942
Stimulus-secretion coupling, 1713
Sting, 668
Stinging insect hypersensitivity, 1194
Stochastic hypothesis, 530
Stokes-Adams attacks, 62
Stokes-Adams-Moragni syndrome, 954
Stomach
  anatomic and functional regions, 1981
  biopsy, 2002
  cancer, 2045-2050, Plate X-3
    adenocarcinoma, 2039, 2045-2050
    carcinoid, 2082
    peptic ulcer disease *versus*, 2038
  drug interactions, 2310-2311
  endoscopic examination, 1994
  gastric acid, 1980-1985
    abnormalities of secretion, 1983-1984
    barrier to infection, 1335
    gastric cancer, 2046
    hypersecretory gastropathy, 2043
    measurement, 2002-2003
    regulation, 1981, 1982
    small bowel bacterial overgrowth, 2060
  gastric analysis, 2002-2003, 2038
  gastric atrophy, 2042
  gastric bezoar, 1979, 2044
  gastric biopsy, 2002
  gastric bypass, 1753, 1876
  gastric emptying, 1978-1979, 2003-2004
    anorexia nervosa, 2030
    gastroesophageal reflux, 2015
    gastroparesis, 2044
  gastric mucus, 1984
  gastric outlet obstruction, 2027, 2040
  gastric polyp, 2045-2046

Stomach—cont'd
  gastric reduction surgery, 2105
  gastric ulcer
    acid secretory values, 2003
    gastric biopsy and cytology, 2002
    upper gastrointestinal endoscopy, 1994
  gastric vagotomy, 2040-2041
  gastric varices, 2166
  gastritis, 2041-2044
    atrophic, 2045
    Helicobacter pylori, 1592-1593
    operative risk, 2263
  gastroenteritis, 1425-1432
    bacterial agents, 1425-1427
    coronavirus, 1502
    coronavirus infection, 1502
    diagnosis, 1430-1431
    diarrhea, 1429-1430
    eosinophilic, 2066-2067
    immunoglobulin A nephropathy, 845
    parasitic agents, 1428-1429
    pathophysiology, 1425
    prophylaxis for traveler's diarrhea, 1432
    rotavirus and Norwalk-like virus, 1519-1522
    Salmonella, 1599
    Staphylococcus aureus, 1548-1549
    treatment, 1431-1432
    Vibrio parahaemolyticus, 1596-1597
    viral agents, 1427-1428
  movement of food, 1978-1979
  normal microflora, 1615
  secondary intraperitoneal infection, 1396
  systemic sclerosis, 1229
  tumors, 2045-2050
  visualization, 2002
Stomatitis, 585
Stomatocyte, 662
Stomatocytosis, 665, 666
Stone clinic effect, 803
Stone disease
  biliary tract stones, 2220-2231
    asymptomatic *versus* symptomatic, 2225
    biliary colic, 2225-2227
    cholecystitis, 2227-2228
    choledocholithiasis, 2228-2230
    cholesterol stones, 2221, 2222
    cholesterolosis, 2230-2231
    classification and composition, 2220, 2221
    Crohn's disease, 2075
    defective bile salt synthesis, 2129
    diagnostic tests, 2224-2225
    epidemiology, 2222-2223
    gallstone pancreatitis, 2230
    hereditary spherocytosis, 665-666
    pathophysiology, 2220-2221
    pigment stones, 2221-2222
    during pregnancy, 2278
    risk factors, 2223-2224
    sickle cell disease, 657, 659
  pancreatic, 2238, 2239, 2240
  renal calculi, 796-805
    autosomal dominant polycystic kidney
      disease, 873
    calcium-containing stones, 797-799
    cystine stones, 799-800
    differential diagnosis, 800
    laboratory and diagnostic testing, 800, 801,
      802
    management, 803-805
    medullary sponge kidney, 875
    obstructive uropathy, 885
    physiology and pathophysiology, 797
    spinal cord injured patient, 1050
    struvite stones, 799
    uric acid stones, 799
    urine calcium, 1744
Stool examination
  acquired immunodeficiency syndrome, 1476
  cholera, 1595
  Clostridium difficile, 1569
  diarrhea, 1431, 2051

Stool examination—cont'd
  giardiasis, 1685
  illness in returned traveler, 1469
  intestinal disorders, 2006
  small bowel malabsorption, 2058-2059
Stop codon, 1722
Storage disorders
  amino acid, 1909-1910
  cholesterol esters, 1898
  glycogen, 1880-1882
  lysosomal, 1911-1920
    Chédiak-Higashi syndrome, 1919
    cystinosis, 1919
    drug-induced lysosomopathies, 1919
    general considerations, 1911-1912
    lipid storage diseases, 1917-1919
    lysosomal physiology, 1911
    mucolipidoses, 1915-1917
    mucopolysaccharidoses, 1912-1915
    treatment, 1919-1920
  monocyte-macrophage abnormalities, 680
  weakness, 1754
Storage pool disease, 611
Stoss treatment, 1954, 1955
Strain 19 vaccine, 1606
Strain pattern, 87
Strawberry gallbladder, 2231
Strawberry tongue
  Kawasaki disease, 1225, 1385
  scarlet fever, 1421
Streptococcal superantigen, 1555
Streptococcal toxic shock-like syndrome, 1384
Streptococcal toxic shock syndrome, 1421,
    1557-1558
Streptococcus
  acquired immunodeficiency syndrome,
    1328-1329
  acute interstitial nephritis, 890
  antibiotic selection, 1347
  brain abscess, 1414
  endocarditis, 226
  group B, 1564
  group C and G *pyogenes*-like, 1564
  infectious gastritis, 2043
  mitral stenosis, 248
  mycotic aortic aneurysm, 299
  nonenterococcal group D, 1564
  normal flora, 1368
  pericarditis, 272
  pharyngitis, 1391-1392
  poststreptococcal glomerulonephritis, 843
  prosthetic valve endocarditis, 230
  respiratory tract infection, 1390
  rheumatic fever, 1256
  Streptococcus intermedius group, 1564
Streptococcus agalactiae, 1433, 1564
Streptococcus bovis, 1564
Streptococcus intermedius group, 1564
Streptococcus pneumoniae
  acquired immunodeficiency syndrome, 1477
  bacterial meningitis, 1402-1403
  chronic bronchitis, 443
  complement deficiency, 1339
  empyema, 507
  lung recipient, 517
  normal flora, 1368
  primary peritonitis, 1396
  respiratory tract infection, 1390
  sickle cell disease, 658
  sinusitis, 1183, 1394, 2308
  spinal epidural abscess, 1418
Streptococcus pyogenes, 1553-1560
  cell structure and extracellular products,
    1554-1556
  cellulitis, 1420
  epidemiology, 1553-1554
  gangrene, Plate VIII-30
  impetigo, 1419
  osteomyelitis, 1433
  peritonsillar abscess, 2306
  pharyngitis, 1392, 1556

Streptococcus pyogenes—cont'd
  poststreptococcal glomerulonephritis, 1559
  rheumatic fever, 1558-1559
  scarlet fever, 1556
  sinusitis, 1394
  soft-tissue infection, 1556-1557
  toxic shock syndrome, 1557-1558
  treatment, 1559-1560
Streptokinase
  activation of plasminogen to plasmin, 540
  cardiac catheterization in ischemic heart
    disease, 113
  deep venous thrombosis, 311
  myocardial infarction, 213
  pulmonary embolism, 503
  shock, 184, 185
  venous thromboembolism, 637
Streptolysin O, 1257, 1555
Streptomycin
  brucellosis, 1605
  effects on kidney, 868
  enterococci resistance, 1561
  glucose-6-phosphate dehydrogenase
    deficiency, 664
  Meniere's disease, 2307
  mycobacterial disease, 1631
  plague, 1610
  tularemia, 1608
  use during pregnancy, 2281
Streptozocin
  effects on kidney, 869
  nephrotoxicity, 584
Streptozotocin, 2243
Streptozyme test, 844
Stress
  amenorrhea, 1757
  angina, 195, 196
  effect on vasopressin release, 1791
  hypertension, 316
  hypogonadism, 1842
  increased catecholamines, 1828
  increased nutrient requirements, 2102
  irritable bowel syndrome, 2056
  long-term modulation of ventricular function,
    46
  neuroendocrinology, 1077
  neutrophilia, 590
  palpitations, 130
  premature ventricular contractions, 149
  skeletal growth, 1716
Stress incontinence, 2291
Stress polycythemia, 588
Stress radiograph, 1164
Stress-shortening-velocity relationships, 42
STRESS trial, 119, 124
Stretch receptor, 45
Striated-muscle antibody, 1157
Striatonigral degeneration, 935
Striatopallidal loop, 991
Stricture
  bile ducts, 2232-2233
    benign extrahepatic, 2232-2233
    primary sclerosing cholangitis, 2201, 2202
  esophageal, 1999-2000, 2018, 2019
    Barrett's esophagus, 2017
    midesophageal, 2017
    upper gastrointestinal endoscopy, 1994
  lye, 1999-2000
  post ischemic colon, 2088
  small bowel bacterial overgrowth, 2060
  ulcerative colitis, 2073
  ureteral, 885
  urethral, 885
Strictureplasty, 2072
Stridor
  croup, 1393
  diphtheria, 1566
  mediastinal abnormality, 511
  parainfluenza, 1494
  supraglotitis, 2306

Stroke, 997-1007
  amnesic syndrome, 1032
  atrial fibrillation, 146
  during cardiac catheterization, 108
  clinical separation of stroke subtypes, 1000-1002
  depression, 1036
  dizziness, 973
  embolism, 1006
  hemorrhagic, 997-998, 1006
  hypertension, 314, 315, 322-323
  ischemic, 998-1000
  laboratory diagnosis, 1002-1004
  parkinsonism, 993
  prevention, complications, and rehabilitation,
    1006-1007, 1054-1055
  respiratory rhythm abnormalities, 1098
  sickle cell disease, 659
  systemic lupus erythematosus, 1093
  thrombotic, 1004-1006
Stroke counts, 104
Stroke index, 110
Stroke Prevention and Atrial Fibrillation II trial,
  134, 640
Stroke volume, 110
  aortic regurgitation, 240
  atrial septal defect, 281
  echocardiography, 97
  ejection fraction, 112
  heart failure, 159
  mitral regurgitation, 250
  pulmonary artery catheterization, 391
Stroke volume index, 391
Stroke work, 112-113
Stroke work index, 110
Stromal cell layer, 531
Stromal cell tumor, 716
Strongyloides stercoralis, 1699, 1700
  acquired immunodeficiency syndrome, 2096
  acute meningitis, 1407
  compromised host, 1388
  diarrhea, 1476
  peritonitis, 2248
Structural protein of coagulation, 538
Structural rhinitis, 1181
Struma ovarii, 1807
Struvite stone, 799, 804
Studies of Left Ventricular Dysfunction,
  157-158, 170, 171
Subacromial bursitis, 1197
Subacute bacterial endocarditis, 844
Subacute combined degeneration, 1080
Subacute cutaneous lupus erythematosus, 1213,
  1291
Subacute sclerosing panencephalitis, 907
Subacute spinal cord compression syndrome, 1012
Subacute thyroiditis, 1807, 1811-1812
Subarachnoid hemorrhage, 1043
  computed tomography, 919
  endocardial hemorrhage with, 1087
  headache, 960
  hemorrhagic stroke, 997
  temporary unconsciousness, 955
  traumatic lumbar puncture *versus,* 904-905
Subarachnoid space, 1405
Subchondral cyst formation, 1168
Subclavian artery
  aberrant right, 291
  aneurysm, 309
  auscultation, 306
  occlusive disease, 1005
Subclavian steal, 1005
Subclinical hypothyroidism, 1811
Subconjunctival hemorrhage, 2305
Subcostal approach in echocardiography, 95
Subcutaneous infection, 1419-1425
  chromoblastomycosis and mycetoma,
    1659-1660
  clostridial, 1575-1576
Subcutaneous nodule
  rheumatic fever, 1257
  sarcoidosis, 1324

Subdeltoid bursitis, 1197
Subdural abscess, 2309
Subdural empyema
  acute meningitis, 1407
  intracranial, 1416-1418
Subdural hematoma, 1043, 1044, 1045
  dementia, 988
  magnetic resonance imaging, 923
Subendothelial deposits, 842, 843
Subendothelium, platelet adhesion, 536
Suberosis, 460
Subluxation, atlantoaxial, 1171, 1172
Submucosa, colonic diverticulum, 2089
Submucosal bronchial glands, 365
Subperiosteal orbital abscess, 2309
Subphrenic abscess, 508
Subpleural blebs, 509
Subpleural emphysema, 439
Substance abuse, 2293-2297
  alcoholism, 2294-2296
    acute meningitis, 1407
    acute pancreatitis, 2233
    alcoholic ketosis, 1865
    carbon tetrachloride poisoning, 2188
    chronic pancreatitis, 2238
    cirrhosis, 2172
    diagnosis, 2197-2198
    hypomagnesemia, 1941
    hypophosphatemia, 1936
    niacin deficiency, 2107
    porphyria cutanea tarda, 1927
    thiamine deficiency, 2106
    weight loss, 1749
  candidiasis, 1661
  cellulitis, 1420
  cocaine, 2296-2297
  hepatitis A virus infection, 2173
  hepatitis B virus infection, 2174
  impotence, 1761
  infective endocarditis, 226, 229-230
  mood disorders, 1036
  narcotics, 2297
  personality disorders, 1039
  renal disease, 853
  tetanus risk, 1572
  tobacco, 2296
    alcohol-tobacco amblyopia, 1081
    alcoholic pancreatitis, 2238
    asthma, 1189
    bladder cancer, 868
    cancer deaths, 550
    carcinogenesis, 548
    chest pain, 126
    chronic obstructive pulmonary disease, 438
    chronic occlusive arterial disease, 308
    coronary artery disease, 200
    coronary artery disease in diabetic patient,
      1869
    coronary artery disease in women, 2271
    development of chronic cough, 407
    esophageal cancer, 2023
    evaluation of respiratory disease, 401-402
    human cytochrome P450 isoforms, 2312
    inflammatory bowel disease and, 2069
    Langerhans' cell granulomatosis, 463
    lung cancer, 486, 725
    nicotine addiction, 2296
    pancreatic cancer, 2242
    polycythemia, 588, 589
    premature ventricular contractions, 149
    squamous cell carcinoma of upper
      aerodigestive tract, 722
    tricuspid regurgitation, 256
    weight loss, 1749
Substance P, 363
Substantia nigra, 990
Substernal goiter, 513
Substrates of neuroendocrine regulation, 1075
Subtotal thyroidectomy, 1806
Subungual melanoma, 1299
Subvalvular aortic stenosis, 235

Succinylcholine, 831
Sucralfate
  interference with oral anticoagulants, 636
  typical medical regimen six months after
    transplantation, 343
Sucrase-isomaltase deficiency, 2068
Sucrose, 2121
Suctioning, secretion clearance and lung
  expansion, 429
Sudan black B fat stain, 481-482
Sudden death, 187-191
  aortic stenosis, 236, 238-239
  congenital aortic stenosis, 287
  diabetic autonomic neuropathy, 1873
  Ebstein's anomaly, 290
  familial hypertrophic cardiomyopathy, 61
  hypertrophic cardiomyopathy, 270
  hypertrophic obstructive cardiomyopathy, 269
  obesity, 1753
  pituitary apoplexy, 1778
  primary pulmonary hypertension, 294
  prosthetic valve problems, 258
  tetralogy of Fallot, 289
  ventricular fibrillation, 153
  Wolff-Parkinson-White syndrome, 142
Sudden unexplained nocturnal death syndrome,
  946
Sudeck's atrophy, 1247
Sugically-induced disorders, 1951
Sugiura procedure, 2167
Sular; *see* Nisoldipine
Sulfacetamide, 663
Sulfacytine, 664
Sulfadiazine
  brain abscess, 1416
  effects on kidney, 868
  glucose-6-phosphate dehydrogenase
    deficiency, 664
  nocardiosis, 1666
  rheumatic fever, 1258
  toxoplasmosis, 1474, 1477, 1678, 1679
Sulfadoxine-pyrimethamine, 2191
Sulfaguanidine, 664
Sulfamerazine, 664
Sulfamethoxazole
  bacterial meningitis, 1411
  chlamydial infection, 1537
  effects on kidney, 868
  hemolysis in glucose-6-phosphate
    dehydrogenase deficiency, 663
Sulfamethoxypyridazine, 664
Sulfanilamide, 663
Sulfapyridine, 663
Sulfasalazine
  Crohn's disease, 2071
  during pregnancy, 2278
  pulmonary toxicity, 479
  rheumatic disease, 1260, 1261-1262
  rheumatoid arthritis, 1208
  ulcerative colitis, 2074
6-Sulfate proteoglycans, 1142
Sulfatide lipidosis, 1918
Sulfatidoses, 1918
Sulfhemoglobin, 351
Sulfinpyrazone, 636
Sulfisoxazole, 664
  chlamydial infection, 1537
  dosage, 1350
Sulfonamides, 1358
  bacterial meningitis, 1411
  brain abscess, 1416
  chlamydial infection, 1537
  Crohn's disease, 2071
  effects on kidney, 868
  glucose-6-phosphate dehydrogenase
    deficiency, 664
  Haemophilus influenzae, 1588
  hemolysis in glucose-6-phosphate
    dehydrogenase deficiency, 663
  hepatic injury, 2191
  induction of acute interstitial nephritis, 889

Sulfonamides—cont'd
  inhibition of folate metabolism, 647
  meningococcal disease, 1580
  nocardiosis, 1666
  during pregnancy, 2278
  pulmonary toxicity, 479
  rheumatic disease, 1260, 1261-1262
  rheumatic fever, 1258
  rheumatoid arthritis, 1208
  toxoplasmosis, 1474, 1477, 1678, 1679
  ulcerative colitis, 2074
  use during pregnancy, 2281
Sulfones, 2191
Sulfonylureas
  diabetes mellitus, 1857
  hypoglycemia, 1875
Sulfosalicylic acid, 567, 743, 761
Sulfur, 2109
Sulfur-containing amino acids, 1908-1909
Sulfur granules, 1664
Sulfuric acid, 834
Sulindac, 1259
  gouty arthritis, 1274
  hepatic injury, 2191
Suloctidil, 2192
Sumatriptan, 962
Summation gallop, 74
Summer-type hypersensitivity, 460
Sunburn, 1306
Sunflower cataracts, 2205
Sunlight
  rickets and osteomalacia, 1951
  vitamin D synthesis in skin, 1719
Sunscreen, 348
Superantigen, 1112, 1127, 1143
Superficial fungal infections, 1307-1312
  candidiasis, 1310-1312
  clinical presentation, 1308-1309
  dermatophyte infection, 1307-1308
  diagnostic procedures, 1309
  Pityrosporum infection, 1309-1310
Superficial migratory thrombophlebitis,
    1317-1318
Superficial nodes, 599
Superficial osteomyelitis, 1436
Superficial spreading malignant melanoma,
    1298-1299, Plate VII-8
Superficial thrombophlebitis, 311, 638
Superinfection, 2210
Superior vena cava syndrome
  aortic dissection, 301
  lung cancer, 488
Superior vena caval obstruction, 511-512
  abnormal jugular venous pulse, 66
  transudative pleural effusion, 507
Superoxide
  aging and, 2283
  lung damage, 373
Superoxide dismutase, 2283
Supinator jerk, 964
Suppression test, 1732
  clonidine, 1740
  hypothalamic-pituitary, 1736-1737
  triiodothyronine, 1739
Suppressor T-cell, 1114
Suppurative gastritis, 2043
Supraclavicular nodes, 598
Supraclavicular systolic murmur, 64
Supraglotittis, 2306
Suprasternal approach in echocardiography, 95
Supratentorial mass lesion, 948
Supravalvular aortic stenosis, 235
Supraventricular arrhythmia
  amiodarone, 138
  myocardial infarction, 223
Supraventricular tachycardia, 141-148
  accelerated atrioventricular junctional rhythm,
    144
  adenosine, 139
  atrial fibrillation, 146-148
  atrial flutter, 144-146

Supraventricular tachycardia—cont'd
  atrioventricular nodal reentrant tachycardia,
    141-142, 144, 145
  digitalis, 138
  ectopic atrial tachycardia, 143-144, 146
  flecainide, 138
  mitral valve prolapse, 254
  multifocal atrial tachycardia, 144, 146
  palpitations, 130
  premature atrial contractions, 141
  sinus tachycardia, 141
  sotalol, 138
  supraventricular tachyarrhythmias, 141, 142, 143
  Wolff-Parkinson-White syndrome, 142-143, 145
Suramin
  African trypanosomiasis, 1689
  onchocerciasis, 1701
  prostate cancer, 720
Surface-connected canalicular system, 536
Surface immunoglobulin, 685
Surface membrane glycoproteins Ib-IX, 536
Surface receptors, 1710
Surfactant, 347
  hypersensitivity pneumonitis, 462
  respiratory defense, 366
Surfactant compounds, 430
Surgery
  acromegaly, 1784
  brain tumor, 1068-1069
  Budd-Chiari syndrome, 2208
  cardiac
    aortic stenosis, 287
    atrial fibrillation after, 146
    atrial septal defect, 282
    coarctation of aorta, 287
    common aortopulmonary trunk, 290
    endocarditis, 233
    hypertrophic cardiomyopathy, 270
    patent ductus arteriosus, 286
    pericardial effusion following, 274
    sternal osteomyelitis after, 1551
    tetralogy of Fallot, 289
    triiodothyronine levels following, 1811
  cholecystitis, 2228
  colon cancer, 2085
  Crohn's disease, 2072
  Cushing's syndrome, 1821
  echinococcal cyst, 2111-2212
  fibrous dysplasia, 1960
  gastric cancer, 2048
  gastroesophageal reflux, 2018
  gastrointestinal complications of acquired
      immunodeficiency syndrome, 2099
  Graves' disease, 1806
  Hirschsprung's disease, 2092
  hyperparathyroidism, 1969-1971
  hypoparathyroidism after, 1931
  increased intracranial pressure, 1084-1085
  infective endocarditis, 233
  insulinoma, 2244
  melanoma, 1299
  neck pain, 971
  obesity, 1753, 2104-2105
  orthopedic
    osteoarthritis, 1268
    rheumatoid arthritis, 1209
  Paget's disease, 1957-1958
  parathyroid, 1969-1970
  Parkinson's disease, 992
  peptic ulcer disease, 2040-2041
  peritonitis, 1402
  preoperative evaluation, 2256-2264
    cardiovascular risk factors, 2257-2260
    endocrine risk factors, 2262
    estimated operative risk, 2256-2257
    gastrointestinal and hepatic risk factors,
      2262-2263
    hematologic risk factors, 2262
    pulmonary risk factors, 2260-2262
    renal risk factors, 2263-2264
  risk associated with, 2256

Surgery—cont'd
  small intestinal malignancies, 2081
  spinal cord injury, 1049
  tissue nematode infection, 1700
  variceal bleeding, 2167
Surgical debridement
  clostridial infection, 1576
  gas gangrene, 1423-1424
  necrotizing fasciitis, 1422
  osteomyelitis, 1435
  synergistic nonclostridial anaerobic
      myonecrosis, 1424
Surgical drainage
  abscess
    anaerobic infection, 1621
    brain, 1416
    liver, 2210
    spinal epidural, 1419
  Caroli's disease, 2233
  furuncle, 1421
  osteomyelitis, 1435
  pericardial effusion, 278
  subdural empyema, 1418
Surgical oncology, 553
Surgical sterilization, 2269-2270
Surgical wound infection, 1480
Susceptibility testing, antimicrobial, 1346
  anaerobic bacteria, 1619-1621
  tuberculosis, 1632
Sustained monomorphic ventricular tachycardia,
    150-151, 224
Sustained ventricular tachycardia with wide QRS
    complex tachycardia, 149-150, 151
SVR; *see* Systemic vascular resistance
Swallow syncope, 953
Swallowing
  achalasia, 2001, 2021-2022
  gastroesophageal reflux, 2015
  manifestations of esophageal disease,
    1998-1999
  movement of food, 1978
  peritonsillar abscess, 2306
Swan-Ganz catheter, 383, 390-395
  adult respiratory distress syndrome, 421
  heart failure, 167
Swan's neck deformity, 1203
Sweat chloride concentration, 481
Sweat test, 938, 2207
Sweating
  autonomic overactivity, 934
  autonomic regulation, 933
  hypoglycemia, 1875
  hypoglycemic coma, 1867
  myocardial infarction, 209
  pheochromocytoma, 322, 1829
  retroperitoneal abscess, 1398
  sarcoidosis, 458
Sweet's syndrome, 1317, 1318-1319
SWIFT trial, 121
Swoon, 955
Swyer's syndrome, 1838
Sycosisbarbae, 1420
Sydenham's chorea, 994-995
syk/ZAP 70 family, 1175
Sylvatic plague, 1610
Symbion Jarvik-7, 186
Sympathectomy
  chronic occlusive arterial disease, 309
  Raynaud's phenomenon, 310, 1227
Sympathetic ganglion blockade, 1227
Sympathetic nervous system, 930, 931
  alimentary motor function, 1977
  bladder, 933
  control of peripheral circulation, 46
  eye, 934
  heart failure, 162
  hypertension, 316
  overactivity in alcohol withdrawal, 934-935
  pancreatic innervation, 2131
  sodium balance, 738-739
  sodium retention in cirrhosis, 819

Sympathomimetics
  arrhythmia, 133
  chronic obstructive pulmonary disease,
     443-444
  during pregnancy, 2277
Symptomatic narcolepsy, 943
Symptomatic seizure, 980
Syncope, 952-957
  aortic stenosis, 236
  cough, 408
  epilepsy *versus,* 981
  hypertrophic obstructive cardiomyopathy, 266
  ischemic heart disease, 197
  mitral valve prolapse, 254
  primary pulmonary hypertension, 294
  pulmonary embolism, 500
  sudden cardiac death *versus,* 188-189
Syndesmophyte, 1170
Syndrome
  acquired immunodeficiency, 1470-1479,
     1533-1534
    acute meningitis, 1407
    adenopathy, 599
    aplastic anemia, 672
    autoimmune hemolytic anemia, 669
    biliary disease, 2202
    brain abscess, 1414
    carcinogenesis, 548
    cardiovascular involvement, 333
    clinical stages, 1471-1472
    clinical syndromes, 1474-1479
    cryptococcosis, 1667
    cryptosporidiosis, 1679
    cutaneous manifestations, 1325-1329
    cyclosporiasis, 1680
    cytomegalovirus infection, 1528
    dementia, 987, 1478
    diagnosis, 1472
    ecthyma, 1420
    epidemiology, 1470-1471
    esophageal ulcerations, 2020
    etiology and pathophysiology, 1470
    evaluation and management, 1472-1474
    fever and rash, 1381
    fever of unknown origin, 1377
    flow cytometry, 1152
    folliculitis, 1420
    gastrointestinal manifestations, 2094-2099
    generalized lymphadenopathy, 599
    gram-negative bacteremia, 1446
    hemophilia, 622
    histoplasmosis, 1655
    hypogonadism, 1843
    isosporiasis, 1680
    meningitis, 1404, 1409
    microsporidiosis, 1680
    nephropathy, 853
    neutropenia, 593
    nocardiosis, 1666
    nontuberculous mycobacterial infection,
      1638, 1639
    nosocomial infection, 1361
    ophthalmic manifestations, 2304-2306
    pericardial effusion, 272
    Pneumocystis carinii pneumonia, 1692-1696
    during pregnancy, 2281
    prevention, 1479
    primary sclerosing cholangitis, 2202
    prognosis and treatment goals, 1479
    prostatic infections, 1463
    retrovirus, 1533-1534
    Salmonella, 1601-1602
    septic arthritis, 1254, 1255
    shigellosis, 1603
    spinal infection, 1013
    syphilis, 1640, 1641
    T-cell function, 1343
    thrombocytopenia, 605
    toxoplasmosis, 1677
    transfusion-associated, 575
    transfusion-transmitted, 575

Syndrome—cont'd
  acquired immunodeficiency—cont'd
    tuberculosis, 1626
    weakness, 1754
    weight loss, 1750
  acute nephritic, 763-764
  acute respiratory distress
    acquired immunodeficiency syndrome, 1475
    acute lung injury, 371-372
    acute pancreatitis, 2237
    with acute respiratory failure, 418
    gram-negative bacteremia, 1449
    mixed venous oxygen saturation, 393
    multiple organ dysfunction syndrome,
      421-423
    pathogenesis, 1341
    pressure-controlled ventilation, 419
    pulmonary edema, 168, 424, 425
    streptococcal toxic shock syndrome, 1558
    transfusion-associated lung injury, 1480
  adrenogenital, 828
  akinetic/rigid, 992
  Alport's, 794, 876-877
  amnesic, 1031-1032
  Angelman's, 1729
  anterior cord, 1048
  anterior spinal artery, 1012
  Anton's, 1033
  Arias,' 2152, 2153
  Asherman's, 1760
  Bartter's
    generation of alkalosis, 839-840
    renal magnesium wasting, 1940
    renal potassium wasting, 828
  basal cell nevus, 1319
  Bazex's, 1317, 1318
  Bernard-Soulier, 536, 603, 611
  Bloom's, 549
  blue rubber bleb nevus, 1320
  Boerhaave's, 2019, 2028
  bronchiolitis obliterans, 517, 522-524
  Brown-Séquard, 1012, 1048
  Budd-Chiari, 2208
    imaging studies, 2140
    liver transplantation, 2219
    oral contraceptives, 2190
  Caplan's, 475, 1204
  carpal tunnel, 1017
    beta$_2$-microglobulin amyloidosis, 1284
    hypothyroidism, 1809
    nerve conduction studies, 915-916
    uremic patient, 1105
  catch-22, 1729
  cauda equina, 1048
  central alveolar hypoventilation, 943
  central cord, 1012, 1047-1048
  central tentorial herniation, 1044
  Chédiak-Higashi, 1919
    chemotactic defects, 1340
    granule abnormalities, 1341
  chest, 658
  chest pain, 101
  chest wall, 410
  chronic fatigue, 1375, 2298-2300
  Churg-Strauss, 465-467, 1220
  congenital long Q-T, 59, 61, 62
  congenital rubella, 2280
  Conn's, 828
  contaminated small bowel, 2129
  conus medullaris, 1048
  Cowden's, 1319
  CREST, 1228, 1293
  cricoid achalasia, 2021
  Crigler-Najjar, 2151-2152, 2153
  cubital tunnel, 915-916
  Cushing's, 1819-1822
    amenorrhea, 1759
    arthropathy, 1247
    cutaneous manifestations, 1323
    dexamethasone suppression test, 1737
    endocrine paraneoplastic syndromes, 583

Syndrome—cont'd
  Cushing's—cont'd
    general appearance, 63
    hypertension, 321-322
    hypokalemia, 829
    insulin resistance, 1862
    mediastinal mass, 513
    medullary thyroid carcinoma, 1816
    obesity, 2103
    plasma cortisol levels, 1740
    screening tests, 1826
    weakness, 1754
  Da Costa's, 131
  Diamond-Blackfan, 674-675
  DiGeorge, 1178, 1342, 1931-1932
  Down
    Hashimoto's thyroiditis, 1811
    hypergonadotropic hypogonadism, 1843
    ostium primum defect, 282-283
  Dressler's, 221-222
    pericarditis, 273
    pleural effusion, 508
  Dubin-Johnson, 2142, 2155, 2157
  Eaton-Lambert, 489
  Ehlers-Danlos, 1287-1289, 1320
  Eisenmenger's, 515
  Ekbom, 1103
  Ellis van Creveld, 280
  empty sella, 1787
  eosinophilia-myalgia, 681, 1234
  Epstein, 603
  erythrocyte fragmentation, 666-667
  euthyroid sick, 1801, 1802-1803
  Evans's, 616
  familial autoimmune endocrine deficiency,
    1846
  familial cholestatic, 2158-2159
  Fanconi's
    aminoaciduria, 879
    chronic lead nephropathy *versus,* 867
    multiple myeloma, 864
    proximal tubule abnormalities, 747, 837,
      881-882
  Felty's
    neutropenia, 593, 679
    rheumatoid arthritis, 1205
    splenomegaly, 601
  fetal alcohol, 280
  Fitz-Hugh-Curtis, 1583, 2248
  fragile-X, 1726
  frequency and dysuria, 763
  frontal lobe, 1032-1033
  functional prepubertal castrate, 1843
  Gardner's
    cutaneous changes and malignancy, 1319
    mesenteric fibromatosis, 2251
    risk for colonic cancer, 2083
    small bowel adenocarcinoma, 2081
  gay bowel, 1429, 1445
  Gerstmann's, 978
  Gilbert's, 2151, 2152, 2153
  Gitelman's, 828
  Goodpasture's, 454, 846-849
    acute glomerulonephritis with hemoptysis,
      775
    autoantibodies, 1155
    immune complexes, 1138
  Gordon's, 832
  Gorlin's, 1319
  Guillain-Barré
    autonomic hyperactivity, 935
    blood pressure control, 1087
    botulism *versus,* 1571
    Campylobacter jejuni infection before, 1591
    complication of influenza, 1491
    F wave, 916
    poliomyelitis *versus,* 1488
    respiratory failure, 1085-1086, 1097
    weakness, 1754
  Hamman-Rich, 452
  hand-foot, 657

Syndrome—cont'd
  hand-foot-mouth, 1489
  Hand-Schuller-Christian, 463
  Harkavy, 465-467
  Heerfordt's, 459
  HELLP, 615, 775, 2274
  hepatopulmonary, 2170
  hepatorenal, 775, 2168-2170
  Hermansky-Pudlak, 611
  high oxygen affinity, 660
  Holt-Oram, 280
  Horner's, 932
    aortic dissection, 301
    lung cancer, 488
    mediastinal mass, 512
    radiation therapy-induced, 1073
  Howell-Evans, 1319
  Hughes-Stovin, 469
  hungry bone, 1936, 1940
  Hunter's, 1912
  Hurler-Scheie, 1912
  Hurler's, 1912
  hyperimmunoglobulin M, 1176, 1343
  hyperinfection, 1403
  idiopathic hypereosinophilic, 681
  inappropriate antidiuretic hormone
    arginine vasopressin secretion, 810
    endocrine paraneoplastic syndromes, 583
    paraneoplastic syndromes, 488-489
    water loading, 1738
  inherited polyposis, 2081
  insulin resistance, 1752, 1862
  irreversible portosystemic, 1102
  irritable bowel, 2055-2056
    abdominal pain, 2035
    celiac sprue *versus*, 2063
    colonic dysmotility, 2007
    diarrhea, 2052
  Jervell and Lange-Nielsen, 62, 153
  Jodbasedow, 1804, 1807
  jugular foramen, 1071
  Kallmann's, 1769, 1841-1842
  Kasabach-Merritt, 614, 2215
  Kearns-Sayre, 62, 1029, 1088
  Kleine-Levin, 943
  Klinefelter's, 1729, 1769
    clinical features, 1844
    gynecomastia, 1764
    Hashimoto's thyroiditis, 1811
    hypergonadotropic hypogonadism, 1843
    impotence, 1762
  Korsakoff's
    amnesic syndrome, 1032
    thiamine deficiency, 2106
  Lambert-Eaton, 1023-1024
    autoantibody, 1075
    peripheral neuropathy *versus*, 1014
  lateral tentorial herniation, 1044
  Laurence-Moon-Biedl
    hypogonadism, 1842
    hypopituitarism, 1776
    obesity, 1752
  Liddle's, 828
  Loffler's, 455
  loin pain-hematuria, 845-846
  Louis-Bar, 1319
  Lowe's, 882, 1911
  Luft's, 1749
  lung involvement, 453
  Lutembacher's, 245, 280
  Lynch, 2083
  Mallory-Weiss, 2019, 2028
  man-in-the-barrel, 951
  Marfan, 1730
    aortic disease, 299
    fibrillin, 1289
    mitral regurgitation, 249
    mitral valve prolapse, 253
    during pregnancy, 2276
    tall stature, 1769
  Maroteaux-Lamy, 1915

Syndrome—cont'd
  McCune-Albright, 1960
  McLeod's, 666
  Meig's, 508
  MELAS, 1029
  MERRF, 996
  middle fossa, 1071
  milkman's, 1950
  Milwaukee shoulder/knee, 1279-1280
  mononeuropathy, 1105
  Morquio's, 1915
  mucocutaneous lymph node, 1385
  Muir-Torre, 1319
  multiple end-organ endocrine deficiency, 1931
  multiple hamartoma, 1319
  multiple organ dysfunction
    adult respiratory distress syndrome, 421-423
    streptococcal toxic shock, 1421
  Munchausen's syndrome-by-proxy, 2027
  myasthenic, 489
  myelodysplastic, 675-676, 690-691
  nail-patella, 877
  nephritic
    anti-neutrophil cytoplasmic
        antibodies-positive glomerulonephritis,
        848
    essential mixed cryoglobulinemia, 857
    immunoglobulin A nephropathy, 845
    poststreptococcal glomerulonephritis, 844
    rapidly progressive glomerulonephritis, 846
  nephrotic, 765-768
    acquired immunodeficiency syndrome
        nephropathy, 853
    amyloidosis, 1282-1283
    clinical manifestations and pathophysiology,
        765-766
    complications, 766-767
    diagnosis and management, 767
    familial Mediterranean fever, 877
    Fanconi's syndrome, 882
    focal glomerular sclerosis, 851-852
    glycosuria, 879
    Henoch-Schönlein purpura, 857
    heroin nephropathy, 853
    hypercholesterolemia, 1894
    hyponatremia, 812
    immunofixation, 568
    lipiduria, 745
    lipodystrophy, 877
    membranoproliferative glomerulonephritis,
        854-855
    membranous nephropathy, 853-854
    mesangial proliferative disease, 851
    minimal change disease, 849-851
    operative risk, 2263
    primary peritonitis, 1396
    sodium balance dysfunction, 820-821
    transudative pleural effusion, 507
  neurologic paraneoplastic, 1071, 1073, 1074
  nocturnal eating (drinking), 944
  nonendocrine paraneoplastic, 583
  non–twenty-four hour sleep-wake, 945
  Noonan's, 1769, 1843
  obesity-hypoventilation, 354, 528
  occipital condyle, 1071
  Ogilvie's, 2079
  Oldfield's, 2083
  Osler-Weber-Rendu
    cutaneous manifestations, 1321
    scleroderma, 1293
  overlap, 1221, 1228
  pacemaker, 139
  paraneoplastic, 582-583
    antibodies, 1158
    arthropathy, 1247
    dementia, 987
    dermatoses, 1316-1319
    lung cancer, 488-489
    myelopathy, 1013
  parasellar, 1071
  Parkinson's-plus, 992-993

Syndrome—cont'd
  Patterson-Kelly, 2020
  perimenstrual, 1077
  Peutz-Jeghers
    cutaneous changes and malignancy,
        1319-1320
    gastric polyp, 2046
    risk for colonic cancer, 2083
    small bowel adenocarcinoma, 2081
  pickwickian, 334, 354
  piriformis, 965
  Plummer-Vinson, 2020
  POEMS, 703
  postcardiotomy, 273
  postcholecystectomy, 2226
  postcoarctation, 287
  posterior column, 1048
  postperfusion, 259, 668
  postpericardiotomy, 259
  postpolio, 1015
  posttraumatic, 1045
  Prader-Labhart-Willi, 1842
  Prader-Willi, 1729
    hypopituitarism, 1776
    obesity, 1752
  preleukemic, 645
  primary antiphospholipid antibody, 1155
  pronator, 1017
  pulmonary-renal, 775
  Ramsay-Hunt, 1527
  red eye, 1963
  Reiter, 1239-1240
    dysuria, 763
    human immunodeficiency virus infection,
        1326
    nongonococcal urethritis, 1441
    septic arthritis *versus*, 1252
    soft tissue swelling, 1165
  renal magnesium-wasting, 1940
  renal phosphate-wasting, 880
  reset osmostat, 815
  resistant ovary, 1760
  restless legs, 784, 944, 1103
  Reye's, 1491
  Richter's, 685
  Riley-Day, 1087
  Romano-Ward, 62, 153
  Rotor's, 2142, 2157-2158
  rubella, 280
  rumination, 2027
  Sanfilippo's, 1914-1915
  Scheie's, 1912
  Schmidt's, 1823-1824, 1838
  scimitar, 282
  Sertoli-cell–only, 1845
  Sézary's, 1331-1332
  short bowel, 2066
  shoulder-hand, 1055, 1247
  Shy-Drager, 935, 992
  sick cell, 812
  sick sinus, 154, 1001
  sinopulmonary-infertility, 1845
  Sipple's, 1829
  Sjögren, 1209-1212
    anti-Ro antibody, 1291
    autoantibodies, 1155
    Fanconi's syndrome, 882
    inflammatory myopathies, 1236
    interstitial lung disease, 453
    neurologic manifestations, 1095
    renal involvement, 891
    systemic sclerosis, 1230
  slow-channel, 1023
  Sneddon's, 1292
  solitary ulcer, 2093
  staphylococcal scalded-skin, 1384, 1421,
      1549, Plate VIII-29
  Steele-Richardson-Olszewski, 992
  Stevens-Johnson, 1313, Plate VII-11
    nongonococcal urethritis, 1441
    vesicular lesions, 1384

Syndrome—cont'd
  stiff-man, 996
  Stokes-Adams-Moragni, 954
  streptococcal toxic shock-like, 1384
  subacute spinal cord compression, 1012
  sudden unexplained nocturnal death, 946
  superior vena cava
    aortic dissection, 301
    lung cancer, 488
  Sweet's, 1317, 1318-1319
  Swyer's, 1838
  systematic inflammatory response, 1445
  tachycardia-bradycardia, 154, 155, 954
  tarsal tunnel, 1017, 1809
  thoracic outlet, 129
  Tietze's, 129, 410
  time zone change, 945
  Tolosa-Hunt, 1063
  Tourette's, 996-997, 1098
  toxic oil, 1234
  toxic parkinsonian, 993
  toxic shock, 1381, 1421-1422
    desquamation, Plate VIII-20
    fever and rash, 1383
    sepsis *versus,* 1450
    skin signs and risk factors, 1423
    staphylococcal, 1421-1422, 1549
    streptococcal, 1557-1558
  Trousseau's, 609, 1317
  tumor lysis, 584, 685
  Turcot's, 2083
  Turner, 1729, 1769
    coarctation of aorta, 286
    Hashimoto's thyroiditis, 1811
    ovarian disease, 1837
  uncal, 1082
  unstable hemoglobin, 660
  upper airway resistance, 526-527, 943
  uremic, 776, 779-880
  urethral, 763, 1455
  urethritis, 1440-1441
  velocardiofacial, Plate IX-1
  Verner-Morrison, 2245
  WAGR, 1729
  Weber-Christian, 1245
  Weil's, 1644-1645
  Werner, 549, 2283
  Williams, W87
  Wiskott-Aldrich, 1178, 1342-1343
    hematopoietic stem cell transplantation, 576
    immunodeficiency, 611
    thrombocytopenia, 603
  Wolff-Parkinson-White, 142-143, 145
    amiodarone, 138
    atrial fibrillation, 148
    Ebstein's anomaly, 289
    hypertrophic cardiomyopathy, 267
    procainamide, 137
  X, 195, 196, 1862
  X-linked fragile-X, 1726
  X-linked hyperimmunoglobulin M, 1176
  XYY, 1843
  Young's, 1845
  Zellweger's, 1907
  Zollinger-Ellison, 2037
    acid secretory values, 2003
    endocrine paraneoplastic syndromes, 583
    gastric acid hypersecretion, 1983
    gastric analysis, 2002
    hypertrophic gastritis, 2043
    reduced pancreatic exocrine secretion, 2134
Synergistic nonclostridial anaerobic myonecrosis, 1424
Synovial effusion, 1162
Synovial fluid, 1161
Synovial fluid analysis, 1161-1163
  complement levels, 1148
  disseminated gonococcal infection, 1584
  infectious arthritis, 1251-1252
  rheumatoid arthritis, 1205

Synoviocyte
  calcium pyrophosphate dihydrate crystal
    phagocytosis, 1277
  rheumatoid arthritis, 1202
Synovitis
  foreign body, 1244
  pigmented villonodular, 1244-1245
Synovium
  osteoarthritis, 1265
  rheumatoid arthritis, 1201
Syphilis, 1640-1644
  acquired immunodeficiency syndrome, 2098
  anal fissure and fistula, 2093
  aortic disease, 303
  aortitis, 302
  granulomatous gastritis, 2043
  meningitis verus, 1409
  neuroarthropathy, 1168
  palmar lesions, Plate VIII-47
  penile chancre, Plate VIII-34
  during pregnancy, 2280
  secondary, Plate VIII-46
  transfusion-transmitted, 575, 576
Syringomyelia, 1012, 1052
Systematic inflammatory response syndrome, 1445
Systemic blood flow, 110
Systemic diseases
  causing dementia, 987
  esophageal motility disorders produced by, 2023
  glomerular involvement, 855-859
  hypogonadotropic hypogonadism, 1842
Systemic lupus erythematosus, 1200, 1212-1218
  alveolar hemorrhage with, 455
  autoantibodies, 1155
  bullous, 1296
  cardiac involvement, 334
  clinical features, 1213-1215
  complement assay, 1147
  cutaneous lesions, 1290
  diagnosis, 1216
  drug-induced lupus syndromes, 1217-1218
  etiology, 1212-1213
  fever of unknown origin, 1377
  incidence and prevalence, 1212
  interstitial lung disease, 453
  laboratory findings, 1215-1216
  multiple cerebral infarct, 989
  neurologic manifestations, 1092, 1093
  neutropenia, 593
  pathogenesis, 1213
  pleural effusion, 508
  during pregnancy, 2279
  renal involvement, 856-857
  self-antigens, 1142-1143
  synovial effusion, 1163
  treatment, 1216-1217
Systemic sclerosis, 1228-1233
  cardiac involvement, 334
  neurologic manifestations, 1092, 1095
  reflux esophagitis, 2023
Systemic vascular resistance, 111
  fetal circulation, 280
  hemodynamic data, 110
  pulmonary artery catheterization, 391
  tetralogy of Fallot, 288
Systole, 72, Plate II-2
Systolic anterior motion of mitral leaflet, 265, 267-268
Systolic ejection murmur, 77, 78
Systolic ejection sounds, 74
Systolic function, 42-43
Systolic heart failure, 180
Systolic hypertension, 312, 315
Systolic murmur, 76-77, 78, 79
  aortic stenosis, 236
  atrial septal defect, 281
  dilated myocarditis, 263-264
  hypertrophic cardiomyopathy, 266
  mitral regurgitation, 251

Systolic murmur—cont'd
  mitral valve prolapse, 253, 254
  tricuspid regurgitation, 256
Systolic pressure measurement, 64

T

T cell, 1108, 1109
  activation, 1113-1114
  acute lymphoblastic leukemia, 683
  basic immunology, 1174-1175
  cell-mediated immunity, 1127
  decreased function during aging, 2285
  HLA restriction of T-cell recognition, 1118
  Hodgkin's disease, 693
  hypersensitivity pneumonitis, 461
  inflammatory myopathies, 1234
  intraepithelial, 1990
  multiple sclerosis, 1008
  Peyer's patches, 1989-1990
  primary disorders, 1342
  respiratory, 367
  rheumatoid arthritis, 1201
  sarcoidosis, 457
  secondary defects, 1343
  shock states, 176
  systemic lupus erythematosus, 1213
  systemic sclerosis, 1228
  tolerance, 1143-1144
T cell leukemia, 1531, 1532
T cell leukemia virus, 548
T cell lymphoma, 682, 695
  chromosomal abnormalities, 544
  cutaneous, 1331-1332
  enteropathy-associated, 2064
  hypercalcemia of malignancy, 1973
  molecular diagnostics, 563
T cell receptor, 1111, 1127, 1174
  antigen binding, 1111
  apoptosis and autoimmunity, 1144
  Southern blot analysis, 560
T cell subsets, 1114
T helper cell, 1114
  adult T-cell leukemia, 1532
  human immunodeficiency virus infection, 1470
  hypersensitivity pneumonitis, 461-462
  inflammatory myopathies, 1234
  Pneumocystis carinii, 1693
  respiratory, 367, 368
  sarcoidosis, 456, 457
T helper cell 1
  differentiation, 1130-1131
  oral tolerance, 1143
  respiratory, 367
T helper cell 2
  differentiation, 1130-1131
  oral tolerance, 1143
  respiratory, 367
t-PA; *see* Tissue plasminogen activator
T-piece weaning technique, 400
T-Score, 1747
T suppressor cell, 1114, 1127
  Graves' disease, 1805
  human immunodeficiency virus infection, 1533
  hypersensitivity pneumonitis, 461, 462
  inflammatory myopathies, 1234
  intraepithelial, 1990
  multiple myeloma, 701
  respiratory, 367, 368
  sarcoidosis, 456
T-tube, 2229, 2230
T-tubule, 38
T wave, 84
  acute pericarditis, 89, 273
  cardiac tamponade, 276
  constrictive pericarditis, 277
  hyperkalemia, 832, 833
  hypokalemia, 829
  ischemic heart disease, 197

T wave—cont'd
  left ventricular hypertrophy, 87
  mitral valve prolapse, 254
  myocardial abnormalities in neurologic
      disease, 1087
  myocardial infarction, 88
  myocarditis, 263
  myopericarditis, 1490
  premature atrial contractions, 141
  pulmonary hypertension, 296
  Q wave myocardial infarction, 211
T1-weighted images, 919
Ta wave, 84
Tabes dorsalis, 1641
Tacaribe virus, 1509
Tachyarrhythmia
  hypertrophic obstructive cardiomyopathy, 266
  mitral valve prolapse, 255
  myocardial infarction, 223
Tachycardia
  acute mitral regurgitation, 252
  acute pancreatitis, 2234
  aortic regurgitation, 244
  atrial
      ectopic, 143-144, 146
      multifocal, 144, 146
      response to carotid sinus massage or
          intravenous adenosine, 134
  atrioventricular nodal reentrant, 134, 141-142,
      144, 145
  atrioventricular reciprocating, 142-143, 145
  gas gangrene, 1423, 1575
  hypoglycemia, 1875
  hypoglycemic coma, 1867
  mitral valve prolapse, 254
  murmur, 76
  myocarditis, 262
  pacemaker-mediated, 139
  pulmonary thromboembolism, 500
  sinus, 141
      dilated cardiomyopathy, 264
      increased automaticity, 132
      myocardial infarction, 223
      palpitations, 130
      response to carotid sinus massage or
          intravenous adenosine, 134
      restrictive cardiomyopathy, 270-271
  supraventricular, 141-148
      accelerated atrioventricular junctional
          rhythm, 144
      atrial fibrillation, 146-148
      atrial flutter, 144-146
      atrioventricular nodal reentrant tachycardia,
          141-142, 144, 145
      ectopic atrial tachycardia, 143-144, 146
      mitral valve prolapse, 254
      multifocal atrial tachycardia, 144, 146
      palpitations, 130
      premature atrial contractions, 141
      sinus tachycardia, 141
      supraventricular tachyarrhythmias, 141, 142,
          143
      Wolff-Parkinson-White syndrome, 142-143,
          145
  thyrotoxicosis, 1804
  ventricular
      automatic implantable cardioverter
          defibrillator, 140
      cardiogenic syncope, 954
      complication of pulmonary artery
          catheterization, 395
      hypertrophic obstructive cardiomyopathy,
          269
      mitral valve prolapse, 254
      myocardial infarction, 180, 223
      nonsustained, 149
      palpitations, 130
      polymorphic, 151-153
      response to carotid sinus massage or
          intravenous adenosine, 134
      sudden death, 187

Tachycardia—cont'd
  ventricular—cont'd
      sustained monomorphic, 150-151
      sustained ventricular tachycardia with wide
          QRS complex tachycardia, 149-150,
          151
Tachycardia-bradycardia syndrome, 154, 155,
    954
Tachygastria, 2025
Tachykinins, 1077
Tachypnea
  diabetic ketoacidosis, 1863
  evaluation of respiratory disease, 402
  gram-negative bacteremia, 1449
  hyperventilation, 355
  mitral stenosis, 245
  patent ductus arteriosus, 285
  pulmonary thromboembolism, 500
  systematic inflammatory response syndrome,
      1445
Tachyzoite, 1676
Tacrine, 2288-2289
Tacrolimus, 2312
  effects on kidney, 870
  lung transplantation, 516
  renal transplantation, 793
Taenia saginata, 1696
Taenia solium, 1696, 1704-1705
Takayasu's arteritis, 311, 470-471, 1224
  aortic obstruction and inflammation, 303-304
  neurologic manifestations, 1092, 1095
Take off pounds sensibly, 2104
Talc granulomatous vasculitis, 470
Tall stature, 1769
Tambocor; *see* Flecainide
TAMI V trial, 122
Tamm-Horsfall glycoprotein, 743, 863
Tamm-Horsfall mucoprotein, 745
Tamm-Horsfall protein, 758-759
  antibacterial defense mechanism, 1456
  inhibition of crystal aggregation, 797
Tamoxifen, 555
  breast cancer, 709, 710
  endometrial cancer, 714
  fibrocystic breast disease, 1850
  hepatic injury, 2191, 2192
  human cytochrome P450 isoforms, 2312
  interference with oral anticoagulants, 636
  medication-induced hypercalcemia, 1928
  retroperitoneal fibrosis, 2250
Tampon-related disease, 1422, 1549
Tangier disease, 1897
Tanner stages of growth, 1770
Tannic acid, 2192
TAP1, 1174, 1175
TAP2, 1174, 1175, 1177
Tapeworm
  intestinal, 1696-1697
  tissue, 1704-1705
Taq polymerase enzyme, 55
Tardive dyskinesia, 995
Target cell, 662, 667, Plate IV-4
Tarsal tunnel syndrome, 1017, 1809
TATA box, 2153
Taurine, 2125
Taxol; *see* Paclitaxel
Tay-Sachs disease, 1919
Teardrop poikilocyte, Plate IV-4
Technetium-99m bis, 103
Technetium-99m imaging, 102-103
  benign hepatic tumor, 2215
  cholestasis, 2156
  Dubin-Johnson syndrome, 2157
  gastric, 2004
  gastrointestinal bleeding, 2012
  ischemic heart disease, 199
  Meckel's diverticulum, 2089
  osteomyelitis, 1434
  pulmonary embolism, 501
  renal scan, 750
Technetium-99m pyrophosphate imaging, 105

Technetium-99m sestamibi imaging
  coronary artery disease, 102-103
  ischemic heart disease, 199
Technetium-99m teboroxime, 103
Technetium-99m tetrofosmin, 103
Technology
  clinical guidelines, 25-26
  economic assessment, 15-16
  medical informatics, 26-29
Teeth, rickets, 881
Tegison; *see* Etretinate
Tegretol; *see* Carbamazepine
Teicoplanin, 1561
Telangiectasia
  lupus erythematosus, 1291
  scleroderma, 1293
  systemic sclerosis, 1230
Temafloxacin, 1359
Temporal arteritis, 311, 959, 1223-1224
  anterior ischemic optic neuropathy, 1059
  glucocorticoid protocol, 1263
  neurologic manifestations, 1092
Temporal artery biopsy, 1223, 1224
Temporal lobe epilepsy, 979
Temporary pacemaker, 139
Temporomandibular joint dysfunction, 2307
Tender-point locations, 1195-1196
Tendinitis, 1168, 1196
Tenex; *see* Guanafacine
Tennis elbow, 1197
Tenormin; *see* Atenolol
Tenosynovitis, 1203
Tension pneumothorax, 510
Tension-time index, 193
Tension-type headache, 959, 962
Teratoma
  incidence, 329
  mediastinal, 513
Terazosin
  hypertension, 325
  urge incontinence, 2293
Terbinafine, 1311
Terbutaline, 479
Terfenadine
  human cytochrome P450 isoforms, 2312
  rhinitis, 1182
Terminal hair, 1755
Tertiary contraction, 1978
Tesla, 389
Testicular cancer, 720-722
  curability with chemotherapy, 552
  gynecomastia, 1764, 1765
  impotence, 1762
Testis, 1838-1846
  age-dependent physiologic changes, 1839-1840
  androgen metabolism, 1838-1839
  assessment of clinical status, 1840
  assessment of hormonal status, 1840-1841
  brucellosis, 1606
  genetic analysis, 1841
  germ cell production, 1839, 1840
  hypogonadotropic syndromes, 1841-1843
  hypothalamus-pituitary axis, 1839, 1840
  mumps, 1496
Testosterone
  amenorrhea, 1759
  congenital adrenal hyperplasia, 1825
  hirsutism, 1756
  hypopituitarism treatment, 1780
  impotence, 1761, 1763
  Leydig cell secretion, 1838
  liver failure, 2171, 2172
  male climacteric, 1844
  normal female levels, 1836
  puberty, 1767
  radioimmunoassay, 1742
  sexual differentiation, 1077
  spermatogenesis, 1839
  stimulation tests, 1840
  treatment of testis disorders, 1845

Testosterone-estradiol-binding globulin, 1838-1839
  gynecomastia, 1765
  Klinefelter's syndrome, 1843
  measurement, 1835
  stimulation tests, 1840
Tetanospasmin, 1572
Tetanus, 1572-1574
Tetanus-diphtheria vaccine, 2255
Tetanus neonatorum, 1573
Tetany, 2106
Tetracyclines, 1356-1357
  acne vulgaris, 1305
  activity against major anaerobes, 1620
  amebiasis, 1683
  antimicrobial mechanisms, 1344
  bacillary angiomatosis, 1474
  balantidiasis, 1691
  brucellosis, 1605, 1606
  chlamydial infection, 1537
  cholera, 1596
  chronic obstructive pulmonary disease, 444
  Dientamoeba fragilis, 1691
  diverticulosis, 2091
  dosage, 1350
  drug-nutrient interactions, 2110
  effects on kidney, 868
  enterococci resistance, 1561
  Fanconi's syndrome induction, 882
  gonorrhea, 1585
  Haemophilus influenzae, 1588
  Helicobacter pylori, 1593
  hepatic injury, 2191
  iliac crest biopsy, 1747
  interference with oral anticoagulants, 636
  leprosy, 1651
  leptospirosis, 1645
  Lyme disease, 1254, 1647
  malaria, 1467
  measurement of bone formation, 1949
  Mycoplasma hominis infection, 1541
  Mycoplasma pneumoniae pneumonia, 1540
  peptic ulcer disease, 2040
  pill esophagitis, 2019
  plague, 1610
  relapsing fever, 1646
  rheumatic disease, 1260, 1262
  rickettsial infection, 1545
  syphilis, 1643
  tropical sprue, 2065
  urethritis, 1441
  use during pregnancy, 2281
Tetrahydrocannabinol, 2028
Tetralogy of Fallot, 288-289
  chest radiography, 91
  second heart sound, 72
Th1 cell, 1114
Th2 cell, 1114
Thalamic aphasia, 976
Thalassemia, 652-656
  beta-thalassemia, 652-656
  neurologic aspects, 1103
  during pregnancy, 2279
Thalassemia intermedia, 654
Thalidomide
  graft-*versus*-host disease, 578
  leprosy, 1651
  refractory discoid lupus lesions, 1292
Thallium, 1020
Thallium-201 imaging, 101-102
  ischemic heart disease, 198-199
  myocardial infarction, 212
Thecal cell, 1832
Theophylline
  asthma, 1190, 1192
  Cheyne-Stokes respiration, 354
  chronic obstructive pulmonary disease, 417, 434, 444
  human cytochrome P450 isoforms, 2312
Therapeutic apheresis, 574
Therapeutic privilege, 12

Therapeutic relationship, 2, 3
Thermal injury
  gram-negative bacteremia, 1446
  hypophosphatemia, 1936
  increased nutrient requirements, 2102
  intravascular hemolysis, 668
  lye, 2019
  nosocomial infection, 1361
Thermocardiac left ventricular assist device, 186
Thermodilution cardiac output, 392-393
Thermodilution method, 110
Thermogenesis, 2103
Thermoregulatory sweat test, 938
Thiabendazole
  hepatic injury, 2191
  Strongyloides stercoralis, 1699
  tissue nematode infection, 1700
Thiamine
  biochemical function, 2105
  comatose patient, 950
  deficiency
    alcoholic patient, 1081, 2106
    dementia, 987
    Wernicke's encephalopathy, 1100-1102
  diabetic polyneuropathy, 1871
  recommended daily dietary allowances, 2115
Thiazide diuretics, 822
  cause of renal potassium wasting and alkalosis, 828
  diabetes insipidus, 1797
  generation of alkalosis, 839
  heart failure, 170
  hepatic injury, 2192
  hypertension, 325, 326
  hyponatremia, 811
  induction of acute interstitial nephritis, 889
  medication-induced hypercalcemia, 1928
  microvascular disease in diabetic patient, 1870
  nephrogenic diabetes insipidus, 884
  pulmonary parenchymal reactions, 476
  pulmonary toxicity, 479
  stone formation reduction, 803
Thiazolsulfone, 663
Thick filament, 39
Thiethylperazine, 2027
Thin basement membrane nephropathy, 877
Thin filament, 39
Thioguanine
  effects on kidney, 869
  hepatic injury, 2192
Thiol-activated cytolysins, 1555
Thiothixene
  disordered thinking, 1041
  schizophrenia, 1042
Thiouracil, 2191
Third-generation cephalosporins, 1354
Third heart sound, 73-74, 75
  aortic regurgitation, 244
  mitral regurgitation, 251
  myocardial infarction, 210
  myocarditis, 262
Third-nerve palsy, 1062-1063
Thirst
  aging and, 2284
  diabetes insipidus, 1793-1794
  diabetic ketoacidosis, 1863
  disorders of urinary concentration, 748
  effects of vasopressin, 809, 1792
  hypernatremia, 814
  hypokalemia, 829
  insulin-dependent diabetes mellitus, 1854
  juvenile nephronophthisis, 875
  nephrogenic diabetes insipidus, 883
  osmoregulatory system, 807
  during pregnancy, 808
  schizophrenia, 1796
Thomsen's disease, 1028, 1086
Thoracentesis, 381-382
  lung cancer, 490
  pleural disease, 506
  pulmonary thromboembolism, 501

Thoracic aorta
  aneurysm, 106, 300
  dissection, 97
Thoracic esophagus, 1978
Thoracic outlet maneuvers, 305, 306
Thoracic outlet syndrome, 129
Thoracic spine
  Paget's disease, 1955
  tuberculosis, 1634, 1635
Thoracolumbar radiculopathy, 1016
Thoracoscopy, 385, 506
Thoracotomy
  lung transplantation, 516
  penetrating injury to heart, 332
Thorax
  inspection and palpation, 67-68, 70, 71
  radiation-induced thyroid carcinoma, 1816-1817
Thorium dioxide, 2249
Thought disorders, 1041-1043
3TC; *see* Lamivudine
Threonine, 1904
Threshold model for decision making, 9
Thrill, 68, 71
  coarctation of aorta, 286
  congenital aortic stenosis, 287
  coronary sinus aneurysm, 291
  mitral stenosis, 246
  patent ductus arteriosus, 285
  pulmonic stenosis, 288
  systolic, 76
  ventricular septal defect, 283, 284
Throat
  abnormal swallowing, 1998
  culture
    fever and rash, 1385
    streptococcal pharyngitis, 1393
  diphtheria, 1566
  movement of food, 1978
  obstructive sleep apnea, 525
  sore, 1392-1393
    acute pharyngitis, 1392
    chronic fatigue, 2298
    common cold, 1391
    epidemic pleurodynia, 1489
    hand-foot-mouth syndrome, 1489
    herpangina, 1488-1489
    infectious mononucleosis, 1529
    influenza, 1490
    Lassa fever, 1510
    Mycoplasma pneumoniae pneumonia, 1539
    peritonsillar abscess, 2306
    rheumatic fever, 1256
    scarlet fever, 1421
    spontaneous pneumomediastinum, 514
    subacute thyroiditis, 1811
    supraglotittis, 2306
    tonsillopharyngitis, 2309
Thrombin, 535
  bovine, 1146
  disseminated intravascular coagulation, 627, 628
  fibrinolysis, 540
  lung repair, 375
  platelet activation, 536
  platelet involvement in thrombin generation, 537
  reactions leading to formation, 537, 539
Thrombin time, 571
  acquired coagulation inhibitors, 630
  disseminated intravascular coagulation, 609, 627
  fibrinogen abnormalities, 625
  hemostatic abnormalities in liver disease, 627
Thromboangiitis obliterans, 308
Thrombocytopenia, 613-617
  acute myelogenous leukemia, 689
  cirrhosis, 627
  evaluation, 569
  gram-negative bacteremia, 1449, 1450
  hemolytic-uremic syndrome, 858

Thrombocytopenia—cont'd
  hemorrhagic fever, 1511
  heparin-induced, 634-635
  hypersplenism, 601
  lymphocytic choriomeningitis virus, 1509
  malaria, 1673
  neonatal cytomegalovirus, 1528
  neurologic aspects, 1104
  petechiae, 603
  during pregnancy, 2279
  pure amegakaryocytic thrombocytopenic
    purpura, 675
  vitamin B$_{12}$ deficiency, 648
  Wiskott-Aldrich syndrome, 1178
Thrombocytopenic purpura
  alloimmune, 616
  immune, 616-617
  pure amegakaryocytic, 675
  thrombotic, 614-615
Thrombocytosis
  Crohn's disease, 2070
  myeloproliferative disorders, 611
  release of cellular potassium, 831
  thrombosis, 609
Thromboembolism
  acute aortic obstruction, 304
  acute pulmonary hypertension, 297
  arterial, 638-641
  candidal, 1663
  cholesterol crystal, 1057
  echocardiography, 97
  heart failure, 174-175
  infective endocarditis, 228
  ischemic stroke, 998-1000
  mesenteric vascular disease, 2086
  mitral stenosis, 246
  myxoma, 330
  primary pulmonary hypertension, 293
  prosthetic heart valve, 261
  pulmonary, 630-638
    acute pulmonary hypertension, 297
    atrial fibrillation, 146
    chest pain, 128
    deep venous thrombosis, 311
    echocardiography, 100
    embolectomy, 503
    heart failure *versus,* 168
    lung scan, 387-388
    nephrotic syndrome, 766
    nosocomial, 1480-1481
    during pregnancy, 2276
    pulmonary angiogram, 388
    pulmonary edema *versus,* 425
    sepsis *versus,* 1451
    wheezing, 1189
  renal artery, 896-897
  risk factors for postoperative, 2261-2262
  stenting, 121
  stroke, 1006
  superficial thrombophlebitis, 638
  transesophageal echocardiography, 100
  venous, 630-638
    clinical features, 631-632
    etiology and pathogenesis, 630-631
    heparin therapy, 634-635
    laboratory features, 632
    oral anticoagulants, 635-637
    thrombolytic therapy, 637-638
Thrombolytic therapy
  activation of plasminogen to plasmin, 540
  angina, 205
  angioplasty after, 121-122
  atrial fibrillation, 640
  cardiac catheterization in ischemic heart
    disease, 113
  cost-utility analysis, 16
  deep venous thrombosis, 311
  myocardial infarction, 212-214
  primary angioplasty *versus,* 122, 123
  pulmonary embolism, 503

Thrombolytic therapy—cont'd
  shock, 182-183, 184, 185
  venous thromboembolism, 632, 637
Thrombomodulin, 537, 538, 539
Thrombophlebitis
  chest wall, 410
  inflammatory bowel disease, 2076
  nosocomial, 1480
  superficial, 311, 638
Thrombopoietin, 535, 1129
Thrombosis, 630-641
  acute aortic obstruction, 304
  angioplasty-induced, 122
  aortic aneurysm, 300
  arterial, 308, 638-641
  Behçet disease, 469
  bleeding disorders, 608-609
  during cardiac catheterization, 108
  chronic pancreatitis, 2241
  coronary, 209, 210
  deep venous, 311
    critical pathway, 21
    diagnosis, 502
    paraneoplastic dermatoses, 1317
    during pregnancy, 2276
    pulmonary embolism, 631
    risk factors for postoperative, 2261-2262
    spinal cord injury, 1049
    superficial thrombophlebitis, 638
  dissection of aorta, 302
  dural venous sinus, 928
  essential thrombocythemia, 688
  extrahepatic portal vein, 2208
  hyperosmolar nonketotic coma, 1866
  hypertrophic obstructive cardiomyopathy, 269
  ischemic stroke, 998-1000
  lupus inhibitor, 629
  mesenteric venous, 2088-2089
  myocardial infarction, 209, 210, 221, 222
  nephrotic syndrome, 766
  osteomyelitis, 1433
  peripheral arterial aneurysm, 309
  plasma coagulation, 570-571
  platelets and platelet function, 568-570
  polycythemia vera, 688
  portal vein, 2089
  during pregnancy, 2276
  primary pulmonary hypertension, 293
  prosthetic heart valve, 258, 261
  pulmonary, 499-504
  pulmonary angiogram, 388
  renal artery, 756, 896-897
  screening tests, 571-572
  superficial thrombophlebitis, 638
  unstable angina, 195
  venous, 311, 630-638
Thrombotic microangiopathy, 858
Thrombotic stroke, 1004-1006
Thrombotic thrombocytopenic purpura, 614-615,
    858
  acute pancreatitis, 2237
  hemolytic anemia, 666
  multiple organ dysfunction syndrome *versus,* 422
  neurologic aspects, 1104
Thromboxane A$_2$, 1141
  multiple organ dysfunction syndrome, 421
  platelet activation, 536
  platelet function, 611
  sepsis, 1448
  unstable angina, 195
  vasoactive effects on pulmonary circulation,
    363
Thrush, 1212, 1310, 1311, 1661
Thumb reflex, 964
Thumbprint sign, 2306
Thymectomy
  myasthenia gravis, 1022
  pure red blood cell aplasia, 675
Thymic cyst, 513, 2310
Thymic hyperplasia, 1022
Thymic hypoplasia, 1342

Thymine, 50
Thymine-adenine thymine-adenine box, 1708
Thymocyte, 1112, 1113
Thymoma, 512-513
  myasthenia gravis, 1022
  pure red blood cell aplasia, 675
  pure white blood cell aplasia, 675
Thymosin, 2182
Thyroglobulin, 1710, 1739, 1797, 1801
Thyroglobulin antibody, 1157
Thyroglossal duct cyst, 2310
Thyroid
  anatomy, 1797, 1798
  biopsy, 1802, 1816
  cancer, 1814-1817
    Hashimoto's thyroiditis, 1811
    pulmonary metastases, 493
    serum calcitonin, 1746
    thyroid biopsy, 1802
  cyst, 2310
  hyperthyroidism
    atrial fibrillation, 146
    cardiovascular involvement, 334
    gynecomastia, 1765
    hypercalcemia, 1928
    hypercalciuria, 798
    impotence, 1762
    nontoxic goiter, 1812
    operative risk, 2262
    physical appearance, 63
    during pregnancy, 2273
    proximal myopathy, 1030
    serum thyroid-stimulating hormone levels,
      1801
    thyroid scan, 1735, 1802
    thyrotoxicosis *versus,* 1804
    weakness, 1754
  hypothalamic-pituitary thyroid system, 1774
  hypothyroidism, 1808-1811
    arthropathy, 1246
    calcium pyrophosphate dihydrate deposition
      disease, 1279
    cardiovascular involvement, 334
    cutaneous manifestations, 1322
    delay in secondary sexual development,
      1768-1769
    dizziness, 974
    hyperprolactinemia, 1785
    impaired hepatic uptake of bilirubin, 2151
    impotence, 1762
    mood disorders, 1036
    operative risk, 2262
    physical appearance, 63
    during pregnancy, 2273
    proximal myopathy, 1030
    serum thyroid-stimulating hormone levels,
      1801
    weakness, 1754
  ultrasound, 1734
Thyroid acropachy, 1246
Thyroid antibody, 1157
  Hashimoto's thyroiditis, 1811
  hypothyroidism, 1809
Thyroid disease, 1797-1817
  acute psychiatric illness, 1803
  arthropathy, 1246
  benign neoplasms, 1813-1814
  cutaneous manifestations, 1322
  dementia, 987
  dysthyroid ophthalmopathy, 1063
  euthyroid hyperthyroxinemia, 1803, 1804
  euthyroid hypothyroxinemia, 1804
  euthyroid sick syndrome, 1802-1803
  goiter, 1812-1813
    euthyroid, 1812-1813
    euthyroid hyperthyroxinemia, 1803
    Hashimoto's thyroiditis, 1811
    substernal, 513
    thyroid-stimulating hormone receptor
      antibodies, 1801
    thyrotoxicosis, 1804

Thyroid disease—cont'd
hypothyroidism, 1808-1811
imaging techniques, 1801-1802
impotence, 1762
invasive techniques, 1802
laboratory tests, 1800-1801
Lambert-Eaton myasthenic syndrome with, 1024
malignancy, 1814-1817
mood disorders, 1036
myasthenia gravis with, 1022
during pregnancy, 2273
thyroid gland anatomy, 1797, 1798
thyroid hormone formation and metabolism, 1797-1799
thyroiditis, 1811-1813
thyrotoxicosis, 1804-1808
L-thyroxine therapy, 1803-1804
Thyroid function tests, 1738-1739, 1800-1801
euthyroid sick syndrome, 1802-1803
goiter, 1813
Thyroid hormone
degradation, 1714
effects on cardiac muscle, 334
formation and metabolism, 1797-1799
low-density lipoprotein clearance, 1891
nuclear receptors, 1713
regulation of albumin synthesis, 2119
synthesis and secretion, 1710, 1713, 1718
thyrotoxicosis, 1804-1808
Thyroid hormone-binding globulin, 1738
Thyroid hormone therapy
Hashimoto's thyroiditis, 1811
hypothyroidism, 1810
thyrotoxicosis, 1807
Thyroid microsomal antigen, 1157
Thyroid receptor protein, 50
Thyroid-stimulating hormone, 1774, 1801
assay, 1738
basal pituitary hormone measurement, 1737
constitutional delay of puberty, 1768
deficiency, 1777
euthyroid sick syndrome, 1802
goiter, 1813
Graves' disease, 1806
gynecomastia, 1765
heart failure, 166
hypopituitarism treatment, 1780
hypothyroidism, 1809
impotence, 1763
nontoxic goiter, 1812
serum levels in thyroid disease, 1801
stimulation test, 1739
subacute thyroiditis, 1811
thyroid hormone formation, 1798
thyroid-stimulating hormone-secreting tumor, 1787
Thyroid-stimulating hormone receptor, 1805
Thyroid-stimulating hormone receptor antibody, 1801
Thyroid-stimulating immunoglobulin, 1739
Thyroid storm, 1451, 1807-1808
Thyroidectomy
Graves' disease, 1806
thyroid carcinoma, 1815
Thyroiditis, 1811-1813
DeQuervain's, 1807
Hashimoto's, 1811
antithyroid antibodies, 1801
autoantibodies, 1155
hypothyroidism, 1808, 1809
thyroid lymphoma, 1816
thyrotoxicosis, 1804
Thyrotoxicosis, 1804-1808
arrhythmia, 133
high-output failure, 160
hyperphosphatemia, 1938
hypokalemic periodic paralysis, 826-827
insulin resistance, 1862
lymphocytosis, 592
during pregnancy, 2273
weight loss, 1749

Thyrotoxicosis factitia, 1807
Thyrotroph cell, 1773, 1774
Thyrotropin-releasing hormone, 1774
regulation of thyroid function, 1799
testing, 1735, 1801
prolactin reserve, 1776
thyroid-stimulating hormone, 1774
Thyroxine
adolescent hypothyroidism, 1772
calcium homeostasis, 1720
corrected concentration, 1738
euthyroid hyperthyroxinemia, 1803, 1804
euthyroid hypothyroxinemia, 1804
formation and metabolism, 1797-1799
goiter, 1813
Graves' disease, 1806
gynecomastia, 1765
hyperthyroxinemia, 1803, 1804
hypothyroidism, 1809
hypothyroxinemia, 1804
impotence, 1763
levels in acute psychiatric illness, 1803
synthesis, 1710
Thyroxine-binding globulin, 1797-1799
euthyroid hyperthyroxinemia, 1803
euthyroid hypothyroxinemia, 1804
measurement, 1800, 1801
Thyroxine-binding prealbumin, 1797
L-Thyroxine therapy
hypopituitarism, 1780
hypothyroidism, 1810
myxedema coma, 1810-1811
thyroid adenoma, 1814
thyroid carcinoma, 1815
thyroid disease, 1803-1804
Tiapamil, 203
Tibia, Paget's disease, 1955, 1956
Tibial nerve, 913-914
Tic, 996-997, 1098
Tic douloureux, 962-963
Ticarcillin, 1352
activity against major anaerobes, 1620
dosage, 1350
intraabdominal infection, 1401
Tick
arbovirus infection, 1514
babesiosis, 1675-1676
Colorado tick fever, 1511-1512
ehrlichiosis, 1545
influence of season and geographic setting, 1381
Lyme disease, 1254, 1646-1648
relapsing fever, 1645-1646
Rocky Mountain spotted fever, 1541
tularemia, 1607
Ticlopidine, 124
angina, 205
human cytochrome P450 isoforms, 2312
inhibitor of cytochrome P450, 2311
Ticrynafen, 2192
Tidal volume
acute respiratory failure, 416
carbon dioxide partial pressure, 834
removal from mechanical ventilation and weaning, 420
ventilated patient, 399
volume-controlled ventilatory mode, 419
Tie sternum, 1950
Tietze's syndrome, 129, 410
Time-gain compensation, 95
Time zone change syndrome, 945
TIMI trial, 121
Timolol
glaucoma, 2302
human cytochrome P450 isoforms, 2312
hypertension, 325
properties, 203
Tin protoporphyrin IX, 2153
Tinea capitis, 1308, 1309, 1311
Tinea corporis, 1308, 1311
Tinea cruris, 1308, 1311, 1422

Tinea manus, 1308, 1309
Tinea pedis, 1308, 1311
Tinea unguium, 1308-1309, 1311
Tinea versicolor, 1309-1310
Tinidazole, 2040
Tinnitus, 974, 2307
TIPS; *see* Transjugular intrahepatic portosystemic shunt
Tissue catabolism, 831
Tissue factor, 373-374, 537, 538
Tissue factor pathway inhibitor, 538, 539
Tissue helminth infections, 1699-1705
cestodes, 1704-1705
nematodes, 1699-1702
trematodes, 1702-1704
Tissue inhibitors of metalloproteinases, 1265
Tissue oxygenation
acute respiratory failure, 414
mixed venous oxygen saturation, 393
Tissue perfusion, 349
hypoxic pulmonary vasoconstriction, 363
multiple organ dysfunction syndrome, 422
Tissue plasminogen activator, 538
after myocardial infarction, 639
cost-utility analysis, 16
fibrinolysis, 540
myocardial infarction, 212, 213, 217
venous thromboembolism, 637
Tissue trematodes, 1702-1704
Tissue tropism, 1334
Titin, 59
Titratable acid excretion, 740, 779
Tizanidine, 997, 1051
To-fro murmur, 79-80
Tobacco use
alcohol-tobacco amblyopia, 1081
alcoholic pancreatitis, 2238
asthma, 1189
bladder cancer, 868
cancer deaths, 550
carcinogenesis, 548
chest pain, 126
chronic obstructive pulmonary disease, 438
chronic occlusive arterial disease, 308
coronary artery disease, 200
diabetic patient, 1869
women, 2271
development of chronic cough, 407
esophageal cancer, 2023
evaluation of respiratory disease, 401-402
human cytochrome P450 isoforms, 2312
inflammatory bowel disease and, 2069
Langerhans' cell granulomatosis, 463
lung cancer, 486, 725
nicotine addiction, 2296
pancreatic cancer, 2242
polycythemia, 588, 589
premature ventricular contractions, 149
squamous cell carcinoma of upper aerodigestive tract, 722
Tobramycin
bacterial meningitis, 1411
cystic fibrosis, 482
dosage, 1349
effect on vestibular function, 972
effects on kidney, 868
enterococci resistance, 1561
respiratory exacerbations in cystic fibrosis, 483
septic arthritis, 1253
use during pregnancy, 2281
Tocainamide, 2192
Tocainide, 138, 476, 479
Todd's paralysis, 981
Toe
chronic pernio, 310
dactylitis, 1241
Togavirus, 1514-1519
Token Test, 903-904
Tolazamide, 2191

Tolbutamide
  diabetes mellitus, 1858
  hepatic injury, 2191
  human cytochrome P450 isoforms, 2312
Tolerance, 1142-1147, 2294
Tolmetin, 1259, 2191
Tolosa-Hunt syndrome, 1063
Toluene, 867
Toluidine blue, 663
Tongue
  abnormal swallowing, 1998
  hypothyroidism, 1809
  leukoplakia, Plate IV-12
  pellagra, 2107
  riboflavin deficiency, 2106
  squamous cell carcinoma, Plate IV-14
Tonic seizure, 979
Tonicity, 806
Tonocard; *see* Tocainide
Tonsil
  peritonsillar abscess, 2306
  tonsillopharyngitis, 2309
Tonsillar diphtheria, 1566
Tonsillar herniation, 1044
Tonsillectomy
  quinsy, 2306
  tonsillopharyngitis, 2309
Tonsillopharyngitis, 2309
Tophaceous gout, 1272, 1275
Topical contraceptive agents, 2270
Topical decongestants, 2308
Topotecan, 702
Toremefene, 710, 711
Torsades de pointes, 135, 151-153
Torsemide, 170, 325
Torsion, omental, 2252
Torulopsis
  normal flora, 1368
  peritonitis, 2248
Total androgen blockade, 719
Total anomalous pulmonary venous connection, 290-291
Total body irradiation
  induction of veno-occlusive disease, 2208
  non-Hodgkin's lymphoma, 698
  toxicity, 579
Total body protein, 2118
Total compliance, 347
Total fasting, 2103
Total hemolytic complement, 1147-1148, 1216, 1339
Total hip replacement, 504
Total iron binding capacity
  hereditary hemochromatosis, 2204
  iron deficiency anemia, 643
  iron overload, 646
  nutritional assessment, 2111
Total lipodystrophy, 1899
Total load, 42
Total lung capacity
  bleomycin-induced pulmonary diseases, 477
  chronic obstructive pulmonary disease, 442
  diaphragm, 358
  interstitial lung disease, 450
  spirometry, 376
Total lymphocyte count, 2111
Total lymphoid irradiation, 341
Total parenteral nutrition, 2112-2115
  acute pancreatitis, 2237
  canalicular cholestasis, 2155
  fatty acid deficiency, 2113
  mineral deficiencies, 2110
  risk of gallstone formation, 2224
  standard formulation, 2117
Total platelet count, 556
Total pulmonary resistance, 110
Total quality management, 18
Total serum amylase, 2144
Total serum bilirubin
  estrogen-related cholestasis, 2157
  hyperbilirubinemia, 2150

Total serum calcium, 1744, 1930
Total solids meter, 742
Total testosterone, 1742, 2171
Total thyroidectomy, 1815
Tourette's syndrome, 996-997, 1098
Toxic cholangitis, 2202-2203
Toxic epidermal necrolysis, 1315, Plate VII-15
Toxic megacolon
  Campylobacter jejuni, 1591
  inflammatory bowel disease, 2076
Toxic nodular goiter, 1807
Toxic oil syndrome, 1234
Toxic parkinsonian syndrome, 993
Toxic renal injury, 866-871
Toxic scarlet fever, 1557
Toxic shock syndrome, 1381
  desquamation, Plate VIII-20
  fever and rash, 1383
  sepsis *versus,* 1450
  skin signs and risk factors, 1423
  staphylococcal, 1421-1422, 1549
  streptococcal, 1557-1558
Toxic sideroblastic anemia, 645
Toxicity
  cardiotoxicity
    amiodarone, 138
    digitalis, 138
  chemotherapeutic agents, 584-585
  digitalis, 138
  hepatotoxicity, 2184-2193
    acetaminophen poisoning, 2188-2190
    acute hepatic injury, 2187-2188
    carbon tetrachloride poisoning, 2188
    chronic liver damage, 2188
    classification of hepatotoxic agents, 2185-2187
    diagnosis, 2193
    herbal remedies and plant toxins, 2192-2193
    medications, 2190-2192
    mushroom and phosphorus poisoning, 2188
    susceptibility of liver to chemical injury, 2185
    treatment, 2193
  megadoses of vitamins, 2108
  nephrotoxicity, 866-871
    cyclosporin A, 794
    diagnostic and therapeutic agents, 868-871
    environmental and occupational agents, 866-868
Toxin
  anion gap acidosis, 837
  botulinus, 1570
  Campylobacter, 1590
  cholera, 1595
  chronic tubulointerstitial nephritis, 891
  clostridial, 1567
  Clostridium difficile, 1568
  diphtheria, 1565
  gonadal, 1844
  Helicobacter pylori, 1592
  hemolytic anemia, 667
  hepatic encephalopathy, 2161, 2162
  Legionella pneumophila, 1623
  megakaryocytic hypoplasia, 614
  myelopathy, 1011
  nosocomial infection, 1362-1363
  pertussis, 1611
  sensorimotor neuropathy, 1020
  staphylococcal, 1549
  tetanus, 1572
  vomiting, 2025, 2026
Toxin-induced sleep disorder, 945
Toxoplasma gondii, 1676-1677
Toxoplasmic retinitis, 2305
Toxoplasmosis, 1676-1679
  acquired immunodeficiency syndrome, 1473, 1474, 1477, 1478
  brain abscess, 1414
  compromised host, 1388
  fever of unknown origin, 1377
  lung transplantation, 518, 520
  during pregnancy, 2281
Toxotere, 710

Trabecular bone, 1714-1715
Trace elements, 2108
Trace metals, 2101, 2110
Tracheal suction, 429
Tracheitis, 1490
Tracheobronchial papillomatosis, 492
Tracheostomy
  acute respiratory failure, 417
  obstructive sleep apnea, 528
  tetanus, 1574
Tracheotomy
  mechanical ventilation, 399
  snoring, 2309
Trachoma, 1535-1536
Traction headache, 958
Traction radiograph, 1164
Tramadol
  chronic fatigue syndrome, 2300
  rheumatic disease, 1260
Trandate; *see* Labetalol
Tranquilizers, 2160
Transaminases
  acute cholecystitis, 2228
  acute fatty liver of pregnancy, 2278
  alcoholic hepatitis, 2196
  amebic liver abscess, 2210
  choledocholithiasis, 2229
  deficiency, 1905
  estrogen-related cholestasis, 2158
  postoperative cholestasis, 2159
Transaortic ventriculomyotomy, 270
Transbronchial biopsy
  acute lung allograft rejection, 521
  cytomegalovirus pneumonia in lung allograft, 518
  cytomegalovirus pneumonitis, Plate VIII-37
  through fiberoptic bronchoscope, 384
Transcellular fluid, 806
Transcellular transport, 1988
Transcortical aphasia, 976
Transcortin, 1819
Transcranial Doppler ultrasound, 929, 1003
Transcription, 50, 1721
  globin genes, 651, 652
  impairment in beta-thalassemia, 654
Transcription factors, 50-51, 542
Transcutaneous electrical nerve stimulation, 2022
Transcutaneous oxygen and carbon dioxide, 396
Transcutaneous pacemaker, 139
Transdiaphragmic pressure, 358
Transducer
  cardiac catheterization, 108-109
  echocardiography, 94
Transection, spinal cord, 1011-1012
Transesophageal echocardiography, 94, 100
  aortic regurgitation, 242
  aortic rupture, 333
  aortic stenosis, 238
  atrial septal defect, 281, 282
  dissection of aorta, 301, 302
  dissection of thoracic aorta, 97
  endocardial cushion defect, 283
  infective endocarditis, 229
  left ventricular assist device, 186
  mitral regurgitation, 251
  myocardial infarction, 212
  myocardial ischemia, 199
  myxoma, 330
  stroke, 1003
  thoracic aortic aneurysm, 300
  ventricular septal defect, 284
Transfer factor, 1188
Transfer ribonucleic acid, 1709
Transferrin
  in alveolar fluid, 367
  hepatic formation, 2120
  iron deficiency, 644
  iron transport, 642
  kwashiorkor, 2101
  nutritional assessment, 2111
  serum protein electrophoresis, 565

Transforming growth factor-alpha, 1720
Transforming growth factor-beta, 1128, 1129, 1131
  calcium homeostasis, 1720
  cardiac growth and hypertrophy, 55
  chronic alcoholism, 2195
  osteoarthritis, 1265
  renal hypertrophy, 860
  tubulointerstitial renal disease, 889
Transfusion
  associated acute lung injury, 1480
  beta-thalassemia, 655
  cold agglutinin disease, 670
  granulocyte, 573-574, 1341
  hypokalemia, 827
  plasma, 573
  platelet, 573
  reactions, 564-576
  sickle cell disease, 658-659
  whole blood and red cell, 572-573
Transfusion-transmitted diseases, 575-576
  babesiosis, 1676
  human immunodeficiency virus transmission, 1471
  malaria, 1672-1673
Transgenic animal, 55
Transgenic mouse, 1145
Transhepatic cholangiography, 2225
Transient global amnesia, 1032
Transient hypogammaglobulinemia of infancy, 1176
Transient hypokalemia, 826-827
Transient ischemic attack
  anticoagulant therapy, 640
  epilepsy *versus,* 981
  risk of stroke, 1001
  thrombosis, 1000
Transient metabolic alkalosis, 840
Transient mild hyperphenylalaninemia, 1905
Transient monocular blindness, 1057-1058
Transient neonatal hypoparathyroidism, 1931-1932
Transient proarrhythmic risk, 135
Transient proteinuria, 761
Transient tyrosinemia of newborn, 1905
Transient vision loss, 2300
Transillumination
  acute maxillary sinusitis, 1394
  sinusitis, 2308
Transjugular intrahepatic portosystemic shunt, 2167
  ascites, 2165, 2166
  Budd-Chiari syndrome, 2208
  cirrhotic ascites, 822-823
  cystic fibrosis, 2207
  hepatopulmonary syndrome, 2170
  hepatorenal syndrome, 2170
Translocation, 1712, 1728
Transluminal extraction catheter, 118, 121
Transmembrane electrical potential, 829
Transpeptidation reaction, 1344
Transplantation
  bone marrow
    acute lymphoblastic leukemia, 683
    acute myelogenous leukemia, 690
    acute renal failure following, 775-776
    aplastic anemia, 674
    beta-thalassemia, 656
    chronic myelogenous leukemia, 687
    lysosomal storage disease, 1920
    multiple myeloma, 702, 865
    myelodysplastic syndrome, 676
    neurologic complications, 1104-1105
    osteopetrosis, 1959
    sickle cell disease, 660
    Wiskott-Aldrich syndrome, 1178
  cardiac, 335-344
    anomalous origin of left coronary artery, 292
    evaluation and medical therapy of heart failure, 335-336

Transplantation—cont'd
  cardiac—cont'd
    function after, 342-343
    future directions, 343-344
    neurologic aspects, 1090-1091
    referral for, 335
    rejection and immunosuppression, 339-342
    selection, 336-339
  Epstein-Barr virus infection, 1529
  formation of immune complexes, 1138
  hematopoietic stem cell, 576-579
  liver, 2217-2220
    neurologic effects, 1102
    vancomycin resistant enterococcal infection, 1562
    veno-occlusive disease following, 2208
  lung, 514-524
    allograft rejection, 520-524
    chronic obstructive pulmonary disease, 445
    complications, 516-520
    cystic fibrosis, 483
    future trends, 524
    immunosuppression, 516
    indications, 514-515
    interstitial lung disease, 452
    outcome, 516
    selection of donor and recipient, 515-516
  lysosomal storage disease, 1919-1920
  pancreatic, 1101-1102
  primary sclerosing cholangitis, 2202
  renal
    allograft dysfunction, 793-794
    chronic renal failure, 791-796
    complications, 794-796
    cytomegalovirus infection, 785
    focal glomerular sclerosis after, 852
    immunosuppression, 792-793
    kidney donor, 791-792
    membranous nephropathy, 854
    multiple myeloma, 865
    myeloma kidney, 703
    neurologic complications, 1106
    recipient, 792
Transporter of antigenic peptides 1 and 2, 1174
Transporter proteins, 1111-1112
Transrectal ultrasound, 717-718
Transseptal approach, 108
Transsphenoidal surgery
  acromegaly, 1784
  Cushing's syndrome, 1821
Transthoracic echocardiography, 94
  atrial septal defect, 281
  endocardial cushion defect, 283
  heart failure, 166
  infective endocarditis, 229
  pulmonary edema, 169
  ventricular septal defect, 284
Transthoracic needle biopsy, 385
  mediastinal mass, 512
  solitary pulmonary nodule, 494
Transthyretin, 1797
Transthyretin amyloidosis, 1284
Transtracheal aspiration, 385
Transudate
  acute pericarditis, 274
  pleural disease, 507
  pleural effusion, 506
  pleural fluid classification, 382
Transvaginal ultrasound, 1835-1836
Transverse myelitis, 1010, 1013
Transverse tubule, 38
Tranylcypromine, 1037, 2191
Trapezioscaphoid space, 1172
Trapidil, 124
Traube's sign, 65, 241
Trauma
  abdominal, 2249
  blunt
    abdominal arteriography, 2033
    cardiac, 332
    pancreas, 2246-2247

Trauma—cont'd
  blunt—cont'd
    thromboangiitis obliterans, 308
    traumatic pericardial disease, 273
  cardiovascular, 332-333
  chronic occlusive arterial disease, 308
  chylothorax, 509
  esophageal, 2018-2019
  head, 1043-1045
    dementia, 988
    endocardial hemorrhage, 1087
    frontal lobe syndrome, 1032
    increased intracranial pressure, 1084
    seizure, 980
  hemophilia A, 619
  hepatic, 2187-2193
    acetaminophen poisoning, 2188-2190
    carbon tetrachloride poisoning, 2188
    clinical aspects, 2187-2188
    medicinal agents, 2190-2192
    mushroom and phosphorus poisoning, 2188
  increased nutrient requirements, 2102
  mechanisms of lung injury and repair, 370-375
  myelopathy, 1011
  osteoarthritis risk, 1264
  pancreatic, 2246-2247
  penetrating
    aortic, 304
    cardiac, 332
    pancreas, 2246
    traumatic pericardial disease, 273
  pericardial disease, 273
  pneumomediastinum, 514
  pneumothorax, 509
  prevention and control of injuries, 2264-2267
  spinal cord, 1045-1053
    classification, 1046-1047
    epidemiology, 1046
    gallstone risk factor, 2223
    mass reflex of autonomic overactivity, 934
    rehabilitation, 1052-1053
    respiratory failure, 1097
    subacute management, 1049-1052
    syndromes, 1047-1049
Traumatic intercostal neuritis, 410
Traveler's infections, 1464-1470
  arboviral and animal-transmitted viral infections, 1465
  Chagas' disease, 1690
  diarrhea, 1432, 1464
  evaluation of problems after international travel, 1469-1470
  helminth infections, 1466
  hepatitis A virus, 2173
  leishmaniasis, 1687
  malaria, 1464-1465, 1672
  pretravel advice, 1466-1469
  protozoan infections, 1465-1466
  rotavirus, 1520
  sexually transmitted disease, 1466
  typhoid, 1465
  viral hepatitis, 1465
Trazodone, 1037
  chronic fatigue syndrome, 2300
  depression in elderly patients, 2289
  hepatic injury, 2191
Treadmill exercise testing, 93
  cardiac rehabilitation, 224
  pulmonary rehabilitation, 436
  thallium-201 imaging, 101
Trematode
  intestinal, 1697-1698
  tissue, 1702-1704
  traveler-related, 1466
Tremor, 993-994
  ethanol withdrawal, 1080
  hepatic encephalopathy, 2160, 2161
  hypoglycemia, 1875
  hypoglycemic coma, 1867
  Parkinson's disease, 989

Tremor—cont'd
  pheochromocytoma, 322
  thyrotoxicosis, 1804
Trendolapril, 325
Treponema carateum, 1644
Treponema pallidum, 303, 1640-1644
  dark-field microscopy, Plate VIII-2
  diarrhea, 1476
Treponema pertenue, 1644
Tretinoin
  acne vulgaris, 1305
  acute myelogenous leukemia, 690
  cancer treatment, 555
  pulmonary toxicity, 478
TRH; *see* Thyrotropin-releasing hormone
Triamcinolone acetonide, 1182
Triaminopteride, 2110
Triamterene, 832
Triatomid insects, 1689-1690
Triazolam, 2312
Triceps jerk, 964
Triceps skinfold, 2111
Trichinella spiralis, 1700, 1702
Trichinosis, 1466, 1702
Trichloroethylene, 866-867
Trichobezoar, 2044
Trichome stain, *Entamoeba histolytica,* Plate
    VIII-52
Trichomonas vaginalis, 1691
  dysuria, 762
  nongonococcal urethritis, 1440
Trichomoniasis, 1442-1443, 1691
Trichomycosis axillaris, 1422
Trichophyton, 1307-1308
Trichorrhexis nodosa, 1907
Trichosporon, 1659
  compromised host, 1388
  serodiagnosis, 1653
Trichuris trichiura, 1696
Tricuspid atresia, 291
Tricuspid regurgitation, 256
  abnormal jugular venous pulse, 66-67
  dilated cardiomyopathy, 264
  infective endocarditis, 229
  nonejection systolic sounds, 75
  pansystolic murmur, 77
  restrictive cardiomyopathy, 271
Tricuspid stenosis, 78, 255-256, 1755
Tricuspid valve, 235
  Ebstein's anomaly, 289-290
  opening snap, 75
  radiographic views, 92
Tricyclic antidepressants, 1037
  anxiety disorders, 1035
  arrhythmia, 133
  cataplexy, 943
  chronic fatigue syndrome, 2300
  depression, 1037
  drug-induced lysosomopathies, 1919
  elderly patient, 2289
  hepatic injury, 2191
  human cytochrome P450 isoforms, 2312
  interference with catecholamine assays, 1740
  multiple sclerosis, 1010
  prophylaxis of migraine, 962
  stress incontinence, 2293
Triethyl tetramine, 2206
Trifluorothymidine, 1526
Triflupromazine, 2027
Trigeminal nerve, migraine, 957
Trigeminal neuralgia, 962-963
Trigger factor in sudden cardiac death, 188
Triggered activity, 132
Triglycerides
  combined hyperlipidemias, 1895-1896
  coronary heart disease, 1888
  digestion and absorption, 1986
  drug-nutrient interactions, 2110
  effects of fasting, 1853
  hydrolysis, 1851
  hyperlipidemia, 1892

Triglycerides—cont'd
  hypertriglyceridemia, 1894-1895
    with elevated cholesterol levels, 1895-1896
    lack of apolipoprotein C, 1898
  lipoproteins, 1885
  metabolism, 1883-1884
  synthesis in liver, 2120
  synthesis of biliary-type lecithin molecules,
    2126
  uremic patient, 786
Triglycine, 1988
Trihexyphenidyl, 992
Triiodothyronine
  calcium homeostasis, 1720
  formation and metabolism, 1797-1799
  goiter, 1813
  Graves' disease, 1806
  hypothyroidism, 1809
  suppression test, 1739
  synthesis, 1710
  toxicosis, 1808
Triiodothyronine-resin uptake test, 1738, 1800
  gynecomastia, 1765
  impotence, 1763
Trilostane, 1822
Trimellitic anhydride, 455, 473
Trimeterene, 170
Trimethaphan, 328
Trimethobenzamide, 2027
Trimethoprim, 1358
  bacterial meningitis, 1411
  dosage, 1350
  drug-nutrient interactions, 2110
  effects on kidney, 868-869
  glucose-6-phosphate dehydrogenase
    deficiency, 664
  hyperkalemia, 832
  inhibition of folic acid metabolism, 1344-1345
  use during pregnancy, 2281
Trimethoprim-sulfamethoxazole
  bacterial prostatitis, 1463
  brucellosis, 1606
  cholera, 1596
  chronic obstructive pulmonary disease, 444
  coccidian parasitic disease, 1679
  cyclosporiasis, 1680
  dosage, 1350
  drug hypersensitivity reaction, 1326
  exanthematous eruption, Plate VII-13
  Haemophilus ducreyi, 1589
  Haemophilus influenzae, 1588
  hepatic injury, 2191
  interaction with cyclosporin, 793
  isosporiasis, 1474, 1680
  Legionella pneumophila, 1624
  nocardiosis, 1666
  Pneumocystis carinii pneumonia, 1473, 1474,
    1694-1695
  prophylaxis in lung transplantation, 518
  shigellosis, 1603
  sinusitis, 1395, 2309
  spontaneous bacterial peritonitis, 2164
  toxoplasmosis, 1473, 1474
  traveler's diarrhea, 1432
  typhoid fever, 1601
  typical medical regimen six months after
    transplantation, 343
  urinary tract infection, 1459-1461
  Whipple's disease, 2065
  Yersinia enterocolitica, 1605
Trimetrexate, 1695
Trimipramine, 1037, 2191
Trinitrotoluene, 663
Triolein breath test, 2145
Triose phosphate isomerase, 663
Tripe palms, 1317, 1319
Tripelennamine, 664
Triple-lumen pulmonary artery catheter, 391
Triple phosphate crystals, 746
Triple product, 193
Triple X female, 1729

Triploidy, 1727, 1728
Trismus, 1573, 2309
Trisomy 21, 1728
  Hashimoto's thyroiditis, 1811
  hypergonadotropic hypogonadism, 1843
  ostium primum defect, 282-283
Trochanteric bursitis, 1197
Trochlear nerve palsy, 1062
Troglitazone, 1858
Troleandomycin, 1191
Tropheryma whippelli, 1101, 1246, 2064
Trophozoite, 1676
  Entamoeba histolytica, Plate VIII-52
  Giardia lamblia, Plate VIII-53
Tropical pulmonary eosinophilia, 1700, 1701
Tropical spastic paraparesis, 1532-1533
Tropical sprue, 2065
Tropomyosin, 51
Tropomyosin gene, 59
Tropomyosin-troponin complex, 39
Troponin
  cytosolic calcium and, 1717
  myocardial infarction, 212
Troponin-C, 39, 59
Troponin-I, 39, 59
Troponin-T, 39, 51, 59
  familial hypertrophic cardiomyopathy, 61
Trousseau's sign, 1932-1933
Trousseau's syndrome, 609, 1317
True aneurysm, 299
True-negative results, 6, 7
True-positive results, 6, 7
Truncus arteriosus, 290
Trypanosoma brucei, 1687-1689
Trypanosoma brucei gambiense, 1687-1689
Trypanosoma brucei rhodesiense, 1687-1689,
    Plate VIII-16
Trypanosoma cruzi, 1689-1690
  achalasia, 2021
  Giemsa stain, Plate VIII-17
  transfusion-transmitted, 576
  traveler's infection, 1466
Trypanosomiasis
  African, 1687-1689
  American, 1689-1690
Trypsin
  absorption of protein, 1987
  acute pancreatitis, 2234
  diagnosis of pancreatic diseases, 2144
  lung damage, 373
Trypsinogen, 1987
Tryptase, 1142
Tryptophan
  drug-nutrient interactions, 2110
  G cell stimulation, 1981
  niacin deficiency, 2107
  related diseases, 1904
Tsetse fly, 1687, 1688
TSH; *see* Thyroid-stimulating hormone
Tsukamoto-French model, 2195
TTP; *see* Thrombotic thrombocytopenic purpura
Tubal ligation, 2269
Tuberculin skin test, 1150, 1629-1630
Tuberculoid leprosy, 1649-1650
Tuberculosis, 1625-1638
  acquired immunodeficiency syndrome, 1472,
    1473, 1474
  Addison's disease, 1823
  after lung transplantation, 520
  characteristics of *Mycobacterium tuberculosis,*
    1625-1626
  chemotherapy, 1630-1633
  clinical spectrum, 1628
  constrictive pericarditis, 277
  dysuria, 762
  empyema, 507
  epidemiology, 1626-1627
  extrapulmonary, 1633-1637
  fever of unknown origin, 1376
  granulomatous gastritis, 2043
  hypercalcemia, 1928

Tuberculosis—cont'd
  impotence, 1762
  joint disease, 1254
  pathogenesis, 1627
  pericarditis, 272
  prevention, 1637-1638
  prostate, 1463
  public health considerations, 1638
  pulmonary, 1628-1630
  pulmonary hypertension, 296
  renal dysfunction, 892-893
  silicosis-related, 475
  skeletal, 1437
  weight loss, 1750
Tuberculous empyema, 1634
Tuberculous meningitis, 1409, 1411-1412, 1636
Tuberculous pericarditis, 1636-1637
Tuberculous peritonitis, 1396, 2248
Tuberculous pleuritis, 1633-1634
Tuberous sclerosis, 1922
Tuboovarian abscess
  anaerobic bacteria, 1618
  clostridial, 1575
Tubular acidification, 740
Tubular maximal reabsorption of phosphate as
          fraction of glomerular filtration rate,
          1745
Tubular proteinuria, 760
Tubular reabsorption
  phosphate, 1745
  proteinuria, 760
  sodium
    cirrhosis, 819
    nephrotic syndrome, 820-821
Tubulointerstitial disease, 888-893
  hematuria, 757
  nephritis and uveitis syndrome, 890
Tubulovillous adenoma, 2086
Tularemia, 1423
Tumor; *see also* Cancer
  adrenal, 1825-1826
  benign
    breast, 708
    bronchial adenoma, 491-492
    cardiac, 329
    cavernous hemangioma, 2215-2216
    colon, 2086
    esophageal, 2023
    gastric, 2050
    small bowel, 2082
    thyroid, 1813-1814
  brain
    computed tomography, 920
    dementia, 988
    depression, 1037
    headache, 960
    magnetic resonance imaging, 923
    neurooncology, 1067-1070
    seizure, 980
    tuberous sclerosis, 1922
  breast, 708
  bronchial adenoma, 491-492
  cardiac, 329-332
  colon, 2082-2086
  cytogenetics, 731
  esophageal, 2023-2024
  fever of unknown origin, 1377
  formation, 540-549
    environmental agents, 548-549
    genetic stability, 549
    multistep genetic pathway, 547-548
    oncogenes, 541-545
    tumor suppressor genes, 545-547
  gastric, 2045-2050
  hepatic, 2212-2217
  Hodgkin's disease, 691-695
  hypercalcemia of malignancy, 1972-1974
  lung, 486-492
  mediastinal, 512-513
  membranous nephropathy with, 854
  mesenteric, 2251-2252

Tumor—cont'd
  neurofibromatosis, 1920-1921
  non-Hodgkin's lymphoma, 695-700
  ovarian, 716, 1838
  pancreatic
    endocrine, 2244-2246
    exocrine, 2242-2244
    fasting hypoglycemia, 1876
    islet cell tumor, 1928
    pancreatic polypeptide secreting tumor,
          2244
  peritoneal, 2249
  pheochromocytoma, 1828-1831
    autonomic hyperactivity, 935
    hypercalcemia, 1928
    hypertension, 322, 1829-1830
    neurofibromatosis, 1921
    weight loss, 1749
  pituitary, 1781-1782
    Cushing's disease, 1786-1787
    gonadotropin-secreting, 1787
    growth hormone-secreting, 1782-1786
    hyperprolactinemia, 1785
    thyroid-stimulating hormone-secreting, 1787
    vasopressin deficiency, 1795
  poorly differentiated carcinoma, 732
  radiation sensitivity of, 553
  renal cell carcinoma, 898-899
  renin-secreting, 321, 829
  response to drug treatment, 552
  retroperitoneal, 2250-2251
  small intestine, 2080-2081
  spinal, 1013
  testicular, 720
    gynecomastia, 1764, 1765
    impotence, 1762
    von Hippel-Lindau disease, 1922
  Wilms,' 899
    curability with chemotherapy, 552
    hypokalemia, 829
Tumor cell burden, 554
Tumor-induced osteomalacia, 1953
Tumor lysis syndrome, 584, 685
Tumor markers
  breast cancer, 708
  cholangiocarcinoma, 2201-2202
  hepatocellular carcinoma, 2213
  lung cancer, 490
  medullary thyroid carcinoma, 1816
  testicular cancer, 720
Tumor necrosis factor, 533
  bacterial meningitis, 1405
  heart failure, 161
  humoral hypercalcemia of malignancy, 1973
  lung injury, 372
  multiple organ dysfunction syndrome, 421
  sarcoidosis, 457
  Shwartzman reaction, 1380
  stimulation of oxygen radicals, 2195
  weight loss in cancer patient, 1750
Tumor necrosis factor-α, 1128, 1129, 1130
  gram-negative bacteremia, 1447, 1448
  psoriasis, 1300
  rheumatoid arthritis, 1201
Tumor necrosis factor-β, 1129, 1130
Tumor-nodes-metastases staging system, 490
  colorectal cancer, 2083
  lung cancer, 725
  squamous cell carcinoma of oral cavity, 723
Tumor plop, 330
Tumor suppressor gene, 541, 545-547
Tumoral calcinosis, 1938, 1952
Turbinate sinusoids, 1181
Turcot's syndrome, 2083
Turkey handler's lung, 460
Turner syndrome, 1729, 1769
  coarctation of aorta, 286
  Hashimoto's thyroiditis, 1811
  ovarian disease, 1837
Twelve-step programs, 2296
24-hour urinary creatinine, 2111

24-hour urinary nitrogen, 2111
24-hour urine collection, 761
Two-dimensional echocardiography, 95, 96
  aortic regurgitation, 242
  aortic stenosis, 238
  atrial septal defect, 281, 282
  chronic cor pulmonale, 446-447
  coarctation of aorta, 286
  constrictive pericarditis, 277
  hypertrophic cardiomyopathy, 267-268
  infective endocarditis, 229
  lower extremity, 307
  Marfan syndrome, 299
  mitral valve prolapse, 254, 255
  myocardial rupture, 219
  myxoma, 330
  pericardial effusion, 275
  tetralogy of Fallot, 289
  tricuspid stenosis, 256
Tylosis, 1319, 2023
Tympanic membrane
  acute otitis media, 1395
  perforation, 2307
Tympanocentesis, 1395, 2307
Tympanomastoidectomy, 2307
Typhoid
  Salmonella typhi, 1600-1602
  serologic diagnosis, 1431
  travel-related, 1465
Typhoidal tularemia, 1608
Typhus
  louse-born epidemic typhus fever, 1544
  scrub, 1545
Tyrosine
  alkaptonuria, 1280
  catecholamines synthesis, 1710
  iodothyronines, 1708
  related diseases, 1904
  thyroid hormone formation and metabolism,
          1797
Tyrosine aminotransferase deficiency, 1905-1906
Tyrosine-based activation motif, 1174, 1175
Tyrosine kinase receptor, 541, 543
Tyrosinemia, 1905-1906
Tzanck smear, 1371
  herpes simplex virus, 1524
  herpesvirus infection, 1439
  impetigo, 1419
  molluscum contagiosum, 1327-1328
  procedure, 1371

U

U wave, 84
Ulceration
  Acanthamoeba, 1684
  Barrett's esophagus, 2017
  Behçet disease, 1243
  chancroid, 1444
  chronic venous insufficiency, 312
  Crohn's disease, 2069, 2070, Plate X-4
  diabetic foot, 1872
  duodenal, 2003
  gastric, 2002, 2003
  genital lesions, 1442
  ischemic foot, 308
  lymphogranuloma venereum, 1535
  mucosal, 784
  peptic ulcer disease, 2035-2041
    acid secretory values, 2003
    Helicobacter pylori, 1592-1593
    operative risk, 2263
  progressive bacterial synergistic gangrene,
          1425
  stasis, 312
  systemic lupus erythematosus, 1214
  Wegener's granulomatosis, 468
  Yersinia pseudotuberculosis, 1611
Ulcerative colitis, 2072-2075
  chronic diarrhea, 2051
  colon cancer *versus,* 2085

Ulcerative colitis—cont'd
colonoscopy, 1996
Crohn's disease *versus,* 2075
cutaneous findings, 1321
diagnosis, 2073, 2074
endoscopic features, Plate X-8
heteropathic arthropathy, 1245-1246
histologic features, Plate X-5
increased risk of cancer, 548
management, 2073-2074
pathologic findings, 2072-2073
pregnancy and, 2278
primary sclerosing cholangitis, 2201
prognosis, 2074-2075
Ulnar nerve
mononeuropathy, 1017
paralysis in leprosy, 1650
Ultimobranchial gland, 1718
Ultrafiltration, glomerular, 737
Ultrafiltration coefficient, 737
Ultralente, 1859
Ultrasound
abdominal, 2033
acute pancreatitis, 2236
appendicitis, 2092
benign strictures of extrahepatic bile ducts,
2232
Budd-Chiari syndrome, 2208
cancer
prostate, 717-718
renal cell carcinoma, 898
testicular, 720
carotid, 929
cavernous hemangioma of liver, 2215
cholangiocarcinoma, 2232
cholestasis, 2156
endocrine evaluation, 1734
endoscopic, 1997
esophageal, 2000
gallstone, 2224, 2226
hepatobiliary tract, 2140
intraabdominal infection, 1399
measurement of bone mineral density, 1748
pancreatic disease, 2146
peripheral arterial aneurysm, 309
pleural, 506
proximal venous thrombosis, 502
pulmonary, 389
renal, 749-750
hematuria, 757
hydronephrosis, 753-754
obstructive uropathy, 886
renal cell carcinoma, 898
stone passage, 800
structural abnormalities of urinary tract,
1457
stroke, 1003
thyroid, 1802
transvaginal, 1835-1836
Ultraviolet light
basal cell carcinoma, 1297
carcinogenesis, 548
photodermatoses, 1306
sensitivity in lupus erythematosus, 1291
tumor formation, 548
Umbilical cord blood, 577
Unbound testosterone, 1742
Uncal syndrome, 1082
Uncinate process, 2129
Unconjugated bilirubin, 2147
Unconjugated hyperbilirubinemia
chronic, 2152-2154
conjugated *versus,* 2150, 2151
diagnosis, 2153-2154
pathophysiology, 2150-2152
treatment, 2154
Underfill theory, 766, 2163
Undernutrition, 1361, 2100-2101
Undulant fever, 1604-1607
Unesterified cholesterol, 2127
Unicuspid aortic valve, 235

Unilamellar vesicle, 2127, 2128
Uniparental disomy, 1729
Unipolar depression, 1036
United Network for Organ Sharing, 791
United States Pharmacopeia Drug Index, 2313
United States Preventive Services Task Force, 2,
25
Univasc; *see* Moexipril
Universal precautions, 1365
during hemodialysis, 790
Unmeasured residue, 2220
Unstable angina, 195, 196
anticoagulant therapy, 639
calcium channel blockers, 204-205
coronary arteriography, 199-200
myocardial revascularization, 206
nitroglycerin and nitrates, 201
prognosis, 208
therapeutic approach, 207
Unstable hemoglobin syndrome, 660
Upper airway obstruction
anaphylaxis, 1193
sarcoidosis, 458
sleep-induced, 527-528
spirometry, 377
Upper airway resistance syndrome, 526-527, 943
Upper esophageal sphincter, 2020-2021
Upper gastrointestinal endoscopy, 1994-1995
gastric cancer, 2047
gastroduodenal diseases, 2002
intestinal obstruction, 2078
Upper gastrointestinal series
abdominal pain, 2033
gastroduodenal diseases, 2002
hypertrophic pyloric stenosis, 2044
small bowel bacterial overgrowth, 2061
small intestinal tumors, 2081
Upper motor neuron deficit, 1015
Upper respiratory tract
infection
immunoglobulin A nephropathy, 845
nosocomial, 1480
otitis media, 2307
sinusitis, 2308
lupus pernio, Plate VII-21
Wegener's granulomatosis, 467, 1222
Upper urinary tract tumor, 899
Upside-down tetraplegia, 1047
Uracil, 50
Urate crystals, 1271
Urate nephropathy, 1273
Urea
glaucoma, 2302
osmolality, 806
prerenal azotemia, 770-771
Urea cycle defects, 1906-1907
Urea reduction ratio, 790
Ureagenesis, 2120
Ureaplasma urealyticum, 1538, 1540-1541
dysuria, 763
eugonadotropic disorders, 1845
nongonococcal urethritis, 1440
normal flora, 1368
Urease
breath urea test, 2003
pyelonephritis, 1456
Uremia, 776
anti-neutrophil cytoplasmic antibodies-positive
glomerulonephritis, 848
chemotactic defects, 1340
hemostatic defect, 611
hyperventilation, 355
impotence, 1761
interstitial lung disease, 452
neurologic complications, 1105-1106
pericarditis, 273
weight loss, 1750
Uremic cardiomyopathy, 784
Uremic encephalopathy, 784
Uremic metabolic acidosis, 831
Uremic serositis, 784

Uremic syndrome, 776, 779-880
Ureter
diversion, 837
intravenous pyelogram, 749
malignant tumor, 899
obstruction
peritoneal mesenteric and omental diseases,
2248
posttransplantation, 794
stricture, 885
Urethra
exam for sexually transmitted disease, 1439
stricture, 885
urodynamic testing, 938
Urethral syndrome, 763, 1455
Urethritis, 1440-1441
dysuria, 763
gonococcal, 1582
pellagra, 2107
Ureaplasma urealyticum, 1540-1541
Urge incontinence, 2291
Urgency
bacterial prostatitis, 1462
urinary tract infection, 1458
Uric acid
calculi, 799, 804
chronic urate nephropathy, 891
crystallization and deposition, 1271
gout and hyperuricemia, 1268, 1269-1270
hyperuricemia, 1268-1276
acute renal failure, 773
after renal transplantation, 795
calcium pyrophosphate dihydrate deposition
disease, 1277
glucose-6-phosphate dehydrogenase
deficiency, 1881
multiple myeloma, 700, 702
Paget's disease, 1956
hyperuricosuria, 799
nephropathy, 775
urolithiathis, 1273
Uricosuric agents, 1275
Uridine diphosphate-glucose, 1880
Uridine diphosphate glucuronosyltransferase,
2128
Uridine-glucose-galactose-1-phosphate-
uridylyltransferase, 1882-1883
Uridine triphosphate, 1880
Urinalysis, 742-744
abdominal pain, 2032
acute renal failure, 771
chronic renal failure, 782
fever of unknown origin, 1379
heart failure, 166
hematuria, 757
hypertension, 318
periodic health examination, 2254
poststreptococcal glomerulonephritis, 844
preoperative medical evaluation, 2256
tubulointerstitial disease, 888
Urinary aldosterone excretion, 1742
Urinary catheterization, 1462
Urinary frequency
bacterial prostatitis, 1462
diabetes insipidus, 1793
frequency and dysuria syndrome, 763
urinary tract infection, 1458
Urinary incontinence
elderly, 2290-2293
hyperosmolar nonketotic coma, 1866
spinal epidural abscess, 1418
Urinary indices, 770
Urinary tract
barrier to infection, 1335
crystal nucleation and stone growth, 797
obstruction, 768, 884-887
tumor, 899
Urinary tract antiseptics, 1359-1360, 1360
antibacterial mechanism, 1345
enterococcal infection, 1563

Urinary tract antiseptics—cont'd
  hemolysis in glucose-6-phosphate
    dehydrogenase deficiency, 663
  hepatic injury, 2191
  interference with catecholamine assays, 1740
  pulmonary parenchymal reactions, 476
  pulmonary toxicity, 478
  use during pregnancy, 2281
Urinary tract infection, 1455-1464
  after renal transplantation, 794
  after stroke, 1007
  autosomal dominant polycystic kidney disease,
    873
  candidiasis, 1664
  chronic renal failure, 781
  clinical symptoms and diagnosis, 1458-1459
  dysuria, 762
  enterococcal, 1562
  epidemiology, 1457-1458
  fever of unknown origin, 1376
  gram-negative bacteremia, 1446
  hematuria, 757
  management, 1459-1462
  microbiology, 1457
  nosocomial, 1363
  pathogenesis, 1455-1456
  pathology, 1456-1457
  during pregnancy, 2281
  prevention, 1462
  prostatitis, 1462-1463
  spinal cord injured patient, 1050
  staphylococcal, 1551
  stone passage complicated by, 800
Urinary urgency
  bacterial prostatitis, 1462
  urinary tract infection, 1458
Urine
  aciduria, 1907
  alkaptonuria, 1280
  aminoaciduria, 879
    dicarboxylic, 879-880
    Fanconi's syndrome, 882
    galactosemia, 1883
    neutral, 879
  bilirubinuria, 2150
  color alterations, 742
  concentration and dilution, 748
  concentration of antimicrobial agents, 1351
  crystal formation, 797
  diabetes insipidus, 1793-1794
  excretion of pyridinium and deoxypyridinium
    crosslinks, 1745
  laboratory and diagnostic tests, 742-748
    acidification, 747
    fractional excretion of sodium, 747
    glomerular filtration rate, 746-747
    microscopic examination of urine sediment,
      744-746
    urinalysis, 742-744
    urinary concentration and dilution, 748
  maple syrup urine disease, 1908
  measurement of hormone concentrations, 1733
  renal concentrating and diluting mechanisms,
    739, 740
  undegraded vasopressin, 1791
  volume in relation to osmolality, 807
Urine 5-hydroxyindoleacetic acid, 1743
Urine 17-hydroxycorticosteroids, 1740
Urine 17-ketosteroids, 1741
Urine acidification, 739-741
  Sjögren syndrome, 1210
  urinary tract infection, 1459
Urine ammonium, 747
Urine amylase, 2145
Urine anion gap, 747, 840
Urine/blood urea nitrogen ratio, 770
Urine calcium, 1968
  bone and mineral disorders, 1744
  crystals, 746
  hypercalciuria, 1744
  primary hyperparathyroidism, 1968

Urine catecholamines, 1740, 1827
  pheochromocytoma, 1830
Urine chloride, 840
Urine citrate, 799
Urine creatinine, 2113
Urine culture
  trichomoniasis, 1691
  urinary tract infection, 1458, 1461
Urine cyclic adenosine monophosphate, 1746
Urine fat, 745, 746
Urine flow
  anuria
    acute tubular necrosis, 772
    obstructive uropathy, 886
    retroperitoneal fibrosis, 2250
  dysuria, 762-763
    bacterial prostatitis, 1462
    hematuria, 757
    Lassa fever, 1510
    urethritis, 1440
    urinary tract infection, 1458
    vulvovaginal candidiasis, 1442
  obstructive uropathy, 884
Urine free cortisol, 1741, 1819, 1826
Urine glucose, 743
Urine hydroxyproline, 1745
Urine lipase, 2145
Urine lipids, 766
Urine monoclonal proteins, 564-568
Urine osmolality, 742
  acute renal failure, 770
  chronic renal failure, 778
  diabetes insipidus, 1794-1795
  nephrogenic diabetes insipidus, 883
  renal concentrating and diluting mechanisms,
    739
  syndrome of inappropriate antidiuretic
    hormone, 489
Urine output
  adult respiratory distress syndrome, 421
  nephrogenic diabetes insipidus, 883
  oliguria
    acetaminophen poisoning, 2190
    acute tubular necrosis, 772
    anti-neutrophil cytoplasmic
      antibodies-positive glomerulonephritis,
      848
    preeclampsia, 2274
    radiocontrast-induced acute renal failure,
      871
    toxicity of nonsteroidal antiinflammatory
      drugs, 870
  polyuria
    after relief of obstruction, 887
    chronic renal failure, 778
    diabetes insipidus, 815, 1793-1794
    diabetic ketoacidosis, 1863
    disorders of urinary concentration, 748
    Fanconi's syndrome, 882
    hypercalcemia, 1929
    hypokalemia, 829
    insulin-dependent diabetes mellitus, 1854
    juvenile nephronophthisis, 875
    nephrogenic diabetes insipidus, 883, 884
    primary hyperparathyroidism, 1967
Urine pH, 742-743
  crystal formation, 797
  proximal renal tubular acidosis, 837
  tests of renal acidification, 747
  uric acid stones, 799
Urine/plasma creatinine ratio, 770
Urine protein, 758-761
Urine protein electrophoresis, 761
Urine sediment
  acute nephritic syndrome, 764
  erythrocytes in, 756
  microscopic examination, 744-746
Urine sodium, 2168
  acute renal failure, 770
  fractional excretion of sodium, 747
Urine tetrahydroaldosterone, 1819

Urine urea nitrogen, 800
Urine uric acid, 799
Urine volume, 739
Urobilinogens, 744, 2128, 2150
Urobilins, 2150
Urodynamic studies, 938, 1066
Urokinase
  activation of plasminogen to plasmin, 540
  deep venous thrombosis, 311
  myocardial infarction, 213
  pulmonary embolism, 503
  venous thromboembolism, 637
Urolithiathis, 1273
Uromodulin, 758-759
Uropathy, obstructive, 753-754, 884-887
Uropontin, 797
Uroporphyrinogen decarboxylase, 1923
Uroporphyrinogen III synthase, 1923
Ursodeoxycholic acid
  bile water production, 2123
  cholesterol gallstones, 2226
  cystic fibrosis, 2207, 2246
  primary biliary cirrhosis, 2200-2201
Ursodiol, 2227
Urticaria
  Churg-Strauss syndrome, 466
  contact, 1304
  drug-induced, 1315-1316
Urticaria pigmentosa, 681
Usual body weight, 2111
Usual interstitial pneumonia, 449
Uterus
  adrenergic responses, 1828
  amenorrhea, 1760
  clostridial infection, 1576
Utilization review, 33
Uveitis, 2075
Uveoparotid fever, 459
Uvulopalatopharyngoplasty, 528
Uvulopharyngopalatoplasty, 2309

V

V segment, 1111
V wave, 37
  cardiac cycle, 72
  jugular venous pulse, 65, 66-67
  mitral regurgitation, 250, 251
  primary pulmonary hypertension, 294
  tricuspid regurgitation, 256
Vaccination
  complement deficiency states, 1339
  human immunodeficiency virus infection,
    1473
  before traveling, 1467-1468
Vaccine
  bacille Calmette-Guérin, 1637-1638
  Borrelia burgdorferi, 1648
  Brucella, 1606
  cholera, 1596
  cytomegalovirus, 1529
  diphtheria, 1567
  encephalitis, 1518-1519
  Haemophilus influenzae type b, 1588-1589
  hepatitis A, 1493
  influenza, 1493
  measles, 1499
  mumps, 1497
  pertussis, 1613
  plague, 1610
  polio, 1492-1493
  rabies, 1506-1507
  Rocky Mountain spotted fever, 1546
  rubella, 1501-1502
  tetanus, 1574
  tularemia, 1608
  typhoid, 1602
VAD regimen, 702
Vagina
  bleeding in endometrial cancer, 713
  exam for sexually transmitted disease, 1439

Vagina—cont'd
  lactobacilli, 1456
  menopause, 2271
  microflora, 1397, 1615
Vaginal discharge
  bacterial vaginosis, 1443
  examination, 1439
  trichomoniasis, 1691
Vaginitis
  anaerobic bacteria, 1618
  candidal, 1661
  dysuria, 762-763
  pellagra, 2107
Vagotomy
  gastric analysis after, 2003
  neurogenic pulmonary edema, 1099
  peptic ulcer disease, 2040-2041
Vagus nerve
  esophageal peristalsis and control of gastric
    emptying, 1977
  integrated pancreatic secretion, 2133
  pancreatic innervation, 2131
Valacyclovir, 1526, 1527
Valine
  disorders of branched-chain amino acid
    metabolism, 1908
  related diseases, 1904
Valley fever, 1655
Valproate, 983
  hepatic injury, 2190, 2191
  prophylaxis of migraine, 962
Valsalva maneuver, 937
Valsalva ratio, 937
Valve area, 97, 111
Valve replacement surgery, 257-261
  aortic regurgitation, 243-244
  aortic stenosis, 239
  mitral regurgitation, 252
  mitral stenosis, 248-249
  pulmonic regurgitation, 257
  reactive pulmonary hypertension, 298
  tricuspid regurgitation, 256
  tricuspid stenosis, 256
Valvotomy, pulmonic stenosis, 288
Valvular ejection sound, 74
Valvular heart disease, 235-262
  aortic regurgitation, 239-245
  aortic stenosis, 235-239
  cardiac catheterization, 108, 109
  dexfenfluramine and, 261
  echocardiography, 100
  fenfluramine and, 261
  interventional cardiac catheterization, 116-125
    approach to specific lesions, 120-121
    background, 116-117
    complications, 122
    coronary angioplasty for acute myocardial
      infarction, 121-122
    devices, 117-120, 121
    pathophysiology, 116
    primary coronary angioplasty, 122
    randomized trials, 117, 118
    referral, 124
    rescue coronary angioplasty, 122
    restenosis, 122-124
  mitral regurgitation, 249-253
  mitral stenosis, 245-249
  mitral valve prolapse, 253-255
  multivalvular, 257
  operative risk, 2260
  penetrating and nonpenetrating injuries, 332
  phentermine and, 261
  during pregnancy, 2276
  prosthetic valves, 257-261
  pulmonic regurgitation, 256-257
  pulmonic stenosis, 256
    with intact ventricular septum, 288
  risk of stroke, 1001
  tricuspid regurgitation, 256
  tricuspid stenosis, 255-256
Van Buchem's disease, 1959

Vancomycin, 1358
  bacterial meningitis, 1411
  brain abscess, 1416
  Clostridium difficile colitis, 1569, 1570
  dosage, 1350
  enterococci resistance, 1561
  furuncle, 1421
  infective endocarditis, 231, 232
  septic arthritis, 1253
  Staphylococcus epidermidis, 1552
  Streptococcus pneumoniae meningitis, 1410
  subdural empyema, 1418
  use during pregnancy, 2281
Vanillylmandelic acid, 930, 1739-1740, 1827, 1830
Vannini-Rizzoli boot, 1053
Variable expressivity in autosomal dominant
  disorders, 1726
Variable number tandem repeats, 578, 1723-1724
Variable surface glycoprotein, 1688
Variant angina, 194
  calcium channel blockers, 205
  continuous ambulatory electrocardiographic
    recording, 94
  coronary arteriography, 199-200
  nitroglycerin and nitrates, 201
  prognosis, 208
  therapeutic approach, 207
Variceal bleeding
  hepatocellular carcinoma, 2213
  portal hypertension, 2165-2168, 2166
  portal vein obstruction, 2208
  primary biliary cirrhosis, 2200
Varicella-zoster virus, 1525-1527
  acquired immunodeficiency syndrome, 1328
  after stem cell transplantation, 579
  compromised host, 1388
  culture, 1369
  esophageal infection, 2019-2020
  pericarditis, 272
  during pregnancy, 2280
Varices
  esophageal
    portal hypertension, 2166
    treatment, 2013-2014
  gastric, 2166
Varicocele, 1845
Varicose bronchiectasis, 484
Varicose veins, 311
  hemorrhoids, 2092-2093
Variegate porphyria, 1926
Vasa recta, 739, 740
Vascor; *see* Bepridil
Vascular adhesion molecule-1, 372
Vascular dementia, 988-989, 2288
Vascular disease
  aortic disorders, 299-304
    aortic aneurysm, 299-300
    aortitis, 302-303
    atherosclerosis, 299
    dissection of aorta, 300-302, 303
    Marfan syndrome, 299
    mycotic aneurysm, 299, 300
    occlusive disease, 304
    syphilis, 303
  chronic tubulointerstitial nephropathy, 892
  complication of systemic cancer, 1072
  diabetes mellitus, 1868-1870
  impotence, 1760, 1761
  intestinal, 2086-2089
  lipoprotein levels, 60
  ocular, 1057-1062
  osteomyelitis resulting from, 1436
  peripheral vascular disease, 304-312
    anticoagulant therapy, 641
    arteritis, 311
    occlusive peripheral arterial disease,
      307-309
    peripheral arterial aneurysm, 309
    peripheral arteries, 305-307
    peripheral veins, 311-312
    vasospastic disorders, 309-311

Vascular disease—cont'd
  radiation therapy-induced, 1073
  retinal, 2302-2304
  systemic sclerosis, 1228
Vascular ejection sounds, 74
Vascular endothelial growth factor, 374
Vascular graft infection, 1551
Vascular headache, 958
Vascular injury
  diabetic glomerulopathy, 860
  Rocky Mountain spotted fever, 1541-1543
Vascular lesion
  chronic gastrointestinal bleeding, 2014
  drug-induced, 2189
Vascular malformation
  angiography, 927
  hemorrhagic stroke, 998
Vascular necrosis, 1218-1226
  alveolar hemorrhage with, 454
  angiocentric immunoproliferative disorders,
    1225
  Churg-Strauss syndrome, 1220
  classification, 1219
  clinical approach, 1225-1226
  giant cell arteritis, 1223-1224
  glomerular involvement, 855-859
  hypersensitivity vasculitis, 1221-1222
  hypokalemia, 829
  Kawasaki's disease, 1225
  microscopic polyarteritis nodosa, 1220-1221
  pathogenesis, 1218-1219
  petechiae, 603
  polyangiitis, 1221
  polyarteritis nodosa, 1219-1220
  primary angiitis of central nervous system,
    1225
  pulmonary, 454
    primary granulomatous, 465-471
  rheumatoid arthritis, 1203
  Sjögren syndrome, 1210
  systemic lupus erythematosus, 1213-1214
  Takayasu's arteritis, 1224
  Wegener's granulomatosis, 1222-1223
Vascular resistance, 46
  patent ductus arteriosus, 285
Vascular shunt infection, 1551
Vascular smooth muscle
  modulation of arterial tone, 47
  pulmonary vessels, 360
Vascular surgery
  complications, 1013
  preoperative evaluation, 2258
Vascular system
  involvement in osteomyelitis, 1434
  mediation by autonomic nervous system,
    931-932
Vascular thrombosis, 794
Vasculitis, 1218-1226
  alveolar hemorrhage with, 454
  angiocentric immunoproliferative disorders,
    1225
  anti-neutrophil cytoplasmic antibodies-positive
    crescentic glomerulonephritis, 847-848
  aspergillosis, 1658
  autoantibodies, 1155
  Behçet disease, 1243
  Churg-Strauss syndrome, 1220
  classification, 1219
  clinical approach, 1225-1226
  compromised host, 1388
  giant cell arteritis, 1223-1224
  glomerular involvement, 855-859
  hypersensitivity vasculitis, 1221-1222
  hypocomplementemia, 1138
  hypokalemia, 829
  intradermal hemorrhage, Plate VIII-45
  Kawasaki's disease, 1225
    anti-neutrophil cytoplasmic antibodies, 1219
    exanthem, 1385
  leprosy, 1650
  leptospirosis, 1644

Vasculitis—cont'd
  leukocytoclastic, 1315
  microscopic polyarteritis nodosa, 1220-1221
  neurologic aspects, 1091
  panniculitis, 1245
  pathogenesis, 1218-1219
  petechiae, 603
  polyangiitis, 1221
  polyarteritis nodosa, 334, 856, 1219-1220
    crescentic glomerulonephritis, 848
    diffuse immune-complex vasculitis, 454
    glucocorticoid protocol, 1263
    microscopic, 1220-1221
    neurologic manifestations, 1092, 1095
  primary angiitis of central nervous system,
    1225
  pulmonary, 454
    primary granulomatous, 465-471
  rheumatoid arthritis, 1094, 1203
  rickettsial infection, Plate VIII-44
  sepsis *versus,* 1451
  Sjögren syndrome, 1210
  systemic lupus erythematosus, 1213-1214
  systemic sclerosis, 1230
  Takayasu's arteritis, 311, 470-471, 1224
    aortic obstruction and inflammation,
      303-304
    neurologic manifestations, 1092, 1095
  temporal arteritis, 311, 959, 1223-1224
    anterior ischemic optic neuropathy, 1059
    glucocorticoid protocol, 1263
    neurologic manifestations, 1092
  Wegener's granulomatosis, 467-468, 469,
    1222-1223
    acute nephritic syndrome, 764
    anti-neutrophil cytoplasmic antibodies, 1219
    crescentic glomerulonephritis, 848
    lung involvement, 453
    neurologic manifestations, 1092, 1095
    renal involvement, 858
Vasectomy, 2269-2270
Vasoactive agents, 294
Vasoactive intestinal polypeptide
  erectile function, 934
  pancreatic exocrine secretion, 2133
  pepsinogen secretion, 1984, 1985
  peristalsis, 1977
  prolactin stimulation, 1775
  VIPoma, 2005, 2245
Vasoactive mediators, 1141
Vasoconstriction
  acute hypertensive retinopathy, 2302
  pheochromocytoma, 1829
  postrenal azotemia, 769
  precapillary pulmonary hypertension, 294, 295
  pulmonary edema, 424
  shock, 176, 177
  unstable angina, 195
Vasodepressor syncope, 952-954
Vasodilation
  nitroglycerin and nitrates, 201
  rhinitis medicamentosa, 2308
Vasodilator Heart Failure Trial I, 171
Vasodilator Heart Failure Trial II, 171
Vasodilators, 138
  achalasia, 2022
  angina, 201, 202, 205
  aortic regurgitation, 243
  atrioventricular reciprocating tachycardia, 143
  autonomic dysreflexia, 1049
  congestive heart failure, 818
  dilated cardiomyopathy, 264
  direct-acting, 173-174
  drug-induced bile duct injury, 2203
  heart failure, 170, 173-174
  hepatic injury, 2192
  human cytochrome P450 isoforms, 2312
  hypertension, 325, 327
  hypertensive emergency, 328
  hypertrophic obstructive cardiomyopathy, 269
  interference with catecholamine assays, 1740

Vasodilators—cont'd
  interference with oral anticoagulants, 636
  ischemic bowel, 2088
  mitral regurgitation, 252, 253
  preeclampsia, 2275
  primary pulmonary hypertension, 295
  pulmonary hypertension, 499
  pulmonary parenchymal reactions, 476
  pulmonary toxicity, 478
  Raynaud's phenomenon, 1227
  uncommon types of sustained ventricular
    tachycardia, 153
Vasogenic cerebral edema, 1405
Vasomotor fibers in nose, 1181
Vasomotor rhinitis, 1181, 2308
Vasomotor tone, pulmonary blood flow, 362-363
Vasoocclusive events in sickle cell disease, 657,
    658
Vasoocclusive mediators, 421
Vasopressin
  aging and, 2284
  biochemistry, 1788-1789
  congestive heart failure, 817
  deficiency, 1777
  diabetes insipidus, 883, 1793-1795
  diverticular bleeding, 2092
  gastrointestinal bleeding, 2012-2013
  heart failure, 160, 161
  hypopituitarism treatment, 1781
  increase after nausea induction, 2025
  nephrogenic diabetes insipidus, 883
  physiology, 1789-1793
  pituitary stimulation tests, 1736
  plasma, 1737-1738
  variceal bleeding, 2167
  vasoactive effects on pulmonary circulation,
    363
  water balance, 739
Vasopressinase, 808, 1791
Vasopressors, 1451
Vasospasm, coronary
  after revascularization surgery, 207
  amrinone, 182
  angioplasty-induced, 122
  coronary arteriography, 200
  myocardial infarction, 209
  variant angina, 194
Vasospastic disorders, 309-311
Vasotec; *see* Enalapril
Vasovagal syncope, 952-954
Vaughn Williams classification of antiarrhythmic
    drugs, 134, 135, 189
VBMCP regimen, 702
Vector deoxyribonucleic acid, 52
Vector in gene therapy, 1732
Vegetables causing occupational asthma, 472
VEGF; *see* Vascular endothelial growth factor
Veillonella, 1368
Vein graft disease, 121
Vellous hair, 1755
Velocardiofacial syndrome, Plate IX-1
Velocity profiles, 98
Vena cava
  inferior
    Budd-Chiari syndrome, 2208
    pulmonary embolism, 638
    venous thromboembolism, 632
    interruption, 504
    superior vena cava syndrome
      aortic dissection, 301
      lung cancer, 488
    superior vena caval obstruction, 511-512
      abnormal jugular venous pulse, 66
      transudative pleural effusion, 507
Venereal Disease Research Laboratory test, 1642
Venezuelan equine encephalitis, 1515, 1517
Venezuelan hemorrhagic fever, 1511
Venlafaxine, 1037, 2289
Veno-occlusive disease
  after stem cell transplantation, 579
  drug-induced, 2189

Veno-occlusive disease—cont'd
  hepatic, 585, 2207-2209
  reocclusion of infarct-related vessel, 214
  retinal vein, 2304, Plate XI-9, Plate XI-10
Venom
  hemolysis, 668
  immunotherapy, 1194
Venous access in pulmonary artery
    catheterization, 390-392
Venous admixture, 352
Venous catheterization with hormone
    measurement, 1735
Venous congestion
  dilated cardiomyopathy, 263
  restrictive cardiomyopathy, 271
Venous disease, 311-312
  calf vein thrombosis, 633
  cortical vein thrombosis, 928
  deep venous thrombosis, 311
    critical pathway, 21
    diagnosis, 502
    paraneoplastic dermatoses, 1317
    during pregnancy, 2276
    prophylaxis, 504
    pulmonary embolism, 631
    spinal cord injury, 1049
    superficial thrombophlebitis, 638
  partial transposition of pulmonary veins, 282
  peripheral vascular disease, 304-312
    anticoagulant therapy, 641
    arteritis, 311
    contraindication to renal transplantation,
      792
    occlusive peripheral arterial disease,
      307-309
    peripheral arterial aneurysm, 309
    peripheral arteries, 305-307
    peripheral veins, 311-312
    vasospastic disorders, 309-311
  portal vein obstruction, 2208-2209
  portal vein thrombosis, 2089
  proximal-vein thrombosis, 631
  pulmonary vein stenosis, 298
  renal vein thrombosis
    acute renal failure, 769
    membranous nephropathy with, 854
    nephrotic syndrome, 766
  total anomalous pulmonary venous connection,
    290-291
  varicose veins, 311
    hemorrhoids, 2092-2093
Venous drainage
  adrenal gland, 1817
  pancreas, 2130
Venous filling time, 305
Venous pressure
  cardiac tamponade, 275
  constrictive pericarditis, 277
Venous return curve, 364
Venous stasis
  chronic venous insufficiency, 312
  thrombosis, 608
Venous thromboembolism, 311, 630-638
  clinical features, 631-632
  etiology and pathogenesis, 630-631
  heparin therapy, 634-635
  laboratory features, 632
  mesenteric, 2088-2089
  oral anticoagulants, 635-637
  perioperative prevention, 2263
  thrombolytic therapy, 637-638
Ventilation
  chemical control, 352
  hypoxic pulmonary vasoconstriction, 363
  mechanical, 396-400
    acute respiratory failure, 416, 418-419, 446
    chronic obstructive pulmonary disease, 417
    endotracheal intubation and tracheotomy,
      399
    gram-negative sepsis, 1452
    initiation, 396-397

Ventilation—cont'd
  mechanical—cont'd
    modes, 397-398
    monitoring ventilatory mechanics, 398-399
    pulmonary edema, 426-427
    respiratory acidosis, 416
    respiratory muscle failure, 359-360
    weaning, 399-400, 420
  neural factors in control, 353
  relationship to perfusion, 349
  during sleep, 525
  unevenness of, 348-349
Ventilation/perfusion lung scan, 502
Ventilation-perfusion mismatching, 349, 413
Ventilation scan, 387-388
Ventilator settings, 397
Ventilatory control studies, 378-379
Ventilatory failure, 359
  neurogenic causes, 1096
  precapillary pulmonary hypertension, 295-296
Ventilatory modes, 397-398
Ventilatory support, 396-400
  acute respiratory failure, 416, 418-419
    with chronic obstructive pulmonary disease,
      446
    weaning, 420
  chronic obstructive pulmonary disease, 417
  endotracheal intubation and tracheotomy, 399
  gram-negative sepsis, 1452
  initiation, 396-397
  modes, 397-398
  monitoring ventilatory mechanics, 398-399
  pulmonary edema, 426-427
  respiratory acidosis, 416
  respiratory muscle failure, 359-360
  weaning, 399-400, 420
Ventricle
  diastolic performance, 43-46
  structure and function, 41-42
  systolic performance, 42-43
Ventricular arrhythmia, 148-153
  abnormal jugular venous pulse, 66
  accelerated idioventricular rhythm, 149, 150
  amiodarone, 138
  antiarrhythmic therapy, 174
  beta-blockers, 138
  flecainide, 138
  lidocaine, 137-138
  mexiletine, 138
  neurologic aspects, 1088
  nonsustained ventricular tachycardia, 149
  polymorphic ventricular tachycardia, 151-153
  premature ventricular contractions, 148-149
  propafenone, 138
  sustained monomorphic ventricular
    tachycardia, 150-151
  sustained ventricular tachycardia with wide
    QRS complex tachycardia, 149-150,
    151
  tetralogy of Fallot, 289
  ventricular fibrillation, 153
Ventricular assist device, 185, 186
Ventricular depolarization, 84
Ventricular fibrillation, 153
  during cardiac catheterization, 108
  hyperkalemia, 833
  myocardial infarction, 223-224
  potassium therapy, 830
Ventricular filling, 37
  constrictive pericarditis, 277
  restrictive cardiomyopathy, 270
  role of pericardium, 271
Ventricular function curve, 158
Ventricular hypertrophy
  chronic cor pulmonale, 446
  echocardiography, 100
Ventricular power output, 43
Ventricular premature contractions, 1942
Ventricular pressure, 44, 112
Ventricular rate, 85

Ventricular septal defect, 283-285
  with aortic regurgitation, 285
  complete transposition of great arteries, 290
  differential diagnosis, 180
  murmur, 77, 79
  precapillary pulmonary hypertension, 296
  pulmonary hypertension, 296
  tetralogy of Fallot, 288-289
  tricuspid atresia, 291
Ventricular septal rupture, 177
  myocardial infarction, 219-220
Ventricular tachyarrhythmia
  mitral valve prolapse, 255
  myocardial infarction, 223-224
Ventricular tachycardia
  automatic implantable cardioverter
    defibrillator, 140
  cardiogenic syncope, 954
  complication of pulmonary artery
    catheterization, 395
  flecainide, 138
  hypertrophic obstructive cardiomyopathy, 269
  mitral valve prolapse, 254
  myocardial infarction, 180, 223
  palpitations, 130
  response to carotid sinus massage or
    intravenous adenosine, 134
  sotalol, 138
  sudden death, 187
  wide QRS complex tachycardia, 150
Ventricular-vascular coupling, 43
Ventriculography
  ischemic heart disease, 113
  mitral valve prolapse, 254
  myocardial infarction, 212
Ventriculomyectomy, 270
Venturi face mask, 429
Verapamil
  angina, 203
  arrhythmias, 138
  atrial fibrillation, 147
  atrial flutter, 146
  cluster headache prophylaxis, 962
  hepatic injury, 2192
  hypertension, 325
  hypertrophic obstructive cardiomyopathy, 269
  interaction with cyclosporin, 793
  multifocal atrial tachycardia, 144
  properties, 204
  prophylaxis of migraine, 962
  sustained ventricular tachycardia and wide
    QRS complex tachycardia, 150
  Wolff-Parkinson-White syndrome, 142
Verbal alexia, 978
Verelan; *see* Verapamil
Verner-Morrison syndrome, 2245
Verruca vulgaris, 1328
Verrucous carcinoma, 723
Vertebral artery occlusion, 1005
Vertebral crush fracture, 1944-1945
Vertebral osteomyelitis, 1433, 1435
Vertebrobasilar artery insufficiency, 2301
Vertigo, 2307
Very low density lipoproteins, 1885-1886
  abetalipoproteinemia, 1897
  atherosclerosis, 1889
  combined hyperlipidemias, 1896
  endogenous hypertriglyceridemia, 1894-1895
  fatty acids, 1851
  hepatic synthesis, 2121
  hyperlipidemia, 1892
  macrovascular disease, 1868
  nephrotic syndrome, 766
  obesity, 1752
  primary biliary cirrhosis, 2200
  uremic patient, 786
Vesicle
  bullous impetigo, 1419
  chickenpox, 1525
  differential diagnosis of fever and rash, 1384
  ecthyma, 1420

Vesicle—cont'd
  genital lesions, 1442
  hand-foot-mouth syndrome, 1489
  herpangina, 1488
  herpes, 1444
  impetigo, 1419
  lipid digestion, 1987
  lymphogranuloma venereum, 1535
  porphyria cutanea tarda, 1927
  Pseudomonas septicemia, 1382
  synergistic nonclostridial anaerobic
    myonecrosis, 1424
  unilamellar, 2127, 2128
Vesicoureteral reflux, 1457
Vesnarinone, 173
VEST survival trial, 171
Vestibular epilepsy, 973
Vestibular eye movement, 1063
Vestibular neuronitis, 972
Vestibular nystagmus, 1064
Vestibular physical therapy, 975
Vestibular system, 971-972
Vestibulocochlear nerve, 973
Vestibuloocular reflex, 947-948, 974
Vibrio, 1593-1598
  cellulitis, 1423
  compromised host, 1388
Vibrio alginolyticus, 1597
Vibrio cholerae, 1594
  acute diarrhea, 1425-1426
  attachment mechanisms, 1446
Vibrio fluvialis, 1598
Vibrio mimicus, 1597
Vibrio parahaemolyticus, 1430, 1596-1597
Vibrio vulnificus, 1423, 1597
Vicious cycle of dyspnea, 432
Vidarabine, 1526
Video-assisted thoracoscopic lung biopsy, 451
Video-assisted thoracoscopic surgery, 385
Videx; *see* Didanosine
Vigorous achalasia, 2022
Villous adenoma of colon, 2086
Villus, 1991, 2057
  mesenteric ischemia, 2087
Vimentin, 731
Vinblastine
  breast cancer, 710
  Hodgkin's disease, 694-695
Vinca alkaloids, 476
  breast cancer, 709, 710
  effects on kidney, 870
  hepatic injury, 2192
  Hodgkin's disease, 694-695
  multiple myeloma, 702
  non-Hodgkin's lymphoma, 698-699
Vincent's angina, 1393
Vincristine
  breast cancer, 709, 710
  effects on kidney, 870
  hepatic injury, 2192
  Hodgkin's disease, 694-695
  multiple myeloma, 702
  non-Hodgkin's lymphoma, 698-699
Vinyl chloride, 548
VIPoma, 2005, 2245
Viracept; *see* Nelfinavir
Viral infection
  acquired immunodeficiency syndrome,
    1327-1328, 1474, 2096
  activation of protooncogenes, 543
  acute pharyngitis, 1392
  adenovirus, 1503-1504
  after renal transplantation, 794-795
  aplastic anemia, 672
  arenavirus, 1508-1511
  cell-mediated immunity, 1132
  cholangitis, 2202
  Colorado tick fever, 1511-1512
  common cold, 1390-1392
  coronavirus, 1502-1503
  culture, 1369-1370

Viral infection—cont'd
  diarrhea, 1427-1428
  differential diagnosis of fever and rash, 1384
  esophageal, 2019-2020
  fever of unknown origin, 1377
  hemophagocytic syndrome, 680
  hepatitis, 2138; *see also* Hepatitis
    acute, 2172-2179
    chronic, 2179-2184
    dialysis-related, 790
    hepatocellular carcinoma, 2212
    during pregnancy, 2277
    travel-related, 1465
  herpesvirus, 1522-1530
    characteristics, 1522-1523
    cytomegalovirus, 1527-1529
    Epstein-Barr virus, 1529-1530
    herpes simplex virus, 1523-1525
    human herpesvirus 6, 1530
    human herpesvirus 8, 1530
    varicella zoster virus, 1525-1527
  Hodgkin's disease, 691
  immune complexes, 1149
  immunocompromised patient, 1387
  measles, 1497-1499
  meningitis, 1488
    clinical manifestations, 1406, 1407
    epidemiology and etiology, 1403-1404
    laboratory investigation, 1406-1408
  mumps, 1495-1497
  myocarditis, 262-263
  nausea and vomiting, 2026
  Norwalk-like virus, 1521-1522
  parainfluenza, 1494-1495
  paramyxovirus, 1494
  parvovirus, 1512-1514
  pericarditis, 272
  picornavirus and orthomyxovirus, 1483-1494
    acute febrile undifferentiated illness, 1487
    acute hemorrhagic conjunctivitis, 1490
    aseptic meningitis, 1488
    characteristics, 1483
    chemoprophylaxis, 1493
    chronic meningoencephalitis, 1490
    classification, 1483-1485
    common cold, 1487
    diagnosis, 1492
    encephalitis, 1488
    epidemic pleurodynia, 1489
    epidemiology, 1484-1485
    exanthems, 1489
    hand-foot-mouth syndrome, 1489
    hepatitis, 1490
    herpangina, 1488-1489
    influenza, 1490-1491
    lymphonodular pharyngitis, 1489
    myopericarditis, 1489-1490
    neurologic complications, 1491
    paralytic poliomyelitis, 1487-1488
    pathogenesis, 1485-1487
    prevention, 1492-1493
    pulmonary complications, 1491
    treatment, 1492
  pleural effusion, 507
  during pregnancy, 2280-2281
  progressive multifocal leukoencephalopathy, 1010
  pure red blood cell aplasia, 675
  rabies, 1505-1508
  respiratory syncytial virus, 1499-1500
  respiratory tract, 1390-1396
  retrovirus, 1531-1534
  rheumatoid factor, 1160
  rotavirus, 1520-1521
  rubella, 1500-1502
  seizure, 980
  septic arthritis, 1255
  Sjögren syndrome, 1210
  subacute thyroiditis, 1811
  travel-related, 1465
  uremic patient, 784

Viral ribonucleic acid, 1473
Viramune; *see* Nevirapine
Virazole; *see* Ribavirin
Virchow's triad, 608
Virginal hypertrophy, 1770
Virilization, 1755, 1756
  Cushing's syndrome, 1820
Virulence factors
  anaerobic bacteria, 1614-1616
  bacterial meningitis, 1405
  chlamydiae, 1535
  Cryptococcus neoformans, 1667
  gram-negative bacteremia, 1446-1447
  Mycoplasma pneumoniae, 1538
  urinary tract infection, 1456
  Vibrio cholerae, 1595
  Vibrio vulnificus, 1597
  Yersinia pestis, 1609-1610
Visceral abscess, 844
Visceral larva migrans, 1700, 1702
Visceral pain, 2030
Visceral peritoneum, 2247
Visceral pleura, 505
Vision loss
  amaurosis fugax, 1057-1058
  Behçet disease, 1243
  disease processes, 1056
Visken; *see* Pindolol
Visual acuity, 2255
Visual evoked responses, 910-911
  multiple sclerosis, 1009
Visual field testing, 2301
Visual hallucination, 1061-1062
Visual impairment, 1033
  amblyopia ex anopia, 1062
  chiasmal, 1060
  elderly, 2287
  hypoglycemia, 1875
  neurologic disorders, 1056-1057
  pheochromocytoma, 1829
  prolactin-secreting pituitary adenoma, 1786
  stroke patient, 1055
Visual loss, 2300-2301
Visual obscurations, 2300-2301
Visual-vestibular interaction testing, 974
Visuospatial behavioral disturbance, 1033
Visuospatial function, 902
Vital capacity
  interstitial lung disease, 450
  Langerhans' cell granulomatosis, 464
  removal from mechanical ventilation and weaning, 420
  respiratory muscle function, 431
Vitamin A
  biochemical function, 2105
  deficiency, 1101, 2105-2106, 2195
  hepatic injury, 2192
  hypervitaminosis A, 2108
  measles therapy, 1499
  megadoses and toxicity, 2108
  primary biliary cirrhosis, 2201
  recommended daily dietary allowances, 2114
Vitamin A analog, 1302
Vitamin B_1
  biochemical function, 2105
  deficiency, 2106
Vitamin B_2
  biochemical function, 2105
  deficiency, 2106
Vitamin B_6
  biochemical function, 2105
  deficiency, 1101, 2107
  drug-nutrient interactions, 2110
  recommended daily dietary allowances, 2115
Vitamin B_{12}
  absorption test for malabsorption, 2007
  bacterial overgrowth, 2060
  biochemical function, 2105
  cellular metabolism, 647
  chronic gastritis, 2043

Vitamin B_{12}—cont'd
  deficiency, 1080, 1101, 2107
    bone marrow, Plate IV-7
    clinical presentation, 647-648
    intestinal disease, 2005
    metabolic myelopathy, 1013
    neurologic aspects, 1103
    thrombocytopenia, 605, 614
  diabetic polyneuropathy, 1871
  drug-nutrient interactions, 2110
  intestinal absorption, 1989
  megaloblastic anemia, 646-647, 649
  recommended daily dietary allowances, 2115
  small bowel malabsorption, 2058
Vitamin C
  beta-thalassemia, 656
  biochemical function, 2105
  cystinosis, 1910
  deficiency, 2107
  glucose-6-phosphate dehydrogenase deficiency, 664
  megadoses and toxicity, 2108
  recommended daily dietary allowances, 2115
Vitamin D
  biochemical function, 2105
  deficiency, 1101, 2106
    Crohn's disease, 2075
    hypocalcemia, 1932
    primary biliary cirrhosis, 2201
    rickets and osteomalacia, 1951
  hypercalciuria, 798
  hypocalcemia, 1934
  intestinal magnesium absorption, 1939
  intoxication, 2108
  metabolic disorders, 1949-1955
  nephrotic syndrome, 767
  osteoporosis, 1947
  recommended daily dietary allowances, 2114
  regulation of intestinal calcium absorption, 1988-1989
  renal osteodystrophy, 1961
  role in calcium metabolism, 1719-1720
  synthesis, 1710
  therapeutic
    renal bone disease, 1964
    rickets or osteomalacia, 1954
  toxicity, 1928
  urine calcium, 1744
  X-linked hypophosphatemic rickets, 880
Vitamin D-binding protein, 1719
Vitamin D-dependent rickets, 1952, 1953
Vitamin D metabolites, 1719
  bone and mineral disorders, 1746
  osteoporosis, 1948
Vitamin E
  abetalipoproteinemia, 1897
  biochemical function, 2105
  deficiency, 1101, 2106
  fibrocystic breast disease, 1849, 1850
  megadoses and toxicity, 2108
  primary biliary cirrhosis, 2201
  recommended daily dietary allowances, 2114
Vitamin K
  antidote to oral anticoagulants, 637
  biochemical function, 2105
  blood clotting factors synthesis, 2120
  deficiency, 625-626, 1101, 2106
    coagulation disorder, 607
  disturbance of prothrombin time, 2135
  drug-nutrient interactions, 2110
  glucose-6-phosphate dehydrogenase deficiency, 664
  hemostatic defects in liver disease, 627
  recommended daily dietary allowances, 2116
Vitamin K epoxidase, 625
Vitamins, 2105-2108
  deficiencies, 2105-2107
    neurologic aspects, 1100
    short bowel syndrome, 2066
  hepatic detoxification, 2122
  parenteral solutions, 2114

Vitamins—cont'd
  small bowel bacterial overgrowth, 2060
  supplementation
    cystic fibrosis, 483, 2246
    diabetic polyneuropathy, 1871
    hemodialysis, 789
  therapeutic use, 2107-2108
Vitiligo, 1155
Vitreous hemorrhage, Plate XI-8
Vitronectin, 1135
Vittaforma, 1680, 1681
Vocal cords
  asthma, 1189
  paralysis, 2309
Vocational rehabilitation, 1052
Voiding cystourethrogram, 938
Voiding dysfunction, 1065-1066
Voltage-dependent ion channels, 58
Voltage-operated gate, 37
Volume depletion
  chronic renal failure, 781
  generation of alkalosis, 839
Volume excess, 424
Volume expansion
  gastrointestinal bleeding, 2010
  gram-negative bacteremia, 1451
  hypotension, 1828
  right ventricular infarction, 178, 220-221
Volume overload
  differential diagnosis, 180
  mitral regurgitation, 250
Volutrauma, 397
Volvulus
  gastric, 2044
  mesenteric hernia, 2251
  radiography, 2078
Vomiting, 2025-2029
  acute cholecystitis, 2227
  acute pancreatitis, 2234
  appendicitis, 2092
  ascites, 2164
  autonomic failure, 935
  bacterial meningitis, 1406
  biliary colic, 2225
  bubonic plague, 1610
  chemotherapy-induced, 581-582
  chronic renal failure, 784
  galactosemia, 1882
  generation of alkalosis, 839
  hepatitis A virus infection, 2173
  hepatocellular carcinoma, 2213
  herpangina, 1488
  hyperemesis gravidarum, 2278
  hypertrophic pyloric stenosis, 2044
  intestinal obstruction, 2077, 2078
  Lassa fever, 1510
  mesenteric panniculitis, 2251
  normotensive renal potassium wasting, 828
  Norwalk virus, 1522
  pancreatic abscess, 1399
  peptic ulcer, 2037
  peritoneal mesenteric and omental diseases,
    2248
  peritonitis, 1398
  pheochromocytoma, 1829
  Rocky Mountain spotted fever, 1543
  rotavirus, 1521
  solitary liver cyst, 2111
  thrombotic thrombocytopenic purpura, 615
Von Hippel-Lindau disease, 1922-1923
Von Recklinghausen's neurofibromatosis,
    1920-1922, 2050
Von Willebrand's disease, 611, 622-624
  factor VIII concentration, 604
  during pregnancy, 2279
Von Willebrand's factor, 538, 622
  activities, 618
  concentration, structure, and function, 569-570
  platelet adhesion, 536, 611
Von Willebrand's factor antigen, 618
VSD; *see* Ventricular septal defect

Vulva
  candidiasis, 1310
  erysipelas, 1420
Vulvovaginitis, 1310, 1441, 1442-1443, 1618
VVI pacemaker, 139

W

WAGR syndrome, 1729
Waist to hip circumference ratio, 1751
Waldenström macroglobulinemia, 703-704
  bleeding problems, 612
  immunoelectrophoresis, 566-567
  plasmacytoid lymphocytes, 595
  renal involvement, 865-866
Walk through angina, 195, 196
Walk-through phenomenon, 126
Wall stress, 159
Wallstent, 120
Warfarin
  after myocardial infarction, 639
  atrial fibrillation, 147, 640
  deep vein thrombosis prophylaxis, 504
  heart failure, 174-175
  human cytochrome P450 isoforms, 2312
  during pregnancy, 2276
  prosthetic heart valve, 258, 640
  prothrombin time, 571
  thrombotic stroke, 1004
  venous thromboembolism, 311, 635-636
Warfarin embryopathy, 636
Warm-reacting antibody hemolytic anemia,
    668-669
Warm-up phenomenon, 126, 143
WAS protein, 1178
Washed red blood cells, 572
Wasp sting, 668
Water
  balance disorders, 805-816
    hypernatremia, 813-816
    hyponatremia, 809-813
    hypothalamic dysfunction, 1776
    principles of osmoregulation, 805-809
  bile water production, 2123-2124
  deprivation test, 1738
  effects of vasopressin, 1792
  excretion in chronic renal failure, 778
  intestinal absorption, 1988
  loss in vomiting, 2028
  metabolism, 739, 740
  replacement in diabetic ketoacidosis, 1864
  restriction
    compulsive water drinkers, 815
    hypotonic hyponatremic syndromes,
      812-813
    serum osmolality, 806
    syndrome of inappropriate antidiuretic
      hormone, 489
  retention
    after cardiac transplantation, 343
    aortic regurgitation, 241
    heart failure, 162-163
Water loading, 1738
Water-soluble vitamins, 789
Waterbrash, 1998-1999
Waterhammer pulse, 65
Waterston-Cooley anastomosis, 289
Watson-Schwartz test, 1926
Waveform, electrocardiographic, 83
Weakness, 1753-1755
  acute aortic obstruction, 304
  acute lymphoblastic leukemia, 682
  aldosterone excess, 1822
  aplastic anemia, 672
  differential diagnosis, 1754
  hyperkalemia, 832
  hypernatremia, 815
  hypokalemia, 829
  hypophosphatemia, 1936
  inflammatory myopathies, 1234

Weakness—cont'd
  Lambert-Eaton myasthenic syndrome,
    1023-1024
  macroglobulinemia, 704
  mitral valve prolapse, 254
  muscle disease, 1024
  muscle phosphorylase deficiency, 1882
  myasthenia gravis, 1022
  myocardial infarction, 209
  peripheral neuropathy *versus*, 1014-1015
  primary hyperparathyroidism, 1966
  primary pulmonary hypertension, 294
  pyogenic liver abscess, 2209
  rheumatoid arthritis, 1204
  rickets, 1949
  sarcoidosis, 458
  spinal epidural abscess, 1418
  systemic lupus erythematosus, 1214
  thiamine deficiency, 2106
  thrombotic thrombocytopenic purpura, 615
  thyrotoxicosis, 1805
  tropical spastic paraparesis, 1532
Weaning from mechanical ventilation, 399-400
Web
  cervical, 2020
  esophageal, 1999, 2020
Weber-Christian syndrome, 1245
Weber's test, 2308
Wechsler Adult Intelligence Scale, 903
Weddellite, 801
Wegener's granulomatosis, 467-468, 469,
    1222-1223
  acute nephritic syndrome, 764
  anti-neutrophil cytoplasmic antibodies, 1219
  crescentic glomerulonephritis, 848
  lung involvement, 453
  neurologic manifestations, 1092, 1095
  renal involvement, 858
Weight
  preventive care guidelines, 2255
  during puberty, 1767-1768
  puberty, 1770
  recommended daily dietary allowances, 2114,
    2117
Weight bearing radiograph, 1164
Weight gain
  constrictive pericarditis, 277
  Cushing's syndrome, 1820
  prolactin-secreting pituitary adenoma, 1786
  puberty, 1770
Weight loss, 1748-1750
  acquired immunodeficiency syndrome, 2095
  acute cholecystitis, 2227
  acute hyponatremia, 811
  acute viral hepatitis, 2177
  adrenal insufficiency, 1876
  after total gastrectomy, 2101
  alpha heavy-chain disease, 704
  anorexia, 2029-2030
  appendicitis, 2092
  ascites, 2164
  benign recurrent intrahepatic cholestasis, 2158
  blastomycosis, 1657
  cancer
    acute lymphoblastic leukemia, 682
    colon, 2085
    esophageal, 2024
    gastric, 2046
    hepatocellular carcinoma, 2213
    intrahepatic cholangiocarcinoma, 2214
    pancreatic, 2242
    small intestine, 2081
  chronic hepatitis, 2180, 2181
  chronic obstructive pulmonary disease, 442
  chronic renal failure, 781, 784, 786
  Crohn's disease, 2069
  effects on lipoproteins, 1890
  eosinophilic enteritis, 2067
  gallstone risk factor, 2223
  glucagonoma, 2244
  heart failure, 169

Weight loss—cont'd
  insulin-dependent diabetes mellitus, 1854
  malabsorption, 2057
  malignant mesothelioma, 510
  mesenteric panniculitis, 2251
  myxoma, 330
  neurohormonal regulation, 1077
  peritoneal mesenteric and omental diseases, 2248
  peritoneal mesothelioma, 2249
  peritonitis, 1398
  primary hyperparathyroidism, 1967
  pyogenic liver abscess, 2209
  sarcoidosis, 458
  somatostatinoma, 2245
  thyrotoxicosis, 1804
  tropical sprue, 2065
  ulcerative colitis, 2073
  VIPoma, 2245
  Whipple's disease, 2064
Weight reduction
  diabetes mellitus, 1856-1857
  diet, 2103
  gastroesophageal reflux, 2018
  hypertension management, 323
  hyperuricemia, 1275-1276
  obesity, 2103-2104
  precapillary pulmonary hypertension, 296
Weight Watchers, 2104
Weil-Felix test, 1544
Weil's syndrome, 1644-1645
Wells-Brookfield viscometer, 567
Wenckebach block, 153
Wenckebach phenomenon, 154, 155
Werdig-Hoffman disease, 1015
Werner syndrome, 549, 2283
Wernicke's aphasia, 975, 976
Wernicke's encephalopathy, 1081
  amnesic syndrome, 1032
  thiamine deficiency, 1100-1102, 2106
West of Scotland Coronary Prevention Study, 1891
Western aphasia battery, 903
Western blot, 52
  detection of autoantibodies, 1156
  human immunodeficiency virus infection, 1472
  infectious disease, 1374
Western equine encephalitis, 1514, 1517
Wet beriberi, 2106
Wet mount, 1370, 1371
  synovial fluid, 1162-1163
  trichomoniasis, 1691
Wheezing, 404, 405
  asthma, 1187
  chronic obstructive pulmonary disease, 442
  differential diagnosis, 407, 1189
  evaluation of respiratory disease, 402
  lung cancer, 488
  pulmonary thromboembolism, 501
Whewellite, 801
Whiff test, 1439
Whipple disease
  arthropathy, 1246
  dementia, 987
  enteropathic arthritis *versus,* 1242
  fever of unknown origin, 1378
  malabsorption, 2064-2065
  neurologic aspects, 1101
Whipple resection, 2243
Whipple triad, 1877
Whipworm, 1696
White blood cell
  abnormal blood cell count, 590-596
    nucleated cells in peripheral blood, 594-596
    quantitative alterations in normal nucleated cells, 590-594
  abnormalities in intestinal disorders, 2005
  abnormalities of phagocytes, eosinophils, and basophils, 678-681
  acute lymphoblastic leukemia, 682-683

White blood cell—cont'd
  automated blood cell analysis, 556
  chronic myelogenous leukemia, 687
  chronic myeloproliferative disorders, 686
  examination of peripheral blood smear, 557
  fecal, 2006
  immune system, 1109
  pure white blood cell aplasia, 675
  source of deoxyribonucleic acid, 51
  urinalysis, 744
  urinary, 744
White blood cell casts, 745
White blood cell count
  acute cholecystitis, 2228
  acute pancreatitis, 2237
  acute pericarditis, 274
  bacterial meningitis, 1407
  bacterial prostatitis, 1463
  choledocholithiasis, 2229
  chronic liver disease, 2136
  Colorado tick fever, 1512
  compromised host, 1388
  human immunodeficiency virus infection, 1473
  mumps, 1497
  Mycoplasma pneumoniae pneumonia, 1539
  nutritional assessment, 2111
  osteomyelitis, 1434
  primary peritonitis, 1399
  synovial fluid, 1162, 1163, 1164
  systematic inflammatory response syndrome, 1445
White clot, 999
White matter, 1011
White pulp, splenic, 600
White thrombus, 638
Whitehead, 1305
Whole blood transfusion, 572
Whole-brain irradiation, 729
Whole chromosome paint, 561, 562
Whole-lung lavage, 456
Whole pelvic radiation, 715
Whooping cough, 1611-1613
Wide QRS complex tachycardia, 149-150, 151
Wiktor stent, 120
Wild measles virus, 1497
Williams syndrome, 287
Wilms' tumor, 899
  curability with chemotherapy, 552
  hypokalemia, 829
Wilson's disease, 2205-2206
  chronic hepatitis, 2180
  hereditary markers, 2138
  irreversible portosystemic encephalopathy, 1102
  liver transplantation, 2219
  osteoarthritis, 1267
Winterbottom's sign, 1688
Winter's formula, 834
Wirsung's duct, 2130
Wiskott-Aldrich syndrome, 1178, 1342-1343
  hematopoietic stem cell transplantation, 576
  immunodeficiency, 611
  thrombocytopenia, 603
Withdrawal, 2294
  alcohol, 1080-1081, 2295-2296
    seizure, 982
    sympathetic nervous system overactivity, 934-935
  cocaine, 2297
  nicotine, 2296
  opiate, 2297
  systemic corticosteroids, 1824
Withholding and withdrawing care, 13
Wolff-Parkinson-White pattern, 89, 90
Wolff-Parkinson-White syndrome, 142-143, 145
  amiodarone, 138
  atrial fibrillation, 148
  Ebstein's anomaly, 289
  hypertrophic cardiomyopathy, 267
  procainamide, 137

Wolman disease, 1898, 1919
Women's health, 2267-2272
  amenorrhea, 1757-1760
    anorexia nervosa, 1769
    hirsutism, 1756
    hypothalamic, 1837
    malabsorption, 2057
    prolactin-secreting pituitary adenoma, 1786
  breast cancer, 706-713
    axillary nodal metastases, 732
    curability with chemotherapy, 552
    hypercalcemia of malignancy, 1973
    incidence and death rates, 550
    neoplastic pericarditis, 272
    oral contraceptives and, 2270
    pulmonary metastases, 493
    risks in benign breast lesions, 1846, 1847-1848, 1849
    screening, 25, 552
    second malignancy, 586
    supraclavicular lymphadenopathy, 598
  cervical cancer, 714-715
  cervicitis, 1441-1442
  Chlamydia trachomatis, 1536
  contraception, 2269-2270
  coronary artery disease, 2271-2272
  dysuria, 762-763
  endometrial cancer, 713-714
  genital examination for sexually transmitted disease, 1439
  gonadal function testing, 1742-1743
  height and weight table, 2112
  hypertension, 313
  mean heights and weights and recommended energy intake, 2117
  menopause, 2270-2271
    insomnia, 947
    osteoporosis, 1946, 1947
    ovarian function, 1833
  oligomenorrhea
    prolactin-secreting pituitary adenoma, 1786
    21-hydroxylase deficiency, 1824
  ovarian cancer, 715-716
    carcinoid tumor, 2082
    peritoneal carcinomatosis, 732
  pelvic inflammatory disease, 1583
  pregnancy, 2272-2282
    acute renal failure, 775
    after renal transplantation, 796
    antibiotic selection, 1348
    arginine vasopressin release, 808
    asthma, 2276-2277
    atrial septal defect, 282
    bacteriuria during, 1457-1458
    cardiovascular disorders, 2276
    chronic hypertension, 2275
    diabetes mellitus, 1873-1874
    dissection of aorta, 301
    endocrine disorders, 2272-2274
    estrogen-related cholestasis, 2158
    gallstone risk factor, 2223
    gestational diabetes, 1856
    gonorrhea, 1583-1585
    hematologic disorders, 2279
    hepatic disorders, 2277-2278
    hyperemesis gravidarum, 2278
    immune thrombocytopenic purpura, 617
    infectious diseases, 2279-2281
    inflammatory bowel disease, 2278-2279
    listeriosis, 1577
    malaria, 1674
    mean heights and weights and recommended energy intake, 2117
    measles, 1498
    neurologic disorders, 2281-2282
    neutrophilia, 590
    oral anticoagulant administration, 636
    parvovirus B19 infection, 1513-1514
    pemphigoid gestationis, 1296
    precautions before international travel, 1468-1469

Women's health—cont'd
 pregnancy—cont'd
  preeclampsia and eclampsia, 2274-2275
  primary hyperparathyroidism, 1968
  recommended daily dietary allowances,
    2114-2115, 2116
  red blood cell mass, 586
  renal disorders, 2274
  rheumatic disorders, 2279
  rhinitis, 1183-1185
  sickle cell disease, 659
  systemic lupus erythematosus, 1217
  thromboembolic disorders, 2276
  thyrotoxicosis, 1808
  toxoplasmosis, 1677
  transient antidiuretic hormone resistance,
    883
  ulcerative colitis, 2074-2075
  vomiting, 2029
 recommended daily dietary allowances,
   2114-2115, 2116
 vaginitis
  anaerobic bacteria, 1618
  candidal, 1661
  dysuria, 762-763
  pellagra, 2107
 violence against women, 2268-2269
Wood dust, 472
Wood units, 111
Wood's light examination
 tinea cruris, 1422
 tuberous sclerosis, 1922
Word blindness, 978
Word retrieval, 975
Work, lung, 347
Work hypertrophy of spleen, 601
Working Formulation, 696
World Health Organization classification of lung
  cancer, 487
Worm infestation, 1696-1706
 brown pigment stones, 2224
 eosinophilia, 1705-1706
 intestinal worms, 1696-1698
 intestinal worms with tissue migratory phases,
   1698-1699
 strictly intestinal worms, 1696-1698
 tissue worms, 1699-1705
 travel-related, 1466
Wound infection
 botulism, 1571-1572
 postoperative, 1363-1364
 surgical, 1480
Wright stain, 1371
 CFU-GEMM, Plate IV-2
 fever and rash, 1385
 granulocyte, Plate IV-6
 hemolytic anemia, 661, 662
 leishmaniasis, 1687
 lymphocyte, Plate IV-5
 plague, 1610
 procedure, 1371
Wrist
 arthritis, 1172
 arthrography, 1164
 rheumatoid arthritis, 1203
 tendinitis, 1197
Wuchereria bancrofti, 1699
Wytensin; *see* Guanabenz

X

X descent, 37
 cardiac tamponade, 275
 constrictive pericarditis, 277
X-linked agammaglobulinemia, 1152, 1175
X-linked cardiomyopathy, 62
X-linked fragile-X syndrome, 1726
X-linked hyperimmunoglobulin M syndrome,
  1176
X-linked hypogammaglobulinemia, 1176

X-linked hypophosphatemic rickets, 880-881
X-linked inheritance, 1726, 1727
X-linked severe combined immunodeficiency,
  1177
X pacemaker, 940
Xanthelasma, Plate VII-19
Xanthogranuloma, 1317, 1318
Xanthogranulomatous pyelonephritis, 755
Xanthoma
 disorder in apolipoprotein A metabolism,
   1897, 1898
 eruptive, Plate VII-18
 hyperlipidemia, 1323-1324
 soft tissue swelling, 1165
Xanthomatosis, cerebrotendinous, 1898
Xanthomonas maltophilia, 480
Xenograft, prosthetic heart valve, 259
Xenon-scan, 387
Xerocytosis, 666
Xeroderma pigmentosum, 549, 1297, 1306
Xerophthalmia, 2105
Xerosis
 human immunodeficiency virus infection,
   1326
 vitamin A deficiency, 2105
Xerostomia, 1209, 1999
XY gonadal dysgenesis, 1838
Xylocaine; *see* Lidocaine
Xylose, 2149
Xylose absorption test, 2006
XYY syndrome, 1843

Y

Y descent, 37
 cardiac tamponade, 275, 276
 constrictive pericarditis, 277
 jugular venous pulse, 65, 66
 pericardial knock, 74
 tricuspid stenosis, 255, 256
Y pacemaker, 940
Yaws, 1644
Yeast artificial chromosome, 1724
Yeast infection
 acquired immunodeficiency syndrome, 1326,
   1328
 azole antifungals, 1654
 Blastocystis hominis, 1476, 1691
 Blastomyces dermatidis, 1657
 Candida, 1310-1312, 1660-1664
  acquired immunodeficiency syndrome,
    1328, 1476
  after renal transplantation, 794
  compromised host, 1388
  continuous ambulatory peritoneal
    dialysis-related peritonitis, 2248
  diabetic patient, 1323
  drug-induced infection, 1313
  endocarditis, 226
  esophageal infection, 2019-2020
  fever, 1383, 1387
  gastric infection, 2043
  genital lesions, 1444
  human immunodeficiency virus infection,
    2094
  lung transplantation, 517, 518, 519-520
  meningitis, 1404, 1409
  odynophagia, 1998
  peritonitis, 1397
  rash, 1383
  serodiagnosis, 1653
  Sjögren syndrome, 1212
  urinary tract infection, 1457
  vaginitis, 762
  vulvovaginal infection, 1442
 Paracoccidioides brasiliensis, 1657
 Pityrosporum, 1309-1310
  acquired immunodeficiency syndrome,
    1326, 1328
  normal flora, 1368

Yellow fever, 1465, 1514-1517
Yersinia, 1609-1611
 acquired immunodeficiency syndrome,
   1476
 antibiotic selection, 1348
 diarrhea, 1427
Yersinia enterocolitica
 appendicitis, 2092
 Crohn's disease, 2070, 2071
Yersinia pestis, 1369
Yo antibody, 1158
Young's syndrome, 1845

Z

Z-disk, 39, 59
Z protein, 2126
Zafirlukast, 1191
Zalcitabine, 1474
Zarontin; *see* Ethosuximide
ZDV; *see* Zidovudine
Zebeta; *see* Bisoprolol
Zellweger's syndrome, 1907
Zenker's diverticula, 2020-2021
Zerit; *see* Stavudine
Zestril; *see* Lisinopril
Zeta globin, 651
Zidovudine
 acquired immunodeficiency syndrome,
   1474
 hepatic injury, 2191
Ziehl-Neelsen stain, 1371
 cryptosporidiosis, 1680
 Cryptosporidium oocyst, Plate VIII-33
 Mycobacterium leprae, 1650-1651
 septic arthritis, 1252
 synovial fluid, 1163
Zileuton, 1191
Zimelidine, 2191
Zinc
 alcoholic cirrhosis, 2172
 deficiency, 2109-2110
 drug-nutrient interactions, 2110
 functions, 2109
 recommended daily dietary allowances, 2115
 sideroblastic anemia, 645
 status after surgery, 2005
 Wilson's disease, 2206
Zinc finger, 50, 1712
Zinc oxide fumes, 473
Zofran; *see* Ondansetron
Zoladex, 710
Zollinger-Ellison syndrome, 2037
 acid secretory values, 2003
 endocrine paraneoplastic syndromes, 583
 gastric acid hypersecretion, 1983
 gastric analysis, 2002
 hypertrophic gastritis, 2043
 reduced pancreatic exocrine secretion, 2134
Zolpidem, 2300
Zona fasciculata, 1817
Zona glomerulosa, 1817
Zona reticularis, 1817
Zone of partial preservation, 1047
Zoonosis
 balantidiasis, 1690-1691
 brucellosis, 1604-1607
 echinococcosis, 2111
 histoplasmosis, 1654
 Lyme disease, 1646
 Pasteurella, 1609
 rabies, 1505-1508
 travel-related, 1465
 tularemia, 1607-1609
Zoster, 1527
Zoxazolamine, 2191
Zygomycetes, 1659
Zymogen granule, 2132, 2234
ZZ phenotype, 2139

✔ *WHEN TO REFER*

Most acute low back pain is self-limited, so persistence of back pain should trigger further diagnostic studies and, if unresolved, a referral to a rheumatologist is indicated. In patients with an established diagnosis of AS, periodic review by a rheumatologist to assess the status of spinal mobility and to evaluate exercise and medical treatments is warranted. Acute exacerbation of focal back pain in a patient with long-standing AS might reflect a spinal fracture with a developing pseudoarthrosis; such a patient should be evaluated by a rheumatologist or spinal surgeon. Neurologic symptoms might reflect impingement or tethering of the spinal cord ("cauda equina syndrome") or instability in the cervical or thoracic spine. Such patients should be referred for a neurosurgical consultation, particularly to a back specialist with experience with AS patients.

✔ *WHEN TO REFER*

Particularly for patients with multisystem disease, referral to a rheumatologist is important for diagnostic confirmation and an initial discussion about what to expect for the natural history of RS and ReA. Similarly, a rheumatologist should be consulted if the institution of NSAID therapy has not brought the synovitis under satisfactory control and a second-line agent is under consideration. For inflammatory eye disease topical corticosteroid drops should suffice, but consultation with an ophthalmologist for initial assessment and outline of a treatment plan is warranted.

used for seronegative oligoarthritis that follows an infection of the gastrointestinal or genitourinary tract. The pathogens implicated in the former are *Salmonella* spp., *Shigella* spp., *Yersinia* spp., and *Campylobacter* spp.; for the latter, *Chlamydia trachomatis* is the main culprit. The term *RS* is appropriate for seronegative oligoarthritis primarily of the lower extremities that occurs in association with at least one of the following: inflammatory eye disease, particularly conjunctivitis; painless oral mucosal ulcers; circinate balanitis; urethritis; and keratoderma blenorrhagica. The synovitis is often accompanied by enthesitis that is evident as Achilles tendonitis or plantar fasciitis (Fig. 200-1). The interval between an antecedent episode of diarrhea and the onset of joint symptoms may be 2 to 3 weeks; if the diarrhea has resolved at the time of presentation, the patient (or referring physician) may not recognize the relevance of the antecedent gastrointestinal tract symptoms and the clinician must seek them specifically.

Diagnostic Approach

The physical examination must be comprehensive and include careful review of mucous membranes, eyes, skin, genitalia, and entheses, as well as the joint examination. Specific examination of the sacroiliac joints should be performed as described earlier. Laboratory tests often reveal mild leukocytosis and anemia, as well as an elevated ESR, but these lack specificity for diagnostic purposes. An elevated serum immunoglobulin A level is commonly seen in postdysenteric ReA. A urinalysis should be performed for possible pyuria. The synovial fluid analysis is inflammatory with a wide range of leukocyte counts and is culture negative. Stool cultures for enteric pathogens should be performed if there are clinical clues to a prior gastrointestinal tract infection, and urethral swabs for *Chlamydia* organisms should be performed if the history suggests a sexually transmitted disease. Radiographs generally reveal only soft tissue swelling in the acute phase of RS, but joint space narrowing and ankylosis can occur if the arthritis enters a chronic phase (Chapter 184).

Differential Diagnosis

The most important entity to exclude is septic arthritis, and demonstration of sterile synovial fluid obtained at joint aspiration is a necessary prerequisite for the diagnosis of RS or ReA. It should be noted that *Salmonella* and *Yersinia spp.* can produce a true septic arthritis as well as trigger ReA, so the synovial fluid cultures are mandatory. The gonococcal arthritis-dermatitis syndrome can mimic RS, involving joints, tendons, skin, and urethral inflammation. In this syndrome the classic skin lesion is a painful pustule, but this is not always present (Chapter 203). The important step is to ensure appropriate cultures of blood and urethral and synovial fluid if there remains any reasonable doubt about a neisserial infection. Other considerations in the differential diagnosis include PsA, and, indeed, the rash of guttate psoriasis can resemble that of keratodermia blenorrhagica on clinical and histologic examination. Nail dystrophy can occur in both conditions but is usually more severe in PsA. Systemic lupus erythe-matosus in boys and men can have articular, cutaneous, and mucosal manifestations, but there are usually other clinical clues such as Raynaud's phenomenon or photosensitivity. If there are clinical grounds for suspicion, an antinuclear antibody (ANA) screen should be performed; the result is negative in patients with RS and ReA.

Management

If an organism is identified on stool or urethral cultures, it is appropriate to institute antibiotic therapy. There is no evidence that antibiotic treatment of postdysenteric ReA alters the natural history, but the course of ReA after chlamydial infection appears to be shortened by antibiotic therapy. *Chlamydia trachomatis* is equally responsive to azithromycin 1 g orally once and to doxycycline 100 mg twice daily for 7 days. The patient's sexual partner should be given treatment concurrently. There is no firm basis for instituting such antichlamydial therapy if there is only circumstantial (and not culture) evidence of *Chlamydia* infection, but this is often instituted empirically to ensure eradication of the organism.

NSAID therapy is the mainstay of managing the joint disease of RS and ReA. Indomethacin up to 200 mg per day in divided doses or diclofenac in similar dosage usually yields prompt improvement and is generally well tolerated in this young adult population. Local intraarticular steroid injections can be of benefit in managing actively inflamed joints, although it has been observed that RS patients are not as responsive to this therapy as are RA patients. For patients who are unresponsive to NSAID treatment, sulfasalazine has been shown to be of benefit, particularly in polyarticular disease. The target dosage is 3 g per day in divided doses, and the medication is well tolerated in most patients. For the small number of patients whose disease remains very active despite these approaches, methotrexate (15 mg per week orally) can be of benefit. The patient should be cautioned to avoid alcohol consumption while taking methotrexate. Education is an important component of the management of the patient with RS, particularly since the genital lesions may raise real concern about sexual transmissibility. The analogy of an allergic reaction to a substance is useful in explaining that the immune response to an infection can trigger arthritis in some individuals. Although the most active phase of synovitis in ReA is often 3 to 4 months in duration, recent studies have highlighted the potential for chronicity, and cautious optimism about the natural history should temper discussion of prognosis.

PSORIATIC ARTHRITIS
Pathophysiology

The frequency of arthritis in patients with psoriasis has been estimated by different studies to be from 7% to 20%. The appearance of joint inflammation in a patient with established psoriasis should raise the possibility of PsA. However, the arthritis can precede the skin lesions, and it may be the family history, the nail dystrophy, or the characteristic pattern of the joint disease that suggests PsA. The pathogenic links between psoriasis and synovitis have not been resolved, although a "reactive" process attributable to cutaneous microbial antigens has been suggested. An association of HLA-B27 with PsA is primarily with sacroiliac involvement in one clinical subset of these patients. PsA does not have the distinctive male predominance that is seen in AS and RS.